18th edition

CECIL

TEXTBOOK
OF
MEDICINE

Edited by

JAMES B. WYNGAARDEN, M.D.

Director, National Institutes of Health,
Bethesda, Maryland

LLOYD H. SMITH, Jr., M.D.

Professor of Medicine and Associate Dean,
University of California, San Francisco, School of Medicine,
San Francisco, California

1988

W. B. SAUNDERS COMPANY

Harcourt Brace Jovanovich, Inc.

Philadelphia/London/Toronto/Montreal/Sydney/Tokyo

W. B. SAUNDERS COMPANY
Harcourt Brace Jovanovich, Inc.

West Washington Square
Philadelphia, PA 19105

Library of Congress Cataloging-in-Publication Data

Textbook of medicine.

Published simultaneously as 1 v. and as a 2 v. set.

Includes bibliographies and index.

1. Internal medicine.   I. Cecil, Russell L.
    (Russell La Fayette), 1881–1965.   II. Wyngaarden,
    James B., 1924–   .   III. Smith, Lloyd H.,
    1924–   .   IV. Title: Cecil textbook of medicine.
    [DNLM: 1. Medicine. WB 100 T354]

RC46.T35 1988   616   86–27980

ISBN 0–7216–1848–0 (single v.)
ISBN 0–7216–1851–0 (set)
ISBN 0–7216–1849–9 (v. 1)
ISBN 0–7216–1850–2 (v. 2)

Acquisition Editor: John Dyson

Designer: Lorraine B. Kilmer

Production Manager: Frank Polizzano

Manuscript Editor: Donna Walker

Indexer: Nancy Guenther

CECIL TEXTBOOK OF MEDICINE

ISBN   0–7216–1848–0   Single Volume
ISBN   0–7216–1849–9   Volume 1
ISBN   0–7216–1850–2   Volume 2
ISBN   0–7216–1851–0   Set

Last digit is the print number: 9   8   7   6

DOSAGE NOTICE

Every effort has been made by the authors, the editors, and the publisher of this book to ensure that dosage recommendations are precise and in agreement with the standards of practice accepted at the time of publication.

However, dosage schedules are changed from time to time in the light of accumulating clinical experience and continuing laboratory studies. This is most likely to occur in the case of recently introduced products.

We urge, therefore, that you check the package information data for the manufacturer's recommended dosage to be certain that changes have not been made in the recommended dose or in the contraindications for administration. In addition, there are some quite serious situations in which drug therapy must be individualized and expert judgment advises the use of a higher dosage or administration by a different route than is included in the manufacturer's recommendations. Throughout the text examples of such instances are indicated by a footnote.

THE EDITORS

ALSO ASSOCIATED WITH THE CECIL TEXTBOOK OF MEDICINE

Review of General Internal Medicine: A Self-Assessment Manual 4th Edition, 1988
Editors: Lloyd H. Smith, Jr., M.D., James B. Wyngaarden, M.D.

The fourth edition of this self-assessment book contains approximately 1200 questions covering all the specialty areas of internal medicine. The answers are linked to the Cecil Textbook of Medicine and to other readily available sources.

Available from W. B. Saunders Company
The Curtis Center
Independence Square West
Philadelphia, Pa. 19106

PREFACE

Medicine is forever mutable. Although certain general principles remain, medical science moves on. Changes in medical practice follow—not in continuous flow, it is true, but nevertheless in rapid sequence. The pace has quickened as we approach the last decade of the twentieth century. New technologies have revolutionized molecular genetics, neurobiology, immunology, cell biology, and structural biology; the application of these disciplines to all branches of the traditional biomedical sciences proceeds apace. The structure of DNA was elucidated only a generation ago. Now it can be confidently predicted that the whole human genome of approximately three billion nucleotide base pairs (the information equivalent to a thousand large telephone books) will be sequenced within the next decade. The language of the new biology has already permeated medicine. Beyond these contributions from the biological sciences, new applications of the physical and mathematical sciences, especially in diagnostic imaging (CT, MRI, PET, sonography) and in the use of the computer, have radically altered medical practice. In such a climate of change medical competence itself is mutable. It must be constantly renewed or else it will erode.

In order to reflect the best in medical practice, a major textbook of medicine must also be constantly renewed. In that spirit this edition of the *Cecil Textbook of Medicine* has been thoroughly revised, the 18th such revision in a span of more than 60 years. Approximately one third of the book is "new" in that different authors have been selected, in this way assuring that their chapters have been completely recast. All other chapters have been revised and updated by their current authors, carefully chosen authorities in their respective subjects. A revised *Cecil* must reflect the problems of the day. As an example, nowhere is this more apparent than in its attention to the acquired immunodeficiency syndrome (AIDS), the most dramatic medical epidemic of our time. In the 17th edition of *Cecil*, this new and baffling syndrome was described in a single chapter of two pages in the section on Diseases of the Immune System. In this current edition are new chapters on "Retroviruses That Cause Human Disease" (R. C. Gallo), "Acquired Immunodeficiency Syndrome" (J. E. Groopman), "AIDS Dementia and Human Immunodeficiency Virus Brain Infection" (R. W. Price), "Cryptosporidiosis" (R. Soave), and "Giardiasis" (D. P. Stevens), as well as expanded descriptions of other disorders that accompany AIDS—Kaposi's sarcoma, pneumocystosis, *Mycobacterium avium-intracellulare* infections, etc. Examples of other chapters reflecting areas of medical progress include "Natriuretic Factors" (P. Needleman) and the expanded treatment of "Slow Virus Infections of the Nervous System." Lyme disease has been transferred from being listed as a form of infectious arthritis and now receives more extensive discussion as a systemic disorder in the section on Spirochetal Diseases. New chapters have been added on "Clinical Decision Making" (S. G. Pauker), "Control of Unintended Injuries and Those Due to Violence" (S. B. Hulley), and "The Health of the Physician" (L. H. Clever). All of these and many other changes throughout the 18th edition, including updated and annotated references, are designed to maintain the traditional theme of *Cecil* as providing "authoritative clinical guidance and a reasoned, scientific basis for the pursuit of medicine."

In this 18th edition the reader will note a major change in format, the first use of color in *Cecil* (other than that of color plates to illustrate specific entities). The introduction of this single additional color is designed to add clarity to headings and figures throughout the book. This innovation is part of a continuing program to make the book more attractive and easier to use.

Cecil not only stands alone; it is also the senior member of an extended family. Four current books are linked to the *Cecil Textbook of Medicine* by design, format, and editorial responsibility. *Cecil Essentials of Medicine* (edited by T. E. Andreoli, C. C. J. Carpenter, F. Plum, and L. H. Smith, Jr.) offers a more abbreviated description of the realm of internal medicine. Designed primarily for the medical student, for whom the authoritative compendium of *Cecil* may sometimes seem formidable, it does not attempt to be complete. Nevertheless it serves as a useful entry guide into the study of medicine. *Review of General Internal Medicine* (edited by the editors of *Cecil*) has appeared in a 4th edition in parallel with this 18th edition of *Cecil*. As before, its 1200 questions and answers are designed to be of general educational benefit as well as to reinforce the value of *Cecil* as a reference text. *Pathophysiology: The Biological Principles of Disease* (edited by L. H. Smith, Jr., and S. O. Thier) gives a more extensive description of the scientific basis of medical practice than can be contained within a book such as *Cecil*, which must devote most of its attention to the practicalities of clinical description, diagnosis, prognosis, and therapy. *Medical Microbiology and Infectious Diseases* (edited by the late A. I. Braude) gives a more extensive description of the world's experience with the infectious and parasitic diseases.

Editing a major textbook is a complex task, as one attempts to balance content, format, style, integration, and innovation. The editors have been privileged to work with an admirable group of colleagues in this shared responsibility. Fred Plum has continued in his role as Editor for Neurologic and Behavioral Diseases. We welcome Thomas W. Smith as our new Consulting Editor for Cardiovascular Diseases. He joins a seasoned team of fellow Consulting Editors: Thomas E. Andreoli (Renal Diseases), Charles C. J. Carpenter (Infectious Diseases), Robert J. Lefkowitz (Therapeutics), John F. Murray (Respiratory Diseases), David G. Nathan (Hematologic and Hematopoietic Diseases), William E. Paul (Immunology), and Marvin H. Sleisenger (Diseases of the Digestive System). The Consulting Editors continually review their respective sections of this complex book and bring us their ideas and expertise concerning modifications. Our special gratitude is extended to the 325 contributors who have written the 543 chapters that collectively comprise this 18th edition. The ultimate value and authenticity of *Cecil* lies not with the editors but with the scholarship and experience that these individual physicians and scientists have brought to this joint enterprise.

"Language is the armoury of the human mind; and at once contains the trophies of its past, and the weapons of its future conquests." The weaponry of language, in Coleridge's image above, does not always come fully burnished in submitted manuscripts. As in the 17th edition, we have been most fortunate to work with seasoned editorial assistants in Bethesda (Margaret Quinlan) and in San Francisco (Judith Serrell), without whose dedication and skill this large project could not have been completed. At W. B. Saunders Company, Lorraine Kilmer, Donna Walker, and Frank Polizzano carried out with experienced professionalism the intricate task of formatting, editing, and assembling the book, made more complex this time by the use of color. The overall editor at the W. B. Saunders Company for this 18th edition of *Cecil* was John Dyson, who has been an invaluable guide, colleague, and good friend. We are deeply indebted to him for his extensive contributions in bringing to completion this 18th edition of a venerable book.

JAMES B. WYNGAARDEN, M.D.
LLOYD H. SMITH, JR., M.D.

CONTRIBUTORS

FRANCOIS M. ABBOUD, M.D.

Professor of Internal Medicine and of Physiology and Biophysics, University of Iowa College of Medicine. Head, Department of Internal Medicine, University of Iowa Hospitals and Clinics, Iowa City, Iowa.

Shock

DAVID H. ALPERS, M.D.

Professor of Medicine and Chief, Division of Gastroenterology, Washington University School of Medicine. Physician, Barnes Hospital; Consultant, Jewish Hospital of St. Louis, St. Louis, Missouri.

Principles of Nutritional Support: Enteral Nutritional Therapy

DAVID F. ALTMAN, M.D.

Associate Clinical Professor of Medicine and Associate Dean, University of California, San Francisco, School of Medicine. Attending Physician and Director, Gastroenterology Clinic, University of California Medical Center, San Francisco, California.

Food Poisoning; Diseases of the Rectum and Anus

WILLIAM J. C. AMEND, Jr., M.D.

Clinical Professor of Medicine and Surgery, University of California, San Francisco, School of Medicine. Attending Physician, Moffitt Hospital, San Francisco, California.

Renal Transplantation

W. FRENCH ANDERSON, M.D.

Chairman, Department of Medicine and Physiology, National Institutes of Health Graduate Program; Adjunct Professor, Graduate Genetics Program, George Washington University, Washington, D.C. Attending and Admitting Physician, Clinical Center, National Institutes of Health, Bethesda, Maryland.

Expectations from Recombinant DNA Research

THOMAS E. ANDREOLI, M.D.

Edward Randall, III Professor and Chairman, Department of Internal Medicine, University of Texas Medical School at Houston. Chief of Medicine, Hermann Hospital; Consultant, M. D. Anderson Hospital, Houston Texas.

Approach to the Patient with Renal Disease; Disorders of Fluid Volume, Electrolytes, and Acid-Base Balance; The Posterior Pituitary

VINCENT T. ANDRIOLE, M.D.

Professor of Internal Medicine and Chief, Infectious Disease Section, Yale University School of Medicine. Attending Physician, Yale-New Haven Hospital, New Haven, Connecticut.

Urinary Tract Infections and Pyelonephritis

CLAUDE D. ARNAUD, M.D.

Professor of Medicine and Physiology, University of California, San Francisco, School of Medicine. Chief, Endocrine Unit, Veterans Administration Medical Center, San Francisco, California.

Mineral and Bone Homeostasis; The Parathyroid Glands, Hypercalcemia, and Hypocalcemia; The Ultimobranchial Cells and Calcitonin

BERNARD M. BABIOR, M.D., Ph.D.

Member, Department of Basic and Clinical Research, Scripps Clinic and Research Foundation. Staff Physician, Division of Hematology-Oncology, Cecil H. and Ida M. Green Hospital of Scripps Clinic, La Jolla, California.

Function of Neutrophils and Mononuclear Phagocytes; Disorders of Neutrophil Function

GEORGE M. BAER, D.V.M.

Chief, Rabies Laboratory, Viral and Rickettsial Zoonoses Branch, Centers for Disease Control, Atlanta, Georgia.

Rabies

GROVER C. BAGBY, Jr., M.D.

Professor of Medicine and Head, Division of Hematology and Medical Oncology, Oregon Health Sciences Center School of Medicine. Acting Chief, Section of Hematology-Oncology, Veterans Administration Medical Center, Portland, Oregon.

Leukopenia; Leukocytosis and Leukemoid Reactions

ROBERT W. BALOH, M.D.

Professor of Neurology, University of California, Los Angeles, UCLA School of Medicine. Staff Physician, UCLA Medical Center and UCLA Neuropsychiatric Institute, Los Angeles, California.

The Special Senses

H. J. M. BARNETT, M.D.

Professor of Neurology, University of Western Ontario. Staff Physician, Clinical Neurological Sciences, University Hospital; The Verschoyle P. Cronyn Scientific Director and Chief Executive Officer of the John P. Robarts Research Institute, London, Ontario, Canada.

Introduction to Cerebrovascular Diseases; Cerebral Ischemia and Infarction; Spontaneous Intracranial Hemorrhage

ROBERT B. BARON, M.D.

Assistant Clinical Professor of Medicine, University of California, San Francisco, School of Medicine. Director of Screening and Acute Care, University of California, San Francisco, Hospitals and Clinics, San Francisco, California.

Protein-Calorie Undernutrition

DAVID W. BARRY, M.D.

Adjunct Professor of Medicine, Duke University School of Medicine. Vice-President of Research, Wellcome Research Laboratories, Burroughs Wellcome Company. Staff Physician, University Hospital, Durham, North Carolina.

Antiviral Therapy

WILLIAM H. BARRY, M.D.

Nora Eccles Harrison Professor of Cardiology, University of Utah School of Medicine. Attending Cardiologist, University of Utah Hospital, Salt Lake City, Utah.

Cardiac Catheterization and Angiography

JOHN G. BARTLETT, M.D.

Professor of Medicine, Johns Hopkins University School of Medicine. Chief, Division of Infectious Diseases, Johns Hopkins Hospital, Baltimore, Maryland.

Lung Abscess; Clostridial Myonecrosis and Other Clostridial Diseases; Pseudomembranous Colitis; Botulism; Tetanus

MICHAEL BARZA, M.D.

Professor of Medicine, Tufts University School of Medicine. Attending Physician, Department of Medicine, Division of Geographic Medicine and Infectious Diseases, New England Medical Center, Boston, Massachusetts.

Diseases Caused by Pseudomonads; Listeriosis; Erysipeloid

DAVID A. BASS, M.D., D.Phil.

Professor of Medicine, Division of Infectious Diseases and Immunology, Bowman Gray School of Medicine of Wake Forest University. Attending Physician in Infectious Diseases, North Carolina Baptist Hospital, Winston-Salem, North Carolina.

Eosinophilic Syndromes

STEPHEN G. BAUM, M.D.

Professor of Medicine, Mount Sinai School of Medicine of the City University of New York. Director, Department of Medicine, Beth Israel Medical Center; Associate Chairman, Department of Medicine, Mount Sinai Hospital, New York, New York.

Mycoplasmal Infections; Adenovirus Diseases

JOHN D. BAXTER, M.D.

Professor of Medicine and of Biochemistry and Biophysics, University of California, San Francisco, School of Medicine. Director, Metabolic Research Unit, and Chief, Section of Endocrinology, Moffitt Hospital, San Francisco, California.

Principles of Endocrinology; Disorders of the Adrenal Cortex

WILLIAM S. BECK, M.D.

Professor of Medicine and Tutor in Biochemical Sciences, Harvard Medical School. Physician and Director, Hematology Research Laboratory, Massachusetts General Hospital, Boston, Massachusetts.

Megaloblastic Anemias

CHARLES E. BECKER, M.D.

Professor of Medicine, University of California, San Francisco, School of Medicine. Head, Division of Occupational Medicine and Toxicology, San Francisco General Hospital, San Francisco, California.

Principles of Occupational Medicine

DONALD P. BECKER, M.D.

Professor of Surgery/Neurosurgery, University of California, Los Angeles, UCLA School of Medicine. Chief, Neurosurgical Service, UCLA Medical Center, Los Angeles, California.

Injuries to the Head and Spine

MICHAEL D. BENDER, M.D.

Associate Clinical Professor of Medicine, University of California, San Francisco, School of Medicine. Chief of Medicine and Director of Medical Education, Peninsula Hospital and Medical Center, Burlingame, California.

Diseases of the Peritoneum; Diseases of the Mesentery and Omentum

PAUL E. BENDHEIM, M.D.

Attending Neurologist and Head, Laboratory of Degenerative Neurologic Diseases, Department of Pathological Neurobiology, New York State Institute for Basic Research, Staten Island, New York.

Creutzfeldt-Jakob Disease

J. CLAUDE BENNETT, M.D.

Chairman and Professor, Department of Medicine, University of Alabama at Birmingham. Physician-in-Chief, University of Alabama Hospitals, Birmingham, Alabama.

Rheumatoid Arthritis

PAUL D. BERK, M.D.

Albert A. and Vera G. List Professor of Medicine and Chief, Division of Hematology, Mount Sinai School of Medicine of the City University of New York. Attending Physician, Mount Sinai Hospital and Bronx Veterans Administration Medical Center, New York, New York.

Erythrocytosis and Polycythemia; Myeloproliferative Disorders

J. THOMAS BIGGER, Jr., M.D.

Professor of Medicine and of Pharmacology, Columbia University College of Physicians and Surgeons. Attending Physician, Presbyterian Hospital in the City of New York; Director, Arrhythmia Control Unit, Columbia-Presbyterian Medical Center, New York, New York.

Cardiac Arrhythmias

DANIEL D. BIKLE, M.D., Ph.D.

Associate Professor of Medicine, University of California, San Francisco, School of Medicine. Co-Director, Special Diagnostic and Treatment Unit, Veterans Administration Medical Center; Attending Endocrinologist, University of California, San Francisco, Hospitals and Clinics, San Francisco, California.

Vitamin D; Osteomalacia and Rickets

J. MICHAEL BISHOP, M.D.

Professor of Medicine and Director, The G. W. Hooper Foundation, University of California, San Francisco, School of Medicine, San Francisco, California.

Oncogenes

ALAN L. BISNO, M.D.

Professor, Department of Medicine, Division of Infectious Diseases, University of Tennessee College of Medicine. Attending Physician, Memphis Regional Medical Center and University of Tennessee Medical Center; Consulting Physician, Baptist Memorial Hospital, Memphis, Tennessee.

Rheumatic Fever

D. MONTGOMERY BISSELL, M.D.

Professor of Medicine, University of California, San Francisco, School of Medicine. Attending Physician, University of California, San Francisco, Hospitals and San Francisco General Hospital Medical Center, San Francisco, California.

Porphyria

DANIEL S. BLUMENTHAL, M.D., M.P.H.

Professor and Chairman, Department of Community Health and Preventive Medicine, Morehouse School of Medicine. Attending Physician, Hughes Spalding Medical Center, Atlanta, Georgia.

Intestinal Nematodes; Angiostrongyliasis

GILES G. BOLE, M.D.

Professor of Internal Medicine, Associate Dean for Clinical Affairs, and Senior Associate Dean, University of Michigan Medical School. Attending Physician, University of Michigan Hospitals; Consultant, Ann Arbor Veterans Administration Hospital, Ann Arbor, Michigan.

Diseases Associated with Arthritis; Miscellaneous Forms of Arthritis; Nonarticular Rheumatism; Synovial Tumors

THOMAS D. BOYER, M.D.

Associate Professor of Medicine, University of California, San Francisco, School of Medicine. Chief of Gastroenterology, Veterans Administration Medical Center, San Francisco, California.

Cirrhosis of the Liver; Major Sequelae of Cirrhosis

PHILIP S. BRACHMAN, M.D.

Professor, Master of Public Health Program, Department of Community Health, Emory University School of Medicine, Atlanta, Georgia.

Anthrax

JEROME S. BRODY, M.D.

Professor of Medicine and Director of Pulmonary Center, Boston University School of Medicine. Staff Physician, University Hospital and Boston City Hospital, Boston, Massachusetts.

Diseases of the Pleura, Mediastinum, Diaphragm, and Chest Wall

PHILIP A. BRUNELL, M.D.

Professor of Pediatrics, The University of Texas Medical School at San Antonio. Attending Physician, Medical Center Hospital and Santa Rosa Medical Center, San Antonio, Texas.

Varicella

JOHN D. BRUNZELL, M.D.

Professor of Medicine, University of Washington School of Medicine. Attending Physician, University Hospital, Seattle, Washington.

The Hyperlipoproteinemias

REBECCA H. BUCKLEY, M.D.

J. Buren Sidbury Professor of Pediatrics and Professor of Immunology, Duke University School of Medicine. Chief, Division of Allergy and Immunology, Department of Pediatrics, Duke University Medical Center, Durham, North Carolina.

Primary Immunodeficiency Diseases

WARD E. BULLOCK, M.D.

Arthur Russell Morgan Professor of Medicine and Director, Division of Infectious Diseases, University of Cincinnati College of Medicine, Cincinnati, Ohio.

Leprosy

PAUL A. BUNN, Jr., M.D.

Professor of Medicine and Head, Division of Medical Oncology, University of Colorado School of Medicine. Head, Division of Medical Oncology, University Hospital, Denver, Colorado.

Paraneoplastic Syndromes; Tumor Markers

DAVID M. BURNS, M.D.

Associate Professor of Medicine, University of California, San Diego, School of Medicine, La Jolla. Medical Director, Department of Respiratory Therapy, Division of Pulmonary and Critical Care Medicine, University of California Medical Center, San Diego, California.

Tobacco and Health

THOMAS BUTLER, M.D.

Associate Professor of Medicine, Case Western Reserve University School of Medicine. Attending Physician, University Hospitals of Cleveland, Cleveland, Ohio.

Typhoid Fever; Shigellosis; Yersinia Infections; Nonsyphilitic Treponematoses; Relapsing Fever

JOEL N. BUXBAUM, M.D.

Professor of Medicine, New York University School of Medicine. Chief, Rheumatology Section, Veterans Administration Medical Center; Attending Physician, Bellevue Hospital, New York, New York.

The Amyloid Diseases

PETER H. BYERS, M.D.

Professor, Departments of Pathology and Medicine (Medical Genetics), University of Washington School of Medicine, Seattle, Washington.

The Marfan Syndrome; The Ehlers-Danlos Syndrome

ANDREI CALIN, M.D.

Consultant Rheumatologist, Royal National Hospital for Rheumatic Diseases, Bath, Ireland.

The Spondyloarthropathies

CHARLES C. J. CARPENTER, M.D.

Professor of Medicine, Brown University Program in Medicine. Physician-in-Chief, Miriam Hospital, Providence, Rhode Island.

Introduction to Microbial Diseases

JOHN P. CELLO, M.D.

Associate Professor of Medicine, University of California, San Francisco, School of Medicine. Chief of Gastroenterology, San Francisco General Hospital Medical Center, San Francisco, California.

Carcinoma of the Pancreas

BRUCE A. CHABNER, M.D.

Director, Division of Cancer Treatment, National Cancer Institute, National Institutes of Health, Bethesda, Maryland.

Principles of Cancer Therapy

ROBERT M. CHANOCK, M.D.

Chief, Laboratory of Infectious Diseases, National Institute of Allergy and Infectious Diseases, National Institutes of Health, Bethesda, Maryland.

Respiratory Syncytial Virus; Parainfluenza Viral Diseases

BAYARD CLARKSON, M.D.

Professor of Medicine, Cornell University Medical College. Chief, Hematology/Lymphoma Service, Department of Medicine, Memorial Hospital for Cancer and Allied Diseases, New York, New York.

The Chronic Leukemias

LINDA HAWES CLEVER, M.D.

Clinical Professor of Medicine, University of California, San Francisco, School of Medicine. Chairman, Department of Occupational Health, Presbyterian Hospital of Pacific Presbyterian Medical Center, San Francisco, California.

The Health of the Physician

RAY E. CLOUSE, M.D.

Assistant Professor of Medicine, Washington University School of Medicine. Assistant Physician, Barnes Hospital, St. Louis, Missouri.

Parenteral Nutrition

CHARLES G. COCHRANE, M.D.

Adjunct Professor of Pathology, University of California, San Diego, School of Medicine. Member, Department of Immunology, Research Institute of Scripps Clinic, La Jolla, California.

Immune Complex Diseases

MARTIN G. COGAN, M.D.

Associate Professor of Medicine and Associate Staff Member, Cardiovascular Research Institute, University of California, San Francisco, School of Medicine. Attending Physician and Medical Director, Acute Hemodialysis Unit, Moffitt-Long Hospitals, San Francisco, California.

Specific Renal Tubular Disorders

ALAN S. COHEN, M.D.

Conrad Wesselhoeft Professor of Medicine, Boston University School of Medicine. Chief of Medicine and Director, Thorndike Memorial Laboratory, Boston City Hospital, Boston, Massachusetts.

Specialized Diagnostic Procedures in the Rheumatic Diseases

JORDAN J. COHEN, M.D.

Professor and Associate Chairman of Medicine, University of Chicago Pritzker School of Medicine. Chairman of Medicine, Michael Reese Hospital and Medical Center, Chicago, Illinois.

Vascular Disorders of the Kidney

LAWRENCE S. COHEN, M.D.

The Ebenezer K. Hunt Professor of Medicine, Yale University School of Medicine. Attending Physician, Yale-New Haven Hospital, New Haven, Connecticut.

Diseases of the Aorta

WILLIAM G. COUSER, M.D.

Professor of Medicine, University of Washington School of Medicine. Head, Division of Nephrology, University Hospital, Seattle, Washington.

Glomerular Disorders

JAMES D. CRAPO, M.D.

Professor of Medicine, Duke University School of Medicine. Chief, Division of Allergy, Critical Care and Respiratory Medicine, Duke University Medical Center, Durham, North Carolina.

Physical, Chemical, and Aspiration Injuries of the Lung

PHILIP E. CRYER, M.D.

Professor of Medicine and Director, Metabolism Division, Washington University School of Medicine. Physician, Barnes Hospital, St. Louis, Missouri.

The Adrenal Medulla and The Sympathetic Nervous System; The Carcinoid Syndrome

RONALD G. CRYSTAL, M.D.

Chief, Pulmonary Branch, National Heart, Lung and Blood Institute, National Institutes of Health, Bethesda, Maryland.

Interstitial Lung Disease

ANTONIO R. DAMASIO, M.D.

Professor and Head of Neurology, University of Iowa College of Medicine. Attending Neurologist, University of Iowa Hospitals and Clinics, Iowa City, Iowa.

Regional Diagnosis of Cerebral Disorders; Focal Disturbances of Higher Functions

RONALD P. DANIELE, M.D.

Professor of Medicine and Pathology, University of Pennsylvania School of Medicine. Attending Physician and Director of the Interstitial Lung Disease Program, Hospital of the University of Pennsylvania, Philadelphia, Pennsylvania.

Asthma

MICHAEL DECK, M.B., B.S.

Professor of Clinical Radiology, Cornell University Medical College. Attending Radiologist, Chief of Neuroradiology, and Vice-Chairman, Department of Radiology, New York Hospital, New York, New York.

Radiologic Imaging of the Neurologic Patient

ANDREW DEISS, M.D.

Associate Professor of Medicine, University of Utah School of Medicine. Associate Chief of Staff for Research and Development, Veterans Administration Medical Center, Salt Lake City, Utah.

Wilson's Disease

VINCENT W. DENNIS, M.D.

Professor of Medicine, Duke University School of Medicine. Chief, Division of Nephrology, Duke University Medical Center, Durham, North Carolina.

Investigations of Renal Function

IVAN DIAMOND, M.D., Ph.D.

Director, Ernest Gallo Clinic and Research Center; Vice-Chairman and Professor, Department of Neurology, and Professor of Pediatrics and Pharmacology, University of California, San Francisco, School of Medicine. Attending Neurologist, University of California, San Francisco, Hospitals, San Francisco General Hospital Medical Center, and Veterans Administration Medical Center, San Francisco, California.

Nutritional Disorders of the Nervous System

CHARLES A. DINARELLO, M.D.

Professor of Medicine and Pediatrics, Tufts University School of Medicine. Physician, New England Medical Center Hospital, Boston, Massachusetts.

Pathogenesis of Fever; The Acute Phase Response

RAPHAEL DOLIN, M.D.

Professor of Medicine, University of Rochester School of Medicine and Dentistry. Head, Infectious Diseases Unit, University of Rochester Medical Center and Strong Memorial Hospital, Rochester, New York.

Enteroviral Diseases

R. GORDON DOUGLAS, Jr., M.D.

E. Hugh Luckey Distinguished Professor in Medicine and Chairman, Department of Medicine, Cornell University Medical College. Physician-in-Chief, New York Hospital, New York, New York.

Immunization; Introduction to Viral Diseases; Influenza; Herpes Simplex Virus Infections

DOUGLAS A. DROSSMAN, M.D.

Associate Professor of Medicine and Psychiatry, University of North Carolina at Chapel Hill School of Medicine. Attending Physician, North Carolina Memorial Hospital, Chapel Hill, North Carolina.

The Eating Disorders

DAVID J. DRUTZ, M.D.

Adjunct Professor of Medicine, University of Pennsylvania School of Medicine. Vice-President, Biological Sciences, Smith Kline & French Laboratories, Philadelphia, Pennsylvania.

Actinomycosis; Nocardiosis; The Mycoses

DAVID T. DURACK, M.B., D.Phil.

Professor of Medicine, Microbiology and Immunology, Duke University School of Medicine. Chief, Division of Infectious Diseases, Duke University Medical Center, Durham, North Carolina.

Pneumococcal Pneumonia; Infective Endocarditis

THEODORE C. EICKHOFF, M.D.

Professor of Medicine, University of Colorado School of Medicine. Director of Internal Medicine, Presbyterian-Saint Luke's Medical Center, Denver, Colorado.

Bartonellosis; Trench Fever; Q Fever; Colorado Tick Fever

RONALD J. ELIN, M.D., Ph.D.

Clinical Professor of Pathology, Uniformed Services University of the Health Sciences School of Medicine. Chief, Clinical Chemistry Service and Clinical Pathology Department, Clinical Center, National Institutes of Health, Bethesda, Maryland.

Reference Intervals and Laboratory Values of Clinical Importance

EDWARD A. EMMETT, M.B., M.S.

Professor and Director, Division of Occupational Medicine, Johns Hopkins Medical Institutions. Staff Physician, Johns Hopkins Hospital; Consulting Physician, Wyman Park Medical Center, Baltimore, Maryland.

Occupational Diseases of the Skin

ANDREW G. ENGEL, M.D.

William L. McKnight-3M Professor of Neuroscience, Mayo Medical School. Attending Physician, St. Mary's Hospital and Rochester Methodist Hospital, Rochester, Minnesota.

Diseases of Muscle and Neuromuscular Junction

JEROME ENGEL, Jr., M.D., Ph.D.

Professor of Neurology and Anatomy, University of California, Los Angeles, UCLA School of Medicine. Attending Neurologist and Chief of Clinical Neurophysiology Laboratories, UCLA Center for Health Sciences and UCLA Neuropsychiatric Institute, Los Angeles, California.

The Epilepsies

STANLEY FAHN, M.D.

H. Houston Merritt Professor of Neurology, Columbia University College of Physicians and Surgeons. Attending Neurologist, Neurological Institute of New York and Presbyterian Hospital in the City of New York, New York, New York.

The Extrapyramidal Disorders

DOUGLAS V. FALLER, Ph.D., M.D.

Assistant Professor, Harvard Medical School. Assistant Physician, Dana Farber Cancer Institute; Assistant in Medicine, Children's Hospital, Boston, Massachusetts.

Diseases of the Spleen

BARRY L. FANBURG, M.D.

Professor of Medicine, Tufts University School of Medicine. Chief of Pulmonary Division, Department of Medicine, New England Medical Center, Boston, Massachusetts.

Sarcoidosis

ANTHONY S. FAUCI, M.D.

Director, National Institute of Allergy and Infectious Diseases, National Institutes of Health, Bethesda, Maryland.

Glucocorticosteroid Therapy

DOUGLAS T. FEARON, M.D.

Professor of Medicine and of Molecular Biology and Genetics, Johns Hopkins University School of Medicine. Director, Division of Molecular and Clinical Rheumatology, Johns Hopkins Hospital, Baltimore, Maryland.

Complement

MARK FELDMAN, M.D.

Professor, Department of Internal Medicine, University of Texas Health Science Center at Dallas. Associate Chief of Staff for Research and Development, Veterans Administration Medical Center, Dallas, Texas.

Peptic Ulcer: Complications

PHILIP J. FIALKOW, M.D.

Professor and Chairman, Department of Medicine, University of Washington School of Medicine. Physician-in-Chief, University Hospital; Attending Physician, Harborview Medical Center, Seattle, Washington.

Clonal Development and Stem Cell Origin of Proliferative Disorders

DANIEL B. FISHBEIN, M.D.

Medical Epidemiologist, Viral and Rickettsial Zoonoses Branch, Centers for Disease Control, Atlanta, Georgia.

Rabies

ALFRED P. FISHMAN, M.D.

William Maul Measey Professor of Medicine, University of Pennsylvania School of Medicine. Attending Physician, Hospital of the University of Pennsylvania, Philadelphia, Pennsylvania.

Pulmonary Hypertension

GARRETT A. FITZGERALD, M.D.

Professor of Medicine and of Pharmacology, Vanderbilt University School of Medicine. Attending Physician, Department of Medicine and S.C.O.R. in Hypertension, Vanderbilt University Medical Center, Nashville, Tennessee.

Prostaglandins and Related Compounds

KATHLEEN M. FOLEY, M.D.

Associate Professor of Neurology and Pharmacology, Cornell University Medical College. Associate Attending Neurologist and Chief, Pain Service, Memorial Sloan-Kettering Cancer Center, New York, New York.

Pain and Its Management

BERNARD G. FORGET, M.D.

Professor of Medicine and Human Genetics; Chief of Hematology Section, Department of Medicine, Yale University School of Medicine. Attending Physician, Yale-New Haven Hospital, New Haven, Connecticut.

Sickle Cell Anemia and Associated Hemoglobinopathies

DAVID W. FRASER, M.D.

President, Swarthmore College, Swarthmore, Pennsylvania. Adjunct Professor of Medicine, University of Pennsylvania School of Medicine, Philadelphia, Pennsylvania.

Legionellosis

F. CLARKE FRASER, Ph.D., M.D.

Professor of Clinical Genetics, Departments of Biology and Pediatrics and the McGill Centre for Human Genetics, McGill University Faculty of Medicine. Medical Geneticist, Montreal Children's Hospital, Montreal, Quebec, Canada.

Genetic Counseling

JOSEPH F. FRAUMENI, Jr., M.D.

Associate Director for Epidemiology and Biostatistics, National Cancer Institute, National Institutes of Health. Adjunct Professor of Epidemiology, Department of Preventive Medicine and Biometrics, Uniformed Services University of the Health Sciences School of Medicine, Bethesda, Maryland.

Epidemiology of Cancer

WILLIAM T. FRIEDEWALD, M.D.

Associate Director for Disease Prevention, National Institutes of Health, Bethesda, Maryland.

Epidemiology of Cardiovascular Disease

GARY D. FRIEDMAN, M.D., M.S.

Assistant Director for Epidemiology and Biostatistics, Division of Research, Kaiser Permanente Medical Care Program, Oakland, California. Associate Clinical Professor of Medicine and of Family and Community Medicine, University of California, San Francisco, School of Medicine, San Francisco; Lecturer in Epidemiology, School of Public Health, University of California, Berkeley, California.

The Preventive Health Examination

JAMES F. FRIES, M.D.

Associate Professor of Medicine, Stanford University School of Medicine, Stanford, California.

Approach to the Patient with Musculoskeletal Disease

LAWRENCE A. FROHMAN, M.D.

Professor of Medicine, University of Cincinnati College of Medicine. Director, Division of Endocrinology and Metabolism, and Director, General Clinical Research Center, University of Cincinnati Medical Center, Cincinnati, Ohio.

Neuroendocrine Regulation and Its Disorders; The Anterior Pituitary

PATRICIA A. GABOW, M.D.

Associate Professor of Medicine, University of Colorado School of Medicine. Director, Medical Services, Denver General Hospital, Denver, Colorado.

Cystic Disease of the Kidney

ROBERT C. GALLO, M.D.

Chief, Laboratory of Tumor Cell Biology, National Cancer Institute, National Institutes of Health, Bethesda, Maryland.

Retroviruses That Cause Human Disease

JEFFREY A. GELFAND, M.D.

Associate Professor, Division of Geographic Medicine and Infectious Diseases, Department of Medicine, Tufts University School of Medicine. Physician, New England Medical Center Hospital, Boston, Massachusetts.

Advice to Travelers

JOHN W. GITTINGER, Jr., M.D.

Professor of Surgery and Neurology and Chairman, Division of Ophthalmology, University of Massachusetts Medical School. Chief of Ophthalmology, University of Massachusetts Medical Center, Worcester, Massachusetts.

Eye Diseases

JOHN H. GLICK, M.D.

Professor of Medicine, University of Pennsylvania School of Medicine; Director, University of Pennsylvania Cancer Center. Attending Physician, Hospital of the University of Pennsylvania, Philadelphia, Pennsylvania.

Hodgkin's Disease

SHERWOOD L. GORBACH, M.D.

Professor of Medicine and Community Health, Tufts University School of Medicine. Attending Physician, New England Medical Center Hospital, Boston, Massachusetts.

Diseases Caused by Non–Spore-Forming Anaerobic Bacteria

JARED J. GRANTHAM, M.D.

Professor of Medicine and Director, Nephrology Division, University of Kansas College of Health Sciences and Hospital School of Medicine, Kansas City, Kansas.

Acute Renal Failure

BRUCE M. GREENE, M.D.

Associate Professor of Medicine, Case Western Reserve University School of Medicine. Associate Chief, Division of Geographic Medicine, University Hospitals of Cleveland, Cleveland, Ohio.

Onchocerciasis

JOSEPH C. GREENFIELD, M.D.

James B. Duke Professor and Chairman, Department of Medicine, Duke University School of Medicine. Chief, Division of Cardiology, Duke University Medical Center, Durham, North Carolina.

Electrocardiography

JAMES H. GRENDELL, M.D.

Assistant Professor of Medicine and Physiology, University of California, San Francisco, School of Medicine. Attending Physician, San Francisco General Hospital Medical Center, San Francisco, California.

Vascular Diseases of the Intestine

JEROME E. GROOPMAN, M.D.

Associate Professor of Medicine, Harvard Medical School. Attending Physician and Chief of Hematology/Oncology, Department of Medicine, New England Deaconess Hospital, Boston, Massachusetts.

Langerhans Cell Granulomatosis; The Acquired Immunodeficiency Syndrome

CARL GRUNFELD, M.D., Ph.D.

Associate Professor of Medicine, University of California, San Francisco, School of Medicine. Co-Director, Special Diagnostic and Treatment Unit, Veterans Administration Medical Center, San Francisco, California.

Pancreatic Islet Cell Tumors

RICHARD L. GUERRANT, M.D.

Professor of Medicine and Head, Division of Geographic Medicine, University of Virginia School of Medicine. Attending Physician, University of Virginia Hospital, Charlottesville, Virginia.

Campylobacter Enteritis; Enteric Escherichia coli Infections

JOHN L. HAMERTON, D.Sc.

Professor of Human Genetics and Pediatrics, University of Manitoba Faculty of Medicine. Scientific Staff, Health Sciences Centre and St. Boniface General Hospital, Winnipeg, Manitoba, Canada.

Chromosomes and Their Disorders

DONALD H. HARTER, M.D.

Benjamin and Virginia T. Boshes Professor of Neurology, Northwestern University Medical School. Attending Neurologist, Northwestern Memorial Hospital, Chicago, Illinois.

Parameningeal Infections

WILLIAM L. HASKELL, Ph.D.

Associate Professor of Medicine, Stanford University School of Medicine, Stanford, California.

Exercise and Health

BARTON F. HAYNES, M.D.

Professor of Medicine and Chief, Division of Rheumatology and Immunology, Duke University School of Medicine, Durham, North Carolina.

Wegener's Granulomatosis and Midline Granuloma

JOHN P. HAYSLETT, M.D.

Professor of Medicine and Chief, Section of Nephrology, Yale University School of Medicine. Attending Physician, Yale-New Haven Hospital, New Haven, Connecticut.

Renal Disease in Pregnancy

LOUIS A. HEALEY, M.D.

Clinical Professor of Medicine, University of Washington School of Medicine. Attending Physician, Virginia Mason Hospital, Seattle, Washington.

Polymyalgia Rheumatica and Giant Cell Arteritis

BERNADINE P. HEALY, M.D.

Chairman, Research Institute, Cleveland Clinic Foundation, Cleveland, Ohio.

Miscellaneous Conditions of the Heart: Tumor, Trauma, and Systemic Disease

DONALD A. HENDERSON, M.D., M.P.H.

Dean and Professor of Epidemiology and International Health, Johns Hopkins School of Hygiene and Public Health, Baltimore, Maryland.

Variola and Vaccinia

ERIK L. HEWLETT, M.D.

Professor of Medicine and Pharmacology and Head, Division of Clinical Pharmacology, University of Virginia School of Medicine. Attending Physician, University of Virginia Hospital, Charlottesville, Virginia.

Diphtheria

J. ALLAN HOBSON, M.D.

Professor of Psychiatry, Harvard Medical School. Principal Psychiatrist, Massachusetts Mental Health Center, Boston, Massachusetts.

Sleep and Its Disorders

EDWARD W. HOLMES, M.D.

Professor of Medicine and Associate Professor of Biochemistry, Duke University School of Medicine. Chief of Metabolism, Endocrinology, and Genetics, Department of Medicine, Duke University Hospital, Durham, North Carolina.

Disorders of Purine Metabolism

LEWIS B. HOLMES, M.D.

Associate Professor of Pediatrics, Harvard Medical School. Pediatrician and Chief, Embryology-Teratology Unit, Massachusetts General Hospital, Boston, Massachusetts.

Congenital Malformations

PHILIP C. HOPEWELL, M.D.

Professor of Medicine, University of California, San Francisco, School of Medicine. Associate Chief of Medical Service, San Francisco General Hospital Medical Center, San Francisco, California.

Critical Care Medicine

DONALD R. HOPKINS, M.D., M.P.H.

Deputy Director, Centers for Disease Control, Atlanta, Georgia.

Dracunculiasis

RICHARD B. HORNICK, M.D.

Professor of Medicine, University of Rochester School of Medicine and Dentistry. Attending Physician, Strong Memorial Hospital, Rochester, New York.

Salmonella Infections Other Than Typhoid Fever; Tularemia; Introduction to Rickettsial Diseases; The Typhus Group; Rocky Mountain Spotted Fever; Other Tick-Borne Rickettsioses; Rickettsialpox; Scrub Typhus

DONALD W. HOSKINS, M.D.

Clinical Associate Professor of Medicine, Divisions of International Medicine and Digestive Diseases, Department of Medicine, Cornell University Medical College. Vice-President of Medical Affairs and Attending Physician in Medicine, Doctors Hospital; Associate Attending Physician, New York Hospital, New York, New York.

Trichinellosis

DAVID S. HOWELL, M.D.

Professor of Medicine and Director of Arthritis Division, Department of Medicine, University of Miami School of Medicine; Medical Investigator, Veterans Administration Medical Center. Attending Physician, James M. Jackson Memorial Hospital, Miami, Florida.

Osteoarthritis; The Painful Shoulder; The Painful Back

R. RODNEY HOWELL, M.D.

David R. Park Professor and Chairman, Department of Pediatrics, University of Texas Health Science Center at Houston. Pediatrician-in-Chief, University Children's Hospital at Hermann; Consultant in Pediatrics, M. D. Anderson Hospital and Tumor Institute; Consultant in Pediatrics, Shriners Hospital for Crippled Children, Houston, Texas.

The Glycogen Storage Diseases; Pentosuria; Essential Fructosuria and Hereditary Fructose Intolerance

STEPHEN B. HULLEY, M.D., M.P.H.

Professor of Epidemiology, Medicine and Health Policy, University of California, San Francisco, School of Medicine. Director, Clinical Epidemiology Program, San Francisco General Hospital Medical Center, San Francisco, California.

Principles of Preventive Medicine; Control of Unintended Injuries and Those Due to Violence

JULIANNE IMPERATO-McGINLEY, M.D.

Associate Professor of Internal Medicine, Cornell University Medical College. Associate Attending Physician, New York Hospital, New York, New York.

Disorders of Sexual Differentiation

WALDEMAR G. JOHANSON, Jr., M.D.

Professor and Chairman, Department of Internal Medicine, University of Texas Medical School at Galveston. Full-time Active Staff Physician, University of Texas Medical Branch Hospitals, Galveston, Texas.

Introduction to Pneumonia; Pneumonia Caused by Aerobic Gram-Negative Bacilli; Recurrent Aspiration Pneumonia

KENNETH P. JOHNSON, M.D.

Professor and Chairman, Department of Neurology, University of Maryland School of Medicine. Attending Neurologist, University of Maryland Hospital, Kernan Hospital for Crippled Children, and Mercy Hospital; Staff Neurologist, Veterans Administration Medical Center, Baltimore, Maryland.

Syphilitic Infections of the Central Nervous System

ALBERT R. JONSEN, Ph.D.

Professor of Ethics in Medicine and Chief, Division of Medical Ethics, Department of Medicine, University of California, San Francisco, School of Medicine, San Francisco, California.

Ethics in the Practice of Medicine

JOHN P. KANE, M.D., Ph.D.

Professor of Medicine and of Biochemistry and Biophysics, University of California, San Francisco, School of Medicine. Attending Physician, University of California Hospitals, San Francisco, California.

The Judicious Diet

ALBERT Z. KAPIKIAN, M.D.

Head, Epidemiology Section, Laboratory of Infectious Diseases, National Institute of Allergy and Infectious Diseases, National Institutes of Health, Bethesda, Maryland.

The Common Cold; Viral Gastroenteritis

MANUEL E. KAPLAN, M.D.

Professor of Medicine, University of Minnesota Medical School. Chief of Hematology/Oncology, Veterans Administration Medical Center, Minneapolis, Minnesota.

Hemolytic Disorders: Introduction; Acquired Hemolytic Disorders

SAMUEL KAPLAN, M.D.

Professor of Pediatrics and of Medicine, University of Cincinnati College of Medicine. Director, Division of Cardiology, Children's Hospital Medical Center, Cincinnati, Ohio.

Congenital Heart Disease

SAMUEL L. KATZ, M.D.

Wilbert Cornell Davison Professor and Chairman, Department of Pediatrics, Duke University School of Medicine, Durham, North Carolina.

Whooping Cough; Measles; Rubella

ALAN S. KEITT, M.D.

Associate Professor of Pathology and Medicine, University of Florida College of Medicine. Director, Hematology Laboratories, Shands Teaching Hospital, Gainesville, Florida.

Introduction to the Anemias; Anemia Due to Bone Marrow Failure

ELLIOTT KIEFF, M.D., Ph.D.

Block Professor of Medicine and Molecular Genetics, University of Chicago Division of Biological Sciences Pritzker School of Medicine. Chief, Section on Infectious Diseases, University of Chicago Hospital, Chicago, Illinois.

Infectious Mononucleosis: Epstein-Barr Virus Infection

BENJAMIN KISSIN, M.D.

Professor Emeritus in Psychiatry, State University of New York Health Sciences Center at Brooklyn, Brooklyn, New York.

Alcohol Abuse and Alcohol-Related Illnesses

SAULO KLAHR, M.D.

Joseph Friedman Professor of Renal Disease and Director, Renal Division, Washington University School of Medicine. Physician, Barnes Hospital; Staff Physician and Consultant in Nephrology, Jewish Hospital of St. Louis, St. Louis, Missouri.

Structure and Function of the Kidneys

JAMES P. KNOCHEL, M.D.

Vice-Chairman and Professor of Internal Medicine, University of Texas Health Science Center at Dallas. Chief, Medical Service, Veterans Administration Medical Center; Senior Attending Physician, Parkland Memorial Hospital, Dallas, Texas.

Disorders Due to Heat and Cold

JUHA P. KOKKO, M.D., Ph.D.

Professor and Chairman, Department of Medicine, Emory University School of Medicine. Chief of Medicine, Emory University Hospital and Grady Memorial Hospital, Atlanta, Georgia.

Chronic Renal Failure

EDWIN H. KOLODNY, M.D.

Professor of Neurology, Harvard Medical School, Boston. Associate Neurologist, Massachusetts General Hospital, Boston; Consultant in Neurology, McLean Hospital, Belmont, Massachusetts.

Gaucher's Disease; Niemann-Pick Disease

HERMES A. KONTOS, M.D., Ph.D.

Professor of Medicine; Chairman, Division of Cardiology; and Vice-Chairman, Department of Medicine, Virginia Commonwealth University Medical College of Virginia School of Medicine, Richmond, Virginia.

Vascular Diseases of the Limbs

STEPHEN M. KRANE, M.D.

Professor of Medicine, Harvard Medical School. Chief of Arthritis Unit, Massachusetts General Hospital, Boston, Massachusetts.

Connective Tissue Structure and Function

RICHARD M. KRAUSE, M.D.

Dean and Robert W. Woodruff Professor of Medicine, Emory University School of Medicine, Atlanta, Georgia.

Streptococcal Diseases

GUENTER J. KREJS, M.D.

Professor and Chairman, Department of Medicine, Karl-Franzens-Universitat, Graz, Austria.

Diarrhea

WILLIAM L. KRINSKY, M.D., Ph.D.

Associate Professor of Epidemiology, Section of Medical Entomology, Yale University School of Medicine, New Haven, Connecticut.

Arthropods and Leeches

DONALD J. KROGSTAD, M.D.

Associate Professor of Medicine and Pathology, Washington University School of Medicine. Co-Director, Microbiology and Serology Laboratories, Barnes Hospital; Assistant Physician, Barnes Hospital and Jewish Hospital of St. Louis, St. Louis, Missouri.

Amebiasis

JAMES P. KUSHNER, M.D.

Professor of Medicine and Chief, Division of Hematology- Oncology, University of Utah School of Medicine. Attending Physician, University of Utah Hospital and Veterans Administration Medical Center, Salt Lake City, Utah.

Normochromic Normocytic Anemias; Hypochromic Anemias

SYLVIA A LACK, M.D.

Director, Chronic Pain Program, Gaylord Hospital, Wallingford. Attending Physician, Gaylord Hospital, Wallingford; World War II Memorial Hospital, Meriden; and Veterans Administration Medical Center, Newington; Consultant in Hospice Care, St. Mary's Hospital, Waterbury, Connecticut.

Care of Dying Patients and Their Families

DAVID J. LANG, M.D.

Professor of Pediatrics, University of Southern California School of Medicine, Los Angeles. Pediatrician-in-Chief and Director of Infectious Diseases, Children's Hospital of Orange County, Orange, California.

Cytomegalovirus Infection

P. REED LARSEN, M.D.

Professor of Medicine, Harvard Medical School. Senior Physician and Director, Thyroid Unit, Brigham and Women's Hospital; Investigator, Howard Hughes Medical Institute, Boston, Massachusetts.

The Thyroid

JOHN LASZLO, M.D.

Professor of Medicine (on leave), Duke University School of Medicine, Durham, North Carolina. Vice-President for Research, American Cancer Society, New York, New York.

Oncology: Introduction

ROBERT B. LAYZER, M.D.

Professor of Neurology, University of California, San Francisco, School of Medicine. Attending Neurologist, University of California, San Francisco, Hospitals and Clinics, San Francisco, California.

Degenerative Diseases of the Nervous System

GERALD M. LAZARUS, M.D.

Milton B. Hartzell Professor and Chairman, Department of Dermatology, University of Pennsylvania School of Medicine, Philadelphia, Pennsylvania.

Panniculitis and Disorders of the Subcutaneous Fat

ROBERT J. LEFKOWITZ, M.D.

James B. Duke Professor of Medicine, Duke University School of Medicine, Durham, North Carolina.

Pharmacologic Principles Related to the Autonomic Nervous System

E. CARWILE LeROY, M.D.

Professor of Medicine, Medical University of South Carolina College of Medicine. Attending Physician, Medical University Hospital, Charleston Memorial Hospital, and Veterans Administration Medical Center, Charleston, South Carolina.

Systemic Sclerosis

BERNARD LEVIN, M.D.

Professor of Medicine, University of Texas Health Science Center at Houston. Attending Physician, M. D. Anderson Hospital and Tumor Institute, Houston, Texas.

Ulcerative Colitis

MICHAEL D. LEVITT, M.D.

Professor of Medicine, University of Minnesota Medical School. Attending Gastroenterologist and Associate Chief of Staff for Research, Veterans Administration Medical Center, Minneapolis, Minnesota.

Pancreatitis

BRIAN J. LEWIS, M.D.

Clinical Professor of Medicine, University of California, San Francisco, School of Medicine. Attending Physician, Cancer Research Institute, University of California, San Francisco, Hospitals and Clinics, San Francisco, California.

Breast Cancer

ROBERT A. LEWIS, M.D.

Associate Professor, Syntex Research, 3401 Hillview Avenue, Paolo Alto, California 94304

Mastocytosis

LAWRENCE M. LICHTENSTEIN, M.D.

Professor of Medicine, Johns Hopkins University School of Medicine. Staff Physician, Good Samaritan Hospital, Baltimore, Maryland.

Anaphylaxis; Insect Sting Allergy

IRIS F. LITT, M.D.

Associate Professor, Department of Pediatrics, Stanford University School of Medicine. Director, Division of Adolescent Medicine, Stanford University Hospital and Children's Hospital at Stanford, Stanford, California.

Adolescent Medicine

JOHN N. LOEB, M.D.

Professor of Medicine, Columbia University College of Physicians and Surgeons. Attending Physician, Presbyterian Hospital in the City of New York, New York, New York.

Polyglandular Disorders

D. LYNN LORIAUX, M.D., Ph.D.

Clinical Director, National Institute of Child Health and Human Development, National Institutes of Health, Bethesda, Maryland.

Hirsutism

DONALD B. LOURIA, M.D.

Professor and Chairman, Department of Preventive Medicine and Community Health, University of Medicine and Dentistry of New Jersey–New Jersey Medical School, Newark, New Jersey.

Trace Metal Poisoning

ROBERT G. LUKE, M.B., Ch.B.

Professor of Medicine, University of Alabama School of Medicine. Director of Nephrology Division, University of Alabama Hospitals, Birmingham, Alabama.

Dialysis

SAMUEL E. LUX, M.D.

Professor of Pediatrics, Harvard Medical School. Chief, Division of Hematology-Oncology, Children's Hospital, Boston, Massachusetts.

Hereditary Defects in the Membrane or Metabolism of the Red Cell

ADEL A. F. MAHMOUD, M.D., Ph.D.

Professor of Medicine and of Molecular Biology and Microbiology, Case Western Reserve University School of Medicine. Attending Physician, University Hospitals of Cleveland, Cleveland, Ohio.

Introduction to Protozoan and Helminthic Diseases; Schistosomiasis

STEPHEN E. MALAWISTA, M.D.

Professor of Medicine and Chief, Section of Rheumatology, Department of Internal Medicine, Yale University School of Medicine. Attending Physician, Yale-New Haven Hospital, New Haven, and Veterans Administration Medical Center, West Haven, Connecticut.

Lyme Disease; Infectious Arthritis

PETER F. MALET, M.D.

Assistant Professor of Medicine, University of Pennsylvania School of Medicine. Attending Physician, Gastrointestinal Section, Department of Medicine, Hospital of the University of Pennsylvania and Veterans Administration Medical Center, Philadelphia, Pennsylvania.

Diseases of the Gallbladder and Bile Ducts

HENRY J. MANKIN, M.D.

Edith M. Ashley Professor of Orthopaedics, Harvard Medical School. Chief of Orthopaedic Service, Massachusetts General Hospital, Boston, Massachusetts.

Bone Tumors

AARON J. MARCUS, M.D.

Professor of Medicine, Cornell University Medical College. Chief, Hematology-Oncology, and Attending Physician, Veterans Administration Medical Center; Attending Physician, New York Hospital, New York, New York.

Hemorrhagic Disorders: Abnormalities of Platelet and Vascular Function

ANDREW M. MARGILETH, M.D.

Professor of Pediatrics, Uniformed Services University of the Health Sciences School of Medicine, Bethesda. Consultant in Pediatrics, Walter Reed Army Medical Center, Washington, D.C.; Bethesda Naval Hospital, Bethesda; and Malcolm Grow U.S. Air Force Medical Center, Camp Springs, Maryland.

Cat Scratch Disease

ALEXANDER R. MARGULIS, M.D.

Professor and Chairman, Department of Radiology, University of California, San Francisco, School of Medicine. Chief of Radiology, University of California, San Francisco, Hospitals and Clinics, San Francisco, California.

Overview of Imaging Techniques and Projection for the Future

HENRY MASUR, M.D.

Professor of Clinical Medicine, George Washington University School of Medicine and Health Sciences, Washington, D.C. Deputy Chief, Critical Care Medicine Department, Clinical Center, National Institutes of Health, Bethesda, Maryland.

Toxoplasmosis; Pneumocystosis

ALVIN M. MATSUMOTO, M.D.

Assistant Professor of Medicine, University of Washington School of Medicine. Attending Physician, Division of Gerontology and Geriatric Medicine, Geriatric Research, Education, and Clinical Center, Veterans Administration Medical Center, Seattle, Washington.

The Testis

RICHARD A. MATTHAY, M.D.

Professor of Medicine and Associate Director, Pulmonary Section, Department of Internal Medicine, Yale University School of Medicine. Associate Director, Winchester Chest Clinic; Co- Director, Medical Intensive Care Unit; and Attending Pulmonologist, Yale-New Haven Hospital, New Haven, Connecticut.

Chronic Airways Diseases; Abnormalities of Lung Aeration

J. BRUCE McCLAIN, M.D.

Associate Professor of Medicine, Uniformed Services University of the Health Sciences School of Medicine, Bethesda, Maryland. Chief, Infectious Disease Service, Walter Reed Army Medical Center, Washington, D.C.

Rat-Bite Fevers; Leptospirosis

T. DWIGHT McKINNEY, M.D.

Professor of Medicine, University of Texas Health Science Center at San Antonio. Attending Physician, Medical Center Hospital and Audie L. Murphy Memorial Veterans Hospital, San Antonio, Texas.

Tubulointerstitial Diseases and Toxic Nephropathies

IRENE MEISSNER, M.D.

Assistant Professor of Neurology, University of Western Ontario. Staff Physician, Clinical Neurological Sciences, University Hospital, London, Ontario, Canada.

Introduction to Cerebrovascular Diseases

RONALD P. MESSNER, M.D.

Professor of Medicine and Director, Section of Rheumatology, University of Minnesota. Attending Physician, University of Minnesota Hospital and Clinics, Veterans Administration Medical Center, and Hennepin County Medical Center, Minneapolis, Minnesota.

Polymyositis

LOUIS H. MILLER, M.D.

Head, Malaria Section, Laboratory of Parasitic Diseases, National Institute of Allergy and Infectious Diseases, National Institutes of Health, Bethesda, Maryland.

Malaria

THOMAS P. MONATH, M.D.

Director, Division of Vector-Borne Viral Diseases, Center for Infectious Diseases, Centers for Disease Control, Public Health Service, Department of Health and Human Services, Ft. Collins, Colorado.

Arthropod-Borne Viral Encephalitides

WILLIAM L. MORGAN, M.D.

Professor of Medicine, University of Rochester School of Medicine and Dentistry. Associate Chairman, Department of Medicine, Strong Memorial Hospital, Rochester, New York.

Clinical Approach to the Patient

DEANE F. MOSHER, M.D.

Professor of Medicine and Physiological Chemistry and Head, Section of Hematology, University of Wisconsin Medical School, Madison, Wisconsin.

Disorders of Blood Coagulation

ARNO G. MOTULSKY, M.D., D.Sc.

Professor of Medicine and Genetics, University of Washington School of Medicine. Attending Physician, University Hospital and Providence Medical Center, Seattle, Washington.

Hemochromatosis; Hereditary Syndromes Involving Multiple Organ Systems

S. HARVEY MUDD, M.D.

Chief, Section on Alkaloid Biosynthesis, Laboratory of General and Comparative Biochemistry, National Institute of Mental Health, Bethesda, Maryland.

Homocystinuria

MAURICE A. MUFSON, M.D.

Professor of Microbiology and Chairman, Department of Medicine, Marshall University School of Medicine. Associate Chief of Staff for Research, Veterans Administration Medical Center; Staff Physician, Cabell Huntington Hospital and St. Mary's Hospital, Huntington, West Virginia.

Viral Pharyngitis, Laryngitis, Croup, and Bronchitis

JOHN F. MURRAY, M.D.

Professor of Medicine, University of California, San Francisco, School of Medicine. Chief of the Chest Service, San Francisco General Hospital Medical Center, San Francisco, California.

Respiratory Diseases: Introduction; Respiratory Structure and Function; Respiratory Failure

BRYAN D. MYERS, M.B.

Professor of Medicine, Stanford University School of Medicine. Acting Chief, Division of Nephrology, Stanford University Hospital, Stanford, California.

Diabetes and the Kidney

DAVID G. NATHAN, M.D.

Robert G. Stranahan Professor of Pediatrics, Harvard Medical School. Physician-in-Chief, Children's Hospital, Boston, Massachusetts.

Introduction to Hematologic Diseases

PHILIP NEEDLEMAN, Ph.D.

Professor and Head, Department of Pharmacology, Washington University School of Medicine, St. Louis, Missouri.

Natriuretic Factors

FRANKLIN A. NEVA, M.D.

Chief, Laboratory of Parasitic Diseases; Member, Section on Clinical Parasitology, Laboratory of Clinical Investigation, National Institute of Allergy and Infectious Diseases, National Institutes of Health, Bethesda, Maryland.

American Trypanosomiasis; Leishmaniasis

CHRISTOPHER J. L. NEWTH, M.B.

Associate Professor of Pediatrics, University of Southern California School of Medicine. Director, Pediatric Intensive Care, Children's Hospital of Los Angeles, Los Angeles, California.

Bronchiectasis; Cystic Fibrosis

ARTHUR W. NIENHUIS, M.D.

Deputy Clinical Director and Chief, Clinical Hematology Branch, National Heart, Lung and Blood Institute, National Institutes of Health, Bethesda, Maryland.

Hemoglobin Synthesis; The Thalassemias

ALAN S. NIES, M.D.

Professor of Medicine and Pharmacology, University of Colorado School of Medicine. Attending Physician, University Hospital, Denver, Colorado.

Principles of Drug Therapy; Interactions Between Drugs; Adverse Reactions to Drugs

CHARLES P. O'BRIEN, M.D., Ph.D.

Professor of Psychiatry, University of Pennsylvania School of Medicine. Chief, Psychiatry Service, Veterans Administration Medical Center, Philadelphia, Pennsylvania.

Drug Abuse and Dependence

ROBERT K. OCKNER, M.D.

Professor of Medicine and Director of Liver Center, University of California, San Francisco, School of Medicine. Chief of Gastroenterology, Moffitt-Long Hospitals, San Francisco, California.

Clinical Approach to Liver Disease; Hepatic Metabolism in Liver Disease; Laboratory Tests in Liver Disease; Approaches to the Diagnosis of Jaundice; Acute Viral Hepatitis; Toxic and Drug- Induced Liver Disease; Chronic Hepatitis

WILLIAM D. ODELL, M.D., Ph.D.

Chairman, Department of Internal Medicine, and Professor of Medicine and Physiology, University of Utah School of Medicine, Salt Lake City, Utah.

Endocrine Manifestations of Tumors: "Ectopic" Hormone Production

JERROLD M. OLEFSKY, M.D.

Professor of Medicine, University of California, San Diego, School of Medicine. Staff, Medical Research Services, Veterans Administration Medical Center, La Jolla, California.

Diabetes Mellitus

SUZANNE OPARIL, M.D.

Professor of Medicine and Associate Professor of Physiology and Biophysics, University of Alabama School of Medicine. Attending Cardiologist, University Hospital, Birmingham, Alabama.

Arterial Hypertension

ERIC A. OTTESEN, M.D.

Staff Physician, Clinical Center, National Institutes of Health, Bethesda, Maryland, and Children's Hospital National Medical Center, Washington, D.C.

Filariasis

CHARLES Y. C. PAK, M.D.

Professor of Internal Medicine, University of Texas Health Science Center at Dallas, Dallas, Texas.

Renal Calculi

FRANK PARKER, M.D.

Professor and Chairman, Department of Dermatology, Oregon Health Sciences University School of Medicine. Staff Physician, Oregon Health Sciences University Teaching Hospital and Veterans Administration Medical Center, Portland, Oregon.

Cutaneous Manifestations of Internal Malignancy; Skin Diseases

STEPHEN G. PAUKER, M.D.

Professor of Medicine and Chief, Division of Medical Information Sciences, Department of Medicine, Tufts University School of Medicine. Chief, Division of Clinical Decision Making, Department of Medicine, New England Medical Center, Boston, Massachusetts.

Clinical Decision Making

WILLIAM E. PAUL, M.D.

Chief, Laboratory of Immunology, National Institute of Allergy and Infectious Diseases, National Institutes of Health, Bethesda, Maryland.

The Immune System: Introduction

HERBERT A. PERKINS, M.D.

Clinical Professor of Medicine, University of California, San Francisco, School of Medicine. Scientific Director, Irwin Memorial Blood Bank, San Francisco, California.

Blood Transfusion

JOSEPH K. PERLOFF, M.D.

Streisand/American Heart Association Professor of Medicine and Pediatrics, University of California, Los Angeles, UCLA School of Medicine, Los Angeles, California.

Diseases of the Myocardium

WALTER L. PETERSON, M.D.

Associate Professor of Medicine, University of Texas Health Science Center at Dallas. Chief, Gastroenterology Section, Veterans Administration Medical Center, Dallas, Texas.

Peptic Ulcer: Medical Therapy; Gastrointestinal Hemorrhage

SIDNEY PHILLIPS, M.D.

Professor of Medicine, Mayo Medical School. Director, Gastroenterology Unit, and Consultant in Gastroenterology, Mayo Clinic, Rochester, Minnesota.

Disorders of Gastrointestinal Motility

THEODORE L. PHILLIPS, M.D.

Professor and Chairman, Department of Radiation Oncology, University of California, San Francisco, School of Medicine. Consulting Physician, University of California, San Francisco, Hospitals and Clinics, Veterans Administration Medical Center, and Mt. Zion Hospital and Medical Center, San Francisco, California.

Radiation Injury

NATHANIEL F. PIERCE, M.D.

Professor of Medicine, Johns Hopkins University School of Medicine; Professor of International Health, Johns Hopkins University School of Hygiene and Public Health, Baltimore, Maryland. Research Coordinator, Global Diarrhoeal Diseases Control Programme, World Health Organization, Geneva, Switzerland.

Cholera

F. XAVIER PI-SUNYER, M.D.

Professor of Clinical Medicine, Columbia University College of Physicians and Surgeons. Director, Division of Endocrinology and Metabolism, and Associate Director, Obesity Research Center, St. Luke's-Roosevelt Hospital Center, New York, New York.

Obesity

FRED PLUM, M.D.

Anne Parrish Titzell Professor and Chairman, Department of Neurology, Cornell University Medical College. Neurologist-in- Chief, New York Hospital–Cornell Medical Center, New York, New York.

Approach to the Neurologic Patient; Disorders of Consciousness and Arousal; The Dementias; Autonomic Disorders and Their Management; Disorders of Motor Function

CHARLES E. POPE II, M.D.

Professor of Medicine, University of Washington School of Medicine. Chief of Gastroenterology, Veterans Administration Medical Center, Seattle, Washington.

Diseases of the Esophagus

RICHARD L. POPP, M.D.

Professor of Medicine and Associate Chairman, Department of Medicine, Stanford University School of Medicine, Stanford, California.

Echocardiography

CAROL S. PORTLOCK, M.D.

Associate Professor of Medicine, Yale University School of Medicine. Staff Physician, Yale-New Haven Hospital, New Haven, Connecticut.

Introduction to Neoplasms of the Immune System; The Non- Hodgkin's Lymphomas; Burkitt's Lymphoma

JEROME B. POSNER, M.D.

Professor of Neurology, Cornell University Medical College. Attending Neurologist and Chairman, Department of Neurology, Memorial Sloan-Kettering Cancer Center, New York, New York.

Pain and Its Management; Nonmetastatic Effects of Cancer on the Nervous System; Disorders of Consciousness and Arousal; Episodic Loss of Motor Function; Disorders of Sensation; Mechanical Lesions of the Spine and Related Structures

RICHARD W. PRICE, M.D.

Associate Professor of Neurology, Cornell University Medical College. Associate Attending Neurologist, Memorial Hospital and New York

Hospital; Associate Member, Memorial Sloan-Kettering Cancer Center, New York, New York.

Introduction to Viral Infections of the Nervous System; Acute Viral Meningitis and Encephalitis; Herpes Virus Infections of the Nervous System; Poliomyelitis; Slow Virus Infections of the Nervous System

BASIL A. PRUITT, Jr., M.D.

Professor of Surgery, Uniformed Services University of the Health Sciences, Bethesda, Maryland. Commander and Director, U.S. Army Institute of Surgical Research, Fort Sam Houston, Texas.

Electric Injury

CHARLES PUTMAN, M.D.

Dean and Vice-Provost for Research and Development, Duke University School of Medicine. Professor of Medicine and Radiology, Duke University Medical Center, Durham, North Carolina.

Radiography of the Heart

THOMAS C. QUINN, M.D.

Senior Investigator, National Institute of Allergy and Infectious Diseases, National Institutes of Health; Associate Professor of Medicine, Johns Hopkins University School of Medicine. Attending Physician, Clinical Center, National Institutes of Health, Bethesda, and Johns Hopkins Hospital, Baltimore, Maryland.

African Trypanosomiasis

CHARLES E. RACKLEY, M.D.

Anton and Margaret Fuisz Professor of Medicine and Chairman, Department of Medicine, Georgetown University School of Medicine. Physician-in-Chief, Department of Medicine, Georgetown University Hospital, Washington, D.C.

Valvular Heart Disease

SAMUEL RAPOPORT, M.D., Ph.D.

Assistant Professor of Neurology, Cornell University Medical College. Assistant Attending Neurologist, New York Hospital, New York, New York.

Neurologic Diagnostic Procedures

ROBERT W. REBAR, M.D.

Professor, Department of Obstetrics and Gynecology, and Head, Section of Reproductive Endocrinology and Infertility, Northwestern University Medical School. Attending Physician, Northwestern Memorial Hospital, Chicago, Illinois.

The Ovaries

FLOYD C. RECTOR, Jr., M.D.

Professor of Medicine and Physiology, University of California, San Francisco, School of Medicine. Staff Physician, University of California Hospitals and Clinics, San Francisco, California.

Obstructive Nephropathy

CHARLES E. REED, M.D.

Professor of Medicine, Mayo Medical School. Consultant in Internal Medicine and Allergic Diseases, Mayo Clinic and Foundation, Rochester, Minnesota.

Drug Allergy

SEYMOUR REICHLIN, M.D., Ph.D.

Professor of Medicine, Tufts University School of Medicine. Chief, Endocrine Division, New England Medical Center, Boston, Massachusetts.

The Pineal

CHARLES T. RICHARDSON, M.D.

Bertha M. and Cecil D. Patterson Professor of Medicine, University of Texas Health Science Center at Dallas. Chief of Staff, Veterans Administration Medical Center, Dallas, Texas.

Gastritis; Peptic Ulcer: Pathogenesis; Zollinger-Ellison Syndrome

RONALD F. RIEDER, M.D.

Professor of Medicine and Director of Hematology, State University of New York Health Science Center at Brooklyn. Attending Physician, Kings County Hospital Center, Brooklyn, New York.

Unstable Hemoglobins; Abnormal Hemoglobins with Altered Oxygen Affinity; Methemoglobinemia and Sulfhemoglobinemia

B. LAWRENCE RIGGS, M.D.

Professor of Medicine, Mayo Medical School. Consultant, Division of Endocrinology and Metabolism, Mayo Clinic and Foundation, Rochester, Minnesota.

Osteoporosis

RICHARD S. RIVLIN, M.D.

Professor of Medicine, Cornell University Medical College. Chief, Nutrition Service, Memorial Sloan-Kettering Cancer Center, and Chief, Nutrition Division, New York Hospital–Cornell Medical Center, New York, New York.

Disorders of Vitamin Metabolism

WILLIAM O. ROBERTSON, M.D.

Professor of Pediatrics, University of Washington School of Medicine. Medical Director, Seattle Poison Center and Washington Poison Network, Children's Orthopedic and Medical Center, Seattle, Washington.

Common Poisonings

RICHARD K. ROOT, M.D.

Professor and Chairman of Medicine, University of California, San Francisco, School of Medicine. Physician-in-Chief, Department of Medicine, University of California, San Francisco, Hospitals and Clinics, San Francisco, California.

The Compromised Host

IRWIN H. ROSENBERG, M.D.

Professor of Medicine, Physiology, and Nutrition, Tufts University School of Medicine. Physician, Tufts–New England Medical Center, Boston, Massachusetts.

Inflammatory Bowel Diseases: Introduction; Crohn's Disease

JOHN ROSS, Jr., M.D.

Professor of Medicine and Head, Division of Cardiology, Department of Medicine, University of California, San Diego, School of Medicine, La Jolla. Attending Physician, University of California Medical Center, San Diego, California.

Cardiac Function and Circulatory Control

RUSSELL ROSS, Ph.D.

Professor of Pathology and Adjunct Professor of Biochemistry, University of Washington School of Medicine, Seattle, Washington.

Atherosclerosis

DAVID A. ROTTENBERG, M.D.

Associate Professor of Neurology, Cornell University Medical College. Associate Attending Neurologist, New York Hospital and Memorial Hospital, New York, New York.

Disorders of Intracranial Pressure

DAVID W. ROWE, M.D.

Associate Professor of Pediatrics, University of Connecticut School of Medicine. Staff Physician, John Dempsey Hospital, University of Connecticut Health Center, Farmington, Connecticut.

Osteogenesis Imperfecta

JOHN W. ROWE, M.D.

Associate Professor of Medicine, Harvard Medical School. Chief of Gerontology, Beth Israel and Brigham and Women's Hospitals, Boston; Director, Geriatric Research Education Clinical Center, Veterans Administration Medical Center, West Roxbury, Massachusetts.

Aging and Geriatric Medicine

ROBERT M. RUSSELL, M.D.

Associate Professor, Tufts University School of Medicine. Attending Gastroenterologist, Tufts–New England Medical Center; Associate Director, USDA Human Nutrition Research Center, Boston, Massachusetts.

Nutrient Requirements; Nutritional Assessment

DAVID C. SABISTON, Jr., M.D.

James B. Duke Professor and Chairman, Department of Surgery, Duke University School of Medicine. Chief of Staff, Duke University Hospital, Durham, North Carolina.

Surgical Treatment of Coronary Artery Disease

R. BRADLEY SACK, M.D., Sc.D.

Professor of International Health, Johns Hopkins University School of Hygiene and Public Health. Staff Physician, Johns Hopkins Hospital and Francis Scott Key Medical Center, Baltimore, Maryland.

The Diarrhea of Travelers

ROBERT A. SALATA, M.D.

Assistant Professor of Medicine, Case Western Reserve University School of Medicine. Attending Physician and Director of the Travelers Clinic, University Hospitals, Cleveland, Ohio.

Brucellosis

SYDNEY E. SALMON, M.D.

Professor of Internal Medicine, University of Arizona College of Medicine. Chairman, Cancer Activities Committee, University Hospital, Tucson, Arizona.

Plasma Cell Disorders

JOHN SALVAGGIO, M.D.

Henderson Professor and Chairman, Department of Medicine, Tulane University School of Medicine. Senior Physician, Charity Hospital at New Orleans; Active Staff, Tulane University Hospital; Consulting Physician, Veterans Administration Medical Center, New Orleans, Louisiana.

Allergic Rhinitis

JAY P. SANFORD, M.D.

Professor of Medicine and Dean, F. Edward Hebert School of Medicine, and President, Uniformed Services University of the Health Sciences. Attending Physician, Walter Reed Army Medical Center and Naval Hospital, Bethesda, Maryland.

Snake Bites

BRUCE F. SCHARSCHMIDT, M.D.

Professor of Medicine, University of California, San Francisco, School of Medicine. Attending Physician, University of California, San Francisco, Hospitals and Clinics and Moffitt- Long Hospitals, San Francisco, California.

Bilirubin Metabolism and Hyperbilirubinemia; Parasitic, Bacterial, Fungal, and Granulomatous Liver Disease; Inherited, Infiltrative, and Metabolic

Disorders Involving the Liver; Acute and Chronic Hepatic Failure and Hepatic Transplantation; Hepatic Tumors

HERBERT H. SCHAUMBURG, M.D.

Professor and Chairman, Unified Department of Neurology, Albert Einstein College of Medicine of Yeshiva University. Attending Neurologist, Bronx Municipal Hospital Center and Montefiore Medical Center, Bronx, New York.

Diseases of the Peripheral Nervous System

ALAN N. SCHECHTER, M.D.

Professor of Biology, Johns Hopkins University, Baltimore; Professorial Lecturer in Biochemistry, George Washington University, Washington, D.C. Chief, Laboratory of Chemical Biology, National Institute of Diabetes and Digestive and Kidney Diseases, National Institutes of Health, Bethesda, Maryland.

Hemoglobin Structure and Function

LAWRENCE R. SCHILLER, M.D.

Clinical Assistant Professor of Internal Medicine, University of Texas Health Science Center at Dallas. Director of Gastrointestinal Research and Associate Attending Physician, Baylor University Medical Center, Dallas, Texas.

Peptic Ulcer: Epidemiology, Clinical Manifestations, and Diagnosis

H. RALPH SCHUMACHER, Jr., M.D.

Professor of Medicine, University of Pennsylvania School of Medicine. Director, Rheumatology-Immunology Center, Veterans Administration Medical Center; Attending Rheumatologist, Hospital of the University of Pennsylvania, Philadelphia, Pennsylvania.

Calcium Crystal Deposition Arthropathies; Relapsing Polychondritis; Multifocal Fibrosclerosis

BENJAMIN D. SCHWARTZ, M.D., Ph.D.

Professor of Internal Medicine, Washington University School of Medicine; Investigator, Howard Hughes Medical Institute. Associate Physician, Barnes Hospital and Jewish Hospital of St. Louis, St. Louis, Missouri.

The Major Histocompatibility Complex and Disease Susceptibility

CHARLES H. SCOGGIN, M.D.

Senior Scientist and Vice-President, Eleanor Roosevelt Institute for Cancer Research; Professor of Medicine, University of Colorado School of Medicine. Staff Physician, University Hospital, Denver, Colorado.

Pulmonary Neoplasms

CHARLES R. SCRIVER, M.D.C.M.

Professor, Departments of Biology and Pediatrics and Center for Human Genetics, McGill University Faculty of Medicine. Physician and Director, Division of Medical Genetics, Montreal Children's Hospital, Montreal, Quebec, Canada.

Hyperaminoaciduria

S. K. K. SEAH, M.D., Ph.D.

Associate Professor of Medicine, McGill University Faculty of Medicine. Attending Physician, Montreal General Hospital; Consulting Physician, Montreal Chinese Hospital, Montreal, Quebec, Canada.

Hermaphroditic Flukes

STANTON SEGAL, M.D.

Professor of Pediatrics and Internal Medicine, University of Pennsylvania School of Medicine. Senior Physician and Director, Division of Biochemical Development and Molecular Diseases, Children's Hospital of Philadelphia; Attending Physician, Hospital of the University of Pennsylvania, Philadelphia, Pennsylvania.

Galactosemia

ROBERT M. SENIOR, M.D.

Professor of Medicine, Washington University School of Medicine. Director, Respiratory and Critical Care Division, Jewish Hospital of St. Louis, St. Louis, Missouri.

Pulmonary Embolism; Fat Embolism Syndrome

F. JOHN SERVICE, M.D., Ph.D.

Professor of Medicine, Mayo Medical School. Consultant in Endocrinology and Metabolism, Mayo Clinic, Rochester, Minnesota.

Hypoglycemic Disorders

RALPH SHABETAI, M.D.

Professor of Medicine and Associate Director of Cardiology, University of California, San Diego, School of Medicine. Chief of Cardiology, Veterans Administration Medical Center, La Jolla, California.

Diseases of the Pericardium

WILLIAM R. SHAPIRO, M.D.

Professor of Neurology, Cornell University Medical College. Attending Neurologist, Memorial Sloan-Kettering Cancer Center and New York Hospital, New York, New York.

Intracranial Tumors

JOHN N. SHEAGREN, M.D.

Professor of Internal Medicine and Associate Dean, University of Michigan Medical School. Chief of Staff, Veterans Administration Medical Center, Ann Arbor, Michigan.

Shock Syndromes Related to Sepsis; Staphylococcal Infections

DEAN SHEPPARD, M.D.

Associate Professor of Medicine, University of California, San Francisco, School of Medicine. Director, Lung Biology Center, San Francisco General Hospital, San Francisco, California.

Occupation Pulmonary Disorders

ROBERT E. SHOPE, M.D.

Professor of Epidemiology, Yale University School of Medicine, New Haven, Connecticut.

Introduction to Arthropod-Borne Viral Diseases; Viral Hemorrhagic Fevers

DONALD H. SILBERBERG, M.D.

Professor and Chairman, Department of Neurology, University of Pennsylvania School of Medicine. Chairman of Neurology, Hospital of the University of Pennsylvania, Philadelphia, Pennsylvania.

The Demyelinating Diseases

SOL SILVERMAN, Jr., M.D., D.D.S.

Professor and Chairman, Division of Oral Medicine, University of California, San Francisco, School of Dentistry. Attending Dentist, Moffitt-Long Hospitals, San Francisco, California.

Oral Medicine

FREDERICK R. SINGER, M.D.

Professor of Medicine, University of Southern California School of Medicine. Associate Program Director, General Clinical Research Center, Los Angeles County/University of Southern California Medical Center, Los Angeles, California.

Paget's Disease of Bone

EDUARDO SLATOPOLSKY, M.D.

Professor of Medicine, Washington University School of Medicine. Director, Chromalloy American Kidney Center; Physician, Barnes Hospital; Consulting Physician, Jewish Hospital of St. Louis, St. Louis, Missouri.

Renal Osteodystrophy

MARVIN H. SLEISENGER, M.D.

Professor and Vice-Chairman, Department of Medicine, University of California, San Francisco, School of Medicine. Chief of Medical Service, Veterans Administration Medical Center; Attending Physician, Moffitt-Long Hospitals, San Francisco, California.

Gastrointestinal Diseases: Introduction; Miscellaneous Inflammatory Diseases of the Intestine

WILLIAM S. SLY, M.D.

Chairman, E. A. Doisy Department of Biochemistry, St. Louis University School of Medicine. Consulting Geneticist, Cardinal Glennon Memorial Hospital for Children, St. Louis, Missouri.

The Mucopolysaccharidoses

LLOYD H. SMITH, Jr., M.D.

Professor of Medicine and Associate Dean, University of California, San Francisco, School of Medicine, San Francisco, California.

Medicine as an Art; Primary Hyperoxaluria; The Hyperphenylalaninemias; Histidinemia; The Hyperprolinemias and Hydroxyprolinemia; Disease of the Urea Cycle; Branched-Chain Aminoaciduria; Disorders of Pyrimidine Metabolism; Phosphorus Deficiency and Hypophosphatemia; Disorders of Magnesium Metabolism

THOMAS W. SMITH, M.D.

Professor of Medicine, Harvard Medical School and M.I.T. Division of Health Sciences and Technology. Chief, Cardiovascular Division, and Senior Physician, Brigham and Women's Hospital; Consultant in Medicine, Massachusetts General Hospital; Consultant in Cardiology, Children's Hospital and Dana Farber Cancer Institute, Boston, Massachusetts.

Approach to the Patient with Cardiovascular Disease; Heart Failure

RALPH SNYDERMAN, M.D.

Adjunct Professor of Medicine, Duke University School of Medicine, and University of California, San Francisco, School of Medicine. Attending Physician, Duke University Hospital, Durham, North Carolina.

Mechanisms of Inflammation and Tissue Destruction in the Rheumatic Diseases; Behcet's Disease

ROSEMARY SOAVE, M.D.

Assistant Professor of Medicine and Public Health, Cornell University Medical College. Assistant Attending Physician, Department of Medicine, New York Hospital–Cornell Medical Center, New York, New York.

Cryptosporidiosis

ROGER D. SOLOWAY, M.D.

Professor of Medicine, University of Pennsylvania School of Medicine. Associate Chief, Gastrointestinal Section, Hospital of the University of Pennsylvania, Philadelphia, Pennsylvania.

Diseases of the Gallbladder and Bile Ducts

NICHOLAS A. SOTER, M.D.

Professor of Dermatology, New York University School of Medicine. Attending Physician, University Hospital, Bellevue Hospital Center, and Manhattan Veterans Administration Hospital, New York, New York.

Urticaria and Angioedema

P. FREDERICK SPARLING, M.D.

Professor of Medicine and Professor and Chairman of Microbiology and Immunology, University of North Carolina at Chapel Hill School of Medicine. Attending Physician in Infectious Diseases, North Carolina Memorial Hospital, Chapel Hill, North Carolina.

Sexually Transmitted Diseases

WALTER E. STAMM, M.D.

Professor of Medicine, University of Washington School of Medicine. Head, Infectious Disease Division, Harborview Medical Center, Seattle, Washington.

Disease Caused by Chlamydiae

ALFRED D. STEINBERG, M.D.

Medical Director, U.S. Public Health Service; Chief, Cellular Immunology Section, Arthritis and Rheumatism Branch, National Institute of Arthritis and Metabolic Diseases, National Institutes of Health. Attending Physician, Clinical Center, National Institutes of Health, Bethesda, Maryland.

Systemic Lupus Erythematosus

DAVID P. STEVENS, M.D.

Associate Clinical Professor of Medicine, Case Western Reserve University School of Medicine. Assistant Physician, University Hospitals, Cleveland, Ohio.

Giardiasis; Other Protozoan Diseases

LYNNE WARNER STEVENSON, M.D.

Assistant Professor of Medicine, University of California, Los Angeles, UCLA School of Medicine, Los Angeles, California.

Diseases of the Myocardium

DANIEL P. STITES, M.D.

Professor and Vice-Chairman, Department of Laboratory Medicine, University of California, San Francisco, School of Medicine. Attending Physician, University of California, San Francisco, Hospitals and Clinics, San Francisco, California.

Diseases of the Thymus

RAINER STORB, M.D.

Professor of Medicine, University of Washington School of Medicine. Member, Fred Hutchinson Cancer Research Center, Seattle, Washington.

Bone Marrow Transplantation

GORDON J. STREWLER, M.D.

Associate Professor of Medicine, University of California, San Francisco, School of Medicine. Clinical Investigator, Veterans Administration Medical Center, San Francisco, California.

Osteonecrosis, Osteosclerosis, and Other Disorders of Bone

WADI N. SUKI, M.D.

Professor of Medicine and of Physiology and Molecular Biophysics, Baylor College of Medicine. Chief, Renal Section, and Senior Attending Physician, Methodist Hospital, Houston, Texas.

Hereditary Chronic Nephropathies

MORTON N. SWARTZ, M.D.

Professor of Medicine, Harvard Medical School. Chief, Infectious Diseases Unit, Massachusetts General Hospital, Boston, Massachusetts.

Bacterial Meningitis; Meningococcal Disease; Infections Caused by Hemophilus Species; Babesiosis

NORMAN TALAL, M.D.

Professor of Medicine and Microbiology, University of Texas Health Science Center at San Antonio. Chief, Section of Clinical Immunology, Audie L. Murphy Memorial Veterans Hospital, San Antonio, Texas.

Sjögren's Syndrome

CLIFFORD TASMAN-JONES, B.Sc., M.B., Ch.B.

Associate Professor of Gastroenterology and Human Nutrition, University of Aukland Medical School. Senior Consultant Physician, Aukland Hospital Board, Aukland, New Zealand.

Disturbances of Trace Mineral Metabolism

ROBERT B. TESH, M.D., M.S.

Associate Professor of Epidemiology, Department of Epidemiology and Public Health, Yale University School of Medicine, New Haven, Connecticut.

Dengue; West Nile Fever; Phlebotomus Fever; Rift Valley Fever; Fevers Caused by Alphaviruses

RICHARD C. THIRLBY, M.D.

Assistant Professor of Surgery, University of Texas Health Science Center at Dallas. Assistant Chief of Surgery, Veterans Administration Medical Center; Attending Surgeon, Parkland Memorial Hospital, Dallas, Texas.

Peptic Ulcer: Surgical Therapy

LEWIS THOMAS, M.D.

Professor, State University of New York at Stony Brook; Professor Emeritus, Memorial Sloan-Kettering Cancer Center, New York, New York.

Medicine as a Very Old Profession

GEORGE TOLIS, M.D., M.Sc.

Auxiliary Professor of Medicine, McGill University Faculty of Medicine, Montreal, Quebec, Canada; Professor of Medicine, University of Crete Medical School. Director, Division of Endocrinology and Metabolism, Hippokrateion Hospital, Athens, Greece.

Nonmalignant Diseases of the Breast

PHILLIP P. TOSKES, M.D.

Professor of Medicine, University of Florida College of Medicine. Director, Division of Gastroenterology, Hepatology and Nutrition, J. Hillis Miller Health Center, Gainesville, Florida.

Malabsorption

GARY J. TUCKER, M.D.

Professor and Chairman, Psychiatry and Behavioral Sciences, University of Washington School of Medicine, Seattle, Washington.

Psychiatric Disorders in Medical Practice

J. BLAKE TYRRELL, M.D.

Clinical Professor of Medicine, University of California, San Francisco, School of Medicine, San Francisco, California.

Disorders of the Adrenal Cortex

JOUNI UITTO, M.D., Ph.D.

Professor of Dermatology, Biochemistry, and Molecular Biology and Chairman, Department of Dermatology, Jefferson Medical College of Thomas Jefferson University. Staff Physician, Thomas Jefferson University Hospital, Philadelphia, Pennsylvania.

Pseudoxanthoma Elasticum

JACK A. VENNES, M.D.

Professor of Medicine, University of Minnesota Medical School, Minneapolis. Staff, University of Minnesota Hospitals and Clinics and Veterans Administration Medical Center, Minneapolis; Consulting Staff, Hennepin County Medical Center, Minneapolis, and St. Paul-Ramsey Medical Center, St. Paul, Minnesota.

Gastrointestinal Endoscopy

FRANCIS WALDVOGEL, M.D.

Professor of Medicine, University of Geneva. Physician-in- Chief, Clinique Medical Therapeutique, University Hospital of Geneva, Geneva, Switzerland.

Osteomyelitis

SUSAN D. WALL, M.D.

Assistant Professor, University of California, San Francisco, School of Medicine. Chief, Abdominal Imaging, Veterans Administration Medical Center, San Francisco, California.

Diagnostic Imaging Procedures in Gastroenterology

PATRICK C. WALSH, M.D.

David Hall McConnell Professor and Director, Department of Urology, Johns Hopkins University School of Medicine. Urologist-in-Chief, James Buchanan Brady Urological Institute, Johns Hopkins Hospital, Baltimore, Maryland.

Diseases of the Prostate

STANLEY J. WATSON, Ph.D., M.D.

Associate Professor of Psychiatry and Associate Director of the Mental Health Research Institute, University of Michigan Medical School, Ann Arbor, Michigan.

The Endorphin Family of Opioid Peptides

HOWARD J. WEINSTEIN, M.D.

Associate Professor of Pediatrics, Harvard Medical School. Associate Physician, Dana Farber Cancer Institute and Children's Hospital, Boston, Massachusetts.

The Acute Leukemias

RICHARD P. WENZEL, M.D., M.Sc.

Professor of Medicine and Preventive Medicine and Director, Division of Clinical Epidemiology, Department of Internal Medicine, University of Iowa College of Medicine. Director, Hospital Epidemiology Program, University of Iowa Hospitals and Clinics, Iowa City, Iowa.

Prevention and Treatment of Hospital-Acquired Infections

CATHERINE M. WILFERT, M.D.

Professor of Pediatrics and Microbiology, Duke University School of Medicine. Staff Physician, Duke University Hospital, Durham, North Carolina.

Foot and Mouth Disease; Mumps

JAMES T. WILLERSON, M.D.

Professor of Medicine and Director, Cardiology Division, University of Texas Health Science Center at Dallas. Chief of Cardiology, Parkland Memorial Hospital, Dallas, Texas.

Sudden Cardiac Death; Angina Pectoris; Acute Myocardial Infarction

RICHARD D. WILLIAMS, M.D.

Professor and Chairman, Department of Urology, University of Iowa College of Medicine. Head of Urology, University of Iowa Hospital; Chief of Urology Section, Veterans Administration Medical Center, Iowa City, Iowa.

Anomalies of the Urinary Tract; Tumors of the Kidney, Ureter, and Bladder

T. FRANKLIN WILLIAMS, M.D.

Director, National Institute on Aging, National Institutes of Health, Bethesda, Maryland.

Management of Common Problems in the Elderly

JOHN WILLIAMSON, B.Sc., M.B., B.S.

Visiting Anaesthetist, Townsville General and Mater Hospitals; Consultant in Diving Medicine, Townsville General Hospital, Townsville, North Queensland, Australia.

Venomous and Poisonous Marine Animals

SIDNEY J. WINAWER, M.D.

Professor of Clinical Medicine, Cornell University Medical College. Attending Physician and Chief, Gastroenterology Service, Memorial Sloan-Kettering Cancer Center, New York, New York.

Neoplasms of the Stomach; Neoplasms of the Large and Small Intestine

MARTIN S. WOLFE, M.D.

Clinical Professor of Medicine, George Washington University School of Medicine and Health Sciences; Clinical Associate Professor of Medicine, Georgetown University School of Medicine. Attending Physician, George Washington University Hospital and Georgetown University Hospital, Washington, D.C.

The Cestodes

SHELDON M. WOLFF, M.D.

Endicott Professor and Chairman, Department of Medicine, Tufts University School of Medicine. Physician-in-Chief, New England Medical Center Hospital, Boston, Massachusetts.

The Febrile Patient; The Vasculitic Syndromes; Polyarteritis Nodosa Group

EMANUEL WOLINSKY, M.D.

Professor of Medicine and Pathology, Case Western Reserve University School of Medicine. Head, Division of Microbiology, Department of Pathology, Cleveland Metropolitan General Hospital, Cleveland, Ohio.

Tuberculosis; Other Mycobacterioses

JERRY WOLINSKY, M.D.

Professor of Neurology, University of Texas Health Science Center at Houston. Attending Neurologist, Hermann Hospital, Houston, Texas.

Subacute Sclerosing Panencephalitis; Neurologic Disorders Associated with Altered Immunity or Unexplained Host-Parasite Alterations

DANIEL G. WRIGHT, M.D.

Associate Professor of Medicine, Uniformed Services University of the Health Sciences; Adjunct Associate Professor of Medicine, George Washington University School of Medicine and Health Sciences. Chief, Department of Hematology, Walter Reed Army Institute of Research, Walter Reed Army Medical Center, Washington, D.C.

Familial Mediterranean Fever

JAMES B. WYNGAARDEN, M.D.

Director, National Institutes of Health, Bethesda, Maryland.

Medicine as a Science; Medicine as a Public Service; The Use and Interpretation of Laboratory-Derived Data; Human Heredity; Inborn Errors of Metabolism; Metabolic Diseases: Introduction; Fabry's Disease; Alcaptonuria; Gout; Acatalasia

LOWELL S. YOUNG, M.D.

Clinical Professor of Medicine, University of California, San Francisco, School of Medicine. Director, Kuzell Institute for Arthritis and Infectious Diseases; Chief, Division of Infectious Diseases, Pacific Presbyterian Medical Center, San Francisco, California.

Antimicrobial Therapy

BARRY L. ZARET, M.D.

Robert W. Berliner Professor of Medicine, Professor of Diagnostic Radiology, and Chief of Cardiology, Yale University School of Medicine. Chief of Cardiology, Yale-New Haven Hospital, New Haven, Connecticut.

Nuclear Cardiology

ELIZABETH J. ZIEGLER, M.D.

Professor of Medicine, University of California, San Diego, School of Medicine, La Jolla. Attending Physician, University of California, San Diego, Medical Center, San Diego, California.

Extraintestinal Infections Caused by Enteric Bacteria

CONTENTS

COLOR PLATES.. XXXV

PART I   MEDICINE AS A LEARNED AND HUMANE PROFESSION.................. 1

PART II   HUMAN GROWTH, DEVELOPMENT, AND AGING......................... 16

PART III   PERSONAL HEALTH CARE AND PREVENTIVE MEDICINE................. 35

PART IV   PRINCIPLES OF DIAGNOSIS AND MANAGEMENT 70

PART V   PRINCIPLES OF HUMAN GENETICS................................ 146

PART VI   CARDIOVASCULAR DISEASES 175

PART VII   RESPIRATORY DISEASES....................................... 390

PART VIII CRITICAL CARE MEDICINE 482

PART IX   RENAL DISEASES 502

PART X   GASTROINTESTINAL DISEASES 656

PART XI   DISEASES OF THE LIVER, GALLBLADDER, AND BILE DUCTS 808

PART XII   HEMATOLOGIC DISEASES 873

PART XIII ONCOLOGY.. 1082

PART XIV   METABOLIC DISEASES.. 1130

PART XV   NUTRITIONAL DISEASES 1204

PART XVI   ENDOCRINE AND REPRODUCTIVE DISEASES....................... 1252

PART XVII DISEASES OF BONE AND BONE MINERAL METABOLISM 1469

PART XVIII INFECTIOUS DISEASES 1523

PART XIX   DISEASES CAUSED BY PROTOZOA AND METAZOA................... 1856

PART XX   DISEASES OF THE IMMUNE SYSTEM............................. 1932

PART XXI   MUSCULOSKELETAL AND CONNECTIVE TISSUE DISEASES 1977

PART XXII NEUROLOGIC AND BEHAVIORAL DISEASES 2053

PART XXIII EYE DISEASE... 2289

PART XXIV SKIN DISEASE.. 2300

PART XXV   OCCUPATIONAL AND ENVIRONMENTAL MEDICINE 2354

PART XXVI LABORATORY REFERENCE RANGE VALUES OF
           CLINICAL IMPORTANCE 2394

(Detailed table of contents begins on the following page)

CONTENTS

COLOR PLATES ... xxxv
PART I   MEDICINE AS A LEARNED AND HUMANE PROFESSION ... 1
PART II   HUMAN GROWTH, DEVELOPMENT, AND AGING ... 16
PART III PERSONAL HEALTH CARE AND PREVENTIVE MEDICINE ... 45
PART IV   PRINCIPLES OF DIAGNOSIS AND MANAGEMENT ... 70
PART V   PRINCIPLES OF HUMAN GENETICS ... 146
PART VI   CARDIOVASCULAR DISEASES ... 173
PART VII RESPIRATORY DISEASES ... 388
PART VIII CRITICAL CARE MEDICINE ... 483
PART IX   RENAL DISEASES ... 509
PART X   GASTROINTESTINAL DISEASES ... 656
PART XI   DISEASES OF THE LIVER, GALLBLADDER, AND BILE DUCTS ... 808
PART XII HEMATOLOGIC DISEASES ... 819
PART XIII ONCOLOGY ... 1082
PART XIV METABOLIC DISEASES ... 1100
PART XV   NUTRITIONAL DISEASES ... 1204
PART XVI ENDOCRINE AND REPRODUCTIVE DISEASES ... 1224
PART XVII DISEASES OF BONE AND BONE MINERAL METABOLISM ... 1366
PART XVIII INFECTIOUS DISEASES ... 1522
PART XIX DISEASES CAUSED BY PROTOZOA AND METAZOA ... 1456
PART XX   DISEASES OF THE IMMUNE SYSTEM ... 1872
PART XXI MUSCULOSKELETAL AND CONNECTIVE TISSUE DISEASES ... 1977
PART XXII NEUROLOGIC AND BEHAVIORAL DISEASES ... 2063
PART XXIII EYE DISEASES ... 2283
PART XXIV SKIN DISEASES ... 2300
PART XXV OCCUPATIONAL AND ENVIRONMENTAL MEDICINE ... 2334
PART XXVI LABORATORY REFERENCE RANGE VALUES OF
          CLINICAL IMPORTANCE ... 2364

CONTENTS

PART I MEDICINE AS A LEARNED AND HUMANE PROFESSION

1 MEDICINE AS AN ART, *Lloyd H. Smith, Jr.* 1
2 MEDICINE AS A SCIENCE, *James B. Wyngaarden* 5
3 MEDICINE AS A PUBLIC SERVICE, *James B. Wyngaarden* 7
4 MEDICINE AS A VERY OLD PROFESSION, *Lewis Thomas* 9
5 ETHICS IN THE PRACTICE OF MEDICINE, *Albert R. Jonsen* 12

PART II HUMAN GROWTH, DEVELOPMENT, AND AGING

6 ADOLESCENT MEDICINE, *Iris F. Litt* 16
7 AGING AND GERIATRIC MEDICINE, *John W. Rowe* 21
8 MANAGEMENT OF COMMON PROBLEMS IN THE ELDERLY, *T. Franklin Williams* 27
9 CARE OF DYING PATIENTS AND THEIR FAMILIES, *Sylvia A. Lack* 31

PART III PERSONAL HEALTH CARE AND PREVENTIVE MEDICINE

10 PRINCIPLES OF PREVENTIVE MEDICINE, *Stephen B. Hulley* 35
11 TOBACCO AND HEALTH, *David M. Burns* 36
12 CONTROL OF UNINTENDED INJURIES AND THOSE DUE TO VIOLENCE, *Stephen B. Hulley* 40
13 THE JUDICIOUS DIET, *John P. Kane* 42
14 EXERCISE AND HEALTH, *William L. Haskell* 45
15 ALCOHOL ABUSE AND ALCOHOL-RELATED ILLNESSES, *Benjamin Kissin* 48
16 DRUG ABUSE AND DEPENDENCE, *Charles P. O'Brien* 52
17 IMMUNIZATION, *R. Gordon Douglas, Jr.* 61
18 THE PREVENTIVE HEALTH EXAMINATION, *Gary D. Friedman* 66
19 THE HEALTH OF THE PHYSICIAN, *Linda Hawes Clever* 67

PART IV PRINCIPLES OF DIAGNOSIS AND MANAGEMENT

20 CLINICAL APPROACH TO THE PATIENT, *William L. Morgan, Jr.* 70
21 CLINICAL DECISION MAKING, *Stephen G. Pauker* 74
22 THE USE AND INTERPRETATION OF LABORATORY-DERIVED DATA, *James B. Wyngaarden* 79
23 OVERVIEW OF IMAGING TECHNIQUES AND PROJECTION FOR THE FUTURE, *Alexander R. Margulis* 82
24 PRINCIPLES OF DRUG THERAPY, *Alan S. Nies* 87
25 INTERACTIONS BETWEEN DRUGS, *Alan S. Nies* 98
26 ADVERSE REACTIONS TO DRUGS, *Alan S. Nies* 102
27 PAIN AND ITS MANAGEMENT, *Kathleen M. Foley and Jerome B. Posner* 104
28 ANTIMICROBIAL THERAPY, *Lowell S. Young* 112
29 ANTIVIRAL THERAPY, *David W. Barry* 124
30 GLUCOCORTICOSTEROID THERAPY, *Anthony S. Fauci* 128
31 PHARMACOLOGIC PRINCIPLES RELATED TO THE AUTONOMIC NERVOUS SYSTEM, *Robert J. Lefkowitz* 133
32 COMMON POISONINGS, *William O. Robertson* 140

PART V PRINCIPLES OF HUMAN GENETICS

33 HUMAN HEREDITY, *James B. Wyngaarden* 146
34 INBORN ERRORS OF METABOLISM, *James B. Wyngaarden* 152

35 EXPECTATIONS FROM RECOMBINANT DNA RESEARCH, *W. French Anderson* 158
36 CHROMOSOMES AND THEIR DISORDERS, *John L. Hamerton* 161
37 CONGENITAL MALFORMATIONS, *Lewis B. Holmes* 169
38 GENETIC COUNSELING, *F. Clarke Fraser* 171

PART VI CARDIOVASCULAR DISEASES

39 APPROACH TO THE PATIENT WITH CARDIOVASCULAR DISEASE, *Thomas W. Smith* 175
40 EPIDEMIOLOGY OF CARDIOVASCULAR DISEASE, *William T. Friedewald* 179
41 CARDIAC FUNCTION AND CIRCULATORY CONTROL, *John Ross, Jr.* 184
42 SPECIALIZED DIAGNOSTIC PROCEDURES 191
   42.1 RADIOGRAPHY OF THE HEART, *Charles E. Putman* 191
   42.2 ELECTROCARDIOGRAPHY, *Joseph C. Greenfield, Jr.* 196
   42.3 ECHOCARDIOGRAPHY, *Richard L. Popp* 201
   42.4 NUCLEAR CARDIOLOGY, *Barry L. Zaret* 207
   42.5 CARDIAC CATHETERIZATION AND ANGIOGRAPHY, *William H. Barry* 211
43 HEART FAILURE, *Thomas W. Smith* 215
44 SHOCK, *Francois M. Abboud* 236
45 CARDIAC ARRHYTHMIAS, *J. Thomas Bigger, Jr.* 250
46 SUDDEN CARDIAC DEATH, *James T. Willerson* 274
47 ARTERIAL HYPERTENSION, *Suzanne Oparil* 276
48 PULMONARY HYPERTENSION, *Alfred P. Fishman* 293
49 CONGENITAL HEART DISEASE, *Samuel Kaplan* 303
50 ATHEROSCLEROSIS, *Russell Ross* 318
51 DISORDERS OF CORONARY ARTERIES 323
   51.1 ANGINA PECTORIS, *James T. Willerson* 323
   51.2 ACUTE MYOCARDIAL INFARCTION, *James T. Willerson* ... 329
   51.3 SURGICAL TREATMENT OF CORONARY ARTERY DISEASE, *David C. Sabiston, Jr.* 337
52 VALVULAR HEART DISEASE, *Charles E. Rackley* 340
53 DISEASES OF THE MYOCARDIUM, *Joseph K. Perloff and Lynne Warner Stevenson* 352
54 DISEASES OF THE PERICARDIUM, *Ralph Shabetai* 362
55 MISCELLANEOUS CONDITIONS OF THE HEART: TUMOR, TRAUMA, AND SYSTEMIC DISEASE, *Bernadine P. Healy* 367
56 DISEASES OF THE AORTA, *Lawrence S. Cohen* 370
57 VASCULAR DISEASES OF THE LIMBS, *Hermes A. Kontos* 375

PART VII RESPIRATORY DISEASES

58 INTRODUCTION, *John F. Murray* 390
59 RESPIRATORY STRUCTURE AND FUNCTION, *John F. Murray* 395
60 ASTHMA, *Ronald P. Daniele* 403
61 CHRONIC AIRWAYS DISEASES, *Richard A. Matthay* 410
62 ABNORMALITIES OF LUNG AERATION, *Richard A. Matthay* 419
63 INTERSTITIAL LUNG DISEASE, *Ronald G. Crystal* 421
64 LUNG ABSCESS, *John G. Bartlett* 435
65 BRONCHIECTASIS, *Christopher J. L. Newth* 438
66 CYSTIC FIBROSIS, *Christopher J. L. Newth* 440
67 PULMONARY EMBOLISM, *Robert M. Senior* 442
68 FAT EMBOLISM SYNDROME, *Robert M. Senior* 450
69 SARCOIDOSIS, *Barry L. Fanburg* 451
70 PULMONARY NEOPLASMS, *Charles H. Scoggin* 457
71 DISEASES OF THE PLEURA, MEDIASTINUM, DIAPHRAGM, AND CHEST WALL, *Jerome S. Brody* 466
72 RESPIRATORY FAILURE, *John F. Murray* 473

PART VIII   CRITICAL CARE MEDICINE

73   CRITICAL CARE MEDICINE, *Philip C. Hopewell* 482

PART IX   RENAL DISEASES

74   APPROACH TO THE PATIENT WITH RENAL DISEASE,
    Thomas E. Andreoli 502
75   STRUCTURE AND FUNCTION OF THE KIDNEYS, *Saulo Klahr* 508
76   INVESTIGATIONS OF RENAL FUNCTION, *Vincent W. Dennis* 520
77   DISORDERS OF FLUID VOLUME, ELECTROLYTES, AND ACID-BASE BALANCE,
    Thomas E. Andreoli 528
78   ACUTE RENAL FAILURE, *Jared S. Grantham* 558
79   CHRONIC RENAL FAILURE, *Juha Kokko* 563
80   TREATMENT OF IRREVERSIBLE RENAL FAILURE 573
    80.1   DIALYSIS, *Robert G. Luke* 573
    80.2   RENAL TRANSPLANTATION, *William J. C. Amend, Jr.* 577
81   GLOMERULAR DISORDERS, *William G. Couser* 582
82   TUBULOINTERSTITIAL DISEASES AND TOXIC NEPHROPATHIES,
    T. Dwight McKinney 602
83   OBSTRUCTIVE NEPHROPATHY, *Floyd C. Rector, Jr.* 614
84   SPECIFIC RENAL TUBULAR DISORDERS, *Martin G. Cogan* 617
85   DIABETES AND THE KIDNEY, *Bryan D. Myers* 624
86   URINARY TRACT INFECTIONS AND PYELONEPHRITIS,
    Vincent T. Andriole 628
87   VASCULAR DISORDERS OF THE KIDNEY, *Jordan J. Cohen* 632
88   RENAL DISEASE IN PREGNANCY, *John P. Hayslett* 634
89   HEREDITARY CHRONIC NEPHROPATHIES, *Wadi N. Suki* 637
90   RENAL CALCULI, *Charles Y. C. Pak* 638
91   CYSTIC DISEASE OF THE KIDNEY, *Patricia A. Gabow* 644
92   ANOMALIES OF THE URINARY TRACT, *Richard D. Williams* 648
93   TUMORS OF THE KIDNEY, URETER, AND BLADDER,
    Richard D. Williams 650

PART X   GASTROINTESTINAL DISEASES

94   INTRODUCTION, *Marvin H. Sleisenger* 656
95   DIAGNOSTIC IMAGING PROCEDURES IN GASTROENTEROLOGY,
    Susan D. Wall 662
96   GASTROINTESTINAL ENDOSCOPY, *Jack A. Vennes* 668
97   ORAL MEDICINE, *Sol Silverman, Jr.* 674
98   DISEASES OF THE ESOPHAGUS, *Charles E. Pope II* 679
99   GASTRITIS, *Charles T. Richardson* 689
100 PEPTIC ULCER 692
    100.1   PATHOGENESIS, *Charles T. Richardson* 692
    100.2   EPIDEMIOLOGY, CLINICAL MANIFESTATIONS, AND DIAGNOSIS,
        Lawrence R. Schiller 696
    100.3   MEDICAL THERAPY, *Walter L. Peterson* 700
    100.4   SURGICAL THERAPY, *Richard C. Thirlby* 703
    100.5   COMPLICATIONS, *Mark Feldman* 706
    100.6   ZOLLINGER-ELLISON SYNDROME, *Charles T. Richardson* 708
101 NEOPLASMS OF THE STOMACH, *Sidney J. Winawer* 709
102 DISORDERS OF GASTROINTESTINAL MOTILITY, *Sidney Phillips* 714
103 DIARRHEA, *Guenter J. Krejs* 725
104 MALABSORPTION, *Phillip P. Toskes* 732
105 INFLAMMATORY BOWEL DISEASES 745
    105.1   INTRODUCTION, *Irwin H. Rosenberg* 745
    105.2   CROHN'S DISEASE, *Irwin H. Rosenberg* 745
    105.3   ULCERATIVE COLITIS, *Bernard Levin* 753
106 VASCULAR DISEASES OF THE INTESTINE, *James H. Grendell* 760
107 NEOPLASMS OF THE LARGE AND SMALL INTESTINE,
    Sidney J. Winawer 766
108 PANCREATITIS, *Michael D. Levitt* 774
109 CARCINOMA OF THE PANCREAS, *John P. Cello* 781
110 FOOD POISONING, *David F. Altman* 784
111 DISEASES OF THE RECTUM AND ANUS, *David F. Altman* 787
112 DISEASES OF THE PERITONEUM, *Michael D. Bender* 790
113 DISEASES OF THE MESENTERY AND OMENTUM, *Michael D. Bender* ... 795
114 GASTROINTESTINAL HEMORRHAGE, *Walter L. Peterson* 796
115 MISCELLANEOUS INFLAMMATORY DISEASES OF THE INTESTINE,
    Marvin H. Sleisenger 800

PART XI   DISEASES OF THE LIVER, GALLBLADDER, AND BILE DUCTS

116 CLINICAL APPROACH TO LIVER DISEASE, *Robert K. Ockner* 808
117 HEPATIC METABOLISM IN LIVER DISEASE, *Robert K. Ockner* 809
118 BILIRUBIN METABOLISM AND HYPERBILIRUBINEMIA,
    Bruce F. Scharschmidt 811
119 LABORATORY TESTS IN LIVER DISEASE, *Robert K. Ockner* 814
120 APPROACHES TO THE DIAGNOSIS OF JAUNDICE, *Robert K. Ockner* .. 817
121 ACUTE VIRAL HEPATITIS, *Robert K. Ockner* 818
122 TOXIC AND DRUG-INDUCED LIVER DISEASE, *Robert K. Ockner* 826
123 CHRONIC HEPATITIS, *Robert K. Ockner* 830
124 PARASITIC, BACTERIAL, FUNGAL, AND GRANULOMATOUS LIVER DISEASE,
    Bruce F. Scharschmidt 834
125 INHERITED, INFILTRATIVE, AND METABOLIC DISORDERS INVOLVING
    THE LIVER, *Bruce F. Scharschmidt* 838
126 CIRRHOSIS OF THE LIVER, *Thomas D. Boyer* 842
127 MAJOR SEQUELAE OF CIRRHOSIS, *Thomas D. Boyer* 847
128 ACUTE AND CHRONIC HEPATIC FAILURE AND HEPATIC TRANSPLANTATION,
    Bruce F. Scharschmidt 852
129 HEPATIC TUMORS, *Bruce F. Scharschmidt* 856
130 DISEASES OF THE GALLBLADDER AND BILE DUCTS, *Peter F. Malet and*
    Roger D. Soloway 859

PART XII   HEMATOLOGIC DISEASES

131 INTRODUCTION, *David G. Nathan* 873
132 INTRODUCTION TO THE ANEMIAS, *Alan S. Keitt* 878
133 ANEMIA DUE TO BONE MARROW FAILURE, *Alan S. Keitt* 884
134 NORMOCHROMIC NORMOCYTIC ANEMIAS, *James P. Kushner* 890
135 HYPOCHROMIC ANEMIAS, *James P. Kushner* 892
136 MEGALOBLASTIC ANEMIAS, *William S. Beck* 900
137 HEMOLYTIC DISORDERS: INTRODUCTION, *Manuel E. Kaplan* 907
138 HEREDITARY DEFECTS IN THE MEMBRANE OR METABOLISM
    OF THE RED CELL, *Samuel E. Lux* 909
139 ACQUIRED HEMOLYTIC DISORDERS, *Manuel E. Kaplan* 917
140 HEMOGLOBIN STRUCTURE AND FUNCTION, *Alan N. Schechter* 925
141 HEMOGLOBIN SYNTHESIS, *Arthur W. Nienhuis* 927
142 THE THALASSEMIAS, *Arthur W. Nienhuis* 930
143 SICKLE CELL ANEMIA AND ASSOCIATED HEMOGLOBINOPATHIES,
    Bernard G. Forget 936
144 UNSTABLE HEMOGLOBINS, *Ronald F. Rieder* 942
145 ABNORMAL HEMOGLOBINS WITH ALTERED OXYGEN AFFINITY,
    Ronald F. Rieder 943
146 METHEMOGLOBINEMIA AND SULFHEMOGLOBINEMIA,
    Ronald F. Rieder 945
147 BLOOD TRANSFUSION, *Herbert A. Perkins* 947
148 FUNCTION OF NEUTROPHILS AND MONONUCLEAR PHAGOCYTES,
    Bernard M. Babior 951
149 DISORDERS OF NEUTROPHIL FUNCTION, *Bernard M. Babior* 957
150 LEUKOPENIA, *Grover C. Bagby, Jr.* 961
151 LEUKOCYTOSIS AND LEUKEMOID REACTIONS, *Grover C. Bagby, Jr.* ... 967
152 CLONAL DEVELOPMENT AND STEM CELL ORIGIN OF PROLIFERATIVE
    DISORDERS, *Philip J. Fialkow* 973
153 ERYTHROCYTOSIS AND POLYCYTHEMIA, *Paul D. Berk* 975
154 MYELOPROLIFERATIVE DISORDERS, *Paul D. Berk* 984
155 THE CHRONIC LEUKEMIAS, *Bayard Clarkson* 988
156 THE ACUTE LEUKEMIAS, *Howard J. Weinstein* 1001
157 INTRODUCTION TO NEOPLASMS OF THE IMMUNE SYSTEM,
    Carol S. Portlock 1007
158 THE NON-HODGKIN'S LYMPHOMAS, *Carol S. Portlock* 1009
159 BURKITT'S LYMPHOMA, *Carol S. Portlock* 1013
160 HODGKIN'S DISEASE, *John H. Glick* 1014
161 LANGERHANS CELL (EOSINOPHILIC) GRANULOMATOSIS,
    Jerome E. Groopman 1022
162 EOSINOPHILIC SYNDROMES, *David A. Bass* 1024
163 PLASMA CELL DISORDERS, *Sydney E. Salmon* 1026
164 DISEASES OF THE SPLEEN, *Douglas V. Faller* 1036
165 BONE MARROW TRANSPLANTATION, *Rainer Storb* 1040
166 HEMORRHAGIC DISORDERS: ABNORMALITIES OF PLATELET AND VASCULAR
    FUNCTION, *Aaron J. Marcus* 1042
167 DISORDERS OF BLOOD COAGULATION, *Deane F. Mosher* 1060

PART XIII   ONCOLOGY

168 INTRODUCTION, *John Laszlo* 1082
169 ONCOGENES, *J. Michael Bishop* 1089
170 EPIDEMIOLOGY OF CANCER, *Joseph F. Fraumeni, Jr.* 1092
171 PARANEOPLASTIC SYNDROMES, *Paul A. Bunn, Jr.* 1097
172 TUMOR MARKERS, *Paul A. Bunn, Jr.* 1099
173 ENDOCRINE MANIFESTATIONS OF TUMORS· "ECTOPIC" HORMONE
    PRODUCTION, *William D. Odell* 1100

174 NONMETASTATIC EFFECTS OF CANCER ON THE NERVOUS SYSTEM,
    Jerome B. Posner 1104
175 CUTANEOUS MANIFESTATIONS OF INTERNAL MALIGNANCY,
    Frank Parker 1107
176 PRINCIPLES OF CANCER THERAPY, Bruce A. Chabner 1113

PART XIV   METABOLIC DISEASES

177 INTRODUCTION, James B. Wyngaarden 1130

Disorders of Carbohydrate Metabolism

178 GALACTOSEMIA, Stanton Segal 1131
179 THE GLYCOGEN STORAGE DISEASES, R. Rodney Howell 1133
180 PENTOSURIA (ESSENTIAL PENTOSURIA), R. Rodney Howell 1135
181 ESSENTIAL FRUCTOSURIA AND HEREDITARY FRUCTOSE INTOLERANCE,
    R. Rodney Howell 1135
182 PRIMARY HYPEROXALURIA, Lloyd H. Smith, Jr. 1136

Disorders of Lipoprotein Metabolism

183 THE HYPERLIPOPROTEINEMIAS, John D. Brunzell 1137
184 FABRY'S DISEASE (GLYCOSPHINGOLIPIDOSIS),
    James B. Wyngaarden 1144
185 GAUCHER'S DISEASE, Edwin H. Kolodny 1145
186 NIEMANN-PICK DISEASE, Edwin H. Kolodny 1147

Inborn Errors of Amino Acid Metabolism

187 HYPERAMINOACIDURIA (WITH A CLASSIFICATION OF THE INBORN
    AND DEVELOPMENTAL ERRORS OF AMINO ACID METABOLISM),
    Charles R. Scriver 1149
188 THE HYPERPHENYLALANINEMIAS, Lloyd H. Smith, Jr. 1155
189 ALCAPTONURIA, James B. Wyngaarden 1157
190 HISTIDINEMIA, Lloyd H. Smith, Jr. 1157
191 THE HYPERPROLINEMIAS AND HYDROXYPROLINEMIA,
    Lloyd H. Smith, Jr. 1158
192 DISEASES OF THE UREA CYCLE, Lloyd H. Smith, Jr. 1158
193 BRANCHED-CHAIN AMINOACIDURIA, Lloyd H. Smith, Jr. 1159
194 HOMOCYSTINURIA, S. Harvey Mudd 1160

Disorders of Purine and Pyrimidine Metabolism

195 GOUT, James B. Wyngaarden 1161
196 OTHER DISORDERS OF PURINE METABOLISM, Edward W. Holmes 1170
197 DISORDERS OF PYRIMIDINE METABOLISM, Lloyd H. Smith, Jr. 1173

Inherited Disorders of Connective Tissue

198 THE MUCOPOLYSACCHARIDOSES, William S. Sly 1174
199 THE MARFAN SYNDROME, Peter H. Byers 1177
200 EHLERS-DANLOS SYNDROME, Peter H. Byers 1178
201 OSTEOGENESIS IMPERFECTA, David W. Rowe 1180
202 PSEUDOXANTHOMA ELASTICUM, Jouni Uitto 1181

Disorders of Porphyrins or Metals

203 PORPHYRIA, D. Montgomery Bissell 1182
204 ACATALASIA, James B. Wyngaarden 1187
205 WILSON'S DISEASE, Andrew Deiss 1188
206 HEMOCHROMATOSIS (IRON STORAGE DISEASE), Arno G. Motulsky 1189
207 PHOSPHORUS DEFICIENCY AND HYPOPHOSPHATEMIA,
    Lloyd H. Smith, Jr. 1193
208 DISORDERS OF MAGNESIUM METABOLISM, Lloyd H. Smith, Jr. 1195

Other Hereditary Disorders

209 FAMILIAL MEDITERRANEAN FEVER, Daniel G. Wright 1196
210 THE AMYLOID DISEASES, Joel N. Buxbaum 1198
211 HEREDITARY SYNDROMES INVOLVING MULTIPLE ORGAN SYSTEMS,
    Arno G. Motulsky 1202

PART XV   NUTRITIONAL DISEASES

212 NUTRIENT REQUIREMENTS, Robert M. Russell 1204
213 NUTRITIONAL ASSESSMENT, Robert M. Russell 1208
214 PROTEIN-CALORIE UNDERNUTRITION, Robert B. Baron 1212
215 THE EATING DISORDERS, Douglas A. Drossman 1215
216 OBESITY, F. Xavier Pi-Sunyer 1219
217 DISORDERS OF VITAMIN METABOLISM: DEFICIENCIES, METABOLIC
    ABNORMALITIES, AND EXCESSES, Richard S. Rivlin 1228
218 DISTURBANCES OF TRACE MINERAL METABOLISM,
    Clifford Tasman-Jones 1241
219 PRINCIPLES OF NUTRITIONAL SUPPORT: ENTERAL NUTRITIONAL THERAPY,
    David H. Alpers 1243
220 PARENTERAL NUTRITION, Ray E. Clouse 1247

PART XVI   ENDOCRINE AND REPRODUCTIVE DISEASES

221 PRINCIPLES OF ENDOCRINOLOGY, John D. Baxter 1252
222 THE ENDORPHIN FAMILY OF OPIOID PEPTIDES: BIOCHEMISTRY, ANATOMY,
    AND PHYSIOLOGY, Stanley J. Watson 1268
223 PROSTAGLANDINS AND RELATED COMPOUNDS, Garret A. FitzGerald 1271
224 NATRIURETIC FACTORS, Philip Needleman 1277
225 NEUROENDOCRINE REGULATION AND ITS DISORDERS,
    Lawrence A. Frohman 1280
226 THE ANTERIOR PITUITARY, Lawrence A. Frohman 1290
227 THE POSTERIOR PITUITARY, Thomas E. Andreoli 1305
228 THE PINEAL, Seymour Reichlin 1313
229 THE THYROID, P. Reed Larsen 1315
230 DISORDERS OF THE ADRENAL CORTEX 1340
   230.1 STRUCTURE AND DEVELOPMENT OF THE ADRENAL CORTEX,
         John D. Baxter 1340
   230.2 SYNTHESIS, CIRCULATION, AND METABOLISM OF ADRENAL
         STEROIDS, John D. Baxter 1341
   230.3 REGULATION OF ADRENAL STEROID PRODUCTION,
         John D. Baxter 1344
   230.4 ACTIONS OF ADRENAL STEROIDS, John D. Baxter 1346
   230.5 LABORATORY EVALUATION OF ADRENOCORTICAL FUNCTION,
         J. Blake Tyrrell 1348
   230.6 ADRENOCORTICAL HYPOFUNCTION, John D. Baxter 1351
   230.7 CUSHING'S SYNDROME, J. Blake Tyrrell 1353
   230.8 MINERALOCORTICOID EXCESS STATES, John D. Baxter 1358
231 DIABETES MELLITUS, Jerrold M. Olefsky 1360
232 HYPOGLYCEMIC DISORDERS, F. John Service 1381
233 PANCREATIC ISLET CELL TUMORS, Carl Grunfeld 1387
234 DISORDERS OF SEXUAL DIFFERENTIATION,
    Julianne Imperato-McGinley 1390
235 THE TESTIS, Alvin M. Matsumoto 1404
236 DISEASES OF THE PROSTATE, Patrick C. Walsh 1421
237 THE OVARIES, Robert W. Rebar 1425
238 HIRSUTISM, D. Lynn Loriaux 1446
239 NONMALIGNANT DISEASES OF THE BREAST, George Tolis 1449
240 BREAST CANCER, Brian J. Lewis 1452
241 POLYGLANDULAR DISORDERS, John N. Loeb 1458
242 THE ADRENAL MEDULLA AND THE SYMPATHETIC NERVOUS SYSTEM,
    Philip E. Cryer 1461
243 THE CARCINOID SYNDROME, Philip E. Cryer 1467

PART XVII   DISEASES OF BONE AND BONE MINERAL METABOLISM

244 MINERAL AND BONE HOMEOSTASIS, Claude D. Arnaud 1469
245 VITAMIN D, Daniel D. Bikle 1477
246 OSTEOMALACIA AND RICKETS, Daniel D. Bikle 1479
247 THE PARATHYROID GLANDS, HYPERCALCEMIA, AND HYPOCALCEMIA,
    Claude D. Arnaud 1486
248 THE ULTIMOBRANCHIAL CELLS AND CALCITONIN, Claude D. Arnaud 1505
249 RENAL OSTEODYSTROPHY, Eduardo Slatopolsky 1507
250 OSTEOPOROSIS, B. Lawrence Riggs 1510
251 PAGET'S DISEASE OF BONE (OSTEITIS DEFORMANS),
    Frederick R. Singer 1515
252 OSTEONECROSIS, OSTEOSCLEROSIS, AND OTHER DISORDERS OF BONE,
    Gordon J. Strewler 1517
253 BONE TUMORS, Henry J. Mankin 1521

PART XVIII   INFECTIOUS DISEASES

Section 1 Introduction

254 INTRODUCTION TO MICROBIAL DISEASES, Charles C. J. Carpenter 1523
255 THE FEBRILE PATIENT, Sheldon M. Wolff 1524
256 PATHOGENESIS OF FEVER, Charles A. Dinarello 1525
257 THE ACUTE PHASE RESPONSE, Charles A. Dinarello 1527
258 THE COMPROMISED HOST, Richard K. Root 1529
259 SHOCK SYNDROMES RELATED TO SEPSIS, John N. Sheagren 1538
260 PREVENTION AND TREATMENT OF HOSPITAL-ACQUIRED INFECTIONS
    Richard P. Wenzel 1541
261 ADVICE TO TRAVELERS, Jeffrey A. Gelfand 1549

Section 2 Bacterial Diseases

Pneumonia

262 INTRODUCTION TO PNEUMONIA, Waldemar G. Johanson, Jr. 1551
263 PNEUMOCOCCAL PNEUMONIA, David T. Durack 1554

264 MYCOPLASMAL INFECTIONS, Stephen G. Baum 1561
265 PNEUMONIA CAUSED BY AEROBIC GRAM-NEGATIVE BACILLI,
    Waldemar G. Johanson, Jr. 1565
266 RECURRENT ASPIRATION PNEUMONIA, Waldemar G. Johanson, Jr. ... 1568
267 LEGIONELLOSIS, David W. Fraser 1570

Streptococcal Diseases

268 STREPTOCOCCAL DISEASES, Richard M. Krause 1572
269 RHEUMATIC FEVER, Alan L. Bisno 1580

Endocarditis

270 INFECTIVE ENDOCARDITIS, David T. Durack 1586

Staphylococcal Infections

271 STAPHYLOCOCCAL INFECTIONS, John N. Sheagren 1596

Bacterial Meningitis, Morton N. Swartz

272 BACTERIAL MENINGITIS 1604
273 MENINGOCOCCAL DISEASE 1611
274 INFECTIONS CAUSED BY HEMOPHILUS SPECIES 1617

Osteomyelitis

275 OSTEOMYELITIS, Francis A. Waldvogel 1622

Whooping Cough

276 WHOOPING COUGH (PERTUSSIS), Samuel L. Katz 1624

Diphtheria

277 DIPHTHERIA, Erik L. Hewlett 1626

Clostridial Diseases, John G. Bartlett

278 CLOSTRIDIAL MYONECROSIS AND OTHER CLOSTRIDIAL DISEASES 1629
279 PSEUDOMEMBRANOUS COLITIS 1632
280 BOTULISM 1633
281 TETANUS 1634

Anaerobic Bacteria

282 DISEASES CAUSED BY NON–SPORE-FORMING ANAEROBIC BACTERIA,
    Sherwood L. Gorbach 1637

Enteric Infections

283 TYPHOID FEVER, Thomas Butler 1641
284 SALMONELLA INFECTIONS OTHER THAN TYPHOID FEVER,
    Richard B. Hornick 1643
285 SHIGELLOSIS, Thomas Butler 1646
286 CAMPYLOBACTER ENTERITIS, Richard L. Guerrant 1648
287 CHOLERA (ASIATIC CHOLERA), Nathaniel F. Pierce 1651
288 ENTERIC ESCHERICHIA COLI INFECTIONS,
    Richard L. Guerrant 1653
289 THE DIARRHEA OF TRAVELERS, R. Bradley Sack 1656

Other Bacterial Infections

290 EXTRAINTESTINAL INFECTIONS CAUSED BY ENTERIC BACTERIA,
    Elizabeth J. Ziegler 1658
291 YERSINIA INFECTIONS, Thomas Butler 1661
292 TULAREMIA, Richard B. Hornick 1664
293 ANTHRAX, Philip S. Brachman 1667
294 DISEASES CAUSED BY PSEUDOMONADS, Michael Barza 1669
295 LISTERIOSIS, Michael Barza 1670
296 ERYSIPELOID, Michael Barza 1673
297 ACTINOMYCOSIS, David J. Drutz 1673
298 NOCARDIOSIS, David J. Drutz 1675
299 BRUCELLOSIS, Robert A. Salata 1676
300 CAT SCRATCH DISEASE, Andrew M. Margileth 1679
301 BARTONELLOSIS, Theodore C. Eickhoff 1681

Diseases Due to Mycobacteria

302 TUBERCULOSIS, Emanuel Wolinsky 1682
303 OTHER MYCOBACTERIOSES, Emanuel Wolinsky 1693
304 LEPROSY (HANSEN'S DISEASE), Ward E. Bullock 1696

Sexually Transmitted Diseases, P. Frederick Sparling

305 INTRODUCTION AND COMMON SYNDROMES 1701
306 GONOCOCCAL INFECTIONS 1706
307 LYMPHOGRANULOMA VENEREUM 1710
308 GRANULOMA INGUINALE (DONOVANOSIS) 1711
309 CHANCROID 1712
310 SYPHILIS 1713

Spirochetal Diseases Other Than Syphilis

311 NONSYPHILITIC TREPONEMATOSES, Thomas Butler 1723
312 RELAPSING FEVER, Thomas Butler 1724
313 LYME DISEASE, Stephen E. Malawista 1726

314 RAT-BITE FEVERS, J. Bruce McClain 1729
315 LEPTOSPIROSIS, J. Bruce McClain 1730

Diseases Caused by Chlamydiae, Walter E. Stamm

316 INTRODUCTION 1732
317 TRACHOMA 1734
318 NEONATAL CHLAMYDIAL INFECTIONS 1735
319 PSITTACOSIS AND RELATED INFECTIONS 1735

Rickettsial Diseases

320 INTRODUCTION, Richard B. Hornick 1737
321 THE TYPHUS GROUP, Richard B. Hornick 1738
322 ROCKY MOUNTAIN SPOTTED FEVER, Richard B. Hornick 1742
323 OTHER TICK-BORNE RICKETTSIOSES, Richard B. Hornick 1745
324 RICKETTSIALPOX, Richard B. Hornick 1745
325 SCRUB TYPHUS, Richard B. Hornick 1746
326 TRENCH FEVER, Theodore C. Eickhoff 1747
327 Q FEVER, Theodore C. Eickhoff 1748

Section 3 Viral Diseases

328 INTRODUCTION TO VIRAL DISEASES, R. Gordon Douglas, Jr. 1750

Viral Infections of the Respiratory Tract

329 THE COMMON COLD, Albert Z. Kapikian 1753
330 VIRAL PHARYNGITIS, LARYNGITIS, CROUP, AND BRONCHITIS,
    Maurice A. Mufson 1757
331 RESPIRATORY SYNCYTIAL VIRUS, Robert M. Chanock 1758
332 PARAINFLUENZA VIRAL DISEASES, Robert M. Chanock 1760
333 INFLUENZA, R. Gordon Douglas, Jr. 1762
334 ADENOVIRUS DISEASES, Stephen G. Baum 1767

Viral Disease of the Gastrointestinal Tract

335 VIRAL GASTROENTERITIS, Albert Z. Kapikian 1768

Viral Infections Caused by Cutaneous Lesions

336 MEASLES (MORBILLI, RUBEOLA), Samuel L. Katz 1772
337 RUBELLA (GERMAN MEASLES), Samuel L. Katz 1776
338 FOOT AND MOUTH DISEASE, Catherine M. Wilfert 1778
339 MUMPS, Catherine M. Wilfert 1778

Diseases Characterized by Herpes-Type Viruses

340 HERPES SIMPLEX VIRUS INFECTIONS, R. Gordon Douglas, Jr. ... 1780
341 CYTOMEGALOVIRUS INFECTION, David J. Lang 1784
342 INFECTIOUS MONONUCLEOSIS: EPSTEIN-BARR VIRUS INFECTION,
    Elliott Kieff 1786
343 VARICELLA, Philip A. Brunell 1788
344 VARIOLA AND VACCINIA, Donald A. Henderson 1791

Diseases Caused by Retroviruses

345 RETROVIRUSES THAT CAUSE HUMAN DISEASE, Robert C. Gallo 1794
346 THE ACQUIRED IMMUNODEFICIENCY SYNDROME,
    Jerome E. Groopman 1799

Enteroviral Diseases, Raphael Dolin

347 INTRODUCTION 1808
348 EPIDEMIC PLEURODYNIA 1810
349 MYOCARDITIS AND PERICARDITIS CAUSED BY ENTEROVIRUSES 1811
350 MUCOCUTANEOUS INFECTIONS CAUSED BY ENTEROVIRUSES 1813
351 ACUTE HEMORRHAGIC CONJUNCTIVITIS 1814

Arthropod-Borne Viral Fevers

352 INTRODUCTION, Robert E. Shope 1814

Undifferentiated Fevers

353 DENGUE, Robert B. Tesh 1816
354 WEST NILE FEVER, Robert B. Tesh 1817
355 PHLEBOTOMUS FEVER, Robert B. Tesh 1817
356 RIFT VALLEY FEVER, Robert B. Tesh 1818
357 FEVERS CAUSED BY ALPHAVIRUSES: CHIKUNGUNYA, O'NYONG-NYONG,
    MAYARO, ROSS RIVER, AND OCKELBO, Robert B. Tesh 1819
358 COLORADO TICK FEVER, Theodore C. Eickhoff 1819

Encephalitides

359 ARTHROPOD-BORNE VIRAL ENCEPHALITIDES, Thomas P. Monath 1821

Viral Hemorrhagic Fevers, Robert E. Shope

360 INTRODUCTION 1829
361 YELLOW FEVER 1830
362 HEMORRHAGIC FEVER CAUSED BY DENGUE VIRUSES 1832
363 TICK-BORNE FLAVIVIRUS DISEASES: KYASANUR FOREST DISEASE AND
    OMSK HEMORRHAGIC FEVER 1833
364 CRIMEAN-CONGO HEMORRHAGIC FEVER 1834

365 HEMORRHAGIC DISEASES CAUSED BY ARENAVIRUSES (ARGENTINE AND
     BOLIVIAN HEMORRHAGIC FEVERS AND LASSA FEVER) 1834
366 AFRICAN HEMORRHAGIC FEVER (MARBURG-EBOLA DISEASE) 1835
367 HEMORRHAGIC FEVER WITH RENAL SYNDROME 1836

Section 4 The Mycoses, David J. Drutz
368 INTRODUCTION 1837
369 HISTOPLASMOSIS 1838
370 COCCIDIOIDOMYCOSIS 1840
371 BLASTOMYCOSIS 1842
372 PARACOCCIDIOIDOMYCOSIS 1843
373 CRYPTOCOCCOSIS 1844
374 SPOROTRICHOSIS 1846
375 CANDIDIASIS (CANDIDOSIS) 1847
376 ASPERGILLOSIS 1850
377 ZYGOMYCOSIS (MUCORMYCOSIS) 1852
378 MYCETOMA (MADUROMYCOSIS) 1853
379 INFECTIONS DUE TO DEMATIACEOUS FUNGI 1854

PART XIX DISEASES CAUSED BY PROTOZOA AND METAZOA

380 INTRODUCTION TO PROTOZOAN AND HELMINTHIC DISEASES,
     Adel A. F. Mahmoud 1856

Section 1 Protozoan Diseases
381 MALARIA, Louis H. Miller 1857
382 AFRICAN TRYPANOSOMIASIS (SLEEPING SICKNESS),
     Thomas C. Quinn 1862
383 AMERICAN TRYPANOSOMIASIS (CHAGAS' DISEASE),
     Franklin A. Neva 1865
384 LEISHMANIASIS, Franklin A. Neva 1869
385 TOXOPLASMOSIS, Henry Masur 1875
386 PNEUMOCYSTOSIS, Henry Masur 1879
387 CRYPTOSPORIDIOSIS, Rosemary Soave 1881
388 GIARDIASIS, David P. Stevens 1883
389 BABESIOSIS, Morton N. Swartz 1884
390 AMEBIASIS, Donald J. Krogstad 1886
391 OTHER PROTOZOAN DISEASES, David P. Stevens 1888

Section 2 Helminthic Diseases

The Cestodes, Martin S. Wolfe
392 INTRODUCTION 1890
393 DIPHYLLOBOTHRIUM LATUM (THE FISH TAPEWORM) 1890
394 TAENIA SAGINATA (THE BEEF TAPEWORM) 1891
395 TAENIA SOLIUM (THE PORK TAPEWORM; HUMAN CYSTICERCOSIS) . 1892
396 HYMENOLEPIS NANA (THE DWARF TAPEWORM) 1893
397 ECHINOCOCCOSIS (HYDATID DISEASE) 1893
398 OTHER, RARER TAPEWORMS 1894
399 TREATMENT OF TAPEWORM INFECTIONS 1894

The Trematodes
400 SCHISTOSOMIASIS (BILHARZIASIS), Adel A. F. Mahmoud 1895
401 HERMAPHRODITIC FLUKES, S. K. K. Seah 1901

The Nematodes
402 INTRODUCTION, Daniel S. Blumenthal 1905

Intestinal Nematodes, Daniel S. Blumenthal
403 STRONGYLOIDIASIS 1905
404 HOOKWORM DISEASE 1906
405 CUTANEOUS LARVA MIGRANS 1907
406 ASCARIASIS 1908
407 TOXOCARIASIS 1908
408 TRICHURIASIS 1909
409 ENTEROBIASIS 1910
410 OTHER ANIMAL NEMATODIASES 1910

Tissue Nematodes
411 TRICHINELLOSIS (TRICHINOSIS), Donald W. Hoskins 1911
412 ANGIOSTRONGYLIASIS, Daniel S. Blumenthal 1913
413 FILARIASIS 1913
     413.1 INTRODUCTION, Eric A. Ottesen 1913
     413.2 LYMPHATIC FILARIASIS, Eric A. Ottesen 1914
     413.3 TROPICAL EOSINOPHILIA, Eric A. Ottesen 1916
     413.4 ONCHOCERCIASIS (RIVER BLINDNESS), Bruce M. Greene 1916
     413.5 LOIASIS, Eric A. Ottesen 1918
     413.6 DRACUNCULIASIS, Donald R. Hopkins 1918
     413.7 OTHER FILARIAL INFECTIONS, Eric A. Ottesen 1919

Section 3 Arthropods and Animal Poisons
414 ARTHROPODS AND LEECHES, William L. Krinsky 1920
415 SNAKE BITES, Jay P. Sanford 1927
416 VENOMOUS AND POISONOUS MARINE ANIMALS, John Williamson 1929

PART XX DISEASES OF THE IMMUNE SYSTEM

417 THE IMMUNE SYSTEM: INTRODUCTION, William E. Paul 1932
418 COMPLEMENT, Douglas T. Fearon 1938
419 PRIMARY IMMUNODEFICIENCY DISEASES, Rebecca H. Buckley .. 1941
420 URTICARIA AND ANGIOEDEMA, Nicholas A. Soter 1948
421 ALLERGIC RHINITIS, John E. Salvaggio 1951
422 ANAPHYLAXIS, Lawrence M. Lichtenstein 1956
423 INSECT STING ALLERGY, Lawrence M. Lichtenstein 1958
424 IMMUNE COMPLEX DISEASES, Charles G. Cochrane 1960
425 THE MAJOR HISTOCOMPATIBILITY COMPLEX AND DISEASE
     SUSCEPTIBILITY, Benjamin D. Schwartz 1962
426 DRUG ALLERGY, Charles E. Reed 1968
427 MASTOCYTOSIS, Robert A. Lewis 1972
428 DISEASES OF THE THYMUS, Daniel P. Stites 1974

PART XXI MUSCULOSKELETAL AND CONNECTIVE TISSUE DISEASES

429 APPROACH TO THE PATIENT WITH MUSCULOSKELETAL DISEASE,
     James F. Fries 1977
430 CONNECTIVE TISSUE STRUCTURE AND FUNCTION, Stephen M. Krane .. 1980
431 MECHANISMS OF INFLAMMATION AND TISSUE DESTRUCTION
     IN THE RHEUMATIC DISEASES, Ralph Snyderman 1984
432 SPECIALIZED DIAGNOSTIC PROCEDURES IN THE RHEUMATIC DISEASES,
     Alan S. Cohen 1993
433 RHEUMATOID ARTHRITIS, J. Claude Bennett 1998
434 THE SPONDYLOARTHROPATHIES, Andrei Calin 2004
435 INFECTIOUS ARTHRITIS, Stephen E. Malawista 2009
436 SYSTEMIC LUPUS ERYTHEMATOSUS, Alfred D. Steinberg 2011
437 SYSTEMIC SCLEROSIS (SCLERODERMA), E. Carwile LeRoy ... 2018
438 SJOGREN'S SYNDROME, Norman Talal 2024
439 THE VASCULITIC SYNDROMES, Sheldon M. Wolff 2025
440 POLYARTERITIS NODOSA GROUP, Sheldon M. Wolff 2028
441 WEGENER'S GRANULOMATOSIS AND MIDLINE GRANULOMA,
     Barton F. Haynes 2030
442 POLYMYALGIA RHEUMATICA AND GIANT CELL ARTERITIS,
     Louis A. Healey 2033
443 POLYMYOSITIS, Ronald P. Messner 2034
444 CALCIUM CRYSTAL DEPOSITION ARTHROPATHIES,
     H. Ralph Schumacher, Jr. 2037
445 RELAPSING POLYCHONDRITIS, H. Ralph Schumacher, Jr. ... 2038
446 OSTEOARTHRITIS (DEGENERATIVE JOINT DISEASE), David S. Howell ... 2039
447 THE PAINFUL SHOULDER, David S. Howell 2041
448 THE PAINFUL BACK, David S. Howell 2043
449 DISEASES WITH WHICH ARTHRITIS IS FREQUENTLY ASSOCIATED,
     Giles G. Bole 2045
450 MISCELLANEOUS FORMS OF ARTHRITIS, Giles G. Bole 2046
451 NONARTICULAR RHEUMATISM, Giles G. Bole 2047
452 SYNOVIAL TUMORS, Giles G. Bole 2048
453 BEHCET'S DISEASE, Ralph Snyderman 2048
454 PANNICULITIS AND DISORDERS OF THE SUBCUTANEOUS FAT,
     Gerald S. Lazarus 2050
455 MULTIFOCAL FIBROSCLEROSIS, H. Ralph Schumacher, Jr., . 2051

PART XXII NEUROLOGIC AND BEHAVIORAL DISEASES

Section 1 Clinical Study of the Patient with Neurologic
          Symptoms
456 CLINICAL STUDY OF THE PATIENT 2053
     456.1 APPROACH TO THE PATIENT, Fred Plum 2053
     456.2 NEUROLOGIC DIAGNOSTIC PROCEDURES, Samuel Rapoport ... 2056
     456.3 RADIOLOGIC IMAGING TECHNIQUES IN THE DIAGNOSIS AND CARE
            OF THE NEUROLOGIC PATIENT, Michael Deck 2058

Section 2 Disorders of Cerebral Function
457 DISORDERS OF CONSCIOUSNESS AND AROUSAL, Fred Plum and
     Jerome Posner 2061

458 SLEEP AND ITS DISORDERS, *J. Allan Hobson* 2077
459 REGIONAL DIAGNOSIS OF CEREBRAL DISORDERS,
    Antonio R. Damasio 2080
460 FOCAL DISTURBANCES OF HIGHER FUNCTION,
    Antonio R. Damasio 2083
461 THE DEMENTIAS, *Fred Plum* 2087
462 PSYCHIATRIC DISORDERS IN MEDICAL PRACTICE, *Gary J. Tucker* 2091

Section 3 Pathophysiology and Management of Major Neurologic Symptoms

463 AUTONOMIC DISORDERS AND THEIR MANAGEMENT, *Fred Plum* 2103
464 THE SPECIAL SENSES, *Robert W. Baloh* 2109
465 DISORDERS OF MOTOR FUNCTION 2124
    465.1 ASTHENIA, FATIGUE, AND WEAKNESS, *Fred Plum* 2124
    465.2 ATAXIA AND RELATED GAIT DISORDERS, *Fred Plum* 2125
    465.3 EPISODIC LOSS OF MOTOR FUNCTION, *Jerome B. Posner* 2127
466 DISORDERS OF SENSATION, *Jerome B. Posner* 2128

Section 4 Alcohol and Nutritional Complications

467 NUTRITIONAL DISORDERS OF THE NERVOUS SYSTEM, *Ivan Diamond* ... 2137

Section 5 The Extrapyramidal Disorders, *Stanley Fahn*

468 PARKINSONISM 2143
469 ESSENTIAL TREMOR (FAMILIAL OR SENILE TREMOR) 2147
470 THE CHOREAS 2147
471 THE DYSTONIAS 2149
472 OTHER EXTRAPYRAMIDAL DISORDERS 2151

Section 6 Degenerative Diseases of the Nervous System, *Robert B. Layzer*

473 HEREDITARY CEREBELLAR ATAXIAS AND RELATED DISORDERS 2152
474 HEREDITARY SPASTIC PARAPLEGIAS 2154
475 HEREDITARY AND ACQUIRED INTRINSIC MOTOR NEURON DISEASES 2154
476 SYRINGOMYELIA 2157
477 THE PHAKOMATOSES 2158

Section 7 Cerebrovascular Diseases

478 INTRODUCTION, *H. J. M. Barnett and Irene Meissner* 2159
479 CEREBRAL ISCHEMIA AND INFARCTION, *H. J. M. Barnett* 2162
480 SPONTANEOUS INTRACRANIAL HEMORRHAGE, *H. J. M. Barnett* 2173

Section 8 Infectious and Inflammatory Disorders of the Nervous System

481 PARAMENINGEAL INFECTIONS, *Donald H. Harter* 2181
482 SYPHILITIC INFECTIONS OF THE CENTRAL NERVOUS SYSTEM,
    Kenneth P. Johnson 2187

Section 9 Viral Infections of the Nervous System

483 INTRODUCTION, *Richard W. Price* 2191
484 ACUTE VIRAL MENINGITIS AND ENCEPHALITIS, *Richard W. Price* 2192
485 HERPES VIRUS INFECTIONS OF THE NERVOUS SYSTEM,
    Richard W. Price 2195
486 POLIOMYELITIS, *Richard W. Price* 2198
487 RABIES, *Daniel B. Fishbein and George M. Baer* 2200
488 SLOW VIRUS INFECTIONS OF THE NERVOUS SYSTEM 2203
    488.1 INTRODUCTION, *Richard W. Price* 2203
    488.2 AIDS DEMENTIA AND HUMAN IMMUNODEFICIENCY VIRUS
          BRAIN INFECTION, *Richard W. Price* 2203
    488.3 CREUTZFELDT-JAKOB DISEASE, *Paul E. Bendheim* 2205
    488.4 SUBACUTE SCLEROSING PANENCEPHALITIS,
          Jerry S. Wolinsky 2206
    488.5 PROGRESSIVE MULTIFOCAL LEUKOENCEPHALOPATHY,
          Richard W. Price 2207

Section 10 Neurologic Disorders Associated with Altered Immunity or Unexplained Host-Parasite Alterations, *Jerry S. Wolinsky*

489 CENTRAL NERVOUS SYSTEM COMPLICATIONS OF VIRAL INFECTIONS
    AND VACCINES 2208
490 REYE SYNDROME 2209
491 NEUROLOGIC COMPLICATIONS IN THE IMMUNOLOGICALLY
    COMPROMISED HOST 2210

Section 11 The Demyelinating Diseases

492 THE DEMYELINATING DISEASES, *Donald H. Silberberg* 2211

Section 12 The Epilepsies

493 THE EPILEPSIES, *Jerome Engel, Jr.* 2217

Section 13 Intracranial Tumors and States of Altered Intracranial Pressure

494 INTRACRANIAL TUMORS, *William R. Shapiro* 2229
495 DISORDERS OF INTRACRANIAL PRESSURE, *David A. Rottenberg* 2235

Section 14 Injury to the Head and Spine, *Donald P. Becker*

496 HEAD INJURIES 2239
497 INJURIES TO THE SPINE 2244

Section 15 Mechanical Lesions of the Spine and Related Structures, *Jerome B. Posner*

498 ANATOMY, PHYSIOLOGY, AND DIFFERENTIAL DIAGNOSIS 2247
499 INTERVERTEBRAL DISC DISEASE 2252
500 NEOPLASMS OF THE SPINAL CANAL 2254
501 INFLAMMATORY DISEASES OF THE SPINAL CANAL 2256
502 VASCULAR DISORDERS OF THE SPINAL CANAL 2257
503 CONGENITAL ANOMALIES OF THE CRANIOVERTEBRAL JUNCTION, SPINE,
    AND SPINAL CORD 2257

Section 16 Diseases of the Peripheral Nervous System, *Herbert H. Schaumburg*

504 INTRODUCTION AND BASIC TERMINOLOGY 2258
505 ANATOMIC CLASSIFICATION OF NEUROPATHY 2259
506 INFLAMMATORY POLYNEUROPATHY (GUILLAIN-BARRE SYNDROME AND
    RELATED DISORDERS) 2260
507 NEUROPATHY ASSOCIATED WITH ENDOCRINE DISEASES 2262
508 HEREDITARY NEUROPATHIES 2264
509 TOXIC NEUROPATHIES 2265
510 MISCELLANEOUS DISEASE-SPECIFIC NEUROPATHIES 2266
511 ACUTE PHYSICAL INJURY AND CHRONIC COMPRESSION-ENTRAPMENT
    NEUROPATHIES 2267

Section 17 Diseases of Muscle (Myopathies) and Neuromuscular Junction, *Andrew G. Engel*

512 GENERAL APPROACH TO MUSCLE DISEASES 2269
513 MUSCULAR DYSTROPHIES 2272
514 MORPHOLOGICALLY DISTINCT CONGENITAL MYOPATHIES 2275
515 INFLAMMATORY MYOPATHIES 2276
516 METABOLIC MYOPATHIES 2277
517 MISCELLANEOUS MYOPATHIES 2283
518 DISORDERS OF NEUROMUSCULAR TRANSMISSION 2284

PART XXIII EYE DISEASES, *John W. Gittinger, Jr.*

519 TRANSIENT VISUAL LOSS 2289
520 CATARACT 2289
521 GLAUCOMA 2290
522 DISC SWELLING AND OPTIC ATROPHY 2292
523 UVEITIS 2293
524 OCULAR INFECTIONS 2294
525 ORBITAL DISEASE AND TUMORS 2295
526 INTRAOCULAR TUMORS 2295
527 EPISCLERITIS, SCLERITIS, AND THE DRY EYE 2296
528 OCULAR VASCULAR DISEASE 2296
529 THE EYE AND MEDICATIONS 2298

PART XXIV SKIN DISEASES, *Frank Parker*

530 INTRODUCTION 2300
531 THE STRUCTURE AND FUNCTION OF SKIN 2300
532 EXAMINATION OF THE SKIN AND AN APPROACH TO DIAGNOSING
    SKIN DISEASES 2306
533 PRINCIPLES OF THERAPY 2314
534 SKIN DISEASES OF GENERAL IMPORTANCE 2318

PART XXV OCCUPATIONAL AND ENVIRONMENTAL MEDICINE

535 PRINCIPLES OF OCCUPATIONAL MEDICINE, *Charles E. Becker* 2354
536 OCCUPATIONAL PULMONARY DISORDERS, *Dean Sheppard* 2356
537 PHYSICAL, CHEMICAL, AND ASPIRATION INJURIES OF THE LUNG,
    James D. Crapo 2365
538 OCCUPATIONAL DISEASES OF THE SKIN, *Edward A. Emmett* 2373
539 RADIATION INJURY, *Theodore L. Phillips* 2375
540 ELECTRIC INJURY, *Basil A. Pruitt, Jr.* 2380
541 DISORDERS DUE TO HEAT AND COLD, *James P. Knochel* 2382
542 TRACE METAL POISONING, *Donald B. Louria* 2385

PART XXVI LABORATORY REFERENCE RANGE VALUES OF CLINICAL IMPORTANCE

543 REFERENCE INTERVALS AND LABORATORY VALUES OF CLINICAL
    IMPORTANCE, *Ronald J. Elin* 2394
    INDEX i

COLOR PLATES

PLATE 1   DIABETES MELLITUS (Part XVI, pages 1360–1381)

PLATE 2   HEMATOLOGIC DISEASES (Part XII, pages 873–1081)

PLATE 3   HEMATOLOGIC DISEASES (Part XII, pages 873–1081)

PLATE 4   LYME DISEASE (Part XVIII, pages 1726–1729)

PLATE 5   PROTOZOAN DISEASES (Part XIX, pages 1857–1890)

PLATE 6   SKIN DISEASES (Part XXIV, pages 2300–2353)

PLATE 7   EYE DISEASES (Part XXIII, pages 2289–2299)

PLATE 8   DISORDERS OF VITAMIN METABOLISM (Part XV, pages 1228–1241)

PLATE 1 DIABETES MELLITUS

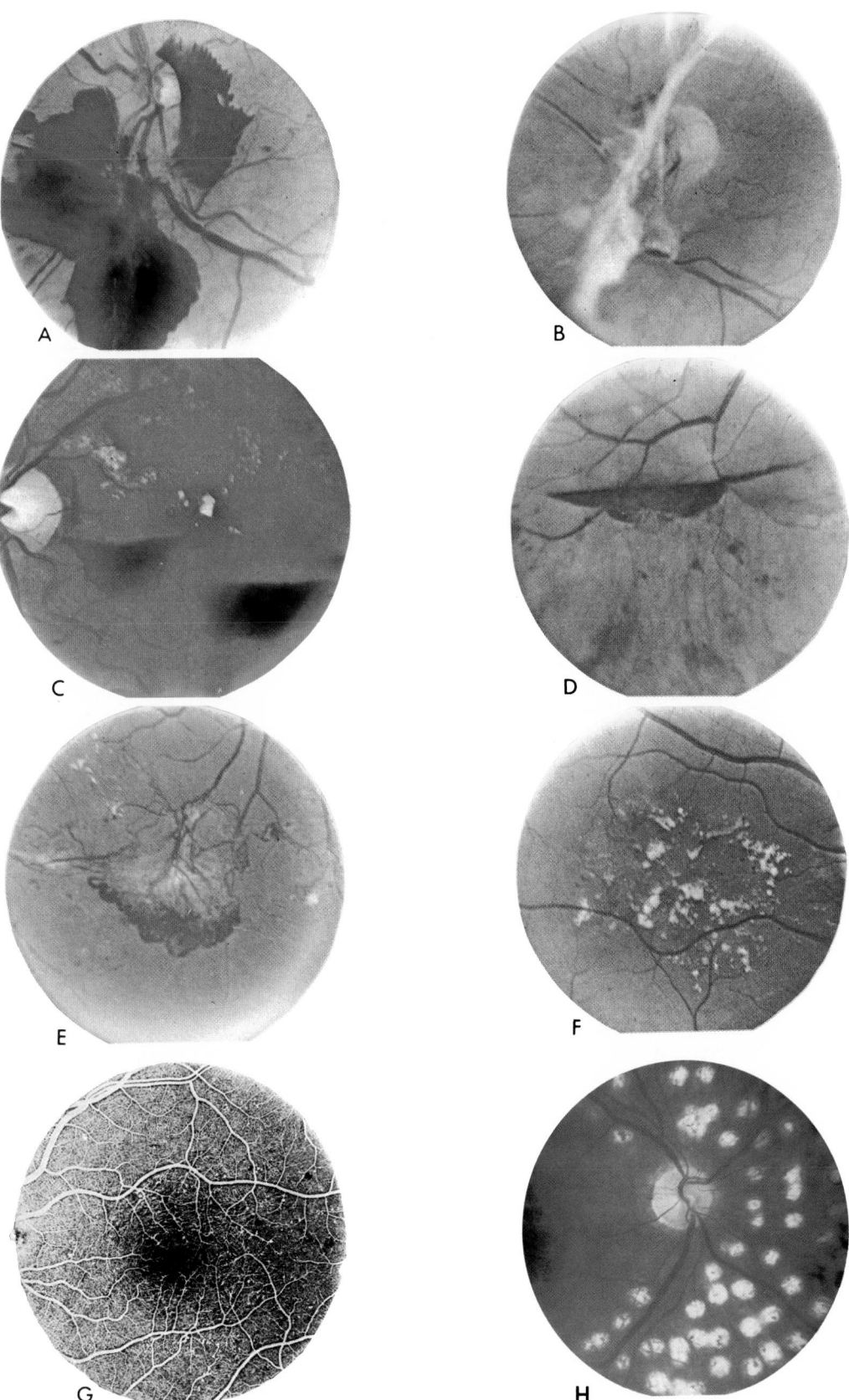

A, Vitreous and preretinal hemorrhage from the disc area secondary to disc neovascularization.

B, Fibrous band resulting from going into a quiescent stage of retinopathy one year after slide *A* was taken. Patient maintained quiescent stage for eight years until he died a cardiac death.

C, Preretinal hemorrhages in region of macula which also has exudates and superficial hemorrhages. Note boat-shaped dependency type of hemorrhage.

D, Preretinal hemorrhage at site of frond of neovascularization. Note the new vessel fan underneath the boat-shaped preretinal hemorrhage. It is these new vessels which rupture spontaneously or with minimal stress.

E, Extensive fan of new vessels with fibrous network elevated forward into vitreous. Feeding vessels come from multiple arteries and veins at the retinal level, the entire process being analogous to an angioma.

F, Characteristic waxy exudates in macular zone accounting for decrease in vision, apparently due to incompetent capillaries and leaking from central areas of rings of waxy exudates where the red blotches are noted.

G, Fluorescein angiography in a diabetic, showing some very fine microaneurysms and some tiny areas of capillary closure but with good parafoveal network of vessels and 20/20 vision. These are early changes of diabetic retinopathy probably not seen on ophthalmoscopy. (Courtesy of Dr. L. Aiello.)

H, Photograph of retina following laser therapy, showing circumscribed areas of destruction and fibrous replacement. (Courtesy of Dr. M. B. Landers, III.)

PLATE 2   HEMATOLOGIC DISEASES

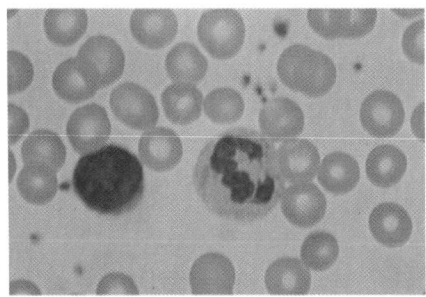

A, Normal peripheral blood smear showing an adult lymphocyte at the left, a mature segmented poly in the center, scattered platelets in the background, and normal appearing red blood cells. Note the normal central one-third pallor of the red cells ($\times$ 1200).

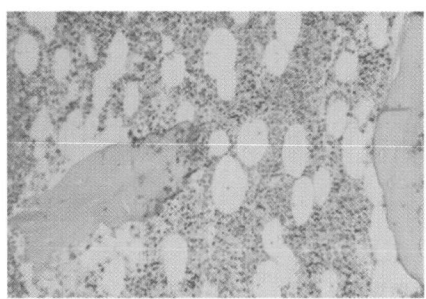

B, Normal bone marrow biopsy, low power. Note the normal fat content, about 50 per cent of the marrow. Normal hematopoietic cells are seen, including scattered megakaryocytes ($\times$ 100).

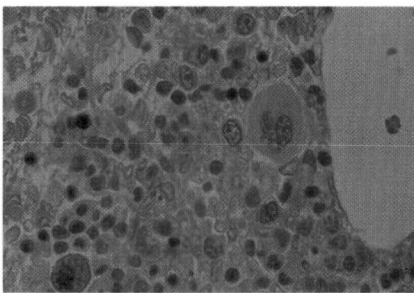

C, Normal bone marrow biopsy, high power. Note the detail of the background megakaryocytes, as well as scattered myeloid and erythroid cells in a ratio of approximately 3:1 ($\times$ 1000).

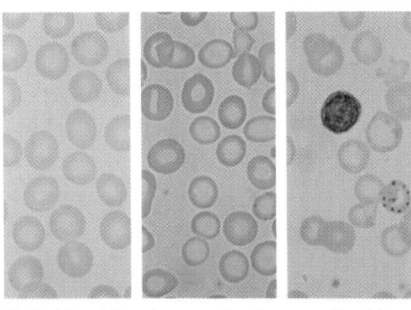

D, Peripheral blood smear showing normal red blood cells (left panel) compared with hypochromic cells of iron deficiency (central panel) or chronic lead poisoning (right panel). In the right panel note the prominent basophilic stippling. The cells are hypochromic as well as macrocytic ($\times$ 1200).

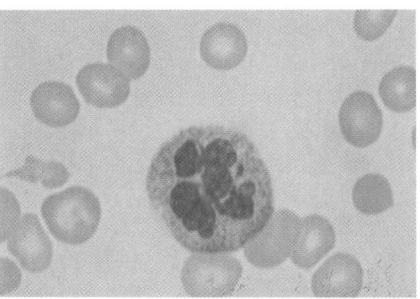

E, Peripheral blood smear showing a gigantic poly (macrocytic hypersegmented poly) in a patient with pernicious anemia. A few macrocytic red cells are noted, along with mild poikilocytes ($\times$ 1200).

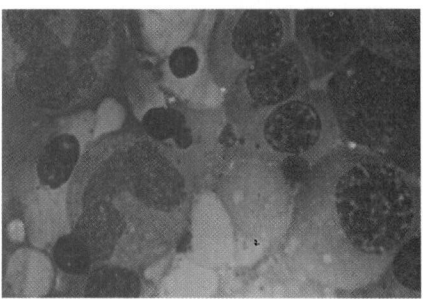

F, Marrow showing megaloblastic findings. Note the megaloblastic erythroid cells, characterized by maturation arrest. Nuclei have open chromatin while the cytoplasm shows early normal hemoglobinization. Several giant metamyelocytes are noted as well.

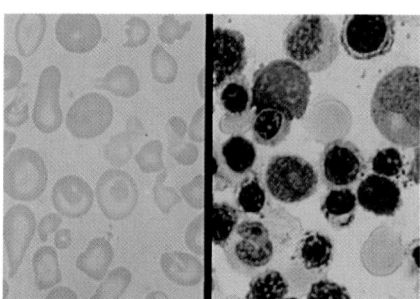

G, Thalassemia major showing marked anisocytosis, poikilocytosis, hypochromia, and target cell formation in the peripheral blood (left panel) and striking erythroid hyperplasia in the right panel, from the bone marrow ($\times$ 1200).

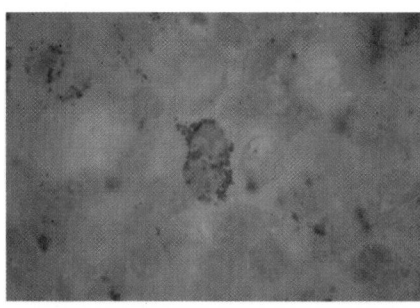

H, Bone marrow smear showing classic ringed sideroblasts. The normoblasts show clumps of iron (hemosiderin) surrounding the nucleus, resulting in a "ring." Physiologically, no more than two or three dots of iron are normally present. Prussian blue stain ($\times$ 1200).

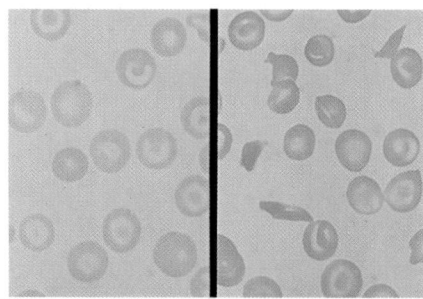

I, Peripheral blood smears from hemoglobin C trait (CA) (left panel) showing target cells and a few spherocytes, and hemoglobin S-C disease (right panel) showing sickled cells as well as target cells and other deformed red cells (x 1200).

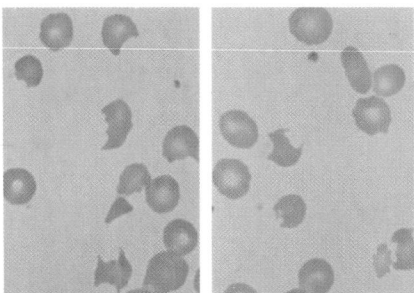

J, Peripheral blood smear from a patient with the hemolytic-uremic syndrome, showing striking schistocytes, also called helmet cells. Note the ragged and deformed red cells caused by rapid intravascular hemolysis due to physical factors ($\times$ 1200).

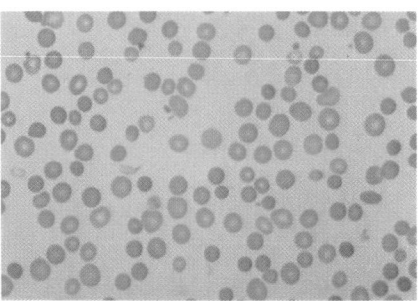

K, Peripheral blood smear from a patient with hereditary spherocytosis showing numerous spherocytes characterized by small size and dense hemoglobin stain. Scattered normal size red cells are also noted, along with occasional larger erythrocytes representing young cells (reticulocytes) ($\times$ 400).

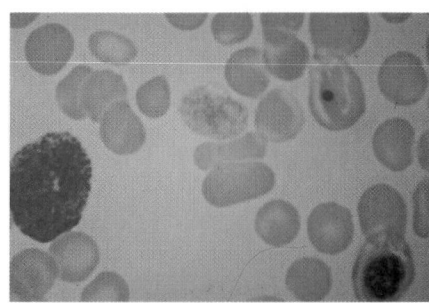

L, Peripheral blood smear showing a Howell-Jolly body in the erythrocyte in the right upper area of the slide. The round, dense granule represents nuclear DNA. At the lower right is a nucleated red cell. A giant platelet is present in the middle of the slide and a basophil is noted in the lower left corner. The patient had an underlying myeloproliferative disorder with a recent splenectomy ($\times$ 1200).

PLATE 3 HEMATOLOGIC DISEASES

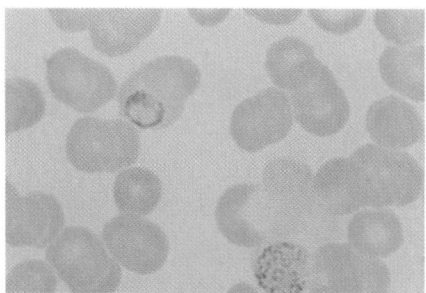

A, Peripheral blood showing malaria parasites within two red blood cells. Note the ringed form in the upper red cell and the numerous parasites in the lower red cell (× 1200).

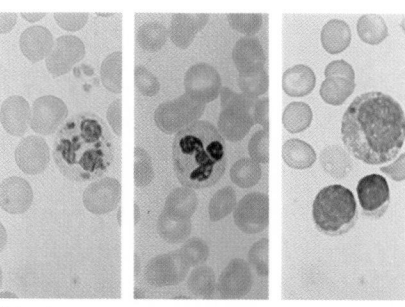

B, Leukocyte inclusions. *Left,* Giant basophilic granules in the Chediak-Higashi anomaly. *Center,* Basophilic inclusions (Döhle's bodies) within immature granulocytes. *Right,* Myelocyte with basophilic granules in Chediak-Higashi syndrome (× 1200).

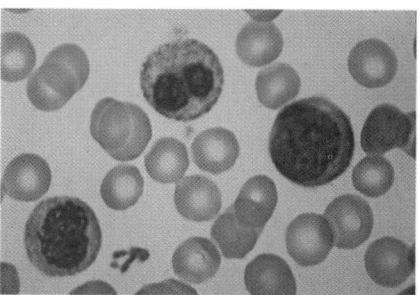

C, Pelger-Huët cells in the peripheral blood of a patient with chronic myeloid leukemia. Note the mature neutrophil in the center with an unsegmented adult poly in the lower left corner. A myeloblast is seen in the right of the slide (× 1200).

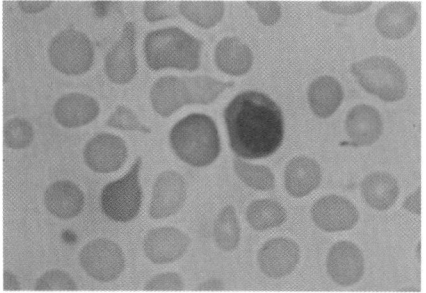

D, Peripheral blood smear showing leukoerythoblastic features, from a patient with myeloid metaplasia. Note the large nucleated red cell along with numerous tear drop–shaped red cells. Polychromatophilia is also present. Not seen in this slide are immature myeloid cells (× 1200).

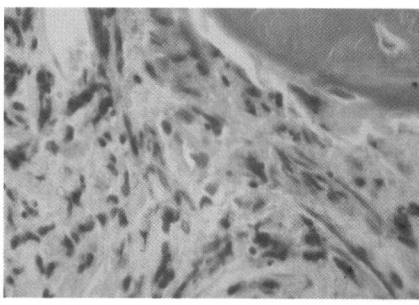

E, Myelofibrosis. Bone marrow biopsy showing intense fibrous tissue and primitive marrow reticulum cells replacing normal bone marrow elements (× 1000).

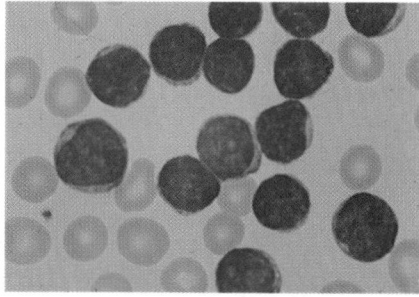

F, Chronic lymphocytic leukemia. Peripheral blood smear showing a majority of small mature-appearing lymphocytes, characterized by clumped nuclear chromatin and a rim of cytoplasm (× 1200).

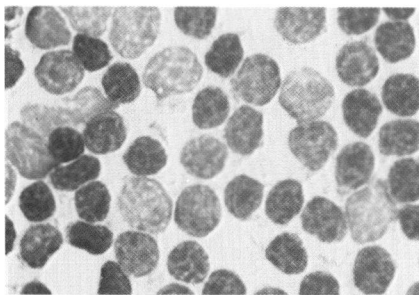

G, Bone marrow. Chronic lymphocytic leukemia showing dense infiltration by small mature-appearing lymphocytes with clumped chromatin and scanty cytoplasm (× 1200).

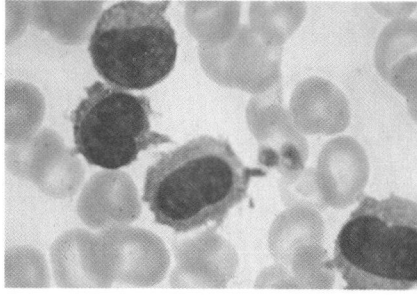

H, Hairy cell leukemia. Peripheral blood showing medium sized lymphoid cells with cytoplasmic strands or "hairs." Nuclei are somewhat immature (light staining) and indented in some of the cells. Indistinct nuclei are evident (× 1200).

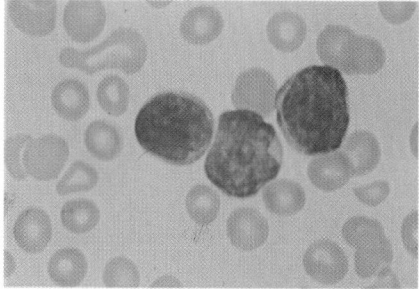

I, Acute lymphocytic leukemia. Peripheral blood showing three lymphoblasts, characterized by small size, immature light staining chromatin pattern, indistinct nuclei, and scanty cytoplasm (× 1200).

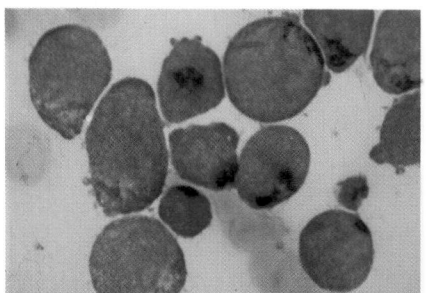

J, Acute myelogenous leukemia. Peroxidase stain showing marked positive activity in the majority of blasts, including the presence of Auer rods (× 1200).

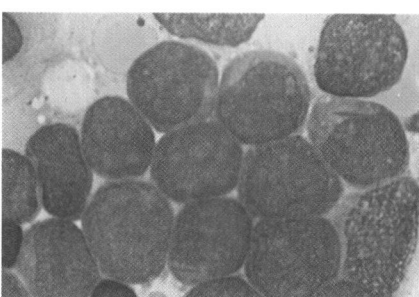

K, Acute myelogenous leukemia. Bone marrow, Giemsa stained, showing myeloblasts, some with prominent Auer rods (× 1200).

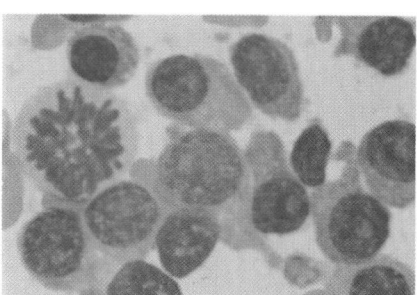

L, Multiple myeloma. Marrow shows a clump of immature plasma cells with eccentric nucleus, prominent nucleoli, and deep blue cytoplasm. A mitosis is present (× 1200).

PLATE 4   LYME DISEASE

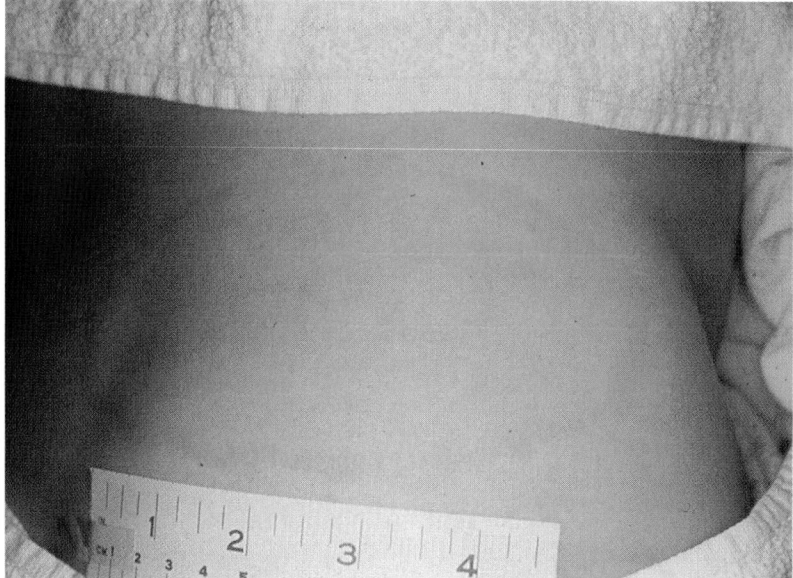

A

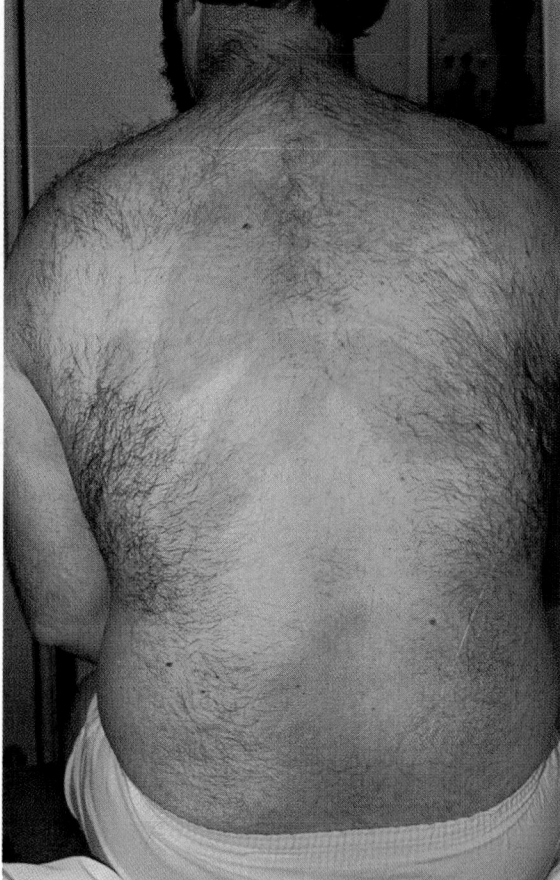

B

Major dermatologic manifestations of Lyme disease.
A, Erythema chronicum migrans (ECM). In a 17-day-old lesion, an
expanding red margin surrounds an area of central clearing. ECM
is the clinical hallmark of Lyme disease.
B, Four days after onset of ECM, this patient has developed secondary
annular lesions; some of their borders have merged. (From Steere
AC, Bartenhagen NH, Craft JE, et al.: The early clinical manifestations
of Lyme disease. Ann Intern Med 99:76–82, 1983.)

PLATE 5.   *See figure on the opposite page.*

A to D show various erythrocyte forms of falciparum or vivax malaria ($\times$ 1500).

A, "Ring forms" of *Plasmodium falciparum.* Note the delicate rings and an erythrocyte containing two organisms.

B, Trophozoite of *Plasmodium vivax.* The red cell is enlarged, Schüffner's dots are seen, and the parasite is large and ameboid.

C, Schizont of *Plasmodium vivax* with at least 18 merozoite nuclei.

D, Gametocyte of *Plasmodium falciparum.* The crescent or banana shape is characteristic.

E, *Trypanosoma rhodesiense* in the peripheral blood. It has a nucleus, posterior kinetoplast, undulating membrane, and flagellum ($\times$ 1500).

F, Spleen smear showing a cell filled with *Leishmania donovani.* The rod-shaped kinetoplast and large round nucleus appear as two adjacent red dots.

G, Methenamine silver nitrate stain of clump of *Pneumocystis* cysts. They appear as black circles against the blue background ($\times$ 800).

H, Stool sample observed by light microscopy, showing a motile *Entamoeba histolytica* moving in a straight line across the field. The ameba contains lucent vacuoles and shows a pseudopod directed to the upper right ($\times$ 500).

(A, C, D, and F are photographs taken by T. C. Jones from the Cornell Parasitology teaching slides; B is from the collection of H. Zaiman, originally photographed by M. Wittner; E and G were provided by R. B. Roberts; H is a photograph of fresh material provided by T. C. Jones.)

PLATE 5   PROTOZOAN DISEASES

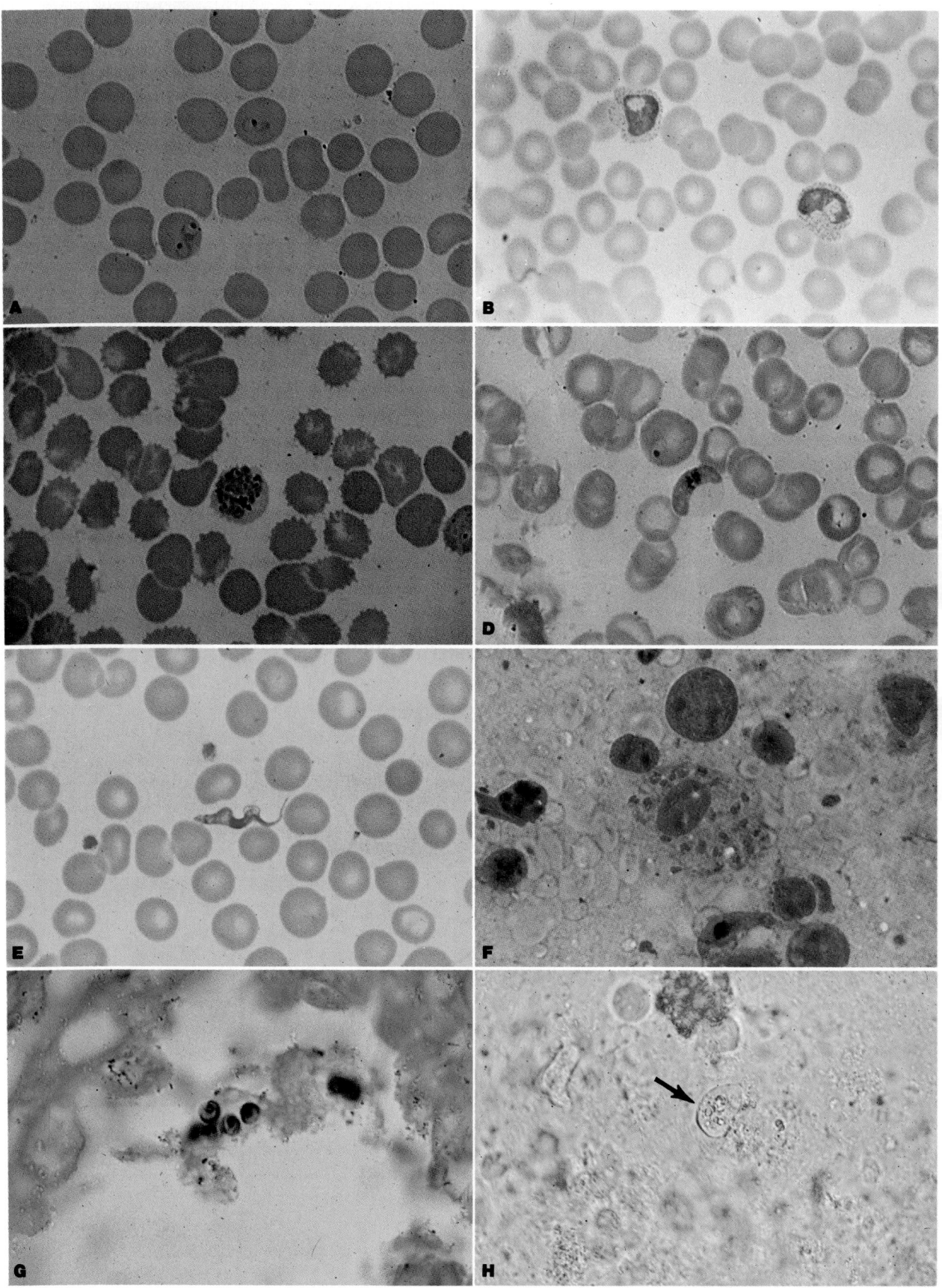

See legend on the opposite page.

PLATE 6   SKIN DISEASES

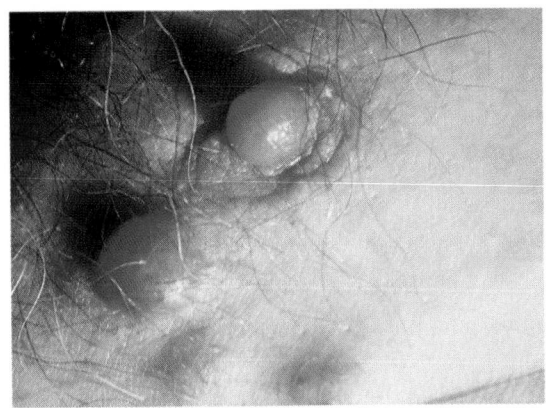

A, Skin metastases. Firm, hard, red nodules.

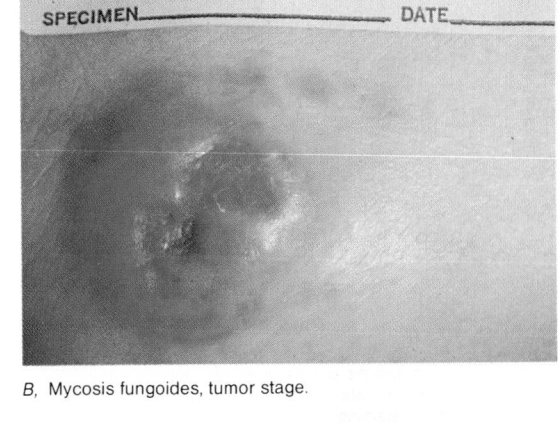

B, Mycosis fungoides, tumor stage.

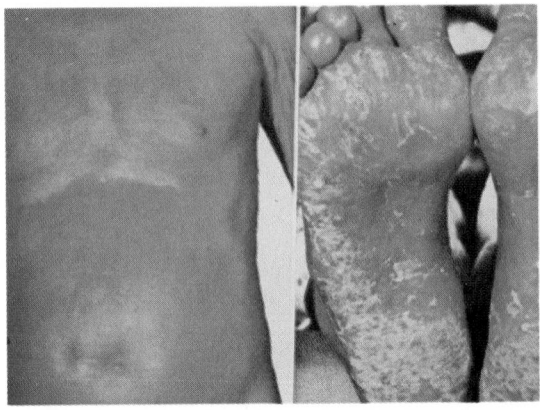

C, Sezary syndrome, exfoliative dermatitis stage.

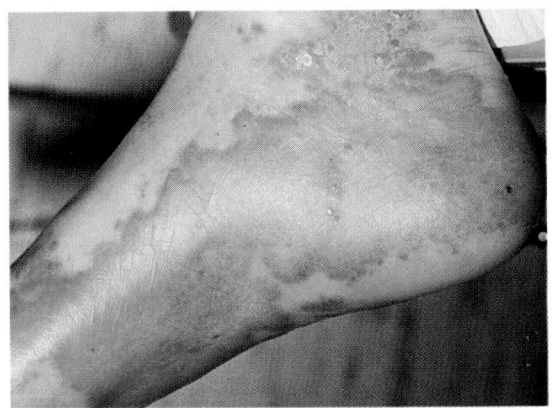

D, Classic Kaposi's sarcoma.

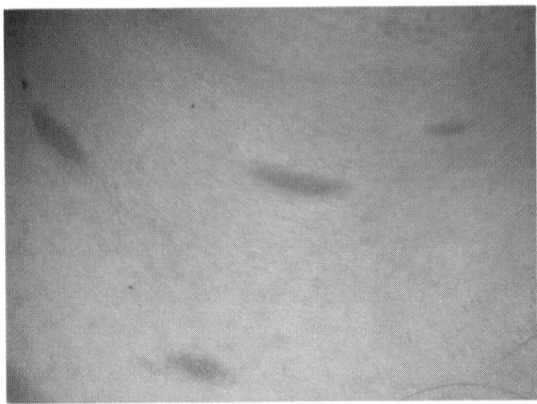

E, Kaposi's sarcoma in AIDS. Red-brown macules, papules, and nodules characteristically appear over the upper body.

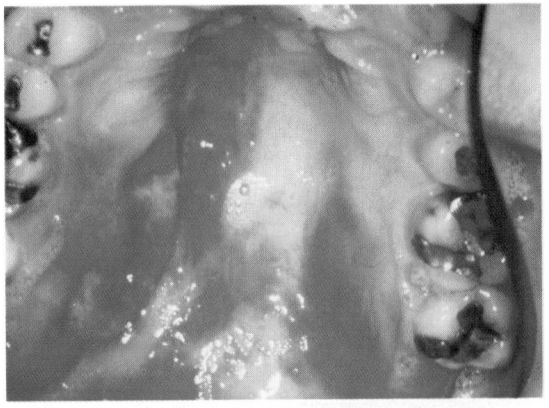

F, Kaposi's sarcoma in AIDS. Involvement of the oral mucosa.

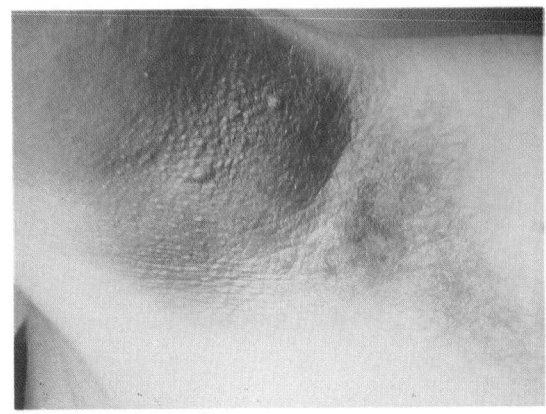

G, Acanthosis nigricans. Axillary lesion.

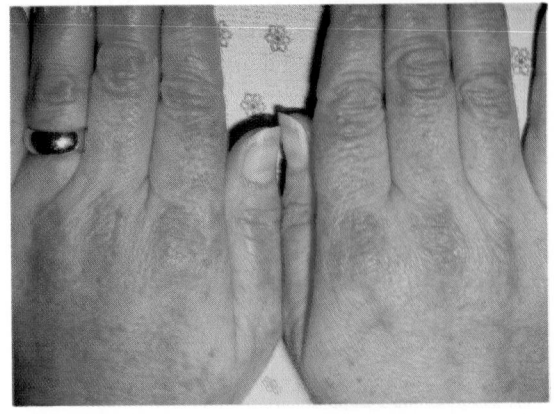

H, Dermatomyositis. Gottron's papules over the knuckles.

PLATE 7   EYE DISEASES

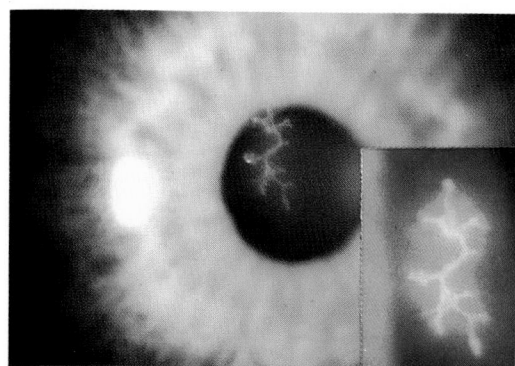

A, *Herpesvirus hominis* corneal epithelial dendrite in diffuse light and (inset) in light passed through a cobalt blue filter after fluorescein staining.

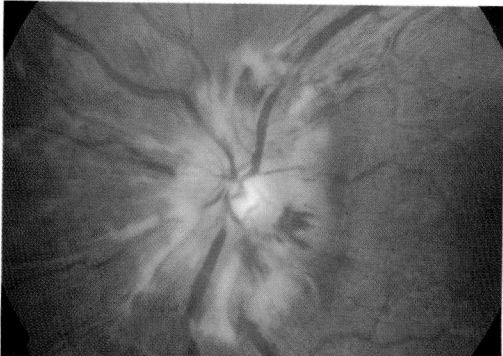

B, Papilledema in a young person. Note disc swelling, hemorrhages, and exudates with preservation of the physiologic cup.

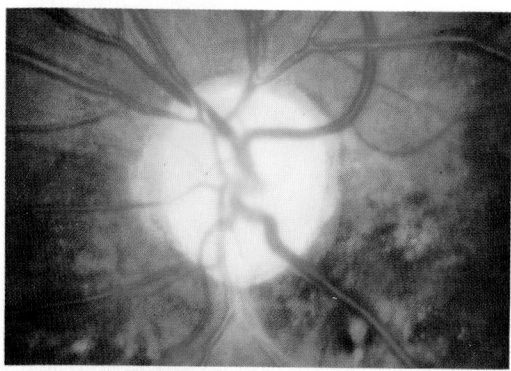

C, Primary optic atrophy in a young black man. The disc is pale, but there is no cupping or gliosis. The glial tissue seen over an inferior arteriole is a normal variant.

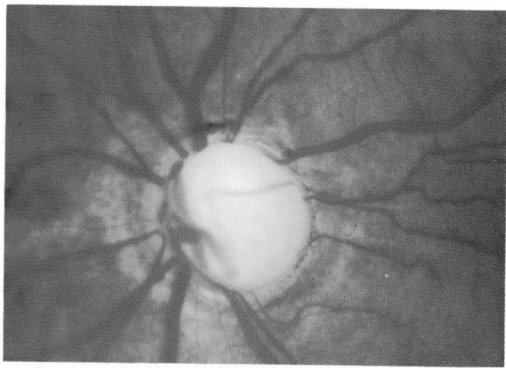

D, Advanced glaucomatous optic atrophy. Vessels curve over the edge of the almost complete cup and disappear into its depths.

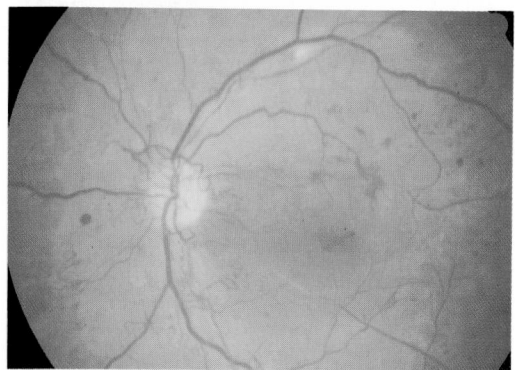

E, Proliferative diabetic retinopathy. Dot and blot hemorrhages appear diffusely, with neovascularization forming at the disc and along the major vascular arcades.

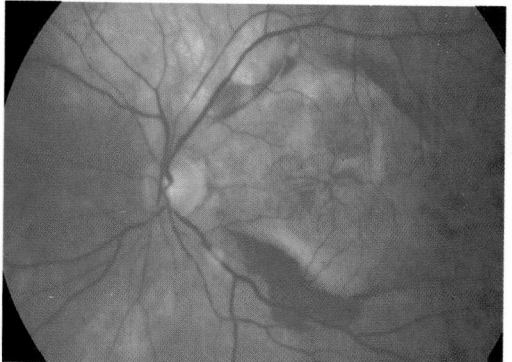

F, Age-related macular degeneration. A neovascular net lies in the macula with surrounding hemorrhage.

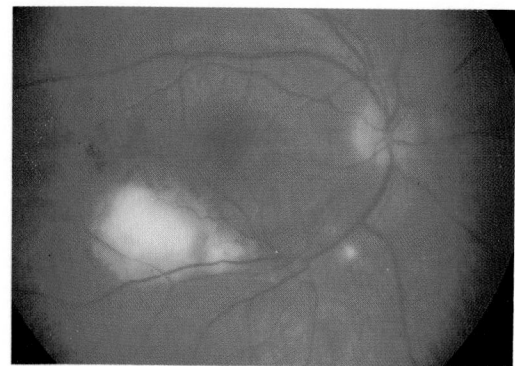

G, Cytomegalovirus retinitis. Hemorrhage and retinal necrosis lie along the inferotemporal vascular arcade.

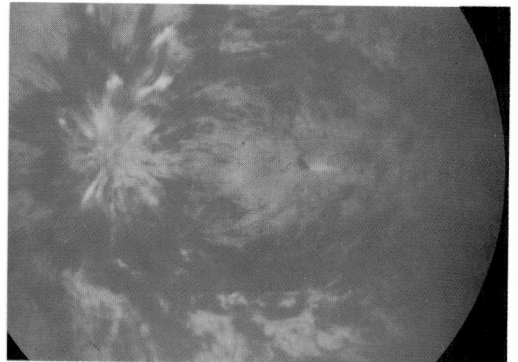

H, Central retinal vein occlusion. Note disc swelling and diffuse hemorrhages.

Photographs taken by Mr. Harry Kachadoorian, C.R.A., University of Massachusetts Medical School, Worcester, Massachusetts

PLATE 8   DISORDERS OF VITAMIN METABOLISM

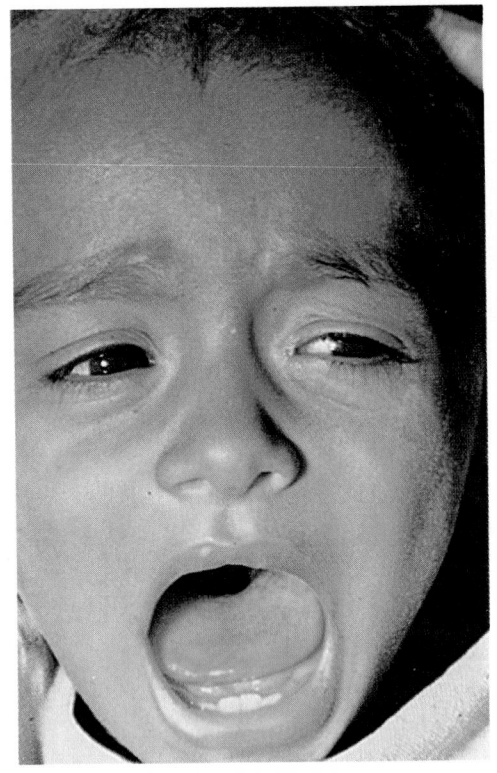

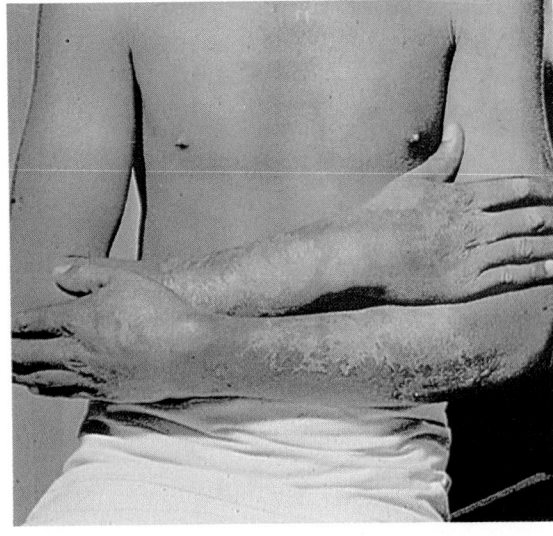

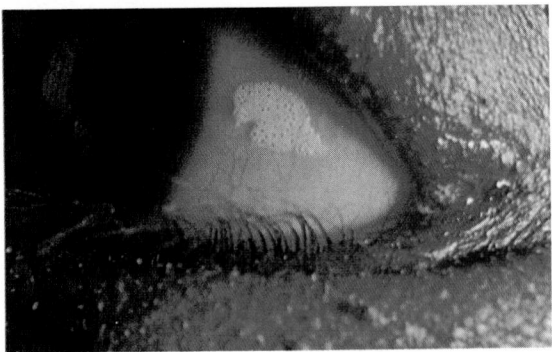

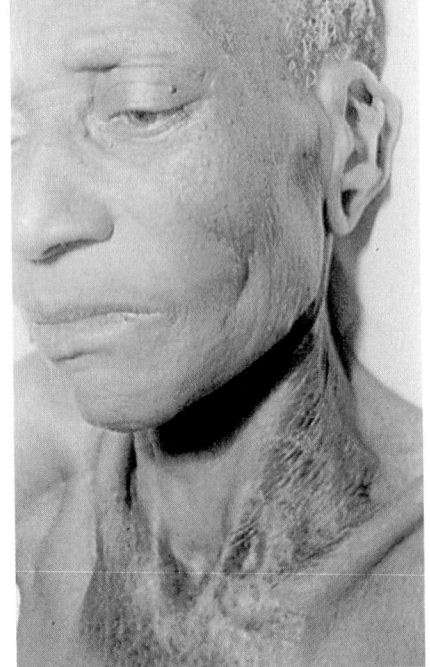

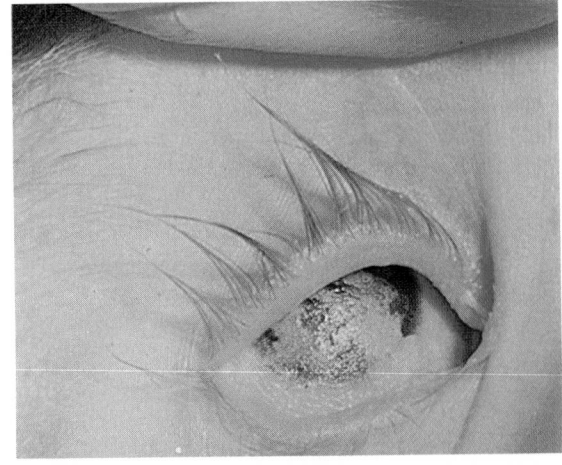

A, Magenta tongue, an abnormality commonly observed in patients with riboflavin deficiency, but probably not completely specific for deficiency of this vitamin. The tongue is purplish red and painful.

B, Early pellagra affecting the arms, resulting from dietary deficiency of niacin. The dermatitis begins with erythema, progresses to blebs and bullae, and in later stages becomes rough, cracked, and brittle, as shown here. Lesions are most prominent in sun-exposed skin but are not necessarily restricted to these areas.

C, Casal's necklace, a broad collar over the neck, is a classic manifestation of pellagra. Skin changes are similar to those shown in *B.*

D, A large, diffuse, foamy Bitot's spot, observed in the conjunctiva of a patient with vitamin A deficiency.

E, Advanced Bitot's spot involving cornea and conjunctiva, producing marked impairment of vision.

(All figures are reproduced from McLaren DS: A Colour Atlas of Nutritional Disorders, with permission from Year Book Medical Publishers.)

PART I

MEDICINE AS A LEARNED AND HUMANE PROFESSION

The *Cecil Textbook of Medicine* is addressed to medical students, residents, fellows, and practitioners of all ages. It deals with the body of knowledge of human disease. In contrast, these introductory essays are presented mainly for those now entering the profession, for students deserve a broader perspective of medicine than is offered by its subject matter alone.

1 MEDICINE AS AN ART
Lloyd H. Smith, Jr.

What is medicine? "Medicine is not a science but a learned profession, deeply rooted in a number of sciences and charged with the obligation to apply them for man's benefit." In this eloquent statement from an earlier edition of this book, Walsh McDermott defined medicine as a human activity undertaken for the benefit of others whether in the area of public health, "statistical compassion," or in the care of the individual patient.

Medicine can also be defined in other terms. It is a mutable body of knowledge, skills, and traditions applicable to the preservation of health, the cure of disease, and the amelioration of suffering. The boundaries of medicine blend into psychology, sociology, economics, and even into cultural heritage. Disease may be encoded in the genome; disease may also be encoded by the deprivations of poverty and ignorance. Medicine must therefore be concerned not only with an abnormal molecule but also with an abnormal childhood. As such it is open ended in a way that is both humbling and exhilarating to those who pursue it as a career.

Medicine is continually changing. The honored verities of one generation become the shopworn shibboleths of the next. Much of what we now so confidently espouse, including that compressed within this edition, will amuse our successors as being remarkably bizarre in its naiveté. Medical competence is based on the continuing pursuit of ever changing concepts. It must be renewed as the substance of medicine itself is transformed.

The practice of medicine is far more than the application of scientific principles to a particular biologic aberration. Its focus is on the patient whose welfare is its continuing purpose. That purpose of medicine is self evident in theory, but more difficult to sustain under the pressures of medical practice. For example, it is tragically easy for the patient to become merely the repository in which a disease or a syndrome has chosen to manifest its particular silhouette. During the training years every physician has subconsciously participated in what might be termed the personification of disease. A case of meningitis is admitted through the emergency room; a

pheochromocytoma will be discussed at Grand Rounds. It is perhaps inevitable that a disease becomes symbolically an entity to the physician who must become familiar with all of its manifestations and guises. In the art of medicine the physician must be the advocate of the patient as well as the adversary of disease. It is the patient who is personified rather than the disease.

THE PATIENT. The description of a patient is simply that of a fellow human being in need of help. The patient comes seeking help because of a problem relating to his or her health. This subjective judgment carries with it disquieting concerns, although these may be unexpressed. Anxiety is present even in the most stoical of patients; this fact must never be forgotten or disregarded by the physician. The patient's anxiety may be specific—for example, in a fear of cancer with all that implies in the public mind concerning pain, degradation, and inexorable death. More often the anxiety is amorphous: fear of loss of independence or employment; fear of failure to meet obligations to one's family or to retain the regard of a loved one; or fear of an inability to maintain a life of dignity and significance. In the rush to crystallize a chief complaint and present illness the physician too often brushes aside these considerations.

The patient presents to the physician on alien and unfamiliar ground—in the structured and artificial setting of an office, a clinic, or a hospital bed. This form of health care of the individual, as opposed to health care in the aggregate, is often described by the unfelicitous phrase "the personal encounter system." Unfortunately it often seems distressingly like confrontation to the patient, who comes after all for comfort, not for encounter. Each human being is unique within a life that is enormously complex—in heredity, early experiences, cultural and psychologic environment, education, opportunities, successes, failures, fantasies, emotional commitments, motivations, and in the adjustments and compromises that serve to cripple or to mature. Living, therefore, is the ultimate personal encounter system. With an extensive and diverse experience the patient comes to the physician with "a problem." A chief complaint is requested. Defenses must be lowered and the emotions that spill out may be distressing. The patient's response must be selective and brief; as a result it is not infrequently distorted, perhaps even misleading.

What does the patient want when coming to see a physician? There are certain common hopes and expectations. Patients want to be listened to, so that their fears and concerns can be fully expressed and the burden shared. They want physicians to be interested in them as fellow human beings in a compassionate but nonjudgmental fashion. They expect professional competence incorporating the best in medical science and technology. They want to be reasonably informed as to the probable cause of their concerns and what the future is likely to hold. They want not to be abandoned. To each patient these desires and expectations vary in relative importance. It is notable that not all patients expect to be cured. These expectations will be further discussed in the light of how the physician should endeavor to meet them.

TRADITIONAL EXPECTATIONS OF PATIENTS. *Patients want to be listened to and understood.* This has been well expressed by Wilfred Trotter, a great English neurosurgeon: ". . . As long as medicine is an art, its chief and characteristic instrument must be human faculty. We come therefore to the very practical question of what aspects of human faculty it is necessary for the good doctor to cultivate. . . . The first to be named must always be the power of attention, of giving one's whole mind to the patient without the interposition of oneself. It sounds simple but only the very greatest doctors ever fully attain it. It is an active process and not either mere resigned listening or even politely waiting until you can interrupt. Disease often tells its secrets in a casual parenthesis. . . ."

Eventually the medical record must be organized in a logical and consistent fashion. But a history rarely unfolds that way. Patients do not divulge their fears in neat paragraphs or in direct responses to a cascade of queries. It is important to let patients tell their own stories. The manner of formulation and expression of symptoms and anxieties may be as informative as the medical data transmitted. The good physician is an attentive listener, with an ear for Trotter's "casual parenthesis."

Patients want physicians to be interested in them as fellow human beings. This interest cannot be that of the unusual "case" of the carcinoid syndrome or of hairy cell leukemia; the center of interest must be the patient as a person. It is difficult for the physician to feign such an interest, for patients are very perceptive, especially during the vulnerability that illness induces. In the practice of medicine the physician will encounter all of the virtues and vices to which mankind is heir. The physician need not be morally neutral in personal judgments, but these must be stringently excluded from professional activities. The response of the physician to human frailty and fallibility should be that of compassion rather than of cynicism, of interest in the infinite variety of human experience rather than of repulsion from its aberrations.

Patients expect professional competence in medical science and technology. The physician must be a scholar both to attain professional competence and to sustain it during times of revolutionary changes in science and technology. All of the other attributes of the good physician will be of little avail in the absence of sound scholarship. Compassion is no substitute for knowing what should be done. The education of the physician and the role of the physician as a scientist will be discussed more fully below.

Patients want to be kept reasonably informed. The physician must listen to and communicate with the patient. Time must be set aside for this. Failure to do so is a serious error, for silence is a form of communication that is usually adverse. The physician should voluntarily answer questions of concern to the patient. The physician must also inform the patient concerning the illness and what it implies. A number of books have been developed to assist in patient education and are often quite effective in translating medical terminology into lay terms. Furthermore, clubs for mutual support and education have been formed by patients who share their common experiences with such chronic disabilities as ileostomies or amputations. Admirable and important as these are, they do not obviate the need for patients to learn from their own physicians about their particular illnesses and what they may mean in and for their future lives. This need extends beyond the legal confines of informed consent, which is now an important issue in medical practice.

Patients want not to be abandoned. Death comes to everyone. There are finite limits to what can be accomplished by medical science and technology in the alleviation of suffering and the prolongation of life. This fact is well known to both patients and physicians. When that limit is reached, the physician often feels powerless and even guilty that no more can be done. As a consequence there is a tendency to withdraw attention and direct it elsewhere. Nothing could be a greater mistake. It is at the margins of medical science that the role of the physician is enhanced. It is here that the art of medicine comes to the forefront in the care of the patient, whether it be by emotional support, relief of pain, small adjustments in medicines or diet, daily conversation and examination, or other methods to show that the patient is still someone of dignity and worth in whom interest has not been lost and for whom hope has not been abandoned. And when no more can be done for the patient it is time to care for the family. It is this caring role rather than the curing role of the physician that is so well described in Ch. 4 by Lewis Thomas. At this stage, as Walsh McDermott has written, "it is up to each of us to follow to the fullest measure the charge laid down long ago for the physician to become himself the treatment."

THE PHYSICIAN. The physician has both chosen and been chosen to enter an arduous and demanding profession, the origins of which stretch back to antiquity. Part priest, part shaman, part mystic, part alchemist, the physician of the past reflected the beliefs and expectations of the time and met a perceived need of fellow men. The history of medicine is part of the heritage of every physician and reflects the cultural history of each society.

The physician enters a profession with established values and traditions of ethical conduct and responsibilities. But each physician, as each patient, is unique. The physician is not a disembodied instrument that can be passively shaped by the profession, but rather a human being with innate strengths and weaknesses that must be recognized in order to meet the expectations of patients and of the profession, not least of which are those standards established for oneself. The qualities of the ideal physician are easy to state but difficult to attain: compassion, sincere interest in one's fellow man, knowledge of human nature, tact, equanimity, sustained scholarship, curiosity, and high ethical standards. Physical and mental vigor might be added to those traits, for the life of the physician is not for the languid or the disengaged. No one has been endowed with or ever fully achieves excellence in all of these qualities. One must first know oneself and judge how one can most closely approach those ideals in one's professional life.

THE EDUCATION OF THE PHYSICIAN. Barriers are encountered at the very beginning in the initial selection for medical school as many seek entry for few positions. Undergraduate education is sometimes distorted and breadth of personal experience curtailed in a grim and often distasteful race for competitive acceptance. This inadvertent feedback inhibition not infrequently results from erroneous conceptions of what may or may not impress admission committees of medical schools. Nevertheless, the phenomenon remains as a concern to all who are interested in the future of our profession. Admission committees of medical schools too often exercise allosteric control over the higher education of those destined to enter our profession.

The Basic Science Years. In the standard curriculum of medical school in the United States two years are largely devoted to the sciences basic to medicine and two years to clinical training. Fortunately there are a number of interesting variations on this thematic progression which diminish its rigidity and permit the student to re-explore basic science after an introductory clinical experience.

In the United States students usually arrive at medical school after an intensive four-year experience at a college or a university. They anticipate a scholarly atmosphere of a graduate school which will prepare them to enter the practice of a profession for which they hold idealistic expectations. Instead they are immediately assailed with a formidable array of "basic sciences" linked to the structure and function of the human organ systems. New facts constitute not so much an intellectual feast as an engorgement. Each discipline is attended by devotees who are passionately persuaded of the seminal role of their segment of science in the future of the profession. This commitment is translated into the basic academic commodity, curricular time, in which these cluttered wares are exhibited. Awed by the dimensionless task, students struggle with uneven success to assimilate and survive, conscious always that their receptor mechanisms are overloaded and of a continuing sense of high output failure. They look forward in hope that subsequent years will reward their endurance in the more congenial atmosphere of the clinic.

This is patently a caricature, as all will recognize. It can be said, as Mark Twain said of Wagner's music, "it is not as bad as it sounds." The quality of basic science in medical schools is often superb; the substance of modern science has a certain grandeur; many faculty members are gifted in imparting a sense of intellectual adventure to their students; finally, many students now arrive at medical school with a mature understanding of one or more of the fundamental disciplines of biology. Nevertheless this caricature contains elements of truth as seen from the perspective of medical students. The central question is not whether basic science is necessary for medical research, since few would deny its importance there, but whether it is relevant in the education of every physician to the degree to which it is currently emphasized. In the real world of patient care, public health, and medical economics, should the student have to struggle with the intricacies of post-transcriptional modifications of messenger RNA, or is this merely a rite of passage prescribed by a science-obsessed faculty? This is a reasonable question and calls for a response other than a simple reference to flexnerian orthodoxy.

A knowledge of the scientific underpinnings of medicine is clearly necessary in order to marshal the basic information required to understand a patient's illness and to be able to reason logically about the problems of diagnosis and therapy. If there were any doubt on that point, it would be quickly dispelled by random perusal of this book. Much of the basic science which seems abstruse and irrelevant today will find its way into clinical practice in the not too distant future. Medical research is only one step removed from patient care.

Beyond the assimilation of scientific information, there is an even more important consideration. Many of you will have most of your professional experience in the twenty-first century. The changes in medical science and technology will be enormous and largely unpredictable. Only the scientific method will remain unaltered as an invaluable instrument with which fallible man can acquire new knowledge and, equally important, debride that which proves fallacious. It is imperative that students learn the scientific method as part of their education if they are to participate critically and effectively in a changing profession. How can this be done? Perhaps the best method is to participate personally, even for a relatively brief period of time, in a research project so that learning comes from first hand experience. If that does not prove practical, one can pursue some scientific topic in depth and write a critical analysis of it. It is important to learn one area of inquiry in great detail, even though it may have to be a limited area, in order to penetrate to its frontier. It is only there that science can be understood as a process rather than as a repository.

The Clinical Years. In his perceptive essay "On Becoming a Clinician," in an earlier edition of this textbook, Paul B. Beeson described many of the disquieting stresses to which the student is subjected on entry into the clinical years. Every medical student will benefit from reading those thoughts from one of America's most distinguished physicians. Most students enter the clinical years with a sense of relief, but it is relief linked with anxieties. Some of these anxieties cluster around the following questions:

How can I cope with the uncertainties of clinical medicine?

What are the boundaries of clinical medicine? How much and what am I supposed to learn?

How will I function in my interactions with patients?

How will I measure up to the expectations of my colleagues?

How will I be able to maintain my own identity as an individual in a profession that so obsessively dominates my time and energy?

Other questions could be formulated. Each student possesses a unique idiotype of anxieties that cannot be purged by platitudes. Each will arrive at personal answers, or more likely at personal accommodations, through experience.

THE UNCERTAINTY PRINCIPLE OF CLINICAL MEDICINE. There is an "uncertainty principle" in medicine as there is in physics. The practice of medicine is inexact and will remain so. If it were not, it would be a science or a technology rather than an art. The measuring instrument is personal and unique. Subjective mensuration defies precision. Who can quantify nausea or the severity of pain? Symptoms may be forgotten, suppressed, or amplified when filtered through the grid of personality. Available data are often indirect, incomplete, or even contradictory. Patients respond in varying fashions to treatment across the range from simple reassurance (which is rarely simple) to surgical or pharmaceutical interventions. Clinical medicine is often based on experience and judgment—which are largely euphemisms for a knowledge of probabilities.

The process of formulating a diagnosis or selecting a therapy is not as arbitrary as it first seems. There are rational means for narrowing the range of diagnostic possibilities: a precise description of symptoms; an accurate and thorough characterization of physical findings; selective laboratory studies to evaluate the functions of organ systems; a synthesis of information to define syndromic patterns; a marshaling of information on etiology and pathogenesis. All of this requires attention to detail, consistency of work habits, and good intellect.

Hypotheses are formed and algorithms branch away from various entry points as new data are obtained which support or fail to support a working diagnosis. This process of clinical reasoning is often best displayed in the Clinicopathologic Conference (CPC). In the absence of certainty, best guesses must be utilized and in making informed guesses, generally dignified as judgments, the clinician actually relies upon subliminal statistics.

Medical decisions based on probabilities are necessary but also perilous. Even the most astute physician will occasionally be wrong. The wise physician will often recognize that a decision is erroneous and discard or modify the hypothesis on which it is based. The best decision may be approached only by successive approximations. Action may have to be taken despite lack of confirmation of a hypothesis (working diagnosis). Chester M. Jones, a noted clinical teacher, used to say: "If you cannot make a diagnosis, make a decision." Despite the remarkable contributions of science and technology, clinical medicine is frequently inexactitude in action. The student entering the clinical years will quickly realize the dangers to the welfare of the patient of dogmatism in clinical practice. The ambiguities and errors that you will encounter in your own experience and observe in the work of others should be an antidote to arrogance. Some errors are inevitable and should not humiliate you, but they should teach humility.

CLINICAL MEDICINE AS A DISCIPLINE WITHOUT BOUNDARIES. The basic sciences are demanding but, as taught in medical schools, they have reasonably defined margins. It is true that these margins are somewhat artificial, since the disciplines of modern biology merge almost imperceptibly into one another. Nevertheless, the educational responsibilities of the medical student can often be designated within the subject material of a lecture course, syllabus, and textbook. Not so in clinical medicine. The student emerges into an open-ended system of bewildering complexity in which science is blurred by sociology; psychology interacts with economics; and traditions and ethical concepts are buffeted by new imperatives. Within this complicated system, the practice of clinical medicine goes forward. The student does not encounter a theoretical discipline to be observed and analyzed in tranquility, but is abruptly thrown into the structured workings of the second largest industry in the United States where the health and even the survival of many people are at stake on a daily basis.

Based on previous educational experiences, students often ask, "How much am I expected to learn in this course?" No one can supply a satisfactory answer. The student stands on the threshold of a learning experience in clinical medicine that will extend over the remainder of an active career as a physician. Learning must have that stretch if the student is to meet the responsibilities of a physician. The course is merely a contrived entry point into that longitudinal experience. More advanced faculty members, medical residents, or even senior students in other rotations in medicine seem remarkably well informed. Yet no single individual has a balanced knowledge in all aspects of medicine. The specialist will often be adept only within a defined subset of medicine, and even the generalist will be uneven in many areas of information. Within this confusing and sometimes overwhelming setting the student must become an independent scholar in medicine—independent in the sense that never again will others outline or circumscribe the subject material.

Most students adapt themselves remarkably quickly to the changed environment of clinical medicine. The new language of the hospital, including its acronymic barbarisms (SOB, PERLA, COPD, etc.), no longer jar the ear, and the concepts of pathophysiology being applied at the bedside awaken latent memories. The student learns that there are habits of thought and clusters of associations so that the physician does not laboriously go back to first principles to meet each new clinical problem. These thought patterns are efficient and useful if they do not gel into medicine by reflex and aphorism. The student learns by listening, participating, observing, arguing, reading, and reflecting. As earlier generations of students have discovered, the intensity of the experience and the special chemistry of confronting the clinical problem of a specific patient serve to fix the information received in one's memory with a vividness far beyond that obtained from even the most brilliant lecture.

Beyond the required participation in clinical rotations, how should the student approach the study of medicine? It would be presumptuous to give a doctrinaire answer. Medical students have usually been seasoned by five or six years of higher education before they begin the study of clinical medicine and during those years have developed their own best methods of learning. In approaching internal medicine, in contrast perhaps to some more circumscribed specialties, it will usually prove most valuable to study in depth the specific problems presented by one's own patients rather than beginning with a systematic approach to cover all of the discipline. In this way one can exploit the intense immediacy of those experiences which, supplemented by conferences, rounds, seminars, conversations, and all of the other ways of learning on the fly, will usually converge to give a broad familiarity with the subject. A share in the responsibility of caring for a patient is a powerful stimulus to learning.

What is the role of the *Cecil Textbook of Medicine* in the learning process? This book attempts to provide the student or the physician with succinct but authoritative summaries about diseases or groups of diseases. Essays written by more than 250 acknowledged experts in their respective fields represent collectively a systematic approach to internal medicine. The chapters are designed to give a basic, lucid, and up-to-date consensus concerning the state of the art in our understanding of specific diseases, but they cannot be all inclusive. Many of the topics discussed within a few pages

have received more extended treatment elsewhere as separate monographs. Each of the subspecialty areas (cardiology, gastroenterology, endocrinology, etc.) is the subject of textbooks similar in size to this one. The student should therefore cultivate the habit of consulting at least some of the carefully selected references that extend the information supplied in this basic text.

In general it is also wise for students to begin reading medical journals early in their study of clinical medicine. In this way a start can be made toward the regular study of current medical literature and also the foundations of one's own medical library can be laid. Each student may have a personal preference. The most frequently read medical journal by students and practitioners is the *New England Journal of Medicine*. It is particularly useful for the student with its CPC, surveys of medical progress, editorial comments on current topics, original articles, and lively correspondence. In this manner the student establishes an early acquaintance with the frontiers of medicine and with its issues, uncertainties, and controversies.

THE STUDENT AND THE PATIENT. One of the student's earliest concerns on entering clinical medicine is how to interact with patients and how to assume the traditional role of a physician. The student is concerned that personal insecurities will impair effective communication with patients in whose care he or she is now called upon to participate. Rarely does this turn out in practice to be a serious problem. The expectations of most patients in the physician-patient interaction, discussed above, are realistic ones. Patients are usually aware of the progression of assigned responsibilities in the student-house staff-faculty team and do not expect omniscience or authoritarianism from the student. Not infrequently the patient forms a special attachment to the student, especially if the student has been perceptive enough to listen in the sense described above by Wilfred Trotter. If the student respects the personal dignity of the patient as a fellow human being, and listens in a sensitive manner, the patient responds with gratitude and returns that respect. Even when patients are initially perceived as hostile or belligerent, the student must maintain equanimity and try to understand the sources of these reactions. Do not allow yourself to be drawn into the flippant cynicism that sometimes passes for sophistication in the subculture of student and house staff training. Francis Peabody's sentient summary is still most apt, "for the secret of the care of the patient is in caring for the patient."

STUDENTS AND THEIR COLLEAGUES. Beginning in the clinical years the relationships of students with their colleagues in medicine undergo a subtle change. No longer are they merely the passive recipients of data and concepts supplied by the faculty through lectures, conferences, syllabi, or laboratories. They are participating with graduated responsibilities in the practice of medicine. A point in the medical history or a question asked by the student may prove decisive in arriving at the solution of a clinical problem. Frequently the most effective teachers of students are the house staff or more advanced students. Students will find many residents to be splendid teachers who not only make them feel at home on the service but also take the extra time to include them in all of the discussions. On most teaching services there is a certain amount of badinage or gamesmanship which enlivens interactions. If this is recognized as such, and not taken too seriously, it can serve to enhance rather than demean the learning experience. As a student you must not hesitate to ask questions or bring up new points of view and must not be intimidated by your current position in this shifting hierarchy. Even the chief medical resident faced similar qualms only a few years ago. But above all, remember that it is the patient's welfare, and not your own ego, that is paramount.

THE PHYSICIAN AS A NONPHYSICIAN. Beginning in the basic science years but exacerbated in the clinical years, students often become concerned about the level of commitment demanded of them. How much of a life that is finite in time and energy must be devoted to medicine? What is the boundary between dedication and obsession? After all one does not really become a physician; one remains a human being who has acquired certain knowledge and skills that allow one to function as a physician during specific periods of time. What should those times be? How and when does one shift roles from being a physician to being a "nonphysician"? This is, of course, a generic question that is as applicable to science, art, business, or any other human activity as it is to medicine.

The student will not readily find an all-embracing answer to this question. Each student will most likely evolve a personal answer and it will be an operational one representing the integral of microcompromises and adjustments made throughout one's subsequent career. The "complete physician," narrowly construed, would be a very poor physician if he were merely an observer rather than a participant in the pageantry of his time. Physicians owe it to themselves, to their families, to society, and to their patients not to become simply skilled but detached automatons. On the other hand, the practice of medicine is not a job but a profession that cannot be sealed off into convenient hours for earning one's living. To attempt to do so smacks of dilettantism. Between these extremes one must decide for oneself where the compromises will be made along the varying border between personal and professional life. Tensions will remain, but properly channeled they can be creative and rewarding.

2 MEDICINE AS A SCIENCE

James B. Wyngaarden

The practice of medicine rests firmly upon a foundation of biologic and behavioral sciences, which in turn trace their evolution to chemistry, physics, mathematics, psychology, anthropology, and epidemiology. During college and medical school years, the physician acquires both an extensive knowledge base in science and a comfortable familiarity with the ways of science. But scientific knowledge is not static. It undergoes continuous remodeling as new discoveries are made and erroneous interpretations are discarded. As a consequence, preservation of professional competence throughout a working lifetime is a daunting challenge. It requires a continuing growth of knowledge, a critical assessment of new hypotheses and scientific advances, and a selective incorporation of the most useful of these into one's own practice.

Advances in biologic science and accompanying technologic developments underlie most of the medical progress of the past half century, which has so remarkably advanced the ability of the physician to intervene in illness. Much of this progress has been in fundamental or "basic" science, conducted in the pursuit of understanding for its own sake. Significant progress has also resulted from research conducted by physician-scientists with a specified clinical goal in mind—for example, the elucidation of a disease mechanism or the critical evaluation of a therapeutic practice. Advances in medicine also continue to occur through serendipity or by astute clinical observations concerning patients or groups of patients and their illnesses. Nevertheless, the only rational approach to finding new methods for prevention or treatment is based on scientific explanations of the causes and mechanisms of disease.

Some years ago, Comroe and Dripps* traced the origins of

---

*Comroe JH, Dripps RD: The top ten clinical advances in cardiovascular-pulmonary medicine and surgery between 1945 and 1975: How they came about. Bethesda, Md., Public Inquiries and Reports Branch, National Heart, Lung, and Blood Institute, National Institutes of Health, 1977.

ten major clinical innovations in cardiovascular and pulmonary medicine in an effort to identify the antecedents of these advances. Over 60 per cent of the enabling discoveries were in the category of basic science; over 40 per cent were the result of research carried out without any particular clinical application in mind. These observations are probably representative of medical progress in general.

The ability to control infections with antibiotics, hypertension with antihypertensive agents, and inflammatory reactions with glucocorticoids represents remarkable advances that have contributed to a lengthening of life expectancy. But the agenda is far from being fulfilled. The major health care problems of our time lie in the continued existence of diseases for which we can as yet do little. Even if the best of contemporary medicine were universally available, cancer would continue to kill, rheumatoid arthritis would continue to cripple, and schizophrenia would continue to render insane. We have no definitive answers for these diseases and for many more the descriptions of which constitute the substance of this book—or else we have what Lewis Thomas has called a "halfway technology," measures capable of modifying and ameliorating illness but not of prevention or cure. Medicine as a science is incomplete. It will remain so, for science itself is by its nature incomplete.

The present bioscientific character of medical practice is a relatively recent development. Throughout most of recorded history, medicine was anything but scientific, being dominated by empiricism and shackled by dogma. Diagnoses were inexact, causes of diseases poorly understood, and therapies frivolous and haphazard. Interventions by physicians consisted of bleeding, purging, cupping, administration of infusions of every known plant and of solutions of every known metal, and prescription of every possible diet—with no scientific foundation for these practices. Nor could there be such a foundation, for the scientific base did not yet exist.

Harbingers of change emerged slowly in the early nineteenth century, as new principles of physics and chemistry were applied to medicine. Physiologists stressed functions of organs and tissues. Its exemplars, especially Claude Bernard (1813–1878), emphasized the experimental method in establishing biologic knowledge and the necessity of basing medical practice in such knowledge. Pathologists, led by Virchow (1821–1902), stressed the critical study of normal and abnormal tissues and the correlation of features of disease with precise anatomic observations. Bacteriologists, with Pasteur (1822–1895) and Koch (1843–1910) in the vanguard, began to identify the microorganisms and to implicate specific organisms in specific diseases—the anthrax bacillus in anthrax, the tubercle bacillus in consumption, the pneumococcus in lobar pneumonia, the streptococcus in puerperal fever. The groundwork for future therapies was being laid by these great Western European scientists, but there was relatively little that physicians could do about most illnesses at the time. Their major contributions were diagnostic, prognostic, and supportive. By correct diagnosis they could advise concerning outcome. By common-sense supportive measures they could provide comfort and maximize opportunities for recovery. But interventions were as likely as not to make things worse. The first edition of Osler's *Textbook of Medicine* in 1892 was revolutionary for its skepticism and its therapeutic nihilism, as this outstanding physician and teacher condemned the majority of nostrums and remedies as useless, even harmful.

Slowly, specific therapies—insulin for diabetes, liver extract for pernicious anemia—or specific immunizations—diphtheria antitoxin, pneumococcic antisera—appeared. But it was not until the decade of 1935 to 1945 that the entry of sulfonamides and penicillin into clinical medicine made curable a large number of previously lethal and untreatable diseases. It is customary to date the beginnings of modern medicine from these relatively recent events.

The language of contemporary biologic science has become

increasingly biochemical. The compositions of organs, tissues, cells, organelles, and membranes have been defined. The biosynthesis and catabolism of hundreds of compounds have been elucidated. The regulation of body processes has been described at progressively finer levels and in chemical language. Many pharmacologic agents are now understood in terms of specific loci and mechanisms of action. The expansion of new knowledge continues at a pace that is bewildering to all but experts in a given field. Current advances are particularly rapid in immunology, molecular and cellular biology, peptide research, and structural biology. A beginning has been made in explaining human behavior in mechanistic terms, as more and more chemical mediators and pharmacologic modifiers are discovered.

We are in a molecular age of basic biologic science. The molecular influence pervades all the traditional disciplines underlying clinical medicine. Approximately 200 inborn errors are now understood in terms of specific missing or abnormal enzymes or other proteins. There are more than 240 known abnormal human hemoglobins, and for each of these the precise structural defect in the DNA of the mutant gene can be defined. Membrane, cytoplasmic, and nuclear receptors for hormones and drugs are exploding upon us, and old as well as new diseases are being defined in terms of receptor abnormalities—for example, type II hypercholesterolemia and nephrogenic diabetes insipidus. Recognition of opiate receptors has led to the discovery of endogenous peptides (endorphins) with analgesic activity. Their localization gives promise of further understanding of the limbic system, affective states, and addictions. The number and function of neurotransmitters has greatly increased, and these and other advances in neuroscience portend exciting developments in understanding how the brain works. DNA sequencing techniques and restriction endonucleases now permit precise identification of the exact structural alteration of the gene in an increasing number of hereditary diseases. The complete sequencing of the human genome is now technically possible; about 0.5 per cent of it has already been done. Gene therapy—both pharmacologic modification of specific gene action and physical replacement of damaged genetic segments—is now possible in experimental systems.

Much of the recent fundamental information in science has been obtained by the process of reductionism—the exploring of details, and the details of details, until all the smallest bits of the structure, or the smallest parts of the mechanism, are exposed to scrutiny. The scientists responsible for our evolving understanding of biologic systems know that the reductionist approach must often precede reconstitutive endeavors. Scientific progress rests on myriads of small observations, tedious measurements, and the findings of investigators asking humble, answerable questions. Instead of reaching for the whole truth, the scientist examines small, defined, and clearly separable phenomena. The pattern of science is a stepwise extension of what came before, with an occasional quantum leap forward through great discovery.

The examples of advances in medical science mentioned above have been largely drawn from the areas of ultrastructure, biochemistry, and molecular biology. In biology these disciplines have arbitrary and porous boundaries: physiology, pharmacology, neurosciences, cell biology, molecular biology, biochemistry, immunology, biophysics—all are in a phase of confluence, and the common language is chemistry. Medicine is not only a branch of applied biology, however. It also subsumes many aspects of psychology, sociology, anthropology, and economics. These disciplines, too long neglected or denigrated as "soft science," are now increasingly recognized as germane to medicine as a discipline and the practice of medicine as a profession.

Critics of the bioscientific strategy of medicine have claimed that the great advances that have dramatically reduced mortality rates consist in the improvement of the environment, the correction of malnutrition, and the control of infectious diseases through immunizations and antimicrobial agents, and that the relevant medical breakthroughs largely occurred before the prodigious expansion of federal support of biomedical science begun in the early 1950's. They contend that the enormous expenditures that have made the United States pre-eminent in biomedical research have produced too little in the way of medical advance to justify their continuation and have instead fostered the development of an extremely costly technology that has had only a minimal effect upon mortality statistics. They propose that the bioscientific strategy of medicine should be replaced by an ecologic strategy for health.

These critics ignore several important realities: (1) A bioscientific strategy for medicine and an ecologic strategy for health are not mutually exclusive, and examples of contributions of both strategies are readily at hand. (2) Major advances have occurred since 1950 that have revolutionized the outlook in individual diseases or disease groups—for example, in Hodgkin's disease, acute lymphocytic leukemia of children, Parkinson's disease, and Wilson's disease. (3) Advances based on the bioscientific strategy have reduced as well as increased health care costs. (4) Such advances have rested in most instances on a deeper and clearer understanding of underlying disease mechanisms. (5) The elucidation of a disease mechanism and the devising of rational therapy usually depend upon the application of basic scientific knowledge to a clinical problem—for instance, the definition of pathways of purine synthesis led to the development of a xanthine oxidase inhibitor (allopurinol) for the control of hyperuricemia and hyperuricaciduria.

The list of human diseases for which there are as yet no definitive measures for prevention or cure is still formidable. Fresh insights into the nature of these diseases are needed. These insights can come only from continued basic research. But the expansion of the knowledge bank of the past quarter century justifies great optimism for the eventual control and cure of major diseases and the possible elimination of premature death from illness.

The practice of medicine is both a science and an art. A skilled physician must have extensive medical knowledge, which is the bedrock of technical competence. In addition, he or she must have judgment, tact, decisiveness, restraint, compassion, interest, time, and other personal qualities of caring and dedication. The science and the art of medicine must remain intimately linked if physicians are to be maximally effective. The student studies the science of medicine first, masters it early, and returns to it frequently. The physician acquires the art of medicine—the skillful application of medical knowledge and judgment in the optimal care of the patient—more gradually and with experience.

THE PHYSICIAN AS A SCIENTIST. Since medicine is derived from a number of sciences relevant to the health of individuals or of groups, physicians must be trained as scientists to utilize these complex disciplines effectively.

To be a scientist, the physician must have more than rote scientific knowledge or even fluency in its particular jargon. Physicians must be conversant with the processes of scientific inquiry—how data are obtained and evaluated; how hypotheses are framed, modified, or discarded; the uses and limitations of inductive reasoning. In short, they must understand science as an intellectual instrument that has been slowly perfected over centuries. Only in this way can they remain attentive to medical progress as a critical and independent participant. Otherwise they will be in danger of being the passive purveyor of medical fashions. Both the spirit and rigor of science are necessary for the physician to become and remain a scholar in medicine. Medical practice itself contains many of the elements of scientific inquiry in the pursuit and evaluation of data (history, physical examination, laboratory studies) and in framing a hypothesis (tentative clinical diagnosis).

As a scientist the physician is the beneficiary of both the fruits of scientific research and of the mental discipline of the scientific method. To a greater or lesser degree the physician also has the opportunity to contribute personally to medical progress. Most medical research is now carried out by teams of participating investigators in elaborately equipped laboratories that utilize the advanced instrumentation and technology of modern science. There is still scope, however, for scientific contributions made by inquiring physicians based on their own experiences in patient care. Much of medical progress has derived from this kind of curiosity in the past. In addition, this form of clinical research, on whatever modest scale it may be engaged in, adds excitement and zest to professional life. As Thomas Hobbes has written: "Desire to know why, and how, curiosity, which is a lust of the mind, that by a perseverance of delight in the continued and indefatigable generation of knowledge, exceedeth the short vehemence of any carnal pleasure."

THE PHYSICIAN AS A HUMANIST. Since the physician deals with fellow human beings in need of help, the patient and the public have every reason to assume that the physician is a humane and caring person as well as a competent practitioner. Yet a crisis of confidence appears to have beset modern medicine.* As the technology and complexity of medicine have increased, medical care has become more institutionalized and its delivery depersonalized. This is a particular risk when many different expert consultants or technologists are called upon to participate each in some segment of a given patient's workup and care. There is a widely held view that the increasingly complex science and technology of medicine are responsible for a decline of compassion in medicine, as though there were something inherently contradictory between science and humanity, between technology and compassion. There is, of course, no reason that scientific knowledge and compassion should be in conflict. Science and technology underlie most of the advances of medicine that enable contemporary physicians to render more effective medical care than their professional forebears were able to offer. Glick even views computed tomography as a technologic advance of extraordinary compassion. Its use has spared patients many more difficult, painful, and dangerous procedures and has permitted definitive diagnoses to be made earlier. Physicians cannot be made more compassionate by downgrading science any more than students can be made more humanistic by study of the humanities. If there is a decline in compassion among physicians, its causes must lie elsewhere. Glick suggests that "the fundamental problems lie for the most part outside the medical establishment, within society as a whole. The physician is largely a reflection of society. . . . Basic human character traits are well developed by the time a student enters medical school." He suggests that the prime examples of humane medicine are to be found in persons in whom service to humanity ranks as a higher priority than personal gratification. That characteristic is a reaffirmation of Hippocrates and of Osler and of every other truly great physician. Its expression is enhanced whenever good science and complex technology are applied for the benefit of the patient by a caring physician or any other personnel who participate in the delivery of medical services to people.

---

*Glick SM: Humanistic medicine in a modern age. N Engl J Med 304:1036, 1981.

3 MEDICINE AS A PUBLIC SERVICE

James B. Wyngaarden

Medicine is a serving profession, one that exists not for its own sake but for the benefit of others. "The responsibilities of medicine are threefold: to generate scientific knowledge and to teach it to others; to use the knowledge for the health of an individual or a whole community; and to judge the moral and ethical propriety of each medical act that directly affects another human being" (McDermott).

We have already discussed the generation of scientific knowledge and the way in which scientific advances continually modify and extend the practice of medicine. In the application of an increasingly technologic medicine, new and sometimes discomfiting issues arise. This chapter will briefly introduce selected issues in the practice of medicine faced by the physician as a member of modern society.

PATTERNS OF MEDICAL PRACTICE. Practitioners who apply medical knowledge for the benefit of patients are of two sorts: those who deal personally with individual patients and those who deal with people as groups. We call the latter activity *community medicine,* which is a component of public health. In community medicine, group membership is usually determined by geographic location or census tract. The members of such a community are not self-selected on the basis of perception of disease; rather, they are identified as members of the community on the basis of other common characteristics, usually location. At any one time a community will comprise many more people who are healthy than who are ill. Important functions of community medicine are the provision of appropriate health services for its members, the continuous surveillance of the population for discovery of individuals in need of care, and the creation of entry points for those so identified. These are large social challenges, as yet imperfectly attained. Marked unevenness in access to and in utilization of physician services remains a problem in most countries. In the United States these problems have been ameliorated but by no means solved by Medicare and Medicaid programs for financing of hospital and physician services. Important though these topics are, they are beyond the scope of this book, which is principally oriented toward the care of the individual patient. By and large the constituency described in this book consists of self-selected patients who consult a physician because of *dis-ease,* i.e., concern about their personal health.

Physicians who render personal medical care do so in a variety of practice patterns, ranging from solo practices to partnerships, to multispecialty groups, to full-time situations in an organized clinic or a medical school faculty, to Health Maintenance Organizations (HMO's) or Independent Practice Associations (IPA's). The traditional doctor-patient relationship, in which the patient identifies a specific physician as his or her own personal doctor, may exist within any of these practice patterns. Many patients want a personal physician who knows them, who is available for first contact and continuing care, and who offers a portal of entry to specialists for those conditions warranting referral. This type of practice, termed "primary care," characterizes activities of general practitioners, family physicians, and general internists, as well as of many pediatricians and obstetricians. Often their services are complemented by nurse-clinicians or physician associates. Physicians who see patients in referral for common conditions that do not require high technology, and who characteristically see them in an office or community hospital setting, are said to be offering "secondary care." Those who manage patients with complex illnesses requiring high technology, or the use of powerful, high-risk drugs or procedures, or specialized knowledge of limited availability, are said to be rendering "tertiary care." University hospitals and many large urban referral hospitals frequently function as "tertiary care centers." But categories of activities are not always clearly separable. Community hospitals and subspecialists often practice a mixture of primary and secondary care medicine. Large teaching hospitals generally offer a full spectrum of services—primary care in their clinics, secondary care as a community referral center, tertiary care for patients who have complex medical problems or who are critically ill.

The provision of continuing comprehensive care has traditionally required a high order of accessibility on the part of the primary care physician. In the following essay, Dr. Thomas eloquently describes the repetitive interruptions of sleep that characterized the nights of his general practitioner father. In recent decades physicians have sought relief from the overwhelming physical and emotional drain of continuous availability with its potentially excessive cost to personal and family life. Solo practitioners arrange to cross-cover each other, partners arrange on-call schedules, and metropolitan physicians often refer nocturnal and weekend patients to emergency rooms. In some group practices, individual doctor-patient relationships have been supplanted by a team approach. These changes in professional mores reflect evolving attitudes on the extent to which compassionate behavior in the practice of medicine should be allowed to dominate a physician's time and personal life. In times past availability was one of the few valuable services an individual physician could offer patients. When no one in the profession had many answers to illness, and treatment consisted largely of evaluation, prognosis, and emotional support, the reassuring presence of the physician constituted in itself the fulfillment of the Hippocratic Oath. As the science and technology of medicine have expanded, no one doctor can any longer be expert in all areas, and the care of the patient, when something is seriously wrong, necessarily becomes a collective effort. The personal interest of each physician continues to be essential, so that there may be a series of satisfying doctor-patient relationships. However, the patient usually wants one doctor as his or her personal advocate, regardless of the extent of sharing of medical responsibility.

THE PATIENT AS A CONSUMER. Some of the traditional and universal expectations of patients have been discussed in the initial essay, "Medicine as an Art." The general trend toward greater consumer awareness has created many new patient expectations. Patients now understand a great deal more about the human body and its disorders than they did a generation ago. As a consequence they expect more detailed information from the physician. Teaching about science and health in grade schools and high schools has improved greatly. Newspapers, magazines, and television regularly inform the public of advances in medicine. Many communities offer health seminars to the general public. Home medical encyclopedias are widely available. The individual has been admonished to take personal responsibility for his or her own health through weight control, dietary discretion, limitation of intakes of saturated fats and of salt, regular exercise, moderation in or abstinence from smoking and drinking, attention to the purity of water and of air, and appropriate diversions from work. These measures are widely accepted as contributing to physical and mental health. For those with chronic illnesses there are primers prepared by voluntary health agencies or the United States Public Health Service. In many instances there are clubs to join, organized about a

diagnosis (e.g., lupus erythematosus clubs) or a procedure (e.g., laryngectomy clubs). One can send a coupon and urine sample to test for diabetes or have one's blood pressure checked at the supermarket. Ethnic groups at increased risk for certain diseases can avail themselves of screening programs for sickle cell disease or Tay-Sachs carrier status. Such measures and others have publicized medical progress and have kindled high expectations for imminent "breakthroughs." Such anticipations are often fanned by an overly exuberant press. All of these factors combine to place increased demands upon the physician to inform in greater detail and to anticipate increasingly sophisticated inquiries from patients and relatives.

The public is also well aware that substantial tax dollars have been spent on medical research and on the production of more physicians since World War II. They have come to view excellent medical care and access to it as birthrights. For the majority of Americans these birthrights have been achieved, but important segments of our society and of many societies throughout the world are still excluded from optimal medical care by poverty, location, or both. For many of those with access to care, the costs have become a preoccupation. The percentage of the American gross national product spent on medical care has risen substantially for two decades and is now about 11 to 12 per cent. In part this reflects the extension of medical care to individuals for whom it was only marginally available in the past. In larger part this reflects the costs of progress in medicine. Drugs are now available to treat conditions that in times past could only be observed. New technologies in medicine permit diagnostic and therapeutic procedures scarcely dreamed of a decade or two ago. The rising costs of medical care are particularly pronounced in circumstances in which partial solutions are much more expensive than the ultimate cure is likely to be. The classic example is poliomyelitis. Current examples include the expensive technology of renal dialysis and transplantation for chronic kidney failure and of coronary bypass surgery and heart transplantation for coronary artery disease. Doctors control many of the expenditures in medical care and therefore must share in the serious concerns about its escalating costs. They decide on hospitalization, order diagnostic studies, prescribe the drugs patients take, or recommend surgery. Control of costs of medical care is a lively topic in the public arena.

The advancing technology of medicine has enabled more and more interventions in the natural course of disease. An increasing number of parts of the body can be replaced by transplanted organs or mechanical substitutes. The term "invasive procedure" has become commonplace in our lexicon. The potential of such procedures for diagnostic information or therapeutic achievement is awesome. Benefits of scientific medicine can now be proffered to patients thought beyond help only several years ago. When all goes well, one is exhilarated by the wonder of the success. But high-risk procedures in high-risk patients cannot always go well. There are unanticipated complexities of disease, adverse biologic responses, genetic differences, flaws of judgment, variations in physicians' skills, mechanical failures. Often the doctor or the hospital or the pharmaceutical company is held responsible, sometimes for events beyond anyone's control.

DEFENSIVE MEDICINE. High-technology medicine has carried with it a lowering of the threshold for litigation on the part of patients when something does go wrong. Some physicians respond by the practice of "defensive medicine." This has at least three components. The first is informed consent. In concept this is unassailable. The patient clearly has the right to have anything that is proposed fully explained in advance, and the right to give or withhold consent. Three or four decades ago informed consent was largely limited to anesthesia and operating permits. Today, informed consent often involves written descriptions of procedures that include explicit accounts of every conceivable misfortune that has ever followed a given diagnostic test, drug therapy, or surgical procedure. Many persons appreciate such candor, but some become frightened and forego needed tests or therapy. Many patients sign forms based on discussions they do not really understand. In such instances the practice clearly is not achieving its intended goals.

Defensive medicine also may extend the medical workup that a prudent physician will perform in a given circumstance. When clinical concern results in an appropriate history, physical examination, and laboratory study, the patient is clearly the beneficiary. But when studies of marginal value are ordered or excessive consultations are requested, solely because of fear of potential litigation, the costs of medical care are driven upward to no good end. Yet physicians are often on the horns of a dilemma, often forced by the perception of their own best interests to exceed what is in the patient's best interest. Experienced physicians who are secure in their knowledge and competence will rely less on extensive studies and wide-ranging consultations than will more apprehensive or tentative doctors.

Defensive medicine also mandates the keeping of more thorough records. In case of challenge to adequacy or competence of care, the written record is the physician's defense. The record should contain all relevant data pertaining to the patient. It should also contain all important data pertaining to the doctor's opinions or conclusions, decisions, prescriptions, actions, and communications. The evolution of thoughts and responses should be clearly discernible from the record. If such entries are recorded at appropriately frequent intervals, an effective reconstruction of events is possible, should the need arise. These are, of course, all benchmarks of good medical practice. But the growing necessity for increasingly detailed documentation has its cost in time. When added to other items of escalating paper work in medical practice, this translates into reduced professional productivity. If defensive medicine benefits the patient, the additional costs may be justified, but in terms of the aforementioned responses the cost-benefit ratio is at present unknown.

PUBLIC ACCOUNTABILITY. The privilege of practicing medicine is increasingly coupled with accountability in the exercise of this stewardship. Private accountability has always been implied in the doctor-patient relationship. The entry of substantial public money into the field of medical care has also brought with it new forms of public accountability and regulation of medical practice.

A profound change is currently under way in the manner in which the private sector is being paid by the federal government for care of elderly and medically indigent patients; the principle of cost reimbursement has been superseded by one of prospective payment. Hospitals are now compensated according to predetermined allowances based on average days of stay and average ancillary charges for each of several hundred diagnosis-related groups into which patients are placed. In addition, peer review organizations have been given considerable power to regulate the system and insure adherence to guidelines concerning admission, early discharge, readmission, or interhospital transfer. Expenses in excess of reimbursement allowances are absorbed by the hospital; savings are banked by the hospital. Funds for graduate medical education have been reduced.

The revisions of federal programs have the dual objective of assuring quality medical care and controlling the rate of growth of the costs of our health care system. Early indications are that hospitals and physicians are making the required adjustments to new conditions, but long-term impacts will not be known for some additional years.

In the final analysis, quality of care depends upon the ability and wisdom of the physician; the adequacy of facilities and equipment; access to safe and effective therapeutic agents; the quality of professional education and training; personal standards of performance, integrity, and dedication; and a resolute self-discipline. The ultimate contract is between the patient and the doctor, and this relationship must be based on mutual trust and mutual respect. Third party participation must not be allowed to supplant that venerable tradition.

4 MEDICINE AS A VERY OLD PROFESSION

Lewis Thomas

I first heard the term "medical ethics" in my childhood, a long time ago. Then, it referred to a small set of unambiguous, nonphilosophical matters worried over only by doctors and their families and related exclusively to money. Doctors who advertised, overcharged their patients, surreptitiously took over the care of patients already being looked after by another doctor, or split fees with other doctors were unethical and that was what the word meant. Doctors who performed abortions were not unethical, they were immoral or criminal, or both. Human experimentation was not unethical because there was no such activity, or perhaps it is better to say that it was not realized, even by practicing doctors, that experiments were performed on patients in the normal course of medical practice.

This was a time ago and medicine has changed a great deal, more than is remembered by most people, changed so much that even those old enough to have lived though the whole period have difficulty in recognizing the connections between the old enterprise and the new one. For, in a certain sense, it is like that: it is as though we gave up altogether one kind of profession called medicine and then took up another one. A long look backward is needed to see the change.

I am just old enough to take that sort of view, first-hand, having been born into a doctor's family during the last decades of the profession's former existence as an applied art, then growing up in a household sustained by that endeavor, then being trained as a doctor at the very turning point when it began to change into something like a science, and finally pursuing a career in the profession which was the result of that evolution. In those years it was easier to shift from one field to another, perhaps because the requirements for deep expertise were less demanding in the absence of so many detailed facts to comprehend. Thus, I had a close professional look at several disciplines along the way: pediatrics, internal medicine, pathology, infectious disease, immunology, and administration. All of these have changed so much in recent years that I cannot imagine people climbing over departmental walls and specialty boards so easily. On the other hand, I do envision a time ahead when the clinical sciences will come to share the same ground in their base of knowledge. Before long, a post-M.D. period of training in internal medicine and molecular genetics might serve to prepare a young graduate for almost any discipline, in the kind of medicine that lies somewhere ahead.

My father began the practice of medicine in 1905. He was a busy and successful general practitioner for most of his life, switching to become a self-trained and self-certified surgeon in his latter years, as was the custom at that time. During all his years in general practice he possessed only small bits of science, used solely for the purpose of diagnosis, and almost no science at all for therapy. What he did, for treating disease, was to "look after" people. This was all he, or anyone else, knew how to do, and it had little to do with technology.

Indeed, if it became known in the small town I grew up in that a doctor had become locally famous for his technical capacity to treat this or that disease, the question of medical ethics was automatically raised by the local establishment. Claims for being able to treat disease were almost, not quite but almost, grounds for being charged with quackery, and usually the charge was warranted. In those days quackery abounded.

Not to say that treatments for illness were not used by doctors, but these were more like gestures of reassurance, sometimes like incantations or amulets. Prescriptions were written in Latin of great complexity for numberless compounds, most of them green and bitter-tasting but without any known biologic properties, issued for all kinds of complaints, but neither my father nor other doctors of this time had any real faith in them. The best that could be said for the treatments was that they did no harm, which, by the way, was considerably more than could be said for the medicine of his father's time, or his grandfather's. I don't recall ever hearing about a suit for malpractice during my father's professional lifetime. The question simply didn't arise. Nobody could possibly have been damaged by the therapy available, even less by omitting it.

The doctors of his generation were mostly passive, and the things they did in their practices were mostly watching and waiting. They had been educated at the end of the first great revolution in medicine, and a large part of their education emerged out of the destruction and abandonment of masses of misinformation which preceding generations of physicians had taken for granted.

For a great many centuries, the technology of therapeutic medicine had been based on something rather like pure guesswork, and anybody's theory stood a good chance of being incorporated into dogma for the generations to follow. It was taken for granted that medicine, to be effective, had to be a strenuous, perilous sort of enterprise, and if things like these were not done the most ordinary kinds of illness would surely end fatally. There was no disease for which a treatment was not recommended. It is sometimes complained by today's medical students that the mountains of reductionist facts to be learned and set in memory are more than the mind can cope with, but the students just before my father's generation had a lot more to complain about. Looking through any textbook of medicine or pediatrics in the last years of the nineteenth century must have caused the learner's heart to sink. Every other page is filled with bizarre, esoteric pieces of therapy, each one to be performed exactly as laid out and learned (since none of them made any intrinsic sense) by rote. Poliomyelitis had to be treated by injections of strychnine, the application of leeches over the spine, the administration by mouth of extracts of belladonna and ergot, potassium iodide, huge doses of mercurial purgatives, faradic stimulation of the muscles, bleeding, and cupping. Meningitis required all these things, plus the spreading of cantharides ointment over the head and spine, strong enough to produce large blisters. Since all patients were treated more or less alike, there were almost no controlled investigations, and chance observations were quickly turned from anecdotes to tradition. Even so esteemed and skilled a pediatrician as Abraham Jacobi wrote in his famous 1896 textbook, concerning erysipelas, "The recovery of a young man observed with such symptoms lately I attribute solely to the large quantities of brandy administered."

Bleeding had been the sovereign therapy throughout the century before my father's entry into practice. The conventional treatment for tuberculosis and rheumatic fever was the removal each day of about a pint of blood, or enough to cause blanching, weakness, faintness, and a palpable weakening of the pulse: early *shock*, in short, facilitated even more by calomel and antimony in doses arranged to produce violent

diarrhea and vomiting. George Washington, by the way, is reported to have been treated for a peritonsillar abscess by the removal of 82 ounces of blood in his last, fatal illness. The point of all this was the doctrine, passed down through the centuries from Galen, that disease—any disease—was caused by the congestion of blood in one organ or another.

Protests against this kind of medicine had been raised as early as the 1830's, and a few observant physicians, here and abroad, took a careful look at what doctors were doing in the treatment of typhoid fever and delirium tremens and realized that they were doing a lot more harm than good. It very slowly dawned on the profession that a great many patients with various illnesses were capable of getting well all by themselves, without any treatment, and that many of the treatments then popular were probably making matters worse, but it took long decades before this kind of medicine was given up. At the same time, a genuine scientific activity, equivalent to the natural history of that day, got underway. Reliable classifications of human disease were constructed, based on careful clinical observations and correlated with the discoveries being made in the emerging field of pathology. Slowly but surely, during the latter part of the nineteenth century, the natural history of disease came to dominate medical education, and the art of making an accurate diagnosis and forecasting the likely outcome of every illness became the highest skill and the indispensable craft of the practicing physician.

This is what the doctors of my father's generation were trained to do. At the same time, largely under the influence of Sir William Osler, they were trained to be skeptical about treating disease. There were a few things they could do, but only a few. Malaria could be treated with quinine, digitalis was used with skill for heart failure, and morphine was the great standby—the most respected of all the drugs in the pharmacopoeia—for pain.

By the time I arrived in medical school in the mid-1930's there had been a few genuine advances, but still only a few: liver extract for pernicious anemia, insulin for diabetes, the early vitamins, immunization against diphtheria and tetanus, antiserum for pneumococcal pneumonia, not much else. I was taught at Harvard Medical School, as my father had been taught at Columbia, that treating disease would be the least of my future responsibilities. The doctor's job was to recognize the nature of disease with precision, so that he could explain to the patient, and to the patient's family, what was happening to him and how it was most likely to turn out.

This task, the explaining of illness, was the most important part of what was then called the art of medicine. It still is. Indeed, it has been a central duty of medicine, justifying all those millennia of the profession's existence, dating all the way back to our origins in shamanism. When you think about it, the first thing a sick person wants to know—and the sicker he is the more urgently he wants to know it—is "What's gone wrong?" And, in the same breath, "What happens next?" "Am I going to live?"

The quality of medicine's answers to these questions, and therefore the very usefulness of the doctor, were always matters of doubt until the great medical reform of the late nineteenth century. By the time of Osler, and in the decades that followed, science became the basis for explanation, and the answers became correspondingly more reliable.

It is easy to see why the mere act of explaining was so important, once you realize what being ill was like in the era before the discovery of antibiotics and the nearly successful conquest of infectious disease. Living was a considerably more chancy enterprise then. If you developed typhoid fever, which was still a common illness in the early years of my father's practice, you knew you were in for two months of constant high fever, deep malaise and debilitation, and the risk at any time of hemorrhage or perforation of the intestine.

You had about one chance in four of dying. If it was lobar pneumonia, which was the most common serious infection when I was a medical student, you had the prospect of dying or recovering spectacularly on your own within a shorter period—two weeks or so. The greatest danger of all, feared by everyone, was tuberculosis. People worried then about TB as they worry now about cancer, but for better reasons; people of all ages died from tuberculosis, and there was nothing at all to be done about it. Rheumatic fever, the cause of rheumatic heart disease, was the first thing to worry about whenever a young child developed a sore throat, and if you didn't worry about this you had to worry about poliomyelitis. The chief cause of insanity, filling the state hospitals of that time, was syphilis of the brain.

It was an enormous relief to be told that you or your family had none of these things the matter, and this was the function of a good doctor. But there was, of course, a lot more to the practice of medicine than simply explaining things.

When I was starting out as an intern, swept off my feet by the new demands for science in treating infectious disease, I used to wonder what my father did to keep so busy in his practice back in the days when there were no sulfonamides, no penicillin, no way of treating anything. Throughout my childhood, the telephone rang all day and all night in our house, and I remember waking up most nights at the sound of my father heaving out of bed and off in the family car on house calls, carrying along his black doctor's bag which contained almost nothing of any real value. There was nothing exceptional about his practice; this is what life was like for all the doctors in town when I was growing up. And yet, there was very little that he could do. He was, by the way, fully aware of this himself, as were his colleagues; he used to complain sometimes that most of the time he felt helpless; he was never really convinced that anything he did made a real difference to the outcome of an illness, in any of his patients, in all his life in medicine.

There is a mystery here, and it is an aspect of medicine that has been forgotten by too many people, doctors and patients alike. Once the nature of the illness had been identified for what it was, and the news conveyed to the patient, several other things happened. First of all, the doctor took on the responsibility for the outcome, for better or worse. And, perhaps most important of all, he stood by. Standing by was, getting down to brass tacks, what the doctor did: he might not have anything much in that black bag, and no magical potions to serve up, and certainly nothing that he could put into or get out of a computer, but he did have his presence, and that made a difference. Sir William Osler used to teach that it could make all the difference in the world: if the doctor understood what was occurring in his patient, and made that understanding available, and made himself available at the same time as a source of hope and strength, these acts of professional skill could turn the tide. I believe these things, even though I do not understand them.

I have one other piece of reminiscence about the medicine of 50 years ago, which has some bearing on the general problem of the future of medicine and medical science. It is this: 50 years ago, just before the profession underwent its transformation and the art began to incorporate science and technology, no one had the ghost of an idea that anything was about to happen. It was taken for granted by my generation that the medicine we were being taught in the year 1935 was precisely the medicine that would be with us for the rest of our lives. We expected nothing to change. If anyone had tried to tell us that the power to control bacterial infections was just around the corner, or that open-heart surgery or kidney transplants would be possible within two decades, or that some kinds of cancer would be cured by chemotherapy, or that there would soon be within reach a comprehensive biochemical explanation, in the most reductionist detail, for

genetics and genetically determined diseases, we would have reacted in blank disbelief. We had no reason to believe that medicine would ever change. We knew that subacute bacterial endocarditis and tuberculous meningitis were always fatal; we regarded schizophrenia as a totally unapproachable and insoluble problem; we believed that mental retardation was an act of nature for which we would never have an explanation, much less a treatment. All this has, of course, changed. Tuberculosis has vanished as a threat to the life of young children. There are so many new clues to the underlying mechanism of neoplasia that it is now a problem to make the right choice of a research line to pursue; senile dementia is out in the open, recognized now as one of the great challenges to medical science in our time.

And so forth. What this recollection tells me is that we should keep our minds wide open to the future. It is going to be different, whatever we think today. And, since change is inevitable, we should be spending more of our thought and energy making sure that the air is right for changes that seem to be in the right direction. This means, from my point of view, which I acknowledge as being self-interested and wholly prejudiced, more science.

We cannot go back to the old days in medicine. We should never allow ourselves to forget the healing property of a physician's presence and we should hang on to this mysterious gift even though we cannot explain it, but we cannot return to the era when that was all there was in medicine. We are nowhere near yet to where we should be; we are beset all around by the imperfections in our profession; we do a lot of things the wrong way and neglect doing essential things we could be doing better; even so, there is no prospect for changing medicine for the better in the years ahead except through science, more and profounder science.

But when people in my position say things like this we are well advised to add a cautionary footnote or two. We are always at risk of sounding like making too many promises, and speaking out of hubris, and we are not as candid as we ought to be about the extent of our ignorance. We are not about to change the world, nor are we in possession of a level of scientific understanding so powerful as to frighten people with what we might do next. We are, I'd say, *pretty* good at using science in medicine, but, thus far, only pretty good.

I wish there were some formal courses in medical school on Medical Ignorance; textbooks as well, although they would have to be very heavy volumes. We have a long way to go.

It is easy, these days, to look ahead. Medicine is being transformed before our eyes, and the power of our technologies for diagnosis and treatment is increasing with every month's new journal.

But I do not foresee any real change in the fundamental responsibility of doctors. Whatever they may gain in the way of technology in the decades ahead, I hope that they will be bound by the same deeply personal obligation to serve their patients. I hope my profession will never lose the memory of this obligation, for it is all we have in the way of historical continuity, the only real link to our professional ancestors.

I remember a short story from real life which illustrates an aspect of the responsibility of doctoring which does not find emphasis in many textbooks of medicine. Some years back I was invited to give a lecture on antibiotics at the annual meeting of a county medical society in a remote part of Mississippi. The audience was almost entirely made up of general practitioners, real country doctors. For the president of the society, a man in his 40's, this meeting was the major event of the year and one of the major occasions in his professional life; he was to be inducted formally into the office of president and had his speech prepared and ready. Just as the meeting began he was handed a note and left the auditorium to take a telephone call. That was the last I saw of him until three hours later, when he came back looking tired and worn out. I knew that he was deeply disappointed to have missed what should have been his own professional triumph, and I asked him what had happened. It was a call from a family of an elderly patient of his who had just died, he said. He felt that he ought to be there, to help the family, and to be useful. He simply had to be there, he said.

This was about 30 years ago, but I've never been able to forget that doctor and his example of good doctoring that evening. It's not quite the same thing as open-heart surgery or curing meningitis, but if I were looking around for a role model for today's medical students to look at very closely, I'd pick that country doctor in the backwoods countryside of Mississippi, if I could find him.

5 ETHICS IN THE PRACTICE OF MEDICINE

Albert R. Jonsen

"The responsibilities of medicine are threefold: to generate scientific knowledge and to teach it to others; to use the knowledge for the health of an individual or a whole community; and to judge the moral and ethical propriety of each medical act that directly affects another human being." With these words, Dr. Walsh McDermott opened his chapter, Medicine in Modern Society, in earlier editions of this textbook. Textbooks of medicine communicate the knowledge that constitutes the science of medicine and explain its application in the art of medicine. The third responsibility, "to judge the moral and ethical propriety of each medical act," is not expounded in the textbooks. Yet no one enters the profession of medicine without becoming vividly aware of its ethical tradition. The science and the art are imparted to students along with implicit ethical imperatives: to seek the patient's benefit, to avoid harm, to be respectful and compassionate, to preserve confidences, and to maintain competence. Medical students see these values embodied in their best professors, although as Louis Lasagna has said, students "may quickly absorb the moral atmosphere around them without questioning it." Physicians praise these values in their best colleagues, past and present. Some physicians fail to honor this ethical tradition; social and financial influences exert counterforces against it. Still, the ideals are clear and their vitality in the behavior of many individual physicians is remarkable.

The current revival of interest in medical ethics was not stimulated by a plague of immorality among physicians. It has not arisen because there is general disdain of, or disagreement about, the general principles of medical ethics. Rather, it has been fostered by a growing awareness on the part of physicians and the public that these general principles often seem inadequate to new situations. In some instances, widely publicized events have dramatized this inadequacy: the "God Committee," which selected patients "of social worth" in the early days of chronic hemodialysis; the Karen Ann Quinlan case; the Willowbrook hepatitis studies. In addition, interested scholars from medicine, philosophy, theology, sociology, and the law have attempted to analyze critically the general principles and to discern how they apply to the contemporary science and practice of medicine. In this way, a new discipline has arisen, sometimes called "bioethics."

Although the issues discussed in this new discipline are compelling, the discussions are necessarily general and abstract. The physician, however, must make decisions about the care of patients; often, those decisions will have ethical implications. The general and abstract must become particular and concrete. It is not enough to have a sincere attitude about, for example, discontinuing life-support systems. It is not sufficient to read a moving essay on allowing the dying "to die in dignity." Attitudes and information must be transformed into choices and practice. When the occasion arises, the ethical problems in the care of a patient must be assessed as skillfully as the patient's medical problem.

Every physician is familiar with the method of organizing clinical information: presenting symptoms and signs, history, physical exam, laboratory data. The competent physician evaluates these elements in seeking a diagnosis and selecting a treatment. A parallel method for reaching an ethical decision can be formulated. In almost any sort of clinical-ethical problem—be it withdrawing treatment, obtaining informed consent, preserving a confidence, or allocating a scarce resource—the facts and values necessary for a careful assessment can be displayed and evaluated under four headings: (1) indications for medical intervention, (2) patient's preferences, (3) patient's quality of life, and (4) external factors. This chapter will briefly explain how these four topics can be helpful in reaching an ethical decision. Thoughtful review of the relevant facts and values can put order into what is often a very confused consideration. Orderly consideration may not, of course, always reach the most suitable conclusion, but it should help avoid the two extremes that often distort clinical-ethical decisions: rash and precipitate action or paralyzing indecision. Both extremes can lead to tragedy for the physician, the patient, the family, and the institution.

INDICATIONS FOR MEDICAL INTERVENTION. Patients approach physicians with the hope of receiving the benefit of improved health or care in illness. The habitual activity of a physician is to gather information from and about the patient and to evaluate it with a view to determining whether or not medical intervention can benefit the patient. Clinical judgment, in which informed and careful estimates are made of the probable benefits and risks of each step in diagnosis and therapy, reflects the primary ethical responsibility of the physician. The most ancient rule of medical ethics is the Hippocratic dictum, "As to diseases, make a habit of two things—to help, or at least to do no harm." This duty manifests the "principle of beneficence," which ethicists designate as one of the fundamental ethical principles. They define it as "the duty to help others further their important and legitimate interests. . . ."

In most encounters between physician and patient, fulfillment of this duty is ethically unproblematic (although it may be medically difficult). Patients can inform the physician of the legitimate interests they wish furthered: they wish their health restored, their pain and symptoms relieved, their disabilities alleviated, their fears allayed. Physicians often respond with actions which have as their goal some specific benefit corresponding to those interests: elimination of meningococci by administration of penicillin G, control of blood pressure of 180/115 by an antihypertensive agent, prevention of the symptoms of celiac sprue by a gluten-restricted diet, and so forth. The interests of the patient and the response of physician center on benefits which reflect the goals of medical intervention: (1) restoration of health, (2) relief of symptoms, (3) restoration of function or maintenance of impaired function, (4) saving endangered life, and (5) supporting the patient by counseling and education. While all of these goals are seldom fully attained, they are the objectives which define the benefits of medicine.

At times, however, it might be asked whether one or another of these benefits is, in truth, a "benefit" for a particular patient. This question may occur to physician or to family in circumstances in which the patient is no longer able to declare his or her own interests. Typical clinical situations in which this sort of problem appears are as follows:

Case 1. A 38-year-old man with AIDS suffers a second episode of *Pneumocystis carinii* pneumonia. He is admitted to the ICU in respiratory failure, becomes hypotensive, acidotic, and septic. He is mentally incompetent. Should he be intubated?

Case 2. A 69-year-old woman has multiple sclerosis, diagnosed 30 years ago. She is now paraplegic and has begun to experience mood disturbance and to show signs of intellectual deterioration. She is brought to the hospital for treatment of pneumonia. Should she be treated?

In these cases, the first important ethical consideration is also the important clinical consideration: what objectives can be achieved by medical intervention? The answer must not be sought in the expected immediate results of some specific clinical intervention, but in those fundamental goals of medicine noted above.

The first formulation of the ethical question must be a realistic assessment of what might be accomplished by intervention (both in terms of the nature of the accomplishment and the probability of its occurrence). In Case 1, the only goal likely to be accomplished is a short prolongation of organic life. This, in and of itself, is not a proper goal of medicine. It is highly questionable that the physician has a duty to sustain and prolong human life when no prospect for any other human function is in view. The duty to prolong life in this sense has no roots in the history of medical ethics; it is an "artifact" of modern intensive care techniques. The physician's ethical obligation to initiate or continue treatment arises from the real probability that treatment will produce genuine benefit to the patient.

In Case 2, several of the goals of medicine can be achieved. Despite the woman's ultimate prognosis, she can be restored to her previous condition and helped in a number of ways. In terms of medical indications, she should be treated. However, her own preferences and the future quality of her life are added considerations. These are treated under the next two headings.

THE PREFERENCES OF THE PATIENT. If benefiting the patient means furthering that person's best interests, the patient's preferences, in general, should determine what constitutes benefit and harm. Individuals are usually the best advocates for their own interests. Recent critics of medicine accuse physicians of "paternalism," of assuming, because of their dominance over patients, the right to judge what is in that person's interest. Certainly, the history of medicine reveals an ethic colored by paternalism. The Hippocratic Oath states, "I will use treatment to help the sick, according to my ability and judgment." The patient's "ability and judgment" are not mentioned. In the past, "compassionate deception" was recommended "for the patient's good." Informed consent is a modern notion. Contemporary medical ethics, in the opinion of some of its proponents, consists almost entirely of the debate over paternalism and autonomy.

Autonomy, the personal liberty to make one's own choices and plan one's own life, is one of the central concepts of ethics. All of us value it highly in our own lives. An ethicist has written, "To respect autonomous agents is to recognize with due appreciation their own considered value judgments and outlooks even when it is believed that their judgments are mistaken."

In the practice of modern physicians, paternalism and autonomy are seldom in stark contrast. Physicians may be deficient in communicating information; often patients' preferences are not elicited or are disregarded. However, most modern physicians consider themselves advisors and, when

important questions arise about diagnosis, prognosis, and therapy, they will inform patients of their options and respect their preferences. The practice of informed consent is growing and the practice of deception waning. Still, there are situations in which serious ethical questions about autonomy must be asked. Two, in particular, occur from time to time in clinical practice: the refusal of recommended treatment believed by the physician to be critical for the patient's well-being, and the decision to treat or not to treat mentally incompetent patients.

Case 3. A 46-year-old woman has all of the indications for coronary angiography. She is known to the physician as timid and fearful. In the office, she is extremely nervous. Her physician fears she may refuse angiography if told the risks. Should she be told?

Case 4. A 54-year-old man, brought to the emergency room, has signs and symptoms strongly indicative of myocardial infarction. He is alert and oriented. He refuses hospitalization and insists on returning home. Should he be restrained?

The physician's anticipation that the patient may refuse recommendations (Case 3) does not justify deception, even though disclosure should be careful and sympathetic. Grounds for this anticipation may be weak. Should the patient suffer an adverse experience about which she was not informed, trust in the physician would be shaken. Deception fails to respect the patient. It undermines confidence in the profession. Should the informed patient actually refuse an intervention, efforts can be made to ascertain the motive and, if it is fear or misunderstanding, to deal with these. Actual refusal by an alert and competent person (Case 4) should be respected once the physician has made serious efforts to assure understanding and to ascertain competence. Similarly, if the woman with multiple sclerosis (Case 2) had no mental deficit, her refusal of treatment for acute disease should be respected.

Autonomy implies competence. Competence consists of the ability to deliberate about information and to draw conclusions: the conclusions need not be "true" or "sensible" or "correct." Clinical evidence of disorientation, confusion, psychosis, or even "peculiar judgments" when metabolic disturbance is suspected can cast doubt on competence. In the absence of clinical evidence of incompetence, it should not be presumed.

Case 5. A 32-year-old man known to his physician as a Jehovah's Witness has been treated for four years for peptic ulcer. He arrives at the hospital bleeding severely and refuses blood. He is lethargic and somewhat disoriented.

Case 6. A 19-year-old college student comes to the infirmary complaining of severe headache, malaise, and stiff neck. She has a fever of 39.4° C, and her pupils are contracted. Spinal fluid shows gram-positive diplococci. She refuses antibiotics but offers no reason.

In Case 4, the refusal of the patient with myocardial infarction to be hospitalized, no solid evidence of incompetence exists. The refusal of hospitalization possibly arises from denial, a common human psychologic mechanism rather than a mark of incompetence. The decision may be foolish and its consequences tragic. But the physician, after attempts at explanation and persuasion, does not bear responsibility for that patient's autonomous choice. Case 5 reveals a patient who is not, at that moment, competent. However, his history verifies long commitment to a doctrine, the consequences of which, it can be presumed, he accepts. His refusal should be respected. The "reasonableness" of that doctrine, in the eyes of others, is irrelevant. Case 6 shows a person who, while appearing oriented, might be presumed incompetent. She has a high fever; she offers no reason for refusal, and the consequences of refusal are certain and serious.

Most ethicists acknowledge that if a person truly is incapable of deciding rationally and freely, a form of limited paternalism is ethical. It involves making judgments in a person's best interest *temporarily*—until such persons are again capable of doing so for themselves. Thus, restraining a person in the hospital whose insistence on leaving appears to arise from a metabolically altered mental state could be justified, but only until the condition clears. However, such paternalism is justified only when there is solid evidence to suspect lack of competence. Vague affirmations, such as "It's his sickness talking," or "She is too emotional to make the right decision," hardly meet this standard. In general, the ethical principle of respect for autonomy requires a physician to formulate a judgment about the best interest of the patient, to offer that judgment to the patient for consideration, and to abide by the patient's considered decision. When the patient lacks ability to express such a decision, the physician should formulate a judgment based upon the best available evidence of that person's preferences: from past experience with the patient, from family and friends, from written directives, and so forth.

QUALITY OF LIFE. The phrase "quality of life" is used when people make judgments about the goodness or satisfaction of the life they are living, or about some part of it. It is a very subjective judgment: one arthritic patient might say, "My life is pretty poor quality. I've a lot of pain and not much mobility."; another might say, "I've got a lot of pain and not much mobility, but I have good quality life, since I can still read and listen to my music." At times it may be quite vague, as when one reads in a chemotherapy research consent form, "This treatment is intended to improve your quality of life; however, any treatment may decrease your quality of life." Doctors and patients alike are interested in life of high quality. In their dealings with each other, that interest dictates efforts to alleviate pain and symptoms, to stop the ravages of disease, and to allay fear and anxiety. Individuals are the best judges of the quality of their own lives. In recent years, however, the phrase has taken on a rather special meaning in medical discussions.

Those discussions often take place about a patient who is severely ill and whose only prospects are a life of pain or extreme limitation. At times, the patient's limitations may not be the result of a current acute illness, but of some other disorder, such as congenital retardation. Again, the patient's life might be one of deprivation or degradation. Still again, the patient may exist in a persistent vegetative state. In such cases, when acute medical intervention is needed, the question may be asked, "Is a life of such quality worth saving?"

The problems raised by this question are extremely complex. In general, several points should be made about the use of "quality of life" as a factor in clinical decisions. First, reports by the person who is living the life should be distinguished from the observations of other parties: the former have a higher claim to validity than the latter.

Second, all quality of life judgments are value judgments. Some of these value judgments can be amply supported by reference to certain manifest facts, such as the perception that someone is in great pain or is depressed. Other value judgments are less dependent on facts and more on personal or social predilections or prejudices, such as disdain for persons of low intelligence, the unproductive, and the unsuccessful. In clinical decisions, the former sort of value judgments legitimately carry considerable weight; the latter, in general, should not be influential (often such "moralistic" attitudes are implicit and have to be uncovered). There are two reasons for this: medicine has long attempted to eliminate moralistic judgments from clinical decisions and to care for suffering persons simply because they are suffering. Reliance on any

such criteria starts one down the slippery slope: the terminally ill are judged worthless, then the mentally ill, then the chronically ill, and so forth. The tragic consequences of this reasoning have marred medicine's history in this century. The less dramatic, but still tragic consequences for patients of certain social and economic status or of certain "unacceptable" life styles have been frequently documented. Quality of life is, then, an extraordinarily subtle notion. Its meaning in clinical decisions must be carefully scrutinized and cautiously applied.

EXTERNAL FACTORS. The three previous themes bear on the well-being, the preferences, and the qualities of the patient as an individual. In addition to these, it is sometimes necessary to consider factors external to the patient. These are the effects created in others' lives or in society by decisions made about the patient. Some of these are burdens: costs incurred by families, institutions, or society; hardships imposed upon relatives; dangers posed to other parties. Some are benefits: relief from hardships, protection of others, teaching and research potential associated with treatment. How are these external factors to be weighed in clinical decisions?

Certain external factors have long been branded as unethical: a physician prolonging useless treatment for profit alone; a family allowing a relative to die for the sake of inheritance. Others have been closely scrutinized and their role in ethical decisions carefully delineated: the use of patients for research purposes, the revealing of confidences for the benefit of others. The general rules are clear in these instances (although their application is often unclear). Except in very special circumstances, patients can be used for research only with their express consent, and, should the research procedure increase their risks, there should be some expectation of compensatory benefit to the patient. Confidences obtained in the course of care must be maintained unless there is well-founded anticipation that, because of lack of that information, notable harm is very likely to come to another party.

The influence of cost of care on clinical decisions is currently being debated. The import of this external factor on clinical decisions must be viewed even more cautiously than quality of life considerations. In principle, it is safe to say that only when patient preferences are unclear or unknown, when likelihood of benefit is low, and when the quality of the expected outcome is poor, the costs of continued care, for the family and for society, may become a legitimate consideration in deciding to forego life-sustaining treatment.

At the level of policy rather than of clinical decision, there may be determinations whether certain classes of patients should receive certain treatments, e.g., persons over or under a given age will not receive chronic hemodialysis; whether certain modalities of treatment will be developed and made available, e.g., a totally implantable artificial heart; whether a preventive modality should be developed in preference to a high-technology therapy. These policies should be designed not only in view of efficiency but also in view of the imperatives of distributive justice, the fair distribution of burdens and benefits throughout a society.

In general, policy determinations should not dictate clinical decisions about particular patients. Policy determinations should be made at that level where authority is properly situated, where public scrutiny can take place, and where information is available. External factors, while important, deserve the lowest priority in ethical decisions about patient care. Only when the objectives of honoring the patient's wishes and providing a benefit to the patient cannot be reasonably met should these factors be considered as important and decisive. Obviously, in any particular case, there will be discussion about the nature of these objectives and the probability of their attainment.

CONCLUSIONS. Ethical positions are neither entirely a matter of private preference nor a matter of general principles.

They are a mixture of preferences, principles, and facts. The mixture is often confused. Since it is the responsibility of the competent practitioner "to judge the moral and ethical propriety of medical acts," the confusion should be dispelled as much as possible. In each difficult case, the ethical perplexity should be clearly stated, the facts carefully discerned, personal prejudices exposed, and the relevant principles thoughtfully examined. This chapter has suggested a method for organizing these elements in view of a clinical decision. However, a method alone will not resolve the problems. Content, in the form of appreciation of ethical values and understanding of ethical principles, must be inserted into the method. Some reading should be done in the now voluminous and valuable literature in medical ethics. Consultation with persons familiar with these issues should be sought. Frank conversation with all involved—the patient, the family, house officers, and nurses—should be promoted. In this way, the practitioner will deserve to be called not only competent but also responsible.

Ad Hoc Committee on Medical Ethics, American College of Physicians: American College of Physicians Ethics Manual. Part I: History of medical ethics, the physician and the patient, the physician's relationship to other physicians, the physician and society. Ann Intern Med 101:129, 1984.

Ad Hoc Committee on Medical Ethics, American College of Physicians: American College of Physicians Ethics Manual. Part II: Research, other ethical issues. Recommended reading. Ann Intern Med 101:263, 2984.

Beauchamp TL, Childress JF: Principles of Biomedical Ethics. 2nd ed, New York, Oxford University Press, 1983. *An excellent systematic treatment, more philosophical than practical, of the basic principles which should underlie medical practice and health care.*

Beauchamp TL, Walters L (eds.): Contemporary Issues in Bioethics. 2nd ed. Encino, CA, Dickenson Publishing, 1982. *A comprehensive anthology of philosophical background and current problems.*

Jonsen AR, Siegler M, Winslade W: Clinical Ethics: A Practical Approach to Ethical Decisions in Clinical Medicine. 2nd ed. New York, Macmillan, 1986. *A practical guide to frequent ethical problems posed to the practitioner; explains the four considerations of medical indications, patient preferences, quality of life, and external factors.*

Reich W (ed.): Encyclopedia of Bioethics. New York, The Free Press-Macmillan, 1978. *An invaluable reference work of comprehensive, concise entries on most of the issues of biomedical ethics.*

Siegler M: Recommended reading in medical ethics. Ann Intern Med 101:268, 1984. *A selection of articles from medical literature on the major ethical problems encountered by the practitioner of internal medicine.*

Walters L (ed.): Bibliography of Bioethics. The Kennedy Institute of Ethics. Washington, DC, Georgetown University, annual. *A comprehensive compilation of citations of English language literature in medical ethics. Issued annually and available as Bioethicsline, a computerized information system of the National Library of Medicine.*

SUMMARY

These introductory essays have been both discursive and eclectic. Medicine is almost boundless in scope as we move toward the last decade of the twentieth century. Although much has changed, there is much that has remained the same in its traditions and common purposes. Eight centuries ago Moses ben Maimon (Maimonides) prayed:

"Grant me an opportunity to improve and extend my training, since there is no limit to knowledge. Help me to correct and supplement my educational defects as the scope of science and its horizon widen day by day. Give me the courage to realize my daily mistakes so that tomorrow I shall be able to see and understand in a better light what I could not comprehend in the dim light of yesterday."

The *Cecil Textbook of Medicine* has been dedicated to furnishing "a better light" for more than half a century. It is a privilege to be associated with this 18th edition of a book that has become an institution in medical education.

JAMES B. WYNGAARDEN AND LLOYD H. SMITH, JR.

PART II

HUMAN GROWTH, DEVELOPMENT, AND AGING

6 ADOLESCENT MEDICINE

Iris F. Litt

The teenager is a psychosocially and physically unique individual, and this uniqueness has important implications for health and health care. In addition to the age-specific features of this period of life, there are significant differences among adolescents, based upon their rates of pubertal development as well as their developmental stages within adolescence. The view of the adolescent from the physical standpoint reveals the importance of stage of pubertal development, rather than chronologic age, as an organizing principle, owing to the wide variability in timing of pubertal events. From a psychosocial perspective, early adolescents, middle adolescents, and late adolescents have many psychosocial and cognitive characteristics shared with others in their own age groups. There is a growing tendency to combine these vantage points and recognize the areas of interaction between pubertal and psychosocial development.

PSYCHOSOCIAL DEVELOPMENT

During adolescence, certain tasks must be mastered if the child is going to evolve into a successful adult in our society. These include the "tasks of adolescence": the process of separation from the protective milieu of the family and, with it, development of independence; incorporation of the physical and emotional effects of pubertal hormonal changes into one's self-concept; development of a clear sexual identity and a sense of sexual adequacy; educational and vocational decision making; and achievement of the capacity for intimacy. Accomplishing these goals may, in actuality, take a lifetime, but the physician caring for adolescents may encounter opportunities to assist in the psychosocial development of the adolescent.

The physician may foster development of independence by encouraging the adolescent to make his or her own appointments, by promising confidentiality when appropriate, by handing the prescription directly to the adolescent patient, rather than to the parent, and so on. Encouraging the parent of a chronically ill adolescent to assign household chores, to provide an allowance, and to allow going to friends' houses for "overnights" may prevent infantilization at the time when adolescents must be allowed to experience their emerging maturity. Failure to do so often results in "acting-out" behavior. One consequence of the stereotype of adolescents as rebellious patients is that physicians may expect them to be noncompliant with prescribed medication. When this stereotype is examined, however, it is found that the incidence of noncompliance is no different among adolescents than among adult patients, in the range of 40 to 50 per cent. The factors associated with noncompliance among adolescents are, however, different. Self-concept is the single most important predictor of compliance: The teenager who has a positive self-image is likely to follow the physician's advice. Moreover, the risk of noncompliance is great with any medication that affects appearance adversely, such as a systemic corticosteroid. The patient's satisfaction, a valid predictor of compliance for adult patients, is also important for the adolescent patient, but, here again, its determinants are different. The satisfied adolescent patient is the one whose privacy is respected, who is afforded the courtesy of confidentiality, and who is informed about the reasons for laboratory testing. Self-concept is also related to the risk of pregnancy during adolescence. Poor self-concept may place the young adolescent girl at increased risk of an exploitative relationship or cause her to lack the confidence to set limits within a sexual relationship. Low self-concept is also associated with poor compliance with oral contraceptives.

Among the many causes of poor self-concept is the timing of pubertal maturation. For males, maturing earlier than the peer group appears to be an advantage, associated with popularity and athletic prowess, whereas a late-maturing male is predisposed to poorer educational performance and lower self-image. For girls, the effects vary with the environmental context; for example, early maturers who remain in a kindergarten-through-eighth grade school exhibit no apparent ill effect from being out of synchrony with their peer group, whereas those early maturers who move to a junior high school have a higher incidence of poor self-image, have a lower grade-point average, and date more. Timing of pubertal development may also influence selection of sports involvement. Early maturing females tend to have more adipose tissue, are more buoyant, and therefore may be channeled into swimming. The late-maturing girl, on the other hand, with her shorter upper to lower body ratio and leaner body may be more likely to become a ballet dancer or runner. An increase in body fat accompanies normal pubertal development in females, who often have difficulty reconciling it with our society's idealized female form of a skinny fashion model. Their dissatisfaction may result in dieting and the risk of nutritional deficiencies. This puberty-associated dieting may be the forerunner of anorexia nervosa in the predisposed individual (see Ch. 13).

The physician may assist the adolescent's development of a healthy sense of sexual identity and adequacy by offering reassurance about the normality of secondary sex characteristics and genitalia during the course of a routine physical examination. This is particularly important when gynecomastia is observed, as this common phenomenon often causes concern to the adolescent male, who is unlikely to have the courage to inquire about it. The female adolescent with asymmetry of her breasts or one who has not gotten pregnant despite having had unprotected intercourse, or the male teenager who has never impregnated his sexual partner, all may be questioning their sexual adequacy and normality. Even more problematic is the male adolescent who has a renal or urologic condition. The separation of reproductive from excretory function and structure may not be known or apparent to the apprehensive patient, though this is often assumed by his physician. A useful method for allaying such fear may be concrete explanations about anatomy and pathogenesis of the condition, prefaced by a comment like the following: "Some other boys who have had this operation have been worried that it may interfere with their ability to have sex. I don't know if you have had this worry, but I want to reassure you that it will not."

COGNITIVE DEVELOPMENT

The issues of counseling and confidentiality in the context of health care delivery to adolescents are complicated by the developmental differences in cognition among them. Piaget classified children and adolescents on the basis of discrete stages of cognitive development (Table 6–1). According to this schema, most early adolescents would be considered to be at the stage of concrete operational thinking, whereas the middle and late adolescent would be more likely to have progressed to the highest stage of development, that of formal operations. This stage is distinguished by the ability to generate hypotheses that may be tested without their actual enactment. Moreover, the person in the stage of formal operations can think abstractly, entertain multiple contingencies simultaneously, and is able to generalize from one situation to another and to consider potential behavioral consequences logically without actually having to experience them. Piaget's static, categoric approach to cognitive development has been challenged. Newer research in the field stresses "trends" in development. For example, the thinking of the younger individual would now be regarded as being more "empirico-deductive" than that of the older adolescent, who is viewed as being more "hypothetico-deductive." Whatever the system used to evaluate cognition, it is important for the physician working with the adolescent patient to be able to assess his or her capacity for understanding the information conveyed and to be able to use it in a manner conducive to improving health status. For example, the adolescent female who is not able to think abstractly may have difficulty adhering to a regimen of oral contraceptives designed to prevent pregnancy. Similarly, truly informed consent to participate in a research project may not be obtainable from an adolescent subject unable to consider hypothetic consequences of his or her decision to participate or not.

PUBERTAL DEVELOPMENT
The Endocrinology of Puberty

The signal that initiates puberty remains elusive but it is known that just prior to puberty there is decreasing sensitivity of the hypothalamus and pituitary to circulating estrogen and testosterone and to the restraining influence of the hypothalamic arcuate neuron gonadotropin-releasing hormone. The latter secretion is a pulsatile secretion and is associated with sleep. The onset of puberty is marked by increased secretion of luteinizing hormone (LH) by the pituitary during sleep in a pulsatile fashion. The amplitude and frequency of LH pulses

TABLE 6–1. PIAGET'S ERAS AND STAGES OF LOGICAL AND COGNITIVE DEVELOPMENT

Era I   (ages 0–2): The era of sensorimotor intelligence
Era II   (ages 2–5): Symbolic, intuitive, or prelogical thought
Era III (ages 6–10): Concrete operational thought
Era IV   (age 11–adulthood): Formal operational thought

increase as puberty progresses. In late puberty, the adult pattern of approximately 12 pulses, evenly distributed over the course of a 24-hour period, is reached. There is a sex difference in gonadotropin secretion during puberty: A dramatic increase in LH levels occurs during early puberty in boys and later in girls. Follicle-stimulating hormone (FSH), on the other hand, rises gradually throughout puberty in boys and manifests an early rise in girls. The effect of the gonadotropin rise in boys is to stimulate testicular production of testosterone. In females, the gonadotropin rise (predominantly involving FSH) stimulates the ovary to produce estradiol, with serum levels rising incrementally as puberty progresses. Cyclic fluctuations in estradiol levels are noted around the time of menarche. Estrone, derived from conversion of estradiol and adrenal androstenedione, reaches its peak at sex maturity rating (SMR) 2 in girls. In boys, both estrone and estradiol (derived from conversion of adrenal and testicular testosterone and androstenedione) contribute to the frequent occurrence (in 30 to 50 per cent) of gynecomastia during SMR 2 and 3. Circulating sex hormones exert a constant or tonic negative feedback upon the hypothalamus in both sexes. The female experiences, additionally, a cyclic positive feedback loop by which increasing levels of circulating estrogens in the follicular phase cause a surge in LH. Sex hormone binding globulin levels fall in males during puberty. As only unbound sex hormones are physiologically active, this results in levels of free testosterone that are more than twice the female level. Prolactin secretion by the pituitary is augmented by estrogen, resulting in higher levels in females than males, peaking between SMR 2 and 3. Prolactin response to thyrotropin-releasing hormone (TRH) stimulation, however, peaks at SMR 4 to 5.

Growth Hormone and Somatomedin-C

Growth hormone is also produced in a pulsatile fashion, during sleep stages 3 and 4 in early puberty. Somatomedins are responsible for the anabolic activity of growth hormone. Somatomedin-C (IGF-1) levels are age dependent and rise in conjunction with advancing development of secondary sex characteristics during puberty. Accordingly, their levels correlate better with stage of sexual maturation than chronologic age.

Physical Growth During Puberty

During puberty, a growth spurt is experienced by every organ system in the body, with the exception of the central nervous system, which remains stable in size, and the lymphoid system, which undergoes involution. The most noticeable changes produced by the pubertal growth spurt are in height, weight, and the secondary sex characteristics.

The pubertal height spurt occurs during midpuberty (SMR 3 to 4) in most individuals, with its peak occurring at an average age of 12 years in girls and 14 years in boys. During this height spurt, males gain 10.3 ± 1.54 cm per year and females gain 9.0 ± 1.03 cm per year. The growth velocity is greater the earlier it occurs. There is an orderly pattern of linear growth, beginning with the foot, followed within six months by the lower leg and then the thigh. Growth of the upper extremity and of the trunk occurs after that of the lower extremity. The later onset of the growth spurt in males than females results in a longer period of prepubertal growth and, hence, longer legs in the former. Assessment of height during puberty should be undertaken using a height velocity curve, which records increments in height per year (Fig. 6–1).

Approximately four months after the peak of leg-length acceleration, there is an increase in the biacromial and biiliac diameters, the former of greater magnitude in males and the latter in females, resulting in characteristic sex differences in adult physiques. At about the same time, the cranial bones

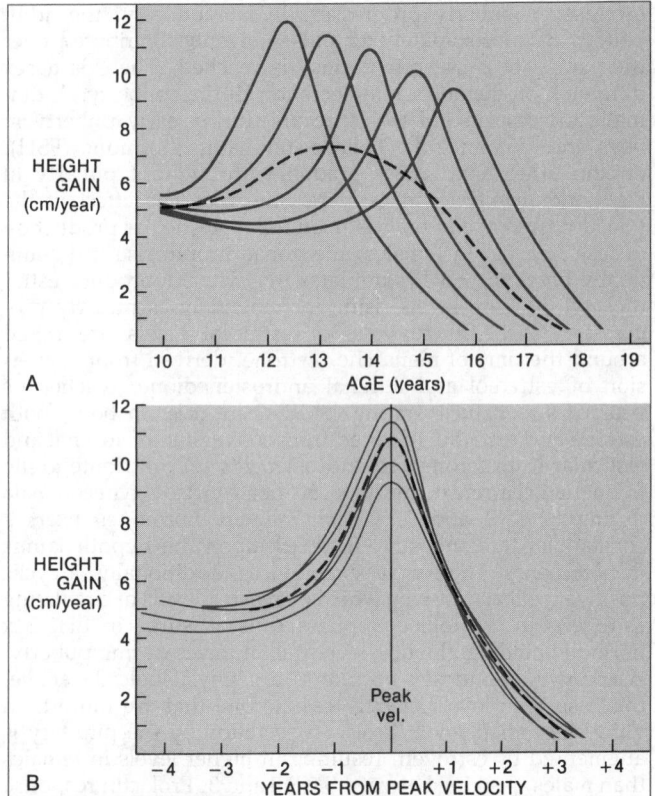

FIGURE 6–1. The relation between individual and mean velocities during the adolescent spurt. *A*, The individual height velocity curves of five boys of the Harpenden Growth Study (solid lines) with the mean curve (dashed) constructed by averaging their values at each age. *B*, The same curves all plotted according to their peak height velocity. (Adapted from Tanner JM: Fetus Into Man. Cambridge, MA, Harvard University Press, 1978, p 12.)

undergo a growth spurt, particularly the jaw, which becomes more prominent, especially in boys. Elongation of the pharynx causes lowering of the hyoid bone. Dentition is another reflection of pubertal development. The cuspids (canines) and first molars of the primary dentition are shed by early adolescence, at which time the permanent cuspids and the first and second premolars erupt in their place. The timing of appearance of the second permanent molar correlates well with that of menarche. The third molars, "wisdom teeth," erupt during late adolescence.

Bone age can be determined from a roentgenogram of the hand, which is compared with standards in an atlas. During puberty, there is close correlation between bone age and stage of sexual maturation (SMR—see below).

Although both sexes experience a weight spurt during puberty, its origin is different in males and females. In males, it is due to increase in muscle mass, and in females, to fat tissue. Eight per cent of body composition is about average fat content in both sexes throughout childhood. At puberty, males experience a loss in fat tissue, whereas it begins to increase in the female and reaches approximately 22 per cent when pubertal growth is complete (SMR 5).

Secondary Sex Characteristics

Estrogen and testosterone have a profound effect on a variety of tissues and organs during puberty. These effects are collectively referred to as secondary sex characteristics. These include voice change, body and facial hair in males, breast development in females, and axillary and pubic hair in both sexes. Of these changes, those that are most consistent in pattern and timing are pubic hair in both sexes and breast development in females. Accordingly, these traits have

formed the basis for categorization of the stages of pubertal development, generally referred to as sex maturity ratings (SMR's).

Stages of Pubertal Development (SMR's): Breast

SMR 1: Childlike. No breast development.
SMR 2: Appearance of a breast bud.
Increase in diameter of the areola. Average age is 11.2 ± 1.6 years.
SMR 3: Enlargement of the breast. Average age is 12.15 ± 1.09 years.
SMR 4: The areola and papilla enlarge to form a mound above the underlying breast tissue. Average age is 13.11 ± 1.15 years.
SMR 5: Adult configuration with areola and underlying breast tissue in same plane. Average age is 14.5 ± 1.6 years.

Stages of Pubertal Development (SMR's): Pubic Hair

SMR 1: Childlike. No pubic hair.
SMR 2: Hair is fine, long, silky, and lightly pigmented. Distributed in the midline, along the separation of the labia majora in females and the base of the phallus in males. Average age is 11.9 ± 1.5 years in females and 12.3 ± 0.8 years in males.
SMR 3: Hair is darker and coarser and begins to curl. It extends upward and laterally. Average age is 12.7 ± 0.5 years in females and 13.9 ± 1.04 years in males.
SMR 4: Adult texture and distributed to cover the mons pubis. Average age is 13.4 ± 1.2 in females and 14.36 ± 1.08 years in males.
SMR 5: Adult texture. Distributed beyond the mons to the medial aspect of the thighs. Average age is 14.6 ± 1.1 years in females and 15.3 ± 0.8 years in males.

Stages of Pubertal Development (SMR's): Male Genitalia

SMR 1: Childlike. Testes average 2 ml in volume.
SMR 2: Scrotal skin begins to redden and thin. Scrotum narrows proximally, testes enlarge, and left testis lowers. Penis begins to lengthen. Mean age is 11.64 ± 1.07 years.
SMR 3: Testes continue to enlarge. Growth of corpora cavernosa penis contributes to widening, as well as lengthening, of penis. Mean age is 12.85 ± 1.04 years.
SMR 4: Further enlargement of testes and penis. Scrotum darkens. The glans becomes prominent. Average age is 13.7 ± 1.02 years.
SMR 5: Testes have reached adult size of approximately 25 ml and weight of 20 gm. Full reproductive capability by this stage. Average age is 15.1 ± 1.1 years.

"Primary" Sex Characteristics

The sine qua non of puberty is attainment of reproductive function. To this end, there is considerable growth of the reproductive organs. As indicated above, this process in the male commences with enlargement of the testes as a result of the growth in size of their seminiferous tubules and the number of Leydig's and Sertoli's cells. The epididymis, seminal vesicles, and prostate enlarge as well. The capacity for ejaculation is achieved approximately one year after testicular growth begins, coincident with appearance of pubic hair (SMR 2). For most, the first ejaculatory episode occurs in the context of masturbation, followed about one year later by nocturnal emissions. The median age for appearance of sperm in the first morning urine sample is 13.5 to 14.5 years. The timing of spermarche is unrelated to other manifestations of puberty, occurring at any SMR from 1 to 5 and antedating the peak height velocity. Although complete reproductive capability is not reached until SMR 5, it is possible for impregnation to occur much earlier. Accordingly, anticipatory guidance about pregnancy prevention should commence during early to middle adolescence for males.

Increasing levels of estrogen during pubertal development lead to endometrial thickening, enlargement of the corpus, and increase in cellular content of actomyosin, creatine phosphokinase (CPK), and adenosine triphosphate (ATP), presumably in preparation for menses and childbirth. Menarche occurs at a mean age of 13.3 ± 1.3 years, although its timing corresponds better with developmental than chronologic age.

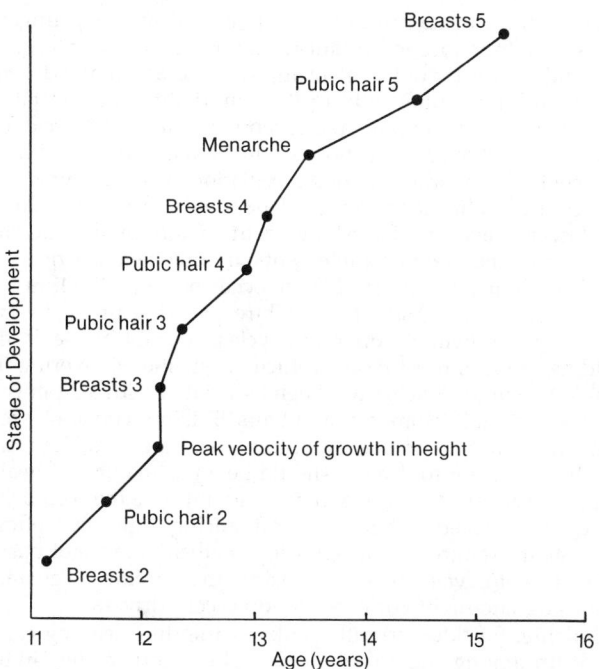

FIGURE 6–2. Sequence of breast and pubic hair development in adolescent girls.

Ten per cent of girls have menarche at SMR 2, 20 per cent at SMR 3, 60 per cent at SMR 4, and the remaining 10 per cent at SMR 5. In addition, there is close concordance between menarche and the peak of the weight velocity curve, which follows by approximately six months the peak of the height velocity curve. The inter-relationships of timing of pubertal events are shown in Figures 6–2 and 6–3. These inter-relationships are useful in the clinical assessment of the young adolescent who is concerned about her failure to begin to menstruate. Regardless of her chronologic age, she should be further evaluated if she is more than one year older than her mother or siblings at the time they experienced menarche, if she is at SMR 5, or if her bone age is 14.5 years or greater. In addition, failure to begin pubertal development by the age of 11 years should be cause for concern. Menarche occurs earlier

in the obese than the lean adolescent female. Moreover, weight loss of as little as 10 per cent of body weight may result in cessation of menstruation, as can vigorous athletic training with or without weight loss. Full reproductive capability is typically reached within a year following menarche, but some adolescents ovulate regularly from the time of menarche, underscoring the need for timely education about pregnancy risk.

HEALTH PROBLEMS OF ADOLESCENTS

The image of adolescents as healthy and therefore not in need of health care has been fostered by a number of factors. Among them is the fact that this age group contributes only 11 per cent of office visits to physicians, the majority for gynecologic or obstetric care or acute injuries. However, data from the National Health Examination Survey of 1966 to 1970 reveal that 20 per cent of presumably healthy 12- to 17-year-olds have previously undiagnosed health problems, the majority of which are related to the rapid growth and maturation that characterize puberty.

Health Problems Related to Puberty

Skeletal System. The marked osseous growth during puberty renders the skeletal system vulnerable at this time. For example, Osgood-Schlatter disease or slipped capital femoral epiphysis and idiopathic scoliosis occur primarily during puberty. Certain neoplasms of osseous origin, such as osteogenic sarcoma, have their peak incidence at this time. Functional problems such as pitcher's elbow or "shin splints" are manifestations of adolescents' propensity for overinvolvement in athletic activities, and fractures are common sequelae of adolescent risk-taking behavior and resultant accidents.

Endocrine System. Failure to achieve puberty at the appropriate time is often the symptom that leads to diagnosis of endocrinopathies, such as pituitary insufficiency, during adolescence. Conversely, syndromes of precocious puberty or exaggerated adrenarche (e.g., hirsutism and acne) may result in discovery at this time of disorders of excess production of hormones (e.g., adrenal hyperplasia or hypothalamic or ovarian tumor). Euthyroid goiter is a common condition of adolescent females and is often the first sign of Hashimoto's thyroiditis.

Gynecologic. Gynecologic problems are common during this age period. They may be the result of previously undiagnosed congenital abnormalities, endocrinopathies, or exposure to oncogenic agents in utero, or they may be acquired as a result of adolescent sexual experimentation.

Primary dysmenorrhea is almost exclusively an adolescent medical problem. One third of adolescent females suffer from severe, incapacitating dysmenorrhea. It is the leading cause of short-term school absence among female teenagers, yet is easily preventable. Intervention is based on suppressing production of prostaglandins $F_{2\alpha}$ and E_2, which are produced in excess by the endometrium of patients with dysmenorrhea. Alternatively, inhibiting ovulation, and thereby the corpus luteum's production of progesterone, which primes the myometrium to the effects of the prostaglandins, will be effective. The first is accomplished through the use of cyclo-oxygenase inhibitors; the second goal is obtained with oral contraceptives. Failure to respond to these approaches should prompt laparoscopy to diagnose possible endometriosis.

Menometrorrhagia also presents special issues when it occurs in this age group. The differential diagnosis can be approached by separating those conditions that are painful from those that are painless (Table 6–2). The most common cause of menometrorrhagia in the adolescent is so-called dysfunctional uterine bleeding. This condition results from the anovulatory cycles following menarche in which estrogen is unopposed by progesterone, causing buildup of proliferative endometrium and its subsequent shedding. Management

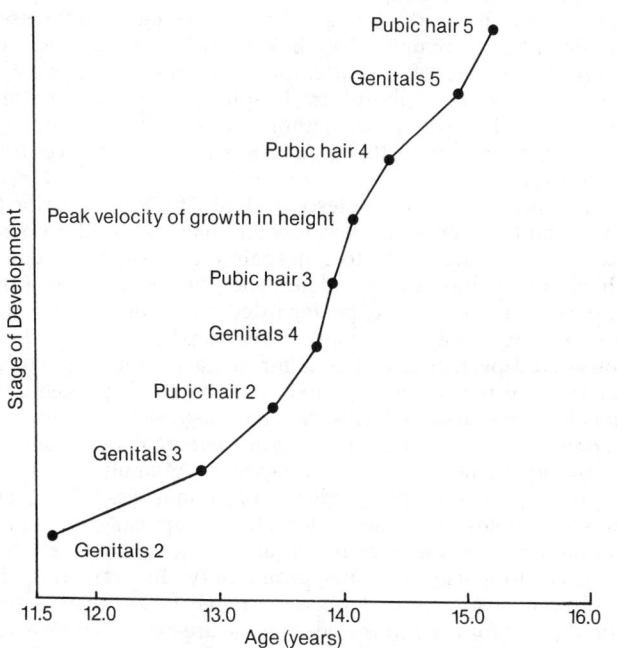

FIGURE 6–3. Sequence of genital and pubic hair development in adolescent boys.

TABLE 6–2. DIFFERENTIAL DIAGNOSIS OF MENOMETRORRHAGIA

Painless	Painful
Systematic	Trauma
Coagulopathy	Threatened abortion
Congenital	Salpingitis
von Willebrand disease	Intrauterine device
Acquired	
Aspirin sensitivity	
Aplastic anemia	
Anticoagulant treatment	
Neoplasm-bone marrow infiltration	
Idiopathic thrombocytopenia	
Endocrine	
Hypothyroidism	
Oral contraceptives—used improperly	
Local	
Gynecologic	
Dysfunctional uterine bleeding	
Neoplasm	

From Litt IF: Menstrual problems during adolescence. Pediatr Rev 4:203, 1983.

of menometrorrhagia in the adolescent includes reassurance (the young patient who develops this problem with her first menstrual period, in particular, will be extremely frightened), cardiovascular support if blood loss has been excessive, and appropriate diagnostic tests (remembering that results of certain of these tests may be altered by the administration of estrogens). Treatment with a combination of high-dose estrogen (for hemostasis) and progestin (to oppose endogenous estrogen effect), as may be found in Enovid (mestranol and norethynodrel), is effective except in cases of pregnancy, trauma, or infection.

Another menstrually associated condition of particular importance in adolescents is toxic shock syndrome (see Ch. 271). Forty-two per cent of cases reported during its peak years of 1980 to 1982 were in this age group.

A number of other gynecologic conditions of adolescents result from sexual experimentation. The reported prevalence of sexual intercourse among American girls between 13 and 19 years of age increases from 10 to 50 per cent and with it an increase in sexually transmitted diseases and pregnancy.

Pregnancy during adolescence continues to be a major problem in the United States, which is distinguished by having the highest rate of any of the developed countries. Close to one-half million 15- to 19-year-olds become pregnant yearly. In addition, over the past two decades, there has been nearly a 200 per cent rise in the number of out-of-wedlock births in this age group, as well as an increase in the number of unmarried adolescents who elect to keep their babies, rather than place them for adoption. Among those under the age of 15 years, the number of births continues to rise, with 30,000 last year. In addition to the psychosocial sequelae of adolescent births (such as adverse educational, vocational, economic, and marital outcomes), those who become pregnant under the age of 15 years are generally at increased risk for obstetric and perinatal complications such as toxemia, postpartum hemorrhage, postpartum infection, and small-for-gestational age and stillborn infants.

Sexually Transmitted Disease (STD). Adolescents have the highest rate of sexually transmitted disease of any age group. The most common of the STDs are gonorrhea and chlamydial infection. Physicians should routinely test for the possible presence of other STDs when one is discovered, treat with the shortest effective methods, including parenteral antibiotics when feasible, and extend confidentiality to contacts.

Violence

Accidents, homicides, and suicides together are responsible for 70 per cent of adolescent deaths. Anticipatory guidance, prevention, and identification and referral of the youngster at risk are therefore important roles for the physician.

Accidents. Although athletic injuries and accidental drowning contribute significantly to their morbidity and mortality, the greatest toll among adolescents is taken by accidents involving motor vehicles. Sixteen- to 19-year-olds constitute 8 per cent of the United States population, yet account for 17 per cent of vehicular fatalities. Passengers in cars driven by adolescents account for 63 per cent of automotive deaths. More male than female adolescents are involved as drivers in fatal accidents, and most of these occur between the hours of 8 P.M. and 4 A.M. Aside from failure to use seatbelts in cars and to wear helmets on motorcycles, alcohol abuse is the leading cause of most motor vehicular fatalities. Lowering the drinking age to 18 years has been associated with a 5 per cent increase in fatal automotive accidents. Talking with adolescent patients about their use of automotive safety devices and alcohol use prior to driving should be a routine part of health care. Moreover, physicians may act to improve the well-being of their teenaged patients by influencing legislative efforts such as those directed at requiring seatbelts in school buses, use of motorcycle helmets, raising the drinking age, and imposing late-night curfews for adolescent drivers.

Suicide. Suicide currently ranks as the third leading cause of death among the 15- to 19-year-old cohort in the United States. Completed suicides are more likely to occur in males, whereas female adolescents are more likely to make uncompleted attempts. Sex differences also exist regarding the method used in the attempt; males are more likely to use violent methods, such as shooting, hanging, or wrist slashing, whereas females are more prone to ingestion of drugs. Chronically ill adolescents are at high risk for suicide, and their own medication may be ingested in the suicide attempt. Alternatively, the medication is often that of the parent with whom the teenager is in conflict. Assessment of the seriousness of the adolescent's suicide attempt becomes crucial to planning following such an act. The physician may be surprised to learn that the youngster who ingested a bottle of antibiotics was actually expecting to die as a result or, conversely, that the one who took a bottle of acetaminophen resulting in admission to the intensive care unit had erroneously thought the substance harmless and was only trying to get some attention from his or her parents. The adolescent who fails in an initial suicide attempt is at increased risk for a subsequent serious one, if the crisis has not been adequately addressed in the interim. Simply attending to the pharmacologic or surgical sequelae of the attempt does little to resolve the underlying conflict. Short-term hospitalization is often effective in providing a secure setting for the teenager and impressing parents with the need to seek help for the contributing problems.

Identification of the adolescent at risk for suicide prior to an attempt presents an even greater challenge to the physician. Mood swings from deep despair to the heights of elation are not uncommon during adolescence, but persistence of the depressed mood should be regarded as a potential sign of trouble. According to Puig-Antich, depression should be considered persistent if it lasts for at least three consecutive hours for three or more periods each week. Expressions of hopelessness and helplessness are also serious signs of depression. Disturbance of eating or sleeping may or may not be found in the depressed adolescent. A family history of depression is a useful predictor of seriousness. Some depressed adolescents may, alternatively, appear perpetually euphoric and may engage in socially self-destructive behavior such as drug use or sexual promiscuity. In evaluating the adolescent suspected of depression, it may be useful to inquire about plans for the future. When none are expressed or when the response is "what does it matter, I won't be here much longer," serious depression is obvious. When there is a suggestion of depression, the physician should not hesitate to inquire if the teenager has ever felt so sad that death was viewed as preferable. If answered in the affirmative, the existence of a suicide plan should be sought and such a patient should be immediately evaluated by a psychiatrist. Such questioning will not prompt suicidal thoughts in a youngster who has not already had them and will be greeted with relief by the one who has.

Substance Abuse

Experimentation with drugs serves a variety of purposes for adolescents in our society. It may symbolize attainment of adult maturity or rejection of parental values, facilitate peer acceptance, reduce stress, and, for some, provide an opportunity to explore the limits of new cognitive abilities through hallucinogenic effects. Intervention strategies for preventing or stopping drug use by adolescents must consider these various developmentally adaptive implications. Since more than 90 per cent of adolescents have experimented with either alcohol or marijuana by the time of high school graduation, the focus of the physician's involvement should be on the functional and physical implications of use rather than on the simple ascertainment of use or non-use.

Overall use of illicit drugs by high school seniors has decreased from a peak of 39 per cent in 1979 to 32 per cent in 1983 (Johnston et al.). Decline of marijuana use to 5.5 per cent is largely responsible for this finding. Declines have also been recorded for use of amphetamine, methaqualone, LSD (lysergic acid diethylamide), barbiturates, tranquilizers, and phencyclidine. Heroin and inhalant use has decreased markedly from their mid 1970's peaks to 1 per cent and 4 per cent, respectively. By contrast, however, cocaine use has doubled and smokeless tobacco is now used by approximately 20 per cent of male adolescents. Other sex differences include the increase in smoking by adolescent females and their 45 per cent lifetime incidence of use of diet pills. Alcohol is the most widely abused substance by this age group, with 93 per cent reporting use at some time and 5.5 per cent citing daily use. The time of greatest risk for initiation of cigarette smoking and alcohol and marijuana use is prior to the age of 20 years. Follow-up studies of adolescent "problem" drinkers demonstrated that one half of the males and one quarter of the females continued to have drinking problems as young adults.

Pubertal growth and development may be adversely affected by the use of drugs during this period of life. That the incidence of menstrual dysfunction resulting from drugs is higher in adolescents than adult women suggests greater vulnerability of the hypothalamic-pituitary-ovarian axis in the young. Heroin appears to block release of gonadotropin-releasing hormone. Amphetamines interfere with stage 4 sleep and may thus impair secretion of gonadotropins in early puberty. Induction of smooth endoplasmic reticulum of the liver by a variety of abused substances, such as opiates, barbiturates and tobacco smoke, has the potential for accelerating metabolism of hormones important for pubertal development, such as estrogens.

Regular use of any drug will eventually diminish the youngster's ability to function appropriately in school, to hold a job, or to operate a motor vehicle. An "amotivational" syndrome has been described in chronic marijuana users who lose interest in age-appropriate behavior.

The "infectious disease" model of prevention has little relevance to the problem of adolescent drug or alcohol abuse, nor are "scare" techniques effective. A more realistic approach is one that anticipates that most adolescents will experiment with some drug at some point and is designed to delay that event as long as possible, to limit the extent of use, and to prevent its use in conjunction with operating a motor vehicle. Presentation of factual information about medical complications of drug use by health professionals appears to have some positive impact. Strategies that enable young adolescents to resist peer pressure to smoke, by the use of trained peer counselors using role-playing techniques, have significantly reduced the onset of smoking in a number of studies.

GROWTH AND DEVELOPMENT

Gross RT, Duke PM: Effects of early versus late physical maturation on adolescent behavior. In Levine MD, Carey WB, Crocker AC, et al. (eds.): Developmental-Behavioral Pediatrics. Philadelphia, W. B. Saunders Company, 1983. *Pubertal development and psychosocial adjustment affect each other. Their interrelationships are well described in this review article.*

Grumbach MM: The neuroendocrinology of puberty. In Krieger DT, Hughes JC (eds.): Neuroendocrinology. Sunderland, Mass., Sinauer Associates, 1980. *The intricacies of neuroendocrine pathways and developmental interrelationship are presented in an easily understood manner.*

Kagan J, Coles R (eds.): Twelve to Sixteen: Early Adolescence. New York, W. W. Norton and Company, 1972. *A series of papers on various psychosocial aspects of adolescent development.*

Litt IF: Adolescent health care. In Green M, Haggerty RJ (eds.): Ambulatory Pediatrics. Edition 3. Philadelphia, W. B. Saunders Company, 1984. *Useful information and suggestions for approaching and screening adolescents in an ambulatory setting.*

Litt IF: Menstrual problems during adolescence. Pediatr Rev 4:203, 1983. *A review of special issues in care of adolescents with menstrual disorders.*

Litt IF, Martin JA: Development of sexuality and its problems. In Levine MD, Carey WB, Crocker AC, et al. (eds.): Developmental-Behavioral Pediatrics. Philadelphia, W. B. Saunders Company, 1983. *Development of sexuality begins at birth and is influenced by a variety of social, psychological and physical factors thereafter. This article reviews the process.*

Marshall WA, Tanner JM: Puberty. In Davis JA, Dobbing J (eds.): Scientific Foundations of Pediatrics. Edition 2. Baltimore, University Park Press, 1974. *A concise, current review of the physiology and endocrinology of puberty with excellent charts and tables.*

Zacharias L, Wurtman RJ: Age at menarche. N Engl J Med 280:868–875, 1969. *The multifactorial influences on menarcheal timing are chronicled.*

DEPRESSION (SUICIDE)

Beck AT, Beck R, Kovacs M: Classification of suicidal behaviors: Quantifying intent and medical lethality. Am J Psychiatry 132:285, 1975. *Useful in the assessment of seriousness of a suicidal attempt in patients of any age.*

Mattsson A: Adolescent depression and suicide. In Friedman SB, Hoekelman RA (eds.): Behavioral Pediatrics. New York, McGraw-Hill Book Company, 1980. *Useful categorization of manifestations of depression in the adolescent.*

Pugh-Antich J, Rabinovich H: Major child and adolescent psychiatric disorders. In Levine MD, Carey WB, Crocker AC, et al. (eds.): Developmental-Behavioral Pediatrics. Philadelphia, W. B. Saunders Company, 1983. *A summary of the psychobiology of adolescent behavioral disorders and their management.*

SUBSTANCE ABUSE

Alan Guttmacher Institute: Teenage Pregnancy: The Problem That Hasn't Gone Away. New York, Alan Guttmacher Institute, 1981. *Summary of statistics relating to adolescent sexual activity, pregnancy, abortion and contraceptive use.*

Jessor R, Jessor SL: Adolescence to young adulthood: A twelve-year prospective study of problem behavior and psychosocial development. In Mednick S, Hornway M (eds.): Longitudinal Research in the United States. New York, Praeger, 1984. *A comprehensive prospective assessment of early psychosocial predictors of drug use during adolescence as well as its implications for adult behavior.*

Johnston LD, O'Malley PM, Bachman JG: Highlights from Drugs and American High School Students, 1975–1983. U. S. Dept. of Health and Human Services, Public Health Service, Alcohol, Drug Abuse and Mental Health Administration, 1984. *A longitudinal study of trends in adolescent drug use.*

Kandel DB, Logan JA: Patterns of drug use from adolescence to young adulthood: 1) Periods of risk for initiation, continued use, and discontinuation. Am J Public Health 74:660, 1984.

7 AGING AND GERIATRIC MEDICINE

John W. Rowe

THE DEMOGRAPHIC IMPERATIVE
The Longevity Revolution

Over the next several decades, the practice of medicine in North America will be increasingly influenced by the health care needs of our rapidly enlarging elderly population. The portion of our population over age 65 years has grown from 4 per cent in 1900 to its current level of 11.6 per cent. As

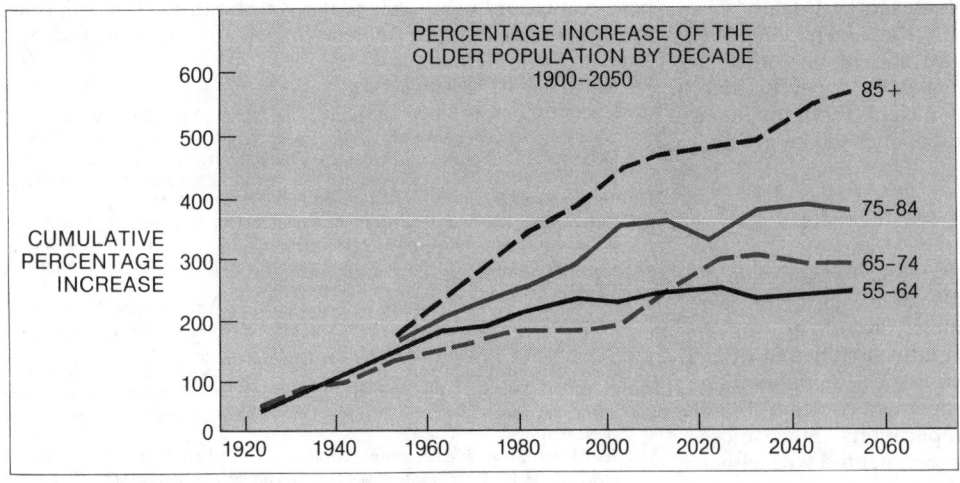

FIGURE 7–1. Past and projected increases in the elderly by decade. (Source: Bureau of the Census, Current Population Reports, Series P-25, No. P52, 1984.)

members of the post World War II "baby boom" age, projections call for a steady rise in the number of elderly in the United States from 25.5 million in 1980 to 64 million in 2030, when one of every five Americans will be 65 years or older. These changes reflect decreased death rates not only in youth and middle age but also in old age: Life expectancy at age 65 has risen from 11.9 years in 1900 to 16.4 years in 1980.

A second demographic shift of major importance is hidden within the general increase in the number of older persons. The elderly population itself is aging rapidly (Fig. 7–1). The longevity revolution has even affected the very old, as the past three decades have brought a 26 per cent reduction in mortality rates in individuals over age 80 in the United States. During the 1980's, it is estimated that the 65- to 69-year-old age group will increase by 13.6 per cent, whereas those 75 to 79 years will increase by 28.8 per cent and those over the age of 85 years will increase by a dramatic 52.4 per cent!

Coupling Longevity with Health

These remarkable improvements in lifespan have focused attention on improving health span and maintaining functional ability in old age. The general health status of older persons is substantially better than is often assumed. Objective health data show a pattern in which vigorous old age predominates. Dependency and institutionalization are the exception rather than the rule, since only 5 per cent of America's elderly reside in nursing homes at any one time. Most community-dwelling older Americans are cognitively intact and fully independent in their activities of daily living.

However, as individuals age they accumulate disabilities and diseases, and doctor visits increase. A substantial portion of community-dwelling elderly report major activity limitations due to chronic conditions. These functional impairments are clearly age related. The proportion of elderly that requires assistance with basic activities increases from approximately 5 per cent at ages 65 to 74 to nearly 12 per cent at ages 75 to 84 to approximately 35 per cent above the age of 85 (Fig. 7–2). Even if one maintains functional independence into old age, the risk of prolonged frailty is still high. For independent persons between the ages of 65 and 70 years, about 60 per cent of the remaining years will be characterized by independence; this proportion falls to 40 per cent at age 85.

Compression of Morbidity

The now familiar mortality curve for a modern aging population (Fig. 7–3C) has beneath it two additional clinically relevant curves, one describing the effect of age on the portion of the population in good health (i.e., morbidity curve, Fig. 7–3A) and another describing the transition of diseased aging

individuals from the asymptomatic to the symptomatic or functionally impaired state (disability curve, Fig. 7–3B).

A major health policy issue relates to the relationship between future changes in morbidity and disability in an aging population. The question is whether we will see a prolongation of dependency (i.e., widening of gap between curves of Fig. 7–3B and C) or whether active life expectancy will increase (i.e., compression of morbidity), as health promotion and disease prevention strategies become increasingly effective and curve 7–3B shifts rightward toward the mortality curve. The initial claim that as mortality declines, morbidity will also decline, has recently been challenged by studies suggesting that the increased lifespan of the oldest old is not accompanied by decreased morbidity and may actually result in more dramatic increases in the need for health care services, unless our understanding of disease in old age, and our capacity to treat it, improve substantially.

BIOLOGIC THEORIES OF AGING
Theories Relating to Alterations in Proteins
Error in Protein Synthesis

This theory holds that age-associated impairments in cellular function result from an accumulation of errors in protein

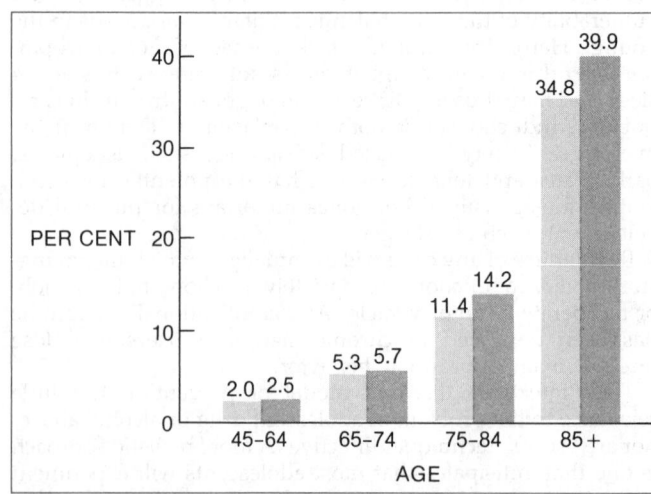

FIGURE 7–2. Percentages of adults, by age group, requiring assistance in basic activities (walking, bathing, dressing, using the toilet, transferring from bed to chair, eating, going outside) and in home-management activities (shopping, chores, meals, handling money) because of chronic disease. Colored bars denote basic activities and gray bars home-management activities.

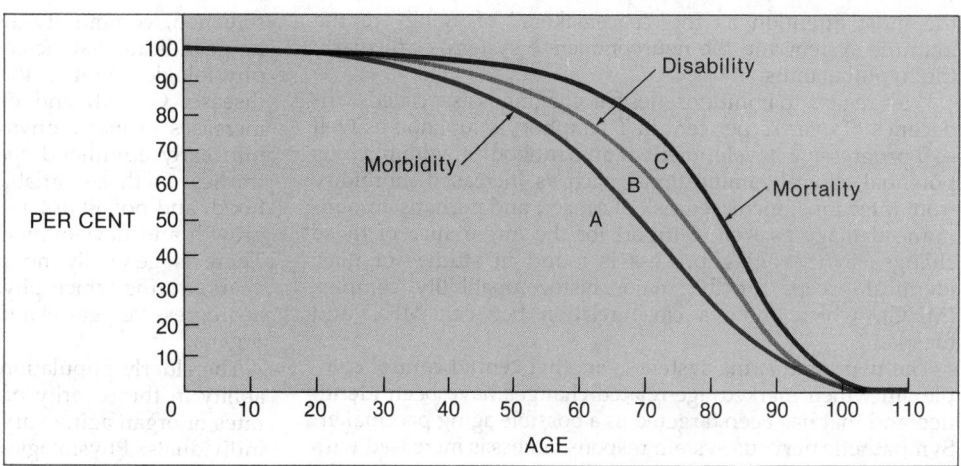

FIGURE 7–3. Mortality (observed), morbidity (hypothetical), and disability (hypothetical) survival curves for females in the United States in 1980.

synthesis. It is reasoned that random errors in DNA, transcription, or translation accumulate with aging to a level that markedly impairs cell function. Substantial basic research in aging over the past two decades has shown that both transcription and translation maintain their fidelity with advancing age and that aging is characterized by a remarkable constancy of the composition of a variety of physiologically important proteins. Specific findings inconsistent with the error catastrophe theory include the facts that aged fibroblasts cultures infected with viruses do not have a decreased virus yield, that newly synthesized enzymes from tissues in the aged are found to contain no synthetic errors, that experimentally induced errors fail to produce an error catastrophe, and that there is no increase in the infidelity of tRNA's with age and no age-related differences in the accuracy of poly(U)-directed protein synthesis. Thus, the error theory is considered by many to be disproven.

Post-translational Modifications (Cross-Linkage Theory)

This theory is based on findings that although transcription and translation are intact with age, *altered* proteins accumulate with advancing age. Thus, post-translational modifications may be important in mediating age-related losses in cell and organ function. A number of physiologically critical enzymes have been shown to undergo post-translational modifications with age, though these changes are by no means universal. One important post-translational modification—glycosylation—appears to be important in age-related development of increasing opacification in crystalline lens protein and eventual development of cataracts. Another modification, increased cross-linking, is central to the major aging modifications in collagen and might have direct clinical consequences for arteriosclerosis and other diseases. Cross-links should not be considered important only in extracellular tissues, since an age-related increase in cross-links has also been shown to occur in DNA. There are a number of criticisms of this theory, including the lack of evidence for varied rates of post-translational change in the same class of molecules in different species despite the remarkable diversity in species specificity of lifespan. Although it is unlikely that post-translational modifications are central to all aging-related biologic decrements, there is general agreement that they may play an important role in the emergence of some clinical consequences of aging.

Altered Protein Turnover

Another aspect of protein chemistry that has attracted substantial gerontologic attention is alteration with age in the *rate* of protein biosynthesis. Although there appears to be no mis-synthesis of proteins with age, many proteins are *produced more slowly* in aged cells than their younger counterparts. Delays have been identified in all of the four major stages of

protein synthesis, including amino acylation of tRNA, initiation, elongation, and termination.

In addition, lysosomal pathways for *elimination* of proteins are substantially altered with age, with some proteins being degraded more quickly than in younger cells and others more slowly. Future experiments involving recombinant DNA techniques to correct modifications in these lysosomal pathways may permit evaluation of the impact of these changes on cell aging.

DNA Damage and Repair Theory

The intact fidelity of protein synthesis with age does not exclude major age-related alterations in DNA, since a substantial portion of DNA is responsible for regulatory rather than synthetic activities. The DNA damage and repair theory focuses on the facts that, throughout life, DNA is constantly damaged and that age-related impairments in the repair mechanisms might be expected to be associated with progressive declines in cellular function. Although modifications in DNA repair capacity with age have been identified, these have generally not been well correlated with lifespan, suggesting either that DNA repair defects are not important in aging or that, to date, investigations have not focused on the critical repair mechanisms.

Free Radical Theory

Free radicals are highly reactive atoms or molecules bearing an unpaired electron, which can cause random damage to structural proteins, enzymes, informational macromolecules, and DNA. In mammals the most important source of free radicals is the reduction of oxygen, with subsequent development of hydrogen peroxide. The free radical theory holds that advancing age is associated with an accumulation of low-level free radical damage, which leads to the physiologic and clinical consequences associated with aging. Normal defense mechanisms against free radical damage include a number of endogenous antioxidants, including selenium-containing glutathione peroxidase, superoxide dismutase, DNA repair mechanisms, and alpha-tocopherol. Preliminary support for this theory rests in studies that indicate that animals whose oxygen consumption is high in proportion to their size have shorter lifespans and that administration of antioxidants results in modest increases in life expectancy. Within primates, the levels of the cellular antioxidant superoxide dismutase correlate well with lifespan. In addition, in lower forms of life, mutations leading to defects in production of free radical quenching enzymes are associated with shorter lifespan.

Organ System Theory (Pacemaker Theory)

This theory holds that certain organs or organ systems decline with advancing age and their loss of function drives the systemic aging process. The organs that have attracted the most attention as the "pacemakers" of aging are the immune system and the neuroendocrine system, particularly the hypothalamus.

With regard to immunosenescence, aging is associated with declines of over 75 per cent in T lymphocyte function as well as a progressive development of autoantibodies, with obvious potential clinical ramifications, such as increased morbidity from infections, increased risk of cancer, and perhaps autoimmune damage as well. Support for the importance of these changes in the aging process is found in studies of mice identical except for the major histocompatibility complex (MHC), which show a close relation between MHC and lifespan.

The neuroendocrine system is another central control complex in which marked age-related changes have been identified and that has been targeted as a possible aging pacemaker. Sympathetic nervous system responsiveness is increased with age, and it has been postulated that this increase might be responsible for a number of age-related changes, such as hypertension, impaired carbohydrate tolerance, and altered sleep architecture. Investigators have also sought to identify the presence of a "death hormone," a substance that is produced in increasing amounts with advancing age and that might regulate the aging process, or perhaps a "Methuselah hormone," which is present in decreasing amounts with advanced age. To date, no firm data are available to support the presence of such substances.

These theories focusing on individual organ systems as major regulators of systemic aging suffer from the weaknesses that not all organisms known to age have well-developed immune or neuroendocrine systems and that such theories would fail to explain the origin of the changes in the pacemaker system itself.

GENETIC ASPECTS OF AGING

Despite the apparent lack of evolutionary value to increases in lifespan beyond the reproductive years, gerontologists have long been attracted to the notion that just as growth and development are clearly regulated by a systematic turning on and off of various genes, so aging might represent a process in which systematic modifications in gene expression result in age-related physiologic and pathologic changes. Several of the theories of aging discussed above are linked by the likelihood that the basic mechanisms of aging—whether they be decreases in the production of antioxidants, impairments in DNA structure or repair, or age-related modifications of protein disposal systems or T lymphocyte function—may all have a genetic basis.

Substantial information exists that supports the view that genetic factors are important to the aging process. There is a remarkable species specificity to lifespan. Within an individual species, the life expectancy of identical twins is more similar than that of nonidentical twins, which in turn is more similar than that of siblings. On a more basic level, recent studies in *Caenorhabditis elegans*, a nematode, have identified mutant varieties with lifespans that exceed normal lifespans by 50 per cent. In some of these strains, the lifespan extension appears to be due to a single gene change. These findings suggest that more intensive genetic approaches are promising avenues for future research in aging.

CLINICAL IMPACT OF THE AGING PROCESS
Distinction Between Successful and Usual Aging

A thorough understanding of age-related physiologic changes that occur in humans, in the absence of disease, is critical to diagnosis and management of disease in old age. These physiologic changes influence the presentation of disease, its response to treatment, and the complications that ensue. Cross-sectional and longitudinal studies in carefully screened, community-dwelling groups across the adult age range indicate that increasing age is accompanied by inevitable physiologic changes that are separate from the effects of disease. Growth and development, characterized by rapid increases in many physiologic functions, generally continue into early adulthood, peaking in the late twenties or early thirties. In those variables that change with age after adulthood, and not all do, a linear decline begins at the end of the growth and development phase and continues into old age. There is generally no pleasant plateau during the middle years, during which physiologic function is stable, but rather a progressive age-related reduction in the function of many organs.

The elderly population is characterized by substantial variability in the severity of age-related physiologic changes, as rates of organ aging vary substantially among healthy elderly individuals. Physiologically, it seems that as individuals become older, they become less like each other. This may be due, in part, to lifestyle differences that confound the effects of aging. For instance, although maximal oxygen consumption has repeatedly been shown to decline with age, studies also indicate that oxygen consumption increases in response to exercise training in older persons, with older master athletes achieving levels higher than those seen in normal young adults. As greater attention is paid to the potential beneficial effects of exercise, diet, smoking cessation, moderation in alcohol intake, and so forth, we may encounter increasing numbers of robust elders who demonstrate *successful aging*, i.e., not only lack of disease, but also physiologic performance only moderately below that of healthy young adults. However, the fact remains that most older adults exhibit another syndrome, that of usual aging, in which the effects of aging per se are mixed with adverse effects of confounding environmental, dietary, or lifestyle factors. Most data in the literature on the physiology of aging exclude diseased individuals and provide a description of usual aging.

Distinction Between Aging and Disease

Since age has an important influence on numerous physiologic variables, and since detection of disease depends upon the determination that an individual is different from what would be expected by virtue of his age, it is important to establish age-adjusted criteria for clinically relevant variables to facilitate differentiation of the physiologic consequences of usual aging from those of concomitant diseases. Such criteria have been in wide clinical use for many years for several clinically important functions. For example, spirometric measures of pulmonary function are commonly expressed as "per cent of expected" for age and body size. Similarly, the validity of an exercise tolerance test as a suitable stress for detection of ischemic heart disease is judged on the basis of age-adjusted achievements of maximum heart rates. Standardized criteria are also available for age-related changes in glomerular filtration rate (GFR) and oral glucose tolerance, although variability of these functions is great among the elderly and individual determinations are required to guide diagnosis or therapy. If measurement of GFR is not available, application of age-related standards of renal function is facilitated by the fact that the age-related decline in creatinine clearance (approximately 10 ml per minute per decade) is balanced by a similar reduction in endogenous creatinine production. Thus, serum creatinine levels remain unchanged in spite of substantially lower GFR's in older patients. Familiarity with age changes in renal function and the hepatic oxidizing system is of particular importance in guiding drug therapy in the elderly (see below).

Interaction of Aging and Disease

There is a wide spectrum of interaction between aging processes and diseases, ranging from a lack of interaction at one extreme to age changes that have direct adverse clinical sequelae. Several specific clinically relevant points along this continuum can be identified.

Physiologic Variables that Do Not Change with Age

Perhaps the most important phenomenon seen in the aged, from a clinical standpoint, is no age-related change at all. Too frequently, clinicians attribute a disability or abnormal physical or laboratory finding to "old age," when the actual cause may be a specific disease process. Often there is no influence of age on the specific variable being evaluated. For example, old patients with low hematocrit values may be incorrectly characterized as having "anemia of old age" and be assured that no diagnostic evaluation or treatment is warranted. Data from several sources clearly indicate that in healthy, community-dwelling elders, there is no age-related change in hematocrit. Thus, a low hematocrit level in an elderly individual cannot be ascribed to normal aging and requires prompt investigation and treatment. Other common clinical measures not strongly influenced by age include fasting blood glucose level, serum electrolyte concentrations, blood pH and carbon dioxide content, and numerous hormone levels, including those of insulin, cortisol, thyroxine, and parathyroid hormone.

Impaired Homeostasis in the Elderly

This category encompasses age-related reductions in the function of numerous organs that place the elderly person at special risk of increased morbidity from coincident pathologic changes in those organs. Although usual age-related declines in physiologic function are not so severe as to result in impairments in function under basal circumstances, these declines are of sufficient magnitude to reduce physiologic reserve and thus to move old individuals closer to the clinical threshold for the emergence of symptoms. Declines in basal immune, renal, and pulmonary function and the declines in glucose tolerance and cardiac function during physiologic stress all place the elderly at risk for earlier emergence or greater severity of clinical disease. This fact can be illustrated with several clinically relevant examples:

1. Aging is associated with significant progressive reductions in the dopamine content of the substantia nigra. These decreases may interact with pathophysiologic changes to account for the increasing prevalence of Parkinson's disease in late life and are also consistent with the well-recognized enhanced susceptibility of older individuals to extrapyramidal side effects of neuroleptic agents.

2. Age-related reductions in pulmonary function are so substantial that healthy individuals in the ninth decade of life frequently have only one half of the pulmonary function of their 30-year-old counterparts. Thus, acute bacterial pneumonias of equal initial severity are much more likely to induce a serious clinical manifestation in the elderly. In addition, the marked decline in immune function with age will also be expressed as an impaired capacity to respond to the infecting agent and a subsequent worsening of the clinical picture.

3. Since usual renal function in older persons may be as much as 40 per cent less than in healthy younger adults, the loss of one kidney due to ureteral obstruction, vascular occlusion, or trauma is more likely to result in a clinically significant reduction in overall renal function in an old patient than in a healthy younger individual.

4. The mortality associated with severe burns increases dramatically with advancing age throughout adulthood (Fig. 7–4). This effect, which reflects the multiple parallel reductions in physiologic function during middle age and early senescence, is apparent well before diseases become highly prevalent and exemplifies the impaired homeostasis associated with the physiologic changes with age.

Altered Presentation of Disease in the Elderly

Age-related alterations in disease presentation have long been recognized as being of major importance to the practice of geriatric medicine. Many diseases occurring in both young and old adults have manifestly different clinical presentations and natural histories, depending upon the age of the individual. These disorders should not be regarded as being either more or less severe in the elderly, but just different. One example is hyperthyroidism. Young individuals often present with agitation, anxiety, an elevated heart rate and blood pressure, hyperactive deep tendon reflexes, complaints of weight loss and irritability, hyperkinesis, and a palpable goiter. In the older person with thyroid hormone levels equally elevated, irritability and hyperkinesis are infrequent and goiter is rare. In addition, deep tendon reflexes may be normal or even hypoactive, and the older patient may present a deactivated clinical picture ("apathetic thyrotoxicosis"). Physicians not familiar with presentation of thyroid hormone excess in the elderly may miss the diagnosis early on, thus permitting the adverse sequelae to persist.

Another disorder that is revealed differently in different

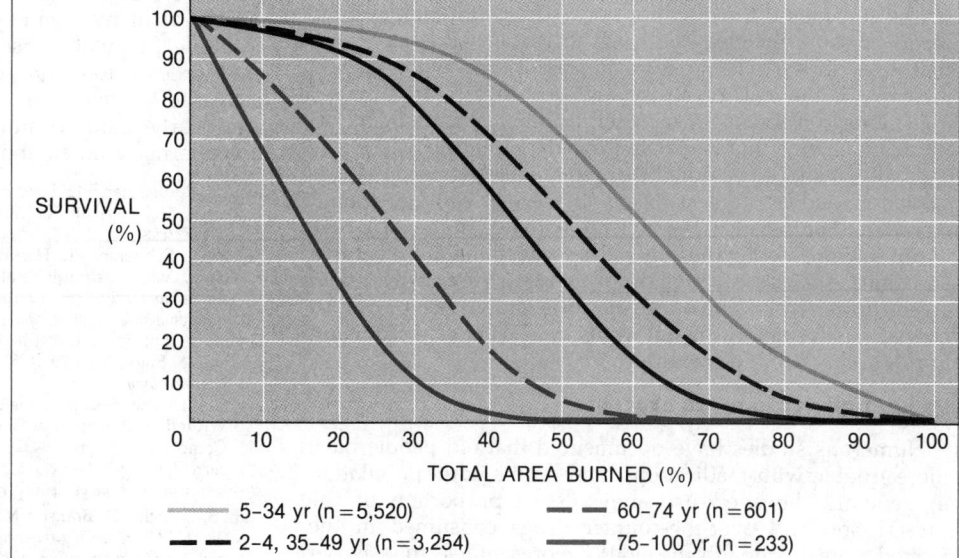

FIGURE 7–4. Survival of patients as a function of the total percentage of body surface burned and age.

age groups is uncontrolled diabetes mellitus. In children and young adults, uncontrolled diabetes is generally manifested as diabetic ketoacidosis. By contrast, the elderly with uncontrolled diabetes will frequently present with hyperosmolar nonketotic coma, with blood glucose levels markedly higher than in ketoacidosis and a relative or absolute lack of circulating ketones. Thus, the elderly may present with obtundation or in coma secondary to markedly high blood osmolality, whereas younger individuals are more likely to present with severe metabolic acidosis, polyuria, or volume depletion or any combination. The physiologic mechanisms underlying these major effects of age on presentation of common diseases remain unexplained.

HEALTH PROMOTION AND DISEASE PREVENTION IN THE ELDERLY

Not many years ago, it would have seemed paradoxical to discuss health promotion and disease prevention for the elderly. Recently, however, this has become an important theme in geriatrics in view of both the remarkable increases in longevity and the awareness that the physiologic and pathophysiologic changes associated with advancing age may be much more reversible than was previously appreciated. This *plasticity* of the aging process is reflected in findings that moderate exercise (30 minutes three times weekly) retards age-related loss of bone mineral content in elderly women, including individuals in their ninth decade of life living in long-term care facilities. Similarly, even though elderly smokers have a much higher risk of cardiac mortality than nonsmokers, quitting smoking late in life is associated with a rapid and sustained reduction in mortality from coronary disease. Clearly, one should not assume that risk factors are necessarily cumulative in their impact or that little is to be gained by altering long-term habits or treating longstanding disorders in the elderly.

A note of caution is required concerning health promotion and disease prevention strategies in the elderly population. Attempts to improve the quality of old age require an understanding of the risk factors for common diseases in the elderly and the efficacy of strategies to decrease the risk of morbidity. Simplistic generalizations of findings in young and middle-aged groups to the elderly are fraught with difficulty. The elderly clearly represent a select group of survivors with physiologic alterations that may influence pathophysiologic processes.

Another aspect of prevention in the care of the elderly is recognition that physiologic or pathologic changes so common in advancing age as to be considered "normal aging" should not be considered to be without risk. Thus, although systolic blood pressure increases with advancing age, it is also clear that rises in systolic pressure are associated with marked increase in the risk of stroke and coronary heart disease. Elevations in blood sugar represent another potentially harmful aging change that is usually considered harmless.

Finally, it should be noted that remarkable beneficial effects can be gained by modest delays in the onset of age-related disorders. For instance, the increase with age in the incidence of hip fracture among the very old is so steep that if preventive strategies, such as calcium supplementation or exercise, delayed clinical expression of osteoporosis for five years, without increasing lifespan, the result would be a 50 per cent reduction in the number of hip fractures.

MEDICATION USE IN OLDER PERSONS

Numerous studies have documented that old people have more trouble with medications than do the adult population in general. The aged use an excessive proportion of the prescription and over-the-counter drugs consumed in the United States. Athough the elderly represent less than 12 per cent of our population, they purchase 25 per cent of the drugs sold in America. This excess consumption of medications is accompanied, not surprisingly, by higher rates of side effects. Of equal importance is that when older people consume the same drugs with the same frequency as the young, toxicity is still more frequent and severe in the elderly. Often, standards for the use of current therapeutic agents were developed in young adults, and simplistic application of these guidelines to the elderly is often hazardous. Rates of adverse drug reaction rise steadily after age 50, and patients over 60 years old are twice as likely to suffer an adverse drug reaction as younger patients. Those over 80 years have a one in four risk of drug intoxication, twice the rate seen in patients under 50 years. Hospital stays are prolonged for all patients with adverse reactions, but older patients remain hospitalized the longest.

This increased toxicity of medication use in the elderly has three components: special vulnerability due to the physiologic effects of aging (drug-age interaction); modification of drug effects by multiple diseases often present in frail elders (drug-disease interaction); and the interactions of a given pharmacologic agent with the other medications, over the counter or prescribed, that the individual is taking (drug-drug interaction).

With regard to drug-age interactions, the changes with aging that occur in hepatic drug oxidation systems and in renal function have their major clinical impact on alterations in the pharmacokinetics of many medications. Several very commonly used medications such as digitalis and aminoglycoside antibiotics are excreted primarily via renal mechanisms and thus have prolonged half-lives in many elderly compared with younger adults, necessitating an adjustment in treatment schedules. These pharmacokinetic considerations are frequently compounded by parallel changes in pharmacodynamics, inasmuch as the tissues of elderly individuals, especially the central nervous system, become more sensitive to some agents with advancing age. Older persons are more sensitive than younger adults to the sedative effects of benzodiazepines and to the analgesic effects of narcotics. The combination of alterations in pharmacokinetics and pharmacodynamics is often further influenced by changes in body composition in the elderly. The average old individual has more fat and less lean body mass per kilogram of body weight than the younger adult. Thus, the volumes of distributions of many agents, such as diazepam, will be altered in the elderly. Similarly, circulating levels of serum albumin fall moderately with age and influence free circulating levels of medications that are highly protein bound, such as phenytoin.

Drug-disease interactions are particularly common in the elderly. It is not uncommon to have five or six major diagnoses exist in as many organ systems of a frail elderly patient. The resulting frequent worsening of one illness by treatment of another leads to disproportionately longer hospital stays and increased frequency of complications. Drug-drug interactions are clearly more common in the elderly in view of the polypharmacy noted above.

Andres R, Bierman EL, Hazzard WR: Principles of Geriatric Medicine. New York, McGraw-Hill Book Company, 1985. *A detailed comprehensive textbook of geriatrics.*

Finch CE, Schneider EL: Handbook of the Biology of Aging. Edition 2. New York, Van Nostrand–Reinhold, 1985. *An encyclopedic reference text, very detailed and well referenced, covering all aspects of aging from plants and nematodes through detailed system-by-system discussions of human aging.*

Greenblatt DJ, Seller EM, Shader RI: Drug therapy: Drug disposition in old age. N Engl J Med 306:1081, 1982. *A useful review of the principles of geriatric pharmacology.*

Hayflick L: Theories of biological aging. *In* Andres R, Bierman EL, Hazzard WR (eds.): Principles of Geriatric Medicine. New York, McGraw-Hill Book Company, 1985, pp. 9–22. *This chapter provides a detailed review of the major current biologic theories of aging, with a good historical review and balanced perspectives of the evidence for and against each theory.*

Katz S, Branch LG, Branson MH, et al.: Active life expectancy. N Engl J Med 309:1218, 1983. *This important paper coined the phrase "active life expectancy" and provides information on the functional capacity of the elderly.*

Rowe JW: Clinical research in aging: Strategies and directions. N Engl J Med

297:1332, 1977. *An overview of the perils, pitfalls and opportunities for clinical gerontologic research.*

Rowe JW: Health care of the elderly. N Engl J Med 312:827, 1985. *A detailed, heavily referenced review of the physiologic changes with age and their clinical influence, with additional updates on several geriatric diseases, including dementia, incontinence, and osteoporosis.*

Rowe JW, Besdine RW: Health and Disease in Old Age. Boston, Little, Brown and Company, 1982. *A concise practical textbook of geriatric medicine for students and practitioners. Emphasis on both normal aging and age-related diseases.*

Salzman C: Clinical Geriatric Psychopharmacology. New York, McGraw-Hill, 1984. *A very concise, practical clinical guide to use of psychotropic medications in the elderly with numerous references and instructive clinical vignettes.*

Schneider EL, Brody JA: Aging, natural death, and the compression of morbidity—another view. N Engl J Med 309:854, 1983. *A detailed update of evidence for and against the compression of morbidity hypothesis.*

8 MANAGEMENT OF COMMON PROBLEMS IN THE ELDERLY

T. Franklin Williams

A physician must approach the care of elderly persons with an informed, comprehensive, balanced perspective about aging itself and about the diseases and disabilities that commonly occur in older people. The previous section has described the physiologic changes that normally occur with aging. From the clinical perspective it is important to keep in mind that most older people are in reasonably good health and, despite some decline in maximum functional ability, can still function well at all ordinary activities. There are many persons in their eighties and nineties who can and do carry on all usual living activities, take long walks, are intellectually sharp with good memories, continue to be sexually active, and most of the time are symptom free. Thus when someone, no matter how old, comes to a physician with a complaint of discomfort or dysfunction, the complaint should not be dismissed as being simply "old age," but should be investigated and treated appropriately.

At the same time, a physician must understand that with increasing age people do accumulate chronic diseases and disabilities. Over the age of 65, 80 per cent have one or more chronic conditions; among the most common are some form of arthritis (present in 40 per cent in national surveys), hearing impairment (30 per cent), and chronic cardiac conditions (20 per cent). One in five persons over the age of 75 may be expected to have diabetes. In those 75 or older, four or more identifiable chronic problems are commonly present.

In addition to recognizing and treating the acute and chronic *diseases* that occur, the physician must give attention to the functional losses, the *disabilities* that are present, and attempt to reverse or minimize them no matter what can or cannot be done about underlying chronic diseases. The ultimate goal of care for elderly persons should be to restore or maintain as much function as possible—to help the patient to maintain as much independence of living, as much of a preferred lifestyle, as possible. Such a rehabilitative approach is an essential part of the therapy.

In those elderly patients who have some irreversible functional losses and thus need regular assistance, an additional part of the plan for care must be identification of who will provide the needed help and where. The extent and quality of family support and the potentials for community or institutional support services must be determined and worked into the overall, ongoing therapeutic program.

SPECIAL FEATURES OF THE WORKUP OF ELDERLY PATIENTS

HISTORY TAKING. Special attention should be given to the history of other (chronic) conditions in addition to the immediate chief complaint and to obtaining additional historical information from close relatives and previous records. An older person, like any patient consulting a physician, is most interested in having the immediate problem addressed and may tend to downplay past history and other chronic but less troubling conditions. It is the interaction of multiple diseases, the necessity to deal simultaneously with these multiple problems, that is one of the distinguishing characteristics of geriatric medicine. A closely related necessity is to obtain complete information on all drugs the patient is taking, both prescribed and over-the-counter medications. The numbers and variety are often astounding, and unfavorable drug interactions commonly contribute to the patient's discomfort and dysfunctions. A good technique is to have the patient (or responsible family member) bring in all the medications the patient is taking, for review, on each office visit.

Certain common functional problems should be explicitly inquired about: any history of falling; any episodes of urinary incontinence; any disturbances in sleep; and any difficulties with vision, hearing, or sexual function.

One must keep in mind the atypical presentations of common acute problems: pneumonia presenting as confusion, acute myocardial infarction as sudden weakness, or an acute abdomen as refusal to eat.

It is a good practice whenever possible to talk with one or more close family members to obtain their observations on the patient's functional status, mood, and daily routines, including intake of food and medicines. Such additional information is absolutely essential if there is evidence of dementia or depression in the patient—in such circumstances the patient may give quite a misleading story. If the patient is living alone (as a third or more of older women are), then it will be desirable or even necessary to have the benefit of observations from a home visit by the physician or by a visiting nurse or social worker.

Any person who has lived 70 years or more will almost always have had previous medical or surgical care, in or out of hospital, and may well have seen several specialists. It should be routine practice, when taking on the care of such a patient (as primary physician or consultant), to obtain summaries or copies of all previous records, including results of all diagnostic tests. Such information should help both in managing current problems and in reducing the extent of further diagnostic tests that are needed. In particularly complex or unclear situations, there should be direct discussion with physicians who have previously seen the patient.

PHYSICAL EXAMINATION. As part of a regular complete physical examination of an older patient, certain features should receive special attention, depending in part on clues from the history. These include evaluation of mobility, of mental status, and of mood. The ability of the patient to move around adequately and the degree of stability in balance and gait can be appraised to a degree from simple observation of the patient as he or she arrives. But because of the commonness of gait and balance disturbances in old people, and in particular if there is any history of falls or near-falls, these characteristics should be explicitly evaluated. The patient should be observed taking a prescribed walk down the corridor, turning and returning. Does each foot carry through a full swing with each step? Is there any limp? Is there any tendency to lean or fall to one side? Is the pace at a usual speed? One should perform the Romberg test and test the patient's ability to maintain balance when purposely given a moderate shove. One should also check for orthostatic hypotension and for any evidence of arrhythmia.

In assessing mental status, it is a good practice to use a standard, short mental status examination as a screening test for any degree of mental impairment and as a benchmark for comparisons on future occasions. Katzman (1986) recommends one of three such tests. Evidence of any degree of mental inadequacy should lead to a thorough investigation of the extent and possible causes of dementia (see below).

Also, in light of the often unrecognized occurrence of depression in older persons, the physician should specifically assess mood. Here, too, short, standardized screening tests are useful—for example, the test developed by Brink et al. (1982).

In light of the frequency of poor eating practices by older persons, particularly those living alone, special attention should be given to any indications of poor nutrition—weight loss, anemia, vitamin deficiency. A careful oral examination is important. Also in light of the frequency of functionally limiting problems, hearing and vision should be adequately tested; joint mobility and muscular strength should be thoroughly evaluated; and the possibility of peripheral neuropathy should be considered.

ASSESSMENT OF FUNCTIONAL STATUS. All aspects of daily functioning should be evaluated by history and physical examinations. Loss of ability to carry out such functions makes the older person dependent on others, at home or in institutional care. These functional characteristics include the usual activities of daily living (ADL): feeding oneself, bathing, dressing, toileting, ambulation, and continence. In addition, the person, particularly if living alone, may need to be able to carry out the "instrumental" activities of daily living (IADL), i.e., those activities necessary for maintenance of the immediate environment: obtaining food, cooking, laundering, housecleaning, transportation, use of telephone, managing medications.

ADDITIONAL DIAGNOSTIC TESTS. The same general principles for choosing diagnostic tests for younger patients should apply in the workup of older patients: The aim is to obtain any information that will help in clarifying the cause of disease or the functional loss, *if* this information will likely lead to effective therapy. The special circumstances that arise more often in older than in younger patients are those in which, because of the other chronic complicating problems, the best judgment may be not to proceed with any form of treatment that may be risky or unpleasant and offers only minimal chance for improvement. Such judgments should be weighed in consultation with the patient and close family before diagnostic procedures are embarked on: If the treatment plans will not be changed by the outcome of the procedure, then it should not be done.

However, because of the tendency, referred to earlier, to dismiss treatable problems of elderly patients as being simply the concomitants of old age, it is important to identify any potentially reversible condition and to use relevant diagnostic aids. An adequate use of diagnostic tests is especially indicated in the common, functionally disabling conditions faced by older people. These are discussed below.

ASSESSMENT OF FAMILY AND COMMUNITY SUPPORTS. A final essential element in the workup of a frail, elderly person, i.e., a patient who may face the necessity of ongoing help with daily activities, is the collection of information about the home environment, the family relationships, the degree of supporting services potentially available, the degree of "burn-out" or exhaustion that may have already occurred, and the availability of home care services and institutional services in the community. A visiting nurse or social worker can be very helpful in obtaining some of these services and in helping to integrate them into an overall plan.

DIAGNOSIS AND MANAGEMENT OF MAJOR COMMON PROBLEMS OF ELDERLY PATIENTS

EPISODES OF ACUTE ILLNESS. Older people with diminished reserves and chronic diseases are more prone to injuries, acute infections (especially respiratory), and other acute illnesses than are younger people, and are also more likely to decompensate at such times. It is a common obser-

vation that an old person, previously mentally competent at home, may become quite confused on admission to the strange environment of a hospital under the stresses of an acute illness. Careful attention must be given to every aspect of the patient's status, looking for the appearance of heart failure, overt diabetes, delirium, or increased risk of falling. Drug regimens should be kept simple and the possibility of deleterious effects of overdosage or drug interactions should be continuously reviewed.

Recovery from an acute illness will also take longer than in a younger person, and there is real risk that the previous functional level may not be regained. As early as possible in an episode of acute illness the older patient should be helped to be up and about, to keep joints supple and muscular strength as intact as possible, to retain or regain urinary continence through use of regular toilet facilities, to dress and feed oneself, and engage in social exchanges in usual ways, i.e., out of bed and dressed. The patient should remain in familiar home surroundings or return there as quickly as possible. Convalescent and rehabilitative efforts should be continued as long as any progress is being made.

DEMENTIA. The loss of mental competence is one of the most common and most distressing of functional disabilities in older persons, affecting about 5 per cent of those over age 65 and 20 per cent of those over age 80. We now know that dementia is *not* a feature of normal aging but instead is due to one or another of several disease processes. The most common form of dementia in old people is that of the Alzheimer's type, accounting for 50 per cent or more of cases. This is a (usually) progressive dementia associated with considerable cerebral atrophy and characteristic pathologic changes in selected regions of the brain, with neurofibrillary tangles within neurons and degenerating plaques at endplates. These damaged neurons are producing far less of the neurotransmitter acetylcholine (and possibly other neurotransmitters also) than normal. With the accumulating evidence that the deficiency in this neurotransmitter is the cause of the failure in mental function, various research efforts are in progress to find ways to achieve more production of acetylcholine (for example, through providing substrate) or to delay its destruction or prolong its effectiveness. Thus far, results are inconclusive.

Other causes of dementia in the elderly include damage from multiple small infarcts or one or more larger infarcts secondary to cerebrovascular disease, metabolic or endocrine disorders such as hypothyroidism and vitamin B_{12} deficiency, brain tumors, brain injury (such as late dementia in professional boxers, which has the same pathologic changes as Alzheimer's disease), Korsakoff's dementia of chronic alcoholism, and the condition known as normal-pressure hydrocephalus. Most importantly, severe depression can present as dementia, reversible with successful treatment of the depression. Indeed, a number of the possible causes are potentially reversible or treatable. Thus it is essential, when confronted by an older person with any signs of dementia, to conduct a thorough differential diagnostic evaluation. This should include comprehensive mental testing to define the extent of the dementia, specific tests for all of the treatable causes, and in most instances, a computed tomographic (CT) scan that can usually identify or exclude infarcts and tumors and can help diagnose normal-pressure hydrocephalus. The finding of cerebral atrophy alone on the CT scan would be consistent with, but not diagnostic of, dementia of Alzheimer's type, inasmuch as a significant degree of atrophy occurs in the normal aging process without loss of mental function.

The physician should be sensitive to the alarm older patients and family members may have at the least sign of any aberration in mentation and should be able to reassure them that "benign forgetfulness" is a common trait at all ages. Benign forgetfulness characteristically is the inability to recall a name or some specific element of a prior experience, when one thinks one should be able to do so. The person can recall many related features of the person or episode and knows precisely what element or name is not being recalled. Usually recall of that element will occur later, unexpectedly. In contrast, a person with progressive dementia will have no recollection of the entire episode, as if it never happened, or can make only feeble, ineffective efforts to reconstruct the identity of the forgotten subject.

If the final diagnosis is dementia of the Alzheimer's type or one of the other irreversible dementias, the physician, nurses, and social workers must treat the family as well as the patient and help them to make the best of a distressing situation. The long-established daily activities of the patient in familiar surroundings should be maintained as much as possible, with avoidance of surprises or new and different decisions to be made. Family members should be helped to understand the disease and also the fact that the patient will likely not understand what is going on. They should be helped to accept the services of home support personnel to assist in the care of the patient—housekeeper, personal care aide, home health aide, or nurse—as needed to help prevent ''burn-out'' on their part; to accept respite care for the patient (temporary full-time care given in the home or a temporary nursing home admission) so that the family members may get away for a vacation or a special occasion; and to accept permanent nursing home care for the patient if this becomes best for everyone. They should be informed of support groups like the Alzheimer's Disease and Related Dementias Association (ADRDA), chapters of which now exist in most larger communities, and should be put in touch with social agencies and legal resources if necessary to help in making various legal and financial arrangements. The physician's involvement in all of these aspects may seem to some to be peripheral to the practice of medicine but in fact is central to the physician's primary goals of maintaining the health and functioning of the patient and the patient's family to the maximum extent possible. In working with problems like these the physician needs the close participation of well-informed nurses and social workers who can take the lead in management of many aspects.

The physician should keep in mind (and the family should be reminded) that any sudden worsening of dementia is not consistent with Alzheimer's disease and is likely a sign of some complicating acute illness.

DEPRESSION. Depressive reactions of varying degrees of severity are more common in elderly persons than has been recognized and warrant more attention in diagnosis and treatment. As a person lives into later years, losses are inevitable—death of family members and friends, usually ''loss'' of job through retirement, usually less income, often loss of some degree of health, less vigor, possibly loss of familiar home environment through moving. Some degree of grief and reactive depression is to be expected in response to such losses, but emotionally healthy older persons will work through such grief and return to their usual level of mood, outlook, and activity. Persistence of depressive symptoms may represent activation of a longer-standing depressed state or appearance of a new disorder.

If depression is suspected, it should be thoroughly evaluated with psychiatric consultation and perhaps treated by therapeutic trials of antidepressant drugs. In severe instances not responsive to drugs, electroshock therapy has been found to be successful in many elderly patients. The use of psychostimulants (methylphenidate, dextroamphetamine) in very introverted patients may be useful as a first, temporary step, preparatory to antidepressant drugs or electroshock therapy.

FALLS. Falling is common as people become older, occurring as often as once a year or more in half of those over age 75. In addition to the accompanying risk of injury—with up to 5 per cent of falls there may be fracture of the hip or arm—one or more falls may lead to such a fear of further falling that an older person will severely limit mobility and activities. Falls are often also a harbinger of other diseases or disabilities; one study in the United Kingdom has reported twice the overall mortality from various causes in the year following a first fall in older people, compared with age- and sex-matched persons who did not fall.

A number of risk factors contribute to the likelihood of falling, and it is typically the multiplicity of such risk factors in the same person that makes falling highly likely, rather than any one of them. These include diminished distant vision, deafness, disturbances in balance, abnormal gait, weakness in the lower extremities, decreased mental status, orthostatic hypotension, depression, and effects of drugs on alertness. All such factors should be searched for and as many as possible corrected as a part of regular preventive care and especially at the time of any fall.

Environmental hazards also contribute to the risk. A home visit by at least one of the professionals should include observation and recommendations for correcting such environmental hazards as poor lighting, rugs that can slide, objects blocking usual walkways, lack of nonslipping strips and handgrips in bathtubs, and lack of handrails on stairs.

A person who has fallen should be thoroughly examined for subtle signs of injury or fracture and for any underlying or associated disease condition, including a new febrile illness, painless myocardial infarction, and stroke. If any such risk factor is present and not fully correctable, the patient should be taught to use a walking aid such as a cane or walker.

URINARY INCONTINENCE. Lack of control of urination is far more common than generally recognized; some studies suggest that up to 50 per cent of older women have this problem. It has been referred to as the ''closet disease'' of old age because of the high frequency of denial of its presence—out of embarrassment or the mistaken view that nothing can be done about it. Older persons living alone may become oblivious to its presence, unaware of the odors that are obvious to visitors. Frequent urinary incontinence, particularly night-time incontinence, by a person living with family is a major cause of caregiver exhaustion and the precipitating reason for their seeking institutional care. Within long-term care institutions, urinary incontinence in a resident means that such a person must be cared for at a skilled nursing or high-intensity intermediate level of care, even if otherwise the person might manage well in a minimal care setting.

For all of these reasons it is important for the physician, in evaluating any older patient, to determine (from patient, family, or visiting nurse) whether the patient has any problem with urinary incontinence and, if so, to conduct a thorough diagnostic workup and, based on the findings, to undertake appropriate treatment. In most instances the problem can be eliminated or controlled.

A good first step in evaluating reported or suspected urinary incontinence is to arrange to have an ''incontinence diary'' kept by the patient or caregiver—a daily record for several days of just when episodes of incontinence occur, roughly how much urine is spilled, the circumstances—while up and about or in bed or while on the way to the bathroom but ''didn't quite make it''—and whether the patient is aware of the episode. In some instances simply keeping such a diary leads a previously careless person to achieve satisfactory control. The diary provides information on the magnitude of the problem and clues to possible causes.

Further workup of the incontinence should proceed from simple to more complex tests, as needed. Urinalysis and culture may indicate a urinary tract infection that, if eliminated, will result in restoration of continence. Observing whether there is any urinary spillage with coughing or straining in the upright position (after adequate hydration) may point to stress incontinence. Catheterization after the patient has attempted to void completely can provide evidence for an obstructed or atonic bladder and overflow incontinence.

The most common cause of urinary incontinence in older people is instability of the detrusor system of the bladder—the loss of normal neurologic inhibiting influences as the bladder fills. The detrusor muscle, if uninhibited, will begin to contract spontaneously when filling has reached relatively small volumes, 150 ml or less, and the patient will find it difficult or impossible to suppress the tendency to void. Unequivocal diagnosis of this condition requires cystometric studies and such should be done when needed; some physicians who are thoroughly familiar with the differential diagnosis of incontinence may choose to use first a trial of therapy for the presumptive diagnosis of instability, once other causes such as those referred to above have been eliminated.

In persons with stress incontinence or detrusor instability, the use of biofeedback and other training exercises has been found to help a number of patients to control this problem. Assuring quick access to a toilet, such as use of a bedside toilet at night, can help a person with detrusor instability reach the toilet in time. If stress incontinence in women is associated with major anatomic changes, e.g., severe uterine prolapse, or when prostatic obstruction in men is the apparent cause, surgical intervention may be indicated.

Drugs with anticholinergic effects are successful in decreasing detrusor instability in some patients; their use is often limited by undesirable anticholinergic effects in other organ systems, such as dry mouth and disturbances in gastrointestinal function. At least theoretically, anticholinergic drugs could worsen dementia of the Alzheimer's type (see above). Efforts have been made to identify drugs of this type whose effects are mainly on the bladder. Oxybutynin has smooth muscle–relaxing as well as anticholinergic effects, and imipramine has at least theoretically useful sympathomimetic and anticholinergic actions.

When overflow incontinence is secondary to a distended, atonic bladder (as with diabetic neuropathy), cholinergic drugs may be helpful.

Even if none of the above approaches is effective, acceptable management of the incontinence may be achieved through use of special waterproof pants with absorbent liners, the use of special absorbent pads on the bed, specially fitted collecting devices in women, and in selected patients the use of intermittent straight catheterization. The use of chronic indwelling catheters is rarely indicated.

PRESSURE ULCERS AND CONTRACTURES. These are unfortunate and for the most part preventable common complications of chronic illness in frail older people. Even a few hours of total immobility, as after a stroke or in the recovery period following surgery, will likely result in pressure damage to the skin and subcutaneous tissues; as little as a day or two of immobility in a joint may lead to contracture formation. Once these problems develop, correcting them is a long, tedious, and expensive process.

Preventive measures for any patient at risk of developing pressure (decubitus) ulcers or contractures should include regular, frequent passive or active movement of joints and turning, assiduous skin care, careful attention to avoiding potential damage from wrinkled bed clothes, and care in lifting, not pulling, a patient while changing his or her position. A patient should be sitting in a chair and also walking as much as possible; while sitting he or she should shift weight at least every 15 to 20 minutes.

Once pressure ulcers have developed, even greater attention should be paid to the preventive practices just described. The ulcer should be kept clean, with scrubbing and soaking three to four times a day; mild antiseptic cleansing solutions such as half-strength povidone are better than stronger agents, which may cause further tissue damage. A good practice is to leave wet-to-dry gauze dressings on the wound. Surgical debridement of any necrotic tissue should be done.

As important as local care of the wound is attention to adequate general nutrition and to the treatment of any systemic disease that may cause a general catabolic response. With good wound care in a patient who is adequately nourished and otherwise well or recovering, ulcers will heal rapidly; the presence of chronic infection elsewhere, or poor nutrition, can thwart the effectiveness of even the best wound care. With large ulcers, once the wound surface is thoroughly healthy, skin grafting may be indicated.

Minor degrees of contractures can often be corrected with regular, frequent, careful stretching exercises, following a regimen established for the patient by a physical therapist. More severe and unresponsive contractures may require surgical correction. Such a step can be valuable and justified if it helps to restore mobility and independence or significantly eases nursing care burdens.

DECISIONS ABOUT LONG-TERM CARE. Elderly persons who acquire chronic, irreversible functional losses must have appropriate ongoing supportive services: The goal should be to substitute help only to the extent necessary, thus preserving the maximum possible degree of independence for the patient.

Often the need for decisions arises at a time of crisis: Already borderline functional capabilities of the older person may have further deteriorated owing to a new condition, e.g., injury, stroke, and so on, or the caregiving spouse or child may become ill or unable to continue the previous extent of care. The physician, in collaboration with other professionals (e.g., visiting nurse, social worker) and the patient and family, must weigh the relative merits and feasibility of maintaining the patient at home with support services or arranging care in a nursing home or intermediate care facility. Most older people strongly prefer to continue living in their familiar home settings, and most families desire to help the patient to stay there. Through thoughtful use of various supportive services—meals on wheels, housekeeper, personal care or home health aides, day programs—it is possible to maintain many such patients at home whose care needs would have equally well justified nursing home admission. The cost of the external supporting services in such instances may be only 50 to 60 per cent as much as the nursing home alternative; the family clearly makes up the difference through their own provision of personal care, meals, and so forth.

These features are discussed here because with the continually growing numbers of very elderly persons in our society there will be major increases in the pressures on our long-term care systems, and physicians will continue to be involved at the critical points of decision making where careful efforts to help stabilize and maintain many patients at home will be most important. Comprehensive geriatric evaluation services are becoming available, as ambulatory or inpatient units, in many settings. They have been shown to be valuable for consultative help at these critical points in the lives of many older people and their families.

CARE OF TERMINALLY ILL ELDERLY PERSONS. "Aging" and "dying" are so often thought of as almost synonymous that the problems of how to approach terminal care and how far to go in heroic or extraordinarily expensive diagnosis and treatment are considered by many to be issues that primarily appear in the care of the aged. The actual picture is somewhat different. Almost all of the circumstances in which inevitable death can be predicted in a fairly short time occur in patients with advanced cancer, at any age. For elderly patients with terminal cancer the same principles of care apply as for younger patients: When patient, family, and the responsible physician have agreed that no further efforts at curative therapy are warranted, the primary goal should be comfort care, avoiding heroics.

Similar decisions can be made in instances in which an older person has had such irreversible loss of mental function that he or she has little, if any, remaining apparent contact with surroundings and communication with others, especially family or nursing personnel. If those who are closest to the patient agree on the hopelessness of further curative or extraordinary treatment, including their view that this is also what the patient would say for himself or herself (or perhaps did say earlier, verbally or in writing, such as in a "living will"), then comfort care should be the practice. In fact, despite frequently expressed views that physicians order too much heroic, expensive care for elderly patients in hopeless situations, one study has found evidence for this in only 10 per cent of instances in two hospitals (and in most of those it was the family that insisted on such efforts); in 90 per cent of the cases everyone involved agreed that putting primary emphasis on comfort care had been appropriately accomplished.

What is comfort care? The precise details will vary with the condition of each individual patient. Overall, the physician should be concerned to see that pain is relieved, that whatever may give the patient enjoyable days (and nights) is done (preferred foods, cleanliness, comfortable positioning, visits by family or friends, outings), and that no diagnostic or treatment efforts are undertaken that may be unpleasant or painful or that will not contribute to comfort. These guidelines do not eliminate all ambiguity: For example, what should the physician decide when confronted with a new infection such as pneumonia in a patient in whom comfort care is the primary goal? If no treatment is given, the patient will likely have several days of very uncomfortable respiratory distress and may or may not survive. Comfort care in this instance would probably include respiratory therapy to help clear the airway and use of an oral antibiotic, avoiding painful injections or intravenous therapy.

Blazer DG: Depression in Late Life. St. Louis, C. V. Mosby, 1982. *A thorough and practically useful presentation of this topic, including information on incidence and prevalence, diagnosis and differential diagnosis, and effective modes of therapy.*

Brink TL, Yesavage TF, Lum O, et al: Screening tests for geriatric depression. Clin Gerontol 1:37, 1982. *A validated, useful screening test for depression in older people.*

Katzman R: Alzheimer's disease (medical progress). N Engl J Med 314:964, 1986. *An excellent summary of current knowledge of pathophysiology, possible causes, diagnosis, and management of this condition, including references to useful screening tests for dementia.*

Radebaugh TS, Hadley E, Suzman R (eds.): Symposium on falls in the elderly: Biological and behavioral aspects. Clin Geriatr Med 1, No. 3, August, 1985. *This NIH symposium covers the many inter-related risk factors contributing to this major cause of disability among older people.*

Resnick HM, Yalla SV: Current concepts: Management of urinary incontinence in the elderly. N Engl J Med 313:800, 1985. *A good summary of our current understanding of this condition and successful approaches to management.*

Rubenstein LZ, Campbell LJ, Kane RL (eds.): Geriatric assessment. Clin Geriatr Med (in press). *With increasing recognition of the value of comprehensive geriatric assessment, this volume provides up-to-date information on when, where, how, and by whom such assessment may best be done.*

9 CARE OF DYING PATIENTS AND THEIR FAMILIES

Sylvia A. Lack

Dying patients need to maintain their self-esteem as their dependency on others increases. Physical distress erodes self-confidence and undermines the ability to make decisions and to give as well as to receive. Good symptom control frees the patient to work on existential and practical matters. Many, regardless of intellectual capability or social class, struggle to answer such questions as the following: "What has been the meaning of my life?" "Am I prepared for death and the life after?" Indeed, faced squarely with the fact of death, physicians are forced to consider such questions for themselves. The resultant unease may be a reason for the subtle withdrawal perceived by many patients.

THE PHYSICIAN AND DEATH

It is natural for a physician to feel unhappy when a patient recognizably deteriorates. One way of responding is to work compulsively against the disease until the patient dies. This is clearly beneficial when there is realistic expectation that the disease can be arrested. This chapter does not focus on the management of such patients, but on care for those *dying* with cancer and other chronic, degenerative illness. When death is inevitable, it is counterproductive to continue fruitless efforts to cure, especially when they only add to the patient's discomfort.

At the end of life the physician's two principal functions of curing disease and relieving suffering can become increasingly incompatible. For those in whom prognostic indicators show little or no prospect of rehabilitation, the caring physician has to shift gears and concentrate on the patient's immediate well-being. This requires an enlarged perspective, including awareness of the needs of the family and the possibilities of home care. Care of the dying, although analytic, is relaxed, with emphasis on listening and availability. Such care must be the best that skilled nursing and medicine can provide, ideally embodying the organizational characteristics found in the hospice movement (Table 9–1). It keeps abreast of developments while at the same time avoiding ineffective therapy.

AVOIDING INAPPROPRIATE TREATMENT

In the dying patient with irreversible underlying disease, the aim of treatment is to make remaining life comfortable and as meaningful and dignified as possible. It is no longer to preserve life at all costs. When cure is no longer possible, disease control and palliation should be considered. When disease escapes control, the emphasis moves to symptom relief and comfort as ends in themselves. What may be appropriate treatment when disease is reversible may be ineffective—and thus poor medical care—in the dying. Cardiac resuscitation, artificial ventilation, intravenous fluids, nasogastric tubes, and antibiotics are all primarily measures for use in acute or acute-on-chronic illness. They assist toward recovery of health or an enjoyable, stable state. Their use in the dying or severely, permanently brain damaged is justified only when specifically directed to providing comfort. The question is not, "to treat or not to treat," but to care enough to select the most appropriate treatment in light of the patient's biologic potential.

No particular type of treatment is in itself inappropriate for any category of patient. Instead, the therapeutic aim should be kept clearly in mind when treatment is employed. Terminal hemorrhage does not mandate blood transfusion, but rather sedation and constant companionship. Terminal pneumonia—if symptomatic—may be treated with antitussives and antipyretics. If these fail to control symptoms, antibiotics may be indicated, but the clinical setting must dictate the choice.

TABLE 9–1. CHARACTERISTICS OF A HOSPICE PROGRAM

1. Coordinated home care—inpatient beds with sufficient administrative autonomy and flexibility to provide intensive personal care.
2. Patient/family regarded as the unit of care.
3. Physician-directed services.
4. Provision of care by an interdisciplinary team.
5. An emphasis on control of symptoms (physical, sociologic, psychologic, spiritual).
6. Services available on a 24-hour-a-day/7-day-a-week/on-call basis, with emphasis on medical and nursing skills—including at-home availability.
7. Utilization of volunteers as an integral part of the interdisciplinary team.
8. Bereavement follow-up.
9. Structured staff support and communications systems.
10. Patient/family acceptance on the basis of health needs, not ability to pay.

COMMUNICATION

The value of good communication cannot be overemphasized. Technical, scientific, and clinical competence is not enough. Those who advocate a conspiracy of silence often convey by action and expression the message they are trying to avoid. It is impossible not to communicate. At a time of increasing uncertainty, the message a patient needs to receive is "You are safe." Only part of this can be said in words:

"One of us will always be available."

"I will be back as often as it takes to get this pain under control."

"Whatever happens, I am going to do all I can to help."

Most of this fundamental communication is nonverbal, transmitted by demonstration and behavior. Normal courtesies are maintained——the handshake, level eye-to-eye contact, a seat taken if at all possible. Greetings include the patient's name and often in this day of fragmented care, a reintroduction of oneself, with a reminder of one's role. Others within hearing range are acknowledged——the neighboring patient and others accompanying the familiar physician.

Once trust is established, a patient will often indicate with a question or statement that he is ready to hear more.

"I don't think I can take this much longer, doctor."

"The wife hopes I'll be home by Christmas? . . . "

"I want to stop chemotherapy; it's not doing me any good."

Total candor is not the only alternative to evasion. No one wants to hear harsh and brutal truths, but almost everyone wants to know what is going on. Words and concepts can be tailored to individual culture, beliefs, fears, frustrations, strengths, and courage. The physician's responsibility is to foster clarity and honesty, but not to force an unwilling patient into realities beyond his capacity to cope psychologically.

SYMPTOM CONTROL

Pain can be a major symptom in the terminal stages of many illnesses, especially cancer. Patients with a diagnosis of cancer frequently wait in a misery of apprehension for pain to start. Since, however, about 50 per cent of cancer patients never develop severe pain, this must be emphasized to such persons. Furthermore, for those who do have severe pain, much can be done to alleviate it, so that optimism and determination are justified. A valid base of trust can be maintained in the area of pain management, despite inability to control the disease process itself. The first mild pain should be taken seriously and controlled. This establishes confidence that the physician does have skills to prevent discomfort. This confidence will be a powerful ally if pain becomes troublesome later in the illness.

The goal of effective control is a pain-free patient with normal affect. The very sick patient may doze when external stimuli are minimal but is able to rouse and be alert to friends, family, and surroundings without drug-induced stupor or euphoria. A normal mental state can be sustained through a three-faceted approach as follows:

1. Identification of the primary cause and exacerbating factors.
2. Maintenance of *continuous* pain relief.
3. Ease of administration.

Narcotics for Selected Terminal Pain

Pharmacologic control of terminal pain is not usually a matter of exotic new techniques, but the correct use of drugs already known. The aim of treatment is to manage pain so that it will not return. Breakthrough or recurring pain erodes confidence while generating anxiety and fear. Constant pain control is achieved through adequate analgesia given at regular, well-timed intervals. This method uses smaller drug doses, minimizes side effects, and allows the dose to be increased as the disease progresses.

In mild pain aspirin or acetaminophen is used; for moderate pain codeine or dextropropoxyphene is effective; for severe pain morphine is the drug of choice. Useful alternatives are hydromorphone and oxycodone. Twycross and Lack (1986) have shown that there is no clinically observable difference between morphine and heroin when given orally in individually optimized doses at regular intervals (Table 9–2).

Meperidine has a two- to three-hour duration of action—rather short for continuous control. Narcotics with longer action are methadone and levorphanol, but these drugs may accumulate in the body, as their half-lives are much longer than their durations of action. In particular, levorphanol

TABLE 9–2. STRONG NARCOTIC ANALGESICS: APPROXIMATE ORAL EQUIVALENTS TO MORPHINE SULFATE

Analgesic	Proprietary Name	Potency Ratio with Morphine Sulfate[1]		Duration of Action (Hours)[2]
Pethidine/meperidine	Demerol	1/8	1/12[3]	2–3
Dipipanone*	in Diconal	1/2	1/3	3–5
Papaveretum	Omnopon, Pantopon	2/3	1/2	3–5
Oxycodone†[4]	in Percodan, Percocet Tylox (capsule) Oxycodyne syrup	1	2/3	3–5
Dextromoramide*	Palfium	2[5]	1.5	2–4
Methadone	Physeptone, Dolophine	3–4[6]	2–3	6–8
Levorphanol	Dromoran, Levo-dromoran	5	3	4–6
Phenazocine*	Narphen	5	3	4–6
Hydromorphone†	Dilaudid	6	4	3–4

*Not available in the United States.
†Not available in Britain.
[1]*Multiply* dose of stated drug by the potency ratio to determine the equivalent dose of morphine sulfate.
[2]Dependent to a certain extent on dose, often longer lasting in very elderly and those with considerable liver dysfunction.
[3]Column of figures in italics refers to approximate potency ratio with *diamorphine* (heroin).
[4]Oxycodone is available in Britain only as oxycodone pectinate suppositories (q.v.).
[5]Dextromoramide—single 5-mg dose is equivalent to 15 mg of morphine (diamorphine, 10 mg) in terms of *peak* effect but is generally shorter acting; overall potency rate adjusted accordingly.
[6]Methadone—single 5-mg dose is equivalent to 7.5 mg of morphine (diamorphine, 5 mg). It has a prolonged plasma half-life, which leads to accumulation when given repeatedly. This means it is several times more potent when given regularly.
(From Twycross RG, Lack SA: Symptom Control and Control of Alimentary Symptoms in Far Advanced Cancer. Edinburgh, Churchill Livingstone, 1986. With permission.)

accumulation in the older patient manifests clinically by the onset of confusion and restlessness several days after starting regular administration.

Narcotics are used when non-narcotics, used correctly, fail to control pain. Some pains are not narcotic responsive. Other methods are sought for tension headache, postherpetic neuralgia, dysesthesia, gastric distention, and muscle spasm. The severity and type of pain guide the choice of analgesic, not the estimate of life expectancy.

Hospice workers have not found narcotic dependence or tolerance to be a practical problem. Addiction, in the popular sense, is rare in patients with no history of drug abuse, despite the widespread use of narcotics for pain control. Drug dependence as defined by the World Health Organization has two components: psychic and physical. Psychic dependence, an overpowering drive to take a drug, occurs in pain patients most commonly after the use of "p.r.n." injections in inadequate dosage. Each request becomes a reminder of the dependence on drugs and the person who administers them. It is preventable by the use of oral narcotics and regular administration. This frees the patient both from the ritual of injections and from continually asking for relief from the presence or threat of pain. With regular analgesia, the self-perpetuating spiral of pain, dependence, and misery is never started. Physical dependence is of little relevance in the patient with limited life expectancy and does not prevent gradual narcotic reduction if the disease goes into remission.

Tolerance is not a problem if the narcotic is precisely adjusted to the degree of pain the patient is experiencing. Patients remain pain free on the same dose for many weeks or months. With the exception of the first few days, when the pain is being brought under control, the total daily dose does not fluctuate unless disease progression increases nociceptive stimuli. The detailed management of cancer pain, both terminal and otherwise, is addressed in Ch. 27.

Unwanted effects should receive prompt management. Constipation is so common that a regular narcotic is never prescribed without concomitant attention to the bowels. Stool softeners, peristaltic agents, and small bowel flushers counteract the antiperistaltic narcotic effect. Nausea and vomiting, which are also initiation side effects and are not universal, can be prevented by the use of a piperazine phenothiazine or haloperidol. Persistent sedation is often due to factors other than the morphine.

Other Factors in Symptom Control

Insomnia is treated resolutely. Night nurses carry a special responsibility for emotional comfort, for discomfort is often worse at night when the patient is alone with his or her pain and fear. The cumulative effect of many sleepless, pain-filled nights is a substantial lowering of the pain threshold.

The therapeutic environment (Table 9–3) is important: light, flowers, art, and, most significantly, caring people.

Physical discomfort looms large in the lives of dying patients, and medicine for the dying must be concerned with smooth sheets, back rubs, relieving constipation, and getting up at night. A person lying in a wet bed is not interested in reassuring words. Patients and families can cope with many

TABLE 9–3. SOME INGREDIENTS OF A THERAPEUTIC ENVIRONMENT FOR THE DYING

Freedom for pets and children to visit
Open visiting at all hours of the day and night
Provision for overnight stays for the family
Arrangements for patient and friends to eat together
Provision of edible food at any time
Nursing and other staffing patterns allowing for interdisciplinary conferences
Mobility for even the bedridden patient to facilitate trips outside and attendance at parties, religious services, concerts, and the like

emotional crises if they are cared for with common sense and professional skills.

There is never a time when "nothing more can be done." Remedies for all the common problems in terminal disease can be compiled. A problem-oriented approach treats each symptom on its own merit. Thus the patient becomes not Mr. Doe with incurable cancer, but Mr. Doe—the man with severe pain for which we can do a great deal. This enables the physician, as part of the team, to approach the patient with an optimistic, realistic attitude. Effective teamwork mandates that the health team gather regularly in conference to work out a coordinated approach.

Inclusion of the family in planning fosters an atmosphere of cooperation and support. If their questions are not answered speedily and satisfactorily, they may stop following their physician's advice and abandon the entire carefully constructed regimen. The attending physician, nurses, and home health aide must also understand the therapy. A visitor's doubts may undermine the positive advantages created by confidence. For the patient, underlying mechanisms are explained in simple terms: "Your shortness of breath is partly due to the illness and partly due to fluid at the base of the right lung. There is some degree of 'waterlogging' throughout the body, particularly in the lungs, and you are slightly anemic—people with your sort of illness often are. I cannot get rid of the underlying tumor—you know that—but this is what we are going to do about the extra fluid. . . ."

The fact that you, the doctor, understand why he or she, the patient, is having trouble is reassuring. No longer is this condition shrouded in mystery. The doctor understands. Treatment options are discussed with the patient, and, if possible, an immediate course of action is decided upon together. Few things are more demeaning to a person's self-esteem than to be disregarded in discussions concerning treatment. The dying have a right to be treated for what they usually are: sane, sensible adults. While it is wise not to promise too much, it is important to reassure the patient that the doctor is going to stand by and do all possible to ensure comfort.

Confidence is crucial to successful symptom management. The patient may resist a drug regimen because of a lifelong habit of never giving in or resorting to drugs. Other reasons for resistance may be fear of constipation, addiction, nightmares, and confusion. Once identified through sensitive inquiry, these fears can be dealt with by discussion, education, and control of unwanted effects. In addition to pressing symptoms such as pain, vomiting, and dyspnea, patients may experience a variety of other discomforts. These include dry mouth, altered taste, anorexia, constipation, frequency, pruritus, cough, and insomnia. Because patients tend to be reluctant to bother their doctor about such symptoms, physicians should inquire about them from time to time.

Bedside assessment precedes treatment. Treatment for the same symptom may vary considerably from patient to patient. In the dying, symptoms are caused by multiple factors, some treatable and some not. Best results are obtained by aggressively dealing with the treatable elements. Instead of attempting *immediately* to relieve the symptom completely, the physician can wear down the problem a little at a time. It is surprising how much can be achieved with determination and persistence. Comprehensive treatment is not limited to the use of drugs. Thus, pruritus is relieved in the majority without resorting to antihistaminic drugs. Application of emollient cream to dry, itching skin several times a day and elimination of soap are frequently sufficient.

Clearly defined medical leadership is vital. Frequent contact with specialist colleagues and readiness to consult with others will assist the physician in the search for symptom relief, but the patient should be discouraged from attending a succession of outpatient clinics.

DYING AT HOME

Although home care is not for all, it is a cost-effective alternative that has historic tradition and has proved to be a well-received option in contemporary communities. Physician availability, information about community resources, 24-hour coverage, and education of family members are crucial issues when keeping someone home to die.

Every family must have a sense of security in order to carry on. Most need professional reassurance, and the home visits of a trusted physician are a great boost to morale. Much discomfort can be assessed and alleviated at the bedside, but not over the phone. In some states, an at-home pronouncement visit is necessary to avoid legal complications. Bereavement counseling can then begin when the death certificate is put aside and the physician inquires:

"Tell me about the last few hours, how have you managed?"

Reassuring the family that "you did well" will help them to overcome feelings of helplessness and guilt.

Change comes quickly in terminal illness and can be planned for by discussion and practical measures, such as a supply of parenteral essentials kept in the home. Common crises include refusal of medication, impaction, disorientation, new pain, and the onset of incontinence or of coma. Poor preparation precipitates premature inpatient admission. Even the best laid plans may prove inadequate, but families often manage if someone who knows the patient is available at any time of the day or night.

Medication regimens should be kept simple to understand and easy to administer, even at the expense of pharmacologic purity. An impossibly complex schedule will not be followed. Short-acting narcotics such as meperidine are rarely satisfactory at home. Similarly, a two-hourly medication regimen is impossible to maintain for long.

THE LAST TWENTY-FOUR HOURS

Careful assessment is still necessary if the patient is to be kept comfortable. Temporary relief from a painful bedsore can be obtained by the application of a local anesthetic gel, which might not be used when life expectancy is longer. A distended bladder can be relieved by catheterization. The sound of rattling secretions can often be diminished by positioning and scopolamine. Pain will not be troublesome at the very end if control has previously been good. There is no final crescendo of pain. Analgesic requirements may decrease. Patients may, however, experience pain even when drowsy. In addition, they may be physically dependent on narcotics.

Withdrawal restlessness may mar their peace if narcotics are stopped. For these reasons it is advisable to continue analgesia by suppository or injection when the patient cannot swallow. At one hospice 60 per cent of patients are able to swallow until a few hours before death and need no change in drug administration. Another 25 per cent require one or two narcotic suppositories; only 15 per cent need an injection. Only one fourth of the original daily dose is needed to prevent withdrawal symptoms, so rigid adherence to the previous schedule is not necessary. Morphine every six to eight hours will usually suffice.

Both staff and relatives are informed that, at this late stage, any injection may be the last. This information may allay in *advance* any lingering fears about "killing the patient":

"She might die just five minutes after you give her the four o'clock injection. How will you feel if that happens? You understand that it would be just a coincidence because she is going to die very soon anyway? We are using injections only to keep her out of pain."

The advent of the modern hospice has done much to raise expectations in both the public and health care professions. We must be wary of replacing one caricature by another—the old image of death as negative and despairing with the new image that "death is beautiful." It does not help to underestimate the problems. Good terminal care is hard work. The very highest standards may be achieved on paper, but this is a futile exercise unless every aspect is tailored to the vagaries of the individual patient and family.

Health and Public Policy Committee, American College of Physicians: Drug therapy for severe, chronic pain in terminal illness. Ann Intern Med 99:870, 1983. *A position paper authoritatively endorsing six principles elaborated by the modern hospice movement over the past 20 years.*

Hinton J: Talking with people about to die. Br Med J 3:25, 1974. *Sixty dying patients comment on their discussions with doctors and nurses, and give their opinions of what degree of truth is desirable. The assumed principle is that the views of dying people count.*

Lack SA: Hospice—a concept of care in the final stage of life. Conn Med 43:367, 1979. *Describes hospice as a specialized health care delivery system, emphasizing the essential administrative characteristics of a program organized to meet the needs of the dying and their families.*

Lasagna L: Heroin: A medical me too. N Engl J Med 304:1539, 1981. *A succinct rationale, with good references, emphasizing why improved terminal pain control in the United States does not require the legalization of heroin.*

Saunders C: Hospice care. Am J Med 65:726, 1978. *The founder traces the origins of the modern hospice movement, correcting some misconceptions in the popular press and defining the position of good terminal management within the mainstream of medicine.*

Twycross RW, Lack SA: Symptom Control and Control of Alimentary Symptoms in Far Advanced Cancer. Edinburgh, Churchill Livingstone, 1986. *More extensive elaboration and detailed discussion of the analytic methods of pain relief and symptom control mentioned in this chapter.*

PART III

PERSONAL HEALTH CARE AND PREVENTIVE MEDICINE

10 PRINCIPLES OF PREVENTIVE MEDICINE

Stephen B. Hulley

In the early part of this century the efforts of preventive medicine were focused on the predominant cause of illness and death at the time, infectious disease. In western countries, governmental provisions to control the spread of disease with modern water and sewage systems complemented the success of the medical profession in putting into practice the developing science of immunization. These programs combined with improved nutrition, better medical care, and other factors to make death from infectious disease an uncommon event (Table 10–1). This remarkable accomplishment has now brought life expectancy to unprecedented levels and has left, as the major causes of death and disability, the noninfectious and chronic diseases. A new set of strategies has evolved to prevent the chief causes of mortality today: coronary heart disease, cancer, stroke, and injury.

Preventive medicine is based on epidemiologic studies that have identified risk factors for these conditions. Many of these risk factors are aspects of individually chosen lifestyles: cigarette smoking (the most important single cause of preventable death) and eating, drinking, and exercising habits. This has changed the nature of the therapeutic relationship. The patient must take on the larger responsibility of making the necessary lifestyle changes, and the physician must now add the role of health counselor to his list of clinical duties.

RISK MODIFICATION

The process of guiding lifestyle change *begins* with serving as a model. A physician who has healthy habits and provides an appropriate environment (prohibiting smoking in the wait-

ing room, for example) has set the stage for successful intervention. The *second step* is to identify the individual characteristics of the patient, testing for the presence of risk factors and exploring motivations for changing, and for not changing, unhealthy habits. The *third step* is to provide a clear message about the scientific facts on the relationship between risk factors and disease, specifying, for example, the nature and extent of the adverse health consequences of cigarettes.

The *fourth step* is to formulate and apply recommendations for change. Behavior modification, an approach to health education with origins in the conditioned response research of Pavlov and Skinner, has five components: (1) involving the patient as a partner in choosing attainable objectives and in making a firm commitment (a written contract may be helpful); (2) adjusting the environment to promote the desired behavior (by not keeping unhealthy food in the home, for example); (3) negatively reinforcing undesired behavior (through criticism or aversive techniques); (4) positively reinforcing desired behavior (through praise or rewards); and (5) involving the family and other social supports. Many clinics include staff with special skills in behavioral medicine, but even in the absence of formal training, physicians can accomplish a great deal just by addressing and lending importance to these activities. In addition to serving as health counselors themselves, physicians can guide the patient's access to other resources for lifestyle changes by providing pamphlets (obtained free from organizations like the American Heart Association) and by referral to appropriate books, support groups, and health professionals.

Whatever the intervention approach, the *fifth step* is a sustained effort to follow up on the risk factor levels. Habits are difficult to change, and health counselors need to have the tenacity and imagination to try a variety of approaches over the years. This does not mean harassing an unwilling or unsuccessful patient. The best health counselors are sensitive to the preferences of their patients and make wise decisions about when to promote recommendations for change and when to leave the patient alone.

TABLE 10–1. ANNUAL MORTALITY RATES AND YEARS OF LIFE LOST PREMATURELY IN THE UNITED STATES IN 1900 AND IN 1980

Causes of Death*	1900 Annual Mortality (rate/100,000)	1980 Annual Mortality (rate/100,000)	Years of Potential Life Lost Before Age 65 by Persons Dying in 1980
Diseases of the heart	137	336	1,636,000
Malignant neoplasms	64	184	1,804,000
Cerebrovascular disease	107	75	280,000
Injuries	83	69	4,487,000
All others	1330	214	2,199,000
Total	1721	878	10,406,000

*The causes of death are the four most common in 1980. The statistics, which are not age adjusted, are subject to the usual inaccuracies of death certificate attribution. The top three causes of death in 1900 were pneumonia and influenza (202/100,000), tuberculosis (194/100,000), and diarrhea and enteritis (143/100,000).

TABLE 10–2. FIFTEEN AREAS OF ENDEAVOR FOR PREVENTIVE MEDICINE ESTABLISHED BY THE U.S. DEPT. OF HEALTH AND HUMAN SERVICES IN 1979

Topics that Are Covered in Chapters of this Section
Smoking and health
Injury prevention
Control of stress and violent behavior
Nutrition
Physical fitness and exercise
Misuse of alcohol and drugs
Immunization

Topics that Are Addressed Elsewhere in this Book
High blood pressure control
Sexually transmitted diseases
Toxic agent control
Occupational safety and health
Surveillance and control of infectious diseases

Topics that Are the Concern of Other Specialties
Family planning
Pregnancy and infant health
Fluoridation and dental health

IMPLICATIONS OF CHRONIC DISEASE PREVENTION

If the entire population were fully successful in the lifestyle changes proposed in this second wave of preventive medicine efforts in the twentieth century, the chief causes of premature death in western countries might become far less common. In addition to further extending life expectancy, the potential reward of fully effective lifestyle intervention is the possibility that most people could live their full lifespan without major illness or disability.

Speculation of this sort is based, in part, on the remarkable decline in mortality observed in the United States over the past 15 years. The chief component of the decline is coronary heart disease, which has decreased more rapidly in the United States than in any other nation (2 per cent per year). It seems reasonable to attribute this, in part, to the changes in lifestyle that are occurring in this country: the substantial decline in the national prevalence of smoking and of inadequately treated hypertension, the decrease in the mean serum cholesterol level, and the movement in the population to become more physically fit.

The extent and thrust of preventive medicine today have been established by formal health goals in 15 areas of endeavor, created in 1979 by the U.S. Department of Health and Human Services (Table 10–2). For each of these topics, there are specific objectives for the nation to achieve by 1990 that address health status, risk factor levels, public and professional awareness, provision of health services, and mechanisms for evaluation. This section of *Cecil Textbook of Medicine* addresses the 7 of the 15 topics that are part of personal health care.

SUMMARY

The emergence of chronic and noninfectious disease as the predominant cause of death and disability in western nations has been accompanied by a growing importance of lifestyle factors as causal agents in health and disease. Among these, cigarette smoking is the single most important modifiable health hazard; excessive use of alcohol, sedentary lifestyle, and improper diet are also important. The clinician's role in preventive medicine still begins with immunization and treatment of such medical conditions as hypertension, but it now extends to health counseling: examining a patient's risk factors, educating the patient, listening to preferences for changing (or not changing) lifestyle, implementing the appropriate behavioral interventions, and following up on the progress of these personal health care strategies over the years.

Freis JR: Aging, natural death, and the compression of morbidity. N Engl J Med 303:130, 1980. *Speculation on the potential ability of lifestyle intervention to postpone chronic disease beyond the normal lifespan of 85 years. See also the response—another viewpoint—in N Engl J Med 309:854, 1983.*

Levy RI: Declining mortality in coronary heart disease. Arteriosclerosis 1:312, 1981. *Analysis of secular trends in heart disease; the United States has the most rapid decline of any nation.*
Martin AR, Coates TJ: A clinician's guide to helping patients change. West J Med. In press (1987). *Practical guidelines in helping patients modify their risks.*
Mason JO, Tolsma DD: Personal health promotion. West J Med 141:772, 1984. *Review of history of lifestyle intervention programs and extent of the current problem.*
Public Health Service, U.S. Dept of Health and Human Services: The 1990 Objectives for the Nation: A mid course review. 1986. *Update on progress in achieving the 1990 objectives.*
U.S. Dept. of Health, Education and Welfare: Healthy People: The Surgeon General's Report on Health Promotion and Disease Prevention. DHEW Publication No. 79–55071, 1979. *Summary of trends in illness and death rates from 1900 to the 1970's.*
U.S. Dept. of Health and Human Services: Promoting Health—Preventing Disease: Objectives for the Nation. DHHS, 1980. *Specific objectives for health promotion and protection in 15 topics, to be achieved by 1990.*

11 TOBACCO AND HEALTH

David M. Burns

Cigarette smoking is the largest preventable public health problem currently existing in the United States. An estimated 300,000 deaths per year, one sixth of the total mortality in the United States, occur prematurely secondary to the smoking habits of the American population.

Tobacco use, both oral and smoking, was introduced to European settlers by the American Indian, and tobacco was one of the main cash crops in revolutionary America. However, the invention of a cigarette-making machine in the 1880's and, around the turn of the century, of matches that could be carried safely resulted in a marked shift in tobacco consumption from predominantly pipes, cigars, and chewing tobacco to predominantly cigarettes. Per capita cigarette consumption in the United States increased from 54 in 1900 to a peak of 4336 in 1963. This dramatic switch to cigarette use was followed some 20 to 25 years later by an equally dramatic rise in deaths from lung cancer. The risks associated with tobacco smoking appear to be closely related to the amount of smoke inhaled. Smokers who have used only pipes or cigars tend not to inhale, and therefore the majority of the health risks are correlated with cigarette consumption (Table 11–1).

In the early part of the century, cigarette smoking was

TABLE 11–1. INCREASED RISKS FOR CIGARETTE SMOKERS

Cardiovascular Disease
Coronary artery disease
Peripheral vascular disease
Aortic aneurysm
Stroke (at younger ages)

Cancer
Lung
Larynx, oral cavity, esophagus
Bladder, kidney
Pancreas

Lung Disorders
Cancer (as noted above)
Chronic bronchitis with airflow obstruction
Emphysema

Complications of Pregnancy
Infants—small for gestational age, higher perinatal mortality
Maternal complications—placenta previa, abruptio placentae

Gastrointestinal Complications
Peptic ulcer
Esophageal reflux

Other
Osteoporotic fractures
Altered drug metabolism

largely a male phenomenon, but in the late 1930's and early 1940's women began to smoke in large numbers. Currently, smoking habits in young adults are similar for the two sexes. The prevalence of cigarette smoking is declining in both men and women in the United States population. In contrast, a major new marketing effort for smokeless tobacco has led to a dramatic resurgence of snuff use, particularly among adolescent males.

CIGARETTE SMOKE

Tobacco smoke is a complex mixture of some 4000 individual constituents. The smoke is a combination of pyrolysis and distillation products distributed between a particulate phase and a gas phase. Tar is the total particulate matter of the smoke once the water vapor and nicotine have been removed and contains the bulk of the carcinogenic effect of whole smoke. The gas phase of the smoke has a number of irritating and ciliotoxic agents, as well as high levels of carbon monoxide (1 to 5 per cent).

FACTORS DETERMINING RISK

The risks due to cigarette smoking are not evenly spread across the smoking population; they vary with differences in individual smoking habits and the presence of other risk factors. For each of the major diseases associated with smoking, the risk increases with the "dose" of smoke to which an individual has been exposed. The risk increases with increasing number of cigarettes smoked per day, depth of inhalation, and duration of the smoking habit. The risk also increases with the younger age at which regular smoking is begun. The risks due to adolescent and preadolescent smoking may be magnified by a vulnerability of the cardiovascular and respiratory systems during growth and maturation.

A given dose of smoke exposure may interact with other personal characteristics or environmental exposures to magnify the risk of disease greatly. Thus, the risks incurred by cigarette smoking in someone with elevated blood pressure or high levels of asbestos exposure are much larger than the risks for smokers without those characteristics. In addition, the presence of smoking-induced disease in one organ system (e.g., chronic obstructive lung disease) may alter the ability to treat or survive a second disease process (e.g., lung cancer).

CARDIOVASCULAR DISEASE

Cigarette smokers have almost twice the risk of nonsmokers of developing a myocardial infarction or dying of coronary heart disease. This relative risk of heart disease is even greater at younger ages, when the incidence of disease would otherwise be very low. The relative risks for sudden death from coronary disease, peripheral vascular disease, and aneurysm of the aorta are even higher. In contrast, cigarette smokers have only a slightly greater risk of developing angina pectoris, and an increased risk of stroke is demonstrable only in smokers at younger ages.

The magnitude of the risk of coronary heart disease associated with cigarette smoking is equivalent to the risks associated with elevated blood pressure or elevated serum cholesterol. The per cent of the population with smoking as a risk factor is substantially larger than the percentage with either elevated blood pressure or elevated serum cholesterol. As a result, *smoking ranks as the largest avoidable cause of coronary heart disease in the American population.*

Cigarette smoking acts as an independent risk factor for coronary heart disease; that is, its effect is not explained by levels of other risk factors. However, when more than one risk factor is present, smoking interacts with the other major risk factors to increase the risk synergistically (Fig. 11–1). The presence of smoking, or of either of the other risk factors, increases the risk by 31 per 1000, compared with the risk of someone with none of the risk factors. The presence of a

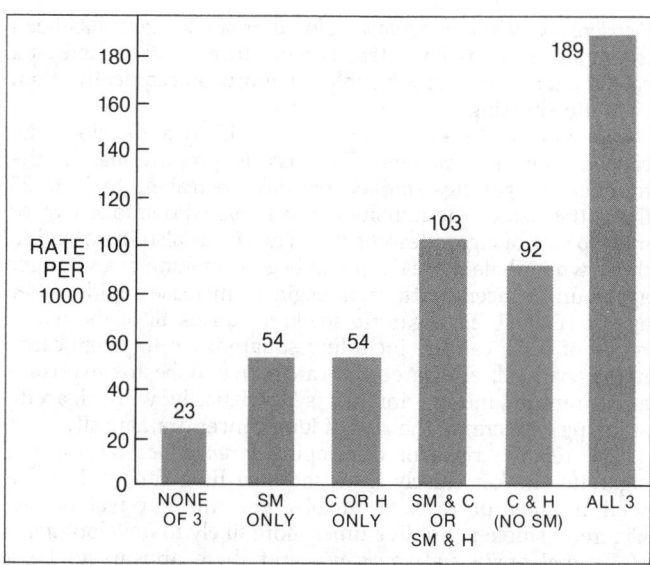

FIGURE 11–1. Major risk factor combinations, 10-year incidence of first major coronary events, men age 30 to 59 at entry, Pooling Project. Risk factor status at entry: Definitions of the three major risk factors and their symbols are hypercholesterolemia (C) = ≥ 250 mg/dl; elevated blood pressure (H) = diastolic pressure ≥ 90 mm Hg; cigarette smoking (SM) = any current use of cigarettes at entry.

second risk factor in someone who smokes results in an increase in risk of 49 per 1000 over the risk when only one risk factor is present, and the addition of a third risk factor increases the risk by 86 per 1000. The actual risk that exists is always greater than the sum of the risks measured independently, suggesting that when multiple risk factors are present they interact to create more disease. This interaction may occur by accelerating the development of atherosclerosis, or it may occur by increasing the likelihood or severity of a myocardial infarction for any given level of atherosclerosis.

Smokers have more atherosclerosis than nonsmokers, particularly in the aorta. Smoking a cigarette results in an increase in heart rate and blood pressure, necessitating a greater myocardial oxygen delivery, while the carbon monoxide in the smoke increases the blood's carboxyhemoglobin level, thus decreasing its oxygen-carrying capacity. Cigarette smoking also increases platelet adhesiveness and lowers the threshold for ventricular fibrillation and may thereby play a role in the acute events surrounding some thrombotic myocardial infarctions.

Cigarette smoking has a more profound effect on the peripheral vascular bed than on the coronary or cerebral vessels. Over 90 per cent of patients with atherosclerotic peripheral vascular disease are cigarette smokers. The cessation of cigarette smoking is a critical therapeutic intervention in these patients; and in those who fail to quit, there is a higher incidence of amputation, and surgical therapy is dramatically less successful.

The risk of coronary heart disease due to smoking is present at all ages beyond 30, but smoking is responsible for a greater proportion of coronary deaths in younger age groups than in older age groups. This risk declines dramatically with the cessation of cigarette smoking. By five years after the last cigarette, the risk in those who had smoked less than one pack per day approximates the risk in lifelong nonsmokers. For those who had smoked more than one pack per day, a small residual risk of coronary heart disease may persist.

CANCER

Lung cancer is the largest cause of death from cancer in men and women (Ch. 70). *Approximately 85 per cent of mortality due to lung cancer is causally attributed to cigarette smoking and is therefore potentially preventable.* No other single agent has been examined in as much detail, is more firmly established as a causal agent, or is responsible for more cancer deaths than cigarette smoking.

Cigarette smokers are ten times more likely to develop lung cancer than nonsmokers. This risk is proportional to the number of cigarettes smoked per day, increasing to 20 to 25 times the risk of the nonsmoker in those who smoke two or more packs of cigarettes per day. The risk is also increased in those who inhale more deeply or began smoking at a younger age. Lung cancer death rates begin to increase rapidly after age 35 (Fig. 11–2). Cigarette smoking causes all of the major types of lung cancer, including squamous cell, adenocarcinoma, oat cell, and large-cell carcinoma. Asbestos exposure and uranium mining interact synergistically with cigarette smoking to increase the risk of lung cancer dramatically.

The relative risks of developing *laryngeal cancer* for the cigarette smoker closely track those of lung cancer, but the total number of cases is smaller and the survival better. Cigarette smokers are five times more likely to develop *cancer of the oral cavity and esophagus*, and there appears to be a synergistic interaction between cigarette smoking and alcohol consumption for cancer of the larynx, oral cavity, and esophagus. Cigarette smoking is also a major contributing factor in *cancers of the bladder, kidney, and pancreas*, and an association between cigarette smoking and *gastric and cervical cancers* has been noted. The use of chewing tobacco or snuff can cause cancers of the cheek or gum. Overall, tobacco consumption is responsible for approximately 30 per cent of the total United States cancer mortality.

Cigarette smoking induces changes in the respiratory epithelium that progress from hyperplasia to dysplasia and even to carcinoma in situ. Tobacco smoke contains a variety of tumorigenic agents, including several that can act as complete carcinogens. In addition, tumor initiators, promoters, and cocarcinogens have been identified in smoke. The impact of these tumorigenic agents may be magnified by the ciliotoxic

agents in the smoke that interfere with the normal clearance mechanisms of the lung and result in a prolonged retention of the carcinogenic agents in the lung.

Cessation of cigarette smoking results in a lessening of the risk of cancer in comparison with the risk to the continuing smoker. The risk for light smokers approximates the risk of the nonsmoker by 10 to 15 years after cessation. Heavy smokers have a residual two- to threefold increased risk that is proportional to their lifetime exposure to smoke.

CHRONIC OBSTRUCTIVE PULMONARY DISEASE (COPD)

Cigarette-induced lung injury is characterized by three overlapping syndromes: cough and mucus hypersecretion, bronchitis with airflow obstruction, and emphysema (see Ch. 61). By age 60 most cigarette smokers have changes in the airways and some degree of pathologic emphysema, but only the minority have symptomatic ventilatory limitation. An increased prevalence of cough can be demonstrated in cigarette smokers by the early teens, and abnormalities in the small airways are present in many smokers by early adulthood. However, it is not clear that either of these changes predicts those who will eventually go on to develop symptomatic chronic airflow limitation.

The cigarette smoking habit is the major predictor in a population for the development of COPD. The prevalence of COPD and risk of death from COPD increase with the number of cigarettes smoked per day and the depth of inhalation, as does the prevalence of chronic cough and sputum production, rate of decline in the measurements of expiratory airflow, and degree of anatomic emphysema.

In contrast to nonsmokers, the majority of cigarette smokers examined at autopsy have some degree of emphysema and hypertrophic changes of the respiratory epithelium. However, only a minority of cigarette smokers manifest clinically significant airflow obstruction. Those who develop chronic airflow obstruction may be a subset of the smoking population identifiable by a rapidly declining FEV_1 early in the course of disease. In any event, it is rare for symptomatic chronic airflow obstruction to develop in anyone who maintained normal measures of expiratory airflow through age 45.

Cessation of cigarette smoking is of some benefit at all preterminal stages of ventilatory impairment. Changes in the small airways and early declines of FEF_{25-75} may reverse within one year of cessation. Cough and sputum production also lessen, and the annual rate of decline in measures of expiratory airflow moderates and approximates the rate of decline in nonsmokers. These changes are probably related to reversal of the chronic inflammatory changes in the large and small airways and the recovery of ciliary function, as there is no evidence that the emphysematous process is reversible.

Lungs of smokers contain increased numbers of alveolar macrophages and polymorphonuclear leukocytes, probably drawn there as part of the inflammatory response to the irritants in the smoke. These cells produce elastase, which is capable of degrading the structural elements of the lung, resulting in a loss of elastic recoil. This destructive process is normally limited by blood-borne antiproteases. However, cigarette smoke contains a number of oxidants that destroy the function of these protective proteins, and the result is an imbalance in the protease-antiprotease system favoring degradation and rupture of alveolar walls.

RISKS FOR WOMEN

There is essentially no protective effect of being female for the risks of developing cancer or chronic lung disease. Much of the premenopausal difference in cardiovascular risk enjoyed by women disappears in those who smoke.

In addition to the risks defined for men, women also incur additional risks related to pregnancy and use of oral contraceptives. Infants of smoking mothers are small for their

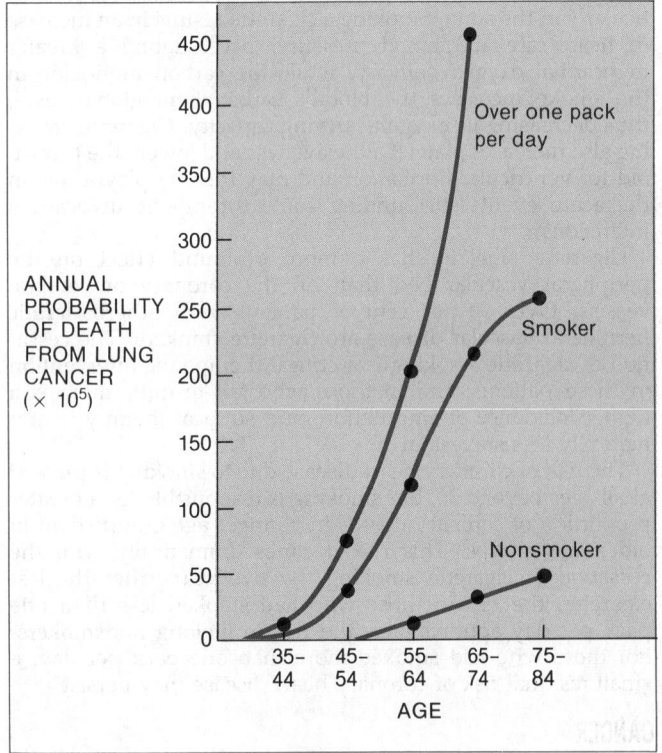

FIGURE 11–2. Annual death rate from lung cancer in nonsmokers, smokers in general, and those who smoke more than one pack per day.

gestational age in weight, length, and head circumference, and they experience a higher perinatal mortality, particularly if other determinants of a high-risk pregnancy are present. The smoking mothers are also at greater risk for the maternal complications of pregnancy, especially placenta previa and abruptio placentae.

Women who smoke and use oral contraceptives are at dramatically increased risk of cardiovascular disease. They are over 30 times more likely to develop a myocardial infarction, and about 20 times more likely to have a subarachnoid hemorrhage, than their nonsmoking peers who do not use oral contraceptives.

INVOLUNTARY SMOKING

Environmental tobacco smoke contains most of the toxic and carcinogenic compounds identified in mainstream smoke; and therefore the question is not whether these agents can cause disease, but rather whether the dose and mode of exposure experienced in involuntary smoking carry a measurable risk. Absorption of smoke constituents from the environment has been documented in both infants and adults, and a number of epidemiologic studies have demonstrated health effects in humans.

Involuntary smoking can cause lung cancer in nonsmokers. The risk is small in comparison to active smoking but is large in comparison to other carcinogenic exposures experienced by the general population. From 500 to 5000 lung cancers per year have been estimated to result from involuntary smoking.

The majority of nonsmokers express annoyance and experience eye and respiratory tract irritation on exposure to smoke. Individuals with pre-existing disease may become more symptomatic on exposure to smoke, particularly those with allergies, and possibly those with chronic heart and lung disease.

Infants of smoking parents have a higher incidence of bronchitis and pneumonia in the first year of life, and the children of smoking mothers experience a developmental lag in lung growth.

CIGARETTES WITH LOW TAR AND NICOTINE

The machine-measured yield of tar and nicotine for the average cigarette smoked by the American population has been steadily declining. Unfortunately this decline in tar yield has not been matched by a proportional drop in the disease risks of smoking these cigarettes. Smokers of lower yield cigarettes have a slightly lower risk of lung cancer than smokers of the high-yield cigarette, but this benefit disappears if they increase the number of cigarettes they smoke per day. There is also a lower prevalence of cough and phlegm, but probably no major impact on the risk of developing cardiovascular disease or chronic airflow obstruction. There are two major reasons why the decline in machine-measured tar and nicotine yield has not been accompanied by a concomitant reduction in biologic effect: (1) Many smokers may compensate for the decline in yield by increasing the number of cigarettes smoked per day, or by inhaling more deeply, thereby negating any possible reduction in smoke exposure "dose." (2) The machine-measured yield may not correspond to the yield when the cigarette is actually smoked. This is particularly true for the very low-yield cigarettes that have vents or channels designed into the filter so that the machine draws very little smoke through the filter. These vents can be occluded by the smoker, or the volume of the puff increased, with a resultant dramatic rise in the yield. For these cigarettes, the measured tar and nicotine yields have almost no relation to either actual yield or biologic potency.

An additional concern is the wide variety of flavoring and other additives that have been used to compensate for the decline in tobacco content. These additives are considered trade secrets and may be added to the cigarette without informing the public of their presence and without any review for toxic effects. These additives represent a major gap in the understanding of the disease risks associated with smoking the modern cigarette.

PEPTIC ULCER DISEASE

Cigarette smokers have a greater incidence of gastric and duodenal ulcers and delayed healing of these ulcers. Smoking also relaxes the esophageal sphincter and may contribute to esophageal reflux.

DRUG METABOLISM AND DIAGNOSTIC TESTS

Several of the constituents of tobacco smoke are capable of inducing hepatic microsomal systems, which then alter the metabolism of other drugs. Theophylline, phenacetin, antipyrine, caffeine, and imipramine are metabolized more rapidly by smokers, and adjustment in the dosage may be required with cessation. Smokers have lower blood levels of vitamins C and B_{12}. Hematocrit and hemoglobin levels, as well as carboxyhemoglobin levels, are elevated in smokers; and smoking is one cause of an elevated red cell volume. Smokers also have small alterations in the other diagnostic tests, including a higher leukocyte count, but these differences are not usually clinically significant for an individual patient.

PIPE AND CIGAR SMOKING

Pipe and cigar smokers who have never smoked cigarettes have a lower risk of cardiovascular disease, lung cancer, and chronic airflow obstruction than do cigarette smokers. They have similar risks of cancer of the upper respiratory tract. These differences are due to the tendency of pipe and cigar smokers not to inhale the more irritating smoke of these forms of tobacco. Cigarette smokers who switch to pipes and cigars do tend to inhale, however, and so it is not clear that switching to a pipe or cigars results in a lowering of the risks for the cigarette smoker.

SMOKELESS TOBACCO USE

The re-emergence of oral snuff use among male adolescents in the last several years has generated substantial public health concern. Smokeless tobacco use can cause cancer of the cheek and gum and gingival recession. It may also increase the risk of other oral cancers, and regular use of snuff can lead to nicotine addiction.

SMOKING BEHAVIOR AND CESSATION

The initiation of regular cigarette smoking occurs almost exclusively during adolescence and early adulthood. The availability of cigarettes and a variety of peer pressures and needs to model adult behavior lead to developing regular smoking behavior, particularly in those adolescents with limited social and academic success. The maintenance of smoking behavior in the adult is conditioned by other factors. The cigarette is used for nonverbal communication, for accentuation of positive feelings, for the reduction of negative feelings, and for coping with stress. An individual may use cigarettes sometimes for stimulation and sometimes for sedation. The result is a pattern of use that builds the cigarette into the way the smoker learns to deal with the world, and the cessation of smoking requires the smoker to give up a major coping mechanism.

Cigarette smoking fulfills all the criteria for an addiction, including a defined withdrawal syndrome. Nicotine almost certainly plays a role in the addictive process, but nicotine alone will not reverse the withdrawal syndrome. Nicotine probably provides a transient pharmacologic stimulus around which the human organism builds a series of psychologic or psychopharmacologic reflexes. These reflexes can be designed to meet the specific needs of an individual, thereby personalizing the cigarette habit. The psychologic and sociologic utility of the smoking behavior may vary qualitatively and quantitatively from individual to individual, and therefore it is not surprising that no single cessation technique will work for all individuals.

The physician can play an important role in cessation. Most smokers say that they would attempt to quit if told to do so by a physician; and, when told, up to one third will actually try to quit.

Successful intervention by the physician to alter smoking behavior requires the acceptance of smoking as a medical problem necessitating both treatment and follow-up. The initial intervention by the physician should consist of the following: asking about the patient's smoking status, reviewing the benefits of quitting, making a firm recommendation to quit, and negotiating an actual quitting date with the patient. Assistance in quitting should be provided through referral to local cessation programs or through provision of self-help materials. Prescription of nicotine gum increases the chances of successful cessation when used in conjunction with some other behavior intervention. Follow-up visits or phone calls also improve the success of cessation attempts, and follow-ups should be scheduled at two weeks after the quit date. Smokers should be encouraged to try to quit "cold turkey" rather than tapering down. A variety of rapid smoking techniques (rapidly smoking several cigarettes to produce adverse symptoms) have been shown to improve cessation rates. Effective intervention by the physician can be delivered in 3 to 5 minutes with 1 to 2 follow-up contacts.

A variety of organizations provide cessation assistance, both in groups and with individual or self-help programs, and these organizations can be located in the telephone directory or by contacting the local heart, lung, or cancer societies.

American Heart Association: Report of the ad hoc committee on cigarette smoking and cardiovascular diseases. Circulation 57:404A, 1978. *A report of the combined experience of the major coronary heart disease incidence studies relating the presence of risk factors to risk of coronary heart disease.*

Fielding JE: Smoking: Health effects and control. N Engl J Med 313:491, 555, 1985. *An overall review of smoking issues.*

Health and Public Policy Committee, American College of Physicians: Methods for stopping cigarette smoking. Ann Intern Med 105:281, 1986. *A review of smoking cessation methods.*

U.S. Dept. of Health and Human Services: The Health Consequences of Smoking: The Changing Cigarette. DHHS Publication No. (PHS) 81–50156, 1981. *A detailed discussion of what is known about low-yield cigarettes and the problems associated with them.*

U.S. Dept. of Health and Human Services: The Health Consequences of Smoking: Cancer. DHHS Publication No. (PHS) 82–50179, 1982. *A review of the evidence on smoking and cancer from the perspective of causality.*

U.S. Dept. of Health and Human Services: The Health Consequences of Smoking: Cardiovascular Disease. DHHS Publication No. (PHS) 84–50204, 1983. *A review of the evidence on smoking and cardiovascular disease.*

U.S. Dept. of Health and Human Services: The Health Consequences of Smoking: Chronic Obstructive Lung Disease. DHHS Publication No. (PHS) 84–50205, 1984. *A review of the evidence on smoking and lung disease.*

U.S. Dept. of Health and Human Services: The Health Consequences of Smoking: Involuntary Smoking. DHHS Publication (CDC) 87-8398, 1986. *A review of the evidence of involuntary smoking.*

U.S. Dept. of Health and Human Services: The Health Consequences of Using Smokeless Tobacco. DHHS Publication No. (PHS) 86–2874, 1986. *A review of the health effects of using snuff.*

12 CONTROL OF UNINTENDED INJURIES AND THOSE DUE TO VIOLENCE

Stephen B. Hulley

Deaths from injury are the fourth most common cause of death in the United States; they number more than 150,000 each year and are the leading cause of death for young and middle-aged people in the age range 1 to 45. The problem is even larger if *nonfatal* injuries, some of which cause permanent disability, are considered: There are several hundred injury-related emergency room visits for every death from injury. One third of all deaths from injury are due to motor vehicles, one third result from other forms of unintended injury (falls are the most common, followed by drowning, fires, and poisoning), and the remaining third are due to violence (homicide and suicide).

Each of these causes of death and disability has risk factors that identify high-risk groups and that are susceptible to physician-mediated efforts to prevent occurrence or recurrence. Yet until recently, injury control has been largely ignored by the medical and public health establishment; it is the sleeping giant of preventive medicine.

THE EPIDEMIOLOGY OF UNINTENDED INJURIES

Motor vehicle fatalities decreased by one third in the 1970's after automobile safety regulations and the 55 mile per hour national speed limit were instituted, but most of the benefit has since been lost as average speeds have returned to higher levels and smaller cars (which have a twofold higher crash fatality rate) have become more prevalent. Deaths due to motor vehicles rise to alarmingly high levels among young adults, particularly males (Fig. 12–1). The impact of this is brought home by the current projection that 1.4 per cent of all 15-year-old boys in the United States will die of an injury before age 25. The most important modifiable risk factors are excessive alcohol intake, which plays a role in half of all fatal crashes, and the failure to observe speed limits and use seatbelts.

Half of all deaths from unintended injury are unrelated to traffic. Falls are the commonest cause (27 per cent of the 49,048 such deaths in 1980), followed by drowning (15 per cent), fire (12 per cent), poisoning (6 per cent), adverse effects of medical care (5 per cent), unintended firearm use (4 per cent), aspiration of food (4 per cent), airplane crashes (3 per cent), machinery accidents (3 per cent), aspiration other than food (3 per cent), electric current (2 per cent), and other less common causes. These deaths tend to have a common pattern of risk factors, including male sex, old age, low income, and alcohol intake.

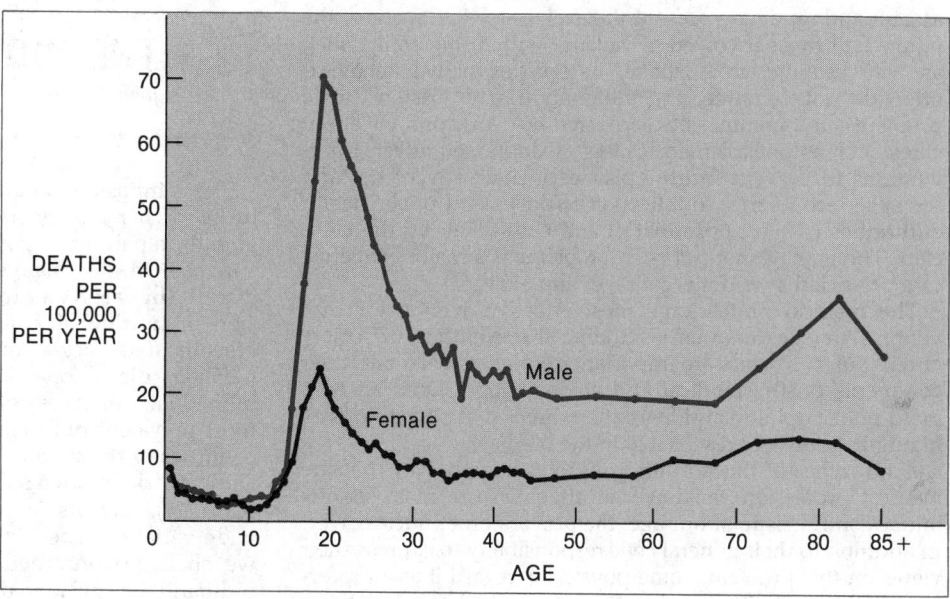

FIGURE 12–1. Age-specific death rates of motor vehicle occupants in the United States in 1976. The very high rates in 16- to 30-year-old males are a major component of the premature loss of life in this country. (From Haddon W, Baker SP: Injury control. In Clark D, MacMahon B [eds.]: Preventive and Community Medicine. Boston, Little Brown & Co, 1981, pp 109–140.)

Implications for Medical Practice

Injury prevention has assumed an important role in the practice of medicine only in the field of pediatrics. Perhaps it has not received more attention in internal medicine because the term "accident" connotes an event that has occurred by chance and is therefore unavoidable. This is far from the case; there are many lifestyle risk factors for injuries that are suitable for intervention with various behavioral techniques. (For this reason, the term "unintended injury" is now preferred over "accident," and the term "motor vehicle crash" over "motor vehicle accident.") The potential for preventing premature death and disability is substantial, and injury prevention advice could become as important in the general practice of medicine as the more familiar interventions on risk factors for cardiovascular disease and cancer.

Advice on preventing *motor vehicle injuries* begins with widely known precepts such as observing the speed limit and using a diagonal-lap or other well-designed seatbelt. From the medical viewpoint, patients should be warned when drugs that impair performance are prescribed, especially those like diazepam that may interact with alcohol. But the most important concern is alcohol itself. The knowledge that a particular patient drinks heavily should prompt a clinician to point out the danger to that individual and to others. Intervention can include counseling on ways to alter alcohol habits and on the use of other drivers, alternative forms of transportation, or different locations for drinking. The alarming motor vehicle crash rate among teenagers can be approached by counseling parents on the rules that they can establish for when and how their teenage children may drive (e.g., curfews for use of the family car). Society plays an important role in these areas—for example, in setting the penalties for drunken driving and for the minimum age for licensing—and physicians can be an important force behind social legislation of this sort.

Injuries due to *falls* in the elderly can be prevented by designing an environment that makes falls less likely (e.g., by providing handrails and night lights and by removing loose rugs) and that reduces the extent of injury should a fall occur (e.g., through avoiding sharp corners and selecting a home without stairs). The clinician should undertake regular tests and appropriate correction of problems with vision and should identify and treat diseases that impair mobility and balance, advising against heavy alcohol use and avoiding drugs that contribute to these problems. Hip fracture has

received less attention than it deserves (there are more than 200,000 each year, involving one of every three women who reach extreme old age, and half of these die or are permanently disabled). White women are at the greatest risk and should receive treatment to retard osteoporosis (Ch. 250). This may include postmenopausal estrogens for some and should always include advice about calcium intake (1000 to 1500 mg per day in the diet or as calcium carbonate supplements), about not smoking (cigarettes are a risk factor for hip fracture), and about being physically active.

Many of the other causes of unintentional injury can be controlled by discussing the role of excess alcohol and other specific risk factors with patients. *Drowning,* for example, can be made less likely by placing barriers between small children and all bodies of water and by instruction in water safety rules. Injury due to *fires* can be reduced by counseling on the dangers of smoking (cigarettes are the commonest cause of fire-related deaths) and on the value of smoke detectors and fire extinguishers.

THE EPIDEMIOLOGY OF INJURY DUE TO VIOLENCE

The homicide rate in the United States has doubled in recent years and now exceeds 20,000 per year. One third of all homicides are between family members, and another third involve people who know each other. In the United States, more than half of all homicides are carried out with handguns. Countries like England, Sweden, and Japan that have strict handgun ownership laws have handgun homicide rates that are 100-fold lower; these countries also have lower overall rates of homicide. It is difficult to estimate the rates of nonfatal injury due to violence (assault, wife beating, rape, and child abuse), but each is undoubtedly far more common than homicide. Suicide rates have increased slightly in recent years, particularly in young men. Almost all forms of violent injury are more common in the male sex and in the socioeconomically disadvantaged, and all are commonly associated with excessive alcohol intake.

Implications for Medical Practice

The medical profession's role in dealing with the death and disability that result from violent behavior begins at an individual level. One focus is on preventing the occurrence (primary prevention) or recurrence (secondary prevention) of violent episodes, and the other is on providing medical, psychiatric, and social service care for the victims. Victims of assault and rape may present themselves for treatment of the injury, but those involved in violence within the family, such as wife beating, child abuse, or self-destructive behavior, often do not volunteer the information. The existence of a problem can sometimes be discovered by gentle probing about clues such as unexplained bruises or depressed affect. Interventions to prevent future episodes include psychiatric and social service referral, notification of police and public health authorities (when appropriate), and counseling by the clinician. The management of such problems is a major challenge to a physician's wisdom, courage, and skill.

The medical profession's most effective avenue for preventing violence may be in guiding the evolution of society and its rules. Doctors are important opinion leaders, and their comments on the medical and epidemiologic facts can help mold public opinion and legislation directed at such things as handgun control and violence in the media.

Approaches of this sort are probably the only way that the medical profession can have an effect on the most serious injury control issue of our age: the prevention of nuclear war. In addition to their general civic responsibility to express their views on this problem, some physicians regard it as a professional responsibility to educate community leaders and acquaintances on medical realities such as the false security of civil defense plans that would be inoperable in the event of a nuclear attack.

SUMMARY

Injuries are the most important cause of premature death and disability in western countries. One third of all deaths from injury are due to motor vehicle crashes, one third to other unintended causes (especially falls), and one third to intentional violence. Interventions designed to prevent each of these sources of injury are a useful and neglected focus for preventive medicine.

Physicians can play a major role in counseling individual patients about lifestyle factors that prevent motor vehicle crash injuries (e.g., avoiding alcohol in excess, using seatbelts, and setting curfews for teenage drivers) and about those that prevent other forms of unintended injuries (e.g., avoiding alcohol in excess and various medical and environmental strategies to prevent falls and osteoporosis). Physicians need to take a greater role in the primary and secondary prevention of injury due to violence. In addition, medical professionals can contribute to the emergence of societal measures dealing with hazards to health that range from drunken driving to nuclear war.

Baker SP, O'Neill B, Karpf RS: The Injury Fact Book. Lexington, Mass., D. C. Heath & Company, 1984. *A fascinating and readable book that comprehensively describes the epidemiology of injury: who is especially at risk and what are the potentially modifiable risk factors.*

Cassel C, McCally M, Abraham H: Nuclear Weapons and Nuclear War: A Source Book for Health Professionals. New York, Praeger Publishers, 1984. *Reports on the medical, biologic, psychologic, and ethical implications by many of the major medical writers on this topic.*

Institute of Medicine: Injury in America. Washington, D. C., National Academy Press, 1985. *The research agenda in the area of injury prevention and control.*

Perry BC: Falls among the elderly: A review of the methods and conclusions of epidemiologic studies. J Am Geriatr Soc 30:367, 1982. *Risk factors and prevention of falls in the elderly.*

Riggs BL, Melton LJ: Involutional osteoporosis. N Engl J Med 314:1676, 1986. *Good review of strategies for preventing osteoporosis.*

Robertson LS: Injuries: Causes, Control Strategies and Public Policy. Lexington, Mass., D. C. Heath & Company, 1983. *Thoughtful discussion of injury control strategies and policy implications.*

Trunkey DD: Trauma. Sci Am 249:28, 1983. *A surgeon's perspective on the epidemiology, prevention, and treatment of injuries.*

13 THE JUDICIOUS DIET

John P. Kane

The composition of an individual's diet and its relationship to his or her energy needs and to special requirements for growth, repair, or response to stress are among the important variables in the maintenance of health or the advent of disease. In Part XV of this book, there is an extensive discussion of nutritional requirements for calories, amino acids, essential fatty acids, minerals, and vitamins. Obviously, a judicious diet is one that meets these requirements for the individual. An excess of calories leads to obesity, one of the most prevalent nutritional disorders found in the developed countries of the world. This is discussed in detail in Ch. 216. Undernutrition can also produce serious impairment of health (Ch. 214). Deficits or excesses of other nutrients lead to a wide variety of specific disorders. In this chapter, however, we shall be concerned with variables within what would ordinarily be considered an adequate diet but that may influence the susceptibility of the individual to four major classes of disease: atherosclerosis, hypertension, cancer, and urolithiasis.

In few areas relevant to health is there so much misinformation and faddism as in the prevailing public arena concerning diets. Billions of dollars are spent in this major national industry to promote an astonishing variety of nostrums and dietary aberrations alleged to maintain holistic health, vitality, and attractiveness, or to reverse the process of disease. By and large, these programs are ingenious but harmless instruments to defraud the credulous. In some cases, however, they either produce harmful dietary abnormalities or delay the patient's seeking effective medical care. Physicians need to be informed about the dimensions of this cultism in order to be able to advise their patients and to participate effectively in the development of controlling public policy.

DIET AND ARTERIOSCLEROSIS

Lipids, primarily free and esterified cholesterol, constitute a major part of atherosclerotic plaques. In current models of atherogenesis, lipids enter the artery wall via plasma lipoproteins. These lipoproteins include low density lipoproteins (LDL), intermediate density lipoproteins (IDL), and, perhaps to a lesser extent, very low density lipoproteins (VLDL). More extensive descriptions of these lipoproteins and of their metabolism are given in Ch. 183. Elevated levels of LDL and IDL are strongly associated epidemiologically with accelerated atherogenesis. For instance, the risk of coronary heart disease in the United States, where the average level of serum cholesterol in an adult male is approximately 230 mg per deciliter, is several-fold higher than in rural Japan, where the average is about 160 mg per deciliter. The atherogenicity of VLDL appears to depend in part on qualitative properties of these lipoproteins. The finding of impaired acceptance of cholesteryl esters by VLDL of hypertriglyceridemic patients with arteriosclerosis suggests that the atherogenic effect may be exerted primarily via impaired retrieval of cholesterol from peripheral sites. An inverse relationship between plasma levels of high density lipoprotein (HDL) cholesterol and risk of coronary heart disease has been noted in a number of epidemiologic surveys, suggesting that total HDL levels may reflect the efficiency of mechanisms involved in the centripetal (retrieval) pathways of cholesterol transport.

The risk of coronary heart disease has been shown to correlate with levels of cholesterol in plasma as low as 180 mg per deciliter. The majority of individuals in industrialized western nations would therefore be expected to benefit from reduction of levels of serum cholesterol, reflecting primarily changes in the content of LDL in plasma. The results of several intervention studies tend to support this contention. Increasing the levels of HDL in plasma in order to increase the mobilization and retrieval of cholesterol might be equally attractive, but no studies of the effect of such an intervention on heart disease have yet appeared.

A single pattern of dietary modification is appropriate for individuals with nearly all types of primary hyperlipidemia (excepting only primary chylomicronemia), as well as for those individuals in the population at large who have less striking elevations of levels of atherogenic lipoproteins. The elements of this "universal" diet will be considered individually.

1. *Reduce body weight to the ideal.* This manipulation primarily induces a marked reduction in elevated VLDL levels. It also effects some reduction in LDL cholesterol levels and may increase HDL cholesterol levels slightly. Maintenance of ideal body weight is the most effective means of forestalling the appearance of type II diabetes, itself a risk factor for atherosclerosis.

2. *Decrease the intake of saturated fat.* This change effects a potent and uniform lowering of LDL cholesterol. The typical American diet contains approximately 40 per cent or more of calories as fat (15 per cent saturated fat). Levels of 30 per cent of calories as fat (8 per cent saturated fat) can be achieved easily, and 20 per cent (5 per cent saturated) is attainable with major modifications of food selection. To achieve the 30 per cent level of dietary fat, fat-rich meats, dairy products, and items such as certain baked goods must be restricted. To achieve the 20 per cent level, major substitution of vegetable protein sources for meats must be made.

When the intake of saturated fats is decreased, there are several possible sources of replacement calories: polyunsaturated fats, monounsaturated fats, or carbohydrates. Major substitution with polyunsaturated fat may result in lower levels of HDL cholesterol and of the principal HDL protein, apolipoprotein A-I. Furthermore, polyunsaturated fatty acids are susceptible to hydroperoxidation, which could lead to generation of free radical chains and perhaps to carcinogenesis. Monounsaturated fats, abundant in certain vegetable oils such as olive oil, do not increase LDL levels and do not hydroperoxidize readily. HDL cholesterol levels are somewhat higher with use of monounsaturates than with diets that are low in total fat. Major substitution of carbohydrate for fat is associated with modest elevations of plasma triglyceride levels in the short term, but these levels return to normal after a period of several months. Strict vegetarians tend to have lower levels of both LDL and HDL than individuals on a typical American diet, but the changes in LDL levels are of much greater magnitude. Furthermore, potentially important differences in composition of HDL are seen, with an increased ratio of phospholipid to cholesterol.

Recently, attention has been drawn to certain features of omega-3 fatty acids, principally eicosapentaenoic and docosahexaenoic acids, contained in marine fish oils. These fatty acids appear to have a unique ability to reduce elevated levels of VLDL and chylomicrons in plasma at doses of 15 to 20 grams per day. Plasma levels of LDL may be decreased modestly in individuals with normal or moderately elevated levels of plasma cholesterol, accompanied by some decrease in HDL cholesterol levels. The marked decreases in plasma triglycerides that occur are due at least in part to inhibition of VLDL secretion. Omega-3 fatty acids moderately reduce formation of thromboxane B_2 in platelets, inhibiting their aggregation and adhesion, an effect that may account in part for the low incidence of arteriosclerotic heart disease in populations for whom temperate and subarctic marine fish are a major food source.

Overall, a major reduction of saturated fat should be made from levels found in Western diets, and carbohydrate should be used in large part to provide the requisite caloric replacement. Small amounts of polyunsaturated fats from plant sources should be used to provide essential fatty acids. The use of fish oils might be considered if hypertriglyceridemia is present.

3. *Decrease the intake of cholesterol.* Reduction of dietary saturated fats automatically eliminates much cholesterol; however, rich sources such as organ meats and egg yolks should be restricted specifically. The effect of restriction of cholesterol on LDL levels varies widely among individuals. This variation appears to reflect two factors: (a) There is an approximately four-fold difference among individuals in the fraction of dietary cholesterol that is absorbed. (b) There are differences in the degree to which dietary cholesterol is capable of suppressing endogenous cholesterogenesis. Lacking metabolic ward studies on a given patient, it must be presumed that reduction of dietary cholesterol is likely to be of benefit. The typical American diet provides 500 mg or more of cholesterol per day, but an intake of 250 to 300 mg per day is relatively easily achieved, and intakes of 100 mg per day can be achieved with more rigorous mixed diets. Strict vegetarian diets contain no cholesterol.

4. *Restrict alcohol.* Alcohol should be limited in all cases to maintain ideal body weight. VLDL secretion is increased dramatically by even limited use of alcohol. Therefore, alcohol should always be restricted in the diet of individuals with elevated serum triglycerides. Increased alcohol intake may be associated with elevated levels of HDL cholesterol, but it is not yet clear whether this change represents subspecies of HDL that participate in centripetal cholesterol transport. No categorical presumption of beneficial effects of alcohol on HDL can yet be made.

5. *Other factors.* Increased dietary fiber appears to have marginal effect on serum lipoprotein levels, though certain sources of fiber, such as oat or wheat bran, appear to reduce LDL levels slightly. In addition, saponins in foodstuffs such as oats may decrease absorption of cholesterol. The ingestion of lecithin, which is widely suggested by health food advocates, also lacks significant effect, as do a number of vitamins and minerals that have been similarly recommended.

Individuals following this judicious dietary regimen usually show reductions of 10 to 15 per cent of plasma cholesterol levels on the basis of reduction of saturated fats. An additional reduction of up to 10 per cent may be achieved by restriction of cholesterol. Based on large epidemiologic studies, it can be roughly estimated that at least a twofold reduction in risk of coronary disease would be expected in the American population if such modifications of lipid levels were uniformly achieved.

DIET AND HYPERTENSION

Essential hypertension has been assumed to result from a constitutional inability to excrete sodium chloride efficiently, because of which calcium ions accumulate in arteriolar smooth muscle cells, increasing their tonicity. Indeed, evidence from cross-transplantation studies in animals and from human renal transplants lends credence to the existence of such a mechanism. Cross-cultural studies also have shown, in the aggregate, convincing positive correlation between blood pressure and intake of salt. More recently, patient populations with essential hypertension have been found to be heterogeneous with respect to renin levels, plasma calcium concentrations, response to individual antihypertensive drugs, and sensitivity to dietary salt. Normotensive individuals and perhaps half of American patients with hypertension do not show a pressor response to increased dietary salt. Thus, justification for the prescription of reduced salt intake appears to be limited to individuals with salt-sensitive hypertension and members of their kindreds. Most Americans consume 10 to 20 grams of salt per day; an intake of 4 grams is a more reasonable goal for individuals in such kindreds. It has been reported, without convincing evidence, that increasing calcium intake can reduce blood pressure. If true, this effect would probably be restricted to a subset of patients. Furthermore, indiscriminate increase in calcium intake could result in augmentation of urinary calcium excretion in individuals with absorptive hypercalciuria (Ch. 90). Thus, no basis yet exists for the general recommendation of increased calcium intake for the prevention of hypertension.

DIET AND CANCER

The consumption of certain major food components is epidemiologically correlated with an increased incidence of some types of cancer. Although the mechanisms of these associations are still largely unknown, a judicious diet at this time involves changes that would be expected to minimize these risks. A number of components that occur in foods naturally or are formed or added during processing are recognized as mutagens in bacterial test systems (Ames test) or as carcinogens or promoters of carcinogenesis in tests in whole animals. Prudence would dictate elimination of these compounds from human consumption to whatever extent is practicable, because definitive studies demonstrating specific risks of these agents in humans may emerge only slowly.

DIETARY FAT. An increased incidence of cancer of the breast, colon, and prostate is epidemiologically related to a high consumption of total fat. Enhancement of chemical carcinogenesis by dietary fat has also been demonstrated in several animal models. Total fat intake correlates best with carcinogenesis at high levels, but polyunsaturated fats appear to be most important at lower levels of intake. Polyunsaturated fats are substrates for hydroperoxidative reactions initiating free radical chains, and therefore they probably should not constitute a major component of the diet. Reduction of total fat intake, with an increased content of complex carbohydrates, is completely compatible with the "prudent" diet for prevention of arteriosclerotic heart disease. In fact, in multination comparisons coronary heart disease and cancer of the breast show a strong correlation.

FIBER. Carcinogens formed in the bowel may play a major role in development of carcinoma of the colon. It has been suggested that increased fiber in the diet, which would decrease the duration of contact of carcinogens with the mucosa, might reduce the risk of cancer. Only minimal epidemiologic support for this view has been forthcoming, and with the possible exception of pentosans from wheat, fiber has not been proven effective in animal models.

ALCOHOL. Alcohol consumption has been found to correlate with risk of carcinoma of the mouth, pharynx, and esophagus. It also appears to be teratogenic in humans and causes congenital malformations, mental dysfunction, and growth retardation in infants born to alcohol-abusing mothers. Alcohol metabolism produces acetaldehyde, which is both mutagenic and carcinogenic, in addition to other mutagenic and carcinogenic compounds.

RELATIONSHIP OF CANCER RISK TO LOW LEVELS OF CHOLESTEROL IN PLASMA. An increased risk of cancer has been associated epidemiologically with very low levels of serum cholesterol. Such an association when present is always weak and tends to be present only in the lowest range of cholesterol levels. Further, in nearly 20 prospective population studies, half have shown no such correlation, especially in those in which sufficient time elapsed between measurement of serum lipids and detection of cancer to minimize the number of pre-existing cancer cases. Furthermore, the risk of colon and rectal cancer is positively correlated with serum cholesterol levels. The correlation of higher levels of cholesterol in plasma with risk of coronary disease is very strong. Thus it appears that dietary modifications directed at lowering the risk of coronary disease should not be abandoned on the premise that a significant increase in the risk of cancer would ensue.

FOOD PREPARATION AND PRESERVATION. Exposure of meats to high temperatures, as in charcoal broiling, may be of importance in oncogenesis because of the formation of compounds with very high carcinogenic potential. In addition to benzo(a)pyrene, several mutagenic pyrolysates formed from amino acids are recognized. Considerable evidence both from epidemiology and from animal studies has linked components of wood smoke in smoked foods to carcinoma of the gastrointestinal tract. Nitrites, used as preservatives in meats, react with a number of natural amines and even certain medications to form nitrosamines, which are mutagenic. This reaction is favored by low pH; hence it proceeds readily in the stomach. Mutagenesis by nitrosamines is readily demonstrated, and clinical observations tend to link nitrites with carcinogenesis of the stomach and esophagus, at least. Vitamin C inhibits the formation of nitrosamines in vitro. Increased intake of this vitamin by the public may account in part for decreases in the incidence of gastric carcinoma observed in recent years. At the present state of our knowledge, restriction of nitrites and nitrosamines in the diet would appear reasonable. This is complicated by the presence of large amounts of nitrates, which can be reduced to nitrites, in certain vegetables that have been overfertilized by growers. The average American ingests about 75 mg of nitrate, 0.8 mg nitrite, and 1 μg of preformed nitrosamines daily.

NATURALLY OCCURRING CARCINOGENS AND MUTAGENS. Several species of *Aspergillus* molds produce aflatoxins, which are among the most potent natural carcinogens. These agents are carcinogenic in a number of animals, chiefly causing carcinoma of the liver. Induction of tumors of colon, lung, and kidney has also been observed. Aflatoxins have been linked strongly to hepatocellular carcinoma in humans in Africa and Asia, probably acting in concert with hepatitis B virus. Aflatoxins have been found chiefly in peanuts, apple products, and grains stored under moist conditions. Efforts to reduce the intake of these agents center on proper storage of foods. Emerging awareness of other naturally occurring mutagens and carcinogens may be expected to lead to an evaluation of their importance in human carcinogenesis. Among these agents are allyl isothiocyanate and the flavonoids quercetin and kaempferol found in many plant sources; hydrazine derivatives found in many mushrooms; safrol of sassafras; the methyl xanthines of coffee, tea, and cocoa; and phorbol esters and pyrrolizidine alkaloids found in herbal teas.

NATURAL INHIBITORS OF CARCINOGENESIS. Some naturally occurring compounds appear to inhibit carcinogenesis by certain agents. Tocopherols, which interrupt free radical chains, are capable of reducing the carcinogenicity of doxorubicin (Adriamycin) and daunomycin and are protective against oxygen radical damage to tissues. Certain indoles found in cruciferous vegetables (broccoli, cabbage, cauliflower, etc.) inhibit the carcinogenicity of benzo(a)pyrene, and substituted isothiocyanates found in these plants inhibit the carcinogenesis induced by polycyclic aromatic hydrocarbons. Higher intakes of retinol and beta-carotene have been correlated with reduced risk of cancer in several studies. This effect should be considered unproven, however, until further evidence is brought forth. Selenium, a cofactor in the reduction of hydroperoxides, also may confer resistance to free radical–mediated carcinogenesis.

DIET AND UROLITHIASIS

Certain general measures that should reduce the risk of urolithiasis are applicable to the general population (also see Ch. 90). Sufficient intake of water to ensure a daily urine volume of 2 to 3 liters is a most important preventive measure and is useful in all forms of urolithiasis. Restriction of dietary purine intake is also desirable because uricosuria can enhance the crystallization of calcium oxalate as well as uric acid stones. Restriction of the intake of red meats, recommended for reduction of saturated fat intake, also tends to reduce the "acid ash" residue of urine, diminishing the urinary excretion of calcium.

Moderate restriction of oxalate intake would appear reasonable in the general population in view of the prevalence of oxalate stones. More stringently reduced intake should be advised for individuals who have had one or more oxalate stones, because the incidence of recurrence tends to be high. The oxalate content is particularly high in rhubarb, spinach, chard, beets, citrus pulp, pecans, peanuts, sweet potatoes, and a number of berries and fruits. Reliable new methods for the determination of oxalate in foods have now led to the availability of lists of oxalate-rich foods for use by the patient. Because calcium in the intestine inhibits the absorption of oxalate, moderate intake of calcium, distributed throughout the day, is probably indicated in the prevention of oxalate urolithiasis. Citrate appears to inhibit the crystallization of calcium with oxalate. Some patients with calcium oxalate urolithiasis have low levels of citrate in urine. Regular intake of citrate-rich, pulp-free fruit juices appears to be a reasonable intervention. In general, restriction of dietary calcium should be limited to patients with hypercalciuria.

SUMMARY

Epidemiologic and experimental data are sufficient to support the following recommendations for dietary modifications among the general populace. Caloric intake should be adjusted to achieve and maintain ideal body weight. Fat intake should be reduced to 30 per cent of total calories (8 per cent as saturated fat) or less, and cholesterol intake to 150 mg, or less, per day. Even moderate use of alcohol should be avoided in individuals with hypertriglyceridemia. Complex carbohydrates should be used to make up the caloric deficits resulting from these changes. Individuals with a predisposition to hypertension should limit salt intake to 4 grams per day. Prudence would also suggest reasonable limitation of charcoal-broiled and smoked foods and foods rich in nitrites or nitrates.

Ames BN: Dietary carcinogens and anticarcinogens: Oxygen radicals and degenerative diseases. Science 221:1256, 1983. *A comprehensive review of mutagens and carcinogens in the diet.*

Ames BN: Food constituents as a source of mutagens, carcinogens, and anticarcinogens. In Knudsen I (ed.): Genetic Toxicology of the Diet. New York, Alan R. Liss, Inc, 1986, pp 3–32. *A discussion of mechanisms by which food constituents can promote or retard the formation of tumors.*

Committee on Diet, Nutrition, and Cancer. Assembly of Life Sciences, National Research Council: Diet, Nutrition and Cancer. National Academic Press, 1982. *A comprehensive evaluation of the roles of dietary components and additives in carcinogenesis.*

Connor WE, Connor SL: The dietary prevention and treatment of coronary heart disease. In Connor WE, Bristow JD (eds.): Coronary Heart Disease: Prevention, Complications, and Treatment. Philadelphia, J. B. Lippincott, 1985, pp 43–64. *A review of principles and practical measures in modification of plasma lipoprotein levels by diet.*

Havel RJ: Dietary regulation of plasma lipoprotein metabolism in humans. Prog Biochem Pharmacol 19:110, 1983. *A discussion of mechanisms underlying dietary effects on lipoproteins.*

MacGregor GA: Sodium is more important than calcium in essential hypertension. Hypertension 7:628, 1985. *A discussion putting forth arguments for the role of salt in hypertension.*

Menkes MS, Comstock GW, Vuilleumier JP, et al.: Serum beta-carotene, vitamins A and E, selenium, and the risk of lung cancer. N Engl J Med 315:1250, 1986. *Epidemiologic evidence relating beta-carotene and vitamin E to a reduced risk of lung cancer.*

Törnberg SA, Holm L-E, Carstensen JM, et al.: Risks of cancer of the colon and rectum in relation to serum cholesterol and beta-lipoprotein. N Engl J Med 315:1629, 1986. *A clinical study demonstrating a positive correlation of serum cholesterol level and risk of cancer in the lower bowel and rectum.*

Willett WC, Stampfer MJ, Colditz GA, et al.: Dietary fat and the risk of breast cancer. N Engl J Med 316:22, 1987. *An important study that confirms high dietary fat as a risk factor, with a useful bibliography of 37 references.*

14 EXERCISE AND HEALTH
William L. Haskell

The biologic and psychologic benefits ascribed to exercise are extremely diverse and vary substantially with regard to scientific documentation of a causal relationship. Some of these benefits have been definitively established and are achievable by anyone who exercises appropriately. Other benefits, frequently promoted by exercise advocates, usually do not occur, and at times inappropriate advice has been given that has placed patients at undue risk for exercise-caused morbidity or mortality. As with many other areas of health promotion, enthusiasm to help others by encouraging them to exercise can easily outstrip the scientific basis for such actions. While the idea that exercise might promote health is not new, many of the details regarding specific health benefits and exercise requirements are still much debated and under investigation.

EXERCISE AND PHYSICAL WORKING CAPACITY

The most effective method of achieving an increase in physical working capacity or "physical fitness" is through a systematic increase in habitual exercise (exercise training). This increase in capacity is an adaptive response by the body to the stress placed on various tissues and biologic functions by the increased metabolic or physical demands of the exercise. If the appropriate type of exercise is performed at the proper intensity, duration, and frequency, sedentary individuals of all ages will achieve significant improvements in physical working capacity. After training, they will be able to exercise at a greater intensity and for a longer duration than before. Also, at the same submaximal exercise intensity they will experience less fatigue. This increase in functional capacity is due to enhanced metabolic capacity of skeletal muscle, increased capacity for substrate and oxygen delivery to the muscle, and changes in autonomic nervous system regulation during exercise.

Increases in physical working capacity often are equated inappropriately with improvements in health status or disease prevention. This is an important and often difficult distinction to make: that while a very high level of physical fitness usually requires good health, an improvement in fitness does not ensure an increase in resistance to disease or a reduction in clinical manifestations. For example, patients with disorders such as emphysema, diabetes, or hypertension can significantly increase their working capacity through exercise without necessarily changing the severity of their disease or their medical prognosis. Becoming more physically fit and improving health status are interrelated but not synonymous.

HEALTH BENEFITS OF EXERCISE

Most of the health-related benefits of exercise appear to result from the increase in metabolism required to provide the energy needed for skeletal muscle contraction. This increase in demand for energy triggers a number of adaptations designed to enhance the efficiency and capacity of the skeletal muscle to perform work and minimize fatigue. Adaptations also occur in those systems that support the increased energy requirements of skeletal muscle, including the nervous, endocrine, cardiovascular, respiratory, and skeletal systems.

CORONARY HEART DISEASE. The area of greatest scientific inquiry regarding the health benefits of exercise has been its potential role in the prevention of coronary heart disease (CHD). In 1952 J. H. Morris and colleagues published data demonstrating that the conductors on double-decker buses in London developed fewer manifestations of CHD than did the less active bus drivers. Since then it has been repeatedly, but not exclusively, demonstrated that men and women who select more active jobs or leisure-time pursuits tend to experience fewer fatal and nonfatal CHD events. While these studies do not demonstrate a cause and effect relationship, the direction of the association is positive and quite consistent, the magnitude of the differences in CHD events is clinically meaningful, and the amount of exercise performed during leisure time associated with lower CHD risk is well within the capacity of most clinically healthy adults. As of yet no randomized trial of adequate design has been performed to determine if an increase in exercise by sedentary adults free of clinically evident CHD on entry into the study would significantly reduce future CHD events.

The six controlled clinical trials so far conducted to evaluate the effects of exercise training on recurrent cardiac events in patients following myocardial infarction have yielded statistically negative results. In three of these six studies, the exercise group tended to have fewer events ($0.05 < p < 0.10$), and in all of the studies the adherence to exercise training was sufficiently poor to raise questions regarding their adequacy as a test of the exercise hypothesis. Thus, no definitive evidence exists to substantiate that an *increase in exercise* will reduce either the primary or the secondary occurrence of CHD clinical events.

There are several mechanisms by which exercise could act to reduce CHD risk. Exercise might maintain or increase oxygen supply to the myocardium by decreasing the progression of atherosclerosis, increasing coronary collateralization, or enlarging the diameter of proximal coronary arteries. Only preliminary evidence has been published documenting that any of these changes occur in humans. Several studies have demonstrated potentially beneficial blood clotting-fibrinolysis activity and altered plasma lipoprotein profiles following training. These changes might improve the coronary blood flow in some individuals.

In contrast to very little evidence for any exercise-induced increase in myocardial oxygen supply, there is unequivocal evidence that endurance exercise training decreases myocardial oxygen demand. This decrease in demand is achieved primarily by a decrease in heart rate at rest and decreases in heart rate and systolic blood pressure during submaximal exercise. These changes are most likely produced by a modification in central nervous system regulation of cardiovascular function (decreased sympathetic and increased parasympathetic drive) and an increase in blood volume, with little, if any, change occurring in intrinsic myocardial function.

CARBOHYDRATE METABOLISM. A potentially important and often unrecognized health benefit of exercise is its effect on carbohydrate metabolism. During large-muscle, dynamic exercise of moderate intensity, the glycogen stored in skeletal muscle is used for the production of energy and becomes partially depleted. For the next 24 to 72 hours this glycogen is replaced by the uptake of glucose from the blood. In addition to this acute effect of increased glucose removal, there also is a more chronic training effect that increases the sensitivity of insulin receptors in skeletal muscle and adipose tissue and thus the rate of glucose removal at any given level of plasma insulin. This "insulin-sparing" effect of endurance exercise training probably decreases long-term insulin production and may reduce the risk of insulin deficiency developing with increasing age.

OSTEOPOROSIS. The bone mineral loss that occurs with aging is accelerated by inactivity, especially bed rest. While exercise will not prevent all of this loss, it appears to provide some benefit. For example, in a survey of 59 postmenopausal women, level of habitual activity was one of the major determinants of bone mass as measured by computerized tomography scanning. In the more active women, arm and leg bone mass was greater after accounting for the effects of age, body weight, and calcium intake. Also, when 18 elderly women exercised 3 times per week for 30 minutes each session, an increase in bone mineral content was observed (2.3 per cent), while 12 women who remained sedentary during this time showed a decrease of 3.3 per cent ($p < 0.005$). These experiences support the use of exercise requiring the movement of body weight against gravity as part of a comprehensive program of osteoporosis prevention.

WEIGHT CONTROL. More physically active individuals tend to weigh less than their sedentary counterparts and at any given body weight have a greater muscle mass. Even though calorie consumption frequently goes up when sedentary people substantially increase their exercise, they usually experience some adipose tissue loss. In addition to the increase in calories expended during the exercise, there is some evidence that *resting metabolic rate* is increased for an extended period after exercise. *Basal metabolic rate* at any given body weight may also increase. For these reasons, exercise, along with proper nutrition, can improve health status by contributing to the maintenance of optimal body composition.

PSYCHOLOGIC STATUS. Many physically active people state that the major health benefit that keeps them exercising is their improved psychologic status. They report less anxiety and depression, more self-confidence, and an increased ability to cope with at-home and job-related stress. How frequently such benefits will occur when sedentary people take up exercise is not known, nor is there any understanding of how to design an exercise program to maximize the positive psychologic effects. Whether or not a biologic basis, rather than just a "situational basis," exists for improvements in psychologic status has not been established. Proposed explanations for a biologic basis are the decrease in circulating catecholamines produced by exercise training and the acute increase in beta-endorphins that occurs during and following vigorous exercise. Regardless of the mechanism, consideration should be given to getting sedentary people up and away from chronic stress-producing environments and having them participate in an exercise of their choice.

OTHER DISORDERS. There are a number of other situations in which patients with an established disease tend to show some clinical improvement if they exercise properly, but there is no good evidence that exercise prevents these disorders. Diseases included in this category are chronic obstructive lung disease (emphysema and bronchitis), mild or labile hypertension, and intermittent claudication. There are no data supporting the notion that exercise prevents any infectious disease. More active people have a greater morbidity and mortality from accidents than would be the case if they remained sedentary!

A Comment on Safety

When recommending exercise for health promotion, one does battle with the proverbial two-edged sword. Inappropriate exercise literally can pose dangers to limbs and life. The most commonly encountered problem is that of musculoskeletal discomfort or injury due to trauma or overuse. Of more severe consequence, but much less frequent, is the precipitation of a major cardiac event, usually ventricular fibrillation. However, the likelihood is remote that exercise will cause a cardiac arrest in individuals without underlying cardiac disease.

There are many other health risks of exercise, but these usually are limited to individuals with established disease (e.g., diabetes, asthma, or renal failure) or occur with very extended or competitive exercise. The most important of these risks is the development of severe heat injury (Ch. 541). The total prevention of these injuries cannot be achieved if adults are to increase their exercise, but the risks can be reduced by proper medical evaluation, individualized exercise recommendations, and improved public education.

MEDICAL EVALUATION

Guidelines vary regarding the type of medical evaluation recommended prior to initiating a health-oriented exercise program. Advice depends on the specific exercise plan to be undertaken, as well as the person's age and clinical status. For sedentary people who plan to undertake a low-level program such as walking, no special medical examination is recommended unless they currently are under treatment for cardiopulmonary, metabolic, or musculoskeletal disorders. Such patients should be evaluated by a physician prior to an increase in exercise. For persons under age 40 who are free of clinically evident cardiopulmonary, metabolic, or musculoskeletal disorders, no special medical evaluation is considered necessary if they also are free of major cardiopulmonary disease risk factors (hypertension, hypercholesterolemia, or cigarette smoking). For persons under age 40 with disease or increased cardiopulmonary risk, and for all people over age 40, it is recommended that they have a medical examination prior to beginning vigorous exercise. Although recommended, but not required, for clinically healthy persons, an electrocardiographic and blood pressure–monitored exercise tolerance test should be included in the medical evaluation of patients with cardiopulmonary, metabolic, or musculoskeletal disorders. Such tests should be symptom limited and monitored by a physician.

IMPLICATIONS FOR MEDICAL PRACTICE

The *type* of exercise that provides the greatest health benefits and permits the greatest increase in energy expenditure with the least fatigue consists of performing rhythmic contractions of large muscles to move the body over a distance or against gravity. Such exercise frequently is referred to as being endurance or "aerobic," since, if it is performed at an intensity that is moderate relative to the person's capacity, most of the resynthesis of high-energy compounds in the muscle is performed in the presence of oxygen. Included in this type of exercise is walking, hiking, jogging or running, cycling, cross-country skiing, swimming, active games and sports, selected calisthenics, and vigorous at-home or on-the-job chores. While very specific activities may be required when training for athletic competition, for health purposes any exercise of this type seems to be of benefit if performed frequently enough at the proper intensity (Table 14–1).

The exercise-induced changes that contribute to health are achieved when the exercise *intensity* is somewhat greater than that usually performed by the individual. This increase intensity or overload causes adaptations that allow the metabolic needs of the muscles during exercise to be more readily met. While exercise intensities that are even slightly greater than that usually performed will produce changes, the usual recommendation is that exercise for optimizing health should be performed at 50 to 75 per cent of the individual's oxygen transport (aerobic) capacity or at 60 to 85 per cent of maximum achievable heart rate during exercise. Using these guidelines, exercise training heart rates for individuals 30 years of age would range from 114 to 162 beats per minute, whereas at age 60 the range would be from 86 to 137 beats per minute. For most people this recommendation produces a substantial intensity overload, since they usually do not exercise at more than about 40 per cent of their aerobic capacity during everyday activities.

The exercise *duration* to be recommended will depend on the person's health or fitness goals and exercise capacity as well as on the type of exercise being performed. One interpretation of the data available on exercise and health is that

TABLE 14–1. THE EXERCISE PRESCRIPTION

Type of Exercise
  Primarily aerobic
  Stretching for flexibility
  Resistance exercise for muscle tone

Intensity
  Moderate relative to capacity (50%–75%)
  Target heart rate = 60%–85% MHR
  Maximum heart rate (MHR) = 220 − age

Duration
  25–45 minutes per session
  Target of 300 kilocalories per session

Frequency
  Daily if intensity <65% MHR and duration <30 minutes
  Every other day if intensity >65% and duration >30 minutes

Session
  Warmup, 3 to 5 minutes
  Conditioning, 15 to 40 minutes
  Cool-down, 2 to 5 minutes

Progression
  Use exercise log
  Keep pulse in target range
  Evaluate every 2–4 weeks or each visit

Warning Signs
  Severe musculoskeletal pain
  Claudication
  Chest pressure/pain, discomfort
  Unusual shortness of breath
  Dizziness, nausea, vomiting

people who do even a little bit of exercise on a regular basis are better off than those who do almost nothing. A reasonable goal seems to be an energy expenditure over usual activities of approximately 300 kilocalories per session with a *frequency* of at least every other day. Most clinically healthy adults have the capacity to expend from 400 to 700 kilocalories per hour while performing activity of moderate intensity; thus they can expend 300 kilocalories in 25 to 45 minutes. Activities meeting this goal include walking or jogging 4 kilometers, cycling or swimming for 30 minutes, or playing several sets of singles tennis lasting for 45 minutes. While lower intensity exercise such as walking or gardening will not produce a large increase in exercise capacity, if performed for longer periods or more frequently, it seems to provide many of the health benefits derived from more vigorous exercise (e.g., facilitates weight control, bone mineral retention, etc.).

SUMMARY

Inactivity does not appear to be the sole cause of any major disease, but a physically active lifestyle improves general health status and retards many of the functional impairments that frequently occur with aging. Success in initiating and maintaining an exercise program is most likely to occur when it is individually designed and takes into account the person's goals, interests, skills, and exercise opportunities, as well as exercise capacity. Instructions should be given to set aside a time for exercise and to fill it with a variety of activities, rather than selecting a single activity as the sole basis for increasing exercise for health purposes. The exercise plan should be convenient to perform, fit within the general lifestyle of the individual, and be considered fun or at least enjoyable. Success at exercise is increased when the individual has acquired the *knowledge* of what is to be done and why, the *confidence* that success can be achieved, and the *patience* to wait for the benefits to accrue.

American College of Sports Medicine: Guidelines for Graded Exercise Testing and Exercise Prescription. 3rd ed. Philadelphia, Lea & Febiger, 1986. *Comprehensive guidelines for the exercise testing and training of healthy persons and patients.*

Paffenbarger RS, Hyde RT, Weng AL, et al: Physical activity, all-cause mortality, and longevity of college alumni. N Engl J Med 314:605, 1986. *Report of major study supporting the relationship between sedentary habits and increased mortality from chronic diseases, especially ischemic heart disease.*

Siscovick DS, Weiss NS, Fletcher RH, et al: The incidence of primary cardiac arrest during vigorous exercise. N Engl J Med 311:874, 1984. *Important conceptual study presenting data on both cardiovascular risk and benefits of vigorous exercise in the general population.*

Vranic M, Lavina H, Lickley A, et al: Exercise and stress in diabetes mellitus. In Davidson JK (ed.): Clinical Diabetes Mellitus: A Problem Oriented Approach. New York, Thieme, 1986, pp 172–205. *Review of exercise effects on glucose metabolism and insulin production and uptake in response to exercise by healthy persons and diabetic patients.*

15 ALCOHOL ABUSE AND ALCOHOL-RELATED ILLNESSES

Benjamin Kissin

About 90 million Americans drink alcoholic beverages in one form or another, some occasionally, some moderately but regularly ("social drinkers"), and some heavily ("heavy drinkers"). About 10 million Americans drink enough to cause difficulties in their personal and/or social adjustment ("problem drinkers"). Of these, about 6 million drink sufficiently, over a long time period, to produce the stigmata of alcohol dependence ("alcoholism").

The medical syndromes associated with alcohol abuse fall generally under four major categories: (1) acute alcohol intoxication, (2) alcohol dependence or "alcoholism," (3) acute alcohol withdrawal syndromes, and (4) medical complications. Alcohol abuse, like the abuse of any other psychoactive drug, is the consequence of the action of a specific pharmacologic agent in a specific individual. The specific clinical syndromes of alcohol abuse derive directly from the pharmacologic effects of ethyl alcohol (ethanol) on body tissues and secondarily from the adaptive responses of the body to excessive exposure to alcohol (tolerance and physical dependence). Alcohol-related illnesses are mainly nutritional in origin and are discussed principally, along with specific organ systems as well, in Chapters 217 and 467.

PHARMACOLOGY OF ETHANOL

ABSORPTION AND METABOLISM. Ethanol is usually ingested in a concentration of 5 per cent (beer), 12 per cent (wine), 20 per cent (reinforced wines), or 43 per cent (86 proof whiskey). The distinctive flavor of different alcoholic beverages is a function of the contained congeners (e.g., higher alcohols, aldehydes), as may also be some complications of heavy drinking (e.g., hangovers). However, the major effects of drinking are due to the content of ethanol itself. Ethanol is rapidly absorbed from the stomach and intestines into the bloodstream, thus accounting for its quick pharmacologic action. It is also rapidly metabolized so that a moderate dose will usually clear from the blood in about one hour. Its absorption and metabolic breakdown make ethanol a fast-acting but short-lasting drug.

Ethanol diffuses rapidly into all aqueous compartments of the body (extracellular and intracellular), so that the blood concentrations of ethanol directly reflect concentrations of the chemical throughout the body. About 10 per cent of the ethanol in the body is directly eliminated by diffusion through the kidneys or lungs, and concentrations in alveolar air and urine can be utilized to estimate blood concentrations. The rest is metabolized in the liver. The rate-limiting element in this sequence is hepatic alcohol dehydrogenase, which, in a 70-kg man, can metabolize about 9.0 grams of ethanol (about three fourths of an ounce of whiskey) per hour. This results in a decrease in the blood level of approximately 15 mg per deciliter per hour. Ingestion of ethanol at a greater rate produces cumulatively rising blood levels.

The conversion of nicotinamide-adenine dinucleotide (NAD) to NADH during the oxidation of ethanol shifts the redox equilibrium and causes metabolic disturbances such as hyperlipidemia and hyperuricemia. Since alcohol dehydrogenase is located almost entirely in the liver, neutral fat deposition (fatty degeneration) occurs in the liver of about 90 per cent of alcoholics.

Alcohol dehydrogenase occurs in various isoenzyme forms, which metabolize ethanol at different rates. Orientals and American Indians tend to have increased hepatic levels of an atypical isoenzyme that metabolizes alcohol unusually rapidly and produces high levels of acetaldehyde. This is thought to produce the characteristic "Oriental flush," a reaction that occurs in about 80 per cent of genetically Mongoloid individuals.

NEUROPHARMACOLOGY. Ethanol is a powerful depressant of the central nervous system with pharmacologic effects similar to those of ether and chloroform. Ethanol is miscible with fats and rapidly enters cell membranes. It is thought that the neuropharmacologic action of ethanol is exercised through neuronal cell membrane effects (1) upon the activation of calcium ion (Ca^{++}), (2) upon the action of the $Na^+ K^+$ ATPase pump, or (3) more directly, through the production of increased fluidity.

Because parts of the brain respond differently to ethanol, its behavioral effects may differ from its neuropharmacologic ones; e.g., the depressant effects of ethanol upon inhibitory control centers may release excitatory behavior. Alcohol tends to depress the brain from above downward, first affecting the cortex, then the limbic system and cerebellum, next the reticular formation, and finally the lower brain stem.

In low doses, alcohol acts both as a stimulant (disinhibitor) and as a relaxant; it is widely used for these effects. The drug is also a euphoriant; perhaps the majority of alcoholics drink mainly for this effect. In larger doses, alcohol is a rapidly acting and potent anxiolytic-analgesic and is frequently taken by agitated individuals to obtain relief.

ACUTE ALCOHOL INTOXICATION

Acute alcohol intoxication occurs infrequently in social drinkers, more frequently in heavy drinkers, and most frequently in problem drinkers and alcoholics. The pattern of aberrant responsiveness is a function of the blood alcohol level (BAL) and of pre-existing tolerance. Alcoholics have a high level of behavioral and physiologic tolerance to ethanol so that they may require blood alcohol levels almost 100 mg per deciliter higher than social drinkers to show comparable impairment. Some alcoholics function adequately with a BAL of 250 mg per deciliter, a concentration at which social drinkers become stuporous (Table 15–1).

Acute alcohol intoxication occurs in two stages. In nontolerant individuals, a BAL of about 100 to 200 mg per deciliter will result in disinhibition and hyperexcitability; with a BAL of above 250 mg per deciliter, stupor and coma usually ensue. Although these two syndromes are part of a continuum, there

TABLE 15–1. BLOOD ALCOHOL LEVELS AND SYMPTOMS

Level (mg/dl)	Sporadic Drinkers	Chronic Drinkers
50 (party level)	Congenial euphoria	No observable effect
75	Gregarious or garrulous	Often no effect
100	Incoordinated	Minimal signs
	Legally intoxicated	
125–150	Unrestrained behavior	Pleasurable euphoria or
	Episodic dyscontrol	beginning incoordination
200–250	Alertness lost → lethargic	Effort required to maintain emotional and motor control
300–350	Stupor to coma	Drowsy and slow
>500	Some will die	Coma

is a sufficient change in symptoms at about the level of 200 to 250 mg per deciliter (depending on individual tolerance) to warrant their separate description.

EXCITATORY STAGE. The social use of alcoholic beverages usually produces a BAL of about 50 mg per deciliter, with a sense of relaxation and of well-being. At levels of 75 mg per deciliter, most individuals tend to feel more relaxed and sociable; a few become garrulous or hostile. At about 100 mg per deciliter, signs of ataxia begin. Coordination and judgment may be impaired at the same time that self-assurance increases. At this level, driving may be hazardous; most state laws define "driving while intoxicated" at a BAL of 100 mg per deciliter or higher.

At BAL's of about 125 to 150 mg per deciliter, behavioral changes occur that usually reflect the underlying personality. Some individuals continue to become more congenial, sociable, and disinhibited; some become hostile and aggressive; and some turn inward and become silent and depressed. Increasing BAL's usually continue to be associated with increasing personality-specific responsivities until the more narcotic effects of ethanol begin to manifest themselves at or about the 200 to 250 mg per deciliter level.

In susceptible persons alcohol may precipitate great agitation and acts of violence. To treat this condition one should give intramuscular benzodiazepines in cautiously increasing doses in order to avoid cumulative narcosis with the alcohol (see below). Individuals who show marked depressive reactions while under the influence of alcohol should be given verbal support until the effects wear off.

DEPRESSANT STAGE. When the BAL rises higher than about 200 to 250 mg per deciliter in nontolerant individuals, and to more than about 300 to 350 mg per deciliter in problem drinkers, the individual passes into a depressant syndrome. This condition requires immediate medical care. BAL's must be taken and evaluated; a single BAL of 300 mg per deciliter should not be interpreted as contravening treatment, since a reservoir of unabsorbed alcohol may be present in the stomach and small intestine. Gastric lavage should be undertaken to reduce this reservoir and to prevent vomiting and pulmonary aspiration. Vital systems must be maintained, with the administration of oxygen, intravenous fluids, and, rarely, ventilatory and circulatory support. Antidotes are ineffective.

HANGOVERS. Ethanol is strongly toxic to both brain and stomach, and its alcohol and aldehyde congeners are even more so, explaining the high incidence of postintoxication malaise, headache, giddiness, tremor, and nausea. These symptoms are generally self limited and respond readily to antacids and aspirin. More serious symptoms occur in more persistent but not yet fully alcoholic drinkers, in whom the so-called "hangover" may actually be an early withdrawal syndrome.

ALCOHOLISM (Alcohol Dependence)

Alcoholism is a drug-dependence syndrome resulting from the prolonged excessive use of ethanol. It is characterized by (1) a "high-risk" individual, (2) the development of self-perpetuating mechanisms producing addiction, (3) a more or less typical clinical course, and (4) specific complications and sequelae. The progressive clinical course is marked by repeated episodes of intoxication followed generally by characteristic withdrawal symptoms.

PREDISPOSING FACTORS. Predisposing factors that contribute to susceptibility to alcoholism may be biologic, psychologic, or social.

Studies of adoptees raised by nonalcoholic foster parents indicate a strong *genetic component* in alcoholics. Upon reaching adulthood, the children of alcoholic biologic parents have a four-fold greater incidence of alcoholism than those of non-alcoholic parents, even where no differences in alcohol consumption exist in the adopting families.

Psychopathology is found more frequently in alcoholics as a group than in nonalcoholics, although it is uncertain which is cause and which effect. The proven occurrence of significant brain damage as a result of prolonged alcoholism lends some weight to the latter argument. Nevertheless, some alcoholics show a characteristic psychologic immaturity, and the reportedly 8 to 10 per cent incidence of major psychoses among alcoholics is significantly higher than the 1 to 2 per cent in the general population. Agitated schizophrenics and manic-depressives not infrequently use alcohol as a means of self-medication. On the other hand, many alcoholics show no evidence of psychologic disturbance prior to the onset of their alcoholism.

Social influences can be the dominant influence in determining the level of drinking. Such factors include sex, ethnicity, religion, nationality, socioeconomic status, occupational subculture, family patterns, and peer pressure. In general, the level of psychopathology in a drug abuser is generally inversely proportional to the acceptability of that form of drug abuse in that individual's subculture. Thus, women alcoholics tend to show more psychopathology than do men, Jewish alcoholics more than Irish, and middle-class heroin addicts more than ghetto addicts.

THE ADDICTIVE CYCLE. Alcoholism (alcohol dependence, alcohol addiction) is the end result of a series of interacting processes that initiate and then perpetuate heavy drinking. The ingestion of alcohol provides temporary gratification of a need for euphoria or temporary relief from some psychologic or physical tension. However, chronic ethanol ingestion induces psychologic and physiologic processes that increase the desire for more alcohol; the substance that satisfies the need paradoxically increases the need.

The sequence in the elaboration of the addictive cycle in alcoholism is (1) primary psychologic dependence, (2) tolerance, (3) physical dependence, and (4) secondary psychologic dependence.

Psychologic Dependence. The first self-perpetuating mechanism is *primary psychologic dependence.* This reflects behavioral conditioning: An action and experience rewarded, either by pleasure or by the relief of pain and discomfort, will be reinforced by every similar succeeding action and experience. Primary psychologic dependence is the cornerstone of the dependency syndrome to all three classes of psychoactive drugs—the depressants, the stimulants, and the hallucinogens. Secondary psychologic dependence develops with the onset of physical dependence and is characterized by the need to drink to prevent withdrawal symptoms.

The combination of these two types of psychologic dependence is translated clinically into the subjective symptoms of *craving,* symptoms manifested as a continuous preoccupation with thoughts of drinking and with an overwhelming desire for alcohol. Craving is especially strong when reinforced by external stimuli such as a bottle of liquor. With long-term abstinence, there is a decline in the manifestations of both types of psychologic dependence, with craving tapering off to a low level after about six months of abstinence and more or less disappearing after about two years. However, craving can be reactivated thereafter by exposure to a strongly stimulating situation, e.g., the bar or tavern previously frequented.

Tolerance. With the continued ingestion of large doses of alcohol, metabolic changes result in an increased tolerance to ethanol. This is manifested clinically as a decreased responsivity to a given dose of alcohol or as the need to ingest a larger dose in order to obtain a desired effect. Tolerance occurs at three physiologic levels.

1. *Metabolic tolerance* results from the increased efficiency of hepatic enzymes breaking down ethanol to its metabolic end-products.

2. *Physiologic or intracellular tolerance* accounts for the major

increase in tolerance to ethanol, reflected in the behavioral and physiologic resistance to high doses of alcohol. The mechanisms of physiologic tolerance are thought to involve intracellular metabolic changes in the central nervous system and may be similar to those for barbiturates and other sedatives but are different from those for the opiates. Thus, individuals tolerant to ethanol show cross-tolerance to barbiturates and vice versa. Also, withdrawal symptoms from either drug can be relieved by administration of the other.

3. *Behavioral tolerance* is considered to be an overall learning response that enables the person to maintain behavioral function while under the influence of ethanol.

Physical Dependence. The same cellular changes that result in physiologic tolerance presumably are responsible for physical dependence. Neurons develop increased excitability to compensate for the depressant effects of chronic alcohol intake. If ethanol levels then drop sharply, a marked increase occurs in central nervous system irritability. The presence of physical dependence on ethanol is expressed by the phenomena of withdrawal.

When a high level of physical dependence develops in alcoholics, withdrawal symptoms become persistent because of the constant rise and fall of the BAL. The alcoholic finds that he is comfortable only while his BAL is rising; a falling BAL is accompanied by distressing withdrawal symptoms. Since quick and effective relief is obtained by alcohol ingestion, withdrawal symptoms become important factors in maintaining drinking behavior. During particularly heavy drinking bouts, severe withdrawal symptoms result whenever the physically dependent alcoholic seeks to stop drinking; this sequence leads to a compulsive pattern of drinking known clinically as *loss of control or inability to abstain*.

CLINICAL COURSE. Problem drinking and alcoholism are progressive syndromes characterized in most instances by repeated episodes of intoxication (in some problem drinkers and in some alcoholics, titration of drinking may conceal such episodes). With the development of physical dependence, the tempo of drinking tends to accelerate, and there is increased evidence of physical, psychologic, and social impairment. Besides developing multiple physical ailments, affected individuals tend to become careless in personal appearance, indifferent to family and social responsibilities, and inadequate at work. The addition of these stresses to already overburdened physiologic and psychologic resources tends further to increase drinking behavior.

An early sign of developing alcoholism is *blackouts*. These are episodes of temporary amnesia occurring during periods of intensive drinking. The amnesia is usually for periods of hours to a day or so, but with prolonged drinking may last up to a week. The syndrome is a characteristic anesthetic effect of alcohol on the brain; it is a precursor to the more chronic forms of brain damage secondary to chronic alcohol abuse.

The acute alcohol withdrawal syndrome occurs episodically after prolonged periods (two to three weeks) of extremely heavy drinking (a fifth of hard liquor daily or its equivalent). It is precipitated either by the cessation of drinking or by a sharp decrease in intake. Many individuals enter treatment for alcoholism after being hospitalized for acute alcohol withdrawal. After a week or so, many of these patients continue to show a low-grade withdrawal syndrome characterized by tremulousness, agitation, and insomnia. This constellation, labeled the *protracted abstinence syndrome*, may persist, to a greater or lesser degree, for up to six months. During this period, the individual is particularly susceptible to the effects of alcohol, since the entire addictive cycle is readily reactivated. Hence it is important with patients hospitalized during acute alcohol withdrawal to be certain that they are adequately detoxified before discharge.

TREATMENT OF ALCOHOL ABUSE. The major goal is to help the patient achieve and maintain total abstinence. The suggestion that treated problem drinkers sometimes may return safely to social drinking has no demonstrated merit and should be discounted. The achievement of abstinence is difficult enough without the interference produced by the reinforcing effects of even small amounts of alcohol. Rehabilitation requires a reconstruction of physical, psychologic, and social adjustment, to help overcome the long-term dependence upon alcohol. Nor is this a short-term affair. The perpetuating mechanisms of the addictive cycle remain very active during the first six months of abstinence and moderately active for the first two or three years of sobriety. The individual in therapy should be encouraged to undertake treatment for at least a two-year period, during which time the necessary physical, psychologic, and social adjustments can occur.

The three most effective treatment modalities for problem drinking and alcoholism are *disulfiram* (Antabuse), *psychotherapy* or counseling, and *Alcoholics Anonymous*. Disulfiram is a slowly excreted, long-acting medication that inhibits the action of acetaldehyde dehydrogenase. Because it is slowly metabolized and slowly excreted, once appropriate blood levels are established by a priming regimen (500 mg daily for one week), each single daily dose of 250 mg will maintain adequate blood levels for the next three or four days. Alcohol in any form is converted by alcohol dehydrogenase to acetaldehyde, but its further degradation is blocked by the action of disulfiram on acetaldehyde dehydrogenase. The piling up in the blood of acetaldehyde, a highly toxic substance, produces prostrating nausea, vomiting, diffuse flushing, and a shocklike reaction. The emergency treatment for the Antabuse-alcohol reaction consists of intravenous fluids and antihistamines. Most alcoholics who have experienced this reaction are careful not to repeat it, and many achieve and maintain abstinence with this drug.

Psychotherapy or the counseling of individuals who are abusing alcohol is directed (1) toward achieving abstinence and (2) toward accomplishing the changes in psychologic and social adjustment necessary to maintain it. Alcoholics Anonymous (AA), an association of ex-alcoholics, provides the companionship of those who have been able to overcome alcohol addiction; it also offers the strong social support and acceptance that alcoholics so often lack and so desperately need. The greatest chance for success in treating an alcoholic lies with continued supportive counseling by the physician plus the patient's participation in AA.

ACUTE ALCOHOL WITHDRAWAL SYNDROMES

Physically dependent alcoholics who go on a lengthy bout of heavy drinking for a period of one or more weeks will, upon reduction or cessation of alcohol intake, develop *acute alcohol withdrawal syndrome* characterized by cortical (behavioral) and beta-adrenergic (autonomic) hyperexcitability. Either pattern may predominate.

DELIRIUM TREMENS. *Delirium tremens* (DT's) represents the most severe type of acute alcohol withdrawal, with marked symptoms of cortical and brain stem hyperexcitability.

The patient in DT's represents an acute medical emergency, since the untreated mortality rate is about 15 per cent, largely from complications such as pneumonia or acute hepatitis. Affected patients are characteristically disoriented, agitated, hallucinating, tremulous, and perspiring. The pulse and respirations are rapid, blood pressure may be high or low, and body temperature is usually elevated. There may be severe muscle cramps because of an associated acute myopathy or generalized paresthesias because of a diffuse polyneuropathy. Nausea and vomiting often signify acute gastritis that induced the reduced alcohol intake and precipitated the acute episode.

The course of fully developed DT's usually follows upon alcohol withdrawal or decline by about three to five days, often after a preceding period of increasing restlessness, tremor, and behavioral agitation. A certain percentage follows upon withdrawal seizures. In untreated or inadequately treated cases, confusion and disorientation may last for several weeks. With adequate treatment, most severe symptoms clear within ten days; lesser ones may last for up to six months.

The specific treatment of delirium tremens involves the substitution of a long-acting drug that is cross tolerant for alcohol. Benzodiazepines are the agents of choice for inducing sedation. Treatment for moderately severe cases consists of diazepam, 25 to 50 mg orally four times daily for the first several days, with gradually tapering doses thereafter. In patients with more severe cases, particularly in those with convulsions, diazepam, 5 to 10 mg intravenously, should be used every one to two hours until the condition is stabilized. Fluids, electrolytes, and thiamine, 100 mg, should be given parenterally. A careful search should be made to detect and treat infection. Good nursing care is essential to provide the necessary physical and psychologic support (Table 15–2).

WITHDRAWAL CONVULSIONS. In *withdrawal convulsions* ("*rum fits*") generalized convulsions occur usually singly but sometimes in short runs or even as status epilepticus following a decline in the BAL. Seizures usually occur in the period of 12 to 48 hours after cessation of drinking. Various causative mechanisms have been suggested for withdrawal seizures, including chronic hypocapnia or hypomagnesemia, but none stand as proved. The attacks usually are without focal features, and consistently focal signs deserve further investigation. Otherwise, computed tomographic (CT) scans of the brain are negative, as are interictal electroencephalographic (EEG) recordings. Treatment consists of stopping the acute convulsions with intravenous diazepam, plus giving a single dose of phenytoin (Dilantin) (see Ch. 493) to prevent immediately recurring seizures. Signs of impending delirium tremens emerge postictally in perhaps one third of cases. "Rum fits" occur only on withdrawal from alcohol; prophylactic, chronic treatment with anticonvulsants is useless.

IMPENDING DELIRIUM TREMENS. The most common clinical manifestation of the acute alcohol withdrawal syndrome is *impending delirium tremens*. Mild-to-moderate symptoms of withdrawal are evident, mainly those associated with beta-adrenergic brain stem discharge. Mild agitation, vasomotor changes, tremors, and insomnia sometimes respond to the alpha-adrenergic drug clonidine, an active antagonist to beta-adrenergic discharge. However, treatment with cross-tolerant benzodiazepines is both more specific and more effective. A mild case may be controlled with 10 to 20 mg of diazepam given orally four times daily for several days. Moderate cases will require up to 20 to 30 mg of the same drug four times daily for a few days, with gradual tapering off over a period of seven to ten days.

ACUTE ALCOHOLIC HALLUCINOSIS. In *acute alcoholic hallucinosis,* auditory hallucinations dominate the clinical picture as opposed to the more common visual hallucinations seen in delirium tremens. In addition, there is characteristically less agitation and tremulousness. Consequently, the clinical picture looks more like that of an acute schizophrenic episode than like that of alcohol withdrawal, and differential diagnosis may be difficult. However, a history of prolonged heavy drinking, followed by a sudden decrease or cessation, reveals the diagnosis. Treatment is the same as for delirium tremens. Recovery may require weeks to a month or more.

ALCOHOL-RELATED ILLNESSES

Medical conditions secondary to prolonged alcohol abuse fall generally into two categories: (1) nutritional diseases caused by dietary insufficiency and (2) diseases caused by the direct toxic effects of ethanol. Because alcoholic beverages provide 7 calories per gram of ethanol, an individual consuming a fifth of 86 proof liquor daily will derive about 2500

TABLE 15–2. TREATMENT OF SEVERE TREMULOUSNESS OR DELIRIUM TREMENS

1. Attempt control by reassurance and observation.

2. Treat systemic problems promptly.

3. Treat uncontrollable agitation: Control with diazepam, 10 mg IV given slowly, followed by 5–10 mg IV, slowly every 15 minutes to induce calmness. Once calm, maintain with diazepam, 5–10 mg IV every 1–4 hours.

4. Continuously supply and balance electrolytes and vitamins, especially thiamine.

calories from alcohol alone. Under such conditions, most alcoholics consume little other food. Since liquor contains no vitamins, minerals, amino acids, or other essential nutritional elements, alcoholics often show marked nutritional deficiencies. Superimposed on this metabolic insufficiency, the direct toxic effect of ethanol produces further damage. Although the diseases secondary to alcohol abuse are generally categorized as either nutritional or toxic, both effects are probably involved in most cases.

Alcohol-related illnesses can involve all organ systems in the body. Table 15–3 indicates alcohol-related illnesses that are due predominantly to the direct toxic effects of prolonged alcohol ingestion and those that are more probably secondary to malnutrition. The effects may be difficult to separate, since most alcoholics are both heavy drinkers and malnourished.

TABLE 15–3. ALCOHOL-RELATED ILLNESSES DUE TO TOXIC AND NUTRITIONAL EFFECTS OF ETHANOL

Organ	Syndromes Due to Toxic Effects	Syndromes Due to Nutritional Effects
Brain	Alcoholic dementia (cortical atrophy)	Wernicke-Korsakoff syndrome (Ch. 467) Cerebellar degeneration Central pontine myelinosis (secondary to electrolyte changes during therapy)
Nerves		Peripheral polyneuropathy (Ch. 305) (thiamine deficiency)
Heart	Alcoholic cardiomyopathy (Ch. 53) Arrhythmia	Beriberi heart disease (thiamine deficiency)
Blood	Leukopenia, anemia, thrombocytopenia	Macrocytic hyperchromic anemia (Ch. 136) (folic acid deficiency)
Gastrointestinal tract	Acute and chronic gastritis (Ch. 99) Acute and chronic pancreatitis (Ch. 108) Carcinoma of the head and neck and of the esophagus	Malabsorption syndrome (Ch. 136) (folic acid deficiency)
Liver	Fatty degeneration Acute hepatitis Laennec's cirrhosis	Laennec's cirrhosis (Ch. 126 to 128)
Metabolic	Hyperlipidemia (Ch. 183) Hyperuricemia (exacerbation of gout)	
Endocrine	Male sexual impairment Increased fetal risk (fetal alcohol syndrome)	
Immune system	Increased susceptibility to infection	
Electrolyte disturbances	Hypocalcemia Hypomagnesemia Hypophosphatemia Acute water intoxication Alcoholic hyperosmolality Alcoholic ketosis	

PROGNOSIS

Prognosis in alcoholism is related to the stage and severity of the disease process. Morbidity and mortality can be divided into two major categories: that directly associated with alcohol abuse and that associated with alcohol-related illness.

PROGNOSIS IN THE ALCOHOLISM SYNDROME. Perhaps the most serious consequences of the alcoholism syndrome are deaths related to alcoholic behavior. It has been estimated that 50 per cent of highway fatalities are caused by drunken driving, with half of the victims alcoholic. Twenty-five per cent of suicides have a history of prolonged alcoholism. In deaths due to drug overdose, alcohol is the associated agent most commonly found. The combined mortality rates of these three behavioral aberrations, together with those associated with alcohol-related medical illnesses, make alcoholism and its behavioral and medical complications the fourth most common cause of death in the United States after heart disease, strokes, and cancer.

Facts belie the generally negative public opinion about the prognosis of alcoholics. In most industrial alcoholism treatment programs where workers are socially stable and (because of the risk to jobs and pensions) well motivated, recovery rates run at the 70 to 80 per cent level. This remarkably high "cure" rate is probably accounted for mainly by early detection when most of the patients are still problem drinkers and have not yet developed the physical and social stigmata of advanced alcoholism. Once the latter develop, success rates seldom exceed 40 to 50 per cent. Early identification and intervention remain the most important steps in the treatment of alcoholism.

PROGNOSIS OF ALCOHOL-RELATED MEDICAL ILLNESSES. The prognosis for specific alcohol-related medical illnesses varies with the nature of the illness and with its severity. Practically no alcohol-related medical illness can be cured if the patient continues to abuse alcohol. The major component of the treatment of alcohol-associated medical illness is the treatment of the underlying alcoholism.

Harper C, Kril J: Brain atrophy in chronic alcoholic patients: A quantitative pathological study. J Neurol Neurosurg Psychiatry 48:211, 1985. *Evidence for common occurrence of cortical and brain stem atrophy in chronic alcoholics.*

Helzer JE, Robins LN, Taylor JK, et al.: The extent of long term moderate drinking among alcoholics discharged from medical and psychiatric treatment facilities. N Engl J Med 312:1678, 1985. *A conclusive demonstration that chronic alcoholics cannot successfully revert to moderate social drinking.*

Kissin B: Medical management of the alcoholic patient. In Kissin B, Begleiter H (eds.): The Biology of Alcoholism. Vol. 5. New York, Plenum Press, 1977. *Description of the role of the family physician in the diagnosis and treatment of alcoholism.*

Mendelson JH, Mello NK: Biologic concomitants of alcoholism. N Engl J Med 301:912, 1979. *A medical progress article reviewing studies dealing with the mechanistic aspects of genetics, metabolism, consequences, behavior, and speculated causes of alcohol addiction.*

Sellers EM, Kalant H: Alcohol intoxication and withdrawal. N Engl J Med 294:757, 1976. *An excellent didactic article dealing with all aspects of acute treatment.*

Thompson WL, John AD, Maddrey WL, et al.: Diazepam and paraldehyde for treatment of severe delirium tremens. A controlled trial. Ann Intern Med 82:175, 1975. *Establishes the clear superiority of diazepam for acute treatment and outlines a clear and effective plan for management.*

16 DRUG ABUSE AND DEPENDENCE

Charles P. O'Brien

Drug abuse is currently a significant problem at every level of our society. It is likely that the average physician will encounter many patients exhibiting behavioral or medical complications of licit or illicit drug use, but the relationship of the symptoms to drugs often goes unrecognized. Early diagnosis, which is critical for effective treatment, is difficult because, at an early stage, patients rarely fit the addict stereotype.

Clinicians have been mainly concerned with *tolerance* and *physical dependence. Tolerance* is the result of a homeostatic process in which the body adapts to the repeated effects of a drug. This adaptation tends to compensate for the pharmacologic effects, with the result that higher doses are required to achieve an effect. With daily dosing, tolerance increases and a state of *physical dependence* can occur. *Physical dependence* is indicated by the presence of a rebound known as a *withdrawal syndrome* that follows interruption of dosing. Withdrawal phenomena tend to be opposite to the effects of the drugs themselves. Thus a drug that produces sedation leads to hyper-reflexia and irritability during withdrawal, and a stimulant withdrawal is followed by weakness and depression.

Behavioral effects are the pivotal diagnostic criteria, however, not simply tolerance and physical dependence. Moreover, with some drugs, *intermittent use* that does not cause tolerance or a withdrawal syndrome may produce behavioral or social consequences that urgently require treatment. *Drug abuse* is therefore defined as a maladaptive pattern of use of any substance that persists despite social, psychologic, or medical consequences. This pattern of use may be intermittent and does not meet the criteria for dependence. *Drug dependence* is a behavioral syndrome that involves compulsive drug taking, neglect of constructive activities, and adverse social effects and *may* include pharmacologic tolerance and physical dependence.

RECOGNITION. Since early diagnosis is so important, the physician should have a high index of suspicion for including drug abuse in the differential diagnosis of any patient. The abuse pattern that presents the most difficulty is that of a successful middle-class adult whose substance abuse is detected incidental to a routine physical examination or during treatment of an unrelated disorder. Invariably, such patients will deny that drug or alcohol abuse is a problem. Physicians must be aware that denial of problems and minimizing of the drug or alcohol use are fundamental aspects of the syndrome. These patients usually will not admit to a problem until it becomes so severe that there is no alternative, by which time, treatment is much more difficult.

The diagnosis of drug abuse or dependence is basically a clinical deduction. The physician should use all of the available information, including the patient's history, information from relatives or the employer, physical examination, and laboratory tests. Blood or urine tests showing the presence of drugs or their metabolites can be useful but also can be misleading. The toxicologic tests, when properly done and confirmed, indicate use within a varying period of time, depending on the drug and its dose. Such tests do not disclose pattern of use or the presence of dependence. Metabolites of some drugs, such as marijuana, remain in the urine for at least several days following a single dose. Thus the tests require interpretation and integration with other clinical information.

Clues discovered on the physical examination include the presence of scars from numerous intravenous injections ("tracks") or the presence of edematous arms and veins that are difficult to find. Chronic sinusitis or a scarred and perhaps perforated nasal septum suggests "snorting" of cocaine, a powerful vasoconstrictor. Frequent injuries due to falls or auto accidents are seen in sedative abusers as well as alcoholics. Infections such as abscesses, hepatitis, respiratory infections, and endocarditis are well-known risks of drug abuse. The most devastating disease associated with drug abuse is the acquired immune deficiency syndrome (AIDS). In the late 1980's, intravenous drug users have become a major reservoir for the AIDS virus (Ch. 346).

Physicians must also be alert to the signs of drug abuse in

order to avoid unwittingly prescribing medications that will perpetuate the dependence. Patients taking sleeping medications, pain medications, or antianxiety agents on a chronic basis may visit several physicians in order to obtain a larger drug supply. Others will deliberately feign illness, particularly pain syndromes. Some will have read textbooks and recite classic descriptions of acute renal calculus, migraine headache, or pancreatitis. Physicians should be particularly wary of patients who ask for a specific medication or who claim to have an "allergy" to nonnarcotic pain medication.

Jaffe J: Drug addiction and drug abuse. In Gilman AG, Goodman LS, Rall TR, et al (eds.): The Pharmacological Basis of Therapeutics. Edition 7. New York, Macmillan, 1985, pp 532–581. *Thorough discussion of pharmacologic and clinical aspects of drug abuse.*

Senay, EC: Substance Abuse Disorders in Clinical Practice. Boston, John Wright, 1983. *Very practical and concise guide to diagnosis and treatment of drug dependence.*

SEDATIVES

Examples of sedatives include the following:

1. Ethanol
2. Barbiturates
3. Meprobamate (Miltown)
4. Glutethimide (Doriden)
5. Diazepam (Valium)
6. Lorazepam (Ativan)
7. Alprazolam (Xanax)
8. Flurazepam (Dalmane)
9. Triazolam (Halcion)

These drugs are central nervous system depressants, and all are capable of producing abuse, tolerance, and physical dependence. Their withdrawal syndromes are generally similar, although the sedatives come from different chemical categories (e.g., alcohol, barbiturate, benzodiazepine). Their effects are additive, and they are often used in combination. This aspect is particularly important in considering interactions with alcohol (Ch. 15) and in treating patients who are dependent on multiple sedatives with different durations of action.

Patterns of Abuse

There are two basic patterns of sedative drug abuse other than that with alcohol: One is produced inadvertently by taking prescription sedatives without proper concern for their potential to produce dependence, and the second involves deliberate use of sedatives to obtain a "high."

PRESCRIPTION SEDATIVES. The problem of improper use of prescription sedatives is a concern to all physicians because these drugs are among the most widely prescribed of all drugs throughout the world. They have legitimate medical uses in the short-term treatment of insomnia, anxiety, and seizure disorders. The chronic use of medication for insomnia, however, often leads to problems because insomnia is merely a symptom. It may signal the presence of an underlying illness, or it may simply require a change in activity patterns, but chronic use of sedatives simply adds a new problem. After daily use for several weeks, tolerance develops, and sleep difficulties may return, often in a modified form. The patient may have become dependent, however, on the daily ingestion of the sedative. If the drug is stopped, a rebound occurs, with the appearance of symptoms worse than those experienced prior to treatment. All sedatives are not equal in their tendency to produce this iatrogenic insomnia. Long-acting benzodiazepines, for example, are unlikely to produce rebound effects at usual doses. Other liabilities are associated with their use, however, such as "hangover" effects, which produce subtle neuropsychologic deficits and may mimic dementia in older persons. On balance, insomnia should not be treated with drugs except for brief periods of time.

Another pattern associated with the prescription of sedatives is that found in the treatment of anxiety. Benzodiazepines (e.g., diazepam, alprazolam) are the most effective medications available for the treatment of anxiety, and they produce relatively less sedation than older medications used for this purpose, such as meprobamate or phenobarbital. Symptoms of anxiety are widespread such that about 15 per cent of all Americans receive a prescription for one of these drugs in a single year. Approximately 6 per cent of the population take benzodiazepines chronically, and this leads to *tolerance* and *physical dependence*. This does not imply *abuse* because the patient may be taking the benzodiazepine for a legitimate anxiety disorder. It does mean, however, that since the patient perceives less sedation, there may be a tendency to increase the dose. It also implies that the patient should be warned about withdrawal symptoms if the drug is terminated abruptly. Occasionally, a patient who allows his prescription to run out is brought to an emergency room because of benzodiazepine withdrawal seizures. Some of these patients are mislabeled as "addicts," even though they have never used more of the antianxiety medication than was ordered. Others, however, become deliberate abusers of sedatives after beginning treatment for anxiety under a doctor's orders and may purposely increase their dose while obtaining medication from several different physicians. Benzodiazepines in general have a relatively low abuse potential, and such cases of deliberate abuse are rare.

DELIBERATE SEDATIVE ABUSE. Sedatives are used at parties by groups of abusers, usually adolescents and young adults, to obtain a "high." The "high" appears to be a form of disinhibition or release and depends partially on the setting in which the drug is taken. As with alcohol, increasing the dose produces depression and eventual loss of consciousness. A dangerous aspect of sedative abuse is that tolerance to the sought-after subjective effects rapidly develops, but tolerance to the depressant effects on the brain stem remains low. As the experienced user increases the dose to obtain a "high," he or she may unexpectedly reach the dose that depresses vital functions and threatens survival.

The most popular deliberately abused sedative over the past 10 to 15 years has been methaqualone (Quaalude), reputed to be an aphrodisiac. Although methaqualone probably does not enhance sexual performance, the drug was so widely abused that the manufacturer withdrew it. Counterfeit versions of methaqualone continue to be available "on the street" in some areas.

Certain benzodiazepines are popular sedatives for abuse and are available for purchase through illicit channels. Diazepam has been popular among abusers, and, more recently, alprazolam has been used by the drug subculture. Although benzodiazepines in general are not preferred drugs of abuse, those with more rapid onset, such as diazepam and alprazolam, may be sought.

Abstinence Syndrome

The withdrawal syndrome following sedative dependence is similar to alcohol withdrawal. Among the sedatives, the syndrome differs in onset, duration, and severity, depending on the dose and duration of action of the drug used and the duration of daily use. The long-acting benzodiazepines, such as diazepam, may have a withdrawal syndrome whose onset is delayed for several days following the termination of the drug. At doses within the therapeutic range, withdrawal symptoms may consist of only mild irritability, complaints of peculiar sensations, diaphoresis, and sleep disturbance accompanied by rebound increases in rapid eye movement (REM) sleep. The symptoms may be similar to the anxiety symptoms for which the drug was initially prescribed. At higher doses, the sedative withdrawal syndrome is more severe and can be life threatening. Major abnormalities include paroxysmal electroencephalographic (EEG) changes, generalized seizures, or a toxic psychosis similar to delirium tremens. During withdrawal from somewhat less, but still high, doses of benzodiazepines (the equivalent of 100 mg of diazepam per day), myoclonic jerking movements without loss of consciousness may be seen. Restlessness, anxiety, tremulousness, and weakness occur, and these are often accompanied by orthostatic hypotension, nausea, cramps, and vomiting. Irritability, anxiety, depressive symptoms, and neuropsychologic deficits may persist for weeks or months.

Treatment

The acute withdrawal syndrome should be considered a serious medical illness usually requiring inpatient treatment. Close monitoring for cardiac arrhythmias or seizures is necessary. Several detoxification techniques are available, each requiring the substitution of a prescribed sedative with cross-tolerance for the drug on which the patient is dependent. The physician should not simply accept the history, but rather determine the level of dependence by giving a test dose of a known sedative, such as diazepam or pentobarbital. If the patient shows no evidence of slurred speech or sedation after a test dose of 20 to 40 mg of diazepam, a higher level of dependence is indicated, and the daily sedative dose should be adjusted accordingly. Gradual detoxification using diazepam can be accomplished over 1 to 3 weeks, although in some treatment centers where diazepam is the object of much drug-seeking behavior and manipulation by patients, phenobarbital is preferred. Patients dependent on both a short-acting sedative, such as alcohol, and a long-acting drug, such as diazepam, should be watched for a biphasic withdrawal. The alcohol withdrawal peaks and subsides during the first week, but the diazepam withdrawal may not be evident until early in the second week. Patients dependent on both an opioid, such as heroin, and a sedative should be maintained on a low dose of methadone until the sedative withdrawal is completed. After detoxification, the patient must be put in a treatment program to prevent recurrence, as described at the end of this chapter.

Hallstrom C, Lader M: Benzodiazepine withdrawal phenomena. Int Pharmacopsychiatry 16:235, 1981. *Description of subtle symptoms of benzodiazepine withdrawal.*

O'Brien CP, Woody GE: Sedative hypnotic and anti-anxiety agents. In Frances AJ, Hales R (eds.): American Psychiatric Association Annual Review, Vol 5. Washington, APA Press, 1986, pp 186–199. *Review of diagnosis, treatment, and prevention of sedative abuse.*

STIMULANTS

Examples of stimulants include the following:

1. Cocaine
2. Dextroamphetamine
3. Methamphetamine
4. Methylphenidate (Ritalin)
5. Phenmetrazine (Preludin)
6. Diethylpropion (Tepanil)

Patterns of Abuse

Cocaine has suddenly become the major drug of abuse in the United States, excluding alcohol, and the problem continues to grow. The enormous profits available to drug dealers have spawned a huge supply system so that despite increased federal efforts, cocaine supplies have increased so rapidly that the price has declined. Not only is cocaine available to a wider audience, especially children, but also its users have developed clever new and efficient ways to administer the drug, increasing its potency and dangerousness.

Until recently, cocaine hydrochloride was available as a white powder through illicit channels in an adulterated form and at a cost so high that only the affluent could afford to use it regularly. The typical mode of administration was

"snorting," which consists of application of the powder to the nasal mucous membranes. Intravenous injection of an aqueous solution was also used, resulting in a more rapid onset and greater likelihood of seizures. However, inhalation of the "free base" alkaloidal form of cocaine has been found to be the most convenient and efficient system for delivering the drug to the brain. A technique for converting the hydrochloride salt into cocaine "free base" using alkalinization and extraction with ether or other organic solvents while heating has become well known because of the devastating fires that sometimes result. During the mid 1980's, this solvent technique has been replaced by a mass-produced solid form of "free base" called "crack." Crack is produced by sodium bicarbonate extraction of cocaine hydrochloride, and the agent can be sold in small, yellow-white lumps for as little as $5 to $10 per dose. When heated in a small pipe, the cocaine vapor can be inhaled, producing a brief and very intense "high." This drug is clearly the *most addicting substance* yet encountered by clinicians. Dependence can be produced very rapidly, perhaps in days and certainly in weeks. Users may administer the drug continuously for several days without eating or sleeping. The widespread availability of "crack", its cheap price, and its proneness to produce dependence have led to problems in all strata of society.

The sought-after effect of cocaine is an intense "high" or euphoria, which is often described in sexual terms but is claimed to be "better than sex." The euphoria may last only a few minutes, depending on the dose and mode of administration. The after-effect is one of depression and craving for more cocaine. During a period of regular cocaine use, the person becomes irritable and suspicious. High doses may result in persecutory delusions or hallucinations, but these are more common with longer acting stimulants such as amphetamines. Families and friends of chronic cocaine users often note personality changes not observed by the users themselves. Alcohol, sedatives, opioids, and marijuana are often taken concurrently to combat the anxiety and irritability experienced by those using cocaine regularly. Users deprived of cocaine experience intense craving, depression, apathy, fatigue, and sleepiness.

Amphetamines have a longer duration of action than cocaine, but many of the effects are similar. These drugs have been used by physicians for a variety of conditions, including weight reduction, narcolepsy, and attention deficit disorder. Amphetamines have not been shown to be of value in weight reduction programs, and their use for all purposes has been curtailed by legal restrictions. Because they produce effects that are mostly pleasant, patients have a tendency to increase the dose of all stimulants and to take them longer than the prescribing physician intended. Tolerance develops rapidly to the stimulant effects of amphetamines, but with higher doses, toxic effects are common. These effects can resemble acute paranoid schizophrenia with delusions and hallucinations. Cessation of amphetamines produces a withdrawal syndrome similar to that after cocaine use and with depressive symptoms that may continue for several months.

The milder stimulants, such as methylphenidate and phenmetrazine, rarely are associated with abuse problems, but they should be prescribed only when specifically indicated and with awareness of their abuse potential.

Pharmacology

Cocaine acts at dopaminergic and other aminergic synapses by blocking reuptake of the neurotransmitter and presumably resulting in enhanced synaptic activity. Systemic effects of cocaine and amphetamine include increased cardiac contraction, increased blood pressure and heart rate, dilated pupils, constriction of peripheral blood vessels, rise in body temperature, relaxation of the bronchial musculature, and increases in central venous pressure, pulmonary arterial pressure, and renal blood flow. Cocaine is an effective topical local anesthetic and vasoconstrictor of mucous membranes. Low doses of stimulants increase alertness and physical and cognitive ability. Stimulants do reduce appetite, but significant tolerance to this effect develops. When stimulants are discontinued, a rebound increase in weight often leaves the person heavier than before the drug was taken.

Heavy users report acute tolerance to the euphorigenic effects of cocaine when the drug is used repeatedly at a single occasion. However, a day or two later, a "high" can again be obtained at approximately the same dose as previously. Tolerance to the respiratory and cardiac stimulatory effects of cocaine does occur. Although abrupt cessation of stimulant use produces a distinct withdrawal syndrome as described above, it is generally limited to *behavioral* evidence of brain dysfunction rather than marked by the development of physical signs. During the excessive periods of sleep seen during withdrawal, the EEG shows increase in the proportion of REM sleep and nightmares may occur. Rarely, withdrawal has been marked by headaches, profuse sweating, muscle cramps, disorientation, and confusion.

Adverse Effects

The most common adverse effect of cocaine use is loss of control, so that a severe dependence syndrome occurs with neglect of all constructive activities. *Acute cocaine toxicity* is dose related and is characterized by sympathomimetic effects, including tachycardia, hypertension, hyperthermia, and arrhythmias, and is followed by seizures, brain stem depression, and cardiorespiratory collapse. Stroke, coma, intracranial vasculitis, myocardial infarction, and sudden death have each been occasionally observed following cocaine binges. At lower doses the acute toxic effects may be marked by a brief period of paranoid behavior with hallucinations. *Acute amphetamine toxicity* is also characterized by excessive sympathomimetic stimulation and more commonly produces grossly paranoid behavior mimicking acute paranoid schizophrenia. There may be stereotyped compulsive behavior, tactile hallucinations consisting of "bugs" crawling under the skin, and visual or auditory hallucinations.

Chronic use of intranasal cocaine commonly causes ulceration or perforation of the nasal septum. Chronic users are typically debilitated and subject to infections as a result of neglect of hygiene, lack of sleep, and poor nutrition. There is evidence of dopamine cell damage in the brains of animals treated chronically with stimulants. This raises the possibility of an increased risk for later development of Parkinson's disease. There are also clinical reports of increased schizophrenic disorders in chronic stimulant users. Chronic cocaine use among pregnant women results in a high incidence of premature, low birth weight, and neurologically abnormal infants.

Treatment

Treatment of the anxiety reactions and irritability produced by cocaine or amphetamines can be accomplished with benzodiazepines. Acute psychotic reactions may require haloperidol if amphetamines are involved, but reactions produced by cocaine are usually self limiting. Withdrawal from stimulant dependence requires a supportive environment and protection from the supply of cocaine. Intense cravings for cocaine are the most prominent of the withdrawal symptoms, and these have been attributed to a state of dopamine depletion in the brain. To reverse these effects, the dopamine receptor agonist bromocriptine has been used experimentally to ease the acute withdrawal. The most difficult aspect of treatment is the prevention of relapse when the patient returns to his or her normal environment and is confronted with opportunities to re-establish the habit. This aspect of treatment is discussed at the end of this chapter.

Ellinwood EH: Amphetamines/anorectics. In Dupont RL, Goldstein A, O'Donnell J (eds.): Handbook on Drug Abuse. National Institute on Drug Abuse, U. S. Government Printing Office, 1979, pp 221–231. *Review of clinical and pharmacologic aspects of stimulant abuse.*

Washton A, Gold MS: Chronic cocaine abuse: Evidence for adverse effects on health and function. Psychiatr Ann 14:733, 1984. *Clear evidence of adverse consequences of chronic cocaine use.*

OPIOIDS

Examples of opioids include the following:

Agonists
1. Morphine
2. Methadone
3. Meperidine (Demerol)
4. Oxycodone (Percodan)
5. Propoxyphene (Darvon)
6. Heroin
7. Hydromorphone (Dilaudid)
8. Fentanyl (Sublimaze)
9. Codeine

Mixed agonist-antagonists
1. Pentazocine (Talwin)
2. Nalbuphine (Nubain)
3. Buprenorphine (Buprenex)
4. Butorphanol (Stadol)

Antagonists
1. Naloxone (Narcan)
2. Naltrexone (Trexan)

Opiates are derivatives of the opium poppy plant, which contains more than 20 alkaloids. Heroin, morphine, and codeine are examples of commonly used *opiates*. Synthetic drugs that act via opiate receptors in the body are called *opioids*. The body also produces peptides that act at these receptors as neurohormones or neurotransmitters and are called *endogenous opioids*.

Patterns of Abuse

Opioid abuse has been a problem in the United States for well over 100 years. The patterns have changed considerably since the turn of the century, when most of the opium-dependent persons were either Civil War veterans or users of patent medicines. At the current time, there are two abuse patterns in this country. The smaller group by far involves patients initially treated by a physician for a legitimate pain problem with opioid drugs. The pain may become chronic, and the dose is increased, usually at the patient's demand. The treatment may have begun with something mild, such as propoxyphene or pentazocine, but it tends to progress to the more potent opioids, such as oxycodone or hydromorphone. Prescriptions may be refilled excessively, and patients may visit more than one physician for medication or may frequent emergency rooms. Such individuals will vehemently deny being addicts; they are just seeking relief of pain. On closer examination, however, they usually turn out to have symptoms of anxiety or depression that are temporarily relieved by opioids.

The second pattern is that of intentional misuse of opioids for their euphoria-producing ability. Intermittent heroin use, primarily among males in the inner city, typically begins during adolescence, and dependence ensues within a year or two of first use. Development in all areas—educational, social, occupational, and even psychosexual—is curtailed by use of heroin. It is not known how many people begin experimenting with heroin and stop using it. Those who continue to use heroin develop tolerance to its euphorigenic effects, continue to increase the dose, and soon find that they must use the drug daily to avoid withdrawal even while chasing that elusive first "high."

Older users tend to introduce younger ones to heroin and to techniques of crime required to support the "habit." Street heroin available in the United States tends to be diluted many times so that there may be an average of only 4 to 10 mg of heroin in a typical 100-mg bag. Furthermore, the heroin on the street at any given time may be more or less potent, depending on the supply and the pressure from law enforcement agencies. Most street heroin users have relatively mild degrees of physical dependence in terms of number of milligrams of heroin or its equivalent in morphine or methadone per day. Heroin-dependent persons, although they insist that they are seeking a "high," actually fear withdrawal and will go to great lengths to obtain sufficient drug to inject themselves one to three times per day.

Some heroin users discover that prescription medications are more reliable than street drugs because the latter have no quality control. Hydromorphone is a very potent opioid that cannot be distinguished from heroin even by experienced users under double-blind conditions. Addicts may visit physicians or emergency rooms and feign pain to obtain opioids. Occasionally, unscrupulous physicians may simply sell prescriptions for whatever the addict requests. A few addicts have had prescription pads printed with their own name and a false Drug Enforcement Agency (DEA) number in an effort to trick pharmacists. Some of the prescription drugs prized on the street are not even the more potent ones. For example, a major problem in some large cities has been pentazocine abuse. The pattern is to obtain tablets of this mixed agonist-antagonist designed for oral use, dissolve the tablets in water under heat, mix them with another drug, such as an antihistamine (tripelennamine), and inject the mixture. Some addicts claim that they prefer the "high" obtained this way to that obtained from heroin. The manufacturer of pentazocine has recently begun supplying the tablets combined with naloxone, an opioid antagonist that is effective parenterally but not orally. Thus if the pentazocine tablets are taken intravenously, the naloxone will counteract the opioid effects, thus frustrating the abuser. Another weak opiate that is abused in combination is codeine. Mixed with glutethimide, a sedative, it is favored by a number of drug abusers.

In recent years, heroin dependence has spread from the inner city to the middle class. The same supply system that distributes cocaine and marijuana also makes heroin available. Some educated and employed persons seeking a "thrill" prefer the effects of heroin. Others learn to use heroin to combat some of the unpleasant anxiety and irritability produced by chronic cocaine use.

Pharmacology

Opioids act at specific receptors that are widely distributed throughout the body in virtually all major organ systems. Since these receptors are heavily represented in the endocrine, cardiovascular, gastrointestinal, and nervous systems, the effects of opioids are many and varied. The potency of individual drugs appears to depend on receptor affinity as well as metabolism. Heroin, for example, is diacetylmorphine, which has high lipid solubility and enters the brain rapidly. It is hydrolyzed to morphine, which is the form active at opiate receptors. Other opioids have similar systemic effects but reach brain receptors less rapidly. The mixed agonist-antagonist drugs, such as pentazocine, butorphanol, and nalbuphine, appear to act as agonists at kappa opiate receptors, but they also act as antagonists at mu (morphine) receptors. Thus, pentazocine can relieve pain on its own but, if given to someone already receiving morphine, will displace the morphine and precipitate withdrawal symptoms. Pure antagonists, such as naloxone and naltrexone, have no opiate-like effects, but they can reverse overdose and precipitate withdrawal if given *after* an opioid and can prevent opiate effects if given *before* the opioid.

After heroin injection, traces of morphine can be found in the urine for about 12 to 48 hours, depending on the dose and the laboratory detection technique. Quinine, a common adulterant of street heroin, persists longer, but it is also found in legal substances such as tonic water. Parenteral injections of morphine or methadone have equal analgesic effects and persist for four to six hours, whereas heroin is three times as potent, and meperidine and codeine are one tenth as potent as morphine. Codeine, meperidine, and methadone remain active when taken orally, and the duration of action of methadone is extended considerably when taken orally. For prevention of withdrawal in dependent persons, methadone remains active for 24 to 30 hours, far longer than its analgesic effect.

Opioids appear to produce analgesia, at least in part, by activation of an endogenous pain control system mediated via opiate receptors. Inhibition of pain sensation occurs at the spinal level as well as within the brain. Opioids are much more effective for clinical pain with anxiety than for experimental pain in research subjects. Opioids produce a reduction in anxiety, some sedation, and a feeling of well-being or euphoria. This effect seems important to their clinical usefulness and to their abuse potential as well. It is this euphoria that is sought by street addicts and that probably leads some medical patients to abuse prescribed opioids.

Tolerance to the euphoric effects of opioids develops rapidly, resulting in a tendency for users to increase their dose, if possible. Only partial tolerance develops to other effects, such as pupillary constriction, inhibition of gastrointestinal contractions, and suppression of anterior pituitary function.

Adverse Effects

Acute opioid overdose occurs when a user inadvertently injects a much higher dose than expected. This also can occur when a previously tolerant person returns to opioid use after a long interval, so that most of his or her tolerance has been lost. Many of the "overdoses" found with street heroin are now thought to have been due to a reaction to some of the adulterants rather than to the opiate. Acute reactions to adulterants, including quinine, allergic reactions, and synergistic interactions among several drugs used simultaneously may produce the *acute heroin reaction*. The syndrome is marked clinically by the rapid development of cyanosis, pulmonary edema, respiratory distress, and altered levels of consciousness progressing to coma. Increased intracranial pressure and occasionally seizures can develop. Fever to 40°C may occur initially and persist for 48 hours in association with leukocytosis. The pupils are usually pinpoint, although dilated, nonreactive pupils may occur with hypoxia or use of multiple drugs. The pathologic picture includes pulmonary congestion and edema and frequently cerebral edema.

Opioids themselves are surprisingly nontoxic even when used in substantial daily doses for many years. There is partial tolerance to their pharmacologic effects on the endocrine system. Thus females on methadone initially are amenorrheic, but the cycle usually returns in 6 to 12 months. Cortisol, luteinizing hormone, and testosterone levels are depressed while the patient is on methadone. Sexual response may be delayed; sperm count and ejaculate volume are reduced. Since street heroin users tend to have frequent periods of partial withdrawal, their endocrine systems are in turmoil. In contrast, a level dose of methadone induces some order, and the effects are reversible when the opioid is terminated. Chronic constipation may persist throughout opioid use.

The major adverse effects of opioid use come from the adulterants found in street drugs and the nonsterile practices typically followed by users. Skin abscesses, cellulitis, and thrombophlebitis are the most frequent complications. Pentazocine injection causes chronic ulcers and sclerosis of muscle in the areas of injection. Septicemia and bacterial endocarditis with involvement of either or both sides of the heart are seen. *Staphylococcus aureus* is frequently the causative agent in right-sided endocarditis. Peripheral and pulmonary embolic phenomena occur.

Viral hepatitis has long been common among intravenous drug abusers owing to the practice of sharing needles during an injection session. In recent years, this illness has been overshadowed by the appearance of AIDS. In 1986, 50 to 60 per cent of patients in methadone programs in some large cities tested positive for HIV antibodies, and it has been suggested that this group is particularly susceptible to the infection because the drugs suppress host resistance. Most of those being treated for AIDS had not previously received treatment for their drug abuse. AIDS not only is becoming a major cause of death among intravenous drug abusers but also threatens the general population because the abusers constitute a major reservoir for the virus.

Among applicants for drug abuse treatment, 75 to 80 per cent of heroin users have significantly abnormal liver function tests. These findings may be related to persistent chronic hepatitis, but alcohol, malnutrition, allergic phenomena, and the toxic effects of adulterants may contribute. Pulmonary complications include pneumonia, abscess, infarct, and tuberculosis. Disseminated extrapulmonary tuberculosis has been reported. Angiothrombotic pulmonary hypertension and granulomatosis result from the intravenous injection of foreign bodies, including talc or cotton. Other complications include nephropathy, local arterial occlusion, phlebitis, mycotic aneurysms, and necrotizing angiitis.

Neurologic complications of street heroin use include transverse myelitis, acute inflammatory polyneuropathy, peripheral nerve lesions, toxic amblyopia secondary to quinine, and muscle disorders, including acute rhabdomyolysis with myoglobinuria and a fibrosing chronic myopathy. Septic states may lead to bacterial meningitis and brain, subdural, and epidural abscesses. Tetanus may result from dirty needles.

Pregnant addicts suffer a high incidence of toxemia and premature deliveries. About 50 per cent of their newborns require treatment of withdrawal symptoms.

Treatment

There are more distinctly different kinds of treatment available for dependence on opioid drugs than for any other type of drug dependence. As with other drugs, the prevention of relapse to drug-seeking behavior is the most difficult aspect, as described later. The treatment of *acute overdose* is effective and straightforward. In any emergency situation in which opioid overdose is suspected, naloxone should be administered, preferably intravenously. The patient will have constricted pupils, and a dose of 0.4 mg of naloxone should cause an increase in pupil size, respiratory rate, and alertness within several minutes. Repeated doses may be necessary if the patient does not respond within several minutes to the first dose. An absent response to naloxone excludes the diagnosis of opioid overdose.

There is virtually no risk in giving naloxone, but the potential benefits mean that it should be tried even in doubtful cases. There are, however, two pitfalls that should be mentioned. One is that not only will naloxone reverse the overdose, but also it will go beyond mere reversal and actually precipitate *withdrawal* symptoms in opioid-dependent persons. To avoid this, the dose of naloxone should be titrated according to the level of consciousness and respiratory rate. The second is that the overdose may recur as the naloxone is metabolized. Naloxone should be titrated via an intravenous drip or repeated every 2 to 3 hours with careful monitoring of vital signs for at least 24 hours.

The opioid withdrawal syndrome varies in severity and duration, depending on the specific drug, dose, and duration of use. The typical heroin-dependent person notes the onset of withdrawal six to ten hours after the last injection. Feelings of drug craving, anxiety, restlessness, irritability, sweating,

rhinorrhea, and yawning develop early. These are followed by dilated pupils, sneezing, piloerection, anorexia, nausea, vomiting, diarrhea, abdominal cramps, bone pains, myalgias, tremors, sleep disturbance, and, very rarely, convulsions or cardiovascular collapse. Untreated, these symptoms peak at 36 to 48 hours and gradually subside over 5 to 10 days. Withdrawal is generally not life threatening, and it has been compared with a severe case of the "flu." There is also a protracted abstinence syndrome consisting of mild symptoms of anxiety, sleep disturbance, and autonomic nervous system instability, which may persist for six months after acute withdrawal. Longer acting opioids, such as methadone, produce an abstinence syndrome that develops more slowly and with less intensity but that persists much longer.

Medically assisted withdrawal is usually accomplished using methadone, beginning with a test dose of 20 mg. If 20 mg has no appreciable effect on the signs and symptoms within one hour, an additional 20 mg can be given. The methadone can be gradually reduced over seven to ten days. An alternative is clonidine, an alpha$_2$-adrenergic agonist/partial agonist, which produces complex central effects that result in reduced central adrenergic outflow. Developed for the treatment of hypertension, clonidine has also been found to reduce many of the signs of autonomic dysfunction during opioid withdrawal. Thus clonidine can be useful in situations in which methadone is not available. Beginning with low doses of 0.1 to 0.2 mg to minimize the possibility of postural hypotension, clonidine can be increased to 1 to 1.5 mg daily in divided doses over four to ten days and then tapered over the next five days.

CANNABIS (Marijuana and Hashish)

Cannabis is not a single drug, but rather a complex preparation containing many biologically active chemicals. Δ-9-Tetrahydrocannabinol (Δ-9-THC) accounts for most of the pharmacologic effects of the complex.

Patterns of Abuse

Cannabis has been used in many societies as a form of folk medicine and for relaxation, but throughout the 1970's, its use increased explosively in the United States. In 1979, more than 50 million Americans reported using the drug at least once, and 9 per cent of high school seniors reported daily use. In the 1980's, the popularity of this drug has declined somewhat, but it is still in widespread use. The vast majority of users smoke marijuana cigarettes or hashish pipes in groups in which the ritual of preparation and sharing is part of the social interaction. Others demonstrate a compulsive pattern of daily use, with lives dominated by the acquisition and use of cannabis.

Pharmacology

Cannabis preparations are three to four times more potent when smoked than when taken orally. After inhalation, effects begin within three minutes, they peak within one hour, and the subject reports feeling "normal" within three hours. There is evidence, however, that psychomotor effects, such as impairment on eye tracking and vigilance tasks, may be evident for up to 11 hours after a single dose.

The acute physiologic effects of cannabis are dose related and include an increase in heart rate, conjunctival vascular congestion, decreased intraocular pressure, bronchodilation, increased airway conductance, and peripheral vasodilation. Dryness of mouth, fine tremors, ataxia, nystagmus, nausea, and vomiting have been noted. Sleep patterns are altered, and orthostatic hypotension occurs infrequently.

Psychoactive effects depend on the dose, route of administration, personality and experience of the user, and the environment in which the drug is used. Enhanced perceptions of colors, sounds, and tastes have been reported. Time seems to pass slowly, and the ability to learn new facts is impaired. There is often some drowsiness and inattentiveness, which may account for some of the poor performance on driving simulators. *Motor vehicular driving performance is definitely impaired by cannabis,* and this may persist for several hours after the period of obvious intoxication. Tolerance and physical dependence have been experimentally demonstrated with regular cannabis use. This is not relevant to the occasional user, but daily heavy users show clinical evidence of withdrawal when deprived of access to cannabis.

Cannabis contains chemicals with unusually high lipid solubility and thus a high affinity for brain tissue. Metabolites persist for several weeks, although their biologic significance is unknown. Urine tests for marijuana can remain positive for more than a week after a dose and even longer in chronic users. Positive urine tests have also been experimentally demonstrated in subjects who simply sat in a small room for several hours where marijuana was being smoked.

Cannabis derivatives have been investigated for their therapeutic potential in several illnesses. The antiemetic effect has been useful to some patients in reducing the nausea produced by cancer chemotherapy. The accompanying psychologic effects have so far limited its usefulness. Glaucoma, convulsive seizures, asthma, and muscle spasticity are other conditions in which a cannabis or a synthetic analogue may eventually prove useful.

Adverse Effects

Most clinicians believe that regular cannabis use by adolescents impairs maturation and often results in poor social and scholastic adjustment. Although there is no way to experimentally demonstrate causality, cannabis use is associated with poor academic performance. Occasional users have fewer problems, but acute panic, paranoid reactions, and frightening distortions of body image are sometimes experienced. Rarely, these reactions are severe enough to require emergency room treatment. Such reactions seem to be more common with higher doses and with oral administration than with smoking, which is easier to titrate. Patients with a history of schizophrenia may be particularly sensitive to adverse consequences of cannabis and should be warned to avoid it.

The cardiac stimulatory effects of cannabis may pose a threat to patients with cardiovascular disease. Chronic smoking of cannabis produces inflammatory changes in the bronchi and sinusitis. Cannabis is carcinogenic experimentally, but clinical studies are confounded by the concurrent use of tobacco by virtually all regular cannabis smokers.

Treatment

The acute anxiety reactions produced by cannabis are seldom severe enough to warrant medical attention. Treatment should be supportive and reassuring, with frequent reminders of the drug-induced nature of the symptoms. Benzodiazepines may be indicated in more severely agitated states. For the chronic heavy user, treatment is much more difficult. Such patients typically insist that treatment is not necessary and they feel no need to stop using cannabis on a daily basis. Meanwhile, they are failing in school or employment. Psychotherapy is unlikely to be of value unless the cannabis consumption can be interrupted. Hospitalization or entrance into a therapeutic community may be indicated, if the patient can be so persuaded. Medication is usually not required to treat withdrawal, and the drug-free patient clears mentally over several weeks. Psychotherapy is often necessary in addition to removing the cannabis.

Marijuana and Health: Report of a Study by a Committee of the Institute of Medicine: Division of Health Sciences Policy. Washington, D.C., National Academy Press, 1982. *Critical review of the published reports of marijuana effects on organ systems and behavior.*

PSYCHEDELICS

Psychedelic drugs include the following:

1. Lysergic acid diethylamide (LSD)
2. Dimethyltryptamine (DMT)
3. Phencyclidine (PCP)
4. Mescaline
5. Psilocybin
6. 5-Methoxy-3,4-methylene dioxyamphetamine (MDMA; "ecstasy")

Many drugs at some dose will produce hallucinations, but the drugs classified here reliably produce distortions in perception or in thinking as a primary effect, even at low dose. This category represents several chemical classes and different mechanisms of action. Phencyclidine, in particular, differs from the others in that it produces, in addition to hallucinations, analgesia and amphetamine-like stimulation.

Patterns of Abuse

Hallucinogenic drugs are among the oldest known psychoactive drugs, having long served as adjuncts to religious practices in some societies. During the 1960's they became well known on college campuses, where they were used in an effort to "gain insight" or experiment in expanding the potential of the mind. Physicians in emergency rooms were frequently called upon to treat young people suffering from "bad trips" or adverse reactions to these sessions. One of the problems with the use of illicit supplies of these drugs is their gross mislabeling. Chemical analysis of samples obtained from street purchases shows that phencyclidine ("angel dust," PCP) and by-products of phencyclidine are often the active ingredient in LSD or psilocybin purchases. Thus users often get unexpected and severe effects. Phencyclidine is available only from clandestine laboratories—hence its purity varies widely. The by-products produced during phencyclidine synthesis may cause severe toxic symptoms.

The use of psychedelics declined in the later 1970's and early 1980's, but the use of PCP has recently shown an upsurge. The typical pattern of psychedelic drug use involves intermittent rather than daily use. Recently, there has been great interest in MDMA, known as "ecstasy." This drug has been reported to facilitate insight and maturation and thus enhance the effects of psychotherapy. A few therapists have supported this notion and encouraged their patients to use MDMA. The drug has never been studied in any organized clinical trial, however, and thus there is no evidence to support these claims. Similar claims were made for LSD in the past, and serious attempts failed to demonstrate scientifically a beneficial effect. Both MDMA and the closely related MDA have been shown to be toxic to serotonergic nerve cells.

Pharmacology

LSD is the most potent psychedelic drug known. The usual illicit street dose is around 200 μg, but doses as low as 20 μg produce psychologic effects in susceptible individuals. Central sympathomimetic stimulation occurs within 20 minutes of oral ingestion and is characterized by mydriasis, hyperthermia, tachycardia, elevated blood pressure, piloerection, increased alertness, and facilitation of monosynaptic reflexes. Nausea and vomiting occasionally occur.

Psychoactive effects of LSD develop within one to two hours. These vary with the subject, dose, setting, expectation, and mood. Perceptions are heightened and may become overwhelming. Afterimages are prolonged and may overlap with ongoing perceptions. There may be a sense of unusual clarity, and one's thoughts may assume extraordinary importance. Time seems to pass slowly, and body distortions are commonly perceived. True hallucinations, usually visual, may occur in susceptible individuals. Mood is highly variable and labile and may range from expansive reactions characterized by euphoria and self-confidence to a constricted reaction marked by depression and panic.

The syndrome begins to clear after 10 to 12 hours, but fatigue and tension may persist for an additional 24 hours. The duration of action of mescaline is about 12 hours and that of psilocybin is 4 to 6 hours. Tolerance develops within three to four days to repeated daily doses of LSD, but recovery is rapid and weekly use of the same dose is possible.

Phencyclidine comes in various forms (powder, liquid, capsule, and tablet) and often is taken inadvertently when the user is expecting something else. It produces a prompt stimulant effect similar to that with amphetamine and usually a feeling of euphoria. Ataxia, slurred speech, nystagmus, and feelings of numbness are common. At higher doses, frightening and bizarre visual hallucinations can arise. There may be hostile or aggressive behavior and amnesia for the episode. With still higher doses, catatonia and coma occur, with the patient's eyes open and the pupils partially dilated. Heart rate and blood pressure are elevated. Tolerance to the stimulant effects occurs, and mild withdrawal symptoms have been observed in daily users.

Adverse Effects

The acute reactions such as panic or psychosis ("bad trip") are the most common complications of psychedelic use. With LSD, these vary in intensity and occasionally have led to suicide or self-injury. Phencyclidine is more likely to produce a severe reaction that results in suicide, often by drowning. Assaults and murders have been attributed to the effects of phencyclidine, and aggressive behavior can occur during the psychotic episode.

Prolonged psychotic episodes sometimes occur after psychedelic use. It is not known whether these can occur only in individuals who have pre-existing tendencies toward psychosis. Many clinicians believe that chronic use or high doses of psychedelics, especially phencyclidine, can produce prolonged psychosis even in healthy individuals.

Overdose resulting in death can occur with phencyclidine. The syndrome can progress rapidly from aggressive psychotic behavior to coma with elevated blood pressure, dilated pupils, muscular rigidity, arrhythmias, and seizures.

Another adverse effect of psychedelic use is known as "flashbacks." These are a brief reappearance of the hallucinations or distortions experienced during the acute ingestion, recurring days or weeks after the last psychedelic dose. "Flashbacks" appear to be more common with heavy use, and they eventually disappear without treatment.

Treatment

The use of medication in an emergency situation with a patient suffering from an unknown drug reaction can be dangerous owing to progression of the street drug effect with further absorption from the gut and to possible drug interactions with any prescribed medications. Thus treatment of acute panic reactions is best accomplished, when possible, by a supportive environment, observation, and reassurance. In severely agitated patients, intramuscularly administered lorazepam or haloperidol can be used. Prolonged psychosis requires hospitalization and treatment with neuroleptics.

Treatment of phencyclidine overdose may require support of vital signs. Gastric lavage with activated charcoal may prevent further absorption of the drug. To enhance the excretion of phencyclidine, acidification of the urine may be accomplished acutely by intravenously administered ammonium chloride, 75 mg per kilogram per day in four divided doses, or ascorbic acid, 500 mg every four hours, with repeated monitoring of blood pH, blood gases, blood urea

nitrogen (BUN), blood ammonia, and electrolytes. If symptoms are mild, cranberry juice and 1 or 2 grams of ascorbic acid given orally four times per day may be sufficient.

Anticholinergic Compounds

Effects in some ways similar to those of psychedelic drugs may be produced by ingestion of the alkaloids *atropine, hyoscyamine, and scopolamine* in their natural forms. These are found in "herbal teas" and a variety of proprietary medications, and several deaths from their use have occurred. Excessive use of *antihistaminic* compounds with anticholinergic effects also occurs. Psychoactive effects are those of an acute toxic delirium with confusion, visual or tactile hallucinations, and amnesia for the episode. Symptoms of the potent peripheral effects of the intoxication include dilated pupils, tachycardia, dry mouth, flushing, and hyperthermia. Treatment is symptomatic and consists of protecting the patient from self-injury, providing fluids, and reducing the fever. Administration of cholinesterase inhibitors and lorazepam intramuscularly may be indicated in severe cases. Phenothiazines are contraindicated because of their anticholinergic effects. Anticholinergic drugs are sometimes sold as hallucinogenics, thus creating a potentially dangerous additive interaction if a phenothiazine is administered in the emergency room to treat a "bad trip."

INHALANTS

Examples of inhalants include the following:

1. Toluene (airplane glue)
2. Gasoline
3. Amyl nitrite
4. Kerosene
5. Carbon tetrachloride
6. Nitrous oxide

Chemicals that are volatile at room temperatures and that produce perceptible changes in brain function when inhaled have been popular among certain groups as a means of producing altered states of consciousness. There are characteristic patterns for each chemical.

Organic solvents, such as toluene, are typically used by children beginning at about age 12. During the 1970's, 10 to 12 per cent of high school seniors reported having tried some inhalant as a drug at least once. The material is usually placed in a plastic bag, and the vapors are inhaled. Dizziness and intoxication are described after several minutes of inhalation. Inhalant abuse also involves the use of aerosol sprays containing fluorocarbon propellants. Prolonged exposure or daily use may result in toxic effects on several organ systems, including cardiac arrhythmias, bone marrow depression, cerebral degeneration, and damage to liver, kidney, and peripheral nerves. Death has occasionally been attributed to inhalant abuse, probably via the mechanism of cardiac arrhythmias, especially accompanying exercise or associated with upper airway obstruction.

Amyl nitrite is a yellowish, volatile, inflammable liquid with a fruity odor. It produces dilation of smooth muscle and has been used in the past for treatment of angina. In recent years, amyl nitrite has been used to enhance orgasm, particularly by male homosexuals. It is sold in the form of room deodorizers and can produce a feeling of "rush," flushing, and dizziness. Adverse effects include palpitations, postural hypotension, and headache progressing to loss of consciousness.

Nitrous oxide, alone or in combination with oxygen, and *halothane* are sometimes used as intoxicants by medical personnel. Compulsive use and chronic toxicity have not been reported, but there are obvious acute dangers of the unauthorized use of such potent agents.

Treatment

Since the effects of solvents are brief, specific acute treatments are generally not indicated. When inhalant use is chronic or associated with other psychiatric diagnoses, specific psychiatric treatment and measures to prevent relapse are indicated.

Lewis JD, Moritz D, Mellis LP: Long term toluene abuse. Am J Psychiatry 138:368, 1981. *Case reports and review of the literature.*

Sharp CW, Brehem ML: Review of Inhalants: From Euphoria to Dysfunction. NIDA Research Monograph Series No. 15, National Institute on Drug Abuse, Rockville, Md. 20857. *Good review of clinical and toxicologic aspects of the spectrum of inhalant problems.*

NICOTINE

The medical consequences of the smoking of tobacco products are covered in many chapters of this book because the effects are so widespread. As the dangers of smoking have become so well known, it has become more apparent that the smoking of cigarettes can produce a very powerful dependence on nicotine. Cessation of smoking may be very difficult even in patients who strongly desire to remain abstinent (Ch. 11).

ILLICIT SYNTHETIC DRUGS (Designer Drugs)

The so-called designer drugs are produced in clandestine laboratories, and they vary in their composition and purity. Fentanyl analogues have been produced that have extremely potent opioid actions and have resulted in overdose deaths. Other attempts at synthesis of opioids have resulted in toxic compounds. A recent example is MPTP, a toxic by-product of botched attempts to synthesize a meperidine (Demerol) analogue, which produces an irreversible Parkinson's syndrome (Ch. 468). Other chemicals recently found in street samples are phenethylamines, which are analogues of amphetamine and various analogues of phencyclidine. In evaluating the drug history of any patient, the physician must remember that those who purchase drugs on the street have no way of knowing what they actually take.

TREATMENT OF DRUG DEPENDENCE

The treatment of drug dependence involves four stages (Table 16–1): acknowledgment, detoxification, pharmacotherapy, and psychiatry.

ACKNOWLEDGMENT OF THE PROBLEM. Rarely does a patient in the early and most treatable phase of drug dependence spontaneously volunteer for treatment. Friends or relatives who observe the signs of a drug problem must confront the patient. Often the family physician is in a good position to notice the problem early and convince the patient to enter treatment. Confrontation is best accomplished when several concerned people approach the patient together in a firm but supportive way. When confronted with evidence of a drug problem, most persons will continue to deny its existence, making persistence necessary.

DETOXIFICATION. The pharmacologic aspects of detoxification were covered in the discussions of specific drug categories. In some cases, hospitalization is mandatory, particularly when there is a large degree of physical dependence. If, however, the drug taking can be interrupted while the individual remains an outpatient, this can be far less expensive and just as effective. "Treatment programs" that advertise a 30-day inpatient treatment of drug dependence are misleading, because the heart of effective treatment is the continued therapy, usually lasting months or years, designed to prevent relapse after the patient returns to work or school. Frequently, the patient has so much cognitive impairment during the detoxification period that he or she retains little of therapy or education provided during this first phase.

PHARMACOTHERAPY. This mode of therapy has been discussed under specific drug categories. For the most part, this involves treatment of specific psychiatric disorders, such as affective disorders or psychosis commonly associated with a particular form of drug dependence. It must be remembered that patients who have abused one drug will have a strong likelihood of abusing a prescribed psychoactive drug. For this reason, antianxiety agents or sedatives should rarely, if ever, be prescribed in the rehabilitation of drug-dependent persons.

Certain pharmacotherapies are directed at the drug-seeking behavior rather than an associated psychiatric disorder. The use of disulfiram (Antabuse) in the treatment of alcoholics is discussed in Ch. 15. Opioid-dependent patients, who have repeatedly relapsed after detoxification, can be transferred from use of illicit drugs to methadone maintenance. The patient can then be maintained on a steady dose of methadone as a substitute for his or her opioid drug of choice. The advantage is that the patient is stabilized owing to the long duration of action of methadone and, if properly managed, experiences no "highs" or "lows." Patients are able to function well on methadone and perform complex tasks competently, including, for those physicians who require this treatment, the practice of medicine. The methadone enables the patient to participate in a rehabilitation program, including psychotherapy. Methadone may involve several years of maintenance and must be used only in authorized programs in which staff have received specialized training.

Naltrexone (Trexan) is a new drug that is a relatively long-acting opioid antagonist. Before receiving this medication, patients must first be thoroughly detoxified, or the naltrexone will precipitate withdrawal. Since naltrexone blocks opiate receptors, the effects of impulsive opioid use are prevented while naltrexone is in the body. This new treatment has been successful in conjunction with a comprehensive rehabilitation program, including a wide range of psychotherapies. The problem is that naltrexone must be taken at least two or three times per week to protect against relapse and it requires strong motivation on the part of the patient to remain opioid free.

PSYCHOTHERAPY. Psychotherapy is generally similar across all classes of drugs. It should be started as early as possible in the treatment program, but it is of little value when the patient is still intoxicated or confused. This treatment is, however, completely compatible with pharmacotherapy, such as psychoactive medication, methadone, naltrexone, disulfiram, or nicotine chewing gum. Such psychotherapy is broadly defined and involves counseling regarding job hunting or legal problems, family therapy, group therapy, individual therapy, all types of behavioral treatments, and self-help programs such as Narcotics Anonymous. The purpose of these treatments is to teach the patient

TABLE 16–1. TREATMENT OF DRUG DEPENDENCE

	Confrontation	Detoxification	Pharmacotherapy	Psychotherapy
Sedatives	S	Diazepam or phenobarbital	Antidepressants as needed	S
Stimulants	I	Not usually needed	Antidepressants or neuroleptics	I
Opioids	M	Methadone or clonidine	Methadone, naltrexone, or antidepressants	M
Cannabis	I	None	Antidepressants as needed	I
Psychedelics	L	None	Neuroleptics as needed	L
Inhalants	A	None	None	A
Nicotine	R	Nicotine gum	None	R

alternate behaviors to drug ingestion and to enable him or her to deal more effectively with problems of living. The general physician often can convince patients to join a specialized treatment program and can collaborate in the medical aspects of the treatment. Severe forms of drug dependence, however, are best managed by a treatment team specially trained in this area of medicine.

Childress AR, McLellan AT, O'Brien CP: Behavioral therapies for substance abuse. Int J Addict 20:947, 1985. *Comprehensive review of behavioral therapies for dependence disorders.*
Woody GE, Luborsky L, McLellan AT, et al: Psychotherapy for opiate addiction: Does it help? Arch Gen Psychiatry 40:639, 1983. *Largest controlled study of psychotherapy in addiction found definite benefits for psychotherapy, and the benefits were greatest for those with significant coexisting psychiatric disorders.*

17 IMMUNIZATION

R. Gordon Douglas, Jr.

Childhood immunizations continue to receive major emphasis as methods of controlling infectious diseases. A standard recommendation for such immunizations is presented in Table 17–1. Detailed immunization recommendations for the common childhood diseases are best secured from two standard references: the current issue of the Red Book of the American Academy of Pediatrics and the Collective Immunization Recommendations by the Advisory Committee on Immunization Practices of the United States Public Health Service.

It is also important to maintain immunizations begun in childhood and to utilize those immunizations primarily intended for adults. The internist must ensure that routine immunizations such as diphtheria-tetanus and influenza are up to date and that adequate records are maintained. He also must recognize special situations that require less commonly used products or booster doses of common immunizing agents.

Both active and passive immunizing agents are available (Tables 17–2 and 17–3). Active immunization, which is most often carried out in anticipation of exposure to a disease, is achieved by using one of the following as immunogens: inactivated virus or viral protein, live attenuated virus, bacterial protein, or bacterial polysaccharides. Live attenuated virus vaccines are associated with greater and more durable immunity than inactivated viral vaccines, but this is achieved at the expense of greater inherent risks. Bacterial proteins and polysaccharides are effective immunogens, but their protective effect is not lifelong.

Passive immunization, which is used for individuals who have recently been or may soon be exposed to a disease, is achieved by using immune globulin (IG), a preparation of pooled human immune globulins that contain specified amounts of antibody against diphtheria, measles, one type of poliovirus, hepatitis A, and hepatitis B. Specific immune globulin preparations are also available, e.g., those against varicella zoster, tetanus, rabies, or hepatitis B. They are obtained from donor pools preselected for high antibody content. Human immune globulins are not associated with a risk of transmitting hepatitis A and B. They are much less likely to evoke hypersensitivity reactions than are immune globulins derived from animals. When using animal-derived antitoxins, intradermal testing for hypersensitivity should always precede their administration.

The physician must consider the risks and benefits to an individual patient when administering a vaccine or immune globulin. With regard to risks, certain general principles must be kept in mind. Hypersensitivity to any vaccine component is a contraindication to use of that vaccine. This is of most

TABLE 17–1. RECOMMENDED SCHEDULE FOR ACTIVE IMMUNIZATION OF NORMAL INFANTS AND CHILDREN*

Recommended Age†	Vaccines‡	Comments
2 mo	DPT-1, OPV-1	Can be given earlier in areas of high endemicity
4 mo	DPT-2, OPV-2	6-wk to 2-mo interval desired between OPV doses to avoid interference
6 mo	DPT-3	An additional dose of OPV at this time is optional in areas with a high risk of polio exposure
15 mo§	MMR, DPT-4, OPV-3	Completion of primary series of DPT and OPV
25 mo§	*Hemophilus* B polysaccharide vaccine	Can be given at 18-23 mo for children in groups who are thought to be at increased risk of disease, e.g., day-care center attendees
4–6 yr**	DPT-5, OPV-4	Preferably at or before school entry
14–16 yr	Td	Repeat every 10 yr throughout life

*From Immunization Practices Advisory Committee, Centers for Disease Control: New recommended schedule for active immunization of normal infants and children. MMWR 35:578, 1986.
†These recommended ages should not be construed as absolute; 2 mo can be 6 to 10 weeks, for example.
‡DPT=diphtheria and tetanus toxoids and pertussis vaccine. OPV = oral, attenuated poliovirus vaccine containing poliovirus types 1, 2, and 3. MMR = live measles, mumps, and rubella viruses in a combined vaccine. Td = Adult tetanus toxoid and diphtheria toxoid in combination, which contains the same dose of tetanus toxoid as DTP or DT and a reduced dose of diphtheria toxoid.
§Simultaneous administration of MMR, DTP, and OPV may be given.
**Up to the seventh birthday.

concern with vaccines grown in eggs, such as measles, mumps, and influenza vaccine. This risk may be assessed by history of ability to eat eggs without adverse effects. Although acute hypersensitivity reactions may also be a theoretic problem with vaccines grown in cell cultures, such reactions are very rare. Hypersensitivity to antibiotics (e.g., neomycin) contained in vaccines is another possible risk. However, penicillin is not used in the manufacture of any vaccine, and information concerning specific components of a vaccine is available in the package insert. Persons with acute febrile illness should not be vaccinated until they recover to avoid additive toxicity and possible diminished response.

Patients with altered immunity or household contacts of such persons should not be given live attenuated virus vaccines because of the risk of disseminated disease. In addition, live attenuated virus vaccines should not be given to pregnant women, except in rare circumstances, because of theoretic risk to the fetus.

Persons receiving live attenuated vaccines should not receive immune globulin or hyperimmune globulin simultaneously, since passively acquired antibody can interfere with the response to such vaccines. Children under 12 months of age should not be given measles, mumps, or rubella vaccines because of possible interference with antibody response by maternal antibody. Several vaccines can be given together without loss of efficacy. For example, influenza and pneumococcal vaccines may be given simultaneously (in different sites), and trivalent oral polio vaccine may be given with combined measles-mumps-rubella vaccine without alteration of antibody responses. Patients receiving intermittent immunosuppressive drugs should be given inactivated vaccines between courses of therapy to maximize antibody responses.

TETANUS. Tetanus toxoid is highly effective and provides long-lasting protection. Antitoxins persist at protective levels, for ten years or more in individuals who have received a full-immunizing series. There are four preparations; tetanus toxoid absorbed (T), tetanus and diphtheria toxoids adsorbed (for adult use) (Td), diphtheria and tetanus toxoids and pertussis vaccine (DTP), and diphtheria and tetanus toxoids adsorbed (for pediatric use) (DT). The aluminum phosphate adsorbed

TABLE 17–2. COMMONLY USED ACTIVE IMMUNIZING AGENTS IN ADULTS

Disease	Type of Material	Preparation	Dosage Schedule*	Other Uses, Comments
Routine use for all adults:				
Tetanus	Bacterial toxoid	Tetanus toxoid combined with diphtheria toxoid, adult type (Td); tetanus toxoid (T)	IM at least every 10 yr	Management of wounds
Diphtheria	Bacterial toxoid	Diphtheria toxoid combined with tetanus toxoid, adult type (Td)	IM at least every 10 yr	Management of contacts of cases of diphtheria
Use in selected populations:				
1. Elderly persons and persons with chronic disease				
Influenza	Inactivated virus	Influenza virus vaccines, trivalent	SC annually	Annual immunization of high-risk individuals: persons with chronic heart or lung disease or other chronic diseases, nursing home residents, age > 65 yr; medical personnel
Pneumococcal disease	Bacterial polysaccharide	Pneumococcal polysaccharide vaccine	SC once	Immunization of high-risk persons over 2 yr of age
2. Postexposure prophylaxis of animal bites				
Rabies	Inactivated virus	Human diploid cell rabies vaccine (HDCV)	Five 1-ml doses	Pre-exposure prophylaxis only in special situations
3. Adolescents and young adults				
Rubella	Live attenuated virus	Rubella virus vaccine, live	SC once	Adolescent and adult females who are unimmunized or who have no serum antibodies; hospital workers
Measles	Live attenuated virus	Measles live vaccine	SC once	Adolescents and young adults who have not had measles and have no serum antibodies to measles or have not received previous live virus vaccine; postexposure protection.
Mumps	Live attenuated virus	Mumps virus vaccine, live	SC once	Prepubertal and adolescent males who have not had mumps or mumps vaccine
4. Special groups				
Hepatitis B	Inactivated virus	Hepatitis B vaccine	Three doses	Persons at high risk of exposure to hepatitis B; health care workers, hemodialysis patient, users of illicit injectable drugs; and other travelers
Poliomyelitis	Live attenuated virus	Poliovirus vaccine, live oral, trivalent (oral polio vaccine, OPV)	Three doses	Not for routine use; IPV for primary immunization of special groups of adults; OPV for boosters in special situations; need for routine booster not established
		Poliomyelitis vaccine (inactivated polio vaccine, IPV)	Three doses	

*IM = Intramuscularly; SC = subcutaneously.

preparations induce more persistent antitoxin titers than fluid forms. DTP and DT are used only for primary immunization and boosters in infants and young children. For all persons over seven years of age, Td is the immunizing preparation of choice because of the increasing frequency of reactions with age to the full dose of diphtheria toxoid contained in DT. T is available for those allergic to diphtheria toxoid. For immunization of individuals not immunized as infants, a series of three doses of Td should be given intramuscularly, the second dose four to eight weeks after the first, and the third, six months to one year after the second. A single booster immunization of Td is recommended for adults every ten years.

Tetanus Prophylaxis in Wound Management. For a clean minor wound, Td is recommended only if the history of tetanus immunization is uncertain, if fewer than three doses had previously been administered, or if it is more than ten years since the last dose. For all other wounds, Td is indicated unless the patient has received three or more doses of toxoid within five years. In addition, for those with such wounds and incomplete or uncertain vaccine status, 250 units of tetanus immune globulin (TIG) should be considered with Td in separate syringes and at separate sites. Adsorbed Td is preferred over fluid toxoid for administration with TIG because of delayed absorption of the toxoid.

DIPHTHERIA. Diphtheria immunizations significantly decrease the occurrence and severity of clinical disease. Protective levels of antibody persist for at least ten years following a primary series or booster doses of diphtheria toxoid. Diphtheria toxoid is combined with tetanus toxoid and pertussis

vaccine (DTP) for use in infants and young children, or with tetanus toxoid (Td), adult type, for use in persons over seven years of age. The diphtheria component in the latter material is only 10 to 25 per cent of that in DTP. A separate diphtheria toxoid is not available in the United States. The primary and booster immunization schedules described for tetanus provide adequate protection against diphtheria.

Diphtheria Immunization for Case Contacts. All asymptomatic, unimmunized close contacts of patients with diphtheria should receive either benzathine penicillin or erythromycin as well as diphtheria toxoid. Since the risk of diphtheria is low in those receiving chemoprophylaxis, diphtheria antitoxin should not be administered. Antitoxin, which is of equine origin, may be useful in therapy of diphtheria. Immediate hypersensitivity reactions occur in 7 per cent and serum sickness in 5 per cent.

INFLUENZA. Influenza epidemics can be expected almost every winter. Immunization efforts are aimed at protecting those at greatest risk of serious illness or death. At highest risk are those with chronic heart or lung disease and residents of nursing homes and other chronic care facilities. At high risk are persons with other underlying conditions, such as asthma, malignancy, and immunosuppressive disorders, those over 65 years of age, and children on chronic aspirin therapy. More than 10,000 deaths have occurred in 18 winters between 1957 and 1986, and on several occasions the number has exceeded 40,000.

Influenza vaccines are composed of highly purified inactivated virus. Whole virion (whole virus) and subvirion (split

TABLE 17–3. PASSIVE IMMUNIZATIONS FOR ADULTS

Disease	Name of Material	Comments and Use
Tetanus	Tetanus immune globulin human (TIG)	Management of tetanus-prone wounds
Diphtheria	Diphtheria antitoxin, equine	Treatment of established disease, high frequency of reactions to serum of nonhuman origin
Rabies	Rabies immunoglobulin, human (RIG)	Postexposure prophylaxis of animal bites
Rubella	Immune globulin, human (IG)	May modify or suppress symptoms but does not prevent infection or viremia
Measles	Immune globulin, human (IG)	Prevention or modification of disease in contacts; not for control of epidemics
Hepatitis A	Immune globulin, human (IG)	Protection of household contacts; control of epidemics; pre-exposure prophylaxis for travelers
Hepatitis B	Immune globulin, human (IG) Hepatitis B immune globulin, human (HBIG)	HBIG for needle stick or mucous membrane contact with HBsAG-positive persons; HBIG for infants born to mothers with HBsAg-positive hepatitis; IG for all other contacts
Herpes zoster/Varicella	Varicella zoster immune globulin (VZIG)	Persons under 15 years of age with underlying disease who have not had varicella and who are exposed to varicella
Erythroblastosis fetalis	Rh immune globulin (RhIG)	Rh-negative women who give birth to Rh-positive infants or who abort
Hypogamma-globulinemia	Immune globulin intravenous	Maintenance therapy
Idiopathic thrombocyto-penic purpura	Immune globulin intravenous	Therapy of acute episodes
Botulism	Monovalent E antitoxin, equine Bivalent A and B antitoxin, equine Trivalent A, B, and E antitoxin, equine	Treatment of botulism trivalent is preferred; most effective is type E
Snakebite	Antivenin, equine (North American coral snake antivenin) Antivenin, equine, Crotalidae, polyvalent	Specific for North American coral snake, *Micrurus fulvius* Effective for viper and pit viper, including rattlesnakes, copperheads, moccasins
Spider bite	Antivenin, equine	Specific for black widow spider, *Latrodectus mactans*, and other members of the genus

virus) preparations are available. In children, split virus vaccines have been associated with fewer side effects than whole virus vaccines, but in adults the vaccines are comparable. Each year vaccine composition is changed to reflect the most recent serotypes circulating in the United States and worldwide. The vaccine is almost always a trivalent vaccine containing two influenza A virus strains, as well as an influenza B virus strain. The protective efficacy against both influenza A and influenza B is about 70 per cent.

A small percentage of subjects will have local reactions consisting of redness and induration, which last 1 to 2 days. Fever and other systemic symptoms occur in only 1 to 2 per cent of subjects, begin 6 to 12 hours after vaccination, and persist for 1 to 2 days. Immediate reactions are extremely rare. In addition to vaccinating those in the highest risk and

high-risk categories, persons such as health care workers and family members capable of nosocomial transmission of influenza to high-risk persons should be vaccinated.

PNEUMOCOCCAL DISEASES. Pneumococcal pneumonia, meningitis, otitis media, and bacteremia occur with increased frequency in persons with sickle cell anemia, anatomic or functional asplenia, agammaglobulinemia, multiple myeloma, renal failure, cirrhosis and alcoholism, or basal skull fractures with cerebrospinal rhinorrhea. Persons with diabetes mellitus or chronic cardiorespiratory, hepatic, or renal disease and persons of increased age may also be at increased risk. Vaccine is intended for individuals who are at high risk.

A 23-valent polysaccharide vaccine containing types (Danish) 1, 2, 3, 4, 5, 6B, 7F, 8, 9N, 9V, 10A, 11A, 12F, 14, 15B, 17F, 18C, 19F, 19A, 20, 22F, 23F, 33F is available. These types have been shown to cause 90 per cent of bacteremic pneumococcal disease in the United States. Antibody responses in healthy persons over two years of age are excellent, and the vaccine has been shown to prevent pneumococcal disease. The duration of immunity is unknown. Mild local side effects occur in 50 per cent of subjects. Booster doses should not be given. Influenza and pneumococcal vaccine can be administered in different sites simultaneously without impairment of immune response or enhancement of side effects.

RABIES. *Postexposure Prophylaxis.* Postexposure rabies immunization should always include both passively administered antibody and vaccine, except for persons who have previously been immunized with rabies vaccine and have a documented adequate rabies antibody titer.

Rabies vaccine (human diploid) (HDCV) is an inactivated vaccine prepared from rabies virus growth in human diploid cell cultures. Rabies immune globulin, human (RIG) is antirabies gamma globulin concentrated from plasma of hyperimmunized human donors; it contains 150 international units (IU) per milliliter.

Following exposure to animals known or suspected to be rabid, five 1-ml doses of HDCV are given intramuscularly. The first dose is given as soon as possible after exposure, and additional doses are given on days 3, 7, 14, and 28 after the first dose.

At the time of the bite and concurrent wtih vaccine, RIG is administered only once at the beginning of antirabies prophylaxis to provide antibodies until the patient responds to vaccination. The dose is 20 IU per kilogram. If possible, up to half the dose of RIG should be thoroughly infiltrated in the area around the wound, and the rest should be administered intramuscularly.

Pre-exposure Immunization. Vaccine may be offered to persons in high-risk groups such as veterinarians, animal handlers, and laboratory workers. For pre-exposure immunization, three 1-ml injections of HDCV are given intramuscularly, one on each of days 0, 7, and 21 or 28. Booster doses should be given every two years for persons with continuing risk of exposure.

Adverse reactions to HDCV include local pain, erythema, swelling, and itching in about 25 per cent of patients, and mild systemic reactions such as headache, nausea, abdominal pain, muscle aches, and dizziness in about 20 per cent. Rare neurologic reactions have been reported; however, causal relationship has not been established.

RUBELLA. All persons should be immune to rubella. Evidence of immunity includes documented proof of having received vaccine or laboratory studies showing immunity, but not a clinical history of disease. All others should be vaccinated, particularly women of childbearing age and susceptible hospital workers, who, if infected, might transmit rubella to pregnant patients. Because of the theoretic risk to the fetus, females of childbearing age should receive vaccine only if they are not pregnant and must understand that they should not become pregnant for three months after vaccination. If a woman who has no immunity to rubella is pregnant, vaccine should be administered in the immediate postpartum period prior to discharge from the hospital. Administration of anti-Rho(D) immune globulin or other blood products is not a contraindication to rubella vaccination. Vaccinating susceptible children whose mothers or other household contacts are pregnant does not present a risk. Vaccination after exposure may not prevent illness, but it is not harmful.

Live attenuated rubella virus vaccine is prepared in human diploid cell cultures. It is available as a monovalent vaccine or in combination with measles (MR) or measles and mumps (MMR) vaccines. A single dose of vaccine induces antibodies in more than 95 per cent of susceptible persons, and vaccine-induced immunity is protective against clinical illness from natural exposure. Although the duration of immunity is not known, it is expected to be long term.

Rash and fever are occasional side effects. Arthralgia and transient arthritis, usually involving the small peripheral joints, may occur in up to 40 per cent of subjects. They generally begin two to ten weeks after vaccination, persist for one to three days, and rarely recur. Allergic reactions have not been associated with this vaccine, and it may be safely administered to persons with allergies to eggs, ducks, and feathers.

MEASLES. All adolescents and adults who have not had measles confirmed by a physician, who do not have laboratory evidence of measles immunity, or who have not been adequately immunized with live measles vaccine when 12 or more months of age should receive vaccine. Persons born prior to 1957 are likely to have been infected naturally and need not be vaccinated. Those vaccinated from 1963 to 1967 may have received inactivated vaccine and should be revaccinated. Persons who received live attenuated vaccine during that period, however, are considered adequately protected. Although established immunity is preferable, live measles vaccine, given within 72 hours of measles exposure, may provide protection.

Live attenuated measles virus vaccine, prepared in chick embryo cell cultures, is available as a monovalent vaccine or in combination with rubella (MR), mumps (MM), or mumps and rubella (MMR). Antibodies that are protective against measles develop in 95 per cent or more of vaccinees. The duration of protective effect, although unknown, appears to be long.

About 5 to 15 per cent of vaccinees will develop fever, beginning about the sixth day after vaccination and lasting up to five days. Transient rashes have been reported rarely. Encephalitis has been reported approximately once for every one million doses administered. No allergic reactions have been associated with the vaccine even among persons with allergies to eggs, chickens, and feathers. Measles vaccine is inactivated by heat and light; it should be stored at 2 to 8°C and protected from light to avoid vaccine failure.

Immune globulin (IG) has been shown to be effective in preventing or modifying measles in a susceptible person exposed less than six days previously. The dose is 0.25 ml per kilogram of body weight. Live measles vaccine can be given after three months. Although effective in individuals, IG should not be used instead of live measles virus vaccine to control epidemics.

MUMPS. Although mumps is generally self-limited, it may be moderately debilitating; and complications involving the central nervous system, including deafness, occur rarely. Orchitis may occur in up to 20 per cent of clinical mumps cases in postpubertal males, but sterility is rare. Susceptible adolescents and adults should be vaccinated against mumps unless otherwise contraindicated. Susceptibility can be determined by documentation of disease by a physician or laboratory or by documented immunization with live mumps vaccine when the subject was 12 months or more of age. Mumps vaccine is not recommended for persons born prior

to 1957, because they are likely to have been infected naturally and generally may be considered immune. Live attenuated mumps virus vaccine, prepared in chick embryo cell cultures, induces antibodies in over 90 per cent of recipients. The duration of immunity is unknown but is probably long lasting. Side effects are very rare and include allergic reactions, rash, and pruritus. No deaths have been reported.

HEPATITIS. Hepatitis B vaccine consists of purified inactivated hepatitis B surface antigen (HBsAg) particles obtained from chronic carriers or HBsAg made by genetically engineered yeast. Most data are available with the older vaccine. It is indicated for persons at high risk of exposure to hepatitis B, such as health care workers exposed to blood or blood products, hemodialysis patients, homosexual males, users of illicit injectable drugs, recipients of certain blood products, certain institutionalized individuals, household or sexual contacts of chronic carriers of HBsAg, and some international travelers. Vaccine is administered intramuscularly in three 20-μg doses at time 0, month 1, and month 6. Vaccine must be given in the deltoid; antibody responses are lower when the vaccine is given in the buttocks. Immunosuppressed and hemodialysis patients should receive 40-μg doses. Doses are one half of this value with the new recombinant vaccine. Efficacy is 80 to 95 per cent up to two years after vaccination. Local reactions and low-grade fever are mild and infrequent. There is no evidence of association with subsequent development of acquired immunodeficiency syndrome (AIDS). There are no contraindications, and there is no risk to those who are carriers or already immune.

Immune globulin (IG) offers effective protection against the clinical manifestations of hepatitis A. When exposure has occurred, 0.02 ml per kilogram of IG is given intramuscularly to persons with close personal contact who have not had hepatitis A. Usually, this means household or day care, but not school, hospital, office, or factory contacts. However, when outbreaks occur that are related to a school or institution, IG may be used to protect contacts. It should be given as early as possible after exposure but may be given up to two weeks thereafter, and protection will be achieved in approximately 80 to 90 per cent of the contacts. It is also useful for pre-exposure prophylaxis for travelers.

For hepatitis B, two preparations are available: IG and hepatitis B immunoglobulin (HBIG). IG produced since 1977 contains anti–hepatitis B antibodies. It may reduce the clinical severity of hepatitis B infection when infection is contracted by the percutaneous or oral route with a small viral inoculum. HBIG is prepared from donor pools preselected for high titer of antibody to hepatitis B (titer >1:100,000). It is recommended for acute exposure following a needle contact or a mucous membrane contact with HBsAg-positive blood. The dose is 0.06 ml per kilogram administered as soon as possible but within 24 hours, and a second dose is administered 25 to 30 days after the first. If HBIG is not available, IG may be given in the same dosage schedule. The first dose (20 μg) of a three-dose vaccine regimen should also be given. For infants born to mothers who are antigen (HBsAG) positive, 0.5 ml, together with hepatitis B vaccine (10 μg), given within 12 hours is recommended. Second and third doses of vaccine should be given at month 1 and month 6. Women at high risk should be screened prenatally for HBsAG. HBIG does not prevent maternal transmission. HBIG may also be used for those with sexual contact with HBsAG-positive persons.

POLIOMYELITIS. The risk of paralytic poliomyelitis is very small in the United States today, but it is important to maintain immunity of the population to prevent further outbreaks.

Routine primary vaccination of adults in the United States is not necessary. Most adults are already immune by virtue of wild-type poliovirus infection or prior vaccination. Vaccine is recommended in the following adults: laboratory workers handling specimens that may contain polioviruses, health care workers who are in close contact with patients who may be excreting polioviruses, and members of communities or specific population groups with disease caused by wild polioviruses. There are no data to substantiate a harmful effect of vaccine on the fetus, but it is advisable to avoid vaccination during pregnancy if possible. Immunocompromised patients, or household contacts of such patients, should not be given vaccine because of their substantially increased risk of vaccine-associated disease. Inactivated vaccine is safe in such patients, although development of protective immune response does not always occur.

Two types of poliovirus vaccines are currently licensed in the United States: oral polio vaccine (OPV) and inactivated polio vaccine (IPV). Both contain all three poliovirus types. The effectiveness of these vaccines is attested to by the dramatic decline in poliomyelitis since their introduction. For primary immunization of normal adults and young children, OPV is preferred because it induces intestinal immunity, is simple to administer, is well accepted by patients, and results in immunization of some contacts. For children it is usually given beginning at two months of age—an exception to the rule that maternal antibody interferes with development of protective antibody following live attenuated virus vaccines.

For adults who were not previously vaccinated, IPV may be considered because the risk of vaccine-associated paralysis following OPV is slightly higher in adults than in children, although it is exceedingly low in both groups. Three doses of IPV should be given at intervals of 1 to 2 months, and a fourth dose at 6 to 12 months after the third. For those who previously received only one or two doses of vaccine, the remaining required doses of either vaccine, regardless of interval, should be given. For those who have had a complete course, a booster dose of OPV may be given for high-risk individuals, but the need for such doses has not been established. Nonimmune parents of infants who are given OPV need not be vaccinated, but there is an exceedingly small risk of OPV-associated paralysis. Therefore, some physicians may wish to give these adults two doses of IPV one month apart or the full series before children receive OPV. If immediate protection is needed, OPV is recommended. IPV has not been associated with serious side effects in the past 20 years.

MENINGOCOCCAL DISEASE. Vaccines against *Neisseria meningitidis* serogroups A, C, Y, and W135 are now available in the United States. Routine vaccination against meningococcal disease is not recommended. The vaccines are reserved to control outbreaks of meningococcal disease caused by one of these serotypes. In the event of an epidemic caused by these serogroups, the population at risk should be identified by some reasonable boundary, and all residents or those at highest risk should be vaccinated. Vaccination should also be considered an adjunct to antibiotic chemoprophylaxis for household contacts of persons with meningococcal disease caused by these serogroups.

Four vaccines are available: monovalent A, monovalent C, bivalent A and C, and multivalent A, C, Y, and W135 combined. They are chemically defined antigens consisting of purified bacterial capsular polysaccharides, each inducing specific serogroup immunity. They have been shown to induce protective antibodies in more than 95 per cent of susceptible persons. A single dose of vaccine is sufficient. Local reactions to the vaccine are infrequent and mild, and serious side effects have not been reported.

HAEMOPHILUS INFLUENZAE **TYPE B DISEASE.** *H. influenza* type B is the most common cause of bacterial meningitis in the United States, occurring mostly among children less than five years of age. In addition, other serious infections occur with this pathogen: epiglottitis, sepsis, cellulitis, septic arthritis, osteomyelitis, pericarditis, and pneumonia. Recently, a vaccine composed of the purified capsular polysaccharide of *H. influenzae* type B has been licensed. Over 90 per cent of children more than two years of age develop protective

levels (0.15 µg per milliliter) of antibody in response to this vaccine.

It is recommended for all children at 24 months of age. For those at high risk, vaccination at 19 months may be considered. At present, insufficient data are available to recommend routine use in older children and adults at high risk of *H. influenzae* type disease.

Mild local reactions lasting less than 24 hours have occurred in up to 50 per cent and systemic or febrile reactions in fewer than 1 per cent. It may be given simultaneously with DTP.

TYPHOID. Routine administration of typhoid vaccine is no longer recommended for persons in the United States. Selective immunization is indicated for persons with intimate exposure to a documented typhoid carrier such as would occur with continued household contact. There is no reason to use typhoid vaccine for persons in areas of natural disaster such as floods or in rural summer camps. The adult dosage is 0.5 ml subcutaneously on two occasions, separated by four or more weeks.

TUBERCULOSIS. An attenuated strain of *Mycobacterium bovis*, bacille Calmette Guérin (BCG), may be protective against infection with *Mycobacterium tuberculosis*. It is not recommended for general use in this country. It is reserved for uninfected persons living in unavoidable contact with an uncontrolled infected person, or for groups with excessive rates of new infection that cannot be controlled by other measures. Excessive rates have been defined as more than 30 cases per 10,000 population.

OTHER DISEASES FOR WHICH ACTIVE IMMUNIZATIONS ARE AVAILABLE. A number of other vaccines licensed in the United States are used only for laboratory or field personnel working with the infectious agent or for other persons with unusual occupational exposure. These include cholera vaccine, smallpox vaccine, plague vaccine, anthrax vaccine, and Rocky Mountain spotted fever vaccine. Live virus vaccines for control of adenovirus types 4, 7, and 21 are available for military but not civilian use. Adenovirus vaccines are not attenuated, but rather produce immunity without disease when introduced into the gastrointestinal tract instead of the respiratory tract, the natural portal of entry.

VARICELLA. Varicella zoster immune globulin (VZIG) is prepared from pooled plasma containing high titers of antibody to varicella virus and is intended primarily for susceptible, immunodeficient children after significant exposure to chickenpox or zoster. VZIG is effective in preventing or modifying varicella infection in immunodeficient patients if administered within 96 hours after exposure. Because of the short supply of VZIG, it is distributed through regional blood centers, and its use is restricted to persons with one of the following illnesses or conditions: leukemia or lymphoma, congenital or acquired immunodeficiency, immunosuppressive treatment, or newborns of mothers who had onset of chickenpox less than five days before delivery or within 48 hours after delivery. In addition, exposure to chickenpox or varicella must have been via household contact, playmate contact, hospital contact, or contact between mother and newborn. The recipient should have a negative or unknown prior history of chickenpox and, for most purposes, be less than 15 years of age, since few patients 15 years of age or more are at risk of infection. The recommended dosage of VZIG is one vial for each 10 kg (22 lb) of body weight, up to a maximum of five vials. Thus, it would be advisable to screen immunodeficient children with a negative or unknown history of chickenpox for antibody to varicella zoster virus when first seen or first hospitalized, to avoid unnecessary administration of VZIG.

ERYTHROBLASTOSIS FETALIS. Rh immune globulin (RhIG) is effective in preventing erythroblastosis fetalis. RhIG is prepared from donors with high Rh antibody titer. It is recommended for Rh-negative women who give birth to Rh-positive infants or who undergo abortion. A single dose should be given within 72 hours after exposure, be it for delivery or abortion. Immunosuppression is transient, and RhIG may be required for Rh-negative women after each birth or abortion.

IMMUNE DEFICIENCY STATES. Intravenous immune globulin offers several advantages over intramuscular preparations: Therapeutic plasma levels can be achieved immediately, and dosage is not limited by muscle mass or bleeding tendencies. Such preparations contain antibodies to most common bacterial and viral pathogens.

Intravenous immune globulin has been shown to be useful in immunodeficiency states and in idiopathic thrombocytopenic purpura (ITP). For prophylaxis in immunodeficiency states, the usual dose is 100 to 200 mg per kilogram monthly. In patients with ITP, a dose of 400 mg per kilogram daily for five days is usual.

BOTULISM. Several preparations of equine antitoxin for passive immunization against *Clostridium botulinum* toxin are available; trivalent containing A, B, and E antitoxins; bivalent A and B; and monovalent E antitoxins. Although the effectiveness of these preparations in treatment is not well established, their use is recommended. The trivalent antitoxin is preferred because of its broader coverage and higher content of antibody. It is available from the Centers for Disease Control. One to three vials of this antiserum should be given intramuscularly as early as possible when botulism is suspected. Twenty per cent of patients will have untoward reactions. Testing for hypersensitivity should always precede its use.

SNAKEBITE. Specific antivenin is effective in neutralizing the systemic effects of snakebite. Two preparations are available: One is polyvalent for snakes of the Crotalidae family, including rattlesnakes, copperheads, moccasins, pit vipers, and vipers; the second is specific for coral snake, *Micrurus fulvius*, bites.

SPIDER BITES. A specific antivenin is highly effective for treatment of systemic effects following bites by the black widow spider, *Latrodectus mactans*, and other members of the genus. The dose is one vial (2.5 ml) intramuscularly.

Hollinger FB, Troisi CL, Pepe PE: Anti-HBs responses to vaccination with a human hepatitis B vaccine made by recombinant DNA technology in yeast. J Infect Dis 153:156, 1986. *Report of duration and magnitude of the antibody responses to new recombinant hepatitis.*

Immunization Practices Advisory Committee, Centers for Disease Control: General recommendations on immunization. Ann Intern Med 98:615, 1983. *Definitions, principles, and routine childhood immunization schedules.*

Immunization Practices Advisory Committee, Centers for Disease Control: Diphtheria, tetanus, and pertussis, guidelines for vaccine prophylaxis and other preventive measures. Recommendation of the Immunization Practices Advisory Committee. Ann Intern Med 103:896, 1985. *Good review of disease and preventive measures.*

Immunization Practices Advisory Committee, Centers for Disease Control: Recommendations for protection against viral hepatitis. Morbidity and Mortality Weekly Report 34:313, 1985. *Summary of nomenclature, risks, vaccine usage, and IG and HBIG usage in hepatitis A, B, non A–non B, and delta.*

Immunization Practices Advisory Committee, Centers for Disease Control: Prevention and control of influenza. Morbidity and Mortality Weekly Report 35:317, 1986. *Presents new strategy for prevention and control of influenza: prioritization of patients.*

Immunization Practices Advisory Committee, Centers for Disease Control: New recommended schedule for active immunization of normal infants and children. Morbidity and Mortality Weekly Report, 35:577, 1986.

18 THE PREVENTIVE HEALTH EXAMINATION

Gary D. Friedman

The primary purpose of preventive health examinations is to maintain or improve health. The rationale is that early detection of disease or of high risk of subsequent disease can lead to treatment or remedial measures that will prevent or postpone morbidity, disability, or mortality.

An "annual physical" for asymptomatic adults was once accepted as good medical practice. In recent years periodic health examinations have become controversial: (1) The costs of a thorough medical history, physical examination, and standard laboratory tests would be enormous if these procedures were annually and universally applied. (2) Many elements of traditional checkups have not been shown to benefit asymptomatic persons. On the other hand, certain simple examination procedures and screening tests can prolong life and prevent disability.

ROUTINE TESTS AND PROCEDURES OF PROVEN OR PROBABLE VALUE IN PREVENTIVE CARE FOR ADULTS. A test is suitable for routine use if it can detect a serious and relatively common disease at an early stage, or at a predisease high-risk stage, when treatment or intervention would be more effective. Furthermore, the test should be relatively economical in terms of both money and professional time. Although controversy continues about some, a few tests or procedures meet these criteria; a few others are of probable value but less universally accepted (Table 18–1).

Routine chest radiographs can now be justified only in settings where tuberculosis is common; they have not proved to be effective in reducing mortality from lung cancer. Although still controversial because of poor sensitivity and specificity, a tonometry test for glaucoma may also be of net benefit. Doubts about tests of probable value revolve primarily around the benefits of treatment compared with the harm of labeling (e.g., mild asymptomatic diabetes mellitus), the high relative frequency and high cost of evaluating false-positive results (e.g., occult blood in the stool), and the low yield of significant disease in the asymptomatic patient (e.g., palpating the abdomen).

ADDITIONAL BENEFITS OF PREVENTIVE HEALTH APPRAISALS. Detecting disease or abnormalities is not the only benefit of the preventive health examination. Negative findings are also of value in the reassurance they provide to the patient, especially if the patient has received what he or she perceives to be a thorough examination. In contemplating cuts in the content of routine checkups, physicians and health care planners must weigh the immediate economic gains against the possible decrease in this reassurance if patients perceive the examinations to be abbreviated or cursory.

A lengthy and thorough examination when a patient is first seen permits collection of baseline data that may be useful when symptoms develop later. For example, an electrocardio-

TABLE 18–1. THE PREVENTIVE HEALTH EXAMINATION

Of Accepted Value	Of Probable Value
Medical History of:	
1. Smoking, particularly cigarettes	1. Postmenopausal uterine bleeding
2. Drinking alcohol to excess	2. Immunization status
3. Failure to wear seatbelts	3. Use of nonmedicinal drugs other than alcohol
	4. Lack of regular physical activity
Physical Examination:	
1. Assessment of obesity	1. Search for cancers or precancerous lesions of the skin, mouth and pharynx, thyroid, abdomen, testes, uterus, prostate, and lymph nodes
2. Measurement of blood pressure	
3. Search for cancer or precancerous lesions of the breast and rectum	
Laboratory or Diagnostic Studies:	
1. Mammography in women at least 50 years of age	1. Hemoglobin or hematocrit
2. Sigmoidoscopy for cancer or polyps	2. Test of stool for occult blood
3. Papanicolaou test for cervical cancer	3. Baseline electrocardiogram
4. Serum cholesterol concentration	4. Blood glucose
5. Serologic test for latent syphilis and a cervical culture for gonorrhea (in individuals at high risk for venereal disease)	5. Tuberculin skin test (in high-risk groups)

gram, recorded when the patient is young and healthy, provides a useful benchmark for evaluating electrocardiograms taken later if chest pain or arrhythmia occurs. Also, the additional time spent in obtaining a medical and social history, examining the patient, and discussing the patient's concerns helps to establish a good doctor-patient relationship. Further, certain valuable information can be obtained during a thorough first examination and need not be sought routinely again. A good example is rheumatic heart disease detected by history and cardiac auscultation.

MULTIPHASIC AND SELECTIVE SCREENING. Screening tests aimed at early disease detection are sometimes offered singly, as in special programs to detect tuberculosis, diabetes mellitus, or breast cancer. Clearly it is more economical and efficient to test for several diseases at a single visit than for single diseases at several visits. Multiphasic screening provides several tests comparatively economically at one patient visit and can be used as part of a periodic health examination. Components of health screening or health examinations may be used for some patients and not others, depending on previous findings, risk characteristics, past medical history, or current symptoms of the patient. For example, once a baseline electrocardiogram has been taken, it need not be repeated at each succeeding health examination unless it initially revealed an abnormality or unless cardiovascular symptoms or indicators of high risk occur. This use of screening tests is known as selective or discriminate screening.

FREQUENCY OF EXAMINATIONS. It is not clear how frequently preventive health examinations, either basic or thorough, should be performed. The physician must strike a balance between excessive costs and low yield of too frequent examinations, and the chance that an important and controllable condition will develop and become irreversible if examinations are not provided often enough. Several sets of recommendations have been made recently based on available evidence and "prudent" judgment (see references). A common theme is that the incidence of most disabling and fatal diseases increases with age. Thus, basic examinations containing essential tests such as blood pressure measurement and breast palpation should increase in frequency from once in several years in the patient's twenties to annually in the fifties or sixties and older. As age advances it is advisable to observe the patient for losses in hearing, vision, and mental functioning as well. Even if losses are irreversible, knowledge

of these limitations will aid in advising the patient and his or her family. Clearly, in our present state of knowledge, clinical judgment must play an important role both in deciding on the frequency of examinations and in selecting examination components for individual patients based on their age, sex, past medical history, and current risk status.

A health examination is of little value without appropriate follow-up, including treatment of early disease if indicated and counseling to encourage favorable changes in risk factors and a healthier lifestyle.

American Cancer Society: Report on the cancer-related health checkup. CA 30:194, 1980. *This is a critical evaluation of methods of early detection of cancer.*

Breslow L, Somers AR: The lifetime health-monitoring program: A practical approach to preventive medicine. N Engl J Med 296:601, 1977. *This review of health examinations contains recommendations that emphasize a changing approach for different age groups and the need for cost-effective preventive measures.*

Canadian Task Force on the Periodic Health Examination (Spitzer W, chairman): The periodic health examination. Can Med Assoc J 121:1193, 1979; 130:1276, 1984; 134:721, 1986. *This is a summary of a thorough review of various components of preventive health examinations and preventive care. The need for a selective rather than a routine approach is emphasized.*

Council on Scientific Affairs, Division of Scientific Activities, American Medical Association: Medical evaluation of healthy persons. JAMA 249: 1626, 1983. *This is a brief compilation of recommendations concerning health examinations at all ages, reviewed in the context of current and previous positions of the American Medical Association.*

Frame PS: A critical review of adult health maintenance. J Fam Pract 22:341, 417, 511; 23:29, 1986. *This is a recently updated and very readable review of major elements of the adult health examination with specific recommendations.*

Medical Practice Committee, American College of Physicians: Periodic health examination: A guide for designing individualized preventive health care in the asymptomatic patient. Ann Intern Med 95:729, 1981. *This review of periodic health examinations provides a diagrammatic summary of recommendations that are viewed as minimal preventive measures to be applied to apparently well asymptomatic individuals at low medical risk.*

19 THE HEALTH OF THE PHYSICIAN

Linda Hawes Clever

Physicians are a curious lot. On the one hand, they have decreased major health risks by not smoking. On the other hand, they usually avoid having immunizations for rubella and hepatitis B, illnesses that can be devastating both to them and to their patients. The purpose of this chapter is to review available data about the lives, deaths, and personal health practices of physicians and to make recommendations about health maintenance activities for physicians.

PHYSICIANS' WORK

Physicians work harder than most people. They work 15 hours per week longer than other professionals; take less vacation time (four weeks per year versus eight weeks per year for most other professionals); and work more years than the general population and therefore have a shorter retirement (3.1 years versus 7.8 years). They also have unique responsibilities and duties.

Demands of Practice

Physicians cite special pressures generated by patients and patients' families. These include unwarranted but firmly held expectations of cure, relief, or certainty. Physicians are disturbed by inflicting pain during diagnostic tests, coping with their own minor or grievous errors, and dealing with dying patients. Physicians feel angry or guilty about work with "difficult" patients or being unable to answer questions. They dislike medical politics, paperwork, and committee work. Public policy changes spawn concerns about preserving the quality of patient care, competition from other physicians and health practitioners, independence, the funding of both research and graduate medical education, and income maintenance. Professional liability casts a long shadow, with a 10 per cent increase per year in medical malpractice suits. The world changes rapidly; morale wavers.

Family and Lifestyle Tensions and Pleasures

It has been said that physicians have one of the few socially acceptable reasons for abandoning a family. The rigors of being "on call" (albeit occurring less frequently now as more physicians enter group and hospital- or institution-based practice) can interfere with family plans. Laser-focus on professional responsibilities leads to muddled values, constricted relationships, and stunted personal growth. Taxing schedules can clash with parenting and squelch creativity. Even reading for pleasure, attending church, and exercise may be squeezed out by the time or priority crunch.

Fairness requires comments on the "other" side. Although continuation of high prestige and income may be uncertain and pressures mount, there are numerous intrinsic pleasures in the medical profession. Making precision diagnoses, teaching, counseling, providing support and motivation, and, indeed, ameliorating suffering, treating disease, and saving lives are noted by physicians to be particularly satisfying. Developing personal relationships with patients and their families and earning a good living have appeal. Working with people during existential crises and dealing with the most private aspects of their lives and bodies provide staggering yet exhilarating experiences.

PHYSICIANS' HEALTH
Overall Mortality

Unfortunately, data about health status of physicians are scattered and rarely provide comparisons with other professionals. It is possible to infer, however, that despite the complexities and challenges of physicians' work and lives, *they are at least as healthy as the general population in most respects.*

Age-specific death rates for physicians are less than those for the white male population in the United States. On the whole, (1) the age-related mortality of male physicians has had a 61 per cent decline since 1929; (2) male physicians had 25 per cent less mortality and female physicians had 16 per cent less mortality than the white United States population compared by age and sex (Goodman study). Firm conclusions about the relative longevity of specialists and nonspecialists await further studies.

Disease-Specific Mortality

TOBACCO-RELATED ILLNESS. About one third of Americans smoke; fewer than 10 per cent of physicians smoke; and fewer than 5 per cent of physicians under 30 years of age smoke. Cigarette smoking is a grave health hazard (Ch. 11). Since physicians have usually smoked less than the general public and smoke far less now, it is not surprising that *smoking-related mortality among physicians is plummeting.* Deaths from lung cancer in male physicians in California halved between 1950 to 1959 and 1970 to 1979; other smoking-related diseases had striking declines (bronchitis, chronic obstructive pulmonary disease, and cancers of the esophagus and mouth). Although the incidence of fatal arteriosclerotic cardiovascular disease among physicians *was* higher than in the general population, it is now lower.

SUICIDES. On the darker side, *early death from suicide* appears to be excessive among physicians. Numbers are impressive for the general population: Suicides account for about 18 deaths per 100,000 in males and about 5 deaths per 100,000 in females. These figures combine to make suicide the eighth commonest cause of death in this country. Despite numerous methodologic problems, some generalizations

about suicide by physicians are warranted. Male physicians probably commit suicide twice as often as the United States white male population. Female physicians take their own lives at a rate slightly more than triple that of white American women who are not physicians. Differences in suicide rates by specialty have not been verified because of inadequate sample size, although there is a suggestion of an increased incidence among psychiatrists. Professionals in other health sciences such as dentistry and pharmacy have substantially higher suicide rates than physicians. Similar results have been found in England and Wales. Overall, however, data are marred by incorrect reporting or under-reporting, small numbers, and inadequate comparison groups by age, sex, and profession. Speculations to explain existing data are plentiful. It is not surprising that physicians may have the same sorts of characteristics that drive others to suicide. These include a variety of family-related markers such as (1) death of a close relative during childhood or thereafter, (2) being single, and (3) excessive or incomplete integration into a family unit. Depression is an extremely important element (see Ch. 462). Other psychiatric diagnoses such as severe personality disorder or psychosis may also be causative. A history of a prior suicide attempt serves as a warning of high suicide risk. Financial problems, poor health, and substance abuse often contribute as well. Special problems that may incline physicians toward suicide include professional isolation, the tensions of training or practice, unrealistic expectations, rifts in relationships, the exhaustion and emotional burdens of patient care, and pre-existing psychiatric vulnerability.

Morbidity

The age-specific death rate of physicians is lower than that of other Americans, but it could be even better if several factors were not in effect. For example, most physicians *do not have their own doctor* who can provide health promotion and surveillance. Fortunately, from the standpoint of risk management, two thirds of physicians in their fifties and above have routine health examinations. Self-treatment, curbstone consultations, and delays because of embarrassment about professional courtesy can impede diagnosis and treatment. Denial may slow care. A pathologic extension of denial is the "physician invulnerability syndrome," which is characterized by the conviction that the personal and family problems, the aggravations, and the diseases that affect others cannot or will not affect the physician. Fear plays an important part in this "syndrome."

Substance Abuse

There is considerable reason for concern about the incidence of alcohol and drug abuse among physicians. Reliable, recent statistics are scarce, however. Past studies have suggested that alcoholism among physicians is at least double that of the general population (see Ch. 15). Current literature supports parity. Drug abuse may be somewhat more prevalent among physicians than other Americans. Regardless of population comparisons, of course, *substance abuse is a deadly problem for physicians, their families, and their patients.* Damage to patients resulting from confusion, inattention, poor judgment, unavailability, or psychomotor deficits often occurs before the physician seeks, or is forced, into care. A substantial majority of physicians in impaired physician rehabilitation programs are under treatment for drug and/or alcohol abuse alone. Automobile and private plane accidents are associated with intoxication, as are family dissolution and substance abuse in children of abusers (see Ch. 16). Although denial seems to play a major role at the inception of addiction ("I won't get hooked; *I'm* not susceptible"), and denial makes therapy more challenging, physicians seem to have a better prognosis, with treatment, than other middle-class substance abusers.

PERSONAL HEALTH PRACTICES OF PHYSICIANS

Many health promotion efforts for adults target smoking cessation, good nutrition, exercise, and moderation of alcohol intake. Immunization for adults is also receiving attention. Seatbelt use has been touted by national agencies, the media, and various professional groups and societies. The exceptional record of physicians in smoking avoidance has already been described, but other health habits seem to be less exemplary. For example, although most physicians report that they are careful about dietary fat, calories, and/or salt, 29 to 58 per cent acknowledge that they are overweight. Thirty-seven to 73 per cent of physicians do not engage in weekly vigorous exercise; indeed, gardening is a favorite recreation. Although moderation in frequency and volume of alcohol consumption is the norm, 13 to 24 per cent of physicians drink daily, and 20 per cent have at least two drinks when they do drink. Up to 10 per cent of physicians may be problem drinkers.

Immunization

By and large, physicians have an abysmal record of immunization for diseases that can affect them or that they can transmit. For example, between only 10 and 31 per cent of rubella antibody–negative physicians who work with children, pregnant women, and other patients receive rubella vaccine. At least 84 per cent of physicians are susceptible to hepatitis B (and, therefore, delta hepatitis), but very few house officers or attending physicians receive hepatitis B vaccine. The incidence of immunization of physicians for tetanus/diphtheria, polio, and influenza is unknown. Since health risks and costs are low, results are favorable, and the professional liability of not being vaccinated is high, wise physicians get vaccinated.

Seatbelt Use

Seatbelt use by physicians is the least well-documented good health habit. In one study, physicians did use seatbelts more often than did attorneys. One might extrapolate from other factors that correlate with seatbelt use (such as educational level, regular visits to a dentist, and nonsmoking) that physicians buckle up more often than others. Such a practice would be felicitous, since (1) many physicians drive hundreds of miles per week; (2) each American has a one in three chance of being disabled by an automobile injury during his or her lifetime; (3) always using a seatbelt can reduce the risk of serious injury or death by greater than one half.

Effects of Good Health Habits by the Physician on Others

Good health practices not only improve the health and lives of physicians themselves but also can affect others as well. As implied above, moderation of alcohol use and eschewing of drug use by physicians can prevent direct harm to patients. Vaccination of physicians can prevent transmission of infectious diseases. Smoking cessation by physicians can even decrease injury to others by reducing side-stream smoke. Of great importance is the observation that *physicians' personal health habits help determine advice that they give to patients.*

TABLE 19–1. SUGGESTIONS TO PHYSICIANS ABOUT GOOD HEALTH

Do:
1. Get help when you need it. Don't deny; don't delay.
2. Fasten your seatbelt—always.
3. Get antibody screening and appropriate vaccination for hepatitis B, tetanus/diphtheria, influenza, rubella, pneumonia, polio, and measles.
4. Practice moderation in diet and alcohol intake.
5. Exercise regularly and sensibly.
6. Engage fully in the pageantry of living in activities with your family, friends, and community.
7. Cultivate your creativity; be interested, not just interesting, and use your sense of humor.
8. Start planning for your retirement 25 to 30 years before your goal.
   a. Feel free to relish your profession, and if you don't, consider important changes.
   b. Get reputable, professional help with financial planning.

Do not:
1. Smoke.
2. Use nonprescribed drugs.
3. Ignore your family and friends in the frenzy of serving others or meeting their demands.
4. Short-circuit your own needs for personal and intellectual growth.
5. Be only a physician—be a person.

Physicians with good health habits (regarding smoking, weight, exercise, and alcohol) are likely to counsel primary prevention; physicians with poor health habits are unlikely to provide any health promotion advice, nor do they even counsel tertiary prevention.

RECOMMENDATIONS

Basically, physicians, in concert with their own physician and family, need to analyze their own health and health behavior (Table 19–1). They need to assess pain and pleasure, risks and benefits. If change is necessary or desirable, a plan needs to be developed. Barriers need to be removed, incentives and rewards incorporated, and progress documented and celebrated.

Clever LH, Arsham GM: Physicians' own health—some advice for the advisors. West J Med 141:846, 1984. *This review article covers a broad spectrum of morbidity and mortality statistics and personal health habits of physicians. It also makes specific recommendations for good health in physicians.*

Goodman LJ: The longevity and mortality of American physicians, 1969–1973. Milbank Mem Fund Q 53:353, 1975. *This paper is a classic because of its statistical methods and breadth and depth of coverage. Sex, age, geography, and medical specialty are analyzed.*

McAuliffe WE, Rohman M, Santangelo S, et al.: Psychoactive drug use among practicing physicians and medical students. N Engl J Med 315:805, 1986. *This well-referenced research paper shows that physicians' use of psychoactive drugs is not too different from that of other professionals. High drug use by younger physicians and poor education of most physicians about drugs and alcohol are a call to action to avoid expanding physician impairment, however.*

Linn LS, Yager J, Cope D, et al.: Health habits and coping behaviors among practicing physicians. West J Med 144:484, 1986. *This thorough and refreshing paper explores the complex, arcane interactions of physicians' health habits and emotional health. It can be a cornerstone of further research and understanding of physicians' behavior.*

Roy A: Suicide in doctors. Psychiatry Clin North Am 8:377, 1985. *Its important topic, incisive commentary, and 44 references make this short paper especially useful.*

PART IV

PRINCIPLES OF DIAGNOSIS AND MANAGEMENT

20 CLINICAL APPROACH TO THE PATIENT

William L. Morgan, Jr.

The scientific basis of medical practice is well established, but only recently has the time-honored *art of medicine* come under scientific scrutiny. Medical educators are now beginning to understand how a physician relates to a patient and are introducing new ways to teach noncognitive skills. Data-gathering skills of interviewing and physical examination can be taught with standardized patients or a videotape. Strategies to select and interpret laboratory tests make the diagnosis of disease more scientific. Problem-oriented records have improved the organization and display of medical information. Understanding the role of a physician enables one to adapt such innovations to medical practice. What follows is a description of the abilities needed by a physician to care for a patient.

A task force of the American Board of Internal Medicine studied clinical competence in internal medicine by analyzing the components of the medical encounter (Tables 20–1 and 20–2). Knowledge, skills, and attitudes are the abilities required of a physician caring for a patient. The major tasks involved in solving a medical problem include data gathering, diagnosis, and patient care.

ABILITIES REQUIRED OF A PHYSICIAN
Noncognitive Abilities

Appropriate attitudes, habits, and interpersonal skills are important abilities needed to develop a positive physician-patient relationship. Without effective attitudes and interpersonal skills, and despite keen intellect and medical knowledge, a physician can fail in relating to and caring for a patient. The physician who is motivated primarily by concern for the patient's welfare is more likely to provide the conditions for an effective relationship. The essence of this rela-

tionship has never been better stated than in Peabody's classic 1927 article: "One of the essential qualities of the clinician is interest in humanity, for the secret of the care of the patient is caring for the patient."

ATTITUDES AND HABITS. Humanistic qualities, the assumption of responsibility, and continuing scholarship are among the major expectations of a physician. Humanistic qualities include integrity, respect, and compassion for the patient. Moral and ethical values are also essential components of clinical competence. Despite patients' psychological handicaps and failure to comply with treatment, the effective physician is sympathetic and nonjudgmental.

The assumption of full responsibility for the care of a patient is a fundamental requirement of the competent physician. This responsibility includes continuing care despite personal inconvenience and emotional demands of the patient. The physician is committed to doing what is best for the patient, and, when necessary, seeks the help of others.

Continuing scholarship is also an essential requirement of an effective physician. Rapid advances in medical sciences, and the resulting diagnostic and therapeutic innovations, make obsolete yesterday's method of medical practice. Each individual learns to recognize deficiencies in knowledge and adopts a plan to keep up with new information. This plan includes reading journals and texts, attending courses and hospital teaching rounds, and undertaking self-study programs. Continuing scholarship requires self-discipline to set aside personal time on a regular basis. An effective way to learn is to pursue knowledge about the disease at the time one sees a patient with a specific illness.

INTERPERSONAL SKILLS. Being able to relate to the patient, to family members, and to others caring for the patient is of particular importance. The ability to communicate well is the basis for effective interpersonal relationships. This communication includes encouraging the patient to share symptoms and personal concerns. One should be aware of nonverbal messages that convey significant information about emotional problems. The physician also has the obligation to transmit information to the patient about the illness itself and about its prognosis and treatment. Competence means communicating well despite intellectual, socioeconomic, and language barriers.

It is a responsibility of the physician to talk with family members, while at the same time respecting patient confiden-

---

TABLE 20–1. ABILITIES REQUIRED OF A PHYSICIAN

Noncognitive abilities
  Attitudes and habits
  Interpersonal skills
  Motor and technical skills
Intellectual abilities
  Knowledge
  Organization
  Synthesis
  Clinical judgment

Modified from American Board of Internal Medicine: Clinical competence in internal medicine. Ann Intern Med 90:403, 1979.

TABLE 20–2. TASKS REQUIRED OF A PHYSICIAN

Data gathering
  Medical history
  Physical examination
  Diagnostic studies
Diagnosis or problem definition
Medical care

Modified from American Board of Internal Medicine: Clinical competence in internal medicine. Ann Intern Med 90:403, 1979.

tiality. Knowing with whom to talk and how much to say requires considerable skill. The competent physician also communicates effectively with others caring for the patient. This interpersonal skill includes the ability to present the patient's problem orally and to transmit information through written orders and the written record.

MOTOR AND TECHNICAL SKILLS. Manual skills are necessary in gathering information from the patient as well as in applying specific treatment. Being able to do a well-ordered and accurate physical examination requires effective motor skills. Diagnostic procedures such as biopsies, sampling of body fluids, or endoscopy also depend on motor and technical skills. Examples of treatment involving these skills include performing minor surgery and using machines for life support. Learning new techniques and continuing to practice them are major requirements for maintaining technical competence.

Intellectual Abilities

Disease is a scientific, impersonal term. *Illness* is personalized and refers to disease in a specific patient. Intellectual skills are directed to the understanding, diagnosis, and theoretical management of disease. Noncognitive abilities deal more with the individual. In approaching a medical problem, the physician begins with relevant medical knowledge and synthesizes the information into an integrated concept. Clinical judgment is used to resolve the problem.

To apply medical knowledge to a patient problem, the physician draws on pertinent medical facts from memory, from clinical experience, and from other sources such as journals, textbooks, and experts. An understanding of pathophysiology helps in anticipating the expected course of the disease. Information derived from the patient, together with medical knowledge, is organized into a logical sequence. Synthesis of organized medical knowledge involves integration of medical facts into practical concepts, which are altered as the patient's condition changes or when new information becomes available. Organization and synthesis of information are important in all tasks of a physician, including data gathering, diagnosis, and planning for study and treatment. The highest level of cognitive ability is clinical judgment, where intellectual skills are called upon to solve problems. The physician makes clinical decisions by discriminating between alternative courses of action. Clinical judgment is used to decide what is of greatest benefit to the patient with the least risk and cost.

TASKS REQUIRED OF A PHYSICIAN

When a patient comes for help, the physician follows a logical series of steps, which are called clinical tasks. The physician first obtains the medical history, does a physical examination, and conducts laboratory studies. Based on this information, an initial diagnosis is made upon which definitive medical care is based.

Data Gathering

MEDICAL HISTORY. The most powerful diagnostic tool of the physician is the interview. By this means, one learns the chronological events and the symptoms of the patient's illness. Diagnostic hypotheses are generated and tested as the patient's history unfolds, resulting in the formulation of the most likely diagnoses at the completion of the interview. These hypotheses are extended, confirmed, or refuted by the subsequent physical examination and diagnostic studies.

The interview has considerable importance beyond "history taking" or the gathering of medical facts. It is the principal means of initiating and developing a relationship with the patient. The interview is a shared experience with goals for both participants. For the patient, the goal is alleviation of distress and restoration of health. The patient must be satis-

fied that the person rendering medical care is not only professionally competent but is also interested in him as an individual. For the physician, the primary objective is to obtain the information needed to understand the illness and to initiate appropriate treatment. This objective is accomplished by demonstrating concern for the patient and by being willing to listen to his personal as well as medical problems. The overt demonstration of concern by the physician will help to build the physician-patient relationship and secure the patient's cooperation.

The most important component of the medical history is the patient's present illness. Here, the interviewer develops a detailed and sequential reconstruction of the symptoms and events contributing to the current illness. The social history is also of considerable importance. The inquiry with interest and empathy into the personal events of the patient's life, while affording the patient time to relate these events, helps to establish a strong physician-patient relationship. Knowledge of the patient's personal circumstances and relationships to others leads to better understanding of his problems and ways of coping with them. More effective planning for the future care of the patient takes place when the limitations imposed on the current life situation are known.

When pursuing information in the interview, the physician begins with open-ended or nondirective questions and concludes with specific questions. Such an approach allows the patient time to respond and to elaborate on his problems. Failure to take time to listen may be interpreted by the patient as a lack of interest on the part of the interviewer and can result in a perfunctory and noninformative interview. To initiate the interview with a series of specific questions may also inhibit the full development of the history. Encouraging the patient to speak freely as the interview proceeds is important, since only the patient can describe what he has been experiencing. On the other hand, the patient does not necessarily understand what the interviewer needs to learn from him. The physician therefore actively pursues the interview in order to develop organization and content. The patient soon learns that events must be dated, sequences established, and symptoms precisely described. Dates and times serve to anchor the history in such a way that relationships between symptoms and events are more clearly understood. Knowledge of disease and clinical syndromes enables the physician to anticipate symptoms the patient does not mention. It is often necessary to intervene in order to clarify terms the patient uses, including medical or quasi-medical terms. Some patients, when asked to tell of their own illnesses, may omit their symptoms altogether and persist in describing only what other doctors said and did. It should be made clear that the interviewer is more interested in learning about the patient's specific symptoms and not the interpretation of those symptoms.

In conducting an effective interview, the physician adapts to the personality of the patient and to limitations imposed by illness. Patients who are especially talkative or who wander from the subject need to be guided back to the pertinent issues. Patients with poverty of associations are encouraged to elaborate on their problems. When an interview becomes primarily a question and answer session, it is likely that the patient is unable to go into detail because of illness or that the interviewer is using poor technique and is therefore missing valuable historical information. In a seriously ill patient, one gives priority to those aspects of the history that appear more relevant to the immediate situation. Other patients, because of the type of disease, may be handicapped in relating their stories. When the interview is limited because of the patient's illness, information is derived from other sources such as family, friends, and previous hospital records. A subsequent interview of the patient at a more opportune time is often valuable.

The appearance and responses of the patient during the

interview are diagnostically helpful. The physical examination begins the moment the patient is seen. One studies the patient's appearance, his emotional state, and his physical and mental limitations. Not only is close attention paid to the overt meaning of what is said, but the interviewer is also alert to nonverbal cues. The physician's own feeling of being uncomfortable, uneasy, or unhappy often reflects the attitude of the patient.

The interview, a powerful diagnostic tool, goes far beyond collecting the facts of illness. Through knowledge and experience, the physician delineates subtle symptoms and interrelationships that are often unrecognized by the patient. A skillful interviewer will uncover personal feelings and circumstances underlying the illness. An interview conducted with sensitivity and concern will help to build a strong relationship between the patient and physician.

PHYSICAL EXAMINATION. A general screening examination is conducted following the interview. This examination is influenced by diagnostic hypotheses developed during the interview which direct the physician to do a more detailed study in the area of suspected abnormality.

Consideration for the patient continues during the physical examination. Privacy is provided for dressing and undressing, and the examination is done with appropriate draping. Both the physician and the patient need to be in a comfortable position throughout the examination in order to apply techniques properly. In certain parts of the examination, the physician tells the patient how to cooperate and forewarns him of any uncomfortable impending maneuver. In general, the examination is done in silence except for necessary instructions to the patient. Talking hinders the physician from concentrating fully on possible underlying abnormalities. The examination is carried out with meticulous care, gentleness, and sensitive attention. One avoids comments or facial expressions that can be misinterpreted by the patient as indicating concern or puzzlement. The physician is also alert to signs of patient fatigue or discomfort.

There are two major principles underlying an efficient physical examination. First, the examination is done by regions; second, there is a well-organized order of examination. To be efficient, one approaches regions sequentially, for example, the head, the neck, the posterior thorax and lungs, the anterior thorax and lungs, and the heart. This type of regional approach also takes into account the comfort of the patient by eliminating the need for frequent shifts in position. One begins with a general survey of each region and then focuses on component parts. If no abnormality is found, the examination is brief but comprehensive. If an abnormality is present, it is studied meticulously, using special maneuvers if necessary. One takes advantage of the symmetry of the human body by comparing one side with the other. In this way, subtle changes are recognized. Small differences in the lung examination, for example, are better detected by cross-comparing symmetrical areas of each lung than by examining each lung individually. Following a prescribed order of examination by regions does not imply a lack of flexibility. The examination varies with the condition of the patient and the type of problem present. Evidence of disease in one area alerts the physician to possible related abnormalities in other areas. If the initial physical examination has not been entirely satisfactory, one does not hesitate to return at a later time to recheck findings when circumstances for reexamination may be more favorable.

Observation is an often neglected technique of great importance. Studying the patient and his surroundings yields helpful diagnostic information. By noting what is on the bedside table, for example, one gains insight into the patient's interests and habits and the support of family and friends. Specifically, one looks for reading materials, cigarettes, and the presence of cards or gifts. When beginning to examine each region, the physician pauses to observe. For example,

an enlarged thyroid gland will readily be seen when a patient extends his neck slightly and swallows; asymmetry of respiratory motion will be more easily observed from the foot of the bed with the patient on his back; and holding an end of a tongue blade lightly at the cardiac apex will magnify the visible impulse of a left ventricular gallop.

The physician learns to do a comprehensive screening examination. Depending on the condition of the patient, the examination will need to be adapted to special circumstances. The patient may be bed-bound and so ill that the examiner requires assistance with positioning. In an acute emergency where an abbreviated physical examination is carried out with deliberate speed, one simultaneously does a brief interview, obtains laboratory work, and initiates treatment. If the patient has a neurologic problem, a complete neurologic examination is done. Regardless of the problem and the condition of the patient, the physician is considerate, systematic, and logical in approach. One keeps in mind diagnostic possibilities, looks for unsuspected disease, and interrelates abnormal findings that may explain the patient's illness.

DIAGNOSTIC STUDIES. Laboratory tests and diagnostic procedures are obtained following the interview and physical examination. A few initial screening tests are usually done to detect unsuspected common entities, such as anemia, diabetes, or chronic renal disease. Studies are discriminatingly chosen to confirm one's impression and are not used in a routine or excessive way to search for unexpected diagnoses. After considering each of the patient's problems, the physician decides which studies are needed, both to confirm the diagnostic impression and to rule in or out other possibilities. If the prevalence of a problem is low and no effective treatment is available, few diagnostic tests are indicated. Laboratory tests and diagnostic procedures are of value not only to help make the diagnosis, but also to assess the severity, course, and prognosis of the disease and to follow the effect of therapy.

When choosing diagnostic studies, the physician begins with those that yield the most comprehensive information and carry the least risk for the patient. The diagnosis frequently becomes apparent with simple tests; more expensive or potentially hazardous studies may not be required. Laboratory tests are often overemphasized. These tests have limitations in accuracy, and there may be errors and misinterpretation of results. The physician's own clinical findings and judgment take precedence in the interpretation of laboratory data.

Potentially hazardous diagnostic or therapeutic procedures require competence on the part of those doing them. Plans for procedures are discussed with the patient, including possible risks. Time is taken to alleviate patient concern and to interpret the results. In carrying out diagnostic studies and treatment, consultant assistance is often required. The physician in charge of the patient takes into account the expert advice of consultants but continues to supervise overall care and makes the ultimate decisions.

Recent research into clinical decision making has been helpful in creating a better understanding of the selection and interpretation of diagnostic tests and procedures. Knowledge of the sensitivity and specificity of diagnostic studies leads to their more rational selection. *Sensitivity* is the probability that a test will be positive when the disease is present. *Specificity* is the probability that the test will be negative when the disease is not present. For example, to exclude the possibility of lupus erythematosus, one chooses a sensitive test such as the antinuclear antibody test. The more specific double-stranded DNA antibody test is ordered to confirm the diagnosis.

Diagnosis or Problem Definition

The physician uses the scientific method in clinical problem solving, as does the investigator in conducting an experiment.

Clinical information is analyzed to develop working hypotheses that are confirmed or refuted by obtaining further information. Problem solving begins at the time the physician initiates the interview. The symptoms and course of the illness lead to the formulation of several diagnostic hypotheses. These diagnostic possibilities direct further questioning of the patient in order to determine which hypothesis best fits the illness. Hypotheses are repeatedly generated and tested during the interview. As the physician completes the interview and physical examination, one or two possibilities usually become more likely and others less likely. With further information, an attempt is made to explain the patient's presenting illness with a single preliminary diagnosis. This goal is often attainable in young patients but seldom in older ones, in whom multiple diagnoses are usually required. One takes into account the likelihood of the disease process in making a preliminary diagnosis. The most common diseases are considered first, particularly those diseases for which specific treatment is available.

Cognitive or intellectual skills are used in formulating a diagnosis. A physician continually refers to knowledge of medical facts and pathophysiology in analyzing information pertaining to the patient's illness. This analysis consists of collecting information and synthesizing it into integrated concepts compatible with known diseases. Abnormal findings are localized anatomically and are interpreted in terms of their structure and function. Clinical judgment is used to weigh the diagnostic possibilities by assigning values to the data in order to arrive at the most likely conclusion. The experienced clinician is able to apply these intellectual processes rapidly and continually while interviewing the patient.

The written record is used to clarify the physician's diagnostic thinking. When there are several diagnostic possibilities explaining the symptoms and events of the present illness, a differential diagnosis is carried out. For each diagnosis considered, the physician weighs information favoring that possibility against information that makes the diagnosis unlikely. Consideration of alternative possibilities in the differential diagnosis is helpful in directing the physician to select diagnostic studies that confirm or exclude each possible diagnosis. In addition to indicating the most likely diagnosis that explains the present illness, the physician lists in descending order of importance all other active problems affecting the patient. This list includes not only specific diseases, but also such problems as the recent loss of a spouse or exposure to environmental toxins. The physician considers all possible factors in the patient's illness, including psychological stresses and underlying conditions that may alter resistance. The functional impact of the illness in terms of its severity and the degree of resulting disability is also taken into account.

Clinical decisions are influenced by policies determined by tradition, by the medical literature, and by the practice of colleagues. These policies may be based on simplistic or even erroneous reasoning. Greater attention needs to be paid to clinical policies that have been shown to be valid. Ongoing investigation of diagnostic reasoning will eventually lead to better understanding of the ways clinicians solve medical problems. The diagnostic thinking of physicians as they interview standardized patients has been studied, and decision analysis has contributed logic theory to problem solving, including the use of probability and decision trees.

Medical Care

The term *medical care* is used rather than the more authoritative *patient management,* because it expresses personal concern and responsibility for all of the patient's problems. In caring for a patient, physician attitudes of integrity, respect, and compassion are particularly important, as is the ability to communicate effectively. In addition, the intellectual skills of the physician are necessary attributes. Up-to-date medical knowledge of pharmacological principles and advances in technology are required. Clinical judgment is used in prescribing drugs, in selecting therapeutic procedures, and in implementing consultant opinions. Knowing when *not* to treat is as important as knowing when to treat. New drugs and procedures are ordered with caution. A full understanding of their potential complications is necessary to be sure that negative side effects do not outweigh possible advantages. To be fully effective, the physician needs the requisite knowledge and skills to treat acute life-threatening illness as well as the supportive staying power to care for the chronically ill patient. One learns to care for patients in a variety of environments: in the office, in the emergency room, in the hospital, by telephone, or when the patient is housebound or in a nursing home.

The care of the patient involves far more than prescribing drugs and completing therapeutic procedures. Attention is paid to the preventive aspects of disease, to the patient's psychological problems, and to conflicts arising from home or place of work. Immunization for infectious disease and advice to avoid smoking and excessive drinking are obvious examples of preventive measures. The patient may need to alter his way of living, if job stress plays a role. Psychiatric or family counseling may help when there are major psychological problems.

Good communication with the patient is required in order to educate him about his illness, its management, and its prevention. A better informed patient will be more motivated to comply with treatment. The ability to communicate well is also needed when dealing with responsible family members and with others caring for the patient. Diabetes mellitus is an excellent example of an illness that requires education and the help of others. The patient needs to understand the disease in order to know why diet is important, why blood sugar levels are high, and why insulin is used. He learns the potential complications and how to prevent them. Nurses help the patient learn to test glucose levels and to use an insulin syringe; dietitians teach a diabetic diet.

In providing excellent care, the competent physician knows how frequently a patient should be seen and how extensive an evaluation is necessary. These decisions require good clinical judgment and a rationale for each action. It is important for the physician to instruct the patient how to obtain medical care at all times, particularly in an acute emergency or when the physician is not available. Above all, the physician demonstrates a continuing personal interest in the patient, is the patient's advocate, and assumes responsibility for all of his health care needs.

THE MEDICAL RECORD

The primary purpose of the medical record is to document the medical experience of the patient. This information is used by those concerned with the patient's current and future care. Legally, it is a public document available to other physicians and to health care providers, to the court by subpoena, and to insurance companies. The medical record varies in format and detail, depending on whether the patient is seen in an ambulatory setting or in the emergency room or is admitted to the hospital.

A major contribution to the organization of the medical record has been the introduction of the problem-oriented method. Of particular importance are the problem list and the problem-oriented progress notes. The medical record of the patient may be organized by combining the traditional format of the history and physical examination with the identification of active problems. If there is a single major problem that is not clearly defined, a formulation is written. The physician gives the reasons for the diagnosis and weighs evidence for and against other diagnostic possibilities. When there are several active problems, these are discussed separately, each with a diagnostic and therapeutic plan.

The problem list is particularly useful when following an

ambulatory patient who has chronic illness and multiple problems. A list of active and inactive problems serves as an index to the record. In this way, problems are summarized and can be quickly reviewed. Problem-oriented progress notes help to organize ongoing clinical information. During the course of an illness, they enable one to easily follow individual problems through the record.

Establishment of the scientific basis of the art of medicine will lead to future clarification of each step of the medical encounter between the patient and physician. The expert clinician's resolution of a problem is not easily understood. Research defining the abilities and tasks of a physician will help to eliminate the dichotomy between the art and science of medicine.

American Board of Internal Medicine: Clinical competence in internal medicine. Ann Intern Med 90:402, 1979. *The major components of the medical encounter are analyzed, which include the abilities required of an internist, the tasks performed to solve a medical problem, the medical illness, and the patient.*

Eddy DM: Clinical policies and the quality of clinical practice. N Engl J Med 307:343, 1982. *A description is given of some of the sources of errors and biases in clinical policy making, with suggested ways to improve the quality of clinical policies.*

Elstein AS, Shulman LS, Sprafka SA: Medical Problem Solving. An Analysis of Clinical Reasoning. Cambridge, Mass., Harvard University Press, 1978. *A detailed, yet readable textbook gives the results of five years of research on medical problem solving and decision making based on the performance of selected internists and students in a variety of experimental situations.*

Griner PF, Panzer RJ, Greenland P: Clinical Diagnosis and the Laboratory. Logical Strategies for Common Medical Problems. Chicago, Year Book Medical Publishers, 1986. *This book provides a review of the scientific approach to selecting and interpreting diagnostic tests and procedures. Preferred diagnostic strategies are given for specific commonly considered clinical problems in adult medicine.*

Kassirer JP, Gorry GA: Clinical problem solving. A behavioral analysis. Ann Intern Med 89:245, 1978. *Tape-recorded interviews of simulated patients by experienced clinicians are studied to determine how hypothesis generation is used in clinical problem solving.*

Morgan WL, Engel GL: The Clinical Approach to the Patient. Philadelphia, W. B. Saunders Company, 1969. *This is a step-by-step guide to interviewing the patient, organizing the physical examination, and handling clinical information, with particular emphasis on how to relate to the patient.*

Weinstein MC, Fineberg HV: Clinical Decision Analysis. Philadelphia, W. B. Saunders Company, 1980. *A detailed quantitative analysis is given of clinical decision making, which includes the use of decision trees and probabilities and the assigning of values to possible outcomes.*

21 CLINICAL DECISION MAKING
Stephen G. Pauker

The primary role of the physician is to make decisions—about what tests to order, about what test results mean, about what drugs to administer, about whether or not to perform surgery. Virtually all medical decisions are made beneath a cloak of uncertainty—about diagnosis, about the effectiveness of therapeutic alternatives, about prognosis. Classic medical education has rarely included a formal approach to decision making in an uncertain world, despite its central position in medical practice. Over the past two decades, normative prescriptive techniques, borrowed from the military and business worlds, have been applied increasingly to medicine.

The benefits of these approaches rest on their explicit nature, on their unyielding requirements for information, and on the ability to ask "What if?" What if this disease were more likely? What if surgery were more effective but also engendered a higher risk? What if the patient is an octogenarian? What if the optimal time for diagnostic testing had passed and the test's sensitivity were therefore diminished? Of course, these approaches also carry significant cost: They are unfamiliar to most physicians, sometimes require extra effort, and always require the decision maker to confront uncertainty and to be explicit about his or her assumptions and data base.

Clinical decision analyses are often confused with clinical algorithms or flow charts, which have gained increasing popularity as media for representing and communicating management strategies. The latter are compact schemata for summarizing a set of rules of "if-then" statements that can lead the clinician down an established management pathway. It would be possible, for example, to translate many of the management strategies in this book into flow charts. Unfortunately, algorithms do not provide a process for creating such rules; they are most often the implicit product of singular or communal experience, although algorithms are sometimes annotated to describe the rationale that underlies them. Indeed, some investigators have used the decision analytic techniques described in this chapter to help formulate algorithms.

THE INTERPRETATION OF DATA

In making a diagnosis, the physician moves continually between two tasks: data gathering and data interpretation. The former task involves identifying potential data elements and deciding which elements to select. The latter task involves modifying a set of hypotheses based on new data elements; those new elements might be drawn from the patient's history, from the physical examination, from laboratory tests, or from the patient's response to diagnostic or therapeutic maneuvers. In each case, however, the new data might suggest new diagnostic hypotheses and almost always will modify the clinician's strength of belief in existing hypotheses. Those beliefs can be most conveniently represented as *probabilities*, the likelihood of each diagnosis on a scale from 0 to 1, which can be manipulated by several basic rules:

1. The probability of a diagnosis being false ($P_{no\ dis}$) equals $(1 - P_{dis})$ where P_{dis} is the probability of the diagnosis.

2. The list of alternative diagnoses must be exhaustive, and the probabilities must sum to 1.0 (thus, one often includes a category "other" in the list of diagnoses).

3. The various hypotheses must be mutually exclusive (thus, if one hypothesis is that diseases a and b coexist, then the explicit hypothesis "diseases a and b" must be included).

4. Among these mutually exclusive diagnoses, the probability that the patient has at least one of several diagnoses equals the sum of their probabilities [thus, $P_{a\ or\ b}$ equals ($P_a + P_b$)].

5. If events are independent, then their joint probability equals the product of the probabilities (thus, $P_{a\ and\ b}$ equals $P_a \times P_b$).

6. If events are dependent, then their joint probability equals the product of the probability of the first (P_a) and the conditional probability of the second, given the first ($P_{b/a}$).

Bayes' Rule

In this context, data are interpreted using Bayes' rule, a relation among probabilities that allows the clinician to modify his or her level of belief in each hypothesis based on incremental data. The technique begins with the probability of each disease before knowledge of the incremental finding. These probabilities are called the *prior probabilities* and are often estimated by the prevalence of each disease. Next, for each disease the *conditional probability* of the incremental finding ($P_{finding/dis_i}$) is specified. Although these probabilities can be combined using the equation for Bayes' rule

$$P_{dis_j/finding} = \frac{P_{dis_j} \times P_{finding/dis_j}}{\sum\limits_{i=1}^{n} P_{dis_i} \times P_{finding/dis_i}}$$

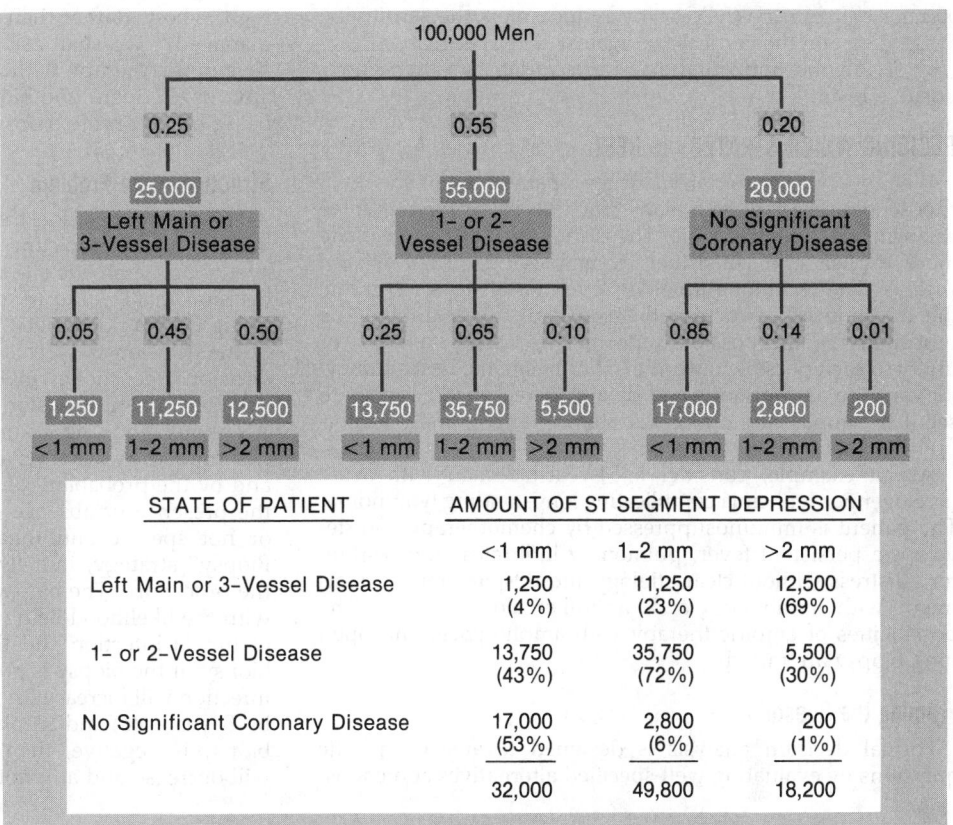

FIGURE 21–1. Cohort flow model of Bayes' rule used to interpret an exercise tolerance test in a 50-year old man with typical angina. Consider a cohort of 100,000 such men: 25 per cent have left main or 3-vessel disease, 55 per cent have 1- or 2-vessel disease, and 20 per cent are free of significant coronary disease. If the conditional probabilities of < 1 mm, 1–2 mm, and > 2 mm of ST depression are as shown and determine how many men from each diagnostic subgroup will have each finding, then of the 1250 + 13,750 + 17,000 (or 32,000) men with < 1 mm of ST depression, 17,000, or 53 per cent, will have no significant coronary disease, 43 per cent will have 1- or 2-vessel disease, and 4 per cent will have left main or 3-vessel disease.

STATE OF PATIENT	AMOUNT OF ST SEGMENT DEPRESSION		
	<1 mm	1–2 mm	>2 mm
Left Main or 3-Vessel Disease	1,250 (4%)	11,250 (23%)	12,500 (69%)
1- or 2-Vessel Disease	13,750 (43%)	35,750 (72%)	5,500 (30%)
No Significant Coronary Disease	17,000 (53%)	2,800 (6%)	200 (1%)
	32,000	49,800	18,200

it is almost always easier to use the tabular form of the technique (Table 21–1) or the cohort flow form (Fig. 21–1).

In the simplest case, the physician considers a single disease and interprets a diagnostic test, which is either positive or negative. In that situation, the probability of a positive test in a patient who has the disease, $P_{positive\ test/dis}$, is called the *sensitivity* of the test, and the probability of a negative test in a patient who does not have the disease, $P_{negative\ test/no\ dis}$, is called *specificity* of the test. The examples in Table 21–1 and Figure 21–1 demonstrate common settings in which implicit test interpretation is fraught with error: (1) In the setting of a low prior probability of disease, a positive finding often does not suggest a very high probability of disease unless the test is extremely specific; and (2) in the setting of a high prior probability of disease, a negative finding often does not suggest a very low probability of disease unless the test is extremely sensitive. Especially in those situations, it would be important to interpret the finding in an explicit and formal manner, using probabilities as described here.

When interpreting several findings, the calculated posterior or revised probabilities based on the first finding become the prior probabilities for interpreting the next finding in a sequential application of Bayes' rule. In such circumstances, the several findings may not be conditionally independent of one another. For example, in the diagnostic evaluation of a patient suspected of having a pulmonary embolism, the chest radiograph and the lung scan are not conditionally independent: In the setting of a normal chest film, a perfusion scan with a segmental defect is far more suggestive of pulmonary embolism than the same scan result in a patient with the radiologic findings of chronic pulmonary disease. In such situations, the probability of the finding must be conditioned on both disease and on the other dependent findings ($P_{finding/dis\ and\ other\ findings}$).

Many findings are innately continuous in nature, e.g., a serum creatine kinase level, the size of the liver, and the size of the left atrium. For a given finding to be positive or negative, one must first establish a *criterion* for defining a positive result. Furthermore, to determine the conditional probabilities of a given finding, one needs a separate *gold standard* to define the presence or absence of each disease. Changing either the gold standard or the test criterion will change the conditional probabilities of the findings. For example, if a positive exercise tolerance test is defined as one with ≥ 1 mm ST depression, then the sensitivity for the diagnosis of coronary disease would be 81 per cent and the specificity would be 85 per cent (see data in Fig. 21–1). On the other hand, if a positive result were defined as > 2 mm ST depression, then the sensitivity would be only 23 per cent but the specificity would be 99 per cent. In general, a more strict criterion (e.g., > 2 mm compared with ≥ 1 mm of ST depression) increases specificity and decreases sensitivity; a more lax criterion increases sensitivity and decreases specificity. The relations among sensitivity, specificity, and the definition of a positive finding are summarized by a *receiver*

TABLE 21–1. USING BAYES' RULE TO INTERPRET A SPUTUM CYTOLOGIC STUDY DEMONSTRATING ATYPICAL CELLS IN A NONSMOKER WITH A PULMONARY NODULE

A Diagnosis	B Prior Probability	C Conditional Probability of Observed Test Result	D Product (Col B times Col C)	E Revised or Posterior Probability (Col E/Sum)
Cancer	0.01	0.40	0.004	0.04
No Cancer	0.99	0.10	0.099	0.96
		Sum =	0.103	

Step 1: List diagnoses in Column A.
Step 2: List prior probabilities in Column B.
Step 3: List conditional probabilities of finding in Column C.
Step 4: Multiply Columns B and C and place products in Column D.
Step 5: Divide each entry in Column D by sum of Column D and place quotients in Column E.

operator characteristic (ROC) curve, which plots the sensitivity, $P_{positive\ result/dis}$, on the vertical axis against $(1 - specificity)$, $P_{positive\ result/no\ dis}$, on the horizontal axis for a variety of criteria for a positive result.

DECIDING WHICH STRATEGY IS BEST

Whenever the physician manages a patient, he or she must choose among alternative plans. Such decisions often involve balancing risks and benefits. These choices often can be made more explicit and consistent by employing formal *decision analysis*. The technique involves seven basic steps: (1) frame the question; (2) structure the problem; (3) determine the probability of the possible outcomes; (4) assign a value or utility to each possible outcome; (5) calculate the best strategy; (6) vary the assumptions and data over reasonable ranges to see if the apparently optimal strategy changes; and (7) interpret the analysis.

As an example, consider a 54-year-old man with acute myelogenous leukemia complicating longstanding lymphoma. The patient is immunosuppressed by chemotherapy and develops a persistent fever, pulmonary infiltrates, and respiratory distress without clear etiology and despite empiric treatment with antibiotics and antituberculosis drugs. The possibilities of empiric therapy with amphotericin and open lung biopsy are raised.

Framing the Question

Formal decision analysis is designed to answer specific questions by evaluating well-specified alternatives and choosing the best. Rather than asking "How should this patient be managed," we shall ask which of three alternatives is best: (1) empiric therapy with amphotericin, (2) conservative therapy, or (3) open lung biopsy with the amphotericin decision being based on the biopsy results.

Structuring the Problem

The typical decision tree contains three basic elements: (1) decision nodes depicting choices, (2) chance nodes depicting events or diagnostic alternatives not under the control of the decision maker, and (3) outcome or terminal nodes summarizing events not explicitly occurring within the time horizon of the decision tree. This problem can be represented by the decision tree shown in Figure 21–2. The three choices are depicted by the decision node at the left. In both the "No Amphotericin" and "Amphotericin" strategies, prognosis is determined by whether or not a fungal infection is present and by the probability of short-term survival, conditioned on the presence or absence of fungal infection and on whether or not specific antifungal therapy is given. In the "Lung Biopsy" strategy, initially there is a chance of dying during the procedure. The biopsy may be either positive or negative, with the likelihood being determined by the prior probability of fungal infection and the sensitivity and specificity of the biopsy. If the biopsy is positive, then the probability of fungal infection will increase (the revised probability being calculated by Bayes' rule) and amphotericin will be administered. If the biopsy is negative, then the probability of fungal infection will decrease and amphotericin will be withheld.

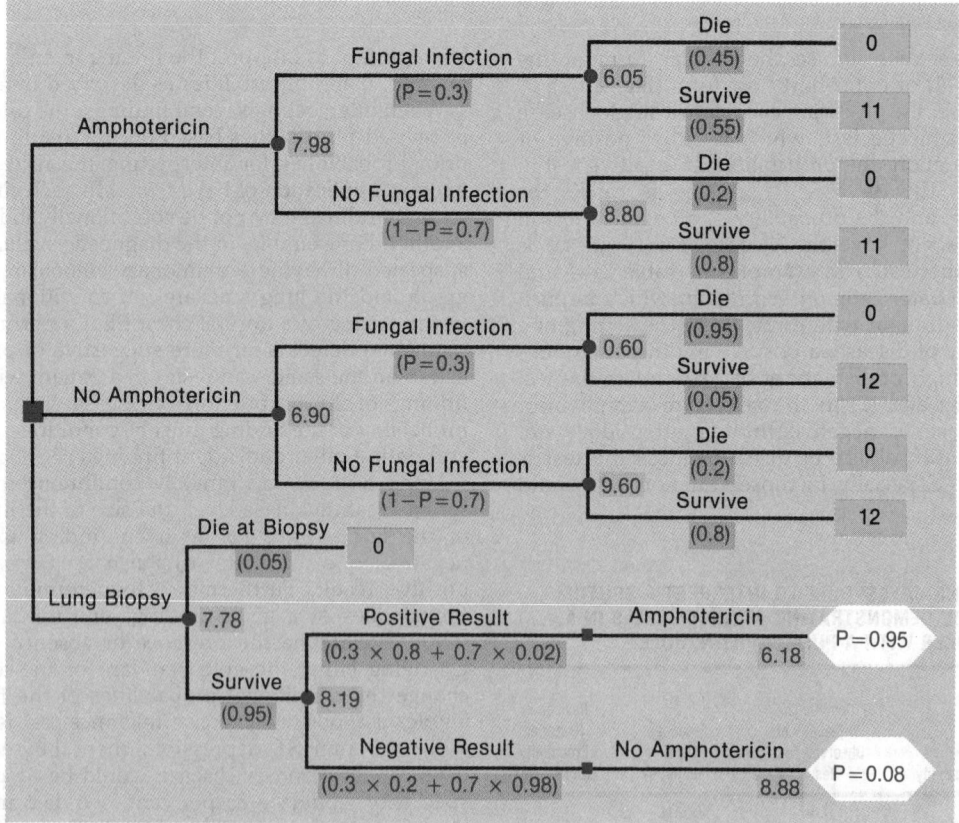

FIGURE 21–2. Decision tree depicting management choices in an immunosuppressed man with fever and pulmonary infiltrates. Decision nodes appear as squares. Chance nodes appear as circles. Outcome or terminal nodes appear as rectangles that contain the assigned utilities (in this case as quality-adjusted months of survival). Probabilities are shown shaded red on each branch of each chance node. The hexagons at the end of the "Lung Biopsy" strategy represent the use of the "No Amphotericin" and "Amphotericin" subtrees (which are used in the first two branches of the main decision node) with the probability of fungal infection being modified to 0.95 and 0.08 after a positive and negative biopsy, respectively, by the application of Bayes' rule. Calculated expected utilities are shown solid red adjacent to each node. The sensitivity of the biopsy is taken as 0.8; the specificity is taken as 0.98. P = Probability of fungal infection.

Determining the Probabilities

In a decision tree, probabilities describe the present state of the patient (e.g., whether or not fungal disease is present) and the patient's prognosis. In both cases, these estimates can be based on the literature or on expert opinion. In either case, the physician uses descriptions of the past experience of other similar patients to predict the current and future state of the patient at hand.

In this case, we estimated the probability of fungal infection to be 30 per cent; we estimated the chance of dying from untreated fungal infection to be 95 per cent and the chance of dying from treated fungal infection to be 45 per cent. If fungal disease is not present, we estimated that the probability of death during this hospitalization to be 20 per cent. We estimated that, in this setting, lung biopsy would be associated with a 5 per cent mortality, a sensitivity of 80 per cent in diagnosing fungal infection, and a specificity of 98 per cent.

Assigning Utilities

The relative value of each possible outcome is summarized on a single consistent scale by a utility. Such scales can be arbitrary (e.g., 0 being the worst outcome and 100 being the best) or can describe the outcomes in identifiable units (e.g., five-year survival, years of life, years of disease-free survival, or even dollars spent). One useful metric can be *quality-adjusted life expectancy*, in which average survival is depreciated by long- and short-term morbidities. If such a metric is used, it is sometimes possible for the patient or the patient's family to contribute to the decision by expressing their attitudes about quality of life.

In this case, we shall use average survival modified by the short-term morbidity of amphotericin therapy. We estimated that survival would be 18 months if the patient achieves a remission of his leukemia but only 3 months if he does not. Because we assumed the chance of remission to be 60 per cent, the average survival for this man, if he survived the acute event, would be 60 per cent × 18 plus 40 per cent × 3, or 12 months. Although many physicians are very conservative in using amphotericin, the literature suggests that death and permanent renal failure are extremely rare complications of that drug; most side effects involve short-term toxicity. We assumed that the average duration of amphotericin therapy would be 2 months and that short-term morbidity would, on average, diminish quality of life during that period to half of what it otherwise would have been. Thus, we subtracted 1 month from the life expectancy to account for this morbidity, yielding a quality-adjusted survival of 11 months if amphotericin is administered. We assigned a utility of 0 to death during this acute illness.

Calculating the Expected Utility

In evaluating a tree, the decision maker follows two basic rules: (1) When facing a choice, select the option with the highest utility or expected utility; (2) when evaluating a chance event, the expected utility is the weighted average of the utilities of its outcomes, with the weights being the respective probability of each outcome. In applying these rules, the decision maker begins at the distal outcome nodes of the tree and sequentially calculates the average or expected utility of each node, moving toward the proximal decision node.

In this case, consider first the top branch of the decision node, the "Amphotericin" strategy. The highest distal chance node describes the short-term consequences of a fungal infection treated with specific antifungal therapy. There is a 0.45 probability of dying (utility 0) and 0.55 probability of surviving (utility 11 quality-adjusted months). The average or expected utility of this chance node is 0.45 × 0 plus 0.55 × 11, or 6.05 quality-adjusted months. Similarly, the expected utility of amphotericin in the absence of a fungal infection (the second distal chance node) is 0.2 × 0 plus 0.8 × 11, or

8.8 quality-adjusted months. The expected utility of the "Amphotericin" strategy is the weighted average of these two expected utilities: 0.3 × 6.05 plus 0.7 × 8.8, or 7.98 quality-adjusted months. In a similar fashion, we calculated the expected utility of "No Amphotericin" to be 6.9 quality-adjusted months.

Next we consider the lowest branch of the main decision node: the "Lung Biopsy" strategy. As depicted at the end of the "Positive" result branch, the expected utility is calculated using the "Amphotericin" subtree, with the probability of fungal infection being increased to 0.95. In that case, the expected utility is 0.95 × 6.05 plus 0.05 × 8.8, or 6.18 quality-adjusted months. Similarly, the expected utility of the "Negative" result branch is calculated with the "No Amphotericin" subtree, with the probability of fungal infection being decreased to 0.08, yielding 0.08 × 0.6 plus 0.92 × 9.6, or 8.88 quality-adjusted months. The weighted average of these expected utilities depends on the probability of a positive result (0.3 × 0.8 plus 0.7 × 0.02, or 0.25). The expected utility of the entire strategy is a weighted average of this result (8.19 quality-adjusted months) and the 5 per cent chance of a procedure-related death (utility 0), providing an expected utility of 7.78 quality-adjusted months.

Performing Sensitivity Analyses

Having calculated the expected utility in the baseline case, we next examine various central assumptions to determine whether reasonable variations in those assumed values will change the conclusions. Such sensitivity analyses initially examine variables one at a time, usually beginning with the "softest" data. Such analyses are often called *one-way sensitivity analyses* (see Fig. 21–3).

Typically, one strategy will be best for all values of the variable below a certain cutoff, and another strategy will be best for all values above that cutoff. The value at which the strategies have equal expected utility is called the *threshold* value for that variable. In addition to finding relevant threshold values, it is often important to examine the magnitude of the differences in expected values of the various strategies. If those differences are very small and potentially clinically insignificant, then the decision may well be a *close call*, and

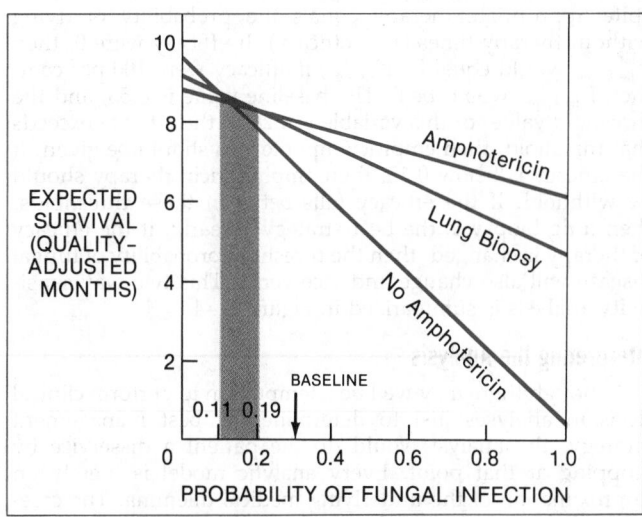

FIGURE 21–3. One-way sensitivity analysis of the effect of changing the probability of fungal infection in the decision tree shown in Figure 21–2. If the probability of fungal infection is zero, then the "No Amphotericin" strategy is best. If the probability of fungal infection is 100 per cent, then empiric amphotericin therapy is best. Lung biopsy is the optimal strategy in the narrow region between the two thresholds (vertical color bar) at 0.11 and 0.19. The baseline value of 0.3 is shown by the arrow.

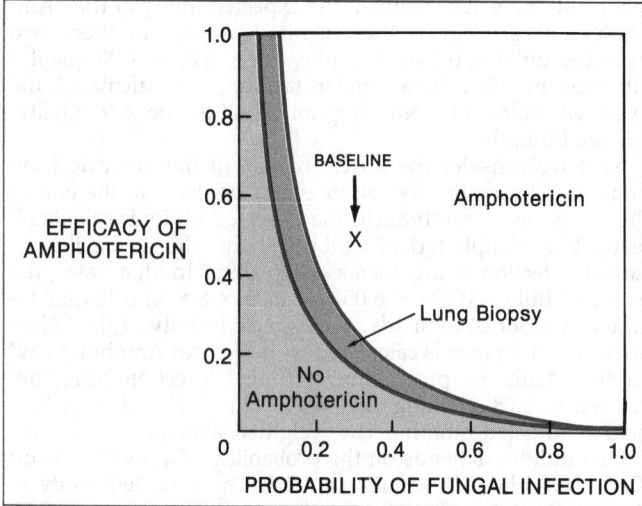

FIGURE 21–4. Two-way sensitivity analysis of the relation between the probability of fungal infection (horizontal axis) and the efficacy of amphotericin (vertical axis). Each combination of values corresponds to a unique point on the graph. All combinations falling in the lighter shaded area correspond to settings in which "no amphotericin" is the best strategy. All combinations falling in the darker shaded area correspond to settings in which "lung biopsy" is best. The baseline values correspond to the bold X, which lies within the settings in which amphotericin is best (indicated by the unshaded area).

there may be relatively little to gain or lose in selecting one management plan over another. With sufficient time and energy or with adequate computational support, the clinician also can examine the effect of simultaneous changes in two or more variables. Such multiway sensitivity analyses are often summarized by decision diagrams that specify the best strategy for each combination of values (see Fig. 21–4).

In this case, the softest piece of data is the likelihood that this patient has a fungal infection. The one-way sensitivity analysis of this variable is summarized in Figure 21–3. Another central variable is the effectiveness of amphotericin in enhancing survival in an immunosuppressed patient known to have fungal disease. We define the *efficacy* of therapy to be $1 - (P_{die/Ampho}/P_{die/No\ Ampho})$. Thus, the probability of dying despite appropriate therapy equals the probability of dying without therapy times $(1 - efficacy)$. If efficacy were 0, then $P_{die/Ampho}$ would equal $P_{die/No\ Ampho}$; if efficacy were 100 per cent, then $P_{die/Ampho}$ would be 0. The baseline value is 0.53, and the threshold value for this variable is 0.28. If the efficacy exceeds that threshold, then empiric amphotericin should be given. If the efficacy is below 0.15, then amphotericin therapy should be withheld. If the efficacy falls between these thresholds, then lung biopsy is the best strategy. Clearly, if the efficacy of therapy is changed, then the threshold probability of fungal disease will also change and vice versa. This two-way sensitivity analysis is summarized in Figure 21–4.

Interpreting the Analysis

Although there may well be a temptation to perform clinical decision analyses just to determine the best management strategy, the analyst would do the patient a disservice by stopping at that point. Every analytic model is merely an approximation of the underlying medical dilemma. The careful analyst must explore the model to discover its limitations. Only then can the clinician have reasonable confidence in its conclusions. One of the central benefits of a clinical decision analysis should be a better understanding of the clinical problem and a delineation of the settings in which the planned strategy is proper.

In this analysis, we see that empiric therapy with amphotericin is appropriate for any patient who has at least a

moderate likelihood (over 20 per cent) of fungal infection. Therapy based on the results of lung biopsy is best only for the narrow wedge of patients falling in the darker shaded region of Figure 21–4. This region would be broadened if lung biopsy had a lower complication rate but would still be limited by the imperfect sensitivity of the test: Some patients with potentially treatable fungal infections would be denied therapy if their biopsy yielded falsely negative results. The major driving force is the surprisingly benign characteristics of amphotericin. Although patients receiving the drug have significant short-term morbidity, very few develop permanent renal insufficiency and even fewer die.

COST-BENEFIT AND COST-EFFECTIVENESS ANALYSIS

The practice of medicine in a world of limited resources sometimes leads the physicians to consider not only what is "best" for the patient but also the resources that such medical care will use. In such contexts, cost-benefit and cost-effectiveness analyses can be used to establish policies. Because those policies may affect the way he or she practices medicine, the physician should understand some of the underlying principles. The basic logic of such analyses is quite similar to that described above; the difference lies in the utility scales that measure the relative worth of the potential outcomes. When resources and societal issues are considered, outcomes are often measured by their economic impact. Economists argue that the magnitude of a cost depends on, among other things, *when* that cost is incurred. Money saved or spent immediately is worth more than money saved or spent in the future. This principle is called the *discounting* of future benefits and costs: Future costs and benefits are diminished by a fixed proportion for each year into the future when such cost and benefits occur. When several different utilities are considered (e.g., survival and economic costs), some analysts argue that all utility scales should be discounted at the same rate; other analysts argue that discounting should be restricted to monetary factors. When considering the economics of medical care, we should be careful to distinguish actual *costs* from *charges*, which may be quite distorted by particular billing practices or insurance plans. We also should consider *indirect costs* (e.g., heating and cleaning in the hospital and even malpractice insurance) and *induced costs* (e.g., the diagnostic evaluation of patients with falsely positive screening test results and even the medical care for treating cancer that develops years later in a patient who is "saved" from tuberculous pneumonia).

In a *cost-benefit analysis*, economic impact is the only utility scale used: All benefits are measured in those terms. Thus, if a strategy increases survival, that benefit is translated into its monetary equivalent: Each year of life saved would be associated with a societal worth, perhaps based on economic productivity. If the benefits minus the costs of a given strategy are positive, the program contributes in the net to society. Presumably, the bigger the difference, the larger the contribution. If the costs of a strategy exceed its benefits, the program should not necessarily be rejected. Society might well wish to underwrite such a program. For example, extending the life of a disabled, elderly nursing home resident might not provide net economic benefit to society, but our ethical values argue strongly against withdrawing care from such individuals.

Because the economic value of life and improved quality of life are difficult to quantify, we often turn to *cost-effectiveness analyses*, in which two separate utility measures are analyzed simultaneously, e.g., monetary costs and years of life saved. The results are expressed as the *ratio* of cost to benefits. That ratio does not measure the overall worth of a single strategy; rather, it is used to compare strategies. Often the strategy that engenders greater resource costs is also the strategy that provides the greater effectiveness. Thus, one usually examines the ratio of the difference in costs to the difference in effectiveness (the *marginal cost-effectiveness ratio*), which might be expressed as additional dollars spent per additional year of life saved or even as additional dollars spent per additional cancer detected. Such analyses rarely tell the decision maker in an absolute sense which strategy is best: They provide only a measure of cost per unit of gain. Some external standard, perhaps established by society, must be applied to decide how much money is too much to spend to gain a year of life. Such analyses can also help when we must choose among alternate uses for a fixed amount of resource, i.e., a budget. When we have only another $100,000 to spend, should we "buy" one heart transplant, five coronary bypass operations, or a year of therapy for 1000 hypertensive men? These are difficult decisions, but physicians must now contribute to the discussion, hopefully in a logical, explicit, and useful way.

Diamond GA, Forrester JS: Analysis of probability as an aid in the clinical diagnosis of coronary-artery disease. N Engl J Med 300:1350, 1979. *Provides data and techniques for the interpretation of exercise testing in the context of various clinical presentations of coronary disease.*

Gottlieb JE, Pauker SG: Whether or not to administer amphotericin B to an immunosuppressed patient with hematologic malignancy and undiagnosed fever. Med Decision Making 1:75, 1981. *The detailed clinical decision analysis that forms the basis for the amphotericin decision model.*

Griner PF, Mayesski RJ, Mushlin AI, et al: Selection and interpretation of diagnostic tests and procedures. Ann Intern Med 94:553, 1981. *Primer on Bayes' rule with many examples.*

Kassirer JP: The principles of clinical decision making: An introduction to decision analysis. Yale J Biol 49:149, 1976. *Conversational introduction to building decision trees for professional football and medicine.*

Kassirer JP, Moskowitz AJ, Lau J, et al.: Decision analysis: A progress report. Ann Intern Med, 106:275, 1987. *Review of the literature and classification of techniques and clinical questions.*

Lusted LB: Introduction To Medical Decision Making. Springfield, Ill., Charles C Thomas, 1968. *One of the first monographs suggesting how probability theory could be applied to medicine.*

McNeil BJ, Keeler E, Adelstein SJ: Primer on certain elements of medical decision making. N Engl J Med 293:211, 1975. *General introduction to Bayes' rule, ROC analysis, and information theory.*

Pauker SG, Kassirer JP: Medical progress: Decision analysis. N Engl J Med, 316:250, 1987. *A tutorial about new techniques.*

Plante DA, Kassirer JP, Zarin DA, et al.: A clinical decision consultation service. Am J Med 80:1169, 1986. *Description of experience using clinical decision analysis in the care of individual patients.*

Raiffa H: Decision Analysis: Introductory Lectures on Choices Under Uncertainty. Reading, Mass., Addison-Wesley, 1968. *The classic introduction to decision theory for business students.*

Weinstein MC, Fineberg HV, Elstein AS, et al.: Clinical Decision Analysis. Philadelphia, W.B. Saunders Company, 1980. *Overall introduction replete with examples.*

22 THE USE AND INTERPRETATION OF LABORATORY-DERIVED DATA

James B. Wyngaarden

The basic workup of a patient begins with the acquisition of information. The experienced clinician will acquire a discerning and sensitive history and perform a thorough physical examination and such laboratory tests as may be necessary to evaluate the general health of the patient, to arrive at a specific diagnosis, to assess the functional status of involved organs, or to provide a basis for monitoring effectiveness of therapy.

Until two decades ago only a few laboratory tests were performed routinely in the workup of a patient. When screening was practiced, the panel of tests was usually limited to hemoglobin (or hematocrit) determination, blood cell counts, urinalysis, stool examination for occult blood, and perhaps a chest x-ray and an electrocardiogram, particularly in adults. Additional tests were ordered only when suggested by the clinical assessment. In this setting an attending physician could evaluate the reasoning process that led a physician in training to order a serum calcium determination or a serum alkaline phosphatase assay. The ordering of laboratory procedures was a consequence of the intellectual discipline of constructing a logical differential diagnosis or of the need to monitor the progress of a patient, e.g., one in diabetic ketoacidosis. Thus it was a vital component of the educational process itself.

In 1966 Thiers published a provocative study comparing the results of a screening battery of 11 tests run by an automated multichannel analyzer with those of tests specifically ordered on the same patients by physicians as part of the admission workup. The screening battery detected twice as many abnormal test results as were uncovered by selective ordering. The most common findings were elevated glucose or uric acid concentrations. Ensuing developments were rapid. Ingenious automated analyzers brought an increasing number and variety of tests within the reach of all practitioners. The cost of such a screening battery fell rapidly until soon one could obtain 12 to 18 test results for no more than the cost of 3 or 4 selected tests run manually a decade earlier.

The inclusion of a panel of chemical tests or enzyme assays of blood (or urine) became a routine component of a basic medical workup. For more than a decade, medical students and resident physicians have been brought up with a dependency upon such screening batteries of chemical measurements. Only a few hospitals resisted the temptation to institute such screening procedures and continued the traditional practice of letting the intellectual evaluation of the patient determine the indications for further laboratory procedures. The pendulum has now begun to swing back, as the limited utility of large panel testing has become more generally recognized. Only a small number of "screening tests" (history, physical examination, stool guaiac test, and blood pressure measurement) have actually been shown to improve the health outcome of asymptomatic outpatients. Admission screening tests, such as a "Chem 12," complete blood count, or sedimentation rate, have a relatively low yield: Fewer than 1 per cent lead to a "new" diagnosis. In fact, fewer than 10 per cent of Chem 12 data are ever used clinically, and as few as 40 per cent of "abnormal" results initiate a follow-up. Furthermore, unnecessary hospitalization has occurred when one laboratory test result of a screening panel was "abnormal" by chance on a statistical basis alone. Whenever 20 procedures are done, whose "normal" range is defined as the central 95 per cent segment, one test result will, on the average, fall outside this range on the basis of chance alone. Statistically, 40 per cent of all Chem 12 panels performed on healthy individuals will result in one "abnormal" result. Repetition of tests showing such aberrant results contributes to the high cost of medical care, but only rarely to the detection of significant dysfunction or disease. As a consequence of this additional experience, some of the larger teaching hospitals have discontinued screening panels. This movement has been accelerated by the exclusion of routine screening procedures from the list of reimbursable expenditures by some third-party payers of medical services.

In order to utilize the results of laboratory tests intelligently (and economically), the physician must be able to evaluate the validity of the test result, understand principles of variation and distribution of values, and integrate the data received from the laboratory with the information acquired from the patient. If the test result deviates from values found in a healthy control population, is the difference trivial, or is it indicative of important dysfunction? Should the test be repeated? How often need a particular measurement be followed up? What additional tests or studies are indicated on the basis of these leads?

The more information the physician has, the more effective the physician should be in caring for the patient. To ensure that this is the result requires knowledge of science and medicine, clinical judgment, and a profound respect for the limitations of the laboratory. One of the best ways of acquiring the constructively critical attitude so essential to the proper evaluation of laboratory data is to work in a laboratory for a while. There is a paradox in the present pattern of medical education: At a time of increasing reliance upon an expanding array of laboratory tests in the practice of medicine, learning experiences in the laboratory have largely been eliminated from the medical curriculum!

SOME LIMITATIONS OF THE LABORATORY

CRITERIA FOR EVALUATION OF LABORATORY METHODS. A trustworthy laboratory test must pass critical evaluations of analytic specificity, sensitivity, accuracy, and precision.

Specificity refers to the detection of the substance in question and no other. It is doubtful that any test is absolutely specific for the substance being measured. There is always some other substance around that is capable of reacting. In biochemical analyses this limitation is most serious in tests dependent upon color development, less in the case of assays dependent upon degradation of the analyte by purified enzymes, and perhaps least in such procedures as atomic absorption spectroscopy.

Sensitivity refers to the ability of the test to detect the substance in question at the required concentrations, namely, those at which the compound exists in body fluids.

Accuracy refers to the quantitative detection of the correct amount of the substance being measured. This property rests upon both specificity and sensitivity. A test may be accurate in the absence of certain interfering drugs, and only in a certain range of values. It may fail this criterion under other conditions.

Precision embodies *repeatability*, the obtaining of the same result on samples analyzed in replicated fashion, and *reproducibility*, representing quality control over time.

THE "LAW OF ERRORS." Early in the nineteenth century, the German mathematician and physicist, Johann C. F. Gauss, introduced the "law of errors." This law states that in repeated measurements of the *same* object or substance, the random component on the errors will be distributed about the mean as a frequency function. This distribution, which is bell shaped, is often called "normal" or "gaussian." Note that the law applies to repeated measurements of the same item. Its extension to a population of those items is justifiable only under certain circumstances, for not all distributions are bell shaped, and not all bell-shaped distributions are gaussian. The matter of distributions will be discussed further below, when we consider the topic of "normal range" of a biologic variable.

SOURCES OF VARIANCE

These include some factors under the control of the clinician, such as the dietary preparation of the patient and the techniques of collection and handling of samples. Reduction of variance to an acceptable minimum requires compulsive attention to every detail of the process.

LABORATORY ERRORS. There is imprecision in every measurement. In tests run by hand, pipetting, timing, reading, and recording errors occur. They are more frequent when technicians are overworked or fatigued. It is common to find greater scatter of results of replicate tests at the end of the day than at the beginning. Technician fatigue can be largely eliminated by automation, but there will always remain the technical limitations of machines and the human error in the preparation of reagents, in the standardization of instruments, and in the copying of test results. The last is not totally avoided by the computer print-out, as even typewriters make misteaks. Quality control varies widely from laboratory to laboratory. Split samples submitted to different laboratories may show surprising disparities in results.

DRUG INTERFERENCE. According to Osler, humans are distinguished from all other members of the animal kingdom by their desire to take drugs. Since many patients do not regard proprietary pain remedies or vitamins as drugs, the physician may obtain a negative drug history unless questions are appropriately phrased. Drugs have great potential for interference with laboratory tests. High-resolution chromatography of urine yields about 300 peaks of ultraviolet-absorbing materials. Two hundred and fifty of these disappear if the "normal subject" abstains from salicylates and vitamins for a few days. Salicylates, vitamins, and many other drugs or their metabolites also produce chromogens that interfere with certain analytic methods employed in automated tests, particularly of the urine.

DISTRIBUTIONS OF VALUES

There is widespread belief among medical students and graduate physicians that if the sample of test results from a healthy population is large enough, the distribution will be "normal" (gaussian); that on this assumption one may justifiably determine a mean value ($\bar{x}$) and its standard deviation (s); that the value, $\bar{x} \pm 2s$, will include the central 95 per cent of all measurements; that this segment of the distribution is the "normal range"; and that values that fall outside this range are by definition "abnormal." These beliefs are erroneous in many instances. The experimental fact is that for about one half of the methods of clinical chemistry, the distribution is smooth, unimodal, and skewed and that $\bar{x} \pm 2s$ does not cut off the desired central 95 per cent. For example, among the distributions of serum calcium, inorganic phosphorus, magnesium, alkaline phosphatase, total proteins, albumin, uric acid, and blood urea, only that of albumin is gaussian. All others are skewed, leptokurtic, or both. In such situations, the value $\pm 2s$ will cut off many more measurements in one tail of the distribution than the other. The uncritical application of principles of normal distributions in situations in which variables are not normally distributed sometimes leads to values of $\bar{x} - 2s$ that are negative, surely a biologic absurdity.

We should discard the notion that the distribution of values in healthy persons is generally gaussian and should avoid estimating the mean and standard deviation for distributions that are nongaussian (see Fig. 22–1).

One can avoid the question of gaussian distribution by use of *nonparametric* methods for estimating the reference range, that is, methods that do not involve any a priori assumption regarding the parental distribution shape except that it is

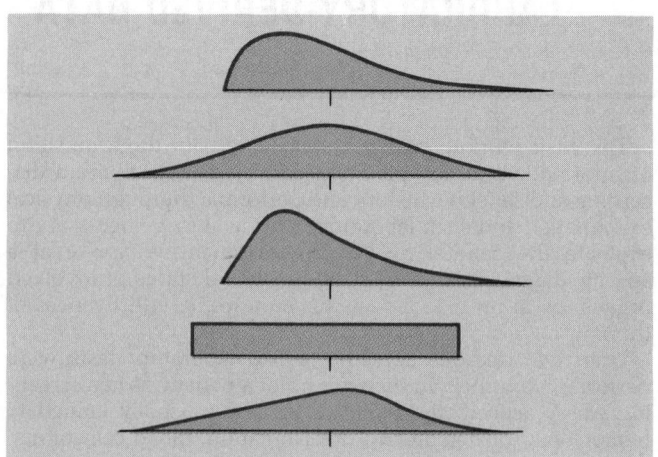

FIGURE 22–1. Five distributions with the same mean and standard deviation ($\bar{x}$ = 4, s = 2.83). From top to bottom: X_4^2, normal, lognormal, rectangular, and mixture of two normals. (From Elveback LR: Mayo Clinic Proc 47:93, 1972, with permission.)

continuous. Two nonparametric methods of normal range estimation are the method of *percentile estimates* with associated nonparametric confidence intervals and the method of nonparametric *tolerance intervals*, which include a specified proportion of the population with a specified probability.

Physicians are familiar with the percentile method of expressing interindividual variation through the use of pediatric growth charts of height and weight. The method avoids the arbitrary distinction of normal and abnormal. It also removes the aura of precision of the standard deviation. The percentile method appropriately fits the real world of nongaussian distributions.

From every laboratory test for which a good normal-value study has been done, the laboratory can report not only the result but also the percentile corresponding to that result and appropriate to the age and sex of the patient under study. With this information the clinician can appreciate just how common or how unusual the test result is. The percentile method is superior to an arbitrary definition of a normal range, such as $\bar{x} \pm 2s$, even in those few cases in which a distribution is gaussian, for it indicates for each test result the relationship of that result to the healthy population. The percentile method is also superior to the definition of the normal range as the range of all observed values in a healthy sample population, for the latter method seriously underestimates any selected segment, e.g., the central 95 per cent, in small samples, and overestimates it in large samples.

The percentile method does not systematically over- or underestimate any selected range, regardless of sample size. If one wishes to cut off the lowest and highest 2.5 per cent, or 5 per cent, one simply orders all values and finds the value that cuts off the desired percentage of observations at either tail of the distribution. Obvious outlier values are discarded. The complete percentile range is readily defined. No assumptions are required about distribution shape except that it is continuous. From the size of the healthy population represented in the distribution, the confidence limits of a given percentile may be ascertained, with known probability, by reference to standard tables. The method should appeal particularly to clinicians who utilize local norms, which are often based on small samples.

THE "NORMAL RANGE." From this discussion, it is clear that "normal range" is an arbitrary and potentially misleading term. By whatever method it is defined, the normal range will exclude observations of the parental distribution of healthy subjects and will very likely include some values of other distributions. What the clinician desires are cut-off points at either end of a distribution that include nearly all values of healthy individuals in the central segment, and very few values of other distributions, i.e., that the numbers of false-positive and false-negative values are both minimized. Ingrained habits will probably lead us to select the central 95 per cent of the parental distribution as "clinical limits," even though there is no magic in this number. Some clinical investigators advocate use of the central 90 per cent.

The term "normal range" has come in for substantial criticism. The connotation of a sharp demarcation between normal and abnormal values is unfortunate and usually erroneous. A value may fall outside the range, $\bar{x} \pm 2s$, or the central 95 per cent segment, on the basis of chance alone. The present consensus is that laboratory results should be interpreted in relationship to "reference intervals" rather than normal ranges. In most instances the quoted reference intervals for a given laboratory test result are the same as the previously published normal ranges, but the term emphasizes the manner in which such intervals are determined, and avoids an assumption of normality or abnormality of the test result. The newer terminology requires the laboratory to describe what it is using as a reference population to generate the interval values.

Influence of Age. The distributions of values of many plasma

TABLE 22–1. PLASMA CHOLESTEROL CONCENTRATIONS ASSOCIATED WITH INCREASED RISK OF CARDIOVASCULAR DISEASE*

Age, yr	Total Cholesterol,* mg/dL		LDL† Cholesterol,* mg/dL		HDL† Cholesterol,‡ mg/dL (Increased Risk)
	Moderate Risk	High Risk	Moderate Risk	High Risk	
Men					
0–14	173	190	106	120	38
15–19	165	183	109	123	30
20–29	194	216	128	148	30
30–39	218	244	149	171	29
40–49	231	254	160	180	29
≥50	230	258	166	188	29
Women					
0–14	174	170	113	126	36
15–19	173	195	115	135	35
20–29	184	208	127	148	35
30–39	202	220	143	163	35
40–49	223	246	155	177	34
≥50	252	281	170	195	36

*Values are adopted from the 75th percentile (moderate-risk) and 90th percentile (high-risk) values obtained by the Lipid Research Clinics.

†LDL indicates low-density lipoproteins; HDL, high-density lipoproteins.

‡The HDL cholesterol values for the lower fifth percentile were taken from the Lipid Research Clinics.

Reprinted from Hoeg JM, Gregg RE, Brewer HB Jr: An approach to the management of hyperlipoproteinemia. JAMA 255:512, 1986. Copyright 1986, American Medical Association.

constituents vary with age in the apparently healthy population. For example, plasma cholesterol concentrations in men, 90 per cent limits, are 216 mg per deciliter in the 20- to 29-year age group and 258 mg per deciliter in the over 50-year age group (Table 22–1).

Influence of Sex. Distributions in men may differ from those in women. For example, in women, cholesterol values analogous to those cited above for men are 208 and 281 mg per deciliter, respectively. Plasma urate concentration values, mean and 90 per cent limits, are 4.9 (2.7 to 7.2) mg per deciliter in men and 4.0 (2.5 to 6.3) mg per deciliter in premenopausal women. Mean serum calcium values in normal men decline 0.0068 mg per deciliter per year from age 20 to age 80. Those of women show no regression against age. This is an important point in the diagnosis of hyperparathyroidism, which is chiefly a disease of the older age group.

Other Influences. These include weight (creatinine values), diet (triglycerides), drugs (diuretics), environment (altitude—hemoglobin), lifestyle (vegetarian diet), habits (alcohol), and the analytic methods themselves.

BIOLOGIC REFERENCE INTERVALS. In a few instances, sufficient data are available to set reference intervals on the basis of risk assessments. For example, Table 22–1 shows reference intervals for total, LDL, and HDL cholesterol in plasma selected on the basis of moderate and high risk, as determined by epidemiologic studies.

Another example concerns urate concentration values. An electrolyte solution with the sodium concentration of plasma is saturated with urate at 6.4 to 6.8 mg per deciliter. In addition, proteins of plasma bind urate equivalent to about 4 per cent of the amount in solution. Values above 7.0 (perhaps 7.2) mg per deciliter represent supersaturation and are associated with increased risk of renal stone and clinical gout. The magnitude of the risk factor increases as urate concentration values rise above 7.0 mg per deciliter. The 95 per cent limits of serum urate values in "healthy" male New Zealand Maoris are 4 to 10 mg per deciliter, and 10 per cent of adult males develop gout. Surely values of serum urate above 7.0 mg per deciliter in this male population cannot be considered "normal," even though they fall within the reference interval as selected by the usual criteria.

DISCONTINUOUS DISTRIBUTIONS. Some traits may be distributed bimodally or trimodally. Such relationships are most likely in families in which there is a monogenetic disease characterized by a chemical abnormality. For example, measurements of galactose-1-phosphate uridyltransferase activity in the families of patients with transferase deficiency galactosemia are distributed trimodally. The effects of two and of one mutant allele are clearly distinguishable from the normal and from each other. Assay values in the three modes are zero, 7.5 to 13.5 units, and 19.5 to 32 units. The intermediate enzyme assay values are found in subjects who are presumed heterozygotes by pedigree analysis. It is common to hear the term "heterozygote value" applied to an enzyme activity value approximately one half of normal. This practice is justifiable only when assay data are combined with pedigree data, for there may be other reasons for a reduced enzyme assay value that have nothing to do with genetics.

An apparently continuous distribution with marked skewing may at times be dissected into two or even three distribution modes by appropriate clinical and pedigree studies. For example, the distribution of plasma cholesterol concentrations in familial hypercholesterolemia displays marked overlap between subjects who are clinically normal and those who are heterozygotes by pedigree analysis. Similarly, there is considerable overlap between heterozygotes and abnormal homozygotes. Only a complete family pedigree permits adequate definition of the range of values in each distribution mode.

THE PHYSICIAN AND THE LABORATORY TEST RESULT

The tables at the end of this book contain values that define the reference intervals for a large number of substances commonly measured in clinical medicine. They represent the best data currently available, but are subject to all the uncertainties discussed above. In some instances more selective data of an age- and sex-matched control population will need to be consulted by the physician.

Clinical judgment will always be required in the interpretation of laboratory data. For example, a blood urea nitrogen (BUN) concentration of 22 mg per deciliter is not a normal value for a patient on a very low protein diet. Also, electrolyte values of sodium at 145 mEq per liter, potassium at 3.5 mEq per liter, chloride at 98 mEq per liter, and CO_2 at 30 mEq per liter may indicate metabolic alkalosis even though all individual values fall within published reference intervals.

Laboratory tests are critical to the diagnosis of disease and management of patients. The physician must know the limits of reliability and usefulness of each test result in the clinical setting of the individual patient. This is particularly true when all deviant test results have returned to normal but the patient is not improving. It is especially when laboratory data provide little or no help that the patient needs a doctor.

Dales LG, Friedman GD, Collen MF: Evaluating periodic multiphasic health checkups: A controlled trial. J Chronic Dis 32:385, 1979. *Only a limited number of screening tests (history or physical examination, stool test for occult blood, and blood pressure) actually improve health outcome of asymptomatic outpatients.*

Dixon RH, Laszlo J: Utilization of clinical chemistry services by medical house staff. Arch Intern Med 134:1064, 1974. *Less than 10 per cent of data obtained from a panel of 12 tests were used clinically.*

Elveback LR, Guillier CL, Keating FR: Health, normality, and the ghost of Gauss. JAMA 211:69, 1970. *Of eight distributions evaluated, only that of serum albumin was "normal" or gaussian.*

Hoeg JM, Gregg RE, Brewer HB, Jr: An approach to the management of hyperlipoproteinemia. JAMA 255:512, 1986. *One of the best examples relating reference intervals to epidemiologic risk factors.*

Keating FR, Jones JD, Elveback LR, et al.: The relation of age and sex to distribution of values in healthy adults of serum calcium, inorganic phosphorus, magnesium, alkaline phosphatase, total proteins, albumin, and blood urea. J Lab Clin Med 73:825, 1969. *A study of the age- and sex-dependency of several constituents of serum. The downward trend to serum calcium values with age in men is particularly noteworthy.*

Korvin CC, Pearce RH, Stanley J: Admissions screening: Clinical benefits. Ann Intern Med 83:197, 1975. *Admission screening tests have a relatively low benefit. Fewer than 1 per cent lead to new diagnoses of significance to the patient.*

Mainland, D: Remarks on clinical "norms." Clin Chem 17:267, 1971. *An excellent*

article explaining the use of nonparametric methods for establishing reference intervals.

Parkerson GR, Eisenson HJ: Association of patient and physician characteristics with follow-up of abnormal laboratory results. J Fam Pract 11:943, 1980. *As few as 40 per cent of abnormal results initiate clinical follow-up.*

23 OVERVIEW OF IMAGING TECHNIQUES AND PROJECTION FOR THE FUTURE

Alexander R. Margulis

HISTORICAL PERSPECTIVE

Radiology has undergone tremendous changes in the post–World War II decades. Progress in technologic developments related to medical imaging has been continuously accelerating, making diagnostic radiology one of the most exciting areas of diagnostic medicine during the last few years. Diagnostic imaging has been and continues to be the direct beneficiary of some of the areas of technology that are most heavily subsidized by governments and industry. Space exploration provided miniaturization of imaging equipment components. Extremely high-resolution television techniques used for space exploration and photographing of the earth's surface and advances in computers and techniques of storage of information have contributed to the development of digital radiography, highly advanced x-ray computed tomography (CT) machines, positron emission tomography, and magnetic resonance imaging. These modalities, although expensive, are eventually cost effective because they significantly reduce invasiveness and permit the performance of many procedures on an outpatient basis. Because of this they have found ready acceptance and have rapidly proliferated, not only in the United States, but throughout the Western world and Japan.

PRESENT STATUS OF RADIOLOGIC IMAGING
Conventional Radiography

The term "conventional radiography" is a misnomer today. Equipment that was considered advanced in the early 1970's is today hopelessly obsolete. Although there have been no breakthroughs in x-ray tube design, the generators and controls have been computerized; the television cameras are smaller and more reliable; and the equipment as a whole has grown more functional and often multipurpose. The highly specialized, extremely expensive rooms used in the past for angiography only are changing, particularly in small hospitals, into rooms that can be used for many different procedures, including digital subtraction fluoroscopy (Fig. 23–1). Even conventional darkrooms are being replaced by daylight developing facilities, which save space, time, and personnel. These trends of saving space, time, and personnel will become even more evident in the future as departments of radiology will have to become smaller and more intensively active and will have to serve inpatients and outpatients with the same equipment over longer hours each day.

As computers improve and the capacity to store data increases, the present halide film will be replaced by laser discs or other similar devices that will significantly reduce the size of filing areas and permit rapid and reliable access to images projected on television monitors. Hard copies will be instantly available in multiple formats similar to x-ray computed tomography.

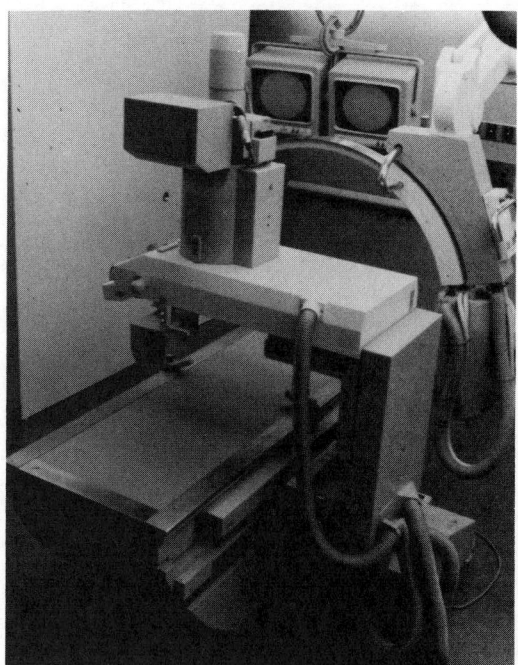

FIGURE 23–1. Photograph of a bi-plane fluoroscopic and radiographic multipurpose room with digital fluoroscopy. Multiple types of procedures are performed in this room: interventional, angiography, biliary procedures (including gallstone removal), gastrointestinal examinations, myelography, etc. Machines of this type, although expensive, are cost efficient because they are in constant use.

As videotaping improves and better resolution is obtained, fluoroscopic information will be recorded on tape and diagnostic frames will be recorded on multiformatted hard copy as the only record. This will result in reduced radiation exposure and eventually in cost saving.

Digital Radiography and Fluoroscopy

Digital subtraction fluoroscopy did not fulfill all the expectations that greeted it when it was introduced at the end of the 1970's. It was expected then that all arteriography would be performed intravenously, noninvasively, with images showing excellent detail. This has not occurred, and angiography still requires that large amounts of iodine-containing contrast media be injected intravenously through catheters advanced into large veins. Even then, owing to breathing or involuntary motion, blurring detracts from the quality of the images. At this time intra-arterial injections of small amounts of contrast medium appear to be the best method for performing digital subtraction angiography (Fig. 23–2). Further improvements in digital subtraction fluoroscopy will probably occur, and eventually it can be expected that most arteriography will be performed with some modification of digital radiography. This is also being facilitated by the continual decrease in price of the equipment.

Computed Tomography

Computed tomography has become an indispensable diagnostic tool in a modern hospital as well as in sophisticated outpatient centers throughout the United States, Canada, most of Western Europe, and particularly Japan. For the last ten years there has been a steady improvement in the quality of images. The speed of scanning, which indirectly also results in better spatial resolution, has come down to 1 second for conventional CT scanners and is in the 50 msec range for the cine CT scanner, an advanced scanner with no moving parts. Computed tomography is today considered to be an excellent method for the examination of the brain (Fig. 23–3) and spine. It is still the modality of choice for the examination of the mediastinum and chest, as well as the abdomen. It is a tomographic examination in the axial plane, but it also allows redisplay of images in any plane (Fig. 23–4). CT numbers accurately reflect the average density of small tissue volume elements and can be used to identify various tissues, fluids, and lesions. Computed tomography is of great advantage in showing tumors, abscesses, ruptures of organs, and accumulation of fluid, with high accuracy. Since the introduction of magnetic resonance imaging, CT has remained the examination of choice for organs in the peritoneal cavity and the alimentary tube, with magnetic resonance imaging rapidly replacing it in most other areas.

Ultrasonography

Diagnostic ultrasonography, or ultrasound, uses a pulse echo device to record reflected waves of a sound beam in two dimensions. The resolution of sonographic images is inferior

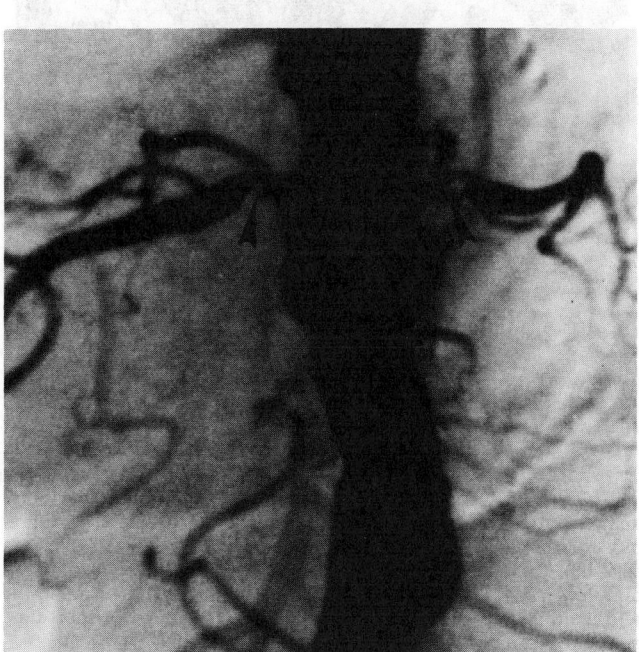

FIGURE 23–2. Intra-arterial digital subtraction aortogram showing bilateral renal artery stenoses (*arrowheads*).

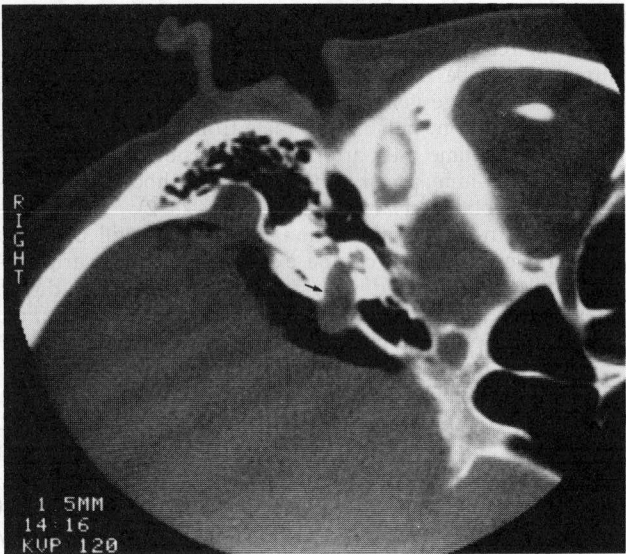

FIGURE 23–3. High resolution axial view computed tomogram showing an acoustic neuroma widening the internal acoustic meatus. The lesion itself (*arrow*) is seen with outstanding detail.

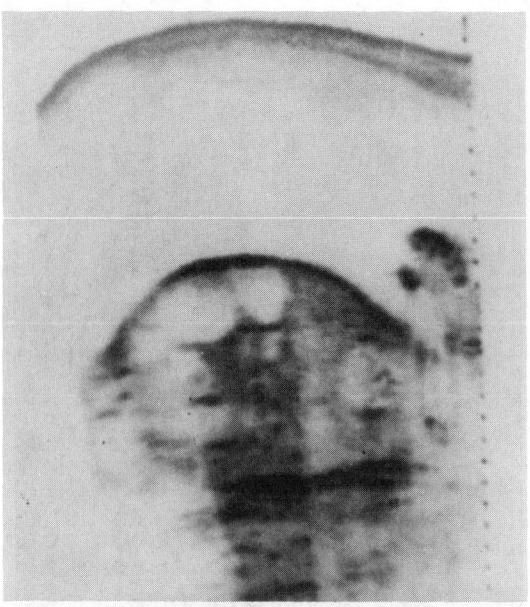

FIGURE 23–5. Multiple dilated loops of small bowel are demonstrated by ultrasound in this fetus with jejunal atresia.

to the image obtained from computed tomography or magnetic resonance. The great advantages of this modality, however, are (1) it is relatively inexpensive, (2) it is rapid, (3) it can produce images in real time, (4) it can obtain images in any plane without revision of format, (5) because of its speed it is ideal for directing certain interventional procedures, and (6) no biologic hazards have been demonstrated within the diagnostic range. It does not depend on ionizing radiation. The disadvantages of the method are that (1) it is highly

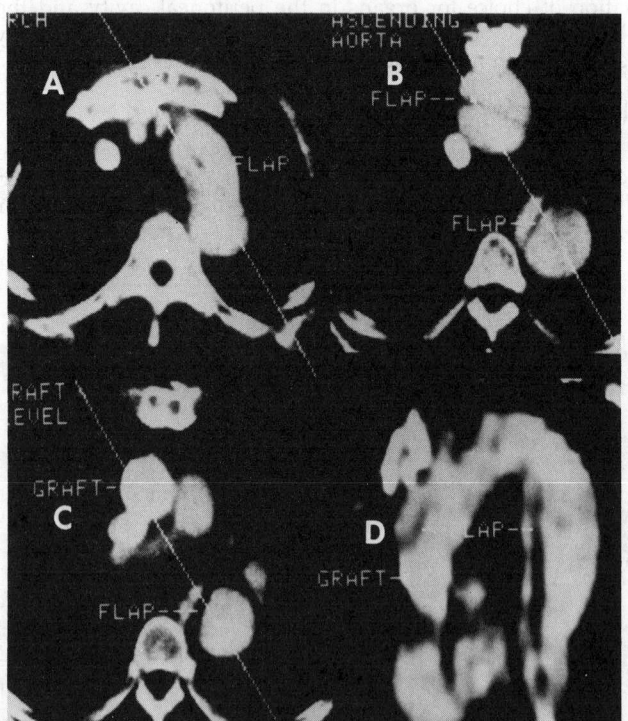

FIGURE 23–4. Dissecting aneurysm of the descending thoracic aorta demonstrated with exquisite detail on dynamic computed tomography reformatted along a plane shown by the dotted line on three axial tomograms at different levels and demonstrated in this illustration under A, B, and C. The flap is seen as a vertical dark line on the reformatted image (D). The Teflon graft was introduced a short time before this examination.

dependent on operator skill, (2) its spatial resolution and resolving power lag behind those of computed tomography and magnetic resonance imaging, and (3) no good contrast media are available at present. In the diagnostic range, ultrasound is of no use in examining the lungs, the brain through the intact skull of an adult, the spine, or areas where there is a great deal of gas. Ultrasound images, however, exceed the quality of CT in asthenic or cachectic individuals. It is currently the method of choice in examining the female pelvis, particularly in obstetrics. An entire field of intrauterine diagnosis of fetal abnormalities by ultrasound has developed, leading also to surgical intrauterine interventions, again guided by ultrasound (Fig. 23–5). Ultrasonography is also of great use in diagnosis of abnormalities of the neonatal brain through the intact skull and in the intraoperative diagnosis of brain abnormalities through open skull flaps.

Magnetic Resonance Imaging

Magnetic resonance imaging (MRI) is a new imaging modality that has been derived from chemical magnetic resonance. For imaging, hydrogen protons give the best images. The strength of the signal will indicate the amount of hydrogen modified by tissue relaxation parameters, T1 and T2. T1, also known as the spin lattice parameter, is dependent on the interaction of other nuclei with hydrogen. T2 depends on the influence of protons on each other. It is also referred to as the spin-spin parameter. The intensity of the signal is also affected by the proton bulk motion effect, which results from the fact that it takes approximately 50 msec for the signal emanating from protons to register. If the protons move through the plane of imaging at a faster rate, the signal will not be recorded. This permits evaluation of speed of flow through blood vessels and visualization of patent blood vessels without contrast media. In addition, the image on MRI is influenced by the technique of acquisition of data. These techniques are so numerous that it is possible to individualize them for given tissue abnormalities and anatomic areas. By applying the right sequence, a great deal of information about the nature of normal and abnormal tissues can be obtained. Magnetic resonance imaging has several characteristics that are advantages when compared with other imaging modalities. Besides giving information about tissue chemistry and metabolic and biochemical data, MRI offers superb resolving power. This is due to contrast resolution that is considerably

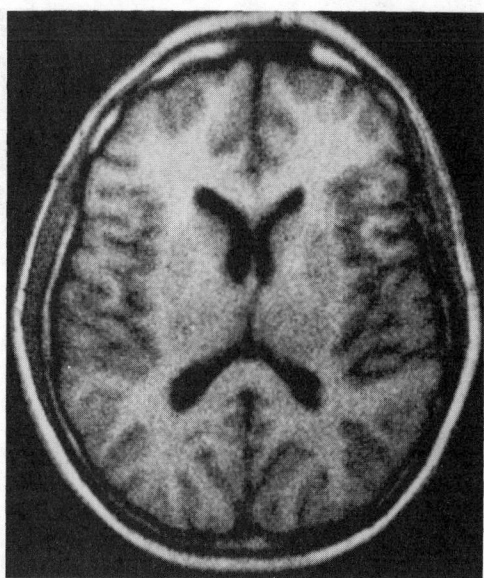

FIGURE 23–6. Axial section through the normal brain with MRI. Notice the excellent demonstration of the ventricles and gray and white matter.

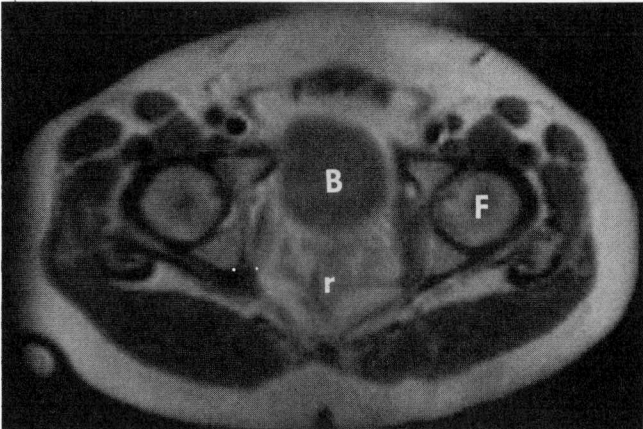

FIGURE 23–8. Axial MRI section through the pelvis of a male. B, Urinary bladder; r, rectum; F, femoral head.

better than that of CT, with spatial resolution becoming comparable to CT. Furthermore, MRI can provide tomographic sections in any desired plane. By exciting section after section while the remagnetization occurs in the original section, multiple simultaneous sections can be obtained in a relatively short time.

Magnetic resonance imaging is already superior to any other imaging modality in the examination of the brain (Figs. 23–6 and 23–7), spinal cord, cancellous bone, the male and female pelvic organs, and the urinary bladder (Figs. 23–8 and 23–9). With the use of surface or specially designed small coils, it is the best method for the examination of large joints (Fig. 23–10). It will probably shortly replace arthrography of the knee, hip, shoulder, and temporomandibular joint. Magnetic resonance imaging has been very successful in the examination of the spine, particularly with the use of surface coils. With

respiratory and electrocardiographic (ECG) gating, it is providing diagnostic images of the heart (Fig. 23–11) and mediastinum of quality unsurpassed by other modalities. It is as valuable in the examination of the liver, particularly in the search for metastases, hepatocellular carcinomas, and hemangiomas. It has advantages over other techniques in the examination of the kidneys. Magnetic resonance imaging does not show calcifications. Magnetic resonance imaging is currently of no value in the examination of the small bowel and its mesentery and has only limited applications in the examination of the pancreas. It is promising in the staging of tumors of the rectum and esophagus. Further drawbacks are relatively slow scanning (in minutes), the expense of the equipment and siting, the large amounts of space necessary for the facility, and the danger of loose metallic objects flying into the machine. Other disadvantages are the inability to examine patients with pacemakers, large metallic prostheses, prosthetic heart valves made with magnetic materials, or freshly introduced vascular magnetic clips or to study patients who are in need of continuous observation and require life-support systems. The drawback of slow scanning by MRI will soon be eliminated by the development of rapid scanning sequences (in seconds), which use different pulses, resulting in reduced flip angles of protons, and imaginative handling of data by the computer.

Magnetic resonance imaging is highly sensitive in detecting disease, but its sensitivity is not matched by specificity. The

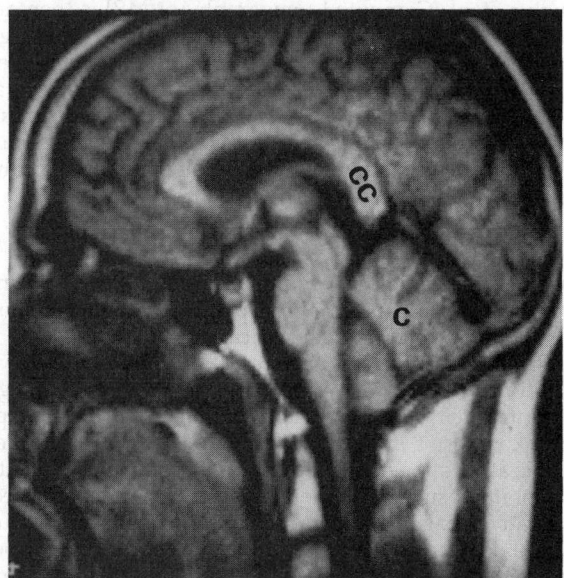

FIGURE 23–7. Sagittal section through the brain with excellent detail showing all the structures through the mid-section. Notice the beautiful demonstration of the gyri, corpus callosum (cc), and cerebellum (c).

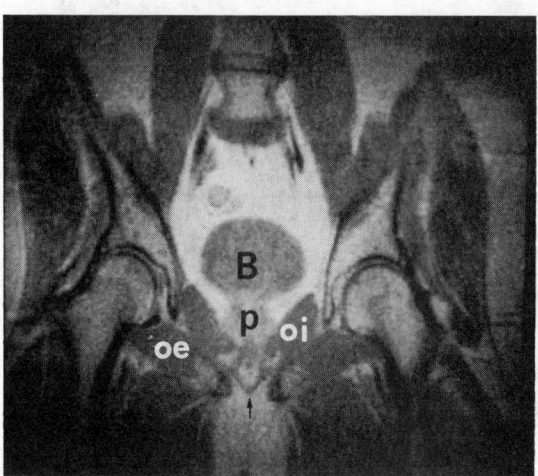

FIGURE 23–9. Coronal section through the pelvis of the male demonstrated in Figure 23–8. B, Bladder; P, prostate; oi, obturator internus muscle; oe, obturator externus muscle; arrow, bulbus spongiosus.

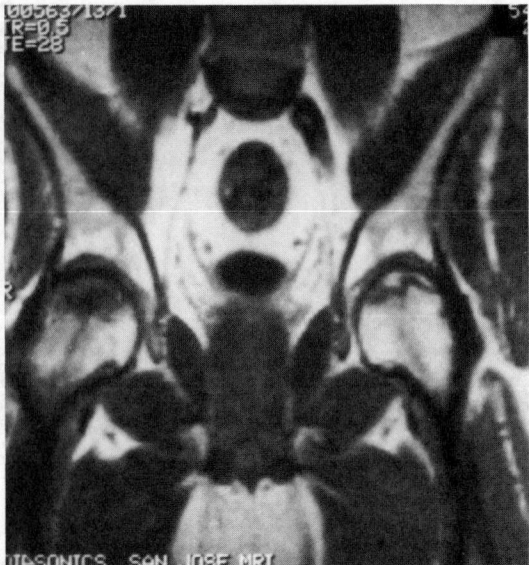

FIGURE 23–10. MRI of bilateral osteonecrosis of the femoral heads. The changes are more advanced on the right.

latter will be improved with the development of paramagnetic contrast media and localized tissue spectroscopy using spectra of multiple elements: ^{31}P, H, ^{19}F, ^{23}Na, ^{15}N, and so on.

The Algorithmic Approach

With many different radiologic modalities, the physician is often in a dilemma as to which examination is indicated and, if several are to be requested, in what order they should be performed. The algorithmic approach offers a logical sequence in which one examination follows the previous one, depending on its results, in order to provide a definitive diagnosis. This approach relies very much on the equipment available as well as on the skills of the operators. It is often linked with local experience and sometimes is tinged with prejudice. The best approach for selecting the proper procedures results from a continuing dialogue between the clinician and radiologist in which the two familiarize each other with the newest developments and experiences. A typical example of an algorithm is in the evaluation of jaundice (Ch. 120). When chemical

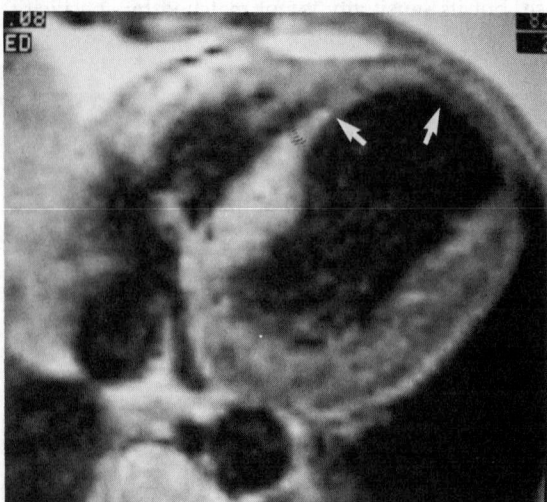

FIGURE 23–11. Gated (ECG) magnetic resonance image at a transverse level through the left ventricle sharply displays the myocardial walls. In this patient with a prior anteroseptal myocardial infarction, the image shows severe thinning of the anterior septum and anterior wall of the left ventricle (*arrows*).

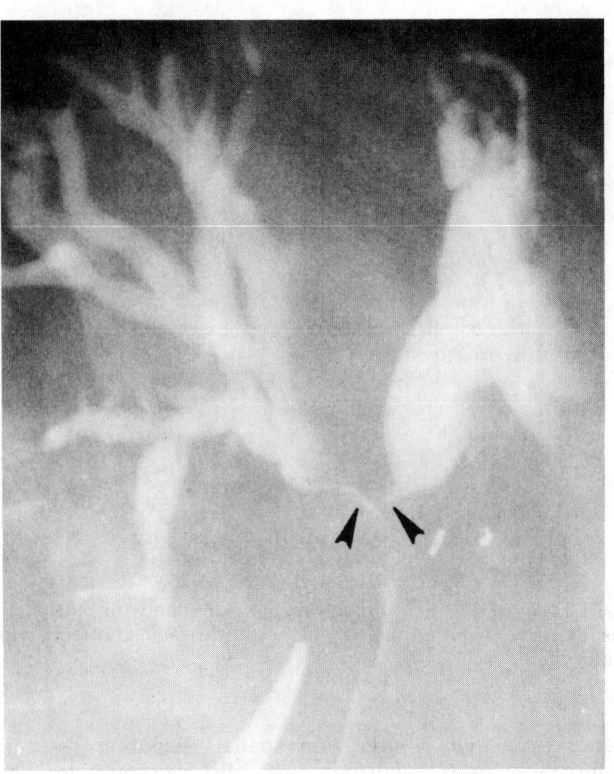

FIGURE 23–12. Percutaneous transhepatic cholangiogram demonstrates high-grade obstructing lesion of the proximal common hepatic duct involving the ductal bifurcation (*arrowheads*). Biopsy demonstrated cholangiocarcinoma.

tests indicate that the jaundice is most likely due to obstruction, the next procedure is ultrasonography (if that capability exists locally) to determine the width of the biliary tree. If the ducts are dilated, and depending on whether the history suggests tumor or stone, either endoscopic retrograde cholangiography (ERC) or percutaneous transhepatic cholangiography is performed. If a stone is found to be obstructing, sphincterotomy is performed by ERC, and if a tumor is seen, either percutaneous transhepatic cholangiography or ERC is performed (Fig. 23–12) with the introduction of drainage through a stent. Computed tomography or MRI is then done for staging of the tumor in order to determine whether surgery is indicated and, if so, whether it is likely to be curative or palliative. For curative surgery, decompression is often valuable. For palliation, an internal stent introduced percutaneously may be all that is necessary. Magnetic resonance imaging has greatly changed many of the previous algorithms as the method is used with increasing frequency.

Financial Considerations

The cost of radiologic equipment has soared; in most hospitals modern imaging equipment has overwhelmed equipment budgets. The sophistication and expense of the equipment necessitate an organized referral system to prevent duplication of equipment and to allow utilization of imaging systems to their best advantage. Noninvasive imaging procedures can result in shorter hospital stays, in avoidance of hospitalization altogether, and in almost complete elimination of exploratory surgery. When surgery is necessary, precise preoperative diagnosis shortens the procedure and reduces the number of complications. Properly utilized and properly distributed imaging systems can enhance outpatient diagnostic capabilities, thus shortening hospital stays and greatly reducing the number of acute care hospitals needed. Interventional radiologic procedures are relatively less invasive than surgical procedures. Their advances have already served in avoiding or shortening hospitalizations and significantly reducing the number of complications and expense of open surgery. The elimination of hospital beds resulting from all these procedures should eventually lead to enormous cost savings.

FUTURE DEVELOPMENTS IN IMAGING

With the continuous advances in the development of computers and television systems, combining increased versatility and decreased cost, diagnostic imaging can expect to make progress in several new directions. It can be expected that the departments of radiology of the future will become totally computerized, integrating into the hospital's general computer system. This means that images themselves as well as reports will be instantly available on television monitors on wards along with laboratory information and information from medical records and pathologic studies. These systems will be expensive but at the same time will be cost effective, saving on personnel, communication, and duration of hospital stay of the patient. Computers will also help to store data correlating clinical information and allowing the most efficient and most rational algorithmic approaches for reaching the correct diagnosis. Computers will therefore help physicians, surgeons, and radiologists to reach the correct, least invasive, and most time-saving sequence of diagnostic studies. Similarly, artificial intelligence based on clinical experience and previous imaging results will also help in selection of the proper techniques, sequences, and planes of imaging for magnetic resonance. This again will result not only in improving clinical results but also in making the use of equipment more cost effective and less traumatic for patients.

These remarkable advances in imaging will increasingly attract the interest and collaboration of other physicians (such as internists, neurologists, ophthalmologists, obstetricians, neurosurgeons, and surgeons) with the radiologist in the field of diagnostic imaging in order to optimize progress through the exchange of experience and ideas. Localized tissue magnetic resonance spectroscopy will provide further advances not only in making imaging yield morphologic information but also in making it possible to follow metabolic processes and specifically identify diseases.

HISTORICAL AND GENERAL REFERENCES

Grigg ERN: The Train of the Invisible Light. Springfield, Ill., Charles C Thomas, 1965. *An extensive, well-illustrated review of the development of roentgenology from its earliest days.*

DIGITAL RADIOGRAPHY AND FLUOROSCOPY

Enzmann DR, Djang WT, Riederer SJ, et al: Digital subtraction angiography: Current status and use of intra-arterial injection. Radiology 146:669, 1983. *A clever technical review of two approaches to digital angiography.*
Foley WD, Milde MW: Intra-arterial digital subtraction angiography. Radiol Clin of North Am 23:293, 1985. *A clear, objective view of the subject.*
Riederer SJ, Kruger RA: Intravenous digital subtraction: A summary of recent developments. Radiology 147:633, 1983. *An extensive summary of multiple approaches with the advantages and disadvantages of each.*

COMPUTED TOMOGRAPHY

Boyd DP: Computerized-transmission tomography of the heart using scanning electron beams. In Higgins CA (ed.): CTT of the Heart: Experimental Evaluation and Clinical Application. Mt. Kisco, N.Y., Futura Publishing Company, 1983. *The author describes an original approach to the generation of a scanning x-ray beam that permits the achievement of cine computed tomography.*
Lee JKT, Sagel SS, Stanley RJ (eds.): Computed Body Tomography. New York, Raven Press, 1982. *A well-illustrated, modern, complete textbook on computed tomography of the body. Particularly good sections on kidney and liver.*
Moss AA, Gamsu G, Genant HK (eds.): Computed Tomography of the Body. Philadelphia, W.B. Saunders Company, 1983. *A large, complete, up-to-date textbook. Particularly good sections on the mediastinum, the digestive tract, and the spine.*

ULTRASONOGRAPHY

Callen PW (ed.): Ultrasonography in Obstetrics and Gynecology. Philadelphia, W.B. Saunders Company, 1983. *A well-illustrated and organized textbook on modern ultrasound applications in the field of obstetrics and gynecology.*

Sarti DA, Sample WF (eds.): Diagnostic Ultrasound. Text and Cases. Boston, G.K. Hall & Company, 1980. *Still the best-illustrated book on ultrasonography, with exquisite illustrations.*

MAGNETIC RESONANCE

Budinger TF, Margulis AR (eds.): Medical Magnetic Resonance Imaging and Spectroscopy: A Primer. Berkeley CA, Society of Magnetic Resonance in Medicine, 1986.
James TL, Margulis AR (eds.): Biomedical Magnetic Resonance. San Francisco, Radiology Research and Education Foundation, 1984.
Margulis AR, Fisher MR: Present clinical status of magnetic resonance imaging. Magnet Res Med 2:309, 1985.
Pykett IL: NMR imaging in medicine. Sci Am 246:78, 1982. *An imaginative, clear, and well-illustrated explanation of the physics and techniques of NMR.*

ECONOMIC DATA AND BENEFITS

Margulis AR, Shea WJ, Jr: Advances in Imaging Technology and Their Impact on Medicine. Mackenzie Davidson Memorial Lecture, April 1986. Forty-fourth Annual Congress of the British Institute of Radiology, Bristol, April 1986.
Newton DR, Witz S, Norman D, et al: Economic impact of CT scanning on the evaluation of pituitary adenomas. Am J Neurol Radiol 4:57, 1983. *A carefully designed study showing the economic benefits of computed tomography in one selected condition where controls were available.*
Norman D, Ulloa N, Brant-Zawadzki M, et al: Intraarterial digital subtraction imaging cost considerations. Radiology 156:33, 1985. *Irrational handling of new technology.*

24 PRINCIPLES OF DRUG THERAPY

Alan S. Nies

Because all patients respond differently to drugs, individualization of drug dosages is required so that therapy will be effective and nontoxic. A basic tenet of clinical pharmacology is that a closer relationship exists between the concentration of drug in the blood and the drug's effect than between drug dose and effect. The relationship between drug concentration and effect has fostered the study of the factors influencing drug movement in the body, a science called pharmacokinetics (Fig. 24–1). Rational drug therapy requires a basic understanding of pharmacokinetic principles that can be applied to patient care. In this way the amount of drug delivered to the target tissue can be controlled within a definable and safe range.

ABSORPTION. When a dose of drug is administered, it must first be absorbed into the systemic circulation to produce its effects. The simplest case is that of the drug's being given intravenously, in which absorption is obviously complete and immediate. For all other routes of administration, there will be a delay in the drug's reaching the circulation, and the absorption may be incomplete. Drug absorption is the only part of the pharmacokinetic process that can be influenced by the physician and the pharmaceutical industry. Most drugs are absorbed by passive diffusion into the circulation from their site of administration. Since the process of diffusion is dependent upon the concentration of drug contacting the absorbing surface, the rate of absorption can be influenced by affecting the rate of dissolution of the dosage form. Depot intramuscular preparations of some drugs (e.g., penicillin, progesterone) slowly release the active drug into tissue fluids, from which it can be absorbed into the circulation. In this way, drug levels in the blood can be maintained by a continuous absorption process for many hours or many days even though the drug is rapidly eliminated from the body. A similar technique can be used for oral drug administration. Long-acting oral preparations can be formulated for drugs with rapid elimination by producing a dosage form that slowly releases the active drug from a matrix. The duration of sustained absorption from an oral preparation, however, is

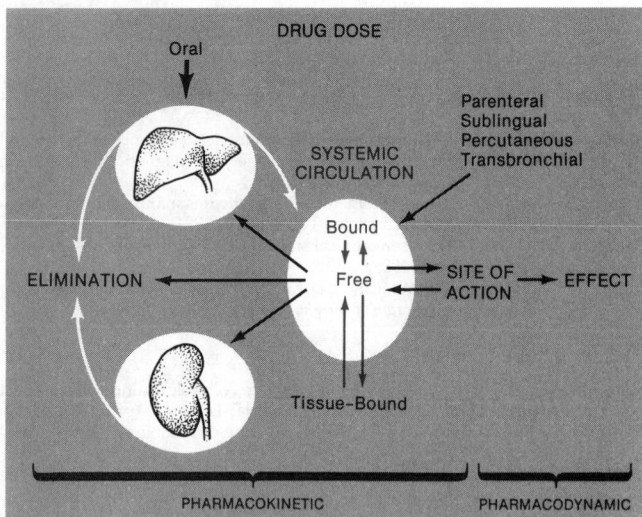

FIGURE 24–1. Drug movement in the body. The variation in effects following a given dose is related to pharmacokinetic and pharmacodynamic factors. The systemic circulation can be sampled to determine the pharmacokinetics.

limited by the gastrointestinal transit time. Drugs that are slowly dissolved and slowly absorbed may be affected by alterations in gut transit time more so than drugs that are rapidly and completely absorbed. An increase in gut motility will lead to a decrease in the extent of absorption of slowly absorbed drugs (such as digoxin), whereas a decrease in motility may actually increase the extent of absorption.

Depending on the drug, absorption can occur from sites other than the gastrointestinal tract, subcutaneous tissue, or muscle. Some lipid-soluble drugs can be absorbed from the skin or through the oral or bronchial mucous membranes. Nitroglycerin can be absorbed percutaneously, buccally, and sublingually. When given as a sublingual tablet or sprayed into the mouth, nitroglycerin is rapidly absorbed into the systemic circulation and produces a transient effect. When applied to the skin, nitroglycerin has a slow but sustained absorption lasting several hours for the ointment or 24 hours with a sustained release patch. The transdermal route also can be used for scopolamine, estradiol, and clonidine. However, most drugs cannot be absorbed well from the skin or oral mucous membrane because of the limited surface utilized for absorption and the solubility characteristics of the drug. Occasionally, percutaneous absorption is an unwanted side effect of drugs (e.g., steroids) applied to the skin to produce topical effects.

The sublingual, transbronchial, and percutaneous routes of absorption have the advantage of delivering the drug directly into the systemic circulation. By contrast, when absorbed by the intestine, the drug enters the portal circulation and is presented to the liver, where a portion of the drug can be eliminated before reaching the systemic circulation (Fig. 24–1). Thus, nitroglycerin can be absorbed readily from the intestine but is rapidly destroyed by the liver so that only a fraction of the orally administered dose reaches the circulation. A similar situation exists for propranolol, in which over half of an orally administered dose is removed by the liver. Hepatic removal during absorption of the drug from the gut is called "first pass" or "presystemic" elimination and, along with poor absorption from the intestine, accounts for the need to give larger oral than parenteral doses of some drugs to achieve equivalent pharmacologic effects. "Oral bioavailability" is the quantitative expression relating the amount of drug reaching the systemic circulation after oral administration to the amount after intravenous administration. Oral bioavailability ranges from 0 per cent (no drug reaches the systemic

circulation) to 100 per cent (all of the ingested dose reaches the systemic circulation). For some drugs, such as lidocaine and morphine, the oral bioavailability is sufficiently low to preclude oral administration. Formulation of oral preparations can affect bioavailability. There are well-documented examples of differences in bioavailability for different brands of the same drug. In addition, sustained-release preparations often show greater interpatient variability in bioavailability than standard formulations of the same drug. For all calculations utilizing the oral dosage, the dosage must be corrected for less than complete bioavailability.

DISTRIBUTION. Once absorbed into the systemic circulation, the drug must distribute throughout the body. If the drug is rapidly administered intravenously, it is first delivered to the well-perfused tissues and only more slowly distributed to less well-perfused tissues. By measuring drug concentrations in plasma at various times after a drug is administered, a curve can be described from which distribution and elimination can be quantified. For example, if 100 mg of lidocaine is given as an intravenous bolus to an adult, the curve in Figure 24–2 results. This curve of lidocaine concentration versus time can be separated into an early distribution phase, during which the drug rapidly disappears from the circulation, and a later elimination phase, during which the drug in the blood is in equilibrium with drug in the tissues and is more gradually eliminated from the body (Fig. 24–2). The effects of most drugs are related to the plasma concentration during the elimination phase. However, whether the plasma concentration of the drug during the distribution phase is predictive of drug effects depends on the particular drug. For a drug such as lidocaine that quickly reaches its sites of action, the initial concentrations shortly after a bolus of drug can produce therapeutic antiarrhythmic effects and toxic effects on the heart or brain. On the other hand, digoxin is an example of a drug that requires time to equilibrate or be transported to its receptors. When given intravenously, digoxin does not produce maximal effects for four to eight hours, during which time the blood levels are falling as the drug equilibrates with tissues. After the equilibration period of eight hours, digoxin concentrations fall more slowly, and only then does the digoxin concentration correlate with the drug's effects.

Apparent Volume of Distribution. The relationship between the amount of drug in the body and the concentration of drug in the plasma is defined as the "apparent volume of distribution" (V_D) of the drug:

$$V_D = \frac{\text{amount of drug in the body}}{\text{concentration of drug in plasma}}$$

The V_D is the "apparent" volume needed to contain the entire amount of drug if the drug were everywhere at the same concentration as in the plasma. The apparent volume of distribution of a drug during the elimination phase can be determined from a graph of the plasma drug concentration versus time by extrapolating the elimination phase back to zero time, giving the C_{P_0} (plasma concentration at time 0), an estimate of the concentration of drug in the plasma that would have been achieved by the intravenous dose of drug if the drug had been distributed throughout the tissues instantaneously. Thus:

$$V_D = \frac{\text{IV dose}}{C_{P_0}}$$

In Figure 24–2, the C_{P_0} for lidocaine is 0.84 mg per liter following a 100-mg dose. The V_D for lidocaine, therefore, is 100 mg ÷ 0.84 mg per liter = 119 liters. The V_D for several drugs are shown in Tables 24–1 and 24–2.

The apparent volume of distribution frequently does not correspond to any given body fluid compartment. For many

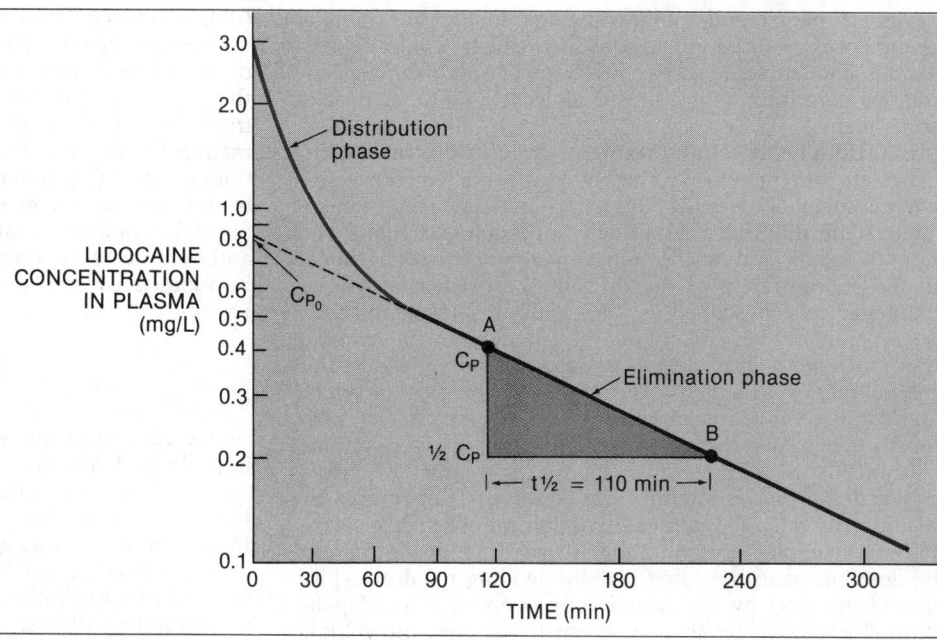

FIGURE 24–2. Lidocaine concentrations on a log scale plotted against time in minutes following a 100 mg bolus given intravenously to a 70-kg person. The C_{P_0} is the concentration of lidocaine in plasma that would be achieved if the dose was distributed instantaneously to the tissues. C_P at point A is twice the concentration of lidocaine at point B. The time between point A and point B is the half-life ($t\frac{1}{2}$).

drugs the V_D is larger than the entire body. For example, digoxin has a V_D of 7 liters per kilogram or about 500 liters in a 70-kg person. When a 0.5-mg dose of digoxin is administered intravenously, it distributes in this "apparent volume" of 500 liters to give a plasma concentration of 1 μg per liter or 1 ng per milliliter. A large apparent volume of distribution is merely an expression of the fact that most of the drug in the body is not in the plasma but is bound to the tissues at a greater concentration than in the plasma. For phenytoin and ethanol the V_D is 0.6 liter per kilogram. Although this figure approximates the value for total body water, it need not be the case that these drugs are distributed only in body water. The V_D is an empirically determined constant that allows one to relate the plasma concentration to the amount of drug in the body and should not be given a physiologic interpretation relating to real body volumes.

LOADING DOSES. One use of the apparent volume of distribution is to calculate the loading dose required to achieve a desired plasma drug concentration. From Figure 24–2 the apparent volume of distribution of lidocaine is 119 liters in a 70-kg person or 1.7 liters per kilogram. In order to establish rapidly a therapeutic plasma lidocaine concentration of 2 mg

per liter, a loading dose of 238 mg (desired concentration × V_D) must be given. After the distribution phase, the loading dose (238 mg) will be contained in an apparent volume of 119 liters, resulting in a plasma concentration of 2 mg per liter. However, because lidocaine and many other drugs can produce toxic effects during the distribution phase, the entire loading dose should not be given in a single bolus; to do so would produce lidocaine concentrations during the distribution phase that would be potentially toxic. The initial high concentrations after a loading dose can be avoided by giving the desired amount of drug in divided doses or as an infusion rather than a bolus. In addition, the loading of drug into the body can be stopped if early signs of drug toxicity occur. If the drug can be given orally, a loading dose may be given that could cause toxicity if given intravenously. Because of the gradual absorption from the intestine, the drug has time to distribute to the tissues during the absorption process, and the very high peak drug concentrations that result from an intravenous bolus do not occur. As an example, the V_D of phenytoin is 0.6 liter per kilogram or 40 liters in a 70-kg adult. To achieve a low therapeutic plasma concentration of 10 mg per liter requires a loading dose of 400 mg. Since phenytoin has an oral bioavailability of 80 to 85 per cent, an oral loading dose of 500 mg will deliver 400 mg to the systemic circulation. The 500 mg of phenytoin can be given safely as a single oral dose even though the 400-mg loading dose given as a bolus intravenously could cause a cardiac arrest. If a patient has an inadequate plasma level, a loading dose can be used to achieve a therapeutic level rapidly. A patient with a phenytoin level of 5 mg per liter can be given a 400-mg phenytoin load (or 500 mg orally) to increase his level by 10 mg per liter to 15 mg per liter.

The estimates of all pharmacokinetic parameters, including the apparent volume of distribution, are derived from an

TABLE 24–1. PHARMACOKINETIC PARAMETERS FOR SOME COMMONLY USED DRUGS

	Cl_r* (ml/min)	Cl_{nr}† (ml/min)	Per Cent‡ Nonrenal	V_D (liter/kg)	$t\frac{1}{2}$ (hours)	Per Cent** Bound
Aminoglycosides	70	3	5	0.3	2–3	<10
Digitoxin	0	3	100	0.6	165	97
Digoxin§	110	40	30	7	36	25
Disopyramide	60	40	40	0.8	6	20–70
Lidocaine	60	800	95	1.7	1.7	70
Lithium	30	0	0	0.6	15	0
Penicillin G	350	35	10	0.2	0.5	65
Phenobarbital	1.5	4	70	0.6	86	50
Procainamide	330	120	30	1.6	3	65
Quinidine	100	200	65	2.5	7	75
Theophylline¶	0	55	100	0.5	7	55

*Cl_r = renal clearance for an adult with a creatinine clearance of 100 ml per minute.

†Cl_{nr} = nonrenal clearance for an adult.

‡Per cent nonrenal is the nonrenal clearance as a percentage of the total clearance.

§The oral bioavailability of digoxin is 65 per cent from the tablet and 95 per cent from the capsule.

¶Aminophylline is 85 per cent theophylline.

**Per cent bound to plasma proteins.

TABLE 24–2. DRUGS SHOWING DOSE-DEPENDENT KINETICS

	Maximal Metabolic Rate	Volume of Distribution
Salicylate	4000 mg/day	0.2–0.6 liter/kg*
Ethanol	8000 mg/hour	0.6 liter/kg
Phenytoin†	700 mg/day‡	0.6 liter/kg

*The volume of distribution of salicylate increases with increasing dose.

†The oral bioavailability of phenytoin is 80 per cent.

‡Some individuals have a lower maximal metabolic rate.

"average" patient and are therefore only first approximations of the doses required in an individual patient. Clinical observations and in some cases, measured plasma drug concentrations give information to the clinician for proper dosage adjustments.

ELIMINATION. *Drug Clearance.* Once in the circulation, drugs are eliminated from the body by two major processes: hepatic metabolism–biliary excretion and renal filtration-secretion into the urine. With a few important exceptions, the rates of hepatic and renal elimination are directly proportional to the concentration of the drug in the plasma, a process mathematically described as "first order." The pharmacokinetic parameter best describing the efficiency of the elimination processes is drug clearance. Drug clearance is defined as the volume of a fluid (usually plasma or blood) from which all drug is removed per unit of time. Clearance is a familiar term to clinicians discussing renal function. Thus creatinine clearance is the volume of plasma that is completely cleared of creatinine per minute and can be directly determined by relating the rate of creatinine excretion into the urine to the plasma creatinine concentration. Renal drug clearances can be determined in the same way by dividing renal excretory rate of the drug by the plasma drug concentration. Hepatic drug clearance is, by analogy to renal clearance, the volume of blood or plasma entirely cleared of drug by the liver and is therefore the rate of removal of drug by the liver divided by the concentration of drug in blood or plasma. Total body drug clearance (Cl) is the sum of all the individual organ clearances, which consists of renal (Cl_r) and nonrenal (Cl_{nr}) clearances. Total drug clearance is the rate of drug elimination by all processes ($\dot{R}$) divided by the plasma concentration (C_p):

$$Cl = \frac{\dot{R}}{C_p}$$

The clearance of drug by the liver and kidney can be influenced by the blood flow to the clearing organ, the binding of drug to the plasma proteins, and the activity of the processes responsible for drug removal, such as hepatic enzyme activity, glomerular filtration rate, and renal secretory processes. In physiologic terms, drug clearance by an organ is the product of organ blood flow (Q) and the fraction of the drug in the blood extracted on a single passage through the organ (E): Cl = QE. The extraction ratio, E, is calculated by dividing the arteriovenous difference in drug concentration ($C_a - C_v$) by the arterial drug concentration (C_a):

$$E = \frac{C_a - C_v}{C_a}$$

Clearance is *independent* of the distribution of drugs in the body (i.e., the V_D), since the eliminating organs "see" and can remove only the drug present in the blood.

Drug Half-Life. Both the clearance and the distribution of drug in the body influence the amount of time necessary to eliminate drug from the body. The proportion of the apparent volume of distribution cleared of drug per unit of time is a constant called the "first order elimination rate constant," or k_e:

$$k_e = \frac{Cl}{V_D}$$

This constant describes the exponential disappearance of drug from the plasma with time during the elimination phase. When plotted on semi-log graph paper, as in Figure 24–2, the exponential elimination phase is a straight line with a slope of k_e. A conceptually more useful term describing the time required to eliminate drug is the drug's elimination half-life

($t\frac{1}{2}$), which is the time required to reduce the plasma concentration of drug (and hence the body load of drug) to half the initial concentration. For drugs with first order elimination, the $t\frac{1}{2}$ is independent of drug concentration. The $t\frac{1}{2}$ is frequently determined graphically as in Figure 24–2, and mathematically the half-life is the natural logarithm of 2 (indicating a reduction of drug concentration by half) divided by the elimination rate constant: $t\frac{1}{2} = \ln 2/k_e = 0.693/k_e$. Since the elimination rate constant is related to both clearance and volume of distribution as independent variables, it can be appreciated that half-life must also be related to these two variables:

$$t\frac{1}{2} = \frac{0.693\ V_D}{Cl}$$

As the apparent volume of distribution increases, the half-life is prolonged for any given drug clearance, since a greater "volume" must be cleared of drug; as clearance increases, half-life shortens for any given V_D. A change in half-life frequently is used as an index of a change in efficiency of drug elimination, but this is true only when the apparent volume of distribution is unchanged. Hepatic, renal, and cardiovascular disease not only can decrease drug clearance but also can alter the apparent volume of distribution. Half-life, being affected by both V_D and Cl, may be affected to a greater or lesser extent than drug clearance, and therefore $t\frac{1}{2}$ may not indicate the degree of abnormality in drug elimination. For example, patients with congestive heart failure have a 50 per cent reduction in the clearance of lidocaine and may, in addition, have a similarly contracted volume of distribution of the drug. Since both Cl and V_D can be reduced by a similar magnitude, the half-life may be unchanged and not give any clue to the abnormal lidocaine clearance and the need for reduced infusion rates to avoid toxicity. (See "Maintenance Doses" below for discussion of the relationship of clearance to steady-state blood concentration.)

For exponential or first order drug elimination, an infinite time is required to eliminate drug entirely from the body. Only half the drug is eliminated in the first half-life, half the remaining drug eliminated in the second half-life, and so forth. Thus, by starting with an effective blood level, which we shall call 100 per cent, 50 per cent will be present after one half-life, 25 per cent after two half-lives, 12.5 per cent after three half-lives, 6.25 per cent after four half-lives, and 3.125 per cent after five half-lives, as shown in Figure 24–3 for lidocaine. For practical purposes, most drugs can be considered to be eliminated completely when less than 10 per cent of the effective concentration remains in the body, requiring three to four half-lives. For lidocaine (Fig. 24–3) this time is about six hours.

DRUG ACCUMULATION. When drug is given as a sustained infusion or in repeated doses, drug accumulates in the body until a steady state is achieved, at which time the amount of drug being administered is equal to the amount of drug eliminated so that body stores and plasma levels remain constant. The time course of drug accumulation, like the time course of elimination, is determined by the drug's elimination half-life, these processes being mirror images of each other (Fig. 24–3). Thus, accumulation to half the ultimate steady state occurs in one half-life, 75 per cent in two half-lives, 87.5 per cent in three half-lives, and 93.75 per cent in four half-lives. For practical purposes, the steady state is considered achieved when 90 per cent of the ultimate accumulation occurs, requiring three to four half-lives. For drugs with short half-lives, accumulation occurs rapidly and loading doses to achieve immediate therapeutic concentrations may not be necessary. For drugs with long half-lives, accumulation occurs slowly and loading doses are frequently required to achieve a therapeutic effect prior to waiting for full accumulation to occur. Regardless of whether a loading dose is given, the

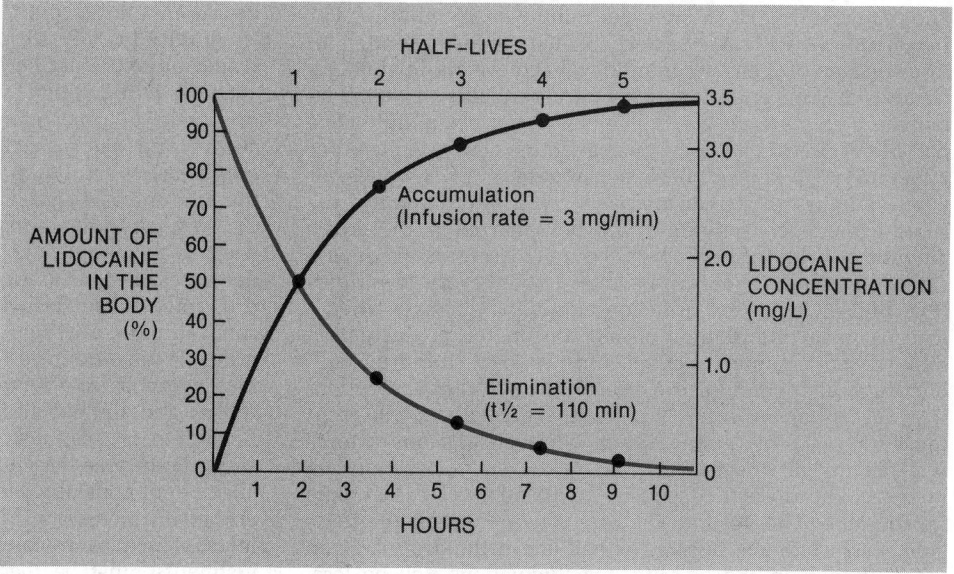

FIGURE 24–3. The accumulation of lidocaine during an infusion of 3 mg per minute and the elimination of lidocaine after the drug is discontinued. Time is indicated in hours and in half-lives and concentration in milligrams per liter. The amount of lidocaine in the body is the percentage remaining after discontinuation of the drug (elimination curve—color) or the percentage of the ultimate steady-state value achieved by the chronic infusion (accumulation curve). The two curves are mirror images of each other.

ultimate steady-state concentration achieved depends only on the maintenance dose and drug clearance. The loading dose only allows one to hasten the approach to a therapeutic concentration of drug. Figure 24–3 shows the accumulation of lidocaine to a steady state during a constant intravenous infusion of 3 mg per minute. The ultimate steady-state plasma level is approached with a half-life of 110 minutes. A loading dose would be required to achieve therapeutic concentrations more quickly.

When a drug is given intermittently, such as procainamide, illustrated in Figure 24–4, the average concentration approaches steady state with the same time course as during a constant infusion. The more frequently doses are given, the smaller the differences between peak and trough plasma concentrations, and the closer the intermittent dosing approximates an intravenous infusion.

Whenever the drug doses or infusion rates are changed, a new steady state will be achieved. The approach to the new steady state also is dependent on the half-life so that three to four half-lives will be required before the plasma concentrations and body stores of drug are at 90 per cent of the new steady state. Therefore, the effects of a dosage adjustment will not be immediate and will not be fully expressed for a time that is dependent on the drug's half-life.

MAINTENANCE DOSES. Steady state is achieved when the rate of drug administration equals the rate of drug elimination. The rate of drug administration is either the infusion rate (I) or the dose per unit time (D/t), and the rate of drug elimination is the product of drug clearance (Cl) and the drug concentration (C_p). Therefore, during a steady-state infusion, $I = ClC_p$, and during intermittent dosing, $D/t = ClC_p$. Note that the steady-state concentrations are independent of the distribution of the drug and are solely dependent on drug clearance and the rate of drug administration. The equations for steady state can be used to calculate the infusion rate or the intermittent dose required to achieve a desired plasma concentration, and, conversely, the plasma concentration at steady state produced by a known infusion rate can be used to calculate drug clearance. With the value for V_D (Table 24–1), half-life can also be calculated from the steady-state data as $0.693 \, V_D/Cl$. For example, in an adult without heart failure or liver disease, the clearance of lidocaine is about 860 ml per minute (Table 24–1). In order to maintain a therapeutic concentration of 3.5 µg per milliliter, an infusion rate of 3 mg per minute must be given: $I = ClC_p = 860$ ml per minute × 3.5 µg per milliliter = 3000 µg per minute = 3 mg per minute. This is the steady-state value illustrated in Figure 24–3. The half-life for lidocaine in this patient is 0.693 (1.7 liters per

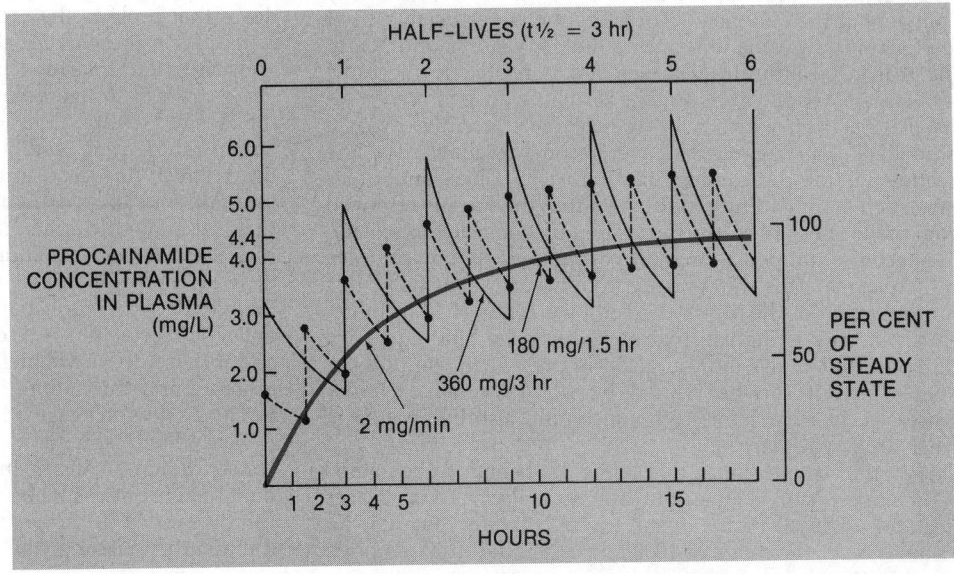

FIGURE 24–4. The accumulation to steady state of procainamide given as an infusion of 2 mg per minute (smooth curve) or intermittent doses of 180 mg per one and one half hours (dashed line) or 360 mg per three hours (solid line). Regardless of the method of administration, the accumulation follows the same time course and requires three to four half-lives to reach 90 per cent of steady state.

kilogram × 70 kg)/0.86 liters per minute = 96 minutes. For procainamide with a clearance of 450 ml per minute, an infusion rate of 2 mg per minute will achieve and maintain a steady-state concentration of 4.4 μg per milliliter: I = 450 ml per minute × 4.4 μg per milliliter = 2 mg per minute. The half-life of procainamide in this patient is 0.693 (1.6 liters per kilogram × 70 kg)/0.45 liters per minute = 172 minutes, or about 3 hours. If procainamide is given intermittently, the same average concentration will be achieved if the entire amount of drug infused over 3 hours (360 mg) is given as a single dose every 3 hours or half that amount every 90 minutes (Fig. 24–4). Obviously, drug concentrations fluctuate when a drug is given intermittently, and the degree of fluctuation depends on the interval between drug doses, the drug half-life, the route of administration, and the speed of absorption. If a dose is given every half-life, the fluctuation will be at most 100 per cent, that is, the blood levels and body stores will fall to half the initial level by the end of the dosage interval. The dose then boosts the blood level back to the initial value. The dose in this case consists of half the body stores, which is lost during the half-life. If the drug is given more often than the half-life, the fluctuations will be less, with the ultimate example being an infusion in which there is no fluctuation. In each case, the drug lost during a dosage interval is replaced by the dose to maintain the steady state. Usually drugs are given at least every half-life to avoid extreme fluctuations of blood levels. Only if very high concentrations are nontoxic or continuously effective plasma levels are not required can a drug be given much less frequently than one half-life. When a dose is given orally, absorption from the gut occurs gradually, and therefore peak concentrations are lower and fluctuations in plasma levels are less than if the same dose were administered as an intravenous bolus. In fact, with sustained-release oral formulations, absorption can be sustained over most of the dosage interval, resulting in minimal fluctuations in plasma levels.

DRUG REMOVAL FOLLOWING OVERDOSE. The principles described above can be used to predict the efficacy of hemodialysis or hemoperfusion in removing drug following an overdose. To be a valuable addition to the therapy of overdose, the drug removal process must make a substantial contribution to overall clearance of the drug and the amount of drug removed must be a significant portion of the body load. Consider the case of a digoxin overdose in an adult producing a plasma digoxin level of 8 ng per milliliter. The body load of digoxin is $V_D \times C_p$ or 500 liters × 8 μg per liter = 4 mg. At a clearance of 100 ml per minute with the hemoperfusion apparatus, the rate of drug removal with a C_p of 8 ng per milliliter is $Cl \times C_p$ = 100 ml per minute × 8 ng per milliliter = 800 ng per minute = 48 μg per hour, or only 1 per cent of the body load. Therefore, hemoperfusion cannot be of significant value in reducing the body stores of digoxin. The reason so little drug is removed is related to digoxin's very large V_D of 500 liters so that very little drug is present in the plasma from which it can be cleared. Recently, digoxin antibodies (Fab fragment) have become available for the treatment of life-threatening digoxin toxicity. These antibodies have such a high affinity for digoxin that the drug is removed from tissue sites, including those areas responsible for toxicity, and becomes trapped as an inactive digoxin-antibody complex in the plasma. This shift of drug from tissue to plasma results in a reduction of the V_D for digoxin by a factor of 10 or more. Thus not only is digoxin toxicity reduced by binding to the antibody, but much more digoxin is present in the plasma, from which it can be cleared by normal renal excretory processes. In theory this technique could also be applied to other drugs with large V_D.

The other circumstance that limits the benefit to be gained by hemoperfusion is when the drug normally has a very large clearance. The clearance of the tricyclic antidepressants, for instance, is in the range of 1000 ml per minute. If a hemoper-fusion apparatus could clear the drug at 100 ml per minute, it would add only 10 per cent to the normal clearance and would therefore not be of substantial value.

DOSE-DEPENDENT PHARMACOKINETICS. For a few drugs, the pharmacokinetics do not follow the rules outlined above, and such drugs are said to have dose-dependent, nonlinear, or saturation kinetics (Table 24–2). For these drugs the amount of drug eliminated is not directly related to the drug concentration (first order), but as the concentration of drug is increased, the relative amount of drug eliminated decreases (i.e., clearance decreases) until a maximal rate of drug metabolism is achieved that is independent of drug concentration, at which point drug elimination is termed zero order. If the amount of drug administered exceeds the maximal metabolic rate for drug elimination, the drug will accumulate indefinitely and very high blood levels will result. Phenytoin is the most important example of a therapeutic agent with dose-dependent kinetics. With phenytoin, clearance is not constant but decreases at increasing dose so that any given increase in dose will result in a disproportionate increase in plasma concentration, and therefore dosage adjustments must be made cautiously. A dose of 300 mg of phenytoin daily may give a plasma level of 8 μg per milliliter, and a dose of 400 mg per day a plasma level of 25 μg per milliliter. Since all patients differ in their ability to eliminate phenytoin, proper dosage adjustments are difficult to predict for an individual patient. In practice, plasma concentration measurements (see below) must be used to establish a proper maintenance dose. High-dose salicylate therapy also behaves in a dose-dependent manner, as does ethanol. However, ethanol is eliminated by zero order kinetics at all doses, and therefore its elimination is much more predictable than that of phenytoin and salicylate, for which the elimination changes from first order to zero order over the therapeutic range.

USE OF PLASMA DRUG CONCENTRATION TO GUIDE THERAPY. The principles outlined above allow the clinician to choose a loading and maintenance dose based on the desired plasma concentration to achieve therapeutic effects and minimize the risk of toxicity. The underlying premise is that following distribution of a dose, the concentration of drug in plasma is in equilibrium with drug at the site of action and therefore is a direct reflection of the drug at the target site (Fig. 24–1).

However, the published pharmacokinetic data on which initial dosage recommendations are based are averages for a population and usually need modification for the individual patient. Dosage adjustment is best accomplished when the therapeutic effects of the drug are readily quantifiable. Thus, antihypertensive drugs can be given in a dose sufficient to lower blood pressure, and oral anticoagulants can be given in doses that prolong the prothrombin time into the therapeutic range. With these drugs the desired effect is the appropriate endpoint, and plasma concentrations of the drug are not necessary for dosage adjustment. For many drugs, however, the desired endpoint is difficult to assess clinically, either because there is no readily quantifiable measurement to assess drug effect or because the disease being treated has an intermittent expression so that the clinician cannot be certain that a therapeutic effect has been achieved. Two good examples are epilepsy and sporadic cardiac arrhythmias, in which drug dosage adjustments are difficult to make with precision. Frequently, therefore, patients with sporadic arrhythmias or epilepsy receive doses of drugs based on the average patient, and if these doses are ineffective or toxic, the drug is deemed a failure and the patient is "resistant" or "intolerant" to the therapy, in which case other drugs are tried.

Dosage adjustment can be aided by using the plasma concentration in cases in which there are no other easily quantifiable endpoints by which the drug's therapeutic effects can be gauged. In order for the plasma concentration to have therapeutic meaning, the drug in plasma must be in equilib-

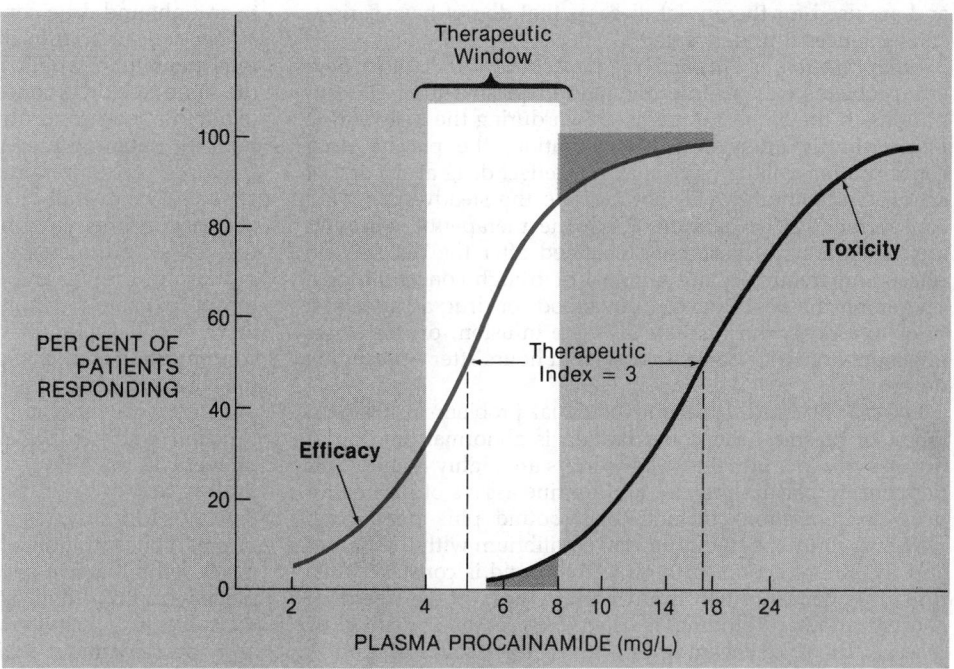

FIGURE 24–5. Population dose-response curves for the antiarrhythmic and acute toxic effects of procainamide. The therapeutic window is the range encompassing most of the therapeutic dose-effect curve and includes less than 10 per cent of the toxic dose-effect curve. The toxic dose divided by the therapeutic dose is the therapeutic index, here shown for 50 per cent of the population. Individual patients may lie anywhere on these curves.

rium with drug at the site of action and the effects must be reversible. If a drug has irreversible effects, such as the effect of aspirin to inhibit platelet aggregation, the plasma level will not correlate with effect. Fortunately, such situations are uncommon.

The sources of variation in drug effects can be divided into pharmacokinetic and pharmacodynamic factors. Those factors that alter the plasma drug concentration resulting from a given dose are the pharmacokinetic variables—absorption, distribution, and clearance. Those factors that alter the response to a given plasma level are the pharmacodynamic variables. If the pharmacodynamic variation among patients is very large, then plasma drug concentrations will not be a helpful guide for therapy. Fortunately, pharmacokinetic factors account for the major variation in response among patients for many drugs, and this variability can be managed with the use of plasma drug level monitoring.

Therapeutic Window. For plasma levels to be a useful guide to therapy, the range of drug concentrations required for optimal therapeutic effects with minimal toxicity must be established. This range is called the "therapeutic window" and is determined experimentally for each drug in a group of patients who are carefully observed for desired and toxic drug effects (Fig. 24–5). The width of the therapeutic window relates to the steepness of the concentration-effect curve and is an index of the pharmacodynamic variability in the population being treated. For procainamide, illustrated in Figure 24–5, the therapeutic window is 4 to 8 mg per liter. The separation between the therapeutic and toxic concentration-effect curves is an index of the toxicity of the drug frequently referred to as the "therapeutic index," which is the toxic dose divided by therapeutic dose. For procainamide the therapeutic index is ~3. With all drugs there is overlap between the therapeutic and toxic ranges. In addition, since the therapeutic window is based on a population of patients, one cannot be certain of the optimal drug concentration for a given patient. Although most patients will achieve a therapeutic effect within the therapeutic range, a few patients require concentrations below or above the range. Similarly, toxicity begins to occur in some patients within the therapeutic window, but the incidence of side effects increases sharply as the therapeutic range is exceeded. Therefore, the plasma concentration cannot be an infallible guide to safe and effective therapy, since it controls only the pharmacokinetic variability and not the

pharmacodynamic variability. It is undoubtedly better, however, than the use of a standard dose that allows for no variability.

Table 24–3 lists some drugs for which therapeutic windows have been established. These drugs have several common characteristics: First, their pharmacologic effects are not readily quantifiable; second, they are used for therapy of serious or life-threatening illness so that therapeutic inefficacy cannot be tolerated; and third, their toxicity is serious, and the therapeutic index is small. Therapeutic windows are not required for drugs that have a very large therapeutic index

TABLE 24–3. THERAPEUTIC WINDOWS

Drug	Therapeutic Range
Cardiovascular Drugs:	
Digitoxin	10–25 µg/liter
Digoxin	0.8–2 µg/liter
Disopyramide	2–6 mg/liter
Flecainide	0.2–1 mg/liter
Lidocaine	1.5–5 mg/liter
Mexiletine	0.5–2 mg/liter
Procainamide	4–8 mg/liter
Quinidine	2–6 mg/liter
Theophylline	8–20 mg/liter
Tocainide	4–12 mg/liter
Antiseizure Drugs:	
Carbamazepine	6–12 mg/liter
Ethosuximide	40–80 mg/liter
Phenobarbital	15–30 mg/liter
Phenytoin	10–20 mg/liter
Valproic acid	50–100 mg/liter
Antibiotics:*	
Amikacin‡	20–40 mg/liter
Carbenicillin	100–300 mg/liter
Gentamicin‡	5–10 mg/liter
Penicillin G†	1–25 mg/liter
Tobramycin‡	5–10 mg/liter
Others:	
Lithium	0.5–1.5 mEq/liter
Nortriptyline	50–150 µg/liter
Salicylate	<300 mg/liter

*Actual concentration required related to minimal inhibitory concentration for infecting bacterium.
†1 mg of penicillin = 1.6 × 10⁶ units.
‡Peak levels.

and are used for therapy of diseases that do not have serious consequences if undertreated.

Interpretation of Plasma Drug Concentrations. TIMING. Several problems exist in interpretation of plasma drug concentrations. If the blood sample is drawn during the distribution phase shortly after drug administration, the plasma drug concentration will be high, may not reflect drug at the site of action, and certainly will not indicate the steady-state drug concentration. The data on which the therapeutic windows are based are concentrations obtained after the distribution phase and frequently are minimal or trough concentrations. Therefore, the best time to draw blood for drug assay is just prior to a dose, during a steady-state infusion, or, for drugs given once or twice daily, at least eight hours after a preceding dose.

PROTEIN BINDING. A second potential problem in interpretation of plasma drug concentration is abnormal binding of drugs to plasma proteins. Many drugs are highly bound (>80 per cent) to plasma protein, and routine assays of plasma for drug concentrations include total (bound plus free) drug. However, only the free drug is in equilibrium with the tissues and the site of action. If the fraction bound is constant, then total drug concentration is an accurate index of the free drug concentration. If binding is altered by other drugs or by disease, then the meaning of a given total concentration of drug will be changed, since a greater proportion of the drug will be unbound. Both liver and kidney disease can alter the protein binding of some drugs (phenytoin, digitoxin, clofibrate, diazoxide, some sulfonamides, valproic acid, and salicylic acid) either by changing the quantity of protein (decreased albumin in liver disease and nephrotic syndrome) or by competition for binding between the drug and endogenous compounds that accumulate in patients with uremia or jaundice. In addition, one drug may compete with another for binding to plasma proteins. Measurement of unbound drug may be required for proper interpretation of the plasma concentration in these circumstances, since if more drug is unbound, the effects or toxicity of any given total plasma concentration will be increased. Unfortunately, most clinical laboratories are not capable of measuring unbound drug concentrations.

Decreased plasma protein binding can also change the kinetics of drug disposition. The volume of distribution will increase because less drug remains in the plasma as the increased free fraction distributes to the tissues. Whether changes in clearance occur with changes in plasma protein binding depends on whether the clearing organ can strip drug from the protein, in which case clearance will not change, since in this circumstance it does not depend on the free drug fraction. However, for many drugs the clearance is restricted to free drug, in which case drug clearance will increase as binding to plasma proteins decreases, since a larger fraction of the total is available for elimination. With these drugs, however, the clearance of *free* drug is unchanged. An unchanged clearance of free drug means that the average plasma free drug concentration will be unchanged at steady state, although protein binding is decreased. However, the total drug concentration will decrease because of the increased drug clearance. Since free drug concentration is not changed and free drug determines the effects of most drugs, the daily dose of drug need not be changed. The best-studied example is that of phenytoin, which is normally >90 per cent bound to plasma albumin. In patients with uremia, phenytoin binding can decrease to 70 per cent so that the unbound fraction increases from 10 to 30 per cent. As a consequence of the increase in free fraction, the apparent volume of distribution of phenytoin increases and clearance increases. The plasma concentration of total phenytoin falls as a result of the increased clearance, but the average free concentration at steady state is unchanged. A therapeutic phenytoin level with 90 per cent protein binding is 10 to 20 mg per liter, corresponding

to an unbound drug concentration of 1 to 2 mg per liter. With 30 per cent unbound, the corresponding therapeutic level of total phenytoin would be 3.3 to 6.7 mg per liter to achieve the same free drug concentration. Obviously, if the goal were to attain a total concentration of 10 to 20 mg per liter with 30 per cent unbound phenytoin, toxicity would result, since the free drug concentration would be threefold higher than therapeutic. The overall pharmacokinetic change resulting from a decrease in phenytoin binding is an unchanged clearance of free drug, an increased clearance of total drug, a lesser increase in the V_D, and a consequent decrease in the half-life to approximately 8 hours from the normal 18 to 24 hours. Since the half-life is shortened but the average free drug concentration is unchanged by the change in phenytoin binding, the total daily dose of phenytoin should be the same in patients with renal failure as in patients with normal renal function, but the drug should be given every 8 hours instead of every 12 to 24 hours to avoid unwanted large fluctuations in drug level.

ACTIVE METABOLITES. A third pitfall in interpretation of the plasma concentration of some drugs is the presence of unmeasured but active or toxic drug metabolites. Propranolol is metabolized to 4-hydroxypropranolol, which has beta-adrenergic–blocking activity. Procainamide is metabolized to *N*-acetylprocainamide, which has antiarrhythmic activity. The importance of active metabolites depends on their intrinsic activity and toxicity and the extent to which they accumulate relative to the parent compound. In situations in which a metabolite accounts for a significant portion of the drug's activity or toxicity, the metabolite must be measured along with the parent drug for proper interpretation.

PHARMACODYNAMIC CHANGES. A final factor altering the interpretation of plasma levels is a physiologic or pathologic change that alters the response to a given plasma concentration. For instance, a change in serum potassium, magnesium, or calcium concentration will alter the toxic concentration-effect relationship for digoxin such that concentrations not usually associated with adverse effects may now be toxic. The development of tolerance to a drug will also distort the relationship of plasma concentration to effect. Tolerance can be defined as a reduction in response to a given concentration of drug at the site of action and has been described for drugs of abuse, particularly opiates. However, with the recent emphasis on drug delivery systems capable of producing constant blood levels of therapeutic drugs over many hours or days, the possibility of tolerance to the beneficial effects of these drugs is worrisome. The tolerance reported with the chronic use of beta-adrenergic agonists for asthma and heart failure may be due to a reduction in the density of beta-adrenergic receptors during chronic agonist stimulation (see Ch. 26). More recently, tolerance to the therapeutic effects of nitroglycerin has been described with the 24-hour transdermal delivery systems.

These alterations in pharmacodynamics of the drug response emphasize the fact that plasma drug concentrations must be interpreted with other clinical and laboratory data that may influence the response to the drug.

ALTERATIONS OF DRUG DOSES IN DISEASE STATES. *Renal Disease.* A decrease in renal function will result in a decreased renal clearance of drugs. Whether a dosage adjustment is required depends on the toxicity of the drug and the importance of renal clearance for drug elimination. If the drug has significant toxicity and the kidney accounts for most of the drug's elimination, then dosage adjustments must be made in patients with renal disease to avoid toxicity. On the other hand, if the drug is nontoxic, dosage adjustment is less critical even if the drug accumulates in patients with renal failure. For instance, penicillin is cleared >90 per cent by the kidneys, but because it is relatively nontoxic, dosage adjustments are not required for low-dose therapy (600,000 to 1,200,000 units per day). However, if massive doses of penicillin are required, then dosage adjustments must be made to avoid penicillin toxicity.

Fortunately, renal drug clearance is closely correlated with the clearance of creatinine even for those drugs that are eliminated by tubular secretion. For this reason, an adjustment of the average drug dose can be calculated from the creatinine clearance. The process is simple: The calculated renal drug clearance is reduced by the same proportion as the reduction from 100 ml per minute in the measured creatinine clearance or the creatinine clearance calculated by the formula:

$$\text{creatinine clearance} = \frac{(140 - \text{age}) \times \text{weight (kg)}}{72 \times \text{serum creatinine (mg/dl)}}$$

for males, with the creatinine clearance for females being 85 per cent of that for males. If the drug is cleared by nonrenal (usually hepatic) mechanisms as well as by renal mechanisms, only the renal clearance (Cl_r) is adjusted; the nonrenal clearance (Cl_{nr}) remains normal. Assuming that the same average plasma concentration (C_p) is desired in patients with renal failure, the dose is adjusted in direct proportion to the change in total clearance, since $Cl \times C_p = \text{dose/time}$. Renal and nonrenal clearances for some drugs are listed in Table 24–1. Consider as an example of this approach the alteration of digoxin dosage in renal failure. The average renal clearance of digoxin is 110 ml per minute at a creatinine clearance of 100 ml per minute; the nonrenal clearance is 40 ml per minute. If the measured creatinine clearance is 50 ml per minute, or half normal, then the renal clearance of digoxin is reduced by a similar fraction; thus, Cl_r (digoxin) = 55 ml per minute in this patient. If the nonrenal clearance is assumed to be unchanged, the total digoxin clearance is $Cl_{nr} + Cl_r = 40 + 55 = 95$ ml per minute in the patient with a creatinine clearance of 50 ml per minute, versus a total digoxin clearance of $40 + 110 = 150$ ml per minute in a patient with normal renal function. The total digoxin clearance is therefore reduced by the fraction $\frac{95}{150}$ and the dose should be adjusted using the same fraction. If the average dose is 0.25 mg per day, this would be decreased to $\frac{95}{150} \times 0.25$ mg = 0.16 mg per day.

These calculations can give only a first approximation of the appropriate dose for an individual patient, since they are based on the average dose for the average patient. In practice, a dose conveniently close to the calculated dose is administered to the patient, and the patient's response and/or plasma drug concentrations are monitored. With the information provided by either the plasma drug concentrations or clinical observations, the dosage can be adjusted.

If the desired plasma concentration is known, one can calculate the dosage directly from the drug clearance, since dose/t = $Cl \times C_p$. For example, an average procainamide concentration of 5 μg per milliliter is desired in a patient with a creatinine clearance of 50 ml per minute. The total procainamide clearance is $\frac{50}{100} \times 330$ (Cl_r) + 120 (Cl_{nr}) = 285 ml per minute. An infusion of 1.4 mg per minute ($Cl \times C_p$) or a dose of 250 mg every three hours will achieve and maintain the desired plasma concentration.

Although drug clearance is the best way to calculate doses for drugs, clearance data are not available for many drugs. For a few drugs, published nomograms are available to guide dosage. It would be preferable, both from a practical and from an intellectual standpoint, to be able to use a more generally applicable method to calculate proper dosage. Two such methods are outlined in the next two paragraphs.

For many drugs, the elimination rate constant (k_e) is known. If the apparent volume of distribution is unchanged in renal disease, then the k_e and Cl are proportional ($k_e = Cl/V_D$) and

the change in k_e can be used to adjust the dose in a manner entirely analogous to the use of changes in clearance to adjust dose. Like clearance values, the elimination rate constant can be expressed as the sum of the rate constants for the separate eliminating organs; thus $k_e = k_{renal} + k_{nonrenal}$. Values for k_r and k_{nr} are listed in Table 24–4. To use these values to adjust dosage in renal insufficiency, the procedure is exactly the same as with the clearance calculations used above. Thus, k_e for amikacin in a patient with normal renal function is 0.31, which is made up of $k_r = 0.3$ and a $k_{nr} = 0.01$. The dose alteration in a patient with a creatinine clearance of 25 ml per minute is calculated as follows: The k_r for the patient is 25/100 $\times$ 0.3 = 0.08. The k_e therefore is $k_r + k_{nr} = 0.08 + 0.01 = 0.09$ versus the normal k_e of 0.31. The dose of amikacin must therefore be reduced to $\frac{0.09}{0.31}$ or 30 per cent of the usual dose per unit time. As can be readily appreciated, the dose of amikacin is reduced almost in proportion to the reduction in creatinine clearance, since the nonrenal elimination is negligible until creatinine clearance is reduced to very low values (i.e., <15 ml per minute). Several other drugs are like amikacin in this regard and are in Group A in Table 24–4. For all these drugs, dosage adjustment can be made by multiplying the usual dose by the fraction of the creatinine clearance remaining in the patient. When the patient has essentially no renal function, then the small k_{nr} may be used to calculate doses as illustrated above. For drugs that have nonrenal elimination that is a substantial fraction (e.g., 20 to 50 per cent) of the total elimination, the dosage reduction in renal insufficiency will be less than the reduction in creatinine clearance and can be calculated as illustrated above. These drugs are in Group B. If the nonrenal elimination is greater than 50 per cent of the k_e, then the dosage usually does not need to be adjusted for changes in renal function. In all cases, the calculations adjust only the average dose, and blood level determinations are required to make final dosage adjustments. This is particularly true if nonrenal elimination may also be reduced, as in liver or cardiac disease.

A final method for estimating the average dose in patients with renal failure is to use the per cent nonrenal elimination determined in normal individuals. These values are listed in Tables 24–1 and 24–4 and are frequently available for drugs even if clearances or elimination rate constants are not. This method uses the nomogram in Figure 24–6, in which creatinine clearance is plotted against the drug clearance as a per cent of normal. The black lines intersecting the black ordinate are for drugs that have a nonrenal elimination of from 0 to 50 per cent in a normal individual. The nomogram is used by drawing a perpendicular line to the creatinine clearance until it intersects the black line corresponding to the drug of interest. The per cent drug clearance can then be read directly from the red ordinate, and the dosage adjusted accordingly. For instance, consider the amikacin example calculated above. Since the per cent nonrenal elimination in a normal individual is ~5 per cent, the clearance values for amikacin fall on the line intersecting the ordinate at 5 per cent in Figure 24–6. The drug clearance as a percentage of normal for a creatinine clearance of 25 ml per minute is ~30 per cent (as indicated by the dotted line), and the dose of this drug in the patient with a creatinine clearance of 25 ml therefore must be 30 per cent normal.

The reduction in dose per unit time can be applied to patient care by giving either the reduced dose at the usual interval or the same dose at a longer interval. By both methods the average plasma level will be the same, but the fluctuations in plasma concentration will be less when the reduced dose is given at the usual intervals.

Loading doses for most drugs used in patients with renal failure need not be adjusted for creatinine clearance because V_D is usually close to normal. However, since the t½ of

TABLE 24–4. THE RENAL ELIMINATION RATE CONSTANTS (k_r), NONRENAL ELIMINATION RATE CONSTANTS (k_{nr}), AND PER CENT NONRENAL ELIMINATION IN A NORMAL INDIVIDUAL FOR SELECTED DRUGS

	k_r (per hour)	k_{nr} (per hour)	Per Cent Nonrenal
Group A (>80% renal)			
Acyclovir	0.2	0.02	10
Amantidine	0.05	0.005	10
Amikacin	0.3	0.01	5
Amoxicillin	0.6	0.1	10
Ampicillin	0.5	0.06	10
Atenolol	0.10	0.005	5
Bretylium	0.07	0.01	15
Carbenicillin	0.5	0.05	10
Cefamandole	0.84	0.04	5
Cefazolin	0.3	0.02	5
Cefoxitin	1.0	0.05	5
Cephalexin	0.7	0.03	5
Cephalothin	1.4	0.03	5
Cephradine	0.5	0.05	10
Colistin	0.3	0.02	10
Flucytosine	0.24	0.01	5
Gentamicin	0.3	0.02	5
Kanamycin	0.3	0.01	5
Methicillin	1.2	0.15	10
Methotrexate	0.07	0.007	10
Moxalactam	0.3	0.02	5
Oxypurinol*	0.03	0.003	10
Penicillin G	1.3	0.1	10
Polymyxin B	0.13	0.02	10
Streptomycin	0.24	0.01	5
Tetracycline	0.07	0.01	10
Ticarcillin	0.6	0.06	10
Tobramycin	0.3	0.01	5
Vancomycin	0.12	0.003	5
Group B (50–80% renal)			
Cefotaxime	0.6	0.28	30
Cephapirin	0.9	0.3	25
Cimetidine	0.27	0.09	25
Dicloxacillin	0.6	0.6	50
Erythromycin	0.30	0.15	35
Ethambutol	0.09	0.09	50
Isoniazid (slow acetylators)	0.12	0.12	50
Lincomycin	0.1	0.06	40
Nadolol	0.03	0.01	25
Nafcillin	0.7	0.5	40
Oxacillin	1.1	0.35	25
Oxytetracycline	0.065	0.015	20
Ranitidine	0.25	0.08	25
Trimethoprim	0.03	0.03	50
Group C (<50% renal)			
Amphotericin B	0.01	0.02	70
Chloramphenicol	0.02	0.3	80
Clindamycin	0	0.25	100
Doxycycline	0.005	0.03	80
Flecainide	0.013	0.03	70
Isoniazid (fast acetylators)	0.1	0.4	80
Mexiletine	0.006	0.06	90
Minocycline	0	0.06	100
Rifampin	0	0.25	100
Sulfamethoxazole	0.01	0.06	85
Tocainide	0.02	0.03	60

*Oxypurinol is the major active metabolite of allopurinol.

renally cleared drugs is prolonged in these patients, drug accumulation during initiation of therapy with maintenance doses will be slower. Because of the slower accumulation, a loading dose may be required in patients with renal failure in order to achieve a therapeutic blood concentration rapidly, whereas patients with normal renal function may not need a loading dose for the same drug. Digoxin, for example, with a half-life of 1.5 days in a patient with normal renal function will accumulate to 90 per cent of steady-state levels in 5 days (3 to 4 half-lives), and many patients need not be loaded, since this accumulation is sufficiently rapid to produce the desired therapeutic effects. On the other hand, in a patient without renal function, digoxin half-life increases to five days. If the anephric patient is begun on the appropriately reduced maintenance dose of digoxin, accumulation to the same steady-state level will take more than 15 days to occur. In this case, a loading dose may be desired to achieve a more rapid effect without waiting for drug accumulation. However, whether or not a loading dose is given, the ultimate steady-state drug concentration will be the same and, as always, depends only on drug dose and drug clearance.

Patients with end-stage renal disease are usually supported with hemodialysis. Dialysis can remove some therapeutic drugs from the circulation and necessitate supplemental dosing to maintain a therapeutic effect. The most important characteristics of the drug that determine the ability of dialysis to remove a significant amount of drug from the body are the V_D, drug binding to plasma proteins, and the nonrenal clearance of the drug. Of these, V_D is the most important parameter, and only if it is less than 1 liter per kilogram can significant amounts of drug be removed by dialysis. Dialysis is also more effective in drug removal if the drug is not highly bound to plasma proteins and is normally cleared primarily by the kidneys. Since clearance of drugs by hemodialysis is limited to a maximum of ~100 ml per minute, drugs that have a relatively small extrarenal clearance (< 400 ml per minute) may have a significant increment in their removal rate during hemodialysis even if they are not normally cleared by the kidney. For instance, aminoglycosides have a small V_D, low binding to plasma protein, and mostly renal clearance and are therefore removed to a significant extent by hemodialysis. Theophylline, although not normally cleared by the kidneys, has a relatively small V_D, a nonrenal clearance of 55 ml per minute, and moderate protein binding and therefore may be sufficiently removed during a three to six hour hemodialysis session to require a modest supplemental dosage. For most drugs that require supplemental therapy after hemodialysis to maintain a therapeutic effect, blood level determinations are available as a guide.

Some drugs form metabolites that are active or toxic and are eliminated by the kidneys. In patients with renal insufficiency, these metabolites may accumulate and produce effects. As an example, procainamide is in part excreted unchanged and in part metabolized to N-acetylprocainamide, which has antiarrhythmic effects and can produce toxicity. The metabolite may achieve concentrations in renal failure that are many-fold higher than the parent drug and can contribute to the antiarrhythmic effects and toxicity of procainamide. Since the concentration of metabolites is not routinely measured by drug assay laboratories, the plasma concentration of parent drug can be misleading. Drugs with renally excreted active or toxic metabolites include (in addition to procainamide) meperidine, propoxyphene, allopurinol, acetohexamide, clofibrate, nitrofurantoin, and nitroprusside. If alternative drugs are available for the treatment of patients with renal insufficiency, it is probably best to avoid these drugs when active or toxic metabolites may accumulate.

Hepatic Disease. Although many drugs are biotransformed by the liver, no quantitative predictor of the degree of abnormality in drug metabolism is available for patients with liver disease. Severe liver disease can result in a decreased metabolic capacity for a large number of drugs. If the indices of the liver's capacity to form proteins (serum albumin level and prothrombin time) are abnormal, then it is probable that drug metabolism will also be abnormal, and the doses of those drugs that are metabolized by the liver should be reduced. Acute liver disease has an inconstant and unpredictable effect on drug metabolism, but, in general, drug metabolism is not as abnormal as with chronic liver disease.

With chronic liver disease, portacaval anastomoses may develop. Not only will this decrease the blood flow to the liver with consequent reduction in clearance of some drugs,

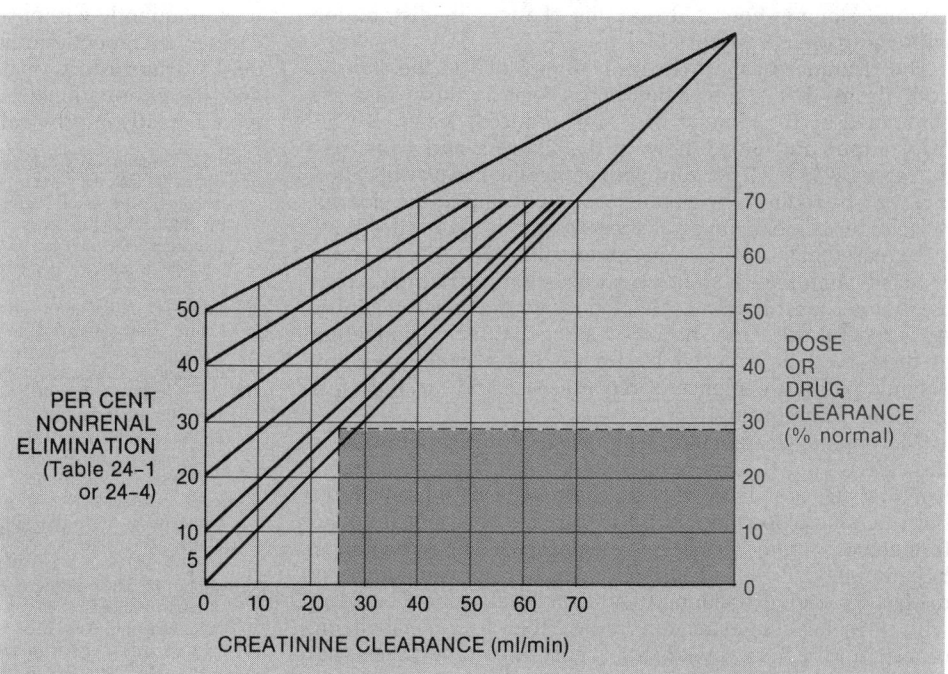

FIGURE 24–6. Nomogram for calculation of drug doses in patients with renal disease. The dose of any drug in a patient with renal disease (as a per cent of normal) is determined by connecting a line from the measured or calculated creatinine clearance to the black line that corresponds to the per cent nonrenal elimination for the drug of interest (from Table 24–1 or 24–4). The point of intersection is then extended to the red axis, where the dose per unit time is read directly. The dotted line indicates that in a patient with a creatinine clearance of 25 ml per minute the dose of amikacin, which normally has 5 per cent nonrenal elimination, must be reduced to approximately 30 per cent of normal.

(Figure labels: PER CENT NONRENAL ELIMINATION (Table 24–1 or 24–4); DOSE OR DRUG CLEARANCE (% normal); CREATININE CLEARANCE (ml/min))

but the portacaval shunting can allow drug absorbed by the gut to pass directly into the systemic circulation and bypass the liver, thereby avoiding the "first pass" or "presystemic" elimination. For those drugs that are largely extracted from the blood by the liver (e.g., propranolol, metoprolol, lidocaine), portacaval shunting will allow a much greater fraction of an orally administered dose to reach the systemic circulation.

Hemodynamic Disorders. Pharmacokinetics can be affected in several ways by disorders of the circulation. Hypotension and poor cardiac output reduce renal blood flow, glomerular filtration rate, and hepatic blood flow. As with primary renal disease, the impairment in renal drug excretion may be estimated by the change in creatinine clearance and dosage adjustments made accordingly. The effects of reduced hepatic blood flow on drug metabolism are highly dependent on the drug. For drugs that are essentially completely cleared from the blood on a single passage through the liver, i.e., when the extraction from blood is close to 100 per cent, a reduction in liver blood flow will reduce hepatic drug clearance proportionately. On the other hand, many drugs that are metabolized are extracted poorly by the liver, and for these drugs a reduction in liver blood flow has relatively little influence on their hepatic clearance. A complicating factor is that circulatory abnormalities also can result in hepatic congestion or tissue hypoxia that can impair hepatocellular function, so that drug metabolism may be reduced during hypotensive states independent of the effects of blood flow on drug delivery to the liver. Therefore, it is difficult to predict the proper dosage of hepatic metabolized drugs in individual patients with circulatory abnormalities. Certainly a drug such as lidocaine that has a very high hepatic clearance will be cleared less well in congestive heart failure or shock, and the maintenance infusion rates must be reduced by about half in these situations to avoid toxicity.

The distribution of some drugs is also affected by hemodynamic changes. For several drugs with large distribution volumes (lidocaine, quinidine, and procainamide), the apparent volume of distribution is decreased in heart failure and shock, and loading doses should also be reduced to avoid toxic plasma concentrations. However, for theophylline, a drug with a relatively small volume of distribution, the apparent volume of distribution is not changed by heart failure. Since data are not available for most drugs, we advise a conservative approach to loading and maintenance doses of toxic drugs in the setting of congestive heart failure or shock, with careful monitoring of the clinical status and plasma levels to guide further dosage adjustments.

USE OF DRUGS IN THE ELDERLY. Elderly persons (over 65 years) comprise 11 to 12 per cent of the United States population, but about 30 per cent of all prescriptions are written for this group of patients. In addition to prescription drugs, 70 per cent of elderly patients regularly use over-the-counter medications, primarily analgesics, compared with only 10 per cent of the general adult population. As an individual ages, changes occur that may affect drug kinetics and drug action. These age-related changes accentuate the normal interindividual variation in drug effects, thus making the elderly the most diverse segment of the adult population in terms of their drug responses. Because of the changes that occur with aging and the large numbers of drugs used in this population, the elderly are also highly susceptible to drug interactions.

The pharmacokinetic changes that may occur in the elderly are related to changes in body composition as well as to changes in function of pharmacokinetically important organs. The changes in gastrointestinal function that occur with aging are a decrease in gastric acid secretion, a decrease in mucosal absorptive surface of the small bowel by about 30 per cent, and a decrease in splanchnic blood flow by about 40 per cent. In spite of these changes, very few studies have shown much effect of aging on drug absorption. This is probably because most drugs are well absorbed and do not require very much of the small bowel for their absorption.

The distribution of drugs may change markedly with aging, probably because lean body mass and total body water decrease as the percentage of total body fat increases. In addition, the plasma concentration of albumin decreases, probably as a result of decreased albumin production by the liver, and this may affect those drugs that are bound to plasma albumin. Alpha$_1$-acid glycoprotein, the major plasma protein that binds basic drugs, is not diminished with aging. Because of the changes in body composition, water-soluble drugs that are not bound to plasma proteins may have a reduced apparent volume of distribution. However, for lipid-soluble drugs, such as many psychotropic agents, the volume of distribution relative to body weight may be increased, probably because of the increased percentage of body weight as fat. For water-soluble, albumin-bound drugs, the changes in distribution with aging are not predictable.

The clearance of many drugs is diminished in the elderly. Both drugs that are metabolized as well as those that are eliminated by the kidneys may have reduced clearance. Cardiac output and blood flow to the kidneys and liver may decrease by 30 to 40 per cent with aging. Glomerular filtration rate may be reduced by as much as 50 per cent in the elderly. Since older persons have a decreased muscle mass, they have a decreased rate of creatinine production. For this reason a reduced creatinine clearance can coexist with a normal serum creatinine concentration as defined for young, healthy adults. As a general rule, one should consider that renal elimination of drugs will be reduced by up to 50 per cent in elderly patients without evidence of renal disease and make dosage adjustments accordingly.

The hepatic clearance of drugs may also be diminished in the elderly, but the interindividual variability in the metabolism of drugs is so large as to preclude any useful predictions. Both hepatic blood flow and the intrinsic ability of the liver to metabolize some drugs may be reduced. The reduction in hepatic blood flow will influence the hepatic elimination of drugs with high extraction ratios, such as lidocaine. For drugs with low hepatic extraction ratios, the drug-metabolizing capacity of the liver appears to be most important. Drugs that are metabolized by the hepatic mixed function oxidase system are more likely to be affected by aging than those drugs that are metabolized by conjugation reactions.

Elimination half-life of many drugs is increased with aging. This is a combination of the effect of changes in the apparent volume of distribution and of changes in metabolic or renal clearance. Frequently, elimination half-life can be prolonged even without changes in drug clearance. This is true with diazepam, which has an increased apparent volume of distribution with no change in metabolic clearance, and this combination of changes produces a prolonged elimination half-life.

The age-related changes that occur with target-organ responsiveness are as important as the changes in pharmacokinetics. There is an increased sensitivity to a variety of drugs. The antianxiety agents and sedative hypnotic agents produce greater degrees of depression of central nervous system function in the elderly than in the young even at the same plasma levels. The hypotensive side effects of many psychotropic drugs are greater in the elderly because of reduced functioning of baroreceptor reflexes. Hemorrhage with anticoagulants is more common in the elderly even with good control of the clotting parameters. These changes in pharmacodynamics require the use of smaller doses of drugs in the elderly, even if the kinetics of the drug are not altered.

The following general principles derive from studies of drugs in the elderly: (1) Drugs that are eliminated by the kidneys will very likely have a reduced clearance, and the doses required to achieve the same blood concentration may be 50 per cent of those required in a young population. (2) Drugs that are eliminated by the liver may be less affected, but for parenterally given drugs such as lidocaine that have high hepatic clearances, the reduction in liver blood flow would be expected to decrease the clearance of the drug. In addition, some individuals may have a reduction in hepatic drug metabolism, and enzyme induction may not occur as readily in the elderly. (3) The sensitivity of target organs to drugs is increased for central nervous system depressants and probably for other drugs as well. Thus, the elderly constitute a population in whom drug use is likely to be marred by enhanced toxicity, and physician awareness of the possibility of altered drug disposition or effects is mandatory. It is a population in which drugs should be used in the lowest effective doses and only in individuals in whom they are absolutely necessary. That this is not commonly done is indicated by the numbers of drugs taken by elderly individ-

uals, frequently without well-defined endpoints or even well-defined therapeutic indications. Frequent reviews of the patient's drug history, including over-the-counter medications, and discontinuation of those drugs that are not necessary would greatly improve medical care for the elderly population.

Benet LZ, Sheiner LB: Design and optimization of dosage regimens: Pharmacokinetic data. In Gilman AG, Goodman LS, Gilman A (eds.): The Pharmacological Basis of Therapeutics. Edition 7. New York, Macmillan, 1985, pp 1663–1733. *This series of tables lists the pharmacokinetic parameters of over 150 drugs with references to the literature. This represents the most concise and complete listing currently available and is the source for some of the data in Table 24–4.*

Bjornsson TD: Nomogram for drug dosage adjustment in patients with renal failure. Clin Pharmacokin 11:164, 1986. *This review of drug elimination in renal disease uses an approach to dosage adjustment similar to the nomogram in this chapter. There is an extensive compilation of over 130 drugs that can be used as a reference for those drugs not in Table 24–1 or Table 24–4.*

Chennavasin P, Brater DC: Nomograms for drug use in renal disease. Clin Pharmacokin 6:193, 1981. *This is a critical review of a variety of published nomograms for determination of creatinine clearance from serum creatinine and for drug dosing in patients with renal disease.*

Gerber JG: Drug usage in the elderly. In Schrier RW (ed.): Clinical Internal Medicine in the Aged. Philadelphia, W.B. Saunders Company, 1982, pp 51–65. *This chapter is an excellent summary of pharmacokinetic principles applied to the elderly patient. The 49 references serve as an entry to the recent literature.*

Reidenberg M: The binding of drugs to plasma proteins and the interpretation of measurements of plasma concentrations of drugs in patients with poor renal function. Am J Med 62:466, 1977. *This review discusses the problems that arise when drug binding to plasma protein is altered by renal disease.*

Wilkinson GR, Shand DG: A physiological approach to hepatic drug clearance. Clin Pharmacol Ther 18:377, 1975. *This article discusses hepatic drug clearance in relation to blood flow, enzyme activity, and plasma protein binding. The concepts are valuable for physiologically oriented individuals.*

25 INTERACTIONS BETWEEN DRUGS

Alan S. Nies

Good medical practice frequently demands treatment with multiple drugs for a single disease in an attempt to maximize therapeutic effects and minimize side effects. When one is treating multiple diseases, the number of coadministered drugs increases, as does the possibility of undesirable interactions occurring between the drugs. Entire textbooks have been written in an attempt to list all of the possible drug interactions. It is obviously impossible for a clinician to remember such lists, and frequently the *clinically important* drug interactions are lost in the midst of large listings of interactions that are based on undocumented case reports, animal experimentation, or theory.

Not all drug interactions that occur are clinically important or even clinically recognized. The reasons for this include the fact that (1) many drugs have such large therapeutic indices that toxicity does not result when there are moderate increases in drug concentration, and thus changes in concentration due to a drug interaction may not be perceived; (2) the disease being treated may not be serious so that a change of drug concentration to less than therapeutic levels may not be easily recognized; (3) many drugs are given without well-defined therapeutic endpoints, making the drug effect difficult to assess, and therefore changes in drug effect will not be recognized; (4) there is a large intersubject variability due to genetic, environmental, and disease factors that may obscure many drug interactions. These comments are not to imply that drug interactions are not important. Drug interactions will be important if the drug has easily recognizable toxicity and a low therapeutic index such that small increases in amount of drug in the body produce significant toxicity. Second, drug interactions will be recognized and important if the diseases that are being controlled with the drug are serious or potentially fatal when undertreated. Third, drug interactions will be recognized if the therapeutic endpoints for the drug are clearly defined or if drug levels are used to maximize therapy for a given drug. Thus major interactions have been reported with anticoagulants and oral hypoglycemics, both of which have easily recognizable toxicity with low therapeutic indices. Drug interactions are reported with antiseizure medication and antiarrhythmic drugs; not only do these drugs have recognized toxicity, but also the diseases being treated become clinically manifest if the amount of drug is inadequate. Drug interactions have also been recognized with cardiac glycosides when blood levels are used to maximize efficacy in some patients.

Clinically important drug interactions are related to either (1) changes in the amount of drug or active metabolite available at the site of action, the so-called pharmacokinetic drug interactions, or (2) changes in drug effect without a change in pharmacokinetics, the pharmacodynamic drug interactions. These latter interactions may result from interactions at a receptor site, from independent actions of two drugs either adding to or counteracting the effects of each other, or from one drug altering the cellular milieu, thus changing the effects of another drug.

PHARMACOKINETIC DRUG INTERACTIONS

These interactions involve the processes of absorption, distribution, renal elimination, and metabolism such that there is a change in the amount of a drug (or an active metabolite) at the site of action. These are the best understood and generally most important drug interactions in clinical medicine. They can be subdivided into those that result in a decreased amount of drug at the site of action and hence a decrease in effect and those that have an increased amount of drug at the site of action and hence an increased effect.

Interactions Resulting in Less Drug Available at the Site of Action

DECREASED ABSORPTION. Since drug absorption generally occurs across the gastrointestinal mucosa by passive diffusion, one drug would not be expected to compete with another for absorption. However, drugs may physically interact in the lumen of the gastrointestinal tract so as to cause decreased absorption. Cholestyramine and colestipol, resins used to bind bile acids and to lower serum cholesterol, can also bind a number of drugs if they are simultaneously present in the gastrointestinal lumen. Thus cholestyramine can diminish the absorption of thyroxin, cardiac glycosides, warfarin, and corticosteroids. It is highly likely that other drugs will also bind to the steroid-binding resins, so that one is advised to view concurrent therapy of these resins with other drugs with caution.

Tetracyclines are potent chelating agents that form insoluble complexes with metal ions such as magnesium, calcium, and aluminum, commonly found in antacids, as well as with iron, with the result that the absorption of tetracycline is reduced. Sucralfate used for peptic ulcer disease has been reported to reduce the absorption of warfarin. Kaolin used to halt diarrhea will effectively inhibit the absorption of some drugs such as lincomycin and digoxin. In addition, drug products may contain "inert" substances that can interact with other drugs. For instance, para-aminosalicylic acid (PAS) contains bentonite (a kaolin-like substance), which can hamper the absorption of coadministered rifampin.

If a drug is susceptible to degradation at acid pH, anything that delays emptying of the stomach, such as a drug with anticholinergic properties, can result in more degradation of the coadministered acid-sensitive drug, e.g., penicillin G or L-dopa, and thus a decrease in the amount of drug absorbed. Conversely, a drug that speeds gastric emptying, such as metoclopramide, can increase the absorption of acid-unstable drugs. With most other drugs only the time course of absorp-

tion is changed so that drug absorption is faster if gastric emptying is enhanced or is slower if gastric emptying is delayed, but the total amount of drug absorbed is unchanged. Whether a change in rate of absorption results in any important clinical effects depends on whether rapid absorption is necessary for drug effect, in which case drug effect will be diminished. Usually, if total absorption is unchanged, then there will not be an important interaction, particularly during chronic administration of drugs.

The pH of the gastrointestinal fluid has little predictable effect on drug absorption. Almost all drugs are absorbed to the greatest extent in the small intestine rather than in the stomach. The classic teaching that acidic drugs, such as aspirin, are best absorbed in the stomach at acid pH because less drug is ionized is untrue. Actually, aspirin is more rapidly absorbed from an alkaline medium, since dissolution is enhanced.

ALTERED DISTRIBUTION. Some drugs reach their site of action via active transport. In this case, drugs can compete with each other for the transport mechanism, and thus one drug can impair the ability of another to reach its site of action. In order to produce blockade of adrenergic activity, the antihypertensive drugs guanethidine, guanadrel, and bethanidine must be actively transported by an amine transport system into adrenergic neurons. This transport system can be interfered with by tricyclic antidepressants, high doses of phenothiazines, and some sympathomimetic amines. Thus coadministration of guanethidine with one of these other compounds will effectively block the antihypertensive effects of guanethidine. This is an undesirable interaction with guanethidine; however, with the antiarrhythmic drug bretylium, sympathetic blockade produces orthostatic hypotension as an unwanted side effect. Bretylium also gains access to adrenergic neurons via the same amine transport system used by guanethidine. Therapeutic advantage can be taken of a drug interaction that blocks access of bretylium to its antiadrenergic site of action. Thus tricyclic antidepressants or ephedrine will reverse bretylium's sympathetic blocking effects but will not affect the direct antiarrhythmic effects of bretylium.

ENHANCED METABOLISM. Several drugs can increase the ability of the liver to metabolize other drugs. Phenobarbital, other barbiturates, phenytoin, rifampin, glutethimide, griseofulvin, ethanol, phenylbutazone, chronic smoking, certain chlorinated hydrocarbons such as lindane and DDT, carbamazepine, and primidone have all been associated with induction of hepatic microsomal, drug-metabolizing enzymes. The amount of enzyme induction that occurs appears to be under genetic control and so not all individuals experience quantitatively similar effects when taking an inducing agent.

Induction of hepatic metabolizing enzymes can affect many drugs. The effects are greatest when the drugs are given orally, because all of the drug must perforce pass through the liver prior to reaching the systemic circulation. Therefore, even for drugs that have a systemic clearance that is largely dependent upon hepatic blood flow, the amount of drug that escapes metabolism on the first pass will be influenced by enzyme-inducing drugs. Some examples of drugs that can have their metabolism induced are oral anticoagulants, quinidine, digitoxin, corticosteroids, low-dose contraceptives, some beta-adrenergic blockers, mexiletine, and theophylline. The induction of corticosteroid metabolism has produced some interesting effects, including (1) inappropriate interpretation of low-dose dexamethasone suppression tests in which the enhanced metabolism of dexamethasone produced by enzyme induction resulted in too low a dexamethasone concentration to inhibit normal steroidogenesis; (2) exacerbation of steroid-dependent asthma; and (3) rejection of a renal transplant by individuals who required steroids and received an enzyme-inducing agent.

Frequently the most critical time comes when the inducing agent is discontinued. At this time the drug-metabolizing activity gradually decreases, and drug toxicity can occur if dosage adjustments are not made of other coadministered drugs. This phenomenon has been described most frequently with induction of warfarin metabolism and resultant warfarin toxicity when the inducing agent is discontinued.

Interactions Resulting in More Drug Available at the Site of Action

ENHANCED ABSORPTION. In general, absorption is not a common process in which drugs can interact to enhance efficacy. One exception is with acid-unstable drugs and enhanced gastric emptying mentioned above. Another potential interaction is with relatively poorly absorbed drugs, such as digoxin, with which absorption occurs throughout the gastrointestinal tract. With such a drug a decrease in intestinal motility could enhance the degree of absorption by prolonging contact with the absorbing mucosa.

ALTERED DISTRIBUTION. Many drugs are bound to plasma proteins, and drug so bound is not available for action at receptors or for distribution throughout the body. In addition, for many compounds only the free drug is available for metabolism or excretion. The drug bound to plasma protein, therefore, acts as an inactive reservoir of drug in the blood. Since drugs can compete with each other for binding to plasma proteins, a potential for interactions exists. Pure plasma protein–binding interactions, however, rarely are clinically significant. The one probable exception to this is the displacement of albumin-bound bilirubin by sulfonamides or salicylates, thus allowing the bilirubin to distribute into the tissues and cause kernicterus in jaundiced infants. With drug/drug interactions, however, when a drug is displaced from plasma protein binding, it will very rapidly distribute into the apparent volume of distribution so that the increase in free drug concentration in the plasma is always considerably less than suggested by experiments in vitro. The larger the apparent volume of distribution, the less of an impact a displacement from protein binding will have. Following the immediate displacement and redistribution of the drug, the free fraction generally is readily available for metabolism or excretion, and the clearance processes in the body will reduce the free drug concentration to that which existed prior to the protein binding interaction (Fig. 25–1). Therefore the effect of such an interaction will be small, transient, and frequently not recognized clinically. The relationship of free drug to total drug, however, will be changed by such drug interactions, and therefore the interpretation of plasma drug assays that measure total drug in blood may have to be altered (see Ch. 24). Some drugs will interact with other drugs by more than one mechanism, and so interactions at protein-binding sites can coexist with interactions at a metabolic site. These dual drug interactions can be clinically important. However, it is not the displacement from protein binding that makes these interactions clinically important but rather the alteration of metabolism that does so. These dual drug interactions include interactions of phenylbutazone and sulfinpyrazone with warfarin and sulfaphenazole with tolbutamide.

Displacement of drugs from tissue-binding sites has only recently been recognized as a situation for drug interactions. Such an interaction would decrease the apparent volume of distribution of the drug and increase the plasma drug concentration. However, if the dose, plasma drug binding, and drug clearance are not altered, the plasma levels will be only transiently elevated, since steady-state plasma concentrations are independent of the apparent volume of distribution. Thus an interaction resulting in only a displacement from tissue stores would not be easily detected. However, as with displacement interactions from plasma protein, drugs can interact at multiple sites. Thus quinidine will displace digoxin from tissue-binding sites, but the persistent elevation in digoxin plasma concentration that results from the interaction is due to quinidine's ability to reduce the clearance of digoxin.

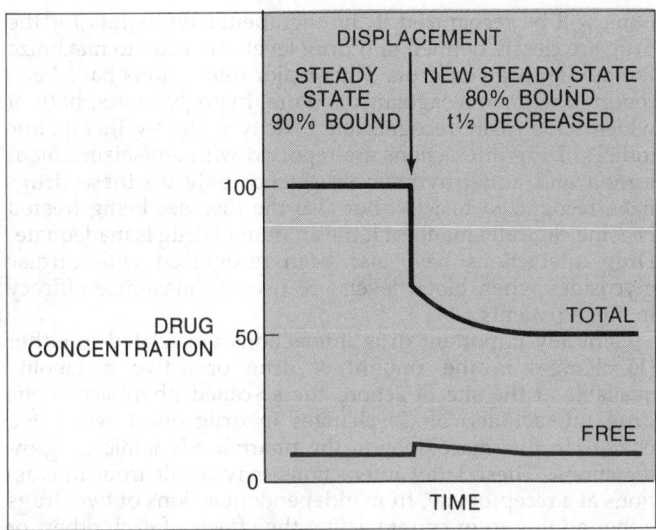

FIGURE 25–1. The effects of altered plasma drug binding on total and free plasma concentrations of the drug. The drug is assumed to be bound 90 per cent to albumin, not bound to tissues, and to have a V_D of 8.5 L. At the arrow an agent is given that displaces the drug from albumin such that binding is reduced to 80 per cent. The expected changes are an immediate increase in free drug concentration by only 40 per cent, with a fall of total concentration to 70 per cent of the initial value. Since the free drug clearance is not altered by this interaction, a new steady state will be achieved with the same free drug concentration and a reduction of total concentration to 50 per cent. For drugs with larger volumes of distribution, i.e., more tissue binding, the immediate increase of free concentration will be even less than in this example, but the ultimate steady-state condition of unchanged free drug concentration and a halving of the concentration of total drug will be the same. (Adapted from Shand et al.: In Handbook of Experimental Pharmacology. Vol 28, No 3, pp 272–314, 1975.)

DECREASED METABOLISM. Inhibition of drug metabolism can have a profound effect on drug disposition, resulting in drug toxicity. Inhibition of the metabolism of one drug by another occurs rapidly, and the enhanced effect or toxicity therefore often occurs shortly after the interaction takes place. Some drugs seem to be rather specific for inhibiting the metabolism of other individual drugs. However, there are a few drugs that can inhibit the metabolism of many drugs. The most commonly used such drug is cimetidine, which can inhibit the metabolism of theophylline, warfarin, diazepam, phenytoin, lidocaine, chlordiazepoxide, propranolol, carbamazepine, digitoxin, imipramine, quinidine, and probably others. The recently approved antiarrhythmic drug amiodarone also appears to be a potent inhibitor of the metabolism of many other drugs, including warfarin, phenytoin, and quinidine. Other important interactions resulting from decreased metabolism are listed in Table 25–1. As with other interactions resulting in an increased amount of drug at the sites of action, the most important examples are drugs that have a low therapeutic index and easily recognized, serious toxicity. The interaction of phenylbutazone or sulfinpyrazone and warfarin is a good example of an important interaction with a complex mechanism. Warfarin exists as R and S stereoisomers, with the S isomer being five times more potent an anticoagulant than the R isomer. Since phenylbutazone and sulfinpyrazone displace warfarin from plasma albumin, the normal occurrence would be for warfarin clearance to be increased by the interaction as more free drug becomes available for metabolism. In fact, this is true for R warfarin, but the metabolism of the more potent S warfarin is inhibited so that unbound S warfarin accumulates, although the total warfarin levels are unchanged or even decreased. It is the increased concentration of unbound S warfarin that results in enhanced anticoagulation.

TABLE 25–1. INHIBITION OF DRUG METABOLISM

Metabolism of	Inhibited by
Phenytoin	Isoniazid (in slow acetylators), chloramphenicol, cimetidine, clofibrate, phenylbutazone, disulfiram, sulfaphenazole, dicoumarol, amiodarone
Tolbutamide	Chloramphenicol, phenylbutazone, clofibrate, sulfaphenazole, dicoumarol
Warfarin	Phenylbutazone, alcohol, disulfiram, allopurinol, cimetidine, disopyramide, sulfinpyrazone, trimethoprim-sulfamethoxazole, metronidazole, amiodarone
Azathioprine, 6-mercaptopurine	Allopurinol
Catecholamines, tyramine	Monoamine oxidase inhibitors
Theophylline	Cimetidine, erythromycin, troleandomycin
Phenobarbital	Valproic acid

In addition to inhibition of hepatic drug metabolism via mixed function oxidase, inhibition of metabolism at other enzyme sites can be important. Thus monoamine oxidase inhibitors can inhibit the metabolism of catecholamines and tyramine at multiple sites, allowing for build-up of these substances and the so-called "cheese reaction" due to enhanced catecholamine release with the ingestion of tyramine-containing foods. Allopurinol inhibits xanthine oxidase, which can be important for the metabolism of azathioprine and 6-mercaptopurine as well as for production of uric acid. If allopurinol is given, much less azathioprine or 6-mercaptopurine is needed for equivalent effects. As discussed above, ethanol can induce hepatic microsomal drug-metabolizing enzymes. However, if ethanol is present, it can also act as an inhibitor of drug metabolism. Thus drugs given to an individual who is intoxicated may have an enhanced effect, whereas drugs given to an individual who has been drinking chronically but is no longer intoxicated may have diminished effect.

DIMINISHED RENAL EXCRETION. Some important drug interactions occur when active transport of one drug across the renal tubule is interfered with by another drug. Most of the reported interactions occur at the acid transport site. Thus probenecid is given to decrease penicillin clearance and thereby increase penicillin blood levels. Phenylbutazone can inhibit the renal clearance of hydroxyhexamide, an active metabolite of acetohexamide, and thereby increase its hypoglycemic effect. Salicylates, phenylbutazone, and probenecid can inhibit the renal elimination of methotrexate and enhance its effect. Drugs can also interact at the renal tubular site for active transport of bases, which is the probable mechanism whereby cimetidine and amiodarone reduce the renal clearance of procainamide.

Quinidine can inhibit the elimination of digoxin into the urine. The exact tubular site at which this interaction occurs is not known, but it is a significant interaction resulting in increased digoxin blood levels and effects. Verapamil and amiodarone also interact with digoxin by inhibiting renal excretion.

Decreased renal excretion of lithium occurs when proximal tubular reabsorption is enhanced. Since lithium and sodium are handled similarly in the proximal tubule, anything that results in more proximal tubular sodium reabsorption will also affect lithium in the same way. Thus dietary salt restriction, salt depletion due to diarrhea, and diuretics acting at more distal segments of the nephron can reduce renal lithium excretion, requiring a reduction in lithium dose. Indomethacin also reduces lithium clearance, probably by enhancing proximal tubular reabsorption of the ion.

PHARMACODYNAMIC DRUG INTERACTIONS

There are numerous examples of drugs interacting with each other at receptor sites or having additive effects by acting at separate sites on cells. Thus vitamin K can inhibit the effects of warfarin. Propranolol can interact with epinephrine by blocking the beta-adrenergic receptors and thus allowing the alpha-adrenergic effects of epinephrine to be unopposed, which can result in severe hypertension. Clonidine has been shown to have its antihypertensive effects in humans inhibited by tricyclic antidepressants. The mechanism for this is not entirely worked out but might be an interaction at an alpha-adrenergic receptor in the brain.

Examples of drugs producing additive effects are also common, such as the negative cardiac inotropic effects of disopyramide adding to the negative inotropic effects of beta-adrenergic blockers, producing heart failure. Two drugs that may affect the eighth cranial nerve, such as ethacrynic acid and aminoglycosides, may produce additional ototoxicity if given together. Drugs that affect neuromuscular function such as curare will have an enhanced effect if given with aminoglycosides, lincomycin, clindamycin, quinidine, or quinine, which also affect neuromuscular function.

One drug may alter the normal homeostatic mechanisms, resulting in a change in the internal milieu and thereby enhancing or diminishing the effect of another drug. The best-studied example of this type of interaction is the effect of diuretics to produce hypokalemia, which enhances the toxicity of cardiac glycosides.

Some drug interactions have not been well characterized, although the interaction is clearly significant. This is true for the interaction of warfarin with clofibrate. Clofibrate has a marked effect to increase the efficacy of warfarin, but there do not appear to be sufficient pharmacokinetic changes to account for this effect even though clofibrate may displace warfarin from plasma protein.

When viewed in perspective, drug interactions are only one of many factors that can alter the response of patients to drugs. Clinicians must be aware of the serious interactions and have well-defined therapeutic goals so that altered amounts or effects of drugs will become evident. The only way to accomplish this is to individualize therapy using effects or plasma drug levels when appropriate. This is particularly important for drugs with low therapeutic indices or during treatment of serious illnesses. Care must be used when a drug regimen is changed in any major way. If an interaction is appreciated, dosage adjustments can be made, and the two drugs often can be used together effectively. Drug interactions are an accepted fact of modern medical practice and should not be ignored, nor should they be overly feared.

Gerber MJ, Tejwani GA, Gerber N, et al.: Drug interactions with cimetidine: An update. Pharmacol Ther 27:353, 1985. *Cimetidine is the most commonly used drug that inhibits the metabolism and/or renal excretion of other drugs. This article reviews the increasing number of drug interactions reported with cimetidine.*

Hansten PD: Drug Interactions. 5th ed. Philadelphia, Lea and Febiger, 1985. *This frequently revised text is a useful compilation of known drug interactions. The interactions listed are referenced, and a estimate of probable clinical significance of the interaction is given.*

McElnay JC, D'Arcy PF: Protein binding displacement interactions and their clinical importance. Drugs 25:495, 1983. *This is a current review that emphasizes the fact that pure binding displacement interactions are unlikely to be of clinical significance.*

Serlin MJ, Breckenridge AM: Drug interactions with warfarin. Drugs 25:610, 1983. *Warfarin is a good model drug to study drug interactions, since its effects are easily measured, and hemorrhage is a readily detectable adverse effect. The several mechanisms of drug interactions affecting warfarin are reviewed with the relevant literature cited.*

Shand DG, Mitchell JR, Oates JA: Pharmacokinetic drug interactions. In Gillette JR, Mitchell JR (eds.): Handbook of Experimental Pharmacology, Vol 28, No 3. Concepts in Biochemical Pharmacology. New York, Springer-Verlag, 1975, pp 272–314. *This is a thorough review of pharmacokinetic mechanisms whereby drugs can interact. It is not a complete listing of potential drug interactions, although many illustrative examples for the various mechanisms are given.*

26 ADVERSE REACTIONS TO DRUGS

Alan S. Nies

Although difficult to quantify, there is little doubt that adverse reactions to drugs constitute an inevitable consequence of modern therapeutics. No drug is devoid of the potential to do harm, and benefit versus risk decisions are made with every decision to start drug therapy. Most ill patients require multiple drugs, and this increases the risk not only of adverse drug reactions but of drug interactions as well. Frequently it is difficult to be certain that an adverse effect is due to an individual drug because of the confounding effects of the underlying disease and the use of multiple drugs.

Studies to determine the incidence of adverse reactions are derived largely from medical services at academic hospitals. The Boston Collaborative Drug Surveillance Program found a 5 per cent incidence of adverse drug reactions, most of which were minor and self limited. Other studies have estimated a higher incidence, particularly in very ill or elderly patients. In a recent study of complications on a medical ward, adverse drug effects were the largest contributor to iatrogenic events, accounting for 42 per cent of all such occurrences. About 18 per cent of patients admitted to the hospital had an adverse drug effect, and 19 per cent of these were life threatening or resulted in serious disability. Drugs implicated in such studies include digitalis, theophylline, nitrates, lidocaine, and other antiarrhythmics, anticoagulants, benzodiazepines, antihypertensives, and antibiotics.

The recent studies do not indicate that the incidence of adverse drug reactions is decreasing. On the contrary, the risk may be increasing as the number of potent drugs available increases. The studies assessing the incidence of drug problems in an academic medical center cannot be generalized to other therapeutic situations such as outpatient clinics, office practices, or community hospitals. Since one of the major determinants of a drug reaction is how ill the patient is and how many drugs he is receiving, it is likely that adverse drug reactions occur much less commonly in situations outside the large general hospital. Also, it is impossible with present data to make a quantitative statement of risk versus benefit of medical therapy. It is clear that adverse reactions cannot be completely prevented even under the best of circumstances. Nonetheless, it is reasonable to continue investigation into ways to assess the risk and to reduce both the incidence and severity of these adverse reactions.

MECHANISMS OF ADVERSE DRUG REACTIONS

Unwanted effects of drugs are due to (1) exaggerated responses to the known desired or unwanted pharmacologic effects of the drug; (2) immunologic reactions to the drug or its metabolites; and (3) toxic effects of a drug or its metabolite. "Idiosyncratic" effects may be due to any of these mechanisms. The extension of the normal pharmacology accounts for most adverse drug effects. However, since these effects are predictable, they often may be avoided or treated by careful dosage adjustment without necessarily discontinuing drug treatment. The immunologically mediated and toxic adverse effects of drugs are less predictable and may be so severe as to require discontinuation of the offending drug. These latter effects are the least well understood, but mechanisms of some of the toxic drug effects have been discovered. Many reactions initially labeled immunologic may be due to other mechanisms. With time the mechanisms of the "idiosyncratic" drug reactions will be determined so that such

reactions may be anticipated or avoided. All organ systems can be affected by drugs, and drug-induced disease should be a consideration in the differential diagnosis of most syndromes that present to an internist.

EXAGGERATED RESPONSES TO DRUGS

Excessive drug effects result from altered pharmacokinetics or altered target-organ response, as discussed in the previous chapters. Thus adverse drug effects are more common in the elderly, in patients with abnormal renal or hepatic function, and in patients receiving other drugs that may result in pharmacokinetic or pharmacodynamic interactions.

An example of a disease exaggerating the unwanted effects of a normally innocuous drug is the reduction in glomerular filtration rate produced by nonsteroidal anti-inflammatory drugs in patients who have activation of their sympathetic nervous system and/or increased plasma renin activity as a result of hepatic, renal, or cardiovascular disease. This adverse effect is a consequence of the same pharmacologic action responsible for the salutary effects of the drug, namely, inhibition of cyclo-oxygenase activity with a reduction in prostaglandin synthesis.

In addition, patients may have genetic abnormalities that make them susceptible to one or another effects of a drug. These genetic differences may be quantitative deviations from the norm or qualitative abnormalities. An example of such quantitative differences is the variability in hepatic drug oxidation that is described by a unimodal frequency distribution. Twin studies have indicated that genetic differences account for much of the variation between individuals in the metabolism of phenytoin, phenylbutazone, warfarin, ethanol, nortriptyline, and salicylate. In addition, several drug metabolic processes are controlled by genes at a single locus, such as slow acetylation of isoniazid, some sulfonamides, and procainamide; deficient parahydroxylation of phenytoin; deficient hydroxylation of debrisoquin; deficient hydroxylation of mephenytoin; deficient N-glucosidation of amobarbital; and deficient hydrolysis of succinylcholine. The excessive drug effects resulting from the genetically determined slow metabolic processes reflect increased drug available at the site of action.

In addition to these quantitative differences in drug metabolism, there are genetic abnormalities that result in qualitatively different responses to drugs. These reactions are due to known properties of the drug that are usually not important but become markedly exaggerated owing to the genetic defect. Thus individuals with a deficiency of the enzyme activity of glucose-6-phosphate dehydrogenase (G6PD) are unable to cope with the oxidative stress produced by some drugs, and hemolysis results. Drugs having this effect include primaquine, aspirin, sulfonamides, nitrofurantoin, sulfones, vitamin K, probenecid, quinidine, and quinine. In a similar manner, genetic deficiency of methemoglobin reductase results in inability to maintain hemoglobin in the ferrous form, resulting in methemoglobinemia upon exposure to some oxidizing drugs such as sulfones, sulfonamides, and nitrites. Likewise certain abnormal hemoglobins may be unstable and result in drug-induced hemolysis or methemoglobinemia. Frequently patients with these "pharmacogenetic" syndromes are unaware that there is any abnormality until they are challenged with a drug that produces the adverse effect.

TOXIC AND IMMUNOLOGIC REACTIONS

Adverse drug reactions in these categories are often lumped together because it is frequently difficult to be certain of the etiology of an individual reaction (Table 26–1). Some reactions that previously were considered to be immunologic have been shown to be toxic.

Toxic reactions include direct effects of a drug on a target organ, such as the nephrotoxicity and ototoxicity produced

TABLE 26–1. "ALLERGIC" DRUG REACTIONS

Type of Reaction	Example (not inclusive)
Definite Immunologically Mediated Syndromes	
1. Immediate hypersensitivity (IgE-mediated) reactions	Penicillin-induced anaphylaxis Insulin-induced wheal and flare
2. Cytotoxic reactions	Drug-induced destruction of formed elements in the blood: Penicillin-induced hemolytic anemia Quinidine- or quinine-induced thrombocytopenia Phenylbutazone-induced granulocytopenia
3. Immune complex–induced vasculitis	Serum sickness–like reactions to penicillin, sulfonamides, and other drugs presenting as fever, rash, palpable purpura, arthralgia, and/or lymphadenopathy
4. Delayed hypersensitivity reactions	Contact dermatitis from topically applied drugs
Possible Immunologically Mediated Syndromes but with Unknown Mechanism	
1. Skin rashes of various types	Many drugs and a variety of skin eruptions
2. Stevens-Johnson syndrome	Sulfonamides, penicillins, phenytoin, phenylbutazone
3. Fever	Antibiotics, quinidine, methyldopa, allopurinol, procainamide
4. Pneumonitis	Loeffler's syndrome
5. Lupus erythematosus–like	Procainamide, hydralazine, isoniazid
6. Hepatic dysfunction	Chlorpromazine-induced cholestasis ? Methyldopa-induced hepatitis
7. Renal dysfunction	Interstitial nephritis from methicillin, furosemide, allopurinol
8. Lymphadenopathy	Phenytoin, sulfonamides

by aminoglycosides. In other cases drugs are metabolized to reactive intermediates that can covalently bind to cellular components, often near the site of metabolism, and produce toxicity. This mechanism is well established for the hepatotoxicity produced by overdoses of acetaminophen. During therapeutic use of acetaminophen the small amount of reactive metabolite formed by oxidative metabolism is rapidly detoxified by interacting with reduced glutathione. With overdose, however, the glutathione is depleted, and the reactive metabolite attacks hepatic macromolecules, resulting in liver damage. Other sulfhydryl-containing compounds such as *N*-acetylcysteine or cysteamine can protect the liver by reducing the amount of toxic metabolite that remains unreacted with a sulfhydryl-containing compound. Other drugs may produce liver disease by somewhat similar mechanisms. Isoniazid-induced hepatitis may result from acetylation to acetylisoniazid that can be hydrolyzed to acetylhydrazine, which can be oxidized to a reactive metabolite. One might expect from this theory that individuals who rapidly acetylate isoniazid would be more susceptible to the hepatotoxicity. However, recent data indicate that the opposite may be true. This apparent discrepancy may be related to observations that rapid acetylators not only form acetylisoniazid rapidly but also quickly convert this metabolite to diacetylisoniazid, which is nontoxic. Slow acetylators, on the other hand, form acetylisoniazid gradually but are much less able to convert it to diacetyliso-

niazid. Consequently, more of the acetylisoniazid is available for hydrolysis to acetylhydrazine and subsequent oxidation to the reactive metabolite. However, there remains considerable controversy regarding the relevance of this theory to the clinical hepatitis that results from isoniazid, and it is clear that other factors, such as the patient's age, are also important.

Hepatocellular damage, such as that produced by methyldopa or halothane, is frequently considered to be immunologically produced. However, it is entirely possible that reactive metabolites could be important for these as well as a variety of other drugs that produce hepatotoxicity on occasion.

Immunologic reactions to drugs account for 5 to 10 per cent of all adverse drug reactions and probably result from the drug or a reactive metabolite combining with a protein to form an antigenic drug-protein complex that stimulates the immune response. Without such a reaction, most drugs, which have a molecular weight less than 1000, would not be able to elicit an immunologic response. The typical immunologic reaction requires a latent period of 10 to 20 days for stimulation of the production of antibodies and activated immune effector cells that cause the allergic reaction. After the initial exposure, however, the allergic reaction will occur with a much shorter or no latent period after re-exposure to the drug. Drug hypersensitivity can produce mediator release, initiate cell lysis, activate the complement system, or activate cellular hypersensitivity reactions.

The most dramatic allergic reaction is anaphylaxis, or IgE-mediated hypersensitivity. Penicillin is the most common drug to produce anaphylaxis, but many other drugs or diagnostic agents (such as Bromsulphalein) can produce this life-threatening reaction. A history of penicillin allergy increases the risk of this reaction occurring, but most (75 per cent) of the 100 to 300 patients dying of penicillin-induced anaphylaxis each year have no history of penicillin allergy. Oral penicillin seems to have a lower incidence of reactions than parenteral penicillin.

Skin testing with penicilloyl polylysine, penicillin G, and penicilloic acid can identify patients at risk for anaphylaxis. Skin tests should be used if there is a history of penicillin allergy and penicillin therapy is considered mandatory. Some day it may be common to skin test all patients who are to receive penicillin, but this is not current practice.

Cytotoxic allergic reactions occur when the drug binds to the surface of a cell and is then attacked by antibody. Penicillin-induced hemolytic anemia is of this type. Immune complexes of drug and antibody may become adsorbed to the cell membrane, resulting in complement-mediated cytotoxicity. Thrombocytopenia and hemolytic anemia due to quinine or quinidine are examples of immune complex–mediated cytotoxicity. Methyldopa-induced Coombs' positivity that occurs in up to 20 per cent of patients on therapy for over six months is of unknown etiology but results in antibodies directed at the Rh loci of the red cell. However, the continued presence of the drug is not necessary for the immune reaction to continue, and the Coombs' positivity only gradually resolves upon discontinuation of the drug.

Circulating immune complexes of drug and antibody can produce serum sickness (see Ch. 420, 431), a vasculitic syndrome produced by deposition of immune complexes. Penicillin, sulfonamides, thiouracil, cholecystographic dyes, phenytoin, and other drugs can cause serum sickness.

Drug-induced lupus syndromes as caused by procainamide, hydralazine, and isoniazid may be associated with circulating immune complexes. In this case the drug or a reactive metabolite may interact with nuclear material to allow formation of antinuclear antibodies. The drug-induced systemic lupus erythematosus (SLE) (see Ch. 436) differs from spontaneous lupus by being uncommon in blacks and by only rarely causing nephritis. The acetylator phenotype also is important in drug-induced lupus. Hydralazine-induced lupus is very uncommon in fast acetylators. Procainamide-induced lupus occurs with smaller doses of drugs and at an earlier time after starting the drug in slow acetylators, although fast acetylators are also at risk.

In addition to the immune phenomena outlined above, many other syndromes are attributed to drug allergy. These include a variety of skin rashes, drug fever, pulmonary reactions, hepatocellular or cholestatic reactions, interstitial nephritis, and lymphadenopathy. For most of these reactions, the exact immune mechanism is unknown. One interesting syndrome that is sometimes classified as immune but may involve other mechanisms as well is that of aspirin sensitivity. In some patients this syndrome resembles IgE-mediated allergy with rhinitis, sinusitis, nasal polyps, and asthma. However, other cyclo-oxygenase inhibitors, such as indomethacin and meclofenamate, also produce asthma in many of these patients, suggesting a possible etiologic role for an arachidonic acid metabolite, such as a leukotriene, rather than an immunologic mechanism. It seems likely that several syndromes of aspirin sensitivity exist.

Some adverse drug reactions mimic anaphylactic reactions but are not immune mediated. Such reactions are due to direct release of mediators by drugs and are called anaphylactoid reactions. Reactions to radiocontrast dyes are of this type. The risk of re-exposure to the dye is unpredictable and skin testing is of no value. If re-exposure is absolutely necessary, pretreatment with steroids and antihistamines is the current practice.

RECOGNITION AND IDENTIFICATION

Adverse drug effects must first be suspected to be recognized. In some situations, the adverse effect mimics the illness being treated (for instance, arrhythmias caused by antiarrhythmic drugs or antibiotic-induced fever). In other instances, the reaction is more obviously drug induced, as is the case with characteristic skin rashes or anticoagulant-induced bleeding. The first confirmation of an adverse reaction is its disappearance with drug withdrawal. In some cases it may be warranted to readminister the putative offending drug cautiously if it is likely that the drug will be required again for therapy. In the case of serious allergic or toxic reactions, however, this may be too dangerous. Tests in vitro are occasionally helpful for drug-induced thrombocytopenia or hemolytic anemia but are not useful for most drug reactions. Skin testing is of value with penicillin, insulin, and horse serum.

Adverse reactions will continue to occur as long as potent drugs are available. Most of the reactions are predictable. The unexpected toxic and immunologic reactions remain a problem that continues to stimulate discussions as to how to detect rare adverse effects. During the process of drug development, reactions occurring less often than 1 per 1000 patients will not be detected. In addition, drugs are developed by testing in patients who have well-defined diseases, are not on many other drugs, are not pregnant, and are usually neither in the pediatric nor the geriatric populations. After approval, however, all patient populations may be exposed to the drug. Therefore, the adverse effects of a new drug frequently are not discovered until after marketing. Different systems exist for early detection of drug reactions after marketing. A major mechanism is an early warning that results from anecdotal reports by practicing physicians to pharmaceutical companies, drug regulatory agencies, or most commonly as letters published in general medical journals. Following the first alerts, a verification mechanism is required. It is in this area that much remains to be learned. Postmarketing surveillance of patients taking drugs will not be effective for uncommon drug reactions unless sample sizes of more than 100,000 patients are followed. Surveys of patients with certain diseases to determine the incidence of use of the drug suspected to have caused the illness (case-control study) may be a more efficient way to detect drug-induced illness for rare adverse effects.

However, the alert practitioner has been and will continue to be the primary individual who makes the initial important observation that often provides the first clue to an unsuspected adverse drug reaction.

Davies DM (ed.): Textbook of Adverse Drug Reactions. Oxford, Oxford University Press, 1977. *This well-referenced book is organized by specific syndromes, with a discussion of the drugs that may cause the syndrome. General problems of detecting and verifying adverse reactions are also discussed.*

Faich GA: Adverse-drug–reaction monitoring. N Engl J Med 314:1589, 1986. *This is a review of the adverse-reaction monitoring program at the FDA and indicates that spontaneous reporting of drug reactions by physicians is critical to providing early warnings of previously unsuspected drug risks.*

Jick H: Adverse drug reactions: The magnitude of the problem. J Allergy Clin Immunol 74:555, 1984. *This report from the Boston Collaborative Drug Surveillance Program is the leading article in a symposium on allergic drug reactions.*

Mitchell JR, Jollow DJ: Metabolic activation of drugs to toxic substances. Gastroenterology 68:392, 1975. *This is a review of adverse drug reactions that result from metabolism of drugs to reactive metabolites that covalently bind to tissue macromolecules.*

Patterson R, Anderson J: Allergic reactions to drugs and biologic agents. JAMA 248:2637, 1982. *Part of the "primer on allergic and immunologic diseases," this short review outlines the mechanisms of immunologic reactions to drugs. The authors provide relevant references and distinguish between allergic reactions for which the immune mechanisms are established and those that are only conjectured to be immunologically mediated.*

Steel K, Gertman PM, Crescenzi C, et al.: Iatrogenic illness on a general medical service at a university hospital. N Engl J Med 304:638, 1981. *This study of a medical service indicates an 18 per cent incidence of iatrogenic illness, of which 42 per cent were drug related.*

27 PAIN AND ITS MANAGEMENT
Kathleen M. Foley and Jerome B. Posner

INTRODUCTION

Pain is the most common symptom for which patients seek medical assistance. To manage pain, the physician must understand its nature—the relationship between its medical, psychologic, and social aspects—and must establish a relationship of mutual trust with the patient. The physician's therapeutic task is twofold: to discover and treat the cause of the pain and to treat the pain itself, whether or not the underlying cause is treatable. Advances in knowledge of the physiology, pharmacology, and psychology of pain perception have led to improved care of patients with both acute and chronic pain (see also Ch. 466), but a lack of generally agreed-upon definitions and classification of pain has hampered communication among physicians. To provide a more common ground for the evaluation and treatment of patients with pain, the International Association for the Study of Pain (IASP) has proposed a working definition: Pain is "an unpleasant sensory and emotional experience associated with either actual or potential tissue damage, or described in terms of such damage." The IASP has also developed a taxonomy of pain syndromes that serves as a universal classification of pain syndromes (see references).

TYPES OF PAIN

Clinically, pain can be classified *temporally* as acute or chronic, *physiologically* as somatic, visceral, or deafferentation, and *etiologically* as medical or psychogenic.

TEMPORAL CHARACTERISTICS. Patients with severe *acute pain* can usually give a clear description of its location, character, and timing. Furthermore, objective signs, particularly of autonomic nervous system hyperactivity, with tachycardia, hypertension, diaphoresis, mydriasis, and pallor are present. The pain is usually self-limited (e.g., postoperative pain, acute traumatic pain). The patient's ability to tolerate acute pain is influenced by the setting of the pain, its duration, and its psychologic significance. Treatment of both the cause of acute pain and the pain itself is usually possible. Pain lasting longer than three months' duration is usually considered *chronic*. In patients with chronic pain, the localization, character, and timing of the pain are often more vague, and because the autonomic nervous system adapts, signs of autonomic hyperactivity disappear. Significant changes occur in the psychologic, social, and functional status of patients with chronic pain, often requiring a multidisciplinary approach to treatment, including pharmacologic, behavioral, and rehabilitative therapeutic approaches.

PHYSIOLOGIC CHARACTERISTICS. *Somatic pain* results from activation of peripheral receptors and somatic efferent nerves, without injury to the peripheral nerves or central nervous system. The pain can be either sharp or dull but is typically well localized and intermittent. *Visceral pain* results from activation of visceral nociceptive receptors and visceral efferent nerves and is characterized as a deep aching, cramping sensation, often referred to cutaneous sites. *Deafferentation or causalgic pain* results from direct injury to peripheral receptors, nerves, or central nervous system. It is typically burning and dysesthetic and often occurs in an area of sensory loss (e.g., postherpetic neuralgia). The autonomic nervous system plays a significant modulatory role in all three types of pain but is most prominent in visceral and deafferentation pain. The somatic and visceral types of pain are readily managed with a wide variety of nonopioid or opioid analgesics, anesthetic blocks, and neurosurgical approaches. In contrast, deafferentation pain responds minimally to nonopioid and opioid analgesics and to anesthetic and neurosurgical procedures.

ETIOLOGIC CHARACTERISTICS. Patients with chronic pain can generally be classified into one of three major etiologic groups, allowing for some overlap. The first group includes patients with chronic pain associated with *structural disease*. Such pain occurs, for example, with rheumatoid arthritis, metastatic cancer, and sickle cell anemia and is usually characterized by prolonged episodes of pain alternating with pain-free intervals or by unremitting pain waxing and waning in severity. Successful treatment of the pain is closely allied with treatment of the disease, but in certain instances treatment of the pain is the only therapeutic goal, e.g., the dying cancer patient with pain. Psychologic factors may play an important role in exacerbating or relieving pain, but analgesic drug therapy is the mainstay of therapy while attempting to treat the underlying disease.

The second group comprises patients who suffer from *psychophysiologic disorders* causing pain. In these patients, structural disease such as a herniated disc or torn ligaments may once have been present but psychologic factors have caused chronic physiologic alterations, such as muscle spasm, which produce pain long after the underlying defect has healed. Typically, such patients are physically inactive and spend much of their time thinking and talking about their pain, often leading to social and emotional isolation. Patients are more impaired by their "chronic illness behavior" than by a defined pathologic condition. They usually respond poorly to analgesic drugs and often suffer from iatrogenic complications, such as adverse drug reactions and ineffective surgical procedures. They use health care resources excessively. Successful treatment can be expected only through a structured rehabilitation program designed to modify pain behaviors and not through medical intervention designed to correct pathologic conditions. Multidisciplinary pain clinics that diagnose and treat intractable pain exist in many centers and should be utilized to evaluate and treat such patients.

Patients of the third group complain of pain that appears to have neither a structural nor a physiologic basis. These patients probably suffer from *somatic delusions*. Such patients usually have serious psychiatric disorders, and the history of the pain is so vague and bizarre and its distribution so unanatomic as to suggest the diagnosis. These patients respond only to psychiatric therapy.

ASSESSMENT OF PAIN

No objective tests (except observing patient behavior) assess the severity of pain or even its presence. Therefore, the physician must accept the patient's report, taking into consideration his or her age, cultural background, environment, and psychologic circumstances known to alter reaction to pain.

A thorough history, general physical examination, and careful neurologic examination are imperative in any patient complaining of pain. The description of the nature and distribution of the pain may be so characteristic (e.g., trigeminal neuralgia or tabetic lightning pains) that it allows no other diagnosis. Inquiry should be made concerning (1) the temporal pattern of pain, (2) its distribution, (3) exacerbating factors, and (4) relieving factors. For example, headache beginning early in the morning before arising suggests increased intracranial pressure, whereas headache occurring late in the day is more suggestive of tension. Back pain and sciatica made worse by sitting or walking suggest disc disease, whereas back pain and sciatica that are worse while the person is in bed indicate intraspinal tumor. Back pain and sciatica exacerbated by cough or sneeze suggest intraspinal disease, whereas similar pain not exacerbated by cough or sneeze is indicative of disease in the pelvis. Pain in the back or legs exacerbated by straight-leg raising suggests disease of the nervous system, whereas a similar pain exacerbated by rotating the hips suggests pelvic or hip disease. All pain is relieved to some extent by distraction and a pleasurable environment and is exacerbated by anxiety or psychologic stress.

A careful psychiatric history, looking particularly for signs and symptoms of depression, should be elicited from all patients. The distinction between pain and suffering should be made by both the physician and the patient. Specifically, physicians should inquire about the degree to which pain has interfered with the patient's activities, whether he or she is having difficulty sleeping, and whether there is a change in appetite or bowel habits. Early morning awakening, anorexia, and constipation are somatic manifestations of depression and may either be caused by chronic pain or exacerbate the effects of the pain.

A general physical examination must be performed. Both the physical and the laboratory examination should begin with the assumption that the site of pathologic change is at the site of pain. The painful areas should be examined for swelling and redness as well as for any obvious deformity. (The pain of herpes zoster usually precedes the rash, and occasionally on examination one may note the faintest reddening of the skin in a dermatomal distribution.) The areas reported as painful should be palpated, the temperature estimated, and points of tenderness sought. (If the site of pain is in a soft tissue, bone, or joint, it should be tender to palpation as well as spontaneously painful.) Joints should be taken through a full range of motion, and the effect of movement on the pain assessed. Nerve trunks going to the extremities should be palpated and stretched by movement of that member (e.g., straight-leg raising: abduction and extension of the arm). Inflamed and compressed nerve roots and nerve plexuses are more painful when stretched. A careful neurologic examination must also be performed. If there are neurologic abnormalities (e.g., weakness, sensory loss, and reflex changes) in the painful part, one can infer that nervous system disease is responsible for the pain. However, the absence of neurologic abnormalities on first examination does not guarantee that the nervous system is free of disease, because the process may simply not have advanced beyond the stage of selectively involving pain pathways. For example, a Pancoast's tumor may cause shoulder and arm pain before other signs of neural involvement, such as Horner's syndrome or motor or sensory loss, appear.

Finally, laboratory examinations are performed. If the site

of disease appears to be in bones or joints, radiographs, computed tomography (CT) scans, or radioisotope scans may localize it. First attention should be paid to the local site of pain, but the physician should be familiar with the common referred patterns of pain (e.g., hip disease commonly causes knee pain, cardiac pain is frequently referred to the ulnar aspect of the arm and forearm, the pain of renal colic may be felt primarily in the groin and testicle, and pain resulting from disease of the throat may be referred to the ear).

Referred pain is pain perceived at a site remote from the source of the disturbance. Usually, referred pain is perceived as cutaneous and is evoked by disease of deep structures innervated by the same dermatome. Referred pain may be associated with cutaneous hyperalgesia and even relieved by procaine injection into the area of referral. When pain is referred to the same dermatome or myotome that innervates the diseased structure (e.g., pain down the medial aspect of the arm [T1-T2] produced by myocardial infarction or angina pectoris), it is often helpful in diagnosis. However, pain is sometimes referred a great distance from the primary site to segments not similarly innervated, and in such cases the mechanism is perplexing (e.g., anginal pain referred to the jaw). Various theories, such as division of the same nerve into deep and superficial branches, release of chemical mediators into the nervous system, and convergence of cutaneous and visceral nerves into a common synaptic pool at the spinal cord, all explain the dermatomal referral of pain but fail to explain pain at remote sites.

MANAGEMENT OF PAIN

Recent advances in pain research provide a scientific rationale that has improved treatment. These include better and more effective use of standard drug therapy (non-narcotic, narcotic, and adjuvant analgesic drugs), the development of new drugs and the use of novel routes of drug administration, more selective anesthetic and neurosurgical approaches, and the integration of behavioral approaches to pain control.

General Principles (Table 27–1)

1. Pain is best managed by treating the underlying disorder (e.g., steroids for giant cell arteritis relieve headache and jaw or temporalis muscle pain promptly; radiation therapy for bone pain caused by cancer is often helpful), but in many patients the pain is chronic and the physician is able neither to treat the underlying disturbances nor to offer specific therapy for that type of pain.

2. Pain should be treated early and promptly. The persistence of untreated pain results in significant psychologic morbidity, most commonly anxiety and depression with a sense of loss of control and hopelessness. Early treatment that provides prompt and continuous pain relief is crucial to prevent further compromise of the patient's emotional resources.

3. Multiple therapeutic approaches, often delivered simultaneously, should be utilized because different treatment modalities may be additive or synergistic when used together rather than separately. For example, combinations of narcotic and non-narcotic analgesics provide greater analgesia than either alone. Nonpharmacologic methods, such as relaxation techniques and cognitive coping skills, coupled with physical therapy and vocational rehabilitation, can often help in selected patients with chronic pain, especially when added to judicious drug therapy.

4. Narcotic drugs should be used with discrimination, but they should not be withheld if alternative therapy is ineffective. Long-term use of narcotics produces tolerance and physical dependence. Tolerance is the term used to describe increasing dose requirements to maintain analgesia. *Physical dependence* means that the signs and symptoms of withdrawal will appear if the narcotic drug is abruptly discontinued.

TABLE 27–1. GUIDELINES FOR THE USE OF ANALGESICS IN PAIN MANAGEMENT

1. Tailor drugs to nature and severity of pain
2. Know the pharmacology of the drug prescribed
   a. Know the duration of the analgesic effect
   b. Know the pharmacokinetic properties of the drug (duration of action and half-life)
   c. Know the equianalgesic doses for the drug and its route of administration (Table 27–2)
3. Adjust the route of administration to the patient's needs using oral, rectal, subcutaneous, intramuscular, intravenous, epidural, and intrathecal routes
4. Administer the analgesic on a regular basis after initial titration of the dose
5. Use drug combinations to provide additive analgesia and reduce side effects, e.g., nonsteroidal anti-inflammatory drugs, antihistamine (hydroxyzine), amphetamine (dextroamphetamine)
6. Avoid drug combinations that increase sedation without enhancing analgesia, e.g., benzodiazepine (diazepam) and phenothiazine
7. For narcotics, anticipate and treat side effects
   a. Sedation
   b. Respiratory depression
   c. Nausea and vomiting
   d. Constipation
   e. Multifocal myoclonus and seizures
8. When using narcotics, watch for the development of tolerance
   a. Switch to an alternate narcotic analgesic
   b. Start with one half of the equianalgesic dose and titrate to pain relief
   c. Use adjuvant analgesics and anesthetic and neurosurgical approaches
9. Prevent acute withdrawal
   a. Taper drugs slowly
   b. Use diluted doses of naloxone (0.4 mg in 10 ml of saline) to reverse narcotic-induced respiratory depression in the physically dependent patient and administer cautiously
10. Do not use placebos to assess pain

These effects should not be confused with psychologic dependence or *"addiction,"* which implies both a craving for the drug for effects other than analgesia and drug abuse behavior. The percentage of patients who actually become psychologically dependent on narcotics when they are given to treat medical illness is unknown, but recent data suggest that psychologic dependence is unusual in patients treated for pain when the pain is later relieved by other means.

5. Psychologic factors play a major role in chronic pain and must be carefully assessed. However, no patient should be diagnosed as having "psychogenic" pain until an exhaustive examination has ruled out structural disease. Depression should be identified and treated, and since the tricyclic antidepressants have analgesic properties as well, they are useful adjuvant analgesic drugs, particularly in patients with neuropathic pain.

6. Placebo effects are important. A positive analgesic response from intramuscular saline indicates only that the patient is a placebo responder. It does not suggest that the pain is unreal or less severe than reported by the patient. Misuse of placebo creates distrust between the patient and the physician and interferes with adequate pain assessment and management. In most clinical studies, up to one third of patients report relief of pain when given a placebo.

Drug Therapy

Analgesic drugs can be divided into three groups: Group I—the non-narcotic analgesics, such as aspirin and acetaminophen and the nonsteroidal anti-inflammatory drugs (NSAID's), act peripherally, probably on pain receptors; Group II—the narcotic agonist and antagonist drugs activate opiate receptors in the central and peripheral nervous systems; and Group III—the adjuvant analgesic drugs are designed for management of symptoms other than pain but produce relief in certain pain states (carbamazepine for trigeminal neuralgia) or potentiate narcotic analgesics. These three groups represent the mainstay of therapy for patients with acute and chronic pain. Effective use of these drugs requires

TABLE 27–2. NON-NARCOTIC ANALGESIC DRUGS

Drug	Indications	Equianalgesic Dose	Starting Dose (mg), Range/24 hr	Comments
Aspirin	Often used in combination with narcotics	650	650	Contraindicated in hepatic and renal dysfunction; avoid during pregnancy, in hemolytic disorders, and in combination with steroids
Acetaminophen	Like aspirin	650	650	
Ibuprofen	Higher analgesic potential than aspirin	ND	200–400	Like aspirin
Fenoprofen	Like ibuprofen	ND	200–400	Like aspirin
Diflunisal	Longer duration of action than ibuprofen; higher analgesic potential than aspirin	ND	500–1000	Like aspirin
Naproxen	Like diflunisal	ND	250–500	Like aspirin

ND = not documented.

an understanding of their pharmacologic characteristics and selection of a particular drug and dose geared to the needs of the individual patient.

NON-NARCOTIC ANALGESICS (Table 27–2). Aspirin, acetaminophen, and the nonsteroidal anti-inflammatory drugs are the first-line agents for the management of mild-to-moderate pain, and in patients with severe pain these drugs potentiate the effects of narcotic analgesics. Non-narcotic analgesics have a ceiling effect, and their long-term use is limited by gastrointestinal and hematologic side effects. The choice and use of these drugs must be individualized, with the patient receiving maximal levels of one drug before another is tried. If pain control is ineffective or the non-narcotic agents poorly tolerated, the use of narcotic analgesics is indicated. In general, the use of narcotics is limited to acute structural or chronic, irreversible structural pain, as in cancer.

NARCOTIC ANALGESICS (Table 27–3). The narcotic analgesics vary in potency, efficacy, and adverse effects. They are classified as agonist or antagonist drugs depending on their ability to bind to the opiate receptors and produce analgesia. The narcotic *agonist* drugs, such as morphine, bind to specific opiate receptors, resulting in analgesia. These

TABLE 27–3. NARCOTIC ANALGESIC DRUGS

Class	Drug	Indications	Equianalgesic Dose (mg)*	Starting Dose (mg) Range/24 hr	Comments
Morphine-like agonist, mild to moderate pain	Codeine	Often used in combination with non-narcotic analgesics	32–65	32–65	Impaired ventilation; bronchial asthma; intracranial pressure
	Oxycodone	Shorter acting; in combination with non-narcotic analgesics, limiting dose escalation	5	5–10	Like codeine
	Meperidine	Shorter acting; biotransformed to normeperidine; toxic metabolite	50	50–100	Normeperidine accumulates with repetitive dosing, causing CNS excitation; not for patients with renal dysfunction or receiving monoamine oxidase inhibitors
	Proproxyphene hydrochloride (Darvon)	Used in combination with non-narcotic analgesics; long half-life; biotransformed to potentially toxic metabolite (norproproxyphene)	65–130	65–130	Propoxyphene and metabolite accumulate with repetitive dosing; overdose complicated by convulsions
Mixed-agonist antagonist	Pentazocine	In combination with non-narcotics, in combination with naloxone to discourage parenteral abuse	50	50–100	May cause psychotomimetic effects, may precipitate withdrawal in narcotic-dependent patients
Morphine-like agonists, moderate to severe pain	Morphine	Lower doses for aged patients; those with impaired ventilation; bronchial asthma; increased intracranial pressure; liver failure	10–60	30–60	Standard of comparison for narcotic-type analgesics
	Hydromorphone (Dilaudid)	Like morphine	1.5–8.0	4–8	Slightly shorter acting high-potency IM dosage form available for tolerant patients
	Methadone (Dolphine)	Like morphine; may accumulate with repetitive dosing, causing excessive sedation	10–20	10–20	Good oral potency; long plasma half-life
	Levorphanol (Levo-Dromoran)	Like methadone	2–4	2–4	Like methadone
	Oxymorphone (Numorphan)	Like morphine IM	1	See "Comments"	Not available orally
	Meperidine (Demerol)	Normeperidine (toxic metabolite) accumulates with repetitive dosing, causing CNS excitation; not for patients with impaired renal function or those receiving monoamine oxidase inhibitors	75–300	Not recommended	Slightly shorter acting; used orally for less severe pain
	Codeine	Like morphine	130–180	See "Comments"	Used orally for less severe pain

*Dose given intramuscularly or by mouth.
IM = intramuscular; CNS = central nervous system.

TABLE 27–4. ADJUVANT ANALGESIC DRUGS

Class	Drug	Indications	Starting Dose (mg), Range/24 hr	Comments
Anticonvulsants	Phenytoin (Dilantin)	Neuropathic pain, acute lancinating type (tic)	100, 100–300	Start with low doses; titrate slowly
	Carbamazepine (Tegretol)	Acute lancinating type (tic)	100, 200–800	Useful in paroxysmal nerve pain
Antidepressants	Amitriptyline, Imipramine	Deafferentation pain, e.g., postherpetic neuralgia	10, 10–150	Start at low dose and titrate slowly; has analgesic properties
Amphetamine	Dextroamphetamine	Somatic and visceral pain, e.g., postoperative	2.5, 10	Additive analgesia in combination with narcotics; reduces sedative effects
Antihistamine	Hydroxyzine	Somatic and visceral pain	25, 100	Additive analgesia in combination with narcotics; antiemetic, antianxiety properties
Phenothiazine	Methotrimeprazine (Levoprome)	Somatic and visceral pain; useful in narcotic-tolerant patients with GI obstruction and pain	10 (IM), 10–40 (IM)	Has antianxiety and antiemetic effects; available only in IM preparation
Steroids	Prednisone	Somatic and deafferentation pain, e.g., inflammatory pain, reflex sympathetic dystrophy	5, 5–60	Anti-inflammatory, antiemetic, analgesic effects
	Dexamethasone		0.5, 0.5–16	

IM = intramuscular; GI = gastrointestinal.

agents are commonly used in the management of chronic pain of structural cause, such as cancer pain. The narcotic *antagonist* drugs block the effect of morphine at its receptor. Included in this category is a group of drugs with analgesic properties referred to as the mixed agonist-antagonist drugs. These drugs are often used in acute postoperative pain management but are of limited use in chronic pain management for several reasons: They produce psychotomimetic effects with increasing doses; only pentazocine is available in oral form and only in combinations with naloxone, aspirin, or acetaminophen; they precipitate withdrawal in narcotic-dependent patients. Effective use of narcotic analgesics requires balancing of the desirable effect of pain relief with the undesirable side effects of nausea, vomiting, mental clouding, sedation, tolerance, and physical dependence. These undesirable effects impose a practical limit on the dose one can give a particular patient.

Much of the difficulty encountered with the clinical use of narcotics arises from individual variation, consisting of differences in response of specific patients to the same drug dose. Thus, although Tables 27–2 to 27–4 can serve as reference points, individualization of drug treatment is the cardinal rule of management. Drugs should be given in sufficient amounts and at time intervals close enough to achieve adequate pain relief. "Weak" narcotics, such as codeine, propoxyphene, and oxycodone, are selected to treat moderate pain. If the pain remains unrelieved, the "strong" narcotic analgesics, such as morphine, hydromorphone, levorphanol and methadone, should be employed. To ensure adequate dosing schedules, one must know the clinical pharmacology of the narcotic analgesics, including their duration of analgesic effect, their half-lives, and the equianalgesic doses for both oral and parenteral routes of administration. For example, the plasma half-lives of the narcotics vary widely and do not correlate with their analgesic time courses. Both methadone, with a half-life of 15 to 30 hours, and levorphanol, with a half-life of 12 to 16 hours, produce analgesia for only 4 to 6 hours. With repeated doses, these drugs accumulate in plasma and can result in excessive sedation and respiratory depression. It is necessary to adjust the dose and schedule, considering both the patient's degree of pain relief and the plasma half-life of the drug when it is introduced.

Knowledge of the equianalgesic doses when a switch is made from one medication to another or from one route of administration to another prevents undermedication. However, cross-tolerance is not complete, and patients tolerant to the analgesic effects of one narcotic can often be given another to provide better analgesia. The usual rule is to begin with one half of the calculated equianalgesic dose of the new drug and increase as required.

Medication should be administered on a regular basis, with the interval between doses based on the duration of the analgesic effect. The pharmacologic objective is to maintain the plasma level of the drug above the "minimal effective concentration for pain relief." The time required to reach steady state after repeated administration depends on the half-life of the drug; full assessment of the analgesic efficacy of a drug regimen may take 24 hours for a drug such as morphine or up to 5 to 7 days for methadone.

Combinations of drugs enable the physician to improve pain relief without escalation of the narcotic dose. Several combinations have been proven effective, including a narcotic plus a non-narcotic (aspirin, acetaminophen, or ibuprofen), a narcotic plus an amphetamine (dextroamphetamine, 10 mg) or a narcotic plus an antihistamine (100 mg of hydroxyzine given intramuscularly). Other drugs such as diazepam and chlorpromazine do not provide additive analgesia and may produce additive sedative effects.

Oral administration of drugs is the most practical route, but the choice must be made according to the needs of the patient. Several alternate methods of drug administration have been developed to maximize pharmacologic effects and minimize the undesirable effects associated with standard methods. The approaches that are most useful in the management of acute or chronic pain with chronic medical illness include slow-release morphine preparations effective for 8 to 12 hours, enabling a full night's rest; continuous subcutaneous and intravenous infusions for patients who are unable to tolerate oral analgesics because of gastrointestinal obstruction or malabsorption and in whom repeated parenteral dosing is difficult because of limited muscle mass or a bleeding diathesis; and epidural and intrathecal narcotic administration via temporary catheters or implanted pumps. This last approach minimizes the distribution of drugs to receptors in the brain stem and cerebral hemispheres, avoids the side effects of systemic administration, and is effective in selected patients with cancer pain who are unable to tolerate the excessive sedation or mental clouding associated with an oral or parenteral route.

Side Effects of Narcotics. Side effects of the narcotic analgesics should be anticipated and treated. *Sedation and drowsiness* vary with the drug dose and may occur after either single or repeated administration. Reducing the individual dose and prescribing it more frequently, switching to a drug with a short plasma half-life (hydromorphone), using an amphetamine (dextroamphetamine, 2 to 5 mg) in combination with the narcotic twice daily, and discontinuing all other sedative drugs are useful approaches to counteract the sedative effects.

Respiratory depression is the most serious adverse effect, but tolerance develops rapidly, allowing prolonged use of narcotics for chronic pain. If respiratory depression occurs, it can be reversed by administering the specific narcotic antagonist naloxone in a dose of 0.4 mg per milliliter. In patients receiving narcotics for prolonged periods who develop respiratory depression, diluted doses of naloxone (0.4 mg in 10 ml of saline) should be infused slowly to reverse the respiratory depression but prevent precipitation of severe withdrawal symptoms. The occurrence of *nausea and vomiting* with one drug does not mean that all narcotics will produce similar symptoms. Changing to an alternate narcotic or using an antiemetic in combination commonly obviates this effect. Tolerance rapidly develops to the emetic effect of narcotics so that after a few days antiemetics often are unnecessary. *Constipation* should be prevented by the provision of a regular bowel regimen, including cathartics, stool softeners, and careful attention to diet. *Multifocal myoclonus* may occur with toxic doses of any narcotic. The most common offender is meperidine because of the accumulation of the active metabolite normeperidine, which can cause seizures. Since the half-life of normeperidine is 16 hours, it may take several days for toxic side effects to clear. Patients should be switched to morphine to control their pain and managed symptomatically for seizures.

Tolerance is common when patients receive narcotic analgesics chronically for pain. The earliest sign is a decrease in the duration of effective analgesia. Increasing the frequency of drug administration of the dose provides improved pain relief. There is no limit to tolerance, and the dose of drug should not be the major concern of the prescribing physician. Adjuvant drugs and anesthetic and neurosurgical methods sometimes help to manage pain in the tolerant patient. These guidelines notwithstanding, the management of pain with narcotic analgesics is difficult and requires meticulous attention by the physician.

ADJUVANT ANALGESICS (Table 27–4). The adjuvant analgesics include several different categories of drugs, including anticonvulsants, phenothiazines, tricyclic antidepressants, antihistamines, amphetamines, and steroids (see Table 27–4). Carbamazepine and phenytoin are useful in the management of patients with some neuropathic pain syndromes, e.g., trigeminal neuralgia. The mechanism of action is through suppression of the spontaneous neuronal firing that commonly occurs with nerve injury. For both drugs, the minimal effective concentration for analgesia is unknown.

Certain phenothiazines have potent analgesic effects. Methotrimeprazine (Levoprome) has an analgesic potential close to that of morphine (15 mg given intramuscularly is equivalent to 10 mg of morphine given intramuscularly). This drug helps manage severe pain in patients tolerant to narcotic analgesics. The tricyclic antidepressants both enhance the analgesic effects of morphine and have independent analgesic properties. Doses of 10 to 75 mg administered orally are used to treat postherpetic neuralgia. The analgesic effects of these drugs occur independently of their antidepressant properties. The antihistamine hydroxyzine and the amphetamine dextroamphetamine are also sometimes helpful adjuvants. Steroids

produce analgesia in patients with acute inflammatory diseases and in patients with tumor infiltration of bone or nerve or both.

Alternate Methods of Pain Control

A variety of nonpharmacologic therapeutic approaches can be used alone or in combination with the analgesic drugs. These include physical therapy, trigger point injections, transcutaneous nerve stimulation, and certain behavioral approaches, all of which should be familiar to general physicians. Technically demanding anesthetic and neurosurgical approaches require consultation with pain experts. Certain guidelines apply to these procedures:

1. Evaluate thoroughly the nature of the pain and the prognosis of the patient's primary disease. Neurolytic nerve blocks and neuroablative and neurostimulatory surgical procedures often yield only temporary relief in patients with chronic pain and are not useful for deafferentation pain. In contrast, patients with cancer pain of somatic origin who are not expected to live for more than several months are excellent candidates for such procedures.

2. Nondestructive procedures, such as transcutaneous electrical stimulation or temporary blocks with local anesthetics, should be tried first.

3. Start with the least destructive procedure. For example, try continuous epidural local anesthetics to manage perineal pain before initiating an intrathecal neurolytic block.

4. Evaluate patients psychologically. If psychologic factors play a major role in the pain, such procedures will not help and will often exacerbate the condition.

5. Inform the patient fully of the potential risks and benefits of the planned procedure.

PHYSICAL THERAPY. Chronic pain is commonly associated with reduced physical activity and splinting or immobilization of the injured body part. A graded exercise program with appropriate use of splints and braces and reactivation of the injured part plays a pivotal role in re-establishing the functional status of the patient. Local rubbing and transcutaneous electrical stimulation for "counterirritation" may help to mobilize the patient with a localized pain. Trigger point injections with either saline or a local anesthetic provide dramatic relief of painful muscle spasm.

BEHAVIORAL THERAPY. Behavioral approaches that often improve the patient's coping mechanism include breathing exercises to increase relaxation, coping strategies to integrate pain symptoms into a functioning lifestyle, and improving control over psychologic factors of anxiety, fear, and demoralization associated with chronic pain.

ANESTHETIC PROCEDURES (Table 27–5). Local anesthetics and injectable neurolytic agents are sometimes useful in managing both acute and chronic pain that occupies a well-defined anatomic site. Sympathetic blocks, for example, often predict the relief that can be expected from sympathectomy in treating causalgia due to peripheral sensory nerve damage. Blocking nerves with short- or long-acting anesthetics determines in a reversible manner whether semipermanent nerve blocks will be effective and what side effects they might have. In some patients, particularly when muscle spasm plays a major role in pain production, repeated temporary blocks produce long-lasting relief of pain. If an anesthetic nerve block has been effective temporarily and then begins to lose its efficacy, neurolytic agents, such as phenol, alcohol, and freezing (cryoanesthesia), can be used to destroy nerve structures. The principal pathologic effect produced by these neurolytic agents is demyelination with secondary nerve degeneration. Because peripheral nerves and roots have overlapping sensory functions, multiple nerves and roots must be blocked to yield adequate pain control. Since such blocks may paralyze as well as anesthetize, they have a limited role in extremity pain and are most useful to treat thoracic and

TABLE 27–5. TYPES OF ANESTHETIC PROCEDURES COMMONLY USED IN CHRONIC PAIN

I. Nerve Blocks	
Peripheral	Pain in discrete dermatomes in chest and abdomen
Epidural	Unilateral lumbar or sacral pain Midline perineal pain Bilateral lumbosacral pain
Intrathecal	Midline perineal pain Bilateral lumbosacral pain
Autonomic	
Stellate ganglion	Reflex sympathetic dystrophy, e.g., frozen shoulder Arm pain
Lumbar sympathetic	Reflex sympathetic dystrophy Lumbosacral plexopathy Vascular insufficiency of the lower extremity
Celiac plexus	Midabdominal pain
II. Continuous Epidural Infusion with Local Anesthetic	Unilateral and bilateral lumbosacral pain Midline perineal pain
III. Chemical Hypophysectomy	Diffuse bone pain
IV. Inhalation Therapy	Generalized pain Incident pain
V. Trigger Point Injection	Focal muscle pain

abdominal pain or perineal and sacral pain in patients with cancer.

Neurolytic agents can be injected into the epidural or intrathecal space as well as into peripheral nerves or roots. However, the limitations of motor weakness and autonomic dysfunction make this technique suitable for only a limited number of patients. Neurolytic blocks find their best use in the management of well-defined localized pain caused by cancer. Their role in managing pain of nonmalignant origin is controversial because they work for only a limited period of time. There is a real risk of adding morbidity without providing pain relief, and they are not effective in managing deafferentation pain.

Blocks of the cervical (stellate ganglion) and lumbar sympathetic chains are most useful in managing limb pain associated with vascular or peripheral nerve injury, as occurs in diabetic peripheral vascular disease and reflex sympathetic dystrophy. Celiac plexus block is the procedure of choice to manage visceral pain from pancreatic carcinoma.

Intermittent or continuous epidural infusions of local anesthetics are useful for temporary relief of chronic pain involving the lumbosacral plexus and sacrum. This approach is most useful to treat an acute exacerbation of chronic cancer pain. The technique does not result in cross-tolerance with opiate analgesia, and it can be appropriately titrated to provide anesthesia without interruption of motor or autonomic function.

Two other anesthetic approaches used to manage diffuse pain include chemical hypophysectomy and intermittent inhalation therapy with nitrous oxide. Chemical hypophysectomy involves the injection of alcohol into the sella turcica under radiologic control. It is used to control pain in patients with widespread bony metastases. Pain relief is reported in 35 to 75 per cent of patients, and many patients experience pain relief independent of whether the pituitary ablation causes tumor regression. Nitrous oxide is used to manage chronic pain in the dying patient, particularly acute incident pain or procedure-related pain. It is administered in oxygen through a non-rebreathing face mask with concentrations ranging from 25 to 75 per cent.

NEUROSURGICAL PROCEDURES (Table 27–6). Pharmacologic procedures requiring neurosurgery include placement of intraventricular, epidural, or intrathecal catheters and im-

planted reservoirs or pumps to infuse agents used to manage selected patients with pain and cancer in whom systemic drugs are either ineffective or associated with excessive side effects. These approaches are not useful in managing non–cancer-related chronic pain problems.

Neurostimulatory procedures are performed by implanting electrodes in or on the desired portion of the nervous system and leading the electrodes to an implanted conductive receiver attached to an external transmitter. The technique allows the patient to control the timing and intensity of the stimulation. Electrical stimulation of the dorsal columns of cervical or thoracic spinal cord sometimes controls bilateral deafferentation pain. Unfortunately, tolerance to the analgesic effect alters long-term usefulness of this procedure. Electrodes are usually placed in the epidural space over the dorsal column rather than directly on the spinal cord, thus reducing the risk of cord damage. Electrical stimulation of the periventricular gray matter of the brain stem also has been used for chronic deafferentation pain, especially if dorsal column stimulation or neurolytic blocks fail. Stimulation is delivered for no longer than 20 to 25 minutes at a time, three or four times a day. Tolerance develops more rapidly with increased use of the stimulator. Both animal studies and observations on human beings indicate that periventricular stimulation is associated with total body analgesia but without a decrease in sensory or motor function. This procedure is still experimental and is available in only a few specialized centers.

Medial thalamic stimulation is used to manage chronic but unilateral intractable pain. Electrodes are placed stereotactically in medial thalamus contralateral to the pain. Stimulation results in localized analgesia. This procedure is used to manage the thalamic pain syndrome, phantom limb pain, and peripheral nerve injury pain, particularly when pain involves the head or neck. About 50 per cent of patients with localized deafferentation pain respond to thalamic stimulation.

In addition to neurostimulatory procedures, portions of the nervous system from peripheral nerves to the cerebral cortex can be lesioned to relieve pain. The most commonly used procedures are dorsal root entry zone lesions and cordotomy. Other procedures have had only limited success and are marked by significant neurologic morbidity. Dorsal root entry zone (DREZ) lesions interrupt the sensory nerve roots as they enter the dorsal horn of the spinal cord. An electrode is introduced for a distance of 2 to 3 mm into the medial sulcus on the dorsal surface of the spinal cord, and a radiofrequency lesion is made. This procedure is most useful in managing

TABLE 27–6. NEUROABLATIVE, NEUROSTIMULATORY, AND NEUROPHARMACOLOGIC PROCEDURES

Site	Neurostimulatory	Neuroablative	Neuropharmacologic
Peripheral nerve	Transcutaneous and percutaneous electrical nerve stimulation	Neurectomy	Local anesthetics
Nerve root		Rhizotomy	Local anesthetics Neurolytic agents*
Spinal cord	Dorsal column stimulation	Dorsal root entry zone lesions Cordotomy Myelotomy	Epidural and intrathecal opiates*
Brain stem	Periaqueductal stimulation	Mesencephalic tractotomy	Intraventricular opiates*
Thalamus	Thalamic stimulation	Thalamotomy	
Cortex		Cingulumotomy Frontal lobotomy	
Pituitary		Trans-sphenoidal hypophysectomy*	Chemical hypophysectomy*

*Procedures restricted for the treatment of chronic cancer-related pain.

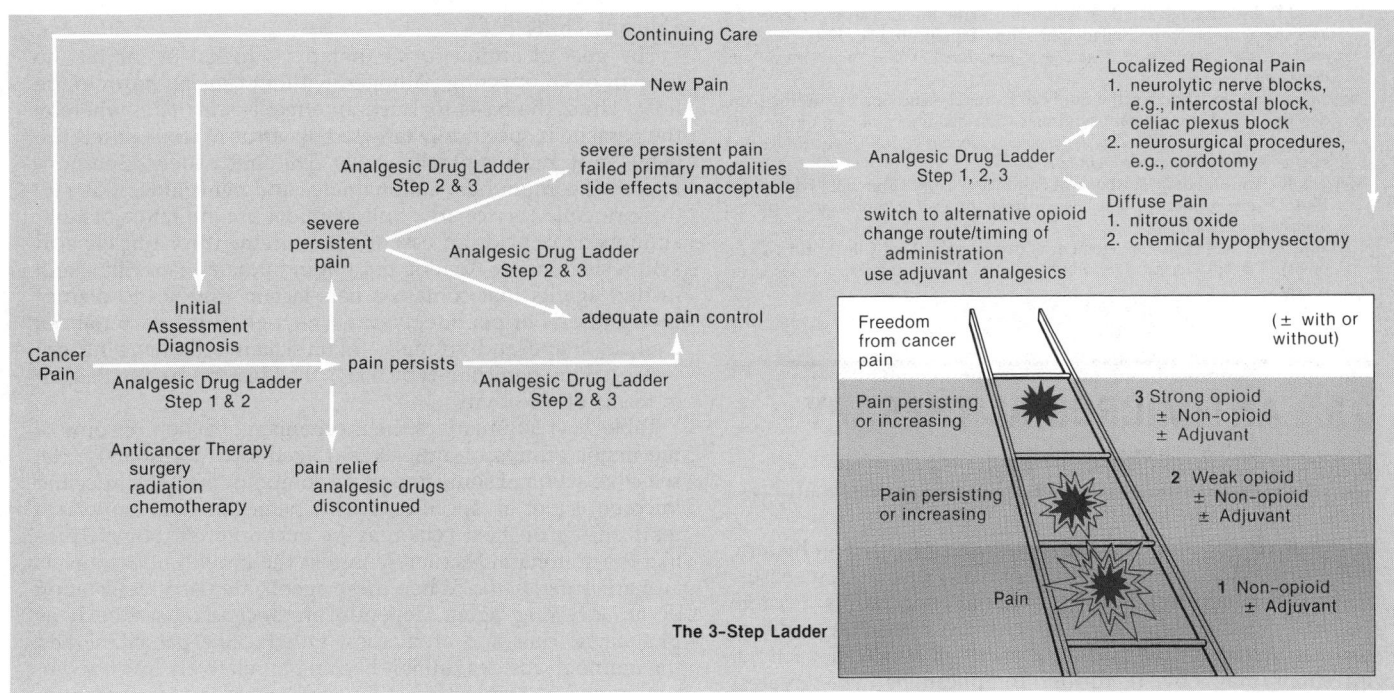

FIGURE 27–1. Algorithm for the management of cancer pain.

the continuous pain of peripheral nerve injury (e.g., post-herpetic neuralgia, avulsions of the brachial or lumbar plexus). It is effective in 50 to 75 per cent of patients so treated. Postoperative complications occur in 20 per cent of patients and consist of ipsilateral clumsiness and weakness, usually transient, of the arm or leg. Cordotomy is the most useful neurosurgical procedure for relief of chronic somatic pain and the most commonly used procedure for the management of patients with localized cancer pain. Cordotomy can be performed as a percutaneous stereotactic radiofrequency procedure or as an open surgical ablation. Because the spinothalamic tract is selectively interrupted, only pain and temperature sensation are lost (on the contralateral side of the body). Cutaneous sensation and motor power remain intact, although some ipsilateral weakness or ataxia occurs transiently in about 20 per cent of patients. Cordotomy is most useful to manage unilateral pain below the neck. Initial pain relief occurs in 90 per cent of patients. This figure drops to 50 per cent at six months and about 40 per cent at the end of one year. One to 2 per cent of postcordotomy patients develop burning dysesthesias (anesthesia dolorosa), which are often as distressing as the original pain. Because of both the limited duration of its effectiveness and the risk of producing deafferentation pain, cordotomy is not indicated for management of chronic nonmalignant pain. Bilateral cordotomy can be performed to manage midline or perineal pain associated with cancer. If performed in the cervical area, bilateral cordotomy risks producing sleep-induced apnea (Ondine's curse). The second risk of bilateral cordotomy is bladder dysfunction. With unilateral cordotomy, 7 to 10 per cent of patients develop mirror pain on the opposite side of the body even when the original pain is relieved. Mirror pain can occur in the absence of a definable lesion in the affected area, and its pathogenesis is unknown. Other neuroablative procedures are rarely used.

Management of Cancer Pain

Figure 27–1 provides an algorithm for the management of cancer pain. It attempts to integrate assessment techniques,

drug therapy, and anesthetic, neurosurgical, and behavioral approaches and stresses continuity of care. Treatment of cancer pain must begin with a careful diagnostic assessment that addresses not only the medical nature of pain but also its psychologic and social components. At the time of assessment, a plan is developed to treat both the cancer, if possible, and the pain itself. If the anticancer treatment is effective, pain relief usually occurs, and the drugs used for analgesia can be discontinued without difficulty. Pain relief begins with analgesic drugs. Incorporated in Figure 27–1 is the World Health Organization's Cancer Pain Relief Program. It proposes an analgesic drug ladder moving from nonopioid drugs alone or in combination with adjuvant drugs through weak opioids to strong opioids. If pain relief is achieved with this program, no further therapy is necessary. In patients with severe, persistent pain not responsive to analgesic drugs or in whom the side effects of the drugs are not tolerated, physicians should first try switching to alternate analgesics or changing the route or timing of drug administration. For example, intrathecal opioids are indicated for relief of pain in patients in whom systemic analgesics produce confusion or excessive sedation.

If the pain is unresponsive to analgesic drugs and is localized (e.g., intercostal pain from tumor infiltration of the chest wall), neurolytic blocks are indicated. If the pain is unilateral and below the waist, cordotomy should be considered. For more diffuse pain unresponsive to analgesics, neurostimulatory procedures, including nitrous oxide inhalation and chemical hypophysectomy, may be considered. Behavioral approaches, which include relaxation techniques, breathing exercises, and cognitive control of pain, serve as adjuvants and should be integrated into the management of patients with chronic pain.

As the algorithm indicates, whatever the techniques of pain management used in patients with cancer, the physician is responsible for delivering continuing care, constantly reassessing both the diagnosis and the treatment to achieve optimum relief of pain and suffering for both patient and family.

Cousins M, Bridenbaugh P (eds.): Neural blockade. In Clinical Anesthesia and Management of Pain. Philadelphia, J.B. Lippincott Co, 1980. *This text describes the commonly used anesthetic procedures in acute and chronic pain management.*

International Association for the Study of Pain: Classification of chronic pain, descriptions of chronic pain syndromes and definitions of pain terms. Pain [Suppl] 3:S1–S225, 1986. *This useful volume contains descriptions of chronic pain syndromes and definitions of pain terms.*

Melzack R, Wall P (eds.): Textbook of Pain. New York, Churchill Livingstone, 1984. *A compendium of the anatomy, physiology, and pharmacology of pain and common pain syndromes.*

Payne R, Foley KM: The management of cancer pain. Med Clin North Am (in press). *A detailed review of the current approach to pain management in the cancer patient.*

28 ANTIMICROBIAL THERAPY

Lowell S. Young

The advent of antimicrobial therapy represented an historic milestone in the cure and control of many infectious diseases. Invariably fatal infections, like bacterial endocarditis, became treatable for the first time. Subsequently, abundant evidence has accumulated that early treatment of localized bacterial infections may obviate further complications. The greatest progress during the modern era of antimicrobial therapy has been in the treatment of acute bacterial infections, although a few chronic diseases such as tuberculosis have become well controlled. New developments offer promise in controlling viral diseases and parasitic infections that are a major burden on much of mankind. There have been some modest developments in the antifungal area as well. Nonetheless, the initial enthusiasm that greeted the introduction of new agents with antibacterial activity has been tempered by a more sobering perspective. Antimicrobial agents are not always innocuous to the host, and their widespread usage appears to have fostered increasing drug resistance throughout the world. The growing complexities of antimicrobial therapy appear to be related to the rapid proliferation of agents of several classes, increasing drug resistance, and a greater recognition of interactions between pharmacologic agents.

SOME DEFINITIONS

The terms *antibiotic*, *antimicrobic*, and *chemotherapeutic agent* have often been used interchangeably to designate defined chemical substances that possess activity against specific microorganisms. Indeed, the earliest definition of an antibiotic was a substance produced in nature by living microbes that inhibited the growth of other microbial organisms at low concentrations. Viewed in this light, antibiotics seem to be a product of evolution and may confer a selective advantage to the producer in a specific ecosystem. Technically, antibiotics differ from chemotherapeutic agents in that the latter represent the products of chemical synthesis, such as the sulfonamide dyes that were subsequently found to have antibacterial activity. Antibiotics in common use, such as penicillins and aminoglycosides, are derived from natural products but from a functional point of view may be considered interchangeable with chemotherapeutic agents. As the development of new antibacterial agents has proliferated, restrictive technical terms have become outdated. For instance, new penicillins, cephalosporins, and aminoglycosides contain synthetic or semisynthetic modifications of existing structures that confer potent new biologic activity. The term *antimicrobic* has been proposed to describe all substances with antimicrobial activity whether of natural or synthetic origin, but its acceptance has been variable.

GENERAL PRINCIPLES

The goal of antimicrobial therapy is to kill or inhibit the growth of an infecting pathogen without causing harm to the host. Thus, the basis for such an effect is *selectivity*, whereby the parasite is specifically targeted by virtue of some difference between it and mammalian cells. The first widely used antimicrobial compounds, sulfonamides and penicillins, illustrate this principle very clearly. Sulfonamides are inhibitors of para-aminobenzoic acid, an essential requirement for nucleic acid synthesis in many bacteria but not in humans. Penicillins and related agents that contain a beta-lactam ring act to disrupt the synthesis of peptidoglycan, which gives the bacterial cell wall its shape and strength. Mammalian cells have no cell wall, making penicillin-type drugs the ideal antibacterial agent in terms of selectivity.

Table 28–1 summarizes the mechanism of action of some of the major groups of antibacterial agents. Unfortunately, the selective action of some important compounds on the infecting microbe is not as specific as with penicillin, and important toxic effects on host cells may be encountered. Some drugs like the sulfonamides merely inhibit the growth of organisms and are *bacteriostatic*. When these agents are used, eradication of an infecting agent depends on host defenses such as phagocytic cells and antibodies. Others, like penicillins and the aminoglycosides, inhibit bacteria at relatively low concentration and at higher (but still usually therapeutic) concentrations can kill them; these are *bactericidal* agents. These designations of a bacteriostatic or bactericidal agent may vary depending on the type of organism: Penicillin G is usually bactericidal for gram-positive cocci but is only static against the enterococcus (*Streptococcus faecalis*), while chloramphenicol is usually bacteriostatic even at very high concentrations but can be bactericidal against *Hemophilus influenzae*. Spectrum refers to range of microorganisms affected by a particular agent, which varies from relatively narrow for low doses of penicillin G to quite broad for large doses of the new cephalosporins. Breadth of spectrum is not necessarily related to mechanism of action.

The interaction between a microbe and therapeutic agent can be complex, and many important variables affect outcome. Intrinsic virulence differs considerably between infecting agents so that the progression of infection ranges from a very indolent tempo to a fulminating course. Host factors influence selection of bactericidal versus bacteriostatic agents and the breadth of spectrum of therapy. The site of infection influences dose and duration of treatment. The proliferation of therapeutic choices compels the physician to obtain in-depth knowledge of any agent prescribed. Treatment can be guided by laboratory studies, but therapeutic choices must be based on knowledge of antimicrobial spectrum, mode of action, pharmacology, toxicity, and all major factors that affect drug activity.

IDENTIFICATION OF THE INFECTING AGENT

It is highly desirable to have the infecting agent identified prior to initiation of treatment, but in most circumstances culture confirmation and tests in vitro of antimicrobial susceptibility will not be available for at least a day. Clinical decision making is usually based on a perception of probabilities and on simple tests, the most important of which is the Gram stain. Even the latter is not necessary in the case of exudative pharyngitis, because the only treatable bacterial causes of the syndrome are hemolytic streptococci and now, rarely, *Corynebacterium diphtheriae*. Other isolates can usually be ignored and therapy with a penicillin initiated. When only a single infecting organism seems likely, therapy with a narrow-spectrum agent is preferable.

TABLE 28–1. MECHANISM OF ACTION OF ANTIMICROBIAL AGENTS

Agent	Site of Action	Effect	Cidal	Static
Penicillins, Cephalosporins	Cell wall	Inhibit cross-linking of peptidoglycan resulting in spheroplast formation	+	Occasionally
Vancomycin	Cell wall	Block transfer of pentapeptide from cytoplasm to cell membrane	+	Occasionally
Polymyxin B, Colistin	Cytoplasmic membrane	Bind phospholipid and disrupt membrane	+	
Aminoglycosides	Ribosome	Bind to 30S ribosomal subunit, thereby inhibiting attachment of messenger RNA; also affect transfer RNA	+	
Tetracyclines	Ribosome	Bind to 30S subunit and inhibit binding of transfer RNA		+
Chloramphenicol	Ribosome	Bind to 50S subunit and inhibit messenger RNA translation	Occasionally	+
Erythromycin, Clindamycin	Ribosome	Inhibit messenger RNA translation	Occasionally	+
Rifampin	Nucleic acid synthesis	Impaired RNA formation by inhibiting DNA-dependent RNA-polymerase	+	Occasionally
Metronidazole	Nucleic acid synthesis	Damages nucleic acid structure	+	
Quinolones	Nucleic acid synthesis	Inhibit DNA gyrase	+	
Sulfonamides	Nucleic acid synthesis	Competitive inhibition of para-amino benzoic acid, thereby blocking formation of thymidine and purines		+

In reality, many infectious processes initially begin as mixed infections: The aspiration of secretions into the lung usually results in the deposition of many types of oral microbes that can lead to pneumonia or lung abscess, or the perforation of an abdominal viscus leads to release of millions of aerobic and anaerobic bacteria into the abdominal cavity. What may survive to be cultured in respiratory secretions or from abdominal drainage may well be the hardiest of bacteria, and not necessarily all of those that were associated with initial infectious morbidity. Not all mixed infectious processes require treatment with broad-spectrum therapy, but the presence of multiple pathogens might explain clinical failure when a mixed infection is being treated and only one component of that infection is being affected by a particular drug regimen.

Initiation of antibiotic therapy prior to obtaining appropriate cultures is perhaps the leading explanation for the failure to document infecting pathogens. On the other hand, the Gram stain or immunofluorescent staining of secretions can identify the cause of infection after treatment is started. Irrespective of when it is done, the Gram stain can provide valuable semiquantitative information about predominant pathogens and can help the clinician decide whether a subsequent culture result can actually be relied upon. For instance, the validity of a sample of respiratory secretions is greatly enhanced by the detection of phagocytic cells such as neutrophils or alveolar macrophages. In contrast, the presence of squamous epithelial cells should be the basis for rejecting the validity of expectorated sputum, since they reflect oropharyngeal contamination. With regard to quantitative evaluation of a potentially infected body fluid, isolation of greater than 10^5 organisms per milliliter has been accepted as establishing the validity of a urine culture result. However, microscopic examination of uncentrifuged urine may still yield an approximate idea of the degree of infection (any organism seen corresponds with 10^5 bacteria per milliliter), as well as the nature of the infection that is taking place in the urinary tract. Isolation of organisms in pure culture from blood or normally sterile body fluids (like spinal fluid) is an unambiguous laboratory result that establishes an infectious etiology. Occasionally, some bloodstream infections are polymicrobial. Some blood culture isolates may be rejected as contaminants. The latter are usually skin flora like corynebacteria or *Staphylococcus epidermidis*. However, repeated isolation of such organisms from blood culture in association with signs of infection calls for careful clinical assessment. *Staphylococcus epidermidis* and corynebacteria can be valid pathogens in immunosuppressed subjects and patients with prosthetic devices.

SUSCEPTIBILITY, RESISTANCE, AND ANTIBACTERIAL SPECTRA

Appropriate antimicrobial therapy is based on the results of laboratory tests and validated by the clinical effect of treatment. Test results and treatment are not always consistent: Patients who have excellent or intact host defenses may recover from infection irrespective of whether the antibiotic they receive has an effect on the infecting agent. Some important pathogens like Salmonella species are very susceptible in vitro to cephalosporin antibiotics, but clinical efficacy has been poor. Nevertheless, in a serious deep-seated or bloodstream infection, laboratory tests do provide an invaluable guide to the selection or adjustment of therapy. Usually a microbe is considered susceptible to an antibacterial agent if it can be inhibited or killed by a concentration of the drug that is realistically achievable at the site of the infection. The levels of drug that must be achieved in the host will vary depending on the site of infection and could be limited by toxic side effects. A common practice is to set the range of susceptibility at or above realistically achievable blood levels, but there are some notable exceptions. For instance, some agents like nalidixic acid or nitrofurantoin are rapidly excreted in the urine, and only very low blood levels are achieved. Low doses of drugs that are effective for some infections are totally inadequate for deep-seated infections. The best example is the relatively low dose of benzyl penicillin G that is required to cure pneumococcal pneumonia, sometimes less than 100,000 units of penicillin per day, which contrasts with the dose of approximately 20 million units per day that may be necessary to treat pneumococcal endocarditis or meningitis. With aminoglycosides the levels for effective therapy of bloodstream infections have been projected to be in the range of 4 to 6 μg per milliliter of gentamicin or tobramycin, and such concentrations are usually accepted as the upper boundary for susceptibility in vitro. However, it is clear that the peak levels of aminoglycosides like gentamicin and tobramycin are sustained for less than an hour. Nonetheless, that time period seems sufficient to achieve rapid killing of many bacterial strains.

Many methods have been introduced to determine the susceptibility of bacteria to antimicrobials in vitro. They have been best standardized for rapidly growing organisms. The most common involve measuring inhibition of growth in a broth medium or the measurement of growth inhibition around an antibiotic-impregnated disk placed on the surface of agar containing the test strain (disk diffusion test). By varying drug concentrations in a series of test tubes or wells, the broth dilution test yields quantitative data on the drug concentration required to inhibit the organism, the minimum inhibitory concentration, or MIC (usually expressed in micrograms per milliliter). Subcultures of broth media make it possible to determine the concentration of drug that kills the test strain—the minimum bactericidal concentration, or MBC. In the disk diffusion test only growth inhibition can be determined, but the diameter of the zone of inhibition usually correlates inversely with the MIC. The two methods give generally similar results (with the disk test being perhaps somewhat easier to perform) and for most infections susceptibility results based on inhibitory measurements are satisfactory. In treating endocarditis, meningitis, and septicemias occurring in immunocompromised hosts, MBC data on infecting isolates are desirable. Bactericidal activity appears to be a requisite for cure of enterococcal endocarditis, as penicillin G or ampicillin inhibits but does not kill this group of organisms. The phenomenon of "tolerance" has also been observed: a wide discrepancy, 32-fold or more, between MIC and MBC. Some investigators believe that strains of staphylococci isolated from endocarditis or osteomyelitis that prove to be tolerant to penicillins or vancomycin should be treated with the addition of gentamicin or rifampin, but this policy remains controversial.

Table 28–2 summarizes the susceptibilities of clinically important gram-positive and gram-negative bacteria in vitro and indicates agents of choice and alternative therapies. The darkened squares (resistant or not indicated) may include drug-pathogen combinations for which clinical evidence fails to support an effect in vitro. Susceptibility testing in vitro is needed because no one agent is predictably effective against all categories of bacteria and because of the increasing incidence and changes in patterns of resistance. There are a few exceptions to this dogma, such as the uniform susceptibility of Group A streptococci to penicillin. On the other hand, relative resistance (intermediate susceptibility) of pneumococci to penicillin G may be increasing, and it is advisable to test blood and cerebrospinal fluid (CSF) isolates.

Antimicrobial resistance may be absolute, in which case increasing the concentration of the agent has no effect, and relative, in which case it may be overcome by dose augmentation. The basis and mechanisms of resistance have become complex, and the simplest approach is to consider (a) the genetic basis for resistance and (b) the actual mechanisms involved. Chromosomal alterations or mutations were the first basis for resistance recognized. These occurred at a relatively predictable rate. Subsequently, a much more common genetic basis has emerged: Plasmids or extrachromosomal DNA elements include R-factors or genetic elements that encode for synthesis of enzymes that functionally inactivate or modify antibiotics. The rapid spread of resistance in some hospital and community settings has been related to acquisition of plasmids by the process of conjugation among gram-negative bacilli and transduction by phages among gram-positive cocci. The mechanisms of resistance are summarized in Table 28–3. The most familiar are the beta-lactamases that hydrolyze to varying degrees agents possessing the beta-lactam ring (penicillins, cephalosporins, monobactams). A great variety of these have been described, occurring in both cocci and bacilli and of both a constitutive and an inducible nature. The latter poses real problems in laboratory diagnosis, as organisms that are initially thought to be susceptible (like Enterobacter species) may harbor inducible enzymes. Beta-lactamases may be of either chromosomal or plasmid origin and are usually responsible for high level resistance that cannot be overcome by dosage escalation. Inactivation can destroy the usefulness of drugs outside the beta-lactam class. A growing number of R-factor–encoded enzymes have been identified that can modify aminoglycosides by the addition of an adenyl, acetyl, or phosphorylating group to hydroxyl or amino groups on the drug structure.

These additions create a sterically altered molecule with ablated or reduced antibacterial activity. Conversely, the design of innovative new antimicrobial agents that prove invulnerable to inactivating enzymes involves further modifications of antibiotic structures that can block the access of inactivating enzymes to target sites. In this sense, the development of new aminoglycosides is analogous to the substitutions that protect the beta-lactam ring from hydrolysis and yield the antistaphylococcal penicillins.

One of the most worrisome mechanisms of resistance involves the ability of bacteria to exclude antimicrobial agents from the cell. Aminoglycosides are actively transported into bacteria, but high-level, multiresistant strains seem to be impermeable to all aminoglycosides. These appear to arise from chromosomal mutation and are selected by aminoglycoside use. The active transport system for aminoglycosides is oxygen dependent. This probably explains the lack of effect of aminoglycosides on anaerobic bacteria, since anaerobic conditions impair the activation of the transport system.

Another type of enzymatic resistance is illustrated by organisms that have acquired a plasmid-encoded "bypass" enzyme that subverts the metabolic block of the sulfonamides.

To have an effect, antibiotics that resist hydrolysis or modification must enter the bacterial cell and reach their target site. Target site alteration explains sudden high-level streptomycin resistance (30S ribosomal subunit) or erythromycin resistance (50S ribosomal subunit). The basis for these changes appears to be chromosomal mutations. A similar basis is postulated for alterations in penicillin-binding proteins, which can result in both low- and high-level resistance.

The indiscriminate use of antimicrobial agents generally favors the emergence of resistance. Antibiotics are not mutagens and do not "create" resistant bacteria. Rather, usage selects for strains that are resistant by virtue of chromosomal mutations or spread of plasmids among the bacterial population. Emergence of resistance during treatment is common with some gram-negative rods such as Serratia and Pseudomonas. This phenomenon must be distinguished from superinfection, whereby a new and usually resistant pathogen becomes a secondary invader. Superinfection may be a consequence of prolonged high-dose therapy and may be avoided by use of narrow-spectrum agents in doses that are not excessive.

PHARMACOLOGIC FACTORS

Laboratory conditions for testing antibacterial agents may differ strikingly from conditions in vivo. In clinical situations the rates of growth of bacteria may be slow, thus affecting the rapidity with which cell wall–active drugs can work. More important, blood and tissue concentrations fluctuate with frequency and method of dosing, and the concentration of drug at the active site of infection may differ from that in body fluids that are more easily sampled. The distribution of agents even within the same class can vary considerably, as they may be metabolized, inactivated, and eliminated by different pathways. Such factors have a crucial effect on the size of doses, the interval between dosing, and possible drug toxicity. Also, the properties of the infecting agent may affect dosing. After exposure of bacteria to an antibiotic, a certain proportion of the population is killed or inhibited and there may be a significant lag time before multiplication of bacteria resumes after the drug concentration falls. This time interval for regrowth has been called the "postantibiotic effect." For different organisms and with different antibiotics, there may be varying postantibiotic effects. Thus, intermittent dosing of agents may be quite feasible if there is rapid killing and a long postantibiotic effect. Some of the more recalcitrant organisms like Pseudomonas regrow rapidly after exposure to antipseudomonal penicillins, and there is very little postantibiotic effect. This argues for more frequent or even continuous dosing, but for the great majority of clinical situations the

TABLE 28–2. SUSCEPTIBILITIES OF CERTAIN BACTERIA TO SELECTED ANTIBIOTICS

Organism	SULFONAMIDES	TRIMETHOPRIM/SULFAMETHOXAZOLE	PENICILLIN G/AMPICILLIN	METHICILLIN/NAFCILLIN/OXACILLIN	CARBENICILLIN/TICARCILLIN	AZLOCILLIN/MEZLOCILLIN/PIPERACILLIN	CEPHALOTHIN/CEPHAPIRIN/CEFAZOLIN	CEFUROXIME/CEFAMANDOLE	CEFOXITIN	CEFOTAXIME/CEFTIZOXIME/MOXALACTAM	CEFTAZIDIME/CEFOPERAZONE/CEFSULODIN	GENTAMICIN/TOBRAMYCIN/SISOMICIN	AMIKACIN/NETILMICIN	POLYMIXIN B/COLISTIN	ERYTHROMYCIN	CLINDAMYCIN	TETRACYCLINES	CHLORAMPHENICOL	VANCOMYCIN	RIFAMPIN	ISONIAZID	NALIDIXIC ACID	METRONIDAZOLE
GRAM POSITIVE																							
Cl. difficile																			1				2
Cl. perfringens			1	3	3	3	3	3	3	3					2		2	3					2
Listeria			1	3	3	3	3	3	3						2	3	3	2	3				
Corynebacterium diphtheriae			1	3	3										1	3	2			2			
Corynebacteria, other																			1	②			
Nocardia	1	1	2		3	3	3			3			3				3	3		3			
Streptococcus			1	3	3	3	3	3	3						2				2				
Str. faecalis			①		3	3						①					3	3	2				
Staph. aureus (pen. sens.)			1	3	3	3	3	3	3	3					2	3		3	3	3			
(pen. resis.)				1			2	2	2	3	3	3	3		3	3		3	2	3			
(meth. resis.)																			1	②			
M. tuberculosis												3	3							①	①		
GRAM NEGATIVE																							
Treponema pallidum			1	3	3	3	3								2		2						
E. coli	3				3	3			3	2	1	1	2	3									
Klebsiella sp.	2						2	2	2	1		1	1	3									
Enterobacter	2									3		2	1	3									
Serratia	2									1		2	1										
Proteus mirabilis	3	1	3		3	3	3	3	3	3	3	1	1										
Providencia												2	1										
Salmonella	2	1	3							3								1					
Shigella	1	2																				3	
Vibrio	2	2															1	3					
P. aeruginosa					②	1					1	1	1	3									
Pseudomonas, other																							
Acinetobacter												2	1										
Campylobacter															1	3	2	2					
Legionella		3													1		3			2			
Hemophilus		2						3		1								1					
N. gonorrhoeae			1					3	2	2													
N. meningitidis			1		3	3				3					2			2		3			
Bacteroides					3	3			2							1		1					1
Brucella	1																1			②			
Yersinia	2																1	2					
Rickettsia																	1	1					

KEY:
- 1 Agent(s) of choice
- 2 Alternative agent
- 3 Usually susceptible
- (blank) Variably susceptible
- (shaded) Resistant or not indicated
- ○ Use in combination

TABLE 28–3. MECHANISMS OF ANTIBACTERIAL RESISTANCE

Antimicrobial Agent	Mechanisms	Representative Organisms
Beta-lactams (penicillins, cephalosporins, carbapenems, monobactams)	Destruction by beta-lactamase	*Staphylococcus aureus* Enterobacteriaceae *Pseudomonas aeruginosa* *Hemophilus influenzae* *Neisseria gonorrhoeae*
	Alteration of penicillin-binding proteins	*Streptococcus pneumoniae* *Staphylococcus aureus*
	Cell wall impermeability	Enterobacter species *Pseudomonas aeruginosa*
Aminoglycosides	Enzymatic modification by N-acetylation, O-phosphorylation, or N-adenylation	*Staphylococcus aureus* Enterobacteriaceae *Pseudomonas aeruginosa* *Streptococcus faecalis*
	Membrane transport O₂ dependent Cell wall impermeability	Anaerobes *Pseudomonas aeruginosa* Serratia species
	Altered 30S ribosome (streptomycin)	*Streptococcus faecalis* Enterobacteriaceae
Chloramphenicol	O-acetylation Cell wall impermeability	*Staphylococcus aureus* Enterobacteriaceae *Pseudomonas aeruginosa*
Erythromycin, clindamycin	Alteration of 23S RNA	*Staphylococcus aureus*
Quinolones	Altered DNA gyrase Cell wall impermeability	Enterobacteriaceae *Pseudomonas aeruginosa*
Tetracyclines	Decreased permeation plus enhanced removal	Enterobacteriaceae
Sulfonamides	Altered dihydrofolate synthetase	*Staphylococcus aureus* Enterobacteriaceae *Neisseria gonorrhoeae*
Trimethoprim	Altered dihydrofolate synthetase Cell wall impermeability Alternate enzymatic pathway	Enterobacteriaceae *Pseudomonas aeruginosa* Enterococci

latter has proved impractical and clinical superiority of continuous dosing has not been established.

Table 28–4 summarizes the recommended doses and some pharmacologic data on most of the commonly used agents. Tissue penetration is linked to serum protein binding. The quantity of drug that diffuses into a site of infection is related to the "peak" or maximum serum concentration of free or unbound drug and the duration that the maximum level is maintained. On the other hand, therapeutic outcome does not always correlate with protein-binding affinity, probably because protein binding is usually easily reversible. Lipid solubility of an antibiotic is another factor affecting tissue penetration and influences the ability of an agent to pass through membranes by nonionic diffusion. Penetration of drug into the spinal fluid is related not only to the drug itself but also to the degree of inflammation in the meninges. Lipid-soluble agents such as chloramphenicol, isoniazid, rifampin, sulfonamides, and metronidazole penetrate spinal fluid well. Aminoglycosides, amphotericin B, and polymyxins do not penetrate well even in the face of inflammation. Penicillins and vancomycin generally penetrate CSF when inflammation is present. Most antibiotics commonly used are excreted primarily through the kidney, but notable exceptions include erythromycin and chloramphenicol. Thus, it may be possible to treat infections of the urinary tract with doses smaller than are required for serious systemic disease, because high urine levels are achieved with most agents. Urine and bile regularly contain higher concentrations of antibiotics than does serum. Penicillins and tetracyclines are concentrated in bile, but aminoglycosides enter bile less well, particularly when liver disease or obstruction is present. Drugs like tetracyclines and clindamycin diffuse readily into bone and have been used successfully in osteomyelitis. Agents that enter prostate tissue well include sulfonamides, trimethoprim, erythromycin, and doxycycline. Some drugs may fail because of pharmacokinetic properties. For instance, amoxicillin is so well absorbed in the small intestine that effective therapeutic levels are usually not achieved in the colon, thereby limiting use for Shigella infections.

Factors besides drug levels per se may limit drug activity. Purulent secretions and high concentrations of calcium and magnesium ions antagonize aminoglycoside activity. Erythromycin and aminoglycosides have markedly diminished activity in acidic environments. Cephalosporins like cephalothin can be metabolized to relatively inactive derivatives, but metabolites of cefotaxime are still quite active.

There is evidence that a high ratio of bactericidal activity in serum (e.g., serum diluted 1:8 or greater possessing a killing effect) against infecting strains is associated with therapeutic success. Such activity may merely reflect the serum concentration required to achieve effective therapy at a site of infection. It should not be assumed that a given dose corrected for weight or body surface area will reliably produce the same levels in all patients. With agents like aminoglycosides that are potentially toxic, therapeutic monitoring is clearly indicated during serious systemic infection. For example, gentamicin peak (postinfusion) levels should exceed 4 μg per milliliter and trough (or "valley") levels should be less than 2 μg per milliliter. Route of administration is important, since orally administered drugs may be poorly absorbed in serious systemic infections. For patients who are in shock, intramuscular or subcutaneous injections should clearly be avoided and all medications should be given intravenously.

MODIFICATION OF DRUG DOSES IN RENAL AND HEPATIC FAILURE

Since the majority of antibiotics are excreted via the kidney, dosage adjustment must be considered in moderate-to-severe renal failure. Many studies have related serum creatinine level or creatinine clearance to degree of dosage modification, and useful nomograms have been derived that may aid in the calculation of dosage. Table 28–4 indicates the agents affected by renal failure and dialysis. Many of these guidelines have been derived by study of patients who are in the "steady state," i.e., patients in renal failure who are on dialysis programs but who may not be infected. Thus, they may not manifest the hemodynamic instability that is often present in patients with serious systemic infection. In unstable patients, there is no substitute for accurate assays of serum or plasma drug concentrations as a guide to appropriate dosing. While dosage modification is indicated in patients with serious renal failure, the initial doses should probably be the same. The

TABLE 28–4. DOSAGE, PHARMACOLOGIC FACTORS, AND ADJUSTMENT IN RENAL AND HEPATIC FAILURE

Class/Agent	Dose Systemic Infection	Oral	Protein Binding (%)	Normal Serum Half-Life (Hrs)	Hepatic Failure	Renal Failure	Serum Levels Affected by Dialysis
Aminoglycosides							
Amikacin	5–7 mg/kg/q8	—	0	2–3	No	Major	Yes
Gentamicin	1.7 mg/kg/q8	—	0	2–3	No	Major	Yes
Netilmicin	1.7 mg/kg/q8	—	0	2–3	No	Major	Yes
Tobramycin	1.7 mg/kg/q8	—	0	2–3	No	Major	Yes
Antifungal Agents							
Amphotericin B	0.7–1 mg/kg/d	—	90	24	No	No	No
Flucytosine	40 mg/kg/q6	Yes	10	3	No	Major	Yes
Ketoconazole	6 mg/kg/d	Yes	98	8	Avoid	No	No
Miconazole	5 mg/kg/q6–8	—	92	2.2	Avoid	No	No
Antituberculous Agents							
Ethambutol	15 mg/kg/d	Yes	10	1.5	No	Major	Yes
Isoniazid	5 mg/kg/d	Yes	10	3	Yes	Minor	Yes
Rifampin	10 mg/kg/d	Yes	70	3	Yes	Minor	No
Cephalosporins							
Cefaclor	7 mg/kg/q6	Yes	20	1	No	Yes	Yes
Cefamandole	30 mg/kg/q6	—	70	1	No	Yes	Yes
Cefazolin	15 mg/kg/q6	—	80	2	No	Major	Yes
Cefotetan	30 mg/kg/q12	—	85	3	No	Major	Yes
Cefoxitin	30 mg/kg/q6	—	70	0.7	No	Yes	Yes
Cephalothin	30 mg/kg/q6	—	70	0.7	Minor	Yes	Yes
Cephalexin	7 mg/kg/q6	Yes	15	1	No	Yes	Yes
Cefoperazone	30 mg/kg/q8–12	—	90	2	Some	Minor	Yes
Cefotaxime	30 mg/kg/q6	—	50	1.2	Some	Minor	Yes
Cefsulodin†	30 mg/kg/q6–8	—	20	1.6	No	Major	Yes
Ceftizoxime	30 mg/kg/q6–8	—	50	1.3	No	Minor	Yes
Ceftriaxone	30 mg/kg/q12–24	—	90	8	No	Yes	Yes
Ceftazidime	30 mg/kg/q8	—	60	2	No	Major	Yes
Moxalactam	30 mg/kg/q8–12	—	50	2	No	Major	Yes
Penicillins							
Amoxicillin	7 mg/kg/q6	Yes	20	1	No	Yes	Yes
Ampicillin	30 mg/kg/q6	Yes	20	1	No	Yes	Yes
Azlocillin	50 mg/kg/q6	—	50	1	Minor	Major	Yes
Carbenicillin	70 mg/kg/q4	—	50	1	Minor	Major	Yes
Cloxacillin	7 mg/kg/q6	Yes	95	0.5	Minor	Minor	Yes
Dicloxacillin	7 mg/kg/q6	Yes	97	0.5	Minor	Minor	No
Methicillin	30 mg/kg/q4–6	—	30	0.5	No	Minor	No
Mezlocillin	50 mg/kg/q6	—	50	1	No	Major	Yes
Nafcillin	30 mg/kg/q4–6	—	90	0.5	Yes	Minor	No
Oxacillin	30 mg/kg/q4–6	—	90	0.5	Yes	Minor	Yes
Penicillin G	0.3–4 million U q4–6h	Yes	60	0.5	No	Yes	Yes
Penicillin V	7 mg/kg/q6	Yes	80	1	No	Minor	Yes
Piperacillin	40 mg/kg/q6	—	50	1	Minor	Major	Yes
Ticarcillin	40 mg/kg/4–6	—	50	1	Minor	Major	Yes
Quinolones							
Ciprofloxacin	10 mg/kg/q12	Yes	30	3	No	Major	Yes
Nalidixic acid	15 mg/kg/q6	Yes	90	1.5	No	Avoid	No
Norfloxacin	6 mg/kg/q12	Yes	15	3	No	Major	Yes
Tetracycline							
Chlortetracycline	7 mg/kg/q6	Yes	50	5	Avoid	Avoid	No
Demeclocycline	7 mg/kg/q12	Yes	50	10	Avoid	Avoid	Yes
Doxycycline	1.5 mg/kg/q12–24	Yes	90	15–20	No	No	No
Minocycline	3 mg/kg/q12–24	Yes	90	15	Avoid	Avoid	No
Oxytetracycline	7 mg/kg/q6–12	Yes	35	8	Avoid	Avoid	No
Tetracycline HCl	7 mg/kg/q6	Yes	50	7	Avoid	Avoid	No
Sulfonamides							
Sulfadiazine	15 mg/kg/q6	Yes	50	3	Avoid	Major	Yes
Sulfamethoxazole	12 mg/kg/q8	Yes	50	6	Avoid	Major	Yes
Trimethoprim (used with above)	2.3 mg/kg/q8–12	Yes	60	10	No	Major	Yes
Sulfisoxazole	15 mg/kg/q6	Yes	50	6	Avoid	Major	Yes
Other Agents							
Aztreonam	30 mg/kg/q8	—	60	2.0	No	Major	Yes
Chloramphenicol	7–15 mg/kg/q6	Yes	30	1.5	Some	Minor	Yes
Clindamycin	7 mg/kg/q6	Yes	90	2.5	Some	Minor	No
Colistin	2 mg/kg/q12	—	0	5	No	Avoid	No
Erythromycin	7 mg/kg/q6	Yes	20	1.5	Some	No	No
Imipenem	7.5 mg/kg/q6	—	15	1	No	Avoid	Yes
Metronidazole	15 mg/kg/q6	Yes	20	8	No	No	Yes
Nitrofurantoin	1 mg/kg/q6	Yes	60	0.3	No	Avoid	No
Polymyxin B	1.5 U/kg/q12	—	0	5	No	Avoid	No
Spectinomycin	30 mg/kg	—	0	2	No	Avoid	No
Vancomycin	7 mg/kg/q6	Yes*	10	6	No	No	No

*Not systemically absorbed.
†Investigational drug in the United States.

timing of the second dose should probably be based on levels anticipated from nomograms, but peak levels after the end of the second dose and third dose should be monitored in order to calculate the next doses. Increased trough concentrations may help to warn of incipient toxicity. As a general principle, many pharmacologic agents are given every three to four half-lives. In renal failure these half-lives are prolonged many-fold. One strategy is to prolong the interval between maintenance doses, which can result in fairly high "peak" or postinfusion levels and rather prolonged (and occasionally subtherapeutic) troughs. Another strategy is to give more frequent doses but to decrease the size of maintenance doses. Subtherapeutic levels may be avoided by the latter tactic, but the approach could be more nephrotoxic (as in the case of aminoglycoside agents). Dialyzable agents are similarly cleared by peritoneal or extracorporeal hemodialysis. Following dialysis a dose approximately two thirds to three quarters of a maintenance dose should be given, depending upon the degree of removal of the antibiotic by dialysis and the timing of the previous maintenance dose.

Several important antibiotics are metabolized in the liver and are partially excreted in the bile. Agents primarily metabolized by the liver include the sulfonamides, chloramphenicol, and tetracycline. There is usually little reason to alter the dose of penicillin, cephalosporins, and aminoglycosides in patients with liver disease. Even with erythromycin, ethambutol, and clindamycin, there is little evidence that dosage reduction is necessary except in severe hepatic failure. For instance, clindamycin should probably be reduced to half-normal doses after two to three days of treatment. Chloramphenicol total dosage should be restricted to 1.5 to 2.0 grams per day (adult) and erythromycin should be reduced to perhaps one half the normal dose after two or three days of treatment. Drugs to be avoided in hepatic failure include sulfonamides and tetracyclines.

COMBINATION ANTIMICROBIAL THERAPY

Use of combinations of antibacterial agents is exceedingly common. The rationale for their use may be summarized as follows: (1) Prior to the identification of pathogens infecting critically ill subjects, combinations offer a broader, more comprehensive antibacterial spectrum than a single agent. (2) Use of a drug combination may eradicate an infection that cannot be cured by a single agent, such as the effect of penicillin on enterococci. Addition of an aminoglycoside or a potentiating agent such as rifampin may result in bactericidal activity at a deep-seated focus of infection, as in endocarditis. (3) Combinations are indicated in the treatment of mixed infections, since not all of the pathogens may be susceptible to a single agent. (4) Combinations may decrease the opportunity for emergence of resistance. This has been documented in tuberculosis. (5) Combinations may interact additively or synergistically against infecting organisms. As a result, there may be an enhancement of antibacterial activity and/or enhanced rate of killing. The latter may lead to more rapid clearing of infection with reduction in duration of therapy. Combinations may permit the use of a lower dosage of one or more components of the regimen, particularly the more toxic component, thereby avoiding undesirable side effects. More rapid killing or greater potency in vivo may be more directly beneficial in patients with impaired host defenses. Some clinical studies suggest an improved clinical response not only when drugs used to treat endocarditis interact synergistically but in sepsis occurring in immunocompromised patients.

The converse of synergism is antagonism between antimicrobial agents. This is best described for combinations of bactericidal plus bacteriostatic agents. Penicillin-type drugs require cell growth to exert their lethal effect. When penicillins are combined with static drugs like tetracycline, only growth inhibition may result. Clinical studies in humans indicate poorer results in treatment of pneumococcal meningitis with penicillin plus tetracycline than with penicillin alone.

Empiric therapy is presumptive or "blind" therapy where clinical severity of likely infection dictates that treatment be started. It is not necessarily combination therapy, as some single agents can still be quite effective. Intelligent choices in the absence of microbiologic information can be made based on the clinical syndrome and the likely infecting pathogen. Epidemiologic factors as well as host factors enter into the decision. The setting in which the patient develops infection or a prior exposure or travel history can be of considerable value. Pneumonias contracted outside of the hospital are usually due to streptococci (and pneumococci) and penicillin-sensitive anaerobes. An "atypical" or diffuse pattern raises the likelihood that community-acquired pneumonia will be better treated with erythromycin than penicillin. Infections that occur in the nosocomial setting or in markedly neutropenic patients should always be initially treated with therapy directed against gram-negative bacilli.

Table 28–5 summarizes recommendations for initial empiric therapy by clinical syndrome.

SPECIFIC ANTIMICROBIAL AGENTS

Table 28–2 summarizes recommended choices of antimicrobial agents for specific infecting agents. The organisms are

TABLE 28–5. INITIAL EMPIRIC THERAPY FOR SERIOUS INFECTION

Syndrome	Qualifying Factors	Recommended Treatment
Septicemia	Immunocompromised Host	
	Neutrophil Count >500 μl	Cephalosporin (cefazolin) + aminoglycoside (gentamicin, tobramycin)
	Neutrophil Count <500 μl	Piperacillin or ceftazidime + aminoglycoside (amikacin, tobramycin)
	Normal Host	
	Urinary source	Ampicillin + gentamicin or third-generation cephalosporin
	Biliary source	Ampicillin + gentamicin or third-generation cephalosporin
	Abdominal or pelvic source	Aminoglycoside + clindamycin or cefoxitin, or broad-spectrum penicillin
	No source	Oxacillin + gentamicin
	Neonate	
	<48 hrs old	Ampicillin + either cefotaxime or ceftriaxone
	>48 hrs old	Ampicillin + oxacillin + aminoglycoside
Meningitis	<6 years	Ampicillin + cefotaxime or ceftriaxone
	>6 years	Ampicillin or penicillin G
Brain Abscess		Penicillin G + cefotaxime or ceftriaxone + metronidazole
Pneumonia	Community acquired	Ampicillin or penicillin G ± erythromycin
	Postinfluenzal	Antistaphylococcal penicillin or cephalosporin
	Postaspiration	Ampicillin or clindamycin
	Nosocomial	Azlocillin or piperacillin + aminoglycoside, or third-generation cephalosporin + aminoglycoside

divided into gram-positive and gram-negative isolates, and antimicrobial agents that are similar are grouped together. Clearly, such a table oversimplifies the appropriate choices for various agents. In some situations, there is no clear-cut agent of first choice, and any member of a class may be appropriate. Differences in pharmacology, cost, and side effects might lead to a selection of one agent in preference to another. There is an increasing divergence in antibacterial spectrum among the newer beta-lactam agents, such as the antipseudomonal penicillins and the third-generation cephalosporins. Among the aminoglycosides, anticipated efficacy may be expressed as follows: While gentamicin and tobramycin remain the most widely prescribed, gram-negative bacilli that are resistant to these agents are more likely to be inhibited by netilmicin and amikacin.

Few oral agents are listed in Table 28–2, but it may be inferred that any of the oral antistaphylococcal agents such as cloxacillin or dicloxacillin could be used to treat mild infections due to penicillinase-producing staphylococci. The spectrum of oral cephalosporins such as cephalexin or cephradine mimics that of cephalothin or cefazolin. In the case of Group A hemolytic streptococci, it would not be necessary to test for susceptibility of these organisms against penicillin G and related penicillins in vitro, since all would be expected to be susceptible. It would, however, be highly desirable if one were to use a penicillin against the Klebsiella species to test that penicillin for susceptibility in vitro; it should probably not be presumed that antibiotics such as piperacillin or mezlocillin will be effective in vitro and in vivo without specific testing. Some agents should always be used in combination to treat serious bloodstream or systemic infections, such as antituberculous therapy (isoniazid plus at least one other agent) or enterococcal sepsis with or without endocarditis (the combination of either a penicillin or a vancomycin with an aminoglycoside). Older agents of the aminoglycoside class such as streptomycin or kanamycin are no longer widely used because their activity is more comprehensively covered by newer drugs (gentamicin and amikacin). The exception to this might be in the conventional therapy of *Mycobacterium tuberculosis*, for which streptomycin is still indicated.

Sulfonamides and Sulfa-Containing Combinations

Sulfonamides were the first chemotherapeutic agents to be introduced into wide clinical use. They are bacteriostatic and previously were quite active against many gram-positive and gram-negative organisms. They are, however, no longer among the first choices for serious systemic infections, the exception being *Nocardia asteroides* infections. Sulfonamides remain effective therapy for coliform organisms causing community-acquired urinary tract infections, but they are unreliable against hospital-acquired microorganisms. More commonly used to treat a wide variety of more serious bacterial infections is the fixed combination (1:5) of trimethoprim and sulfamethoxazole. Synergism in vitro against many enteric bacteria can be demonstrated with this combination, yet trimethoprim is a highly active agent itself. A major argument in favor of continued use of the fixed combination is that it may reduce the likelihood of the development of resistance to one component in the pair. Trimethoprim/sulfamethoxazole is usually active against enteric bacteria and *H. influenzae* (including most penicillinase-producing strains), and it has been effective in parasitic infections such as *Pneumocystis carinii* pneumonia. The diffusion of trimethoprim into prostate fluid makes it a useful agent in prostatic infections. Central nervous system penetration is good. The oral preparation is well absorbed, although a parenteral form is available for patients in whom gastrointestinal absorption may be erratic. Occasional side effects include neutropenia and all of the dermal and systemic hypersensitivity reactions that have been well associated with sulfonamides.

Penicillin G and Related Agents

The primary spectrum of penicillin G (benzyl penicillin) is gram-positive, with such organisms as *Streptococcus pyogenes*, *Streptococcus pneumoniae*, and *Streptococcus viridans* remaining exquisitely susceptible. Procaine penicillin is readily administered intramuscularly, and because of slow absorption, dosing of 600,000 units every 12 hours remains effective therapy for pneumococcal pneumonia. Benzathine penicillin is a long-acting (two to three weeks) agent that is slowly released after intramuscular injection and provides therapeutic levels for streptococcal pharyngitis and some forms of syphilis and prophylactic effect against acute rheumatic fever. For oral use in mild respiratory infections, phenoxymethyl penicillin (V) is acid stable and preferable to penicillin G. In large doses penicillin G is still effective against *Neisseria meningitidis*, most *N. gonorrhoeae*, and anaerobic organisms including Clostridium species, but usually not against strains of *Bacteroides fragilis*. Against enterococci, penicillin G or ampicillin should be used in combination with an aminoglycoside such as streptomycin or gentamicin. Ampicillin may be preferable in the treatment of Salmonella, central nervous system infections due to Hemophilus strains, and *Listeria monocytogenes*. When used in large doses, penicillin G or ampicillin is effective against a few gram-negative organisms, most notably *Proteus mirabilis* (but not other Proteus species). Penicillin G and related penicillins should not be used against the great majority of coagulase-producing staphylococci, most of which now produce beta-lactamases.

Antistaphylococcal Penicillins

The antistaphylococcal penicillins are beta-lactamase–stable and relatively narrow in spectrum. Parenteral preparations include methicillin, nafcillin, and oxacillin. There is little choice among this category of agents in terms of antistaphylococcal activity. There may be some differences in side effects, with methicillin possibly associated with more hypersensitivity nephritis and oxacillin with a greater incidence of abnormal serum elevations of hepatic enzymes. When used in appropriate doses, the central nervous system penetration is probably adequate to treat meningitis. The oral antistaphylococcal agents should not be used to treat serious infections, but mild or moderately severe infections may respond to dicloxacillin or cloxacillin. Combination of antistaphylococcal penicillins with an aminoglycoside or rifampin has been recommended for refractory staphylococcal infections or when the isolates demonstrate tolerance. *Staphylococcus epidermidis* may produce beta-lactamase like most coagulase-positive *Staphylococcus aureus*. However, serious infections like prosthetic valve endocarditis are better treated with vancomycin plus rifampin or an aminoglycoside.

Broad-Spectrum Penicillins and Related Compounds

Although ampicillin and amoxicillin are technically classified as broad-spectrum penicillins, the extended spectrum really only includes *Escherichia coli*, *H. influenzae*, Salmonella, and Shigella species. Even then, amoxicillin should not be used orally for Shigella infections because excellent absorption from the upper gastrointestinal tract results in subtherapeutic levels in the lower gut. Other penicillins like carbenicillin, ticarcillin, mezlocillin, azlocillin, or piperacillin are notable for their activity against *Pseudomonas aeruginosa*, most Proteus species, and anaerobic pathogens such as *Bacteroides fragilis*. On a weight basis, carbenicillin and ticarcillin have relatively weak antipseudomonal activity and so must be used in considerably larger doses than most penicillins, in the range of 18 to 30 grams a day for adults (200 to 400 mg per kilogram). The large sodium load given with such doses may aggravate congestive failure and cause electrolyte abnormalities. While these antipseudomonal penicillins are important agents for serious infections, emergence of resistance and variable stability to beta-lactamases has led to the tendency to combine these agents with an aminoglycoside. They are quite active against the coccal organisms that ampicillin usually inhibits, but none of these agents should be used against coagulase-positive staphylococci. The combination of a beta-lactamase inhibitor (clavulanate) with amoxicillin or ticarcillin confers stability to staphylococcal penicillinase and broadens coverage of some gram-negative bacilli. Other potential uses of extended-spectrum penicillins include treatment of infection caused by Acinetobacter species, Listeria, and a variety of anaerobes. Like the antistaphylococcal penicillins, their half-life is relatively short, but protein binding is low. Thus, frequent dosing at four- to six-hour intervals is usually necessary. Newer antipseudomonal penicillins such as mezlocillin, azlocillin, or piperacillin are augmented in their antipseudomonal activity, in the case of the latter two approximately six- to eight-fold by weight in comparison to carbenicillin when organisms are tested at low inoculum concentrations. On the other hand, the tendency has been to use smaller doses of these more potent penicillins in order to avoid the side effects associated with large doses of carbenicillin. The result is that no clear-cut clinical differences have been found between these agents when they are used in combination with aminoglycosides. Some of these newer penicillins, such as mezlocillin and piperacillin, have variable activity against Klebsiella species and must be tested prior to use.

Newer compounds that possess a beta-lactam nucleus (and thus are related to the penicillins) include (1) imipenem, an agent with very broad activity against gram-positive and gram-negative bacteria; and (2) monobactams, such as aztreonam or carumonam.* These latter compounds are entirely devoid of activity against gram-positive bacteria, but, like the third-generation cephalosporins, they are potent agents for treatment of gram-negative bacillary infections.

Cephalosporins

Cephalosporins are structurally related to penicillins, yet there are major differences in activity between these agents in vitro and in vivo. The first cephalosporins, such as cephalothin, cephaloridine, and cefazolin, were effective against penicillinase-producing staphylococci as well as pneumococci and streptococci (except enterococci). Additionally, they offered good activity against several important gram-negative pathogens such as E. coli, Klebsiella, and Proteus mirabilis. Despite activity in vitro, they are not effective against Salmonella and Shigella and do not penetrate the blood-brain barrier. The enormous popularity of these agents appears related to a low incidence of side effects, fairly broad coverage against community-acquired respiratory and urinary tract pathogens, and the availability of both oral and parenteral dosing. Nevertheless, these compounds have not been considered the agents of choice for any serious systemic infections. They have been successfully used to treat patients with a history of mild penicillin-type reactions, such as rash, but not urticaria or anaphylaxis. With the development of newer cephalosporins the principal advantages of these older compounds (often referred to as "the first generation") have been in the prophylactic surgical usage and relatively greater activity against penicillinase-producing Staphylococcus aureus.

The so-called "second-generation" cephalosporins offer a few improvements over cephalothin and cefazolin. Cefoxitin is a compound with fairly consistent activity against B. fragilis. Cefamandole and cefuroxime lack the anaerobic spectrum of cefoxitin but have modestly improved activity against some gram-negative organisms not inhibited by the first generation, such as H. influenzae and Enterobacter species. Oral agents include cefaclor, which has greater activity against penicillinase-producing H. influenzae than cephalexin.

The newest cephalosporins (often referred to as "third generation"), or structurally related compounds such as moxalactam, a 1-oxy-beta-lactam, have markedly enhanced activity against enteric bacteria as well as variable coverage of P. aeruginosa. These compounds are stable against the beta-lactamases of H. influenzae and N. gonorrhoeae and cross the blood-brain barrier in sufficient concentrations to offer effective therapy for gram-negative meningitis (with perhaps the exception of P. aeruginosa infection). Among the agents shown to be effective in gram-negative central nervous system infections are cefotaxime, moxalactam, ceftazidime, and ceftriaxone. Several of these agents have a much longer half-life than first-generation cephalosporins, permitting dosing intervals of 8 to 12 hours. In the case of one agent, ceftriaxone, once-a-day dosing has been possible in some infections because of an eight-hour half-life. The antipseudomonal activity of these compounds is variable; nonetheless, newer antipseudomonal cephalosporins like cefsulodin* and ceftazidime represent some of the most potent antipseudomonal agents introduced into clinical practice, and these compounds appear to be significantly safer than aminoglycosides. Table 28–6 summarizes the relative properties of these agents, as well as selected comments. As a general rule, the increased activity against gram-negative pathogens is also coupled with relatively diminished activity against gram-positive cocci. While the gram-positive, particularly antistaphylococcal, coverage of these agents may be satisfactory for initial therapy, serious staphylococcal disease as well as pneumococcal infection is better and certainly more economically treated with older beta-lactam agents (e.g., oxacillin, penicillin G, respectively). These agents are also not without serious untoward effects, including the triggering of disulfiram reactions, inhibition of platelet adhesiveness, and hypoprothrombinemia. In many patients with community-acquired and mild to moderately severe nosocomial infections, third-generation cephalosporins offer the potential of effective single-agent therapy. The results in immunocompromised hosts suggest that these compounds may still be more efficacious when combined with aminoglycosides.

Chloramphenicol

Chloramphenicol is an oral or parenterally administered drug whose spectrum makes it useful for a wide variety of bacterial and rickettsial infections. The antibacterial spectrum includes gram-positive organisms such as streptococci and staphylococci, but the agent has not been considered to be one of the more potent antistaphylococcal compounds. It is usually bacteriostatic except against H. influenzae, against which it is bactericidal. Many enteric organisms are inhibited by chloramphenicol, but Pseudomonas strains are usually resistant. Important therapeutic uses include typhoid fever, central nervous system infections, anaerobic infections, intraocular infections, and serious rickettsial infections. Against B. fragilis, it remains one of the most useful agents. On the other hand, chloramphenicol has been associated with severe hematologic toxicity. In the great majority of individuals receiving courses in excess of one week of chloramphenicol, there is a dose-dependent inhibition of erythropoiesis. Some patients, estimated at 1 in 50,000, have developed irreversible aplastic anemia following oral or parenteral dosing. While it remains a highly effective agent in selected situations, there are now a number of very reasonable alternatives to chloramphenicol. The unpredictability of the hematologic toxicity should lead physicians to reserve this agent for serious infections in which there are major indications for avoiding alternative drugs.

---

*Investigational drug in the United States.

*Investigational drug in the United States.

TABLE 28–6. THIRD-GENERATION CEPHALOSPORINS AND RELATED COMPOUNDS

Agent	Protein Binding (%)	Peak Serum Levels (μg/ml) After 1 gm I.V.	Half-Life (Hours)	Comments
Aztreonam*	60	50	2	No activity vs. gram-positive organisms
Cefmenoxime*	77	40	1	Weak antipseudomonal activity
Cefoperazone	90	125	2.1	Primary excretion is biliary with little dose adjustment in renal failure
Cefotaxime	38	40	1.1	Good CNS penetration but weak antipseudomonal activity
Cefsulodin*	30	65	1.5	Primarily antipseudomonal activity, not much else
Ceftazidime	20	70	1.9	Potent antipseudomonal activity
Ceftizoxime	30	75	1.4	Potent gram-negative activity except for Pseudomonas
Ceftriaxone	85	140	8.0	Very long half-life, good CNS penetration, but poor antipseudomonal activity
Imipenem	15	50	0.9	Broad gram-positive and gram-negative activity
Moxalactam	50	60	2.3	Good anaerobe coverage but associated with coagulopathy.

*Investigational drug in the United States.
CNS = central nervous system.

The Tetracyclines

Tetracyclines inhibit a wide range of gram-positive and gram-negative bacteria as well as Mycoplasma species, but they are not agents of choice for any serious bacterial infections. Their activity against gram-positive organisms is static, and the results do not appear to approach those obtained with bactericidal agents. Gram-negative coverage includes E. coli and Klebsiella species, but there are major gaps in their spectrum, including Pseudomonas, Serratia species, and other serious nosocomial pathogens. Tetracycline may be useful in urinary tract infections, rickettsial infections, mycoplasmal infections, and the prophylaxis or treatment of traveler's diarrhea (caused by toxigenic E. coli). Older preparations such as chlortetracycline or oxytetracycline have been supplanted by tetracycline HCl, minocycline, or doxycycline. The last-named two preparations have certain pharmacologic advantages, including less frequent dosing, and doxycycline may be used in renal failure.

Erythromycin

This is the most commonly available member of the class of macrolide antibiotics. Traditionally, erythromycin has been regarded as an agent of second choice for streptococcal and staphylococcal infections, to be used in those patients with history of serious penicillin allergy. In this regard, erythromycin remains a useful agent, but its primary appeal in recent years has been its clinical efficacy against several important new causes of infection such as Mycoplasma, Legionella, Chlamydia, and Campylobacter species. Against all of these pathogens, erythromycin can be considered the agent of choice. In serious respiratory infections, erythromycin should be administered parenterally, but this use is associated with high incidence of phlebitis. The compound is one of the safest of all antimicrobials, but mild gastrointestinal disturbances are common. Several oral preparations are available, but none seems clinically superior.

Clindamycin and Lincomycin

Clindamycin and lincomycin mimic some of the spectrum of erythromycin. Their major advantage over erythromycin is greater activity against anaerobes, particularly B. fragilis. Nonetheless, the antianaerobic spectrum of these compounds is not complete. In the treatment of intra-abdominal infections these agents are usually combined with aminoglycosides for gram-negative coverage. A major problem with clindamycin therapy has been antibiotic-associated diarrhea and pseudomembranous colitis. The incidence and severity of this complication vary, and the problem is not always associated with clindamycin. The development of gastrointestinal symptoms on treatment should be a warning to discontinue use of these agents.

Metronidazole

Metronidazole has long been used for the therapy of trichomoniasis, amebiasis, and giardiasis. Subsequently, it has been found to be a highly effective and bactericidal agent against many anaerobic pathogens, including B. fragilis. It is available in both oral and parenteral forms and must be considered the therapy of choice for B. fragilis infections involving deep-seated foci such as heart valves and the central nervous system. Many infections involving anaerobes are mixed processes that also involve aerobic organisms. Because it is almost exclusively active against anaerobic pathogens, metronidazole is usually combined with other antimicrobials. The drug must be metabolized to its active form. Its excellent distribution, rapid bactericidal activity, and penetration in "closed spaces" are appealing characteristics, but it also has the potential of inducing disulfiram reactions and potentiating the effects of warfarin (Coumadin). There is concern about metronidazole's carcinogenicity in animals and mutagenicity in bacteria. These effects have not been demonstrated in humans, but it seems wise to restrict this agent to use in severe infections.

Rifampin

Rifampin is a semisynthetic derivative of rifamycin B and has been used principally for the therapy of tuberculosis. It is one of the most potent and effective antituberculous agents available, with a spectrum that includes both M. tuberculosis and atypical organisms. It has been found to be very active against the wide variety of gram-positive and gram-negative organisms, including staphylococci (both coagulase-positive and coagulase-negative) and Legionella species. The compound is one of the few that has been effective in terminating meningococcal carrier state, and it inhibits methicillin-resistant staphylococci. The principal drawback to the use of rifampin is that almost all microorganisms have the ability to develop resistance rapidly. Therefore, even in tuberculosis this drug must be combined with another active agent. It seems useful as an adjunct to other antibacterial agents, such as in combination with antistaphylococcal penicillins to treat "tolerant" strains in endocarditis and meningitis. It inhibits methicillin-resistant staphylococci but is best used with vancomycin. Another potential advantage has been excellent penetration into phagocytic cells. A disadvantage, however, is its potent ability to induce enzymes that decrease the half-life of a number of other pharmacologic agents, including steroids, sulfonylureas, and digitoxin.

Vancomycin

Initially developed during an intense search for agents active against coagulase-producing staphylococci, this agent developed a reputation for efficacy as well as toxicity to the eighth cranial nerve and to renal function. More modern preparations of vancomycin do not appear to be strongly associated with these side effects. Indeed, the compound has been used effectively to treat serious infections in patients with renal failure because it is not significantly excreted by the kidneys; prolonged bactericidal activity results from widely spaced doses. The spectrum includes not only *Staphylococcus aureus*, but also *Staphylococcus epidermidis*, *Staphylococcus faecalis* (enterococci), and Corynebacteria species. Vancomycin has not been considered an agent of primary choice for *Staphylococcus aureus* but is an effective alternative in the penicillin-allergic patient. In prosthetic valve endocarditis caused by *Staphylococcus epidermidis*, it is often considered the agent of choice in combination with rifampin or gentamicin or both.

Aminoglycosides

Aminoglycosides are rapidly bactericidal against most of the clinically important gram-negative bacilli, including enteric bacteria and *P. aeruginosa*. Most isolates of *Staphylococcus aureus* are also inhibited by aminoglycosides. The initial compounds of this series, like streptomycin, were also shown to be effective against *M. tuberculosis*, and in combination with a penicillin, either streptomycin or gentamicin offers the best available therapy for deep-seated enterococcal infections. Older agents like streptomycin, neomycin, and kanamycin are considerably less useful today because they appear to be relatively more toxic or have been supplanted by agents with greater activity against *P. aeruginosa*. The contemporary aminoglycosides include gentamicin, tobramycin, netilmicin, and amikacin. The last two compounds offer some advantages in that they are stable to inactivation by some of the plasmid-encoded enzymes that acetylate, adenylate, or phosphorylate the older agents. Thus, amikacin or netilmicin may be preferred to treat infections caused by gentamicin- or tobramycin-resistant strains, but susceptibility testing in vitro is necessary because some isolates may be resistant to all agents within this class. Rapid bactericidal effect and good distribution except for the central nervous system make these highly desirable compounds for the treatment of serious systemic gram-negative infections. Unfortunately, aminoglycosides are toxic to renal function, can cause eighth cranial nerve (both cochlear and vestibular function) and renal damage, and occasionally manifest curare-like effects. Pharmacologically, there is a narrow range between the therapeutic levels achievable by dosing every 8 to 12 hours and levels that are associated with toxicity. Aminoglycoside therapy should be closely monitored by frequent blood level determinations in treating serious infections, when large doses are used for prolonged courses. These agents are either additive or often synergistic with beta-lactam compounds against pathogens such as *P. aeruginosa*, Serratia species, and other gram-negative rods. For immunocompromised hosts, aminoglycosides remain an important component of therapy, usually as part of a combination with a beta-lactam agent. Aminoglycosides do not penetrate well into the central nervous system or bone and are not absorbed via the oral route. They are perhaps overused as topical agents and in that setting the rapid emergence of resistance has been documented. For prophylaxis in colonic surgery, older aminoglycosides like neomycin or kanamycin may suffice in regimens that transiently suppress the growth of aerobic bowel flora.

Spectinomycin also belongs to the aminoglycoside class and is used exclusively for the treatment of gonorrhea when penicillin-type agents have failed. Such antigonococcal activity is shared by other members of the class.

Polymyxin, Colistin (Polymyxin E)

Polymyxin B and colistin (polymyxin E) are closely related cationic polypeptide detergents that bind to the lipoproteins of many gram-negative outer cell membranes. They are rapidly bactericidal in vitro, particularly against *P. aeruginosa* and enteric rods except Proteus species and Serratia. These agents are without effect against gram-positive organisms. Resistance has rarely emerged on therapy. Because of poor clinical results and nephrotoxic potential, the use of these compounds has decreased markedly. Lack of clinical efficacy could be due to properties of poor diffusion and rapid binding to tissues.

Quinolones

The quinolone group of agents includes older compounds like nalidixic acid and newer, more active agents such as ciprofloxacin,* norfloxacin, and ofloxacin.* Nalidixic acid has few modern uses and may be regarded as a urinary antiseptic for suppression of chronic infection. The newer quinolones have very broad activity against both gram-positive and gram-negative organisms (including Mycoplasma and Legionella) and can be administered orally. Their use is best defined for urinary tract infection and, depending on pharmacology, for respiratory and bone infection. Quinolone therapy for serious systemic infections requires additional study.

Urinary Antiseptics

Mandelamine, nitrofurantoin, and nalidixic acid are agents that are effective only in urinary tract infections, and usually as suppressive therapy in chronic infections. Resistance to some of these compounds may emerge rapidly. They may be useful in situations where the goal is suppression rather than a cure because of unremediable anatomic abnormalities. Gastrointestinal side effects have been commonly associated with each of these preparations. Additionally, the optimum antibacterial effect of mandelamine is at urine pH of less than 5.0, so that additional acidification of the urine with acidic substances is required for efficacy.

DURATION OF THERAPY

There are no easy formulas for determining duration of therapy, although a practical guide is treating for two to four days after defervescence and resolution of signs of infection. The site of infection, host factors, the nature and antimicrobial susceptibility of infecting organisms, the severity of infections, and the response to treatment should be taken into consideration. For bloodstream infections not accompanied by endocarditis or bone involvement, 10 to 14 days is a usual course of treatment. Most respiratory infections are adequately treated in the same interval. Uncomplicated meningitis caused by the meningococcus or pneumococcus is probably adequately treated by seven to ten days of high-dose parenteral penicillin G. Endocarditis, deep-seated bone infections, and infections involving prostheses require a minimum four- to six-week course of treatment but in some cases more. It is important to remember that signs of inflammation, particularly pulmonary infiltration, may persist long after infecting organisms are killed or contained by host defenses, and delayed resolution of lung infiltrates is not uncommon. On the other hand, deep-seated infections like endocarditis and osteomyelitis may have to be treated for periods long after subsidence of signs of infection. Thus, the decision to continue or stop treatment at the end of an appropriate interval must be based on the thorough clinical examination and careful reasoning. Patients with impaired host defenses may require longer therapy than those individuals who are basically healthy. A single dose of an effective antimicrobial agent may be adequate to cure lower urinary tract infection involving the bladder, but a much longer duration, on the order of several weeks, is required to ensure therapeutic success in treatment of intrarenal infection.

---

*Investigational agents.

FAILURE TO RESPOND TO TREATMENT

One of the most important clinical dilemmas is the persistence of fever and other manifestations of infection after a course of costly and potentially toxic therapy has been started. At the same time that every component in antimicrobial therapy is being reassessed, an alternative explanation for fever, pain, and inflammation must also be sought. For instance, tumors or hypersensitivity reactions can incite febrile reactions. Usually, an interval of two to five days is necessary in order to judge the efficacy of treatment. At that point, the following are indicated: (1) Assessing the accuracy of the diagnosis of infection; (2) determining if the drug selection is appropriate, and particularly if the dose and mode of administration are responsible for the lack of success of therapy; and (3) searching for (a) presence of anatomic abnormalities, (b) foreign body, (c) undrained abscess, (d) infarction of tissue, (e) development of superinfection, (f) emergence of resistance, or (g) presence of a simultaneous infectious process that is not being treated by antibacterial therapy. If these are unrevealing, a noninfectious origin of fever or drug reaction should be considered.

In the severely immunosuppressed host, fever and signs of infection may persist despite appropriate therapy. In these patients clinical failure of drug treatment is more realistically regarded as host failure; if any improvement is possible in this difficult situation, it usually correlates with improvement in underlying disease or the immunologic status of the host. If an infection is documented and responds poorly to initially prescribed treatment, then a change to an alternate regimen is indicated. If signs and symptoms progress or new complications appear in spite of seemingly appropriate treatment, a change in therapy is indicated as well as a search for superinfection or an undiagnosed process such as a viral or fungal infection. One of the greatest clinical dilemmas is presented by the patient in whom drug fever or a hypersensitivity reaction is suspected but in whom discontinuing treatment could be dangerous. In such individuals, it is usually prudent to give alternative medication rather than stop antibacterial therapy.

ANTIBIOTIC TOXICITY AND UNTOWARD REACTIONS

A large proportion of drug reactions is related to antimicrobial agents. As many as 10 per cent of patients receiving penicillins and sulfonamides experience some type of toxic or hypersensitivity reaction. These reactions can be fatal, as in the anaphylaxis associated with penicillin or the aplastic anemia due to chloramphenicol. Table 28–7 summarizes some of the major untoward reactions to antibiotics. The majority of toxic reactions are, however, short lived and reversible. Nephrotoxicity secondary to aminoglycosides may be averted by careful therapeutic drug monitoring. A commonly recognized complication of antibiotic therapy is diarrhea and/or pseudomembranous colitis. This is due to bowel overgrowth by C. difficile, which elaborates an exotoxin that is responsible for symptoms. Discontinuation of antibiotic therapy will usually lead to resolution of treatment, but some patients require vancomycin or metronidazole.

Besides anaphylaxis, other hypersensitivity reactions include fever, hemolytic anemia, serum sickness, and a wide variety of dermal reactions that include rash and exfoliation. When serious infection is being treated, mild hypersensitivity reactions may be suppressed by a variety of symptomatic medications. Manifestations of hypersensitivity such as rash may fade despite continued treatment, as is common with ampicillin. The decision to continue therapy in the face of such reactions must be based on severity of infection and the lack of reasonable alternatives. Another issue of great clinical importance that is not fully resolved is the potential cross-reactivity between penicillins and cephalosporins. However, the great majority of patients who have only rash following exposure to penicillin, ampicillin, or related penicillins can be safely treated with cephalosporin compounds. The immediate hypersensitivity-type reactions such as anaphylaxis, wheezing, and urticaria should be carefully noted. Patients with a history of immediate reactions to penicillin should not be rechallenged with cephalosporins unless they have life-threatening infections and can be observed under close medical supervision.

MAJOR ANTIBIOTIC DRUG INTERACTIONS

An increasing number of interactions have been reported between antimicrobials, or antimicrobials and other pharmacologic agents that seriously ill patients may be receiving. Some of these are summarized in Table 28–8. Some noteworthy examples include the induction of hepatic enzymes by rifampin, which may hasten the metabolism of other anti-

TABLE 28–7. UNTOWARD EFFECTS OF SOME ANTIMICROBIAL AGENTS

Target	Agent	Mechanism	Manifestation
Endocrine	Ketoconazole	Altered steroid synthesis	Gynecomastia
	Sulfonamides	Block iodine uptake	Goiter
Gastrointestinal	All agents, esp. ampicillin, clindamycin	(1) Altered bowel flora	Diarrhea
		(2) Exotoxin of *Clostridium difficile*	Pseudomembranous colitis
	Isoniazid, rifampin, tetracyclines	Hepatocellular necrosis	Hepatitis
	Neomycin	Villous damage	Malabsorption
Hematologic	Chloramphenicol	(1) Protein synthesis inhibition	Reversible anemia, leukopenia
		(2) Idiosyncratic	Aplastic anemia
	Carbenicillin, others	Inhibition of platelet aggregation	Bleeding
	Moxalactam	Impaired prothrombin synthesis	Bleeding
	Penicillins, many others	Impaired leukopoiesis, thrombopoiesis	Neutropenia, thrombocytopenia
	Sulfonamides	G-6-PD deficiency	Hemolytic anemia
Kidney	Aminoglycosides, polymyxins	Tubular damage	Renal failure
	Amphotericin	Tubular damage	Hypokalemia, renal failure
	Carbenicillin	Na-K exchange	Hypokalemia
	Penicillins	Interstitial nephritis	Renal failure
	Sulfonamides	Tubular crystallization	Renal failure
Nervous System	Aminoglycosides	(1) Damage to hair cells of Corti	Deafness
		(2) Vestibular damage	Vertigo
		(3) Neuromuscular blockade	Respiratory arrest
	Isoniazid	Pyridoxine antagonism	Neuropathy
	Penicillins, cephalosporins	Cortical irritation	Seizures
	Polymyxins	Neuromuscular blockade	Respiratory arrest
Pulmonary	Nitrofurantoin	Interstitial inflammation	Fibrosis
Skin	Tetracyclines	Bind to dermal structures	Photosensitivity
	Penicillins, sulfonamides, tetracyclines, others	Allergic reactions	Rash, serum sickness, erythema multiforme

TABLE 28–8. IMPORTANT ANTIBIOTIC DRUG INTERACTIONS

Antimicrobial Agent	Interacting Drug	Result
Amphotericin B	Curariform drugs	Increased curare-like effect
Aminoglycosides	Neuromuscular blockers (i.e., tubocurarine, pancuronium)	Additive blockade
	Diuretics: ethacrynic acid, furosemide	Increased ototoxicity
	Antibiotics: amphotericin B	Increased nephrotoxicity
	Carbenicillin/ticarcillin (other penicillins)	Inactivation, resulting in reduced activity
Ampicillin/Amoxicillin	Allopurinol	Rash
Cephalosporins (cefamandole, cefoperazone, moxalactam)	Alcohol	Disulfiram reaction
Chloramphenicol	Warfarin	Decreased warfarin metabolism and inhibition of vitamin K–producing gut bacteria, thus increasing prothrombin time
	Phenytoin	Decreased phenytoin metabolism levels
	Oral hypoglycemic agents	Increased hypoglycemia
Isoniazid	Warfarin, phenytoin	Increased risk of toxicity by decreased drug metabolism
	Disulfiram	Psychosis
	Rifampin, para-aminosalicylic acid	Additive hepatotoxicity
	Oral contraceptives	Decreased contraceptive effect
Metronidazole	Alcohol	Disulfiram-like reaction (nausea)
	Disulfiram	Psychosis
Nalidixic Acid	Warfarin	Increased prothrombin time
Polymyxins	Curariform drugs	Increased curare-like effect
Quinolones	Theophylline	Increase quinolone blood levels
Rifampin	Warfarin, phenytoin	Decreased warfarin, phenytoin effect
	Isoniazid	Additive hepatotoxicity
	Methadone	Withdrawal symptoms
	Oral contraceptives	Decreased contraceptive effect
	Steroids	Decreased steroid effect
Sulfonamides	Procaine	Decreased sulfonamide effect
	Hypoglycemic agents	Hypoglycemia
	Warfarin, phenytoin	Displace drugs from protein-binding sites causing increased warfarin and phenytoin effects
Tetracyclines	Antacids, oral iron	Decreased tetracycline absorption

biotics or drugs. An unexplored area of drug interactions is that which may involve more than two agents. Penicillins like ampicillin or carbenicillin gradually inactivate aminoglycosides like gentamicin in renal failure, when a long half-life for both types of drugs provides opportunity for complexing between the two classes of agents. While this effect is not apparent when patients have normal renal function, the net effect in patients in renal failure is effectively to lower the levels of circulating aminoglycosides and penicillin.

USE OF TOPICAL ANTIBIOTICS

Topical antibiotics or antiseptics have been commonly applied to burns and open wounds, and they are often incorporated into irrigants. A few studies suggest that topical agents can suppress bacteria in burn wounds and reduce sepsis originating from this source. Some topical antiseptics, such as those that contain iodine, are probably too toxic to inflamed tissues and their local application should be discouraged. Topically applied antibiotics can provide only surface suppression of microbial flora. They also provide ample opportunity for development of resistance, since large numbers of organisms may be present on injured skin. Antibiotics in irrigants may be irritating, may be absorbed in large quantities so as to cause increased toxicity, and may offer little advantage over irrigation per se.

Bennett WM, Aronoff GR, Morrison G, et al.: Drug prescribing in renal failure: Dosing guidelines for adults. Am J Kidney Dis 3:155, 1983. *A highly practical guide to antibiotic dose reduction in renal failure.*
Garrod LP, Lambert MP, O'Grady F: Antibiotics and Chemotherapy. London, Churchill-Livingstone, 1981. *Succinct text oriented to microbiologists, but with much information useful to clinicians.*
McGowan JR Jr: Antimicrobial resistance in hospital organisms and its relationship to antibiotic use. Rev Infect Dis 5:1033, 1983. *An important subject exhaustively reviewed.*
Medical Letter: Choice of antimicrobial drugs. Med Lett Drugs Ther 26:19, 1984. *A somewhat conservative but practical compendium of "drugs of choice" and alternative agents for most pathogens.*
Neu HC: Relation of structural properties of beta-lactam antibiotics to antibacterial activity. Am J Med 79(Suppl 2A):2, 1985.

Siegenthaler WE, Bonetti A, Luthy R: Aminoglycoside antibiotics in infectious diseases. Am J Med 80(Suppl 6B):2, 1986. *Succinct summary of this group of agents, which remain important in modern antimicrobial chemotherapy.*
Young LS: Empirical antimicrobial therapy in the neutropenic host. N Engl J Med 315:580, 1986. *Summarizes, with relevant references, the debate over the merits of combination antimicrobial therapy versus the use of a single agent for empiric treatment of immunocompromised hosts.*

29 ANTIVIRAL THERAPY
David. W. Barry

Advances in our knowledge of basic virologic replicative mechanisms have led to the discovery of a number of new antiviral agents within the past decade. This chapter reviews clinical experience with these agents and examines the criteria to be considered before any new therapy is established as safe and effective. Only those agents that have withstood the tests of time and scientific scrutiny will be described.

Some antiviral agents have been available for over 20 years. Certain fundamental principles of viral infections prevent direct extrapolation from knowledge gained from antibacterial therapy. Viruses are obligate intracellular parasites and must divert normal host cell metabolism into providing the constituents for the reproduction of new viral particles. Thus the effectiveness of any antiviral drug will depend not only on its ability to penetrate mammalian cell membranes but also on its capacity to inhibit viral-directed metabolic functions and viral replication. In addition, in some instances, viral deoxyribonucleic acid (DNA) or viral ribonucleic acid (RNA)–directed cDNA may be integrated into the human genome, where it cannot be attacked by any known agent or process. Limited success has been achieved with agents that appear to inhibit viral replication from this genomic template. Furthermore, host immune function has a greater influence on the outcome of viral than bacterial infections in humans. Finally, the influence of intracellular metabolism and replication has slowed, complicated, or prevented the establishment of the relationship between the sensitivity of the virus to a drug in vitro, achievable serum levels of the agent, and its ability to cure an infection.

Evaluation of the effectiveness of antiviral agents is difficult because a number of virus infections are self-limited or mild, with virus replication often well past its peak by the time the physician is consulted. Therapeutic intervention will therefore usually occur simultaneously with the rising tide of the body's own defenses, and a "placebo effect" is prominent in mild and self-limited illnesses. Even in the case of acquired immunodeficiency syndrome (AIDS) or chronic hepatitis B infection, the clinical course is so variable that, as with milder infections, any study on the effectiveness of an antiviral that is not double blind and placebo controlled must be regarded with skepticism.

CHEMOTHERAPEUTIC AGENTS
Herpesvirus Infections

The earliest examples of successful antiviral chemotherapy have been the treatment of superficial infections of the eye caused by herpesviruses. Details of therapy may be found in the ophthalmologic literature, and only certain pharmacologic aspects of the treatment of these viral infections will be discussed here. The majority of the agents found to be effective in the treatment of herpetic keratitis interfere with viral DNA synthesis. Some, such as trifluorothymidine, idoxuridine, and cytosine arabinoside, are relatively toxic when given systemically because they also interfere with DNA replication in rapidly dividing host cells such as myelocytes and lymphocytes. However, when they are given topically in the eye, only minimal amounts are absorbed. Others, such as adenine arabinoside, acyclovir, and interferon, have much more limited toxicity even when given systemically. The final selection of an antiherpes keratitis agent will thus depend on such factors as local tolerance, allergic reactions, observed or potential drug resistance, rapidity of healing, depth of corneal ulceration, and the cost of the drug.

IDOXURIDINE. The first effective antiherpes drug to be developed was idoxuridine, also known as 5-iodo-2'-deoxyuridine or IUDR. It is an analogue of deoxythymidine and is chemically related to trifluorothymidine, which will be discussed later. The action of IUDR results in part from its inhibition of thymidine kinase but more significantly from its inappropriate incorporation into viral or host cell DNA and its formation of false base pairs with guanine rather than adenine. When given in the usual regimen of one drop of a 0.1 per cent aqueous solution in the affected eye every hour, IUDR will cure 75 to 90 per cent of patients with the milder or "dendritic" form of herpes keratitis. A 0.5 per cent ointment is also available. Unfortunately, IUDR cures a lower percentage (40 to 50 per cent) of patients with the more severe "geographic" ulcers. It appears to be relatively ineffective in patients who have deeper disease involving the corneal stroma or the uveal tract. Some patients are intolerant of or allergic to the drug and develop bothersome edema and erythema of the periorbital tissue. Resistance to the drug in vivo and in vitro develops fairly rapidly. As with all other antiherpes agents, IUDR does not eradicate "latent" virus when the organism is in a metabolically inactive state and when herpes nucleic acid may be integrated with host cell DNA. Thus, recrudescent infections are common (approximately 50 per cent will recur within two years) and add credence to the pessimism concerning complete cure of herpes infections.

Comparable success has not been obtained in systemic use of IUDR. For a number of years IUDR was used to treat herpes encephalitis but critically controlled studies showed

that it was not effective. Accordingly, IUDR should not be used for this purpose; in addition, systemic toxicity predisposes the patient to serious superinfection and bleeding. Its use topically, even combined with dimethylsulfoxide, in the treatment of various cutaneous herpes and zoster infections has produced unimpressive results.

ADENINE ARABINOSIDE. Another nucleoside analogue that has been shown to be effective in the treatment of herpetic keratitis is adenine arabinoside, also known as vidarabine, ara-A, or Vira-A. It is phosphorylated intracellularly, and the triphosphate noncompetitively inhibits viral DNA polymerase more efficiently than host cellular DNA polymerase. The 3 per cent ophthalmic ointment applied every three hours has been associated with cure rates of keratitis higher than with IUDR. Like IUDR, it is ineffective against stromal and uveal tract disease. It is also the first drug shown to have some activity in herpes simplex encephalitis, lowering the mortality rate from 70 per cent to approximately 30 to 40 per cent. Some survivors were left with severe and permanent neurologic residua, and its effectiveness was obvious only in those patients who were not stuporous or comatose when therapy was initiated. Its use in this illness has been supplanted by acyclovir (see below). Multicenter studies have demonstrated that intravenous ara-A can also significantly reduce the high mortality rate in disseminated neonatal herpes simplex infections if administered early. As with herpes encephalitis, some survivors are left with significant sequelae. Intravenous ara-A has also been shown to produce some clinical improvements, including the prevention of visceral complications, in immunocompromised patients with cutaneous herpes zoster, although the overall clinical improvement was not dramatic. To produce these benefits, the drug must be given within 72 hours of infections, and conflicting data exist showing that the clinical benefit is seen only in younger (<35 years of age) or older (>38 years of age) individuals.

Treatment of other viral infections has met with varying success. Ara-A has some beneficial influence on the biochemical markers of chronic active hepatitis, but the degree and permanence of these changes are more impressive when it is given with prolonged courses of interferon, although toxicity is increased. It does not appear to be effective in preventing or curing cytomegalovirus pneumonia.

Ara-A also has a number of significant disadvantages, the first of which is its relative insolubility. Often an adult's daily dose (10 to 15 mg per kilogram intravenously) must be given in 2 or more liters of fluid—a potential hazard in patients with encephalitis, who often have significantly elevated intracranial pressure. In addition, the drug is rapidly deaminated to the relatively ineffective hypoxanthine arabinoside. Because of its insolubility and almost immediate deamination, the drug must be given as a continuous infusion over 12 to 24 hours, a cumbersome dosing schedule to maintain. Maximal levels of less than one fourth to one third of the inhibitory dose in vitro for most herpesviruses are achieved in the serum, an observation that must not necessarily engender newer concepts of intracellular micropharmacokinetics in order to explain the apparent clinical activity of the drug. The phosphorylated analogue (ara-AMP) is considerably more soluble, but clinical trials showed it to be ineffective in herpes encephalitis, possibly because it must be dephosphorylated before it can enter infected cells. At high doses, ara-A suppresses the bone marrow, although considerably less than cytosine arabinoside. Higher dosage regimens have been associated with tremors, hyperexcitability, and seizures. These reactions are more common in patients with compromised renal or hepatic function and is likely the result of higher blood and tissue levels. Like IUDR, it is not effective when applied topically to oral or genital herpetic lesions.

TRIFLURIDINE. Trifluridine, also known as trifluorothymidine, TFT, or Viroptic, is, like IUDR, an analogue of deoxythymidine. It is suitable only for topical use in the treatment of herpetic keratitis (one drop of a 1 per cent solution every two hours). When given intravenously, TFT induces significant bone marrow suppression, but applied topically in the eye, it produces only minimal adverse reactions, primarily mild stinging and burning in a low percentage of patients. Its major advantage is a higher cure rate than that for IUDR, and possibly ara-A, in herpetic keratitis. It is significantly better than IUDR for both dendritic and geographic ulcers and has also proved effective in those cases clinically or virologically resistant to either IUDR or ara-A. The drug has also shown some promise in certain adenovirus infections of the eye. It is not effective when applied topically to cutaneous lesions such as those of herpes genitalis or herpes labialis.

ACYCLOVIR. The next effective antiherpes agent to be developed was the acyclic nucleoside 9-(2-hydroxyethoxymethyl) guanine, also known as acyclovir, acycloguanosine, or Zovirax. It is similar in structure to guanosine but only half the ribose ring is present, yielding an ''acyclic'' structure. Its wide therapeutic index is based upon its selectivity as a substrate for virus-specified thymidine kinase. Normal host cell thymidine kinase does not effectively utilize acyclovir as a substrate. Herpesvirus-specified thymidine kinase converts acyclovir to its monophosphate, which is then transformed by cellular enzymes to di- and triphosphates. The triphosphate is both an inhibitor of and a substrate for herpesvirus-specified DNA polymerase. Because it does not contain a 3' carbon, its incorporation into viral DNA selectively stops virus replication. The cellular α-DNA polymerase in infected cells is also inhibited by the triphosphate, but only at concentrations several-fold higher than those that inhibit the viral-specified DNA polymerase. Since acyclovir is preferentially taken up and converted to its active form by herpesvirus-infected cells, it has a low toxic potential for normal, uninfected cells.

Experiments in vitro have shown acyclovir to be effective against herpes simplex types I and II, varicella-zoster virus, and Epstein-Barr virus, but less potent against cytomegalovirus. Intravenous regimens of 5 to 10 mg per kilogram every eight hours produce peak serum levels of 4 to 15 μg per milliliter. If the solubility of the drug in renal tubular fluid (2.5 mg per milliliter at 37°C) is exceeded, through rapid infusion, poor hydration, or coexistent renal failure, tubular obstruction can occur and lead to usually reversible renal failure. The drug penetrates into the cerebrospinal fluid moderately well (~50 per cent of serum levels) and the inhibitory concentrations for herpes simplex, varicella-zoster, and Epstein-Barr viruses range from ~0.01 to 2 μg per milliliter. Intravenous acyclovir has been shown to be effective in the treatment of mucocutaneous herpes infections and in varicella-zoster infections in normal as well as immunocompromised patients. It is more effective than ara-A in the treatment of herpes encephalitis and as effective as ara-A in herpes neonatalis. Although there are suggestions of efficacy in acute and chronic mononucleosis, additional studies are required to define its therapeutic index in these illnesses. It does not appear to be effective in cytomegalovirus infections. Acyclovir has limited absorption from the gastrointestinal tract (15 per cent), yet a regimen of 200 to 400* mg every four hours has been shown to ameliorate genital herpes infections. Most striking is the fact that 200 mg taken orally two to five times per day effectively prevents the appearance of recurrent genital lesions. Like IUDR, ara-A, and TFT, it is very effective when applied topically to the lesions of herpes keratitis.

DHPG. The agent 9-1(1,3-dihydroxy-2-propoxymethyl) guanine (DHPG)† is a very close analogue of acyclovir and has shown great usefulness in the treatment of cytomegalovirus (CMV) infections. The presence of a 3' carbon allows it to be phosphorylated very efficiently, by metabolic processes yet to be identified, in CMV-infected cells. Most CMV isolates are inhibited in vitro by levels of 1 to 5 μg per milliliter. It is also active against herpes simplex virus and varicella-zoster virus, but its use in these infections is limited because it has significantly greater toxicity than acyclovir in these infections. Although it produces severe and usually irreversible damage to spermatogenic tissue in animals and men, careful dose titration has permitted successful treatment of CMV retinitis and gastroenteritis, primarily in AIDS patients. Retinal lesions from CMV usually recur shortly after DHPG has been discontinued, often necessitating persistent treatment for as long as the patient remains severely immunocompromised. It is the only drug known to eliminate CMV from the pneumonic lesions of bone marrow transplant recipients. Unfortunately, this has not been associated with an improved clinical outcome.

Poxviruses

METHISAZONE. One of the earliest chemotherapeutic agents to demonstrate anti-DNA virus activity was 1-methylisatin-3-thiosemicarbazone, also known as thiosemicarbazone, methisazone, or Marboran.* In the early 1960's it was found to have a wide antiviral spectrum in vitro, most impressively against variola, the virus that caused smallpox. Several prophylactic studies conducted during that decade showed a reduction in secondary attack rates among household contacts of smallpox cases. Methisazone did not significantly decrease the mortality rate in those who did develop the disease, nor was it effective in acute smallpox infections.

With the worldwide eradication of smallpox over the past two decades, this drug has seen little use. Nevertheless, methisazone is probably effective in treating complications of smallpox vaccination such as vaccinia gangrenosa, vaccinia necrosum, and generalized vaccinia, particularly when used in conjunction with vaccinia immune globulin. Smallpox vaccination has virtually disappeared, except in the military, and thus little use for this drug is expected in the future.

Influenza

AMANTADINE. One of the most significant advances in anti-RNA virus therapy was the development of amantadine, also known as Symmetrel. A drug with an odd, birdcage-like structure, it was first found to have antiviral activity in the early 1960's. In tissue culture, influenza A viruses, but not influenza B viruses, are inhibited by amantadine. Drug resistance can be induced fairly readily in vitro, although the clinical significance of this observation has yet to be established. The gene determining resistance has been linked with that governing the matrix protein. Amantadine appears to inhibit either viral penetration or viral uncoating within the cell by as yet undefined mechanisms. The concentration required to inhibit 50 per cent of the virus in tissue culture (ID_{50}) ranges between 0.1 and 6 μg per milliliter; the ID_{100} is often closer to 25 μg per milliliter. After a single oral dose of 2.5 to 4.0 mg per kilogram (roughly equivalent to the usual adult dose of 200 mg per day) peak serum levels of 0.3 to 0.5 μg per milliliter are attained. Significant concentration (10- to 60-fold) occurs in both mouse and human lung tissue. Amantadine has a very long half-life (20 to 24 hours) and two to three days are required before a steady state is reached. Eventually 90 to 99 per cent is excreted unchanged in the urine, and thus very significant dose reductions must be made in patients with compromised renal function.

Amantadine taken prophylactically provides protection rates against influenza infection in the range of 70 to 90 per cent (similar to that observed following the inoculation of influenza vaccines). At the usual therapeutic and prophylactic

---

*Exceeds manufacturer's recommended dosage.
†Investigational agent.

*Experimental drug available from Burroughs Wellcome Company.

dose of 100 mg twice a day, amantadine will induce adverse reactions in 10 per cent or more of recipients. These reactions are generally more frequent and more severe in older individuals, who need most to be protected from influenza. Fortunately, these reactions are generally not severe and consist most often of mild agitation, confusion, mental depression, and insomnia. Adverse reactions are more common or more prominent when the patient is also taking antihistamines, but those of amantadine alone are not greater than those of antihistamines alone. Overdosages associated with blood levels above 1.5 µg per milliliter have led to severe central nervous system reactions, including coma and convulsions.

Amantadine also appears to be active against influenza when given orally. This efficacy, however, is more difficult to define, and the difference in the rates of significant clinical improvement between drug- and placebo-treated groups is often marginal. Sophisticated tests, such as those measuring frequency-dependent compliance, have shown that the duration of the diminished pulmonary function that occurs for a number of weeks after influenza may be markedly shortened by the use of amantadine during acute illness. Whether amantadine is effective in the treatment of primary influenza pneumonia has not been established. An analogue, rimantadine, which has been used in some European countries and has been studied in the United States, is reported to have a better therapeutic toxic ratio than amantadine.

Respiratory Syncytial Virus

RIBAVIRIN. Convincing and consistent results of double-blind, placebo-controlled studies of ribavirin (1-β-D-ribofuranosyl-1,2,4,-triazole-3-carboxamide), also known as Virazole, have become available. This analogue of guanosine or inosine appears to inhibit inosine monophosphate dehydrogenase and thus interferes with the de novo synthesis of guanine nucleotides necessary for viral replication. Ribavirin is converted by cellular enzymes to ribavirin triphosphate (RTP). RTP also inhibits GTP-dependent capping of the 5' end of viral mRNA's. It is active against a broad spectrum of RNA and DNA viruses in vitro, although precise levels of sensitivity are dependent on the cell substrate employed in the assays. When given in doses of 333 mg every eight hours for ten days, ribavirin is effective in the treatment of Lassa fever. Although clinical studies of ribavirin in herpes and influenza infections have yielded inconclusive or mixed results, the use of continuous or semicontinuous aerosolized ribavirin (20 mg per milliliter in water) for a minimum of three days ameliorated the course of respiratory syncytial virus infection in children. Few adverse reactions were noted, although oral dosages* of 600 to 1200 mg per day for 5 to 14 days have been associated with reversible depressions in red cell counts and elevations of bilirubin. This anemia appears to be caused in part by the accumulation of RTP within erythrocytes, which cannot efficiently cleave the phosphate moieties and allow exit of the molecule from the cell. The half-life of ribavirin in erythrocytes is therefore much prolonged (approximately 40 days), and erythrocytes heavily ladened with RTP have a significantly shortened survival. Higher doses of ribavirin are also directly marrow suppressive. Loading doses of 1200 mg t.i.d., followed within a few days by a regimen of 300 mg b.i.d., yield serum levels of 6 to 15 µmol (and cerebrospinal fluid levels of 7 to 11 µmol). Hemolytic anemia is said not to occur if serum levels of ribavirin are kept below 20 µmol, although several patients required transfusions when this regimen was used over an eight-week period. Ribavirin is also mutagenic, tumorigenic, and teratogenic, and thus additional experience must be gained before a precise therapeutic index can be determined, particularly in infections requiring higher or more prolonged dosing regimens.

---

*Oral use not recommended by the manufacturer. Approved for aerosol administration only.

Human Immunodeficiency Virus

AZIDOTHYMIDINE. This compound is also known as AZT, zidovudine, Retrovir, Compound S, and BW509U. It is identical to thymidine with the exception that an azido (N_3) group has been substituted for a hydroxyl group in the 3' position of the sugar moiety. AZT is monophosphorylated by cellular thymidine kinase, then di- and triphosphorylated by other as-yet-unidentified cellular enzymes. The triphosphate form inhibits retroviral reverse transcriptase at concentrations 100-fold less than those required to inhibit cellular DNA polymerase. Because of the azido in the 3' position, it is also a DNA chain terminator. Many aerobic gram-negative bacteria and most animal and human retroviruses are inhibited by low concentrations (<0.5 µg/ml) of AZT, and animal studies have shown positive therapeutic and prophylactic effects in these infections.

Clinical studies in humans have shown that the drug is well absorbed (60 to 70 per cent) following oral administration, has a half-life of approximately one hour, has low (30 per cent) serum binding, is excreted primarily in the inactive glucuronidated form, and penetrates well into the CNS, with CSF concentrations averaging about 50 per cent of simultaneous serum concentrations. A double-blind, placebo-controlled study showed that AZT could ameliorate most of the clinical and immunologic manifestations of severe HIV infections, including the incidence of opportunistic infections and deaths, over a six-month observation period. The dosage used in the study was 250 mg by mouth every four hours, but a number of patients required dose reduction because of marrow suppression. AZT causes a macrocytic anemia secondary to inhibition of DNA replication in red and white cell precursors. The severity of the anemia is directly proportional to the degree of pre-existing impairment in the patient's marrow reserve. AZT also caused a moderate incidence of nausea and headaches in these patients.

Additional studies are required to determine the full therapeutic profile of this drug. Such studies would include its use in milder manifestations of HIV infection as well as its use with other agents, such as acyclovir (with which it is synergistic in vitro), interferon, colony stimulating factor, and other immunostimulants.

BIOLOGIC AGENTS

INTERFERON. The most prominent and perhaps the most promising biologic agent used for the therapy of virus infections is interferon. This protein has a molecular weight of approximately 20,000. It is a natural compound produced by many types of cells, particularly lymphocytes, in all vertebrate and possibly invertebrate species, but its activity is fairly species specific. In tissue culture, it is effective against a wide variety of viruses if the cells have been treated with interferon before virus is added to the medium. The mechanism of action of interferon is still being elucidated, but it appears to act by interfering with translation functions once the virus has entered the cell. Interferon has an extremely high specific activity of approximately 1 billion units per milligram of protein (1 unit of interferon = the amount required to reduce viral plaques in tissue culture by 50 per cent). It is produced by infecting human lymphocytes, lymphoblasts, or fibroblasts with a virus or exposing them to a chemical inducer. The cells respond by releasing interferon into the medium, and the material is then purified by a number of complex chemical steps. Alternatively, the gene for interferon production can be inserted in bacteria, allowing for large-scale and efficient production of this complex protein.

Unfortunately, the early promise of interferon in the potential treatment of a host of viral infections has been eclipsed by its toxicity or the appearance of chemical antivirals with a better therapeutic index. It is effective in the topical treatment of herpes keratitis, but numerous other effective agents are available, although it may somewhat enhance their effectiveness. Sprayed intranasally, interferon partially attenuates the symptoms of experimental rhinovirus infections, but bothersome nasal congestion and bleeding associated with a dense submucosal accumulation of lymphocytes preclude its clinical use to prevent upper respiratory viral infections. High-dose interferon (up to 5.1×10^5 units per kilogram) is effective in limiting the severity and progression of both herpes zoster and varicella infections in immunocompromised patients, but the common adverse reactions of fever, lassitude, prostration, and myalgias render it clearly less useful than other agents, such as acyclovir. Parenteral interferon can lower or ablate the serum markers of chronic hepatitis B infection, but the permanence and clinical significance of these changes will remain unclear until additional long-term studies are completed.

The most impressive activity of interferon is in the treatment of infection caused by human papillomaviruses. These agents cause juvenile laryngeal papillomas, which can cause severe and debilitating illness in children, and they also cause genital warts (condyloma acuminatum). Daily doses of 1 to 5 million units per square meter of body surface area induce significant lesion reduction or disappearance in the majority of patients. Additional studies will determine the duration of permanence of these remissions. Some of the more common adverse reactions diminish with long-term therapy, but less common ones, such as hypotension and hepatic and cardiac damage, can be severe. Therefore, only patients with the most severe forms of papillomavirus infections are suitable candidates for long-term interferon therapy.

IMMUNE GLOBULINS. Purified globulins have been used as "postexposure prophylaxis" for viral illness for a number of years. Such "prophylaxis" is in reality treatment of the viral infection before it is clinically manifest. Since antibodies cannot enter cells, they are effective only when the virus is circulating in the blood or when the newly formed viruses are spreading through interstitial fluid rather than via direct cell-to-cell contact. Antibodies may also exert their effect by attaching to a cell that has a viral antigen expressed on its surface, allowing complement and/or lymphocytes to destroy the infected cell. Serum prepared from patients convalescing from the illness to be treated, or serum selected to contain high titers of antibody to the virus to be treated, usually produces the best clinical results. The dosage to be given is often expressed in terms of volume (milliliters per kilogram). This is somewhat misleading, because the appropriate dose will be a factor not only of the volume of the serum preparation but also of the concentration of antibody within it. In some instances, this has been standardized.

Human globulin has been shown to be effective in several clinical situations. These include measles, rabies, and hepatitis A and B. Discussion and schedules of globulin therapy are provided under the individual topics. As newer chemical antivirals become available, the importance of these biologics that do not affect replicating viruses will wane.

Barry DW, Blum MR: Antiviral drugs: Acyclovir. In Turner P, Shand DG (eds.): Recent Advances in Clinical Pharmacology. New York, Churchill Livingstone, 1983, pp 57–80. *A review of preclinical and clinical studies of acyclovir.*

Bauer DJ: The Specific Treatment of Virus Diseases. Lancaster, United Kingdom, MTP Press Ltd., 1977. *This book contains an excellent review of the principles of antiviral chemotherapy. Excellent analysis of clinical data relating to methisazone.*

Bean B, Braun C, Balfour HH: Acyclovir therapy for acute herpes zoster. Lancet 2:118, 1982. *Intravenous acyclovir was effective in these normal patients, but crystalluria can occur if infusions are given too rapidly.*

Bryson YJ, Dillon M, Lovett M, et al.: Treatment of first episode of genital herpes simplex virus infection with oral acyclovir. N Engl J Med 308:916, 1983. *This double-blind, placebo-controlled study demonstrated good efficacy with minimal side effects.*

Collaborative DHPG Treatment Study Group: Treatment of serious cytomegalovirus infections with 9-(1,3-dihydroxy-2-propoxymethyl) guanine in patients with AIDS and other immunodeficiencies. N Engl J Med 314:801, 1986. *Those with retinitis did well. Those with pneumonia did poorly.*

Evans AS (ed.): Viral Infections of Humans. New York, Plenum Medical Book Company, 1976. *The most complete text on the epidemiology, pathophysiology, diagnosis, and therapy of viral infections.*

Fields BF (ed.): Virology. New York, Raven Press, 1985. *This impressive tome covers all aspects of virology, including recent data on the pathophysiology of virus infections as well as chemotherapeutic inhibition of replicative processes.*

Galasso, GJ, Merigan TC, Buchanan RA (eds.): Antiviral Agents and Viral Diseases of Man. 2nd ed. New York, Raven Press, 1984. *This book reflects the status of antiviral chemotherapy in 1984.*

Goepfert H, Sessions RG, Gutterman JU, et al.: Leukocyte interferon in patients with juvenile laryngeal papillomatosis. Ann Otol Rhinol Laryngol 91:431, 1982. *Clear demonstration of the activity of interferon in this viral-induced "proliferative" disease.*

Hall CB, McBride JT, Gala CL, et al.: Ribavirin treatment of respiratory syncytial viral infection in infants with underlying cardiopulmonary disease. JAMA 254:3047, 1985.

Heidelberger C, King DH: Trifluorothymidine. Pharmacol Ther 6:427, 1979. *Excellent review of this drug by its originator.*

Hirsch MS, Swartz MN: Antiviral agents. N Engl J Med 302:903, 949, 1980. *This concise review contains up-to-date information on antivirals, particularly acyclovir and interferon.*

McCormick JB, King IJ, Webb PA, et al.: Lassa fever: Effective therapy with ribavirin. N Engl J Med 314:20, 1986.. *Clear reduction in mortality if therapy begun within the first week of illness.*

Oxford JS, Drasar FA, Williams JD: Chemotherapy of Herpes Simplex Virus Infections. New York, Academic Press, 1977. *This book thoroughly examines drugs affecting double-stranded DNA virus replication.*

Whitley RJ, Alford CA, Hirsch MS, et al.: Vidarabine versus acyclovir therapy in herpes simplex encephalitis. N Engl J Med 314:144, 1986. *This study showed the superiority of acyclovir in decreasing death rate as well as incidence of neurologic sequelae.*

Whitley RJ, Nahmias AJ, Soong SJ, et al.: Vidarabine therapy of neonatal herpes simplex virus infections. Pediatrics 66:495, 1980. *Demonstration of the activity of ara-A in neonatal herpes.*

Whitley RJ, Soong SJ, Dolin R, et al.: Early vidarabine therapy to control the complications of herpes zoster in immunosuppressed patients. N Engl J Med 307:971, 1982. *This article contains the results of a multicenter, double-blind study, which showed the effectiveness of ara-A in herpes zoster.*

Yarchoan R, et al.: Administration of 3'-azido-3'-deoxythymidine, an inhibitor of HTLV-III/LAV replication, to patients with AIDS or AIDS-related complex. Lancet 1:575, 1986.

30 GLUCOCORTICOSTEROID THERAPY

Anthony S. Fauci

In 1949, Hench and coworkers reported marked clinical improvement in patients with rheumatoid arthritis treated with cortisone. During the next 30 years glucocorticosteroids became a major factor in the successful chemotherapy of a wide range of diseases, particularly those in which inflammation or immunologically mediated phenomena played a prominent role. However, these agents have proved a mixed blessing, for glucocorticosteroid therapy is also marked by a high incidence of deleterious and often devastating side effects. Perhaps as much as with any therapeutic agents, the use of corticosteroids requires an appreciation of the toxic as well as the beneficial effects of these drugs, since the one is almost invariably associated with the other. An understanding of the mechanisms of action as well as of the advantages and disadvantages of different glucocorticosteroids, and their treatment regimens, is essential for the physician to exercise appropriate clinical judgment in their use.

BIOCHEMISTRY AND PHARMACOLOGY. Cortisol (hydrocortisone) is synthesized endogenously from cholesterol via pregnenolone and progesterone. Approximately 95 per cent of the endogenous cortisol in the circulation is bound to plasma proteins, particularly to a specific corticosteroid-binding globulin (CBG or transcortin); a lesser amount is bound to albumin. Cortisol is rapidly removed from the circulation with a plasma half-life of approximately 90 minutes. Cortisol is rapidly metabolized in a number of tissues, especially the liver. Less than 2 per cent of the cortisol produced is excreted in the urine unchanged. The active moiety of cortisol is the

11-betahydroxyl group. Exogenously administered compounds such as cortisone and prednisone, which are 11-keto compounds, lack glucocorticosteroid activity until they are converted in vivo into the corresponding 11-betahydroxyl compounds cortisol and prednisolone. This reaction occurs chiefly in the liver. Patients with serious impairment of liver function should be given prednisolone instead of prednisone in order to ensure availability of the active compound.

There are a number of synthetic analogues of cortisol in clinical use today. These differ in their plasma half-life, relative anti-inflammatory potency, and salt-retaining potency (Table 30–1). Among them, cortisone and cortisol have the highest sodium-retaining potency. For this reason, these agents are rarely the steroids of choice in situations requiring long-term administration, except as replacement therapy in adrenal insufficiency. Certain cortisol analogues such as dexamethasone are much less susceptible than cortisol to metabolic degradation. Thus, their plasma half-lives are longer, contributing to their greater relative anti-inflammatory potency.

MECHANISMS OF GLUCOCORTICOSTEROID ACTION. Most, if not all, of the cellular and tissue responses to glucocorticosteroids are initiated via the common denominator of an intracellular glucocorticosteroid receptor, which is present in virtually every mammalian tissue. Exogenously administered glucocorticosteroids are thought to penetrate the cell membrane and bind with high affinity, but reversibly, to this receptor. The hormone-receptor complex then migrates to the cell nucleus and binds to nuclear protein. The association of the steroid-receptor complex with nuclear DNA modulates gene expression. Specific mRNA's then code for proteins that are thought to be responsible for the expression of the glucocorticosteroid effect. The predominant protein induced by glucocorticoids is lipocortin, which is a potent inhibitor of phospholipase A_2. Certain cases of resistance to steroid therapy have been associated with receptor defects, particularly in the refractoriness of some patients with acute lymphoblastic leukemia to glucocorticosteroid therapy.

The effects of glucocorticosteroids subsequent to receptor binding, are complex. Glucocorticosteroids are most often administered for their anti-inflammatory and immunosuppressive effects (the use of these agents as tumoricidal drugs in various chemotherapeutic protocols is discussed in Ch. 176). They are also occasionally administered to stabilize the cardiovascular system, as in hypotensive states arising from sepsis or other causes of cardiovascular collapse. Their efficacy in these latter situations is controversial. Proposed mechanisms of their efficacy in shock include a vasoconstrictive effect on the capillary bed either directly or via potentiation of the action of alpha-adrenergic agents, an increase in cardiac contractility and cardiac output, maintenance of capillary wall integrity, and prevention of tissue breakdown.

Another clinical use of glucocorticosteroids is in the treatment of brain edema, particularly that resulting from brain tumors. The precise mechanisms by which steroids work in this setting are unclear. In situations in which vascular permeability is altered, steroids may act by maintaining vascular integrity, as also postulated in shock. In situations in which brain edema occurs in the presence of an apparently intact vasculature, the mechanisms of steroid effect are even more speculative. However, in these situations the effects are probably related, at least in part, to a decrease in the accumulation of sodium in the tissue edema.

Glucocorticosteroids are also administered therapeutically to ameliorate certain types of hypercalcemia, such as that associated with sarcoidosis and certain neoplasms. The therapeutic effect is related to an increase in renal excretion of calcium and a decrease in calcium absorption from the gastrointestinal tract.

The mechanisms whereby glucocorticosteroid administration results in anti-inflammatory and immunosuppressive effects are also complex. Glucocorticosteroids cause a rapid (four to six hours after administration) but transient lymphocytopenia and monocytopenia, not by lysis and destruction of cells, as in certain animal models, but by a redistribution of cells out of the circulation into other lymphoid compartments, which renders the cells less accessible to sites of inflammation and immune reactivity. In steroid-induced lymphocytopenia, thymus-derived (T) lymphocytes are more markedly depleted than bone marrow-derived (B) lymphocytes; similarly, within the T lymphocyte population, certain subsets of cells are more markedly affected than others. This has potential clinical relevance, since certain immunologically mediated diseases express abnormalities predominantly of specific subpopulations of cells. On the other hand, steroid administration results in a neutrophilia by mobilizing neutrophils from the bone marrow reserve, prolonging the circulating half-life of these cells, and blocking the free migration of these cells out of the circulation into inflammatory and other extravascular sites. One mechanism of this blockage of cell migration is interference with the initial adherence of neutrophils to the microvasculature endothelium. In addition, steroids may block the interaction of various chemotactic factors with neutrophils. Glucocorticosteroid administration also causes a profound eosinopenia. Although the mechanisms of this effect are unknown, the eosinophils are thought to be redistributed out of the circulation similarly to lymphocytes following steroid administration. Furthermore, in vivo and in vitro, glucocorticosteroids interfere with chemotaxis of eosinophils.

Besides affecting the movement and circulatory kinetics of inflammatory and immunologically competent cells, glucocorticosteroids can also have direct effects on their functional capabilities. These include effects of cell activation, proliferation, and differentiation; generation and release of cell products; levels of mediators of inflammation and immune reactions, as well as the response of certain cell types to such mediators; phagocytosis; antigen processing; cytotoxic effector functions; and several others. Various cell types may be selectively sensitive or resistant to the effects of steroids on one or another functional capability. Steroid sensitivity of different cell types also may vary, depending on the stage of activation of the cell. The direct effect of glucocorticosteroids on the functional capability of a cell usually requires higher sustained concentrations of hormone than does their effect on the traffic of the cell.

Of the two major circulating phagocytic cells in humans, the monocyte is much more sensitive to direct suppression of its functional capabilities by steroids than the neutrophil. This has clinically relevant implications, since the monocyte is one of the focal cells in the formation of granulomas, which are quite sensitive to the suppressive effects of glucocorticosteroids. Granulomatous *hypersensitivity* diseases are generally responsive to steroid therapy, whereas infectious diseases such as tuberculosis and certain fungal diseases that are characterized by granulomatous reactions are prone to exacerbation and relapse during high-dose glucocorticosteroid therapy.

TABLE 30–1. COMPARISON OF COMMONLY USED GLUCOCORTICOSTEROID PREPARATIONS

Compound	Equivalent Potency (mg)	Sodium-Retaining Potency	Plasma Half-Life (minutes)
Cortisone	25	2+	30
Hydrocortisone (cortisol)	20	2+	90
Prednisone	5	1+	60
Prednisolone	5	1+	200
Methylprednisolone	4	0	180
Triamcinolone	4	0	300
Dexamethasone	0.75	0	200

Although many antibody and immune complex–mediated diseases are treated with glucocorticosteroids, the antibody-forming cells (B lymphocytes and plasma cells) are relatively resistant to the suppressive effects of these agents. Extremely high doses of drug are required to suppress antibody production by B cells and their progeny. The beneficial effects of steroids in antibody and immune complex–mediated diseases are most likely through indirect effects on the inflammatory response subsequent to the binding of antibody or deposition of immune complexes. At least one of the mechanisms of therapeutic efficacy of glucocorticosteroids in certain of the autoimmune hemolytic anemias and other cytopenias is blockage of the clearance of antibody-coated cells by the reticuloendothelial system.

Glucocorticosteroids are used extensively and beneficially in the treatment of asthma and immediate hypersensitivity allergic conditions. The precise mechanisms responsible are not well understood. Although glucocorticosteroids cause a circulating eosinopenia, the precise role of the eosinophil in allergic and asthmatic reactions is unclear. Glucocorticosteroids have very little effect on serum IgE levels or on the early-phase components of immediate hypersensitivity (Type I) immunologic reactions, although they do alter the late-phase components. In certain systems, glucocorticosteroids induce an increase in intracellular cyclic adenosine monophosphate (cAMP), which in turn is associated with a decrease in release of certain mediators of inflammation. Corticosteroids also decrease the biosynthesis of prostaglandins and leukotrienes, most likely by inducing the synthesis of lipocortin, which inhibits the activity of membrane phospholipase A_2, thus decreasing the availability of arachidonic acid for subsequent conversion by the cyclo-oxygenase and lipoxygenase pathways. Although corticosteroids do not protect animals against histamine-induced shock, several days of steroid treatment can decrease the histamine content of certain tissues. Furthermore, corticosteroids inhibit IgE-mediated release of histamine from human basophils after prolonged incubations. Finally, glucocorticosteroids suppress the expression of lymphocyte surface receptors for the Fc portion of IgE as well as the glycosylation of IgE-binding factors.

TREATMENT OF DISEASE STATES WITH GLUCOCORTICOSTEROIDS. Diverse disease states, with widely differing causes and pathophysiologic mechanisms, have been treated effectively with corticosteroids. These include disorders requiring merely physiologic or replacement doses of the hormone, such as adrenal insufficiency, as well as diseases of suspected or proven inflammatory and/or immunologic mediation, which require pharmacologic doses of drug. These diseases include the connective tissue disorders, particularly systemic lupus erythematosus, rheumatoid arthritis, acute rheumatic fever, dermatomyositis and polymyositis, and mixed connective tissue disease; several of the vasculitides; the idiopathic nephrotic syndrome; severe asthma; various hypersensitivity and allergic states; prophylaxis and treatment of organ transplant rejection; noninfectious granulomatous diseases such as sarcoidosis; autoimmune hemolytic anemia and the immunologically mediated cytopenias; a wide range of dermatologic and ophthalmologic conditions; and several others. Corticosteroids have proven effective in the amelioration of brain edema but have been inconsistent in septic shock and as adjunctive therapy to antibiotics in infections such as tuberculous meningitis.

From the standpoint of the physician, the critical issue is usually not whether the steroid will have a beneficial effect, but the choice of the most appropriate therapeutic regimen in a given patient at a specific phase of a particular disease.

DESIGN OF GLUCOCORTICOSTEROID THERAPEUTIC REGIMENS. The number of possibilities for different steroid regimens is enormous. To facilitate the proper choice, certain fundamental issues must be addressed. The first and most obvious is whether the disease is serious enough to warrant glucocorticosteroid therapy. A closely related question is whether the disease necessitates long-term administration of the drug for a reasonable therapeutic effect to be realized. For example, in mild asthma that is relatively well controlled on bronchodilators, or rheumatoid arthritis that is well managed on nonsteroidal anti-inflammatory agents, there is little question that administration of glucocorticosteroids would ameliorate symptoms even more. However, the required long-term use of even low doses of steroids militates strongly against their use in such situations. On the other hand, one would not hesitate to administer even massive doses (1 gram of methylprednisolone per dose) for limited periods of time in disorders such as status asthmaticus and acute organ transplant rejection. In clinical situations in which it is generally agreed that glucocorticosteroid therapy will be necessary for more than a brief time, other issues must be addressed by the physician. These include consideration of patient disposition to known toxic side effects of steroid therapy such as diabetes mellitus, peptic ulcer, psychiatric difficulties, osteoporosis (older individuals), exacerbations of underlying infections such as tuberculosis, and other potential hazards. If this is the case, alternative therapeutic regimens or modification of the steroid regimen (alternate-day therapy as opposed to daily therapy) to lessen the incidence of such side effects must be considered.

Local Versus Systemic Therapy. In some clinical situations, local glucocorticosteroid therapy that delivers high concentrations of drug directly to the involved site is much preferable to systemic administration of drug. Typical examples are certain dermatologic conditions such as contact dermatitis, in which steroid-containing creams and ointments can be applied directly. However, if a large enough area is exposed to the steroid for a sufficient amount of time, absorption can be great enough to result in systemic effects. Other examples of local administration include topical conjunctival administration of corticosteroids for a variety of ocular conditions as well as steroid enemas for ulcerative proctitis. The latter situation is especially prone to systemic absorption of drug, since denuded mucous membrane is exposed to the hormone.

One of the most important advances in the development of glucocorticosteroid agents has been inhaled aerosol steroids used in the treatment of bronchial asthma. In patients with steroid-dependent asthma, inhalants such as beclomethasone sprayed into the airways via the mouth in doses of two inhalations (100 μg) three to four times per day have allowed a reduction of systemic steroid dosage—and in some individuals, discontinuation of systemic steroid therapy—while controlling symptoms in large numbers of patients. Nasal instillation of aerosol steroids has also proved effective in certain cases of allergic rhinitis.

Type of Agent Employed. Although relatively few glucocorticosteroid preparations are used by clinicians, several factors must be considered in the choice of a steroid agent. A steroid preparation that possesses little or no mineralocorticoid activity is generally preferred in order to avoid the sodium-retaining side effects. Among the commonly used preparations, cortisol (hydrocortisone) has the greatest degree of mineralocorticoid activity. One of the major uses of this agent is in replacement therapy for adrenal insufficiency. Most normal adults secrete about 20 mg of endogenous cortisol per day, and so adults with nearly complete adrenal insufficiency (Addison's disease) require approximately 20 mg of hydrocortisone per day in a single or divided dose. The mineralocorticoid effect is desirable in this situation. In fact, an additional mineralocorticoid (usually fludrocortisone, 0.1 mg per day) is generally administered to the addisonian patient. Hydrocortisone is also indicated in stress situations such as severe trauma and extensive surgical procedures in patients who are or have recently been receiving glucocorticosteroid therapy and may be relatively addisonian (see below).

Among the commonly employed glucocorticosteroids, dexamethasone and methylprednisolone have the least sodium-retaining properties, while prednisone and prednisolone exhibit a slight to moderate degree, significantly less than hydrocortisone (Table 30–1).

Ever since the development of synthetic glucocorticosteroids, great effort has been made to develop agents that are potent and long acting but relatively nontoxic. Unfortunately, as a general rule, there is a correlation between duration of plasma half-life, potency, and toxic side effects. For example, dexamethasone is longer acting, more potent, and associated with greater deleterious side effects than the more commonly used prednisone. From a strictly anti-inflammatory or immunosuppressive standpoint, it would be desirable to administer a high dose of a long-acting agent at frequent intervals for an extended period of time in order to induce and maintain disease remission. However, the toxic side effects of such a regimen render it unacceptable except under the most extraordinary circumstances. In situations such as in the chronic connective tissue diseases, it is more appropriate to employ a short-acting agent such as prednisone in a single dose in the morning or on alternate days. Shorter acting agents are essential for the construction of long-term regimens that closely mimic the normal diurnal cortisol cycle. What then is the indication for a potent long-acting agent such as dexamethasone? Although there are no absolute indications, dexamethasone is generally considered to be the steroid of choice in clinical situations in which sustained high levels of potent glucocorticosteroids are desirable for limited periods of time, as in brain edema.

Dose and Dose Interval of Glucocorticosteroid Administration. BURST OR INTERMITTENT THERAPY. Examples of common, relatively minor ailments for which "burst" or intermittent administration of glucocorticosteroids is employed are poison ivy and poison oak dermatitis. Patients are generally given 60 mg of prednisone for two to three days, followed by rapid tapering of drug by 10-mg decrements over several days until complete discontinuation of therapy. On this regimen, there is little danger of complications. There are other situations that call for short periods of "massive" doses of glucocorticosteroid. Some of the most common are treatment of acute organ transplant rejection and of septic shock. The efficacy of such regimens is clearly documented for organ transplant rejection, in which methylprednisolone is given in doses of several grams per day for a limited time (usually three to five days), followed by conversion to more standard regimens of 60 to 100 mg of prednisone, which is then tapered according to the individual clinical situation. Methylprednisolone is generally employed for the burst therapy because of its relatively low sodium-retaining activity and high potency. Such brief courses of massive-dose steroid therapy have also been used in some cases of acute deterioration in certain connective tissue diseases, particularly systemic lupus erythematosus with active nephritis. The efficacy of such an approach is not certain at this time.

DAILY GLUCOCORTICOSTEROID THERAPY. The most commonly employed regimen for inflammatory and immunologically mediated diseases is the administration of prednisone on a daily basis either as a single dose in the morning or in divided doses over the day. A given dose of a relatively short-acting agent such as prednisone is more potent in its anti-inflammatory and immunosuppressive properties when administered in daily divided doses. Divided dose therapy is also attended by a greater incidence of complications, particularly suppression of the hypothalamic-pituitary-adrenal (HPA) axis. Administration of the same total amount of drug in a single dose on alternate days provides less anti-inflammatory and immunosuppressive effect but also produces significantly fewer toxic side effects. Ideally, a short-acting agent should be administered in a manner that closely mimics the normal diurnal cortisol cycle—namely, peak levels of cortisol early in the morning (6 to 8 A.M.), with tapering off by mid to late afternoon so that the low levels late at night release the pituitary gland from feedback inhibition and permit secretion of adrenocorticotropic hormone (ACTH). The therapeutic aim is to deliver the hormone in a bolus without interrupting the normal feedback mechanisms and thus without disrupting the normal pattern of steroid levels. Persistence of supraphysiologic or pharmacologic levels of hormone late in the day likely accounts for the toxic "tissue" effects and surely accounts for the suppression of the normal HPA cycle seen with divided dose administration of glucocorticosteroids.

Virtually all therapeutically effective regimens of daily divided dose glucocorticosteroid will have some of these effects. Even single daily doses as low as 15 to 20 mg per day of prednisone will cause both toxic tissue effects and HPA axis suppression. Because of its longer plasma half-life, a single dose of dexamethasone will likely have the same deleterious side effects as an equivalent anti-inflammatory dose of prednisone given in divided doses over the day. Since most of the complications of glucocorticosteroid therapy are dose, dose interval, and time related, one should administer the smallest possible dose in the least toxic dose interval over the shortest period of time sufficient to control disease activity. It is inappropriate to initiate steroid therapy in a patient with a flagrantly active inflammatory disease by administering a low dose of a short-acting drug (prednisone) in a single daily dose or on alternate days in order to avoid toxic side effects. It is just as inappropriate to allow a patient whose disease has been put into remission by high doses of divided daily prednisone to remain on that regimen for an inordinate period of time.

Since the diseases that are treated with glucocorticosteroids are heterogeneous and of varying severity, it is difficult to set strict rules for drug administration. However, there can be general and flexible guidelines. For example, if a patient presents with an inflammatory or hypersensitivity disease that is quite active, one should initiate therapy with prednisone at a dose of at least 1 mg per kilogram per day in up to three divided doses. Although this is a potentially toxic regimen if administered over an extended period of time, it may be essential in order to induce a remission of disease. A less aggressive therapeutic regimen may fail while still subjecting the patient to side effects. Once remission has been attained, attempts should be made to taper to the least toxic regimen, with the ultimate goal of completely discontinuing the drug if possible. A common mistake is to leave the patient on the regimen that induced remission while the toxic side effects go unnoticed for some time. Once clinical remission is induced, the divided daily dose can gradually be consolidated into a single daily dose of the same total amount. If remission is maintained, the daily dose can gradually be tapered while monitoring closely for symptoms of disease exacerbation, adrenal insufficiency, or withdrawal (see below). Tapering is continued to the lowest possible dosage that can maintain remission or until the drug is discontinued. Adjunctive therapy with, e.g., nonsteroidal anti-inflammatory drugs for connective tissue diseases, or disodium cromoglycate in asthma, often facilitates the tapering schedule. The advantage of converting from daily divided doses to a single daily dose is that the normal diurnal cortisol cycle can be closely mimicked, which will better acclimate the body to the ultimate discontinuation of therapy. One of the most effective regimens for a smooth tapering of glucocorticosteroid therapy is to convert from a daily divided dose to a single daily dose to an alternate-day administration and ultimately to complete discontinuation (see below).

ALTERNATE-DAY GLUCOCORTICOSTEROID THERAPY. Many inflammatory diseases can be maintained in clinical remission by alternate-day glucocorticosteroid therapy. The rationale is to deliver at regular intervals (every 48 hours) a dose of a short-acting steroid that will maintain the suppression of disease activity while avoiding the toxic side effects associated with single daily dose or divided daily dose regimens. The drug is administered in a single dose in the morning at a time when the normal endogenous cortisol level is at its peak, with maximal feedback suppression of ACTH secretion already occurring. By evening, the administered drug is no longer present in the circulation and the HPA axis will secrete ACTH, which in turn will stimulate the secretion of endogenous cortisol the following morning, when the patient will not be receiving exogenous hormone. In this way, the normal endogenous cortisol levels will maintain the patient's homeostatic function on the "off" day of exogenous steroid. The following day the drug is again administered, and the pharmacologic effect is apparently sufficient to maintain the disease in clinical remission.

It may be necessary to initiate exogenous hormone therapy on a daily basis or even in divided doses to induce remission of an active inflammatory process. However, once the process is adequately suppressed, doses of steroid as widely spaced as 48 hours may be adequate to maintain the disease in remission.

The logistics of conversion from a daily to an alternate-day steroid regimen are difficult. Two common pitfalls are attempting to accomplish the conversion too rapidly and failing to give a sufficient amount of drug on the "on" day. On the basis of the plasma half-life of prednisone, the highest practical single dose that one could administer on an alternate-day basis without suppressing the cortisol cycle on the "off" day is 120 mg. In actual practice, however, 80 to 100 mg is probably maximal. Clearly, a short-acting agent must be used, since administration of a long-acting agent such as dexamethasone on alternate days is intrinsically contradictory. Thus, if a patient is receiving 60 mg of prednisone per day, the daily dose is gradually tapered to 40 or 50 mg per day. At this point, the dose on the ultimate "on" day is immediately doubled to 80 or 100 mg. The dose on the ultimate "off" day is gradually tapered by 5- to 10-mg decrements over several cycles until it reaches 20 mg, and then by 2.5-mg decrements until the patient is receiving no drug that day. The rapidity with which the dosage is tapered on the "off" day varies considerably among patients and depends on the underlying disease and the tolerance of the patient to the tapering process. The judicious use of nonsteroidal anti-inflammatory agents during the tapering process can often prove most helpful. Once the patient has reached a true alternate-day regimen, the dose on the "on" day is maintained for variable periods of time, depending upon individual patient factors, and then it, too, can be tapered to the lowest possible dose required to maintain remission, which may be complete discontinuation of therapy. Although not every patient who requires glucocorticosteroids will be maintained on an alternate-day regimen, such a regimen should be attempted when possible.

ACTH VERSUS GLUCOCORTICOSTEROIDS. There is no convincing evidence that ACTH is superior to glucocorticosteroids in the treatment of any disease. Furthermore, glucocorticosteroids are preferable to ACTH for a number of reasons. ACTH must be injected, whereas glucocorticosteroids can be administered orally. The ACTH effect depends on the stimulation of release of variable amounts of cortisol from the adrenal gland, whereas the dose of administered glucocorticosteroid can be precisely controlled. In addition, ACTH stimulates other hormones, such as androgens and mineralocorticoids, which may have undesirable side effects. Also, administration of ACTH may result in hyperpigmentation.

APPROACH TO HPA AXIS SUPPRESSION. One of the most disputed topics in glucocorticosteroid therapy is the duration of steroid administration that will result in HPA axis suppression. A closely related topic is the duration of HPA axis suppression following cessation of steroid therapy. It is virtually impossible to identify the shortest period of therapy or the smallest dose at which clinically significant suppression

of the HPA axis will occur. The most conservative estimates will be given here.

Patients who have received the equivalent of 30 mg of prednisone per day for more than a week should be considered to have sustained suppression of the HPA axis. This may be asymptomatic except under conditions of severe stress. In patients who have been exposed to high doses of glucocorticosteroids daily over a prolonged period of time, as much as 12 months may be required following cessation of therapy before normal hormonal response to stress returns. If patients who are suspected of HPA axis suppression are to be subjected to severe stress such as a major surgical procedure, they should receive parenteral hydrocortisone in doses of 100 mg every four to six hours during surgery and for several days thereafter, depending on the recovery period.

It is possible to determine the integrity of the HPA axis in a patient who has recently received glucocorticosteroid therapy. The standard test is to administer 50 units of ACTH as a constant intravenous infusion over six to eight hours and measure the resulting rise in plasma cortisol. Alternatively, synthetic ACTH (beta 1-24 ACTH) can be given as a rapid intravenous infusion (250 µg), with measurement of plasma cortisol at 30 minutes and one hour after injection. In patients with normal adrenal glands, plasma cortisol levels should rise to at least 30 µg per milliliter.

Once glucocorticosteroid therapy has been withdrawn, recovery from suppression of the HPA axis is a gradual process, the rate of which varies considerably among patients. There are no proven manipulations to hasten this process. Hypothalamic-pituitary function returns before adrenocortical function. The use of ACTH has not been proved to hasten recovery of HPA function. Conversion to alternate-day steroid therapy prior to withdrawal generally leads to a less symptomatic recovery, but it does not hasten the process. Suppression of the HPA axis can be associated with a diverse array of symptoms.

WITHDRAWAL SYNDROMES. Withdrawal from glucocorticosteroid therapy may result in both subjective and objective manifestations of adrenal suppression. Features of withdrawal may include lethargy, weakness, anorexia, nausea, fever, arthralgia, orthostatic hypotension with syncope, hypoglycemia, weight loss, and desquamation of the skin. The entire symptom complex may relate to HPA axis suppression, for which replacement therapy is indicated. However, exacerbation of certain underlying diseases may manifest similar symptoms. It is essential for the physician to monitor the patient closely, with appropriate diagnostic measures aimed at determining disease activity as well as integrity of the HPA axis. If the patient manifests HPA axis suppression, reinstitution of glucocorticosteroid therapy with more gradual withdrawal is indicated.

A number of patients may manifest a physical or psychologic dependence on glucocorticosteroids and yet have neither exacerbation of underlying disease nor suppression of normal HPA function. If the dependence is psychologic, appropriate counseling and encouragement are indicated. However, physical dependence may exist in the face of normal HPA function, since the tissues may have been acclimated to high levels of glucocorticosteroids for such a period of time that, despite "normal" levels of cortisol, the patient experiences symptoms of steroid deprivation. Under these circumstances, reinstitution of physiologic doses of a short-acting drug such as prednisone, followed by a more protracted tapering period, may be indicated. Finally, certain patients may manifest biochemical evidence of HPA axis suppression without evidence of exacerbation of underlying disease and without symptoms.

COMPLICATIONS OF GLUCOCORTICOSTEROID THERAPY. The major limiting factor in the use of glucocorticosteroid therapy is the wide array of deleterious side effects that may occur. The frequency and severity of glucocortico-

TABLE 30–2. COMPLICATIONS OF GLUCOCORTICOSTEROID THERAPY

Central nervous system	Endocrinologic
Pseudotumor cerebri	Suppression of HPA axis
Psychiatric disorders	Growth failure
Musculoskeletal	Secondary amenorrhea
Osteoporosis with spontaneous	Metabolic
fractures	Hyperglycemia and unmasking of
Aseptic necrosis of bone	genetic predisposition to
Myopathy	diabetes mellitus
Ocular	Nonketotic hyperosmolar states
Glaucoma	Hyperlipidemia
Cataracts	Alterations of fat distribution
Gastrointestinal	(typical cushingoid appearance)
Peptic ulceration	Fatty infiltration of the liver
Intestinal perforation	Drug interactions (decreased
Pancreatitis	anticoagulant effect of ethyl
Cardiovascular and fluid balance	biscoumacetate)
Hypertension	Fibroblast inhibition
Sodium and fluid retention	Inhibition of wound healing
Hypokalemic alkalosis	Subcutaneous tissue atrophy
Hypersensitivity reactions	(striae, purpura, ecchymosis)
Urticaria	Suppression of host defenses
Anaphylaxis	Immunosuppression, anergy
	Effects on phagocyte kinetics and
	function
	Increased incidence of infections

Baxter JD, Rousseau GG: Glucocorticoid Hormone Action. New York, Springer-Verlag, 1979. *An excellent book with comprehensive and sophisticated coverage of basic mechanisms of glucocorticoid action. One of the outstanding works on steroid hormone action, with contributions by recognized leaders in the field.*

Dixon RB, Christy NP: On the various forms of corticosteroid withdrawal syndrome. Am J Med 68:224, 1980. *An excellent, lucidly written discussion of corticosteroid withdrawal syndromes, with use of case presentations as example.*

Fauci AS: Alternate-day corticosteroid therapy. Am J Med 64:729, 1978. *Concise editorial discussion on usefulness and limitations of alternate-day glucocorticosteroid therapy.*

Fauci AS, Dale DC, Balow JE: Glucocorticosteroid therapy: Mechanisms of action and clinical considerations. Ann Intern Med 84:304, 1976. *An extensive review of mechanisms of action of glucocorticosteroids as they relate to therapeutic efficacy in the treatment of inflammatory and immunologically mediated diseases. Practical outlines of the design and modification of therapeutic regimens.*

Kehrl JH, Fauci AS: The clinical use of glucocorticoids. Ann Allergy 50:2, 1983. *An updated review article on the theoretic and practical aspects of the use of corticosteroids in clinical medicine.*

Thorn GW: Clinical considerations in the use of corticosteroids. N Engl J Med 274:775, 1966. *This superb article remains the classic treatise on the rational use of corticosteroid therapy.*

Udelsman R, Ramp J, Gallucci WT, et al.: Adaptation during surgical stress. A reevaluation of the role of glucocorticoids. J Clin Invest 77:1377, 1986. *An updated article establishing that the permissive actions of physiologic glucocorticoid replacement are both necessary and sufficient to tolerate surgical stress.*

Zora JA, Zimmerman D, Carey TL, et al.: Hypothalamic-pituitary-adrenal axis suppression after short-term, high-dose glucocorticoid therapy in children. *This updated study firmly establishes that short-term, high-dose glucocorticoid therapy produces only transient suppression of the hypothalamic-pituitary-adrenal axis.*

steroid-related complications are directly related to the dose, duration, and schedule of therapy. Although all the complications listed in Table 30–2 have been amply documented, the direct cause-effect relationship between drug administration and complications has not been equally convincing for each of the complications. For example, there is a high incidence of spontaneous peptic ulcer in certain diseases that are treated with glucocorticosteroids, particularly rheumatoid arthritis. In addition, other gastrointestinal irritants such as the nonsteroidal anti-inflammatory agents are often administered concomitantly with the steroid. In the absence of adequately controlled studies, it is difficult to determine whether glucocorticosteroids increase the incidence of peptic ulceration. Also, daily administration of steroid is associated with an increase in infectious disease complications. Several diseases that are treated with steroids, such as lymphoid malignancies and systemic lupus erythematosus, have defects of host defense. These act synergistically with the steroid-induced compromise of host defenses to result in an increased incidence of opportunistic infections. On the other hand, patients with asthma who are treated with steroids do not seem to have an increased incidence of infections. This may be related to the otherwise normal host defenses of these patients as well as to the low doses of steroid usually employed. By contrast, osteoporosis and cataracts are commonly and directly related to glucocorticosteroid therapy.

Questions often arise about the effects of steroid therapy on delayed cutaneous hypersensitivity responses. This effect is variable and dose related. Generally, patients receiving less than 80 mg of prednisone on alternate days have intact delayed cutaneous hypersensitivity. By contrast, patients receiving daily steroid will generally become anergic if the dose is 15 mg of prednisone or greater, with the onset of anergy usually within days after initiation of therapy. Following cessation of therapy, if all other factors involved in delayed hypersensitivity are intact, responses generally return within ten days to two weeks.

Glucocorticosteroids are not considered to increase teratogenic risk among newborns of mothers who receive steroids during pregnancy. However, such infants should be monitored for adrenal insufficiency during the neonatal period. Also, since glucocorticosteroids are excreted in breast milk, inhibition of endogenous steroid production as well as growth suppression can occur in infants who are breast fed by mothers receiving the hormone.

31   PHARMACOLOGIC PRINCIPLES RELATED TO THE AUTONOMIC NERVOUS SYSTEM

Robert J. Lefkowitz

ORGANIZATION AND PHYSIOLOGY OF THE AUTONOMIC NERVOUS SYSTEM

The autonomic nervous system regulates the functions of smooth muscle, the heart, and glands. It is composed of two major divisions, termed sympathetic and parasympathetic, which are anatomically, physiologically, and biochemically quite distinct. Activation of the sympathetic system leads to the classic "flight or fight" responses of tachycardia, increased force of cardiac contraction, vasoconstriction, mydriasis, bronchodilation, and hyperglycemia. Parasympathetic nervous activity results in a situation better exemplified by "an old man sleeping after dinner," with slow heart rate, noisy respirations (caused by bronchial constriction), meiosis, and saliva running out of the corner of his mouth. Auscultation of the abdomen would reveal loud bowel sounds.

Anatomically, the *sympathetic nervous system* is composed of pathways that originate from neurons with cell bodies in the "thoracolumbar" segments of the spinal cord. These preganglionic neurons synapse in the sympathetic ganglia with postganglionic neurons, which in turn innervate end-organs, including vascular, gastrointestinal, and genitourinary smooth muscle and the heart.

By contrast, the *parasympathetic pathways* originate from neurons that have their cell bodies in the "craniosacral" portions of the neuraxis, including the midbrain, the medulla, and the sacral portions of the spinal cord. Preganglionic fibers synapse in peripheral ganglia that are in general closer to innervated organs than is the case with the sympathetic system.

Communication between neurons in the autonomic nervous system, and between neurons and effector cells, is mediated by chemicals called neurotransmitters. Acetylcholine encodes communication between preganglionic and postganglionic neurons in both the sympathetic and parasympathetic nervous systems. Norepinephrine is generally the neurotransmitter at sympathetic postganglionic nerve endings, whereas acetylcholine is the transmitter at parasympathetic postganglionic nerve endings.

The *adrenal medulla* is anatomically and functionally analogous to the sympathetic ganglia. Its chromaffin cells are innervated by typical preganglionic fibers. The major product of the adrenal medulla is epinephrine, which is secreted into the bloodstream. Epinephrine has many of the same biologic activities as the sympathetic neurotransmitter norepinephrine. Because of the strong analogies and the concerted physiologic functioning of the sympathetic system and the adrenal medulla in situations such as stress or fright, these two components are often considered a unified "sympathoadrenal system."

NEUROTRANSMITTERS. A great deal is known about the biochemical basis of neurotransmission as mediated by norepinephrine in the sympathetic and acetylcholine in the parasympathetic system. Several discrete processes have been identified and elucidated. These include the mechanisms of (1) biosynthesis of transmitter in nerves, (2) storage of transmitter within granules in sympathetic and parasympathetic nerve endings, (3) release of transmitter at synapses, (4) interaction of transmitter with receptors on effector cells, and (5) termination of transmitter activity by reuptake and/or metabolizing processes.

There is a great diversity of physiologic autonomic effects and, because so much is known about neurotransmitter function, therapeutic interventions that modify autonomic function are among the most rational and important at the physician's disposal. For both the sympathetic and parasympathetic nervous system an understanding of the basic organization and physiology permits predictions of not only therapeutic but also adverse effects of a wide variety of drugs. The purpose of this chapter is to delineate the general principles underlying pharmacologic approaches that modify autonomic nervous system function. Although examples are provided, the reader is referred to other chapters for details of dosage, administration, and specific indications of individual drugs in disease states.

Each of the processes described above, including biosynthesis, uptake and storage in granules, release, receptor binding, and degradation of neurotransmitters, is susceptible to pharmacologic manipulation. A much wider variety of therapeutic interventions is possible in the sympathetic system than in the parasympathetic system, and these are summarized in Figure 31–1.

For the parasympathetic system the major clinical interventions involve drugs that act as agonists or antagonists at postsynaptic muscarinic receptors. Agents are also available that, by inhibiting the destruction of acetylcholine, lead to cholinergic agonist effects at postsynaptic receptors (cholinesterase inhibitors). Botulinum toxin appears to cause neuromuscular blockade by blocking release of acetylcholine from cholinergic nerves.

ADRENERGIC AND CHOLINERGIC RECEPTORS

Of the therapeutic interventions indicated in Figure 31–1, the most important relate to drugs that stimulate or block the postsynaptic receptors for adrenergic and cholinergic neurotransmitters. The concept that there are specific receptor molecules that mediate the effects of hormones has been popular throughout most of this century. This hypothesis has gained additional support over the past decade from radioligand binding studies, which have permitted the direct identification of these sites in cells with radioactively labeled drugs. Some of these receptors have been purified, and their

genes have been cloned, leading to elucidation of their complete primary amino acid sequences.

Any discussion about receptors depends on certain essential pharmacologic concepts. Adrenergic receptors are the cellular sites at which catecholamines or related drugs are initially bound. The binding of drugs with adrenergic receptors induces changes in the receptors, which then lead to a series of events in the cell, resulting in the characteristic physiologic effects of the drug. Thus adrenergic receptors are recognition sites on the plasma membrane that transduce the interaction of catecholamines with the cell into a physiologic response. Agonist drugs are those capable of inducing a response. A "full" agonist causes a maximal response, whereas a "partial" agonist causes a qualitatively similar response of lesser magnitude. An "antagonist" is a drug that interacts with the receptor but elicits no response on its own. However, by occupying the receptor an antagonist may reduce the effect of an agonist. The "intrinsic activity" of a drug is a measure of its maximal effect. The intrinsic activities of full agonists are defined to be 1.0, whereas those of antagonists are 0. Partial agonists have intrinsic activities greater than 0 but less than 1.

The interaction of a drug with a receptor involves the notion of affinity or potency. Affinity is a measure of the avidity or tightness with which a drug combines with a receptor. The greater the affinity of a drug for a receptor, the lower the concentration of the drug necessary to occupy any specified fraction of the receptors. The affinity of a drug is unrelated to its intrinsic activity. Thus some drugs may have very great affinity for a receptor but virtually no intrinsic activity, e.g., potent antagonists.

ALPHA- AND BETA-ADRENERGIC RECEPTORS. Modern concepts concerning adrenergic receptors, the sites of action of epinephrine and norepinephrine, have their origin in the work of Raymond Ahlquist in 1948. He suggested that there were two main classes of adrenergic receptors, which he termed alpha and beta. This demarcation was based on the relative potencies of several agonist drugs for stimulation of physiologic responses in several tissues. The two major patterns observed were epinephrine>norepinephrine>>isoproterenol (alpha) and isoproterenol>epinephrine>norepinephrine (beta). He suggested that two distinct types of adrenergic receptors (alpha and beta) mediated responses displaying distinct potency series. Virtually all adrenergic responses fell into one or the other category. Table 31–1 lists some typical alpha and beta receptor–mediated adrenergic responses.

Although alpha- and beta-adrenergic receptors were originally defined by their agonist potency series, highly specific antagonists were subsequently developed, such as propranolol for the beta-adrenergic receptors and phentolamine for the alpha receptors. Refinements in the classification of adrenergic receptors have occurred over the past three decades with the realization that there are subtypes of both alpha- and beta-adrenergic receptors. For the beta-adrenergic receptors these were originally distinguished based on relative potencies of epinephrine and norepinephrine. Thus at $beta_1$-adrenergic receptors, such as those mediating positive inotropic effects in the heart, epinephrine and norepinephrine are of similar potency. By contrast, at $beta_2$-adrenergic receptors, such as those found in vascular and bronchial smooth muscle, epinephrine is much more potent than norepinephrine.

$Beta_1$- and $beta_2$-adrenergic receptors both appear to function by mediating stimulation of the plasma membrane-bound enzyme adenylate cyclase. The cyclic adenosine monophosphate (cAMP) generated in response to such stimulation leads to phosphorylation of key target proteins by cAMP-dependent protein kinases. Alteration in the functioning of such proteins as a result of phosphorylation presumably then leads to the

FIGURE 31–1. Therapeutic interventions in the peripheral adrenergic nervous system. Abbreviations: ACH = acetylcholine; DBH = dopamine beta hydroxylase; DOPA = dihydroxyphenylalanine; NE = norepinephrine; MAO = monoamine oxidase. (1) Competitive antagonism of nicotinic cholinergic receptors on postganglionic neuron in autonomic ganglia, e.g., trimethaphan. (2) Inhibition of transmitter (norepinephrine) synthesis, e.g., alpha methyl-p-tyrosine. (3) Drugs that enter the normal biosynthetic pathway and are transformed into "false neurotransmitters," e.g., alpha-methyldopa→ →alpha-methylnorepinephrine. (4) Drugs that prevent the storage of transmitter in granules by inhibiting transport across storage granule membrane, e.g., reserpine. (5) Drugs that deplete transmitter from granules by displacement, e.g., guanethidine. (6) Drugs that inhibit the release of norepinephrine, e.g., bretylium. (7) Drugs that deplete neuronal norepinephrine by blocking the amine transport system of the neuronal membrane, e.g., cocaine or imipramine. Another major mechanism for the termination of norepinephrine action is by metabolism by catechol-o-methyl transferase. (8) Inhibition of metabolic destruction of transmitter, e.g., monoamine oxidase inhibitors. Relation of enzyme inhibition to therapeutic effects not clear, e.g., pargyline. (9) Indirectly acting agonists that displace norepinephrine from storage granules, e.g., tyramine, amphetamine (solely indirect), ephedrine, and metaraminol (also have direct actions). (10) Blockade of postsynaptic alpha receptors (e.g., phentolamine, phenoxybenzamine, prazosin) or beta receptors (propranolol). (11) Agonists that occupy postsynaptic receptors and mimic the effect of the neurotransmitter, e.g., isoproterenol (beta), phenylephrine (alpha). (12) Presynaptic alpha-adrenergic receptors. Although agonists and antagonists that specifically act through these receptors are not in general use, some adverse effects of other drugs, e.g., tachycardia after phentolamine administration, may be due to occupancy of these receptors. (13) Inhibition of breakdown of cyclic AMP by phosphodiesterase, e.g., aminophylline.

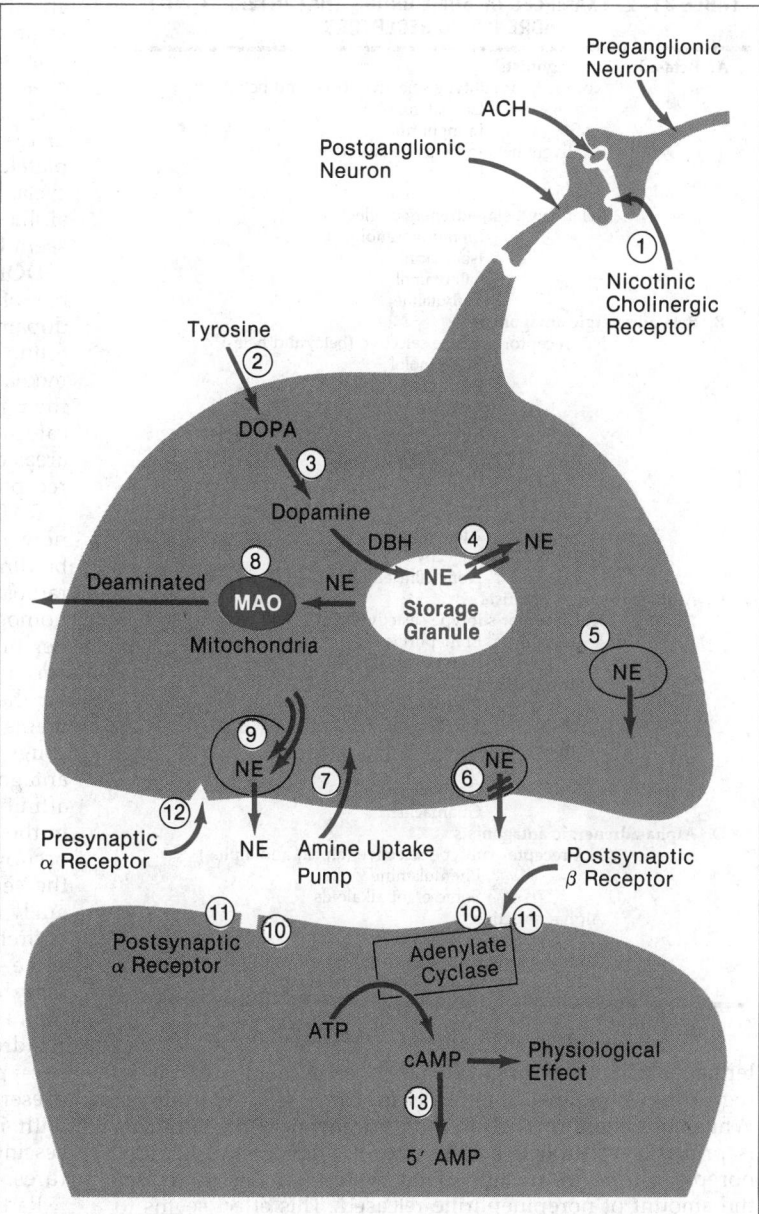

characteristic physiologic or pharmacologic effects of beta-adrenergic drugs.

A number of agonist and antagonist drugs showing preferential selectivity (affinity) for beta₁- or beta₂-adrenergic receptors are known, and some of these are summarized in Table 31–2. Many drugs show no preference for one or the other receptor subtype. The clinical use of these drugs is discussed below. The beta-adrenergic receptor subtypes in various tissues are listed in Table 31–2.

Alpha-adrenergic receptor subtypes are even more distinct than the beta receptor subtypes, differing not only in pharmacologic specificity but also in biochemical mechanism of action. Alpha₁ or typical "postsynaptic" alpha receptors are found, for example, in vascular smooth muscle, where they mediate the vasoconstrictor effect of sympathetic nerve stimulation. Pharmacologically, such alpha₁ receptors are characterized by their very high affinity for certain alpha antagonists such as prazosin and phenoxybenzamine. Typical alpha-adrenergic agonists such as phenylephrine and methoxamine stimulate these alpha₁ receptors quite effectively. Although the molecular mechanisms mediating alpha₁-adrenergic receptor effects are not clearly understood at present, a distinct signaling system appears to be involved. This leads to the hydrolysis of polyphosphoinositides to two second messengers, inositol trisphosphate and diacylglycerol. Inositol trisphosphate leads to the release of intracellular calcium from intracellular stores, whereas diacylglycerol activates the ubiquitous enzyme protein kinase C.

A second major subclass of alpha-adrenergic receptors,

TABLE 31–1. SOME EXAMPLES OF ADRENERGIC RECEPTOR–MEDIATED RESPONSES

Beta₁-adrenergic receptors
  Heart—positive inotropism
  Adipose tissue—lipolysis
Beta₂-adrenergic receptors
  Vascular smooth muscle—relaxation
  Bronchial smooth muscle—relaxation
Alpha₁-adrenergic receptors
  Vascular smooth muscle—contraction
Alpha₂-adrenergic receptors
  Platelets—aggregation
  Presynaptic nerve terminal—inhibition of norepinephrine release
  Postsynaptic—vascular smooth muscle contraction, some vascular beds

TABLE 31–2. EXAMPLES OF SOME DRUGS THAT INTERACT WITH ADRENERGIC RECEPTORS

A. **Beta-adrenergic agonists**
    Not receptor subtype selective (beta$_1$ and beta$_2$)
        Isoproterenol
        Epinephrine
    Relatively beta$_1$-adrenergic selective
        Norepinephrine
        Dobutamine
    Relatively beta$_2$-adrenergic selective
        Metaproterenol
        Isoetharine
        Salbutamol
        Terbutaline

B. **Beta-adrenergic antagonists**
    Not receptor subtype selective (beta$_1$ and beta$_2$)
        Propranolol
        Alprenolol
        Timolol
        Pindolol
        Oxprenolol
        Nadolol
    Relatively beta$_1$ selective
        Metoprolol
        Atenolol
    Relatively beta$_2$ selective
        None clinically available

C. **Alpha-adrenergic agonists**
    Not receptor subtype selective (alpha$_1$ and alpha$_2$)
        Epinephrine
        Norepinephrine
    Relatively alpha$_1$ selective
        Phenylephrine
        Methoxamine
    Relatively alpha$_2$ selective
        Clonidine
        Guanabenz
        Guanfacine

D. **Alpha-adrenergic antagonists**
    Not receptor subtype selective (alpha$_1$ and alpha$_2$)
        Phentolamine
        Some ergot alkaloids
    Alpha$_1$ selective
        Prazosin
    Alpha$_2$ selective
        None clinically available

termed alpha$_2$, was originally discovered to play a role in regulating norepinephrine release from nerve terminals. While norepinephrine release from adrenergic nerve terminals is primarily controlled by the rate of firing of the neuron, norepinephrine in an autoinhibitory fashion acts to reduce the amount of norepinephrine released. This effect seems to be mediated by alpha-adrenergic receptors (since it is blocked by classic alpha-adrenergic antagonists) that have distinct pharmacologic characteristics and are possibly located on presynaptic sites on the nerve ending itself. Stimulation of these receptors by norepinephrine in the synaptic cleft serves to reduce the amount of norepinephrine released by subsequent nerve impulses.

In recent years alpha-adrenergic receptors with pharmacologic properties virtually identical to the "presynaptic" receptors described above have been found in a variety of "postsynaptic" locations, e.g., the platelet. In addition, alpha$_2$-adrenergic receptors play a distinct role in mediating effects on smooth muscle contraction in some vascular beds. Because alpha$_2$-adrenergic receptors may be found in both pre- and postsynaptic locations, it seems preferable to use the designations alpha$_1$ and alpha$_2$ rather than the earlier terminology of "presynaptic" and "postsynaptic" alpha receptors. Physiologic effects of alpha$_1$ and alpha$_2$ receptor stimulation are summarized in Table 31–1.

A variety of drugs demonstrate selective affinity for alpha$_2$ receptors. Among agonists the most notable examples are clonidine and related drugs. Yohimbine, a plant alkaloid antagonist, also is somewhat selective for alpha$_2$ receptors. The classic alpha-adrenergic antagonists phentolamine and the ergot alkaloids are not selective and possess comparable affinity for alpha$_1$ and alpha$_2$ receptors. Subtype selectivity of some alpha-adrenergic drugs is listed in Table 31–2.

In several model systems such as the platelet, stimulation of alpha$_2$-adrenergic receptors inhibits the enzyme adenylate cyclase. The resultant reduction in cellular cAMP levels mediates the alpha-adrenergic effect in question—in this case, platelet aggregation. It is not yet known whether adenylate cyclase inhibition is the common biochemical basis of all alpha$_2$-adrenergic effects. Alpha$_1$-adrenergic effects do not seem to involve modification of adenylate cyclase activity.

DOPAMINE RECEPTORS. Catecholamines are also capable of interacting with a third class of receptors termed dopamine receptors. Peripheral dopaminergic receptors are found in the renal and mesenteric vasculature, where they mediate vasodilation. These receptors are characterized by their relatively higher affinity for dopamine than for other catecholamines. Dopamine receptors are also found in certain areas of the brain, such as the corpus striatum. Dopaminergic receptors will not be considered further in this chapter.

RADIOLIGAND BINDING STUDIES. Direct methods are now available to measure adrenergic receptors by radioligand binding techniques. These techniques involve the use of radiolabeled drugs to tag the receptors in whole-cell or cell-homogenate preparations. Such studies have provided a number of insights of clinical relevance. These methods permit very precise and direct measurement of the affinities of drugs for the various adrenergic receptor subtypes. Such measurements indicate that even for presumably "subtype" selective drugs, the "selectivity" is only relative. Thus a beta$_1$ selective antagonist such as metoprolol has only 10- to 50-fold higher affinity for beta$_1$ receptors in the heart than for beta$_2$ receptors in the lung. As the dose of such a compound is raised, it will occupy increasing numbers of beta$_2$ as well as beta$_1$ receptors; the selectivity therefore is not absolute. Thus, it is not generally possible to block the beta$_1$ receptors in the heart and entirely spare the beta$_2$ receptors in the lung. By contrast, some alpha$_1$ receptor selective antagonists such as prazosin may have as much as 10,000-fold higher affinity for alpha$_1$ than for alpha$_2$ receptors.

Adrenergic receptor subtypes are distinct molecular entities—proteins—the pharmacologic properties of which are preserved even through extensive purification. In analogy with isoenzymes, they may represent "isoreceptors," possessing relatively subtle differences in their molecular structures.

Radioligand binding studies have also documented the wide distribution of binding sites throughout the central nervous system that have properties identical to the beta$_1$ and beta$_2$ and alpha$_1$ and alpha$_2$ receptor binding sites present in the peripheral nervous system. In most cases the physiologic role of these "central" adrenergic receptors is not known. It is, however, clear that alpha$_2$-adrenergic receptors in the vasomotor center act to decrease sympathetic outflow and hence sympathetic tone. This is possibly a major site of action of clonidine, an antihypertensive alpha$_2$ agonist.

PHYSIOLOGIC REGULATION OF RECEPTORS. Adrenergic receptors are subject to a wide variety of modulating influences that regulate their numbers and binding properties. For example, chronic exposure of beta receptors to high concentrations of agonists leads to a decrease in the number of beta-adrenergic receptors and a decrease in their efficiency for stimulating adenylate cyclase. The result is a decrease in beta-adrenergic responsiveness often termed *desensitization*. Similar findings have been documented for certain alpha-adrenergic receptors. This may explain the decreased responsiveness of asthmatics to chronically administered beta-agonist bronchodilators. Antagonists do not cause such desensitization effects. Indeed, hypersensitization may occur when receptors are chronically occupied by antagonists. Under such circumstances the number of receptors on cells may increase with the potential for supersensitivity when the antagonist drug is discontinued. (See below for discussion of "propranolol withdrawal syndrome.")

In certain animal models the number of beta receptors may be increased in hyperthyroidism. This provides one possible mechanism for the salutary effect of propranolol in relieving the hyperadrenergic symptoms of hyperthyroidism.

ACETYLCHOLINE RECEPTORS. Most of the principles discussed in relation to receptors for the sympathetic nervous system also apply to receptors for the parasympathetic system. Receptors for acetylcholine appear to be of two major types defined in terms of affinities for interaction with a variety of selective antagonists. The cholinergic receptors present on autonomic effector cells are of one major type termed "muscarinic" cholinergic receptors. These receptors are blocked by muscarinic antagonists such as atropine and stimulated not only by cholinergic agonists such as carbachol but also by drugs that prolong the effect of acetylcholine by blocking its hydrolysis.

The second major type of receptor for acetylcholine is termed "nicotinic" and mediates the effects of the neurotransmitter in autonomic ganglia (sympathetic and parasympathetic) as well as at neuromuscular junctions. The cholinergic receptors of the autonomic ganglion are blocked by antagonists such as hexamethonium or trimethaphan. These nicotinic receptors can be distinguished from the nicotinic receptors of skeletal muscle, which are selectively blocked by antagonists such as decamethonium. Thus there are in effect two subtypes of nicotinic receptors. These are sometimes referred to as N_1 (autonomic ganglia) and N_2 (neuromuscular junction).

The various types of cholinergic receptors have also been studied by ligand binding techniques. The different types of receptors appear to be distinct biochemical entities subject to regulation by excessive stimulation (tolerance or desensitization) as well as other factors.

Nicotinic receptors appear to function by regulating Na^+ conductance and consequent depolarization. By contrast, muscarinic cholinergic receptors may function by inhibiting adenylate cyclase in analogy with the alpha$_2$-adrenergic receptors that inhibit adenylate cyclase in the platelet.

SYMPATHOMIMETIC AMINES

In addition to the various amines that act directly on adrenergic receptors, there are several drugs that appear to act indirectly by causing the release of endogenous catecholamines from nerve terminals. Their pharmacologic effects are therefore similar to those of norepinephrine or epinephrine, i.e., they cause beta-adrenergic stimulation of the heart and alpha-adrenergic mediated vasoconstriction. These drugs include metaraminol, mephentermine, and ephedrine. Since these drugs work by causing secretion of endogenous transmitter, their prolonged use is associated with tachyphylaxis resulting from depletion of transmitter stores.

The most important therapeutic effects of epinephrine and norepinephrine are due to their actions on the heart and smooth muscle. Isoproterenol, epinephrine, and norepinephrine all have strong positive inotropic and chronotropic effects caused by interaction with cardiac beta receptors. In addition, epinephrine and norepinephrine generally have a vasoconstrictor effect (vascular alpha receptors), whereas isoproterenol is a strong and selective vasodilator by virtue of its interaction with vascular beta$_2$ receptors but not with vasoconstrictor alpha receptors. Since epinephrine can also combine with the beta$_2$ receptors, it may also cause vasodilation under certain circumstances. These catecholamines, as well as several related agents such as dopamine and dobutamine, may be used to stabilize the circulation in some forms of shock (see Ch. 44 for details).

Beta-adrenergic sympathomimetic amines may also be used to increase cardiac rate and improve atrioventricular conduction in patients with heart block. Alpha agonists such as metaraminol may be used to elevate blood pressure transiently to revert paroxysmal atrial tachycardia to normal sinus rhythm by provoking a reflex vagal discharge that may slow the heart rate. Their use in such circumstances should always be by slow intravenous infusion with careful monitoring of blood pressure.

Adrenergic agonists used in the treatment of hypertension include clonidine and guanabenz, which are relatively selective alpha agonists that appear to have primarily a central nervous system site of action. Rapid discontinuation of antihypertensive treatment with clonidine has occasionally been reported to be associated with marked rebound hypertension. This syndrome may be associated with transient elevations in catecholamine release, and hence alpha-adrenergic antagonists may be of use in its treatment.

A major application of beta-adrenergic agonists is in the treatment of asthma. Epinephrine by injection and isoproterenol by inhalation have long been used to achieve bronchodilation by stimulation of beta$_2$-adrenergic receptors. In recent years a number of beta$_2$ selective agonists have been developed. These include isoetharine, terbutaline, salbutamol, and metaproterenol. These agents have the advantage of causing somewhat less beta$_1$-adrenergic receptor stimulation and hence have less tendency to cause tachycardia for any given level of beta$_2$ stimulation (bronchodilation).

Adverse side effects are often a predictable consequence of the interaction of adrenergic agonists with adrenergic receptors of similar specificity in organs other than those in which specific therapeutic effects are sought. Some examples include tachycardia with bronchodilators and ectopic rhythms after inotropic or vasopressor agents.

ADRENERGIC ANTAGONISTS

BETA-ADRENERGIC BLOCKERS. Beta-adrenergic antagonists are among the most widely used drugs in the practice of medicine. As with adrenergic agonists, both therapeutic and adverse effects of beta-adrenergic antagonists are readily understood in terms of their competitive occupancy of beta-adrenergic receptors. Propranolol is the prototypic example of a beta antagonist. Propranolol and a number of related compounds also possess a direct "membrane stabilizing," "local anesthetic, or quinidine-like" effect, which gives them additional utility in the treatment of certain arrhythmias. These direct membrane effects can be dissociated from beta-blocking properties by the fact that the receptor blocking effects reside largely in the (−) stereoisomer, whereas the membrane effects are present equally in both the (+) and (−) stereoisomers. These membrane effects also appear to require somewhat higher blood concentrations.

Some, but not all, beta blockers also possess intrinsic sympathomimetic properties; i.e., they have intrinsic activities greater than 0. This means they are weak "partial agonists." Several of the earliest beta-adrenergic antagonists such as dichlorisoproterenol possessed such activity to an extent that markedly limited their therapeutic utility. Propranolol does not possess intrinsic sympathomimetic effects; it is a pure antagonist. Of the commonly used beta blockers, only pindolol and acebutolol have significant intrinsic sympathomimetic effects.

Propranolol is readily absorbed from the gastrointestinal tract, but much of the compound is immediately extracted from the portal circulation by the liver. There is marked patient-to-patient variability in hepatic metabolism, which leads to great differences in plasma drug concentrations at any given dose. An important metabolite of propranolol, 4-OH propranolol, is very active biologically, although it has a shorter half-life. Most of the propranolol in the circulation is bound to plasma proteins.

In normal persons the half-life of propranolol is quite short. The usual dosage range is 40 to 320 mg per day, with great variations observed in the dose required for optimal effects.

Propranolol has generally been administered orally four times daily because of its short half-life. However, especially in the treatment of hypertension, twice-a-day dosage is adequate. In contrast to the hepatic metabolism and short plasma half-life of propranolol and metoprolol is the renal excretion of atenolol and nadolol in largely unchanged form. As a result, these drugs are eliminated from the plasma much more slowly, which may permit once-a-day dosage.

It is believed that abrupt withdrawal of propranolol may be followed in some patients by a transient period of "supersensitivity" to catecholamines. This is especially important in patients with ischemic coronary artery disease. This phenomenon has been called the "propranolol withdrawal syndrome" and may be manifested by arrhythmias, angina, and myocardial infarction. The existence of such a syndrome and the possible basis for such supersensitivity is controversial. Experimental work in animals and humans indicates that propranolol therapy may be associated with an increase in beta receptor number in certain tissues. Many physicians prefer to taper the dosage of propranolol rather than to stop it abruptly, especially in patients with coronary artery disease.

Propranolol has equal affinity for beta$_1$- and beta$_2$-adrenergic receptors. The same is true of timolol, alprenolol,* oxprenolol,* and pindolol. In recent years several antagonists have been developed that have relative selectivity for the beta$_1$ receptors in the heart. The first of these, practolol, led to a variety of ocular, dermatologic, and other adverse effects that precluded its use in humans. More recently several other agents such as metoprolol, atenolol, and tolamolol* have become available and seem to possess some beta$_1$ selectivity. The indications for and clinical pharmacology of metoprolol are similar to those of propranolol. The potential advantage of such agents is the decreased tendency to provoke bronchospasm in susceptible subjects compared with propranolol (see below). Table 31–3 compares the important properties of several of the beta-adrenergic receptor-blocking drugs.

There are several major indications for the use of beta-adrenergic antagonist agents. In general, all of the agents have similar activities regardless of selectivity or partial agonism.

Angina. The salutary effect appears to be due primarily to a reduction of myocardial oxygen consumption as a consequence of decreased pulse rate, myocardial contractility, and, in hypertensive patients, blood pressure. Propranolol is one of the mainstays of medical therapy in many patients, and its effects may be additive with those of nitrates.

Hypertension. Beta blockers have become a very important part of antihypertensive therapeutic programs. They are used either as first-line monotherapy or often added as a second drug to a diuretic. Despite their proven efficacy, the mode of action of the drugs remains uncertain and may be related to decreased cardiac output, decreased renin release, central nervous system mechanisms, or other effects. These drugs are particularly effective in combination with a peripheral

vasodilator such as hydralazine, since the reflex and possibly deleterious cardiac stimulation evoked by the vasodilator is blocked by the beta antagonist. Another positive feature of propranolol as an antihypertensive drug is that it is generally well tolerated, which is important when chronic therapy and patient compliance are required, as in hypertension.

Arrhythmias. Antiarrhythmic effects of beta blockers are the result of both beta receptor blockade and quinidine-like effects. The drug is most useful in situations in which ectopic rhythms caused by excess catecholamines (e.g., pheochromocytoma) or digitalis are involved. (See also "Hyperthyroidism," below.) In emergency situations propranolol can be administered intravenously in doses that are a small fraction of the usual oral dose.

Hyperthyroidism. Certain manifestations of hyperthyroidism such as hyperdynamic circulation, palpitations, and tremors mimic a "hyper–beta-adrenergic" state and may reflect alterations in the beta receptors themselves. These symptomatic manifestations are often dramatically improved by beta-adrenergic antagonists. A particular indication is in the circumstance of "thyroid storm" with difficult-to-control metabolic (e.g., hyperthermia) and cardiovascular (e.g., paroxysmal atrial fibrillation with rapid ventricular response) complications. Digitalis may be particularly ineffective in treating the rapid ventricular response to atrial arrhythmias in such patients, and beta blockers are often uniquely useful. This is one circumstance in which propranolol administration in the presence of congestive heart failure is not contraindicated, since it may reverse the underlying cause (very rapid arrhythmia).

Other Uses. Beta antagonists have also been found useful in circumstances in which ventricular outflow is compromised by hypertrophy and transient increases in cardiac contractility such as hypertrophic cardiomyopathy and tetralogy of Fallot. In addition, propranolol is used for prophylaxis of migraine.

Also, some beta blockers are used after myocardial infarction, since they have been shown to decrease the incidence of both reinfarction and sudden death.

Several other uses, such as benign familial tremor, are promising but currently still under investigation. The beta blocker timolol is used topically for the treatment of open-angle glaucoma.

Beta blockers are also used in the symptomatic treatment of certain of the manifestations of pheochromocytoma. However, they should never be used in the absence of concomitant alpha-adrenergic blockade, since marked hypertension may result.

Side Effects. The adverse effects of beta blockers, like their therapeutic actions, are largely consequences of their competitive occupancy of beta-adrenergic receptors. These include depression of cardiac contractility resulting from loss of normal sympathetic support with precipitation of previously latent or incipient congestive heart failure; worsening or precipitation of high degrees of heart block; and bronchoconstriction caused by blockade of bronchial beta$_2$-adrenergic receptors in susceptible individuals. When bronchoconstric-

---

*Investigational drug for this purpose.

TABLE 31–3. PROPERTIES OF SOME BETA-ADRENERGIC RECEPTOR–BLOCKING DRUGS

Drug	Relative Potency (Propranolol = 1)	Relative Beta$_1$ Selectivity	Intrinsic Sympathomimetic Activity	Membrane-Stabilizing Activity	Plasma Half-Life (hrs)
Acebutolol	0.3	+	+	0	3–4
Atenolol	1	+	0	0	6–9
Metoprolol	1	+	0	0	3–4
Nadolol	1	0	0	0	14–24
Pindolol	6	0	+++	+	3–4
Propranolol	1	0	0	++	3.5–6
Timolol	6	0	0	0	3–4

tion occurs, the usual beta-agonist bronchodilators may be ineffective owing to the very high affinity of propranolol for beta-adrenergic receptors. In such circumstances, drugs such as aminophylline, which dilate airway smooth muscle without the need for beta receptor interactions, are particularly useful.

In diabetics requiring insulin, propranolol may, in rare cases, cause or worsen hypoglycemia by interfering with beta-adrenergic–mediated hyperglycemic counter-regulatory mechanisms. It may also mask those symptoms of hypoglycemia that are mediated by beta-adrenergic stimulation, such as tachycardia or pupillary dilation. The presence of incipient congestive heart failure, heart block or impaired cardiac conduction, history of bronchoconstriction, or brittle diabetes may represent contraindications to the use of beta-adrenergic antagonists.

Other reported adverse effects with beta blockers include lethargy, depression, lightheadedness, and mild diarrhea.

ALPHA-ADRENERGIC ANTAGONISTS. Alpha-adrenergic blockers are used much less frequently than are the beta antagonists. Until recently the two most commonly employed agents have been phentolamine and phenoxybenzamine. Phentolamine is a classic rapidly reversible (i.e., "competitive") antagonist, whereas phenoxybenzamine is an irreversible ("noncompetitive") alpha-adrenergic antagonist. Thus, after occupancy of alpha receptors by phenoxybenzamine, a stable covalent bond forms between the drug and some portion of the receptor by an alkylation mechanism. This may lead to a very prolonged duration of action.

The major indication for these two drugs is in patients with known or suspected pheochromocytoma. As described in Ch. 242, phentolamine may be used in diagnosing pheochromocytoma, in which its injection leads to a marked drop in blood pressure. This potentially hazardous maneuver is only rarely indicated. Both phenoxybenzamine and phentolamine are used to prevent the hypertension of pheochromocytoma, for which they represent highly specific therapy. They are particularly useful in the perioperative period, when large fluctuations of serum catecholamines may occur (Ch. 242). Other than in patients with pheochromocytoma, non–subtype selective alpha antagonists such as phentolamine do not appear particularly useful in the treatment of hypertension.

Adverse effects of alpha antagonists such as phentolamine include nasal stuffiness, orthostatic hypotension, tachycardia, positive inotropic effects, and worsening angina. These effects may be explained, at least in part, by the observation that phentolamine is very potent not only at postsynaptic vascular alpha$_1$ receptors, which mediate smooth muscle contraction, but also at presynaptic alpha$_2$ receptors. Blockade by phentolamine of the alpha$_2$ receptor–mediated autoinhibitory effect of endogenous norepinephrine leads to increased release of norepinephrine in the heart. This increased concentration of norepinephrine causes enhanced stimulation of beta-adrenergic receptors, resulting in positive inotropic and chronotropic effects.

Prazosin is a highly selective alpha$_1$ antagonist that is useful in the treatment of hypertension. It exerts its major antihypertensive effect by reversible blockade of postsynaptic alpha$_1$ receptors. Prazosin is the most potent alpha$_1$-blocking drug currently available. In marked contrast to phentolamine, prazosin is an extremely weak antagonist of alpha$_2$ receptors both in physiologic studies and in direct radioligand binding experiments. This may explain why prazosin is apparently more effective as an antihypertensive agent than non–subtype selective alpha-adrenergic blocking drugs such as phentolamine. The very weak affinity of prazosin for alpha$_2$ receptors presumably accounts not only for its relatively better antihypertensive effect but also in part for the absence of certain adverse effects that are characteristically seen with non–subtype selective alpha blockers (see above). First, tachycardia is uncommon with prazosin. Since it is so weak in blocking alpha$_2$ receptors, enhanced norepinephrine release would not be expected. Second, since enhanced "norepinephrine overflow" from sympathetic nerves does not occur with prazosin, beta-adrenergic stimulation of renin secretion is absent and plasma renin concentrations do not generally rise with prazosin as they do with other alpha-adrenergic antagonists. Also, prazosin would not be expected to block the alpha$_2$ receptors, which are conjectured to inhibit renin release.

Another use of prazosin is in the management of patients with severe and intractable congestive heart failure. The beneficial hemodynamic changes are due to a combination of decreased mean arterial pressure (decreased "afterload") and decreased venous tone leading to decreased venous return (decreased "preload") (see Ch. 43).

In addition to the agents discussed above, a number of other drugs not normally thought of as "alpha blockers" have significant alpha-adrenergic antagonist potency. In particular, phenothiazines such as chlorpromazine and butyrophenones such as haloperidol are relatively potent alpha blockers. This may explain why hypotension is encountered with these drugs.

CHOLINERGIC DRUGS

ANTAGONISTS. Postganglionic parasympathetic cholinergic receptors are of one major type termed muscarinic. The major clinical muscarinic antagonist is atropine, one of the oldest drugs in medicine. Scopolamine is a closely related alkaloid.

Atropine blocks the effects of the parasympathetic nervous system on smooth muscle, cardiac muscle, and various glandular cells. Because atropine blocks the cardiac actions of the vagus nerve it increases the rate of firing of the sinoatrial node and facilitates conduction through the atrioventricular node. Accordingly atropine can be used in the treatment of atrioventricular block or sinus bradycardia, as for example in the setting of myocardial infarction or after digitalis excess. The drug is generally used intravenously or subcutaneously in such circumstances.

Atropine and less purified preparations of belladonna alkaloids also reduce gastrointestinal motility and gastric secretion and may be useful in symptomatic treatment of peptic ulcer disease.

As with the adrenergic antagonists, adverse effects of atropine are largely extensions of the therapeutic effects of receptor blockade. These include dry mouth, urinary retention, constipation, and blurred vision. Large doses may cause hallucinations, marked agitation, dilated pupils, and dry skin. In cases of severe atropine poisoning anticholinesterases such as physostigmine are quite effective (see below).

CHOLINERGIC AGONISTS. The actions of administered acetylcholine-like drugs are due to their interaction with both muscarinic receptors (parasympathetic effectors) and nicotinic receptors (autonomic ganglia). Because of its rapid inactivation by acetylcholinesterase, acetylcholine itself is not effective systemically. Several synthetic esters of choline are more resistant to hydrolysis and are therefore of greater therapeutic utility. Methacholine (acetyl-beta-methylcholine) and bethanechol have purely muscarinic effects, whereas carbamylcholine is both nicotinic and muscarinic. Such drugs have limited therapeutic applications. They are used occasionally, for example, in cases of postoperative urinary retention.

ANTICHOLINESTERASES. Inhibition of cholinesterases by inhibitors that bind reversibly to the active site of the enzyme leads to a competitive decrease in the rate of hydrolysis of acetylcholine, thus raising the concentration of the neurotransmitter at nicotinic and muscarinic receptors. Several such drugs are physostigmine, a naturally occurring alkaloid, and the synthetic agents neostigmine, pyridostigmine, and edrophonium. These agents may be used for their nicotinic actions in the treatment of myasthenia gravis (see Ch. 518). Because edrophonium is so short acting, it may be used intravenously to help determine if myasthenia gravis is actually present (marked improvement in symptoms) but is not used therapeutically in this disease. These drugs may also be used for their muscarinic actions to treat paralytic ileus or postoperative urinary retention.

Another application is in the treatment of paroxysmal atrial tachycardia, either alone or in conjunction with carotid sinus massage to stimulate the vagal fibers to the heart. Edrophonium is generally used for this purpose.

Several organophosphorous agents such as diisopropyl fluorophosphate (DFP) and parathion are used in insecticides and are potent *irreversible* inhibitors of cholinesterases. They appear to act by phosphorylation of the active site of the enzyme. Cases of poisoning result from absorption of the agent through the skin or gastrointestinal tract or by inhalation. Symptoms may have a subtle onset with signs of excess cholinergic stimulation, i.e., salivation, hyperhidrosis, pupillary constriction and muscle twitching, and nausea. A relatively specific antidote, pralidoxime, reactivates the enzyme by removing the phosphate group. Atropine is generally used acutely to relieve symptoms.

GANGLIONIC BLOCKERS

Ganglionic blockers competitively antagonize the nicotinic effect of acetylcholine in the autonomic ganglia. They have limited therapeutic applications at present. Because tonic sympathetic nerve outflow to vasculature is reduced after ganglionic blockade, these agents reduce blood pressure. Examples are hexamethonium* and trimethaphan. They are potent drugs and when administered by slow intravenous infusion can be used to titrate the blood pressure in hypertensive emergencies and aortic dissection. As expected, they have a variety of severe side effects that limit their therapeutic utility. These include postural hypotension, ileus, urinary retention, and, at high infusion rates, respiratory arrest.

Frishman WH: Beta-adrenoceptor antagonists: New drugs and new indications. N Engl J Med 305:500, 1981. *A detailed review of the pharmacodynamics and pharmacokinetics of all the commonly available beta blockers.*

Lefkowitz RJ, Caron MG, Stiles GL: Mechanisms of membrane receptor regulation: Biochemical, physiological and clinical insights derived from studies of the adrenergic receptors. N Engl J Med 310:1570, 1984. *An overview of physiologic and pathophysiologic factors found to regulate adrenergic receptor binding sites.*

Yusuf S, Peto R, Lewis J, et al.: Beta blockade during and after myocardial infarction: An overview of the randomized trials. Prog Cardiovasc Dis 27:335, 1985. *The basis for the use of beta-adrenergic receptor blockers to reduce post–myocardial infarction morbidity and mortality.*

*Investigational drug for this purpose.

32 COMMON POISONINGS

William O. Robertson

DEFINITION. Man's chemical environment was recognized as a threat to health long before the birth of Christ. Well-documented outbreaks of occupational mercury and lead "poisonings" had been recorded and preventive measures implemented by 200 B.C. The Middle Ages saw arsenic poisoning employed as a political weapon. More recent times have seen increasing recognition of industrial toxins, "accidental poisoning" in childhood, purposeful overdoses in adults, adverse reactions to drugs, and environmental hazards for us all. The common theme is entrance of an exogenous chemical into an organism and subsequent disruption of its metabolism. The term "poison" has undergone quantitative redefinition so that now such ubiquitous substances as table salt and drinking water are firmly established as being "poisonous." Finally, the host-organism itself has contributed to a better comprehension of the word "poison," as genetic

variability has been recognized to determine the impact of a given molecule in such hereditary disorders as phenylketonuria, glucose-6-phosphate dehydrogenase deficiency, and others. As man's understanding of life has expanded, the connotation of poisoning has undergone substantial evolution.

ETIOLOGY. Approximately 1.2 million chemical entities had been identified and coded by 1950; the number had risen to more than 4.3 million by 1976. By 1987, the number will exceed 10 million. Although not all of these compounds have been marketed, many new organic compounds have appeared in the home and the workplace. For example, available formulations of pesticides have increased fifty-fold over the past 30 years. Moreover, manufacturing processes have released additional compounds (e.g., dioxins) into the workplace or the environment with capabilities of serving as poisons.

New chemical techniques have permitted prompt and complete identification of poisonings and have uncovered the causes of such diverse entities as Minamata disease (teratogenesis consequent to methyl mercury), an outbreak of ascending paralysis affecting more than 4000 with more than 400 deaths in Iraq (also caused by methyl mercury), the "gray syndrome" in premature infants (caused by chloramphenicol), mesotheliomas induced by asbestos, and an epidemic of angiosarcoma of the liver among industrial workers (caused by vinyl chloride). Nevertheless, many unknowns remain and justify careful prospective monitoring of industry, of the home, and of the environment.

INCIDENCE. Over the past 25 years progressively more reliable data have been gathered about deaths from poisonings, the leading agents, and the number of such deaths attributable to each among children less than five years old and among the overall population (Table 32–1). Although concerns for infants and toddlers prompted the creation of our nation's Poison Center Network, deaths from poisoning among that group have plummeted over the past 30 years; these children were, fortunately, greatly under-represented in 1984, accounting for only 2.2 per cent of poisoning deaths despite the fact that their "accidental ingestions" account for 61 per cent of the 900,513 human exposures summarized by the National Data Collection System of the American Association of Poison Control Centers. Among adults precise data

TABLE 32–1. DEATHS DUE TO ACCIDENTAL POISONING IN THE UNITED STATES, 1982

	All Ages	Under 5 Years	5–44 Years	45+ Years
Total: Solids and Liquids	3474	67	2295	1112
Medications	2862	41	2000	821
Analgesics, antipyretics	1171	16	835	282
Opiates	559	2	501	56
Sedatives, hypnotics	141	0	99	52
Psychotropic drugs	265	7	171	87
Other central nervous system (CNS) drugs	216	1	188	27
Other drugs	1375	24	865	486
Nondrugs	612	26	295	291
Alcohol	412	0	199	213
Paints, solvents, and cleaning agents	84	8	50	26
Pesticides	29	5	12	12
Corrosives, caustics	27	5	4	18
Foods, plants	7	0	4	3
Others	53	8	26	19
Gases and vapors	1259	37	707	515
Carbon monoxide	1022	21	584	417

Data from National Safety Council: Accident Facts. Chicago, National Center for Health Statistics, 1985.

are more difficult to retrieve. Incomplete data attest that a minimum of 12,000 deaths occur annually as a result of suicide by poisoning.

EPIDEMIOLOGY. There are significant differences in the epidemiology of poisonings among children under five years of age compared with the remainder of the population. With adults, occupational and industrial exposures, suicide gestures or attempts, and homicides depend upon host factors and environmental settings as well as involved chemicals. In contrast, among children under five, host and environmental factors are less variable. In the United States, occurrences peak at 24 to 32 months of age, and more male than female children are involved; poisonings happen most frequently between 11 A.M. and 12 noon or between 5 and 6 P.M. and in places of easiest exposure—the kitchen, the bedroom, and the bathroom. In addition, illness in the family or "life stress situations" increase the likelihood of accidental ingestion.

PREVENTION. Avoiding exposure to the toxin is the ultimate precaution; among adults, a variety of approaches have been employed—some with obvious effectiveness, others without. For example, the use of mercury in the felting process of hats has been outlawed since 1941; that source of mercury poisoning has disappeared in the hatting industry. Beryllium has been excluded from fluorescent light bulbs, and that source of exposure no longer exists. Similarly, where arsenic has been eliminated from pesticidal preparations and where naphthylamine has been eliminated from the rubber industry, human illness has been avoided. Some of these steps have resulted from legislative processes; others are the result of voluntary activity on the part of industry or an aware public.

Among children some approaches have also proved effective; others are without much evidence of success. For example, efforts directed at altering toddlers' exploratory behaviors in family settings have not proved effective. In contrast, the use of safety caps on medicine bottles had important consequences. For the ten-year period between 1959 and 1969, almost 100 deaths occurred annually from accidental salicylate poisoning in children under five; in 1978, only 12 such deaths were reported. Several variables have been cited as definitely contributory: (1) the manufacturers' voluntary reduction of the number of tablets as well as of the amount of aspirin per bottle; (2) the introduction of a favorable flavor to the "baby aspirin" as an attractive alternative to larger tablets; (3) programs of professional and public education; (4) the appearance of acetaminophen as a rival to aspirin, with its subsequent capture of 30 per cent of the analgesic-antipyretic market, and more recently, their replacement by still newer nonsteroidal anti-inflammatory drugs (NSAID's); and (5) the mandated use of safety caps or child-resistant containers. All have had an impact, but current professional opinion holds that safety caps have contributed approximately 60 per cent of the variance. As safety caps have subsequently been applied to other prescription products and dangerous household items such as petroleum distillates and caustics, their impact has been felt there also. Unfortunately, safety caps may have a negative effect among the geriatric population, among whom as many as 50 per cent cite them as contributing to their lack of compliance in taking prescribed medications.

Since 1953, more than 500 poison centers have been established across the country to provide professionals and patients with ingredient information, toxic potentials, and treatment alternatives. Initially, the FDA's National Clearinghouse of Poison Control Centers was intended to serve as the coordinating unit; it also provided technical information to centers. In recent years, several microfiche systems—particularly "Poisondex" (Micromedex, Denver)—have been developed to catalogue product information and to outline management approaches; they are capable of storing information on more than 300,000 products in a limited space and in an easily retrievable manner. Moreover, such microfiche systems avoid

filing errors and permit updating of information on a quarterly basis. With recent advances in computer technology—e.g., hard disk drives, laser processing, and so forth—these data systems are now available on self-contained personal computer packages.

Over the years the American Association of Poison Control Centers has served to produce educational material aimed at preventing poisoning, to establish standards for the operation of poison centers, to conduct self-assessment examinations for those staffing poison centers, and to implement a nationwide program aimed at regionalizing the poison center network. More recently, the American Academy of Clinical Toxicology and the American Board of Medical Toxicology have been developed to serve as the specialty society and certifying body, respectively, to further the academic and professional goals of physicians involved in such programs.

DIAGNOSIS. The diagnosis of an accidental (or a purposeful) poisoning can be made only if considered; this is true for either the adult or child with unexplained signs or symptoms. Once the possibility of poisoning is entertained, a careful search is made for a possible container and its label or for a solid medication form and its drug-identifying imprint; next, the toxic potential of the substance can be verified from existing information or by contacting the nearest poison center. Often the presenting clinical signs and symptoms are so characteristic as to permit diagnosis—i.e., the hyperventilation (following vomiting) of acute salicylism, the extrapyramidal manifestations of phenothiazine reactions. Sometimes diagnostic confirmation can be established by the patient's response to a specific antidote, e.g., naloxone. On other occasions, analysis of specimens of body fluids—blood, urine, vomit, gastric contents, or stool—is necessary for diagnosis. As a generalization, "routine toxic screens" have proved to be of relatively little value in the child and are decried by many experts as inaccurate, confusing, and not helpful in the adult. Where the history or the environment provides a lead to the potential toxins, modern technology is proving increasingly useful. In the absence of such leads, helpful results are admittedly scarce.

Particularly helpful to toxicologists have been the Consumer Product Act of 1970 and the Commission Coordinating Safety Packaging Regulations, which have promulgated adequate labeling of hazardous substances across the country. *The label on the container is the single most useful information in accidental poisonings.* In the absence of a label, generic information about ingredients of household, industrial, and pharmaceutical products is available from a poison center or from a particularly useful textbook: Clinical Toxicology of Commercial Products. The information on the prescription bottle, on the package insert, or from the imprint of the solid medication form (such imprints exist on virtually all tablets and capsules) is equally important and ought to be diligently pursued.

Once the ingested poison has been identified, the problem remains to determine its potential for harm in the particular patient. That potential depends upon the amount and form ingested, the toxicity of the agent, the time lapse involved, and a variety of host factors. The amount ingested can sometimes be estimated by observers or by determining the amount of material remaining in the container. The toxicity of a particular poison can be assessed by reference to known data on human experiences, to animal LD50's, and to derivative "minimal lethal doses." One must be particularly cautious about overinterpreting LD50's or animal studies; in many instances the results are not transferable to the human. A toxicity rating has proved useful in estimating the degree of risk to the patient (Table 32–2).

In recent years, toxicologic analysis of body fluids has assumed an increasingly significant role in the diagnosis and management of poisoning, but it remains a relatively small one. Technical developments perfecting chemical analysis by mass spectrophotometry, gas-liquid chromatography, and

TABLE 32–2. TOXICITY RATING*

Rating	Probable Lethal Dose	
	mg/kg	*For 70-kg Man*
6—Super toxic	<5	A taste <7 drops
5—Extremely toxic	5–50	7 drops to 1 tsp
4—Very toxic	50–500	1 tsp to 1 oz
3—Moderately toxic	500 mg–5 grams	1 oz to 1 pint
2—Slightly toxic	5–15 grams	1 pint to 1 quart
1—Practically nontoxic	>15 grams	>1 quart

*From Gosselin RE, Hodge HC, Smith RP: Clinical Toxicity of Commercial Products. 5th ed. Baltimore, Williams & Wilkins Company, 1984.

spin resonance now allow toxic screening for a variety of poisons from minuscule amounts of body fluids. Commercial laboratories as well as a number of hospital, public health, and university laboratories provide qualitative and quantitative analyses for sedatives, narcotics, psychotropics, heavy metals, pesticides, and other compounds, all of which enable a speedy and accurate diagnosis. Nevertheless, such determination (e.g., specifying the type and amount of barbiturate in the blood) often does not alter management of the patient. Thus, in instances of barbiturate overdose, measurements of blood gases and pH prove more effective in coping with the clinical problem than does the quantitative determination of barbiturate level. Notable exceptions occur when specific quantification is critical in deciding on therapy—e.g., the use of acetaminophen blood levels and the Matthews-Rumack nomogram in deciding on the use of its antidote (*N*-acetylcysteine) before clinical signs or symptoms of illness appear, or the use of the serum salicylate concentration and the Done nomogram in determining the need for therapy in acute salicylate ingestion; and the value of the serum iron concentration along with clinical signs and symptoms in contemplating chelation therapy with desferrioxamine for iron poisoning. So too, identifying the presence of methyl alcohol or ethylene glycol can be critical in therapeutic management. Regardless of these several exceptions, the point remains that historical and clinical features plus the routinely available laboratory tests are usually paramount. Assisting the physician are a number of texts listed at the end of this chapter.

TREATMENT. Even before the ingested (or inhaled) substance has been identified and its toxic potential determined, first aid measures and supportive care ought to be initiated. Subsequent efforts are directed toward (1) preventing absorption of the substance; (2) curtailing its conversion in the body to its active form or hastening its conversion to an inactive one; (3) neutralizing or counteracting its clinical effect; and (4) enhancing its excretion from the body. In the majority of instances instituting measures to enable the patient to tolerate the temporary impact of the toxin and then to recuperate on his or her own remains the most effective course of action and often prevents subsequent poisonings as a result of overzealous treatment.

Supportive Measures. Prompt attention to supportive measures before a crisis has arisen, is, in fact, usually the single most critical element in managing the overdosed patient. The airway must be maintained, ventilation assured, cardiac output sustained, peripheral vascular collapse avoided, convulsions controlled, and hypertension and increased intracranial pressure lowered. Physical and chemical options ought to be carefully reviewed in advance of the patient's arrival if possible. Life support mechanisms can tide the patient over a period of compromised function as a result of anesthesia, an accidental overdose, or the purposeful induction of "barbiturate coma." But those measures must be carefully planned, carried out by skilled personnel, and monitored in detail if optimal benefit is to be achieved.

Prevention of Absorption. This is best accomplished in the conscious child or adult by *induction of emesis* as opposed to gastric lavage. Although gastric lavage has a tradition in

emergency medicine, its yield of ingested material falls short of the returns by emesis. Moreover, despite improved emergency transport systems, there are significant time delays in delivering the patient to a health care facility where lavage can be undertaken. During that time, significant absorption takes place. By contrast, efforts to induce vomiting can be initiated in the home—particularly if syrup of ipecac is available there. If not, it is readily obtained from local pharmacies, 24-hour corner groceries, emergency vehicles, and neighbors. One should administer 15 ml to a child or 15 to 30 ml to an adult together with 200 to 300 ml of any fluids—water, soft drinks, milk, or juices—and wait 10 to 15 minutes with an appropriate receptacle for vomiting to occur. If no vomiting ensues in 20 minutes, one should repeat the initial dose of syrup of ipecac and administer more fluids. If no syrup of ipecac is available, one should try gagging the patient but should be prepared for failure; one should then encourage the patient to drink 30 to 45 ml of liquid dishwashing detergents (anionic or nonionic but *not* cationic detergents) together with 240 ml of fluid. If the patient has already arrived in the emergency room, apomorphine can be used. It proves effective in four to five minutes but results in a drowsy patient despite use of naloxone. In all circumstances one should avoid table salt as an emetic agent; its use can compound the problem with acute hypernatremia. One should always avoid emesis in the comatose or convulsing patient or in the patient who has ingested a caustic. Syrup of ipecac proves effective in acute phenothiazine ingestions, but not in the face of chronic overdose; any form of emesis is maximally effective in the first one to one and a half hours after ingestion; seldom is it useful after two to three hours' delay.

Gastric lavage, using a large-bore tube and 1000 to 3000 ml of half-strength saline as the rinse, together with terminal instillation of activated charcoal, is the only option for the unconscious patient. In patients over two years of age, concomitant use of a cuffed endotracheal tube is indicated to avoid aspiration. Despite the fact that most toxins are absorbed rapidly and thus escape delayed evacuation efforts, on occasion substantial portions of ingested agents have been recovered, especially in suicidal patients who have consumed poisons that delay gastric emptying, slow intestinal motility, or depress overall body function. In those instances attempts at evacuation are recommended, but cannot be expected to be effective in more than one of five patients.

Activated charcoal can be used to complement either of the measures discussed above, but not with syrup of ipecac until after emesis has occurred. The large surface area of charcoal permits significant adsorption of the toxin, precluding its absorption from the gut. Given by mouth or via nasogastric tube in amounts of 5 to 15 times the amount of the ingested toxin, activated charcoal has diminished absorption by as much as 50 per cent with significant therapeutic benefits. Recent pharmacologic research supports the contention that absorption may be prevented by early intervention with charcoal, but equally importantly, finds that excretion of those compounds that are recycled via the gastrointestinal tract can be significantly increased by repetitive oral instillation of activated charcoal.

Cathartics, laxatives, enemas, and *colonic irrigations* are "heroic" measures devoid of evidence of effectiveness; in fact, cathartics can increase the rate of absorption of some barbiturates.

Inhibition of metabolism of a potential toxin to its active form or conversion to an inactive form is an option and, when feasible, may prove beneficial. For example, methyl alcohol becomes active only after it is converted to formaldehyde and formic acid; administering ethyl alcohol to the patient takes advantage of substrate competition (it is favored over methyl alcohol by the enzymatic processes involved), permitting significant reduction in the rate of metabolism of methyl alcohol and resulting in diminished formation of formaldehyde and formic acid, which in turn can be more easily scavenged by existent metabolic processes.

In other instances, enhancement of enzymatic activity may *activate* a toxin. For example, pretreatment of the pregnant woman and fetal liver with phenobarbital will enhance conjugation of bilirubin, but such pretreatment augments the conversion of carbon tetrachloride to its deleterious metabolite.

Chelating agents also limit the entry of certain toxins into metabolic pathways and augment excretion of the inactivited material. This approach has been particularly useful in poisonings by heavy metals—treatment of arsenic, mercury, and lead with dimercaprol (BAL), D-penicillamine, and edetate (EDTA), respectively. Similarly, desferrioxamine is useful in both acute and chronic iron poisoning.

Specific antidotes to counteract the effects of specific toxins are limited to a few compounds, but when one exists its usefulness is great. Paramount is the example of naloxone, an opiate derivative, which, when administered in adequate amounts (often *considerably more* than the recommended 0.4 mg) to a patient with heroin overdose, results in patient's sitting up and talking within 20 seconds! Administered to the nonoverdosed patient, naloxone is devoid of any action, thus constituting a unique example of an antagonist drug without any agonist effects. Most other antidotes have agonist as well as antagonist effects. Common examples of such antidotes include atropine for organophosphate and carbamate insecticide poisoning, methylene blue for methemoglobinemia, nitrites plus thiosulfate for cyanide ingestion, N-acetylcysteine for acetaminophen overdoses, and diphenhydramine for phenothiazine-induced extrapyramidal reactions. In addition, recent advances in immunology have resulted in the use of portions of antibodies ("Fab" fragments) to "neutralize" the clinical effects of overwhelming digoxin poisonings. Introduced as Digibind, this antidote is still limited in its availability; the nearest Poison Center should be contacted for available details. Moreover, monoclonal antibodies to various toxins are being developed for possible clinical use—either via injection into the patient or by being affixed to perfusion columns.

Enhancing elimination of a toxin can be accomplished by several mechanisms. For example, in carbon monoxide poisoning, use of 100 per cent oxygen by ventilatory mask has both theoretic and practical benefit. In instances of phencyclidine ingestion, continuous gastric lavage, taking advantage of "ion trapping" of the recycled phencyclidine via the gastric mucosa, is reported to be effective. Ion trapping is also employed in acute salicylate poisoning via alkalinization of the urine. In the kidney tubule, free salicylate molecules ionize in the presence of an alkaline medium and are not resorbed, thus being "captured" in the urine and excreted into the bladder. In contrast, amphetamine (a weak base) is captured in the kidney tubule by acidifying the urine with ascorbic acid or ammonium chloride. In general, forced osmotic diuresis, particularly chemical diuresis with common diuretics (e.g., furosemide), is of little or no benefit in enhancing the excretory processes.

By contrast, *dialysis* and *hemoperfusion* have proved to be effective therapeutic tools, although not as effective as had been initially believed. For example, a decade ago many patients with barbiturate overdose were subjected to extracorporeal or peritoneal dialysis; today, less than 1 in 300 such patients is so treated. If renal shutdown has occurred, as in mercury poisoning, dialysis will prove lifesaving, although it is unlikely to augment excretion of the mercury molecule. Exceptions do exist, as in dialysis for ethylene glycol overdoses. Hemoperfusion and lipid dialysis both serve as effective mechanisms in eliminating specific offending substances from the body, e.g., ethchlorvynol. To be effective, a significant proportion of the total body toxin must be present in the blood and must not be tightly bound to serum protein. For many compounds, such as digoxins, tricyclic antidepressants,

and phenothiazines, these conditions are not met, and dialysis and hemoperfusion do little to reduce the total body burden of toxin. Knowledge of the "apparent volume of distribution" of a compound permits prediction of the usefulness of dialysis or hemoperfusion (see Ch. 80.1).

Occasionally, still other techniques, such as *exchange transfusions* in boric acid or iron poisoning, may be useful. So-called gut lavage, a virtually continuous through-and-through rinse of the bowel via instillation of large amounts of physiologic fluids into the intestine through a nasogastric tube, has been reported effective in paraquat overdoses when no alternatives exist. Careful consideration of the metabolic pathways of the involved substance combined with empiric evidence of previous outcomes serves as the best guide for management.

Treatment of Specific Common Poisonings. In addition to the general principles of treatment discussed above, a few common poisonings warrant specific mention.

Aspirin (salicylate) poisoning formerly accounted for 20 per cent of ingestions among children under five years of age; today, it is responsible for only 1 to 2 per cent. However, it remains a concern for all age groups—particularly because of its widespread use as a potential suicidal agent among the elderly. Acute ingestions in excess of 100 mg per kilogram of body weight deserve induction of emesis; aspirin leads to rapid metabolic acidosis in children under four years of age and to initial respiratory alkalosis in the adult. Both groups vomit; this permits early detection and helps in differentiation from acetaminophen ingestion. Alkalinizing the urine proves remarkably effective with the single acute ingestion; one should consult the Done nomogram for prognosis. The administration of intravenous $NaHCO_3$ (3 mEq per kilogram of body weight) to young children usually proves effective in raising urine pH above 7.0. A later second or third dose of approximately one half of that amount may be necessary to sustain alkalinization of the urine and thereby promote ionization and reduce reabsorption of salicylate. The use of acetazolamide to alkalinize the urine should be avoided; its mechanism of action also accelerates transport of salicylate into the central nervous system (CNS). Urinary elimination of the salicylate moiety removes the cause of the acidosis—a far more effective approach to therapy than treatment of the systemic acidosis itself. In the adult, initial blood pH may be elevated; nonetheless, it is the urine pH that is critical to monitor. In general, additional potassium administration is necessary only for the chronically intoxicated patient or later in the course of acute intoxications in adults. Occasionally dialysis may be warranted, but ordinarily general supportive measures prove sufficient. Chronic overdoses are far less responsive to any specific interventions, but supportive treatment can be crucial.

Acetaminophen has captured 30 per cent of today's analgesic-antipyretic market; liquid formulations are being augmented by solid preparation forms, some of which are in "extra strength" dosages. In Britain, acetaminophen has been a particularly popular suicidal substance; management is often complicated by the fact that no significant symptoms may appear until after irreversible liver damage has occurred. If recognized early—preferably less than 12 hours and certainly less than 24 hours after ingestion—determination of the serum level and comparison of it against standards on the Matthews-Rumack nomogram permit an appropriate decision about the possible use of an antidote, either N-acetylcysteine or methionine (both sulfhydryl donors). Both appear to enter into metabolic pathways via glutathione mechanisms and to preclude the formation of an epoxide derivative of acetaminophen that binds covalently to liver macromolecules, resulting in liver cell destruction. An intravenous preparation of the antidote is available that is strongly favored and widely used in Britain; it ought to be available in the United States soon. Currently, only an oral form is available in the United States, and its use presents difficulties because of associated emesis.

Of special note is the apparent diminished susceptibility to toxicity in the preadolescent compared with the adult.

Significant overdoses of *anticholinergic substances* in various forms (e.g., tricyclic antidepressants, atropine, antihistamines, phenothiazines, jimson weed) produce fever, flushing, widely dilated pupils, and CNS signs and symptoms varying from somnolence and coma to delirium and seizures. Each of these specific drugs may also produce additional specific symptoms by other mechanisms—e.g., diphenhydramine hydrochloride (Benadryl) occasionally results in extrapyramidal reactions; tricyclic antidepressants cause cardiac arrhythmias. For this class of drugs, physostigmine is available both as a diagnostic agent and as a therapeutic substance; because administration of physostigmine may itself induce seizures in 15 to 20 per cent of treated patients, its use has declined significantly. The dose is 0.5 mg administered slowly intravenously for the child under five and 1 to 2 mg for the adult, repeated as often as necessary to control seizures. Today, however, most centers rely on diazepam treatment instead. In all instances atropine should be immediately available during physostigmine infusion, and Valium also ought to be available should a convulsion occur. Tricyclic antidepressant overdoses are now numerically the most serious of prescription medicine hazards. These are best approached by using diazepam (Valium) or phenobarbital to control seizures, by maintaining a blood pH above 7.45 to prevent tachyarrhythmias either by administering $NaHCO_3$ or by controlled ventilation in the obtunded patient, and by use of conventional cardiac drugs should arrhythmias ensue.

Acute petroleum distillates (hydrocarbons) cause their most significant damage as a function of their initial action on the lungs via aspiration; such aspiration occurs at the time of ingestion or inhalation. Both in laboratory animals and in humans, large amounts of various petroleum distillates have been consumed and retained without development of any signs or symptoms save for odoriferous eructations ("smelly burps") and diarrhea. As a general rule, neither lavage nor induction of emesis is indicated in such ingestions unless some additional toxin (e.g., parathion) has been dissolved in the hydrocarbon. When such is the case, induction of emesis has supplanted gastric lavage as the treatment of choice. When pulmonary aspiration has occurred, supportive measures are introduced; antibiotics and steroids are widely used but without much evidence of effectiveness.

Carbon monoxide (see Ch. 537) ranks high as a contributor to common poisonings, suicides, and accidental deaths. The mechanism of action involves acute interruption of both oxygen transport and oxygen metabolism, with a rapid cessation of life functions. Prompt recognition of exposure and removal of the patient from the contaminated environment are essential. Hastening of excretion of carbon monoxide by administration of oxygen and consideration of hyperbaric oxygen treatment are currently the hallmarks of management.

Caustic compounds, including acids and alkalis, appear to exert their toxic effects largely via alterations of pH and their consequences on the gastrointestinal tract. Experimental evidence suggests that the damage done by alkalis is complete within 30 seconds after exposure; that done by acids may be somewhat slower to appear. Current recommendations of management are avoidance of major efforts to empty the gastrointestinal tract, neutralization of the offending compound by the administration of a protein-containing substance (such as milk), and careful assessment of the esophagus for the possibility of acute burns. This last point frequently necessitates esophagoscopy because the presence or absence of burns in the mouth proves nonpredictive of the status of the esophagus. In addition to concerns about the acute situation—managed by dilatation, steroids, and antibiotics—much interest now focuses on follow-up for 20 to 40 years because of a significantly increased risk of carcinoma of the esophagus.

Cyanide has gained its deserved reputation for toxicity by its ability to inhibit oxygen utilization at the level of the cell via cytochrome oxidase inhibition; severe metabolic acidosis can occur almost instantaneously. Most exposures are occupational; occasional exposures are the result of homicidal efforts, particularly associated with capsule tampering, and rare consequences are found subsequent to l-mandelonitrile-β-glucuronic acid (Laetrile) administration or nitroprusside overdose. As soon as cyanide poisoning is suspected, administration of nitrite—via a 3 per cent solution intravenously or amyl nitrite inhalation—is crucial. It converts hemoglobin to methemoglobin, which selectively binds cyanide. This is followed by administration of sodium thiosulfate to convert cyanide to the less toxic thiocyanate. Recent experience in Europe suggests the use of dicobalt edetate may be even more effective—but avoidance is the goal.

Drugs of abuse haunt the profession, the emergency room, and our society. Were the offending agent easily identified with certainty—e.g., heroin—the immediate remedy would be obvious—naloxone. Such instances are almost nonexistent; more than 90 per cent of what is bought and sold "on the street" is not what it has been represented to be. Even imprinted capsules have been counterfeited in efforts to "con" the buyer. In other instances the basic ingredient has been "cut" with an inert substance or "laced" with some other psychoactive substance. Enormous geographic variations seem to exist across the country, with phencyclidine ("angel dust," PCP) being particularly popular in Los Angeles and Detroit, Ritalin in Seattle, and heroin and cocaine ("crack") in New York.

The laboratory may be helpful in instances of opiate overdose but is of virtually no value for lysergic acid diethylamide (LSD) or PCP (see Ch. 466). As a consequence, symptomatic management predominates; the unconscious or convulsing adult may routinely be approached as a potential heroin addict, an alcoholic, or a hypoglycemic individual; the hyperactive, "spacey" patient prompts consideration of PCP, LSD, and related sympathomimetic agents (amphetamine, phenylpropanolamine, etc), as well as recreational cocaine or psychosocial decompensation. Supportive measures may include monitoring, restraints, sedatives (diazepam is "customary"). succinylcholine, hydration, and ventilatory and cardiac measures. As a generalization, the acute management proves far more successful than treatment of the underlying problem, but efforts ought to be directed at the latter, as it provides the only true solution to the basic problem.

Ethyl alcohol (see Ch. 467) is mentioned here to stress its ubiquity and the epidemiologic point that it is remarkably prevalent as a cause of admission to hospital for children, with both purposeful and accidental ingestions, as well as a cause of birth defects among newborns. Also, ethyl alcohol augments the potential toxicity of a number of other compounds, such as diazepam.

Halogenated hydrocarbons (including chlorinated insecticides such as chlorophenothane, or DDT) serve as a source of a myriad of occupational, industrial, and pharmacologic exposures. Almost invariably lipid soluble, most are readily absorbable by the gastrointestinal tract, the respiratory epithelium, or the skin. Fortunately, most are metabolically rather stable compounds within the human organism; thus reproduction of still more hazardous metabolites is minimized. Nonetheless, many of the compounds gain access to fat storage deposits or neural tissue and cause both central and peripheral nervous system symptoms. For some (e.g., 2,3,7,8-tetrachlorodibenzodioxin, or dioxin) there are concerns about long-term toxicity and teratogenicity. Treatment modes include elimination of subsequent exposures, attempts to retrieve unabsorbed quantities from the gastrointestinal tract, and general supportive measures in response to symptoms.

Iron salts ($FeSO_4$, Fe gluconate) represent a hazard confined almost exclusively to children who "accidentally" consume prenatal tablets. To date, virtually no cases of acute poisoning have been reported in adults. While initial reports of a 50 per cent mortality rate were greatly inflated (instead it hovers at approximately 1 per cent), iron poisoning typifies the problem of the "unsuspected toxin" about which parents, parent surrogates, and physicians may be uninformed. When ingestions are known to exceed 50 to 60 mg per kilogram or when serum levels (taken three to six hours after ingestion) exceed 400 to 500 µg per deciliter, observation and chelation with desferrioxamine ought to be seriously considered, particularly if clinical symptoms such as upper abdominal pain, nausea, and vomiting are present. Management of the acute ingestion calls for prompt gastric emptying and instillation of a 5 per cent solution of sodium bicarbonate into the stomach in an attempt to minimize absorption of the resultant ferrous carbonate compound. More serious overdoses have prompted heroic measures, including surgical extirpation of ingested tablets and attempts at exchange transfusion. To date, studies have documented no serious consequences from ingestion of iron as a component of children's chewable vitamin preparations.

Methanol and *ethylene glycol* present significant problems of metabolic acidosis in clinically poisoned patients. Diagnosis is often considered following discovery of an unexplained anion gap. These compounds both depend upon alcohol dehydrogenase for their metabolism. The current approach to therapy takes advantage of this situation and provides ethanol (5 to 10 grams per hour intravenously) as a competitive inhibitor of toxin metabolism—thus slowing the formation of toxic metabolites, formaldehyde, and formic acid from methanol, or glycoaldehyde and glycolic, glyoxylic, and oxalic acids from ethylene glycol, to rates of formation permitting these products to be disposed of by ordinary metabolic or excretory pathways. By contrast, for large overdoses hemodialysis may be required to eliminate the offending toxin.

Organophosphate and carbamate insecticides can both prove exquisitely toxic in minute amounts. The mechanism of action involves inhibition of acetylcholine metabolism via cessation of cholinesterase function. Prompt recognition of symptoms secondary to acute exposure can prove lifesaving. Detecting symptoms secondary to chronic exposure (e.g., peripheral neuropathy) can serve to eliminate much patient distress and employee unhappiness. In general, acute distress is ushered in via excessive secretions in the upper airway, with respiratory distress, diffuse muscular weakness, nausea, vomiting, and collapse. Treatment requires prompt and repeated administration of large amounts of atropine for both types of poisoning. Pralidoxime (2PAM) is also strongly recommended to assist in the rejuvenation of cholinesterase levels. Introduced in large measure as a "safer" replacement for DDT these compounds have been responsible for large numbers of acute poisonings but, as far as can be determined, are yet to be implicated in carcinogenicity, teratogenicity, or chronic liver disease.

Paraquat (and its associated congeners) is a particularly popular and effective herbicide. While controversy rages about the consequences of environment exposures, no controversy exists on the issue of acute, purposeful overdoses; they are devastating. Paraquat is a harsh gastrointestinal irritant that also inhibits renal function; its most destructive impact is on the respiratory tract, where it inhibits superoxide dismutase and kills via "oxygen toxicity." Current approaches to therapy favor such dramatic efforts as "gut lavage," with some suggestion that hemoperfusion might be warranted. However, overdoses are likely to be lethal.

Theophylline and its congeners have been recognized as inducing seizures, cardiac arrhythmias, and occasional deaths in overdose situations. More recently, "therapeutic misadventures" have been recognized; inadvertent overdoses, alterations of theophylline metabolism by viral infections and nutritional variations, and the tendency to use theophylline in large quantities for relatively minor illnesses all increase the

likelihood of such occurrences. Beta blockers can be used in managing the clinical symptoms of overdose—particularly the associated anxiety and tachycardia—but should not be used in asthmatic individuals. Children seem more resistant to the serious side effects than do adults, but occasionally both groups may have to be considered for hemoperfusion. Peritoneal and extracorporeal hemodialysis have both been reported to be ineffective.

Although ingestions of *plants and plant elements* constitute the single most frequent reason for telephoning poison centers, the overall problem is best put in perspective by Fraser's analysis of Britain's most recent 20-year experience with poisonings:

Plants are the most overrated poisons of childhood. In earlier decades there were occasional deaths, most caused by the umbelliferae (particularly hemlock water dropwort) and the solanaceae (various nightshades). From 1958 to 1977 there were three deaths, and in one the role of the ingestion in the child's demise is doubtful. The others were caused by hemlock and by *Amanita phalloides* (death cup), both in children aged five and nine. Laburnum is frequently cited as the most toxic and commonly fatal poisonous plant in both children and adults, but there appears to be no report this century of childhood poisoning death. One adult death in unusual circumstances has been recorded.

CONCLUSION. Chemical hazards have always been a way of life. Today their numbers continue to escalate. But modern technology permits both identification and quantification of minuscule amounts of some toxins—uncovering, for example, tamperings with cyanides. As a consequence, the physician is well advised to add possible poisoning to the differential diagnosis for any unexplained collection of signs or symptoms in a patient of any age. Moreover, unless the physician is confident of the timeliness and completeness of his or her understanding about a specific item, additional consultation is strongly advised.

Arena J, Drew RH: Poisoning: Chemistry, Symptoms and Treatment. 5th ed. Springfield, Ill., Charles C Thomas, 1986. *Derived from years of experience and leadership in the poisoning field, this book is well organized, carefully edited, and readable, with a remarkable collection of cases and common sense.*

Dreisbach RH, Robertson WO: Handbook of Poisoning. 12th ed. Los Altos, Calif., Lange Publishing Company, 1987. *This pocket-sized book is both comprehensive and concise. Up-to-date and always helpful to review for omissions in one's approach, it proves particularly valuable to the primary care physician.*

Goldfrank LR, Flomenbaum N, Lewin N, et al.: Toxicologic Emergencies. 3rd ed. Norwalk, CT, Appleton-Century-Crofts, 1986. *Probably the most clinically relevant and readable of all the texts available, it summarizes a remarkable amount of experience in readily retrievable form—and in a format aimed at anticipating the reader's needs.*

Gosselin RE, Hodge HC, Smith RP: Clinical Toxicology of Commercial Products. 5th ed. Baltimore, Williams & Wilkins Company, 1984. *Long established as the "bible" of the field, this compendium provides a concise overview of poisoning issues, as well as a thorough and well-edited clinical description of approximately 50 generic poisonings. It has a comprehensive listing of trade-name entities and generic items in household and commercial product fields. Authoritative the world over.*

Haddad LM, Winchester JF: Clinical Management of Poisoning and Drug Overdose. Philadelphia, W. B. Saunders Company, 1983. *A recent book with contributions chiefly by American experts, this is currently the most comprehensive text for the recognition and clinical management of poisoning.*

Klaassen CD, Amdur MD, Doull J: Toxicology: The Basic Science of Poisons. 3rd ed. New York, Macmillan, 1986. *This text constitutes the "compleat" basic science approach for the toxicologist. With 42 contributors and critical editing, the final product covers the field from salt to water to radiation.*

Proudfoot A.: Diagnosis and Management of Poisoning. Oxford, Blackwell Scientific Publications, 1982. *Stemming from the extensive experience of Edinburgh's Regional Poison Center, this clinically oriented manual ought to prove of special benefit to physicians seeking instantaneous updates on management concepts.*

Journals: Virtually any clinical journal may prove the source of a fascinating case report or a valuable review in the field of poisoning. Lancet, JAMA, N Engl J Med, and the traditional medical and pediatric specialty journals are particularly valuable resources. In the more limited field of clinical toxicology the following are of note: (1) Veterinary and Human Toxicology: The official journal of the American Association of Poison Control Centers and the American Academy of Clinical Toxicology, always updating the clinical field. (2) The American Journal of Emergency Medicine, published by W. B. Saunders Company. (3) Clinical Toxicology: A blend of industrial, environmental, and accidental cases appears here, together with results of bench research. (4) Emergency Medicine: A controlled circulation journal particularly noted for "The Toxic Emergency," a monthly contribution of Donald Kunkel. (5) Medical Toxicology: Newly published, focuses on definitive reviews and is worldwide in perspective.

PART V
PRINCIPLES OF HUMAN GENETICS

33 HUMAN HEREDITY

James B. Wyngaarden

The appreciation of genetic factors as arbiters of human disease is a relatively recent development in medical history. Scattered references to inheritance of biologic characteristics may be found in the records of several millenia, including the frequently cited Talmudic exemption from circumcision of males born into families of bleeders, but discernible patterns of hereditary transmission were recognized first in the eighteenth and nineteenth centuries. In the 1750's Maupertuis described the autosomal dominant inheritance of polydactyly. The essential features of X-linked inheritance of hemophilia were described in the early 1800's by several writers and the pattern formally outlined by Nasse in 1820. The pattern of inheritance now recognized as autosomal recessive was described by Adams in 1814, and the biologic consequences of consanguinity first reported by Bemiss in 1857. In 1876, Galton introduced the twin method of separating effects of heredity from those of environment; later he initiated quantitative studies of polygenic inheritance.

Genetics as an experimental science owes its origins to Gregor Mendel and his cross-breeding of garden peas, tall and short, yellow seed and green seed, round seed and wrinkled seed. From these studies Mendel derived concepts of dominant and recessive traits, hereditary factors (which we now call *genes*), alternative factors (*alleles*), true breeding plants with two identical factors (*homozygotes*), and nontrue breeding plants with alternative factors (*heterozygotes*). His experiments led to the formulation of laws of *unit inheritance* (that "factors" retain their identity from generation to generation and do not blend in the hybrid), of *segregation* (that two members [alleles] of a single pair of factors [genes] are never found in the same gamete but always segregate), and of *independent assortment* (that members of different pairs of genes [nonalleles] assort to gametes independent of one another). These laws, formulated in 1865, had almost no immediate impact on biologic thought, but they are now cornerstones of genetics. They were rediscovered about 1900 by several workers independently and first applied to human disease by Sir Archibald Garrod in his concept of "inborn errors of metabolism" in 1908.

In 1944 Avery and his associates at the Rockefeller Institute established that the hereditary information in the transforming principle of pneumococci resided in its deoxyribonucleic acid (DNA). From that date onward DNA has been considered the basic material of the gene. In 1953 Watson and Crick proposed a molecular model for the structure of DNA, consisting of two polynucleotide strands twisted together in a double helix with the purine and pyrimidine bases facing inward and attached to each other, binding the two chains. This model offered a rational structure for replication of DNA and for storage of hereditary information within sequences of purine and pyrimidine bases.

This structure has since been established by x-ray crystallography. The genetic code, namely the precise triplet sequences of purine and pyrimidine bases in the structural gene that specify the individual amino acids of a polypeptide chain, was discovered by Nirenberg in 1961.

The amount of DNA in each human cell is sufficient to code for approximately 1 millon polypeptides of average length. Estimates of the number of structural genes in humans range from 50,000 to 100,000; large amounts of DNA constitute noncoding sequences whose function is as yet obscure. Only a small number of structural genes has been identified. In the most recent update of his catalogue of *Mendelian Inheritance in Man*, McKusick lists phenotypic variations or diseases of 1906 established genetic loci, thus implying that at least that many genes have undergone mutation so as to cause human disease or polymorphism. In humans, hereditary information is distributed in 23 pairs of chromosomes—22 pairs of autosomes and one pair of sex chromosomes ($X + Y$, male; $X + X$, female)—plus the unpaired "mitochondrial chromosome" (see below).

Genetics is concerned with the study of hereditary variations. Most of these variations are not harmful; indeed, they confer a distinct biologic advantage by enabling the species to adapt to changing environments. When variations are extreme and impair the health, fitness, or reproductive capacity of the individual, we consider them diseases. These extreme variations are of three principal types: (1) chromosomal aberrations, (2) single-gene differences that exhibit mendelian patterns of inheritance, and (3) polygenic disorders, in which two or more, often multiple, genes each contribute to the characteristic in question. Examples of the first two categories are relatively easy to recognize. They are discussed in Ch. 34 and Ch. 36. Many genetic diseases are dependent upon environmental factors for their expression, e.g., phenylalanine ingestion in phenylketonuria or milk ingestion in galactosemia. Other hereditary diseases are kept in abeyance by specific environmental factors: Scurvy is an inborn error of metabolism (absence of the hepatic enzyme that converts L-gulonolactone to L-ascorbic acid in man, monkey, and guinea pig) kept in remission by vitamin C; metabolic cretinism is foiled in its expression by the administration of thyroid hormone. The greatest difficulty in sorting out the relative importance of genetic and environmental influences is encountered with common diseases. In disorders such as rheumatoid arthritis, essential hypertension, and coronary artery disease, genetic influences are important but hard to identify in specific biochemical terms. In most polygenic disorders, genetic factors are multiple and still beyond definition.

The pace of genetic advance across the full spectrum of molecular biology to human heredity is currently very rapid. The revolution in biology of the past three decades is increasingly molding medical science and practice. New insights into the genetic control of the immune response (see Ch. 425) are explaining disease susceptibilities and facilitating organ and tissue transplantation. Susceptibility to cancer is being explained by the interplay between oncogenes, antioncogenes and environmental exposures (see Ch. 169). As additional genetic mechanisms are disclosed, they will illuminate more and more human diseases and from time to time suggest new avenues of therapy.

THE FAMILY HISTORY. A careful family history is indispensable in the assessment and understanding of hereditary disease. The interviewer should ascertain whether anyone in the family has had a condition similar to that of the patient, and whether this condition or any other "runs in the family." Particularly in the case of rare disorders one should inquire whether the parents are related, and, if this is not known, whether they or their families came from the same village or community and whether their forebears may have intermarried. Since some disorders are more common in certain ethnic groups than in others, the ethnic origin of the parents should also be elicited.

The rarer the recessive disorder in a specific population, the greater is the likelihood of parental consanguinity. Tay-Sachs disease is relatively rare in non-Jews, in whom the gene frequency is low, but a high proportion of non-Jewish parents of Tay-Sachs children are consanguineous. By contrast, Tay-Sachs disease is relatively common in Jews of eastern European origin, in whom the gene frequency is relatively high. In parents of Jewish children with Tay-Sachs disease in the United States the frequency of consanguinity is only slightly higher than in the general population.

Certain ethnic backgrounds increase the likelihood of certain diagnostic possibilities while decreasing that of others. Thalassemia is chiefly a disorder of people of the Mediterranean region and of Southeast Asia, familial Mediterranean fever is a disorder of Armenians and Sephardic Jews, acatalasia is a disease of Japanese and Koreans, and gout is very common among the Maori. By contrast, cystic fibrosis is rare in blacks, phenylketonuria is uncommon in Jews, and sickle cell anemia does not occur in Caucasians.

PEDIGREE ANALYSIS. The chief method of study of an inherited disease in humans is the observation of its pattern of distribution in kindreds, i.e., of its pedigree pattern. The construction of a pedigree pattern begins with the individual first detected, who is referred to as the proband, index case, or propositus (female=proposita). The pedigree pattern allows one to judge whether the distribution conforms to mendelian principles of segregation and assortment and thus represents single-factor inheritance. Patterns that do not conform to mendelian principles may represent polygenic traits in which a number of genes each contributes a minor effect. Valid pedigrees depend on accurate and extensive information about the kindred. This information is likely to be more reliable when based on observer detection than when based on memory.

MONOGENIC DISORDERS. Disorders caused by single mutant genes show one of four simple (mendelian) patterns of inheritance: (1) autosomal dominant, (2) autosomal recessive, (3) X-linked dominant, or (4) X-linked recessive. Dominant traits are those expressed in the heterozygote (as well as in the homozygote or hemizygote). Recessive traits are those expressed in the homozygotes (or hemizygotes) but silent in the heterozygote. The terms *dominant* and *recessive* refer to the phenotypic expression of the trait, not to the expression of the gene. Thus it is incorrect to speak of a dominant or recessive gene. A gene is either expressed or not expressed. Whether the trait is considered dominant or recessive often depends upon the level of observation. Sickle cell anemia is a recessive trait, i.e., it requires a double dose of the abnormal gene for expression at the clinical level. Nevertheless, the sickle gene is expressed in single dose as well, giving rise to carriers with SA hemoglobin. Recessive traits are *codominant* when viewed biochemically at the level of the gene product.

With few exceptions, each of the approximately 1900 mendelian diseases is rare. The overall population frequency of monogenic disorders is about 10 per 1000 live births, com-

TABLE 33–1. PREVALENCE OF SELECTED MONOGENIC DISORDERS AMONG LIVEBORN INFANTS*

Disorder	Estimated Prevalence
Autosomal Dominant	
Familial hypercholesterolemia	1 in 500
Polycystic kidney disease	1 in 1250
Huntington's disease	1 in 2500
Hereditary spherocytosis	1 in 5000
Marfan's syndrome	1 in 20,000
Autosomal Recessive	
Sickle cell anemia	1 in 625 (U.S. blacks)
Cystic fibrosis	1 in 2000 (Caucasians)
Tay-Sachs disease	1 in 3000 (U.S. Jews)
Cystinuria	1 in 7000
Phenylketonuria	1 in 12,000
Mucopolysaccharidoses (all types)	1 in 25,000
Glycogen storage disease (all types)	1 in 50,000
Galactosemia	1 in 57,000
Homocystinuria	1 in 200,000
X-linked	
Duchenne muscular dystrophy	1 in 7000
Hemophilia	1 in 10,000

*Data assembled from Galjaard, Carter, and Motulsky.

prising about 7 per 1000 dominants, about 2.5 per 1000 recessives, and about 0.4 per 1000 X-linked conditions (see Table 33–1).

If a particular disease shows a mendelian pattern of inheritance, its pathogenesis, no matter how complex, must be due to a single abnormal protein molecule. For example, in sickle cell disease, such seemingly unrelated disturbances as hemolytic anemia, painful crises, nephropathy, vascular occlusions, and *Salmonella* osteomyelitis are all physiologic consequences of a single missense mutation, resulting in a single amino acid substitution in the β-globin chain. When two or more phenotypic characters are controlled by a single gene, that gene is said to have *pleiotropic* effects.

AUTOSOMAL DOMINANT TRAITS. Autosomal genes are those genes situated on chromosomes other than the X or Y. When there are two alleles, A and a, at a locus, three possible genotypes exist: AA, Aa, and aa. Genotypes AA and aa are *homozygotes*; Aa is a *heterozygote*.

Dominant traits are fully manifest in the presence of a gene in the heterozygous state, i.e., when only one abnormal gene (*mutant allele*) is present and the corresponding partner allele on the homologous chromosome is normal. Figure 33–1 shows

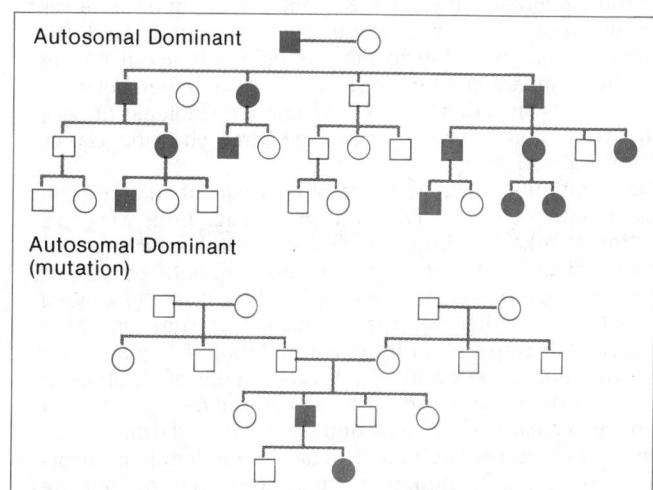

FIGURE 33–1. Pedigrees of autosomal dominant traits. In the lower pedigree the normal parents of the affected individual suggest the possibility of a new mutation. Solid symbols indicate those affected. (For details see text.)

a typical pedigree of transmission of an autosomal dominant trait. The following features are characteristic: (1) Each affected individual has an affected parent (unless the condition arose by a new mutation in a germ cell that formed the individual); (2) an affected individual will bear, on average, an equal number of affected and unaffected offspring; (3) males and females will be affected in equal numbers; (4) each sex can transmit the trait to male and female offspring (i.e., male-to-male transmission is possible); (5) normal children of an affected individual will have only normal offspring; and (6) when the trait does not impair viability or reproductive capacity, there will be *vertical* transmission of the trait through successive generations.

Most autosomal dominant disorders show two additional characteristics that are not seen in recessive disorders: (1) marked variability in severity, or *expressivity*, and (2) delayed age of onset. Dominant traits in humans often exert only mild effects. Occasionally the expression of the abnormal gene is so weak that a generation appears to be skipped because the carrier of the abnormal gene is clinically normal. When this is the case, the trait is said to be *nonpenetrant*. When a gene of a dominant trait exists in the homozygous state, the effect may be very severe, perhaps lethal. Examples are common in animals in which experimental matings can be constructed, but rare in humans, because matings of two affected heterozygotes are exceptional. One example is homozygous familial hypercholesterolemia. Others possibly include achondroplasia and Osler-Weber-Rendu syndrome. Delayed age of onset is seen in Huntington's disease and adult polycystic kidney disease. These disorders do not become manifest clinically until adult life, even though the mutant gene has been present since conception.

In every autosomal dominant disease some affected persons owe their disorder to a new mutation rather than to an inherited allele. Since a reasonable estimate of the frequency of mutation is of the order of 5×10^{-6} mutations per gene per generation, and since a dominant trait requires a mutation in only one of the parental gametes, one would expect that about 1 in 100,000 newborn persons would possess a new mutation at any given genetic locus. Many mutations will be silent or will involve a recessive function and not be manifest in a single gene dose. However, others will cause a defective gene product that gives rise to a dominant trait.

The percentage of patients with dominant disorders that represents a new mutation is inversely proportional to the effect of the disease upon *biologic fitness*, i.e., survival to adult life, and reproductive capacity. If a dominant mutation produces early death or absolute infertility, genetic transmission is impossible, and all cases represent new mutations. In tuberous sclerosis, the severe mental retardation reduces biologic fitness to about 20 per cent of normal, and the proportion of cases due to new mutations is about 80 per cent. In dominant conditions such as familial hypercholesterolemia, in which there is no reduction in biologic fitness, virtually all cases have a family pedigree showing classic vertical transmission

New mutations appear to be more frequent in the germ cells of fathers of relatively advanced age. Both Marfan's syndrome and achondroplastic dwarfism display such "paternal age effect." Fathers of sporadic cases of both conditions are an average of five to seven years older than the general population of fathers or than fathers who transmit these syndromes because of an inherited mutation. Diagnosis of a new mutation must exclude low expressivity of the trait in the carrier parent and also mistaken paternity.

The molecular basis of most of the more than 900 autosomal dominant disorders is obscure. Because in a dominant disorder expression of the mutation in only 50 per cent of the gene product may be sufficient to cause disease, the mutations are likely to involve two classes of proteins: (1) those that regulate complex metabolic pathways, such as membrane receptors as in familial hypercholesterolemia, and (2) key nonenzymic or structural proteins, such as hemoglobin or collagen, or a membrane protein as in hereditary spherocytosis.

In contrast to recessive disorders, in which an enzyme deficiency is the rule, defective enzymes are only rarely found in dominant disorders. Deficiencies of *Cl-esterase inhibitor* in hereditary angioedema and of *uroporphyrinogen-1 synthetase* in acute intermittent porphyria are exceptions to this general rule.

AUTOSOMAL RECESSIVE DISORDERS. Autosomal recessive conditions are clinically apparent only in the homozygous state, i.e., when both alleles at a particular genetic locus are mutant alleles. Figure 33–2 shows a typical pedigree of an autosomal recessive trait. The following features are characteristic: (1) The parents are clinically normal; (2) only siblings are affected; (3) males and females are affected in equal proportions; (4) if an affected individual marries a homozygous normal person, none of the children will be affected but all will be heterozygous carriers; (5) if an affected individual marries a heterozygous carrier, one half of the children will be affected, and the pedigree pattern will superficially suggest a dominant trait; (6) if two individuals who are homozygous for the same mutant gene marry, all of their children will be affected; (7) if both parents are heterozygous at the same genetic locus, one fourth of their children will be homozygous affected, one fourth will be homozygous normal, and one half will be heterozygous carriers of the same mutant gene; and (8) the less frequent the mutant gene is in the population, the greater is the likelihood that the affected individual is the product of consanguine parents.

In actual practice, unless the kinship is very large, the ratio of affected to unaffected sibs is frequently greater than one in four. Inclusion of probands in the enumeration loads the results in favor of the trait. In a sibship of 100 or even 10 the loading factor is not pronounced. However, in all ascertainable one-child sibships the involvement is 100 per cent, in two-child sibships it is 67 per cent (when the fundamental probability is 50 per cent), in three-child sibships it is 57 per cent, and so on. In small sibships a correction must be made for *bias of ascertainment*. The simplest method is to exclude the proband from the calculation and to determine the proportion of affected children among the remaining sibs.

In most autosomal recessive conditions the clinical presentation tends to be more uniform than in dominant diseases, and the onset is often early in life. Recessive disorders are commonly diagnosed in childhood. Approximately 800 well-established recessive traits have been recognized in humans, and in over 250 of these the mutant enzyme or other protein has been identified.

A *completely* recessive disease is one in which the heterozygote is clinically normal. When some features of the disease are detectable in the heterozygote, the disease is sometimes said to show *intermediate inheritance*, or to be *incompletely recessive* or *incompletely dominant*. The ambiguity of these terms

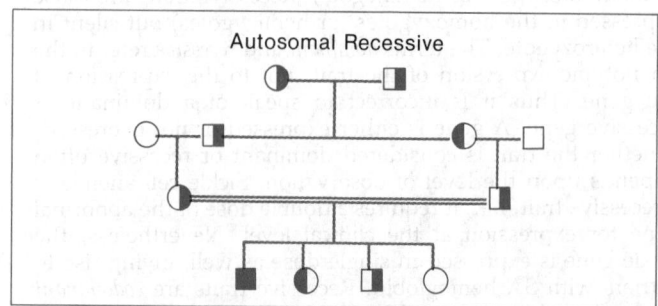

FIGURE 33–2. Pedigree of autosomal recessive trait. Note that both parents are heterozygous. One sib is affected, two are carriers, and one is normal. Double line (═══) indicates that parents are related by descent (first cousins).

from classic genetic studies of phenotypes is further emphasized by results of different methods of detection of gene effects. In many instances of completely recessive inheritance, refined biochemical observations enable the recognition of the trait in the clinically normal heterozygote. An example is Tay-Sachs disease, in which clinically normal parents and some sibs can be shown to be heterozygotes by assay of hexosaminidase A in leukocytes. Because of its importance in genetic counseling the detection of healthy heterozygous carriers of genes that in the homozygous state cause overt disease is one of the most significant aspects of medical genetics. Since by definition a dominant trait is one that is detectable in the heterozygous state, Tay-Sachs disease (and many others) is recessive when the clinical phenotype is considered and dominant when the biochemical phenotype is determined.

In pure form a recessive disease requires the inheritance of identical mutant genes from both parents. When the mutant genes are rare, the likelihood that any two unrelated parents are carriers for the same defect is small. Inheritance of two different mutant genes derived from the same locus gives rise to *heteroallelic compounds*. Individuals with Hb SC disease are genetic compounds who have inherited a different abnormal β-globin gene from each parent. Genetic compounds are also known in cystinuria, phenylketonuria, certain of the mucopolysaccharidoses, "homozygous" familial hypercholesterolemia, and several other disorders.

If the parents of a child with a recessive disorder have a common ancestor who carried a mutant gene, then the likelihood that two of the descendants would each have inherited the gene becomes relatively great. The less frequent the gene, the stronger is the likelihood that an affected individual has resulted from a consanguine mating. First cousins share, on the average, one eighth of their genes. When two first cousins marry, an offspring has, on the average, one sixteenth of the loci homozygous for a gene derived from a common ancestor. In general, offspring of first-cousin mating are slightly more likely to have congenital malformations, as well as mental defects and metabolic diseases, than are children born to unrelated parents.

Increased frequency of consanguinity will not be observed if the recessive disease is common. Sickle cell anemia, phenylketonuria, cystic fibrosis, and Tay-Sachs disease are examples in which the carrier (heterozygote) state is frequent in certain populations and in which consanguinity is usually not present in the parents. Increase in consanguinity would also not be expected in dominant or X-linked traits or genetic compounds.

A high percentage of recessive disorders involves abnormalities of enzyme proteins. In most reactions the normal maximal enzyme activity is greatly in excess of catalytic requirements; i.e., the concentration of a substrate is usually maintained at a point well below saturation for the enzyme that metabolizes it. Hence a reduction to 50 per cent of normal activity in a heterozygote does not impair the health of the carrier, whereas a total or near total deficiency may result in a serious inborn error of metabolism. These conditions are discussed in Ch. 34.

X-LINKED INHERITANCE. Diseases or traits that result from genes located on the X chromosome are termed X-linked. Since the female has two X chromosomes, she may be either heterozygous or homozygous for the mutant gene, and the trait may exhibit recessive or dominant expression. The male has only one X chromosome and therefore is *hemizygous* for X-linked traits. Males can be expected to express X-linked traits regardless of their recessive or dominant behavior in the female. Thus, the terms X-linked dominant or X-linked recessive refer only to expression of the trait in females.

Since males transmit their X chromosome only to daughters, an important feature of X-linked inheritance is the absence of male-to-male transmission. Affected males transmit the trait to all of their daughters and none of their sons.

Since the female carries two X chromosomes in each cell, it might be expected that the concentrations of proteins determined by genes on the X chromosome would be twice that of males who carry only one X chromosome per cell. This is not the case, and the explanation is provided by the process of X-inactivation first proposed by Mary Lyon, and often termed the *Lyon hypothesis*. In all adult female cells only one of the X chromosomes is genetically active. Early in differentiation one of the X chromosomes becomes inactive and forms the *Barr body*. Inactivation is random so that for each cell there is an equal probability that the paternally or maternally derived X chromosome will be inactivated. Once one of the two X chromosomes is inactivated, the same X chromosome remains inactive throughout all subsequent cell divisions. Thus, on the average one half of the cells of a female will express the X chromosome of her father, and one half of her mother: In this respect the normal female is a mosaic. If one of the X chromosomes carries a mutant gene, the probability is that the mutant phenotype will be expressed in one half of her cells. However, this statistical probability may be disturbed in at least two ways: (1) Since inactivation of one of the X chromosomes occurs early in development and is random, some females may by chance have many more cells that carry an active X chromosome derived from one parent than from the other; and (2) if one of the X chromosomes carries a mutant gene that confers a metabolic disadvantage upon cells with that mutation, these cells may survive less frequently during development, and the female offspring may have cells that carry predominantly or exclusively the active X chromosome without the mutation.

Over 120 loci have been identified on the human X chromosome, and many have been mapped to specific regions on the long or the short arm of the chromosome.

X-Linked Dominant Traits. This mode of inheritance (Fig. 33–3) is uncommon. Its characteristic features are as follows: (1) Females are affected about twice as often as males, (2) heterozygous females will transmit the trait to both sexes with a frequency of 50 per cent, (3) hemizygous affected males will transmit the trait to all of their daughters and none of their sons, and (4) the expression is more variable and generally less severe in heterozygous females than in hemizygous affected males. Examples of X-linked dominant inheritance include the Xg(a⁺) blood group, vitamin D-resistant (hypophosphatemic) rickets, and pseudohypoparathyroidism.

Some rare X-linked dominant disorders occur only in the heterozygous female, because the condition is lethal in the hemizygous affected male. Additional characteristics of this form of inheritance are as follows: (1) An affected mother will transmit the trait to one half of her daughters (heterozygotes), and (2) an increased frequency of abortions occurs in affected women, the abortions representing affected male fetuses. Examples of disorders that appear to fit this mode of inheritance include incontinentia pigmenti, focal dermal hypoplasia, orofaciodigital syndrome, and hyperammonemia caused by ornithine transcarbamylase deficiency.

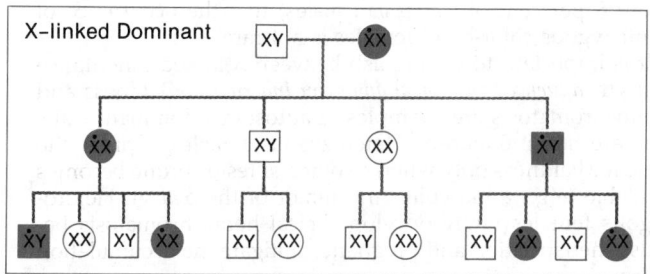

FIGURE 33–3. Pedigree of dominant X-linked trait. The X chromosome bearing the abnormal gene is designated by a small dot.

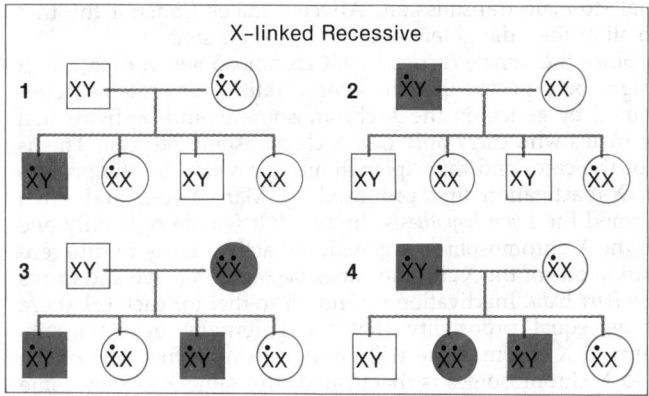

FIGURE 33–4. Pedigrees of X-linked recessive trait. The X chromosome bearing the abnormal gene is designated by a small dot. Affected individuals are indicated by solid squares (males) and circles (females). Pedigree 1 is commonly observed; pedigree 4 is rare.

X-Linked Recessive Traits. This mode of inheritance (Fig. 33–4) is relatively common. Its characteristic features are as follows: (1) The disorder is fully expressed only in the hemizygous affected male. (2) Heterozygous females are usually normal; occasionally they may exhibit mild features of the disorder; rarely they may be almost as severely affected as the hemizygous affected male (this variability is attributed to the probability that a disproportionate percentage of *normal* X chromosomes of the heterozygous female may have been inactivated early in development [see "Lyon hypothesis," above]). (3) On average, a heterozygous female will transmit the trait to one half of her sons (hemizygous affected), but the other half will be normal. (4) On average, one half of daughters of a heterozygous female will be carriers and one half will be normal. (5) All daughters of an affected male married to a normal female will be carriers, and no sons of such a union will be affected (no father-to-son transmission). (6) In the rare event of the union of an affected male and a heterozygous female, one half of daughters will be homozygous affected and one half will be heterozygous carriers; one half of sons will be hemizygous affected (maternal inheritance) and one half will be normal. Thus in this situation, one half of all offspring will be affected. (7) If the trait is rare, parents and relatives will be normal except for male relatives in the female line; e.g., on average, one half of maternal uncles will be affected. This "uncle and nephew" pattern gives rise to an *oblique* pedigree pattern, in contrast to the vertical pattern of autosomal dominant conditions and the horizontal pattern of autosomal recessive conditions.

Examples of X-linked recessive conditions include hemophilia A, Duchenne form of muscular dystrophy, the Lesch-Nyhan syndrome, glucose-6-phosphate dehydrogenase deficiency, and Fabry's disease. In several of these, e.g., Duchenne muscular dystrophy and Fabry's disease, heterozygous females may exhibit mild or even moderately severe forms of the disease. Color blindness is also an X-linked inherited trait, but it is sufficiently frequent (occurring in about 8 per cent of Caucasian males) that the occurrence of homozygous color-blind females is not rare.

It is important to distinguish between X-linked inheritance and *sex-influenced autosomal dominant inheritance.* Baldness and hemochromatosis are examples of autosomal dominant traits that are sex influenced. Heterozygous females express the gene for baldness only when a source of testosterone becomes available (e.g., a masculinizing tumor of the ovary). Heterozygous females rarely develop clinical hemochromatosis because menstruation and pregnancy mitigate the accumulation of iron.

Y-LINKED INHERITANCE. A gene on the Y chromosome will be transmitted through the father to all of his sons and none of his daughters. The only genes currently known to be located on the Y chromosome are those that determine "maleness" and an antigen that influences graft rejection.

POLYGENIC INHERITANCE. Most phenotypic traits are determined by the collaboration of many genes at different loci rather than by single gene effects. Polygenic inheritance is suggested for traits that show continuous variation in the form of a normal distribution curve. Height and intelligence are examples of polygenic traits in which the extremes of the distribution are not necessarily considered abnormal. Parents and offspring, and on average siblings also, have 50 per cent of their genes in common. Second-degree relatives share on average one fourth of all genes $(\frac{1}{2})^2$, and third-degree relatives (cousins) share one eighth $(\frac{1}{2})^3$. Thus as the degree of relation becomes more distant, the probability of inheriting the same combination of genes is reduced, and the degree of resemblance is likely to be less.

Many of the common chronic diseases of adults (such as essential hypertension, diabetes mellitus, hyperuricemia, hypercholesterolemia, coronary artery disease, and schizophrenia) and the common birth defects of children (such as cleft palate and lip and congenital heart disease) that tend to run in families fit best into the category of *multifactorial genetic disease.* This category should be suspected when the pedigree of a disease does not support inheritance in a simple dominant or recessive manner. In multifactorial genetic disease there is both a polygenic component and an environmental component of causative factors. In the population at large there are *risk* genes present in low frequency. If in any one individual there is a particularly large number of risk genes, the latent disorder becomes overt. When an individual inherits just the right combination of risk genes, he or she passes beyond a "risk threshold" at which environmental factors may determine the expression and severity of disease (Fig. 33–5). In order for another family member to develop the same disease, that individual would have to inherit the same or nearly similar combination of genes. The likelihood of such an occurrence is clearly greater in first-degree than in more distant relatives. The chances of any relative's inheriting the right combination of risk genes also decrease as the number of genes required for the expression of a given trait increases. Elegant and complex mathematical models have been advanced for polygenic-multifactorial disease, but these should not obscure the fact that each of the risk genes must express itself, like any other gene, by way of a specific biochemical product. Eventually the vague concept of genetic susceptibility of polygenic inheritance must yield to the basic premise that genes control the synthesis of specific proteins with specific functions.

The hypothesis of polygenic components in the inheritance of multifactorial disease has been given a potential mechanistic basis by the demonstration that as many as 28 per cent of all gene loci may contain polymorphic alleles that vary among

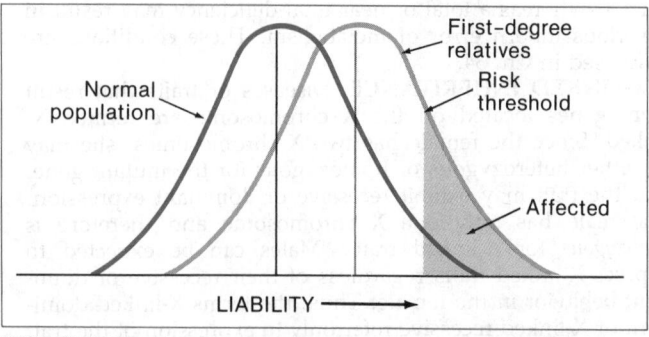

FIGURE 33–5. Diseases that conform to a polygenic multifactorial model of inheritance lead to an increased prevalence of disease among the relatives of affected individuals. This increased prevalence is most evident among first-degree relatives.

individuals. Such a large degree of variation in normal genes provides basis for variation in genetic predisposition with which other genetic or environmental factors can interact. To date genetic loci most prominently associated with disease susceptibility are those composing the major histocompatibility (MHC) locus or human leukocyte antigen (HLA) system. The HLA system consists of four distinct but closely linked, highly polymorphic loci situated on the short arm of chromosome 6. These loci as ordered on the chromosome are HLA-A, HLA-C, HLA-B, and HLA-D/DR. The A, B, C, and DR loci are defined serologically; the D locus controls lymphocyte (LD) antigens detectable by the mixed lymphocyte reaction (MLR). The D and DR (D-related) loci are closely linked but may not produce identical antigens. The products of these genes are proteins that are found on the surface of body cells and that enable an individual's immune system to distinguish its own cells (self) from those of someone else (nonself). Each HLA locus in the population consists of multiple alleles, each of which produces an immunologically distinct protein. HLA-A has at least 20 alleles, HLA-B has at least 42, C has at least 8, D has at least 12, and DR has at least 10 identified thus far. The inheritance of certain alleles predisposes to the development of certain diseases, in some instances when the individual is exposed to a particular environmental challenge. For example, the frequency of B27 allele in the white population is approximately 8 per cent. In patients with ankylosing spondylitis the frequency of B27 is over 90 per cent. In Australian aborigines and black Africans the B27 antigen is virtually absent and the frequency of ankylosing spondylitis is sharply reduced. A Caucasian with the B27 antigen is approximately 120 times more likely to develop ankylosing spondylitis than one who does not posses the antigen; the increased liability among Japanese with the B27 antigen is 300 times. Reiter's syndrome may follow an infection of the bowel or urinary tract with *Shigella*, *Salmonella*, or *Yersinia* organisms. No less than 20 per cent of B27-positive individuals with *Shigella* infections will develop Reiter's syndrome. Other disease associations of the HLA system are discussed in Ch. 425.

Multifactorial or polygenic inheritance must not be confused with *genetic heterogeneity*. Hypercholesterolemia and hyperuricemia behave as multifactorial traits when viewed at the population level. At the family level, however, it is sometimes possible to identify a single locus that is mainly responsible for the disease in that family. Examples include familial hypercholesterolemia, an autosomal dominant trait present in about 5 per cent of subjects with premature myocardial infarctions, which in single-gene dosage produces atherosclerosis in the absence of any extraordinary environmental factor; or hypoxanthine-guanine phosphoribosyltransferase deficiency, an X-linked recessive trait present in about 0.5 per cent of subjects with gout, which in the hemizygous state produces marked purine overproduction without any relationship to obesity or alcohol consumption.

MITOCHONDRIAL INHERITANCE. Each mitochondrion contains several circular chromosomes that code for certain ribosomal and transfer ribonucleic acids (RNA's) and for 13 polypeptides involved in oxidative phosphorylation, the chief function of the mitochondrion. The mitochondrial code differs from that of nuclear DNA and that of any contemporary prokaryote; it is similar to that of bacteria. Mitochondrial inheritance is exclusively matrilineal. Lebar's optic atrophy and certain myopathies associated with "ragged-red fiber" disease are thought to involve mitochondrial inheritance.

GENE FREQUENCY. The distribution of a mutant gene in the general population may be calculated on the basis of the Hardy-Weinberg equation. If the frequency of a particular gene A is p, then that of its alternative allele is $(1 - p) = q$. There will be three genotypes in the population: Those who are homozygous AA, those who are heterozygous Aa, and those who are homozygous aa. In a randomly mating popu-

lation the frequencies of these genotypes will be in the proportion p^2(AA), 2pg(Aa), and q^2(aa). An important consequence of this distribution is that irrespective of the initial frequency of the genes A and a in the population, the proportion of the three genotypes will tend to remain constant in succeeding generations, provided that there is no difference in biologic fitness of any of the genotypes. If there is unequal viability or fertility among the three genotypes, or if mating is not random, the frequency calculations require considerable correction, and in small populations major changes in gene frequency can occur on the basis of chance alone.

If the frequency of a recessive disease in a particular population is known, the frequency of heterozygous carriers and of the abnormal gene can be calculated. Thus for a recessively inherited disease aa (q^2) with a frequency of 1 per 10,000 (e.g., albinism), the frequency of the gene a (q) will be 1 per 100, and that of heterozygous carriers will be $2 \times p \times q = 2 \times 99/100 \times 1/100 =$ approximately 1 in 50. Thus, in this particular example there will be 200 clinically unaffected carriers of the abnormal gene for every affected individual. Table 33–1 lists the frequency of several inherited diseases. Cystic fibrosis, a recessively inherited disease, has a prevalence in the white population of about 1 per 2500 (q^2); thus the frequency of the gene (q) is 1 in 50 and of heterozygous carriers is approximately 1 in 25, or 4 per cent of the white population. A similar calculation with respect to sickle cell anemia among United States blacks ($q^2 = 1/625$) yields a frequency of heterozygous carriers of 1 in 12.5, or 8 per cent of the United States black population.

The frequency of most genes in the population is relatively stable. When a gene is rare and severely disadvantageous, the rate of its introduction into a population by spontaneous mutation is balanced by the rate of elimination of the disadvantageous gene by natural selection. The frequency of the disadvantageous gene, however, can be stabilized at a high level if the heterozygotes are slightly favored (increased biologic fitness) and leave a greater number of progeny than either homozygote. When a rare form of a species is present at a frequency that cannot be maintained by recurrent mutation alone, a *balanced polymorphism* is said to exist. Usually this means that the rarer of two allelic forms occurs with a frequency of at least 1 per cent of the population. When this is found, *heterozygote advantage* should be suspected. An example of such a balanced polymorphism is the increased resistance of individuals heterozygous for the sickle cell trait to falciparum malaria. Although persons with sickle cell disease (homozygotes, SS hemoglobin) often die before they can reproduce, and thus remove the sickle cell gene from the population, the prevalence of heterozygotes (SA hemoglobin) may nevertheless reach 40 per cent in certain West African populations. Death from falciparum malaria is much less frequent in carriers of the sickle cell trait than in noncarriers, and thus the heterozygote does have an advantage. Whether the extraordinary frequency of heterozygotes for the sickle gene in West Africa is due entirely to differential mortality or in part to differential fertility is uncertain, but this example suffices to illustrate that the effects of genes can be assessed only in relation to a particular environment. In most instances, however, a distinct advantage for the heterozygote of a polymorphic trait (of which there are many; see Ch. 34) cannot be demonstrated, and the possibility exists that certain polymorphic traits are genetically neutral.

The term *genetic load* has been used to describe the total genetic disability of a population. It comprises both a *mutational load*, based on recurrent mutation of a normal gene to a lethal or sublethal gene, and a *segregational load*, resulting from segregation of the harmful gene from advantaged heterozygotes, as in the example of sickle cell heterozygotes discussed above. Each individual has been estimated to have three to eight genes, which, if homozygous instead of heterozygous, would be lethal. The relative contribution of the segregational and mutational loads to the total genetic load is uncertain.

THE HUMAN GENE MAP. Over 1780 autosomal loci are known, on the basis mainly of characteristic patterns of inheritance of alternative forms of a particular trait. Some chromosomal mapping information is available for over 30 per cent of these loci. In addition, over 120 loci have been assigned to the X chromosome, and about an equal number are suspected but unproved.

Assignment of a locus to a specific chromosome is based on a variety of methods: (1) study of linkage of traits in large families with multiple alleles at two loci; (2) co-segregation of specific proteins and single chromosomes in clones from somatic cell hybrids; (3) DNA-RNA in situ hybridization; (4) deductions from amino acid sequences of proteins; (5) deletion mapping or gene dosage effects; (6) induction of microscopically detectable chromosomal change by adenovirus; (7) DNA/cDNA molecular hybridization in solution or "Cot analysis" of somatic cell hybrids containing a small number of human chromosomes; (8) DNA restriction endonuclease techniques; and (9) chromosomal aberrations.

About 68 per cent of gene assignments have been made on the basis of somatic cell hybridization studies (method 2, above), about 22 per cent on the basis of linkage of traits in families (method 1), and about 20 per cent from in situ hybridization studies (methods 3 and 7). (Many loci have been mapped by two or more methods.)

Some interesting observations have emerged. Structural genes for enzymes that catalyze sequential steps in a metabolic pathway are as a rule not located on the same chromosome. Thus, whereas in bacteria the enzymes for sequential metabolic steps are often determined by linked genes, thus assuring coordinate regulation of activity, the situation in humans is quite different. This finding accords with the lack of evidence for coordinate regulation of enzyme activity, or for an operon-like organization of structural genes, in eukaryotic cells. Even the subunits of polymeric proteins may be coded by genes on different chromosomes. The genes for the α chains of hemoglobin are on chromosome 16, whereas that for the β chain is on chromosome 11. Lactate dehydrogenase is an example of an enzymic protein that is constituted by subunits coded by genes on different chromosomes: LDH-A by a gene on chromosome 11, LDH-B by one on chromosome 12.

When the location of a gene is known, physicians can use the concept of gene linkage to predict which individual in a given family will be affected by a given trait. For example, the locus for the gene specifying the Rh blood group factor and the locus for the gene producing one form of the dominant trait, hereditary elliptocytosis, occur in close proximity on chromosome 1. Thus, if a subject with hereditary elliptocytosis transmits the anomaly to an offspring, the offspring will usually inherit the allele that is present at the Rh locus on the chromosome. If the Rh allele on this chromosome happens to be a rare one in the population (such as r'), one can assume that whichever offspring inherits the r' allele at the Rh locus will also inherit the abnormal allele at the elliptocytosis locus.

Carter CO: Monogenic disorders. J Med Genet 14:316, 1977. *An estimate of birth frequencies of selected genetic conditions.*

Cavalli-Sforza LL, Bodmer WF: The Genetics of Human Populations. 2nd ed. San Francisco, W. H. Freeman and Company, 1978. *An authoritative textbook of human genetics.*

Galjaard H: Genetic Metabolic Diseases. Early Diagnosis and Prenatal Analysis. Amsterdam, Elsevier/North Holland Biomedical Press, 1980. *An 850-page book on hereditary disorders, about one third of which is devoted to methods and results of prenatal diagnosis.*

McKusick VA: The anatomy of the human genome. Am J Med 69:267, 1980. *An excellent discussion of the basis and significance of the assignment of more than 350 genes to specific chromosomes, with a catalogue of assignments up to mid 1980.*

McKusick VA: Human Genetics. 2nd ed. Englewood Cliffs, N.J., Prentice-Hall, 1969. *An excellent introductory survey of human genetics.*

McKusick VA: Mendelian Inheritance in Man. 7th ed. Baltimore, Johns Hopkins University Press, 1986. *A catalogue of autosomal dominant, autosomal recessive, and X-linked phenotypes, with brief descriptions and literature references for each.*

Motulsky AG: Frequency of sickling disorders in U.S. blacks. N Engl J Med 288:31, 1973. *Gives estimated prevalence of all sickling disorders in the population (HB SS disease, Hb SC disease, and Hb S-β thalassemia).*

Vogel F, Motulsky AG: Human Genetics: Problems and Approaches. 2nd ed. Berlin, Springer-Verlag, 1986. *A superb and up-to-date treatment of human genetics.*

34 INBORN ERRORS OF METABOLISM

James B. Wyngaarden

The inspired concept of inborn errors of metabolism, developed by Archibald Garrod in the first decade of this century, marks the birth of biochemical genetics. Garrod's studies of alcaptonuria, pentosuria, albinism, and cystinuria led to the proposal of a new category of diseases in which a block in a metabolic pathway arises from an inherited deficiency of a specific enzyme. This concept was proved in 1948 when Gibson found a deficiency of NADH-dependent methemoglobin reductase in recessive methemoglobinemia. This was soon followed by the discovery in 1952 by Cori and Cori of a deficiency of glucose-6-phosphatase in von Gierke's disease, in 1953 by Jervis of phenylalanine hydroxylase deficiency in phenylketonuria, and in 1956 by LaDu of homogentisic acid oxidase deficiency in alcaptonuria as originally predicted by Garrod. By 1987 deficiencies of over 215 different enzymes have been associated with hereditary disease. Of even greater importance in the history of genetics was the remarkable insight in Garrod's hypothesis that the primary action of a gene is to control the synthesis of a specific enzyme. Decades later Beadle (1945) independently proposed the one gene–one enzyme hypothesis anticipated by Garrod.

In 1949 Pauling, Itano, and associates observed that sickle cell hemoglobin exhibited abnormal electrophoretic behavior and introduced the concept of *molecular disease*, in which a structural alteration in a macromolecule accounted for a specific functional change that was responsible for a disease state. In 1953 Ingram demonstrated the substitution of a single amino acid residue in the β-chain of sickle cell hemoglobin, confirming the concept of molecular disease and initiating an ever-lengthening series of findings of structural alterations in macromolecules that result from gene mutations. For a time "missing" enzyme diseases and hemoglobinopathies were thought to represent distinct categories of disease, perhaps representing defects of control and structural genes, respectively. More sensitive techniques have disclosed low levels of residual activity of the deficient enzyme in many inborn errors of metabolism. In some cases the mutation has affected a critical portion of the enzyme, radically reducing its catalytic activity; in others the mutation has rendered the enzyme highly unstable. In the case of erythrocytes that lack a nucleus and cannot continue to synthesize new protein, enzyme lability results in low enzyme activity values in the older cells. In several instances amino acid sequence studies of enzymes have disclosed single amino acid substitutions analogous to the defect in sickle hemoglobin. Thus many inborn errors of metabolism are molecular diseases in which the *primary* defect lies in the genetic specification of the protein.

Although most of the well-defined inborn errors of metabolism are inherited as recessive conditions, in principle any human phenotype showing mendelian genetics must be based on a specific variant or missing protein. Thus not only autosomal and X-linked recessive but also autosomal and X-linked dominant conditions may be expressed through abnormal proteins. Examples in which a mutant protein has been identified include autosomal recessive, alcaptonuria (homogentisic acid oxidase); X-linked recessive, Lesch-Nyhan syndrome (hypoxanthine–guanine phosphoribosyltransferase); autosomal dominant, acute intermittent porphyria (uroporphyrinogen I synthetase). No example of an X-linked dominant condition in which the mutant protein has been identified can be cited as yet. In one condition of this category, vitamin D–resistant (hypophosphatemic) rickets, a defect in phosphate transport is suspected but the membrane carrier has not been identified. The concept of inborn errors of metabolism has broadened considerably since first propounded by Garrod. A reasonable definition would include any condition of clinical significance that shows a mendelian mode of inheritance, but in practice the term is restricted to conditions that have recognizable biochemical manifestations.

A mutant protein that cannot be detected by functional assay may nevertheless retain immunologic reactivity. However, in some instances no protein can be detected by functional or immunologic means. In the terminology of microbial genetics, the former class of mutants is frequently called CRM(+) ("krim" positive) and the latter CRM(−). The presence of CRM(+) material suggests that the genetic defect is due to a mis-sense mutation with a consequent amino acid substitution that destroys the activity but not the antigenicity of the mutant enzyme. In most cases in which mutant enzymes have been studied, cross-reactive material has been detected. However, in the Lesch-Nyhan syndrome only 1 CRM(+) mutant has been found among 14 studied. At the pseudocholinesterase locus, 17 CRM(+) mutants and 18 CRM(−) mutants have been recognized. A CRM(−) reaction does not prove that no protein is present; the protein may be so altered that both enzyme function and immunologic reactivity have been lost.

Mutation does not necessarily result in loss of enzyme activity. Several examples of increased activity are known. The best examples are three types of phosphoribosylpyrophosphate synthetase overactivity associated with purine overproduction and gout. In one there is a 2.5-fold increase in enzyme activity per molecule; in another, excessive activity is a reflection of diminished affinity for normal intracellular nucleotide inhibitors; in a third, the overactivity results from an increased affinity for ribose 5-phosphate, a substrate of the reaction. All of these changes reflect alterations of enzyme structure. Some of the clinical conditions in which an abnormality of a specific protein has been observed are listed in Tables 34–1 and 34–2. Others include deficiencies of peptide hormones, abnormalities of binding proteins (receptor diseases) and of epidermal proteins, and defects in transmembrane transport (e.g., cystinuria). Chromosome mapping data exist for many inborn errors. Some examples are given in Table 34–3.

ETIOLOGY. The etiology of an inborn error of metabolism is a mutant gene. If the amino acid sequence of the mutant protein is known, it is possible to deduce the nature of the mutation from the genetic code. The human variant of glucose-6-phosphate dehydrogenase, G6PD Hektoen, differs from normal G6PD in a single amino acid substitution, HIS →TYR. This substitution corresponds to a mutation from GTA(or G) to ATA(or G) in a codon in the structural gene for G6PD. Most of the amino acid sequence information of human mutant proteins has been obtained from studies of red blood cell proteins, such as hemoglobin and G6PD. At least four types of mutations can be discerned by this approach: deletions, duplications, mis-sense mutations, and frame-shift mutations.

Another type of mutation, the non-sense mutation, has also been demonstrated in humans, using DNA restriction enzyme analysis and DNA sequencing techniques. The partial nucleotide sequence of β-globin mRNA isolated from a unique patient with homozygous β°-thalassemia disclosed a replacement of an adenine by a uracil in the codon for position 17. This changed the RNA codon from AAG to AUG, a termination codon. As a result a nonfunctional partial β-chain, only 16 amino acids long, was synthesized. Hb McKees-Rock represents another example of mutation of an amino acid codon to a terminator codon, but in this case the β-globin is shortened by only two amino acids and is functional.

DNA cloning techniques permit direct study of the altered DNA sequence in many human mutations, even those that involve genes that code for quantitatively minor proteins, such as most enzymes. These recent developments are discussed in Ch. 35.

PATHOGENESIS OF GENETIC DISEASE. The consequence of a mutation will depend on the function normally served by the product of the gene. Mutations in genes for rRNA or tRNA would very likely affect protein synthesis generally and might be incompatible with life. No such mutations have been identified in mammalian systems, although they are known in bacteria.

Defects involving nonenzymic proteins undoubtedly account for a large number of genetic diseases, but relatively few have been defined biochemically. The hemoglobinopathies are an exception. Over 580 hemoglobin variants are now known. A few additional examples exist. In one of these, the ZZ variant of α-1-antitrypsin deficiency, two amino acid substitutions (mis-sense mutations) in α-1-antitrypsin lead to the production of a modified protein that is not susceptible to normal post-translational processing. As a consequence carbohydrate residues are not added to the protein in the normal manner, and the defective glycoprotein accumulates in liver cells, possibly because the altered molecule cannot be secreted. Other examples in which a specific mutant protein has been identified, although the precise molecular alteration has not yet been defined, include the abnormal plasma membrane receptor in familial hypercholesterolemia, the abnormal cytoplasmic androgen receptor in the complete form of testicular feminization, an abnormal insulin in familial hyperproinsulinemia, and an abnormal protein called dynein in the microtubules of cilia in Kartagener's syndrome.

The largest number of known inborn errors of metabolism involves deficiencies of enzymes that catalyze discrete steps in biosynthetic or catabolic sequences. The consequences of metabolic blocks depend upon the function of the affected sequence and the properties of the affected substrates. In some conditions the disease is manifested by the inability to form a specific product, as in the failure of melanin production in one form of albinism. In others, accumulation of the precursor of a blocked reaction results in toxicity or in a storage disease. In phenylketonuria the block in phenylalanine hydroxylase results in accumulation of phenylalanine and overproduction of toxic phenylketone products. Deficiencies of various catabolic enzymes explain the progressive tissue accumulations in the mucopolysaccharidoses and sphingolipidoses. In some enzyme deficiencies, disease results from failure to modify another protein. For example, in some types of Ehlers-Danlos syndrome collagen polypeptide synthesis is normal but enzymes essential in cross-linking are deficient, with the result that fragile collagen is produced.

Polymorphism. Many proteins exist in two or more forms in the population. These multiple forms are the result of multiple genes (*alleles*) at the same genetic locus. If the most common allele at a given locus accounts for fewer than 99 per cent of the alleles in the population, *polymorphism* is said to occur. By definition, when polymorphism exists at a genetic locus, at least 2 per cent of the population must be heterozygous at that locus. Table 34–4 lists selected proteins for which polymorphism has been demonstrated electrophoretically. Many of these genetically determined variations in protein structure are unassociated with clinical disease.

Polymorphism appears to be very common. As many as 28 per cent of genetic loci coding for enzyme and other proteins of erythrocytes and serum show multiple alleles in the population, but this figure may be as low as 2 per cent of loci of

TABLE 34—1. DISORDERS IN WHICH DEFICIENT ACTIVITY OF A SPECIFIC ENZYME HAS BEEN DEMONSTRATED IN HUMAN BEINGS*

Condition	Enzyme with Deficient Activity	Condition	Enzyme with Deficient Activity
Acatalasia	Catalase	Hemolytic anemia	Glucose-6-phosphate dehydrogenase
Acid phosphatase deficiency	Acid phosphatase	Hemolytic anemia	Glucose phosphate isomerase
Acyl CoA dehydrogenase deficiency	Acyl CoA decarboxylase	Hemolytic anemia	Glutathione peroxidase
Adrenal hyperplasia I	20,22 Desmolase	Hemolytic anemia	Glutathione reductase
Adrenal hyperplasia II	3-β-Hydroxysteroid dehydrogenase	Hemolytic anemia	Glutathione synthetase
Adrenal hyperplasia III	Steroid cytochrome P450-21-hydroxylase	Hemolytic anemia	Hexokinase
		Hemolytic anemia	Phosphoglycerate kinase
Adrenal hyperplasia IV	11-β-Hydroxylase	Hemolytic anemia	Pyrimidine 5'-nucleotidase
Adrenal hyperplasia V	17-α-Hydroxylase	Hemolytic anemia	Pyruvate kinase
Albinism	Tyrosinase	Hemolytic anemia	Triosephosphate isomerase
Alcaptonuria	Homogentisic acid oxidase	Histidinemia	Histidine:ammonia lyase
Aldosterone deficiency I	18-Hydroxylase (corticosterone methyl oxidase I)	HMG-CoA lyase deficiency	3-Hydroxy-3-methylglutarate-CoA lyase
Aldosterone deficiency II	18-OH-Dehydrogenase	Homocystinuria I	Cystathionine beta-synthase
Alpha-methylacetoaceticaciduria	β-Ketothiolase	Homocystinuria II	N(5,10)-Methylenetetrahydrofolate reductase
Anemia, megaloblastic	Dihydrofolate reductase		
Apnea, drug-induced	Pseudocholinesterase	4-Hydroxybutyricaciduria	Succinic semialdehyde dehydrogenase
Argininemia	Arginase	Hydroxyprolinemia	Hydroxyproline oxidase
Argininosuccinic aciduria	Argininosuccinate lyase	Hyperalaninemia	β-Alanine-α-ketoglutarate aminotransferase
Aspartylglycosaminuria	Special hydrolase (AADG-ase)		
Ataxia, intermittent	Pyruvate decarboxylase	Hyperammonemia I	Ornithine transcarbamylase
Carnosinemia	Carnosinase	Hyperammonemia II	Carbamyl phosphate synthetase
Cerebrotendinous xanthomatosis	Mitochondrial 26-hydroxylase	Hyperammonemia III	N-Acetylglutamate synthetase
Cholesteryl ester deficiency (Norum-Gjone disease)	Lecithin cholesterol acyltransferase (LCAT)	Hyperglycerolemia	ATP:glycerol phosphotransferase
		Hyperglycinemia, ketotic I	Propionyl CoA carboxylase, α subunit
Citrullinemia	Argininosuccinate synthetase	Hyperglycinemia, ketotic II	Propionyl CoA carboxylase, β subunit
Coproporphyria	Coproporphyrinogen III oxidase	Hyperglycinemia, nonketotic form	Glycine formiminotransferase
Crigler-Najjar syndrome	Glucuronyl transferase	Hyperlysinemia	Lysine-α-ketoglutarate reductase
Cystathioninuria	γ-Cystathionase	Hyperprolinemia I	Proline oxidase
2,8-Dihydroxyadenine nephrolithiasis	Adenine phosphoribosyl transferase	Hyperprolinemia II	δ-1-Pyrroline-5-carboxylate dehydrogenase
Disaccharide intolerance I	Invertase		
Disaccharide intolerance II	Invertase, maltase	Hypoglycemia	Glycogen synthase
Disaccharide intolerance III	Lactase	Hypophosphatasia	Alkaline phosphatase
Ehlers-Danlos syndrome, type VI	Collagen lysyl hydroxylase	Ichthyosis, X-linked	Steroid sulfatase
Ehlers-Danlos syndrome, type VII	Procollagen peptidase	Immunodeficiency disease	Adenosine deaminase
Ehlers-Danlos syndrome, type IX	Lysyloxidase	Immunodeficiency disease	Purine nucleoside phosphorylase
Ethanolaminosis	Ethanolamine kinase	Immunodeficiency disease	Uridine monophosphate kinase
Fabry's disease	α-Galactosidase A	Intestinal lactase deficiency (adult)	Lactase
Farber's lipogranulomatosis	Ceramidase	Isovaleric acidemia	Isovaleryl CoA dehydrogenase
Formiminotransferase deficiency	Formiminotransferase	Ketoacidosis, infantile	Succinyl CoA:3-ketoacid CoA-transferase
Fructose intolerance	Fructose-1-phosphate aldolase "B"		
Fructose-1,6-diphosphatase deficiency	Fructose-1,6-diphosphatase	Krabbe's disease	Galactocerebroside β-galactosidase
Fructosuria	Hepatic fructokinase	Lactic acidosis, congenital	Dihydrolipoyl dehydrogenase
Fucosidosis	α-L-Fucosidase	Lactosyl ceramidosis	Neutral β-galactosidase
Galactokinase deficiency	Galactokinase	Leigh's necrotizing encephalomyelopathy	Pyruvate carboxylase
Galactose epimerase deficiency	Galactose epimerase	Lesch-Nyhan syndrome	Hypoxanthine-guanine phosphoribosyl transferase
Galactosemia	Galactose-1-phosphate uridyl transferase		
Gangliosidosis, G$_{M1}$, type I or infantile	β-Galactosidase A,B	Lipase deficiency, congenital	Lipase (pancreatic)
Gangliosidosis, G$_{M1}$, type II or juvenile	β-Galactosidase A,B	Lipoprotein lipase deficiency (type I hyperlipoproteinemia)	Lipoprotein lipase
Gangliosidosis, G$_{M2}$ (Tay-Sachs disease)	β-Hexosaminidase A	Lysine intolerance	L-Lysine:NAD-oxidoreductase
Gangliosidosis, G$_{M2}$, juvenile	β-Hexosaminidase A	Male pseudohermaphroditism	Testicular 17,20-desmolase
Gangliosidosis, G$_{M2}$, adult	β-Hexosaminidase A	Male pseudohermaphroditism	Testicular 17-ketosteroid dehydrogenase
Gangliosidosis, G$_{M2}$ (Sandhoff's disease)	β-Hexosaminidase B		
Gangliosidosis, G$_{M3}$	UDP-N-acetyl-galactosaminyl transferase	Male pseudohermaphroditism	Steroid 5α-reductase
		Mannosidosis	α-Acid-mannosidase
Gaucher's disease	Acid β-glucosidase	Maple sugar urine disease	Branched-chain keto acid decarboxylase
G6PD deficiency (favism, primaquine sensitivity, etc.)	Glucose-6-phosphate dehydrogenase	Metachromatic leukodystrophy I	Arylsulfase A (cerebroside sulfatase)
Glutaric aciduria I	Glutaryl-CoA dehydrogenase	Methemoglobinemia	NAD-methemoglobin reductase
Glutaric aciduria II	Acyl-CoA dehydrogenase	Methionine adenosyl transferase deficiency (hypermethioninemia)	Methionine adenosyl transferase
Glutathionemia	γ-Glutamyl transferase		
Glycogen storage disease Ia	Glucose-6-phosphatase	β-Methyl crotonyl glycinuria I	β-Methyl crotonyl-CoA carboxylase
Glycogen storage disease Ib	Glucose-6-phosphate translocase	Methylmalonic aciduria I (vitamin B$_{12}$-unresponsive)	Methylmalonic CoA mutase
Glycogen storage disease II	α-1,4-Glucosidase		
Glycogen storage disease III	Amylo-1, 6-glucosidase	Methylmalonic aciduria II (vitamin B$_{12}$-responsive)	5'-Deoxyadenosyl transferase
Glycogen storage disease IV	Amylo-(1,4 to 1,6)-transglucosidase		
Glycogen storage disease V	Muscle phosphorylase	Mitochondrial myopathy	NADH-CoA reductase
Glycogen storage disease VI	Liver phosphorylase	Mucolipidoses II and III	N-Acetylglucosamine-1-phosphotransferase
Glycogen storage disease VII	Muscle phosphofructokinase		
Glycogen storage disease VIII	Liver phosphorylase kinase	Mucolipidosis IV	Ganglioside neuramindase
Gout, primary	Hypoxanthine-guanine phosphoribosyl transferase	Mucopolysaccharidosis IH (Hurler's)	α-L-Iduronidase
		Mucopolysaccharidosis IS (Scheie's)	α-L-Iduronidase
Gout, primary	PP-ribose-P synthetase (increased)	Mucopolysaccharidosis II (Hunter's)	Sulfo-iduronidase sulfatase
Granulomatous disease, X-linked	NADPH oxidase ?	Mucopolysaccharidosis IIIA (Sanfilippo's)	Heparan sulfate sulfatase
Gynecomastia, familial	Aromatase (elevated)		
Hemolytic anemia	Adenosine triphosphatase	Mucopolysaccharidosis IIIB (Sanfilippo's)	N-Acetyl-α-D-glucosaminidase
Hemolytic anemia	Adenylate kinase		
Hemolytic anemia	Aldolase A	Mucopolysaccharidosis IIIC	Acetyl-CoA:alpha glucosaminide N-transferase
Hemolytic anemia	Diphosphoglycerate mutase		
Hemolytic anemia	γ-Glutamylcysteine synthetase	Mucopolysaccharidosis IIID	N-Acetyltransglucosamine-6-sulfate sulfatase

TABLE 34–1. DISORDERS IN WHICH DEFICIENT ACTIVITY OF A SPECIFIC ENZYME HAS BEEN DEMONSTRATED IN HUMAN BEINGS* Continued

Condition	Enzyme with Deficient Activity	Condition	Enzyme with Deficient Activity
Mucopolysaccharidosis IVA (Morquio's)	Galactosamine-6-sulfate sulfatase	Prolidase deficiency	Prolidase
Mucopolysaccharidosis IVB	β-Galactosidase	Protoporphyria	Heme synthetase (ferrochelatase)
Mucopolysaccharidosis VI (Maroteaux-Lamy)	Arylsulfatase B	Pulmonary emphysema, or cirrhosis	α-1-Antitrypsin
Mucopolysaccharidosis VII	β-Glucuronidase	Pyridoxine-dependent infantile convulsions	Glutamic acid decarboxylase
Multiple carboxylase deficiency, late-onset	Biotinase	Pyrimidinemia	Dihydropyrimidine dehydrogenase
Multiple carboxylase deficiency (several forms)	Holocarboxylase synthetase	Pyruvate carboxylase deficiency	Pyruvate carboxylase
		Refsum's disease	Phytanic acid α-oxidase
Myeloperoxidase deficiency with disseminated candidiasis	Myeloperoxidase	Renal tubular acidosis with deafness	Carbonic anhydrase B
Myopathy	Myoadenylate deaminase	Rickets, vitamin D dependent	25-Hydroxycholecalciferol 1-hydroxylase
Myopathy, lipid	Carnitine palmitoyl transferase I or II	Saccharopinuria	Saccharopine dehydrogenase
Niemann-Pick disease, A and B	Sphingomyelinase	Sarcosinemia	Sarcosine dehydrogenase complex
Niemann-Pick disease, C	Cholesterol esterification defect	Sialidosis	α-Neuraminidase
Ornithinemia with gyrate atrophy	Ornithine ketoacid aminotransferase	Sulfite oxidase deficiency	Sulfite oxidase
Orotic aciduria I	Orotate phosphoribonyl transferase and orotidine-5' phosphate decarboxylase	Sulfite oxidase and xanthine dehydrogenase deficiency	Molybdenum cofactor
		Thyroid hormonogenesis, detect in, II	Iodide peroxidase
Orotic aciduria II	Orotidylic decarboxylase	Thyroid hormonogenesis, defect in, IV	Iodotyrosine dehalogenase (deiodinase)
Oxalosis I (glycolic aciduria)	Alanine: glyoxylate aminotransferase		
Oxalosis II (glyceric aciduria)	D-Glyceric dehydrogenase	Trimethylaminuria	Trimethylamine oxidase
5-Oxoprolinuria (pyroglutamic aciduria)	Glutathione synthetase	Trypsinogen deficiency	Trypsinogen
		Tyrosinemia I	Para-hydroxyphenylpyruvate oxidase
Pentosuria	L-Xylulose reductase	Tyrosinemia II (Richner-Hanhart syndrome)	Tyrosine transaminase
Phenylketonuria I	Phenylalanine hydroxylase	Urocanase deficiency	Urocanase
Phenylketonuria II	Dihydropteridine reductase	Valinemia	Valine transaminase
Phenylketonuria III	Dihydrobiopterin synthetase	Wernicke-Korsakoff syndrome	Transketolase
Porphyria, acute hepatic	Porphobilinogen synthetase	Wolman's disease	Acid lipase
Porphyria, acute intermittent	Uroporphyrinogen I synthetase	Xanthinuria	Xanthine oxidase
Porphyria, congenital erythropoietic	Uroporphyrinogen III cosynthase	Xanthurenic aciduria	Kynureninase
Porphyria cutanea tarda	Uroporphyrinogen decarboxylase	Xeroderma pigmentosum	Ultraviolet-specific endonuclease
Porphyria variegata	Protoporphyrinogen oxidase	Xylosidase deficiency	Xylosidase

*Based upon McKusick VA: Mendelian Inheritance in Man. 7th ed. Baltimore, Johns Hopkins University Press, 1986, pp xxxi–xxxvi, with modifications.

the more abundant proteins of the cell. An average individual is demonstrably heterozygous at 7 per cent of loci. Since only about one third of base changes alter the charge of a protein, each individual may actually be heterozygous at as many as 20 per cent of loci.

At most genetic loci (e.g., the gene for β-globin) one standard allele accounts for the vast majority of alleles in the population, and alternative alleles are rare. At other loci, no single allele occurs with sufficient frequency to be designated as standard or normal. The α-chain of haptoglobin, a plasma protein, represents one such extreme example of genetic polymorphism. In this instance all polymorphic forms of haptoglobin appear to function equally in hemoglobin bind-

ing. Polymorphisms represent conspicuous examples of human biochemical diversity.

Genetic Heterogeneity. When two or more mutations produce identical or closely similar clinical syndromes, *genetic heterogeneity* is said to exist. In some instances the mutations may be at different loci (*nonallelic* genes), whereas in others they may occur in different portions of the same locus (*allelic* genes). Hemophilia can be caused by a mutation at either of two distinct loci on the X chromosome, one leading to a deficiency of factor VIII (classic hemophilia) and the other to a deficiency of factor IX (Christmas disease). By contrast, the multiple variants of G6PD, over 315 as of 1986, represent different structural gene mutations at a single locus. A striking example of both allelic and nonallelic heterogeneity is hereditary methemoglobinemia, which can be produced by at least ten different mutations at three distinct loci: two at the locus for the α-chain of hemoglobin, three at the locus for the β-chain, and at least five at the locus for NADH methemoglobin reductase.

In view of the multiple alleles that occur at virtually all genetic loci, persons who appear to be homozygous for a genetic trait may actually have inherited different abnormal alleles from each parent. Such individuals are said to be *genetic compounds*. The clinical syndrome in a genetic compound may be intermediate in severity and manifestations between the syndromes produced by homozygosity for either allele. A classic example is hemoglobin SC disease, which results when an offspring inherits a Hb S gene (β-6$^{glu \to val}$) from one parent and a Hb C gene (β-6$^{glu \to lys}$) from the other. Another is the mucopolysaccharide storage disease resulting from inheritance of one gene for Hurler's disease (severe) and one for Scheie's disease (mild). In both these examples the severity is intermediate between the diseases associated with the respective homozygous states. Table 34–5 lists selected inherited diseases for which genetic compounds have been demonstrated.

TABLE 34–2. SOME DISORDERS IN WHICH A DEFICIENCY OF A PLASMA PROTEIN HAS BEEN DEMONSTRATED IN HUMAN BEINGS

Condition	Plasma Protein
Afibrinogenemia	Fibrinogen
Agammaglobulinemia, X-linked	IgA, IgG
Agammaglobulinemia, selective IgA	IgA
Agammaglobulinemia, selective IgG	IgG
Analbuminemia	Albumin
Atransferrinemia	Transferrin
Complement deficiency states, selective C1q, C1r, C1s, C2, C3, C4, C5, C6, C7, C8	C1q, C1r, C1s, C2, C3, C4, C5, C6, C7, C8
Factor VII deficiency	Factor VII
Factor X (Stuart factor) deficiency	Factor X
Fibrin-stabilizing factor deficiency	Factor XIII
Hageman trait	Factor XII
Hemophilia A	Factor VIII
Hemophilia B	Factor IX
Hereditary angioedema	C1-inhibitor
Hypoprothrombinemia	Factor II
Parahemophilia	Factor V
PTA deficiency	Factor XI

PTA = plasma thromboplastin antecedent.

TABLE 34–3. METABOLIC DISEASES THAT HAVE BEEN MAPPED TO SPECIFIC AUTOSOMES*

Disease	Chromosome†
Disorders of carbohydrate metabolism	
Glycogen storage disease, Type II (Pompe's disease)	17
Galactosemia	9p
Galactokinase deficiency	17q
Galactose-4-epimerase deficiency	1p
Disorders of amino acid metabolism	
Classic phenylketonuria (phenylalanine hydroxylase deficiency)	1p
Atypical phenylketonuria (dihydropteridine reductase deficiency)	4
Argininosuccinic aciduria	7
Citrullinemia	9
Transcobalamin II deficiency	9q
Tetrahydrofolate methyltransferase deficiency	1
Disorders of lipoprotein and lipid metabolism	
Familial lecithin:cholesterol acyltransferase deficiency	16q
Disorders of lysosomal enzymes	
Mucopolysaccharidosis, Type VI (Maroteaux-Lamy syndrome)	5
Mucopolysaccharidosis, Type VII (β-glucuronidase deficiency)	7
Fucosidosis	1p
Mannosidosis	19
Wolman's disease and cholesteryl ester storage disease	10
Lysosomal acid phosphatase deficiency	11p
Metachromatic leukodystrophy	22q
Sandhoff's disease	5q
Tay-Sachs disease	15q
Generalized gangliosidosis	3
Disorders of steroid metabolism	
Adrenogenital syndrome (steroid 21-hydroxylase deficiency)	6p
Disorders of purine and pyrimidine metabolism	
Adenine phosphoribosyltransferase deficiency	16
Adenosine deaminase deficiency	20q
Nucleoside phosphorylase deficiency	14q
Disorders of metal metabolism	
Hemochromatosis	6p
Disorders of the blood and blood-forming tissues	
Glucosephosphate isomerase deficiency	19
Hexokinase deficiency	10
Triosephosphate isomerase deficiency	12p
Elliptocytosis	1p
Sickle cell anemia and all other β-chain variants	11p
Hemoglobin Constant Spring and all other α-chain variants	16p
α-Thalassemias	16p
β-Thalassemias	11p
Disorders of immune and other defense systems	
C2 deficiency	6p
C3 deficiency	19p
C4 deficiency	6p

*Modified from McKusick VA: Am J Med 69:267, 1980.
†These numbers indicate the chromosome that carries the particular locus. The chromosome arm is indicated when known: p = short arm; q = long arm.

TREATMENT OF INBORN ERRORS OF METABOLISM.

Treatment of the patient with an inherited disorder depends upon accurate diagnosis and an understanding of the pathophysiology of the disease, including an appreciation of the interaction of genetic and environmental factors. Well-known examples are phenylketonuria, which predisposes to toxic reactions to dietary phenylalanine, and G6PD deficiency, which predisposes to hemolysis following ingestion of fava beans, during the course of acute viral hepatitis and infectious mononucleosis, or after administration of certain drugs, including aspirin and phenacetin. In such instances control of environmental factors may mitigate or neutralize the effect of the genetic change.

The balance of this chapter will be devoted to a discussion of forms of treatment of value in specific hereditary disorders.

Dietary Restriction of Substrate. Dietary restriction will often reduce the excessive substrate that accumulates behind a metabolic block. A general reduction in protein intake will prevent brain damage in disorders of the urea cycle associated with ammonia intoxication, including argininosuccinicaciduria and citrullinemia. A diet low in phenylalanine is effective in preventing growth and mental retardation in phenylketonuria, if started soon after birth. A fructose-free diet controls the symptoms of hereditary fructose intolerance resulting from deficiency of fructose-1-phosphate aldolase. Similarly, a diet that is virtually galactose free will avert brain damage and cataract formation in children with galactokinase or galactose-1-phosphate uridyl transferase deficiency.

Replacement of the Deficient End-Product. A metabolic block may also result in a critical shortage in the product of the reaction or later products of the sequence. Replacement may alleviate the deficiency state. Goiter resulting from a block in thyroxine production can be treated and cretinism prevented by replacement of thyroid hormone. In the adrenogenital syndromes, corticosteroid administration supplies the missing hormone, corrects the disordered steroidal secretory pattern, and leads to remission of the clinical manifestations. In orotic aciduria, administration of uridine supplies the pyrimidines needed for hematopoietic functions and corrects the macrocytic anemia, and also suppresses orotic acid synthesis and urolithiasis.

TABLE 34–4. SOME PLASMA PROTEINS AND CELLULAR ENZYMES THAT EXHIBIT ELECTROPHORETICALLY DETECTABLE POLYMORPHISMS*

Protein	Locus Name
Plasma proteins	
Haptoglobin (α-chain)	Hp α
Transferrin	Tf
Vitamin-D binding protein	Gc (for group-specific component)
Ceruloplasmin	Cp
α-1-Antitrypsin	Pi (for protease inhibitor)
α-1-Acid glycoprotein	Oro (for orosomucoid)
β-2-Glycoprotein I	—
Properdin factor B	Bf
Complement	
Second component	C2
Third component	C3
Fourth component	C4
Sixth component	C6
Enzymes	
Pancreatic amylase	AMY₂
Cholinesterase	E₂
Red blood cell enzyme	
Acid phosphatase 1	ACP₁
Adenosine deaminase	ADA
Adenylate kinase	AK₁
Carbonic anhydrase 2	CA₂
Diaphorase (NADPH-dependent)	DIA₂
Esterase D	ESD
Galactose-1-uridyltransferase	GALT
Glucose-6-phosphate dehydrogenase	Gd
Glutamic pyruvic transaminase	GPT
Glutathione peroxidase	GPX
Glutathione reductase	GSR
Glyoxalase I	GLO
Peptidase A	PEPA
Peptidase C	PEPC
Peptidase D	PEPD
Phosphoglucomutase 1	PGM₁
Phosphoglucomutase 2	PGM₂
Phosphogluconate dehydrogenase	PGD
Uridine monophosphate kinase	UMPK
White blood cell enzymes	
Aconitase (soluble)	ACON₈
Cytidine deaminase	CDA
α-L-Fucosidase	αFUC
α-Glucosidase	αGLUC
Glutamic-oxaloacetic transaminase (mitochondrial)	GOT_M
Hexokinase 3	HK₃
Malic enzyme (mitochondrial)	ME_M
Phosphoglucomutase 3	PGM₃

*From Giblett ER: Ann Rev Genet 11:13, 1977.

TABLE 34–5. INHERITED METABOLIC DISEASES FOR WHICH GENETIC COMPOUNDS HAVE BEEN DEMONSTRATED*

α-1-Antitrypsin deficiency
Cystinosis
Cystinuria
"Homozygous" familial hypercholesterolemia (LDL receptor-internalization defect)
Galactosemia (galactose-1-phosphate uridyltransferase deficiency)
Gaucher's disease (glucocerebrosidase deficiency)
Glucosephosphate isomerase deficiency
Hemoglobin α-chain variants
Hemoglobin β-chain variants
Hurler-Scheie syndrome (α-L-iduronidase deficiency)
Iminoglycinuria
Metachromatic leukodystrophy (cerebroside sulfatase deficiency)
Hereditary methemoglobinemia (NADH dehydrogenase deficiency)
Phenylketonuria (phenylalanine hydroxylase deficiency)
Pseudocholinesterase deficiency
Pyruvate kinase deficiency

*Modified from McKusick VA: Am J Hum Genet 25:446, 1973.
LDL = low density lipoprotein; NADH = reduced form of nicotinamide adenine dinucleotide.

Depletion of Storage Substances. In some hereditary disorders the clinical consequences result from accumulation of stored materials in the tissues, and removal of the excess material may ameliorate the effects of the genetic lesion. Removal of stored copper in Wilson's disease by penicillamine and of excess iron in hemochromatosis by frequent phlebotomy illustrates this approach. Use of uricosuric agents to deplete the body of uric acid in tophaceous gout and of cholestyramine to reduce serum cholesterol levels in familial hypercholesterolemia are additional examples.

Use of Metabolic Inhibitors. When a toxic metabolite accumulates because of a metabolic error, it may be possible to control its production by use of an appropriate metabolic inhibitor. Allopurinol inhibits xanthine oxidase and controls uric acid production in gout and 2,8-dioxyadenine production and renal stone formation in patients with homozygous adenine phosphoribosyltransferase deficiency. Clofibrate, which inhibits synthesis or release of glyceride from the liver, reduces blood lipid levels to normal in type III hyperlipoproteinemia.

Amplification of Enzyme Activity. Many enzyme proteins require cofactors for biologic activity. In some inborn errors the mutation affects the ability of the apoenzyme to combine with its cofactor. In other genetic disorders there is a metabolic defect in the conversion of a precursor vitamin to its active cofactor form. In both situations administration of the appropriate cofactor may increase the catalytic activity of the apoenzyme. Pyridoxine (vitamin B_6) is a cofactor for cystathionine synthetase. In more than one half of patients with homocystinuria caused by deficient synthetase activity, administration of large doses of pyridoxine partially overcomes the block in homocysteine metabolism. Similarly the ketoacidosis of some patients with methylmalonicaciduria is corrected by treatment with pharmacologic doses of vitamin B_{12}, and the clinical and hematologic abnormalities of patients with hereditary dihydrofolate reductase deficiency are corrected by administration of small doses of 5-formyltetrahydrofolate, which bypasses the metabolic block (replacement of deficient endproduct).

Phenobarbital and certain other drugs increase production of smooth endoplasmic reticulum and of certain of its enzymes, including NADPH-cytochrome C reductase, cytochrome P-450, and several drug-hydroxylating enzymes. Administration of phenobarbital to patients with unconjugated hyperbilirubinemia in a variant of the Crigler-Najjar syndrome or with Gilbert's syndrome may reduce plasma bilirubin levels following induction of hepatic glucuronyltransferase.

Replacement of Mutant Protein. Direct replacement of the missing protein is an attractive approach to the treatment of recessively inherited diseases. Greater success has been achieved in deficiencies of nonenzymic than of enzymic proteins. Examples include replacement of gamma globulin in agammaglobulinemia, of albumin in analbuminemia, and of factor VIII in hemophilia. In each of these cases, the deficient gene product is a plasma protein. The metabolic and immunologic defects of patients with adenosine deaminase deficiency are transiently corrected by infusion of irradiated erythrocytes containing normal levels of adenosine deaminase.

Much less success has attended efforts to replace missing enzymes that normally function within cells. Enzyme infusions have been attempted in the mucopolysaccharidoses, Gaucher's disease, Tay-Sachs disease, and Pompe's disease, but therapeutic benefits are unproved. The lysosomal storage diseases are perhaps the best candidates for treatment by administration of exogenous enzyme, for cells have highly specific mechanisms for taking up exogenous proteins and delivering them to lysosomes. However, the exogenous protein must bind to a specific recognition site on the plasma membrane of the target cell so that it can be selectively internalized. Enzymes have been coupled covalently to other molecules for which tissues contain receptors, on the theory that in this manner the enzyme might be conveyed to the lysosomes along with the primary ligand. This type of experimental work holds promise for the future.

Modifying the Mutant Protein. Many proteins can be modified by the addition of subgroups. For example, sickle cell hemoglobin can be carbamylated by cyanate at the valine in position 1 of the β-chain, which then blocks the hydrophobic bonding of the normal val-1 to the mutant val-6 of β-globin of Hb S, thereby preventing sickling in vitro. Severe toxic reactions, such as peripheral neuropathy, sharply limit the clinical usefulness of cyanate therapy in patients with sickle cell disease. Nevertheless, this approach holds promise for the future.

Organ Transplantation. Allotransplantation of the organ in which the deficient enzyme is normally synthesized has been attempted in a variety of inherited diseases. The greatest experience has involved renal transplantation, which has been performed in Alport's syndrome, renal amyloidosis, cystinosis, Fabry's disease, Gaucher's disease, oxalosis, and some other conditions. The results in most instances have paralleled those of renal transplantation for other forms of end-stage renal disease. There has been no evidence of reactivation of the renal lesion in patients with Alport's syndrome, or of development of cystinosis or Fabry's disease in the transplanted kidneys. Amyloidosis has recurred in the graft on rare occasions. By contrast severe recurrent oxalosis has developed in a number of transplanted kidneys, and end-stage renal failure resulting from oxalosis is not now considered an indication for renal transplantation. Patients with Fabry's disease have developed measurable levels of the missing enzyme, ceramide trihexosidase, in plasma following renal transplantation, and there have been a few long-term survivals. Nevertheless, renal transplantation in patients with inborn errors of metabolism should be limited to replacement of failed kidneys. Results do not warrant use of renal transplantation primarily for enzyme replacement.

Transplantation of allogenic marrow has successfully corrected a number of immunodeficiency states, including lymphopenic hypogammaglobulinemia (Swiss type), Wiskott-Aldrich syndrome, and severe combined immunodeficiency disease.

Liver transplantation has been successful in cases of hepatic failure from Wilson's disease, α-1-antitrypsin deficiency, and homozygous familial hypercholesterolemia. Heart transplantation has been employed in many cases of hereditary cardiomyopathy.

Surgical removals also play a role in certain hereditary disorders. Examples include splenectomy in hereditary spherocytosis and colectomy in preventing neoplastic transformation in polyposis of the colon. Also, surgery offers a quick and permanent cure for polydactyly as well as for certain other dominantly inherited defects.

Genetic Engineering. The use of recombinant DNA technology in the diagnosis and treatment of inborn errors is discussed in Ch. 35.

Giblett ER: Genetic polymorphisms in human blood. Ann Rev Genet 11:13, 1977. *A review of polymorphic protein in blood, including alloantigens of red and white blood cells and plasma proteins, and electrophoretic variants of plasma and cellular components.*

McKusick VA: Phenotypic diversity of human diseases resulting from allelic series. Am J Hum Genet 25:446, 1973. *An analytical review of different disorders that can result from series of mutations involving the same gene.*

Stanbury JB, Wyngaarden JB, Fredrickson DS, et al. (eds.): The Metabolic Basis of Inherited Disease. 5th ed. New York, McGraw-Hill Book Company, 1983. *Authoritative discussions of all inborn errors of metabolism for which there is a substantial body of metabolic or biochemical information.*

35 EXPECTATIONS FROM RECOMBINANT DNA RESEARCH

W. French Anderson

Over the past dozen years, a revolution has occurred in DNA research, variously referred to as recombinant DNA technology, genetic engineering, molecular cloning, gene splicing, or biotechnology. The new DNA research is beginning to make a major impact on clinical medicine in four major areas: (1) understanding of the molecular basis of human (particularly genetic) diseases, (2) prenatal diagnosis, (3) production of human biologic products, and (4) gene therapy. Categories 1 to 3 are already a reality, whereas human gene therapy is fast approaching that status.

THE MOLECULAR BASIS OF HUMAN DISEASES

Although the human diseases studied by recombinant DNA techniques at present are the genetic diseases, the power of this technology is beginning to be felt in many other areas of human physiology and pathophysiology. All living processes are ultimately controlled by genes. Therefore, as genes are "cloned" (i.e., isolated) and as their products (which can be obtained in large amounts once the gene is cloned; see below) are studied both in vitro and in vivo, more is learned about the reactions that the genes govern. The result is that the normal physiology of a process becomes better understood. An example is the regulation of the hematopoietic system. As the genes for various growth factors and cytokines are obtained and their products made available for study (e.g., granulocyte-macrophage colony-stimulating factor, [GM-CSF], erythropoietin, interleukin-2 [Il-2], and so forth), a much clearer understanding is emerging on how proliferation and differentiation are controlled in the bone marrow. Another example is the immune system, in which the genes for the various cell surface receptors (e.g., Il-2 receptor, T-cell receptor, and so on) are being cloned and analyzed.

It is the genetic diseases, however, that have primarily benefited from the recombinant DNA revolution. Most studied are the thalassemias and hemoglobinopathies (see Ch. 142, 143). A decade ago the genetics of beta-thalassemia was extremely confusing. There were various clinical classifications to account for the range of severity seen. It was assumed that there must be different genotypes and that many patients were probably genetic compounds. Now, most of the genotypes that can produce beta-thalassemia have been sequenced, and the mechanisms underlying the various beta-zero and

beta-plus thalassemias have been elucidated (see Ch. 142). Not only has this information led to a better comprehension of the thalassemia syndromes, but also it has made prenatal diagnosis and genetic counseling much more accurate. Similar progress in the understanding of a number of other genetic diseases is under way.

PRENATAL DIAGNOSIS

Prenatal diagnosis can be used for the detection of a number of genetic diseases; see, for example, the discussion in the chapter on sickle cell anemia (Ch. 143). Recombinant DNA technology has greatly expanded the accuracy, range, and safety of this procedure. Previously, it was necessary to obtain the gene product in sufficient amounts to be detectable by biochemical methods. For example, in the prenatal diagnosis of beta-thalassemia, fetal blood would be sampled at around 18 weeks of gestation (either by fetoscopy or placental aspiration), with a 5 per cent fetal mortality rate. Globin chains would then be fractionated. Analysis of fetal DNA, on the other hand, can be carried out on a small number of amniotic cells (with a fetal mortality rate of only 0.3 per cent) or from chorionic villi (with a fetal loss of 4 per cent but with the distinct advantage of making a diagnosis as early as 9 to 10 weeks of gestation).

There are a number of techniques that can be used to analyze fetal DNA for single-gene disorders. First is the straightforward method of restriction endonuclease mapping. A restriction enzyme cuts DNA at a specific short (4- to 6-nucleotide) sequence. If a genetic disorder alters the sequence recognized by a restriction enzyme, digestion of the fetal DNA with that enzyme provides an immediate diagnosis. Unfortunately, there are only a few situations in which this technique is applicable (e.g., sickle cell anemia). A second procedure is to make a linkage analysis with a restriction fragment length polymorphism (known as RFLP) (see Ch. 34). This approach will become increasingly valuable as sufficient RFLP's are located to make a roadmap of the entire human genome. Finally, a procedure that promises to be extremely valuable is the use of oligonucleotide probes that are specific for individual mutations. In theory, every genetic disease could be detected directly by hybridizing a normal and "mutant" oligonucleotide probe to a sample of fetal DNA.

It is clear that the new technology will revolutionize prenatal diagnosis. What is uncertain is how long it will take to transfer these sophisticated procedures from research laboratories to routine clinical use.

HUMAN BIOLOGICS PRODUCED BY BIOTECHNOLOGY

Genetic engineering is currently being used by biotechnology companies to produce large quantities of previously unavailable human biologics (usually peptides or proteins). What products are being made? Why these products? How are they being made? How good are they?

The first human proteins produced by the new technology are now being evaluated in clinical trials: Insulin, growth hormone (GH), and α and β interferon have been licensed by the United States Food and Drug Administration (FDA); gamma interferon, interleukin-2 (Il-2), and tumor necrosis factor (TNF) are under study. In each case, they were chosen because of the importance of the protein in treating specific human disease states (either established: insulin, GH; or postulated), the commercial market expected for the compound, and the ability to apply recombinant DNA techniques to synthesize large quantities of the human protein in bacteria (or in yeast or other cells) inexpensively.

The Technology

A gene is a sequence of nucleotides in DNA that code for a product. In order to get a bacterium (the most common biologic "factory" in use at present) to produce a human protein, it is necessary to obtain a DNA copy of the protein—in other words, to obtain a piece of double-stranded DNA that carries the precise sequence of nucleotides that code for the protein. This DNA is then inserted into a bacterial plasmid—a circle of naturally occurring nonchromosomal DNA that replicates freely in the cytoplasm of a bacterium. Any gene (bacterial, plant, animal, or human) that is inserted into the plasmid with the correct control signals can, in theory, be transcribed and translated into protein within the bacterium. The synthesized protein can then be purified from the bacterial cells.

There are a number of ways to acquire a human gene suitable for engineered protein production in bacteria. One procedure is to sequence a portion of the human protein of interest and then, by using the genetic code, determine the DNA sequence that would give the known amino acid sequence. Then a segment of DNA one and one half to several dozen nucleotides long is chemically synthesized (longer DNA molecules are very difficult to synthesize and purify) that will be exactly complementary to a portion of the expected sequence of the messenger RNA (mRNA). "Exactly complementary" means that the DNA "probe" will have T (thymine) where the mRNA has an A (adenine), a C (cytosine) where the mRNA has a G (guanine), and so forth. This DNA probe can be tagged with radioactivity and then be used to find (by hybridization) the desired mRNA in extracts of the appropriate human cells. The mRNA is isolated, purified, and shown to be capable of being translated in vitro to give the predicted human protein. This mRNA is then transcribed into full-length complementary (or copy) DNA, called cDNA, by the enzyme reverse transcriptase. The resulting DNA is an exact code of the mRNA for the human protein. It can now be made double stranded (by the action of other enzymes) and inserted into a bacterial plasmid along with the appropriate control signals.

Several requirements must be met in order to obtain large quantities of human proteins in bacteria. The human gene must be attached within the plasmid to a bacterial control signal that will be switched on at a high level. Several such "promoter" regions are used, including those from the lactose operon, from the bacteriophage lambda, and so on. Second, other regulatory signals (for example, a binding site so that the transcribed RNA will attach to and be translated by ribosomes) must be present adjacent to the human gene. Third, any hard-to-handle portion of DNA (for example, nucleotides producing a leader sequence of amino acids or an intervening sequence) should be removed, since bacteria are not equipped to carry out many of the post-transcriptional and post-translational modifications that eukaryotic cells can perform. Fourth, the human protein must be protected from proteinases within the bacterium.

How good are these biologically engineered human proteins? They should be perfectly acceptable for administration to patients. In most cases, they should be pure and contain no infectious contaminants or animal antigenic material. However, unless purified extensively, they might contain clinically relevant amounts of bacterial antigenic substances. In addition, since some products isolated directly from the body have a number of biologic compounds bound to them, the clinical effect of a "pure" engineered product (e.g., albumin) might be somewhat different from that of the natural product.

The Next Products

What human biologics are now under development? Those being prepared for human trials fall into four broad categories; vaccines, blood components, neurohormones, and diagnostics.

VACCINES. The first recombinant DNA vaccine approved by the FDA (July 1986) for clinical use was that for hepatitis B. Specific vaccines for influenza and malaria are in clinical trials. Potential vaccines for a number of other diseases are currently in preparation, e.g., leprosy, tuberculosis, typhoid, acquired immunodeficiency syndrome (AIDS), and so forth. This new generation of vaccines should be superior to those in use today. A precise portion of the antigenic surface of a virus or a parasite can be selected and the DNA complement to this moiety prepared. Since a bacterial control signal will transcribe any sequence of DNA attached to it, the DNA coding for just the antigenic site desired can be inserted into bacteria for large-scale production of material. Or the DNA could be inserted into, for example, vaccinia in order to take advantage of a well-characterized vaccination agent. It appears to be possible to prepare highly specific vaccines by this approach.

BLOOD COMPONENTS. Several different types of blood components are being prepared for clinical trials.

Clotting Factors. The genes for factor VIII, von Willebrand's factor, and factor IX have been obtained. Human protein C has also been cloned.

Albumin. The great demand for albumin as a plasma expander has resulted in a major effort to produce human albumin in bacteria. The advantages of engineered albumin (besides increased availability and decreased cost) should be that there will be no risk of hepatitis, AIDS, or other infectious contamination.

Thrombolytic Agents. Blood clots are a major cause of death and disabling diseases in the United States. Consequently, readily available clot-specific thrombolytic agents would be clinically useful. Biotechnology is being employed to isolate the genes for, and to engineer the production of, tissue-type and urokinase-type plasminogen activators. These proteins should be superior to the currently available agents, urokinase and streptokinase. Considerable progress has been made toward bringing tissue plasminogen activators to market.

Biologic Response Modifiers. Besides the family of interferons, Il-2, and TNF, which are under active clinical investigation, other cytokines (Il-1, GM-CSF, human granulocyte CSF, and so forth) are undergoing engineered production. Considerable effort is under way to identify other factors, particularly a molecule that would stimulate the earliest pluripotent stem cell. Major advances in clinical manipulation of the immune system are expected when the genes of the major histocompatibility complex and the immunoglobulin gene families are more fully understood.

NEUROHORMONES. This complex group includes a large number of hormones, various neuropeptides, and the neurotransmitters with their receptors. Insulin and growth hormone are already being tested clinically; peptides from the pro-opiomelanocortin family should be available shortly.

DIAGNOSTICS. Since viruses consist of sequences of DNA or RNA with a coat, diagnostic techniques that would rapidly and accurately identify the presence of specific viruses in body tissues or fluids by using DNA probes are being developed.

OTHER AREAS. Finally, two other areas need to be mentioned. A further understanding of oncogenes and their role in cancer should lead to the development of drugs or antibodies that could be used to inhibit specific steps in the pathway leading from a normal to a malignant cell. Second, the tremendous potential of recombinant DNA research to produce useful new agricultural plants and improved farm animals should have a large effect on the food supply of the world.

GENE THERAPY

By gene therapy is meant the insertion of a normal gene into the appropriate cells of a patient in such a way that the exogenous gene produces a product that will cure, or at least ameliorate, the genetic defect. For some genetic conditions (specifically those caused by a single gene mutation that produces a defective product that can be isolated), gene therapy should be a beneficial therapeutic procedure in the future.

The Technology of Gene Therapy

It is now possible by the use of recombinant DNA technology to isolate specific normal genes from the DNA of human tissue. A gene can be isolated if it can be recognized, and it can be recognized if the protein product that it makes can be isolated. The defective product in many genetic diseases is a protein (e.g., an enzyme in many of the inborn errors of metabolism; beta-globin in sickle cell anemia or Cooley's anemia). In a manner similar to that described above in the section on human biologics, a DNA probe can be synthesized. With this probe it is possible to locate the gene in human DNA, isolate (i.e., clone) it, and purify it. Any gene can be cloned once a probe for the gene exists.

The cloned gene can be inserted into cells in any one of a number of ways. The three most commonly used techniques are (1) microinjecting directly into a cell's nucleus, (2) forming a calcium phosphate precipitate of the DNA and then incubating tissue culture cells with this precipitate, and (3) inserting the gene into a nonpathogenic virus and infecting cells with this recombinant virus. All three procedures have been used successfully to insert cloned genes into cells growing in tissue culture. By far, the most efficient procedure at present is the use of retrovirus-based vectors carrying exogenous genes.

Vectors derived from retroviruses possess several advantages as a gene delivery system. First, up to 100 per cent of cells can be infected and can express the integrated viral (and exogenous) genes. Second, as many cells as desired can be infected simultaneously. Third, under appropriate conditions, the DNA can integrate as a single copy at a single, albeit random, site. Finally, the infection and long-term harboring of a retroviral vector usually does not harm cells. Several retroviral vector systems have been developed; those projected for human use are constructed from the Moloney murine leukemia virus. Evidence obtained from studies with experimental animals and in tissue culture indicates that retroviruses can be used as a reasonably efficient delivery system.

The next question is, what target cell to use? At present, the only human tissue that can be used effectively for gene transfer is bone marrow. No other cells (except, perhaps, skin cells) can be extracted from the body, grown in culture to allow insertion of exogenous genes, and then successfully reimplanted into the patient from whom the tissue was taken. In the future, as more is learned about how to package the DNA and to make it tissue specific, the intravenous route would be the simplest and most desirable. However, attempting to give a foreign gene by injection directly into the bloodstream is not advisable with our present state of knowledge, since the procedure would be enormously inefficient and there would be little control over the DNA's fate.

Studies are considerably more advanced with bone marrow than skin cells as a recipient tissue for gene transfer. Bone marrow consists of a heterogeneous population of cells, most of which are committed to differentiate into red blood cells, white blood cells, platelets, and so on. Only a small proportion (0.1 to 0.5 per cent) of nucleated bone marrow cells are stem cells (that is, blood-forming cells that have not yet differentiated into specific cell types and that divide as needed to maintain the marrow population). In gene therapy, it would be these stem cells that would be the primary target.

Initial Disease Candidate for Gene Therapy

For many years, clinical investigators thought that the human genetic diseases most likely to be the initial ones successfully treated by gene therapy would be the hemoglobin abnormalities (specifically, beta-thalassemia) because these disorders are the most obvious ones carried by blood cells, and bone marrow is the easiest tissue to manipulate outside the body. Regulation of globin synthesis, however, is unusually complicated. Not only are the embryonic, fetal, and adult globin chains carefully regulated during development, but also the subunits of the hemoglobin molecule are coded by genes on two different chromosomes. To understand the regulatory signals that control such a complicated system and to develop means for obtaining controlled expression of an exogenous (i.e., inserted by gene therapy) beta-globin gene will take considerably more research effort. It now appears that the most likely gene to be used in the first experiments on human gene therapy is adenosine deaminase (ADA), the absence of which results in severe combined immunodeficiency disease (in which children have a greatly weakened resistance to infection and cannot survive the usual childhood diseases).

ADA deficiency has a number of features that make it an ideal initial candidate.

1. The disease can be cured by infusion of normal bone marrow cells from a histocompatible donor. Selective replication of the normal marrow cells appears to take place. This observation offers hope that defective bone marrow can be removed from a patient, the normal ADA gene inserted into a number of cells through gene therapy, and the treated marrow reimplanted into the patient, where it may have a selective growth advantage. If selective growth occurs, elimination of the patient's own marrow would not be necessary. If, however, corrected marrow cells have no growth advantage over endogenous (i.e., the patient's own untreated) cells, then partial or complete marrow destruction (either by irradiation or by other means) may be required in order to allow the corrected marrow cells an environment favorable for expansion. The latter situation (which will probably be necessary in most other genetic diseases) would require much greater confidence that the gene therapy procedure would work before a clinical trial should be undertaken.

2. Experience with mismatched bone marrow transplantation has demonstrated poor results for ADA deficiency. There is not a good alternative therapy for patients without a matched donor.

3. The entire pathophysiology of the disease appears to be confined to the lymphoid population of the marrow. Therefore, successful treatment of these cells should be curative.

4. Regulation of the inserted gene does not need to be precise, since individuals with levels of 5 to 5000 per cent of normal ADA activity are relatively symptom free.

Ethics

The ethics of gene therapy in humans has been discussed for many years. Essentially all observers have stated that they believe that it would be ethical to insert genetic material into a human being for the sole purpose of medically correcting a severe genetic disorder in that patient—in other words, somatic cell gene therapy. Attempts to correct a patient's reproductive cells (i.e., germ line gene therapy) or to alter or improve a "normal" person by gene manipulation (i.e., enhancement or eugenic genetic engineering) are controversial areas. However, somatic cell gene therapy for a patient suffering a serious genetic disorder would be ethically acceptable if carried out under the same strict criteria that cover other new experimental medical procedures. The techniques now being developed by clinical investigators for human application are for somatic cell, not germ line, gene therapy.

What criteria should be satisfied prior to the time that somatic cell gene therapy is tested in a clinical trial? Three general requirements are that it should be shown in animal studies that (1) the new gene can be put into the correct target cells and will remain there long enough to be effective; (2) the new gene will be expressed in the cells at an appropriate level; and (3) the new gene will not harm the cell or, by extension, the animal. These criteria are very similar to those required prior to the use of any new drug, therapeutic procedure, or surgical operation. The requirements simply state that the new treatment should get to the area of disease, correct it, and do more good than harm.

Although retroviruses have many advantages for gene transfer, they also have disadvantages, which lead to questions about safety. One problem is that they can rearrange their own structure, as well as exchange sequences with other retroviruses. There is a built-in safety feature with the mouse retroviral vectors now in use, however; these mouse structures have a very different sequence from known primate retroviruses, and there appears to be little or no homology between the two. Therefore, it should be possible, with continuing research, to build a safe retroviral vector.

Even with a "safe" vector, however, the problem of insertional mutagenesis remains. Since a retroviral vector incorporates into the genome randomly, it may inactivate an important gene or, worse, activate an oncogene. It is uncertain how great a danger this problem poses. As with any new clinical protocol, the total expected benefit for the patient must be weighed against potential risks. Ultimately, local institutional review boards and the National Institutes of Health, the latter through its Working Group on Human Gene Therapy, must decide if a given protocol is ready for human application.

Present Capabilities

What is the present capability for transferring a functional gene into an intact animal in a manner that has potential clinical application? Encouraging results have been obtained in mice as well as in nonhuman primates and sheep.

Several laboratories have successfully carried out a bone marrow transplantation (BMT)/gene transfer protocol in mice. A neomycin resistance gene (carried by a retroviral vector) has been transferred into murine bone marrow cells, followed by the reinsertion of the treated marrow cells into lethally irradiated mice. After several months, the fully reconstituted animals were shown still to carry a functioning neomycin resistance gene in their bone marrow and peripheral blood cells. Analysis demonstrated that, in some animals, all the blood cell lineages contained the active gene.

It has been more difficult to obtain expression of a human gene in vivo in mice. However, when a retroviral vector was built in which the human ADA gene was regulated by a primate (SV40) promoter, excellent expression of the human gene could be obtained in primate cells in culture. T and B cells isolated from patients with ADA deficiency were shown to produce normal human ADA after insertion of the ADA gene. When a protocol similar to the mouse BMT/gene transfer procedure was carried out in nonhuman primates using the primate-promoted ADA vector, several monkeys were found to carry and express the human ADA gene in a small number of their blood cells several months after treatment. These results offer encouragement that retroviral vectors may soon be sufficiently developed to be used in a clinical trial of gene therapy.

There are some genetic diseases that might be most optimally treated in utero rather than waiting until after birth, when some irreversible damage may already have occurred. Recent experiments in fetal sheep suggest that, at least in this animal model, a gene can be inserted into fetal blood cells that have been removed and then reinfused during midpregnancy. The gene (in this case, the neomycin resistance gene previously studied in mice) is active and continues to function for at least several months after the birth of the lamb. Thus, in utero gene therapy is a theoretic possibility.

What still needs to be done? First, the efficiency of the BMT/gene transfer should be improved. Although positive selective pressure may take place in patients with ADA

deficiency, there is no assurance that the inserted ADA gene will be adequately expressed in stem cells as well as in mature T and B cells. Therefore, the more efficient the gene transfer procedure is, the higher is the likelihood that the patient will be helped. Second, the procedure should be shown to be reproducible. Only a few animals have been studied up to this point. Third, the safety of the procedure should be verified. Do the animals develop a viremia? Is there any indication that the vector has spread from the bone marrow to other cells (including germ cells)? Are there any signs of a malignancy or other pathologic condition?

Overview

It now appears that effective delivery-expression systems are becoming available that will allow reasonable attempts at somatic cell gene therapy. The first clinical trials will probably be carried out within the next couple of years. The initial protocols will be based on treatment of bone marrow cells with retroviral vectors carrying a normal gene. Patients severely debilitated by having no normal copies of the gene that produces the enzyme ADA are the most likely first candidates for gene therapy.

Gene therapy is a procedure with enormous potential. It should, in the future, provide a cure for hereditary diseases caused by a single gene defect. It is even possible that the germ line might be corrected so that the children of a patient will also be free from disease. This would be, indeed, a powerful therapeutic tool. But some claims made about the potential of genetic engineering in humans are highly unlikely. Patients with multigenic diseases, in which the genes as well as the intracellular products involved are unknown, will not be candidates for gene therapy for a long time to come, if ever. Likewise, characteristics such as personality and intelligence are probably outside the realm of this technique's potential. Only traits produced by identifiable single genes can be approached by genetic engineering. Of course, if, as now seems the case, some very widespread pathologic conditions (namely, lipid deposition in vessels to produce atherosclerosis) are influenced by identifiable individual genes, then gene therapy might have a far wider application than currently visualized.

The power to cure a genetic defect is an awesome one. But the goal of biomedical research is, and has always been, to alleviate human suffering. Gene therapy, with proper safeguards imposed by society, is a logical part of that effort.

Anderson WF: Prospects for human gene therapy. Science 226:401, 1984. *This review summarizes the medical, technical, and ethical issues involved in human gene therapy.*
Parkman R: The application of bone marrow transplantation to the treatment of genetic diseases. Science 232:1373, 1986. *This recent review places gene therapy in the context of present-day treatment of genetic disorders, particularly bone marrow transplantation.*
Walters L: The ethics of human gene therapy. Nature 320:225, 1986. *This commentary surveys the social issues related to gene therapy.*
Weatherall DJ: The New Genetics and Clinical Practice. 2nd ed. 2. Oxford, Oxford University Press, 1985. *This well-written, easy-to-follow, small volume describes the clinical implications of recombinant DNA technology.*

36 CHROMOSOMES AND THEIR DISORDERS

John L. Hamerton

Cytogenetics is the study of the chromosomes and their behavior as it relates to transmission of the genetic material from parent to offspring. Errors in chromosome behavior and structure are the cause of a wide range of clinical syndromes.

Humans have 46 chromosomes, which consist of 22 pairs

of homologous chromosomes (identical in regard to morphology and constituent gene loci) and one pair of sex chromosomes (X and Y), one partner of each pair being derived from the mother and one from the father. The genes are arranged along the chromosomes in linear order, each gene having a precise position or *locus*. Genes that have their loci on the same chromosome are said to be *linked*, or more precisely, to be *syntenic*. Alternate forms of a gene that occupy the same locus are called *alleles*. Any one chromosome bears only a single allele at a given locus, although in the population as a whole there may be multiple alleles, any one of which can occupy that specific locus.

CELL DIVISION

The number of chromosomes found in somatic cells is constant and is termed the diploid (2n) number. Each gamete, however, has only half the *diploid* number and is said to be *haploid* (n). In order to maintain this regularity two types of cell division occur: *mitosis*, which is the cell division occurring in somatic tissues during growth and repair, and *meiosis*, which is the specialized form of cell division occurring during the formation of the gametes.

MITOSIS. The function of mitosis is the distribution and maintenance of the continuity of the genetic material in every cell of the body. This process consists of a number of different phases, which results in an equal distribution of the chromosomes to the two daughter cells. The cell cycle has four stages: mitosis or M, G_1, S, and G_2. The G_1 phase follows mitosis, during which RNA and protein synthesis occurs. S is the period during which DNA replication takes place and the DNA content of the cell doubles, and G_2 is the period

during which energy requirements for cell division are built up and any repair of errors in DNA synthesis takes place.

MEIOSIS (Fig. 36–1). This process occurs only during the formation of the gametes and results in four daughter cells, each with the haploid number of chromosomes. In males each primary spermatocyte forms four functional spermatids that develop into sperm, while in females each oocyte forms only one ovum, the remaining products of meiosis being nunfunctional polar bodies.

The first division of meiosis consists of an extremely long and complex *prophase* during which DNA replication occurs. This is divided into a number of stages during which crossing over and reassortment of genetic material occur. Initially the chromosomes are apparently single threads that begin to shorten and thicken. This is followed by the commencement of pairing of homologous chromosomes (*synapsis*). After pairing is completed, the chromosomes continue to shorten and are now known as *bivalents*, which are held together only at specific points (*chiasmata*). At this stage of prophase each homologous chromosome can be seen to be visibly doubled (two chromatids) so that each bivalent, which continues to shorten and thicken, consists of four chromatids.

The end of prophase is marked by the disappearance of the nuclear membrane and the formation of a spindle, heralding entry into *metaphase* of the first meiotic division. The bivalents are arranged on the equatorial plate of the spindle as a result of a series of complex chromosome movements. The homologous centromeres are undivided at this point and lie opposite each other on the equatorial plate (co-orientation). As soon as this process is complete, the paired homologues separate and move to opposite poles (*anaphase*). The cell then proceeds to the second meiotic division. This is essentially a mitotic

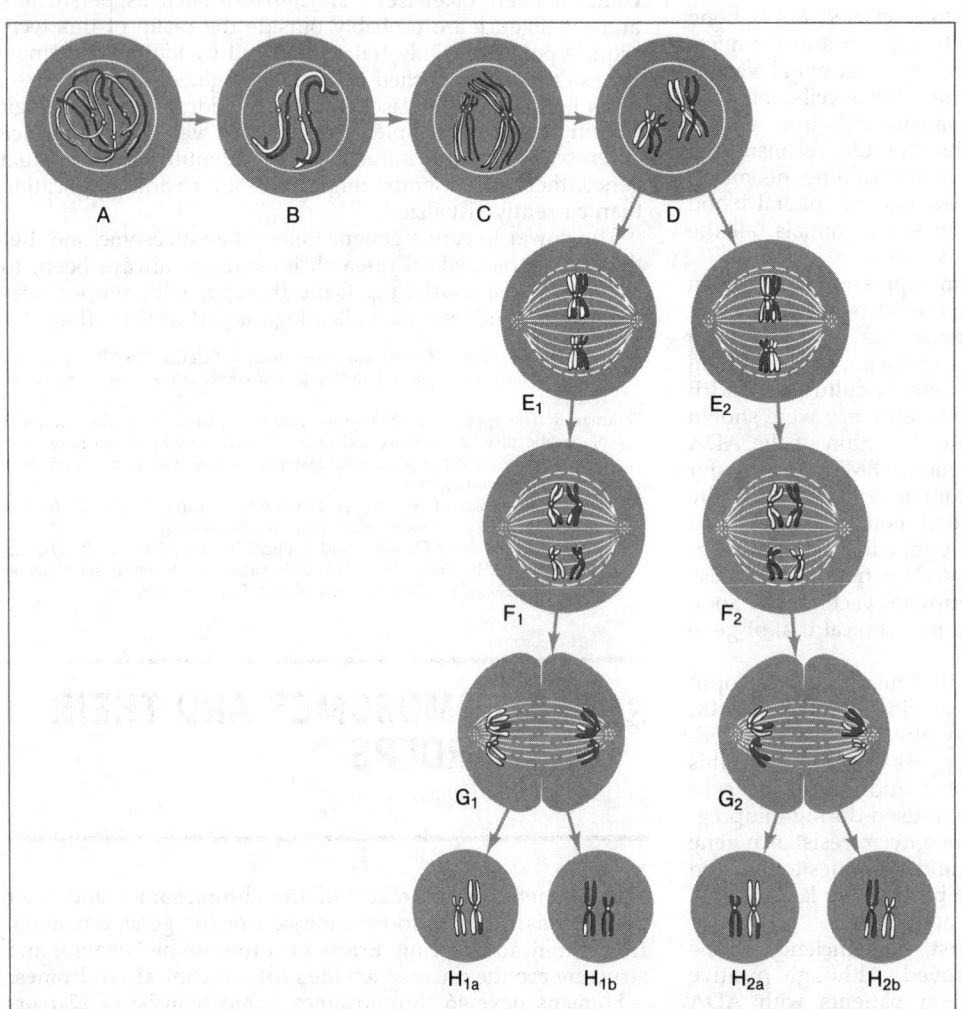

FIGURE 36–1. The stages of the first division of meiosis. Paternal and maternal chromosomes are shown in red and white, respectively. A to D, Stages of prophase. E to G, Metaphase 1 to anaphase 1. H1 to H2, Daughter cells with haploid number of chromosomes prior to entering the second division of meiosis. Note the chromosome exchanges that have taken place.

division in which the chromosomes have already doubled so that there is no need for DNA synthesis. In addition, the genetic material has undergone exchange at meiosis I so that the sister chromatids are not genetically identical.

The major consequences of meiosis are threefold: (1) the halving of the chromosome number; (2) the co-orientation of the bivalents on the metaphase plate, which ensures the regular distribution of the chromosomes to the daughter cells; and (3) the independent assortment of genetic material that results both from genetic crossing over and from the random assortment of the maternal and paternal homologues to the two daughter cells in meiosis I.

Two processes are fundamental to meiosis: chromosome pairing, which results in formation of the bivalents, and chiasma formation. Chiasmata have two main functions: They are the points on the chromosomes at which genetic crossing over takes place, and they serve to maintain bivalent association throughout the prophase and metaphase. Meiosis thus ensures genetic variability as a result of random segregation of the parental homologous chromosomes and the exchange of genetic material by crossing over between nonsister chromatids.

METHODS FOR THE PREPARATION OF CHROMOSOMES

Since nondividing chromosomes cannot be analyzed, dividing cells are required for chromosome analysis. The cell type most commonly used is the mitogenically stimulated peripheral blood lymphocyte. Skin fibroblasts, bone marrow cells, amniotic fluid cells, and chorion villus cells are also used for special tests. Dividing cells are accumulated at metaphase. Colcemid added to the culture medium toward the end of the culture period is most commonly used to accomplish this. The cells are then subjected to hypotonic treatment, followed by fixation and spreading on microscope slides. The slides are then stained.

Staining techniques may result in either a nonbanded or a banded appearance of the chromosomes. Most laboratories today use one of several banding techniques, since this results in a great deal of additional information.These methods provide a means for the precise identification of an extra or missing chromosome and the precise localization of breakpoints in chromosome rearrangements (Fig. 36–2).

Recent developments have resulted in the expansion of the number of visible bands from between 200 and 300 to between 1000 and 2000. This allows the recognition of small deletions and duplications. Most laboratories today work with chromosomes in which between 400 and 800 bands can be recognized.

HUMAN CHROMOSOME NOMENCLATURE

The 46 human chromosomes consist of three types designated by the position of the centromere or primary constriction. These are metacentric, submetacentric, and acrocentric, depending upon whether the position of the centromere is median, submedian, or terminal. Now that each individual chromosome pair can be recognized, the chromosomes are numbered from 1 to 22 in descending order of length. In the female the two sex chromosomes, designated X chromosomes, are identical, while in the male the two sex chromosomes, designated X and Y, are morphologically different.

Chromosome Variants

This term refers to consistent minor chromosome changes often involving the short arms of the acrocentric chromosomes, the long arm of the Y chromosome, or the constitutive heterochromatin near the centromere of chromosomes 1, 9, and 16. These have little obvious clinical significance but may be useful as genetic markers. They occur much more frequently in the population than do major chromosome abnormalities, and they often segregate in families in a mendelian manner. Recent studies suggest that about 70 per cent of newborn infants carry one or more variant chromosomes.

Nomenclature

The nomenclature used to describe the chromosomes, chromosome bands, chromosome variants, and chromosome rearrangements is given in detail in ISCN (1985). A shorthand notation is used to describe the chromosome complement of an individual. In this notation the number of chromosomes

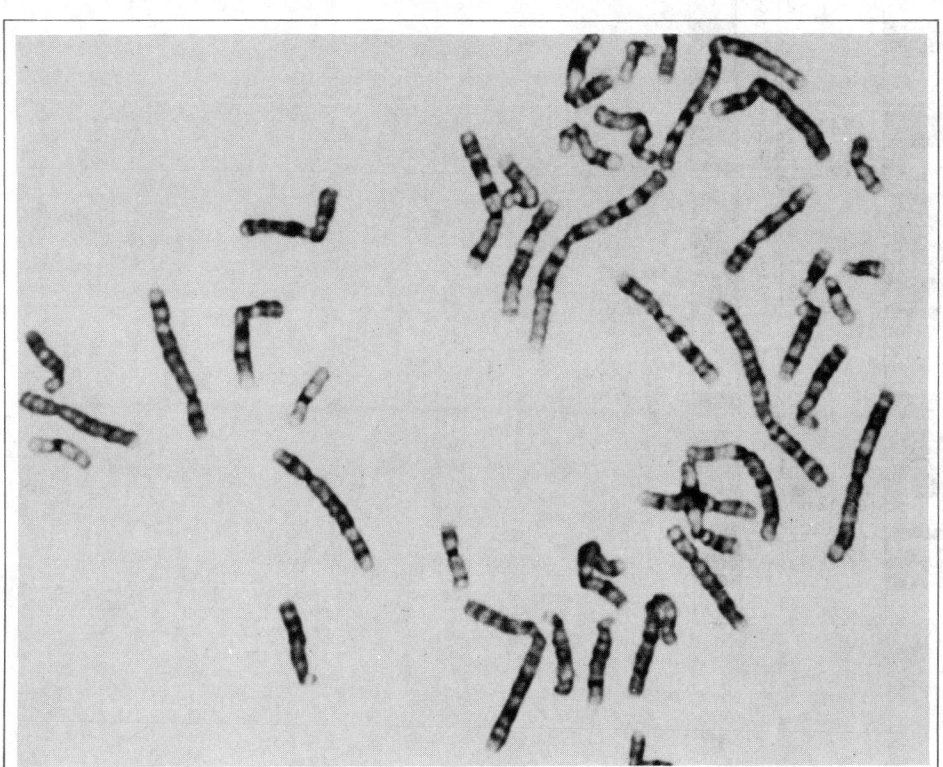

FIGURE 36—2. Human chromosomes at mitotic metaphase. G-banding, approximately 550 band stage. (Courtesy of Dr. H. S. Wang.)

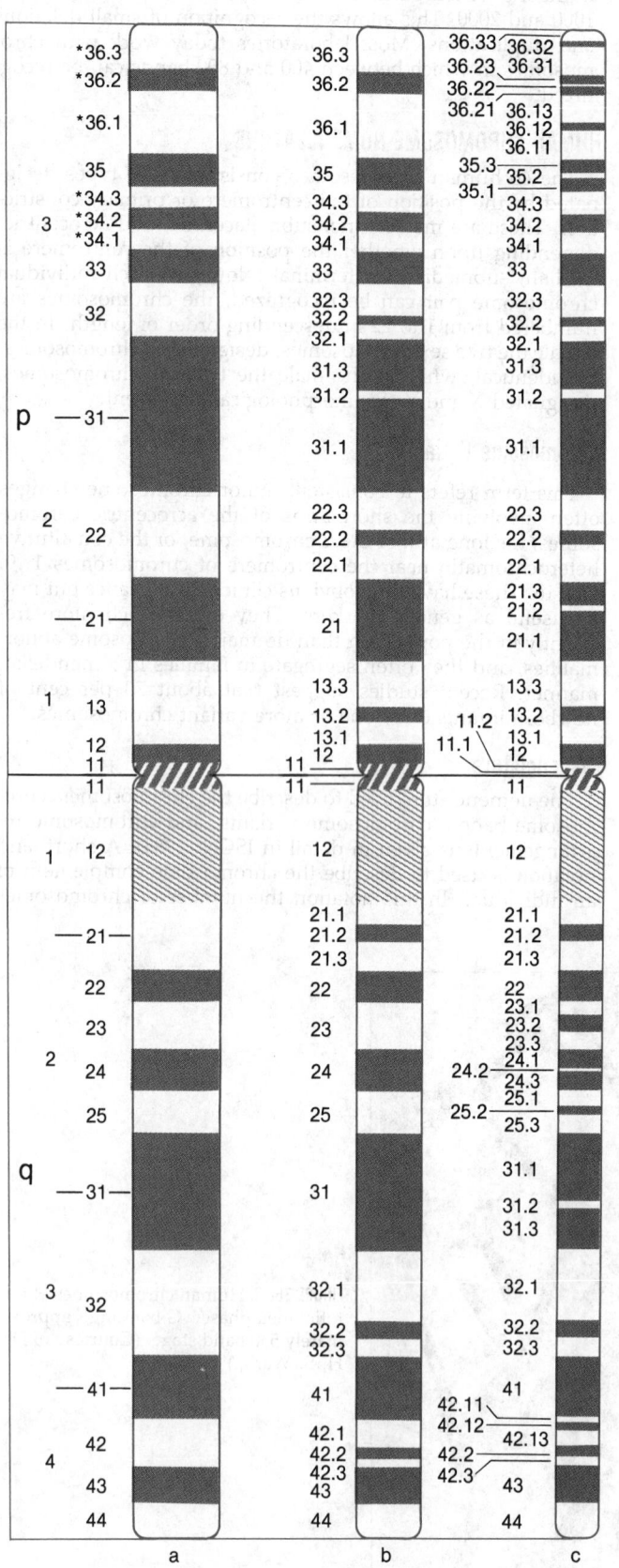

FIGURE 36–3. Human chromosome 1. Idiogram showing chromosome bands at different resolutions. *a*, Approximately 400 bands; *b*, 550 bands; *c*, 850 bands. The band nomenclature and subdivision are according to the internationally agreed system (ISCN 1985).

is specified first, followed by the listing of the sex chromosomes. Thus a normal female karyotype is designated 46,XX and a normal male karyotype 46,XY. Any deviations from a normal karyotype are written after the sex chromosomes. An individual autosome is referred to by its number, its short arm by the letter "p," and its long arm by the letter "q." A "+" or "−" sign written after the p or q indicates an increase (+) or decrease (−) in the length of the arm. When written before a designated chromosome the sign indicates that the chromosome is extra (+) or missing (−).

Examples: 46,XY,18q− describes a male with 46 chromosomes, including one chromosome 18 whose long arm is diminished in length.

47,XX,+21 describes a female with 47 chromosomes, including an extra chromosome 21 in addition to the 46 chromosomes of the normal karyotype.

A diagrammatic representation of the human chromosome 1 showing differing degrees of chromosome banding is given in Figure 36–3.

CHROMOSOME ABNORMALITIES

Chromosome abnormalities can be divided into two classes: abnormalities of number and of structure.

Abnormalities of Chromosome Number. These arise from nondisjunction, that is, from *the failure of two homologous chromosomes in the first division of meiosis or of two sister chromatids in mitosis or the second division of meiosis to pass to opposite poles of the cell* (Fig. 36–4). Nondisjunction results in cells with abnormal chromosome numbers. If these cells are gametes, fertilization will result in a zygote with an abnormal chromosome number. If nondisjunction occurs during an early cleavage division of a zygote, then a chromosome mosaic may result. This is an individual with two or more cell lines

TABLE 36–1. EXAMPLES OF CHROMOSOME ABNORMALITIES DUE TO NONDISJUNCTION IN HUMANS

Sex Chromosomes	Autosomes†
47,XXY (Klinefelter's syndrome) *46,XY/47,XXY	21-trisomy (47,XX or XY, +21)
47,XYY	13-trisomy (47,XX or XY, +13)
47,XXX	18-trisomy (47,XX or XY, +18)
45,X (Turner's syndrome) *45,X/46,XX (ovarian dysgenesis)	21-monosomy (45,XX or XY, −21)

*Examples of chromosome mosaics due to nondisjunction or chromosome loss during an early cleavage division.

†In describing a chromosome abnormality the words "trisomy" and "monosomy" refer simply to an additional or missing chromosome.

differing in chromosome complement. Table 36–1 gives examples of chromosome abnormalities resulting from nondisjunction.

Abnormalities of Chromosome Structure. These result from chromosome breakage and reunion. When a chromosome breaks it can rejoin in its old form (restitution) or it can rejoin with another broken chromosome (reunion). Reunion leads to a structural rearrangement that can be *balanced* or *unbalanced*. If it is balanced the amount of genetic material is presumed to be identical to that found in a normal cell, and there is a simple rearrangement of the distribution of this material. Types of balanced rearrangements include the balanced reciprocal translocation, robertsonian translocations, and inversions. Balanced chromosome rearrangements do not usually lead to any clinical change. If the rearrangement is unbalanced this indicates loss or gain of chromosome material.

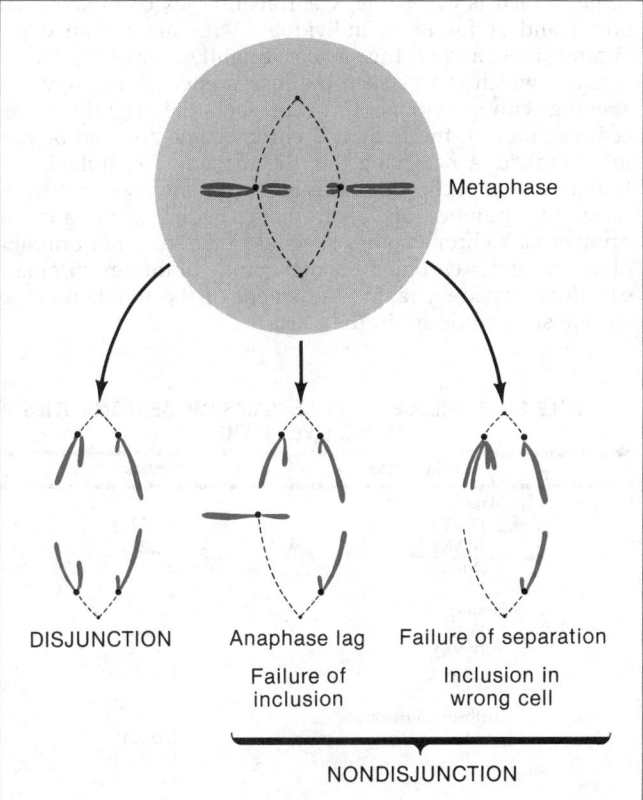

FIGURE 36–4. Diagram illustrating chromosome disjunction and two types of nondisjunction—anaphase lagging and failure of separation. (From Hamerton JL: Human Cytogenetics, Vol 1. New York, Academic Press, 1971.)

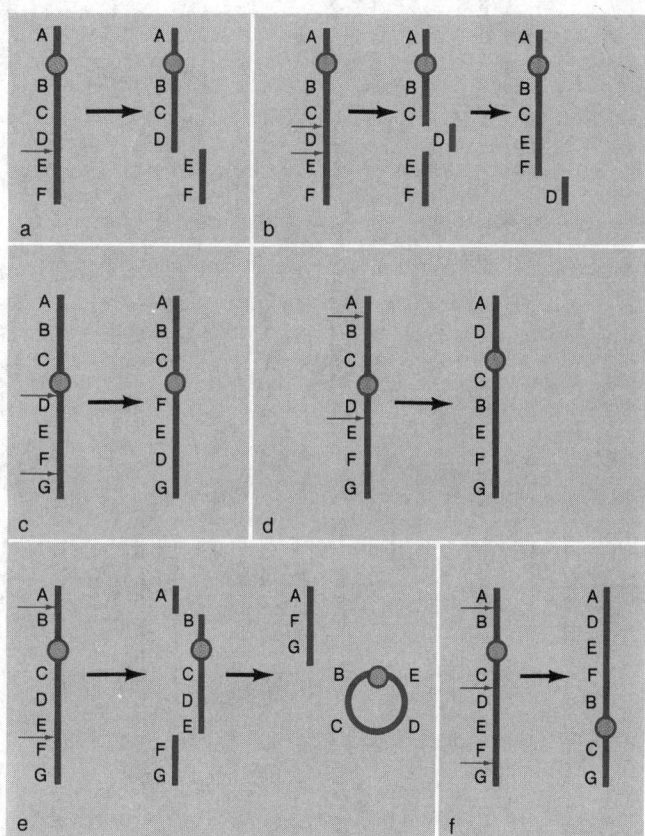

FIGURE 36–5. Types of chromosome rearrangement: *a,* terminal deletion; *b,* interstitial deletion; *c,* paracentric inversion; *d,* pericentric inversion; *e,* ring chromosome; *f,* segmental shift. (From Hamerton JL: Human Cytogenetics, Vol 1. New York, Academic Press, 1971.)

Loss includes a deficiency or a deletion. Gain includes a duplication. Such unbalanced rearrangements will usually result in changes in the clinical phenotype.

CHROMOSOME DELETION. Deletion is the loss of a chromosome segment following chromosome breakage. Deletions may be terminal or interstitial or result in ring chromosomes (Fig. 36–5*A*, *B*, and *E*).

INVERSIONS (Fig. 36–5*C* and *D*). These result from two chromosome breaks and inversion of the intervening segment and can be detected only by chromosome banding studies that show a changed banding sequence. Inversions result in disturbances in chromosome pairing and in the formation of unbalanced as well as balanced gametes.

BALANCED RECIPROCAL TRANSLOCATION (Fig. 36–6). This results from exchange of chromosome segments between nonhomologous chromosomes. An individual carrying such a rearrangement will have a higher frequency of abnormal gametes as the result of a disturbance in chromosome pairing at meiosis. Such individuals will themselves have a balanced chromosome complement and be clinically normal, but they may have a high risk of having congenitally malformed children and/or spontaneous abortions. Normal children may also be born, and such persons require careful genetic counseling.

ROBERTSONIAN TRANSLOCATION. This is a specific type of unequal reciprocal translocation that occurs between acrocentric chromosomes, resulting in the formation of a new metacentric chromosome from two acrocentric chromosomes. Such rearrangements may be important in the transmission of Down's syndrome when one of the chromosomes involved is chromosome 21, the other usually being chromosome 14.

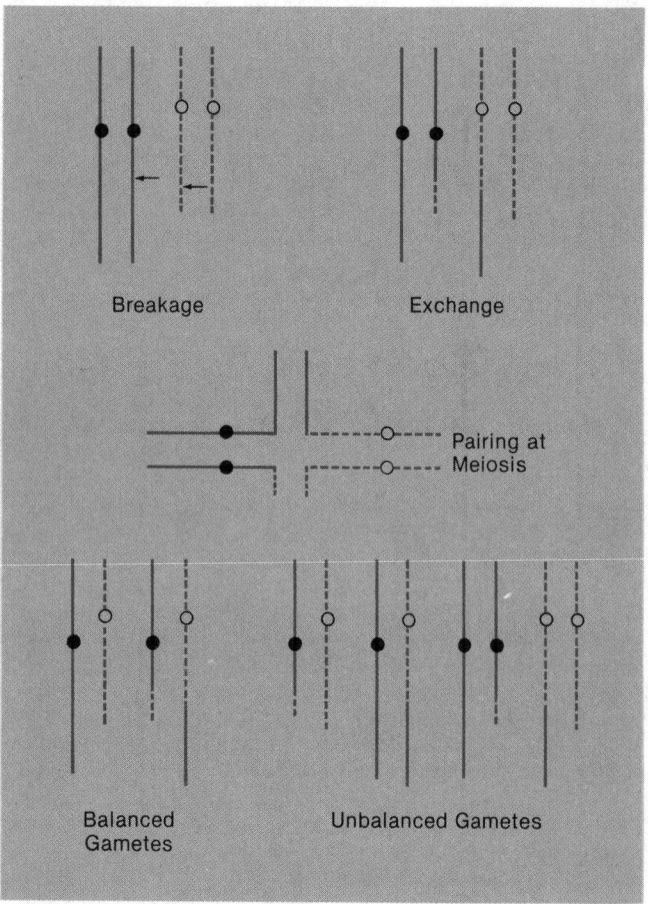

FIGURE 36–6. Consequences of reciprocal translocation. Note both balanced and unbalanced gametes are possible as a result of segregation of the exchanged chromosomes.

POPULATION CYTOGENETICS

Chromosome abnormalities form a significant component of the deleterious genetic load carried by the human population. About 6 per 1000 newborn babies have a major chromosome abnormality that may result in some degree of morbidity or mortality at some time during life. The frequency of the different types of chromosome abnormalities found when large numbers of newborn infants are screened is shown in Table 36–2.

Chromosome abnormalities found among infants at birth are, however, only a very small proportion of the total load of chromosome abnormalities seen at conception. The majority of these are lethal or sublethal and are lost during gestation as either very early abortions or failure of implantation (monosomies, and so on), or as recognized abortions and perinatal deaths. This group includes most trisomies, triploids (3n), and tetraploids (4n). A significant proportion of infants dying in the perinatal and neonatal periods have been shown to have a major chromosome abnormality. About 50 per cent of all embryos and fetuses spontaneously aborted have a chromosome abnormality, and about 6 per cent of stillborn infants and those dying in the perinatal period have abnormal chromosomes.

In addition to the large amount of data on newborn babies and spontaneous abortions, there are now data on large numbers of mothers who have received amniocentesis because of a maternal age of 35 and over. A recent study of over 50,000 amniocenteses shows that, overall, about 2 per cent of the fetuses in midtrimester pregnancies in mothers aged 35 and above have a chromosome abnormality.

SEX CHROMATIN

There are two types of sex cromatin that can be seen in somatic cells: (1) the interphase chromocenter, which represents the genetically inactivated and condensed X chromosome, which is called the X chromatin (sex chromatin, Barr body) and is found in individuals with more than one X chromosome; and (2) the smaller, brightly fluorescing chromocenter, which can be seen by fluorescence microscopy after staining with quinacrine; this represents the brightly fluorescent segment of the human Y chromosome and can be seen in all individuals carrying this chromosome. In diploid cells, the number of X chromosomes is always one greater than the maximum number of X chromatin bodies seen, and the number of Y chromosomes is equal to the maximum number of fluorescent Y chromatin bodies. Study of the sex chromatin can thus provide a rapid assessment of the numbers of sex chromosomes present in the cells.

TABLE 36–2. FREQUENCY OF CHROMOSOME ABNORMALITIES AMONG LIVE BIRTHS*

Sex Chromosomes	Frequency
Male	
47,XYY	1:1022
47,XXY	1:1022
Other	1:1277
Female	
45,X	1:9586
47,XXX	1:958
Other	1:2739
Autosomal trisomics	
+D	1:18984
+E	1:8136
+G	1:802
Balanced structural	1:517
Unbalanced structural	1:1675
Total	1:167

*Based on 54,952 babies: 35,779 males, 19,173 females.

TABLE 36–3. COMMON SEX CHROMOSOME ABNORMALITIES

Chromosome Complement	Eponym	X Chromatin	Frequency (live birth)	Phenotype
Males 47,XXY	Klinefelter's syndrome	Positive	1:1000	Often tall, eunuchoid males with hypogonadism, feminine distribution of hair, gynecomastia, testicular atrophy after puberty with hyalinized tubules, Leydig cell hyperplasia, often low IQ. May have psychosocial difficulties (see Ch. 235).
47,XYY	—	Negative	1:1000	Often no phenotype abnormalities; usually tall to very tall. May have psychosocial problems.
Females 45,X and other variants of the X chromosome and mosaics	Turner's syndrome or ovarian dysgenesis	Negative or positive	1:10,000	These patients have ovarian dysgenesis with webbing of neck, short stature (< 153 cm). Often congenital heart disease, skeletal defects, and renal anomalies. This is Turner's syndrome. Other patients may have ovarian dysgenesis without webbing of the neck and with much less frequent somatic anomalies. Invariably they are of short stature (< 153 cm) (see Ch. 237).
47,XXX	None	Double	1:1000	This is extremely variable. Often no phenotypic abnormalities but may be mentally retarded or may have psychosocial problems. Often fertile although may be infertile.

Late-replicating X chromosomes can be identified by autoradiography using tritiated thymidine or by the incorporation of 5-bromodeoxyuridine (BUDR) into DNA in place of thymidine, followed by staining with a dye that differentiates between BUDR and thymidine (the Hoechst-BUDR technique). It is now known that the condensed, late-replicating X chromosomes are genetically inactivated. This inactivation is a random process that may affect either the maternal or the paternal X chromosome at random, occurs early in embryogenesis, and remains fixed for a given cell lineage (Lyon's hypothesis).

The clinical significance of this phenomenon is best demonstrated in females heterozygous for a gene carried by the X chromosome. Such females will have two types of somatic cells in their bodies, one in which the normal allele is inactivated and the other in which the abnormal allele is inactivated. Thus studies on clones of cells (colonies of cells derived from a single progenitor) may allow differentiation between the active and inactive X chromosome and the identification of carrier females. Examples of diseases in which carrier detection has been based on this phenomenon include the Lesch-Nyhan syndrome, Fabry's disease, testicular feminization syndrome, and mucopolysaccharidosis type II (Hunter's syndrome).

Clinical Cytogenetics

Sex Chromosomes

The major features of a few common sex chromosome abnormalities are summarized in Table 36–3. Other sex chromosome abnormalities include the rare females with four or five X chromosomes, as well as males with multiple X and Y chromosomes. Such individuals are usually mentally retarded and may have somatic anomalies. Individuals with various degrees of chromosome mosaicism have also been reported, most frequently as variants in Klinefelter's syndrome or Turner's syndrome.

Autosomes

The clinical features of the three best known autosomal trisomies are listed in Table 36–4.

Other autosomal trisomies in fetuses surviving to term include trisomies 8, 9, and 22. All other autosomes have been reported as trisomic among spontaneous abortions. The advent of banding techniques has greatly widened the scope of chromosome pathology, and numerous examples of chromosome imbalance resulting from deletion or duplication of chromosome material have been reported. Such chromosome imbalance results in dysmorphic features and often developmental and mental retardation.

INDICATIONS FOR CHROMOSOME STUDY

Chromosome abnormalities result in a significant amount of clinical pathology, and chromosome studies should be initiated to rule out this etiologic factor in a patient when a recognizable chromosome syndrome is suspected; in patients with two or more unexplained major congenital malformations involving different systems possibly combined with the presence of minor malformations; and in patients with unexplained developmental or mental retardation. Certain cases of abnormal sexual development, leukemia, and certain solid

TABLE 36–4. THREE BEST-KNOWN AUTOSOMAL TRISOMIES

Chromosome Complement	Eponym	Frequency (live birth)	Phenotype
21-Trisomy (47,XX, + 21 47,XY, + 21)	Down's syndrome Mongolism	1:700	Typical facial appearance, epicanthic folds, oblique palpebral fissures, broad bridge of the nose, protruding tongue, open mouth, square-shaped ears, flattened facial profile. Invariable mental retardation, muscular hypotonia, and often congenital heart disease (Fig. 36–7).
18-Trisomy (47,XX, + 18 47,XY, + 18)	Edwards' syndrome	1:8000	Full-term infants of low birth weight with severe mental and motor retardation. Usually have a prominent occiput and frequently occurring facial abnormalities, including micrognathia, a Grecian nose, low-set and malformed ears, cleft lip and palate. Flexion deformities of fingers are often severe. Mental retardation is often severe. They are sublethal, and survival for more than a few months is rare.
13-Trisomy (47,XX, + 13) 47,XY, + 13	Patau's syndrome	1:20,000	Usually low birth weight infants of full-term gestation with a typical facial appearance, including a broad nose, hypertelorism, microphthalmia, anophthalmia, often with coloboma, and micrognathia. They are usually microcephalic, ears are low-set and malformed, and there is a large broad and bulbous nose. There are often flexion deformities and frequent polydactyly and syndactyly. Survival is usually very short.

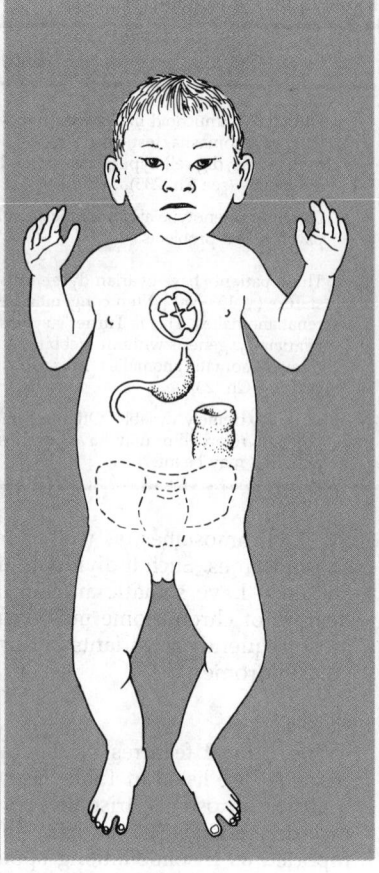

Growth failure

Mental retardation

Flat occiput

Dysplastic ears

Many "loops" on finger tips

Simian crease

Medial axial triradius

Unilateral or bilateral absence of one rib

Intestinal stenosis

Umbilical hernia

Dysplastic pelvis

Hypotonic muscles

Big toes widely spaced

Broad flat face

Slanting eyes

Epicanthus

Short nose

Small and arched palate

Big wrinkled tongue

Dental anomalies

Short and broad hands (clinodactyly)

Congenital heart disease

Megacolon

FIGURE 36–7. Clinical findings in trisomy 21. (From Vogel F, Motulsky AG: Human Genetics: Problems and Approaches. Berlin, Springer-Verlag, 1986.)

tumors associated with congenital malformations and known to be associated with specific chromosome abnormalities (aniridia, Wilms' tumor, retinoblastoma) require chromosome studies. Chromosome banding is mandatory to identify the chromosome involved as well as to rule out possible structural changes not detectable by other means.

Chromosome Breakage Syndromes

Three diseases are commonly associated with unrepaired chromosome breaks. These are Fanconi's anemia (FA), ataxia-telangiectasia (AT), and Bloom's syndrome (BS). These are so characterized because in addition to their typical clinical features they share the propensity to chromosome breakage that can be seen in cultured cells and that commonly occurs with several times the frequency observed in normal individuals. Each of these diseases is inherited as an autosomal recessive condition. Two of these conditions are associated with congenital malformations (BS and FA), and all three have an increased frequency of malignancy. This may be the consequence of alterations in DNA repair process.

Sister chromatids can be differentially stained by a modification of the Hoechst-BUDR technique. This permits the identification of exchanges between sister chromatids. Such sister chromatid exchanges (SCE) occur with an increased frequency in BS and in normal individuals may be increased as the result of exposure to chromosome-damaging agents.

Heritable Fragile Sites

Chromosome breakage is usually random; however, some individuals may exhibit breakage or a nonstaining chromosome region (chromosome gap) at a specific site in a significant proportion of metaphases. In many cases such sites may be induced by the use of folate-deficient culture medium, although a few sites are folate insensitive. These specific sites, known as fragile sites, may represent alterations in the DNA

and are often heritable. While most fragile sites are not associated with disease or other clinical problems, the fragile site at Xq28 is known to be associated with one common form of X-linked mental retardation among males.

PRENATAL DIAGNOSIS

The diagnosis of chromosome abnormalities at midtrimester gestation is now a routine procedure for certain pregnancies. It involves the aspiration of a small sample of amniotic fluid (amniocentesis), culturing of the fetal cells contained in the fluid, and determination of the karyotype of these cells and thus of the fetus. The major indications for the use of this technique for the detection of chromosome abnormalities are: (1) Maternal age—usually offered to all mothers over the age of 35 at the time of delivery; (2) presence of a parental chromosome abnormality—if one parent is a balanced translocation carrier and particularly if the translocation was detected as the result of the previous birth of a clinically abnormal infant; (3) previous trisomy—those cases in which the mother has previously had a trisomic infant or possibly in which she is known to have had a previous instance of spontaneous abortion in which the abortus was karyotyped and shown to be trisomic; and (4) abnormal levels (high or low) of alpha-fetoprotein.

The safety and reliability of amniocentesis as a diagnostic technique have now been well established by numerous studies, and it is generally accepted that amniocentesis increases the risk of miscarriage by between 0.5 and 1 per cent above the inherent risk for that individual without intervention. Other risks of the test, including fetal and maternal morbidity, are negligible. In competent hands the test has been shown to have a near 100 per cent reliability for the detection of chromosome abnormalities.

Recently, direct transcervical aspiration of chorionic villi (chorionic villus sampling, or CVS) has been used for prenatal diagnosis, and several randomized, controlled trials of CVS compared with genetic amniocentesis (GA) are in progress in different countries. These trials will determine whether CVS is as safe, accurate, and reliable as GA. If it is found to be an acceptable alternative, then the diagnosis of chromosome abnormalities may be moved from the second to the first trimester of pregnancy.

DeGrouchy J, Turleau C: Clinical Atlas of Human Chromosomes. 2nd ed. New York, John Wiley & Sons, 1984. *A review of chromosomal syndromes with numerous illustrations and references.*

Hamerton JL: Population cytogenetics: A perspective. In Adonolfi M, Baron P, Giarnelli F, et al. (eds): Pediatric Research: A Genetic Approach. London, Heineman Medical Books, 1982. *Deals with frequency of chromosome abnormalities in populations.*

ISCN: An International System of Human Cytogenetic Nomenclature. Birth Defects Original Article Series 21:1–116. New York, March of Dimes, 1985. *The basic handbook of nomenclature rules for human chromosomes including high-resolution banding.*

Vogel F, Motulsky AG: Human Genetics: Problems and Approaches. 2nd ed. Berlin, Springer-Verlag, 1986. *A detailed treatise on human genetics from both a basic and a clinical viewpoint. Numerous references. Chapter 2 deals extensively with human cytogenetics.*

Yunis JJ: The chromosomal basis of human neoplasia. Science 221:227, 1983. *A review of our current knowledge about chromosome abnormalities and gene mapping in relation to human tumors.*

37 CONGENITAL MALFORMATIONS

Lewis B. Holmes

INCIDENCE

Two per cent of newborn infants have serious malformations, most of which are compatible with survival. Many additional malformations, such as genitourinary, vertebral, and heart defects, are identified during childhood and the teenage years. Many adults with congenital malformations are unaware of the significance of these problems for their health or the potential significance for their unborn children.

ETIOLOGIES

The recognized causes of malformations include genetic abnormalities, environmental factors, and the combined effects of mutant genes and environmental factors, i.e., multifactorial inheritance (Table 37–1). Multifactorial inheritance is the most common of these etiologies. However, at least 40 per cent of all malformations cannot be explained. One example of a cause that is neither environmental nor genetic is a vascular abnormality. Occlusion of blood vessels during development has been postulated to cause intestinal atresia and hydranencephaly; absence of vessels and abnormal persistence of vessels have been observed in absence of the radius and absence of the tibia.

A few hereditary malformations have been shown to be due to biochemical abnormalities, such as a deficiency of 5α-reductase in individuals with pseudovaginal perineoscrotal hypospadias, an autosomal recessive disorder characterized by ambiguous genitals. An abnormal alpha-2 chain in type I collagen has been identified in skin fibroblasts from a woman with type I osteogenesis imperfecta, a skeletal dysplasia inherited as an autosomal dominant trait (see Ch. 201).

In multifactorial inheritance, clinical studies of human and laboratory examples have shown that several genes (including major genes) are involved, as well as environmental factors such as maternal influences, uterine factors, the season of the year, and socioeconomic class. Most individuals with a malformation attributed to multifactorial inheritance are the only affected members of their families. However, affected individuals have an increased risk of having affected sibs or affected

children. The recurrence risk is usually between 1 and 10 per cent, which is 10 to 40 times greater than the incidence of the malformation in the general population.

About 0.6 per cent of newborn infants have a major chromosome abnormality, but many do not survive to the adult years. Down's syndrome results from the most common trisomy, and survival of most affected newborns to the adult years is now expected. In trisomy 21, the associated chromosome abnormality in 95 per cent of the cases, the extra chromosome comes from the mother 75 per cent of the time. Since women over age 35 now are having a smaller portion of all pregnancies, 80 per cent of the infants with Down's syndrome are being born to women of less than 35 years.

Common sex chromosome abnormalities, such as 47,XYY and 47,XXX, are usually not associated with any congenital malformations. Boys with 47,XXY (Klinefelter's syndrome) may have abnormal physical features that are evident in the teenage years. Girls with the 45,X (Turner's) syndrome are usually recognized in infancy because of associated lymphedema, webbed neck, heart defects, and short stature or in the teenage years because of failure of puberty to occur spontaneously.

CLINICAL RELEVANCE

The following examples illustrate the potential significance of a malformation to the affected adult and his or her children.

Relevance to the Health of the Affected Person

CONGENITAL ABSENCE OF ONE KIDNEY. About 1 in 700 infants has unilateral renal agenesis. Most affected individuals are asymptomatic. However, they have an increased risk of structural malformations of the ureter, such as ureteropelvic junction stricture, and associated infections, hypertension, and so forth. The affected female may have a bicornuate uterus or absence of the half of the uterus on the same side as the renal aplasia. Affected males may have absence of the vas deferens on the same side. Parents with unilateral renal

TABLE 37–1. RECOGNIZED ETIOLOGIES OF MALFORMATIONS PRESENT IN ADULTS

	Examples
1. Genetic abnormalities	
a. Single mutant gene	
i. Autosomal dominant trait	Polycystic kidney disease, adult type Polysyndactyly
ii. Autosomal recessive trait	Mohr's syndrome (oro-facial-digital syndrome, type II)
iii. X-linked dominant trait	Telecanthus-hypospadias (BBB) syndrome
iv. X-linked recessive trait	Metacarpal 4-5 fusion
b. Chromosome abnormalities	
i. Trisomy of autosomes	Down's syndrome
ii. Interstitial deletion	Aniridia-Wilms' tumor
iii. Sex chromosome abnormalities	45,X (Turner's syndrome); 47,XXY (Klinefelter's syndrome)
2. Environmental factors	
a. Uterine factors	Amniotic band syndrome
b. Intrauterine infection	Congenital rubella syndrome
c. Drugs	Fetal hydantoin syndrome
3. Genetic plus environmental factors (multifactorial inheritance)	Heart defects
	Cleft lip and/or palate
	Hypospadias
	Pyloric stenosis
	Hirschsprung's disease

agenesis have an increased risk of having infants with either the same malformation or bilateral renal agenesis, which is fatal.

BRACHYDACTYLY, TYPE E. Owing to premature closure of epiphyses, persons with this autosomal dominant disorder have short hands and feet with a variable pattern of shortening of the first, fourth, and fifth metacarpals and metatarsals and distal phalanges of the thumb and great toe. They also have a mild-to-moderate degree of shortness of stature. Severe hypertension is often a problem in the affected teenager and young adult. This cause of the hypertension has not been determined.

BRANCHIO-OTO-RENAL SYNDROME. The person with this autosomal dominant disorder has a pattern of malformations that includes malformed ears, preauricular tags, preauricular sinus, and branchial cleft sinus. The mildly affected adult is often not diagnosed until a more severely affected child is born. The affected adult may have significant hearing loss or renal hypoplasia.

KLIPPEL-FEIL SYNDROME. The person with fusion or hemivertebrae of one or more cervical vertebrae usually has a short neck, limited rotation of the head, a low hairline, and a webbed neck. Common associated problems include hearing loss, heart defects, Sprengel's deformity, and genitourinary anomalies, such as aplasia of mullerian structures.

POLYCYSTIC KIDNEY DISEASE. The affected individual with the adult form has an increased risk of having cerebral aneurysms and pancreatic cysts. Prenatal diagnosis using DNA probes is now possible.

Relevance to Increased Risk of Having Affected Children

MULTIFACTORIAL INHERITANCE. The adult with one of the common malformations attributed to this process has an increased risk of having an affected child. For malformations that show an altered sex ratio, the sex of the affected parent is important in determining the risk of having an affected child (Table 37–2). In general, the parent of the less frequently affected sex has a greater risk of having affected children. For example, *intestinal aganglionosis* (Hirschsprung's disease) is much more common in males than females, but the affected female has a much greater risk of having affected children (Table 37–2).

With early surgical closure and better treatment of the associated hydrocephalus and urinary tract infections, males and females with *spina bifida* (myelomeningocele) are surviving to adult years and often have normal intelligence. Both affected males and females may be fertile. The affected adult has an increased risk of about 3 per cent that each child will have a neural tube defect.

HYPERTELORISM. The mother who has a broad bridge of the nose and hypertelorism* has an increased risk of having severely malformed sons. For example, the female who carries the X-linked gene for the telecanthus-hypospadias (BBB) syndrome will show only hypertelorism, but sons who inherit this gene have a severe malformation syndrome that may include hypertelorism, broad nasal bridge, cleft lip and palate, heart defects, imperforate anus, hypospadias, and mental deficiency. Mothers with the autosomal dominant disorder known as the Opitz-Frias (or G) syndrome also have hypertelorism and a broad bridge of the nose. Their affected sons and daughters have at birth aspiration due to a laryngotracheoesophageal cleft, stridor, and associated malformations such as cleft lip, heart defects, hypospadias (males), and imperforate anus. Unfortunately, the physical feature of broad nasal bridge and hypertelorism is nonspecific and the risk for the woman with no affected children cannot be determined.

MENTAL RETARDATION. There are many causes of mental retardation. The mildly retarded woman without strik-

*Hypertelorism can be determined most precisely from an anteroposterior radiograph that shows an increased bony interorbital distance.

TABLE 37–2. RISK OF AFFECTED CHILDREN FOR PARENT WITH MALFORMATION ATTRIBUTED TO MULTIFACTORIAL INHERITANCE

Malformation	Risk of Affected Child (per cent)	Prevalence of Condition in General Population (per cent)
1. Intestinal aganglionosis (Hirschsprung's disease)	2.0	0.02
2. Hypospadias	6.0	0.8
3. Club foot	1.4	0.13
4. Congenital hip dislocation	4.3	0.8
5. Ventricular septal defect	4.0	0.2
6. Pyloric stenosis	4 (affected father) 13 (affected mother)	
7. Cleft palate	6.2	0.3
8. Spina bifida (meningomyelocele)	3.0	0.14

ing physical abnormalities may be a carrier of significant and relatively common genetic abnormalities that give her an increased risk of having severely affected sons. Two examples are the fragile-X syndrome and the Coffin-Lowry syndrome. The fragile-X syndrome is a common cause of mental retardation, mild facial abnormalities, and sometimes macroorchidism in males. The affected female may show mosaicism for the marker X chromosome, an abnormality of the distal portion of the long arm of the X chromosome that can be identified in cytogenetic studies only if special media and processing are used. The woman who has the X-linked gene for the Coffin-Lowry syndrome shows only mild mental retardation, short stature, short and hyperextensible hands, and tufted distal phalanges. The affected male is much more severely affected, with severe mental deficiency, short stature, stiff joints, coarse facial features, pectus carinatum, and large, soft hands.

PRENATAL DIAGNOSIS

The techniques used most often for diagnosing malformations in the fetus are cell culture of amniocytes removed at 16 to 18 weeks of gestation, assay for alpha-fetoprotein (AFP) in the amniotic fluid and maternal serum, and ultrasound imaging. Early amniocentesis is now offered at 12 to 14 weeks of pregnancy at some medical centers. Parents who have previously had a child with trisomy 21 have a 1 per cent risk of recurrence regardless of the mother's age. To rule out this possibility amniocentesis for chromosome analysis is offered. For the woman who has previously had a child with anencephaly or spina bifida, prenatal diagnosis includes amniocentesis to measure the level of AFP and ultrasound imaging for hydrocephalus, the cranial defect in anencephaly, and the spinal defect in meningomyelocele. If the level of AFP is elevated, a neural tube defect is confirmed by an increase in the level of acetylcholinesterase in the amniotic fluid. Both the amniocytes removed at amniocentesis and the chorionic villi removed transcervically at 9 to 11 weeks of gestation can be used to identify chromosome abnormalities, hemoglobinopathies, and metabolic disorders in the fetus. Limb malformations, such as absent radius, ectrodactyly, hydrocephalus, and bilateral renal agenesis, can be investigated with ultrasound imaging. However, the accuracy of this method of prenatal diagnosis is not known.

Prenatal screening for neural tube defects is now available as an option in prenatal care. Serum AFP is measured in the mother at 16 to 18 weeks of pregnancy. The pregnant woman with an elevated serum level of AFP on two occasions should have prenatal studies, including amniocentesis for AFP and acetylcholinesterase and ultrasound imaging. Errors in diagnosis result from incorrect gestational age and alterations in the range of normal values in obese women and in women with diabetes mellitus. Elevations in AFP also occur in twin pregnancies, intrauterine death, and other malformations such as esophageal atresia, omphalocele, and hereditary nephrosis. A skin-covered neural tube defect, such as a lumbar meningocele, will be missed in prenatal screening with serum AFP. In general, prenatal AFP screening is most effective if carried out by individuals who are experienced in identifying the causes of false-positive and false-negative values and who educate the parents initially about the steps involved and the benefits and accuracy of the testing.

FETAL SURGERY

Catheters have been introduced to relieve malformations that cause obstruction of the flow of urine or of cerebrospinal fluid. This approach is experimental. One major problem is to identify an abnormality early enough to permit intervention before the fetus has suffered irreversible damage, such as the lung hypoplasia that is a cause of death in infants with oligohydramnios from urinary tract obstruction. Another problem is that the fetus in whom only hydrocephalus or urinary tract obstruction is visible by ultrasound may have multiple malformations that will be apparent only after birth.

PREVENTION OF MALFORMATION

Pregnant women with several different medical diseases or exposures have an increased risk of having children with birth defects. If the patient is informed of this risk before conception or soon after conception, these risks can be either lessened or eliminated. These efforts at prevention require special efforts in education, as most women receive routine prenatal care too late to benefit from counseling. Specific opportunities in prevention include the following:

CHRONIC ALCOHOLISM. Exposure of the fetus to high maternal levels of alcohol causes growth retardation before and after birth, microcephaly, brain malformations, mental deficiency, a characteristic pattern of craniofacial features, and at times other malformations, such as vertebral anomalies and spina bifida (fetal alcohol syndrome). The lower the level of exposure, the less the risk of damage to the fetus. If the pregnant woman decreases her alcohol consumption at any time in pregnancy, it is beneficial to the fetus, although a decrease before or soon after conception is the most beneficial.

DIABETES MELLITUS. The woman with insulin-dependent diabetes mellitus is two to three times more likely to have a child with serious malformations than the nondiabetic woman. The malformations include spina bifida, anencephaly, heart defects, vertebral and genitourinary malformations, and multiple malformations. The risk of having a malformed infant correlates inversely with the quality of control of her disease, glucose metabolism in particular, very early in pregnancy. The lower the level of glycosylated hemoglobin before or soon after conception, the lower her risk of having a malformed child.

MATERNAL PHENYLKETONURIA (PKU). Children with PKU identified at birth through neonatal screening for metabolic diseases will have normal development and intelligence if the dietary treatment (low phenylalanine, low protein) is begun soon after birth. The diet is usually discontinued in the early school years. However, successfully treated females with PKU who are no longer on the diet have a risk of over 90 per cent that any pregnancy will either end in a spontaneous abortion or result in a child with microcephaly and mental deficiency, and often heart defects as well. The risk of damage to the fetus correlates with the blood level of phenylalanine in the mother. If the woman with PKU resumes the low-phenylalanine diet before conception she has her best chance of having a normal child. If the diet is resumed in the first trimester, as soon as she knows she is pregnant, the child is less severely damaged than if no dietary treatment is used during pregnancy. Unfortunately, many young women with PKU are not aware of their risk of having children with serious birth defects.

Bergsma D (ed.): Birth Defects Compendium. 2nd ed. New York, Alan R. Liss, Inc., 1979. *An up-to-date, brief summary on all common birth defects.*
Briggs GG, Freeman RK, Yaffe SJ: Drugs in Pregnancy and Lactation. 2nd ed. Baltimore, Williams & Wilkins Company. *A summary of current information on the potential teratogenic effect of many common exposures.*
Jacobs PA, Glover TW, Mayer M, et al.: X-Linked mental retardation: A study of 7 families. Am J Med Genet 7:471, 1980. *A thorough study of this very common hereditary cause of mental deficiency in affected males and carrier females.*
Lenke RR, Levy HL: Maternal phenylketonuria and hyperphenylalaninemia. N Engl J Med 303:1202, 1980. *The results of an international survey of the teratogenic effect of PKU in the pregnant woman and the attempts at prevention.*
Reeders ST, Zerres K, Gal A, et al.: Prenatal diagnosis of autosomal dominant polycystic kidney disease with a DNA probe. Lancet 2:6, 1986. *The report of this new development.*
Report of the U.K. Collaborative Study on Alpha-Fetoprotein in Relation to Neural-tube Defects. Amniotic-fluid alpha-fetoprotein measurement in antenatal diagnosis of anencephaly and open spina bifida in early pregnancy. Lancet 2:651, 1979. *A summary of the findings in the U.K. Collaborative Study of using maternal AFP screening to detect fetuses with spina bifida and anencephaly.*
Smith DW: Recognizable Patterns of Human Malformation. 3rd ed. Philadelphia, W.B. Saunders Company, 1982. *A thorough tabulation of recognized malformation syndromes.*
Temtamy SA, McKusick VA: The Genetics of Hand Malformations. New York, Alan R. Liss, Inc., 1978. *The best source of information on malformations of the hands, arms, and legs.*

38 GENETIC COUNSELING
F. Clarke Fraser

Genetic counseling is the process whereby patients and their families are helped to deal with a problem created by the occurrence, or potential occurrence, of a disorder in the family that they think may have a genetic basis. The need for genetic counseling starts with one or more questions. "My child is born with Nevererdofit syndrome. What caused it? Will it happen again? Should we stop having children?" "My grandfather has developed Huntington's disease. Might I get it?" "I have fallen in love with my cousin. Would our children all be malformed or mentally retarded?" "I volunteered for a screening program and they say I have the gene for Tay-Sachs disease. What harm will it do?" "I am 35 years old and I read that I should have a test that will make sure my baby will be normal. Should I?"

In many cases the genetic principles underlying the answers to such questions are simple and should be in the repertoire of every physician. Some cases require more sophisticated calculations or special tests and can be referred to a genetic counselor. The answers may depend not only on genetic principles but also on complex social and ethical issues that will require several interviews and perhaps the effort of both the family physician and the genetic counselor to resolve.

DIAGNOSIS

The first step in the counseling process is to confirm, or establish, the diagnosis (Fig. 38–1). This may already have been done, or it may require special tests (karyotype, carrier detection tests, and so forth). Do not ignore the family history, which may sometimes be an aid to diagnosis. Genetic heterogeneity (see Ch. 34) may confound the issue and require special tests to be done on the patient or family members. In

FIGURE 38–1. Map of the genetic counseling process. It begins with a question, raised by the advent of a child with a ? genetic disorder, other aspect of the family history, etc. There must be a diagnosis (Dx), which may depend on information from clinicians, syndromologists, x-ray studies, laboratory tests, dermatoglyphics, cytogenetics, and the family history (FH). To answer the question usually requires estimating a probability (P), using information from the family history, cytogenetics, the literature, the mendelian principles, and Bayesian calculations. Following informative and supportive counseling (often influenced by social, moral, economic, and family pressures) the counselee may reach a decision either to refrain from reproduction or to go ahead. Both of these may require appropriate referral. If the "GO" decision results in a recurrence, further counseling may be required. Follow-up of the counselee and the extended family may result in reentry into the process. Asterisks indicate where the physician can play an important role. (Reprinted with permission from Nora JJ, Fraser FC: Medical Genetics: Principles and Practice. 3rd ed. Philadelphia, Lea and Febiger, 1988.)

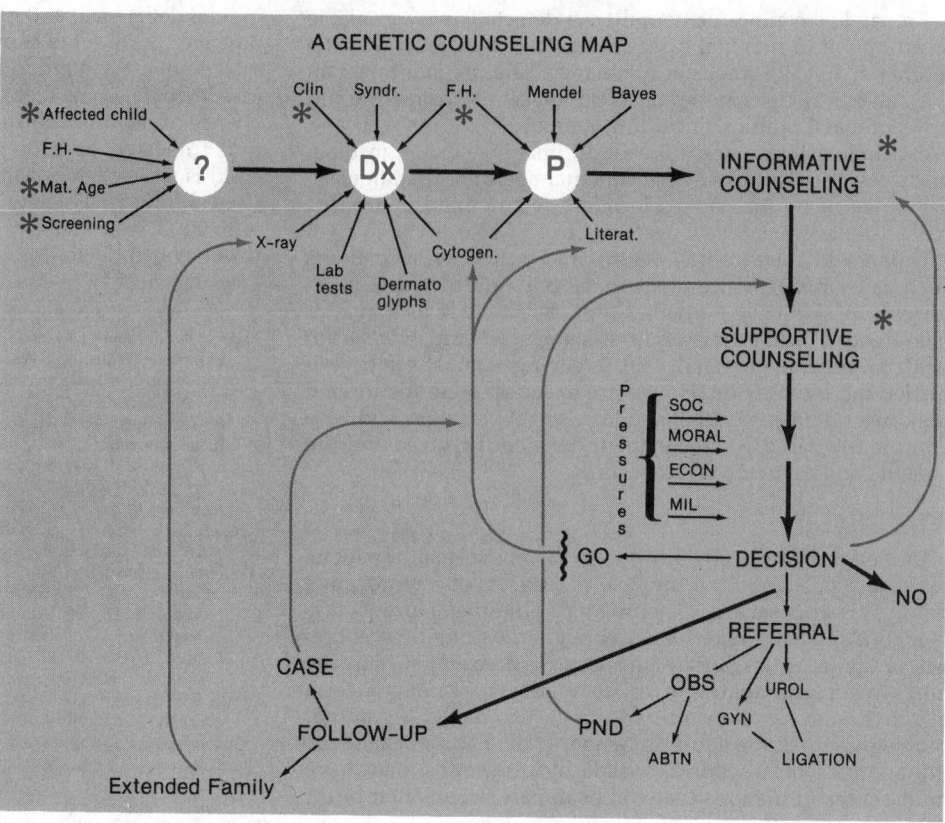

A GENETIC COUNSELING MAP

some cases, a specific diagnosis cannot be reached and the counseling must be done on an "either-or" basis—an unsatisfactory situation, but informed uncertainty is better than erroneous certainty.

ESTABLISHING "P"

The next step is to derive the probability, P, of the event that concerns the counselee, usually a risk of recurrence. Prerequisite to this is a carefully taken *family history*, which will serve not only as the basis for calculating P but also as a screening procedure that may pick up additional warning signals relevant to the counselee (this function applies also to the routine family history taken as part of the workup of any patient). A near relative with a neural tube defect may make the counselee eligible for prenatal diagnosis even though the condition for which she was referred does not. A sib or parent with non–insulin-dependent diabetes mellitus puts the counselee at increased risk for this disease; this raises the question of early detection tests and preventive measures. The same applies to most common, familial disorders, including hypertension, early coronary disease, the common neoplasms, and the common psychoses.

If the disease is known to have a *mendelian basis*, P can often be calculated on the basis of the known mode of inheritance (see Ch. 33). In some cases bayesian algebra can be used to improve the precision of the estimate by using additional family information. For instance, if a man's parent has Huntington's disease, which has a variable age of onset, the man had a 50 per cent chance of inheriting the gene at conception, but the longer he lives, free of the disease, the more likely it is that he did not inherit the gene. Similarly, for a woman who had a 50 per cent chance of inheriting the gene for hemophilia from her mother, the chance that she did inherit it diminishes with each unaffected son she bears. The precise probability can be calculated for the specific family situation. If the calculations tax the mathematical abilities of the physician, a genetic counselor can be consulted.

The rapid advances in mapping the human genome (Ch. 33) and particularly the use of DNA markers (RFLP's) are making it possible, in an increasing number of diseases, to identify carriers of mutant genes either before onset of the disease (e.g., Huntington's chorea) or prenatally (e.g., hemoglobinopathies, cystic fibrosis of the pancreas).

Diseases that do not fit the mendelian rules of family segregation often fit the expectations for *multifactorial inheritance*, particularly if they are known to be common (1 in 1000 or so) and familial. For these conditions the risk increases with the genetic proximity to an affected relative and with the number of affected relatives. Empiric estimates of average risks are available for counselees of varying degrees of relationship to the affected individual, and these can be modified upward or downward, according to the numbers of affected and unaffected relatives, by formulae based on the assumption of multifactorial inheritance.

Empiric estimates of risk must also be used for *chromosomal disorders*. We know the frequencies of liveborn trisomics at various maternal ages (see Ch. 36) and the probability of a recurrence after having had one.

Estimating risks for carriers of balanced chromosomal rearrangements is more difficult. One can derive the theoretic ratios of balanced to unbalanced offspring, but actual segregations are usually not random, and the question of whether theoretically possible unbalanced products will be viable or nonviable complicates the issue. Both segregation ratios and viability will vary with the length and position of the rearranged segments, and it is difficult to obtain enough data for any one rearrangement to derive segregation ratios. The genetic counselor can use a combination of general principles and empiric knowledge to obtain an estimate of the risk but must recognize the uncertainties involved.

Finally, there is the uncomfortably large group of disorders, particularly those involving mental retardation and dysmorphic features, for which the risk of recurrence is unknown. It may be as high as 1 in 4, for an as yet unrecognized autosomal recessive syndrome, or less than 1 per cent for an unrecognized environmental teratogen. Since unrecognized autosomal recessive syndromes will, one hopes, be in the minority (unless these is parental consanguinity), the risk in such cases will average out as low.

INFORMATIVE COUNSELING

Once P has been established as precisely as possible, we pass on to the stage of "informative counseling"—imparting the prognosis, probability of recurrence, and reproductive options to the counselee or counselees.

The processes by which families reach their reproductive decisions are complex, variable, and not well understood. Odds seem more easily appreciated than percentages, and the term "chances" does not have the opprobrious overtones of "risks." A statement such as, "if 20 couples who have had a baby like John each have another baby, on the average one of them would be like John and 19 would not," is easier to understand and less threatening than "the risk of your next baby's being affected is 5 per cent." Make sure they understand that the odds are the same for each child, and that (when the odds are one to three, for example), if they have one affected child, it does not mean that the next three will be normal.

Imparting the information may be relatively simple if the risk is so low as to be reassuring, and the nature of the disorder is well known to the counselees, who may have firsthand experience with it, or if the risk and burden are so high that no further reproduction is contemplated. It is in the intermediate group, who must decide on various reproductive options, often complicated by a host of social, ethical, economic, and family pressures, that genetic counseling may be most helpful.

SUPPORTIVE COUNSELING

This process involves helping the family to choose, among the various options, the one that is best for their own particular set of circumstances. Obviously, informative and supportive counseling go on together and are separated only for didactic purposes.

Who should do the counseling may depend on the local scene. If the physician knows the family best and the genetics is simple, the physician may be the most suitable counselor. If the genetics and the reproductive options are complex, the genetic counselor may be the appropriate resource. Often the two can work together in helping the family to reach an informed and responsible decision.

Parents often tend to ignore the numerical risk and focus on the burden; they may work toward a decision by trying out, in their imagination, various scenarios and selecting the "least-lose" option that they could live with. The risk of recurrence may, in this process, be incorporated into the burden. The "1" in the odds may loom large even if the denominator is quite big, particularly if the counselee is a pessimist. "No matter how big the n is in the 1 in n odds, the 1 never goes away."

The process of deciding may take some time, and the counselees may need several sessions with a counselor, as new issues or questions come up. Throughout this time, the counselor acts as both a source of information and a sounding board, trying to steer an understanding and supportive course between paternalistic directiveness ("with that high a risk, you shouldn't have children") and Olympian detachment ("It's your decision; don't ask me to make it for you.").

REFERRAL

Having reached a decision, the counselee or counselees may require referral—for tubal ligation (fallopian or vas deferens), artificial insemination, prenatal diagnosis, or care during the next pregnancy.

PRENATAL DIAGNOSIS

Prenatal diagnosis has changed the face of genetic counseling, since, for a growing number of conditions, it can change odds to certainty. It behooves the physician to know what categories of disorder are eligible, and although he or she cannot be expected to keep up with the latest additions to the list, it is at least possible to establish rapport with a clinical genetics center where this information can be found.

Techniques used in prenatal diagnosis include visualization by ultrasound examination or, less frequently, x-ray. Ultrasound will detect structural malformations such as anencephaly and overt spina bifida, renal agenesis, polycystic kidney disease, and exomphalos. As techniques improve, the array of detectable defects increases, and it is now possible to detect a remarkable number of disorders, including cleft lip, cleft palate, various heart malformations, microphthalmia, and some types of short-limb dwarfism. Fetoscopy permits direct examination, blood sampling, and even skin or muscle biopsy, although the risk of miscarriage may be as high as 5 per cent, even in experienced hands.

Amniotic fluid can be obtained by amniocentesis at 12 to 14 weeks of gestation, with a risk of fetal damage or induced miscarriage that seems well below 1 per cent in experienced hands. The cells can be cultured for karyotyping or biochemical studies. The fluid can be examined for alpha-fetoprotein, hormones (adrenogenital syndrome), intestinal enzymes (imperforate anus), or other appropriate chemicals. Techniques for chorionic biopsy are now becoming available that will allow examination of cells with the same genotype as the fetus as early as 8 to 10 weeks of gestation, permitting earlier diagnosis and, if necessary, termination of pregnancy. This along with the increasing array of conditions that can be diagnosed prenatally, will exacerbate the problems, both ethical and practical, involved in deciding what conditions and what circumstances justify the procedure. Genetic counselors tend to be nondirective, assuming that the parents (presumably well informed and conscientious) are in the best position to balance the burden of caring for an affected child against that of the guilt and suffering of a midtrimester abortion. They tend to draw the line, however, at prenatal diagnosis for nonpathologic conditions, and in particular the determination of sex for reasons of social preference.

The physician's main responsibility would seem to be to ensure that prospective parents at risk are aware that prenatal diagnosis is possible. The desire to practice good preventive medicine may be reinforced by the risk of litigation in cases in which parents have a child affected by some serious condition for which prenatal diagnosis is available and were not told about it. The main indications to be kept in mind are the following:

1. Maternal age: in most centers 35 or more at the expected time of birth.
2. Neural tube defect in a previous child, in the counselee, or in a first-degree relative. The risk of recurrence in a child or sib ranges from 1.5 to 10 per cent, depending on the frequency in the general population, and the risk for a nephew or niece is close to 1 per cent. Neural tube defects in this context include spina bifida occulta if there are multiple vertebral defects or spinal dysraphism. The advisability of maternal serum screening for neural tube defects by alpha-fetoprotein determination is a complex question, which must be answered for each population, depending on the frequency of neural tube defects and the availability of adequate laboratory, amniocentesis, and genetic counseling resources.
3. Chromosomal rearrangement in a parent. Couples who have had two or more spontaneous abortions deserve karyotyping, as about 1 in 20 will be found to carry a balanced chromosome rearrangement.

4. Sex determination, when the mother is at risk for being a carrier of an X-linked disorder not amenable to prenatal diagnosis.

5. A growing list of inborn errors of metabolism and other mendelian disorders, including the hemoglobinopathies. The dramatic advances in molecular genetics are rapidly expanding the number of such conditions (see Ch. 34 and 35).

6. Structural anomalies detectable by ultrasound, x-radiography, or, possibly, fetoscopy.

In most centers the number of positive diagnoses is about 2 per cent of the total number of cases, and the main benefit is to relieve anxiety and to allow couples who would otherwise refrain from having children, because of their high risk, to go ahead, without fear of the disorder in question.

FOLLOW-UP

The final stage in the genetic counseling process is the follow-up. As with any patient, follow-up is advisable to keep track of the results. The content of the informative counseling should be summarized in a letter, and a telephone call or note a few months later will establish whether the information has been understood, whether new questions have arisen, or whether new circumstances have changed the odds.

It may also be necessary to follow up the extended family. Often the discovery that a couple is at risk for a genetic disorder means that other family members are at risk, particularly in the case of autosomal dominant and X-linked disorders.

In diseases for which treatment is available, such as Wilson's disease or multiple polyposis of the colon, early detection in high-risk relatives is vitally important. Often, it may be possible to test individuals known by pedigree analysis to be at risk for carrier status. The hemoglobinopathies, glucose-6-phosphate dehydrogenase (G6PD) deficiency, Duchenne muscular dystrophy (creatine kinase levels), hemophilia (factor VIII clotting versus antigenic activity), and Tay-Sachs disease are examples. Cystic fibrosis will soon be on the list.

Good preventive medicine requires that these relatives be informed of their risks. This may require some ingenuity to avoid breaches of confidence. Sometimes a key family member will take on the role of genetic advocate, or an approach through the family doctor may solve the problem. One way or another, one strives to avoid the tragedy of an affected child, born to parents whose family history placed them at increased risk, and who bitterly demand, "Why didn't somebody tell me?"

Bergsma D: Birth Defects Compendium. 2nd ed. New York, Alan R. Liss, 1979. *A useful compilation of descriptive and etiologic data on dysmorphic syndromes and other birth defects.*

Brock DJH: Early diagnosis of fetal defects. Cur Rev Obstet Gynaecol 2:165, 1982. *A review of prenatal diagnosis.*

Capron AM, Lappé M, Murray RF (eds): Genetic counselling: Facts, values, and norms. Birth Defects 20:1, 1979. *A multiauthored volume on the concepts, psychology, ethics, and legal issues in genetic counseling.*

Fraser FC: Taking the family history. Am J Med Genet 34:585, 1963. *A discussion of family history-taking at various levels from routine office to research.*

Fraser FC, Nora JJ: Genetics of Man. Philadelphia, Lea and Febiger, 1986. *A textbook oriented toward medical students.*

Lippman-Hand A, Fraser FC: Genetic counseling—the postcounseling period. II. Making reproductive choices. Am J Med Genet 4:73, 1979. *The third in a series of articles on the psychodynamics of genetic counselees.*

McKusick V: Mendelian Inheritance in Man. 7th ed. Baltimore, The Johns Hopkins University Press, 1986. *An exhaustive catalogue of disorders showing mendelian inheritance.*

39 APPROACH TO THE PATIENT WITH CARDIOVASCULAR DISEASE

Thomas W. Smith

Common to the care of all patients with cardiovascular disease is a data base on which sound diagnostic and therapeutic decisions can be made. This chapter outlines an approach to cardiovascular data collection that emphasizes general principles and strategies and is intended to complement the more specific consideration of disease entities in the chapters that follow. One of the endlessly fascinating aspects of medicine is that each patient presents to the physician a unique story of his or her past history and present illness. Textbook descriptions of disease therefore convey at best a set of findings that the author regards as typical but that never quite fit in detail the findings present in any one individual patient. Hence, an open mind is essential during the evaluation of each patient so that diagnostic possibilities are not overlooked or prematurely discarded.

A dazzling array of diagnostic tests is now available for the evaluation of patients with evident or suspected cardiovascular disease. Sensitivity and specificity are known, or can be estimated, for each method under a given set of clinical circumstances. Redundancy must be avoided to achieve a favorable cost:benefit ratio (e.g., radionuclide ventriculography will often yield information regarding ventricular function that can be obtained from a two-dimensional echocardiogram, and both methods may be superfluous if the patient undergoes left ventriculography as part of a cardiac catheterization procedure). The emerging discipline of decision analysis (see Ch. 21) should help in formulating strategies in the development of an adequate cardiovascular data base.

Although accurate diagnosis is a key element in patient care, prognosis is also vitally important to the patient and often to the physician, who must formulate a program of treatment. Information over and above that needed to establish a diagnosis is typically required to allow an accurate prediction of outcome. This exercise in probability statistics is challenging and deserves careful attention as an essential component of the comprehensive care of the patient.

COMPONENTS OF THE CARDIOVASCULAR WORKUP

The three essential components of the clinical data base are the history, physical examination, and laboratory studies. Although this sequence of data acquisition will typically be followed, the value of returning to the bedside (often repeatedly) to refine the assessment of historical information and physical findings as the workup progresses cannot be overstated.

History

The cardinal symptoms of cardiovascular disease are listed in Table 39–1. *Dyspnea* and the related items in the first line are discussed in detail in Ch. 43. Historical information is particularly important in distinguishing among heart failure, pulmonary disease (including pulmonary emboli), metabolic disturbances producing acidosis, and anxiety as factors causing dyspnea. The nature of onset and duration of symptoms, relation to position, and precipitating and alleviating factors all provide important clues to the underlying pathophysiologic process.

Fatigue and *weakness* are common to many physical and emotional disease states and are nonspecific; nevertheless, it is important to record quantitative information in the history (e.g., flights of stairs or distance on level ground that the patient can manage) for current and future reference. *Cough,* initially dry and irritative, is a common early manifestation of elevated left-heart filling (and hence pulmonary venous) pressures. *Hemoptysis* should be characterized in regard to color and nature of admixture of blood and sputum to help distinguish between pulmonary (e.g., bronchitis, pulmonary infarction) and cardiac causes (e.g., pulmonary edema, hemorrhage from loss of bronchial vein integrity, as in mitral stenosis). *Cyanosis* is discussed in Ch. 43.

Chest pain should be characterized in terms of location, quality, course of onset and offset, duration, and precipitating and alleviating factors. Pain due to ischemic heart disease is considered in Ch. 51.1. Pericardial pain is more likely to be left sided, sharp in character, and related to breathing and position. Pleuritic pain also tends to be localized and sharp and is related to breathing or coughing. Chest wall pain is often long lasting and associated with tenderness to pressure applied at the trigger area.

Palpitation refers to an awareness of the heart beat, usually occurring in response to a change in cardiac rhythm or rate or by increased contractile force. It is a common anxiety-related symptom in patients without heart disease. Awareness of irregularity of the heart beat is more closely correlated with cardiac rhythm disturbances. *Dizziness* and *syncope* are frequent manifestations of cardiac arrhythmias and demand careful evaluation, often with 24-hour electrocardiographic (ECG) monitoring. These symptoms also occur as a consequence of orthostatic hypotension due to reduced blood volume, vasodilator drugs, or autonomic dysfunction. Obstruction to venous return from any cause will also predispose

TABLE 39–1. CARDINAL SYMPTOMS OF CARDIOVASCULAR DISEASE

Dyspnea, orthopnea, paroxysmal nocturnal
   dyspnea, wheezing
Fatigue, weakness
Cough, hemoptysis
Cyanosis
Chest pain
Palpitations, dizziness, syncope
Edema
Pain in extremities with exertion
   (claudication)

to these symptoms. *Claudication* refers to pain or an uncomfortable sensation of tiredness, usually in calf and/or thigh muscles, that occurs in response to exertion and is relieved by rest. This common symptom of peripheral arterial insufficiency is further discussed in Ch. 57.

Edema refers to swelling, usually of a dependent part of the body, due to retention of excess fluid. It is typically maximal in the feet at the end of the day and resolves, at least partially, by morning. Local factors such as deep venous disease predispose to unilateral edema. Patients confined to bed usually accumulate fluid in the sacral area.

The Physical Examination

Five elements constitute the cardiovascular physical examination. These are

1. Physical appearance
2. Venous pressure and pulse contours
3. Arterial pressure and pulse contours
4. Movement of the heart
5. Auscultation

PHYSICAL APPEARANCE. This is important in assessing the nature and severity of heart disease and also in providing clues to systemic diseases that affect the heart. Important cardiac problems are frequently encountered in patients with Marfan's syndrome, Turner's syndrome, Down's syndrome, the pickwickian syndrome, scleroderma, and thyroid disease, all of which are often recognizable on the basis of careful inspection of the patient's appearance. The funduscopic examination yields important information with regard to hypertension, diabetes mellitus, and sometimes infective endocarditis (Roth's spots). Cheyne-Stokes respirations are often seen in patients with advanced heart failure. Sometimes a highly specific cardiac diagnosis can be made on the basis of the physical appearance, such as the association of atrial septal defect with the bony abnormalities of the upper extremity which constitute the Holt-Oram syndrome. Cyanosis and clubbing of the fingertips indicate right-to-left shunting in patients with congenital heart disease.

VENOUS PRESSURE AND PULSE. Both external and internal jugular veins require careful inspection: external for estimation of mean right atrial pressure and internal for wave form as well as pressure. Figure 39–1 illustrates the typical features of the normal jugular venous pulse and indicates the terminology applied to the various aspects of this wave form. The A wave reflects right atrial contraction and occurs immediately prior to the carotid arterial pulse and first heart sound. The X descent occurs with right atrial relaxation and continues with early right ventricular contraction. The C wave, often superimposed on the beginning of the A wave, coincides with the carotid pulse itself. The V wave in the normal jugular venous pulse represents passive right atrial filling behind a closed and competent tricuspid valve. The Y descent reflects sudden termination of the V wave with right ventricular relaxation and opening of the tricuspid valve. The X descent is normally the more evident of the two declining phases of the jugular venous pulse. These phenomena are best noted with the patient so positioned that the top of the venous column can be observed throughout the cardiac cycle. Estimation of the central venous pressure is accomplished by estimating its height in centimeters above the sternal angle of Louis, adding 5 cm to allow for the normal relation of the right atrium to the external chest wall. Normal venous pressure varies from 5 to 10 cm of H_2O. The A wave tends to be accentuated in disease states characterized by reduced right ventricular compliance, tricuspid stenosis, or rhythm disturbances in which the atrium contracts against a closed tricuspid valve ("cannon" A waves). Tricuspid insufficiency produces systolic or regurgitant waves that obliterate the normal jugular

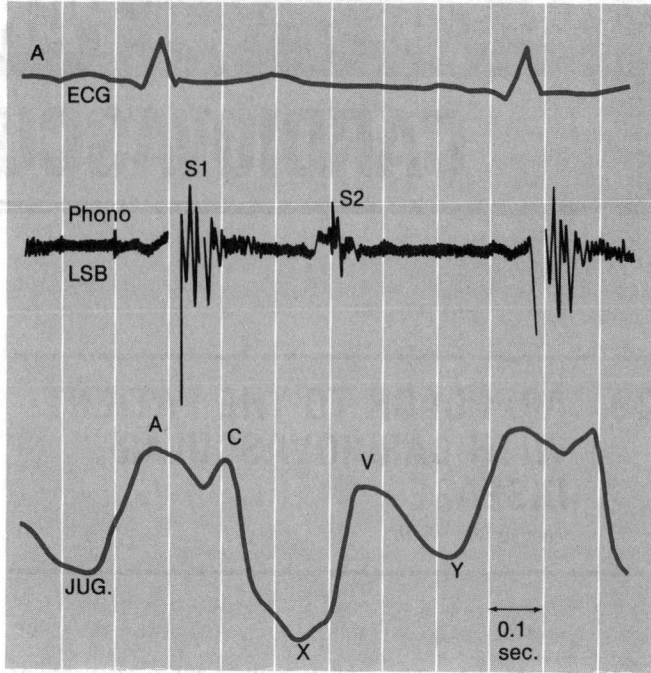

FIGURE 39–1. Normal jugular venous pulse.

venous V waves. Abnormalities associated with pericardial disease are discussed in Ch. 54.

ARTERIAL PRESSURE AND PULSE. Examination of the arterial pulse yields critically important information regarding the cardiovascular system. Arterial pressure should always be measured in both arms because of the unexpected discrepancies that are encountered in disease states or that are occasionally due to congenital anomalies. Use of a cuff of appropriate size is essential, and the arterial blood pressure should be recorded in both supine and standing position to assess volume status and the adequacy of reflex vasoconstrictor responses. Pulsus paradoxus refers to a decrease in systolic blood pressure of greater than 10 mm Hg on inspiration and is a typical feature of pericardial tamponade.

The carotid arteries provide the most direct reflection of cardiac activity because of their central location in proximity to the left ventricle and aorta. The amplitude of the carotid pulse is typically increased under circumstances associated with higher cardiac output, including fever, anemia, hyperthyroidism, and arteriovenous fistulas. The regularity (or lack thereof) indicates disturbances of rhythm or hemodynamics as in pulsus alternans. The wave form of the arterial pulse yields clues regarding runoff from the aorta, as in aortic insufficiency or arteriovenous fistula; a bisferiens quality is often present in aortic insufficiency and should be distinguished from the spike-and-dome contour encountered in patients with hypertrophic cardiomyopathy with obstruction (i.e., hypertrophic subaortic stenosis). The volume of the carotid pulse is typically reduced in heart failure and in mitral or aortic stenosis. Peripheral arterial pulses other than the carotid pulses should be felt and compared, with particular attention to a pulse delay at the femoral artery as a manifestation of coarctation of the aorta. Patients with claudication should have their lower extremity pulses examined both at rest and with exercise, since the latter maneuver will often accentuate asymmetries.

MOVEMENT OF THE HEART. Observation, palpation, and percussion are the traditional means for physical examination of cardiac movements. Inspection of the precordium will reveal asymmetries that serve as clues to chronic cardiac hypertrophy, particularly in congenital disease. The partial left lateral decubitus position is optimal for observation as well as palpation of the left ventricle in most patients. Diffuse left parasternal cardiac movement is often best appreciated with the heel of the palm, whereas higher frequency events (S$_1$, ejection clicks, S$_2$, opening snap, and thrills) are best felt with firm pressure and the tactile use of the fingertips. Precordial movements should be described at the apex, left parasternal area, and the right and left second intercostal spaces. The normal tapping impulse of the left ventricular apex is replaced by a more diffuse and sometimes dyskinetic impulse in patients with cardiac enlargement from a variety of causes. Displacement of the left ventricle is typically downward and to the left with cardiomegaly. Systolic overload with concentric hypertrophy increases the duration of the apex impulse and can be distinguished from the hyperdynamic impulse accompanying volume overload lesions, such as mitral or aortic insufficiency. Right ventricular enlargement produces a left parasternal systolic lift that is occasionally mimicked by the anterior motion of the heart with systolic expansion of the left atrium in the presence of severe mitral insufficiency. Pulmonary hypertension may be accompanied by a palpable pulmonary artery segment in the second left interspace and by a palpable pulmonic component of the second sound (P$_2$). Prominent third or fourth heart sounds can often be palpated as well as heard.

Thus, with the data gleaned from physical appearance, the venous and arterial pulse characteristics, and cardiac motion properties, the experienced clinician is armed with substantial information about cardiac anatomy and physiology before employing the stethoscope.

AUSCULTATION. Satisfactory cardiac auscultation requires a stethoscope that fits the ears snugly but comfortably and has the shortest tubing consistent with convenient use. The examination should be carried out in a quiet area, which sometimes requires moving the patient to a more suitable place when ambient noise levels are excessive. A systematic approach, as in all facets of physical examination, is important. Apart from the most obvious and dramatic auscultatory events, one generally hears only what one listens for. Beginning at the apex, the timing and nature of the first and second heart sounds are determined. Separable components of these events should be carefully noted. If the first sound has more that one component, S$_4$, asynchronous closure of mitral and tricuspid valves, and ejection clicks must be distinguished. Higher frequency transient systolic and diastolic sounds are listed in Table 39–2 and should be listened for explicitly. Murmurs should be identified and characterized, using the diaphragm to distinguish high-frequency events and the bell for lower frequency sounds. The examination should include listening with the patient sitting and leaning forward, supine,

and in the left lateral decubitus position. Standing, exercising, isometric handgrip, and the Valsalva maneuver will be important in specific circumstances, as outlined in the chapters that follow.

The plethora of sophisticated laboratory examinations now available should refine, rather than render obsolete, physical diagnostic skills. Every opportunity should be taken to review physical findings with the additional insights provided by noninvasive and invasive laboratory studies.

Laboratory Studies

Laboratory studies of patients with cardiovascular disease run the gamut from routine examinations (chest radiograph, electrocardiogram) that should be performed on virtually every patient being evaluated to highly sophisticated techniques that would be appropriate for specific individual subsets of patients. Remarkable progress in the past decade in noninvasive techniques now permits adequate evaluation of many patients without need for cardiac catheterization. Nevertheless, catheterization and angiography are essential components of the cardiovascular workup in most patients with advanced valvular or coronary artery disease.

ELECTROCARDIOGRAM. The standard 12-lead electrocardiogram remains a cornerstone of the clinical cardiologic evaluation. Although vectorcardiography and other more sophisticated approaches have their proponents, the standard 12-lead ECG remains a highly cost-effective screening test. It is reviewed in detail in Ch. 42.4. Detailed clinicopathologic correlations accumulated over two generations provide a wealth of background information. The most important applications are in assessment of cardiac arrhythmias, in which analysis of the P wave and the QRS complex, and their temporal relation to each other, forms the basis for the definition and clinical diagnosis of cardiac rhythm disturbances. Existence and location of myocardial ischemia and infarction represent other important components of the information inherent in the ECG. Right and left ventricular hypertrophy patterns, as well as right and left atrial abnormalities, are well described. Characteristic electrocardiographic findings are frequently important in the assessment of congenital heart disease.

The 12-lead electrocardiogram augmented with a standard exercise protocol is important in the assessment of ischemic heart disease (see Ch. 51.1). Both establishment of coronary artery obstructive disease and useful prognostic information are available from this study. Risk stratification in patients who have had myocardial infarctions is heavily dependent upon the exercise ECG. The predictive accuracy of the exercise ECG examination for coronary artery disease in specific patient subsets is well defined. It is important not only to classify ST-segment depression but also to assess duration of exercise, maximum heart rate achieved, time of onset of ST-segment depression, and time of resolution. A decrease in blood pressure during exercise correlates closely with advanced three-vessel or left main coronary artery obstructive disease. As in all such examinations, the diagnostic and predictive accuracy is dependent on the population of patients studied, and false-positive exercise ECG results are relatively commonly encountered in women, especially from populations with a low predicted incidence of obstructive coronary artery disease.

Assessment of symptoms of palpitations, dizziness, and syncope now rests heavily on the 24-hour (Holter) ECG. This approach is essential in the evaluation of cardiac arrhythmias and of response to antiarrhythmic drug regimens. Recent technical advances permit the assessment of transient ST-segment and T-wave changes reflecting myocardial ischemia, findings of particular value in the assessment of patients with variable threshold or "silent" ischemia.

CHEST RADIOGRAPH. This is a component of virtually every cardiovascular evaluation. Important findings are re-

---

TABLE 39–2. SYSTOLIC AND DIASTOLIC SOUNDS

Systolic
Early
 Ejection sounds (aortic, pulmonary)
 Systolic ejection clicks (mitral apparatus)
 Opening click of aortic valve mechanical prosthesis
Mid to late
 Mitral valve clicks (prolapse)

Diastolic
Early
 Opening snaps
 Early third sound of pericardial constriction or mitral regurgitation
 Opening click of mitral valve mechanical prosthesis
 "Tumor plop" of atrial myxoma
Mid
 Third heart sound or gallop (S$_3$)
 Summation gallop (S$_3$ + S$_4$)
Late (presystolic)
 Fourth heart sound (S$_4$)

viewed in Ch. 42.1. Chest radiography always supplements, rather than replaces, physical examination, since both approaches yield complementary information. Current practice usually limits the radiographic examination to the posteroanterior and lateral views. Echocardiography yields more accurate and specific information regarding individual chamber sizes. Evidence of calcification of cardiac structures should be sought on the chest radiograph, although fluoroscopic examination is generally more sensitive for this purpose.

ECHOCARDIOGRAPHY. This noninvasive technique uses high-frequency sound waves that reflect from cardiac structures, permitting the imaging of cardiac anatomy and motion. The technique is considered in detail in Ch. 42.3. Two-dimensional echocardiography has largely replaced the conventional M-mode display, although the latter provides superior quantitative details regarding wall thickness and chamber dimensions. This examination is now standard in the assessment of ventricular function and valvular abnormalities.

The Doppler method has rapidly gained acceptance and yields important additional information on intracardiac blood flow, shunts, and valvular stenosis and regurgitation. In selected patients, echocardiographic information, together with full clinical assessment, will permit valvular surgery without prior cardiac catheterization. Echocardiography is diagnostic in cases of left atrial myxoma, mitral valve prolapse, and hypertrophic cardiomyopathy. It is frequently useful for visualization of vegetations on heart valves in patients with infective endocarditis. Pericardial fluid and tamponade are routinely assessed by echocardiography, which is also useful in guiding pericardiocentesis.

RADIONUCLIDE STUDIES. These tests involve injection of radioisotopes into the circulation with detection by special instrumentation. One of the most useful of these techniques is radionuclide ventriculography, also referred to as gated blood pool scanning. Technetium 99m (^{99m}Tc) bound to albumin stays in the blood pool and permits imaging of the size and contractile function of cardiac chambers. Special applications include detection of intracardiac shunts by "first pass" methods. Most commonly, the technique is used to assess left and right ventricular function by measurement of end-systolic and end-diastolic dimensions, permitting evaluation of regional wall motion and the derivation of values for right and left ventricular ejection fractions.

Scanning with radioactive thallium (^{201}Tl) permits assessment of myocardial perfusion. The radioisotope is injected at maximum exercise and localizes in cardiac muscle as a function of coronary flow; areas of diminished myocardial perfusion are visualized as "cold" spots on the myocardial image. Viable but ischemic myocardium subsequently fills in with more homogeneous ^{201}Tl distribution, whereas previous infarction produces a persistent cold spot.

Scanning with ^{99m}Tc pyrophosphate is used to visualize areas of myocardial necrosis and is useful in evaluation of patients with suspected myocardial infarction when other studies are equivocal. These techniques are discussed in detail in Ch. 42.4.

CLINICAL APPLICATION. The safety of noninvasive techniques tempts the clinician to overutilize them, since no physical harm is likely to result and some incremental information is often obtained. Cost-effectiveness considerations must be kept in mind, however, and the use of these tests must be orchestrated so that the essential clinical decisions can be made without unnecessary cost and inconvenience to the patient. In particular, noninvasive test information will often be superfluous if the patient is destined to undergo complete evaluation by cardiac catheterization and angiography.

CARDIAC CATHETERIZATION. This invasive approach provides information on intracardiac and vascular pressures and flows. Gradients across stenotic valves and great vessels can be measured and systemic and pulmonary blood flows

quantified. Contrast agents can be injected selectively to define the anatomy of cardiac chambers, coronary vessels, and pulmonary and peripheral vessels. The technique of cardiac catheterization and angiography is considered in detail in Ch. 42.5. This diagnostic approach will usually be employed when a cardiac surgical procedure is under consideration.

Other applications of cardiac catheterization include electrophysiologic studies with pacing and mapping procedures to evoke and localize the source of cardiac rhythm disturbances. Endomyocardial biopsy is now a standard technique for the assessment of transplant rejection, unexplained cardiomyopathy, suspected myocarditis, suspected infiltrative diseases such as cardiac amyloidosis, or doxorubicin cardiotoxicity.

Cardiac catheterization procedures form the basis for therapeutic interventions, including percutaneous transluminal coronary angioplasty, or ablative procedures, such as those under development for the management of patients with Wolff-Parkinson-White syndrome refractory to drug therapy.

Although cardiac catheterization involves substantial expense and a small but finite risk of morbidity and mortality, this approach remains indispensable in the assessment of a wide array of cardiac problems that remain unsolved after complete noninvasive assessment. A frequent problem is the adult patient with a chest pain syndrome consistent with angina pectoris but with a negative or equivocal exercise electrocardiogram. Such patients may be severely disabled by these symptoms and attendant anxiety. Even though coronary artery surgery may not loom as a likely therapeutic approach, coronary arteriography can be of substantial value, especially when normal coronary anatomy is found, directing the diagnostic evaluation in more productive directions and restoring a previously incapacitated patient to full activity.

ELEMENTS OF A COMPLETE CARDIOVASCULAR DIAGNOSIS

Coordinated use of the history, physical examination, and laboratory studies will permit a full diagnosis to be established in nearly all patients, including the following five elements:

1. Etiology of the cardiovascular problem
2. Anatomic abnormalities, including quantification to the extent possible
3. Physiologic status, including pressures, flows, and relevant gradients
4. Functional capacity (see Table 39–3)
5. Prognosis

Diagnostic Strategies

The most appropriate approach to a patient with suspected cardiovascular disease will depend on the age and clinical presentation of the patient. A systolic ejection murmur at the base in a healthy teenager with an otherwise normal clinical evaluation, including ECG and chest radiograph, should ordinarily constitute adequate grounds for reassurance and avoidance of more elaborate studies. In an elderly patient with a systolic ejection murmur at the base, slow-rising carotid arterial pulses, and symptoms suggesting possible aortic stenosis, however, the chest radiograph, electrocardiogram, and echocardiogram with Doppler study will be necessary, at a minimum, to determine whether further and more aggressive evaluation is warranted.

Since prevention is a highly desirable goal in cardiovascular medicine, certain diagnostic tests may be warranted in individual patients even in the absence of specific symptoms. In addition to careful history and physical examination, serum cholesterol measurements will be appropriate in many patients, especially those with a family history of coronary artery disease, to assess risk and to guide therapeutic intervention. Use of exercise electrocardiography in sedentary, middle-aged individuals who are contemplating an exercise program remains controversial; many physicians would advocate this procedure, especially if the patient has risk factors for coronary artery disease.

TABLE 39–3. A COMPARISON OF THREE METHODS OF ASSESSING CARDIOVASCULAR DISABILITY

Class	New York Heart Association Functional Classification	Canadian Cardiovascular Society Functional Classification	Specific Activity Scale
I	Patients with cardiac disease but without resulting limitations of physical activity. Ordinary physical activity does not cause undue fatigue, palpitation, dyspnea, or anginal pain.	Ordinary physical activity, such as walking and climbing stairs, does not cause angina. Angina with strenuous or rapid or prolonged exertion at work or recreation.	Patients can perform to completion any activity requiring ≥ 7 metabolic equivalents, e.g., can carry 24 lb up eight steps; carry objects that weight 80 lb; do outdoor work (shovel snow, spade soil); do recreational activities (skiing, basketball, squash, handball, jog/walk 5 mph).
II	Patients with cardiac disease resulting in slight limitation of physical activity. They are comfortable at rest. Ordinary physical activity results in fatigue, palpitation, dyspnea, or anginal pain.	Slight limitation of ordinary activity. Walking or climbing stairs rapidly, walking uphill, walking or stair climbing after meals, in cold, in wind, or when under emotional stress, or only during the few hours after awakening. Walking more than two blocks on the level and climbing more than one flight of ordinary stairs at a normal pace and in normal conditions.	Patient can perform to completion any activitiy requiring ≥ 5 metabolic equivalents but cannot and does not perform to completion activities requiring ≥ 7 metabolic equivalents, e.g., have sexual intercourse without stopping, garden, rake, weed, roller skate, dance fox trot, walk at 4 mph on level ground.
III	Patients with cardiac disease resulting in marked limitation of physical activity. They are comfortable at rest. Less than ordinary physical activity causes fatigue, palpitation, dyspnea, or anginal pain.	Marked limitation of ordinary physical activity. Walking one to two blocks on the level and climbing more than one flight in normal conditions.	Patient can perform to completion any activity requiring ≥ 2 metabolic equivalents but cannot and does not perform to completion any activities requiring ≥ 5 metabolic equivalents, e.g., shower without stopping, strip and make bed, clean windows, walk 2.5 mph, bowl, play golf, dress without stopping.
IV	Patient with cardiac disease resulting in inability to carry on any physical activity without discomfort. Symptoms of cardiac insufficiency or of the anginal syndrome may be present even at rest. If any physical activity is undertaken, discomfort is increased.	Inability to carry on any physical activity without discomfort—anginal syndrome *may be* present at rest.	Patient cannot or does not perform to completion activities requiring ≥ 2 metabolic equivalents. *Cannot* carry out activities listed above (Specific Activity Scale, Class III).

Reproduced by permission of the American Heart Association, Inc., from Goldman L, et al: Comparative reproducibility and validity of systems for assessing cardiovascular functional class: Advantages of a new specific activity scale. Circulation 64:1227, 1981.

There is no simple formula for defining the data base that is adequate for clearance of patients for noncardiac surgery. A simple, informal stress test of walking up one or more flights of stairs to observe the presence or absence of dyspnea or chest discomfort will often obviate the need for more expensive and elaborate formal exercise testing. When extensive procedures such as peripheral vascular surgery or abdominal aortic aneurysm resection are contemplated in older patients with known or suspected coronary artery disease, aggressive diagnostic work-up, sometimes including cardiac catheterization and coronary arteriography, may be necessary because of limitations imposed by vascular disease on exercise electrocardiography or other approaches to assessment of cardiac reserve requiring exercise stress.

Perloff JK: Physical Examination of the Heart and Circulation. Philadelphia, W. B. Saunders Company, 1982. *A pocket-sized compendium of up-to-date information, well illustrated and referenced.*

40 EPIDEMIOLOGY OF CARDIOVASCULAR DISEASE

William T. Friedewald

Cardiovascular diseases have been the major health problem and the leading cause of death in the United States for several decades. The various statistics defining the magnitude of the problem are staggering. Estimates suggest that over 60 million people have some form of cardiovascular disease. In 1985, 981,000 people died of cardiovascular diseases, which accounted for 47.3 per cent of all deaths. This problem also ranks as the leading reason for social security disability, limitation in physical activity, and hospital bed use, accounting for 46 million bed days in 1984. In 1982 it was estimated

that cardiovascular diseases carried a direct health expenditure cost of $48 billion and additional indirect costs of $54 billion.

COMPONENTS OF CARDIOVASCULAR DISEASE

Cardiovascular disease is a general diagnostic category consisting of several separate diseases. One component, congenital heart disease, occurs at a rate of approximately 7 per 1000 live births, leading in 1983 to 6100 deaths, 3500 of which occurred before the age of one year. Another component, rheumatic heart disease, has had a dramatic 90 per cent decline over the last 40 years in the age-adjusted death rate (Table 40–1). Although 1.6 million people still have the disease, with approximately 6100 deaths in 1985, it has become a minor contributor to the overall cardiovascular disease problem. Coronary heart disease and cerebrovascular disease continue to be the major components of cardiovascular disease. Each year an estimated 1.25 million heart attacks occur (of which 800,000 are first attacks), leading to 534,000 deaths in 1985. Ten per cent of men and 3.3 per cent of women aged 45 to 64 years have overt coronary heart disease, and over the age of 65, these percentages increase to 13.4 in men and 9.4 in women. Cerebrovascular disease is found in 1.7 per cent of men (1.4 per cent of women) between the ages of 45 and 64 and 5.6 per cent of men (5.8 per cent of women) aged 65 and older, with 152,000 deaths due to this cause in 1985.

CARDIOVASCULAR DISEASE MORTALITY

These diseases have not always been the major health problem of the United States. In 1900 the five leading causes of death were (1) pneumonia and influenza combined, (2) tuberculosis, (3) diarrhea, enteritis, and ulceration of the intestines, (4) diseases of the heart, and (5) intracranial lesions of vascular origin. These categories all had rates greater than 100 per 100,000 population. By 1940, only two disease categories still had rates greater than 100 per 100,000: diseases of the heart and cancer and other malignant tumors. The infectious diseases had, to a large extent, been controlled, and

TABLE 40–1. AGE-ADJUSTED DEATH RATES* FOR MAJOR CARDIOVASCULAR DISEASES AND ALL OTHER CAUSES OF DEATH COMBINED IN THE UNITED STATES, 1905 TO 1985

Year	All Causes	All Causes Except Cardiovascular Diseases	Total	Cardiovascular Diseases Coronary Heart Disease	Cerebrovascular Diseases	Rheumatic Heart Disease
1905	1673.5	1315.9	357.6	NA	134.4	NA
1915	1443.4	1072.6	370.8	NA	123.3	NA
1925	1299.9	920.5	379.4	NA	114.2	NA
1935	1165.8	777.9	387.9	NA	94.4	NA
1945	947.4	556.9	390.5	NA	85.4	18.4
1955	764.6	368.5	396.1	200.0	83.0	11.2
1960	760.9	367.4	393.5	214.6	79.7	9.6
1965	739.0	364.8	374.2	215.8	72.7	7.4
1970	714.3	368.0	346.3	200.4†	66.3	6.3
1975	630.4	337.0	293.4	170.1†	53.7	4.8
1980	585.8	325.4	260.4	149.8	40.8	2.6
1985	545.3‡	316.6	228.7	127.3	33.1	1.8

*Rate per 100,000 population age adjusted to the United States population, 1940.
†Comparability ratio applied to convert rate to level comparable to rates for 1980 and 1985.
‡Estimated.
NA = not available.

their mortality rates have continued to fall to the present. The "epidemic" of cardiovascular disease, especially coronary heart disease had begun. By 1963, the mortality rate from coronary heart disease reached a peak; there has been a progressive and steady decline since then (Fig. 40–1). Despite the continued magnitude of the coronary heart disease problem, the focus recently has been on this dramatic reversal. Not only is the percentage of decline large, but also the impact on the total number of deaths in the United States is large and has led to an increase in life expectancy. In fact, the recent rate of improvement in life expectancy compares with that seen in the 1940's, when tuberculosis and other infectious diseases were being controlled. In 1983 a 45-year-old person could, on the average, expect to live 3.3 years longer than would have been expected in 1963. Estimates suggest that 45 per cent of this declining total mortality rate is due to the decline in coronary heart disease. The decline in death due to cerebrovascular disease, though even more impressive with a 63 per cent decrease since 1950, has been less of a contributing factor because it is less prevalent.

Declines in coronary heart disease mortality have been greater in younger adults, but there has been a remarkable uniformity among blacks and whites and among men and women. Despite some early doubts when the reversal in rates was beginning, this decline in coronary mortality is real and not artifactual. It cannot be explained by (1) problems in trend measurement, such as a shift in classifying deaths as due to

some other disease, (2) the waning of periodic respiratory epidemics that can contribute to the death of many patients with coronary heart disease, or (3) the depletion of the pool due to other causes of death in people expected to be susceptible to coronary heart disease. In addition, the decline has been too steep and long lasting to be reasonably explained by a simple random, temporary downturn. Determining precisely when the true decline began is complicated by these factors, but the increasing rate most likely changed to a decline beginning in the mid 1960's, perhaps somewhat earlier in women.

Data from other countries during the same period offer a perspective on understanding the United States rates. The multinational data in Figure 40–2 are for coronary heart disease death rates averaged over the four ten-year age groups for men 35 to 74 years of age. These data are not comparable to the age-adjusted rates in the table, but they still offer an important perspective for comparing the changes over time. During the period 1969 to 1978, among the 27 countries compared, the United States had the largest decrease in its coronary heart disease mortality rate and moved from second to eighth in rank. During this period, four other countries (Australia, New Zealand, Canada, and Israel) also had significant declines, whereas several others (e.g., Scotland and Northern Ireland) had increases despite having had initially high rates. Although the large absolute difference in rates by country in any given year might suggest that the genetic

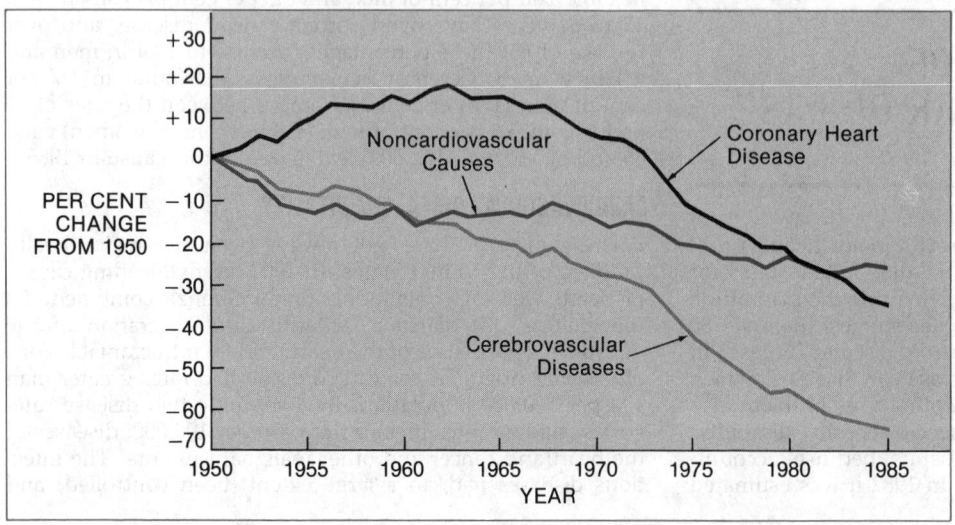

FIGURE 40–1. Per cent change in age-adjusted death rates for coronary heart disease, cerebrovascular diseases, and noncardiovascular causes of death in the United States, 1950 to 1985. (Source: Vital Statistics of the United States, National Center for Health Statistics.)

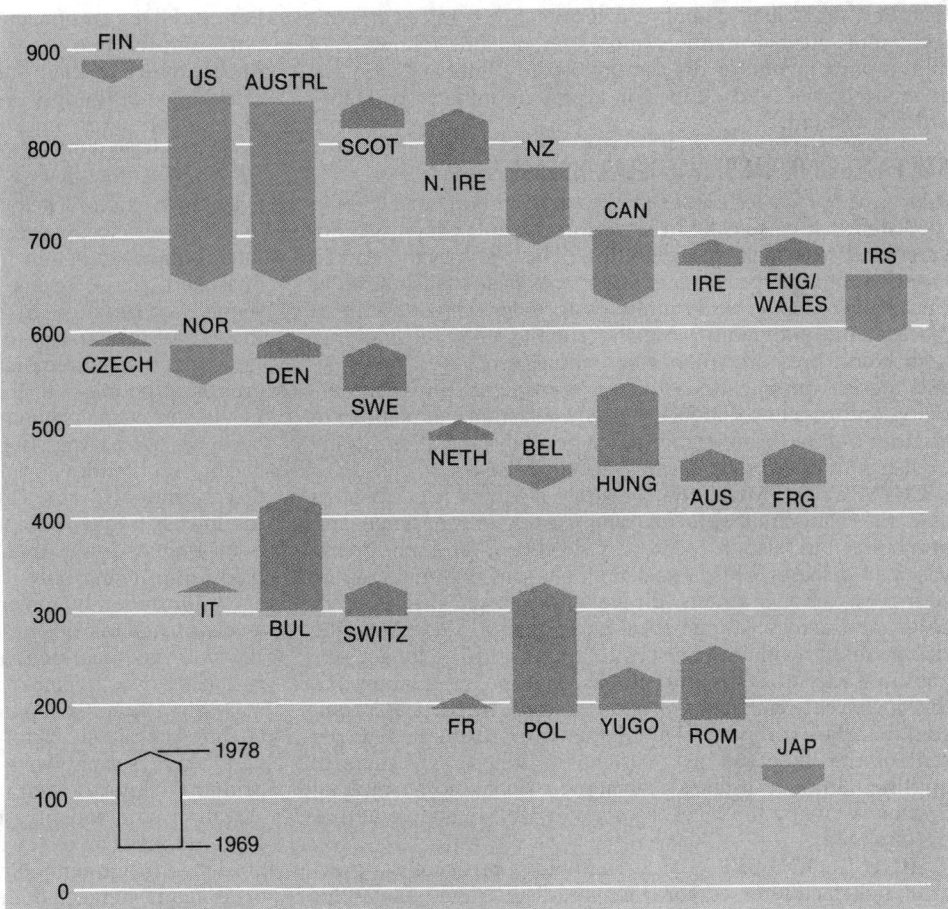

FIGURE 40—2. Coronary heart disease mortality rates per 100,000 population for men ages 35 to 74 by country (1969 to 1978). (Source: World Health Organization, World Health Statistics Annual, 1970 . . . 1981.)

differences among the populations account for this range, the large changes within a country over time demonstrate that regardless of genetic factors, the disease process can be significantly modified. Identification of the factors specifically responsible for these changes has proved to be difficult. Although the relative contributions of prevention efforts versus improved treatment modalities or improved general health measures have not been distinguishable, all most likely have contributed.

ATHEROSCLEROSIS AND CARDIOVASCULAR DISEASE

The major pathologic process leading to disease of the heart and blood vessels is atherosclerosis, with hypertension either a contributing or a primary problem. Atherosclerosis in its most malignant and rare form begins in early childhood and becomes rapidly manifest as clinical coronary heart disease or sudden death in adolescence. The more common and highly prevalent form begins to develop in adolescence and slowly progresses over several decades, gradually occluding the arterial lumen and eventually manifesting clinically as a stroke, angina pectoris, claudication, myocardial infarction, or, most devastatingly, as sudden death. Although the factors that may lead to an acute clinical event, such as arterial spasm, acute thrombosis, or embolism, are not completely understood, the underlying, if not immediate, problem is predominantly atherosclerosis.

Laboratory and clinical research efforts continue in the search for the underlying cause or causes of atherosclerosis, examining those factors that may initiate the process as well as those that may cause the milder, highly prevalent, presumed early forms of the disease (i.e., fatty streaks on the arterial surface) to progress in many individuals to the more serious, complicated, and obstructing form of the disease. Other research efforts are concentrating on the later, but still

preclinical, stages of the process, searching for improved and more quantitative diagnostic techniques. Meanwhile, epidemiologic research efforts have made and continue to make major contributions to both prevention and treatment approaches to the cardiovascular disease problem through identification of personal and environmental characteristics that markedly increase an individual's probability of developing specific cardiovascular diseases.

RESEARCH IN CARDIOVASCULAR DISEASE

The research approach that has been repeatedly used in several large observational studies of cardiovascular disease is exemplified by the Framingham Heart Study, begun in 1948 in a relatively small town in Massachusetts. A sample (5209 men and women aged 30 to 62) of the total population agreed to be part of this study, undergoing thorough examinations every two years, with intense follow-up for the development of both fatal and nonfatal diseases. This population has remained under close scrutiny continuously since originally recruited and examined over the two-year period from 1948 to 1950. Similar studies have been performed in other groups in the United States, as well as around the world. In Tecumseh, Michigan, 8624 men and women, in Evans County, Georgia, 3102 men and women, in Albany, New York, 1913 male civil servants, and in Chicago, Illinois, 1264 male gas company employees and 1983 male employees of the Western Electric Company were recruited and observed over several years. The critical elements of these studies have been the (1) inclusion of relatively large numbers of people to allow for important and sufficiently powerful subsample analyses, (2) enrollment of participants by methods that would make them reasonably representative of the total population from which they were recruited, (3) careful determination of all the variables (such as height, blood pressure, smoking and dietary histories, and blood chemical determinations) in a standardized, reproducible manner, and (4) meticulous follow-up of all the participants for the development of fatal and nonfatal events recorded and defined in a predetermined and standardized fashion.

RISK FACTORS IN CARDIOVASCULAR DISEASE

From these United States studies and others worldwide, a consistent list of so-called risk factors for subsequent cardiovascular disease has been identified. These risk factors can be grouped into two broad categories: *unmodifiable* (such as older age, male gender, and family history of premature heart disease) and potentially *modifiable* (such as cigarette smoking, high blood pressure, high blood cholesterol level, diabetes, and the less prognostic factors of overweight, physical inactivity, and psychosocial factors). These factors can be used to identify clearly those in the population who are at especially high risk of developing cardiovascular disease.

CIGARETTE SMOKING. Cigarette smoking is established as a risk factor not only for lung cancer, emphysema, and bronchitis but also for coronary, cerebral, and peripheral vascular disease. This association has been seen in many countries, among widely different ethnic groups, in both sexes, and across various adult age groups. In addition, the risk increases with heavier cigarette use and the longer one has smoked. Equally important has been the observation that this increased risk falls rapidly over time when people quit smoking. For coronary heart disease, approximately 40 per cent of the increased risk is removed within five years of quitting, although it takes several more years of nonsmoking to achieve finally the level associated with someone who has never smoked.

HIGH BLOOD PRESSURE. High blood pressure is a powerful risk factor for cerebrovascular disease, as well as for coronary heart disease and the atherosclerotic process directly. An estimated 58 million people have high blood pressure, defined as a level equal to or greater than 140 mm Hg systolic or 90 mm Hg diastolic or as being on a regimen of antihypertensive medications. An important result of the epidemiologic studies was the observation that the relationship between blood pressure and cardiovascular risk was not only a positive one (a higher blood pressure resulted in a higher disease rate) but also a smooth one (there was no sharp breakpoint in the curve such that below a certain blood pressure level the risk remained constant or became nonexistent). Thus, the lower the blood pressure, within reasonable physiologic limits, the lower the level of risk. These observations prompted several important intervention trials, which have now clearly established the value of aggressively treating elevated blood pressure.

BLOOD CHOLESTEROL LEVELS. A clear and positive relationship between blood cholesterol levels and subsequent coronary heart disease has repeatedly been demonstrated. Later information refined the nature of this association but did not weaken it. Cholesterol in the plasma is transported by the lipoproteins. The cholesterol level associated with the low density lipoprotein (LDL) fraction was seen to be positively correlated with coronary heart disease, whereas the cholesterol associated with the high density lipoprotein (HDL) was negatively correlated (the higher the level, the lower the risk). These initial observations have been verified in several different populations and were shown to be independent of each other, as well as of other known risk factors. As with blood pressure and cardiovascular disease risk, for both LDL cholesterol and HDL cholesterol, the curve is smooth (in the populations studied, there was no breakpoint in the curve observed). The evidence regarding HDL, though more recent than that for LDL, supports a powerful role for HDL in coronary heart disease risk and may explain some of the difference in risk between men and women, with women having average levels of HDL higher than men. The ratio of LDL to HDL, an efficient method of combining the information from the two separate measures, has been shown to be more predictive than either measure alone. The appropriate clinical use of the mix of LDL, HDL, and/or LDL:HDL values must await more information and experience. Information from over 350,000 American men screened for eligibility in the Multiple Risk Factor Intervention Trial demonstrated that even down to and below levels of total blood cholesterol of 182 mg per deciliter the risk continues to fall off. Recent intervention studies in hypercholesterolemic men have demonstrated that lowering blood cholesterol levels lowers subsequent coronary heart disease morbidity and mortality and the rate of progression of coronary atherosclerosis.

Each of these three risk factors alone can be used to separate groups of people into those at high or low risk. But as these risk factors occur simultaneously in individuals, the risk range becomes even larger (Fig. 40–3). Based on the Multiple Risk Factor Intervention Trial screenee data, the coronary heart disease mortality rate (1.6/1000 screenees) for nonsmokers in the lowest tertile of diastolic blood pressure, and cholesterol is nine times lower than the rate (14.6/1000) for the highest risk group, using only these three variables. As can be seen, age uniformly remains one of the most powerful factors at all levels of risk, as does male gender, with women realizing a 10- to 20-year differential before attaining the same level of risk as men with similar risk factors.

OBESITY. Initial epidemiologic data identified obesity as an important risk factor for coronary heart disease. Subsequent analyses, however, suggested that obesity was not a primary risk factor, but rather that it acted indirectly through elevation of blood pressure and of blood cholesterol levels. More recent analyses of the data from the Framingham Heart Study, with longer follow-up of people in the cohort, have once again suggested that obesity is indeed a primary risk factor that acts independently of these other factors. Clinically, the resolution of this issue of primary versus secondary causation is somewhat irrelevant. Weight reduction should lower the risk of coronary heart disease, whether it acts through a lowered blood pressure and/or cholesterol level or as a lowered risk factor itself.

DIABETES. Diabetes is a powerful and independent risk factor for cardiovascular disease, which remains the major cause of death in diabetic persons. An important remaining issue is whether an elevated blood glucose level is responsible for the observed higher rate of cardiovascular disease and, if it is, whether lowering or, preferably, normalizing the glucose level will lower the risk. Regardless of the answers, for the present the important observation is that diabetic individuals are at higher risk of cardiovascular disease, and thus careful attention should be paid not just to the blood glucose level and its control, but also to the other risk factors that may coexist in a given patient and additionally elevate the risk.

PHYSICAL INACTIVITY. An association between a less active lifestyle and increased risk of coronary heart disease has been shown in multiple longitudinal and cross-sectional studies in such diverse groups as London transit workers, United States longshoremen, and United States college graduates. However, studies establishing a clear cause-and-effect relationship have not been forthcoming. One of the major problems in the randomized studies investigating this question has been adherence to the prescribed exercise regimen. Another problem is that as people begin an exercise program, other factors change as well. Overweight people tend to lose weight; HDL cholesterol levels rise; the diet tends to change; and those individuals who are cigarette smokers frequently stop smoking. Although these covarying factors make the scientific evaluation of physical exercise as an isolated risk factor difficult, they tend to favor the recommendation of a prudent exercise program because of the multiple healthful consequences of such activity.

Other risk factors for cardiovascular disease have been

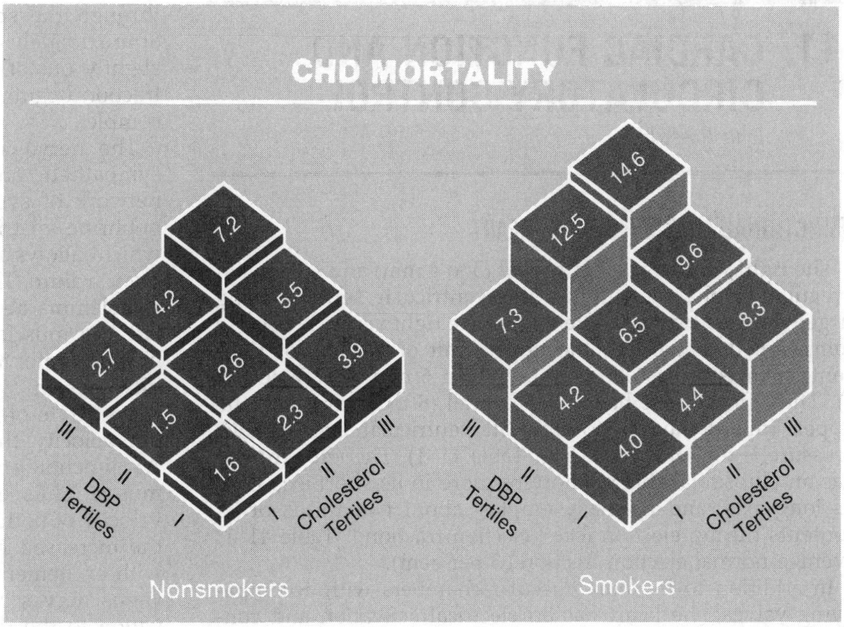

FIGURE 40–3. Age-adjusted CHD mortality rates/1000 screenees for the Multiple Risk Factor Intervention Trial among smokers and nonsmokers for cholesterol tertiles (I = ≤ 196, II = 197–228, III = ≥ 229) and diastolic blood pressure (DBF) tertiles (I = ≤ 79, II = 80–87, III = ≥ 88).

identified in single or multiple studies, but further information is needed to establish them as independent, important prognostic factors.

RISK FACTORS AFTER MYOCARDIAL INFARCTION. After surviving a myocardial infarction, the primary risk factors become those related to the infarct itself and the damage to myocardial tissue. As part of the Coronary Drug Project clinical trial, 2789 post–myocardial infarction patients were given usual medical care and observed over a period of five years. The most powerful factors increasing risk in this group were persistent resting electrocardiographic abnormalities (namely ST segment depression and ventricular conduction defects), use of diuretics, a higher (and therefore more activity-restrictive) New York Heart Association functional classification, and a higher heart rate. Although the traditional risk factors, such as cigarette smoking and elevated blood cholesterol levels and blood pressure, remained prognostic, they were weaker factors overshadowed now by primary damage to the myocardium. In addition, with sudden death as the initial clinical presentation of cardiovascular disease in approximately one quarter of patients, it is obviously important to establish effective prevention modalities before the onset of clinical disease. Much current myocardial infarction research is focusing on therapeutic approaches that seek to minimize the extent of myocardial damage or even prevent the development of the infarct entirely. Nonetheless, the greatest potential for continuing and accelerating the decline in cardiovascular disease rates rests with prevention or treatment of the factors that lead to clinical presentation of disease and more profoundly of the factors that lead to or accelerate the atherosclerotic process.

CHANGES IN RISK FACTORS. Significant changes have occurred nationally in the major modifiable risk factors. In 1965, 52 per cent of men aged 20 or greater were cigarette smokers. In 1983 that figure had dropped to 35 per cent (age adjusted). For women the change has been modest, falling from 34 per cent in 1965 to 30 per cent in 1983. From 1965 to 1983, consumption of tobacco fell from 11.5 to 6.6 pounds per capita. In 1971 and 1972 only 16.5 per cent of people with high blood pressure (defined as a level equal to or greater than 160 mm Hg systolic or 95 mm Hg diastolic or as being on a regimen of antihypertensive medication) were effectively controlled. By the late 1970's, this figure had increased to 34 per cent. During this same period, visits to a physician for high blood pressure increased by 35 per cent. In addition,

salt sales fell from 2.2 pounds per capita in 1972 to 1.4 in 1985. Average blood cholesterol levels in men fell from 217 mg per deciliter in the period between 1960 and 1966 to 211 in the late 1970's. Annual per capita consumption of several foods changed over the 20-year period from 1964 to 1984. Vegetable fat and oil consumption rose from 32.5 to 48.1 pounds, whereas that of animal fats and oils fell from 18.3 to 13.5 pounds; butter use fell from 6.9 to 5.0 pounds, and the number of eggs eaten fell from 322 to 264 per person per year. These impressive changes clearly demonstrate that the United States public can and will modify lifestyle behavior and suggest that additional gains in the prevention of the cardiovascular diseases can be made.

Food Consumption, Prices and Expenditures, 1964–1984. Economic Research Service, U.S. Department of Agriculture. Statistical Bulletin No. 736, December 1985. *A collection of tables on the food system, marketing, nutrition, and demand for food in the United States.*

Goldman L, Cook EF: The decline in ischemic heart disease mortality rates: An analysis of the comparative effects of medical interventions and changes in lifestyle. Ann Intern Med 101:825, 1984. *An interesting attempt at quantification of the relative contribution of lifestyle and treatment factors on the decline in coronary heart disease mortality.*

Gordon T, Garcia-Palmieri MR, Kagan A, et al.: Differences in coronary heart disease in Framingham, Honolulu and Puerto Rico. J Chronic Dis 27:329, 1974. *A valuable comparison of the relationship between risk factors and subsequent coronary heart disease in three geographically and ethnically diverse populations.*

Grundy SM, Ad Hoc Committee to Design a Dietary Treatment of Hyperlipoproteinemia: Recommendations for the Treatment of Hyperlipidemia in Adults: A Joint Statement of the Nutrition Committee and the Council on Atherosclerosis of the American Heart Association. Arteriosclerosis 4:445A, 1984. *A succinct review of the hyperlipidemias and hyperlipoproteinemias with treatment recommendations and 265 references.*

Health, United States, 1985. U.S. Department of Health and Human Services, Public Health Service, National Center for Health Statistics. DHHS Publication No. (PHS) 85–1232, December 1985. *A frequently updated report presenting national data on morbidity and mortality, health delivery costs, and prevention programs with detailed tables.*

The Joint National Committee on Detection, Evaluation, and Treatment of High Blood Pressure: The 1984 Report of the Joint National Committee on Detection, Evaluation, and Treatment of High Blood Pressure. Arch Intern Med 144:1045, 1984. *A succinct and authoritative review of the major clinical issues involving high blood pressure with a list of key references.*

Kaplan NM, Stamler J: Prevention of Coronary Heart Disease: Practical Management of the Risk Factors. Philadelphia, W.B. Saunders Company, 1983. *A concise, informative, and readable summary of the current information on the risk factors for coronary heart disease.*

Proceedings of the Conference on the Decline in Coronary Heart Disease Mortality. U.S. Department of Health, Education, and Welfare, Public Health Service. DHEW Publication No. (NIH) 79–1610, 1979. *A careful review of the issues bearing on the decline with a useful appendix.*

World Health Statistics Annual 1970–1985. World Health Organization. *International vital statistics and population data in tabular form by country.*

41 CARDIAC FUNCTION AND CIRCULATORY CONTROL

John Ross, Jr.

FUNCTIONAL ANATOMY OF THE HEART

The right ventricle is thin walled (3 to 4 mm) and somewhat irregular in shape, with the interventricular septum being largely formed by the left ventricle. The right ventricle is more compliant than the left, the upper limit of normal for right ventricular end-diastolic pressure being 6 mm Hg (Table 41–1). The left ventricle has a thicker wall (8 to 9 mm), and the upper limit of normal for the left ventricular end-diastolic pressure is higher (12 mm Hg, Table 41–1). The left ventricle has an ellipsoidal shape, shortens more in its short axis than its long axis, and normally empties about two thirds of its contents during ejection (see "ejection fraction," Table 41–1, average normal ejection fraction 65 per cent).

In addition to its four muscular chambers with accompanying valves, the heart has an electrical activation and conduction system, an autonomic neural supply, and a coronary circulation. The three main coronary arteries divide into lesser branches and eventually send small, penetrating vessels directly into the myocardium to supply a very dense capillary network. During coronary vasodilation, approximately one capillary per muscle cell provides a rich blood supply to the heavily working myocardium.

The electrical subsystem includes the sinoatrial (SA) node, comprising special pacemaker cells with continuous phase 4 depolarization, and the atrioventricular (AV) node, which exhibits delayed or decremental conduction, allowing atrial depolarization to precede ventricular depolarization by approximately 140 msec and atrial contraction thereby to serve as a "booster pump" for filling the ventricles. From the AV junction (or node) the electrical impulse rapidly spreads through the specialized His-Purkinje conduction system in approximately 40 msec to reach the ventricles, which contract slightly out of phase (left before right), left ventricular contraction beginning about 50 msec after the onset of the QRS complex.

The nervous subsystem supplying the heart consists of sympathetic and parasympathetic divisions. There is a rich network of sympathetic nerve terminals containing norepinephrine distributed throughout the atria and ventricles, which allows reflex regulation of the contractility of the myocardium. The beta-adrenergic receptors on the myocardial sarcolemma also permit circulating catecholamines to stimulate the muscle during stress. The sympathetic nerves also heavily innervate the SA node and AV junction, where increases in sympathetic tone increase the heart rate (enhanced rate of phase 4 depolarization) and improve conduction velocity, thereby decreasing conduction time through the AV junction and improving synchronicity of the ventricular muscle. Thus, enhanced strength of contraction and increased velocity of both muscle contraction and relaxation accompany the increased heart rate during sympathetic stimulation, as with excitement or exercise. Parasympathetic fibers from the vagus nerves containing acetylcholine provide heavy innervation to the right and left atria, the SA node, and the AV junction, but there are few parasympathetic nerve terminals in the ventricles or the conduction system below the AV junction. Activation of the parasympathetic system has a slowing effect on the SA node (reduced rate of phase 4 polarization) and slows conduction through the AV junction, providing reciprocal neural control with the sympathetic nervous system. The contractility of atrial muscle is depressed by parasympathetic stimulation, but there is minimal effect on the ventricles because of their sparse innervation by this branch of the autonomic nervous system.

Unlike skeletal muscle, cardiac muscle can regulate its contractility, or inotropic state. The force of cardiac muscle contraction, as well as its velocity is normally regulated in large part by the amount of free calcium (Ca^{++}) that is released by the action potential. Events associated with arrival of the action potential at the myocyte trigger release of calcium from the sarcoplasmic reticulum; calcium then binds to a subunit of troponin on the actin filament, causing a conformational change that uncovers the active site and allows a tension-generating bond to occur between actin and myosin. More calcium allows more sites to bind. *Between* contractions, the sarcoplasmic reticulum (together with subsarcolemmal binding sites) rapidly and actively sequesters calcium, so that the level at the myofilaments falls below that required for the actin-myosin interaction. Calcium enters the cell during phase 2 of the action potential and is extruded against an electrical and chemical gradient by an ATP-driven sarcolemmal calcium pump and by a 3:1 sodium for calcium exchange mechanism across the sarcolemma, which is driven mainly by the sodium gradient generated by the sodium/potassium ATPase membrane pump. Myocardial contractility is normally increased by catecholamines, which stimulate the beta receptors and augment intracellular cyclic adenosine monophosphate (AMP), which leads to increased calcium influx during the action potential. Increasing extracellular calcium also augments myocardial contractility.

A variety of mechanisms stimulate myocardial contractility in the failing heart. Digitalis, by inhibiting membrane sodium/potassium ATPase, causes an increase of intracellular sodium, which decreases the sodium gradient, thereby leading to increased intracellular calcium and enhanced contractility. Beta-adrenergic agonist drugs such as dobutamine are used to treat the acutely failing heart as well. Some newer positive inotropic agents (e.g., amrinone and milrinone) act largely by inhibiting phosphodiesterase, leading to increased intracellular cyclic AMP, and other new drugs are under study that may directly affect calcium influx during the action

TABLE 41–1. PRESSURES AND VOLUMES IN THE NORMAL HEART

Pressures
  Left sided
    1. Left atrial pressure (normal mean pressure ≤ 12 mm Hg)
    2. Left ventricular pressure
      a. Peak systolic pressure (same as aorta)
      b. Maximum dP/dt (1200–3500 mm Hg/sec)
      c. Left ventricular end-diastolic pressure (normal ≤ 12 mm Hg)
    3. Aorta
      a. Systolic pressure (wide normal range, usually 100–150 mm Hg in adults)
      b. Diastolic pressure (wide normal range, usually 60–90 mm Hg in adults)
  Right sided
    1. Right atrial pressure (normal mean pressure ≤ 6 mm Hg)
    2. Right ventricular pressure
      a. Peak systolic pressure (normal 15–30 mm Hg)
      b. Right ventricular end-diastolic pressure (normal ≤ 6 mm Hg)
    3. Pulmonary artery
      a. Systolic pressure (normal 15–30 mm Hg)
      b. Diastolic pressure (normal 4–12 mm Hg)
Volumes
  Left sided (at rest)
    1. Left ventricular end-diastolic volume (normal 70–100 ml/m²)
    2. Left ventricular end-systolic volume (normal 25–35 ml/m²)
    3. Stroke volume (wide normal range, usually 40–70 ml/m²)
    4. Ejection fraction (stroke volume divided by end-diastolic volume [normal 0.55–0.80])
Time-related measurements
    1. Heart rate (wide normal range, usually 60–100 beats/minute)
    2. Cardiac index (2.5–4.2 liters/min/m²)
Resistances
    1. Systemic vascular resistance (770–1500 dynes sec cm⁻⁵)
    2. Pulmonary vascular resistance (20–120 dynes sec cm⁻⁵)

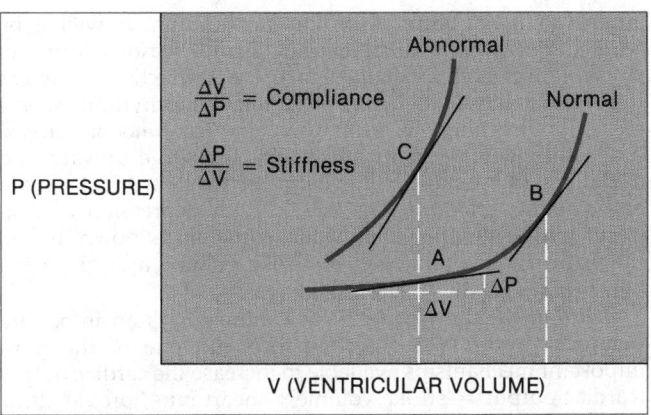

FIGURE 41–1. Diastolic pressure-volume curves of left ventricle under normal conditions and in the presence of severe ventricular hypertrophy (abnormal). Note the nearly exponential shape of the curves. The stiffness at any point on the normal curve ($\Delta P/\Delta V$) is shown by a tangent. Notice that ventricular stiffness increases (tangent A to tangent B) with ventricular filling to a larger ventricular volume. The stiffness of two ventricular chambers can be compared at a common volume, and comparison of the stiffness of the normal with that of the abnormal (hypertrophied) ventricle shows that the latter is markedly increased (tangent A versus tangent C). Compliance is the inverse slope ($\Delta V/\Delta P$) of the curve, and therefore the abnormal ventricle has a markedly reduced compliance. (Adapted from West JB (ed): Best & Taylor's Physiological Basis of Medical Practice. 11th ed. Baltimore, Williams & Wilkins Co., 1985).

potential or increase the sensitivity of the myofilaments to calcium.

DIASTOLIC PROPERTIES OF THE HEART. A major feature of cardiac muscle is its intrinsic stiffness while at rest. Unlike skeletal muscle, which, when isolated from its bony supports, can be overstretched easily, cardiac muscle at first stretches readily but then, when stretched further while in the relaxed state, it reaches an elastic limit, giving a much steeper relation between length and resting tension at long muscle lengths than in skeletal muscle. Thus, there is intrinsic stiffness within the walls of the ventricles, particularly the left ventricle, which tends to prevent overdistension with sudden changes in the venous return to the heart.

This property of heart muscle results in a nearly exponential relation between cardiac volume and pressure wherein small changes in volume produce large pressure changes as the ventricle is further filled beyond the upper limit of normal for left ventricular end-diastolic pressure (Fig. 41–1). Thus, the slope of this relation or chamber stiffness ($\Delta P/\Delta V$) increases as the ventricle is filled, and compliance ($\Delta V/\Delta P$) falls. Of course, when an abnormal chamber, such as a hypertrophied left ventricle, is compared with a normal chamber at the same cardiac volume, the entire diastolic pressure-volume relationship is shifted upward and steepened (Fig. 41–1), and the abnormal chamber is said to be stiffer or less compliant than normal. Even in chronically dilated hearts (as in the normal heart), it does not appear possible to stretch sarcomere lengths much beyond 2.2 μm, so that the heart never appears to operate on a descending limb of the sarcomere length-tension relation.

Although emphasis is often placed on a description of the systolic function of the heart, a greater appreciation of the importance of the diastolic properties of the heart has developed in recent years. A thick, hypertrophied ventricle with decreased compliance causes increased resistance to filling. This frequently leads to atrial dilation and hypertrophy in order to maintain the atrial contribution to ventricular filling. The importance of this contribution is apparent in patients with severe hypertrophy caused, for example, by aortic stenosis or hypertrophic obstructive cardiomyopathy. Loss of an

appropriately timed atrial contraction (as with atrial fibrillation) often results in marked exacerbation of the left-heart failure. In these patients, during sinus rhythm the left ventricular end-diastolic pressure is markedly elevated owing to a large A wave, whereas mean diastolic pressure, which is reflected back through the pulmonary veins into the lungs, is maintained at a lower level. When atrial contraction and the A wave "kick" are lost, however, there is an increase in mean left atrial and pulmonary venous pressures in an attempt to maintain the same level of end-diastolic pressure and cardiac output. This frequently leads to disabling dyspnea.

CARDIAC CONTRACTION AND ITS REGULATION

DETERMINANTS OF CARDIAC PERFORMANCE. There are four major determinants of the performance of both ventricles; the discussion will be focused primarily on the left ventricle, however.

1. Preload
2. Afterload
3. Contractility
4. Heart rate

The Preload. This refers to the loading condition on the heart at the end of diastole, which is primarily set by the venous return to the heart. In isolated heart muscle, it is defined as the force stretching the resting muscle to a given length prior to contraction. In the intact heart, it is less easily defined. Estimates of preload include measurements of the ventricular end-diastolic volume or the end-diastolic pressure (although the two are not linearly related, Fig. 41–1), and in acutely ill patients, it may be convenient to measure the ventricular "filling pressure" (the mean right or left atrial pressure, or the pulmonary artery wedge pressure) as an index of the preload. Within limits, as the preload increases, there is an increase in cardiac performance manifested by an increase in systolic pressure development or the volume of blood ejected. This represents the ascending limb of the familiar Frank-Starling relationship.

This overall relationship is often referred to as a ventricular function curve (Fig. 41–2). Some measure of cardiac performance, such as the stroke volume or stroke work (stroke volume × arterial pressure) is plotted as a function of some measure

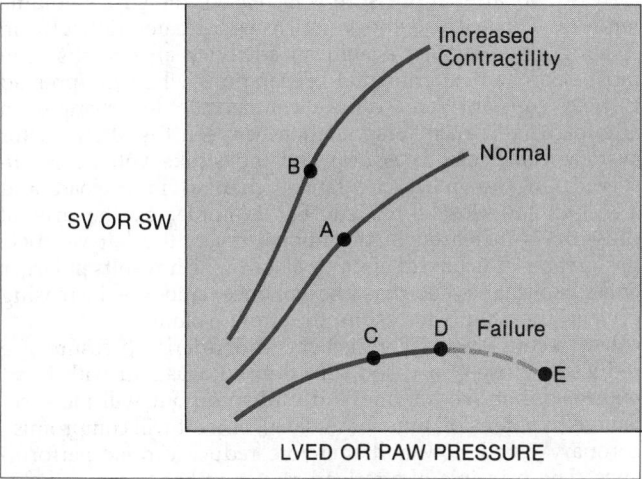

FIGURE 41–2. Left ventricular function curves relating the left ventricular filling pressure to ventricular performance expressed as stroke volume (SV) or stroke work (SW). The filling pressure can be expressed as either the left ventricular end-diastolic (LVED) pressure or the pulmonary artery wedge (PAW) pressure. Curves indicate normal, increased, or depressed ventricular contractility. Points A and B show the effects of a positive inotropic drug, which increases ventricular performance while reducing the filling pressure. See text for further discussion.

of the preload, such as the filling pressure or the end-diastolic pressure. The concept of the ventricular function curve is important, since it allows an objective assessment of the contractility of the ventricles. For example, the normal ventricle has a steep function curve, relatively small changes in end-diastolic pressure producing large changes in performance, whereas the failing ventricle has a downwardly displaced and flattened curve (Fig. 41–2). Such curves can permit a comparison between subjective signs or symptoms and objective measurements. Since the failing left ventricle operates near the peak of its ventricular function curve, the combination of a high filling pressure and low cardiac output (Fig. 41–2, point D) explains the clinical picture of dyspnea and fatigue (see Ch. 43).

An important distinction must be made between the right atrial pressure, which represents the filling pressure of the right ventricle and can be estimated from the jugular veins, and the left atrial pressure, which is the filling pressure of the left ventricle. The mean left atrial pressure can be assessed from the mean pulmonary artery (or "capillary") wedge pressure, often measured by a flow-directed balloon catheter. In manipulating the volume status of the acutely ill patient, except in cases of isolated right ventricular failure, it is preferable to measure the left ventricular filling pressure, because the failing left ventricle usually has a more important role in determining arterial pressure and the forward cardiac output.

The Afterload. Afterload refers to the load against which the ventricle must contract when it ejects blood. In isolated heart muscle, it can be accurately defined as the load (or force) resisting shortening after the muscle is stimulated to contract. In the intact heart, afterload is often estimated as the systolic arterial pressure. A better measure of the afterload is the systolic wall stress, which can be related to the systolic pressure, heart size, and wall thickness through the simplified Laplace relation:

$$\sigma = \frac{PR}{2h}$$

in which σ = wall stress or force/cross-sectional area, P = intraventricular pressure, R = radius of chamber (radius of curvature of the wall), and h = wall thickness.

The effect of afterload on performance is relatively straightforward. As arterial pressure is increased, the stroke volume tends to fall because the ventricle has greater difficulty in ejecting blood against a higher load. Such an effect is seen most clearly in experimental preparations when the preload is held constant (and cannot compensate for changes in afterload), and an inverse relation between the afterload (or systolic ventricular pressure) and the stroke volume is observed. In the intact circulation, changes in preload and afterload are closely related. For example, as the arterial pressure is increased in the normal heart, the left ventricle has greater difficulty in ejecting blood, which results in larger end-systolic and end-diastolic volumes, and the increasing preload then tends to restore the stroke volume.

If systemic vascular resistance and arterial pressure are reduced by use of a vasodilator drug in a patient with heart failure, the stroke volume and cardiac output will increase. Severe hypotension must be avoided, since it will compromise coronary blood flow and therefore reduce cardiac performance. The principle of afterload reduction has become one of the most important concepts in the therapy of both acute and chronic heart failure.

Contractility. The inotropic state, or contractility, refers to the vigor of contraction of heart muscle and is best defined in isolated heart muscle as an increased velocity and extent of shortening when the loading conditions (preload and afterload) do not change. Contractility is altered under normal conditions primarily by reflex release of norepinephrine from adrenergic nerve terminals in the myocardium, as well as by adrenal release of catecholamines during various forms of stress. Drugs such as digitalis increase contractility, whereas hypoxia, ischemia, acidosis, and certain antiarrhythmic agents reduce contractility. In terms of ventricular function curves, drugs that increase contractility shift the curve upward and to the left, increasing stroke volume or stroke work at a given end-diastolic pressure (Fig. 41–2). With depression of contractility, the ventricular function curve shifts down and to the right, with a reduction in stroke volume at a given left ventricular end-diastolic pressure (Fig. 41–2).

Heart Rate. The frequency of contraction is an important determinant of cardiac performance and one of the most important mechanisms available to increase the cardiac output (cardiac output = stroke volume × heart rate), provided the venous return is increased (see below). Increased heart rate has a modest positive inotropic effect, increasing the velocity and extent of shortening while reducing the duration of contraction. During the response to moderate exercise, when the venous return increases, a higher heart rate is mainly responsible for the change in cardiac output, since the increase in stroke volume is relatively small.

The level of the heart rate may be an important indicator of the cardiovascular status of an individual patient. For example, in a patient with acute failure who has a sinus tachycardia of 140 beats per minute, the marked reduction in stroke volume is compensated for by the tachycardia in order to maintain an acceptable cardiac output. Other factors that can raise the resting heart rate must also be considered, including fever, anemia, thyrotoxicosis, and anxiety.

ASSESSMENT OF CARDIAC PERFORMANCE. Quantitative indices of cardiac performance can be measured in the cardiac catheterization laboratory or in critical care units. For reference, normal pressures, cardiac volumes, cardiac output, and vascular resistance are listed in Table 41–1. Volume measurements are normalized to allow interpatient comparison by dividing by the body surface area (square meters), obtained from a standard table based on height and weight. The maximum value of the first derivative of left ventricular pressure during isovolumetric systole (dP/dt) is sometimes used as a measure of contractility. One very useful index of ventricular function is the ejection fraction, which is the stroke volume divided by the end-diastolic volume. A normal ejection fraction of the left ventricle is 0.55 or greater, and in severe heart failure the ejection fraction may be reduced to less than 0.20.

As discussed above, *ventricular function curves* (Fig. 41–2) are often employed to demonstrate changes in inotropic state, whereas changes in preload move the ventricle up and down on a *single* curve. Experimentally, they are produced by progressive infusions of fluid, whereas in the clinical setting often only two points on a curve are available, before and after an intervention.

When two ventricular function curves are compared, they generally are compared at the same level of mean arterial pressure, since, as discussed above, the stroke volume of the ventricle is changed by altered afterload. Hence, decreased afterload would shift the relation between stroke volume and filling pressure upward, and increased afterload would shift the relation downward. In heart failure, such an effect caused by increased blood pressure is sometimes represented as an apparent "descending limb" of function. In such a setting, the preload reserve is exhausted and increased arterial pressure will result in movement from point D to E (Fig. 41–2), whereas lowering the afterload would move the ventricle from E to D, improving stroke volume and cardiac performance.

Venous return and cardiac output curves can be used to represent cardiocirculatory responses under experimental conditions, and although venous return curves cannot be performed in humans, they allow insight into the highly important role of the venous return. The heart behaves as a demand pump, ejecting whatever blood is returned to it under normal conditions, and only in heart failure or when filling is impaired (as in constrictive pericarditis) does the heart itself become the limiting factor for cardiac output. Therefore, the return of blood to the heart (the venous return), which is regulated by a number of mechanical, neural, and humoral factors, through its influence on preload is a key determinant of cardiac performance under normal conditions.

In A.C. Guyton's analysis, cardiac function is represented by a cardiac output curve that intersects a venous return curve at any given-state condition (Fig. 41–3). Noncardiac factors that influence the venous return include the volume of blood in the vascular bed (transfusion shifts the venous return curve upward, whereas bleeding shifts it downward). The position of the venous return curve is also affected by neurohumoral factors, increased sympathetic tone shifting the venous return curve upward and to the right and vice versa; venoconstriction produced by increased sympathetic tone also displaces blood from the peripheral circulation toward the central (cardiopulmonary) circulation, whereas decreased tone to the veins causes pooling of blood in the peripheral circulation. With this framework, changes in *both* cardiac performance and peripheral circulatory regulation (venous return) can be represented as they influence the cardiac output. Positive inotropic interventions, decreased afterload, and other factors shift the cardiac output curve upward, and opposite effects, including heart failure, shift it downward (Fig. 41–3).

The importance of venous return can be illustrated by the response to electrical cardiac pacing to increase the heart rate, a response in which myocardial contractility is increased. Since no significant effects on the peripheral circulation occur, no change in the cardiac output is observed. This response occurs because the normal heart operates near the flat portion of the normal venous return curve (near the point of venous

collapse), and therefore even though the cardiac output curve is shifted upward, the venous return curve is unchanged, and there can be no alteration of the cardiac output (Fig. 41–3, point A to B). The response to exercise using this diagram is discussed subsequently under integrated responses.

REGULATION OF MYOCARDIAL OXYGEN CONSUMPTION

The heart is almost entirely supplied with energy from ATP and creatine phosphate produced by aerobic metabolism, and for practical purposes, the total energy expenditure of the normal heart can be equated with its oxygen consumption. The myocardial oxygen consumption ($\dot{M}\mathrm{V}_{O_2}$) of the left ventricle can be determined using the Fick principle as the product of its coronary blood flow and the arteriovenous oxygen difference, calculated using blood samples from an artery and from the coronary sinus. Since the heart is a continuously active organ, its oxygen consumption is high relative to other organs, and the $\dot{M}\mathrm{V}_{O_2}$ of the normal human left ventricle at rest is approximately 6 to 8 ml per minute per 100 grams.

The determinants of the $\dot{M}\mathrm{V}_{O_2}$ of the heart (most of which is used by the left ventricle) consist of the basal oxygen consumption, which supplies energy for cell maintenance processes including the calcium and sodium pumps, protein synthesis, and so on. The remainder of the oxygen expenditure is controlled by the type of activity that the heart is called upon to perform. The determinants of $\dot{M}\mathrm{V}_{O_2}$ are

1. Basal oxygen requirements
2. Systolic pressure (or wall stress)
3. Heart rate
4. Myocardial contractility (inotropic state)
5. Wall shortening against a load (related to cardiac work)

Systolic pressure, heart rate, and *contractility* are the major determinants of $\dot{M}\mathrm{V}_{O_2}$, whereas shortening of the wall utilizes relatively less oxygen. There is a nearly linear relation between systolic pressure development by the left ventricle and $\dot{M}\mathrm{V}_{O_2}$, and with the Laplace equation, this relation can also be expressed as systolic wall stress versus $\dot{M}\mathrm{V}_{O_2}$. Thus, as systolic pressure doubles, the $\dot{M}\mathrm{V}_{O_2}$ of the left ventricle approximately doubles. There is also a nearly linear relationship between heart rate and the $\dot{M}\mathrm{V}_{O_2}$ and, again, an approximate doubling of the $\dot{M}\mathrm{V}_{O_2}$ occurs as the heart rate increases twofold. If the heart rate and systolic pressure are held constant and a positive inotropic agent is administered, a rather marked increase in $\dot{M}\mathrm{V}_{O_2}$ can be demonstrated, associated with a pronounced increase in the velocity of shortening and some increase in the extent of myocardial fiber shortening. It is possible that this extra energy expenditure is related, at least in part, to increased oxygen use by the calcium sequestration mechanism of the sarcoplasmic reticulum. Decreased contractility of the myocardium has been shown to cause a reduction of $\dot{M}\mathrm{V}_{O_2}$.

The oxygen cost of myocardial fiber shortening against a load is relatively low. This is exemplified by experiments in which the systolic arterial pressure was elevated while the cardiac output and heart rate were held constant, and a marked stimulation of $\dot{M}\mathrm{V}_{O_2}$ was produced, whereas if the cardiac output was increased over a wide range while the arterial pressure and heart rate were constant, only small changes in $\dot{M}\mathrm{V}_{O_2}$ occurred. These findings indicate a high oxygen cost of "pressure work" and a relatively low oxygen cost of "volume work." The importance of heart rate and systolic pressure has resulted in the use of simplified indices of $\dot{M}\mathrm{V}_{O_2}$, such as the heart rate × blood pressure (the "double product"). In clinical studies, this provides a means of estimating the effect of an antianginal drug (such as a beta blocker) on cardiac oxygen requirements during exercise.

The fact that myocardial energy expenditure, expressed as $\dot{M}\mathrm{V}_{O_2}$, is closely linked to mechanical cardiac performance

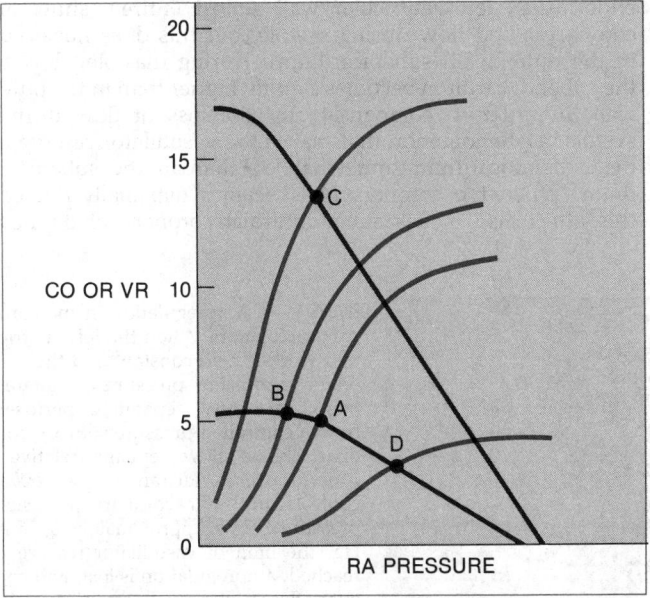

FIGURE 41–3. Relationship between the filling pressure of the heart, expressed as the right atrial (RA) pressure, and either cardiac output (CO) or venous return (VR). Venous return curves are represented as an inverse relation between the cardiac output or venous return and the right atrial pressure; the lower curve represents normal conditions and the upper curve shows the effect of marked sympathetic stimulation during exercise. The series of cardiac output curves shows a positive relation between right atrial pressure and cardiac function. Any steady-state condition is represented by the intersection of these two curves. Shown are normal conditions (A), electrical pacing of the heart (B), severe exercise (C), and heart failure (D). See text for further discussion.

carries important implications in various disease states. For example, in valvular heart disease, chronic mitral regurgitation places a large volume overload on the heart due to the low impedance backward leak into the left atrium. In this condition, the systolic left ventricular pressure is not elevated, and since the left ventricle is performing extra "volume work," the $\dot{M}O_2$ of the left ventricle is not significantly increased. Therefore, in the absence of coronary artery disease, oxygen supply-demand imbalance and angina pectoris are rarely seen in chronic mitral regurgitation. In contrast, in patients with aortic stenosis, the high left ventricular systolic pressures with elevated $\dot{M}O_2$ of the entire chamber can lead to reduction of coronary vasodilator reserve. Therefore, subendocardial ischemia with angina pectoris is quite common in aortic stenosis, particularly during exercise or when left ventricular failure is beginning to occur, even in the absence of coronary artery disease. Of course, in chronic coronary artery disease, during exercise virtually all of the major determinants of $\dot{M}O_2$ are augmented, and in the presence of a stenosed coronary artery with impaired vasodilator reserve, coronary blood flow cannot keep pace with enhanced oxygen demands, and regional myocardial ischemia with angina pectoris occurs (see Ch. 51.1).

REGULATION OF CORONARY BLOOD FLOW

In keeping with the high energy requirements of the normal myocardium, coronary blood flow is relatively high, averaging 60 to 90 ml per minute per 100 grams in the normal human left ventricle when an individual is at rest. Extraction of oxygen by the heart is the highest of any organ, so that little additional oxygen extraction can occur during stress. This means that changes in oxygen demand of the heart are met chiefly by alterations in oxygen supply through changes in coronary blood flow, reflected by a nearly linear positive relation between the $\dot{M}O_2$ and the coronary blood flow. Although cardiac metabolism is the main determinant of coronary blood flow, several additional factors can be of importance:

1. $\dot{M}O_2$
2. Coronary perfusion pressure
3. Systolic compression
4. Alpha-adrenergic tone to the coronary arteries (or exogenous vasoconstrictors)
5. Vasodilators (epinephrine, exogenous vasodilator substances)

Since the $\dot{M}O_2$ is influence by each of the major determinants of cardiac performance, coronary blood flow is altered in the appropriate direction. There is evidence that release of the ATP metabolite adenosine, a potent coronary vasodilator, is involved in some of the responses of the coronary blood flow to altered cardiac performance and metabolism, although a number of other stimuli to vasodilation (such as decreased PO_2, decreased pH, and increased K^+ during enhanced metabolic activity) may also be important.

Under normal conditions, the mean coronary perfusion pressure is not a major determinant of coronary blood flow, except as it affects the systolic arterial pressure and therefore the $\dot{M}O_2$. Of course, on a moment-to-moment basis, the phasic pattern of coronary blood flow to the left ventricle shows a slow fall during diastole as the aortic pressure falls, as well as a sharp drop during systole as the squeezing action of the left ventricular wall compresses the intramural vessels and shuts down coronary blood flow, particularly to the subendocardial layers. However, the mean flow has been shown to be independent of the mean coronary perfusion pressure within certain limits, a phenomenon termed "autoregulation." Studies in which the coronary arteries are perfused *separately* from the aorta show that between mean coronary perfusion pressures of about 60 mm Hg and 150 mm Hg coronary blood flow is maintained constant, provided that the $\dot{M}O_2$ of the heart does not change (Fig. 41–4). When the coronary perfusion pressure drops below 60 mm Hg, the coronary bed reaches the limit of autoregulation and tends to become fully dilated; at that point, perfusion pressure becomes the major determinant of coronary blood flow, and flow will drop as pressure falls below that value with an exponential relation between pressure and flow typical of a passive blood vessel (Fig. 41–4). Obviously, in coronary artery disease the coronary perfusion pressure can become extremely important, since the perfusion pressure beyond an area of stenosis may be relatively low.

Systolic compression of coronary vessels in the inner (subendocardial) left ventricular wall almost entirely shuts off coronary blood flow during systole, but this does not occur in the outer wall (subepicardium). During diastole, flow to the subendocardium becomes slightly higher than in the outer wall, in order to compensate for the loss of flow during systole, a phenomenon that makes the vasodilator reserve in the subendocardium somewhat *less* than in the subepicardium. When the coronary bed becomes maximally dilated, this effect also makes subendocardial coronary blood flow

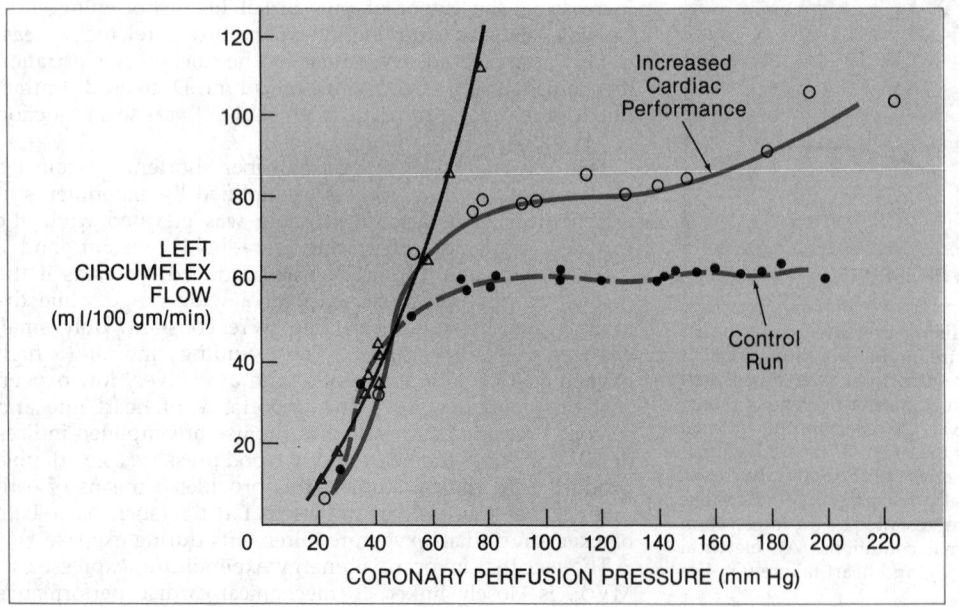

FIGURE 41–4. Autoregulation in the coronary circulation. When the left ventricular work is held constant and the coronary perfusion pressure is altered (coronary artery separately perfused from a controlled pressure source), coronary blood flow remains relatively constant over a wide range (*closed circles*, control run). At a coronary perfusion pressure below approximately 60 mm Hg, the limit of vasodilator reserve is reached, autoregulation is lost, and coronary flow is directly determined by the coronary perfusion pressure. The pressure-flow relation then falls on a curve of maximum vasodilation (passive pressure-flow curve of a distensible blood vessel, *open triangles*). Coronary blood flow is regulated at a higher level when cardiac performance and hence $\dot{M}O_2$ are increased (*open circles*, increased cardiac performance). (Adapted from West JB (ed): Best and Taylor's Physiological Basis of Medical Practice. 11th ed. Baltimore, Williams & Wilkins Co., 1985).

highly dependent upon the time available for diastolic perfusion. For example, if heart rate increases under such circumstances, systolic time per minute is increased at the expense of diastolic time, and coronary flow will fall. This can occur in coronary artery disease, when, during exercise, the heart rate increases and coronary blood flow consequentially falls beyond an area of coronary stenosis (decreased oxygen supply), in the face of increased oxygen demands. Beta-adrenergic blockade is often used to treat angina pectoris in this setting (Ch. 51.1).

Alpha-adrenergic constrictor influences on the coronary vascular bed have been demonstrated. Although such an effect is of relatively minor significance under normal conditions, under certain circumstances of reflex activation it can be of great significance. There is recent evidence that under conditions of exercise-induced ischemia, alpha-adrenergic coronary vasoconstrictor tone exists and can be reduced by vasodilators or by alpha-adrenergic blockade.

A variety of substances can relax the smooth muscle of coronary arteries, including nitroglycerin and calcium channel blockers, and these are used to treat angina due to coronary artery spasm, as well as exercise-induced angina pectoris. Certain prostaglandins and agents such as vasopressin and ergonovine are coronary vasoconstrictors.

REGULATION OF THE PERIPHERAL CIRCULATION

The heart pumps blood sequentially through the pulmonary and systemic circulations. Throughout the circulation, the small arterioles provide the main site for vascular resistance regulation. The normal distribution of peripheral blood flow at rest is shown in Figure 41–5. There is a wide variability in cardiac output distribution and in oxygen extraction by various organs; for example, the kidneys have a high blood flow (20 per cent of the cardiac output) and a low oxygen extraction, whereas the coronary circulation has a lower flow but a much higher oxygen extraction (Fig. 41–5). The large conduit arteries have a high velocity of blood flow (aorta = 31 cm per second), whereas in the capillaries, the enormous total cross-sectional area results in marked slowing of blood flow (0.05 cm per second), allowing exchange of metabolites. The veins contain 75 to 80 per cent of the total blood volume in the circulation and serve a capacitance function, i.e., as a blood volume reservoir.

The general organization of the systemic circulation is such that the arterial bed serves as a pressure reservoir from which the circulations to the various organs operate in parallel (Fig. 41–5). Thus, each organ takes the blood supply that it requires by regulating its *local* vascular resistance primarily on the basis of metabolic needs (autoregulation, as discussed earlier for the coronary circulation), whereas the *total* peripheral vascular resistance (TPVR) is primarily controlled by cardiovascular reflexes and maintains the pressure in the arteries. Thus, the blood pressure, which equals the product of the cardiac output and the TPVR (blood pressure = cardiac output × TPVR), is protected by the reflexes. For example, during exercise the vascular resistance in exercising skeletal muscles decreases markedly, and despite the increase in cardiac output, the blood pressure might fall were it not for a reflex increase in vascular resistance in nonexercising muscles and certain other areas.

REFLEX NEURAL CONTROL. The autonomic nervous system and certain neurohumoral factors maintain circulatory homeostasis through regulation of the heart rate, myocardial contractility, vascular tone in the arterioles and small veins, and the blood volume (discussed in a subsequent section).

The high-pressure baroreceptors, which sense stretch in the walls of arteries, are located in the carotid sinuses and aortic

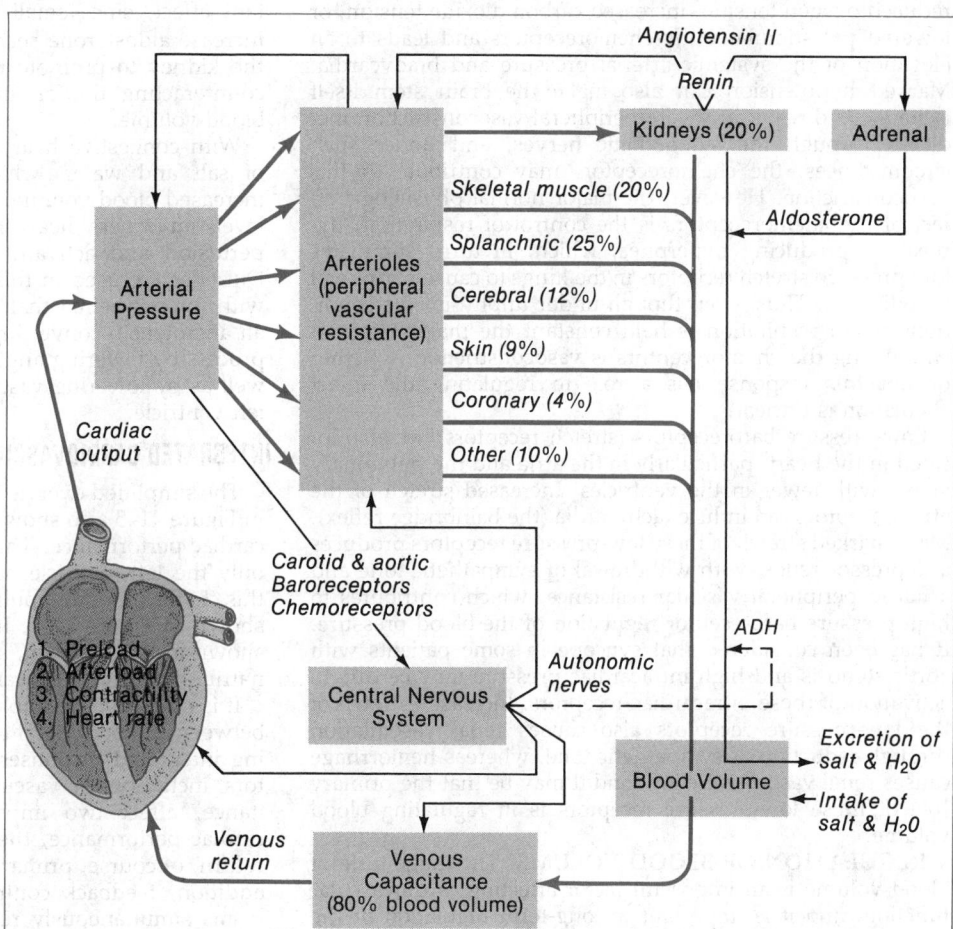

FIGURE 41–5. Schematic representation of the circulatory system. See text for details.

arch. They increase their afferent impulse traffic when the blood pressure rises, and vice versa, and these nerve impulses pass through the cardiovascular regulatory centers in the medulla, which alter the relative magnitude of efferent vagal and sympathetic impulses. For example, as arterial pressure is increased, the enhanced impulse traffic stimulates the vagus to slow the heart rate and simultaneously inhibits the cardioaccelerator center. Simultaneously, the vasoconstrictor center is also inhibited, reducing sympathetic tone to the peripheral arterioles and also lowering venous tone. Thus, the reduced peripheral vascular resistance and venous return, together with the slowed heart rate, lower the increased blood pressure toward its previous level. With a decrease in blood pressure, as with moderate bleeding, this reflex arc would reduce vagal tone and enhance sympathetic tone, both of which would cause the heart rate to increase, which, together with increased myocardial contractility and venous tone, would increase the cardiac output, whereas increased arteriolar tone would enhance peripheral vascular resistance. All of these factors would rapidly restore the lowered blood pressure toward its previous level. With a significant drop in blood pressure, reflex release of catecholamines from the adrenal glands also occurs.

Reflex control of the heart and circulation is also under the influence of higher brain centers, as when marked emotional stress activates the sympathetic nervous system. Such central stimulation, as well as reflex activation of the sympathetic nervous system via receptors in the exercising skeletal muscle, produce the marked sympathetic stimulation of exercise. At rest, there appears to be little sympathetic tone affecting heart rate or myocardial contractility, and the heart rate is primarily under the control of parasympathetic influences.

Chemoreceptors lying in the carotid bodies near the carotid bifurcation and in the aortic arch respond to changes in pH, P_{CO_2}, and P_{O_2}. When ventilation is controlled experimentally, reduced oxygen tension, increased carbon dioxide tension, or lowered pH stimulates the chemoreceptors and leads to an elevation of the systemic arterial pressure and bradycardia. Marked hypotension can also make the brain stem itself ischemic and result in severe peripheral vasoconstriction mediated through the sympathetic nerves, and under such circumstances, the chemoreceptors may contribute to this vasoconstriction. However, the major normal physiologic effect of the chemoreceptors is the control of respiration, hypoxemia producing hyperpnea, which, in turn, stimulates low-pressure stretch receptors in the lungs to cause peripheral vasodilation. Thus, even though under unphysiologic conditions when respiration is held constant the major effect of stimulating the chemoreceptors is vasoconstriction, whether or not this response has a role in regulating the intact circulation is unclear.

Low-pressure baroreceptors (stretch receptors) are also located in the heart, particularly in the atria and the pulmonary veins, with fewer in the ventricles. Increased stretch of the atrial receptors can induce tachycardia (the Bainbridge reflex). More marked stretch of these low-pressure receptors produces a depressor reflex, with withdrawal of sympathetic tone and a fall in peripheral vascular resistance, which contributes to high-pressure baroreceptor regulation of the blood pressure. It has been considered that syncope in some patients with aortic stenosis and high intracardiac pressure may be due to activation of these intracardiac receptors. Increased stretch of the low-pressure receptors also causes renal vasodilation through reduction of sympathetic tone, whereas hemorrhage causes renal vasoconstriction, and it may be that the primary role of these low-pressure receptors is in regulating blood volume.

REGULATION OF BLOOD VOLUME. The magnitude of blood volume is an important factor affecting cardiovascular function, and it is important in long-term regulation of the blood pressure. Some of the factors involved in the maintenance of extracellular fluid and blood volume are listed on the right-hand side of Figure 41–5. Loss of fluid volume occurs primarily through the kidneys, whereas sweating, respiratory, and gastrointestinal losses are less important (except during extreme conditions). Since approximately 20 per cent of the resting cardiac output passes through the kidneys, they provide an ideal location for regulating sodium and water balance. In addition, the hypothalamic osmoreceptors that regulate thirst and antidiuretic hormone (ADH) secretion are of great importance. Since these subjects are discussed in detail in Ch. 77, only selected cardiovascular factors are mentioned here.

An increase in blood volume, as might occur by increased intake of salt and water, would increase the cardiac output. This, in turn, would tend to raise arterial pressure and renal perfusion and thus augment urine output, which would then decrease blood volume back toward normal. Atrial receptors sensitive to stretch are responsible for vasodilating reflexes to the kidneys, as mentioned, and atrial receptors also reflexly stimulate the central nervous system to diminish the secretion of ADH. These factors would tend to increase the output of urine and sodium excretion. A decrease in effective blood volume would have opposite effects.

An additional highly important control mechanism for the regulation of arterial pressure and blood volume is the renin-angiotensin system (see Ch. 47). Reduction in renal perfusion (reduced pressure and flow) is sensed by the juxtaglomerular apparatus, which releases renin, whereas increased effective blood volume shuts off the stimulus for renin release. (This response forms the basis for alterations in sodium intake and volume as provocative tests for altering renin levels.) Renin enzymatically promotes the formation of angiotensin I from a precursor in the bloodstream, which is then converted to angiotensin II by the converting enzyme. Angiotensin II is a powerful vasoconstrictor, but this may not be its most important effect, since small subpressor doses of angiotensin II increase aldosterone secretion. Aldosterone, in turn, acts on the kidney to promote retention of salt and water, thereby counteracting the original stimulus of decreased effective blood volume.

With congestive heart failure, there is increased retention of salt and water, which leads to edema formation and increased blood volume. There may be increased aldosterone levels in severe heart failure secondary to reduced renal perfusion and activation of the renin-angiotensin system. Diuretics are used in this setting, and in severe heart failure with hyponatremia that is unresponsive to diuretics, use of an angiotensin-converting enzyme inhibitor may reverse this process by lowering angiotensin II and aldosterone levels, as well as by lowering vascular resistance and afterload on the left ventricle.

INTEGRATED CARDIOVASCULAR RESPONSES

The simplified overview of the circulatory system illustrated in Figure 41–5 also shows the four factors directly influencing cardiac performance. These factors affect performance of not only the left ventricle but also the right ventricle, although this chamber and the pulmonary circulation are not separately shown in Figure 41–5. In addition, a number of factors not shown in this diagram, such as the prostaglandins and atrial natriuretic factor, also can affect overall circulatory function.

It is important to emphasize the significance of interactions between the peripheral circulation and the heart in considering integrated responses. Certain peripheral circulatory factors, including the vascular resistance and the venous capacitance, affect two important mechanical determinants of cardiac performance, the preload and the afterload. Venous return, of course, primarily determines the cardiac output. In addition, feedback control by neurohumoral reflex mechanisms simultaneously regulates both the heart and the peripheral circulation.

CHANGES IN VENOUS RETURN. Changing from the supine or sitting to a standing position causes venous blood to pool in the distensible veins of the abdomen and lower extremities, leading to an immediate drop in the venous return and cardiac output and in the blood pressure. However, prompt action of cardiovascular reflexes via the baroreceptor mechanism causes an increase in vascular resistance, tending to restore the blood pressure toward normal, and further stimulates restoration of the cardiac output by sympathetic reflexes, which enhance the heart rate and the contractility of the myocardium. A more marked stimulus, the Valsalva maneuver, which is useful in the physical diagnosis of heart murmurs, causes a marked decrease in the venous return to the heart because of the abrupt elevation of intrathoracic pressure, and after 15 to 20 seconds, the associated drop in blood pressure produces reflex tachycardia and increased myocardial contractility. During this phase of the maneuver, cardiac murmurs associated with blood flow across a narrowed valve, such as that of aortic stenosis, diminish in intensity because of the reduced cardiac output, whereas the murmur associated with hypertrophic cardiomyopathy increases owing to the reduced heart size and increased contractility.

Vasodilator drugs that have a considerable venodilating effect, such as nitroglycerin and nitroprusside, can have different effects on the cardiac output in the normal circulation and in congestive heart failure. Thus, in the normal circulation the cardiac output falls with nitroprusside, since the venous return curve is shifted downward as blood volume is displaced from the central circulation and pooled in the peripheral veins (decreased effective blood volume), whereas during cardiac failure, the associated unloading of the left ventricle by the arteriolar-dilating action of this drug releases blood from the central circulation, which counterbalances the drug's venodilator effect; therefore, the venous return curve is not shifted downward, and the marked shift upward of the cardiac output curve owing to reduced afterload results in an increased cardiac output (Fig. 41–3, D to A).

It is also important to note that certain chronic cardiac conditions can limit the venous return to the heart because of impaired cardiac filling. These include chronic constrictive pericarditis and restrictive cardiomyopathy.

CHANGES IN HEART RATE. The lack of effect on cardiac output of changing heart rate by electrical pacing over a wide range has been previously discussed (see Fig. 41–5). But the usual increases in heart rate that occur as a component of cardiocirculatory reflex responses are ordinarily accompanied by increased myocardial contractility, venoconstriction, and an increased cardiac output. Below a certain level of heart rate, as in complete heart block with a ventricular rate of 40 beats per minute, the resting cardiac output may not be maintained, since the stroke volume is maximal (preload reserve fully utilized) and the ventricular output becomes rate limited. In addition, with marked resting tachycardia (approaching 200 beats per minute or more), as in paroxysmal atrial or ventricular arrhythmias, the available diastolic filling time is shortened because of the increased number of contractions per minute, and inadequate ventricular filling leads to a fall in the cardiac output. The loss of an appropriately timed atrial contraction in some dysrhythmias may further contribute to inadequate cardiac filling.

EXERCISE. Many mechanisms can come into play to cause the increased cardiac output that accompanies normal exercise. In individuals with some degree of physical training, the heart rate is lowered both at rest and with exercise, and during low levels of exercise, increased stroke volume, combined with a mild increase in heart rate, augments the cardiac output. With marked exercise, as sympathetic stimulation and circulating catecholamine levels increase, the increased venous return causes further utilization of the Frank-Starling mechanism, and the stroke volume is further enhanced as

increased myocardial contractility augments the ejection fraction. However, the most important cardiac mechanism allowing a very high cardiac output during intense exercise in such individuals is augmented heart rate, which may reach 180 beats per minute or higher. Increased myocardial contractility combines with decreased total peripheral vascular resistance (caused by marked vasodilation in the exercising muscles) to shift the cardiac output curve upward (Fig. 41–5).

In addition, increased sympathetic tone shifts the venous return curve upward, and it is steepened by decreased venous and arteriolar resistance (Fig. 41–5). Therefore, the intersection of the venous return and cardiac output curves occurs at a markedly increased cardiac output, with only a mild elevation of the right atrial pressure (Fig. 41–5, point C). Thus, both peripheral and circulatory adaptations are involved in the exercise response.

Braunwald E (ed.): Heart Disease: A Textbook of Cardiovascular Medicine. 2nd ed. Philadelphia, W.B. Saunders Company, 1984, pp 409–466. *Up-to-date review of cardiac performance from the cellular level to the intact heart. Also includes the pathophysiology of heart failure.*
Guyton AC: Circulation Physiology: Cardiac Output and Its Regulation. Philadelphia, W.B. Saunders Company, 1963. *Classic text on the importance of venous return and the relationship between venous return and cardiac output.*
Ross J Jr: Cardiac function and myocardial contractility: A perspective. J Am Coll Cardiol 1:52, 1983. *Current concepts concerning left ventricular function under normal and abnormal loading conditions, including heart failure and valvular heart disease.*
West JB (ed.): Best and Taylor's Physiological Basis of Medical Practice. 11th ed. Baltimore, Williams & Wilkins Company, 1985, pp 207–262. *Basic physiology text that assumes little advanced knowledge. Pathophysiologic examples are concerned with cardiac function, circulatory control, myocardial oxygen consumption, and coronary circulation.*

42 SPECIALIZED DIAGNOSTIC PROCEDURES

42.1 Radiography of the Heart

Charles E. Putman

The standard posteroanterior (PA) and lateral chest radiographs are the most frequently used imaging procedures in evaluating the heart. The examination is simple to perform and requires relatively inexpensive equipment and very little technical expertise. The advantages of chest radiographs in the evaluation of the cardiac patient are as follows: (1) an experienced observer may detect significant abnormalities not available by other noninvasive methods; (2) recognized abnormalities may be followed, and response to therapy can be documented; and (3) results are easily reproducible, and the radiograph provides a reliable comparative index to changing pathology or alteration of normal cardiovascular function.

TECHNIQUE

There is considerable variation in the configuration of the normal cardiac silhouette. The two most important factors influencing cardiac size and shape are (1) thoracic cavity dimensions and symmetry of the musculoskeletal structure and (2) intrathoracic pulmonary pressure. As the diaphragm descends during normal inspiration, the heart will become smaller and more vertical and conversely during expiration the heart will be larger and more transverse. If the radiograph is exposed during a Valsalva maneuver, there will be a decrease in heart size because of decreased venous return secondary to increased intrathoracic pressure. Variation of technical factors from one examination to another may be responsible for misinterpretation of cardiac dimensions.

INTERPRETATION

To evaluate the cardiovascular status adequately, a systematic approach to reading the standard PA and lateral radiographs is necessary (Figs. 42–1 and 42–2). In addition to evaluating the heart, one should study the great vessels, the pulmonary vascularity, the pleura, the bones, the abdominal viscera, and the extrathoracic structures that may provide useful clues to diagnosis. It is necessary to know which chambers and vascular structures contribute to the cardiac boundaries in the two standard views (Figs. 42–1 to 42–4). When there is suggestive evidence of heart disease, two additional views, the right and left anterior oblique views, may be obtained (Figs. 42–5 and 42–6). These four radiographs are called "the cardiac series" and are usually obtained following the swallowing of barium sulfate to outline and distend the esophagus. Encroachment on the esophageal column by enlarged or displaced cardiac chambers can then be more easily ascertained and the appropriate differential diagnosis facilitated. The value of these views in defining specific cardiac pathology is illustrated in Figures 42–7 to 42–10.

HEART SIZE. Cardiac enlargement is the single most important observation in the suspect cardiac patient, and yet it can be a difficult assessment from the chest radiograph. Various measurements of heart size have been suggested, but the most reliable is a nomogram published by Ungerleider and Gubner. A series of tables indicates predicted normal transverse cardiac diameter for adults of various heights and weights. In actual practice, these tables are rarely used, and instead the cardiothoracic ratio is employed. This measurement is determined by dividing the maximal transverse diameter of the heart by the maximal transverse diameter of the thorax on the PA radiograph. The normal cardiothoracic ratio averages 0.45, but values up to 0.55 may be seen in normal subjects with a greater than average stroke volume. Measurements from the chest radiographs (Figs. 42–1 and 42–2), like other measurements in medicine, are only statisti-

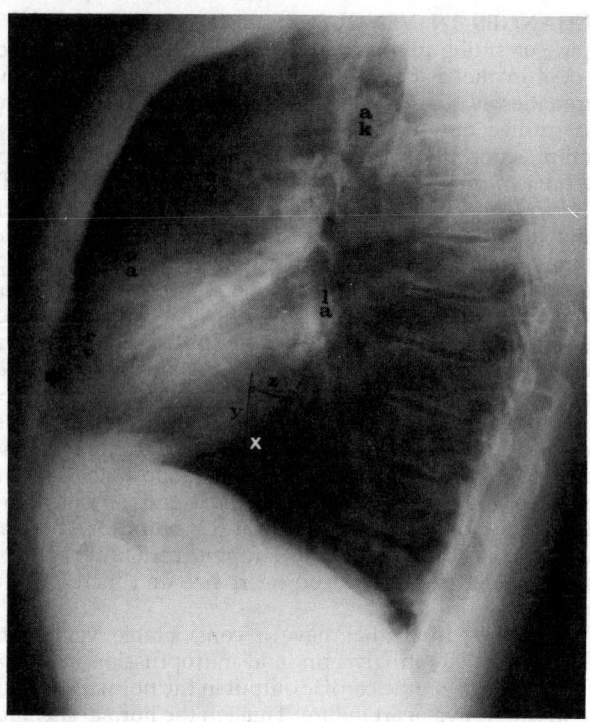

FIGURE 42–2. Normal lateral view. x = The crossing point between the inferior vena cava and the posterior border of the left ventricle; y = distance from point x, 2 cm cephalad along the inferior vena cava; z = posterior dimension of the left ventricle (according to Hoffman and Rigler), which should be smaller than 1.8 cm. Other abbreviations are as in Figure 42–3. Arrow points to the removal position of the subpericardial fat line (very close to the sternum).

cally reliable when applied to subgroups and are therefore less consistent for a given individual. Radiographic cardiac measurements are most meaningful when they can be compared with measurements from previous radiographs of similar quality and technique. Solitary chamber enlargement without cardiomegaly is usually better delineated by the electrocardiogram or echocardiogram than by the radiograph.

PULMONARY VESSELS. Following the determination of cardiac size and chamber predominance, an evaluation of the pulmonary vessels allows for a more precise differential diagnosis. There are four basic patterns of abnormal pulmonary circulation identified by the standard radiograph. Certain groups of diseases may be identified on the basis of (1) decreased flow, (2) increased flow, (3) increased pulmonary resistance, or (4) pulmonary venous hypertension. Each has a specific radiographic pattern that allows for discrimination.

With *decreased pulmonary flow* (e.g., tetralogy of Fallot) there is a decrease in size of the central and peripheral vessels. *Increased pulmonary flow* is indicative of high output states (e.g., hyperthyroidism) or more commonly of left-to-right shunts (e.g., atrial septal defect). With small shunts, no abnormality may be detected by the standard radiograph. Larger shunts cause enlargement and tortuosity of the central and peripheral vessels (Fig. 42–7). Increased pulmonary resistance or *pulmonary arterial hypertension* is identified by dilatation of the central vessels and narrowing or attenuation of the peripheral vessels. *Pulmonary venous hypertension* is a more common hemodynamic state and is usually due to mitral stenosis or left ventricular failure. In upright humans 60 to 70 per cent of the blood flow normally goes to the lower portion of the chest. This can be appreciated on the standard PA radiograph by visualizing larger vessels at the lung bases than in the upper zones of the lung. Pulmonary venous hypertension produced by increased resistance distal to the pulmonary capillaries causes distention and recruitment of upper lobe vessels because of diversion of blood from the constricted

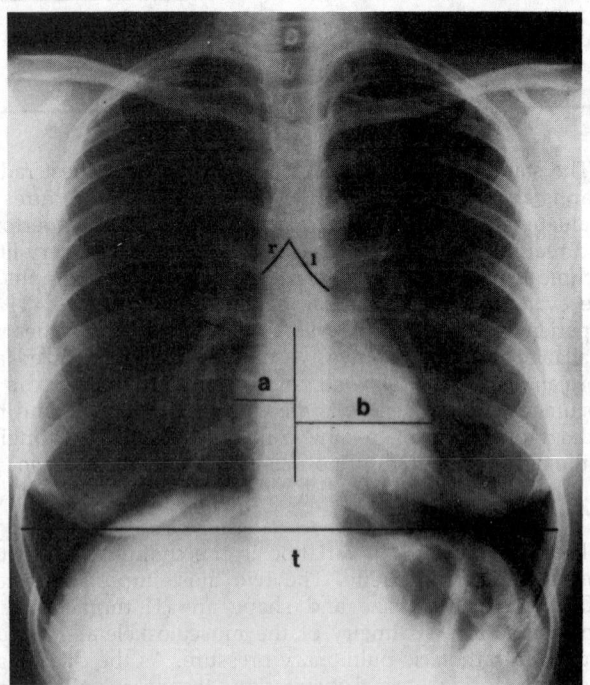

FIGURE 42–1. Normal PA view: a = Transverse diameter of the heart to the right of the midline; b = transverse diameter of the heart to the left of the midline; t = transverse diameter of the thorax; l = lower margin of the left stem bronchus; r = lower margin of the right stem bronchus. The measurements of the right descending pulmonary artery (*arrow*) are 10 to 15 mm for males and 9 to 14 mm for females. The maximal normal angle between the two bronchi is 75 degrees for adults in deep inspiration. The cardiothoracic ratio = a + b/t.

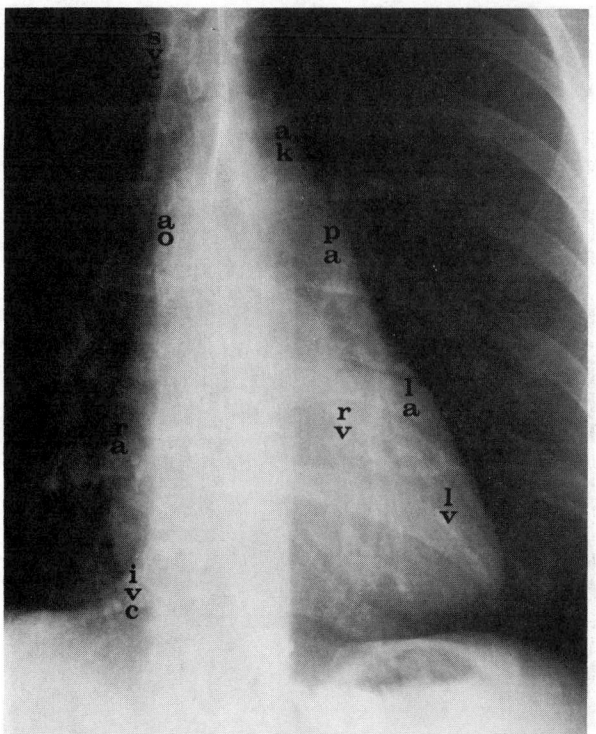

FIGURE 42–3. PA view of the chest with barium in the esophagus. The major border-forming cardiovascular structures are marked as follows: ak = aortic knob (the arch joining the transverse and descending portions of the thoracic aorta); pa = pulmonary artery (the pulmonary trunk); la = left atrium; lv = left ventricle; rv = right ventricle (left lateral border); ivc = inferior vena cava; ra = right atrium; ao = ascending aorta; svc = superior vena cava.

lower zones. Radiographically, this produces an equalization of vascular caliber between the upper and lower lobes. As left atrial pressure increases, upper lobe vessels become larger than lower lobe vessels (Fig. 42–11A). The ability of the radiograph to detect these subtle changes in left atrial pressure is an adequate indication to obtain chest radiographs period-

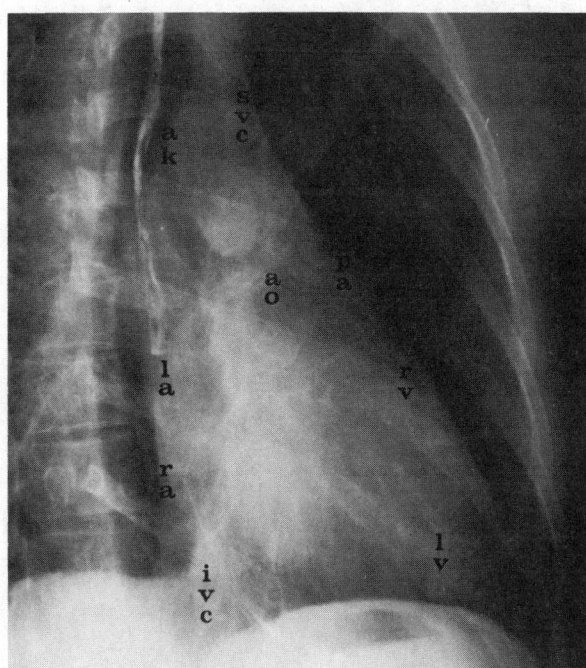

FIGURE 42–5. Forty-five degree right anterior oblique (RAO) view with barium in the esophagus. Abbreviations are as in Figure 42–3.

ically in patients who are prone to heart failure, e.g., the hypertensive patient.

HEART FAILURE. Other radiologic signs of incipient congestive heart failure may not be so obvious. When the pulmonary venous pressure exceeds 20 mm Hg, fluid will begin to accumulate in the interstitium of the lung. Radiographically, this is detected by the appearance of Kerley's B lines (edema of interlobular septa), which are thin horizontal reticular lines seen most often in the costophrenic angles (Fig. 42–11B). Also, the hilar structures may be indistinct and the peripheral vessel margins hazy. As the pulmonary venous pressure exceeds 30 mm Hg, alveolar edema and pleural effusion appear—classic radiographic signs of congestive heart failure.

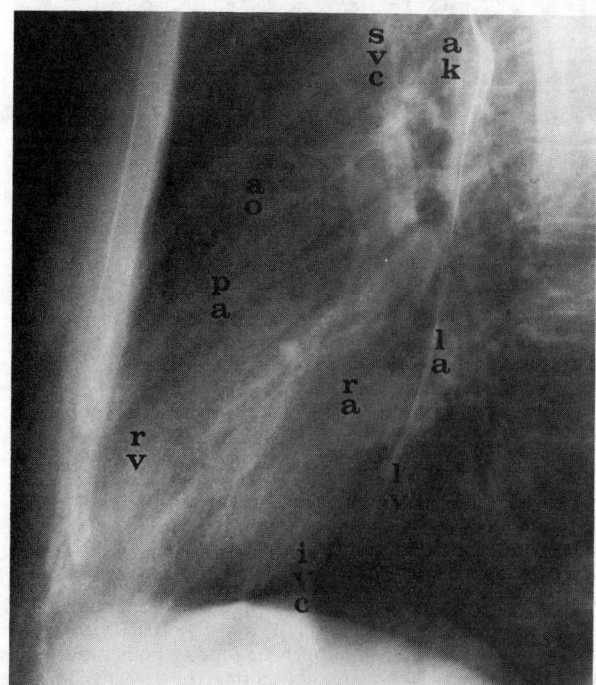

FIGURE 42–4. Left lateral view of the chest with barium in the esophagus. Abbreviations are as in Figure 42–3.

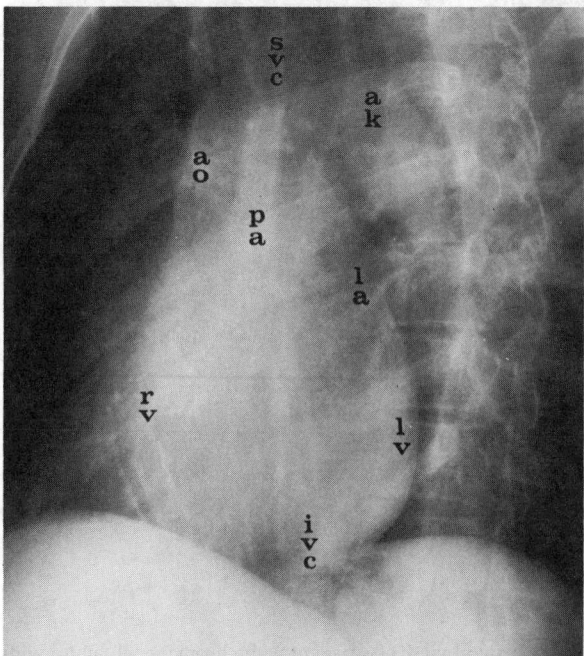

FIGURE 42–6. Sixty degree left anterior oblique (LAO) view without barium in the esophagus. Abbreviations are as in Figure 42–3.

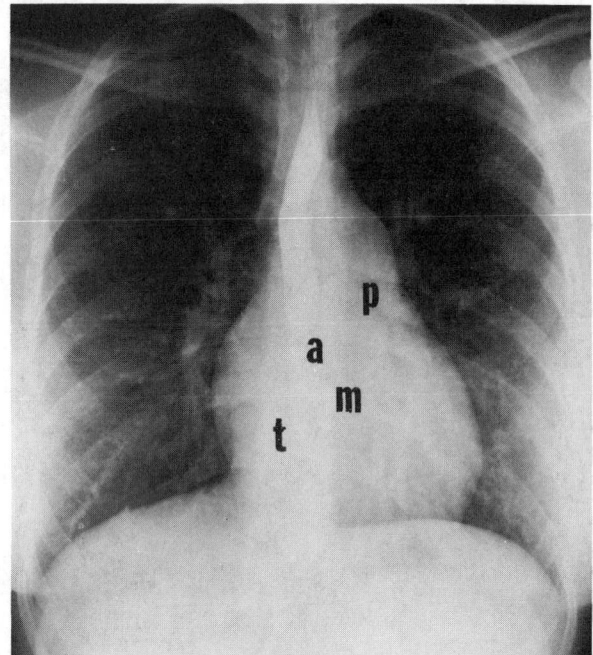

FIGURE 42–7. PA view of a patient with secundum atrial septal defect showing bilateral increase in pulmonary vascularity, right-sided cardiomegaly, marked dilatation of the pulmonary trunk, and an inconspicuous aortic knob. There is no deviation of the barium-filled esophagus or double density to suggest left atrial enlargement. The four cardiac valve positions are marked as follows: a = aortic valve; m = mitral valve; p = pulmonic valve; t = tricuspid valve.

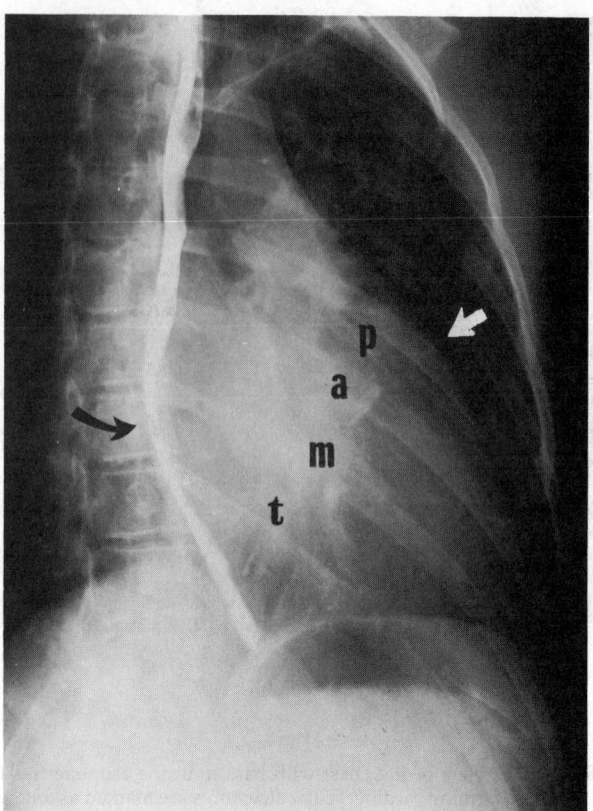

FIGURE 42–9. RAO view of a patient with mitral stenosis. Note that the barium-filled esophagus is deviated posteriorly by the enlarged left atrium (*curved arrow*). The right ventricular enlargement presents as an anterior bulge along the upper cardiac border (*straight arrow*). The four cardiac valve positions in this view are designated as in Figure 42–7.

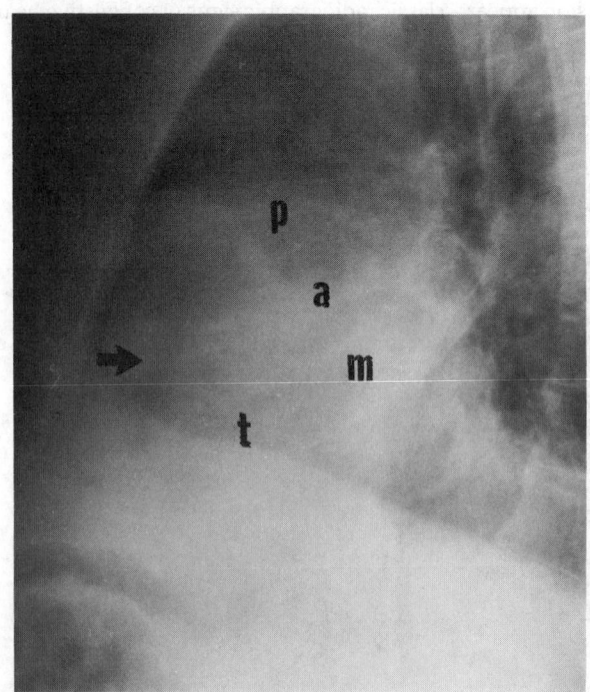

FIGURE 42–8. Lateral view of a patient with chronic renal failure with a large pericardial effusion showing marked posterior displacement of the subepicardial fat line (*arrow*). The four valve positions are marked in the same manner as in the PA view (Fig. 42–7).

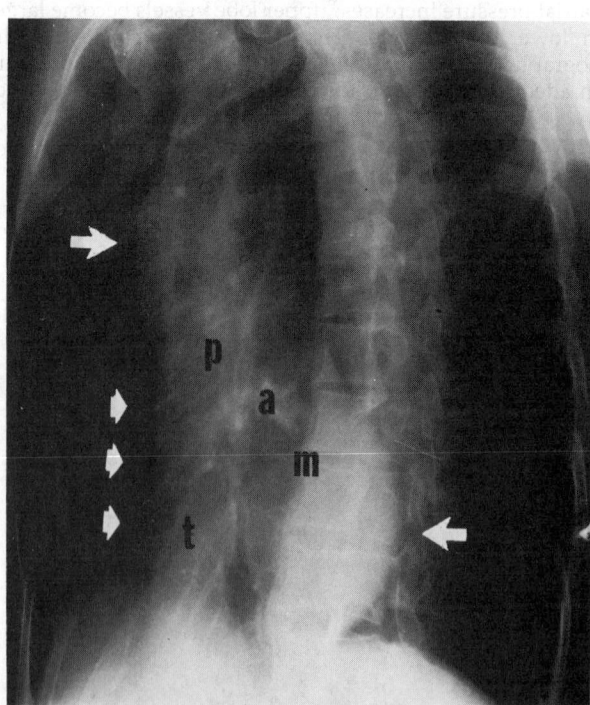

FIGURE 42–10. LAO view of a patient with aortic valve stenosis. The four valve positions are labeled as in Figure 42–7. Heavy aortic valve calcification is visible (a). The upper long arrow points to the post-stenotic dilatation of the ascending aorta. The hypertrophied left ventricle is marked by the lower long arrow posteriorly. The three short arrows point to the left anterior cardiac border formed by the normal right ventricle.

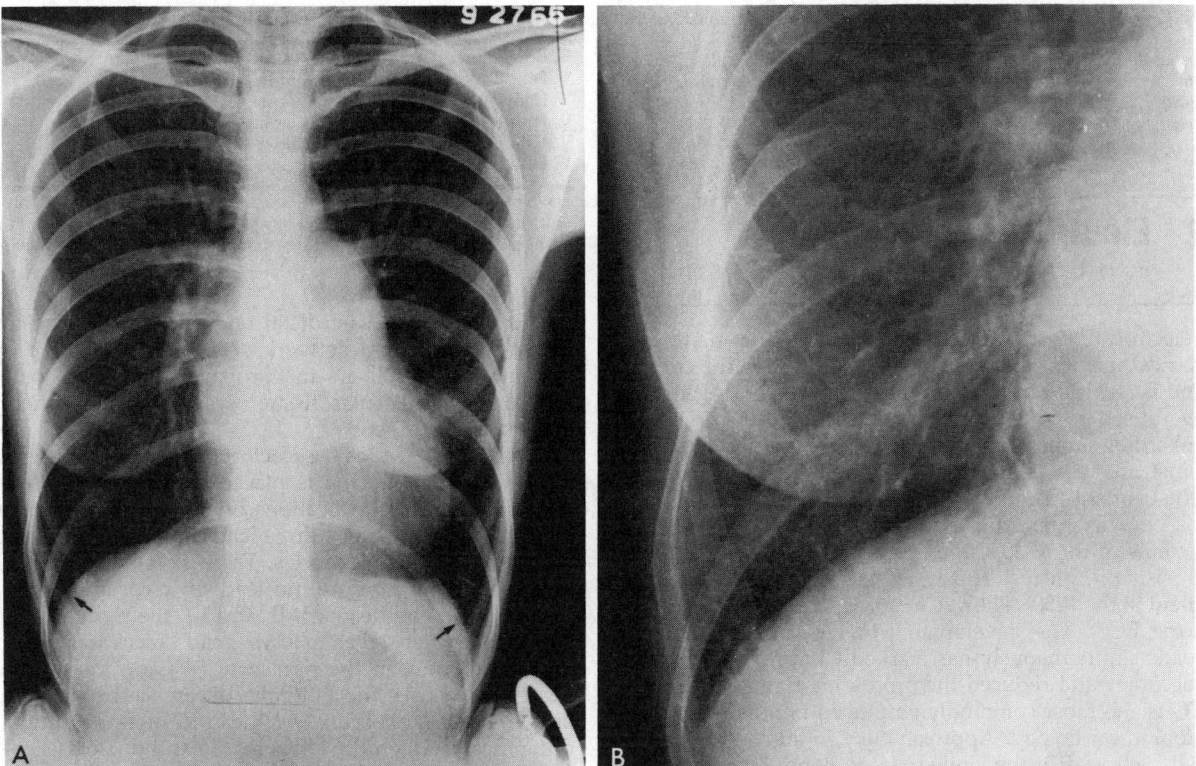

FIGURE 42–11. Patients with severe mitral stenosis. *A*, PA view shows striking redistribution of pulmonary blood flow. Note dilatation of upper and central vessels and constriction of lower and peripheral vessels. Arrows indicate Kerley's B lines in both costophrenic sulci. *B*, Magnified view of the right lower lung zone, showing multiple distinct Kerley's B lines.

PERICARDIAL EFFUSION. A large heart does not always imply heart failure but may be indicative of pericardial effusion. A rapidly enlarging cardiac silhouette without evidence of pulmonary venous congestion strongly suggests pericardial fluid accumulation, especially if of the "water-bottle" configuration. A more definitive radiographic sign of pericardial effusion is the inward displacement of the subepicardial fat line (Fig. 42–8; compare with Fig. 42–2).

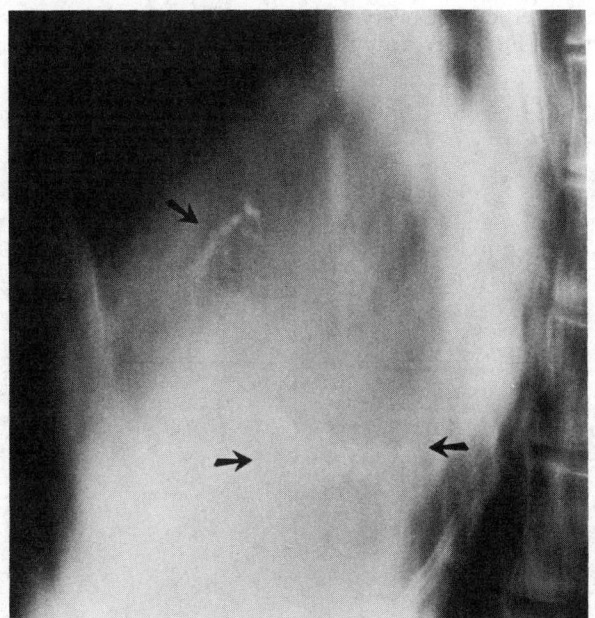

FIGURE 42–12. Lateral tomogram of a patient with severe calcific mitral stenosis. The heavily calcified mitral valve is indicated by the two opposing arrows. The upper arrow points to a heavily calcified anterior descending coronary artery.

FLUOROSCOPY. Fluoroscopy, the technique for visualizing the body structures in real time using a continuous x-ray beam and projecting the image on a recording device such as a television monitor, is a technique commonly applied to evaluate dynamic function of various organ systems. Occasionally it may clarify questionable abnormalities depicted on the standard two- or four-view radiographs of the heart. Pulsation and calcification are better evaluated by fluoroscopy than by static films. Pericardial calcification is curvilinear and is usually seen in the anterior portion of the cardiac shadow. Valvular calcifications are usually seen as multiple dense opacities in the respective valve regions (Figs. 42–10 and 42–12). Myocardial calcification, following myocardial infarction, is linear in distribution and usually occurs at the cardiac apex. Fluoroscopy can reveal faint calcifications in the coronary vessels (Fig. 42–12), which always signify atherosclerosis.

Decrease in cardiac pulsations is suggestive of pericardial effusions, constrictive pericarditis, cardiomyopathy, or generalized cardiac failure. Localized decrease in cardiac motion may be seen in myocardial infarction, and paradoxical movement may be indicative of a ventricular aneurysm. However, regional myocardial contraction abnormalities may not be reliably demonstrated by fluoroscopy. Echocardiography has become the method of choice in this context. Increased cardiac motion on fluoroscopy may indicate hyperthyroidism, hypertension, anemia, or aortic insufficiency.

An accurate assessment of the standard radiograph in the evaluation of the suspect or known cardiac patient will depend on an understanding of normal anatomy and physiology, and an appreciation of the reliability and limitations of the radiographic image. Accurate and skillful radiographic interpretation requires a thorough knowledge of the clinical history and physical findings, as well as of radiographic signs.

Chen JT: The plain radiograph in the diagnosis of cardiovascular disease. Radiol Clin North Am 21(4):609–623, 1983. *This article is the most comprehensive review of the conventional radiograph in evaluation of the cardiovascular system. The bibliography accompanying this paper is current and thorough.*

Colley RN, Capp MP, Lester RG, et al.: Plain Film Diagnosis of Cardiovascular Disease. Syllabus Set 14, Copyright American College of Radiology, 1979. *This is an excellent syllabus and self-evaluation text encompassing all aspects of the interpretation of conventional radiographs. A broad spectrum of cardiac cases is presented, always emphasizing the correlation of the radiographic abnormalities with pertinent clinical, laboratory, and electrocardiographic data.*

TABLE 42–1. POSITION OF CHEST LEADS

V_1 Fourth intercostal space (ICS) at the right sternal border
V_2 Fourth ICS at the left sternal border
V_3 Halfway between V_2 and V_4
V_4 Fifth ICS at the left midclavicular line
V_5 Fifth ICS at the left anterior axillary line
V_6 Fifth ICS at the left midaxillary line

When several sequential ECG's are to be obtained, e.g., in the coronary care unit, it is important to mark the location of the chest electrodes to minimize changes in the waveform resulting from variation in electrode placement.

42.2 Electrocardiography

Joseph C. Greenfield, Jr.

The electrocardiogram (ECG) is a graphic representation of the electrical activity generated by the heart during the cardiac cycle and is recorded from the body surface. In 1903, Wilhelm Einthoven used a string galvanometer to record the first EKG (Elektrokardiogramm, Ger.) Shortly thereafter, a clinically useful instrument was manufactured by the Cambridge Scientific Instrument Company. Following the pioneering work of Frank N. Wilson and his associates in the development of lead systems in the 1930's, the ECG became standardized. It now consists of 12 leads. The availability of the direct-writing instrument in the 1950's allowed a rapid increase in the routine use of the ECG. The development of recorders that obtain three leads simultaneously has markedly improved the diagnostic accuracy and reduced the processing time. At present, the ECG is the most commonly employed noninvasive diagnostic tool in cardiology. Approximately 75 million ECG's are recorded each year in the United States alone.

ELECTROPHYSIOLOGY. Cardiac muscle may be conveniently divided into specialized conducting tissue and nonspecialized myocardial tissue. While all myocardial cells possess the potential for electrical activity, the rate and pattern of depolarization and subsequent repolarization differ markedly in different regions of the heart. Some cells of the specialized conducting tissue possess the potential for spontaneous depolarization, a process termed automaticity.

The electrical activity of all myocardial cells is made possible by the presence of ionic gradients maintained across the membranes of individual cells. The concentration of intracellular potassium is approximately 30 times greater than its extracellular concentration, and it is the diffusion of this ion out of the cell that results in a resting transmembrane potential of approximately -90 mV in the fully repolarized state. The extracellular sodium concentration is approximately 15 times greater than its intracellular concentration, and the rapid influx of this ion into the cells results in the usual process of rapid cellular depolarization. When cells are partially depolarized to less than -55 mV, however, the sodium channels in the cell membrane are no longer operative, and a slower depolarization process may occur that predominantly involves calcium ions.

Myocardial activation normally begins with the spontaneous calcium-dependent depolarization of cells within the sinoatrial (SA) node located at the junction of the right atrium and superior vena cava. The impulse then propagates in a wavelike fashion through the atrial myocardium to the atrioventricular (AV) node located in the lower portion of the interatrial septum. Conduction through the AV node primarily involves the calcium-dependent process of depolarization and is delayed owing to membrane properties of nodal cells. The membrane properties in the proximal and distal segments of the AV node vary such that conduction in the proximal segment is slow and may occur with decrement, whereas conduction in the distal segment is more rapid.

The impulse is rapidly transmitted through the bundle of His, which then bifurcates into the narrow right bundle branch (RBB) and the fibers that become the left bundle branch (LBB). The LBB divides further into two main collections of fibers forming the anterior (superior) and posterior

(inferior) fascicles. The distal portion of the specialized conducting system is a network of smaller fibers, the Purkinje system, which delivers the propagated impulse to the nonspecialized ventricular tissue, resulting in a synchronized myocardial contraction.

LEAD SYSTEMS. Five electrodes are used in the standard ECG lead system. One is placed on each of the four limbs and one at different locations on the anterior chest wall (in instruments that record three leads simultaneously, there are six separate chest electrodes; Table 42–1). The right leg electrode functions as a ground lead. In recording the standard frontal plane limb leads, I, II, and III, the right arm, left arm, and left leg are used as follows: Lead I measures the potential difference between the right arm $(-)$ and the left arm $(+)$. Lead II measures the potential difference between the right arm $(-)$ and the left leg $(+)$. Lead III measures the potential difference between the left arm $(-)$ and the left leg $(+)$. This is the original bipolar lead configuration designed by Einthoven. The other three frontal plane leads, aV_R, aV_L, and aV_F, are constructed using a modified central terminal of Wilson, which augments the voltage output, hence the prefix aV. The exploring electrode, placed on the right arm (aV_R), left arm (aV_L), and left leg (aV_F), functions as a positive unipolar lead. The relationship among the six frontal plane leads is shown in Figure 42–13. The six chest leads also function as positive unipolar leads, using the central terminal as the reference point. The ECG leads are displayed in sequence, beginning with lead I, II, and III, followed by aV_R, aV_L, and aV_F, and then the chest leads from V_1 through V_6. A normal ECG recorded in this manner is illustrated in Figure 42–14.

The ECG is recorded on a paper chart, using a standard paper speed of 25 mm per second. The paper is marked with a light vertical line every millimeter (0.04 second) and a heavy vertical line every 5 mm (0.20 second). The paper also has

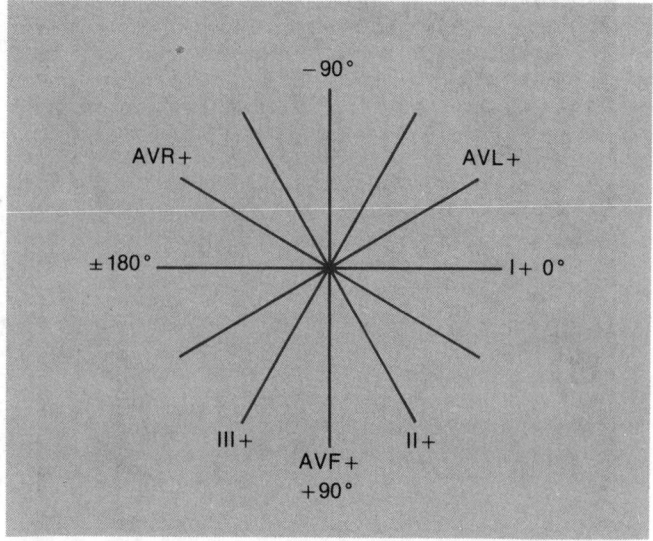

FIGURE 42–13. The limb leads are used to form a hexaxial reference system for the frontal plane. The axis of each lead is separated by approximately 30 degrees from the axes of the two adjacent leads.

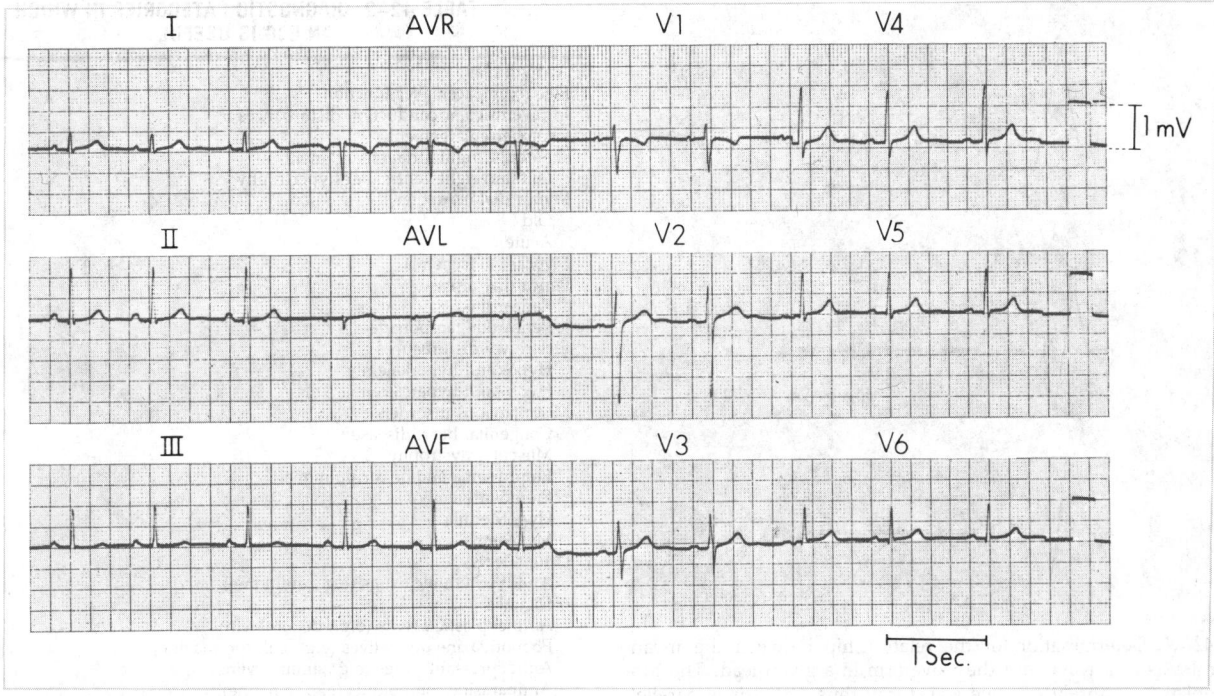

FIGURE 42–14. Normal electrocardiogram; the three leads in each column or lead set are recorded simultaneously.

horizontal lines separated by 1 mm and a dark horizontal line every 5 mm. Vertical deflection is calibrated in terms of voltage so that 10 mm equals 1.0 mV.

WAVEFORMS. The waveforms and intervals of the ECG are shown in Figure 42–15. The P wave is the electrical activity recorded during atrial depolarization and, in the normal ECG, precedes ventricular depolarization. The QRS complex occurs during ventricular depolarization. The Q wave is the initial downward deflection, the R wave is the initial upward deflection, and the S wave is the second downward deflection. A second upward deflection or a third downward deflection is defined as R' or S', respectively. A Q, R, and S may not be present in each lead; e.g., if the entire lead is negative, it is termed a QS wave. The time from the onset of the P wave to the beginning of ventricular depolarization is the PR interval; normally the range is 0.12 to 0.20 second. The QRS duration is normally less than 0.10 second. The T wave is inscribed during the period of ventricular repolarization. The electrical activity during atrial repolarization is usually masked by the QRS complex. The interval from the end of ventricular depolarization to the beginning of the T wave is termed the ST segment. The interval from the onset of ventricular depolarization to the end of the T wave is the QT interval. This interval is a function of rate. A small deflection following the T wave is the U wave; the precise origin of this waveform is unknown.

LEARNING ELECTROCARDIOGRAPHY. There are two general approaches to learning electrocardiography: (1) the pattern recognition method and (2) the spatial vector approach. In the former, the student memorizes the multiple normal and abnormal waveforms for each lead and gains the necessary expertise through experience in interpreting a large number of ECG's with clinical correlation. This technique is used by all experienced electrocardiographers, and illustrations of this approach are provided in the legends of Figures 42–18 to 42–22. In the spatial vector approach, popularized by R. P. Grant, the waveform is reduced to a vector representing the magnitude and direction of the mean electrical forces of P, QRS, and T. Using this technique, the student can quickly learn to define the normal ECG and the major abnormalities. This approach is based on the fact that the magnitude of a wave in any lead is a function of the relationship between the electrical axis of the heart and that lead (Fig. 42–16). From the hexaxial reference system of the six frontal plane leads illustrated in Figure 42–13, the spatial vector approach can be used to obtain the mean frontal plane axis for the normal electrocardiogram (Fig. 42–14). The QRS complex is upright (positive) in lead I; thus the mean axis must be between +90 degrees and −90 degrees—i.e., on the positive side of a line perpendicular to lead I. Since the QRS complex is also positive in leads II and III, the axis must be between +30 and +90 degrees. Since the mean QRS complex is slightly negative in lead aV$_L$, the mean QRS vector is approximately +70 degrees. A similar determination then can be made for P and T waves. In the frontal plane, the mean P vector should be between 0 and +80 degrees, and the mean QRS and T vectors should lie between −30 and +90 degrees. A mean QRS vector more negative than −30 degrees is considered left-axis deviation and more positive than +90 degrees is defined as right-axis deviation. The angle between the mean QRS and T vectors in the frontal plane should be less than 80 degrees. Application of the spatial vector tech-

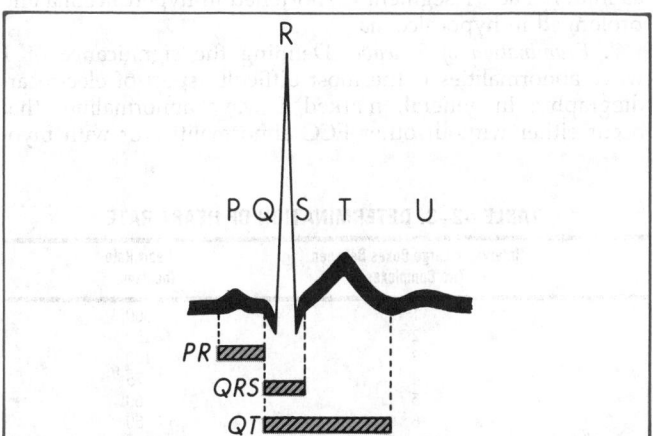

FIGURE 42–15. The ECG waveforms and intervals (horizontal bars) are illustrated. For description, see text.

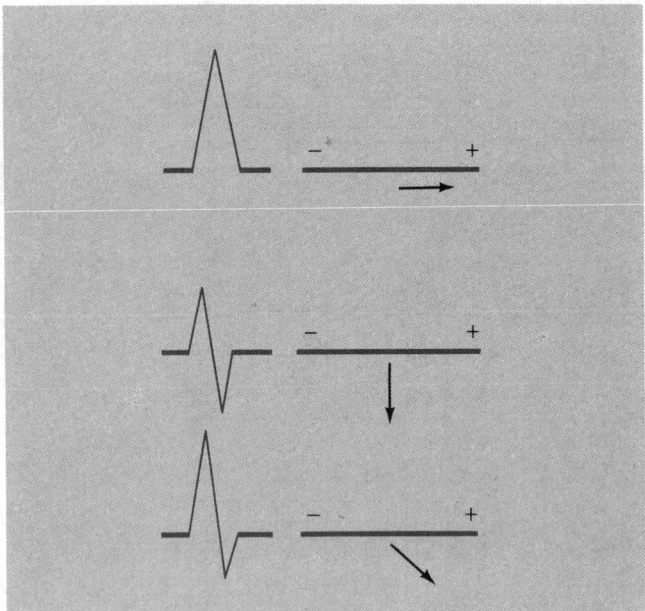

FIGURE 42–16. Determination of the relationship between the mean electrical axis of a wave and the waveform in a given lead. The top row depicts an entirely positive waveform; thus, the axis is parallel to the lead. In the second row the waveform is biphasic and the summation of the positive and negative parts is zero. In this instance, the mean electrical axis of the wave is perpendicular to the lead. (Note that the arrow could be drawn in the opposite direction and still be perpendicular to the lead.) In the third row, a biphasic waveform is shown in which the majority of the area is positive. The mean electrical axis is roughly at a 45-degree angle to the lead.

nique to the transverse plane is somewhat more difficult, since the six precordial leads do not define a precise reference system. An estimate of the vector can be obtained by noting when the waveforms make their transition from a negative to a positive deflection. In a normal ECG, the QRS transition is between V$_2$ and V$_5$, and the T wave makes its transition before the QRS. The next step is to determine the direction of the initial 0.04 second vector of the QRS. It is this portion of the QRS that defines the presence of myocardial infarction. The initial 0.04 second vector should lie between 0 and +90 degrees in the frontal plane; outside this range it suggests myocardial infarction (see Fig. 42–19). The direction of the terminal 0.04 second vector is used to aid in the diagnosis of ventricular conduction abnormalities (see Fig. 42–21).

APPROACH TO INTERPRETING AN ECG. The diagnostic categories in which an ECG may be useful are outlined in Table 42–2. In interpreting an ECG, it is important to develop a routine so that each aspect of the recording is carefully analyzed. Since the waveforms of the ECG are influenced to a certain extent by the age and body habitus of the patient, this information should be available to the electrocardiographer. The following eight sequential steps are necessary for proper ECG interpretation.

1. *Quality of the ECG recording.* This includes proper standardization (Fig. 42–17), lead placement (Fig. 42–18), and identification of significant artifact. The student must learn to evaluate the quality of the recording and not interpret an inadequately recorded ECG. Serious misdiagnosis can result if the quality of the ECG is ignored.

2. *Measurements.* The heart rate can be estimated adequately by employing the method outlined in Table 42–3. The amplitude, duration, and intervals of the various waveforms are usually measured in the standard frontal plane limb leads. Abnormality of the QRS duration, PR interval, and QT interval also is determined in these leads. Proper measurement of the waveforms is enhanced by simultaneous recording of three

TABLE 42–2. DIAGNOSTIC CATEGORIES IN WHICH AN ECG IS USEFUL

Arrhythmias	+ +
Electronic pacemaker function	+ +
Intraventricular conduction disturbances	+ +
Chamber enlargement	
Left and right atrial enlargement	+
Left and right ventricular hypertrophy	+
Myocardial infarction	
Old	+
Acute	+
Myocardial ischemia	+
Pericardial disease	
Pericarditis	±
Pericardial tamponade	±
Electrolyte disturbances	
Hypo- and hyperkalemia	+
Hypo- and hypercalcemia	+
Miscellaneous disorders	
Congenital heart disease	±
Muscular dystrophy	±
Emphysema and/or cor pulmonale	±
Pulmonary emboli	±
Hypothermia	±
Myxedema	±
Drug effects	
Antidysrhythmic drugs (e.g., quinidine)	±
Digitalis	±
Antineoplastic agents (e.g., doxorubicin)	±
Phenothiazine derivatives (e.g., chlorpromazine)	±
Antidepressant drugs (e.g., amitriptyline)	±
Antiparasitic compounds (e.g., emetine)	±

The symbols indicate the necessity for ECG to establish diagnosis:
+ + ECG is essential for diagnosis.
 + ECG is important for diagnosis.
 ± ECG may be useful for diagnosis.

leads, since the inter-relationships between the waveforms can be easily seen. The QT interval must be corrected for heart rate. The corrected QT interval (QT$_c$) is given by Bazet's formula:

$$QT_c = \frac{QT}{\sqrt{RR \text{ interval (seconds)}}}$$

and should be between 0.33 and 0.47 second.

3. *Determination of rhythm.*

4. *Examination of P wave.* Determine if atrial enlargement (see Fig. 42–20) or intra-atrial block is present.

5. *Examination of QRS.* Determine if myocardial infarction (Fig. 42–19), ventricular hypertrophy (Fig. 42–20), or ventricular conduction defect (Fig. 42–21) is present.

6. *Examination of ST segment.* Determine if subendocardial (Fig. 42–22) or epicardial (Fig. 42–19) injury is present; abnormal displacement of the ST segment is defined by convention as injury. The ST segment is shortened in hypercalcemia and prolonged in hypocalcemia.

7. *Examination of T wave.* Defining the significance of T wave abnormalities is the most difficult aspect of electrocardiography. In general, marked T wave abnormalities that occur either without other ECG abnormalities or with myo-

TABLE 42–3. DETERMINATION OF HEART RATE

Interval in Large Boxes Between Two Complexes	Heart Rate (beats/min)
1	300
2	150
3	100
4	75
5	60
6	50

The ECG recording paper is marked vertically by light lines; every fifth line is heavily marked. The time increment separating two heavy lines (one large box) is 0.20 second. To determine the rate rapidly, note the interval between two complexes and estimate the rate from this table.

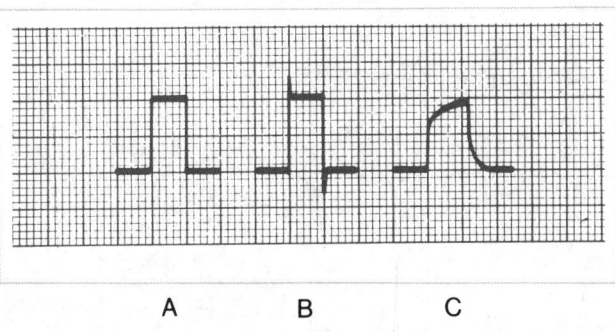

FIGURE 42–17. In *A*, a correct standardization having a true square wave response is illustrated. *B* represents a standardization obtained from an instrument in which the response is underdamped; the amplitude of the waves will be spuriously enhanced. In *C*, the recorder is overdamped, resulting in both a spuriously decreased amplitude and an increased width of the waveform.

A B C

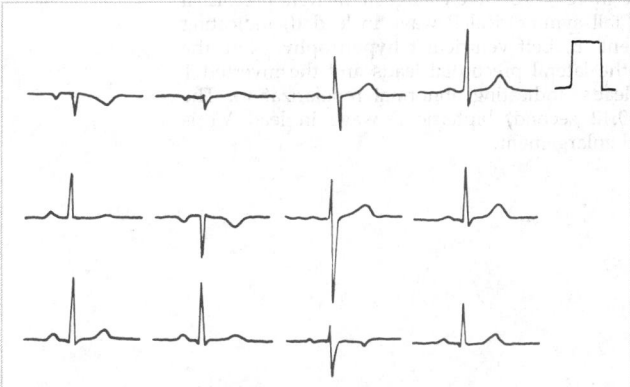

FIGURE 42–18. Two examples of incorrect lead placement from the same patient illustrated in Figure 42–14. Both the left and right arm leads and chest leads V1, 2, 3 are reversed. Reversal of the arm lead results in a mirror image recording of lead I and is easily recognized, since the P wave is negative. If missed, a spurious diagnosis of lateral wall infarction may be made. Reversal of the right precordial leads may result in an incorrect diagnosis of either right ventricular hypertrophy or posterior wall infarction.

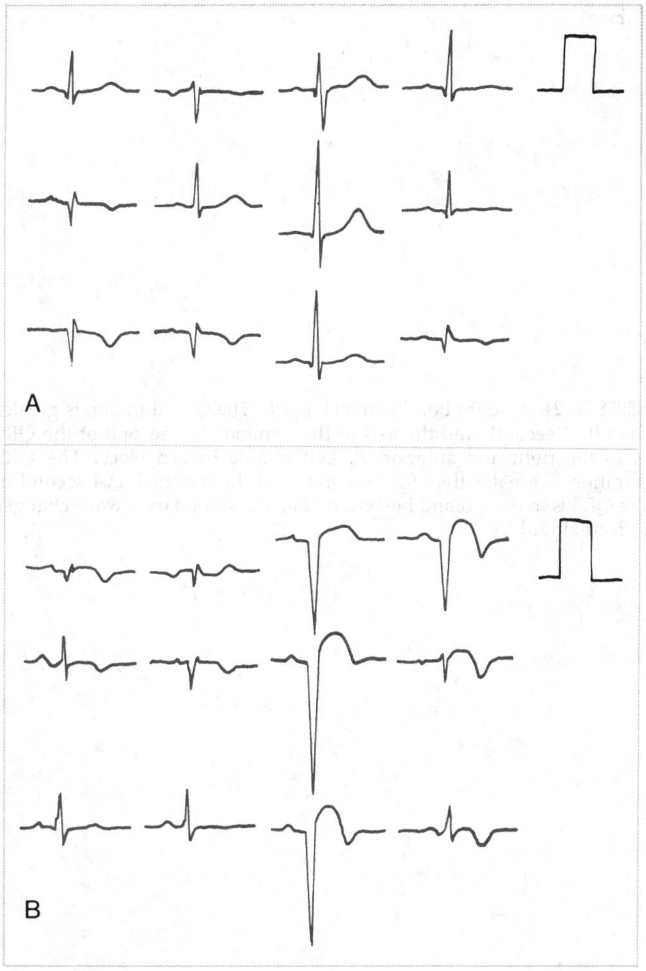

FIGURE 42–19. The ECG lead sets are recorded in the same sequence as in Figure 42–14. *A*, Inferior and posterior infarction. Note the abnormal superiorly and anteriorly directed initial forces, i.e., significant Q waves in leads II, III, and AVF, and a broad R wave in V1. Note the concomitant negative T waves in the same frontal plane leads (inferior ischemia). *B*, Anterolateral myocardial infarction. The initial forces are posterior and to the right, i.e., extensive Q waves in leads I, AVL, and V1 through V4. Also note the concomitant ST segment elevation (epicardial injury) and T wave inversion (anterior ischemia) in the precordial leads, indicating that the myocardial infarction is probably acute.

A

B

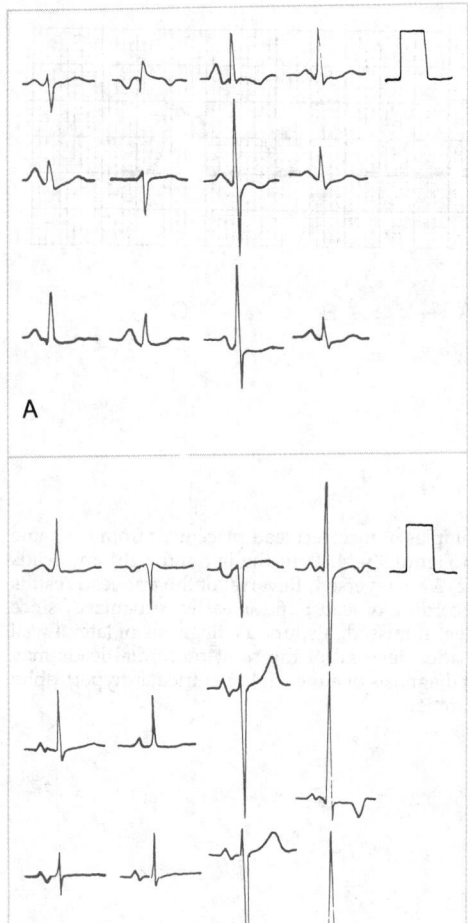

FIGURE 42–20. *A*, Right ventricular hypertrophy. The mean frontal plane axis is to the right, and there is excessive voltage in the right precordial leads. Also note the tall symmetrical P wave in lead II, indicating right atrial enlargement. *B*, Left ventricular hypertrophy. Note the excessive voltage in the lateral precordial leads and the inverted T waves in the same leads, indicating abnormal repolarization. The wide (greater than 0.12 second) biphasic P wave in lead V1 is indicative of left atrial enlargement.

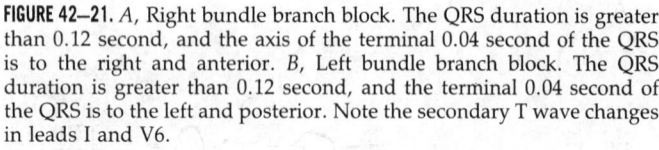

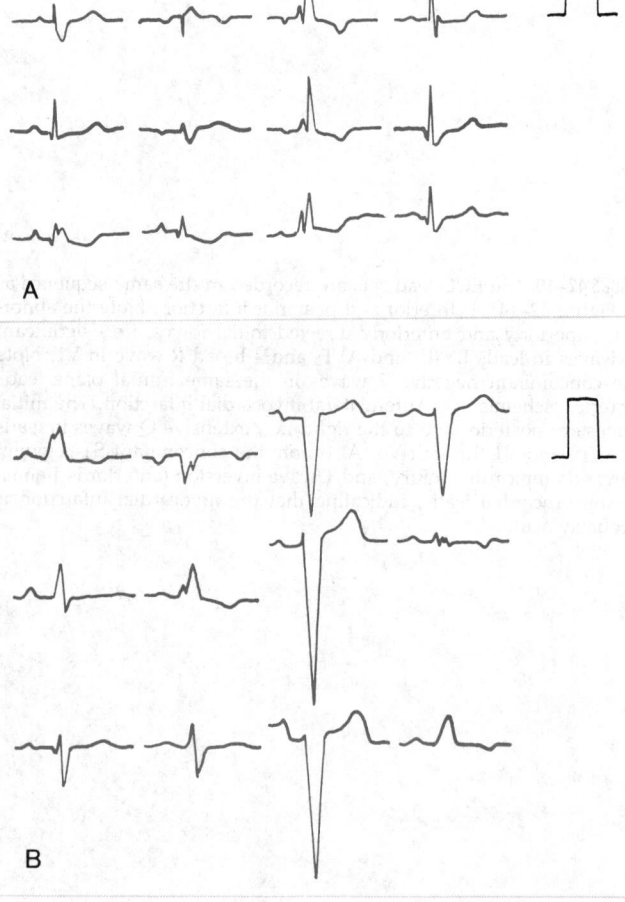

FIGURE 42–21. *A*, Right bundle branch block. The QRS duration is greater than 0.12 second, and the axis of the terminal 0.04 second of the QRS is to the right and anterior. *B*, Left bundle branch block. The QRS duration is greater than 0.12 second, and the terminal 0.04 second of the QRS is to the left and posterior. Note the secondary T wave changes in leads I and V6.

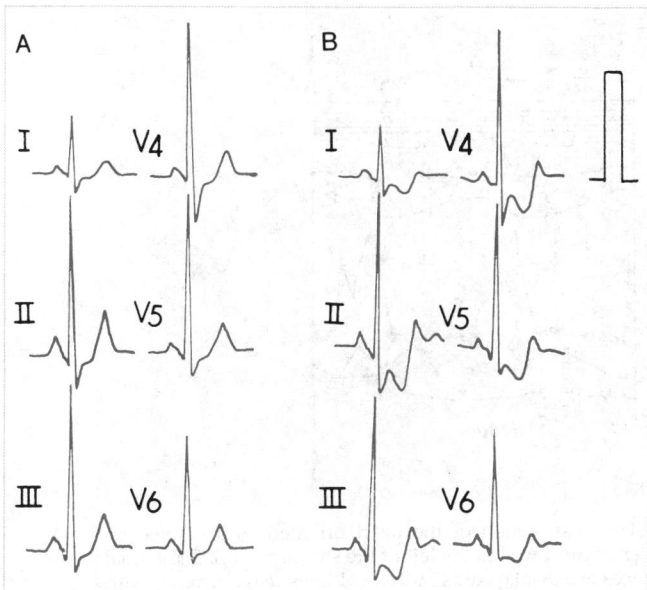

FIGURE 42–22. Recording obtained (*A*) prior to and (*B*) during an exercise test. Note the depression and downward sloping of the S-T segment wave during exercise. This is a typical pattern of subendocardial injury.

enhancing the diagnosis of myocardial infarction, conduction defects, and ventricular hypertrophy.

A further refinement of this approach is body surface mapping, in which multiple precordial leads are obtained and a computer is utilized to generate a continuous body surface map of the change in electrical potential during depolarization and repolarization. These techniques are still in the experimental stage, but ultimately may prove to be important in obtaining the maximal information available from the electrical activation of the heart.

The ECG stress test is a widely used physiologic technique designed to assess the ability of the coronary circulation to deliver oxygen at a rate commensurate with the metabolic needs of the myocardium. Because myocardial metabolism is almost entirely aerobic, an inadequate increase in coronary flow quickly results in ischemia of the inner layers of the heart. The concomitant ST segment changes have been empirically defined as subendocardial injury. The characteristic ST segment response is a flat (square wave) or downward-sloping ST segment of 0.1 mV or greater measured 0.08 second after the end of the QRS complex (Fig. 42–22).

Chou TC, Helm RA: Clinical Vectorcardiography. 2nd ed. New York, Grune & Stratton, 1974. *Complete coverage of vectorcardiography.*

Lipman BS, Massie E, Kleiger RE: Clinical Scalar Electrocardiography. 6th ed. Chicago, Year Book Medical Publishers, 1973. *Excellent general text covering all phases of electrocardiography.*

Marriott HJL: Practical Electrocardiography. 7th ed. Baltimore, Williams & Wilkins, 1983. *A comprehensive description of electrocardiography.*

42.3 Echocardiography

Richard L. Popp

PULSED REFLECTED ULTRASOUND

Echocardiography includes a family of diagnostic procedures that use ultrahigh-frequency sound waves to record the structure of the heart, and the blood flow velocities within the heart, throughout the cardiac cycle. Sound frequencies in the range of 1 to 10 million cycles per second, or megaHertz (MHz), are transmitted from a piezoelectric crystal along a carefully defined path within the thorax. A transducer is placed on the chest wall, and a short burst of ultrasound is transmitted through the chest and into the underlying cardiac structures. The transducer then acts as a sound receiver until the next pulse. At each interface of materials with differing acoustic impedance, part of the sound is reflected or refracted and the remaining sound energy is further transmitted for subsequent acoustic reflection. The acoustic reflecting interfaces oriented perpendicular to the path of sound travel produce reflected sound that is received by the transducer on the chest wall as an "echo" of the transmitted sound. The location of each reflecting surface relative to the transducer can be calculated from the known velocity of sound in tissue and the elapsed time between sound transmission and reception of the echo. This series of depth readings is displayed on an oscilloscope for each pulse of sound, as shown in Figure 42–23. The strength of each echo is indicated by the brightness of the signal on the display device. Blood within the heart chambers usually gives signals of low amplitude that are not displayed. This "brightness-modulated" (B-mode) record of the reflecting interfaces is the building block for both two-dimensional (2D) and time-motion (M-mode) echocardiography.

One thousand pulses per second are created with typical instruments used clinically. A high sampling rate facilitates tracking motion of cardiac structures, yet there is usually enough time for the sound to return from even the most distant reflectors before the next pulse. Sequentially directing

cardial infarction are defined as ischemic or primary T wave changes (Fig. 42–19). T wave abnormalities that occur with conduction defects or ventricular hypertrophy are spoken of as secondary. Abnormal T waves are seen in hypertrophy (Fig. 42–20). The T waves also are important in the diagnosis of drug effects and electrolyte abnormalities.

8. *Comparison with patient's previous ECG's.* It is extremely important to compare a new tracing with a previous electrocardiogram for two reasons: (1) although the ECG may still be within the normal range, significant changes may have occurred since the previous record; and (2) a comparison allows the electrocardiographer to date specific abnormalities and may have important therapeutic implications.

COMPUTER INTERPRETATION OF THE ECG. The development of algorithms to process and interpret ECG's has progressed to the point that, at present, there are several acceptable programs available for routine clinical use. Although these programs are helpful in decreasing processing time, they must be viewed as an assist device to the electrocardiographer and not as a replacement.

OTHER RECORDING TECHNIQUES. Several of the other ECG recording techniques and their uses are described in Table 42–4.

The vectorcardiogram (VCG) is used to obtain a true orthogonal lead system (XYZ leads) so that the cardiac dipole is in the center of the chest. The most commonly employed lead system was devised by E. Frank. It is time consuming to record a VCG properly, and for this reason the VCG has not been generally accepted in clinical medicine. The VCG is primarily beneficial in teaching electrocardiography and in

TABLE 42–4. DIAGNOSTIC USES OF OTHER ECG RECORDING TECHNIQUES

Vectorcardiograms: old myocardial infarction, ventricular hypertrophy, ventricular conduction abnormalities
Body surface mapping: precise definition of instantaneous depolarization and repolarization—primarily experimental at present
Exercise electrocardiography: transient subendocardial or transmural injury
Ambulatory monitoring: arrhythmias, transient subendocardial injury
Transtelephone monitoring: arrhythmias, pacemaker function
His bundle recordings: arrhythmias and conduction defects
Esophageal leads: arrhythmias

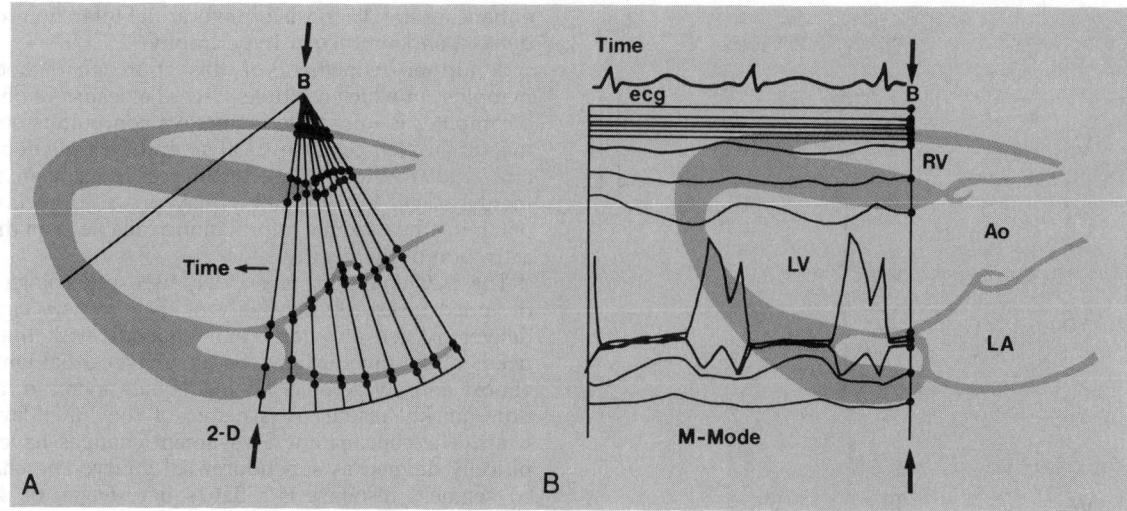

FIGURE 42–23. *A,* A schematic two-dimensional (2-D) image of a cross-section of the heart oriented as displayed by echocardiography. The sound transducer is located on the anterior chest wall to the left of the sternum, at B. Sequential sound pulses and the returning echoes from reflecting interfaces are displayed as individual lines (*large arrows*), with dots of light defining the loci of reflectors. B = brightness-modulated display. Many such lines, accumulated over 1/60 to 1/15 second, make up a single 2-D image. *B,* A schematic time-motion (M-mode) echocardiogram produced by tracing out the location of structures moving during the cardiac cycle under a stationary sound transducer. As in *A,* the transducer on the chest wall creates a B-mode (B, *arrows*) display of sequential pulses and traces the motion pattern of each echo-producing interface. The M- and W-shaped patterns represent the anterior and posterior mitral valve leaflets, respectively. Ao = Aorta; ecg = electrocardiogram; LA = left atrium; LV = left ventricle; RV = right ventricle. (Modified from Popp RL, Rubenson DS, Tucker CR, et al: Echocardiography: M-mode and two-dimensional methods. Ann Intern Med 93:844, 1980.)

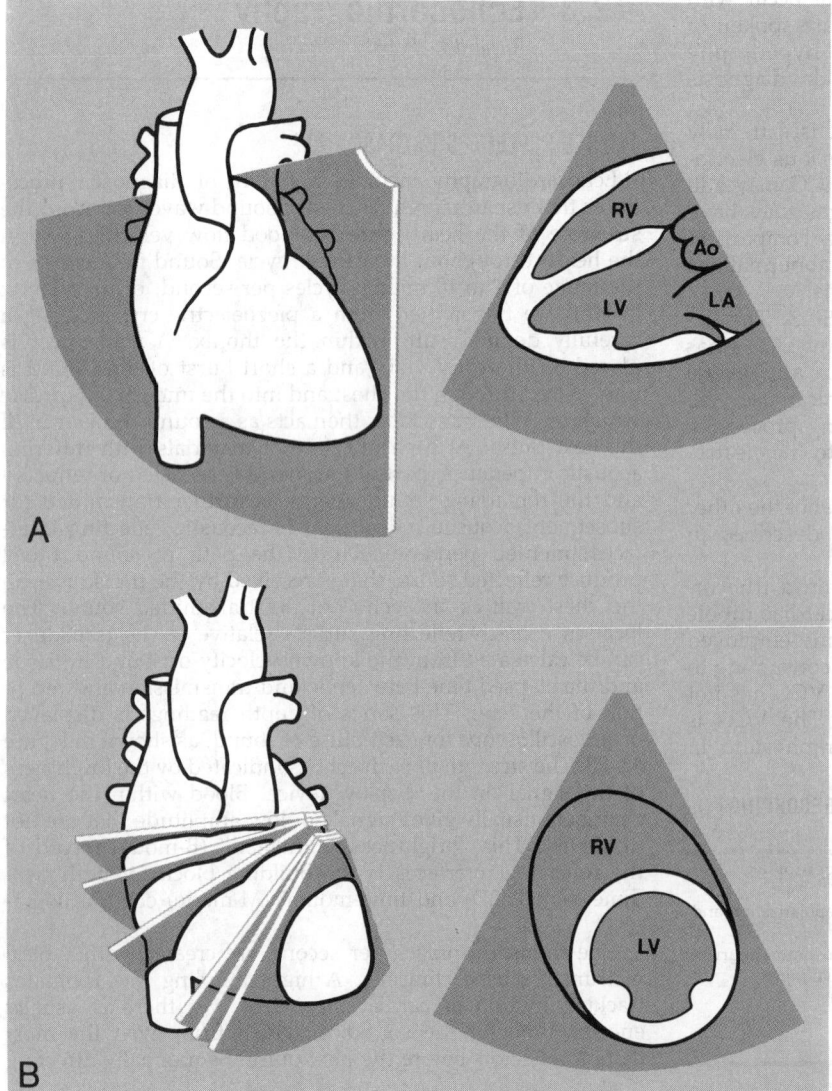

FIGURE 42–24. Schematic illustration of some standard 2-D imaging planes used for clinical cardiac studies. *A,* Parasternal transducer position, with the imaging plane oriented parallel to the long axis of the left ventricle (LV) and intersecting a portion of the right ventricular outflow tract (RV), aortic root (Ao), and left atrium (LA). *B,* Transducer position as in *A,* but the imaging planes (six illustrated) are oriented parallel to the left ventricular short axis.

Illustration continued on opposite page

the sound beam along a given path, usually a pie-shaped sector of a circular plane, for each successive pulse produces a two-dimensional map of the structures underlying the transducer, called a two-dimensional (2D) echocardiogram (Fig. 42–23). Clinical instruments sweep the sound beam through an arc of 60 to 90 degrees, by electronic or mechanical means, to create an imaging plane for visualizing a cross-section of the heart. Thus each 2D ultrasonic image is made up of multiple individual lines of sound reflection information. Depending on the basic pulse repetition rate, the time required for a single sound pulse to travel round trip through the thorax, and the number of such pulses per 2D image, 15 to 60 individual 2D image frames per second are available for interpretation. The images usually are presented on a digital scan converter that interpolates data between the scan lines and gives the impression of watching the heart in motion. The standardized examination provides multiple 2D cross-sectional planes through all parts of the heart using specific transducer locations, as shown in Figure 42–24. The dynamic three-dimensional structure of the heart can be understood by mentally assembling these multiple slices. An electrocardiogram is included as a reference signal in these studies.

A single direction of the sound beam, within the 2D image, may be selected for special attention and very high sampling rate. In this case, a given sound beam direction is repeatedly sampled, and the motion along the path of the sound beam is displayed with respect to time. The usual display is on an oscilloscope or strip chart recorder and is called a time-motion, T-M, or M-mode echocardiogram (right panel, Fig. 42–23). This method of recording is especially useful for identifying precise timing of motion of cardiac structures, such as valves, with respect to the electrocardiogram, phonocardiogram, or

Doppler echocardiogram (to be described below). Historically, the M-mode echocardiogram was the first to be used.

Normal or abnormal patterns of cardiac chamber size and connection, wall thickness, wall motion, valve structure, and valve motion all are well assessed by echocardiographic study (Figs. 42–25 and 42–26). It is the method of choice for visualizing many abnormal structures, such as vegetations of infective endocarditis, intracardiac tumors, mural thrombi, and pericardial fluid.

During acute and chronic ventricular ischemia and acute infarction, the echocardiographic images accurately show the extent of myocardial thinning and segmental akinesis or dyskinesis. Exercise-induced segmental abnormalities may be observed as well. The acute complications of myocardial infarction that may be detected by imaging and Doppler echocardiography include pericardial effusion with or without cardiac tamponade, flail mitral leaflet (ruptured papillary muscle), acute mitral regurgitation of papillary muscle dysfunction, acute ventricular septal defect, myocardial rupture with pseudoaneurysm formation, infarct expansion producing true aneurysm, and right ventricular infarction.

Echocardiographic imaging also may be performed "invasively," as when transesophageal transducers are used or during thoracotomy with direct application of the transducer to the epicardium. These approaches produce superb images owing both to lack of sound scattering in the thorax and to the feasibility of using very high-frequency (5 to 10 MHz) ultrasound, which has high physical resolution but poor soft tissue penetration. Intravenous injections of many fluids, such as physiologic saline solution, contain myriad microbubbles of gas, which may be visualized by echocardiography as they travel through the right side of the heart. The gas does not

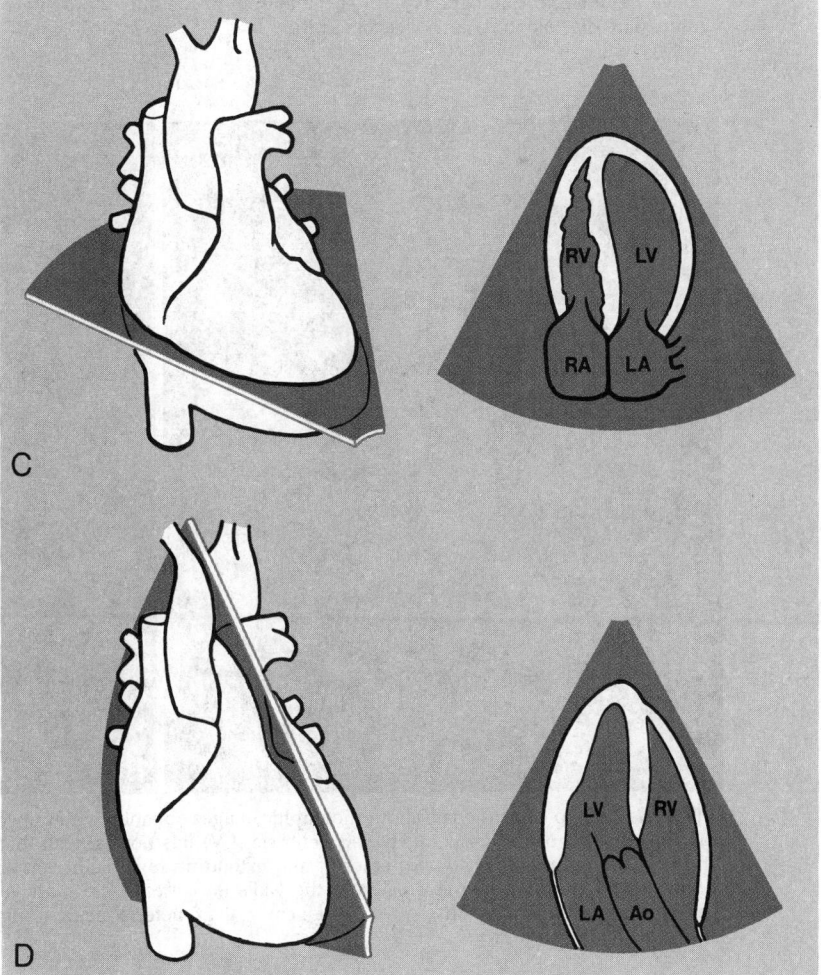

FIGURE 42–24 Continued C, Apical transducer position, with the imaging plane oriented to show the four main chambers of the heart (4-chamber view). The 2-D image is displayed relative to the transducer so that the cardiac apex is shown near the transducer. RA = right atrium. D, Transducer position as in C, but the imaging plane is oriented parallel to the left ventricular long axis, as in panel A. (Redrawn from Popp RL, Fowles RE, Coltart DJ, et al.: Cardiac anatomy viewed systematically with two-dimensional echocardiography. Chest 75:579, 1979.)

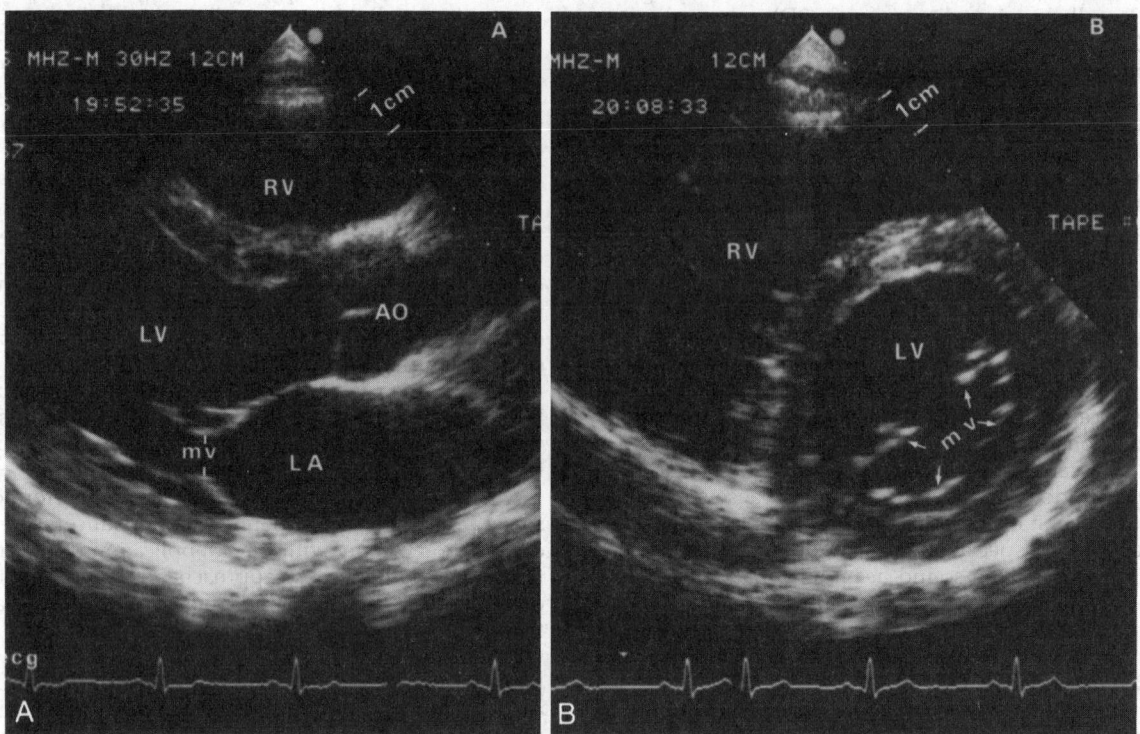

FIGURE 42–25. Two-dimensional echocardiographic images of a normal heart. Panels *A* and *B* were obtained with transducer positions and imaging plane orientations as shown in Figure 42–24*A* and *B*, respectively. Abbreviations as in Figure 42–24. mv = Mitral valve leaflets. (Note depth calibration scale at 1-cm intervals along right margin of each image.) The electrocardiograms (ecg) at the bottom of the panels are interrupted to indicate the timing of each image frame (late diastole in *A*, early diastole in *B*).

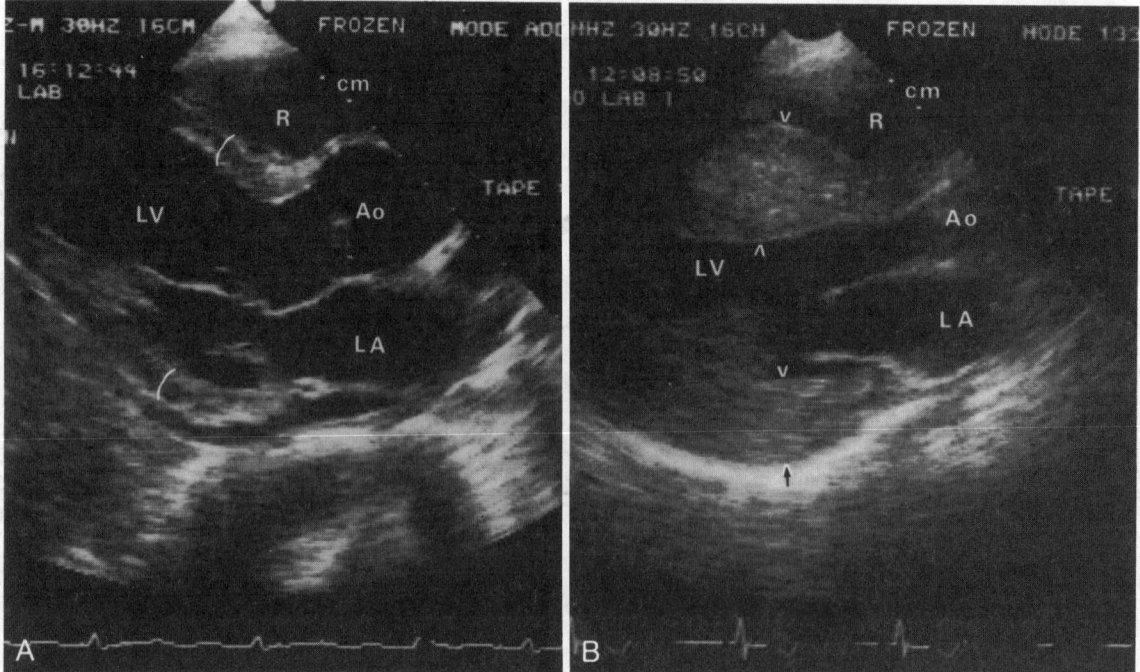

FIGURE 42–26. Two-dimensional echocardiographic images obtained with transducer position and image plane orientation as shown in Figure 42–24*A*. *A*, The left ventricle (LV) has normal wall thickness (white brackets). A relatively echo-free space posterior to the lower bracket, and extending toward the left atrium (LA), represents a small pericardial effusion. *B*, The LV cavity is small and the walls (*arrowheads*) are massively thickened in a patient with concentric hypertrophic cardiomyopathy. Ao = Aorta; cm = centimeter scale; R = right ventricle.

pass through the pulmonary capillary bed, so if microbubble echoes are seen immediately in the left side of the heart, one may assume an intracardiac shunt is present, and a delayed appearance implies an intrapulmonary shunt. Direct intra-aortic or intracoronary injection of various contrast agents has been used in attempts to visualize coronary perfusion areas of the left ventricle and experimentally to assess washout rates with altered coronary flow.

DOPPLER ULTRASOUND

Sound energy is transmitted as a series of compression-rarefaction waves with a given periodicity or wave frequency. Sound reflected from stationary surfaces has the same basic frequency as the transmitted sound, as shown in Figure 42–27. However, if the reflector or reflectors are moving relative to the direction of sound transmissions, the sequential interaction of the compression-rarefaction waves with the reflector results in a change in the frequency of the sound, as shown in Figure 42–27. This frequency shift is the Doppler effect, and it enables calculation of the velocity of the reflector if one knows the originally transmitted frequency, the received frequency, the speed of sound in the medium (soft tissues), and the angle between the sound beam and the direction of the moving reflectors. The moving column of blood, with its cells and fluctuations in spatial distribution of cells, is the source of the Doppler frequency shift measured by echocardiography. An indicator of the beam direction undergoing Doppler frequency analysis is superimposed on the 2D image to help orientation and facilitate placing the beam in the general direction of flow. Fortunately, the change in frequency obtained with clinical instruments is in the audible range, so one may optimally match the direction of the sound beam with the direction of the blood flow by adjusting the transducer while listening to the signal. A beam-to-flow angle of zero degrees is desirable, since the calculated velocity is a function of the cosine of this angle ($\cos 0° = 1$), but an angle of up to 20 degrees produces underestimation of velocities of up to only 6 per cent.

Blood flow toward or away from the transducer produces an increase or decrease in sound frequency, respectively, so both the velocity and the direction of the blood are measurable. These signals are usually displayed with velocites calculated from received Doppler shifted frequencies plotted versus time. The velocity spectrum is arranged above or below a baseline to convey information on flow direction, as shown in Figures 42–28 and 42–29.

Pulsed wave (PW) Doppler echocardiography is performed with pulses of ultrasound as described above, and frequency analysis is possible for sound returning from any given distance from the transducer. Thus, a signal received during systole from the left atrium and indicating high-velocity flow directed into the atrium from the ventricle signifies mitral regurgitation. This technique has proved especially valuable in locating intracardiac shunts, such as atrial or ventricular septal defects (Fig. 42–28) and patent ductus arteriosus. Since the product of the mean flow velocity (centimeters per second) and cross-sectional flow area (square centimeters) is volumetric flow (cubic centimeters per second), flow within the pulmonary artery or left ventricular outflow tract, or across the tricuspid or mitral valves, can be estimated. Comparison of flows across the pulmonary artery and aorta give an estimate of shunt flow across the septal defects, for example. Measurement of cardiac output by this method is useful clinically; however, the procedure is technically demanding.

PW methods provide spatial resolution but have limited velocity resolution because of the physical-mathematical constraints of sampling periodically. This trade-off is the opposite of that with continuous wave (CW) Doppler echocardiography, which uses one transducer to transmit, and another to receive, reflected sound continuously. CW Doppler methods have no spatial resolution within the path of the beam but can display frequency shifts corresponding to very high flow velocities. A major series of applications of Doppler echocardiography derives from the relationship of measured velocities to corresponding drops in pressure within the heart or vascular system. A cardiac valve stenosis presents an obstacle to flowing blood, which results in an increased velocity through the area of obstruction. This convective acceleration is the major factor producing a drop in pressure (ΔP, or pressure gradient) across the stenosis. The pressure difference can be accurately estimated instantaneously by CW Doppler echocardiography from the maximum flow velocity (V) achieved ($\Delta P = 4V^2$), as first shown by Holen and coworkers (1976). The ability to obtain intracardiac and intravascular pressure information noninvasively has been a significant advance in the capabilities of echocardiography. Many patients with aortic or mitral stenosis or both now have adequate preoperative hemodynamic assessment on the basis of clinical features and echocardiography only. The method for calculating instantaneous and mean pressure drops across a stenotic aortic valve is shown in Figure 42–29.

The pressure drop across a stenotic valve is dependent on both the valve area and the blood volume crossing the valve per unit of time. Aortic valve area is accurately estimated by applying the Gorlin formula (see Ch. 42.5) using Doppler ultrasound–derived values for ejection time, stroke volume, and pressure gradient. Alternatively, one may calculate the flow per beat (see above) from the mean flow velocity and

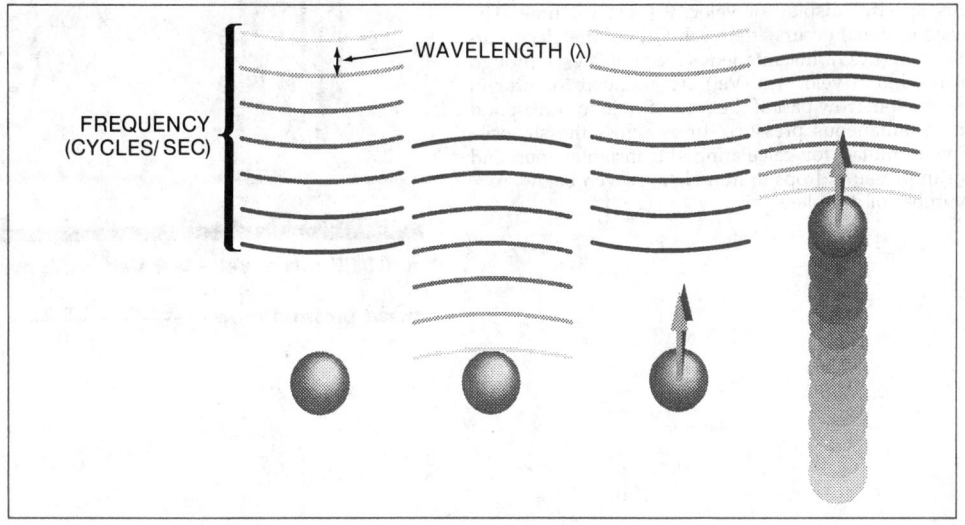

FIGURE 42–27. Schematic diagram of the Doppler principle as applied in echocardiography. From left to right: Sound waves of a given frequency (cycles/sec) and wave length (λ) are transmitted into the chest. Sound reflected from a stationary target has the same frequency as that transmitted. Sound directed toward a moving target will interact with the reflector and alter the frequency of the returning sound by a factor related to the speed of the moving target, the original sound frequency, and the angle of interception of the two.

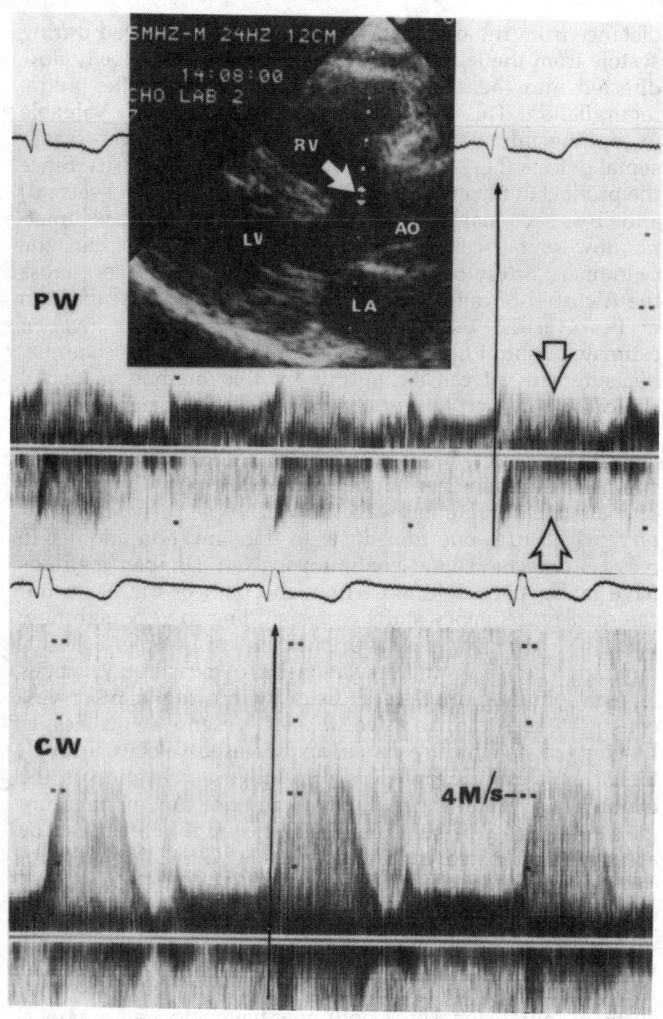

FIGURE 42–28. Methods of displaying a Doppler echocardiographic study in a patient with ventricular septal defect. The black panel above is a 2-D image taken with transducer position and image plane orientation as in Figure 42–24*A*. The white arrow points to the sample volume indicator for pulsed-wave (PW) Doppler ultrasound analysis. This illustration is from a patient with a large defect of the septum between the right ventricle (RV) and left ventricle (LV). The white panels below are spectral displays of the Doppler ultrasound signals in a patient with a small ventricular septal defect. The PW record indicates a frequency shift (*open arrows*) from the area of the sample volume (above), which occurs in systole after the onset of the electrocardiographic QRS (*long arrow*). The continuous-wave (CW) record indicates high-velocity (>4 M/s) flow somewhere along the dotted line shown above. The systolic pressure difference between the right and left ventricles can be calculated from the CW signal as shown in Figure 42–29. The location of the signal origin is defined by PW, while the CW signal defines high-flow velocity quantitatively but is ambiguous regarding signal locus. Other abbreviations as in Figure 42–23.

FIGURE 42–29. Continuous-wave Doppler ultrasound recording of aortic outflow velocities from a patient with aortic stenosis. The transducer is at the apex, so flow toward the aorta is registered below the baseline in this spectral display of velocity (M/s) vs. time. The systolic signal occurs after each QRS of the electrocardiogram (ECG). Instantaneous (vertical lines a through e) maximum velocities (Vel) are assumed to occur in the most narrow part of the stenosis and to correspond to instantaneous pressure drops across the stenosis. The formulae for calculating the instantaneous and mean pressure drops in mm Hg are given below. n = Number of samples.

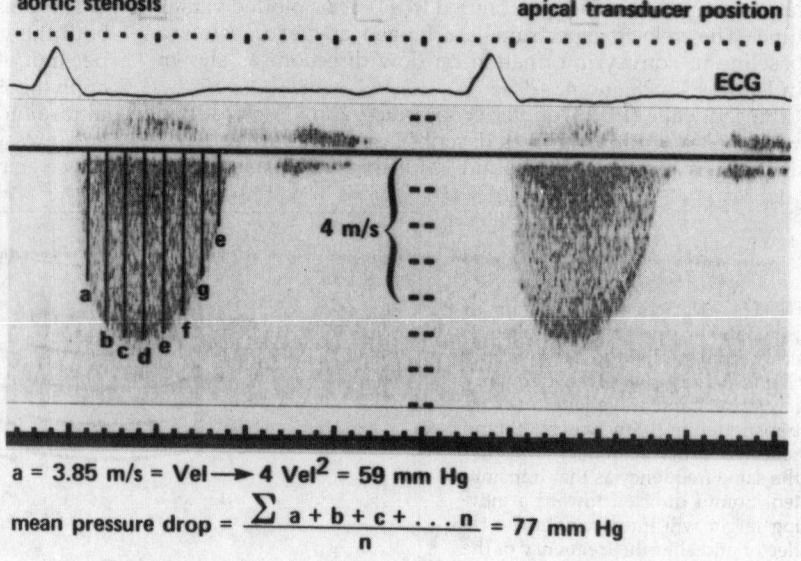

$$a = 3.85 \text{ m/s} = \text{Vel} \longrightarrow 4\,\text{Vel}^2 = 59 \text{ mm Hg}$$

$$\text{mean pressure drop} = \frac{\sum a + b + c + \ldots n}{n} = 77 \text{ mm Hg}$$

cross-sectional area of the left ventricular outflow tract immediately below the stenotic valve and assume this same flow is represented by the product of the mean flow velocity within, and the cross-sectional area of, the stenotic valve. The outflow tract flow velocity, outflow tract area, and aortic valve flow velocity are obtainable, permitting calculation of the aortic valve area. This method is reliable even when aortic regurgitation is present. It is fortuitous that the time required for the pressure drop across the mitral valve to reach one half of the maximum level is directly related to the valve area at virtually all clinically relevant flows. Thus mitral valve area may be accurately calculated from data developed by Holen and colleagues (1977) without the necessity for measuring stroke volume.

Recording the velocity of blood flowing across a narrow orifice between any two chambers or cardiovascular loci permits calculation of the absolute pressure level in one chamber if the pressure in the other chamber is known. For example, the systolic pressure difference between the right ventricle and right atrium can be calculated from the velocities recorded from tricuspid regurgitant flow. The sum of jugular venous or right atrial pressure and the atrioventricular pressure difference is the right ventricular systolic pressure. The prevalence of tricuspid regurgitation detectable by Doppler echocardiography sufficient to perform this calculation ranges from over 90 per cent (in normal subjects) to 80 per cent (in patients with cardiomyopathy and pulmonary hypertension). This concept is useful in assessing ventricular pressures in ventricular septal defect and is under investigation for several conditions. Quantitating the pressure gradient across prosthetic valves and assessing the central or perivalvular origin of regurgitant prosthesis leaks noninvasively are major advances because the alternative of catheter placement to get similar information may require trans-septal catheterization of the left side of the heart or direct left ventricular puncture.

Advancing microprocessor technology for high-speed processing of ultrasonic echoes has permitted superposition of flow direction and velocity information, obtained from Doppler frequency shift analysis throughout the imaging field, upon the 2D image itself. The velocity data are coded in color and shade for direction and velocity, respectively, and are presented as a color velocity map within the cardiac chambers of the 2D image at frame rates of 12 to 30 per second. This flow velocity tomographic image is similar to angiographic projectional images in that it gives the appearance of blood moving normally or abnormally across the valves and within the chambers. Clinical instruments generally provide standard 2D, M-mode, PW, and CW Doppler audio and spectral displays as well as the color flow velocity images.

Echocardiography has some advantages over competing imaging technologies. These include no risk from ionizing radiation, portability of equipment, noninvasive imaging, high imaging rate, no requirement for contrast injection, and generally low cost for the study. Its disadvantages include poor-quality images in 5 to 20 per cent of various patient groups and lack of complete quantitative data from most clinical laboratories.

Feigenbaum H: Echocardiography. 3rd ed. Philadelphia, Lea & Febiger, 1986. *This encyclopedic text is useful for the neophyte as well as the advanced student. Its strength in discussion of M-mode and 2D methods is not quite matched in areas discussing Doppler ultrasound.*

Hatle L, Angelsen B: Doppler Ultrasound in Cardiology. 2nd ed. Philadelphia, Lea & Febiger, 1985. *The most authoritative text on this subject. The chapters on the physics of blood flow and Doppler analysis are excellent. The comprehensive illustrations of pathologic and normal flow velocity patterns are superb. Much of the information included is not published elsewhere.*

Holen J, Aaslid R, Landmark K, et al.: Determination of pressure gradient in mitral stenosis with a non-invasive ultrasound Doppler technique. Acta Med Scand 199:455, 1976. *The classic work describing the clinical use of the relationship between maximum blood velocity detected by Doppler ultrasound and pressure gradient calculated from the velocity.*

Holen J, Aaslid R, Landmark K, et al.: Determination of effective orifice area in mitral stenosis from non-invasive ultrasound Doppler data and mitral

flow rate. Acta Med Scand 201:83, 1977, *Original description of the pressure half-time method for estimation of mitral orifice area using Doppler ultrasound.*

Popp RL, Macovski A: Ultrasonic diagnostic instruments. Science 210:268, 1980. *A more detailed discussion of the instrumentation for producing ultrasonic images than given in this chapter.*

42.4 NUCLEAR CARDIOLOGY

Barry L. Zaret

Nuclear cardiology is based upon the ability of externally placed instruments to detect, define, and quantify radiation emanating from cardiac structures following injection of a radioisotope. The utility of nuclear procedure for defining pathophysiologic, prognostic, and diagnostic phenomena in cardiac patients has been established. The procedures can be safely repeated and are suitable for both imaging and biodistribution studies. Changes in cardiac function, cardiac blood volume, myocardial perfusion, and metabolism can be evaluated routinely.

CARDIAC PERFORMANCE

At present, a major clinical application of nuclear cardiology is in the assessment of global and regional cardiac performance. This is achieved with radionuclides that remain within the intravascular space during the period of study. Computer technology is critical for appropriate measurement. Cardiac performance can be assessed in two general ways: during the first pass of the isotope through the central circulation or following its equilibration in the cardiac blood pool. First-pass radionuclide angiocardiography is completed within 30 seconds following intravenous injection of a technetium-99m compound. There is temporal and anatomic segregation of the radioactive bolus during its first transit through the central circulation. Thus it is possible to make concomitant measurements of right and left ventricular function without concern that radioactivity present in one ventricle is interfering with the analysis of the other. Analysis of time-activity curves generated from the respective ventricular regions allows determination of ventricular ejection fraction (Fig. 42–30). Count rates emanating from a cardiac chamber are proportional to the volume of the chamber. In addition to analysis of ejection fraction, rates of ventricular filling and emptying, and ventricular volumes, quantitative and qualitative assessments of regional wall motion can be made from the same data (Fig. 42–31).

The alternative and more widely used approach to assessing cardiac performance involves complete equilibration of the radionuclide within the intravascular space. Physiologic signals are introduced that convert the conventional static imaging procedure into a dynamic assessment of cardiac function. To obtain this goal, technetium-99m is bound to the patient's own erythrocytes. The technetium-99m label remains evenly distributed throughout the intravascular blood volume for several hours. With the use of the electrocardiogram, nuclear data are segregated according to the time of their occurrence within the cardiac cycle. The R wave peak corresponds to maximal (end-diastolic) radioactivity. Data are summed over several hundred cardiac cycles, and composite data are quantified and displayed as sequential 10- to 50-msec points, which together define a representative cardiac cycle. The ventricular volume curve derived from these data is suitable for direct measurement of ejection fraction, rates of filling and ejection, and ventricular volumes. The data also may be displayed as a series of images that, when projected in cinematic format, provide a direct visual assessment of the regional contraction patterns of the heart (Fig. 42–32). Newly developed computer techniques now make it possible also to quantify regional motion accurately.

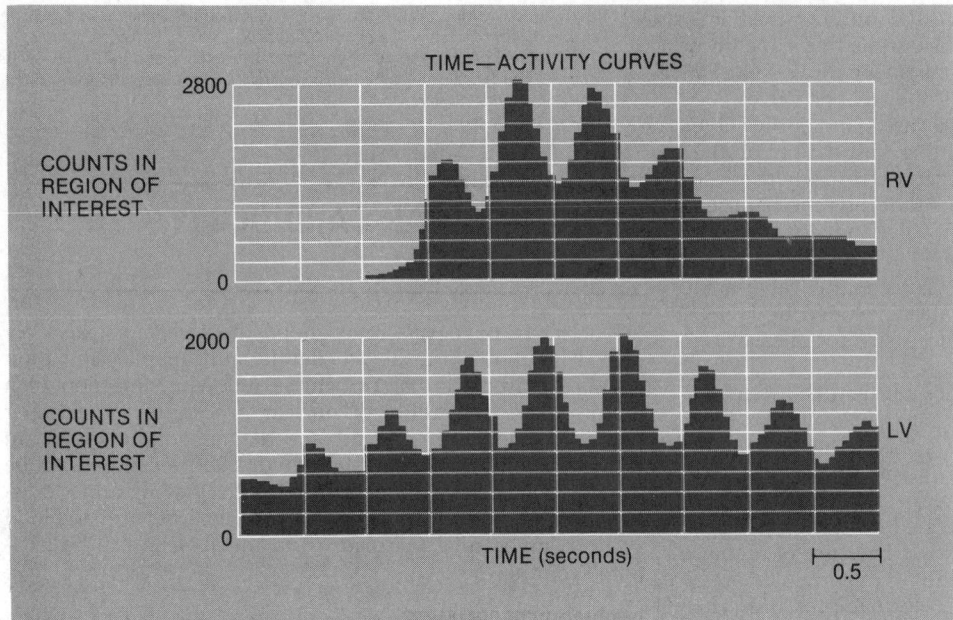

FIGURE 42–30. Right ventricular (RV) and left ventricular (LV) time-activity curves obtained at 20 frames per second with the computerized multicrystal scintillation camera. Analysis of these time-activity curves allows determination of ventricular ejection fraction. (Redrawn from Berger HJ, et al.: Semin Nucl Med 9:275, 1979.)

Both first-pass and equilibrium techniques can be employed to study cardiac performance under conditions of rest and exercise. Data may be accumulated during supine, semisupine, or upright bicycle exercise. Often critical data concerning cardiovascular status emerge only when the patient is evaluated during stress. The normal response to exercise involves an augmentation in the pump function of both ventricles. Normal ventricular reserve generally is defined as an increase in ejection fraction of each ventricle of at least 5 per cent (in absolute ejection fraction units) and the presence of normal regional wall motion. Abnormal exercise ventricular reserve may be encountered in a variety of pathophysiologic conditions involving coronary artery disease and intrinsic myocardial, valvular, and congenital heart disease.

The study of cardiac performance employing nuclear techniques has been particularly useful in patients with coronary artery disease. The ejection fraction is the single best clinical indicator of global ventricular pump performance. This index is of major prognostic importance in patients with coronary artery disease, either immediately following myocardial infarction or in the chronic stable phase of disease. Analysis of the ventricular ejection fraction is based upon radioactivity counts taken over the entire cardiac cycle. It is not dependent upon geometric assumptions concerning ventricular shape or ventricular volume. In coronary artery disease, particularly following myocardial infarction, asymmetric contraction patterns are common. In these ischemic ventricles, cavitary shapes frequently cannot be approximated by idealized geometric models. Consequently, in coronary artery disease, ejection fraction is measured most accurately by the nuclear approach. Using portable equipment, it is possible to study cardiac performance at the bedside of the acutely ill in coronary and intensive care units. Such studies have demonstrated substantial abnormalities in the functioning of the ischemic left ventricle during the acute phase of myocardial infarction. Abnormalities of both left and right ventricles can be identified. Right ventricular infarction occurring in the course of inferior wall infarction has been identified and further defined. The important negative prognostic impact of functional left ventricular aneurysm formation during acute anterior infarction has been defined. Assessment of regional and global function also is an important means of evaluating the effect of thrombolytic therapy for acute infarction.

Abnormalities of ventricular performance are found in approximately 85 per cent of patients with coronary artery disease studied during exercise stress. Myocardial ischemia is reflected in abnormal ventricular reserve. Abnormal responses of the ejection fraction may be encountered in a variety of conditions, but the development of new regional abnormalities of wall motion is quite specific for coronary artery disease. Abnormal exercise performance has important prognostic implications, particularly following infarction.

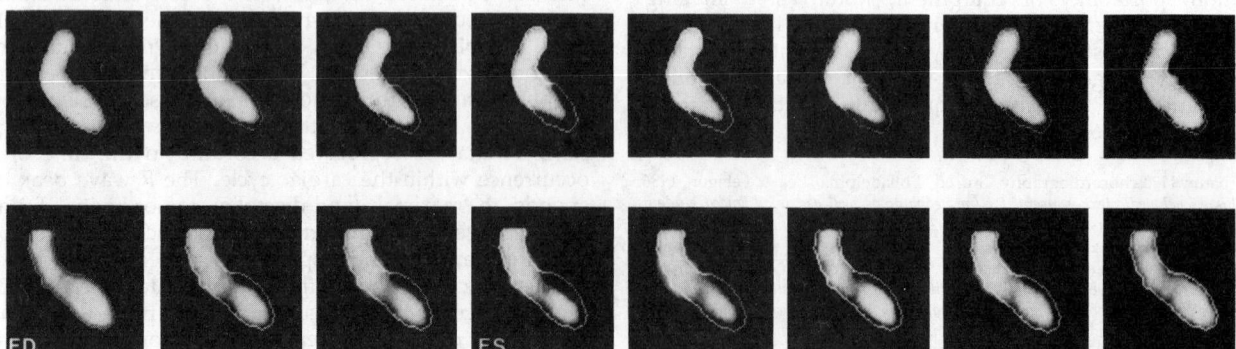

FIGURE 42–31. Selected serial 50-millisecond left ventricular images obtained throughout the cardiac cycle shown superimposed over the end-diastolic perimeters. The first frame in each series represents end-diastole (ED) and the fourth frame end-systole (ES). The upper row of images was obtained at rest and the lower row during maximal bicycle exercise in a patient with coronary artery disease. The two series are displayed at the same heart rate. Regional wall motion is normal at rest. However, inferoapical hypokinesis is present during exercise. (Reproduced from Berger HJ, et al.: Semin Nucl Med 9:275, 1979.)

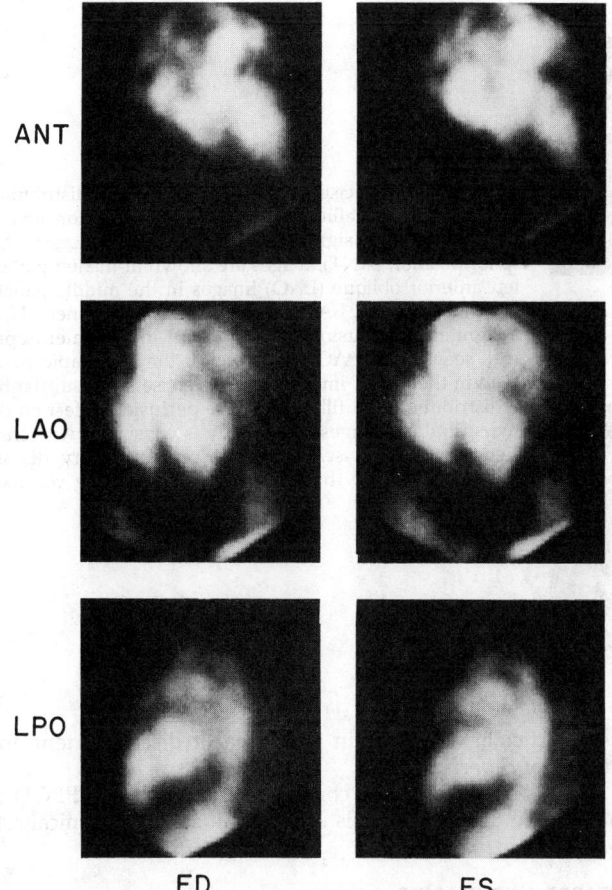

ED   ES

FIGURE 42–32. Gated cardiac blood pool studies obtained in the anterior (ANT), 45-degree left anterior oblique (LAO), and left posterior oblique (LPO) positions. End-diastolic images (ED) are shown on the left and end-systolic (ES) on the right. Note that radioactivity is present throughout the entire cardiac blood pool. A large anteroapical left ventricular aneurysm is appreciated in all three positions. Note that in the LAO position image the left ventricle is the posterior cardiac structure and the right ventricle the anterior structure. These are separated by the interventricular septum, which is displayed as an area devoid of radioactivity. (Reproduced from Berger HJ, et al.: Radiol Clin North Am 18:441, 1980.)

Radionuclide assessment of ventricular performance may also be employed in the evaluation of patients with valvular disease at rest or exercise. Resting measurement of cardiac function provides important preoperative prognostic data and may also be of value in defining the physiologic significance of valvular lesions such as mitral regurgitation. For example, normal left ventricular function in a patient with severe mitral regurgitation would imply a primary valvular problem, whereas severe ventricular dysfunction would suggest secondary mitral regurgitation resulting from diffuse myocardial disease. Assessment of performance under hemodynamic stress may help define the advent of irreversible damage in valvular heart disease. This is particularly important in aortic regurgitation, in which irremediable change in left ventricular function is frequently present by the time valve surgery is considered.

Assessment of ventricular performance is critical to the understanding and treatment of congestive heart failure. Knowledge of the degree of impairment in ventricular performance has prognostic and therapeutic relevance. In addition, an important group of patients with primary diastolic dysfunction (normal systolic function and impaired measures of diastolic filling) has been defined. Such patients require other than conventional therapy for heart failure.

Radionuclide studies also have been employed in the evaluation of myocardial function in patients with lung disease in which the major hemodynamic burden falls on the right ventricle. Right ventricular performance can probably be evaluated best with the first-pass technique. Abnormalities in right ventricular performance have been noted at rest and during exercise in patients with chronic obstructive pulmonary disease and have been related to the degree of impairment in ventilatory performance. Pharmacologic interventions may modify abnormal right ventricular performance.

These techniques also have been utilized for long-term studies assessing cardiac therapy. A prototype example has been the application of first-pass radionuclide angiocardiography for the serial assessment of ventricular function in patients receiving the antineoplastic agent doxorubicin. Use of this agent has been limited by the frequent development of a drug-induced cardiomyopathy. Serial measurement of cardiac ejection fraction during the course of therapy has led to a set of guidelines of dosage and schedule that help avert cardiotoxicity.

In addition, left-to-right shunts can be detected and quantified during performance of the first-pass radionuclide angiocardiogram. With this technique, a time-activity curve is generated from a region in the lung field. In the presence of a shunt, early recirculation is detected. The curve can be deconvoluted so that the major components can be quantified and the pulmonic-systemic blood flow ratios determined.

MYOCARDIAL PERFUSION IMAGING

Myocardial perfusion imaging utilizes radionuclides that traverse the myocardial capillary system and enter the myocardial cell. The radionuclide currently employed for these studies is thallium-201. This tracer is considered a potassium analogue, since its distribution generally mirrors that of intracellular potassium. Thallium-201 is produced in the cyclotron and has a physical half-life of approximately 72 hours. After intravenous injection it is rapidly extracted and distributed within the myocardium according to regional myocardial blood flow and regional cellular viability. Recently, a new group of technetium-99m perfusion tracers has been developed. These compounds are now being investigated actively; in the future, they may replace thallium.

At rest, the normal myocardial perfusion image demonstrates homogeneous uptake in the left ventricular wall with a central area of decreased activity corresponding to the left ventricular cavity. In approximately 20 per cent of normal persons, there is a region of decreased uptake at the cardiac apex corresponding to a normal relative thinning of this portion of the left ventricle. Abnormal image patterns will demonstrate a zone of decreased myocardial perfusion as a region of relatively decreased radionuclide uptake. Images are obtained in multiple positions. This is necessary to confirm the presence of a defect and define its location. The normal right ventricle is not visualized at rest because of its smaller mass compared with that of the left ventricle.

In the resting state, abnormalities usually represent either acute or remote myocardial infarction. However, studies have also demonstrated perfusion defects at rest in patients with unstable angina or coronary spasm (either spontaneous or induced by ergonovine maleate) or, rarely, in patients with severe obstructive coronary disease in the absence of clinical evidence of acute ischemia. Defects are noted with high sensitivity during the early hours of acute myocardial infarction. Within the first six hours, virtually all infarcts may be identified. After 24 hours, sensitivity falls to 80 to 90 per cent.

In most patients with coronary artery disease without previous infarction, myocardial perfusion patterns appear normal at rest. This is to be expected, since from a pathophysiologic standpoint coronary blood flow is relatively uniform at rest, even in the presence of severe coronary obstruc-

EXERCISE

REDISTRIBUTION

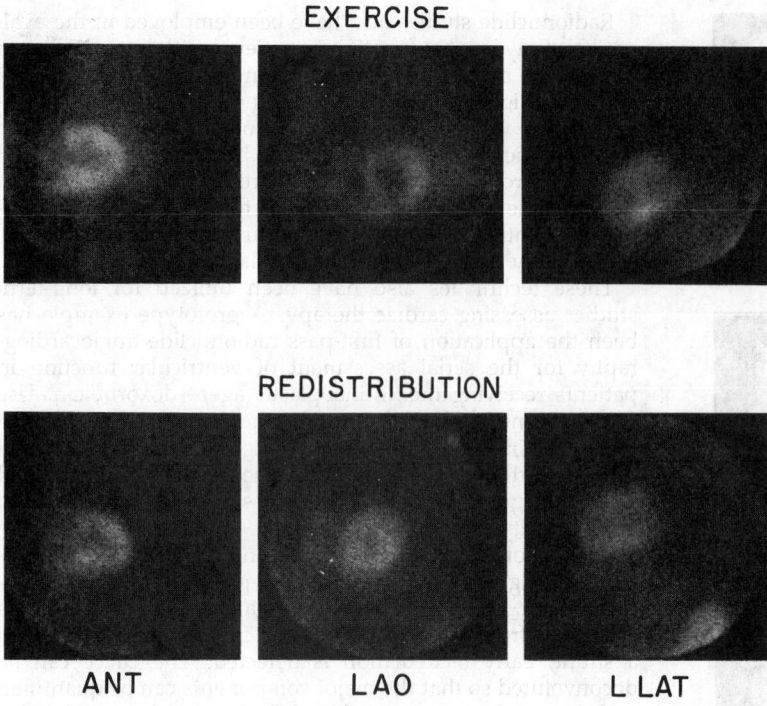

ANT   LAO   L LAT

FIGURE 42–33. Exercise (upper panels) and redistribution (lower panels) thallium-20l myocardial perfusion images in a patient with significant coronary artery disease. Anterior position (ANT) images are shown in the left panels, left anterior oblique (LAO) images in the middle panels, and left lateral (L LAT) images in the right panels. Note a significant perfusion defect present in the anteroseptal wall seen in the LAO image and in the anteroapical wall seen in the L LAT image during exercise, with substantial redistribution and filling in of the perfusion defect on the redistribution images. This study is consistent with transient myocardial ischemia and coronary artery disease involving at least the left anterior descending coronary artery.

tion. The major physiologic abnormality in coronary disease is diminished coronary vascular reserve. Therefore, to detect perfusion abnormalities in coronary disease it is necessary to study patients under conditions of increased myocardial blood flow. Most work has employed exercise as an appropriate stress. Thallium 201 is injected at peak exercise, and imaging is begun within ten minutes after injection. Since thallium is rapidly extracted by myocardium, it can be injected during the period of maximal heterogeneity of regional myocardial blood flow, and its distribution will reflect this heterogeneity. Comparison of images obtained immediately following exercise with those obtained following a redistribution phase two to four hours after exercise allows definition of transiently ischemic zones (Fig. 42–33). Defects present on exercise but not at redistribution are most consistent with transient ischemia; defects that are unchanged are most consistent with previous infarction and scar; and defects that are present at redistribution but are markedly increased during exercise are most consistent with transient ischemia superimposed upon the scar. The overall sensitivity of this technique for detecting significant ischemic disease is approximately 80 per cent. The specificity of the technique is excellent. This technique is of greatest value diagnostically in patients with equivocal exercise electrocardiograms, abnormal baseline electrocardiograms, or suspected false-positive or false-negative conventional exercise tests. Both imaging with the patient at rest and exercise/redistribution studies have been of value in evaluating thrombolysis and reperfusion. Exercise studies also have been of value in assessing prognosis following infarction and in evaluating patients after coronary angioplasty.

An alternative means of stress perfusion imaging involves use of the coronary vasodilator, dipyridamole. Thallium myocardial distributions following dipyridamole provide data comparable to those noted with exercise. However, with pharmacologic stress, evaluation is based upon differences in flow without implying ischemia, whereas with exercise, evaluation is based upon heterogeneity of flow, generally associated with ischemia.

Thallium planar imaging is becoming increasingly quantitative. Computer techniques now provide objective definition of the presence and extent of defects as well as quantification of regional tracer washout kinetics. Kinetic analysis has added a new dimension to diagnostic and functional assessment,

with particular relevance in definition of disease extent and efficacy of reperfusion.

Single photon emission computed tomography (SPECT) of thallium studies currently is under evaluation. Its clinical role awaits further definition.

INFARCT-AVID IMAGING

An additional radionuclide approach involves definition of acute myocardial infarction and regions of acute myocardial necrosis. This is performed with "infarct-avid" radiotracers, which bind selectively to regions of acute infarction. The current agent for this procedure is technetium-99m stannous pyrophosphate, although recent research suggests that radiolabeled antimyosin antibody also may be employed. With this technique, acute infarcts are visualized as regions of increased radionuclide uptake. The mechanism of abnormal pyrophosphate accumulation appears to be related to regional calcium deposition, as well as binding to denatured proteins. Pyrophosphate uptake also is dependent upon sufficient residual blood flow to allow entry of the radioactive tracer.

The infarct zone can be visualized within 24 to 48 hours of the onset of infarction. Maximal visualization generally occurs from 48 to 72 hours after the infarct. Images usually are not positive within the first 24 hours unless thrombolysis has occurred. Images generally are no longer positive seven to ten days after the infarct. From the standpoint of diagnosis, pyrophosphate imaging appears to be a sensitive means of detecting acute myocardial infarction as well as extension of the infarct. Sensitivity is less in patients with nontransmural compared with transmural infarction. Pyrophosphate infarct imaging is most valuable in patients presenting several days after infarction when other studies are equivocal or nondiagnostic.

POSITRON TOMOGRAPHY

This technique involves imaging and quantification of the intracardiac distribution of positron-emitting radionuclides. By virtue of the types of radionuclides available and the instrumentation employed, this technique has provided new insight into metabolism and coronary flow. Since carbon-11 is a positron emitter, a variety of biologically active compounds can be radiolabeled and used for imaging. These include fatty acids, receptor ligands, and neurotransmitters. Although still primarily research in nature, these studies offer great potential for ultimate clinical application. Because of the cost involved and general need for an on-site cyclotron, this technique currently remains experimental and localized to only a few centers.

In addition to positron studies, additional metabolic studies have been obtained using conventional imaging. Studies to date have focused on radioiodinated fatty acids and their analogues.

Berman DS, Garcia EV, Maddahi J, et al.: Thallium-201 myocardial perfusion scintigraphy. In Freeman LM (ed.): Freeman and Johnson's Clinical Radionuclide Imaging. New York, Grune & Stratton, 1984, pp 479–536. *A detailed clinical and technologic explication of myocardial perfusion imaging.*

Pohost GM, Higgins CB, Morganroth J, et al. (eds.): New Concepts in Cardiac Imaging: 1986. Chicago, Year Book Medical Publishers, 1986. *This book contains detailed chapters on perfusion imaging, equilibrium blood pool studies, and positron emission tomographic studies. The contrasting efficacy of other imaging approaches is also outlined in other chapters in this volume.*

Zaret BL, Berger HJ: Techniques of nuclear cardiology. In Hurst JW (ed.): The Heart. 6th ed. New York, McGraw-Hill Book Company, 1986, pp 1809–1858. *A comprehensive review of current clinically relevant aspects of nuclear cardiology with 255 individual references cited.*

42.5 Cardiac Catheterization and Angiography

William H. Barry

Cardiac catheterization provides a unique, comprehensive, and quantitative assessment of cardiac structure and function. As facilities have become more widely available and the risks have decreased, there has been a progressive tendency to employ catheterization in the diagnosis and management of patients with heart disease. With the development of additional techniques such as bedside hemodynamic monitoring, intracardiac electrophysiologic testing, endomyocardial biopsy, and percutaneous transluminal coronary angioplasty, it is increasingly important for the internist to understand the indications, capabilities, and risks of cardiac catheterization.

INDICATIONS FOR CARDIAC CATHETERIZATION AND ANGIOGRAPHY

In general, cardiac catheterization and angiography are performed when the history, physical examination, and noninvasive studies have provided insufficient information to allow a definitive decision about diagnosis or treatment. The accuracy of noninvasive evaluation has increased remarkably recently, because of the greatly improved sensitivity and specificity of two-dimensional echocardiography combined with Doppler procedures, radionuclide ventriculography, thallium 201 myocardial perfusion scintigraphy, and fast computed atrial tomographic (CAT) and magnetic resonance imaging (MRI) scanners. Therefore, cardiac catheterization is performed most frequently to quantify the severity of disease present and to determine whether the patient is a candidate for surgical intervention. In Table 42–5 are shown the diagnoses of a typical series of patients referred for cardiac catheterization. As can be seen, the vast majority of patients undergoing this procedure have coronary artery disease, with patients having valvular disease a distant second. In Table 42–6 are listed the usual indications for cardiac catheterization and coronary angiography in patients with coronary artery disease or valvular heart disease.

TECHNIQUES AND THEIR HAZARDS

ARTERIAL AND VENOUS ACCESS. Two basic approaches are used for insertion of catheters into arteries and veins. The first involves incision of the skin overlying the vessel, dissection of the vessel free of surrounding tissue, and incision of the vessel with direct insertion of the catheter. This method is usually reserved for the brachial artery or antecubital vein. The advantage of this technique is that one has direct access to the vessels, so that they may either be tied off (vein) or repaired (brachial artery) after completion of the catheterization procedure. This procedure decreases the likelihood of hematoma formation. The disadvantages of the technique are that an incision is required in the skin, increasing the patient's discomfort in the postcatheterization period, and that there is a significant (2 to 3 per cent) incidence of thrombosis of the brachial artery. For these reasons, and because it requires a longer time to perform, this technique is less commonly employed than the percutaneous method. However, it may be preferred in patients with severe atherosclerotic disease of the aorta or iliofemoral arteries.

In the Seldinger technique, an artery or vein is punctured percutaneously with a needle, and a thin, flexible guide wire is then inserted through the needle into the vessel and advanced up the vessel. The needle is withdrawn over the wire, and then a catheter may be inserted directly over the wire, or a short arterial or venous sheath may be inserted, using a dilator, over the wire and into the vessel to provide access. The percutaneous technique is employed most frequently for the femoral artery and vein, the axillary artery, or the subclavian or internal jugular vein. This technique is relatively simple, and no sutures are required. The disadvantage is that one does not have direct control of the vessels after withdrawal of the catheters or sheaths, and control of postcatheterization bleeding may be more difficult than with the direct-approach. Patients must therefore be relatively immobile at least four to six hours. At present, the percutaneous femoral approach in which the femoral artery and femoral vein are punctured is most commonly utilized for cardiac catheterization.

Because of potential hemostasis problems after the procedure, elective cardiac catheterization is usually not performed if the prothrombin time is greater than 18 seconds. To decrease the risk of thrombosis during the catheterization procedure, heparin is frequently used for catheterization of the left side of the heart. The anticoagulant effect of heparin is usually reversed with protamine at the termination of the procedure, before the final withdrawal of the sheath or catheter. The main risks of arterial or venous puncture and subsequent catheter manipulation are thrombosis of the vessel, hemorrhage, cerebrovascular accident, and myocardial infarction induced by clot from the tip of the catheter or dislodgment of atherosclerotic material. Table 42–7 summarizes the incidence of complications during cardiac catheterization and coronary angiography. Catheterization of the left side of the heart generally carries a much higher risk than catheterization of the right side of the heart because of the ability of the lung vascular bed to filter out thrombi. Angiography carries a higher risk than simple pressure measurements of the left side of the heart because of the additional catheter manipu-

TABLE 42–5. DIAGNOSES OF 562 PATIENTS CONSECUTIVELY STUDIED

Coronary Artery Disease (CAD)	Valvular Disease	CAD and Valvular Disease	Cardiomyopathy	Normal Persons	Congenital Heart Disease	Miscellaneous
62.6%	16.7%	6.0%	5.9%	6.4%	1.4%	0.9%

Adapted from Barry WH, et al.: Cathet Cardiovasc Diagn 8:401, 1979.

TABLE 42–6. POSSIBLE INDICATIONS FOR CARDIAC CATHETERIZATION AND ANGIOGRAPHY

Suspected Coronary Artery Disease

1. Angina, especially if:
   unstable
   refractory to treatment
   strongly positive treadmill ECG
   young person with positive
   family history

2. After acute myocardial infarction,
   if:
   angina
   positive treadmill result

3. In selected patients suspected to
   have "silent" ischemia
   occupational hazards
   strong family history of
   infarction/sudden death

4. Patients with ischemic
   cardiomyopathy and congestive
   heart failure (CHF)

5. In patients with high risk (age, diabetes, lipid disorder) prior to major
   noncardiac surgery; in patients at risk for coronary artery disease in
   whom cardiac surgery is planned.

Suspected Valvular Disease

1. Aortic stenosis
   angina
   syncope
   CHF

2. Aortic regurgitation
   CHF
   angina
   progressive cardiac
   enlargement

3. Mitral stenosis*
   CHF refractory to digitalis
   and diuretics
   Recurrent emboli with
   atrial fibrillation

4. Mitral regurgitation
   CHF
   Progressive cardiac
   enlargement

Additional Miscellaneous Indicators

   Congenital heart disease
   Pericardial disease
Other: Percutaneous transluminal coronary angioplasty
   Electrophysiologic study
   Biopsy
   Hemodynamic monitoring

*Operation may be performed without catheterization if diagnosis is certain.

TABLE 42–7. COMPLICATIONS OF CARDIAC CATHETERIZATION AND ANGIOGRAPHY*

Complication	Incidence (%)
Death	0.14
Myocardial infarction	0.07
Cardiovascular accident	0.07
Arrhythmia	0.56
Vascular complications	0.57
Other	0.41
TOTAL	1.82

*Data on 53,581 patients.
Adapted from Kennedy JW: Complications associated with cardiac catheterization and angiography. Cathet Cardiovasc Diagn 8:5, 1982.

catheterization of the right and left sides of the heart, all the pressures within the heart are measured, with the usual exception of the left atrial pressure. The pulmonary capillary "wedge" position, in which a segment of the pulmonary arterial tree is occluded either with the catheter tip or with a small balloon attached to the end of a catheter (a flow-directed Swan-Ganz type of catheter), gives a pressure that resembles closely the true left atrial pressure (Fig. 42–34). Normally, the diastolic pressure of the pulmonary artery is very close to the mean wedge pressure. However, in patients with tachycardia or with increased pulmonary vascular resistance, pulmonary artery end-diastolic pressure may be significantly higher than the mean wedge pressure. The normal values for intracardiac pressures are given in Ch. 41.

In addition to the average pressures, the shape and magnitude of the waveforms frequently contain diagnostic information. For example, in mitral regurgitation there is a large v wave in the left atrial or pulmonary artery wedge pressure recording (Fig. 42–35). A large v wave in the right atrial pressure tracing indicates tricuspid insufficiency. Simultaneous pressures are usually measured in the pulmonary wedge position and left ventricle to quantitate mitral valve function. A pressure gradient in diastole between the pulmonary wedge pressure and left ventricular diastolic pressure is seen, for example, in mitral stenosis (Fig. 42–36). Left ventricular and aortic pressures are measured simultaneously to assess aortic valve function.

Comparison of pressures in different chambers can be very useful. In patients with pericardial constriction, there is equalization of the right atrial and the pulmonary artery wedge pressures, and the mean right atrial pressure is greater than one third of the right ventricular systolic pressure. Measure-

lation, selective placement of the catheters within the coronary arteries, and use of angiographic contrast solution, especially in patients with more severe cardiac diseases.

PRESSURE MEASUREMENTS. Measurement of intracardiac pressure is an essential part of the cardiac catheterization procedure. Pressures are measured by attaching the end of the fluid-filled catheter to an external pressure transducer. The pressure waveform transmitted through the fluid-filled catheter deforms a pressure-sensitive diaphragm in the transducer, which changes the resistance of an electrical circuit and allows recording of the pressure waveform as voltage signals. Phasic pressure waveforms up to 12 Hz may be recorded with this technique (Fig. 42–34). During routine

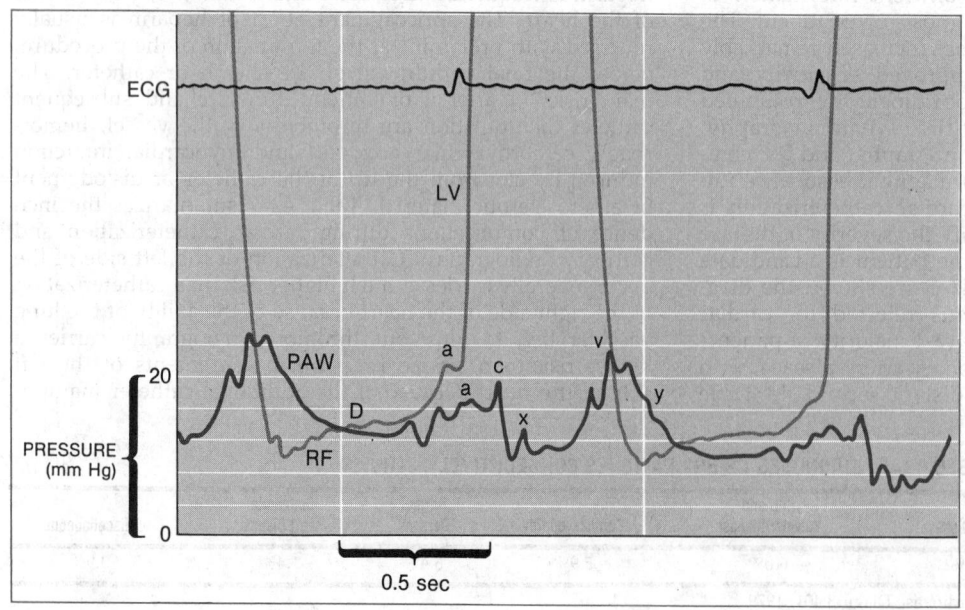

FIGURE 42–34. Simultaneous pulmonary artery wedge (PAW) pressure and left ventricular pressure (LV) in a normal patient. RF = Rapid LV filling; D = diastasis of LV filling; a = atrial contraction pressure wave. Note the delay of the PAW pressure relative to LV pressure.

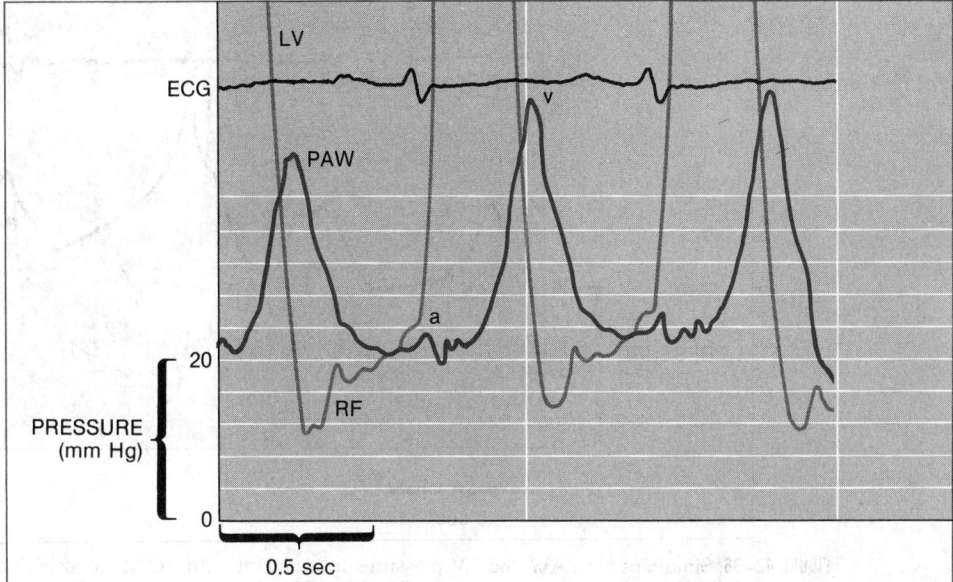

FIGURE 42–35. Simultaneous PAW and LV pressures in a patient with severe mitral regurgitation. Note large v wave, with rapid y descent.

ment of intracardiac pressures during exercise or pacing stress may also provide useful information. For example, patients with mitral stenosis or mitral insufficiency may have relatively normal resting pressures but abnormally high pulmonary artery wedge pressures with exercise. Patients with coronary artery disease may have normal left ventricular diastolic pressures at rest, which elevate markedly during the stress of pacing tachycardia owing to ischemic left ventricular dysfunction.

MEASUREMENT OF CARDIAC BLOOD FLOW. Another important part of cardiac catheterization is measurement of cardiac output. In the Fick method, oxygen consumption is measured by collecting all expired air over a three-minute period into a bag and determining the oxygen content in the expired air. This allows determination of oxygen consumption in milliliters per minute. Collection of samples from the pulmonary artery (mixed venous sample) and a systemic artery allows determination of the arteriovenous (A-V) oxygen difference. If the value for hemoglobin concentration in the blood is known, this allows calculation of the milliliters of blood that had to flow through the lungs to acquire the amount of oxygen consumed. (See bottom of page.)

Cardiac output may be normalized by dividing by body surface area (m^2) and expressed as cardiac index. The determined cardiac output by the Fick technique is most accurate when the cardiac output is low and thus the A-V oxygen content difference is large. In patients with intracardiac shunts, correction for the shunt must be made. This occurs most commonly in adult patients with atrial septal defects or ventricular septal defects with a left-to-right shunt. The pulmonary artery saturation in these conditions is elevated relative to the true mixed venous saturation, which is most closely approximated by the superior vena cava saturation. Standard methods for quantification of left-to-right and right-to-left intracardiac shunts exist.

Another method commonly used for measurement of cardiac output is dye dilution, in which indocyanine green dye is injected in a peripheral vein, with continuous sampling of the dye concentration from a peripheral artery. The cardiac output is calculated as $\dfrac{i}{c \times t}$, where i is the quantity of indicator injected, c is the average arterial concentration of the indicator during its first pass, and t is the total duration of the dye concentration curve in the arterial blood. The product of c and t is easily measured as the area under the first-pass curve determined by planimetry. The error of the dye dilution indicator curve is greatest in patients with extremely low outputs or with mitral or aortic regurgitation. The dye curve is also distorted by the presence of intracardiac shunts and in fact may be used in certain circumstances to diagnose the presence and direction of an intracardiac shunt. The indicator dye curve output is most accurate in patients with high cardiac output and a narrow A-V oxygen difference.

The thermodilution method is another dilution indicator method; in this case, the indicator is not dye, but cold saline injected into the right atrium. Temperature changes are detected with a thermistor in the pulmonary artery. The advantages of the thermodilution method are that it is relatively unaffected by mitral and aortic regurgitation and that it may be repeated frequently to measure serial outputs. It is influenced by respiration, by the presence of shunts that increase pulmonary flow, and by the presence of tricuspid regurgitation. At the presence time, the Fick method is most commonly employed in the cardiac catheterization laboratory, and the thermodilution method is most commonly utilized in intensive care unit settings where patients are being monitored with catheters in the right side of the heart.

From measurements of cardiac output and pressure gradients across vascular beds, the systemic and pulmonary vascular resistances may be calculated. Elevations in systemic vascular resistance are important in patients with chronic congestive heart failure and may identify those patients who will respond favorably to vasodilator therapy. Pulmonary vascular resistance is frequently elevated in patients with severe left ventricular failure and elevated wedge pressures, in patients with mitral valve disease, in patients with left-to-right shunts, and always in patients with primary pulmonary hypertension. Measurement of changes in pulmonary and

$$\text{Cardiac output (liters/min)} = \frac{\text{oxygen consumption (ml O}_2\text{/min)}}{\text{A-V O}_2\text{ difference (ml O}_2\text{/liter blood)}}$$

$$\text{A-V O}_2 \text{ difference (ml O}_2\text{/liter blood)} = 13.9 \times \text{hemoglobin (gm/dl)} \times (\% \text{ sat A} - \% \text{ sat V})$$

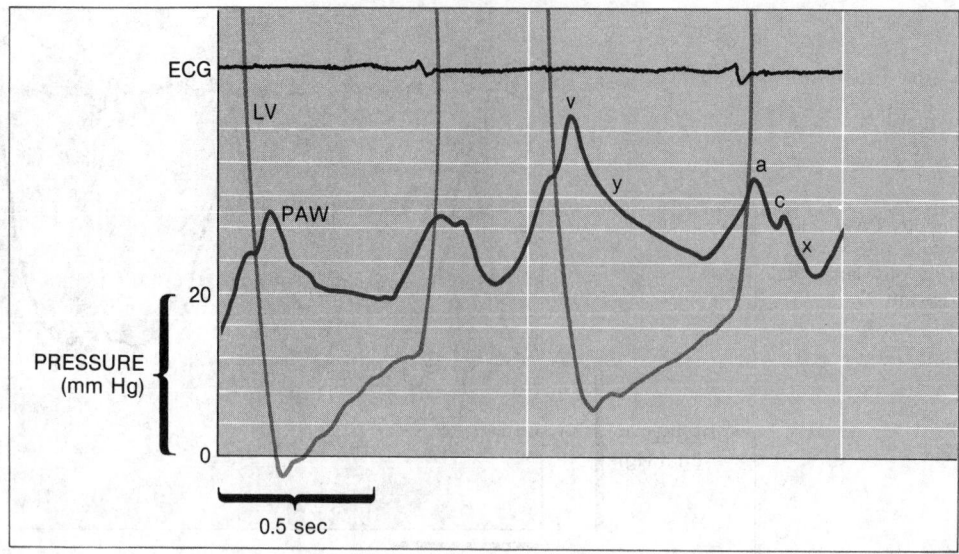

FIGURE 42–36. Simultaneous PAW and LV pressures in a patient with mitral stenosis. Notice slow y descent, and the large gradient throughout diastole between PAW and LV diastolic pressures. The actual mitral valve area (M.V.A.) may be estimated as:

$$M.V.A. = \frac{\text{diastolic mitral flow (ml/sec)}}{38\sqrt{\text{diastolic pressure gradient}}}$$

Thus, for a given M.V.A., the pressure gradient across the valve goes up as the *square* of mitral valve flow. This explains why the PAW pressure rises so markedly with increased cardiac output and hence increased mitral valve flow. Increased heart rate shortens diastolic time, and hence increases the mitral valve flow rate per unit of diastolic time at any given cardiac output.

systemic vascular resistances and in cardiac outputs and pressures before and after administration of vasodilator drugs may be helpful in guiding treatment of patients with specific disorders and is frequently employed, in the catheterization laboratory setting.

Measurement of pressure gradients across the aortic, mitral, tricuspid, or pulmonic valve allows estimation of valve area utilizing the Gorlin formula (see Fig. 42–36). The calculated valve area may differ significantly from the true value, particularly in situations of very low cardiac output or valvular insufficiency. Nevertheless, this measurement is often useful in guiding surgical interventions.

ANGIOGRAPHY. During routine cardiac catheterization, left ventriculography and coronary angiography are commonly performed. In left ventriculography, contrast material is injected into the left ventricular chamber and cineangiographic filming is performed at 30 to 60 frames per second. Ejection fraction is determined as the fraction of end-diastolic ventricular volume ejected each systole. In patients with mitral or aortic regurgitation, the angiographic regurgitant volume can be estimated by comparing the angiographic stroke volume and the forward stroke volume determined by the Fick method. However, because of frequent inaccuracies in absolute volume measurements by angiographic methods, the degree of regurgitation is usually graded on a simple 1+ to 4+ scale. In patients with coronary artery disease, segmental contraction abnormalities are frequently present, and these may be quantified by a variety of regional indices of left ventricular performance.

Adverse effects of left ventriculography include a negative inotropic effect due to calcium binding by the contrast agent and an intravascular volume–expanding effect due to hyperosmolality of the contrast material. The myocardial depressant effects of contrast agents are usually not a problem unless left ventricular function is severely compromised. In these patients, the risks of left ventriculography may be reduced by using nonionic, non–calcium-binding contrast agents or by use of digital image enhancement techniques that permit use of a small volume of contrast material, or both.

Injection of dye into the aortic root allows assessment of the degree of aortic insufficiency, and right ventricular contrast injection allows assessment of the tricuspid valve. Pulmonary angiography may be performed to assess the pulmonary vasculature and to detect presence of pulmonary emboli.

Coronary cineangiography is performed by injecting a contrast agent selectively into the right or left main coronary ostia and filming at 30 frames per second. The degree of coronary artery obstruction in multiple views is assessed by measuring the percentage of narrowing of the artery at the site or sites of obstruction or by determining the percentage of area of stenosis by video densitometric measurements. The presence and location of collateral vessels to partially or totally occluded coronary segments are also determined. In patients with no or only minor coronary artery narrowings, but with a suggestive history of chest pain, ergonovine may be infused intravenously to precipitate coronary artery spasm, which then can be documented angiographically.

Insertion of a catheter into the coronary tree may precipitate coronary occlusion by provoking spasm, by dislodging thrombus, or by dissecting the arterial wall. With current techniques, however, these complications are rare (see Table 42–6). Recent developments (nonionic contrast material, smaller high-flow catheters, and digital coronary angiographic image enhancement techniques) can be expected to decrease further the risk of this procedure.

Barry WH, Grossman W: Cardiac catheterization. In Braunwald E. (ed.): Heart Disease. Philadelphia, W.B. Saunders Company, 1984.

Cowley MJ. Vetrovec GW, Di Sciascio G, et al.: Coronary angioplasty of multiple vessels: Short term outcome and long term results. Circulation 73:1314, 1985. *Representative report of current success rate and complications.*

Grossman W: Cardiac Catheterization and Angiography. Philadelphia, Lea & Febiger, 1980. *Excellent comprehensive text on catheterization and angiography.*

Kennedy JW: Complications associated with cardiac catheterization and angiography. Cathet Cardiovasc Diagn 8:5, 1982. *Excellent description of type and incidence of complications.*

Rahimtoola SH, Zipes DP: Consensus statement of the state of the art of electrophysiological testing in the diagnosis and treatment of patients with cardiac arrhythmias. Circulation, April 1987. *Summary of current status of invasive electrophysiologic testing.*

43 HEART FAILURE

Thomas W. Smith

The heart generates the motive force to satisfy the metabolic needs of tissues by delivery of blood containing oxygen and nutrients. The minute-to-minute adjustments in the distribution of the cardiac output according to physiologic priorities (e.g., muscular exercise, heat loss, and digestion) require a complex regulatory system that must also serve to protect vital organs such as the heart and brain when cardiac output is compromised.

The normal or failing heart, in terms of its structure and function, may be examined as a pump, as a muscle, or as a component of the circulatory system. This chapter will address aspects of heart failure common to the various disease entities discussed in subsequent chapters.

GENERAL ASPECTS

The term *heart failure* is generally used as a synonym for myocardial failure, emphasizing the impaired performance of the heart as a muscle and as a pump. It also provides a rationale for medical treatment. Subsequent chapters deal with syndromes in which the cause of circulatory compromise lies elsewhere, such as in abnormalities of the heart valves or pericardium or inappropriate heart rates.

Imbalance between circulatory demands and cardiac response sets the stage for the syndrome of heart failure. Volume overload is generally tolerated better than pressure overload. Aortic or mitral insufficiency produces *volume* overload that may be tolerated for years without overt heart failure; *pressure* overload from aortic stenosis, in contrast, usually results in much earlier onset of heart failure. Gradually developing overloads are accommodated better than acute overloads. Thus, gradually developing chronic mitral regurgitation is often present for years without signs of failure, whereas acute mitral regurgitation from a ruptured chorda tendinea can precipitate life-threatening pulmonary edema.

The myocardium adapts quite differently to volume and pressure loads. Volume overloads typically produce dilation followed by hypertrophy; pressure overloads characteristically elicit concentric hypertrophy until late in the natural history when dilation supervenes. Primary myocardial disease usually results in both dilation and hypertrophy.

Precipitating stresses (see Table 43–2) often tip the balance of the compromised heart toward decompensation and constitute important items for therapeutic attention.

CLINICAL CATEGORIES OF HEART FAILURE

Types of heart failure are often categorized according to five features: duration (acute or chronic), initiating mechanisms, the ventricle primarily affected, the clinical syndrome, and the underlying physiologic derangements.

Acute Versus Chronic Heart Failure

The clinical manifestations of heart failure often begin insidiously and progress gradually into a chronic state. Alternatively, onset may be abrupt, as after myocardial infarction.

Compensatory mechanisms in both acute and chronic heart failure include increased systemic vascular resistance and redistribution of blood flow. However, these adaptive mechanisms in acute and chronic heart failure differ quantitatively and sometimes also in direction. For example, *acute* distention of the left atrium generally promotes a sodium-poor diuresis, whereas *chronic* distention of the left atrium elicits salt and water retention.

Initiating Mechanisms

Each initiating mechanism has its own distinctive characteristics. For example, the symptoms and signs that evolve in rheumatic heart disease differ from those of hypertensive heart disease, whereas both have a different natural history from that of cor pulmonale. Even a single etiology, arteriosclerosis, may have distinctly different consequences, depending on the size and location of affected vessels: Progressive narrowing and gradual occlusion of distal branches of the coronary arteries may be so covert that shortness of breath and fatigue may be misinterpreted as the general physical decline of advancing age. In contrast, abrupt closure of a major coronary artery may result in myocardial necrosis followed by an acute low output state or by progressive chronic heart failure.

Left Versus Right Heart Failure

One ventricle bears the brunt of many disease processes and fails before the other. Because of the prevalence of cardiac disorders that overload or damage the left ventricle, heart failure most often begins with that ventricle. Breathlessness is the most common presenting symptom and is a direct consequence of elevated left ventricular filling pressure and pulmonary congestion. When the right ventricle fails, systemic venous congestion and peripheral edema predominate. Left ventricular failure is the most common cause of right ventricular failure, and breathlessness may improve as right ventricular output falls and pulmonary congestion diminishes.

The mechanism by which left ventricular failure causes the right ventricle to fail is not clear. Pulmonary hypertension secondary to left ventricular failure may contribute, but the degree of pulmonary hypertension is often insufficient to constitute a formidable burden on the right ventricle. Interdependence of the two ventricles, with failure of shared muscle in the ventricular septum, may also contribute. How often right ventricular failure causes left ventricular failure is still a matter of debate, complicated by the high frequency of independent and unrelated left ventricular disease in elderly patients with right ventricular failure.

The combination of left and right ventricular (biventricular) failure, with elevated filling pressures of both ventricles causing pulmonary and systemic venous hypertension, is known as "congestive heart failure." This term implies reduced effort tolerance, breathlessness, distended neck veins, hepatic engorgement, and peripheral edema.

Backward Versus Forward Heart Failure

"Backward failure" refers to elevated cardiac filling pressures and attributes to the consequent venous congestion a critical role in the evolution of the syndrome of heart failure. "Forward failure" refers to decreased cardiac output and inadequate perfusion of organs. This distinction has limited clinical usefulness and has largely been replaced by more specific consideration of ventricular filling pressures and cardiac output.

High Versus Low Output Failure

The separation into "high" and "low" output failure distinguishes certain clinical manifestations, rather than causes, of myocardial failure. It serves: (1) to distinguish a type of myocardial failure ("high output failure") in which the circulation remains brisk and the extremities tend to remain warm despite elevated venous pressures and a lower cardiac output than existed prior to the onset of heart failure; (2) to emphasize that the cardiac output and the circulatory adjustments during heart failure are conditioned by the state that existed prior to heart failure; and (3) to relate etiology to typical clinical features of heart failure. In regard to this last point, the more common causes—arteriosclerosis, hypertension, myocardial disease, valvular disease, and pericardial disease—tend to produce low output states; other, less common causes, including hyperthyroidism, Paget's disease of bone, anemia, beriberi, and arteriovenous fistula, tend to be associated with high output states. The essence of cardiac failure, however, remains the inability of the heart to increase its output appropriately in relation to demand.

Congestive Failure Versus Congested State

Elevated volume of the circulation, with preserved ventricular function, characterizes the "congested state." It is commonly encountered in intensive care facilities, where vigorous volume infusions are often used to combat systemic hypotension. It is encountered on a chronic basis in severe anemia and chronic renal insufficiency and less often in Paget's disease or beriberi. In these situations, venous hypertension results from expanded intravascular volume, rather than from impaired myocardial contractile state.

In time, myocardial failure may supervene but may then be difficult to detect on clinical grounds alone, because the hyperkinetic circulation tends to persist and the congestion may be only modestly increased. Cardiac catheterization, however, discloses an inadequate increase in cardiac output for the increment in oxygen uptake during exercise. Identification of the transition from a "congested state" to "congestive heart failure" is of greater theoretic than practical importance, since correction of inciting factors and administration of diuretics are effective in both situations.

SUBCELLULAR BASIS FOR CONTRACTION

Cardiac contraction is initiated by depolarization of the sarcolemmal membrane, which activates slow calcium channels that undergo a transient increase in calcium permeability. The resulting calcium influx triggers the release of a much larger amount of calcium from the sarcoplasmic reticulum with consequent sarcomere shortening; the sarcoplasmic reticulum then resequesters calcium to turn off myofilament interaction, permitting myocardial relaxation.

Contractile force in heart muscle is generated by interactions among contractile proteins in repeating units (sarcomeres) that compose the individual muscle fibers (myofibrils). Within each sarcomere, the contractile proteins are arranged in thick filaments consisting of myosin and thin filaments consisting of actin and the modulator proteins troponin and tropomyosin. Interaction of calcium with one of three proteins composing troponin initiates the contractile process by removing a troponin-tropomyosin–induced inhibition of thick and thin filament interaction.

Changes in the length of heart muscle during contraction and relaxation are explained by the sliding filament hypothesis. During contraction, the thin actin filaments are propelled past the myosin thick filaments by force generated by ATP-dependent movement of cross-bridges consisting of the head portion of the myosin molecule. As the muscle shortens, the cross-bridges disengage and then engage other sites with a ratchet-like action. Depending on the number of cross-bridges that interact at a given time, different tensions will be developed. Uptake of cytosolic calcium by the sarcoplasmic reticulum allows cross-bridge disengagement and relaxation to occur. Abundant mitochondria generate energy for the contractile machinery by oxidative phosphorylation fueled by free fatty acids and, to a lesser extent, glucose.

For the sarcomere, as for the whole heart (see Preload, below), the tension developed during contraction is directly related to its end-diastolic length. Stretching to permit optimal thick and thin filament overlap increases the ability of individual contractile elements to develop force. There are still many uncertainties regarding molecular details of the contractile process, and much is still to be learned about cardiac

"success" as an essential background against which to examine basic mechanisms in cardiac "failure."

PATHOPHYSIOLOGIC INTERPLAY

Because of their location, structure, and function, the heart and lungs operate as a functional unit. The continuity of the muscle that surrounds the ventricular chambers, the shared ventricular septum, and the encasing pericardium ensure coordinate function, yet each ventricle functions as a separate muscular pump with its own atrial booster pump. In the normal heart, at least 50 per cent of the ventricular end-diastolic volume is ejected with each beat. Although many properties of ejection are inherent in the architecture and physiology of cardiac muscle, adaptability to changing metabolic needs is provided by a superimposed set of neurohumoral adjustments that modulate cardiac contractility.

Each ventricle has its own capacity to withstand and repair the stresses imposed by normal and abnormal function. The two ventricles also have different designs in keeping with their different physiologic functions. Before birth, both ventricles bear similar pressure loads. After birth, the right ventricular work load decreases as pulmonary arterial pressure falls, and the durability of right ventricular performance thus tends to exceed that of the left ventricle. These prospects are enhanced by the greater prevalence of diseases that compromise the left side of the heart and its blood supply.

ASSESSMENT OF CARDIAC PERFORMANCE

In terms of its performance, the heart may be assessed as a pump, as a muscle, or as a component of the circulatory system. Hemodynamic pressure and flow measurements characterize its behavior as a pump. Principles of muscle mechanics are used to describe its behavior as a muscle. Its adequacy as a component of the circulatory system is reflected in the consequences of reduced cardiac output, redistribution of blood flow, organ hypoperfusion, and pulmonary or systemic venous congestion.

Heart as a Pump: Hemodynamics

By the time overt heart failure is apparent, a variety of mechanisms operate to compensate for its diminished performance. Despite an inappropriately low cardiac output, the blood pressure at rest tends to remain normal or even increases.

CARDIAC OUTPUT. In response to peripheral demands, a complex set of control mechanisms modulates heart rate and the extent of stretch and shortening of myocardial fibers and, hence, the stroke volume and the cardiac output (stroke volume times heart rate). Three principal variables determine the stroke volume (Table 43–1): preload, afterload (resistance to ventricular emptying during systole), and the contractile state of the heart. For practical purposes, three of the principal determinants of cardiac output—preload, afterload, and heart rate—are readily measured. Contractile (inotropic) state remains difficult to assess in quantitative terms. Ejection fraction is commonly used as an index (albeit impure) of contractile state, and the maximum rate of pressure rise during the isovolumetic phase of systole (dP/dt) is a useful measure.

Relationships among these determinants vary with the state of the heart and circulation. Thus when contractility is impaired, stroke output and cardiac output tend to be maintained by ventricular dilation (Frank-Starling mechanism), limiting the value of cardiac output as a measure of inotropic state to experimental circumstances in which preload, afterload, and heart rate can be held constant.

Indicator-dilution techniques are useful for the bedside determination of cardiac output. In resting adults, the normal range is between 2.5 and 3.6 liters per minute per square meter of body surface area. Decreased cardiac output at rest occurs only in advanced stages of cardiac impairment. A

TABLE 43–1. TERMS USED TO DESCRIBE DETERMINANTS OF CARDIAC PERFORMANCE

Term	Relation to Cardiac Function
Afterload	Resistance that the ventricle must overcome during systole in order to eject the stroke volume. The two major determinants are aortic impedance (see below) and left ventricular volume.
Energetics	Generally determined as myocardial oxygen consumption. For any contractile state, the wall tension developed and maintained during contraction represents the major mechanical determinant of oxygen consumption. An increase in myocardial wall tension occurs in heart failure as filling pressure increases and the ventricle dilates, thereby increasing the energy cost of contraction (see Fig. 43–3).
Impedance (during ejection)	Instantaneous relationship between rate of change in aortic pressure and aortic blood flow. The aortic input impedance reflects the forces external to the heart that impose a load on the left ventricle, including stiffness of aortic wall. Determined primarily, but not exclusively, by total peripheral vascular resistance to runoff from the arterial tree. Normal peripheral resistance is approximately 1500 dynes · sec/cm^{-5} or 15 peripheral resistance units (also known as Wood's units).
Inotropic state	A measure of contractility.
Preload	Rigorously, stretch of myocardial fibers at end-diastole; commonly used as a synonym for venous return to the heart or end-diastolic volume.

blunted cardiac output response to exercise occurs much earlier. Supine exercise in normal subjects should increase the cardiac output by at least 600 ml per minute for each 100-ml increment in oxygen consumption; lower values indicate reduced cardiac performance. In heart failure the arteriovenous oxygen difference is abnormally wide, resulting chiefly from the low oxygen content of venous blood returning to the heart. Oxygenation of blood in the lungs remains nearly normal until pulmonary vascular congestion becomes sufficiently severe to create ventilation-perfusion mismatch with effective shunting, or abnormal diffusion barriers to oxygen transport.

During exercise, cardiac output normally increases as a linear function of oxygen consumption, although for any level of exercise the cardiac output tends to be lower in the upright position. Increases in cardiac output in the upright posture are accomplished principally by increases in heart rate rather than in stroke volume. In heart failure, cardiac output is particularly dependent on heart rate, both at rest and during exercise.

VENTRICULAR END-DIASTOLIC PRESSURE AND VOLUME (PRELOAD). Impaired systolic ventricular emptying leads to an increase in the end-systolic residual volume of blood in the ventricle, predisposing to an increase in end-diastolic volume. Since this is inconvenient to measure or monitor, ventricular end-diastolic pressure is customarily followed for clinical purposes on the premise that a change in pressure is effected by a change in ventricular volume. Exceptions occur, however, including structural changes in the myocardium (fibrosis, edema, and hypertrophy) and pericardial constriction that cause disproportionate rises in end-diastolic pressure relative to volume. Acute ischemia also produces transient reduction in left ventricular compliance. Conversely, in some states of chronic volume overload, compliance increases so that increased volumes are accommodated at end-diastole with relatively modest pressure increases.

A left ventricular end-diastolic pressure greater than 12 to 15 mm Hg is abnormal. The corresponding upper limit for the right ventricle is 6 to 10 mm Hg. It is straightforward to estimate the right ventricular end-diastolic pressure by measuring the central venous pressure. In the absence of mitral

obstruction or increased pulmonary vascular resistance, pulmonary arterial diastolic pressure approximates left ventricular end-diastolic pressure. Pulmonary capillary wedge pressure or diastolic pressure measured with a Swan-Ganz catheter is widely used in intensive care settings to monitor left ventricular filling pressures.

To summarize, the performance of heart muscle depends on two essential components: fiber length (Frank-Starling mechanism) and inherent contractility (inotropic state). The normal heart autoregulates to maintain cardiac output. The variables involved are preload, afterload, contractility, and heart rate. With chronic overloading, the heart undergoes dilation, hypertrophy, or both.

PRELOAD. According to the Frank-Starling mechanism, an increase in end-diastolic volume (preload) results in more forceful contraction with enhancement of ventricular emptying and stroke volume. A unique ventricular function curve exists for each state of contractility (Fig. 43–1). The curve for a failing ventricle is shifted downward and flattened such that stroke volumes are reduced despite abnormally high end-diastolic volumes or pressures. The elevated filling pressures are responsible for congestion and edema in the venous beds leading to the failing ventricle.

In the normal heart, the Frank-Starling mechanism serves to match the stroke outputs of the two ventricles. In heart failure, this mechanism plays the additional role of helping to support the cardiac output.

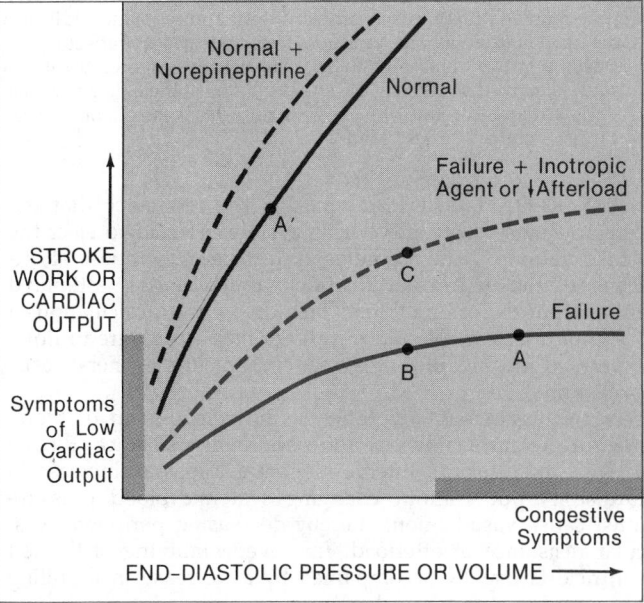

FIGURE 43–1. Schematic diagram demonstrating the relationship between ventricular end-diastolic pressure or volume and cardiac index in a normal and a failing heart. The normal left ventricle increases its stroke output as preload (often measured clinically as pulmonary capillary wedge pressure) increases, moving up the ascending limb of the curve until reserve is exhausted. In heart failure, the ventricular function curve is displaced downward and to the right. An increase in contractility, as after administration of norepinephrine or digitalis, displaces the curve to the left; i.e., a larger stroke output is accomplished at any given filling pressure. A and A' represent the operating points at rest of a hypothetical patient with heart failure and of a normal person, respectively. Reduction of physical activity allows the failing heart to meet the demands of the metabolizing tissues. Treatment of heart failure by a reduction in preload (e.g., with a diuretic or a vasodilator acting predominantly on the venous bed) causes a shift from point A to B on the same ventricular function curve. Administration of a positive inotropic agent or a vasodilator producing afterload reduction will shift the curve as shown, resulting in improvement of the circulatory state in the direction shown by a shift from point A to C.

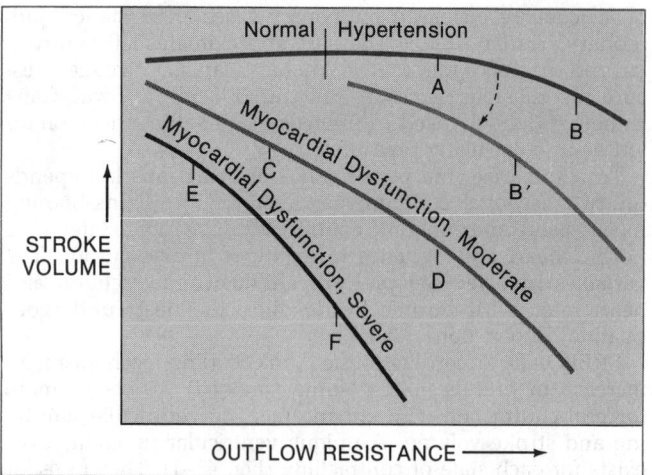

FIGURE 43–2. Relation of left ventricular stroke volume to systemic outflow resistance in normal and diseased hearts. A family of curves may be described, depending on the severity of the myocardial disease. If cardiac function is normal, a rise in resistance results in hypertension, since cardiac output remains fairly constant. Heart failure in a hypertensive patient could be shown by a move to either point B, a high resistance with normal function, or point B', which represents a shift to a slightly depressed ventricular function curve. When myocardial dysfunction is more severe, as shown by the lower two curves, blood pressure is no longer directly determined by resistance, since stroke volume and resistance are inversely related. Consequently, arterial pressure may be similar at points E and F despite marked differences in cardiac output and resistance. It is also apparent that a reduction in outflow resistance will not affect significantly the stroke volume of the normal ventricle. However, it can produce a marked increase in the stroke volume of the failing ventricle (F →E). (Adapted from Cohn JN, Franciosa JA: Vasodilator therapy of cardiac failure. N Engl J Med 297:27, 1977.)

AFTERLOAD. Afterload refers to the resistance that the ventricle must overcome during systole in order to eject the stroke volume. It incorporates all factors that oppose shortening of the ventricular fibers. In practice, it is estimated either from the arterial blood pressure or from calculation of systemic vascular resistance (ratio of blood pressure to flow, expressed in units of dynes $\cdot$ sec/cm^{-5} or in peripheral resistance units).

In the assessment of patients, the relationship of blood pressure to cardiac output and peripheral resistance (P/Flow = R) is quite useful. Interventions that cause an increase in cardiac output without changing systemic blood pressure must cause vasodilation, thereby decreasing peripheral vascular resistance or afterload. Improved emptying of the left ventricle is usually accompanied by a decrease in its filling pressure (pulmonary wedge or diastolic pressure).

If preload and contractility remain constant, increasing afterload in the normal heart tends to decrease both the extent and the speed of contraction to a minor extent. Reduction in afterload has the opposite effects. Within broad physiologic limits, the normal ventricle maintains a relatively constant stroke volume as afterload is increased (Fig. 43–2). The impaired ventricle responds quite differently, with progressive diminution in its ability to eject blood against a given afterload as the severity of myocardial dysfunction advances. Figure 43–2 illustrates the rationale for afterload reduction in the management of heart failure.

CONTRACTILITY (INOTROPIC STATE). Modulation of sympathetic nervous activity provides the major component of short-term adjustment of contractile state in the normal heart and also mediates increases in heart rate and venous tone. Unlike the Frank-Starling mechanism, the increase in force and velocity of contraction is accomplished without any increase in fiber length (end-diastolic volume). Contractility does not limit the output of the normal heart. By contrast,

the failing heart is limited in its myocardial performance, as indicated by displacement of the ventricular function curve, which is shown in Figure 43–1.

An objective index of myocardial contractility that could be measured independent of myocardial fiber length would be useful (1) to assess the effects on the myocardium of interventions such as the administration of digitalis or other inotropic agents; (2) to determine serial changes in inotropic state in an individual during the evolution of heart failure and in response to treatment; and (3) to compare the inotropic state in different individuals. However, distinction between the effects of loading conditions and intrinsic contractility is difficult because of the strong influence of loading on hemodynamic measurements. Changes in preload or afterload can modify ventricular performance greatly without affecting intrinsic inotropic state. Since conventional hemodynamic measurements do not take heart size into account, comparisons of contractility in hearts of different size are difficult to interpret.

Ejection Fraction. This term denotes the fraction of the right or left ventricular end-diastolic volume ejected per beat. It is useful as an integrative measure of contractility and is determined by contrast ventriculography, by gated radionuclide imaging, or by echocardiography. The normal left ventricular ejection fraction ranges from 0.56 to 0.78. A reduced ejection fraction in a patient with normal valves and a dilated ventricle strongly suggests decreased contractility, particularly in the absence of increased afterload. Abnormalities of regional myocardial function are often evident in the pattern of ventricular contraction demonstrated by these techniques.

Other Techniques. Simultaneous graphic recording of the electrocardiogram, phonocardiogram, and carotid arterial pulse contour provides another noninvasive means of assessing cardiac function. This approach does not readily distinguish between inotropic state and other determinants of cardiac performance, and interpretation is greatly complicated by disturbances in conduction or the presence of valvular disease. Accurate measurement of dP/dt can be accomplished at cardiac catheterization and provides a measure of contractile state less subject to the influence of loading conditions than most other approaches.

CHRONIC COMPENSATORY MECHANISMS. In chronic heart failure compensatory mechanisms include tachycardia, increased contractility due to sympathetic nervous activity, dilation, and hypertrophy. The increase in sympathetic activity is a mixed blessing, since it tends to increase systemic vascular resistance in addition to its salutary effects on cardiac output by increasing the heart rate and inotropic state.

Heart Rate. Chronic tachycardia characterizes decompensated heart failure. The increase in rate stems in part from cardiac reflexes stimulated by distention of structures at the venoatrial junctions (Bainbridge reflex). Tachycardia is, in terms of energy, an expensive way to support the cardiac output, and it is possible to precipitate heart failure by inducing sustained tachycardia.

Dilation. Progressive ventricular dilation typically occurs with the transition from compensation to overt failure. Dilation may serve as a useful compensatory mechanism for a time via the Frank-Starling relationship, but with progressive disease it ultimately becomes inadequate to maintain stroke output or does so only at the cost of markedly elevated filling pressures.

Mechanisms contributing to the inability of the dilated heart to maintain adequate function include (1) ultrastructural changes with slippage of sarcomeres during progressive dilation; as a result, they are not stretched to generate optimal contractility; and (2) increased wall tension (law of Laplace, Fig. 43–3) resulting in increased myocardial oxygen consumption; a corollary is that in contrast to the normal heart, in which the wall tension decreases in the course of systole, wall tension tends to remain high in the dilated heart. Thus chronic

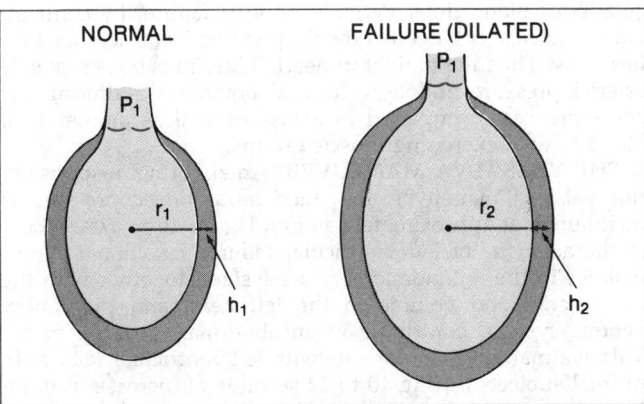

FIGURE 43–3. Laplace relationship applied to the dilated heart. The tension developed in the wall of the heart during systole (T) is a directional force that is proportional to the product of the mean pressure that the wall is supporting (P) and the mean radius (r). Dilation of the heart ($r_2 > r_1$) at the same pressure ($p_1 = p_2$) increases wall tension ($T_2 > T_1$). Should the wall become thinner during dilatation, the wall stress would increase as the cross-sectional area of myocardium (h) decreased (equation 2). The use of wall force (equation 3), which is proportional to the pressure and volume of the chamber, eliminates considerations of chamber size and shape and of the thickness of the myocardial wall.

$$
\begin{aligned}
\textit{Wall tension} &= \text{Force per circumferential length of myocardium} \\
&= \frac{P \cdot \pi r^2}{2\pi r} \tag{1} \\
&= \frac{P \cdot r}{2} \\
\textit{Wall stress} &= \text{Force per cross-sectional area of myocardium} \\
&= \frac{P \cdot \pi r^2}{2\pi r h} \tag{2} \\
&= \frac{P \cdot r}{2h} \\
\textit{Wall force} &= \text{Pressure} \cdot \text{cross-sectional area of chamber} \\
&= P \cdot r^2 \tag{3}
\end{aligned}
$$

dilation has important limitations as a compensatory mechanism in cardiac failure.

Hypertrophy. Sustained abnormal pressure or volume loads lead to an increase in ventricular mass. This involves increased protein synthesis and perhaps decreased degradation in response to mechanical overload or dilation. The stimulus for hypertrophy appears to involve an increase in wall stress and possibly in the energy requirements of a chronically dilated heart with elevated filling pressures.

The hypertrophy pattern depends on the nature of the load. Chronic volume overloading leads to increased total mass as the chamber size enlarges, but wall thickness changes little ("eccentric" hypertrophy). By contrast, chronic exposure to increased pressure (e.g., systemic hypertension or aortic stenosis) leads to a "concentric" hypertrophy pattern in which end-diastolic volume remains unchanged but wall thickness increases.

Abnormal electrical conduction patterns can interfere with the normal, smoothly coordinated contraction pattern of the normal heart, as can myocyte loss with focal or diffuse fibrosis. Ischemic myocardial damage may lead to hypertrophy and remodeling of residual muscle because the geometry of the abnormal ventricle causes it to operate at a mechanical disadvantage and also because normal muscle must work, and expend energy, in moving and stretching adjacent damaged muscle or scar.

In early or mild hypertrophy, muscle mass and capillary vessels increase proportionately, preserving the nutritive and contractile properties of the myocardium. With progressive hypertrophy, additional sarcomeres are laid down, wall thickness increases, and ventricular wall stress tends to be maintained at a normal level despite increased cavity pressure, as

indicated in equation 2, Figure 43–3. This process ultimately exacts a price, however, since increased wall thickness often leads to increased wall stiffness (reduced compliance), thus necessitating a disproportionate rise in filling pressure to maintain adequate end-diastolic ventricular volume. This leads to elevated pulmonary or systemic venous pressures, which contribute to symptoms of dyspnea or peripheral edema. In addition, beyond a certain point, coronary flow reserve diminishes and contractile function declines. Thus, once unremitting hypertrophy begins, the myocardium has embarked on the road to overt failure.

Despite the depressed contractile state associated with later stages of hypertrophy, circulatory function is maintained for a time by the combination of increased muscle mass, dilation, and augmented sympathetic drive. With continuing loss of myocardial contractility, or loss of muscle cells (e.g., from ischemic or inflammatory processes), circulatory compensation can no longer be maintained. The typical clinical and hemodynamic manifestations of congestive heart failure then emerge as cardiac output fails to meet demands and filling pressures increase.

Heart as a Muscle

Consideration of the ventricular performance of the failing heart usually centers on the contraction phase. Events during diastole, however, influence ventricular compliance and hence filling pressures, as well as the subsequent contraction and the energy supply for contraction and relaxation.

RELAXATION AND DISTENSIBILITY. Diastolic filling of the ventricle depends on the time available (a function of heart rate), the timing and properties of atrial systole, and the diastolic properties of the ventricle. Relaxation of cardiac muscle is an energy-requiring process (see above) that is quite vulnerable to adenosine triphosphate (ATP) depletion caused by ischemia. Although heart failure per se does not necessarily impair ventricular relaxation, associated processes of hypertrophy, fibrosis, and ischemia may reduce chamber distensibility and further increase filling pressures. This problem can be particularly severe in hypertrophic cardiomyopathy and in diseases such as amyloidosis that markedly reduce left ventricular diastolic compliance.

ENERGETICS. The heart depends on aerobic metabolism for its supply of energy, the bulk of which is spent to support contraction. The major determinants of oxygen consumption of the heart include the interrelated components of rate, ventricular pressure, volume, work, wall tension, and contractile state. The time integral of systolic tension relates closely to myocardial oxygen consumption, whereas fiber shortening has a minor effect on myocardial oxygen consumption.

The cellular and biochemical basis for heart failure remains unsettled. It is generally agreed that there are no consistent defects in energy metabolism or in protein synthesis and turnover. Current investigation is centered on excitation-contraction coupling and mechanisms that control calcium homeostasis.

Compensatory mechanisms in advanced heart failure tend to increase myocardial oxygen requirements by several mechanisms, including increased preload due to salt and water retention and enhanced sympathetic drive with consequently increased afterload, contractility, and heart rate. Increased preload and afterload are also the result of activation of the renin-angiotensin-aldosterone system.

Heart as Component of the Circulatory System

With loss of cardiac reserve and onset of overt heart failure, peripheral mechanisms are called upon to sustain blood pressure and cardiac output.

VENOUS HYPERTENSION. As the ejection fraction falls and the ventricle fails to empty properly during systole, the volume of unexpelled blood increases with an accompanying increase in diastolic pressure in the ventricles and in the atrium and proximal veins. Other elements that contribute to the venous hypertension include (1) increased tone in venous capacitance vessels; (2) blood volume expansion as a consequence of renal sodium and water retention; and, on occasion, (3) incompetence of mitral or tricuspid valves with regurgitation of blood from ventricle to atrium as the valve becomes incompetent from intrinsic valvular disease, papillary muscle dysfunction, ventricular dilation, or inadequate closure during an arrhythmia.

PERIPHERAL MECHANISMS TO SUSTAIN BLOOD PRESSURE AND CARDIAC OUTPUT. To sustain and distribute the cardiac output, and to maintain systemic arterial pressure, important peripheral mechanisms are activated.

In the normal circulation, the cardiac output doubles in response to a four- or fivefold increase in total body oxygen consumption. When functional impairment is such that the cardiac output cannot keep pace with peripheral demands, blood flow is redistributed to defend vital areas such as the brain and heart. The autonomic nervous system participates in this modulation of the circulation and contributes also to activation of mechanisms that mediate the retention of sodium and water.

Peripheral vasoconstriction and tachycardia characterize the common forms of heart failure. However, despite a generalized increase in sympathetic nervous activity, norepinephrine stores in the heart muscle are depleted because of its enhanced turnover rate. Pharmacologic agents such as reserpine or guanethidine, which further deplete cardiac catecholamine stores, aggravate heart failure, as do beta-adrenergic antagonists such as propranolol.

The contribution of the parasympathetic nervous system to the control of heart rate and baroreceptor activity is impaired in heart failure, but therapeutic consequences of these phenomena are not yet clear.

Peripheral Vasoconstriction. Peripheral arteriolar and venous constriction, mediated in large part by increased sympathetic nervous activity, is an important compensatory mechanism in heart failure that has both positive and negative consequences, as noted earlier. The second regulatory system that contributes to elevated peripheral vascular resistance is the renin-angiotensin system (see Ch. 47). The extent to which accumulation of sodium and water in the arteriolar wall contributes to increased arteriolar resistance is as yet unclear.

Venoconstriction augments venous return by facilitating the return of blood to the central veins, increasing central venous pressure and hence preload. The principal determinant of elevated filling pressures, however, is the inability of the failing ventricle to eject the venous return.

Redistribution. Maintenance of oxygen and substrate delivery to brain and myocardium during states of limited cardiac output requires diversion of flow from skin, kidneys, splanchnic viscera, and skeletal muscle. This redistribution of blood flow initially occurs during activity or stress as cardiac output fails to increase sufficiently to meet the increment in metabolism; in severe heart failure, redistribution operates also at rest. The redistribution of blood flow to essential beds depends on the balance among sympathetic innervation, renin-angiotensin system activity, and local metabolism. The vasculature of skin, kidney, splanchnic beds, and skeletal muscle is richly innervated. Furthermore, these tissues have relatively low metabolic rates, permitting sympathetic nervous and angiotensin II–mediated vasoconstriction to override local vasodilator effects of metabolites. By contrast, the circulations to brain and myocardium are less subject to alpha-adrenergically mediated vasoconstrictor influences because these organs, with their high oxygen consumption, produce metabolic dilator substances that offset increased sympathetic tone.

Under normal physiologic circumstances, exercise with the attendant need for heat dissipation induces an increase in cutaneous blood flow. Patients in heart failure, by contrast, fail to increase cutaneous flow despite this increased need for heat loss. Thus the patient in heart failure preserves systemic arterial pressure and flow to vital organs by suffering the consequences of impaired heat loss as well as limitation of blood flow to exercising muscle groups.

THE VALSALVA MANEUVER. An abnormal response to the Valsalva maneuver, in which intrathoracic pressure is maintained at approximately 40 mm Hg for 10 to 12 seconds, is characteristic of left ventricular failure. Functional abnormalities in the autonomic nervous system, together with the expanded blood volume in the left heart and pulmonary venous system, contribute to an abnormal response to the Valsalva maneuver in patients with left ventricular failure. In normal subjects during 10 to 12 seconds of increase in intrathoracic pressure to 40 mm Hg, there is a characteristic decrease in blood pressure and pulse pressure and increase in heart rate; at cessation of straining, the blood pressure, pulse pressure, and bradycardia tend to overshoot. By contrast, in the presence of left ventricular failure there is a "square wave" response of blood pressure. Blood pressure increases at the onset of straining, stays elevated throughout the maneuver, and decreases abruptly to baseline after the maneuver with no overshoot; there is little, if any, change in pulse pressure, and tachycardia is absent. The blunting of reflex changes results from the absence of stroke output or arterial pulse pressure changes during the phase of reduced venous return, and hence no reflex changes are elicited.

SALT AND WATER RETENTION. As overt heart failure develops, there is typically a decrease in renal blood flow and glomerular filtration rate, with an associated redistribution of renal blood flow. These changes contribute to the sodium and water retention that characterizes heart failure, but the nature and extent of the response differ according to the severity of heart failure, as discussed subsequently under diuretics. Hemodynamic abnormalities are undoubtedly involved in activating the renin-angiotensin-aldosterone system both via direct effects on the kidney and via indirect effects stemming from activation of mechanoreceptors in the distended left atrium. Recognition of the role of hyperaldosteronism in the genesis of sodium and water retention has resulted in the development of aldosterone antagonists as useful adjuncts in the therapy of heart failure.

Sweat and saliva are sodium poor in patients with decompensated heart failure. Antidiuretic hormone (arginine vasopressin) levels tend to be elevated in heart failure and may contribute to elevated systemic vascular resistance, but probably are not important in salt or water retention.

An increase of about 10 to 20 per cent in circulating blood volume contributes to maintenance of cardiac output and perfusion of vital organs in moderate-to-severe heart failure, augmenting ventricular end-diastolic volume and thereby tending to improve ventricular performance. The resulting elevation of filling pressure, however, promotes edema formation by raising venous and capillary pressures proximal to the failing ventricle. By the time the circulating blood volume has increased by 20 per cent, the extravascular fluid volume may well have increased by a factor of two.

Exercise Testing

On the premise that the circulatory function of the heart has failed when it can no longer provide sufficient oxygen and nutrients to satisfy metabolic needs, graded treadmill or bicycle exercise testing has been used investigatively to determine maximum total body oxygen uptake (aerobic capacity). The endpoint of fatigue generally coincides with the point at which aerobic metabolism can no longer meet tissue demands and lactate production begins (anaerobic threshold). This approach has also been used to assess quantitatively the effects of therapeutic interventions for the treatment of heart failure.

CLINICAL MANIFESTATIONS OF HEART FAILURE

The signs and symptoms of heart failure depend on which ventricle has failed and the severity and duration of failure. The clinical picture in left ventricular failure is dominated by *symptoms* of pulmonary congestion and edema. By contrast, right ventricular failure is dominated by *signs* of systemic venous congestion and peripheral edema. Weakness, fatigue, and effort intolerance are common to right or left ventricular failure as well as biventricular failure.

Left Ventricular Failure

The symptom of breathlessness predominates in the patients with left ventricular failure and varies with position and activity. Noteworthy physical signs are most evident in the heart, the lungs, or respiratory control mechanisms.

DYSPNEA. Dyspnea (breathlessness) during limited exertion is typically the earliest symptom of left heart failure and is usually associated with an increased rate of breathing (tachypnea). Although many details of the physiologic basis for the sensation of dyspnea remain unclear, some aspects of the etiology of respiratory symptoms from pulmonary congestion deserve consideration. Since the bronchial capillaries drain for the most part via the pulmonary veins, congestion tends to develop in alveolar and bronchial vascular networks simultaneously. Interstitial edema surrounding pulmonary capillaries appears to stimulate juxtacapillary receptors known as J-receptors, which in turn elicits a reflexly mediated pattern of rapid and shallow breathing. At the same time, bronchial congestion stimulates mucus production, and the distended bronchial capillaries may rupture, with resulting cough and hemoptysis. Bronchial mucosal edema causes increased resistance in small airways, producing wheezing and respiratory distress known as cardiac asthma. The increased work of moving fluid-laden, noncompliant lungs must be accomplished in the face of decreased blood flow to respiratory muscles and also increased diffusion barriers to oxygen exchange across the alveolar-capillary interface, contributing to respiratory muscle fatigue and the sensation of dyspnea.

In any event, the symptom of dyspnea in left heart failure clearly relates to the increase in blood volume and interstitial fluid content of the lungs at the expense of air. Ventilation increases, and the awareness of dyspnea becomes more severe as minute ventilation approaches the maximal ventilatory capacity.

ORTHOPNEA. Dyspnea that occurs soon after lying flat (and is relieved by sitting up) is known as orthopnea. The pathophysiologic basis for orthopnea is the increase in venous return from the lower extremities and splanchnic bed to the lungs in the recumbent position, together with the reabsorption of peripheral edema that accumulates during the day. Orthopnea is a relatively reliable marker for left ventricular failure, whereas the dyspnea associated with chronic lung disease or musculoskeletal disorders is not typically aggravated by lying flat. Patients usually learn to avoid dyspnea of this sort by sleeping with the head and thorax on two or more pillows. In advanced heart failure, orthopnea may be so severe as to cause the patient to sleep upright in a chair. An orthopneic cough has the same significance as orthopnea and is presumably the consequence of venous congestion and edema, as discussed previously. Patients with left heart failure may also complain of precordial distress in the supine position that is difficult to distinguish from symptoms caused by myocardial ischemia.

NOCTURIA. In early heart failure, limitation of renal blood flow with upright activity during the day gives way to more normal renal perfusion and diuresis while supine at night. This causes nocturia, a common early symptom of incipient heart failure.

PAROXYSMAL NOCTURNAL DYSPNEA. Severe respiratory distress may arouse the patient from sleep. Relief is urgently sought by sitting up and often by finding an open window. Such episodes are caused by marked exacerbations of pulmonary vascular congestion and edema during supine sleep. Blunting of the respiratory center response to sensory input from the lungs during sleep, together with increased venous return, allows pulmonary venous congestion and edema to accumulate and trigger the alarming episode of breathlessness.

ACUTE PULMONARY EDEMA. In an episode of acute left ventricular failure, pulmonary venous and capillary pressure can increase abruptly to levels exceeding plasma oncotic pressure, with consequent rapid accumulation of edema fluid in the interstitial spaces and alveoli. Interstitial pulmonary edema leads to an increase in respiratory rate (see foregoing discussion) and tends to produce alveolar hyperventilation and respiratory alkalosis. However, when free fluid enters the alveoli and bronchioles, respiratory acidosis may occur owing to an intolerable increase in the work of breathing. Hypoxemia also occurs commonly because of imbalances between alveolar ventilation and alveolar blood flow (ventilation-perfusion mismatch or "shunting").

Symptoms of pulmonary edema may begin with a nonproductive cough, with wheezing, or with frank dyspnea. Apart from tachypnea and possibly evidence of underlying heart disease on physical examination, few physical signs may be present initially. Later, as free fluid accumulates in distal airways, rales become audible at the lung bases and extend upward accompanied by rhonchi as the episode progresses. In severe acute pulmonary edema, the patient is typically pale, sweating, cyanotic, gasping for breath, and sometimes producing pink or blood-tinged frothy sputum.

HEMOPTYSIS. Rust-colored sputum containing heart failure cells (alveolar macrophages containing hemosiderin) sometimes occurs in severe chronic left heart failure and is seen with particular frequency in patients with advanced mitral stenosis. Frankly bloody sputum should suggest the possibility of pulmonary infarction, but expectoration of substantial quantities of blood can also occur as a consequence of rupture of engorged bronchial capillaries in patients with severe chronic left heart failure, including that caused by uncorrected mitral stenosis.

CHEYNE-STOKES RESPIRATION. Advanced heart failure may be accompanied by periodic breathing with alternate periods of apnea and hyperventilation. Due to slowing of the circulation time from lungs to brain, the arterial P_{O_2} reaches its peak and the arterial P_{CO_2} its nadir during apnea. At this time alveolar gas tensions are exactly opposite. During hyperpnea the alveolar P_{O_2} reaches its peak and the alveolar P_{CO_2} its nadir. Thus, changes in arterial blood gases are responsible for the cyclic ventilation, which in turn causes the changes in alveolar gas tensions. As would be expected from this delay of the normal negative feedback loop, the longer the circulation time, the longer are the cycles of hyperventilation and apnea. The neurologic changes of advanced age predispose to Cheyne-Stokes breathing, as does cerebrovascular disease.

Physical and Laboratory Signs of Left Heart Failure

The patient with decompensated left heart failure is generally tachypneic, pale, dusky, and sweaty. The handshake is cold because of peripheral vasoconstriction, and tachycardia is present. The pulse pressure is usually narrow, often with a modest increase in diastolic pressure. The neck veins are not distended if the left ventricle alone has failed.

THE HEART. Cardiac enlargement is often evident with inspection, percussion, and palpation of the apical impulse and is confirmed by radiographic examination, although this finding is more typical of valvular or primary myocardial disease than of ischemic heart disease. With increased left heart filling pressure pulmonary venous pressure increases and the pulmonary arterial pressure must also increase. The pulmonic component of the second heart sound (P_2) therefore tends to increase in intensity. In the presence of left ventricular dilation, papillary muscle dysfunction, or both, the mitral valve leaflets may fail to appose properly, resulting in mitral incompetence.

Gallop Rhythm. The presence of a protodiastolic third heart sound (S_3 gallop) in an adult with heart disease usually signifies the presence of heart failure. The timing of the normal first and second sounds and the abnormal third sound, in conjunction with an increased heart rate, results in the characteristic cadence of the gallop rhythm. The third heart sound occurs in early diastole coincident with rapid ventricular filling. The S_3 gallop appears to be produced by vibrations of the ventricular walls as the rapidly inflowing blood is abruptly arrested. A third heart sound is a normal finding in children and in young adults.

Presystolic gallop rhythms result from the atrial contribution to ventricular filling. The atrial or S_4 gallop is characteristic of decreased ventricular compliance and typically results from left ventricular hypertrophy or ischemia rather than from myocardial dysfunction or failure. When a patient with an audible fourth heart sound develops overt heart failure, a third sound may appear, causing a quadruple rhythm. If the heart rate is sufficiently rapid or the PR interval is prolonged, S_3 and S_4 may merge, producing a summation gallop. The presence of a summation gallop has the same clinical implication as other protodiastolic (S_3) gallop rhythms.

Pulsus Alternans. The presence of alternating strong and weak beats (the fundamental rhythm remaining regular) usually signifies advanced heart failure. Pulsus alternans can be detected by palpation or by sphygmomanometry and often follows an atrial or ventricular premature beat for several cycles. Mechanical alternans of this sort is only rarely associated with electrical alternans. Pulsus alternans has been attributed to a severe disturbance of excitation-contraction coupling, the detailed pathophysiology of which is unclear.

THE LUNGS. The sequence of pulmonary findings with advancing left heart failure has been described in the foregoing section on acute pulmonary edema.

THE ELECTROCARDIOGRAM. Electrocardiographic abnormalities result from underlying cardiac disease, therapeutic agents (e.g., digitalis), or both and yield little information regarding the functional status of the heart.

RADIOLOGIC ASPECTS. The chest radiograph is usually quite helpful in the diagnosis and assessment of left ventricular failure (see Ch. 42.1). The cardiac silhouette is typically, but not invariably, enlarged and may assume telltale configurations that are determined by the underlying disease process. In contrast to normal, the pulmonary vasculature is prominent in the upper lung zones, reflecting pulmonary venous hypertension and redistribution of blood flow because of encroachment upon the lower lung vessels by edema and possibly fibrosis. Enlarged hilar shadows and prominent septal lines, particularly near the costophrenic angles (Kerley's B lines), are typical findings. Alveolar edema results in a generalized clouding of the lung fields but can occur in focal or patchy distributions that are difficult to distinguish from pneumonia. Pleural effusions sometimes occur in predominantly left-sided heart failure but are more characteristic of biventricular failure. Interstitial and alveolar edema may lessen or disappear with onset of right ventricular failure. A widened superior vena cava shadow suggests right ventricular failure and systemic venous congestion.

PULMONARY FUNCTION TESTS. The course of left ventricular failure, including the response to treatment, can be followed by consecutive determinations of vital capacity, although this practice has been largely supplanted by other approaches in recent years. With interstitial pulmonary edema, expiratory flow rates at low lung volumes are reduced and distal airways tend to close prematurely during expiration, trapping gas within the lungs and disturbing the normal relation of ventilation to perfusion. This produces a widening of the alveolar-arterial P_{O_2} difference and a decrease in arterial P_{O_2} due to venous admixture. Arterial oxygen saturation is typically nearly normal, however, unless intrinsic lung disease is present. The arteriovenous oxygen content difference increases with decreasing cardiac outputs as tissue extraction of oxygen becomes more complete. Systemic arterial P_{CO_2} remains normal or low unless ventilation is compromised in the course of pulmonary edema. Endotracheal intubation and assisted ventilation may be indicated if progressive carbon dioxide retention is documented by serial blood gas measurements.

Right Ventricular and Biventricular Failure

CLINICAL MANIFESTATIONS. Isolated right ventricular failure is uncommon in adults and is usually a consequence of cor pulmonale secondary to intrinsic lung disease or, on occasion, chronic volume overload from a congenital atrial septal defect. Right ventricular failure is encountered most often as a complication of left ventricular failure. In the presence of elevated right heart filling pressures, neck veins are distended and fill from below. Hepatic enlargement and tenderness to gentle palpation result from passive congestion, and compression causes further distention of the neck veins (hepatojugular reflux). In the presence of biventricular failure, signs of right ventricular failure may dominate, but the presence of dyspnea and rales should suggest additional left ventricular failure. Accompanying low cardiac output results in signs of increased sympathetic nervous activity and of organ hypoperfusion. It should be remembered that a critically lowered cardiac output from any cause sufficient to produce metabolic acidosis will occasion hyperventilation in defense of acid-base balance, and this must be distinguished from the tachypnea of left heart failure.

Advanced right-sided or biventricular failure may be associated with anorexia, weight loss, and malnutrition ("cardiac cachexia"). Digitalis excess, high doses of diuretics, and electrolyte disturbances often contribute to the genesis of this manifestation of end-stage heart failure.

Cyanosis. Cyanosis is caused by 5 or more grams per 100 ml of unoxygenated hemoglobin in the subpapillary venous plexus of the skin. This occurs in right heart failure because the congested venules contain blood from which considerable oxygen has been extracted because of the slow flow. This is typically accompanied by relatively normal arterial P_{O_2} values unless intrinsic lung disease or intracardiac shunting is present. Cyanosis is usually absent in left heart failure unless caused by a complication (e.g., pneumonia) or by pulmonary edema.

Abnormal Heart and Lungs. Although dyspnea accompanying left ventricular failure may be partially relieved by onset of right ventricular failure, some dyspnea usually persists, together with tachypnea and basal rales. Tricuspid valvular insufficiency commonly accompanies severe right ventricular dilation and failure and contributes to systemic venous engorgement. The murmur of tricuspid insufficiency is distinguished from that of mitral insufficiency by its location (lower left border of sternum), by its tendency to increase during inspiration, and by associated physical signs, such as hepatic pulsation and systolic waves in the jugular venous pulse. Doppler echocardiography greatly assists in the assessment of this problem. Pleural effusion, often unilateral, is more common in right-sided or biventricular than in isolated left ventricular failure.

Systemic Venous Congestion. Elevation of systemic venous pressure is a sine qua non of right heart failure. Responsible mechanisms include (1) the inability of the failing ventricle to eject the venous return without abnormally high filling pressures, causing (2) an increase in the volume of blood in the large systemic veins; and (3) increased venomotor tone resulting from increased sympathetic nervous system activity.

Increased systemic venous pressure is responsible for the hepatomegaly, occasional splenomegaly, and peripheral edema that characterize decompensated right ventricular failure. Usually less apparent are the associated congestion and edema of the gastrointestinal tract.

Pressure in the jugular venous system, a useful index of right atrial pressure, may be estimated from the height of the column of blood distending the cervical veins. The cervical veins are normally flat in the upright posture in the absence of raised intrathoracic pressure, whereas in right heart failure they are prominent and distended. The wave form of venous pulsation is usually best appreciated from inspection of the right internal jugular vein, adjusting the angle of the patient's upper body to bring out the top of the venous pressure column. Tricuspid insufficiency distorts the normal venous pulse by producing a systolic or C-V wave that has no counterpart in the normal jugular venous pulse. Occasionally, compression over the liver is necessary to display the increased blood volume in the venous system, but the examiner must avoid being misled by venous distention from involuntary expiration against a closed glottis (Valsalva's maneuver).

Liver. The liver is typically enlarged and tender in right heart failure. If the onset is acute, right upper quadrant pain may result from constraint of the swollen liver by its tight capsule. Splenomegaly is uncommon except in prolonged passive congestion of the liver, and pain or tenderness of the spleen should raise the question of superimposed systemic embolization and splenic infarction.

Early congestion of the liver may cause modest increases in the concentrations of hepatic enzymes such as alkaline phosphatase in serum, and increases in serum bilirubin may occur. Hyperbilirubinemia from this cause usually consists of a combination of conjugated and unconjugated bilirubin. Frank jaundice is uncommon unless hepatic congestion is associated with longstanding pulmonary congestion or pulmonary infarction.

Hypoglycemia may occur if cardiac output is severely compromised and hepatic congestion is marked and protracted. This is attributed to depletion of liver glycogen stores and increased formation of lactic acid from glucose induced by hypoxia.

Repeated and prolonged episodes of right heart failure with reduced hepatic blood flow and elevated venous pressures can cause atrophy and centrilobular necrosis of liver cells and can lead to extensive fibrosis ("cardiac cirrhosis") that is difficult to distinguish from posthepatitic cirrhosis. Hepatic failure with precoma or coma is a rare, preterminal complication of this sequence of events.

Extracellular Fluid Compartments. The fluid compartments of the body are normally maintained constant by neurohormonally mediated interplay among intake (governed by thirst and appetite), exchanges of fluid and electrolytes (governed by passive and active transport mechanisms), and excretion (regulated primarily by the kidneys). In heart failure, excessive retention of sodium and water by the kidneys results in an isosmotic expansion of extracellular fluid, including the circulating blood volume. In mild heart failure, retention of sodium and water may serve to expand the blood volume to sustain venous return and the forward output of the failing heart through the Frank-Starling mechanism. However, retention of salt and water only exacerbates pulmonary and systemic congestion and edema when the myocardium can no longer respond positively to increased filling pressure and volumes.

The distribution of excess extracellular ("third space") fluid varies among patients. Under the influence of gravity, edema accumulates in the feet and ankles of ambulatory patients but shifts to the sacral region in the bedridden patient. Localization occurs in areas of low tissue pressure, such as the back of the ankle. Colloid osmotic pressure and the integrity of the lymphatic system also influence extracellular fluid distribution.

Peripheral Edema. Dependent edema developing over the course of the day and subsiding by morning is a characteristic feature of right heart failure. It is a direct consequence of elevated systemic venous pressure and is typically preceded by a gain in weight. Persistent edema is accompanied relatively frequently by complications such as low-grade cellulitis, and the combination of edema and sluggish venous flow predisposes to deep venous thrombosis and pulmonary embolism.

Pleural Effusion. The infrequency of hydrothorax in isolated right ventricular failure dictates that the association of pleural effusion and cor pulmonale should lead one to search for another cause, such as pulmonary infarction. It is, however, common in biventricular failure. Hydrothorax results from impaired removal of isotonic fluid from the pleural space because of elevated venous pressures in both the pulmonary and the systemic circulations, compromising transcapillary exchange of water at the pleural surface and also impeding lymphatic drainage. Hydrothorax contributes to dyspnea reflexly, probably by stimuli from lungs and chest wall, as well as by displacing ventilated lung tissue from the relatively fixed volume of the thoracic space. Pulmonary embolism and infarction may contribute to pleural effusion in two ways: by transit of fluid from the infarcted area of the lung and to the pleural space or by aggravation of heart failure.

Ascites. The presence of free fluid in the abdominal cavity is a late manifestation of right heart failure, usually associated with systemic venous hypertension, peripheral edema, and hydrothorax. It is commonly encountered in the setting of tricuspid valve disease or chronic constrictive pericarditis. Elevated pressures in portal and hepatic veins and in the systemic veins draining the peritoneum contribute to the formation of ascites, but renal retention of sodium and water is a prerequisite. It may contribute to anorexia and can cause abdominal discomfort or pain in patients with severe right ventricular failure.

Pericardial Effusion. Patients with chronic heart failure commonly have increased amounts of fluid in the pericardial sac that can be demonstrated echocardiographically. Only rarely, however, does it accumulate to an extent that produces further hemodynamic compromise (tamponade).

Anasarca. Advanced and protracted right ventricular failure without adequate treatment can cause edema fluid to accumulate throughout the body, most conspicuously in subcutaneous tissues as well as abdominal and thoracic cavities. Face and arms are typically spared until the preterminal stages of failure. This clinical picture occurs rarely in the present era of potent diuretics.

Gastrointestinal Tract. Systemic venous hypertension leads to edema of the bowel wall. These changes interfere with absorption of drugs or foods only when heart failure is severe, but reduced bioavailability of furosemide and perhaps other drugs can occur under these circumstances. In severe congestive heart failure, anorexia, nausea, and vomiting may occur from reflex, central, local, or drug-induced causes. Protein-losing enteropathy can occur in the setting of severe right heart failure.

Brain. Nonspecific complaints, including headache and insomnia, are common in heart failure and are usually attributable to some diminution of cerebral blood flow and triggering mechanisms such as dyspnea that contribute to insomnia. Neurologic or behavioral aberrations are more frequent when the burdens of a limited cardiac output are superimposed on antecedent neurologic disease (e.g., cerebrovascular disease or prior stroke) or on personality disorder. Irritability, restlessness, and limited attention span are associated with severe congestive heart failure. Stupor and coma supervene when cardiac output is critically reduced.

Kidney. Oliguria occurs with decompensation in isolated right or left heart failure but is more prominent in the latter or in biventricular failure. The urine is sodium poor but has a relatively high specific gravity (1.020 to 1.030). Prerenal azotemia is common, particularly in the presence of intrinsic renal disease or after vigorous diuresis. Azotemia with high urine specific gravity is characteristic of heart failure (and dehydration) and stands in contrast to the low specific gravity expected with renal insufficiency due to intrinsic renal disease. Blood urea nitrogen is typically elevated out of proportion to serum creatinine. Proteinuria is common but does not usually exceed 1 gram per day.

Other Manifestations. In chronic severe congestive heart failure, weakness and gradual loss of tissue mass are frequent concomitants and may progress to cachexia. At this late stage, the patient is usually suffering from anorexia and often gastrointestinal symptoms and electrolyte disturbances as well. Although organ hypoperfusion and congestion play an important part in this syndrome, the physician must maintain vigilance to avoid additional contributions from overvigorous use of digitalis and diuretics.

Anxiety. This is a common feature of cardiac disease by the time the heart fails. Manifestations of anxiety may be difficult to distinguish from symptoms of the underlying cardiac disorder because of the nonspecific nature of complaints such as breathlessness. Symptoms related to hyperventilation as well as palpitations may contribute to the patient's anxiety by reinforcing the impression that organic heart disease is present. The physician must proceed with the separate assessment of organic and psychosomatic aspects of the disease process, recognizing that a careful history and physical examination, together with judicious use of noninvasive diagnostic methods, will usually establish the extent to which organic heart disease is responsible for the patient's symptoms.

CLINICAL MANAGEMENT OF HEART FAILURE
General Approaches

The management of congestive heart failure includes three general types of approaches. The first is removal of the underlying cause. This is the first priority in all cases and includes measures such as surgical correction of valvular lesions or congenital malformation. It also includes medical treatment of hypertension or infective endocarditis when present.

The second approach consists of removal of precipitating causes of heart failure. Frequently the initial development or exacerbation of heart failure is related not to worsening of the underlying cardiac condition but rather to a superimposed stress. Typical factors that can precipitate overt congestive heart failure, apart from changes in the status of the heart itself, are listed in Table 43–2.

The third set of measures, treatment of clinical manifestations of heart failure, will occupy the remainder of this chapter. This approach may in turn be divided into three categories, as summarized in Table 43–3:

1. Measures to improve the contractile performance of the heart.
2. Measures to reduce cardiac work.
3. Measures to control excessive retention of salt and water.

As listed in Table 43–3, several therapeutic entities are available in each category. Cardiac glycosides and sympathomimetic agents constitute the principal drugs that enhance the pumping performance of the failing heart. In addition, placement of a pacemaker may improve pumping performance either by supporting a more appropriate heart rate or by restoring atrial augmentation of ventricular filling if synchronous atrioventricular contraction can be achieved (see Ch. 45).

Reduction of the work load of the failing heart can be accomplished by physical and emotional rest, by appropriate

TABLE 43–2. PRECIPITATING OR EXACERBATING FACTORS IN CONGESTIVE HEART FAILURE

Increased demand:
  Anemia
  Fever
  Infection
  Fluid overload
  Increased dietary salt intake
  High environmental temperature
  Renal failure
  Hepatic failure
  Thyrotoxicosis
  Arteriovenous (A-V) shunt (Paget's disease of bone)
  Respiratory insufficiency
  Emotional stress
  Pregnancy
  Obesity
Arrhythmias
Pulmonary embolism
Ethanol ingestion
Thiamin deficiency
Uncontrolled hypertension
Poor compliance with therapeutic regimen
Drugs
  Beta-adrenergic blockers
  Antiarrhythmic drugs (e.g., disopyramide)
  Salt-retaining drugs
    Steroids
    Nonsteroidal anti-inflammatory agents

treatment of obesity, and by vasodilator therapy. Under specific circumstances, assisted circulation with the intra-aortic balloon pump can usefully contribute to this goal.

Finally, control of the excessive retention of salt and water is approached by instituting a low-sodium diet and the use of diuretic drugs. Under some circumstances, mechanical removal of fluid will be of value.

These measures are customarily applied in a stepwise fashion, as outlined in detail in Table 43–4.

Strategy of Heart Failure Management

The many etiologies and degrees of severity of heart failure demand an individualized approach to each patient. Nevertheless, certain general principles apply to the management of various subsets of patients. It is usually not appropriate to institute specific therapeutic measures until symptoms of overt heart failure occur—that is, until the patient makes the transition from functional class I to class II. The first approach in all instances will include judicious limitation of activity, advising the patient to avoid physical exertion that produces undue dyspnea or exhaustion. The degree of restriction should be tailored to the severity of heart failure. It is important not to limit activity so severely that skeletal muscle deconditioning, rather than the underlying cardiac problem,

TABLE 43–3. MEASURES IN THE MANAGEMENT OF CONGESTIVE HEART FAILURE

A. Improve pump performance of the failing ventricle
  1. Cardiac glycosides (digoxin)
  2. Sympathomimetic drugs (dopamine, dobutamine)
  3. Other positive inotropic drugs (amrinone)
  4. Pacemaker for bradycardia or loss of atrioventricular synchrony
B. Reduction of cardiac work load
  1. Rest (physical and emotional)
  2. Correction of obesity
  3. Vasodilator drugs
  4. Assisted circulation (e.g., intra-aortic balloon counterpulsation)
C. Control salt and water retention
  1. Limit dietary sodium intake
  2. Diuretics
  3. Mechanical removal of fluid
    a. Thoracentesis
    b. Paracentesis
    c. Dialysis
    d. Phlebotomy

TABLE 43–4. STEPS IN THE MANAGEMENT OF CHRONIC CONGESTIVE HEART FAILURE

Steps	Functional Class II	III	IV
A	*Restrict physical activity:* Limit competitive sports and heavy labor	Reduce work schedule; rest periods during day	Limit to house and finally to bed and chair
B	*Dietary sodium restriction:* Eliminate salt shaker and heavily salted foods	Eliminate salt in cooking and at table (Na intake ~ 1.2 to 1.8 grams)	As in III, plus low-sodium foods (Na intake <1 gram)
C	*Diuretics:* Thiazide or low-dose loop diuretic	Loop diuretic (progressive doses); consider adding distally acting (K-sparing) diuretic	Loop diuretic with distally acting (K-sparing) and/or thiazide diuretic
D	*Digitalis glycosides:* Conventional maintenance doses ⟶		Dose to maintain serum level in 1.5 ng/ml range
E		*Vasodilators:* Hydralazine and isosorbide dinitrate *or* captopril	Intravenous nitroprusside
F			*Other inotropic drugs (intravenous):* Dopamine, dobutamine, amrinone
G			*Consider cardiac transplantation Thoracentesis, paracentesis Dialysis Assisted circulation (e.g., intra-aortic balloon pump)*

becomes the limiting factor in the patient's activity. Physical activity should, however, be markedly restricted in the setting of acute decompensation of chronic heart failure, a situation in which hospitalization will generally be advisable.

Diuretics or cardiac glycosides may be added in early class II, with the choice of one or both based on the balance between risk and expected benefit. In many cases, modest doses of digoxin and a mild diuretic such as thiazide will restore the patient to an essentially asymptomatic state. Dietary sodium restriction may be limited to avoidance of heavily salted foods and the use of the salt shaker at the table. Special low-sodium foods are expensive and can be so unpalatable as to impair nutrition.

When symptoms persist or evolve on the simple regimen outlined above, intensification of the diuretic regimen is usually the next step. Depending upon the etiology of the heart failure, vasodilators may be instituted in late class II or class III failure. Problems such as mitral regurgitation will be particularly amenable to successful treatment with vasodilators, as discussed below.

As the severity of heart failure advances, increased restriction of physical activity is usually necessary, and patients will often require rest periods during the day as class III symptoms evolve. When patients remain symptomatic during ordinary activity on a program that includes digitalis, loop diuretics, and vasodilators, hospitalization is often advisable to search for precipitating causes and to consider the possibility of more aggressive approaches. In patients who have progressed to functional class IV, hospitalization will usually be advisable and the use of intravenous sympathomimetic agents can be considered, as well as optimization of the vasodilator, diuretic, and cardiac glycoside regimens. In younger patients who meet appropriate criteria, cardiac transplantation should also be considered at this time.

During episodes of decompensation, the hazards of deep venous thrombosis and pulmonary embolism must be guarded against, and the use of minidose heparin (see Ch. 57) is a relatively safe and effective approach during hospitalization. At these times, emotional as well as physical rest is important, and anxiety-provoking situations should be carefully avoided. Marked anxiety or insomnia may be treated with benzodiazepines such as diazepam or the shorter-acting agent triazolam.

DIET. Rigid salt restriction can usually be avoided until diuretics are no longer capable of controlling the accumulation of salt and water. Water intake will, in general, not require specific restriction unless dilutional hyponatremia supervenes.

OXYGEN. Patients with hypoxia, and certainly those with pulmonary edema, will benefit from oxygen inhalation, conveniently given by nasal prongs at 4 to 6 liters per minute. In general, supplemental oxygen is worthwhile whenever the arterial oxygen saturation falls below 90 per cent. This will be a particularly effective way of reducing right ventricular afterload, since oxygen is a potent pulmonary arteriolar vasodilator.

PHYSICAL REMOVAL OF FLUID. The availability of potent diuretics limits the need for thoracentesis or paracentesis, but these procedures may be important diagnostically when the accumulation of fluid in serous cavities is not readily explained on the basis of heart failure alone. Pulmonary embolism, for example, is a relatively common cause of pleural effusion, and a diagnostic thoracentesis will often provide critically important information leading to this diagnosis. Drainage of pleural or ascitic fluid should be carried out slowly, at a rate of not more than about 1500 ml per hour, and the total quantity of fluid removed on any single occasion should not exceed about 1500 ml because of the risk of fluid shifts from the vascular to the extravascular compartment, with consequently inadequate ventricular filling pressures. Particular caution is required in patients (such as those with aortic stenosis or hypertrophic cardiomyopathy) who have reduced ventricular compliance and require high ventricular filling pressures to maintain adequate stroke volume.

Acute Pulmonary Edema

Acute pulmonary edema is a medical emergency in which the immediate therapeutic goals are to (1) improve oxygenation; (2) reduce venous return (preload); (3) reduce anxiety; and (4) treat causal and precipitating factors. Placement of flow-directed pulmonary artery (Swan-Ganz) and arterial lines for monitoring of pressures and arterial blood gases will often be advisable. The patient is placed in a trunk-up, legs-down posture and given humidified 100 per cent oxygen, by positive pressure mask if possible. Vital signs are monitored frequently, and an intravenous cannula is inserted for secure intravenous access. Arterial blood gas, blood urea nitrogen (BUN) or creatinine, electrolyte, and complete blood count measurements are obtained at once. An electrocardiogram and chest radiograph (taken with a portable machine if necessary) should also be obtained, and electrical conversion of supraventricular or ventricular tachyarrhythmias should be considered if present and if not due to digitalis excess.

Morphine given intravenously (2 to 10 mg, repeated every 10 to 15 minutes) will reduce venous return and allay anxiety; naloxone should be available in case of respiratory depression. Nitroglycerin given sublingually or possibly intravenously will further reduce venous return; nitroprusside given intravenously may be used if the blood pressure is adequately maintained and afterload reduction is desirable. Furosemide should be given intravenously in a 20- to 40-mg dose and repeated in increasing doses as necessary to achieve a diuresis. Aminophylline, 250 to 500 mg given slowly intravenously (5.6 mg per kilogram), will be useful to relieve bronchospasm and promote diuresis but can exacerbate sinus or ectopic tachycardias.

If severe respiratory distress persists, tourniquets applied to three of four extremities and rotated every 15 to 20 minutes may be of value. If respiratory acidosis (pH of 7.10 or less) or severe hypoxemia (P_{O_2}<50 mm Hg) persists, endotracheal intubation and controlled positive pressure ventilation should usually be instituted. Phlebotomy or hemodialysis deserves consideration in refractory cases. Digitalis has a secondary role in this clinical setting, except occasionally in the management of supraventricular tachyarrhythmias. Superimposed hypotension and low cardiac output states are considered in Ch. 44. Concurrently, vigorous attention should be directed to the identification and management of precipitating factors (Table 43–2).

Digitalis Glycosides

Cardiac glycosides have been used in the management of heart failure for more than 200 years and remain the only drugs currently available for long-term ambulatory use that have a positive inotropic effect. The unusually narrow therapeutic-toxic ratio of cardiac glycosides renders them particularly difficult to use, and the clinician should have a detailed understanding of the actions and pharmacokinetics of one drug of this class, such as digoxin. Because digoxin has supplanted almost entirely the use of other cardiac glycosides in the United States, the discussion will focus on this agent.

BASIC MECHANISM OF CARDIAC GLYCOSIDE ACTION. A consensus exists that the sequence of events leading to the positive inotropic effect of digitalis on both normal and failing cardiac muscle is as summarized in Figure 43–4. The digitalis glycosides bind to the extracellular facing aspect of NaK-ATPase, the enzyme constituting the "sodium pump" that moves sodium and potassium across cell membranes against their respective concentration gradients. The complete

amino acid sequences of the alpha and beta subunits of the enzyme are known. When a cardiac glycoside binds to the alpha subunit, that individual sodium pump unit is completely inhibited. When a fraction of NaK-ATPase sites on a cardiac myocyte are occupied, intracellular sodium concentration tends to rise. Through the mechanism of sodium-calcium exchange, this leads in turn to augmentation of the intracellular calcium content. Since calcium constitutes the trigger that leads to the contractile event, the increase of intracellular calcium stores (up to a point) enhances the contractile state of both normal and failing myocardium.

The electrophysiologic toxicity commonly observed with excessive doses of digitalis is probably due to the same fundamental mechanism of sodium pump inhibition. At higher doses and myocardial concentrations of the drug, impairment of sodium and potassium transport leads to characteristic disturbances of impulse formation and conduction, as discussed below. It is likely that intracellular calcium overload contributes to the cardiotoxicity of the digitalis glycosides, at least under the circumstances that have been studied experimentally.

ELECTROPHYSIOLOGIC EFFECTS. Table 43–5 summarizes the major electrophysiologic effects of digitalis on the heart. Most of the antiarrhythmic effects of digitalis are the results of its actions at the level of the atria and atrioventricular junction. These effects are largely mediated by increased vagal tone, rather than by direct effects of cardiac glycosides, although the latter can be documented at the upper end of the dose range. Of particular importance in the management of supraventricular tachyarrhythmias is the tendency of digitalis to lengthen the refractory period and to slow conduction in the atrioventricular node. At toxic doses and blood levels, digitalis enhances sympathetic nerve traffic to the heart, thus increasing the propensity to ectopic impulse formation at atrial, atrioventricular junctional, and ventricular levels.

HEMODYNAMIC EFFECTS. The positive inotropic action is a direct effect of digitalis on cardiac myocytes in isolated muscle as well as the intact heart. Endogenous norepinephrine stores are not necessary to permit expression of this effect. A useful way to appreciate the effect of digitalis on the intact circulation is by consideration of the ventricular function curves shown in Figure 43–1. In contrast to diuretics, which

TABLE 43–5. EFFECTS OF DIGITALIS ON CARDIAC ELECTROPHYSIOLOGY

Property	Effect
Pacemaker Automaticity	
S-A node	→ ↓ (↑, after atropine or toxic doses)
Purkinje fibers	↑
Excitability	
Atrium	→*
Ventricle	variable*
Purkinje fibers	↑*
Membrane Responsiveness	
Atrium	variable* (↓, after atropine)
Ventricle	↓ (toxic doses)
Purkinje fibers	↓ (toxic doses)
Conduction Velocity	
Atrium, ventricle	↑ (slight)*
A-V node	↓
Purkinje fibers	↓
Effective Refractory Period	
Atrium	↓ (↑, after atropine)
Ventricle	↓
A-V node	↑
Purkinje fibers	↑*

Key: The arrows indicate the direction, not the magnitude, of the changes indicated: ↑, increased; ↓, decreased; →, no significant change.

*Decreased with high or toxic doses of digitalis.

From Moe GK, Farah AE: Digitalis and allied cardiac glycosides. In Goodman LS, Gilman A (eds.): The Pharmacological Basis of Therapeutics. 5th ed. New York, The Macmillan Company, 1975, p 661.

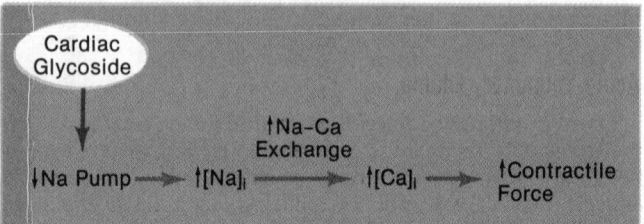

FIGURE 43–4. Schematic representation of the mechanism of inotropic action of cardiac glycosides. Binding of digitalis to NaK-ATPase inhibits this enzyme and hence the active outward transport of Na$^+$ across the myocardial cell membrane. Na$^+$ pump inhibition leads to increased intracellular Na$^+$ ([Na]$_i$) content and activity, which in turn alters Na-Ca exchange with consequent increase in Ca influx, decrease of Ca efflux, or both. The resulting increase in intracellular Ca ([Ca]$_i$) is presumed to mediate the observed increase in myocardial contractile force.

reduce preload and shift the circulatory state to the left along a given ventricular function curve, a positive inotropic agent will shift the entire curve upward and to the left toward the normal curve. Since contractility does not limit cardiac output in the normal circulation, digitalis would not be expected to change output in normal subjects. This is the case. As soon as the contractile state becomes limiting, however, digitalis will increase cardiac output and lower filling pressures of both the right and the left ventricles. Thus, cardiac glycosides are of clinical value in patients with congestive heart failure in the presence or absence of supraventricular tachyarrhythmias such as atrial fibrillation or atrial flutter. Although opinion is less uniform regarding patients in sinus rhythm, recent studies have documented benefit in the majority of patients who have dilated, failing ventricles with poor systolic function. These patients must be carefully distinguished from those with relatively noncompliant ventricles and elevated filling pressures, but normal ejection fractions at rest, who are unlikely to benefit. Thus, patients who are most likely to benefit are those having cardiomegaly with impaired systolic contraction, often accompanied by S_3 gallops. There is no convincing evidence of desensitization or tolerance to the cardiac effects of digitalis, and the positive inotropic effects are sustained over periods of months and years in patients with congestive heart failure.

To summarize, as pathologic processes, such as ischemia, volume or pressure loads, or primary myocardial disease, lead to reduced contractility, compensatory mechanisms emerge. Elevated end-diastolic pressure and volume will augment ventricular performance through the Frank-Starling mechanism. Sympathetic tone will tend to increase, thus enhancing contractile state, and the process of ventricular hypertrophy will generate additional contractile elements. Each of these mechanisms, however, exacts a price. Excessive elevation of filling pressures results in pulmonary or peripheral edema. Excessive sympathetic tone results in tachycardia and inappropriately increased peripheral vascular resistance as well as increased myocardial oxygen consumption. With the progression of underlying cardiac disease, the compensatory mechanisms will ultimately fail, or the consequences of these mechanisms will become limiting (for example, with emergence of pulmonary edema). Administration of cardiac glycosides under these circumstances will enhance myocardial contractility, decreasing the dependence of the circulation on compensatory mechanisms and providing improved cardiac reserve. Improved ventricular function will yield a higher cardiac output at any given ventricular filling pressure. With the alternative therapeutic modalities now available, there is little virtue in giving cardiac glycosides to the point of toxicity. Rather, conventional doses (see below) resulting in serum digoxin concentrations not exceeding 1.5 to 1.7 ng per milliliter appear to yield the best risk-benefit ratio.

PHARMACOKINETICS, BIOAVAILABILITY, AND DOSAGE CONSIDERATIONS. Summarized in Table 43–6 are the important pharmacokinetic variables and dosage ranges for cardiac glycosides in current clinical use. The values cited are averages, and individual variation is to be expected.

Digoxin. This is the most widely used preparation in the United States, particularly in hospitalized patients. Its virtues include flexibility of route of administration and intermediate duration of action. Digoxin is excreted exponentially (i.e., first-order kinetics) with a half-life of about 36 hours in young, healthy, normal subjects. In older patients with cardiac disease but without nitrogen retention, a half-life of 48 hours represents a more appropriate first approximation. Such patients will excrete approximately one third of body stores daily, for the most part in unchanged form, although about 10 per cent of patients excrete substantial quantities of the inactive metabolite dihydrodigoxin, which arises through bacterial biotransformation in the gut lumen. The excretion of digoxin by the kidney is directly proportional to glomerular filtration rate (and hence creatinine clearance) and is relatively independent of the rate of urine flow in patients with intact renal function. Clearance may decrease somewhat in patients with prerenal azotemia. There is also evidence for some secretion of the drug at the renal tubular level.

Therapy can be instituted in patients without urgent indications by starting the daily maintenance dose without a loading dose. This results in stable plateau concentrations of the drug in four to five excretory half-lives, or about one week. In patients with severe renal impairment, the half-life of the drug is prolonged to as much as four to five days, and steady-state levels are reached on a daily maintenance regimen only after three to four weeks.

Digoxin is extensively bound to tissues (large volume of distribution), and the drug is consequently not effectively

TABLE 43–6. PHARMACOLOGY OF CARDIAC GLYCOSIDES

Agent	Gastrointestinal Absorption	Onset of Action* (minutes)	Peak Effect (hours)	Average Half-Life†	Principal Metabolic Route (Excretory Pathway)	Average Digitalizing Dose		Usual Daily Oral Maintenance Dose ‖
						Oral‡	Intravenous§	
Ouabain	Unreliable	5–10	½–2	21 hours	Renal; some gastrointestinal excretion	—	0.30–0.50 mg	—
Deslanoside	Unreliable	10–30	1–2	33 hours	Renal	—	0.80 mg	—
Digoxin	55%–75%¶ (Lanoxicaps 90%–100%)	15–30	1½–5	36–48 hours	Renal; some gastrointestinal excretion	1.25–1.50 mg	0.75–1.00 mg	0.25–0.50 mg††
Digitoxin	90%–100%	25–120	4–12	4–6 days	Hepatic#; renal excretion of metabolites	0.70–1.20 mg	1.00 mg	0.10 mg
Digitalis leaf	About 40%	—	—	4–6 days	Similar to digitoxin	0.80–1.20 g	—	0.10 g
Lanatoside C	10%–40%	—	—	Similar to digoxin	Renal	10 mg	—	0.5–1.5 mg
Gitalin**	—	—	—	4–6 days	Similar to digitoxin	6 mg	—	0.25–1.25 mg
Acetyldigitoxin	About 70%	20–30	8–10	Similar to digitoxin	Similar to digitoxin	2.0–3.0 mg	1.4–1.6 mg	0.1–0.2 mg

Modified from Smith TW: Drug Therapy: Digitalis glycosides. N Engl J Med 288:719, 1973.

*For intravenous dose.

†For normal subjects (prolonged by renal impairment with digoxin, ouabain, and deslanoside and probably by severe hepatic disease with digitoxin and digitalis leaf).

‡Divided doses over 12 to 24 hours at intervals of 6 to 8 hours.

§Given in increments for initial subcomplete digitalization, to be supplemented by further small increments as necessary.

‖ Average for adult patients without renal or hepatic impairment; varies widely among individual patients and requires close medical supervision.

¶For tablet form of administration (may be less in malabsorption syndromes and in formulations with poor bioavailability).

#Enterohepatic cycle exists.

**Gitalin is a mixture of cardiac glycosides, the principal one of which is digitoxin.

††Approximately 20 per cent lower maintenance doses are required if gel solution in capsules (Lanoxicaps) is used.

removed from the body by hemodialysis. Lean body mass should be used for purposes of dosage calculation. Infants and children absorb and excrete digoxin much as do adults, although secretion at the renal tubular level may be somewhat more important in prepubertal patients.

An important interaction between digoxin and quinidine has been described, leading to a substantial increase in steady-state serum digoxin levels (averaging about twofold) when conventional quinidine doses are added to a maintenance digoxin regimen. Increases in the serum digoxin level are also observed when verapamil or amiodarone are given concurrently.

Bioavailability of digoxin in the standard tablet formulation is 55 to 75 per cent. The higher estimate is usually used in converting oral to intravenous doses. A recently marketed preparation in which digoxin is dissolved in an encapsulated gel gives higher bioavailability, requiring a slight adjustment in the standard maintenance doses, as noted in Table 43–6. Previously marketed preparations with poor bioavailability properties are no longer available in the United States, thanks to appropriate controls imposed by regulatory agencies.

The maintenance digoxin dose required to replace daily losses will vary from about 37 per cent of the body content in patients with normal renal function to 14 per cent in patients with essentially no renal function. The latter figure is an average, however, and some patients will require substantially more or less than the maintenance dose that would be predicted by the 14 per cent figure. A useful approximation of daily per cent of loss of digoxin from the body is given by the following expression:

$$\text{Per cent daily loss} = 14 + \frac{C_{Cr} \text{ in ml/min}}{5}$$

Useful nomograms have been developed for loading and maintenance doses of digoxin, but it is important that these be used only as first approximations and that the patient be followed closely until a stable steady state is reached. Adjustments subsequently will be required with changes in renal function, related either to intrinsic renal disease or to altered renal perfusion due to cardiac disease.

Digitoxin. This cardiac glycoside is the least polar and the most slowly excreted of the cardiac glycosides in common use. It is the principal constituent of the whole leaf of the digitalis plant. Gastrointestinal absorption of digitoxin is virtually complete. The drug binds avidly to serum albumin, and only about 3 per cent of the drug circulates in the free, pharmacologically active state at conventional doses and serum levels. It thus differs substantially from digoxin, which is only about 23 per cent bound to plasma proteins at usual doses. Because of the high degree of serum protein binding, renal clearance of digitoxin is minimal and the drug is metabolized to a variety of poorly defined derivatives, presumably in the liver. Some enterohepatic cycling occurs in the case of digitoxin but is not important for digoxin. The half-time for digitoxin excretion averages about five to six days and is not appreciably affected by altered renal function.

Standard pharmacology texts give details of pharmacokinetics of other glycosides such as deslanoside and ouabain, which are rarely used at present in the United States.

DIGITALIS USE IN CONGESTIVE HEART FAILURE. The therapeutic use of digitalis in patients with normal sinus rhythm is complicated by the lack of any easily measurable therapeutic endpoint, such as that provided by the ventricular rate in patients with atrial fibrillation. Digitalis is of value in patients with symptoms and signs of heart failure due to ischemic cardiomyopathy, valvular disease, hypertensive heart disease, many types of congenital heart disease, and dilated cardiomyopathies and in some patients with cor pulmonale and overt right ventricular failure. The drug is of no demonstrated benefit in isolated mitral stenosis with normal sinus rhythm unless right ventricular failure is present. Sim-

ilarly, little benefit can be expected in patients with pericardial tamponade or constrictive pericarditis. The latter disease states are all characterized by mechanical limitations to cardiac function, rather than by impairment of myocardial contractility. In hypertrophic cardiomyopathy with an obstructive element, digitalis may in fact be deleterious if left ventricular contractility increases and produces greater outflow obstruction. As noted previously, patients with symptoms of dyspnea on exertion due to high diastolic filling pressure from decreased ventricular compliance, but with well-preserved ejection fractions, are unlikely to benefit from digitalis if sinus rhythm is present.

The prophylactic use of digitalis in patients with diminished cardiac reserve who are expected to undergo a major stress such as surgery remains controversial. Many clinicians prefer to withhold digitalis until a specific indication arises.

The use of digitalis in the management of supraventricular rhythm disturbances is considered in Ch. 45. The drug is potentially dangerous in patients with Wolff-Parkinson-White syndrome.

INDIVIDUAL SENSITIVITY TO DIGITALIS. Table 43–7 lists factors that influence the sensitivity of individual patients to digitalis. These are factors intrinsic to the patient, rather than factors that influence *apparent* sensitivity, such as alterations in drug bioavailability or in the excretion pattern of the drug.

Electrolyte and Acid-Base Disturbances. Potassium depletion increases the likelihood that patients will develop digitalis toxicity. Hypokalemia has a primary arrhythmogenic effect of its own and also tends to increase cellular binding of digitalis glycosides. Potassium depletion must be guarded against carefully in patients on potassium-wasting diuretics. Magnesium depletion also predisposes to digitalis toxicity and is a common concomitant of diuretic therapy. Elevated serum calcium levels may enhance ventricular automaticity and may also predispose to digitalis toxicity.

Acid-base disturbances appear to exert their effects largely through shifts in serum potassium concentration, and the acid-base disturbances per se usually have little effect within the range commonly encountered clinically.

Drug Interactions. Several drugs, including cholestyramine, colestipol, and neomycin, decrease absorption of orally administered digoxin, as do nonabsorbable antacids and Kaopectate. Quinidine, verapamil, and amiodarone all increase steady-state serum digoxin levels.

Type and Severity of Underlying Heart Disease. The most important factor influencing individual digitalis sensitivity is the type and severity of underlying heart disease. Otherwise healthy subjects are remarkably tolerant of large doses of digitalis, and toxicity typically manifests itself as disturbances of atrioventricular conduction rather than life-threatening tachyarrhythmias. In patients with advanced heart failure or severe focal ischemia, however, the therapeutic ratio of digi-

TABLE 43–7. FACTORS INFLUENCING INDIVIDUAL SENSITIVITY TO DIGITALIS

Type and severity of underlying cardiac disease
Serum electrolyte derangement
  Hypokalemia or hyperkalemia
  Hypomagnesemia
  Hypercalcemia
  Hyponatremia
Acid-base imbalance
Concomitant drug administration
  Anesthetics
  Catecholamines and sympathomimetics
  Antiarrhythmic agents
Thyroid status
Renal function
Autonomic nervous system tone
Respiratory disease

talis is remarkably low, and these patients may experience potentially life-threatening toxicity at doses and serum levels no more than twice the optimal amount.

Digitalis and Coronary Artery Disease. The effects of digitalis on myocardial oxygen consumption, and therefore its use in patients with ischemic heart disease, depend primarily on the prior state of the ventricle. In the normal-size ventricle, the enhanced contractile state may modestly increase oxygen consumption. If failure and ventricular dilation are present, however, digitalis administration will tend to reduce cardiac dimensions and thereby reduce wall tension (Laplace's relation) such that myocardial oxygen consumption may not increase or may even be reduced. It is important, therefore, to assess carefully the state of ventricular function prior to instituting digitalis therapy in patients with ischemic disease.

The role of digitalis therapy after acute myocardial infarction remains controversial. Other measures are generally preferable in the management of mild congestive heart failure in this setting. When symptoms and signs of overt left ventricular failure persist despite optimal use of diuretics, digitalis may be added at about 75 per cent of the usual loading dose. The loading dose should be given over a period of 18 to 24 hours with close monitoring of cardiac rhythm. It is customary to use digoxin in the presence of atrial fibrillation, which is typically a manifestation of heart failure in patients with acute myocardial infarction.

Some evidence suggests that patients may experience excess mortality when maintained on digitalis in the long-term following acute myocardial infarction, but most studies indicate that the mortality trends are accounted for by baseline variables such as greater severity of heart failure, rather than a deleterious effect of conventional doses of digoxin.

Advanced Age. It is unlikely that advanced age per se has an independent adverse effect on digitalis tolerance, but the reduced renal and pulmonary functions that attend advanced age require appropriate consideration.

Renal Failure. Factors influencing digitalis absorption and elimination, as well as rapid shifts in electrolytes with hemodialysis, predispose to digitalis toxicity. It is wise to leave an extra margin of safety in digitalis doses in managing these patients.

Thyroid Disease. Hyperthyroidism tends to reduce the response of patients to digitalis, whereas hypothyroidism increases the likelihood of digitalis toxicity. The failure of a patient with atrial fibrillation to respond to standard doses of digoxin with appropriate slowing of the heart rate should raise the question of occult thyrotoxicosis.

Pulmonary Disease. It is generally agreed that patients with chronic pulmonary disease, and especially with acute respiratory insufficiency, experience an increased frequency of digitalis intoxication. This may be related both to the underlying lung disease and hypoxia and to the sympathomimetic drugs that these patients often receive. It should be assumed that patients with a variety of pulmonary diseases may be sensitive to the arrhythmogenic effects of conventional doses and serum levels of cardiac glycosides.

SERUM DIGITALIS CONCENTRATIONS. Assay of serum digoxin concentration is routinely performed in most clinical laboratories, usually with the radioimmunoassay technique. There is a relatively constant ratio of serum or plasma to myocardial digoxin concentration, and thus the clinical effect of digoxin is directly related to the serum level. Nevertheless, there is considerable overlap in serum levels between patients with and without evidence of toxicity. Thus, serum concentration data must always be interpreted in the overall clinical context. Mean serum digoxin concentrations in groups of patients without evidence of toxicity, and with an expected therapeutic effect, average 1.4 ng per milliliter. Doubling the digoxin dose in a patient on a steady-state regimen can be expected to double the serum concentration when a new steady state is reached.

Serum digitoxin concentrations average about tenfold higher than those of digoxin because of the binding of digitoxin to serum proteins.

The upper limit of the "therapeutic" range for digoxin is usually taken as about 2.0 ng per milliliter, but patients with supraventricular tachyarrhythmias, including atrial fibrillation and atrial flutter, may require appreciably higher levels to gain adequate control of the ventricular response and may tolerate these higher levels with no evidence of toxicity. Conversely, unusually sensitive patients may experience toxicity at serum levels as low as 1.0 ng per milliliter. It is not necessary to monitor serum digoxin levels routinely in patients who are doing well on standard maintenance doses of the drug. Serum levels may be of use, however, in the assessment of unexpected responses to therapy, including lack of the expected therapeutic response (Is the patient taking the drug?) or in situations in which digitalis toxicity is suspected (for example, multifocal ventricular premature beats in a patient with overt congestive heart failure who is taking digoxin).

DIGITALIS TOXICITY. At the cellular level, exposure to excessive levels of cardiac glycosides causes increased automaticity and decreased conduction. These abnormalities are reflected in a broad array of rhythm disturbances that are often difficult to distinguish from those caused by underlying heart disease.

Sinus Node and Atrium. Slowing of the sinus rate in patients with congestive heart failure is largely mediated by improved cardiac function and withdrawal of elevated sympathetic tone. Sinus rate is not a very useful indicator of digitalis effect, since it will tend to remain rapid in the presence of fever, infection, anemia, thyrotoxicosis, or a variety of other conditions that predispose to sinus tachycardia. At high toxic doses, digitalis can cause direct depression of sinus node automaticity, or more likely sinoatrial exit block, which will produce bradyarrhythmias.

Atrioventricular Node. The effective refractory period of the atrioventricular (AV) node is prolonged by digitalis, chiefly through increased vagal activity. In addition, the conduction velocity through the AV junction is reduced. As digoxin doses are increased, first-degree block (PR interval > 0.20 second) may appear, followed by second-degree AV block of the Mobitz type I or Wenckebach variety (see Ch. 45). With still higher doses, complete AV dissociation and third-degree block can occur. A typical manifestation of digitalis toxicity in the presence of atrial fibrillation is AV dissociation, often accompanied by increased automaticity of pacemakers in the AV junction. This causes regularization of a previously irregular ventricular rate.

His-Purkinje System. Digitalis-induced increase in the automaticity of cells in the His-Purkinje system is a relatively common manifestation of digitalis excess and is responsible for rhythm disturbances, including ventricular premature beats, ventricular bigeminy, and ventricular tachycardia. Table 43–8 shows the approximate relative incidence of rhythm disturbances most commonly produced by digitalis.

Clinical Manifestations of Digitalis Toxicity. GASTROINTESTINAL SYMPTOMS. Anorexia, nausea, and vomiting are common consequences of digitalis toxicity. Unfortunately, these are present prior to the onset of rhythm disturbances in only about 50 per cent of cases.

NEUROLOGIC SYMPTOMS. Headache, fatigue, malaise, disorientation, confusion, delirium, and seizures can occur, and visual symptoms, including disturbances of color vision, are well known. In fact, the gastrointestinal symptoms actually arise from the effects of digitalis on the chemoreceptor trigger zone in the medulla rather than as a result of direct irritation of the gastrointestinal system.

MASSIVE CARDIAC GLYCOSIDE OVERDOSE. Suicidal or accidental digitalis overdose can produce the entire array of typical cardiac arrhythmias, including refractory ventricular fibrilla-

TABLE 43–8. RELATIVE INCIDENCE OF CARDIAC ARRHYTHMIAS ATTRIBUTED TO DIGITALIS TOXICITY IN 14 STUDIES (926 PATIENTS)

Rhythm Disturbance	Number of Arrhythmias	Per Cent of Patients with This Arrhythmia
Ventricular ectopic rhythms	567	62
AV block	314	34
1°	91	
3°	82	
Atrial arrhythmias	248	27
Sinoatrial arrhythmias	106	11
AV dissociation	92	10
AV junctional rhythms	138	15

AV = atrioventricular.

Data from Fisch C, Stone JM: Recognition and treatment of digitalis toxicity. In Fisch C, Surawicz B (eds): Digitalis. New York, Grune & Stratton, 1969, pp 162–173, with permission.

tion. In addition, hyperkalemia is sometimes encountered owing to interference with sodium and potassium transport across cell membranes throughout the body. This must be taken into account in considering the use of potassium supplements in cases in which massive toxicity may occur.

Treatment of Digitalis Intoxication. The most important element of successful treatment is early recognition that a cardiac rhythm disturbance is due to digitalis toxicity. For many of the most common manifestations, such as occasional ventricular premature beats, first-degree AV block, or atrial fibrillation with a slow ventricular response, temporary withdrawal of the drug with electrocardiographic monitoring (if indicated) until the arrhythmia has disappeared will constitute adequate management. The maintenance dose should then be adjusted to prevent recurrence. Arrhythmias that impair cardiac function because of rates that are too rapid or too slow, or those that suggest the possibility of progression to more malignant arrhythmias, require more aggressive management. Ventricular tachycardia due to digitalis toxicity requires immediate vigorous treatment. Bradyarrhythmias, including sinus bradycardia, sinoatrial arrest, or exit block, and atrioventricular block of second or third degree can sometimes be treated effectively with atropine, 0.5 to 1.0 mg given intravenously. Pervenous electrical pacing should be instituted if atropine is not rapidly effective.

POTASSIUM. Potassium repletion is useful in the treatment of ectopic tachyarrhythmias when hypokalemia is present or when the serum potassium level is in the low normal range. Potassium must be given with caution in other circumstances because of the risks of hyperkalemia, particularly in the presence of renal impairment or of conduction disturbances.

PHENYTOIN AND LIDOCAINE. These are the most useful drugs in the treatment of ectopic rhythm disturbances caused by digitalis. They tend to have minimal adverse effect on sinoatrial or AV conduction. Phenytoin* is given in a dose of 100 mg by slow intravenous infusion, repeated every five minutes until onset of toxicity or control of the arrhythmia, followed by an oral maintenance dose of 400 to 600 mg per day if control of the rhythm disturbance is achieved. Lidocaine is given intravenously in 100-mg bolus doses every three to five minutes, followed by a maintenance intravenous infusion of 15 to 20 µg per kilogram of body weight per minute, as required to maintain control of the rhythm disturbance and to avoid neurologic signs and symptoms.

PROPRANOLOL. Beta blockade has been useful in the treatment of some arrhythmias caused by digitalis excess but tends to decrease conduction as well as myocardial contractility and therefore is not widely used in this setting.

QUINIDINE AND PROCAINAMIDE. These drugs carry a risk of depression of sinoatrial and atrioventricular node function and can also depress myocardial contractility. Other agents are usually preferable for use in digitalis toxicity.

*This use is not listed in the manufacturer's directive.

DIRECT CURRENT (DC) COUNTERSHOCK (also see Ch. 45). This is generally inadvisable in the presence of digitalis intoxication because it may evoke severe arrhythmias in this setting. However, it must occasionally be used when other methods have been ineffective in the presence of a life-threatening arrhythmia. Risk is decreased when lower energy levels are employed, and careful titration of dose is essential. In general, ventricular tachycardia will convert easily at an energy level of 25 watt-seconds or less. Cardioversion is generally a benign procedure in patients without digitalis-induced rhythm disturbances.

STEROID-BINDING RESINS, HEMODIALYSIS, AND HEMOPERFUSION. These techniques have not been demonstrated to be effective in the management of advanced digitalis intoxication and are not recommended. Hemodialysis may be of value in controlling the serum potassium level in patients with refractory hyperkalemia.

DIGOXIN-SPECIFIC ANTIBODIES. Purified Fab fragments of digoxin-specific antibodies have recently been released for treatment of advanced digitalis toxicity of sufficient severity to be potentially life threatening. More than 400 patients have now been treated, with a high degree of efficacy and with no major adverse side effects. This approach is recommended for patients in whom conventional measures are not rapidly effective.

Diuretics

Salt and water retention with consequent expansion of the intravascular and interstitial compartments is a sine qua non of chronic congestive heart failure and accounts for many of the common signs and symptoms. Elimination of excess salt and water is an essential goal in management of heart failure.

Two stages characterize diuretic use: first, the elimination of accumulated excess fluid; and second, maintenance of optimal "dry" weight. Care of patients in the hospital typically focuses on elimination of excess fluid, which is facilitated by the controlled salt intake and limited activity of hospitalized patients. Maintenance of optimal fluid balance out of hospital requires adjustments in the context of the individual patient's diet and activity. A sound approach is the use of the mildest diuretic program that is consistent with maintenance of appropriate fluid balance and a salt intake that promotes a nutritious diet. Severe sodium restriction is usually unnecessary except in very severe congestive heart failure. Overly rigorous restriction of sodium intake, together with use of potent diuretics, is a well-known formula for impaired renal function, oliguria, and prerenal azotemia, particularly in the elderly.

CONTROL OF SODIUM BALANCE. The key role of diuretics in management of heart failure relates to the central role of the kidney as a target of many of the neurohumoral and hemodynamic changes that occur in heart failure. Reduced cardiac output causes activation of the renin-angiotensin system in the kidney, with consequent reduction in renal blood flow and increased glomerular filtration fraction, leading to increased resorption of salt and water by the proximal tubule. Elevated plasma angiotensin II levels contribute to increased systemic vascular resistance and increase aldosterone release from the adrenal. Increased renal sympathetic nerve activity also tends to reduce renal blood flow and to release renin from the macula densa, as well as directly augmenting sodium resorption along other segments of the nephron. Intrarenal blood flow redistribution contributes to the formation of relatively concentrated urine. Plasma vasopressin levels are frequently elevated in patients with heart failure, causing further limitation of free water clearance. Together with the increase in thirst of patients with advanced heart failure, this leads to a hyponatremic state that is a particularly ominous prognostic sign in heart failure.

Diuretics intervene in the pathophysiology of heart failure by reducing the reabsorption of sodium and its accompanying

TABLE 43–9. PROPERTIES OF DIURETIC DRUGS

Diuretic	Brand Name	Principal Site and Mechanism of Action	Effects on Urinary Electrolytes	Effects on Blood Electrolytes and Acid-Base Balance	Extrarenal Effects	Usual Dosage*	Drug Interactions
Thiazides and Related Compounds							
Chlorothiazide	Diuril	*Distal tubule:*	↑ Na^+	↓ Na^+, particularly in elderly patients	↑ Glucose	500–1000 mg, IV or p.o.	Efficacy reduced by prostaglandin inhibitors
Hydrochlorothiazide	Hydrodiuril	Enhance NaCl reabsorption and ↓ Ca^{++} excretion	↑ Cl^-	↓ Cl, ↑ HCO_3— mild metabolic alkalosis	↑ LDL/triglycerides (may be dose related)	25–100 mg/day	Reduces renal clearance of lithium
Trichlormethiazide	Metahydrin		↑ K^+			2–8 mg/day	
Chlorthalidone	Hygroton		↑ H^+	↑ Uric acid		25–100 mg/day	
Metolazone	Zaroxolyn		↑ Mg^{++} ↓ Ca^{++}	↑ Ca^{++}		5–10 mg/day	Synergistic effects on NaCl and K^+ excretion with loop diuretics
Indapamide	Lozol	Smooth muscle vasodilator *Proximal tubule:*			Extrarenal effects less marked with indapamide	2.5–5 mg/day	
Acetazolamide	Diamox	Carbonic anhydrase inhibitor	↑ Na^+, ↑ K^+ ↑ HCO_3^-	Metabolic acidosis	↑ Ventilatory drive ↓ Intraocular pressure	250–500 mg/day	May be useful in alkalemia due to other diuretics
Osmotic Diuretics							
Mannitol	Osmitrol	*Proximal tubule* (primarily)	↑ Na^+, ↑ Cl^-	↑ Extracellular volume transiently	↓ Intracranial pressure	50–200 grams/day, IV	May enhance loop diuretic effectiveness by maintaining GFR
Glycerol	Glyrol		↑ H_2O		↓ Intraocular pressure	1–1.5 grams/kg, p.o.	
Loop Diuretics							
Furosemide	Lasix	*Thick ascending limb of loop of Henle:* Inhibition of Na/K/Cl cotransport	↑↑ Na^+	Hypochloremic alkalosis (↑ HCO_3^-)	Acute: ↑ Venous capacitance	20–600 mg/day, p.o. or IV	Tubular secretion delayed by competing organic acids (renal failure) and some drugs
Bumetanide	Bumex		↑↑ Cl^-		↑ Systemic vascular resistance	0.5–40.0 mg/day	
Piretanide†			↑ K^+ ↑ H^+ ↑ Mg^{++},Ca^{++}	↓ K^+, ↓ Na^+, ↓ Cl^- ↑ Uric acid (less than thiazide)	Chronic: ↓ Cardiac preload	6–20 mg/day	Effectiveness reduced by prostaglandin inhibitors
Ethacrynic Acid	Edecrin	↑ Renin, AII; ↑ PG's			Ototoxicity	50–150 mg/day	
Indacrinone				Uricosuric potency depends upon ratio of ± enantiomers in final drug			Additive ototoxicity with aminoglycosides Excessive hypotension may occur in patients treated chronically with diuretics and begun on ACE inhibitors
Potassium-Sparing Diuretics							
Spironolactone	Aldactone	*Aldosterone antagonist*	↑ K^+ ↑ Na^+ ↑ Cl^- ↑ HCO_3^-	↑ K^+, particularly in patients with ↓ GFR; metabolic acidosis	Gynecomastia Antiandrogen effects	25–200 mg/day	Useful adjunct to therapy with K^+-wasting diuretics
Canrenone							
Triamterene	Dyrenium	*Inhibit Na^+/H^+ exchanger:*				100–300 mg/day	Triamterene with indomethacin may cause abrupt ↓ GFR
Amiloride	Midamor	Primary effect is in distal nephron				5–10 mg/day	Triamterene may cause renal calculi

*Route of administration is p.o. except as noted.
†Investigational drug.
AII = Angiotensin II; PG = prostaglandin; GFR = glomerular filtration rate; LDL = low density lipoproteins; ACE = angiotensin-converting enzyme inhibitor.

anions, as well as water, by the renal tubule. The four major classes of diuretics in current clinical use are summarized in Table 43–9. Each of these agents affects renal tubular function in a distinct way, and each tends to produce a characteristic set of abnormalities in electrolyte patterns, fluid balance, and acid-base homeostasis. The more potent the diuretic, the greater the potential risk for severe and sometimes life-threatening disturbances of electrolyte and acid-base balance.

THIAZIDES. Because of their effectiveness by oral administration, their predictable effects, and their relative freedom from toxicity, thiazide diuretics are very commonly used in the management of heart failure. The thiazide diuretics include several agents with chemical and pharmacologic similarities. The prototype is chlorothiazide. Chlorthalidone and metolazone are heterocyclic compounds that share the basic benzothiadiazine nucleus. All of these drugs inhibit sodium chloride reabsorption in the distal tubule. This effect is not dependent upon the weak carbonic anhydrase inhibitory

activities common to most of these drugs. By inhibiting sodium chloride transport in the distal tubule, dilution of tubular fluid is prevented and delivery of solute and water to the hydrogen- and potassium-secreting sites in the collecting duct is enhanced. Calcium reabsorption is also promoted by the thiazides, probably by enhancement of calcium entry into epithelial cells of the distal tubule and perhaps by mild volume depletion as well.

The thiazides are useful in the initial management of mild-to-moderate congestive heart failure. Their utility is limited, however, by avid solute reabsorption in the more proximal nephron segments. Thiazides are largely ineffective when the glomerular filtration rate is less than 30 ml per minute. They are often useful in the treatment of refractory edema in combination with loop diuretics, as discussed subsequently.

Potentially troublesome side effects include potassium depletion, hyperuricemia, glucose intolerance, and plasma lipid elevations, as discussed below. Care must be taken to avoid gastric and small bowel irritation from the potassium chloride supplements that are often required in conjunction with thiazide diuretics.

CARBONIC ANHYDRASE INHIBITORS. Related to the thiazides are the carbonic anhydrase inhibitors, of which acetazolamide is the only agent currently available. This drug results in urinary sodium and bicarbonate losses until the plasma bicarbonate level falls to the point at which renal tubular bicarbonate reabsorption (both proximal and distal) exceeds the filtered load of bicarbonate. Thus, these agents tend to have a transient effect. The sodium and potassium loss accompanying bicarbonate excretion is moderate, but acetazolamide may be of value in patients with high serum bicarbonate levels, as may occur in cor pulmonale or metabolic alkalosis. The presence of metabolic acidosis, e.g., from renal failure or hepatic failure, constitutes a contraindication to its use.

LOOP DIURETICS. These agents are the most potent diuretics in common clinical use and are capable of inducing a natriuresis of up to 20 per cent of the filtered load of sodium for limited periods. They are of particular value in three situations: in acute pulmonary edema, used intravenously; in severe or refractory heart failure; or when renal function is impaired. Ethacrynic acid is chemically different from furosemide and its analogues but appears to share a similar set of pharmacologic properties. These diuretics act to inhibit the Na/K/2 Cl transport system that is responsible for solute reabsorption in the thick ascending limb of the loop of Henle. Each of these drugs is secreted into the tubular lumen by the organic acid secretory pathway, and their effects may therefore be delayed or decreased by exogenous (e.g., probenecid) or endogenous (organic anion accumulation in uremia) competitive inhibitors of the transporter.

Gastrointestinal absorption of furosemide, the most commonly used of the loop diuretics, is variable, with an average bioavailability of 60 per cent. This is substantially diminished when the drug is given with meals. Congestive heart failure appears to decrease absorption of both furosemide and bumetanide. The nonsteroidal anti-inflammatory drugs, including aspirin, tend to blunt the natriuretic response to all of the loop diuretics.

The loop diuretics in general produce systemic hemodynamic changes that precede and are presumably unrelated to the degree and extent of diuresis they induce. Acute administration of furosemide causes a rapid increase in venous capacitance, with a consequent decline in cardiac filling pressures. This effect is accompanied by an increase in plasma renin activity that can produce an appreciable rise in systemic vascular resistance. These effects on the peripheral vasculature tend to plateau in the lower dose range at about a 20-mg intravenous dose of furosemide. Although the loop diuretics are potent inhibitors or Na/K/2 Cl cotransport, this process is not clinically important outside the kidney, except in the cochlea, where it is thought to account for the eighth nerve toxicity that is seen with loop diuretics, particularly ethacrynic acid. The ototoxicity of loop diuretics is synergistic with that of aminoglycoside antibiotics.

Bumetanide and piretanide tend to have higher bioavailability and greater potency than furosemide and may be slightly less ototoxic. Other differences among these closely related compounds appear to be small and probably clinically unimportant.

An important advantage of the loop diuretics is their rapid onset of action, with a diuretic response typically appearing within a few minutes of intravenous administration.

ORGANOMERCURIAL DIURETICS. With the availability of potent oral diuretics, these agents are no longer part of the contemporary management of heart failure.

POTASSIUM-SPARING DIURETICS. Two groups of drugs fall into this class: (1) the aldosterone antagonists; and (2) the direct inhibitors of sodium permeability in the collect-

ing duct. The aldosterone antagonist most frequently used is spironolactone, although canrenoate and canrenone have essentially identical effects. The aldosterone antagonists compete with the native hormone for cytoplasmic receptors in responsive cells, ultimately reducing sodium reabsorption. Therapeutic efficacy of these agents is limited when used alone, but they are often useful in combination with other potent diuretics.

Amiloride and triamterene are structurally related compounds that inhibit sodium uptake in collecting duct epithelial cells by blocking sodium-hydrogen exchange. A principal effect of these drugs is to reduce renal potassium secretion, which may be useful in concert with the action of potassium-wasting compounds such as the thiazides and loop diuretics, but which may lead to clinically important hyperkalemia, particularly in patients with renal failure. The potassium-sparing diuretics tend to cause a mild metabolic acidosis. In patients with chronic obstructive pulmonary disease, these agents may be preferred to diuretics that enhance renal hydrogen losses and secondarily reduce ventilatory drive. Apart from causing hyperkalemia, these drugs are relatively benign. Spironolactone can cause troublesome gynecomastia.

OSMOTIC DIURETICS. These agents are rarely of use in the management of heart failure, but it should be remembered that radiographic contrast dyes are filtered by the glomerulus and act as osmotic diuretics, increasing urinary loss of salt and water. This volume-contracting effect can be important in fragile patients, such as those with severe aortic stenosis. An important characteristic of osmotic diuresis is its ability to maintain urine flow even at very low glomerular filtration rates, as occur in hypotension or dehydration.

COMBINED DIURETIC REGIMENS. Combined use of diuretics in patients with heart failure is usually considered for two main reasons: to avoid electrolyte disturbances that occur with the isolated use of a powerful agent such as a loop diuretic, especially in chronic therapy; and to augment salt and water excretion in the face of refractory edema. A third possible indication is the avoidance of ototoxicity from large doses of loop diuretics.

Combined use of potassium-sparing diuretics with a more proximally acting agent such as a thiazide or a loop diuretic constitutes a common practice. The potassium-sparing diuretics limit potassium and hydrogen loss induced by diuretics that act more proximally.

The combination of a loop diuretic with a thiazide often results in a synergistic augmentation of salt and water excretion. This combination of agents is capable of producing marked intravascular volume depletion and electrolyte disturbances. Potassium wasting can be severe, and serum potassium levels require close monitoring. In general, this combination of diuretics should be initiated in a hospital setting, with careful regulation of the regimen on an outpatient basis with weight measurements taken daily and frequent checks of serum electrolyte and creatinine levels.

COMPLICATIONS OF DIURETIC THERAPY. Problems complicating diuretic therapy include intravascular volume depletion and hypotension from overly vigorous diuresis; hyponatremia, often due to prolonged diuretic therapy with inadequate sodium intake and often with excessive water intake; hypokalemia from the use of thiazides or loop diuretics, or both, with inadequate potassium supplementation, predisposing to digitalis intoxication; hyperkalemia from potassium-sparing diuretic administration and potassium supplements; metabolic alkalosis with or without potassium depletion; hyperuricemia secondary to thiazide or loop diuretic administration; magnesium depletion, often occurring in parallel with potassium losses; and increased serum low density lipoproteins and triglyceride levels in patients receiving thiazides.

As a final comment, many patients treated for congestive heart failure spend a period of weeks developing the excessive fluid accumulation that characterizes this disease state; there is little virtue and much potential harm in attempting to correct this problem in an unduly short period of time. In general, in the absence of acute pulmonary edema, a reasonable goal (even in the era of DRG's) is about 1 kg of fluid loss per day.

Vasodilators

Cardiac function has a strong dependence on the resistance and capacitance properties of the peripheral vascular bed. Thus, vasodilator therapy in heart failure is designed to reduce the preload or afterload, or both, of a failing ventricle by relaxing vascular smooth muscle in the periphery. This approach to the management of heart failure improves survival in patients with continuing symptoms of heart failure who are taking digitalis and diuretics. This approach is an addition to, rather than a substitute for, use of cardiac glycosides and diuretics.

PRINCIPLES OF VASODILATOR THERAPY. As summarized in Figure 43-2, the normal ventricle is able to respond to increased afterload with an increase in the force of contraction such that there is little, if any, change in stroke volume until extreme elevations in afterload are encountered. As the ventricle fails, the relationship between afterload and stroke volume shifts downward and to the left so that a relatively modest change in outflow resistance causes a substantial alteration in stroke volume. This constitutes both a pathophysiologic problem and a therapeutic opportunity. The opportunity follows from the uniform increase in peripheral vascular resistance observed in untreated patients with decompensated congestive heart failure. Activation of the sympathetic nervous system and of the renin-angiotensin system accounts for most of the increase in peripheral resistance. These responses of the peripheral vascular system to a perceived decrease in cardiac output have survival value under conditions of hemorrhage or dehydration by redirecting the cardiac output to essential beds, including the brain and coronary circulation. Since congestive heart failure was presumably not an evolutionary pressure, it is not surprising that these primitive mechanisms for the defense of blood flow to vital organs prove maladaptive in the patient with chronic congestive heart failure.

As illustrated in Figure 43-1, the failing heart responds to a reduction in afterload by shifting its ventricular function curve toward normal, although the inotropic state remains unchanged. An attractive feature of afterload reduction is the ability to increase cardiac output without increasing preload or myocardial oxygen consumption.

VASODILATOR AGENTS. In the following discussion, primary consideration is given to vasodilator therapy for left ventricular failure, although the failing right ventrical will also benefit from reduced pulmonary vascular resistance. The most potent afterload-reducing agent in the pulmonary circulation is oxygen; there is, as yet, no drug that reliably exerts a preferential afterload-reducing effect in the pulmonary circulation.

The action of vasodilator drugs is described in terms of effects on the venous bed (preload) or the arteriolar bed (afterload). Table 43-10 summarizes data on the vasodilators in current clinical use in the management of heart failure.

Venous Dilators. These reduce the vascular smooth muscle tone in the systemic venous bed, increasing its capacitance and shifting blood volume from the arterial to the venous side of the circulation. Thus, patients with pulmonary vascular congestion and edema due to high left heart filling pressures will obtain symptomatic relief, limited only by the necessity to maintain a level of preload that results in an adequate forward cardiac output. The most selective agents for this purpose are the nitrates, including nitroglycerin and the longer-acting orally administered compounds, such as isosorbide dinitrate. Many investigators believe that much or most of the clinical benefit of vasodilator use derives from the venous dilator component. In chronic congestive heart failure,

TABLE 43-10. MAJOR VASODILATOR DRUGS*

Drug	Mechanism of Action	Venous Dilating Effect (Preload Reduction)	Arteriolar Dilating Effect (Afterload Reduction)	Usual Dosage	Comments
Nitroglycerin	Direct	+ + +	+	10–100 μg/min, IV 5–20 mg, transdermal 0.4 mg, s.l.	Tolerance may be a problem with sustained continuous use. May be used sublingually to control acute increases in left atrial pressure.
Isosorbide dinitrate	Direct	+ + +	+	5–20 mg q. 2 hr, s.l. 10–60 mg q. 4 hr, p.o.	Improved survival shown in chronic CHF when used with hydralazine.
Nitroprusside	Direct	+ + +	+ + +	5–150 μg/kg/min IV; usual dose, 50–75 μg/kg/min	Used IV only. Drug is light sensitive. Hazard of thiocyanate or cyanide toxicity with prolonged high doses.
Hydralazine	Direct	0	+ + +	10–75 mg q. 6 hr p.o.	Sustained benefit in heart failure not shown when used as sole vasodilator.
Phenoxybenzamine	Alpha-adrenergic blockade (nonselective)	+ +	+ +	10–20 mg q. 8 hr p.o.	Current use is limited.
Phentolamine	Alpha-adrenergic blockade (nonselective)	+ +	+ +	5 mg q. 4–6 hr IV	Current use is limited.
Prazosin	Alpha-adrenergic blockade (alpha₁ selective)	+ + +	+ +	1–5 mg q. 6 hr p.o.	Extra caution required with initial doses. Tolerance requires dosage adjustments.
Trimazosin†	Alpha-adrenergic blockade and undetermined mechanism	+ + +	+ +	50–450 mg b.i.d., p.o.	Investigational use only.
Captopril	Angiotensin converting enzyme inhibitor	+ + +	+ +	6.25–25.0 mg q. 6–8 hr, p.o.	Approved by F.D.A. for use in chronic CHF. Acute renal failure can occur with initial doses; initiate use with extra caution. Avoid potassium-sparing diuretics.
Nifedipine	Calcium channel blockade	+	+ +	10–30 mg q. 6 hr, p.o. 10–40 mg q. 6 hr, p.o.	Negative inotropic effect may be unmasked in severe CHF.

*All of these agents may cause severe hypotension, and special caution is required with initial use, particularly in patients with severe congestive heart failure. Heart rate changes with all agents listed are usually minor unless a hypotensive response elicits reflex tachycardia; prazosin can cause bradycardia with initial use.

†Investigational drug.

CHF = congestive heart failure; F.D.A. = Food and Drug Administration.

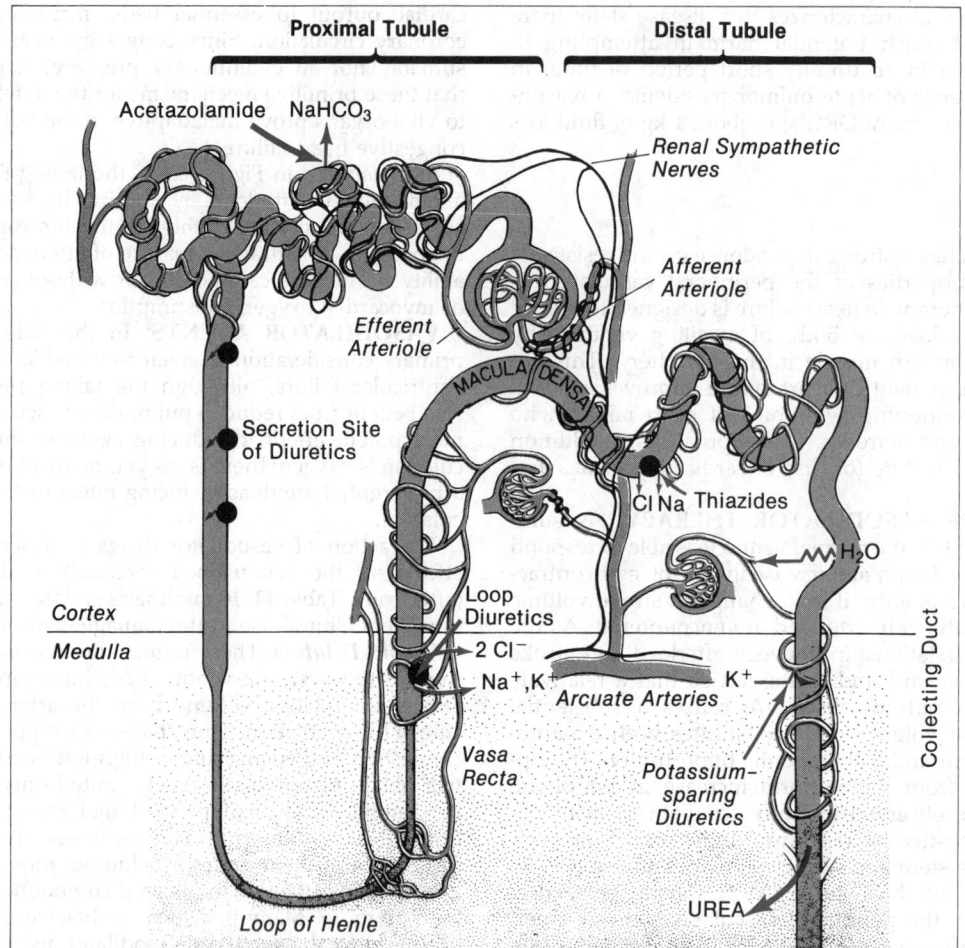

FIGURE 43—5. Sites of diuretic action in the mammalian nephron. Fluid resorption across the proximal tubule accounts for approximately two thirds of the resorption of filtered sodium and H_2O. Neuronal, hormonal, and hemodynamic factors, both extrinsic and intrinsic to the kidney, affect the volume and content of urine formation by altering the rate of formation of glomerular filtrate, thereby altering the balance of Starling forces between the proximal tubule and postglomerular peritubular capillaries. Agents that alter the rate of formation of glomerular filtrate, such as angiotensin-converting enzyme inhibitors, may enhance the delivery of solute and water to more distal segments of the nephron that are sensitive to diuretics. Nonsteroidal anti-inflammatory drugs may diminish the glomerular filtration rate, thus reducing the flow of urine to distal diuretic-sensitive portions of the nephron. A reduction in systemic blood pressure, or in renal artery pressure distal to the stenotic arterial lesion, below that necessary for formation of glomerular filtrate will render the kidney refractory to any diuretic. With the exception of the osmotic diuretics that are freely filtered at the glomerulus, most diuretics reach their site of action along the nephron after being secreted into the tubular lumen by the organic anion secretory transport system of the straight proximal tubule (pars recta).

About one third of the glomerular filtrate arrives at the descending limb of Henle's loop; no active transport of solute occurs here, although the tubular epithelium is highly permeable to water, which leaves the nephron for the increasingly hyperosmotic medullary interstitium. Most of the solute transport responsible for maintaining the hypertonicity of the medullary interstitium occurs in the water-impermeable thick ascending limb of Henle's loop. Here, a NaK cotransport system in the luminal membrane is coupled to the uptake of two chloride ions, a process dependent upon the electrochemical driving force for sodium generated by the NaK-ATPase on the basolateral membrane of these cells. This Na/K/2 Cl cotransport system on the luminal membrane of the tubular cells is the site of action for the loop diuretics (furosemide, bumetanide, and ethacrynic acid). Inhibition of cation transport by loop diuretics prevents the normal generation of the hypertonic medullary interstitium, thus reducing the osmotic gradient for free water clearance of ADH-sensitive tubular cells in the collecting duct, and also delivers large amounts of solute and water to the distal nephron, thus overwhelming distal Na^+ and Cl^- resorption sites.

The thick ascending limb approaches its own glomerulus as it re-

enters the cortex and passes between the afferent and efferent arterioles to form the juxtaglomerular apparatus (JGA), the tubular contribution to which is termed the macula densa. Loop diuretics may directly stimulate the release of renin by the JGA, an action that may contribute to the extrarenal vascular effects of these drugs. The distal convoluted tubule begins beyond the macula densa. Na^+ and Cl^-, as well as other ions (e.g., Ca^{++}) are resorbed in this segment. The thiazide diuretics and related drugs inhibit NaCl resorption in this segment, although the mechanism is unknown; they also enhance Ca^{++} resorption by tubular cells in this segment. Salt resorption by this distal, water-impermeable portion of the nephron allows the formation of a dilute urine, hence the term "cortical diluting segment." Thiazide-induced inhibition of NaCl resorption in this segment therefore may lead to hyponatremia, particularly when accompanied by elevated ADH levels and increased thirst.

The cortical collecting duct actively resorbs NaCl via an aldosterone-sensitive mechanism. This leads to increased net resorption of Na^+ into cells and hence to a lumen negative potential difference that favors the secretion of K^+ and H^+ ions. This is why increased Na^+ concentrations and high flow rates in the cortical collecting duct, as after loop or thiazide diuretic administration, leads to enhanced passive K^+ secretion. Anti-aldosterone drugs, such as spironolactone, competitively inhibit aldosterone's binding to its receptor, thereby limiting Na^+ permeability by the apical membrane and reducing K^+ secretion.

As illustrated, the blood supply to each nephron is derived from several sources. The afferent arteriole that enters the glomerulus is richly innervated with sympathetic nerve endings, particularly as it enters the glomerulus at its vascular pole within the juxtaglomerular apparatus. Increased sympathetic discharge to the kidney results in increased net NaCl resorption even in the absence of changes in glomerular hemodynamics. Elevated efferent sympathetic activity, as is often seen in decompensated congestive heart failure, would be expected to result in avid retention of solute due to reduced renal perfusion, increased renin release, and enhanced tubular resorption of solute. Dopamine is a potent renal vasodilator and may directly affect tubular epithelia to reduce NaCl resorption, thus acting as a natriuretic agent. Exogenously administered dopamine, particularly when infused at rates of 5 μg per kilogram per minute, may be a useful adjunct to diuretic therapy in selected patients with advanced CHF.

administration of agents that preferentially dilate the arteriolar bed without a preload-reducing component, such as minoxidil and hydralazine, fail to show sustained benefit.

Arteriolar Dilators. These reduce left ventricular afterload and tend to redistribute blood flow among organ beds in ways that are, unfortunately, not always predictable. The improvement in blood flow to exercising skeletal muscle is relatively limited. Nevertheless, the forward stroke output of the left ventricle is delivered with a lower wall tension, such that myocardial oxygen consumption is favorably affected. The most selective agent routinely used in obtaining an afterload-reducing effect is hydralazine.

The balanced vasodilators exert an effect on both preload and afterload through a generalized relaxing effect on vascular smooth muscle. The prototype short-acting agent of this kind is nitroprusside. This agent has found widespread application in the management of acute heart failure states, including acute pulmonary edema. Used with care, it can also improve the circulatory state of patients with combined hypotension and low forward output, provided that adequate arterial pressure can be maintained by the use of volume loading or inotropic drugs or both. The tendency of nitroprusside to reduce systemic arterial pressure is offset to a considerable extent by the increased stroke output. The unloading effect of nitroprusside is most helpful when the left ventricular filling pressures are maintained in the vicinity of 15 mm Hg, which may require administration of intravenous fluids. An important advantage of nitroprusside in intensive care unit settings is its short duration of action, permitting minute-to-minute titration of the circulatory state.

A regimen frequently employed to obtain a balanced vasodilator effect is hydralazine and nitrates, often given as the long-acting oral preparation isosorbide dinitrate. In an important multicenter study (Cohn, 1986), the protocol randomly assigned patients who were symptomatic while taking digitalis and diuretics to hydralazine with isosorbide dinitrate, to prazosin, or to placebo. The group treated with hydralazine and nitrates showed a 38 per cent mean reduction in mortality during the initial year of treatment, and the improved survival was sustained to the three-year point. The prazosin-treated group showed no significant difference from the placebo group.

The angiotensin-converting enzyme inhibitor captopril is now available as a balanced vasodilator for the management of patients with advanced heart failure. Multicenter trials have demonstrated sustained improvement in symptoms and exercise tolerance, although a study designed to examine the issue of survival has not yet been completed. Many clinicians find that captopril provides a relatively simple and controllable approach to vasodilator therapy, and it is the vasodilator of choice in many centers. Special care is required in administering initial doses of captopril, which can produce severe hypotension and renal failure. In general, the initial dose should not exceed 6.25 mg, and institution of therapy for patients with advanced heart failure is best carried out in the hospital.

Only about one half of patients who appear to be reasonable candidates for vasodilator use in advanced heart failure can tolerate the drugs initially, and only half of that group (or 25 per cent of the total) still show demonstrable benefit at the end of three months. Although these figures may be improved by careful selection of patients and judicious use of available agents, the fact remains that many patients with advanced heart failure are unable to tolerate vasodilators, chiefly because of postural hypotension.

Refractory Heart Failure

Therapeutic advances have left in their wake a subset of patients with marked impairment of ventricular function (often with left ventricular ejection fractions in the 10 to 20 per cent range) who survive but are severely symptomatic on maximal tolerated doses of digitalis, diuretics, and vasodilators. Those aged 50 years or less who meet additional relevant criteria (including preserved function of other organ systems, no elevation of pulmonary vascular resistance, no glucose intolerance, no active infection) may deserve consideration of heart transplantation after detailed explanation of the potential risks and benefits of this procedure. This procedure now has relatively widespread application since the advent of cyclosporine for immunosuppression, and more than 50 centers in the United States now have active programs. Survival exceeds 50 per cent at 5 years in larger series, compared with an expected mortality well in excess of 50 per cent at 12 months in patients treated by conventional means, and functional recovery is often gratifying.

Treatment of acute decompensation using intravenous beta-adrenergic or dopaminergic agonists, or both, is covered in Ch. 44. Longer-term use of orally active adrenergic drugs has proved disappointing because of rapid development of tolerance and cannot be recommended. Intermittent use of intravenous dobutamine for ambulatory patients with severe heart failure is under investigation, as are several phosphodiesterase inhibitor drugs, including amrinone, milrinone,* and enoximone,* that have both vasodilator and positive inotropic properties related to enhancement of cyclic adenosine monophosphate levels in vascular smooth muscle and myocardium. Although symptoms are improved in some patients treated with these investigational agents, evidence of improved survival is lacking. The artificial heart has been developed sufficiently for placement in several patients, but results to date have been disappointing because of unsolved thromboembolic problems.

---

*Investigational drug.

ACKNOWLEDGMENT: The author is indebted to Alfred P. Fishman, M.D., the author of this chapter in the seventeenth edition, for his valuable advice regarding the structure and content of the sections of this chapter dealing with general aspects, categories, pathophysiology, and clinical findings in heart failure. Ralph A. Kelly, M.D., has made major contributions to the coverage of diuretics, including Figure 43–5.

Berger BE, Warnock DG: Clinical uses and mechanisms of action of diuretic agents. In Brenner BM, Rector FC (eds.): The Kidney. Philadelphia, W. B. Saunders Company, 1986, pp 433–455. *A compact summary of clinically relevant information as stated in the title.*

Braunwald E, Mock MB, Watson JT (eds.): Congestive Heart Failure. New York, Grune & Stratton, 1982. *A series of informative monographs covering all aspects of heart failure, originally presented at an NIH-sponsored conference intended to summarize the current state of the art.*

Captopril Multicenter Research Group: A placebo-controlled trial of captopril in refractory congestive heart failure. J Am Coll Cardiol 2:755, 1983. *A well-designed controlled trial demonstrating improved clinical state and effort tolerance among 92 patients with heart failure refractory to digitalis and diuretics randomized to additional treatment with placebo or the angiotensin-converting enzyme inhibitor captopril, which was subsequently approved by the United States Food and Drug Administration for the indication of congestive heart failure.*

Cohn JN, et al.: Effect of vasodilator therapy on mortality in chronic congestive heart failure: Results of a VA cooperative study. N Engl J Med 314:1547, 1986. *Random assignment of 642 men with heart failure on digitalis and diuretics (which were continued) to additional placebo, prazosin, or hydralazine and isosorbide dinitrate. At a mean follow-up of 2.3 years, this study showed improved survival (risk reduction of 34 percent) among patients treated with hydralazine and nitrates. Mortality in the prazosin-treated group was indistinguishable from that in the group receiving placebo. Overall mortality, as expected, was high (36 to 47 per cent at three years). Additional useful references on vasodilator therapy in heart failure are cited.*

Colucci WS, Wright RF, Braunwald E: New positive inotropic agents in the treatment of congestive heart failure: Mechanisms of action and recent clinical developments. N Engl J Med 314:290, 349, 1986. *This two-part review article covers the stated subjects well, with a clinical emphasis.*

New Concepts in the Mechanisms and Treatment of Congestive Heart Failure. Am J Cardiol 55:1A, 1985. *This symposium, chaired by J. N. Cohn, includes up-to-date discussions of current problems in the study of heart failure. Epidemiology is well summarized by W. McF. Smith.*

Smith TW (ed.): Digitalis Glycosides. Orlando, Fla., Grune & Stratton, 1986. *This 348-page book summarizes available information on all aspects of the basic and clinical pharmacology, clinical use, and toxicity problems related to the cardiac glycosides.*

Smith TW, Braunwald E: The management of heart failure. In Braunwald E (ed.): Heart Diseases. 3rd ed. Philadelphia, W. B. Saunders Company, 1987. *A detailed consideration of general and specific aspects of congestive heart failure management with 562 references.*

44 SHOCK

*François M. Abboud**

Shock is a complex clinical syndrome that demands vigilant medical attention, careful hemodynamic monitoring, and thorough understanding of the basic principles of circulatory control and of the pharmacology of cardiac and vasoactive drugs. This chapter covers the basic principles of *circulatory control* as they relate to the shock syndrome, the *cellular mechanisms* involved in the pathogenesis of shock, and the *therapy* of shock.

DEFINITION. Shock, regardless of cause, is a failure of the circulatory system to maintain cellular perfusion and function. This results in cellular membrane dysfunction, abnormal cellular metabolism, and eventually cellular death.

CAUSES. Table 44–1 lists the most common clinical situations associated with decreased cardiac output, hypotension, decreased tissue perfusion, capillary endothelial injury, and cellular damage.

CLINICAL PICTURE. The classic clinical presentation is one of a patient who is hypotensive (with a systolic blood pressure of 90 mm Hg or less); has a tachycardia with a thready pulse; is hyperventilating; has cold, clammy, cyanotic skin; and has a dulled sensorium ranging from agitation to stupor or coma. The patient is frequently oliguric, with a urinary output of less than 20 ml per hour.

This clinical picture is not always present, and the recognition of the subtle or early presentation of shock may be crucial. For example, a patient may have a "normal" blood pressure (i.e., 110/70), but this may actually represent "relative hypotension" if the patient has a history of hypertension. Early shock may be indicated only by unexplained agitation or tachycardia in the absence of cardiovascular collapse. Some patients with septic shock may initially present with warm hyperperfused extremities (so-called warm shock) due to abnormal peripheral vasodilatation.

Frequently, the clinical findings follow a progressive pattern as shock evolves from the early compensated phase to the advanced stages (Table 44–2). In addition, the signs and symptoms of the underlying precipitating disease are present, e.g., severe pain of acute myocardial infarction or dissecting aneurysm, visible bleeding, burn, peritonitis, sepsis, or trauma.

PATHOPHYSIOLOGY AND STAGES OF SHOCK. The basic elements in the pathogenesis of shock are portrayed in Figure 44–1.

Stage I: Compensated. Hypotension may be caused either by a fall in cardiac output or by vasodilatation. The fall in cardiac output and hypotension trigger compensatory mechanisms, which restore arterial pressure and blood flow to the more vital organs such as brain and heart. Symptoms and signs are minimal, and appropriate intervention is most effective.

Stage II: Decompensated. In this stage, the compensatory mechanisms to maintain perfusion of vital organs are insufficient. Evidence of decreased cerebral perfusion may be

*The author acknowledges the assistance of David W. Ferguson in the revision of this chapter.

TABLE 44–1. CAUSES OF SHOCK AND INITIATING MECHANISMS

I. **Decreased intravascular volume**
   A. Acute hemorrhage (e.g., gastrointestinal bleeding, retroperitoneal bleeding, ruptured aortic aneurysm, hemoptysis, hemothorax, trauma)
   B. Excessive fluid loss
      1. Vomiting (intestinal or pyloric obstruction)
      2. Severe diarrhea, sweating, and dehydration
      3. Excessive urine (e.g., diabetes mellitus, diabetes insipidus, excessive diuretics, diuretic phase of acute renal failure)
      4. Peritonitis, pancreatitis, splanchnic ischemia, intestinal obstruction, and gangrene
      5. Trauma and extensive muscle injury
      6. Burns
   C. Vasodilatation (relative hypovolemia)
      1. Neurogenic: drug induced (e.g., anesthesia, ganglionic and adrenergic blockers, overdoses such as barbiturates, poisons); nervous system damage (e.g., spinal cord injury, cerebral vascular accident, severe dysautonomia)
      2. Metabolic, toxic, or humoral vasodilatation: septicemia (gram-negative endotoxemia or gram-positive bacteremia); acute adrenal insufficiency, anaphylactic reaction

II. **Cardiac**
   A. Acute myocardial infarction
   B. Myocarditis, myocardial depression (hypoxia, acidosis, septic shock, myocardial depressant factors [MDF], drugs, hypoglycemia), severe low-output failure
   C. Acute valvular insufficiency, myocardial rupture, septal perforation
   D. Arrhythmias: severe bradycardia, tachycardia, and fibrillation
   E. Mechanical compression or obstruction
      1. Pericardial effusion or tamponade
      2. Positive pressure ventilation, tension pneumothorax
      3. Pulmonary embolism
      4. Ball-valve thrombus or atrial myxoma

III. **Microcirculatory endothelial injury and aggregation of corpuscles**
   A. Anaphylaxis
   B. Disseminated intravascular coagulation
   C. Burns, septic shock, trauma

IV. **Cellular membrane injury**
   A. Septic shock
   B. Anaphylaxis
   C. Ischemia, prolonged hypoxia, pancreatitis, tissue injury

apparent from the mental state of the patient; decreased renal perfusion may reduce urinary output, and patients with coronary artery disease may experience myocardial ischemia. The external appearance of the patient also reflects excessive sympathetic discharge, with cyanosis, coldness, and clamminess of the skin. The majority of patients are recognized in this phase, and rapid aggressive intervention to restore cardiac output and perfusion of the tissues may reverse the shock syndrome.

Stage III: Irreversible. Excessive and prolonged reduction of tissue perfusion leads to significant alterations in cellular membrane function, aggregation of blood corpuscles, and "sludging" in the capillaries. The vasoconstriction that has taken place in the less vital organs in order to maintain blood pressure is now excessive and has reduced flow to such an extent that cellular damage occurs.

Arterial pressure continues to fall progressively to a critical level at which the perfusion of vital organs is reduced. Critical impairment of renal perfusion leads to acute tubular necrosis. Ischemia of the gastrointestinal tract leads to necrotic damage

TABLE 44–2. CLINICAL FINDINGS AT VARIOUS STAGES OF SHOCK

Stages	I Compensated*	II Decompensated	III Irreversible
Arterial blood pressure	N or ↓	↓	↓↓
Heart rate	↑	↑↑	↑↑ → ↓↓
Pulse pressure	↓	↓↓	↓↓↓
Cardiac output	↓	↓↓	↓↓↓
Respiratory rate	N	↑	↑↑ → ↓↓
Mental status	Anxiety	Obtunded	Coma
Urinary output	N or ↓	↓↓	Anuria
Skin	Cool	Mottled	Cold, cyanotic

*N = no change. A high cardiac output and warm skin may be present in septic shock.

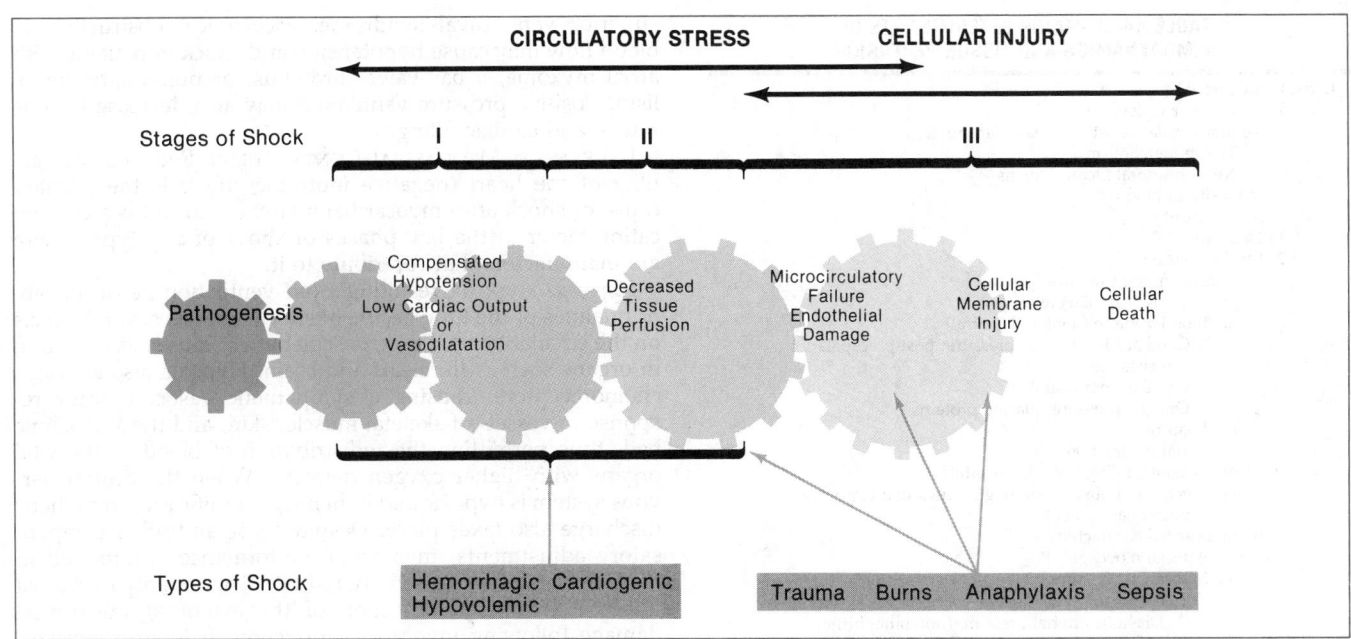

FIGURE 44–1. Pathophysiology of shock.

of the mucosa and absorption into the circulation of bacteria and toxic bacterial products that have detrimental effects on other organs and may lead to generalized endothelial damage with disseminated intravascular coagulation. Bacterial toxins react with neutrophils and cause the release of vasodilator polypeptides that contribute to the fall in arterial pressure. The severe acidosis resulting from anaerobic metabolism also contributes to vasodilatation. The decreased perfusion pressure of the coronary vessels, particularly in patients with coronary disease, results in reduction of myocardial perfusion, which in turn decreases myocardial contractility and creates a vicious cycle as the decreased contractility causes further decrements in arterial blood pressure. Hypoxia impairs reflex neurogenic circulatory adjustments that help in maintaining arterial pressure. Damage to the capillary endothelium leads to loss of fluid and protein through the capillaries, with exacerbation of hypovolemia and hypotension. Damage to cellular membranes from ischemia leads to leakage of lysosomal enzymes and intracellular ions, to progressive reduction in high energy phosphate reserves, and to cellular destruction.

CIRCULATORY CONTROL IN SHOCK

Major Determinants of Tissue Perfusion

The major determinants of hemodynamics and tissue perfusion are listed in Table 44–3. Perfusion of any organ depends upon systemic arterial pressure (which is the driving force for blood to flow through all organs), the resistance offered by the vasculature of that organ, and the patency of nutritional capillaries. Systemic arterial pressure is in turn determined by cardiac output and the resistance of the total vascular tree. Vascular resistance is predominantly a function of the radius or caliber of blood vessels. Vascular caliber is influenced by neurogenic, humoral, and myogenic factors that regulate the tone of vascular smooth muscle. Thus blood flow to any one organ depends on cardiac function and on vascular muscle tone and caliber in all the arterial tree as well as in the organ itself. The determinant of exchange of substrates and metabolites with the tissues is the microcirculation. A patent nutritional capillary network is the critical interface between the circulation and the cell.

This discussion deals with cardiac, vascular, and microcirculatory factors.

CARDIAC FACTORS. Cardiac output is the product of heart rate and stroke volume. A rate of 70 beats per minute and a stroke volume of 70 ml per beat give a cardiac output of approximately 5 liters per minute, an amount more than sufficient to deliver 250 ml of oxygen per minute to all the tissues. This consumption of oxygen reflects metabolic needs at rest. A drop in cardiac output below 2 liters per minute per square meter is an indication of severe shock.

Heart Rate. Tachycardia usually increases cardiac output, but a marked increase in heart rate may limit cardiac diastolic filling time and result in a low cardiac output and arterial blood pressure. For example, ventricular tachycardia or rapid atrial fibrillation in a patient with recent myocardial infarction causes a reduction in cardiac output and arterial pressure that, if uncorrected, could result in cardiogenic shock. Immediate treatment to restore heart rate is essential. In considering the treatment of tachycardia in shock, one has to be cautious in avoiding treatment of a "compensatory tachycardia" often seen in patients with fever, anemia, sepsis, hemorrhage, or severe hypovolemia. Tachycardia is often an appropriate reflex circulatory adjustment to maintain cardiac output.

Extreme bradycardia may also cause a low output and hypotension. Sinus bradycardia and atrioventricular block are often seen immediately following myocardial infarction and should be reversed if they contribute to hypotension.

Stroke Volume. A decrease in stroke volume may be caused by (1) a decrease in cardiac filling, (2) a decrease in myocardial contractility, or (3) an increased afterload (Fig. 44–2).

DECREASE IN CARDIAC FILLING PRESSURE. The amount of blood filling the ventricles at the end of diastole is the "preload," and it regulates the subsequent contraction and stroke volume (Starling's law of the heart). Although there are many factors that determine preload, such as the rate and duration of filling, ventricular compliance, and venous tone, a most important determinant is total blood volume. Reduction in blood volume may be either absolute or relative to the capacity of the vascular tree. Absolute reductions in blood volume are apparent when blood or fluids are lost, causing a hypovolemic state leading to hypovolemic shock. This is seen in hemorrhage (either external or internal bleeding), excessive vomiting, diarrhea, burns, renal loss of fluids such as in diabetes mellitus or diabetes insipidus, excessive diuresis, and exces-

TABLE 44–3. MAJOR DETERMINANTS OF HEMODYNAMICS AND TISSUE PERFUSION

I. Systemic arterial pressure
 A. Total vascular resistance
  1. Total arteriolar resistance, vascular muscle tone
   a. Tissue metabolism
   b. Neurohumoral factors, toxins
  2. Viscosity of blood
 B. Cardiac output
  1. Heart rate
  2. Stroke volume
   a. Cardiac filling pressure (preload)
    i. Venous (vascular) tone
    ii. Blood volume (total and central)
     Capillary hydrostatic pressure: post-precapillary resistance
     Capillary permeability
     Oncotic pressure, plasma proteins
    iii. Posture
    iv. Atrial contraction
    v. Diastolic filling time (heart rate)
    vi. Mechanical obstruction (e.g., pericardial tamponade, pulmonary embolus)
   b. Myocardial contractility
    i. Arterial blood pH, P_{O_2}
    ii. Myocardial O_2 supply:
     Increase supply:
      ↑ Diastolic arterial pressure (norepinephrine, dopamine)
      Capillary diffusion
      Coronary dilatation (nitroglycerin, dopamine, metabolites)
     Decrease supply:
      ↓ Diastolic arterial pressure (isoproterenol, vasodilators)
      Coronary artery disease, myocardial infarction
      Hypoxia, anemia
    iii. Myocardial O_2 demand
     Increase demand:
      ↑ Cardiac size (pulmonary wedge pressure)
      ↑ Afterload (systolic arterial pressure, impedance)
      ↑ Contractility (norepinephrine, dopamine, isoproterenol) and heart rate
     Decrease demand:
      ↓ Cardiac size
       ⎰ Digitalis, ↑ ejection fraction
       ⎱ Venodilatation (nitroprusside, nitroglycerin, phentolamine)
       ⎰ Diuretics
      ↓ Afterload, impedance (vasodilators)
      ↓ Contractility and heart rate
    iv. Humoral factors
      Catecholamines
      Myocardial depressant factors
    v. Drugs
      Increase norepinephrine, dopamine, isoproterenol, digitalis
      Decrease propranolol, anesthetics
   c. Afterload
    i. Arterial blood pressure, vascular impedance
    ii. End-diastolic cardiac wall tension
    iii. Severe aortic stenosis
II. Organ vascular resistance
 A. Occlusive arterial disease
 B. Local arteriolar resistance
 C. Local venular resistance
 D. Viscosity of blood
III. Patency of nutritional capillaries
 A. Precapillary sphincter tone
 B. Intracapillary aggregation of corpuscles
 C. Capillary endothelial integrity

sive perspiration without fluid replacement. Internal losses of fluid occur in peritonitis, pancreatitis, intestinal obstruction with extravasation of fluid, splanchnic ischemia with bowel necrosis and gangrene, fractures with extensive muscle trauma, hemothorax, and hemoperitoneum.

Relative decreases in blood volume occur when there is loss of vascular tone because of the administration of anesthetics or ganglion blockers, after spinal cord injury, and in patients with neuropathy or autonomic insufficiency. Pooling of blood thus results in a decrease in cardiac filling pressure. Compression of the heart may also prevent its filling, as is seen during pericardial tamponade, in tension pneumothorax, or in the

superior vena caval syndrome. Mechanical obstruction to blood flow may cause hypotension and shock in patients with atrial myxoma, a ball-valve thrombus, or pulmonary embolism. Positive pressure ventilation may also decrease venous return and cardiac filling.

DECREASE IN MYOCARDIAL CONTRACTILITY. Reduced contractility of the heart (negative inotropic effect) is the primary cause of shock after myocardial infarction, and it is a complicating factor in the late phases of shock of any type. There are many factors that contribute to it.

Hypoxia. Hypoxia resulting from ventilation-perfusion abnormalities of the lung occurs in shock and has several effects on the circulation. A direct, vascular effect causes vasodilation in organs such as the heart and brain. Hypoxia also activates chemoreceptors, causing a sympathetic vasoconstrictor response in vessels of skeletal muscle, skin, and the splanchnic bed, thus permitting the redistribution of blood to the vital organs with higher oxygen demand. When the central nervous system is hypoxic and ischemic, a significant sympathetic discharge also takes place. Despite these and other compensatory adjustments, myocardial performance is impaired in the presence of decreased arterial P_{O_2}. The severity of arterial hypoxia is often a reflection of the extent of myocardial damage following myocardial infarction. It is an important, potentially reversible cause of depression of myocardial contractility.

Acidosis. Acidosis results from anaerobic metabolism with release of lactate, from decreased renal perfusion with accumulation of organic acids, and possibly from hypoventilation of certain pulmonary segments, leading to respiratory acidosis. Acidosis reduces myocardial contractility and the vasoconstrictor response to various neurohumoral factors.

Myocardial Ischemia and Perfusion Pressure. Myocardial performance depends on perfusion of the ischemic myocardium, which is determined to a great extent by the level of arterial diastolic pressure. The fall in arterial pressure during hemorrhagic or hypovolemic shock in patients with coronary artery disease may cause myocardial ischemia. Restoration of arterial pressure is critical to preservation of myocardial function. In the presence of coronary artery disease, resistance to flow is due largely to structural changes in the vessel wall, and vasomotor tone is minimal because of excessive accumulation of vasodilator metabolites downstream from the site of coronary narrowing. Thus arterial pressure becomes the determinant of perfusion of the ischemic segment through collateral vessels or across a narrowing or a plaque.

Increased Myocardial Oxygen Demand Relative to Supply. Although oxygen supply to the ischemic myocardium is in-

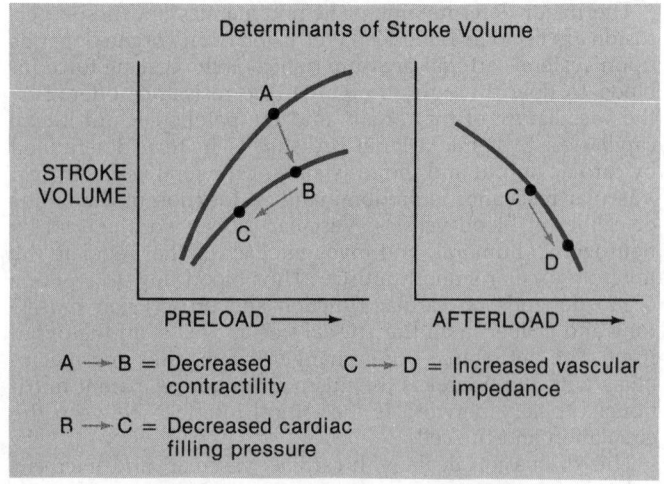

FIGURE 44–2. Determinants of stroke volume.

creased by increasing arterial pressure, hypertension is detrimental, as it increases myocardial work and oxygen demand. Conversely, hypotension decreases myocardial work and oxygen needs, but it also reduces myocardial perfusion as mentioned above. Judicious restoration of arterial pressure is necessary.

Increased cardiac size is associated with increased myocardial wall tension, which causes greater myocardial oxygen consumption. Drugs such as isoproterenol may increase myocardial oxygen demand out of proportion to the associated increase in coronary flow.

Other Factors that Depress Contractility. Drugs such as the barbiturates may depress cardiac output by a direct effect on the myocardium. More frequently, myocardial depression occurs from suppression of the adrenergic drive with propranolol, ganglion-blocking drugs, catecholamine depleters such as reserpine or guanethidine, or high spinal anesthetics, or with such conditions as spinal cord injury or an intracranial lesion involving the medullary centers. These interventions not only depress myocardial contraction but also decrease peripheral vascular tone.

Myocardial depressant factors may be released from damaged cells in various organs during shock from burns, pancreatitis, septicemia, or hemorrhage, and add an element of myocardial depression. Oxygen free radicals generated during ischemia and reperfusion may cause significant myocardial depression.

INCREASE IN AFTERLOAD. To eject the stroke volume the ventricle has to generate enough force to oppose the end-diastolic wall tension, the arterial pressure, and the vascular impedance. In severe heart failure with high ventricular end-diastolic pressure, cardiomegaly, and very low cardiac output, a vasodilator agent that decreases afterload by reducing vascular impedance and cardiac size may increase stroke volume.

VASCULAR FACTORS. These determine the resistance to blood flow and transcapillary exchange. Resistance to flow of blood is determined by the viscosity of blood and by the length and the cross-sectional area of the vessels. The cross-sectional area is the most important component, because the calculated resistance is inversely proportional to the fourth power of the radius of the vessels. The radius is in turn determined by the tone of vascular smooth muscle in the wall of the vessels. Vascular smooth muscle tone is modulated by neurogenic influences mediated primarily through the sympathoadrenal system and by circulating humoral and local metabolic factors.

Neurogenic Control. Sympathoadrenal discharge to the circulatory system is regulated by medullary neurons in the vasomotor center. Activity of these neurons is modulated by afferent neural impulses originating in various receptors located in strategic areas around the body. Important among these receptors are arterial and cardiac baroreceptors, chemoreceptors, somatic receptors in skeletal muscle, and thermal receptors. Activities originating in various parts of the central nervous system (cerebellum, fastigial and vestibular nuclei, and hypothalamus) also impinge upon the vasomotor center to modulate its output. Activation of cardiac sensory receptors, particularly those in the left ventricle, during volume expansion and stretch of the myocardium, inhibits sympathoadrenal activity. Conversely, reduction in the stretch of these ventricular receptors during hypovolemia and hemorrhage release the sympathoadrenal efferent activity to cause reflex tachycardia and vasoconstriction, to restore arterial blood pressure, and to release renin. The arterial baroreceptors, activated by a rise in blood pressure, suppress sympathoadrenal tone; conversely, during hypotension they increase sympathoadrenal drive and restore arterial pressure.

Severe hypoxia, often associated with shock from any cause, activates the chemoreceptor reflex and causes an increase in sympathoadrenal drive. The reduction of central or cardiopulmonary blood volume and arterial pressure during hemorrhage activates the cardiopulmonary reflex and the arterial baroreceptor reflex simultaneously, and the two reflexes are synergistic with respect to the final sympathetic efferent activity. Similarly, the combined activation of the arterial baroreceptor reflex by hypotension and the chemoreceptor reflex by hypoxia results in a significant synergistic effect on the ventilatory response as well as the circulatory sympathetic drive.

Conversely, there may be situations in which reflex responses have competing effects. This may occur, for example, when cardiac receptors are activated following acute myocardial infarction by the dyskinetic bulge of the left ventricle, while the arterial baroreceptors are inactivated because of hypotension. In the experimental preparation the inhibitory influence of the bulging left ventricular wall on the sympathetic outflow predominates and overrides the arterial baroreflex, preventing vasoconstriction and thus causing a decrease in the afterload of the damaged left ventricle. Teleologically, this effect may be beneficial, as it will tend to decrease left ventricular work following its acute insult.

There have been few studies of the effects of endotoxin on neurocirculatory reflexes. An increase in baroreceptor activity for any level of arterial blood pressure has been reported in endotoxemia, a situation that would tend to inhibit sympathoadrenal tone, and might explain in part the decreased vascular resistance often seen in septic shock.

Humoral Factors. The release of hormones such as renin, vasopressin, steroids, prostaglandins, and kinins is partly mediated through the sympathoadrenal system and cardiovascular mechanoreceptors and partly through direct and indirect cellular effects of toxins, ischemia, and antigens in various organs. These hormones have direct cardiovascular and renal effects and indirect effects on central or peripheral adrenergic transmission.

RENIN-ANGIOTENSIN. A fall in arterial blood pressure or an increase in sympathoadrenal sympathetic discharge to the kidney causes the release of renin. The resulting formation of angiotensin causes peripheral vasoconstriction, maintains arterial pressure, stimulates the release of aldosterone to retain sodium and water, and has an intrarenal effect on tubular sodium reabsorption that also permits greater sodium and water retention and preserves blood volume during hypotensive states.

VASOPRESSIN. This important water-retaining and constrictor hormone is released from the posterior pituitary primarily in response to increases in osmolality and may also play a role in the circulatory control in shock. Its release is reduced by stretch of the left atrial receptors during hypervolemia or by stretch of the arterial baroreceptor during hypertension; conversely, during hemorrhage and systemic hypotension, or when patients are on cardiopulmonary bypass, the blood levels of vasopressin increase significantly. Thirst and the release of vasopressin may be induced by a central nervous system action of angiotensin.

KININS. A variety of potent vasodilator polypeptides is formed by the action of certain proteolytic enzymes on plasma protein precursors. Bradykinin serves as the prototype for this class of endogenous peptides. Their major physiologic role may be the local regulation of blood flow and function of such organs as the salivary gland, pancreas, and kidney. In pathophysiologic states, kinins are believed to play a part in the hyperemia associated with inflammation and as vasodilators in hypotension produced by anaphylactic reactions. Renal kinins may cause diuresis and natriuresis.

SEROTONIN AND HISTAMINE. Serotonin released from platelets and histamine released from mast cells during anaphylaxis or during complement activation in shock may play an important role in regulating local vascular tone and capillary permeability.

PROSTACYCLIN AND THROMBOXANE A_2. Prostaglandins may be released in various organs during ischemia and may contribute to the reactive hyperemia and vasodilatation. The prostaglandin endoperoxides formed in platelets and in blood vessels are pivotal in the synthesis of two potent substances with opposing effects on the formation of thrombi. Prostacyclin, a powerful vasodilator and inhibitor of platelet aggregation, is synthesized in the vascular wall, mostly in the endothelial layer, from endoperoxides. In the platelets, however, endoperoxides are converted to thromboxane A_2, which causes vasoconstriction and platelet aggregation. In shock, damage to endothelial cells may inhibit synthesis of prostacyclin; in addition, platelets may release thromboxane A_2, causing intravascular platelet aggregation, clumping, and vasoconstriction.

ENDORPHINS. β-Endorphin and adrenocorticotropin are stored in the pituitary gland and secreted concomitantly under stress. β-Endorphins may contribute directly or indirectly to myocardial depression in shock. Studies in endotoxin (E. coli) shock and hemorrhagic shock in animals indicate that the specific opiate antagonist, naloxone, rapidly reverses the hypotension primarily through a positive inotropic effect on the heart. Naloxone has minimal cardiovascular effects in the absence of shock. The beneficial effect of synthetic steroids in experimental shock may be caused by suppression of β-endorphins. It is difficult, however, to demonstrate a convincing beneficial effect of either naloxone or steroids on humans in shock.

Local Autoregulatory Adjustment of Blood Vessels. Blood vessels have an intrinsic ability to regulate vascular tone and thereby maintain blood flow over a wide range of perfusion pressures. This property is referred to as the autoregulatory capacity for blood flow and is independent of systemic neurogenic influences or humoral factors. Different vascular beds vary with respect to their ability to maintain blood flow. The cerebral, coronary, and renal circulations are most potent. Thus during a fall in arterial pressure, vasodilatation of the cerebral, coronary, and renal vasculatures maintains blood flow and oxygen delivery to the brain and heart as well as sodium and water balance. Although a myogenic response intrinsic to the smooth muscle may explain the phenomenon, accumulation of tissue metabolites following a transient period of ischemia may also cause vasodilatation and restore blood flow. The specific mediator of metabolic vasodilatation is not known, but it is likely that a combination of changes in oxygen, carbon dioxide, and hydrogen ions and other cations, in osmolality, in the amount of adenosine compounds, and in Krebs cycle intermediates and other metabolites released in the immediate environment of blood vessels contributes to adjustments in vascular tone.

MICROCIRCULATION AND TRANSCAPILLARY EXCHANGE. Perhaps the most critical aspect of the pathogenesis of shock takes place at the level of the microcirculation. Delivery of a significant amount of blood to an organ does not guarantee that all the segments of that organ and all capillaries are perfused appropriately.

Intraorgan Blood Flow Distribution. Adequate tissue perfusion depends on blood flow through vascular channels in which diffusion between the blood and tissues can occur. These are referred to as nutritional capillaries, as contrasted with nonnutritional vessels that do not permit capillary exchange. The latter are also referred to as arteriovenous shunts, although there may be little anatomic evidence for the existence of such shunts. An example of the importance of the intraorgan redistribution of blood flow is observed in myocardial infarction, in which an increase in coronary blood flow may not increase perfusion to the infarcted segment. Under some circumstances a coronary vasodilator might redistribute flow away from ischemic into nonischemic regions.

Similarly, intraorgan blood flow distribution may be critical in the kidney. Acute tubular necrosis associated with shock may reflect a reduction in glomerular filtration in the outer cortex because of a localized increase in vascular resistance in

this region and a selective reduction in blood flow. Interventions that alter total renal blood flow can produce significant redistribution of flow within the kidney; for example, renal vasoconstriction following adrenergic discharge tends to shunt blood away from the outer cortex, whereas renal vasodilators such as furosemide shunt blood toward the outer cortical nephrons.

Pre- and Postcapillary Resistance. The *precapillary sphincters* regulate the patency of nutritional or "exchange" capillaries. The tone of those spincters may be modulated by neurohumoral factors that contribute to the circulatory adjustments in shock. The metabolic products at the local tissue level are important determinants of the patency of these sphincters, which regulate the total capillary surface area and in turn determine the intravascular-extracellular fluid and solute exchange. The capillary hydrostatic force driving fluid out of the capillaries into the extracellular space is dependent on the ratio of post- to precapillary resistances. In hypovolemic or hemorrhagic shock, the fall in arterial pressure causes activation of the sympathoadrenal system, constriction of precapillary resistance vessels, and a fall in capillary hydrostatic pressure, facilitating movement of fluids from the extracellular into the intravascular space. This partially restores intravascular volume. Hematocrit and viscosity of blood and plasma oncotic pressure fall. The decline in plasma oncotic pressure may be partially corrected by rapid synthesis of new proteins. However, with persistent hypotension and ischemia, the vasoconstrictor response of precapillary resistance vessels becomes less pronounced because of tissue acidosis while resistance of *postcapillary* vessels (venules) increases. This creates a situation in which more fluid is lost from the vascular to the interstitial space. Thus, *venular resistance* and the reactivity of venules to the various vasoactive agents involved in shock become important. Venules may even be *relatively* more reactive than precapillary resistance vessels to catecholamines, which activate constrictor alpha receptors. This differential effect in favor of postcapillary vasoconstriction also further increases hydrostatic pressure and intravascular fluid loss. One might consider the administration of a venodilating drug in late stages of shock, in which failure of the microcirculation is a predominant factor.

Capillary Permeability and Oncotic Pressure. Colloidal osmotic pressure is a major determinant of intravascular volume. Albumin (molecular weight 69,000) is the main osmotically active protein in plasma. The balance between colloidal osmotic pressure and capillary hydrostatic pressure determines the balance between intravascular and extracellular fluid spaces. A significant degree of hypovolemia and hemoconcentration may take place either because of excessive capillary hydrostatic pressure from an increase in the ratio of post- to precapillary resistance or because of a reduction in plasma protein and consequently reduction of plasma oncotic pressure. Reduction of plasma protein occurs as a result of increased capillary permeability and loss of plasma protein from the intravascular to the extracellular space. The balance between oncotic and hydrostatic pressures is also an important determinant of the level of pulmonary edema and is critical in the management of the shock lung syndrome. Plasma oncotic pressure should be restored through careful selection of the type of fluid to be used in volume replacement. Fluids containing crystalloids may be undesirable, as these further decrease the oncotic pressure. Administration of blood or colloids may be more appropriate to reduce pulmonary edema if pulmonary venous (or wedge) pressure is low. If there is increased vascular permeability in the lung because of damage to pulmonary capillaries, only a fall in hydrostatic pressure reduces pulmonary interstitial fluid. Positive end-expiratory pressure or an increase in oncotic pressure does not help.

Shock resulting from increased vascular permeability, as in anaphylactic shock or snake venom poisoning, is characterized by a dramatic reduction of plasma volume. Hematocrit rises sharply and oncotic pressure drops. This increase in capillary permeability may be partly related to release of histamine, metabolites, or humoral factors that alter endothelial permeability.

Intravascular Hemagglutination and "Blood Sludging." Erythrocytes, leukocytes, and platelets undergo agglutination to a variable degree in association with the shock syndromes in thermal burn, sepsis, trauma, and perhaps even hemorrhage. These aggregates may cause obstruction of capillaries as well as arterioles. The precipitating events are numerous. They may include platelet aggregation by catecholamines; damage to endothelial lining of small blood vessels and capillaries with subsequent fibrin deposition and accumulation of microthrombi; hypoxia increasing the rigidity of red cells; oxygen free radicals generated by endothelial cells or neutrophils; and release of vasoactive peptides and anaphylatoxins as a result of complement activation. These may cause additional damage to endothelial cells and increase the tone of precapillary sphincters, leading to further reduction in tissue perfusion and cellular injury.

Disseminated intravascular coagulation is a syndrome often seen in shock, particularly from gram-negative septicemia. The syndrome causes renal cortical necrosis, generalized ischemic damage of multiple organs, consumption of coagulation factors, and bleeding, and may also contribute to the pathogenesis of shock lung.

Shock Lung. Pathologic studies of the lungs in patients dying from shock may reveal marked capillary dilatation, pulmonary edema, alveolar hemorrhages, massive pulmonary vascular congestion and hyaline membrane formation, atelectasis, superimposed bronchial pneumonia, and, if the patient survives for weeks or months after the initial injury, pulmonary fibrosis. Shock affects the lung by producing endothelial damage in the vast capillary bed or precapillary arterioles. Microaggregates of platelets, polymorphonuclear leukocytes, and red cells block capillaries, destroy capillary endothelial cells by releasing hydrolytic enzymes and/or superoxide radicals, and eventually cause the increased capillary permeability that is responsible for the pulmonary interstitial edema seen in shock. The trigger for aggregation of neutrophils in the lung is not clear. Complement is a likely candidate; C5a produced with the activation of complement may cause white cells to aggregate in the lung. One must also keep in mind the role of lymphatic drainage. Lymph flow is greatly increased in the very early stages of shock, and patients dying in hemorrhagic shock may have a widely distended pulmonary lymphatic system filled with proteinaceous material.

The decrease in pulmonary blood flow may also interfere with production of surfactant. Lack of surfactant reduces the patency of alveoli and perpetuates leakage of fluid across pulmonary arterioles. Pulmonary venular constriction in response to tissue hypoxia may also contribute to pulmonary capillary congestion. It is also possible that with cerebral ischemia and hypoxia, neurogenic influences on the lung may cause a differential increase in venular resistance and increase capillary hydrostatic pressure and permeability. During *Pseudomonas* infusions in animals, there may be a direct effect of the endotoxin on capillary permeability, although sometimes a delayed response suggests an immune reaction with release of serotonin, contributing to pulmonary edema. Regardless of its cause, the damage to pulmonary capillary endothelium in shock perpetuates both the resistance to blood flow and systemic hypoxia and accelerates cellular death.

CELLULAR AND BIOCHEMICAL FACTORS IN SHOCK

OXYGEN-HEMOGLOBIN (Hb) AFFINITY. Arterial blood with normal hemoglobin and oxygen saturation of 90 per cent at a P_{O_2} of 100 mm Hg carries close to 20 ml of oxygen per deciliter to the tissues. The mixed venous blood has an oxygen saturation of 75 per cent at a P_{O_2} of 40 mm Hg and contains 15 ml of oxygen per deciliter. The normal arteriovenous oxygen difference is 5 ml per deciliter. The extraction of oxygen from Hb by the tissues is not complete and depends to a large extent on the affinity of oxygen to Hb, i.e., the shape of the oxygen-Hb dissociation curve. Hydrogen ions (Bohr effect), carbon dioxide, and 2,3-diphosphoglyceric acid (2,3-DPG) cause greater dissociation of oxygen from Hb because of their preferential affinity for reduced hemoglobin. The concentration of 2,3-DPG in red cells results from a side reaction of glycolysis and increases during anemia, hypoxia, and acidosis. A drop in hemoglobin, hypoxia, and acidosis may thus be partly compensated for by a shift of the oxygen dissociation curve to the right, favoring greater delivery of oxygen to the tissues at the same P_{O_2}. This compensatory mechanism, in addition to the increase in cardiac output, provides for better oxygenation as extraction of oxygen from the oxygen reserve in venous blood increases. In certain tissues, however, such as the myocardium, extraction of oxygen at rest is already large, and any additional oxygen demand or a decrease in oxygen-Hb dissociation such as in alkalosis requires greater delivery of oxygen, i.e., higher coronary blood flow.

In shock, the pH, carbon dioxide, and 2,3-DPG levels are changing, and one cannot calculate oxygen extraction from values of P_{O_2} because the shape of the oxygen dissociation curve cannot be predicted accurately. It is preferable to measure oxygen content or saturation of venous and arterial blood; if saturation is lower than predicted from values of P_{O_2}, one can deduce that there is a shift of the dissociation curve to the right, and vice versa. Overzealous correction of acidosis with bicarbonate may, through the Bohr effect on Hb affinity for oxygen, actually reduce oxygen delivery to the tissues. Hypophosphatemia reported during hyperalimentation may decrease 2,3-DPG and oxygen delivery.

CELLULAR STRUCTURE AND FUNCTION IN SHOCK. Survival of aerobic cells depends on availability of substrates and oxygen to the mitochondria, which provide most of the high-energy phosphate needs of the cell and utilize most of the available oxygen in the process. During oxidative phosphorylation, 36 moles of adenosine triphosphate (ATP) are produced per mole of glucose, whereas in the anaerobic state, glycolysis provides only 2 ATP molecules during the breakdown of 1 glucose molecule. Synthesis of ATP from adenosine diphosphate (ADP) is associated with the most active state of respiration in mitochondria (state 3 respiration) and is determined by cell energy demands. In addition to oxidative phosphorylation and ATP synthesis, mitochondria bind and accumulate calcium. This function determines calcium availability for other intracellular organelles and thereby regulates biochemical processes of contractile events, as in cardiac or vascular muscle.

Two processes may lead to cellular death. One is a marked inhibition of the electron transport system caused by severe ischemia or anoxia or by administration of cyanide or actinomycin A. This process leads to depletion of ATP, and the electron microscopic appearance of cells undergoing that type of death does not show any calcium phosphate accumulation in the mitochondria, presumably because of inhibition of the energy-dependent calcium transport mechanism. The other type of cell death is initiated by an injury to the cell membrane caused by activation of complement, or by antigen-antibody reaction, or by administration of certain polyenes, such as amphotericin B, or certain bacterial or microbiologic products, such as phospholipases or antitoxin. This type of cellular membrane damage is generally characterized by the precipitation of calcium phosphate in mitochondria, presumably because active processes requiring ATP are preserved until late stages and calcium can be transported into mitochondria.

Several structural changes take place in cellular membranes in shock. The earliest manifestation consists of swelling of the cell associated with an increase in intracellular sodium and clumping of nuclear chromatin, followed by dilation of the endoplasmic reticulum. In this phase the cell membrane is unstable, and "blebs" may appear at the surface. The mitochondria will then begin to swell, and electron-dense clumps of flocculent material will appear within them. As the swelling of the mitochondria continues, Ca^{++} may or may not accumulate in them, depending on the type of cellular damage. The process of cell death becomes irreversible, lysosomes begin to disappear, and finally the cell is converted to a mass of debris, with large inclusions resembling myelin.

One can relate the sequence of structural changes in the cellular membranes to specific biochemical changes. Initially there is probably an increase in cellular permeability for sodium and water causing cellular swelling, followed by increased sodium-potassium ATPase activity in an attempt to drive sodium out of the cell. Increased membrane ATPase activity might eventually lead to depletion of ATP and cyclic adenosine monophosphate (AMP), the latter leading to alteration of cellular responses to insulin, glucagon, catecholamines, and other hormones. For example, the effect of insulin on glucose uptake in muscle of animals that have been subjected to hemorrhagic shock is reduced. The unresponsiveness to insulin in peripheral tissues may be one of the reasons for hyperglycemia following injury or in shock. There is also a decrease in ATP, particularly in liver in early shock and in most other organs in late shock. It is difficult to determine the critical level of ATP necessary for cellular function, but it is believed that as long as there is ADP and oxygen, and substrate is provided, ATP generation can be resumed within minutes if mitochondrial structure is preserved. The organs that are most seriously affected in shock include, in descending order, the liver, kidneys, muscle, and lung.

MITOCHONDRIAL FUNCTION. Hypoxia may reduce the rate of ATP synthesis by mitochondria, but it does not cause significant damage to mitochondrial membrane functions unless it is severe, sustained, or associated with ischemia, which also reduces the availability of other substrates. In fact, adaptation to hypoxia appears to take place such that when mitochondria are isolated from animal tissues after the animals have been exposed to brief periods of hypoxia (at a Po_2 of 30 to 40 mm Hg), their capacity to respire and synthesize ATP in vitro is enhanced. In contrast to hypoxia, hemorrhagic and endotoxin shock reduce calcium transport by mitochondrial membranes, particularly in organs that become ischemic; state 3 respiratory activity and ATP synthesis and mitochondrial ATPase activity are inhibited, and finally mitochondrial damage ensues. The mechanism by which ischemia and endotoxins induce mitochondrial damage is not known. Whether such mitochondrial changes are direct effects of deprivation of vital substrates or are secondary to release of lysosomal enzymes, changes in intracellular pH, or other changes in cellular ionic environment with accumulation of metabolites is not apparent.

Glucocorticoids may exert a protective effect on mitochondrial function in endotoxemia in rats. Very large doses of glucocorticoids completely protect the mitochondria when rats are given a lethal dose (LD) 60 of endotoxin. The protective effect is not apparent, however, when an LD 90 is given. One may summarize the mitochondrial effects by saying that hypoxia by itself triggers some adaptive mechanisms that tend to increase respiratory activity if oxygen and ADP become available. In contrast, ischemia and endotoxemia can induce significant mitochondrial damage that heralds cellular death.

THE LYSOSOMAL THEORY. Lysosomes are cytoplasmic granules that contain a variety of potent hydrolytic enzymes bound in a latent form. These enzymes are capable of hydrolyzing a wide variety of both natural and synthetic substances and can digest all intra- and extracellular macromolecules if they are released from their membranes. When released from the organelles, either inside or outside the cell, as a consequence of certain forms of cellular injury, they may contribute to the pathogenesis or the propagation and perpetuation of shock. They are most active at an acid pH, which would make them potentially more destructive in the setting of hypoxia and shock.

Numerous morphologic and biochemical observations implicate the lysosomal enzymes in the perpetuation of shock, but at this time the evidence for their primary involvement is not convincing. In organs such as liver, spleen, and intestine, the lysosomes enlarge and lose their granules during the early phases of shock. This is associated with a decrease in the total activity of lysosomal hydrolases in tissues and a corresponding increase in activity in the soluble fraction of the tissue homogenate. This indicates a loss of lysosomal membrane integrity in vivo. The lysosomes obtained from animals in shock demonstrate an enhanced release of enzymes in vitro. A reduction in lysosomal membrane integrity has also been observed in animals after administration of endotoxin. In several animal studies the levels of hydrolases found in blood, lymph, or serum seem to correlate with severity of shock.

The appearance of a *myocardial depressant factor* or factors (MDF) in shock, although still controversial, may be an indirect manifestation of the effect of lysosomal enzymes. In experimentally induced pancreatitis and in a variety of other shock states, plasma MDF activity closely parallels lysosomal hydrolases in the plasma. It has been suggested that pancreatic ischemia associated with shock results in the release of lysosomal and other enzymes within the pancreas. These enzymes act on an endogenous substrate to yield a peptide with low molecular weight and MDF activity, which is then released into the circulation. The resulting myocardial depression maintains the state of low cardiac output and sustains shock.

Another indication of the involvement of MDF has been the reproducibility of the shock syndrome with infusion of lysosomal hydrolases in animals. These animals demonstrate the hypotension, circulatory collapse, and pathologic changes in the tissues that are seen in other experimental forms of shock.

Other suggestive evidence of the involvement of MDF has been the responsiveness of certain animals in shock to large amounts of corticosteroids. In vitro, corticosteroids stabilize the lysosomal membranes and prevent their lysis. Treatment with steroids suppresses circulating serum levels of lysosomal hydrolases in a variety of shock states.

Endotoxemia is associated with increased levels of serum hydrolases, but in vitro the endotoxins do not increase the lysis of lysosomes. It has been suggested that endotoxins may cause the formation of a lysosomal releasing factor, LRF, through activation of the alternative as well as the classic complement pathways. Activation of complement in fresh human serum has been found to generate a factor (LRF) that stimulates human polymorphonuclear leukocytes to release their lysosomal enzymes. This factor has many of the properties of human C5a.

COMPLEMENT ACTIVATION IN SHOCK. The complement system consists of a series of discrete plasma proteins that are present as inactive precursors until they are activated by highly specific biochemical reactions (see Ch. 418). Activation of the complement system results in the cleavage of several low molecular weight vasoactive peptides from the complement molecules. These peptides in turn have a wide variety of significant biologic effects. For example, during the activation of C2, a cleavage product occurs that has kinin-like activity, which then can significantly influence capillary permeability. Two other activation peptides, C3a and C5a, release histamine from mast cells, have chemotactic activity, and constrict vascular smooth muscle. Another fragment, C3b, acts as an opsonin and facilitates phagocytosis. Polymorphonuclear leukocytes may be attracted chemotactically through activation of esterases on their surface and may release their lysosomal enzymes if the concentration of the complement reaction product C5a is large enough. Platelets may have an increase in their procoagulant activity, and endothelial cells may contract. In addition to the direct and indirect effects of the fragments of activated complement on cells, their aggregation as decamolecular complexes on the surface of the cell membranes causes cellular destruction. The expressions of all these effects are increased capillary permeability; increased leukocyte accumulation and infiltration; release of lysosomal enzymes; and activation of intravascular coagulation factors. Clinically, these result in such entities as glomerulitis, necrotizing vasculitis, the Shwartzman reaction, thrombocytopenia, and other manifestations of microcirculatory collapse and intravascular plugging seen in prolonged shock and in endotoxemia.

Although the side effects of complement activation in shock are detrimental, leading to cellular death, the fundamental biologic activities of the complement components are beneficial in enhancing phagocytosis and mediating the inflammatory response to local infection or irritation, in the vital neutralizing of viruses, and, finally, in modulating the immune response.

OXYGEN FREE RADICALS. Oxygen free radicals generated during ischemic reperfusion of myocardium may contribute significantly to myocardial depression and injury. They include superoxide anion, hydrogen peroxide, and hydroxyl radicals, which are produced in vascular endothelium and neutrophils by the degradation of membrane phospholipids and the subsequent metabolism of arachidonic acid or by the conversion of xanthine dehydrogenase to xanthine oxidase and subsequent oxidation of hypoxanthine.

The unpaired electron in these radicals may react with any cellular component, but particularly with unsaturated fatty acids and sulfhydryl amino acids, and cause cellular damage. The scavengers of oxygen radicals, such as superoxide dismutase and catalase, and the competitive antagonist of xanthine oxidase, allopurinol, have proved protective against myocardial injury in different animal models. The clinical documentation of the relative importance of these factors and the effectiveness of their elimination awaits further experimentation in humans.

TREATMENT OF SHOCK

GENERAL PRINCIPLES. There are five main goals in the management of the patient in shock: (1) rapid recognition of the shock state, (2) correction of the initiating insult (e.g., pericardiocentesis, defibrillation, hemostasis, antibiotics), (3) correction of the secondary consequences of the shock state (e.g., hypovolemia, acidosis, hypoxemia, disseminated intravascular coagulation), (4) maintenance of the function of vital organs (e.g., cardiac output, arterial pressure, urinary output), and (5) identification and correction of aggravating factors. All five goals are approached simultaneously. The prognosis of a patient in shock is determined in part by the etiology of the shock state (e.g., hypovolemic traumatic shock in a young, healthy adult carries a mortality of less than 20 per cent in many centers, while cardiogenic shock due to massive anterior infarct carries a mortality of more than 70 per cent even in the most aggressive medical center). Prognosis is also affected by the duration of shock and consequent secondary organ dysfunction and by the speed of recognition and appropriateness of medical intervention.

A key element in the therapy of a patient in shock is hemodynamic monitoring.

PATIENT MONITORING. Management of the patient in shock requires accurate and serial measurements of heart rate and rhythm, respiratory rate and adequacy of gas exchange, systemic blood pressure and cardiac filling pressures, cardiac output and tissue perfusion indices, and end-organ function (mental status, urine output, liver function, etc.).

1. *The electrocardiogram* permits serial assessment of cardiac rate and rhythm and promptly detects serious arrhythmias such as premature ventricular beats, ventricular tachycardia or fibrillation, third-degree heart block, serious sinus bradycardia, and atrial arrhythmias. In addition, serial 12-lead ECG's may allow an indirect assessment of the severity of myocardial ischemia.

2. *Arterial blood gases and pH.* These should also be monitored routinely. Correction of acidosis and hypoxia is essential in management of early phases of shock.

3. *Central venous and Swan-Ganz catheters.* The monitoring of central venous pressure provides an index of the status of absolute and relative blood volume and of the need for fluid replacement. The catheter should be inserted through the antecubital or external jugular vein; only if the physician is experienced should it be introduced through the subclavian or internal jugular vein. Central venous pressure obtained with the catheter advanced to the superior vena cava is normally between 5 and 8 mm Hg, but it should be elevated to 10 mm Hg if one is to expect an adequate cardiac output in patients in shock. Central venous pressure reflects the filling pressure of the right ventricle and hence is an adequate indicator of cardiac filling pressure *only* in patients who have no underlying cardiac or pulmonary disease and are not on a mechanical ventilator. The central venous pressure is probably adequate only for the initial management of young adults suffering from traumatic hypovolemic shock. In the patient with known or suspected cardiac or pulmonary disease, or in whom management includes the use of positive pressure ventilation, state of the art management requires the use of a Swan-Ganz catheter to measure pulmonary capillary wedge pressure as an indicator of left ventricular filling pressure. In addition, the Swan-Ganz catheter allows serial assessment of cardiac output and provides a route for oximetric studies.

The filling pressure of the left ventricle can be estimated from measurement of the "pulmonary capillary wedge" pressure with a Swan-Ganz balloon-tip catheter. A triple-lumen thermodilution catheter is introduced intravenously with or without fluoroscopy but with electrocardiographic monitoring. Its tip is advanced to the pulmonary artery; the balloon is inflated with air, and it can be floated to a wedge position in one of the pulmonary arteries. The recorded pressure downstream from the inflated balloon is the "pulmonary capillary wedge" pressure, and the appearance of the left atrial pressure wave form on the oscilloscope confirms the position of the catheter tip. The wedge pressure reflects left ventricular end-diastolic pressure, but a discrepancy between the two may occur if there is severe mitral stenosis or left atrial tumors. If for some reason one is unable to get the wedge pressure, the pulmonary artery diastolic pressure may be a useful index of the wedge pressure.

The Swan-Ganz catheter has been modified to include an extra lumen that allows measurement of right atrial pressure simultaneously with the wedge pressure. Another modification includes a temperature sensor device at the tip that allows detection of changes in temperature following injection of cold dextrose in the right atrium, and the temperature dilution curve obtained with the temperature sensor provides an estimate of cardiac output. Further modifications of the Swan-Ganz catheter allow the continuous monitoring of intracardiac electrocardiogram and of oxygen saturation in blood and introduction of a pacing wire through a right ventricular port.

The Swan-Ganz catheter is expensive, and complications such as arrhythmias, sepsis, or pulmonary infarction may accompany its use. Nevertheless, it is a very important tool for monitoring patients in shock and for providing important data for judicious administration of fluids and sympathomimetic amines. The catheter should probably be removed within 72 hours after its insertion to avoid sepsis or pulmonary infarction and should not be left continuously in the "wedged" position. The normal wedge pressure is 12 mm Hg, but it often needs to be raised to 15 or 20 mm Hg in shock in order to maintain adequate organ perfusion unless there is pulmonary edema.

A discrepancy between right atrial and left atrial pressures may occur in patients with acute myocardial infarction, sepsis, or trauma when a high left atrial or pulmonary capillary wedge pressure may be accompanied by a low right atrial pressure, and under those circumstances monitoring right atrial pressure alone may lead to excessive administration of fluids. Conversely, patients with pulmonary disease, pulmonary embolism, pulmonary hypertension, and right ventricular infarction have relatively high levels of right atrial pressure compared with the pulmonary capillary wedge pressure, and avoidance of fluids under those circumstances may deprive the patient of important therapy. In addition to providing information on pressure, the triple-lumen Swan-Ganz catheter provides proximal and distal ports for sampling of right atrial and pulmonary arterial blood for oximetry to rule out a left-to-right intracardiac shunt. The sampling of "mixed venous" (pulmonary arterial) and systemic arterial blood to measure the oxygen content allows the estimation of cardiac output, since output equals oxygen consumption divided by arteriovenous oxygen difference. The use of a thermodilution catheter permits serial direct measurements of cardiac output by the thermodilution technique. At least three consecutive samples of thermodilution curves with less than 10 per cent variance should be averaged.

4. *Urinary catheter.* This allows the routine hourly measurement of urinary output. A decline in urinary output to less than 20 ml per hour is an indication of inadequacy of arterial pressure and renal perfusion. It is a sensitive index of progress of the shock syndrome and reflects the effectiveness of management. The most frequent cause of oliguria in shock is hypovolemia. Fluid deficits are often underestimated, particularly in the presence of sepsis. If oliguria persists despite adequate administration of fluid and elevated wedge pressure, diuretic therapy may be necessary to avoid acute renal tubular necrosis, which complicates prolonged hypotension.

5. *Arterial catheterization for arterial pressure monitoring.* Patients with severe or persistent hypotension and shock in whom it is difficult to measure blood pressure with the sphygmomanometer are candidates for intra-arterial pressure monitoring. There is often a discrepancy between intra-arterial pressure measurements and cuff pressure. There may be a low or even no recordable arterial pressure by the cuff technique when intra-arterial pressure by cannulation is normal or even at times slightly elevated. This discrepancy may result from severe peripheral vasoconstriction and low output and pulse pressure. Since the sphygmomanometric measurement of arterial pressure in shock may be erroneously low, it is advisable to palpate the femoral artery in the groin to get a better index of the strength of the pulse pressure and to introduce an arterial cannula for monitoring arterial pressure before administering vasopressors or resorting to counterpulsation. An arterial cannula also allows the frequent determination of blood gases and pH. The radial, brachial, or femoral arteries may be cannulated. The radial artery is the preferred site for cannulation with the lowest complication rate. Brachial or femoral arterial cannulation is preferred in patients who are severely hypotensive, who are on large doses of vasoactive drugs, who are markedly vasoconstricted, and in whom the radial artery is difficult to palpate.

6. *Cardiac output.* Measurement of cardiac output by thermal or dye dilution techniques is used for management of selected patients or for evaluation of new therapeutic regimens. The mixed venous blood oxygen content may be used as an index of total body perfusion. Within certain limitations, one can estimate the effectiveness of total body perfusion and delivery of oxygen to tissues by monitoring oxygen content of mixed venous or pulmonary arterial blood. The assumptions are that total body oxygen consumption is constant or does not change drastically and that arterial oxygen content is high and does not vary significantly. An arteriovenous oxygen difference of 6 ml per deciliter or more indicates poor tissue perfusion.

MANAGEMENT. *General Measures.* Management consists of primary therapy, directed at the underlying insult, and secondary therapy, directed at consequences of the shock state. Patients in shock may be in pain and frightened. They should be reassured and put in a horizontal position with legs slightly elevated, unless this position is uncomfortable or causes shortness of breath. In that case, they should be allowed to be in the most comfortable position. Pain should be relieved with morphine sulfate intravenously, preferably in small repeated doses of 2 to 5 mg; if side effects occur, such as hypotension, cold clammy skin, bradycardia, nausea, and vomiting, atropine may provide some relief. Another analgesic, meperidine, 50 to 100 mg, may be given intravenously. Intravenous fluid and monitoring of various functions should begin promptly to guide further therapy. Oxygen, norepinephrine, or dopamine may be initiated while the cause of shock is determined. Reversible factors that decrease cardiac output and cause hypotension should be corrected promptly (i.e., tension pneumothorax, marked acidosis or alkalosis, cardiac tamponade).

CORRECTION OF HYPOVOLEMIA. Hypovolemia may occur in any type of shock whether or not it is associated with external signs of blood or fluid loss. If there is no evidence of actual fluid or blood loss, there may be a significant shift of fluid from the intravascular to extracellular space because of increased capillary permeability and endothelial damage. This may occur in any vascular bed, but more specifically in the splanchnic and the pulmonary vasculature. In any shock syndrome associated with decreased tissue perfusion, fluid may also shift intracellularly because of changes in cellular membrane permeability and increased intracellular sodium and water. Fluid replacement is essential for restoration of cardiac output. Without an adequate filling pressure, there will not be an adequate cardiac output. The administration of potent cardiotonic drugs in the presence of hypovolemia and low cardiac filling pressure may be ineffective and may potentially aggravate the clinical condition rather than improve it. On the other hand, these drugs increase cardiac output significantly if left ventricular end-diastolic pressure and volume are adequate.

If the patient has cardiogenic shock or if there are signs of pulmonary congestion or edema, one should insert a Swan-Ganz balloon catheter into the pulmonary artery or pulmonary arterial wedge position for measurements of pulmonary artery diastolic pressure or pulmonary capillary wedge pressure. If pulmonary artery diastolic or pulmonary artery wedge pressure is less than 15 mm Hg, one should give 100 ml of Ringer's lactate, saline, or dextran every 10 to 15 minutes. If perfusion improves and wedge pressure remains less than 15 mm Hg, one should continue infusion at the same rate, trying to achieve a pressure between 15 and 20 mm Hg. If perfusion of tissues is unchanged or worse, if wedge pressure increases above 20 mm Hg, or if there are signs of pulmonary congestion, one should stop volume expansion. Improvement in tissue perfusion is evaluated by examining the degree of cyanosis, clamminess of the skin, level of arterial blood pressure, and urinary output, as well as the sensorium and alertness of the patient, blood gases, and pH.

If a Swan-Ganz catheter is not available or if pulmonary artery diastolic pressure or wedge pressure cannot be obtained, insertion of a central venous catheter is a helpful guide for administration of fluids. If central venous pressure is less than 10 mm Hg, one should expand volume until arterial pressure and tissue perfusion return to satisfactory levels, central venous pressure is between 10 and 15 mm Hg, or pulmonary congestion develops. Central venous or pulmonary capillary wedge pressures should be measured with careful reference to a constant point marked on the chest at the level of the right atrium or the phlebostatic axis. Patients who are on respirators or are receiving positive pressure assistance or positive pressure ventilation will have an abnormally elevated pressure. Under those circumstances, the filling pressure should be recorded at the time the respirator is transiently disconnected.

Treatment for hemorrhagic hypotension is with blood replacement, but while waiting for typing and cross-matching, the patient should be given saline or Ringer's lactate. The effects of these fluids are transient, because the crystalloids will rapidly leave the intravascular space. A more effective treatment might include colloids that stay longer in the circulation and increase oncotic pressure. This is particularly important when patients have manifestations of the shock lung syndrome, when extensive endothelial damage and interstitial edema are suspected, or when patients are chronically ill or malnourished and have hypoalbuminemia. Under those circumstances, dextran or mannitol, albumin, or plasma would expand blood volume. The excretion of dextran or mannitol by the kidney will increase oncotic pressure in Bowman's capsule and create a favorable hydrostatic-oncotic pressure gradient across the glomerulus, facilitating filtration even at low arterial pressure. If arterial pressure is not rapidly restored or oliguria persists despite administration of diuretics such as furosemide in conjunction with fluid replacement, then there might be danger of overexpansion of plasma volume and accentuation of pulmonary edema.

Development of pulmonary edema is closely correlated with the gradient between plasma oncotic and pulmonary artery wedge pressure, which reflects the capillary hydrostatic pressure in the lung. Plasma oncotic pressure of normal adults is approximately 25 mm Hg whereas pulmonary wedge pressure is 10 to 12 mm Hg. Capillary filtration takes place normally in the lung despite a low hydrostatic and a relatively high oncotic pressure, because of the equally high interstitial oncotic pressure in the lung. Plasma oncotic pressure may fluctuate. After 12 hours of bed rest, for example, it declines markedly. If oncotic pressure remains significantly higher (>8 mm Hg) than pulmonary capillary hydrostatic pressure, the risk of pulmonary edema is negligible; but if oncotic pressure is only 1 to 3 mm Hg higher than pulmonary wedge pressure, the patient is at high risk for pulmonary edema.

Types of Fluid. Isotonic saline solution contains 140 mEq of sodium and 140 mEq of chloride, whereas Ringer's lactate solution has 130 mEq of sodium, 4 mEq of potassium, 108 mEq of chloride, and 28 mEq of lactate. Lactate and acetate are converted to bicarbonate and maintain the alkalinity of the blood. When large volumes of fluid are administered, isotonic saline causes a dilution acidosis, which can be avoided if Ringer's lactate is used.

Human serum albumin comes in two concentrations, 5 grams per deciliter, which is the usual dose used, or 25 grams per deciliter salt-poor albumin. The 25 grams per deciliter solution is necessary only in the presence of severe hypoalbuminemia. An alternative is purified plasma protein, which is free of hepatitis virus contamination but has some contamination with vasoactive substances such as prekallikrein activator, causing the Food and Drug Administration to express concern about its use. Both albumin and purified plasma protein are expensive. They cost between $70 and $300 per 500 ml and represent a significant strain on blood donor programs. They should not be used indiscriminately.

There are two types of dextran: dextran 40 with 40,000 molecular weight and dextran 70 with approximately 70,000 molecular weight. Dextran 70 comes in a 6 per cent solution, and dextran 40 comes in a 10 per cent solution. Dextran 70 maintains vascular volume for up to 24 hours. While dextran 40 volume expansion lasts only a few hours owing to rapid

renal clearance, the effective volume expansion is nearly twice as great as that of an equal volume of infused 5 per cent albumin or dextran 70. Dextran solutions cost one third to one half as much as albumin. If given in amounts exceeding 1 liter, they may cause serious side effects, including platelet dysfunction and abnormalities in bleeding and coagulation, the nature of which are not clearly defined, and occasional anaphylactoid reactions. Approximately 5 per cent of patients receiving dextran have had such reactions, but very few of these are fatal. It should probably be avoided in patients with hypofibrinogenemia and bleeding dyscrasias.

With dextran 40 there is an incidence of acute renal failure, presumably because the rapid filtration of the low molecular weight dextran into the urine is accompanied by maximal reabsorption of the filtered salt and water, leading to a high intratubular concentration with an increase in intratubular viscosity and possibly physical occlusion of the renal tubule by dextran precipitates. This does not seem to occur with dextran 70 because it is filtered at a much slower rate owing to its molecular size.

Another colloid is hydroxyethyl starch or hetastarch, which maintains volume expansion almost twice as long as dextran 40 and has fewer side effects. It interferes minimally with coagulation, it has a very mild anaphylactoid effect, and its cost is one third that of albumin. New synthetic oxygen-carrying compounds are currently under investigation for use in the setting of acute hemorrhagic shock.

CORRECTION OF HYPOXIA. Oxygenation of the patient and interpretation of serial blood gases require the use of high-flow oxygen delivery systems, where the delivery system supplies the entire inspired gas mixture. The currently used high-flow systems include intubation with mechanical ventilation or T-tube devices, or tight-fitting face masks making use of the Venturi principle. These systems deliver a fixed inspired oxygen concentration ($F_{I_{O_2}}$), allow careful titration of oxygen as a drug, and permit the calculation of alveolar-arterial oxygen gradients that require a constant $F_{I_{O_2}}$. Low-flow systems (such as nasal prongs or simple face masks) do *not* deliver the entire inspired gas mixture, and hence the $F_{I_{O_2}}$ varies with the rate and depth of ventilation. While more comfortable, these low-flow systems are much less accurate.

Adequacy of the airway should be assessed in any patient in shock. If the patient is obtunded and cannot protect his or her airway, intubation with a cuffed endotracheal tube is essential. Occasionally the use of positive pressure respirators to improve gas exchange is necessary. Positive pressure ventilation may simultaneously decrease the venous return by increasing intrathoracic pressure and thereby perpetuate and aggravate a low-output state. Also, 100 per cent oxygen by mask may lead to toxic changes in the lung if continued more than a few hours. Thus when a respirator is required, the preferred approach is to select an $F_{I_{O_2}}$ of 50 per cent and to increase the $F_{I_{O_2}}$ and employ positive pressure only if needed to achieve a P_{O_2} of about 70 mm Hg.

CORRECTION OF ACIDOSIS. If arterial blood pH is less than 7.3 and respiratory acidosis has been ruled out, it is advisable to give 1 ampule of sodium bicarbonate intravenously (50 mEq per 50 ml). If the arterial blood pH is less than 7.2, 2 ampules may be administered and values repeated for further therapy in 15 to 30 minutes. Overcorrection of acidosis to alkalosis may decrease oxygen delivery to tissues by shifting the oxyhemoglobin dissociation curve to the left. Serial assessment of arterial blood gases permits careful titration of $NaHCO_3$. There is a risk of pulmonary edema with large volumes of $NaHCO_3$.

TREATMENT OF ARRHYTHMIAS. Arrhythmias, particularly after myocardial infarction, may limit cardiac output and perpetuate shock.

Sustained ventricular tachycardia may be treated first with intravenous lidocaine in a bolus of 1.5 to 2.0 mg per kilogram; if there is associated hypotension or any evidence of hemodynamic deterioration, synchronized electrical countershock should be used immediately. Ventricular fibrillation should be treated immediately with countershock. If the first or second shock is unsuccessful, the patient must receive closed chest massage, mouth-to-mouth respiration, and possibly intravenous sodium bicarbonate before again attempting electrocardioversion. In patients who fail to respond to adequate doses of lidocaine and have recurrent refractory ventricular fibrillation or tachycardia, bretylium tosylate in a bolus dose of 5 mg per kilogram of body weight is the next preferred agent.

Accelerated idioventricular rhythm is seen frequently in patients with myocardial infarction, particularly in those with diaphragmatic infarction. The rate is slightly faster than sinus rhythm, and a period of sinus bradycardia seems to favor the development of this arrhythmia. This is usually a benign rhythm and does not require therapy unless it degenerates into rapid ventricular tachycardia.

Supraventricular arrhythmias (atrial tachycardias, flutter, fibrillation, or junctional rhythms) should generally be treated pharmacologically with calcium channel blockers (e.g., verapamil), beta blockers (e.g., propranolol), or digitalis glycosides. But if the rhythm persists or there is an associated hypotension or hemodynamic deterioration, synchronized countershock therapy should be utilized. Sinus bradycardia, if severe (less than 40 beats per minute), can contribute to hypotension. It is commonly associated with inferior infarction, and, if accompanied by frequent premature ventricular beats, restoration of a more rapid sinus rhythm can eliminate them. Atropine is most effective intravenously in incremental doses of 0.4 mg to 2 or 3 mg. If bradycardia persists and hypotension or other signs of hypoperfusion are evident, electrical pacing should be instituted.

Conduction disturbances such as atrioventricular block carry a variable prognosis. The conduction disturbance that occurs with inferior infarction has a better prognosis than that associated with anterior infarction. It generally occurs early, is associated with sinus bradycardia, and may be caused by a temporary reflex increase in vagal tone to the conduction system or by atrioventricular nodal ischemia with only localized necrosis of this discrete structure. In anterior wall infarction heart block is related to ischemic damage of the three fascicles of the conduction system, which results from a more extensive degree of necrosis and is associated with higher mortality. Patients with inferior infarction benefit from temporary electrical pacing if they do not respond to atropine, whereas those with anteroseptal infarction generally require a permanent pacemaker, and the correction of the electrical disturbance may not alter their prognosis.

Treatment of Sepsis. Both gram-negative and gram-positive organisms have been associated with septic shock (see Ch. 259). In gram-negative septicemia, *E. coli* is the predominant organism, and infections with *Klebsiella-Aerobacter* (enterobacter) groups are not uncommon; endotoxin is an important factor in the pathogenesis of this syndrome. Gram-positive infections without endotoxemia, such as in pneumococcal pneumonia, *Staphylococcus aureus* infections, or streptococcal bacteremia, may cause shock. Chronic alcoholism is a common associated illness among these patients. The toxic shock syndrome, a complication of *S. aureus* infection most commonly associated with tampon usage in women, is discussed in Ch. 271.

The characteristic hemodynamic abnormality in septic shock (whether gram-positive or gram-negative) is a marked decrease in peripheral vascular resistance; cardiac output may be increased, normal, or decreased. In contrast, in cardiogenic shock cardiac output is low and peripheral resistance is normal, increased, or occasionally decreased, and in hypovolemic shock cardiac output is low and peripheral resistance is increased. The treatment of septic shock includes the aggressive treatment of the infection with antibiotics and drainage of any abscesses. Although cardiac output may be normal or high, it may be insufficient to meet metabolic needs of the tissues. An absolute or relative decrease in intravascular volume requires fluid administration. Crystalloids or colloids are given to restore and raise central venous pressure to levels of 10 to 15 mm Hg or pulmonary wedge pressure to 20 mm Hg. In these patients who have marked peripheral vasodilation in the face of arterial hypotension, a potent peripheral vasoconstricting agent such as norepinephrine may be the agent of choice if correction of intravascular volume fails to provide adequate arterial blood pressure.

Use of Steroids. The use of steroids in shock remains controversial. If used, they are given early and in large doses. Their potential beneficial effect appears to be related primarily to their action on cellular membranes. Steroids interact with biomembranes and probably become incorporated within their bilayer structures. A stabilizing effect on biomembranes has been demonstrated in vitro in studies of lysosomes isolated from animals treated with these agents. These lysosomes acquire a resistance to lysis in vitro. Apparently this beneficial action of corticosteroids is not related to their glucocorticoid properties. For example, testosterone is another potent membrane-stabilizing agent. The reason for the continued question concerning the effectiveness of corticosteroids is that the consequences of membrane stabilization by corticosteroids in vivo are not really known. Experimental studies in animals subjected to septic, endotoxin, or hemorrhagic shock indicate improved survival with administration of corticosteroids. In shock, considerable damage to the microcirculation may be attributed to membrane interactions between platelets, polymorphonuclear leukocytes, and endothelium. Activation by the bacteria of the alternative complement pathway with the release of various peptides may favor platelet aggregation with endothelium and leukocytes, clot formation, and obstruction of the microcirculation. Corticosteroids may prevent these membrane interactions in vivo. Steroids may also prevent the pituitary release of β-endorphins, which may cause myocardial depression. Animals pretreated with cortisone or naloxone (β-endorphin antagonist) exhibit an impressive resistance to endotoxin-mediated shock. Use of corticosteroids in doses of 30 mg per kilogram of methylprednisolone as early as possible in patients with septicemia and hypotension may be justifiable (but see also Ch. 30). The extension of the use of corticosteroids to patients with cardiogenic shock is unwise. There is evidence that malignant arrhythmias develop after the administration of corticosteroids to such patients, and the incidence of ventricular aneurysms may be increased.

It is claimed that corticosteroids have significant cardiovascular effects with possible alpha receptor blocking activities, but pharmacologic studies indicate that the steroids have little, if any, significant direct cardiovascular action; they may augment the action of catecholamines, but they do not block alpha receptors.

Sympathomimetic Amines. These drugs are used to increase cardiac output through their cardiotonic effect and to redistribute blood flow to vital organs by their selective vasoconstricting action; by virtue of these two effects, they raise arterial pressure and allow perfusion of ischemic regions, particularly in the myocardium, through collateral vessels. There are two potential problems with their use. If arterial pressure is elevated significantly, the hypertension may be detrimental, as it increases myocardial work and oxygen demand. Thus judicious elevation of arterial pressure to levels between 110 and 120 mm Hg systolic pressure would be reasonable. One cannot predict the optimal arterial pressure necessary to perfuse the coronaries in any particular patient because one does not know the severity of coronary disease and its extent, or the extent of myocardial reserve that would allow the heart to cope with a slight increase in afterload induced by the rising arterial pressure. Nevertheless, hypotension, particularly following myocardial infarction, should be corrected and arterial pressure maintained. The second potential problem with these drugs is their vasoconstricting effect; however, some vasoconstriction can be beneficial if it occurs in nonvital organs and if it is associated with increased cardiac output. This combination of effects raises arterial pressure and improves perfusion of vital organs. Therefore the proper use of sympathomimetic amines in shock requires a thorough knowledge of their cardiovascular effects. Their action depends upon their affinity for various types of adrenergic receptors (see Ch. 31).

ADRENERGIC RECEPTORS. The adrenergic receptors may be classified as alpha or beta receptors with respect to their cardiovascular action. The alpha receptors are predominantly in blood vessels and mediate vasoconstriction. The beta receptors are present in the blood vessels as well as the myocardium. Activation of the beta-1 receptors in myocardium causes an increase in myocardial contractility and in heart rate, whereas activation of beta-2 receptors in blood vessels causes vasodilation. The same catecholamine may activate both alpha and beta receptors, depending on dose and the organ in which it is acting (Table 44–4). The sympathomimetic amines that are available clinically include norepinephrine, epinephrine, dopamine, isoproterenol, phenylephrine, and dobutamine. The relative actions and potencies of these agents are summarized in Tables 44–5 and 44–6.

NOREPINEPHRINE. Norepinephrine increases myocardial contractility by activating beta-1 receptors and thus may increase cardiac output. In blood vessels it activates primarily alpha, or vasoconstricting, receptors. The magnitude of its effect on alpha receptors varies from one organ to another. It is a very potent vasoconstrictor in skin, muscle, and splanchnic beds, whereas in the coronary vessels it activates the beta-2 receptors as well as the alpha receptors; and because there is a paucity of alpha receptors in the coronary vessels in contrast to other vascular beds, the drug causes vasodilatation of the coronaries.

It offers several distinct advantages in the treatment of shock. It increases cardiac output and redistributes blood flow away from the extremities and toward the heart and brain and increases arterial pressure, which in turn increases coronary flow to ischemic myocardium. It should be administered intravenously through an indwelling catheter to avoid the risk of extravasation, which results in necrosis of subcutaneous tissues. Two ampules of Levophed (4 mg base per ampule) may be dissolved in 500 ml glucose and water and an infusion started at a very low rate to determine the smallest dose necessary to maintain arterial pressure between 100 and 120 mm Hg, which should provide adequate perfusion to the heart, brain, and kidney (unless the patient was hypertensive or has extensive arteriosclerotic disease). A dose of 4 μg per minute may occasionally be adequate; however, many patients require up to 40 μg per minute; and in general if such doses are necessary to maintain pressure, prognosis is poor. The average dose is between 10 and 15 μg per minute. If hypoxia, hypovolemia, and acidosis have been corrected, the lack of response to norepinephrine is probably an indication of significant myocardial damage. Norepinephrine may be the preferred agent in the management of profound hypotensive septic shock.

TABLE 44–5. RELATIVE ADRENERGIC POTENCIES

Amine	Alpha (Vascular)	Beta-1 (Cardiac)	Beta-2 (Vascular)
Norephinephrine	+ + + +	+ + +	+
Epinephrine	+ + +	+ + + +	+ +
Dopamine	+ +	+ + + +	+ +
Isoproterenol	0	+ + + +	+ + + +
Phenylephrine	+ + + +	0	0
Dobutamine	+	+ + + +	+ +

DOPAMINE. This is a naturally occurring precursor of norepinephrine. Its cardiovascular effect depends on its dose and the type of receptor that it activates. When given in low doses, less than 3 μg per kilogram per minute, it has a vasodilator action in the renal, mesenteric, cerebral, and coronary vessels because of activation of dopaminergic (DA) receptors. DA-1 postsynaptic receptors mediate vasodilatation and DA-2 presynaptic receptors prevent the release of endogenous norepinephrine. In doses of 3 to 10 μg per kilogram per minute, it increases myocardial contractility and cardiac output through the activation of beta-1 receptors. In larger doses of more than 20 μg per kilogram per minute, it causes vasoconstriction through activation of alpha-adrenergic receptors of arteries and veins in most vascular beds. Thus this drug may redistribute blood flow away from the extremities and toward the kidney, gut, heart, and brain; however, it may be necessary to give large doses to maintain arterial pressure and coronary blood flow, particularly following myocardial infarction; these large doses tend to oppose the beneficial vasodilator effects in some vascular beds. Dopamine may cause nausea and vomiting and increased cardiac irritability in some patients.

EPINEPHRINE. Epinephrine activates myocardial beta-1 receptors and vasoconstrictor alpha receptors in most vessels except in skeletal muscle and coronary vessels, where it activates beta-2 receptors when administered in low doses. It increases cardiac output but redistributes flow away from the kidney and splanchnic circulations toward skeletal muscle. Given in a dose range from 2 to 30 μg per minute intravenously, its effect on the redistribution flow is not optimal, and its effect on arterial pressure is only modest because of its vasodilator effect in skeletal muscle.

ISOPROTERENOL. Isoproterenol is a synthetic sympathomimetic amine that activates primarily vascular beta-2 receptors, causing vasodilatation, and myocardial beta-1 receptors, increasing cardiac output. The magnitude of the vasodilator effect of isoproterenol varies in different vascular beds, depending on the density of beta-2 receptors and the affinity of the drug for them. The major vasodilator action of isoproterenol is in skeletal muscle beds.

This drug is not recommended in either cardiogenic or septic shock. In cardiogenic shock, isoproterenol significantly increases myocardial oxygen requirement, and, despite the increase in coronary flow, the ischemic region of the myocardium may be hypoperfused as indicated by increased lactate production. Its use should be limited to the treatment of atropine-resistant complete heart block in an attempt to maintain an idioventricular rhythm and hemodynamic stability until more definitive therapy with pacing can be carried out.

TABLE 44–4. ADRENERGIC RECEPTORS

Receptor Type	Site	Action
Beta-1	Mycocardium	↑ Atrial and ventricular contraction
	Sinoatrial node	↑ Heart rate
	Atrioventricular	↑ Atrioventricular conduction
Beta-2	Arterioles	Vasodilation
	Lung	Bronchial dilation
Alpha	Arterioles	Vasoconstriction
	Venules	
	Veins	

TABLE 44–6. RELATIVE INITIAL HEMODYNAMIC EFFECTS

Amine	Heart Rate	Arterial Pressure	Cardiac Output	Systemic Resistance
Norepinephrine	↑	↑ ↑	↑ →	↑ ↑
Epinephrine	↑	↑	↑	↑ →
Dopamine	↑	↑	↑	↑ →
Isoproterenol	↑	↓ →	↑	↓
Phenylephrine	→	↑	→ ↓	↑ ↑
Dobutamine	→	→	↑	→

Isoproterenol may prevent the recurrence of ventricular tachycardia associated with the long QT syndrome and presenting as "torsades de pointes." The usual dose of isoproterenol is 2 to 20 μg per minute.

DOBUTAMINE. Dobutamine is a synthetic sympathomimetic amine that has predominant beta-1 activity. In contrast to dopamine, dobutamine has much less alpha-vasoconstricting activity but equal positive inotropic effects. Thus, in equal inotropic doses, dobutamine tends to lower the pulmonary capillary wedge pressure while dopamine tends to increase it. Dobutamine is also reported to have a lower incidence of cardiac arrhythmias. In experimental models of canine infarction, the administration of dobutamine results in significantly smaller infarcts compared with dopamine, possibly owing to the intracardiac release of norepinephrine produced by dopamine. Thus, especially in the setting of acute myocardial infarction with low output but no significant hypotension, dobutamine may be a preferred agent over dopamine for improvement in the cardiac output.

One can summarize the use of sympathomimetic amines by saying that the goal is to attain an arterial pressure adequate to perfuse the kidney, the ischemic myocardial segment, and the brain without overloading the left ventricle. The drug used should redistribute blood flow toward the more vital organs and away from skin and muscle for the optimal utilization of the limited cardiac output in shock. Finally, the drug should also have an inotropic action, and drugs such as methoxamine and phenylephrine, which cause arterial vasoconstriction only by activating alpha receptors without stimulating the heart, should be avoided. With these goals in mind, norepinephrine, dopamine, and dobutamine should be chosen in the management of shock.

Vasodilator Therapy in Shock. The beneficial effects of vasodilator therapy are (1) to decrease myocardial oxygen demands by decreasing preload or cardiac filling pressure and cardiac size and decreasing afterload by decreasing arterial pressure and arterial impedance, and (2) to dilate microcirculatory vessels.

The effectiveness of vasodilators (nitroprusside, nitroglycerin, phentolamine, or hydralazine) is impressive in the acutely failing heart following myocardial infarction without shock and with an elevated left ventricular end-diastolic pressure or capillary wedge pressure over 20 to 25 mm Hg; but the presence of *hypotension* should be a contraindication to the use of this therapy alone. Under these circumstances one may have to use a vasodilator drug along with norepinephrine or dopamine.

REDUCTION IN PRELOAD. One can reduce oxygen demand of the myocardium by decreasing cardiac volume in patients who have a high filling pressure. Reduction in cardiac size decreases myocardial wall tension, which is a major determinant of myocardial oxygen requirements. It may be achieved by administration of diuretics or venodilator drugs, which reduce filling pressure by pooling blood in the peripheral veins. The goal of "venodilator therapy" is to decrease preload and cardiac size and not to decrease arterial blood pressure. This effect is desirable as long as cardiac filling pressure does not drop excessively, causing a drop in cardiac output. In some patients with severe pulmonary congestion and high cardiac filling pressure with systemic arterial hypotension, it may be necessary to combine vasodilator therapy with another drug that will cause selective arteriolar vasoconstriction in certain organs and will increase peripheral vascular resistance and raise and maintain arterial pressure, such as dopamine or norepinephrine.

REDUCTION IN AFTERLOAD. This is a beneficial effect of the vasodilators, because it will decrease the arterial impedance against which the left ventricle ejects its blood; thus cardiac output improves. This is desirable as long as it is not associated with a significant reduction in systemic arterial diastolic pressure, particularly in patients who are normotensive or

have borderline hypotension. The dose of vasodilator drug must be adjusted so that it will not cause a significant reduction in diastolic arterial pressure. Any drop in arterial pressure by more than 10 mm Hg should be avoided, and the diastolic pressure should certainly not be allowed to decrease below 65 mm Hg. Reduction in afterload is ideal in patients with chronic severe congestive failure with high filling pressure, pulmonary congestion, and low cardiac output, but without a significant reduction in arterial pressure. Patients with cardiomyopathy but without coronary artery disease may be the best candidates for this therapy.

Neither a vasodilator alone nor propranolol, which also reduces myocardial oxygen demand, has a place in the management of cardiogenic hypotension following myocardial infarction. The elimination of the cardiotonic effect of the normal sympathetic drive by propranolol may significantly impair cardiac output and precipitate failure. If the patient has continuing pain and *a normal or elevated blood pressure,* despite administration of narcotics, morphine or meperidine, and nitroglycerin, administration of propranolol might then be considered.

MICROCIRCULATORY VASOCONSTRICTION AND ALPHA RECEPTOR BLOCKERS. In some patients, despite prolonged administration of dopamine or norepinephrine, tissue perfusion is not improved. The reason may be that myocardial infarction or cellular damage is extensive. It is also possible that constriction of microcirculatory vessels may be preventing perfusion of exchange capillaries. The alpha receptor blocker phentolamine has a specific effect on vasoconstricting alpha receptors and does not block beta receptors in the myocardium. Thus the cardiotonic effect of sympathomimetic amines is not prevented, yet vasoconstricting effects at the microcirculatory level are antagonized. Phentolamine has a greater inhibitory effect on alpha receptors in venules and veins than in arterioles, and its dilator action may therefore be greater in veins than in arterioles. This effect calls for a note of caution, because rapid relaxation of large veins may abruptly lower cardiac filling pressure if the patient is hypovolemic. For this reason, it is essential to ascertain that the patient has received adequate amounts of fluid before giving phentolamine.

NITROPRUSSIDE. This is a very effective vasodilator drug that causes relaxation of veins to decrease preload and some relaxation of arterioles to decrease arterial impedance. It may be started intravenously at a dose of 16 μg per minute and increased to 200 μg per minute with constant monitoring of arterial and cardiac filling pressures. Occasionally larger doses have been necessary. Prolonged administration may lead to thiocyanate toxicity.

NITROGLYCERIN. This is also a very effective vasodilator with predominant effects on the venous system and lesser effects on arteriolar resistance vessels. When given as an intravenous infusion of 15 to 100 μg per minute, it reduces preload and is useful in congestive heart failure complicating acute myocardial infarction, particularly when the wedge pressure is high and the arterial pressure is normal. Intravenous nitroglycerin may also cause coronary vasodilatation and improve subendocardial flow.

In cardiogenic shock with arterial hypotension and an elevated pulmonary artery wedge pressure, the combination of intravenous nitroglycerin and dopamine may be appropriate.

Other vasodilator drugs, such as hydralazine, which primarily exert an action on the arterioles, would not be very effective in reducing cardiac size and myocardial oxygen demand, and may be detrimental in causing a significant reduction in arterial blood pressure.

DIGITALIS. It is advisable not to use digitalis in patients in cardiogenic shock due to acute myocardial infarction even if there is evidence of pulmonary congestion and an elevated pulmonary artery wedge pressure. In the setting of acute myocardial infarction it may increase myocardial irritability.

In addition, the renal excretion of digoxin may be impaired because of decreased renal perfusion and arterial blood pressure.

Mechanical Ventricular Assistance and Surgical Treatment in Cardiogenic Shock. Intra-aortic balloon counterpulsation may be beneficial in cardiogenic shock. The balloon is introduced into the aorta at the end of a catheter inserted through the femoral artery via surgical cutdown or percutaneously via the Seldinger technique. It is inflated during early diastole and is collapsed during systole. This sequence decreases afterload during ejection and increases coronary perfusion pressure and coronary flow during diastole. Improvement of the hemodynamic status has been observed, but because a large number of patients with myocardial infarction and shock have extensive coronary artery disease, the long-term survival is still disappointing. Balloon counterpulsation appears to be of greatest potential benefit in support of patients who have seriously compromised hemodynamics after myocardial infarction, are refractory to medical management, and are candidates for a surgical procedure. This mechanical assistance sustains the hemodynamics during cardiac catheterization and coronary arteriography in preparation for surgery. Emergency revascularization surgery or infarctectomy, which has been carried out in some centers, has not been uniformly encouraging. Two complications of myocardial infarction require surgical intervention and carry a reasonable prognosis; these are ruptured papillary muscle and interventricular septal perforation. In both, there is decreased ejection from the left ventricle and a fall in arterial pressure. Attempts to increase systemic arterial pressure with drugs exaggerate the regurgitation or the left-to-right shunt. In these circumstances, selective lowering of arterial systolic pressure with intra-aortic balloon counterpulsation is ideal, as it will facilitate ejection and reduce mitral regurgitation or left-to-right shunt. A significant reduction in afterload and vasodilatation may also be achieved with drugs such as nitroprusside or nitroglycerin, but the associated fall in diastolic pressure may extend the myocardial ischemia. Surgical management, as soon as it is feasible and safe, should be the course to pursue. Severe papillary muscle dysfunction or papillary muscle rupture (the posterior more frequently than the anterior) may cause significant left ventricular failure, and the surgical replacement of the mitral valve has been satisfactory, particularly in patients with good myocardial function. Patients with a perforation of the ventricular septum have congestive failure in association with the sudden appearance of a pansystolic murmur, often accompanied by a thrill. Clinically, it is often impossible to differentiate this condition from a ruptured papillary muscle. The demonstration of a left-to-right shunt by cardiac catheterization or radionuclide angiography confirms the diagnosis. Rupture of the septum should be treated surgically, preferably six to eight weeks after infarction, so that the margins of the defect can have sufficient scar tissue to permit surgical closure with relative ease.

Abboud FM, et al.: Reflex control of the peripheral circulation. Prog Cardiovasc Dis 18:371, 1976; and Abboud FM, Thames MD: Interaction of cardiovascular reflexes in circulatory control. In Shepherd J, Abboud F (eds.): Handbook of Physiology. Bethesda, Md., American Physiological Society, 1984, pp 675–753. *These are reviews of factors that regulate peripheral vascular resistance (neural, humoral, local, and metabolic). The characteristic behavior of different vascular beds and various vascular segments is described. The role of cardiac sensory receptors, arterial baroreceptors, and chemoreceptors in the reflex control of the circulation is also described. Circulatory adjustments to various stressful conditions, including hypotension, acute myocardial infarction, and hypoxia, in animals and in humans are discussed.*

Berne R: The coronary circulation. In The Handbook of Physiology, Section 2: The Cardiovascular System. Bethesda, Md., American Physiological Society, 1979, pp 873–952. *This is a thorough review of the factors that regulate coronary blood flow, with emphasis on the potential metabolic determinants and interplay between local metabolic control and neurogenic control.*

Chaudry IH: Cellular mechanisms in shock and ischemia and their correction. Am J Physiol (Regulatory Integrative Comparative Physiology 14) 245:R117, 1983. *This is a review that deals specifically with cellular and subcellular alterations in shock. The potential mechanisms responsible for mitochondrial abnormalities, for alterations in cellular nucleotide levels, for the reduction in transmembrane potential, and for the increase in sodium-potassium ATPase activity are discussed. The depression of the reticuloendothelial system phagocytic activity and the release of lysosomal enzymes are also mentioned. The therapeutic attempts to restore cellular integrity by providing specific substrates are reviewed briefly, with emphasis on the proven effectiveness of ATP MgCl₂ as an adjunct therapy in restoring cellular function and improving survival rates in experimental shock.*

Goldberg LI: Dopamine—clinical uses of an endogenous catecholamine. N Engl J Med 291:707, 1974; and Goldberg LI, Rajfer SI: Dopamine receptors: Applications in clinical cardiology. Circulation 72:245, 1985. *These are reviews of the cardiovascular and renal actions of dopamine, of its hemodynamic effects in humans, and of its effectiveness in the treatment of shock. The action of dopamine is contrasted with that of other sympathomimetic amines. A regimen for its use in shock and its adverse effects are described.*

Goldfarb RD, Glenn TM: Regulation of lysosomal membrane stabilization via cyclic nucleotides and prostaglandins—the effects of steroid and indomethacin, pp 147–166. *The authors review data that suggest a significant change in the integrity of myocardial lysosomes during myocardial ischemia and propose that intramyocardial lysosome stability can be positively correlated with myocardial cyclic AMP/cyclic guanosine monophosphate (GMP) ratio. Furthermore, intramyocardial cyclic AMP concentration was negatively correlated with prostaglandin A and E concentrations. In that study, indomethacin treatment decreased myocardial prostaglandin A and E concentration approximately 60 per cent following coronary arterial ligation. One might conclude that myocardial infarction induces synthesis and release of prostaglandins, which, in turn, induce alterations in intramyocardial cyclic nucleotide ratio such that release of lysosomal enzymes is promoted. In a section of the monograph entitled* Therapeutics of Shock and Trauma *(pp 199–322), several authors review different approaches considered at the experimental stage. These include the use of dibutyryl cyclic AMP; a comparison of methylprednisolone and hydrocortisone in the treatment of shock patients (double-blind study suggesting that methylprednisolone may have a more beneficial effect); the use of calcium channel blockers in the treatment of shock, particularly after myocardial infarction, which may have a direct cellular effect that could be beneficial independently of changes in perfusion; the use of the antiproteolytic enzyme aprotinin in endotoxin shock, which preserves the phagocytic function of the reticuloendothelial system (aprotinin antagonizes serine endopeptidases and thus prevents the conversion of prekallikrein to kallikrein and consequently the conversion of kininogen to kinin) and protects the integrity of the capillaries and prevents aggregation of leukocytes in endotoxin shock.*

Lefer AM, Schumer W (eds.): Molecular and Cellular Aspects of Shock and Trauma. New York, Alan R. Liss Inc, 1983. *This volume represents the proceedings of a USA-Japan Binational Conference on this topic held in June, 1982. New concepts in cellular and metabolic aspects of shock and their therapeutic implications were reviewed. Following are brief comments on some of the article.*

Lefer AM: Pharmacologic and surgical modulation of myocardial depressant factor (MDF) formation and action during shock, pp 111–123. *This is a review of the chemical properties and the formation as well as the pathophysiology of MDF. There are no specific antagonists to MDF, and the author reviews the means of prevention of its formation and some of the pharmacologic approaches to counteracting its action.*

The Cell in Shock. Proceedings of a Symposium on Recent Research Developments and Current Clinical Practice in Shock. The Upjohn Company, April, 1976. *Several important concepts are reviewed. For example:* Baue AE: Mitochondrial function in shock, pp 11–15. *This article reviews Dr. Baue's research on the cellular events that may take place during shock and ischemia. A sequence of cellular membrane damage, mitochondrial dysfunction, and lysosomal breakdown is discussed.* Trump BF: The role of cellular membrane systems in shock, pp 16–19. *This is a detailed analysis of the sequential structural changes that occurs in cells in shock correlated with biochemical changes.* Goldstein IM: Lysosomes and their relation to the cell in shock, pp 30–34. *The potential role of lysosomal enzymes in cellular destruction in endotoxin shock is reviewed. The mechanisms of lysosomal enzyme release from human leukocytes, microtubule assembly, and membrane fusion induced by a component of complement are reviewed. A lysosomal releasing factor, or LRF, sharing many of the components of human C5a, appears to stimulate human polymorphonuclear leukocytes to release lysosomal enzymes selectively.* Müller-Eberhard HJ: The significance of complement activity in shock, pp 35–38. *This is a brief review of the complement system, its activation, and its role in the release of vasoactive peptide, which may contribute to the syndrome of shock.*

The Organ in Shock. Proceedings of the Second Symposium on Recent Research Developments and Current Clinical Practice in Shock. The Upjohn Company, April, 1977. *The following are brief comments on some of the articles:* Mela LM: Oxygen's role in health and shock, pp 8–15. *Dr. Mela reviews the membrane alterations induced by ischemic cell injury that are characteristically different in each organ, reflecting the particular organ's most delicately balanced plasma membrane functions. The author emphasizes that hypoxia alone does not induce inhibition in mitochondrial activity, whereas ischemia does.* Ayres, SM: The shock lung, pp 24–31. *The role of lymphatics, capillary permeability, and arteriovenous shunts in the pathogenesis of the shock lung syndrome is reviewed, and the structural and functional changes in the lungs are discussed.* Mueller HS: The heart and oxygen transport, pp 38–49. *This is a review of the treatment of coronary shock in patients with acute myocardial infarction. A careful survey of the hemodynamic changes and of survival in response to various catecholamines, and intra-aortic balloon counterpulsation, is described. Emphasis is placed on the early recognition and aggressive management of patients with incipient ventricular failure to improve survival rate. Caution regarding the use of vasodilators in patients who have low systolic blood pressure is expressed, and potential use of intra-aortic balloon counterpulsation coupled with an aggressive work-up and surgical approach to severe cardiogenic shock unresponsive to medical management is discussed.*

Werns SW, Shea MJ, Lucchesi BR: Free radicals and myocardial injury: Pharmacologic implications. Circulation 74:1, 1986. *The authors review the growing evidence that oxygen free radicals generated during ischemia and reperfusion may contribute significantly to myocardial depression and injury. The mechanisms for generation of these oxygen free radicals and their removal by therapeutic interventions are discussed. The potential clinical implications are important in view of the more aggressive management of acute myocardial infarction with thrombolytic therapy and the frequently noted post-reperfusion myocardial depression and arrhythmias.*

Ziegler EJ, McCutchan JA, Fierer J, et al.: Treatment of gram-negative bacteremia and shock with human antiserum to a mutant *Escherichia coli.* N Engl J Med 307:1225, 1982. *This is a randomized controlled trial of human J5 antiserum in patients with gram-negative bacteremia and shock. The antiserum was prepared by vaccinating healthy men with heat-killed E. coli J5 mutant, which lacks lipopolysaccharide-oligosaccharide side chains so that the core (which is nearly identical to that of most other gram-negative bacteria) is exposed for antibody formation. The antiserum reduced death substantially.*

45 CARDIAC ARRHYTHMIAS

J. Thomas Bigger, Jr.

Optimal management of cardiac arrhythmias requires knowledge of their (1) mechanism, etiology, and natural history and (2) effect on the hemodynamic state. Before selecting therapy, the physician should thoroughly assess the patient's physical, psychologic, and biochemical state. The chosen treatment, whether drugs, devices, or surgery, must be monitored closely for its initial and continued effectiveness and for adverse effects. In this chapter we will discuss mechanisms, electrocardiographic (ECG) recognition, and management of cardiac arrhythmias.

ANATOMIC CONSIDERATIONS

Normal Specialized Impulse-Generating and Conducting System

SINUS NODE. The sinus node is situated on the right anterolateral margin of the junction between the superior vena cava and the right atrium. The node surrounds a large central artery arising from the right (55 per cent) or left circumflex coronary artery (45 per cent). Two types of special muscle fibers are found in the node: P (pacemaker) and T (transitional) cells. P cells are small (diameter of 5 to 10 microns) ovoid or stellate cells that have a low density of mitochondria, sarcoplasmic reticulum, and myofibrils, suggesting a lack of contractile function. P cells occur in tight clusters and attach only to other P cells or T cells; intercellular attachments are sparse, correlating with the slow conduction found in the sinus node.

T cells are intermediate in size, structure, and cellular organization between P cells and ordinary atrial myocardium. T cells may attach either to P cells or to working myocardial cells. Perinodal T cells surround the sinus node and presumably serve both to organize impulses leaving the node and to hinder access of premature ectopic atrial impulses.

INTERNODAL TRACTS. Three internodal tracts connecting the sinus node to the atrioventricular (AV) node have been described: anterior, middle, and posterior. The *anterior internodal tract* also connects to the left atrium via the interatrial bundle of Bachmann. The three internodal tracts are widely separated in the interatrial septum but converge above and behind the AV node.

Internodal tracts contain working atrial cells interspersed with large cells that resemble ventricular Purkinje cells. Because internodal pathways are difficult to trace by serial microscopic sections, some doubt their presence or functional significance. Internodal tracts continue to function in high extracellular K$^+$ concentrations, a property that has been used to demonstrate their functional continuity and preferential internodal conductivity.

ATRIOVENTRICULAR NODE. The AV node lies beneath the endocardium of the right atrium near the septal leaflet of the tricuspid valve and immediately anterior to the ostium of the coronary sinus. The AV node artery usually arises from the right coronary artery. In the central portion of the AV node, the myocytes form tangled swirls with ample interconnections. Ultrastructurally, cells in the mid AV node resemble the sinus node T cells. Toward the distal end of the AV node, myocytes palisade into linear arrays as they form the bundle of His.

The region between the ostium of the coronary sinus and the posterior margin of the AV node is richly supplied by cholinergic ganglia. Retronodal chemoreceptors may trigger vagal reflexes during ischemia of the posterior wall of the heart. These reflexes can produce marked bradycardia, peripheral vasodilatation, nausea, sweating, and salivation.

THE HIS-PURKINJE SYSTEM. The AV bundle (bundle of His) is a thick, cable-like structure, about 15 mm in length, that emerges from the anterior, inferior border of the AV node (Fig. 45–1). The bundle of His penetrates the central fibrous body and courses to the crest of the muscular interventricular septum, where it divides into left and right bundle branches. The His bundle is the only normal route for AV conduction. Damage to the AV bundle can cause AV conduction delay or block. The His bundle is generously supplied with arterial blood from the anterior and posterior descending coronary arteries; therefore, extensive coronary disease is required to produce ischemic damage.

The left bundle branch is a broad sheet of fibers that cascade under the noncoronary cusp of the aortic valve and down the left side of the interventricular septum. The left bundle branch connects first with myocardium in the septum and near the papillary muscles, causing early activation of these regions.

The right bundle branch emerges from the bundle of His and courses down the right side of the interventricular septum to make its first connections with ventricular myocardium near the base of the anterior papillary muscle. From here, the peripheral branches of the right bundle spread up the interventricular septum and the free wall of the right ventricle.

The terminal Purkinje fibers form extensive interconnected lacy networks on the endocardial surface of both ventricles. In human hearts, no cells of the Purkinje type can be identified in the outer two thirds of the ventricular walls. Purkinje cells are large—15 to 30 mm in diameter and 20 to 100 mm in length. The nucleus is round and centrally located in the cell, and Purkinje fibers contain fewer myofibrils and mitochondria than working ventricular muscle. External to the sarcolemmal basement membrane is a thick surface coat of negatively charged glycoproteins that function in Ca^{++} binding and exchange. Intercalated discs are well developed in Purkinje fibers and provide low-resistance pathways for current flow and for diffusion of K$^+$.

Function of the Specialized Impulse-Generating and Conducting System

The normal heart beat begins in the sinus node and spreads slowly through the perinodal fibers to reach specialized atrial tracts and ordinary atrial muscle (Fig. 45–1). The specialized atrial tracts transmit the cardiac impulse rapidly from the sinus node to the AV node and to the left atrium. The cardiac impulse slows dramatically in the AV node, accounting for most of the PR interval in the ECG. Conduction accelerates tremendously in the His bundle, and excitation of the bundle branches and peripheral Purkinje fibers occurs with blazing speed. The great mass of ordinary ventricular muscle is activated almost simultaneously over much of its endocardial surface. Then, activation spreads from endocardium to epicardium to complete cardiac excitation.

FIGURE 45–1. The anatomy and characteristic action potentials of the specialized impulse-generating and conducting system of the heart. *A*, A diagram of the conduction system of the heart. SAN = Sinoatrial node; AVN = atrioventricular node; HB = bundle of His; RBB = right bundle branch; LBB = left bundle branch; PF = Purkinje fiber. *B*, Typical action potentials from the sinus node (SN), atrium (AT), atrioventricular node (AVN), Purkinje fiber (PF), and ventricular muscle (VM). *C*, Relationship of deflections in the His bundle (HB) electrogram to depolarization of the sites shown in *B* and to the electrocardiographic deflections. Depolarization of the lower atrial septum (A), bundle of His (H), and ventricular septum (V) is recorded in the bipolar His bundle electrogram. The H deflection partitions the P-R interval into two subintervals: the A-H interval, representing atrioventricular nodal conduction, and the H-V interval, which measures conduction to the His-Purkinje system. (From Braunwald E.: Heart Disease: A Textbook of Cardiovascular Medicine. Philadelphia, W. B. Saunders Company, 1980.)

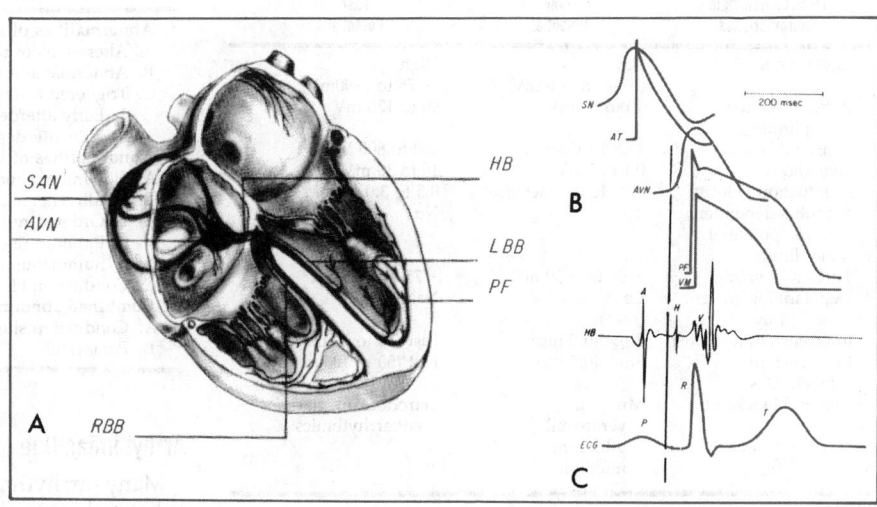

BRIEF REVIEW OF CARDIAC CELLULAR ELECTROPHYSIOLOGY

Resting Potentials

The sarcolemma of cardiac cells is a hydrophobic phospholipid bilayer. Protein molecules cross the entire width of the membrane, provide hydrophilic channels, and permit hydrated cations or anions to cross the sarcolemma. Ion-selective channels and energy-dependent ion pumping establish transmembrane gradients of Na^+ and K^+ that determine the resting voltage difference of about -80 to -90 mV across the sarcolemma, the *resting transmembrane voltage* (Vm).

Action Potentials

When cardiac cells activate, a complex sequence of voltage changes occurs as a function of time and membrane ionic currents. Figure 45–2 diagrams the four phases of a Purkinje

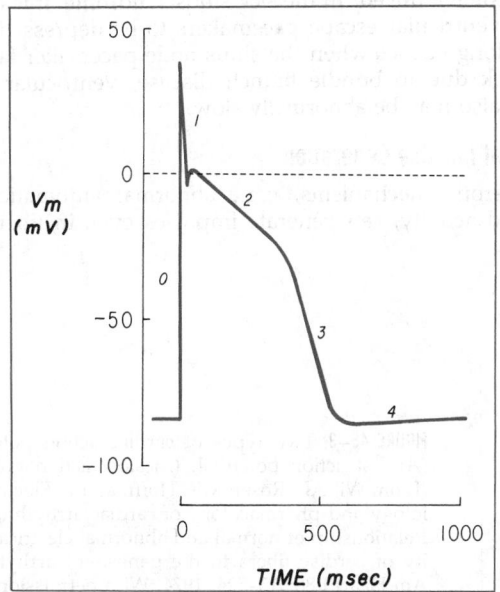

FIGURE 45–2. The cardiac action potential of a Purkinje fiber has five distinct phases: rapid depolarization (0), early repolarization (1), the plateau (2), rapid repolarization (3), and diastole (4). (From Braunwald E.: Heart Disease: A Textbook of Cardiovascular Medicine. Philadelphia, W. B. Saunders Company, 1980.)

fiber *action potential*. Sinus and AV nodal cells have a slowly rising phase 0 and lack distinct phases 1, 2, and 3 (Fig. 45–1). Many cells hold a steady level of transmembrane voltage during phase 4, whereas automatic fibers in the sinus node and His-Purkinje spontaneously depolarize during this period and can initiate impulses that propagate to the rest of the heart.

The ionic basis for cardiac action potentials is still a subject of debate and active study.

Overdrive Suppression

In the normal heart, P cells in the sinus node depolarize and overdrive subsidiary pacemaker cells in the atrial specialized tracts, coronary sinus region, or His-Purkinje system. The faster subsidiary pacemakers are overdriven, the more Na^+ enters the cell per unit of time. As the $[Na]_i$ increases, the activity of the Na^+/K^+ exchange pump becomes more electrogenic, i.e., the ratio of the Na^+ out to K^+ in will increase, hyperpolarizing the cell and counteracting pacemaker activity. If the dominant pacemaker stops, there will be a pause in rhythm. However, as the $[Na]_i$ is pumped out, outward pump current will decline until spontaneous depolarization resumes. As the pump current declines, firing rate in the subsidiary pacemaker will increase gradually, producing the well-known "warmup" behavior.

Fast and Slow Responses

Cardiac action potentials are classified as *fast* or *slow* responses (see Table 45–1). The *fast response* (Fig. 45–3) is generated by intense inward [Na]; has a large, fast-rising phase 0; propagates rapidly; and has a large safety factor for conduction. Working myocardial cells in the atria, ventricles, and Purkinje fibers have fast responses. The *slow response* has a slowly rising phase 0, propagates slowly, and has a low safety factor for conduction (Fig. 45–3). Cells in the sinus node, pectinate muscles, AV node, and AV rings have slow responses. Depolarization in slow-response fibers is due to slow inward current (i_{si}) carried by Ca^{++} and, to a lesser extent, Na^+ ions.

Refractoriness

The concept of refractoriness is used to explain the pathogenesis of many arrhythmias and the mechanism of action of antiarrhythmic drugs. The effective refractory period, the minimum interval between two propagating responses, is

TABLE 45–1. COMPARISON OF SLOW AND FAST ACTION POTENTIALS

Electrophysiologic Characteristics	Slow Potential	Fast Potential
Resting potential	Low (−40 to −70mV)	High (−75 to −90mV)
Action potential amplitude	40 to 80 mV	90 to 120 mV
Phase 0 $\dot{V}$ max	1 to 10 V/sec	200 to 800 V/sec
Overshoot	0 to 15 mV	10 to 30 mV
Conduction velocity	0.01 to 0.1 meter/sec	0.5 to 3.0 meter/sec
Stimulus-dependent action potential amplitude	Yes	No
Threshold voltage	−50 to −30 mV	−75 to −65 mV
Depolarizing current carried by	Ca^{++} (Na^+)	Na^+
Ionic current activates	Slow (0.5 msec)	Fast (10 to 20 msec)
Ionic current inactivates	Slow (0.5 msec)	Fast (50 to 100 msec)
Channel blocked by	Mn^{++}, La^{+++}, verapamil, diltiazem, nifedipine	Tetrodotoxin, class 1 antiarrhythmics

TABLE 45–2. MECHANISMS RESPONSIBLE FOR CARDIAC ARRHYTHMIAS

I. Abnormalities of impulse generation
  A. Alterations of normal automaticity
  B. Abnormal automaticity
  C. Triggered activity
    1. Early afterdepolarizations
    2. Late afterdepolarizations
II. Abnormalities of impulse conduction
  A. Slowing of conduction and block
  B. Unidirectional block and re-entry
    1. Ordered re-entry
    2. Random re-entry
    3. Summation and inhibition
  C. Conduction block, electrotonus, and reflection
III. Combined abnormalities of impulse generation and conduction
  A. Conduction showed by phase 4 depolarization
  B. Parasystole

closely linked to action potential duration in fast-response fibers because recovery from inactivation in the Na^+ channel closely parallels repolarization. However, in sinus and AV nodal cells (slow responses), refractoriness can outlast full repolarization so that the effective refractory period is much longer than the action potential duration.

Responsiveness and Conduction

The term *membrane responsiveness* describes the response of a cardiac fiber to a stimulus. Changes in the maximum rate of depolarization during phase 0 (Vmax) provide an index of changes in availability of the Na^+ current. In cardiac Purkinje fibers and other fast-response fibers, Vmax is strongly dependent on Vm at the instant of excitation; as soon as the fiber is fully repolarized, it is fully responsive. In slow-response fibers, responsiveness does not return until well after repolarization is complete. There is a considerable safety factor for conduction in fast-response fibers; Vmax must be reduced to less than one half of normal before conduction velocity decreases. The safety factor is much lower in slow-response fibers so that premature impulses are likely to experience substantial conduction delay or block.

MECHANISMS OF CARDIAC ARRHYTHMIAS

An arrhythmia is an abnormality of rate, regularity, or site of origin of the cardiac impulse or a disturbance in conduction that causes an abnormal sequence of activation. Arrhythmias may arise because of alterations in impulse generation, impulse conduction, or both (Table 45–2).

Arrhythmias Due to Abnormalities of Impulse Generation

Many arrhythmias arise because of either depressed or enhanced normal automaticity. Abnormal automaticity and triggered activity also are important mechanisms for arrhythmogenesis.

ALTERED NORMAL AUTOMATICITY. Only a few cardiac cell types develop normal automaticity: sinus node, internodal tracts, fibers near the ostium of the coronary sinus, distal AV node, and the His-Purkinje system.

Sinus Node. The rate of firing in the sinus node can be altered by autonomic activity or intrinsic disease. Increased vagal activity can slow or stop sinus node pacemakers by increasing membrane K^+ conductance of P cells. Increased sympathetic traffic to the sinus node causes sinus tachycardia.

Purkinje Fibers. Augmented automaticity due to increased sympathetic nerve activity in the His-Purkinje system is a common cause of human arrhythmias. Atrioventricular junctional pacemakers can fire faster than a normal sinus node because of selective traffic on sympathetic nerves, local release of catecholamines, or enhanced responsiveness of beta-adrenergic receptors. In addition, vagal and autonomic activity can increase together; the vagus slows sinus rate and AV conduction, whereas sympathetic traffic increases the firing rate in the His-Purkinje system.

In diseased hearts, automaticity in the His-Purkinje system may become reduced. In the sick sinus syndrome, it is typical for the ventricular escape pacemakers to be depressed, producing long pauses when the sinus node pacemaker fails. In AV block due to bundle branch disease, ventricular pacemakers also may be abnormally slow.

Abnormal Impulse Generation

Numerous mechanisms, e.g., abnormal automaticity or triggered activity, can generate impulses even in fibers that

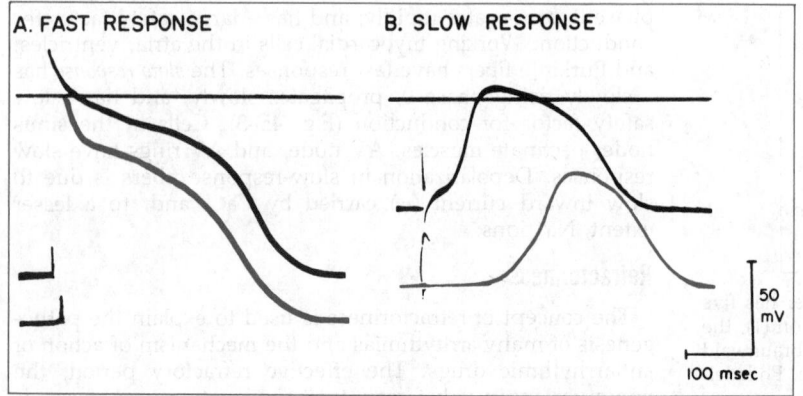

FIGURE 45–3. Two types of cardiac action potentials: (A) fast action potential, (B) slow action potential. (From Wit AL, Rosen MR, Hoffman BF: Electrophysiology and pharmacology of cardiac arrhythmias. II. Relationship of normal and abnormal electrical activity of cardiac fibers to the genesis of arrhythmias. Am Heart J 88:515–524, 1974. With permission of the publisher.)

A. FAST RESPONSE   B. SLOW RESPONSE

50 mV

100 msec

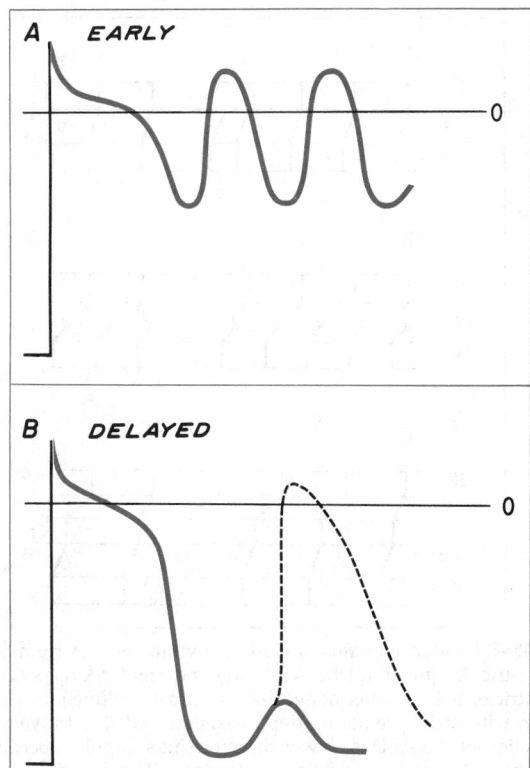

FIGURE 45–4. After-depolarizations and triggered activity. *A*, Early after-depolarization. Repolarization of the Purkinje fiber is interrupted by two secondary depolarizations, which can activate adjacent fibers and cause arrhythmias, e.g., torsades de pointes. *B*, Delayed after-depolarizations. After full repolarization, the Purkinje fiber depolarizes. If the after-depolarization reaches threshold voltage, a propagating response can occur. (From Bigger JT: Electrophysiology for the clinician. Euro Heart J 5(Suppl B):1–9, 1984.)

are incapable of normal automaticity, e.g., ordinary atrial or ventricular muscle cells.

ABNORMAL AUTOMATICITY. Abnormal automaticity refers to spontaneous diastolic depolarization in depolarized cells. Purkinje fibers, atrial cells, and ventricular cells can show spontaneous diastolic depolarization and repetitive automatic firing when their resting Vm is reduced to -60 mV or below. Abnormal automaticity is seen in Purkinje fibers depolarized by acute myocardial infarction. Abnormal automaticity and repetitive firing can be evoked in normal atrial or ventricular cells by applying depolarizing current. Abnormal automaticity is not readily suppressed by overdrive pacing.

TRIGGERED ACTIVITY. Repetitive firing in heart muscle can be caused by triggered activity. Triggered activity is *not* a form of automaticity but is capable of producing a sustained tachyarrhythmia. Two primary mechanisms can initiate triggered activity: early afterdepolarizations and delayed afterdepolarizations (Fig. 45–4).

Early Afterdepolarizations. Early afterdepolarizations are secondary depolarizations that occur before repolarization is complete, often from the action potential plateau (Fig. 45–4). Experimentally, early afterdepolarizations have been produced in cardiac Purkinje fibers by stretching or crushing, hypoxia, cooling, low $[K]_o$, high $[Ca]_o$, catecholamines, and chemicals and drugs (such as veratrine, aconitine, quinidine, sotalol, or N-acetylprocainamide). Torsades de pointes (see below) in humans is thought to be the counterpart of triggered activity due to early afterdepolarizations.

Delayed Afterdepolarizations. A delayed afterdepolarization is a secondary depolarization occurring after full repolarization has been achieved but is dependent on a prior action potential (Fig. 45–4). Delayed afterdepolarizations can reach threshold

and cause a single premature depolarization or trigger a series of impulses. Delayed afterdepolarizations can be induced easily by digitalis in the His-Purkinje system and with more difficulty in specialized atrial or ordinary ventricular cells. Some of the digitalis-induced ventricular tachycardias in humans have characteristics that resemble triggered activity produced by digitalis in isolated tissue preparations. In the atria, coronary sinus, and mitral valve, delayed afterdepolarizations and triggered activity can be caused by catecholamines.

Arrhythmias Caused by Abnormalities of Impulse Conduction

Re-entry seems to be a common cause of cardiac arrhythmias in humans, particularly paroxysmal supraventricular tachycardia and constantly coupled ventricular premature depolarizations. Re-entrant arrhythmias usually are started by an initiating premature depolarization, i.e., are self-sustained but are not self-initiated. To start re-entry, one-way conduction block must occur and there must be an anatomic or functional "barrier" that forms a circuit (Fig. 45–5). In addition, the path length of the re-entrant circuit must be greater than the wavelength of the cardiac impulse (wavelength = conduction velocity × refractory period). For re-entry to occur, conduction must be very slow, refractoriness very short, or both. Re-entry has been demonstrated in anatomic loops (e.g., rings of Purkinje fibers) and around anatomic obstacles (e.g., scars). Re-entry occurring in unbranched bundles or sheets of cardiac muscle has been given specialized names, e.g., reflection or leading circle re-entry.

Re-entry can be subdivided into random and ordered forms. In random re-entry, the cardiac impulse conducts over circuits that change their location and size as a function of time, e.g., atrial and ventricular fibrillation. In ordered re-entry, the circuit for re-entrant activity is relatively constant.

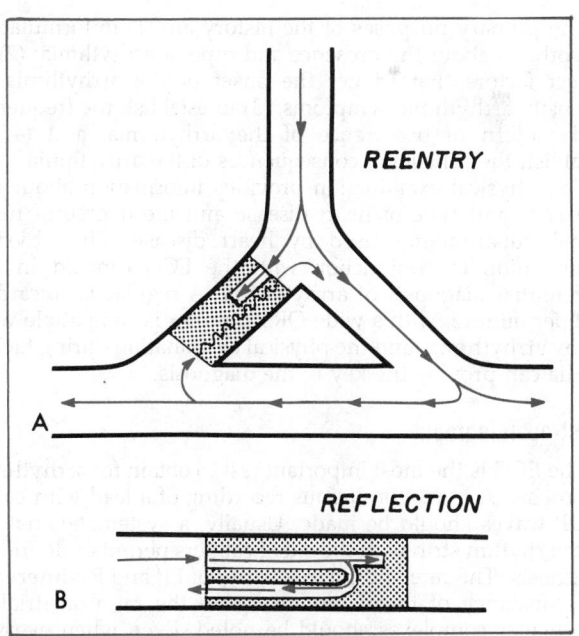

FIGURE 45–5. Two models of re-entry according to Schmitt and Erlanger. *A*, Diagram showing a loop of cardiac fibers that could represent either a terminal branch of a Purkinje fiber ending on ventricular muscle or a loop of the Purkinje syncytium. In this case, one-way block and slow conduction permit re-entry. *B*, A linear strand of cardiac muscle showing a depolarized zone in a portion of its cross section. One-way block occurs in the depolarized zone, permitting the propagating impulse to reflect back in the direction from which it came. (From Braunwald E.: Heart Disease: A Textbook of Cardiovascular Medicine. Philadelphia, W. B. Saunders Company, 1980.)

LEADING EDGE RE-ENTRY. Re-entrant excitation can be initiated in vitro by premature stimulation in small, thin pieces of normal atrium that contain no anatomic obstacles of loops of tissue. Conduction is slowed because activation occurs when the tissue is partially refractory. Block occurs in some regions because of local differences in refractory periods. The pathway for re-entrant activity can stabilize and be sustained.

Cranefield PF: The Conduction of the Cardiac Impulse. Mount Kisco, NY, Futura Publishing Company, 1975. *A monograph that reviews the concepts of fast and slow action potentials and their role in the genesis of re-entrant cardiac arrhythmias.*

Fozzard HA, Haber E, Jennings RB, et al. (eds.): The Heart and Cardiovascular System: Scientific Foundations. New York, Raven Press, 1986. *The section on cardiac electrophysiology and arrhythmias contains detailed reviews of current knowledge and thought on the electrophysiology of the heart, the genesis of cardiac arrhythmias, and the epidemiology of human arrhythmias. Other sections contain excellent reviews of the embryology, anatomy, and pathology of the heart. Profusely illustrated and exhaustively referenced.*

Hackel DB: Anatomy and pathology of the cardiac conducting system. In Edwards JE, Lev M, Abell MA (eds.): The Heart. Baltimore, Williams & Wilkins Company, 1974, pp 232–247. *A concise description of the normal anatomy and pathology of the conduction system.*

Noble D: The Initiation of the Heartbeat. London, Oxford University Press, 1979. *An account of cardiac electrophysiology for medical students and clinicians who are unfamiliar with electronics and mathematics. The most difficult concepts of cardiac excitation are explained clearly and concisely. Selective references to the classic papers on electrophysiology.*

DIAGNOSTIC APPROACHES TO CARDIAC ARRHYTHMIAS

The history, physical examination, 12-lead electrocardiogram, 24-hour continuous electrocardiographic recordings, exercise tests, intermittent electrocardiographic recorders, and clinical electrophysiologic studies are the primary tools used in the diagnosis of cardiac arrhythmias. Decisions about treatment may require other laboratory studies to define better the etiology of heart disease, other aspects of the functional status of the heart, e.g., left ventricular function or perfusion, or function of other organ systems.

History and Physical Examination

The primary purposes of the history are (1) to formulate a hypothesis about the presence and type of arrhythmia; (2) to detect factors that trigger the onset of the arrhythmia or intensify arrhythmic symptoms; (3) to establish the frequency and pattern of occurrence of the arrhythmia; and (4) to establish the functional consequences of the arrhythmia.

The physical examination provides information about the presence and type of heart disease and the degree of functional impairment caused by heart disease. The physical examination in conjunction with the ECG can aid in the differential diagnosis of arrhythmias. A regular tachycardia, 150 per minute, with a wide QRS complex is compatible with many arrhythmias and the physical examination during tachycardia can provide the key to the diagnosis.

Electrocardiography

The ECG is the most important test to obtain for arrhythmia diagnosis. A long, continuous recording of a lead with clear-cut P waves should be made. Usually, a systematic analysis of the rhythm strip with the aid of calipers permits a definitive diagnosis. The rate and the regularity of PP and RR intervals, the constancy of the PR interval, and the ratio of atrial to ventricular complexes should be noted. Even when every P wave and QRS complex is identified, the ECG pattern may be compatible with more than one diagnosis. Ladder diagrams are helpful for displaying the possibilities in an unequivocal manner (Fig. 45–6).

Carotid Sinus Pressure

Taking ECG rhythm strips during carotid sinus pressure is a valuable bedside maneuver for diagnosis of cardiac arrhythmias. Carotid massage activates a reflex arc that increases the

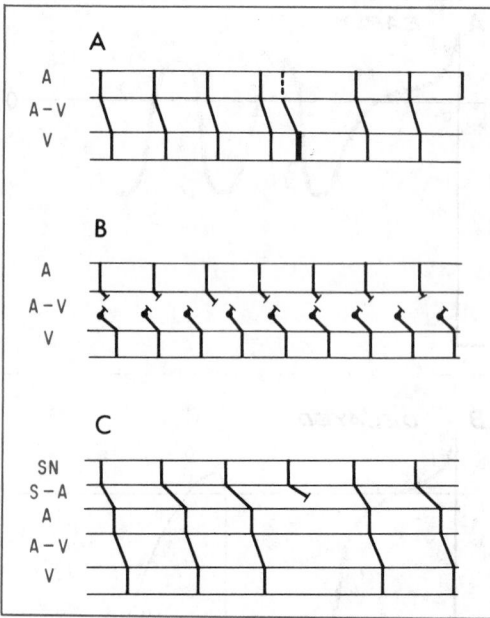

FIGURE 45–6. Ladder diagrams of cardiac rhythm. A = Atrium; A-V = atrioventricular junction (the A-V node and His-Purkinje system); V = ventricle; SN = sinus node; S-A = sinoatrial junction. *A,* Sinus rhythm with atrial premature depolarization (APD). Atrioventricular conduction of the APD is slower than for sinus impulses because the atrioventricular node is partially refractory. The broad line in the ventricular tier indicates aberrant ventricular conduction of the APD, which occurs because the premature impulse arrives during the relative refractory period of the His-Purkinje system. *B,* Atrioventricular junctional rhythm. The A-V junctional automatic rhythm captures the ventricles but shows retrograde block. The sinus node controls the atria, but the sinus impulse finds the A-V node refractory and is blocked; i.e., there is interference between the sinus and junctional rhythm. *C,* Type I (Wenckebach) sinoatrial block. The sinus impulse travels through the perinodal junctional tissues with increasing delay until block finally occurs. (From Braunwald E.: Heart Disease: A Textbook of Cardiovascular Medicine. Philadelphia, W. B. Saunders Company, 1980.)

vagal traffic to the heart. The most important use of carotid sinus pressure is to aid in the analysis of rapid, regular tachycardia when P waves are not clearly apparent. The responses of various arrhythmias to carotid sinus massage are listed in Table 45–3.

Carotid sinus pressure carries significant risks, particularly in older patients, i.e., syncope, convulsions, stroke, prolonged asystole, or ventricular tachyarrhythmias. In patients with digitalis toxicity, carotid sinus pressure may provoke malignant ventricular arrhythmias.

Special Procedures to Detect Atrial Activation

All of the P waves must be identified to make rhythm analysis reliable. P waves can be detected using special lead placement, e.g., the Lewis lead, esophageal electrograms, or transvenous bipolar catheter electrodes.

Ambulatory Electrocardiographic Recording

In 1961, Holter described the technique of ambulatory ECG recording. A light, portable tape recorder makes continuous 24-hour ECG recordings while the patient performs his or her usual daily activities and records activities and symptoms in a diary. The primary uses of ambulatory ECG recordings in individual patients are listed in Table 45–4.

INTERMITTENT RECORDERS. When symptoms occur only occasionally, intermittent recorders permit monitoring lasting from a few days to many weeks, even though the ECG recordings are brief (seconds to minutes). The recorders may be attached to the patients continuously or intermittently.

TABLE 45–3. EFFECT OF CAROTID SINUS PRESSURE ON TACHYARRHYTHMIAS

Arrhythmia	Response to Carotid Sinus Pressure
Sinus tachycardia	1. Gradual slowing during massage, gradual speeding after massage
Paroxysmal supraventricular tachycardia (AV nodal)	1. No effect or 2. Abrupt conversion to sinus rhythm or 3. Slight slowing
Paroxysmal supraventricular tachycardia (anomalous AV connection)	1. No effect or 2. Abrupt conversion to sinus rhythm or 3. Slight slowing
Nonparoxysmal supraventricular tachycardia	1. No effect or 2. Atrioventricular block, slowed ventricular rate or 3. Gradual slowing of ventricular rate (rare)
Atrial flutter	1. Atrioventricular block, slowed ventricular rate or 2. No effect or 3. Atrial fibrillation
Atrial fibrillation	1. Atrioventricular block, slowed ventricular rate or 2. No effect
Ventricular tachycardia	1. No effect or 2. Atrioventricular dissociation

AV = atrioventricular.

Hard-Wired Recorders. Intermittent recorders of the "hard-wired" type are continuously attached to the patient by electrodes and cables. Patients activate these recorders by pressing a switch. Some units have 40 to 100 seconds of electronic memory and sample the ECG continuously, replacing old data with new. When activated, 30 to 60 seconds of ECG prior to patient activation are recorded. Data are retrieved from "hard-wired" systems either by direct playback or by telephonic transmission.

Intermittently Attached Recorders and Telephonic Transmission. These devices are typically about the size and shape of a radiopaging unit. The patient applies ECG leads when symptoms occur. Units with memory can store one to three ECG samples for subsequent telephone transmission. Com-

TABLE 45–4. INDICATIONS FOR LONG-TERM CONTINUOUS ECG RECORDINGS

I. **Detect and quantify arrhythmias or conduction defects in patients with symptoms** (e.g., syncope or other central nervous system symptoms, palpitations, or angina pectoris)
II. **Quantification of arrhythmias, conduction defects, or ischemia in patients with predisposing conditions**
   A. Sick sinus syndrome
   B. Pre-excitation syndromes
   C. AV conduction defects
   D. Pacemaker malfunction
   E. Mitral valve prolapse
   F. Long QT syndrome
   G. Post myocardial infarction
   H. Angina pectoris
   I. Hypertrophic or dilated cardiomyopathy
   J. Heart failure
III. **Evaluate activity**
   A. For potential to cause arrhythmias or conduction defects
   B. To evaluate ischemia during activity
IV. **Evaluate therapy**
   A. Antiarrhythmic drug treatment
   B. Fad diets
   C. Drugs with adverse cardiac effects
   D. Pacemakers
   E. Automatic implantable cardioverter defibrillator
   F. Surgery
      1. Ischemia or arrhythmias after coronary artery bypass graft surgery
      2. Pre-excitation after division of anomalous AV connection
      3. AV conduction after surgical division or catheter ablation of the His bundle

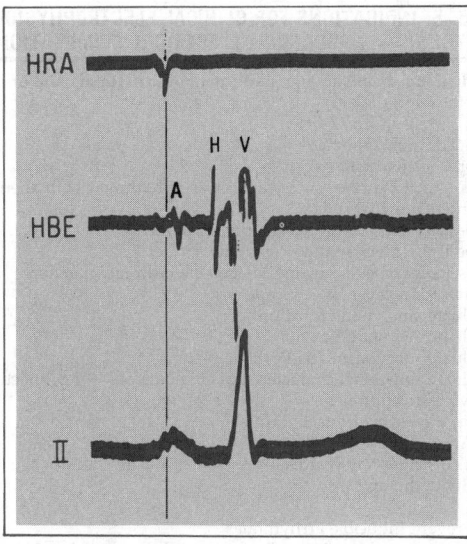

FIGURE 45–7. Intracardiac recordings. A high right atrial bipolar electrogram (HRA), His bundle bipolar electrogram (HBE), and tracing from lead II of the electrocardiogram. A = Atrial depolarization; H = depolarization of the His bundle; V = depolarization of the upper ventricular septum. The P-A interval represents intra-atrial conduction time (upper to lower atrium); A-H represents atrioventricular nodal conduction; and H-V represents the His-Purkinje conduction time. The thin vertical line correlates the onset of atrial activation in the three recordings. (From Braunwald E.: Heart Disease: A Textbook of Cardiovascular Medicine. Philadelphia, W. B. Saunders Company, 1980.)

mercial services provide immediate evaluation of the ECG transmission. Transmissions are acted on in accordance with the instructions of the patient's physician.

Intracardiac Recording and Stimulation (Endocardial Electrical Stimulation)

Over the past 20 years, intracardiac recording and stimulation have developed as a diagnostic and therapeutic tool for the management of human cardiac arrhythmias. Local electrical activity can be recorded from the portions of the heart that are electrically silent on the body surface ECG, e.g., sinus node, His bundle, right bundle branch, left bundle branch, and selected sites in the right or left ventricle. The sequence and time of activation of atria and ventricles can be mapped and AV conduction can be partitioned into AV nodal and His-Purkinje components (see Fig. 45–7). Recordings from selected sites are used with pacing and programmed stimulation sequences to evaluate automaticity, conduction, refractoriness, and the causes of arrhythmias in intact humans. These techniques not only have enhanced our understanding of arrhythmias and conduction defects but also have improved our ability to select and evaluate therapy. Some of the major clinical uses of electrophysiologic studies are listed in Table 45–5.

Bigger JT Jr, Reiffel JA, Coromilas J: Ambulatory electrocardiography. In Platia EV (ed.): Nonpharmacologic Management of Cardiac Arrhythmias. Philadelphia, J. B. Lippincott Company, 1986, pp 36–61. *A comprehensive review of the technology, indications, and clinical uses of ambulatory electrocardiography. Liberally illustrated and referenced.*

Horowitz LN, Josephson ME, Kastor JA: Intracardiac electrophysiologic studies as a method for the optimization of drug therapy in chronic ventricular arrhythmias. Prog Cardiovasc Dis 23:81, 1980. *Gives the details of electrophysiologic methods for evaluating drug therapy of malignant ventricular arrhythmias.*

Josephson ME, Seides SF: Clinical Cardiac Electrophysiology: Techniques and Interpretations. Philadelphia, Lea & Febiger, 1979. *A detailed description of the techniques of clinical electrophysiology and the interpretation of the findings. Intended for the internist and clinical cardiologist without an extensive background in cardiac electrophysiology.*

Morganroth J: Ambulatory Holter electrocardiography: Choice of technologies and clinical uses. Ann Intern Med 102:73, 1985. *A concise review of the current status of ambulatory electrocardiography.*

TABLE 45–5. INDICATIONS FOR CLINICAL ELECTROPHYSIOLOGICAL STUDIES—ENDOCARDIAL ELECTRICAL STIMULATION

I. **To evaluate mechanism, site, and extent of arrhythmia and/or conduction defect**
   A. Sick sinus syndrome
   B. Pre-excitation syndrome
   C. Supraventricular tachycardia
   D. Distinguish between supraventricular arrhythmias with aberration and ventricular arrhythmia
   E. Type I AV block with bundle branch block
   F. Type II AV block with normal QRS
   G. Bifascicular block occurring in acute myocardial infarction

II. **To search for a cause for syncope**
   A. Evaluate sinus node function
   B. Evaluate AV node function
   C. Evaluate function of His-Purkinje system
   D. Evaluate functional characteristics of anomalous AV connections
   E. Provoke arrhythmias
      1. Supraventricular tachycardia
      2. Atrial flutter or fibrillation
      3. Ventricular tachycardia

III. **To evaluate therapy**
   A. Drug therapy
      1. Prevent inducible arrhythmias
      2. Measure conduction and refractoriness in anomalous AV connections
      3. Evaluate adverse effects
         a. Sinus node function
         b. AV node function
         c. His-Purkinje system
         d. Effect on device function
   B. Surgical therapy
      1. Preoperative endocardial catheter mapping
         a. Location of anomalous AV connections
         b. Location of VT circuit
         c. Need for concomitant pacemaker implantation
      2. Postoperative evaluation
         a. Presence of anomalous AV connections
         b. Arrhythmia inducible
   C. AICD therapy
      1. Preoperative evaluation
         a. Determine that VT or VF is inducible
         b. Determine that VT or VF is drug resistant
         c. Determine need for concomitant pacemaker implantation
      2. Intraoperative evaluation
         a. Determine quality of right or left ventricular sensing electrograms
         b. Determine quality of patch electrograms for the probability density function
         c. Determine defibrillation thresholds
         d. Induce clinical arrhythmia to test sensing and termination of ventricular arrhythmias by the AICD
      3. Postoperative evaluation
         a. Induce VT or VF to test the performance of the AICD
         b. Acquaint the patient with the symptoms during AICD discharge
   D. Pacemaker therapy
      1. Evaluate condition for suitability for pacemaker therapy
         a. Supraventricular tachycardia—reciprocation in the AV node
         b. Supraventricular tachycardia—reciprocation in anomalous AV connections
      2. Determine the information needed to select pacemaker type and parameters

IV. **To apply ablation therapy**
   A. Posterior septal anomalous AV connections
   B. AV node
   C. Ventricular tachycardia

AICD = automatic implantable cardioverter defibrillator; VT = ventricular tachycardia; VF = ventricular fibrillation.

SPECIFIC CARDIAC ARRHYTHMIAS

Clinically, cardiac arrhythmias are classified by their presumed site of origin, i.e., atrial, AV junctional, or ventricular, and as premature complexes, bradycardia, or tachycardia. It would be desirable to use the precise mechanism to classify cardiac arrhythmias, but this is impossible because we do not know the precise mechanism of many arrhythmias. For some arrhythmias, e.g., the ventricular arrhythmias, prognostic significance can be assigned with reasonable precision. When this is the case, a prognostic classification is useful for guiding decisions about management. In this section, we will use a classification based on the site of origin and rate as the framework in which to discuss the definition, pathophysiology, electrocardiographic diagnosis, significance, and management of each arrhythmia. The emergency and chronic treatments of cardiac arrhythmias are outlined in Tables 45–6 and 45–7.

ATRIAL ARRHYTHMIAS
Sinus Rhythm

ECG DIAGNOSIS. Sinus rhythm is recognized in the ECG by a normal atrial rate and P wave vector, i.e., an upright P wave in leads III and aV_F. The PR interval is normal in classic sinus rhythm. In adults, sinus rates below 60 or 50 per minute are called sinus bradycardia and those above 100 per minute, sinus tachycardia. Heart rate changes synchronized with breathing are called sinus arrhythmia and are caused by changes in autonomic nervous activity. Sinus arrhythmia is more pronounced in children and young adults than the elderly. Marked sinus arrhythmia can be difficult to distinguish from sinoatrial block or ectopic atrial rhythms.

CLINICAL FEATURES. Resting heart rate in sinus rhythm varies with age: from 130 to 160 per minute in infants to 50 to 100 per minute in adults. Sex, temperature, emotion, effort, and neurohumoral factors also influence sinus rate. The maximum heart rate during exercise varies from almost 200 per minute in healthy young persons to less than 140 per minute in the elderly. Many drugs increase or decrease the sinus rate, usually by interacting with autonomic mechanisms.

MANAGEMENT. Sinus bradycardia is treated only when symptomatic. When acute and symptomatic sinus bradycardia is due to increased vagus nerve activity, heart rate can be increased by intravenous (IV) atropine injection. Rarely, IV isoproterenol infusion may be needed. Chronic symptomatic sinus bradycardia is an indication for an electronic pacemaker. Treatment of sinus tachycardia is based on the cause, usually non-cardiac.

Atrial Premature Depolarizations

Atrial premature depolarizations (APD's) arise in the atria outside the sinus node. Atrial premature depolarizations occur in normal and diseased hearts. In heart disease, APD's herald sustained arrhythmias such as atrial flutter, atrial fibrillation, or paroxysmal supraventricular tachycardia.

ECG DIAGNOSIS. Atrial premature depolarizations typically have premature P waves, abnormal P wave morphology, and a prolonged PR interval. Early APD's can be difficult to see because the P wave is superimposed on the T wave. In addition, APD's can block the AV node discharge to produce pauses that can be misinterpreted as a sinus pause or sinoatrial block. Usually, APD's reset the sinus node so that the sum of the pre- and post-extrasystolic PP intervals is less than two sinus cycles (see Fig. 45–8). If sinus reset does not occur because the APD occurs late or the perinodal refractory period is long, a compensatory pause will occur. An APD can conduct aberrantly, causing the QRS complex to be wide and bizarre like a ventricular premature depolarization (see Fig. 45–9). Aberrant conduction occurs when APD's activate one of the bundle branches, usually the right, during its relative refractory period. Left bundle branch block aberrancy implies an abnormality in the left bundle branch (see Fig. 45–9).

MANAGEMENT. The objectives of treating APD's are to control symptoms or prevent sustained symptomatic arrhythmias. In patients with normal hearts, treatment should be focused on general hygienic measures; rest and reducing the use of tobacco, alcohol, or caffeine often reduce the frequency of APD's. In some patients with intermittent, sustained atrial arrhythmias, APD's should be treated with digitalis or class I, II, or IV antiarrhythmic drugs to prevent sustained arrhythmias.

TABLE 45–6. EMERGENCY TREATMENT OF CARDIAC ARRHYTHMIAS

Arrhythmia	Usual First Treatment	Other Effective Treatments	Comments
Atrial fibrillation	Digitalis	Cardioversion; propranolol; acebutolol; verapamil	If hypotensive due to rapid ventricular rate, cardiovert. Avoid propranolol or verapamil in patients with heart failure or hypotension. Avoid digitalis or verapamil in Wolff-Parkinson-White syndrome.
Atrial flutter	Cardioversion	Digitalis; verapamil; propranolol; acebutolol; rapid atrial pacing	Very large doses of digitalis, e.g., 4–6 mg, often are required to achieve AV block in atrial flutter.
Paroxysmal supraventricular tachycardia (AV nodal)	Vagal maneuvers; verapamil	Digitalis; propranolol; acebutolol; procainamide	Do not treat wide QRS complex tachycardia with verapamil unless the diagnosis of PSVT is certain. Use cardioversion for PSVT with hypotension.
Paroxysmal supraventricular tachycardia (anomalous AV connection)	Vagal maneuvers; verapamil	Cardioversion	If the RP interval suggests anomalous AV connection, an electrophysiologic study should be considered.
Sick sinus syndrome	Pacemaker	Digitalis; pacemaker plus class I antiarrhythmic drug	Digitalis usually improves atrial tachyarrhythmias without aggravating sinus bradycardia or AV block.
Nonparoxysmal AV junctional tachycardia	Stop digitalis	Potassium; observation	If the arrhythmia is caused by digitalis toxicity and serum K+ is low, digitalis should be stopped and potassium should be given.
Sustained ventricular tachycardia	Cardioversion	Lidocaine; procainamide	If ventricular tachycardia is well tolerated, intravenous lidocaine or procainamide can be tried.
Ventricular fibrillation	Cardioversion		Lidocaine or bretylium tosylate or propranolol may be helpful when ventricular fibrillation recurs several times immediately after cardioversion.
Digitalis toxic atrial tachycardia with block or ventricular tachycardia	Lidocaine; phenytoin	Potassium	Avoid cardioversion or bretylium tosylate, which may precipitate ventricular fibrillation.
Digitalis toxic asystole or AV block	Pacemaker	Fab fragments of digoxin-specific antibodies; dialysis	If associated with malignant hyperkalemia, these rhythms are always fatal unless treated promptly with Fab fragments of digoxin-specific antibodies.

PSVT = paroxysmal supraventricular tachycardia.

TABLE 45–7. CHRONIC TREATMENT OF CARDIAC ARRHYTHMIAS

Arrhythmia	Usual First Treatment	Other Effective Treatments	Comments
Atrial fibrillation	Digitalis	Class I antiarrhythmic drug and digitalis; digitalis and propranolol; digitalis and verapamil	Class I antiarrhythmic drugs are used to maintain sinus rhythm; propranolol, acebutolol, or verapamil is used as an adjunct to control ventricular rate in atrial fibrillation
Atrial flutter	Class I antiarrhythmic drug	Digitalis; propranolol; verapamil	—
Paroxysmal supraventricular tachycardia (AV nodal)	Digitalis	Class IC antiarrhythmic drug; propranolol	—
Paroxysmal supraventricular tachycardia (anomalous AV connection)	Class IC antiarrhythmic drug	Class IA antiarrhythmic drug	Surgical ablation is preferable if patient also has atrial fibrillation with rapid ventricular response, if the anomalous AV connection has a short refractory period, or if the patient is noncompliant or has adverse effects from drugs.
Sick sinus syndrome	Pacemaker	Pacemaker and digitalis; pacemaker and class I antiarrhythmic drug	With the arrhythmias effectively treated, prognosis is determined by the severity of associated heart disease
High-grade AV block	Pacemaker		No drugs are needed.
Symptomatic ventricular premature depolarizations	Class I antiarrhythmic drug	Beta blocker	For benign and potentially malignant ventricular arrhythmias, class IC drugs are the most effective and usually have the lowest incidence of adverse effects. When heart failure is present, disopyramide and flecainide are relatively contraindicated.
Symptomatic unsustained ventricular tachycardia	Class I antiarrhythmic drug	Beta blocker	Class IC drugs are the most effective and usually have the lowest incidence of adverse effects. When heart failure is present, disopyramide and flecainide are relatively contraindicated.
Sustained ventricular tachycardia	Class I antiarrhythmic drug	Class III antiarrhythmic drug	Treatment must be guided by a method with proven high predictive accuracy, e.g., endocardial electrical stimulation. A common sequence of drugs is class IA → class IA + class IB → class IC → class III. If drugs fail or cannot be evaluated, an implantable cardioverter defibrillator usually is the best treatment. In selected cases, surgical excision of the arrhythmogenic tissue is the best choice.

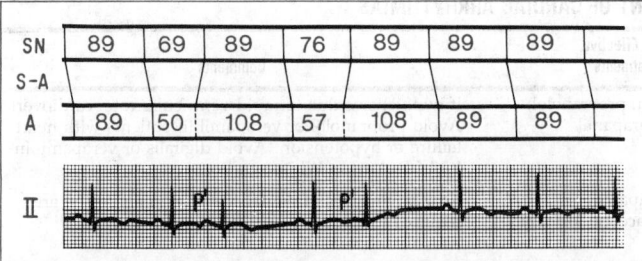

FIGURE 45–8. Atrial premature depolarization (APD). The ladder diagram correlates with the events in the lead II electrocardiographic strip below. SN = Sinus node; S-A = junctional tissues between sinus node and atrium; A = atrium. The time intervals in the ladder diagram are given in msec × 10⁻¹ (e.g., 89 represents 890 msec). The third and fifth P waves are APD's (P'). These P' waves are premature and inverted. The P'-R interval is prolonged, and QRS duration is normal. The APD's capture the sinus node and reset it; therefore, the pause following APD's is less than compensatory. (From Braunwald E.: Heart Disease: A Textbook of Cardiovascular Medicine. Philadelphia, W. B. Saunders Company, 1980.)

Paroxysmal Supraventricular Tachycardia

ECG DIAGNOSIS. Typically, paroxysmal supraventricular tachycardia (PSVT), also known as paroxysmal atrial or nodal tachycardia and reciprocating AV nodal tachycardia, has the following electrocardiographic features: a regular, rapid rate of 150 to 230 per minute; QRS complex duration less than 100 msec; and an abnormal P wave in a fixed relationship to each QRS. The P wave often is superimposed on the T wave or the QRS complex. Paroxysmal supraventricular tachycardia starts abruptly, usually started by an atrial or ventricular premature depolarization. Often, the atrial rate in PSVT will be about 180 per minute. The rate of PSVT is often faster in infants and children, in the Wolff-Parkinson-White (WPW) syndrome, and in thyrotoxicosis. The rate of PSVT is likely to be slower when AV node disease or certain drugs are present. The RR intervals in typical PSVT are extremely regular except for the first or last few cycles of an episode. Carotid sinus massage either has no effect on PSVT or terminates it. In the presence of AV nodal disease or drugs that depress nodal conduction, e.g., digitalis or verapamil, fixed 2:1 AV block or AV Wenckebach can occur during PSVT.

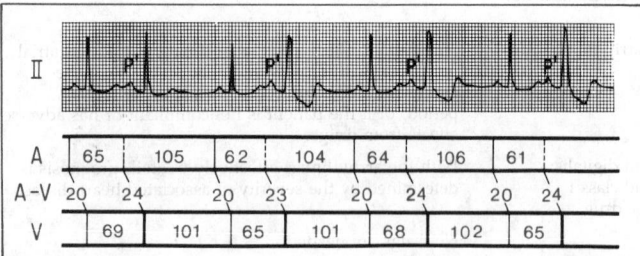

FIGURE 45–9. Atrial premature depolarizations (APD's) with aberrant conduction. The ladder diagram depicts the events in the lead II electrocardiographic strip above. A = Atrium; A-V = atrioventricular node and His-Purkinje system; V = ventricle. Time intervals are in msec × 10⁻¹ (65 represents 650 msec). APD's are represented by dashed lines in the atrial tier; the wide QRS complexes are represented by a wide bar in the ventricular tier. APD's occur in a bigeminal pattern. The even (ectopic) P waves (P') are premature and have configurations slightly different from the odd P waves. Although the P-P' interval is relatively long (>600 msec), the P'-R interval is also prolonged, and the QRS complex following each P' is aberrant (left bundle branch block configuration)—a pattern of aberration suggesting bundle branch disease. Note that the QRS complex after the longest P-P' interval (second QRS) is least aberrant. (From Braunwald E.: Heart Disease: A Textbook of Cardiovascular Medicine. Philadelphia, W. B. Saunders Company, 1980.)

The QRS complexes may be wide owing either to a preexisting wide QRS or to aberrant conduction of the rapid atrial rhythm, resembling ventricular tachycardia. If atrioventricular dissociation can be documented, the rhythm originates in the subatrial location and is not PSVT. His bundle electrography can differentiate between PSVT and ventricular tachycardia (Fig. 45–10).

The mechanism of PSVT is often AV nodal re-entry initiated by an APD. In the WPW syndrome, the PSVT is re-entrant, using the anomalous AV connection in the retrograde direction and the AV node in the antegrade direction (see Fig. 45–11).

Nonparoxysmal atrial tachycardia probably is due to ectopic automaticity or triggered activity in the atrium. Atrial tachycardia with AV block suggests digitalis toxicity, particularly if the atrial rate is slow.

CLINICAL FEATURES. PSVT occurs in normal as well as diseased hearts. Attacks of PSVT begin abruptly, cause palpitations, and may also end abruptly after a period of time. The patient may learn maneuvers that are likely to stop the tachycardia, e.g., cough, Valsalva's maneuver, or facial immersion. The hemodynamic effects of PSVT vary tremendously and depend on rate and underlying mechanical reserve of the heart. When the rate of PSVT is rapid, e.g., 180 to 220 per minute, systemic arterial pressure usually falls and diastolic filling pressures rise in both ventricles, even in persons without heart disease. Prolonged and rapid supraventricular tachycardia is likely to cause marked salt and water retention.

MANAGEMENT. Either vagal maneuvers (e.g., Valsalva's maneuver or carotid sinus massage) or verapamil is effective in about 90 per cent of the episodes. When PSVT causes hypotension or heart failure, DC cardioversion should be used. For prevention of recurrences of PSVT due to AV nodal re-entry, digitalis usually is tried first. If digitalis fails, potent class I antiarrhythmic drugs (see below, Specific Antiarrhythmic Drugs, and Tables 45–9 to 45–11) are quite effective. Surgical interruption (see Table 45–16) of the anomalous AV conduction pathway may be preferred to drugs in the WPW syndrome with recurrent symptomatic tachyarrhythmias.

Atrial Flutter

ECG DIAGNOSIS. Typically, atrial flutter has the following electrocardiographic features: a rapid atrial rate, 250 to 350 per minute; a narrow QRS complex; and a ventricular rate of about 150 per minute, i.e., 2:1 AV conduction ratio (see Fig. 45–12). In atrial flutter, the baseline of the ECG has a characteristic sawtooth or undulating appearance best seen in leads II, III, and aV_F. An AV conduction ratio greater than 2:1 suggests AV node disease or drug effect. Rarely, atrial flutter will conduct to the ventricles with a 1:1 ratio, resulting in a ventricular rate of about 300 per minute and hemodynamic collapse. The QRS complex usually is normal during atrial flutter but may be wide owing to pre-existing bundle branch block.

CLINICAL FEATURES. Atrial flutter usually signifies either intrinsic heart disease or adverse extrinsic influences on the heart. Atrial flutter is associated with scarred atria due to rheumatic heart disease, coronary heart disease, or primary myocardial disease. In addition, atrial flutter is associated with atrial enlargement, e.g., in interatrial septal defect, mitral or tricuspid stenosis or regurgitation, or chronic ventricular failure. Atrial flutter occurs in toxic or metabolic conditions that affect the heart, e.g., thyrotoxicosis, alcoholism, or beriberi, or when the pericardium is inflamed or infiltrated, e.g., with pneumonia or bronchogenic carcinoma. In all these conditions, atrial flutter is much less common than atrial fibrillation. Atrial flutter tends to be unstable, either reverting to sinus rhythm or converting to atrial fibrillation. Probably because the atria contract vigorously in atrial flutter, systemic emboli are less common than during atrial fibrillation.

MANAGEMENT. The best choice for the acute treatment

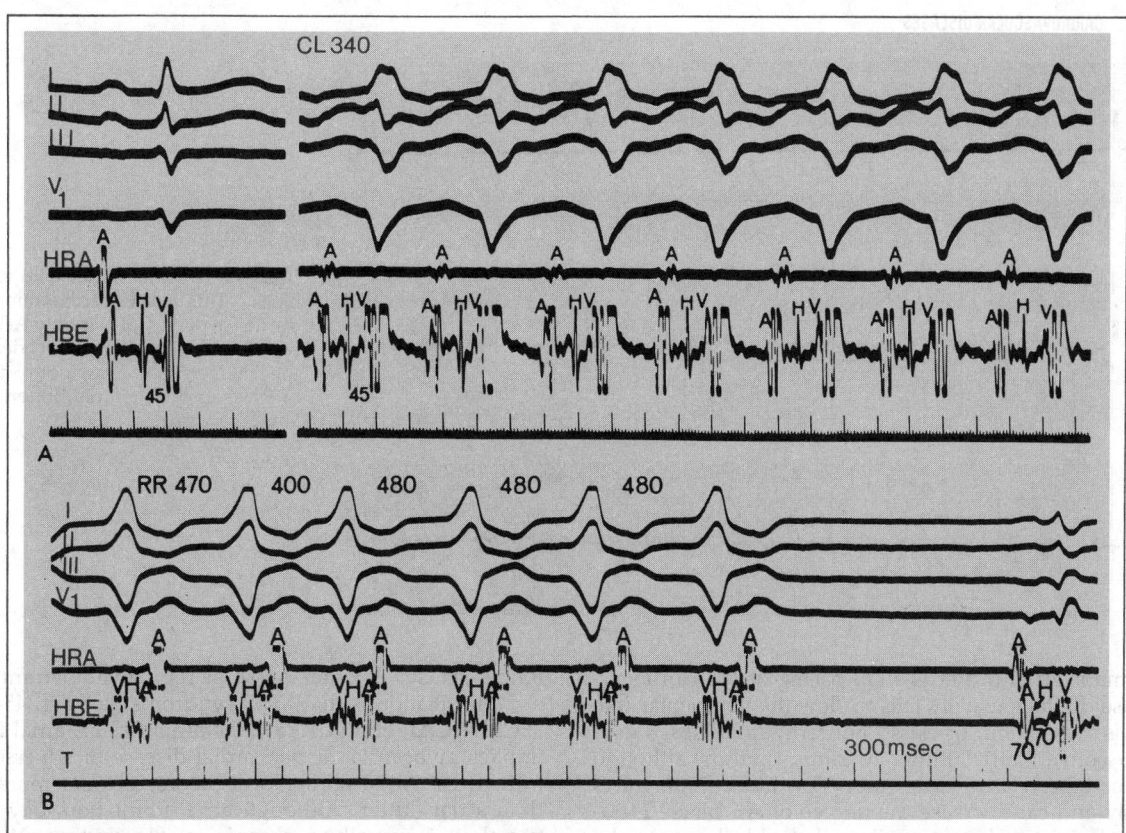

FIGURE 45–10. His bundle recording in regular tachycardia with a wide QRS complex. *A,* Supraventricular tachycardia. The left panel is a record taken during sinus rhythm; the QRS is normal. The right panel is a record taken during tachycardia; a left bundle branch block pattern is present. The normal H-V interval in the His bundle electrogram (HBE) indicates that the rhythm is supraventricular tachycardia with aberrant conduction. *B,* Ventricular tachycardia. The last six depolarizations of a tachycardia and the first of sinus rhythm are shown. A left bundle branch block pattern is present during the tachycardia. In the His bundle electrogram, the ventricles depolarize (V) before the bundle of His (H), indicating that the rhythm is ventricular tachycardia. Ventriculoatrial conduction shows a stable 1:1 pattern. (From Caracta AR, Damato AN: Significance of His bundle electrocardiography. In Fowler NO (ed.): Cardiac Diagnosis and Treatment. 2nd ed. New York, Harper and Row, 1976, pp 979–1008.)

FIGURE 45–11. Mechanism of supraventricular tachycardia utilizing an accessory pathway. The upper panel demonstrates an electrocardiogram recorded in a patient with Wolff-Parkinson-White syndrome during straight atrial pacing and the introduction of a premature atrial beat. The first five beats are preceded by a stimulus artifact (S); a short P-R interval and a wide QRS complex indicate the presence of pre-excitation. Following the introduction of a premature beat, a narrow QRS tachycardia is initiated. The events underlying this supraventricular tachycardia are diagrammatically shown in the lower panels. During sinus rhythm (A), fusion is present owing to conduction over the A-V node (AVN) and the accessory pathway (AP). In B, an atrial premature depolarization blocks the accessory pathway and conducts with delay over the A-V node, thus dissociating the activity of the normal and accessory pathways. In C, the impulse conducting through the ventricle travels retrograde over the accessory pathway and re-enters the atrium, establishing a tachycardia. D demonstrates schematically the re-entry circuit underlying supraventricular tachycardia resulting from re-entry confined to the A-V node.

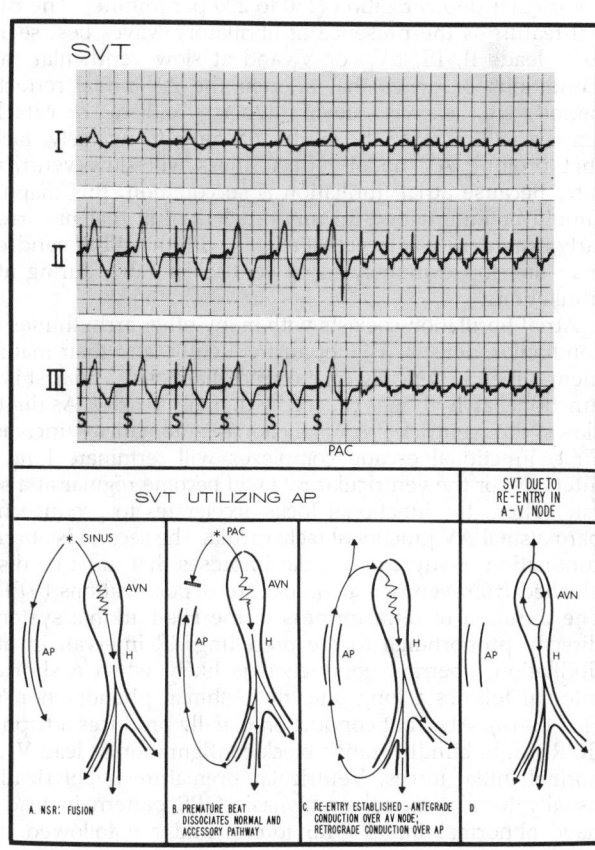

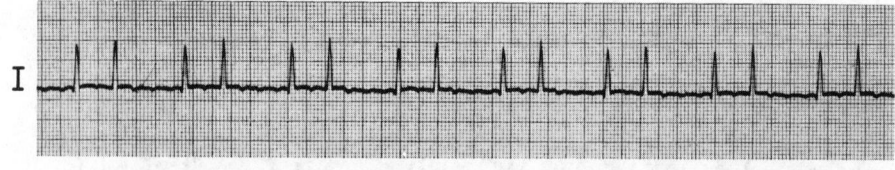

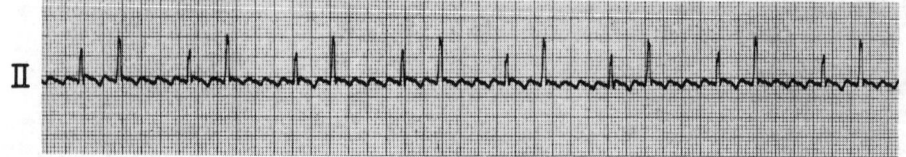

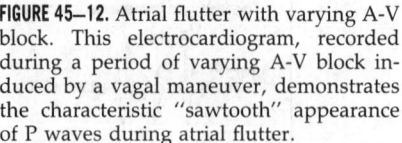

FIGURE 45–12. Atrial flutter with varying A-V block. This electrocardiogram, recorded during a period of varying A-V block induced by a vagal maneuver, demonstrates the characteristic "sawtooth" appearance of P waves during atrial flutter.

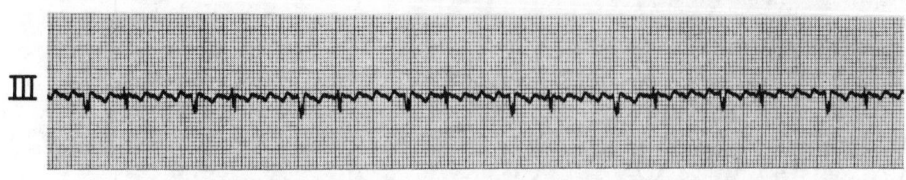

of symptomatic atrial flutter is atrial pacing or DC cardioversion because digitalis usually fails to slow the ventricular rate and digitalis, verapamil, or class I antiarrhythmic drugs usually fail to convert atrial flutter to sinus rhythm, although quinidine or other class I drugs may slow atrial flutter rates dramatically and can increase the degree of AV block. Intravenously administered verapamil or beta blockers can be useful temporizing measures to control heart rate while arrangements are made for DC cardioversion. A class I antiarrhythmic drug with or without digitalis is the usual treatment to prevent recurrence of atrial flutter.

Atrial Fibrillation

ECG DIAGNOSIS. Atrial fibrillation has the following features: absence of P waves; irregular atrial activity at a rate of 350 to 600 per minute; and rapid, irregularly irregular ventricular depolarization (150 to 200 per minute). The cardinal feature is the presence of fibrillatory waves best seen in ECG leads II, III, aV_F, or V_1 and at slow ventricular rates. Conditions or drugs that shorten the AV nodal refractory period, e.g., exercise, fever, hyperthyroidism, or catecholamines will increase the ventricular rate. Conversely, factors that prolong AV nodal refractoriness will slow ventricular rate. Because atrial fibrillation is so common, this diagnosis should be entertained for any rapid rhythm that has irregularly irregular RR intervals. Patients with the WPW syndrome may develop extremely rapid ventricular rates during atrial fibrillation.

Atrial fibrillation coexists with many other arrhythmias and conduction defects. Two occur frequently, and their management depends critically on a correct diagnosis. The first is AV junctional arrhythmias caused by digitalis toxicity. As digitalis slows the ventricle, AV junctional automaticity increases. First, junctional escape complexes will terminate long RR intervals, or the ventricular rate will become regular at a slow rate. Then, the junctional focus accelerates to produce nonparoxysmal AV junctional tachycardia. The second is aberrant conduction of supraventricular impulses that must be distinguished from ventricular premature depolarizations (VPD's). The duration of refractoriness in the His-Purkinje system is directly proportional to the preceding RR interval. In atrial fibrillation, aberrant conduction is likely when a short RR interval follows a long one, the Ashman phenomenon (see Fig. 45–13). Aberrant conduction usually produces a triphasic (RSR') right bundle branch block configuration in lead V_1 and normal initial forces. Ventricular premature depolarizations usually have a mono- or biphasic QRS pattern in lead V_1, have abnormal initial QRS forces, and are followed by a longer pause. Another cause of repetitive aberrant QRS's in atrial fibrillation is the WPW syndrome (see Fig. 45–14).

CLINICAL FEATURES. Like atrial flutter, atrial fibrillation implies myocardial or pericardial disease or adverse extrinsic influences. Atrial fibrillation is about 20 times more common than atrial flutter. Although atrial fibrillation may be paroxysmal, it is usually a chronic, stable rhythm. When atrial fibrillation occurs abruptly in patients with serious heart disease, the consequences may be dramatic, e.g., disconcerting palpitations, pulmonary edema, or angina pectoris. If the ventricular rate is well controlled with digitalis, atrial fibrillation may cause little hemodynamic impairment and is compatible with decades of uneventful survival. As with atrial flutter, atrial fibrillation occurs in many etiologic forms of heart disease. Chronic atrial inflammation and lack of effective atrial contraction promote left atrial thrombi and increased risk for systemic emboli. Atrial fibrillation may occur as an isolated arrhythmia in patients without heart disease or any other systemic illness. This condition has been called "lone atrial fibrillation."

MANAGEMENT. The objective of treating acute atrial fibrillation is to slow the rate. For symptomatic hypotension, immediate cardioversion is indicated. Usually, rate is controlled with IV digoxin (see Table 45–11). Verapamil or beta-blocking drugs are useful adjuncts for achieving rate control but can aggravate heart failure or cause hypotension. Digitalis and verapamil are best avoided in patients with the WPW syndrome because they can increase the ventricular rate and trigger ventricular fibrillation.

Multifocal Atrial Tachycardia

ECG DIAGNOSIS. The ECG features of multifocal atrial tachycardia are frequent APD's, often occurring in runs that

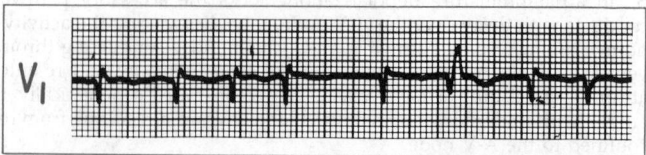

FIGURE 45–13. Aberrant conduction in atrial fibrillation (the Ashman phenomenon). The sixth QRS complex has a right bundle branch appearance. Note that this complex ends a long R-R–short R-R sequence and that its initial forces are similar to those of the other QRS complexes. These features suggest aberrant conduction of a supraventricular impulse. (From Braunwald E.: Heart Disease: A Textbook of Cardiovascular Medicine. Philadelphia, W. B. Saunders Company, 1980.)

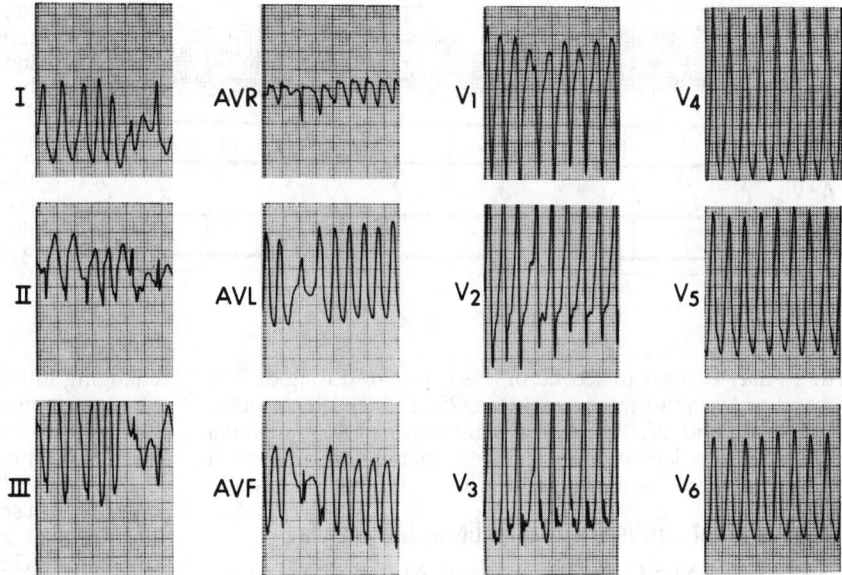

FIGURE 45–14. Atrial fibrillation in the Wolff-Parkinson-White syndrome. The electrocardiogram demonstrates the irregularly irregular response associated with anomalous-appearing QRS complexes resulting from atrial fibrillation with rapid conduction over the accessory pathway to the ventricle.

TG M79212

have dramatically different P wave morphology and marked variability in PP interval.

CLINICAL FEATURES. This rhythm occurs in patients with decompensated or overtreated chronic obstructive pulmonary disease. These patients often have severe derangement of arterial blood gases and electrolytes and are being treated aggressively with theophylline or catecholamines or both.

MANAGEMENT. Multifocal atrial tachycardia is resistant to digitalis therapy. Therapy is directed at improving ventilation and eradicating infection to improve arterial blood gases. The dose of bronchodilators may need to be reduced as well. Verapamil can be used to control the arrhythmia while the other medications are adjusted.

Sinoatrial Block

ECG DIAGNOSIS. Impulses generated in the sinus node may conduct slowly or block in the junction between the sinus node and atrium. First-degree sinoatrial (SA) block, i.e., a delay in conduction from sinus node to the atrium, cannot be recognized in the standard ECG but can be identified by electrophysiologic studies. Second-degree SA block can be diagnosed electrocardiographically. Type I second-degree SA block is recognized by Wenckebach periodicity of the PP intervals (see Fig. 45–15). In type II second-degree SA block, the PP interval suddenly lengthens to a value almost precisely

twice that of the usual PP interval. Third-degree SA block causes atrial arrest.

CLINICAL FEATURES. Sinoatrial block indicates intrinsic sinus node disease, electrolyte disturbance, or an adverse drug effect, most often digitalis. Class I antiarrhythmic drugs also cause SA block in patients with pre-existing sinus node dysfunction.

Sick Sinus Syndrome. The sick sinus syndrome is characterized by intrinsic inadequacy of sinus node pacemaking or conduction failure between the sinus node and the rest of the atrium, or both. In the bradycardia-tachycardia syndrome, recurrent supraventricular tachyarrhythmias alternate with sinus bradycardia or subatrial bradyarrhythmias or both. Conduction disturbances are common in the atria, AV node, bundle branches, and ventricles, but ventricular ectopic activity is rare.

Symptoms in sick sinus syndrome may be intermittent, varied, and difficult to correlate with ECG changes. Syncope, dizziness, and palpitations are common, probably because these symptoms are used for case finding and diagnosis. Congestive heart failure or angina can be aggravated. Cerebral thromboembolism is common in the bradycardia-tachycardia syndrome. Treatment of atrial fibrillation in the sick sinus syndrome can cause severe bradycardia. A temporary ventricular pacemaker should be used when attempting to convert atrial fibrillation with slow ventricular rate.

MANAGEMENT. Persistent, symptomatic sinus bradycardia is an indication for pacemaker therapy. Digitalis can be used to control the atrial tachyarrhythmias and, contrary to expectation, usually does not aggravate coexistent bradyarrhythmias. After pacemaker implantation, class I antiarrhythmic drugs can be used to control tachyarrhythmias. Symptoms can be improved with pacemaker therapy in the bradycardia-tachycardia syndrome, but cerebral thromboembolism continues. The prognosis of effectively treated sick sinus syndrome is determined by the associated heart disease.

ATRIOVENTRICULAR JUNCTIONAL ARRHYTHMIAS
Atrioventricular Junctional Premature Depolarizations

ECG DIAGNOSIS. Atrioventricular junctional premature depolarizations are much less common than either atrial or ventricular premature depolarizations. Typical ECG features are an abnormally premature or absent P wave and a premature QRS complex with a normal configuration. The position of the premature P wave (P') is critical to the diagnosis.

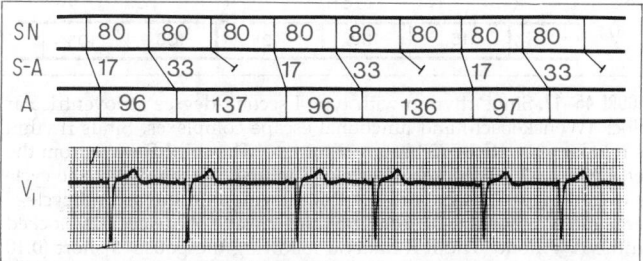

FIGURE 45–15. Second-degree sinoatrial block, type I (Wenckebach). The ECG shows periodicity of the P waves and QRS complex. The PR is constant. This pattern is consistent with a constant sinus node rate of 75 per minute (sinus cycle length = 800 msec) with 3:2 sinoatrial shock. The sinoatrial conduction times are assumed. (From Braunwald E.: Heart Disease: A Textbook of Cardiovascular Medicine. Philadelphia, W. B. Saunders Company, 1980.)

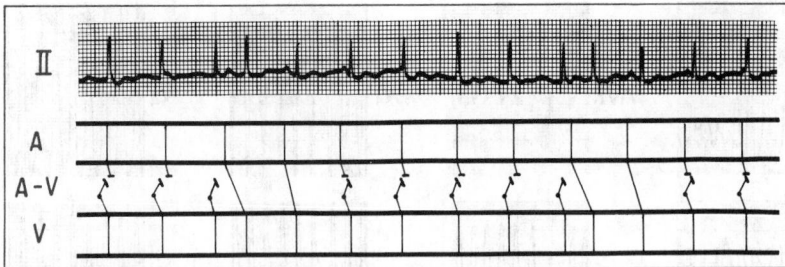

FIGURE 45–16. Nonparoxysmal atrioventricular junctional tachycardia with atrial capture of the ventricles. Two independent rhythms coexist: sinus tachycardia at 107 beats per minute and atrioventricular junctional tachycardia at 115 beats per minute. Sinus rhythm always controls the atria. The ventricles are usually controlled by the A-V junctional focus, because its rate is faster. When time relationships are appropriate, atrial depolarizations propagate through the A-V junction and capture the ventricles. (From Braunwald E.: Heart Disease: A Textbook of Cardiovascular Medicine. Philadelphia, W. B. Saunders Company, 1980.)

The P' may occur 0.10 second or less before or during or 0.20 second or less after the premature QRS. The P' is inverted in leads II, III, and aV_F. The clinical significance of AV junctional premature depolarizations is similar to that of nonparoxysmal AV junctional tachycardia (see below).

Nonparoxysmal Atrioventricular Junctional Tachycardia

ECG DIAGNOSIS. Nonparoxysmal AV junctional tachycardia is caused by enhanced automaticity in the AV junction. The junctional focus depolarizes at a rate between 70 and 130 per minute (see Fig. 45–16). The QRS complex usually is normal or slightly aberrant. If the AV junctional focus captures the atria, the retrograde P may be positioned 0.10 second or less in front of the QRS, simultaneous with the QRS, or 0.20 second or less after the QRS. This arrhythmia often is associated with AV nodal conduction impairment and AV dissociation. The atrial rhythm may intermittently capture the junctional focus and ventricle (see Fig. 45–16).

CLINICAL FEATURES. Nonparoxysmal AV junctional tachycardia has great significance because it is associated specifically with acute inferior myocardial infarction, digitalis toxicity, acute carditis (e.g., viral myocarditis or acute rheumatic fever), or surgical trauma.

MANAGEMENT. Treatment should be focused on the underlying condition, e.g., myocarditis or digitalis toxicity. In acute inferior myocardial infarction, and after open heart surgery, nonparoxysmal AV junctional tachycardia is usually transient and requires no therapy. In digitalis toxicity, this arrhythmia should prompt intensive management of toxicity.

Atrioventricular Block

ECG DIAGNOSIS. Atrioventricular block is classified as first, second, and third degree. First-degree AV block, i.e., a prolonged PR interval, is caused by conduction delay in the AV node. Second-degree AV block is subdivided into type I (AV nodal) and type II (His-Purkinje). Type I second-degree AV block has characteristic Wenckebach periodicity, i.e., the PR interval prolongs with each cycle until a P wave fails to conduct to the ventricles (see Fig. 45–17). The longest RR interval is less than twice the shortest RR interval. Type II second-degree AV block is recognized by the sudden failure of a P wave to conduct to the ventricles without previous lengthening of the PR interval. Type II AV block nearly always occurs in patients with bundle branch disease, and the site of block is distal to the AV node.

In third-degree AV block, sinus or some other atrial rhythm controls the atria, whereas the ventricles are controlled by an independent AV junctional or ventricular pacemaker. The QRS usually is prolonged, and the ventricular rate is between 35 and 50 per minute.

CLINICAL FEATURES. First-degree AV block produces no symptoms but may cause the first heart sound to be soft because the AV valves almost close before ventricular contraction. Second-degree AV block usually causes no symptoms unless the ventricular rate becomes very slow. It may be possible to discern second-degree AV block by characteristic pulse intervals, intermittent, prominent "A" waves, and

changing intensity of the first heart sound. In complete heart block with sinus rhythm, the pulse is slow, full, and regular; intermittent cannon "A" waves occur in the jugular venous pulse; and the first heart sound varies in intensity.

MANAGEMENT. First-degree AV block requires no treatment. Type I second-degree AV block usually resolves without the need for a temporary pacemaker. When type I block is caused by a chronic AV junctional disease, block can progress slowly to complete AV block. Type II second-degree AV block usually results from chronic bundle branch disease and often progresses to complete heart block. Chronic, symptomatic second- or third-degree AV block should be treated with an implanted pacemaker.

VENTRICULAR ARRHYTHMIAS
Ventricular Premature Depolarizations (VPD's)

ECG DIAGNOSIS. The QRS is premature, wide, and often bizarre in appearance; the ST segment and T wave are opposite in direction to the QRS complex; and no premature P wave precedes the premature QRS complex (see Fig. 45–18). As the impulse leaves its ectopic site of origin, it activates the ventricle in an abnormal sequence, accounting for the striking QRS-T changes. Typically, the VPD is followed by a fully compensatory pause, i.e., the RV interval, and the VR interval is equal to two RR intervals in sinus rhythm (see Fig. 45–18). Ventricular premature depolarizations may be *interpolated* between two successive sinus complexes. "Concealed" retrograde conduction of the interpolated VPD into the AV node causes the PR interval of the subsequent sinus complex to prolong. Certain patterns of VPD's have special names. When every other QRS is a VPD, the pattern is termed *bigeminy*; a

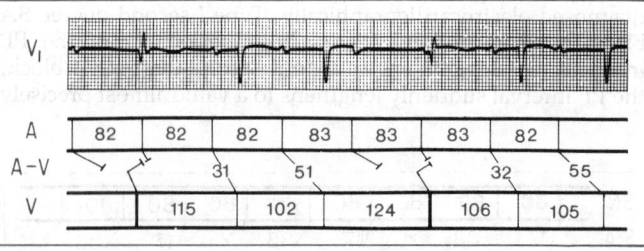

FIGURE 45–17. Sinus rhythm with type I second-degree atrioventricular block (Wenckebach) and junctional escape complexes. Sinus rhythm is regular at a rate of 73 beats per minute. The third P wave from the left begins a 3:2 Wenckebach cycle. The first P-R interval of the cycle is quite long (0.31 sec), and the P-R increment in the second cycle is large (an additional 0.20 sec). The third P wave of the cycle is blocked in the A-V node. The P-R interval following the pause is short (0.10 sec), and the QRS complex is aberrant; this is a junctional escape complex. The tracing demonstrates both impaired conduction and enhanced automaticity in the A-V junction. Type I A-V block nearly always occurs in the A-V node, and A-V junctional escape complexes are presumed to arise in the bundle of His or the most proximal portions of the bundle branches. (From Braunwald E.: Heart Disease: A Textbook of Cardiovascular Medicine. Philadelphia, W. B. Saunders Company, 1980.)

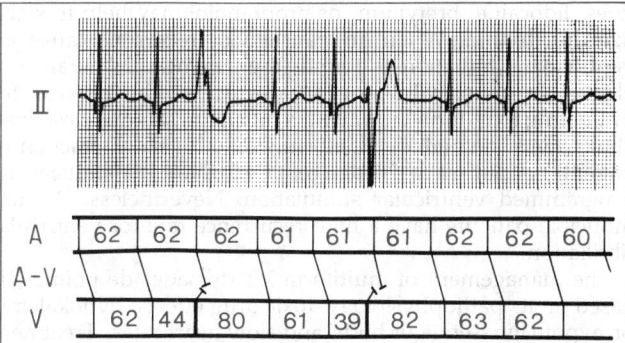

FIGURE 45–18. Multiformed ventricular premature depolarizations. The third and sixth QRS complexes are VPD's with strikingly different configurations. Also, the coupling interval of the two VPD's differs by 50 msec. Such a difference in configuration may be due either to a different site of origin or to a difference in the sequence of ventricular activation from the same site of origin. (From Braunwald E.: Heart Disease: A Textbook of Cardiovascular Medicine. Philadelphia, W. B. Saunders Company, 1980.)

VPD every third QRS is termed *trigeminy*; and two successive VPD's are termed a *pair* or a *couplet*.

CLINICAL FEATURES. Infrequent VPD's are commonly found even in young persons, and VPD frequency increases with age. Although sporadic VPD's in persons with normal hearts do not seem to affect outcome adversely, VPD's confer significant risk of subsequent cardiac death in persons with heart disease. When VPD's are caused by drug toxicity, e.g., digitalis, quinidine, or tricyclic antidepressants, lethal rhythm disturbances may ensue unless the drug is discontinued. A strong association exists between myocardial infarct size and the frequency of VPD's in acute myocardial infarction, and a weak association exists between poor left ventricular function and frequency of VPD's during recovery.

MANAGEMENT. The most important issue in the treatment of VPD's is the selection of patients for treatment. In general, only symptomatic VPD's need treatment, and class IC or class II antiarrhythmic drugs (see Table 45–9) are the first choices for treatment of benign and potentially malignant ventricular arrhythmias. Intravenously administered lidocaine or procainamide is usually used to treat VPD's occurring immediately after myocardial infarction or cardiac surgery.

Ventricular Tachycardia

ECG DIAGNOSIS. The most prevalent definition of ventricular tachycardia (VT) is three or more VPD's in succession at a rate of 100 per min or greater. Ventricular tachycardia may be unsustained, i.e., last less than 15 to 30 seconds, or sustained (see Fig. 45–19). In a tachycardia with wide QRS complexes, two findings strongly suggest VT: *ventricular captures* and *fusion complexes*. Sinus impulses may capture the ventricle during VT, producing either a normal QRS (ventricular capture) or a QRS intermediate in contour between normal and the QRS of ventricular tachycardia (fusion complex). Sustained VT can be difficult to distinguish from supraventricular arrhythmias with a wide QRS complex. A His bundle recording can easily distinguish between these two possibilities (Fig. 45–10).

CLINICAL FEATURES. Unsustained VT nearly always occurs in patients with heart disease, most often in those with coronary heart disease. After myocardial infarction, about 10 per cent of patients have VT detected by a single 24-hour continuous ECG recording. Patients with class III or IV heart failure have a 40 to 50 per cent prevalence of VT in a 24-hour ECG. Most episodes of VT in either setting are brief, i.e., three to five consecutive VPD's, and asymptomatic yet increase the risk of dying two- to fourfold. Sustained VT is rare

and has a poor prognosis. As with other tachyarrhythmias, the severity of symptoms in sustained VT is related primarily to the rate of the tachycardia and left ventricular function. Sustained VT is prone to deteriorate into ventricular fibrillation (Fig. 45–19).

MANAGEMENT. The management of symptomatic, unsustained VT is the same as that described above for VPD's. Sustained VT in chronic heart disease is treated acutely with IV lidocaine or procainamide, if the patient is hemodynamically stable, or by DC cardioversion, if unstable (Fig. 45–19). Baseline studies should include 48 hours of continuous ECG recording, exercise testing, and endocardial electrical stimulation. The drug-dose finding and long-term management of these patients should be guided by rigorous methods with high predictive accuracy. The standard method is endocardial electrical stimulation. A programmatic noninvasive approach using 24-hour continuous ECG recordings and exercise tests also can be used. The usual sequence for drug testing is class IA (e.g., quinidine or procainamide), IA plus IB (e.g., quinidine and mexiletine), IC (e.g., encainide or flecainide), and finally III (amiodarone). If an effective drug is not found, an implantable defibrillator is usually the best treatment. In selected cases, surgery is the best choice.

Accelerated Idioventricular Rhythm

ECG DIAGNOSIS. Accelerated idioventricular rhythm (AIVR) is defined as three or more consecutive QRS complexes of ventricular origin with a rate between 50 and 100 per minute (see Fig. 45–20). Fusion QRS complexes often begin or end an episode of AIVR.

CLINICAL FEATURES. Accelerated idioventricular rhythm occurs in about 30 per cent of patients during the course of either inferior or anterior acute myocardial infarction. Accelerated idioventricular rhythm frequently follows coronary reperfusion. This rhythm is usually asymptomatic and therefore needs no treatment. The incidence of ventricular fibrillation and hospital mortality is not increased in patients who have AIVR.

Ventricular Parasystole

ECG DIAGNOSIS. Ventricular parasystole is an automatic rhythm in the His-Purkinje system that competes with sinus

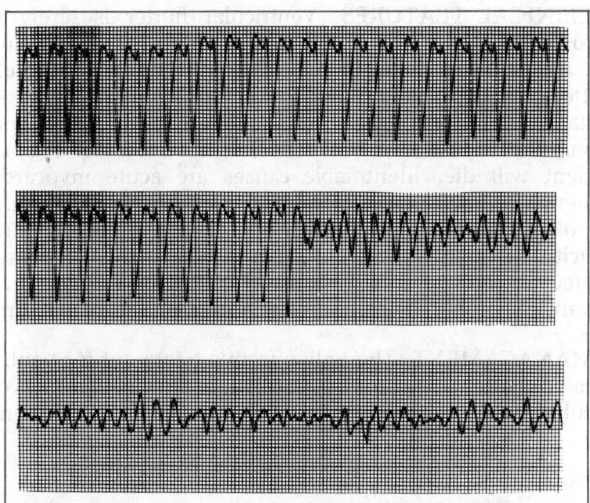

FIGURE 45–19. Ventricular tachycardia and ventricular fibrillation. Three continuous strips from lead V4 of a Holter electrocardiograph. The top strip shows ventricular tachycardia at 214 cycles per minute—an unusually rapid rate for ventricular tachycardia. Ventricular fibrillation begins in the middle strip and continues on the bottom strip. Note the irregularity in amplitude and period of deflections recorded during ventricular fibrillation. (From Braunwald E.: Heart Disease: A Textbook of Cardiovascular Medicine. Philadelphia, W. B. Saunders Company, 1980.)

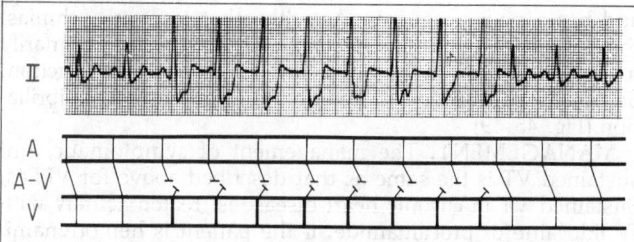

FIGURE 45–20. Accelerated idioventricular rhythm. Sinus rhythm at 88 cycles per minute is interrupted by a rhythm with wide QRS complexes at 95 cycles per minute. Note that the P-R interval progressively shortens at the onset of the ventricular rhythm and that sinus rhythm continues unperturbed by the ventricular rhythm (atrioventricular dissociation). After eight QRS complexes of ventricular rhythm, sinus rhythm resumes. (From Braunwald E.: Heart Disease: A Textbook of Cardiovascular Medicine. Philadelphia, W. B. Saunders Company, 1980.)

rhythm. Parasystole has two cardinal features: variable coupling of VPD's and a common denominator for interectopic intervals. Entrance block removes the parasystolic focus from the suppressant influence of the sinus impulses, permitting a stable automatic rhythm to emerge; the ectopic focus will activate the ventricle every time it fires unless the ventricle is refractory (Fig. 45–20).

CLINICAL FEATURES. Parasystole often is resistant to antiarrhythmic drug therapy, and untreated patients seem to have a good prognosis.

Ventricular Flutter and Fibrillation

ECG DIAGNOSIS. The electrocardiographic diagnosis of ventricular flutter is made when the ventricular tachyarrhythmia has large sinusoidal or zigzag QRS's and the rate is between 240 and 280 per minute. Multiform VT, or torsades de pointes, is recognized by the periodic twisting of the points of the QRS complexes (see Fig. 45–21). Ventricular fibrillation is recognized in the ECG by the absence of QRS complexes and T waves and the presence of low-amplitude baseline undulations that are variable in both amplitude and periodicity (see Fig. 45–19).

CLINICAL FEATURES. Ventricular flutter is rarely recorded, because it is unstable and tends to convert to sinus rhythm or, more often, to ventricular fibrillation. Ventricular flutter or fibrillation is catastrophic. Cardiac pumping ceases instantly, the patient loses consciousness, and, if cardiopulmonary resuscitation is not started within a few minutes, the patient will die. Identifiable causes are acute myocardial ischemia or infarction; marked electrolyte disturbances, e.g., hypokalemia; marked hypothermia; electrocution; and drug toxicity. Most victims of ventricular fibrillation who are resuscitated do *not* have one of these conditions but do have advanced coronary atherosclerosis and poor ventricular function.

MANAGEMENT. The only effective treatment for ventricular fibrillation is prompt defibrillation. In most cases, ventricular fibrillation will not recur after defibrillation. When it

does, lidocaine, bretylium, or propranolol may help to stabilize the rhythm. When no transient or reversible cause for ventricular fibrillation is found (e.g., myocardial infarction, electrolyte abnormality, or drug toxicity), the process for evaluating long-term treatment is much the same as described above for sustained VT. Unfortunately, a smaller fraction of patients, about 60 to 70 per cent, will have VT induced by programmed ventricular stimulation. Nevertheless, the uninducible patients have a high recurrence rate for ventricular fibrillation.

The management of multiform VT (torsades de pointes) is based on its pathophysiology: toxic drug effects, hypokalemia or hypomagnesemia or both, and slow heart rates. Treatment may include avoidance of class I antiarrhythmic drugs, ventricular pacing, reducing the level of the culprit drug, repletion of electrolytes, and catecholamine or magnesium sulfate infusion.

PROGNOSTIC CLASSIFICATION OF VENTRICULAR ARRHYTHMIAS. Table 45–8 outlines the classification of ventricular arrhythmias as determined by the presence of heart disease, left ventricular function, and arrhythmia characteristics. Prognosis is an important basis for deciding whom to treat and how to sequence the treatment choices.

Bigger JT Jr, Reiffel JA: Sick sinus syndrome. Ann Rev Med 30:91, 1979. *A comprehensive review of the human sinus node dysfunction. Liberally referenced.*

Marriott HJL: Practical Electrocardiography. Baltimore, Williams & Wilkins Company, 1983. *A textbook designed to emphasize the simplicities of the ECG, provide only those concepts that make everyday ECG interpretation more intelligible, and provide illustrations and discussion of all-important ECG patterns. Excellent for learning or reviewing the ECG patterns of arrhythmias.*

Zipes DP: Specific Arrhythmias: Diagnosis and treatment. In Braunwald E (ed.): Heart Disease: A Textbook of Cardiovascular Medicine. Philadelphia, W. B. Saunders Company, 1984, pp 683–743. *Detailed description of the clinical features, electrocardiographic recognition, and treatment of cardiac arrhythmias. Contains 48 figures and 375 references.*

ANTIARRHYTHMIC DRUGS

Classification of Antiarrhythmic Drugs

Antiarrhythmic drugs have been classified according to their mechanisms of action into four classes (see Table 45–9). One could think of digitalis as having class V drug action, i.e., a strong cholinergic action that can repolarize stretched or damaged atrial cells and thereby speed conduction. Digitalis glycosides slow conduction in the AV node, tending to abolish re-entrant rhythms that use that structure.

Use-Dependent Block of Ionic Channels—An Antiarrhythmic Action

Many antiarrhythmic drugs act on ionic channels in the sarcolemma. Class I antiarrhythmic drugs block the Na^+ channel so that ionic conductance falls to zero until the drug dissociates from the channel. Most class I drugs bind to open or inactivated channels; drug-associated channels have slow or incomplete reactivation. Drug binding and Na^+ channel blockade increase with rate, producing *use-dependent block*. If the association and dissociation of drug from the Na^+ channel both are rapid, use-dependent block will attain a steady state after a few action potentials, and if the interval between action potentials is reasonably long, little block will persist at the

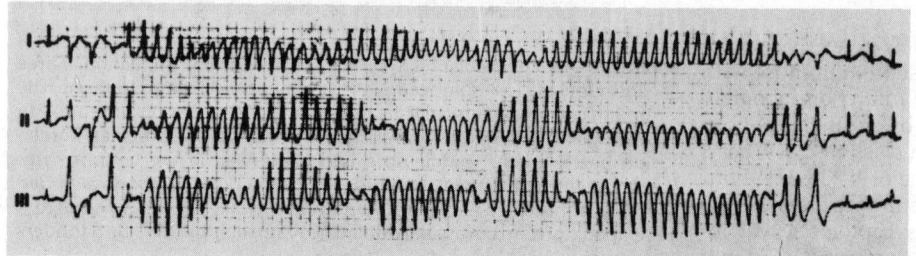

FIGURE 45–21. Torsades de pointes. Sinus rhythm associated with a long Q-T interval is present at the beginning and at the end of this rhythm strip. Sinus rhythm is interrupted by a rapid wide QRS tachycardia. Note that during the tachycardia, the direction of the points of the QRS complex appears to revolve around an imaginary isolelectric line. (From Krikler DM, Curry DVL: Br Heart J 38:118, 1976. With permission of the British Heart Journal and authors.)

TABLE 45–8. PROGNOSTIC CLASSIFICATION OF VENTRICULAR ARRHYTHMIAS

	Benign	Potentially Malignant	Malignant
Risk for sudden death	Very low	Moderate	High
Clinical presentation	Palpitations; detected by routine examination	Palpitations; detected by routine examination or screening	Palpitations; syncope; cardiac arrest
Heart disease	Usually absent	Present	Present
Cardiac scarring and/or hypertrophy	Absent	Present	Present
VPD frequency	Low to moderate	Moderate to high	Moderate to high
Paired VPD and/or unsustained ventricular tachycardia	Absent	Common	Common
Sustained ventricular tachycardia	Absent	Absent	Present
Hemodynamic effects of arrhythmia	Absent	Absent; mild	Moderate; severe

VPD = ventricular premature depolarization.

The characteristics listed in this table are typical and do not represent the full range of observations. For example, benign ventricular arrhythmias can be frequent and, occasionally, repetitive.

time of the next action potential upstroke. If dissociation is slow, use-dependent block will require many action potentials to develop fully, and a significant degree of block will remain at the time of each action potential upstroke.

SPECIFIC ANTIARRHYTHMIC DRUGS

This section gives a brief summary of the pharmacology and indications for each antiarrhythmic drug. This information is supplemented by information given in tables; Table 45–10 gives pharmacokinetic data for the drugs, and Table 45–11 gives information on dosing and on contraindications, precautions, and adverse effects.

Class IB Antiarrhythmic Drugs

LIDOCAINE. Lidocaine is a local anesthetic used frequently, since the early 1960's, for the intravenous treatment of ventricular arrhythmias in the intensive care unit setting because of two major advantages: It reaches a steady state rapidly after starting or changing the dose, and it lacks significant adverse hemodynamic effects.

Pharmacology. Lidocaine prevents re-entrant rhythms, decreases automaticity in Purkinje fibers, and increases the ventricular fibrillation threshold. Lidocaine has an intense depressant action on depolarized tissues, but almost none on normal cardiac cells. The drug has a negligible effect on the ECG. Lidocaine shortens the effective refractory period (ERP) of the His-Purkinje system. It has no significant effect on the autonomic nervous system.

Indications. Lidocaine is used only for ventricular arrhythmias, particularly those caused by acute myocardial infarction, open heart surgery, and digitalis intoxication. Lidocaine is relatively ineffective for ventricular arrhythmias in chronic coronary heart disease or cardiomyopathy.

Pharmacokinetics. Lidocaine is administered intravenously and, rarely, intramuscularly. Plasma lidocaine concentration dynamically follows the hepatic blood flow. About 70 per cent of lidocaine in the plasma is bound to alpha$_1$-acid glycoprotein,

an acute phase reactant. At a given total plasma concentration, the free concentration will fall as the alpha$_1$-acid glycoprotein increases in the first few days after infarction or surgery.

MEXILETINE. Mexiletine is a new orally active local anesthetic that is similar to lidocaine chemically and electrophysiologically.

Pharmacology. Mexiletine has an antiautomatic effect on Purkinje fibers and depresses phase 0 of fast action potentials more than lidocaine. It shortens the action potential duration and refractoriness of Purkinje fibers and ventricular muscle cells. Mexiletine has little effect on the ECG.

Indications. Like lidocaine, this drug is not indicated for atrial arrhythmias, and its efficacy is less than the class IA or class IC antiarrhythmic drugs for ventricular arrhythmias. In chronic coronary heart disease or cardiomyopathy, the drug is about 60 per cent effective in controlling unsustained ventricular arrhythmias.

PHENYTOIN. Phenytoin* is an anticonvulsant drug that is electrophysiologically very similar to lidocaine and has no significant effect on the ECG. Phenytoin has complex central autonomic actions that decrease efferent traffic on cardiac sympathetic nerves in digitalis toxicity. Phenytoin has no peripheral cholinergic or beta-adrenergic–blocking activity.

Indications. Phenytoin is used to treat paroxysmal atrial flutter or fibrillation, supraventricular arrhythmias, and ventricular arrhythmias caused by digitalis but is ineffective for the common atrial arrhythmias, e.g., atrial flutter, atrial fibrillation, and PSVT. Phenytoin is effective against ventricular arrhythmias after acute myocardial infarction or open heart surgery, but lidocaine is easier to use. Plasma concentrations above 10 µg per milliliter are effective for reducing ventricular arrhythmias in the year after myocardial infarction. Phenytoin, like other class I antiarrhythmic drugs, is relatively ineffective against recurrent, drug-resistant VT in patients with chronic coronary heart disease.

Pharmacokinetics. The enzymes that metabolize phenytoin can saturate at antiarrhythmic plasma concentrations, causing plasma concentration to rise sharply to toxic levels. Phenytoin should not be infused because its alkaline pH causes severe phlebitis.

TOCAINIDE. Tocainide is an orally effective analogue of lidocaine that has cardiac electrophysiologic effects almost identical to those of lidocaine and has almost no effects on the ECG. In addition, it is well tolerated hemodynamically.

Indications. Tocainide is indicated for the oral treatment of ventricular arrhythmias. The drug is similar to mexiletine in its efficacy, i.e., it controls about 60 per cent of the chronic unsustained ventricular arrhythmias. There is about a 70 per cent concordance between the responses to IV lidocaine and oral tocainide.

TABLE 45–9. CLASSIFICATION OF ANTIARRHYTHMIC DRUGS ACCORDING TO THEIR MECHANISM OF ACTION

Class	Action	Drugs
I. Sodium channel blockade		
A.	Minimal phase 0 depression Slow conduction 0 to 1+ Shorten repolarization	Lidocaine; mexiletine; tocainide
B.	Moderate phase 0 depression Slow conduction 2 + Prolong repolarization	Quinidine; procainamide; disopyramide
C.	Marked phase 0 depression Slow conduction 4 + Little effect on repolarization	Encainide; flecainide
II. Beta-adrenergic blockade		Propranolol; acebutolol
III. Prolong repolarization		Amiodarone; bretylium; sotalol
IV. Calcium channel blockade		Diltiazem; verapamil

*This use of phenytoin is not listed in the manufacturer's directive.

Text continued on page 270

TABLE 45–10. PHARMACOKINETIC PROPERTIES OF ANTIARRHYTHMIC DRUGS

Drug	Volume of Distribution (liters/kg)	Half-time of Elimination (hr)	Bioavailability (%)	Major Route of Elimination	Protein Binding (%)	Effective Plasma Concentration (μg/ml)
Digoxin	10.0	24–72	50–80	Kidney	25	>0.0008
Lidocaine	1.0	1–3	—	Liver	70	1.5–5
Mexiletine	9.5	8–14	80–90	Liver	60	0.7–2.0
Phenytoin	0.7	18–30	60–80	Liver	90	8–20
Tocainide	3.0	10–14	80–90	Kidney; liver	10	6–15
Disopyramide	0.8	7–9	75–90	Kidney	Dose dependent	2–5
Procainamide	2.0	3–6	75–85	Kidney; liver	15	4–20
Quinidine	2.5	5–9	70–80	Liver	90	2–6
Encainide	4.0	1–3	20–40	Liver	80	—
Flecainide	10.0	13–30	>90	Kidney; liver	40	0.2–1.0
Acebutolol	1.2	2–4	35–45	Kidney; liver	25	—
Propranolol	4.0	3–6	20–50	Liver	>90	0.04–0.9
Amiodarone	60.0	500–1000	30–40	Liver	>95	0.5–2.5
Bretylium	6.0	8–12	20–30	Kidney	5	—
Diltiazem	5.5	2–6	40–50	Liver	75	0.5–2.0
Verapamil	4.0	4–10	10–35	Liver	90	0.1–0.2

TABLE 45–11. DOSING AND ADVERSE EFFECTS OF ANTIARRHYTHMIC DRUGS

	Usual IV Dose		Usual Oral Dose				
	Loading	Maintenance	Loading	Maintenance	Contraindications	Precautions	Adverse Effects
Digoxin							
Tablets 0.125, 0.25, 0.5 mg	—	—	0.5–1.00 mg p.o., followed by 0.125–0.375 mg p.o. in 6–8 hr	0.125–0.375 mg p.o. once a day	Hypersensitivity to the drug	Reduce dose in renal insufficiency; hypokalemia, hypomagnesemia, and hypercalcemia predispose to digitalis toxicity; may accelerate the ventricular response to atrial flutter or fibrillation in Wolff-Parkinson-White syndrome; may worsen outflow obstruction in HOCM; serum digoxin concentration increased by quinidine and verapamil; absorption may be increased by some antibiotics; use cautiously with beta blockers or calcium channel antagonists in atrial fibrillation	Ventricular arrhythmias, including ventricular tachycardia; accelerated junctional rhythms; atrial tachycardia with AV block; AV dissociation; progression of AV block
Lanoxicaps capsules 0.05, 0.1, 0.2 mg	—	—	—	0.1–0.3 mg p.o. once a day			Anorexia; nausea, vomiting; visual disturbances; weakness
IV 2-ml ampule, 0.25 mg/ml	0.5–1.00 mg IV, followed by 0.125–0.375 mg IV in 6–8 hr		—	—	—		
Pediatric preparation 1-ml ampule, 0.1 mg/ml	0.015–0.030 mg/kg IV, followed by 0.005–0.010 mg/kg/day (age dependent)		—	—			
Lidocaine							
IV	50–100 mg IV over 2–5 min; may repeat 50 mg after 5 min	10–40 μg/kg/min	—	—	Known hypersensitivity to local anesthetics of the amide type; patients with Stokes-Adams syndrome or with severe degrees of sinoatrial, AV, or intraventricular block in the absence of a pacemaker	Accumulation in heart failure, in hepatic or renal insufficiency, or after prolonged infusions; reduce dosage in children and elderly patients; safety in malignant hyperthermia not established; cimetidine and propranolol increase plasma lidocaine concentration	Bradycardia, hypotension, and cardiovascular collapse
IM	300 mg IM		—	—			Drowsiness; confusion; dizziness; respiratory depression and arrest; vomiting; visual disturbances; convulsions; twitching; unconsciousness; allergic reactions secondary to lidocaine sensitivity

TABLE 45–11. DOSING AND ADVERSE EFFECTS OF ANTIARRHYTHMIC DRUGS *Continued*

	Usual IV Dose		Usual Oral Dose		Contraindications	Precautions	Adverse Effects
	Loading	*Maintenance*	*Loading*	*Maintenance*			
Mexiletine Capsules 150, 200, 250 mg	—	—	400 mg p.o.	200–400 mg p.o. q. 8 hr	Cardiogenic shock; pre-existing second- or third-degree AV block in the absence of a pacemaker	Patients with first-degree AV block, sinus node dysfunction, intraventricular conduction abnormalities, hypotension, heart failure, liver disease; may worsen arrhythmias; mexiletine levels increased by cimetidine; use cautiously in patients with a history of seizures, hypotension, heart failure, or liver disease	GI distress; light-headedness; tremor; coordination difficulties; diplopia; paresthesia; confusion
Phenytoin* Tablets 100 mg	—	—	Day 1, 400 mg Day 2, 300 mg Day 3, 300 mg (1000 mg total)	100 mg p.o. t.i.d.; 200 mg p.o. b.i.d.	History of hypersensitivity to hydantoin products; sinus bradycardia, sinoatrial block, second- or third-degree AV block; Stokes-Adams syndrome	Use cautiously in presence of hypotension and myocardial depression; may worsen arrhythmias; discontinue if skin rash develops; may cause hypoglycemia; multiple drug interactions; may be associated with congenital malformations	Hypotension and bradycardia with rapid IV injection Nystagmus, ataxia, slurred speech; Stevens-Johnson syndrome; sensory neuropathy; lymphadenopathy; pancytopenia; megaloblastic anemia; gingival hyperplasia; hyperglycemia; hypocalcemia
Extended capsules 100 mg	—	—	—	300 mg or 400 mg p.o. q. day			
IV 2-ml ampules, 50 mg/ml 5-ml ampules, 50 mg/ml	100 mg IV q. 5 min to a maximum of 1000 mg	—	—	—			
Tocainide Tablets 400, 600 mg	—	—	—	400–800 mg p.o. q. 8 hr	Hypersensitivity to this drug or to local anesthetics of the amide type; second- or third-degree AV block in the absence of a pacemaker	May cause blood dyscrasias, pulmonary fibrosis, pneumonitis; may aggravate heart failure or worsen ventricular arrhythmias; may accelerate the ventricular response in atrial fibrillation; accumulates in severe renal or hepatic insufficiency	Nausea, vomiting; light-headedness; dizziness; tremor; diplopia; paresthesia; confusion; *agranulocytosis*; thrombocytopenia; hypoplastic anemia
Disopyramide Capsules 100, 150 mg	—	—	300 mg p.o.	100–200 mg p.o. q. 6 hr	Cardiogenic shock; pre-existing second- or third-degree AV block in the absence of a pacemaker; congenital QT prolongation; known hypersensitivity to the drug	*Use cautiously with left ventricular dysfunction*, sick sinus syndrome, bundle branch block, or AV block; prior digitalization suggested for atrial flutter or fibrillation to prevent increase in ventricular rate; may precipitate myasthenia crisis, glaucoma, or urinary retention; may cause hypoglycemia; serum level may be lowered by phenytoin	*Heart failure;* worsening of arrhythmias; AV block; hypotension; may cause significant prolongation of QRS and QT intervals *Urinary retention;* dry mouth; constipation; blurred vision; impotence; cholestatic jaundice; fever; thrombocytopenia; granulocytopenia; gynecomastia
Norpace CR (controlled release) 100, 150 mg	—	—	—	200–400 mg p.o. q. 12 hr			
Procainamide HCl Tablets, capsules 250, 375, 500 mg	—	—	1 gm p.o.	500–1250 mg p.o. q. 3–4 hr	Second- or third-degree AV block unless a pacemaker is present; torsades de pointes; lupus-like syndrome; hypersensitivity to the drug	Reduce dosage in renal insufficiency; may accelerate the ventricular response in atrial fibrillation or atrial flutter; may exacerbate myasthenia gravis	Hypotension; worsening of ventricular arrhythmias; myocardial depression; AV block
Procainamide SR (sustained release) 250, 500, 750, 1000 mg	—	—	—	1000–3000 mg p.o. q. 6–8 hr			

*This use of phenytoin is not listed in the manufacturer's directive.

TABLE 45–11. DOSING AND ADVERSE EFFECTS OF ANTIARRHYTHMIC DRUGS *Continued*

	Usual IV Dose		Usual Oral Dose		Contraindications	Precautions	Adverse Effects
	Loading	*Maintenance*	*Loading*	*Maintenance*			
Procainamide HCl for IV use	100 mg injected q. 5 min IV for 7–10 doses or 20 mg/min infusion IV for 40–60 min	20–80 μg/kg/min	—	—			*Lupus-like syndrome;* GI distress; *agranulocytosis;* hemolytic anemia; fever; thrombocytopenia; rash; myalgia; hallucinations, psychosis
Quinidine sulfate Tablets 100, 200, 300 mg	—	—	—	200–500 mg p.o. q.i.d.	Hypersensitivity to quinidine; complete AV block; complete bundle branch block or other severe intraventricular conduction defects exhibiting marked QRS widening; myasthenia gravis; arrhythmias due to digitalis toxicity	May accelerate the ventricular response to atrial flutter or atrial fibrillation; *concurrent use with digoxin will increase plasma digoxin levels;* drugs that increase hepatic drug-metabolizing enzymes decrease the plasma concentration of quinidine; may worsen heart failure; test dose recommended because of idiosyncratic response; may require change in oral anticoagulant dose	Hypotension; worsening of ventricular arrhythmias; asystole; may increase AV or bundle branch block; may cause significant prolongation of QRS and QT intervals; *syncope; torsades de pointes*
Quinidine Extentabs (sustained release) 300 mg	—	—	—	300–600 mg p.o. q. 8–12 hr			
Quinidine gluconate 330 mg (200-mg quinidine base)	—	—	—	330–660 mg p. o. q. 8 hr			*Diarrhea;* nausea; *thrombocytopenia;* hemolytic anemia; granulocytopenia; fever; visual disturbances; hypersensitivity reaction; cinchonism; rash
Quinidine polygalacturonate 275 mg (200-mg quinidine base)	—	—	—				
Encainide* Tablets 25, 35, 50 mg	—	—	—	25–50 mg p.o. t.i.d.	Second- or third-degree AV block or right bundle branch block with associated hemiblock unless a pacemaker is in place; cardiogenic shock; known hypersensitivity	May worsen sinus node dysfunction; increases pacing thresholds; may suppress ventricular escape rhythms; reduce dose with renal insufficiency; cimetidine increases encainide serum concentration	*New or worsened ventricular tachycardia or ventricular fibrillation;* second- or third-degree AV block Dizziness, vertigo; visual disturbances; headache; leg cramps
Flecainide Tablets 100 mg	—	—	—	100–200 mg p.o. b.i.d.	Second- or third-degree AV block or right bundle branch block with associated hemiblock unless a pacemaker is in place; cardiogenic shock; known hypersensitivity to the drug	May worsen sinus node dysfunction; increases pacing thresholds; may suppress ventricular escape rhythms; avoid concurrent administration of disopyramide or verapamil	*New or worsened ventricular tachycardia or ventricular fibrillation* in patients with sustained ventricular arrhythmias; *heart failure;* second- or third-degree AV block Dizziness; *visual disturbances;* dyspnea; hepatic dysfunction; blood dyscrasias
Acebutolol Capsules 200, 400 mg	—	—	—	200–600 mg p.o. q. 12 hr	Severe sinus bradycardia; second- and third-degree AV block; overt cardiac failure; cardiogenic shock	Exacerbation of angina may occur or myocardial infarction may occur following abrupt withdrawal; may mask symptoms of hypoglycemia or hyperthyroidism; cautious use in renal insufficiency or with concurrent alpha-adrenergic or catecholamine-depleting drugs	Congestive heart failure; bradycardia; hypotension; increase in AV block Fatigue; headache; dizziness; arterial insufficiency; bronchospasm; impotence

*Investigational drug.

TABLE 45-11. DOSING AND ADVERSE EFFECTS OF ANTIARRHYTHMIC DRUGS *Continued*

| | Usual IV Dose | | Usual Oral Dose | | Contraindications | Precautions | Adverse Effects |
	Loading	*Maintenance*	*Loading*	*Maintenance*			
Propranolol							
Tablets 10, 20, 40, 60, 80, 90 mg	—	—	—	10–160 mg p.o. q. 6 hr*	Cardiogenic shock; sinus bradycardia; second- or third-degree AV block; asthma; congestive heart failure	Exacerbation of angina may occur or myocardial infarction may occur following abrupt withdrawal; may mask symptoms of hypoglycemia or hyperthyroidism; may cause severe sinus bradycardia following termination of tachycardia; may worsen hypertension in pheochromocytoma unless used with an alpha-adrenergic–blocking drug	Congestive heart failure; bradycardia; increase in degree of AV block; hypotension
Inderal LA capsules 80, 120, 160 mg	—	—	—	One daily*			Bronchospasm; arterial insufficiency; Raynaud's phenomenon; mental depression; sleep disturbances; weakness; impotence; disorientation; memory loss; blood dyscrasias
IV 1-mg ampule	1–3 mg, at rate ≤ 1 mg/min	—	—	—			
Amiodarone							
Tablets 200 mg	—	—	800–1600 mg per day for 1–3 weeks; 600–800 mg per day for 4 weeks	400 mg per day	Severe sinus node dysfunction; marked sinus bradycardia; second- or third-degree AV block; history of syncope due to bradycardia unless a pacemaker is in place	Raises serum digoxin concentration; potentiates the effect of oral anticoagulants; increases levels of quinidine, procainamide, phenytoin; may potentiate bradycardia or AV block when used with beta blockers or calcium antagonists; may worsen arrhythmias	Sinus bradycardia *Pulmonary fibrosis;* interstitial pneumonitis; corneal microdeposits; photosensitivity; blue-gray pigmentation; hypo- and hyperthyroidism; *hepatic injury;* nausea, vomiting; anorexia; constipation; tremor; malaise; gait disturbance; *peripheral myopathy or neuropathy*
Bretylium tosylate							
IV 50 mg/ml	5–10 mg per kg IV	1 mg/min infusion or 5–10 mg/kg IV q. 6 hr	—	—	—	*Severe hypotension may occur in patients with fixed cardiac output;* may aggravate digitalis toxicity; reduce dosage in renal insufficiency	*Hypotension, especially postural hypotension;* transient hypertension and increased frequency of ventricular arrhythmias
IM	5–10 mg per kg IM	—	—	—			Nausea and vomiting, usually with rapid IV infusion; increased sensitivity to catecholamines
Diltiazem							
Tablets 30, 60 mg	—	—	—	30–90 mg p.o. q. 6–8 hr	Sick sinus syndrome; second- or third-degree AV block in absence of a ventricular pacemaker; systolic BP < 90 mm Hg	Cautious use in renal or hepatic insufficiency; additive effects on AV conduction when used with digitalis or beta blockers	Bradycardia; hypotension; AV block Edema; headache; nausea; dizziness; rash; abnormal hepatic enzymes
Verapamil							
Tablets 80, 120 mg	—	—	—	80–160 mg p.o. q. 6–8 hr	*Severe left ventricular dysfunction;* hypotension or cardiogenic shock; sick sinus syndrome (except with a pacemaker); second- or third-degree AV block; concurrent intravenous beta blockers and intravenous verapamil; known hypersensitivity to verapamil	Reduce oral dose with hepatic dysfunction; avoid use with disopyramide; use cautiously with renal insufficiency, beta blockers, quinidine, or severe HOCM; will raise serum digoxin level; *may accelerate ventricular response in atrial flutter or fibrillation in the presence of an accessory AV connection;* may potentiate activity of neuromuscular blocking agents	Hypotension; AV block; heart failure; bradycardia; asystole (with IV use); *severe hypotension or ventricular fibrillation when given IV to patients with ventricular tachycardia* Peripheral edema; headache; elevation of liver function test values; constipation
IV formulation 5 mg vials 10-mg vials	5–10 mg IV over 2–5 min; after 30 min, 10 mg IV if needed	—	—	—			

*Dose and interval depend on indication.

IV = intravenous; HOCM = hypertrophic obstructive cardiomyopathy; GI = gastrointestinal.

Class IA Antiarrhythmic Drugs

DISOPYRAMIDE. Disopyramide suppresses normal automaticity in Purkinje fibers and depresses phase 0 of the action potential and conduction in the atria and ventricles. Disopyramide may be somewhat more potent than quinidine in increasing atrial or ventricular refractoriness but seems less potent in the His-Purkinje system. Therapeutic concentrations cause little change in heart rate or PR or QT intervals and increase the QRS duration by about 25 per cent. It increases the ERP in the atrium and ventricle, but not in the AV node or His-Purkinje system. Disopyramide has a prominent anticholinergic action that counteracts its direct effects on the sinus and AV nodes.

Indications. Disopyramide is indicated for the oral treatment of symptomatic, unsustained ventricular arrhythmias. It also will terminate attacks of PSVT and will decrease the frequency of recurrences. It is about as effective as quinidine for preventing recurrence of atrial fibrillation after cardioversion. Disopyramide prolongs the refractory period of anomalous AV connections and can control arrhythmias in the WPW syndrome.

PROCAINAMIDE. Procainamide has been used since the 1950's for treatment of atrial and ventricular arrhythmias. The cardiac electrophysiologic effects of procainamide are similar to those of disopyramide and quinidine. It suppresses automaticity in cardiac Purkinje fibers, slows the phase 0 depolarization in fibers with fast action potentials, and delays repolarization and increases refractoriness in the atrium, His-Purkinje system, and ventricle. Procainamide produces a small increase in the PR and QT intervals in the ECG and produces a 20 to 30 per cent increase in the QRS duration at therapeutic plasma concentrations. In addition, procainamide increases slightly the ERP of the atrium, has little effect on the refractoriness of the AV node, and prolongs the conduction time and refractoriness of the His-Purkinje system slightly in humans. Procainamide has no significant anticholinergic or alpha-adrenergic–blocking properties.

Indications. Procainamide is indicated for the treatment of atrial fibrillation, atrial flutter, PSVT, premature ventricular depolarizations, and ventricular tachycardia. It can suppress digitalis-induced toxic ventricular arrhythmias, but lidocaine or phenytoin is a better choice.

Pharmacokinetics. Procainamide is biotransformed in the liver to N-acetylprocainamide (NAPA). In the steady state, the plasma NAPA concentrations can equal or exceed those of the parent drug. NAPA is qualitatively different electrophysiologically from procainamide; it has a weak effect on phase 0 depolarization and a pronounced effect on action potential duration and refractoriness, a class III action. NAPA is eliminated by the kidney and can accumulate to toxic levels when renal or congestive heart failure is present.

QUINIDINE. Quinidine, an alkaloid derived from the bark of the cinchona tree, has been used for the treatment of atrial and ventricular arrhythmias since the 1920's.

Pharmacology. Quinidine has powerful direct effects on most types of cardiac cells and has significant anticholinergic and alpha-adrenergic–blocking activity. Quinidine has little effect on the automaticity of normal sinus nodes but can markedly depress abnormal sinus nodes. It substantially decreases automaticity of normal cardiac Purkinje fibers but has little effect on abnormal automaticity. Quinidine increases atrial and ventricular pacing and fibrillation thresholds; depresses phase 0 of atrial, ventricular, and Purkinje cells; and delays repolarization and increases the ERP of atrial, ventricular, and Purkinje cells. In humans, quinidine causes a small increase in heart rate and in the PR, QRS, and QT intervals in the ECG and usually prolongs the HV interval slightly.

Indications. Quinidine is indicated for the chronic treatment of atrial flutter or fibrillation, PSVT, and symptomatic ventricular arrhythmias. For symptomatic benign or potentially malignant ventricular arrhythmias, the quinidine dose is titrated until symptoms are controlled and unsustained VT is 90 or more per cent suppressed. Quinidine is selected for malignant arrhythmias if it renders them uninducible by programmed ventricular stimulation or if it abolishes unsustained VT from Holter recordings.

Class IC Antiarrhythmic Drugs

ENCAINIDE. Encainide is a class IC antiarrhythmic drug that became available for use in the United States in 1987. Encainide has little effect on the normal sinus node but can depress abnormal sinus nodes. It decreases spontaneous phase 4 depolarization in Purkinje fibers and markedly depresses phase 0 in fast-response cardiac cells. Encainide slows conduction substantially and shortens the ERP in the atrium, the ventricle, and the His-Purkinje system. In humans, chronic oral encainide prolongs the refractory periods on the atrium, ventricle, and anomalous AV connections. It increases the AH and HV intervals and the PR, QRS, and QT intervals in the ECG. The increase in QRS duration is greater than that caused by class IA drugs. Encainide has two active metabolites, O-demethylencainide (ODE) and 3-methoxy-O-demethylencainide (MODE). The metabolites have more potent electrophysiologic effects and longer elimination half-times than encainide. Encainide is notable for minimal myocardial depression in patients with poor left ventricular function.

Indications. At the present time, encainide is indicated only for the treatment of symptomatic ventricular arrhythmias. However, it has been shown to be extremely effective against PSVT in the WPW syndrome, and it is being investigated for its effectiveness against atrial flutter and fibrillation and AV nodal re-entrant tachycardia.

FLECAINIDE. Flecainide is a new class IC antiarrhythmic drug that has little effect on the normal sinus node but can depress abnormal sinus nodes. It decreases spontaneous phase 4 depolarization in Purkinje fibers and markedly depresses depolarization in fast-response cardiac cells. The drug slows conduction substantially in the atrium, the ventricle, and the His-Purkinje system. Flecainide shortens repolarization in the atrium, the ventricle, and the His-Purkinje system. In humans, flecainide prolongs the refractory periods of the atrium, ventricle, and anomalous AV connections. It increases the AH and HV intervals and the PR and QRS intervals in the ECG. The increase in QRS duration is much greater than that seen with class IA drugs. Flecainide can aggravate left ventricular dysfunction.

Indications. Flecainide is indicated for symptomatic, unsustained VT and frequent VPD's and for life-threatening arrhythmias, such as sustained VT. Flecainide is not currently indicated for atrial arrhythmias, but early studies suggest that, like encainide, it will have an important role in the future.

Class II Antiarrhythmic Drugs

PROPRANOLOL. Propranolol was the first beta blocker approved in the United States and has been on the market more than 20 years. Of the many beta-adrenergic–blocking drugs now approved for use, only acebutolol, propranolol, timolol, and esmolol are approved for the treatment of arrhythmias, and only propranolol, timolol, and metoprolol are indicated to reduce cardiovascular mortality after myocardial infarction. There are many significant differences among the beta-adrenergic–blocking agents in terms of cardioselectivity, intrinsic sympathomimetic action, electrophysiologic effects, and pharmacokinetics.

Pharmacology. Beta blockers decrease automaticity in the sinus node and His-Purkinje systems when it is enhanced by sympathetic influences but have little effect when catecholamines are absent. Propranolol has little effect on phase 0 depolarization of cardiac fibers at low concentrations. At high concentrations, i.e., 1000 to 3000 ng per milliliter, phase 0 depolarization is depressed. Propranolol shortens, whereas other beta blockers can prolong, action potential duration in atrial, ventricular, and particularly His-Purkinje cells; these effects are unrelated to beta-blocking activity. In humans, propranolol and other beta blockers increase the ERP of the AV node, a major antiarrhythmic effect but have little effect on atrial or ventricular refractoriness.

Indications. Propranolol is indicated for supraventricular arrhythmias, particularly those induced by catecholamines or those associated with the WPW syndrome or thyrotoxicosis; for symptomatic APD's; and for control of the ventricular rate in atrial flutter or fibrillation. It is also indicated for ventricular arrhythmias caused by catecholamines. Propranolol or another beta blocker is often chosen for the treatment of symptomatic but benign VPD's.

Class III Antiarrhythmic Drugs

AMIODARONE. Amiodarone is a benzofuran derivative, 37 per cent iodine by weight, originally developed as a smooth muscle relaxant and coronary vasodilator to treat angina pectoris. In 1986, amiodarone was approved by the United States Food and Drug Administration (FDA) as a last-resort treatment for malignant ventricular arrhythmias. There have been no controlled studies of its efficacy.

Pharmacology. Amiodarone substantially prolongs action potential duration and ERP in atrium, ventricle, and Purkinje fibers (a class III action). Amiodarone slows sinus rate by a direct effect. Under laboratory conditions, amiodarone can have a substantial class I effect. In humans, amiodarone slows the sinus rate, and it increases the PR and QT intervals in the ECG, with less effect on the QRS. In addition, it increases the atrial, AV nodal, and ventricular refractory periods and prolongs the HV intervals.

Indications. Amiodarone is indicated only for treatment of recurrent ventricular fibrillation or recurrent, hemodynamically unstable, sustained VT that has not responded to documented adequate doses of other antiarrhythmic drugs or when alternative agents cannot be tolerated. Treatment must be assessed by a method with high predictive accuracy. Endocardial electrical stimulation is the method of choice. About 20 per cent of patients with inducible VT can be rendered uninducible, and these patients do very well. In another 40 to 50 per cent, the VT rate slows enough to prevent significant symptoms during sustained VT. In this group, recurrences of VT are not reduced much but usually are not fatal. Patients who have inducible symptomatic, sustained VT after being loaded with amiodarone should be considered for some alternate treatment. Because of the serious nature of the arrhythmias for which amiodarone is indicated and the unpredictable time course of effect, amiodarone should be started in a monitored hospital setting.

BRETYLIUM TOSYLATE. Bretylium is a postganglionic adrenergic neuron blocker approved for intramuscular or intravenous use as an antiarrhythmic drug.

Pharmacology. Bretylium causes marked lengthening of the action potential duration and ERP of ventricular muscle and Purkinje fibers (class III action). It is selectively taken up in peripheral adrenergic nerves and causes the acute release of norepinephrine; later, it produces chemical sympathectomy, preventing the norepinephrine release during nerve action potentials. Bretylium has no significant effect on phase 0 depolarization or conduction (i.e., it has no class I action), but it does increase the ventricular fibrillation threshold. Bretylium does not depress myocardial performance but can cause severe postural hypotension by interfering with the efferent limb of the baroreceptor reflex arc.

Indications. Bretylium is indicated for the therapy and prophylaxis of ventricular fibrillation and for the treatment of life-threatening ventricular arrhythmias, e.g., sustained VT, that have failed to respond to first-line antiarrhythmic drugs, e.g., lidocaine. Use of bretylium should be restricted to intensive care units. Ventricular fibrillation usually responds within minutes, whereas the full effect on unsustained VT and VPD's takes hours.

Class IV Antiarrhythmic Drugs

VERAPAMIL. Verapamil is a papaverine derivative long used as a coronary vasodilator. Later, its calcium channel–blocking properties were discovered, and in 1981 it was approved for treatment of angina pectoris and supraventricular arrhythmias.

Pharmacology. Verapamil slows spontaneous firing in isolated sinus node preparations; the effect is less marked in vivo because of reflex sympathetic nervous activity by peripheral vasodilation. Verapamil decreases normal automaticity in Purkinje fibers and abolishes delayed afterdepolarizations and triggered activity in experimental digitalis toxicity. It prolongs refractoriness and conduction in the AV node by blocking Ca^{++} channels. This action accounts for the ability of verapamil to terminate and prevent PSVT. Verapamil can abolish experimental VT due to slow potentials. In addition, it can delay ischemic injury and prevent arrhythmogenic electrophysiologic effects caused by transient ischemia. Verapamil also has alpha-adrenergic–blocking properties. In humans, verapamil slows the heart rate and increases the PR interval without any change in the QRS and QTc.

Indications. Intravenous verapamil is indicated for a rapid conversion of PSVT to sinus rhythm (see Table 45–11). The quick effectiveness of verapamil has made it a drug of first choice in emergency rooms and offices. Verapamil should not be given to patients with wide QRS tachycardias until the rhythm is *proven* to be PSVT.

Verapamil can provide temporary control of rapid ventricular rate in atrial fibrillation. A 5- to 10-mg IV dose of verapamil will slow the ventricular rate about 20 per cent for 15 to 30 minutes while a more permanent treatment is being established. Verapamil can be used orally to prevent PSVT or help to control the ventricular rate in atrial flutter or fibrillation.

Bigger JT Jr, Hoffman BF: Antiarrhythmic Drugs. In Gilman AG, Goodman LS, Rall TW, et al. (eds.): The Pharmacological Basis of Therapeutics. 7th ed. New York, The Macmillan Company, 1985, pp 748–783. *A concise summary of the pharmacology and clinical use of antiarrhythmic drugs. Selectively referenced.*

Siddoway LA, Roden DM, Woosley RL: Clinical pharmacology of old and new antiarrhythmic drugs. Cardiovasc Clin 15:199, 1985. *A discussion of the pharmacodynamics, pharmacokinetics, drug interactions, and clinical use of antiarrhythmic drugs. Extensively referenced.*

ELECTRICAL DEVICES IN THE MANAGEMENT OF CARDIAC ARRHYTHMIAS

Temporary or permanent cardiac pacemakers and DC cardioversion or external defibrillation are well-established forms of electrical therapy. In 1985, an automatic implantable cardioverter defibrillator was approved by the FDA.

Cardiac Pacemakers

Permanent pacemakers were first implanted in the 1960's, and over the ensuing 25 years, the pacemaker industry has matured, providing highly sophisticated and diverse products for the management of bradyarrhythmias, and, to a lesser extent, tachyarrhythmias. About 100,000 pulse generators are implanted each year in the United States, about one half of the world's pacemaker implants. There are approximately 500,000 patients with pacemakers living in the United States.

INDICATIONS FOR CARDIAC PACING. The joint report of the American College of Cardiology and American Heart Association grouped pacemaker use into three classes: I, definitely indicated; II, possibly indicated; and III, not indicated (see Table 45–12). Pacing is indicated for bradycardia

TABLE 45–12. DEFINITE INDICATIONS FOR IMPLANTED PACEMAKER

A. Complete heart block, permanent or intermittent, with any one of the following complications:
1. Symptomatic bradycardia
2. Congestive heart failure
3. Conditions that require treatment with drugs that suppress ventricular escape rhythms
4. Asystole ≥ 3 seconds or ventricular rate <40 per minute
5. Mental confusion that clears with pacing
B. Patients with complete heart block or advanced second-degree AV block that persists after myocardial infarction
C. Chronic bi- or trifascicular block with intermittent complete heart block or type II second-degree AV block associated with symptomatic bradycardia
D. Sinus node dysfunction with documented symptomatic bradycardia
E. Hypersensitive carotid sinus syndrome with recurrent syncope and asystole >3 seconds provoked by minimal carotid sinus pressure
F. Symptomatic supraventricular tachycardia that does not respond to medical treatment

TABLE 45–13. CODE FOR PACEMAKER MODES

Chamber Paced	Chamber Sensed	Mode of Response
V = Ventricle	V = Ventricle	I = Inhibited
A = Atrium	A = Atrium	T = Triggered
D = Double (atrium and ventricle)	D = Double (atrium and ventricle)	D = Double (atrium triggered and ventricle inhibited)
	O = None	R = Reserve
		O = None

with complete heart block or advanced second-degree AV block with symptoms such as transient dizziness, light-headedness, near syncope or syncope, marked exercise intolerance, or congestive heart failure. Asymptomatic conditions that are definite indications are permanent high-grade AV block after myocardial infarction or surgical repair of congenital heart disease, or complete heart block with a ventricular rate of less than 40 per minute.

LEAD PLACEMENT. More than 90 per cent of permanent pacing leads are placed via cephalic, subclavian, or external jugular veins. Most transvenous leads are stainless steel, multifilament, helical coil wires insulated with polyurethane or silicone rubber. These leads are small, steerable, and fracture resistant. Leads are anchored by tines or a screw-in arrangement at their tips. Both unipolar and bipolar electrodes are commonly used. For simple ventricular pacing, one lead is placed in the right ventricular apex. For dual chamber pacing, a second lead is placed in the right atrium.

PULSE GENERATORS. Modern pacemaker generators weigh 40 to 50 gm, are powered by lithium batteries that last seven to 10 years, and have circuitry for sensing intracardiac electrograms. Pacemakers can be interrogated to evaluate the pulse generator or reprogrammed to meet changing requirements. Multiprogrammability provides flexibility in obtaining diagnostic information and individualizing the pacemaker prescription.

MODES OF CARDIAC PACING. Pacemaker modes are expressed in the three- or five-letter notation proposed by the Inter-Society Commission for Heart Disease Resources. Table 45–13 shows the first three letter codes. The three letters indicate the chamber paced, the chamber sensed, and the response to sensing. The fourth and fifth positions describe programmable and antitachycardia features and are used less frequently.

SELECTION OF THE PACEMAKER MODE. Selection of the appropriate pacemaker has become more complex as options have become more diverse. Table 45–14 summarizes common selections, considering the atrial rhythm and status of AV and VA conduction.

Rate-Responsive Pacing. Many patients who would benefit from heart rate increase during exercise have relative contraindications for DDD pacing (see footnote, Table 45–14), e.g., inadequate sinus node function of atrial fibrillation. Rate-responsive pacing can be provided by sensing activity with a piezoelectric accelerometer mounted in the pulse generator case. Heart rate can be increased by as much as 90 per minute, i.e., from 60 at rest to 150 during exercise. Cardiac output and the patient's ability to perform daily activities also increase.

COMPLICATIONS. Transvenous implants are associated with cardiac perforation, arrhythmias, infection, thrombosis, emboli, and lead pipe fracture or displacement. Thoracotomy carries the risk of general anesthesia, bleeding, infection,

postoperative respiratory compromise, and late threshold increases. With either route of implantation, the pulse generator may erode through the skin. Pacemakers can be inhibited by intense magnetic fields such as large telephone transformers, microwave devices, diathermy, cautery, antitheft devices, and certain types of motors, e.g., electric razors. Unipolar pacemakers may be inhibited by local myopotentials.

The "pacemaker syndrome" was first defined as light-headedness or syncope related to long cycles of AV asynchrony that occurred during VOO or VVI pacing. The definition also includes (1) episodic weakness or syncope associated with alternating AV synchrony and asynchrony; (2) inadequate cardiac output associated with continued absence of AV synchrony or with fixed asynchrony (persistent VA conduction); and (3) the patient's awareness of beat-to-beat variation in vascular pulsation.

PACEMAKER FOLLOW-UP. Implanted pacing devices require careful follow-up. Regular transtelephonic monitoring permits early detection of battery depletion. At the present time, the principal problem in pacemaker follow-up is the

TABLE 45–14. INDICATIONS FOR PACING MODES

	Atrial Rhythm		
AV Conduction	Normal	Bradycardia	Bradycardia-Tachycardia
Normal	None indicated	AAI	AAI
AV block; normal VA conduction time	VDD, DDD	DDD, DVI	DVI, VVI
AV block; prolonged VA conduction time	DVI	DVI	DVI

AAI: Fixed-rate atrial pacing occurs unless inhibited by sensed atrial depolarizations. This mode can be used for patients with symptomatic sinus node dysfunction and normal AV conduction.

VDD: Ventricular pulses are delivered when atrial depolarization is sensed and inhibited when ventricular depolarization is sensed. The VDD mode is used when adequate atrial rates and sensing are present, along with high-grade AV block and normal VA conduction. VDD pacing provides atrial augmentation of ventricular filling and avoids the pacemaker syndrome but is contraindicated for patients with supraventricular tachyarrhythmias.

DVI: Both chambers are paced at a preselected rate and AV interval. Pacing is inhibited by ventricular, but not atrial, activity. The DVI mode is used when synchronous AV contraction is needed in patients with symptomatic atrial bradycardia. The pacing rate does not increase during exercise. DVI pacing is contraindicated in patients who have supraventricular tachyarrhythmias.

DDD: Both atria and ventricles are paced and sensed. The atrial or ventricular pacemaker pulses are inhibited when either atrial or ventricular premature activity is detected. When atrial activity is sensed, a ventricular pulse is provided. This mode of pacing provides synchronous AV contraction over a wide range of heart rates. DDD pacemakers are adaptive: totally inhibited in sinus rhythm with normal AV conduction; AAI pacing during sinus bradycardia with normal AV conduction; VDD pacing during sinus rhythm with impaired AV conduction; DVI pacing during sinus bradycardia with impaired AV conduction. DDD pacemakers are contraindicated in patients with persistent or frequently occurring atrial tachyarrhythmias and those with long VA conduction times who can develop pacemaker-mediated reciprocating tachycardia.

VVI: This mode can be used for any symptomatic bradyarrhythmia. The VVI mode is contraindicated in patients who have had the pacemaker syndrome (see text), those with congestive heart failure, or in those who need rate-responsive pacing.

diversity of pacemaker models and methods for interrogating pacemaker function.

DC Cardioversion

DC cardioversion was introduced in 1962 and has become a mainstay in the management of cardiac arrhythmias. Cardioversion depolarizes all or most of the heart, interrupts re-entrant circuits, and terminates arrhythmias. It is effective for atrial fibrillation, atrial flutter, PSVT, ventricular tachycardia, or ventricular fibrillation. Drug-resistant arrhythmias, e.g., atrial flutter, may respond readily to DC cardioversion. Because of its speed, cardioversion is preferable to drug therapy for arrhythmias that adversely affect hemodynamics, such as rapid atrial arrhythmias, sustained ventricular tachycardia, or ventricular fibrillation. Elective cardioversion is indicated for atrial fibrillation of recent onset (< 6 months) to control symptoms and hemodynamic abnormalities and to lower the risk of systemic embolism.

LIMITATIONS AND CONTRAINDICATIONS. Chronic atrial fibrillation, i.e., that greater than 6 to 12 months in duration, is so likely to recur after cardioversion that digitalis therapy may be preferred. Contributing causes, e.g., hyperthyroidism, pericardial inflammation, pulmonary thromboembolism, chronic obstructive pulmonary disease, or alcohol abuse, should be controlled before cardioversion; otherwise, atrial fibrillation is likely to recur. Sinus rhythm is difficult to maintain after cardioversion of atrial fibrillation in patients with heart failure or large left atria (> 45 mm in diameter by echocardiography). In the bradycardia-tachycardia syndrome, cardioversion often produces inadequate rhythms and atrial fibrillation usually resumes within a few hours. Cardioversion is contraindicated for arrhythmias caused by digitalis intoxication because it can precipitate ventricular fibrillation.

ANTICOAGULATION. Despite the lack of controlled evaluation, most patients who have been fibrillating for more than three weeks are treated with anticoagulants before cardioversion, particularly those with (1) a history of embolization, (2) a prosthetic mitral valve, (3) an enlarged left atrium, or (4) congestive heart failure. The prothrombin time is kept at 2.5 times the normal value with warfarin for about three weeks before and a week after cardioversion.

RESULTS. The immediate results of cardioversion are excellent (Table 45–15). The main long-term problem is reversion to atrial fibrillation. Class I antiarrhythmic drugs decrease the

chance of recurrence of atrial fibrillation one year after cardioversion from about 75 to 50 per cent.

COMPLICATIONS. Few complications attend technically excellent cardioversion. Occasionally, transient SA or AV block or ventricular arrhythmias occur immediately after DC shock, especially when digitalis dosage is excessive. In the sick sinus syndrome, the sinus may fail to resume control of cardiac rhythm after cardioversion. Atropine, isoproterenol, and/or external pacing usually will maintain the patient until a temporary transvenous pacemaker can be inserted. Occasionally, worsening heart failure or frank pulmonary edema occurs within a few hours after cardioversion. The cause of this syndrome is unknown. Elevation of myocardial creatine kinase after DC cardioversion is rare.

Automatic Implantable Cardioverter Defibrillator

The first automatic implantable defibrillator (AID), a device that responded only to ventricular fibrillation, was implanted in 1980. The first automatic implantable cardioverter defibrillator (AICD) was implanted in 1982. This unit detects and cardioverts ventricular tachycardia as well as providing defibrillation.

INDICATIONS. The AICD is recommended for patients who have had a documented episode of life-threatening ventricular tachyarrhythmia or cardiac arrest not associated with the acute phase of myocardial infarction. In addition, patients should have inducible ventricular tachycardia or ventricular fibrillation unsuitable for drug or surgical therapy.

IMPLANTATION. The electrode systems are implanted via a thoracotomy. The 292-gram power unit is implanted subcutaneously in an abdominal pocket. During implantation, defibrillation thresholds and detection of ventricular tachycardia/fibrillation are tested extensively to ensure proper function. The AICD usually lasts 18 to 24 months or 100 discharges.

The device monitors the ECG continuously. When ventricular tachycardia of fibrillation is detected and verified, the AICD charges its capacitors and delivers a 20- to 30-joule pulse.

FOLLOW-UP. The AICD is a complex device that requires careful follow-up. Potential problems with the device include (1) depletion of the battery, (2) lead breakage or migration, (3) inappropriate discharges, (4) infection, and (5) skin erosion. After implantation, a magnet test should be performed every two months to evaluate the device and reform the capacitors.

Between 1980 and the end of 1986, more than 1000 AID or AICD units were implanted. Follow-up reveals a one-year cardiovascular mortality of about 10 per cent and a sudden death rate of about 2 per cent. Although the device is complex and expensive, it is highly effective for selected patients with malignant ventricular arrhythmias.

DeSilva RA, Graboys TB, Podrid PJ, et al.: Cardioversion and defibrillation. Am Heart J 100:881, 1980. *A thorough review of the history, theory, and practice of cardioversion and defibrillation.*

Echt DS, Armstrong K, Schmidt P, et al.: Clinical experience, complications, and survival in 70 patients with the automatic implantable cardioverter/defibrillator. Circulation 71:289, 1985. *A description of a large experience with the implantable defibrillator. Provides an excellent perspective on the current use of the device.*

Frye RL, Collins JJ, DeSanctis RW, et al.: Guidelines for permanent cardiac pacemaker implantation, May 1984. J Am Coll Cardiol 4:434, 1984. *A report of a task force to review cardiac pacing. The report defines current indications for cardiac pacing and makes recommendations about the selection of devices for treatment of specific clinical problems. This report is used as a standard by the medical profession, regulatory agencies, and reimbursement sources.*

Mirowski M: The automatic implantable cardioverter-defibrillator: An overview. J Am Coll Cardiol 6:461, 1985. *A review of the concepts, evolution, clinical use, and follow-up of the automatic implantable cardioverter defibrillator by the originator of the device.*

Parsonnet V, Bernstein AD: Pacing in perspective: Concepts and controversies. Circulation 73:1087, 1986. *A perspective on cardiac pacing. Provides a concise view of the history, development, current practice, and future directions in cardiac pacing.*

TABLE 45–15. ENERGY FOR CARDIOVERSION/DEFIBRILLATION

Arrhythmia	Recommended Initial Energy* (joules)	Comments
Atrial flutter	50	100% conversion; most will convert with about 25 joules.
Atrial fibrillation	200	85–95% conversion; a few patients may require 300–400 joule DC shocks to cardiovert.
Paroxysmal supraventricular tachycardia	100	100% conversion
Ventricular tachycardia	50	90–95% conversion; 80% will convert with <10 joules, but a few need 100 joules or more.
Ventricular fibrillation	300–400	90–95% defibrillation; many will convert at 200 joules or below, but time is of the essence in successful defibrillation.

*An energy level with a high probability of converting the arrhythmia

TABLE 45–16. SURGERY FOR CARDIAC ARRHYTHMIAS

Arrhythmia	Operative Approach
Atrial fibrillation	Ablation of AV node and implantation of a pacemaker; left atrial exclusion (highly experimental)
Ectopic atrial focus	Excision of the focus after accurate mapping
PSVT (Pre-excitation)	Surgical division of anomalous AV connection
PSVT (AV nodal)	Partial catheter ablation of AV node; division of His bundle and implantation of pacemaker
Ventricular tachycardia (coronary heart disease)	Endocardial resection guided by mapping
Ventricular tachycardia (arrhythmogenic right ventricular dysplasia)	Simple ventriculotomy; isolation of arrhythmic site
Ventricular tachycardia (after repair of tetralogy of Fallot)	Resection of infundibulectomy scar
Multiform ventricular tachycardia (long QT syndrome)	Left stellate ganglionectomy

PSVT = paroxysmal supraventricular tachycardia.

SURGICAL TREATMENT OF CARDIAC ARRHYTHMIAS

The objective of arrhythmia surgery (Table 45–16) may be (1) to remove the arrhythmic focus, (2) to interrupt a re-entrant pathway, or (3) to prevent the ventricles from responding to supraventricular tachyarrhythmias. For surgery to be seriously considered, the arrhythmia must pose significant risk to life or interfere substantially with the quality of life.

Supraventricular Arrhythmias

INTERRUPTION OF THE BUNDLE OF HIS. Atrial flutter and fibrillation can be palliated by interruption of the His bundle and implantation of a ventricular pacemaker when drug therapy cannot control ventricular rate. The need for such surgery has diminished with the advent of beta-adrenergic blockers, verapamil, and catheter ablation.

Catheter Ablation. Recently, a catheter technique for His bundle ablation has been found to be safe and effective. With the use of fluoroscopy, a multielectrode catheter is placed so as to record the bundle of His depolarization. Then, one or more large energy shocks are delivered to the electrode (cathode) that records the largest His bundle depolarization. Shocks can be repeated until AV conduction is interrupted.

REMOVAL OF AUTOMATIC FOCI. Automatic or tiny re-entrant ectopic foci can be excised or ablated. The key to removal or ablation is accurate localization by epicardial and/or endocardial activation mapping.

INTERRUPTION OF RE-ENTRANT PATHWAYS. Surgery is very effective for paroxysmal supraventricular tachycardia (PSVT) that uses an anomalous AV connection as an essential portion of the circuit or for atrial fibrillation with rapid ventricular response in the Wolff-Parkinson-White syndrome. Preoperative electrophysiologic studies delineate the mechanism of PSVT, the site of the accessory AV connection, and the route of cardiac excitation during PSVT. During operation, the anomalous AV connection or connections are located precisely using cardiac stimulation and epicardial or endocardial mapping during sinus rhythm, ventricular pacing, and PSVT. Traditionally, division of anomalous AV connections is done on cardiopulmonary bypass with the atrium open. More recently, dissection and cryoablation have been used successfully without cardiopulmonary bypass. Centers with major programs obtain cure rates of greater than 85 per cent with surgical mortalities of less than 1 per cent. These results usually make surgery a better choice than drug treatment.

Sustained Ventricular Tachycardia

VENTRICULAR ANEURYSMS. The largest surgical experience has been gathered in patients with recurrent, sustained ventricular tachycardia (VT) and coronary heart disease; most of these patients have left ventricular aneurysms, two- or three-vessel disease, and severely impaired left ventricular function. The rate of VT tends to be slow and easily induced and can be mapped during electrophysiologic studies. Accurate preoperative endocardial maps are critical because adequate maps are often impossible to obtain at surgery. At surgery, the arrhythmogenic tissue is removed or ablated with a cryoprobe. Map-guided excision, isolation, or cryoablation is about 80 per cent effective in controlling sustained VT during one to three years of follow-up. However, the perioperative mortality is about 15 to 20 per cent, primarily because of advanced coronary disease and severity of left ventricular dysfunction.

ARRHYTHMOGENIC RIGHT VENTRICULAR DYSPLASIA. Patients who have VT due to right ventricular arrhythmogenic dysplasia usually can be cured by an incision across the dysplastic area that shows the latest activation in sinus rhythm and earliest activation during VT. Small areas of dysplasia can be excised, and large areas can be isolated if simple incision is not feasible.

TETRALOGY OF FALLOT. Ventricular tachycardia occurs rarely in patients who have had total repair of tetralogy of Fallot. Epicardial excitation mapping at surgery shows that VT arises in the right ventricular infundibular scar and scar resection effects a cure.

LONG QT SYNDROME. Patients with the congenital form of the long QT syndrome can have recurrent attacks of malignant, multiform VT of the torsades de pointes type. These rhythms are associated with cardiac arrest and sudden cardiac death. Unequal sympathetic nerve traffic to the heart is part of the explanation for the heterogeneous electrophysiologic condition of the ventricles. Excision of the left stellate ganglion markedly reduces the mortality rate in high-risk patients with the congenital long QT syndrome.

Cox JL, Gallagher JJ, Cain MM: Experience with 118 consecutive patients undergoing operation for the Wolff-Parkinson-White syndrome. J Thorac Cardiovasc Surg 90:490, 1985. *A review of a large, successful experience with surgery for anomalous AV connections.*

Cox JL: The status of surgery for cardiac arrhythmias. Circulation 71:413, 1985. *A perspective on surgery for both supraventricular and ventricular arrhythmias.*

Klein GJ, Guiraudon GM: Surgical therapy of cardiac arrhythmias. Cardiol Clin 1:323, 1983. *A summary of present and future concepts that form the basis for surgical treatment of cardiac arrhythmias.*

46 SUDDEN CARDIAC DEATH
James T. Willerson

DEFINITION AND FREQUENCY. The definition of *sudden cardiac death* used in this chapter is the sudden cessation of effective cardiac contraction resulting from ventricular tachycardia-fibrillation or asystole. Sudden cardiac death claims approximately 1200 lives daily in the United States. It is the leading cause of death among men between the ages of 20 and 60, and approximately 25 per cent of patients dying suddenly have had no previously recognized symptoms of heart disease. Sudden cardiac death among women is approximately one fourth as frequent as among men.

ETIOLOGY AND PATHOGENESIS. Important data regarding the individual who suffers sudden cardiac death come from the Seattle Heart Watch study. During a six-year period of 1710 episodes of ventricular fibrillation, there were 346 long-term survivors. Cobb has shown that most instances of sudden cardiac death are not related to identifiable acute myocardial infarcts, which were detected by electrocardiography in only 19 per cent of patients hospitalized after resuscitation from ventricular fibrillation. Nevertheless, the majority of individuals resuscitated have extensive coronary artery disease, including 75 per cent with multivessel involvement. Patients experiencing cardiac arrest without concomitant acute myocardial infarcts have a considerably higher incidence of recurrent sudden death in the next two years than do those with acute infarcts. The annual recurrence rate is approximately 30 per cent for those within acute infarcts.

It seems likely that the most critical etiologic factor is electrophysiologic instability related to chronic ischemic heart disease, cellular damage associated with cardiomyopathy, or chronic severe valvular heart disease. Since the frequency of recurrence of sudden death is high in those with chronic ischemic heart disease without acute infarcts, it is important to protect such patients with antiarrhythmic agents and, when appropriate, also with coronary artery revascularization and/ or an internal cardiac defibrillator, or "antitachycardiac" pacemaker.

Most patients experiencing sudden death have chronic ischemic heart disease or chronic myocardial scarring and ventricular dysfunction. However, sudden death from ventricular arrhythmias occurs in some individuals with mitral valve prolapse, in some with left ventricular outflow obstruction, including valvular aortic stenosis and asymmetric septal hypertrophy, and in some with hereditary prolongation of the QT interval with or without associated deafness. Sudden death also occurs in individuals with various cardiomyopathies, in those with chronic valvular insufficiency and myocardial dilatation and/or hypertrophy, in those with cardiac tamponade, in some young athletes while they are exercising, and in an occasional individual suddenly aroused or frightened by an external event. Sudden death from a ventricular arrhythmia may also occur in the Wolff-Parkinson-White syndrome; in those with advanced atrioventricular block without pacemakers, or with diffuse conduction system disease ("sick sinus syndrome"); and in severe electrolyte alterations, including hypokalemia, hyperkalemia, and hypercalcemia. Drug overdose, particularly with cardiac glycosides, may also be a cause for sudden cardiac death. Additional causes for sudden death or death within a few hours that do not initially involve the heart include intracerebral or subarachnoid hemorrhage, pulmonary emboli, severe drug overdose, hypoxia associated with chronic obstructive lung disease or lung injury, dissecting aortic aneurysms, and rupture of an aortic aneurysm.

In order to reduce the frequency and risk of sudden death in susceptible individuals, at least two additional developments are needed: (1) better means to identify those at risk and (2) better understanding of mechanisms involved in ventricular tachycardia or fibrillation in susceptible patients. Although most patients who experience sudden death have heart disease, the risk factors for atherosclerosis do not singly or in combination identify a subset of patients prone to sudden death. The mechanism of sudden death is ordinarily ventricular fibrillation.

IDENTIFICATION OF HIGH-RISK PATIENTS. In patients with acute infarction, certain types of ventricular premature beats are considered precursors of ventricular fibrillation. In coronary care units, more than seven ventricular premature beats per minute, multiform ventricular premature beats, ventricular premature beats occurring on or close to the apex of the T wave, and runs of two or more ventricular premature beats are considered potential harbingers of ventricular tachycardia or fibrillation. These "malignant ventricular premature beats" are ordinarily suppressed by pharmacologic agents such as lidocaine. However, some patients with acute myocardial infarcts have ventricular tachycardia or fibrillation without precursor ventricular arrhythmias. Moreover, there is a relationship between recurrent ventricular tachycardia or fibrillation and the overall size of myocardial infarcts, such that patients with large infarcts may have recurrent ventricular (and supraventricular) arrhythmias.

In patients with chronic ischemic heart disease, only advanced grades or complex ventricular premature beats and the presence of important ventricular dysfunction predict sudden cardiac death. The frequency of sudden death and of ventricular premature complexes increases with age. In addition, the frequency of ventricular premature beats increases in relationship to the extent of ventricular damage from earlier myocardial infarcts. Ventricular ectopic activity is often more frequent and complex in patients with multivessel coronary artery disease than in those with only single-vessel involvement. Therefore, a knowledge of the extent of coronary disease and of ventricular dysfunction may be useful in predicting the risk of sudden death. Specifically, patients with a left ventricular ejection fraction of 40 per cent or less and (1) frequent ventricular premature beats (≥ 8 per hour) and/or (2) complex ventricular premature beats have a several-fold increased risk of sudden death in the initial six months after myocardial infarction. An increased risk has also been claimed for patients demonstrating repetitive ventricular beating following ventricular stimulation. Dynamic myocardial scintigraphic characterization of ventricular function at rest and during submaximal exercise in patients with acute infarction before hospital discharge may identify those most at risk for future coronary events. Increasing in popularity are techniques that determine the efficacy of a particular antiarrhythmic regimen prior to hospital discharge in patients at risk, including electrophysiologic studies in a cardiac catheterization laboratory, which test individual vulnerability for sustained ventricular arrhythmias while the patient is on and off selected antiarrhythmic agents. This approach is important because merely administering an antiarrhythmic agent to a patient with the hope of preventing sudden death is often not successful. Schaffer and Cobb (1975) reported that 73 per cent of 64 patients with recurrent ventricular fibrillation were receiving antiarrhythmic therapy at the time of sudden death. This information emphasizes the need to select and optimize antiarrhythmic therapy for the individual patient. It is also important to realize that antiarrhythmic agents, particularly quinidine and procainamide (Pronestyl), given in normal doses to the patient with a prolonged QT interval, may cause life-threatening ventricular arrhythmias, including a ventricular tachycardia known as *torsade de pointes*. In addition, each of the available antiarrhythmic agents has a certain incidence of causing ventricular ectopic beats ("proarrhythmic effect") even when given at normal doses.

PREVENTION OF SUDDEN DEATH. Beta blockers without intrinsic sympathomimetic activity have been shown to reduce mortality from cardiac events in selected patients in the months to years after myocardial infarction. Left stellate ganglionectomy may also reduce the risk of sudden deaths in patients with hereditary prolongation of the QT interval and recurrent ventricular tachycardia and/or fibrillation. However, it is critically important that we develop an improved understanding of mechanisms that initiate and sustain life-threatening ventricular arrhythmias in patients in diverse clinical settings. Unanswered questions include the following: Do platelet aggregation and subsequent thromboxane A_2 and/or serotonin release play a role in leading to sudden death in patients with coronary artery disease but without identifiable acute myocardial infarction? Are the important ventricular arrhythmias that develop with acute myocardial ischemia related primarily to re-entrant mechanisms or to increased ventricular automaticity resulting in part from variations in regional concentrations of potassium or catecholamines, from alterations in autonomic nervous system activity, from alterations in adrenergic receptor numbers or affinity, or from local accumulation of phospholipid degradation products? It is important to determine why some individuals with chronic congestive heart failure and others with chronic cardiomegaly and ventricular dysfunction are at risk of sudden death from ventricular arrhythmias. It is not clear at present whether increased triglyceride uptake and the inability of injured myocardial cells to metabolize long-chain fatty acids contribute to the ventricular arrhythmias of ischemic heart disease. Specific myocardial cellular mechanisms associated with increased risk of ventricular arrhythmias need to be elucidated, as does the role of psychologic stress in the initiation of ventricular arrhythmias in humans.

Extensive efforts are being made to develop more effective means of correcting recurrent and life-threatening ventricular arrhythmias. New antiarrhythmic agents are being developed and tested but still unavailable is one or more agents with (1) marked efficacy against ventricular and supraventricular arrhythmias, (2) few or no important side effects, and (3) the need for relatively infrequent administration, i.e., once per day. Amiodarone has proved to be useful in the control of recurrent ventricular tachycardia when other antiarrhythmic agents have failed, but there is a relatively high risk of important side effects, including pneumonitis and pulmonary fibrosis, in patients treated with this agent. Surgical resection of ventricular sites of ectopic impulse formation has been successfully utilized following epicardial and endocardial "activation mapping" in the treatment of patients with sustained ventricular tachycardia. Surgical revascularization has been successful in reducing mortality from ventricular dysrhythmias in selected patients with extensive coronary artery stenoses. Mirowski has developed an implantable automatic defibrillator capable of identifying and then spontaneously discharging and converting ventricular tachycardia-fibrillation to sinus rhythm. This device is useful in allowing prompt conversion of life-threatening ventricular arrhythmias when adequate control is not provided by antiarrhythmic agents and the patient is clearly at risk for sudden death. Implantable, programmable pacemakers capable of sensing and correcting ventricular tachyarrhythmias by rapid and brief pacing have also been developed and are alternative methods for treating high-risk patients.

Bigger JT Jr., Fleiss JL, Kleiger R, et al.: The relationships among ventricular arrhythmias, left ventricular dysfunction, and mortality in the 2 years after myocardial infarction. Circulation 69:250, 1984. *A thorough review of these relationships.*

Cobb LA, Baun RS, Alvarez H III, et al.: Resuscitation from out-of-hospital ventricular fibrillation: 4 year follow-up. Circulation 51, 52(Suppl III):III, 1975. *A follow-up of patients following resuscitation from sudden death.*

Doyle JT, Kannel WB, McNamara RM, et al.: Factors related to the suddenness of death from coronary disease: Combined Albany-Framingham Studies. Am J Cardiol 37:1073, 1976. *An epidemiologic study of factors involved in sudden death.*

Hoffman BF, Dangman KH: The role of antiarrhythmic drugs in sudden cardiac death. J Am Coll Cardiol 8:104A, 1986. *A thorough description of the relative advantages and disadvantages of antiarrhythmic agents.*

Horowitz LN, Harken AH, Kastor JA, et al.: Ventricular resection guided by epicardial and endocardial mapping for treatment of recurrent ventricular tachycardia. N Engl J Med 302:589, 1980. *Aggressive but effective surgical techniques for abolishing ventricular rhythm disturbances are described.*

Kannel WB, Doyle JT, McNamara PM, et al.: Precursors of sudden coronary death: Factors related to incidence of sudden death. Circulation 51:606, 1975. *A review of risk factors related to sudden death.*

Lown B: Sudden cardiac death: The major challenge confronting contemporary cardiology. Am J Cardiol 43:313, 1979. *A thorough review of this subject.*

Mirowski M, Reid PR, Mower MM, et al.: Termination of malignant ventricular arrhythmias in man with an implanted defibrillator. N Engl J Med 303:322, 1980. *The development of an implantable defibrillator is described.*

Mukharji J, Rude RE, Poole K, et al.: Risk factors for sudden death after acute myocardial infarction: Two-year follow-up. Am J Cardiol 54:31, 1984. *Patients with recent myocardial infarction and left ventricular ejection fractions < 40 per cent and > 8 ventricular beats per hour are at increased risk of sudden death.*

Willerson JT: Prevention and control of ventricular arrhythmias (editorial). N Engl J Med 303:332, 1980. *A review of the prevention and control of sudden death.*

47 ARTERIAL HYPERTENSION

Suzanne Oparil

DEFINITION

Arterial hypertension is defined as elevated arterial blood pressure (BP). Since BP in the general population falls on a gaussian curve of normal distribution, it is not possible to define with precision the limits of "normal" BP. In addition, the BP of a given individual varies widely over time, depending on many variables, including sympathetic activity, posture, state of hydration, and skeletal muscle tone. Accordingly, any definition of hypertension must be arbitrary. The Joint National Committee on Detection, Evaluation and Treatment of High Blood Pressure recommends the scheme shown in Table 47–1 for the diagnosis of hypertension in patients aged 18 years or older. The diagnosis of hypertension in adults is made when the average of two or more diastolic BP measurements on at least two subsequent visits is 90 mm Hg or higher or when the average of multiple systolic BP readings on two or more subsequent visits is consistently greater than 140 mm Hg (Table 47–2). The patient should be clearly informed that a single elevated reading does not constitute a diagnosis of hypertension but is a sign that further observation is required (Table 47–3).

Essential, or primary, hypertension is arterial hypertension of unknown cause. Over 95 per cent of all cases of arterial hypertension are in this category.

Secondary hypertension is arterial hypertension of known cause. Fewer than 5 per cent of all cases of systemic hypertension are in this category. The importance of identifying patients with secondary hypertension is that they sometimes may be cured by surgery or can be easily controlled by specific medical treatment. Thus the morbidity and mortality of potentially ineffective empiric medical therapy can be avoided and the cumulative cost of medical treatment reduced. The most common causes of secondary hypertension are summarized in Table 47–4.

Benign hypertension is a descriptive term for uncomplicated hypertension, usually of long duration and mild-to-moderate severity. Benign hypertension may be primary or secondary.

Malignant hypertension is the syndrome of markedly elevated BP (diastolic BP usually > 140 mm Hg) associated with papilledema. Accelerated hypertension is the syndrome of markedly elevated BP associated with hemorrhages and exu-

TABLE 47–1. CLASSIFICATION OF BP

Range (mm Hg)	Category*
Diastolic	
< 85	Normal BP
85–89	High normal BP
90–104	Mild hypertension
105–114	Moderate hypertension
≥ 115	Severe hypertension
Systolic, when diastolic BP is < 90	
< 140	Normal BP
140–159	Borderline isolated systolic hypertension
≥ 160	Isolated systolic hypertension

*A classification of borderline isolated systolic hypertension (systolic BP, 140 to 159 mm Hg) or isolated systolic hypertension (systolic BP, > 160 mm Hg) takes precedence over a classification of high normal BP (diastolic BP, 85 to 89 mm Hg) when both occur in the same person. A classification of high normal BP (diastolic BP, 85 to 89 mm Hg) takes precedence over a classification of normal BP (systolic BP, < 140 mm Hg) when both occur in the same person.

Reprinted with permission from The 1984 Report of the Joint National Committee on Detection, Evaluation, and Treatment of High Blood Pressure. Arch Intern Med 144:1045, 1984.

TABLE 47–2. FOLLOW-UP CRITERIA FOR FIRST-OCCASION MEASUREMENT

Range (mm Hg)	Recommended Follow-Up*
Diastolic	
< 85	Recheck within 2 yr
85–89	Recheck within 1 yr
90–104	Confirm promptly (not to exceed 2 mo)
105–114	Evaluate or refer promptly to source of care (not to exceed 2 wk)
≥ 115	Evaluate or refer immediately to a source of care
Systolic, when diastolic BP is < 90	
< 140	Recheck within 2 yr
140–199	Confirm promptly (not to exceed 2 mo)
≥ 200	Evaluate or refer promptly to source of care (not to exceed 2 wk)

*If recommendations for follow-up of diastolic and systolic BP's are different for those aged 18 years or older, the shorter recommended time period supersedes and a referral supersedes a recheck recommendation.

Reprinted with permission from The 1984 Report of the Joint National Committee on Detection, Evaluation, and Treatment of High Blood Pressure. Arch Intern Med 144:1045, 1984.

dates (grade 3 Kimmelstiel-Wilson [K-W] retinopathy). If untreated, accelerated hypertension presumably progresses to a malignant phase. Both the accelerated and the malignant types of hypertension are associated with widespread degenerative changes in the walls of resistance vessels. They are usually characterized by extreme BP elevations, sudden onset, a fulminant course, and evidence of severe, generalized vascular damage, including grade 3 or 4 K-W retinopathy, hypertensive encephalopathy, hematuria, and renal dysfunction. Malignant hypertension is usually fatal unless treated promptly and vigorously. If BP can be controlled, prognosis depends on the state of renal function.

Complicated hypertension is the descriptive term for arterial hypertension of any etiology in which there is evidence of cardiovascular damage related to the BP elevation. Hypertensive complications commonly include stroke, congestive heart failure, renal failure, myocardial infarction, and arterial aneurysm.

Labile hypertension, sometimes referred to as prehypertension or the hyperkinetic heart syndrome, is a descriptive term for intermittent hypertension in which some BP measurements are elevated and some are normal in the untreated patient. Patients with labile hypertension tend to maintain pressures that are above average for the general population and are at greater risk of cardiovascular morbidity and mortality than the general population. As a group, these patients

TABLE 47–3. FOLLOW-UP CRITERIA FOR SECOND-OCCASION MEASUREMENT

Range (mm Hg)	Recommended Follow-Up*
Diastolic	
< 85	Recheck within 2 yr†
85–89	Recheck within 1 yr
≥ 90	Evaluate or refer promptly to a source of care
Systolic, when diastolic BP is < 90	
< 140	Recheck within 1 yr
≥ 140	Evaluate or refer promptly to a source of care

*If recommendations for follow-up of diastolic and systolic BP's are different for those aged 18 or older, the shorter recommended time period supersedes and a referral supersedes a recheck recommendation.

†Rechecking within one year is recommended for persons at increased risk of progressing to higher BP's, including family history of hypertension or cardiovascular event, weight gain or obesity, black race, use of an oral contraceptive, and excessive ethanol consumption.

Reprinted with permission from The 1984 Report of the Joint National Committee on Detection, Evaluation, and Treatment of High Blood Pressure. Arch Intern Med 144:1045, 1984.

TABLE 47–4. CAUSES OF SECONDARY HYPERTENSION

Systolic and diastolic hypertension
Renal vascular disease
Renal parenchymal disease
Renin-secreting tumors
Syndromes of mineralocorticoid excess
  Primary aldosteronism
  Overproduction of 11-deoxycorticosterone (DOC), 18-OH DOC, and other mineralocorticoids without accompanying defects in steroid synthesis
  Congenital adrenal hyperplasia
  Ingestion of licorice of carbenoxolone
Pheochromocytoma
Oral contraceptives
Pregnancy
Coarctation of the aorta
Cushing's syndrome
Hyperparathyroidism
Acromegaly
Increased intracranial pressure
Open heart surgery

Isolated systolic hypertension
Aging
Decreased peripheral vascular resistance
  Arteriovenous shunts
  Paget's disease of bone
  Beriberi
Increased cardiac output
  Anemia
  Thyrotoxicosis
  Aortic valvular insufficiency

manifest increased cardiac output, more rapid heart rate, and higher left ventricular ejection rate than either the normotensive population or the population of patients with stable hypertension. The proportion of such patients who go on to develop sustained hypertension and secondary vascular damage varies from 10 to 70 per cent in published series.

ETIOLOGY

Pathophysiologic factors that have been implicated in the genesis of essential hypertension include increased sympathetic nervous system activity, overproduction of an unidentified sodium-retaining hormone, chronic high sodium intake, increased or "inappropriate" renin secretion, deficiencies of various vasodilatory substances such as prostaglandins, congenital abnormalities of the resistance vessels, and unknown genetic factors. It is likely that essential hypertension represents a collection of diseases or syndromes with distinct pathophysiologic features. The most common etiologies of secondary hypertension are summarized in Table 47–4. The neurohumoral and circulatory abnormalities that are responsible for these forms of hypertension are discussed below.

INCIDENCE AND PREVALENCE

More than 60 million persons in the United States have hypertension. The prevalence of hypertension is higher among blacks than whites, and it increases with age in all groups (Fig. 47–1). The reason for the increased prevalence of hypertension among blacks is unclear, but it has been variously attributed to heredity, greater salt intake, and greater environmental stress. The rise in BP over time in a population is related to both aging and the level of BP: The higher the BP, the greater the rate of change in pressure over time. Hypertension is more common in men than in women up to approximately age 50; after that time, hypertension is more common in women (Fig. 47–1). The reason for the increased prevalence of hypertension in postmenopausal women is unknown.

PATHOGENESIS
Essential Hypertension

HEMODYNAMICS. Elevation of BP results from any disturbance of the circulation that increases cardiac output or

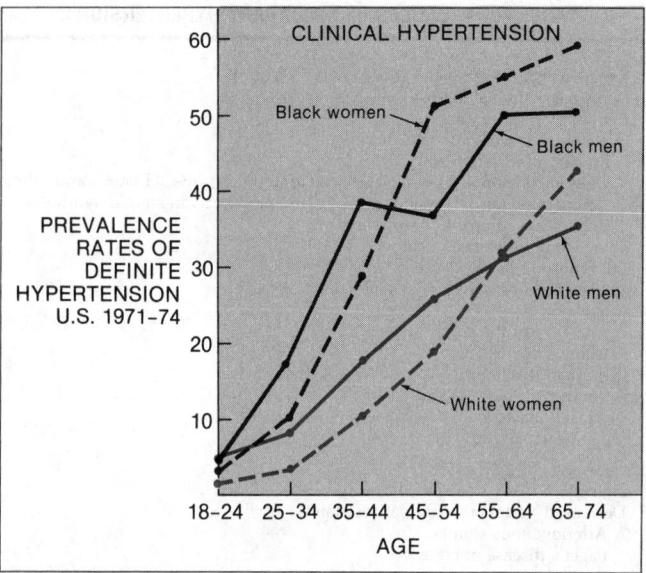

FIGURE 47–1. The prevalence of hypertension in the United States defined as a systolic blood pressure of at least 160 mm Hg or a diastolic blood pressure of at least 95 mm Hg. (From Health and Nutrition Examination Survey, 1971–1974. Source: Advance Data, Vital and Health Statistics of the National Center for Health Statistics, No. 1, October 18, 1976.)

total peripheral resistance, or both. Increases in total peripheral resistance elevate both systolic and diastolic pressures. Cardiac output is elevated early in the course of essential hypertension. Patients with hypertension of recent onset show a pattern of increased cardiac output, tachycardia, increased dp/dt, and venoconstriction, with normal or even low peripheral vascular resistance at rest. In contrast, patients with longstanding established hypertension usually have a slightly decreased cardiac output and increased peripheral vascular resistance. Thus, increased cardiac output plays a role in the initiation of essential hypertension, and elevated peripheral resistance is more important in its maintenance. Longitudinal studies of untreated hypertensive patients have documented a fall in cardiac output, due mainly to a decrease in stroke volume, and an increase in total peripheral resistance over time.

The elevation in cardiac output seen in persons with labile hypertension has been related to increased sympathetic nervous system function with enhanced venoconstrictor tone and a resultant redistribution of blood volume from the periphery to the cardiopulmonary segments (central redistribution of blood volume). Central blood volume, the volume of blood in the heart and lungs, is generally normal or increased in the presence of decreased total blood volume in these patients. Further, forearm venous distensibility is diminished in untreated patients with essential hypertension, indicating that venoconstrictor tone is increased.

AUTONOMIC FUNCTION. The autonomic nervous system is involved in both the initiation and the maintenance of elevated arterial pressure in essential hypertension. In patients with early hypertension, both parasympathetic and sympathetic control mechanisms are abnormal. The tachycardia, increased cardiac output, increased dp/dt, and venoconstriction characteristic of these patients are due to a combination of diminished resting parasympathetic inhibition and enhanced sympathetic stimulation. These patients have elevated plasma renin and norepinephrine levels and enhanced vascular responses to stress as a consequence of their increased sympathetic activity. The concentration of norepinephrine in cerebrospinal fluid from patients with essential hypertension is higher than in healthy normal volunteers, suggesting that noradrenergic pathways in the central nervous

system are hyperactive in persons with essential hypertension.

Patients with essential hypertension have an exaggerated pressor response to stress and an exaggerated depressor response to relaxation. Blood pressure falls during sleep, meditation, and other states of relaxation and rises during isometric exercise and the stress of mental arithmetic in these patients to a greater extent than in normotensive control subjects. The impressive fall in BP that is frequently seen when a hypertensive patient is removed from the home environment and brought into the hospital suggests that environmental stress exacerbates hypertension. The increased prevalence of hypertension in urban populations compared with rural groups and the occurrence of age-related rises in BP in societies with changing value systems but not in those with a stable social structure provide evidence for a psychogenic contribution to essential hypertension. Stress presumably mediates its pressor effect through the sympathetic nervous system.

HUMORAL CONTROL OF PRESSURE AND VOLUME. *Renin-Angiotensin System.* Renin is a proteolytic enzyme that is synthesized, stored, and secreted mainly in the kidney, but also in brain and blood vessel walls. Renin cleaves its glycoprotein substrate, angiotensinogen, to produce angiotensin I (Fig. 47–2). Angiotensin I is a decapeptide prohormone that is activated by conversion to the octapeptide angiotensin II via angiotensin-converting enzyme. Angiotensin II is a potent vasoconstrictor and stimulator of aldosterone synthesis and secretion. It also has pressor and dipsogenic effects through actions on the central nervous system and on facilitation of norepinephrine release from sympathetic nerve terminals. Angiotensins I and II are destroyed in peripheral capillary beds by a number of enzymes, the angiotensinases.

Kallikrein-Kinin System. The kallikrein-kinin system is involved in the maintenance of BP by control of regional blood flow and water and electrolyte excretion. Kinins are potent vasodilator and natriuretic peptides released from inactive precursors, the kininogens, by the kininogenases, a group of serine proteases that includes the plasma and glandular kallikreins. The kinins are rapidly inactivated in the circulation, suggesting that, rather than producing systemic vasodilatation, their physiologic role is to maintain regional blood flow and, in the case of the kidney, to influence sodium excretion. One of the kinin-inactivating enzymes, kininase II, also catalyzes the conversion of angiotensin I to II (Fig. 47–2). Thus, the same enzyme generates a vasoconstrictor peptide (angiotensin II) and hydrolyzes a vasodilator/natriuretic peptide (bradykinin). Kallikrein in the luminal plasma membrane of the distal tubule catalyzes the formation of kinins that effect a natriuresis by (1) inhibiting sodium transport in the distal nephron, (2) causing renal vasodilatation, and (3) altering the osmotic gradient of the renal medulla.

The kallikrein-kinin system also alters renal blood flow and sodium handling indirectly by effects on the renin-angiotensin-aldosterone system and on renal prostaglandins (Fig. 47–3). Kallikrein stimulates renin release and activates inactive renin. Further, kinins stimulate the synthesis of vasodilator prostaglandins, probably by activation of phospholipase A_2 and increased release of arachidonic acid. Part of the vasodilator effect of the kinins is mediated through the release of prostaglandins. Conversely, angiotensin, aldosterone, and prostaglandins, as well as arginine vasopressin (AVP), can stimulate the release of renal kallikrein and perhaps the intrarenal formation of kinins.

Both reductions and elevations in urinary kallikrein excretion have been described in patients with various forms of hypertension. Whether these abnormalities in kallikrein excretion are etiologically related to the hypertension is uncertain.

Prostaglandins. Prostaglandins (PG) in kidney and blood vessel walls participate in BP regulation through both their

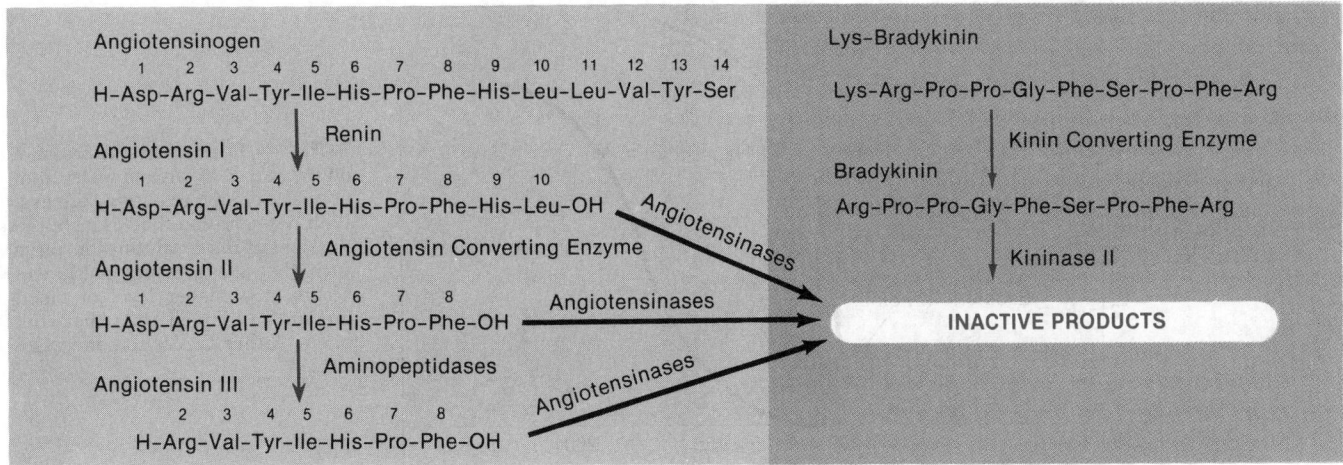

FIGURE 47–2. Biochemistry of the renin-angiotensin system and its interaction (via converting enzyme or kininase II) with the kallikrein-kinin system.

intrinsic effects and their interactions with other vasoregulatory systems. Prostaglandins stimulate the kallikrein-kinin and renin-angiotensin systems, and prostaglandin production is stimulated by both bradykinin and angiotensin II (Fig. 47–3). The antihypertensive effects of the prostaglandins predominate over their pressor effects, since intravenous administration of their precursor, arachidonic acid, generally lowers BP, whereas indomethacin, which inhibits prostaglandin production, tends to exacerbate hypertension.

Prostaglandins oppose the vasoconstrictor effects of a number of humoral agents. Prostaglandins E_2 and I_2 decrease the release of norepinephrine during sympathetic nerve stimulation and reduce the vasoconstrictor effect of infused norepinephrine. Further, prostaglandins whose synthesis is stimulated by angiotensin II attenuate the vasoconstrictor effects of angiotensin II.

Prostaglandins, principally PGE, which are found in high concentrations in the renal medulla, act as local vasodilators and powerful natriuretic agents. It has been proposed that the prostaglandins operate in concert with the kallikrein-kinin system to maintain renal blood flow and facilitate natriuresis, thus opposing those factors that elevate BP through intrarenal mechanisms.

Prostaglandin metabolism may be altered in patients with essential hypertension. Urinary excretion of PGE_2 is often depressed in essential hypertension but not in hypertension secondary to aldosterone excess or renovascular disease, suggesting that reduction of renal PGE_2 synthesis in essential hypertension may be a primary abnormality rather than a secondary response to the elevated BP. These data, coupled with the observation that renal kallikrein-kinin activity is often

reduced in essential hypertension, are consistent with the interpretation that these local renal hormones regulate systemic BP and vascular resistance through control of renal blood flow and sodium excretion.

Arginine Vasopressin. Arginine vasopressin (AVP), the mammalian antidiuretic hormone, has pressor effects that are mediated by direct actions on vascular smooth muscle and by indirect actions on the brain, including resetting of the baroreceptor. Levels of AVP in plasma and urine are elevated in patients with renovascular hypertension and in a subset of patients with essential hypertension. Whether AVP plays an etiologic role in the hypertension or represents a marker of other neurohumoral abnormalities remains to be determined.

Atrial Natriuretic Peptides. Mammalian atria synthesize, store, and release into the circulation peptides with potent diuretic, natriuretic, and vasorelaxant properties. The atrial natriuretic peptides inhibit the action of endogenous vasoconstrictors and reduce aldosterone synthesis. These properties suggest that the atrial natriuretic peptides may be physiologic regulators of sodium, volume, and pressure homeostasis or may play a role in the pathogenesis of hypertension, or both. Plasma levels of atrial natriuretic peptide in patients with untreated essential hypertension are two- to eightfold greater than those in control normotensive subjects. The mechanism by which circulating atrial natriuretic peptide levels are elevated in hypertensive subjects likely involves a combination of increased left atrial stretch secondary to systemic hypertension and increased right atrial stretch secondary to volume expansion.

RENAL SODIUM HANDLING. Hemodynamic, neural, and humoral factors all participate in the control of volume

Figure 47–3. A schematic representation of the interactions of the renal kallikrein-kinin, renin-angiotensin, and prostaglandin systems. Solid lines represent stimulation or conversion, and dotted lines inactivation or inhibition. LBK = Lysylbradykinin; BK = bradykinin; ACE = angiotensin-converting enzyme. (From Smith MC, Dunn MJ: Renal kallikrein, kinins and prostaglandins in hypertension. In Brenner BM, Stein JH (eds): Contemporary Issues in Nephrology. Vol. 8. New York, Churchill Livingstone, Inc., 1981, by permission.)

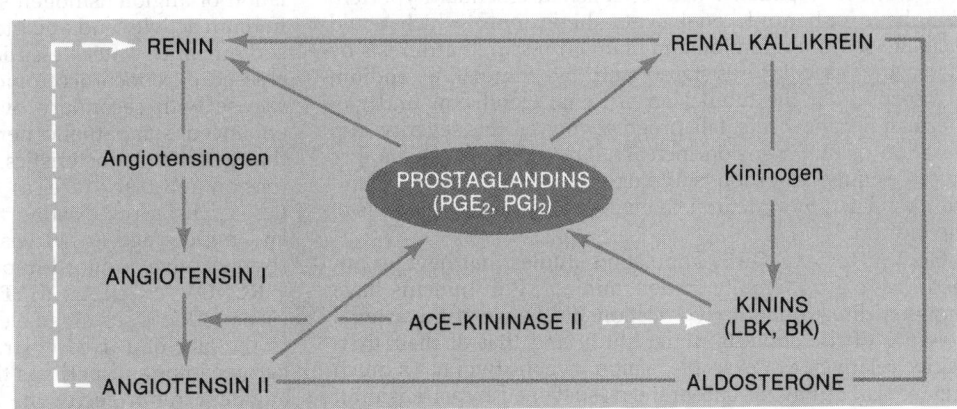

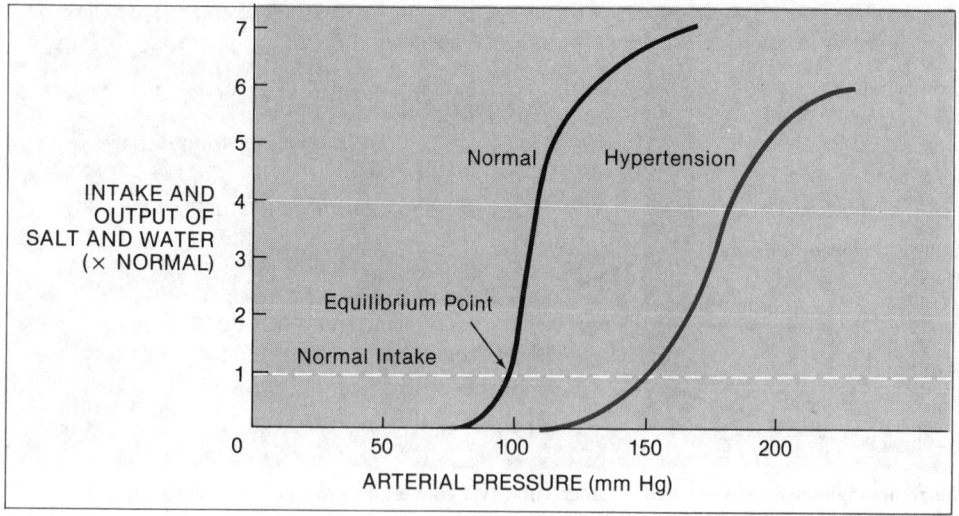

FIGURE 47—4. Effect of arterial pressure on the output of salt and water from normal and hypertensive kidneys. With hypertension there is a shift to the right of the renal function curve such that the pressure natriuresis occurs at a higher level of blood pressure. (Adapted from the work of Dr. Arthur C. Guyton and associates.)

and pressure homeostasis by regulating renal sodium handling. The normal kidney plays an important role in maintaining intravascular volume and arterial BP. It responds to increments in perfusion pressure by increasing sodium and water excretion, thus reducing intravascular volume and restoring arterial pressure to normal levels (Fig. 47–4). Normally, sodium intake and output are balanced at a mean perfusion pressure of 100 mm Hg. An alteration in this relationship, such that higher perfusion pressures are needed to produce a natriuresis, would facilitate the development and maintenance of hypertension. A variety of neurohumoral factors, intrinsic and extrinsic to the kidney, can influence the relationship between perfusion pressure and sodium excretion. Intrinsic factors include angiotensin II, prostaglandins, and kinins; extrinsic factors include circulating catecholamines, AVP, aldosterone, and sympathetic nervous activity. In addition, a kidney subjected to elevated pressure over time develops structural changes that limit its ability to excrete sodium and water in response to increases in pressure.

A defect in the excretion of salt and water may be central to the pathogenesis of many, if not all, forms of hypertension. Animal models provide evidence that changes in the renal circulation due to increased sympathetic nervous system activity favor salt and water retention and the genesis of hypertension. Renal denervation delays the development of hypertension in these models. Renal abnormalities have also been demonstrated in patients with essential hypertension. In patients with established uncomplicated essential hypertension, renal blood flow tends to be reduced in the presence of a normal or slightly reduced glomerular filtration rate. Alterations in renal blood flow and tubular function in uncomplicated essential hypertension usually result from reversible arteriolar vasoconstriction rather than from fixed structural changes. Many patients with established essential hypertension have enhanced renal sympathetic tone, which could facilitate sodium retention and blunt a pressure natriuresis by increasing vascular resistance and by stimulating sodium reabsorption at the tubular level. Renal blood flow and glomerular filtration rate fall progressively as the severity and duration of hypertension increase. These functional changes are consequences of longstanding elevations in pressure and can be related to structural changes in resistance of vessels of the kidney.

GENETIC FACTORS. Population studies that have examined the role of heredity in determining BP in humans have shown a direct quantitative relationship between the arterial pressure of the subjects under study and that of their first-degree relatives. For example, a monozygotic twin has a much greater risk of having borderline or sustained hypertension if his or her twin has either condition. To date, no specific set of BP-regulating genes has been identified, nor have genetic markers that permit early detection of individuals at risk for developing hypertension been characterized.

Hypertensive Crisis

Approximately 1 per cent of hypertensive patients enter an accelerated phase characterized by severe hypertension and necrotizing arteriolitis, leading to progressive end-organ damage that may be irreversible if the hypertension is untreated. Hypertensive crisis is a medical emergency; left untreated, the five-year mortality rate is 100 per cent. This syndrome can result from essential hypertension or from hypertension secondary to any cause, except coarctation of the aorta, and is particularly common in patients with renovascular hypertension. The triggering mechanism for the development of arteriolar lesions has been related to the absolute level or rate of rise of arterial pressure, the presence of disseminated intravascular clotting in association with microangiopathic hemolytic anemia, or activation of the renin-angiotensin system. Whatever the initiating mechanism, the syndrome is perpetuated by deposition of fibrin in arteriolar walls, which in turn leads to retinopathy, renal damage, and increased renin release.

Secondary Hypertension

ORAL CONTRACEPTIVE–INDUCED HYPERTENSION. Approximately 5 per cent of women who use oral contraceptives experience the new onset of hypertension, which resolves with withdrawal of oral contraceptive therapy. Mechanisms by which oral contraceptives may precipitate hypertension in a genetically susceptible host include stimulation of angiotensinogen synthesis with secondary increases in renin activity and angiotensin II generation, increased renal sodium and water retention, increased cardiac output, increased adrenocorticotropic hormone (ACTH) synthesis and release with secondary overproduction of aldosterone, and enhanced sympathetic nervous system activity. It is likely that genetic characteristics, such as family history of hypertension and black race, as well as environmental characteristics, such as pre-existing and occult renal disease, obesity, and middle age (> 40 years), increase susceptibility to oral contraceptive–induced hypertension.

RENOVASCULAR HYPERTENSION. Renovascular disease produces sustained elevation of circulating renin activity. In the face of a fixed obstruction to perfusion, the intrarenal baroreceptor and perhaps the macula densa are stimulated to augment renin secretion. Angiotensin and aldosterone are increased secondarily, resulting in sodium and water retention, but because of a block in the feedback loop proximal to the intrarenal baroreceptors, renin production cannot be turned off. In renovascular hypertension, renin levels are elevated primarily and aldosterone levels secondarily. Elevated circulating angiotensin II and aldosterone levels are primarily responsible for BP elevation early in the course of renovascular hypertension, and increased sodium and water retention and enhanced sympathetic nervous system activity play dominant roles in the maintenance of hypertension in the chronic phase of the syndrome. Deficiencies of antihypertensive factors, such as prostaglandins and renomedullary neutral lipid, may also contribute to the pathogenesis of this form of hypertension.

Any lesion that obstructs either large or small renal arteries can cause renovascular hypertension. The most common and clinically important of these are intrinsic lesions of the large vessels, because they can be physically removed and the hypertension either cured or ameliorated. Atherosclerotic disease is found in two thirds of patients with renovascular hypertension; fibrous or fibromuscular disease, in one third. Patients with atherosclerotic renal artery lesions tend to be older and to have higher systolic BP measurements and more frequent extrarenal arterial disease than patients with essential hypertension and are more likely to develop target-organ damage. Patients with fibromuscular disease tend to be younger and predominantly female and are less likely to develop cardiovascular complications. Prognosis is generally worse in atherosclerotic disease than in fibromuscular disease.

PRIMARY ALDOSTERONISM. Primary aldosteronism is the most common of the syndromes of mineralocorticoid excess. Despite its low prevalence in hypertensive populations (< 1 per cent), the syndrome has received much attention because it can be easily suspected by the finding of depressed serum potassium levels and can frequently be cured by surgery.

Primary aldosteronism is a syndrome of hypertension associated with hypokalemia, suppressed plasma renin activity, and increased aldosterone production in which the other abnormalities result from the relatively autonomous secretion of aldosterone. Autonomous production of aldosterone is associated with excessive salt and water retention, which leads to an increase in effective blood volume and suppression of renin release. Since mineralocorticoid production is not angiotensin dependent, the feedback loop is interrupted, and excessive mineralocorticoid production continues. Renin is therefore suppressed, and the level of aldosterone is elevated. Hypokalemia is a direct consequence of the effects of aldosterone on the renal tubule, but the pathogenesis of the hypertension remains poorly understood. Increases in plasma volume have been described but are inconstant findings. Hemodynamic studies suggest that increased peripheral resistance is important in maintaining the hypertension.

PHEOCHROMOCYTOMA. Pheochromocytoma is a rare but important cause of surgically curable hypertension. Although it accounts for less than 0.5 per cent of all cases of hypertension, diagnosis is critical because pheochromocytomas may be malignant, the hypertension may be severe and refractory to conventional antihypertensive treatment, and patients with unrecognized pheochromocytoma are subject to hypertensive crises during anesthesia and angiography and following administration of drugs such as guanethidine and the ganglion blockers.

Pheochromocytoma is a tumor of neural crest origin that produces sustained or paroxysmal hypertension by releasing catecholamines, usually a combination of norepinephrine and epinephrine, into the circulation. Ninety per cent of pheochromocytomas are located in the adrenal medulla, and 10 per cent of these are bilateral. The remaining 10 per cent are scattered in the distribution of autonomic tissue. Fifteen per cent of all pheochromocytomas are malignant. These are generally slow growing and resistant to radiation therapy. They usually metastasize to lymph nodes, liver, lung, and bone. Malignant pheochromocytomas and their metastases may or may not be functional. Pheochromocytomas are common in patients with neurocutaneous syndromes such as von Recklinghausen's disease and in families with the syndromes of multiple endocrine adenomatosis. Patients with pheochromocytoma have an increased incidence of neuroectodermal tumors, including brain tumors.

DIAGNOSIS
Initial Evaluation

The initial evaluation of the hypertensive patient is designed to establish the diagnosis of arterial hypertension, grade its severity, determine the need for treatment, and assess the likelihood of a secondary cause for the hypertension. The Joint National Committee on Detection, Evaluation, and Treatment of High Blood Pressure has published guidelines for the detection, follow-up, and stepped-care therapy of hypertensive patients.

BLOOD PRESSURE MEASUREMENT. The accurate and reproducible measurement of BP by the cuff technique is the most critical part of the diagnostic evaluation. On the initial visit, the BP should be taken after the patient has been seated comfortably for at least five minutes with his or her arm bared. Constriction of the upper arm by a rolled sleeve should be avoided, as it distorts the BP measurement. Two or three measurements should be taken at each visit, and at least two minutes should be allowed between readings. Proper cuff size is critical to accurate BP measurement. The width should be about two thirds the width of the arm (15 cm in most adults), and, more important, the bladder cuff should be long enough to circle the arm. Falsely elevated readings can be obtained when the bladder is too short, and the error is magnified if the cuff is also too narrow. Mercury manometers are preferred, but aneroid manometers can be used if they are standardized frequently against a mercury manometer.

To obtain an accurate systolic pressure, the cuff should be inflated rapidly to at least 30 mm Hg above the systolic pressure, as determined by palpation of the radial artery. This inflation is necessary to avoid underestimating the pressure because of the auscultatory gap, an unexplained disappearance of Korotkoff's sounds for some interval between systole and diastole. The systolic reading is taken as the level of pressure at which clear Korotkoff's sounds are heard with each heart beat. The diastolic reading is taken at the level both when sounds become muffled (Korotkoff phase IV) and when sounds disappear (phase V). Both readings should be recorded. It is not known whether the level of muffling or of disappearance is a more accurate reflection of the intra-arterial diastolic pressure, so selection of one over the other as the clinical measurement of diastolic pressure is a matter of convenience and reproducibility.

The use of home BP recordings by either the patient or another person in the household or the use of 24-hour ambulatory BP recordings, or both, is useful, particularly in monitoring patients with labile hypertension, anxious patients whose BP readings tend to be falsely elevated in the doctor's office, and patients whose doses of antihypertensive medications need to be adjusted frequently. Home recordings should be taken at various times of day, in various positions, and during periods of stress and relaxation in order to assess the effects of diurnal variations in hormones, posture, and emotional state of BP. Standard sphygmomanometers and stethoscopes are appropriate for this purpose; most automated indirect BP measuring devices are inaccurate and should not be used. The patient's skill at BP measurement should be tested at frequent intervals by a professional.

Selection of Patients for Evaluation for Secondary Hypertension

Once a diagnosis of stable hypertension has been established, the need for antihypertensive treatment should be assessed, and, where indicated, diagnostic evaluation for secondary causes of hypertension should be undertaken. In view of the rarity of secondary causes of hypertension and the high cost and risk of elaborate diagnostic studies, the routine pretreatment workup should be limited to defining the severity of the hypertension and to identifying its complications and associated cardiovascular risk factors. All of the secondary causes combined account for less than 5 per cent of the adult hypertensive population, but since some patients with secondary hypertension are potentially curable, diagnostic evaluation is warranted in selected patients. These include the following:

1. Those in whom routine history, physical examination, or routine laboratory data suggest a specific secondary cause.
2. Those who are younger than 30 years of age, since they have the greatest prevalence of correctable secondary hypertension.
3. Those in whom drug therapy is inadequate or unsatisfactory.
4. Those whose BP has suddenly worsened.

MEDICAL HISTORY. A careful, complete history should be obtained and a physical examination should be performed in all hypertensive patients before therapy is started. The medical history should include any previous history of hypertension, including prior and current antihypertensive treatment; a history of factors regarded as predisposing to hypertension, including excessive salt intake, the use of oral contraceptives or other estrogen preparations, stressful occupation, and a family history of hypertension and its complications; evidence of hypertensive complications, including congestive heart failure, coronary artery disease, renal dysfunction, and stroke; and a history of other cardiovascular risk factors, including diabetes, obesity, cigarette smoking, and lipid abnormalities. A history of weakness, muscle cramps, and polyuria suggests hypokalemia and the possibility of hyperaldosteronism; a history of headaches, palpitations, or hyperhidrosis suggests pheochromocytoma.

PHYSICAL EXAMINATION. The physical examination should include two or more BP measurements, at least one of which is obtained in the standing position; funduscopic examination for hypertensive retinopathy; careful examination of the cardiovascular system for evidence of congestive heart failure, cardiomegaly, myocardial dysfunction, and peripheral vascular disease; examination of the abdomen for bruits; auscultation over all scars for evidence of arteriovenous fistulas; and a careful neurologic examination for the stigmas of stroke.

LABORATORY EVALUATION. Pretreatment laboratory tests can be restricted to those generally performed as part of a routine medical checkup; hematocrit, urinalysis, creatinine or blood urea nitrogen levels, serum potassium levels, chest film, and electrocardiogram. Other tests, which can be obtained as part of most automated blood chemistry batteries, such as the blood glucose, serum cholesterol, and serum uric acid levels, are helpful in assessing other cardiovascular risk factors and can be used as a baseline for monitoring the effects of antihypertensive treatment. Serial electrocardiograms and echocardiograms may be useful in assessing the effects of hypertension and antihypertensive treatment on the heart.

Hypertensive Crisis

Patients with accelerated hypertension usually present with hypertension encephalopathy, rapidly progressive renal insufficiency, or acute left ventricular failure. Hypertensive encephalopathy is characterized by the rapid onset of confusion, headache, visual disturbances, seizures, and, in severe cases, somnolence and even coma. Increased intracranial pressure with papilledema occurs, presumably resulting from failure of autoregulation of cerebral blood flow with breakthrough vasodilatation and secondary extravasation of intravascular contents. Death from a cerebrovascular accident frequently occurs if the hypertension is untreated, but the encephalopathy usually clears rapidly following successful antihypertensive treatment. Renal damage secondary to necrotizing arteriolitis results in proteinuria, hematuria, and azotemia. Assuming that the blood pressure can be controlled, the presence of renal damage at the time of diagnosis has prognostic significance. The five-year survival of treated patients with grade IV retinopathy and azotemia is 23 per cent and that of nonazotemic patients, 64 per cent.

Evaluation of Patients for Secondary Causes of Hypertension

ORAL CONTRACEPTIVE–INDUCED HYPERTENSION. The diagnosis of oral contraceptive–induced hypertension can be made by documenting the onset of hypertension de novo during contraceptive therapy and the resolution of the hypertension upon drug withdrawal. This form of hypertension usually begins during the first year of oral contraceptive administration.

Oral contraceptive–induced hypertension can, in part, be prevented by avoiding use of these agents in women who are at high risk. Evidence of thromboembolic disease or chronic hypertension of any cause is an absolute contraindication to use of oral contraceptives. A family history of hypertension and a personal history of pre-existing or occult renal disease or of pregnancy complicated by hypertension are relative contraindications to oral contraceptive use. Women over 35 years of age, particularly if obese, should be cautioned about the increased risk of developing hypertension while ingesting oral contraceptives. Such patients should be followed closely: BP measurement and a funduscopic examination should be performed and an interval history obtained on several occasions during the first year of treatment and at yearly intervals thereafter.

RENOVASCULAR HYPERTENSION. Patients most likely to have renovascular hypertension include those with hypertension of abrupt onset, especially in the young or in those in late middle age; those with malignant hypertension or sudden acceleration of benign hypertension; and those who have failed to respond to medical therapy. Generally, these patients have moderately severe to severe fixed diastolic hypertension. The presence of an upper abdominal bruit, particularly one that is systolic-diastolic or continuous in timing, is high pitched, and radiates laterally from the midepigastrium, is strongly suggestive of functionally significant renal artery stenosis. Such bruits have been described in one half to two thirds of patients with surgically proved renovascular hypertension. Because of the cost of the diagnostic evaluation for renovascular hypertension, diagnostic study should be reserved for patients with one or more of the characteristics discussed above.

Screening tests, including the rapid-sequence or hypertensive intravenous pyelogram (IVP), abdominal ultrasonography, and pharmacologic screening with a converting enzyme inhibitor, have some role in the preliminary evaluation of patients for renovascular hypertension, particularly in those in whom the index of suspicion for the syndrome is low. The lack of specificity of these screening procedures limits their usefulness, however, so that, in patients in whom the index of suspicion of renovascular hypertension is high, it is reasonable to move directly to definitive diagnostic testing, which generally requires hospitalization.

Definitive diagnosis of functionally significant renal artery stenosis is made by a combination of *selective renal angiography*

TABLE 47–5. ANTIHYPERTENSIVE AGENTS THAT INHIBIT RENIN RELEASE

Agent	Trade Name
Beta-adrenergic–blocking agents	
Propranolol	(Inderal)
Metoprolol	(Lopressor)
Nadolol	(Corgard)
Atenolol	(Tenormin)
Timolol	(Blocadren)
Acebutolol	(Sectral)
Combined alpha- and beta-adrenergic–blocking agent	
Labetalol	(Normodyne)
Sympatholytic agents	
Alpha-methyldopa	(Aldomet)
Clonidine	(Catapres)
Guanabenz	(Wytensin)
Reserpine	(Serpasil)
Guanethidine	(Ismelin)
Ganglion-blocking agent	
Trimethaphan camsylate	(Arfonad)

and differential renal vein renin measurement. Renal angiography is needed to define the anatomy of the stenotic renal artery in order to plan the approach to revascularization. Documentation of the functional significance of an anatomic lesion requires demonstration of increased renin production by the involved kidney. When renin activity in the venous effluent from the involved kidney is 1.5 or more times that of the uninvolved side and when the uninvolved side can be shown not to produce renin, the probability of improvement in BP after renal revascularization is approximately 90 per cent. Stimulation of renin release with provocative maneuvers—such as tilting, salt deprivation, or administration of vasodilators, diuretics, or converting enzyme inhibitors—has been shown to enhance selectively renin release from the affected kidney. Converting enzyme inhibitors increase the renal vein renin ratio in patients with hypertension secondary to unilateral renal artery stenosis by two mechanisms: lowering BP and blocking feedback inhibition of renin release by angiotensin II. A convenient regimen is administration of 25 mg of captopril p.o. two to four hours before the procedure. The diagnosis of surgically remediable renal artery stenosis can be missed when renal vein sampling is performed in the unstimulated state or when renin-suppressing antihypertensive drugs (Table 47–5) are not discontinued prior to study. False-positive lateralization secondary to excess stimulation of renin release has not been reported.

PRIMARY ALDOSTERONISM. The diagnosis of primary aldosteronism should be considered in patients with refractory hypertension, particularly those with spontaneous or diuretic-induced hypokalemia. A normal plasma potassium value on screening does not rule out the diagnosis of primary aldosteronism. Many (7 to 38 per cent) patients with primary aldosteronism have intermittently normal plasma potassium values, particularly if dietary sodium is restricted or potassium supplementation is given. In a recent prospective study of 80 patients with primary aldosteronism, all of whom were referred for evaluation because of spontaneous hypokalemia, diuretic-induced hypokalemia, and/or refractory hypertension, only 73 per cent had spontaneous hypokalemia (serum potassium level < 3.5 mEq per liter on a normal sodium intake) and only 86 per cent had provoked hypokalemia (serum potassium level < 3.5 mEq per liter on a high sodium intake for three days) (Table 47–6). More than one half of patients in this series developed moderately severe hypokalemia (serum potassium level < 3.0 mEq per liter) while on usual diuretic therapy. Thus, although reliance on serum potassium measurements in screening would cause the diagnosis of primary aldosteronism to be missed in about one fourth of patients, hypokalemia does provide an important clue to the presence of primary aldosteronism. Approximately 50 per cent of hypertensive patients with unprovoked hypokalemia have primary aldosteronism, whereas less than 0.5 per cent of those with normal plasma potassium levels have the syndrome. When hypokalemia is observed, the concomitant measurement of urinary potassium excretion when the patient is not taking diuretics is valuable in distinguishing primary aldosteronism from other causes. Inappropriate potassium wastage (> 40 mEq per 24 hours) is seen in primary aldosteronism with hypokalemia, but not in hypokalemia of other causes.

The best single test for identifying patients with primary aldosteronism is the measurement of aldosterone excretion after three days of salt loading (Table 47–6). Under these conditions, most patients with primary aldosteronism have aldosterone excretion rates of greater than 14.0 μg per 24 hours. There is little or no overlap with the range of values obtained in normal subjects or in patients with essential hypertension. Measurements of plasma renin activity and plasma and urinary aldosterone levels obtained under uncontrolled dietary conditions are not useful in screening for primary aldosteronism, and plasma renin measurements made under conditions of stimulation (sodium restriction, diuretic administration, and upright posture) are inadequate to rule out the diagnosis of primary aldosteronism.

Adenoma Versus Hyperplasia. Once a presumptive diagnosis of aldosterone excess is made, additional procedures are needed to differentiate between adrenal adenoma—or, rarely, carcinoma—and bilateral adrenal hyperplasia as sources for the hormone. A solitary adrenal cortical adenoma is the cause of primary aldosteronism in 60 to 85 per cent of cases; bilateral adrenal cortical hyperplasia is the cause in the remaining 15 to 40 per cent. Aldosterone-producing adenoma is generally associated with more severe hypertension, more extreme aldosterone elevation and renin suppression, and more marked electrolyte imbalance than hyperplasia. The distinction is important in guiding therapy, as patients with adrenal adenomas can have their hyperaldosteronism and

TABLE 47–6. SENSITIVITY AND SPECIFICITY OF VARIOUS SCREENING TESTS FOR PRIMARY ALDOSTERONISM[a]

Test	Standard	Sensitivity (no. of patients)	Specificity (no. of patients)
Serum potassium[b]	Spontaneous (< 3.5 mEq/liter)	0.73 (58/80)	0.94 (66/70)
Serum potassium[c]	Provoked (< 3.5 mEq/liter)	0.86 (70/80)	0.96 (67/70)
Plasma renin activity[d]	Suppressed (< 2.0 ng/ml/hr)	0.64 (51/80)	0.83 (58/70)
Aldosterone excretion rate[c]	Nonsuppressible (> 14 μg/24 hr)	0.96 (77/80)	0.93 (65/70)
Plasma aldosterone concentration[c]	Nonsuppressible (> 22 ng/dl)	0.72 (31/43)	0.91 (31/34)

[a]Sensitivity = percentage of subjects with disease who have positive results. Specificity = percentage of subjects without disease who have negative results. Standards for aldosterone excretion rate and plasma aldosterone concentration represent the upper 95 per cent range of values obtained in subjects with essential hypertension.
[b]Normal sodium intake for three to five days.
[c]High sodium intake for three days.
[d]Low sodium intake for four days.
Reprinted with permission from Bravo EL, Tarazi RC, Dustan HP, et al.: The changing clinical spectrum of primary aldosteronism. Am J Med 74:641–651, 1983.

hypertension cured by unilateral adrenalectomy, whereas those with bilateral hyperplasia often remain hypertensive even after both adrenal glands are removed.

Several techniques are available for localizing aldosterone-producing adenomas. Computed tomography (CT) scanning can resolve adrenal tumors that are more than 1.0 cm in diameter and has a localizing accuracy of 75 per cent for aldosteronomas. In patients with suspected bilateral adrenal cortical hyperplasia, the CT scan reveals either bilateral adrenal enlargement or normal-appearing glands. Computed tomographic scans have largely replaced ¹²⁵I-19-iodocholesterol scintiscans in the diagnostic evaluation of patients with primary aldosteronism. Computed tomographic scanning offers several practical advantages over radioisotope studies, including immediate availability of results, lower absorbed radiation doses, greater convenience for the patient, and greater availability to the physician. Direct adrenal vein sampling by percutaneous catheterization, with measurement of adrenal venous aldosterone levels, is the most accurate (90 per cent accuracy in experienced hands). Elevated values with a less than twofold difference between sides suggest bilateral hyperplasia; aldosterone-producing adenomas generally result in a more than tenfold difference between sides. Adrenal venography, although accurate in localizing adrenal tumors, is no longer in general use because of the high incidence (5 to 10 per cent) of retroperitoneal and intra-adrenal hemorrhage.

In summary, when biochemical findings suggest the presence of an aldosterone-producing adenoma, an adrenal CT scan should be performed and can be considered diagnostic if an adrenal mass is clearly identified. If the results of the CT scan are inconclusive, adrenal venous sampling for aldosterone is indicated.

PHEOCHROMOCYTOMA. The most common signs and symptoms of pheochromocytoma include unusually labile hypertension; symptomatic paroxysms of hypertension and tachycardia characterized by "spells" with headache, palpitations, sweating, pallor, and hypertension; accelerated hypertension, hypertension refractory to conventional therapy; hypermetabolism and weight loss; abnormal carbohydrate metabolism; and pressor responses to induction of anesthesia or antihypertensive treatment. Most patients with pheochromocytoma are symptomatic, so it is legitimate to use symptoms and physical signs in screening patients for the tumor. Biochemical tests need to be performed only in patients who have clinical evidence of the disorder.

Diagnosis of pheochromocytoma requires the demonstration of increased concentrations of catecholamines or their metabolites, or both, in plasma or urine and the localization of a tumor via CT scanning, radionuclide techniques, or angiography. Measurements of 24-hour urinary excretion of VMA (3-methoxy-4-hydroxymandelic acid) and of metanephrine and normetanephrine are the most commonly used screening tests for pheochromocytoma because of their low cost, simplicity, and general availability. Assay of plasma catecholamines offers advantages over measurement of urinary catecholamines or metabolites, or both, in that it eliminates the unreliability inherent in 24-hour urine collections and artifacts secondary to interference from drugs and angiographic contrast media. Measurement of plasma catecholamines is more reliable than 24-hour assessment of urinary metanephrines or VMA, or both, in screening for pheochromocytoma as long as appropriate precautions are taken in obtaining plasma samples. Patients must be resting and the stress of venipuncture avoided by insertion of an indwelling catheter 20 to 30 minutes before sampling. Plasma catecholamine levels are usually enormously elevated in patients with pheochromocytoma compared with controls with essential hypertension (Fig. 47–5). In contrast, urinary metanephrine and VMA values in patients with pheochromocytoma

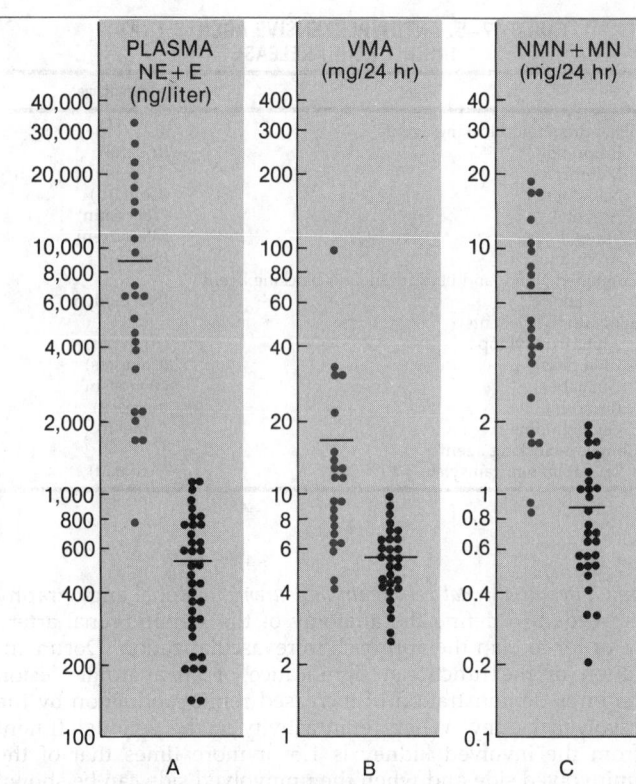

FIGURE 47–5. *A,* Plasma norepinephrine (NE) and epinephrine (E) measured at rest in patients with (*red circles*) and without (*black circles*) evidence of pheochromocytoma. All but 1 of the 23 patients with pheochromocytoma had plasma catecholamine values greater than the highest value in patients without pheochromocytoma. *B* and *C,* Twenty-four hour urinary vanillylmandelic acid (VMA) and total metanephrines (NMN + MN) collected on the same day as blood drawing for the determination of plasma catecholamines in patients depicted in *A.* (Reprinted, with modifications, from Bravo EL, et al.: Circulating and urinary catecholamines in pheochromocytoma. N Engl J Med 301:684,1979.)

show substantial overlap with the range of values obtained in patients with essential hypertension.

The sensitivity and specificity of plasma catecholamine assays in the diagnosis of pheochromocytoma can be enhanced by repeating the assays after administration of clonidine or pentolinium. In normal subjects or patients with essential hypertension, stimulation of central alpha-adrenergic receptors with clonidine or administration of a ganglion blocker suppresses plasma norepinephrine by blunting central sympathetic outflow. These agents have no effect on plasma norepinephrine levels in patients with pheochromocytoma, in whom circulating norepinephrine levels depend on autonomous release from the tumor. Interestingly, both groups show similar reductions in BP and heart rate, measured with the patient supine, after administration of these agents, suggesting that catecholamines secreted by the tumor are not responsible for the maintenance of hypertension in patients with pheochromocytoma. The clonidine and phentolamine suppression tests are useful adjunctive procedures to rule out pheochromocytoma in hypertensive patients with suggestive symptoms and borderline resting catecholamine values. Caution must be employed in the use of the clonidine suppression test in patients who are being maintained on antihypertensive treatment, as serious hypotensive reactions have been reported in that group.

Once a presumptive diagnosis of pheochromocytoma has been made by demonstrating elevations in plasma catecholamine levels or by a positive clonidine or phentolamine suppression test, localization studies are indicated. In most cases the tumor can be localized by adrenal CT scanning. For the 10 per cent of pheochromocytomas that are smaller than the resolving power of the CT scan (1.0 cm in diameter) or are located outside the adrenal glands, other means of localization are required. The guanethidine analogue ^{131}I-metaiodobenzylguanide(^{131}I-MIBG) is useful in imaging pheochromocytomas that are undetectable by CT scan. False-negative results have been reported with both CT and ^{131}I-MIBG scans. In such cases, selective arteriography or differential venous catheterization with measurement of regional plasma-catecholamines, or both, may help in localizing the tumor. These procedures are associated with appreciable risk to the patient, so they are indicated only if the scans are negative.

TREATMENT
General Considerations

The goal of antihypertensive therapy is to reduce excess cardiovascular morbidity and mortality due to hypertension. In any given patient, the decision to initiate therapy is governed by the extent of the BP elevation and the presence or absence of cardiovascular complications or additional cardiovascular risk factors, or both. Antihypertensive treatment is indicated in patients with diastolic BP measurements of 95 mm Hg or higher and in those with lesser elevations (90 to 94 mm Hg) who are at high risk of developing cardiovascular morbidity or mortality. The high-risk group includes patients with target-organ damage, diabetes mellitus, and/or other major risk factors for coronary artery disease. The initial goal of therapy is to lower diastolic BP to levels less than 90 mm Hg with minimal adverse effects. A reasonable further goal is the lowest diastolic BP consistent with safety and tolerance. An effort should be made to correct other cardiovascular risk factors in all hypertensive patients.

In patients with moderate-to-severe hypertension, even partial BP reduction has been shown to decrease cardiovascular morbidity. Therefore, in these patients, a more limited therapeutic goal may be accepted if side effects are intolerable at doses necessary to achieve normal BP. For patients with diastolic BP readings in the range of 90 to 94 mm Hg who are otherwise at low risk, an initial trial of nonpharmacologic therapy with careful BP monitoring should be carried out. If the diastolic BP remains higher than 90 mm Hg despite nonpharmacologic therapy, use of antihypertensive drugs should be considered, although controlled clinical trials have not demonstrated a clear benefit from effective antihypertensive treatment in this subset of patients.

Antihypertensive treatment is probably indicated in isolated systolic hypertension, since pharmacologic therapy has recently been shown to be well tolerated and effective in lowering BP in this group. Patients with systolic pressures greater than 160 mm Hg are generally considered to deserve treatment. The efficacy of such treatment in reducing cardiovascular morbidity and mortality has yet to be demonstrated, however.

Nonpharmacologic Therapy

Modifications in diet and lifestyle are generally more difficult to achieve than the administration of antihypertensive medication, so they should be considered adjuncts to drug therapy in hypertension. However, since the behavioral modifications useful in hypertensive persons are not costly and are generally beneficial in promoting good health, their gradual introduction should be attempted in all hypertensive patients. Institution of such measures in patients already on antihypertensive treatment may obviate the need for medical therapy or reduce the dosage requirements for adequate control.

Dietary sodium restriction is the most efficacious of all nonmedical measures in the treatment of hypertension. Moderate restriction of salt intake (to 4 to 6 grams per day) lowers BP and potentiates the antihypertensive effect of diuretics in hypertensive subjects. Conversely, a high sodium intake (15 to 20 grams per day) may overcome the antihypertensive effect of diuretics. An additional benefit of moderate sodium restriction is protection from diuretic-induced hypokalemia: In the sodium-restricted subject, less sodium is delivered to the distal exchange site and kaliuresis is minimized. Moderate sodium restriction can be effected by the simple and tolerable measures of not adding salt to food during preparation or at the table, avoiding dairy products, and avoiding processed foods to which salt is added as the preservative. Salt substitutes in which sodium is replaced with potassium are useful in hypertensive patients who do not have renal dysfunction. This form of dietary therapy should be attempted in all hypertensive subjects and may enhance the ease of control with conventional antihypertensive therapy.

Restriction of caloric intake in order to control obesity produces substantial decrements in BP, even if ideal body weight is not achieved. There appears to be a causal relationship between obesity and hypertension, and obesity may be a risk factor for coronary artery disease, independent of hypertension. In addition, obesity is an important marker for susceptibility to hypertension in the young: Body weight and weight gain are associated with the development of hypertension in children. Since caloric and sodium restriction and a reduction in saturated fats and cholesterol can easily be combined, a dietary approach to the treatment or prevention of hypertension and atherosclerotic disease has great appeal. Weight reduction should be an integral part of therapy for all obese persons (> 115 per cent of ideal weight) with hypertension. The practical problem with such an approach is widespread nonadherence to weight reduction regimens.

Dietary calcium supplementation lowers BP in some patients with essential hypertension. The mechanism of this effect is uncertain but has been related to calcium-induced natriuresis. The magnitude of this effect and the risk/benefit ratio of adding calcium to the diet are currently under investigation. Until more complete data are available, it is premature to advocate dietary calcium supplementation as a general therapeutic measure in hypertensive patients.

Reduction of alcohol consumption may be useful in the management of hypertension, since ingestion of more than 2 ounces of alcohol per day is associated with an increased prevalence of hypertension. *Coffee* has not been found to have such a deleterious effect. *Cigarette smoking* can elevate BP, but when a hypertensive patient stops smoking, BP does not usually change appreciably. The failure of smoking cessation to lower BP has been attributed to concomitant weight gain.

Relaxation techniques and other methods designed to minimize psychogenic stress have been explored in the treatment of hypertension. The theoretic basis for this approach is the observation that excess mental stress may raise the BP in humans, presumably via activation of the sympathetic nervous system. Reports on the antihypertensive efficacy of techniques of behavior modification, such as yoga, biofeedback, and meditation, have been mixed. Various relaxation and biofeedback therapies or combinations of such treatments may produce modest BP reduction in selected groups outside the laboratory for as long as one year. However, controlled studies with longer periods of follow-up are needed before these techniques can be recommended for widespread application in the treatment or prevention of hypertension. Other means of reducing stress, such as enforced vacations or job changes and the use of sedatives and tranquilizers, have not been systematically evaluated.

The role of exercise in the prevention and treatment of hypertension has not been adequately assessed. Studies in small groups of hypertensive patients have shown that BP is lowered significantly (mean of 14/10 mm Hg) after physical training. The numbers of patients studied and the duration of follow-up in these studies are inadequate to determine whether the beneficial effects of exercise are reproducible and sustained. The potential benefits of exercise include a relaxation effect and weight loss.

Pharmacologic Therapy

Ideally, therapy should be tailored to correct the specific disturbance responsible for initiating or maintaining elevated BP. Patients in whom hypertension is associated with elevated or suppressed plasma renin activity, increased cardiac output, increased effective intravascular volume, or enhanced sympathetic tone may be candidates for individualized therapy aimed at the specific abnormality. In practice, however, detailed characterization of hormone patterns and hemodynamics in most patients with essential hypertension is not feasible and adds little to the efficacy of drug therapy.

The empiric selection of antihypertensive medication is directed toward a variety of goals. Treatment should be inexpensive, long acting, effective over the long term, and associated with minimal side effects. It should control systolic and diastolic hypertension whether the patient is supine or upright, without impairing postural regulation of BP. Expensive and complicated drug regimens are frequently associated with poor compliance and treatment failure, particularly when they disturb sexual function, mood, or alertness.

In recent years, considerable attention has been devoted to improving compliance with antihypertensive regimens. Improved education of the patient, with direct involvement of patients in their own care by having them measure and record their own BP, has been shown to improve control. Instituting treatment early in the course of the disease, when BP measurements are minimally elevated and target-organ damage has not developed, helps to ensure compliance because sim-

pler, less costly drug regimens with fewer associated adverse effects can be used. Other new approaches, such as simplifying diagnostic evaluations to minimize cost and inconvenience to the patient and using ancillary personnel in routine management and education of the patient, are beneficial in improving adherence of the patient to antihypertensive therapy.

Appropriate utilization of currently available drugs will permit adequate control of BP in most (80 to 90 per cent) patients. The guiding principle of antihypertensive treatment in ambulatory patients is to control BP using the simplest regimen possible (fewest drugs in the lowest doses administered over the most convenient dosage schedule). This is usually implemented by a stepped-care program, in which therapy is started with a small dose of a single drug and the dose of that drug is increased until either the BP is controlled or the maximal therapeutic dose is achieved. Additional drugs are then added, one at a time, in increasing doses until the BP is controlled. An example of such a stepped-care regimen is given in Figure 47–6. Alternative regimens can be used as required, based on the patient's experience and preferences. In patients who present with moderately severe to severe hypertension, it may be desirable to initiate treatment with more than one agent, because it can be predicted that a single agent will not be adequate to control the BP. It is generally advisable to see the patient once every one to two weeks while the BP is being titrated downward and once every three to four months once the BP is controlled. This interval is thought to be necessary to reinforce the need for compliance, to assess the patient for side effects of the medication, and to titrate the dosage of antihypertensive drugs. Recommended dose ranges for individual drugs are listed with each agent in Tables 47–7 and 47–8.

TABLE 47–7. DIURETICS

Generic Name	Trade Name (manufacturer)	Adult Dosage (mg/day)	Duration (hr)	Dispensing Unit (mg)
Benzothiadiazine Diuretics				
Thiazides				
Chlorothiazide	Diuril (MSD)*	250–500	6–12	250, 500
Hydrochlorothiazide	Esidrix (CIBA)	25–50	12–18	25
	HydroDIURIL (MSD)			50
	Oretic (Abbott)			
Bendroflumethiazide	Naturetin (Squibb)	5–20	18–36	2.5, 5.0
				10
Benzthiazide	Aquatag (Tutag)	25–50	12–18	50
	Diucen (Central)			
	Edemex (Savage)			
	Exna (Robins)			
	Lemazide (Lemmon)			
Cyclothiazide	Anhydron (Lilly)	1–2	18–24	2
Hydroflumethiazide	Saluron (Bristol)	25–50	18–24	50
Methyclothiazide	Aquatensen (Wallace)	2.5–10.0	24–48	5.0, 2.5
	Enduron (Abbott)			
Polythiazide	Renese (Pfizer)	2–4	24–48	1, 2, 4
Trichlormethiazide	Metahydrin (Merrell Dow)	2–4	24–48	2
	Naqua (Schering)			4
Indapamide	Lozol (USV Pharmaceutical)	2.5–5.0	18–24	2.5
Phthalimidines				
Chlorthalidone	Hygroton (USV Pharmaceutical)	25–50	24–72	25, 50, 100
	Chlorthalidone (Parke-Davis)			25, 50
	Thalitone (Boehringer Ingelheim)			
Metolazone	Zaroxolyn (Pennwalt)	2.5–5.0	12–24	2.5, 5.0, 10.0
	Diulo (Searle)			2.5, 5.0, 10.0
Quinazolines				
Quinethazone	Hydromox (Lederle)	50–100	18–24	50
Loop Diuretics				
Furosemide	Lasix (Hoechst-Roussel)	20–1,000	3–6	20, 40, 80
Ethacrynic acid	Edecrin (MSD)	50–400	3–6	25, 50
Bumetanide	Bumex (Roche)	0.5–2.0	1–4	0.5, 1.0
Potassium-sparing Diuretics				
Spironolactone	Aldactone (Searle)	50–100	3–6	25, 50, 100
	Spironolactone (Parke-Davis)			25
Triamterene	Dyrenium (SKF)*	50–100	3–6	50, 10
Amiloride	Midamor (MSD)	5–10	24	5

*MSD = Merck Sharp & Dohme; SKF = Smith Kline & French.

TABLE 47–8. ANTIHYPERTENSIVE DRUGS IN AMBULATORY TREATMENT OF HYPERTENSION

Generic Name	Trade Name (manufacturer)	Adult Maintenance Dose (mg/day)	Frequency of Administration (times/day)	Duration of Action (hr)
Sympatholytic Agents				
Centrally acting alpha-adrenergic agents				
Methyldopa	Aldomet (MSD)†	250–2000	2	6–12
Clonidine	Catapres (Boehringer Ingelheim)	0.2–0.8	2	6–12
Guanabenz	Wytensin (Wyeth)	8–64	2	8–12
Reserpine and rauwolfia alkaloids	Serpasil (CIBA)	0.1–0.25	1	24
Beta-adrenergic–blocking agents				
Propranolol	Inderal (Ayerst)	40–640	2	6–12
Metoprolol	Lopressor (CIBA)	100–450	2	12
Atenolol	Tenormin (ICI)	50–100	1	24
Nadolol	Corgard (Squibb)	40–320	1	24
Timolol	Blocadren (MSD)	20–60	2	6–12
Pindolol	Visken (Sandoz)	10–60	2	6–12
Acebutolol	Sectral (Wyeth)	400–1200	1 or 2	12–24
Alpha-adrenergic–blocking agent				
Prazosin	Minipress (Pfizer)	2–20	2 or 3	3–6
Mixed alpha- and beta-adrenergic–blocking agent				
Labetalol	Normodyne (Schering) Trandate (Glaxo)	200–800	2	3–6
Ganglion-blocking agent				
Mecamylamine	Inversine (MSD)	25	2	12–24
Peripherally acting sympatholytic agent				
Guanethidine	Ismelin (CIBA)	10–300	1	24
Direct Vasodilators				
Hydralazine	Apresoline (CIBA)	20–300	2 or 3	6
Minoxidil	Loniten (Upjohn)	5–100	1 or 2	up to 72
Converting Enzyme Inhibitors				
Captopril	Capoten (Squibb)	75–450	3	4–8
Enalapril	Vasotec (MSD)	5–40	1 or 2	12–24
*Calcium Channel–Blocking Agents**				
Nifedipine	Procardia (Pfizer)	30–120	3 or 4	6–8
Diltiazem	Cardizem (Marion)	90–240	3 or 4	6–8
Verapamil	Isoptin (Knoll) Calan (Searle)	240–480	3 or 4	6–8

*These agents have not been approved by the Food and Drug Administration (FDA) for the treatment of hypertension.
†MSD = Merck Sharp & Dohme.

STEP 1. Agents that should be considered as initial therapy include thiazide diuretics, beta-adrenergic blockers, and converting enzyme inhibitors (Fig. 47–6). Any of these agents given as monotherapy will control BP in the majority of patients with mild to moderate hypertension with a minimum of adverse effects.

Thiazide diuretics have been used as initial therapy in all of the major clinical trials of antihypertensive treatment. Advantages of these agents include efficacy in almost all classes of hypertensive patients, low cost, convenient dosing schedules, and potentiation of other antihypertensive drugs. Disadvantages include induction of electrolyte imbalance (hypokalemia and hypomagnesemia) with associated ventricular ectopic activity; hypercholesterolemia and hypertriglyceridemia, which enhance the tendency to develop atherosclerosis; hyperglycemia; and hyperuricemia, which may precipitate gout (Table 47–9). Despite these disadvantages, diuretics are the preferred step 1 agent in volume-dependent forms of hypertension, in blacks, and in older patients.

The beta-adrenergic blockers are preferred step 1 agents in patients with a hyperdynamic circulatory state (indicative of increased sympathetic activity) and in patients with coronary artery disease, as they have proved useful in heart attack prevention. Disadvantages of beta blocker therapy include exacerbations in obstructive pulmonary disease, asthma, and peripheral vascular insufficiency; fatigue; sexual dysfunction; bradycardia; and hypertriglyceridemia and reductions in high density lipoprotein (HDL) cholesterol.

The converting enzyme inhibitors may prove to be advantageous as step 1 agents in patients with renin-dependent hypertension. When given as monotherapy to unselected patients with essential hypertension, captopril restores BP to normal in approximately 50 per cent of cases; the remainder

require addition of a diuretic or of a diuretic and beta-adrenergic blocker to achieve satisfactory BP control. Superior results may be obtained with the newer, more potent converting enzyme inhibitors, such as enalapril and lisinopril.* Advantages of converting enzyme inhibitors as step 1 therapy include paucity of subjective adverse effects and an absence of metabolic effects. Disadvantages include high cost and the lack of efficacy in patients whose hypertension is not renin dependent, including blacks and those with volume-dependent forms of hypertension.

STEP 2. Patients whose BP is not controlled with a step 1 drug require the addition of a second agent. Figure 47–6 summarizes therapeutic options frequently used at step 2. Step 2 agents should be added in small doses initially; then the dose should be increased until BP is controlled, the patient experiences adverse effects of the treatment, or the maximal dose is reached.

STEP 3. If step 2 therapy is inadequate in controlling BP, a third agent should be added. Figure 47–6 summarizes therapeutic options frequently used at step 3.

STEP 4. If the third step of therapy is ineffective, an additional agent that has a different mechanism of action should be added. Figure 47–6 summarizes therapeutic options frequently used at step 4.

Once BP is controlled on a stable dosage of antihypertensive drugs, fixed-dose combination tablets may be substituted in order to simplify the patient's regimen and reduce medication costs. Use of fixed-dose combination tablets provides the convenience of taking several drugs in a single tablet but has several disadvantages. The durations of action of the various components are frequently different, and the dosages may

---
*Investigational agent.

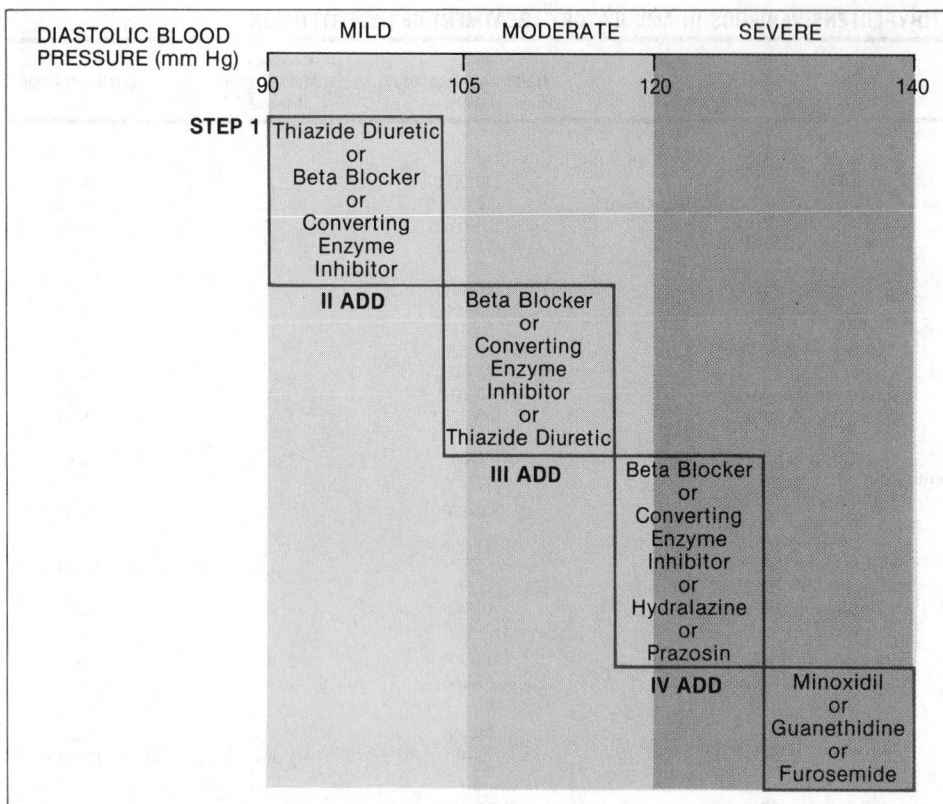

FIGURE 47–6. General antihypertensive ("stepped care") regimen.

not be appropriate for the patient's needs. The fixed-dose ratio precludes the adjustment of doses of constituent drugs to suit requirements of the individual patient.

"Step-down" therapy, or reduction of drug dosages, may be attempted in patients whose BP has been controlled for longer than one year. Administration of the lowest maintenance dose of therapy consistent with adequate BP control has the advantages of minimizing cost and adverse effects of treatment. Downward titration of doses or withdrawal of antihypertensive medications should be carried out only under careful medical supervision.

Systolic Hypertension in the Elderly

Elderly patients with rigid aortas have decreased baroreceptor responsiveness and are highly susceptible to postural hypotension when antihypertensive treatment is started. This susceptibility can be minimized by beginning with very small doses of drug and increasing dosage slowly. It has been recommended that diuretic treatment begin with half the usual starting dose, since small volume losses may give rise to large falls in pressure. Vasodilators, in small doses, are favored as second agents rather than sympatholytic drugs because the latter frequently cause central nervous system depression and may exacerbate postural hypotension.

Hypertensive Crisis

The goal of treatment in hypertensive crisis is to lower the BP as rapidly as possible to levels adequate to arrest progressive end-organ damage without causing hypoperfusion. Table 47–10 lists the antihypertensive drugs most commonly used in the management of hypertensive crisis, with recommended doses and common adverse effects. Intravenous furosemide should be administered along with these agents to assist in controlling BP and to prevent complicating fluid retention. The drug of choice in hypertensive crisis is sodium nitroprusside because it is almost always effective, has a very rapid onset of action, and has an antihypertensive effect that can be regulated precisely if monitoring facilities are available.

Secondary Hypertension

ORAL CONTRACEPTIVE–INDUCED HYPERTENSION. All patients who become hypertensive while on oral contraceptive treatment should have the drug withdrawn immediately. A treatment algorithm for such patients is outlined in Figure 47–7.

RENOVASCULAR HYPERTENSION. In general, the approach to patients with renovascular hypertension is to attempt revascularization with percutaneous transluminal angioplasty at the time of diagnosis in those with anatomically favorable lesions. If angioplasty is initially unsuccessful in dilating a lesion, or if restenosis occurs, the procedure can be repeated. If repeat angioplasty is unsuccessful, surgical revascularization should be attempted in patients with favorable lesions who can tolerate the procedure, particularly those whose BP is controlled even with medical treatment or whose renal function is deteriorating. In patients with anatomically unfavorable lesions, those who are not surgical candidates, and those whose BP can be controlled on antihypertensive drugs, medical treatment is indicated. Reliance on medical treatment is greater in patients over 50 years of age who have atherosclerotic renal artery disease and overt extrarenal vascular disease than in younger patients with fibromuscular disease. The relative efficacy of medical, percutaneous angioplastic, and surgical treatment of renovascular hypertension has never been rigorously evaluated in a randomized, controlled prospective study, so it is difficult to make firm recommendations about which therapeutic modality should be chosen for a given patient with this syndrome.

Percutaneous Transluminal Angioplasty. Dilatation of the renal artery is technically successful in 60 to 70 per cent of patients with atherosclerotic disease and 90 per cent of those with fibromuscular disease. Complete occlusion of the renal artery and bilateral renal artery stenosis have been successfully treated with transluminal angioplasty, as have the fibrotic, scarred lesions of renal transplant arterial stenosis and stenosis at the site of previous renal arterial repair. In contrast, atherosclerotic lesions located at the ostium of the renal artery

TABLE 47–9. ADVERSE DRUG EFFECTS

Drugs	Side Effects	Precautions and Special Considerations
Diuretics*		
Thiazides and related sulfonamides	Hypokalemia, hyperuricemia, glucose intolerance, hypercholesterolemia, hypertriglyceridemia, and sexual dysfunction	May be ineffective in renal failure; hypokalemia increases digitalis toxicity; and hyperuricemia may precipitate acute gout
Loop diuretics	Same as for thiazides	Effective in chronic renal failure; cautions regarding hypokalemia and hyperuricemia same as above; and hyponatremia may be found, especially in the elderly
Potassium-sparing agents	Hyperkalemia	Danger of hyperkalemia in patients with renal failure
Amiloride hydrochloride	Sexual dysfunction	—
Spironolactone	Gynecomastia, mastodynia, and sexual dysfunction	—
Triamterene	—	—
Adrenergic Antagonists		
Beta-adrenergic blockers†	Bradycardia, fatigue, insomnia, bizarre dreams, sexual dysfunction, hypertriglyceridemia, decreased high-density lipoprotein cholesterol	Should not be used in patients with asthma, chronic obstructive pulmonary disease, congestive heart failure, heart block (greater than first degree), and sick sinus syndrome; use with caution in patients with diabetes and peripheral vascular disease
Central-acting adrenergic inhibitors	Drowsiness, dry mouth, fatigue, and sexual dysfunction	
Clonidine	—	Rebound hypertension may occur with abrupt discontinuance
Guanabenz	—	Same as for clonidine
Methyldopa	—	May cause liver damage and positive direct Coombs' test
Peripheral-acting adrenergic inhibitors	Sexual dysfunction and nasal congestion	—
Guanadrel sulfate	Orthostatic-hypotension and diarrhea	Use cautiously in elderly patients because of orthostatic hypotension
Guanethidine monosulfate	Same as for guanadrel	Same as for guanadrel
Rauwolfia alkaloids	Lethargy	Contraindicated in patients with a history of mental depression; use with caution in patients with a history of peptic ulcer
Reserpine	Same as for rauwolfia alkaloids	Same as for rauwolfia alkaloids
Alpha$_1$-adrenergic blocker		
Prazosin hydrochloride	"First-dose" syncope, orthostatic hypotension, weakness, and palpitations	Use cautiously in elderly patients because of orthostatic hypotension
Combined alpha and beta-adrenergic blockers		
Labetalol hydrochloride‡	Asthma, nausea, fatigue, dizziness, and headache	Contraindicated in cardiac failure, chronic obstructive pulmonary disease, sick sinus syndrome, and heart block (greater than first degree); use with caution in patients with diabetes
Vasodilators		
Vasodilators	Headache, tachycardia, and fluid retention	May precipitate angina in patients with coronary heart disease
Hydralazine hydrochloride	Positive antinuclear antibody (without other changes)	Lupus syndrome may occur (rare at recommended doses)
Minoxidil	Hypertrichosis, ascites (rare)	May cause or aggravate pleural and pericardial effusions
Angiotensin-Converting Enzyme Inhibitors		
Angiotensin-converting enzyme inhibitors	Rash and dysgeusia (rare)	Can cause reversible acute renal failure in patients with bilateral renal arterial stenosis; neutropenia may occur in patients with autoimmune collagen disorders; and proteinuria may occur (rare at recommended doses)
Calcium Channel–Blocking Agents§		
Calcium channel–blocking agents	Headache, hypotension, and dizziness	—
Diltiazem hydrochloride	Nausea	Use with caution in patients with congestive heart failure or heart block
Nifedipine	—	—
Verapamil hydrochloride	Flushing, edema, and constipation	Same as for diltiazem

*See Table 47–7 for a list of these drugs.
†Sudden withdrawal of these drugs may be hazardous in patients with heart disease.
‡This drug has not been approved by the Food and Drug Administration (FDA).
§These agents have not been approved by the FDA for the treatment of hypertension.
Modified from The 1984 Report of the Joint National Committee on Detection, Evaluation, and Treatment of High Blood Pressure. Arch Intern Med 144:1045, 1984.

TABLE 47–10. ANTIHYPERTENSIVE DRUGS FOR PARENTERAL ADMINISTRATION IN MANAGEMENT OF HYPERTENSIVE CRISIS

| | Dosage | | | | |
| | | Intravenous | | | |
Drugs	Intramuscular (mg*)	Single Dose (mg*)	Continuous Infusion (μg/kg/min)*	Onset of Action	Adverse Effects
Direct Vasodilators					
Sodium nitroprusside (Nipride)†	—	—	0.5–10	Instantaneous	Nausea, vomiting, muscle twitching, apprehension, sweating, thiocyanate intoxication
Diazoxide (Hyperstat)	—	50–100 at 5 to 10-min intervals until satisfactory BP response is achieved	Rarely used	3–5 min	Tachycardia, palpitations, flushing, headache, nausea, vomiting, aggravation of angina or congestive heart failure or both, hyperglycemia, hyperuricemia, hypotension
Hydralazine (Apresoline)	10–40 at 30-min intervals until satisfactory BP response is achieved	10–20‡ at 30-min intervals until satisfactory BP response is achieved	Rarely used	Intramuscularly, 30 min; intravenously, 5–10 min	Tachycardia, palpitations, flushing, headache, vomiting, aggravation of angina or congestive heart failure or both
Sympathetic Blocking Drugs					
Ganglion-blocking agents					
Trimethaphan camsylate (Arfonad)	—	—	4–90	5–10 min	Urinary retention, paralytic ileus, paralysis of pupillary reflex and accommodation of eye, dry mouth, orthostatic hypotension
Central nervous system–active agents					
Methyldopate hydrochloride (Aldomet ester)	—	250–500§; may be repeated at 6-hr intervals	—	2–3 hr	Drowsiness
Alpha-receptor–blocking agents					
Phentolamine (Regitine)†	5–15	5–15 (rapid injection essential)	—	Instantaneous	Tachycardia, flushing
Labetalol	—	50 (over a 1-min period)	3 to a total dose of 200 mg in malignant hypertension; 300 mg in pheochromocytoma	Instantaneous	Postural dizziness with or without postural hypotension; paradoxical pressor responses have been reported; nausea, vomiting, scalp tingling, burning in throat and groin

*Start with the smallest dose shown. Subsequent doses and intervals of administration should be adjusted according to the blood pressure response.

†Start infusion slowly and adjust rate according to response to BP. Constant surveillance is mandatory. Concentration of solution can be adjusted according to patient's fluid requirements.

‡The total dose should be contained in a volume of at least 20 ml, and the solution should be administered from a 20- or 50-ml syringe. Blood pressure should be monitored continuously while the injection is being made. Rate of injection should not exceed 0.5 ml per minute. To avoid hypotension, the injection should be stopped frequently when the BP is falling.

§Diluted up to 100 ml and injected during a 30- to 60-minute period.

Modified from The 1984 Report of the Joint National Committee on Detection, Evaluation, and Treatment of High Blood Pressure. Arch Intern Med 144:1045, 1984.

respond poorly to balloon dilatation, and angioplasty should not be attempted in patients with such lesions.

Complications of percutaneous transluminal angioplasty, including occlusion of the renal artery secondary to intimal dissection or thrombosis, renal artery perforation, retroperitoneal bleeding, and balloon rupture, are uncommon. Many of these complications require emergency surgery, however, so renal angioplasty should be done only with the backup of a vascular surgeon. Hypotension immediately after angioplasty can be a problem, particularly in patients who have had severe hypertension or who have been maintained on large doses of antihypertensive drugs up to the time of angioplasty. Special attention should be given to keeping these patients well hydrated.

Long-term results of transluminal dilatation for renal artery stenosis, as assessed by vessel patency and effect on BP, are promising. Approximately 85 per cent of patients with technically successful angioplasties show sustained improvement in BP control. Life-table analysis gives a cumulative success rate of 81 per cent for a three-year period: The cure rate (diastolic BP < 90 mm Hg with no medication) is 20 per cent; the improvement rate (diastolic BP < 100 mm Hg with decreased medication) is 65 per cent. Cure rates and improvement rates in fibromuscular disease are greater than in atherosclerotic disease.

In summary, percutaneous transluminal dilatation of the renal artery offers advantages over renovascular surgery that include lower cost, morbidity, and mortality; greater ease of documenting results by recording pressures across the stenosis before and after dilatation; and ease of repetition if restenosis occurs. Disadvantages include technical failure in 10 to 20 per cent of cases due to inability to pass through the stenosis or inability to dilate the artery when very firm lesions or ostial lesions are present.

Renovascular Surgery. In most published series, the overall surgical cure rate of patients with hypertension secondary to unilateral renal artery stenosis is 40 to 50 per cent; the improvement rate is approximately 50 per cent, and the failure rate is 10 per cent. Results in patients with fibromuscular disease are better than in those with arteriosclerotic disease, and morbidity and mortality rates are lower in the former group. Results in unilateral disease are better than in bilateral disease. Preoperative duration of hypertension is also an important predictor of the outcome of renovascular surgery. Approximately 80 per cent of patients who have had hypertension for less than five years before surgery, but only 25 per cent of those who have had hypertension for more than five years, show a favorable BP response. Recently, improved results (1 to 2 per cent mortality and low morbidity rates) in renovascular surgery have been attributed to sophisticated

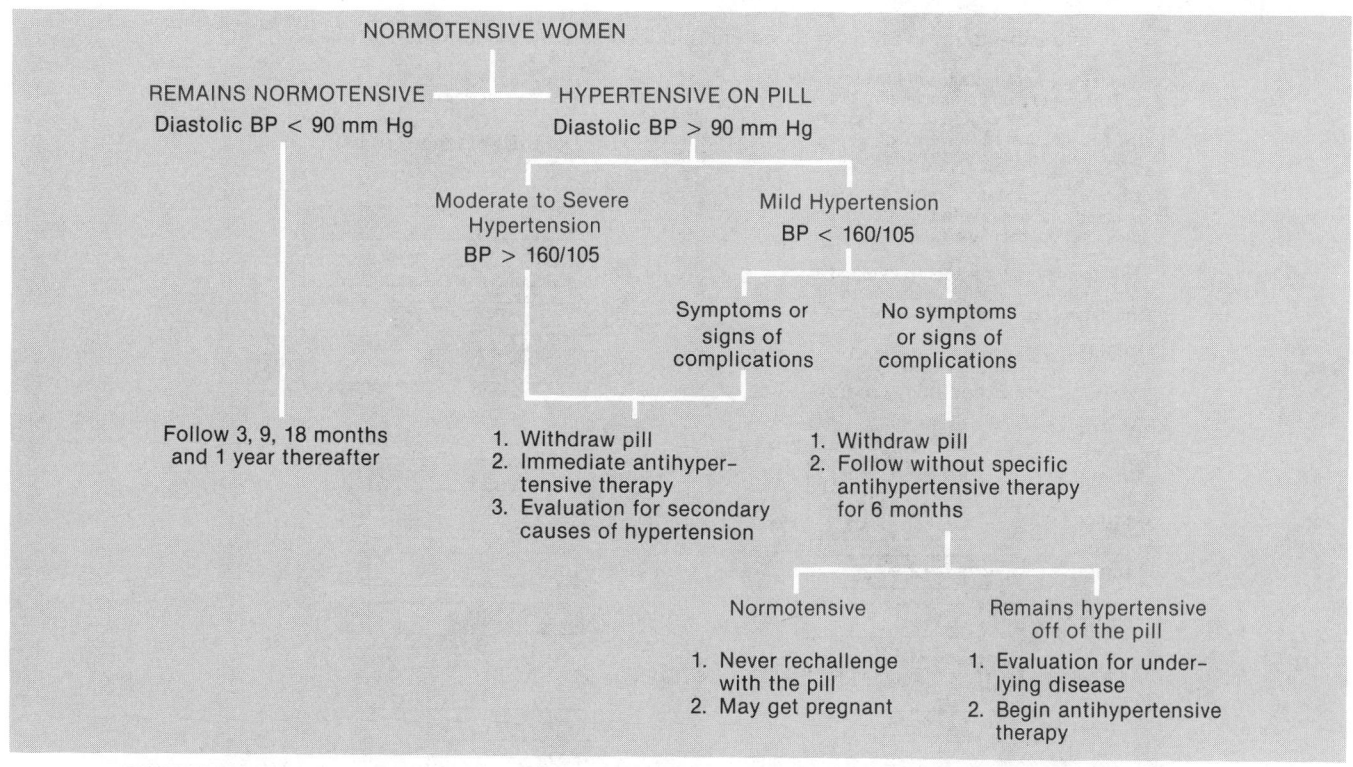

FIGURE 47—7. Diagnosis and management of oral contraceptive pill hypertension. (Reprinted with permission from The Journal of Reproductive Medicine 15:205, 1975.)

preoperative screening, preoperative correction of coexisting coronary or cerebrovascular disease, and employment of methods of revascularization, such as hepatorenal, splenorenal, or ileorenal bypass or autotransplantation, that obviate operation on a severely diseased aorta.

In summary, the noninvasive nature, low cost, and low morbidity of percutaneous renal angioplasty make it the procedure of choice in the initial approach to patients with renovascular hypertension and disease confined to the renal artery. Renovascular surgery should be reserved for those patients who are not candidates for angioplasty or for those whose artery cannot be successfully dilated because of the particular lesions present.

Medical Treatment. Converting enzyme inhibitors administered alone or in combination with a diuretic are effective in controlling BP while sparing renal function and maintaining negative sodium balance in patients with renovascular hypertension secondary to unilateral renal artery stenosis. These regimens are simple and well tolerated and represent the medical treatment of choice in most patients with renovascular hypertension. Converting enzyme inhibitors induce acute, reversible renal failure in a subset of patients with renovascular hypertension: those with bilateral renal artery stenosis or renal artery stenosis in a solitary kidney, whether native or allograft, or those with unilateral renal artery stenosis and severe parenchymal disease in the contralateral kidney. This form of reversible renal insufficiency is a consequence of impairment in the autoregulation of glomerular filtration secondary to blockade of the intrarenal renin-angiotensin system in the presence of reduced renal artery perfusion pressure. This explanation assumes that there is (1) enhanced intrarenal angiotensin II production under conditions of impaired renal perfusion and (2) a preferential constrictor effect of angiotensin II on the efferent arteriole, causing enhanced postglomerular vascular tone, thus maintaining an effective filtration pressure and glomerular filtration rate. Autoregulation of glomerular filtration rate, which is dependent on an intact

intrarenal renin-angiotensin system, is lost when a converting enzyme inhibitor is administered.

Careful monitoring of renal size and function is mandatory in patients who are undergoing medical treatment for renovascular hypertension even if BP control is satisfactory. Deterioration of renal function and loss of renal mass can occur rapidly in patients with atherosclerotic disease who are treated medically. Progressive loss of renal mass, presumably related to parenchymal ischemia due to progression of the renal artery lesion, is common in medically treated patients with renovascular hypertension and does not appear to be related to BP control. Significant reduction in renal length is the most sensitive index of loss of renal mass. Serial (every three to six months) estimates of renal size, as by intravenous pyelography (IVP) or ultrasonography, are important in the follow-up of patients who are being treated medically for renovascular hypertension.

PRIMARY ALDOSTERONISM. The treatment of choice for hypertension secondary to an aldosterone-producing adenoma is unilateral adrenalectomy. In 70 to 80 per cent of cases, surgery restores both blood pressure and electrolytes to normal levels. Administration of spironolactone in doses of 200 to 400 mg per day for four to eight weeks can be used to predict the response to surgery: If spironolactone restores the BP to normal, a good surgical result can be expected; but if BP is unaffected by spironolactone, surgery is not likely to be successful.

Occasionally, the syndrome of primary aldosteronism is caused by adrenal carcinoma. The treatment of choice in this case is surgery, particularly if there is no evidence of metastasis. Alternatively, pharmacologic therapy—including aldosterone antagonists (spironolactone) and inhibitors of steroid biosynthesis, such as aminoglutethimide (Cytadren or trilostane) or the adrenolytic agent o,p'-DDD—can be used.

In patients with bilateral adrenal hyperplasia, remission of hypertension after bilateral total adrenalectomy occurs in only 18 to 35 per cent of cases. Chronic spironolactone administra-

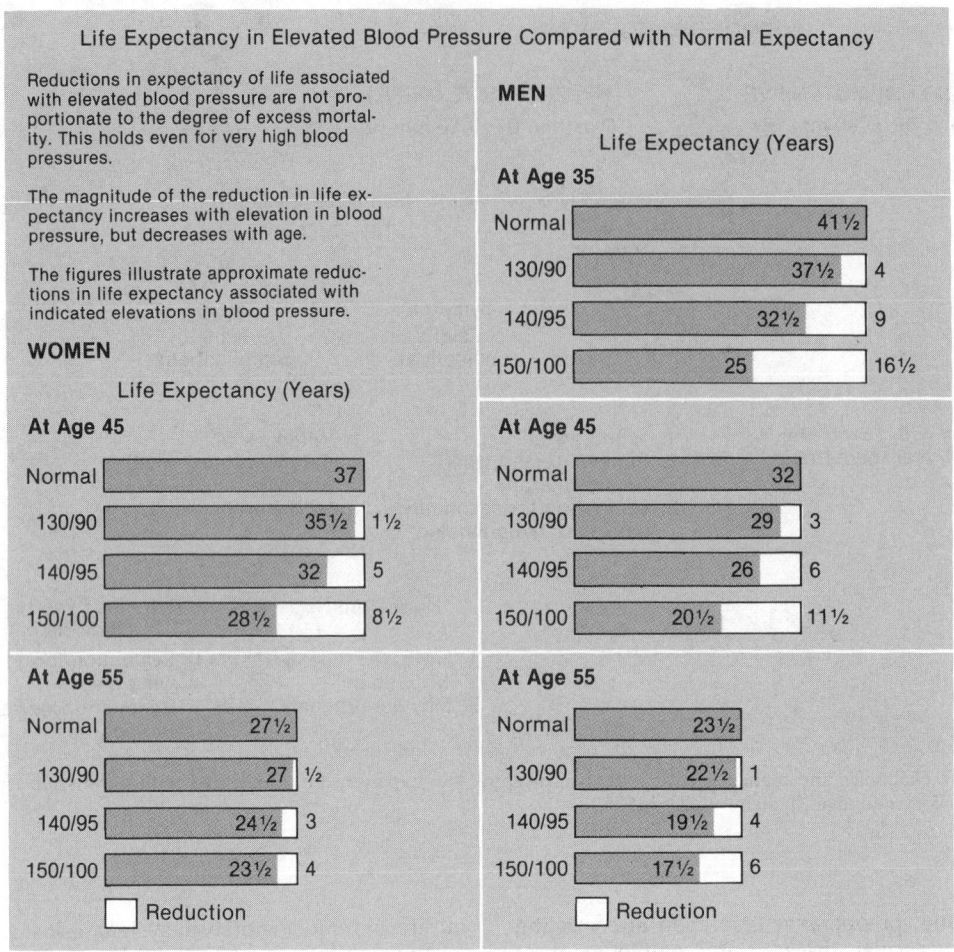

FIGURE 47—8. Life expectancy table. Normal means 120/80 mm Hg or less. (From Metropolitan Life Insurance Company: Blood Pressure: Insurance Experience and Its Implications, New York, Metropolitan Life Insurance Co., 1961.)

tion in doses greater than 200 mg per day is effective in controlling hypertension in these patients. The adverse effects of the drug, including nausea, vomiting, gynecomastia, impotence, hirsutism, and intermenstrual bleeding, limit its chronic use. In patients who are intolerant of spironolactone, amiloride may be an appropriate substitute.

PHEOCHROMOCYTOMA. Treatment of pheochromocytoma is surgical unless the tumor is metastatic or the patient is inoperable for other reasons. Patients should be prepared with alpha-adrenergic–blocking agents (phenoxybenzamine, prazosin, or labetalol) for one to two weeks before surgery to block the pressor effects of circulating norepinephrine and expand intravascular volume.

If surgery cannot be performed, patients can be managed medically with alpha-and beta-adrenergic blockers or the new combined alpha- and beta-adrenergic antagonist labetalol. Alpha-methylparatyrosine (Demser) inhibits tyrosine hydroxylase, the rate-limiting enzyme in catecholamine biosynthesis, thus reducing catecholamine production by the tumor and secondarily lowering BP. The many adverse effects of alpha-methylparatyrosine, including sedation, diarrhea, galactorrhea, anxiety, tremulousness, and crystalluria, limit its clinical usefulness.

PROGNOSIS

The excess mortality associated with hypertension is related mainly to cardiovascular disease and cerebral hemorrhage. Natural history studies in the era prior to the development of antihypertensive therapy showed that the mean age of onset of hypertension was the early 30's and the mean survival was 20 years. Thus life expectancy in hypertensive subjects was shortened by 15 to 20 years on the average. Survival was shorter for men (20 per cent surviving for 20 years) than for women (50 per cent surviving for 20 years) (Fig. 47–8). Further, subjects with hypertension of early onset and with more severe hypertension had shorter life expectancies. The prognosis for women was thought to be better because of their lower incidence of coronary artery disease and accelerated hypertension. Despite the variable rate of progression of hypertensive vascular disease, the average hypertensive pa-

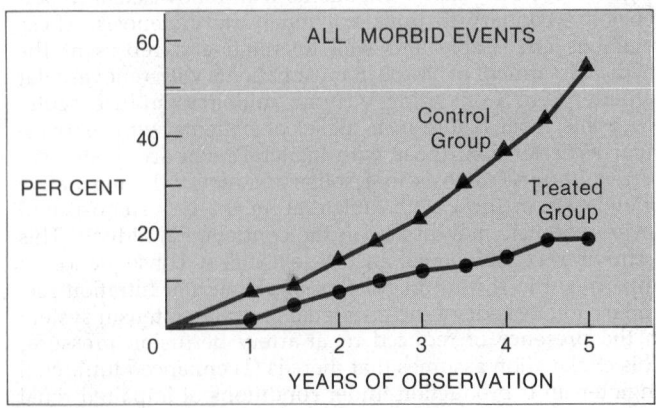

FIGURE 47—9. Life-table analysis, comparing the percentage of incidence of cardiovascular complications over a five-year period in controls versus treated patients with initial diastolic blood pressure between 90 and 114 mm Hg. (From Freis ED: VA Cooperative Study: JAMA 213:1143, 1970. Copyright 1970, American Medical Association.)

tient was free of symptoms and vascular complications for most of the duration of the syndrome.

The cardiovascular complications of hypertension include stroke secondary to cerebral hemorrhage or thrombosis, coronary artery disease with associated angina pectoris and acute myocardial infarction, left ventricular hypertrophy, congestive heart failure, aortic dissection, renal insufficiency, and peripheral vascular disease with intermittent claudication.

Controlled studies have demonstrated that effective antihypertensive treatment reduces the incidence of cardiovascular complications. In the Veterans Administration Cooperative Study, a randomized, double-blind prospective clinical trial in 523 male patients whose initial diastolic pressures ranged from 90 to 129 mm Hg, treatment with a combination of hydrochlorothiazide, reserpine, and hydralazine caused a sharp reduction in the incidence of stroke, congestive heart failure, accelerated hypertension, and renal failure. Although antihypertensive treatment did not significantly reduce the incidence of myocardial infarction or sudden death, there was a trend suggesting fewer fatal myocardial infarctions in treated subjects. Life-table analysis of these results indicates that over a five-year period the risk of developing a serious cardiovascular complication was reduced from 55 to 18 per cent by treatment (Fig. 47–9). The reduction in cardiovascular morbidity was related to the level of diastolic BP that was attained with treatment: Partial control of BP resulted in partial reductions in cardiovascular morbidity and mortality.

More recently, controlled trials in patients with mild hypertension (diastolic BP of 90 to 104 mm Hg) have uniformly shown that control of BP with antihypertensive drugs protects against stroke, left ventricular hypertrophy, congestive heart failure, and progression to more severe hypertension. Two studies, the Hypertension Detection and Follow-up Program (HDFP) and the Australian National Trial, demonstrated a benefit of antihypertensive therapy in reducing fatal and nonfatal coronary events. By contrast, a clear benefit from effective antihypertensive treatment has not been demonstrated in the subset of patients with a diastolic BP of 90 to 94 mm Hg. For that reason and because of concerns about the toxicity of antihypertensive agents, pharmacologic treatment of patients with mild hypertension is not always recommended.

Bravo EL, Tarazi RC, Gifford RW, et al.: Circulating and urinary catecholamines in pheochromocytoma: Diagnostic and pathophysiologic implications. N Engl J Med 301:682, 1979. *Comparison of the value of measuring plasma catecholamines versus urinary excretion of catecholamine metabolites in the diagnosis of pheochromocytoma. Plasma catecholamine measurement is a much more sensitive and specific diagnostic procedure than the measurement of urinary catecholamine metabolites.*

Bravo EL, Tarazi RC, Dustan HP, et al.: The changing clinical spectrum of primary aldosteronism. Am J Med 74:641, 1983. *A prospective study of 80 patients with primary aldosteronism (70 with adenoma and 10 with hyperplasia) that demonstrated that (1) measurements of serum potassium concentration and plasma renin activity are inadequate screening tests; (2) excessive aldosterone production measured as urinary aldosterone excretion rate after three days of salt loading is highly sensitive and specific for identifying patients with primary aldosteronism; and (3) the most accurate localizing procedure for adrenal adenoma is selective adrenal venous sampling for plasma aldosterone concentration.*

Genest J, Koiw E, Kuchel O: Hypertension. 2nd ed. New York, McGraw-Hill, 1983. *A comprehensive textbook that covers all aspects of the pathophysiology of systemic hypertension in animals and in humans.*

Hypertension Detection and Follow-up Program Cooperative Group: The effect of treatment on mortality in "mild" hypertension. N Engl J Med 307:976, 1983. *Evidence of significantly reduced five-year mortality in patients with mild hypertension and no evidence of end-organ damage treated with stepped care in special clinics compared with those treated according to usual community standards. These findings were interpreted as supporting a recommendation that in patients with mild hypertension, treatment should be considered early, before end-organ damage occurs.*

Kaplan NM: Clinical Hypertension. 4th ed. Baltimore, Williams & Wilkins Company, 1986. *A comprehensive textbook that covers the pathogenesis, diagnosis, and treatment of all forms of clinical hypertension.*

The 1984 Report of the Joint National Committee on Detection, Evaluation, and Treatment of High Blood Pressure. Arch Intern Med 144:1045, 1984. *Detailed recommendations for the diagnosis and pharmacologic and nonpharmacologic treatment of systemic hypertension.*

Oparil S, Haber E: The renin-angiotensin system. N Engl J Med 291:389, 1974. *A detailed and authoritative review of the biochemistry and physiology of the renin-angiotensin system.*

Oparil S, Katholi RE: Humoral control of the circulation. In Garfein OB (ed.): Cardiovascular Physiology: A Review. New York, Academic Press (in press). *A review of the hormonal and neural mechanisms that control normal cardiovascular homeostasis. It provides a useful basis for understanding the perturbations that occur in systemic hypertension.*

Veterans Administration Cooperative Study Group on Antihypertensive Agents: Effects of treatment on morbidity in hypertension: I. Results in patients with diastolic blood pressures averaging 115 through 129 mm Hg. JAMA 202:1028, 1967. *Demonstration that male hypertensive patients with diastolic blood pressure averaging 115 mm Hg or above represent a high-risk group in which hypertensive therapy exerts a significant beneficial effect.*

Veterans Administration Cooperative Study Group on Antihypertensive Agents: Effects of treatment on morbidity in hypertension: II. Results in patients with diastolic blood pressure averaging 90 through 114 mm Hg. JAMA 213:1143, 1970. *Demonstration that treatment of male patients with mildly elevated blood pressure is more effective in preventing congestive heart failure and stroke than in preventing the complications of coronary artery disease and that the degree of benefit of treatment is related to the level of prerandomization blood pressure.*

48 PULMONARY HYPERTENSION

Alfred P. Fishman

The pulmonary circulation is a highly distensible, low-resistance vascular bed interposed between the systemic veins and the systemic arteries. Its major function is gas exchange with ambient air. It differs from the circulation to other organs in that it is perfused by the entire output of the right ventricle (the cardiac output) and from the systemic circulation in that it lacks elaborate mechanisms for regulating blood pressure. Because of its large capacity, its great distensibility, and its low resistance, the pulmonary circulation is not prone to become hypertensive. When pulmonary hypertension does occur, it is usually secondary to cardiac or pulmonary disease. Only on rare occasion is "primary" or "unexplained" pulmonary hypertension encountered. Nonetheless, although uncommon, "primary" pulmonary hypertension is of considerable theoretic interest for the understanding of the clinical picture, natural history, and management of uncomplicated pulmonary hypertension.

The normal pulmonary hemodynamics of adults residing at sea level and at altitude are indicated in Table 48–1. Because of the passive nature of the pulmonary vascular bed, the pulmonary arterial pressure—particularly in hypertensive states—must be assessed with respect to the pulmonary blood flow (cardiac output). For a cardiac output of 5 to 6 liters per minute, the normal pulmonary arterial pressure at sea level is about 20 mm Hg systolic and 12 mm Hg diastolic, with a mean of about 15 mm Hg; the same level of blood flow is asssociated with higher pressures at altitude. Pulmonary arterial pressures also tend to increase somewhat with age.

Pulmonary hypertension is a colloquialism for pulmonary *arterial* hypertension. Unless otherwise stipulated, the term refers to *chronic* pulmonary hypertension. Acute pulmonary hypertension occurs most often clinically as a result of pulmonary embolism or the adult respiratory distress syndrome. This chapter will be confined to the chronic states.

Criteria for pulmonary hypertension depend on the altitude: In the resting individual at sea level, a *mean* pulmonary arterial pressure greater than 19 to 20 mm Hg establishes the diagnosis; the corresponding limit at altitude is higher—at about 15,000 feet, a *mean* pulmonary arterial pressure greater than 25 mm Hg signifies pulmonary hypertension. Pulmonary hypertension is important only if it imposes a heavy burden on the right ventricle. Thus mild pulmonary hypertension is clinically insignificant because it can be well tolerated by the right ventricle for a lifetime. However, mild pulmonary hy-

TABLE 48–1. REPRESENTATIVE VALUES AT REST FOR THE NORMAL PULMONARY CIRCULATION AT SEA LEVEL AND AT ALTITUDE

	Sea Level	14,900 ft
Pulmonary arterial pressure (mm Hg, systolic/diastolic, mean)	20/12, 15	38/14, 25
Cardiac output (liters/min)	6.0	6.0
Cardiac index (liters min/m², body surface area)	3.1	3.1
Left atrial pressure (mm Hg)	5.0	5.0
Pulmonary vascular resistance (R units*)	0.1†	0.2

*R units express calculated resistance in terms of $\frac{\text{mm Hg}}{\text{ml/sec.}}$. To convert to C.G.S. units (dynes · sec · cm^{-5}), the value in R units is multiplied by 1328.

†Based on the data in this table, at sea level, R $= \frac{15 - 5}{6000/60} = 0.1$ R units.

pertension at rest generally signifies higher levels during exercise or upon exposure to a pulmonary vasoconstricting stimulus, e.g., hypoxia. Not infrequently, pulmonary hypertension remains subclinical until an explanation is sought for unanticipated right ventricular failure. This is so because the normal right ventricle can handle comfortably a moderate afterload; e.g., it can generate systolic pressures of about 50 mm Hg. It can also cope with heavier work loads if allowed time to hypertrophy. However, when inordinate loads are imposed, e.g., pulmonary arterial pressures approximating systemic arterial pressures, it is destined to fail. Moreover, at high levels, hazards other than ventricular failure often supervene, including a propensity to syncope, precordial pain, and sudden death.

Pulmonary *venous* hypertension is a different entity with respect to etiology, pathogenesis, clinical manifestations, and management. It is said to exist when pulmonary venous or left atrial pressure exceeds 12 mm Hg; this limit applies to altitude as well as to sea level. In the normal pulmonary circulation an acute increase in pulmonary venous pressure to the range of 20 to 30 mm Hg increases the risk of pulmonary edema. The same levels are less threatening when sustained chronically, as in mitral valve disease, presumably by thickening of the walls of the fluid-exchanging vessels in the lungs. However, in these individuals, a further increment in venous pressure—as by exercise or infusions—topples them into pulmonary edema.

THE NORMAL PULMONARY CIRCULATION
Structure

In the normal adult, the small muscular arteries and arterioles constitute the "resistance" vessels. In the adult at sea level, these vessels are thin-walled and sparsely equipped with muscle; in the fetus and in the native resident at altitude, the muscle is thicker and more extensive. In contrast to the pulmonary circulation, the normal bronchial circulation is minute but capable of undergoing remarkable proliferation in congenital heart disease and in pulmonary disorders involving local suppuration and fibrosis.

Hemodynamics

Because of the low resistance and high distensibility of the pulmonary vascular bed and the pulsatile nature of pulmonary blood pressure, the large pulmonary blood flow is accomplished by only a small drop in mean pressure between the pulmonary artery and the left atrium (Table 48–1). The mean pressure difference is ordinarily about 5 to 10 mm Hg.

Calculated pulmonary vascular resistance has become a popular tool for assessing the state of the normal and abnormal pulmonary circulation and for detecting pulmonary va-

soconstriction or vasodilation. Unfortunately, interpretation in terms of vasomotor activity can be clouded by passive changes that occur when pulmonary vascular blood pressures, or flow, or both are changing. For example, exercise normally elicits a passive decrease in resistance due to distention of open vessels and recruitment of vessels that were previously closed. Also, clinical short-cuts, such as the substitution of pulmonary arterial pressure for the pressure drop between pulmonary artery and left atrium, deprive the calculation of any physiologic meaning, although it may still suffice in pulmonary hypertensive states as an empiric tool. Finally, since the calculation involves a ratio, interpretation in terms of clinical significance can become highly subjective. For example, a decrease in calculated pulmonary resistance involving a drop in pulmonary arterial pressure in conjunction with an increase in cardiac output (while heart rate and left atrial and systemic blood pressures remain unchanged) would seem preferable for the welfare and favorable prognosis of a patient to the same decrease in resistance brought about by an increase in cardiac output, an unchanged pulmonary arterial pressure, and tachycardia.

A large increase in cardiac output, i.e., three times that at rest, increases pulmonary arterial pressure in the normal lung by only a few millimeters of mercury. But after restriction of the pulmonary vascular bed by disease or surgery, lesser increments in pulmonary blood flow elicit more striking increases in pulmonary arterial pressure.

The role of increase in the pulmonary blood volume is much more subtle and less susceptible to measurement. The normal pulmonary blood volume is about 500 ml, approximately 100 ml of which is in the pulmonary capillaries. Expansion of the pulmonary blood volume limits the distensibility of the pulmonary circulation and decreases the capability for avoiding sizable increments in pulmonary arterial pressure by recruiting new vessels. The pulmonary blood volume expands as cardiac output increases and during systemic vasoconstriction.

Although autonomic nerves supply the pulmonary vascular tree, they are far less effective in mediating vasoconstriction or vasodilation than are local stimuli. Indeed, hypoxia acting within the lungs is the most powerful mechanism for eliciting pulmonary vasoconstriction, particularly if reinforced by a concomitant acidosis. The mechanism by which hypoxia exerts its local pressor effect is unknown. Hypercapnia also exerts a pressor effect, presumably by way of the local acidosis that it generates.

CLINICAL MANIFESTATIONS

As indicated above, most cases of pulmonary hypertension are secondary (Table 48–2). As a rule, in these pulmonary hypertensive states, the clinical picture is dominated by the signs and symptoms of the underlying disease, which also shapes the natural history, prognosis, and response to treatment. The clinical entity of "primary pulmonary hypertension," in which the heart and lungs are not etiologically related to the pulmonary hypertension, is described subsequently.

SECONDARY PULMONARY HYPERTENSION

As causes of secondary pulmonary hypertension, heart or lung diseases dominate in numbers. Less impressive in number but of great clinical importance because of the potential for prevention and cure on the one hand and catastrophe on the other is pulmonary thromboembolic disease. Heart disease exerts its effects by increasing pulmonary blood flow or pulmonary venous pressure. In contrast, lung disease and thromboembolic disease cause pulmonary hypertension by increasing resistance to blood flow, albeit by different mechanisms.

TABLE 48–2. CLASSIFICATION OF CHRONIC PULMONARY (ARTERIAL) HYPERTENSION

I. **Secondary**
   A. Cardiac Disease
     1. Acquired disorders of the left side of the heart causing pulmonary venous hypertension
       Left ventricular failure
       Mitral valve disease
       Left atrial myxoma
       Decrease in left ventricular compliance
     2. Congenital heart disease
       Pre-tricuspid
       Post-tricuspid
   B. Occlusive Pulmonary Vascular Disease
   C. Respiratory Disorders
     1. Interstitial fibrosis
     2. Obstructive airways disease
     3. Combined fibrosis, emphysema, and chronic bronchitis
     4. Alveolar hypoventilation despite normal lungs
     5. Adult respiratory distress syndrome
     6. Multiple systemic diseases
II. **Primary**

Cardiac Disease

Acquired disorders of the left side of the heart and certain types of congenital heart disease often lead to pulmonary hypertension.

ACQUIRED DISORDERS OF THE LEFT SIDE OF THE HEART. Left ventricular failure is the outstanding cause of pulmonary hypertension. It is also the most common cause of right ventricular failure. Rarely is the level of pulmonary hypertension sufficient to account for the right ventricular failure. The discrepancy is usually attributed to concomitant failure of the muscle in the ventricular septum.

Myocardial disorders and lesions of the mitral and aortic valves are the most common left ventricular disorders leading to pulmonary hypertension. Occasional instances also occur of constrictive pericarditis, which compromises primarily the compliance of the left ventricle, thereby increasing its end-diastolic pressure. All first raise pulmonary venous pressure, which, in turn, evokes an increase in pulmonary arterial pressure that is necessary to maintain antegrade flow. How this automatic adjustment is accomplished is unclear. But, in time, three types of morphologic changes appear: (1) occlusive intimal and medial changes in pulmonary *precapillary* vessels as well as in pulmonary venules and veins; (2) perivascular interstitial edema, which not only contributes directly to the increase in resistance to blood flow but also stimulates perivascular fibrosis; under the influence of gravity, the vascular and perivascular changes are most marked in the dependent portions of the lungs; and (3) occlusion of small pulmonary vessels by emboli or thrombi; especially in states of slowed systemic blood flow, emboli are much more apt to arise from thrombi in the veins of the extremities than from the right side of the heart. Depending on the reversibility of the vascular and perivascular lesions, surgical relief of the pulmonary venous hypertension, as by mitral valve commissurotomy or replacement, generally reduces the pulmonary arterial pressure.

CONGENITAL HEART DISEASE. At term, pulmonary arterial pressure approximates aortic pressure and is generally about 70/40, with a mean of 50 mm Hg. After birth, the combination of closure of the ductus arteriosus and pulmonary vasodilation causes pulmonary arterial pressure to fall rapidly to about one half of systemic levels. Thereafter, a gradual drop usually brings pulmonary arterial pressures to normal adult values in one to four weeks.

Congenital defects that produce left to right shunting of blood within the heart or between the great vessels are commonly associated with pulmonary arterial hypertension. But acute left to right shunts per se do not produce appreciable pulmonary hypertension in normal lungs unless flow is mas-

sive, i.e., at least three times greater than normal. Therefore, even though the increase in pulmonary blood flow produced by the left to right shunt is often the cardinal initiating element in this type of pulmonary hypertension, important contributing factors are the degree of arterial hypoxemia and the duration of the hemodynamic abnormalities. The interplay of these mechanisms leads to occlusive pulmonary vascular changes that, depending on the congenital defect, preferentially damage pulmonary vascular intima or media and inflict different degrees of pulmonary vascular injury. Not infrequently, as the hemodynamic abnormalities persist, the anatomic changes in the pulmonary resistance vessels take over as the dominant mechanism in sustaining the pulmonary hypertension and in determining its reversibility.

It was noted above that the pulmonary vascular lesions in pulmonary arterial hypertension are somewhat variable. However, sustained increases in pulmonary arterial pressure and arterial hypoxemia are generally associated with medial hypertrophy, whereas large pulmonary blood flows usually elicit intimal proliferation. Once pulmonary hypertension becomes chronic, distinctions between pressure and flow effects on the vascular wall tend to blur. In addition, as the pulmonary hypertension approaches systemic levels, various consequences of necrotizing arteritis supervene, including plexiform and angiomatoid lesions. Congenital defects in which pulmonary hypertension persist from birth also seem to interfere with the normal involution of the pulmonary resistance vessels so that the characteristic thin-walled resistance vessels of the normal adult lung fail to evolve. To complicate matters further, atherosclerotic lesions in the pulmonary hypertensive circulation and local thrombi or emboli add a final hypertensive element to the occlusive pulmonary vascular processes.

Important differences exist with respect to the natural history of pulmonary hypertension caused by "pre-tricuspid" congenital defects (e.g., secundum atrial septal defect) on the one hand and "post-tricuspid" congenital defects (e.g., ventricular septal defect) on the other. These are described elsewhere in this volume.

Occlusive Pulmonary Vascular Disease

The causes of secondary pulmonary hypertension due to occlusive vascular disease vary with geography. In the United States and Europe, extensive obliteration of the pulmonary arterial tree by pulmonary emboli is a common cause. In other parts of the world, other etiologies predominate. Thus, in Egypt, where schistosomiasis is endemic, pulmonary vascular disease caused by mechanical obstruction and hypersensitivity reactions is not uncommon. Elsewhere, filariasis is considered to be an important cause of pulmonary hypertension. In the United States, sickle-cell disease, the most common cause of pulmonary vascular thrombosis, rarely causes pulmonary hypertension. Several types of cancer, notably choriocarcinoma, can embolize the pulmonary circulation after the tumor has invaded the liver or the inferior vena cava.

Another important, but less common, cause of obliterative pulmonary vascular disease is the connective tissue disorders, such as systemic lupus erythematosus. Although it is generally held on morphologic grounds that connective tissue disorders of the lungs favor large, rather than small, vessels, recent improvements in the sensitivity and diversity of serologic testing for autoimmune disorders have lent credence to the proposition that connective tissue disorders may affect the small pulmonary vessels more often than previously believed.

The common denominator in pulmonary hypertension due to chronic obliterative pulmonary vascular disease is amputation and occlusion of large segments of the pulmonary circulation, abetted by pulmonary vasoconstriction largely attributable to systemic arterial hypoxemia. Early in the course of embolic pulmonary vascular disease, systemic arterial hypoxemia is mild and contributes little of the pulmonary arterial hypertension. Preterminally, however, as the right ventricle fails, the role of the "anatomic venous admixture," or "shunt," increases considerably as the oxygen content of blood returning to the lung decreases because of the slowed circulation and greater oxygen extraction in peripheral tissues.

In patients who have chronic pulmonary hypertension secondary to pulmonary emboli, two different types of pathogenetic sequences can usually be identified: (1) *clinically detectable* thromboembolic disease originating in systemic veins that is either progressive, overlooked, or neglected, and (2) a syndrome of "multiple pulmonary emboli" that is covert and mimics primary pulmonary hypertension in its clinical expression and natural history. In the latter type, precapillary vessels throughout the lung are partially or totally occluded by organized clots. Since the lesions are microscopic, only lung biopsy or autopsy can distinguish multiple pulmonary emboli from primary pulmonary hypertension. Although the possibility exists that the multiple pulmonary "emboli" are in reality multiple pulmonary thrombi secondary to widespread endothelial damage, by the time the nature of the disorder is recognized, scarring has occurred and the practical implications for management are no different from those of primary pulmonary hypertension.

Usually management involves antithrombotic therapy, occasionally supplemented by surgical elimination of the veins from which the emboli originate. Much less amenable to medical or surgical interventions are the covert multiple pulmonary emboli, in which the source and occurrence of pulmonary emboli are inapparent during life.

Tachypnea is a hallmark of pulmonary emboli. It persists during sleep and is generally associated with tachycardia. This pattern of rapid, shallow breathing is indistinguishable from that arising from stiffened lungs of any cause, e.g., interstitial pulmonary edema. And, by analogy with pulmonary interstitial edema, vagal afferent impulses arising from juxtacapillary (J) receptors and irritant receptors are generally believed to be responsible. The result of the rapid, shallow breathing is alveolar and dead space hyperventilation that, in turn, decreases the Pco_2 in arterial blood and alveolar gas and widens the alveolar-arterial difference in Po_2. Indeed, the combination of arterial hypoxemia, hypocapnia, and a widened alveolar-arterial gradient for Po_2 suggests pulmonary emboli.

Since there is no obstructive disease of the airways to cloud the clinical picture, right ventricular enlargement secondary to pulmonary hypertension is manifested in pure form (see Primary Pulmonary Hypertension).

The "gold standard" for detecting pulmonary emboli is selective, high-resolution pulmonary angiography. However, even this paragon is not perfect, especially in detecting multiple pulmonary emboli of minute vessels. More expedient, but far less certain, are lung scans that have great consistency when normal in excluding pulmonary emboli and, when abnormal, in pinpointing areas of the lungs to be explored by selective angiography. By the time the characteristic chest radiograph of pulmonary hypertension has evolved, angiography and lung scans are rarely of much help in distinguishing healed multiple pulmonary emboli from primary pulmonary hypertension. But, on occasion, they do settle the issue by disclosing one or more organized clots in the pulmonary arterial tree. Right-sided heart catheterization is often done to determine the level of the pulmonary arterial hypertension, to confirm that pulmonary wedge pressures are normal, to assess the state of right ventricular performance, and to test the efficacy of pulmonary vasodilator agents.

Once pulmonary hypertension has been established in the patient with thromboembolic disease, it is generally irreversible. Therefore, preventive measures, directed at the source of emboli, hold more promise than treatment. The medical and surgical approaches to thromboembolic disease are described elsewhere in this volume.

As symptomatic measures, oxygen-enriched inspired mixtures are often helpful in relieving breathlessness, in enhancing cerebration, in relieving arterial hypoxemia, and, thereby, in decreasing the level of pulmonary hypertension. However, unless arterial hypoxemia is marked, the drop in pulmonary arterial pressure during oxygen breathing is rarely striking, and it is usually unclear whether the slight relief in pulmonary arterial pressure is due to a decrease in cardiac output or to pulmonary vasodilation. Almost invariably, once the diagnosis is entertained or established, anticoagulation is initiated even if a search for the sources of emboli proves fruitless. The investigation and treatment are rarely more than gestures, because the pulmonary disease is usually too far advanced for impressive improvement to occur or for the downhill course of the disease to be arrested. Pulmonary vasodilators have not proved to be a reliable form of therapy.

Other forms of secondary obliterative pulmonary vascular disease are usually equally difficult to manage unless a reversible component can be identified, as in a connective tissue disorder that responds to steroids. The lessons learned from pulmonary embolic disease are the importance of prevention and early intervention to control or eliminate the systemic venous (rarely cardiac) source of clots to the lungs.

Respiratory Disorders

Respiratory disorders elicit pulmonary hypertension in different ways: widespread interstitial fibrosis and/or inflammation in the vicinity of the minute pulmonary vessels, by encroaching upon vascular lumens, thereby limiting their distensibility and amputating peripheral segments of the pulmonary vascular tree; obstructive airways disease by causing arterial hypoxemia; conglomerate fibrosis, emphysema, and chronic bronchitis by a combination—in varying proportions—of distorting, encasing, and occluding large segments of the pulmonary vascular tree and promoting vasoconstriction of the pulmonary resistance vessels by inducing alveolar hypoxia and arterial hypoxemia.

INTERSTITIAL FIBROSIS. Familiar examples of this category are sarcoidosis, asbestosis, and radiation fibrosis. Lymphangitic spread of carcinoma within the lungs can produce the same functional effect.

The clinical picture is generally dominated by dyspnea and tachypnea; cough is rarely a prominent feature. The chest radiograph is particularly diagnostic in disclosing a widespread pattern that is consistent with either interstitial fibrosis or infiltration, or both. Corticosteroids are usually the main hope in therapy, often in conjunction with enriched oxygen mixtures. Oxygen therapy holds little promise for relieving pulmonary hypertension unless appreciable arterial hypoxemia is present at rest.

OBSTRUCTIVE AIRWAYS DISEASE. Chronic bronchitis and emphysema ("chronic obstructive lung disease, or COPD") is the most common cause of pulmonary hypertension and cor pulmonale. Even though chronic bronchitis and emphysema generally coexist, it is the chronic bronchitis that is predominantly responsible for the alveolar hypoxia and the low Po_2, high Pco_2, and resultant low pH that lead to pulmonary hypertension. Emphysema per se probably does predispose to pulmonary hypertension by amputating segments of the pulmonary vascular bed. But emphysema does not cause pulmonary hypertension, even when rarefaction of the lungs is extensive, because ventilation-perfusion relationships are not severely deranged as in chronic bronchitis. Cystic fibrosis provides another illustration of the importance of chronic obstructive airways disease in evoking pulmonary hypertension. Here, as in chronic bronchitis, the basic mechanism is persistent alveolar hypoxia, arterial hypoxemia, and, to a lesser extent, respiratory acidosis resulting from ventilation-perfusion abnormalities.

The indiscriminate use of "COPD" to designate the spectrum of obstructive airways disease, without distinguishing between predominant bronchitis and predominant emphysema, tends to promote ambiguity with respect to perceptions of the natural history of this group of diseases. In essence, pulmonary hypertension (often leading to cor pulmonale) is encountered in two different settings: episodically in the "pink puffer" during an acute respiratory infection and chronically in the "blue bloater," with periodic exacerbations during an acute respiratory infection. In the "blue bloater" the course of the pulmonary hypertension is inexorably progressive. It is noteworthy that in the patient first seen during a bout of respiratory failure, clinical distinction between a "pink puffer" and a "blue bloater" is often impossible. However, after recovery from the acute episode, distinction is usually quite simple.

One of the cardinal signs of pulmonary hypertension is right ventricular enlargement. However, recognition of right ventricular enlargement may be difficult in obstructive airways disease because of hyperinflation and cardiac rotation. Right ventricular failure often is accompanied by striking cyanosis, unexplained drowsiness or inappropriate behavior, distended neck veins, warm hands, suffused conjunctivas, hepatomegaly, and edema of the extremities. Right ventricular gallops (S_3 and S_4) are generally present, and the murmur of tricuspid insufficiency can often be elicited. Not only is the liver generally displaced downward by the low diaphragm, but it is also enlarged and tender to gentle pressure over the abdomen. Hepatomegaly is invariably associated with distended neck veins and often with peripheral edema. Once suspicion is raised that the clinical picture of right ventricular failure stems from ventilation-perfusion abnormalities, an arterial blood sample will confirm that the P_{O_2} is low ($P_{O_2} < 40$ to 50 torr), the P_{CO_2} is high ($P_{CO_2} > 50$ torr), and respiratory acidosis is present. Such arterial blood gas tensions are rare in left ventricular failure unless the patient is in frank pulmonary edema. The chest radiograph is often more helpful in detecting right ventricular enlargement retrospectively than during right ventricular failure.

Electrocardiographic evidence of right ventricular enlargement is also often equivocal in patients with bronchitis and emphysema because of rotation and displacement of the heart, widened distances between electrodes and the cardiac surface, and the predominance of dilation over hypertrophy in the cardiac enlargement. Indeed, if right ventricular enlargement is apparent, it can be assumed that the degree of cardiomegaly is severe.

Because of these limitations, it is not surprising that standard electrocardiographic criteria for right ventricular enlargement apply in about only one third of patients with chronic bronchitis and emphysema who have right ventricular hypertrophy at autopsy. Consecutive changes in the electrocardiogram are often more useful than a single electrocardiogram in detecting right ventricular overload due to pulmonary hypertension. As the arterial P_{O_2} drops to distinctly subnormal levels (e.g., below 60 to 70 torr while awake), T waves tend to become inverted, biphasic, or flat in the right, precordial leads (V_1 to V_3), the mean electrical axis of the QRS shifts 30 degrees or more to the right of the patient's usual axis, ST segments become depressed in leads II, III, and aVF, and right bundle branch block (incomplete or complete) often appears. These changes tend to reverse as arterial oxygenation improves.

In the patient with bronchitis and/or emphysema in whom pulmonary hypertension has been elicited or aggravated by a bout of bronchitis or pneumonia, the goal of therapy is to maintain tolerable levels of arterial oxygenation while waiting for the upper respiratory infection to subside. If the pulmonary hypertension is acute, modest enrichment of inspired air with oxygen, as by 28 per cent oxygen delivered by a Venturi mask, generally suffices to relieve arterial hypoxemia and to restore pulmonary arterial pressures toward normal. Considerable improvement may also be accomplished even in the individual who has chronic pulmonary hypertension by sustained (virtually continuous) breathing of oxygen-enriched air that restores arterial P_{O_2} to nearly normal values.

Once the right ventricle has failed, cardiotonic agents must be used cautiously beause of the threat of arrhythmias posed by arterial hypoxemia and respiratory acidosis. Moreover, after adequate oxygenation has been achieved, the need for digitalis and diuretics often decreases, since the hemodynamic burden on the right ventricle (i.e., the pulmonary arterial hypertension) decreases. Even though each episode of acute hypoxia and acidosis seems to elicit about the same increment in pulmonary arterial pressure, each bout of pulmonary hypertension appears to leave behind a slightly higher level of pulmonary hypertension after recovery.

Arterial blood gas composition is the therapeutic compass to the control of pulmonary hypertension in obstructive airways disease. The degree of hypoxia is usually underestimated by conventional practice for blood sampling, since hypoxemia is regularly more marked during sleep than during waking hours. In managing ambulatory patients, serial determinations of the hematocrit may serve as a practical clue to the occurrence of covert arterial hypoxemia. However, once right ventricular failure has set in, there is no substitute for determining arterial P_{O_2} and P_{CO_2} as a guide to therapy. Ensuring the return of arterial oxygenation toward normal is much more vital than is the administration of cardiotonic measures. When respiratory infection has triggered the episode of pulmonary hypertension, a vital strategy for achieving a lasting improvement in arterial oxygenation is the administration of an appropriate antibiotic. While awaiting the salutary effects of antibiotic therapy, attention is paid to hydration, to postural drainage, and to adequate alveolar ventilation. The management of respiratory acidosis is described elsewhere in this volume.

Phlebotomy was once popular as an ancillary measure because of the prospect that increased blood viscosity contributes importantly to the pulmonary hypertension. This practice has fallen into disuse. Polycythemia is rarely severe enough to be a serious problem in cor pulmonale that is associated with bronchitis and emphysema.

Vasodilators have recently been tried in various types of secondary pulmonary hypertension, including that due to obstructive airways disease. The agents tried are the same as those outlined for primary pulmonary hypertension and their efficacy is far less impressive or predictable. To date, the most reliable approach to pulmonary vasodilation in obstructive arterial hypoxemia is enriching inspired air with oxygen.

CONGLOMERATE FIBROSIS, EMPHYSEMA, AND CHRONIC BRONCHITIS. Pulmonary hypertension is uncommon in uncomplicated silicosis or tuberculosis. By contrast, in patients in whom smouldering, long-standing tuberculosis or conglomerate, massive fibrosis has shrunk and distorted the lungs, pulmonary hypertension is virtually the rule. The likelihood of pulmonary hypertension (and cor pulmonale) is enhanced by chronic pleurisy, fibrothorax, or excisional surgery, which exert their effects by a combination of anatomic restriction of the vascular bed and disturbances in gas exchange. Of all of these derangements, the disturbances in gas exchange are most susceptible to relief. Although these combinations are generally complicated, the principles of management are those outlined above for obstructive airways disease. Unfortunately, therapeutic triumphs are uncommon, because of the fixed anatomic changes.

ALVEOLAR HYPOVENTILATION IN PATIENTS WITH NORMAL LUNGS. In those individuals who develop net alveolar hypoventilation even though their lungs are normal, as in those with ventilation-perfusion abnormalities, the common pathogenetic denominators are alveolar hypoxia and arterial hypoxemia, often reinforced by respiratory acidosis. The global alveolar hypoventilation in individuals with normal lungs generally originates in either an inadequate ventilatory drive in subtle upper airways obstruction, as in the sleep apnea syndromes, or in an ineffective chest bellows. Among the disorders associated with global alveolar hypoventilation are residual paralyses of respiratory muscles, unresponsive respiratory "centers," kyphoscoliosis, and extreme obesity. The corresponding clinical syndromes are considered elsewhere in this volume.

The clinical manifestations are detemined by the etiology and pathogenesis; the occurrence of pulmonary hypertension depends on the development of alveolar hypoxia sufficient to evoke arterial hypoxemia. Early in the disorder, when arterial hypoxemia (and hypercapnia) is minimal, cyanosis may appear only during exercise, as the ventilation fails to keep pace with the increased metabolic demand. Alternatively, as in the sleep apnea syndromes, arterial hypoxemia and hypercapnia may become appreciable only during sleep. Regardless of the underlying cause, an upper respiratory infection often topples the subject into acute respiratory failure and severe pulmonary hypertension.

For the patient in combined respiratory and cardiac (right ventricular) failure, the highest priority is to improve oxygenation. Success with this strategy results in a decrease in pulmonary arterial pressures, thereby relieving the overburdened right ventricle. Recently, potent but short-acting pulmonary vasodilators, such as prostacyclin, have been advocated for urgent relief of right ventricular overload. But, in this category of patients, pharmacologic therapy is rarely needed because of the efficiency of the oxygen therapy in promoting pulmonary vasodilation.

ADULT RESPIRATORY DISTRESS SYNDROME. In this disorder, pulmonary hypertension is quite common, occasionally in conjunction with pulmonary venous hypertension secondary to fluid overload but more often as a consequence of mechanical influences exerted by pulmonary edema and atelectasis operating in conjunction with respiratory acidosis. This concomitant disorder requires no special treatment, since it follows the course of the illness, decreasing spontaneously as the patient recovers.

MULTIPLE SYSTEM DISEASES. Pulmonary hypertension is occasionally caused by the pulmonary arterial lesions of connective tissue diseases, notably lupus erythematosus, scleroderma, and dermatomyositis. However, the most common cause of pulmonary hypertension in systemic disorders is sarcoidosis, not only because this disorder is more prevalent than the connective tissue disorders but also because of the proclivity of the parenchymal lesions for the vicinity of the small pulmonary arteries and arterioles.

PRIMARY (UNEXPLAINED) PULMONARY HYPERTENSION

Definition

Primary pulmonary hypertension is a synonym for "unexplained" pulmonary arterial hypertension. It is also a diagnosis of exclusion. As a rule, pulmonary veno-occlusive disease (see below) is not included under the rubric of primary pulmonary hypertension because, although unexplained in etiology, its pathologic features and pathogenetic mechanisms are different and usually quite distinctive.

The clinical diagnosis of primary pulmonary hypertension rests on three different types of evidence: (1) clinical, radiographic, and electrocardiographic manifestations of pulmonary hypertension; (2) demonstration by right-heart catheterization of the typical hemodynamic constellation of abnormally high pulmonary arterial pressures and pulmonary vascular resistance in association with a normal pulmonary wedge pressure and a nearly normal cardiac output; and (3) inability to attribute the pulmonary hypertension to a disorder of the heart, lungs, or systemic circulation.

With respect to corroborating the clinical diagnosis, the pathologist is most helpful in proving that the cause of the pulmonary hypertension is as obscure after death as it was during life. Unfortunately, the idea of a pathognomonic vascular lesion—notably the "plexiform" lesion—has not been rewarding on three accounts: (1) Primary pulmonary hypertension seems to be the final common pathway for multiple unknown etiologies; (2) the vascular lesions have been shown by biopsy and at autopsy to be quite heterogeneous; and (3) plexiform lesions probably represent a healed pulmonary arteritis and are diagnostic of one type of primary pulmonary hypertension if other causes of plexiform lesions can be excluded.

GENERAL FEATURES. Primary pulmonary hypertension is an uncommon disorder and, at autopsy, is responsible for about 1 per cent of all causes of cor pulmonale. A total of about 1000 cases have been reported.

After puberty, females predominate, most strikingly between 10 and 40 years of age. Before puberty, no sex difference is discernible. Consequently, the paradigmatic patient with primary pulmonary hypertension is a young woman in the prime of life without discernible cause for symptoms. This fact is sometimes useful in the clinical differentiation between primary pulmonary hypertension and pulmonary thromboembolic disease, which, unless preceded by a predisposing disease, trauma, or intervention, favors men, particularly in their later years.

Until recently, virtually all reports of primary pulmonary hypertension dealt with sporadic cases. About 25 families have now been identified in which the disease seems to be hereditary. The question has been raised whether detailed histories would demonstrate that some sporadic cases are actually familial.

Over the years, evidence has accumulated that primary pulmonary hypertension may be the end result of diverse etiologies, ranging from incomplete involution of the fetal circulation to autoimmunity, diet, and drugs (Table 48–3). The diversity of potential causes complicates management. In addition, they confuse descriptions of natural history. Thus, although the paradigm cited above indicates death within two to three years, several instances now exist of much longer life spans. Moreover, occasional instances are known of regression of the disease, most notably during the subsidence of the epidemic of primary pulmonary hypertension associated with the ingestion of the anorectic agent Aminorex in Europe between 1967 and 1970.

Pathology

The seat of the disease is the small pulmonary arteries (between 40 and 100 μ in diameter). The obliterative lesions are diverse, affecting one or more layers of the small muscular arteries and arterioles. In some instances, medial hypertrophy predominates; in others, combinations of inflammation and fibrosis coexist. The "classic" picture of concentric intimal fibrosis, necrotizing arteritis, and plexiform lesions encountered in the Aminorex epidemic is far from the rule. Pathologists can usually distinguish with confidence the obliterated vessels of primary pulmonary hypertension from those of multiple pulmonary emboli. An important basis for this distinction is the *concentric* pattern of the fibroelastosis that obliterates the vascular lumens in primary pulmonary hypertension and the *eccentric* fibroelastosis that follows organization of venous clots after pulmonary embolization. But these differences are not absolute.

Pathophysiology

The hemodynamic hallmarks of primary pulmonary hypertension studies at rest are well known: a high pulmonary arterial pressure in association with a nearly normal cardiac output and a normal left atrial (pulmonary wedge) pressure.

TABLE 48–3. SUGGESTED ETIOLOGIES FOR PRIMARY PULMONARY HYPERTENSION

Etiology	Comment
Autoimmune mechanisms	Especially in young women, associated with Raynaud's phenomenon and collagen diseases, such as disseminated lupus erythematosus, rheumatoid arthritis, progressive systemic sclerosis, polyarteritis nodosa, and dermatomyositis.
Persistence of fetal pulmonary vascular bed	A distinct syndrome in neonatal life that is questionably related to the adult syndrome.
Dietary pulmonary hypertension	Suggested by an outbreak of primary pulmonary hypertension related to an anorectic agent, Aminorex. Only 2% of those who ingested the drug developed pulmonary hypertension, suggesting individual predisposition. Pulmonary hypertension (with different vascular lesions) also produced experimentally by ingesting seeds of leguminous plant *Crotalaria spectabilis*.
Sustained vasoconstriction	A classic suggestion which is difficult to accept as initiating mechanism; more likely a contributing factor.
Combined portal and pulmonary hypertension	Common denominator suggested by occurrence of pulmonary hypertension in some patients with hepatic cirrhosis. Also related to mechanism of dietary pulmonary hypertension.
Multiple pulmonary emboli	Once considered to be the major cause of primary pulmonary hypertension. May still be difficult to distinguish on clinical grounds but can almost always be distinguished morphologically.
Familial pulmonary hypertension	Although familial instances do occur, and individual susceptibility has been demonstrated in some instances, the connecting links between inherited defect or predisposition and clinical disease are unclear.

As a result of this constellation, calculated pulmonary vascular resistance is high, generally leading to the logical conclusion that the resistance vessels, i.e., the small muscular arteries and arterioles, are the predominant sites of vascular obstruction. During exercise, as cardiac output increases, pulmonary arterial pressures increase; the increments in pressure in the pulmonary hypertensive circuit are generally much more striking than in the normotensive pulmonary circulation.

Most protocols using pulmonary vasodilators currently center on the response to rest and exercise. Several clinical and hemodynamic changes are sought as desirable endpoints:

1. Improvement in exercise tolerance. This increase in physical capacity is usually accompanied by an increase in cardiac output and presumably improved distribution of blood flow to peripheral organs and tissues.

2. A decrease in the level of pulmonary arterial hypertension, both at rest and during exercise.

3. A decrease in calculated pulmonary vascular resistance. Although this goal is often attained in acute experiments, its clinical value is doubtful unless an increase in cardiac output (with minimal increase in heart rate) occurs in conjunction with a decrease in pulmonary arterial pressure.

4. Agents that relax pulmonary vessels also usually cause vasodilation if they gain access to the systemic circulation, thereby unloading the left ventricle and calling into play the systemic baroreceptors. As a result, pulmonary blood volume and pressure may fall even though systemic arterial pressures remain virtually unchanged.

It remains to be learned if pulmonary vasodilation will promote long-term survival, even though there now seems to be little doubt that an increase in cardiac output, and the accompanying redistribution of systemic blood flow, can provide symptomatic relief.

Clinical Picture

In its early stages, the disease is difficult to recognize. In the sporadic case, the first clue is often an abnormal chest radiograph or electrocardiograph indicative of right ventricular hypertrophy. But these are late manifestations: By the time that these changes appear, pulmonary hypertension is moderate to severe and generally longstanding. Initial complaints, particularly easy fatigability and chest discomfort, are often dismissed except during the course of an epidemic, as that associated with Aminorex, or in familial pulmonary hypertension. Direct determination of pulmonary circulatory pressures by cardiac catheterization is currently the only way to prove the diagnosis.

When the disease is advanced, dyspnea, particularly during exercise, is common. Many patients are tachypneic and complain of nondescript chest pain as well as breathlessness. Other common symptoms are weakness, fatigue, and effort syncope. In time, right-sided heart failure develops. On rare occasion, an enlarged pulmonary artery causes hoarseness because of compression of the left recurrent laryngeal nerve.

Patients with severe pulmonary hypertension seem prone to sudden death. Thus, death has occurred unexpectedly during normal activities, cardiac catheterization, and surgical procedures, and after the administration of barbiturates or anesthetic agents. The mechanisms for sudden death are not clear.

On physical examination, the jugular venous pulse usually shows a prominent "a" wave. Right ventricular hypertrophy causes a cardiac thrust along the left sternal border, and a distinct impulse is palpable over the region of the main pulmonary artery. The pulmonic component of the second sound is markedly accentuated, the second heart sound is narrowly split, and an ejection click is heard in the pulmonic area. Often a fourth heart sound emanating from the hypertrophied right ventricle is heard at the lower left sternal border. In some patients an ejection murmur is audible at the pulmonic area; as pulmonary arterial pressures approximate systemic arterial levels, the murmur of pulmonary valvular insufficiency often appears.

Right ventricular failure is accompanied by jugular venous distention and a gallop (S_3); inspiration intensifies the gallop. The liver becomes enlarged and tender and a hepatojugular reflux can be elicited; in time dilation of the failing right ventricle leads to tricuspid insufficiency manifested by a holosystolic murmur, best heard in the fourth interspace to the left of the sternum, which increases in intensity during inspiration. The liver develops expansile pulsations synchronous with the heart beat. Hydrothorax and ascites are uncommon even in the face of hepatomegaly and peripheral edema.

In the early stage, the chest radiograph is generally normal. Later it shows cardiac enlargement in association with enlargement of the pulmonary trunk while the peripheral pulmonary arterial branches are attenuated; the lung fields appear oligemic. Although fullness of the central pulmonary arterial trunks and peripheral "pruning" are distinctive, appearances vary somewhat from patient to patient in accord with the level and pace of the pulmonary hypertension and the age of the patient. The electrocardiogram almost always shows some evidence of right ventricular enlargement and usually of right atrial enlargement. Radiographic evidence of right ventricular enlargement usually becomes overt only late in the course of the pulmonary hypertension.

Lung scans and angiography help to exclude multiple pulmonary emboli. Rarely do these procedures prove to be more enlightening than the standard chest radiograph.

The results of cardiac catheterization are consistent with diffuse obliterative disease of the pulmonary arterial tree: Pulmonary arterial hypertension is associated with a normal pulmonary wedge pressure and a normal, or nearly normal, cardiac output (see Pathophysiology). Cardiac catheterization is most valuable in excluding known causes of pulmonary arterial hypertension and in screening the response of the pulmonary circulation to vasodilator agents.

Diagnosis

The diagnosis of primary pulmonary hypertension rests on two pillars: (1) the detection of pulmonary hypertension, and (2) exclusion of known causes of high pulmonary arterial pressure. The history is of utmost importance. Before categorizing pulmonary hypertension as "primary" or "unexplained," due regard must be paid to the predilection of primary pulmonary hypertension for young women, its occasional familial occurrence, associated signs and symptoms of connective tissue disorders (e.g, Raynaud's phenomenon), and, above all, the likelihood of pulmonary thromboembolism. Pulmonary function tests are useful in excluding diffuse pulmonary disorders, paricularly interstitial fibrosis and granuloma. The value of cardiac catheterization in eliminating acquired or congenital heart disease has been indicated above. But even after these procedures, distinction is often not possible, particularly between primary pulmonary hypertension and pulmonary arterial hypertension secondary to multiple pulmonary emboli. Theoretically, this distinction is of great importance because of the possibility of intervening therapeutically in thromboembolic disease by using anticoagulants, inferior vena caval or common femoral vein ligation, or even pulmonary embolectomy. Unfortunately, by the time pulmonary hypertension is recognized, the anatomic lesions are generally so far advanced that the likelihood of arresting or reversing the obliterative pulmonary vascular disease in either disorder is exceedingly slim.

Treatment

GENERAL FEATURES. The aim of treatment in primary pulmonary hypertension is to decrease pulmonary arterial pressure, preferably in conjunction with an increase in cardiac output. By this combination, the afterload on the right ventricle will decrease and organ blood flow will improve. In recent years, attempts have been made to identify pulmonary vasodilators that, by decreasing pulmonary vascular resistance, will provide symptomatic relief and prolong life.

To aid in pursuing this goal, the National Heart, Lung, and Blood Institute has established a national registry by which experiences with the disease and with the use of pharmacologic agents can be shared. To date, about 200 patients have satisfied the criteria for inclusion in the registry. Although the data have not yet been analyzed in detail, enough information is already on hand to underscore the difficulties in evaluating therapy: (1) The natural history of primary pulmonary hypertension is inconsistent, probably in keeping with the diverse etiologies that can elicit pulmonary hypertension. (2) Instances are being reported of long-term survival without vasodilator therapy. (3) Unless documented by morphologic studies, i.e., lung biopsy or autopsy, secondary pulmonary hypertension—notably multiple pulmonary emboli and less often vasculitis—can masquerade clinically as primary pulmonary hypertension. (4) All vasodilators, except those destroyed during a single pulmonary circulation (currently acetylcholine and prostacyclin), cannot be administered so that they act solely on the pulmonary circulation; as a corollary, all run the risk of troublesome side effects on the heart and systemic circulation. (5) For both acute and chronic administration, optimal therapeutic doses are difficult to establish. (6) Criteria for efficacy in acute studies are inconsistent; many rely almost entirely on a drop in calculated pulmonary vascular resistance even though pulmonary arterial pressure usually remains unchanged and the work of the right ventricle increases. (7) Symptomatic improvement after the acute administration of a presumed pulmonary vasodilator is most closely related to an increase in cardiac output. (8) The acute response to a pulmonary vasodilator is not a reliable predictor of the chronic response. Because of these reservations, optimism for the use of pulmonary vasodilators in primary pulmonary hypertension remains cautious. The ideal would still be prevention (as in thromboembolic disease) or treatment according to etiology (e.g., corticosteroids for interstitial granulomas due to sarcoidosis).

Despite these general caveats and uncertainties, pulmonary vasodilator therapy continues to be tried in the hope that individual patients will respond. The pulmonary vasodilators currently in use are summarized in Table 48–4. Not shown are acetylcholine and prostacyclin, both of which have been used to assess the potential for pulmonary vasodilation. Although promising as agents for testing and for acute reduction of right ventricular overloading, neither is as yet available for chronic administration. Nor is oxygen listed, since it is only apt to cause pulmonary vasodilation if arterial hypoxemia coexists with pulmonary hypertension.

DIRECTLY ACTING DRUGS. Two agents in this category are currently in wide use to test acutely for responsiveness: nitroprusside and hydralazine.

Nitroprusside. Nitroprusside elicits vasodilation in both arteries and veins. It is ideal for acute testing, but cannot be administered chronically. Sublingual nitroglycerin has been tried for chronic administration of a nitrate. However, its effectiveness as a chronic pulmonary vasodilator has not been documented. Instead, when nitroprusside given intravenously does produce pulmonary vasodilation, oral therapy with long-acting nitrates is usually begun, using a combination of isosorbide dinitrate, which primarily causes venodilatation, and hydralazine, an alpha-adrenergic blocker, which acts primarily on the arterial resistance vessels (arterioles). The effectiveness of the isosorbide in this combination is conjectural.

Hydralazine. This agent is currently very much in vogue. It exerts its vasodilator effect predominantly on vascular smooth muscle, much more on arterioles than on veins. It also increases cardiac output, both by a positive inotropic effect and by tachycardia; the latter seems to originate centrally as well as peripherally in response to the drop in systemic arterial pressure that the drug produces. When used in the treatment of systemic hypertension, the incidence of side effects is high but many can be avoided, or eliminated, by concurrent administration of a beta-adrenergic antagonist, e.g., propranolol. Although experience with this agent in treating primary pulmonary hypertension is limited, enthusiasm is high.

Side effects have not been reported despite its high potential for evoking circulatory upsets. Noteworthy is the observation that during chronic hydralazine therapy, pulmonary arterial pressure remains high even though pulmonary vascular resistance drops, both at rest and during exercise, and even though the patients feel better and can do more. The basis for the sustained pulmonary hypertension is the concomitant increase in cardiac output. Unexplained is the increase in oxygen consumption during hydralazine therapy, possibly related to cutaneous vasodilatation and heat loss, a property that hydralazine shares with other cutaneous vasodilators.

DRUGS ACTING ON ADRENERGIC RECEPTORS. Two agents in this broad category are still quite popular: isoproterenol and phentolamine.

Isoproterenol. Isoproterenol is a powerful sympathomimetic amine that acts on beta receptors everywhere, leaving alpha receptors virtually unaffected. Its predominant effects are on the heart and the smooth muscle of vessels and bronchi. Intravenous administration raises the cardiac output because of the chronotropic and inotropic effects of the drug coupled with the increase in venous return effected by peripheral vasodilation. Sublingual or oral administration is unreliable. Its effectiveness as a pulmonary vasodilator has been remarkably unpredictable and inconsistent.

Phentolamine. Phentolamine (Regitine) in doses of 100 to 200 mg per day acts primarily on vascular smooth muscle to

**TABLE 48–4. SOME VASODILATOR DRUGS CURRENTLY USED
IN THE MANAGEMENT OF PRIMARY PULMONARY HYPERTENSION***

	Mechanism of Action	Acute Testing	Usual Maintenance Therapy	Major Side Effects; Comments
Nitroprusside	Directly on vascular smooth muscle; relaxes both systemic arteries and veins.	10 μg/min IV, increasing by 10 μg/min every 4 min until systemic systolic < 95 torr or PA† systolic > 10 torr over control (max 60 μg/min).	Hydralazine 10 mg every 6 h, increasing up to 50 mg every 6 h, + isosorbide dinitrate 10 mg every 6 h, increasing up to 50 mg every 6 h.	Systemic vasodilation and hypotension, cyanide toxicity at high concentrations. Half-life of a few minutes.
Hydralazine	Directly on vascular smooth muscle, presumably via prostacyclin production; greater dilator effect on arterioles than on veins; myocardial stimulant.	10 mg IV repeated once after 10 min. Resting hemodynamics followed by exercise 20 min later.	Hydralazine, start with 10 mg every 6 h, increase to 50–75 mg every 6 h.	Flushing, nasal congestion, conjunctivitis, CNS† stimulation, drug fever, muscle cramps. Lupus-like syndrome at doses of 200–400 mg/day. Side effects lessened by gradual increase in dosage. Surprisingly few side effects reported as yet in treating primary pulmonary hypertension.
Isoproterenol	Beta-adrenergic agonist; relaxes vascular smooth muscle when tone is high; increases venous return to heart; positive inotropic and chronotropic effects.	1 μg/min IV and increasing by 1 μg/min until heart rate > 120/min or PA systolic > 10 torr over control, up to maximum dose of 5 μg/min.	Isoproterenol (sublingual) 10 mg every 4 h, increasing up to 20 mg every 3 h. Terbutaline 5 mg tid.	Palpitation, tachycardia, flushing, cardiac arrhythmias exceedingly common.
Phentolamine	Alpha-adrenergic blocker; dilates both systemic arterioles and large veins; positive inotropic effect.	0.5 mg/min IV to a maximum of 10 mg.	Phentolamine 25 mg every 6 h, increasing to 50 mg every 3 h while awake. Phenoxybenzamine 10 mg daily, increasing by 10 mg every 4 days to a maximum of 40 mg daily. Prazosin 2 mg tid, increasing up to 5 mg tid.	Tachycardia, cardiac arrhythmias, angina, gastrointestinal stimulation.
Nifedipine§	Interferes with calcium fluxes in vascular smooth muscle.	10 mg sublingually repeated once after 15 min. Exercise 15 min later.	Nifedipine 50 mg bid.	Systemic vasodilation and hypotension; flushing, rhythm disturbances; dysesthesias, peripheral edema; currently the most popular vasodilator agent for empiric trial (without hemodynamic testing).

*Based on a table developed by a working group as part of suggested protocols for use by centers for primary pulmonary hypertension, recently established by the National Heart, Lung, and Blood Institute. Members of this working group were Drs. Edward H. Bergofsky (chairman), Michael Beaven, Alfred P. Fishman, Michael Heymann, John T. Reeves, Lynne M. Reid, and Marvin A. Sackner. (Reprinted with permission from Fishman AP [ed.]: Update: Pulmonary Diseases and Disorders. New York, McGraw-Hill Book Company, 1982.)

†PA = pulmonary arterial; CNS = central nervous system.

‡Some clinics prefer the calcium channel blocker diltiazem, up to 30 mg 3 times daily, for oral maintenance therapy.

§This use of nefedipine is not listed in the manufacturer's directive.

cause vasodilation; this direct effect is supplemented by a modest degree of blockade of sympathetic nervous activity and of antagonism to circulating catecholamines; higher doses elicit the full picture of alpha-adrenergic blockade, including marked gastrointestinal side effects. Its use has not been uniformly successful.

Quinazoline Derivatives. Prazosin also acts predominantly as an alpha-adrenergic blocking agent on vascular smooth muscle. It resembles nitroprusside in its effects on the systemic arterial and venous circulations. However, it has been reported to become increasingly ineffective during prolonged administration.

DRUGS THAT BLOCK CALCIUM TRANSPORT. The designation *calcium blocker* or *calcium antagonist* refers to a heterogeneous group of agents of different structural, pharmacologic, and electrophysiologic properties. The agents currently receiving the most clinical attention as potential pulmonary vasodilators are nifedipine and diltiazem. Of the two, nifedipine is the more popular. Verapamil, once used extensively, has fallen into disuse, largely because of its undesirable negative inotropic effect.

*Nifedipine.** Nifedipine is a synthetic agent that is unrelated to other vasoactive or cardiotonic drugs. It is a potent, long-

acting systemic vasodilator that has grown increasingly popular for the treatment of coronary vasospasm. No myocardial depressant effects have been demonstrated, nor does it seem to possess antiarrhythmic properties. In an experimental model of pulmonary hypertension in the dog, it was judged more effective than either verapamil or diltiazem. It is now the agent of choice for empiric therapy when hemodynamic trials of the various pulmonary vasodilators are not feasible as a preliminary.

OTHER AGENTS. Diazoxide has proved during the past few years to have too many untoward side effects to warrant the risk of using it, particularly because more manageable agents, like nifedipine, are available. Captopril has also proved disappointing, and its use has fallen off.

Arachidonic Acid Metabolites. Enthusiasm is currently high about the effectiveness of prostacyclin (PGI$_2$) in evoking pulmonary vasodilation in patients with primary pulmonary hypertension. This agent seems to have several attractive features: (1) It is a powerful relaxant of increased pulmonary vascular tone, i.e., it is a potent vasodilator; (2) it reduces pulmonary vascular resistance in a dose-dependent way so that dosage can be titrated to achieve maximal pulmonary vasodilation without undue systemic side effects, e.g., headache, nausea, flushing, and vomiting; (3) adverse effects stop when the infusion stops; and (4) it seems to indicate whether

*This use is not listed in the manufacturer's directive.

there is a vasoconstrictive element to the pulmonary hypertension that other pulmonary vasodilators might affect.

Among its disadvantages are (1) it is an investigational drug only available in a form fit for intravenous use, and (2) in some patients, it is ineffective or even increases pulmonary vascular resistance. Until the agent becomes widely available for clinical trials, this promising drug cannot be fully assessed.

HEART-LUNG TRANSPLANTATION. Many patients with primary pulmonary hypertension are unresponsive to pulmonary vasodilator therapy. Young individuals threatened by syncope and incapacitated by right ventricular failure are candidates for heart-lung transplantation. A few patients with primary pulmonary hypertension seem to have undergone this procedure successfully. However, organs for transplant are in short supply. In a few patients with primary pulmonary hypertension, continued infusion of prostacyclin for two months to two years has helped to tide over candidates for transplantation.

Prognosis

The diagnosis of primary pulmonary hypertension carries with it a poor prognosis. Although death usually occurs within a few years after the onset of symptoms, instances of long-term survival do occur. Exceptions to the rule of a short and fatal course were also reported in the Aminorex epidemic in patients in whom the drug was stopped. At present, there is no specific treatment for primary pulmonary hypertension. Pulmonary vasodilators have, in some patients, improved exercise tolerance and the quality of life but have not yet been shown to prolong life. Neither anticoagulants nor corticosteroids have been of value. The cause of death is generally right ventricular failure. In some patients, sudden death terminates the illness.

PULMONARY VENO-OCCLUSIVE DISEASE

In a few patients with unexplained pulmonary arterial hypertension the disease appears to originate in progressive obstruction of pulmonary veins. Characteristically, anatomic lesions in the pulmonary veins predominate, but pulmonary arteries and arterioles are also involved. The etiology is unknown, but the obstructive venous lesions seem attributable to thrombosis after local injury, possibly secondary to a viral infection.

When the pulmonary hypertension is suspected to originate distal to the pulmonary capillary bed, mitral valve disease or myocardial dysfunction, or even left atrial myxoma, has the greater likelihood of being the cause than does primary pulmonary venous obstruction. More esoteric etiologies for the pulmonary venous hypertension to be excluded are congenital atresia of pulmonary veins and coexistent phlebitis of systemic and pulmonary veins.

Predominantly children and young adults are affected, but the age range has been from infancy to 48 years. There seems to be no sex difference. Although hints exist of possibly related familial cardiac disorders, the patients are too few to do more than raise suspicion of a familial or common environmental cause.

Clinical suspicion of this disorder generally arises when a patient with congested and edematous lungs, consistent with occult mitral valvular disease or left ventricular failure, proves to have a normal mitral valve and left ventricle. However, this stereotype is not always encountered and some patients have carried the diagnosis of primary pulmonary arterial hypertension until autopsy disclosed the characteristic pulmonary venous lesions.

The cardinal signs are dyspnea and fatigue or exertion in conjunction with evidence of pulmonary hypertension, particularly radiologic evidence of postcapillary pulmonary hypertension without evidence of an increase in left atrial pressure. Pleural effusions are common. Cyanosis, syncope,

hemoptysis, and finger clubbing have been inconsistent findings.

Cardiac catheterization discloses a high pulmonary arterial pressure, often with a normal pulmonary wedge pressure. The low wedge pressure has been attributed to discontinuities and channels of high resistance between the pulmonary capillaries and the pulmonary and bronchial venous channels so that wedging interrupts all sources of flow distal to the area blocked by the catheter. A few lung biopsies have been done during life.

Both lungs are involved, but the venous lesions may be more marked in one region than in another. As a rule, the pulmonary arteries as well as the pulmonary veins are affected, but the lesions are different. Most striking are the morphologic changes in the pulmonary veins and venules, which are narrowed or occluded by fibrous tissue; up to 95 per cent of the veins and venules may be affected, but complete occlusion is uncommon. Bronchial veins and bronchopulmonary anastomoses share in the occlusive process. Hypertrophy in the walls of the pulmonary arteries may be also quite striking, whereas the pulmonary capillary bed is generally unaffected. Thrombi in the pulmonary arteries are common. The lungs show congestion, edema, and focal fibrosis, which may become extensive.

Management has been disappointing, since the lesions are generally irreversible. The usual duration after recognition ranges from a few weeks in infants to several years in adults, with seven the maximum.

Bjornsson J, Edwards WD: Primary pulmonary hypertension: A histopathologic study of 80 cases. Mayo Clin Proc 60:16, 1985. *Describes the histologic features that seem to form the morphologic substrate for the increase in pulmonary vascular resistance that characterizes primary pulmonary hypertension.*

Fishman AP: Pulmonary circulation. In Fishman AP, Fisher A (eds.): Handbook of Physiology: The Respiratory System, Vol I. Bethesda, Md., American Physiological Society, 1986, pp 93–165. *A comprehensive survey of the regulation of the pulmonary circulation, particularly useful as a background for considering pathogenesis of clinical pulmonary hypertension. Emphasis is placed on the concept of pulmonary vascular resistance, the interpretation of pulmonary wedge pressures, and the identification of pulmonary vasomotor activity.*

Fishman AP: Pulmonary thromboembolism: Pathophysiology and clinical features. In Fishman AP (ed.): Pulmonary Diseases and Disorders. New York, McGraw-Hill Book Company, 1980, pp 809–826. *A succinct account of pulmonary thromboembolic disease that calls special attention to the category of multiple pulmonary emboli.*

Fishman AP, Pietra GG: Primary pulmonary hypertension. Ann Rev Med 31:421, 1980. *A review of current understanding of primary pulmonary hypertension with special emphasis on etiology. Comprehensive bibliography.*

Groves, BM, Rubin LJ, Frosolono MF, et al: A comparison of the acute hemodynamic effects of prostacyclin and hydralazine in primary pulmonary hypertension. Am Heart J 110:1200, 1985. *Interest in this comparison for those using pulmonary vasodilator agents lies in the hypothesis that hydralazine, which can be taken orally, exerts its effects by way of prostacyclin, for which no oral form is yet available.*

Higenbottam T, Wheeldon D, Wells F, et al: Long-term treatment of primary pulmonary hypertension with continuous intravenous epoprostenal (prostacyclin). Lancet 1:1046, 1984. *This paper describes the first of now seven patients, unmanageable by oral vasodilators, who were treated by continous infusion of prostacyclin for months up to two years. After one year of continuous self-administration of prostacyclin intravenously, the patient remained greatly improved.*

Reitz BA, Wallwork JL, Hunt SA, et al: Heart-lung transplantation: Successful therapy for patients with pulmonary vascular disease. N Engl J Med 306:557, 1982. *Initial successful experiences with heart-lung transplantation are described, including three patients with primary pulmonary hypertension.*

Rubin LJ, Peter RH: Oral hydralazine therapy for primary pulmonary hypertension. N Engl J Med 302:69, 1980. *Hydralazine taken orally (50 mg q 6 hours) by four patients increased cardiac output and exercise tolerance, leaving pulmonary arterial pressure unchanged; heart rate increased in all. Although calculated vascular resistance fell in each instance, the hemodynamic burden of the right ventricle was unchanged. Clinical improvement was probably related to increased cardiac output.*

Trell E: Benign, idiopathic pulmonary hypertension. Acta Med Scand 193:137, 1973. *Two cases of unusually long duration of idiopathic pulmonary hypertension (about 27 and 40 years, respectively) are presented and discussed with respect to others reported in the literature. No autopsy or biopsy findings.*

Voelkel NF, Reeves JT: Primary pulmonary hypertension. In Moser KM (ed.): Pulmonary Vascular Diseases. New York, Marcel Dekker, 1979, pp 573–628. *Excellent clinical and physiologic review of current understanding of primary pulmonary hypertension against a background of a large personal experience with both this disorder and the pulmonary hypertension of high altitude.*

Wagenvoort CA, Wagenvoort N: Pathology of Pulmonary Hypertension. New York, John Wiley & Sons, 1977. *Splendid morphologic treatise on primary* pulmonary hypertension based on years of collecting pathologic material, careful analysis, and intriguing extrapolations from morbid anatomy to etiology and clinical syndromes.

Weir EK, Reeves JT: Pulmonary Hypertension. Mt. Kisco, NY, Futura Publishing Company, 1984. A collection of papers that summarize the current understanding of pulmonary hypertension and its various subsets. Considerable emphasis on management.

49 CONGENITAL HEART DISEASE

Samuel Kaplan

Congenital diseases of the heart occur in about 8 to 10 of 1000 live births. The spectrum of severity varies widely. One fourth to one third are symptomatic in the first year of life, frequently as neonates. In others, such as in patients with a functionally normal bicuspid aortic valve, the lesion may remain silent throughout life. With the development of palliative or radical surgical treatment, another large group has evolved that was treated during infancy or childhood and has reached adult life. Accordingly, adults with congenital heart disease fall into several groups: Some have anomalies with a natural history for long survival, others have had successful palliative or "curative" surgery in childhood, and still others have had lesions that were mild in childhood but have increased in severity in adult life (e.g., aortic stenosis).

Etiology

The cause is usually unknown in individual patients. The etiology of congenital heart disease is thought to be multifactorial, primarily due to an interaction between genetic predisposition and intrauterine environmental factors. It is estimated that congenital heart disease is associated with chromosomal abnormalities in 5 per cent of cases and with single mutant genes and environmental factors in 3 per cent each. Among *chromosomal abnormalities* the prevalence of congenital heart disease is about 50 per cent in trisomy 21 (Down's syndrome), 95 per cent in trisomy 18, 90 per cent in trisomy 13, and 35 per cent in Turner's (XO) syndrome. Among *single mutant gene* disorders (autosomal dominant or recessive or X-linked phenotypes), the more frequent syndromes in which the heart is involved are hypertrophic cardiomyopathy and the syndromes of Noonan and Holt-Oram. Numerous *environmental factors* have been implicated. Women who contract rubella during the first trimester of pregnancy may give birth to infants with pulmonic stenosis (especially pulmonary artery branch stenosis), persistent patent ductus arteriosus, and less often other defects. Other viruses have also been implicated, but the evidence that they produce congenital heart disease is not so strong. These include cytomegalovirus, coxsackievirus, and herpesvirus. Among drugs implicated in congenital heart disease are the anticonvulsants, especially phenytoin and trimethadione, and lithium salts (with an apparent predilection for atrioventricular valve disease, especially Ebstein's malformation of the tricuspid valve), progesterone, warfarin, and amphetamines. The offspring of diabetic women are at greater risk for a variety of congenital heart diseases. Patent ductus arteriosus is more frequent in children born at high altitudes. It is estimated that about one half of the offspring of alcoholic mothers have congenital heart disease, usually left to right shunts.

Counseling

Parents of children with congenital heart disease are concerned about the cause and about the possibility of recurrence in future pregnancies. This concern is greatest when the child is first born or the baby succumbs during the neonatal period. An explanation should be offered about the known causes of congenital heart disease and guilt feelings allayed. The prevalence of congenital heart disease in a second infant is 2 to 5 per cent. Although this figure is higher than in the general population, it is still quite low and parents should be supported if they decide to have another child. When congenital heart disease has recurred in two siblings, the prevalence is higher in a third pregnancy (estimated to be 20 to 25 per cent). Many women with congenital heart disease who had corrective surgery during childhood have reached childbearing age. The prevalence of congenital heart disease in their children ranges from 3 to 16 per cent. Recurrence risks are low in the offspring of fathers with congenital heart disease.

Circulatory Shunts

Pathophysiology

MAGNITUDE AND DIRECTION. Factors that determine the magnitude and direction of intra- and extracardiac shunts are the size of the defect, pressure differences between the cardiac chambers or vessels, and resistance to ejection produced by outflow obstruction, as well as the ratio of systemic to pulmonary vascular resistance. Since normal systemic vascular pressures and resistances greatly exceed those in the pulmonary circuit, flow across small defects (such as ventricular septal defects) is from left to right but is limited in magnitude by the small opening. When the defect is large and nonrestrictive, peak systolic pressures in the ventricles are virtually identical, so that the direction and magnitude of flow are regulated by outflow resistance. If systemic vascular resistance significantly exceeds that in the pulmonary circuit with large defects (in the absence of pulmonic stenosis), torrential left to right shunts are present. The magnitude of the shunt is decreased as pulmonary vascular resistance approaches that in the systemic circuit, and it is bidirectional or right to left with continued increase of pulmonary resistance. When severe pulmonic stenosis is present, resistance to right ventricular ejection virtually equalizes peak systolic pressures in both ventricles so that flow across ventricular defects is right to left or bidirectional. A major determinant of direction and magnitude of shunting at the atrial level is the diastolic distensibility of the ventricles. Flow, frequently torrential, is from left to right, since the thin-walled right ventricle is easily filled even though atrial pressures are equal and low.

PULMONARY HYPERTENSION. This complication (see Ch. 48), common in congenital heart disease, results from increased pulmonary blood flow and/or resistance. Torrential pulmonary blood flow (as in secundum atrial septal defects) can be accommodated by the pulmonary circulation without increase in pressure. Pulmonary hypertension develops frequently in the presence of large defects at the ventricular level or communications between the aorta and pulmonary arteries. In infants and small children with these defects, "hyperkinetic" pulmonary hypertension is present. This term refers to a vasoactive pulmonary bed that undergoes vasodilation in response to oxygen or tolazoline. These agents reduce the level of pulmonary arterial pressure by pulmonary vasodilation even though pulmonary blood flow increases. Hyperkinetic pulmonary hypertension is uncommon in adults but is seen in some with secundum atrial septal defects. Generally, pulmonary vascular disease is present in adults, so that pulmonary vascular resistance is greatly increased even when pulmonary blood flow is not excessive (see Eisenmenger's Syndrome below). The status of the pulmonary vascular bed determines the clinical picture, prognosis, and feasibility of surgical treatment of intra- and extracardiac shunts. The goal of management is to prevent the development of severe pulmonary vascular changes by surgical ablation of the shunt. This implies serial measurements of pulmonary and systemic pressures and resistances, especially in infants and toddlers with large ventricular or aortopulmonary defects.

Right to Left Shunts

PULMONARY BLOOD FLOW AND SYSTEMIC DESATURATION. Right to left shunts are characteristically associated with arterial oxygen desaturation. The degree of desaturation is determined by pulmonary blood flow and the magnitude of right to left shunt. When effective pulmonary blood flow is markedly reduced (as in tetralogy of Fallot), systemic venous blood is ejected preferentially through the ventricular septal defect into the left ventricle and aorta, so that arterial oxygen saturation is severely reduced and cyanosis is obvious. On the other hand, right to left shunts may be associated with markedly increased pulmonary blood flow (as in transposition of the great arteries). In this situation pulmonary venous blood is almost fully saturated so that systemic arterial saturation is only moderately decreased. Cyanosis is not as intense in the latter group of patients, but they suffer from volume loading and failure of the left ventricle.

ARTERIAL HYPOXEMIA. *Cyanosis,* a dusky purple color of the skin but especially the mucous membranes and nail beds, is due to reduced hemoglobin in the arterial blood from right to left shunts. Clinical cyanosis may not be evident until the arterial oxygen saturation is below 85 per cent (normal is 94 to 98 per cent). *Clubbing* of fingers and toes is common, especially when arterial hypoxemia is marked. This sign may appear in childhood (beyond the age of one year) and is progressive. When arterial oxygen saturation returns to normal (at rest and during exercise), as occurs after surgical correction, clubbing regresses and even severe forms disappear within two to three years after operation.

Polycythemia results from adaptation of the hemopoietic system to the anoxic stimulus. This compensatory mechanism increases arterial oxygen content. When the hematocrit exceeds 65 to 70 per cent, blood viscosity increases so that the patient is at risk for intravascular thrombosis. Thrombi may develop in any organ system but are more frequent in the cerebral circulation (generally in the dural sinuses and cerebral veins) and pulmonary arteries. Dehydration increases the risk of intravascular thrombosis. Headaches are common in severely polycythemic patients (see Eisenmenger's Syndrome, below). The combination of iron deficiency anemia and polycythemia is not well tolerated. There is greater risk for intravascular thrombosis, and iron therapy is required even though this results in a further elevation of hematocrit. Severely polycythemic patients have a delicate balance between intravascular thrombosis and bleeding from coagulation defects. The more frequent abnormalities associated with a bleeding diathesis are a combination of thrombocytopenia, accelerated fibrinolysis, hypofibrinogenemia, prolonged prothrombin time, and prolonged partial thromboplastin time.

BRAIN ABSCESS AND PARADOXICAL EMBOLUS. Brain abscess occurs in older children and adults. Predisposing factors include previous occlusive microcirculatory disease from thrombosis or emboli. Clinical recognition may be difficult because the onset is insidious, symptoms are vague, and fever is low grade. In others, the onset is more acute, with headache, seizures, and localized neurologic signs that are dependent on the size and site of the abscess and the presence of increased intracranial pressure. The diagnosis is established with computed axial tomography or magnetic resonance imaging or both. Treatment is with antibiotics, generally followed by surgical drainage. In patients with right to left shunts, venous blood bypasses the lungs so that emboli arising from systemic veins enter the systemic circulation directly to occlude an artery anywhere in the body, especially the brain. This complication is rare.

SHUNT LESIONS
Atrial Septal Defect

Atrial septal defects occur more frequently in females and are designated according to their site in the septum. The most common are in the region of the fossa ovalis (*ostium secundum defect*) and are among the most prevalent congenital cardiac anomalies in adults. A less frequent variety (*sinus venosus defect*) occupies the upper part of the atrial septum and is closely related to the entry of the superior vena cava. This structure receives one or more anomalously draining pulmonary veins, usually from the right lung. (The *ostium primum defect* is discussed under Endocardial Cushion Defect, below).

The principal factors that determine the magnitude of the left to right shunt are the size of the defect, the relative compliance of the cardiac chambers, and the vascular resistances in the pulmonary and systemic circulations. If the defect is moderate or large (>2 cm in diameter in an adult), the greater distensibility of the right atrium and ventricle and the low pulmonary vascular resistance allow an abundant left-to-right shunt. On the other hand, in infancy the relatively thick and less compliant right ventricle limits the magnitude of left to right shunts. Large defects with torrential left to right shunts produce right atrial and ventricular enlargement, which encroaches on the left-sided chambers. Pulmonary pressures and resistances are generally normal. In the unusual instances in which they are elevated, the pulmonary circulation remains vasoactive, so that pressures and resistances return to normal after surgical ablation of the shunt. Those with severe pulmonary vascular disease are described under Eisenmenger's Syndrome.

DIAGNOSIS. Although symptoms are trivial and physical signs subtle, the diagnosis is usually made during childhood. However, many escape detection in the first decade of life and are recognized in later years only because of effort dyspnea and fatigue. Superimposed coronary artery disease or systemic hypertension can cause the left ventricle to be less distensible, favoring the development or worsening of these symptoms because of a further increase in left to right shunt and right volume overload. In some instances the presence of the defect is first appreciated when pulmonary hypertension develops with persistence of a torrential left to right shunt. The advent of atrial arrhythmias, fibrillation, flutter, or paroxysms of supraventricular tachycardia is not well tolerated. These events increase in frequency beyond the fourth decade. Some patients with an uncomplicated atrial septal defect are recognized for the first time because of an abnormal "routine" chest roentgenogram.

In children failure to gain weight is common but by no means the rule. The characteristic physical appearance is that of a thin child with nearly normal height and a gracile habitus. Generally, adults have a normal physical appearance, but again some are thin and gracile. The jugular venous pulse shows "a" and "v" waves of equal heights because the atria are in free communication. Dominant "a" waves suggest the presence of pulmonary hypertension, and dominant "v" waves are associated with tricuspid regurgitation. Right ventricular volume overload results in an easily palpable left parasternal lift. The importance of this sign cannot be overemphasized, and in some the dilated pulmonary artery is palpated in the second left interspace. The soft ejection systolic murmur, seldom accompanied by a thrill, is best heard at the upper left sternal edge and is produced by increased blood flow into the pulmonary artery. A loud murmur is widely transmitted to the chest anteriorly and posteriorly, especially in slightly built patients. The murmur is preceded by an accentuated first heart sound and sometimes by a pulmonic ejection sound. The auscultatory hallmark is the easily audible, widely split second heart sound. This split is virtually fixed in all phases of respiration and during the Valsalva maneuver. When the defect is large, a mid-diastolic murmur is audible at the lower left sternal edge and is produced by extravagant flow across the tricuspid valve. An early diastolic murmur of pulmonary regurgitation may accompany pulmonary hypertension, but this is rare.

The *electrocardiogram* shows right axis deviation and right ventricular hypertrophy (generally rsR¹ in right precordial leads). This pattern is due to terminal depolarization of the hypertrophied right ventricular outflow tract. Less frequent findings include tall P waves (because of right atrial enlargement), complete right bundle branch block, a prolonged PR interval, and Wolff-Parkinson-White syndrome. Supraventricular arrhythmias may be detected in untreated adults or many years after surgical closure of the defect. These consist of atrial fibrillation or flutter, paroxysmal atrial tachycardia, and multiple premature atrial contractions. Left axis deviation usually denotes the presence of an ostium primum atrial defect but is seen occasionally in secundum defects. Another rare finding is a normal electrocardiogram.

The *chest roentgenogram* is often distinctive, especially in adults. Varying degrees of cardiac enlargement are due to dilatation of the right atrium and ventricle, which displaces the normal or relatively small left-sided chambers posteriorly. The large pulmonary trunk contrasts with the smaller aortic knob, which is especially notable on the posteroanterior view. The primary branches of the pulmonary artery are enlarged and the vascularity increased toward the periphery of both lung fields.

Echocardiography not only is diagnostic but also is useful in excluding other suspected anomalies. In uncomplicated secundum atrial defects the right ventricular end-diastolic dimension is increased and the ventricular septal motion is flat or paradoxical. Real-time two-dimensional echocardiograms define the location and size of the defect and also confirm the significant enlargement of the right atrium. The deformity of the ventricular septum resulting from right ventricular volume overload is recognized, and its encroachment into the left ventricular cavity is visualized. Flow disturbance across the interatrial septum can be detected by measurements based on the Doppler principle. The pulmonary and aortic flows can be estimated by two-dimensional echo and Doppler techniques, and the difference between these flows represents the shunt volume. *Mitral valve prolapse* may be associated with secundum atrial septal defects and in many instances the suspicion is raised by the echocardiogram. Since various criteria are used for the echo diagnosis of mitral valve prolapse, caution should be exercised in the diagnosis of combined atrial septal defect and mitral valve prolapse. It is probable that the association has been overestimated.

There is an ongoing debate about whether *cardiac catheterization* is indicated in all patients. Physical examination supplemented by the electrocardiogram and chest roentgenogram usually suggests the diagnosis. This can be confirmed by visualizing the site of the defect by echocardiography and estimating the pulmonary-systemic flow ratio. However, this view is not held universally and some prefer to confirm the shunt by demonstration of a step-up in oxygen concentration between the vena cava and the right atrium, to define the site of entry of pulmonary veins, and to measure the level of pulmonary arterial pressure and resistance. The study should be undertaken in the adult in whom pulmonary hypertension or coexisting coronary artery disease is suspected.

NATURAL HISTORY. The vast majority of secundum atrial septal defects are recognized and treated surgically during childhood or adolescence. Spontaneous closure does occur, but this is usually prior to the age of about three years. Although life expectancy is shortened, adult survival is the rule and some live to an advanced age. Pregnancy is usually well tolerated, especially in women who were asymptomatic prior to pregnancy.

COMPLICATIONS. After the age of 40 years complications are frequent, and most patients who survive beyond the age of 60 years show symptoms of effort dyspnea and fatigue. Death may be unrelated to the defect, but when a relationship exists cardiac failure is the most common cause. Heart failure may be due to right ventricular failure alone or may be intensified by a dilated tricuspid valve ring with resultant

incompetence. The prevalence of atrial arrhythmias increases after the fourth decade and may precipitate heart failure, especially when the ventricular response is rapid in the presence of a large shunt. Coronary artery disease or systemic hypertension may result in a less distensible left ventricle, which favors an increase in left to right shunting. Pulmonary hypertension may be due to the high pulmonary blood flow or may progress to a state in which pulmonary and systemic vascular resistances are virtually identical and the shunt is abolished or reversed (see Eisenmenger's Syndrome). Infective endocarditis is rare in isolated lesions.

TREATMENT. Treatment is surgical ablation of the shunt, especially when the pulmonary systemic flow ratio exceeds 2:1. This is preferably accomplished between the ages of about three and four years, when the surgical risk is minimal. In these young patients the right ventricular dimension returns to normal. Surgical treatment in older children and adolescents usually improves the size of the right-sided chambers, but they may not return to normal. When the operation is performed in adults, patchy fibrosis of the chronically volume-loaded right ventricle persists, as does some degree of right ventricular dilatation. These residua may explain the blunted chronotropic response during exercise, with resultant decreased cardiac output and decreased working capacity. Nevertheless, patients in the fifth, sixth, or even seventh decade with high pulmonary blood flow and low resistance benefit from surgical repair, which can be done with a comparatively low risk. Defects in older patients can be closed surgically despite moderate pulmonary hypertension and cardiac failure, provided there is still a significant left to right shunt. Operation is contraindicated when pulmonary vascular resistance is greatly elevated so that the shunt is abolished or reversed. Late-onset arrhythmias occur in fewer than 5 per cent, 10 to 20 years after surgery. The commonest are atrial flutter, atrial fibrillation, paroxysmal supraventricular tachycardia, and frequent premature atrial contractions. Less frequent arrhythmias are sick sinus syndrome, junctional tachycardia, and complete heart block.

Lutembacher's Syndrome

This condition consists of a secundum atrial septal defect with acquired mitral stenosis. Obstruction to left ventricular inflow aggravates the left to right shunt across the atrial septum. Atrial fibrillation is common. A prominent jugular "a" wave is visible because left atrial pressure is transmitted to the right atrium and the systemic venous return. Physical findings resemble those described under secundum atrial septal defects. Auscultatory findings of mitral stenosis are present but may not be obvious. The echocardiogram is diagnostic in that signs of mitral stenosis are superimposed on right ventricular volume overload. Patients with this condition derive great symptomatic relief after intracardiac repair.

Endocardial Cushion Defect

The embryonic endocardial cushions contribute to the development of the mitral and tricuspid valves and to the growth and convergence of the atrial and ventricular septa. Maldevelopment during this stage of cardiac morphogenesis results in varying degrees of complex malformations involving the atrioventricular valves and the atrial and ventricular septa. The *ostium primum defect* is situated in the lower portion of the atrial septum overlying both the mitral and tricuspid valves. A cleft in the anterior leaflet to the mitral valve is usual, and the tricuspid valve is frequently thickened but otherwise normal. The ventricular septum is intact functionally. *Common atrioventricular canal* (complete endocardial cushion defect) consists of a common defect of both the intra-atrial and intraventricular septa with a single atrioventricular valve. This valve, common to both ventricles, has an anterior and posterior leaflet with a lateral leaflet in each ventricle. This anomaly is relatively common in patients with Down's syndrome. *Transitional forms* are intermediate between atrioventricular canal and ostium primum defects.

OSTIUM PRIMUM DEFECTS. Ostium primum defects may be associated with recurrent lower respiratory tract infections with or without congestive heart failure during infancy and early childhood. However, the majority are asymptomatic and are recognized because of the murmur of mitral incompetence. In others, the degree of mitral regurgitation is trivial. The physical signs resemble those of ostium secundum defects with superimposed mitral regurgitation. The electrocardiogram is distinctive in that there is a superior counterclockwise frontal plane axis (left axis deviation), varying degrees of right ventricular hypertrophy (rsR^1 is common), and sometimes voltage criteria for left ventricular hypertrophy because of mitral regurgitation. The chest radiograph simulates an ostium secundum atrial septal defect. The echocardiogram is also characteristic, showing enlargement of both right ventricle and right atrium, a low lying atrial septal defect, and a cleft in the anterior mitral leaflet. The mitral valve apparatus is displaced so that the anterior mitral leaflet encroaches upon the left ventricular outflow. Cardiac catheterization demonstrates the left to right atrial shunt, the level of pulmonary arterial pressure, and the degree of mitral valve incompetence. Left ventriculography shows the characteristic "goose-neck" deformity produced by the abnormal position of the mitral valve. Surgical treatment is advised during infancy or childhood with the purpose of obliterating the left to right shunt and alleviating mitral valve incompetence. In adult life, many years after surgery, atrial arrhythmias may occur as described under secundum atrial septal defect. In addition, a small number of patients have progressive mitral valve incompetence that may require mitral valve replacement.

COMPLETE ATRIOVENTRICULAR CANAL. Congestive cardiac failure, significant elevation of pulmonary artery pressures, and resistances and intercurrent pulmonary infections are common during infancy. At that time surgical treatment is undertaken to attempt to prevent progression of these complications. Without treatment, survival of these patients to adolescence and adult life is usually associated with the development of severe pulmonary vascular disease (see Eisenmenger's Syndrome, p 316) or congenital obstruction to right ventricular outflow, which limits pulmonary blood flow.

Ventricular Septal Defect

The commonest form of congenital heart disease is an isolated ventricular septal defect. Perimembranous defects are the most frequent (Fig. 49–1). The magnitude of the shunt depends on the size of the defect and status of the pulmonary vascular bed. A small defect limits the size of the left to right shunt so that cardiac chambers are normal in size and pulmonary arterial pressures and resistances remain within normal limits. Large defects are associated with a marked increase in pulmonary blood flow, as well as varying degrees of elevation of pulmonary arterial pressures and resistance. In these instances pulmonary vascular disease may be progressive, so that systemic and pulmonary vascular resistances are virtually equal (Eisenmenger's syndrome) (see Ch. 42.5).

SMALL VENTRICULAR SEPTAL DEFECTS. Spontaneous closure of the defect is frequent, especially in the first year of life, and is estimated to occur in more than one half of instances. If the defect does not close spontaneously within the first three years of life, it is likely that the clinical condition will remain unchanged. These patients are generally asymptomatic and have a normal heart size. A systolic thrill may be palpable at the lower left sternal edge and is accompanied by a harsh, loud pansystolic murmur that is widely distributed but loudest at the site of the thrill. The electrocardiogram and chest roentgenogram are normal. Generally these defects are too small to be visualized by two-dimensional echocardio-

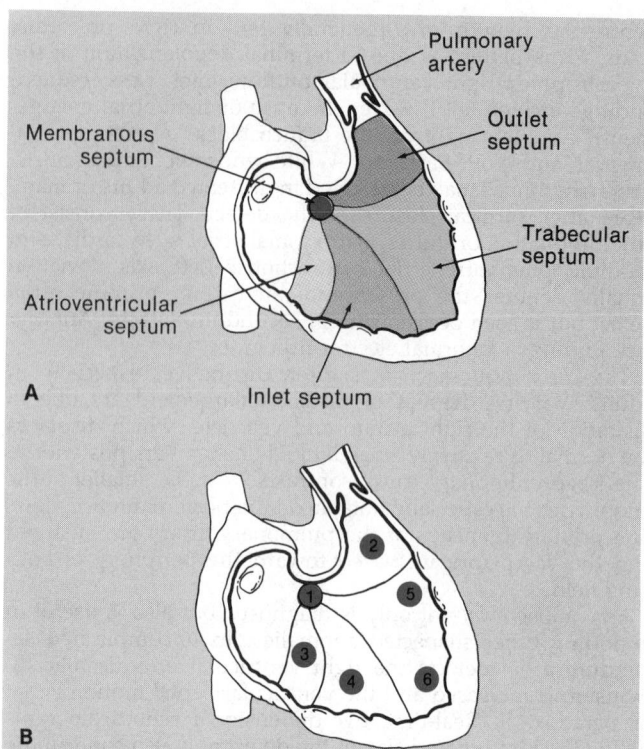

FIGURE 49–1. Diagrams of the right side of the ventricular septum. Anterior portions of the right ventricle and atrium have been removed, as has the tricuspid valve. *A,* Subdivisions of the ventricular septum. *B,* Locations of ventricular septal defects (VSD). 1. Perimembranous VSD (most common type). 2. Subpulmonic VSD (also known as infundibular, conal, or outlet VSD). 3. Atrioventricular canal VSD. 4, 5, and 6. Muscular VSD's in various parts of the septum; defects may be single or multiple. VSD's may extend to adjacent parts of the septum so that perimembranous VSD's may involve the inlet, trabecular, or outlet septum. The tricuspid valve may straddle the defect (rare in isolated VSD). Malalignment of the ventricular septum with override of a semilunar valve is unusual in isolated VSD and is more frequent with tetralogy of Fallot, double outlet ventricles, and truncus arteriosus and in some patients with transposition of the great arteries.

grams, although turbulence is recorded in the right ventricle by the Doppler principle, especially in the outflow tract. It is now believed that spontaneous closure of a small ventricular septal defect may also occur in early adult life. This notion is based on the fact that congenital ventricular septal defects are seldom found in older adults. Sometimes the development of an ejection click heralds a course that in a few years is associated with complete disappearance of all abnormal auscultatory findings when the defect is completely closed. Uncomplicated small ventricular septal defects do not require surgical closure, and the only treatment is prophylaxis against infective endocarditis.

LARGE VENTRICULAR SEPTAL DEFECTS. Large defects with unrestricted flow from the left to the right ventricle and into the pulmonary vascular bed are common in early life and rare in adults. These defects are associated with increased pulmonary vascular pressure and resistance. Furthermore, volume loading of the left heart may lead to superimposed left ventricular failure. Symptoms are present during infancy, especially between the ages of two and six months, and are produced by congestive cardiac failure, poor physical development, and recurrent pulmonary infections. These infants may respond to anticongestive measures. If this improvement is maintained, especially beyond the age of one year, the defect frequently decreases in size, with continuing clinical improvement. However, in a significant number response to therapy is not maintained, physical development remains poor, and signs of pulmonary hypertension persist. In these instances surgical closure of the defect is indicated, since the mortality rate from surgery is acceptably low and soon after operation there is a growth spurt when heart failure and pulmonary hypertension regress.

Clinical improvement in some babies with a large ventricular septal defect may be due to the development of *acquired pulmonic stenosis*, which limits pulmonary blood flow. Generally, right ventricular outflow tract obstruction is due to infundibular hypertrophy and is progressive. During infancy or early childhood the clinical course changes in that signs of heart failure improve and heart size decreases because pulmonary blood flow is limited by the pulmonic stenosis. Right ventricular pressure rises to approximate that of the left ventricle, with resultant right to left shunting and cyanosis. The clinical picture resembles that of tetralogy of Fallot (see below).

VENTRICULAR SEPTAL DEFECT WITH AORTIC REGURGITATION. The ventricular septal defect is usually small or moderate in size and its presence is known from infancy. During childhood or adolescence aortic valve regurgitation occurs because of prolapse of the right or, at times, the noncoronary cusp. The clinical picture is extremely variable, from the asymptomatic child with a small left to right shunt and trivial aortic regurgitation to the symptomatic young adult with congestive cardiac failure, angina pectoris, massive cardiomegaly, and florid aortic regurgitation. The latter patient requires surgical closure of the defect and relief of aortic regurgitation; this generally requires aortic valve replacement. The asymptomatic patient with mild regurgitation needs to be observed closely. Some believe that closure of the ventricular defect will prevent further prolapse of the aortic valve. Others recommend simultaneous aortic valvuloplasty prior to the development of significant valvular regurgitation and left ventricular dysfunction.

VENTRICULAR SEPTAL DEFECT WITH LEFT VENTRICULAR–RIGHT ATRIAL SHUNT. The atrioventricular septum is divided by the insertions of the tricuspid valve and the mitral valve. The insertion of the tricuspid valve is below that of the mitral. Thus, this area is common to the right atrium and left ventricle, and a defect in this area allows shunting from the left ventricle directly into the right atrium. In others the defect is below the tricuspid valve and is associated with an abnormal tricuspid septal leaflet. The physical signs simulate those of an isolated small to moderate ventricular septal defect. If the shunt is above the tricuspid valve, cardiac catheterization demonstrates a left to right shunt at the atrial level that may be confused with an atrial septal defect; this issue is resolved by the fact that the physical signs are not compatible with an atrial septal defect and left ventriculography demonstrates direct opacification of the right atrium from the left ventricle. This condition should be treated surgically.

OTHER DEFECTS ASSOCIATED WITH VENTRICULAR SEPTAL DEFECTS. *Patent Ductus Arteriosus.* In some instances the murmurs of both lesions are audible, so that a continuous murmur is present at the upper left sternal edge and a holosystolic murmur is heard at the lower left sternal edge. However, in many patients the physical findings are dominated by either the ventricular defect or the patent ductus arteriosus. Echocardiography combined with the Doppler technique is helpful in the diagnosis, disclosing shunting at the ventricular level as well as a patent ductus arteriosus. Left ventriculography demonstrates the ventricular septal defect, and aortography is necessary to confirm the associated ductus arteriosus if this structure is not entered directly by the catheter from the pulmonary artery.

Secundum Atrial Septal Defect. In patients with a ventricular septal defect and an ostium secundum atrial septal defect, the clinical picture is usually dominated by the ventricular defect.

This combination of defects is more likely to be present during infancy and may result in torrential pulmonary blood flow, pulmonary hypertension, and congestive heart failure. The defects are recognized by echocardiography and, if uncontrolled by medical measure, are both treated surgically during the same procedure.

Coarctation of the Aorta. Signs of coarctation of the aorta usually dominate, and sometimes the signs of ventricular septal defect are erroneously attributed to the collateral circulation associated with coarctation.

Communications Between the Aorta and Pulmonary Arteries

PATENT DUCTUS ARTERIOSUS. Persistent patency of the ductus arteriosus is more frequent in females, in premature babies, in infants born at high altitude, and in infants whose first trimester of intrauterine life is complicated by maternal rubella. The aortic end of the ductus is opposite the origin of the left subclavian artery, and the vessel enters the pulmonary artery, usually at its bifurcation.

The hemodynamic effects of a patent ductus arteriosus depend on the size of the communication, the length of the ductus, and the resistance relationships between the systemic and pulmonary circulations. Generally, the flow through the ductus is small to moderate so that pulmonary arterial pressures and resistances remain normal. These patients usually are asymptomatic, and the only abnormal physical sign is a typical continuous murmur. This murmur, sometimes accompanied by a thrill, is heard best at the upper left sternal edge, rises to a peak in late systole, continues without interruption through the second sound, and wanes during the course of diastole. Larger shunts with a significant aortic runoff result in a wide pulse pressure and a "waterhammer" or bounding arterial pulse. The left atrium and ventricle enlarge to accommodate the increased pulmonary blood flow, and this is recognized by a lateral and downward displacement of the apical impulse, which is lifting in character. The typical continuous murmur is still present, but in addition an apical mid-diastolic murmur may be audible because of increased flow across the mitral valve. When pulmonary arterial pressure and resistance rise to systemic levels, flow across the ductus is limited. In patients with pulmonary hypertension effort dyspnea is common, the wide pulse pressure disappears, and right ventricular enlargement is prominent. The auscultatory findings are dominated by those produced by pulmonary hypertension in that the typical continuous murmur disappears and is replaced by a short systolic murmur frequently preceded by an ejection click, a booming second heart sound due to loud pulmonic valve closure, and sometimes an early diastolic murmur of pulmonic valve incompetence. Occasionally the shunt through the ductus is reversed so that the descending aorta is perfused with desaturated pulmonary arterial blood. This results in cyanotic lower extremities with clubbing of the toes and normal color and shape of the fingers and fingernails.

The *electrocardiographic findings* are normal when the ductus is small. Moderate or large flows result in left ventricular hypertrophy. In the presence of severe pulmonary hypertension right ventricular hypertrophy dominates. The *chest roentgenogram* is normal if the flow is small. With larger flows the heart is enlarged because of left atrial and left ventricular prominence, the pulmonary arterial trunk and aorta are enlarged, and there is pulmonary plethora. With the development of severe pulmonary hypertension, heart size decreases, there is prominence of the right ventricle and especially the main pulmonary artery, and the size of the aorta may not be increased. In older patients the ductus may calcify. The *echocardiogram* defines and identifies the degree of chamber enlargement and visualizes the ductus. Evidence of continuous flow is recorded using the Doppler technique from the ductus arteriosus and the major pulmonary arteries.

Surgical correction is advisable by division of the ductus. In the adult with a large left to right shunt and normal pulmonary vascular resistance surgery is also advised. Extensive calcification of the ductus increases the surgical risk, but surgery should still be advised if the shunt is large. Occasionally, an adult is seen with a small, hemodynamically insignificant patent ductus. The decision of surgical treatment for these patients must take into account that they are at risk for infective endocarditis, but on the other hand they may remain asymptomatic and some may experience spontaneous closure of the defect. Thus individual judgment is required in these patients.

AORTIC-PULMONARY SEPTAL DEFECT. This rare anomaly consists of a communication between the ascending aorta and the pulmonary arterial trunk. The defect is generally large and associated with a torrential pulmonary blood flow and pulmonary hypertension. Congestive cardiac failure is common during infancy and childhood. In the absence of severe pulmonary hypertension the signs are dominated by a wide pulse pressure, cardiomegaly, a systolic murmur at the left and right upper sternal edges, and occasionally a continuous murmur. The electrocardiogram generally shows biventricular hypertrophy, although isolated left or right dominance may be present. Roentgenographic examination of the chest defines the degree of cardiomegaly and shows prominence of the pulmonary artery and ascending aorta, as well as pulmonary plethora. The echocardiogram is helpful in defining the presence of two semilunar valves (which excludes the diagnosis of truncus arteriosus) and shows a normal relationship of a large aorta and pulmonary artery. The diagnosis is confirmed by aortography. The hemodynamic effects are measured at the same time by cardiac catheterization. These defects usually require surgical correction.

TRUNCUS ARTERIOSUS. A single arterial trunk supplies the systemic, pulmonary, and coronary circulations. Both ventricles eject blood through a ventricular septal defect into the single trunk. The number of semilunar valve cusps varies from two to six, and in most patients pulmonary arteries arise from the ascending portion of the truncus proximal to the origin of the innominate artery. When the major source of pulmonary blood flow is from aortopulmonary collateral arteries, the condition is considered to be pulmonary atresia with ventricular septal defect (previously known as truncus arteriosus type IV or pseudotruncus arteriosus).

In the majority the pulmonary blood flow, pressure, and resistance are greatly increased, so that signs of heart failure appear in infancy. Cyanosis is minimal or absent. The heart is usually enlarged, the precordium is hyperdynamic, a systolic ejection murmur sometimes preceded by a click is audible along the left sternal edge, and the second heart sound is loud and generally single. Occasional patients survive infancy because of the development of severe pulmonary vascular disease, which limits pulmonary blood flow. The clinical picture in these patients simulates that of Eisenmenger's syndrome. Incompetence of the truncal valve or, less frequently, stenosis of this valve may complicate the picture at any age. The diagnosis is confirmed by cardiac catheterization and angiocardiography. Since rapid deterioration is frequent during infancy, surgical treatment is advised, at which time the ventricular septal defect is closed, the pulmonary arteries are detached from the truncus, and a conduit is inserted from the right ventricle to the pulmonary arteries.

Communication Shunts Between the Aortic Root and the Right Heart

CORONARY ARTERIAL FISTULA. A fistulous branch, most frequently from the right coronary artery, enters the right atrium or right ventricle and occasionally the pulmonary trunk. The right coronary artery becomes massively dilated. Although the volume of shunt from the coronary artery to the right heart is variable, it is usually small. The diagnosis is suspected when an atypically located continuous precordial murmur is heard. The electrocardiogram and chest roentgenogram are normal. Studies using the Doppler technique demonstrate the site of entry of the fistula: The diagnosis is confirmed with an aortic root injection of contrast material that demonstrates the large, tortuous right coronary artery and its site of entry into the right heart. Surgical treatment is advised.

CONGENITAL ANEURYSMS OF THE SINUSES OF VALSALVA. The usual aneurysm involves the right or noncoronary sinus, which begins as a blind pouch or diverticulum. The aneurysms may remain as unruptured diverticula but usually enter the right ventricle or right atrium. Patients with these aneurysms are generally asymptomatic and the left to right shunt is small. The diagnosis is suspected because of an atypically located continuous murmur and confirmed by injection of contrast material into the ascending aorta. Surgical treatment is advisable even in asymptomatic patients. Acute rupture of a large aneurysm in a previously healthy young adult produces a dramatic clinical picture. This is characterized by sudden onset of dyspnea, chest pain, brisk arterial pulses, and a loud continuous murmur. Cardiac failure with pulmonary edema supervenes rapidly. The electrocardiogram shows left or combined ventricular hypertrophy. The chest roentgenogram shows cardiomegaly with prominent vascular markings due to pulmonary arterial overcirculation and prominent pulmonary veins and signs of pulmonary edema. The diagnosis is confirmed by two-dimensional echocardiography and Doppler methods, supplemented by cardiac catheterization and aortography. Surgical correction is urgently indicated in acute rupture.

ANOMALOUS ORIGIN OF THE LEFT CORONARY ARTERY FROM THE PULMONARY TRUNK. The right coronary artery originates normally from the aorta, and the left coronary artery receives blood from intercoronary anastomoses so that blood flow in the left coronary artery drains *into* the pulmonary trunk. Thus left ventricular myocardial perfusion is significantly compromised. Generally symptoms are present within the first few months of life because of myocardial infarction, congestive cardiac failure, and mitral valve incompetence due to papillary muscle dysfunction. About 15 per cent of patients with this anomaly reach adult life because of exuberant intercoronary anastomoses, which may produce a continuous murmur. The electrocardiogram is important because signs of anterior and anterolateral myocardial infarction are present in a relatively young person. The chest roentgenogram shows cardiomegaly with dominance of the left ventricle. The origin of the left coronary artery from the aorta cannot be demonstrated by echocardiography. The diagnosis is confirmed by selective right coronary arteriography, which demonstrates the dilated right coronary artery, the intercoronary anastomoses, and opacification of the left coronary artery from these anastomoses as it enters the pulmonary artery. Reconstitution of normal coronary flow from the aorta to the left coronary artery is advised, although in many instances fibrosis of the left ventricle has resulted in permanent damage to ventricular function.

Pulmonary Arteriovenous Fistula

Fistulous communications between the pulmonary arteries and pulmonary veins may be multiple, small, and diffuse in both lungs or large and relatively localized. Hereditary hemorrhagic telangiectasia (Rendu-Osler-Weber syndrome) with angiomas of the buccal and nasal mucous membranes, gastrointestinal tract, and liver is present in about one half of patients or other members of their family. Desaturated pulmonary arterial blood flows through the fistula and enters the pulmonary vein without oxygenation. When total flow across the fistulous communications is significant, left atrial and left ventricular blood is desaturated, resulting in cyanosis and digital clubbing. Pulmonary arterial pressure remains normal because the flow across the fistula is at low pressure and resistance; cardiomegaly is unusual and heart failure uncommon. Hemoptysis may occur and is sometimes massive. Recurrent epistaxes and gastrointestinal bleeding are features of hereditary hemorrhagic telangiectasia. Transitory central nervous symptoms, including dizziness, vertigo, speech disturbances, visual aberrations, motor weakness, and convulsions, may result from paradoxical emboli, cerebral thromboses, or abscess. Findings on auscultation of the chest may be normal; in others soft systolic or continuous murmurs are audible anywhere in the chest. The electrocardiogram is usually normal. Roentgenographic examination of the chest shows the presence of large fistulas only. Selective pulmonary arteriography is diagnostic and visualizes the site, extent, and distribution of the fistulas. Large localized fistulous communications are treated surgically by lobectomy or wedge resection. Smaller communications may be obliterated by embolization; these emboli are introduced selectively through a strategically placed catheter in the branch of the pulmonary artery that feeds the fistula. Successful treatment is usually followed by disappearance of symptoms, although in some there is postoperative growth of small previously unrecognized fistulas and recurrence of symptoms.

OBSTRUCTIVE LESIONS WITH OR WITHOUT SHUNTS
Tetralogy of Fallot

The tetralogy of Fallot comprises a combination of four defects consisting of (1) right ventricular outflow tract obstruction (pulmonic stenosis), (2) ventricular septal defect, (3) overriding of the aorta above the ventricular defect, and (4) right ventricular hypertrophy. The pulmonic stenosis is usually a combination of obstruction at the valve as well as in the right ventricular outflow. The pulmonary arterial trunk may be short and smaller than normal, and there may be branch stenosis. The pulmonic valve is often bicuspid, may have a small ring, and occasionally is the only site of obstruction. Infundibular stenosis is produced by the anteriorly displaced hypoplastic infundibular (conal) septum. Occasionally, right ventricular outflow is completely obstructed (pulmonary atresia) and pulmonary blood flow is maintained by a patent ductus arteriosus and/or collateral flow via aortopulmonary collaterals. The ventricular septal defect is generally large, approximating the size of the aortic orifice; involves, but is not limited to, the membranous septum; and is related to the right and posterior aortic cusps. The ascending aorta is displaced anteriorly (dextraposed), and the aortic arch is to the right in about 20 per cent.

The severity of right ventricular outflow tract obstruction determines the hemodynamics and therefore the clinical picture. Severe obstruction is common, pulmonary blood flow is decreased, and blood is shunted from the right ventricle across the ventricular defect into the aorta. This right to left shunt results in systemic hypoxemia manifested as marked cyanosis, digital clubbing, and polycythemia. When obstruction to right ventricular outflow and a ventricular septal defect coexist without right to left shunting, the condition is known as acyanotic tetralogy of Fallot.

In severe cases, *cyanosis* is present from birth. In others, this finding develops in infancy, generally before the first birthday. The absence of cyanosis in the neonatal period is related to maintenance of pulmonary blood flow via a patent ductus arteriosis, which closes spontaneously in the first few months of life. Cyanosis increases in intensity progressively during the first years and is associated with poor physical development. *Dyspnea* with exertion is usual.

Hypoxic ("blue") spells occur primarily in infants with hypoxemia. These spells consist of a sudden onset of dyspnea, restlessness, increased cyanosis, gasping respirations, and syncope. They are associated with a further decrease of arterial PO_2 and a reduction of an already compromised pulmonary blood flow. These frightening episodes are treated by placing the child in a knee-chest position and by administering oxygen and intravenous bicarbonate if acidemia develops. The frequency and severity of these episodes can be reduced by oral propranolol. However, surgical treatment is generally indicated to increase pulmonary blood flow and thus relieve the hypoxemia.

Squatting is common in children with hypoxemia, who may assume this position to relieve dyspnea associated with exertion. Physical activity is usually resumed within a few minutes. Squatting decreases the magnitude of right to left shunt by increasing systemic vascular resistance and pulmonary blood flow. Adults seldom squat because they know the limitation of their exercise tolerance and discontinue physical activity before arterial PO_2 is significantly decreased.

Physical examination confirms the presence of delayed growth and development, cyanosis, and clubbing. Characteristically, the heart size is normal but the apical impulse is tapping owing to right ventricular hypertrophy. The systolic murmur, sometimes accompanied by a thrill, is produced by the right ventricular outflow tract obstruction. Auscultatory findings are variable; the systolic murmur, which is loudest at the upper left sternal edge but is widely transmitted, may be ejection in type or pansystolic. The murmur is less intense when the obstruction is severe. Aortic blood flow is increased, and this may result in an early ejection click. The second heart sound is single, produced by aortic valve closure, and pulmonic valve closure is generally inaudible. In rare instances a systolic and diastolic murmur may be audible in any part of the chest, anteriorly or posteriorly, and is produced by bronchial collateral flow to the lung or rarely by a patent ductus arteriosus. This auscultatory finding is frequent with pulmonary atresia.

Roentgenographically the heart size is normal, with a rounded, elevated cardiac apex likened to a wooden shoe (coeur en sabot). There is a concavity in the region of the main pulmonary artery, and the pulmonary vasculature is diminished. The aorta is large and arches to the right in 20 per cent. The *electrocardiogram* shows right axis deviation and right ventricular hypertrophy. Sometimes the P wave is tall and peaked. *Echocardiography* demonstrates the major intracardiac abnormalities. Echocardiographic examinations show the large ventricular septal defect, the degree of aortic override, and thick right ventricle; the right ventricular outflow tract obstruction may be visualized or inferred from Doppler turbulence in this area. The echocardiogram also helps to distinguish tetralogy of Fallot from other anomalies that may closely simulate this condition, namely, double outlet right ventricle with pulmonic stenosis, arterial transposition with pulmonic stenosis and ventricular septal defect, and a group of complex cardiac malformations consisting primarily of single ventricle and pulmonic stenosis.

These abnormalities are also excluded by *cardiac catheterization and angiocardiography*, and these tests are essential for surgical management. Cardiac catheterization confirms that the peak systolic pressures in both ventricles are virtually identical and that there is a significant gradient across the right ventricular outflow. The degree and direction of shunting at the ventricular level are also demonstrated. Arterial oxygen saturation is decreased and at rest is usually between 75 and 85 per cent. Selective right ventriculography identifies the site or sites of right ventricular outflow tract obstruction, the narrowed pulmonic valve ring, the presence of abnormalities of the pulmonary arterial trunk, and any stenoses of the pulmonary arterial branches (Fig. 49–2). In patients with pulmonary atresia, the anatomy of pulmonary blood flow is complex. Although there may not be filling of the main pulmonary artery, a central confluence of left and right intrapulmonary arteries may be present. Left ventriculogra-

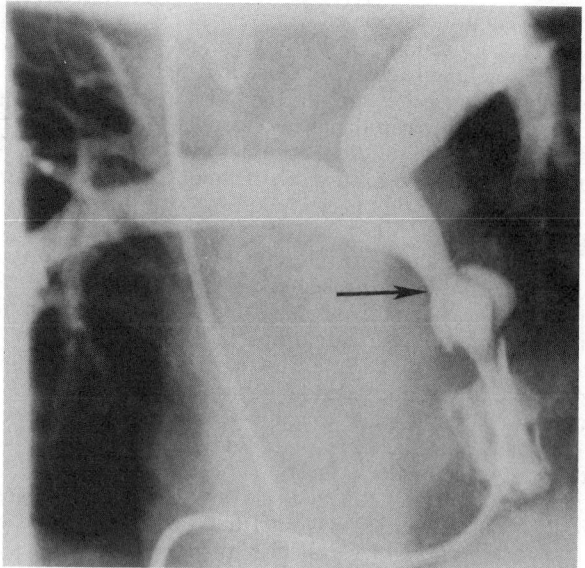

FIGURE 49–2. Cineangiograms in tetralogy of Fallot. Contrast injected in outflow of the right ventricle showing subvalvular obstruction, pulmonary valve stenosis with small annulus (*arrow*), and supravalvular stenosis with short pulmonary arterial trunk.

phy shows the position and size of the ventricular septal defect and the presence of an overriding aorta. In a few instances, a large coronary artery courses over the right ventricular outflow; preservation of this artery during surgical repair is essential. *Surgical treatment* is usually advised during infancy or childhood. The type of surgical procedure and its timing are still controversial. Infants with severe anoxemia in the first few months of life are frequently treated with a systemic to pulmonary arterial shunt to augment pulmonary arterial blood flow. Beyond the age of one to two years correction of the defect is advised, at which time any previous systemic to pulmonary shunt is taken down. Older children should have surgical correction of the anomaly because they are generally symptomatic. In all groups surgical correction is more difficult when there is severe deformity of the right ventricular outflow, including a small pulmonic valve ring. The surgical procedure consists of closure of the ventricular septal defect and relief of obstruction by infundibular resection and/or pulmonic valvotomy. Right ventricular outflow may need to be enlarged.

Ebstein's Anomaly of the Tricuspid Valve

This abnormality consists of an abnormal tricuspid valve that is displaced into the right ventricular cavity so that portions of the valve leaflet are attached to the right ventricular wall rather than to the atrioventricular ring. The portion of the right ventricle proximal to the tricuspid valve is thin, functions as an extension of the right atrium, and is known as "atrialized right ventricle." Leaflets of the tricuspid valve are generally redundant and frequently incompetent. The right atrium is large and an atrial septal defect or patent foramen ovale may be present. Increased right atrial pressure, as from tricuspid regurgitation, results in a right to left shunt across the atrial septum and cyanosis of varying degrees. Pulmonary blood flow is decreased.

Ebstein's anomaly in adults varies considerably in severity, so that many patients have active and productive lives, but survival beyond age 50 years is unusual. Symptoms vary in intensity, and with mild anomalies the only complaint is fatigue. Cardiac arrhythmias are frequent and generally supraventricular, the commonest being attacks of paroxysmal atrial tachycardia. The precordium is quiet to palpation. Auscultation reveals a systolic murmur, sometimes accompanied by a thrill over most of the anterior left chest, and third and fourth heart sounds are audible, resulting in triple or quadruple rhythms. A diastolic murmur is frequent, appears to be superficial, and may mimic a pericardial friction rub. Other auscultatory findings include multiple systolic ejection clicks and an opening snap of the tricuspid valve. The *electrocardiogram* shows right bundle branch block, tall and/or broad P waves, and a prolonged PR interval. Wolff-Parkinson-White syndrome (usually type B) is present in some. *Roentgenographic examination* shows a variable heart size; in extreme instances massive cardiomegaly is present because of great enlargement of the right atrium (Fig. 49–3). The outflow portion of the right ventricle is sometimes visible in the region usually occupied by the pulmonary artery in the posteroanterior view. The pulmonary vasculature is normal to decreased, and the aorta is small. The *echocardiogram* shows significant delay in tricuspid valve closure and an increased amplitude of motion of the tricuspid valve. The large right atrium and the displaced tricuspid valve can also be visualized. Surgical treatment should be advised in symptomatic patients, especially those with progressive cyanosis. Therapy consists of tricuspid valvuloplasty or valve replacement and ablation of the anomalous pathways between the atrium and ventricle in patients with Wolff-Parkinson-White syndrome and supraventricular tachycardia.

Tricuspid Atresia

In this condition there is no communication between the right atrium and right ventricle so that the entire systemic venous return enters the left heart through a defect in the intra-atrial septum. The left ventricle ejects blood into the normally related aorta and through a ventricular septal defect into the pulmonary arteries. If these vessels are transposed,

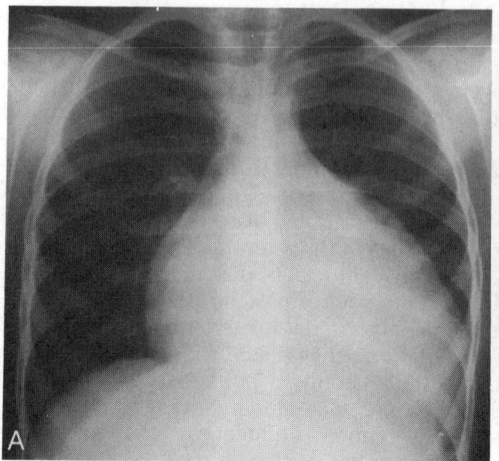
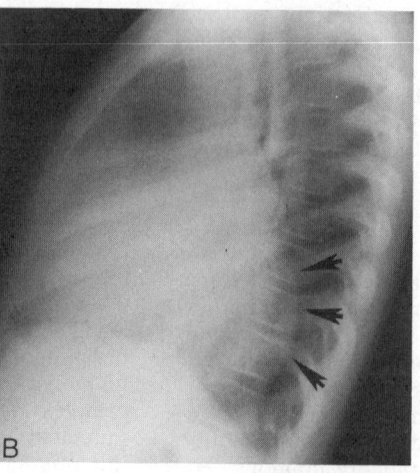

FIGURE 49–3. Chest roentgenograms in Ebstein's anomaly of the tricuspid valve. *A,* Posteroanterior view showing globular cardiac silhouette with narrow waist simulating pericardial effusion. *B,* Left anterior oblique view showing marked cardiomegaly due to massive right atrial enlargement, which extends posteriorly (*arrows*) and also encroaches on the anterior clear space.

the aorta arises from a hypoplastic right ventricle that fills from a ventricular septal defect. These patients have a marked increase in pulmonary blood flow and pressure so that heart failure and minimal cyanosis are common in infancy. Survival usually depends upon pulmonary arterial banding to limit pulmonary arterial flow. When the great arteries are normally related, the right ventricle can be minute and associated with marked pulmonic stenosis or atresia. In these patients pulmonary blood flow is derived from a patent ductus arteriosus or collateral bronchial flow. In other instances the left ventricle ejects its blood through a ventricular septal defect into a small right ventricle and then into the pulmonary artery.

Symptoms are usual during infancy and with decreased pulmonary blood flow consist of cyanosis, anoxemia, and poor physical development. Minimal cardiac enlargement is present, and the systolic ejection murmur along the left sternal edge is nonspecific. Left axis deviation with left ventricular hypertrophy is usual, and these *electrocardiographic findings* in the presence of cyanosis suggest the diagnosis. *Roentgenograms* of the chest show pulmonary undercirculation but are otherwise nonspecific. The *echocardiogram* confirms absence of the tricuspid valve, delineates the size of the small right ventricle, confirms the presence of a large left ventricle, and identifies the presence or absence of transposition of the great arteries. Most infants with decreased pulmonary blood flow require enlargement of the intra-atrial septal defect to ensure easy communication between the two atria as well as a systemic to pulmonary shunt. In later years more radical surgery is undertaken with anastomosis of the right atrium to the pulmonary artery and closure of the intra-atrial septal defect. This procedure effectively separates pulmonary and systemic blood flows, abolishes cyanosis, and improves exercise tolerance. A similar procedure is also used in patients who had pulmonary arterial banding during infancy.

Single Ventricle

Atrial blood empties through two separate atrioventricular valves or a common valve into a single ventricle from which the aorta and pulmonary artery arise. Associated cardiac abnormalities are present, but their nature varies considerably. The most frequent ones are transposition of the great arteries, pulmonic stenosis, and aortic origin from a rudimentary outlet chamber. The clinical picture depends on the nature of the associated anomalies. If pulmonic stenosis is severe, cyanosis and anoxemia dominate. In the absence of pulmonic stenosis pulmonary blood flow and vascular resistance are increased. The clinical picture is then dominated by congestive heart failure. Although these malformations are complex, surgical palliation is undertaken. In the presence of pulmonic stenosis the blood flow is increased with a systemic pulmonary shunt. On the other hand, high pulmonary blood flow is treated with a pulmonary arterial band. In later years, a surgical connection is established between the right atrium and pulmonary artery, and the atria are partitioned so that systemic venous return flows into the pulmonary artery and pulmonary venous return is ejected from the single ventricle into the aorta. When the aorta arises from a rudimentary chamber, systemic flow is dependent on an unobstructed communication between the single ventricle and the rudimentary chamber. This communication (the bulboventricular foramen) may narrow, resulting in a variable but often significant subaortic gradient. This complication may occur at any time, even postoperatively, and produces cardiomegaly and heart failure.

Inflow Obstruction to the Left Ventricle

Conditions of inflow obstruction are grouped together since they result in high pulmonary venous pressure with potential pulmonary edema. The lesions may occur anywhere from the insertion of the pulmonary veins into the left atrium to the area of the mitral valve. They are extremely rare abnormalities. *Pulmonary vein stenoses* at their site of entry into the left atrium are difficult to treat surgically or by balloon angioplasty. *Cor triatriatum* consists of a diaphragmatic partition of the left atrium. The upper portion receives the pulmonary veins, and the distal portion communicates with the mitral valve or through an atrial septal defect into the right atrium. The opening in the diaphragm is generally small so that symptoms are present in early life. The condition is surgically correctable by excision of the diaphragm and closure of associated atrial septal defects. A *supravalvular ring* above the mitral valve produces a similar clinical picture. *Congenital mitral stenosis* may be due to marked abnormality of the mitral valve apparatus, which includes fused, thickened mitral valve leaflets with short chordae, or the valve may have a parachute deformity in which the leaflets are also abnormal but the chordae converge and insert into a single papillary muscle.

Hypoplastic Left Heart Syndrome

Varying degrees of underdevelopment of the left side of the heart coexist, including marked underdevelopment of the left ventricle and atrium, and stenosis or atresia of the aortic and mitral orifices with hypoplasia of the ascending aorta. This complex malformation is a significant cause of cardiovascular death in the neonatal period. Attempts at surgical management have not been standardized.

OBSTRUCTIVE AND REGURGITANT LESIONS
Pulmonic Stenosis with Intact Ventricular Septum

Obstruction to right ventricular outflow can be valvular, subvalvular, supravalvular, or a combination of obstructions at these sites. Valvular obstruction, the most common variety, results from varying degrees of commissural fusion so that the deformed valve appears domelike. Dysplastic thick valve leaflets are less common and may accompany Noonan's syndrome (see Ch. 211). Subvalvular obstruction usually accompanies severe valvular stenosis, is due to infundibular hypertrophy, and occasionally is seen as an isolated abnormality with a normal pulmonic valve. Pulmonary arterial branch stenosis may be isolated or may occur at multiple sites and may be associated with supravalvular stenosis. These peripheral lesions are a feature of congenital rubella.

The hemodynamic consequences of valvular pulmonic stenosis are produced by the severity of obstruction. When the right ventricular outflow gradient is between 50 and 80 mm Hg the obstruction is considered to be moderate; pressures below and above that range are considered mild and severe, respectively. Pulmonary arterial pressure is normal or low. The arterial oxygen saturation is normal except when the obstruction is severe (sometimes with suprasystemic right ventricular pressure). Poor right ventricular compliance with or without an increase in right ventricular end-diastolic pressure increases right atrial pressure and may result in right to left shunting across the intra-atrial septum.

Symptoms are usually absent when the obstruction is mild or moderate, but when it is severe, effort dyspnea may be present. The physique is frequently normal, and some patients appear robust. When the stenosis is *mild*, the venous pressure is normal and the heart is not enlarged. A systolic murmur of varying intensity with midsystolic peaking is heard best at the upper left sternal edge and is preceded by a pulmonic ejection click. The second heart sound may be normal, but the pulmonic component is frequently delayed and of normal intensity. The electrocardiogram is normal or shows signs of minimal right ventricular hypertrophy. The chest *roentgenogram* shows prominence of the pulmonary arterial trunk because of poststenotic dilatation, but the heart size and pulmonary vasculature are normal. Echocardiography shows the domed stenotic valve. When pulmonic stenosis is *moderate*, the venous pressure may be normal or slightly elevated, with a prominent "a" wave in the jugular pulse. A right ventricular parasternal lift is palpable and may be accompanied by a systolic thrill at the upper left sternal edge. The systolic murmur, frequently preceded by an ejection sound, is accentuated in late systole. The second heart sound is split with a delayed and diminished pulmonic component. Electrocardiographic evidence of right ventricular hypertrophy is usual, sometimes with a prominent spiked P wave. The chest roentgenogram shows a normal or mildly enlarged heart, prominence of the pulmonary arterial trunk, and normal pulmonary vasculature. The abnormal valve is visualized by echocardiograms.

In *severe* pulmonic stenosis cyanosis may be present, owing to a small cardiac output or a right to left shunt across the intra-atrial septum. A large presystolic "a" wave is usual in the jugular venous pulse and the increased venous pressure may be transmitted to the liver, resulting in a presystolic pulsation. The heart is moderately or greatly enlarged, with a conspicuous parasternal right ventricular lift. The systolic ejection murmur is usually loud, frequently accompanied by a thrill, and audible maximally at the upper left sternal edge, but it may radiate widely over the entire precordium and into the neck and back. The murmur is accentuated in late systole, frequently encompasses the aortic component of the second heart sound, and may be preceded by an ejection sound. The pulmonic component of the second heart sound is either inaudible or soft and very late. The electrocardiogram shows gross right ventricular hypertrophy with tall P waves attributed to right atrial enlargement. The chest roentgenogram confirms the cardiac enlargement, prominence of the right ventricle and atrium, poststenotic dilatation of the pulmonary artery, and pulmonary vasculature that is either normal or decreased. The echocardiogram demonstrates systolic doming of the stenotic leaflets into the dilated pulmonary arterial trunk. In the presence of significant obstruction, the right ventricular wall is thick, the right atrium is enlarged, and the intra-atrial septum bows toward the left. The degree of obstruction is quantified with Doppler techniques by applying a modified Bernoulli equation using peak velocity of flow ($P = 4V^2$, where P = pressure gradient and v = peak flow velocity).

Cardiac catheterization demonstrates the pressure gradient across the pulmonic valve and determines the degree of severity. Selective right ventriculography visualizes the site and nature of the obstruction. During ventricular systole contrast material is seen as a jet through the domed stenotic valve. Subvalvular hypertrophy, which may intensify the obstruction, is also demonstrated by this method.

The clinical course of patients with mild obstruction is usually good, and progression of the disease is unusual, especially in adolescence and adult life. Many with moderate obstruction also do well, although their progress needs to be evaluated at regular intervals, especially during childhood. Progression of the obstruction is detected clinically by the change in character of the murmur, which becomes accentuated in late systole. Also, the width of the splitting of the second heart sound increases as the right ventricular pressure rises. These signs are associated with an increase in the severity of the electrocardiographic signs of the right ventricular hypertrophy.

Two options are now available for treatment of moderate to severe obstruction. These consist of surgical valvotomy or balloon valvuloplasty. There is a long experience with surgical treatment, and children with isolated pulmonic stenosis generally do well for many years after valvotomy. This is due to immediate decrease in right ventricular pressure after valvotomy. Pulmonic valve incompetence after surgery is usually mild, presents as a short early diastolic murmur, and is generally of no clinical significance. Recurrence of obstruction

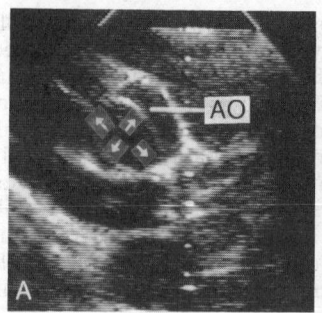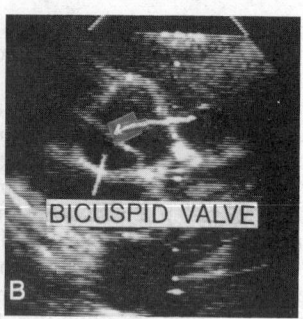

FIGURE 49–4. Short axis echocardiogram of bicuspid aortic valve. *A*, Open valve orifice during systole (*arrows*). *B*, Competent bicuspid valve during diastole. Arrow points to line of apposition of valve leaflets.

after surgery is extremely rare. The results of surgery in adults with severe obstruction may not be uniformly good. Right ventricular dysfunction may persist despite relief of the gradient, and this has been attributed to a poorly compliant right ventricle due to persistent hypertrophy and fibrosis. Pulmonic valvuloplasty for valvular stenosis is accomplished by a balloon catheter inserted percutaneously. Rapid inflation and deflation of the balloon placed across the valve annulus significantly increase the size of the valve orifice. When the valve is not dysplastic and greatly thickened, valvuloplasty is the treatment of choice in many institutions. Patients who have had this new form of treatment are at present being observed to determine whether the initial reduction of gradient is maintained over many years, and whether valvuloplasty produces significant pulmonic valve regurgitation.

Bicuspid Aortic Valve

This condition is said to occur in about 2 per cent of the population. The valve consists of two commissures and two cusps, one of which is generally larger. The bicuspid aortic valve may have normal function so that there is no systolic gradient across the valve and during diastole the valve remains competent. This normal function may continue throughout life, and the bicuspid valve may be found only incidentally at necropsy. In others, abnormality of the aortic valve can be suspected during examination of teenagers or young adults. These findings relate to minor degrees of valvular obstruction and/or incompetence. The auscultatory findings consist of short, soft systolic murmurs heard at the upper right sternal edge. An early aortic ejection click, which precedes the murmur, excludes an innocent murmur. In others, the systolic murmur may be followed by a short, high-pitched early diastolic murmur of aortic incompetence. The diagnosis may be confirmed by echocardiography, which demonstrates only two aortic leaflets (Fig. 49–4).

The natural course of bicuspid aortic valves is variable. In some, the valve may function normally for many decades and produce no abnormal clinical signs. In others the valve leaflets become thickened, fibrotic, and calcified, so that clear signs of aortic stenosis of varying severity develop during early or midadult life. In others, there is eversion or prolapse of one of the aortic cusps, resulting in progressive aortic regurgitation that can become severe. A bicuspid aortic valve is particularly susceptible to infective endocarditis, which may convert a benign lesion into one associated with acute severe aortic regurgitation.

Congenital Valvular Aortic Stenosis

See Ch. 52 for a discussion of this lesion.

Subvalvular Aortic Stenosis (Discrete)

Obstruction to left ventricular outflow is produced by a fibrous membrane situated just below the aortic valve. The membrane is a collar-like structure extending from the intraventricular septum and involving the anterior mitral leaflet.

The high-velocity jet of blood flowing through the obstructed area during ventricular systole impinges on the aortic valve, which results in fibrous thickening and incompetence of the valve. The clinical picture simulates that of valvular aortic stenosis with important exceptions. An aortic ejection sound is usually absent, and the murmur occupies the whole of systole. This condition is frequently mistaken for a ventricular septal defect or mitral incompetence. Mild forms of obstruction may coexist with other lesions, especially a ventricular septal defect. This obstruction may be unrecognized at the time of surgical closure of the ventricular septal defect, and the obstruction may progress over the ensuing years. A useful differential sign is the presence of an early diastolic murmur of aortic valve incompetence, which is a common finding when the obstruction is moderate or severe. Laboratory findings simulate those described under valvular aortic stenosis. However, the echocardiogram is diagnostic in that the discrete membrane is visualized. Cardiac catheterization and angiocardiography are undertaken to measure the severity of obstruction and to outline the membrane by left ventriculography or aortography if the aortic valve is incompetent. Indications for surgery are liberalized, since continued damage to the aortic valve should be prevented. Excision of the membrane gives immediate good results, but complications include damage to the anterior mitral leaflet with resultant regurgitation or conduction abnormalities, including complete heart block from trauma to the intraventricular septum. Furthermore, there may be recurrence of obstruction from regrowth of the membrane.

A rarer form of subaortic stenosis is a long, narrow fibromuscular channel frequently associated with hypoplasia of the aortic ring. This disease is more frequent in childhood and is difficult to treat surgically because relief of obstruction may require enlargement of the aortic valve ring. In extreme cases a valve-bearing conduit is inserted between the left ventricle and the aorta.

Hypertrophic Cardiomyopathy

See Ch. 53.

Supravalvular Aortic Stenosis

The obstruction may be localized to a segmental hourglass-shaped narrowing immediately above the aortic sinuses. Beyond the area of obstruction the aorta may be normal in diameter or show varying degrees of tubular hypoplasia, frequently involving the ascending aorta but occasionally extending for a varying length along the course of the aorta, even to its bifurcation. Aortic valve leaflets may be thickened, with resultant mild aortic regurgitation. During systole the aortic valve leaflets may impinge upon the orifices of the coronary arteries so that coronary flow is impaired; this may be further aggravated by the coronary arteries themselves, which can be enlarged and tortuous but have a narrow lumen. Supravalvular aortic stenosis is frequently associated with the *Williams syndrome*, consisting of typical facies (broad, prominent forehead, flattened bridge of the nose, epicanthal folds, and long upper lip), mild mental retardation, and low-pitched voice; children with this syndrome are particularly friendly and converse easily. In the absence of the Williams syndrome, supravalvular aortic stenosis occurs sporadically and is sometimes familial. Pulmonary arterial branch stenosis may coexist. Carotid and brachial arterial pulses may be asymmetric, with more conspicuous pulses on the right side. This finding has been attributed to preferential flow into the innominate artery. Other components of the clinical picture simulate those described under valvular aortic stenosis. Echocardiography visualizes the ascending aorta, identifies the area of obstruction, and defines the degree of aortic hypoplasia. Cardiac catheterization and angiocardiography determine the severity of the obstruction, visualize the anatomy of the aorta and the ob-

struction, and demonstrate severity of pulmonary arterial branch stenosis, if present. Surgical treatment to relieve the obstruction is advised when the gradient is severe. However, surgical treatment is complicated, especially when the transverse and thoracic aortae are markedly hypoplastic.

Coarctation of the Aorta

Narrowing of the aortic lumen may occur at isolated or multiple sites in the aorta. By far the commonest site of discrete obstruction is just distal to the origin of the left subclavian artery. The lesion is more frequent in males and is also seen in patients with Turner's (XO) syndrome. Associated cardiac malformations are frequent, the commonest being a bicuspid aortic valve, congenital aortic stenosis with or without incompetence, ventricular septal defect, and lesions of the mitral valve with or without valvular regurgitation. Extensive collateralization usually develops, especially from branches of the subclavian, internal mammary, superior intercostal, and axillary arteries. These vessels join the intercostal arteries of the descending aorta and inferior epigastric branches of the femoral arteries, which allow channels for arterial blood to bypass the area of coarctation. These collateral vessels can become enormously enlarged and tortuous by early adult life.

Children and young adults are generally asymptomatic. However, hypertension may develop in the arteries above the coarctation and may be associated with epistaxis and throbbing headaches. Other symptoms include leg fatigue, complaints of cold extremities, and occasionally intermittent claudication. Beyond the second decade coarctation may be discovered by the finding of brachial arterial hypertension during routine physical examination. The methods of presentation in adults include infective endocarditis, usually involving the aortic valve, and rupture of the aorta or dissecting aneurysm may occur especially in the 20's and 30's. The site of rupture is either in the proximal aorta or in an aneurysm in the area of coarctation. Cerebral vascular disease with resultant cerebral hemorrhage or infarction may result from complications of hypertension or from the rupture of an aneurysm, usually of the circle of Willis. Hypertension and associated atherosclerosis of the coronary circulation may result in congestive cardiac failure, sometimes preceded by acute myocardial infarction. Pregnancy is usually well tolerated, especially if hypertension is controlled. However, the risk of aortic rupture is increased especially toward the end of the third trimester.

Classic signs of aortic coarctation are the disparity in pulsations and blood pressures of the arms and legs. The bounding pulses of the arms and carotid vessels contrast with the weak, delayed, or absent femoral and/or distal arterial pulses in the legs. Also, the blood pressure in the arms exceeds that in the legs. This applies especially to the systolic reading, and there is a further rise of systolic blood pressure in response to exercise. If the systolic arterial pressure in the right arm exceeds that of the left arm by more than 30 mm Hg, the left subclavian artery is involved in the coarctation. Collateral arterial circulation may be visible but is usually palpable, especially in the back, at the angles of the scapulae and in the axillae. Murmurs are variable in location, quality, and intensity. The usual is a precordial midsystolic murmur heard best at the left sternal edge, but it may be loudest in the back between the scapulae. Additional systolic or sometimes continuous murmurs are audible over the anterior or posterior chest and are produced by flow through the large, tortuous collateral arteries. The *electrocardiogram is* usually normal during childhood and adolescence. In adults, varying degrees of left ventricular hypertrophy are present. *Roentgenographic* examinations during childhood may not be striking. However, prominence of the left ventricle occurs thereafter and during adult life. The heart may be moderately enlarged. Notching of the inferior border of the ribs from collateral vessels is common. This may be unilateral if one of the subclavian arteries arises below the area of coarctation. Poststenotic dilatation of the descending aorta is usual and is demonstrated by a barium esophagram, and the prominent left subclavian artery produces a shadow in the left mediastinum. *Echocardiography* visualizes the area of coarctation, the large left subclavian artery, poststenotic dilatation of the descending aorta, and associated intracardiac anomalies, especially those of the aortic valve. These associated anomalies are confirmed by cardiac catheterization and selective left ventriculography and angiography. Coarctectomy is advised, preferably in early childhood between ages three and five years.

Pulmonic Valvular Regurgitation

Isolated congenital pulmonic valve regurgitation is rare and seldom produces symptoms; an early diastolic murmur at the upper left sternal edge is the only abnormal sign. However, pulmonic valvular regurgitation may accompany other conditions such as those associated with severe pulmonary hypertension or after surgical transection of the pulmonic valve ring for the treatment of severe obstruction of the right ventricular outflow.

Absence of Pulmonic Valve

Absence of the pulmonic valve is a congenital anomaly in which pulmonic valve leaflets are virtually absent. Although the lesion may be isolated it is usually associated with other defects, especially tetralogy of Fallot or isolated ventricular septal defect.

Vascular Rings and Other Aortic Arch Anomalies

The more common anomalies are double aortic arch, right aortic arch with left ligamentum arteriosum, origin of the right subclavian artery from the thoracic aorta distal to the left subclavian artery, anomalous origin of the innominate or left carotid arteries, and anomalous left pulmonary artery, which arises from the elongated pulmonary trunk and courses between the trachea and the esophagus. The clinical picture is extremely variable, and in many instances there are no symptoms. Tracheal compression, especially during infancy, produces respiratory distress with wheezing and a brassy cough. Dysphagia may occur in older patients. Surgery is advised in symptomatic patients to relieve the tracheal and esophageal compression.

THE TRANSPOSITIONS
Transposition of the Great Arteries

In this condition the aorta arises from the right ventricle and the pulmonary artery from the left ventricle. Systemic venous return is to the right atrium, and pulmonary venous return is to the left atrium. Systemic venous blood flows through the tricuspid valve into the right ventricle and is ejected into the aorta. Pulmonary venous blood flows from the left atrium through the mitral valve into the left ventricle and is ejected into the pulmonary artery. Thus, the circulations are parallel. Survival is dependent on mixture of blood through the foramen ovale, a ventricular septal defect, or patency of the ductus arteriosus. This condition is a common malformation that occurs predominantly in males, with symptoms in the neonatal period or soon thereafter.

ISOLATED "SIMPLE" TRANSPOSITION OF THE GREAT ARTERIES. In this malformation the ventricular septum is intact. Mixing of systemic and pulmonary blood occurs primarily from bidirectional shunting across the foramen ovale. This condition produces symptoms and signs of anoxemia in the neonate, is suspected in an otherwise normal neonate who is cyanotic and tachypneic, and is verified by echocardiography, which demonstrates the abnormal origin of the great arteries, as well as the fact that the aorta is usually anterior to the pulmonary artery. Emergency balloon atrial septostomy that ruptures the foramen ovale allows greater mixing at the atrial level and decompresses the left atrium. Generally, these babies do well for many months, until surgical treatment is undertaken, usually between the ages of 6 and 12 months. Currently, there is debate about the preferred method of surgical treatment. There has been greater experience with intra-atrial redirection of venous return so that systemic venous blood flows into the left ventricle and is ejected out the pulmonary artery; pulmonary venous return flows through the tricuspid valve and is pumped by the right ventricle into the aorta. Immediate results are excellent, but concern has been expressed about late onset of supraventricular arrhythmias (especially bradyarrhythmias and sick sinus syndrome) and about right ventricular failure and pulmonary edema, since this ventricle is ejecting blood into the aorta. Because of these concerns, the arterial switch operation was developed whereby the origins of the great arteries are transected and the pulmonary artery is connected to the stump of the vessel arising from the right ventricle and the aorta to the left ventricle with implantation of the coronary arteries into the new aorta.

TRANSPOSITION OF THE GREAT ARTERIES WITH VENTRICULAR SEPTAL DEFECT. When the septal defect is small, the clinical picture is similar to that of simple transposition, and many of these small defects close spontaneously. If the ventricular septal defect is large and nonrestrictive, significant mixing of blood occurs and symptoms are frequently delayed. The clinical picture is dominated by signs of congestive cardiac failure with minimal cyanosis. In the untreated state there is progressive pulmonary hypertension with severe pulmonary vascular disease. Treatment is required during infancy, and a number of options are available for surgical treatment. The greatest experience has been with a staged procedure. Pulmonary arterial banding is done during infancy to restrict pulmonary blood flow and prevent the onset of pulmonary vascular disease. In later years, usually during childhood, the second stage is undertaken, in which the pulmonary artery is debanded and transected, the ventricular septal defect is closed so that the left ventricle ejects blood into the aorta, and a conduit is placed from the right ventricle to the transected pulmonary artery (*Rastelli procedure*). Another option consists of the arterial switch operation as described above.

TRANSPOSITION OF THE GREAT ARTERIES WITH PULMONIC STENOSIS. The importance of this condition is that it may closely simulate the clinical picture produced by tetralogy of Fallot. The condition generally requires an aortic pulmonary shunt during infancy to increase pulmonary blood flow and relieve the symptoms of anoxemia. In later years the Rastelli procedure is undertaken.

Double Outlet Right Ventricle

In this malformation both the pulmonary artery and the aorta arise from the right ventricle, and the only outlet from the left ventricle is a ventricular septal defect. The clinical picture simulates a large, uncomplicated ventricular septal defect with pulmonary hypertension. The echocardiogram is diagnostic in that there is discontinuity between the anterior mitral leaflet and the aorta, since the latter structure arises from the right ventricle. Uncontrollable heart failure and pulmonary hypertension are frequent during infancy so that pulmonary arterial banding is usually required. In later years, generally during childhood, the Rastelli operation is advised. Double outlet right ventricle may be complicated by pulmonic stenosis when the condition simulates that described under Tetralogy of Fallot.

Corrected Transposition (L Transposition of the Great Arteries)

This condition consists of *ventricular inversion* and transposition of the great arteries. Systemic venous blood enters a normal right atrium, flows through a mitral valve into the left ventricle, and is ejected into the pumonary artery. Pulmonary venous blood flows from the left atrium through a tricuspid valve into the right ventricle and is ejected into the aorta. If the condition is uncomplicated, blood flow and hemodynamics are normal. However, associated anomalies are usual, such as ventricular septal defect, pulmonic stenosis, left atrioventricular valve (tricuspid) anomalies, including an Ebstein-like malformation of this valve, and atrioventricular conduction abnormalities—frequently complete atrioventricular block. The clinical picture is dominated by the associated lesions. The chest roentgenogram may suggest the abnormal origin of the great arteries in that the ascending aorta occupies the upper left border of the cardiac silhouette in the posteroanterior view. Since ventricular inversion is present, the electrocardiogram may show absent q waves in leads I and V_6, initial q waves in III, aVF, and V_1, and prominent T waves in the right precordial leads. During surgical treatment the bundle of His may be injured because it is located abnormally, so that complete heart block may occur. In others, significant regurgitations via the Ebstein-like tricuspid valve requires valve replacement.

Anomalous Pulmonary Venous Connection

The anomalous pulmonary venous return may be partial or total. *Partial anomalous pulmonary venous return* simulates the clinical picture produced by a secundum atrial septal defect. In fact, one of these forms is the sinus venosus defect.

TOTAL ANOMALOUS PULMONARY VENOUS CONNECTION. The site of entry of the pulmonary veins may be supradiaphragmatic (into a left superior vena cava or vertical vein, coronary sinus, right superior vena cava, or right atrium) or infradiaphragmatic (portal vein, hepatic veins, or inferior vena cava). Thus, there is no connection between the pulmonary vein and the left atrium. Generally the pulmonary veins converge to form a single trunk, which then enters the systemic venous circulation. Varying degrees of pulmonary venous obstruction are present and depend on the length of the common pulmonary venous trunk before its entry into the systemic vein as well as localized areas of obstruction.

The clinical picture is variable. In some instances, especially those of infradiaphragmatic connection, pulmonary edema and cyanosis are present in the neonatal period or soon thereafter. When there is a large intra-atrial communication and obstruction to pulmonary venous return is moderate, symptoms occur in later infancy and the clinical picture is dominated by congestive cardiac failure. When pulmonary venous obstruction is absent and there is a large communication between the right and left atria, symptoms may be delayed until early childhood and very occasionally adolescence. The clinical picture of these patients simulates that produced by a large left to right shunt at the atrial level.

The *electrocardiogram* reflects the hemodynamic state so that symptomatic infants have marked right ventricular hypertrophy with prominent P waves. Chest *roentgenograms* in neonates with pulmonary venous obstruction are characterized by pulmonary edema with a normal heart size. In older infants the heart is large and pulmonary overcirculation evident. In older children with pulmonary venous connection to the left superior vena cava, the cardiac silhouette has the appearance of a snowman or figure 8. The supracardiac shadow is produced by marked dilatation of the left superior vena cava, innominate vein, and right superior vena cava. The *echocardiogram* shows signs of right volume overload, and sometimes a common venous trunk is visualized. *Cardiac catheterization* demonstrates the severity of pulmonary hypertension, and

pulmonary arteriograms show return of contrast material to the pulmonary veins and their anomalous site of insertion into the systemic venous system. Surgical treatment is indicated when the common pulmonary venous trunk is anastomosed to the left atrium, the atrial septal defect closed, and the anomalous connection to the systemic venous system obliterated. Results of surgical treatment have been good, with greatest risk in symptomatic neonates.

CARDIAC MALPOSITION

Knowledge of the position of the heart as well as the location (situs) of abdominal viscera aids in defining the nature of these anomalies. Roentgenography of the abdomen helps identify abdominal situs by localizing the position of the stomach bubble and other abdominal structures, but many viscera cannot be visualized by this method alone. Generally, atrial and visceral situs are related; if the viscera are normally located, the atria have a normal position. In abdominal situs inversus, the left atrium is usually to the right and the right atrium to the left. Location of the atria is further and more accurately assessed by evaluation of the tracheobronchial air column on chest roentgenogram. A normal tracheobronchial tree with an epiarterial bronchus on the right indicates normal atrial situs, and this finding is independent of the position of the heart.

Dextrocardia

The heart is in the right chest, and the cardiac apex points to the right. Associated abdominal situs inversus (mirror-image dextrocardia) in adults is usually associated with a normally functioning heart. However, poorly motile cilia may result in sinusitis and bronchiectasis (Kartagener's syndrome). Dextrocardia may be discovered by physical examination when the heart sounds are more clear in the right chest or accidentally on a routine chest film. The electrocardiogram demonstrates the mirror image so that the P, QRS, and T are inverted in lead I; aV_R and aV_L are the reverse of normal, and the right precordial leads resemble those usually recorded from the left chest. *Isolated dextrocardia* with abdominal viscera in normal position (situs solitus) is invariably associated with various combinations of severe cardiac malformations, the commonest being ventricular inversion, single ventricle, pulmonic stenosis, abnormalities of the atrioventricular valves, and anomalies of systemic and pulmonary venous return.

Isolated Levocardia

Isolated levocardia is accompanied by varying degrees of anomalous position of abdominal viscera (heterotaxia) so that situs inversus is partial or complete. Severe cardiac malformations are usual, including various combinations of anomalies of systemic and pulmonary venous return, common atrioventricular canal, pulmonic stenosis or atresia, defects of the atrial and ventricular septa, and single ventricle.

Mesocardia

Mesocardia is the term used when the heart is centrally located in the chest or the cardiac silhouette on roentgenogram is toward the right chest. The cardiac anatomy is normal with normal relationships of the cardiac chambers, venous return, and origin of the great arteries. Cardiac malformations are usually absent.

Asplenia Syndrome

This condition is characterized by absence of the spleen, undefinable situs of the abdominal viscera (situs ambiguus), bilateral *right-sidedness*, and complex, severe cardiac malformations. Bilateral right-sidedness is identified by bilateral trilobed lungs with bilateral epiarterial bronchi. In the majority the liver is located centrally so that the liver edge is palpable across the entire upper abdomen. The stomach is located on the right in about half the patients, and varying degrees of malrotation of the small bowel are present. Both atria have the morphologic characteristics of the right atrium. Common cardiovascular anomalies include total anomalous pulmonary venous connection, transposition of the great arteries, pulmonic stenosis or atresia, complete atrioventricular canal, single ventricle, and dextrocardia. The condition is suspected in a deeply cyanotic male infant with dextrocardia and a centrally placed liver. Howell-Jolly and Heinz bodies in the peripheral red blood cells are suggestive of asplenia, but these findings are not conclusive. Infants with asplenia are susceptible to severe intercurrent infections so that continued antibiotic prophylaxis has been suggested as a preventive measure. Aortopulmonary shunts during infancy are indicated when severe anoxemia is present owing to pulmonic stenosis, and right atrial-pulmonary shunts (Fontan) are advised in later years.

Polysplenia Syndrome

The features of this condition are multiple splenic masses (two or more), ambiguous abdominal situs, and *bilateral left-sidedness*; while cardiovascular abnormalities are frequent, they are generally not as complex as in the asplenia syndrome. The lungs are bilobed and epiarterial bronchi are absent. The liver is frequently located centrally in the upper abdomen, and the stomach is right- or left-sided. Malrotation of the bowel is common. Both atria have the morphologic features of the left atrium. The hepatic segment of the inferior vena cava is frequently absent so that systemic venous return is by way of the azygos vein. The cardiac apex points to the left in the majority. Pulmonary venous return may be normal, arterial transposition is present in only a minority, and pulmonic stenosis is unusual. The cardiac malformations are generally associated with left to right shunts at atrial or ventricular levels.

THE ADULT WITH "UNCURED" CONGENITAL HEART DISEASE

Strategies of management of symptomatic patients with congenital heart disease have changed recently so that the majority are treated during infancy or early childhood. Many adolescents and adults now exist who have trivial lesions, have remained asymptomatic, and have lived a normal lifestyle. Other patients have anomalies that are silent until adult life. Palliative surgery may have been undertaken in another group who have remained relatively well and have now approached adult life. Another cohort of patients who may not have had surgical treatment during early life develop progressive pulmonary hypertension during childhood, and in adult life their lesions are associated with severe pulmonary vascular disease. This section discusses these groups of patients.

VENTRICULAR SEPTAL DEFECTS. A significant number of patients seen in pediatric cardiac clinics have trivial shunts across a small ventricular septal defect. They remain asymptomatic throughout the growing years, and as adults the only abnormal physical sign is a long, harsh systolic murmur, which may be accompanied by a thrill and is heard best at the lower left sternal edge. It is unusual to see such patients beyond the age of 40 years so that it has been assumed that many of these defects close spontaneously. While the defect remains, these patients are at risk to develop infective endocarditis and occasionally aortic regurgitation or discrete subaortic stenosis.

VALVULAR PULMONIC STENOSIS. Generally, asymptomatic children with mild pulmonic stenosis (resting peak right ventricular pressure less than one half of systolic systemic pressure) do not require surgical treatment. There is no consensus about the course of untreated mild to moderate pulmonic stenosis. The generally held belief, however, is that

progressive increase in severity is unusual, especially if the patient is beyond the age of 12 years. This optimistic view also applies to those who had a valvotomy during childhood, which relieved the obstruction. Restriction of physical activity is not required, pregnancy is well tolerated, and, although infective endocarditis of the pulmonic valve is not common, prophylaxis is advisable at the time of risk for this complication.

CONGENITAL COMPLETE HEART BLOCK. Fetal echocardiography may be prompted by the recognition of intrauterine bradycardia, and this test unmasks the presence of complete atrioventricular (AV) block. This study is especially important during pregnancy of mothers with connective tissue disease, such as systemic lupus erythematosus, since the offspring are at greater risk for complete AV block. It is suggested that antinuclear antibodies of the IgG category cross the placenta and damage the fetal conduction system. This occurs in mothers whose disease is active but also when there are no overt clinical manifestations and only positive serologic evidence is present. In about 70 per cent of children with complete AV block the lesion is isolated, and the remainder have associated complex cardiac malformations, such as ventricular inversion or single ventricle. Familial complete AV block is well recognized. Adolescents and adults with isolated congenital complete AV block are usually asymptomatic, but it is not possible to predict episodes of syncope. The pulse rate is inappropriately slow for age. The large stroke volume and vasodilatation produce jerky pulses, systolic hypertension, and cardiomegaly. Cannon waves may be visible in the jugular venous pulse. The first heart sound varies in intensity and may be followed by a nonspecific systolic ejection murmur. The diagnosis is confirmed by the electrocardiogram, in which there is no constant relationship between the P waves and QRS complexes. Usually the QRS is of normal duration, which suggests that the site of the lesion is above the bundle of His. Marked ventricular slowing may be recorded by continuous, 24-hour electrocardiographic monitoring, especially during sleep. It is not known whether there is any relationship between the slow ventricular rates during sleep and the prognosis. Since patients with congenital complete AV block have been observed in late adult life, there is a generally held view that the prognosis is good. However, the lesion is not benign, in that complications may occur at any time and are not predictable. Syncope is an indication for implantation of a permanent pacemaker. Decisions about treatment in asymptomatic patients are more difficult. The demonstration of ventricular tachycardia or fibrillation during continuous electrocardiographic monitoring or graded exercise testing is an indication for pacemaker implantation. There remains a group of asymptomatic patients in whom treatment is not standardized, including those with premature ventricular contractions during and after exercise, extreme nocturnal bradycardia, and ventricular depolarization initiated from a focus low in the bundle of His.

EISENMENGER'S SYNDROME. This syndrome is associated with marked elevation of pulmonary vascular resistance with reversed or bidirectional shunt, which is intracardiac or between the aorta and pulmonary arteries. Thus, pulmonary vascular disease is the hallmark of this syndrome, and the site of the shunt is incidental. Medial hypertrophy of pulmonary arteries and arterioles is present and is associated with cellular, fibrotic, and fibroelastic intimal reactions, and in more severe forms plexiform lesions encroach into the lumen of the vessel. These changes in the pulmonary vascular bed are directly related to pulmonary arterial pressure. Extension of muscle into the peripheral arteries occurs when pulmonary hypertension is still associated with increased pulmonary blood flow. With progressive vascular disease, a reduction in the number of small arteries may precede obliterative pulmonary vascular disease.

Historically these patients are frequently symptomatic during infancy and early childhood because of congestive cardiac failure, poor physical development, and recurrent lower respiratory tract infections. As pulmonary vascular resistance rises, the left to right shunt decreases so that symptoms improve. These children may lead nearly normal lives, but their stamina is limited and mild exertional cyanosis is evident. In early adult life there is progressive anoxemia with intensification of cyanosis, digital clubbing may be extreme, and polycythemia increases. Progressive decrease in effort tolerance develops over many years, culminating in congestive cardiac failure in early or mid-adult life. Other symptoms include hemoptysis, angina pectoris attributed to right ventricular ischemia, syncope, and palpitations from premature atrial or ventricular contractions. Jugular venous pressure is increased, with a prominent "v" wave in the presence of complicating tricuspid valve regurgitation. Hepatomegaly and marked dependent edema with ascites are usual with heart failure. The heart size is increased to a variable extent, greatest when there are shunts at the atrial level and when there is complicating tricuspid and/or pulmonic valve incompetence. The precordium is active with a right ventricular heave along the left sternal edge. Pulmonary arterial pulsations and the second heart sound may be palpable at the upper left sternal edge. The systolic murmur varies in intensity and is frequently initiated by a pulmonic ejection click. The second heart sound is booming, single, or narrowly split in ventricular shunts, but wide, fixed splitting may be audible in isolated atrial shunts. Signs of pulmonary and/or tricuspid valve regurgitation are superimposed when there is dilatation of these valve rings secondary to pulmonary hypertension or right ventricular failure. The *electrocardiogram* shows marked right ventricular or biventricular hypertrophy with prominent P waves. Complete right bundle branch block may be present, especially when the shunt is at the atrial level. In others the electrocardiogram is influenced by the underlying anomaly (e.g., single ventricle, ventricular inversion, etc.). The *chest roentgenogram* confirms the degree of cardiomegaly. The pulmonary trunk is enlarged with prominence of the primary divisions, which diminish in caliber in the peripheral branches. The *echocardiogram* helps to identify the anatomy of the underlying intracardiac or extracardiac malformation. *Cardiac catheterization* is undertaken when the diagnosis cannot be established by clinical findings and noninvasive studies. One of the purposes of catheterization is to determine whether the pulmonary vascular bed is vasoactive, as indicated by a fall in pulmonary artery pressure and resistance during the breathing of 100 per cent oxygen. Another major indication is to exclude the presence of left ventricular inflow lesions, which result in elevation of pulmonary venous pressure and secondary pulmonary hypertension. Angiocardiography carries a small increased risk because the contrast medium may produce a fall in systemic vascular resistance and increased right to left shunting with a further fall in systemic arterial saturation.

Polycythemia may become extreme, and when the hematocrit exceeds 70 per cent excruciating headaches may occur. These are difficult to treat but do respond to repeated venesection. This treatment should not be undertaken lightly, since reduction of red cell count and blood volume is not tolerated. Heart rate and blood pressure are monitored during the procedure. Small aliquots of blood ($\pm$ 30 ml) are removed and immediately replaced with a similar volume of fresh frozen plasma or human albumin. Repeated venesection results in iron deficiency anemia so that daily oral iron replacement is essential. The usual goal is to reduce the hematocrit to between 55 and 60 per cent. *Hemoptysis* occurs from rupture of pulmonary vessels or is due to pulmonary arterial thrombosis or embolism. This symptom is usually limited to adult life, blood loss is not excessive, and symptomatic treatment is all that is needed. However, hemoptysis can be life threatening if associated with hypotension, an increase in the degree

of hypoxemia, and the development of acidemia. Long-term anticoagulation is not indicated. *Syncope and sudden death* cannot be predicted, but patients with Eisenmenger's syndrome between the ages of about 20 and 40 years are at risk. The mechanism is not clear but has been attributed to arrhythmias, probably ventricular tachyarrhythmias, which result in hypotension and an increase in right to left shunting. *Pregnancy* is not well tolerated and sudden death has been reported during the third trimester or in the postpartum period.

Treatment. Surgical treatment of the cardiac anomaly is contraindicated because these patients succumb to the effects of pulmonary vascular disease. Palliation has been successful in the presence of transposition of the great arteries, ventricular septal defect, and severe pulmonary vascular disease; the procedure involves redirection of the venous return (as described under Transposition of the Great Arteries), but the ventricular defect is not closed. The experience with transplantation of the heart and lungs is still small and follow-up is short, but this therapy is being watched with interest, since patients with progressive symptoms are at great risk of dying. Drugs have been used to attempt to manipulate pulmonary and systemic vascular resistance to reduce the right to left shunt; generally the results have been disappointing.

COMPLEX CARDIAC MALFORMATIONS. When pulmonic stenosis is an important part of the anomaly, surgical aortopulmonary shunting is undertaken during infancy or childhood to alleviate hypoxemia. In others with torrential pulmonary blood flow and pulmonary hypertension, pulmonary arterial banding is undertaken in infancy to prevent progressive pulmonary vascular disease. Many have now reached adolescence or adult life with normal or low pulmonary vascular resistance. These patients are candidates for operation using the Fontan principle (direct anastomosis of the right atrium to the pulmonary artery).

THE ADULT WITH SURGICALLY "CURED" CONGENITAL HEART DISEASE

Surgical treatment for extracardiac anomalies has been undertaken for four decades, and 30 years have elapsed since the introduction of surgical procedures for intracardiac congenital malformations. Immediate results after operation continue to be excellent, even dramatic, but it is now recognized that complications may develop many years after surgery.

INTRA-ATRIAL SURGERY. Many anomalies may be treated by an approach through the right atrium. These include atrial septal defects of all types, endocardial cushion defects, transposition of the great arteries, and total anomalous pulmonary venous connection. Frequently isolated ventricular septal defects are closed surgically transatrially and the defect (especially the more common perimembranous defect) is approached through the tricuspid valve and the shunt obliterated. Persistent *conduction disturbances* may occur immediately after operation or appear for the first time many years later. These consist of supraventricular arrhythmias (atrial flutter or fibrillation, paroxysmal supraventricular tachycardia, and junctional rhythm), sick sinus syndrome, or varying degrees of atrioventricular block. These rhythm disturbances occur even when there is complete anatomic correction of the abnormality. The treatment of these abnormalities in conduction is similar to the treatment of these arrhythmias of any cause. The *function of the right ventricle* and competence of the tricuspid valve have also been of concern especially in transposition of the great arteries.

INTRAVENTRICULAR SURGERY. Right ventriculotomy is the approach used in most patients who require intraventricular surgery. The more common lesions treated this way include some forms of ventricular septal defect, tetralogy of Fallot with or without pulmonary atresia, and various forms of transposition of the great arteries. Some of these complications may be reduced in future years, since earlier operation is being advised, especially in some patients with tetralogy of Fallot.

Conduction Disturbances. Permanent complete heart block from intraoperative trauma to the conduction system has decreased to a point where it is no longer a major problem soon after operation. *Bifascicular block* (left anterior hemiblock with complete right bundle branch block) may occur from intraoperative trauma to the bundle of His and its branches. These patients usually remain well for many years after operation, but the conduction abnormality may progress to complete AV block. Bifascicular block does not require treatment. *Sudden unexpected cardiac arrest* may occur many years after operation. While this catastrophe may occasionally occur from complete AV block, more frequent mechanisms are ventricular tachyarrhythmias and deterioration into ventricular fibrillation. The risk of ventricular tachycardia is higher in patients who have multiple unifocal or multifocal premature ventricular contractions at rest. Bursts of ventricular tachyarrhythmia may be recorded during 24-hour electrocardiographic recording or unmasked during or immediately after graded exercise testing. While these arrhythmias may occur in patients who have had adequate relief of right ventricular outflow tract obstruction and in whom the ventricular defect is closed, there appears to be greater risk when residual defects are present, such as severe pulmonic stenosis, persistent large shunts across the ventricular septum, and right ventricular aneurysms. Significant residual defects should be treated by reoperation, and the ventricular arrhythmia may be abolished by excision of arrhythmogenic right ventricular aneurysms. Medical treatment of the ventricular tachycardia is indicated and although there is a choice of many drugs, phenytoin (Dilantin) has been used with particular success.

Reconstruction of the Right Ventricular Outflow Tract. Treatment of extreme forms of tetralogy of Fallot, especially pulmonary atresia, and many forms of transposition of the great arteries with pulmonic stenosis or previous arterial banding, requires a prosthesis to establish continuity between the right ventricle and the pulmonary artery. During the last decade the most frequently used prosthesis consisted of a Dacron tube with an aortic valve bearing a porcine heterograft. The durability of this prosthesis is unpredictable, since recurrence of obstruction may occur anywhere along its length from narrowing of the anastomotic sites or from development of an exuberant neointima that encroaches on the lumen of the Dacron tube. Because of these complications, a human valve bearing aortic or pulmonary homografts is being used with greater frequency.

Congenital Aortic Stenosis. See above.

Valvular Pulmonic Stenosis. See above.

Coarctation of the Aorta. It is now common practice to advise surgical treatment of coarctation of the aorta in preschool years. One of the reasons for earlier operation is the notion that late-onset complications will be reduced. These complications in adult life have been related to recurrence of hypertension, progressive atherosclerosis, myocardial infarction, and cerebral vascular accidents. It is therefore advisable that patients who have had previous coarctation therapy be followed carefully so that treatment can be instituted, especially for hypertension, prior to the onset of some of these complications.

Adams FH, Emmanouilides GC: Moss' Heart Disease in Infants, Children and Adolescents. 3rd ed. Baltimore, Williams and Wilkins, 1983. *The standard comprehensive text on all aspects of congenital heart disease.*

Fontan F, Deville C, Quaegebeur J, et al.: Repair of tricuspid atresia in 100 patients. J Thorac Cardiovasc Surg 85:647, 1983. *Evolution of the principles for treatment of tricuspid atresia. These principles are also applicable to many complex cardiac malformations.*

Garson A, Nihill MR, McNamara DG, et al.: Status of the adult and adolescent after repair of tetralogy of Fallot. Circulation 59:1232, 1979. *Long-term results are evaluated with emphasis on complications in the adult.*

Giuliani ER, Fuster V, Brandenberg RO, et al.: Ebstein's anomaly. Mayo Clin Proc 54:163, 1979. *Clinical features and natural history are reviewed in a lucid manner.*

Goldberg SJ, Allen HD, Sahn DJ: Pediatric and Adolescent Echocardiography. 2nd ed. Chicago, Year Book Medical Publishers, 1980. *A comprehensive handbook describing the M-mode, two-dimensional, and Doppler features of congenital cardiac malformations.*

Kirklin JW, Barratt-Boyes BG: Cardiac Surgery. New York, John Wiley and Sons, 1986. *Comprehensive analyses of combined clinical experiences from two respected pioneers in all aspects of cardiac surgery, especially congenital heart disease.*

Krongrad E: Prognosis for patients with congenital heart disease and postoperative intraventricular conduction defects. Circulation 57:867, 1978. *A useful guide to mechanisms, prognosis and treatment.*

Liberthson RR, Boucher CA, Strauss HW, et al.: Right ventricular function in adult atrial septal defect. Am J Cardiol 57:56, 1981. *This preoperative and postoperative assessment has important clinical applications relative to the defects of preoperative right ventricular dysfunction and pulmonary hypertension on the expected result from operation.*

Meyer RA: Echocardiography. In Adams FH, Emmanouilides GC (eds.): Moss' Heart Disease in Infants, Children and Adolescents. 3rd ed. Baltimore, Williams and Wilkins, 1983, pp 58–82. *Up-to-date, concise, and well illustrated. Discusses anatomic features as well as cardiac performance.*

Perloff JK: The Clinical Recognition of Congenital Heart Disease. 3rd ed. Philadelphia, W.B. Saunders Company, 1986. *A book that focuses on the anatomic and physiologic derangements in congenital heart disease, setting the stage for an understanding of the history, physical signs, electrocardiogram, chest roentgenogram, and echocardiogram. All age groups are dealt with.*

Rabinovitch M: Pulmonary hypertension. In Adams FH, Emmanouilides GC (eds.): Moss' Heart Disease in Infants, Children and Adolescents. 3rd ed. Baltimore, Williams and Wilkins, 1983, pp 669–692. *Up-to-date information on quantitative structural analysis of the pulmonary vasculature bed in congenital heart disease.*

Roberts WC: Adult Congenital Heart Disease. Philadelphia, F.A. Davis Company, 1987. *The specific focus is on adults with congenital heart disease. Natural history and surgical treatment are considered.*

50 ATHEROSCLEROSIS

Russell Ross

Atherosclerosis is responsible for the majority of cases of myocardial and cerebral infarction and thus represents the principal cause of death in the United States and western Europe. Atherosclerosis is the descriptive term for thickened and hardened lesions of the medium and large muscular and elastic arteries. It is a lipid-rich lesion, in contrast with arteriosclerosis, which is the generic term used for thickened and stiffened arteries of all sizes. Other forms of arteriosclerosis include focal calcific arteriosclerosis (Mönckeberg's arteriosclerosis) and arteriolosclerosis, a disease of small vessels.

The lesions of atherosclerosis occur within the innermost layer of the artery, the intima, and are largely confined to this region of the vessel. The lesions are generally eccentric and, if they become sufficiently large, can occlude the artery and thus the vascular supply to a tissue or organ, resulting in ischemia or necrosis. If this occurs, it often leads to the characteristic clinical sequelae of myocardial infarction, cerebral infarction, gangrene of the extremities, or sudden cardiac death.

THE NORMAL ARTERY

The normal artery consists essentially of a tube lined on its luminal aspect by a continuous layer of endothelium and on its outer aspect by loose connective tissue containing fibroblasts and smooth muscle cells, which package an intermediate layer of pure smooth muscle cells that are bound together in such a manner that, by working with the elastic laminae and the collagen and proteoglycans that surround the cells, the smooth muscle cells contract and maintain the tonus of the artery wall as the blood flows through with each systole and diastole.

The lining cells of the artery, the endothelium, represent the interface with the cells of the blood. It is at this interface that different blood cell types can interact with the endothelium and, under appropriate circumstances, lead to the development of lesions of atherosclerosis. These cells are the platelet, the monocyte, and the lymphocyte. Their potential roles in atherogenesis will be discussed below.

THE LESIONS OF ATHEROSCLEROSIS

The two principal forms of atherosclerosis are the early lesion, or fatty streak, and the advanced lesion, or fibrous plaque, which can become an advanced complicated lesion.

The Fatty Streak

The fatty streak is the most common and ubiquitous lesion of atherosclerosis. It occurs at all ages and in Western society is present at birth in some infants and is common in young children. The lesions of atherosclerosis are confined principally to the intima. Initially, the fatty streak appears to contain a single cell type, a foam cell that consists of macrophages filled with lipids, principally in the form of cholesteryl esters. These macrophages are derived from blood-borne monocytes that are chemotactically attracted into the artery wall, where they develop into the foam cells. As the fatty streak enlarges, it does so by continuing attachment and migration of monocytes into the intima with their consequent development into macrophages. Subsequently, smooth muscle cells appear to migrate into the intima from the media and also begin to accumulate lipid and take on the appearance of foam cells. As the fatty streak becomes larger and more advanced, it contains varying numbers of smooth muscle cells mixed together with the predominant lipid-filled macrophages. Fatty streaks can be found in young individuals at the same anatomic sites that are later occupied by advanced lesions, as well as at sites where they may either regress and disappear or remain as fatty streaks throughout life.

The Fibrous Plaque

The fibrous plaque is also located in the intima and characteristically leads to the eccentric thickening of the artery

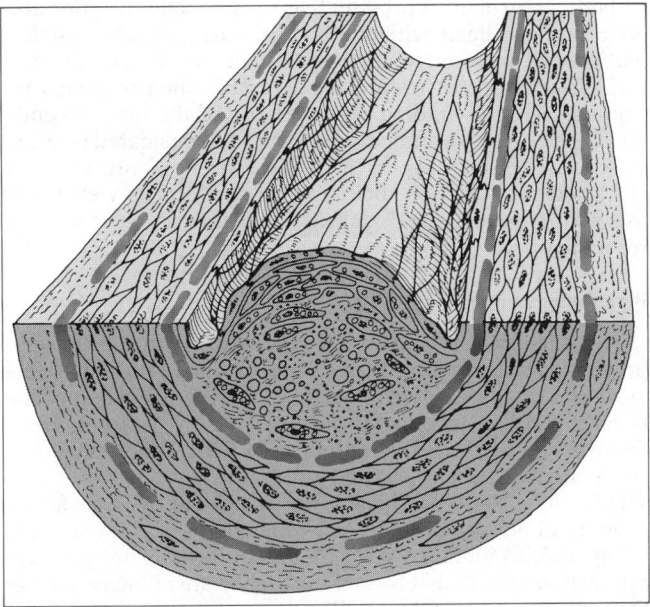

FIGURE 50–1. The *fibrous plaque*, which characteristically consists of numerous proliferated smooth muscle cells together with macrophages and variable numbers of lymphocytes. In this diagram, the fibrous plaque is covered by an intact endothelial monolayer and contains a fibrous cap of smooth muscle cells. These smooth muscle cells lie in a dense connective tissue matrix that covers a deeper collection of smooth muscle cells and macrophages, both of which may contain numerous lipid droplets and take the form of foam cells mixed together with variable numbers of lymphocytes. These collections of cells lie in a mixture of connective tissue matrix and free extracellular deposits of lipid. The fibrous plaque usually intrudes into the lumen owing to its proliferative nature. This diagram represents only in general terms the relative appearance of such a lesion.

that often results in occlusion of the lumen. The fibrous plaque is typically covered at its luminal aspect by a thickened cap of dense connective tissue containing a special form of flattened, pancake-shaped smooth muscle cell that has formed the dense collagenous matrix in which it is embedded. Beneath this cap, the lesion is highly cellular and contains large numbers of smooth muscle cells, some of which may be full of lipid droplets. It also contains numerous macrophages, many of which take the form of foam cells, together with variable numbers of T and B lymphocytes. These collections of cells usually overlie a deeper area of necrotic foam cells and debris. This necrotic area sometimes becomes calcified and often may contain cholesterol crystals. (Figure 50–1 details the cellular composition of a fibrous plaque.)

The Complicated Lesion

The complicated lesion is a fibrous plaque that has undergone extensive degeneration and often calcification. It may contain ulcerations, cracks, and fissures, which serve as sites for platelet adherence, aggregation and thrombosis, and subsequent organization. When this occurs, thrombosis may result in sudden occlusion of the artery.

Morbid Anatomy of the Lesions

Fatty streaks are flat lesions that often appear as yellow discolorations on the surface of the artery but seldom intrude into the lumen and thus cause no clinical sequelae. The fibrous plaques and complicated lesions are raised lesions that are often pearly gray in appearance but may be discolored when associated with erythrocytes and thrombi.

Localization of the Lesions

The arteries most commonly involved with atherosclerosis are the aorta; the femoral, popliteal, and tibial arteries; the coronary arteries; the internal and external carotid arteries; and the cerebral arteries.

In the aorta, the abdominal portion is commonly involved with lesions of atherosclerosis at an earlier age, and, as in the thoracic aorta, lesions most commonly form around orifices of branches and bifurcations of the artery. There is a greater incidence of atherosclerotic lesions in the leg arteries, whereas they are relatively rare in the vessels of the upper limbs. Atherosclerosis of the smaller arteries, particularly those of the legs and the coronary arteries, is more common in cigarette smokers or in individuals who have glucose intolerance.

Coronary atherosclerosis is most prominent in the main stems of the coronary arteries, particularly in the segments closest to the ostia of the coronary vessel. The degree of luminal narrowing in the coronary arteries can be variable; however, atherosclerosis is generally present in the epicardial segment of the vessels, whereas the intramural coronary arteries are generally spared. Typically, after coronary bypass surgery, the perianastomotic site of the bypass is often (30 per cent of the time) involved in the development of a new lesion of atherosclerosis.

The carotid and cerebral arteries generally have a patchy distribution of the lesions of atherosclerosis, which often first appear at the base of the brain in the carotid, basilar, and vertebral arteries.

The pulmonary arteries are generally spared of lesions of atherosclerosis, except in association with pulmonary hypertension.

RISK FACTORS

The risk factor concept evolved from epidemiologic studies of the incidence of coronary artery disease conducted in the United States and in Europe. Prospective studies demonstrated a consistent association of characteristics observed in apparently healthy individuals with the subsequent incidence of coronary artery disease in the same individuals. These studies demonstrated an association between an increase in the concentration of plasma lipoproteins, principally low density lipoprotein (LDL) and thus plasma cholesterol (see Ch. 183), and the rate of occurrence of new events of coronary artery disease. Also observed was an increased incidence of the disease in relation to cigarette smoking, hypertension, clinical diabetes, age, male sex, obesity, stress and particular personality characteristics (denoted as type A), and genetic factors. Because of these associations, each of these characteristics was termed a risk factor for atherosclerosis (see Ch. 40). At least three independent predictors of risk for individuals within a population are valuable in anticipating increased incidence of atherosclerosis. These are hyperlipidemia, cigarette smoking, and hypertension.

Hyperlipidemia

There is a clear association between chronic hypercholesterolemia and increase in incidence of ischemic heart disease. The Framingham Study demonstrated this association, particularly in men between the ages of 20 and 40. When the plasma cholesterol levels are greater than 220 mg per deciliter, there is a marked increase in the relative incidence of myocardial infarction, which is most easily demonstrated in individuals with familial hypercholesterolemia. The range of normality is not entirely clear in defining cholesterol and triglyceride levels for a given population as they relate to increased risk of ischemic heart disease. However, in the United States, 220 mg per deciliter is considered to be the upper limit of normal for the plasma cholesterol level (although this is probably too high), which increases from birth through young adulthood until the age of approximately 50 in men and to somewhat older ages in women. Similarly, there is an age-related increase in plasma triglyceride levels. Triglyceride is associated with increases in very low density lipoproteins (VLDL), whereas elevation in plasma cholesterol level is generally associated with increase in LDL.

Abnormal accumulation of lipoproteins in the plasma can occur from overproduction, from deficient removal, or from a combination of these abnormalities. There are numerous forms of genetically derived hyperlipoproteinemias that are either monogenic or polygenic. Perhaps more common are forms of hyperlipoproteinemia that are secondary to other disease, such as diabetes, renal disease, alcoholism, hypothyroidism, and the dysglobulinemias, or to treatment with corticosteroids or estrogens (see Ch. 183).

HOMOZYGOUS FAMILIAL HYPERCHOLESTEROLEMIA. Patients with homozygous familial hypercholesterolemia (FH disease) represent one of the best demonstrations of the capacity of hypercholesterolemia to induce the cellular changes that lead to atherogenesis. Although FH disease is much rarer than the secondary hyperlipoproteinemias or other forms of genetic hyperlipidemia, we know a great deal about its course in humans and in an animal model, the Watanabe heritable hyperlipidemic rabbit, as well as diet-induced hypercholesterolemia in the nonhuman primate. In the case of genetic hyperlipidemia, the plasma cholesterol and LDL levels are inordinately high owing to faulty or missing LDL receptors. When LDL is bound to its normal receptor, it suppresses the activity of the rate-limiting enzyme for cholesterol synthesis, HMG-CoA-reductase. In individuals with FH disease, the liver and peripheral cells continue to synthesize large amounts of cholesterol because absent or faulty receptors fail to generate a feedback inhibitory signal and cholesterol synthesis goes on unabated. Under these conditions, plasma cholesterol levels reach 500 to 1000 mg per deciliter or higher, and rampant atherosclerosis develops, with advanced occlusive lesions. This can occur at very young ages, and myocardial infarcts have been described in young children with this disease.

TREATMENT OF HYPERCHOLESTEROLEMIA. The Lipid Research Clinic Trials have demonstrated that it is beneficial to lower plasma levels in patients with chronic elevations of LDL. These studies showed that the decrease in plasma cholesterol levels can be correlated with a reduction in the incidence of myocardial infarction and thus atherosclerosis. Premature ischemic heart disease is usually associated with hypercholesterolemia, particularly when levels of plasma cholesterol are greater than 260 mg per deciliter. When this occurs, the incidence of atherosclerotic disease can be as high as fivefold greater than for individuals with plasma cholesterol levels below 220 mg per deciliter.

Hypertriglyceridemia is usually associated with increases in VLDL in the plasma, which may be complicated by increases in cholesterol as well. Patients with increased VLDL levels who come from families with familial combined hyperlipidemia are at increased risk for atherosclerosis, whereas those with elevated VLDL levels from families with monogenic familial hypertriglyceridemia are not at increased risk. Increased VLDL levels can increase the risk of atherosclerosis if it accompanies other risk factors, such as diabetes mellitus or cigarette smoking.

It is important to examine all patients over the age of 20 for hyperlipidemia, particularly if they have a family history of premature ischemic heart disease. This is best done by measuring the concentrations of cholesterol and triglyceride in plasma after an overnight fast. Cholesterol levels above 250 mg per deciliter or triglyceride levels above 200 mg per deciliter, or both, are indicative of hyperlipidemia, requiring attention and therapy, the first step of which should be dietary intervention. Such patients should be brought to normal weight if this is excessive and maintained on a diet low in saturated fat and cholesterol. Those with hypertriglyceridemia should limit or eliminate intake of alcohol. In general, reduction of intake of calories, cholesterol, and saturated fat is the best approach to begin with in most patients. Severe hyperlipidemia with cholesterol levels in excess of 350 mg per deciliter or triglyceride levels in excess of 400 mg per deciliter, or both, is usually representative of a genetic disorder and often first manifests with xanthomas. Such patients' families, particularly first-degree relatives, should also be examined.

If dietary approaches are unsuccessful, then regimens including bile acid–binding resins or one of the more recently developed lipid-lowering drugs should be considered (see Ch. 183). Use of such agents is dependent not only on their efficaciousness, but on their long-term effects as well. Their use before puberty and during pregnancy is currently not recommended.

High Density Lipoprotein (HDL)

In epidemiologic studies, elevations of high density lipoprotein particles in the plasma are inversely related to the incidence of atherosclerosis and its sequelae. Elevation of the HDL cholesterol level is "protective" against ischemic heart disease; conversely, the individuals with abnormally low levels of HDL are at increased risk.

HDL has been postulated to participate in transfer of cholesterol out of cells. Women generally have elevated HDL levels prior to menopause. If their HDL level is decreased in association with diabetes or obesity, they are at increased risk for ischemic heart disease. Regular strenuous exercise, decreased cigarette smoking, and diet rich in some fish oils (eicosapentaenoic acid) are associated with increased HDL levels, although the basis for the increase is poorly understood.

Cigarette Smoking

Cigarette smoking is one of the most common risk factors associated with increased incidence of atherosclerosis, and when it is reduced or eliminated, the risk of developing the disease decreases. Stroke, myocardial infarction, and intermittent claudication are common in male cigarette smokers, who, together with female smokers, show an increased incidence of symptoms associated with atherosclerosis. In addition to atherosclerosis of the large coronary arteries, cigarette smokers characteristically have occlusive disease of the leg arteries. There is a mean increase of approximately 70 per cent in the death rate and a three- to fivefold increase in the risk of ischemic heart disease in males who smoke more than one pack of cigarettes per day, compared with nonsmokers.

Sudden death is frequently associated with cigarette smoking, and of particular importance is the observation that cessation of cigarette smoking leads within a year to reduction of the risk of the sequelae of atherosclerosis to levels of that of nonsmokers. The basis for atherosclerosis in cigarette smokers is not well understood.

Glucose Intolerance and Diabetes Mellitus

Both insulin-dependent and non–insulin-dependent diabetics show at least a twofold increase in the incidence of myocardial infarction, compared with nondiabetics. Younger diabetics have a marked increase in the risk of atherosclerosis and thus of ischemic heart disease, and diabetic women appear to be even more prone than diabetic men. Gangrene of the lower extremities is one of the principal sequelae of atherosclerosis in diabetics. It is not clear what factors are responsible for the increased incidence of atherosclerosis in diabetes.

Hypertension

Elevation in blood pressure is an important risk factor associated with increased incidence of atherosclerosis and is of particular importance since this is a factor that is easily diagnosed and highly treatable. The risk of atherosclerosis and its sequelae increases progressively with increase in blood pressure, and when the blood pressure exceeds 160 mm Hg systolic and 95 mm Hg diastolic in middle-aged men the risk is five times greater than in normotensive men with blood pressure of 140 mm Hg systolic and 90 mm Hg diastolic or less. The increase in diastolic pressure may be more important than that in systolic pressure in both hypertensive men and women. After the age of 50, hypertension may be more important as a risk factor in predicting increased incidence of atherosclerosis than hypercholesterolemia. Recent intervention studies of individuals with hypertension have demonstrated that a reduction of diastolic pressure levels below 105 mm Hg can significantly reduce the incidence of symptomatic cerebrovascular disease, ischemic heart disease, and congestive heart failure in men (see Ch. 47). When multiple risk factors are present, including hypertension, it is particularly important to treat the hypertension, since it is the most easily accessible and treatable aspect of this disease process.

Obesity

When body weight is greater than 20 per cent above the norm, there is an increased risk of ischemic heart disease. Obesity may particularly accelerate atherosclerosis in individuals below the age of 50. Obesity is generally associated with hypertriglyceridemia, hypercholesterolemia, glucose intolerance, and hypertension.

Physical Activity

There are many and conflicting studies related to the value of increased physical activity in reducing the incidence of ischemic heart disease. The Framingham Studies suggest that sedentary individuals are more susceptible to atherosclerosis and to sudden death than individuals who maintain an active lifestyle. It has been suggested that increased physical activity may elevate the level of high density lipoprotein. Appropriately supervised physical training can improve exercise performance in patients with angina due to ischemic heart disease.

Genetic Factors

Clearly, genetic factors are critical in atherosclerosis. The best example of this is the increased incidence of atherosclerosis in individuals with homozygous familial hypercholesterolemia and familial combined hyperlipidemia. Other risk factors, such as hypertension and diabetes mellitus, can also be inherited, and it is possible that protective factors, such as increased high density lipoprotein, may also be inherited, although the latter is not well understood. As a consequence, family history must be included in assessing the risk for a given individual.

THE PATHOGENESIS OF THE LESIONS OF ATHEROSCLEROSIS

The lesions of atherosclerosis as they occur in the intima of the artery essentially consist of three biologic entities. First and foremost of these is an increase in the number of intimal smooth muscle cells, together with an accumulation of macrophages and variable numbers of lymphocytes. The increased number of smooth muscle cells is responsible for the second entity, the formation of large amounts of connective tissue matrix containing collagen, elastic fibers, and proteoglycans. The third entity, lipid, accumulates within the smooth muscle cells and the macrophages and in many instances causes them to develop into foam cells. Lipid also accumulates within the surrounding connective tissue matrix. Thus the advanced lesions of atherosclerosis represent the culmination of a usually longstanding proliferative disease process in which it becomes important to understand the basis for the proliferation of smooth muscle, accumulation of macrophages, formation of new connective tissue, and accumulation of lipid.

The Response to Injury Hypothesis of Atherosclerosis

During the past decade, it has been possible to develop a hypothesis that takes into account most of what is known concerning risk factors, the biology of the artery wall, the cells involved, and the biologic processes that may result in the lesions of atherosclerosis.

The response to injury hypothesis of atherosclerosis suggests that some form of "injury" affects the lining endothelial cells. The injury may alter the functional characteristics of the endothelium, leaving the endothelium morphologically intact. Thus endothelial injury could alter the permeability of the endothelium, its nonthrombogenic character, its ability to form vasoactive substances and growth factors, and its capacity to regenerate. At the other extreme, endothelial injury may lead to endothelial cell-cell disjunction and endothelial retraction, exposing the underlying connective tissue or accumulated foam cells, such as macrophages, that form the first and ubiquitous lesion of atherosclerosis, the fatty streak.

In hypercholesterolemic animals, including nonhuman primates, swine, rabbits, and rats, the first change that occurs in the artery wall is a chemotactic attraction of circulating monocytes, which increasingly adhere to the surface of the endothelial cells in clusters located throughout the arterial tree. These adherent monocytes migrate on the surface of the endothelium, penetrate between endothelial junctions, localize subendothelially, accumulate lipid, and become intimal foam cells. The accumulation of these intimal monocytes that become converted to lipid-laden macrophages represents the initial lesion of atherosclerosis, the fatty streak. These fatty streaks expand by continued attraction and accumulation of monocytes in the artery. They also expand by migration of some smooth muscle cells from the underlying media into the intima, where they localize beneath the accumulated macrophages and also accumulate lipid.

With increasing time, level, and duration of hypercholesterolemia, a second series of changes occurs in the endothelial cells in which endothelial cell-cell junctions separate and endothelial cells retract, particularly at anatomic sites such as branches and bifurcations of the artery, where the flow characteristics of the blood may make the endothelium more susceptible to injury. If the endothelial cells retract and expose the underlying foam cells in the fatty streaks at the sites, then the exposed macrophages or connective tissue, or both, can be thrombogenic and induce platelets to adhere. Within one to two months, sites where mural thrombi have formed become loci of increased migration and proliferation of smooth muscle cells that accumulate and form large amounts of connective tissue matrix. Thus sites of platelet adherence and aggregation subsequently become sites of intimal smooth muscle proliferation.

At other anatomic sites, the endothelium may remain intact, but the fatty streak will expand by the continued attraction and accumulation of monocytes. Over a longer period of time, those areas that maintain an intact endothelial cover also appear capable of developing into a fibrous plaque.

Numerous investigations have attempted to determine what factors are responsible for the migration and proliferation of smooth muscle cells into the intima. Growth factors able to induce smooth muscle cell migration and proliferation can be formed and secreted by several cells. Of particular importance is the capacity of platelets to release growth factors and of activated macrophages to release the same as well as other types of growth factors. The growth factors that may play a critical role in atherogenesis include platelet-derived growth factor (PDGF), a potent growth factor for mesenchymal connective tissue cells such as fibroblasts and smooth muscle; fibroblast growth factor (FGF), an angiogenic agent; epidermal growth factor (EGF), an agent capable of stimulating the growth of epithelial cells; and transforming growth factor beta (TGF-beta), a factor that may act in an inhibitory fashion or, in other circumstances, synergistically with PDGF.

PDGF is a potent mitogen that, at nanogram and picogram levels, can induce cells such as those of smooth muscle to multiply and to form new connective tissue. Platelet-derived growth factor can be derived from platelets, from activated macrophages, and from appropriately stimulated or "injured" endothelial cells. Thus, if endothelial injury occurs, appropriate opportunities may be present for the release of mitogens

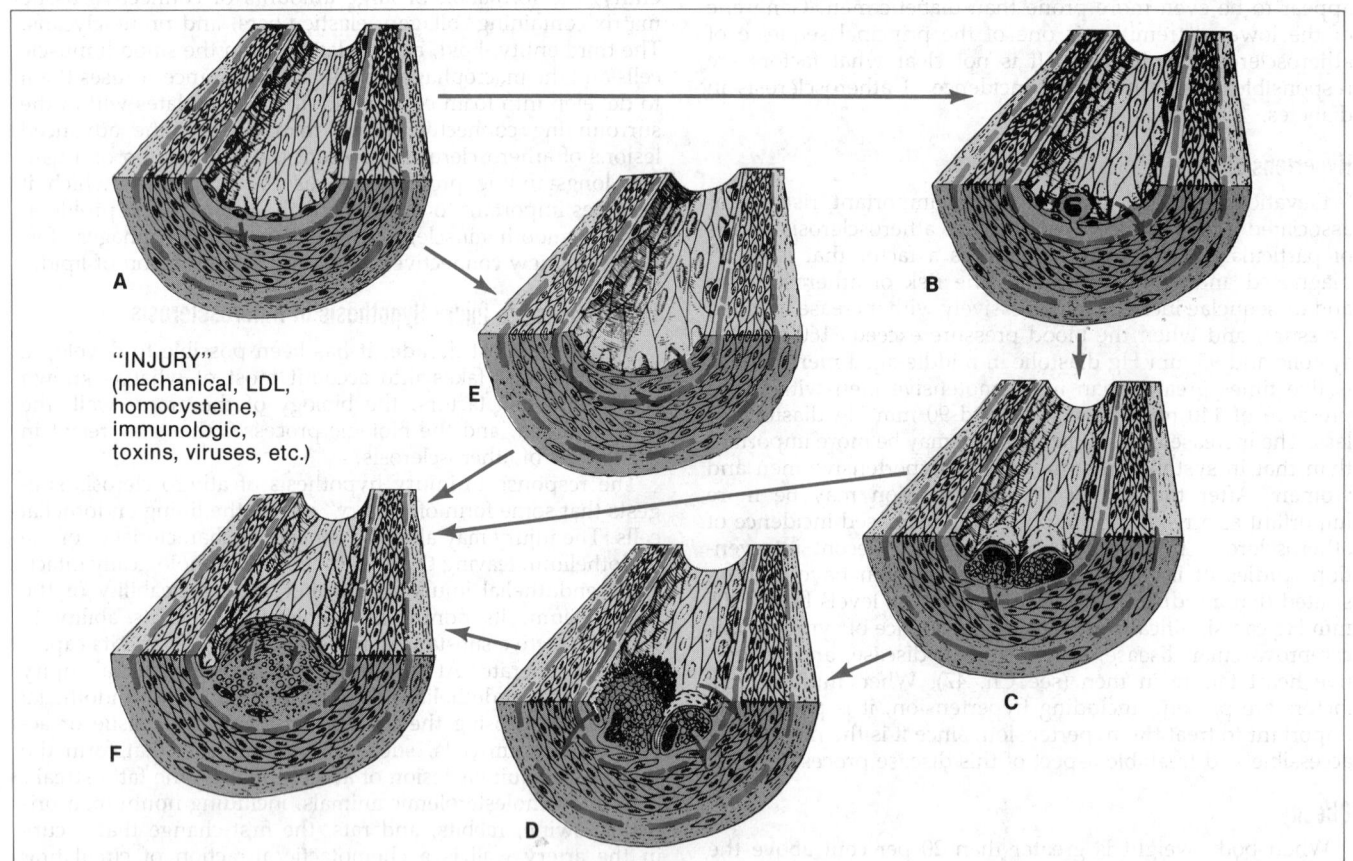

"INJURY"
(mechanical, LDL,
homocysteine,
immunologic,
toxins, viruses, etc.)

FIGURE 50-2. Endothelial injury: The response to injury hypothesis. Advanced intimal proliferative lesions of atherosclerosis may occur by at least two pathways. The pathway demonstrated by the clockwise (long) arrows to the right has been observed in experimentally induced hypercholesterolemia. Injury to the endothelium (A) may induce growth factor secretion (*short arrow*). Monocytes attach to endothelium (B), which may continue to secrete growth factors (*short arrow*). Subendothelial migration of monocytes (C) may lead to fatty streak formation and release of growth factors such as platelet-derived growth factor (PDGF) (*short arrow*). Fatty streaks may become directly converted to fibrous plaques (*long arrow* from C to F) through release of growth factors from macrophages or endothelial cells or both. Macrophages may also stimulate and or injure the overlying endothelium. In some cases, macrophages may lose their endothelial cover and platelet attachment may occur (D), providing three possible sources of growth factors—platelets, macrophages, and endothelium (*short arrows*). Some of the smooth muscle cells in the proliferative lesion itself (F) may form and secrete growth factors such as PDGF (*short arrows*).

An alternative pathway for development of advanced lesions of atherosclerosis is shown by the arrows from A to E to F. In this case, the endothelium may be injured but remained intact. Increased endothelial turnover may result in growth factor formation by endothelial cells (A). This may stimulate migration of smooth muscle cells from the media into the intima, accompanied by endogenous production of PDGF by smooth muscle as well as growth factor secretion from the "injured" endothelial cells (E). These interactions could then lead to fibrous plaque formation and further lesion progression (F). (Reproduced by permission from Ross R: The pathogenesis of atherosclerosis—an update. N Engl J Med 314:496, 1986.)

such as PDGF from all three cells. Such growth factor release may be related to increased incidence of atherogenesis in experimental animals. There is also some suggestion that smooth muscle cells, once they have been induced to proliferate in the artery wall, may in themselves be capable of expressing the gene for PDGF and of secreting this growth factor so that they may, in effect, stimulate themselves in an autocrine fashion to continue the proliferative response.

The response to injury hypothesis of atherogenesis suggests that the "injury" to the endothelium results in cellular changes that lead to a modified form of inflammation in which monocytes and lymphocytes enter the artery wall and the monocytes become macrophages that can secrete growth factors, act as scavenger cells, and accumulate lipid and become foam cells. The fatty streak then becomes converted into a smooth muscle proliferative lesion, or fibrous plaque, and probably does so by local release within the artery of growth factors derived from activated macrophages, injured endothelium, and/or platelets that may interact with the artery wall at sites where the protective cover of the endothelium may be altered. These changes are diagrammatically shown in Figure 50–2, which suggests how the lesions of atherosclerosis may form.

The response to injury hypothesis also offers an opportunity to consider means of preventing and intervening in the formation of the lesions of atherosclerosis. Clearly, alteration in lifestyle habits, including changes in dietary habits and alteration of risk factors associated with increased incidence of atherosclerosis, could be potentially important in preventing these cellular changes from occurring and possibly in inducing lesion regression.

Regression of Atherosclerosis

In experimental animals the fatty streak is clearly capable of regressing and disappearing entirely if hypercholesterolemic animals are placed on a normocholesterolemic regimen for a sufficient period of time. There is some evidence to suggest that fatty streaks can also regress in humans, based upon examination of individuals who decreased their dietary intake of lipids and atherogenic foods. Fibrous plaques, or complicated lesions in humans may also be partially reversible, based upon angiographic studies. It is not yet clear how far a lesion must progress before it becomes irreversible. Cessation of cigarette smoking is associated with decreased risk, and this in combination with treatment of hypertension, dietary intervention, treatment of diabetes mellitus, and removal, where possible, of other associated causes may be important in inducing regression of the lesions of atherosclerosis. More remains to be learned concerning this approach to reversing the disease process.

Prevention of atherosclerosis, rather than treatment, has to be the principal goal for all patients. In consideration of the association between hyperlipidemia and increased atherosclerosis, and with recognition of the decline in the death rate in the United States from premature ischemic heart disease, it becomes increasingly important to understand that early detection of risk and approaches toward change in dietary habits and in lifestyles are important in the prevention of atherosclerosis in individuals who may potentially be at increased risk. It is important to detect those who may be at increased risk on a familial basis, who may be hypertensive, who are cigarette smokers, or whose dietary habits could be altered with a resultant reduction in risk. Treatment of hypertension, as well as advice regarding diet, cigarette smoking, and exercise, can be valuable adjuncts to helping a patient deal with these problems. Pharmacologic treatment of hyperlipidemia should be limited to individuals at risk who do not respond adequately to dietary management. The long-term value of antiplatelet drugs and, potentially in the future, of drugs that may affect growth factor activity could be of importance in reducing the incidence of atherosclerosis and the long-term sequelae of this disease process.

Brown MS, Goldstein JL: How LDL receptors influence cholesterol and atherosclerosis. Sci Am 251:158, 1984. *A discussion of how LDL receptor interactions control cholesterol metabolism.*

Gordon T, Castelli WP, Hjortland MC, et al.: Diabetes, blood lipids, and the role of obesity in coronary heart disease risk for women. The Framingham Study. Ann Intern Med 87:393, 1977.

Gordon T, Castelli WP, Hjortland MC, et al.: High density lipoprotein as a protective factor against coronary heart disease. The Framingham Study. Am J Med 62:707, 1977. *These two papers represent epidemiologic studies that relate the role of several of the principal risk factors to atherosclerosis and indicate the potential protective effect of HDL in atherosclerosis.*

Report of the Working Group of Arteriosclerosis of the National Heart, Lung, and Blood Institute. Vol. 2. Department of Health, Education and Welfare (National Institutes of Health) Publication No. 82–2035. Washington, D.C., Government Printing Office, 1981. *This represents an overview of a large number of individuals who have examined both the epidemiology and the nature of the lesions of atherosclerosis.*

Ross R: The pathogenesis of atherosclerosis—an update. N Engl J Med 314:488, 1986.

Ross R, Glomset JA: The pathogenesis of atherosclerosis. N Engl J Med 295:369, 1976. *These two papers review the anatomic structure of the artery wall, lesions of atherosclerosis, and the potential roles of the cells in atherosclerosis. They provide a hypothesis for how atherogenesis may come about.*

Steinberg D: Lipoproteins and atherosclerosis: A look back and a look ahead. Arteriosclerosis 3:283, 1983. *A discussion of the role of lipoproteins and atherosclerosis that highlights many of the important questions.*

51 DISORDERS OF CORONARY ARTERIES

51.1 Angina Pectoris
James T. Willerson

Angina pectoris is the clinical term used to describe chest pain resulting from a relative oxygen deficiency in heart muscle. Angina occurs when oxygen demand exceeds oxygen supply. Most individuals with angina pectoris have underlying atherosclerotic coronary artery disease, but angina may also develop in some patients with ventricular hypertrophy, left ventricular outflow obstruction, severe aortic valvular regurgitation or stenosis, cardiomyopathy, or dilated ventricles in whom coronary artery stenoses are not present. The explanation for the development of angina in these circumstances is that under certain conditions even normal coronary arteries may not adequately supply hypertrophied, dilated, or failing heart muscle with oxygen. In some circumstances, a limited coronary vasodilator reserve may also explain angina pectoris, especially in some patients with left ventricular outflow obstruction (valvular aortic stenosis and idiopathic hypertrophic subaortic stenosis) or ventricular hypertrophy or both. Normal individuals do not develop angina, probably because the heart is protected from an important imbalance in oxygen delivery by other factors that limit physical activity, such as dyspnea and fatigue.

The predisposing pathologic alteration in coronary arteries ordinarily responsible for angina is atherosclerosis. Severe narrowing of the lumen of coronary arteries results in a decreased ability to deliver oxygen to areas supplied by the involved vessels. Consequently, under conditions of exercise, cold exposure, or emotional stress, or after eating, angina may develop. This is most easily understood by recalling that the primary determinants of oxygen demand in the heart are heart rate, contractile state, and wall tension. Emphasis upon relative oxygen demand makes it easier to understand why some individuals with valvular heart disease and associated ventricular hypertrophy develop angina even in the absence of coronary artery disease. Systolic pressure development is relatively costly in terms of oxygen utilization, and, together with ventricular hypertrophy and increased wall tension, is an important factor in the development of angina in patients with valvular aortic stenosis and without coronary artery stenoses. However, a limited coronary vasodilator reserve is also a factor. Development of angina in individuals with marked pulmonary hypertension may be the result of increased right ventricular pressure and hypertrophy.

Angina pectoris may also develop in individuals with severe volume overload of the ventricle, including those with aortic or mitral regurgitation. "Volume work" results in a smaller increase in oxygen demand than "pressure work" until important cardiac dilatation occurs. At this point, increased oxygen demand may not be met because of reduced diastolic coronary perfusion pressure. The presence of angina pectoris in patients with aortic regurgitation is often an ominous prognostic sign.

Angina may also occur because of extracardiac influences. In particular, severe anemia or carbon monoxide exposure limits the capacity of the blood to carry or release oxygen and may result in angina under conditions that the subject would otherwise tolerate well. Increases in systemic arterial pressure and consequent dilatation of the heart may result in angina pectoris. Increases in heart rate or contractile state, such as occur with hyperthyroidism, pheochromocytoma, or exogenous administration or endogenous release of catecholamines, may also result in angina pectoris.

Primary decreases in coronary blood flow and myocardial oxygen delivery, such as occur with progressive atherosclerosis, partial coronary artery thrombosis, coronary arterial spasm or transient platelet aggregation, may also lead to angina pectoris. Similarly, increases in coronary artery tone associated with platelet aggregation and the release of humoral mediators, such as thromboxane or serotonin or both, may interact with intrinsic narrowing in coronary luminal diameter to decrease coronary flow and oxygen delivery and result in angina. With primary decreases in coronary blood flow, there is no necessary association between symptoms and exertion, and the majority of the anginal episodes occur at rest. These patients usually have little change in heart rate or blood pressure prior to the onset of pain, or the pain occurs first and is followed only later by an increase in blood pressure or heart rate. Continuous electrocardiographic monitoring may document transient ST segment change with the onset of pain, either ST segment elevation indicating transmural ischemia or ST depression when subendocardial ischemia occurs. Alternatively, ST segment alterations may occur in the absence of chest pain, emphasizing the presence of *silent ischemia* in some patients with primary decreases in myocardial oxygen delivery and angina at rest.

PATHOPHYSIOLOGY. Angina occurs most commonly in circumstances in which regional myocardial oxygen demand exceeds oxygen availability. This occurs when myocardial oxygen demand is increased by (1) an increase in intramyocardial systolic tension resulting from increases in blood pressure, cold exposure, congestive heart failure, ventricular hypertrophy, or left ventricular outflow obstruction; increases in intramyocardial systolic tension are directly proportional to blood pressure and the radius of the ventricle (Laplace's rule); (2) an increase in heart rate, such as occurs with exercise or emotion; and (3) an increase in the contractile state of the myocardium, such as occurs during physical effort, with catecholamine administration, with fright, or with the use of certain pharmacologic interventions that increase inotropy and myocardial oxygen demand more than they increase myocardial oxygen delivery. Rest generally relieves angina that occurs with effort, emotion, or exercise. Nitroglycerin also relieves angina, typically within three to five minutes. The beneficial effect of nitroglycerin is related to its ability to dilate medium-sized penetrating coronary vessels and thus improve coronary blood flow and its distribution to the subendocardial ischemic region or regions and to its ability to dilate systemic veins so that venous return to the heart and

ventricular end-diastolic volume are reduced, thereby reducing wall tension and oxygen demand.

CLINICAL DIAGNOSIS. Angina is typically described as a substernal or left precordial chest discomfort that is perceived as a "tightness" or "heaviness" ("like a weight on my chest") or as "a pressure." On occasion, the pain may radiate into the neck; it often radiates down the ulnar aspect of the left arm. It is typically produced by effort, exercise, emotion, or cold exposure or occurs after a large meal is eaten; it is relieved by rest or nitroglycerin. As mentioned earlier, it may also occur at rest as an expression of progressive atherosclerosis (more than 70 per cent luminal diameter narrowing), partial coronary artery thrombosis, coronary artery spasm, and/or platelet aggregation with the release of humoral mediators that increase coronary vascular resistance at sites of severe coronary arterial stenosis. Some patients do not describe their angina in typical terms but refer to it as "a hurt," "a little discomfort," or "a sharp pain." Others note the pain only in atypical locations, including the jaw, the teeth, the forearm, or the back. Some describe their angina as beginning in the epigastric region and radiating up into the chest. Finally, some patients have *silent* angina. Ten to 20 per cent of patients with both diabetes mellitus and coronary artery disease have silent angina, and in those with acute myocardial infarcts, 10 to 20 per cent are silent (painless) infarcts. Many patients after cardiac transplantation do not perceive angina even though coronary artery atherosclerosis occurs in the coronary arteries of the transplanted heart.

Left or right ventricular dysfunction may develop even with transient ischemic episodes. This may explain the dyspnea or orthopnea, paroxysmal nocturnal dyspnea, tachycardia, and alterations in blood pressure, including hypotension, that occur with some episodes of angina. Further, some patients develop transient murmurs of mitral or tricuspid regurgitation because of papillary muscle dysfunction occurring as a consequence of the ischemic process; acute mitral insufficiency may also contribute to the development of transient left ventricular failure during angina. Typically, left ventricular end-diastolic pressure rises during angina; this is a consequence of a reduction in ventricular compliance and, in some instances, possibly of incomplete relaxation of the ventricular muscle leading to increased left atrial and pulmonary venous pressures and the development of dyspnea, orthopnea, and pulmonary congestion during myocardial ischemia. Palpation of the precordium during an episode of angina may reveal a dyskinetic impulse. Auscultation may identify a third heart sound and rales or a murmur of mitral insufficiency. Occasionally, patients develop paradoxical splitting of their second heart sounds. The murmur of papillary muscle dysfunction reflects mild-to-moderate mitral regurgitation and is classically a mid to late systolic murmur, but it may be holosystolic.

Noncardiac problems may also cause chest pain, including peptic ulcer disease, pancreatitis, cholecystitis, esophageal reflux or spasm, and primary pulmonary abnormalities such as pneumonia, pulmonary embolism with infarction, atelectasis, and spontaneous pneumothorax. Other causes of chest pain that must be differentiated from angina pectoris are the pain of dissecting aortic aneurysm, musculoskeletal chest pain, and the pain that occurs with herpes zoster, which may develop before skin lesions occur.

CLINICAL CLASSIFICATION OF ANGINAL SYNDROMES. Table 51–1 lists the various coronary artery syndromes that should receive specific attention. Segregation of patients with coronary artery disease into the various anginal syndromes is useful diagnostically, therapeutically, and prognostically. Patients with stable angina usually have angina with effort or exercise or during other conditions in which myocardial oxygen demand is increased. This often occurs in a predictable manner and is usually relieved promptly by rest or nitroglycerin. However, some of these patients have angina

TABLE 51-1. ANGINAL SYNDROMES OF PATIENTS WITH CORONARY ARTERY DISEASE

Stable angina pectoris
Unstable angina pectoris (crescendo angina, angina at rest, and angina of recent onset)
Variant angina pectoris (Prinzmetal's angina)
Acute myocardial infarction

at variable levels of effort and, on occasion, also at rest, suggesting that intermittent increases in vascular smooth muscle tone and decreases in coronary blood flow contribute to the development of angina. Thus, in patients with stable angina, there may be a spectrum of pathophysiologic mechanisms responsible for angina leading to effort or emotion-related angina but also for angina occurring occasionally at lesser effort and even at rest.

Increasingly frequent angina with chest pain produced by less effort or provocation and occurring in a crescendo pattern is generally termed *unstable angina pectoris*. Patients with the initial development of angina at low levels of activity or at rest should probably be included in this category. Individuals with unstable angina pectoris often have pain at rest, and the pain may last for longer periods of time and be more difficult to relieve. Unstable angina should be considered a medical emergency and warrants hospitalization and evaluation of the patient for acute myocardial infarction.

Variant angina pectoris (Prinzmetal's angina) is defined as chest pain at rest in association with ST segment deviation (ordinarily ST segment elevation, but ST segment depression may also occur depending on the size of the coronary vessel in which spasm occurs) without preceding increase in heart rate or blood pressure. The mechanism of variant angina is coronary artery spasm shown by coronary arteriography often to involve large and medium-sized vessels with transmural myocardial blood flow distribution. As the chest pain disappears, the ST segment deviation resolves in association with relief of the coronary spasm. In most patients, many more episodes of ST segment deviation than of chest pain occur; therefore, continuous recording of multilead electrocardiograms is recommended for patients with this abnormality. In those circumstances in which the coronary artery spasm is prolonged, acute myocardial infarction, important ventricular arrhythmias, heart block, or death may occur.

Ten to 20 per cent of patients with Prinzmetal's angina have angiographically normal coronary arteries; this further emphasizes the role of spasm in the pathophysiology of variant angina. The most common arteriographic pattern is significant single-vessel stenosis involving the proximal portion of either the right or the left anterior descending coronary artery. However, any pattern of coronary artery disease may be seen. Although variant angina pectoris attributable to coronary spasm occurs as a specific syndrome, there is also speculation that spasm may be a factor in more patients with stable and unstable angina pectoris than previously realized and that it may contribute to the variable threshold angina found in some of these patients.

It is not clear which pathophysiologic factors are most important in the conversion of stable angina to the various anginal syndromes mentioned above. However, current interest centers on the role of platelet aggregability, hemorrhage into atherosclerotic plaques, increases in local vascular concentrations of thromboxane, serotonin, and histamine, and relative decreases in prostacyclin, tissue plasminogen-activating factor, and/or endothelial relaxing factor concentrations at the site of coronary arterial intimal injury or atherosclerotic plaque or both.

DIAGNOSTIC TESTS. An association of the chest pain with exercise, effort, and emotion and of relief with rest or nitroglycerin is presumptive evidence that the chest pain represents angina pectoris. In addition, certain diagnostic maneuvers, such as carotid sinus pressure or the Valsalva maneuver, may help to determine the etiology of chest pain. Both these maneuvers slow the heart rate and reduce the blood pressure as a consequence of increased vagal and reduced sympathetic tone.

One may also use certain tests to provoke angina. In particular, exercise testing on a bicycle or on a treadmill is often used for this purpose. The patient exercises at graded loads, starting from low and progressing to higher ones. Blood pressure and heart rate are monitored throughout, and multilead electrocardiograms (ECG) are obtained prior to, during, and toward the end of each exercise level (continuous multilead monitoring of the electrocardiogram is preferable). An exercise test result is positive if typical angina develops and/or if the test is associated with ST segment deviation of 1 mm or greater, flat or downsloping, 0.08 second after the ST junction. There are both false-positive and false-negative exercise test results, however. Particularly in women, false-positive results occur in up to 20 to 30 per cent of patients. False-positive results may also occur in patients with electrolyte abnormalities, in patients taking digitalis, and in those with ventricular hypertrophy, conduction abnormalities (including left or right bundle branch block), or ST-T wave abnormalities prior to the onset of exercise. In addition, in some patients with anatomically important coronary artery stenoses, diagnostic ECG changes do not occur with stress. The incidence of false-negative results with adequate exercise tests and multilead ECG analysis is at least 10 to 15 per cent. Additional hemodynamic and clinical variables monitored during the exercise testing are heart rate, systolic blood pressure, exercise work load achieved, and the development of frequent or complex ventricular ectopic beats. Angina that develops during exercise at a relatively low heart rate and blood pressure and/or at a low work load or a reduction in systolic blood pressure with exercise generally indicates more extensive and physiologically important coronary artery stenoses and a poorer prognosis with medical therapy. Prominent ST segment depression (≥ 3 mm) developing at low or moderate exercise work loads often identifies more extensive coronary artery stenoses or a significant left main coronary artery stenosis or both. Frequent or complex ventricular ectopic beats occurring during exercise may subsequently be adequately suppressed by a beta blocker or a slow channel calcium antagonist.

Additions to the standard exercise ECG include the use of selected nuclear cardiology tests. One approach uses a myocardial perfusion agent such as thallium 201, which is injected at the peak of exercise. Myocardial scintigraphic images are obtained immediately thereafter. Regions of relative perfusion deficit observed during exercise that are normal at rest three to four hours later are generally indicative of physiologically significant coronary artery stenoses. When a maximal exercise effort is achieved, thallium 201 myocardial scintigraphy with tomographic imaging has a 90 per cent sensitivity and specificity in the noninvasive detection of anatomically important (≥ 70 per cent luminal diameter narrowing) coronary artery stenoses.

An alternative approach is to label the patient's red blood cells in vivo with technetium 99m pertechnetate or to inject intravenously a radionuclide such as technetium-labeled albumin or technetium pertechnetate and obtain a radionuclide ventriculogram (RVG) at rest and at each level of exercise. With either approach, one may measure global and segmental ventricular performance at rest and at each exercise level and determine directly whether alterations in regional wall motion, ventricular volumes, or global ejection fraction occur. In individuals without important coronary artery stenoses or myocardial disease, ventricular ejection fraction increases with exercise, but in those with physiologically important coronary artery stenoses, and particularly those with multivessel disease, the ventricular ejection fraction usually decreases with exercise. Similarly, in the patient with physiologically important coronary artery stenoses, left ventricular end-systolic volumes increase rather than decrease, and segmental wall motion abnormalities may develop. With a maximal exercise effort, the sensitivity of RVG in detecting physiologically important multivessel or proximal coronary stenoses is approximately 90 per cent. However, the specificity is only approximately 50 per cent, since patients with myocardial and valvular heart disease may also demonstrate ventricular dysfunction at rest or with exercise or both.

CORONARY ARTERIOGRAPHY. Coronary arteriography is the most reliable diagnostic test currently available to detect anatomically important coronary atherosclerosis and to estimate the extent of such disease. Resting coronary blood flow is not decreased, but effort-related increases in coronary blood flow may be reduced by coronary artery luminal narrowing of 50 per cent or greater. Resting coronary blood flow may be reduced by luminal diameter narrowing of greater than 70 per cent. However, there are sometimes discrepancies between the apparent anatomic severity of a coronary artery stenosis and its physiologic significance; thus, exercise testing with or without the scintigraphic assessments may be important in evaluating the physiologic significance of apparently anatomic important coronary artery stenoses.

A subset of patients with angina has normal coronary arteriograms but objective evidence of myocardial ischemia by ECG criteria or by lactate production during rapid pacing or by both. This pattern occurs in some patients with ventricular hypertrophy or systemic arterial hypertension or both, and in others with no obvious underlying cardiovascular disease.

Indications for coronary arteriography in patients with angina vary. A widely accepted clinical indication is the presence of limiting angina in the patient on a good medical regimen. However, some practitioners also use coronary arteriography to evaluate young patients (those less than 40 years of age) who have had previous acute myocardial infarcts. Others use coronary arteriography and left ventricular catheterization to evaluate the cause of congestive heart failure in patients in whom the etiology is not clear. Radionuclide ventriculography and echocardiography with Doppler may also be used for this purpose, especially to characterize regional and global ventricular function, to exclude sizable ventricular aneurysms, to identify valvular regurgitation and to estimate its severity, and to detect intracardiac shunt lesions. Coronary arteriography may also be used to help resolve the etiology of undiagnosed chest pain that is limiting or frightening for the patient. In general, however, coronary arteriography is reserved for patients selected as potential candidates for coronary artery surgery or precutaneous transluminal coronary angioplasty (PTCA) because of symptomatic angina pectoris.

MANAGEMENT. The therapeutic approach to patients with angina pectoris can be medical or surgical. These alternatives are not mutually exclusive, since many patients continue to take long-acting nitrates, propranolol, a calcium antagonist, or combinations of these agents following coronary artery revascularization or PTCA. In addition, one does everything possible to correct underlying risk factors, such as smoking, systemic arterial hypertension, hypercholesterolemia, overweight, major stress, and emotional conflicts, and to encourage proper amounts of exercise, especially in younger individuals. Control of multiple risk factors, especially discontinuing smoking and reducing serum cholesterol concentrations, has a beneficial effect in reducing subsequent mortality risks; and in experimental animals with hypercholesterolemia and coronary artery stenoses, reductions in serum cholesterol may be associated with some regression of coronary artery plaques.

Patients with angina pectoris should be encouraged to carry nitroglycerin with them. Nitroglycerin (0.3 to 0.5 mg) should be taken sublingually when angina develops in order to prevent it from becoming severe; if one nitroglycerin tablet is ineffective, a second should be taken. In addition, the patient should sit or lie down in order to help relieve the pain. If the angina is not relieved by two or three nitroglycerin tablets and rest, the individual should go to the hospital for further evaluation, specifically concerning the possibility that he or she is having an acute myocardial infarct. Nitroglycerin may also be taken prophylactically prior to engaging in activities the individual knows will produce angina, i.e., before physical effort, sexual intercourse, or an emotional experience that cannot be avoided. Nitroglycerin tablets should be replaced every 6 to 12 months, since they deteriorate. One needs to be certain that important reductions in blood pressure or increases in heart rate do not occur following the administraton of nitroglycerin, because under these circumstances coronary flow to the vulnerable myocardium may actually decrease.

Long-acting nitrates may also be used. The effectiveness, proper dosage, and route of administration are subjects of controversy. However, isosorbide dinitrate may be taken sublingually or orally, and it exerts an effect similar to that of nitroglycerin for 40 to 60 minutes after its administration. Nitroglycerin ointment is also an effective long-acting agent in most patients. It is generally applied to a small area of the chest as a thin film. The nitrate preparations in common use today are described in Table 51–2. Over time, many individuals develop a tolerance to the hemodynamic effects from the nitrate preparations, such that the same dose of nitrate is much less effective or even ineffective. The cellular biochemical alterations responsible for tolerance to nitrates are not yet elucidated, but less frequent administration of a particular nitrate and mixing the nitrates so that one might rely on

TABLE 51–2. NITRATE PREPARATIONS USED IN THE TREATMENT OF ANGINA PECTORIS

Preparation	Dosage	Duration of Effect	Frequency of Administration
Sublingual nitroglycerin	0.3–0.5 mg	15–30 min	For individual episodes
Sublingual or chewable isosorbide dinitrate	2.5–10 mg	30 min to 1 hr	May be used instead of nitroglycerin
Oral isosorbide dinitrate (Isordil)	5–30 mg	2 hr	Every 2 to 3 hr while the patient is awake
Oral isosorbide dinitrate (Tembid), longer-acting preparation	40 mg	6–8 hr	Every 6–8 hr
Pentaerythritol tetranitrate (Peritrate)	10–40 mg	3–4 hr	Every 3–4 hr
Oral	80 mg	8–10 hr	Every 8–10 hr
Sustained-release oral nitroglycerin (Nitro-Bid)	2.5–6.5 mg	6 hr	Every 6 hr
Nitroglycerin ointment	Thin film on 1 to 2 inches over small area of anterior chest	4–6 hr	Every 4–6 hr
Nitroglycerin patches (sustained-release)	5–20 mg	More than 6 hr	Every 12–24 hr

Modified from Willerson JT, Hillis LD, Buja LM: Ischemic Heart Disease: Clinical and Pathophysiological Aspects. New York, Raven Press, 1982, p 189.

TABLE 51–3. BETA-ADRENERGIC ANTAGONISTS

Name	Beta-Blockade Potency Ratio (Propranolol—1.0)	Cardioselective*	Usual Therapeutic Dose Range (mg/day)	Elimination Half-life	Route of Excretion
Propranolol	1.0	0	80–480	3.5–6.0 hr	Urine
Timolol	6.0	0	5–40	4–5 hr	Urine
Oxprenolol†	0.5–1.0	0	40–360	2 hr	Urine
Sotalol†	0.3	0	80–480	5–13 hr	Urine
Metoprolol	1.0	+	100–800	3–4 hr	Urine
Pindolol	6.0	0	2.5–30.0	3.4 hr	Urine
Atenolol	1.0	+	100–400	6–9 hr	Approximately 40% of unchanged drug in urine
Alprenolol†	0.3	0	200–800	2–3 hr	Urine
Acebutolol	0.3	+	400–800	8 hr	Uncertain

*Seen only at low dosage.
†Investigational drug.
Reproduced with permission from Hillis LD, Firth BG, Willerson JT: Manual of Clinical Problems in Cardiology. 2nd ed. Boston, Little, Brown and Company, 1984, p 285.

nitroglycerin paste during the night hours and a long-acting nitrate, such as isosorbide dinitrate, during the day help to reduce the likelihood of tolerance.

The second major group of agents used to control angina comprises the beta-adrenergic–blocking drugs (Table 51–3). Beta-adrenergic blockers decrease heart rate and blood pressure responses to exercise and usually reduce the frequency of angina related to exercise or effort. They also decrease the inotropic response to exercise in normal hearts but may actually improve global and segmental left ventricular contractility for any particular exercise effort in patients with important coronary artery stenoses. The most common contraindications to the use of beta blockers are congestive heart failure, bradycardia, bronchospastic lung disease, and insulin-requiring diabetes. Second- or third-degree heart block is also a contraindication to the use of beta blockers. Relatively cardioselective beta blockers (such as metoprolol and alprenolol)* that exert their effects on heart rate and blood pressure rather than on bronchial dilatation are alternatives. However, at higher dosages, the relatively selective beta blockers exert a nonspecific beta-blocking effect.

The use of "slow channel" calcium antagonists, such as nifedipine, verapamil, or diltiazem, is gaining in popularity (Tables 51–4 and 51–5). These agents reduce calcium entry into myocardial and vascular smooth muscle cells. This effect results in a reduction in vascular contractility and vascular resistance. These agents are effective in treating patients with vasospastic angina (Prinzmetal's angina), but they are also useful in treating patients with stable angina pectoris. Some calcium antagonists decrease myocardial contractility and atrioventricular conduction (verapamil and diltiazem), so they must be used with caution in patients with congestive heart failure, bradycardia, or atrioventricular (AV) conduction blocks, but they do not augment bronchoconstriction and thus may be of particular benefit as an alternative to beta blockers for those with bronchospasm and chronic obstructive lung disease. Nifedipine decreases systemic vascular resis-

tance, and therefore, clinically apparent reductions in cardiac contractility are usually not evident. Nifedipine does not decrease AV conduction. Thus, nifedipine is safer to administer to patients with bradycardia, heart failure, or AV conduction abnormalities. The effect of nifedipine in decreasing systemic vascular resistance is often associated with a reflex increase in heart rate that may preclude giving nifedipine (Procardia) to the patient with tachycardia.

Many patients are given long-acting nitrates, beta blockers, and/or calcium antagonists concomitantly. Continuing angina at low levels of effort is generally considered an indication for coronary arteriography and, when appropriate, coronary artery revascularization or PTCA.

Carefully supervised and individually developed physical training and exercise programs are also appropriate for patients with stable angina. The major benefit of training appears to be to improve the hemodynamic response to exercise, including reducing heart rate and blood pressure changes for any given exercise effort. Exercise training may also improve skeletal muscle performance at any given blood flow, thus contributing to improved effort tolerance in patients with coronary artery disease. Whether exercise programs increase collateral coronary blood flow is controversial.

Pain relief occurs following complete bed rest in 90 per cent of patients with unstable angina. Patients who continue to have pain while at bed rest are given nitrates initially orally, sublingually, and/or topically. If angina at rest recurs or angina at low levels of effort persists, a slow channel calcium antagonist (nifedipine, verapamil, or diltiazem) should be administered. In the patient with a well-maintained blood pressure and heart rate who has continuing angina at rest or at a low level of effort and in whom coronary artery spasm (Prinzmetal's angina) is not believed to be the pathophysiologic mechanism, a beta blocker may be administered. In the patient believed to have coronary artery spasm, i.e., those having chest pain at rest with transient ST segment elevation during the episode of pain and without a preceding increase in heart rate or blood pressure, calcium antagonists should be used instead of a beta blocker. If angina at rest persists or recurs,

*Investigational drug.

TABLE 51–4. PHARMACOLOGIC EFFECTS OF THE CALCIUM CHANNEL BLOCKERS

	Heart Rate		Conduction SA Node	Conduction AV Node	Myocardial Contractility	Peripheral Vasodilator	Cardiac Output	Coronary Blood Flow	Myocardial O₂ Demand
	Acute	Chronic							
Diltiazem	↓	↓	↓	↓	↓	↓	V	↑	↓
Nifedipine	↑	↑	—	↑	↓	↓↓	↑	↑↑	↓
Verapamil	↓	↓	↓	↓	↓↓	↓↓	V	↑	↓

↓ = decrease; ↑ = increase; — = no change; V = variable effect.
Modified from Packer M, Frishman WH: Calcium Channel Antagonists in Cardiovascular Disease. East Norwalk, CT, Appleton-Century-Crofts, 1984, p 13.

TABLE 51–5. CLINICAL USE OF CALCIUM CHANNEL BLOCKERS

	Dosage		Onset of Action		Therapeutic Plasma Concentration	Metabolism	Excretion
	Oral	*I.V.*	*Oral*	*I.V.*			
Diltiazem	30–90 mg q 6–8 hr	75–150 µg/kg (10–20 mg)	< 30 min	< 10 min	50–200 ng/ml	Deacetylation N-demethylation O-demethylation	60% fecal
Nifedipine	10–40 mg q 6–8 hr	5–15 µg/kg	< 20 min	< 5 min (3 min sl)	25–100 ng/ml	A hydroxycarboxylic acid and a lactone with no known activity	20–40% fecal 50–80% renal
Verapamil	80–120 mg q 6–12 hr	150 µg/kg (10–20 mg)	< 30	< 5 min	80–300 ng/ml	N-dealkylation N-demethylation Major hepatic first pass effect	15% fecal 70% renal

sl = sublingual.

Reproduced with permission from Packer M, Frishman WH: Calcium Channel Antagonists in Cardiovascular Disease. East Norwalk, CT, Appleton-Century-Crofts, 1984, p 8.

intravenous nitroglycerin is begun. In selected patients with angina at rest despite the therapy outlined above, intra-aortic balloon counterpulsation may be utilized. The equivalent of one to four aspirin per day has been shown to reduce the risk of death and myocardial infarction for up to two years after the development of unstable angina. If pain relief does not occur with bed rest and the use of appropriate drugs, the risk of subsequent myocardial infarction, sudden death, or important ventricular arrhythmias is increased.

Coronary arteriography is generally recommended in patients with unstable angina pectoris once the pain is controlled and a myocardial infarct is excluded. In the patient in whom angina at rest recurs despite a good medical regimen, cardiac catheterization and coronary arteriography become almost mandatory. This approach is recommended because 10 to 15 per cent of patients with this syndrome have significant (≥50 per cent stenosis) main left coronary artery disease; in these patients, coronary artery bypass surgery has been shown to prolong their lives. Approximately 10 per cent of patients with unstable angina have no angiographic evidence of significant coronary artery stenoses. Thus, in 25 per cent of these patients, the angiographic findings help to provide a therapeutic approach. In the remaining patients, identifying the location and extent of coronary artery disease is helpful prognostically, and in the patient with continuing angina at rest, the arteriographic findings allow the physician to consider coronary bypass surgery or angioplasty (PTCA).

Subsequently, in those patients in whom angina is controlled medically and in whom there are no coronary angiographic findings requiring revascularization, exercise testing is usually performed. Submaximal exercise tests are often obtained within four to ten days after the angina is controlled, followed several weeks later by a more vigorous exercise test. Patients with continuing angina or objective evidence of intermittent myocardial ischemia at low levels of activity despite a good medical regimen and those with significant three-vessel coronary artery stenoses and depressed left ventricular function (left ventricular ejection fraction, or LVEF <50 per cent) usually undergo coronary artery revascularization, either by coronary artery bypass grafting or by PTCA.

Variant angina is generally treated with nitrates or calcium antagonists or both, including nifedipine, verapamil, or diltiazem. Calcium antagonists appear to be particularly successful in reducing the frequency of episodes of coronary artery spasm. Direct coronary artery surgery and coronary angioplasty have not been as successful in these patients as in those with more typical angina pectoris, although these therapeutic approaches are used in patients with important underlying coronary artery stenoses in whom one cannot obtain symptomatic relief of the angina. One report (Bertrand, 1980) suggests that plexectomy coupled with coronary artery revas-

cularization may be more successful than revascularization by itself.

DIRECT CORONARY ARTERY SURGERY. Large groups of patients now have undergone direct coronary artery surgery in the form of saphenous vein or internal mammary artery bypass grafting (see Ch. 51.3). These surgical procedures result in relief or reduction in the frequency of angina for months to years after the procedure in the majority of patients. For patients with significant left main coronary artery stenoses and/or three-vessel stenoses and impaired left ventricular function, improved survival has been documented following coronary artery revascularization. The best results from coronary artery surgery are obtained in (1) patients with "limiting angina" who are on a medical regimen and who have important proximal coronary artery narrowing but good distal vessels and (2) patients in whom the most important obstructing lesions can be bypassed completely with coronary revascularization. Recent evidence also suggests that the internal mammary artery graft represents the best surgical revascularization because of its durability and effectiveness.

Graft occlusion during the first year in most reported series varies from 10 to 12 per cent. Only a small additional percentage of grafts occlude during the second and third years. However, coronary artery surgery is a palliative procedure, and most patients redevelop angina months to years after the procedure. The most common reason for redevelopment of angina is progression of the intrinsic coronary artery disease. Incomplete revascularization may also be a cause for persistent angina or angina that develops soon after surgery. Graft occlusion and relatively inadequate revascularization with limited increases in coronary blood flow in grafted arteries subsequently are additional reasons for unfavorable results.

Grafted vessels may develop progressive atherosclerosis over time. This occurs most commonly in patients with hypercholesterolemia, in those with diabetes mellitus, and in those with important distal vascular disease such that coronary graft flow is reduced. Native coronary arteries proximal to the site of insertion of coronary artery bypass grafts may develop an accelerated pattern of atherosclerosis following coronary artery surgery. It is almost certainly beneficial to control serum cholesterol concentrations and correct all other risk factors as thoroughly as possible to provide the best opportunity for a prolonged period of coronary graft patency. The administration of aspirin preoperatively or within a few hours of the surgical procedure also appears to be useful in protecting the patency of the coronary artery bypass grafts.

There is a risk of perioperative myocardial infarction, but the frequency with which this occurs is controversial. If the electrocardiogram is used to document the frequency of perioperative infarction, estimates range from 1 to 10 per cent. However, if myocardial scintigraphic techniques are used, the incidence is approximately twice as high. This discrepancy probably reflects "non–Q wave" infarcts not detected by the electrocardiogram.

In addition to the subjective relief of angina that usually occurs for months to years following coronary artery revascularization, some patients also have objective improvement in ventricular function, both at rest and during exercise.

CORONARY ARTERY ANGIOPLASTY. Gruentzig introduced direct coronary artery dilatation with a balloon catheter (PTCA) for proximal coronary artery lesions. This procedure provides a means to increase luminal diameter in selected patients. Important complications occur relatively infrequently. Nevertheless, this procedure should be performed only with facilities available for subsequent direct coronary artery surgery, should that be necessary. Experienced surgeons have a success rate in carefully selected patients of greater than 80 per cent, with less than a 10 per cent risk of acute myocardial infarction or need for emergency coronary artery revascularization. The ideal coronary lesions for PTCA are those with moderately tight proximal stenoses over a short segment and without severe calcification or branch vessel involvement. Left main coronary lesions are not considered suitable for PTCA. Patients are generally pretreated with platelet-active agents (aspirin* and dipyridamole*) and a calcium antagonist in an attempt to reduce the risk of coronary artery spasm during and immediately following angioplasty. Approximately 30 per cent of patients develop restenosis of the dilated coronary artery in the initial six months following the procedure; thus, close follow-up with exercise testing and imaging assessments is important.

PROGNOSIS. There is extreme variance in symptoms and progression of coronary artery stenoses among patients. In some, angina may remain stable for many years. However, approximately 25 per cent of men and 12 per cent of women with angina can expect a myocardial infarct within 5 years. In the population over 55 years of age, the overall 5-year survival rate is 75 per cent for those with stable angina pectoris.

The prognosis of patients with chronic ischemic heart disease is related directly to the location and extent of physiologically important coronary artery stenoses and to left ventricular function. Patients with significant three-vessel coronary stenoses have an expected annual mortality of 6 to 8 per cent; if they also have had a previous myocardial infarction, the mortality rate is increased. On the other hand, patients with significant single-vessel coronary artery disease have an annual mortality rate on medical therapy of approximately 2 to 3 per cent. Patients with main left coronary artery disease equal to or greater than 70 per cent luminal diameter narrowing have a prognosis similar to those with severe three-vessel coronary disease. In fact, most patients with left main coronary artery disease have extensive additional coronary artery stenoses. Survival is also reduced in patients with left ventricular ejection fractions lower than 40 per cent and in those with frequent and complex ventricular ectopy and left ventricular dysfunction. As noted earlier, patients with significant multivessel coronary stenoses, impaired left ventricular function, and objective evidence of myocardial ischemia at relatively low work loads also have a reduced survival with medical therapy.

---

*Investigational uses.

Brensike JF, Levy RI, Kelsey SF, et al.: Effects of therapy with cholestyramine on progression of coronary arteriosclerosis: Results of the NHLBI Type II Coronary Intervention Study. Circulation 69:313, 1984. *A beneficial effect from lowering serum cholesterol values on progression of coronary arteriosclerosis is suggested by these data.*

Folts JD, Crowell EB, Rowe GG: Platelet aggregation in partially obstructed vessels and its elimination with aspirin. Circulation 54:365, 1976. *This study suggests that intermittent platelet aggregation can decrease coronary blood flow in narrowed canine coronary arteries.*

Hillis LD, Braunwald E: Myocardial ischemia. N Engl J Med 296:971, 1977. *A thorough review of myocardial ischemia.*

Hirsh PD, Hillis LD, Campbell WB, et al.: Release of prostaglandins and thromboxane into the coronary circulation in patients with ischemic heart disease. N Engl J Med 304:685, 1981. *Patients with unstable angina have increased transcardiac concentrations of thromboxane occurring in temporal association with unstable angina, thereby suggesting a possible role for platelet aggregation and the release of thromboxane in the pathophysiology of this syndrome.*

Johnson SM, Mauritson DR, Corbett JR, et al.: Double-blind, randomized, placebo-controlled comparison of propranolol and verapamil in the treatment of patients with stable angina pectoris. Am J Med 71:443, 1981. *In 18 patients with exertional angina, propranolol and verapamil were each effective.*

Kannel WB, Feinleib M: Natural history of angina pectoris in the Framingham Study: Prognosis and survival. Am J Cardiol 29:154, 1972. *Of 303 patients with angina followed long term, the mortality averaged about 5 per cent per year in men and 2 to 3 per cent per year in women.*

Maseri A, Severi S, DeNes M, et al.: "Variant" angina: One aspect of a continuous spectrum of vasospastic myocardial ischemia. Am J Cardiol 42:1019, 1978. *Vasospastic angina can occur in the presence of extremely variable degrees of coronary atherosclerosis and in any phase of ischemic heart disease.*

Roberts WC: The coronary arteries and left ventricle in clinically isolated angina pectoris: A necropsy analysis. Circulation 54:388, 1976. *Postmortem findings regarding coronary artery disease and ventriculographic abnormalities in patients with angina pectoris.*

Truett J, Cornfield J, Kannel WB: A multivariate analysis of the risk of coronary heart disease in Framingham. J Chronic Dis 20:511, 1967. *Detailed analysis of risk factors involved in the acquisition of coronary artery disease.*

Willerson JT, Hillis LD, Winniford M, et al.: Speculation regarding mechanisms responsible for acute ischemic heart disease syndromes. J Am Coll Cardiol 8:245, 1986. *Speculations regarding the etiologies for unstable angina and coronary artery spasm.*

51.2 Acute Myocardial Infarction

James T. Willerson

Myocardial infarction is the term used to describe irreversible cellular injury and necrosis occurring as a consequence of prolonged ischemia. Infarction may occur secondary to coronary occlusion, major reduction in blood flow to certain regions of heart muscle, or an insufficient increase in coronary blood flow relative to regional oxygen demand during periods of severe stress. In almost every instance, some degree of narrowing of coronary artery luminal diameter resulting from coronary atherosclerosis exists, but there are exceptions. Acute myocardial infarcts may also result from coronary artery dissection, coronary emboli, coronary artery spasm, vasculitis, anomalous origin of one of the coronary arteries from the pulmonary artery, and congenital coronary arteriovenous fistula.

The pathogenesis of coronary atherosclerosis is considered in detail in Ch. 50 and in brief in Ch. 51.1.

RISK FACTORS FOR CORONARY ARTERY DISEASE. Several epidemiologic studies have established that hyperlipidemia, especially hypercholesterolemia, constitutes a major risk factor predisposing to the development of premature atherosclerosis. Approximately one third of survivors of acute myocardial infarction at an age less than 60 years have some form of hyperlipidemia, defined as serum cholesterol and/or triglyceride levels above the ninety-fifth percentile for the control population. Other factors associated with an increased risk of development of coronary atherosclerotic disease include systemic arterial hypertension, smoking, lack of regular physical activity, and emotional stress. Risk factors are discussed more extensively in Ch. 40 and 50.

MECHANISMS OF ACUTE MYOCARDIAL INFARCTION. Acute myocardial infarction occurs primarily in patients with significant coronary artery disease (Fig. 51–1). In such patients, the primary determinants of vulnerability to acute myocardial infarction include (1) prolonged increases in myocardial oxygen demand under conditions in which increases in oxygen delivery cannot occur because of significant coronary artery disease (included are prolonged and marked increases in heart rate, contractility, and myocardial wall tension) or (2) primary decreases in oxygen delivery to the

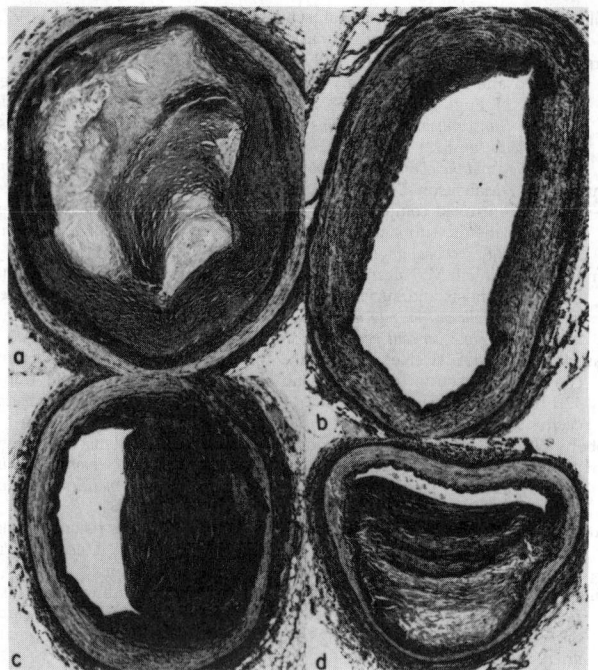

FIGURE 51–1. Sections of coronary arteries at sites of maximal narrowing in a 54-year-old woman who died suddenly at home. She had angina pectoris. *a,* Right coronary artery 3 cm from the aortic ostium. The lumen is more than 90 per cent obstructed. *b,* Left main coronary artery. *c,* Left circumflex coronary artery in the first 1 cm. *d,* Left anterior descending coronary artery 3 cm from the bifurcation of the left main coronary artery. These sections demonstrate the extent of coronary artery disease that may be present in an individual patient. (From Roberts WC: Circulation 48:1161, 1973. Reproduced by permission of The American Heart Association, Inc.)

myocardium. The latter may be caused by (1) coronary artery thrombosis, (2) coronary artery spasm, (3) hemorrhage into an atherosclerotic plaque, and (4) systemic arterial hypotension (coronary artery perfusion is dependent on mean and diastolic aortic blood pressure).

Several clinicopathologic studies of patients with fatal ischemic heart disease and clinical evaluations in patients with evolving acute myocardial infarcts have established that approximately 90 per cent of "Q wave infarcts" (usually transmural myocardial infarcts) are caused by proximal coronary artery occlusion by a thrombus. The coronary thrombosis generally occurs at a tight stenosis and often in association with hemorrhage into an ulcerated atherosclerotic plaque. In contrast, only about 30 per cent of "non–Q wave infarcts" (usually subendocardial myocardial infarcts) have an occlusive coronary thrombus in the infarct-related artery. Instead, most of these patients have significant multivessel coronary artery stenoses and a low-flow state, possibly associated with microthrombosis due to platelet aggregation at sites of severe coronary artery stenosis.

In a clinicopathologic study of 100 episodes of acute ischemic heart disease, the incidence of acute coronary occlusion was 61 per cent (57 in situ thrombi, 2 thromboemboli, and 2 isolated plaque hemorrhages), including 90 per cent for transmural infarcts, 35 per cent for subendocardial infarcts, and 11 per cent for multifocal microinfarcts associated with clinical acute coronary insufficiency syndromes (Buja and Willerson). The incidence of plaque erosion or rupture with coronary thrombus formation was 68 per cent for infarcts of age three weeks or less but decreased to 20 per cent with older infarcts, probably because organization and healing made identification of these lesions more difficult. Other investigators, using serial section techniques, have described a higher incidence (usually over 90 per cent) of plaque erosion

and rupture associated with major plaque hemorrhage and acute coronary artery thrombosis. Potential causative factors for plaque rupture include hemodynamic trauma, inflammatory or chemical injury to coronary artery endothelium and subendothelial tissue, increased intraplaque pressure resulting from infiltration of blood or other mechanisms, and coronary vasospasm. Factors to be considered in the development of coronary artery thrombosis are platelet aggregation; local increase of catecholamines; autonomic neural influences; and local alterations in fibrinolytic systems related to potential decreases in prostacyclin, tissue plasminogen-activating factor, and/or endothelial relaxing factor at sites of coronary artery stenosis and endothelial injury and to increases in thromboxane A_2 and serotonin released from aggregating platelets and/or infiltrating white blood cells at the same sites. Local increases in thromboxane A_2 and serotonin promote platelet aggregation and potentially are capable of altering coronary artery tone dynamically by increasing coronary vascular resistance, thereby decreasing coronary blood flow.

It also seems plausible that coronary artery thrombosis may develop without plaque disruption in severely stenotic coronary arteries. Experimental studies in canine models show increased coronary vascular resistance and reduced reflow in the necrotic or severely damaged subendocardium after 90 to 120 minutes of coronary artery occlusion. Coronary collateral flow may sometimes compensate for acute coronary thrombosis so that no important myocardial necrosis results. It seems likely that variations in the extent of generalized coronary atherosclerosis and of coronary collateral flow may influence the extent and location of acute infarction subsequent to acute coronary thrombosis.

Sudden cardiac death syndromes and acute myocardial infarction are usually separate entities with differing pathogenesis, since the majority of patients resuscitated from sudden death do not develop evidence of important myocardial infarction. Sudden cardiac death usually is caused by a primary ventricular arrhythmia, usually ventricular tachycardia or fibrillation, often produced by an acute ischemic event but not involving major coronary thrombosis, or it may be caused by ventricular ectopy occurring against a background of chronic coronary artery disease and ventricular scarring, but not necessarily triggered by acute myocardial ischemia.

RECOGNITION OF ACUTE MYOCARDIAL INFARCTS.
History. The history is of the utmost importance in the recognition of acute myocardial infarction. Typically, the chest pain is severe and usually lasts until the patient receives analgesic medication from a physician. The pain is ordinarily described as being substernal or left precordial and as a "heaviness" or "tightness," or "like a weight on my chest," and is often associated with nausea and diaphoresis. The chest pain may radiate to the back, the neck, the jaw, or the left arm, particularly down its ulnar aspect. Occasionally, the pain may exist only in the back, the jaw, the left arm, or the neck. Chest pain in patients with acute myocardial infarcts generally lasts longer than 30 minutes and is typically the most severe pain an individual has experienced. Many patients have unstable angina pectoris for hours to days prior to their acute myocardial infarcts; by contrast, 10 to 20 per cent of patients have "silent," i.e., painless or relatively painless, infarcts. Painless infarction is noted with special frequency in diabetic patients and following cardiac transplantation.

Physical Examination. GENERAL. Patients with small myocardial infarcts, particularly non–Q wave infarcts, may not have detectable abnormalities on physical examination. At the other extreme, patients with more than 40 per cent irreversible cellular damage to the left ventricle often develop severe left ventricular failure with pulmonary edema and cardiogenic shock.

INSPECTION AND PALPATION. The findings depend on the extent of the myocardial damage. Most patients are in obvious discomfort. They are often diaphoretic, pale, and extremely anxious. Those with extensive damage develop a reduction in systemic arterial blood pressure ranging from mild to severe. Cardiogenic shock is defined as hypotension resulting from extensive myocardial damage with evidence of inadequate systemic perfusion, such as cool skin, mental confusion, and oliguria. Patients with extensive myocardial necrosis may also have an alternating force of their pulse (pulsus alternans). Most patients have frequent ventricular premature beats.

Patients with second- or third-degree atrioventricular block may have intermittent cannon A waves in their jugular venous pulse. Patients with atrial fibrillation lack an A wave and have an irregular pulse. Patients with right ventricular failure usually have an increased jugular venous pressure.

AUSCULTATION. Fourth heart sounds are almost invariably heard, and all the heart sounds are usually soft. When the mitral valve apparatus is damaged, a new murmur of mitral insufficiency may be audible. These murmurs have variable auscultatory characteristics and may occur in mid to late systole or be holosystolic. Acute mitral insufficiency occurs most commonly in patients with inferior, lateral, or subendocardial myocardial infarcts. Patients with inferior myocardial infarcts and structural damage to the tricuspid valve may develop tricuspid insufficiency. Rupture of the interventricular septum occurs most commonly in patients with acute anterior myocardial infarcts. Murmurs resulting from ventricular septal defects are located along the lower left sternal border and are holosystolic. They may radiate toward the cardiac apex. Acute interventricular septal defects are often associated with a systolic thrill along the left sternal border. The distinction between a holosystolic murmur caused by acute mitral insufficiency and a ruptured septum is not always clear on physical examination.

Third heart sounds may occur in patients with ventricular filling pressures of 15 mm Hg or greater (ventricular failure) or in those with at least moderately severe mitral insufficiency. The second heart sound is paradoxically split in some patients with left ventricular failure, in some with left bundle branch block, and in some during chest pain. The pulmonic closure sound is increased in intensity in patients with pulmonary hypertension resulting from left ventricular failure. Pericardial friction rubs are detected in less than 10 per cent of patients with acute myocardial infarcts. Patients with audible pericardial friction rubs are ordinarily those with the largest Q wave infarcts. If large pericardial effusions develop, heart sounds may be distant and the jugular venous pressure is elevated. Cardiac tamponade results in shock, pulsus paradoxus, distant heart sounds, and an elevated jugular venous pressure. Bibasilar or more extensive moist rales develop in patients with left ventricular failure. Pulmonary edema occurs with extensive myocardial infarction and in patients with myocardial ischemia superimposed on extensive myocardial infarction. Evidence of reduced peripheral perfusion accompanied by clear lungs and an elevated jugular venous pressure should raise the question of extensive right ventricular infarction in the patient with an inferior myocardial infarct.

Electrocardiographic Diagnosis. The electrocardiogram (ECG) provides an excellent means for recognition of acute Q wave myocardial infarction (Figs. 51–2 to 51–4). The characteristic sequence of ECG alterations with Q wave infarction is as follows: (1) the initial development of prominent, peaked T waves in the ECG leads, representing sites of epicardial injury; (2) the development of hyperacute ST segment elevation; and (3) the development of significant Q waves, i.e., of 0.04 second in duration, and/or loss of more than 30 per cent of the amplitude of the R wave (Fig. 51–2). The rate of evolution of these ECG changes is variable; they may occur in minutes or may be delayed for several hours. Some patients with acute myocardial infarcts have relatively normal electrocardiograms in the first few hours after the event. Problems in using the ECG to identify acute myocardial infarction are

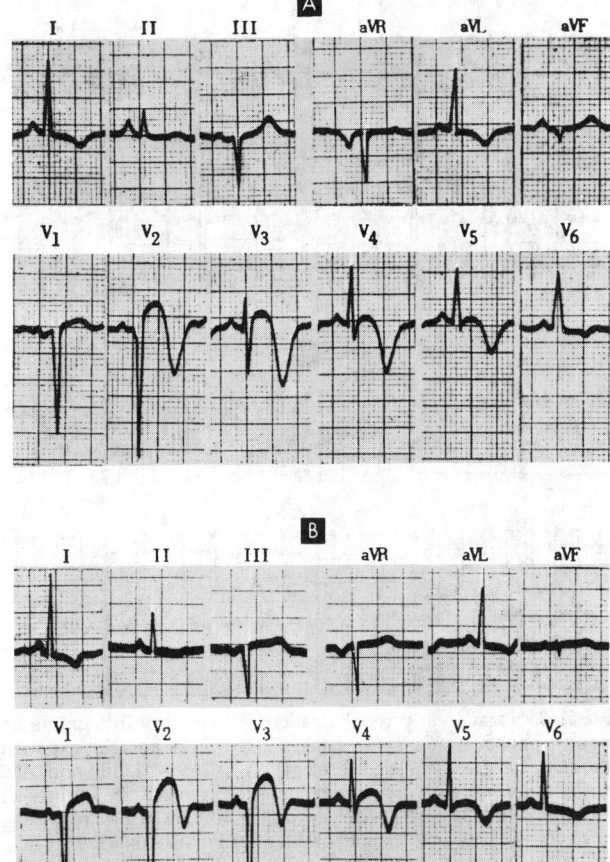

FIGURE 51–2. Acute anteroseptal myocardial infarction. Panel *A* was obtained on the day of hospitalization and demonstrates inverted T waves in V$_2$ through V$_5$ and a Q wave in V$_2$. Panel *B* was obtained three days later and shows further evolutionary changes compatible with an acute anteroseptal myocardial infarction. (Reproduced by permission from Lipman BS, Massie E, Kleiger RE: Clinical Scalar Electrocardiography. 6th ed. Chicago, Year Book Medical Publishers, 1979.)

as follows: (1) In patients with left bundle branch block, acute anterior myocardial infarcts are not recognized by the ECG; (2) in patients with previous Q wave infarction, recognition of new injury can be difficult; and (3) in individuals in whom rapid ECG evolution occurs, it may not be possible to differentiate old from new myocardial infarction. ST segment elevation may also occur (1) with normal early repolarization (Fig. 51–3); (2) with transient myocardial ischemia, as in Prinzmetal's angina or with ischemia in an area of previous myocardial damage; (3) in some individuals with chronic ventricular aneurysms; (4) transiently, following electrical cardioversion; (5) in the anterior precordial ECG leads in patients with left bundle branch block; (6) in patients with left ventricular hypertrophy; and (7) in some patients with hyperkalemia.

In contrast to the usefulness of the ECG in the recognition of Q wave myocardial infarcts, the ECG does not allow one to recognize acute non–Q wave myocardial infarction with certainty. The ECG demonstrates ST depression and T wave inversion with non–Q wave myocardial infarction; the only evolution is a return toward baseline. Unfortunately, subendocardial ischemia, ventricular hypertrophy, rapid heart rates, emotional influences, electrolyte alterations, and the use of certain medications, including cardiac glycosides, may produce the same ECG changes. Indeed, bizarre T wave altera-

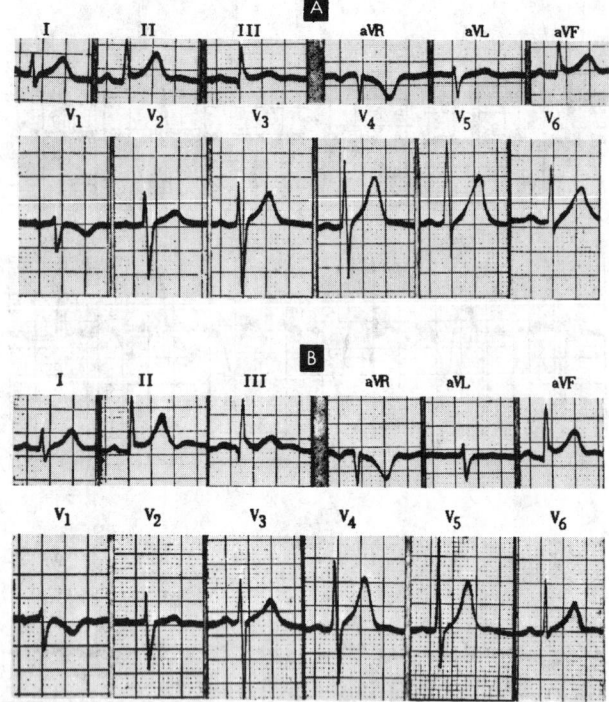

FIGURE 51–3. Normal early repolarization. The electrocardiograms obtained in panels A and B were taken two weeks apart in a patient without heart disease. The ST elevation in leads II, III, and AVF represent normal early repolarization. (Reproduced by permission from Lipman BS, Massie E, Kleiger RE: Clinical Scalar Electrocardiography. 6th ed. Chicago, Year Book Medical Publishers, 1979.)

tions occur sometimes in patients with intracranial hemorrhage. The only useful rule in the ECG recognition of non–Q wave myocardial infarction is that the deeper the ST segment depression and the longer it lasts, the more likely the presence of myocardial infarction.

Serum Enzyme Changes. Currently, the preferred enzymatic technique for detection of myocardial infarction is the measurement of creatine kinase (CK) and in particular the "myocardial specific" CK-MB isoenzyme measured by spectrophotometric, fluorometric, or radioimmunoassay technique. CK-MB increases in the sera of patients approximately 2 to 4 hours after acute myocardial infarction, peaks within 12 hours with small or reperfused infarcts and between 16 and 24 hours with large or non-reperfused infarcts, and often returns to normal within 24 to 36 hours after the event. Radioimmunoassay measurement of alterations in serum myoglobin concentration allows slightly earlier recognition of acute myocardial infarction, but at present there is no means to distinguish between myoglobin release from the heart and from the skeletal muscle when both are injured. Radioimmunoassay measurement of alterations in the serum concentration of the light chain of myosin may also allow a relatively early recognition of acute myocardial infarction. In the past, serial serum measurements of glutamic-oxaloacetic transaminase (SGOT), lactic dehydrogenase (LDH), or the LDH isoenzymes were used to recognize acute myocardial infarction.

Myocardial Scintigraphy. The use of radionuclide scintigraphic techniques to recognize acute myocardial infarction has gained in popularity (see Ch. 41.4). These techniques allow one to see the region or regions of acute myocardial infarction (infarct-avid imaging techniques) or to identify areas of severely decreased myocardial perfusion (cold spot imaging techniques). The prototype infarct-avid imaging agent is technetium 99m stannous pyrophosphate. This agent accumulates in irreversibly damaged myocardium one to five days after infarction; its sensitivity in the detection of acute infarction of

3 grams or larger is greater than 90 per cent when tomographic imaging is utilized. Thallium 201 is the perfusion imaging agent of choice at present. When used within 12 hours after acute infarction, its sensitivity is approximately 90 per cent. The extent of the initial ^{201}Tl defect and the volume of pyrophosphate uptake after acute myocardial infarction have prognostic significance; the larger the volume of pyrophosphate uptake or of the ^{201}Tl perfusion defect, the poorer the in-hospital prognosis. Finally, one may employ technetium-labelled red blood cells to evaluate the impact of acute myocardial infarction on regional and global ventricular function, using "dynamic myocardial scintigraphy." This technique allows one to measure or identify ventricular ejection fraction, ventricular volumes, regional wall motion, left-to-right shunts (i.e., ventricular septal defects), ventricular aneurysms, and valvular insufficiency, including mitral or tricuspid regurgitation.

DIFFERENTIAL DIAGNOSIS. The differential diagnosis of acute myocardial infarction theoretically includes every cause of chest pain, cardiac arrhythmia, and heart failure. Important diagnostic considerations are (1) unstable angina pectoris, (2) variant (Prinzmetal's) angina, and (3) dissecting aortic aneurysm. Less common as difficult diagnoses to exclude, but still sometimes important to differentiate, are (1) peptic ulcer disease, (2) pancreatitis, (3) cholecystitis, (4) pulmonary embolic disease, (5) spontaneous pneumothorax, (6) pericarditis, and (7) pneumonitis. Careful attention to the history and physical examination and the proper use of

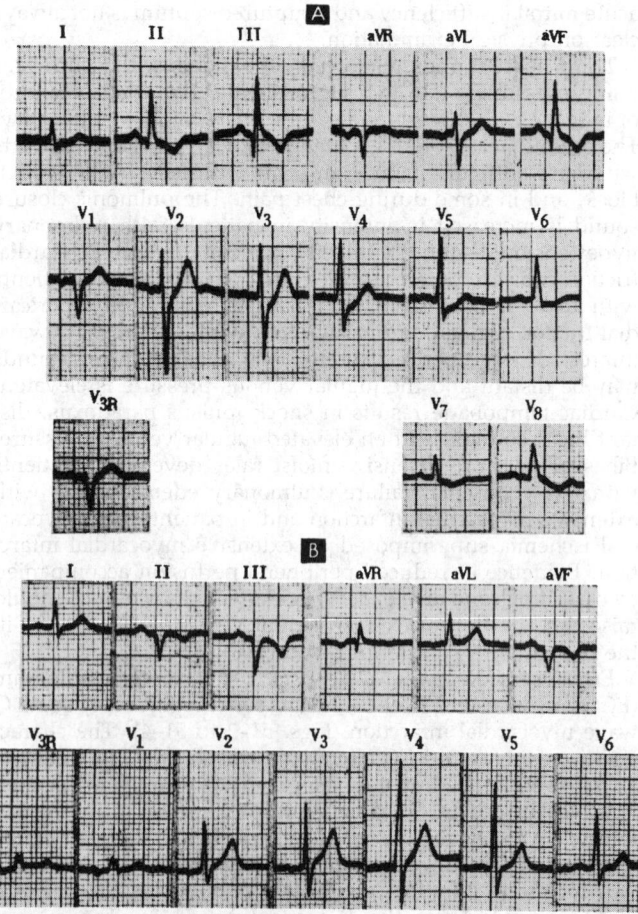

FIGURE 51–4. A true posterior myocardial infarct (panel B). Panel A contains the ECG of a middle-aged male eight hours following the onset of severe chest pain. Panel B demonstrates the ECG 72 hours later, at which time prominent R waves have developed in precordial leads V₁ and V₂. Panel B also demonstrates an acute inferior transmural myocardial infarct.

relevant blood tests, electrocardiograms, and myocardial scintigraphy usually allow one to make the proper diagnosis.

COMPLICATIONS OF ACUTE MYOCARDIAL INFARCTS. *Mechanical Complications.* Patients with cardiogenic shock as a consequence of extensive left ventricular damage occurring with acute myocardial infarction have a poor prognosis. Cardiac assistance devices such as intra-aortic balloon counterpulsation have reduced mortality slightly in patients with acute myocardial infarcts and cardiogenic shock, particularly when coupled with coronary artery revascularization or ventricular aneurysmectomy. However, the extent of myocardial damage is generally so severe that a majority of these patients still succumb.

An important complication of acute myocardial infarction is infarct extension or expansion. Approximately 10 per cent of patients extend their myocardial infarcts within the first five days. The incidence is slightly higher for those with anterior Q wave infarcts and those with subendocardial ischemia or non–Q wave infarction or both at hospital admission, and the consequences of infarct extension for patients in these groups are more serious. The incidence of infarct extension is approximately twice as high when assessed by laboratory methods as by clinical symptoms alone. Infarct expansion (dilatation of the infarct region secondary to stress-and-strain relationships) may be associated with worsening ventricular function and increased morbidity and mortality.

Other mechanical problems that may complicate acute myocardial infarction include papillary muscle dysfunction or rupture with consequent acute mitral regurgitation, and the development of a ventricular septal defect. Rupture of an entire papillary muscle is ordinarily fatal within minutes to hours owing to massive mitral regurgitation, which results in severe left ventricular failure and cardiogenic shock. Rupture of one head of a papillary muscle may be tolerated for longer periods of time, allowing clinical evaluation and occasionally surgical correction. Partial or complete rupture of a papillary muscle occurs in less than 5 per cent of patients with acute infarction. Dysfunction of a papillary muscle occurs more commonly when ischemia or infarction of the papillary muscle prevents proper coaptation of the mitral leaflets, causing mitral regurgitation. Patients with papillary muscle dysfunction generally have milder left ventricular failure and are responsive to medical intervention. Patients who develop acute mitral insufficiency usually do so within one to seven days after acute myocardial infarction.

Rupture of a portion of the ventricular septum is usually associated with a holosystolic murmur and systolic thrill along the left sternal border. Ventricular septal defects develop in about 1 per cent of patients with acute myocardial infarcts and often result in right and left ventricular failure. They may occur within hours or as late as 10 to 12 days following infarction. If ventricular failure is severe, one must consider emergency surgical correction even though surgical mortality rates are highest within the first month after myocardial infarction. Afterload reduction using intra-aortic balloon counterpulsation or pharmacologic means, or both, may benefit patients with ventricular septal defects or mitral regurgitation occurring acutely after myocardial infarction.

Ventricular aneurysms usually develop within hours of myocardial infarction and may enlarge over subsequent weeks or months. If sizable, they may result in congestive heart failure. They may also be associated with ventricular arrhythmias or with mural thrombosis and systemic embolization. Left ventricular endocardial thrombi can be demonstrated in at least 50 per cent of patients with ventricular aneurysms at autopsy.

Right ventricular infarction develops occasionally in patients with inferoposterior myocardial infarction. Occasionally, right ventricular involvement may be sufficient to cause systemic hypotension with low pulmonary capillary wedge and left ventricular filling pressures. Alternatively, extensive right ventricular infarction may simulate a large pericardial effusion and cardiac tamponade. Recognition is important, since proper therapy includes fluid administration, which is not usually employed in the hypotensive patient with a dominant left ventricular infarct. Right ventricular infarction may also lead to tricuspid valvular insufficiency secondary to papillary muscle dysfunction.

Arrhythmias and Heart Block. More than 90 per cent of patients develop ventricular premature beats in the first 72 hours after acute myocardial infarction. Ventricular premature beats can be suppressed by pharmacologic intervention in most patients. However, in those with large infarcts, they may be difficult to suppress, and death may occur because of medically refractory arrhythmias.

Various types of atrioventricular and intraventricular blocks (see Ch. 45) may occur as a consequence of acute myocardial infarction. First-degree heart block is common with acute inferior infarction, and as an isolated finding, it is not a cause for concern. Second-degree heart block of the Mobitz I type (Wenckebach block) also occurs following acute inferior infarction. It is usually transient, and even if it progresses to complete heart block, it is usually only temporary. Temporary pacemaker insertion is indicated only in patients with Mobitz I block who have slow ventricular rates resulting in syncope, congestive heart failure, angina pectoris, or ventricular arrhythmias. Mobitz II heart block occurs most often as a consequence of anterior myocardial infarction. The level of block is located below the atrioventricular junction within the ventricle. Mobitz II block should be treated with a pacemaker as soon as it is recognized. Permanent pacing is indicated in such patients at a later date.

Complete heart block may develop abruptly or follow either of the two forms of second-degree heart block described above. Complete heart block complicating acute anterior myocardial infarction is often permanent and usually requires permanent pacing. It often coexists with other signs of a large infarct, and the subsequent prognosis is poor. Complete heart block after inferior myocardial infarction is ordinarily only transient, and temporary ventricular pacing almost always suffices.

Acute left bundle branch block ordinarily develops as a consequence of a large anterior myocardial infarction. The risk of complete heart block in patients who develop left bundle branch block with acute infarction is approximately 40 per cent, and many physicians elect to insert a temporary pacemaker prophylactically. The acute development of right bundle branch block is not a reflection of infarct size and does not necessarily indicate a high risk of complete heart block. Bilateral bundle branch block (left-axis deviation and right bundle branch block, right-axis deviation and right bundle branch block, or first-degree atrioventricular block and left bundle branch block) that develops acutely after myocardial infarction indicates a large infarct and a relatively poor prognosis with a high risk of complete heart block. These patterns develop most commonly with anterior infarction, and temporary pace-makers should be inserted. Many patients who develop acute bilateral bundle branch block die as a consequence of a low-output state. Those patients who survive and have even transient atrioventricular block in the hospital should be paced permanently.

Other Complications. Other complications of acute myocardial infarction include (1) pericarditis, (2) pulmonary emboli, (3) lower extremity venous thrombosis, (4) systemic arterial embolization, (5) rupture of the heart, (6) Dressler's syndrome, and (7) the shoulder-hand syndrome. Pericarditis is evident clinically in 7 to 15 per cent of patients with acute infarcts. However, a higher percentage have transient pleuritic chest pain, which itself may indicate pericarditis. Pericarditis generally occurs with transmural infarcts of at least moderate size. Pericarditis may be recognized by auscultation of a pericardial friction rub, but the majority of patients with pericarditis in this setting do not have rubs. The pain of pericarditis must be distinguished from the pain of persistent angina. Anticoagulation should be avoided (if possible) in patients with pericarditis in order to minimize the risk of hemorrhagic pericardial effusion.

Pulmonary embolism is treated with heparinization followed by longer-term anticoagulation; lower extremity venous thrombosis is treated similarly. Systemic embolization is generally due to a mural thrombus developing in the damaged left ventricle, and when it occurs, anticoagulation is indicated. The visualization of a left ventricular thrombus in a patient soon after anterior myocardial infarction should also result in the administration of anticoagulants.

Rupture of the heart occurs one to ten days following infarction and is the cause of death in 2 to 15 per cent of fatal cases. Rupture is most common in patients with systemic arterial hypertension and following an initial anterior infarct. The classic clinical clue indicating myocardial rupture is "electromechanical dissociation," in which electrical activity persists without detectable blood pressure or pulse. When rupture occurs, death is ordinarily so rapid that surgical intervention is not possible. An occasional patient, however, may develop a slow leak of blood into the pericardial space, and clotting of blood may serve to compress and partially seal the tear in the heart. This may allow emergency pericardiocentesis and an attempt at surgical repair. Untreated survivors of a sealed-off rupture typically develop "false aneurysms" of the left ventricle; the "false aneurysms" have a high risk of rupture and should be repaired surgically.

Dressler's syndrome is characterized by pericarditis and pericardial effusion, pleural effusion, and often fever two weeks to nine months after myocardial infarction. The etiology of this syndrome is not clear. It is treated with aspirin or indomethacin. If these agents are unsuccessful, steroids usually relieve the chest pain, suppress the fever, and result in the ultimate disappearance of the effusions.

The shoulder-hand syndrome, of rare occurrence, consists of the development of pain and stiffness in the left shoulder or hand and vasomotor changes sometimes associated with muscle atrophy. Typically, it occurs several weeks to months after the infarct. It is believed that prolonged immobilization and bed rest used to treat patients with acute myocardial infarction in the past may have been responsible for the development of this problem.

ESTIMATION OF INFARCT SIZE. Accurate measurements of the extent of reversible and irreversible cellular damage are helpful. Such measurements should be relatively noninvasive, ideally should be applicable early in the patient's clinical course, should be capable of being repeated with reasonable frequency, should provide measurements of the extent of damage with various types of infarcts, and should be available generally. No perfect measurement of infarct size or of the extent of ischemic damage exists at present, but there are many promising developments. Included among these are (1) enzymatic indices of infarct size, including, most importantly, measurement of creatine kinase enzyme release from the heart; (2) electrocardiographic estimates of the extent of ischemic injury, including precordial electrocardiographic mapping to identify the extent of QRS alterations; (3) scintigraphic measurements of infarct size, including infarct-avid and cold spot techniques (see above); (4) dynamic myocardial scintigraphy to estimate abnormalities of global and segmental ventricular function, using either first-pass or equilibrium studies; and (5) two-dimensional echocardiography. Each of these techniques has its limitations, but each also provides important information concerning location or relative size of infarcts. For the scintigraphic measurements, it is necessary to use three-dimensional estimates of the extent of myocardial damage; tomographic cameras are available that provide three-dimensional estimates of infarct size and of the extent

of perfusion defects and also allow estimates of global and regional ventricular function.

EVALUATION OF VENTRICULAR FUNCTION IN PATIENTS WITH MYOCARDIAL INFARCTS. Invasive and noninvasive techniques have been developed to allow more precise characterization of ventricular function in patients with reduced systemic arterial blood pressure and uncertain left ventricular functional status in order to assess the need for volume replacement, diuresis, or inotropic support. A flow-directed catheter, such as the Swan-Ganz catheter, allows measurement of left ventricular filling pressure without entering a systemic artery or the left ventricle. This balloon-tipped, flow-directed catheter may be placed in the pulmonary artery from a systemic vein. One positions the Swan-Ganz catheter in the pulmonary artery, either with the aid of fluoroscopy or with continuous pressure monitoring to identify the characteristic right atrial, right ventricular, and pulmonary artery pressures. Once the catheter is in the pulmonary artery, the balloon is partly inflated, allowing the measurement of pulmonary capillary wedge pressure. In the absence of mitral valve or pulmonary venous disease, the mean pulmonary capillary wedge pressure approximates the left ventricular end-diastolic or filling pressure. Measurements of left ventricular filling pressure with the Swan-Ganz catheter differentiate between hypotension because of hypovolemia and hypotension resulting from left ventricular failure. Cardiac output may also be measured. Patients with acute myocardial infarction and shock often benefit from an indwelling arterial cannula inserted to allow measurement of arterial pressure and moment-to-moment monitoring of pressure changes.

TREATMENT. Patients with proven or suspected acute myocardial infarction should be admitted to a coronary care unit, where their heart rate and rhythm are monitored continuously. In patients evaluated within the first three hours of the onset of symptoms with acute anterior Q wave myocardial infarcts, with new Q wave infarcts and previous myocardial infarction, or with new Q wave infarcts in a low-output state, thrombolytic therapy should probably be administered. Thrombolytic therapy (tissue plasminogen-activating factor, streptokinase, or urokinase) may be given intravenously or directly into the infarct-related coronary artery. When given intravenously four to five hours after the onset of symptoms suggestive of myocardial infarction, tissue plasminogen-activating factor appears superior to streptokinase in achieving thrombolysis. Successful thrombolytic therapy within the first one to two hours after the infarct appears to reduce infarct size, preserve segmental ventricular function, and reduce mortality in patients with anterior Q wave infarcts, in patients with previous infarcts, and in some patients in a low-output state. However, 20 to 30 per cent of patients develop rethrombosis of the infarct-related artery after successful thrombolytic therapy initially, despite the administration of heparin in the initial three to four days followed by warfarin or platelet-active agents (aspirin and dipyridamole) thereafter. Rethrombosis is most likely to occur in patients with the most severe, persistent residual coronary artery stenoses of the infarct-related artery.

Currently, it is not clear whether percutaneous transluminal coronary angioplasty (PTCA) should be used to dilate the infarct-related artery following thrombolytic therapy in an effort to reduce the risk of reocclusion. Future studies will probably identify a severity of residual coronary artery stenosis after thrombolytic therapy that would benefit from PTCA to prevent reocclusion of the infarct-related artery.

More than 90 per cent of patients with acute myocardial infarction have ventricular ectopy, which often requires pharmacologic suppression. Since many of the important complications of acute myocardial infarction occur in the first 96 hours after the event, it is advisable to keep patients in a coronary care unit for this period. Complete bed rest is recommended initially, followed by gradual mobilization of patients who are clinically stable. Emotional stimulation and strenuous physical effort are to be avoided. Chest pain during the initial 24 hours after the infarct is usually treated with narcotics, usually intravenous morphine or meperidine; thereafter, recurrent chest pain believed to represent angina is usually treated with nitrates, and a calcium antagonist, buffered aspirin, and/or beta blockers are used if angina persists. Recent data suggest that in-hospital infarct extension is reduced in patients with non–Q wave infarcts by the calcium antagonist diltiazem. Angina that recurs frequently at minimal activity despite nitrates, calcium antagonists, and/or beta blockers is often treated with a constant intravenous infusion of nitroglycerin. If this is unsuccessful, intra-aortic balloon counterpulsation may be used for temporary control of the angina. However, if this aggressive effort is required to control angina, one also prepares the patient for coronary arteriography, and if the coronary anatomy is suitable, PTCA or coronary artery revascularization is usually performed.

Two points of caution regarding persistent or recurrent angina at rest or at minimal effort in patients with acute myocardial infarction should be emphasized. One needs to determine that intermittent coronary spasm is not responsible for angina that occurs at rest. This determination may be accomplished by obtaining 24-hour multilead ECG monitoring, which allows identification of ST segment shifts (usually elevation) with and without anginal episodes. Such findings unassociated with preceding alterations in blood pressure or heart rate are presumptive evidence of coronary artery spasm or platelet aggregation or both at the site or sites of a severely narrowed coronary artery, causing further phasic reductions in coronary blood flow. Recurrent coronary spasm is treated with nitrates or calcium antagonists, or both, rather than with a beta blocker. Aspirin (one to four 300-mg tablets per 24 hours) may reduce the risk of reinfarction in patients with continuing angina at rest or at low levels of activity (unstable angina) after myocardial infarction. One also needs to be certain that recurrent chest pain after myocardial infarction is not due to pericarditis (which is usually treated with indomethacin or salicylates) or to some noncardiac problem such as atelectasis, pneumonia, pulmonary embolic disease, pancreatitis, peptic ulcer disease, or cholecystitis.

During the initial few hours after acute myocardial infarction, oxygen is usually administered by face mask or nasal cannula. Vital signs are checked frequently, chest pain is relieved with narcotics, and sedatives are provided as necessary. Reassurance that the chest pain will be relieved and that survival is likely is important. Specific complications of the acute myocardial infarction are recognized using the clinical criteria described earlier and the methods described in more detail later in this chapter. Anticoagulants are not administered uniformly to patients with acute myocardial infarction. Some physicians use low-dose heparin to prevent the post–myocardial infarction complications related to prolonged bed rest and restricted activity. Patients with documented left ventricular thrombi after infarction, those with embolic events, and those treated with thrombolytic therapy usually receive heparin for several days, followed by warfarin or platelet-active agents or both. Anticoagulants are relatively contraindicated in the very elderly, in patients with severe hypertension, bleeding diatheses, and peptic ulcer disease, and in those who develop pericarditis. Anticoagulants administered to patients with pericarditis complicating acute myocardial infarction may result in large hemorrhagic pericardial effusions and pericardial tamponade.

Smoking is prohibited in the coronary care unit; subsequently, one attempts to convince the patient to discontinue smoking altogether. The patient with an uncomplicated myocardial infarction is allowed to use a bedside commode, but those with shock, severe heart failure, or frequent and recurrent angina use a Foley catheter or bedpan. Stool softeners and laxatives are administered to prevent fecal impaction and to prevent the patient from straining to defecate.

Patients are allowed regular diets with the following exceptions: Extremes of hot or cold beverages are avoided in the first two or three days, salt restriction is provided for those with important heart failure, low-cholesterol diets are often used, and certain calorie and carbohydrate restrictions are provided for obese and diabetic patients, respectively, Diabetic patients receiving insulin are treated with regular insulin for the initial several days after their infarct.

Patients with uncomplicated myocardial infarction are usually discharged from the coronary care unit after three to four days to an "intermediate care" or "step down" unit. Such areas should be able to monitor heart rate and rhythm for several additional days. Most physicians begin a gradual rehabilitation program that encourages patients to be up in a chair several times a day beginning on approximately day 3 and to walk in their rooms and short distances outside their rooms by five to eight days after myocardial infarction. Patients with complications such as severe congestive heart failure, shock, important arrhythmias, or recurrent angina at rest or at low levels of effort remain in the coronary care unit until they are stable.

Some physicians recommend relatively early discharge from the hospital, even by seven or eight days after the event for patients with uncomplicated myocardial infarcts. Other physicians feel that 10 to 12 days in the hospital are indicated even for those with uncomplicated mycoardial infarcts. Patients with complicated myocardial infarctions remain in the hospital longer. Once at home, patients are gradually rehabilitated so that by four to six weeks they return to work and a more normal lifestyle. Resumption of sexual activity and mild exercise is allowed at approximately four weeks after myocardial infarction for asymptomatic patients. Angina that develops with minimal-to-moderate effort requires medical therapy with long-acting nitrates and, when appropriate, with a beta blocker or a calcium antagonist. Patients who continue to have symptoms at moderate or less effort while on good medical regimens should undergo coronary arteriography and should be considered for coronary artery revascularization. Patients, with their physicians' help, should also be encouraged to correct all risk factors, including overweight, hypercholesterolemia, cigarette smoking, and emotionally difficult circumstances. They should also be encouraged to get appropriate amounts of exercise in the future, but the exact type, duration, and level of effort should be guided by a physician. In addition, three recent studies have demonstrated that the beta-adrenergic antagonists timolol, metoprolol, and propranolol reduce mortality and the risk of reinfarction in selected patients with myocardial infarction when administered within a few hours to a few days after the myocardial infarction and continued for periods ranging from 90 days to 3 years. These beta blockers appear most protective in older patients, in those with larger and anterior infarcts, in patients with transient evidence of heart failure, and in patients with several previous infarcts. More work is needed to identify specific patients most likely to benefit from beta blocker therapy, but it appears that beta-adrenergic blockers have the potential to reduce mortality in patients with recent myocardial infarction considered to be at relatively higher risk for future coronary events. More recently, data have been provided to suggest that aspirin therapy (one 300-mg tablet) after infarction also reduces the risk of subsequent coronary events, especially in patients with well-preserved ventricular function, in patients following their initial myocardial infarction, and in patients with non–Q wave infarcts.

Protection of Ischemic Myocardium and Containment of Infarct Size. There has been considerable interest in the possibility that one may limit infarct size with pharmacologic or physiologic interventions that reduce myocardial oxygen demand, increase myocardial oxygen delivery (increase coronary blood flow), reduce inflammatory processes, reduce or retard lysosomal enzyme release, or alter metabolism or calcium influx in such a way as to prevent cell death. In experimental animals, pharmacologic interventions that increase coronary blood flow to the ischemically injured tissue (particularly the subendocardial region) have been effective in reducing the enzymatic, ECG, and morphologic indices of the size of experimentally induced myocardial infarction. Containment of infarct size depends on pharmacologic intervention within the first six hours after infarction. Beyond that time, some interventions are less successful or ineffective. In experimental animals, certain interventions may increase infarct size. This group includes those interventions that (1) increase myocardial oxygen demand, (2) divert coronary blood flow from the ischemic tissue, (3) reduce systemic arterial pressure and thereby coronary perfusion pressure, (4) alter myocardial metabolism in a detrimental manner, or (5) primarily decrease oxygen availability. In particular, the administration of isoproterenol or the development of hypotension, hypoglycemia, hypoxemia, and rapid heart rates results in an increase in infarct size in experimental animal models. Some of the interventions capable of limiting infarct size in experimental animal models are listed in Table 51–6.

Whether pharmacologic or physiologic interventions other than early thrombolytic therapy are capable of limiting infarct size in patients with acute myocardial infarction is at present unknown. In the future, continuing attention will probably be directed to determining the influence of thrombolytic therapy and selected pharmacologic interventions used together in reducing infarct size and preserving segmental and global left ventricular function.

PROGNOSIS. *In Hospital.* Most patients with acute myocardial infarction have an uncomplicated course. Some patients, however, develop life-threatening complications during the first one to two weeks, and others die (Table 51–7). In the early 1970s, 50 per cent or more of patients died prior to reaching the hospital; these deaths were due to ventricular arrhythmias that developed in the initial seconds or minutes following the onset of chest pain. Optimal emergency ambulance systems have achieved a 25 to 30 per cent reduction in the incidence of death prior to hospitalization in patients with

TABLE 51–6. INTERVENTIONS CAPABLE OF LIMITING INFARCT SIZE IN EXPERIMENTAL ANIMAL MODELS

1. Interventions that reduce myocardial oxygen demand and myocardial work
   a. Beta blockers
   b. Calcium antagonists (nifedipine, verapamil, or diltiazem)
   c. Circulatory assistance (intra-aortic balloon counterpulsation)
2. Interventions that increase coronary blood flow to the damaged myocardium
   a. Nitrates (nitroglycerin)
   b. Calcium antagonists
   c. Hyperosmotic agents (hypertonic mannitol)*
   d. Hyaluronidase
   e. Corticosteroids
   f. Circulatory assistance
3. Agents that decrease inflammation, alter immunologic mechanisms, stabilize lysosomal membranes, and/or directly protect myocardial cells and sarcolemmal membranes
   a. Hyaluronidase
   b. Corticosteroids†
   c. Hypertonic agents (hypertonic mannitol)*
   d. Glucose, potassium, and insulin
   e. Cobra venom
   f. Calcium antagonists
   g. Phospholipase inhibitors
   h. Anti-inflammatory agents

*Effective for approximately one hour after experimental coronary occlusion when serum osmolality is increased by 30 to 40 mOsm.
†Given in modest dosage and only once or twice.

Table 51–7. POTENTIAL LIFE-THREATENING COMPLICATIONS OF ACUTE MYOCARDIAL INFARCTION

Ventricular arrhythmias (ventricular tachycardia, ventricular fibrillation, or asystole)
Extremely rapid atrial arrhythmias in association with extensive myocardial infarction (atrial flutter or atrial fibrillation)
Heart block (second- or third-degree types)
Marked bradycardia
Loss of atrial contribution to cardiac contraction (atrioventricular junctional rhythm)
Infarction $\geq$ 40 per cent of left ventricle
Extensive right ventricular infarction
Acute ventricular septal defects
Acute and severe mitral regurgitation
Severe pulmonary edema
Rupture of the heart
Systemic and/or pulmonary emboli

acute myocardial infarction and sudden cardiac arrest syndromes.

Overall mortality in patients with acute myocardial infarction who reach the hospital ranges from 3 to 30 per cent depending upon the population studied. In general, patients with anterior infarction have a higher mortality than patients with inferior infarction; this appears to be related to greater loss of left ventricular muscle with anterior infarcts.

Patients can be divided into groups with differing prognosis on the basis of initial hemodynamic measurements. Those without left ventricular failure and with a mean systolic arterial pressure of greater than 100 mm Hg, an average cardiac index greater than 2.5 liters per minute per square meter, and a normal pulmonary capillary wedge pressure (or pulmonary artery diastolic pressure) have relatively low mortality rates, i.e., approximately 3 to 12 per cent. Similarly, patients with left and right ventricular ejection fractions greater than 48 per cent have a relatively low in-hospital mortality risk. If death occurs in patients in these groups, it is generally from a ventricular arrhythmia, from later infarct extension, or from a mechanical complication such as myocardial, septal, or papillary muscle rupture. Patients with cardiogenic shock, including hypotension with systolic arterial pressures less than 90 mm Hg, with decreased peripheral perfusion without a reversible cause, with reduced cardiac index (less than 2.0 liters per minute per square meter), and with an increased pulmonary capillary wedge or pulmonary diastolic pressure (greater than 25 mm Hg) have a mortality of greater than 70 per cent. Those with clinical evidence of left ventricular failure and a normal or elevated systemic arterial pressure have an expected mortality rate of 5 to 30 per cent. Patients with left ventricular ejection fractions less than 40 per cent have substantially increased mortality risk in-hospital and following hospital discharge.

Following Hospital Discharge. Long-term mortality risks after recovery from an initial myocardial infarct are related to the presence of ventricular arrhythmias, the extent of myocardial damage, the presence or absence of additional myocardium at risk, and the age of the patient. Patients with left ventricular ejection fractions of 40 per cent and less are at increased risk for future coronary events and sudden deaths. Patients with eight or more ventricular premature beats per hour, coupled ventricular premature beats, and runs of ventricular tachycardia are also at increased risk of sudden death. Patients with both a left ventricular ejection fraction of 40 per cent or less and frequent or complex ventricular premature beats as defined above have an 11 times greater risk of sudden death in the ensuing six months than patients without these clinical characteristics. In addition, patients developing ST depression of 1 mm or greater or a reduction in their left ventricular ejection fraction or an increase in their left ventricular end-systolic volume at low levels of exercise prior to hospital discharge have an increased risk for new coronary events (new myocardial infarct, unstable angina, new or worsening heart failure, and sudden death) in the subsequent eight months. Similarly, patients developing reversible thallium 201 perfusion defects at low levels of exercise also are at increased risk for future coronary events. Finally, patients with previous anterior Q wave and non–Q wave infarcts also have an increased risk of subsequent myocardial infarction in the months following hospital discharge.

With regard to the patients described above, medical therapy should be developed as appropriate for the individual patient. However, when medical therapy does not prevent angina at rest, low-level exercise-induced angina, ECG changes, reductions in left ventricular ejection fractions, increases in left ventricular end-systolic volumes, or reversible perfusion defects, then cardiac catheterization with subsequent coronary revascularization should be considered.

Beta Blocker Heart Attack Study Group: The beta-blocker heart attack trial. JAMA 246:2073, 1981. *This study established the potential value of propranolol in reducing postinfarct mortality in patients.*

Buja LM, Willerson JT: Clinicopathologic correlates of acute ischemic heart disease syndromes. Am J Cardiol 47:343, 1981. *Detailed postmortem pathophysiologic correlates of anatomic and clinical relationships.*

Corbett J, Dehmer GJ, Lewis SE, et al.: The prognostic value of submaximal exercise testing with radionuclide ventriculography following acute myocardial infarction. Circulation 64:535, 1981. *This study demonstrates the prognostic value of submaximal exercise testing coupled with dynamic myocardial scintigraphy in predicting prognosis for patients after their myocardial infarcts. The scintigraphic data added substantially to the ability to predict future prognosis; measurements of alterations in ventricular function at rest and during exercise were more sensitive in predicting future prognosis than were ECG changes alone.*

Gibson RS, Watson DD, Craddock GB, et al.: Prediction of cardiac events after uncomplicated myocardial infarction: A prospective study comparing predischarge exercise thallium-201 scintigraphy and coronary angiography. Circulation 68:321, 1984. *Thallium 201 myocardial scintigraphy with submaximal exercise at hospital discharge following myocardial infarction may be used to identify patients at risk for future ischemic heart disease complications.*

Gruppo Italiano per lo Studio Della Streptochinasi Nell'infarto miocardico (GISSI): Effectiveness of intravenous thrombolytic treatment in acute myocardial infarction. Lancet 1:397, 1986.

Hjalmarson A, Herlitz J, Malek I, et al.: Effect on mortality of metoprolol in acute myocardial infarction. Lancet 2:823, 1981. *The beneficial influence of metoprolol on mortality risk in patients with recent myocardial infarction is demonstrated in this study.*

The I.S.A.M. Study Group: A prospective trial of intravenous streptokinase in acute myocardial infarction (I.S.A.M.): Mortality, morbidity, and infarct size at 21 days. N Engl J Med 314:1465, 1986. *This study provides data suggesting that intravenously administered streptokinase reduces infarct size when given to patients soon after myocardial infarction.*

Kennedy JW, Ritchie JL, Davis KB, et al.: Western Washington randomized trial of intracoronary streptokinase in acute myocardial infarction. N Engl J Med 309:1312, 1983. *Data suggest that mortality is reduced by successful thrombolytic therapy in patients with acute anterior Q wave infarcts.*

Maseri A., L'Abbate A, Baroldi G, et al.: Coronary vasospasm as a possible cause of myocardial infarction: A conclusion derived from the study of "preinfarction" angina. N Engl J Med 299:1271, 1978. *An interesting suggestion that coronary artery spasm may play a role in the pathogenesis of acute myocardial infarcts.*

Norwegian Multicenter Study Group: Timolol-induced reduction in mortality and reinfarction in patients surviving acute myocardial infarction. N Engl J Med 304:801, 1981. *This study provides evidence that timolol reduces the mortality risk and the likelihood of reinfarction when it is given chronically to patients after myocardial infarction.*

O'Neill W, Timmis G, Bourdillon P, et al.: A prospective, randomized clinical trial of intracoronary streptokinase versus coronary angioplasty for acute myocardial infarction. N Engl J Med 314:812, 1986. *Coronary angioplasty is an effective means of achieving thrombolysis acutely after myocardial infarction and also reduces the risk of postinfarction angina and protects regional ventricular function better than thrombolytic therapy alone.*

Rothkopf M, Boerner J, Stone M, et al.: Detection of myocardial infarction extension by CK-B radioimmunoassay. Circulation 59:268, 1979. *The frequency with which in-hospital extension of acute myocardial infarcts occurs is described in this study.*

The TIMI Study Group: Thrombolysis in myocardial infarction (TIMI Trial): Phase I findings. N Engl J Med 312:932, 1985. *Intravenously-administered tissue plasminogen-activating factor is superior to streptokinase in achieving thrombolysis when given approximately five hours after the event.*

Wackers FJ, Busemann S, Samson G, et al.: Value and limitations of thallium-201 scintigraphy in the acute phase of myocardial infarction. N Engl J Med 295:1, 1975. *A description of the advantages and limitations of a "cold spot" imaging technique, thallium-201 myocardial scintigraphy, in infarct recognition.*

Willerson JT, Parkey RW, Bonte FJ, et al.: Technetium stannous pyrophosphate myocardial scintigrams in patients with chest pain of varying etiology. Circulation 51:1046, 1975. *The applications and usefulness of an infarct-avid myocardial imaging technique, technetium 99m stannous pyrophosphate, in the recognition of acute myocardial infarcts are described.*

51.3 Surgical Treatment of Coronary Artery Disease

David C. Sabiston, Jr.

The development of coronary artery bypass grafts (CABG) has made a remarkable impact upon the management of ischemic heart disease. Each year some 800,000 patients in the United States survive an acute myocardial infarction, and approximately 175,000 undergo CABG. Complete relief of anginal pain is achieved in more than two thirds of patients following operation, and the life expectancy is increased in specific groups.

The *natural history* of coronary atherosclerosis is important in selecting therapy, since many factors are of prognostic significance. These include the number of coronary arteries involved, the severity of the lesions, the status of left ventricular function, and the presence of associated cardiac or systemic disorders. The prognosis of patients with angina is adversely affected by a familial history of coronary artery disease, cigarette smoking, hypertension, diabetes, and obesity.

SELECTION OF PATIENTS FOR SURGICAL THERAPY. Surgical management is usually indicated in patients with chronic stable angina in whom medical therapy has failed and in whom it is desirable to provide the highest likelihood of relief of myocardial ischemia. Moreover, CABG improves survival in those with left main coronary lesions as well as in patients with proximal left anterior descending (LAD) disease as a part of two-vessel disease and those with a positive exercise test for ischemia with two- or three-vessel disease (Table 51–8). Patients with left ventricular dysfunction also show improvement in wall motion following CABG. *Medical therapy* is better than or equal to surgical management in patients without evidence of myocardial ischemia and in those with one- or two-vessel disease without proximal LAD lesions, since long-term survival is not appreciably different.

In the selection of patients for CABG, noninvasive radionuclide angiocardiography is useful in assessment. This rapid, safe, and relatively simple technique makes possible an objective evaluation of ventricular function, including end-systolic and end-diastolic ventricular volumes, ejection fraction, cardiac output, and left ventricular wall motion. These parameters may be determined both at rest and during exercise. Patients with significant coronary artery disease may have essentially normal values at rest, but deterioration of cardiac function follows exercise. Thallium scans also quantify ventricular function and demonstrate abnormalities of wall motion. These techniques demonstrate the type, location, and extent of myocardial perfusion abnormalities and are often predictive of the role of CABG. Many now consider these techniques more reliable than exercise electrocardiography.

Coronary arteriography is essential in the selection of patients for CABG. Diseased vessels to be grafted should have a

TABLE 51–8. MEDICAL VERSUS SURGICAL MANAGEMENT OF PATIENTS WITH CHRONIC STABLE ANGINA

Surgical management better than medical therapy for
1. Relief of myocardial ischemia
2. Improving long-term survival in
   Left main coronary artery disease
   Three-vessel disease
   Proximal left anterior descending disease (part of two-vessel disease)
   Positive exercise test for ischemia in two- or three-vessel disease
3. Symptoms and pharmacologic therapy of ischemia
4. Left ventricular dysfunction due to myocardial ischemia

Adapted from Rahimtoola SH: A perspective on the three large multicenter randomized clinical trials of CABG for chronic stable angina. Circulation 72(Suppl V):123, 1985.

reasonable lumen (1.0 to 1.5 mm in diameter) and evidence of distal runoff indicative of a patent peripheral coronary bed. However, vessels that do not opacify distally may be found at operation to be patent. Both cardiac catheterization and noninvasive radionuclide arteriography provide helpful data for assessment of ventricular function. Certain features are apt to be associated with an increased surgical risk, including cardiomegaly, low ejection fraction (below 25 per cent), an increased left ventricular volume, large arteriovenous oxygen difference (greater than 6 volumes per cent), and an elevated left ventricular end-diastolic pressure. However, the presence of any one or a combination of these abnormalities does not necessarily represent a contraindication to operation or preclude a successful postoperative result.

Left ventricular *aneurysms* may follow myocardial infarction and are hazardous both for the paradoxical dilatation during systole, which makes the heart more inefficient, and as a source of systemic arterial emboli. These aneurysms may also be the site of electrical instability and may incite refractory dysrhythmias. Patients with aneurysms may also have coexisting valvular disease, which may further increase surgical risk.

Patients with *unstable angina* may be candidates for urgent CABG. Some patients can be managed by intensive pharmacologic therapy, but CABG may be preferable if the anginal pain is not rapidly controlled. Moreover, it has been shown in several series that patients with unstable angina initially treated by medical therapy ultimately require CABG. This fact became clear in the Coronary Artery Surgery Study (CASS), in which more than one third of patients ultimately required CABG. In a recent study of 100 consecutive patients with atypical angina on the coronary care unit, relief of anginal pain could not be obtained despite the use of intravenous nitroglycerin, propranolol, and nifedipine, and therefore CABG was performed. In this group, 52 had a myocardial infarction (6 hours to 30 days prior to operation) and 75 had serious disease as exhibited by either left main or three-vessel coronary disease or an ejection fraction less than 45 per cent. The operative mortality was only 4 per cent, and survival at one year was 90 per cent, showing that the procedure can be done in severely ill patients with superior results (Rankin, 1984).

Acute myocardial infarction may be associated with several complications requiring surgical therapy. An acquired ventricular septal defect (VSD) occurs in 1 to 2 per cent of patients with myocardial infarction, and the prognosis is poor, the survival being only 20 per cent at two months without operation. Surgical closure is indicated in nearly all patients, and it is preferable to allow healing of the infarct to permit the edges of the defect to become fibrotic and enable a better operative repair. Intractable cardiac failure may appear early and may require urgent operation. Multiple VSD's are present in approximately a third of these patients and should be carefully sought. The defects are generally closed with a plastic prosthesis, and CABG may be necessary to improve coronary blood flow. If early operation is mandatory, the results are less favorable than in patients able to survive for several weeks and undergo an elective procedure.

SURGICAL PROCEDURES. The techniques for CABG have progressively improved since the first use of a saphenous vein bypass graft for coronary disease in 1962 (Sabiston). Originally, most patients had autologous vein grafts, but the use of the internal mammary artery graft has dramatically increased in the past several years owing to improved long-term patency. It is preferable to use one or both internal mammary arteries in nearly all CABG procedures with venous grafts as necessary. It is important that the internal mammary artery be dissected with a sufficient pedicle of tissue to preserve the vasa vasorum and thus the blood supply of the arterial wall. Extracorporeal circulation is used with moderate *total body hypothermia*, and the temperature of the heart is

further lowered by infusion of a potassium solution at 4°C to produce cardioplegia. To maintain a myocardial temperature of 10 to 15°C, cold saline or ice slush topically surrounds the heart. Intracoronary injection of potassium solution eliminates cardiac contraction and further reduces myocardial metabolism to a very low level. The motionless heart and bloodless operative field are ideal for performing the best coronary anastomoses. The use of very fine, monofilament sutures, often placed with the use of magnifying lenses, has been helpful in achieving long-term patency. Comparative data also show that *all* major coronary arteries with significant stenoses should be grafted. In addition, branches of the primary vessels are also frequently bypassed beyond significant stenoses. Approximately four grafts are currently inserted in the average patient.

The *surgical mortality* for CABG varies in accordance with the severity of the disease. The CASS randomized multicenter evaluation study sponsored by the National Institutes of Health (1975 to 1979) demonstrated a very low mortality in patients considered good risks. For those with Class I and Class II angina, who are less than 65 years of age, who do not have a history of congestive heart failure or previous CABG, and who have an ejection fraction greater than 35 per cent, the surgically treated group had an annual mortality for single-, double-, and triple-vessel disease of 0.8, 0.8, and 1.2 per cent, respectively, compared with an annual mortality in medically managed patients of 1.1, 0.6, and 1.2 per cent, respectively. In more recent series, the surgical mortality in patients undergoing CABG who do not have significant associated cardiac conditions is generally 1 per cent or less. In addition, attention must be given to the fact that medical therapy has also improved with greater utilization of agents such as nitrates, beta blockers, and calcium channel blockers.

POSTOPERATIVE MANAGEMENT. A number of postoperative problems may arise in patients following CABG and require prompt diagnosis and immediate therapy. Adequate oxygenation is essential, and ventilatory support should be assessed by blood gas Po_2, Pco_2, and pH. The cardiac output should be maintained at a normal level by continuous monitoring of central venous pressure, systemic arterial pressure, the electrocardiogam, and urinary output. Should the *low cardiac output syndrome* develop, dopamine, dobutamine, and other agents should be employed as necessary. In many patients, the pulmonary artery diastolic pressure, as well as left atrial pressure, should be continuously monitored through an indwelling catheter placed at operation. Cardiac dysrhythmias occur and may require the use of appropriate drugs, pacing, or electrical cardioversion. Temporary pacing wires should be placed at operation.

Certain special complications occur following CABG, such as perioperative myocardial infarction (2 to 5 per cent), and cause hypotension and cardiac conduction defects. Most postoperative infarctions are limited and only occasionally are associated with serious clinical symptoms. Cardiac dysrhythmias and pericarditis usually respond well to appropriate medication. A serious postoperative complication (about 1 per cent) is *mediastinitis*, which should be managed aggressively with open drainage and, in some instances, by placement of pedicle grafts.

RESULTS. In nearly all series, relief of pain is complete in approximately two thirds of patients following CABG, with pain in the remainder of patients being much improved. Early assessments at rest and at exercise show improvement of left ventricular function in the first week following CABG. Although CABG does not prevent subsequent myocardial infarction, if such occurs, the infarcts are smaller and have fewer untoward effects.

In all series following CABG, *graft patency* is critical to long-term prognosis. Approximately 85 per cent of patients have patent anastomoses at one year, with an attrition rate in the general range of 2 per cent annually. In one large series, the patency rate of saphenous vein grafts followed for five years or longer was 47 per cent, whereas that of the internal mammary artery grafts during the same period was 90 per cent (Lytle). Therefore, use of the internal mammary artery graft is indicated in nearly all patients.

The role of platelets and platelet inhibitors in the long-term patency of coronary grafts is of major significance, and long-term administration of aspirin and dipyridamole is clearly effective in reducing graft occlusion. Postoperatively, dipyridamole* should be given at a dose of 75 mg three times a day and aspirin* at a dosage of 325 mg three times a day orally and should be continued indefinitely.

Late graft changes include intimal fibrosis, which reduces luminal caliber or may produce complete obstruction. The graft may also thrombose, and this is generally the cause of early failure. In addition, technical difficulties at the site of the anastomosis, such as kinking, can produce obstruction. A distinctive *fibrous proliferation* also occurs. The basic atherosclerotic process may progress in the coronary arteries, and in one series followed one to four years postoperatively with repeat coronary arteriography, 55 per cent of the original lesions proximal to the graft progressed and 14 per cent of the ungrafted vessels showed progression (McLaughlin).

REOPERATION. Should the symptoms of angina pectoris reappear and coronary arteriography provide evidence that there is either occlusion of previous grafts or an increase in the severity of the original disease, consideration may be given to reoperation. Although the technical procedure is somewhat more difficult, favorable results can nevertheless be predicted in the majority of patients. In one series of 1000 consecutive patients undergoing reoperation, the surgical mortality declined from 5 per cent early in the series to 2 per cent. During the same time, the number of grafts placed at the second operation increased from 1.4 to 2.3 (Loop). The five-year actuarial survival for patients was 89 per cent and was affected by the extent of disease and preoperative level of ventricular performance.

PERCUTANEOUS TRANSLUMINAL CORONARY ANGIOPLASTY. Gruentzig introduced percutaneous transluminal coronary angioplasty (PTCA) in 1977, and it has since become an increasingly useful procedure for patients with coronary artery disease. During the past decade, this technique has assumed an important role in the management of both *chronic myocardial ischemia* and *acute myocardial infarction*, especially in association with the intracoronary administration of thrombolytic agents. Tissue plasminogen activator (TPA), which is a recombinant human tissue-type plasminogen activator and is associated with minimal toxic reactions, can be given with favorable results. Although originally PTCA was reserved for patients with early symptoms, single-vessel disease, short segmental stenoses, and favorable anatomy, on the basis of wider use, the indications have increased to include more severe disease and multiple lesions. Current estimates indicate that some 70,000 PTCA procedures are being done annually. Better guide wires, angioplastic catheters, larger balloons (3.5 mm), and greater experience have been responsible for this escalation and for an 80 to 90 per cent success rate. In approximately 5 per cent of patients, clinical deterioration occurs, with evidence of ischemia, angina, and ST segment changes. Appropriate intervention with pharmacologic agents, as well as further attempts to open stenotic lesions, is indicated, but emergency CABG may be necessary. If symptoms reappear several days to weeks later, such may be due to coronary arterial spasm and may be relieved by calcium channel–blocking agents. If symptoms continue, coronary arteriography should be repeated, with determination of whether a further angioplastic procedure is indicated or if CABG is needed. Following PTCA, patients should be given platelet-inhibiting drugs, including dipyridamole* and aspirin,* indefinitely.

LONG-TERM SURVIVAL. The results of several randomized studies on the effect of CABG are available. The first convincing evidence that CABG improved longevity in patients with myocardial ischemia was the Veterans Administration Cooperative Study of patients with significant lesions of the *left main coronary artery*. The data showed that the survival of surgically treated patients at 3½ years was 88 per cent, whereas in those treated medically the survival was 65 per cent (Takaro). For patients with *three-vessel disease*, surgical management has generally been associated with increased survival, most impressively in the European Prospective Randomized Coronary Surgery Study. An eight-year follow-up in this series showed that patients managed surgically have an 89 per cent survival compared with 80 per cent for those managed medically. In the CASS Study, the survival at five years was 94 per cent in surgically managed patients compared with 82 per cent among those medically managed. The figures at the end of eight years were 92 per cent and 77 per cent, respectively (Rahimtoola).

---

*This use is not listed in the manufacturer's directive.

Austin EH, Odlham HN Jr, Sabiston DC Jr, et al.: Early assessment of rest and exercise following coronary artery surgery. Ann Thorac Surg 35:159, 1983. *In this study, significant improvement in left ventricular performance in patients following CABG was demonstrated at one week.*

Beller GA, Gibson RS, Watson DD: Radionuclide methods of identifying patients who may require coronary artery bypass surgery. Circulation 72 (Suppl V):V-9, 1985. *An excellent review of patient selection for CABG. The role of radionuclide technique in determining the type, location, and extent of coronary perfusion abnormalities as well as the status of myocardial performance in patients with angina pectoris.*

Chesbro JH, Clements IP, Fuster V, et al.: A platelet-inhibitor-drug trial in coronary-artery bypass operations: Benefit of perioperative dipyridamole and aspirin therapy on early postoperative vein-graft patency. N Engl J Med 307:73, 1982. *An excellent randomized study demonstrating the value of aspirin and dipyridamole maintaining long-term patency of coronary artery bypass grafts.*

Crean PA, Waters DD, Bosch X, et al.: Angiographic findings after myocardial infarction in patients with previous bypass surgery: Explanations for smaller infarcts in this group compared with control patients. Circulation 71:693, 1985. *A careful study of a series with myocardial infarction and CABG compared with controls. Those with CABG had smaller and less significant infarctions.*

Fuster V, Chesbro JH: Role of platelets and platelet inhibitors in aortocoronary artery vein-graft disease. Circulation 73:227, 1986. *Recent confirmatory evidence for use of platelet inhibitors to improve long-term graft patency.*

Gold HK, Fallon JT, Yasuda T, et al.: Coronary thrombolysis with recombinant human tissue-type plasminogen activator. Circulation 70:700, 1984. *The role of this relatively nontoxic and effective fibrinolysin is discussed.*

Jones RH, Floyd RD, Austin EH, et al.: The role of radionuclide angiocardiography in the preoperative prediction of pain relief and prolonged survival following coronary artery bypass grafting. Ann Surg 197:743, 1983. *An evaluation of the usefulness of radionuclide angiocardiography (RNA) in the selection and prognosis of patients with coronary artery disease. Calculations comparing the maximal increase in survival and complete pain relief, using multiple criteria known to provide prognostic information, showed that the exercise response on RNA is the single most important variable in selection of therapy.*

Loop FD, Lytle BW, Gill CC, et al.: Trends in selection and results of coronary artery reoperations. Ann Thorac Surg 36:380, 1983. *A large series of patients undergoing reoperation for myocardial revascularization are studied. Emphasis is placed upon the fact that the mortality is now relatively low, despite the technical difficulties encountered in some of these procedures. The results are quite favorable.*

Lytle BW, Loop FD, Cosgrove DM, et al.: Long-term (5 to 12 years) serial studies of internal mammary artery and saphenous vein coronary bypass grafts. J Thorac Cardiovasc Surg 89:248, 1985. *In this series of patients, the markedly improved patency rate of internal mammary grafts was clearly demonstrated compared with that of saphenous vein grafts.*

McLaughlin PR, Berman ND, Morton BC, et al.: Saphenous vein bypass grafting. Changes in native circulation and collaterals. Circulation 51–52(Suppl 1):66, 1975. *A carefully performed study of the continuing changes that occur in the coronary circulation after an initial diagnosis of stenotic atherosclerotic coronary disease. It emphasizes the need for continuing attention toward prevention of the basic process in addition to surgical therapy.*

Pryor DB, Harrell FE Jr, Lee KL, et al.: A study demonstrating the improving prognosis in medically treated patients with coronary artery disease. Am J Cardiol 52:444, 1983. *This study emphasizes that the mortality from coronary artery disease has decreased during the past decade and cannot be explained solely on the basis that less severe patients are being evaluated but is due at least in part to the decrease in mortality from coronary artery disease.*

Rackley CE: Advances in Critical Care Cardiology. Philadelphia, F. A. Davis Company, 1986. *An updated monograph of recent advances in the management of patients with acute cardiac problems. Appropriate diagnostic tests, together with a spectrum of medical therapy, transluminal coronary angioplasty, and CABG, are each thoroughly presented. There are notable discussions of the role and appropriate use of various cardiac pharmacologic agents, emergency procedures for myocardial ischemia, and the management of cardiac dysrhythmias.*

Rahimtoola SH: A perspective on the three large multicenter randomized clinical trials of CABG for chronic stable angina. Circulation 72(Suppl V):123, 1985. *A comparative review by an outstanding cardiologist of the three large and well-publicized multicenter clinical trials of CABG for chronic stable angina.*

Rankin JS, Newman GE, Muhlbaier LH, et al.: The effects of coronary revascularization on left ventricular function in ischemic heart disease. J Thorac Cardiovasc Surg 90:818, 1985. *A review of a series of patients with severe coronary artery disease and depressed myocardial function. CABG not only reverses exercise-induced ischemic ventricular dysfunction but can also have a similar effect on resting ventricular performance. Despite the fact that over 80 per cent of the patients in the study were New York Heart Association (NYHA) Stage IV, the mortality was 2.2 per cent.*

Rankin JS, Newman JR Jr, Califf RM, et al.: Clinical characteristics and current management of medically refractory unstable angina. Ann Surg 200:457, 1984. *A unique series of seriously ill patients, all on the coronary care unit, with refractory unstable angina who underwent CABG with excellent rate of survival.*

Sabiston DC Jr: The coronary circulation. The William F. Rienhoff, Jr. Lecture. Johns Hopkins Med J 134:314, 1974. *A review of the anatomic, physiologic, and pathologic aspects of the coronary circulation. The data presented are based upon experimental and clinical findings in the normal and pathologic coronary circulation and their relationships to surgical management. The first patient treated with a saphenous vein bypass graft for coronary artery disease in 1962 is described.*

Shearn DL, Brent BB: Coronary artery bypass surgery in patients with left ventricular dysfunction. Am J Med 80:405, 1986. *A study of a series of patients with poor left ventricular ejection fractions (less than 45 per cent) managed by CABG. Significant improvement in global left ventricular ejection fraction and regional left ventricular systolic function was demonstrated.*

Takaro T, Hultgren HN, Lipton MJ, et al.: Circulation 54(Suppl 3):107, 1976. *A randomized study showing definite superiority for long-term survival of surgical over medical therapy in patients with significant lesions of the left main coronary artery.*

Varnauskas E: Survival, myocardial infarction, and employment status in a prospective randomized study of coronary bypass surgery. Circulation 72(Suppl V):V, 1985. *A long-term report of the European Coronary Surgery Study Group indicating improved longevity in patients treated surgically as opposed to those managed medically. An eight-year result of survival is reported, together with five-year results on recurrent myocardial infarction and employment status of patients undergoing CABG compared with randomized controls.*

52 VALVULAR HEART DISEASE

Charles E. Rackley

The clinical manifestations of valvular heart disease result from either stenosis or incompetence of cardiac valves, or both. These mechanical disturbances lead to either pressure or volume overload on the affected chambers. The most frequently involved cardiac chamber in valvular heart disease is the left ventricle, which compensates for chronic volume or pressure overload with dilatation and hypertrophy. Myocardial oxygen requirements are related to the increased mechanical work and hypertrophy of the myocardium. In the advanced stage of valvular heart disease, myocardial decompensation, a reduction in cardiac output, and decreased coronary perfusion can impair oxygen delivery despite increased myocardial oxygen demands.

Although rheumatic heart disease remains prevalent in the temperate climates of the world, control of streptococcal infections in the United States has reduced the incidence of rheumatic fever and subsequent rheumatic heart disease. Today mitral valve prolapse is the most common valvular abnormality. A bicuspid aortic valve is the most common cause of aortic stenosis, but calcification of the degenerative aortic valve is recognized with increasing frequency in the aging adult.

Recognition of a heart murmur on physical examination is the usual means of initially diagnosing valvular heart disease. Thus, the clinical examination remains important for detection of valvular heart disease, recognition of cardiac deterioration, and assessment of follow-up status. The noninvasive technologies of electrocardiography, chest radiography, echocardiography, radionuclide angiography, and stress testing play an important role in assessing the impact of valvular heart disease on cardiac function and determining the timing of operative intervention. Cardiac catheterization continues to be important in the accurate measurement of gradients across stenotic valves, evaluation of left ventricular function, and recognition of concomitant coronary artery disease. In recent years advances in echocardiography have resulted in more accurate assessment of valvular orifice size, and catheterization is reserved to confirm impressions and to identify underlying coronary artery disease.

GENERAL APPROACH TO THE PATIENT WITH VALVULAR HEART DISEASE

History

The patient with valvular heart disease usually recalls a history of a heart murmur, and therefore the first recognition of the murmur may be helpful in establishing the etiology. Although cardiac murmurs are frequent in healthy, physically active children and adolescents, congenital valvular etiologies are often recognized at birth. Detection of a heart murmur in early adulthood often suggests a rheumatic basis, whereas development of the murmur in later years is often due to the degenerative changes in valvular structure. In addition to ascertaining the earliest detection of the heart murmur, the physician should carefully assess the patient's physical activities and note the initial onset of dyspnea or fatigue. The physician's interpretation of the patient's symptoms dictates the appropriate timing of noninvasive and invasive cardiac studies as well as the decision for surgical correction.

Physical Examination

The physical examination of the patient with valvular heart disease should be performed in the standard manner. Particular attention should be paid to the vital signs. Fever should raise the possibility of infective endocarditis. Palpation of the peripheral pulse may indicate stenosis or incompetence of the aortic valve. The habitus can suggest Marfan's syndrome as well as other heritable disorders of connective tissue. Funduscopic examination can demonstrate subtleties in arterial pulsations in aortic incompetence or the characteristic hemorrhages or Roth's spots in infective endocarditis. Careful attention to the vessels in the neck can reveal abnormalities in venous pulsation reflecting right ventricular failure or tricuspid stenosis or incompetence. Carotid arteries reveal pulsatile abnormalities and transmitted bruits from the aortic valve.

Cardiac examination must include inspection, palpation, percussion, and auscultation. These maneuvers should be performed with the patient both in the sitting and in the recumbent positions. Auscultation at the apex, left sternal border, and pulmonic and aortic areas should be performed with the patient in the sitting, recumbent, and left lateral decubitus positions as well as after mild exercise. The remainder of the examination consists of documenting fluid retention, such as hepatic enlargement, ascites, and peripheral edema.

Laboratory Studies

Electrocardiogram

The electrocardiogram can provide information on atrial and ventricular enlargement. Left atrial enlargement is recognized by a prominent, prolonged, notched P wave in leads II, III, and aV_L, as well as in lead V_1. Left ventricular hypertrophy increases QRS voltage as well as ST-T wave abnormalities. Right ventricular hypertrophy produces right-axis deviation of the QRS complex as well as ST-T wave changes in leads V_1 and V_2. Atrial fibrillation often develops in the course of valvular heart disease from enlargement of the left atrium.

Chest Radiograph

Standard posteroanterior and lateral chest films provide information on heart size and chamber enlargement as well as evidence of pulmonary venous and arterial hypertension. Chest radiographs are useful in the follow-up of patients with valvular heart disease to detect changes in cardiac dimensions and alterations in pulmonary vascularity.

Echocardiography

Because of technical improvements, echocardiography has become a major noninvasive tool in the assessment of valvular heart disease. Valvular anatomy, pressure gradients, chamber dimensions, wall thickness, and ventricular function can be precisely assessed and quantitated using modern echocardiography. Valvular motion, calcification, orifice size, and the presence of infective endocarditis can all be determined with this technology.

Radionuclide Imaging

Radionuclide techniques can provide information on cardiac function, valvular incompetence, and the cardiac response to exercise. The imaging capability is particularly useful in evaluating the function of the right ventricle as well as tricuspid valve integrity. The response of the left ventricle to exercise is increasingly used to identify the earliest possible time for surgical correction of valvular abnormalities.

Exercise Testing

Standard exercise testing can be used to assess exercise capacity as well as document symptoms of dyspnea and fatigue. The test is useful in the initial and follow-up evaluations of patients with valvular heart disease to detect deterioration in cardiac performance.

Cardiac Catheterization

Cardiac catheterization remains a definitive procedure in the evaluation of valvular heart disease but, despite the improvements in techniques, is still limited by the number of times patients can tolerate this procedure. Objectives for cardiac catheterization are (1) to identify the underlying valve lesions, (2) to assess ventricular function, (3) to evaluate the anatomy of the coronary arteries, (4) to recognize any additional cardiac lesions, and (5) to assess the performance of prosthetic heart valves.

AORTIC STENOSIS
Etiology and Pathology

Aortic stenosis (Table 52–1) can result from a congenital abnormality, rheumatic fever, or degeneration with calcification in the aging patient. A bicuspid valve is the most common congenital abnormality, and invariably there is a raphe in one of the cusps that indicates failure of the commissure to develop. Rarely, a unicuspid valve can be present at birth. Although the bicuspid valve may not be initially stenotic, fibrosis and thickening lead to eventual reduction of the orifice size with calcification. Rheumatic fever produces scarring of the leaflet margins, and there is eventual fusion of the commissures with calcification. More than 50 per cent of adults with aortic stenosis will be found to have a bicuspid valve, but fibrosis and calcification may make it difficult to determine whether the valve is bicuspid or tricuspid. In the aging patient with degenerative aortic stenosis, calcium deposits usually develop in the sinuses and annulus, whereas the margins of the leaflets remain free.

In any of the conditions producing hemodynamic stenosis of the aortic valve, the systolic hypertension in the ventricular chamber is compensated by concentric hypertrophy of the myocardial wall. As myocardial failure develops from depression of the contractile state, dilatation of the ventricle will occur. Fibrosis of the myocardium also occurs. Myocardial oxygen consumption remains high owing to the elevation of systolic pressure within the left ventricle and the increase in left ventricular mass. Thus, significant aortic stenosis creates conditions in which high myocardial oxygen demands are inadequately supported by reduced oxygen supply, which leads to subendocardial ischemia. Eventually, with a decline in the inotropic state of the myocardium, the ventricle dilates and the ejection fraction is decreased below the normal range. Further elevation of the left ventricular end-diastolic pressure results in pulmonary venous hypertension The increased myocardial oxygen demands in aortic stenosis with the underperfused subendocardial myocardium can produce arrhythmias, chest pain, and even sudden death. In adults there may be coexistent coronary artery disease, which further contributes to myocardial ischemia.

Clinical Features

Chest pain, syncope, and heart failure are the characteristic symptoms of aortic stenosis, even though a gradient across the valve can exist for years before the patient develops symptoms. Children with a severe gradient can suddenly develop symptoms, whereas in adults the increase in mortality occurs later in the course of the disease.

The anginal chest discomfort is exertional and indistinguishable from that of ischemic heart disease. Approximately 50 per cent of patients with aortic stenosis who are above the age of 40 years will have underlying coronary artery disease whether exertional chest pain is present or not. Syncope can be an initial symptom of aortic stenosis and is probably related to the same mechanism as the chest pain, that is, critical reduction in myocardial oxygen supply with increased demands. Orthostatic syncope can result from the inability of the cardiac output to increase with abrupt assumption of the upright position, whereas exertional syncope is further aggravated by peripheral vasodilatation unaccompanied by an increase in cardiac output. Arrhythmias due to myocardial ischemia can also contribute to syncope and sudden death. When aortic stenosis is found at autopsy, approximately 15 per cent of the patients will have died suddenly without previous symptoms.

Heart failure in aortic stenosis generally reduces life expectancy to less than two years, whereas patients with syncope or angina may survive, on the average, two to five years. With calcification of the aortic valve, hemolytic anemia due to destruction of red cells can develop; furthermore, patients with aortic stenosis have an increased incidence of gastrointestinal bleeding resulting from angiodysplasia. Finally, patients with aortic stenosis are susceptible to infective endocarditis.

Physical Examination

In aortic stenosis, the typical physical findings include a delay in the upstroke of the peripheral pulse, a diamond-shaped crescendo-decrescendo systolic murmur, and hypertrophy of the left ventricle. The peripheral pulse is diminished in amplitude, delayed in upstroke, and prolonged owing to sustained ejection across the aortic valve (pulsus tardus et parvus). The changes in the peripheral pulse are caused by a reduction in the systolic pressure and a gradual decline in diastolic pressure. The harsh murmur is often transmitted to the carotid vessels, and a palpable thrill develops with a substantial gradient across the aortic valve.

Since the contour of the heart does not become enlarged with concentric hypertrophy, there may be no visible abnormalities on examination of the chest. However, the apical impulse of the pressure-overloaded ventricle may be sustained

TABLE 52–1. AORTIC STENOSIS

Etiology	Physiology	Symptoms	Physical Examination	Electrocardiogram	Chest	Echocardiogram	Catheterization	Medical Therapy	Surgical Therapy
Congenital Rheumatic Degenerative	LV* pressure overload LV hypertrophy Decreased LV compliance	Chest pain Syncope Heart failure	Delayed arterial pulse wave Aortic thrill Diamond-shaped aortic area, left sternal border and apex	LV hypertrophy	Normal cardiac size Poststenotic dilatation of ascending aorta	Anatomy of aortic valve/calcium Number of cusps LV wall thickness EchoDoppler estimate of valvular gradient Valvular area	Valvular gradient LV function Valvular area Coronary anatomy Mitral lesions	Endocarditis prophylaxis	Symptoms Gradient >50 mm Hg Valvular area <0.8 cm²

*LV = left ventricular.

even though localized. When the ventricle dilates owing to myocardial failure, there is lateral displacement of the impulse, which becomes more diffuse. Detection of palpable systolic vibrations over the primary aortic area, with the patient in the sitting position during full expiration, often correlates with a gradient across the aortic valve of more than 40 mm Hg. An atrial (S₄) gallop is usually audible, and an ejection click may be heard along the left sternal border. The aortic second sound becomes diminished, except in calcific stenosis of the elderly, in which the margins of the leaflets usually maintain their mobility. The diamond-shaped ejection murmur develops after the first sound, peaks in mid- and late systole, and disappears before the second heart sound. If an ejection click is present, the murmur develops immediately after the click and can sometimes be erroneously identified as a holosystolic murmur. The murmur is most intense over the aortic area and along the left sternal border, but in the elderly patient, the musical quality of the murmur can sometimes be loudest at the apex. The intensity in the apical area can be confusing and may make it difficult to distinguish this murmur from that of mitral regurgitation. A faint diastolic blow is often audible along the left sternal border, since the severely stenotic valve may have a mild degree of incompetence.

Laboratory Studies

Electrocardiogram

Left ventricular hypertrophy is the most common finding on the electrocardiogram, with an increase in QRS amplitude and ST-T changes of a strain pattern. Left-axis deviation can develop as well as conduction disturbances and left bundle branch block. As the left ventricle becomes noncompliant, there may be enlargement of the left atrium with a negative P wave in lead V₁. Because of myocardial fibrosis, Q waves can develop in the precordial leads, but these as well as the ST-T wave abnormalities are indistinguishable from underlying coronary artery disease.

Chest Radiograph

The heart size remains unchanged in the early phase of aortic stenosis, since hypertrophy does not increase the cardiothoracic ratio. There may be poststenotic dilatation and prominence of the ascending aorta. Calcification is often present but may require fluoroscopy for confirmation. Development of heart failure will enlarge the left ventricle and cause pulmonary congestion. Since a bicuspid aortic valve is sometimes associated with coarctation of the aorta, rib notching should always be sought on the chest film.

Echocardiogram

The echocardiogram can demonstrate thickening of the aortic leaflets, determine the number of leaflets, detect calcification of the valves, and reveal left ventricular wall thickness and function. Two-dimensional echocardiography can give an estimated size of the aortic orifice, and the Doppler technique can assess accurately the systolic pressure gradient across the valve. Thus, available echocardiographic techniques can provide accurate diagnosis and assessment of aortic stenosis (Fig. 52–1).

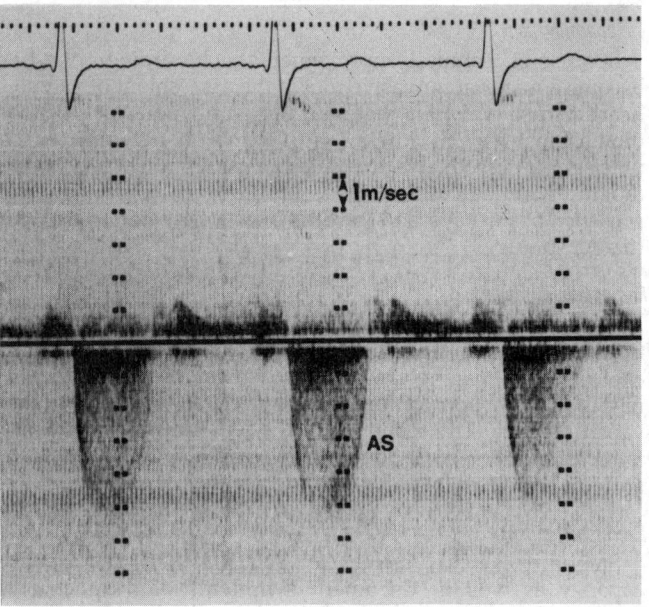

FIGURE 52–1. Continuous wave Doppler recording from the ascending aorta in a patient with severe aortic stenosis. The peak velocity is approximately 5 m/sec. Utilizing the modified Bernoulli equation, a peak instantaneous gradient across the aortic valve of 100 mm Hg can be calculated. Peak-to-peak gradient at catheterization was 80 mm Hg.

Cardiac Catheterization

The pressure gradient across the aortic valve can be accurately measured with simultaneous measurements of left ventricular and aortic pressures. A decline in cardiac output will be associated with a reduced pressure gradient across the valve, and the valvular area will tend to be overestimated when the cardiac output is reduced and only the pressure gradient is analyzed.

The size of the normal aortic orifice is 2.5 to 3 cm², and mild stenosis develops when the orifice is reduced to 0.75 to 1.5 cm². Moderate stenosis is present when the valvular size is less than 0.75 cm² and severe stenosis when the valvular area is less than 0.5 cm². Surgery is usually advised when the aortic valve gradient is greater than 50 mm Hg or the valve area is less than 0.8 cm². Left ventricular angiography is helpful in determining the presence of mitral regurgitation. With the information available from echocardiography, cardiac catheterization may be primarily indicated for coronary arteriography, since 50 per cent of patients over the age of 40 years will have underlying coronary artery disease.

Differential Diagnosis

In children, valvular aortic stenosis has to be differentiated from congenital forms of both supra- and infravalvular lesions. In hypertrophic cardiomyopathy with obstruction, the systolic ejection murmur is similar to that of valvular aortic stenosis, but the peripheral pulse is hyperdynamic with a rapid upstroke and a double-notch or bisferious contour compared with the delayed upstroke observed in valvular stenosis. With rupture of the chordae or papillary muscle, acute mitral regurgitation may produce a harsh systolic murmur. This murmur can be transmitted to the left atrial wall and aorta, resulting in a palpable and audible "aortic" murmur. However, the murmur of acute mitral regurgitation transmitted into the aortic area is holosystolic rather than midsystolic. A systolic ejection murmur accompanies significant aortic regurgitation and is generally caused by turbulence of the large stroke volume across the aortic valve.

Medical Therapy

Prophylaxis with antibiotics is indicated for dental, genitourinary, and gastrointestinal procedures in the asymptomatic patient to reduce the likelihood of infective endocarditis. Prophylaxis should be routine throughout life in a patient with a stenotic or prosthetic valve. For dental and respiratory tract procedures, an adult should receive penicillin V, 2.0 gm orally one hour before, then 1.0 gm six hours later. For patients unable to take oral medications, 2 million units of aqueous penicillin G given intravenously (IV) or intramuscularly (IM) 30 to 60 minutes before a procedure and 1 million units 6 hours later may be substituted. For patients with prosthetic valves, ampicillin, 1.0 to 2.0 gm given IM or IV, plus gentamicin, 1.5 mg per kilogram given IM or IV, is recommended one-half hour before a procedure, followed by 1.0 gm of oral penicillin V six hours later. Alternatively, the parenteral regimen may be repeated once eight hours later. For patients allergic to penicillin, erythromycin, 1.0 gm, should be given orally one hour before the procedure, then 500 mg six hours later; or for parenteral administration, vancomycin, 1.0 gm, should be given IV slowly over one hour, starting one hour before, without a repeat dose. For genitourinary or gastrointestinal tract procedures, ampicillin, 2.0 gm given IM or IV, plus gentamicin, 1.5 mg per kilogram given IM or IV, is given one-half to one hour before a procedure, and a follow-up dose is administered eight hours later. For minor or repeated procedures, amoxicillin, 3.0 gm orally, is recommended one hour before a procedure and 1.5 gm six hours later. In children, appropriately reduced doses for each of these programs should be used.

If the patient with aortic stenosis develops a supraventricular tachycardia, digitalis and an antiarrhythmic drug may be necessary to slow the ventricular response. Development of chest pain warrants catheterization to evaluate underlying coronary artery disease, but the use of nitrates should be undertaken with great caution, since arterial pressure may fall and further reduce coronary blood flow. Since life expectancy is reduced when aortic stenosis becomes symptomatic, chest pain, syncope, or heart failure warrants appropriate studies and consideration for surgery.

Surgical Therapy

In children with aortic stenosis, surgery may be considered before the development of symptoms. If the pressure gradient is high, valvuloplasty can sometimes be performed before calcification has developed. The operative mortality for aortic valve replacement is 2 to 3 per cent and is less than 5 per cent if coronary bypass surgery is also performed. Even if heart failure has developed, surgery with prosthetic valve replacement can improve ventricular function. A mechanical valve will require long-term coagulation, but the porcine valve can be utilized in older patients or in those in whom anticoagulation is contraindicated. Currently, the porcine valve will usually last ten years or longer before deterioration in adults, but it is not recommended in children or adolescents. If indicated, coronary bypass surgery should also be performed at the time of valve replacement. The ten-year survival of combined aortic valve replacement and coronary revascularization approaches 55 per cent. Late cardiac events occur at a rate of approximately 6 per cent per year and include throm-

boembolic neurologic insults, myocardial infarction, congestive heart failure, endocarditis, bleeding, peripheral thromboembolism, and reoperation.

AORTIC REGURGITATION
Etiology and Pathology

Aortic regurgitation (Table 52–2) can be caused by disease conditions that render the aortic leaflets incompetent or affect the ascending aorta with dilatation of the annulus of the aortic valve. Rheumatic fever produces scarring and fibrosis of the valvular margins. Myxomatous degeneration of the aortic cusp can lead to incompetence. Hypertension, as well as arteriosclerosis, can be associated with scarring of the aortic valve and mild incompetence. Congenital lesions, such as bicuspid aortic valve, are predominantly stenotic, but scarring and calcification can result in associated incompetence as well. An aneurysm of the sinus of Valsalva may be associated with a ventricular septal defect as well as aortic regurgitation.

Conditions that affect the ascending aorta and produce valvular incompetence include syphilis, heritable disorders of connective tissue, arthritic diseases, and cystic medial necrosis of the aorta. In syphilis, the granulomatous process can result in calcification of the aorta, extreme dilatation, and ostial narrowing of the coronary arteries. Myxomatous degeneration of the aortic valve occurs in Marfan's syndrome. Ankylosing spondylitis, rheumatoid arthritis, and Reiter's syndrome are arthritic conditions that can cause aortic root dilatation and aortic cusp thickening. Cystic medial necrosis and aortic ectasia can produce extreme dilatation of the aorta with secondary aortic regurgitation. Aortic regurgitation can result from dissection of the aorta, perforation of the valve with infective endocarditis, rupture of a sinus of Valsalva, and mechanical complications of a prosthetic aortic valve.

Physiology

Aortic regurgitation imposes a volume overload on the left ventricle. Although the end-diastolic pressure may be normal or slightly elevated in the early phases, progressive regurgitation will elevate the end-diastolic pressure and dilate the chamber by slippage of myocardial fibers, sarcomere replication, and myocardial hypertrophy. These compensatory mechanisms support a large left ventricular stroke volume, which is often achieved with an ejection fraction above 50 per cent.

The systolic ejection of a large stroke volume into the high-impedance area of the systemic circulation increases the systolic pressure. Systolic wall stress or afterload can be maintained within the normal range by hypertrophy of the myocardium, but myocardial oxygen demand is significantly increased. A progressive decline in aortic diastolic pressure due to regurgitation of blood into the left ventricle can reduce coronary blood flow and thus create conditions for subendocardial ischemia in severe chronic aortic regurgitation.

The gradual volume overload of chronic aortic regurgitation can be tolerated for years before the inotropic state of the myocardium deteriorates. Eventually, the declining ejection fraction and inotropic state, along with limits to the dilatation hypertrophy mechanism, cause marked elevation of the left ventricular filling pressure with pulmonary venous capillary congestion.

Left ventricular hemodynamics in acute aortic regurgitation, compared with those in chronic aortic regurgitation, are immediately disturbed, since the regurgitant volume may be imposed on a normal end-diastolic volume. Under such circumstances, sudden incompetence of the aortic valve can severely elevate the left ventricular filling pressure, since the acute dilatation of the left ventricle is limited. With such rapid regurgitation through the aortic valve, the mitral valve may close prematurely, and the aortic diastolic murmur may persist beyond the diminished first heart sound.

TABLE 52–2. AORTIC REGURGITATION

Etiology	Physiology	Symptoms	Physical Examination	Electrocardiogram	Chest	Echocardiogram	Catheterization	Medical Therapy	Surgical Therapy
Chronic									
Rheumatic fever	Chronic volume overload	Fatigue	Wide arterial pulse pressure	LV hypertrophy and strain	Enlarged LV	Valvular anatomy	Contrast from aorta to LV	Preload and after load reduction	LV systolic echo dimension >55 mm
Connective tissue disorders	LV* dilatation	Dyspnea	Enlarged LV		Dilated aorta	Aortic root size	LV function		
Hypertension, atherosclerosis	LV hypertrophy	Edema	Diastolic aortic murmur			Enlarged LV		Diuretics	Ejection fraction <50%
Syphilis			Systolic ejection murmur			Mitral valve fluttering		Digitalis	
Cystic medial necrosis			Third sound			LV function			
Aortic ectasia			Apical diastolic rumble						
Congenital heart disease									
Acute									
Endocarditis	Acute LV diastolic pressure and volume overload	Pulmonary edema	Loud diastolic musical murmur	LV strain	Pulmonary edema	Valvular anatomy	Contrast from aorta to LV	Preload and afterload reduction	Urgent surgery
Aortic dissection			Right and left sternal border radiation with thrill		Normal heart size	Aortic size and intimal flap	Aortic and intimal flap		
Ruptured sinus of Valsalva			Soft S$_1$ and third sound						
Prosthetic valve			Continuous murmur if rupture into right side of heart						

*LV = left ventricle or ventricular.

Clinical Course

Since the volume overload of aortic regurgitation is well tolerated, patients may remain asymptomatic for long periods of time. The patient may be aware of prominent precordial activity as well as exaggerated pulsation of the carotid arteries. Diffuse sweating patterns and vague abdominal discomfort are less frequent symptoms. The accelerated development of angina, heart failure, or sudden death within several years has been observed in patients with a pulse pressure greater than 140/40 mm Hg and left ventricular enlargement demonstrated on electrocardiography or chest radiograph. Dyspnea, orthopnea, and paroxysmal nocturnal dyspnea result from impaired left ventricular contractility in pulmonary venous hypertension. Although tachycardia may impair ventricular function, the shortened diastolic filling period can be beneficial in reducing the duration of the aortic regurgitation. Chest pain and syncope are infrequent symptoms. Chest pain is often associated with underlying coronary artery disease, and syncope is usually attended by arrhythmias.

With acute aortic regurgitation, pulmonary edema is often the presenting manifestation. Severe chest pain suggests aortic dissection when acute aortic incompetence develops.

Physical Examination

In aortic regurgitation, the physical findings reflect the large left ventricular stroke volume into the systemic circulation and the rapid diastolic run-off into the left ventricle. The peripheral pulse is characteristically bounding, and additional manifestations of the wide pulse pressure include head bobbing, pulsation of the retinal arterioles, bounding carotid pulse, pistol shot sounds over the femoral arteries, a to-and-fro murmur elicited from the femoral artery with slight compression of the stethoscope, and capillary pulsations in the nail beds. With connective tissue and arthritic diseases that produce aortic regurgitation, there may be characteristic changes in habitus, such as the musculoskeletal type in Marfan's syndrome and kyphosis of the thoracic spine in ankylosing spondylitis.

The precordium is hyperdynamic with a laterally displaced apical impulse. The auscultatory hallmark is the high-pitched, blowing, decrescendo diastolic murmur heard best along the left sternal border while the patient is in the sitting position during full expiration. As the regurgitation becomes more severe, a diastolic rumble or Austin Flint murmur due to vibration of the anterior leaflet of the mitral valve in the regurgitant jet may be audible at the apex. If the ascending aorta is dilated, the diastolic murmur may be heard along the right sternal border as well. With extreme left ventricular dilatation, mitral regurgitation can produce an apical systolic murmur, and heart failure is attended by a ventricular gallop at the apex.

With acute aortic regurgitation due to disruption of an aortic leaflet or dissection dilating the aortic annulus, the diastolic murmur may be harsh with palpable vibrations along the left sternal border. A perforated or prolapsed aortic leaflet, as well as the detached aortic intima from dissection, can generate prominent musical qualities in the diastolic murmur.

Laboratory Studies

Electrocardiogram

The electrocardiogram typically reveals left ventricular hypertrophy with increased QRS voltage amplitude and ST-T wave changes of the strain pattern. With acute aortic regurgitation, the hypertrophy may be absent, and the ST-T wave changes can indicate myocardial ischemia.

Chest Radiography

Significant cardiomegaly usually attends chronic aortic regurgitation, with the increase in size due to dilatation of the left ventricle. The ascending aorta is often prominent. Calcium in the aortic valve or annulus is best appreciated by fluoroscopy, but calcification of the ascending aorta caused by syphilis can be detected on the chest film. Left ventricular failure will be accompanied by pulmonary congestion and venous prominence.

Echocardiogram

Echocardiography has become the most useful noninvasive tool to recognize anatomic abnormalities of the aortic valve and to assess dimensions of the annulus and ascending aorta. The intensity of the regurgitant flow can be appreciated by the vibrations of the anterior mitral leaflet, and the echo-Doppler technique can estimate the severity of the regurgitation. Left ventricular chamber dimensions and wall thickness permit calculation of end-diastolic volume and hypertrophy. Finally, an end-systolic dimension of 55 mm has been proposed by several investigators to represent the limit of surgically reversible dilatation of the left ventricle so that aortic valve replacement should be performed before this chamber size is exceeded. Additional clinical experience has challenged the validity of the 55-mm systolic limit, since postoperative reduction in chamber size remains variable. Thus, echocardiographic studies of left ventricular dimensions and function are important in evaluation, follow-up, and timing for aortic valve replacement in aortic regurgitation.

Exercise Testing

Although exercise capacity can be measured and followed periodically in patients with aortic regurgitation, exercise testing is best clinically used in combination with radionuclide angiography. A reduction in exercise ejection fraction by 5 per cent or more is considered by some an indication for surgery even in the absence of symptoms.

Cardiac Catheterization

Cardiac catheterization can confirm the presence of aortic incompetence when contrast material injected into the aorta regurgitates into the left ventricle. The primary clinical indications for catheterization are to recognize coexisting lesions, such as mitral regurgitation, and to detect coronary artery disease. Dimensions of the aortic annulus and the ascending aorta will be useful for the choice of a prosthetic device in the operative procedure.

Differential Diagnosis

In the evaluation of a diastolic murmur along the left sternal border, aortic insufficiency is far more common than pulmonic insufficiency. The pulsatile characteristics of the peripheral circulation can be helpful in differentiating an aortic from a pulmonic origin of the diastolic murmur. In systemic hypertension, accentuated tambour qualities of the second heart sound can sometimes suggest mild aortic regurgitation, but the level of the diastolic blood pressure can be helpful in distinguishing incompetence from reverberations of the second sound. Any condition that causes aortic stenosis through immobility of the valve leaflets is often accompanied by some degree of aortic regurgitation.

Medical Therapy

Antibiotic prophylaxis is indicated for the prevention of endocarditis. When symptoms of heart failure develop, vasodilating agents such as hydralazine, prazocin, or nifedipine may be beneficial, but benefits are rarely maintained. Thus, the use of digitalis, diuretics, and afterload-reducing agents is primarily of short-term benefit in aortic regurgitation.

Surgical Therapy

A major clinical decision in aortic regurgitation is the timing of aortic valve replacement before irreversible dilatation of the left ventricle has developed. The echocardiographic dimensions and evidence of reduced left ventricular function are now being utilized to advise valve replacement before symptoms of heart failure have developed. Even after heart failure has developed, patients still improve clinically after aortic valve replacement. Valve replacement can be undertaken with a mortality of less than 3 to 5 per cent. The type of prosthetic valve will depend on the patient's age and the ability to be anticoagulated. In aortic dissection, there may also be replacement of the ascending aorta, since acute regurgitation requires intervention.

MITRAL STENOSIS

Etiology and Pathology

Rheumatic fever remains the predominant cause for mitral stenosis (Table 52–3). Calcification of the mitral valve annulus in the elderly patient can occasionally cause hemodynamic obstruction. Space-occupying lesions, such as left atrial myxoma, or thrombus formation can rarely obstruct the mitral valve. The characteristic pathologic change in rheumatic fever is fibrosis and scarring, particularly at the margins of the valve. This process can also extend into the chordae, with shortening and fusion. Eventually, fibrotic and destructive changes lead to calcification of the valve, and pulmonary hypertension with thickening of the pulmonary veins and capillaries, along with intimal and medial proliferation of the pulmonary arteries, occurs. With longstanding mitral stenosis and pulmonary hypertension, right ventricular hypertrophy and fibrosis develop.

Physiology

The hemodynamic abnormalities in mitral stenosis result from obstruction of diastolic blood flow into the left ventricle. The normal cross-sectional area of the mitral valve ranges from 4 to 6 cm², and turbulence of diastolic flow occurs when the valvular orifice is reduced below 2 cm². Increased demands for cardiac output, such as in exercise or fever, may be necessary to produce the diastolic murmur when the mitral valve orifice is reduced to 1.5 to 2 cm². In the second stage of progressive reduction in the mitral orifice size, a diastolic gradient develops between the left atrium and left ventricle under resting conditions when the valvular area is 1.5 to 1 cm². In the advanced stage, mitral orifice size is less than 1 cm², and left atrial and pulmonary hypertension becomes significant. The pulmonary capillary pressure often exceeds 20 to 25 mm Hg, and this leads to significant pulmonary arterial hypertension, pressure overload on the right ventricle, and compensatory hypertrophy of the right ventricle. Although the cardiac output can be maintained until the late stage of severe mitral stenosis, exercise will not produce a normal increase in cardiac output owing to impaired diastolic filling. Another hemodynamic complication in chronic mitral stenosis is atrial fibrillation due to left atrial enlargement. Atrial fibrillation and the increased ventricular response can aggravate hemodynamic abnormalities by reducing the diastolic filling period and leading to further elevation of pressure in the lungs.

Clinical Features

The average age at which rheumatic fever occurs is 10 to 12 years, and generally there is a 10-year period before the murmur of mitral stenosis can be detected. Mitral stenosis affects females more than males, and symptoms usually develop between the ages of 25 and 30 years. In temperate zones, mitral stenosis can accelerate in childhood, with severe hemodynamic impairment by the age of 10 to 12 years. Dyspnea is the most common symptom secondary to pulmonary venous hypertension and can be precipitated by any

TABLE 52–3. MITRAL STENOSIS

Etiology	Physiology	Symptoms	Physical Examination	Electrocardiogram	Chest	Echocardiogram	Catheterization	Medical Therapy	Surgical Therapy
Rheumatic Myxoma Calcification Congenital	Pressure overload LA* and pulmonary veins	Dyspnea Fatigue Palpitations Hemoptysis	Loud S₁ Opening snap Diastolic rumble Signs of pulmonary hypertension: RVH* ↑ P₂ Diastolic blow	Broad, notched P wave in lead II	Enlarged LA Prominent pulmonary veins	Square wave of EF slope of mitral valve Estimation of gradient and orifice size	Elevated PA* wedge pressure and normal LV diastolic pressure	Dental prophylaxis Digitalis for atrial fibrillation Warfarin (Coumadin)	Symptoms Valvular area <1.0 cm²

*LA = left atrium; RVH = right ventricular hypertrophy; PA = pulmonary arterial.

circumstance that increases cardiac output, such as exercise or febrile conditions. Paroxysmal atrial fibrillation can precipitate symptoms by increasing the ventricular rate. As the stenosis progresses, patients experience symptoms with minimal effort or at rest. With longstanding mitral stenosis and chronic pulmonary hypertension, the compensatory thickening of the pulmonary capillaries can protect the lungs from extravasation of fluid despite severe elevations of pulmonary pressure.

Systemic embolization resulting from underlying atrial fibrillation and left atrial thrombus development can also be a manifestation of mitral stenosis. Females can become symptomatic in the second trimester of pregnancy, when the blood volume increases significantly and elevates pulmonary pressures. As the blood volume diminishes late in the third trimester, the symptoms may slightly improve. With severe enlargement of the left atrium and infringement on the mainstem bronchus, persistent cough may develop. Hemoptysis can result from rupture of small vessels in the bronchi due to longstanding venous hypertension. Infective endocarditis can complicate mitral stenosis at any stage, but this generally occurs when mitral regurgitation is present as well.

Physical Examination

The classic physical findings of mitral stenosis are an accentuated first sound at the apex, an opening snap, and a diastolic rumble. If the condition is severe, the diminished peripheral pulse and blood pressure reflect a reduced left ventricular stroke volume. Patients may display typical "mitral facies" with florid congestion of the cheeks. The distended neck veins indicate right ventricular failure with secondary tricuspid regurgitation. If tricuspid stenosis coexists with mitral stenosis, a prominent *a* wave may be observed in the jugular vein.

Inspection of the precordium may reveal activity along the left sternal border, indicating right ventricular enlargement and pulmonary hypertension. On palpation, the accentuated first sound, the opening snap, and the diastolic rumble can sometimes be felt at the apex. With significant right ventricular dilatation, the left ventricular apical impulse may be displaced laterally, and the right cardiac border may be percussed to the right of the sternum. The opening snap can vary from 0.04 to 0.10 second after the second sound at the apex. The higher the left atrial pressure, the closer the opening snap to the second heart sound (S_2), and thus the S_2-OS interval indicates the severity of the mitral stenosis. The opening snap is a high-pitched sound and is heard best with the patient in the left lateral decubitus position. The opening snap can sometimes be appreciated at the base of the heart but must be differentiated from a split pulmonic second sound. The diastolic rumble at the apex is a low-pitched murmur following the opening snap. If sinus rhythm is present, there will be presystolic accentuation due to atrial contraction. Since the murmur of mitral stenosis may be faint in the early stages, to complete the physical examination, the patient should exercise by performing sit-ups or hopping on one foot to increase the heart rate. With the increased flow across the mitral valve, the diastolic rumble may be more easily detected.

The diastolic murmur of pulmonic insufficiency should be sought along the left sternal border, but this can be difficult to distinguish from aortic regurgitation. A widened systemic pulse pressure favors aortic versus pulmonic insufficiency with mitral stenosis. Rarely, tricuspid stenosis can simultaneously occur with the mitral stenosis. The murmur of tricuspid stenosis is heard along the lower left sternal border and is greatly accentuated with inspiration. Finally, some degree of mitral incompetence often accompanies mitral stenosis and will produce an apical systolic murmur of varying intensity.

Laboratory Studies

Electrocardiogram

The electrocardiographic changes of mitral stenosis include left atrial enlargement and right ventricular hypertrophy due to pulmonary hypertension. Characteristic notching and prolongation of the P wave are most prominent in leads II, III, and aV_F. The terminal portion of the P wave is usually negative in lead V_1. Right-axis deviation and an increased amplitude of the R wave in V_1 are evidence of right ventricular hypertrophy.

Chest Radiograph

Radiographic evidence of mitral stenosis includes left atrial enlargement, pulmonary venous hypertension, and right ventricular prominence. The enlarged left atrium produces a double contour along the right cardiac silhouette, as well as straightening of the left cardiac border due to the large left atrial appendage. This change produces elevation of the left mainstem bronchus. The pulmonary venous hypertension redistributes the blood flow to the apices of the lungs, with a reduction in blood volume of the lower lung. Pulmonary arterial hypertension renders the hilar arteries more prominent. Kerley's B lines due to fibrosis and lymphatic engorgement appear as transverse linear densities at the lung bases above the diaphragm.

Echocardiogram

The echocardiogram is the most accurate noninvasive technique for detection of mitral valve stenosis and is recognized by the characteristic square wave motion of the E to F slope of the valve during diastole. The concordant movement of anterior and posterior mitral valve leaflets is one of the cardinal echocardiographic findings in mitral stenosis. Calcification produces additional echoes from the stenotic valve. The two-dimensional echo can accurately measure the diastolic area of the mitral valve, and the echoDoppler technique can estimate the pressure gradient across the valve, as well as left atrial and left ventricular dimensions, and provide an assessment of left ventricular function. Thrombus or a myxoma in the left atrium will produce multiple echoes during diastolic filling.

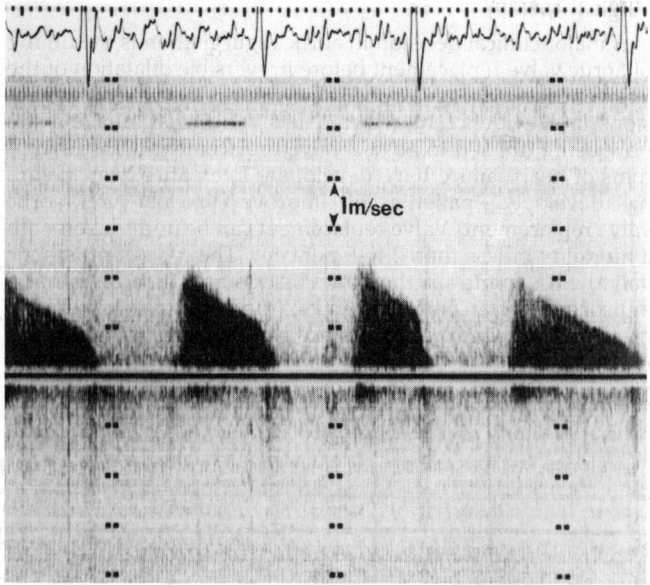

FIGURE 52–2. Continuous wave Doppler echocardiogram of mitral valve flow in a patient with mitral stenosis and atrial fibrillation.

Exercise Testing

Treadmill or bicycle exercise testing can establish aerobic capacity and the degree of exercise impairment. These observations can be useful in following the young patient with mitral stenosis during the early stages of the disease. The response of the heart rate to exertion and early symptoms of fatigue or dyspnea can be documented with an exercise test.

Cardiac Catheterization

Hemodynamic confirmation of mitral stenosis requires measurement of the diastolic pressure gradient across the mitral valve. Left atrial pressure can be obtained directly through trans-septal puncture or as reflected in the pulmonary capillary wedge pressure and recorded simultaneously with the left ventricular pressure. The Gorlin formula (see Ch. 42.5) permits calculation of the mitral orifice size based on the diastolic flow derived from the forward cardiac output and the simultaneous pressure gradient across the valve. The mitral valve gradient can vary from 5 to 25 mm Hg. In an individual without symptoms, mitral valve area can range from 1.5 to 2.0 cm². In those exhibiting symptoms with usual activity, valvular size may be 1.5 cm² or less, and patients with marked limitations usually have an orifice size less than 1.0 cm². Sometimes, a minimal mitral valve gradient is obtained under resting circumstances, but exercise can markedly increase pulmonary pressures to the level of heart failure. At the time of catheterization, associated valve lesions should be assessed, such as mitral regurgitation, aortic stenosis, and aortic regurgitation. If the patient is above 40 years of age, coronary arteriography should also be performed.

Differential Diagnosis

Several cardiac conditions can be confused with the symptoms and physical findings of mitral stenosis. A left atrial myxoma can produce dyspnea or syncope with an opening snap and a diastolic rumble. Primary pulmonary hypertension in young women can be associated with dyspnea and an accentuated pulmonic second sound, but other auscultatory findings are lacking. An atrial septal defect can mimic mitral stenosis with an accentuated first sound, opening snap, and diastolic rumble. However, the accentuated first sound is due to tricuspid valve closure, the opening snap is a split pulmonic second sound, and the diastolic rumble is created by flow across the tricuspid valve.

Medical Therapy

Medical therapy is directed at reducing the incidence of rheumatic fever, prophylaxis for infective endocarditis, control of atrial fibrillation with a rapid ventricular response, and anticoagulation for thromboembolic phenomena. The patient should continue on rheumatic fever prophylaxis until he or she is 30 years of age.

Since atrial fibrillation can aggravate and precipitate symptoms of pulmonary congestion, digitalis should be administered to control ventricular response. Anticoagulation on a chronic basis should be considered in all patients with mitral stenosis and atrial fibrillation. If the patient develops pulmonary edema with atrial fibrillation, cardioversion should be attempted. Ideally, the patient should be anticoagulated two weeks prior to elective cardioversion for atrial fibrillation. Quinidine should be started two days before the elective procedure, and if digitalis has been administered, this may be discontinued one day prior to the cardioversion. If cardioversion is successful, the patient should remain on long-term anticoagulation and quinidine therapy. For thromboembolic phenomena from the left atrium, anticoagulation is indicated. For acute embolism to the extremities or abdomen, surgical embolectomy may be beneficial.

Although considered experimental at present, valvuloplasty via catheter is being performed in selected patients with mitral stenosis, particularly in children or in young women desiring to become pregnant at a later date.

Surgical Therapy

The decision for surgery is based on the development of symptoms of pulmonary congestion during activity or at rest. In addition to pulmonary congestion, recurrent atrial fibrillation with aggravation of pulmonary congestion, thromboembolic phenomena, and hemoptysis can be indications for surgery. Mitral commissurotomy remains the procedure of choice with a pliable mitral valve without calcification or mitral regurgitation and carries an operative mortality of less than 1 per cent. This procedure should be considered particularly for the young female who has a desire for pregnancy. Sometimes commissurotomy can be performed before the development of significant symptoms. Patients may benefit for 5 to 20 years after commissurotomy, but if symptoms occur at a later time, mitral valve replacement may be required. Mitral valve replacement carries an operative mortality of 2 to 3 per cent. The type of mitral valve depends on the age of the patient as well as the circumstances for anticoagulation in a young female. The porcine valve can be inserted without the need for chronic anticoagulation but may require replacement after 10 years. If the valve is calcified or if the patient has had a previous commissurotomy, a prosthetic device is preferred. When there is a contraindication to anticoagulation, as in the aging patient, the porcine valve can be inserted.

Anticoagulation and antibiotic prophylaxis are required in patients with a prosthetic valve. Should atrial fibrillation persist with a rapid ventricular response, digitalis will still have to be administered. Long-term complications of prosthetic mitral valves, such as thrombus formation, infection, and mechanical dysfunction, are estimated to occur at a rate of 1 to 2 per cent per year. Thromboembolism occurs at a rate of 3 per cent per year with a mechanical mitral valve, whereas with the porcine valve, the incidence is 1 to 2 per cent per year.

MITRAL REGURGITATION
Etiology and Pathology

Mitral valve prolapse has now become the leading cause of mitral regurgitation (see next section), although rheumatic heart disease remains an important cause of mitral regurgitation (Table 52–4). Connective tissue disorders, coronary artery disease, annular calcification, and any condition producing left ventricular dilatation can create incompetence of the mitral valve. Several congenital cardiac conditions, such as partial atrioventricular (AV) canal, corrected transposition of the great arteries, and isolated cleft of the mitral valve seen with the ostium primum atrial septal defect, can be associated with mitral valve regurgitation.

Acute mitral regurgitation can result from sudden disruption of the normal function of the mitral valve apparatus. Ruptured mitral valve chordae from endocarditis, myxomatous degeneration of the valve, or trauma can produce sudden mitral regurgitation. Acute myocardial infarction can rupture the papillary muscle, and infective endocarditis can perforate the mitral valve leaflet or the chordae. Mechanical disturbances with a prosthetic mitral valve can lead to mitral incompetence.

Physiology

Incompetence of the mitral valve apparatus during systolic ejection permits regurgitation into the left atrium and pulmonary veins. The extent of the hemodynamic abnormalities imposed on the left ventricle and the left atrium is influenced by the chronic or acute nature of the valvular disturbance as well as the pre-existing functional state of the left ventricle. In chronic mitral regurgitation, a volume overload is imposed on the left ventricle, and the size of the regurgitant volume

TABLE 52–4. MITRAL REGURGITATION

Etiology	Physiology	Symptoms	Physical Examination	Electrocardiogram	Chest	Echocardiogram	Catheterization	Medical Therapy	Surgical Therapy
Chronic									
Prolapse	LV volume overload	Initially asymptomatic	Holosystolic apical murmur	LV hypertrophy	Enlarged LV	Enlarged LV and LA	Contrast from LV to LA	Afterload reduction	Symptoms
Rheumatic		Fatigue	Decreased S₁		Enlarged LA		LA v wave	Diuretics	LV echo
Coronary artery disease	LV dilatation and hypertrophy	Dyspnea	Third sound			Mitral valve anatomy		Digitalis	Diastolic dimension >60 mm†
Annular calcification	LA* enlargement								
Connective tissue disorder									
LV* dilatation									
Prosthetic valve									
Acute									
Ruptured chordae	Pressure overload LA and pulmonary veins	Acute pulmonary edema	Harsh holosystolic murmur radiating into back	No change Acute myocardial infarction	Normal LV and LA dimension	Abnormal mitral valve apparatus	Massive LA regurgitation	Preload and afterload reduction	Surgery may be urgently required
Ruptured papillary muscle			Third sound		Pulmonary edema		Large v wave		
Perforation of leaflet	No change in LV dimension						Normal-sized LA		
Prosthetic valve									

*LV = left ventricle, ventricular; LA = left atrium atrial.
†Proposed.

will determine the increase in the end-diastolic volume. Systolic regurgitation into the left atrium produces a prominent v wave, which accentuates the normal filling of the left ventricle from the pulmonary venous inflow. With chronic mitral regurgitation, distensibility of the left atrium and pulmonary veins and increased compliant properties of the left ventricle permit rapid ventricular diastolic filling. As a result of the increased atrial and ventricular compliance, mean left atrial pressure and left ventricular end-diastolic pressure often remain within the normal range in chronic mitral regurgitation.

In *chronic mitral regurgitation,* the large total left ventricular stroke volume maintains the forward stroke volume despite the regurgitant volume into the left atrium. Total left ventricular output may reach six times the normal forward cardiac output. Left ventricular hypertrophy accompanies the increased left ventricular end-diastolic volume. Eventually, the contractile properties of the left ventricular myocardium decline, and the end-systolic volume is abnormally increased. The ejection fraction declines, even though the value may remain near the normal range in the early stage of left ventricular decompensation. An increase in the end-systolic volume elevates the pressure and wall stress values beyond those that can be attributed solely to changes in wall thickness or hypertrophy. This occurrence has been designated as a mismatch in afterload and preload. Even though the deterioration of the contractile state of the left ventricle may gradually elevate the left ventricular end-diastolic pressure, in rare instances the left atrium enlarges to such dimensions that ventricular end-diastolic and left atrial pressures remain normal, as encountered in the giant left atrium syndrome.

In coronary artery disease, mitral regurgitation results from abnormalities of posterior wall motion and papillary muscle function. Ischemia of the papillary muscle has been proposed as a mechanism, and disturbances in posterior wall motion are usually present with mitral regurgitation. When the residual scar after myocardial infarction exceeds 20 per cent of the total surface area of the ventricle, compensatory dilatation of the left ventricle is often attended by some degree of mitral regurgitation.

Severe dilatation of the left ventricle from either a primary volume overload or a secondary myocardial decompensation will eventually result in mitral regurgitation. Dilatation of the left ventricular chamber displaces the papillary muscles so that coaptation of the leaflets is impaired during systolic ejection. Conditions producing ventricular dilatation are further aggravated by depression of the contractile state, and the left ventricular hemodynamic abnormalities primarily reflect myocardial failure with an additional overload on the ventricle.

In *acute mitral regurgitation,* a sudden pressure overload is imposed on the left atrium and pulmonary veins from the left ventricular regurgitant volume. This pressure overload is intensified by the inability of the left atrium and left ventricle to dilate suddenly. The v wave in the left atrium may be as high as 60 to 70 mm Hg, resulting in acute pulmonary edema.

Clinical Features

When mitral regurgitation results from primary defects in the mitral apparatus, significant enlargement of the left ventricle develops, but the patient may remain symptom free with normal exercise tolerance. Since pulmonary venous hypertension and congestion are not features of mitral regurgitation in the early phase, fatigue due to reduced forward cardiac output is a more frequent symptom than dyspnea. Gradual impairment of the contractile state is attended by further enlargement of end-systolic and end-diastolic volumes and elevation of the left ventricular end-diastolic and left atrial pressures. Atrial fibrillation commonly develops when the left atrium enlarges and further aggravates heart failure.

In coronary artery disease, significant mitral regurgitation is usually accompanied by symptoms of impaired left ventricular function, such as dyspnea, fatigue, and orthopnea. This condition is sometimes designated as the ischemic cardiomyopathy syndrome. In acute syndromes of mitral regurgitation, pulmonary edema is often the initial presentation because of the suddenly imposed pressure and volume overload on the left atrium and pulmonary venous system.

Physical Examination

The typical physical finding of mitral regurgitation is the apical holosystolic murmur, but the intensity, variation during the ejection phase, and radiation over the precordium are influenced by the underlying mechanism. The peripheral pulse can sometimes be rapid in upstroke with a short duration because of the abbreviated systolic ejection time, since a large volume of blood is regurgitated into the left atrium. The precordium may reveal a diffusely hyperdynamic impulse, and the first heart sound at the apex is diminished. The characteristic holosystolic murmur radiates into the axilla and often to the left sternal border. A protodiastolic or ventricular gallop sound is frequently audible and may be followed by an early diastolic rumble due to the large inflow of blood from the left atrium. When mitral regurgitation is caused by left ventricular dilatation and depression of the contractile state, the systolic murmur may be mid-, late-, or holosystolic. Under these circumstances, the systolic murmur is usually grade II/VI or less and is accompanied by a left ventricular (S₃) gallop sound.

In acute mitral regurgitation due to rupture of the mitral valve apparatus, the murmur is harsh, grade III or IV/VI, and accompanied by a palpable thrill at the apex.

Laboratory Studies

Electrocardiogram

In chronic mitral regurgitation, the electrocardiogram will show evidence of left ventricular dilatation and hypertrophy with increased QRS voltage and ST-T wave changes in the lateral precordial leads. Left atrial enlargement will produce a negative P wave in lead V_1, but atrial fibrillation often develops in the late stages. When coronary artery disease is the etiology of mitral regurgitation, there is often evidence of an inferior or posterior wall myocardial infarction.

Chest Radiograph

Left ventricular enlargement due to the volume overload can be appreciated from the standard chest film. Left atrial enlargement will cause a prominence along the right sternal border, but the pulmonary venous pattern may show no abnormalities until heart failure and venous congestion have developed.

Echocardiogram

The echocardiogram can define the anatomy of the mitral valve apparatus as well as left atrial and left ventricular chamber dimensions and function. Calcification of the valve leaflets and the annulus can be recognized. Depression of left ventricular ejection fraction and increases in end-diastolic and end-systolic dimensions are observed in secondary causes of mitral regurgitation with heart failure. With acute mitral regurgitation, a flail leaflet, ruptured chordae, or nidus of infection with infective endocarditis can sometimes be identified by the echocardiogram. The echoDoppler technique can assess the intensity of the regurgitant jet into the left atrium. Finally, left ventricular end-diastolic and end-systolic dimensions have been used to identify the optimal time for mitral valve replacement before significant and irreversible myocardial deterioration has taken place.

Exercise Testing

The standard exercise tests and radionuclide angiography can quantify functional capacity and document early deterioration in patients with mitral regurgitation.

Cardiac Catheterization

Left ventriculography confirms mitral regurgitation by demonstrating systolic regurgitation of contrast material into the left atrium. Although the magnitude of the regurgitation can be quantified, the mechanism is not always apparent from left ventriculography. Left ventricular end-diastolic and end-systolic dimensions can be utilized to calculate ejection fraction, left ventricular mass, wall stress, and regurgitant volume per beat into the left atrium. The difference between the angiographic left ventricular stroke volume—that is, the end-diastolic volume minus the end-systolic volume on left ventriculography—and the forward stroke volume, calculated from the Fick or thermodilution methods, yields the regurgitant stroke volume per beat across the mitral valve. Coronary artery disease and the wall motion abnormalities contributing to disturbance in mitral valve function can also be confirmed at catheterization. The prominent v wave of mitral regurgitation can be recorded in the left atrium or the pulmonary capillary wedge pressure tracing. In acute mitral regurgitation, dimensions of the left ventricle and left atrium may be normal, but the regurgitant v wave can rise to 60 to 70 mm Hg. Cardiac catheterization can also detect coexistent lesions in the aortic valve. Since the left ventricular ejection fraction may be misleading maintained in the normal range despite deterioration of the contractile state, additional assessment of

the contractile state is important in all causes of mitral regurgitation. Calculation of end-systolic wall stress from pressure, volume, and wall thickness dimensions has proved useful in recognizing early deterioration of the contractile state in mitral regurgitation.

Differential Diagnosis

A holosystolic murmur identifies mitral regurgitation, even though the mechanism may not be apparent. Tricuspid regurgitation can cause a holosystolic murmur at the lower left sternal border, but inspiration accentuates the murmur more than in mitral regurgitation. If the murmur is not holosystolic, conditions such as aortic stenosis could be considered, along with papillary muscle dysfunction and mitral valve prolapse. In calcific aortic stenosis of the elderly patient, the murmur may sometimes be more prominent in the apex and may be confused with that of mitral regurgitation. A ventricular septal defect also causes a harsh holosystolic murmur at the lower left sternal border, but this generally radiates to the right of the sternum, compared with the axillary radiation of the murmur in mitral regurgitation.

Medical Therapy

In the early phase of mitral regurgitation without symptoms, only antibiotic prophylaxis is warranted. The same antibiotic program as described in the mitral stenosis should be administered to these patients. When atrial fibrillation develops, digitalis is indicated to slow the ventricular response. Afterload-reducing agents, such as nitrates and antihypertensive drugs, have been found useful in maintaining the forward stroke volume in mitral regurgitation. Once heart failure develops, diuretics and inotropic agents are required, but major consideration should be given to surgery.

Surgical Therapy

The operative mortality of mitral valve replacement in mitral regurgitation has remained higher than the 2 to 3 per cent in mitral stenosis and for the symptomatic patient may range from 5 to 10 per cent. In the past, surgery has been delayed until patients develop symptoms, but the advanced symptomatic stage and depressed left ventricular function contribute to high operative mortality rates. When the ejection fraction falls below 20 per cent, operative mortality for mitral valve replacement may be as high as 25 per cent. Therefore, surgery should be considered before the patient becomes extremely symptomatic. An echocardiographic diastolic dimension greater than 60 mm has been proposed as a predictor for mitral valve replacement. In the selection of the optimal prosthetic device, the patient's age, underlying condition, and circumstances for anticoagulation must be considered. The mechanical prosthetic valve in the mitral position is more likely to develop thrombotic material than in other locations, so anticoagulation must be maintained. Any contraindication to anticoagulation warrants consideration of a porcine valve. Thromboembolism in patients with mechanical valves who are on anticoagulation occurs at a rate of 3 per cent per year, and for preoperative functional classes I through III, there is a yearly mortality rate of 3 per cent over a ten-year follow-up period. With a porcine valve, the rate of thromboembolism is lower but may reach 1.5 per cent per year.

MITRAL VALVE PROLAPSE
Etiology and Pathology

Although an isolated systolic click has been regarded as benign for decades, echocardiography has identified prolapse of the mitral valve in as many as 5 per cent of the adult population. A variety of synonyms include the midsystolic click–late systolic murmur, click murmur syndrome, and Barlow's syndrome. Pathologic findings include myxomatous degeneration of the valve and redundancy of the valve leaflets. These changes can also involve the chordae as well as the mitral valve. Although the underlying mechanism is still incompletely understood, these changes in the mitral valve are seen with several connective tissue diseases, including Marfan's syndrome and osteogenesis imperfecta, and sometimes with coronary artery disease. The syndrome occurs most frequently in women in early adulthood and can also be found in families.

Physiology

The abnormalities of mitral valve prolapse can affect both anterior and posterior leaflets, but the posterior leaflet is most frequently involved. With the onset of ventricular systole, normal closure of the mitral valve takes place, but redundancy of the leaflets results in further upward motion of the valve into the left atrium. Sudden cessation of the valvular motion is thought to generate the click, and the lack of proper positioning of the two leaflets results in the systolic regurgitant murmur in mid- and late systole. Occasionally, both the anterior and posterior leaflets prolapse, and in extreme conditions, there can be extensive prolapse of both leaflets in the absence of a click or murmur. In a small number of patients, progressive degenerative changes in the valve or rupture of the chordae or both can produce severe mitral regurgitation.

Clinical Features

The majority of patients with mitral valve prolapse remain asymptomatic, but a spectrum of symptoms can be encountered. Symptoms include palpitations, fatigue, chest pain, orthostatic changes, and psychologic aberrations. Frequently, symptoms fail to correlate with the prominence of the physical findings and the extent of mitral regurgitation. Circulatory studies on changes in tilting, along with heart rate and blood pressure response changes, have lead to a diagnosis of dysautonomia in certain of these patients. In 10 to 15 per cent of affected individuals, palpitations may become frequent, and in a smaller number there may be progressive mitral regurgitation. Infective endocarditis occurs with a slightly higher incidence than in the normal population. Sudden deaths associated with this syndrome have been sporadically reported.

Physical Findings

Patients are often female, with a thin habitus and a narrow anteroposterior chest diameter. The principal findings are the early to midsystolic click and a mid- or late systolic murmur. The timing of the click as well as the characteristics of the murmur can vary widely. Often the murmur is crescendo and decrescendo, but it can be sustained in its frequency. The click or the murmur may be present alone, and not infrequently, both click and murmur are absent. The click and the murmur are influenced by the dimensions of the ventricle, and maneuvers that decrease ventricular filling, such as standing and the Valsalva maneuver, will result in movement of the click closer to the first sound, followed by early onset of the murmur. Conditions that increase filling of the ventricle, such as the squatting maneuver, can delay the onset of the click and the murmur.

Laboratory Studies

Electrocardiogram

The electrocardiogram may reveal a variety of T wave and ST segment changes, along with atrial or ventricular ectopic beats. Most commonly, the T wave is slightly inverted in the inferior and lateral precordial leads, and occasionally there is associated ST segment depression. Rarely, QT prolongation with deep coving of the T wave is seen in the precordial leads. Runs of premature beats, both from the atrium and the

ventricle, can be recorded by Holter monitoring. Frequently, symptoms do not correlate with the frequency and occurrence of cardiac ectopic activity.

Chest Radiograph

The habitus is asthenic; the chest has a narrow anteroposterior diameter, and the cardiac silhouette is elongated.

Echocardiography

The echocardiogram is the diagnostic technique of choice for mitral valve prolapse. In one form, late systolic prolapse of the posterior leaflet resembles an inverted question mark. In the second form, there may be prolapse of the posterior leaflet throughout the systolic ejection phase with a hammock type of configuration. The echocardiographic findings of prolapse can be recognized in the absence of the click and the murmur. At other times, the click and murmur cannot be confirmed by echocardiographically evident prolapse of the leaflet. The standard for diagnosis of mitral valve prolapse is the two-dimensional echo, which can define the plane of the mitral annulus and demonstrate extension of the mitral valve leaflets beyond the annulus into the left atrium.

Exercise Testing

Stress testing can aggravate or precipitate cardiac irritability in these patients. Furthermore, the exercise test can document the patient's fatigue and musculoskeletal symptoms, which often are at variance with the echocardiographic findings.

Cardiac Catheterization

Although left ventriculography has been the standard invasive method for documenting redundancy and prolapse of the mitral leaflets, the precision of echocardiography has obviated the necessity of catheterization in the majority of patients with prolapse. Atypical chest discomfort sometimes requires coronary arteriography to exclude coronary artery disease. Wall motion abnormalities have been recognized on the ventriculogram, but these do not correlate with coexisting abnormalities in the coronary arteries. Prolapse of the tricus-

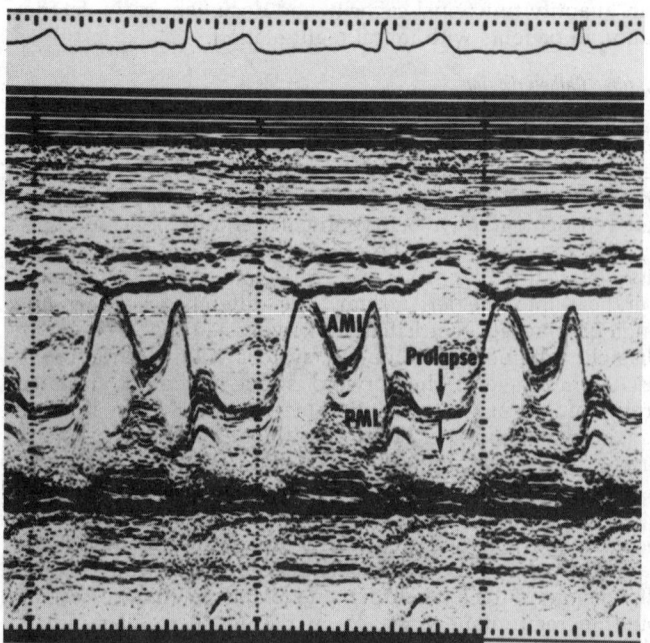

FIGURE 52–3. M-Mode echocardiogram of a patient with mitral valve prolapse. Note the systolic posterior motion of the anterior (AML) and posterior (PML) mitral valve leaflets.

pid valve can also occur. With mitral valve prolapse in connective tissue disorders, there may be associated aortic regurgitation.

Differential Diagnosis

The mid- and late systolic murmur, as well as the crescendo-decrescendo qualities of mitral valve prolapse, can be similar to the murmur of regurgitation in papillary muscle dysfunction. In coronary artery disease or hypertrophic cardiomyopathy with obstruction, the crescendo-decrescendo murmur may be similar to that of mitral valve prolapse. However, the harsh intensity of the murmur is much louder with the hyperdynamic contraction of hypertrophic cardiomyopathy. Maneuvers that increase the murmur of mitral valve prolapse intensify the murmur of cardiomyopathy with obstruction even more. However, in the latter condition, the murmur is often holosystolic. If ventricular irritability is present, the intensity of the murmur of hypertrophic cardiomyopathy with obstruction will be much louder in the post-extrasystolic beat.

Treatment

The majority of patients with mitral valve prolapse require no treatment. Ventricular ectopy and symptoms of palpitations can be effectively managed with beta-blocking drugs. However, the fatigue in these patients can sometimes be aggravated with beta blockade. In patients with the prolonged QT interval or syncope, treatment with an antiarrhythmic is warranted. Infrequently, control of ectopy may be difficult despite the use of standard antiarrhythmic agents.

Infective endocarditis is a potential problem in these patients. Originally, all patients were advised to have antibiotic prophylaxis. Statistical studies now suggest that only those patients with an audible click and murmur should be treated with antibiotic prophylaxis. Patients with prolapse demonstrated on echocardiography without a click or murmur may be at no greater risk than the normal population. When mitral regurgitation becomes progressive with chamber enlargement or with ruptured chordae, mitral valve replacement may be necessary. Mitral valve reconstruction and mitral valve annuloplasty are preferred by some surgeons to total valve replacement. Fortunately, for the majority of patients, reassurance and conservative follow-up constitute the best treatment.

TRICUSPID STENOSIS

The most common cause of stenosis of the tricuspid valve remains rheumatic fever, but this condition is invariably associated with involvement of left-sided valves by the same rheumatic process. Rare conditions such as carcinoid tumor, endocardial fibroelastosis, and right atrial myxoma can create stenosis or obstruction of the tricuspid valve. Tricuspid stenosis causes right atrial hypertension and elevated systemic venous pressure. Stenosis of the tricuspid valve may serve as a protective mechanism for the pulmonary vascular bed in patients with mitral stenosis. Symptoms of tricuspid stenosis are dyspnea and fatigue, but the pulmonary manifestations of mitral stenosis can diminish with the development of significant stenosis of the tricuspid valve. Pulsations in the neck veins and peripheral edema develop.

Physical examination reveals a prominent, often giant, a wave in the neck veins caused by the vigorous atrial contraction against the stenotic valve. The diastolic murmur is heard best along the left lower sternal border and is presystolic if sinus rhythm is present or midsystolic with atrial fibrillation. The murmur increases prominently with inspiration, but an opening snap is barely heard. Since mitral stenosis is usually concurrent, the auscultatory maneuvers must specifically locate the tricuspid stenosis murmur. If tricuspid stenosis is the dominant hemodynamic lesion, pulmonary hypertension and

right ventricular hypertrophy will not be detected on the physical examination.

The electrocardiographic finding is a tall, tented P wave in leads II, III, and aV$_F$ with absence of right ventricular hypertrophy. The chest radiograph should reveal a large right atrium without prominence of the pulmonary arteries. The echoDoppler technique may detect and assess the gradient across the tricuspid valve. If cardiac catheterization is performed simultaneous catheters must be placed in the right atrium and the right ventricle for accurate detection of the pressure gradient. Respiratory variations will introduce inaccuracies in a pull-back tracing across the tricuspid valve. Treatment consists of antibiotic coverage. If surgery is performed for lesions in the left side of the heart, correction of the tricuspid lesion can also be undertaken.

TRICUSPID INSUFFICIENCY

Tricuspid insufficiency is, most commonly, secondary to right ventricular dilatation and hypertrophy. Tricuspid regurgitation can rarely result from infective endocarditis, trauma, prolapse, or congenital heart disease such as atrial septal defect or Ebstein's anomaly. Symptoms of tricuspid regurgitation are those of hepatic congestion or peripheral edema.

On physical examination, atrial fibrillation is commonly present and large cv waves can be detected in the jugular veins. The murmur is holosystolic along the left sternal border and increases with inspiration. The electrocardiogram often reveals atrial fibrillation without other significant features. The chest film will demonstrate a prominent right atrium and ventricle. The echocardiogram can document prolapse of the tricuspid leaflets as well as a nidus of infection or disruption of a chorda. Contrast-echo and echoDoppler techniques can accurately detect and assess the amount of tricuspid regurgitation. Therapy usually consists of treatment of conditions leading to right ventricular failure. Should surgery be performed for left-sided lesions, the tricuspid valve can be inspected. Often the leaflets are anatomically normal, and annuloplasty is indicated rather than valve replacement. If the tricuspid valve is replaced, along with insertion of mitral and aortic prostheses, mortality remains high at 20 per cent.

PULMONIC REGURGITATION

Regurgitation of the pulmonic valve is most invariably secondary to severe pulmonary hypertension, which can be caused by mitral stenosis, chronic lung disease, or pulmonary emboli. Inflammatory diseases and endocarditis can sometimes render the pulmonic valve incompetent, and previous surgery for congenital heart disease may create pulmonic regurgitation. The murmur (Graham Steell) is typically a high-pitched diastolic blow along the left sternal border similar to that in aortic regurgitation. No characteristic electrocardiographic changes are found, but the chest radiograph will often demonstrate a prominent pulmonary artery. The echoDoppler technique may detect turbulence in the pulmonary outflow tract. Cardiac catheterization is useful only to exclude aortic regurgitation as a cause of the diastolic murmur. Treatment consists of management of pulmonary hypertension with medical agents or occasionally with mitral valve surgery.

PULMONIC STENOSIS

Stenotic lesions of the pulmonic valve are almost always caused by congenital malformations (see Ch. 49). Rarely, hypertrophic cardiomyopathy can involve the right side of the heart with obstruction of the right ventricular outflow tract.

AORTIC VALVE DISEASE

Currie PJ, Seward JB, Reeder GS, et al.: Continuous wave Doppler echocardiographic assessment of severity of calcific aortic stenosis: A simultaneous

Doppler catheter correlative study in 100 adult patients. Circulation 71:1162, 1985. *A comparison of noninvasive and invasive estimates of aortic pressure gradients.*

Hoshino PK, Gaasch WH: When to intervene in chronic aortic regurgitation. Arch. Intern. Med 146:349, 1986. *A thorough review of noninvasive and invasive indications for the timing of aortic valve replacement in aortic regurgitation.*

Rackley CE, Edwards JE, Wallace RB, et al.: Aortic valve disease. In Hurst JW (ed.): The Heart. 6th ed. New York, McGraw-Hill Book Company, 1985, p 729.

Wood P: Aortic stenosis. Am J Cardiol 1:553, 1958. *A classic description of aortic stenosis.*

MITRAL VALVE DISEASE

Nishimura RA, McGoon MD, Shub C, et al.: Electrocardiographically documented mitral valve prolapse: Long term follow-up of 237 patients. N Engl J Med 313:1305, 1985. *A large clinical review with noninvasive criteria, for early mitral valve replacement.*

Rackley CE, Edwards JE, Karp RB: Mitral valve disease. In Hurst JW (ed.): The Heart. 6th ed. New York, McGraw-Hill Book Company, 1985, p. 754.

Rappaport E: Natural history of aortic and mitral valve disease. Am J Cardiol 36:221, 1975. *A ten-year follow-up of the stenotic and regurgitant lesions of the aortic and mitral valves.*

VALVE SURGERY

Cohn L, Allred E, Cohn L, et al: Early and late risk of mitral valve replacement. J Thorac Cardiovasc Surg 90:872, 1985. *A large review of the morbidity and mortality in porcine valve prostheses and prosthetic disc valves.*

Ivert TSA, Dismukes WE, Cobbs CG, et al.: Prosthetic valve endocarditis. Circulation 69:223, 1984. *An extensive review of a large series on prosthetic valve endocarditis.*

Magilligan DJ, Lewis JW, Tilley B, et al.: The porcine bioprosthetic valve twelve years later. J Thorac Cardiovasc Surg 89:499, 1985. *An extensive experience with the porcine prosthetic valve.*

53 DISEASES OF THE MYOCARDIUM

Joseph K. Perloff and Lynne Warner Stevenson

"Cardiomyopathy" means heart (cardio) muscle disease (myopathy). The term is appropriately applied to disorders characterized by *primary* involvement of ventricular myocardium. The cardiomyopathies are best classified according to their anatomic and pathophysiologic types as dilated, hypertrophic, or restrictive (Table 53–1, Fig. 53–1). In each category, the cause or causes may or may not be known.

DILATED CARDIOMYOPATHY

DEFINITION AND GENERAL DESCRIPTION OF FINDINGS. Dilated cardiomyopathy is characterized by an increase in left ventricular or biventricular internal dimensions without an appropriate increase in septal and free wall thicknesses. The essential physiologic impairment is in systolic function (depressed contractility).

Certain *general pathophysiologic principles* apply. Injured myocytes do not regenerate but are replaced by connective tissue. Hypertrophy of remaining cells does not adequately compensate for the loss of contractile elements. Ventricular volumes increase as ejection fractions fall, and the ventricles progressively dilate, especially the left. Stroke volume is initially maintained despite depressed ejection fraction, and compen-

TABLE 53–1. PATHOPHYSIOLOGIC CLASSIFICATION OF THE CARDIOMYOPATHIES

1. Dilated
2. Hypertrophic
   a. Asymmetric (eccentric)
   b. Symmetric (concentric)
3. Restrictive (nondilated, nonhypertrophic)
   a. Increased septal wall thickness
   b. Normal septal wall thickness

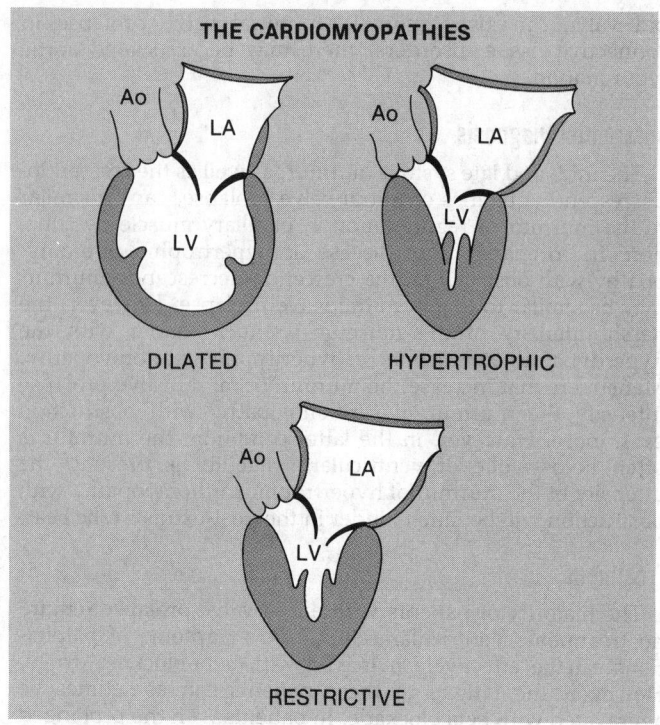

FIGURE 53–1. Schematic illustrations of dilated, hypertrophic, and restrictive cardiomyopathies. (Modified from Roberts WC, Ferrans VJ: Pathologic anatomy of the cardiomyopathies. Human Pathol 6:287, 1975. Reprinted with permission from W. B. Saunders Co.)

satory tachycardia may help maintain cardiac output. This state of compensated systolic dysfunction is usually replaced by decompensated heart failure in which cardiac output is critically limited. The development of atrioventricular valve regurgitation adds to the hemodynamic burden and further depresses cardiac output. Hypervolemia and peripheral vasoconstriction contribute additionally to net ventricular overload.

Two major threats confront the chronically afflicted patient, namely, progressive hemodynamic deterioration and sudden death. An insidious decrease in exercise tolerance is followed by frank exertional dyspnea, orthopnea, and paroxysmal nocturnal dyspnea. Both ventricles are usually involved, but the clinical manifestations of left ventricular failure generally predominate. The risk of sudden death is primarily the result of ventricular electrical instability—ventricular tachycardia or ventricular fibrillation. However, sudden death may also be due to systemic emboli from the left side of the heart or to pulmonary emboli.

On *physical examination*, the arterial pulse may be rapid (compensatory tachycardia) with a relatively small pulse pressure and pulsus alternans. The jugular venous pulse exhibits elevated A and V waves with preserved X and Y descents until the advent of tricuspid regurgitation, which increases the V wave and blunts the X descent. Precordial palpation identifies a displaced left ventricular impulse. Auscultation detects third and fourth heart sounds. Systolic murmurs originate from mitral and tricuspid regurgitation. Occasional patients have disproportionate right ventricular failure (peripheral edema, ascites, and painful hepatic congestion). An enlarged, tender liver exhibits an hepatic pulse that mirrors the jugular venous pulse.

The *electrocardiogram* may show nothing more than nonspecific ST-T wave abnormalities, but occasionally Q wave "infarct patterns" are present and are believed to reflect myonecrosis. Left bundle branch block is relatively frequent in chronic idiopathic dilated cardiomyopathy, but Chagas' disease is most commonly manifested by right bundle branch block.

The *chest roentgenogram* reveals varying degrees of cardiomegaly and pulmonary venous congestion. The increase in heart size principally reflects dilatation of the ventricles, although the atria are enlarged as well.

Two-dimensional echocardiography identifies increased internal dimensions of the ventricles at end-diastole, normal or reduced septal and free wall thicknesses, and depressed ventricular function. Although global hypokinesis is the rule, regional wall motion abnormalities occur and are believed to reflect zones of injury caused by a cardiotropic myonecrotic virus. Doppler echocardiography establishes the presence and degree of atrioventricular valve regurgitation. Technetium 99m radionuclide imaging sheds light on abnormal ventricular function and wall motion. The depressed response to exercise can be studied by technetium-99m scintigraphy and stress echocardiography. Magnetic resonance imaging provides refined morphologic information and, together with two-dimensional echocardiography, serves to identify left ventricular endocardial thrombi.

INCIDENCE. Over 10,000 deaths and 100,000 annual hospital admissions in the United States are attributed to dilated cardiomyopathy annually. Current estimates exceed 140 cases per million population per year, a threefold higher incidence than in 1970. The apparent increase probably reflects enhanced awareness and diagnostic accuracy.

ETIOLOGY, PATHOGENESIS, AND PATHOLOGY. The dilated cardiomyopathies are caused by primary myocardial injury that results in depressed systolic function and progressive ventricular dilatation. Table 53–2 lists most of the etiologic categories.

Myocardial inflammation—myocarditis—can be infectious or noninfectious. The majority of cases of dilated cardiomyopathy are believed to represent sequelae of myocarditis, generally infectious. Myocarditis, defined as inflammatory infiltrates and myocardial cell necrosis, is due to direct tissue invasion by the offending infectious agent, to an autoimmune process, or to toxins elaborated by an infectious organism. Every major type of infectious agent has been implicated as causative (Table 53–2), although with widely divergent incidence. In western Europe and the United States, infectious myocarditis is most commonly due to viruses, especially enteroviruses.

TABLE 53–2. ETIOLOGIC CLASSIFICATION OF THE DILATED CARDIOMYOPATHIES

I. **Idiopathic**
II. **Inflammatory**
   A. Infectious
      1. Viral
      2. Bacterial
      3. Mycobacterial
      4. Parasitic
      5. Rickettsial
      6. Spirochetal
      7. Fungal
   B. Noninfectious
      1. Autoimmune diseases
      2. Peripartum
      3. Hypersensitivity reactions
      4. Transplantation rejection
III. **Toxic**
   A. Ethyl alcohol
   B. Chemotherapeutic agents
   C. Elemental compounds
   D. Catecholamines
IV. **Metabolic**
   A. Nutritional
   B. Endocrinologic
   C. Electrolyte abnormalities
V. **Familial cardiomyopathy**
   A. Neuromyopathic
      1. Progressive muscular dystrophy
      2. Myotonic muscular dystrophy
      3. Friedreich's ataxia
   B. Hereditary dilated cardiomyopathy

The most convincingly documented cause of human myocarditis is coxsackievirus group B infection. Experimental murine coxsackievirus B3 infection results in an initial phase of active intramyocardial viral replication and cell necrosis during which physical exercise or immunosuppressive agents enhance replication of the virus and reinforce tissue injury. In the next phase, virus is not detectable in the myocardium. Instead, there is a population of thymus-derived lymphocytes apparently sensitized to myocytes. This phase of myocardial inflammation is believed to reflect immunologic virus-induced myocardial cellular injury caused by cytolytic thymus-derived T lymphocytes—immunopathic myonecrosis. Reduction of the offending lymphocyte population appears to coincide with a decrease in late myocyte injury. Infected animals may recover, die, or progress to a late third stage in which the dilated heart contains little or no inflammation but large areas of fibrosis.

The lymphocyte infiltration and myocyte necrosis of human viral myocarditis are found in the left and right ventricles and may be present in the atria as well. There is reason to believe that the left ventricle—the relatively high-pressure systemic chamber—responds more adversely to viral myocarditis than the less stressed right ventricle, which is a low-pressure, low-resistance pump.

Extensive lymphocytic infiltration and myocardial necrosis often occur in the absence of symptoms. It is likely, therefore, that many cases of primary myocarditis initially escape clinical detection. In the late phase of the natural history, active inflammatory cell infiltration is absent or nearly so. Chronic dilated cardiomyopathy is then characterized by the presence of areas of fibrosis interwoven among shrunken or hypertrophied myocytes. At this stage, the designation *idiopathic dilated cardiomyopathy* is commonly applied because thorough clinical evaluation fails to identify a specific cause in more than 80 per cent of patients so afflicted. Nevertheless, an association between myocardial inflammation initiated by cardiotropic viruses and the subsequent development of dilated cardiomyopathy is persuasive, as argued earlier.

In South America, up to 15 per cent of the rural population have primary myocardial injury due to infection by *Trypanosoma cruzi* (Chagas' disease). Chagas' cardiomyopathy is characterized by an acute tissue invasive phase followed by a chronic phase of extensive myocardial fibrosis believed to be the result of a lymphocyte- or an antibody-mediated autoimmune reaction. Chronic chagasic injury not only affects myocytes (with a peculiar propensity to cause apical left ventricular aneurysm) but also has a predilection for specialized tissues and for cardiac parasympathetic ganglia (denervation).

Noninfectious inflammation of the myocardium occurs with systemic diseases of connective tissues (autoimmune disorders), such as systemic lupus erythematosus. Of the *toxic agents* that directly injure ventricular myocardium, ethyl alcohol, or ethanol, is the commonest and has been implicated in at least 10 per cent of patients with dilated cardiomyopathy. The undesirable acute effects of ethyl alcohol on the myocardium are masked by the beneficial effects of peripheral vasodilatation and the positive inotropic response to released catecholamines, but ethanol in the autonomic blockaded heart causes a significant decrease in contractility. Both ethanol and acetaldehyde (its first metabolite) in sufficient concentrations can severely affect myocardial metabolism. Alcoholic cardiomyopathy is attributed to the toxicity of ethanol and acetaldehyde on the myocardial cell. In addition to the effects of ethyl alcohol and its metabolites, constituents of the brew may also depress contractility. Cobalt added to beer to stabilize foam is a case in point. In the beriberi heart disease of chronic alcoholics, high-output heart failure of thiamine deficiency is imposed upon the depressed myocardium of alcoholic cardiomyopathy. In addition, there is a positive epidemiologic association between excessive alcohol ingestion and systemic hypertension. An important clinical aspect of alcoholic cardiomyopathy is its reversibility, at least initially. However, pathologic studies late in the natural history reveal myocardial cell necrosis with replacement fibrosis.

A host of other toxic substances and drugs reportedly cause myocardial injury either as a result of excessive exposure or as idiosyncratic responses. Catecholamine excess may cause myonecrosis, and doxorubicin (Adriamycin) and other anthracycline chemotherapeutic agents are additional examples. The structural changes in response to anthracycline antitumor agents are dose related. Doxorubicin rarely results in acute heart failure and only occasionally produces acute arrhythmias and conduction disturbances. About 2 to 5 per cent of patients receiving 500 mg of the drug per square meter slowly develop overt heart failure, but over one half of patients have abnormal responses to exercise and exhibit histologic changes on endomyocardial biopsy. The microscopic pattern of doxorubicin-induced myocardial injury is characterized by the gradual appearance of vacuolar degeneration, myofibrillar loss, and juxtaposition of disrupted cells among normal cells.

The distinct clustering of *peripartum cardiomyopathy* in the last month of gestation and especially in the first three postpartal months supports the contention that the disorder is unique to pregnancy. Incidence has been estimated at from 1 in 3000 to 1 in 15,000 confinements. Myocardial inflammation is sufficiently frequent to warrant the designation "myocarditis," but the inflammation is not infectious. Despite diligent search, no role of cardiotropic viruses has been established. The peripartal myocardial injury is believed to result from an autoimmune reaction triggered by release of myocyte antigens from the late-term pregnant uterus.

Metabolic derangements that adversely affect systolic function and result in dilated cardiomyopathy include endocrinopathies, trace element deficiencies, and electrolyte abnormalities. In diabetes mellitus, systolic dysfunction with ventricular dilatation may be unrelated to large- or small-vessel coronary artery disease. Dilated heart failure in hyperthyroidism principally reflects pre-existing impairment of contractile reserve made clinically overt by the hypermetabolic state. An analogy is the high-output state of beriberi (vitamin B_1 deficiency) in chronic alcoholics. In classic Asian beriberi, however, dilated heart failure is due to thiamine deficiency per se in individuals without myocardial depression from other causes. Teenagers who excessively consume processed foods deficient in thiamine may suffer from heart failure provoked by heavy exercise. Although the principal initial physiologic effect of thiamine deficiency is on the peripheral circulation, persistent deficiency may lead to dilated cardiomyopathy. Abnormal regulation of carnitine, a cofactor in mitochondrial fatty acid metabolism, has also been associated with dilated heart failure.

A number of *electrolyte disorders* may aggravate pre-existing abnormalities of myocardial contractility. If the availability of calcium is inadequate, ejection fraction falls, as in patients receiving large transfusions of blood preserved with citrate, which chelates calcium, or in patients with hypoparathyroidism. Hypophosphatemia leads to inadequate stores of high-energy phosphate compounds, as in alcoholism, diabetes, and hyperalimentation. Magnesium, a cofactor for thiamine-dependent reactions and for sodium-potassium adenosine triphosphatase (ATPase), may be depleted by impaired gastrointestinal absorption or increased renal excretion(diuretics).

A number of heredofamilial *neuromyopathic disorders* are associated with dilated cardiomyopathy. Examples include X-linked, slowly progressive muscular dystrophy (Becker's dystrophy), certain patients in the late stages of Duchenne's dystrophy, Friedreich's ataxia, and the childhood form (but not the adult form) of myotonic muscular dystrophy.

DIAGNOSIS. Dilated cardiomyopathy should be suspected in relatively young patients who present with cardiac enlargement, congestive heart failure, systemic emboli, and ventricular arrhythmias. Chest pain indistinguishable from myocar-

dial infarction (myonecrosis caused by the cardiotropic virus) sometimes accompanies acute myocarditis, but the mechanism of chest pain occasionally associated with chronic dilated cardiomyopathy is unclear. The diagnosis of dilated cardiomyopathy hinges on firm exclusion of pre-existing or coexisting heart disease. Cardiac catheterization has given way to noninvasive diagnostic procedures (see earlier) except for the exclusion of ischemic cardiomyopathy (coronary artery disease) in older patients, especially males.

If dilated cardiomyopathy presents sufficiently early in its course (persistent myocardial inflammation), throat and stool cultures and viral titers should be secured and serially compared. Up to 50 per cent of patients with clinical myocarditis have evidence of recent coxsackievirus B infection, especially types 1 to 5. Myocardial inflammation has been identified by gallium 67 scintigraphy, but more specifically by endomyocardial biopsy from the right ventricular septum. Biopsy positivity depends largely on when in the natural history the specimen is secured.

TREATMENT AND PROGNOSIS. Dilated cardiomyopathy confronts us with four major therapeutic concerns: the potential presence of ongoing myocardial injury, the hemodynamic state of the dilated heart, the threat of systemic emboli, and the risk of ventricular arrhythmias.

During the tissue-invasive stage of acute myocarditis, immunosuppressive agents provoke viral replication and are therefore proscribed. The majority of patients who present with active myocardial inflammation do so after the acute tissue-invasive stage. Attempts at pharmacologic suppression of persistent myocardial inflammation require documentation of the presence of inflammation. Although immunosuppression for biopsy-proven myocarditis in human subjects remains controversial, experience with cardiac transplant patients teaches us that immunosuppressive therapy can be lifesaving. Many patients with virally induced myocarditis improve during treatment with prednisone and azathioprine, and relapses have occurred after discontinuing immunosuppression. Whether or not immunosuppression is used, clinical status improves in up to one half of patients with biopsy-proven myocarditis. Not surprisingly, even patients who clinically improve usually have persistent abnormalities of ventricular systolic function. The grim prognosis of peripartum cardiomyopathy, coupled with evidence of noninfectious myocardial inflammation, argues for treatment with immunosuppressive agents, even though the relatively high incidence of spontaneous improvement is a confounding variable. If resolution occurs within six months after delivery, prognosis is good, although one half of such women have recurrences during subsequent pregnancies. Alcoholic cardiomyopathy often responds dramatically to abstention even after patients have become significantly symptomatic. Benefits previously attributed to strict bed rest in patients with dilated cardiomyopathy were largely the result of forced abstinence from ethyl alcohol. Continued ethanol consumption is associated with an inexorable deterioration and a three-year mortality of up to 80 per cent. Abstention should be undertaken in hospital so compliance can be assured, diet monitored, and arrhythmias controlled.

Doxorubicin (Adriamycin) cardiotoxicity is generally irreversible and is the cause of death in over 60 per cent of patients so afflicted. Careful monitoring during doxorubicin therapy minimizes the risk. Potential cardiomyopathy in response to doxorubicin can be identified by radionuclide angiography, two-dimensional echocardiography, or endomyocardial biopsy. Patients without additional cardiac risks are best studied after 450 mg per square meter of drug administration. Although a decline in ejection fraction at rest or with exercise arouses legitimate concern for myocyte damage, the frequency of false-positivity mandates that damage be confirmed by endomyocardial biopsy before therapy is withdrawn. Cardiotoxicity of doxorubicin is related not only to peak levels but also to cumulative dose. Toxicity is reduced by slow infusion rates.

In the treatment of the depressed hemodynamic state of dilated cardiomyopathy, digitalis glycosides have little to offer, and in fact toxicity is believed to be increased. Because the most disabling symptoms are due to circulatory congestion rather than to inadequate systemic perfusion, the establishment and maintenance of minimal ventricular filling pressures are critical to symptomatic control. Early in the natural history, this end can be achieved by empiric diuretic and vasodilator therapy adjusted according to symptomatic response. Should symptoms of circulatory congestion persist, especially in the face of relative systemic hypotension or declining renal function, hospitalization for insertion of a flotation catheter permits hemodynamic monitoring to seek a more effective regimen of diuretics and vasodilators.

The use of beta blockade in chronic dilated cardiomyopathy is seemingly contradictory and remains controversial. The theoretic benefit of reducing myocardial oxygen demand in the failing ventricle by beta-blocking agents has not been established by clinical trials. Some patients experience improvement in symptoms and ejection fraction, whereas in others serious decompensation ensues.

The risk of systemic emboli in dilated cardiomyopathy prompts use of long-term oral anticoagulants, which are obligatory if an endocardial thrombus announces itself as a systemic embolus or if a thrombus is found prior to embolization during noninvasive imaging. Systemic emboli arising from intracardiac thrombi occur in up to 30 per cent of patients with dilated cardiomyopathy, and pulmonary emboli are not uncommon.

The risk of ventricular arrhythmias is closely coupled with clinical and hemodynamic deterioration, but ventricular arrhythmias appear to be an independent variable in early mortality. Although patients with symptomatic ventricular tachycardia should be treated with antiarrhythmic agents, the value of such treatment for asymptomatic ventricular arrhythmias has not been established.

Prognosis of idiopathic dilated cardiomyopathy depends largely, but not exclusively, on the clinical and hemodynamic stages of the natural history at the time of presentation. Patients who are New York Association Class III or IV have a one-year mortality approaching 50 per cent and a five-year mortality of over 90 per cent. The lower the ejection fraction and cardiac index and the higher the left ventricular filling pressure, the higher the mortality. The above therapeutic recommendations may have dramatic impact on symptoms, but mortality remains high, although vasodilator therapy appears to reduce mortality in patients with mild symptoms. Hemodynamic failure and its complications account for only 50 to 70 per cent of mortality. Sudden death remains a major threat that is not convincingly reduced by antiarrhythmic agents, including amiodarone.

Cardiac transplantation has been performed in a total of more than 2500 patients, over one half of whom had primary dilated cardiomyopathy. The current one-year post-transplantation survival is 80 per cent, with a five-year survival of 60 per cent for patients on prednisone and cyclosporin immunosuppression. Limitation in donor availability restricts access to cardiac transplantation, and postoperative infection and rejection remain major causes of morbidity and mortality. Up to one third of candidates die before transplantation can be performed.

Dec GW, Palacios IF, Fallon JT, et al.: Active myocarditis in the spectrum of acute dilated cardiomyopathies: Clinical features, histologic correlates, and clinical outcome. N Engl J Med 312:885, 1985. *A series of 27 patients with dilated cardiomyopathy of recent onset in which biopsy-proven myocarditis and subsequent improvement were frequent, whether or not immunosuppressive drugs were given.*

Fowles RE, Mason JW: Role of cardiac biopsy in the diagnosis and management of cardiac disease. Prog Cardiovasc Dis 27:153, 1984. *This review includes a description of the biopsy procedure, the histology of many cardiomyopathies, and general indications for biopsy.*

Gillum RF: Idiopathic cardiomyopathy in the United States, 1970–1982. Am Heart J 111:752, 1986. *The discussion focuses on the difficulties in estimating the incidence of dilated cardiomyopathy and the apparent increase in incidence over the past ten years.*

Johnson RA, Palacios I: Dilated cardiomyopathies of the adult. N Engl J Med 307:1051, 1119, 1982. *An extensive review of the etiologies and diagnosis of dilated cardiomyopathies.*

Kantrowitz NE, Bristow MR: Cardiotoxicity of anti-tumor agents. Prog Cardiovasc Dis 27:195, 1984. *The review discusses the possible pathogenesis of cardiotoxicity and a strategy for monitoring cardiac injury.*

O'Connell JB, Costanzo-Nordin MR, Subramanian R, et al.: Peripartum cardiomyopathy: Clinical, hemodynamic, histologic, prognostic characteristics. J Am Coll Cardiol 8:52, 1986. *Characterization and prognosis of 14 patients who developed peripartum cardiomyopathy despite good general health and prenatal care. The relatively high incidence of myocarditis is documented and discussed.*

O'Connell JB, Henkin RE, Robinson JA, et al.: Gallium-67 imaging in patients with dilated cardiomyopathy and biopsy-proven myocarditis. Circulation 70:58, 1984. *Sixty-eight patients underwent gallium scans and endomyocardial biopsies. The study disclosed the sensitivity but lack of specificity of gallium imaging in diagnosing myocarditis.*

Perloff JK: Neurological disorders and heart disease. In Braunwald E (ed.): Heart Disease. 3rd ed. Philadelphia, W.B. Saunders Company, 1987. *A comprehensive review of the interplay between systemic neuromuscular disorders and cardiac involvement.*

Regan TJ: Alcoholic cardiomyopathy. Prog Cardiovasc Dis 27:141, 1984. *A comprehensive review of the pathogenesis, preclinical course, and prognosis of alcoholic cardiomyopathy.*

Reyes MP, Lerner AM: Coxsackie myocarditis—with special reference to acute and chronic effects. Prog Cardiovasc Dis 27:373, 1985. *A comprehensive review of the murine model of myocarditis and its relation to myocarditis in human subjects.*

THE HYPERTROPHIC CARDIOMYOPATHIES

DEFINITION. This category of disorders is represented grossly by asymmetric (eccentric) or symmetric (concentric) hypertrophy of the left ventricle in the absence of another cardiac or systemic disease capable of producing left ventricular hypertrophy (Table 53–1). In the asymmetric variety, the septum is disproportionately thick relative to the left ventricular free wall beneath the mitral annulus (Fig. 53–2). In the symmetric variety, the septum and left ventricular free wall are of equal thickness. Ventricular cavity size is normal or reduced in both types.

ETIOLOGY. Just over one half of patients with hypertrophic cardiomyopathy have clear evidence of genetic transmission, usually an autosomal dominant trait. Sporadic occurrences may represent new mutations, reduced penetrance in first-degree relatives, autosomal recessive transmission, or nongenetic occurrence. Biochemical determinants in the pathogenesis are not firmly established but have focused on two inter-related hypotheses—the proposed intrauterine links between myocyte development and norepinephrine stimulation and/or excess intracellular calcium.

PATHOLOGY. Genetic hypertrophic cardiomyopathy is characterized by two gross morphologic and two histologic features. The gross morphologic features are asymmetric septal hypertrophy and a catenoid ventricular septal configuration (Fig. 53–2). The most typical histologic feature—cellular disarray—is significantly more common (95 per cent of patients) and quantitatively considerably more extensive in hypertrophic cardiomyopathy than in other cardiac disorders or in normal subjects. In its proper clinical and pathologic context, extensive septal cellular disarray remains an important marker of genetic hypertrophic cardiomyopathy. The second histologic feature—thick-walled intramural coronary arteries with narrow lumens—occurs in more than three fourths of patients with genetic hypertrophic cardiomyopathy, especially in the ventricular septum. The pathogenetic and clinical significance of the thickened intramural coronary arteries is unresolved.

PHYSIOLOGY. Characterization of the physiologic derangements in genetic hypertrophic cardiomyopathy sets the stage for an understanding of the clinical manifestations, diagnosis, and treatment. The principal physiologic features include a hypercontractile left ventricular free wall (enhanced

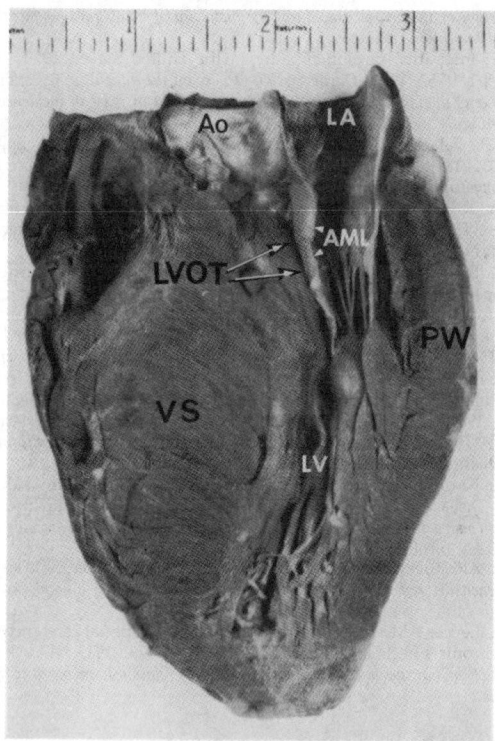

FIGURE 53–2. One of Teare's original cases of "asymmetrical hypertrophy of the heart." The ventricular septum (VS) is substantially thicker than the left ventricular posterior wall (PW). The cavity of the left ventricle (LV) is much reduced. The base of the ventricular septum bulges into the left ventricular outflow tract (LVOT) adjacent to the anterior mitral leaflet (AML). Ao = Aorta; LA = left atrium. (From Teare D: Asymmetrical hypertrophy of the heart in young adults. Br Heart J 20:1, 1958, with permission. Labels superimposed.)

systolic function), prolonged left ventricular isovolumetric relaxation (impaired diastolic function), hypocontractile ventricular septum, and left ventricular cavity obliteration. Normal ventricular contraction consists of an isovolumetric phase that occupies about 10 per cent of systole and an ejection phase with fiber shortening that occupies 80 to 90 per cent of systole. In genetic hypertrophic cardiomyopathy, a third phase is added. High-velocity ejection is completed in the first 60 to 80 per cent of systole, following which the cavity

obliterates and the myocardium contracts isometrically. Thus, hypertrophic cardiomyopathy is characterized by enhanced systolic function, a prolonged and abnormally powerful isometric contraction phase followed by prolonged left ventricular isovolumetric relaxation (impaired diastolic function).

Classic genetic hypertrophic cardiomyopathy is accompanied by a singular physiologic feature that continues to generate lively interest and considerable controversy—the left ventricular to aortic dynamic pressure gradient (Fig. 53–3). Entrapment of the catheter tip during cavity obliteration spuriously elevates the recorded systolic pressure within the left ventricle. However, a true gradient has been ascribed to narrowing of the left ventricular outflow tract by the thick base of the ventricular septum, coupled with systolic anterior motion of the anterior mitral leaflet, which is usually accompanied by mitral regurgitation. Although the term "hypertrophic obstructive cardiomyopathy" is applied in this setting, it has been argued that neither the gradient nor systolic anterior motion of the anterior mitral leaflet is justifiably equated with the presence of true obstruction. The earlier term "idiopathic hypertrophic subaortic stenosis" has fallen out of use because hypertrophic cardiomyopathy is not necessarily so characterized, even though the disorder first came into prominence because of the systolic pressure difference across the subaortic portion of the left ventricular outflow tract.

The gradient is "dynamic," a term that calls attention to its lability and to its response to certain physical and pharmacologic interventions (Fig. 53–3). Interventions that reduce left ventricular internal dimensions (cavity size) intensify the gradient and vice versa. The gradient increases during the straining phase of Valsalva's maneuver; during prompt standing, especially from the squatting position; following the compensatory pause after a premature beat; and in response to isotonic exercise, tachycardia, digitalis, isoproterenol, amyl nitrite, and nitroglycerin. The gradient decreases during the overshoot phase of Valsalva's maneuver, during Muller's maneuver, upon squatting, in response to isometric exercise (handgrip), and in response to beta-adrenergic blockade or alpha-adrenergic stimulation. In patients with significant gradients, administration of inotropic drugs or volume-depleting diuretics can be accompanied by sudden and serious deterioration.

CLINICAL MANIFESTATIONS. The symptomatically overt disease typically becomes manifest in young adults (mid third decade), but it is not uncommon for patients to present after 60 years of age. In infants, the disorder announces itself

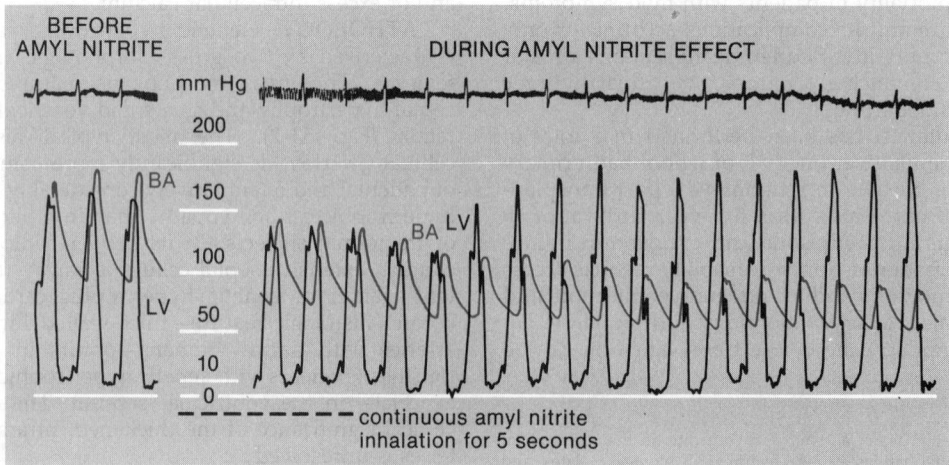

FIGURE 53–3. Tracings from a patient with asymmetric hypertrophic cardiomyopathy. The control tracing shows no outflow gradient. Amyl nitrite induced a peak LV-BA systolic gradient of 100 mm Hg. Observe the initial parallel fall in both left ventricular (LV) and brachial arterial (BA) pressures with subsequent divergence. (From Marcus FI, Perloff JK, De Leon AC: The use of amyl nitrite in the hemodynamic assessment of aortic valvular and muscular subaortic stenosis. Am Heart J 68:468, 1964, with permission.)

as a murmur and marked congestive failure, with the majority of afflicted babies dying before their first birthday. In adults, the clinical picture varies from incapacitating symptoms to asymptomatic relatives who exhibit few or no manifestations of illness except on echocardiography. It is dramatic but not uncommon for the disease to declare itself as syncope or sudden death in previously healthy young persons engaged in strenuous exertion. The commonest cluster of symptoms consists of dyspnea, fatigue, chest pain (similar to, if not identical with, angina pectoris), and syncope. The most prevalent symptom is dyspnea, which is intensified by exertion and which is a reflection of high end-diastolic and pulmonary venous pressures (left ventricular diastolic dysfunction). Symptoms are unrelated to the presence or degree of the left ventricular outflow gradient. Clinical deterioration is typically slow with two major exceptions—sudden death or the onset of atrial fibrillation. Loss of coordinated atrial contraction in the face of impaired left ventricular diastolic distensibility results in acute dyspnea (sudden increase in end-diastolic and pulmonary venous pressures).

In older subjects, chest pain coupled with electrocardiographic Q waves (see later) prompts a diagnosis of atherosclerotic coronary artery disease, which may coexist. However, symptoms resembling angina pectoris occur in relatively young patients without extramural coronary artery disease.

Cerebral symptoms vary from lightheadedness to frank syncope and are not strictly analogous to the cerebral symptoms in discrete aortic valve stenosis. Patients sometimes feel faint in the upright position (promptly corrected by lying down) or in response to physical exercise. Occasional patients report such a history for years without apparent clinical deterioration. Signs of cerebral hypoperfusion may in part reflect a fall in cardiac output due to physical interventions that decrease left ventricular cavity size and left ventricular filling. Arrhythmic syncope is ominous and heralds sudden death (see below).

The *physical examination* in asymptomatic patients without systolic gradients is unimpressive except for a relatively prominent left ventricular impulse and a fourth heart sound. The jugular venous pulse may exhibit a prominent A wave (increased force of right atrial contraction) that does not reflect pulmonary hypertension, but instead is a response to impaired distensibility of the right ventricular cavity caused by massive thickening of the ventricular septum. The increase in velocity of left ventricular ejection is reflected in the brisk rate of rise of the systemic arterial pulse while the blood pressure remains normal (small waterhammer pulse). Twin peaking results from a mid- to late-systolic trough, a feature better recorded than palpated. Precordial palpation sometimes detects a relatively uncommon but more characteristic *triple* apical impulse composed of double systolic movement coupled with presystolic distention. A systolic thrill may be present at the apex and toward the lower left sternal edge in patients with left ventricular outflow gradients, but the thrill corresponds more closely to mitral regurgitation than to the severity of the pressure gradient. Auscultation detects a prominent apical fourth heart sound, a normal first sound, and at the left base a second sound that is usually normally split, sometimes narrowly split or single, and occasionally paradoxically split. Despite the increased velocity of left ventricular ejection, aortic ejection sounds are sufficiently exceptional to call the diagnosis of hypertrophic cardiomyopathy into question. Systolic murmurs in patients with left ventricular outflow gradients represent combinations of midsystolic murmurs caused by increased velocity of ejection and a longer, if not holosystolic, apical murmur caused by mitral regurgitation. The murmur is typically loudest at the apex, with radiation into the axilla or to the left lower sternal edge, less prominently to the base, and seldom into the neck. The systolic murmur is important less because of its presence than because of the diagnostic significance of its response to

TABLE 53–3. EFFECTS OF BEDSIDE PHYSICAL INTERVENTIONS ON THE SYSTOLIC MURMUR OF ASYMMETRIC HYPERTROPHIC CARDIOMYOPATHY

Increased Intensity of Murmur
  Dynamic exercise
  Straining phase of Valsalva's maneuver
  Prompt standing after squatting
Decreased Intensity of Murmur
  Release (overshoot) phase of Valsalva's maneuver
  Squatting
  Isometric exercise (handgrip)

physical and pharmacologic interventions (Table 53–3). Third heart sounds occur in the presence of mitral regurgitation and are occasionally followed by brief after-vibrations that create the auscultatory impression of a short mid-diastolic murmur. A high-frequency early diastolic murmur of aortic regurgitation makes the diagnosis of hypertrophic cardiomyopathy doubtful.

Normal *electrocardiograms* are confined to a minority of asymptomatic patients. The tracings are almost invariably abnormal in symptomatic patients with left ventricular outflow gradients. P wave morphology generally reflects a left atrial abnormality alone, but occasionally together with a right atrial configuration. The PR interval is often short but only rarely in conjunction with evidence of pre-excitation, even when the short PR interval is accompanied by initial force slurring reminiscent of delta waves. Atrial fibrillation, the commonest sustained supraventricular rhythm disturbance, is not associated with accelerated atrioventricular conduction.

Prominent Q waves occur in upwards of 50 per cent of cases. The Q waves tend to be abnormal because of their depth rather than their duration. The Q waves have been ascribed to abnormal electrophysiologic properties in areas of cellular disarray. Electrocardiographic evidence of left ventricular hypertrophy is common but not invariable and is reflected in the increased voltage and ST segment and T wave abnormalities. Giant T wave inversions in mid to left precordial leads imply *apical* hypertrophic cardiomyopathy.

In the *chest roentgenogram*, enlargement of the left atrium is relatively common, especially when mitral regurgitation coexists. Dilatation of the left atrium is most conspicuous when mitral regurgitation is accompanied by atrial fibrillation. Left ventricular size and contour range from normal to a prominent convex silhouette projecting to the left, inferior and posterior. The aortic root is typically inconspicuous, and calcification of aortic valve or mitral apparatus is absent.

The echocardiogram is the mainstay of the *laboratory diagnosis* of hypertrophic cardiomyopathy, providing virtually all necessary clinical diagnostic information. The cardinal echocardiographic features of genetic hypertrophic cardiomyopathy are disproportionate thickness of the ventricular septum with a septal/posterior left ventricular wall ratio of 1.5:1 or more, a small left ventricular cavity, and exaggerated contractility of the left ventricular free wall with a relatively hypocontractile ventricular septum. Two-dimensional echocardiography establishes the location and extent of disproportionate septal thickness and occasionally shows on real-time imaging a ground-glass appearance of the septum believed to be related to cellular disarray. Systolic anterior motion of the anterior mitral leaflet, an important feature of the echocardiogram in the presence of left ventricular outflow gradients, is almost invariably accompanied by mitral regurgitation established by Doppler interrogation. Doppler echocardiography is pivotal in establishing the patterns of left ventricular ejection and in characterizing the abnormal diastolic properties of the left ventricle (impaired relaxation).

Technetium 99m gated radionuclide ventriculography identifies the thickness of the ventricular septum, the relative motions of septum and free wall, and the left ventricular cavity size in diastole and systole. Magnetic resonance imaging, with its capability of recording in multiple planes, provides refined morphologic information.

Prior to noninvasive imaging (especially echocardiography), *cardiac catheterization* provided the standards for the clinical diagnosis of hypertrophic cardiomyopathy. The systemic arterial pulse pressure fails to increase in the beat ending the compensatory pause after a premature ventricular contraction. The significance of recorded differences in systolic pressure between left ventricular cavity and aortic root is still debated. The subaortic gradient, like the systolic murmur, is reinforced by pharmacologic interventions that reduce left ventricular cavity size (Table 53–3, Fig. 53–3), and the gradient, like the murmur, decreases in response to interventions that increase left ventricular cavity size. Left ventriculography reveals a relatively small, angulated chamber in diastole, with systolic cavity obliteration and mitral regurgitation. In older patients with chest pain, selective coronary angiography is necessary to resolve the issue of coexisting atherosclerotic artery disease.

An important variation on the foregoing theme is the excessive *concentric* hypertrophic cardiomyopathy occasionally found in mildly hypertensive elderly patients. Two-dimensional echocardiographic features include severe concentric left ventricular hypertrophy, reduced left ventricular cavity size, enhanced systolic emptying with cavity obliteration, and impaired diastolic function.

TREATMENT. Hypertrophic cardiomyopathy cannot be prevented, but echocardiographic identification of clinically occult disease in first-degree relatives is desirable and sets the stage for genetic counseling. Certain proscriptions are important, such as sudden, strenuous, or isometric exercise or the use of digitalis glycosides, beta-adrenergic stimulants, or nitrates, all of which reduce left ventricular cavity size and may significantly enhance symptoms. Prophylaxis for infective endocarditis is necessary when mitral regurgitation accompanies hypertrophic cardiomyopathy.

Treatment falls into two broad categories: first, relief of symptoms (especially dyspnea and chest pain); and second, control of arrhythmias. A prime pharmacologic objective is to improve abnormal left ventricular relaxation and to enhance diastolic filling. Beta-adrenergic blockade has been a keystone of medical therapy in this regard. The largest clinical experience has been with propranolol. Dyspnea and angina pectoris respond favorably, the latter more so than the former. Disappointing, however, is the long-term capability of propranolol in maintaining its beneficial effects. Only a minority of patients experience long-term improvement, and an increase in dosage is often accompanied by unacceptable side effects. Calcium channel blockers, especially verapamil, are important therapeutic alternatives. Nifedipine is less effective, and data on diltiazem are currently inadequate to provide a basis for judgment. Intravenous verapamil is capable of decreasing the left ventricular outflow gradient with maintenance of cardiac output. The mechanism of action is believed to be enhancement of left ventricular diastolic filling and a decrease in left ventricular systolic function in response to reduced myocardial uptake of calcium. Verapamil improves exercise capacity and relieves symptoms during short- and long-term therapy in patients who previously experienced inadequate symptomatic relief with beta receptor–blocking agents. The most serious adverse effects of verapamil are electrophysiologic, namely, atrioventricular dissociation, Wenckebach periods, or sinus arrest. Verapamil administration can also be accompanied by postural hypotension and pulmonary congestion, the latter generally requiring cessation of administration. Because of these adverse effects, the drug should be used with caution or not at all in patients with significant abnormalities of atrioventricular conduction or sinus node function or in patients with low systemic systolic blood pressure or clinical evidence of increased pulmonary venous pressure. Because the adverse electrophysiologic effects of verapamil

are dose related, a reduction in dose sometimes permits continuation of the drug.

The foregoing therapeutic recommendations are also applicable to the mildly hypertensive elderly patient with symptomatic *concentric* hypertrophic cardiomyopathy (see earlier). In this setting, abnormal diastolic function and excessive systolic emptying are favorably influenced by beta antagonists and calcium channel blockers and are aggravated by conventional therapy with inotropic agents or vasodilators.

Antiarrhythmic therapy in genetic hypertrophic cardiomyopathy deals chiefly with atrial fibrillation or ventricular arrhythmias. Atrial fibrillation is properly regarded as a medical emergency and should be electrically cardioverted without delay (even before preconversion treatment with intravenous heparin) to circumvent the serious hemodynamic sequelae following loss of the atrial contribution to ventricular filling. Amiodarone (see below) is the most efficacious drug for maintaining sinus rhythm. Because of the relatively long interim between initial amiodarone administration and its sustained pharmacologic effect, heparin administration is advisable during that interval.

Ventricular arrhythmias are relatively common in hypertrophic cardiomyopathy and are represented by uniform or polymorphic premature ventricular beats occurring singly or repetitively. Because ventricular tachycardia and fibrillation are believed to be the chief causes of sudden death, antiarrhythmic suppression is pivotal. Treatment with conventional agents such as quinidine, disopyramide, or mexiletine has been disappointing, and propranolol-induced relief of angina pectoris and dyspnea has not been accompanied by a significant reduction in ventricular arrhythmias. The potentially malignant ventricular arrhythmias that prevail in genetic hypertrophic cardiomyopathy are essentially unknown in the hypertrophic cardiomyopathy of Friedreich's ataxia, whether asymmetric or concentric, and septal cellular disarray has not been found at necropsy in Friedreich's disease. Accordingly, the electrical instability inherent in cellular disarray may be the fundamental cause of ventricular arrhythmias in genetic hypertrophic cardiomyopathy. Amiodarone suppresses ventricular tachycardia in this setting, and long-term use of the drug may favorably influence the risk of sudden death.

Surgery is a therapeutic option in markedly symptomatic patients who do not respond satisfactorily to medical management. The most widely used operation is transaortic ventricular septal myotomy-myectomy, which consists of excising a portion of the hypertrophied septum. Surgery reduces or abolishes the left ventricular outflow gradient as well as the mitral regurgitation and appears to prevent progression of hypertrophy, although the operative risk is 5 to 10 per cent. Mitral valve replacement, a less desirable and seldom applied alternative, also eliminates the left ventricular outflow gradient and the mitral regurgitation. Because the symptoms in hypertrophic cardiomyopathy are not correlated with the presence or magnitude of the left ventricular outflow gradient, operation is believed to exert its beneficial effects for unestablished reasons that are apart from the reduction in gradient. Late postoperative progression to left ventricular dilatation and failure—dilated cardiomyopathy—is a serious and not exceptional sequel.

PROGNOSIS. Except for the infant with clinically overt hypertrophic cardiomyopathy in the first year of life, the natural history is usually characterized by slow progression. The most ominous threat is sudden death, which often occurs during exercise in persons who were previously clinically well. There is no necessary relationship between prognosis and the presence or degree of the left ventricular outflow gradient. Atrial fibrillation, however, is a poor prognostic eventuality accompanied by congestive heart failure and the risk of systemic embolization. Infective endocarditis is a complication related chiefly to the presence of mitral regurgitation. The transition of hypertrophic cardiomyopathy to dilated cardiomyopathy usually, but not necessarily, proceeds after septal myotomy-myectomy (see earlier). Less commonly, progressive left ventricular dilatation and failure occur as part of the natural history and have been ascribed to myocardial infarction with or without extramural atherosclerotic coronary artery disease.

In women of childbearing age, the prognosis accompanying pregnancy is good despite a number of undesirable hemodynamic variables during the course of gestation, labor, and delivery. The increases in cardiac output and left ventricular diastolic volume during pregnancy reduce the left ventricular outflow gradient, but the fall in systemic resistance counteracts this effect. Supine compression of the inferior vena cava by the gravid uterus impedes venous return, reduces left ventricular volume, and augments the left ventricular outflow gradient. Accordingly, pregnant patients with hypertrophic cardiomyopathy are advised to avoid the supine position toward term and during labor. A number of conflicting variables come into play during labor. Adrenergic stimulation associated with pain and stress, together with the Valsalva maneuver (bearing down), increases the left ventricular outflow gradient, but the rise in central blood volume during active uterine contraction has the opposite effect. The rapid decline in blood volume during the puerperium reduces left ventricular internal dimensions and intensifies the outflow gradient.

Criiey JM, Siegel RJ: Has "obstruction" hindered our understanding of hypertrophic cardiomyopathy? Circulation 72:1148, 1985. *A concise, informative editorial summarizing the controversy regarding obstruction to left ventricular outflow in patients with asymmetric hypertrophic cardiomyopathy.*

Maron BJ, Merrill WH, Freier PA, et al.: Long-term clinical course and symptomatic status of patients after operation for hypertrophic subaortic stenosis. Circulation 57:1205, 1978. *Late results of operation were reviewed in 124 patients with hypertrophic cardiomyopathy. Surgical technique, operative risk, and short-term and long-term outcomes are reviewed.*

Maron BJ, Nichols PF, Pickle LW, et al.: Patterns of inheritance in hypertrophic cardiomyopathy: Assesment by M-mode and two-dimensional echocardiography. Am J Cardiol 53:1087, 1984. *This important paper focuses on the mode of inheritance of hypertrophic cardiomyopathy in 367 relatives from 70 families.*

Maron BJ, Roberts WC, Epstein SE: Sudden death in hypertrophic cardiomyopathy: A profile of 78 patients. Circulation 65:1388, 1982. *No morphologic or hemodynamic variable was characteristic of patients with hypertrophic cardiomyopathy and premature sudden death or cardiac arrest. The implication is an arrhythmogenic cause.*

McKenna WJ, Oakley CM, Krikler DM, et al.: Improved survival with amiodarone in patients with hypertrophic cardiomyopathy. Br Heart J 53:412, 1985. *The control of ventricular arrhythmias with amiodarone was associated with significantly improved survival, suggesting that the cause of sudden death is arrhythmogenic and that amiodarone may prevent death in patients with hypertrophic cardiomyopathy and ventricular tachycardia.*

Perloff JK: Pathogenesis of hypertrophic cardiomyopathy. In Goodwin JF (ed.): Heart Muscle Disease. Lancaster, England, MTP Press Ltd., 1985, pp 7–22. *Pathogenesis is dealt with in light of anatomic, physiologic, and clinical features of hypertrophic cardiomyopathy. The catecholamine hypothesis is elaborated.*

Rosing DR, Idanpaan-Heikkila U, Maron BJ, et al.: Use of calcium channel blocking drugs in hypertrophic cardiomyopathy. Am J Cardiol 55:185B, 1985. *An important long-term drug study dealing with 227 patients treated with verapamil. A policy regarding drug administration is recommended, and the beneficial and adverse effects are reviewed.*

Topol EJ, Traill TA, Fortuin NJ: Hypertensive hypertrophic cardiomyopathy of the elderly. N Engl J Med 312:277, 1985. *Excessive concentric left ventricular hypertrophic cardiomyopathy with reduced cavity size, enhanced systolic emptying, and impaired diastolic function was identified in elderly patients with mild systemic hypertension. Diagnostic and therapeutic implications are underscored.*

Wigle ED: Hypertrophic cardiomyopathy: A 1987 viewpoint. Circulation 75:311, 1987. *An editorial that takes the form of an excellent review of hypertrophic cardiomyopathy.*

THE RESTRICTIVE CARDIOMYOPATHIES

DEFINITION. Restrictive cardiomyopathies, the least common of the three major categories (Table 53–1), are characterized by a *primary* abnormality of *diastolic* ventricular function (impediment in filling) with normal or nearly normal systolic function (contraction). The term "restrictive cardiomyopathy" is not appropriately applied when the primary derangement

TABLE 53–4. ETIOLOGIES OF THE RESTRICTIVE CARDIOMYOPATHIES

I. Myocardial
  A. Infiltrative
    1. Amyloid
    2. Sarcoid
    3. Hemochromatosis
    4. Glycogen storage diseases
    5. Hurler's disease
    6. Fabry's disease
  B. Noninfiltrative
    1. Idiopathic
    2. Radiation
    3. Scleroderma
II. Endomyocardial
  A. Endomyocardial fibrosis
  B. Idiopathic hypereosinophilic syndrome

is systolic function associated with variable degrees of diastolic impairment (late-stage dilated cardiomyopathy, for example). Nor is the term properly used to characterize the impaired diastolic function secondary to cardiac hypertrophy (hypertrophic cardiomyopathy, see above). In the restrictive cardiomyopathies, there is little or no increase in end-diastolic or end-systolic dimensions of either ventricle—hence the designation "nondilated, nonhypertrophic cardiomyopathy" or "congestive heart failure with normal systolic function." Restrictive cardiomyopathy functionally resembles constrictive pericarditis.

Myocardial stiffness refers to those effects that reflect changes in each unit of muscle, in contrast to *chamber stiffness*, which refers to changes in muscle mass rather than in unit of muscle. Chamber stiffness can be increased while myocardial stiffness is normal (left ventricular hypertrophy), whereas in restrictive cardiomyopathy, chamber stiffness is closely coupled to myocardial stiffness. Myocardial stiffness can be impaired for a host of reasons, many of which are shown in Table 53–4.

Infiltrative Restrictive Cardiomyopathies (Table 53–4)

AMYLOIDOSIS. Amyloid heart disease is the paradigm of the infiltrative cardiomyopathies. Classification of amyloidosis remains imprecise, although the hallmark of tissue injury in typical cardiac amyloidosis is replacement of normal contractile elements by interstitial deposits. The gross appearance of the heart in primary amyloidosis is occasionally normal, but the myocardium is characteristically firm, rubbery, and noncompliant, with ventricular cavities that are normal to small (Fig. 53–4). Histologically, insoluble fibrillar proteins are deposited in the interstitium of all four chambers. Primary amyloidosis also involves the pericardium and cardiac valves (especially atrioventricular) and infiltrates the sinus node in about 50 per cent of cases. Deposition of amyloid in the walls of intramural coronary arteries and arterioles is almost invariable and is held responsible for myocardial ischemia.

The pathophysiologic mechanisms of disturbed ventricular function and the clinical manifestations of cardiac amyloidosis are understood in light of certain morphologic details. *Interstitial* infiltration impairs diastolic function, leaving systolic function initially normal or nearly so. Systolic function is sometimes well preserved despite advanced amyloid deposition, although with progressive replacement of contractile elements, systolic function is reduced. Impaired ventricular distensibility results in elevated filling pressure and in a rise in pulmonary and systemic venous pressures analogous to constrictive pericarditis.

Biventricular circulatory congestion, the commonest overt clinical feature of cardiac amyloidosis, often presents as congestive heart failure of unknown cause. Right-sided congestion is typically dominant, with peripheral edema and occasionally ascites more evident than orthopnea and nocturnal dyspnea, which are usually absent or nearly so. Angina pectoris occurs in approximately one third of patients (amyloid

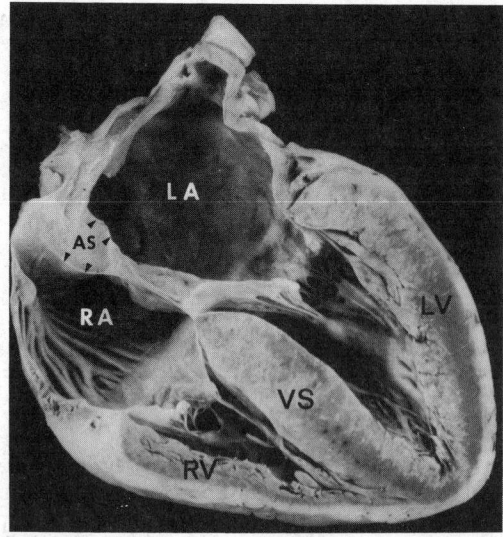

FIGURE 53—4. Pathologic specimen of a typical amyloid heart with thick, infiltrated ventricular septum (VS), left (LV) and right (RV) free walls, and atrial septum (AS). RA, LA = Right and left atria. (Courtesy of Dr. William Edwards, Mayo Clinic, Rochester, Minnesota.)

involvement of the coronary arteries; see above). Impaired atrioventricular conduction occurs in about 35 per cent of cases, with bundle branch block and atrial fibrillation less prevalent. Upwards of a third of patients experience orthostatic hypotension, lightheadedness, or syncope; sudden death is comparatively common.

Physical examination reveals peripheral edema without orthopnea or rales. The arterial pulse is normal or small. Pulsus alternans is usually absent because systolic function is relatively well preserved. The elevated jugular venous pulse is often visible only when the patient sits bolt upright, and it resembles the jugular pulse in constrictive pericarditis, including Kussmaul's sign. The left ventricular impulse is normal in location or only moderately displaced to the left, and its systolic movement is, as a rule, normal. Auscultation detects a soft first heart sound (PR interval prolongation), no murmur or soft systolic murmurs of atrioventricular valve regurgitation, and a third but not a fourth heart sound. Hepatomegaly is common, and ascites is occasionally present.

The electrocardiogram shows left atrial or right atrial P wave abnormalities and varying degrees of atrioventricular block. Abnormal infranodal conduction takes the form of left anterior fascicular block or isolated right or left bundle branch block. QRS voltage is characteristically low. Poor R wave progression or QS deformities in right precordial leads are believed to reflect myocardial replacement with amyloid.

In the chest roentgenogram, cardiac size and configuration are normal, including the atria, but in later stages, moderate cardiac enlargement reflects increased left ventricular internal dimensions. Radiologic signs of pulmonary venous congestion are almost invariable, and pleural effusions are common. Pericardial calcium is conspicuous by its absence.

Echocardiography, especially two-dimensional imaging, is the best means of identifying early cardiac amyloid infiltration and in gauging its subsequent progression. The early asymptomatic phase is manifested on echocardiography by a mild-to-moderate increase in left ventricular and/or right ventricular wall thicknesses. A useful and distinctive, but by no means invariable, feature of advanced cardiac amyloidosis is the granular sparkling appearance of the myocardium on two-dimensional real-time imaging. Avid myocardial pyrophosphate uptake is an important feature of advanced cardiac amyloidosis, and technetium-99m pyrophosphate myocardial scintigraphy is a safe, useful, and relatively specific diagnostic intervention in the proper clinical context. Endomyocardial

biopsy remains the definitive means of identifying amyloid deposits in the heart, but the combination of circulatory congestion and a relatively small heart, together with the above features on electrocardiography, echocardiography, and technetium pyrophosphate myocardial scintigraphy, goes far in establishing the diagnosis without recourse to myocardial biopsy.

The treatment of cardiac amyloidosis is supportive, usually ineffective, and occasionally inadvertently harmful. Progression cannot be arrested, and regression of tissue deposits is unknown. Overzealous use of diuretics reduces left ventricular filling pressure and relieves symptoms of circulatory congestion, but at the expense of an obligatory and undesirable fall in cardiac output. Digitalis sensitivity should be underscored not only because of the proarrhythmic effects of the glycoside but also because of its effect on already depressed sinus node and atrioventricular (AV) node function. Also to be considered is the inability of the sinus node to act as an effective pacemaker following pharmacologic or electroconversion in patients with atrial fibrillation. A right ventricular endocardial pacemaker for high-degree heart block may be less than ideally effective because of amyloid deposits at the site of electrode implantation. Nitroglycerin for angina pectoris reinforces the orthostatic hypotension believed to be caused by amyloid infiltration of the autonomic nervous system or of the systemic resistance vessels.

SARCOIDOSIS. Primary cardiac involvement occurs when granulomas preferentially infiltrate the cephalad portion of the ventricular septum and the atrioventricular junction and His bundle. The left and right ventricular free walls, endocardium, pericardium, and rarely the cardiac valves or intramural coronary arteries may also be involved. Clinically overt myocardial infiltration occurs in about 5 per cent of patients with proven sarcoidosis, although myocardial granulomas are found in approximately 25 per cent of such patients at necropsy. Granulomatous myocardial infiltration is initially interstitial and is functionally reflected by impaired diastolic filling with normal or nearly normal systolic function. Injury of contractile elements with fibrous replacement subsequently results in impaired systolic function. Relevant to this discussion is the restrictive phase of sarcoid cardiomyopathy (increased ventricular filling pressure with pulmonary and systemic venous congestion), although pulmonary hypertension, high-degree heart block, and papillary muscle dysfunction are important features of the cardiac response to sarcoidosis. An elevated mean jugular venous pressure with tall but equal A and V waves and brisk X and Y descents is a feature of myocardial restriction and reflects biventricular restrictive cardiomyopathy or, less commonly, sarcoid involvement of the pericardium (effusion or constriction). On physical examination, a right ventricular impulse is inconspicuous or absent, and auscultation detects a prominent third heart sound due to rapid ventricular filling. The echocardiogram identifies impaired diastolic ventricular function without increased thicknesses of ventricular free walls and septum and initially with relatively well-preserved systolic function and comparatively little increase in ventricular end-diastolic dimensions. Echocardiography is useful in establishing myocardial restriction and in excluding a confounding pericardial effusion, but ultrasonic imaging is not sensitive in delineating functionally significant noncalcific pericardial constriction. Endomyocardial biopsy does not sample the most likely sites of cardiac involvement (see earlier). Perfusion imaging with thallium-201 is sometimes useful in detecting segmental defects of sarcoid infiltration of the myocardium. Increased myocardial uptakes of technetium-99m pyrophosphate and gallium have been reported in myocardial sarcoidosis.

Prognosis from the cardiac point of view reflects not only the restrictive cardiomyopathy but also the risks of ventricular arrhythmias, high-degree heart block, and pulmonary hypertension (see earlier). Steroid administration has been advocated for the treatment of patients with biopsy-proven myocardial sarcoidosis. Sarcoid granulomas in the heart are reportedly more responsive to steroids than granulomas in other organs, although the myocardial granulomas may be replaced by connective tissue, with aneurysmal thinning of the ventricular wall.

HEMOCHROMATOSIS. Iron is stored normally as ferritin in reticuloendothelial cells, but with the iron overload of hemochromatosis, the proportion of hemosiderin (an insoluble granular aggregate) to ferritin increases, and storage is chiefly in parenchymal cells, where it is potentially harmful. Impaired diastolic ventricular function (restrictive cardiomyopathy) reflects the presence of iron within myocardial cells prior to significant myocyte injury or fibrous replacement. During this stage, ventricular internal dimensions and systolic function are normal or nearly so despite increased thickness of the infiltrated ventricular septum and ventricular free walls. Myocyte disruption and replacement fibrosis subsequently result in impaired systolic function. Clinical manifestations depend upon where in this natural history a given patient falls. Progressive diastolic dysfunction with rising ventricular filling pressure is symptomatically expressed as effort dyspnea, right-sided failure may dominate the clinical picture. During the myocardial restrictive phase of hemochromatosis, the arterial pulse and blood pressure are normal, there is an increased mean jugular venous pressure with elevated A and V waves and brisk X and Y descents, a normal left ventricular impulse, and a prominent third heart sound. When systolic dysfunction supervenes, the physical signs resemble those of dilated cardiomyopathy (see earlier). In either case, hepatic enlargement may be due to the hemochromatosis per se and not to the passive congestion of restrictive cardiomyopathy.

The echocardiogram initially shows a nondilated, concentrically thick left ventricle with evidence of diastolic dysfunction but normal or nearly normal ejection fraction. Endomyocardial biopsy provides a tissue diagnosis and sheds light on the degree of iron deposition, on myocyte integrity, and on the presence and degree of myocardial fibrosis.

Heart failure need not be progressive but may respond to iron depletion therapy if initiated when cardiac muscle cells are viable and when there is relatively little myocardial fibrosis. The corollary to this observation is that prevention of myocardial fibrosis is achieved when early recognition of myocardial infiltration with iron is effectively treated by phlebotomy.

GLYCOGEN STORAGE DISEASE. Restrictive cardiomyopathy is commonest in type II (Pompe's disease), in which the glycogen within cardiac muscle cells is biochemically normal but present in excessive amounts. There is dramatic thickening of the ventricular septum and of right and left ventricular free walls with reduced cavity size and markedly impaired diastolic distensibility. Pompe's disease is always fatal, usually within the first two years of life. The electrocardiogram is unique, exhibiting a remarkable increase in QRS amplitude, together with a short PR interval. Two-dimensional echocardiography in clinical context is virtually diagnostic.

FABRY'S DISEASE. In this X-linked inborn error of metabolism, deficiency of the lysosomal enzyme α galactosidase leads to progressive deposition of glycosphingolipids in cardiac muscle, resulting in an increase in mass and myocardial restriction. The disease is relatively benign until the second or third decade, but cardiovascular involvement may lead to early death.

HURLER'S SYNDROME. This autosomal recessive disorder is the prototype of the mucopolysaccharidoses, which result from defects in the degradation of complex carbohydrates and mucopolysaccharides. Hurler's cells laden with mucopolysaccharide moities are found in the myocardial interstitium, together with interstitial fibrosis, imparting to the myocardium its characteristic firm consistency and resulting in reduced diastolic distensibility (restrictive cardiomyopathy). Approximately a third of deaths in Hurler's syndrome result from congestive heart failure, but it is difficult clinically to isolate the effects of myocardial involvement per se from the effects of infiltration of mitral and aortic valves and from the ischemic effects of infiltration of the coronary arteries and the sequelae of systemic hypertension. Survival into the early teens is exceptional.

Noninfiltrative Restrictive Cardiomyopathies

IDIOPATHIC RESTRICTIVE CARDIOMYOPATHY. This term applies the clinical and hemodynamic findings of restrictive heart disease in the absence of a morphologic cause. Ventricular cavity size is normal or nearly so, ventricular septal and wall thicknesses are increased little, if at all, and microscopic study, including histochemical stains, may show nothing more than mild interstitial fibrosis. Echocardiographic, hemodynamic, and angiographic evaluations disclose reduced diastolic distensibility, elevated filling pressures, and normal global systolic function. Relatively normal ventricular cavity size contrasts with marked biatrial dilatation in response to reduced ventricular compliance and atrioventricular valve regurgitation, especially tricuspid. Atrial fibrillation is not uncommon, and high-degree heart block often requires a permanent pacemaker. The chief differential diagnosis is noncalcific constrictive pericarditis. An abnormal jugular venous pulse, peripheral edema, and ascites reinforce that impression. At biventricular catheterization, slight but distinct differences in the filling characteristics of right and left ventricles favor restrictive cardiomyopathy, but the distinction is often imprecise. Magnetic resonance imaging is a diagnostic step forward in identifying the absence, presence, or degree of pericardial thickening and may distinguish idiopathic restrictive cardiomyopathy from noncalcific constrictive pericarditis. The clinical course may be protracted even in the presence of chronic atrial fibrillation and high-degree heart block, provided a permanent pacemaker is inserted. Inotropic agents such as digoxin are not beneficial in light of normal or nearly normal systolic ventricular function. Calcium antagonists (verapamil) or beta-adrenergic blockers have been recommended to improve diastolic distensibility and prolong diastolic filling time, but the efficacy of these drugs is unproven.

IRRADIATION RESTRICTIVE CARDIOMYOPATHY. Restrictive physiology develops disproportionately in the more exposed anterior right ventricle, which exhibits interstitial fibrosis. The differential diagnosis between irradiation restrictive cardiomyopathy and radiation injury to pericardium (thickening, effusion, and occasionally tamponade) is important.

SCLERODERMA HEART DISEASE. Insidious interstitial myocardial fibrosis may result, at least initially, in restrictive cardiomyopathy. Hemodynamically significant pericardial effusion is exceptional.

Endomyocardial Restrictive Disease (Table 53–4)

ENDOMYOCARDIAL FIBROSIS. This disorder accounts for 15 to 25 per cent of deaths due to heart disease in equatorial Africa and is encountered, but less often, in South America and Asia and more recently in western Europe and the United States. In the left ventricle, there is involvement of the posterior mitral leaflet with varying degrees of mitral regurgitation. Thrombi overlie the endocardial lesions. The outflow portion of the left ventricle and the anterior mitral leaflet are spared. In the right ventricle, there is dense endocardial fibrous thickening of the inflow tract and apex, with involvement of papillary muscles and chordae tendineae causing varying degrees of tricuspid regurgitation. The outflow tract of the right ventricle is uninvolved. Functional derangements consist of impaired diastolic filling and atrioventricular valve regurgitation with relatively well-preserved systolic function.

In the presence of intractable biventricular failure and atrioventricular valve regurgitation, surgical resection of the fibrous endocardium, together with valve replacement, is a therapeutic option.

THE IDIOPATHIC HYPEREOSINOPHILIC SYNDROME. In this disorder, signs and symptoms of organ involvement, especially heart and nervous system, are accompanied by persistent eosinophilia of 1500 eosinophils per cubic millimeter for at least six months or death before 6 months with lack of evidence of recognized causes of the eosinophilia despite meticulous evaluation. It has been persuasively argued that the idiopathic hypereosinophilic syndrome and endomyocardial fibrosis (see above) are the same disease at different stages of development. The capability of the eosinophil or its contents to cause tissue damage (the Gordon phenomenon) has been known for over 50 years and is held responsible for the primary damage to ventricular endocardium. Platelet thrombi form over the denuded endocardium with an evolution that ultimately results in pathologic findings indistinguishable from those described earlier in endomyocardial fibrosis. Rigorous treatment directed at lowering the eosinophil count (prednisone alone or with hydroxyurea) appears to alleviate clinical manifestations of myocardial restriction, stabilizing and perhaps reversing the cardiac disease and favorably influencing survival.

Cueto-Garcia L, Tajik AJ, Kyle RA, et al.: Serial echocardiographic observations in patients with primary systemic amyloidosis; Smith TJ, Kyle RA, Lie JT: Clinical significance of histopathologic patterns of cardiac amyloidosis. Mayo Clin Proc 59:547, 589, 1984. *Two comprehensive articles that deal with the pathology and serial echocardiographic diagnoses of cardiac amyloidosis.*

Dabestani A, Child JS, Henze E, et al.: Primary hemochromatosis: Anatomic and physiologic studies characteristic of the cardiac ventricles and their responses to phlebotomy. Am J Cardiol 54:153, 1984. *Clinically occult cardiac involvement was identified by echocardiography and equilibrium blood pool imaging. Therapeutic phlebotomy ameliorated or reversed the deleterious effects of cardiac iron deposition if initiated prior to irreversible connective tissue replacement.*

Fauci AS, Harley JB, Roberts WC, et al.: The hypereosinophilic syndrome. Ann Intern Med 97:78, 1982. *This comprehensive National Institutes of Health conference deals with clinical, pathophysiologic, and therapeutic considerations in the hypereosinophilic syndrome and with the relationship of the disorder to endomyocardial fibrosis.*

Siegel RJ, Shah PK, Fishbein MC: Idiopathic restrictive cardiomyopathy. Circulation 70:165, 1984. *This form of cardiomyopathy is characterized chiefly by elevated left and right ventricular filling pressures, normal global ventricular systolic function, and normal or nearly normal ventricular septal and wall thicknesses and internal dimensions in the absence of specific infiltrative disorders or of diseases of pericardium or coronary arteries.*

Silverman KJ, Hutchins GM, Bulkley BH: Cardiac sarcoid: A clinicopathologic study of 84 unselected patients with systemic sarcoidosis. Circulation 58:1204, 1978. *An extensive study of the pathology of sarcoid involvement of the heart with clinical correlations.*

Stewart JR, Fajardo LF: Radiation-induced heart disease: An update. Prog Cardiovasc Dis 27:173, 1984. *An informative review of the pathology, physiology, pathogenesis, diagnosis, treatment, and prevention of radiation-induced heart disease.*

54 DISEASES OF THE PERICARDIUM

Ralph Shabetai

Diseases of the pericardium typically present in one or more of three clinical forms: acute pericarditis, pericardial effusion, and pericardial constriction. Pericardial involvement may progress from inflammation to effusion and then constriction, or it may present as effusion or constriction without clinical evidence of preceding inflammation.

ETIOLOGY

The pericardium may be involved in a large number and variety of diseases. The most important are listed in Table

TABLE 54–1. MAJOR CAUSES OF PERICARDIAL DISEASE

1. Inflammation	
Virus	
Coxsackie (usually B)	(E)
Echo	(E)
Other	
Bacterial	
Pneumococcus	(E)
Staphylococcus	(E,C)
Meningococcus	(E,C)
Mycobacterium tuberculosis	(E,C)
Hemophilus influenzae	(C)
Other	
Fungus	
Histoplasma capsulatum	(E,C)
Other	
Other living organisms	
Parasites	(E)
Protozoa	(E)
Nonliving agents	
Trauma	(E,C)
Radiation	(E,C)
Chemical	
Chemotherapeutic agents	
2. Idiopathic	
(Many may be viral, but unproven)	(E,C)
3. Neoplastic	
Secondary to carcinoma of	
Lung	(E,C)
Breast	(E,C)
Other	
Lymphoma	(E)
Primary	
Mesothelioma	(E)
Other	
4. Metabolic	
Chronic renal disease	
Associated with dialysis	(E)
End-stage uremia	(E)
Myxedema	(E)
Chylopericardium	(E)
Hypoalbuminemia	(E)
5. Myocardial injury	
Myocardial infarction	
Acute	
Dressler's syndrome	(E)
Congestive heart failure	(E)
6. Trauma	(E,C)
Postpericardiotomy syndrome	(E)
Postoperative	(C)
7. Connective tissue disorders and hypersensitivity	
Acute rheumatoid fever	
Rheumatic arthritis	(C)
Systemic sclerosis	
Lupus erythematosus	
Drugs	
Procainamide	
Others	
8. Congenital	
Absence of left pericardium	
Partial	
Complete	
Cyst	
Other	

(E) = effusion common; (C) = constrictive pericarditis common.

54–1. Pericardial disease may be asymptomatic, but may also cause dramatic symptoms and signs.

The clinical syndromes of pericardial disease are listed in Table 54–2.

INFECTIONS WITH LIVING AGENTS. *Virus Infection.* Many viruses may cause pericarditis; the common offenders are listed in Table 54–1. The number of cases of idiopathic pericarditis that are caused by preceding viral infection is unknown.

Bacterial Infection. Bacterial pericarditis is still important, although the spectrum has altered. Pneumococcal pericarditis, once a frequent complication of pneumonia, is now rare, whereas infection by staphylococci, fungi, and exotic organisms is more common, especially in persons at either extreme

TABLE 54–2. CLINICAL SYNDROMES OF PERICARDIAL DISEASE

Dry, fibrinous pericarditis
   Usually acute (R)
Lax pericardial effusion
   Chronic effusive
Cardiac tamponade (R)
Constrictive pericarditis
   Subacute
   Chronic
Effusive-constrictive pericarditis

(R) = Relapse or recurrence common.

of age and in the immunologically compromised host. Meningococcal pericarditis may be a manifestation of either direct infection or hypersensitivity.

Tuberculosis. Tuberculous pericarditis is less common now that tuberculosis is better controlled and treated. Pulmonary tuberculosis may be present, but often pericardial effusion is an isolated manifestation. *Mycobacterium tuberculosis* can be recovered from only one third of effusions. Even pericardial biopsy findings are not uniformly positive. Commonly, the diagnosis is presumptive and based on circumstantial evidence, such as a positive skin test result or a history of recent contact.

Hemophilus influenzae infection is an important cause of constrictive pericarditis in children.

Fungal Infection. In an otherwise normal population fungal pericarditis is uncommon, but infection with *Histoplasma capsulatum* should be considered in patients who reside in the Ohio Valley. Similarly, coccidioidomycosis should be considered in patients who have been in the San Joaquin Valley of California.

PERICARDIAL INFLAMMATION CAUSED BY NONLIVING AGENTS. *Trauma.* Blunt and sharp trauma is an important cause of pericarditis and may lead to pericardial effusion with or without tamponade and ultimately to constrictive pericarditis. Common examples of acute trauma include gunshot and knife wounds. Impact against a steering wheel, explosions, and crushing are the major causes of blunt injuries.

Radiation. The pericardium may be exposed to considerable injury when radiotherapy is employed to treat neoplasia, for example, Hodgkin's disease and lung or breast neoplasms. The latent period between radiation and clinical pericardial disease may extend for many years.

PERICARDIAL DISEASE IN METABOLIC DISORDERS. *Renal Disease.* Pericardial disease continues to be one of the more frequent major complications of chronic dialysis and may cause cardiac tamponade. Fortunately, constrictive pericarditis is rare. The etiology is not understood: It may be a manifestation of end-stage renal disease, but the process of dialysis itself may be responsible in whole or in part.

Myxedema. Pericardial effusion may occur and accounts in part for apparent cardiomegaly on chest radiograph; it may also contribute to the low voltage and T wave inversion that, in addition to sinus bradycardia, characterize the electrocardiogram. Pericardial effusion may contain cholesterol crystals.

CHYLOPERICARDIUM. Chylopericardium, a pericardial collection of fluid bearing a large quantity of chyle may be idiopathic but often follows surgical or other trauma of the thoracic duct.

MYOCARDIAL INFARCTION. Acute dry, fibrinous pericarditis can be detected in about one third of patients with acute myocardial infarction. Autopsy evidence is more common. Acute pericarditis early in the course is often a contiguous inflammation over the infarction but may also represent reaction to myocardial injury. Rupture of an infarction, aneurysm, or pseudoaneurysm creates greater or lesser degrees of hemopericardium, the former usually ending fatally.

In some patients, pericarditis (often accompanied by effusion) occurs in the weeks or months following acute myocardial infarction. This syndrome (Dressler's) is thought to be a delayed autoimmune reaction and is often recurrent.

CONNECTIVE TISSUE DISORDERS. Pericardial reaction may occur in virtually all of these disorders. Acute pericarditis is a constituent of rheumatic pancarditis but does not progress to constriction. On the other hand, subacute constrictive pericarditis can occur in rheumatoid arthritis. Pericarditis is an important manifestation of lupus erythematosus, both spontaneous and induced by drugs such as procainamide, and can cause tamponade.

HEART FAILURE. In patients with fluid retention, small pericardial effusion may be seen by echocardiography.

CONGENITAL LESIONS AND CYSTS. Partial absence of the pericardium produces a striking abnormality on the chest radiograph. Pericardial cysts are more frequent. They are filled with clear fluid, and most often occupy the right cardiophrenic angle, although they may occupy atypical locations. They are benign and usually produce no symptoms.

ACUTE (FIBRINOUS) VIRAL OR IDIOPATHIC PERICARDITIS

SYMPTOMS. Findings are often preceded by generalized malaise and fever. The chief symptom is chest pain, which may be either sharp or crushing. Frequently, the pain is precordial but may shift to the left side, simulating pleurisy. Characteristically, the pain is relieved by sitting up and exacerbated by deep inspiration. Thus, pericardial pain has features that may suggest either myocardial ischemia or pleural inflammation. Referral of pain to the right trapezius ridge is a specific but uncommon sign of its pericardial origin.

CLINICAL FINDINGS. *Pericardial Friction Rub: The Pathognomonic Sign of Pericardial Inflammation.* Classically, the rub has components accompanying atrial systole, ventricular systole, and ventricular diastole (see LMSB line, Fig. 54–1). Commonly, the rub is biphasic and must be distinguished from to-and-fro murmurs. When it is monophasic, it must be differentiated from systolic murmurs. It is typically superficial and scratchy, and although it may be widely distributed over the precordium, it is usually most apparent at the left sternal edge. Appreciation is enhanced by firm pressure with the diaphragm of the stethoscope. Changes in posture and the respiratory cycle may alter the intensity. Pericardial friction rubs are often transient and should be sought frequently when pericarditis is suspected. They must be distinguished not only from cardiac murmurs but also from mediastinal crunch due to air in the mediastinum, crepitations from surgical emphysema, and artifacts produced by movement of the skin against the stethoscope.

LABORATORY FINDINGS. *Electrocardiogram.* The typical findings of pericarditis are shown in Figure 54–2. ST segment elevation, although common, is not invariably present, depression of the ST segment being usual in leads aV_R and V_1. Depression of the PR segment, although highly specific, is less common than ST segment elevation.

On a single tracing and without clinical information, ST segment elevation cannot always be distinguished from the early repolarization normal variant or from the early stage of acute myocardial infarction. In the latter, evolution of the pattern in serial tracings is helpful. In acute pericarditis, the ST segment returns to baseline without inversion of the T wave (which may occur later if pericarditis becomes chronic), whereas in acute myocardial infarction, T wave inversion typically occurs before the ST segment becomes isoelectric.

Other Laboratory Findings. The erythrocyte sedimentation rate is elevated and there is variable leukocytosis. Viral titers may confirm the origin of the illness but are seldom performed in clinical practice. Gallium radioisotope scanning may display the epicardium, but this expensive test is required only in exceptional cases. Plasma levels of cardiac enzymes may be elevated, but this determination need not be made routinely.

DIAGNOSIS. The diagnosis can usually be made reliably from symptoms and signs. When any of the conditions listed

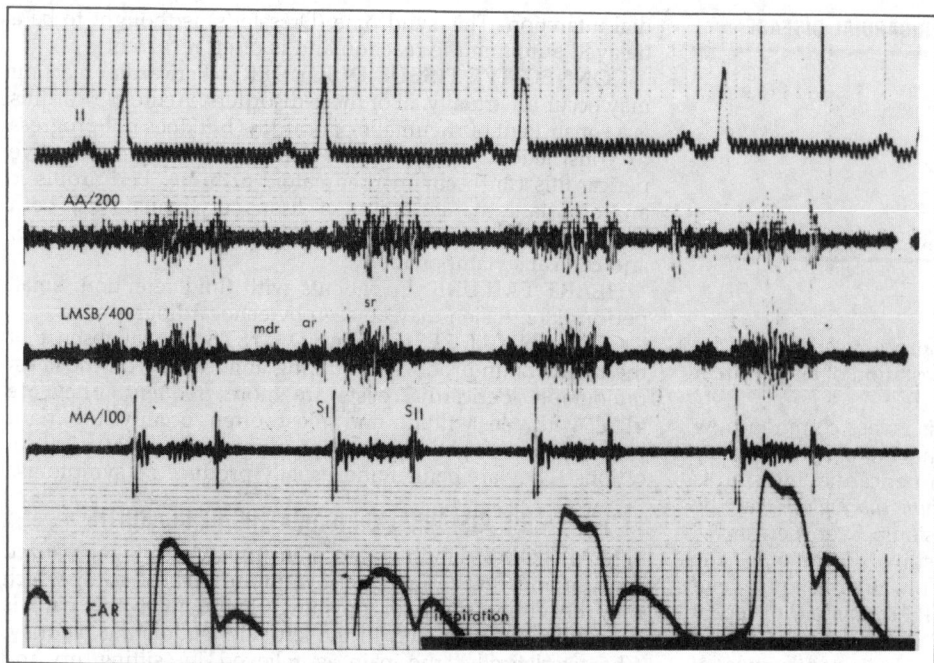

FIGURE 54–1. Phonocardiography of pericardial friction rub. AA = Aortic area; LMSB = left mid-sternal border; MA = mitral area. Note the three-component rub heard along the left mid-sternal border. Numbers refer to filter settings. (Reproduced by permission from Spodick DH: Am Heart J 81:114, 1971.)

in Table 54–1 is suspected, the symptoms and signs of pericarditis should be specifically sought and the diagnosis confirmed by electrocardiography. When the pain simulates that of pleurisy, pneumonia or pulmonary infarction must be considered. When it is retrosternal and crushing, myocardial infarction must be ruled out. On occasion, other major causes of chest discomfort, such as acute pulmonary embolism or dissection of the aorta, need to be considered.

CLINICAL COURSE, PROGNOSIS, AND MANAGE-MENT. Commonly, this is a self-limiting disease. However, its natural history is seldom observed, as it usually responds rapidly to treatment with nonsteroidal anti-inflammatory agents such as indomethacin (25 to 50 mg three to four times a day) or ibuprofen. Even aspirin is often satisfactory. Resistant cases may require steroid treatment—for instance, prednisone, starting with 75 mg a day and rapidly tapering to the minimum dose that suppresses symptoms and signs.

Detectable pericardial effusion occurs in a small proportion of cases and may progress to cardiac tamponade. Similarly, acute pericarditis may rarely lead to chronic constrictive pericarditis.

Recurrent Pericarditis. Perhaps the most troublesome of all complications is frequent recurrence over a period of years. The patient is greatly disturbed by the frequent occurrence of disabling pain, and when steroidal agents must be used for resistant cases, their side effects may become significant.

PERICARDIAL EFFUSION

LAX PERICARDIAL EFFUSION. Pericardial effusions that do not raise intrapericardial pressure more than 3 or 4 mm Hg do not cause symptoms. The physical findings are variable and frequently do not provide valuable clinical clues. Pericardial effusion should be strongly suspected in the setting of acute pericarditis if the cardiopericardial silhouette is enlarged on the chest radiograph. A previous radiograph showing a normal-sized silhouette is particularly helpful. The diagnosis can be made with certainty by echocardiography (Fig. 54–3).

PERICARDIAL EFFUSION COMPLICATING ACUTE PERICARDITIS. When echocardiograms are performed routinely in acute pericarditis, effusion is found in a considerable proportion of cases. However, in clinical practice, echocardiography is not required if the heart size remains normal, there is no evidence of cardiac tamponade or myocarditis, and the findings subside within 48 to 72 hours after beginning treatment. Myocarditis should be suspected when depolarization changes, such as left or right bundle branch block, or conduction abnormalities develop and when a third heart sound is audible. In such cases, echocardiography is often

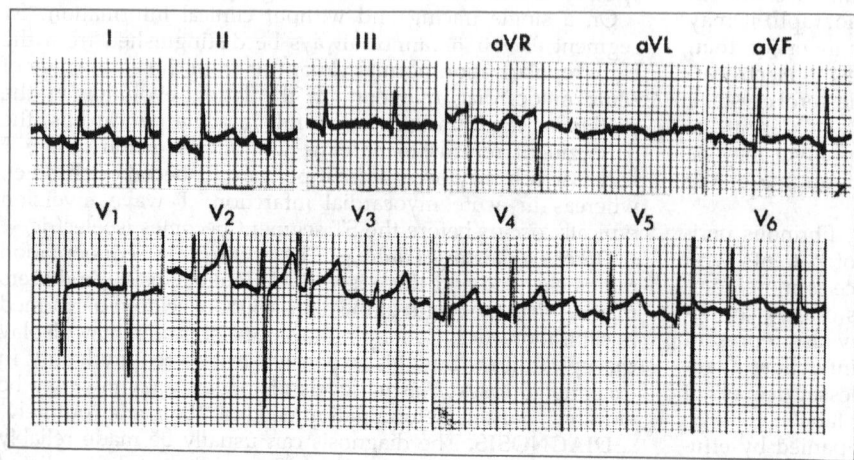

FIGURE 54–2. ECG from a case of acute pericarditis. Note the ST segment elevation in leads I, II, aVF and V_4 to V_6 and ST segment in leads aVR and V_1. (From Shabetai R: The Pericardium. New York, Grune & Stratton, 1980.)

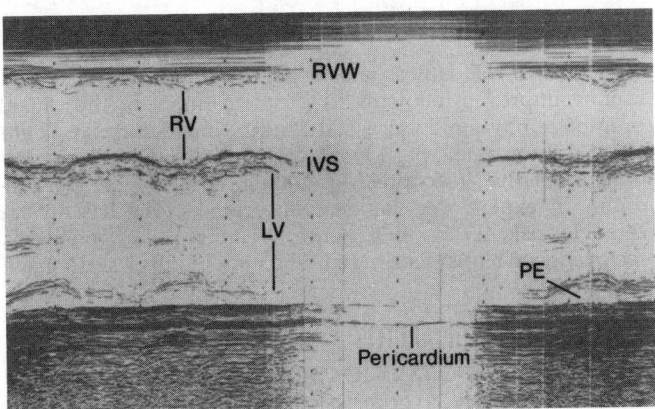

FIGURE 54–3. M = mode echocardiogram of moderate pericardial effusion. RVW = Right ventricular free wall; RV = cavity of right ventricle; IVS = interventricular septum; LV = left ventricular cavity; PE = pericardial effusion. The pericardial echo is identified in the middle of the photo, where other less echo-dense structures have been damped.

useful in distinguishing cardiac chamber enlargement from pericardial effusion.

ETIOLOGY OF PERICARDIAL EFFUSION. The causes of pericardial effusion are indicated in Table 54–1. Pericardial effusion must always be considered in patients who have or are likely to have one of these disorders, but especially when there is or has been evidence of acute pericarditis or when there is circulatory compromise. When the patient has a possible cause of cardiac tamponade or constrictive pericarditis, pericardial disease must be ruled out before attributing circulatory abnormalities to heart disease.

PERICARDIOCENTESIS. When the venous pressure is normal, systemic arterial hypotension is absent, and the

etiology of pericardial effusion has been established with reasonable certainty, pericardiocentesis is seldom needed. On the other hand, if the clinician suspects or diagnoses purulent effusion, or cardiac tamponade that is not responding satisfactorily to medical treatment, removal of pericardial fluid via a needle or open drainage becomes necessary. In a smaller fraction of cases, pericardiocentesis is required to establish a tissue or bacteriologic diagnosis. In such instances, the relative merits of the less traumatic and less expensive pericardiocentesis, versus surgical drainage, must be weighed against local experience and preference and the relative importance of pericardial biopsy in establishing the diagnosis.

Lax pericardial effusions have minimal hemodynamic effects, but when large and chronic, as, for example, in idiopathic chronic effusive pericarditis, a number of clinicians recommend surgical drainage.

CARDIAC TAMPONADE

ETIOLOGY AND PATHOPHYSIOLOGY. Pericarditis of virtually any cause may be associated with pericardial effusion, and virtually any pericardial effusion can progress to cardiac tamponade. The important causes are indicated in Table 54–1. The pathophysiology is illustrated in Figure 54–4, taken from cardiac catheterization data from a patient with severe cardiac tamponade.

Normal pericardial pressure is subatmospheric (Fig. 54–4F) and approximates pleural pressure. When pericardial effusion rapidly accumulates, pericardial pressure rises abruptly because of the limited capacity of the parietal pericardium to stretch acutely (Fig. 54–4D). A few hundred milliliters accumulating rapidly can generate intrapericardial pressures in excess of 20 mm Hg, whereas a slowly developing effusion may assume gigantic proportions with only minimal elevation of intrapericardial pressure. In clinical practice, cases may be encountered anywhere between these two ends of the spectrum.

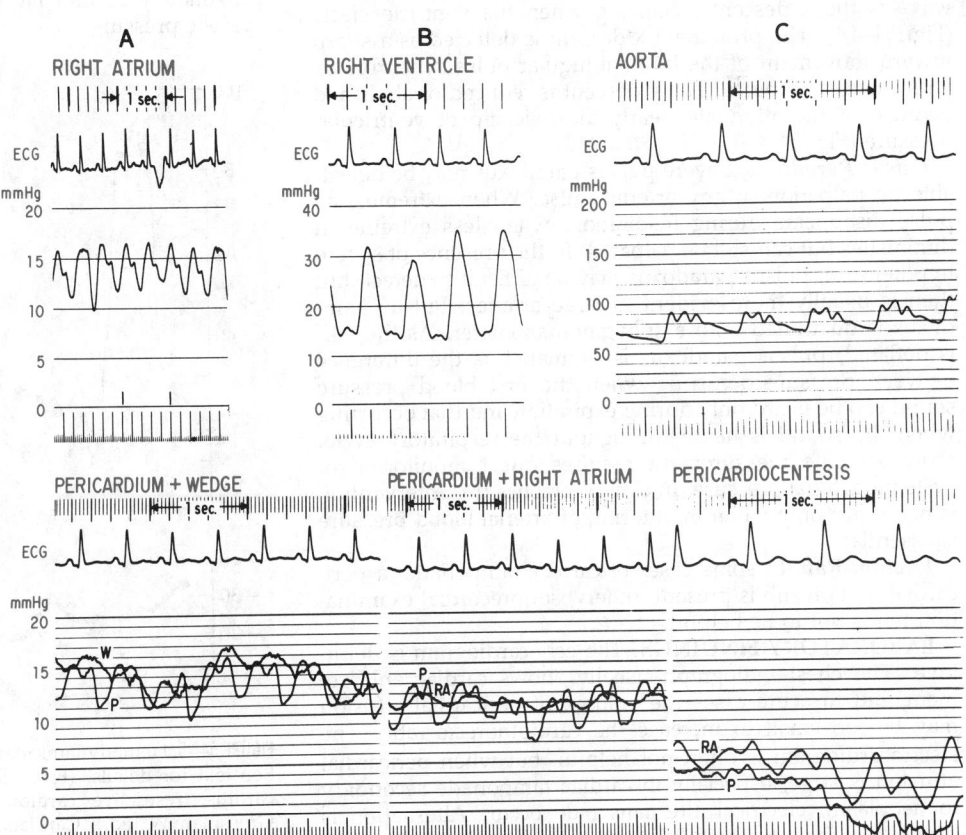

FIGURE 54–4. Hemodynamic data from a patient with cardiac tamponade. See text for discussion.

If effective circulation is to be maintained, systemic venous pressure must rise to equal intrapericardial pressure to maintain venous return. Figure 54–4E indicates equilibration of right atrial and pericardial pressure. Unless the pre-existing left ventricular diastolic pressure was higher than pericardial pressure during cardiac tamponade, this pressure also must rise to the same level to maintain filling of the left ventricle. Figure 54–4 A to E shows equally elevated pulmonary wedge, right atrial, right ventricular diastolic, and intrapericardial pressures. During inspiration the normal inspiratory drop of systemic venous pressure is maintained (Fig. 54–4A), but the normal systemic arterial systolic and pulse pressure drop is exaggerated during inspiration (Fig. 54–4C). The latter finding is termed pulsus paradoxus. Systemic arterial hypotension is absent (Fig. 54–4C) in mild-to-moderate cardiac tamponade. Surgical causes such as trauma or rupture of the heart or the aorta into the pericardium are usually associated with profound hypotension. In medical cases, cardiac output is often reduced to the range shown in Figure 54–4, but in surgical cases still lower cardiac outputs are often observed.

CLINICAL FINDINGS. The chief component in recognizing tamponade is thinking of it. Cardiac tamponade must be considered whenever evidence suggesting heart disease or heart failure develops in a patient who may reasonably be suspected of a disorder listed in Table 54–1. In extreme cases consciousness may be impaired, and arterial blood pressure may drop to shock levels. Frequently there is oliguria, because cardiac tamponade, and the resulting drop in cardiac output and blood pressure, is a powerful stimulus for sodium retention by the kidney. Pericardial pain may or may not be present; often there is a sensation of fullness of the chest and sometimes frank dyspnea.

Venous Pressure. Important evidence of cardiac tamponade includes abnormal jugular venous pulses. The venous pressure is elevated, usually considerably so, unless there is concomitant acute blood loss or severe dehydration. The right atrial (and therefore the jugular) pulse is monophasic, the normal inspiratory drop is maintained, and the predominant wave is the x descent, occurring when the ventricle ejects (Fig. 54–4A). The prominent x descent is detected as a sharp inward movement of the internal jugular pulse synchronous with the carotid pulse. The y descent is reduced or abolished because of the attenuated early diastolic dip of ventricular pressure (Fig. 54–4B).

Pulsus Paradoxus. Severe pulsus paradoxus may be detectable by palpation of any arterial pulse. When extreme, the pulse disappears during inspiration; when less extreme, it diminishes but can still be palpated. In the presence of severe hypotension, pulsus paradoxus may be difficult to detect, but then is usually more evident in large arteries. Pulsus paradoxus is quantified with a sphygmomanometer. As the cuff is deflated, pulsus paradoxus is estimated as the difference between pressure occurring when the first blood pressure sound can be heard only during expiration and that occurring when the sound is heard throughout the respiratory cycle. More accurate measurement requires direct monitoring of systemic arterial pressure. In clinical practice this intervention is necessary only when monitoring of arterial blood pressure is essential.

Friction Rub. In some cases of cardiac tamponade, a pericardial friction rub is present; otherwise, precordial examination tends not to be helpful.

LABORATORY FINDINGS. The echocardiogram is definitive. The chest radiograph usually shows cardiac enlargement, but in acute cases the volume of pericardial effusion may be too small to increase the cardiothoracic ratio. The electrocardiogram is often not helpful, but when pericardial effusion is large, especially in cardiac tamponade secondary to neoplasm, electrical alternans may occur. Alternation is usually confined to the QRS complex; more specific for pericardial effusion, but less common, is alternation of P, QRS, and T waves.

TREATMENT. Unless tamponade is mild or moderate and rapidly improves following medical treatment of the cause, prompt removal of pericardial fluid is mandatory. In acute cases only a small portion of the fluid need be removed, because of the steep pressure-volume curve of the pericardium. In experienced hands, pericardiocentesis has an acceptable risk. When experience is limited, tamponade is recurrent, or biopsy is needed, subxiphoid surgical drainage is preferred.

CONSTRICTIVE PERICARDITIS

DEFINITION AND ETIOLOGY. Constrictive pericarditis produces thickening, fibrosis, and often calcification of the pericardium with restriction of the diastolic filling of the ventricles. The most common causes are listed in Table 54–1. In the United States and western Europe, constrictive pericarditis most often is idiopathic, secondary to neoplasm or radiation, post-traumatic, or due to connective tissue disease. Tuberculosis and pyogenic infection are less common causes than they used to be. More subacute and fewer chronic cases are therefore seen, and heavy calcification of the pericardium is less frequent.

PATHOPHYSIOLOGY. The pathophysiology and hemodynamics are shown in Figure 54–5 from the study of a stock car driver with post-traumatic pericarditis. Panel A shows pressures recorded simultaneously from both ventricles. In early diastole there is a prominent dip of pressure, and in mid and late diastole the pressure forms a plateau. The two plateaus are elevated and equal. During early diastole, ventricular filling is faster than normal, signified by the early diastolic dip, at the end of which cardiac volume reaches the limit set by the rigid pericardium. The ventricular diastolic pressures are then elevated but do not rise through the remainder of diastole, signifying absence of further ventricular filling. Elevation of left ventricular diastolic pressure to approximately 20 mm Hg causes elevation of right ventricular systolic pressure.

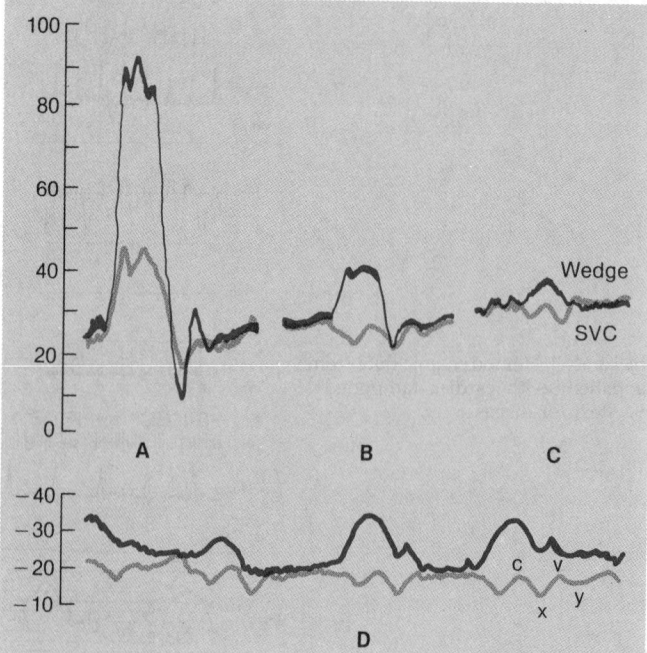

FIGURE 54–5. Hemodynamic data from a case of constrictive pericarditis. See text for details. (From Shabetai R: Profiles of constrictive pericarditis, restrictive cardiomyopathy and cardiac tamponade. In Grossman W [ed.]: Cardiac Catheterization and Angiography. 2nd ed. Philadelphia, Lea & Febiger, 1980.)

Panel B shows simultaneous pressure records from the right ventricle and right atrium. In contradistinction to cardiac tamponade, right atrial pressure is biphasic, showing a prominent x descent with ventricular ejection and prominent y descent coincident with the early diastolic dip of ventricular pressure. The y descent can be recognized at the bedside as a sharp inward movement of the jugular pulsation out of phase with the carotid pulse. Respiratory variation is absent. Panel C shows simultaneous pulmonary wedge and superior vena cava pressures, confirming equilibration of filling pressures on the two sides of the heart. Panel D shows pressures simultaneously recorded from the pulmonary artery and the pulmonary wedge position. In late diastole all cardiac pressures equilibrate around 20 mm Hg.

CLINICAL FINDINGS. Elevation of the filling pressure of the left side of the heart causes dyspnea and pulmonary congestion, which in severe cases is evident on the chest radiograph. Elevated filling pressure of the right side of the heart causes peripheral edema; hepatic enlargement, congestion, and dysfunction; and frequently ascites.

When ventricular filling is suddenly checked at the end of the early diastolic pressure dip, a loud third heart sound ("pericardial knock") is frequently audible. The apex beat may not be palpable, or there may be systolic retraction. Ascites is often prominent in relation to peripheral edema. The liver is usually enlarged and pulsatile. When present, palmar erythema, spider angiomas, and mild jaundice testify to severe, chronic hepatic congestion.

The abnormally small ventricular end-diastolic volume reduces stroke volume even when systolic function is well maintained, as it usually is.

LABORATORY FINDINGS. By chest radiography, the heart is normal in size to moderately enlarged. In chronic cases, particularly those associated with tuberculosis, calcification may be seen in the pericardium. The electrocardiogram usually shows T wave inversions and frequently a wide, notched P wave due to chronic elevation of left atrial pressure. In longstanding cases, atrial fibrillation often supervenes. Liver function test results are abnormal, and hypoalbuminemia may be compounded by protein-losing enteropathy.

Echocardiography. The echocardiogram is less helpful than in pericardial effusion. Sometimes increased thickness of the pericardium can be detected, especially if there is a small effusion. The cardiac walls move abruptly in early diastole and are stationary throughout middle and late diastole, corresponding with the hemodynamic alterations. Motion of the interventricular septum is often abnormal.

Other Imaging Techniques. The thickened pericardium is more adequately visualized by computerized tomography, which at present is the imaging technique of choice for chronic constrictive pericarditis. Magnetic resonance imaging promises to be as good or better.

DIAGNOSIS. Systemic venous congestion not explained by heart failure or other causes should suggest the possibility of constrictive pericarditis, especially when one of the etiologies listed in Table 54–1 is present or suspected. Although nonspecific systolic murmurs are common, murmurs of predominant valvular heart disease are absent.

When patients present with massive edema and liver dysfunction, the most common erroneous diagnosis is cirrhosis of the liver. This major error can be avoided by examination of the venous pressure in the neck. When the venous pressure is elevated, anasarca is generally due to cardiac or pericardial, not hepatic, causes.

Pericardial effusion may produce a large "water-bottle" heart on chest radiograph. Constrictive pericarditis may produce only minimal enlargement but may be detectable by calcification of this pericardium. Cardiac imaging shows normal systolic function and normal cardiac valves. The ventricles are often small and fill rapidly in early diastole but not at all for the remainder of diastole. This finding, together with

increased thickness of the pericardium, establishes the diagnosis.

Restrictive cardiomyopathy is a disease of heart muscle (see Ch. 53) that mimics constrictive pericarditis. Characteristically, however, left ventricular diastolic pressure exceeds that on the right. In some cases, endomyocardial biopsy and occasionally exploratory thoracotomy are needed to establish the correct diagnosis.

TREATMENT. For the vast majority of patients, the treatment of choice is pericardiectomy. The patient may be prepared by modest diuresis. With modern techniques of cardiopulmonary bypass, especially in cases that are not too far advanced, the operation yields gratifying clinical improvement; full benefit may not be evident for about six months.

Engel PH: Echocardiographic findings in pericardial disease. *In* Fowler NO (ed.): The Pericardium in Health and Disease. Mt. Kisco, NY, Futura Publishing Company, 1985. *An up-to-date, well-written discussion.*

Klopfenstein HS, Schuchard G, Wann LS, et al.: The relative merits of pulsus paradoxus and right ventricular diastolic collapse in the early detection of cardiac tamponade. An experimental echocardiographic study. Circulation 71:829, 1985. *Describes the correlation between hemodynamics and echocardiographic abnormalities in cardiac tamponade.*

Shabetai R: The Pericardium. New York, Grune & Stratton, 1980. *A comprehensive monograph dealing with the normal pericardium and pericardial diseases.*

Shabetai R, Fowler NO, Fenton JC, et al.: Pulsus paradoxus. J Clin Invest 44:1882, 1965. *An experimental study of the mechanisms of pulsus paradoxus.*

Spodick DH: Pathogenesis and clinical correlations of the electrocardiographic abnormalities of pericardial disease. Cardiovasc Clin 8:201, 1977. *A well-illustrated and complete account of theory and clinical application.*

55 MISCELLANEOUS CONDITIONS OF THE HEART: TUMOR, TRAUMA, AND SYSTEMIC DISEASE

Bernadine P. Healy

CARDIAC TUMORS

Tumors of the heart and pericardium are uncommon, and as a cause of clinical cardiac disease they are especially rare. Consecutive autopsy studies suggest that primary tumors of the heart are seen in only 1 in 2000 postmortem examinations; tumors secondary to metastases are roughly 20 times more frequent than primary lesions. A number of factors have made cardiac tumors a more visible current medical problem. With improved medical diagnostic technology, we are more apt to recognize both primary and secondary cardiac tumors; and with better therapy, patients with metastatic neoplasms live longer, increasing the likelihood for the heart to develop secondary cancers.

In part because of their relative rarity as a cause of clinical heart disease, cardiac tumors often go unrecognized. A general awareness of the pathophysiology of the heart afflicted with tumor and the ways in which it so often mimics more common forms of heart disease is essential to diagnosis and recognition of options for therapeutic intervention.

Primary Tumors of the Heart

Primary tumors of the heart are almost always benign and are considerably less common than tumors secondary to metastatic disease. The myxoma, of endocardial origin, is overwhelmingly the most common and best known of the primary cardiac tumors. Less common is the rhabdomyoma, a benign congenital tumor of myocardium most often seen in children. The sarcoma is the predominant malignant form of primary heart tumor and includes a variety of types, such as rhabdomyosarcoma, angiosarcoma, and fibrosarcoma. Among these tumor types, the myxoma is of greatest clinical importance in terms of relative frequency, tendency to produce symptoms, and ease of diagnosis and therapy.

The cardiac myxoma has been recognized as a pathologic entity for several hundred years, occurring with an incidence of about 0.03 per cent at autopsy. Myxomas are typically solitary, smooth-surfaced, globular tumors, which vary in size from 1 to 8 cm (average 5 cm), and most are pedunculated. In about 90° per cent of cases they occur in the left atrium; most of the rest occur in the right atrium. They are attached to the interatrial septum in the region of the fossa ovalis. Clinical presentation is related to location of the tumor, as well as to the presence of a pedicle. Larger myxomas, generally over 3 cm in diameter, are more apt to be symptomatic. The presence of a pedicle, allowing the myxomas to move about in the cardiac chambers, also correlates with symptomatology.

Myxomas occur most frequently (75 per cent) in women and usually manifest with symptoms in persons between the ages of 35 and 60 years. Because myxomas are most commonly located in the left atrium, signs and symptoms of cardiac dysfunction are usually referable to left-sided cardiac disease. The most common clinical cardiac problem is congestive heart failure, present in roughly half of patients, and often the heart failure is paroxysmal and precipitated by positional change, such as lying down. Other signs include chest pain, murmurs of mitral stenosis or regurgitation or both, syncope, and arrhythmias (including atrial fibrillation, often paroxysmal in nature). Other, noncardiac manifestations of atrial myxomas include systemic or pulmonary embolism, fever, malaise, arthralgias, and hematologic abnormalities suggestive of chronic infection. With these clinical manifestations, it is not surprising that atrial myxomas often have been misdiagnosed as rheumatic mitral valve disease, infective endocarditis, fever of unknown origin, or connective tissue disease. Indeed, cardiac myxomas may be viewed as the "great simulators"; their correct clinical diagnosis is among the most challenging in internal medicine.

Some of the challenge and error in the clinical recognition of cardiac myxomas has been diminished by the advent of improved noninvasive techniques. Echocardiography, particularly two-dimensional study, readily identifies atrial tumors and has virtually eliminated the need for invasive contrast angiography. Radionuclide ventriculography (gated blood cardiac scan) will also identify a moving filling defect within the cardiac chambers and can be used in making the diagnosis of intracavitary tumor. Once the diagnosis of cardiac myxoma has been made, the only treatment is surgical excision. Undiagnosed atrial myxomas are often fatal, but when considered, are readily detected and, once detected, straightforwardly treated and virtually always cured.

Secondary Tumors of the Heart

The heart may be a target for secondary tumor invasion. Cancer has been reported to involve the heart in anywhere from 5 to 20 per cent of patients with metastatic malignant disease, with an apparent increase in reported involvement of the heart in recent years. Almost any type of primary neoplasm may involve the heart. Malignant melanomas are among the most common solid tumors that spread to the heart. Cardiac lesions occur in 40 to 50 per cent of patients with metastatic disease, and as a group, melanomas constitute approximately 3 per cent of all cardiac metastases. Leukemias frequently infiltrate the heart, with microscopic invasion evident in approximately half of patients. Other tumors that frequently metastasize to the heart include carcinomas of the lung, breast, and thyroid, the lymphomas, and the sarcomas, including Kaposi's sarcoma. Carcinomas of the lung and breast, because of their relative frequency among malignan-

cies, together account for approximately 50 per cent of the secondary tumors of the heart.

What is most striking about cardiac invasion by metastatic tumor is that it is so often clinically silent, despite what may be extensive disease. The clinical manifestations of cardiac metastases are myriad and generally reflect the anatomic site of invasion. Congestive heart failure, cardiac arrhythmias, and signs of pericardial constriction are among the most common clinical manifestations of cardiac metastases. Myocardial ischemia and infarction may also result from coronary compression or invasion. Although most cardiac metastases are diagnosed post mortem, they may be clinically detected by a variety of means. When a malignant pericardial effusion is present, cytologic examination of pericardial fluid readily provides diagnosis. Identification of a mass in one or more cardiac chambers or of an irregularity in chamber contour or wall thickness may be accomplished by cross-sectional cardiac echocardiography, radionuclide ventriculography, or invasive contrast angiography. Pathologic examination is necessary, however, to identify tumor type. Unlike treatment for myxomas, surgery for primary or secondary malignancies of the heart is generally ineffective. The major role for cardiac surgery is to obtain tissue for pathologic diagnosis or to alleviate mechanical obstruction. Radiotherapy and chemotherapy are utilized, depending on tumor type.

CARDIAC DISEASE SECONDARY TO CANCER THERAPY. Cardiac disease or dysfunction may also occur as a consequence of chemotherapy and radiotherapy and may obscure even further the diagnosis of metastatic tumors of the heart. Many of the antineoplastic drugs, particularly doxorubicin (Adriamycin), produce a dose-dependent toxicity that leads to a dilated congestive cardiomyopathy. Doxorubicin causes a characteristic degeneration of the myocyte that can be detected by myocardial biopsy. Radiotherapy may also produce dose-dependent cardiac damage to all three layers of the heart. Pericarditis and pericardial effusions are most common, but fibrosis of the myocardium and of mural and valvular endocardium may occur. Prevention is the best therapy for radiation- and drug-induced cardiac damage, which is generally irreversible.

CARDIAC TRAUMA

Trauma is a major cause of morbidity and mortality in our society, and tragically it often affects those who are otherwise healthy. Cardiac trauma results from either a penetrating object or a nonpenetrating blunt assault on the thorax. Death may immediately occur as a result of asystole, ventricular fibrillation, or exsanguination. Those who survive long enough for transport to a hospital pose immediate diagnostic and therapeutic challenges.

Penetrating wounds of the heart are believed to be fatal in over 90 per cent of instances, with most patients never reaching medical attention. Stab and gunshot wounds may lacerate any portion of the heart. Pericardial laceration with cardiac tamponade or exsanguination is most common, usually in conjunction with rupture of some portion of the myocardium. Because of their anterior location, the right ventricle and pulmonary outflow tract are particularly susceptible. Valve lacerations leading to incompetence and coronary injuries leading to ischemia or infarction, or both, are of particular importance for survivors, who may be left with residual lesions.

The diagnosis of cardiac trauma in the setting of a penetrating wound of the thoracic cavity is not always straightforward. Patients usually present acutely with hypotension due either to cardiac tamponade or to hemorrhage. The diagnosis is assumed when profound hypotension is present in the setting of a penetrating mediastinal wound with or without an object in or near the cardiac silhouette. In this setting, emergency thoracotomy, preferably in an operating room, is virtually always necessary for both diagnosis and therapy. The wisdom of performing a diagnostic pericardiocentesis has been challenged, as false-negative readings may result from local clot formation. Pericardiocentesis may be necessary, however, to stabilize a patient with cardiac tamponade prior to emergency thoracotomy. Once the diagnosis of trauma has been made and cardiac surgical repair initiated, the survival rate may be as high as 70 per cent.

Nonpenetrating trauma to the chest cavity may also cause a similar range of cardiac injuries requiring emergency thoracotomy. Unlike penetrating wounds, however, physical evidence of trauma to the chest wall may be minimal or even absent, and the severity of chest wall trauma does not correlate with likelihood or extent of cardiac injury. Among the most common causes of cardiac trauma are steering wheel injuries to the sternum. Others include sports activities, industrial accidents, and personal assaults. The myocardium is the major site of injuries, which may range in severity from mild myocardial contusion to rupture of the ventricle or interventricular septum. Pericardial laceration, valve disruption, coronary artery thrombosis, or great vessel rupture, particularly of the ascending aorta, may also occur.

Diagnosis is difficult, since symptoms are often absent or misleading. Symptoms of chest pain similar to that associated with myocardial infarction are the most frequent. Cardiac arrhythmias and hypotension may also signal cardiac injury in the proper setting. Survivors of myocardial injury may develop false aneurysms with their usual complications. Early and late cardiac arrhythmias (atrial or ventricular) may be caused by myocardial contusions, and the electrocardiographic abnormalities may include those of myocardial infarction or acute pericarditis. Serum enzyme assays (creatine kinase, MB fraction) and echocardiography are helpful in making the diagnosis, and if coronary compromise is suggested, cardiac catheterization with coronary angiography would be appropriate. Treatment depends on the extent of cardiovascular compromise. Pain and arrhythmias alone are treated similarly to those of acute myocardial infarction, except that anticoagulants should be strictly avoided. Thoracotomy is necessary if there are signs of myocardial rupture or pericardial tamponade. Late complications, such as valvular or interventricular septal rupture or false aneurysms of the heart or aorta, require surgical correction.

CARDIAC MANIFESTATIONS OF SYSTEMIC DISEASE

The heart may be afflicted secondarily by a variety of systemic conditions and diseases. The most frequent cardiac manifestations of systemic disease are those common disorders that primarily involve the vascular system and produce cardiac dysfunction by virtue of increased volume or pressure load on the heart or interruption in blood flow to the myocardium. Systemic hypertension, whether essential, renal, or endocrine in cause, often leads to cardiac hypertrophy and heart failure. Atherosclerosis is a systemic vascular disease with the heart as a prime target. Less common are the anemias, which produce a volume load and at times hypoxic insult to the heart, leading to congestive heart failure. In addition to these widely recognized disorders, there are several systemic diseases that secondarily involve the heart in a distinctive fashion. Examples of these disorders include the connective tissue diseases (e.g., systemic lupus erythematosus [SLE], progressive systemic sclerosis and polyarteritis nodosa); endocrine-humoral disorders (thyroid disease, pheochromocytoma, and metastatic carcinoid); and systemic infiltrative disease (amyloidosis).

CONNECTIVE TISSUE DISEASES. Although the connective tissue diseases may affect the heart only secondarily, the cardiac disorder may dominate the clinical course. In systemic lupus erythematosus, the endocardium, myocardium, and pericardium all are potential targets. A fibrinous pericarditis is a common cardiac lesion and frequently produces clinical symptoms. Fibrofibrinous thrombotic lesions may develop on the surface of the cardiac valves (a condition termed Libman-Sacks endocarditis) and are usually clinically silent. On occasion this endocarditis may lead to significant mitral or aortic valve dysfunction. Myocarditis may occur but is an infrequent result of SLE. Coronary arteritis and thromboembolism may also develop, and in patients with corticosteroid-treated lupus, in particular, there may be accelerated coronary atherosclerosis.

Progressive systemic sclerosis (PSS) or scleroderma may produce cardiac dysfunction by means of its effect on the myocardium. Focal fibrosis and necrosis of myocardium may lead to a picture of dilated congestive cardiomyopathy. Morphologic and clinical evidence now suggests that the etiology of the myocardial disease in PSS is small vessel coronary spasm, causing ischemia, i.e., a Raynaud's phenomenon of the coronary arteries. Polyarteritis nodosa may cause a focal or a diffuse coronary arteritis, with formation of coronary thrombosis or aneurysm or both. The latter may lead to myocardial ischemia or infarction and, combined with systemic hypertension, to congestive heart failure. Cardiac manifestations of the connective tissue diseases are diagnosed and treated with the standard technology and methods used for valvular, myocardial, pericardial, or coronary disease. Therapy also includes the immunosuppressive drugs used for treatment of the systemic diseases.

ENDOCRINE-HUMORAL DISORDERS. Thyroid disease has long been known to target the heart. Thyroid hormone increases oxygen consumption and metabolic rate, has a direct inotropic and chronotropic effect on the heart, and has been shown to have a direct trophic effect on the myocardium, inducing a physiologic pattern of hypertrophy. The major clinical manifestation of thyroid hormone excess is a hyperkinetic heart and circulation. Other symptoms include a variety of arrhythmias (atrial fibrillation, in particular), and, with severe disease, congestive heart failure may develop. Although less common, hypothyroidism may produce an idiopathic dilated cardiomyopathy, but its etiology is obscure. More often, hypothyroidism causes bradycardia and pericardial effusions. The latter may contain cholesterol crystals, a finding believed to be characteristic of a myxedema-associated effusion. Identification of the basis for these cardiac disorders is confirmed by abnormal serum thyroxine levels. Thyroid hormone levels should be obtained routinely in patients with idiopathic atrial fibrillation and in those with heart failure of obscure etiology.

Pheochromocytomas, which are chromaffin cell tumors, produce norepinephrine and, to a varying degree, epinephrine, which may cause systemic hypertension as well as induce direct myocardial toxicity. Autopsy studies have shown focal myocardial contraction band necrosis and fibrosis in as many as 50 per cent of patients with this tumor. Similar lesions may be produced in experimental animals with catecholamine infusions and are believed to relate to norepinephrine-induced calcium overload. Although this tumor may cause cardiomyopathy, it is exceedingly rare.

CARDIAC AMYLOIDOSIS. This disorder may be primary but occurs most often secondary to systemic conditions, including multiple myeloma, systemic amyloidosis, familial Mediterranean fever, and aging. Amyloid may infiltrate myocardium and coronary arteries, and less often the cardiac valves, and typically causes increased myocardial mass and focal fibrosis. The latter leads to decreased myocardial compliance and ultimately congestive heart failure—a picture that may simulate hypertrophic or restrictive cardiomyopathy. Cardiac amyloid deposits may also affect the conduction system of the heart, causing a variety of arrhythmias. The diagnosis of cardiac amyloid is confirmed by myocardial biopsy. Therapy for the cardiac dysfunction of amyloidosis is the standard treatment for arrhythmias or heart failure or both. A proclivity to digitalis toxicity, possibly related to conduction system infiltration by amyloid, should be considered when treating heart failure in these patients.

Doherty NE, Siegel RJ: Cardiovascular manifestations of systemic lupus erythematosus. Am Heart J 110:1257, 1985. *A review article summarizing present information on the clinical and morphologic aspects of the heart in systemic lupus erythematosus.*

Follansbee WP, Curtiss EI, Medsger TA, et al.: Physiologic abnormalities of cardiac function in progressive systemic sclerosis with diffuse scleroderma. N Engl J Med 310:142, 1984. *Description of cardiac dysfunction in patients with PSS, showing by noninvasive techniques the relationship of circulatory disturbances to ventricular dysfunction.*

Frazee RC, Mucha P Jr, Farnell MB, et al.: Objective evaluation of blunt cardiac trauma. J Trauma 26:510, 1986. *A review of the cardiovascular consequences of blunt chest trauma, describing CK-MB elevations, arrhythmias, and ventricular dysfunction as assessed by echocardiography in a wide range of cardiac injuries.*

McDonnell PJ, Mann RB, Bulkley BH: Involvement of the heart by malignant lymphoma: A clinicopathologic study. Cancer 49:944, 1982. *A clinicopathologic study of the cardiovascular manifestations of lymphomatous involvement of the heart and a general review of the range of malignant tumors of the heart and how they cause cardiac dysfunction.*

Morkin E, Flink IL, Goldman S: Biochemical and physiologic effects of thyroid hormone on cardiac performance. Prog Cardiovasc Dis 25:435, 1983. *An in-depth and current review of the effect of thyroid hormone on the normal heart and its role in disease.*

Salcedo EE, Adams KV, Lever HM, et al.: Echocardiographic findings in 25 patients with left atrial myxoma. J Am Coll Cardiol 1:1162, 1983. *Describes the use of echocardiography to diagnose myxomas noninvasively.*

Schrader ML, Hochman JS, Bulkley BH: The heart in polyarteritis nodosa: A clinicopathologic study. Am Heart J 109:1353, 1985. *A clinicopathologic study of the heart in polyarteritis nodosa and a review of the literature.*

Skhvatsabaja LV: Secondary malignant lesions of the heart and pericardium in neoplastic disease. Oncology 43:103, 1986. *A review of clinical and laboratory data in 240 patients with metastatic tumors of the heart and pericardium, focusing on clinical symptoms and diagnosis.*

56 DISEASES OF THE AORTA

Lawrence S. Cohen

The aorta is vital to the proper functioning of every organ system in the body. The coronary arteries are the first arteries to arise from the aorta, followed by vessels of the head and central nervous system and then the gastrointestinal, renal, and genitourinary arteries. Disease in any segment of the aorta, therefore, can have profound consequences upon bodily function. The aorta is susceptible to four major disease processes: *aneurysm, dissection, arteriosclerotic occlusive disease,* and *aortitis.*

At its origin the aorta is approximately 3 cm in diameter. The ascending aorta is approximately 5 cm in length, coursing in a left-to-right direction in the same ejection axis as the left ventricle. The aortic arch is also approximately 5 cm in length and takes an upward, posterior, and leftward direction, terminating along the left border of the thoracic vertebrae. The aortic arch lies entirely within the superior mediastinum. The descending thoracic aorta is contained in the posterior mediastinum. It is a bit narrower than the ascending aorta and is approximately 20 cm in length. It runs to the diaphragm at the level of the twelfth thoracic vertebra and supplies the arteries to the spinal cord. The abdominal aorta is the continuation of the thoracic aorta, ending at the level of the fourth lumbar vertebra. The average length is 15 cm, with an average diameter of 2 cm at its origin and a slightly smaller diameter at its lower end.

ANEURYSM

Definition

An aneurysm is a widening of a vessel involving the stretching of fibrous tissue within the media of the vessel. A true aneurysm is a widening of the vessel, whereas a false aneurysm represents a localized rupture of the artery with sealing over by clot or adjacent structures. The natural history of aneurysms is to enlarge. Not only does the etiologic process tend to continue and progress but also the law of Laplace is a factor. As described by Laplace, the tension in the wall of a spherical chamber enclosing a fluid under pressure is related to this pressure under which the fluid is kept and the radius of curvature of the containing vessel. As the radius increases so does wall tension. Hence, enlargement of the vessel begets more enlargement.

It is convenient to classify aneurysms according to etiology, morphology, and location. Arteriosclerosis is the most common cause of aneurysms. Other causes are cystic medial necrosis, trauma, and infection, including syphilis. Rarer causes are rheumatic aortitis, Takayasu's syndrome, temporal arteritis, and relapsing polychondritis. Marfan's syndrome is characterized by cystic medial necrosis (Ch. 199). In some forms of Ehlers-Danlos syndrome, rupture of blood vessels, including the aorta, may occur. Aneurysms can be classified into three morphologic types: (1) fusiform, in which the aneurysm encompasses the entire circumference of the aorta and assumes a spindle shape; (2) saccular, in which only a portion of the circumference is involved and in which there is a neck and an asymmetric outpouching of the aneurysm; and (3) dissecting, in which an intimal tear permits a column of blood to dissect along the media of the vessel. This is often called a dissecting hematoma. Location is a further way to classify aneurysms. Aneurysms involve (1) the ascending aorta, including the sinuses of Valsalva; (2) the aortic arch; (3) the descending thoracic aorta, originating just distal to the left subclavian artery, and (4) the abdomen, most commonly distal to the renal arteries.

The most proximal portion of the ascending aorta comprises the sinuses of Valsalva. Aneurysms in this location are usually congenital in origin. Most involve either the right sinus or the right portion of the noncoronary sinus. Aneurysms of the sinus of Valsalva are often silent until they rupture into the right side of the heart, usually the right ventricle or right atrium. This event may occur spontaneously or may be a consequence of infective endocarditis. Other causes of aortic sinus aneurysm are Marfan's syndrome, syphilis, or infective endocarditis. Aneurysms of the ascending aorta may be arteriosclerotic, but cystic medial necrosis with or without other features of Marfan's syndrome is more common. Syphilis was once a common cause of ascending aortic aneurysm but has all but disappeared as an etiology. The more distal the aortic location of the aneurysm, the more likely it is to be arteriosclerotic.

Clinical Manifestations

Clinical manifestations of aneurysms of the thoracic aorta (other than rupture) are due to compression, distortion, or erosion of surrounding structures. Pain is the most common symptom. Pain in a gradually enlarging aneurysm is insidious and may be described as boring and deep. Increasing intensity of pain is an ominous sign and may presage impending rupture.

Aortic valve regurgitation may be associated with aneurysms of the ascending aorta. Distortion of the aortic annulus and separation of the aortic valve cusps accounts for the regurgitation. If regurgitation occurs rapidly, the clinical consequences can be dramatic, with the patient developing acute pulmonary edema. Many patients will develop a murmur of aortic regurgitation gradually and may be relatively asymptomatic. Aneurysms of the transverse aortic arch are less common than are aneurysms in other sites. The consequences of such aneurysms are often formidable, since the innominate and carotid arteries arise from the transverse aortic arch. In addition, the arch is contiguous with other vital structures such as the superior vena cava, pulmonary artery, trachea, bronchi, lung, and left recurrent laryngeal nerve. Symptoms may include dyspnea, stridor, hoarseness, hemoptysis, cough, or chest pain.

The most common site of an aneurysm of the thoracic aorta is between the origin of the left subclavian artery and the diaphragm. Arteriosclerosis is the most common cause, with age, hypertension, and probably smoking contributing as risk factors. One factor in the pathogenesis of aneurysms of the descending aorta may be the immobility of the aorta at this site and the unique stresses imposed on the aorta immediately distal to the left subclavian artery. Distortion of the architecture in this area may result in sufficient turbulence to cause elastic tissue degeneration, accelerated arteriosclerosis, and localized dilatation.

Pain from descending thoracic aortic aneurysm is often intrascapular but can vary considerably. Hoarseness may occur from stretching of the left recurrent laryngeal nerve. Hemoptysis may occur owing to leakage into the left lung. Thoracic aortic aneurysms, like those of the abdominal aorta, threaten life by potential rupture. They are rarely complicated by thrombosis or embolism. Thoracoabdominal aneurysms involve the celiac, superior mesenteric, and renal arteries. Fortunately, they are not common, for they represent a great challenge to the vascular surgeon. Although some are caused by cystic medial necrosis, most are of arteriosclerotic origin and occur in older men.

The most common form of aneurysm is the abdominal aortic aneurysm. The prevalence of this aneurysm at autopsy is in the 1 to 3 per cent range but is even more common in men over 60. Its frequency in men outnumbers that in women by 6:1. Almost all of these aneurysms are below the renal arteries. Most are of arteriosclerotic origin, but trauma, infection (including syphilis), and arteritis make up a small fraction. A fortunate feature of these aneurysms is their accessibility on physical examination. A mass that pulsates in all directions may well be an aneurysm, whereas a pulsation in one direction only is usually a transmitted pulsation through an overlying visceral mass. Rupture of an abdominal aneurysm is the greatest threat and may lead to a rapid demise because of shock and hypotension. Other less acute symptoms may also occur. Pain in the lower back is a sign of enlargement of the aneurysm and at times is a warning of impending rupture. Almost all abdominal aortic aneurysms are lined with clot or have ulcerated plaques. Embolization of atherothrombotic material may lead to a variety of symptoms, ranging from digital infarction to anuria from a shower of emboli to the kidneys.

The likelihood of rupture increases with increasing aortic aneurysm size. Sixty to 80 per cent of patients with lesions 7 cm or larger die of rupture, and 95 per cent of patients with lesions over 10 cm die of aneurysm rupture. The risk of rupture in aneurysms 5 cm or less is considerably lower. Given these data, general guidelines about surgical repair have emerged. Aneurysms associated with aortic thrombosis or distal embolic events should be repaired promptly. Aneurysms suspected of rupture or acute expansion should be treated surgically immediately. Although there are differences of opinion concerning when elective repair of asymptomatic aneurysms should be undertaken, once the aneurysm exceeds 5 cm in diameter, the prognosis on continued medical management becomes increasingly guarded.

Diagnosis

Palpation is usually the first step in diagnosing abdominal aneurysms. Ultrasound imaging is an excellent technique to confirm the diagnosis, as it is noninvasive, inexpensive, and accurate to within 2 to 3 mm of aneurysm size when compared with the findings at surgery. Computed tomographic (CT) scanning utilizing contrast material is equal in effectiveness to ultrasound in the detection and sizing of abdominal aortic aneurysms. Often lumbar spine x-ray films will clearly outline the walls of an abdominal aortic aneurysm if there is calcium in the walls. Aortography, either arterial or venous with digital subtraction, may not reflect the true size of the aneurysm; an extensive laminated clot may reduce the lumen.

Joyce JW: Aneurysmal disease. In Spittell JA Jr (ed.): Clinical Vascular Disease. Philadelphia, F. A. Davis Company, 1983, pp 89–101. *A concise summary of aneurysmal disease, including management guidelines for aneurysms in all aortic locations.*

Spittell JA Jr: Abdominal aortic aneurysms. Hosp Pract 21:105, 1986. *This is a short, well-illustrated practical management update. Modern diagnostic tools are discussed, and management strategies are reviewed.*

MARFAN'S SYNDROME

Patients with Marfan's syndrome (see Ch. 199) develop both aortic aneurysm and aortic dissection. Myxomatous degeneration of valve leaflets may also occur. The mitral valve cusps may be involved. The chordae tendineae may elongate or rupture, predisposing to mitral valve prolapse, or flail mitral valve with mitral regurgitation. Regurgitation at either the mitral or the tricuspid valve may be the most prominent finding in certain patients. However, the most commonly affected tissue is the aorta. The aorta enlarges, beginning with the sinuses of Valsalva. The enlargement most often extends to the innominate artery, although at times the entire aorta may be involved in what has been referred to as annuloaortic ectasia. Aortic dilation may begin as early as the fifth year of life or as late as the sixth decade.

Aortic regurgitation may occur secondary to participation of the aortic root in the development of an aortic aneurysm. Dissection of the aortic root may lead to acute aortic regurgitation. Dilation of the pulmonary artery is common.

Diagnosis

Dilation of the aortic root is easily measured by echocardiography. Two-dimensional echocardiography shows the classic flask-shaped dilation of the aorta extending from the aortic valve to the innominate artery (Fig. 56–1). Echocardiography may also be used to demonstrate the major complications of aortic root dilation, dissection of the aorta, and aortic regurgitation. The echocardiogram has also helped in defining the optimal time for operative intervention.

Therapy

It is now generally agreed, although not absolutely proven, that beta blockade may inhibit the pace of aortic dilation.

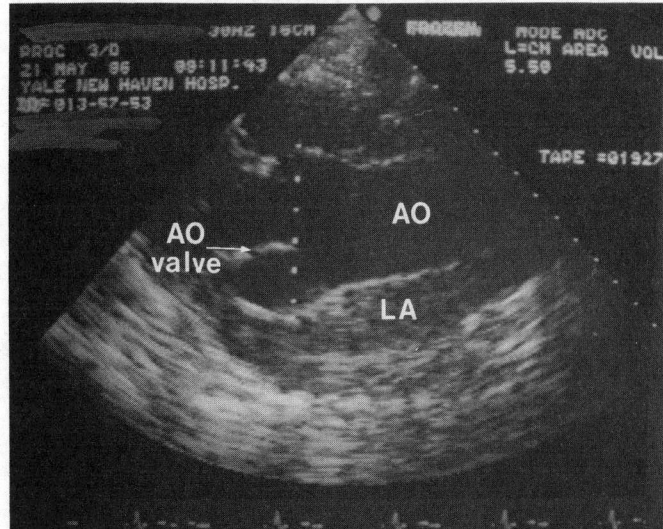

FIGURE 56–1. Echocardiogram, long axis parasternal view of a patient with Marfan's syndrome. The sinuses of Valsalva are flared and the aortic root is dilated.

Therefore, it is appropriate to obtain serial echocardiograms in patients thought to have Marfan's syndrome. When incipient dilation of the aorta is recognized, institution of a beta blocker may be warranted. By diminishing the velocity with which the left ventricle ejects blood, the forces on the weakened aortic wall may be lessened.

Complications of aneurysms in the ascending aorta account for more than 90 per cent of deaths from the Marfan's syndrome. The likelihood of both aortic dissection and aortic regurgitation increases as the size of the aortic root increases. Operation in the face of an acute dissection is fraught with considerable hazard. Therefore, prophylactic operation is recommended if the aortic root enlarges to 6 cm on echocardiography. The operation most commonly utilized for patients with the Marfan's syndrome is replacement of the ascending aortic aneurysm with a composite tube graft that includes a prosthetic valve at its proximal end. The coronaries are anastomosed to the sides of the tube graft. The aneurysm is wrapped around the tube graft to help establish hemostasis. The overall hospital mortality of the procedure is 2 per cent (Gott and colleagues). Although it may seem radical to recommend aortic replacement to a patient who may be asymptomatic, the adverse prognosis of the patient with Marfan's syndrome whose aorta dilates to greater than 6 cm in diameter probably warrants this recommendation.

Gott VL, Pyeritz RE, Magovern GJ Jr, et al.: Surgical treatment of aneurysms of the ascending aorta in the Marfan syndrome. N Engl J Med 314:1070, 1986. *The results of ascending aorta replacement with a composite graft in 50 consecutive patients with Marfan's syndrome are reported. Because of the unfavorable natural history of Marfan's syndrome, the authors recommend prophylactic repair when the aneurysm reaches a diameter of 6 cm.*

Halpern BL, Char F, Murdoch JL, et al.: A prospectus on the prevention of aortic rupture in the Marfan syndrome with data on survivorship without treatment. Johns Hopkins Med J 129:123, 1971. *This is one of the first articles to advocate the prophylactic use of beta blockers in patients with the Marfan's syndrome in order to prevent further dilation and dissecting aneurysm.*

DISSECTING ANEURYSM OF THE AORTA

The incidence of aortic dissections is not known exactly, but it is estimated that approximately 2000 acute cases occur in the United States each year.

Classification of aortic dissection is based upon duration and anatomic location of the dissection. Dissection is considered acute if it occurred within two weeks, and chronic if it occurred more than two weeks, prior to the institution of therapy.

Aortic dissection is more commonly classified by site of the intimal tear and extent of dissecting hematoma. In type I and type II dissections, the intimal tear is in the ascending aorta, usually within a few centimeters of the aortic valve. In type I aneurysms, the dissecting hematoma extends and involves at least the aortic arch and often the descending aorta as well. Type II aneurysms involve the ascending aorta only. Type III aneurysms are characterized by an intimal tear in the descending aorta, usually immediately distal to the left subclavian artery. The dissecting hematoma usually propagates distally but at times may extend in a retrograde manner to the aortic arch (Fig. 56–2).

Etiology

The most consistent etiologic factor in aortic dissection is hypertension. Other conditions are associated with dissection in the absence of hypertension. Marfan's syndrome has been discussed. There is a peculiar association between pregnancy and dissection. It is postulated that hormonal changes during pregnancy may alter the composition of the aorta and make it more susceptible to rupture. Stresses and strains of labor may also be a factor.

Valvular aortic stenosis, particularly that due to a bicuspid valve, is associated with dissection. Turbulence established beyond the stenotic valve increases lateral forces, thereby enhancing the likelihood of an intimal tear and development

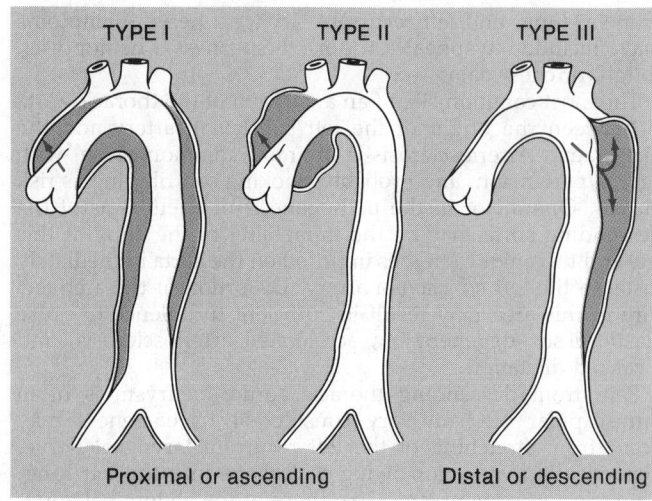

FIGURE 56–2. Classification of dissecting aneurysms of the aorta. (Modified from DeBakey.)

of a dissection. The association between coarctation of the aorta and dissection is well known. The years of proximal aortic hypertension prior to repair of the coarctation may establish the conditions that ultimately lead to aortic dissection. In addition, there is a high incidence of bicuspid aortic valves in patients with coarctation of the aorta. Before the advent of antimicrobial agents, syphilitic aortitis was the most common cause of aortic dissection. It is now unusual. Trauma may be a cause of dissecting aneurysm. Other unusual etiologies are the Ehlers-Danlos syndrome and relapsing polychondritis.

Pathogenesis

Aortic dissection begins most frequently in an intimal tear in the ascending aorta a short distance above the aortic valve. The primary tear is often referred to as the *entry intimal tear*. The *re-entry* or *secondary tear* occurs more distally. The basic pathologic condition resides in the underlying media, the chief supporting layer of the aorta. Most tears are transverse or circumferential, reflecting the direction of the muscular fibers of the media.

The two key ingredients of aortic dissection are arterial hypertension and medial degeneration. In any given patient, one or the other of these abnormalities may be the more important. Many patients with Marfan's syndrome or the Ehlers-Danlos syndrome develop dissecting aneurysms without ever developing hypertension. Alternatively, individuals with longstanding hypertension may develop dissection without any apparent specific weakness of the aortic medial wall. Additional factors in the pathogenesis of aortic dissections are the anatomy and motion of the heart and great vessels themselves. The heart beats an average of 70 times per minute, over 80,000 times per day and over 35 million times per year. The heart is not absolutely fixed in place but is limited in its anterior-posterior movement by the sternum and vertebral column, respectively. Its motion is both side to side and twisting as it ejects blood into the ascending aorta. This produces a flexing stress in the ascending aorta and contributes to the frequency of ascending aortic dissections. The descending aorta becomes fixed distal to the left subclavian artery, accounting for the alternative predilection for dissection to occur at that site. Once an intimal tear occurs, the dissecting hematoma is propagated through the weakened medial wall. The forces that continue the propagation are the arterial pressure and the pulse wave properties (dp/dt) of left ventricular ejection. Some dissecting hematomas will rupture back into the aortic lumen at a distal site. Rupture may also occur externally into the pericardial or pleural space.

Clinical Manifestations

Pain is often excruciating and may occur primarily in the anterior chest. It may migrate to the back as the dissecting hematoma works it way down the aorta. Patients sometimes describe an accentuation of the pain with each heart beat suggesting the driving force of the pulse wave. Pain may occur in the neck, jaw, or teeth if the aortic arch is involved. Less common symptoms are syncope, stroke, paraplegia, or loss of pulses in any of the extremities. Rarely, a dissection may be clinically silent and be suggested only by an abnormal roentgenogram. If aortic regurgitation occurs owing to the dissection, patients may develop congestive heart failure. A diastolic murmur is usually present in these circumstances, although the duration of the murmur may be relatively short if the filling pressure in the left ventricle rises rapidly because of the acute nature of the regurgitation. Such murmurs may be heard commonly along the right sternal border.

The clinical presentation and physical findings in patients with aortic dissection are determined by the course taken by the dissecting hematoma. (1) Loss of any pulse can occur as the circulation to any major artery arising from the aorta may be compromised. (2) Aortic regurgitation may result from disruption of the supporting structures of the aortic valve. (3) Neurologic symptoms may occur if the head and neck vessels are compromised by the dissection. Paraplegia may occur owing to loss of blood supply to the spinal cord. A number of other physical findings may be seen in patients with aortic dissection. These include Horner's syndrome due to compression of the superior cervical ganglion, vocal cord paralysis and hoarseness due to pressure against the recurrent laryngeal nerve, superior vena cava syndrome, pulsating neck masses, dyspnea due to tracheal or bronchial compression, hemorrhagic pleural effusion, myocardial infarction if the hematoma dissects retrograde across a coronary ostium, and symptoms and signs of mesenteric infarction. Persistent fever has also been described.

Diagnosis

Time is often of utmost importance in management. Once the patient is stabilized, aortography should not be delayed. Routine laboratory tests do not generally add much to the diagnosis. Leukocytosis is a common but nonspecific finding.

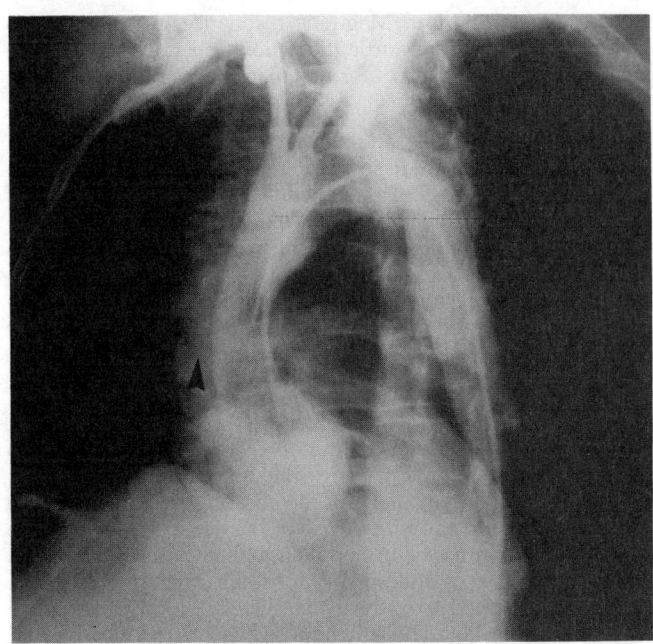

FIGURE 56–4. Aortic root angiogram in the left anterior oblique projection. The black arrowhead demonstrates the false lumen caused by the aortic dissection.

A chest roentgenogram may be normal but will often show widening of the aortic shadow (Fig. 56–3). Aortic angiography is the definitive procedure, yielding precise information necessary for proper management. The extent of the dissection, the entry and re-entry sites, the competence or degree of regurgitation of the aortic valve, and aortic branch vessel involvement can all be ascertained (Fig. 56–4).

The differential diagnosis of a patient with chest or back pain, pulmonary edema with a new murmur of aortic regurgitation, any acute neurologic syndrome, or sudden loss of pulse in an extremity should include aortic dissection.

Computed tomography with the use of contrast material is also highly accurate in demonstrating aortic dissection, although it is not always possible to perform this examination rapidly. Two-dimensional echocardiography does not necessitate the use of contrast agents or ionizing radiation and is easily performed. False-negative and false-positive diagnoses remain a problem with this procedure, but it is nevertheless useful (Fig. 56–5). Echocardiography can detect the presence

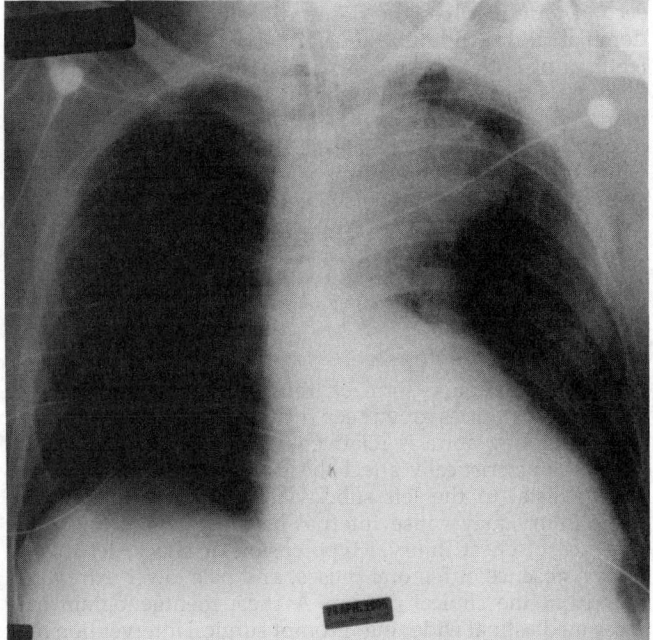

FIGURE 56–3. Chest roentgenogram of a patient with a dissecting aneurysm demonstrating marked enlargement of the aortic arch and descending aorta.

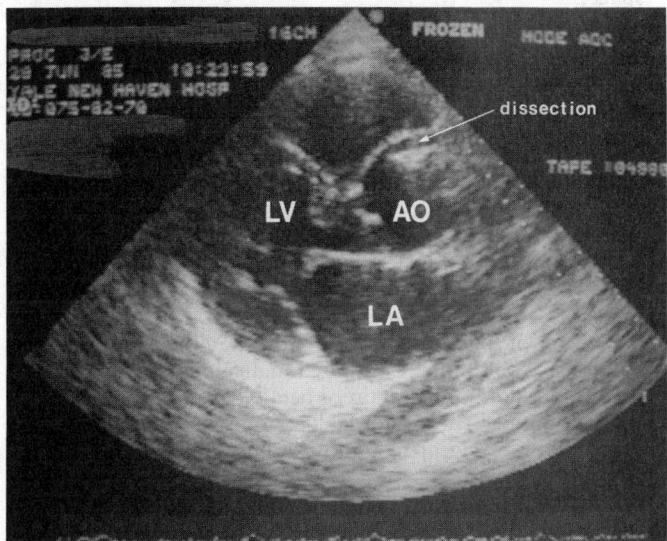

FIGURE 56–5. Echocardiogram, long axis parasternal view of a patient with dissecting aneurysm. The dissection arises in the proximal aortic root. LV = Left ventricle; AO = aortic root; LA = left atrium.

of aortic regurgitation. Magnetic resonance imaging is also capable of diagnosing aortic dissection and does not require the use of contrast agents for vascular imaging.

Prognosis

In untreated aortic dissection, the prognosis is poor. Approximately 20 per cent of patients die in 24 hours, 60 per cent in 2 weeks, and 90 per cent in 3 months. The principal cause of death is not the initial intimal tear but is related to the effects of propagation of the dissecting hematoma. Progressive aortic regurgitation may occur if the hematoma dissects in a retrograde direction. Rupture into the pericardial or pleural space is often a fatal complication.

Treatment

Prompt diagnosis and institution of therapy are critical to the success of treatment. Since the most important known factors in the propagation of the dissecting hematoma are hypertension and the rate of rise of the aortic pressure pulse (dp/dt), efforts must be undertaken to alter both of these. An intravenous drip of sodium nitroprusside is started, and the infusion is titrated to reduce the systolic blood pressure to 100 to 120 mm Hg. The infusion rate can usually be started at 1 μg per kilogram per minute. Simultaneously, propranolol should be given in intermittent intravenous boluses of 0.5 to 1.0 mg until the heart rate is in the range of 60 beats per minute. When possible, an intra-arterial line to measure blood pressure accurately and a central venous line or Swan-Ganz catheter should be utilized. Once the patient's blood pressure and other hemodynamic and clinical features are stable, aortography should be performed. Computed tomographic scanning or echocardiography may be of some diagnostic aid at this stage while awaiting aortography.

Operative intervention is usually indicated if the dissection involves the ascending aorta, as in Types I and II aneurysms. These aneurysms are unstable and pose the threat of retrograde dissection, rupture, severe aortic regurgitation, or fatal pericardial tamponade. This type of acute dissection can be corrected surgically with a mortality rate in the range of 20 per cent. Type III aneurysms that involve the distal or descending aorta can generally be treated medically. If the patient's condition stabilizes, drug therapy can be continued into the chronic phase. Surgical intervention for the patient with a Type III aneurysm is indicated if there is evidence of increasing size of the dissecting hematoma, impending rupture, inability to control pain, or bleeding into the pleural space.

The operative approach must be flexible and individualized. For patients with ascending aortic dissection and involvement of the annulus or root, it is often necessary to replace the entire aortic root and aortic valve with a composite conduit, which is attached proximally to the aortic annulus and distally to the aorta after obliteration of the false lumen. The coronary ostia are then reimplanted into the tubular graft. If the ascending aorta is involved but the sinuses of Valsalva are spared, operative repair consists of resection of the aneurysmal portion with replacement by a synthetic tubular graft. This same technique applies for descending aortic dissections. In all cases, the false lumen is obliterated. Management and follow-up of patients initially treated either surgically or medically is the same. Continued meticulous control of blood pressure and administration of beta blockers to control dp/dt are warranted. The systolic blood pressure should be kept below 130 mm Hg at rest and the heart rate below 72 beats per minute at rest.

Cooke JP, Safford RE: Progress in the diagnosis and management of aortic dissection. Mayo Clin Proc 61:147, 1986. *This is an excellent short article that concentrates on the available diagnostic studies in patients with aortic dissection.*

Eagle KA, Quertermous T, Kritzer GA, et al.: Spectrum of conditions initially suggesting acute aortic dissection but with negative aortograms. Am J Cardiol 57:322, 1986. *This study defines the differential diagnosis of aortic dissection, discusses the frequency of false-negative aortographic findings, and contrasts the clinical features of patients with and without dissection.*

Roberts WC: Aortic dissection: Anatomy, consequences, and causes. Am Heart J 101:195, 1981. *A well-illustrated review of aortic dissection with emphasis on pathologic findings.*

Slater EE, DeSanctis RW: The clinical recognition of dissecting aortic aneurysm. Am J Med 60:625, 1976. *The clinical, roentgenologic, and laboratory findings in 124 patients with dissecting aneurysm of the aorta are discussed. Patients with dissections of the proximal aorta were younger and had a higher incidence of Marfan's syndrome, cystic medial necrosis, anterior chest pain, pulse deficits, neurologic compromise, aortic regurgitation, and congestive heart failure. Back pain, hypertension, and atherosclerosis characterized patients with distal dissection.*

Wheat MW Jr: Acute dissecting aneurysms of the aorta: Diagnosis and treatment—1979. Am Heart J 99:373, 1980. *The author, a surgeon, presents arguments for vigorous medical therapy in order to control hypertension and rate of pressure development in the aorta.*

MISCELLANEOUS FORMS OF AORTITIS AND THE AORTIC ARCH SYNDROME

Arteritis

A number of inflammatory processes can involve the aortic arch and its major branches. Aortic arteritis, no matter what the etiology, may cause narrowing or occlusion of the major arch vessels. Blood supply to the areas supplied by the innominate artery, the left common carotid artery, and the left subclavian artery may be impaired. Symptoms may include transient ischemic attacks, syncope, disorders of vision or speech, claudication of the upper extremities or of the muscles of the jaw, decreased pulses in the neck and upper extremities, or symptoms of basilar artery insufficiency. As a group, these entities are called the aortic arch syndrome. They include aortitis due to syphilis, tuberculosis, giant cell arteritis, polyarteritis nodosa, Takayasu's syndrome, or dissecting aneurysm. Kawasaki's mucocutaneous lymph node syndrome may cause an aortitis, but the coronary arteries are the principal vessels involved. Giant cell arteritis may cause the aortic arch syndrome in addition to temporal and ophthalmic artery disease.

Takayasu's arteritis may be a more specific form of aortitis. Initially it was thought that the arteritic process was limited to the aortic arch and its branches. Subsequent studies have demonstrated that the arteritis is not confined to these areas. Three varieties are now recognized. In one type, the involvement is localized to the aortic arch and its branches. The second type involves the descending thoracic aorta and abdominal aorta without the arch. The third type contains features of both. There is a preponderance of females with "pulseless disease." Although early reports were more common in Japan, increasing numbers of patients are being recognized in the United States. The presence of hypertension with absent pulses in the upper extremities has caused this syndrome to be called reversed coarctation.

Lupi-Herrera E, Sanchez-Torres G, Marcushamer J, et al.: Takayasu's arteritis: Clinical study of 107 cases. Am Heart J 93:94, 1977. *A review of Takayasu's arteritis involving 107 patients. This entity is not limited to Asian patients. It is a nonspecific inflammatory process affecting the aorta and its main branches.*

TRAUMATIC AORTIC DISEASE

The most common form of trauma to the aorta is due to deceleration injuries, often seen in automobile accidents. Since the descending aorta is relatively immobile, deceleration injuries characteristically affect the portion of the aorta immediately distal to the left subclavian artery. Nonpenetrating aortic injury may cause internal bleeding with no external evidence of chest injury. Hypotension or shock, left hemothorax, absence of femoral pulses, and pale lower extremities round out the clinical picture. A chest roentgenogram may show mediastinal widening. Prompt surgical intervention may be life saving.

57 VASCULAR DISEASES OF THE LIMBS

Hermes A. Kontos

VASCULAR DISEASES OF THE LIMBS CAUSED BY ABNORMAL RESPONSES OF VASCULAR SMOOTH MUSCLE
Raynaud's Phenomenon and Disease

DEFINITION. Raynaud's phenomenon is a syndrome manifested by attacks of pallor and cyanosis of the digits in response to cold or to emotion. As the attack abates, these color changes are replaced by redness. When the disorder is primary, it is called Raynaud's disease, when it is secondary to another disease or cause, it is called Raynaud's phenomenon.

ETIOLOGY AND INCIDENCE. Raynaud's disease is the most common cause of Raynaud's phenomenon, accounting for 60 per cent of patients with this disorder. The cause of Raynaud's disease is unknown. Although it can begin at any age, it becomes clinically manifest most commonly between the ages of 20 and 40 years. Raynaud's disease is much more common in women than in men. Two theories have been advanced to explain its occurrence. Raynaud believed that it is caused by increased sympathetic nerve activity. However, measurements of the sympathetic nerve traffic in the median nerve failed to show differences between patients with Raynaud's disease and normal individuals. Lewis discovered that attacks of Raynaud's phenomenon could be induced after interruption of the sympathetic nerves. He concluded that the cause of the disorder was a fault in the arterial wall that rendered the vessels hyper-responsive to the vasoconstrictive effects of cold. He ascribed the vasospastic attacks to spasm of the digital arteries as a result of this hypersensitivity. Little is known about the defect in the vessel wall, which renders the vessel hypersensitive to cold. The circulation of the digits of patients with Raynaud's disease is not hypersensitive to infused norepinephrine. Also, determination of the arteriovenous concentration differences of norepinephrine and epinephrine across the hand showed that there was no excessive release of catecholamines from the hands of patients with Raynaud's disease. More recently, accelerated destruction of platelets and release of agents such as serotonin or thromboxane A_2 have been proposed as causing vasoconstriction in some patients with Raynaud's phenomenon. It is not known whether platelet destruction is the cause of spasm in such patients or a consequence of it.

In a recent study, 26 per cent of patients with the variant type of angina pectoris were found to have migraine, and 24 per cent were found to have Raynaud's phenomenon. This suggested that some patients with Raynaud's phenomenon may have a generalized defect that predisposes arteries in many regions to vasospasm. An association of Raynaud's phenomenon with idiopathic pulmonary hypertension has also been reported. This association may reflect a very high level of peripheral vascular tone secondary to the severe reduction in cardiac output.

Secondary Raynaud's phenomenon is observed frequently as a manifestation of the diseases listed in Table 57–1.

In the presence of arterial obstruction, vasoconstrictive stimuli that normally do not cause clinical manifestations result in more severe reduction in blood flow and may cause Raynaud's phenomenon.

Raynaud's phenomenon is very often associated with connective tissue diseases; it is particularly frequent in scleroderma. Almost all patients with scleroderma develop Raynaud's phenomenon at some time during the course of their illness. A distinctive syndrome consisting of calcinosis, Raynaud's phenomenon, abnormal esophageal motility, sclerodactyly, and telangiectasia (CREST syndrome) is recognized. Raynaud's phenomenon may be the presenting manifestation in connective tissue diseases and may precede the appearance of other manifestations by several years. The presence of abnormal nail fold capillaries in patients with Raynaud's phenomenon has predictive value for the future development of scleroderma. Structural changes in the vessel wall that limit flow and increase the sensitivity to vasoconstrictive influences appear to account for the frequent occurrence of Raynaud's phenomenon in these diseases. Vascular injury may also result from repetitive minor occupational trauma or from a severe exposure to cold, as in frostbite. Consequent hypersensitivity to cold causes Raynaud's phenomenon.

Neurogenic lesions cause Raynaud's phenomenon because of irritation of sympathetic nerves and consequent vasoconstriction. Intense or sustained vasoconstriction caused by drugs may also result in Raynaud's phenomenon, as in 3 to 6 per cent of patients taking beta-adrenergic receptor–blocking drugs. Propranolol is the main offender. These drugs block a beta-adrenergic vasodilative mechanism in the digits and may also enhance the vasoconstrictive effects of norepinephrine.

Intravascular aggregation or coagulation of blood elements may obstruct the vessels and cause ischemia and Raynaud's phenomenon.

PATHOPHYSIOLOGY. The pallor during the attack of Raynaud's phenomenon is explained by intense vasoconstriction or spasm of the digital arteries. This results in severe reduction in blood flow. In a later stage of the attack, the vasoconstriction becomes less severe, and the capillaries and veins are partially filled with blood whose hemoglobin becomes markedly deoxygenated. This accounts for the cyanosis. Upon rewarming, cyanosis is replaced by an intense red color associated with reactive hyperemia. Between attacks, blood flow to the digits is usually reduced, especially in patients who have trophic changes, but may be normal in some patients. In those patients without trophic changes, blood flow to the hand during maximum vasodilation is the same as in normal individuals, but it is severely reduced in those with trophic changes, a reflection of structural changes in the blood vessels.

TABLE 57–1. CAUSES OF SECONDARY RAYNAUD'S PHENOMENON

1. Occlusive arterial disease
   a. Arteriosclerosis obliterans
   b. Buerger's disease
   c. Arterial embolism
   d. Vasculitis
   e. Arterial thrombosis
2. Connective tissue diseases
   a. Scleroderma
   b. Rheumatoid arthritis
   c. Systemic lupus erythematosus
3. Vascular injury
   a. Repetitive minor occupational trauma, as in pneumatic hammer operators, pianists, or typists
   b. Frostbite
4. Neurogenic causes
   a. Thoracic outlet compression by cervical rib, by scalenus anticus muscle, or in hyperabduction syndrome
   b. Carpal tunnel syndrome
   c. Sympathetic causalgia
   d. Spinal cord diseases
5. Drugs or exposure to chemicals
   a. Ergotamine
   b. Ergotism
   c. Methysergide
   d. Polyvinyl chloride
   e. Beta-adrenergic receptor blockers
6. Intravascular coagulation or aggregation
   a. Cryoglobulinemia
   b. Cold agglutinins

PATHOLOGY. In the early stages of the disease, the digital blood vessels are histologically normal. In longstanding cases, the intima becomes thickened, and the media may be hypertrophied. In severe progressive cases, complete obstruction from thrombosis may occur, and gangrene of the tips of the digits may ensue.

CLINICAL MANIFESTATIONS. The onset of Raynaud's disease is usually gradual. The patient notices an occasional mild and short-lasting attack during winter. Over succeeding years, the severity and duration of the attacks may increase. A wide variation in severity is present. Most commonly, the attacks are provoked by exposure to cold. In some patients, attacks are also precipitated by emotion. The attacks may be terminated by rewarming, or they may abate spontaneously. Between attacks, in a warm environment, the patient is asymptomatic, and physical examination shows no abnormalities. Some patients, however, complain of chronically cold hands and feet, and they may have cold fingers with cyanosis on examination. In a typical attack of Raynaud's phenomenon, the digits become pale. Usually, all digits are affected symmetrically. The pallor is sharply demarcated at the level of the metacarpophalangeal joints, a reflection of spasm of the digital arteries. At a later stage during the attack, pallor is replaced by cyanosis. The patient may have feelings of coldness, numbness, and occasionally pain. Upon rewarming, the cyanosis is replaced by intense redness, and the patient may feel tingling or throbbing. Most commonly, only the hands are affected. Frequently, both hands and feet are affected. Rarely, the nose, cheeks, ears, and chin are affected also.

Atypical attacks are not infrequent. In these, the involvement of the digits may be asymmetric, with only one or two digits being affected. In some cases, only a portion of the digit is affected. In these instances, the most severely affected portion of the digit is the most distal one. Thus, one may see pallor of the fingertip or of the terminal phalanx of one digit. In other cases, more than one phalanx may be involved.

In severe, progressive cases, trophic changes may occur after a few years of involvement. The hair may disappear from the dorsal aspect of the digits. The nails grow more slowly and become brittle and deformed. The skin becomes atrophic, thin, and tight (sclerodactyly). Ulcerations may develop at the fingertips or around the nail bed. These heal slowly and may become infected. They are extremely painful, especially at night. When they heal, they leave characteristic small, pitted scars.

DIAGNOSIS. The diagnosis of Raynaud's phenomenon can usually be made on the basis of the history of vasospastic attacks in the digits, precipitated by cold and relieved by warming. In atypical cases or when the patient's description of the attack is not clear, provocation of an attack may be helpful. This may be done by immersing the hands in water at a temperature of 10 to 15°C. Whole-body exposure to cold is more successful in provoking attacks. A negative result does not exclude Raynaud's phenomenon.

In typical cases, Raynaud's phenomenon is easily distinguished from acrocyanosis, but when involvement is atypical, the differentiation may be more difficult. Distinguishing features include the following: The color changes in Raynaud's phenomenon are episodic, whereas in acrocyanosis they are sustained. Pallor is not a prominent feature of acrocyanosis. Cyanosis is the more typical color change, whereas in Raynaud's disease digital pallor is characteristic. In Raynaud's disease, only the digits are involved, whereas in acrocyanosis the color changes usually involve the whole hand or foot and sometimes even more proximal portions of the limbs. In Raynaud's disease the skin of the palms is usually dry, whereas in acrocyanosis it is wet and clammy with sweat. Finally, acrocyanosis rarely causes trophic changes and ulcerations.

Obstruction of major arteries from arteriosclerosis, angiitis, embolism, or thrombosis may lead to color changes in the digits that simulate Raynaud's phenomenon. The distinction is made by the demonstration of changes in arterial pulses and by the fact that the color changes in these disorders are likely to be confined to one limb rather than be symmetric. Arteriography, which demonstrates the arterial lesion, is helpful. However, secondary Raynaud's phenonenon may be superimposed upon any of these diseases. In Raynaud's phenomenon, Doppler velocity studies show patent arteries and sharply peaked blood flow velocity patterns in the digits. Arteriography shows normal major arteries and diffuse spasm of the digital arteries.

The distinction of Raynaud's disease from secondary Raynaud's phenomenon is based mainly on the exclusion of disorders known to cause secondary Raynaud's phenomenon. The exclusion of obstructive arterial disease is discussed above. Connective tissue disorders, particularly scleroderma, are excluded by the absence of arthralgias or arthritis, alterations of esophageal motility, and the absence of a pulmonary oxygen diffusion defect. The presence of a normal sedimentation rate and the absence of circulating autoantibodies, such as antinuclear antibodies, provide additional reassurance. A careful occupational history is necessary to exclude Raynaud's phenomenon secondary to minor repetitive trauma. A history of drug ingestion or exposure to chemicals is helpful in identifying drug-induced Raynaud's phenomenon. Neurologic disorders can be recognized by their somatic neurologic manifestations. Thoracic outlet compression syndromes can be excluded by the appropriate maneuvers. The presence of intravascular agglutination or coagulation of the blood elements may be suspected if, in the presence of cyanosis, the blood cannot be expelled from vessels by pressure, and when there are isolated areas of redness as the attack abates during rewarming. Confirmation is obtained by demonstrating the cold agglutinins or cryoglobulins in the patient's blood.

PROGNOSIS. The prognosis of patients with Raynaud's disease is good. There is no mortality associated with the disease and morbidity is low, it is generally limited to loss of portions of digits as a result of ulcerations. In approximately 50 per cent of patients with Raynaud's disease, the disorder improves and may disappear completely after several years. In only a fraction of 1 per cent of patients is amputation necessary. Approximately 15 per cent of patients with Raynaud's phenomenon eventually develop a connective tissue disorder, particularly scleroderma.

The prognosis in secondary Raynaud's phenomenon depends on the course of the primary disorder. In scleroderma, the prognosis is unsatisfactory, particularly when the disease has caused digital ulcerations.

TREATMENT. Management of patients with Raynaud's phenomenon must be tailored to the individual needs of the patient, taking into consideration the frequency and severity of the attacks (Table 57–2). All patients benefit from reassur-

TABLE 57–2. TREATMENT OF RAYNAUD'S PHENOMENON

Frequency and Severity of Vasospastic Attacks	Suggested Treatment
1. Rare or mild attacks	Protective measures, cessation of smoking, and no drug therapy
2. Frequent or severe attacks without trophic changes	Protective measures and calcium antagonists
3. Frequent attacks with trophic changes but no open ulcers	Protective measures plus calcium antagonists or oral reserpine plus liothyronine
4. Frequent attacks with active, painful ulcers	Intravenous PGE_1, intra-arterial reserpine followed by calcium antagonists; or reserpine plus liothyronine

TABLE 57–3. SOME DRUGS USEFUL IN THE TREATMENT OF RAYNAUD'S PHENOMENON

1. Calcium antagonists
   a. Nifedipine*
   b. Diltiazem*
2. Alpha-adrenergic receptor blockers
   a. Phenoxybenzamine*
   b. Tolazoline
   c. Prazosin*
3. Drugs that interfere with sympathetic nerve activity
   a. Reserpine*
   b. Guanethidine*
   c. Alpha-methyldopa*
4. Vasodilators
   a. PGE_1*
   b. PGE_2*
   c. PGI_2*
   d. Nitroglycerin (topical)*
5. Miscellaneous
   a. Liothyronine*

*Investigational drug for this purpose.

ance and protective measures against exposure to cold. The patients should limit the duration of exposure to cold to the greatest extent possible. They should wear heavy clothing, protecting not only the hands and feet but also the face and trunk, especially when there is a cold wind, this is important because exposure to cold of other portions of the body may reflexly induce vasoconstriction in the digits and precipitate Raynaud's phenomenon. When prolonged exposure to cold is unavoidable, the use of electrically powered or solid fuel–powered hand and foot warmers is advisable. These patients should be taught to recognize and terminate attacks by returning promptly to a warm environment, placing their hands in warm water, or using a warm-air hairblower to warm their hands rapidly. Smoking causes cutaneous vasoconstriction; therefore, tobacco smoking is contraindicated in Raynaud's phenomenon. The use of induced vasodilation by placing the hands in warm water (43°C) has been reported to raise skin temperature and minimize the severity of attacks of Raynaud's phenomenon. Biofeedback to teach patients to raise skin temperature voluntarily has been shown to limit the duration and frequency of vasospastic attacks, but its effect is nonspecific because it is also seen in control patients who received no such treatment and in those in whom biofeedback is used to teach relaxation.

The simple measures outlined above usually suffice for patients with infrequent or mild attacks. When Raynaud's phenomenon is more frequent or more severe, and especially when it has resulted in trophic changes or ulcerations, these measures need to be supplemented by drugs. The aim of drug therapy is to induce vascular smooth muscle relaxation, thereby relieving spasm, raising resting blood flow, and limiting the degree of ischemia during attacks. The drugs most frequently used in treating patients with Raynaud's phenomenon are shown in Table 57–3. For most patients, the drug of choice is a calcium antagonist. Nifedipine* has been found to be effective in several well-controlled, double-blind studies. The drug is administered at a dose of 10 to 20 mg three or four times daily. Diltiazem,* at a dose of 60 mg three or four times daily, may be substituted, if nifedipine is not well tolerated or if it causes side effects. In one study of very severely affected patients, verapamil was found not to be effective.

Reserpine* is the best-studied drug among the group that interferes with the function of the adrenergic nervous system. It is administered by mouth in doses of 0.1 to 0.5 mg daily. In cases in which ulcerations have developed, it may be given intra-arterially in a dose of 0.5 to 1 mg, dissolved in saline and administered into the brachial or radial artery by slow infusion over several minutes. The drugs in this group may

also be administered by means of tourniquet-controlled intravenous injection (Bier's block). The administration by the last two routes gives a much higher local concentration and largely avoids systemic side effects.

In controlled trials, nitroglycerin* ointment or topical prostaglandin E_2* (PGE_2) has been found effective in Raynaud's phenomenon. The topical application of these drugs is advantageous because their local relaxant action is not counteracted by reflex vasoconstriction, secondary to changes in blood pressure that may occur when they are given systemically.

Prostaglandin E_1* (PGE_1) or prostacyclin* (PGI_2) administered intravenously has a beneficial effect in patients with Raynaud's phenomenon. These drugs can be given by constant intravenous infusion in a dose of 6 to 10 ng per kilogram per minute for a few hours or up to three days. It is reported that the beneficial effect outlasts this therapy by several weeks.

A novel but effective way of inducing vasodilation in the digits is via the iatrogenic induction of hyperthyroidism by the administration of sodium liothyronine* (triiodothyronine), 75 µg daily. The resultant hypermetabolism elicits thermoregulatory reflex cutaneous vasodilation. The combination of triiodothyronine and reserpine has been found to be most effective.

Preganglionic sympathectomy to eliminate vasoconstrictor tone may have a beneficial immediate result, but the longterm results are disappointing. The duration of benefit is limited by regeneration of the nerves. If sympathectomy is contemplated, it is advisable to try sympathetic blockade with local anesthetics to verify a beneficial result. A recently devised technique that involves surgical stripping of the palmar and digital arteries to bring about a local sympathectomy may also be tried, but its results have not been fully evaluated.

Coffman JD, Davis WT: Vasospastic diseases: A review. Prog Cardiovasc Dis 18:123, 1975. *A comprehensive, well-referenced review of vasospastic diseases.*

Cohen RA, Coffman JD: β-Adrenergic vasodilator mechanism in the finger. Circ Res 49:1196, 1981. *Demonstration of a beta-adrenergic, humorally activated, vasodilative mechanism in the arteriovenous anastomoses of the human finger. Blockade of this mechanism may explain the occurrence of Raynaud's phenomenon in patients taking beta-adrenergic receptor–blocking drugs.*

Fagius J, Blumberg H: Sympathetic outflow to the hand in patients with Raynaud's phenomenon. Cardiovasc Res 19:249, 1985. *Demonstration that sympathetic nerve activity in patients with Raynaud's phenomenon under baseline conditions and during maneuvers that increase sympathetic nerve traffic does not differ from that in normal controls. The results do not support the theory that Raynaud's disease is caused by increased sympathetic nerve activity.*

Harper FE, Maricq HR, Turner RE, et al.: A prospective study of Raynaud's phenomenon and early connective tissue disease. Am J Med 72:883, 1982. *This study of capillaries of the nail fold shows that the presence of capillary abnormalities in patients with Raynaud's phenomenon may have predictive value for the future development of scleroderma.*

Kontos HA, Wasserman AJ: Effect of reserpine in Raynaud's phenomenon. Circulation 39:259, 1969. *An analysis of the effects of reserpine given intraarterially and orally on hand blood flow in patients with Raynaud's disease. It also contains evidence against the hypothesis that defective catecholamine metabolism may account for Raynaud's disease. Beneficial results from oral administration of reserpine are also presented.*

Miller D, Waters DD, Warnica W, et al.: Is variant angina the coronary manifestation of a generalized vasospastic disorder? N Engl J Med 304:763, 1981. *Provocative study showing high incidence of migraine and Raynaud's phenomenon in patients with variant angina, suggesting the possibility that we may be dealing with a generalized vasospastic disorder.*

Smith CR, Rodeheffer RJ: Treatment of Raynaud's phenomenon with calcium channel blockers. Am J Med 78 (Suppl 2B): 39, 1985. *Concise consideration of the pathophysiology of Raynaud's phenomenon and review of available evidence concerning the effectiveness of treatment with calcium antagonists.*

Acrocyanosis

DEFINITION. Acrocyanosis is a rare disorder characterized by persistent cyanosis of the skin of the hands and, less commonly, of the feet associated with reduced skin temperature.

ETIOLOGY. Acrocyanosis is a primary disorder of unknown cause. It is much more common in women than in

---

*Investigational drug for this purpose.

*Investigational drug for this purpose.

men. The onset of the disease is usually in young adults or middle-aged persons. The high incidence of the disease among patients with psychiatric disorders is of unknown significance.

PATHOPHYSIOLOGY. The smaller precapillary vessels (arterioles) are abnormally constricted, causing reduction in blood flow and accounting for cyanosis and reduced skin temperature. The veins are secondarily dilated. Constriction of the arterioles occurs under normal environmental conditions and becomes more pronounced on exposure to cold because of increased sensitivity of these vessels to the effects of cold. An important feature of acrocyanosis is the reduced venous tone. No venous obstruction is present. These features can be demonstrated by elevating the involved limb and eliminating the blue color or intensifying the blue color by placing the limb in a dependent position and overfilling the veins.

CLINICAL MANIFESTATIONS. Patients with acrocyanosis have persistent blue discoloration of the hands. Less commonly, the feet are also involved. In some cases, the blue color extends to more proximal portions of the limbs. The skin is cold, and the palms are wet and clammy from sweat. No pallor is usually present. In some cases, there may be spots of pallor surrounded by confluent cyanosis. The blue color is intensified by exposure to cold, and it is converted into purplish or red color by exposure to heat. There are few accompanying symptoms. The patient has feelings of coldness and, occasionally, numbness. Ulcerations and other trophic changes are distinctly unusual. Patients with acrocyanosis seek medical advice either because they are frightened or because the cyanosis is cosmetically unappealing.

DIAGNOSIS. The distinction between acrocyanosis and Raynaud's phenomenon is discussed above in the section on Raynaud's phenomenon. Differentiation from cyanosis secondary to arterial obstruction can be made on the basis of normal pulses, by the bilateral and symmetric occurrence of acrocyanosis, and, if necessary, by the angiographic verification of absence of obstruction. The limitation of the cyanosis to the hands and feet, the improvement in a warm environment, and the absence of reduced arterial blood saturation distinguish acrocyanosis from generalized, systemic cyanosis.

TREATMENT. Since acrocyanosis is a benign disease, no drug therapy is usually required. Reassurance and protection from cold usually suffice. In some cases, cosmetic considerations or unusually severe symptoms may necessitate drug therapy. In these cases, the same drugs that are useful in Raynaud's phenomenon may be tried.

Lewis T, Landis EM: Observations upon the vascular mechanism in acrocyanosis. Heart 15:229, 1930. *Classic description of the clinical features of acrocyanosis. Evidence is presented showing that the disease is the result of an abnormal responsiveness of the smaller blood vessels.*

Livedo Reticularis

DEFINITION. Livedo reticularis is a reticular, bluish discoloration of the skin of the extremities that produces a lacy, irregular appearance outlining central areas of normal-appearing skin. The etiology is not known. The disorder usually begins in young individuals before age 20 to 30 years. It is equally common in men and women but more often symptomatic in women.

PATHOLOGY. Proliferative lesions of the arterioles of the skin with perivascular infiltration have been described. In some cases, there may be thrombosis of arterioles leading to cutaneous infarction and ulceration. Similar changes are seen in the veins.

PATHOPHYSIOLOGY. The mechanism of livedo reticularis is presumed to be similar to that of acrocyanosis, namely, constriction of arterioles followed by stasis and dilation of capillaries and veins. The latter are filled with desaturated blood. The reticular appearance of livedo reticularis reflects

the anatomic arrangement of the affected vessels. It is believed that the bluish areas represent the arborizations of peripheral capillaries from central penetrating arterioles. Blood flow is faster in the central regions closer to the penetrating arteriole, whereas the more distant areas have lower flow, with consequent stasis and cyanosis.

CLINICAL MANIFESTATIONS. Patients seek medical attention for cosmetic reasons or because they are frightened by the bluish discoloration. The lower extremities are involved more often than the upper extremities. The patient usually has no symptoms. In some cases, there may be paresthesias or a feeling of coldness. The bluish discoloration becomes more intense on exposure to cold and may disappear in a warm environment. Ulcerations occur rarely; when they do, they appear in winter and heal in summer.

TREATMENT. In most cases no treatment is required. Protection from cold and abstinence from tobacco are useful. In severe cases, drugs useful in the treatment of Raynaud's phenomenon, such as nifedipine and reserpine, may be tried.

Feldaker M, Hines EA, Kierland RR: Livedo reticularis with ulcerations. Circulation 13:196, 1956. *Report of the clinical and pathologic features of 18 patients with livedo reticularis with ulcerations. A brief review of the earlier literature is included.*

Erythromelalgia (Erythermalgia)

DEFINITION. Erythromelalgia is a disorder manifested by episodes of erythema accompanied by increased skin temperature and by pain involving the feet and, less commonly, the hands. It may be primary or secondary to other disorders. These include obstructive arterial disease, polycythemia, and hypertension. There is no sex predilection, and the disease may occur at any age. It is occasionally hereditary.

PATHOPHYSIOLOGY. The symptoms of erythromelalgia are dependent on skin temperature. Rise in skin temperature above a certain level causes the manifestations. In each person this critical point is fairly constant. Vasodilation and consequent hyperemia are the usual causes of the rise in skin temperature. However, an increased blood flow is not essential, since once symptoms have been induced by heat, they may continue even though blood flow is reduced to zero with a cuff inflated above the systolic pressure levels. These features suggest that the cause of the disorder is abnormal sensitivity of the cutaneous pain fibers to heat or tension from the dilated blood vessels.

CLINICAL MANIFESTATIONS. The onset of the disease is gradual. With progression, the frequency and duration of the attacks become more pronounced. Eventually, symptoms may become almost continuous and cause total disability. During an attack the patient complains of burning pain, usually in the feet and, less commonly, in the hands. The pain is usually located in the balls of the feet and in the tips of the toes and in the corresponding parts of the hands. Pain is aggravated by dependency and ameliorated by elevation of the limbs. Exposure to heat aggravates the disorder, whereas cold provides relief. Trophic changes, ulcerations, and gangrene are rare.

DIAGNOSIS. Peripheral neuropathy may cause burning pain simulating erythromelalgia. The pain may be accompanied by cutaneous vasodilation. The detection of the associated sensory and motor manifestations of peripheral neuropathy should help distinguish this condition from erythromelalgia. Arteriosclerosis obliterans or thromboangiitis obliterans may also produce localized burning pain and redness. The alterations in the arterial pulses and the absence of high skin temperature distinguish these conditions from erythromelalgia. Vascular damage from prolonged exposure to cold, as after frostbite, may simulate erythromelalgia. In these cases, the condition is more persistent, and the history of cold exposure should help make the distinction possible.

TREATMENT. Avoidance of exposure to heat, particularly dry heat, prevents attacks of erythromelalgia. Elevation of the extremity and application of cold may terminate an attack. Aspirin, 0.5 gram orally, relieves the pain in many cases. The response is sometimes so striking that it is of diagnostic value. Vasoconstrictive agents, such as methysergide or epinephrine, or beta-adrenergic blocking agents, such as propranolol, have been reported to be effective in some patients. In secondary cases, treatment of the primary disorder may alleviate the attacks.

Babb RR, Alarcon-Segovia D, Fairbairn JF: Erythermalgia: Review of 51 cases. Circulation 29:136, 1964. *Description of the features of primary and secondary erythromelalgia based on a study of a large number of patients.*

Lewis T: Clinical observations and experiments relating to burning pain in the extremities, and to so-called "erythromelalgia" in particular. Clin Sci 1:175, 1933. *A classic paper with detailed clinical descriptions of the manifestations of erythromelalgia. The paper also presents clinical investigations pertinent to the pathogenesis of the disease.*

VASCULAR DISEASES OF THE LIMBS CAUSED BY DAMAGE FROM COLD

Immersion Foot (Trench Foot)

DEFINITION AND ETIOLOGY. Immersion foot is characterized by vascular damage resulting from prolonged exposure of the extremities to cold by wearing wet socks or wet footwear. Usually, the exposure is for several days at about 0°C. Dependency of limbs and immobility, as well as conditions that lead to general debility (lack of sleep and starvation), are contributory factors. The condition occurs primarily in soldiers at war.

Immersion foot has been described in survivors of shipwrecks, who were immobilized in crowded small craft for prolonged periods of time, and exposed to wetness and cold. Maceration of the skin with sea water and secondary infection also contribute.

PATHOPHYSIOLOGY. This condition results from vascular injury. The initial effect of cold is to cause vasoconstriction. Loss of heat is facilitated by moisture. The resultant ischemia causes tissue and vascular injury with increased endothelial permeability. There is extensive extravasation of protein and fluid. As a result, there may be increased hematocrit, sludging, and further aggravation of ischemia.

PATHOLOGY. Little is known about the earliest pathologic change in the blood vessels in immersion foot. Most of the available information has been obtained from advanced cases with extensive vascular injury and gangrene. In these cases, the small arteries exhibit periarterial fibrosis and thickening and may be occluded. The veins show perivenous fibrosis, inflammatory reaction, and hemorrhage. The nerves may also be affected. In cases of immersion foot at relatively high temperatures, hyperhydration of the plantar stratum corneum may be the only finding.

CLINICAL MANIFESTATIONS. Three successive stages, each with distinct clinical manifestations, are recognized. During exposure to the wet, cold environment, there is vasoconstriction. The involved extremity becomes pale and cool, and the patient has paresthesias and a feeling of coldness. A second hyperemic stage follows. Patients are observed most commonly during this stage, because this is when they seek attention. The involved extremity is red, hot, and edematous. There may be pain or paresthesias. The swelling may be aggravated by heat and by placing the limb in a dependent position. Subsequently, blebs appear, filled with serous or hemorrhagic fluid. Hemorrhages may occur into the skin and subcutaneous tissue. This stage may persist for several days. In severe cases, gangrene may supervene. The condition may be complicated by lymphangitis, cellulitis, and thrombophlebitis. Mild cases or those treated early may recover after this second hyperemic phase. In other cases, a third late vasospastic phase occurs in which there is increased sensitivity to cold and typical secondary Raynaud's phenomenon, with excessive sweating, pain, and paresthesias of the lower extremities. This phase may persist for years.

TREATMENT. If the patient is seen in the initial vasoconstrictive phase, bed rest with the extremity in the horizontal position and a warm environment are necessary. During the hyperemic phase, the extremity should be placed at heart level and kept cool to diminish edema. Local care to keep the foot dry and clean should be instituted to avoid infection. Control of pain may require analgesics or narcotics. Sympathectomy may be helpful in the hyperemic stage and also in preventing the late vasospastic phenomena.

Abramson DI, Lerner D, Shumacker HB, et al: Clinical picture and treatment of the later stage of trench foot. Am Heart J 32:52, 1946. *Clinical report based on the study of 633 patients with trench foot. Emphasis is placed on the late sequelae of the disorder.*

Frostbite

DEFINITION AND ETIOLOGY. Frostbite results from freezing of the tissues and consequent vascular injury. In most cases, frostbite occurs during prolonged exposure to temperatures below 0°C. Other environmental factors also play a role, such as high wind and humidity. Predisposing factors include vascular disease, inadequate clothing, lack of acclimatization, and general debility.

PATHOPHYSIOLOGY. Tissue damage results from cold-influenced vasoconstriction. Freezing causes water crystal formation in cells and dehydration. Endothelial damage with increased permeability to protein ensues, causes edema, and further contributes to stasis and eventual thrombosis.

PATHOLOGY. The vessels show endothelial swelling and vacuolization and proliferative changes. Subsequently, there are inflammatory reactions and atrophic changes in the skin.

CLINICAL MANIFESTATIONS. Initially, the patient notices a prickling sensation followed by numbness. The skin becomes bloodless and appears white and cold. This is followed by redness, swelling, and increased temperature. Blisters may form 24 to 48 hours after thawing. They are filled with either serous yellow or hemorrhagic fluid. There may be hemorrhages under the nail beds. Necrosis and gangrene may supervene. The subsequent course may be similar to that of sudden arterial occlusion, including ischemia and gangrene. Spontaneous amputation may require several weeks or months. After an attack of frostbite, the affected extremities may remain sensitive to cold for a period of time or permanently, and secondary Raynaud's phenomenon may occur.

TREATMENT. Frostbite should be treated with immediate rewarming. If frostbite affects deep tissues, rewarming should be done with water at 40 to 44°C. Muscular exercise of the involved limb and massage should be avoided, because they tend to increase edema and pain. If pain is severe, it should be treated with analgesics or narcotics. After the tissues have thawed, the exposed parts should remain at room temperatures. Vesicles should be left untouched, and the limb should be left exposed, without dressings. Antibiotic therapy should be used if infection is present. Sympathectomy has been reported to be beneficial in the initial stages as well as in preventing the delayed sequelae of frostbite.

Washburn B: Frostbite. N Engl J Med 266:974, 1962. *Comprehensive consideration of the clinical features, pathology, diagnosis, prevention, and treatment of frostbite.*

Chilblain (Pernio)

DEFINITION. Chilblain is an inflammatory condition of the skin of the extremities induced by cold and characterized by erythema, itching, and ulceration. The cause is unknown. It is more common in cold, damp climates, as in England, than in the United States. Women are affected more commonly than men. In most patients, the disease begins before the age of 20 years.

PATHOLOGY. In chronic cases, the lesions consist of angiitis with intimal proliferation, thickening of the arterial wall, and perivascular infiltration with lymphocytes and polymorphonuclear leukocytes. There may be necrosis of the adipose tissue and chronic inflammatory infiltrates in the subcutaneous tissue.

CLINICAL MANIFESTATIONS. Both acute and chronic forms of the disease are recognized. The typical patient is a young woman who, in the winter, notices bluish-red discoloration and edema of the skin of the lower limbs associated with burning and warmth. The lesions are persistent and are associated with itching. They generally last from 7 to 10 days and then clear up, sometimes leaving residual pigmentation of the skin. In severe cases, the lesions may become hemorrhagic, or blebs may appear. Infection may supervene.

With repeated exposure to cold, susceptible persons may develop chronic lesions. These are erythematous, ulcerative, and hemorrhagic lesions that begin as raised, red areas 0.5 to 1 cm in diameter. These lesions are then transformed into blebs and finally ulcerate. Healing occurs in the summer, leaving a permanently pigmented region.

DIAGNOSIS. Acute chilblain is distinguished from other forms of dermatitis by its characteristic distribution and by its relationship to cold. Chronic chilblain needs to be distinguished from erythema induration and erythema nodosum. Erythema induratum of Bazin is caused by *Mycobacterium tuberculosis*. If the infection is active, the differential diagnosis may be made by the microscopic demonstration or culture of bacteria. Erythema induratum affects the upper part of the legs more frequently than the lower part. The lesions are more nodular, deeper, and infiltrative. They are also more permanent, whereas those of chronic chilblain clear up in the summer. Erythema nodosum is a more acute process, and it is usually associated with a systemic reaction, consisting of fever, malaise, and arthralgias. There is no seasonal association.

TREATMENT. In mild cases, protection from cold, local application of anti-inflammatory ointments, avoidance of scratching, and cessation of smoking are usually sufficient. In more severe cases, drugs that have been found useful in the treatment of Raynaud's phenomenon, such as reserpine, may be effective.

Eskell J: Reserpine in the treatment of chilblains. Practitioner 189:792, 1962. *Report of a controlled clinical trial of reserpine in patients with chilblain showing excellent benefit.*

Lynn RB: Chilblains. Surg Gynecol Obstet 99:720, 1954. *Concise description of the clinical and pathologic features of chilblain.*

VASCULAR DISEASES OF THE LIMBS CAUSED BY ORGANIC ARTERIAL OBSTRUCTION

Arteriosclerosis Obliterans

DEFINITION. Arteriosclerosis obliterans consists of segmental arteriosclerotic narrowing or obstruction of the lumen in the arteries supplying the limbs.

ETIOLOGY AND INCIDENCE. The etiology of arteriosclerosis in general is discussed in another chapter (see Ch. 50).

Arteriosclerosis obliterans is the commonest cause of arterial obstructive disease of the extremities. The disease becomes clinically manifest usually between the ages of 50 and 70. It is unusual in individuals younger than 30 years of age. Men are affected more often than women. The lower limbs are involved much more frequently than the upper limbs. The most commonly affected vessel is the superficial femoral artery. The distal aorta and its bifurcation into the two iliac arteries and the popliteal artery are the next most frequent sites of involvement. The presence of diabetes mellitus influences arteriosclerosis obliterans in a number of important ways. In diabetics, arteriosclerosis obliterans is likely to be more progressive. This is reflected in a much higher incidence of intermittent claudication in diabetics. The disease affects arterial vessels of smaller caliber and more distally located vessels more frequently than in nondiabetics. The incidence of involvement of vessels below the knee with arteriosclerosis obliterans in diabetics is considerably higher than in nondiabetics.

PATHOLOGY. The lesions of arteriosclerosis obliterans are typical atheromatous plaques involving the intima of the arteries. As a rule, there is superimposed thrombus formation. The media of the vessels shows degenerative changes. Calcification of the media is frequent and may take the form of a ringlike arrangement, as in Monckeberg's sclerosis. Medial calcification is twice as frequent in diabetics as in nondiabetics. These arteriosclerotic lesions are segmental, and they are typically multiple. Weakening of the media may give rise to aneurysmal dilation of the involved artery. Such arteriosclerotic aneurysms are most common in the popliteal fossa or in the femoral artery below the inguinal ligament. They may be filled with thrombi.

PATHOPHYSIOLOGY. The arterial obstruction or narrowing causes reduction in blood flow during exercise or at rest. Clinical symptoms are caused by the consequent ischemia. The most important feature of the stenosis in determining ischemia is the cross-sectional area of the stenotic segment. Because the vascular bed of the extremities generally has a high resting vascular tone and, therefore, a large capacity for vasodilation, a moderate degree of stenosis can be compensated fully by downstream dilation. Stenoses that decrease the cross-sectional area of the vessel by less than 75 per cent do not usually affect resting blood flow. When the prevailing flow rates are high, as in exercise, decreases of 60 per cent or more in cross-sectional area are required before a reduction in flow occurs. Vasodilation in response to ischemia is the result of the action of local mechanisms. These include myogenic mechanisms related to reduction in intravascular pressure or metabolic mechanisms due to release of vasodilative metabolites from the ischemic tissues. These local mechanisms compete with neurogenic mechanisms that, when activated, cause vasoconstriction. Increased sympathetic activity, as from exposure to cold, may, therefore, induce ischemia in the presence of an arterial obstructing lesion.

The presence or absence of ischemia in the face of severe arterial stenosis or obstruction is frequently determined by the degree of development of collateral circulation. Some collateral vessels are present in the normal limb but are not used until obstruction takes place. They open up immediately after an acute arterial occlusion. Others take several weeks or months to become fully developed. Little is known about the responsiveness of collateral vessels. They are subject to neurogenic vasoconstriction from the action of adrenergic nerves. They dilate in response to increased blood pressure, resulting in improved collateral blood flow.

CLINICAL MANIFESTATIONS. The symptoms of arteriosclerosis obliterans are intermittent claudication, pain at rest, and trophic changes in the involved limb. Intermittent claudication denotes pain that develops in a limb on exercise and disappears when the patient rests. The pain is usually described as a cramp or a tightness or as severe fatigue of the exercising muscles. The amount of exercise necessary to induce the pain is usually constant for any given patient. The pain is usually bilateral. In some patients, the pain disappears by slowing the pace of walking without complete cessation of exercise. The location of the pain is distal to the arterial obstruction. The most frequently affected muscles are those of the calf, because of the high frequency with which the femoral artery is involved. The muscles of the lower part of the back, the buttocks, the thigh, and the foot may also be affected.

Pain at rest occurs when a pronounced reduction in resting blood flow is present. It is a sign of severe disease. The pain may be localized to one or more toes, or it may have a stocking-type distribution. The character of the pain is usually burning or gnawing. It is generally worse at night. It is improved by placing the limb in a dependent position and by cooling. There may be associated coldness and numbness, together with cyanosis or pallor of the extremity.

Examination discloses reduced or absent arterial pulses distal to the obstruction. There may be bruits audible over the aorta or its branches. These may be systolic, or they may be continuous. In advanced cases, examination may reveal signs of ischemia. The skin temperature may be abnormally low, or there may be pallor or cyanosis. Ischemic damage may cause persistent reddish or reddish-blue discoloration. There may be trophic changes, including a dry, scaly, and shiny skin. The hair may disappear, and the toenails may become brittle, ridged, and deformed. There may be ulcerations or gangrene. The ischemic ulcers are usually at pressure points and may be inflamed and painful.

Leriche's syndrome refers to isolated aortoiliac disease, which produces a fairly characteristic clinical picture. There is intermittent claudication of the low back, buttocks, and thigh or calf muscles. There is atrophy of the limbs and pallor of the skin of the feet and legs. Impotence may also be present. Arterial pulses in the legs are absent, they may be present but weak in the femoral arteries. Systolic bruits may be audible over the femoral arteries and lower abdomen.

Arteriosclerotic aneurysms may occur, and present as pulsatile, expansible masses in the popliteal fossa or in the femoral artery below the inguinal ligament. These may cause symptoms by pressure on adjacent structures, and, occasionally, by embolism of peripheral vessels or by hemorrhage into the tissues.

DIAGNOSIS. The diagnostic approach to the patient with arteriosclerosis obliterans should be directed at establishing the site of the arterial obstruction, its severity, the degree of ischemia, and the adequacy of the collateral circulation. Palpation of the arterial pulses and auscultation of bruits usually suffice to determine the presence and site of arterial obstruction. Trophic changes and alterations in skin color and temperature indicate ischemia. The latter, as well as the adequacy of the collateral circulation, can be further ascertained by determining the blood pressure at the ankle at rest and during exercise. Several tests may be helpful. With the patient in a warm environment, so that vasoconstrictor tone is low, the leg is raised to a 45-degree angle while the patient is supine. The color of the plantar surface of the foot is observed. Pallor during this test is indicative of severe arterial insufficiency. Venous and capillary filling times can be measured when the patient shifts from the recumbent to the sitting position. Ordinarily, delay in flushing by more than 20 to 30 seconds indicates inadequate collateral circulation. The systolic blood pressure in the dorsalis pedis or posterior tibial arteries can be determined with the use of a Doppler velocitometer at rest as well as during exercise. Ordinarily, this pressure should not be lower than 90 per cent of the level of systolic pressure in the brachial artery. In the presence of severe ischemia, pressures may fall to very low levels. As a rule, pressures less than 30 mm Hg indicate ischemia of sufficient severity to cause gangrene.

The confirmation of arterial obstruction is carried out by arteriography, which is essential to establish the exact anatomy of the arterial vessels and to determine the advisability of surgery.

Arterial embolism is usually distinguishable from arteriosclerosis obliterans because of the sudden onset of the ischemic manifestations and the usually unilateral involvement. Intermittent claudication may occur in severe anemia, in venous disease, and in muscle phosphorylase deficiency (McArdle's syndrome). These conditions are distinguished from arteriosclerosis obliterans by the presence of normal pulses. Ergotamine or methysergide toxicity may cause severe vasospasm, which may affect the large arteries and diminish pulses. The history of drug ingestion may help distinguish these from arteriosclerosis obliterans. In difficult cases, angiography shows the generalized vasospasm and absence of segmental obstructions. A number of conditions of nonvascular nature, such as arthritis and lumbar disc disorders, may cause pain in the limbs and may be confused with intermittent claudication. The presence of normal pulses and other manifestations of these diseases distinguishes them from arteriosclerotic obliterans. In diabetics, ulcerations may be present as a result of diabetic neuropathy. The cause of these ulcers may be difficult to ascertain in the presence of arteriosclerosis obliterans.

TREATMENT. Patients with arteriosclerosis obliterans without evidence of ischemia should be treated medically. Limitation of physical activity, avoidance of tobacco smoking (which causes vasoconstriction), and a regular exercise program are advisable. The treatment of hyperlipidemia, if present, may prevent development of new arteriosclerotic lesions. The control of diabetes, if present, is required. Patients should maintain the skin of the affected limbs clean, dry, and soft and protect it from cold and trauma. Infections and trauma should be attended to promptly. There is no evidence that vasodilative drugs are effective in the treatment of arteriosclerosis obliterans. In fact, they may be harmful under certain circumstances by lowering arterial blood pressure and reducing collateral blood flow or by diverting blood to proximal healthy areas, thereby reducing the perfusion pressure in the more distal portions of the limb. Pentoxifylline, 400 mg administered orally three times daily, has been shown in controlled trials to prolong the duration of exercise and the distance the patient is able to walk prior to the onset of claudication. The drug acts by increasing red cell membrane deformability, thereby reducing effective blood viscosity.

Surgical treatment is advisable when ischemia is present, or if intermittent claudication seriously interferes with the patient's activities. Surgery involves either endarterectomy of the stenotic artery or a bypass operation. Bypass can be performed with either a vein graft or synthetic material. Vein grafts are preferred because of the lower incidence of thrombosis. It is essential that the presence of patent vessels below the obstruction be ascertained before the grafting procedure is carried out. Axillofemoral or femorofemoral grafts for aortoiliac disease have been successful. The larger the size of the vessels grafted, the higher the rate of successful restoration of blood flow.

Percutaneous transluminal angioplasty offers an attractive alternative to surgery in the treatment of arteriosclerosis obliterans. It is simple, has low morbidity, and is less costly than surgery. In this technique, the segmental stenosis or obstruction is dilated by suddenly inflating a balloon introduced into the artery at the site of the lesion by percutaneous catheterization. High success rates and good long-term rates of patency of the dilated vessels have been reported. Angioplasty is more successful in larger vessels, when the stenotic segment is relatively short and when the vessel is not completely occluded.

If the anatomy of the disease makes surgery impossible and ischemic manifestations are present, bed rest is essential. The affected extremity should be kept in a slightly dependent position at 20 to 30 degrees below horizontal, and direct application of heat should be avoided. The limb is best kept warm by placing it under a cradle, under which the temperature is regulated below 38°C. Analgesics or narcotics may be required to control pain. Ulcers should be kept clean with warm saline soaks and debrided. Appropriate antibiotics should be used if infection is present. Intra-arterial administration of PGE_1,* may be beneficial in patients with gangrene or ulceration in whom surgery is not possible. Amputation may be necessary to arrest advancing gangrene. The level of amputation is chosen by the presence of warm, viable tissue having normal color.

Long-term anticoagulants are of questionable value. Fibrin-

---

*Investigational drug for this purpose.

olytic therapy with intravenous streptokinase is reported to be helpful in a few patients with recent onset of the disease.

Preganglionic lumbar sympathectomy may be performed as an acute intervention to treat ischemic manifestations of arteriosclerosis obliterans. Before surgery, it must be demonstrated that the interruption of sympathetic nerves is likely to cause improvement in the circulation of the limb. This is done by inducing temporary sympathetic blockade with local anesthetics. This is essential, especially in diabetics in whom peripheral neuropathy may have already produced spontaneous sympathectomy. Sympathectomy does not influence the long-term prognosis of intermittent claudication.

PROGNOSIS. Arteriosclerosis obliterans in the absence of diabetes is a slowly progressive disease. No significant deterioration may be detected for several years. In the presence of diabetes, the disease tends to progress more rapidly, and the prognosis is less satisfactory. The location of obstructing lesions also influences the prognosis. When the lesions are in larger arteries, the probability of successful surgical intervention or percutaneous angioplasty is higher, and the prognosis is better. Frequently arteriosclerosis obliterans is only one of the manifestations of a generalized arteriosclerotic process. Mortality results from arteriosclerotic involvement of other vascular beds, such as the coronary or the cerebral circulation, with death from myocardial infarction or stroke.

Coffman JD: Intermittent claudication and rest pain. Physiologic concepts and therapeutic approaches. Prog Cardiovasc Dis 22:53, 1979. *A comprehensive, well-referenced consideration of the clinical features, diagnosis, and treatment of arteriosclerosis obliterans.*

Freiman DB, Spence R, Gatenby R, et al.: Transluminal angioplasty of the iliac and femoral arteries: Follow-up results with anticoagulation. Radiology 141:347, 1981. *Transluminal angioplasty for the treatment of obstructive disease of the iliac and femoral arteries. Excellent results are reported in 192 patients.*

Porter JM, Culter BS, Lee BY, et al.: Pentoxifylline efficacy in the treatment of intermittent claudication: Multicenter controlled double-blind trial with objective assessment of chronic occlusive arterial disease patients. Am Heart J 104:66, 1982. *A controlled trial of pentoxifylline in patients with intermittent claudication demonstrating objectively improved exercise tolerance.*

Schadt DC, Hines EA, Juergens JL, et al.: Chronic atherosclerotic occlusion of the femoral artery. JAMA 175:937, 1961. *A long-term follow-up study showing slow progression of arteriosclerosis obliterans.*

Thromboangiitis Obliterans (Buerger's Disease)

DEFINITION. Thromboangiitis obliterans is an obstructive arterial disease caused by segmental inflammatory and proliferative lesions of the medium and small arteries and veins of the limbs.

ETIOLOGY. The cause of thromboangiitis obliterans is unknown. Almost all patients with this disease are moderate or heavy smokers, particularly of cigarettes. Many show cutaneous hypersensitivity to intradermally injected tobacco products. There is a high prevalence of HLA-A9 and HLA-B5 antigens in affected persons. An autoimmune mechanism is suggested by a study of cellular and humoral immune responses of 39 patients with thromboangiitis obliterans. Lymphocytes from 77 per cent of these patients exhibited cellular sensitivity to human type I and type III collagen, both of which are constituents of the vascular wall. In addition, approximately 50 per cent had significant levels of anticollagen antibodies in their blood. By contrast, normal controls and patients with arteriosclerosis obliterans had considerably lower levels of cellular sensitivity to collagen and no circulating anticollagen antibodies.

INCIDENCE. Thromboangiitis obliterans is a disease mostly of young males. The disease begins most frequently between the ages of 20 and 40 years, and the ratio of men to women affected varies from 9:1 to as high as 75:1. There is a high prevalence of the disorder in Israel, the Orient, and in India as compared with the United States and Western Europe, suggesting the possibility of a genetic predisposition. The disease has been occasionally reported to occur in familial form.

PATHOLOGY. The disease affects small and medium-sized arteries and veins in segmental fashion. Acute lesions are manifested by proliferation of the intima and thrombosis. There is inflammatory infiltration with polymorphonuclear leukocytes, lymphocytes, and giant cells of all coats of the artery or vein, extending into the thrombus. The media remains intact. Calcium or cholesterol deposition does not occur. These lesions are distinguished from those of arteriosclerosis obliterans because of the more cellular thrombus, the preservation of the media, and the inflammatory infiltration of all coats of the vessel. Older lesions become less cellular, and eventually they may be transformed into a dense scar. Typically, in any one vessel, lesions of varying ages are seen.

CLINICAL MANIFESTATIONS. The typical patient with thromboangiitis obliterans is a young man who smokes cigarettes heavily, has manifestations of ischemia of the extremities, and has a history or evidence of superficial thrombophlebitis. Common presenting complaints are Raynaud's phenomenon with digital ulcerations or pain from ischemia. Pain in thromboangiitis obliterans may be of several types. The most frequent is pain at rest in one or more digits. This pain may be accompanied by manifestations of ischemia, such as color or temperature changes of the skin. This type of pain may be a forerunner of ulceration or gangrene. In the presence of these trophic lesions, there may be localized pain that is aching in character and more severe at night. Another type of pain may occur along the course of the inflamed blood vessels. Ischemic neuropathy may result and cause a paroxysmal, shocklike pain, which may follow the distribution of sensory nerves. Paresthesias may accompany this type of pain. Typical intermittent claudication occurs commonly in the lower extremities. It most often occurs in the arch of the foot because of involvement of the vessels of the leg and sparing of the femoral and iliac arteries. Some patients have intermittent claudication of the forearm or hand. Sensitivity to cold with paresthesias and the development of secondary Raynaud's phenomenon are common. Migratory superficial thrombophlebitis is manifested by the development of inflamed, tender, red segments of the superficial veins, which subside over a period of several weeks.

Physical examination discloses impaired arterial pulsations in the more distal portions of the limbs, such as the radial, ulnar, dorsalis pedis, and posterior tibial arteries. The more proximal arteries are normal, a finding that contrasts with arteriosclerosis obliterans. There may be cyanosis or pallor or persistent redness in the digits, and associated changes in temperature may be noted. Postural changes in color are also common. Gangrene or ulcerations of the digits may be present in both upper and lower extremities. Edema of the foot is common. Occasional patients have involvement of visceral arteries with stenosis or occlusion of mesenteric, coronary, cerebral, or renal arteries and manifestations of ischemia of these organs.

DIAGNOSIS. The diagnosis of thromboangiitis obliterans should be entertained when there is evidence of ischemia of the extremities from arterial occlusive disease in association with migratory superficial thrombophlebitis. The age and sex of the individual and the involvement of the upper extremities are additional helpful characteristics. Arteriography may be helpful in disclosing segmental multiple occlusions of the medium-sized and small arteries associated with collateral vessel visualization. The larger arteries are generally spared, a finding that also helps distinguish the disorder from arteriosclerosis obliterans. Final confirmation may be obtained only from biopsy material of an early lesion and histologic demonstration of the characteristic inflammatory and proliferative lesion of the disease.

PROGNOSIS. Thromboangiitis obliterans is not usually life threatening except in rare individuals in whom the visceral arteries are involved. The disease, however, results in disability and amputation of the extremities in a high percentage of cases. It is generally more rapidly progressive than arteriosclerosis obliterans, especially in individuals who refuse to stop smoking.

TREATMENT. Cessation of tobacco smoking is essential. Continuation of smoking results in a progressive course. If the patient stops smoking, new lesions do not develop or they develop more rarely. The approach to the patient with thromboangiitis obliterans is generally the same as that of patients with advanced arteriosclerosis obliterans. It consists of conservative measures, including protection from cold, local care in the event of ulceration or gangrene, and eventually amputation, if these lesions occur. Sympathectomy is tried frequently and may be effective, at least temporarily, if vasospasm is a prominent feature. Vasodilative drug therapy can be tried in cases of Raynaud's phenomenon with ulcerations, but its effectiveness is questionable.

Adar R, Papa MZ, Halpern Z, et al.: Cellular sensitivity to collagen in thromboangiitis obliterans. N Engl J Med 308:1113, 1983. *An important study showing high incidence of cellular sensitivity to collagen and the presence of circulating anticollagen antibodies in patients with thromboangiitis obliterans. The results have profound implications concerning the etiology of the disease and offer possible means of differentiating it from arteriosclerosis obliterans.*

McKusick VA, Harris WS, Ottesen OE, et al.: Buerger's disease: A distinct clinical and pathologic entity. JAMA 181:5, 1962. *A concise and thoughtful consideration of the clinical features, arteriographic findings, and histopathology of 30 cases with Buerger's disease.*

Sudden Arterial Occlusion

DEFINITION. Sudden arterial occlusion may result from obstruction of an artery of the extremity by embolism or by thrombosis in situ. The clinical manifestations are the result of the consequent ischemia.

ETIOLOGY. The major cause of sudden arterial occlusion is arterial embolism. The heart is the most frequent source of emboli in this syndrome. Emboli may arise from thrombi in the left atrium in the presence of atrial fibrillation or mitral valve disease, usually mitral stenosis. Emboli may also arise from mural thrombi from a myocardial infarction or in the presence of a cardiomyopathy. Septic emboli may arise from vegetations from the mitral or aortic valves in the presence of bacterial endocarditis. Less commonly, emboli may arise from an arteriosclerotic plaque in more proximal parts of the arterial tree or from aneurysms. In rare cases, the embolus may arise from the venous side and enter the arterial tree via a patent foramen ovale (paradoxical embolism). More rarely, the embolus consists of calcium fragments from a calcified valve leaflet, cholesterol crystals from an arteriosclerotic plaque, or foreign materials such as a bullet.

Sudden arterial thrombosis occurs in about 10 per cent of the cases of arteriosclerosis obliterans. The condition is rare in thromboangiitis obliterans or in polyarteritis nodosa. Acute arterial thrombosis may occur in conditions in which the coagulability of the blood is increased in the presence of normal vessels, such as in polycythemia vera or in cryoglobulinemia. Rarely, arterial thrombosis may occur in the presence of normal vessels in infections such as septicemia, pneumonia, peritonitis, tuberculosis, ulcerative colitis, and other debilitating diseases. Trauma from penetrating wounds, as from arterial puncture or catheterization, may cause arterial occlusion.

PATHOLOGY. The structure of emboli that arise from thrombi in the heart or from aneurysms is the same as that of the parent thrombi. Emboli lodge in an artery and obstruct the vessel. There may be extension of the thrombus distally by further clotting of the blood. The fate of the embolus varies. In some cases it may become organized and finally be recanalized, and in other cases it may become fragmented and the fragments may lodge in more distal vessels.

PATHOPHYSIOLOGY. The sudden arterial occlusion causes reduction of blood flow to the more distal portions of the limb and consequent ischemia. There have been suggestions that vasoactive agents released from the emboli, such as serotonin from platelets, may cause contraction of vascular smooth muscle in more distal portions of the vascular tree and result in vasospasm that further aggravates ischemia. The severity and extent of ischemia depend on the size of the vessel occluded and on the extent of collateral circulation. The larger the occluded vessel, the more likely it is that severe ischemia would result.

CLINICAL MANIFESTATIONS. Sudden arterial occlusion causes the abrupt onset of severe pain accompanied by manifestations of ischemia in about half the patients. In the remainder, the onset is gradual with either mild pain or numbness and paresthesias. Pain is present in about 75 per cent of the cases. There may be muscular weakness or outright paralysis. A saddle embolus of the aortic bifurcation causes abdominal pain, nausea, and vomiting and may result in a shocklike state.

Examination of the patient discloses diminished or absent pulses distal to the occlusion. Evidence of ischemia is present with low skin temperature and pallor or cyanosis or a combination of the two. If the occluded artery is superficial, the site of lodgment of the embolus may be identified as a tender region. The subsequent course depends on the adequacy of the collateral circulation. If this is adequate, gradual improvement occurs. Otherwise, gangrene supervenes.

DIAGNOSIS. The diagnosis of sudden arterial occlusion is usually relatively easy in the patient who has the acute onset of pain and ischemia of an extremity. If the cause is an embolus, its source may be evident. Rarely, patients with acute thrombophlebitis of the iliac and femoral veins may have feeble or absent arterial pulses and show manifestations resembling those of ischemia from an arterial embolus. In these cases, the demonstration of the feeble pulse and the presence of distended veins and pronounced edema help make the differentiation possible.

PROGNOSIS. The outcome of acute arterial obstruction depends on the size of the vessel affected, the age of the patient, the extent of the collateral circulation, and the timing of therapeutic intervention. When a large artery is occluded, the prognosis is poor without surgical treatment. In older patients with pre-existing arterial occlusive disease, the prognosis is poor because of obstruction of multiple vessels, including collateral vessels.

TREATMENT. The goal of therapeutic intervention is the removal or dissolution of the thrombus and re-establishment of patency of the occluded artery. This goal can be achieved by surgical embolectomy or by thrombolytic therapy. Urgent embolectomy is the preferred method of treatment when a large artery is occluded, such as with a saddle embolus of the bifurcation of the aorta. When smaller vessels are occluded and the thrombus is not easily accessible or when the patient's general condition does not permit surgical intervention, intravenous or intra-arterial streptokinase or urokinase may be given, if there are no contraindications for their use. Streptokinase is given intravenously as a bolus of 250,000 IU, followed by an infusion of 100,000 IU per hour. The infusion is continued for 72 hours. Intra-arterial administration can be used instead, in a dose of about one tenth of the intravenous dose; it can be coupled with angioplasty. Thrombolytic therapy is followed by conventional anticoagulants. The success rate of thrombolytic therapy is critically dependent on how early it is administered after the onset of symptoms. It is more effective for thrombotic lesions than embolic ones. Streptokinase or urokinase cannot be safely followed by surgery because of the danger of bleeding from the arteriotomy. The choice of therapy, therefore, must be carefully considered.

If neither therapeutic approach can be used, the patient should be treated conservatively. The patient should be placed at rest. The limb should be placed in a slightly dependent position under a cradle whose temperature is controlled at 30 to 35°C. Anticoagulation with heparin should be started as soon as possible to prevent extension of the thrombus and to prevent formation of additional emboli. If vasospasm is prominent, lumbar sympathectomy may be tried to reduce vasomotor tone and improve blood flow to the limb.

When a patient is treated by conservative medical measures, he or she should be followed closely for evidence of deterioration. If this occurs, immediate surgical intervention and embolectomy should be attempted. The results of embolectomy depend, to a large extent, on the timing of intervention. Therefore, surgery should not be delayed longer than a few hours. If therapy fails, gangrene may supervene, and amputation may become necessary.

Haimovici H: Peripheral arterial embolism. Angiology 1:20, 1950. *Detailed consideration of the clinical features of the arteries of the limbs based on study of 330 cases.*

Hargrove WC, Barker CF, Berkowitz HD, et al.: Treatment of acute peripheral arterial and graft thromboses with low-dose streptokinase. Surgery 92:981, 1982. *A report of good results from the use of intra-arterial streptokinase for the treatment of acute arterial thrombosis.*

Hinton RC, Kistler JP, Fallon JT, et al.: Influence of etiology of atrial fibrillation on incidence of systemic embolism. Am J Cardiol 40:509, 1977. *A study of the pathology of arterial embolism in 333 patients with atrial fibrillation. The paper emphasizes that the risk of embolism is independent of the cause of atrial fibrillation.*

VASCULAR DISEASES OF THE LIMBS CAUSED BY ABNORMAL COMMUNICATION BETWEEN ARTERIES AND VEINS

Arteriovenous Fistula

DEFINITION. Arteriovenous fistula is an abnormal direct communication between an artery and a vein.

ETIOLOGY. Arteriovenous fistulas in the limbs may be congenital or acquired. Congenital fistulas are usually multiple, acquired ones are usually single. The most common type is iatrogenic, created to carry out renal dialysis. Acquired arteriovenous fistulas may also result from trauma caused by penetrating wounds or surgical procedures.

PATHOPHYSIOLOGY. The low resistance of the direct communication between artery and vein results in a high arterial inflow into the vein, with a resultant increase in venous pressure. The elevated venous pressure causes engorgement of the vein and distention and may lead to the production of varicose veins. In the region of the fistula, blood flow is high, whereas more distal portions are deprived of capillary blood flow and may show ischemia and trophic changes.

Large fistulas cause a reduction in systemic vascular resistance and impose a burden on the heart because of the associated increase in cardiac output. Total blood volume may be increased. Left ventricular failure may eventually result.

PATHOLOGY. In the region of the fistula the veins become thickened, whereas the artery undergoes thinning and loss of elastic and muscular fibers in the media.

CLINICAL MANIFESTATIONS. The patient may be totally asymptomatic, and the discovery of the fistula may be accidental. In other cases, there may be pain in the location of the fistula, edema, varicosities, and asymmetry in the size of the limbs. In some cases, the presenting symptoms may be those of cardiac decompensation with dyspnea on exertion, palpitations, and orthopnea. Examination of the involved limb reveals tortuous, dilated, superficial veins and venous pulsation at the site of the fistula. The temperature of the skin may be high, and distal portions of the limb may show ischemic changes. A bruit or a thrill may be heard over the fistula during systole. At other times, a continuous bruit may be present. The extremity may be swollen, or the girth of the limb may be increased because of hypertrophy of the soft tissues. Temporary compression of the artery proximal to the fistula causes immediate increase in systemic vascular resistance and leads to reflex decrease in heart rate (Branham's sign), a change that may be helpful diagnostically.

DIAGNOSIS. When the fistula is superficial and large, the diagnosis can be made easily. If this is not possible from the physical examination, arteriography should be attempted for a definitive diagnosis. The oxygen saturation of the venous blood from the involved limb is higher than that of its contralateral part, and this comparison may be helpful in making the diagnosis.

TREATMENT. The treatment of choice is surgical intervention with closure of the fistula and re-establishment of the continuity of the involved artery and vein. If such restoration is not possible, ligation of the artery or vein or both may be necessary, but this may lead to arterial or venous insufficiency of the limb. In some cases, the fistula involves an anomalous artery. In this case, the ligation of the artery and the obstruction of the veins by the injection of sclerosing solutions may give a satisfactory result. It may not be practical to treat surgically patients with multiple fistulas. In these cases, conservative measures consisting of local care, relief of pain, and wearing elastic bandages may be helpful. If the fistula is inoperable and cardiac decompensation is present or threatened, amputation may be necessary.

Nickerson JL, Elkin DC, Warren JV: The effect of temporary occlusion of arteriovenous fistulas on heart rate, stroke volume, and cardiac output. J Clin Invest 30:215, 1951. *A classic study of the systemic hemodynamic effects of arteriovenous fistulas in a large number of patients.*

Rossi P, Carillo FJ, Alfidi RJ, et al.: Iatrogenic arteriovenous fistulas. Radiology 111:47, 1974. *A comprehensive review of 154 cases of iatrogenic arteriovenous fistulas. The paper provides a good review of the literature.*

Glomus Tumor (Glomangioma)

DEFINITION. Glomangioma, or glomus tumor, is a benign tumor of the glomus body.

PATHOLOGY. The glomus tumor is an encapsulated structure consisting of a hypertrophied arteriovenous anastomosis. The tumor varies in size from 0.5 to 2.5 cm in diameter. It can be found in various parts of the upper and lower extremities but is most frequently located in the nail beds.

CLINICAL MANIFESTATIONS. The most common symptom is severe burning pain in the location of the tumor. The pain may precede the appearance of the tumor. Pain may occur spontaneously, or it may be precipitated by exposure to heat or cold. Occasionally, the tumor is exquisitely sensitive to touch, and even the slightest pressure from contact with clothing may cause severe pain. Severe disability and atrophy of the limb from disuse may occur secondary to fear of pain. Examination of the involved area shows a reddish, purplish, or bluish mass that is sharply demarcated. At times, the tumor may not be easily visible or palpable. In this case, pressure with the head of a pin may help identify the location of the tumor. When it is located under the nail bed, the nail and the phalanx may be visibly deformed, thereby giving a clue to the location of the tumor.

TREATMENT. The glomus tumor is a benign tumor. Surgical excision results in complete relief without recurrence.

Cooke SAR: Misleading features in the clinical diagnosis of the peripheral glomus tumour. Br J Surg 58:602, 1971. *The clinical manifestations of glomus tumor are described based on the study of 24 cases.*

DISEASES OF THE VEINS OF THE LIMBS

Thrombophlebitis and Deep-Vein Thrombosis

DEFINITION. Thrombophlebitis refers to venous thrombosis with accompanying inflammation of the venous wall. For important practical reasons, superficial thrombophlebitis is distinguished from deep-vein thrombosis. Superficial thrombophlebitis does not cause embolic complications, but deep-vein thrombosis is a frequent cause of pulmonary embolism.

PATHOLOGY. Thrombi in veins consist mostly of red cells with a few platelets held together with fibrin. They propagate in the direction of the bloodstream by extension of the thrombotic process. They attach to the wall of the vein at one end, while the more proximal end floats freely into the lumen of the vessel. This is the portion that is commonly broken off and travels to the lungs. Varying degrees of inflammatory reaction of the venous wall may be present. Venous thrombosis may exist in the absence of inflammation, as is the case in some patients with malignancy. This is referred to as "phlebothrombosis." In most cases, however, inflammation and thrombosis coexist. The disorder may start as a pure thrombotic process, and inflammation usually occurs secondary to the presence of the thrombus.

INCIDENCE. Deep-vein thrombosis is a common disorder. It is more common in women than in men. All races seem to be affected equally, at least in civilized countries. The incidence of the disease increases with advancing age. The disease is very common in hospitalized patients. Approximately one third of the patients over age 40 who have undergone major surgery or have had an acute myocardial infarction develop deep-vein thrombosis. The incidence is even higher after certain operations such as repair of hip fractures or prostatectomy. Patients with thrombotic strokes have an equally high incidence of deep-vein thrombosis. This occurs almost exclusively in the paralyzed limb.

Superficial thrombophlebitis occurs most commonly in patients with varicose veins, possibly as a result of minor trauma. It is also frequent after pregnancy. A migratory type of superficial thrombophlebitis also occurs in patients with thromboangiitis obliterans.

PATHOGENESIS. Venous stasis, injury to the venous wall, and a hypercoagulable state are the three main factors that lead to venous thrombosis. In most cases, more than one of these factors are present, and their effect may be cumulative. The combination of venous stasis and changes in the clotting mechanism of the blood accounts for the increased incidence of deep-vein thrombosis in pregnancy and during administration of oral contraceptives. Venous stasis is the major factor in the development of venous thrombosis in patients with heart disease, in paralyzed patients, in patients undergoing major surgery, in those who have varicose veins, and in healthy individuals after long trips. Increased viscosity, leading to stasis, and alterations in the clotting factors of the blood account for the high incidence of polycythemia vera. Patients with familial deficiencies of certain anticlotting factors are susceptible to recurrent thrombophlebitis. These include deficiencies of antithrombin III, protein S, protein C, and heparin cofactor II. Injury to the venous wall may result from administration of certain vasoconstrictive or chemotherapeutic agents, or it may result from infectious agents. Patients with malignancies may have migrating thrombophlebitis, which has been attributed to low-grade activation of intravascular coagulation.

CLINICAL MANIFESTATIONS. The presence of superficial thrombophlebitis is usually easily ascertained by finding the inflamed vein. This may be apparent as a red, tender cord. By contrast, deep-vein thrombosis frequently causes few distinctive clinical features, about one half of patients with deep-vein thrombosis are asymptomatic. The first manifestation of deep-vein thrombosis may be the occurrence of pulmonary embolism. Pain in the region of the thrombosed veins at rest or only during exercise and edema distal to the obstructed veins are the usual symptoms of deep-vein thrombosis. Examination of the patient may disclose several helpful manifestations. Edema or pitting of the malleolar fossa may be present and may cause loss of the normal concavity of that portion of the leg. There may be a difference between the two legs in the circumference of the calf. A difference in maximal circumference in excess of 1.4 cm in men and 1.2 cm in women is highly suspicious. The temperature of the skin may be increased as a result of the inflammatory reaction, and palpation may disclose the thrombosed veins in the calf or in the popliteal fossa. There may be tenderness to palpation. Increased resistance or pain on voluntary dorsiflexion of the foot (Homans' sign) may be present. A useful sign is the presence of tenderness on inflation of a blood pressure cuff around the calf. Most normal individuals tolerate this without pain up to pressures of 160 to 180 mm Hg.

Thrombosis of the iliac and femoral veins usually presents with a characteristic clinical picture consisting of rapidly advancing swelling of the entire limb. The thrombosed vein may be tender if it extends below the inguinal ligament. Collateral distended veins may be present in the upper thigh. In some cases, secondary ischemia may occur as a result of the very high venous pressure that impedes arterial inflow. Cyanosis of the toes and even gangrene may occur under these circumstances.

Thrombosis of the subclavian vein may result in swelling of the upper extremity, and collateral veins may be present. In axillary thrombosis, a similar clinical picture occurs; the thrombosed vein may be felt in the axilla. A history of walking on crutches or sleeping in a sitting position on a bench with the arms behind the backrest may be helpful. Thrombosis of the superior vena cava causes increased venous pressure in the neck and face with distention of the neck veins in the upper part of the chest.

In septic thrombophlebitis, there may also be systemic manifestations of infection, such as fever, chills, and leukocytosis. In cases in which septic phlebitis begins from infected needles or catheters, an inflamed, tender cord may appear at the site of the venipuncture.

DIAGNOSIS. Ileofemoral thrombophlebitis is usually easily recognized by the rapid swelling of the entire limb, engorged collateral veins in the thigh, and signs of inflammation, such as increased skin temperature.

By contrast, in the majority of cases of deep-vein thrombosis involving the calf, popliteal area, and thigh, the clinical picture is not sufficiently distinctive to allow diagnosis with a high degree of confidence. Confirmation of the diagnosis must be provided by resorting to one or more of a number of diagnostic tests. The most commonly employed tests are the following:

X-ray Venography. Venography is one of the most accurate means of making the diagnosis of deep-vein thrombosis. The test involves the injection of a contrast medium into the venous system, which has been previously emptied of blood by gravity. The test relies on finding a filling defect or a sharp cutoff, indicating the presence of occluding thrombus in the vein. The test may result in inflammatory reaction followed by thrombosis in a few cases. It is sensitive and highly specific, for these reasons, venography is considered the "gold standard" in the diagnosis of deep-vein thrombosis.

Radionuclide Venography. This test is similar to x-ray venography except that instead of contrast medium, a radioisotope, such as ^{99m}Tc-macroaggregated albumin, is injected in a foot vein. External scanning detects venous obstruction and the presence of collateral circulation. In another variation of the technique, ^{99m}Tc-labeled red cells from the patient's own blood are injected intravenously, and a blood pool scan is obtained. The sensitivity and specificity of the technique are somewhat less than those of x-ray venography. The technique is probably better in detecting venous thrombosis in the thigh than in the calf.

Radioisotope-labeled Fibrinogen. This test consists of intravenous administration of fibrinogen labeled with ^{125}I and the subsequent incorporation of the radioactive material into the thrombus. The accumulation of radioactivity is detected by external counting. This test detects an active thrombophlebitis, it may be negative in cases in which the active process has stopped but thrombi exist in the veins. The reliability of the test depends on the location of the thrombus. It is of little use in detecting pelvic thrombi because of the high background due to the bladder and iliac arteries. It is most useful in detecting thrombosis of the calf. Another disadvantage is that it requires one or two days for a sufficient number of counts to build into the thrombosed vein for detection. This test is, therefore, most useful in longitudinal screening of high-risk populations.

Liquid Crystal Thermography. This test relies on the detection of small increases in skin temperature as a result of the venous inflammation. The test is easy to perform. It has high sensitivity but relatively low specificity. It can be a useful adjunct to ultrasonography or impedance plethysmography for monitoring patients at risk.

Ultrasonography. This test utilizes the Doppler principle to detect venous obstruction. Thus, during various maneuvers that alter venous flow, such as deep inspiration, Valsalva's maneuver, or leg compression, the ultrasonogram may detect the presence of obstructed veins. The disadvantages of the technique are that a high degree of stenosis is necessary for the test result to be abnormal and that it does not distinguish between occlusion from external pressure and occlusion by thrombus. Also, the result may be negative if an effective collateral circulation has developed. The test is most sensitive for thrombosis of the veins above the knee.

Impedance Plethysmography. This test detects alterations in blood volume of the extremities by detecting changes in the electrical impedance of the tissues. The test is carried out during respiratory maneuvers or during alterations in blood flow by occluding the limb with a pneumatic pressure cuff. Like ultrasonography, this test requires significant proximal obstruction for positive results. The reported sensitivity and specificity of the last two tests are high (over 90 per cent).

Choice of Tests. The choice of tests to be performed depends to a large extent on their availability. If all are available, it is preferable to use first ultrasonography and impedance plethysmography and resort to venography only if the results of these are inconclusive. The radioactive fibrinogen test and thermography should be reserved for screening of patients at high risk.

DIFFERENTIAL DIAGNOSIS. A number of conditions that cause localized pain or edema in the lower extremities may be confused with deep-vein thrombosis. A ruptured popliteal synovial membrane or cyst (Baker's cyst) may simulate most of the manifestations of venous thrombosis. The diagnosis can be suspected if there is a history or physical findings of arthritis of the knee joint. The diagnosis may be confirmed by an arthrogram revealing the entry of dye from the joint into the calf muscles. Rupture of the calf muscles may cause pain, tenderness, and edema and may simulate thrombophlebitis. The diagnosis can be made from the history of strenuous or unusual exercise, the presence of ecchymosis from extravasated blood, and the palpation of a hematoma. Sometimes the patient reports an audible snap during the activity when the pain first occurred. The differential diagnosis is important because anticoagulants are contraindicated in this condition. A severe muscle cramp may cause pain and swelling for a considerable period of time. Other manifestations of thrombophlebitis are, however, lacking in this situation. The pain of a lumbar disc may be localized in the calf. There are no other manifestations of venous thrombosis,

however, and there may be neurologic findings to identify the cause of the pain. Lymphedema is recognized by its slower and gradual onset and the absence of signs of inflammation and of collateral veins. Finally, cellulitis may be confused with superficial thrombophlebitis.

COMPLICATIONS. Pulmonary embolism is a frequent and serious complication of deep-vein thrombosis. About 80 to 90 per cent of pulmonary emboli arise in the deep veins of the lower limbs. Although deep-vein thrombosis may begin frequently in the veins of the calf, it is only when the thrombosis extends above the knee that serious pulmonary embolism occurs.

About 5 per cent of patients with deep-vein thrombosis develop venous insufficiency with stasis dermatitis (postphlebitic syndrome). This is more likely to occur in those with more proximal venous obstruction. A rare complication of iliofemoral thrombophlebitis is venous claudication, in which the patient develops pain on exercise which is relieved by rest, as in arterial occlusive disease.

PROPHYLAXIS. Prophylactic therapy against deep-vein thrombosis should be attempted in high-risk patients (Table 57–4). The exact regimen used must take into consideration the risk of deep-vein thrombosis and consequent pulmonary embolism and the potential risk of hemorrhagic complications from the prophylactic therapy. Low-dose heparin is currently the most commonly used prophylactic technique. For surgical patients, this consists of administration of 5000 units of heparin subcutaneously 2 hours before surgery and then every 8 or 12 hours until the patient is ambulatory. This method is effective in reducing the incidence of deep-vein thrombosis and pulmonary embolism in patients subjected to a variety of surgical procedures. It is also effective in reducing the incidence of deep-vein thrombosis in patients following acute myocardial infarction, but it is not known whether there is also a reduction in the incidence of pulmonary embolism. Low-dose heparin has been shown to be ineffective in patients undergoing surgery for hip fracture and hip replacement, and its effectiveness has not been established in urologic procedures. Higher dose heparin adjusted to give an activated partial thromboplastin time (APTT) in the upper limits of the therapeutic range has been reported to be more effective than low-dose heparin. In addition, the administration of dihydroergotamine mesylate, 0.5 mg subcutaneously, together with low-dose heprin, is more effective in preventing deep-vein thrombosis than heparin alone in surgical patients. Warfarin and other similar drugs are also effective in protecting patients from thromboembolism during a variety of surgical techniques. Low molecular weight dextran given on the day of surgery and at suitable intervals thereafter has been reported in most cases to give favorable results. There is a risk of fluid overload, and, to a lesser extent, hemorrhagic complications. This method can be used in instances in which there is a high risk of bleeding from anticoagulants. Drugs that interfere with platelet aggregation, such as aspirin and other nonsteroidal anti-inflammatory agents, have not been

TABLE 57–4. PREVENTION OF VENOUS THROMBOEMBOLISM

Representative Patient Groups	1. Medical patients without predisposing factors on short bed rest 2. Young patients without predisposing factors undergoing brief (<1 hr) general surgical procedure	1. Medical patients with predisposing factors or on prolonged bed rest 2. Middle-aged or old patients without predisposing factors undergoing general surgical procedure longer than 1 hr	1. Patients with hip fracture 2. Patients undergoing extensive orthopedic or pelvic surgery 3. Middle-aged or old patients with predisposing factors or with previous venous thrombosis undergoing general surgical procedure longer than 1 hr
Approximate Incidence of Venous Thrombosis	5%	20–40%	50–70%
Approximate Incidence of Pulmonary Embolism	Almost zero	5%	10%
Suggested Prophylaxis	None	Low-dose heparin or intermittent pneumatic compression	Warfarin, low-dose heparin plus either intermittent pneumatic compression or dihydroergotamine; or higher dose heparin

shown convincingly to be effective as prophylactic agents. In patients in whom anticoagulation is contraindicated, such as patients with neurosurgical procedures, it is prudent to use conservative means of prophylaxis. These include early ambulation, elastic stockings, and external periodic calf compression. The external compression devices have been reported to be effective. There are no risks associated with their use; the only negative aspect is low patient acceptance during prolonged use, because they are uncomfortable or cumbersome.

TREATMENT. Antocoagulation is not necessary for the treatment of superficial thrombophlebitis. Local measures, sometimes coupled with administration of anti-inflammatory drugs, such as indomethacin, suffice to bring about healing and relief of symptoms.

Full anticoagulation is the preferred treatment for deep-vein thrombosis. Heparin is preferred for initiation of treatment because of its immediate action, whereas warfarin-type drugs may not become fully effective for a considerable period of time. Heparin inhibits coagulation by binding and activating antithrombin III, an inhibitor of activated factor X. Heparin is best administered by constant infusion. Initially a bolus of 5000 units is given intravenously, followed by constant infusion of 750 to 1000 units per hour. The dose is adjusted by monitoring the APTT so that a level about two times the normal control is achieved. APTT is checked four to six hours after the initial bolus and once a day thereafter. An alternative method is intermittent intravenous administration of 5,000 to 10,000 units every four to six hours. If no suitable veins are found, heparin may be administered subcutaneously in a dose of 15,000 to 30,000 units every 12 hours. After five days of heparin therapy, oral warfarin at a dose of 10 to 15 mg daily is given until the one-stage prothrombin time (PT) is one and one half to two times the normal level. Subsequently, a daily maintenance dose is administered to maintain the PT at the desired level. Warfarin brings about anticoagulation by decreasing the level of factors II, VII, IX, and X. Many drugs interact with warfarin. Some of them potentiate its action and others inhibit it. If the patient requires other drug therapy while on warfarin, each drug should be carefully screened for potential interaction. If bleeding occurs in the course of heparin therapy, its effect can be counteracted by administration of 1 mg of protamine per 100 units of heparin. If bleeding develops in the course of warfarin treatment, the patient should receive vitamin K₁ intramuscularly to reduce PT to the therapeutic range (0.25 to 1.0 mg usually suffices). If bleeding is serious, blood or fresh frozen plasma may be necessary.

Thrombolysis with fibrinolytic agents, such as streptokinase or urokinase, administered intravenously in patients with deep-vein thrombosis has been shown to achieve more complete dissolution of the thrombus and better preservation of the venous architecture than conventional anticoagulants. These drugs act by causing activation of plasminogen to plasmin, thereby causing dissolution of the thrombus. Steptokinase is administered intravenously as an initial bolus of 250,000 to 500,000 IU, followed by an infusion of 100,000 IU per hour for 24 to 72 hours. The effectiveness of the drug diminishes after the first 24 hours. Urokinase is less likely to cause anaphylactic reactions, but it is more expensive. It is given in a dose of 4400 IU per kilogram as a bolus, followed by an infusion of 4400 IU per kilogram per hour for the same duration as streptokinase. Thrombolytic therapy is the preferred method of treatment of patients with iliofemoral or subclavian-axillary vein thrombosis. In patients with more distal deep-vein thrombosis, the high effectiveness of heparin and its lower rate of hemorrhagic complictions render this the preferred method of treatment.

In patients in whom anticoagulation is contraindicated, simple measures—elevation of the extremity and local heat—should be used. When the risk of pulmonary embolism is low, as is the case of deep-vein thrombosis limited to the calf, these measures suffice. In patients with deep-vein thrombosis extending above the knee, in whom the risk of pulmonary embolism is high, implantation of an inferior vena caval filter or ligation of the inferior vena cava may also be considered. This form of therapy should also be used when anticoagulation needs to be terminated because of complications, when recurrent thromboembolism occurs in the presence of adequate anticoagulation, and when septic thromboembolic disease not controlled by antibiotics is present.

Bed rest should be continued until local signs of inflammation, including tenderness and edema, subside. After 7 to 15 days the patient is allowed to walk wearing elastic stockings. If no discomfort occurs, resumption of full activity is allowed one to two weeks later. Anticoagulation for three months is usually sufficient to prevent recurrence of deep-vein thrombosis.

Coon, WW: Epidemiology of venous thromboembolism. Ann Surg 186:149, 1977. *A detailed, well-referenced consideration of the epidemiology of venous thrombosis.*

Moser KM, Fedullo PF: Venous thromboembolism, three simple decisions (part 1). Chest 83:117, 1983. *A practical, well-reasoned approach to the prophylaxis and treatment for venous thrombosis is presented.*

Mudge M, Hughes LE: The long term sequelae of deep vein thrombosis. J Surg 65:692, 1978. *A report of long-term follow-up of patients who had evidence of venous thrombosis after surgery. The sequelae of venous thrombosis are described.*

The Multicenter Trial Committee: Dihydroergotamine-heparin prophylaxis of postoperative deep-vein thrombosis. JAMA 251:2960, 1984. *A multicenter investigation showing that the combination of dihydroergotamine and heparin is superior in preventing deep vein thrombosis in surgical patients to heparin or dihydroergotamine alone.*

Painter TD: Thrombophlebitis: Diagnostic techniques. Angiology 31:386, 1980. *Comprehensive consideration of the diagnostic techniques for venous thrombosis.*

Shafer KE, Jaffe AS: Thrombolytic therapy: Current and potential uses. Drug Ther 13:95, 1983. *A concise consideration of the uses of thrombolytic agents.*

Sharma GVRK, Cella G, Parisi AF, et al.: Thrombolytic therapy. N Engl J Med 306:1268, 1982. *Detailed consideration of the use of streptokinase and urokinase in vascular thrombosis.*

Wessler S, Gitel SN: Low-dose heparin: Is the risk worth the benefit? Am Heart J 98:94, 1979. *A review of the use of low-dose heparin for prophylaxis against venous thrombosis.*

Wessler S, Gitel SN: Warfarin: From bedside to bench. New Engl J Med 311:645, 1984. *A concise consideration of the mechanism of action and clinical uses of warfarin in thrombotic disease.*

Varicose Veins

DEFINITION. Varicose veins are prominent, abnormally distended, and tortuous veins.

INCIDENCE. Approximately 20 per cent of adults develop varicose veins. A familial history is present in 15 per cent of patients. They are more common in women than in men by a factor of 5 to 1. Most women date the onset of varicose veins from the time of pregnancy. The veins of the lower extremities are most frequently affected because of the effects of gravity on venous pressure.

ETIOLOGY. Congenitally absent or defective valves are a recognized cause of varicose veins in early life. Varicose veins may develop secondary to sustained elevations of venous pressure from obstruction of the veins. The cause of the obstruction may be thrombosis secondary to thrombophlebitis or external pressure, as is the case in pregnancy, ascites, and tumors. However, in most affected individuals, no clearly identifiable cause or precipitating factor can be found. The possibility of a genetically determined structural defect in the venous wall has been suggested. Individuals with varicose veins in the lower extremities have been found to have increased venous distensibility and reduced amounts of collagen and hexosamine in the wall of unaffected veins. In the face of such a generalized defect, a sustained elevation in venous pressure from the effects of gravity in the lower extremities or from other factors may lead to stretching of the walls and, finally, to incompetence of the valves and overdistention of the veins. An association of varicose veins with hemorrhoids and diverticulosis of the bowel suggests the possibility that increased intra-abdominal pressure during bowel movements may play a role in their pathogenesis.

CLINICAL MANIFESTATIONS. Most patients are asymptomatic, especially in the early stages of the disease. They may seek attention because the dilated, tortuous varicosities are cosmetically unappealing. In some cases, aching in the lower extremities and edema, especially after prolonged standing or exercise, may be present. The edema usually subsides overnight. When the communicating veins are incompetent, symptoms are more common. Prolonged venous insufficiency leads to the postphlebitic syndrome, with sustained edema, induration, and fibrosis. Eventually, trophic changes with brownish discoloration of the skin and ulceration may result. Ulcers usually occur above the medial malleolus. An incompetent communicating vein may be identified in the vicinity of the ulcer. The arterial pulses are normal, and no evidence of ischemia is present.

DIAGNOSIS. Clinical inspection suffices to make the diagnosis. The Trendelenburg test can identify the presence of defective valves and incompetent communicating veins. With the patient recumbent, the leg is elevated to empty the veins, and a tourniquet is then applied to occlude the superficial veins. The patient is instructed to resume the erect position, and the tourniquet is released. If the venous valves are incompetent, the veins immediately become distended as a result of the back flow. If two tourniquets are applied, the distention of the veins in the intervening portion of the limb identifies the presence of incompetent communicating veins. The patency of the deep venous system can be examined by venography. It is prudent to exclude other causes of edema, such as congestive heart failure and renal disease.

PROGNOSIS. The prognosis of uncomplicated superficial varicose veins is excellent. The postphlebitic syndrome, once established, is usually progressive and resistant to treatment.

TREATMENT. Simple measures usually suffice to treat uncomplicated varicose veins. These consist of frequent periods of rest with elevation of the limbs, external pressure with elastic stockings or bandages, and avoidance of obstruction of the veins by garments, such as girdles. In more severe or advanced cases, ligation and stripping of the saphenous veins or injection of sclerosing solutions may become necessary to prevent the postphlebitis syndrome. An injection/compression technique in which the sclerosing solution is injected into a vein emptied of blood, followed by compression by external pressure, is simple, cheap, and effective. It is widely used in Europe. When stasis ulcers are present, local care with warm, wet dressings is necessary. If infection is present, local and systemic antibiotics may be administered. If considerable fibrosis is present, it may be necessary to excise the entire area and carry out skin grafting to eliminate ulceration.

Beresford SSA, Chant ADB, Jones HO, et al.: Varicose veins: A comparison of surgery and injection/compression sclerotherapy Lancet 1:921, 1978. *A five-year follow-up comparing the effects of surgery and injection/compression sclerotherapy for varicose veins.*

Hobbs JT: The Treatment of Venous Disorders: A Comprehensive Review of Current Practice in the Management of Varicose Veins and Post-thrombotic Syndrome. Philadelphia, J. B. Lippincott Company, 1977. *A well-written, comprehensive consideration of the clinical features, diagnosis, and treatment of varicose veins and post-thrombotic syndromes.*

DISEASES OF THE LYMPHATIC VESSELS OF THE LIMBS
Lymphangitis

DEFINITION. Lymphangitis is an inflammation of the lymphatic vessels. It is usually of bacterial origin.

ETIOLOGY. In most cases the responsible infective agent is the hemolytic streptococcus or *Staphylococcus aureus*, coagulase-positive. The bacteria gain access to the lymphatics via local trauma or from ulcerations. In many instances no identifiable portal of entry can be found. Infection spreads from the lymphatics to the regional lymph nodes.

PATHOLOGY. Various stages of inflammation are found in the subcutaneous tissue and regional lymph nodes.

CLINICAL MANIFESTATIONS. The local manifestation of lymphangitis consists of a red streak that appears at the site of initial entry of the infective organism and extends to the regional lymph nodes. The latter are swollen and tender. There may be a surrounding area of cellulitis. Systemic accompaniments of infection may constitute the presenting manifestations.

DIAGNOSIS. The local manifestations of lymphangitis and the accompanying system reaction are usually sufficient to make the diagnosis. Leukocytosis with predominance of polymorphonuclear leukocytes may be present. Confirmation is obtained by culturing the organism from the portal of entry or from the subcutaneous tissues. Acute lymphangitis may be difficult to distinguish from a generalized cellulitis or from thrombophlebitis.

PROGNOSIS. With treatment the prognosis is good when one is dealing with an initial attack in an otherwise normal limb. In the case of recurrent attacks, lymphedema may develop and residual increase in the girth of the limb may occur.

TREATMENT. This consists of systemic administration of the appropriate antibiotics. In addition, surgical drainage of the focus of infection is important. Supportive measures, including rest and elevation of the infected limb and local warm, wet dressings, are also helpful. The use of elastic support hose may be necessary for a period of several weeks to prevent lymphedema. In recurrent cases, the causes of secondary lymphedema should be sought.

Schinger A, Martin WJ, Spittell JA: Acute lymphangitis and cellulitis. Minn Med 48:191, 1965. *Concise consideration of the clinical features, diagnosis, and treatment of lymphangitis.*

Lymphedema

DEFINITION. Lymphedema refers to edema from accumulation of lymph secondary to obstruction to its flow.

ETIOLOGY AND INCIDENCE. Lymphedema can be primary or secondary. The most frequent type of primary lymphedema is simple congenital lymphedema, which is not familial and is present at birth. A congenital familial form (Milroy's disease) is inherited as an autosomal dominant trait. Another hereditary form is associated with Noonan's syndrome in about 15 per cent of cases. Lymphedema praecox becomes manifest in puberty and is associated with congenital hypoplasia of the lymphatics. A late form may become manifest in middle age.

Primary lymphedema is more common in women. Most cases are manifest at birth or become apparent before age 40. A syndrome characterized by yellow nails, recurrent pleural effusion, and lymphedema is believed to be secondary to multiple lymphatic abnormalities in the areas involved. A familial syndrome consisting of recurrent intrahepatic cholestasis and lymphedema is probably due to defective hepatic lymphatic vessels as well as those in the extremity.

Secondary lymphedema results most commonly from trauma. It commonly results from surgical removal of lymph nodes and from fibrosis secondary to radiation following surgery for cancer. Lymphoma or metastatic carcinoma involving the lymph nodes may also cause obstruction to the flow of lymph and lymphedema. Filarial infection in the tropics is a cause of secondary lymphedema.

PATHOLOGY. In cases of congenital lymphedema there is absence or hypoplasia of the lymphatic vessels. In secondary lymphedema there are numerous small, irregular lymphatics, together with tortuous and sometimes greatly enlarged varicose lymphatic vessels.

CLINICAL MANIFESTATIONS. Typically, lymphedema begins gradually with an enlargement of the involved limb without other manifestations. The swollen extremity is soft and pitting. The edema subsides at night. With time, the skin becomes thickened and cannot be raised into a fold, and the edema becomes more persistent. The lower extremities are involved most often. In about half the patients the edema is unilateral. Superimposed lymphangitis and cellulitis may occur, and in longstanding cases lymphangiosarcoma may develop.

DIAGNOSIS. The diagnosis of lymphedema may be confirmed with a radioisotope lymphogram. ^{99m}Tc-labeled rhenium sulfur colloid or ^{99m}Tc-labeled antimony trisulfide colloid is injected in the web spaces of the foot. The ilioinguinal region is scanned 30 and 60 minutes later. In lymphedema, the uptake of isotope by the lymph nodes is reduced, whereas in edema due to venous obstruction it is greater than normal owing to increased lymph flow. The precise diagnosis of the type of lymphedema is made by lymphangiography. Contrast medium is injected directly into a lymphatic vessel in the foot, or a water-soluble contrast agent is injected intracutaneously and taken up by the lymphatics. By this technique, a distinction can be made between absence or hypoplasia of the lymphatic vessels on one hand, which characterizes congenital lymphedema, and the hyperplasia and numerous small lymphatics, which characterize secondary lymphedema, on the other.

PROGNOSIS. Primary lymphedema is usually a slowly progressive disorder, not easily amenable to treatment. The prognosis of secondary lymphedema depends on the cause. In cases in which it results from infection, it can be effectively managed by treatment with antibiotics.

TREATMENT. In primary lymphedema this is aimed at keeping the limb as free of edema as possible to prevent fibrosis and secondary infection. Frequent elevation of the limb, the use of elastic stockings, and the administration of diuretics may be useful. In cases not controlled by these simple measures, benzopyrones have been reported to be useful. These drugs break down protein by activating macrophages; hence, they reduce viscosity and facilitate the flow of lymph. Surgery may be tried in advanced cases to remove subcutaneous tissue and to induce new lymph vessel formation. Anastomosis of small lymphatic vessels with veins by microsurgery has been reported to give good results in some cases.

Allen EV, Ghormley RK: Lymphedema of the extremities: Etiology, classification and treatment; report of 300 cases. Ann Intern Med 9:516, 1935. *Comprehensive consideration of the clinical features of primary and secondary lymphedema in a large series of cases.*

Browse NL: The diagnosis and management of primary lymphedema. J Vasc Surg 3:181, 1986. *A concise account of the diagnosis and management of primary lymphedema.*

Browse NL, Stewart G: Lymphoedema: Pathophysiology and classification. I Cardiovasc Surg 26:91, 1985. *An up-to-date description of the pathophysiology and classification of lymphedema.*

Partsch H, Wenzel-Hora BI, Urbanek A: Differential diagnosis of lymphedema after indirect lymphography with iotasul. Lymphology 16:12, 1983. *Description of the usefulness of indirect lymphangiography using a water-soluble contrast medium for the differential diagnosis of lymphedema.*

Pillar NB: Lymphoedema, macrophages and benzopyrones. Lymphology 13:109, 1980. *Discussion of the role of macrophages in lymphedema. The effectiveness of benzopyrones in this disease is ascribed to activation of macrophages.*

PART VII

RESPIRATORY DISEASES

58 INTRODUCTION

John F. Murray

Respiration includes all the processes that contribute to O_2 uptake and CO_2 elimination. The lungs are the major organs of gas exchange, but the nose, oropharynx, extrapulmonary airways, brain, spinal cord, nerves, thoracic cage, respiratory muscles, lymph nodes and vessels, and cardiovascular system are also involved. Thus respiratory diseases, literally interpreted, include a large variety of abnormalities arising in all the different structures concerned with gas exchange. In general, a more limited definition applies, and respiratory diseases are considered to include disturbances of the air passages, lungs, pleura, chest wall, muscles of respiration, and mediastinum (excluding the heart, systemic vessels, and esophagus).

Acute respiratory diseases are probably the most common afflictions of humankind and are responsible for more absences from school and work than any other type of illness. Chronic respiratory diseases, particularly emphysema and bronchitis, are second only to cardiovascular diseases as causes of disability payments. Cancer of the lung kills more persons each year than any other kind of malignancy. Because of the remarkable incidence of these and other respiratory diseases, it is important that all physicians, not just internists and chest specialists, be well versed in the clinical manifestations and methods of diagnosis, treatment, and prevention of the most common disorders. The material concerned with respiratory diseases here and elsewhere in the book is intended as a primer of necessary knowledge with which to recognize and to treat the major respiratory diseases; additional information is available in the references cited at the end of each chapter.

Patients with respiratory disease often seek medical attention because they have at least one of three cardinal manifestations: *cough* (including its derivative hemoptysis), *chest pain*, and *dyspnea*. These are nonspecific and sometimes trivial abnormalities, but the frequency with which they are associated with serious underlying thoracic disease means that the complaints must always be considered carefully and often become the focus of diagnostic evaluations. Because of the clinical importance of cough, chest pain, and dyspnea, the mechanisms, special features, and diagnostic approach to each symptom are briefly reviewed in the following pages. Further information can be found under the headings of the specific diseases in which the sensations occur.

COUGH

Healthy persons seldom cough, their scant bronchial secretions, although constantly being produced, are imperceptibly carried up the tracheobronchial system by the action of cilia and, after reaching the pharynx, swallowed. Coughing is an essential defense mechanism that protects the airways from the adverse effects of inhaled noxious substances and also serves to clear them of retained secretions. Patients recognize that coughing indicates an abnormality, and this symptom is the second most common reason given for seeking medical advice.

MECHANISM. Coughing may be produced voluntarily, but more often it results from reflex stimulation. Extrathoracic cough receptors are located in the nose, oropharynx, larynx, and upper trachea. Intrathoracic rapidly adapting irritant receptors, which cause cough, are located in the epithelium of the lower trachea and large central bronchi, which are the air passages from which coughing is effective in clearing secretions or removing foreign material. Depending on which cough receptors are activated, afferent stimuli travel to the brain via the trigeminal, glossopharyngeal, superior laryngeal, or vagus nerves. Efferent pathways include the recurrent laryngeal nerves, to cause closure of the glottis, and the corticospinal tract and peripheral nerves, to cause contraction of the thoracic and abdominal musculature. The cough reflex begins with a deep breath followed by glottic closure, relaxation of the diaphragm, and contraction of the expiratory muscles. Collectively, these acts generate a positive pressure of 100 to 300 mm Hg within the thorax, which is suddenly released when the glottis opens. During cough, the *volume*-rate of flow out of the lungs (liters per second) is only slightly greater than or the same as it is during a forced expiratory maneuver, a fact that is not always appreciated. However, because the positive pressure in the pleural space is higher than the luminal pressure in the trachea and central bronchi, a pressure difference is created that causes the posterior membranous portion of the airway walls to fold inward and nearly to obliterate the lumen. By this means, the *linear* velocity of airflow through the narrowed channels (centimeters per second) is markedly increased, and a shearing force is created that dislodges secretions and particles from the mucosal surface.

PRODUCTIVE COUGH. The daily quantity of bronchial secretions produced by a normal person is not known, but it is sufficiently small to be removed by mucociliary action alone, and coughing and expectoration are not required. Secretions can accumulate in the tracheobronchial system in the presence of one or more of the following abnormalities: excessive production, altered physical properties, and deficient clearance. Thus, productive cough, which clears retained secretions from the airways, is an important defense mechanism and one of the hallmarks of acute and chronic inflammatory conditions of the lungs and airways. Patients who are unconscious, intubated, or for other reasons cannot cough must have their tracheobronchial secretions removed by suctioning to prevent the complications of atelectasis and/or bronchopulmonary infection.

NONPRODUCTIVE COUGH. In addition to the cough that serves an expectoration function, another type of cough—an irritative phenomenon—is encountered frequently. The stimulus may be mechanical, chemical, thermal, or inflammatory, including reactions from infection. There is increasing evidence that alteration of the surface epithelium of the major airways, into which the terminal filaments of irritant receptors are inserted, exposes the receptors more directly or somehow sensitizes them to the effects of stimulants; the cough reflex thus becomes hyper-reactive, and coughing occurs in response to ordinarily innocuous stimuli. When the causes of chronic cough are analyzed, asthma often heads the list. Indeed, chronic nonproductive cough, especially at night, may be the sole presenting complaint of patients who subsequently prove to have bronchial asthma.

COMPLICATIONS. Coughing seems to provoke more coughing. Paroxysms of coughing, as in pertussis, may terminate in vomiting, which seems to break the cycle. Paroxysmal attacks may also terminate in syncope. The mechanism of *cough syncope* is uncertain, but the effects of increased intrathoracic pressure on venous return, cardiac output, and blood flow to the brain are believed to play a role. At times, severe coughing attacks have continued to the point of utter exhaustion. The muscular force developed during coughing may be sufficient to cause occasional fractures of ribs (*cough fractures*) and even compression fractures of vertebral bodies.

DIAGNOSTIC APPROACH. It is difficult to generalize about a condition as common but as varied as coughing. Obviously, many episodes of coughing are innocent and transient. The essential first step in evaluating a patient complaining of cough is to obtain a thorough history with particular attention to the following aspects: (1) acute or chronic, (2) productive or nonproductive, (3) character, (4) time relationships, (5) type and quantity of sputum, and (6) associated features. A specific diagnosis of the cause of chronic intractable cough can be made by history alone in the majority (80 per cent) of patients.

An acute cough is usually associated with viral laryngotracheobronchitis but may signify other bronchopulmonary infections. Less commonly, acute episodes of coughing may be the chief manifestation of the inhalation of various immunologic or irritative substances. A chronic cough is the diagnostic hallmark of chronic bronchitis but also occurs in asthma, tuberculosis, bronchiectasis, and bronchogenic carcinoma. The frequency with which chronic bronchitis and bronchogenic carcinoma coexist, both being a complication of cigarette smoking, has led to the important axiom that *any change in the character or pattern of a chronic cough warrants immediate diagnostic evaluation, with special attention directed toward the detection of bronchogenic carcinoma.*

A productive cough usually implies an underlying inflammatory process, often infectious, whereas a nonproductive cough signifies a mechanical or other irritative stimulus. The character of the cough may be described as "brassy" from major airways involvement or "barking" or "croupy" from laryngeal disease. Paroxysmal coughing with "whoops" is characteristic of pertussis. A cough that occurs mainly at night may accompany congestive cardiac failure; one occurring at meals suggests esophagogastric disease, such as hiatal hernia or diverticulum; and the cough of severe bronchitis or bronchiectasis is often worse upon awakening because of pooling of secretions during sleep. Each of these patterns tends to recur repeatedly under similar circumstances.

A description of the secretions produced in association with cough is diagnostically useful. Foul-smelling sputum indicates anaerobic infection, as in lung abscess or necrotizing pneumonia. Abundant frothy saliva-like sputum is a well known but rare symptom of bronchoalveolar carcinoma. Pink foamy sputum, which is often voluminous, indicates pulmonary edema. In pneumococcal pneumonia, the classic rust-colored or "prune juice"-colored sputum may be observed. The chronic production of copious purulent sputum with intermittent blood streaking, especially on change of postures, is an important clue to bronchiectasis.

The associated features of coughing episodes are of considerable clinical importance: wheezing—a disorder with obstruction to airflow such as asthma; stridor—involvement of the pharynx–larynx–extrathoracic trachea; fever and chills—acute infection; weakness and weight loss—tuberculosis or other chronic infection or malignancy; and recurrent pneumonias—bronchiectasis, foreign body, or obstructing tumor. In view of the importance of cigarette smoking in the pathogenesis of cough, a careful smoking history is crucial to the evaluation of cough.

Physical examination may reveal signs of pulmonary involvement that provide clues to the specific diagnosis. Regardless of the presence or absence of physical findings, evaluation of significant cough entails roentgenographic examination of the chest. When indicated, simple pulmonary function tests will demonstrate abnormalities of airflow and/or lung volumes. In patients whose routine spirometric tests are normal, bronchial provocation studies are indicated. Appropriate studies of sputum, especially culture and cytology, are often the easiest and most direct way of establishing a diagnosis. Fiberoptic bronchoscopy or other special diagnostic tests are sometimes needed.

TREATMENT. The ideal treatment of cough is elimination of its underlying cause. This is possible in most kinds of bronchopulmonary infections by suitable antimicrobial treatment of the responsible microorganism. Cessation of cigarette smoking nearly always eliminates the cough of chronic bronchitis. Disabling, irritative nonproductive cough may be suppressed by an antitussive drug such as codeine, 15 mg every six hours. In contrast, productive cough should not be suppressed because retention of secretions impairs the distribution of inspired air, which worsens gas exchange, and promotes the development of atelectasis and secondary infection. Adequate hydration, not overhydration, is traditionally recommended, although its effect on pulmonary secretions is difficult to substantiate. Expectorants and ultrasonic aerosols have not been shown to be beneficial. When secretions are difficult to raise because of their physical properties and/or ineffective coughing, respiratory physical therapy with postural drainage and percussion may be helpful and a trial is warranted.

HEMOPTYSIS

Regardless of whether the sputum is grossly bloody or merely blood streaked, the expectoration of any blood whatsoever denotes hemoptysis. Patients with chronic bronchitis may produce faintly blood-tinged sputum from time to time, but apart from this exception every patient with hemoptysis deserves a thorough diagnostic workup. A substantial proportion of all patients who expectorate bloody sputum have a serious disease; approximate figures indicate bronchogenic carcinoma 20 to 30 per cent; bronchiectasis 20 to 30 per cent; bronchitis 10 to 20 per cent; and other inflammatory disorders, including tuberculosis, 10 to 20 per cent. Other conditions that may present with hemoptysis include pulmonary embolism, mitral stenosis, pulmonary arteriovenous fistula, and Goodpasture's syndrome. All series include an appreciable number (5 to 15 per cent) of undiagnosed cases despite complete investigation.

DIAGNOSTIC APPROACH. The amount of expectorated blood may vary widely, from slight streaking of sputum to massive exsanguinating hemorrhage. The patient may not be aware of the pulmonary origin of the bleeding and often states that the blood "welled up" in his or her throat. For this reason, patients with true hemoptysis may seek the services of an otolaryngologist. Although it is always wise to examine the nasopharynx thoroughly, it is rare that hemoptysis is due to lesions in the upper respiratory tract.

Bleeding of esophageal, gastric, or duodenal origin may be confused with bleeding from the respiratory tract. Hematemesis can usually be differentiated from hemoptysis by the presence of symptoms of gastrointestinal involvement such as nausea and vomiting, a history of peptic ulcer disease or alcoholism, or signs of cirrhosis. Prompt endoscopy will settle the issue in doubtful cases.

Historical and physical examinations may provide clues to the underlying cause of hemoptysis but are seldom diagnostic. Chest roentgenograms, which should be obtained in all patients complaining of hemoptysis, may reveal evidence of old or new inflammatory lesions, probable malignancies, or vascular abnormalities. At times, the underlying lesion may be obscured by the densities caused by the presence of blood itself. Once the bleeding has stopped, however, intra-alveolar blood usually clears within a week so that delayed roentgenographic examinations are often helpful. Routine laboratory evaluation should include a complete blood count and tests to exclude a coagulopathy. It is useful to collect and measure the quantity of blood coughed up.

Virtually every patient with significant hemoptysis should undergo bronchoscopy to determine the site of bleeding and its cause. If bleeding is brisk, the earlier this is done the better. Even if the cause cannot be ascertained during the initial examination, it is important to determine from which bronchus the blood is coming; this is absolutely necessary in patients bleeding massively who are being considered for surgery, but it is also extremely difficult because the tracheobronchial system contains so much blood that it is frequently impossible to identify a bleeding point. The fiberoptic bronchoscope is often used in patients with hemoptysis, but many experts prefer the rigid scope because its larger lumen permits easier aspiration of blood and, when necessary, control of bleeding by packing.

If surgical treatment is a consideration, the origin of the bleeding must be identified each time hemoptysis occurs. Even if a lesion is obvious on chest roentgenographic examination, the patient may be bleeding from an occult site. Similarly, even if a source of blood has been identified on a previous occasion, the blood may come from a different abnormality next time.

TREATMENT. Fortunately, intrapulmonary bleeding usually stops spontaneously. Until it does, the patient should be kept with the affected lung, from which the bleeding is occurring, in the dependent position; the airways should be kept free of blood—coughing may suffice but suction may be necessary; and strong sedatives, which abolish cough, should be avoided, but mild sedatives, to relieve anxiety, are often advisable. A thoracic surgeon should be notified about the problem, and an endotracheal tube and suction apparatus must be ready at the bedside. If massive bleeding suddenly occurs, the tube can be inserted blindly into the right main bronchus and the balloon inflated to separate the two lungs and keep the blood confined to one of them. If circumstances permit, it is even better to put a balloon catheter, under bronchoscopic guidance, into a lobar or segmental bronchus to isolate the blood to as small a region of lung as possible. Blood transfusions are given according to the usual clinical guidelines of quantity of blood lost, hematocrit, blood pressure, pulse rate, and urine output.

After the bleeding stops, the patient should be investigated as outlined to determine the cause of the hemorrhage as well as the extent and severity of the underlying disease(s). Then, in consultation with a thoracic surgeon, a rational decision can be made concerning the need for and likelihood of success of an operation. Ordinarily, localized lesions (e.g., bronchial adenoma or sequestration) are resected and generalized lesions (e.g., widespread bronchiectasis or multiple fistulas) are left alone. However, there is considerable clinical ground between these two extremes and each patient must be considered individually.

An even more difficult problem is the selection of patients with "massive" hemoptysis for emergency pulmonary resection, usually lobectomy but occasionally pneumonectomy. Part of the problem lies in defining what actually constitutes "life-threatening" hemorrhage. Emergency resection in the presence of bleeding from relatively localized, chronic conditions (e.g., broncholithiasis) produces good results; in contrast, in patients hemorrhaging from acute parenchymal infections (e.g., lung abscess), there is a high incidence of postoperative complications. Patients who bleed massively from bronchogenic carcinomas or extensive benign lesions that are nonresectable are particularly difficult; the method of bronchial or intercostal arterial catheterization and embolization with Gelfoam to occlude the bleeding site has been tried with some success in these patients.

CHEST PAIN

Various types of chest pain are extremely common. Chest pain is one of the most frequent symptoms that cause the sufferer to seek medical attention. Because there is no clear relationship between the intensity of the discomfort and the importance of its underlying cause, all complaints of chest pain must be considered carefully. Pain that is virtually diagnostic because of its typical pattern of onset, location, and relation to effort and to respiratory movements is found in pleurisy, intercostal neuritis, costochondral disease, and disorders of the chest wall. The location and character of pain from myocardial ischemia are also characteristic but may be simulated by the pain of acute and chronic pulmonary hypertension. Occasionally, chest pain is elusive and difficult to diagnose, but it must always be taken seriously. A *meticulous history* is essential in evaluating chest pain. From the patient's story alone, a differential diagnosis can be formulated that serves as the basis for subsequent examinations.

MECHANISM. The anatomy, physiology, and biochemistry of pain in the body are reviewed in Ch. 466. Chest pain is no different from other types in that receptors and afferent pathways transmit a stimulus to the central nervous system, where that stimulus is perceived as pain. However, the capacity of various intrathoracic structures to serve as a source of pain differs. The lung parenchyma and the visceral pleura covering it are insensitive to ordinarily painful stimuli. In contrast, pain often accompanies involvement of the parietal pleura, the major airways, the chest wall, the diaphragm, or the mediastinal structures, including the heart. The mechanism of pain in myocardial ischemia is unknown, but the actuating event is clearly an imbalance between myocardial oxygen supply and demand. The pain of pericarditis may be in part related to involvement of the adjacent pleura, thus accounting for the striking respiratory component of what is primarily a cardiac disease. Pain in the esophagus is provoked by stimulation of receptors from acid reflux or muscle spasm.

PLEURAL PAIN. Pleurisy, or acute inflammation of the pleural surfaces, usually causes chest pain that has several distinctive features. The pain is restricted in distribution rather than diffuse, is nearly always on one side or the other, and tends to be distributed along the intercostal nerve zones. Pain from diaphragmatic pleurisy is often referred to the shoulder and side of the neck. The most striking and important characteristic of pleural pain is its clear relationship to respiratory movements. The pain may be variously described as "achy," "sharp," "burning," or simply a "catch," but whatever its designation, it is typically worsened by taking a deep breath, and coughing or sneezing causes intense distress. Patients with pleurisy frequently also complain of dyspnea because the aggravation of their pain during inspiration makes them conscious of every breath. Movement of the trunk, including bending, stooping, or even turning in bed, increases pleural pain, and patients usually find and remain in the position in which movements of the affected region are most restricted.

The rapidity of development of pleural pain provides a clue to its cause. An immediate onset attends pulmonary embolism or spontaneous pneumothorax, a slower but still acute onset over a few hours, especially with fever and cough, accompanies pneumonia, finally, a gradual onset over days or even weeks, often associated with features of chronic illness such as weakness and weight loss, suggests tuberculosis or malignancy.

INTERCOSTAL NEURITIS. The distribution and superficial and knifelike quality of the pain of intercostal neuritis may resemble pleural pain and, sometimes, may even be mistaken for myocardial ischemia. Usually, the pain of intercostal neuritis is worsened by vigorous respiratory movements such as coughing, sneezing, and straining but, unlike pleurisy, not by ordinary breathing. A neuritic origin may be suggested by the presence of lancinating or electric shock sensations unrelated to movements, and hyperalgesia or anesthesia over the distribution of the affected intercostal nerve provides further confirmatory evidence.

COSTOCHONDRAL DISEASE. Pain localized to the costosternal cartilaginous junctions may be confused with other, more serious causes of chest pain. The discomfort is usually described as dull with a gnawing, aching quality; there is little if any relationship to respiratory or other movements, although the pain may be most noticeable when the patient is lying in bed at night. The diagnostic key lies in the fact that there is tenderness to palpation that is clearly localized to one or more of the costal cartilages. There may be redness, swelling, and enlargement of the costal bridges (*Tietze's syndrome*), but the frequency of these is overemphasized. The most common sites of costosternal perichondritis are the second, third, and fourth cartilages, but any part of the large and complex cartilaginous shield along the central and lower portions of the anterior thoracic cage may be involved.

DISORDERS OF THE CHEST WALL. The system of joints, muscles, and fasciae involved in movements of the thoracic wall is complex. Because these structures are in constant motion throughout a person's life, it is surprising that "rheumatic" pains of the chest do not occur more frequently than they do. Fibrositis of the muscle-bone attachments may simultaneously involve the chest wall and other parts of the skeleton. Similarly, spondylitis of the thoracic spine may have its rib cage component, and many less definable skeletal disorders may produce discomfort in the chest. Localized pain in the thoracic cage may be related to unusually severe exercise or motion of the involved area. At times, the abnormality appears to be spontaneous, although even in these cases it is possible that pain was delayed in onset after either injury to the muscles of the chest wall or fractures of ribs during minor trauma or an unnoticed episode of coughing.

PULMONARY HYPERTENSION. The pain of pulmonary hypertension may simulate the pain of myocardial ischemia in its substernal location, its pattern of radiation, and its crushing or constricting quality. This type of pain may occur in patients with acute pulmonary hypertension from multiple and/or massive pulmonary emboli or in patients with chronic pulmonary hypertension from vasculitis or mitral stenosis. The mechanism of the pain is unknown, but it is believed to differ in the acute and chronic varieties. In the former it is related to sudden distention of the main pulmonary artery and stimulation of mechanoreceptors, and in the latter to an imbalance between the oxygen supplied to and utilized by the pressure-overloaded right ventricle. Although substernal pain related to the sudden onset of pulmonary hypertension is a well-recognized complication of pulmonary embolism, more commonly emboli cause pain in the lateral part of the chest that is typically pleuritic in character whether or not they produce pulmonary infarction.

MYOCARDIAL ISCHEMIA. Among the most important types of chest pain is that of myocardial ischemia, which is usually caused by coronary artery atherosclerosis (see Ch.

51). These attacks are provoked by an imbalance, which may be transient or permanent, between the supply of and demand for oxygen by the ventricular myocardium. Ischemic pain spans a continuum of severity from angina pectoris on the one hand to myocardial infarction on the other. Typical anginal pain is induced by exercise, heavy meals, and emotional upsets, the pain is usually described as a substernal "pressure," "constriction," or "squeezing" that, when intense, may radiate to the neck or down the ulnar aspect of one or both arms. Variant or Prinzmetal's anginal pain is similar in location and quality to typical angina pectoris but occurs in cycles at rest rather than during stressful episodes. Both typical and variant types of angina pectoris are relieved by coronary vasodilatory drugs such as nitroglycerin. Typical angina also decreases with rest or removing the inciting stress. In contrast, the pain of myocardial infarction, although similar in location and character to anginal pain, is usually of greater intensity and duration, is not alleviated by rest or by nitroglycerin, may require large doses of opiates, and is often accompanied by diaphoresis, nausea, hypotension, and arrhythmias. Although patients are often short of breath during attacks of myocardial ischemia, and myocardial infarction may induce severe pulmonary edema, the pain itself is neither related to breathing nor affected by respiratory movements.

OTHER SOURCES. Pericarditis causes pain that is usually pleuritic in nature but may be steady and substernal, typically, the pain is worse while the patient is recumbent or lying on the left side. Dissecting aneurysm of the aorta is associated with severe, unremitting anterior chest pain that often radiates through to the back or into the abdomen. A deep substernal pain may result from esophageal reflux or spasm or from spontaneous mediastinal emphysema. Finally, psychogenic disorders may be associated with various forms of chest pain, the most common of which is a substernal tightness or aching sensation that may last from 30 minutes to several days. The pain may vary somewhat in intensity from time to time, and the ancillary features of myocardial infarction and a respiratory component are absent.

DIAGNOSTIC APPROACH. The approach to the general problem of the diagnosis of chest pain varies according to how seriously ill the patient is when first seen. Patients with acute chest pain who are gravely ill, as evidenced by hypotension, intense dyspnea, profuse diaphoresis, agitation, and restlessness, are usually evaluated first in the emergency room. The chief diagnostic considerations in this common clinical complex are myocardial infarction, pulmonary embolism, and dissecting aneurysm, less likely possibilities are tension pneumothorax, pericardial tamponade, and ruptured esophagus. An initial tentative diagnosis can usually be made from the results of careful historical and physical examinations, supplemented by an electrocardiogram and chest roentgenograms. Except when the electrocardiogram reveals clear evidence of acute myocardial ischemia, definitive diagnosis depends on the results of later studies such as ventilation-perfusion lung scans, pulmonary angiography, aortography, serial enzyme determinations, and coronary artery catheterization.

Patients with less severe chest pain may present during an episode of pain or afterward. Again, a detailed history of the character and behavior of the pain provides the best guide for the selection of subsequent diagnostic studies. Most patients will require an electrocardiogram, ideally taken during an episode of pain, and chest roentgenograms; then, based on the results of these examinations, diagnostic evaluation proceeds as needed for the particular entities under consideration.

TREATMENT. The treatment of chest pain depends on its cause. Anginal pain responds to coronary artery vasodilator drugs, whereas myocardial infarction usually requires opiates, often in large doses. Pleural pain responds to analgesics, given as required. However, pleurisy in association with pneumonia may be alleviated by anti-inflammatory drugs such as indomethacin; in refractory cases, intercostal nerve block is needed. For costochondral and other types of chest wall pain, mild analgesia, reassurance, and time usually suffice; rapid relief can be obtained, when necessary, by injection of local anesthetic agents into the involved area.

DYSPNEA

When healthy persons undertake a steadily increasing amount of physical activity, they will eventually become aware of their breathing; the exercise required to provoke this sensation depends on their physical fitness. If they increase the level of activity even further, the awareness will increase as the sensation becomes progressively more unpleasant; if they stop exercising, the feeling will quickly disappear. The sensation experienced by normal subjects during physical exertion is aptly described as "shortness of breath" but not as dyspnea. The term dyspnea implies that the awareness is disproportionate to the stimulus and, moreover, that the sensation is abnormally uncomfortable. Many patients will describe their breathing discomfort as "breathlessness," but many others will complain only of "tightness," "choking," "inability to take a deep breath," "suffocating," and simply "can't get enough air." Thus dyspnea is difficult to define precisely and it is impossible to quantify. As with the evaluation of chest pain, a thorough history is required to explore all the vagaries of this elusive symptom.

MECHANISM. It is impossible to find a common mechanism for what appears to be the same or similar sensation of difficulty in breathing that may occur in respiratory, cardiac, erythropoietic, metabolic, and psychogenic disorders. Dyspnea in patients with respiratory diseases is believed to have a reflex origin and thus must begin with stimulation of receptors in one or more of the organs concerned with breathing. There are three types of intrapulmonary receptors (stretch, irritant, and C-fibers, which include the J- and probably other receptors), each of which has its afferent pathway to the central nervous system in the vagus nerve. There are also receptors in the muscles and tendons that participate in breathing, and chemoreceptors are situated in systemic arteries and the brain. The theory of "length-tension inappropriateness" postulates that misalignment of muscle spindles in the respiratory musculature serves as the genesis of dyspnea. Perhaps the best explanation is that dyspnea is the subjective perception of the intensity of the stimuli that are generated by *all* the receptors activated during or in association with the act of breathing.

PATTERNS. Dyspnea occurs with many underlying conditions and in several different patterns. Some of these are sufficiently characteristic to warrant separate designations. Episodes of breathlessness that wake patients from a sound sleep are called *paroxysmal nocturnal dyspnea;* these are most often observed in patients with chronic left ventricular failure but may also occur in patients with chronic pulmonary diseases because of pooling of secretions, gravity-induced decreases in lung volumes, or sleep-induced increases in airflow resistance. *Orthopnea,* or the onset or worsening of dyspnea on assuming the supine position, like paroxysmal nocturnal dyspnea, is found in patients with heart disease and occasionally in patients with chronic lung disease. The inability to assume the supine position (instant orthopnea) is particularly characteristic of the rare condition of paralysis of both hemidiaphragms. *Platypnea* denotes dyspnea that occurs in the upright position and *trepopnea* the even rarer form of dyspnea that develops in either the right or left lateral decubitus position. Both the terms *hyperpnea,* an increase in minute volume, and *hyperventilation,* an increase in alveolar ventilation in excess of carbon dioxide production, indicate that ventilation is increased above normal. However, neither term carries any implication about the presence or absence of dyspnea.

DIAGNOSTIC APPROACH. The differential diagnosis of the dyspneic patient begins with a careful history. In patients with chronic respiratory or cardiac disease, dyspnea initially develops only during physical activity, and the amount of exertion required to provoke the symptom relates in a general way to the severity of the underlying condition. Sudden episodes of dyspnea, unrelated to physical activity, typically occur with pulmonary embolism, spontaneous pneumothorax, and anxiety; the acute attacks in each of these disorders characteristically remit, but bouts of breathlessness may recur with varying severity.

The results of historical and physical examinations, routine blood tests, electrocardiography, and chest roentgenography nearly always indicate whether the dyspneic patient is suffering from a respiratory, cardiac, hematologic, renal, or hepatic abnormality. Special diagnostic studies are often then required to determine what specific kind of disease is present. Measurements of lung volumes, expiratory flow rates, and diffusing capacity, studies during exercise, and noninvasive tests of cardiac function are particularly valuable in three difficult clinical situations: (1) differentiating between dyspnea of cardiac and pulmonary origin and, if abnormalities of both systems coexist, as is often the case, estimating the severity of each; (2) identifying the presence of either pulmonary vascular obstructive disease or diffuse pulmonary infiltrative disorders in dyspneic patients whose routine studies, including chest roentgenograms, are normal; and (3) helping to establish, by ruling out significant cardiorespiratory abnormalities, that dyspnea in a given patient is psychogenic in origin (a diagnosis that is always tenuous).

TREATMENT. Unlike cough, for which there are effective antitussives, and pain, for which there are powerful analgesics, there is no category of medications for relief of dyspnea. Cure or alleviation of dyspnea depends on recognizing its origin and treating the basic abnormality. In acute reversible conditions, the dyspnea subsides along with improvement of its underlying cause. In chronic cardiac and pulmonary disorders, sufficient physical exertion will continue to provoke dyspnea, but even in these conditions rehabilitation programs can be used to enable patients to increase their physical activity up to the maximum of the limits imposed by their disease.

CONCLUSION

This introduction to the three most common and important symptoms of *all* diseases of the respiratory system is meant to supplement the material presented not only in the remainder of Part VII but also elsewhere in the book. Acute infections of the upper and lower respiratory tract caused by viruses, bacteria, fungi, protozoa, and helminths are discussed in Parts XVIII and XIX. Systemic diseases in which the lungs may be involved are also discussed elsewhere: Wegener's granulomatosis (Ch. 441), eosinophilic syndromes (Ch. 162), and the "collagen diseases" (Ch. 429 to 455). Various abnormalities of the pulmonary circulation, exclusive of pulmonary embolism, and pulmonary edema, an important disorder (not disease) of the lungs, are discussed chiefly in Part VI.

Adelman M, Haponik EF, Bleeker ER, et al.: Cryptogenic hemoptysis: Clinical features, bronchoscopic findings and natural history in 67 patients. Ann Intern Med 102:829, 1985. *Review of workup and outcome in patients with hemoptysis and no initial diagnosis; known causes discussed as well.*

Altose MD: Assessment and management of breathlessness. Chest 88(suppl):77S, 1985. *Brief but thorough discussion of current theories about the mechanisms of dyspnea.*

Schneider RR, Seckler SG: Evaluation of acute chest pain. Med Clin North Am 65:53, 1981. *Comprehensive description of pain arising from different organs within the thorax; 75 references.*

Stulbarg M: Evaluating and treating intractable cough. Medical Staff Conference, University of California, San Francisco. West J Med 143:223, 1985. *Excellent review of the pathophysiology, causes, diagnosis, and management of intractable cough; 49 references.*

59 RESPIRATORY STRUCTURE AND FUNCTION

John F. Murray

Respiration can be defined as "those processes concerned with gas exchange between an organism and its environment." This definition, which emphasizes that the chief function of the respiratory system is *gas exchange*, is sufficiently comprehensive to apply to all animals, ranging from simple one-celled protozoa to infinitely more complex mammals. In human beings, the basic processes leading to gas exchange, or the uptake of O_2 and the elimination of CO_2, are usually separated into four functional subdivisions:

1. *Ventilation*—the movement of air from outside to inside the body and the distribution of air within the tracheobronchial system to the gas exchange units of the lungs.

2. *Diffusion*—the movement of O_2 and CO_2 across the alveolar-capillary membrane between the gas in alveolar spaces and the blood in pulmonary capillaries.

3. *Perfusion*—the flow of mixed venous blood through the pulmonary arterial circulation, distribution of the blood to the capillaries of the gas exchange units, and removal of the blood from the lungs through pulmonary veins.

4. *Control of breathing*—the regulation of ventilation, usually in accordance with changing metabolic demands.

VENTILATION

Air moves from outside the body into the gas exchange units of the lungs because contraction of the muscles of respiration normally generates sufficient force to expand the lungs and chest wall and to overcome the resistance and inertia in the system. Accordingly, the volume of gas that reaches the individual gas exchange units is determined by the mechanical properties of the lung parenchyma, airways, and chest wall, and by the force provided by the muscles of respiration (or by a mechanical ventilator).

The amount of air that enters the lung with each breath is called the *tidal volume*. When the lungs are fully expanded, the amount of gas they contain is called the *total lung capacity*. The maximal volume of gas that a person can exhale from total lung capacity is called the *vital capacity*, and the amount of gas remaining in the lungs at the end of maximal expiration

is called the *residual volume*. Another important static lung volume is the *functional residual capacity*, which is the volume of gas in the lungs at the end of a normal breath. The relationships among these different lung volumes, which vary in different disorders and which will be frequently referred to, are shown in Figure 59–1.

Static Properties

Both the lungs and chest wall are elastic structures. This means that they can be distended and, when the distending force is removed, they recoil back to their resting volumes. Although the lungs and chest wall are similar in this respect, they differ considerably in their respective resting volumes when there is no expanding force.

The elastic properties of isolated lungs are shown by the dashed line in Figure 59–1. The slope of the line, or the change in volume (ΔV) for a given change in pressure (ΔP), is known as the compliance of the lungs. This curve demonstrates that (1) the lungs collapse almost completely when there is no distending pressure, (2) the slope of the volume-pressure curve is relatively steep at low lung volumes (i.e., as the lungs are beginning to inflate, their compliance is high), and (3) at high lung volumes, the curve flattens (compliance decreases) so that little increase in volume results from a large increase in pressure. The elastic forces of the lungs originate within the tissues that are being stretched, particularly those containing elastin and collagen, and from the surface tension of the film of *surfactant* that lines the air-liquid interface of alveolar spaces. The static properties of the isolated chest wall (including the diaphragm and abdominal contents that must be displaced during breathing) are shown by the solid light red line in Figure 59–1. The chest wall is a compressible and distensible structure that contains an appreciable volume in its resting state. To decrease the volume of the thorax, a force must be applied to overcome the tendency of the chest wall to resist compression and recoil back to its resting position. Conversely, to increase the volume of the thorax, the applied force must overcome the elastic forces in the chest wall that also cause it to recoil back to its resting position.

It is useful conceptually to consider the behavior of the lungs and chest wall separately, but obviously they function together. Because their action is coupled by the pleural pressure that keeps each lung expanded against the chest wall, the lungs and chest wall ordinarily change their volumes by exactly the same amount. Thus the pressures required to change the volume of the respiratory system are obtained by simply adding the separate pressures necessary to inflate the

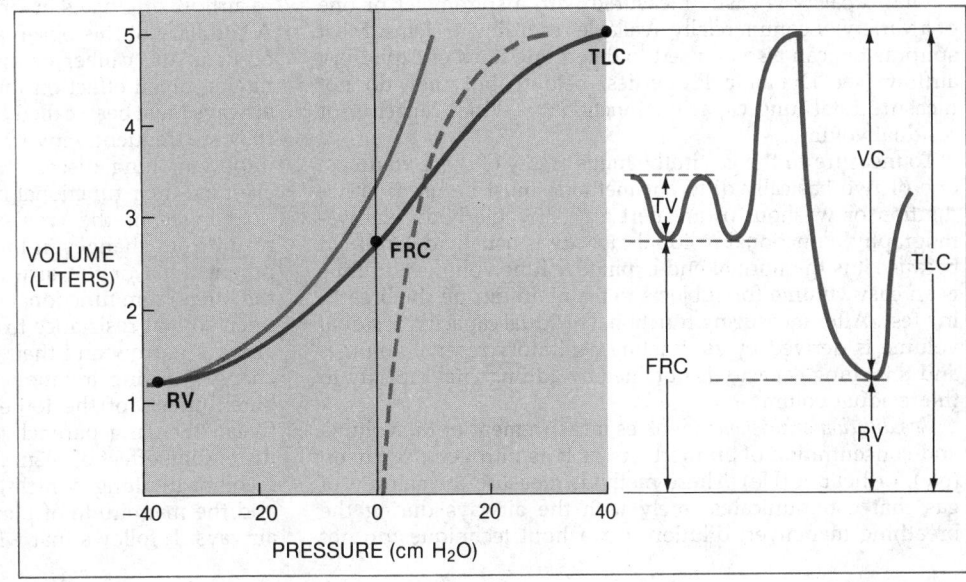

FIGURE 59–1. Schematic representation of the volume-pressure relationships of the chest wall (*solid light red line*), lungs (*dashed light red line*), and chest wall and lungs combined (*solid dark red line*). Total lung capacity (TLC) occurs when the lungs are fully expanded, and residual volume (RV) is the amount of gas remaining in the lungs at the end of a maximal expiration. Functional residual capacity (FRC) occurs at that volume at which the recoil pressures of the chest wall and lung are equal and opposite (i.e., the distending pressure = 0 cm H_2O). On the right is a spirometric tracing (volume-time) of the breathing maneuvers of the person whose pressure-volume curves are on the left. TV = Tidal volume; VC = vital capacity.

lungs and chest wall to a given volume. The solid line in Figure 59–1 indicates the pressure that must be produced by contraction of the respiratory muscles, or by a mechanical ventilator, to inflate or deflate both the lungs and chest wall. Figure 59–1 also shows that functional residual capacity is the volume at which the inward recoil force of the lungs is equal and opposite to the outward recoil force of the chest wall; in other words, functional residual capacity is that volume at which the net force of the respiratory system is zero.

During inspiration, the force developed by the contracting muscles of inspiration meets progressively increasing (inward) recoil forces from the combined expansion of the lungs and chest wall. Furthermore, because shortening muscle fibers generate progressively less force, inspiration finally ceases at that volume (total lung capacity) at which the weakening inspiratory muscle forces can no longer overcome the increasing forces required to expand the lungs and chest wall. Similarly, during expiration, the net force developed by the contracting muscles of expiration meets progressively increasing (outward) recoil forces from the chest wall. In children and young adults, expiration ceases at that volume (residual volume) at which the decreasing expiratory muscle forces can no longer overcome the increasing forces required to compress the chest wall. In older persons, residual volume is governed mainly by factors that regulate the caliber and patency of peripheral airways; thus even though the expiratory muscles are capable of further compression of the thorax, emptying is prevented by airway closure and trapping of gas in the lungs.

Vital capacity, or the volume between total lung capacity and residual volume, is determined by the factors that influence maximum inspiration and expiration, i.e., the balance of forces generated by the muscles of respiration and by the mechanical properties of the lungs and chest wall combined. Changes in these variables explain the characteristic changes in lung volumes that occur in patients with the respiratory disorders discussed in subsequent chapters.

Lung volumes also vary among healthy persons according to their age, sex, and physical structure (especially height). Because body build varies slightly from one ethnic group to another, it is important to have normal data that pertain to the population being studied. Measured volumes are usually expressed as both the observed value and the percentage of the predicted mean value for a normal subject of the same age, sex, and height. Measured values should not be considered abnormal unless they are clearly outside the range of values likely to be found in normal persons (100 per cent ± 20 per cent for vital capacity and 100 per cent ± 25 per cent for total lung capacity, residual volume, and functional residual capacity).

Vital capacity is easily measured with a spirometer or one of a variety of commercially available recording systems. Most spirometers can also be used to determine rates of expiratory airflow (see Dynamic Properties, below), but they do not measure total lung capacity, functional residual capacity, or residual volume.

To measure *all* the gas in the lungs at any of these volumes, one of two basically different methods must be used: either dilution or washout of an inert gas or whole body plethysmography. Functional residual capacity is usually determined because it is the normal end-expiratory lung volume and thus is an easy volume for subjects to maintain during the breathing test. After measuring functional residual capacity, residual volume is derived by subtracting expiratory reserve volume, and total lung capacity is obtained by adding vital capacity to the residual volume.

Gas dilution or washout involves measurement of the volume and concentration of an inert gas such as nitrogen (N_2), neon (Ne), or helium (He). These methods measure the amount of gas that communicates freely with the airways during the breathing maneuver; dilution or washout techniques do not detect gas trapped beyond closed (or very narrowed) airways and in poorly communicating regions, like bullae.

Body plethysmography involves placing the subject in the plethysmograph, a large airtight box resembling a telephone booth, and having him or her breathe through a mouthpiece in which a shutter can be closed to stop the flow of air. When the subject attempts to pant against the closed shutter, the volume of the thorax and gas in the lungs expands and contracts, which changes the pressure measured inside the mouthpiece. Movement of the thorax also changes the pressure in the box by compressing and expanding the gas surrounding the subject. From application of Boyle's law, which states that the pressure times the volume of a gas is constant if temperature remains the same, the volume of gas in the thorax can be calculated. The body plethysmograph measures all the gas present during the breathing maneuver, including that in freely communicating airspaces *and* any that may be trapped behind poorly communicating airways or in closed spaces (pneumothorax).

In normal subjects, measurements of functional residual capacity by dilution (or washout) and plethysmographic techniques are virtually identical. In contrast, in patients with airways obstruction or bullous disease, the communicating volume may be considerably less than the plethysmographic volume and the difference is a measure of the noncommunicating (sometimes called trapped) volume.

Dynamic Properties

To cause air to flow from outside the body into the gas exchange units, a muscular (or other mechanical) force must be exerted to overcome not only the elastic recoil properties of the lungs and chest wall but also their resistive and inertial properties. In contrast to distensibility, which is not affected by the rate of movement, the forces required to offset resistance and inertia are markedly influenced by the velocity of airflow. Except in a few patients (e.g., those with severe obesity), inertial forces are ordinarily small and usually ignored, thus only those factors affecting airways resistance need be considered in detail.

Resistance to airflow is affected chiefly by the caliber of the air passages. Although the diameter of each successive generation of airways decreases, the combined total cross-sectional area at any level increases steadily throughout the tracheobronchial tree from the main bronchi to the peripheral airways. This means that airways resistance progressively decreases and that most of the resistance of the human tracheobronchial tree resides in large airways: direct measurements reveal that between 50 and 80 per cent of total resistance to airflow originates in airways *greater than* 2 mm in diameter. A corollary of this observation is that substantial changes can occur in the caliber of the small peripheral airways without having much effect on total airways resistance. Hence, small airways have been called the lung's "quiet zone," and because they are frequently involved early in the evolution of clinically important lung disease, special tests have been devised to examine their functional behavior.

Changes in the cross-sectional area of airways can also result from changes in lung volume and diseases of the lung parenchyma or the airways themselves. During inflation of the lungs from functional residual capacity, airways are pulled open so that resistance to airflow decreases; during deflation, airways narrow and their resistance increases. Airway caliber changes during inflation and deflation because of the combined effects of the tethering action of the attachments between the lung parenchyma and small bronchioles and the distending effect of pleural pressure on larger airways. Elastic recoil of the lung, which governs the pull of the attachments and the magnitude of pleural pressure, affects the size of all airways. It follows that when elastic recoil is decreased, as in patients with emphysema, airways are narrowed and resistance is increased, this mechanism accounts for much of the airflow obstruction found in patients with emphysema.

Airway narrowing can also result from bronchospasm, edema of the mucosal lining, and secretions within the lumen. Also, changes in the viscosity and density of the inspired gas affect airways resistance, and gas mixtures of different densities are sometimes used to study the dynamic properties of the tracheobronchial system.

Resistance to airflow can be measured in a body plethysmograph; however, this procedure has limited clinical usefulness. Fortunately, the important dynamic properties of the respiratory system can be assessed by several readily available tests of airways function. The simplest and most widely used of these is the forced expiratory volume in one second (FEV_1), expressed as a ratio of the forced vital capacity (FVC), or FEV_1/FVC (Fig. 59–2). To perform the FVC maneuver, the subject inhales fully and then exhales as rapidly and completely as possible. In normal persons, the FVC equals the vital capacity from a slow or nonexpulsive maneuver, but in patients with airways obstruction, vigorous expiration may cause airways to narrow and close prematurely so that the FVC may be less than the vital capacity; the magnitude of the difference between the two values is an indication of the amount of air trapped behind compressed airways. The FEV_1/FVC decreases with age in normal persons after reaching adulthood and is usually higher in women than in men at all ages.

Additional measurements of airways behavior besides the FEV_1 can be obtained from the FVC maneuver (Fig. 59–2): several derivatives of time such as the $FEV_{0.5}$ and FEV_3 (the subscript denoting the number of seconds after beginning expiration at which the expired volume is measured), the maximal expiratory flow rate (MEFR or often $MEFR_{200-1200\ ml}$, indicating that the flow rate was measured between expired volumes of 200 and 1200 ml), and the maximal mid-expiratory flow rate (MMFR or often $MMFR_{25-75\%}$, indicating that the rate

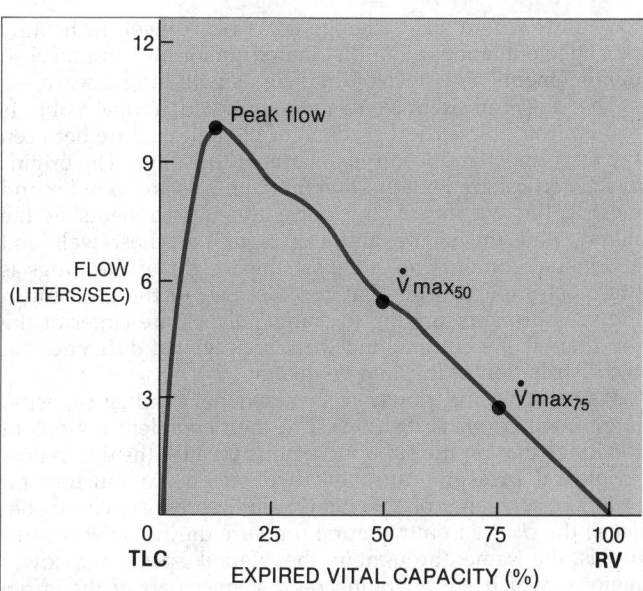

FIGURE 59–3. Typical forced expiratory flow-volume tracing of a normal adult man showing points of peak flow, maximal flow at 50 per cent expired vital capacity ($\dot{V}max_{50}$) and maximal flow at 75 per cent expired vital capacity ($\dot{V}max_{75}$). TLC = total lung capacity, RV = residual volume. (From Smith LH, Thier SO: Pathophysiology. The Biological Principles of Disease. Philadelphia, W. B. Saunders Company, 1981.)

was measured between expired volumes of 25 and 75 per cent of the FVC). None of these has any particular advantage over the FEV_1 except that the MMFR is less dependent on the effort exerted by the subject than the other variables and reflects the flow properties of small as well as large airways.

Another way of examining the events during an FVC maneuver is by recording flow against volume instead of volume against time, which provides a maximal expiratory flow–volume curve (Fig. 59–3). From these records, maximal flow rates at any given fraction of the expired vital capacity, usually 50 per cent ($\dot{V}max_{50}$) or 75 per cent ($\dot{V}max_{75}$), can be determined and reported as the percentage of the predicted values for a subject of the same age, sex, and body size. The early portion of the maximal expiratory flow–volume curve, which includes peak flow, is determined by the effort exerted by the subject and is thus called the effort-*dependent* segment; the later portion is less influenced by effort and is called the effort-*independent* segment or that part of the curve during which expiratory airflow limitation occurs. Additional effort does not increase expiratory airflow (i.e., maximal velocity is limited), because "choke points" develop in those airways in which the velocity of airflow has increased to equal the speed at which pressures will propagate along the airways. Because events recorded in the effort-independent portion of the flow-volume curve require less cooperation and understanding by the subject, they are more reproducible than those in the effort-dependent portion.

Maximal expiratory flow-volume curves can also be recorded after a few breaths of 79 per cent He and 21 per cent O_2 (He-O_2) as well as after breathing room air (79 per cent N_2 and 21 per cent O_2). Although much has been learned about the behavior of the airways by comparing the curves obtained with the two gas mixtures, these tests have not proved as reliable as originally believed in detecting disease localized to peripheral (small) airways.

Distribution of Ventilation

During the movement of air from outside the body into the lungs during inhalation, the airstream is partitioned as it flows through the branching airways to the terminal respira-

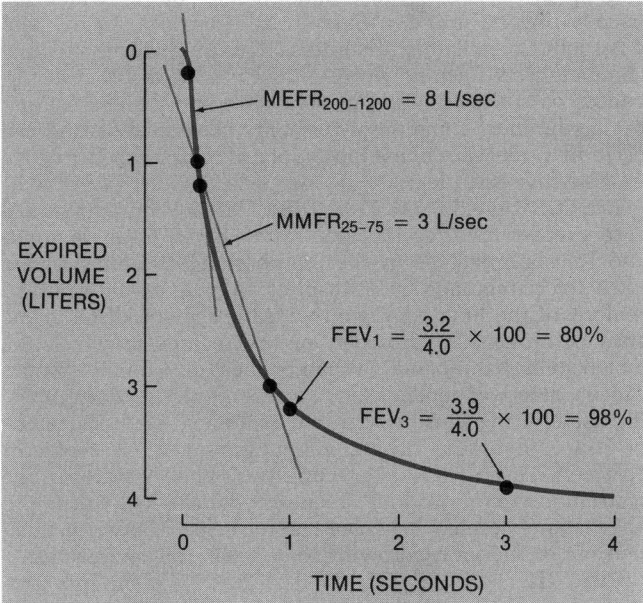

FIGURE 59–2. Schematic representation of a normal forced vital capacity (FVC) maneuver (expired volume against time, *heavy red line*) and the derivation of several variables commonly used to evaluate airways obstruction. $MEFR_{200-1200}$ = maximal expiratory flow rate, measured between expired volumes of 200 and 1200 ml, $MMER_{25-75}$ = maximal mid-expiratory flow rate, measured between 25 and 75 per cent of the total FVC, FEV_1 = forced expiratory volume in one second, expressed as percentage of total FVC, FEV_3 = forced expiratory volume in three seconds, expressed as percentage of total FVC.

tory units where gas exchange takes place. Even in healthy persons ventilation is not distributed uniformly, and marked derangements may develop in patients with lung disease.

The unevenness of ventilation found in normal subjects results from the vertical gradient of pleural pressure between the uppermost and lowermost parts of the lungs. The origins of the vertical gradient in different mammals are complex and include the weight of the lungs, their attachments at the hilum, and the shape and effects of the chest wall and abdominal contents, in humans, the weight of the lungs is the most important determinant. Because of the gradient in the pressure surrounding the lungs, alveoli are larger at the top than at the bottom, and there are regional differences in the distribution of inspired ventilation.

When breathing slowly from functional residual capacity, more inspired air is distributed to the dependent regions of the lungs than to the superior regions because the differences in pleural pressure cause the two regions to function on different segments of the same volume-pressure curve. Because the *change* in intrapleural pressure during quiet breathing is the same throughout the pleural space, the lower regions, which are operating on a steeper part of the curve and thus receive more volume for the same pressure change, inflate more than the upper regions. When inspiration continues to total lung capacity, alveoli at the top and bottom of the lungs inflate to nearly the same size because both regions are functioning on the flat portion of the volume-pressure curve even though the pleural pressure difference persists. When the rate of inspiratory airflow increases, as during exercise, the distribution of ventilation becomes more uniform than it is at rest.

During expiration, pleural pressure surrounding the most dependent portion of each lung becomes positive; this causes airways in that region to close. As expiration continues, airway closure progresses from the lowermost regions up the lungs, involving more and more airways. Regional differences in the distribution of ventilation can be examined by the test of closing volume (Fig. 59–4). After labeling alveolar gas by one of two methods (bolus or resident gas techniques), gas concentration measured at the mouth during the subsequent exhalation varies according to the sequence of regional emptying and occurs in four phases. Phase I reflects the composition of gas from the tracheobronchial system and contains none of the label; the concentration rapidly rises during Phase II as alveoli containing the label begin to empty, a near-plateau is evident in Phase III as alveoli throughout the entire lung deflate; finally, the plateau terminates abruptly with a steep rise in concentration during Phase IV. Closing volume is the junction between Phases III and IV and is that volume at which airways in the dependent regions of the lung begin to close, accordingly, the rising concentration of the label in the subsequent expirate indicates the progressively increasing contributions from the preferentially labeled alveoli in the upper regions of the lung.

Because an increase in closing volume reflects premature closure or narrowing of airways, an increase in closing volume occurs in patients with lung disorders in which the caliber of peripheral airways is decreased from either decreased elastic recoil (e.g., in emphysema) or abnormalities of the airways themselves (e.g., in bronchitis or asthma). Furthermore, increases in closing volume have been detected in asymptomatic patients, usually smokers, and may be an early manifestation of lung disease. In addition, examination of the slope of Phase III is useful because it provides a sensitive measure of the adequacy of the distribution of ventilation. Well-ventilated units fill and empty more completely and rapidly than poorly ventilated units, this means that the concentration of the label will be lower in the better-ventilated regions that empty early during exhalation than in the poorly ventilated regions. Thus, the more uneven the distribution of ventilation within the lung, the steeper the slope of Phase III.

Other tests of the distribution of ventilation utilize the gamma ray–emitting properties of certain radioactive gases, chiefly ^{133}Xe, which are nontoxic and can be detected after inhalation in low concentrations by external counters. The distribution of ventilation can be assessed during a breath hold at end-inspiration after a single breath of ^{133}Xe or at intervals during its elimination by normal breathing after the lung has been labeled uniformly by rebreathing ^{133}Xe from a closed system.

Abnormalities of Ventilation

Lung diseases that cause abnormalities of ventilation are usually divided into two different categories: restrictive and obstructive ventilatory disorders. This classification is not completely satisfactory because it ignores the fact that disturbances of the distribution of ventilation are the earliest and by far the most common abnormality of ventilation and can occur in the absence of manifestations of coexisting obstructive or restrictive disorders.

DISTURBANCES OF DISTRIBUTION. Whenever a disease process involves the lung parenchyma or airways unevenly, abnormalities in the distribution of ventilation are likely to occur because more inspired gas will reach the normal regions of the lung compared with the regions distal to the sites of bronchial narrowing, or the regions in which the distensibility is impaired. Whether these functional changes can be detected depends on the extent and severity of the disease and the sensitivity of the test being used. The slope of Phase III of the closing volume maneuver is the most commonly used test for detecting early abnormalities in the distribution of ventilation. Frequency dependence of compliance is an extremely sensitive test for distribution of ventilation but is seldom used owing to its technical complexities.

RESTRICTIVE VENTILATORY DISORDERS. The term *restrictive ventilatory disorder* denotes a pattern of abnormalities in lung function. The word "restrictive" is employed to indicate a restriction of or limitation to the amount of gas within the lungs. Thus restrictive ventilatory disorders are characterized by reductions in lung volumes (Table 59–1). The hallmark of restriction is a decreased vital capacity, but because this change also occurs in obstructive ventilatory disorders, it is important to exclude the presence of airways obstruction (see Obstructive Ventilatory Disorders, below) or

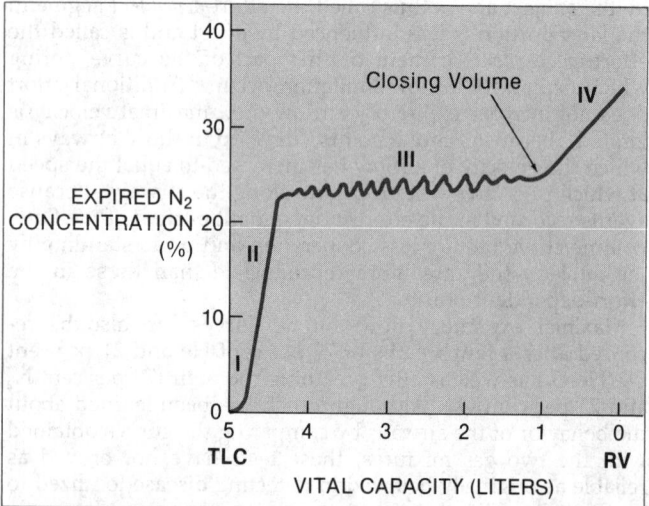

FIGURE 59–4. Representative tracing of expired nitrogen (N₂) concentration after taking a single breath of 100 per cent oxygen. An explanation of the four numbered phases (I, II, III, IV) is provided in the text. TLC = total lung capacity; RV = residual volume. (From Smith LH, Thier SO: Pathophysiology: The Biological Principles of Disease. Philadelphia, W. B. Saunders Company, 1981.)

TABLE 59–1. CHARACTERISTIC CHANGES IN LUNG VOLUMES AND TESTS OF AIRWAYS RESISTANCE IN PATIENTS WITH RESTRICTIVE AND OBSTRUCTIVE VENTILATORY DISORDERS*

Test	Restrictive	Obstructive
Vital capacity	Decreased	Decreased or normal
Residual volume	Decreased	Increased
Total lung capacity	Decreased	Normal or increased
RV/TLC	Normal or slightly increased	Markedly increased
FEV$_1$/FVC	Normal or increased	Decreased
MMFR	Normal or decreased	Decreased
Slope of phase III	Normal or increased	Increased

*Abbreviations: RV/TLC = residual volume to total lung capacity ratio; FEV$_1$/FVC = forced expiratory volume in one second to forced vital capacity ratio; MMFR = maximum mid-expiratory flow rate.

to demonstrate the presence of reductions in other lung volumes, particularly total lung capacity.

Many components of the lungs, chest wall, and respiratory control system determine the amount of gas that can be breathed into the lungs. Accordingly, restrictive ventilatory disorders can develop in diseases that (1) affect the chest wall or respiratory muscles (kyphoscoliosis, myasthenia gravis), (2) cause infiltrations in the lung parenchyma or airspaces (diffuse interstitial fibrosis, pulmonary edema), (3) involve the pleura (pleural thickening), (4) occupy space within the thorax (tumors, effusions, cardiac enlargement), and (5) occur after lung resection (pneumonectomy).

OBSTRUCTIVE VENTILATORY DISORDERS. The term *obstructive ventilatory disorder* denotes the constellation of abnormalities that result from limitation of expiratory airflow, regardless of its cause. Because the functional disturbances depend on the presence of increased airways resistance, obstructive ventilatory disorders are detected mainly by tests of the behavior of the respiratory system under dynamic conditions (Table 59–1). The FEV$_1$/FVC test is the most widely used, but tests of maximal flow-volume relationships are being used increasingly in the *early* diagnosis of airways obstruction, especially when the obstruction is situated in peripheral airways.

Obstructive ventilatory disorders are found in patients with asthma, bronchitis, emphysema, advanced bronchiectasis, or other diseases that cause narrowing of the tracheobronchial system. When the term "obstructive" was originally employed, it was not possible to differentiate among these various entities, so they were lumped together in the nonspecific category of chronic obstructive pulmonary disease. Now, however, it is possible by means of specialized tests of lung function to sort out the various diseases that cause airways obstruction, even when they coexist; the characteristic features of asthma, chronic bronchitis, and emphysema are described in subsequent chapters.

DIFFUSION

Diffusion can be defined as the movement of molecules from a region of higher to one of lower concentration; accordingly, diffusion tends to eliminate differences in concentration within the various regions accessible to the molecules. Diffusion is a passive process that results from the kinetic motion of the molecules, and no extra energy is required. In the lungs, O_2 moves by diffusion from alveolar gas into pulmonary capillary blood; similarly, in the peripheral tissues, O_2 moves by diffusion from capillary blood into neighboring cells. Carbon dioxide also moves by diffusion but usually in the direction opposite to that of O_2. Both O_2 and CO_2 undergo chemical reactions in the bloodstream at the start and finish of their journeys between the lungs and the peripheral tissues; O_2 reacts solely with hemoglobin, and CO_2 reacts in part with hemoglobin and in part to form bicarbonate.

Diffusing Capacity

The diffusing capacity of the lungs or any gas indicates the quantity of that gas that diffuses across the alveolar-capillary membrane per unit time in response to the difference in mean pressures of the gas within the alveolus and pulmonary capillary. Most inert gases (e.g., N_2) diffuse across the air-blood barrier so rapidly that the amount taken up by the lungs is not detectably limited by the diffusibility of the gas and the properties of the lungs and blood but is determined solely by the solubility of the gas and the volume of tissue and blood into which it can dissolve. This phenomenon enables use of highly soluble gases like acetylene, dimethyl ether, or nitrous oxide to measure lung tissue volume and pulmonary capillary blood flow.

The only two gases that can be used to measure the diffusing capacity of the lungs are O_2 and CO. Because of their unique ability to combine with hemoglobin, both have to diffuse across the alveolar-capillary membrane in large quantities to saturate the available hemoglobin at the gas pressure prevailing in the alveoli. Thus it may not be possible for complete equilibrium to occur before the hemoglobin-containing red blood cells leave the pulmonary capillaries and gas transfer ceases. Of the two gases, CO is much more widely used for the measurement of diffusing capacity than O_2 because of the ease and convenience of applying the various CO tests and because CO uptake is always diffusion limited. In contrast, O_2 uptake is not limited by diffusion (i.e., is not a test of diffusing capacity) in normal subjects except during heavy exercise or while breathing low concentrations of O_2.

Two general types of tests using CO are available that involve either a breath-holding maneuver (single-breath method) or continuous rebreathing (steady-state methods). These two methods yield systemically different results, largely because neither technique summarizes accurately the events taking place in the 100,000 gas exchange units of the lung, in each of which P_{CO} varies according to the ventilation and blood flow to the unit. Despite this shortcoming, measurements of pulmonary diffusing capacity have provided useful empiric information concerning the function of the lungs in healthy persons and patients with lung diseases.

The quantity of CO that will diffuse in a known period of time from alveolar gas into capillary blood and combine with hemoglobin in response to a given pressure difference between gas and blood depends on (1) the solubility and diffusibility of CO in each layer of the air-blood barrier, (2) the surface area and thickness of the barrier, and (3) the rate of the chemical reaction between CO and hemoglobin within red blood cells. Because the solubility and diffusibility of CO are physical characteristics that presumably do not change under ordinary circumstances, the two chief components of diffusing capacity are the area and thickness of the alveolar-capillary membrane available for diffusion (D_M) and the pulmonary capillary blood volume (Vc), both of which can be derived by performing several measurements of diffusing capacity (DL_{CO}) with the subject breathing gas mixtures of different concentrations of CO and O_2.

Normal values for CO-diffusing capacity depend chiefly on the person's lung volume and therefore closely correlate with body size, especially height. Approximately half the total resistance to diffusion of CO from alveolar gas to capillary blood resides in the membrane compartment and the other half in the chemical reaction that takes place in the pulmonary capillary blood volume. Accordingly, changes in the hemoglobin concentration have a calculable effect on total CO diffusion that should be taken into account when establishing the predicted "normal" value for a patient with anemia or polycythemia.

Diffusing capacity is normally higher in the supine than the erect posture because position changes the volume of blood in pulmonary capillaries, and at high compared with low lung volumes because inflation recruits alveolar-capillary surface. When blood flow to the lung increases, as in muscular exercise, capillary blood volume also increases owing to recruitment of previously nonperfused capillaries and dilatation of others; these phenomena account for the progressive increase in DL_{CO} during increasingly strenuous levels of exercise. Similarly, the elevated pulmonary arterial pressures encountered in persons who live at high altitudes also recruit capillaries, increase capillary blood volume, and cause an increase in "normal" DL_{CO}. For unexplained reasons (possibly genetic), natives of high altitudes have higher DL_{CO} values than sojourners fully acclimatized to the same altitude.

Abnormalities of CO-Diffusing Capacity

On the basis of the physiologic principles that govern the diffusion of CO, it can be inferred that DL_{CO} may increase or decrease in patients with various cardiopulmonary disorders that affect the membrane, the capillary blood volume, or both. When tests of diffusing capacity were first used to study patients with various forms of lung disease, it was assumed that abnormalities of gas transfer would result from thickening of the air-blood barrier by a pathologic process that lengthened the pathway for diffusion of gases; this concept led to the formulation of what became widely known as the *alveolar-capillary block syndrome*. The "block" meant that the distance CO molecules had to travel from gas to blood was increased and, in turn, that extra time was required for diffusion to reach equilibrium across the air-blood barrier. Now it is known that the importance of alveolar-capillary block has been greatly exaggerated because a decreased diffusing capacity is not a satisfactory cause for arterial hypoxia, especially in patients at rest; when a low Po_2 occurs, it is nearly always attributable to a ventilation-perfusion abnormality, or less often to a right-to-left shunt.

Pulmonary vascular disorders, such as pulmonary emboli and pulmonary vasculitis, that affect (directly or indirectly) the pulmonary capillary bed decrease DL by decreasing capillary blood volume. Similarly, DL_{CO} is reduced in patients with infiltrative disorders of the interalveolar septum that obliterate or destroy capillaries. This is the usual mechanism underlying reduction of DL_{CO} in patients with sarcoidosis, diffuse interstitial fibrosis, berylliosis, or collagen diseases of the lung.

Changes in the characteristics of the membrane account for a decreased DL_{CO} in patients with diseases in which some form of intra-alveolar filling process has occurred and the air-to-blood diffusion pathway is actually lengthened: pneumonia, pulmonary edema, alveolar proteinosis. A decrease in both membrane and blood volume components produces a low DL_{CO} in patients with disorders associated with removal or destruction of lung tissue, such as resectional surgery or emphysema.

An increase in DL_{CO} results occasionally from an increase in capillary blood volume secondary to hemodynamic changes in the pulmonary circulation: an increase in pulmonary arterial or left atrial pressures, as in congestive heart failure, or an increase in pulmonary blood flow, as in atrial septal defect. The DL_{CO} is sometimes increased in patients with bronchial asthma during an attack, but the cause of this change is not known.

PERFUSION

The pulmonary circulation delivers blood in a thin film to the gas exchange units so that O_2 uptake and CO_2 elimination can occur. The physiologic determinants of pulmonary blood flow are analogous to those of ventilation in that the total volumes of ventilation and blood flow must be adequate to meet metabolic needs, and the distribution of both must be such that proportionate amounts of inspired fresh air and incoming mixed venous blood are delivered to individual gas exchange units. Ventilatory volume is controlled by the factors that regulate breathing (see below), whereas the volume of blood flowing through the lungs is determined mainly by the extrapulmonary mechanisms that govern cardiac output.

Distribution of Pulmonary Blood Flow

Pulmonary blood flow is not distributed uniformly throughout the lungs but is normally greatest in the dependent regions where pulmonary arterial pressure is highest and, conversely, is least in the superior regions where pulmonary arterial pressure is lowest. In the upright subject under resting conditions, the apices of the lungs are barely perfused and considerably more blood flows, even allowing for differences in the amount of lung tissue, to the basilar regions. The presence of nonuniform blood flow, which is not matched by comparable changes in ventilation, leads to important differences between regions of the lung in their defense capabilities and efficiency of gas exchange.

Regional blood flow is also governed by local factors, the most important of which is vasoconstriction secondary to alveolar hypoxia. As a consequence, blood flow is redistributed away from poorly ventilated gas exchange units and the matching of ventilation and perfusion is preserved.

Distribution of pulmonary blood flow can readily be measured by injecting radioactive substances, such as ^{125}I-albumin aggregates or ^{133}Xe dissolved in saline, and then detecting their location in the lung with an external counter system. Abnormalities in the volume and distribution of pulmonary blood flow may result from diseases that involve the blood vessels themselves (emboli, vasculitis, emphysema), from compression of blood vessels (tumors, cysts), or from vasoconstriction of blood vessels (alveolar hypoxia secondary to local abnormality of ventilation).

Other Functions

The pulmonary circulation has important functions besides providing blood flow for continuous gas exchange: (1) it acts as a filter of virtually the entire venous drainage; (2) it supplies substrates for the nutrition and metabolic needs of the lung, including the synthesis of surfactant; (3) it serves as a reservoir of blood for the left ventricle; (4) it affects endocrine function by modifying the pharmacologic properties of a variety of circulating substances; and (5) it provides a large surface area for the absorption and filtration of liquids and solutes.

CONTROL OF BREATHING

The respiratory system must maintain gas exchange during periods of stress, such as exercise and other forms of increased metabolic needs. The O_2 consumption may increase more than ten-fold from rest to strenuous exercise; over this range, arterial Po_2 remains remarkably constant. The correspondence between the volume of ventilation and the demands for O_2 uptake and CO_2 elimination results from the responsiveness of three reasonably well-characterized receptor systems that interact to regulate breathing in normal persons and patients with a variety of disease states: (1) receptors in the airways and lung parenchyma, (2) peripheral chemoreceptors, and (3) central chemoreceptors. Nerve impulse traffic from these receptors is integrated and modulated in the medulla with impulses arising from higher centers in the brain. The medulla can be viewed as the main headquarters for initiating, processing, and relaying messages concerning breathing to other parts of the body via nervous pathways. Some of the resulting medullary neural activity may reach the cerebral cortex and evoke conscious perception of breathing (i.e., the symptom of dyspnea); other impulses may travel through efferent pathways in the autonomic nervous system to the lungs and other organs; still other impulses may descend in the spinal cord to be processed with afferent impulses from peripheral nerves at different cord segments before finally being transmitted to the muscles of respiration and other effectors.

Abnormalities of Control of Breathing

Variations, usually increases, in the rate and depth of breathing occur in patients with many common clinical disturbances such as fever, metabolic diseases, or psychiatric disorders. Several frequently used drugs (e.g., aspirin, antidepressants, and alcohol) also affect ventilation. *Hyperventilation* occurs when ventilation increases out of proportion to CO_2 production and arterial P_{CO_2} decreases; *hypoventilation* is the converse. *Hyperpnea* signifies an increase in the rate and depth of breathing, such as occurs during exercise, but carries no implication concerning arterial P_{CO_2} values. It should be emphasized that a decrease in the O_2 pressure (P_{O_2}) of arterial blood has several causes. In contrast, the pressure of CO_2 (P_{CO_2}) is governed simply by the relationship between CO_2 production ($\dot{V}_{CO_2}$) and CO_2 elimination by alveolar ventilation ($\dot{V}$alv):

$$P_{CO_2} = k\dot{V}_{CO_2}/\dot{V}alv$$

Because alveolar ventilation normally changes to keep pace wth CO_2 production, for practical purposes abnormal arterial P_{CO_2} values can always be interpreted as indicating hyper- or hypoventilation.

Abnormalities of the control of breathing can result from excitation of intrapulmonary receptors (pulmonary embolism, pneumonia, asthma), depression of peripheral chemoreceptors (natives of high altitudes, sedative drugs, severe chronic bronchitis), stimulation of peripheral chemoreceptors (drugs such as doxapram), depression of central chemoreceptors (sedative drugs, obesity, myxedema, neurologic disorders), and stimulation of central chemoreceptors (drugs such as aspirin, irritative neurologic lesions). Special tests of the ventilatory response to breathing gas mixtures with increased CO_2 or decreased O_2 and a test that determines the pressure developed during the first 0.1 second of breathing against a closed mouthpiece ($P_{0.1}$) help in defining the physiologic derangements among these disorders.

GAS EXCHANGE

The end-product of respiration is gas exchange, which in human beings consists of maintaining the values for P_{O_2} and P_{CO_2} in arterial blood within normal limits. As stated previously, respiration consists of ventilation, including the distribution of inspired air throughout the tracheobronchial system, diffusion, blood flow, including the distribution of mixed venous blood throughout pulmonary capillaries, and the control of breathing. Each of these contributes in a unique way to gas exchange such that an impairment in one process cannot be compensated for by improvement in another.

Ambient air consists primarily of N_2 and O_2 with varying amounts of water vapor. As air is inhaled, it is warmed to body temperature and fully saturated with water vapor (P_{H_2O} $37°$ C = 47 mm Hg); the addition of water vapor has the effect of diluting the inspired mixture of N_2 and O_2 and reduces their respective pressures proportionately. During gas exchange in the alveoli, more O_2 is removed than CO_2 is added; this causes the volume of each respiratory unit to decrease slightly and raises the concentration and pressure of N_2 slightly. When ventilation and perfusion are each uniformly distributed to various units (Fig. 59–5), "ideal" conditions for gas exchange exist and there is no difference between the P_{O_2} values in (mean) alveolar gas and arterial blood. The alveolar-arterial P_{O_2} difference is an important measure of the uniformity of matching of ventilation and perfusion. The difference is derived from a direct measurement of the arterial P_{O_2}, which is subtracted from alveolar P_{O_2} ($P_{A_{O_2}}$) calculated according to the following equation:

$$P_{A_{O_2}} = P_{I_{O_2}} - P_{A_{CO_2}} \left[F_{I_{O_2}} + \frac{1 - F_{I_{O_2}}}{R} \right]$$

where $P_{I_{O_2}}$ = P_{O_2} of inspired gas, $P_{A_{CO_2}}$ = alveolar P_{CO_2} (usually assumed to equal arterial P_{CO_2}), $F_{I_{O_2}}$ = fractional concentration of O_2 in inspired gas, and R = respiratory exchange ratio (often assumed to equal 0.8).

However, gas exchange in healthy lungs is not perfect because there is a small (5 to 10 mm Hg) alveolar-arterial P_{O_2} difference, which occurs because of the normal presence of a slight nonuniformity in the distribution of ventilation with respect to perfusion and a small right-to-left shunt. It is also noteworthy that the sum of the pressures of the individual gases in mixed venous blood is less than the total atmospheric pressure. Because the tissues and spaces of the body are in approximate equilibrium with venous blood, these structures are also subatmospheric. The "suction" serves to keep the lung expanded against the chest wall and to cause the reabsorption of gas from tissue spaces (e.g., a pneumothorax).

Abnormal Gas Exchange

Measurements of arterial P_{O_2} and P_{CO_2} and calculations of the alveolar-arterial P_{O_2} difference are reliable guides to the overall adequacy of respiration. In determining whether or not an abnormalitiy is present, it must be remembered that normal values for P_{O_2}, but not P_{CO_2}, vary with age and that both P_{O_2} and P_{CO_2} are influenced by the altitude at which the subject is living. There are five physiologic mechanisms known to cause arterial hypoxia, defined as a decrease below normal of arterial P_{O_2}: (1) hypoventilation, (2) decreased diffusion, (3) ventilation-perfusion imbalance, (4) right-to-left shunting of blood, and (5) breathing air (or a gas mixture) with a low P_{O_2}. Except for a few uncommon clinical examples, such as breathing air with its P_{O_2} reduced by combustion of O_2 and addition of smoke or suffocation, item 5 can be ignored. Items 1 to 4 can be separated, at least for practical clinical purposes, by analyzing the values from a given blood specimen and a few easy tests.

HYPOVENTILATION. The simplest disturbance of gas exchange occurs when not enough fresh air is breathed into alveolar spaces to raise pulmonary capillary P_{O_2} to normal levels and to allow CO_2 to leave the bloodsteam. Although arterial P_{CO_2} may theoretically increase in patients with other disturbances of gas exchange (ventilation-perfusion abnormalities and right-to-left shunts), for clinical purposes an elevated value should be interpreted as indicating alveolar hypoventilation.

Pure hypoventilation is a relatively uncommon clinical event. When it is found, depression of the central nervous system resulting from anesthetic agents or other sedative drugs is the usual cause. More commonly, hypoventilation occurs in association with other disturbances of oxygenation. When these coexist, they can be recognized by the fact that the decrease in arterial P_{O_2} is more than can be accounted for by the increase in arterial P_{CO_2}.

IMPAIRED DIFFUSION. Decreased diffusion, from either loss of pulmonary capillaries or thickening of the air-blood barrier, does not usually cause important alveolar-arterial P_{O_2} differences *at rest*. Thus abnormalities of diffusion can be ignored in patients with arterial hypoxia whose blood specimens are obtained while they are resting. In contrast, impaired diffusion is one of the two major causes of severely worsening hypoxia during exercise (right-to-left shunting of blood is the other). Regardless of the cause of the diffusing impairment, under resting conditions there is sufficient time to allow gas transfer to reach equilibrium between gas and blood. However, during exercise, cardiac output and the velocity of blood flow through pulmonary capillaries increase; thus the time for gas transfer is reduced and alveolar-end-capillary P_{O_2} differences may occur.

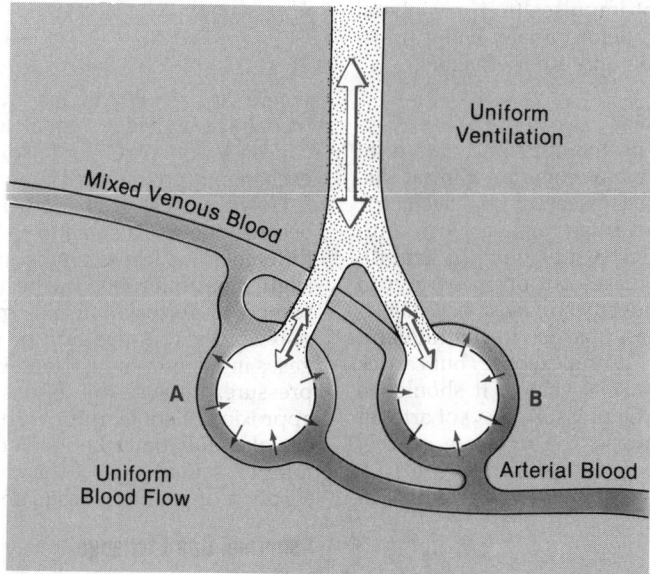

FIGURE 59–5. Schematic representation of gas exchange in an idealized two-compartment model of the lung in which there is uniform distribution of ventilation and blood flow. (Adapted from Comroe JH Jr, et al.: The Lung: Clinical Physiology and Pulmonary Function Tests. 2nd ed. Chicago, Year Book Medical Publishers, 1962. Reprinted by permission from the authors and Year Book Publisher, Inc.)

	A	B	A + B	Units
Alveolar ventilation	2.4	2.4	4.8	L/min
Pulmonary blood flow	3.0	3.0	6.0	L/min
Ventilation-perfusion ratio	0.8	0.8	0.8	
Mixed venous P_{O_2}	40	40	40	mm Hg
Mixed venous S_{O_2}	75	75	75	per cent
Mixed venous P_{CO_2}	46	46	46	mm Hg
Alveolar P_{O_2}	101	101	101	mm Hg
Arterial P_{O_2}	101	101	101	mm Hg
Arterial S_{O_2}	97.5	97.5	97.5	per cent
Arterial P_{CO_2}	40	40	40	mm Hg
Alveolar-arterial P_{O_2} difference	0	0	0	mm Hg

VENTILATION-PERFUSION MISMATCHING. Because the distributions of inspired air and pulmonary blood flow in normal lungs are neither uniform nor proportionate to each other, a slight ventilation-perfusion imbalance exists in healthy persons. Moreover, increased (above normal) mismatching of ventilation and perfusion is by far the most common cause of arterial hypoxia encountered clinically. Virtually all forms of lung disease are associated with a detectable ventilation-perfusion abnormality.

When a unit is underventilated relative to its perfusion (i.e., has a low ventilation-perfusion ratio), O_2 uptake by that unit must decrease so that the P_{O_2} of its end-capillary blood is lower than normal; P_{CO_2} tends to increase but cannot rise above the value in mixed venous blood (Fig. 59–5). Thus the process affects values for P_{O_2} more than P_{CO_2}. Furthermore, in those units that are overventilated owing to a redistribution of inspired air, the high ventilation-perfusion ratio causes P_{O_2} to increase and P_{CO_2} to decrease. But there is an important difference in the effects of these changes in pressures on the actual quantities (contents) of O_2 and CO_2 in the capillary blood leaving units with high ventilation-perfusion ratios. Given the shapes of the respective dissociation curves, O_2 content is not appreciably increased but CO_2 content is decreased. Thus increasing ventilation with respect to perfusion in some regions corrects the tendency to CO_2 retention that would otherwise exist but does not correct the hypoxia caused by low ventilation-perfusion relationships in other units. Another invariable consequence of a ventilation-perfusion abnormality is an increase in the alveolar-arterial P_{O_2} difference.

RIGHT-TO-LEFT SHUNTING. A small right-to-left shunt of blood is found in normal persons, and shunts of considerable magnitude may occur in patients with pulmonary disease. A right-to-left shunt may be visualized as a pathway(s) through which mixed venous blood flows from the right to the left side of the heart without having contacted functioning gas exchange units along the way. Thus there is a continuous admixture of venous blood that has flowed through the abnormal pathway with arterialized blood from normal pathways in the lungs. Arterial hypoxia and an increased alveolar-arterial P_{O_2} difference occur that vary in severity with the magnitude of the shunt and its O_2 content. Right-to-left shunts may occur through intracardiac communications in patients with congenital heart disease. In patients with lung disease, although shunts may be extremely large, they seldom occur through abnormal vascular channels such as pulmonary arteriovenous fistulas; instead, they are caused by blood perfusing normal vessels in regions of lung that are atelectatic or in which alveoli are filled with edema fluid, pus, or blood; in either case, because gas transfer is impossible, a shunt occurs.

The consequences of a right-to-left shunt are similar to those of a ventilation-perfusion imbalance owing to basic similarities between the two disturbances. A shunt can be viewed as an extreme ventilation-perfusion abnormality in which there is perfusion but *no* ventilation at all. It is impossible to differentiate between a ventilation-perfusion disturbance and a right-to-left shunt while the subject is breathing ambient air; therefore the effects of both are combined and designated as venous admixture or a "shunt-like" effect. The two causes of hypoxia can be separated by giving the patient 100 per cent O_2 to breathe and measuring arterial Po_2 after all the N_2 has been washed out of the lungs. When a ventilation-perfusion abnormality exists, the N_2 is replaced by O_2 and all the blood perfusing the lungs equilibrates at a high Po_2 (approximately 600 mm Hg); in this way 100 per cent O_2 is said to "correct" a ventilation-perfusion disturbance. In contrast, in the presence of a right-to-left shunt, the admixture of mixed venous blood continues despite breathing 100 per cent O_2 and arterial hypoxia persists. In fact, the alveolar-arterial Po_2 difference in patients with a right-to-left shunt is higher during breathing of 100 per cent O_2 compared with room air, whereas the opposite occurs in patients with ventilation-perfusion inequalities.

Significance of Arterial Blood Gas Values

The availability of accurate rapid analyzers for measuring Po_2, Pco_2, and pH has been one of the major clinical advances of the last 25 years. Virtually the entire therapeutic approach to patients with acute and chronic respiratory failure is dictated by the presence and magnitude of blood gas and pH abnormalities (see Ch. 72). Every physician should know the mechanisms of arterial hypoxia and how to differentiate them, because it is important clinically whether a patient's hypoxia results from hypoventilation, impaired diffusion, ventilation-perfusion mismatching, or right-to-left shunting. Evaluating the course and prognosis of the lung disease, determining the need for and outcome of therapy, and assessing disability, operability, and the limits of resection in patients considered for pulmonary surgery all depend to some extent on the findings of blood gas analysis. Thus all physicians who care for patients must become familiar with the technique of arterial puncture and must know how to interpret the results of blood gas analysis.

EXERCISE

Tests of pulmonary function are customarily performed with the subject seated at rest. The results of these studies provide useful information about the functional abnormalities that characterize common and important pulmonary diseases. Occasionally, the results of routine tests are perfectly normal in symptomatic patients, usually those with exertional dyspnea. In these circumstances, tests during exercise may reveal severe functional disturbances that lead to further evaluation and a diagnosis of either pulmonary vascular or parenchymal infiltrative diseases. Exercise tests are also essential to document the presence of and mechanisms underlying disability.

Cotes JE: Lung Function. 4th ed. Philadelphia, J. B. Lippincott Company, 1979. *Good textbook of pulmonary physiology.*

Hyatt RE: Expiratory flow limitations. J Appl Physiol 55:1, 1983. *Concise and understandable explanation of the wave-speed theory of expiratory flow limitation.*

Jones NL, Campbell EJM: Clinical Exercise Testing. Philadelphia, W. B. Saunders Company, 1982. *Comprehensive survey of and instructions for exercise testing.*

Murray JF: The Normal Lung: The Basis for Diagnosis and Treatment of Pulmonary Disease. 2nd ed. Philadelphia, W. B. Saunders Company, 1986. *Review of normal anatomy, pulmonary physiology, and structure-function correlations.*

Roussos C, Macklem PT (eds.): The Thorax, Parts A and B. New York, Marcel Dekker, Inc., 1983. *Extremely thorough, authoritative discussion of the interrelationships among the thorax, lungs, and respiratory muscles in health and disease.*

Torre-Bueno JR, Wagner PD, Saltzman HA, et al.: Diffusion limitation in normal humans during exercise at sea level and simulated altitude. J Appl Physiol 58:989, 1985. *Elegant study of the effects of diffusion limitation in normal persons.*

Wilson AF (ed.): Pulmonary Function Testing: Indications and Interpretations. Orlando, Fla., Grune & Stratton, 1985. *Good summary of pulmonary function testing; well referenced.*

60 ASTHMA
Ronald P. Daniele

DEFINITION AND PREVALENCE. Asthma is a disorder that is characterized by increased responsiveness of the trachea and bronchi to various stimuli, resulting in widespread narrowing of the airways. These changes are reversible either spontaneously or as a result of therapy. The currently accepted definition does not specify a cause or causes, identify unique clinical or pathologic features, or mention immunologic mechanisms. It does describe, however, the fundamental abnormality that is common to all asthmatic patients—reversible hyper-responsiveness of tracheobronchial smooth muscle.

Most asthmatic patients are diagnosed by a triad of episodic symptoms: wheezing, cough, and dyspnea. Characteristically, these signs and symptoms are highly variable in severity and duration. They may run the gamut from being completely absent for days, months, and even years to being protracted and unresponsive to outpatient therapy (status asthmaticus).

Asthma may afflict as many as 5 per cent of the population in the United States. In over half the cases it is diagnosed between ages 2 and 17 years, and in this group it is the leading cause of disease and disability. About one third of asthmatic patients are first diagnosed after 30 years of age.

CLASSIFICATION. Patients with asthma may be separated into two clinical groups, extrinsic and intrinsic (Table 60–1). Extrinsic asthma is characterized by childhood onset, seasonal variation, and a well-defined allergic history to a variety of inhaled allergens (atopy). The extrinsic form accounts for less than 10 per cent of all patients. Intrinsic asthma usually begins after the age of 30 and tends to be perennial and more severe; status asthmaticus is more common in this group. By definition, in intrinsic asthma an allergic etiology cannot be identified. More than 80 per cent of asthmatic patients have clinical features that are common to both groups, but for purposes of discussion each will be discussed separately.

PATHOLOGY. Most descriptions of the pathologic features of asthma come from patients dying in status asthmaticus. In these cases, the lungs are markedly distended and fail to collapse owing to the occlusion of most bronchi by thick, tenacious plugs of mucus, which often extend to the terminal bronchioles. Histopathologic hallmarks include bronchial smooth muscle hypertrophy, mucosal edema, thickening of the basement membrane, and inflammatory cells in submucosal tissue, particularly eosinophils. The lung parenchyma is

TABLE 60–1. CLASSIFICATION OF ASTHMATIC PATIENTS

Extrinsic*	Intrinsic*
Known external allergens	No known external allergens
Positive immediate skin tests	Negative skin tests
IgE raised in 50–60% of subjects	IgE normal or low
Onset usually in childhood or early adult life	Onset usually (but not invariably) in older adults
Intermittent asthma	More continuous asthma
Other allergies (hay fever and eczema) often present (54%)	Other allergies uncommon (7%)
Family history of multiple allergies (asthma, hay fever, eczema) common (50%)	Family history of multiple allergies less common (20%)

*Blood and sputum eosinophilia common in *both* groups.

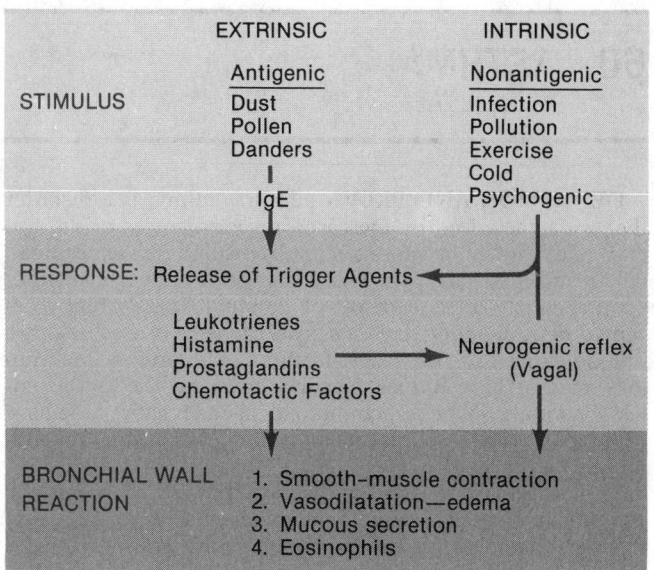

FIGURE 60–1. Dual pathways involved in the pathogenesis of bronchial constriction. (Adapted from Fishman AP [ed.]: Pulmonary Diseases and Disorders. New York, McGraw-Hill Book Company, 1980.)

remarkably spared with no evidence of fibrosis or destruction of the alveolar septa. Unexpectedly, similar abnormalities have been found in asthmatic patients dying from other causes who were presumably symptom free prior to death. The presence of mucous plugs in the small airways (less than 2 mm) of these patients may explain some of the persistent functional abnormalities (reduced midmaximum expiratory flow rate [MMEF] and increased alveolar-arterial difference for Po_2) found even in asymptomatic patients.

PATHOPHYSIOLOGY OF EXTRINSIC ASTHMA. In extrinsic asthma, the sequence of events after sensitization leading to the pathologic features described above is shown in Figure 60–1. Inhaled allergens interact with specific IgE antibodies that are fixed to mast cells that line the tracheobronchial tree. Mast cells (and possibly basophils) that are sensitized with IgE are primed to respond to specific allergens when cell-bound IgE is bridged by divalent allergen. This membrane event signals mast cells to secrete a variety of mediators by two processes. First, preformed mediators con-

tained in metachromatic granules of mast cells are released by a process of exocytosis. Important examples of preformed mediators include histamine, eosinophilic factors of anaphylaxis (ECF-A), and neutrophil chemotactic factor (NCF). In the second process, unstored mediators, such as slow-reacting substance of anaphylaxis (SRS-A) (now called the leukotrienes), platelet activating factors (PAF), and prostaglandins (PGD_2 and $PGF_{2\alpha}$), are synthesized and secreted by mast cells within minutes after antigen stimulation. Some of the properties and functional characteristics of these mediators are summarized in Table 60–2. For a more extensive discussion of mast cell structure and function, the reader is referred to Ch. 427.

Two advances have extended our knowledge of the role of mediators in asthma: the elucidation of the arachidonic acid metabolic pathways and the characterization and synthesis of SRS-A, which proved to be a group of compounds called leukotrienes. Leukotrienes, as well as prostaglandins, are synthesized from the 20-carbon unsaturated fatty acid, arachidonic acid (Fig. 60–2). Arachidonic acid is derived from cell membrane phospholipids by the action of phospholipases and may be converted by cyclo-oxygenase to prostaglandins and thromboxanes. A second pathway that is catalyzed by 5-lipoxygenase leads to the formation of 5-hydroperoxyeicosatetraenoic acids (5-HPETE) and then to an unstable intermediate, leukotriene A_4 (LTA_4). LTA_4 may then be converted to leukotriene B_4, a potent chemotactic factor for eosinophils and neutrophils. Alternatively, LTA_4 may be transformed by several cell types (mononuclear cells and basophils) into leukotriene C_4 by the enzymatic addition of glutathione (S-glutamylcysteinylglycine). Leukotriene C_4 may undergo further conversion to leukotriene D_4 (S-cysteinylglycine) by enzymatic removal of glutamine and then by removal of glycine to leukotriene E_4 (S-cysteine). SRS-A is composed of the cysteinyl-containing leukotrienes (LTC_4, LTD_4, and LTE_4), of which LTD_4 is the most potent bronchoconstrictor (Table 60–2). The leukotrienes are a thousand times more potent on a molar basis than histamine or $PGF_{2\alpha}$ and exert their effect predominantly in the small or distal airways. In asthmatic patients, allergens induce the release of leukotriene C_4, D_4, and E_4 from the lung tissue in amounts that correlate well with their capacity to induce bronchial contraction.

Secretion of primary mediators described in Table 60–2 apparently initiates the release of secondary mediators, such as serotonin, prostaglandins, and possibly kinins. Serotonin

TABLE 60–2. MEDIATORS IN THE ATOPIC INFLAMMATORY RESPONSE

Mediator	Molecular Characteristics	Source	Function
Histamine	Beta-imidazolylethylamine MW* = 111	Mast cells, basophils, preformed and stored in granules	Increases vascular permeability, bronchial smooth muscle contraction (H_1 type) ↑ cyclic AMP in mast cells (H_2 type) ↑ mucous secretion
Slow-reacting substance of anaphylaxis (SRS-A) Leukotrienes C_4 (LTC_4) LTD_4 LTE_4	Polyunsaturated substituted C-20 fatty acids MW ≈ 625 ≈ 500 ≈ 425	Mast cells, eosinophils, mononuclears, lung cells? (not preformed)	Increases vascular permeability, bronchial smooth muscle contraction
Eosinophil chemotactic factors of anaphylaxis (ECF-A)	Tetrapeptides (Val/Ala-Gly-Ser-Glu), MW ≈ 360–390, and acid peptides	Mast cells, basophils, preformed and stored in granules	Attracts eosinophils
Neutrophil chemotactic factor (NCF)	Structure ? MW > 750,000	Mast cells, basophils, lung tissue, preformed and stored	Attracts neutrophils
Platelet-aggregating factors (PAF)	Phospholipids 1-0-alkyl-2-acetyl-sn-glyceryl-3-phosphorylcholine MW ≈ 520–550	Neutrophils, ? mast cells, basophils, other lung cells? (not preformed)	Aggregates platelets and release of other mediators (serotonin, PG)
Prostaglandins (PG)	Polyunsaturated C-20 fatty acids, MW ≈ 350	Mast cells, basophils, platelets, other lung cells? (not preformed)	↑ cyclic AMP PGE_1, PGE_2—dilate smooth muscle PGD_2, $PGF_{\alpha2}$—contracts smooth muscle Release of PG probably stimulated by other mediators

*MW = molecular weight.

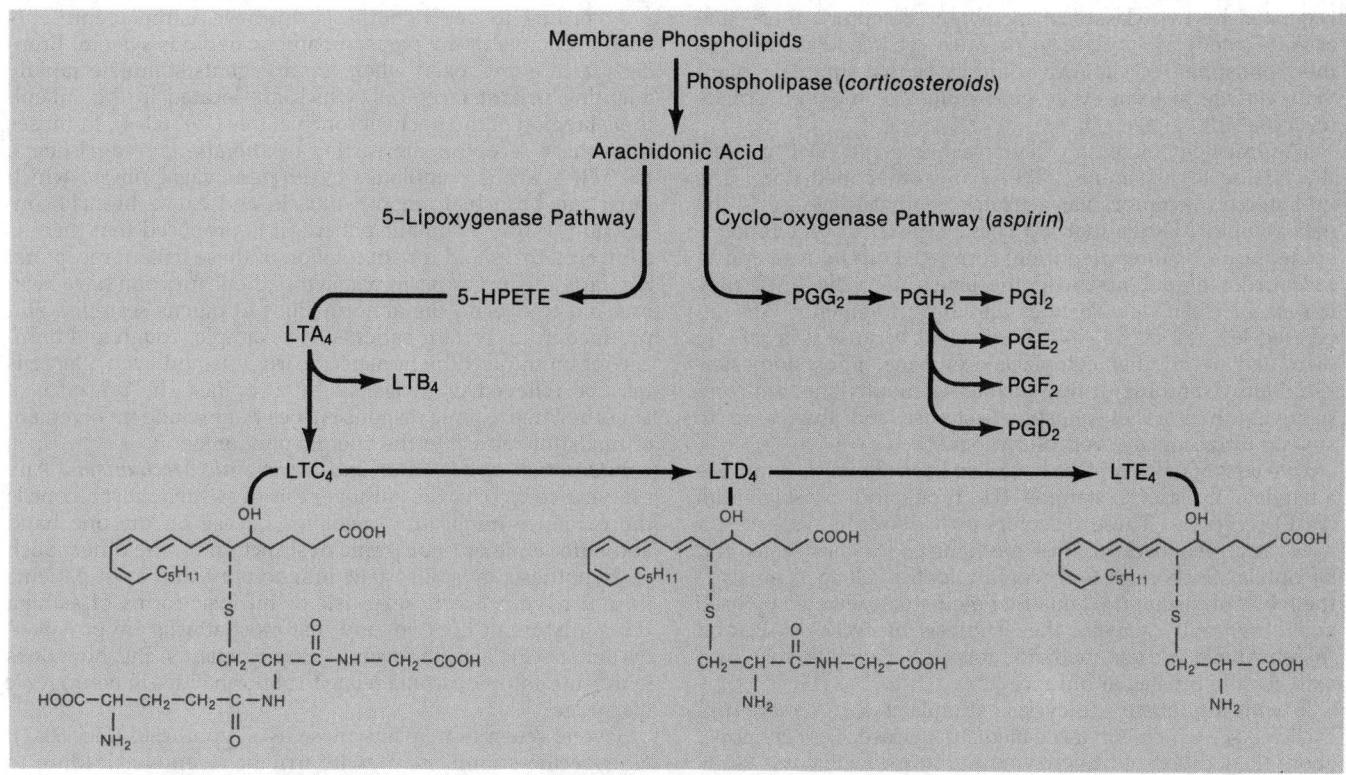

FIGURE 60–2. Arachidonic acid metabolic pathways. The figure depicts major prostaglandin (PG) products of the cyclooxygenase pathway. Also shown are the structural formulas of the three leukotrienes that constitute slow-reacting substance of anaphylaxis and that are generated through the lipoxygenase pathway. It is noteworthy that corticosteroids inhibit the phospholipases involved in synthesis of arachidonic acid. Aspirin inhibits the cyclooxygenase pathway. Not shown in the figure are thromboxanes that are derived from PGH$_2$.

constricts bronchial smooth muscle directly but may also induce bronchoconstriction by stimulating irritant receptors (see below). Prostaglandins of the E series (PGE$_1$ and PGE$_2$) are potent dilators of airways and blood vessels. Although the lung is a major site for their production, the principal cell types involved are not defined.

The effects of these mediators may be viewed as two waves of an inflammatory response: The first is an immediate serous transudation caused by increased capillary permeability. The second occurs hours to days after antigen stimulation and involves the accumulation of inflammatory cells (*late-onset asthmatic response*).

In more than one half of asthmatic patients inhalation of specific allergens causes an immediate bronchoconstriction that resolves within minutes to hours and then recurs six to ten hours later. This *late-onset response* of the airways is thought to be associated with an accumulation of neutrophils, platelets, and eosinophils in the bronchial mucosa and submucosa. The reaction is initiated by mast cell (and basophil) degranulation and release of mediators, including leukotriene B$_4$, other eicosanoids, and eosinophil and neutrophil chemotactic factors. The arrival of neutrophils appears to elicit the infiltration of mononuclear cells in the submucosa, which may persist for several days. An appreciation of late-onset reactions is reshaping our thinking about asthma: It is not solely a syndrome of brief and reversible airways obstruction but also a disease involving a progressive, multistage inflammatory response. The identification of late-onset responses also has important therapeutic implications because they are poorly managed by standard bronchodilator therapy (beta$_2$ drugs and methylxanthines) (see below).

The eosinophil and neutrophil appear to play prominent roles in the late-onset reaction, especially in their capacity to inflict injury. Granular constituents derived from the eosino-phil, particularly major basic protein, and the secretion of oxygen free radicals can injure bronchial epithelial cells, rendering the mucosa more permeable to allergens and possibly lowering the threshold of underlying irritant receptors.

Mast Cell Receptors—Intracellular Regulation. As shown in Figure 60–3, secretion by mast cells and basophils is

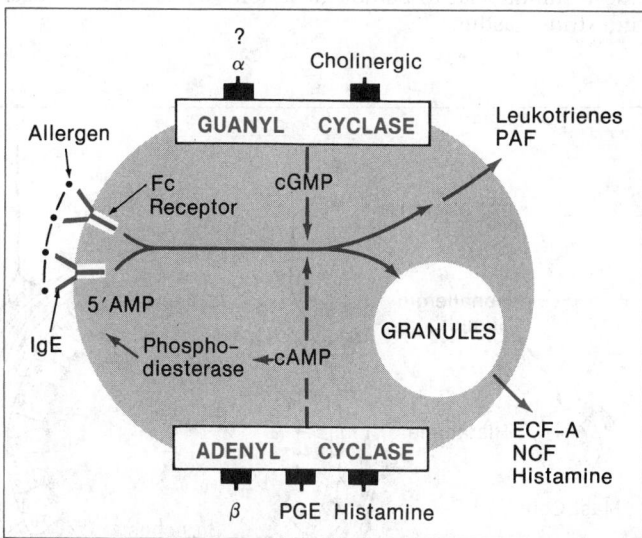

FIGURE 60–3. Membrane receptor interactions involving allergen-IgE and agonists that result in the stimulation of cyclic AMP or cyclic GMP and modulation of mediator release from mast cells and basophils. (From Fishman AP [ed.]: Pulmonary Diseases and Disorders. New York, McGraw-Hill Book Company, 1980.)

regulated by two classes of membrane receptors: those that activate adenylate cyclase to produce cyclic adenosine-3',5'-monophosphate (cyclic AMP); and those that stimulate guanylate cyclase to form cyclic guanosine-3',5' monophosphate (cyclic GMP).

The transient increase of cytoplasmic cyclic AMP inhibits the release of histamine, SRS-A, and other mediators. The best-studied receptor that activates adenylate cyclase is the beta receptor. Drugs that are beta agonists (isoproterenol > epinephrine > norepinephrine) correlate both in dose and in rank order of potency with the levels of cyclic AMP they induce in isolated leukocytes and lung fragments. The increased level of cyclic AMP is transient because it is rapidly degraded by another cytoplasmic enzyme, phosphodiesterase. Methylxanthine drugs, such as aminophylline, are competitive inhibitors of phosphodiesterase and thus tend to sustain intracellular levels of cyclic AMP.

Two additional receptors have also been shown to stimulate adenylate cyclase: histamine (H_2 type) and prostaglandin (PGE) receptors. These receptors provide some evidence for a negative feedback control mechanism for mast cells and basophils. Such receptors would allow a cell to "perceive" the levels of histamine (and other mediators) secreted by itself and other cells, activate the synthesis of cyclic AMP, and thereby limit further mediator release. A similar role may exist for the prostaglandin receptor.

In contrast, guanylate cyclase stimulates the formation of cyclic GMP, which enhances mediator release. Less is known about the location of this enzyme and its associated receptors. However, a cholinergic receptor has been identified whereby acetylcholine stimulates the production of cyclic GMP.

According to a current hypothesis, the balance between the inhibitory (cyclic AMP) and excitatory (cyclic GMP) messenger molecules regulates mediator release. It has been proposed that asthma results from a partial blockade of beta receptor, leading to an imbalance of these regulatory molecules.

The elucidation of the mechanisms of mediator release in asthma has greatly extended our understanding of bronchospasm and provides a more rational basis for therapy. Nevertheless, most attacks of asthma are not precipitated by allergens.

INTRINSIC ASTHMA—PATHOPHYSIOLOGIC MECHANISMS. In intrinsic asthma, reversible airways obstruction is caused by a variety of stimuli that are nonantigenic and seemingly unrelated. Nonetheless, as shown in Figure 60–1, these stimuli lead to pathologic lesions similar to those seen in extrinsic asthma.

According to one hypothesis, intrinsic asthma represents an abnormality of the parasympathetic nervous system. Bronchospasm is provoked when certain agents stimulate rapidly adapting irritant receptors, which are located in the subepithelial region of the tracheobronchial tree (Fig. 60–4). Impulses from these receptors are carried by the afferent vagal fibers; the reflex arc is completed by efferent vagal fibers, which innervate bronchial smooth muscle and cause bronchoconstriction. In the asthmatic patient, it is proposed that there is a lowered threshold for stimulation of these irritant receptors. Similarly, disturbances in parasympathetic function have been invoked to explain the abnormalities in mucus secretion and production. In certain patients, for example, cough and bronchospasm induced by nonspecific irritants and even allergens may be relieved or abolished by atropine. The presence of abnormal neurogenic responses does not exclude involvement of mediator release in the allergic phenomenon.

Interaction of Mediator and Neurogenic Mechanisms. Any unifying concept of the pathogenesis of asthma must reconcile the evidence implicating mediator release on the one hand and autonomic or neurogenic dysfunction on the other. Such an hypothesis must also take into account that most patients do not have primarily extrinsic or intrinsic forms of asthma but a mixture of the two, and that most attacks are provoked by nonspecific stimuli, even in atopic patients. But how does extrinsic or atopic asthma relate to abnormalities in neurogenic discharge?

Several schemes may link these two hypotheses (Fig. 60–4). Nonspecific stimuli may excite irritant receptors, leading to bronchospasm by way of efferent vagal pathways. Allergen-antibody complexes may stimulate mast cells, releasing mediators that might have a direct action on smooth muscle as well as an indirect effect by stimulating irritant receptors and thereby producing bronchospasm. Alternatively, both nonspecific irritants and allergen-antibody interaction might stimulate mediator release from mast cells. Certain mediators, such as histamine and serotonin, are potent stimulants of irritant receptors. By such a scheme, stimuli may induce bronchospasm by direct action of mediators on smooth muscle or by indirect action that operates via neurogenic reflexes, or by both mechanisms.

The late-onset reactions may also be involved in the interaction between mediator release and neurogenic stimuli. An important feature of the late-onset response is an increase in airway hyper-reactivity. It is likely that the infiltration of the bronchial mucosa with inflammatory cells and continued release of mediators further stimulate irritant receptors. Late-

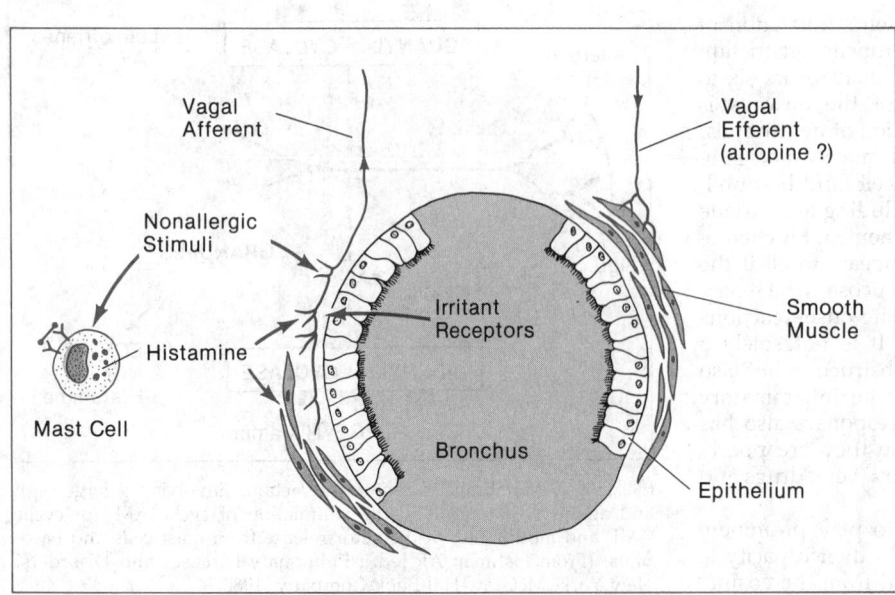

FIGURE 60–4. Possible interactions between mediators and neurogenic reflexes in the elicitation of bronchial smooth muscle contraction in asthma. Also indicated in the figure is one potential site of action for anticholinergic drugs in asthma.

onset reactions are caused not only by allergic stimuli but also by certain nonallergic provocative stimuli discussed below (e.g., viral infection and pollutants).

Nonallergic Provocative Stimuli. One of the most important nonspecific irritants is *respiratory tract infection*, particularly by viral agents. Both lower and upper respiratory infections may initiate or aggravate bronchospasm. This is not due to a hypersensitivity to the infecting agents, but is thought to result from the capacity of viral agents to lower the threshold for stimulation of irritant receptors.

Airborne pollutants may play a role in the pathogenesis of asthma. In "Tokyo-Yokohama asthma" and in "New Orleans asthma," a high density of air pollutants was found to have initiated or aggravated wheezing and dyspnea in asthmatic patients as well as in certain previously asymptomatic individuals who were later shown to have *hyperirritable* airways. Air pollutants (e.g., ozone) are thought to increase hyper-reactivity of bronchial smooth muscle by stimulating irritant receptors in the tracheobronchial tree.

A variety of *occupational dusts and fumes* may provoke asthmatic attacks in susceptible individuals. The onset of wheezing, cough, or dyspnea may be related to the working hours. More commonly, however, symptoms are not closely linked to occupation but may be delayed for several hours until after the patient has left the work place. Important diagnostic clues include a cyclic pattern in which symptom-free periods occur during weekends or vacations. Both allergic and irritant stimuli are thought to be involved in occupational asthma. A more extensive discussion of occupational asthma is contained in Ch. 536.

In some patients, *hyperpnea, laughing,* or *exercise* may also induce bronchoconstriction. Moreover, the inhalation of *cold air* may initiate or intensify bronchospasm. There are two hypotheses to explain how bronchospasm is induced by such diverse ventilatory maneuvers: One implicates mainly heat transfer from the respiratory tree; the other proposes that it is respiratory water loss, resulting in an increase in the osmolarity of the epithelial lining fluid. When all other variables are controlled, the major determinant is the volume of air that is to be warmed and humidified on inspiration. Heat and water loss occurs as the minute ventilation increases in response to exercise. This loss is independent of whether minute ventilation is voluntary or the result of exercise. Although it is unsettled regarding which mechanism is predominantly involved in exercise-induced asthma, both the inhalation of cold air and an increase in the osmolarity of lining fluid cause mediator release as well as stimulate vagal efferent pathways. Cromolyn or beta$_2$ drugs or both may blunt or prevent symptoms when given by inhalation prior to exercise. Measures that humidify and warm inhaled air, such as cold weather masks, are also helpful.

In about 10 per cent of asthmatic patients, a peculiar triad exists of *bronchospasm, nasal polyps,* and *sensitivity to aspirin.* Ingestion of aspirin, indomethacin, aminopyrine, or yellow food additives (e.g., tartrazine yellow) may induce severe bronchospasm, urticaria, and even hypotension. Interestingly, these patients are sensitive to acetylsalicylic acid but not to sodium salicylate. The reaction is not immunologic but appears related to an abnormality in prostaglandin metabolism, which is unmasked by these drugs. The arachidonic acid pathways may provide a clue to this abnormality (Fig. 60–2). In certain asthmatic patients, ingestion of aspirin or indomethacin, known inhibitors of cyclo-oxygenase, may divert arachidonic metabolism toward the lipoxygenase pathway and the production of spasmogenic leukotrienes.

Least understood are the *psychologic factors* that influence the asthmatic patient. It is thought that emotional stress influences bronchomotor tone, rendering it more susceptible to irritant and allergic stimuli.

Bronchospasm is usually induced by nonspecific stimuli that presumably involve nonimmunologic pathways. Allergic asthma also has a background of hyper-reactivity to nonspecific stimuli, and this abnormality may persist long after atopy disappears.

CLINICAL MANIFESTATIONS. In most patients, an asthma attack begins with a nonproductive cough and wheezing, usually followed by a tightness in the chest and dyspnea. In a minority of patients, cough may be the most conspicuous and even sole manifestation of the attack. Attacks frequently occur at night and during sleep. They usually do not last for more than several hours and resolve spontaneously or with therapy. The end of an attack is often heralded by a change to a productive cough with expectoration of mucous plugs and casts.

Physical findings of airway obstruction include prolonged expiration and wheezing in both phases of respiration. In more severe attacks, increasing dyspnea may be associated with a diminution of wheezing. This may lead to a silent chest, an especially serious finding that suggests impending respiratory failure. Severe attacks are also associated with lung hyperinflation, causing an increase in the anteroposterior diameter of the chest wall and the finding of hyper-resonance and low diaphragms on chest percussion. Important physical findings in gauging the severity of the attack are the patient's use of accessory respiratory muscles, sternocleidomastoid retractions, and the appearance of pulsus paradoxus. Cyanosis is a late and unreliable sign.

LABORATORY FINDINGS. A wet preparation of sputum of many asthmatic patients contains spiral casts (Curschmann's spirals), eosinophils, and Charcot-Leyden crystals. The presence of sputum and blood eosinophilia is suggestive of the diagnosis of asthma but does not distinguish between extrinsic and intrinsic types.

Arterial blood gases should be obtained only in patients experiencing severe asthmatic attacks or prolonged attacks that are unresponsive to bronchodilator therapy. Hypoxemia is invariably present during an acute attack and, when mild to moderately severe, is usually associated with a decrease in the arterial P_{CO_2} and an increase in arterial pH. Hypocapnia and respiratory alkalosis are due to increased alveolar ventilation. Respiration may be stimulated by increased chemical drive (when Pa_{O_2} is less than 60 torr), but neurogenic reflexes (irritant and stretch receptors) are probably more important. Determination of arterial blood gases is important for two reasons. First, the degree of hypoxemia generally reflects the degree of mismatching of ventilation to perfusion ($\dot{V}/\dot{Q}$) and thus gives some objective measure of the severity of airways disease. Second, a *normal* or increased Pa_{CO_2} signals severe airway obstruction and impending respiratory failure.

Chest roentgenograms may demonstrate lung hyperinflation, usually without parenchymal infiltrates. However, in patients with severe disease, roentgenograms should be scrutinized for (1) infiltrates suggesting a respiratory infection; (2) atelectasis or collapse of a segment or lobe, implicating mucous plugging of a bronchus; and (3) the presence of pneumothorax or pneumomediastinum.

Pulmonary function tests are important in assessing the severity of an attack and the response to bronchodilator therapy and in providing objective information about the resolution of disease. Pulmonary function tests may also be used to define hyperirritable airways in an asymptomatic asthma patient by provoking increases in airway resistance with aerosolized doses of histamine or methacholine, which would have no effect in normal individuals. In addition, the degree of airway hyper-responsiveness, as measured by these challenge tests, may give a more precise assessment of the severity of asthma. Pulmonary function tests may also identify patients with exercise-induced asthma.

During the acute attack, airway narrowing decreases the forced expiratory volume in one second (FEV$_1$), the maximal midexpiratory flow rates (MMF), and the peak expiratory flow rates. When the FEV$_1$ is less than 25 per cent of predicted (e.g., <1.0 liter), it is often accompanied by other signs of severe disease (e.g., pulsus paradoxus). All lung volumes are affected in an acute attack. There is a decrease in vital capacity (VC), with large increases in residual volume (RV), functional residual capacity (FRC), and total lung capacity (TLC). The peak expiratory flow rate (PEFR) is a particularly useful measurement because it is easy to perform repeatedly and does not require the patient to do the entire forced expiratory maneuver. The devices available for such measurements are small and convenient and may be kept in the home so that patients can produce daily records of their airway function.

Signs and symptoms are not entirely reliable in assessing the severity of an asthma attack or the optimal response to therapy. For example, in patients whose symptoms remit and signs of wheezing disappear, FEV_1's may be 40 to 60 per cent of normal and residual volumes greater than 200 per cent of predicted. Moreover, in patients whose attack has resolved for weeks or months, maximal midexpiratory flow rates may remain abnormal. The latter test emphasizes that the peripheral airways (less than 2 mm in diameter) are "silent" zones where considerable airway disease and obstruction may exist without signs or symptoms. These considerations have important therapeutic and clinical implications because the tendency for asthmatic attacks to recur seems to depend on the degree of residual disease. Also, a subpopulation of patients may have disease that exists predominantly in peripheral airways.

During symptom-free periods, skin tests or specific serum IgE antibodies (RAST test) may be useful in demonstrating hypersensitivity to suspected allergens. The use of RAST avoids the risk of sensitization or anaphylaxis and the need to interrupt medication. When compared with skin testing, however, it does not improve on specificity or sensitivity. Moreover, a positive skin test does not necessarily mean that exposure to the same allergen will produce respiratory symptoms. Newer inhalational tests may be more precise in identifying offending agents, including those that are implicated in occupational asthma and late-onset asthmatic responses. Use of these tests should be restricted to atypical patients in whom usual approaches are insufficient to establish a causative role for inhaled antigens.

DIFFERENTIAL DIAGNOSIS. Recurrent bronchospasm may occur in other diseases such as congestive heart failure, pulmonary embolism, and chronic bronchitis (see Ch. 61). There is usually little difficulty in distinguishing bronchospasm of congestive heart failure, since it is associated with other signs of underlying cardiac dysfunction. Distinguishing features of recurrent pulmonary emboli include pleural pain and effusions, signs of venous disease in the lower extremities, and characteristic findings on radioisotope lung scans and arteriography. Episodic and reversible wheezing may occur in patients with chronic bronchitis. In these patients, however, a persistent and productive cough exists in a setting of hyperirritable airways. Bronchospasm usually responds to bronchodilator therapy.

TREATMENT. Management of the asthmatic patient may be divided into two phases: treatment of the acute episode and maintenance therapy. The major classes of drugs will be reviewed as a background for recommendations on their optimal use in the treatment of asthma.

Sympathomimetic Drugs. Epinephrine has direct beta-adrenergic action but also stimulates alpha receptors. Its usefulness is limited by its actions on the heart, its restrictive use by inhalational and parenteral administration, and its short duration of action. Epinephrine is used in the treatment of acute asthmatic attacks and for this purpose is usually given in adults subcutaneously (0.2 to 0.5 ml of a 1:1000 solution). Tolerance develops after repeated use.

Isoproterenol has a potent selective beta-adrenergic effect. It is not absorbed orally, it has a relatively short duration of action, and certain patients may become refractory to its effects. Isoproterenol is usually administered by inhalation.

There are two types of beta-adrenergic receptors: Beta$_1$ agonists are cardiac stimulants (e.g., tachycardia); beta$_2$ agonists relax bronchial smooth muscle and blood vessels. The potential for selective beta$_2$ activity has led to the generation of new beta agonists with reduced cardiac side effects. These include the resorcinols, such as *metaproterenol* and *terbutaline*. The advantages of these agents are rapid onset of action, the potential for oral administration, and longer duration of action. Both agents are available in the United States for parenteral, oral, and aerosol administration. Skeletal muscle tremors are the main side effect. Newer agents with similar advantages but apparently even greater beta$_2$ selectivity are now available in the United States (e.g., *albuterol*). The use of beta$_2$ agents has replaced the use of older, less specific drugs such as ephedrine.

The administration of beta$_2$ drugs, such as albuterol, has a number of advantages when used by the inhalational compared with the oral route. These include a rapid onset of action, fewer systemic side effects (skeletal muscle tremors), and preservation of beta$_2$ selectivity. When given by mouth, beta$_2$ drugs have a longer duration of action but lose beta$_2$ selectivity.

Because at least one third of asthmatic patients use metered dose inhalers incorrectly, it is important for physicians to ascertain personally that their patients learn proper inhalational techniques to insure adequate delivery of the drug (e.g., beta$_2$ agonists, beclomethasone).

Methylxanthines. Methylxanthines were once thought to cause smooth muscle relaxation by their action on the cytoplasmic enzyme phosphodiesterase. At the therapeutic doses currently used, however, tissue concentrations result in little (about 10 per cent) inhibition of phosphodiesterase. Other possible mechanisms of action of the methylxanthines are the enhancement of diaphragmatic contractility and the blocking of adenosine receptors, which may also play a role in bronchoconstriction. The recommended therapeutic concentration of *theophylline* in plasma is between 10 and 20 μg per milliliter. Because of considerable variation in metabolism of the drug, maintenance doses may range between 500 and 5000* mg per day. Thus, when theophylline preparations are used alone, blood levels should be determined to establish the proper dosage. When levels exceed 20 μg per milliliter, anorexia, nausea and gastrointestinal upset, and central nervous system irritability may occur. Newer timed-release preparations show promise of achieving more stable blood levels, reducing side effects, and permitting twice-a-day administration. Patients with congestive heart failure and liver disease usually require lower maintenance dosages; smokers may require higher doses.

Corticosteroids. Why corticosteroids are so effective in the treatment of asthma remains unclear. They stabilize cellular lysosomal membranes, reduce cellular stores of histamine and SRS-A, and restore the responsiveness of leukocytes and airway smooth muscle to beta agonists. Interestingly, corticosteroids do not inhibit the release of mediators or influence their effect on target cells. Their main action may be to inhibit the late cellular inflammatory response. Nonetheless, steroids are important therapeutic agents in patients whose symptoms cannot be controlled with optimal combinations of bronchodilator therapy or whose disease becomes progressively severe and life threatening.

The onset of action, whether the drug is given intravenously or orally, occurs at about six hours. Thus, patients whose disease is severe enough to require intravenous steroids should continue to receive optimal doses of bronchodilator

---

*This dose exceeds manufacturer's maximum recommended dose.

therapy. Patients who require maintenance steroid therapy should receive a short-acting drug, such as *prednisone*, in a single morning dose, and the course of therapy should be as short as possible to reduce pituitary adrenal suppression. Because of reduced side effects, alternate-day administration is preferable, and the dose should be tapered as rapidly as possible. Patients receiving corticosteroid therapy should be monitored for complications such as ulcer disease, reactivation of tuberculosis, hypertension, diabetes, and cataracts.

Some synthetic steroids, such as *beclomethasone diproprionate*, can be delivered by inhalation. When doses are between 400 and 1200 μg (8 to 24 puffs daily),* there is minimal systemic absorption. Side effects include oropharyngeal candidiasis and exacerbation of rhinitis, nasal polyposis, and atopic dermatitis. Inhaled steroids are usually used to withdraw patients from long-term systemic steroids. In this situation, it is important to watch for signs of adrenal insufficiency. Inhaled steroids are used to prevent asthmatic symptoms; they should not be used to treat acute attacks because they can worsen symptoms.

The Cromones. *Disodium cromoglycate* is believed to reduce the release of chemical mediators by its action on the mast cell or basophil membrane. It is not a bronchodilator, and it does not have anti-inflammatory or antihistaminic effects. Thus, it is a prophylactic drug and is not to be used during an acute asthmatic attack. In fact, inhalation of the drug may initiate or aggravate bronchospasm. Metered dose inhalers (two puffs or 2 mg every four to six hours), which are now available in the United States, are easier to use and permit more effective delivery of cromolyn sodium than inhalation of the dry powder by turbo-inhaler (Spinhaler). Response or failure of response to cromolyn sodium is unpredictable. For example, not only patients with extrinsic asthma but also a significant number of patients with mixed or intrinsic asthma, particularly those with exercise-induced bronchospasm, may benefit from the drug. In patients who respond to the drug, it may be possible to reduce or eliminate the use of corticosteroids. Because of its low frequency of toxicity and side effects, a trial of therapy with cromolyn sodium should be carried out in patients with moderate-to-severe asthma in whom conventional bronchodilator therapy has been inadequate. Proper evaluation of the drug requires a four- to eight-week course of therapy.

Anticholinergic Agents. Atropine is one of the oldest treatments in asthma but has been all but abandoned because of its untoward side effects. Interest, however, has been rekindled in atropine-like drugs because of new insights into neurogenic mechanisms involving the vagal reflexes (Fig. 60–4) and the development of a congener of atropine (*ipratropium*), which is a nonabsorbable aerosol and remarkably free of side effects. Ipratropium may be useful as an adjunct to current therapy and of value to patients whose predominant symptom is chronic bronchitis or cough.

Calcium Antagonists. Another group of investigational drugs are the calcium antagonists. The translocation of calcium from the external medium or cell stores into the cytosol is a fundamental signal in the stimulation of mast cell and mucous gland secretion and smooth muscle contraction. With the aim of blocking this signal, calcium antagonists (*verapamil* and *nifedipine*) have been given by mouth or inhalation to asthmatic patients to alleviate bronchoconstriction. Some benefit has been achieved in patients with exercise-induced asthma, but the exact role of these agents in the management of asthma is unclear.

Management of the Acute Asthmatic Attack. There is no simple recipe for the management of the asthmatic patient. Each therapeutic program must be tailored to the patient. The following comments are meant to be general guidelines.

For patients with mild attacks, one drug may suffice. Therapy may begin with a theophylline preparation or a beta$_2$ sympathomimetic amine or both. Theophylline may be started at dosages (200 mg) that produce few or no side effects. If this is inadequate, the addition of a beta$_2$ sympathomimetic amine, preferably by inhalation (metered dose inhaler), may be effective with relatively low doses of theophylline. There is an additive effect when a beta-adrenergic agent is combined with theophylline. Thus, when used together, therapeutic doses and side effects of either agent may be reduced.

In the treatment of asthma, therapy should be guided by objective evidence (e.g., pulmonary function tests) rather than relying solely on the resolution of symptoms or signs. The measurement of FEV$_1$ or PEFR is appropriate and can be performed in the physician's office or at home (PEFR).

If asthma becomes progressively more severe or if the patient does not respond adequately to therapy after several hours of observation, then the patient should be hospitalized. Aminophylline may then be given by continuous intravenous infusion. The initial recommended dosage for adult patients is a loading dose of 5.6 mg per kilogram given over 15 to 30 minutes, followed by a continuous infusion of 0.9 mg per kilogram per hour for smokers, 0.6 mg per kilogram per hour for nonsmokers, and 0.3 mg per kilogram per hour for severely ill patients (e.g., congestive heart failure, pneumonia, and liver disease). Maintenance doses must also be reduced ($\simeq$ 0.3 mg per kilogram per hour) for patients taking certain drugs, such as cimetidine or triacetyloleandomycin, which interfere with hepatic microsomal enzymes. After 36 hours, theophylline levels should be measured. If patients have recently received theophylline, then the loading dose should be decreased (50 to 75 per cent) or eliminated to avoid toxic levels and a continuous infusion begun. Patients should also receive controlled oxygen therapy and physiotherapy to relieve bronchial secretions. Fluids are given by mouth or intravenous infusion to correct dehydration if present. Electrolyte imbalance, particularly hypokalemia, should be corrected. Tranquilizers and sedatives must be avoided.

If the patient remains unresponsive or the attack becomes more severe, then the patient must be hospitalized and treated with corticosteroids, with continuation of full dosages of bronchodilator therapy. The correct dosage for intravenous corticosteroids is unsettled. One regimen recommends 2 mg per kilogram of methylprednisolone sodium succinate initially, followed by 1 to 2 mg per kilogram every four to six hours. When clinical signs and objective evidence indicate that the patient is responding to therapy, usually after 48 to 72 hours, then steroids may be converted to oral preparations. Sixty mg of prednisone may be started as a single morning dose. If the patient continues to improve, it may be reduced by 5 mg every third or fourth day.

In some patients it may not be possible to withdraw steroids. In this situation, the following approaches may be tried: maintenance with the lowest possible dose given on alternate days, a trial of cromolyn therapy, or conversion to aerosolized steroids. It is important that the latter two agents should be started only after there has been an optimal therapeutic response for the acute attack.

Long-term Management. Maintenance therapy should be based on similar clinical and objective criteria as in treating the acute attack. For example, outpatient spirograms should be used routinely in following the patient. Also, the patient should be convinced as to the chronicity of the disease and dissuaded from adjusting or stopping medication when symptoms abate. Asthma should not be treated symptomatically.

It is also important to identify specific precipitating or triggering factors, including allergic and nonallergic stimuli. A thorough history may allow elimination of offending agents from the environment or occupation. Other underlying conditions such as chronic sinusitis should be carefully evaluated (e.g., sinus roentgenograms). The successful medical or sur-

---

*This dose exceeds manufacturer's maximum recommended dose.

gical treatment of chronic sinusitis may have a dramatic impact on the treatment of asthma.

Immunotherapy with extracts of allergens may benefit certain allergic patients. This form of therapy, however, is just beginning to be established on firm scientific grounds.

Patients with late-onset asthmatic responses may not be adequately managed on maintenance bronchodilator therapy alone (beta$_2$ drugs and aminophylline). Beta$_2$ bronchodilators and theophylline are not effective in preventing or reversing the late-onset reactions. In contrast, corticosteroids inhibit as well as reverse the inflammatory response of the late-onset reaction. Cromolyn sodium is useful strictly because it is a prophylactic agent. Thus, the use of cromolyn sodium or steroids (by mouth or inhalation) or both may be necessary for successful long-term maintenance therapy of late-onset asthma. A trial of immunotherapy may also benefit this group of patients.

PROGNOSIS. There are about 9 million patients with asthma in the United States, and several thousand deaths per year are attributable to the disease. Statistics concerning the long-term prognosis of asthma are as variable as the disease. For example, the percentage of childhood asthma reported to persist until adult life varies from 26 to 78 per cent. Also, it is generally held, without good data, that adult asthma improves or disappears with age. Taken together, the evidence supports Osler's adage that "asthmatics pant their way into old age."

Anderson SD: Issues in exercise-induced asthma. J Allergy Clin Immunol 76:763, 1985. *A review of the pathophysiologic mechanisms involved in exercise-induced asthma. It contrasts the evidence implicating heat versus water loss as the primary stimuli for this phenomenon.*

Barnes NC, Costello JF: Mast-cell–derived mediators in asthma: Arachidonic acid metabolites. Postgrad Med 76:140, 148, 1984. *A clear and concise summary of a difficult subject dealing with arachidonic acid metabolic pathways. It describes how leukotrienes and prostaglandins are generated within the lung and their potential role in bronchoconstriction.*

Cherniack RM: Chronic and acute asthma: Key to successful management. Postgrad Med 75:87, 1984. *A practical review of management strategies for acute and chronic asthma.*

Kaliner MA: Hypotheses on the contribution of late-phase allergic responses to the understanding and treatment of allergic diseases. J Allergy Clin Immunol 75:311, 1985. *A current and concise review of the pathophysiologic events involved in the late-onset asthmatic reactions. It also discusses the clinical implications and the drugs that are efficacious in reversing or preventing late-onset reactions.*

McFadden ER Jr, Feldman NT: Asthma: Pathophysiology and clinical correlates. Med Clin North Am 61:1229, 1977. *A review that summarizes the correlations between manifestations and pulmonary function abnormalities.*

Morris HG: Mechanisms of action and therapeutic role of corticosteroids in asthma. J Allergy Clin Immunol 75:1, 1985. *A review of our current understanding of the mechanisms of action of corticosteroids in inhibiting the inflammatory response in asthma. It also identifies current indications, efficacy, and side effects of systemic and topical steroids that are used in the therapy of bronchial asthma. It contains an extensive bibliography.*

Nadel JA, Barnes PJ: Autonomic regulation of the airways. Ann Rev Med 35:451, 1984. *Reviews the sympathetic and parasympathetic innervation of the airways with particular reference to how they modulate smooth muscle tone and mucosal gland secretion. It also presents evidence implicating autonomic dysfunction in asthma.*

Sheppard D: Mechanisms of bronchoconstriction from nonimmunologic environmental stimuli. Chest 90:584, 1986. *A brief review that discusses the general mechanisms by which diverse inhaled agents cause bronchoconstriction by nonimmunologic mechanisms.*

Weinberger M, Hendeles L: Current concepts: Slow-release theophylline: Rationale and basis for product selection. N Engl J Med 308:760, 1983. *A review of the therapeutic strategies for theophylline. It also contains details on drug preparations and their doses.*

Woolcock AJ, Yan K, Salome CM, et al.: What determines the severity of asthma? Chest 87:209S, 1985. *A good discussion of epidemiologic and clinical factors that are considered to influence the severity of asthma.*

61 CHRONIC AIRWAYS DISEASES*

Richard A. Matthay

CHRONIC BRONCHITIS AND EMPHYSEMA

Chronic generalized airway disorders that are not the direct result of a "specific" bronchopulmonary disease are discussed in this chapter. Common to most of these diseases is chronic airways obstruction, caused most frequently by a diffuse involvement of peripheral (small) airways or, more rarely, by localized obstruction of central (large) airways. The designation *chronic obstructive pulmonary disease (COPD)* is an imperfect, although widely utilized, term, since it includes several specific disorders with different clinical manifestations, pathologic findings, therapy requirements, and prognoses.

Four *diffuse* airway disorders are examined in this chapter: simple chronic bronchitis, asthmatic bronchitis, chronic obstructive bronchitis, and emphysema. Some classifications include all of these entities in the broad term COPD. Moreover, various combinations of these disorders coexist; for instance, patients often have chronic obstructive bronchitis as well as emphysema. *Localized* airway obstruction, above and below the tracheal bifurcation, is discussed in a separate section of this chapter.

DEFINITIONS OF TERMS. Unfortunately, *chronic bronchitis* has been used variably to refer to a simple smoker's cough or, as in the British literature, to severe COPD. In this discussion, chronic bronchitis will be considered "simple," "obstructive," or "asthmatic" to reduce ambiguity. It is useful clinically to differentiate between the extremely common simple chronic bronchitis and the less common but often devastating form, chronic obstructive bronchitis. These two entities will therefore be described in separate sections.

Simple chronic bronchitis, a syndrome characterized primarily by a chronic productive cough, is the result of low-grade exposure to bronchial irritants in an individual without hyperreactive airways. This syndrome is associated with enhanced mucous secretion, reduced ciliary activity, and impaired resistance to bronchial infection. Simple chronic bronchitis is defined in clinical terms: (1) excessive production of mucus; (2) presence of symptoms, largely cough, on most days for at least three months annually during two or more successive years; and (3) exclusion of bronchiectasis, tuberculosis, or other causes of these symptoms. The term does not describe the underlying process, which may vary widely. The patient population ranges from those who are asymptomatic except for a morning "cigarette cough" productive of mucus in small amounts (*simple chronic bronchitis*) to patients with a severe disabling condition manifested by increased resistance to airflow, hypoxia, and often hypercapnia (*chronic obstructive bronchitis*). Chronic obstructive bronchitis, which develops in a relatively small proportion of individuals with simple chronic bronchitis, results in irreversible narrowing of air-

---

*Portions of this chapter were rewritten from the 17th edition of *Cecil Textbook of Medicine*, with permission from Benjamin Burrows.

TABLE 61–1. FEATURES OF THE EMPHYSEMATOUS AND BRONCHIAL TYPES OF COPD

	Emphysematous (Type A)	Bronchial (Type B)
Clinical features		
Dyspnea	Insidious onset, slowly progressive	Often noted first only during chest infections
Sputum	Usually scant and mucoid	Often copious and purulent
Weight loss	Often marked	Usually slight or absent
Chronic cor pulmonale with heart failure	Infrequent until terminal stages of the disease	Common
Chest examination	Quiet chest (except slight wheeze at end expiration), marked hyperinflation	Noisy chest, slight hyperinflation
Chest radiograph	Hyperlucent, overinflated lung; often regional attenuation of vessels	Often evidence of old inflammatory disease
Physiologic tests		
Total lung capacity	Increased	Normal or slightly decreased
Residual volume	Markedly increased	Moderately increased
Lung compliance, static	Increased	Near normal
Lung compliance, dynamic	Normal or slightly low	Very low
Lung recoil	Markedly reduced	Variable
Inspiratory airways resistance	Normal	Increased
Diffusing capacity	Markedly reduced	Variable
Arterial P_{O_2}	Slight reduction at rest; usually falls with exertion	Often very low at rest; variable change with exertion
Arterial P_{CO_2}	Usually normal or low	Often chronically elevated
Resting pulmonary artery pressure	Normal or slightly elevated at rest; increases with exertion	Often markedly elevated at rest
Cardiac output	Often low	Usually near normal

ways. Because the obstruction is in bronchioles and bronchi 2 mm or less in diameter, the term *small airways disease* has been used.

Exposure to bronchial irritants in individuals with hyperreactive or "twitchy" airways can lead to bronchospasm (i.e., bronchial smooth muscle constriction), frequently accompanied by excessive mucous production and edema of bronchial walls. Recurrent episodes of symptomatic bronchospasm are called *asthma* (discussed in Ch. 60). The present discussion must consider bronchospasm, since a degree of reversible airways obstruction often accompanies other reactions to inhaled noxious agents. In fact, episodic airways obstruction is common in individuals with chronic bronchitis. This combination, called *asthmatic bronchitis*, may closely resemble classic asthma. The term *chronic asthmatic bronchitis* is applied in patients with persistent airways obstruction, a chronic productive cough, and a major problem of episodic bronchospasm.

Emphysema, another lung response to noxious stimuli, is characterized by abnormal, permanent enlargement of airspaces distal to the terminal bronchioles, accompanied by destruction of their walls, and without obvious fibrosis. The alterations of emphysema cause reduction in lung elastic recoil, which permits excessive airway collapse upon expiration and leads to irreversible airflow obstruction.

These definitions are not mutually exclusive; there is considerable crossover between the emphysematous (type A) and bronchial (type B) findings listed in Table 61–1. For example, most individuals with emphysema also have a chronic productive cough. It may be difficult to determine the relative importance of emphysema and chronic obstructive bronchitis, with obliteration of small airways. Accordingly, general terms such as *chronic obstructive pulmonary disease (COPD)* have been used to describe this clinical syndrome.

PATHOPHYSIOLOGY OF AIRWAYS OBSTRUCTION.
Airways obstruction denotes slowing of forced expiration. As outlined in Ch. 59, the speed of forced expiration is determined primarily by three factors: intrinsic resistance of the airways, compressibility of the airways, and lung elastic recoil. Reduced maximum expiratory flow (Vmax) results from high airways resistance, reduced lung recoil, and/or excessive airways collapsibility.

In general, a low FEV_1/FVC^* ratio is indicative of airflow obstruction; the amount of reduction in FEV_1 itself establishes the severity of the obstruction (Fig. 61–1). Some prefer to use

$FEF_{25-75\%}$, the average flow over the middle half of a forced expiration.

Actual Vmax values can be measured, commonly at 50 per cent or 75 per cent of the forced expired volume ($Vmax_{50\%}$ or $Vmax_{75\%}$, respectively*). $Vmax_{75\%}$ has become popular in epidemiologic studies because it appears to be more sensitive than the FEV_1.

In clinical practice, FEV_1 is used more widely because it is easy to measure, is quite reproducible, has a relatively narrow normal range, and tends to reflect the clinical severity of disease.

A variety of physiologic abnormalities are associated with obstructive airways disorders (also discussed in Ch. 59). Increased venous admixture and hypoxemia develop owing to ventilation and perfusion mismatching. Unless there is an increase in overall ventilation, this mismatching also may lead to increased physiologic dead space and hypercapnia. Carbon dioxide retention is likely when airways obstruction is severe, respiratory muscle fatigue occurs, and the drive to breathe is depressed. Air trapping and an increase in residual volume develop because obstructed airways tend to close prematurely during a maximal exhalation. In emphysema, total lung capacity may be enhanced as well. The pulmonary diffusing capacity measurement is usually reduced in emphysema owing to loss of functioning alveolar capillary membrane surface area.

Because of the large total cross-sectional diameter of the small airways, marked alterations are required to produce discernible changes in the FEV_1 values. Several potentially more sensitive tests have been proposed to detect mild abnormalities of the small airways: closing volume, helium response of the maximal expiratory flow volume (MEFV) curve, and frequency dependence of compliance. These tests are specific for small airways abnormalities, but clinical application has not been established yet.

Burrows B: An overview of obstructive lung disease. Med Clin North Am 65:455, 1981. *This is the lead article of an 11-chapter symposium on obstructive lung diseases. The entire symposium is recommended reading and an excellent source of original references.*

Fishman AP: The spectrum of chronic obstructive disease of the airways. In

---

*FEV_1 = forced expiratory volume in one second; FVC = forced vital capacity; FEF = forced expiratory flow.

---

*Because use of these symbols has caused confusion, it has been suggested that $Vmax_{50\%}$ and $Vmax_{75\%}$ be expressed as $FEF_{50\%}$ and $FEF_{75\%}$, respectively. Moreover, $Vmax_{75\%}$ as defined herein has sometimes been reported as $Vmax_{25\%}$, the 25% referring to the portion of the FVC remaining when the flow measurement is made.

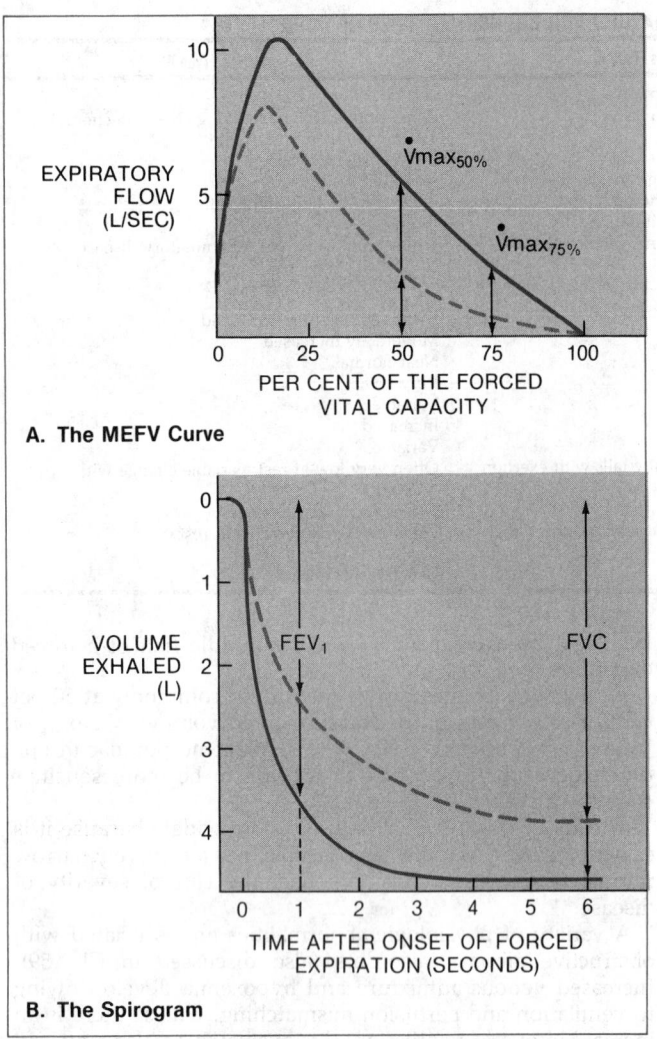

A. The MEFV Curve

B. The Spirogram

FIGURE 61–1. Solid lines are used to show a normal maximum expiratory flow-volume (MEFV) in *A* and a normal spirogram in *B*. Broken lines indicate typical curves for a patient with mild airways obstruction. Measurements of the forced vital capacity (FVC), the forced expiratory volume at one second (FEV_1), and forced flow rates at 50 per cent and 75 per cent of the FVC ($\dot{V}max_{50\%}$ and $\dot{V}max_{75\%}$) are depicted as vertical lines. (Adapted from Burrows B: Chronic airways disease. Cecil Textbook of Medicine. 17th ed.)

Fishman AP (ed.): Pulmonary Diseases and Disorders. New York, McGraw-Hill Book Company, 1980, p 458. *A concise, clearly written description of the different types of airways obstructive disorders and how they overlap.*

Snider GL, Kleinerman J, Thurlbeck WM, et al.: The definition of emphysema. Am Rev Respir Dis 132:182, 1985. *Up-to-date, succinct statement of the definition, anatomic subtypes, and clinical diagnosis of emphysema.*

Thurlbeck WM: The anatomical pathology of chronic airflow obstruction. Curr Pulmonol 4:1, 1982. *A good discussion of the pathologic conditions associated with airways obstruction.*

Simple Chronic Bronchitis and Asthmatic Bronchitis

PREVALENCE AND PATHOGENESIS. "Simple chronic bronchitis" refers to a productive cough that persists for at least three months of the year for two consecutive years. It affects 10 to 25 per cent of the adult population. Cough with sputum production is more common in men than in women and more common in persons over the age of 40 than in younger individuals. All forms of chronic bronchitis are strongly linked to cigarette smoking. Thus, a large proportion of cigarette smokers, particularly those over age 45, have simple chronic bronchitis. Some occupations involving dust (e.g., handling grain and mining) are associated with an abnormally high incidence of chronic bronchitis, even after statistics are corrected for smoking habits. Few individuals

with simple chronic bronchitis consult a physician, and then the visit is usually prompted by acute or recurrent respiratory tract infections or wheezing in addition to chronic cough. *Chronic asthmatic bronchitis* tends to develop in elderly individuals, most commonly in smokers. Three direct effects of inhaling bronchial irritants cause chronic bronchitis: (1) stimulation of mucous secretion in the airways, (2) impaired mucous clearance due in part to interference with ciliary activity, and (3) lowered resistance to bronchopulmonary infection due to disturbed alveolar macrophage function. Cough develops owing to accumulation of secretions. As a result of bacterial colonization by organisms usually found in the nasopharynx, normally sterile bronchi now harbor organisms.

Although cigarette smoking is the most important of the identifiable causal factors, not all smokers develop mucus hypersecretion and no more than 15 to 20 per cent develop airflow obstruction. Little is known about the reasons for the variable susceptibility to hypersecretion and airflow obstruction in smokers or why reversible airways obstruction develops in many patients with chronic bronchitis. Retention of secretions may be a major factor in some instances. Immunologic factors and other mediators of bronchoconstriction may play a role, since some patients have subacute or chronic bronchospasm resembling classic asthma.

PATHOLOGY. Enlargement of mucous glands in the large airways, the most characteristic abnormality, is primarily due to increased numbers of their constituent cells (hyperplasia) rather than to enlargement of cells (hypertrophy). Retained bronchial secretions and variable degrees of inflammatory changes in the bronchial walls also are identified. Narrowing or obliteration of some small airways, increased mucus in these airways, and scattered centrilobular emphysema may be found, even though clinically significant obstruction is absent. Since asymptomatic smokers may have similar small airways and emphysematous changes, it is unclear whether these alterations are related to simple chronic bronchitis except through a common association with cigarette smoking.

CLINICAL MANIFESTATIONS. When the disease is mild, *cough* occurs on arising or usually after smoking the first cigarette of the day. The cough is productive of a small amount of mucoid sputum and occurs most regularly in the winter months. As the severity increases, the patient coughs throughout the day, symptoms are present throughout the year, sputum volume increases, and episodes of severe coughing develop. Near the end of a severe paroxysm of coughing, wheezing may occur, probably owing to cough-induced bronchospasm. Lying down may induce wheezing, which is probably caused by retained secretions, for cough often provides relief.

Symptoms associated with purulent sputum, suggesting overgrowth of bacteria, may reappear after a viral respiratory infection. *Haemophilus influenzae* and *Streptococcus pneumoniae* may be present, but sputum cultures usually show normal nasopharyngeal flora.

Bacterial organisms probably represent secondary pathogens rather than being the primary cause of these exacerbations of symptoms. During exacerbations, various degrees of bronchospasm also may develop, blurring the distinction between such episodes and asthma. Whereas *blood-streaked sputum* is noted occasionally, severe or repeated hemoptysis may indicate a more serious entity, such as pulmonary neoplasm.

The sputum may become chronically purulent as the disorder progresses, and the term *mucopurulent bronchitis* may be applied to this stage of the disease. Rarely, drug-resistant organisms (e.g., *Pseudomonas aeruginosa*) are identified on sputum cultures, especially if the patient has received multiple antibiotics.

In mild disease, physical examination may be normal. As the disease advances, variable coarse crackles, which may clear or change location with coughing, and scattered wheezes are heard. A forced expiratory maneuver often induces a wheeze or a paroxysm of coughing.

If reversible airway obstruction is present, the patient may resemble the typical asthmatic person, with wheezing and slowing of forced expiration as prominent features.

LABORATORY FINDINGS. The chest radiograph, blood counts, and differential smear are all normal in the uncomplicated case. Leukocytes and a mixed flora of organisms are noted on sputum examination. Although spirometry often shows some slowing of forced expiration, flow rates may be normal in simple bronchitis. Individuals with *chronic asthmatic bronchitis* may have severe airways obstruction even between acute attacks. During episodes of bronchospasm in patients with asthmatic bronchitis, functional abnormalities are more severe, and both blood and sputum eosinophilia may be present.

COURSE AND PROGNOSIS. In patients with simple chronic bronchitis, symptoms may fluctuate widely. Increased cigarette use, inclement weather, and acute respiratory infections all tend to enhance cough and sputum production. Cessation of smoking in mild cases usually leads to disappearance of symptoms. A slight reduction in ventilatory function is common in simple chronic bronchitis, but progressive respiratory insufficiency does not necessarily develop.

The long-term outcome of patients with asthmatic bronchitis has not been studied extensively. Some patients may become asymptomatic for years after an initial excellent response to therapy, whereas others require progressively more medication to control bronchospasm. Progress to irreversible airways obstruction occurs in at least a few patients despite good medical management.

DIFFERENTIAL DIAGNOSIS. A persistent, productive cough not attributable to an upper respiratory tract disorder, an allergic reaction of the airways, a specific endobronchial disease, or parenchymal lung disease justifies the diagnosis of chronic bronchitis. Exclusion of a parenchymal lesion requires a chest radiograph. Moreover, a careful upper airway examination should be done, and physical findings, such as a persistent, localized wheeze, must be sought to identify a localized airways disorder. Cystic fibrosis must be excluded in children and in young adults who have severe symptoms of chronic bronchitis (see Ch. 66). In addition, in individuals with one of the immotile cilia syndromes, symptoms of chronic bronchitis may be noted (see Ch. 65).

When there is no identifiable source of chronic bronchial irritation, the diagnosis of simple chronic bronchitis should be made with caution. Sputum and blood eosinophilia should be sought in a nonsmoking patient whose symptoms are associated with exposure to allergens or in a patient with episodes of combined wheezing and dyspnea. Asthmatic bronchitis, which may respond to bronchodilators or corticosteroids, is suggested by high eosinophil levels.

Bronchoscopy and even bronchography or a computed tomography (CT) scan may be indicated to rule out an endobronchial lesion or localized bronchiectasis in patients with severe or repeated hemoptysis or with physical findings suggesting localized disease. In the routine case, these procedures are not indicated.

Severe mucopurulent bronchitis may be difficult to distinguish from bronchiectasis. In fact, in persons with severe bronchitis, the bronchi may show mild, diffuse, cylindric dilatation. Saccular bronchiectasis is suggested by (1) repeated pneumonias in the same lung zone, (2) honeycombed areas on the chest radiograph, and (3) recurrent hemoptysis. Bronchography provides an accurate diagnosis, but this invasive procedure is usually indicated only if resection of the bronchiectatic area or areas is considered. Otherwise, there is little difference in therapy for mucopurulent bronchitis and bron-

chiectasis. Computed tomography of the chest has been used successfully to diagnose localized and diffuse bronchiectasis.

TREATMENT. Cigarettes and any other bronchial irritants should be removed initially, since this step alone may relieve the symptoms. If the symptoms persist after maximal effort to avoid provoking factors, the following measures are applied.

Antibiotic Therapy. Infection is considered present when the patient is producing a noneosinophilic purulent sputum. A seven- to ten-day course of tetracycline or ampicillin (1 gram daily in divided doses) or double-strength sulfamethoxazole-trimethoprim (one tablet twice daily) should be administered. Failure of this antibiotic therapy to clear the sputum warrants a sputum culture and sensitivity test. Successive doses of different antibiotics should be avoided, since this may lead to resistant flora. Therapeutic failure generally is due to inadequate drainage of the airways more often than to an improper choice of antibacterial drugs.

The antibiotic may have to be changed on the basis of drug susceptibility studies when resistant organisms are cultured from the sputum. (For severe purulent exacerbations, penicillin has proved to be inadequate therapy.)

Bronchodilators. The bronchodilator agents are the mainstays for managing bronchospasm associated with simple chronic bronchitis and for control of any reversible component of COPD. They are also useful in conjunction with bronchial hygiene therapy, described below. Both of the main classes of bronchodilators, the methylxanthines and the beta-adrenergic agonists, help to relieve bronchospasm and to prevent recurrent attacks. The inhaled route of administering beta-adrenergic drugs is usually more effective and rapid in relieving bronchospasm than the oral route. Patients must be carefully instructed, however, in the proper technique for utilizing inhalers. Inhaled atropine may exhibit a combined beneficial effect of reducing copious amounts of sputum and partially relieving bronchospasm in the person with severe bronchitis. The principles and details for therapeutic application of these agents are described in Ch. 60.

Corticosteroids. When significant airways obstruction persists or recurs in the patient with asthmatic bronchitis in spite of maximal therapy with bronchodilators, corticosteroids are indicated. If the patient is ambulatory, modest doses (e.g., 20 to 40 mg of prednisone per day) are administered for several days and then tapered to the lowest dose that will sustain improvement. Often, improvement is rapid, and the drug can be discontinued in seven to ten days. Thereafter, a short "burst" of corticosteroids is used to treat occasional relapses. In some patients, tapering corticosteroids leads to recurrence of symptoms. In these individuals, the dose should be maintained as low as possible to relieve bronchospasm and to prevent recurrent attacks. Alternate-day single-dose corticosteroids should be used if possible.

Once bronchospasm has been relieved and a maintenance dose of corticosteroid achieved, an inhaled, poorly absorbed preparation such as beclomethasone should be added. This medication is inhaled from a pressurized container, two to four puffs (100 to 200 μg) two to four times daily, depending upon the preparation. The inhaled agent may permit reduction in the maintenance dose of corticosteroid without recurrence of bronchospasm. When significant bronchospasm is present, inhaled corticosteroid agents should be avoided, since this medication may aggravate bronchoconstriction and fail to reach the distal airways. For some patients, premedication with an inhaled bronchodilator (e.g., a beta-adrenergic agent) may relieve airway irritation and permit successful use of inhaled corticosteroids. In general, inhaled corticosteroids replace 7.5 to 10 mg per day of oral prednisone.

After the addition of an inhaled agent, the dose of oral prednisone should be reduced slowly (over several months) to avoid adrenal insufficiency in a corticosteroid-dependent patient who has received months or years of systemic medication. In up to 30 per cent of patients, oropharyngeal candidiasis occurs owing to inhaled corticosteroids. This condition responds, however, to specific therapy and rarely requires discontinuation of the inhaled preparation. Nasal symptoms, previously controlled by oral prednisone, may recur, requiring reinstitution of oral agents.

Bronchial Hygiene. These measures are designed to clear retained bronchial secretions. Deep breathing followed by deliberate coughing is the most important maneuver. Sputum production may be more effective if the most involved lung regions are in the superior position (postural drainage) and chest percussion and vibration are applied.

Bronchial hygiene measures may be better tolerated and more effective if the patient is premedicated with an inhaled bronchodilator and then inhales a bland mist to loosen secretions. Although some patients are convinced of its efficacy, objective benefits of bland mist therapy have been difficult to establish. Because patients' reactions to this therapy vary, only measures that prove effective should be continued, since the full program is uncomfortable and time consuming.

To avoid inspissation of secretions, patients should be encouraged to keep well hydrated. Intravenous fluids may be required for acute exacerbations. Although the efficacy of expectorant medications has not been established, some authorities recommend 10 to 12 drops of a saturated solution of potassium iodide three times daily. This program is associated with a high rate of side effects, some severe; yet, it does seem effective in some patients. Cough syrups and lozenges have little effect on the viscosity of bronchial secretions, but they may relieve a "tickle" in the throats of many persons with bronchitis. Cough sedatives should be used only for acute episodes of a severe, nonproductive cough and are otherwise contraindicated.

Treatment of Severe Exacerbations. Severe exacerbations of asthmatic bronchitis can be life threatening, particularly when associated with severe airways obstruction. The approach to status asthmaticus outlined in Ch. 60 is appropriate, although the patient with asthmatic bronchitis may require more attention to bronchial hygiene measures to clear secretions than does the person with classic asthma.

Anthonisen NR, Manfreda J, Warren CPW, et al.: Antibiotic therapy in exacerbations of chronic obstructive pulmonary disease. Ann Intern Med 106:196, 1987. *Double-blind placebo controlled trial that reports significant benefit from antimicrobial therapy during exacerbations of chronic bronchitis.*

Burrows B: Irreversible airways obstruction and asthma. Pract Cardiol 8:69, 1982. *This article presents in more detail views concerning the overlap of reversible and irreversible airways obstructive diseases.*

Burrows B, Lebowitz MD, Barbee RA, et al.: Interactions of smoking and immunological factors in relationship to airways obstruction. Chest 84:657, 1983. *This paper presents evidence that chronic asthmatic bronchitis may result from an interaction of the irritant effects of smoking and immunologic factors.*

Iafrate RP, Massey KL, Hendeles L: Current concepts in clinical therapeutics: Asthma. Clin Pharmacol Ther 5:206, 1986. *A good review of the use of bronchodilators and corticosteroids in reversible airways diseases.*

IPPB Trial Group: Intermittent positive pressure breathing therapy of chronic obstructive pulmonary disease. Ann Intern Med 99:612, 1983. *This study establishes that there is no significant benefit in positive pressure breathing over other modalities of delivering bronchodilators.*

Sachs FL: Chronic bronchitis. In Pennington JE (ed.): Respiratory Infections: Diagnosis and Management. New York, Raven Press, 1983, p 113. *Comprehensive review of the etiologic role and need for therapy of respiratory infection during exacerbations of chronic bronchitis.*

Chronic Obstructive Bronchitis and Emphysema

PREVALENCE AND PATHOGENESIS. As a major cause of chronic disability in older individuals, chronic obstructive bronchitis and emphysema (COPD) rank only behind heart disease and schizophrenia in the United States. Chronic obstructive pulmonary disease is the fifth leading cause of death in the United States, and there has been a 22 per cent increase in the death rate from this condition over the past 20 years. Approximately 65,000 individuals die yearly from COPD in the United States, one half of the number dying annually from lung cancer.

Emphysema is common and increases with age. It is present at autopsy in approximately 65 per cent of adult men and 15 per cent of adult women. The prevalence of emphysema is strongly related to cigarette smoking.

Chronic obstructive pulmonary disease is usually diagnosed between ages 55 and 65. The greater incidence in men than in women most likely reflects the lower incidence of smoking in women in earlier decades. Recent trends, however, show that more teenage girls than boys are starting to smoke. Thus, in several decades COPD may be as common or more common in women.

Smoking. Patients with COPD have some combination of chronic obstructive bronchitis and pulmonary emphysema, both of which are closely associated with cigarette smoking. The chronic, progressive destruction of the alveolar structures characteristic of emphysema is thought to occur because of an imbalance between the proteases (proteolytic enzymes) and antiproteases in the lower respiratory tract. According to this concept, proteases, particularly neutrophil (PMN) elastase and possibly elastases in pulmonary alveolar macrophages (PAM's), work unimpeded to destroy alveolar structures and their elastin network. Cigarette smokers have increased numbers of PAM's, and PMN's are recruited into their lungs so that increased numbers of both cell types are recoverable on bronchoalveolar lavage. Recruitment of PMN's into the lungs may occur as a result of the elaboration of chemotactic factors by PAM's stimulated by cigarette smoke. Moreover, smoke components can cause elastase to be released by PMN's by inducing cytotoxic reactions and by stimulating secretion from viable cells. Macrophages exposed to cigarette smoke in vitro or in vivo increase secretion of an elastase-like enzyme. This potential for a greatly increased protease (primarily elastase) burden must be counteracted by the antiprotease defense system of the lungs.

The protease-antiprotease theory of the pathogenesis of emphysema has received further support from the recognition that patients with severe (homozygous phenotype) alpha$_1$-antitypsin deficiency have markedly reduced levels of serum alpha$_1$-antitrypsin and progressive panacinar emphysema. As might be expected, patients with severe alpha$_1$-antitrypsin deficiency have little or no alpha$_1$-antitrypsin in their lower respiratory tracts when studied by bronchoalveolar lavage. Nor do they have alternate antiprotease protection against neutrophil elastase.

Cigarette smokers without alpha$_1$-antitrypsin deficiency also show reduced elastase inhibitory capacity, compared with nonsmokers, because of inactivation of alpha$_1$–proteinase inhibitor (alpha$_1$-PI). Chemical oxidation of alpha$_1$-PI by material in cigarette smoke is postulated as a major cause of the observed decrease in elastase inhibitory capacity. Smoking may interfere with elastin repair mechanisms, as documented by studies both in vivo and in vitro.

Severe genetic deficiency of serum alpha$_1$-antitrypsin occurs in 0.5 to 2 per cent of patients with COPD. Typically, in such individuals, emphysema is likely to develop by age 40 in smokers and by age 60 in nonsmokers. Presumably, prolonged exposure to irritants, primarily cigarette smoke, further reduces lung antiprotease defenses and induces low-grade inflammation and destructive changes in the parenchyma of the lungs.

The protease-antiprotease hypothesis of the pathogenesis of emphysema does not readily explain all of the observations in experimental and human emphysema. For instance, experimental enzyme-induced emphysema is panacinar rather than centrilobular, the more common type in humans with chronic airflow obstruction. Moreover, it does not explain the predominant localization of centrilobular emphysema to the upper lung zones or of panacinar emphysema to the lung bases or of paraseptal emphysema to the regions beneath the pleura and adjacent to fibrous septa. There is a close relationship between slowing of forced exhalation and cigarette smoking. The average heavy smoker has a 40 to 45 ml per year decline in FEV_1, whereas the average nonsmoking adult shows a decline of only 20 to 25 ml per year. Nonsmokers with alpha$_1$-antitrypsin deficiency have approximately an 80 ml per year decline in FEV_1; cigarette smokers with this deficiency have approximately a 150 ml per year decline. When individuals with alpha$_1$-antitrypsin deficiency stop smoking, this excess rate of decline in FEV_1 ceases. Nevertheless, the average effect of cigarette smoking alone does not explain the more severe reduction in FEV_1 noted in patients with COPD. Moreover, why is it that only a minority of smokers develop clinically significant COPD? Some individuals may be particularly susceptible for various reasons: respiratory disorders in childhood, intercurrent respiratory infections, or genetic factors, for example.

Can COPD be detected early by screening lung function in young to middle-aged adults? Longitudinal studies are attempting to identify susceptible cigarette-smoking individuals with an excessive rate of decline in pulmonary function throughout adult life. The hypothesis is that the individual who will develop COPD later in life should be identifiable by age 40 because he or she will show at least a mild ventilatory abnormality by then. There is no direct evidence yet, however, that any physiologic test applied early in life identifies the individual who will develop disabling COPD.

Alpha$_1$-Antitrypsin Deficiency. A deficiency in serum antiproteolytic activity associated with a susceptibility to COPD has been noted in several families. The protease inhibitor, or "Pi," phenotype of the subject determines the serum's trypsin inhibitory capacity. Two M genes (Pi MM phenotype) are present in normal individuals. When only Z genes are present (Pi ZZ phenotype), serum alpha$_1$-antitrypsin levels are severely reduced (< 50 mg per deciliter), and the alpha$_1$-antitrypsin that is present in plasma is less effective in inhibiting neutrophil elastase than alpha$_1$-antitrypsin in individuals with the Pi MM phenotype. Deficiency of alpha$_1$-antitrypsin is transmitted as an autosomal recessive trait. This antiproteolytic deficiency, present in approximately 1:4000 of the population, is associated with hepatitis in infancy and the development of emphysema in the third, fourth, and fifth decades. Present in 3 to 5 per cent of the population, the heterozygous state (Pi MZ phenotype) is associated with a moderately reduced serum antiproteolytic activity, but no predilection for developing an excess of respiratory disorders. Several other Pi genes have been identified (of which S is the most common), but only the Z gene clearly leads to COPD. In Ch. 125, the hepatic manifestations of alpha$_1$-antitrypsin deficiency are discussed.

PATHOLOGY. Alveolar wall destruction with a nonuniform pattern of airspace enlargement is the basic abnormality in emphysema. The orderly appearance of the acinus and its components is disturbed and may be lost, as airspaces are fewer in number but enlarged. In centrilobular emphysema, the process is most severe in the central portion of the lobule, whereas in panacinar emphysema the defect occurs uniformly throughout the acinus. Both centrilobular and panacinar emphysema may be noted in the same lung. In severe centrilobular emphysema, the entire acinus ultimately may become involved. Centrilobular emphysema generally is the most common form of emphysema in patients with chronic airflow obstruction.

In large airways, inflammation is noted in and around air passages, with narrowing of the lumina, impaction of mucus, and obliterative changes. Small airways abnormalities usually are not obvious on cursory examination and require careful morphometric studies.

CLINICAL MANIFESTATIONS. Dyspnea is usually the predominant complaint, but some patients consult a physician initially because of cough, wheezing, recurrent respiratory infections, or, occasionally, weakness or weight loss. Patients may date the onset of chronic symptoms to an acute respiratory infection. In some, shortness of breath is present only during acute exacerbations.

A productive cough is usually present, associated with a thick or "sticky" sputum varying widely in quantity. Copious amounts of purulent sputum production, coupled with a severe cough, are noted by some patients.

The physical examination may be normal relatively early in the illness (FEV_1 >1.0 liter). Auscultation of the chest may reveal rhonchi, or the chest may be quiet, particularly in patients with extensive emphysema. Wheezing, which may be absent on quiet breathing, can often be heard on forced exhalation. As the disease progresses, marked hyperinflation with low diaphragms and a reduced area of cardiac dullness are common. After minimal exertion or even at rest, labored breathing, at times through pursed lips, may be noted. Patients tend to lean forward on their elbows when sitting, assuming a stooped posture, while using accessory muscles of respiration. Cyanosis and dependent edema may be noted.

Occasionally, patients first seek medical attention when signs of right heart failure due to cor pulmonale appear. In such cases, the FEV_1 is likely to be below 1 liter and the arterial Po_2 below 45 mm Hg. The pulmonary hypertension in these patients with COPD and cor pulmonale is most closely related to the severity of hypoxemia.

Table 61–1 shows features of relatively distinctive COPD clinical syndromes and their associated underlying pathologic conditions. These two clinical types of COPD, emphysematous (type A) and bronchial (type B), represent extremes of presentation; most individuals, if followed chronically, develop a mixture of findings from the type A and type B groups. Type A patients, described as "pink puffers," often hyperventilate, maintaining a normal or nearly normal arterial O_2 tension and CO_2 tensions. In contrast, type B patients, "blue bloaters," often have a low arterial O_2 tension, high CO_2 tension, cyanosis, and right-sided congestive heart failure. The "blue bloater" syndrome may also result from disordered breathing during sleep, a common problem in patients with COPD.

LABORATORY FINDINGS. The routine blood count and differential study are normal except for erythrocytosis in some COPD patients with hypoxemia. When eosinophilia is found, a reversible (asthmatic-bronchitic) component of the disease should be suspected.

Early in the disease, the chest radiograph may be normal; however, in severe emphysema, lung hyperinflation and an increased retrosternal airspace, with flattening of the diaphragms and regional attenuation of blood vessels, are usually noted. Frank bullae outlined by hairline margins are present in some cases. The chest radiograph should not be the sole basis for the diagnosis of COPD, for individuals with perfectly normal lung function may have radiographic findings typical of the disease. Chest CT can be used to determine the presence of emphysema and to quantify its severity with reasonable accuracy.

Persistent reduction in forced expiratory flow rates is the most typical finding in COPD. Two lung volume measurements, the residual volume and the residual volume/total lung capacity ratio, are elevated. Ventilation-perfusion mismatch and nonuniformity of ventilation are also typical findings, whereas arterial hypoxemia and physiologic shunting vary among patients. When the diffusing capacity is very depressed and the total lung capacity is clearly elevated, emphysema is likely to be extensive.

Ventilation and perfusion lung scans should be interpreted cautiously when pulmonary emboli are suspected. These scans reveal the uneven ventilation and perfusion typical of COPD. Areas of diminished perfusion may be mistaken for pulmonary emboli. Accordingly, when pulmonary embolism is suspected in a patient with COPD, a pulmonary angiogram is often required for definitive diagnosis.

The electrocardiogram tends to be normal, particularly early in the course of the disease. Later, the axis is shifted to the right, and there are early R waves in the precordial leads V_1 and V_2 and net negative electrical forces in leads V_5 and V_6. Especially during exacerbations, peaked P waves ("p pulmonale") are present. Unfortunately, these changes do not correlate well with pulmonary artery hypertension and cor pulmonale. The presence of R waves over the right precordium is the most reliable indication of cor pulmonale.

COURSE AND PROGNOSIS. Initially, there is a variable response to bronchodilator therapy, dependent upon the degree of bronchospasm. Thereafter, the disease progresses slowly, with an annual average decrement in FEV_1 of 50 to 75 ml. Because the variability in FEV_1 may be greater than the true annual decline, a follow-up of several years is required to determine the rate of loss of lung function. If the patient stops smoking, cough and sputum production may cease. However, most other symptoms progress gradually.

In terms of absolute FEV_1, patients are dyspneic upon moderate exertion when the value is 1.2 to 1.5 liters; they are forced to be relatively sedentary at 1.0 liter; and they are often invalids when the FEV_1 is 500 ml or less. As the FEV_1 drops below 1 liter, severe arterial hypoxemia, hypercapnia, and cor pulmonale often are evident.

Median survival varies considerably. Despite initially very low FEV_1 values, some individuals live 12 to 15 years. Generally, however, when the FEV_1 is more than 1.2 liters, patients survive about ten years; when the FEV_1 is 1.0 liter, survival is approximately five years; and when the FEV_1 is less than 700 ml, survival is about two years. Signs of a poor prognosis include a resting tachycardia, severe arterial hypoxemia or hypercapnia or both, and evidence of cor pulmonale. If a patient resides at altitudes higher than 3500 feet, longevity is reduced.

Increased cough and dyspnea are hallmarks of periodic worsening of the disease. Symptoms characteristically occur after an acute respiratory infection and may be accompanied by bronchospasm. Such exacerbations in patients with severe COPD may be life threatening and may lead to acute respiratory failure as well as right heart failure. The latter occurs secondary to pronounced increases in pulmonary artery pressure and pulmonary vascular resistance, which, in turn, are due primarily to hypoxic pulmonary vasoconstriction.

DIFFERENTIAL DIAGNOSIS. Three criteria are required to diagnose COPD: (1) The FEV_1 must be reduced, and this reduction must be proportionately more than any lowering in the FVC (i.e., both the FEV_1 per cent predicted and the FEV_1/FVC ratio must be depressed); (2) in spite of intensive, prolonged medical treatment, this slowing of forced expiration must persist; and (3) other bronchopulmonary disease that might explain the observed physiologic abnormalities must be excluded. Sufficient evidence for the last criterion generally includes absence of extensive parenchymal abnormalities on the chest radiograph and absence of any signs of upper airway obstruction, such as neck mass, stridor, or narrowing of the upper airway on chest radiograph. Irreversibility of the obstructive ventilatory defect may be more difficult to establish. This is discussed further in the treatment section.

Assessing the relative contribution of emphysema and intrinsic airway changes can also be difficult. Emphysema is usually severe when the diffusing capacity is very depressed and the chest radiograph shows hyperlucent lungs with attenuation of the vascular markings. In contrast, if the diffusing capacity is normal or nearly normal, extensive emphysema is unlikely. Esophageal balloon measurements, which are required to assess lung elastic recoil (the best guide to the severity of emphysema), are seldom justified as part of the clinical evaluation.

If there is a family history of emphysema or if an emphysema type of COPD develops at an early age, a homozygous alpha$_1$-antitrypsin deficiency should be considered. Suspicion is heightened when the patient is a nonsmoker or a woman or when the chest radiograph shows a bibasilar distribution of emphysematous changes. Laboratory confirmation is provided by almost complete absence of alpha$_1$-globulin, by a markedly reduced serum trypsin inhibitory capacity, and, most specifically, by demonstrating a pattern of a pure Z phenotype on crossed immunoelectrophoresis of the serum.

TREATMENT. The following are therapeutic goals in patients with COPD: (1) to relieve the portion of airway obstruction that is reversible; (2) to control cough and sputum production; (3) to eliminate and prevent airway infections; (4) to increase exercise tolerance to the maximum allowable at the individual's level of physiologic deficit; (5) to control remedial disease complications, such as arterial hypoxemia and cardiovascular problems; (6) to avoid smoking and other airway irritants, narcotics and sedatives, and noncritical surgery, all of which aggravate the disease; and (7) to relieve the anxiety and depression that are often present in the patient with COPD.

In spite of treatment, most patients with severe COPD show progressive ventilatory deterioration; yet, therapy should not be withheld. A comprehensive therapeutic program can reduce symptoms, decrease the frequency of hospital admissions, prevent premature death, and permit patients to lead a more active and satisfying life.

A formal rehabilitation program using a team approach is effective. Nevertheless, good results also can be obtained by a dedicated individual physician assisted, perhaps, by an office nurse who can help patients with physical therapy and bronchial hygiene measures.

Initial Treatment. During the initial visit, it is impossible to predict with certainty the degree of reversibility of airway obstruction in a patient with COPD. Therefore, all patients should be considered as having potentially reversible disease. Bronchodilators should be administered according to tolerance, as outlined in the therapy for asthmatic bronchitis and asthma. Smoking should be discontinued and other bronchial irritants avoided. As mentioned in the therapy for simple chronic bronchitis, bronchial hygiene measures and, when indicated by purulent mucous production, antibiotics should be used. Diuretics should be given when heart failure is present. In addition, the Pneumovax vaccine and yearly administration of the influenza vaccine are indicated.

The effects of this initial therapy both on symptoms and on pulmonary function test results should be determined and adjustments made in medication to minimize side effects. Apparently ineffective measures (e.g., postural drainage that leads to no symptom relief or sputum production) should be discontinued. Next, if further reversibility of the disease is considered possible, a three- to four-week trial of corticosteroids can be initiated. Several findings suggest that corticosteroids may help: (1) provide a more than 20 per cent improvement in FEV_1 after acute inhalation of a bronchodilator; (2) provide a similar increase in FEV_1 after several days or weeks of intensive bronchodilator therapy; (3) a history of acute attacks of wheezing not precipitated by exertion or of marked fluctuation in symptoms; (4) a noisy chest or wheeze upon auscultation; (5) sputum or blood eosinophilia; (6) provide any evidence of atopy, such as a history of hay fever, positive results in allergy skin tests, or an elevated level of serum IgE; (7) associated nasal polyps or vasomotor rhinitis; (8) a normal pulmonary diffusing capacity; or (9) provide normal chest film except for hyperinflation.

Generally, 20 to 40 mg of prednisone daily is given for three to four weeks, and spirometry tests are used to assess the efficacy of this medication. Other bronchodilators are continued at full doses. When improvement is noted, the corticosteroid dose should be tapered to the lowest maintenance dose possible, as outlined for asthmatic bronchitis. If there is no significant improvement in FEV_1 (e.g., > 20 per cent), corticosteroids should be tapered slowly and discontinued.

Maintenance Therapy. Frequently, objective improvement (i.e., increase in FEV_1) cannot be demonstrated with bronchodilator therapy. Yet, oral theophylline, combined with an inhaled beta-adrenergic agent, is recommended to prevent superimposed bronchospasm. In COPD, theophylline can (1) enhance respiratory muscle function, in both the fatigued and the nonfatigued state; (2) augment right and left ventricular systolic pump function while decreasing pulmonary artery pressures and pulmonary vascular resistance (potentially helpful in patients with cor pulmonale); and (3) in some patients, reduce dyspnea. The beta-adrenergic agents also improve biventricular systolic pump performance and decrease pulmonary vascular resistance. Whether any of these potentially salutary effects are additive or synergistic when oral theophylline is administered in conjunction with beta-adrenergic agents has not been established.

Aerosolized adrenergic agents also are used (1) to relieve acute attacks of dyspnea; (2) prior to exposure to known bronchial irritants, such as cold air; or (3) as a regular part of a bronchial hygiene program.

If a patient with COPD shows improvement in airflow rates (particularly FEV_1) with bronchodilators or adrenocortical hormones, these agents should be maintained as in asthmatic bronchitis. Those with a productive cough, retained secretions, or repeated episodes of bronchopulmonary infection should be treated with the same measures as described for simple chronic bronchitis. In addition, some other forms of treatment are uniquely applicable to patients with COPD.

Physical Therapy. Exercise has not been shown to improve lung function, but it may enhance cardiovascular fitness and train skeletal muscles to function more efficiently, thus increasing exercise tolerance. Accordingly, unless contraindicated by an underlying cardiac abnormality, progressively increasing exercise (usually walking) should be prescribed. In most cases, the program can be recommended directly by the physician, but if the patient is severely disabled, a trained physical therapist can initiate an appropriate exercise program. Arterial blood gas levels should be obtained at rest and exercise prior to instituting a vigorous exercise program, particularly if the FEV_1 is less than 1 liter. Supplemental oxygen should be used during exercise if the patient becomes severely hypoxemic.

Although breathing exercises probably do not alter the usual breathing pattern of patients with COPD, occasionally they are recommended to encourage diaphragmatic breathing. Perhaps it is more useful and more realistic to teach patients slow, deep breathing as a quicker, more effective method for relieving dyspnea rather than rapid, shallow "panic" breathing. Breath holding should be avoided during exertion. Many authorities now recommend inspiratory muscle training by breathing against a graded resistor, but mechanical devices, intermittent positive pressure breathing (IPPB) machines, and emphysema belts are of unproven value.

Oxygen Therapy. In some individuals with COPD, there are clear indications for home oxygen therapy. One indication is development of severe exertional hypoxemia (PaO_2 < 40 mm Hg) in patients who respond to supplemental oxygen therapy with an increase in exercise tolerance. A second indication is found in patients with severe, persistent arterial hypoxemia at rest (PaO_2 < 55 mm Hg) accompanied by secondary signs of hypoxemia after all other therapeutic measures have been exhausted and the patient has completely recovered from exacerbation of the disease. Both continuous oxygen therapy and that spanning 12 to 15 hours per day prolong survival, but continuous therapy (i.e., 10 to 24 hours per day) is associated with longer survival. To raise the PaO_2 to the necessary 60 to 80 mm Hg usually requires 1 to 3 liters of oxygen per minute via nasal prongs.

Since patients may become habituated to this therapy and

thus increase their invalidism, oxygen should not be prescribed solely for episodes of dyspnea.

Environmental Control. All patients with severe COPD should be cautioned to avoid high altitudes and should reside at altitudes below 4000 feet. Supplemental oxygen may be required for those with severe hypoxemia when they travel by air. A change in residence may be indicated in patients who live in areas with heavy air pollution.

Cold winter climates are avoided by some patients who find relief in either warm desert climates or warm, humid regions. No specific climate has been shown to alter the overall course of the disease. Accordingly, the economic and social hardships of a move should be weighed carefully against the potential symptomatic benefit provided by relocation to a more agreeable climate. Before moving, the patient should spend a trial period in the new climate to assess symptomatic benefit.

Treatment of Edema and Cor Pulmonale. Even in the absence of frank right-sided congestive heart failure, pedal edema is common and control is usually obtained with small doses of diuretics. Ankle edema associated with cor pulmonale is more difficult to control, but oxygen combined with diuretics often will suffice. Digitalis is useful for enhancing right ventricular function only if there is concomitant left heart failure; accordingly, digitalis should be reserved for combined right and left heart failure. Phlebotomy is not required in most oxygen-treated patients but may transiently relieve central nervous system symptoms, especially when the hematocrit is above 60 per cent.

Treatment of Hypercapnia. Chronic hypercapnia is common in late stages of COPD, but it requires no therapy. However, during exacerbations, blood gases must be monitored closely for severe respiratory acidosis, and all narcotics, sedatives, and tranquilizers should be avoided. In patients with stable chronic hypercapnia, mechanically assisted ventilation and respiratory stimulants are unnecessary.

Surgical Therapy. In the absence of significant emphysema (e.g., manifested by a moderate-to-severe reduction in diffusing capacity), bullectomy may benefit patients with large bullae compressing normal or nearly normal lung. Careful, detailed preoperative evaluation is required to select suitable operative candidates.

Supportive Measures. Careful, detailed education of the patient regarding the nature of the disease is essential. The significance of symptoms such as purulent sputum production, potential side effects of medication, and therapeutic goals should be explained. A prompt, prearranged treatment plan should be discussed with the patient for intercurrent exacerbations.

Above all, within the limits of respiratory impairment and within the constraints of therapy, these patients should be encouraged to live active lives with daily exercise. Some patients benefit from vocational rehabilitation and occupational therapy.

Replacement Therapy in Severe Alpha₁-Antitrypsin Deficiency Emphysema. Chronic, weekly replacement therapy with intravenous alpha₁-antitrypsin concentrate of normal plasma has been undertaken at the National Heart, Lung and Blood Institute in individuals with severe alpha₁-antitrypsin deficiency. Serum alpha₁-antitrypsin was elevated to levels likely required for effective antielastase protection of the lungs (average post-therapy level achieved, 130 mg per deciliter; average pretherapy level, 31 mg per deciliter). Alpha₁-antitrypsin levels after bronchoalveolar lavage increased in these individuals to about 60 per cent of normal, associated with an equivalent restoration of functional antineutrophil elastase activity. Moreover, the incidence of adverse reactions was limited to a transient postinfusion fever in less than 1 per cent of the patients.

Recently, recombinant DNA methodology has been used to produce alpha₁-antitrypsin. The future may bring widespread clinical application of this potentially less expensive material in patients with the Pi ZZ phenotype. When only mild airways disease is present, this therapy will re-establish the lung antineutrophil elastase defenses and protect the alveolar walls from elastolytic attack.

Treatment of Exacerbations. Antibiotics, increased bronchodilator medications, and even corticosteroids often are indicated for acute exacerbation. Immediate hospitalization is indicated for severe hypoxemia, increasing carbon dioxide tension, or congestive heart failure. Ch. 43 and 72 outline the management of decompensated cor pulmonale and acute respiratory failure, respectively. The same management utilized in patients with status asthmaticus is indicated in COPD patients with superimposed refractory bronchospasm.

Anthonisen NR: Hypoxemia and O₂ therapy. Am Rev Respir Dis 126:729, 1982. *A quality review of the British and American studies establishing that oxygen therapy prolongs life in patients with hypoxemic COPD.*

De Marco FJ Jr, Wynne JW, Block AJ, et al.: Oxygen desaturation during sleep as a determinant of the "blue and bloated" syndrome. Chest 79:621, 1981. *One of several papers by this group of investigators proposing that sleep-related breathing disorders are important in COPD patients.*

Higgins MW, Keller JB: Estimating your patient's risk of COPD. J Respir Dis 4:97, 1983. *This paper discusses the use of routine spirometric testing to detect subjects who are at high risk of developing clinically significant airways obstructive disease.*

Janoff A: Elastases and emphysema: Current assessment of the protease-antiprotease hypothesis. Am Rev Respir Dis 132:417, 1985. *Reviews ten years of progress in elucidating the pathogenesis of emphysema.*

Petty TL (ed.): Chronic Obstructive Pulmonary Disease. 2nd ed. New York, Marcel Dekker, 1985. *Comprehensive statement on all aspects of COPD.*

Snider GL (ed.): Emphysema. Clin Chest Med 4:327, 1983. *Quality monograph emphasizing the pathology and pathogenesis of emphysema.*

LOCALIZED AIRWAY OBSTRUCTION

Extrinsic compression of airways, intraluminal obstruction, and diseases of the airways themselves all can cause localized airway obstruction. Signs and symptoms depend upon location of the obstruction, whether it is partial or complete, variable or fixed. The discussion of localized lesions is divided into obstructions above and below the bifurcation of the trachea.

Obstruction Above the Tracheal Bifurcation

PARTIAL OBSTRUCTION. Stridor, frequently accompanied by inspiratory retraction of the intercostal spaces, is the principal finding in partial obstruction above the main (tracheal) carina. On both forced inspiration and forced expiration, airflow rates are reduced, and there may be a characteristic appearance to the MEFV curve. As shown in Figure 61–2, the site and nature of the obstruction determine the findings on spirometry. When the obstruction is severe, hypoxemia and hypercapnia may result owing to reduced overall ventilation.

Among the intrinsic airway diseases that can cause partial airway obstruction are (1) tonsil and adenoid enlargement, especially in young children; (2) stenosing lesions secondary to trauma; (3) neoplasms or granulomatous processes (e.g., sarcoidosis, fungi) involving the hypopharynx, larynx, vocal cords, or trachea; (4) bilateral paralysis of the vocal cords; (5) spasm or edema of the larynx; or (6) inflammation in several locations—the pharynx (e.g., peritonsillar abscess), the larynx (e.g., croup), or the trachea (e.g., diphtheria). An enlarged thyroid, a paratracheal neoplasm, or a mediastinal infection can cause extrinsic compression of the airway. An artificial airway, tracheostomy, or surgical repair is indicated when the primary cause of the obstruction cannot be eliminated.

COMPLETE OBSTRUCTION. Rapid asphyxiation results unless complete obstruction above the main carina is relieved promptly. There is a pathognomonic presentation with absent airflow at the mouth in spite of both inspiratory efforts and inspiratory retraction of the intercostal muscles. Aspiration of poorly chewed food (so-called "café coronary") is the most common cause of acute obstruction. If a sharp blow to the

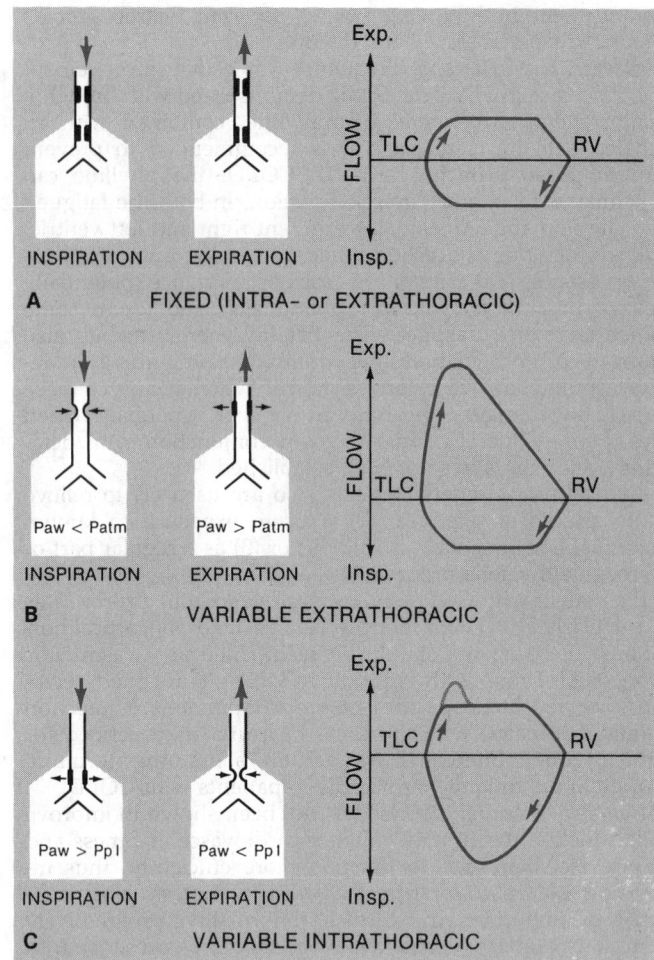

FIGURE 61–2. Airways obstruction above the carina may produce characteristic flow-volume abnormalities, depending on the type and site of obstruction. *A*, If the obstruction is fixed, both inspiratory and expiratory flows will be decreased whether the obstruction is intrathoracic or extrathoracic (for purposes of illustration, obstruction is shown in both locations). Note that this pattern is usually seen when the obstruction is at the level of the thoracic inlet. *B*, When a variable obstruction is extrathoracic in location, the airway narrows during inspiration when airway pressure (Paw) is less than atmospheric (Patm) and inspiratory flow is diminished. Expiratory flows are often limited but to a lesser extent. *C*, When a variable obstruction is intrathoracic in location, airway pressure is less than pleural pressure (Ppl) during expiration, and expiratory flow is diminished. Inspiratory flows are often limited but to a much lesser extent. (Reproduced with permission from Burrows B, et al.: Respiratory Disorders—A Pathophysiologic Approach. 2nd ed. Copyright 1983 by Year Book Medical Publishers, Inc., Chicago.)

back fails to dislodge the obstructing material, forced pressure is applied to the epigastrium—the *Heimlich maneuver*.

When the glossopharyngeal structures fall back in some obese individuals, complete obstruction of the upper airway occurs. Local abnormalities in the hypopharynx may also cause complete upper airway obstruction, resulting in disordered breathing, especially during sleep. Frequent awakening, a troubled sleep, and somnolence are characteristic. This clinical picture, often confused with the pickwickian syndrome and other forms of sleep disorders, is discussed in Ch. 458.

Obstruction Below the Tracheal Bifurcation

PARTIAL OBSTRUCTION. A primary neoplasm, compressing or growing into an airway, is the most common cause of obstruction below the bifurcation of the trachea.

Other causes include aspiration of foreign bodies, acute or chronic inflammatory lesions of the bronchi, and compression of bronchi by enlarged hilar lymph nodes or mucous plugs. A localized expiratory wheeze over the site of obstruction and hyperinflation of the lung distally are characteristic. Spirometry may be normal or only mildly abnormal because airflow from the remaining lung is unimpaired; yet, other tests will show nonuniformity of ventilation. A ventilation lung scan may reveal an area of diminished airflow. Bronchoscopy usually provides a definitive diagnosis, and treatment is directed at the cause of obstruction.

Infection and perhaps an abscess may develop with partial bronchial obstruction because of impaired secretion clearance from the distal lung. Partial obstruction of the proximal bronchus should be suspected in patients with recurrent infections in the same lung zone, slow resolution of pneumonia, or a lung abscess.

COMPLETE OBSTRUCTION. "Obstructive atelectasis" is a condition due to absorption of air into the bloodstream from lung distal to a complete obstruction. This condition is discussed in Ch. 62 under Atelectasis. Complete occlusion of a bronchus and resultant obstructive atelectasis may develop with progression of any of the above-mentioned causes of partial obstruction.

Heimlich HJ: A life-saving maneuver to prevent food-choking. JAMA 234:398, 1975. *The original report on a new standard method to remove aspirated food from the airway.*

Loughlin GM, Taussig LM: Upper airway obstruction. Semin Respir Med 1:131, 1979. *This is an excellent review of upper airways obstructive disorders in infants and children.*

Miller RD: Obstructing lesions of the larynx and trachea: Clinical and pathophysiologic aspects. In Fishman AP (ed.): Pulmonary Diseases and Disorders. New York, McGraw-Hill Book Company, 1980, p 490. *An excellent review of the causes, consequences, and treatment of tracheolaryngeal obstruction.*

62 ABNORMALITIES OF LUNG AERATION*

Richard A. Matthay

LOCALIZED HYPOAERATION (ATELECTASIS)

Atelectasis, or reduced aeration of the lung, is present in many bronchopulmonary disorders and assumes a variety of forms. A total loss of ventilation to a lung region (i.e., with total airway collapse) leads to a shunt wherein blood traversing this region fails to participate in gas exchange and behaves as if it were moving directly from the right to the left side of the heart. Accordingly, total atelectasis causes an "absolute" shunt. In contrast to the "shuntlike" effect of increased venous admixture present in most bronchopulmonary diseases, inhalation of 100 per cent oxygen does not fully correct the "absolute shunt."

TYPES OF ATELECTASIS AND THEIR PATHOGENESIS. *Obstructive atelectasis* is a condition of alveolar collapse that develops within a few hours after obstruction of an airway distal to the tracheal bifurcation. The collapse develops because gas in the lung behind the obstruction is slowly absorbed into the bloodstream. If the lung is filled with oxygen-rich gas rather than ambient air, the alveoli collapse more rapidly. Nitrogen in ambient air is poorly soluble, whereas oxygen is rapidly absorbed into the bloodstream. As a result, high inspired oxygen tensions encourage the development of atelectasis behind obstructing mucous plugs.

Contraction atelectasis occurs when fibrotic changes in a local area of the lung increase its recoil. Contraction, or shrinkage, of the involved lung, rather than complete airlessness, results.

Patchy atelectasis develops throughout the lung owing to alveolar instability in adult and infant (newborn) respiratory distress syndromes.

A large pneumothorax, pleural effusion, or other space-occupying lesion in the thorax can increase intrapleural pressure, causing a portion of the lung to decrease in volume. This *compression atelectasis* is more appropriately called *relaxation atelectasis* because the atelectasis results from the tendency of the lung to recoil when the distending forces are relaxed. As small airways close in the affected region because of marked relaxation atelectasis, any air remaining distally is absorbed into the bloodstream.

Although its pathologic significance is unclear, *platelike atelectasis* may be visible on the chest radiograph. This condition is characterized by horizontal radiopaque streaks, usually in the lung bases. Commonly associated with poor lung aeration, these streaks are seen when the patient has been unable to breathe deeply for a sustained period or when the diaphragm is elevated, such as after intra-abdominal surgery.

CLINICAL MANIFESTATIONS. The chronicity and extent of the process determine the physiologic and clinical consequences of atelectasis. When the obstruction evolves slowly, typical of bronchial neoplasms, usually few or no symptoms develop and hypoxemia is minimal. In contrast, profound dyspnea and severe hypoxemia often develop after acute collapse of a large section of the lung. As blood-flow through the nonventilated lung diminishes over several hours, symptoms and hypoxemia lessen. The acute picture typically includes development of obstructive atelectasis due to aspiration of a foreign body or due to retention of secretions (which may develop in the postoperative period).

The type of atelectasis determines the physical findings. In obstructive or contraction atelectasis, the physical findings depend upon the amount of lung involved. In major atelectasis, the trachea and mediastinum shift to the affected side, the diaphragm is elevated, and the involved hemithorax is smaller and shows less respiratory motion than the unaffected side. Patchy atelectasis is associated with findings like those of the respiratory distress syndrome reviewed in Ch. 72. The underlying condition (e.g., pleural effusion, pneumothorax, space-occupying lesion) determines the findings in relaxation atelectasis. Platelike atelectasis is primarily a chest radiographic diagnosis without distinctive abnormalities on physical examination.

DIAGNOSIS, TREATMENT, AND OUTCOME. The chest radiograph confirms the presence of atelectasis. When obstructive atelectasis is suspected, bronchoscopy is required to establish the etiology; it may be possible to remove the occluding material through the bronchoscope. However, a bronchogenic neoplasm should always be considered when obstructive atelectasis is present and the patient is not severely ill.

Treatment is directed at the underlying disorder in nonobstructive forms of atelectasis.

When relaxation atelectasis is relieved (e.g., by insertion of a chest tube for a large pneumothorax), the lung usually returns to normal. However, obstructive atelectasis often is accompanied by secondary complications, such as infection, which lead to abscess formation, localized bronchiectasis, and fibrosis. Moreover, after prolonged collapse, the affected lung may fail to re-expand after the obstruction is removed. The *middle lobe syndrome* provides a typical sequence of events. In this syndrome, the middle lobe bronchus in the right lung usually has been compressed by large hilar lymph nodes in tuberculosis or other granulomatous lung diseases. Even after the lymph nodes finally decrease in size, the affected lung fails to expand fully, there are often bronchiectatic changes, and the lobe may be a site of recurrent or chronic infection. Although less common, the same sequence of events may

---

*Portions of this chapter were rewritten from the 17th edition of *Cecil Textbook of Medicine* with permission from Benjamin Burrows.

occur in other lung regions. The involved lung may have to be resected if recurrent pneumonia, chronic suppuration, or repeated episodes of hemoptysis develop.

LOCALIZED HYPERAERATION

BLEBS AND BULLAE. Blebs are small collections of gas that are entirely enclosed within the visceral pleura. The gas resides between the multiple leaves of the visceral pleura rather than within the lung itself. Blebs are the uncommon result of dissection of air from the lung interstitium into the lung septa and thence into and between the layers of visceral pleura. Blebs are not clinically important except on the rare occasions that they rupture and cause a spontaneous pneumothorax. Sometimes blebs are visible on the plain chest radiograph, particularly in the lung apex; they are more easily seen when there is a pneumothorax and partial collapse of normal surrounding lung.

Bullae are larger airspaces in the parenchyma of the lung (> than 1 cm in diameter) that are associated with destruction. A bulla denotes severe, localized emphysema causing the formation of a large airspace. Bullae may occur with several different types of emphysema and are common in patients with chronic obstructive bronchitis and emphysema. Individuals without any generalized obstructive airways disorder and without diffuse emphysema also may develop bullae.

Bullae are commonly located in the apices of the lungs and are often multiple. A lack of an endothelial lining distinguishes bullae from cysts. Moreover, on the chest radiograph, bullae have "hairline" (thin) margins and, unlike cysts, are usually irregularly shaped, are frequently trabeculated, and rarely contain fluid.

When they become large enough to compromise the function of the remaining normal lung and cause shortness of breath, bullae are clinically important. However, like blebs, when small, they are of little significance, unless they rupture and lead to a pneumothorax.

A difficult clinical problem may be to ascertain whether dyspnea is secondary to diffuse emphysema of the lungs or to bullae (observed on the chest radiograph). Surgery may be indicated in the latter case, but it is contraindicated in the former. Ventilation-perfusion radionuclide lung scans, computed tomography (CT) scans, and pulmonary angiograms may be necessary to make this distinction and to evaluate the state of the remaining lung. As a rule, unless there is associated generalized obstructive airways disease, bullae that occupy less than half a hemithorax are not associated with severe dyspnea and significant functional impairment. Moreover, unless there is diffuse disease, severe slowing of expiratory airflow is unusual, even with very large bullae. An ideal surgical candidate has moderate-to-severe dyspnea, bullae that fill most of a hemithorax, only mild slowing of flow rates on forced expiration, good perfusion of normal remaining lung on lung scan and pulmonary angiogram, and no evidence of significant emphysema (e.g., the diffusing capacity measurement is normal or only moderately reduced, and lung compliance studies are normal).

The diagnosis is usually made by the sound chest radiograph; however, on physical examination, a tympanitic percussion sound and reduced breath sounds may be noted over very large bullae. The radiolucency of a very large bulla of the chest film may be mistaken for a pneumothorax.

BRONCHOGENIC CYSTS. Bronchogenic cysts may occur in the mediastinum or within the lung parenchyma. These congenital malformations can be differentiated from bullae by their epithelial lining. On the chest radiograph, mediastinal cysts are seen as masses in the hilar, paraesophageal or paratracheal, and, most commonly, subcarinal region. In the parenchyma, these cysts are most commonly in the lower lobes and are usually filled with a proteinaceous material until they may become infected and communicate with the bronchial tree. They may have thin, even paper-thin, walls. During early development, acquired lung cysts often have relatively thick walls; later even those resulting from lung abscesses often have very thin walls that simulate bullae.

Large cysts may cause respiratory symptoms in young children, but adults with these large lesions are usually asymptomatic, and the chest radiographic abnormality tends to be an incidental finding. In the differential diagnosis, mediastinal cysts must be distinguished from other mediastinal masses. Lung cysts must be differentiated from acute lung abscesses, cavitated carcinomas, and cystic bronchiectasis. Frequently, thoracotomy and resection of the lesion are required to obtain a specific diagnosis, although chest CT combined with needle aspiration has been useful for diagnosis and drainage.

Only when they have a bronchial connection (communication) do bronchogenic cysts manifest as abnormalities in lung aeration. Although often partially filled with fluid, they may appear as airspaces when there is a bronchial communication. Infection in fluid-filled cysts is unusual and may require that they be removed surgically after a course of antibiotics. Cysts containing air often can be distinguished from bullae by their regular outline, lack of trabeculation, and the presence of a fluid level. Distinguishing bronchogenic cysts in the lung from thin-walled cavities secondary to granulomatous infections, prior abscesses, prior pulmonary infarcts, and squamous cell carcinomas may be more difficult.

BRONCHOPULMONARY SEQUESTRATION. In *bronchopulmonary sequestrations* of the intralobular type, cystic lesions may be identified. This sequestration is caused by abnormal budding in the tracheobronchial tree of the early embryo. The involved area is most often in the bases of the lungs posteriorly, and the affected lung region is nonfunctional. On the chest radiograph, involved areas are opaque.

Only when there is a bronchial communication do aircontaining cysts develop, and in such situations secondary infection is the prime concern. These lesions are asymptomatic and are incidental chest radiographic findings unless infection develops. An aortogram that shows an abnormal vascular supply distinguishes a sequestration from a simple cyst. The arterial supply to some sequestrations arises at least partially from below the diaphragm. Surgical excision is the only treatment.

THE UNILATERAL HYPERLUCENT LUNG. Swyer-James or Macleod's syndrome, a rare disorder, is generally discovered on chest radiograph. Increased translucency of one hemithorax is noted owing to diminished vascular markings in the lung on that side. On the inspiration chest radiograph, the affected lung is usually not hyperinflated. However, air trapping has been described, and an expiration chest radiograph may show hyperinflation of the affected lung relative to the other uninvolved lung and shift of the mediastinum to the unaffected side. Extensive bronchitis and bronchiolitis are usually noted on biopsy. These abnormalities likely date from childhood. In fact, in some children the condition develops six months to five years after viral bronchiolitis, and there is a history of some such incidence in more than half of the patients. Dyspnea, a productive cough, and occasionally hemoptysis may occur.

At bronchoscopy, there is no obstruction of the main bronchi. But bronchography shows irregular dilatation of the bronchi to the fifth order, with failure to fill the peripheral airways, and an appearance characteristic of bronchiolar obliteration. Patency of the pulmonary artery on the angiogram differentiates Swyer-James syndrome from pulmonary artery stenosis or atresia. On the affected side, the lung scan shows reduced ventilation and perfusion. Pulmonary function test findings are variable and usually include some evidence of airways obstruction and an increase in residual volume, suggesting air trapping. Severe expiratory obstruction of airflow is uncommon.

Resection is not indicated, and treatment is limited usually to managing infection.

Allison RS, Chirnside AM: Pulmonary sequestration: A review of 12 cases. NZ Med J 596:381, 1983. *Well-written, complete coverage of the types, presentation, and management of pulmonary sequestration.*

Boushy SF, Kohen R, Billig DM, et al.: Bullous emphysema: Clinical, roentgenologic and physiologic study of 49 patients. Dis Chest 54:327, 1968. *A good description of the range of manifestations seen with pulmonary bullae.*

Hamilton CR Jr, Ballinger WF II, Cader G: The unilateral hyperlucent lung syndrome. Bull Johns Hopkins Hosp 123:222, 1968. *A good review of this unusual syndrome.*

Primrose WR: Spontaneous pneumothorax: A retrospective review of etiology, pathogenesis, and management. Scott Med J 29:15, 1984. *Succinct, up-to-date review of spontaneous pneumothorax.*

Proto AV, Tocino I: Radiographic manifestations of lobar collapse. Semin Roentgenol 15:117, 1980. *A comprehensive review of chest radiographic features of lobar collapse.*

Rodgers BM, Harman PK, Johnson AM: Bronchopulmonary foregut malformations—the spectrum of anomalies. Ann Surg 203:517, 1986. *A review of the various foregut malformations, including both bronchogenic cysts and sequestration, complete with ultrasound and CT images and a quality bibliography.*

Wagner RB, Johnston MR: Middle lobe syndrome. Ann Thorac Surg 35:679, 1983. *The etiology, pathophysiology, and therapy of this syndrome are up to date.*

63 INTERSTITIAL LUNG DISEASE

Ronald G. Crystal

General Description

The interstitial lung diseases (ILD) are a heterogeneous group of diffuse inflammatory disorders of the lower respiratory tract. The term "interstitial lung disease" refers to the fact that the interstitium of the alveolar walls is thickened, usually by fibrosis. While this is true, the ILD are also characterized by derangements of the epithelial and endothelial cells of the alveolar walls and, in many cases, of the small airways and/or blood vessels of the lung parenchyma.

There are many disorders associated with ILD. In some, the ILD is the only manifestation; in others it is a part of a systemic disorder. The natural history of many of the ILD is one of slowly progressive loss of the functional alveolar-capillary units, often eventuating in respiratory insufficiency and death. Because of their insidious nature and the nonspecificity of the accompanying symptoms, such as dyspnea on exertion or a nonproductive cough, the ILD may go undiagnosed and untreated until large numbers of alveolar-capillary units become scarred and irrevocably lost.

These disorders are inflammatory diseases; the bulk of the damage to the lung parenchyma is caused by activated inflammatory cells that have accumulated in the alveolar structures. The diagnosis, staging, and treatment of the ILD require defining the character and intensity of the inflammation in the lung and the derangements of the alveolar structures caused by the inflammation.

Anatomy

The lower respiratory tract is composed of alveoli, grapelike units branching off the terminal bronchioles, and the vascular network of pulmonary arterioles, capillaries, and venules that bring blood to and from the lung (Fig. 63–1). The walls of the alveoli are lined by a single layer of epithelial cells resting on a thin, continuous basement membrane. Ninety-five per cent of the alveolar surface is covered by type I epithelial cells, with the remainder by type II epithelial cells, the cell that produces the surfactant, material that prevents alveolar collapse. Underneath the epithelial basement membrane is the alveolar interstitium, a region containing fibroblasts and supporting connective tissue matrix composed of collagen, elastic fibers, proteoglycans, and various glycoproteins. The pulmonary capillaries form a branching network of tubes lined by a single layer of endothelial cells resting on their own basement membrane. The capillaries weave through the interstitium such that the capillary basement membrane often abuts the epithelial basement membrane beneath the type I epithelial cells. It is at these sites that air and blood are in closest approximation and where gas exchange takes place.

The normal alveolar wall is thin (5 to 10 μm wide) compared with the space occupied by air (200 to 300 μm). In the ILD, the walls are thickened severalfold and the space for air is correspondingly less. The derangements that accompany the thickening of the alveolar walls in the ILD can be conceptualized in two groups (Fig. 63–2). In the distortion form of derangement, typified by sarcoidosis and the early phases of hypersensitivity pneumonitis, the alveolar walls are deformed by the accumulation of inflammatory cells in the interstitium, altering the normal architecture. Because there is little injury to the normal structures, this form of derangement is often reversible if the process causing the distortion is eliminated.

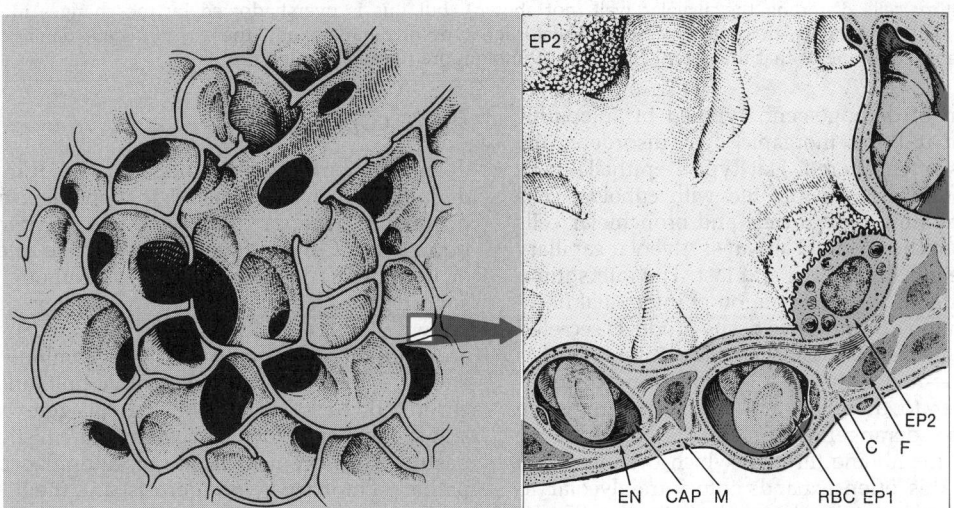

FIGURE 63–1. Structure of the normal lower respiratory tract. *Left*, Representation of a low-power view of the distal lung; the terminal bronchiole is shown but the pulmonary artery and vein are omitted. *Right*, Representation of a high-power view of an alveolus; the cut surface demonstrates the type I (EP1) and type II (EP2) epithelial cells, endothelial cells (EN), basement membranes (M), red blood cells (RBC) in the capillaries (CAP), fibroblasts (F), and connective tissue (C). Inflammatory cells are not shown. (Reprinted with permission from Crystal RG, Bitterman PB, Rennard SI, et al.: Interstitial lung diseases of unknown cause: Disorders characterized by chronic inflammation of the lower respiratory tract. N Engl J Med 310:154, 1984.)

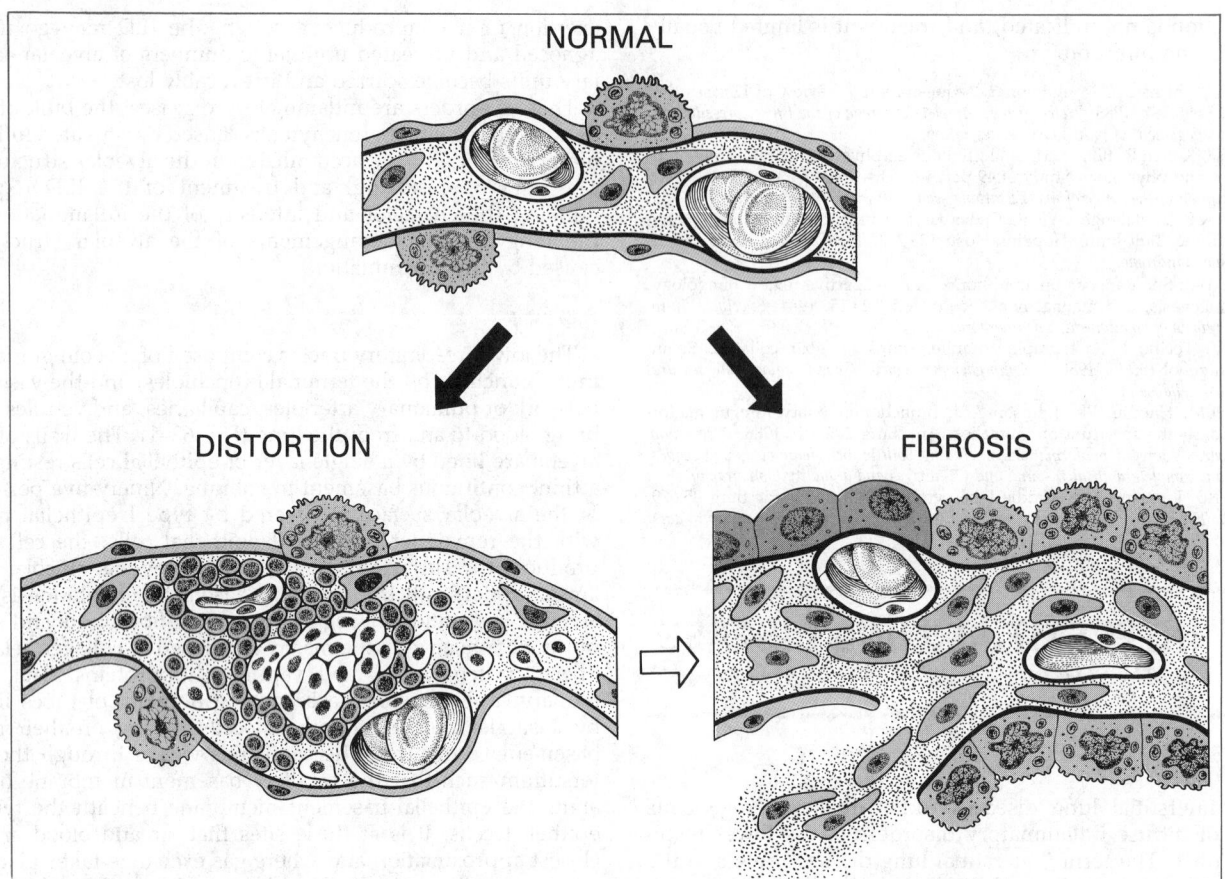

FIGURE 63–2. Typical forms of derangement of alveolar structures in the interstitial lung disorders. *Top*, Schematic of a cut surface of the normal alveolar wall. Shown are the type I and II epithelial cells, endothelial cells lining the capillaries, basement membranes, fibroblasts, and interstitial connective tissue. The few inflammatory cells normally present are not shown. *Lower left*, Schematic of a similar view of the alveolar wall deranged by the distortion caused by the accumulation of inflammatory cells. The example used is that of sarcoidosis, in which T lymphocytes, macrophages, and granulomas (massed accumulations of differentiated macrophages) distort the normal alveolar walls. *Lower right*, Schematic of a similar view of the alveolar wall deranged by fibrosis. The example used is that of idiopathic pulmonary fibrosis. In contrast to the distortion type of derangement, in which there is little damage and change in the lung parenchyma, in the fibrotic form of derangement the type I cells are injured, leaving denuded basement membrane. In some areas, the interstitial contents protrude into the airspace, causing intra-alveolar fibrosis. Note that some of the injured type I cells have been replaced by the type II cells and bronchiolar cells that have migrated down from the airways. Capillaries are injured; the basement membranes are thickened; there are expanded numbers of fibroblasts; and the density of connective tissue is increased. In the fibrotic type of derangement, there are also inflammatory cells distorting the alveolar wall (not shown), but this is overshadowed by the changes in normal parenchymal components. In some cases of the distortion type of derangement, there is sufficient damage to the parenchymal components that the derangements shift into a more fibrotic-type picture.

In the fibrosis form of derangement, typified by idiopathic pulmonary fibrosis and the inorganic dust disorders, the epithelial surface is often altered: Flat type I epithelial cells are lost, and the surface is repopulated with cuboidal cells derived from proliferating type II cells and bronchiolar cells migrating down from the terminal airways. Alveolar capillary endothelial cells are usually injured and lost. The interstitium is thickened with edema and proliferation of interstitial fibroblasts and accumulation of connective tissue products secreted by the fibroblasts, particularly collagen. The interstitium is scarred and fibrotic—hence the term "fibrotic lung disease" is also used to refer to these ILD. In the more aggressive forms of fibrosis-type derangements, there are breaks in the epithelial basement membrane through which the interstitial contents protrude; this often expands into intra-alveolar fibrotic masses called "intra-alveolar buds." As the fibrotic form of ILD progresses, the alveolar-capillary units become less distinguishable, and the lung parenchyma takes on the appearance of "end-stage lung" characterized by masses of fibrotic tissue interspaced with cystic areas representing the remnants of alveoli and dilated terminal bronchioles.

Epidemiology

The epidemiology for most of the ILD is not carefully defined, but it is estimated that in the United States their prevalence is approximately 20 to 40 per 100,000 of the population. Conventionally, the ILD are categorized as those of unknown and known etiology. Although there are more subcategories of ILD of known etiology than those of unknown etiology, in terms of total numbers of patients, more are of unknown etiology. The most common ILD of unknown etiology (Table 63–1) are idiopathic pulmonary fibrosis (IPF), chronic ILD associated with the collagen-vascular disorders, and sarcoidosis. Much less common are histiocytosis-X, Goodpasture's syndrome, chronic eosinophilic pneumonia, idiopathic pulmonary hemosiderosis, and the ILD associated with the pulmonary vasculitides. The other ILD of unknown etiology are very rare, with far fewer than 1000 cases of each reported in the world literature.

The ILD of known etiology are most commonly due to the inhalation of inorganic dusts, particularly crystalline silica, asbestos, and coal dust (Table 63–2), the hypersensitivity

TABLE 63–1. INTERSTITIAL LUNG DISEASES (ILD) OF UNKNOWN ETIOLOGY*

- Idiopathic Pulmonary Fibrosis (IPF)
- Sarcoidosis
- ILD Associated with the Collagen-Vascular Disorders
  Rheumatoid arthritis
  Progressive systemic sclerosis
  Systemic lupus erythematosus
  Polymyositis/dermatomyositis
  Sjögren's syndrome
  Mixed connective tissue disease
  Ankylosing spondylitis
  Histiocytosis-X
  Goodpasture's Syndrome
  Idiopathic Pulmonary Hemosiderosis
  Chronic Eosinophilic Pneumonia
  Lymphocytic Infiltrative Disorders
  Immunoblastic lymphadenopathy
  Lymphocytic interstitial pneumonitis
  Pseudolymphoma
  ILD Associated with Pulmonary Vasculitides
  Wegener's granulomatosis
  Lymphomatoid granulomatosis
  Churg-Strauss syndrome
  Systemic necrotizing vasculitides ("overlap" vasculitides)
  Hypersensitivity vasculitis
  Inherited Disorders
  Familial idiopathic pulmonary fibrosis
  Neurofibromatosis
  Tuberous sclerosis
  Hermansky-Pudlak syndrome
  Niemann-Pick disease
  Gaucher's disease

ILD Associated with Pulmonary Airway Disease
  Bronchocentric granulomatosis
  Bronchopulmonary aspergillosis
Lymphangioleiomyomatosis
Alveolar Proteinosis
ILD Associated with Liver Disease
  Chronic active hepatitis
  Primary biliary cirrhosis
ILD Associated with Bowel Disease
  Whipple's disease
  Ulcerative colitis
  Crohn's disease
Weber-Christian Disease
Amyloidosis
Hypereosinophilic Syndrome
Pulmonary Veno-occlusive Disease
ILD Caused by Failure of Other Organs
  Chronic left ventricular failure
  Chronic left-to-right intracardiac shunt
  Chronic renal disease with uremia
Graft-versus-Host Disease
Recovery Phase of Adult Respiratory Distress Syndrome

*Disorders indicated with "●" are the most common ILD of unknown etiology.

pneumonitides (diseases caused by the repeated inhalation of organic dust—Table 63–3), and the drug-induced ILD (Table 63–4). Much less frequent are the ILD resulting from paraquat, radiation, the sequelae of known infectious agents, and the inhalation of gases, aerosols, chemical dusts, fumes, and vapors (Table 63–5). Occasionally, however, large populations develop ILD when exposed to a single agent at one time, such as occurred in Bhopal, India, in 1984 when methyl isocyanate was released into a crowded urban area.

Differential Diagnosis

The initial problem in assessing ILD is to differentiate it from other disorders that may also present with symptoms of respiratory deficiency and diffuse infiltrates on the chest radiograph (Table 63–6). In general, pulmonary edema, high-flow states, hemorrhage, and aspiration pneumonitis can be easily differentiated from the ILD by history and physical examination. The major problem is in ensuring that the patient does not have an infection or malignancy, diagnoses that require an appropriate evaluation of specimens from the lower respiratory tract for the presence of infectious agents or malignant cells, respectively. In some cases, such as HIV infection or filarial infestation, serologic studies are necessary.

The diagnosis of a specific ILD is made by a combination of historical, physical examination, blood, urine, roentgenographic, physiologic, scintigraphic, and bronchoscopic criteria. In addition, unless an agent of known etiology is apparent (e.g., long-term asbestos exposure), it is mandatory to evaluate the disease by morphologic means, usually by open lung biopsy. The only exception to this rule is when the ILD is in clear association with a systemic disorder (e.g., a collagen-vascular disease, Goodpasture's syndrome) in which the diagnosis can be made by evaluation of organs other than the lung.

Pathogenesis

The ILD are inflammatory disorders in which most of the derangements of the alveolar walls, including the fibrosis, are mediated by the accumulated inflammatory and immune effector cells. The inflammation, usually referred to as the "alveolitis" of the disease, not only involves the alveoli, but often involves the walls of small airways and sometimes the pulmonary blood vessels. The critical importance of the alveolitis is simply stated: Although dysfunction of the alveolar-capillary units causes the symptoms and impairment of the patient, it is the alveolitis that causes the derangements of the alveolar-capillary units, resulting in their dysfunction and eventual loss as gas-exchanging units (Fig. 63–3).

INITIATION OF THE ALVEOLITIS. Although it is not clear what initiates the inflammation in the ILD of unknown etiology, many of the processes that maintain the alveolitis are understood. For example, in idiopathic pulmonary fibrosis, alveolar macrophages, activated by immune complexes, release neutrophil-specific chemotactic factors that attract blood neutrophils to the lung. In contrast, in sarcoidosis, activated lung T lymphocytes release a monocyte-specific chemotactic factor that modulates the accumulation of blood monocytes in the alveolar structures.

For the disorders of known etiology, the causative agent most commonly activates the inflammatory cells that are normally present, which, in turn, propagate the alveolitis. Alternatively, the causative agent may directly injure the alveolar walls, and the resulting deranged tissue initiates the inflammation. For example, bleomycin, an antineoplastic drug, can injure lung parenchyma cells and by unknown mechanisms induce the formation of an alveolitis.

CHARACTER OF THE ALVEOLITIS. The inflammatory component of the ILD is defined by the number, type, and state of activation of the effector cells composing the alveolitis. The differences in the form and extent of the derangements

TABLE 63–2. INHALED INORGANIC DUSTS THAT CAUSE INTERSTITIAL LUNG DISEASE*,†

Silica (variants of SiO_2)
- Crystalline silica ("silicosis")
  Amorphous
Silicates
- Asbestos ("asbestosis")
  Talc (hydrated Mg silicates; "talcosis")
  Kaolin (china clay, hydrated aluminum silicate)
  Diatomaceous earth (Fuller's earth, aluminum silicate with Fe and Mg)
  Nepheline (hard rock containing mixed silicates)
  Aluminum silicates (sericite, sillimanite, zeolite)
  Portland cement
  Mica (principally K and Mg aluminum silicates)
Carbon (with or without crystalline silica)
- Coal dust ("coal worker's pneumoconiosis")
  Graphite ("carbon pneumoconiosis")
Metals
  Beryllium ("berylliosis")
  Aluminum ("aluminosis")
    Powdered aluminum ("aluminum lung")
    Bauxite (aluminum oxide; "Shaver's disease")
  Barium (powder of baryte or $BaSO_4$; "baritosis")
  Iron ("siderosis")
  Tin ("stannosis")
  Antimony (oxides and alloys)
  Mixed dusts
    Hematite (mixed dusts of iron oxide, silica and silicates; "siderosilicosis")
    Mixed dusts of silver and iron oxide ("argyrosiderosis")
  Hard metals
    Titanium oxide
    Tungsten, titanium, hafnium, niobium, cobalt, and vanadium carbides
    Cadmium
Rare earths (cerium, scandium, yttrium, lanthanum)
$CuSO_4$ neutralized with hydrated lime (Bordeaux mixture; "vineyard sprayer's lung")

*The most common inorganic dust–induced interstitial lung diseases are indicated with "●".
†Disorders given a specific name are indicated in quotes in parentheses; others are referred as "(name of the dust) pneumoconiosis."

TABLE 63–3. INHALED ORGANIC DUSTS THAT CAUSE INTERSTITIAL LUNG DISEASE*

Disorder	Causative Agent†
• Farmer's lung	*M. faeni, T. vulgaris, A. fumigatus, T. candidus*
• Humidifier lung, air conditioner lung	*T. vulgaris, T. candidus,* thermotolerant bacteria, protozoa, *Penicillium* species, *Naegleria gruberi*
• Bird breeder's disease‡	Avian proteins, feathers
Maple bark stripper's lung	*Cryptostroma corticale*
Cheese worker's lung	*A. clavatus, Penicillium caseii*
Malt worker's lung	*A. clavatus, A. fumigatus*
Sequoiosis	*Aureobasidium pullulans, Graphium* species
Paprika splitter's lung	*Mucor stolonifer*
Wheat weevil disease	*Sitophilus granarius*
Suberosis	*Penicillium frequentans*
Bagassosis	*T. sacchari*
Mushroom worker's lung	*M. faeni, T. vulgaris*
Pituitary snuff lung	Porcine and bovine proteins
Wood-pulp worker's disease	*Alternaria* species
Sauna-taker's disease	*Aureobasidium* species
Detergent worker's lung	*Bacillus subtilis*
Lycoperdonosis	*Lycoperdon bovista*
Rodent handler's disease	Serum and urine constituents
Dry rot disease	*Merulius lacrymans*
Wood-dust worker's lung	Unknown
Furrier's lung	Unknown
New Guinea lung	*Saccharomonospora irridis*
Coptic disease (mummy unwrapper's disease)	Antigens associated with mummy wrappings
"Summer type" disease	*Cryptococcus neoformans* §*Cephalosporium* species §*Streptomyces albus* §*Bacillus subtilis*

*The most common interstitial lung disorders caused by inhaled organic antigens are indicated with "•".

†M. = *Micropolyspora*; T. = *Thermoactinomyces*; A. = *Aspergillus*.

‡Includes pigeons, parakeets, budgerigars, turkeys, chickens, and ducks.

§Hypersensitivity pneumonitis has been described in association with these agents, in circumstances in which no common name has been given to the disorder.

to the lower respiratory tract in these disorders are defined by the sum of these characteristics.

In the normal lung there are approximately 80 inflammatory cells per alveolus. Most (greater than 80 per cent) are alveolar macrophages, phagocytic cells derived from blood monocytes. The remainder are lymphocytes, mostly T cells, but with a

TABLE 63–4. DRUGS THAT CAUSE INTERSTITIAL LUNG DISEASE

Antineoplastic Agents	Cardiovascular Drugs	Anti-inflammatory Agents
Azathioprine	Hydralazine	Gold salts
Bleomycin	Procainamide	Phenylbutazone
Cyclophosphamide	Beta blockers	Beclomethasone
Methotrexate	(propranolol,	Naproxen
Nitrosoureas	practolol, pindolol,	
Carmustine (BCNU)	acebutolol)	**Oral Hypoglycemic**
Lomustine (CCNU)	Tocainide	**Agents**
Semustine (methyl-CCNU)	Amiodarone	Chlorpropamide
	Reserpine	Tolbutamide
Chlorozotocin (DCNU)		Tolazamide
Melphalan	**Central Nervous**	
Busulfan	**System Drugs**	**Miscellaneous**
Chlorambucil	Phenytoin	Penicillamine
6-Mercaptopurine	Carbamazepine	Allopurinol
6-Thioguanine	Chlorpromazine	Cromolyn sodium
Mitomycin C	Imipramine	Hydrochlorothiazide
Procarbazine	Amitriptyline	Mineral oil
Uracil mustard	Methylphenidate	Intravenous drugs
Zinostatin	Dantrolene	containing
	Mephenesin	particulate material
Antibiotics		Silicon used for tissue
Nitrofurantoin	**Ganglionic Blocking**	augmentation
Penicillins	**Agents**	
Sulfonamides	Mecamylamine	
Erythromycin	Hexamethonium	
Tetracycline	Pentolinium	
Isoniazid		
para-Aminosalicylic acid		
Niridazole		

TABLE 63–5. OTHER AGENTS KNOWN TO CAUSE INTERSTITIAL LUNG DISEASE

Paraquat
Radiation
Sequela of Known Infectious Agents

Bacteria	*Mycoplasma*
Mycobacteria	*Legionella pneumophila*
Fungi	Parasites
Viruses	

Inhaled Agents Other Than Inorganic or Organic Dusts
Gases

Oxygen	Sulfur dioxide
Oxides of nitrogen	Methyl isocyanate
Chlorine gas	

Aerosols

Aspiration pneumonia	Pyrethrum (a natural insecticide)
Fats	Toluene diisocyanate
Oils	

Chemical dusts
  Synthetic fibers (Orlon, polyesters, nylon, acrylic)
  Bakelite
  Vinyl chloride, polyvinyl chloride powder
Fumes
  Oxides of Zn, Cu, Mn, Cd, Fe, Mg, Ni, Se, Sn, Sb, V, and brass
  Diphenylmethane diisocyanate
  Trimellitic anhydride
Vapors
  Hydrocarbons
  Mercury
  Thermosetting resins

small number of B cells. Polymorphonuclear leukocytes are rare in the normal lung, although small numbers do accumulate with a long history of cigarette smoking. As a general rule, alveolar macrophages and T and B lymphocytes are not activated in the normal lung. Immunoglobulins are present in the normal lower respiratory tract (IgG > IgA >> IgM), as are most complement components. Macromolecules that defend against inflammatory injury, including antiproteases and antioxidants, are also present.

Active, untreated ILD are generally characterized by a marked increase in the number of inflammatory cells in the alveolar walls and on the alveolar epithelial surface. Commonly, this increase in numbers of effector cells is also characterized by a shift in their relative proportions. Different patterns of alveolitis are generally referred to by the cell types that are most abundant. For example, when the inflammation is dominated by neutrophils and macrophages it is referred to as a neutrophil-macrophage alveolitis. The alveolitis patterns most frequently observed in ILD are a macrophage-dominant alveolitis, a lymphocyte-macrophage alveolitis, and

TABLE 63–6. DISORDERS INVOLVING THE LOWER RESPIRATORY TRACT THAT CAN BE CONFUSED WITH INTERSTITIAL LUNG DISEASE*

Pulmonary Edema
Neoplasms
  • Leukemic infiltration
  • Lymphoma
  • Lymphangitic spread of carcinoma
    Multiple metastases
    Primary pulmonary malignancy
Infections
  • Viruses†
    Fungi
    Bacteria‡
  • Mycobacteria
  • Parasites§
  • Mycoplasma
    Psittacosis
    Q fever
Pulmonary Hemorrhage
Aspiration

*Disorders frequently confused with the ILD are indicated with "•".

†Of the viruses known to involve the lung—influenza, cytomegalovirus (CMV), varicella zoster, and measles—HIV are most commonly confused with ILD.

‡Particularly *Legionella*.

§*Pneumocystis* and filarial disease are commonly mistaken for ILD.

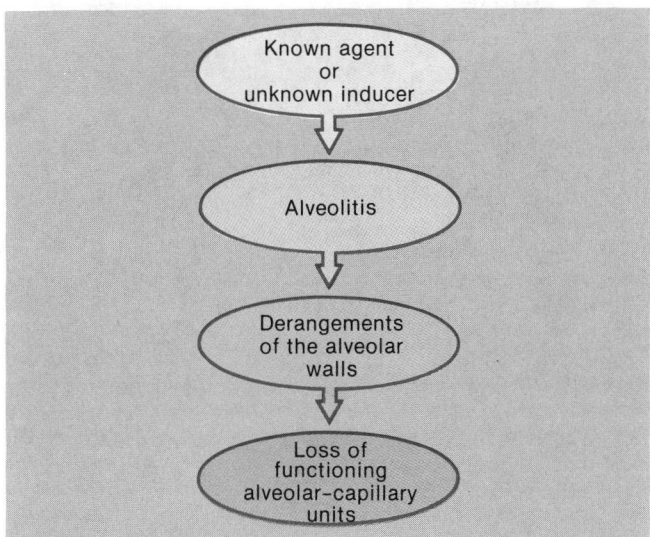

FIGURE 63–3. Pathogenesis of the interstitial lung diseases of unknown and known etiology. In both groups, the inflammation (alveolitis) is responsible for the bulk of the derangements of the alveolar walls. In some disorders, the deranged wall components may accelerate the alveolitis by recruiting additional inflammatory cells. In the disorders of known etiology, the causative agent may directly damage the alveolar structures, which, in turn, initiates and/or accelerates the alveolitis.

a neutrophil-macrophage alveolitis. Eosinophils play a role in the alveolitis of many ILD but rarely dominate it. Subcategories of the common alveolitis patterns have also been described. For example, the granulomatous lung disorders, sarcoidosis and berylliosis, are characterized by a T-helper cell macrophage alveolitis, while chronic hypersensitivity pneumonitis is usually characterized by a T-suppressor/cytotoxic cell macrophage alveolitis, sometimes including neutrophils.

In addition to the numbers and types of inflammatory cells present, the consequences of the alveolitis critically depend on the state of activation of these cells. The simple presence of the inflammatory cells in the alveolar structures distorts the alveolar walls but usually is not damaging. When activated, however, some inflammatory cells can injure the alveolar walls, particularly sensitive type I epithelial cells and capillary endothelial cells. If the alveolitis is self limiting, or if it is suppressed by therapy before the injury becomes too severe, the architecture of the lower respiratory tract can be re-established and normal lung function restored. If, however, the injury is extensive, with fibroblast proliferation and collagen deposition, the normal architecture of the affected alveolar-capillary units can never be fully re-established. Therapeutic success in treating ILD means suppression of the alveolitis and thus prevention of further loss of alveolar-capillary units.

DISTORTION AND FIBROSIS. Whether the derangements to the alveolar walls take the form of distortion and/or fibrosis is dictated by the characteristics of the alveolitis. Importantly, while the distortion type of derangement is usually reversible if the inflammation is suppressed, the consequences of the fibrosis form of derangement are commonly sufficient to prevent a return to the normal architecture.

Accumulation of sufficient numbers of any type of inflammatory cells results in some distortion of the tissue. However, this form of derangement is most important when the inflammation involves lymphocytes and macrophages, such as when there is an accumulation of activated T-helper lymphocytes that direct the formation of granuloma. Together, the T cells and masses of macrophages distort the normal architecture but usually do not cause permanent damage.

The fibrosis form of derangement is characterized by injury to parenchymal components, together with the accumulation of fibroblasts and their secreted connective tissue products. The neutrophil is the most damaging of all inflammatory cells by virtue of its highly reactive oxygen metabolites that are toxic to the parenchymal cells and its connective tissue-specific proteases that can damage the interstitial collagens and basement membranes. Injury to the epithelial basement membrane has profound consequences because the epithelial cells no longer have a surface upon which to migrate, making it impossible to reconstruct a normal alveolar surface. The eosinophil can also injure lung parenchymal cells and connective tissue, but on a per cell basis it is far less potent than the neutrophil. Activated human alveolar macrophages release toxic oxidants and thus can be cytotoxic to normal lung parenchymal cells. The macrophage also mediates the accumulation of fibroblasts and the connective tissue that characterizes the fibrosis type of derangement to the alveolar walls. The fundamental problem is the accumulation of fibroblasts in the alveolar walls. Since fibroblasts are major producers of collagen, the consequence of an increase in fibroblast numbers is an accumulation of collagen in the alveolar interstitium. As a result, the alveolar wall is thickened and scarred and has decreased compliance. The macrophage mediates the accumulation of fibroblasts by releasing exaggerated amounts of at least three mediators, platelet-derived growth factor, fibronectin, and alveolar macrophage-derived growth factor. Platelet-derived growth factor, a product of the *c-sis* oncogene, attracts fibroblasts and is a potent stimulus for fibroblasts to begin traversing the cell cycle. Fibronectin, a 440,000-dalton glycoprotein, attracts fibroblasts, attaches them to the extracellular matrix, and stimulates them to enter the cell cycle. The alveolar macrophage–derived growth factor, an 18,000-dalton protein, induces the fibronectin-primed fibroblasts to continue through the cell cycle and proliferate.

Clinical Features

HISTORY. Occasional patients are detected as having ILD because a routine chest radiograph is noted to be abnormal, but most come to medical attention because of symptoms related to the chest. All ILD are characterized by abnormalities in the transfer of oxygen from air to blood secondary to slowly progressive derangement of the lower respiratory tract. The initial symptoms are those of insufficient oxygen transfer, such as *fatigue* and *breathlessness with exertion*. These symptoms are often initially denied by the patient or are attributed to being "out of shape" or "overweight" or to a prior chest infection, usually a viral syndrome. As the disease progresses, the dyspnea becomes more apparent and eventually is felt at rest. In contrast to cardiac-induced dyspnea, paroxysmal nocturnal dyspnea and orthopnea are rare, as are platypnea and trepopnea. Nonproductive cough, pleuritic pain, and hemoptysis are less common presenting complaints. Early in the disease, chest pain is rare, although later, when pulmonary hypertension develops, substernal discomfort may be noted.

The history also plays an important role in the diagnosis of the type of interstitial disease. Since a large number of agents cause ILD, a careful exposure history is essential in order to determine not only the agents to which the patient has been exposed, but also the circumstances, intensity, and duration of exposure. Exposure to agents that cause ILD may be found in nonclassic situations. For example, silicosis has been described in workers involved in the manufacture of pencils, furniture, and tombstones; talcosis in the manufacture of rubber condoms; and hypersensitivity pneumonitis in office buildings where the offending organic antigen was located in the air conditioning system.

The lack of a history of exposure to a known agent that causes interstitial disease is very important to diagnosing the ILD of unknown etiology. For example, pulmonary sarcoidosis is very difficult to separate from berylliosis unless there is a negative history of beryllium exposure. Likewise, idiopathic pulmonary fibrosis is difficult to diagnose if an exposure history is unavailable or if there is a clear history of sufficient exposure to one or more agents that cause ILD. Some ILD of unknown etiology are associated with diseases that often involve other organs, such as the collagen-vascular disorders, primary biliary cirrhosis, and Wegener's granulomatosis, which may be suspected from the history.

PHYSICAL EXAMINATION. The chest expansion is typically reduced, reflecting the reduced total lung capacity of individuals with ILD. Most have fine, crackling inspiratory and expiratory rales, heard best at the posterior lung bases. These rales have a characteristic sound, described as "Velcro-like" (i.e., the sound of unwrapping a blood pressure cuff) or like the sound of rubbing hair together. Coarse rales, wheezing, and rhonchi are occasionally heard. As the disease progresses, these patients may be tachypneic at rest, but unlike emphysema victims, they do not use the accessory muscles of respiratory and do not assume the posture of placing their hands on their thighs to "fix" the upper body to assist in respiration.

Early in the disease, examination of the heart is normal. Later, an accentuated P_2 reflects mild pulmonary hypertension. Eventually, obvious evidence of pulmonary hypertension is noted, including a right ventricular heave. Patients with ILD rarely develop frank right-sided failure with liver enlargement and peripheral edema, presumably because they die from the complications of insufficient oxygen delivery before the right ventricle deteriorates.

Clubbing of the fingers and sometimes the toes is common in ILD, particularly in idiopathic pulmonary fibrosis and asbestosis. Cyanosis occurs, but usually very late in the disease. Other physical findings in ILD are those associated with problems with oxygen transport (e.g., left ventricular failure, central nervous system signs) and those characteristic of associated diseases (e.g., the rash of systemic lupus erythematosus, the skin changes of scleroderma).

LABORATORY STUDIES. No blood test is diagnostic for one ILD, and the intensity and character of the alveolitis are not reflected in the blood. The hemoglobin and hematocrit are usually normal despite associated hypoxemia, and the white blood cell count and differential usually bear no relationship to the alveolitis. In most ILD, the sedimentation rate is elevated.

A patient with suspected ILD should have routine blood screening tests for hematologic, liver, renal, and muscle abnormalities and collagen-vascular disorders. Other blood tests directed toward specific diseases may be ordered as the workup proceeds and specific disease is suspected. For example, serologic tests for antibodies against organic antigens are ordered only in the context of suspected hypersensitivity pneumonitis and anti–basement membrane antibodies only when there is suspected Goodpasture's syndrome.

Rheumatoid factor and antinuclear antibodies are occasionally present in low titer and do not necessarily indicate the presence of an underlying collagen-vascular disorder. Plasma immunoglobulins may be elevated, but this finding is usually nonspecific. Except in those circumstances in which the disease is systemic (e.g., sarcoidosis, a collagen-vascular disorder), other screening blood studies are generally normal.

The electrocardiogram (ECG) is usually normal in ILD except for evidence of pulmonary hypertension. As the loss of alveolar-capillary units progresses, the ECG demonstrates a pattern of right atrial and ventricular strain. The hypoxemia of ILD may exacerbate coexisting coronary heart disease, evoking arrhythmias and evidence of coronary insufficiency, particularly with exercise.

RADIOGRAPHIC STUDIES. The posteroanterior and lateral chest films play a major role in establishing the diagnosis of ILD, although 5 to 10 per cent of patients with biopsy-proven disease have a normal chest film. A ground-glass

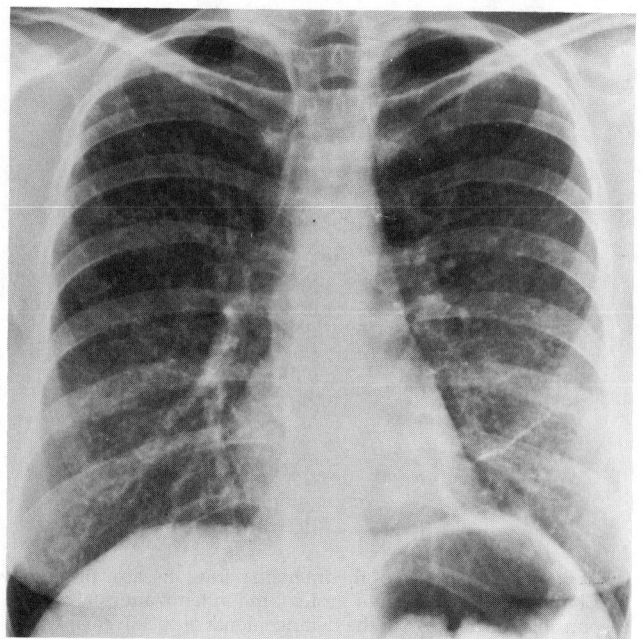

FIGURE 63–4. Chest radiograph of a patient with idiopathic pulmonary fibrosis, typical of the radiographic findings of many interstitial lung diseases. There is a diffuse reticulonodular infiltrate throughout the lung fields, most prominent at the bases. The heart and pleura are normal.

pattern may be seen early in the disease. More typically, the chest radiograph demonstrates a diffuse, finely nodular, reticular, or reticulonodular pattern usually more prominent at the bases (Fig. 63–4). As the disease evolves, the pattern becomes coarser, with cystic areas appearing and, finally, a honeycomb pattern. Initially the pulmonary arteries appear normal, but in the later stages of ILD evidence of pulmonary hypertension may be present.

A definitive diagnosis of a specific ILD can never be made by the chest radiograph alone. However, certain radiographic patterns are characteristic of specific diseases or groups of diseases and thus are very helpful in establishing a diagnosis. For example, some ILD are also characterized by hilar and/or paratracheal lymph node enlargement, while others manifest pleural disease.

Except for rare circumstances, radiographic studies other than the routine chest film have little use in the evaluation of ILD. Oblique films, tomography, bronchography, and angiography are occasionally used to evaluate localized lesions on a background of ILD but usually are difficult to interpret. At present, computerized axial tomographic (CT) scans of the chest are not used in the evaluation of these patients except in the circumstance in which questionable pleural lesions are being evaluated.

PULMONARY FUNCTION TESTS. The classic physiologic alterations in ILD include reduced lung volumes (vital capacity, total lung capacity), reduced diffusing capacity, and a normal or supranormal ratio of forced expiratory volume in 1 second to forced vital capacity. In some ILD, sensitive tests such as flow-volume curves and maximum flow-static recoil curves can detect mild limitation of airflow. Measurement of static lung compliance demonstrates decreased lung volumes for a given transpulmonary pressure, and an increased maximal transpulmonary pressure, i.e., very high negative pressures (relative to the atmosphere), must be generated to open the fibrotic alveoli.

Arterial blood gases typically show mild hypoxemia; carbon dioxide retention is rare, even late in the course of the disease. Patients with ILD tend to hyperventilate and have a reduced P_{CO_2} and compensated respiratory alkalosis, mostly as a result of an increase in respiratory rate. The drive to hyperventilate is not due to hypoxemia or abnormalities in acid-base status but rather to the subjective sense of dyspnea or from an increased stimulation of the respiratory center from neural signals arising in the deranged lung parenchyma. With exercise, the arterial P_{O_2} drops, while the P_{CO_2} remains constant. The loss of alveolar-capillary bed in ILD and hence the limitation of cardiac output seriously impair oxygen delivery and thereby markedly limit the exercise tolerance of these patients. This leads to their propensity to suffer hypoxic damage to vital organs. The arterial pH is usually normal in ILD, but it can fall with exercise as a consequence of oxygen deprivation of muscles, which then resort to anaerobic metabolism.

At rest, the hypoxemia of ILD results from abnormal matching of pulmonary ventilation and perfusion. With exercise, however, an apparent "diffusion block" also contributes. It was originally thought that this resulted from a limited oxygen diffusion through the thickened alveolar walls, but it is now recognized to be due to red blood cells passing through the functioning pulmonary capillaries too rapidly to permit full saturation of hemoglobin. In rare instances, some of the hypoxemia of ILD results from shunts, either in the lung parenchyma or through a patent foramen ovale in the setting of pulmonary hypertension.

The loss of pulmonary capillary bed in ILD is associated with pulmonary hypertension, first with exercise only and later at rest. The pulmonary hypertension is thought to result from mechanical reasons (e.g., the loss of pulmonary capillary bed) and not from hypoxia-induced vasoconstriction or from local mediators. Right ventricular end-diastolic pressure rises late in the disease, but this rarely leads to frank right-sided failure.

SCINTIGRAPHIC STUDIES. Conventional ventilation and perfusion scans usually demonstrate diffuse abnormalities. The perfusion scans show multiple subsegmental areas of impaired perfusion. The normal, upright individual has limited blood flow to the upper lobes at rest. The perfusion scan in ILD, however, shows a redistribution of perfusion to the upper lobes resulting from the loss of pulmonary capillary bed and developing pulmonary hypertension. The ventilation scan shows multiple subsegmental areas of reduced ventilation. Comparison of the perfusion and ventilation scans demonstrates numerous areas of ventilation and perfusion mismatch. The presence of numerous perfusion defects limits the usefulness of these techniques in evaluation of patients with ILD with suspected pulmonary emboli. In such circumstances, pulmonary angiography is mandatory.

Gallium-67 scans are used to evaluate the alveolitis of ILD. Whereas the normal lung parenchyma takes up little gallium-67, ILD with an active alveolitis demonstrate positive gallium-67 lung scans with either a diffuse or a patchy pattern (Fig. 63–5). A high density of activated alveolar macrophages is thought to play a major role in the lung uptake of gallium-67 in these patients.

BRONCHOSCOPIC STUDIES. Most patients with suspected ILD are evaluated by fiberoptic bronchoscopy to rule out neoplastic or infectious disease. In selected patients (see below), transbronchial biopsy can be carried out at the same time.

The technique of bronchoalveolar lavage can be used to sample the inflammatory cells constituting the alveolitis. To accomplish this, the bronchoscope is wedged into a distal bronchus, and aliquots of sterile saline are used to recover the inflammatory cells and epithelial lining fluid of the lower respiratory tract. In normal individuals, 80 per cent or more of the recovered cells demonstrate alveolar macrophages, with the remainder being lymphocytes (almost all T lymphocytes). Polymorphonuclear leukocytes are normally very rare. In patients with ILD, the pattern of alveolitis is reflected by the cells recovered by lavage. For example, in pulmonary sarcoidosis, the proportions of T cells may be 30 to 60 per cent,

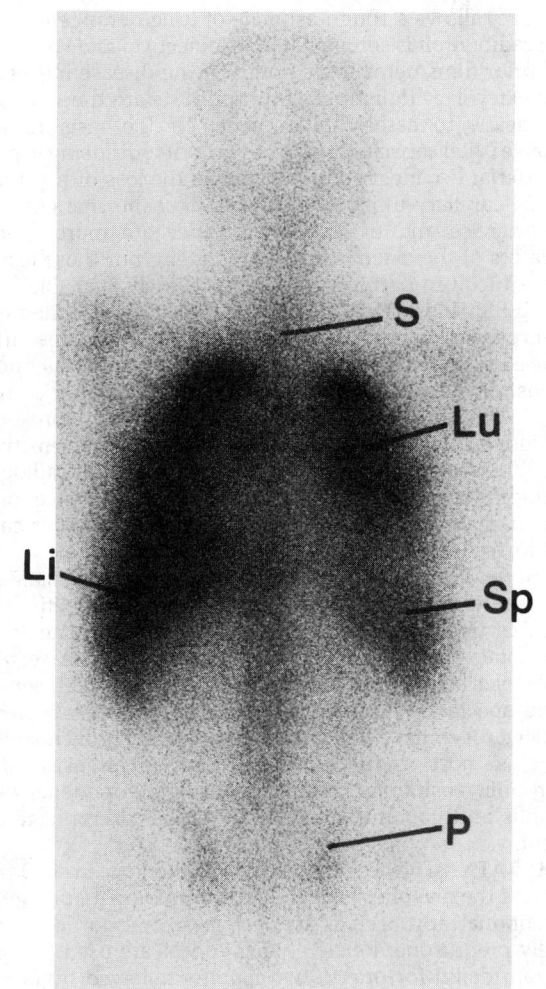

FIGURE 63–5. Gallium-67 scan of a patient with sarcoidosis. There is diffuse uptake of the isotope throughout the lung parenchyma (Lu). Structures that normally take up gallium-67 are also seen, including the spine (S), liver (Li), spleen (Sp), and pelvis (P).

while in idiopathic pulmonary fibrosis, the proportion of neutrophils is greater than 10 per cent. The diagnostic usefulness of bronchoalveolar lavage has not been established, but it can help to orient the clinician to the category of alveolitis that is present. Furthermore, because alveolar macrophages are phagocytic and ingest foreign materials present in the lung parenchyma, bronchoalveolar lavage can also be used to help diagnose specific agents that cause ILD, including inorganic dust diseases.

BIOPSY. The diagnosis of many ILD depends upon pathologic studies of lung parenchyma. The method of choice is the open lung biopsy, usually performed in the right middle lobe or lingula in an area of "average" disease as judged by the chest film. Transbronchial biopsy through the fiberoptic bronchoscope is useful for diagnosing sarcoidosis, but for most other ILD the samples are too small for a definitive diagnosis to be made.

Staging and Therapy

A patient with ILD should be evaluated to assess the contribution of the disease to his functional impairment. The activity of the disease process should be independently assessed. Once both are known, rational decisions can be made concerning prognosis and therapy.

ASSESSMENT OF IMPAIRMENT. The consequences of ILD are assessed by history, chest radiograph, and lung function testing. A careful history of the patient's sensation of breathlessness, combined with an estimate of exercise tolerance, allows a rough estimate of lung derangement. The chest radiograph is somewhat more objective, and comparison with prior films helps to determine if the disease has become more extensive. Pulmonary function tests are the most accurate means to assess impairment. Of the tests routinely available, vital capacity, total lung capacity, diffusing capacity, and arterial Po_2 most accurately gauge the loss of functioning alveolar-capillary units. Measurements of the changes in Po_2 with exercise and of static compliance are more sensitive indicators of the extent of the impairment, but these tests are more difficult to perform and are not widely available.

ASSESSMENT OF ACTIVITY. Alveolitis is confined to the lower respiratory tract, so that its character or extent is difficult to measure directly. Circulating immune complexes and angiotensin-converting enzyme have been suggested as measures of the alveolitis in idiopathic pulmonary fibrosis and sarcoidosis, respectively, but neither test is very sensitive or specific. Likewise, attempts to correlate the chest radiograph or lung function tests with morphologic evidence of the alveolitis have been disappointing, and thus neither can be used to accurately evaluate the alveolitis.

Open lung biopsy, bronchoalveolar lavage, and *gallium-67 scanning* are the best present methods to stage alveolitis. Open biopsy is the most accurate method but is very rarely performed more than once in the course of the disease. Bronchoalveolar lavage and gallium-67 scanning are both sensitive to and specific for the alveolitis, but neither has been fully validated for routine clinical use. At this time, bronchoalveolar lavage is most useful for evaluating the intensity of the neutrophil, eosinophil, and lymphocyte components of the alveolitis and gallium-67 scanning for the macrophage component.

THERAPY. The principal aim of therapy in ILD is to suppress the alveolitis. For the ILD of unknown etiology, the conventional approach is to treat with oral corticosteroids, usually prednisone. Relatively high doses are used (1 mg per kilogram daily) for one to two months followed by tapering doses over two to three months to maintenance levels (0.25 mg per kilogram daily), which are continued for varying periods of time. The corticosteroids are generally given once daily; it is not known if alternate-day regimens are equally effective. There has never been a large controlled trial of corticosteroids in any ILD, but some patients with ILD respond to corticosteroids in a fashion that cannot be explained by spontaneous remission. "Successful" therapy does not necessarily mean improvement in pulmonary function, chest radiograph, or subjective symptoms, since severely damaged alveoli are lost forever. In this context, successful suppression of the alveolitis usually means no further loss of alveoli. If improvement does occur, it likely results from suppression of the contribution of the inflammation itself to the derangements of the alveolar structures.

If the disease stabilizes, the corticosteroids are usually tapered. If the deterioration restarts after a period of quiescence, corticosteroids are often restarted, but their efficacy under these circumstances is limited. A variety of cytotoxic and other anti-inflammatory drugs have also been used in the treatment of the ILD of unknown etiology, but there has been no controlled series to demonstrate their efficacy.

For the ILD of known etiology, the initial treatment is to remove exposure to the causative agent. If the inflammation persists months after removal from the known agent, the patients are usually treated in a similar fashion to ILD of unknown etiology. The exception to this rule is in most of the pneumoconioses, for which no therapy is used.

In all ILD, attention should be given to prompt treatment of lung infections. Bronchodilators are sometimes used in mid to late course in these diseases to help mobilize secretions. Oxygen therapy, particularly with exercise, is often used as the patient reaches the late stage of ILD, but its efficacy in increasing the lifespan of these patients is unproven.

INTERSTITIAL LUNG DISEASES OF UNKNOWN ETIOLOGY

The ILD of unknown etiology represent the majority of all cases of ILD. Although of unknown etiology, each represents a specific entity with distinct features (Table 63–1). The best understood ILD of unknown etiology are idiopathic pulmonary fibrosis and sarcoidosis.

Idiopathic Pulmonary Fibrosis (IPF)

CLINICAL MANIFESTATIONS. IPF, the "classic" fibrotic lung disease, is characterized by a neutrophil-alveolar macrophage alveolitis and progressive scarring of alveolar-capillary units. In the past IPF was sometimes called the Hamman-Rich syndrome, but this designation is not generally used now. Typically, IPF presents in middle age, but all age groups can be affected. The sex distribution is equal. Patients present with dyspnea on exertion and/or a dry cough, often following a viral illness. Fever is rare. Physical examination demonstrates dry, bibasilar rales, often associated with clubbing of the fingers and sometimes of the toes. The chest radiograph typically shows a diffuse reticulonodular infiltrate most prominent at the bases without hilar or pleural abnormalities. Some patients have various "autoimmune" abnormalities that likely represent nonspecific epiphenomena. Circulating immune complexes are common. Pulmonary function tests are typical for ILD, with reduced volumes and diffusing capacity. Routine tests of airflow are normal, but sensitive tests reveal mild airflow limitation, an observation that correlates with morphologic evidence of narrowing of small airways. Patients with IPF have mild resting hypoxemia that drops significantly with physical activity. Typically, a resting Po_2 of 80 torr will fall to 50 torr with exercise equivalent to walking up one flight of stairs. Ventilation and perfusion studies reveal diffuse patchy abnormalities with mismatching of air and blood. The gallium-67 scan usually shows a diffuse uptake of isotope throughout the lung parenchyma, and bronchoalveolar lavage reveals an alveolitis pattern dominated by neutrophils and macrophages, with fewer numbers of lymphocytes and eosinophils. The epithelial lining fluid of the lower respiratory tract contains elevated levels of IgG, immune complexes, and neutrophil products, including collagenase and myeloperoxidase. Open lung biopsy shows a diffuse alveolitis that is patchy in its intensity. There is marked derangement of the alveolar walls with a fibrosis type pattern, including denudation of the epithelial basement membranes; replacement of the type I epithelial cells by type II epithelial cells and bronchiolar cells; loss of capillaries; and expansion of the interstitium with edema, increased fibroblast numbers, and masses of deranged collagen fibers. The epithelial basement membranes have holes through which the interstitial fibrosis extends into the airspaces.

The clinical course of IPF is characterized by progressive loss of alveolar-capillary units, with eventual respiratory failure and death an average of five years after the onset of symptoms. Occasional patients have a rapidly progressive course; others may live for ten or more years. IPF is associated with a higher than expected incidence of lung carcinoma, myocardial infarction, and pulmonary embolism.

DIFFERENTIAL DIAGNOSIS. Although the term "IPF" suggests that the diagnosis is one of exclusion, its features are so characteristic that the diagnosis is usually not difficult. Most confusion comes in separating ILD associated with the collagen-vascular disorders, which are systemic diseases, whereas IPF is compartmentalized to the lung. To exclude the ILD of known etiology that can mimic IPF, it is mandatory to take a careful history of past exposures to agents that can cause ILD. An open lung biopsy is necessary for diagnosis, but IPF cannot be diagnosed using morphologic criteria alone. While the biopsy features of IPF fit the morphologic categories of "usual interstitial pneumonitis (UIP)," "desquamative interstitial pneumonitis (DIP)," or, more commonly, a mixture of UIP and DIP, these features are not specific for IPF and can be found in other ILD of both known and unknown etiology.

PATHOGENESIS. IPF likely results from uncontrolled inflammatory processes that ensue after any of a variety of insults to the lower respiratory tract of susceptible individuals. There is likely an inherited susceptibility to this disease, but links to a specific genetic locus have not been made. The neutrophil-macrophage–dominated alveolitis, the first known manifestation of IPF, may be driven by immune complexes of unknown origin formed within the lower respiratory tract. The immune complexes are probably associated with enhanced lung B cell immunoglobin production, with at least some of the immunoglobulins directed against local self-antigens. These immune comlexes activate alveolar macrophages to release neutrophil-specific chemotactic factors that continuously recruit neutrophils to the alveolar structures. The neutrophils damage the alveolar walls by releasing toxic oxygen radicals and proteases. IPF macrophages spontaneously release exaggerated amounts of platelet-derived growth factor, fibronectin, and alveolar macrophage–derived growth factor and thus expand the numbers of fibroblasts, resulting in fibrosis of the alveolar walls.

STAGING AND THERAPY. The degree of lung damage in IPF is determined by history, chest radiograph, and pulmonary function testing. The intensity of the alveolitis of IPF can be gauged by gallium-67 scanning and bronchoalveolar lavage, with particular emphasis placed on the intensity of the neutrophil component of the alveolitis. Conventional therapy is use of corticosteroids, usually as lifelong therapy. Approximately 10 to 20 per cent of IPF patients improve with corticosteroids, particularly if the disease is detected early, before the alveolitis causes significant abnormalities. The second line of therapy is either the addition of massive doses of methylprednisolone sodium succinate (Solu-Medrol) (2 grams IV once weekly) or oral cyclophosphamide (1.5 mg per kilogram daily). Either approach helps suppress the alveolitis, but their long-term efficacy is unknown.

Sarcoidosis

Sarcoidosis (Ch. 69) is a multisystem granulomatous disease of unknown etiology characterized in affected organs by a T-helper lymphocyte–mononuclear phagocyte inflammatory process, noncaseating granulomata, and derangement of normal tissue architecture. While most organs can be affected by sarcoidosis, the lower respiratory tract is the site that most commonly causes morbidity and mortality. Pulmonary sarcoidosis is characterized by sharply circumscribed granulomata in the alveolar, bronchial, and vascular walls, composed of tightly packed cells derived from the mononuclear phagocyte system. In addition, the alveolar walls are deranged in a fashion similar to IPF, but much less so. Significant interstitial fibrosis occurs in 20 to 25 per cent of patients. Sarcoidosis is described in detail in Ch. 69 and will not be discussed further here.

ILD Associated with the Collagen-Vascular Disorders

All collagen-vascular disorders are associated with ILD. In most cases the collagen-vascular disorder is apparent before lung involvement is noted, but occasionally the ILD develops first and the other characteristic systemic signs and symptoms appear later. In either case, these disorders are frequently confused with IPF.

RHEUMATOID ARTHRITIS (Ch. 433). The ILD associated with rheumatoid arthritis include (1) an IPF-like disorder, (2) Caplan's syndrome (rheumatoid arthritis associated with coal worker's pneumoconiosis), (3) pulmonary parenchymal rheumatoid nodules, (4) pulmonary arteritis, and (5) apical fibrobullous disease. A few patients with rheumatoid arthritis have been described with dyspnea, severe irreversible airway obstruction with hyperinflation, and morphologic evidence of obliterative bronchiolitis. While some of this terminal airway disease may be related to penicillamine therapy, it may represent another manifestation of rheumatoid arthritis in the lung parenchyma.

The IPF-like disorder is by far the most common pulmonary manifestation of rheumatoid arthritis. Approximately 25 per cent of chest radiographs of patients with rheumatoid arthritis show interstitial changes, and the diffusing capacity is reduced in 50 per cent of all patients. In most cases the lung disease is much milder than IPF. The pathogenesis of the ILD is unknown but assumed to be the consequence of the same processes that affect the joints. The alveolitis is similar to IPF, but the neutrophil component is much less evident. There is no relationship between the extent of disease and the titer of the rheumatoid factor. Most cases of ILD associated with rheumatoid arthritis do not need to be treated. If treatment is instituted, guidelines similar to those for IPF are used. Gold salts, a common therapy for rheumatoid arthritis, can also induce ILD. There is no way to distinguish between gold salt– and rheumatoid arthritis–induced ILD, except that the gold-induced disease may reverse when the drug is discontinued.

PROGRESSIVE SYSTEMIC SCLEROSIS (PSS) (Ch. 527). The most common form of ILD associated with PSS is similar to IPF. The incidence of ILD among patients with PSS is very high; at autopsy, morphologic changes are found in 90 per cent and radiographic evidence of ILD is found in 30 to 40 per cent of patients. PSS patients with the CREST syndrome (calcinosis, Raynaud's phenomenon, esophageal involvement, sclerodactyly, and telangiectasia) rarely develop ILD. The ILD associated with PSS is generally indolent, but if it becomes symptomatic, the four-year survival rate is about 50 per cent. Although PSS is considered to be a connective tissue disorder with fibrosis as its main feature, patients with the ILD associated with PSS have an alveolitis, albeit milder than that of IPF. Gallium-67 scans are often positive. For most patients, the alveolitis is dominated by macrophages, but neutrophils and sometimes lymphocytes play a role. The ILD associated with PSS is associated with a higher than normal incidence of bronchogenic carcinoma, particularly bronchoalveolar cell carcinoma.

Occasional patients with PSS develop an ILD characterized by pulmonary hypertension with relatively less disease of the alveolar-capillary units. Morphologically, there is thickening of the pulmonary arteries with fibrosis and some inflammation. Many of these patients develop rapidly progressive respiratory failure.

The pathogenesis of the ILD associated with PSS is unknown. The therapeutic guidelines are unclear, although patients with progressive disease usually are treated in a similar fashion to those with IPF. Penicillamine has been suggested as an alternative therapy, but its efficacy is unproven.

SYSTEMIC LUPUS ERYTHEMATOSUS (SLE) (Ch. 436). The common manifestations of SLE in the lung include pleurisy with or without effusion, atelectasis, or acute pneumonitis. Less frequently, SLE manifests as uremic pulmonary edema, diaphragmatic dysfunction, parenchymal hemorrhage, or chronic ILD. Most cases of chronic ILD have pulmonary features similar to IPF, together with the systemic findings of SLE. Rarely, ILD associated with SLE can also present with a lymphocytic alveolitis similar to Sjögren's syndrome, a disorder similar to idiopathic pulmonary hemosiderosis, or a hypersensitivity vasculitis–like picture. Together, the incidence of acute and chronic pulmonary involvement in SLE is less than 20 per cent of all cases of SLE, and chronic ILD occurs in less than 5 per cent. Chronic ILD can appear insidiously or follow the acute pneumonitis of SLE, a severe illness characterized by fever, tachypnea, radiographic evidence of patchy or diffuse infiltrates, and hypoxemia. The pathogenesis of the ILD associated with SLE is thought to result from the deposition of circulating immune complexes in the alveolar walls. Therapy is usually with corticosteroids, but specific treatment guidelines have not been established. SLE can be associated with pulmonary infections, and this must be distinguished from ILD before corticosteroid therapy is started.

POLYMYOSITIS/DERMATOMYOSITIS (Ch. 443). The incidence of ILD in polymyositis/dermatomyositis is 5 to 10 per cent. Of all the collagen-vascular disorders, a higher proportion of patients who develop the ILD associated with polymyositis/dermatomyositis develop the ILD before the other systemic manifestations of the disease. The ILD is similar to IPF, but its pathogenesis is unclear. Patients are usually treated with corticosteroids, but methotrexate has been suggested as alternative therapy.

SJÖGREN'S SYNDROME (Ch. 438). Approximately 3 per cent of patients with Sjögren's syndrome develop ILD that manifests as either a mild IPF-like disease or, more commonly, a disorder with a lymphocyte-dominant alveolitis, similar to the lymphocytic infiltration of other organs in these patients. This lymphocytic form of ILD can be mild to severe and can undergo transformation to a lymphocytic malignancy, an event that is invariably fatal. Therapy of either ILD associated with Sjögren's syndrome is controversial; corticosteroids, immunosuppressive agents, and no therapy have all been advocated.

MIXED CONNECTIVE TISSUE DISEASE (Ch. 437). Up to 80 per cent of patients with this systemic disorder have ILD. The lung disease is usually IPF-like. Pulmonary hypertension is common and can occur without significant parenchymal involvement. Therapy is usually with corticosteroids with or without cytotoxic agents.

ANKYLOSING SPONDYLITIS (Ch. 434). Lung disease, manifested as chest wall restriction and upper lobe fibrobullous disease, occurs in about 1 per cent of patients with ankylosing spondylitis. Most patients are asymptomatic, but colonization with organisms such as *Aspergillus* or atypical mycobacteria is common, and hemoptysis and pneumothorax occur in the late stages of the disease. While HLA-B27 is strongly associated with ankylosing spondylitis, it is not common in those patients with the associated ILD. The morphology of the ILD is IPF-like, together with localized destruction of alveolar walls and bullae. There is no known therapy.

Histiocytosis-X

Histiocytosis-X (HX) (Ch. 161), also called "primary pulmonary histiocytosis" and "eosinophilic granuloma," is a fibrotic-destructive disorder of the lower respiratory tract associated with an intense mononuclear phagocyte–dominant alveolitis. HX is grouped with the other proliferative disorders of the mononuclear phagocyte system, such as Letterer-Siwe and Hand-Schüller-Christian disease. In adults, HX is primarily a lung disease, although bone, skin, and central nervous system manifestations do occur. At least 50 per cent of all patients have chronic symptoms, and the disease can be fatal. More than 1000 cases have been reported; most new patients are 20 to 40 years of age and there is an equal sex distribution. Almost all patients with HX have been cigarette smokers.

The patient with HX presents with a nonproductive cough, dyspnea on exertion, or chest pain. Spontaneous pneumothorax occurs in 10 per cent of cases; fever, weight loss, hemoptysis, and wheezing are occasionally noted. Bone involvement is present in a minority of patients. Posterior pituitary involvement with diabetes insipidus is unusual, as are skin lesions. Physical examination commonly reveals decreased breath sounds and rales. The chest radiograph shows upper and midzone small, irregular nodules superimposed

on a delicate cystic pattern. The costophrenic angles are usually clear, and the pleura and hila are normal. Pulmonary function tests show a mixed restrictive-obstructive pattern with reduced lung volumes, reduced diffusing capacity, airflow limitation, and hypoxemia that worsens with exercise.

Definitive diagnosis is made by open lung biopsy. The disease is focal but poorly demarcated. There are sites of intense alveolitis dominated by alveolar macrophages and Langerhans cells. Gallium-67 scans are negative or only mildly positive. Bronchoalveolar lavage reveals a macrophage-dominant alveolitis and the Langerhans cells can be detected in lavage by ultrastructure and the T6 monoclonal antibody. The pathogenesis of this rare entity is discussed in Ch. 161. The lung disease in adults is considered untreatable.

Goodpasture's Syndrome

Goodpasture's syndrome (Ch. 81) is characterized by diffuse pulmonary hemorrhage, ILD, glomerulonephritis, and circulating antiglomerular basement membrane (anti-GBM) and anti–alveolar basement membrane (anti-ABM) antibodies. It is assumed that the anti-GBM and anti-ABM antibodies are identical and cross-react with identical components in the kidney and lung basement membranes. Goodpasture's syndrome can be mimicked by SLE, Wegener's granulomatosis, and the systemic necrotizing vasculitides. In the appropriate clinical setting, the diagnosis of Goodpasture's syndrome is straightforward but does require (1) demonstration of the circulating antibodies, (2) characteristic linear deposits of immunoglobulin along the glomerular basement membrane, and (3) demonstration that the antibodies (either those circulating or those eluted from the kidney) are specific. It is usually not necessary to obtain lung tissue to make the diagnosis, but the diagnosis can be confirmed by histologic and immunofluorescence study of lung tissue obtained by transbronchial biopsy.

Almost all of the anti–basement membrane antibodies in Goodpasture's syndrome are IgG, but IgA anti-GBM, and anti-ABM antibodies have been described in the setting of pulmonary hemorrhage and glomerulonephritis. The basement membrane antigen(s) against which the antibodies are directed is thought to be a portion of type IV (basement membrane) collagen that is somehow unmasked in the kidney and lung.

Goodpasture's syndrome occurs mostly in young men. In most cases, evidence of alveolar hemorrhage precedes the clinical evidence of renal disease. Hemoptysis occurs in almost all cases, tends to be recurrent, and occasionally is massive and life threatening. In such cases, death is from asphyxiation. Anemia is almost always present. The chest radiograph reveals interstitial and alveolar infiltrates. The patchy infiltrates due to the hemorrhage often clear, but the interstitial markings, reflecting chronic ILD, often remain. Histologic findings include alveolar hemorrhage, hemosiderin-laden macrophages, focal areas of alveolitis, and interstitial fibrosis. Linear deposits of IgG can be detected in the alveolar walls.

Spontaneous remissions of Goodpasture's syndrome can occur but are rare. Therapy generally consists of corticosteroids, cytotoxic agents, and plasmapheresis.

Idiopathic Pulmonary Hemosiderosis (IPH)

IPH is a rare disorder of unknown cause characterized by alveolar hemorrhage, iron deficiency anemia, transient parenchymal infiltrates on the chest radiograph, and ILD. The disease is most common in individuals less than 20 years of age, but adult cases are seen. The disease is occasionally found in families, but a genetic basis has not been proven. IPH is compartmentalized in the lung and must be distinguished from Goodpasture's syndrome, Wegener's granulomatosis, SLE, and the vasculitides.

The patient with IPH presents with repetitive acute episodes of dyspnea, cough with hemoptysis, and fever. Iron deficiency anemia is common. The chest radiographs associated with these acute episodes reveal transient infiltrates, a miliary pattern, or massive confluent shadows. On this background of intermittent episodes, a chronic ILD develops with increasing dyspnea, rales, clubbing, and pulmonary hypertension. While the childhood form of the disease is aggressive, with a mean survival of about three years, adult IPH tends to be more insidious. Lung function tests are typical for ILD, but the diffusing capacity may be falsely high owing to increased uptake of the carbon monoxide (used as the test gas) by free hemoglobin in the lung parenchyma. Hemosiderin-laden macrophages in sputum or lavage fluid suggest prior parenchymal hemorrhage. In the appropriate clinical setting, when there are no detectable anti-GBM antibodies, a definitive diagnosis of IPH can be made with an open lung biopsy revealing focal hemorrhage, a macrophage-dominant alveolitis with hemosiderin-positive macrophages, and typical findings of ILD. The pathogenesis of this disorder is unknown. Corticosteroids are generally used to treat the acute episodes and the chronic ILD, but there is no evidence regarding their efficacy.

Chronic Eosinophilic Pneumonia (CEP)

CEP is a chronic ILD characterized by cough, dyspnea, malaise, fever, night sweats, weight loss, variable degrees of blood eosinophilia, and a chest film revealing peripheral, nonsegmental, nonmigratory infiltrates. Hilar adenopathy rarely occurs. Asthma accompanies CEP in 50 to 60 per cent of cases. High proportions of eosinophils are sometimes recovered in sputum or by lavage. A very high sedimentation rate is common, and elevated levels of IgE during acute episodes have been described. The histologic findings of CEP include a diffuse alveolitis dominated by eosinophils and macrophages with fewer numbers of neutrophils and lymphocytes. Eosinophilic abscesses, multinucleated giant cells, angiitis of small pulmonary vessels, and interstitial fibrosis are common.

Although the stimulus to the accumulation of the eosinophils in the lung is unknown, the eosinophil can damage the cells and matrix of the alveolar walls through its release of toxic oxygen radicals, collagenase, and major basic protein, a highly charged polypeptide associated with the eosinophil granules.

An open lung biopsy is required to make a definitive diagnosis. However, because CEP usually responds dramatically to corticosteroids, a tentative diagnosis is often made on clinical grounds only without biopsy confirmation and corticosteroid therapy is instituted. In some patients, the disease is only partly suppressed by corticosteroids, and long-term treatment is required.

Lymphocytic Infiltrative Disorders

This is a group of rare, diffuse ILD characterized by infiltration of the alveolar structures by cells of the lymphocyte series. Most patients present with cough and dyspnea, occasionally with fever. All of the lymphocyte infiltrative disorders of lung can progress to frank lymphoma.

Immunoblastic lymphadenopathy (also called angioimmunoblastic lymphadenopathy) is a systemic disorder, usually of elderly individuals, characterized by generalized lymphadenopathy hepatosplenomegaly, and variable amounts of ILD. The disease has no known etiology, but associations with drugs have been reported, including antibiotics and phenytoin. A skin rash is observed in one third of cases; there may be a coexistent collagen-vascular disorder or hemolytic anemia. There are polyclonal increases in serum immunoglobulins. The alveolar structures exhibit a pleomorphic alveolitis representing all levels of lymphocyte differentiation. Diagnosis is usually made by lymph node biopsy. The disease can remit spontaneously, but patients die from progressive respiratory failure, infection, or malignancy. There is a variable response to therapy with corticosteroids and/or cytotoxic agents.

Lymphocytic interstitial pneumonitis is limited to the lung. The signs and symptoms are typical for an insidious, slowly progressive ILD. It is most common in women in their 40's, but it is observed in males and all age groups. The chest radiograph characteristically shows diffuse reticulonodular infiltrates. Most patients have dysproteinemias. Hyper- and hypogammaglobulinemia have been described, and an association with Sjögren's syndrome is common. The diagnosis is made by an open lung biopsy revealing diffuse parenchymal infiltration with mature lymphocytes, plasma cells, and immunoblasts. Granulomas are sometimes observed. Because the infiltrating cells may form germinal centers, the disease is sometimes called "pseudolymphoma." The prognosis of lymphocytic interstitial pneumonitis is variable, and some patients progress to end-stage lung disease or lymphoma. Treatment is with corticosteroids and/or immunosuppressive agents.

ILD Associated with Pulmonary Vasculitis

Many of the systemic vasculitides result in ILD as a consequence of a pulmonary vasculitis causing a secondary alveolitis and derangements of the alveolar structures.

Wegener's granulomatosis is a granulomatous vasculitis of the upper and lower respiratory tracts and glomerulonephritis (Ch. 441). There is a limited form of the disease without clinically apparent renal disease. All patients have pulmonary involvement, but only one third have symptoms related to the lungs. Airway involvement is common. The parenchymal lung disease can appear as discrete nodules and/or diffuse ILD; either can undergo necrosis and cavity formation. Hemoptysis, cough, sputum production, dyspnea, and pleuritic pain are common. Lung function tests reveal a mixed restrictive-obstructive pattern. Diagnosis is usually made by open lung biopsy. Untreated disease is usually fatal, but with cyclophosphamide therapy long-term survival is the rule.

Lymphomatoid granulomatosis is a systemic vasculitis involving the lung, skin, central nervous system, and kidneys. The lung is always affected, but involvement of other organs is variable. In the lung, the walls of the blood vessels are infiltrated with typical and atypical lymphocytes together with some granulomata, and there is associated ILD. A mild form of lymphomatoid granulomatosis has been described ("benign lymphocytic angiitis and granulomatosis"). The disease is most common in middle age. There are multiple, fleeting nodular densities on the chest film; occasionally there are diffuse infiltrates. Death is usually due to parenchymal destruction with sepsis and occasionally due to massive hemoptysis. The diagnosis is usually established by biopsy of the lung or skin. The lung disease often responds to corticosteroids and cyclophosphamide, but the central nervous system lesions do not. Lymphoma occurs in about 10 per cent of cases.

The *Churg-Strauss syndrome* ("allergic angiitis and granulomatosis") (Ch. 439) is a form of systemic necrotizing vasculitis that almost always involves the lung, unlike classic polyarteritis nodosa, which rarely does. The pulmonary manifestations, consisting of asthma and diffuse infiltrates, often precede systemic involvement by one or two years. An allergic history is common. An elevated sedimentation rate and total eosinophil count are common. The systemic vasculitis involves skin, heart, and gastrointestinal tract. Diagnosis is made by open lung biopsy, which shows a granulomatous vasculitis with eosinophilic infiltration, a secondary diffuse alveolitis, interstitial granulomata, and fibrosis. Treatment is the same as for the other pulmonary vasculitides.

"Hypersensitivity vasculitis" represents a heterogeneous group of vasculitides whose development is thought to be related to sensitization to antigens such as drugs or serum proteins. Skin involvement is most common; most cases do

not involve the lung. When they do there is a small-vessel polymorphonuclear leukocyte vasculitis with fibrinoid necrosis and secondary ILD. Diagnosis is usually made by skin biopsy, and the disorder is often self limiting. A similar disorder can occur in association with mixed cryoglobulinemia or Henoch-Schonlein purpura.

Inherited Disorders

There is a small group of rare ILD that are clearly inherited. Almost all are autosomal dominant disorders, although the autosomal recessive disorders Hermansky-Pudlak syndrome, Niemann-Pick disease, and Gaucher's disease may rarely be associated with interstitial lung disease.

FAMILIAL IDIOPATHIC PULMONARY FIBROSIS. This is a chronic, usually fatal autosomal dominant disorder identical to IPF. Symptoms usually begin in the fifth or sixth decade, but the disease can be manifested earlier. Some of the asymptomatic children of affected family members have evidence of a mild alveolitis yet with normal lung function, suggesting that the disease begins with an alveolitis.

NEUROFIBROMATOSIS (Ch. 477). Von Recklinghausen's disease is an autosomal dominant disorder characterized by pigmented skin lesions and neurofibromas of the peripheral and central nervous systems. In 10 to 20 per cent of adult cases there is a coexisting ILD and/or bullous lung disease. The ILD has histologic features similar to those of IPF, but it is not known whether it responds to similar therapies.

TUBEROUS SCLEROSIS (Ch. 477). This is a hamartomatous autosomal dominant disorder involving the central nervous system, skin, kidneys, eyes, bones, heart, and, in 1 per cent of patients, the lungs. Although the hamartomatous "tumors" are composed of various cell types in most affected organs, in the lung they are composed only of smooth muscle cells. The accumulation of smooth muscle cells in the alveolar interstitium causes ILD, together with parenchymal destruction. Unlike most ILD, there is little alveolitis. The chest radiograph shows diffuse infiltrates and honeycombing, and lung function tests show a mixed pattern with a dominant obstructive pattern. Pneumothorax is common. There is no known therapy.

ILD Associated with Pulmonary Airway Disease

This term refers to disorders in which the ILD is likely secondary to a primary airway disease. It is unclear if there are many such diseases or only one. The characteristic lesions are necrotic granulomata in the bronchial walls, with the bronchiolar lumens filled with palisading epithelioid cells, cellular debris, and polymorphonuclear leukocytes. There are usually a diffuse alveolitis and nongranulomatous fibrosis-type derangements of the alveolar walls. Approximately one third have asthma, blood eosinophilia, mucus plugging, fungal hyphae identifiable in the airways, and positive sputum cultures for *Aspergillus* organisms. These patients are usually referred to as having "*bronchopulmonary aspergillosis*" (see Ch. 376). It is unclear, however, whether the fungus is a primary cause of the disease or represents a secondary process.

The remaining two thirds of patients, referred to as having "*bronchocentric granulomatosis*," do not have asthma, microscopic evidence of fungi, or blood eosinophilia. The disease can present in an insidious manner or as an acute febrile illness. The chest film usually shows nodular or mass lesions; diffuse infiltrates are seen in about 20 per cent of cases. Lung function tests demonstrate a mixed obstructive-restrictive pattern. Corticosteroids are usually the therapy of choice.

Lymphangioleiomyomatosis

This is a rare disease of women, usually of childbearing age, characterized by the proliferation of benign but atypical smooth muscle cells in walls of the lymphatics of the lower respiratory tract, pleura, mediastinum, and retroperitoneum.

Although it is an ILD characterized by thickening and derangements of the alveolar walls, there is very little inflammation present. Eventual destruction of the alveolar walls is common. The clinical findings include dyspnea, recurrent unilateral or bilateral chylous pleural effusions, pneumothorax, hemoptysis, and occasionally peritoneal chylous effusions. The chest radiograph has a characteristic reticulonodular pattern on a background of diffuse cystic changes, similar to that seen in histiocytosis-X. Lung function tests reveal a mixed obstructive-restrictive pattern. An open lung biopsy is required to make the diagnosis. It has been theorized that the disease results from an abnormal response to estrogens, and thus oophorectomy, progesterone, and tamoxifen therapy have all been tried in these patients. There is no proven efficacy of such therapies, and the disease is almost always fatal, usually within 10 years of diagnosis.

Alveolar Proteinosis

In this disorder the alveoli are filled with a periodic acid–Schiff (PAS)–positive lipid and protein-rich granular material. There may be an accompanying mononuclear cell alveolitis and fibrosis-type derangements of the alveolar walls. Although of unknown etiology, alveolar proteinosis can be associated with silicosis, hematologic malignancies, bronchogenic cyst, and mycobacterial and fungal diseases of the lung. Why this material accumulates in the alveoli is unknown but is speculated to result from the breakdown of cells in the lower respiratory tract, from the overproduction of substances normally secreted into the alveolar spaces (e.g., surfactant), from increased transudation of plasma proteins, or from decreased alveolar clearance mechanisms.

The disease usually begins insidiously with dyspnea as the initial symptom. The chest radiograph has a characteristic diffuse, finely nodular alveolar filling pattern. Lung function tests show decreased lung volumes and diffusing capacity. There is usually hypoxemia secondary to pulmonary blood shunting by filled alveoli. Open lung biopsy is usually required for the diagnosis. However, in the appropriate clinical setting, bronchoalveolar lavage recovery of the typical material, together with transbronchial biopsy evidence of alveoli filled with PAS-positive material, is usually diagnostic. Alveolar proteinosis can be fatal but can also spontaneously resolve. The recommended therapy is massive whole lung lavage under general anesthesia. Corticosteroid therapy has no proven use and may lead to the development of opportunistic infections.

Miscellaneous Other ILD of Unknown Etiology

There are several ILD of unknown etiology that are reasonably well defined but so rare that there is little information available concerning their pathogenesis and no apparent guidelines relating to their staging and therapy. These are included by list in Table 63–1 but will not be discussed individually here.

INTERSTITIAL LUNG DISEASE OF KNOWN ETIOLOGY

Approximately 135 agents are known to cause ILD, but together they are responsible for only one third of all cases of ILD. In terms of numbers of patients that come to medical attention, the most important agents are crystalline silica, asbestos, coal dust, organic dusts of the *Micropolyspora* and *Thermoactinomyces* genera and those derived from avian proteins, some antineoplastic drugs, nitrofurantoin, and hyperoxia.

Inhaled Inorganic Dusts

ILD resulting from the chronic inhalation of an inorganic dust is called a "pneumoconiosis" (see Table 63–2). The most common are silicosis, asbestosis, and coal worker's pneumoconiosis. The common pneumoconioses are all characterized by fibrosis-type derangements of the lower respiratory tract.

There are several important principles relevant to understanding the pneumoconioses. (1) The dusts themselves cause little damage to the lung parenchyma; it is the inflammatory response to the dusts that causes the loss of functional alveolar-capillary units. (2) A number of defense mechanisms prevent such dusts from reaching the alveoli, and others remove most dusts that might reach the lower respiratory tract. Just because an individual has been exposed to an inorganic dust does not mean that the dust has necessarily caused ILD. (3) Abnormalities on a chest radiograph consistent with exposure to an inorganic dust do not prove that the individual has a functionally significant ILD. (4) These chronic disorders result from the inhalation of high concentrations of inorganic dusts over many years; i.e., history of a brief exposure sometime in the past is not sufficient evidence to implicate a particular dust. (5) No known therapy has proven efficacy for any pneumoconiosis; current "treatment" for all pneumoconiosis is permanent removal from inhalation of the causative agent. (6) Many individuals exposed to inorganic dusts also have a history of chronic cigarette smoking; this must be taken into account when evaluating these patients. (7) Physical evidence of the inorganic dust in the lung is useful but not critical in making the diagnosis of a common pneumoconiosis (silicosis, asbestosis, coal worker's pneumoconiosis) as long as the chronic exposure history is very clear and unambiguous. For the other inorganic dusts, however, biopsy evidence is required to make a definitive diagnosis. (8) While the miners and millers of these inorganic dusts represent the "classic" exposure situations, inorganic dust materials are widely used in manufacturing. A careful occupational history is required or the exposure history may be missed. *Coal worker's pneumoconiosis, silicosis, asbestosis,* and *berylliosis* are described in Ch. 536 on Occupational Lung Disease.

Inhaled Organic Dusts

The repeated inhalation of certain organic dusts (see also Ch. 536) causes a granulomatous ILD called *"hypersensitivity pneumonitis"* or *"extrinsic allergic alveolitis."* The term "hypersensitivity pneumonitis" is reserved for those ILD caused by organic dusts derived from living sources. A large number of organic dusts have been implicated (Table 63–3), but the most common are the thermophilic organisms of the *Micropolyspora* and *Thermoactinomyces* groups and those derived from avian proteins.

The nomenclature relating to hypersensitivity pneumonitis is confusing because the "name" of the disease usually refers to the situation of exposure (e.g., "maple bark stripper's disease," "humidifier lung") even though the organic dusts causing different "diseases" may be identical. For example, *Thermoactinomyces vulgaris* can cause "farmer's lung," "humidifier lung," and "mushroom worker's lung." The most common exposure situations are farmers exposed to moldy hay, individuals exposed to organic antigens growing in humidifiers and air conditioners, and bird breeders, particularly those raising pigeons. The other exposure situations are varied, and the list is ever expanding (Table 63–3).

Classically, four to six hours after inhalation of the antigen, a sensitized individual develops acute symptoms of hypersensitivity pneumonitis, including fever, cough, dyspnea, and malaise. The chest film at this time shows diffuse parenchymal infiltrates, and lung function tests demonstrate decreased lung volumes, decreased diffusing capacity, mild airflow limitation, and hypoxemia. If the individual is removed from the antigen exposure, there is gradual improvement in symptoms, the chest film, and lung function tests over a 24-hour period. If the exposures are few, there are few sequelae other than the acute episodes. However, in some individuals, for unknown

reasons, repetitive exposure leads to a chronic ILD characterized by lymphocyte-macrophage alveolitis occasionally mixed with neutrophils. Initially, the derangements are of the distortion type, with lymphocytes and granulomata in the alveolar walls. Later, however, there are fibrotic changes, including intra-alveolar fibrosis. Rarely, the chronic form develops in an insidious manner without the acute episodes.

The diagnosis of hypersensitivity pneumonitis is made in the context of a history of exposure to a known causative antigen, the presence of ILD, the presence of antigen-specific antibodies in the blood, and an open lung biopsy demonstrating the characteristic morphology. The gallium-67 scan is usually positive, and bronchoalveolar lavage shows a lymphocyte-macrophage alveolitis, mixed with neutrophils when the exposure has been recent. When the history is typical, a biopsy is not necessary to make the diagnosis, but there must be a clear demonstration of the acute symptoms four to six hours after inhalation of the antigen.

The mechanisms by which sensitization to these organic dusts causes either the acute or chronic disease are unknown. T lymphocytes, the majority of which have suppressor/cytotoxic surface markers, are associated with the alveolitis. The T cells in the lung and blood are sensitized to the offending antigen. Besides the circulating antigen-specific immunoglobulins, there are increased levels of IgG and IgM in the lower respiratory tract. However, there is no evidence that the immunoglobulins play a role in the pathogenesis of the disease, and immune complexes have not been convincingly demonstrated in the lower respiratory tract. One of the confusing aspects of this disease is that, although many exposed individuals become sensitized to the organic antigen (as manifest by the presence of antigen-specific antibodies in the blood), only a very small proportion will develop either the acute or chronic symptoms of hypersensitivity pneumonitis.

The prognosis of chronic hypersensitivity pneumonitis is not clear. In those with farmer's lung, there is a 10 per cent mortality over six years, with an additional 30 per cent having significant functional impairment. Management of hypersensitivity pneumonitis is directed toward removing the patient from the source of antigen and suppressing the alveolitis, usually with corticosteroids.

Drug-Induced ILD

Drug-induced ILD are disorders in which the lower respiratory tract is structurally and/or functionally deranged as a result of a pharmacologic agent. The list of drugs reported to cause ILD is large (Table 63–4) and includes acute, subacute, and chronic ILD. Drug-induced ILD can be serious and sometimes fatal, but they are usually effectively treated simply by recognizing the disorder and discontinuing the responsible drug.

It is generally assumed that many of the drug-induced ILD are "hypersensitivity" reactions, but proof of an immune basis for these diseases is circumstantial at best. In many cases, it is thought that the drug injures the lung parenchyma in some fashion to initiate an alveolitis that propagates the injury.

Typically, the acute and subacute forms of drug-induced ILD present with respiratory decompensation following a prodrome of fever and cough. At this time there are usually increased heart and respiratory rates, dry rales, and, occasionally, cyanosis. The chest radiograph shows a patchy or diffuse reticulonodular infiltrate that can be confused with pulmonary edema. Pleural effusions are common. Blood studies often show eosinophilia and arterial hypoxemia and hypocarbia. Lung function tests are typical for ILD, and the gallium-67 scan is often positive. Open lung biopsy demonstrates parenchymal cell injury, edema of the alveolar wall, fibrin in the airspaces, and a patchy lymphocyte-macrophage alveolitis, sometimes mixed with neutrophils and/or eosinophils. In some cases, the course is rapidly downhill, requiring mechanical ventilation and oxygen administration. The disease is usually reversible if the drug is discontinued but can be fatal if this is not done early in the course.

One major area of confusion in conceptualizing and categorizing the drug-induced ILD disorders has resulted from the use of the term "pulmonary infiltration with eosinophilia (PIE) syndrome" to describe patients receiving drugs who develop an acute or subacute disorder characterized by blood eosinophilia and parenchymal infiltrates on the chest film. However, the PIE syndrome is far from diagnostic as a drug-induced ILD. Many nondrug-associated ILD of both known (e.g., acute beryllium-induced disease) and unknown etiology (e.g., IPF, sarcoidosis) can be associated with blood eosinophilia, and tropical pulmonary eosinophilia caused by filarial infestation presents in an identical manner. In addition, there is no evidence that the blood eosinophilia has any relevance to the pathogenesis of the disease in the lung. Thus, most clinicians have abandoned the concept of the "PIE syndrome" and simply think of these disorders as part of the spectrum of ILD in which the presence of blood eosinophilia is a helpful, but not definitive, clue to the diagnosis.

The chronic form of drug-induced ILD is much more insidious and difficult to associate with a drug as the etiologic agent. Fever is less common, and patients usually present with typical ILD. Occasionally there is blood eosinophilia. Because of the insidious nature of the chronic form of drug-induced ILD, many clinicians use lung function tests, particularly measuring the diffusing capacity, to follow patients on drugs commonly associated with the development of ILD. The gallium-67 scan is usually positive. Open lung biopsy usually shows a lymphocyte-macrophage alveolitis with mixed numbers of polymorphonuclear leukocytes. The derangements are fibrosis-type, often with intra-alveolar fibrosis. Unlike the acute and subacute forms of the drug-induced ILD, the chronic form often persists after the drug is discontinued. The reasons why this occurs are not clear, but it is likely that the injury to the parenchyma has been sufficient to establish a chronic alveolitis that propagates the disorder in the absence of the initial stimulus. In such cases, therapeutic strategies are directed toward suppressing the alveolitis, usually with corticosteroids.

ANTINEOPLASTIC AGENTS. *Bleomycin*-induced disease is common; up to 10 per cent of patients receiving bleomycin develop some ILD and 1 per cent die from the ILD. Toxicity from this agent occurs in both acute and chronic forms and is potentiated by concomitant therapy with oxygen or irradiation. *Busulfan* lung disease occurs in 2 to 3 per cent of those receiving the drug. The disease is chronic, usually takes at least one year of therapy before it appears, and usually does not respond to withdrawal of the drug or to corticosteroids. *Methotrexate*-induced ILD can appear in acute or chronic form. Leucovorin or corticosteroids are not protective, but recovery is common once the drug is stopped. There are increasing numbers of reports of ILD induced by the *nitrosoureas*. The incidence of toxicity is about 1 per cent and occurs two months to three years after initiation of therapy. *Procarbazine* causes an acute ILD with pleural effusions, peripheral eosinophilia, and an eosinophilic alveolitis. Although *cyclophosphamide* is used to treat many ILD of unknown etiology, it can rarely cause acute or chronic ILD. Several other antineoplastic agents are reported to cause ILD but very rarely.

ANTIBIOTICS. ILD induced by *nitrofurantoin* is a common adverse drug reaction, occurring in both acute and chronic forms. The acute form, five to ten times more frequent than the chronic form, occurs in sensitized individuals within one month of reinstituting treatment. The disease almost always clears when the drug is discontinued. The chronic disease occurs following 6 to 12 months of therapy. Approximately 60 per cent have positive antinuclear antibodies. The prognosis is good once the drug is stopped, but permanent loss of lung function is common, and approximately 10 per cent die from the disease. The ILD caused by other antibiotics are also mostly acute disorders and are very rare.

CARDIOVASCULAR DRUGS. *Hydralazine* and *procainamide* induce an acute ILD similar to that associated with systemic lupus erythematosus (SLE). In contrast to spontaneously occurring SLE, which is common in blacks and females, the ILD produced by both of these drugs occurs more commonly in whites and affects a significant number of males. Most affected individuals have serum antinuclear antibodies. The disease usually disappears when the drug is stopped. Other drugs that can cause a similar syndrome include isoniazid, phenytoin, and allopurinol. Increasingly, ILD has been observed in association with amiodarone, a useful antiarrhythmic agent. The ILD is usually dose dependent and self limiting but can be chronic even after the drug has been discontinued. The beta blockers can cause chronic ILD, but rarely. The disease is insidious and IPF-like but often associated with fibrosis elsewhere in the body.

OTHER DRUGS. *Gold salts* can induce ILD after one to six months of therapy and can be difficult to distinguish from the ILD associated with rheumatoid arthritis. The disease is thought to represent a hypersensitivity reaction. *Mineral oil*-induced ILD, sometimes called "lipoid pneumonia," results from the aspiration of mineral oil used as nose drops or ingested as a laxative. The open lung biopsy demonstrates a typical picture of lymphoid cells, lipid-laden macrophages, and fibrosis. With an appropriate history, however, the diagnosis can be made by recovering lipid-laden macrophages by bronchoalveolar lavage. The intravenous use of drugs meant for oral use can cause ILD by virtue of the presence of particulate material in the drugs, including talc, starch, maltose, or quinine. The disease is usually chronic and characterized by foreign-body granulomatous reactions affecting pulmonary capillaries.

Many other drugs are known to cause acute and/or chronic ILD, and the list is ever expanding. Because these disorders are all potentially curable if the drug is stopped, it is critical to have a high index of suspicion of drug-induced disease whenever confronted by a patient with ILD.

Other Agents Known to Cause ILD

Beyond inorganic dusts, organic dusts, and drugs, the most important known causes of ILD are paraquat, radiation, the sequelae of prior infectious processes, hyperoxia, and chronic aspiration pneumonia. The others are very rare and mostly represent anecdotal case reports (see Table 63–5).

PARAQUAT. Poisoning with the herbicide paraquat can occur with oral, parenteral, aerosol, or dermal exposure. Paraquat is available in granules, aerosols, and liquid concentrates; ingestion of the liquid either by accident or by suicidal intent is the most common means of paraquat poisoning. Paraquat is an extremely potent cause of parenchymal derangement and fibrosis and consequent respiratory insufficiency. As little as one teaspoon of the concentrate can be fatal. The disease is usually acute, but chronic cases have been described. In the acute cases, dyspnea, fever, fatigue, and gastrointestinal complaints follow one to five days after poisoning. Mouth, pharyngeal, and esophageal ulcerations are common following oral ingestion. Diffuse radiographic changes of ILD are quickly followed by rapidly progressive respiratory failure, usually requiring ventilatory support. Open lung biopsy reveals a neutrophil-macrophage alveolitis and alveolar wall derangements typical of ILD, but very severe. In addition to interstitial fibrosis, intra-alveolar fibrosis is common. In these acute cases, there is a rough correlation between plasma levels of paraquat and survival. If the plasma paraquat concentration eight hours after ingestion is greater than 1200 μg per liter, death is inevitable. In addition to these acute cases, intermittent low-dose skin exposure may be hazardous and lead to a chronic ILD.

Paraquat causes ILD by virtue of its propensity to be taken up by parenchymal cells of the lower respiratory tract, where it generates toxic oxygen radicals sufficient to damage the normal parenchymal components severely. There is a secondary alveolitis that further injures the parenchyma and mediates the development of fibrosis-type derangements. Treatment of paraquat poisoning is mostly supportive. Attempts should be made to remove the paraquat (gastric lavage with bentonite, Fuller's earth, or charcoal, followed by charcoal hemoperfusion). Since hyperoxia accelerates paraquat-induced injury, oxygen concentrations should be kept as low as possible. Antioxidant therapy (e.g., vitamin E) has been suggested, but its efficacy is unknown. In chronic cases, corticosteroids are usually used to suppress the alveolitis.

RADIATION. ILD resulting from thoracic irradiation is a common sequela of radiotherapy of breast, lung, or esophageal carcinoma and lymphoma and is potentiated by the concomitant use of antineoplastic drugs known to cause ILD. Radiation-induced lung disease is described in Ch. 539.

SEQUELA OF KNOWN INFECTIOUS AGENTS. All types of infections of the lower respiratory tract may occasionally result in significant injury and fibrosis. Usually, the ILD remains localized to the site of infection and does not progress after eradication of the infectious agent. A typical example is the localized upper lobe scars left by mycobacterial infection. ILD has been described following *Mycoplasma* infection as well as *Legionella* pneumonia, and there are scattered reports of viral infections causing a progressive ILD. Tropical pulmonary eosinophilia due to chronic microfilarial infestation is a subacute ILD (see Ch. 413.3) and can evolve into a chronic ILD.

INHALED AGENTS OTHER THAN INORGANIC OR ORGANIC DUSTS. These agents include gases, aerosols, chemical dusts, fumes, and vapors. Most are rare causes of ILD, and there is little information available concerning pathogenesis, clinical course, staging, or therapy. Most are acute disorders that reverse when the agent is removed unless significant injury to the parenchyma has occurred.

The most common gas causing ILD is *oxygen.* The inhalation of high concentrations of oxygen over several days often causes parenchymal lung damage, particularly in the setting of acute respiratory failure in the intensive care situation (see Ch. 72). Oxygen toxicity can also be chronic. In contrast, the inhalation of gases such as the oxides of nitrogen, chlorine gas, and sulfur dioxide almost always cause only acute injury; if the patient survives the initial insult and respiratory failure, there are rarely any sequelae. In contrast, many of the survivors of methyl isocyanate exposure develop chronic fibrosis-type ILD.

Aerosols are particles of liquid suspended in a gas. The most common examples of ILD due to aerosol inhalation are the acute and chronic ILD resulting from aspiration of gastric contents (see Ch. 537) and the aspiration of mineral oil. Exposure to aerosols of cooking oils, pyrethrum (a neutral insecticide used in commercial and household products), and toluene diisocyanate has also been implicated as a cause of ILD.

ILD due to the inhalation of chemical dusts such as synthetic fibers, bakelite, and vinyl chloride and polyvinyl chloride powder are probably hypersensitivity-type disorders similar to those associated with the repeated inhalation of organic dusts from living sources. Little is known about the clinical course of these disorders. ILD have also followed the inhalation of various fumes and vapors (Table 63–5).

Basset F, Ferrans VJ, Soler P, et al.: Intraluminal fibrosis in interstitial lung disorders. Am J Pathol 122:443, 1986. *Overview of the patterns of fibrosis in the interstitial lung disorders.*

Crystal RG, Bitterman PB, Rennard SI, et al.: Interstitial lung diseases of unknown cause: Disorders characterized by chronic inflammation of the lower respiratory tract. N Engl J Med 310:154, 235, 1984. *A useful review of the interstitial lung disorders of unknown etiology.*

Crystal RG, Ferrans VJ: Reactions of the interstitial space to injury. In Fishman AP: Pulmonary Diseases and Disorders. New York, McGraw-Hill (in press). *General concepts of the processes that derange the alveolar walls.*

Crystal RG, Gadek JE, Ferrans VJ, et al.: Interstitial lung disease: Current concepts of pathogenesis, staging, and therapy. Am J Med 70:542, 1981. *Overviews the current concepts of the pathogenesis of the interstitial lung disorders and emphasizes the current approaches to staging and therapy.*

Davis WB, Crystal RG: Chronic interstitial lung disease. In Simmons DH (ed.): Current Pulmonology, Vol V. New York, John Wiley and Sons, 1984, pp 347–473. *Reviews the recent observations in each of the interstitial lung disorders.*

Fanburg BL (ed.): Sarcoidosis and Other Granulomatous Diseases of the Lung. New York, Marcel Dekker, 1983. *A good general review of sarcoidosis.*

Keogh BA, Crystal RG: Alveolitis: The key to the interstitial lung disorders. Thorax 37:1, 1982. *Summarizes the importance of alveolitis in the interstitial disorders.*

Morgan WKC, Seaton A: Occupational Lung Diseases. 2nd ed. Philadelphia, W. B. Saunders Company, 1984. *Overall summary of the interstitial lung disorders resulting from the inhalation of inorganic dusts.*

Rom WN (ed.): Environmental and Occupational Medicine. Boston, Little, Brown and Company, 1983. *Well-referenced text detailing known environmental causes of interstitial lung disease.*

Schoenberger CI, Crystal RG: Drug induced lung disease. In Isselbacher KJ, Adams RD, Braunwald E, et al. (eds.): Harrison's Principles of Internal Medicine. Update IV, New York, McGraw-Hill Book Company, 1983, pp 49–74. *Details the pathogenesis and clinical findings in all of the drug-induced interstitial lung disorders.*

64 LUNG ABSCESS
John G. Bartlett

DEFINITION. Lung abscess literally means a collection of pus within a destroyed portion of the lung; thus there are numerous possible causes of such a lesion (Table 64–1). As used clinically, however, the term lung abscess refers to a pulmonary infection with parenchymal necrosis, generally caused by bacteria other than mycobacteria. Lung abscesses are usually solitary, but occasionally multiple discrete lesions are observed. Numerous small abscesses confined to a given region of the lung are sometimes referred to as "necrotizing pneumonia." Because they share a common pathogenesis, there is considerable overlap among aspiration pneumonia, lung abscess, and necrotizing pneumonia, and each of these may lead to and coexist with an empyema (a collection of pus within the pleural space).

ETIOLOGY. As indicated in Table 64–1, many different underlying processes can lead to the formation of a lung abscess. By far the most important are necrotizing pulmonary infections and, of these, anaerobic bacteria are responsible for

TABLE 64–1. CLASSIFICATION OF LUNG ABSCESS

I. Necrotizing infections
   A. Pyogenic bacteria (*Staphylococcus aureus, Klebsiella,* mixed anaerobes, *Nocardia asteroides*)
   B. Mycobacteria (*Mycobacterium tuberculosis, M. kansasii,* and *M. avium-intracellulare*)
   C. Fungi (*Coccidioides immitis, Histoplasma capsulatum*)
   D. Parasites (*Entamoeba histolytica, Paragonimus westermani*)

II. Cavitary infarction
   A. Bland embolism
   B. Septic embolism (*Staphylococcus aureus, Candida*)
   C. Vasculitis (Wegener's granulomatosis, periarteritis)

III. Cavitary malignancy
   A. Bronchogenic carcinoma
   B. Lymphoma
   C. Metastatic malignancies

IV. Other
   A. Infected cysts, bullae, or sequestration
   B. Necrotic conglomerate lesions (silicosis, coal miner's pneumoconiosis)

Adapted from Hirschmann JV, Murray JF: Pulmonary and lung abscess. In Petersdorf RG, et al. (eds.): Harrison's Principles of Internal Medicine. 10th ed. New York, McGraw-Hill Book Company, p 1532.

the majority. These organisms account for essentially all "putrid" lung abscesses and nearly all that have been classified as "nonspecific" or "primary." Most of these infections involve multiple bacterial species, which may include aerobic organisms. The dominant bacteria are *Fusobacterium nucleatum*, *Bacteroides melaninogenicus*, *B. intermedius*, peptostreptococcus, aerobic streptococci, and microaerophilic streptococci.

Pneumonia, particularly cases caused by *Staphylococcus aureus* and *Klebsiella pneumoniae*, may also be complicated by abscess formation. Less frequent but well-documented agents of lung abscess include *Streptococcus pyogenes* (group A beta-hemolytic streptococci), *S. pneumoniae* (especially type 3), *Streptococcus milleri*, *Hemophilus influenzae* (type B), *Pseudomonas aeruginosa*, *Pseudomonas pseudomallei* (melioidosis), *Actinomyces* (actinomycosis), *Legionella*, *Nocardia*, *Paragonimus westermani* (lung fluke), and *Entamoeba histolytica* (amebiasis). Enteric gram-negative bacilli other than *K. pneumoniae* may cause lung abscess, but this occurs almost exclusively in debilitated patients with severe associated medical-surgical conditions. Necrotizing alveolitis is a separate entity diagnosed by microscopic examination and usually caused by *Pseudomonas aeruginosa*; sometimes these microabscesses coalesce to form radiographically detectable cavities.

INCIDENCE AND PREVALENCE. The incidence of primary lung abscess has decreased substantially since the pre-chemotherapeutic era. Nevertheless, most large academic centers encounter 10 to 30 cases annually.

EPIDEMIOLOGY. Most lung abscesses, and nearly all involving anaerobic bacteria, involve the normal flora of the oropharynx. Abscesses involving *S. aureus* or gram-negative bacilli are more likely to be nosocomial in origin. Amebic lung abscess results from the direct extension of an hepatic abscess through the diaphragm into the lung. *Nocardia* causes lung abscess almost exclusively in immunocompromised hosts, especially in recipients of corticosteroids. Septic pulmonary emboli commonly lead to multiple solitary abscesses in noncontiguous sites and are usually caused by *S. aureus*, anaerobic bacteria, or *P. aeruginosa*; hematogenous abscesses are most often found in intravenous drug abusers with tricuspid valve endocarditis, patients with infected indwelling cannulas. Lung abscesses due to *Paragonimus westermani* and melioidosis are usually acquired in the Far East or Indonesia.

PATHOGENESIS. The formation of an anaerobic lung abscess nearly always involves two coexisting abnormalities: (1) periodontal sepsis such as gingivitis or pyorrhea, which provides the inoculum, and (2) aspiration, which provides access to the lung parenchyma. The usual causes for aspiration are those that compromise consciousness and the gag reflex, such as alcoholism, drug addiction, general anesthesia, seizure disorder, sedative use, or neurologic disorders. Other factors predisposing to aspiration include dysphagia resulting from esophageal disorders or neurologic deficits; disruption of the usual mechanical barriers as with nasogastric intubation, tracheostomy, or nasogastric feeding tubes; or pharyngeal anesthesia as seen with dental procedures or surgery involving the upper airway. Most healthy persons periodically aspirate small inocula from the upper airways, but these are readily cleared by the normal cough reflex and other pulmonary defense mechanisms without deleterious consequences. Patients who develop aspiration pneumonia and lung abscesses presumably do so because of the relatively large inocula of bacteria and failure of the usual protective mechanisms.

The initial lesion is pneumonitis, or "aspiration pneumonia," that typically involves dependent pulmonary segments, e.g., those favored by gravitational flow. The dependent pulmonary segments in patients who aspirate in the recumbent position are the superior segments of the lower lobes or posterior segments of the upper lobes. Aspiration in the upright or semi-upright position favors involvement of the basilar segments of the lower lobes. Patients who have a

defined period of known or probable aspiration demonstrate with sequential radiographs that 7 to 14 days are usually required for the appearance of a typical air-fluid level on chest radiograph.

CLINICAL MANIFESTATIONS. Patients with anaerobic abscesses tend to have indolent symptomatology with medical complaints dating for two or more weeks before presentation. The usual symptoms are fever, malaise, cough, sputum production, and pleuritic pain. The frequent observation of weight loss and anemia provides testimony to the chronicity of the infection. There may be "chilliness," but frank rigors are rare and their presence suggests organisms other than anaerobes. The cough often becomes more productive at the time of cavitation, and it is at this time that the patient is most likely to note the onset of putrid sputum, which is considered diagnostic of anaerobic infection. Putrid sputum is found in 60 per cent of patients with a confirmed anaerobic etiology. Many patients will also note an unusually noxious taste to sputum. Most patients have a history of compromised consciousness or other risk factors for aspiration, and many have gingival crevice disease. Nevertheless, about 10 per cent of patients with anaerobic lung abscesses have no identifiable predisposing condition. Occasional patients with anaerobic lung abscesses are edentulous; the incidence of underlying bronchogenic neoplasms seems particularly high in this group. Patients with lung abscesses due to *S. aureus*, gram-negative bacilli, and amebae usually have a more fulminant course, with the precipitous onset of symptoms. Other features that may be noted in this group include chills, the lack of putrid discharge, and the absence of the usual associated findings. The physical findings in the early phases of disease are those of pneumonia, with or without a pleural effusion. At a later stage there may be amphoric or cavernous breath sounds, pleural effusions are common, and approximately 25 per cent of patients have an associated empyema.

DIAGNOSIS. The diagnosis of lung abscess is usually established with a chest radiograph showing a parenchymal infiltrate with a cavity containing an air-fluid level (Fig. 64–1). The differential diagnosis of this roentgenographic finding is included in Table 64–1. Certain roentgenographic features may provide clues to the presence of an infected cyst, bulla, or sequestration. Massive pulmonary fibrosis with necrosis from occupational exposure is usually distinctive. A loculated empyema with an air-fluid level may be differentiated from lung abscess with computerized tomography.

Studies for an etiologic agent are often hampered by the limitations of bacteriologic analysis of expectorated sputum. These specimens are useful in detecting mycobacteria, pathogenic fungi, and parasites, and they may be used for cytologic studies. However, routine aerobic cultures often give erroneous results, and they are not valid for meaningful anaerobic culture owing to the universal presence in oral secretions of anaerobes that contaminate the specimen during passage through the upper airways. Blood cultures are useful, primarily for patients with infections involving *S. aureus* or gram-negative bacilli, but most patients with anaerobic abscesses do not have bacteremia. Pleural fluid is a valuable culture source for both aerobic and anaerobic bacteria in any patient with an empyema, so that thoracentesis should be performed before treatment is begun. For most patients with anaerobic pulmonary infections restricted to the pulmonary parenchyma, the preferred specimen source is from a transtracheal aspiration or from a fiberoptic bronchoscopy utilizing a double-lumen catheter with a distal occluding plug combined with quantitative cultures. Each requires specimen collection prior to institution of antibiotic therapy. In most cases of anaerobic abscesses, the etiologic agents will not be defined and the therapeutic regimen will be selected empirically. Bronchoscopy, which used to be performed routinely in patients with lung abscesses, is now usually restricted to patients who fail to respond to antibiotic treatment or who

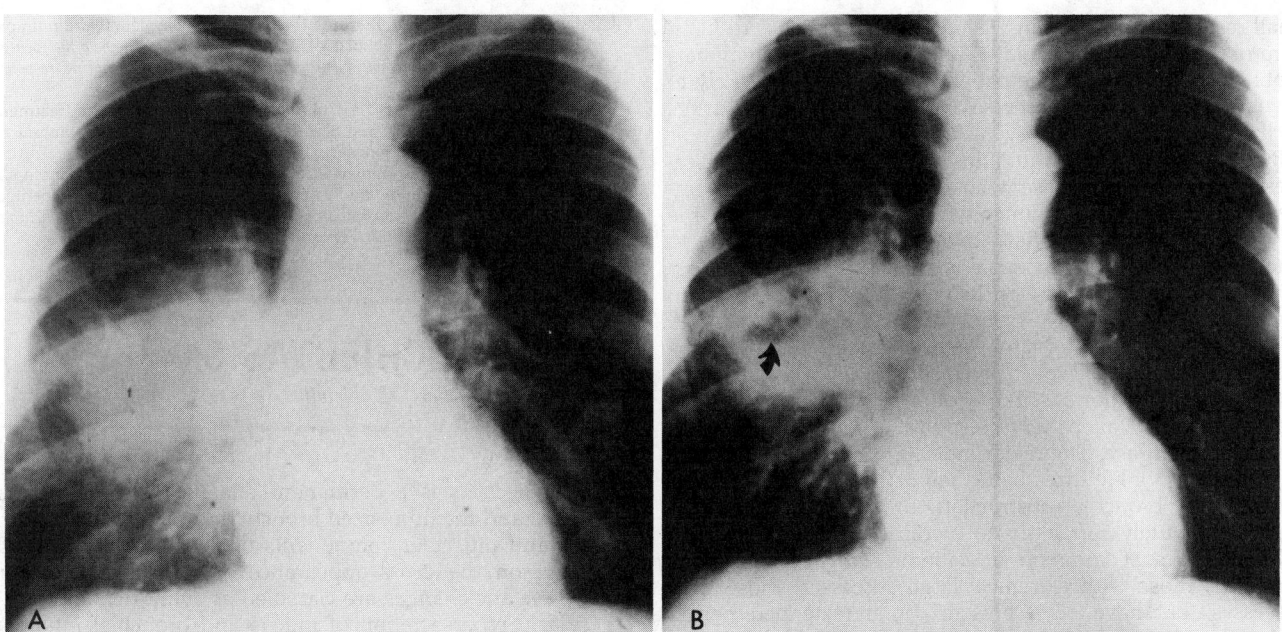

FIGURE 64–1. Chest radiographs of a 55-year-old alcoholic man. The first film (*A*) shows pneumonitis involving the superior segment of the right lower lobe, a common segment for aspiration pneumonia. The second radiograph (*B*), taken one week later, shows cavitation with an air-fluid level as indicated by the arrow. A transtracheal aspirate yielded *F. nucleatum, B. melaninogenicus,* and anaerobic streptococci. The final diagnosis was aspiration pneumonia with progression to lung abscess due to anaerobic bacteria.

have an atypical clinical presentation. Major concerns are a cavitating neoplasm, an obstructing tumor, or a foreign body.

TREATMENT. Obviously, treatment of lung abscess will depend on the underlying cause. For those due to infection, the most important facets of the treatment program are the administration of appropriate antibiotics and adequate drainage of any associated empyema. Physiotherapy with postural drainage should be utilized when possible; however, this must be done with considerable caution in patients with large lung abscesses because of the possibility of spillage of purulent contents with extensive involvement of other lobes.

The drugs of choice for the treatment of abscesses caused by aerobic pyogenic microorganisms, *M. tuberculosis,* fungi, and *Entamoeba histolytica* are reviewed in detail elsewhere in this volume. For aspiration-related lung abscess involving anaerobic bacteria, the three antimicrobial regimens recommended are penicillin, clindamycin, or penicillin plus metronidazole. Penicillin has traditionally been regarded as the favored drug on the basis of its long, well-established track record. There is considerable variation in the dosage recommendations, but most authorities recommend doses of 10 to 20 million units per day. This is continued until the patient is afebrile and clinically improved, at which time treatment is changed to intramuscular or oral penicillin using penicillin G, penicillin V, ampicillin, or amoxicillin in doses of 500 to 750 mg four times daily. Some authorities suggest an arbitrarily selected total duration of treatment of three to six weeks, whereas others continue treatment until the chest radiograph changes have cleared or there is only a small stable residual lesion. The latter criterion commonly requires two to four months or longer but may be necessary to prevent relapses.

Clindamycin is active against most penicillin-resistant anaerobes that are found in 20 to 25 per cent of cases, including many or most strains of *B. melaninogenicus, B. fragilis, B. ruminicola,* and *B. ureolyticum.* Some regard clindamycin as the preferred agent for all lung ascesses due to anaerobic bacteria; others advocate it only for patients who fail to respond to penicillin, have a contraindication to penicillin, or have a serious infection with a fulminant course. The usual regimen is 600 mg given intravenously every six to eight hours until the patient is afebrile and clinically improved,

followed by 300 mg orally four times daily. An alternative regimen is penicillin G (above doses) combined with metronidazole (2 gm orally per day in two to four divided doses). Metronidazole is active against nearly all clinically important anaerobes, but penicillin must be added owing to the probable importance of aerobic and microaerophilic streptococci. The necessity to treat the aerobic components of mixed aerobic-anaerobic infections is controversial, but this is generally advocated for patients who are seriously ill or fail to respond to clindamycin. In selecting regimens for these mixed infections, it is important to note that most penicillins are equally effective against oral anaerobes. These include penicillin G, penicillin V, ampicillin, amoxicillin, carbenicillin, and piperacillin. However, antistaphylococcal penicillins, such as nafcillin or oxacillin, are considered inferior and unacceptable. Cephalosporins are considered nearly equivalent to penicillins in terms of in vitro activity, although the clinical experience is much more limited than it is with penicillin or clindamycin.

Patients with lung abscesses involving *S. aureus* should be treated with a penicillinase-resistant penicillin or a first-generation cephalosporin. Vancomycin is the preferred agent for methicillin-resistant strains of *S. aureus.* This agent or clindamycin may be used for patients with a contraindication to beta-lactam antibiotics. Penicillin G is the preferred agent for infections involving group A beta-hemolytic streptococcal infection. Antibiotic selection for infections involving gram-negative bacilli requires in vitro sensitivity data. This usually consists of an aminoglycoside combined with an expanded spectrum penicillin such as ticarcillin for *P. aeruginosa* or an aminoglycoside combined with a cephalosporin for *Enterobacteriaceae.* Sulfonamides are preferred agents for *Nocardia* infections.

The expected response to antimicrobial agents is subjective improvement with decreased fever within 3 to 7 days and elimination of fever within 7 to 14 days. The putrid odor of the sputum, when initially present, usually resolves in three to ten days. Radiographic response is delayed; in fact, there is often extension of the infiltrate and increased cavity size or new cavity formation during the first week. Chest radiographs should be followed at two- to three-week intervals with the expectation that infiltrates will clear and that there will be a small residual scar or a thin-walled cyst. Compliance to long-term oral regimens of antibiotics among outpatients may be a problem, particularly in the patient population most likely to develop primary lung abscesses and with expensive drugs such as clindamycin.

Bronchoscopy is indicated in patients with an atypical presentation and in those who fail to respond to recommended antimicrobial regimens. The major purpose of the procedure is to differentiate cavitating neoplasms and to detect underlying lesions, such as bronchogenic neoplasms, bronchostenosis, or a foreign body. It may also be used to facilitate drainage. Other considerations in patients who fail to respond include alternative infectious and noninfectious causes of roentgenographic changes, the use of alternative antibiotics, and the possibility of an empyema requiring drainage. Nearly all patients respond to antibiotics and do not require surgery. The major indications for surgery are an uncontrollable or life-threatening hemorrhage, a bronchogenic neoplasm, a bronchial obstruction, or a lung abscess that proves absolutely refractory to medical treatment. Medical failures are most common in patients with an obstructed bronchus, those with extremely large abscesses, those with abscesses that have been present for an extended period before the institution of treatment, and those with infections involving certain bacteria such as gram-negative bacilli. The usual surgical procedure is lobectomy. Patients with prohibitive operative risks may benefit from percutaneous drainage, but care must be taken to avoid contamination of the pleural space.

PROGNOSIS. The natural course of lung abscesses was best studied in the prechemotherapeutic era. Treatment at that time was nearly equally divided between conservative management using postural drainage and supportive care, and surgery. The mortality rate was about 33 per cent in both groups. An additional third of patients developed a chronic debilitating disease or suffered recurrent symptoms. The technique of resectional surgery was developed at about the time penicillin became available, and the relative merits of these two approaches as the primary therapeutic modality were widely debated. During the past two decades, however, the majority of patients have been treated with antibiotics alone, including those with "delayed closure" (i.e., the persistence of a cavity demonstrated by a chest radiograph at four to six weeks after the initiation of antibiotic therapy), because most of these cavities eventually resolve if the antibiotics are continued long enough. The mortality rate for aspiration-related lung abscess is currently reported at 5 to 6 per cent. Findings that herald a relatively poor prognosis include (1) large cavity size, particularly cavities greater than 6 cm in diameter, (2) prolonged symptoms prior to presentation, especially symptoms for over six weeks, (3) necrotizing pneumonia characterized by multiple small abscesses in contiguous segments, (4) patients who are elderly, debilitated, or immunologically compromised, (5) abscesses associated with bronchial obstruction, and (6) abscess due to aerobic bacteria, including *S. aureus* and gram-negative bacilli.

PREVENTION. The major preventive measures are factors used to reduce the incidence or magnitude of aspiration, appropriate care of periodontal disease, early treatment of pneumonia, and adequate courses of antimicrobials to prevent relapses.

Bartlett JG: Lung abscess. Johns Hopkins Med J 150:141, 1982. *The literature is reviewed, including a summary of bacteriologic studies, treatment guidelines, and prognosis.*

Bartlett JG, Gorbach SL, Tally FP, et al.: Bacteriology and treatment of primary lung abscess. Rev Respir Dis 109:510, 1974. *The authors report their experience with lung abscesses using transtracheal aspiration to define the infecting flora.*

Hagan JL, Hardy LD: Lung abscess revisited. A survey of 184 cases. Ann Surg 197:755, 1983. *Update on the surgical point of view concerning lung abscess; 11 per cent were operated on.*

Landay MJ, Christensen EE, Bynum LJ, et al.: Anaerobic pleural and pulmonary infections. Am J Roentgenol 134:233, 1980. *The authors review the roentgenographic features of anaerobic pleuropulmonary infections, including response to antibiotic treatment.*

Snow N, Lucas A, Horrigan TP: Utility of pneumonotomy in the treatment of cavitary lung disease. Chest 87:731, 1985. *A description of the procedure and results with percutaneous drainage.*

Stark DD, Federle MP, Goodman PC, et al.: Differentiating lung abscess and empyema: Radiography and computed tomography. Am J Roentgenol 141:163, 1983. *Nice demonstration that computed tomography is extremely useful in this important differential diagnosis.*

65 BRONCHIECTASIS

Christopher J. L. Newth

Bronchiectasis is a permanent dilatation of one or more proximal and medium-sized bronchi due to destruction of the elastic and muscular components of the bronchial wall. Depending on the gross appearance of the dilated segment, bronchiectatic changes are classified as cylindric, varicose, or saccular. Hypersecretion of mucus and bronchial inflammation secondary to recurrent infections cause the clinical expression of the disease.

PREVALENCE

Bronchiectasis was once a common disease, but effective vaccines for pertussis and measles and better antibiotics for tuberculosis and bacterial pneumonia have all but removed these conditions as precursors. Most new cases of this now rare disease have some predisposing genetic cause, with cystic fibrosis (Ch. 66) responsible for about half the cases. Sporadic events such as adenovirus infections still account for some bronchiectasis, as may congenital lesions (e.g., bronchomalacia), aspiration of gastric contents and foreign bodies, tumors, and external compression (by impairing mucociliary clearance and enhancing the chance of necrotizing infection of the bronchial wall).

PATHOLOGY

Bronchiectatic segments show dilated lumina filled with suppurative material and inflamed, often necrotic, mucosal surfaces. The infection extends into the bronchial wall, disrupting smooth muscle and elastic tissue. The ciliated columnar epithelium is replaced by nonciliated cuboidal cells or fibrous tissue, resulting in localized dilatation and eventually traction as a result of peribronchial scarring. *Cylindrical* (fusiform) bronchiectasis is mild bronchial dilatation with mucous plugging that is usually managed conservatively. *Varicose* bronchiectasis is a more advanced stage characterized by moderate dilatation and distortion of bronchi that resemble varicose veins. *Saccular* (cystic) bronchiectasis, which usually involves proximal (central) bronchi, is the most advanced form. The most common sites of involvement are the posterior basilar segments of the lower lobes, presumably because of the lack of gravitational drainage. The middle lobe of the right lung is also predisposed owing to angulation of the lobar bronchus at its takeoff; the presence of peribronchial lymph nodes at its origin, which may be involved in a number of pathologic processes; and the relative lack of collateral ventilation. Upper lobe bronchiectasis is most commonly secondary to tuberculosis or lung abscess.

CLINICAL MANIFESTATIONS

Bronchiectasis usually begins in childhood. In most cases, symptoms occur before the age of four years, and the majority are diagnosed within the first two decades of life.

The classic form of bronchiectasis is characterized by chronic cough with production of copious amounts of putrid sputum, fetid breath, emaciation, severe secondary bacterial pneumonias, repeated episodes of hemoptysis, cyanosis, digital clubbing, and reduced life expectancy. This presentation is now seldom seen, and bronchiectasis is more likely to be a manifestation of a systemic disorder than of a local pulmonary process. The most usual symptom now is a chronic productive cough that may be more distressful when the patient is recumbent owing to pooling of secretions. The amount and type of sputum produced vary markedly, but it is generally more voluminous and purulent during intercurrent infections. Frank hemoptysis is now uncommon, but blood-streaked sputum is present frequently. There are recurrent bouts of pneumonia, which usually involve the same pulmonary segment or lobe when the bronchiectasis is localized. Exertional dyspnea, clubbing, fatigue, and malaise may be noted in patients with extensive disease. The most characteristic finding on physical examination is persistent, moist, coarse rales over the area involved. If the disease is widespread, there may be generalized wheezing, evidence of air trapping, and progression to cor pulmonale, as in other forms of chronic obstructive pulmonary disease. *Sinusitis* is a frequent companion to diffuse bronchiectasis, but *secondary amyloidosis* and *metastatic abscesses* are now rare complications.

DIAGNOSIS

Bronchiectasis should be suspected in any patient with a chronic productive cough, particularly if there is intermittent blood streaking or increased purulence of the sputum. Knowledge of a precursor event or a genetic error that predisposes to bronchiectasis, or documentation of recurrent pneumonias (particularly those involving the same lobe or segment), should arouse suspicion further. The differential diagnosis for patients with chronic cough and sputum production includes foreign body aspiration, chronic bronchitis, tuberculosis, and chronic lung abscess.

The diagnosis of bronchiectasis depends on demonstrating the abnormal anatomy of the bronchial tree. This is usually accomplished radiologically. *Plain chest films* may be normal or may show only patchy infiltrates, bronchial crowding, or evidence of bronchial thickening, such as "tram tracks" and ring shadows. In advanced cases of saccular bronchiectasis, the diagnosis may be apparent from the presence of multiple cystic lesions with or without fluid levels. *Computed tomography* (CT) is an accurate screening device for bronchiectasis and is all that is required to confirm the diagnosis in most cases.

Bronchography is the definitive procedure with which to establish the diagnosis, determine the extent of involvement, and describe the distribution of lesions. However, because of its potential complications, it is indicated only in patients who are likely candidates for surgery. Bronchography should not be performed until exacerbations of cough, sputum production, and pulmonary infection have been thoroughly treated, since reversible changes that are similar to those of bronchiectasis may occur in the bronchi during this period.

Magnetic resonance imaging is sensitive for mucus impaction and peribronchial edema, but there is little experience with this technique in bronchiectasis.

Bronchoscopy does not establish the diagnosis of bronchiectasis but is useful for detecting conditions that cause obstruction and determining the source of bleeding and secretions.

Pulmonary function studies show a range of abnormalities depending on the extent and severity of disease. There is a correlation between the number of involved segments and the overall impairment of lung function. Regional ventilation-perfusion mismatch can be documented early by hypoxemia and radionuclide scan. In the later stages of diffuse bronchiectasis, the vital capacity is reduced, with marked airflow obstruction and airtrapping.

TABLE 65–1. DIAGNOSTIC FEATURES OF FAMILIAL BRONCHIECTASIS

Disorder	Clinical Findings	Laboratory Tests
Cystic fibrosis (Ch. 66)	Pancreatic insufficiency Mucoid *Pseudomonas* strain Obstructive azospermia Infertility	Sweat chloride
Immotile cilia syndrome	Infertility, sinusitis, otitis media +/− dextrocardia in Kartagener's syndrome	Electron microscopy of cilia Absent mucociliary clearance Immotility in living cells (nasal, sperm)
Alpha$_1$-antitrypsin deficiency	Emphysema, cirrhosis	Serum alpha$_1$-antitrypsin, Pi typing
IgG deficiency (Ch. 419)	Recurrent infections	Quantitative Ig IgG subclass
IgA deficiency (Ch. 419)	Autoimmune phenomena Atopy	Quantitative Ig
Williams-Campbell syndrome	Disease restricted to chest	Bronchographic expiratory collapse of proximal bronchi
Neutrophil deficiencies (Ch. 149)	Recurrent infections +/− thrombocytopenia +/− pancreatic disease	Blood smear Differential leukocyte count, NBT test*
Complement deficiencies (Ch. 418)	Recurrent infections	C3 levels, CH50 determination

*NBT = nitroblue tetrazolium dye.

Sputum culture often grows normal flora and, less commonly, *Streptococcus pneumoniae, Haemophilus influenzae,* and anaerobes. Patients with mucoid strains of *Pseudomonas aeruginosa* should be tested for cystic fibrosis. *Aspergillus* may grow in asthmatic patients with bronchiectasis secondary to bronchopulmonary aspergillosis.

Unless there has been an obvious predisposing event, all patients should be investigated for one of the familial causes of bronchiectasis (Table 65–1).

TREATMENT

The underlying anatomic defects are irreversible, so medical therapy is aggressively directed toward controlling symptoms and limiting or preventing progression of disease. Basic supportive measures include postural drainage to mobilize secretions, hydration, bronchodilators for patients with bronchospasm (and as an aid to ciliary clearance of mucus), discontinuation of smoking, and treatment of associated sinusitis. Expectorants are of questionable value. Antimicrobials are indicated for infectious exacerbations manifested by increased cough, blood streaking, and purulent sputum production. Progressive dyspnea, malaise, and weight loss may also indicate an infectious exacerbation. The choice of antibiotic should be guided by the results of sputum culture. However, these cultures often grow "normal flora," and in this circumstance ampicillin is appropriate for empiric use. Trimethoprim-sulfamethoxazole or tetracycline is usually adequate for those patients who have a contraindication to penicillins. A course of antibiotics may require from one to three weeks to achieve the desired therapeutic effect. Long-term courses and inhaled delivery of antibiotics have not been proved effective in the management of bronchiectasis with the sole exception of that occurring in cystic fibrosis. Oxygen should be used for hypoxia during an acute exacerbation and on a domiciliary basis for those with chronic respiratory insufficiency. Influenza vaccines should be administered annually.

Resectional surgery, once a mainstay of treatment, is now seldom indicated because (1) patients with mild symptoms usually respond well to medical therapy, (2) those with severe symptoms usually have extensive disease with many segments involved and limited pulmonary reserve, and (3) many patients with bronchiectasis frequently have a systemic disorder, and although their bronchiectasis may appear well localized initially, new sites of involvement develop later. The major indication for resectional surgery is localized disease that responds poorly to medical management, particularly in young patients with illness sufficient to impair their ability to live a normal life. Segmental resection or lobectomy in these patients may be curative. A now rare indication is massive hemoptysis from an aneurysmal vascular deformity in a bronchiectatic cavity. Embolization of bronchial arteries can be a successful (though usually only palliative) procedure in patients with significant hemoptysis who cannot tolerate pulmonary resection.

PROGNOSIS

Progression within involved segments is common, but extension to previously normal segments is unusual unless the underlying disease is a generalized process that predisposes the entire bronchial system (Table 65–1). As a general rule, patients with familial bronchiectasis have a tendency to improve during the second and third decades of life and may remain relatively stable with decreased pulmonary symptoms and good quality of life. There is, however, a reduced life expectancy.

Cochrane GM: Chronic bronchial sepsis and progressive lung damage. Br Med J 290:1026, 1985. *A concise review with 39 references, outlining current theory, research, and therapy.*

Davis PB, Hubbard VS, McCoy K, et al.: Familial bronchiectasis. J Pediatr 102:177, 1983. *A well-referenced review of the familial syndromes that lead to recurrent infections and bronchiectasis.*

Ellis DA, Thornley PE, Wightman AJ, et al.: Present outlook in bronchiectasis: Clinical and social study and review of factors influencing prognosis. Thorax 36:659, 1981.

Grenier P, Maurice F, Musset D, et al.: Bronchiectasis: Assessment by thin-section CT. Radiology 161:95, 1986. *A prospective study correlating CT with bronchography. The authors conclude that CT is a reliable, noninvasive method for detection and assessment of bronchiectasis.*

66 CYSTIC FIBROSIS

Christopher J. L. Newth

Cystic fibrosis (CF) is an autosomal recessive disease affecting both eccrine and exocrine gland function. Cystic fibrosis is characterized by elevated levels of sodium and chloride in sweat and by abnormally viscid secretions from mucous glands leading to chronic pulmonary disease in most and pancreatic insufficiency in 85 per cent, along with other manifestations (Table 66–1). It is the most common lethal genetic disease of the white population in the United States.

The abnormal gene (which is known to lie on chromosome 7) has a carrier rate of about 5 per cent in Caucasians, resulting in an incidence of CF of 1 per 1600 to 2000 births (compared with 1 per 17,000 in blacks and 1 per 100,000 in Asians). There is no test for heterozygotes for the CF gene, who are clinically normal. The disease is recognized in most patients prior to adolescence; rarely, the diagnosis may not be made until the third or fourth decade of life.

PATHOGENESIS

Obstruction and dilatation of glands and their ducts occur secondary to abnormal mucous clearance, which is presumed to be caused by the unknown basic biologic defect. However, no primary abnormalities of the mucoproteins secreted, of ciliary function, or of host defenses (including cell-mediated, humoral, and secretory immunity) have been demonstrated.

Although morphologically normal, the sweat glands in CF have defective tubular reabsorption of electrolytes or water or both, resulting in a striking increase in the levels of sodium and chloride in the sweat. Similar abnormalities have not been found in the secretions of other glands, with the exception of the submaxillary salivary glands.

CLINICAL MANIFESTATIONS

The major medical problems encountered in adolescents or young adults with CF are disorders of the tracheobronchial tree, the pancreas, and the gastrointestinal tract (Table 66–2). There are no abnormalities in the respiratory tract at birth; the earliest changes are hypertrophy of bronchial glands and metaplasia of goblet cells. Meconium ileus at birth, which occurs in about 10 to 15 per cent of CF patients, is the earliest common manifestation. The pulmonary problems increase and dominate the clinical picture as the patient gets older, whereas problems with malabsorption seem to decline.

Chronic pulmonary disease characterized by chest deformity, clubbing, and bronchiectasis is present in 97 per cent of adults with CF and is the major cause of morbidity and mortality. Pulmonary function tests show mixed obstructive and restrictive disease, with the obstructive element being dominant in most patients. The serial measurement of FEF 25–75 appears to be the most sensitive index of pulmonary decline. A sudden change, particularly in female adolescents, is a very serious

TABLE 66–1. CLINICAL MANIFESTATIONS OF CYSTIC FIBROSIS

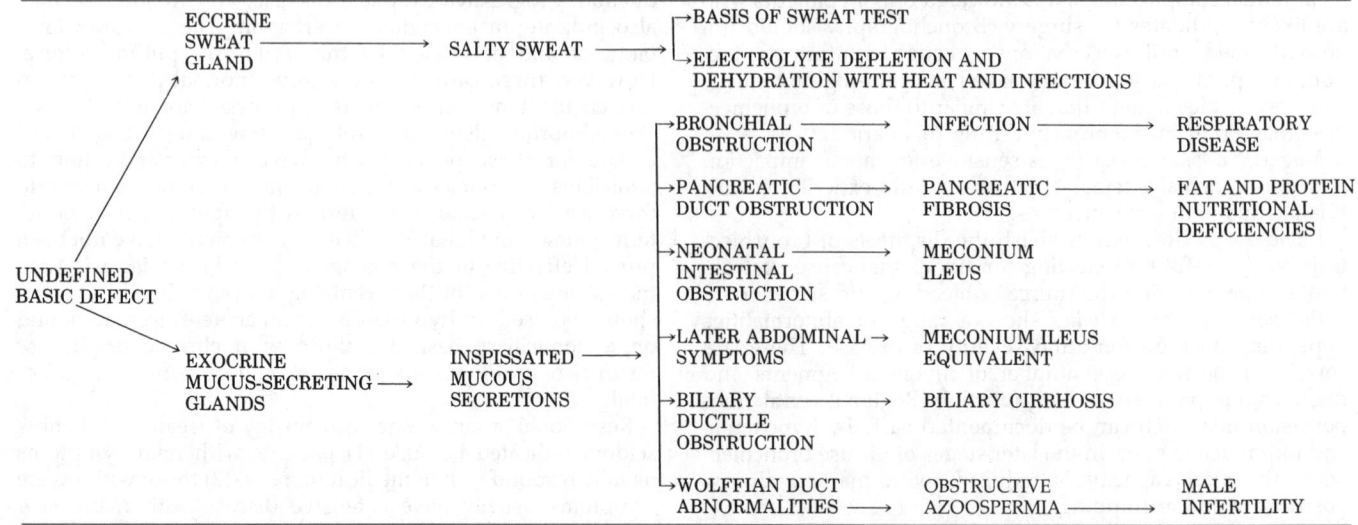

TABLE 66–2. CLINICAL MANIFESTATIONS OF CYSTIC FIBROSIS IN ADOLESCENTS AND ADULTS*

Clinical Feature	Percentage
Pulmonary disease	97
Hemoptysis	60
Pneumothorax	16
Nasal polyps	48
Cirrhosis	5
Heat prostration	5
Intestinal obstruction	21
Meconium ileus equivalent	24
Intussusception	5
Pancreatic insufficiency	95
Glucosuria	8

*Modified from di Sant'Agnese PA, Davis PB: Cystic fibrosis in adults. Am J Med 66:121, 1979.

sign. The respiratory disease is characterized by recurrent flareups of chronic bacterial bronchitis and bronchopneumonia, terminating in respiratory failure and death. The chronic bacterial infection is due primarily to mucoid strains of *Pseudomonas aeruginosa*. *Staphylococcus aureus*, which is present in about 50 per cent of adult patients, is rarely implicated in acute pulmonary complications. *Pseudomonas cepacia* occurs in the sputum of 5 to 10 per cent of patients with CF and is associated with a more rapid decline of pulmonary function. In adults with CF, minor hemoptysis occurs in 60 per cent, massive hemoptysis in 7 per cent, and pneumothorax in 16 per cent. Half of the adults with this disease have nasal polyps, but usually they are not obstructive. Over 70 per cent of patients die with cor pulmonale; the appearance of right ventricular failure usually means death within two years.

Pancreatic exocrine insufficiency occurs in 85 to 90 per cent of patients with CF. This results in deficient enzymatic hydrolysis of fats and proteins (Ch. 104). The salivary amylase allows normal carbohydrate metabolism. Malabsorption of fat may be associated with deficiencies in essential fatty acids such as linoleic acid and the fat-soluble vitamins (A, D, E, and K). Patients with residual pancreatic exocrine function tend to have better pulmonary function and probably a better prognosis. Pancreatic function may decline with age in those patients born without malabsorption.

Cystic fibrosis may also affect the small bowel, liver, bile ducts, and male reproductive organs. Intestinal obstruction secondary to meconium ileus may occur at birth. Later, distal small bowel obstruction, or "meconium ileus equivalent," occurs in about 20 per cent of older patients and is presumably related to inspissation of mucofeculent material. Patchy biliary cirrhosis may result in hepatic enlargement and rarely may progress to severe portal hypertension with varices. The incidence of cholelithiasis is increased owing to lithogenic bile rich in cholesterol. Diabetes mellitus occurs in about 10 per cent of adults, associated with decreased levels of insulin and glucagon secondary to pancreatic destruction The diabetes is relatively easy to control, and ketoacidosis is rare. Puberty, skeletal maturity, and the pubertal growth spurt are delayed in the majority of adolescents. Men are usually infertile owing to reduced vasa deferentia function, and women, although able to conceive despite having an abnormal cervical mucus, frequently develop secondary amenorrhea as they deteriorate clinically. Pregnancies can be carried to term in most cases, with a 2.5 per cent risk of the infant's having CF.

DIAGNOSIS

Cystic fibrosis is diagnosed in nearly 80 per cent of patients in the first three years of life. The diagnosis should be suspected in any adolescent or young adult presenting with chronic bronchopulmonary disease and pancreatic insufficiency or obstructive azoospermia. For diagnosing CF, a quantitative pilocarpine iontophoresis sweat test should be performed in a laboratory with established expertise. At least 100 mg of sweat should be collected, and the results should be confirmed with a second test. Elevated sodium and chloride concentrations in sweat, exceeding 60 mEq per liter in children and 70 mEq per liter in adults, are diagnostic of CF.

Prenatal tests are available for the homozygous condition, but their reliability has not yet been established. In the first four to six weeks of life, when it is difficult to obtain sufficient sweat for testing, high serum concentrations of immunoreactive trypsin may prove to be diagnostic and can be used for routine newborn screening. Early detection of CF by such screening has not yet been shown to increase the long-term survival but does decrease morbidity in the first two years of life.

TREATMENT

An increasingly large number of patients with CF survive into adulthood, and an additional small number of patients with previously undiagnosed CF are identified in young adulthood. The major source of morbidity in later life is pulmonary disease. Vigorous pulmonary toilet is basic, and good bronchial clearance can be obtained with a combination of chest physical therapy, active coughing, and exercise. Patients should be encouraged to pursue any form of exercise within their capacity. About 50 per cent of adult patients have bronchial hyper-reactivity. Aerosols of bronchodilators in normal saline are sometimes partially effective. In occasional cases, airflow can be improved by oral corticosteroids without any evidence of worsening of the bronchopulmonary infection.

Antimicrobial agents are particularly important in the therapy of CF lung disease. Chronic antistaphylococcal therapy can be given orally for years without evidence of drug resistance or complications. Antipseudomonal agents are essential for acute exacerbations of bronchial infections and intermittent bouts of pneumonia. These infections generally remain localized in the lungs; bacteremia, empyema, and extrapulmonary spread are unusual. The initial treatment of *Pseudomonas aeruginosa* infection in adolescents and adults is most commonly a combination of intravenous tobramycin and ticarcillin. Subsequent modification should be based on the results of sputum cultures and in vitro sensitivity tests. Aerosolized antibiotics directed against *Pseudomonas aeruginosa* have been found efficacious in both acute and chronic bronchopulmonary exacerbations. When the bronchopulmonary exacerbation is due to *Pseudomonas cepacia*, the antimicrobial choice is usually extremely limited.

Most patients with pancreatic insufficiency can be maintained on a normal diet with supplemental pancreatic enzymes. The preferred agents are enteric-coated microsphere pancreatic enzyme preparations, such as Pancrease and Cotazym-S, given in doses of five to seven capsules per meal. The concomitant use of sodium bicarbonate or H_2-receptor antagonists (cimetidine, ranitidine) may also improve the fat and protein absorption, since the efficacy of pancreatic enzymes is markedly increased at higher intraluminal pH levels.

"Meconium ileus equivalent" can usually be treated with enemas or nasogastric suction. Surgery is necessary on rare occasions. The administration of increased amounts of pancreatic enzymes may reduce the frequency of this complication. The lithogenicity of the bile can be reversed with appropriate pancreatic enzyme replacement. No treatment is available for the hepatic or vas deferens abnormalities. Nocturnal oxygen therapy is being evaluated to determine if prevention of arterial oxygen desaturation during sleep decreases cardiopulmonary morbidity and prolongs survival. The psychosocial aspects of this disease are formidable, and, where possible, patients should be cared for by special units so that their manifold problems can be dealt with by staff experienced with their management.

PROGNOSIS

About half of the patients with CF in the United States live to be 20 years of age. In areas where patients are cared for by special units, such as those supported by the Cystic Fibrosis Foundation and National Institutes of Health (NIH), 50 per cent survive to at least 25 years of age, with males doing much better than females.

Factors associated with a better prognosis in CF are the male sex, maintenance of appropriate weight, single-system (gastrointestinal or pulmonary) involvement at presentation, and a normal chest radiograph within the first year of presentation. Preservation of pancreatic exocrine function is likely to be a good prognostic factor.

Beaudat A, Bowcock A, Buchwald M, et al.: Linkage of cystic fibrosis to two tightly linked DNA markers: Joint report from a collaborative study. Am J Hum Genet 39:681, 1986. *Two DNA markers (MET and D758) have been discovered which flank the CF locus on chromosome 7. The finding of these probes has implications for diagnosis as well as for final characterization of the CF gene itself.*

Di Sant'Agnese PA, David PB: Cystic fibrosis in adults. Am J Med 66:121, 1979. *An excellent review of the clinical aspects of CF as the disease is seen by the internist in the adolescent and adult patient.*

Estivill X, Farrall M, Scambler PJ, et al.: A candidate for the cystic fibrosis locus isolated by selection for methylation-free islands. Nature 326:840, 1987. *Description of a novel technique for honing in on the site of the abnormal gene responsible for cystic fibrosis.*

Kuzemko JA: Evolution of lung disease in cystic fibrosis. Lancet 1:448, 1983. *This article describes an interesting hypothesis that circulating pancreatic proteases may play a role in lung injury in CF, to be followed by superinfections with bacteria and/or viruses.*

Moss AJ: The cardiovascular system in cystic fibrosis. Pediatrics 70:728, 1982. *An extensive review, with 135 references, concerning the cardiovascular findings in CF, with special emphasis on the importance of cor pulmonale as a complication.*

Rodman HM, Doershuk CF, Roland JM: The interaction of two diseases: Diabetes mellitus and cystic fibrosis. Medicine 65:389, 1986. *The occurrence of diabetes mellitus in cystic fibrosis (approximately 15 per cent of CF patients over age 18) does not seem to affect the rate of progress of the disease.*

Spier S, Rivlin J, Hughes D, et al.: The effect of oxygen on sleep, blood gases, and ventilation in cystic fibrosis. Am Rev Respir Dis 129:712, 1984. *A study demonstrating the beneficial effect of nocturnal oxygen on sleep quality and on the arterial oxygen desaturation that occurs during REM sleep in CF. The hypoventilation that occurs in this sleep state was not made clinically worse.*

Wilcken B, Chalmers G: Reduced morbidity in patients with cystic fibrosis detected by neonatal screening. Lancet 2:1319, 1985. *An Australian study that documents the reduction in morbidity in the first two years of life in patients detected by neonatal immunoreactive trypsin screening by a dried blood spot method.*

67 PULMONARY EMBOLISM

Robert M. Senior

DEFINITION

Pulmonary embolism is the impaction of material into branches of the pulmonary arterial bed. Although they may completely prevent blood flow, most pulmonary emboli do not produce necrosis of lung parenchyma ("pulmonary infarction") because (1) a dual circulation (bronchial and pulmonary) supports lung parenchymal tissue, and (2) exchange of oxygen and carbon dioxide can occur directly between the tissue and alveolar gas. Most pulmonary emboli are blood clots ("thromboemboli"); much more rarely, neoplastic cells, fat droplets (Ch. 68), air bubbles, exogenous materials (such as talc and corn starch particles in intravenous drug abusers), or pieces of intravenous catheters and catheter introducers occlude pulmonary vessels. The ensuing discussion deals with pulmonary thromboembolism.

PATHOGENESIS

Pulmonary embolism is a complication of venous thrombosis: That is, emboli come from thrombi in peripheral veins, principally the deep veins of the lower extremities and pelvis

(Ch. 57), and "travel" through the circulation to the pulmonary artery. In fact, in 70 per cent of patients with pulmonary thromboembolism, coexisting thrombi can be found in the deep veins of the thighs or pelvis. In the remaining cases, it is presumed that the emboli either come from other sites that escape detection or represent the entire thrombus that originated in the lower extremities. Thrombosis of superficial veins of the lower extremities does not lead to pulmonary thromboemboli, and thrombosis confined to deep veins in the leg distal to the popliteal vein infrequently leads to pulmonary thromboemboli. The renal veins can be a source of thromboemboli, particularly in patients with the nephrotic syndrome, but thromboemboli in nephrotic patients do not necessarily arise only from the renal veins. Pulmonary thromboemboli seldom originate in veins of the upper extremities, head or neck, but they may arise from mural thrombi in the right side of the heart. Venous thromboemboli may be trapped in the right atrium or ventricle, from which they embolize to the lungs intact or fragment in the heart and shower the lungs with emboli at one time or at different times.

Venous thrombosis can be attributed to one or more of the following: stasis of blood, increased tendency for blood to coagulate, and endothelial injury. Many clinical situations have been associated with risk of proximal deep venous thrombosis (Table 67–1), but, practically speaking, most are associated with decreased blood flow in lower extremity veins due to immobilization, elevated systemic venous pressure, extrinsic pressure on pelvic and lower extremity veins, intraluminal venous blockage from previous venous thrombosis, or decreased venous tone.

Pulmonary embolism occurs in 1 to 2 per cent of patients over age 40 following general surgery. The incidence is higher (5 to 10 per cent) with orthopedic surgery of the hip or knee. The risk associated with surgery is increased by advanced age, obesity, a lengthy operative period, underlying malignancy, pre-existent venous disease, prolonged bed rest after surgery, and postoperative infection. Venous stasis due to immobilization is probably a major reason for venous thrombosis associated with surgery, but other factors come into play: increased blood coagulability associated with release of tissue thromboplastin and exposure of subendothelium, postoperative decreased blood fibrinolytic activity, and vessel damage, particularly in surgery of the lower extremities or pelvis.

TABLE 67–1. CLINICAL RISK FACTORS FOR VENOUS THROMBOSIS AND PULMONARY THROMBOEMBOLISM

Common:
Surgical and nonsurgical trauma, including burns
Orthopedic injuries and procedures
Age over 50
Malignancy
Immobilization (bed rest, stroke, prolonged travel, and so forth)
Congestive heart failure
Previous deep venous thrombosis
Pregnancy, particularly in the puerperium and after cesarean section
Estrogen therapy
Obesity (?)

Uncommon:
Acquired
  Systemic lupus erythematosus
  Inflammatory bowel disease
  Nephrotic syndrome
  Persistent thrombocytosis
  Polycythemia vera
  Paroxysmal nocturnal hemoglobinuria
Inherited
  Hemocystinuria
  Antithrombin III deficiency
  Protein C deficiency
  Protein S deficiency
  Dysfibrinogenemia

Cancers of the lung, breast, and abdominal viscera have a strong association with venous thromboembolism, and the thromboembolism may antedate clinical recognition of the malignancy. Factors released from tumors may increase blood coagulability, decrease fibrinolytic activity, and alter endothelial surfaces. Malignancies also predispose to deep venous thrombosis by leading to venous stasis through immobilization and surgical interventions. Prolonged bed rest from any cause and paralysis resulting from stroke are also associated with a high incidence of venous thrombosis. Pulmonary embolism is commonly found at autopsy in patients who die of congestive heart failure.

In pregnancy, multiple factors predispose to venous thrombosis: (1) venous stasis induced by compression on pelvic veins, increased intra-abdominal pressure, and hormonal relaxation of vascular smooth muscle; (2) altered blood rheologic properties; and (3) increased concentrations of factors in the coagulation cascade (fibrinogen, factors VII, VIII, IX, and XII), with concomitant reductions in antithrombin III and fibrinolytic activity. There may be an increased risk of thromboembolism during pregnancy, but there is clearly an increased risk in the puerperal period, particularly after cesarean section. Estrogen therapy has been associated with an increased incidence of venous thrombosis, and the risk appears related to the dose, but the precise degree of increased risk and the mechanisms involved are not certain. Multiple possibilities have been considered, including reduction in antithrombin III concentration, decreased plasminogen activator level, increased platelet aggregability, increased blood viscosity, and increased distensibility of peripheral veins leading to venous stasis.

When pulmonary embolism occurs without an obvious predisposing factor, hereditary conditions involving decreased antithrombotic proteins (antithrombin III, proteins C and S) or deficient plasminogen activators should be considered (Ch. 167).

INCIDENCE

Pulmonary embolism is a major cause of morbidity and death. The annual incidence in the United States has been estimated at approximately 600,000. About one third of the episodes are fatal, with nearly all of the fatalities either sudden (within one hour of onset) or undiagnosed during life. In approximately half of the people who die, there is serious underlying disease apart from venous thrombosis. Autopsy studies have reported pulmonary emboli as a major cause of death (10 to 20 per cent of all hospital deaths and 15 per cent of postoperative deaths). The incidence of fatal pulmonary embolism in hospitalized patients may be declining. In one medical center, autopsy-documented fatal pulmonary embolism fell from 9.3 per cent to 3.8 per cent over a recent ten-year period. Interestingly, during the same years, there was a concomitant increase, from 4 per cent to 12.3 per cent, in the percentage of adult patients given anticoagulant therapy.

PATHOPHYSIOLOGY

Pulmonary emboli produce respiratory and hemodynamic responses that reflect the extent of pulmonary vascular obstruction, the time elapsed since embolization, and the presence or absence of pre-existent heart or lung disease.

HYPERPNEA AND ALVEOLAR HYPERVENTILATION. Acute pulmonary embolism stimulates ventilation. The increase in minute ventilation, manifested clinically by increased respiratory rate, usually offsets the increased physiologic dead space produced by obstruction of the pulmonary vascular bed, so that the arterial P_{CO_2} (Pa_{CO_2}) does not rise. On the contrary, the Pa_{CO_2} typically falls below 35 mm Hg, indicating that hyperpnea does not occur solely to preserve a normal Pa_{CO_2}. Similarly, alveolar hyperventilation is not due to hypoxemia, as it occurs even when arterial oxygenation is

normal, and it cannot be abolished with supplemental inspired oxygen. The stimulus for alveolar hyperventilation is unknown but presumably involves reflexes initiated from the pulmonary parenchyma in the area of the obstructed vessel. A reduction of Pa_{CO_2} below baseline may occur even among those with chronic hypercapnia. Although a lower than normal Pa_{CO_2} is usual, the Pa_{CO_2} rises in individuals who cannot increase their minute ventilation adequately to compensate for the increased physiologic dead space—for example, in those with neuromuscular disease, those receiving controlled mechanical ventilation, or those with severe pleuritic pain. The Pa_{CO_2} may also rise when there is massive embolization that confines pulmonary blood flow to a severely reduced portion of the pulmonary vascular bed.

HYPOXEMIA. A decrease in arterial oxygen tension (Pa_{O_2}) is common in acute pulmonary embolism. The mechanisms are complex. Ventilation-perfusion ($\dot{V}a/\dot{Q}$) inequality seems to be the predominant mechanism early in the course of pulmonary embolization, with intrapulmonary shunting the dominant cause after 48 hours. Regional bronchoconstriction, atelectasis, and pulmonary edema are postulated as the anatomic basis for these physiologic defects. If cardiac output fails to keep up with metabolic demands, as is common with massive pulmonary embolism, mixed venous oxygen saturation falls and accentuates the effects of abnormal $\dot{V}a/\dot{Q}$ and intrapulmonary shunting. If pulmonary hypertension develops and there is a patent foramen ovale, blood may be shunted from right to left within the heart, another factor causing arterial hypoxemia.

PULMONARY HYPERTENSION AND ACUTE COR PULMONALE. Pulmonary thromboembolism is the most common cause of acute pulmonary hypertension. The rise in pulmonary arterial pressure results primarily from mechanical blockage of the pulmonary vascular bed. Vasoconstrictive reflexes and mediators may also contribute. The rise in mean pulmonary arterial pressure tends to match the extent of blockage of the pulmonary arterial tree, but in patients without pre-existing cardiac or pulmonary disease, mean pulmonary arterial pressure is usually below 20 mm Hg, unless pulmonary vascular obstruction exceeds 50 per cent. Pressures of 20 to 40 mm Hg occur only with 50 to 75 per cent obstruction. The pressure seldom goes above 40 mm Hg because the normal right ventricle is incapable of generating higher pressures. A mean pulmonary arterial pressure above 40 mm Hg indicates chronic right ventricular hypertrophy secondary to recurrent pulmonary emboli or other diseases. When a sudden and marked increase in pulmonary vascular resistance causes the mean pulmonary arterial pressure to approach 40 mm Hg, several events occur. Right ventricular diastolic pressure, right atrial pressure, and systemic venous pressure all increase. The cardiac index falls below 2.5 liters per minute per square meter, and systemic hypotension and other clinical signs of hemodynamic distress appear.

PATHOLOGY

Most episodes of acute pulmonary embolism involve multiple emboli. Both lungs are affected about two thirds of the time. Lower lobe vessels are involved more often than upper lobe vessels, and the right lung is affected more often than the left. Emboli in the main branches of the right or left pulmonary arteries are seen in only a small percentage of patients. A large embolus obstructing the main pulmonary artery or straddling the pulmonary artery bifurcation (so-called "saddle embolus") is uncommon even in fatal acute pulmonary embolism. When a thromboembolus is poorly organized, it is apt to fragment in passage through the heart and is thus more likely to impact in smaller vessels than are organized thromboemboli.

The likelihood that emboli will cause pulmonary infarction is determined by the size of the vessel involved, by the extent of obstruction, by the potential for delivery of bronchial arterial blood flow, and by the adequacy of ventilation to the lung tissue supplied by the blocked pulmonary artery. Occlusions of segmental arterial vessels or smaller branches are more likely to lead to infarction than are emboli lodged in larger vessels. Infarction is also more likely in the setting of elevated pulmonary capillary pressure from any cause—hence the frequency of infarction in patients with congestive heart failure—but otherwise healthy individuals can develop pulmonary infarcts. Histologically, pulmonary infarction is characterized by intra-alveolar hemorrhage and necrosis of alveolar walls, but little inflammation. Cavitation rarely develops without coexisting pulmonary infection or an infected thrombus, although it has recently been reported in the adult respiratory distress syndrome without associated infection.

CLINICAL MANIFESTATIONS

The clinical features of pulmonary embolism can be diverse and confusing and range from no symptoms to sudden death. Occasionally, the principal manifestations are fever, arrhythmias, or refractory congestive heart failure. Usually, however, the presentations are not obscure. Three clinical patterns predominate: (1) sudden dyspnea with no physical findings but tachypnea; (2) sudden pleuritic chest pain and dyspnea accompanied by findings consistent with pleural effusion and pulmonary consolidation; and (3) sudden apprehension, chest discomfort, and dyspnea, with findings of acute cor pulmonale (accentuated pulmonic closure sound in the second left interspace, right ventricular lift, jugular venous distention) and systemic hypotension. It is this last pattern that may culminate in death within a few minutes.

The type of pattern that develops depends upon the extent of pulmonary arterial tree blockage, whether there is pre-existing cardiopulmonary disease, and whether pulmonary infarction occurs. Severe disturbances in pulmonary and systemic hemodynamics seldom occur unless there is extensive vascular obstruction or pre-existent heart or lung disease. Pleuritic pain and signs of pulmonary consolidation and pleural effusion indicate that embolization involves one or more peripheral pulmonary arterial branches. Large discrepancies may exist between the severity of embolization and symptoms. Some patients with massive embolization may appear remarkably comfortable, whereas others with minimal embolization may show great distress.

The most common symptoms of pulmonary embolism are *dyspnea* and *chest pain*, each occurring in more than 80 per cent of patients (Table 67–2). *Tachypnea* is the most common sign. *Hemoptysis*, on the other hand, often considered typical, is not common. Its absence, therefore, is not evidence against pulmonary embolism. Similarly, deep venous thrombosis of the lower extremities is seldom clinically apparent.

DIAGNOSIS

Although the history and physical examination are the means by which the diagnosis of pulmonary embolism is suggested, a diagnosis that rests on clinical grounds alone is often incorrect. The differential diagnosis of pulmonary embolism can encompass many disorders, but principally those leading to acute shortness of breath, substernal or pleuritic chest pain, hemoptysis, and hemodynamic collapse. Thus, at times the possibility of pulmonary embolism must be distinguished from asthma, the hyperventilation syndrome, pneumothorax, pulmonary edema, a fractured rib, herpes zoster before the appearance of vesicles, pleurodynia, pleuritis due to collagen vascular diseases, pneumonia, empyema, bronchiectasis, bronchogenic carcinoma, acute myocardial infarction, pericarditis, dissecting aortic aneurysm, esophageal rupture, and upper abdominal processes such as acute cholecystitis. Several features point away from the diagnosis of pulmonary embolism: (1) the absence of a precipitating factor for deep venous thrombosis, (2) recurrent chest pain in the

TABLE 67–2. SYMPTOMS AND SIGNS IN 327 PATIENTS WITH PULMONARY EMBOLI

Symptoms*	Per Cent	Signs*	Per Cent
Chest pain	88	Respirations above 16/min	92
Pleuritic	74	Rales	58
Nonpleuritic	14	S_2P† increased	53
Dyspnea	84	Pulse above 100/min	44
Apprehension	59	Temperature above 37.8°C	43
Cough	53	Diaphoresis	36
Hemoptysis	30	Gallop	34
Sweats	27	Phlebitis	32
Syncope	13	Edema	24
		Murmur	23
		Cyanosis	19

*Apprehension, syncope, increased pulmonic component of the second heart sound, gallop, diaphoresis, murmur, and cyanosis occurred more often with massive emboli (angiographically at least two lobar arteries obstructed), whereas hemoptysis and pleuritic pain were more often present with submassive emboli.

†S_2P = intensity of the pulmonic component of the second heart sound.

(From Bell WR, Simon TL, DeMets DL: The clinical features of submassive and massive pulmonary emboli. Am J Med 62:355, 1977, with permission.)

same location, (3) pleuritic chest pain of more than one week's duration that is increasing in severity, (4) pleuritic chest pain with negative findings on the chest radiograph, (5) hemoptyis of greater than 5 ml with negative findings on the chest radiograph, (6) pericardial friction rub, (7) purulent sputum, and (8) spiking fever in excess of 39°C lasting more than one week.

DIAGNOSTIC STUDIES. When pulmonary embolism is suspected, confirmation of the diagnosis depends upon establishing that there is intravascular obstruction to pulmonary arterial blood flow. The definitive means of making the diagnosis is by pulmonary arteriography; however, a high degree of certainty can also be achieved with ventilation-perfusion scanning. Other approaches to visualizing the pulmonary circulation (digital subtraction pulmonary arteriography) and novel methods of directly visualizing intrapulmonary blood clots (radioisotopically labeled platelets or monoclonal antibodies that recognize fibrin but not fibrinogen) are under development and may prove useful in the future.

Arterial blood gas measurements, the electrocardiogram, the chest radiograph, and thoracentesis may help in the evaluation of patients suspected of having pulmonary embolism, either by pointing toward or pointing away from diagnoses with which pulmonary embolism can be confused, but these studies lack specificity and therefore cannot be used in place of imaging the pulmonary circulation. Many efforts have been made to develop blood tests with specificity for the diagnosis of pulmonary embolism. None has been found useful.

Arterial Blood Gases. Typically in pulmonary embolism, there is a reduction in Pa_{O_2} and a concomitant reduction in Pa_{CO_2}. In patients with arteriographically proved acute pulmonary embolism who do not have previous cardiopulmonary disease, Pa_{O_2} values are less than 50 mm Hg in 13 per cent, 50 to 59 mm Hg in 19 per cent, between 60 and 80 mm Hg in 55 per cent, and greater than 80 mm Hg in 13 per cent. Even in those with a normal Pa_{O_2}, there is an increased alveolar-arterial oxygen difference, reflecting reduced efficiency of alveolar gas exchange. A Pa_{O_2} less than 50 mm Hg is confined to those with greater than 50 per cent occlusion of major pulmonary arterial branches; however, in individuals with underlying cardiopulmonary disease, less severe degrees of pulmonary vascular obstruction can be associated with severe hypoxemia. Arterial blood gas abnormalities have no specificity for pulmonary embolism (similar abnormalities occur in conditions with which pulmonary embolism is confused). Similarly, a normal Pa_{O_2} does not exclude pulmonary embolism.

Electrocardiogram. The main value of the electrocardiogram is to help exclude acute myocardial infarction. The most common finding in pulmonary embolism is sinus tachycardia. With emboli that provoke a substantial rise in pulmonary arterial and right-sided cardiac pressures, patterns of S_1, Q_3, T_3, inverted T waves in leads V_{1-3}, right ventricular strain, right-axis deviation, right bundle branch block, and atrial arrhythmias may occur. These changes, when they occur, are apt to be transient, lasting a few minutes or hours, disappearing as the pulmonary arterial pressure returns toward normal.

Chest Radiograph. A normal chest radiograph is uncommon in acute pulmonary embolism, but the usual radiographic findings are nonspecific: elevation of one of the hemidiaphragms with basilar atelectasis, infiltrates, and unilateral pleural effusion. Cardiac dilatation, dilatation of the main branches of the pulmonary artery, and zones of oligemia may occur with massive embolization. Besides lacking specificity, the chest radiograph shows a poor correlation with pulmonary arteriographic findings. Parenchymal densities tend to be in the lower lung fields, pleural based, and triangular and are commonly associated with pleural effusions. These densities usually represent extravasated blood rather than infarcted tissue. In summary, the principal value of the chest radiograph is to help exclude other possible diagnoses.

Thoracentesis. Pleural effusions, usually unilateral, are common with pulmonary embolism. The fluid is most often an exudate and is often hemorrhagic (but has a low hematocrit).

Ventilation-Perfusion Lung Scans. Isotopic scans of pulmonary perfusion ("Q̇" scans) provide a sensitive, safe means of assessing regional pulmonary blood flow and therefore have proved of great value in the diagnosis of pulmonary embolism. They can be performed alone or in combination with isotopic scans of ventilation. The combination of scans ("V̇/Q̇ scans") increases the specificity of the Q̇ scan. Ventilation-perfusion lung scanning has become the accepted means of initially assessing the patient suspected of pulmonary embolism. The strategy of using these scans is summarized in Figure 67–1.

A perfusion scan requires intravenous administration, with the patient supine, of technetium 99m–labeled particles of macroaggregated albumin or albumin microspheres, followed by scanning of the thorax with a gamma camera in six views (anterior, posterior, right and left lateral, and right and left posterior oblique). The particles, which are slightly larger in diameter than the cross-section of the precapillary vessels of the pulmonary circulation, are injected into a peripheral vein, flow through the peripheral and central venous circulation, the right side of the heart, and the main pulmonary arteries, and finally lodge in precapillary vessels, where they remain for hours and can be externally imaged. The standard dose of particles blocks less than 0.2 per cent of the pulmonary precapillary vessels in the normal pulmonary vascular bed. For a ventilation scan, the patient inhales and then rebreathes air containing a trace of radioactive gas, usually xenon[133]. The procedure involves obtaining images on the initial breath, at equilibration (about five minutes later), and during the washout of the tracer, beginning when the patient is returned to breathing room air. Typically, the ventilation scan is done from only one view (posterior) and for technical reasons is best done before the perfusion scan. Besides xenon[133], two other isotopes are gaining usage for ventilation scanning: (1) krypton[81m], which has the advantage over xenon[133] of enabling the scan to be obtained in the same views and at the same time as the perfusion scan, with minimal radiation exposure, and (2) technetium[99m] diethylene triamine penta-acetate in aerosols, which is more convenient from the standpoint of stability of the preparation and ease of handling.

A normal perfusion scan eliminates the diagnosis of pulmonary embolism. A normal scan reveals a homogeneous distribution of isotopic activity with an image that conforms to the anatomic shape of the lungs. In the presence of a pulmonary embolus, the radiolabeled particles are prevented from reaching vessels distal to the embolus, and the scan shows one or more perfusion defects in the image. The sensitivity of the perfusion lung scan to pulmonary arterial obstruction is excellent, as obstruction of vessels 3 mm in diameter or more leads to defects. Perfusion defects may show some resolution within a few days, but substantial abnormalities commonly persist for several weeks and may be present even a year later.

Defects on perfusion lung scans are interpreted in conjunction with the chest radiograph. Defects that do not have a corresponding abnormality on the chest radiograph are scored by number and size for the probability of pulmonary embolism (Table 67–3). Single segment-sized defects and defects smaller than segments carry low probability (less than 10 per cent) for pulmonary embolism, whereas multiple defects that are segmental or larger carry a substantially higher probability for pulmonary embolism. Perfusion defects that have corresponding abnormalities on the chest radiograph are called indeterminate, although some evidence indicates that a perfusion defect can be assigned a probability of embolus score based upon its size relative to the radiographic abnormality.

TABLE 67–3. VENTILATION-PERFUSION LUNG SCANS: FREQUENCY OF EMBOLISM BY ARTERIOGRAPHY*

Interpretation	Scan Patterns	Frequency (%)
Normal	Normal perfusion	0
Low probability	Matching defects Small subsegmental defects with mismatch (Q̇ defects smaller than chest roentgenogram abnormalities)	Less than 10
Intermediate probability	Single segmental defect with mismatch Multiple segmental defects with mismatch and match (Q̇ defects same size as chest roentgenogram abnormalities)	20–30
High probability	Multiple segmental or lobar defects with mismatch (Q̇ defects larger than chest roentgenogram abnormalities)	~90

*When perfusion scans are done without ventilation studies, the frequencies are lower.

(Adapted from Biello DR, Mattar AG, McKnight RC, et al.: Ventilation-perfusion studies in suspected pulmonary embolism. Am J Roentgenol 133:1033, 1979.)

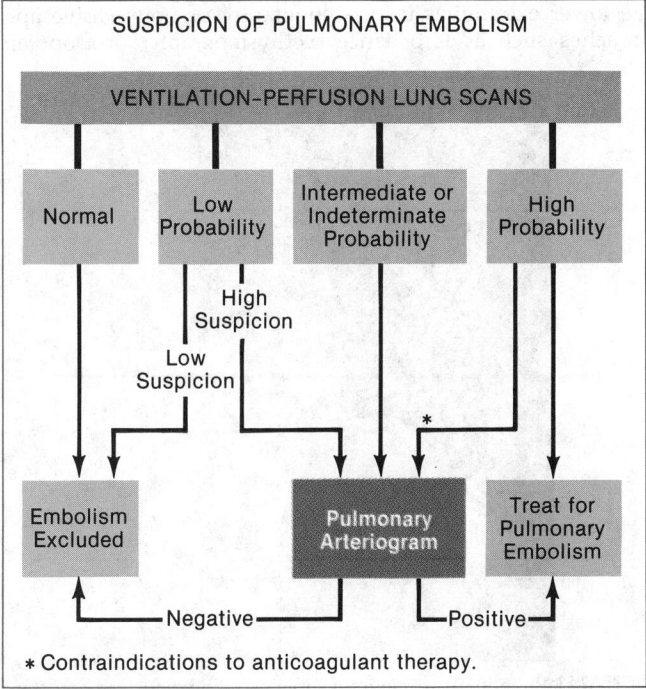

FIGURE 67–1. Ventilation-perfusion lung scanning in the evaluation of the patient suspected of having pulmonary embolism.

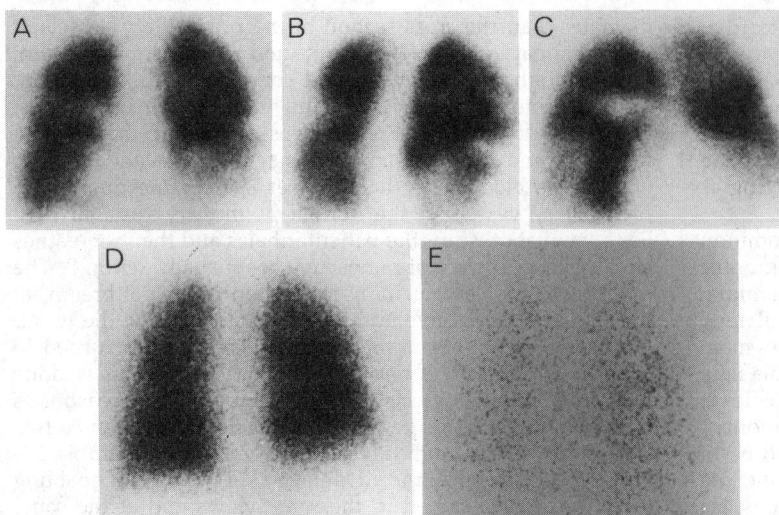

FIGURE 67–2. Selected views of ventilation-perfusion lung scans in a 60-year-old man who experienced sudden, severe shortness of breath 14 days after a suprapubic prostatectomy. The perfusion scans—(A) posterior, (B) right posterior oblique, and (C) left posterior oblique—show multiple segmental defects, whereas the ventilation scans are normal—(D) at equilibrium, (E) 1 minute of washout. This combination of scan findings indicates a high probability of pulmonary embolism and with the clinical setting is sufficient to make the diagnosis of pulmonary embolism. (Courtesy of Dr. Keith C. Fischer.)

The limitation of the perfusion scan is nonspecificity. Besides emboli, perfusion defects can be caused by lesions that compress pulmonary vessels, by increased pulmonary vascular resistance, by regional alveolar hypoxia, and by regional loss of pulmonary parenchyma, as in pulmonary emphysema. In practice, obstructive lung disease is the most common clinical condition causing perfusion defects that are not due to pulmonary embolism. Even in patients with known obstructive lung disease, perfusion scans are indicated when pulmonary embolism is suspected because they serve as a guide to selective angiography when the procedure is indicated.

Ventilation lung scans increase the specificity of perfusion scans for pulmonary emboli because pulmonary emboli do not usually disrupt regional ventilation as much as regional blood flow, unlike other causes of perfusion defects, especially obstructive lung disease. Ventilation scans may indicate the preservation of ventilation when there are perfusion defects ("V̇/Q̇ mismatches"), the loss of ventilation when there are perfusion defects ("V̇/Q̇ matches"), and delays of washin or washout indicative of obstructive lung disease. V̇/Q̇ mismatches establish a higher probability of pulmonary emboli than perfusion defects alone (Table 67–3). With some patterns of V̇/Q̇ mismatch, the diagnosis of pulmonary embolism can be made with virtual certainty (Fig. 67–2). Matched V̇/Q̇ defects are less likely to represent pulmonary embolism, but pulmonary embolism is not excluded. At large institutions, approximately 25 per cent of V̇/Q̇ studies are interpreted as being either normal or of high probability for pulmonary embolism.

Pulmonary Arteriography. *Pulmonary arteriography is the definitive test for the diagnosis of pulmonary embolism.* It involves insertion of a catheter into the pulmonary artery, usually by a percutaneous approach through one of the femoral veins. After the catheter is advanced at least as far as the right or left mainstem branch of the pulmonary artery, or more selectively into lobar or segmental branches, the contrast medium is injected and films are taken in rapid sequence. Radiographic images—supine, oblique, or lateral views—are examined for filling defects (Fig. 67–3) in branches of the pulmonary artery; these establish the diagnosis of pulmonary embolism. Abrupt terminations ("cut offs") of pulmonary arterial branches also point toward that diagnosis, although less definitely. The filling defects or cutoffs should be present in vessels of at least 2 to 3 mm in diameter. Other types of abnormalities, including delayed filling and diminished number of small vessels, are not diagnostic. Once a diagnosis of pulmonary embolism is made, the study is terminated. A negative study has rarely been proved wrong. Arteriography should be done promptly after the onset of symptoms, but it is doubtful that there will be major changes within a few days in most cases.

Pulmonary arteriography is indicated when scans are indeterminate or demonstrate an intermediate probability of pulmonary embolism. Arteriography is also warranted in the following circumstances: (1) when V̇/Q̇ scans suggest a high probability of pulmonary embolism but there are concerns about using anticoagulation therapy, (2) before using thrombolytic agents, (3) when there are clear-cut contraindications to anticoagulation therapy so that other forms of treatment will be needed, and (4) when there is an apparent failure of anticoagulation therapy and surgical treatment is being contemplated. When scans are interpreted as indicating a low probability of pulmonary embolism, a decision regarding arteriography should be guided by clinical suspicion. Thus, in patients in whom the possibility is high on the basis of clinical and laboratory tests, arteriography should be done. In approximately 10 per cent of these patients, an arteriogram will be positive. Clearly, therefore, a low probability V̇/Q̇ scan is not equivalent to an exclusion of pulmonary embolism. Indeed, some clinicians contend that pulmonary arteriography should be done routinely upon finding a low probability scan regardless of the strength of the clinical impression of pulmonary embolism. An approach to reduce the need for pulmonary arteriography has been to investigate the veins of the lower extremities using venography or noninvasive approaches such as impedance plethysmography or Doppler

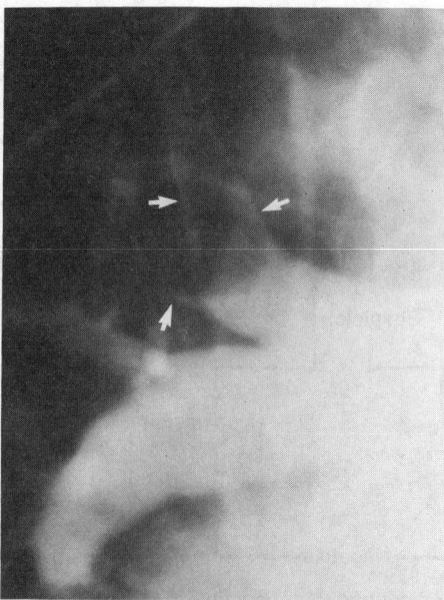

FIGURE 67–3. Pulmonary arteriogram showing filling defects in branches of the right pulmonary artery, indicative of pulmonary embolism. (Courtesy of Dr. Noah Susman.)

study. It is argued that a positive study of the extremity veins indicates the need for the same anticoagulant therapy necessary to treat pulmonary embolism and that a negative study of a lower extremity vein, along with a low-probability V̇/Q scan, excludes pulmonary embolism. While this concept has some merit, one must remember that in 30 per cent of patients with proven pulmonary emboli, studies of lower extremity veins are negative.

Many experts in this field believe that pulmonary arteriography is underutilized because physicians have concerns about the safety of the procedure. Pulmonary arteriography for the diagnosis of pulmonary embolism has proved very safe. In large series, the risk of a serious complication is 1 to 2 per cent and of death, about 0.25 per cent. The deaths have occurred almost exclusively in people with severe pulmonary hypertension who were given large amounts of contrast media.

THERAPY

Nearly all patients with acute pulmonary embolism who survive long enough to have the diagnosis confirmed will survive the acute episode. Accordingly, the primary goal of therapy is to prevent a recurrence that might be fatal. Additional goals are to reduce the morbidity of the acute episode and to prevent chronic pulmonary hypertension.

The overall therapeutic approach is summarized in Figure 67–4. The cornerstone of therapy is the use of anticoagulant drugs, since most patients with acute pulmonary embolism are hemodynamically stable and do not have a contraindication to anticoagulants. Patients who are treated with therapeutic doses of anticoagulants for an appropriate period seldom have a recurrence of pulmonary embolism, and fatal recurrences are rare indeed. Thrombolytic therapy accelerates restoration of pulmonary blood flow and normal pulmonary hemodynamics and therefore is the initial therapy for massive pulmonary embolism that has produced hemodynamic instability. When anticoagulants and thrombolytic agents are contraindicated or prove ineffective, therapy consists of interruption of the inferior vena cava, combined with pulmonary embolectomy in patients with hemodynamic instability.

Supportive measures can reduce the morbidity of the acute episode and on occasion are essential to tide the patient through a period of hemodynamic crisis. These include sup-plemental oxygen to correct hypoxemia, analgesics for pleuritic pain, and hemodynamic and ventilatory support.

ANTICOAGULANT THERAPY. Anticoagulant therapy prevents future embolization by preventing the formation of new deep venous thrombi and the propagation of residual thrombi in the deep venous system. During anticoagulant therapy, pulmonary emboli and residual deep venous thrombi either organize or undergo dissolution or both. Anticoagulation does not, however, hasten resolution of the thromboemboli within the lungs.

Table 67–4 presents a regimen for the use of anticoagulant agents. Heparin is the initial therapy because its effect is immediate. It may also be a more effective antithrombotic agent than warfarin. Heparin, an acidic glycosaminoglycan obtained from pig intestinal mucosa or beef lung, accelerates the inhibitory effect of antithrombin III upon the coagulation enzymes, thrombin, and Factors IXa, Xa, XIa, and XIIa. In patients who are suspected of having pulmonary embolism, an intravenous bolus of heparin (5000 units) should be given while diagnostic studies are under way, unless there is intracranial bleeding, intracranial lesions predisposed to bleed, or active internal bleeding, all of which are absolute contraindications to heparin.

Heparin is usually administered intravenously by continuous infusion. Intermittent intravenous injection and subcutaneous injection are alternative means of administration, but a higher incidence of bleeding complications may occur with intermittent injection, and it is difficult to establish the correct dose with the subcutaneous route. The risk of recurrent venous thromboembolism is low if the activated partial thromboplastin time is maintained 1.5 to 2 times the control (about 25 seconds beyond the control) at all times. Accordingly, this is the goal of therapy. The usual daily dose is 25,000 to 50,000 units. Heparin therapy should be monitored particularly closely during the first few days after the thromboembolic event, as the heparin requirements are greatest then.

The most common and most serious complication of heparin therapy is bleeding. The risk of bleeding may be more closely related to risk factors, such as trauma, recent surgery, recent invasive procedures, and the inhibition by heparin of platelet function, than to the absolute anticoagulant effect produced by the drug. Thrombocytopenia may also complicate therapy and cause bleeding. Approximately 10 per cent of patients exhibit platelet counts less than 100,000 per cubic millimeter

FIGURE 67–4. The therapy of pulmonary embolism.

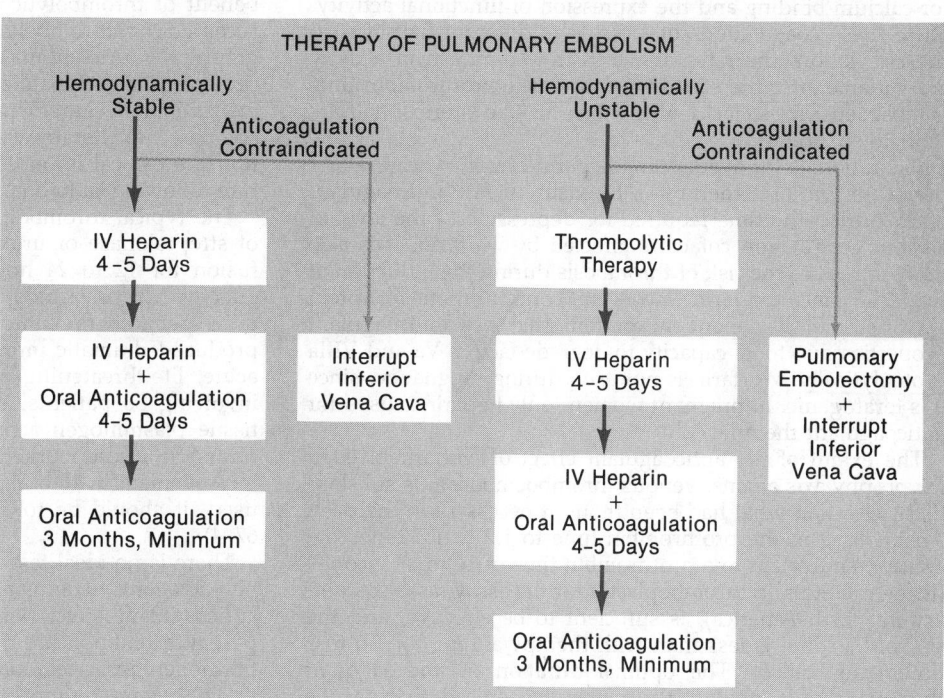

THERAPY OF PULMONARY EMBOLISM

Hemodynamically Stable → IV Heparin 4–5 Days → IV Heparin + Oral Anticoagulation 4–5 Days → Oral Anticoagulation 3 Months, Minimum

Anticoagulation Contraindicated → Interrupt Inferior Vena Cava

Hemodynamically Unstable → Thrombolytic Therapy → IV Heparin 4–5 Days → IV Heparin + Oral Anticoagulation 4–5 Days → Oral Anticoagulation 3 Months, Minimum

Anticoagulation Contraindicated → Pulmonary Embolectomy + Interrupt Inferior Vena Cava

TABLE 67–4. GUIDELINES FOR ANTICOAGULANT THERAPY WITH HEPARIN AND WARFARIN IN PULMONARY EMBOLISM

Embolism Suspected	Embolism Confirmed
Obtain baseline APTT,* PT,* and platelet count and give heparin bolus (5000–10,000 units) IV* Order diagnostic test: ventilation-perfusion lung scan or pulmonary arteriogram	Give loading dose of heparin (5000 units) and start constant IV infusion at approximately 1000 units/hr Monitor APTT at 4–6 hr and thereafter until the APTT is stabilized between 1.5 and 2.0 times control value Monitor platelet count while administering heparin Start warfarin by day 4 or 5 by instituting the estimated daily maintenance dose (usually 4–10 mg) After at least 7–10 days of heparin therapy and 4–5 days of joint therapy, stop heparin and check PT four hours later Maintain PT off heparin at 1.2 to 1.5 times control or pretreatment value (using rabbit brain thromboplastin) Maintain full-dose anticoagulation for at least 3 mo in patients without continuing risk factors, longer in others

*APTT = activated partial thromboplastin time; PT = one-stage prothrombin time (1.2 times control performed with rabbit brain thromboplastin is roughly equal to 2.0 times control with human brain thromboplastin); IV = intravenous.
(Adapted from Hyers TM, Hull RD, Weg JG: Antithrombotic therapy for venous thromboembolic disease. Chest 89:26S, 1986, with permission.)

during heparin therapy; there seems to be no correlation between this complication and the type of heparin used. The thrombocytopenia, which appears to have an immunologic basis, seldom occurs until after several days of therapy. A rare complication of heparin-induced thrombocytopenia is thrombosis, mainly of arteries. With long-term administration, heparin can cause accelerated osteoporosis.

After four to five days of heparin therapy, oral anticoagulation is begun with *warfarin*. Both agents are continued together for four to five days, after which the heparin is discontinued. Warfarin acts in the liver to inhibit the gamma-carboxylation of specific glutamic acid residues in several vitamin K–dependent coagulation cofactors: II, VII, IX, and X (Ch. 167). These gamma-carboxyglutamic acids are required for calcium binding and the expression of functional activity. Since these coagulation cofactors have different half-lives in the circulation, the rates at which they diminish in activity are variable after the start of therapy. The prothrombin time is most sensitive to factor VII, which has the shortest half-life (four to six hours).

The rationale for overlapping heparin therapy with the first period of warfarin therapy is to ensure a full anticoagulant effect during the time required for depression of the level of all four coagulation cofactors affected by warfarin. It is also done to reduce the risk of thrombosis during the induction of warfarin, since warfarin lowers the concentration of protein C, a vitamin K–dependent protein that has anticoagulant properties due to its capacity to degrade factors Va and VIIIa proteolytically. Warfarin is not used during pregnancy, since it is teratogenic. In pregnant women, only heparin is used for anticoagulant therapy.

The extent of the anticoagulant effect of warfarin needed for prophylaxis against venous thromboembolism is substantially less than what had been thought necessary in the past. An increase in the prothrombin time to 1.2 to 1.5 times the control, equivalent to a prothrombin time of 14 to 17 seconds (using rabbit brain thromboplastin for the assay, as is customary in North America), is sufficient to be effective, and the risk of bleeding is less than with therapy aiming for 1.5 to 2 times the control. The optimal duration of anticoagulant therapy is not known. It is generally advised to continue therapy for at least three months in all patients, to extend therapy as long as identifiable risk factors are resolving, and to give therapy indefinitely to patients in whom an increased risk for deep venous thrombosis is permanent.

THROMBOLYTIC THERAPY. Thrombolytic agents, by dissolving pulmonary emboli and thrombi in the deep venous system, can alleviate the hemodynamic disturbances caused by pulmonary emboli, eliminate the source of further emboli, and perhaps diminish postphlebitic complications in the lower extremities. Two thrombolytic agents, streptokinase and urokinase, have been used for a number of years. A third, tissue-type plasminogen activator (TPA), is currently in use in limited trials and should be generally available soon.

Streptokinase and *urokinase* convert circulating endogenous plasminogen to plasmin, a potent serine protease that dissolves fibrin. Urokinase cleaves plasminogen to plasmin directly, whereas streptokinase forms a complex with plasminogen, allowing expression of plasminogen's normally hidden active site, which then cleaves other plasminogen molecules to plasmin. At equivalent dosage, streptokinase is considerably cheaper than urokinase, but, unlike urokinase, it can produce febrile and allergic reactions. Plasmin formed by either agent lyses the fibrin clot in pulmonary emboli, but unfortunately it also cleaves other molecules in the circulation, including fibrinogen and factors V and VIII, and it leads to consumption of circulating plasmin inhibitors, in particular alpha 2-antiplasmin. Thus, besides solubilizing pulmonary emboli and deep venous thrombi, these agents can solubilize hemostatic plugs where they are important, such as at incisional sites, and can reduce hemostatic competence generally. *Tissue-type plasminogen activator*, which has been used widely in trials for acute coronary occlusion, has shown dramatic thrombolytic effects on pulmonary emboli in a small number of patients. It has the advantage of expressing little activity in the absence of fibrin.

These thrombolytic agents restore pulmonary arterial pressure and pulmonary perfusion toward normal faster than does heparin, but their use seems to result in no improvement in mortality or in pulmonary perfusion, compared with heparin, a few weeks after the acute episode. There is also no difference between thrombolytic agents and anticoagulants in the rate of recurrence of pulmonary embolism. Thrombolytic therapy appears to offer only an immediate short-term advantage over heparin, but studies do not exclude a life-saving benefit of thrombolytic therapy in some patients. It is now accepted that thrombolytic therapy should be given for angiographically proven massive pulmonary embolism that has produced hemodynamic instability. There may be better normalization of pulmonary capillary blood flow after a year compared to therapy with heparin only, but this is of questionable clinical importance, since pulmonary impairment is rare following pulmonary emboli in either case.

The typical thrombolytic regimen involves a loading dose of streptokinase or urokinase, followed by a continuous infusion for 12 to 24 hours, but other regimens may be as effective. In one study, a single bolus of urokinase, 15,000 units per kilogram into the right atrium over 10 minutes, produced dramatic improvements in 12 of 14 patients with acute, life-threatening pulmonary emboli. In another study involving 36 patients, short-term infusions of recombinant tissue plasminogen activator (50 to 90 mg over two to six hours) produced marked clot lysis in 24 patients and objective improvement in 10 others. Whatever thrombolytic regimen is used, it should be followed by anticoagulant therapy (Fig. 67–4).

There is no ideal test for monitoring patients given thrombolytic agents. The usual approach is to document either an anticoagulant effect (lengthening of the prothrombin time, partial thromboplastin time, or thrombin time) or evidence of fibrinogen/fibrin degradation (decreased fibrinogen concentration or increased titers of fibrin degradation products) or both.

Because these agents digest substrates besides fibrin in pulmonary emboli, proof that a thrombolytic agent has exerted some effect by these tests does not, however, prove an effect upon pulmonary emboli. Nor is it possible to use results from these tests to titrate the dose. On the other hand, clinical effectiveness is usually apparent from improvement in the patient's cardiopulmonary status.

Because thrombolytic agents may start or aggravate bleeding, they are absolutely contraindicated when there is active internal bleeding or within a few months of stroke, neurologic or ophthalmologic surgery, or head injury. They are relatively contraindicated within ten days of major surgical procedures or biopsies of internal organs or arteriographic studies, during pregnancy and the first ten days postpartum, and in a variety of medical states associated with increased risk of bleeding, such as severe hypertension. In the patient who is critically ill from pulmonary emboli, however, the danger of bleeding must be weighed against the potential benefits and the risks of alternate forms of therapy.

VENA CAVAL INTERRUPTION. The principal reasons for interruption of the inferior vena cava are (1) absolute contraindications to anticoagulant therapy (active internal bleeding and recent central nervous system lesions that are bleeding or are predisposed to bleed), (2) severe internal bleeding that develops during therapeutic anticoagulation, and (3) recurrent emboli despite adequate anticoagulation. Infrequently, vena caval interruption is necessary for septic embolism, after pulmonary embolectomy, or after massive embolization of such severity that further embolization might well be fatal. In the last-noted situation, anticoagulation therapy is used as well.

Like anticoagulation therapy, interruption of the vena cava is only preventive against future emboli. It does not promote resolution of emboli already in the lungs, and it does not alleviate the hemodynamic effects of emboli. In addition, it may not provide permanent protection against pulmonary embolism, since collateral veins bypassing the interruption can enlarge and provide other routes for thromboemboli to reach the lungs. Since most bleeding during anticoagulant therapy is not life threatening and can be controlled by reduction in anticoagulant dosage, a conservative approach is advised regarding the interruption of the vena cava. Similarly, recurrence of pulmonary embolism after anticoagulation therapy is begun should not be taken as an automatic indication for vena caval interruption. Unless massive embolism is documented angiographically, anticoagulation therapy should be continued, with maximal effort made to ensure an adequate anticoagulant effect at all times. As noted above, fatal pulmonary embolism is rare during therapeutic anticoagulation.

Methods of vena caval interruption include ligation or clipping, which must be done with the patient under general or spinal anesthesia, and the use of umbrellas or filters, which are inserted percutaneously through jugular or femoral veins with the patient under local anesthesia. Except in the case of septic embolism, percutaneous devices are preferred.

PULMONARY EMBOLECTOMY. Pulmonary embolectomy is rarely performed and is limited to patients with massive pulmonary emboli involving pulmonary arteries shown to be accessible on pulmonary angiography, with hypotension and end-organ (brain and kidney) dysfunction despite maximal medical support, and in whom there are contraindications to thrombolytic therapy or in whom thrombolytic therapy has proved ineffective. Few patients meet these conditions and survive long enough to have surgery. The surgical mortality for emergency pulmonary embolectomy is at least 25 per cent. In contrast, elective surgery for symptomatic, unresolved pulmonary emboli in large branches of the pulmonary artery has proved effective and reasonably safe. The procedure for chronic emboli, which amounts to an endarterectomy for removal of organized thromboemboli, can improve functional status, reduce pulmonary arterial pressure, and normalize pulmonary arterial perfusion and arterial oxygenation.

PROGNOSIS

The majority of deaths from pulmonary embolism occur either too quickly for therapy to be given or because the condition is not recognized. If pulmonary embolism goes untreated, survival is only 70 per cent, with death occurring as a result of recurrent thromboembolism within a few weeks of the first episode. In contrast, among those individuals in whom a diagnosis is made and therapy begun, 92 per cent survive and do so without sequelae. Among those few individuals who do not survive despite therapy, two thirds of the deaths are due to associated critical diseases. In those in whom death is due to pulmonary embolism, systemic hypotension is usually present at the onset of the episode, and pulmonary vascular obstruction is usually greater than 75 per cent. Even when hypotension and acute cor pulmonale are present at the onset of acute pulmonary embolism, however, it does not necessarily mean a fatal outcome. Clinical signs of massive embolization can subside quickly, presumably because vascular obstruction decreases as a result of fragmentation or remodeling of the emboli or because pulmonary vasoconstrictive reflexes and mediators dissipate. The presence of pulmonary infarction has no effect on survival.

In less than 1 per cent of those who survive acute pulmonary thromboembolization, the emboli persist and result in a chronic syndrome of exertional dyspnea, pulmonary hypertension, right ventricular enlargement, and right ventricular failure. Individuals presenting with this syndrome usually have a history that contains clues to recurrent episodes of pulmonary embolism and to conditions predisposing to venous thromboembolic disease.

PREVENTION

Several therapeutic regimens reduce the risk of deep venous thrombosis and by doing so reduce the risk of pulmonary thromboembolism. These regimens—which include early ambulation, low-dose subcutaneous heparin, low-dose warfarin, dextran, external pneumatic calf compression, and gradient elastic stockings—are easy to use, have minimal complications, and require essentially no laboratory monitoring. The most thoroughly proven regimen, low-dose subcutaneous heparin (5000 units twice daily), is effective for (1) general surgery patients with high-risk features (over age 40, obese, previous deep venous thrombosis or previous pulmonary embolism, current malignancy, and complex surgery), (2) patients undergoing urologic or gynecologic surgery (excluding procedures for gynecologic malignancies), and (3) patients with congestive heart failure and those recovering from acute myocardial infarction. Low-dose subcutaneous heparin is not effective for prophylaxis of deep venous thrombosis in patients with traumatic hip fracture. In that situation, low-dose warfarin or pneumatic compression should be used. Because there is some risk of bleeding with low-dose heparin, it should not be used in patients having intracranial or eye surgery or in those who have suffered spinal cord trauma. For these situations, pneumatic compression is a satisfactory, safe alternative. Prophylaxis for deep venous thrombosis should be given wider usage because it is the only way that a substantial reduction in fatal pulmonary embolism will be achieved.

Bounameaux H, Vermylen J, Collen D: Thrombolytic treatment with recombinant tissue-type plasminogen activator in a patient with massive pulmonary embolism. Ann Intern Med 103:64, 1985. *Describes dramatic resolution of life-threatening pulmonary embolism within a few hours after a bolus of tissue-type plasminogen activator delivered through a catheter placed in the right ventricle.*

Consensus Development Panel: NIH Consensus Development Conference Statement on the Prevention of Venous Thrombosis and Pulmonary Embolism. JAMA 256:744, 1986. *Summarizes current views about prophylactic therapy for deep venous thrombosis and concludes that such therapy is effective and should be used more widely.*

Dismuke SE, Wagner EH: Pulmonary embolism as a cause of death. JAMA 255:2039, 1986. *Reports a declining incidence of massive fatal pulmonary embolism in a university hospital between 1966 and 1980, coincident with an increased use of anticoagulants.*

Goldhaber SZ (ed.): Pulmonary Embolism and Deep Venous Thrombosis. Philadelphia, W. B. Saunders Company, 1985. *Detailed reviews of various aspects of pulmonary embolism.*

Goldhaber SZ, Markis JE, Meyerovitz MF, et al.: Acute pulmonary embolism treated with tissue plasminogen activator. Lancet 2:886, 1986. *Reports angiographic improvement in 34 of 36 patients, which was marked in 24, within six hours after receiving recombinant human tissue-type plasminogen activator intravenously.*

Heim CR, Des Prez RM: Pulmonary embolism: A review. Adv Intern Med 31:187, 1986. *Summarizes clinical aspects of pulmonary embolism.*

Hirsh J: Venous thromboembolism: Prevention, diagnosis and treatment. Chest 89:369S, 1986. *Articles on the management of pulmonary embolism.*

Huet Y, Lemaire F, Brun-Buisson C, et al.: Hypoxemia in acute pulmonary embolism. Chest 88:829, 1985. *Using the multiple inert gas technique to analyze alveolar gas exchange, this study shows that the mechanisms for hypoxemia in pulmonary embolism change during the course of the illness.*

Hyers TM (ed.): Symposium on pulmonary embolism and hypertension. Clin Chest Med 5:383, 1984. *Articles on various aspects of venous thromboembolism.*

Hyers TM, Hull RD, Weg JG: Antithrombotic therapy for venous thromboembolic disease. Chest 89:26S, 1986. *Describes how to use anticoagulants in the management of venous thrombosis and pulmonary embolism.*

Petitprez P, Simmoneau G, Cerrina J, et al.: Effects of a single bolus of urokinase in patients with life-threatening pulmonary emboli: A descriptive trial. Circulation 70:861, 1984. *Twelve of 14 patients with massive pulmonary embolism had rapid clinical improvement shortly after receiving one large dose of urokinase delivered in the right atrium over 10 minutes.*

Shafer KE, Santoro SA, Sobel BE, et al.: Monitoring activity of fibrinolytic agents: A therapeutic challenge. Am J Med 76:879, 1984. *Reviews the fibrinolytic system, mechanisms of fibrinolysis, and methods for monitoring therapy with fibrinolytic agents.*

68 FAT EMBOLISM SYNDROME

Robert M. Senior

DEFINITION

Fat embolism syndrome refers to the constellation of clinical manifestations that may develop when fat droplets impact in the pulmonary microvasculature and other microvascular beds, especially in the brain. The principal clinical features of fat embolism syndrome are respiratory failure, cerebral dysfunction, and petechiae.

CLINICAL SETTING

Fat embolism syndrome occurs almost exclusively as an early complication of traumatic fractures of the pelvis and of long bones, particularly the shaft of the femur. Delays in stabilization of fractures and periods of systemic hypoperfusion after trauma increase the risk of the syndrome. The syndrome develops in 2 to 25 per cent of persons with fresh long bone fractures, depending on criteria for the diagnosis and selection of patients at risk. In contrast, it rarely follows elective orthopedic surgery on long bones, even though fat droplets can be found routinely in the venous blood draining the operative sites. Other rare settings for fat embolism include massive soft tissue injury, severe burns, conditions associated with fatty liver, osteomyelitis and conditions causing bone infarcts such as sickle cell hemoglobinopathy, and prolonged corticosteroid therapy.

DIAGNOSIS

There are no laboratory tests that are diagnostic of fat embolism syndrome. Specifically, looking for the presence of fat droplets in the blood, urine, and sputum is not helpful in making the diagnosis, as droplets may not be present in patients who clearly have fat embolism syndrome but may be found after traumatic fractures in patients without evidence of the syndrome. The diagnosis is based on the presence of at least one of the following features within the first 72 hours after traumatic fracture: (1) otherwise unexplained dyspnea, tachypnea, arterial hypoxemia, and diffuse alveolar infiltrates on chest radiograph; (2) otherwise unexplained confusion or other signs of cerebral dysfunction, and (3) petechiae over the upper half of the body, including the axillae, conjunctivae, and oral mucosa. Further support for the diagnosis is provided by fluffy retinal exudates and hemorrhages and unexplained fever. The diagnosis is definite if all three criteria are present. The diagnosis is unlikely if the signs and symptoms first begin more than 72 hours after the injury. In this situation, pulmonary edema from massive fluid replacement, aspiration, sepsis, pneumonia, or venous thromboembolism is a more probable cause of respiratory distress.

PATHOGENESIS

The specific cellular mechanisms leading to fat embolism syndrome are not fully understood, but it is clear that the syndrome is not simply a consequence of mechanical obstruction of small vessels by fat droplets. An important aspect of the pathogenesis appears to be endothelial injury caused by fatty acids released from impacted fat droplets by lipoprotein lipase, with ensuing increased microvascular permeability and fluid leakage into interstitial spaces. Some data suggest that individuals who have had fat embolism syndrome after trauma have abnormalities of carbohydrate and lipid metabolism, increased capillary fragility, and abnormal neurohumoral responses to stress and are distinguishable by these characteristics from individuals with comparable trauma who did not develop fat embolism syndrome.

The fat droplets found in small vessels are from the trauma site. As the first microvascular bed encountered by fat droplets in the venous circulation, the lungs bear the brunt of fat embolization. Presumably, fat emboli in other organs, especially the brain, reach those sites by passing through the pulmonary microvasculature or through right-to-left shunts in the heart.

Although the effects of fatty acids upon endothelium appear to be important in the mechanism of lung injury, the pathogenesis of respiratory failure may be more complex in some cases. Other tissue components besides fat may be liberated from fracture sites, and these as well as the injured pulmonary endothelium may activate the clotting, complement, and contact systems. Thus, the pathogenesis of lung injury may be multifactorial, as in other forms of the adult respiratory distress syndrome, involving thrombosis, mediators of inflammation, and products of inflammatory cells.

Hypoxemia explains brain dysfunction in many cases, but not all. In some fatal cases, cerebral symptoms reflect direct brain injury, with many fat emboli and associated hemorrhage and necrosis. Moreover, patients with comparable hypoxemia from causes other than fat embolism syndrome seldom have brain dysfunction, and occasional patients with fat embolism syndrome have neurologic features that precede hypoxemia or are disproportionate to the degree of hypoxemia.

The reason for petechiae is not known, although in some patients there may be thrombocytopenia and disseminated intravascular coagulation. There is also no explanation for the striking localization of the petechiae to the pectoral regions and conjunctivae.

THERAPY

Management of fat embolism syndrome is supportive and usually consists primarily of ensuring good arterial oxygenation. Supplemental oxygen is given to maintain the arterial oxygen tension in the normal range, 75 to 90 mm Hg. If endotracheal intubation and ventilatory support are necessary, positive end-expiratory pressure may reduce the need for high concentrations of inspired oxygen. Restricting fluid intake and even giving diuretics, if systemic perfusion can be maintained, may minimize fluid accumulation in the lungs.

The role of corticosteroids is controversial; there is no clear-cut evidence that they are helpful.

In patients with acute long bone fractures, the risk of fat embolism syndrome is reduced by prompt surgical stabilization of the fractures and by correcting or preventing decreased systemic perfusion. In addition, administration of corticosteroids at a high dose for a short period (7.5 mg per kilogram of methylprednisolone intravenously at six-hour intervals for three days) seems to prevent development of the syndrome.

PROGNOSIS

The mortality from fat embolism syndrome is 10 per cent or less and thus is clearly much lower than the 50 per cent or greater mortality for most causes of the adult respiratory distress syndrome. Even severe respiratory failure seldom leads to death. In one report of 54 cases, there was not a single fatality from the syndrome, although severe hypoxemia was common during the acute stages.

Guenter CA, Braun TE: Fat embolism syndrome: A changing prognosis. Chest 79:143, 1981. *This study emphasizes that with modern respiratory care, death from post-traumatic fat embolism is unusual.*

Peltier LF: Fat embolism: An appraisal of the problem. Clin Ortho Rel Res 187:3, 1984. *Reviews clinical investigations of the source and composition of post-traumatic fat emboli and the pathogenesis of fat embolism syndrome.*

Rosen JM, Braman SS, Hasan FM, et al.: Nontraumatic fat embolization: A rare cause of new pulmonary infiltrates in an immunocompromised patient. Am Rev Resp Dis 134:805, 1986. *Describes fatal fat embolism syndrome in a patient with lymphoma who was receiving high-dose corticosteroid therapy.*

Schonfeld SA, Ployongsang Y, DiLisio R, et al.: Fat embolism prophylaxis with corticosteroids: A prospective study in high-risk patients. Ann Intern Med 99:438, 1983. *This study presents persuasive evidence for the efficacy of steroids in prevention of post-traumatic fat embolism syndrome.*

69 SARCOIDOSIS

Barry L. Fanburg

DEFINITION

Sarcoidosis, a multisystem granulomatous disease, begins most frequently in people between 20 and 40 years old. The etiology is unknown, but alterations in the immune system are clearly involved in its pathogenesis. Organ involvement is usually asymptomatic, and the disease most frequently regresses spontaneously, but it may progress to a more chronic state of fibrosis with severe functional impairment of various organs. No natural animal models of sarcoidosis have been discovered.

EPIDEMIOLOGY AND GENETICS

Sarcoidosis occurs with similar manifestations world wide, but its incidence differs strikingly, from 0.04 per 100,000 in Spain, for example, to 64 per 100,000 in Sweden. The reported numbers are susceptible to considerable error based upon procedures for evaluation, but large unexplained differences in prevalence clearly exist. The majority of cases occur during adulthood, but sarcoidosis is also present in the pediatric population.

The disease has been reported to be transmissible in experimental animals, but this work still has not been rigorously tested for confirmation. Sarcoidosis is not contagious in humans.

Familial occurrences have been reported in approximately 200 instances, but no specific patterns of parent-child or sibling relationships have emerged. Sarcoidosis has been reported in twins, with a preponderance of monozygotic over dizygotic twins. The disease seems not to be linked with specific human leukocyte antigen (HLA) types.

IMMUNOLOGY

A postulated schema for the immunopathology of sarcoidosis is presented in Figure 69–1. The macrophage most likely initiates the cellular response of sarcoidosis, possibly in response to some unknown presenting antigen. Various factors released by the macrophage, such as interleukin-1, cause accumulation and proliferation of helper T lymphocytes. Factors secreted by the lymphocytes attract and immobilize other inflammatory cells. In addition, B lymphocytes are stimulated to produce increased amounts of immunoglobulins, and fibroblasts are stimulated to proliferate.

As a result of these various immunologic interactions (1) inflammatory cells proliferate in the affected organ (forming the granuloma), (2) cutaneous delayed hypersensitivity responses to common antigens are depressed, and (3) immune globulins are synthesized and circulate in excess. In addition, circulating immune complexes may be present; high levels of serum antibodies to common environmental antigens such as *Mycoplasma pneumoniae* and various viruses frequently occur; antibody responses to immunization may be exaggerated; and circulating rheumatoid factor, antinuclear antibody, and autoantibodies to T lymphocytes may be present.

Intradermally injected extracts of homogenized tissue of involved organs from patients with sarcoidosis are capable of producing a delayed inflammatory reaction in patients with sarcoidosis. This antigen that causes the so-called *Kveim-Siltzbach reaction* has not been purified, and the basis for its response has not been defined. The reaction differs from a cutaneous delayed hypersensitivity reaction in that it takes four to six weeks to develop and then persists for several months.

CLINICAL PRESENTATION

Sarcoid lesions may develop in almost any organ system so that the clinical presentation is quite varied (Fig. 69–2). In fact, "silent" granulomas are frequently present in multiple organs. Most characteristically, the patient is asymptomatic, but the disease is detected by an abnormal chest radiograph, usually showing bilateral symmetric hilar adenopathy often associated with paratracheal adenopathy (Fig. 69–3) and/or reticulonodular parenchymal infiltrates. Patients with sarcoidosis may also present with hilar and paratracheal adenopathy in association with some combination of acute peripheral arthritis, uveitis, and erythema nodosum (the so-called acute sarcoidosis or Loeffgren's syndrome). Except for Loeffgren's syndrome, significant constitutional symptoms other than those of fatigue are unusual in sarcoidosis. When anorexia, weight loss, and fever are present, other diseases should be strongly considered.

Lungs

The lungs are the most frequently involved organ, and pulmonary symptoms, when present, include dyspnea on exertion, nonproductive cough, and wheezing. Dyspnea is usually caused by fibrotic or granulomatous pulmonary parenchymal disease, but it may also result from granulomatous obstruction of upper airways. Granulomas in the nose may cause nasal congestion and in the larynx may result in hoarseness. Hemoptysis is rare in sarcoidosis but may occur from an associated mycetoma in advanced cavitary sarcoidosis. Acute dyspnea secondary to a pneumothorax also occasionally develops in patients with more advanced fibrotic pulmonary disease. Pleural involvement has been reported but is unusual.

Skin

Erythema nodosum may be associated with sarcoidosis as a secondary vasculitic reaction. Sarcoid granulomas also occur directly in the skin to produce a variety of small, asymptomatic

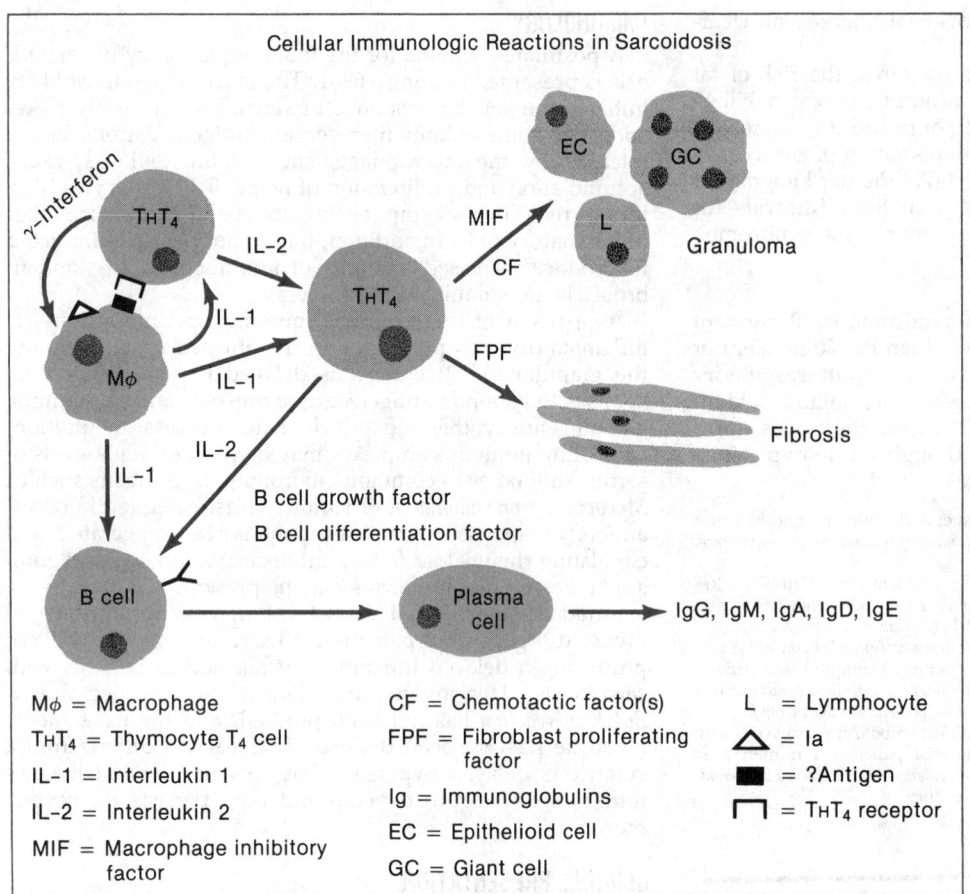

Cellular Immunologic Reactions in Sarcoidosis

Mφ = Macrophage
THT4 = Thymocyte T4 cell
IL-1 = Interleukin 1
IL-2 = Interleukin 2
MIF = Macrophage inhibitory factor

CF = Chemotactic factor(s)
FPF = Fibroblast proliferating factor
Ig = Immunoglobulins
EC = Epithelioid cell
GC = Giant cell

L = Lymphocyte
△ = Ia
■ = ?Antigen
⊓ = THT4 receptor

FIGURE 69–1. Immunologic abnormalities associated with sarcoidosis.

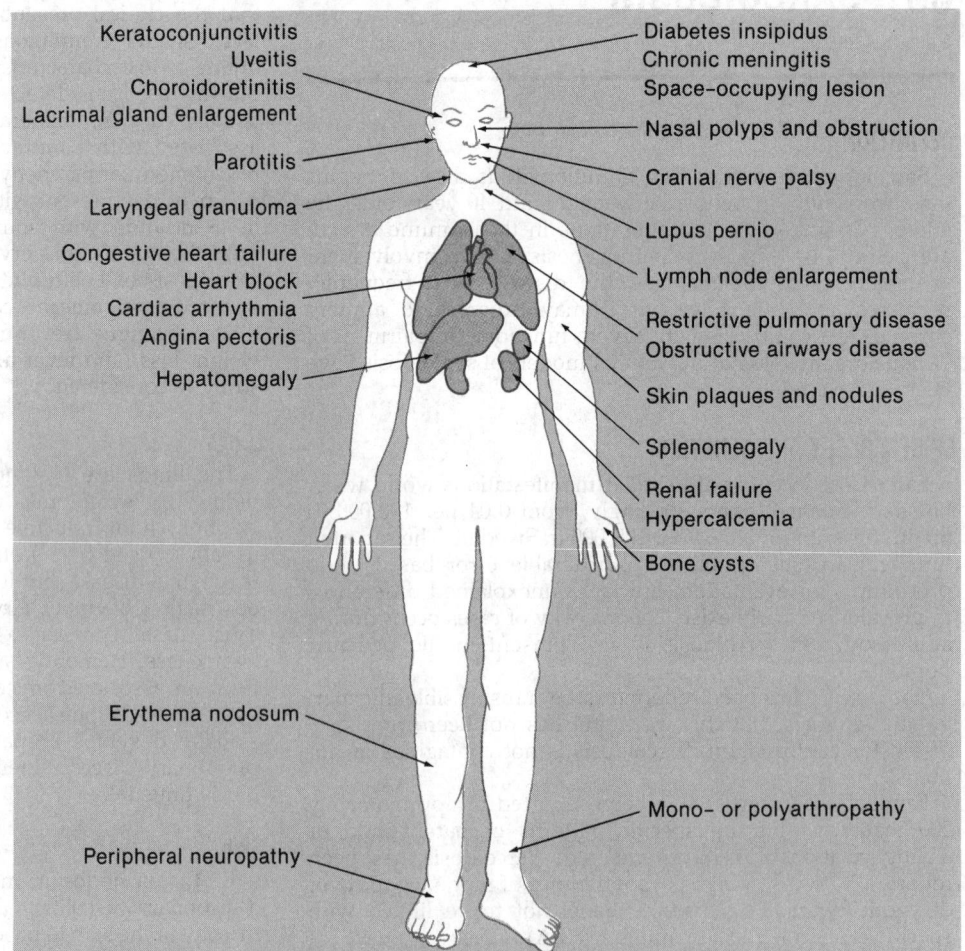

FIGURE 69–2. Organ abnormalities associated with sarcoidosis.

Keratoconjunctivitis
Uveitis
Choroidoretinitis
Lacrimal gland enlargement
Parotitis
Laryngeal granuloma
Congestive heart failure
Heart block
Cardiac arrhythmia
Angina pectoris
Hepatomegaly

Diabetes insipidus
Chronic meningitis
Space-occupying lesion
Nasal polyps and obstruction
Cranial nerve palsy
Lupus pernio
Lymph node enlargement
Restrictive pulmonary disease
Obstructive airways disease
Skin plaques and nodules
Splenomegaly
Renal failure
Hypercalcemia
Bone cysts

Erythema nodosum

Mono- or polyarthropathy

Peripheral neuropathy

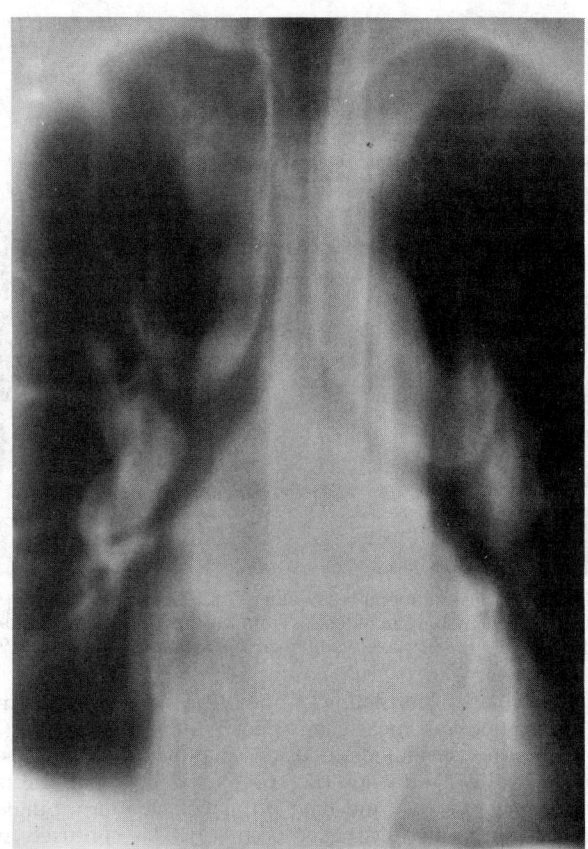

FIGURE 69–3. Tomogram of chest showing hilar and paratracheal adenopathy. (From Murray JF, Nadel J: Textbook of Respiratory Medicine. Philadelphia, WB Saunders Company, 1987.)

macular and papular lesions that are present either superficially or more deeply in the dermis. *Lupus pernio*, consisting of violaceous plaques over the nose, cheeks, and ears, is the most commonly described skin lesion. It may be disfiguring. Granulomas may also occur in scar tissue.

Eyes

Ophthalmologic lesions most commonly consist of inflammation of the uveal tract, but involvement of the conjunctiva, retina, and lacrimal glands may also occur. These lesions may produce nonspecific ocular symptoms of visual impairment and discomfort; chronic lesions may progress to blindness. Anterior uveitis in combination with parotitis and facial nerve palsy has been referred to as *Heerfordt's syndrome*.

Nervous System

Almost any portion of the neurologic system may be involved by sarcoidosis, and the diagnosis may prove difficult. The most common cranial nerve to be involved is the facial nerve, but any cranial nerve may be affected. Disease of the optic nerve may result in papilledema. Palsies of the ninth and tenth cranial nerves manifest as dysphagia, absent gag reflex, and vocal cord paralysis, and disease of the eighth cranial nerve occurs as deafness, tinnitus, and vertigo. Mono- or polyneuropathy of peripheral nerves causes sensory loss, paresthesias, or motor weakness. Meningitis produced by sarcoidosis is usually insidious in presentation and chronic in its course. Diabetes insipidus results from involvement of the hypothalamus or posterior pituitary gland. Granulomas of the brain may produce a space-occupying lesion and cause headaches, seizures, or focal symptoms. Rarely, personality changes have been observed, and the total constellation of findings resulting from multiple areas of involvement of the nervous system by sarcoidosis may bewilder the diagnostician.

Heart

Although cardiac granulomas are often present on autopsies of patients with sarcoidosis, symptomatic cardiac involvement is unusual. Granulomatous or fibrotic cardiac lesions resulting from sarcoidosis may cause congestive heart failure, heart block, arrhythmias (often ventricular), angina pectoris, ventricular aneurysm, recurrent pericardial effusion, or sudden death. Since these abnormalities may also be due to other causes, it may be difficult to prove a relationship to sarcoidosis. Cor pulmonale is an infrequent presentation, occurring usually in association with advanced pulmonary fibrosis, but there has been the rare report of pulmonary hypertension without severe restrictive lung disease.

Kidneys

Granulomas of the kidneys are usually infrequent and asymptomatic. When kidney failure occurs, other lesions such as pyelonephritis, nephrocalcinosis, and hyalinization of various kidney structures are present. The kidneys may be severely and irreversibly damaged by calcium nephropathy caused by altered calcium metabolism that produces hypercalcemia and hypercalciuria. Symptoms of kidney failure may be the predominant feature of sarcoidosis in these cases. Sarcoid lesions can enzymatically activate vitamin D precursors to 1,25-dihydroxycholecalciferol, thereby increasing intestinal absorption of calcium. The result may be hypercalcemia and hypercalciuria, with renal damage from nephrocalcinosis and recurrent nephrolithiasis.

Musculoskeletal System

Bones, joints, and muscles are frequently involved in sarcoidosis. Bone changes are found most commonly in chronic cases and are particularly common in blacks with chronic skin disease. The phalanges, metacarpals, and metatarsals are the bones most frequently involved. Osteoporosis, cystic or reticulated changes, and external manifestations of digital deformation and dystrophic nails may be present. Joints are usually spared destructive changes except in the vicinity of bone lesions.

Arthritic changes may also manifest acutely by mono- or polyarthralgias or arthritis of the larger joints, such as the ankles, knees, wrists, or elbows. The associated symptoms may be migratory and usually recede with no residual deformities. Although, like the liver, muscles frequently contain asymptomatic granulomas, acute myositis or chronic myopathy with associated muscular enzyme abnormalities are uncommon findings in sarcoidosis. Gout may complicate sarcoidosis, presumably owing to overproduction of purines in widespread granulomas.

Miscellaneous

Although diffuse granulomas may be present, clinical manifestations of liver, gastrointestinal, or pancreatic disease are very unusual. Similarly, clinical evidence for involvement of the endocrine and reproductive systems is rare. As noted earlier, posterior pituitary and hypothalamic involvement may result in diabetes insipidus. Hypopituitarism from anterior pituitary disease occurs very rarely and, when present, is associated with diabetes insipidus. Alteration in fertility by sarcoidosis has not been described. Peripheral lymph nodes, in contrast to hilar nodes, are seldom more than moderately enlarged and usually go unnoticed by the patient. Although the spleen is moderately enlarged in 5 to 10 per cent of patients, gross enlargement that causes discomfort and predisposes to rupture occurs rarely. Thrombocytopenia is occasionally present and may be associated with hypersplenism.

PHYSICAL FINDINGS

Physical findings in the chest in sarcoidosis are often normal despite radiographic abnormalities that may be extensive.

Fever is absent, except with Loeffgren's syndrome. Other physical findings usually relate to granulomatous or fibrotic involvement of a specific organ system. Skin lesions may be readily apparent or found only with careful examination. Subcutaneous or muscle nodules may be identified. Slit-lamp examination may be necessary to demonstrate ocular lesions. Lymph nodes are often palpable but usually only moderately enlarged. As noted above, hepatosplenomegaly may be present. Digits may be deformed by bone lesions, and the nails may be dystrophic in cases of chronic disease. Acute arthritic changes may be apparent, in particular in association with erythema nodosum, and must be differentiated from associated gout.

ROUTINE LABORATORY STUDIES

Routine laboratory evaluation may reveal lymphopenia, hyperglobulinemia, hypercalcemia, and/or hypercalciuria. The platelet count is rarely decreased. It is unusual for the sedimentation rate to be significantly elevated, except with Loeffgren's syndrome. Liver function tests may be moderately abnormal, and, in particular, alkaline phosphatase levels may be elevated. With complications of the disease, the expected but nonspecific changes in arterial blood gases and serum chemistries accompany respiratory or renal failure, respectively. Cerebrospinal fluid examination may show nonspecific pleocytosis and increased protein in meningitis caused by sarcoidosis.

DIFFERENTIAL DIAGNOSIS

The differential diagnosis of sarcoidosis depends largely upon the clinical presentation of the patient. With hilar lymphadenopathy, lymphoma is most frequently considered; with pulmonary parenchymal disease, a wide variety of diffuse interstitial diseases must be considered (Ch. 63). Tuberculosis and other granulomatous pulmonary infections must always be ruled out. Eosinophilic granuloma is another diagnostic possibility, particularly when diabetes insipidus is present. Exposure to beryllium may produce disease very similar to sarcoidosis. Pulmonary sarcoid nodules raise the possibilities of primary or metastatic tumor. Conglomerate lesions with hilar retraction or eggshell calcification of lymph nodes may be confused with silicosis. Hypercalcemia in sarcoidosis raises the question of a number of metabolic or malignant disorders, especially primary hyperparathyroidism (Ch. 247). Arthritis or arthralgia associated with sarcoidosis may be confused with acute rheumatic fever or gout. The isolated finding of granulomas on biopsy of various tissues raises the possibilities of foreign body reactions, fungal or tubercular infections, and malignancy associated with granulomatous reactions. Granulomas occurring only in the liver may result in confusion between granulomatous hepatitis and sarcoidosis. The presence of granulomas in the intestinal wall may suggest Crohn's disease. Finally, renal and hepatic impairment or cardiac abnormalities occurring in sarcoidosis may be caused by more common co-existing diseases rather than by sarcoidosis itself.

RADIOLOGIC EVALUATION

Radiologic evaluation of the chest is particularly useful in sarcoidosis, since the disease is so often asymptomatic and so often involves the thorax. Radiologic abnormalities that occur in sarcoidosis have been arbitrarily classified as follows: Grade 0—absence of abnormal radiographic findings; Grade 1—lymph node enlargement without pulmonary parenchymal abnormalities; Grade 2A—combination of lymph node and diffuse pulmonary parenchymal disease; Grade 2B—diffuse parenchymal disease without lymph node enlargement; and Grade 3—radiographic changes indicating more chronic disease with pulmonary fibrosis ("honeycombing" or hilar retraction). The most frequent parenchymal abnormality is re-

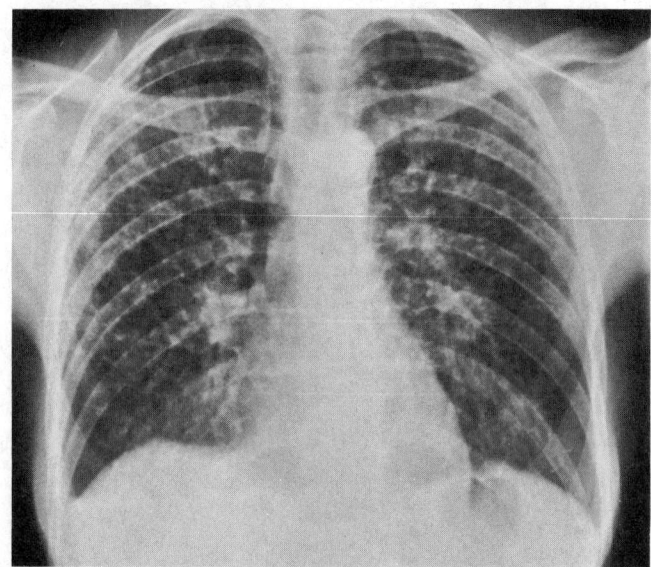

FIGURE 69–4. Chest radiograph showing typical reticulonodular appearance of parenchymal sarcoidosis. (From Murray JF, Nadel J: Textbook of Respiratory Medicine. Philadelphia, WB Saunders Company, 1987.)

ticulonodularity, consisting of fine linear densities and small, irregular nodules measuring 3 to 5 mm in diameter (Fig. 69–4). Large, conglomerate lesions may be present in association with hilar retraction (Fig. 69–5). Parenchymal infiltrates are at times "fluffy" and have an alveolar pattern. Single or multiple large nodules may occur and be confused with tumor. Small nodules may cause a miliary pattern suggestive of tuberculosis.

A large variety of other changes may be present on the radiograph. Pleural effusion occurs rarely in sarcoidosis. Mediastinal or hilar lymph nodes may show eggshell calcification. In addition to bullous changes, true cavities may be present that, at times, contain mycetomas. Lobar atelectasis may be caused by intrabronchial granulomas, and postobstructive bronchiectasis may be present. In addition to the more common locations in the short tubular bones of the hands and feet, lytic or sclerotic bone lesions may occur in the ribs.

Computed tomographic (CT) scans can demonstrate lymphadenopathy more clearly and, in particular, can detect anterior mediastinal and subcarinal lymph nodes that have gone

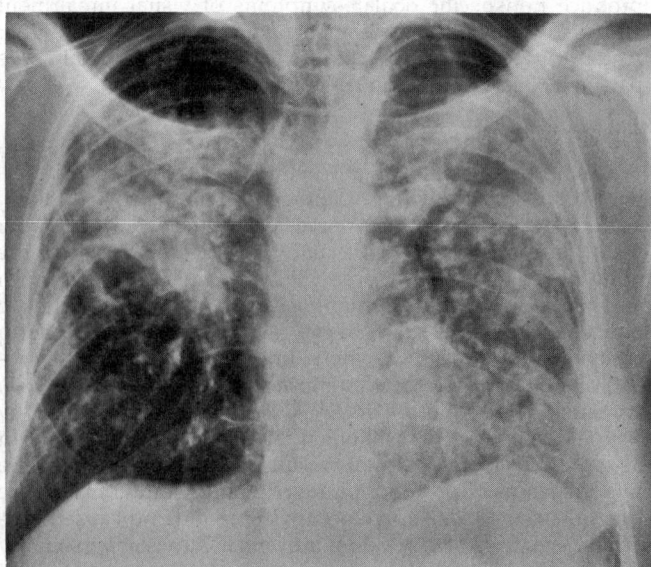

FIGURE 69–5. Chest radiograph showing large conglomerate lesions associated with hilar retraction. (From Murray JF, Nadel J: Textbook of Respiratory Medicine. Philadelphia, WB Saunders Company, 1987.)

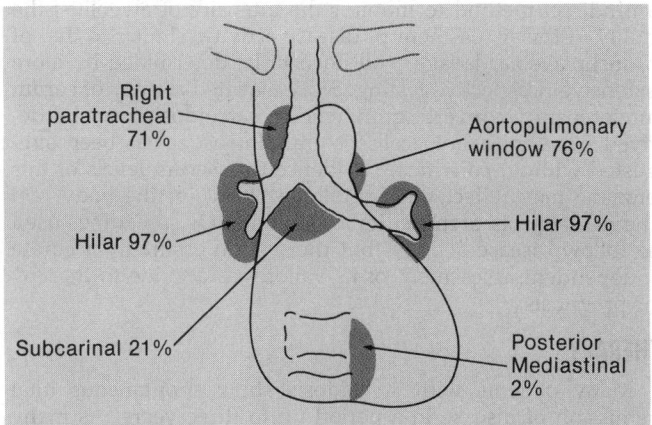

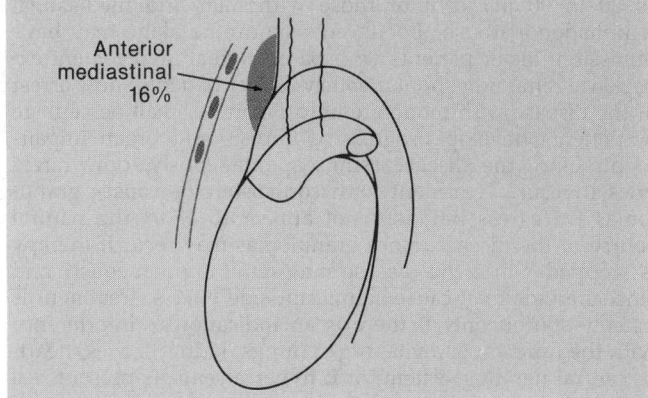

FIGURE 69–6. Schematic representation of CT detection of thoracic lymphadenopathy in sarcoidosis.

undetected on conventional films of the chest (Fig. 69–6). This examination, however, is needed in only a limited number of patients with sarcoidosis.

PHYSIOLOGIC CHANGES

The most common pulmonary physiologic changes occurring in sarcoidosis are decreases in vital capacity and diffusing capacity. Although useful in determining the extent of functional impairment at the onset and in following the course of the disease, physiologic changes do not correlate well with symptoms or radiologic abnormalities. At times pulmonary function studies are totally normal despite radiologic evidence of pulmonary disease. Conversely, functional abnormalities, especially of diffusing capacity, may be present when the lung parenchyma appears normal radiographically. Evidence of airway disease may also be present, and, at times, this is the predominant feature of sarcoidosis, causing confusion with asthma. An elevation in arterial P_{CO_2} is unusual, but moderate arterial hypoxemia may be present. As with other interstitial diseases, arterial hypoxemia often worsens with exercise.

APPROACH TO DIAGNOSIS

With a very typical presentation (i.e., bilateral symmetric hilar and paratracheal lymphadenopathy in an asymptomatic patient 20 to 40 years of age or in one with erythema nodosum, uveitis, and arthralgias), the clinical diagnosis of sarcoidosis can be made with a high degree of certainty by physicians familiar with this disease (Table 69–1). In all other cases in which the diagnosis is less clear, further support must be obtained by examination of biopsy material.

Diagnosis by Biopsy

Typical sarcoid granulomas consist of whorls of epithelioid cells surrounding multinucleated giant cells, which may or may not contain inclusion bodies (Fig. 69–7). Mononuclear

TABLE 69–1. FEATURES CONSIDERED IN THE DIAGNOSIS OF SARCOIDOSIS

Primary
1. Clinical and radiologic presentation
2. Biopsy material showing granuloma, but no mycobacterial, fungi, or refractile material

Secondary
1. Anergy to skin tests
2. Positive Kveim-Siltzbach reaction (infrequently performed)
3. Significant elevation of serum angiotensin I–converting enzyme with exclusion of other obvious diseases associated with elevation (i.e., Gaucher's disease, leprosy, and so on)

Current Research Modalities
1. Evaluation of cells obtained by bronchial lavage
2. Gallium-67 scanning

cells are present at the periphery of the granulomas, and various amounts of fibrosis and/or hyalinization are present throughout the tissue. True caseation does not occur. The histologic appearance, even when typical, is always nonspecific. To strengthen the diagnosis of sarcoidosis, infectious agents and foreign bodies must be excluded by special stains, cultures, and examination under polarized light.

What tissue should be examined by biopsy? In the absence of specific skin lesions, transbronchial biopsy of the lung is usually most specific, since rarely, if ever, will nonspecific granulomas be found (in contrast to liver or lymph nodes). Approximately 60 per cent of patients with sarcoidosis show granulomas on transbronchial lung biopsy even if their chest radiographs are normal; this number increases to 85 to 90 per cent when there is a parenchymal abnormality on chest radiograph. If the transbronchial biopsy yields negative findings but a high suspicion of sarcoidosis exists and there is obvious parenchymal disease on the chest radiograph, a repeat transbronchial biopsy may be justified. Other reasonable approaches at this juncture of evaluation include mediastinoscopy or, at times, open lung biopsy.

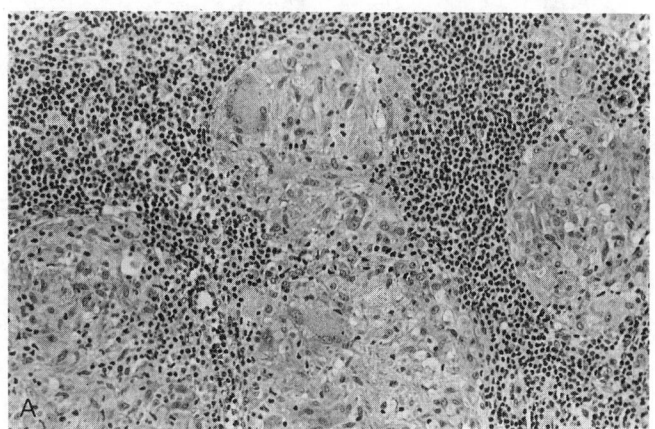

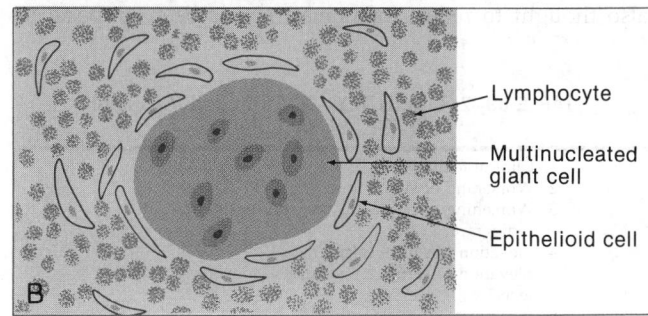

FIGURE 69–7. Typical histologic appearance of granuloma of sarcoidosis with accompanying schematic representation.

Blind conjunctival, lacrimal gland, or gingival biopsies are frequently not rewarding in the absence of overt disease at these locations. When these organs are involved, however, the yield is high. Biopsies of skin lesions are particularly useful, since they may show granuloma and, in association with other findings, may provide an easy diagnosis, if foreign body granuloma can be excluded. Biopsy of identifiable subcutaneous or muscle lesions also may be diagnostic. Biopsy of lesions of erythema nodosum shows a nonspecific panniculitis or vasculitis and therefore is not useful. Other localized lesions, such as those of the pharynx or larynx, require direct biopsy for diagnosis. Diagnosis by biopsy sometimes becomes problematic for neurologic disease caused by sarcoidosis when other tissues do not provide a positive diagnosis, since the involved tissue is often not easily accessible.

Other Available Tests

The Kveim-Siltzbach test lacks precision, and the required antigen is not readily available. It is therefore rarely used. Anergy to delayed hypersensitivity skin test antigens is a frequent finding but is obviously not diagnostic of sarcoidosis. Similarly, characterization of cells obtained by bronchial lavage and the use of gallium-67 scanning of the lungs are not in themselves diagnostic of sarcoidosis, although abnormalities consistent with that diagnosis may be found. For this reason, and because of cost and radiation exposure, these last two tests are not justified currently for diagnosis in clinical practice.

Serum angiotensin I–converting enzyme activity is often elevated in sarcoidosis, but a number of other diseases may be similarly associated with its increased activity (i.e., miliary tuberculosis, leprosy, Gaucher's disease). If these diseases can be readily excluded, measurement of this enzyme may be useful. This is the case when the primary diagnostic considerations are lymphoma and sarcoidosis, since angiotensin I–converting enzyme activity is not increased in lymphoma. Elevations of other proteolytic enzymes in serum, such as lysozyme and thermolysin-like metalloendopeptidase, have been evaluated but are not yet commonly used for diagnostic purposes.

ACTIVITY OF DISEASE

Sarcoidosis may remit spontaneously; the concept of "activity of disease" is therefore useful when considering therapeutic strategies (Table 69–2). "Activity of disease" is very difficult to define, since occult granulomatous lesions may exist throughout many tissues of the body. Clinical findings provide some indication of activity of disease, but often in a nonquantitative and imprecise way, especially when the patient is relatively asymptomatic. Radiologic and pulmonary function study changes also may be helpful in assessing "activity of disease." Bronchoalveolar lavage to measure the percentage of lymphocytes as a reflection of parenchymal inflammation has been advocated. A high percentage of lymphocytes has been referred to as high-intensity alveolitis, denoting a poorer prognosis, but this approach has not gained wide acceptance. Gallium-67 scanning of the lung, which is also thought to reflect inflammation, has been proposed as

an indirect method to monitor the intensity of alveolitis; the utility of this assessment of disease activity, similar to that of bronchoalveolar lavage, will need to be determined by more extensive prospective testing. Since elevated activity of serum angiotensin I–converting enzyme in sarcoidosis may be derived from epithelioid cells or granulomas, it has been suggested without convincing evidence that serum levels of this enzyme may reflect the granuloma "load" of the body. On the basis of this premise, its measurement is sometimes used to follow disease activity, but there is no assuredly accurate independent assessment of its validity as a guide to therapy or prognosis.

THERAPY

Many patients with sarcoidosis show spontaneous total remission of disease in a period up to three years. As many as 80 to 90 per cent of those with hilar and mediastinal lymphadenopathy or Loeffgren's syndrome alone may have remission; fewer patients with parenchymal involvement experience remission spontaneously. Other patients show arrest of the disease with moderate fibrosis, and a small percentage of patients develop progressive fibrosis and organ impairment. Once the disease remits spontaneously, only rarely does it recur. Treatment with corticosteroids causes granulomas to regress but does not appear to affect the natural course of the disease, since granulomas may recur if therapy is stopped. Since the disease may remit spontaneously and since steroids may cause significant side effects, treatment is usually started only if there is an indication of interference with the function of a vital organ (lungs, kidneys, eyes, heart, or central nervous system) or if hypercalcemia is present. All patients with sarcoidosis should be followed carefully so that therapy can be started as soon as deterioration of organ function has been detected.

Prednisone is usually the drug of choice for the treatment of sarcoidosis. The usual starting dose is 30 to 40 mg per day, but at times a schedule of 50 to 60 mg every other day is used for initial therapy. A response in terms of symptoms or radiologic findings should be seen within two to four weeks. The steroid dose should be tapered after several weeks, and the eventual maintenance dose should be the lowest one that is effective in maintaining the response that is being followed (see below). Often 10 to 15 mg of prednisone every other day, a dose that has a low risk of side effects, will suffice. Attempts to stop therapy may be tried after several months, but evidence of disease activity (symptoms, chest radiographic abnormalities, or worsening of pulmonary function) may recur, and prednisone may have to be restarted.

What are the best parameters to follow as indicators of disease activity? As noted earlier, measurements of disease activity are imprecise. Certainly, clinical symptoms should be assessed carefully, and chest radiographic and pulmonary function changes often give indication of disease activity. However, both radiographic abnormalities and pulmonary function changes correlate poorly with clinical parameters. Serum angiotensin I–converting enzyme levels are easily obtained and may provide clues to activity, but tests such as bronchial lavage and gallium-67 scanning are still largely experimental. Failure of response may indicate irreversible fibrosis, a situation in which steroid therapy causes more potential risk than benefit.

All of the usual side effects associated with steroid therapy may occur in patients treated for sarcoidosis (Ch. 30). The dose can usually be reduced sufficiently, however, so that infection with opportunistic organisms occurs rarely. Cosmetic problems of weight gain and fluid accumulation are often the most bothersome side effects. More difficult decisions about steroid therapy arise when there are associated disorders, such as diabetes mellitus, that may be exacerbated by these agents. Since tuberculin skin tests will become positive in patients with sarcoidosis who contract tuberculosis,

---

TABLE 69–2. CURRENTLY ACCEPTED INDICATORS OF "ACTIVITY" OF SARCOIDOSIS

1. Clinical features
2. Worsening of symptoms
3. Worsening of pulmonary function tests/chest radiograph
4. Elevation of serum calcium level
5. Elevation of serum angiotensin I–converting enzyme level?
6. Gallium scanning positivity?
7. Evidence of alveolitis on bronchial lavage?

appropriate prophylaxis or treatment should be given when the tuberculin skin test is positive or converts to positivity.

Topical steroids have been used for dermatologic and ophthalmologic lesions, and chloroquine and methotrexate have been used for sarcoidosis of the skin. Indomethacin and other nonsteroidal anti-inflammatory agents may be useful for arthritis occurring in Loeffgren's syndrome. Aerosolized steroids approved for use in the United States have not been effective for pulmonary sarcoidosis, but other aerosolized preparations are being tried in Europe. Sarcoidosis that manifests with bronchoconstriction does not respond well to conventional bronchodilator therapy other than steroids. It remains to be determined whether avoidance of sunlight will significantly influence calcium metabolism in sarcoidosis.

Bascom R, Johns CJ: The natural history and management of sarcoidosis. Adv Intern Med 31:213, 1986. *This is an excellent general review of this controversial area, with 138 references.*

Crystal RG, Roberts WC, Hunninghake GW, et al.: Pulmonary sarcoidosis: A disease characterized and perpetuated by activated lung T-lymphocytes. Ann Intern Med 94:73, 1981. *A good review of immunologic features in sarcoidosis.*

Delaney P: Neurologic manifestations in sarcoidosis, review of the literature with a report of 23 cases. Ann Intern Med 87:336, 1977.

Fanburg BL: Sarcoidosis and Other Granulomatous Diseases of the Lung. New York, Marcel Dekker, 1983. *A comprehensive textbook covering both clinical and experimental aspects of sarcoidosis.*

James DG, Williams WJ: Sarcoidosis and Other Granulomatous Disorders. Philadelphia, W. B. Saunders Company, 1985. *Another good monograph with an extensive review of all phases of sarcoidosis. Excellent clinical descriptions and comprehensive references.*

Roberts WC, McAllister HA Jr, Ferrans VJ: Sarcoidosis of the heart: A clinicopathologic study of 35 necropsy patients (Group I) and review of 78 previously described necropsy patients (Group II). Am J Med 63:86, 1977.

Rockoff SD, Ronatagi PK: Unusual manifestations of thoracic sarcoidosis. Am J Radiol 144:513, 1985. *A comprehensive coverage of radiologic features of sarcoidosis.*

Venet A, Hance AJ, Saltini C, et al.: Enhanced alveolar macrophage-mediated antigen-induced T-lymphocyte proliferation in sarcoidosis. J Clin Invest 75:293, 1985. *Further information about immunologic abnormalities in sarcoidosis.*

70 PULMONARY NEOPLASMS

Charles H. Scoggin

The lung can be involved in a variety of neoplasms (Table 70–1). Bronchogenic carcinoma accounts for over 90 per cent of all lung tumors. The major management questions of lung cancer are the following: Is the tumor resectable? Is the tumor small cell lung cancer? Other tumors may metastasize to the lung. Benign tumors of the lung are infrequent compared with malignant tumors.

BRONCHOGENIC CARCINOMA

Lung cancer, a primary neoplasm arising within the airways, is a frequent and important neoplasm. In the United States it is the leading fatal neoplasm of men and women. In 1985 approximately 135,000 cases of lung cancer were diagnosed in the United States, and approximately 110,000 people died of the cancer. The medical care of patients with lung cancer in the United States is estimated to cost more than $10 billion annually, approximately 1.5 per cent of the national health care expenditure. Lung cancer is strongly associated with the use of tobacco products, particularly with cigarettes. Although surgery or radiation therapy may lead to eradication of tumors in a small number of patients, the majority of people with lung cancer will have advanced disease at the time of diagnosis and will die of the disorder within one year of its detection. Determining the cell type and the stage of the disease is important in the clinical management of lung cancer, since these factors will affect treatment and prognosis. Four types of tumors account for 95 per cent of all lung

TABLE 70–1. WORLD HEALTH ORGANIZATION CLASSIFICATION OF LUNG TUMORS

I. Epithelial tumors
  A. Benign
    1. Papillomas (squamous cell and "transitional")
    2. Adenomas (includes pleomorphic and monomorphic)
  B. Dysplasia, carcinoma in situ
  C. Malignant
    1. Squamous cell carcinoma (epidermoid carcinoma)
    2. Small cell carcinoma
    3. Adenocarcinoma (includes acinar, papillary, bronchiolar, alveolar, and solid with mucus formation)
    4. Large cell carcinoma (giant cell and clear cell)
    5. Adenosquamous carcinoma
    6. Carcinoid tumor
    7. Bronchial gland carcinomas (includes adenoid cystic and mucoepidermoid carcinoma)
    8. Others
II. Soft tissue tumors
III. Mesothelial tumors
  A. Benign mesothelioma
  B. Malignant mesothelioma
IV. Miscellaneous tumors
  A. Benign
  B. Malignant
    1. Carcinosarcoma
    2. Pulmonary blastoma
    3. Malignant melanoma
    4. Malignant lymphoma
    5. Others
V. Secondary tumors
VI. Unclassified tumors
VII. Tumor-like lesions
  A. Hamartoma
  B. Lymphoproliferative lesions
  C. Tumorlet
  D. Eosinophilic granuloma
  E. "Sclerosing hemangioma"
  F. Inflammatory pseudotumor
  G. Other

malignancies: squamous cell (epidermoid), adenocarcinoma (including alveolar cell), large cell (also known as large cell anaplastic), and small cell lung cancer. Small cell lung cancer is distinguished from other types of lung cancer because it often shows a clinical response to chemotherapy.

Incidence and Prevalence

No population group is exempt from lung cancer. Lung cancer is the leading cause of cancer-related death of men in 28 developed countries of the world. In 1986 lung cancer surpassed breast cancer as the leading cause of death from cancer in women in the United States. The worldwide incidence of lung cancer is anticipated to continue to increase owing to the spread of the use of cigarettes, particularly in the Third World.

Lung cancer as a major health problem is a phenomenon of the twentieth century. In 1912, only 374 cases of primary lung neoplasms had been reported in the world's medical literature. There is little doubt that the exposure to cigarette smoke and other carcinogens accounts for the rapid increase in the occurrence of lung cancer.

The exact incidence of each type of lung cancer is difficult to determine. Squamous cell carcinoma is thought to be the most frequent form of the tumor (30 to 35 per cent of all cases), followed by adenocarcinoma, large cell carcinoma, and small cell carcinoma. Adenocarcinoma may be the most frequent lung cancer of women currently, but there is evidence that small cell lung cancer may soon surpass it.

Lung cancer occurs principally between the ages of 45 and 75 years. All histologic types of lung cancer in men peak at approximately 70 to 74 years of age. In women adenocarcinoma peaks at an earlier age than in men (50 to 59 years).

Epidemiology

CIGARETTE SMOKING. About 80 to 90 per cent of all cases of lung cancer are caused by smoking cigarettes (see also Ch. 11 and 170). It is estimated that there are 50 million smokers in the United States. Cigarette smoking causes cancer in humans and experimental animals in a dose-dependent manner. Consumption of cigarettes is commonly quantitated as number of packs smoked per day and number of years smoked ("pack years"). A person who has smoked two packs per day for 20 years (40 pack years) has a 60- to 70-fold increased risk of developing lung cancer compared with a person who has never smoked. Because the duration of smoking is strongly associated with risk of lung cancer, the incidence and death rate from lung cancer are highest in the older age groups. Other factors that are important are depth of inhalation and tar and nicotine content of cigarettes.

Decreased smoking of cigarettes is associated epidemiologically with a declining incidence of lung cancer. A reduction in the prevalence of smoking among men in Sweden, Australia, Canada, and the United States has resulted in a reduction or slowing of deaths from lung cancer in men. A lag phase of about 20 years exists between an increase in cigarette smoking in a particular population and a rise in deaths from lung cancer. This lag is reflected in the current rise in deaths, from lung cancer among women of the United States, among whom there was an increase in cigarette consumption in the 1950's. A similar phenomenon is thought to account for increasing occurrence of lung cancer among Japanese men.

Passive inhalation of cigarette smoke may also be a risk factor for lung cancer. It is estimated that 4700 nonsmoking Americans died in 1985 from bronchogenic cancer due to passive smoking. Sidestream smoke has a higher concentration than mainstream smoke of carcinogens such as nitrosamines, naphthalene, and benzopyrene.

OCCUPATIONAL ASSOCIATIONS. Occupational exposures also increase the incidence of lung cancer: uranium (in miners), haloethers (such as dichloromethyl ether and chloromethyl methyl ether), arsenical fumes, isopropyl oil, nickel, metallic iron, iron oxide, and beryllium. Asbestos exposure in nonsmokers is associated with a four to fivefold increased incidence of lung cancer. Asbestos and radon gas probably act as cocarcinogens with cigarette smoke. Smoking increases the risk of bronchogenic cancer 80- to 90-fold in persons also exposed to asbestos. Radon gas exposure may also occur as an environmental pollutant in heavily insulated homes. As many as 12 per cent of homes in the United States may contain unhealthy levels of radon gas. Chronic inflammation of the lung, such as from interstitial fibrosis and areas of scarring, is associated with the occurrence of adenocarcinoma. Certain genetic determinants, such as levels of aryl hydrocarbon hydroxylase, may also be important.

Pathogenesis

CELL OF ORIGIN. The development of lung cancer is a multistep process. The pulmonary endodermal cell seem to be the common stem cell of origin of all lung cancer cell types. Because it demonstrates certain amine precursor uptake and decarboxylation (APUD) properties, small cell lung cancer has been hypothesized to arise from Kulchitsky's cell. There is no direct evidence to support this hypothesis, however.

CIGARETTE SMOKE. Cigarette smoke contains many carcinogens in both the gaseous and the particulate phases. Nitrosamines and other compounds are thought to be important in the gaseous phase. Carcinogens in the particulate phase include benzopyrene and related polycyclic aromatic hydrocarbons, nitrosonornicotine, polonium, and arsenic. Reduction in particulate factors correlates with decreased incidence of lung cancer. A 20 per cent reduction in risk of lung cancer has been associated with a 50 per cent reduction in tar delivery in cigarettes in the United States, Canada, and other countries.

CELLULAR CHANGES. In the natural history of bronchogenic cancer, bronchial epithelial cells first become cytologically abnormal. At this stage, they are not malignant nor are they invariably predictive of the eventual development of malignancy. The next step is carcinoma in situ, i.e., carcinomatous changes localized above the basement membrane and productive of no symptoms. The next change is epidermal invasion by tumor cells, followed by metastasis of the tumor. In situ tumors are indolent and slow growing. As malignancy progresses, so too does the rapidity of tumor spread.

CELLULAR EVENTS. Three aspects of the cellular events that attend the transformation of normal bronchial epithelial cells to malignant cells are important: (1) damage to cellular deoxyribonucleic acid (DNA); (2) alteration in cellular oncogene expression; and (3) tumor-derived factors that stimulate cellular division.

Cigarette smoke, ionizing radiation, and chemical carcinogens damage cellular DNA, in part through inducing chromosomal deletions and rearrangements and point mutations. The most widely recognized chromosomal abnormality seen in lung cancer is a deletion of genetic material in the 3p14 to 23 region in the malignant, but not the normal, cells of patients with small cell lung cancer. Activation of oncogenes appears to be a common event in bronchogenic carcinoma (Ch. 169). Expression of members of both the *ras* and the *myc* oncogene families has been found in lung tumor cells, in contrast to normal lung cells. Another important factor is the production of so-called autocrine growth factors by lung cancer cells. Cultured small cell lung cancer cells secrete growth factors into their media. This is thought to account for their decreased requirement for serum growth factors. One such factor is bombesin/gastrin–related peptide. These growth factors stimulate cell division constantly. They may be of future clinical importance in that monoclonal antibodies to bombesin/gastrin–related peptide inhibit tumor growth of cells in culture and in experimental animals.

Clinical Manifestations

SYMPTOMS OF LUNG CANCER (Table 70–2). Most patients with lung cancer have some symptoms that cause them to seek medical attention. A typical patient will present with pulmonary complaints such as cough, hemoptysis, and weight loss. Only 5 to 15 per cent of patients are asymptomatic when discovered to have bronchogenic carcinoma.

Some Characteristics of Specific Tumors. Squamous cell, or epidermoid, carcinoma usually begins as a central lesion that tends to invade locally. The patient often presents with symptoms referable to the airways, such as cough, dyspnea, or hemoptysis. It may also invade the chest wall, diaphragm, or mediastinum. Unlike other primary lung neoplasms, squamous cell tumors may cavitate.

Adenocarcinoma usually begins as a peripheral lesion. It is more aggressive than squamous cell carcinoma. Symptoms at the time of diagnosis often reflect invasion of lymph nodes, pleura, or the other lung or metastasis to other organs, such as the central nervous system or adrenal glands. *Bronchioloalveolar carcinoma*, a special subtype of adenocarcinoma, usually accounts for no more than 1 to 5 per cent of primary lung neoplasms. Bronchioloalveolar carcinoma often manifests as

TABLE 70–2. CLINICAL MANIFESTATIONS OF LUNG CARCINOMA

1. Due to primary lesions

Cough	Wheezing
Dyspnea	Weight loss
Hemoptysis	Fever
Sputum	Pneumonia

2. Due to local extension

Chest pain	Dysphagia
Hoarseness	Pericardial effusion
Superior vena cava syndrome	Pleural effusion
Pancoast's syndrome	Diaphragm paralysis
Horner's syndrome	

3. Extrapulmonary manifestations (see Table 171–1, p 1097)

a solitary pulmonary nodule (approximately 60 per cent) but may also appear as a localized infiltrate or area of lobar consolidation mimicking infection. *Large cell carcinoma* usually manifests as a bulky peripheral mass.

Small cell lung cancer should be carefully distinguished from non–small cell lung cancer, from which it differs both in biologic features and in clinical manifestations (Table 70–3). Small cell lung cancer commonly begins as a central tumor, but 70 to 90 per cent of patients have disease outside the original hemithorax at the time of detection. Because of its propensity to metastasize and to produce paraneoplastic syndromes, small cell lung cancer is usually symptomatic for three months or less before diagnosis. In contrast, symptoms associated with squamous cell carcinoma appear, on the average, eight months before the diagnosis is made, and up to 25 per cent of patients with adenocarcinoma are asymptomatic at presentation. The severity of symptoms is also an important prognostic factor, particularly in small cell lung cancer. The more severe the tumor symptoms, the worse the prognosis.

Symptoms Referable to the Chest. Most patients with bronchogenic carcinomas present with symptoms referable to the chest, sometimes reflecting the area of lung involved. Central or endobronchial tumors can manifest as dyspnea, cough, hemoptysis, wheezing, or pneumonitis with fever and purulent sputum. Even small tumors may cause a disproportionately high degree of dyspnea. Hemoptysis, a common complaint, is more frequent in non–small cell lung cancer, since small cell lung cancer is often submucosal in location without ulceration into the airway itself. Peripheral tumors may manifest as chest pain due to pleural or chest wall involvement.

Spread to thoracic lymph nodes is common in lung cancer, especially in small cell lung cancer. Regional spread to hilar and mediastinal nodes may cause dysphagia due to esophageal compression, hoarseness because of recurrent laryngeal nerve compression, Horner's syndrome due to sympathetic nerve involvement, and elevation of the hemidiaphragm from phrenic nerve compression. Superior sulcus, or Pancoast's, tumor may involve the brachial plexus, resulting in a C7–T2 neuropathy with pain, numbness, and weakness of the arm.

Cardiac involvement is seen at autopsy in 20 to 25 per cent of patients with small cell lung cancer but less frequently in non–small cell lung cancer. Clinical findings of cardiac involvement are arrhythmias, cardiomegaly, and pericardial effusion with pericardial friction rub. Cardiac tamponade may occur.

Systemic Symptoms. Constitutional symptoms of anorexia, weight loss, and generalized weakness are common in lung cancer. Patients may also have fever without obvious infection.

Tumors that obstruct the superior vena cava cause the superior vena cava syndrome: swelling of the head and neck, breast enlargement, and prominence of the superficial veins of the thorax. Bronchogenic carcinoma, particularly small cell lung cancer, may demonstrate extrathoracic spread to other organ systems. Metastasis to the spinal cord causes spinal cord pain and symptoms of cord compression. Pain may precede weakness and sensory changes by days. Metastasis to the liver may cause pain, chemical dysfunction of the liver, and biliary obstruction. Metastasis to the bone may result in pain or bone marrow invasion.

Paraneoplastic Syndromes. Paraneoplastic syndromes are remote effects of tumor. They are described in detail in Ch. 173, 174, and 175, to which the reader is referred. They lead to metabolic and neuromuscular disturbances unrelated to the primary tumor, metastases, or treatment. Paraneoplastic syndromes may be the first sign of the tumor or of tumor recurrence. They do not necessarily indicate that a tumor has spread. Paraneoplastic syndromes often respond to treatment of the primary tumor. Osteoarthropathy associated with lung cancer is seen in up to 30 per cent of patients with lung cancer but is rare in patients with small cell lung cancer. Manifestations include digital clubbing and painful periosteal inflammation. Periosteal elevation usually involves the long bones. It may be confused with certain forms of arthritis, including rheumatoid arthritis. Endocrinologic manifestations are well recognized in bronchogenic carcinoma. Up to 10 per cent of epidermoid tumors secrete humoral factors resulting in hypercalcemia and hypophosphatemia. Metastasis to the adrenal glands may rarely result in adrenal insufficiency. Other endocrinologic manifestations, most common with small cell lung cancer, include Cushing's syndrome due to production of adrenocorticotropic hormone (ACTH), hyperpigmentation from production of melanocyte-stimulating hormone (MSH), and rarely the "somatostatinoma syndrome," which consists of vomiting, abdominal pain, diarrhea, mild diabetes, and cholelithiasis. Patients with lung cancer develop the syndrome of inappropriate antidiuretic hormone secretion (SIADH) in 10 to 15 per cent of cases (Ch. 173). Neuromyopathic manifestations of lung cancer are rare (< 1 per cent) but may dominate the clinical picture when they occur (Ch. 174). Such manifestations include the Eaton-Lambert syndrome (seen in small cell lung cancer), polymyositis, subacute cerebellar degeneration, spinocerebellar degeneration, and peripheral neuropathies. Nonbacterial (marantic) endocarditis, migratory thrombophebitis (Trousseau's syndrome), and disseminated intravascular coagulation as complications of malignancy are described in Ch. 171.

PHYSICAL FINDINGS OF LUNG CANCER. Physical examination often does not reflect either the presence of lung cancer or the state of the disease. Digital clubbing may be found in up to 12 per cent of patients and gynecomastia in 5 to 7 per cent of patients (the latter most frequently associated with large cell anaplastic cancer). Acanthosis nigricans may be found with adenocarcinoma, and hyperpigmentation of the palms and soles may be seen with squamous cell carci-

TABLE 70–3. COMPARISON BETWEEN NON–SMALL CELL LUNG CANCER AND SMALL CELL LUNG CANCER

	Small Cell Lung Cancer	Non–Small Cell Lung Cancer
Cytopathology	Scant cytoplasm; indistinct nucleoli	Large amount of cytoplasm; prominent nucleoli
Cytogenetics	Deletion 3p14→23	No known specific chromosomal alteration
Biochemistry and Hormone Production	Multiple enzymes and hormones (neuron-specific enolase, creatinine kinase BB, L-dopa decarboxylase, ACTH, bombesin, ADH, somatostatin, MSH)	Ectopic hormone production rare; paraneoplastic syndromes less common than in small cell lung cancer
Clinical Presentation	Hemoptysis rare; most patients symptomatic at presentation; usually metastatic at presentation	Hemoptysis common, symptoms less frequent at time of presentation; dissemination at presentation less common than in small cell carcinoma
Treatment		
Surgery	Seldom, if ever, indicated	Primary hope for cure
Radiation	Limited role; palliation and perhaps prophylaxis of CNS metastasis	Palliation, possible cure
Chemotherapy	Main treatment (up to 80 per cent response)	Effect on survival undetermined

ACTH = adrenocorticotropic hormone; ADH = antidiuretic hormone; MSH = melanocyte-stimulating hormone; CNS = central nervous system.

noma (Ch. 175). Obstruction of the superior vena cava may cause superior vena cava syndrome. Examination of the head may disclose the presence of Horner's syndrome, i.e., a unilaterally constricted pupil, enophthalmos, narrowed palpebral fissure, and loss of sweating on the same side of the face. Endobronchial obstruction may result in a localized wheeze detected during physical examination of the chest. Lobar collapse may result in an area of decreased breath sounds and dullness to percussion. Decreased movement of a hemidiaphragm may occur as a consequence of phrenic nerve compression. Liver metastasis may cause hepatic enlargement or nodularity. Weakness, altered reflexes, and decreased sensation may be found in patients with tumors metastatic to the central nervous system.

Diagnosis of Bronchogenic Carcinoma

The diagnosis of lung cancer requires detecting the tumor, establishing its cell type, and defining the stage of the malignancy. Determining cell type is important because it guides the approach both to staging and to treatment.

THE CHEST RADIOGRAPH. The presence of lung cancer is usually suggested by abnormalities on the chest radiograph. The most frequent finding is a mass in the lung field. Lesions usually cannot be detected if they are < 5 to 6 mm. Tumors occur in the right lung more than in the left (3:2) and in the upper lobes more than in the lower lobes. Secondary manifestations seen on chest radiograph include lobar collapse, pleural effusion, pneumonitis, elevation of the hemidiaphragm, hilar and mediastinal adenopathy, and erosion of ribs or vertebrae due to metastases. Alveolar cell cancer can manifest as a localized infiltrate mimicking pneumonia.

HISTOLOGIC DIAGNOSIS. When lung cancer is suspected, the next step in evaluation after the chest radiograph should be that of obtaining tissue specimens for histologic examination. The diagnostic yield of sputum cytologic evaluation will depend upon the adequacy of the specimen, the expertise of the cytologist, the type of tumor, and the number of specimens examined (three to four specimens are considered adequate). Sputum cytologic study is more likely to be negative in patients with small cell lung cancer than in those with non–small cell lung cancer. A negative sputum study should never be regarded as conclusive evidence for absence of carcinoma.

Bronchoscopy is important both for determining if a tumor is present and for obtaining tissue for histologic diagnosis. The combination of bronchial brushing and forceps biopsy is positive 90 to 93 per cent of the time with tumors located in proximal airways. Bronchial washings are less successful (approximately 80 per cent positive). For lesions than are not proximal enough in the airways for direct visualization, transbronchial biopsy with fluoroscopic guidance may be utilized. Yield of histologic diagnosis is 25 per cent for tumors less than 2 cm in diameter and 65 per cent for larger lesions. Transbronchial needle aspiration can also be employed. Peripheral lesions can be aspirated using a transthoracic needle with guidance by multiplane fluoroscopy or chest computerized tomography (CT). Success rates as high as 95 per cent have been reported. Pneumothorax is the major complication. Contraindications to pulmonary biopsy include pulmonary hypertension, hypoxemia with carbon dioxide retention, and a bleeding diathesis.

If a diagnosis is not established by cytologic study of the sputum, bronchoscopy, or needle biopsy, thoracotomy may be necessary. The decision to undertake thoracotomy should be a reasoned one, weighing the importance to the patient of making the diagnosis against other factors such as age or other complicating illness.

In some circumstances, a histologic diagnosis can be made by biopsy of metastatic sites such as liver, lymph nodes, bone, or bone marrow. When the pleural space is involved with

tumor, combined thoracentesis and pleural biopsy will provide a diagnostic yield of up to 90 per cent.

SCREENING STUDIES. Screening studies for early stages of lung cancer, using chest radiographs alone or in combination with sputum cytology, have been proposed for cigarette smokers who are 45 years of age or older. Early detection leads to higher resectability rate and longer survival from time of diagnosis (80 to 85 per cent five-year survival). Mass screening has not been shown to have an overall benefit, however, in decreasing mortality from lung cancer. Yearly sputum studies and chest radiographs may be reasonable in smokers over 45 years, particularly if they have been exposed to cocarcinogens such as asbestos or radon gas. Use of hematoporphyrin derivatives that accumulate in neoplastic tissue and are visible with fluorescent bronchoscopy is being explored as an adjunct to early diagnosis of lung cancer. Carcinoembryonic antigen (CEA), neural peptides, and neurogenic enzymes are not currently useful in detecting lung tumor, its metastases, or its recurrence.

Staging of Lung Cancer

Lung cancers are staged first for location (anatomic staging) and then for the patient's ability to withstand various treatments aimed at curing the tumor or increasing life expectancy (physiologic staging). Staging for non–small cell lung cancer differs from that for small cell lung cancer.

NON–SMALL CELL LUNG CANCER. For non–small cell lung cancer, the first and most important decision is whether or not the tumor is operable. Routine staging to exclude inoperable patients has increased survival of patients undergoing surgical resection of lung cancer. Table 70–4 lists a widely used tumor, node, and metastasis (TNM) system for classifying lung cancer.

Patients with stages I and II are considered candidates for surgical resection. Certain patients with stage III cancer may be candidates for surgery with postoperative irradiation of the mediastinum. Surgical resection of N2 disease is controversial. Detection of mediastinal lymph node involvement with cancer is best determined by mediastinoscopy for tumors in the right hemithorax. Tumor assessment of the left hemithorax requires an anterior exploration (Chamberlain procedure). Transbronchial and percutaneous needle aspiration is sometimes used to evaluate hilar lymph nodes. Size alone cannot be used to judge whether or not mediastinal lymph nodes are involved with metastatic cancer; however, enlarged nodes in the presence of known bronchogenic carcinoma argues strongly for metastatic disease. Computerized tomographic scanning of the chest is useful in excluding the presence of other tumors in the chest. In addition, scanning of the adrenal glands can be useful in determining if adrenal enlargement, possibly due to metastases, is present. Routine bone scan, CT scanning, liver scan, and bone radiographs are not recommended unless physical examination or history suggests that these organs are involved.

SMALL CELL LUNG CANCER. Small cell lung cancer has often metastasized at the time of diagnosis; the TNM system has not proved to be useful. Small cell lung cancer is defined as either limited or extensive (Table 70–5). Limited disease is confined to one hemithorax, with or without involvement of mediastinal lymph nodes. Spread of disease beyond this point is extensive. In addition, performance status is also an important prognostic factor. Survival correlates with degree of symptoms and functional impairment.

Treatment of Bronchogenic Carcinoma

NON–SMALL CELL LUNG CANCER. Both surgery and radiation therapy may benefit patients with non–small cell lung cancer, but chemotherapy remains experimental. Newer modalities such as laser bronchoscopy may lead to sympto-

TABLE 70–4. TNM CLASSIFICATION OF LUNG CANCER

Primary Tumor (T)

TX:	Tumor present as determined by presence of malignant cells in bronchopulmonary secretions, but not radiographically or bronchoscopically visible; no evidence of primary tumor
T0:	No evidence of primary tumor
T1S:	Carcinoma in situ
T1:	Tumor 3 cm or less surrounded by lung or visceral pleura, but without evidence of invasion proximal to lobar bronchus at bronchoscopy
T2:	Tumor more than 3 cm or tumor invading visceral pleura or associated with obstructive pneumonitis or atelectasis; involving less than entire lung; at broncoscopy, proximal extent of visible tumor must be within a lobar bronchus or at least 2.0 cm distal to carina
T3:	Tumor of any size with direct extension into chest wall, diaphragm, or mediastinal pleura or pericardium without involving heart, great vessels, trachea, esophagus, or vertebral body; also includes superior sulcus tumors and tumor in main bronchus within 2 cm of carina but not involving carina
T4:	Tumor of any size invading mediastinum or involving heart, great vessels, trachea, esophagus, vertebral body, or carina or presence of malignant pleural effusion.

Nodal Involvement

N0:	No demonstrable metastasis to regional lymph nodes
N1:	Metastasis to peribronchial or the ipsilateral, or both, hilar lymphnodes, including direct extension
N2:	Metastasis to ipsilateral mediastinal lymph nodes and subcarinal lymph nodes
N3:	Metastasis to contralateral mediastinal lymph nodes, contralateral hilar lymph nodes, ipsilateral or contralateral scalene or supraclavicular lymph nodes

Distant Metastasis (M)

M0:	No (known) distant metastasis
M1:	Distant metastasis present—specify site(s)

Stage Grouping

Occult carcinoma	TX	N0	M0
Stage 0	T1S	Carcinoma in situ	
Stage I	T1	N0	M0
	T2	N0	M0
Stage II	T1	N1	M0
	T2	N1	M0
Stage IIIa	T3	N0	M0
	T3	N1	M0
	T1–3	N2	M0
Stage IIIb	Any T	N3	M0
	T4	Any N	M0
Stage IV	Any T	Any N	M1

matic improvement by relieving endobronchial obstruction and may have a role in the treatment of carcinoma in situ.

Surgery. Surgical resectability of lung cancer is determined in large measure by the extent of lymph node metastasis. Patients with stage I and stage II non–small cell lung cancer (Table 70–4) should be treated with surgical resection aimed at cure. Patients with stage III disease characterized by ipsilateral intranodal mediastinal lymph node involvement may benefit from surgical resection of the primary and involved lymph nodes. Intranodal disease is defined as tumor completely confined within the capsule of the mediastinal lymph nodes. These patients should also receive postoperative mediastinal irradiation. Patients with superior sulcus tumors that have not metastasized to mediastinal lymph nodes or systemically should be treated with preoperative irradiation and en bloc resection. Irradiation is usually given as 3000 rads in ten treatments, followed in three to six weeks by surgical resec-

TABLE 70–5. TWO-STAGE CLASSIFICATION FOR SMALL CELL LUNG CANCER

Limited Diseases (30%)
1. Primary tumor confined to hemithorax
2. Ipsilateral hilar lymph nodes
3. Ipsilateral and contralateral supraclavicular lymph nodes
4. Ipsilateral and contralateral mediastinal lymph nodes
5. Pleural effusion

Extensive Disease (70%): More advanced than limited
1. Metastasis in the contralateral lung
2. Distant metastasis (brain, bone, liver, etc.)

tion. En bloc surgical resection of tumors that have invaded the chest wall, but have not metastasized systemically or to the mediastinal lymph nodes may be of benefit. Surgical resection of both superior sulcus and chest wall tumors is associated with increased surgical mortality compared with other less extensive surgical resections of lung cancer.

Limited resection of tumors yields results comparable to more extensive surgical procedures. In general, lobectomy is recommended. Even less extensive procedures, such as lobar segment and wedge resection, are usually reserved for patients with peripheral lesions or limited pulmonary function.

Approximately 40 per cent of patients with non–small cell lung cancer undergo thoracotomy, with an overall five-year survival from 10 to 35 per cent. At the time of thoracotomy, 75 per cent of patients undergo tumor resection with the aim at cure. The overall survival of patients resected for cure varies according to histopathologic type of tumor: squamous cell carcinoma, 37 per cent; adenocarcinoma, 27 per cent; large cell undifferentiated carcinoma, 27 per cent; and bronchoalveolar, 56 per cent. Stage of the tumor is also an important determinant of surgical survival: stage I, 54 per cent; stage II, 35 per cent; and stage III without systemic or mediastinal lymph node metastasis, 19 per cent.

Pulmonary function is another very important factor in the evaluation of patients for surgery. Forced vital capacity greater than 2 liters and a forced expiratory volume in the first second (FEV_1) of greater than 50 per cent of the forced vital capacity predict that a patient can tolerate the consequences of pneumonectomy. Radionuclide scanning has generally replaced differential spirometry as a method of assessing the lung to be resected for its contribution to overall respiration.

Elderly patients should not be excluded from consideration for resection of tumor. The most limiting factor of survival in this age group is not age, but the tumor. Bronchogenic carcinoma is a highly aggressive tumor in the elderly. Average life expectancy of patients with untreated tumor is eight months. This compares with an average life expectancy in the United States of 11.1 and 14.8 years, respectively, for men and women aged 70 years. Elderly patients carefully selected for surgery have a five-year survival of 35 to 42 per cent.

Radiation Therapy. Most non–small cell lung cancers are responsive to radiation treatment. Radiation therapy is indicated in patients with stage III disease without metastases or in stage I or stage II patients who refuse surgical treatment. A consistently small but reproducible group of patients with disease in the chest alone benefit from radiation treatment aimed at cure. Patients with operable lung cancer may have a five-year survival rate with radiation therapy alone of up to 21 per cent. Treatment is generally 5500 to 6000 rads by either split course or continuous fraction irradiation. Acute esophagitis is a common complication. Patients receiving irradiation of a lung for cure of cancer may develop radiation pneumonitis; therefore, patients must have pulmonary function equivalent to that necessary to tolerate pneumonectomy.

Most tumors will respond to irradiation by decreasing in size; however, treatment of patients with nonresectable non–small cell lung cancer with irradiation has been disappointing in prolonging survival.

Postoperative mediastinal irradiation is recommended in patients who have undergone resection and who have intranodal lymph node involvement, but preoperative and postoperative adjuvant radiotherapy for T2 and T3 tumors has not been shown to be beneficial and may even be detrimental. The single exception appears to be superior sulcus, or Pancoast's, tumor.

TREATMENT OF PATIENTS WITH DISSEMINATED NON–SMALL CELL LUNG CARCINOMA. Seventy per cent of patients with non–small cell lung cancer have unresectable disease at the time of diagnosis or thoracotomy. In such patients, irradiation and other forms of palliative treatment are very important.

Radiation. Irradiation effectively decreases tumor size to reduce endobronchial obstruction and to re-expand the atelectatic lung. Important intrathoracic complications may respond to irradiation: the superior vena cava syndrome, 80 to 90 per cent; hemoptysis, 84 per cent; cough 60 per cent; and atelectasis, 23 per cent. Radiation therapy may also palliate bone pain and cerebral metastases.

Chemotherapy. A response rate of 30 to 40 per cent in non–small cell lung cancer has been achieved with cisplatin regimens, especially in combination with etoposide (VP-16) and/or mitomycin-C. This should not be regarded as routine therapy. Substantive improvement in symptoms and survival remains to be proved. Potential benefit to the patient must be weighed against chemotherapy-induced side effects. The effectiveness of combined modalities such as chemotherapy plus radiotherapy or chemotherapy plus surgery is still unproved.

SMALL CELL LUNG CANCER. The median survival of untreated small cell lung cancer from the time of diagnosis is 2.8 months. Less than 1 per cent of untreated patients will survive five years. The treatments of choice for small cell lung cancer are chemotherapy and radiation. Surgical resection has little, if any, role, because at the time of detection the tumor has usually spread beyond the limits of surgical removal. For example, the mean survival with radiotherapy alone (284 days) is statistically greater than the mean survival with surgical treatment (199 days), although it remains very low.

Chemotherapy. Small cell lung cancer is highly responsive to chemotherapy. Moderately intensive therapy with three agents is usually given initially in an attempt to eradicate the tumor. The use of additional drugs beyond three is associated with a disproportionate increase in side effects compared with benefit. Examples of currently employed regimens are cyclophosphamide, methotrexate, and lomustine (CCNU); cyclophosphamide, doxorubicin, and vincristine; and cyclophosphamide, doxorubicin, and etoposide (VP-16). These regimens appear to be approximately equal in producing responses and long-term survival. Objective responses usually occur within 6 to 12 weeks after initiation of treatment. The effective length of treatment is yet to be established. Most protocols involve treatment for 12 months or less. Alternating non–cross-resistant combinations of drugs and using intensive therapy with autologous bone marrow transplantation have not been shown to increase survival. Combined modalities of irradiation and chemotherapy may be of use in limited disease, although this is yet to be conclusively proved.

Most chemotherapy regimens produce a greater than 80 per cent response rate in all patients. Complete response, defined as absence of any evidence of residual tumor, is seen in greater than 50 per cent of patients with limited disease and 20 per cent of patients with extensive disease. This results in a median survival of about 14 months in patients with limited disease and 7 months in patients with extensive disease. Twelve to 15 per cent patients with limited disease will survive 6 to 11 years.

Aggressive chemotherapy produces complications and symptoms in all patients. All experience anemia and leukopenia. Opportunistic infection is an important complication. Approximately 60 per cent of neutropenic patients experience febrile episodes. Herpes zoster occurs in 8 to 12 per cent of patients with small cell lung cancer treated with chemotherapy. Other complications include nausea, vomiting, alopecia, hemorrhagic cystitis, mucositis, electrolyte imbalance, possible cardiotoxicity, and peripheral neuropathy. A long-term complication of chemotherapy for small cell lung cancer is a secondary malignancy: leukemia, lymphoma, and other neoplasms. Risk appears to increase with intensity of drug dosage and the number of drugs utilized. Finally, patients successfully treated for small cell carcinoma are still at risk for non–small cell carcinoma.

Radiation Therapy. Radiation therapy is of proven benefit in controlling bone pain, spinal cord compression, superior vena cava syndrome, and bronchial obstruction. More than 90 per cent of patients have been reported to have palliation of symptoms due to brain metastases. The use of radiation therapy in combination with chemotherapy is controversial and should be reserved for experimental studies.

Prophylactic Cranial Irradiation. Although chemotherapy has increased the survival of patients with small cell lung cancer, this survival has been accompanied by an increased risk of relapse in the central nervous system. The cumulative risk of central nervous system metastases at two years may be as high as 80 per cent. This risk is reduced to about 3 to 12 per cent with the use of prophylactic cranial irradiation. Unfortunately, this decreased rate of brain metastasis is not associated with increased survival. Prophylactic cranial irradiation is generally reserved for patients who have achieved a complete response to chemotherapy, but even in these patients the benefit in terms of increased survival is slight. In all other patients cranial irradiation should be used when central nervous system metastases are diagnosed. Most patients who survive long term exhibit memory loss, confusion, ataxia, loss of vision, and dysphonia. This encephalopathy is probably a complication of cranial irradiation with a possible contribution by chemotherapy as well.

OTHER CONSIDERATIONS IN THE TREATMENT OF LUNG CANCER. *Bone Metastasis.* Metastasis of lung cancer to bone most frequently cause pain, but pathologic fracture may also occur. Bone involvement is best detected by bone scan, although large lesions will be visible radiographically. Pain can usually be palliated by radiation to the involved areas.

Hypercalcemia. Hypercalcemia is one of the most important complications of lung cancer. Serum calcium values in excess of 12 mg per deciliter are considered life threatening. Treatment is aimed at lowering the serum calcium level. Treatment of hypercalcemia is discussed in detail in Ch. 247.

Central Nervous System Metastasis. Metastases from lung cancer to the central nervous system usually cause symptoms in proportion to their size and location. Corticosteroids are effective in relieving acute symptoms of increased intracranial pressure in about 75 per cent of patients. Doses of 8 to 12 mg of dexamethasone should be acutely administered. Osmotic agents given to reduce intracranial pressure, such as a 20 per cent solution of mannitol intravenously, may be useful in treating cerebral herniation. Acute control of increased pressure should be followed by radiation therapy.

Pleural Effusion. Malignant pleural effusion frequently complicates bronchogenic carcinoma. It is exudative in nature. The diagnosis is made by cytologic examination of the fluid and by pleural biopsy. Effusions complicated by dyspnea or pain should be drained. If the fluid recurs, obliteration of the potential pleural space should be accomplished by introducing a sclerosing agent. This is best performed by insertion of a chest tube to drain the effusion completely, followed by the instillation of 1 gram of tetracycline dissolved in 100 ml of normal saline and 50 ml of 1 per cent Xylocaine into the chest through the tube. The tube should then be clamped and the patient turned into different positions to distribute the sclerosing fluid along the pleural surface. The tube is then allowed to drain until the amount of fluid over a 12- to 14-hour period is 100 ml or less. Malignant pleural effusions with pH less than 7.0 are associated with a very poor prognosis.

Weakness and Weight Loss. Weight loss, muscle weakness, and difficulty in eating are frequent and distressing manifestations of lung cancer. The pathophysiology of weight loss in lung cancer is poorly understood but can be partially explained by altered carbohydrate and protein metabolism and the release of toxic factors into the circulation. The use of aggressive nutritional support in lung cancer patients in whom traditional forms of treatment have been ineffective is of limited value and may even be adverse.

Cough and Dyspnea. Reversible causes of cough and dyspnea, such as bronchospasm, bronchitis, and pneumonitis, should be excluded. The mainstays of cough control are narcotic cough suppressants. Narcotics and tranquilizers used in low dosages may produce remarkable relief of severe dyspnea. When clearance of large airway secretions becomes difficult, patients may "rattle" when they breathe (so-called "death rattle"). This is particularly distressing to family members. In patients who are terminally ill, scopolamine, 0.4 to 0.6 mg subcutaneously every four hours as necessary, will tend to dry up secretions and relax the smooth muscle of the airways. It is preferred to atropine, since the former is a central nervous system depressant, in contrast to atropine, which is a stimulant.

Pain. The therapeutic goal of managing pain, the most common symptom of advanced lung cancer, should be not only its relief but also its prevention. Narcotics should be taken every four hours around the clock to prevent the patient from awakening with pain. There is no single optimal dosage schedule for narcotics. Most patients have their pain controlled with 30 mg of morphine, or its equivalent, given orally on a four-hour basis. Patients, families, and those caring for the patient should be counseled that tolerance and addiction do not present a real clinical problem in patients with advanced lung cancer. The most common adverse side effects of narcotic treatment are constipation and nausea, which must preferably be prevented, but treated aggressively if they appear.

Patients who have been treated for lung cancer with apparent success continue at risk for a second primary lung cancer, or "metachronous" tumor. Such tumors can be of identical or different histologic pattern from the first primary tumor. Metachronous tumors occur in 1 to 3 per cent of patients with lung cancer. Treatment is determined by the same factors that affect other primary lung tumors, however, the physiologic impact of treatment of the first primary cancer may limit surgical resection or radiation dosage.

Filderman AE, Shaw C, Matthay RA: Lung cancer part 1: Etiology, pathology, natural manifestations, and diagnostic techniques. Invest Radiol 21:80, 1986. *Particularly good for summarization of roentgenographic manifestations of primary pulmonary malignancies.*

Ginsberg RJ, Feld RJ (eds.): IV World Conference on Lung Cancer. Chest 89:314S, 1986. *Comprehensive summaries of epidemiologic, diagnostic, and therapeutic aspects of lung cancer.*

Greco FA, Johnson DH, Hainsworth JD, et al.: Chemotherapy of small-cell lung cancer. Semin Oncol 12:31, 1985. *Summarizes current approaches to treatment of small cell lung cancer.*

Iannuzzi MJ, Scoggin CH: Small cell lung cancer: state of the art. Am Rev Respir Dis 134:593, 1986. *Focuses on clinical and investigational aspects of small cell lung cancer.*

Klastersky J, Sculier JP: Chemotherapy of non–small-cell lung cancer. Semin Oncol 12:38, 1985. *Specific discussion of issue of use of chemotherapy for treatment of non–small cell lung cancer. Contains information relevant to the decision on whether to offer treatment beyond surgery and radiotherapy.*

Marini N, McCormack P: Therapy of stage III (non-metastatic) lung cancer. Semin Oncol 10:95, 1983. *Reviews treatment of superior sulcus (Pancoast's) tumor.*

Peh SB Jr, Wernly JA, Aki BF: Lung cancer—current concepts and controversies. West J Med 145:52, 1986. *This medical progress article considers a variety of controversial methods and alternatives for management of patients with lung cancer, including classification, staging, radiotherapy, chemotherapy, and palliation.*

Risk NW: Selection of patients with non–small-cell lung carcinoma for surgical resection. West J Med 143:636, 1985. *Review of criteria for determining which patients should and should not receive consideration for surgical resection.*

Whang-Peng J, Bunn PA, Kao-Shan CS, et al.: A nonrandom chromosomal abnormality, del 3p(14–23), in human small cell lung cancer (SCLC). Cancer Genet Cytogenet 6:119, 1982. *Description of a chromosomal abnormality found in small cell lung cancer.*

Woolner LB, Fontana RS, Cortese DA, et al.: Roentgenographically occult lung cancer: Pathologic findings and frequency of multicentricity during a 10 year period. Mayo Clin Proc 54:453, 1984. *Details of the problem of occurrence of new primary tumor in patients treated for lung cancer.*

OTHER MALIGNANCIES OF THE LUNG
Carcinoid Tumors

These tumors, sometimes termed "bronchial adenomas," are in fact distinct entities with different clinical courses and histologic manifestations. Three types are recognized: bronchial carcinoids, cylindromas, and mucoepidermoid tumors. Tumors may manifest with endobronchial obstruction or hemoptysis. Carcinoid tumors, including bronchial carcinoids, are considered in Ch. 243.

Scheithauer BW, Carpenter PC, Block B, et al.: Ectopic secretion of a growth hormone–releasing factor: Report of a case of acromegaly with bronchial carcinoid tumor. Am J Med 76:605, 1984. *Reviews different extrapulmonary manifestations of bronchial carcinoid tumors.*

Primary Lymphoma of the Lung

Hodgkin's disease and non-Hodgkin's lymphoma are discussed in Ch. 158 and 160. Such lymphoma may arise in the lymph nodes of the chest or within the lung itself. Patients with tumor involving the lung may present with weight loss, fever, cough, or pleuritic chest pain. Pleural effusion may be an initial or complicating manifestation.

Non-Hodgkin's tumors arising within the parenchyma of the lung are often discrete masses with or without hilar and mediastinal lymph node enlargement. An intrathoracic Hodgkin's tumor mass may cavitate or compress the bronchial tree to cause atelectasis or postobstructive pneumonitis. A common differential diagnosis of hilar adenopathy is that between lymphoma and sarcoidosis (Ch. 69). Enlargement of anterior mediastinal lymph nodes suggests lymphoma, as this is an unusual region of lymphadenopathy in sarcoidosis.

Other lymphoproliferative disorders that involve the lung are pseudolymphoma and lymphocytic interstitial pneumonitis. Pseudolymphoma appears as a nodular lesion, whereas lymphocytic interstitial pneumonitis manifests as a diffuse infiltrate. The diagnosis is made by histologic examination of lung biopsy specimen. Distinguishing between benign disease and true pulmonary lymphoma may be difficult. Some patients who initially present with an apparently benign lymphoproliferative disorder later develop malignant lymphoma. The development of hilar or mediastinal lymphadenopathy suggests the presence of malignancy.

The diagnosis of lymphoproliferative disorders of the lung depends upon histologic examination of tissue obtained by bronchoscopy, transbronchial biopsy, mediastinoscopy, or thoracotomy.

The treatment of Hodgkin's and non-Hodgkin's lymphomas of the lung is by the use of radiation or chemotherapy as would be employed for nonpulmonary lymphoma (Ch. 158 and 160). Pseudolymphoma can be removed by surgical resection. No established treatment for lymphocytic interstitial pneumonitis exists, although chemotherapy has been attempted.

Colby TV, Carrington CB: Pulmonary lymphomas: Current concepts. Pathol Annu 14:884, 1983. *Presents criteria for and classification of pulmonary lymphoid lesions.*

Uncommon Primary Lung Malignancies

Cylindromas are the second most common tumors of the trachea and bronchi. (The most common tumors are bronchogenic carcinomas.) The tumors arise from the mucous glands of the bronchial epithelium. The most common symptoms are airway obstruction and cough. Men and women are equally affected, and the age of occurrence ranges from 30 to 65 years. The diagnosis is made by bronchoscopy and biopsy. Treatment is by surgical resection, although cure may be difficult owing to the tumor's propensity to metastasize.

Mucoepidermoid tumors also arise from the bronchial mucous glands and usually manifest in persons between the ages of

40 and 55. The diagnosis is made by the bronchoscopic finding of a polypoid endobronchial mass, followed by biopsy. Treatment is by surgical resection, with a better prognosis than with cylindroma. *Carcinosarcoma*, an unusual tumor, contains both malignant epithelial elements and sarcomatous changes. It may occur as a peripheral mass or as an endobronchial lesion. Treatment is by surgical resection. *Pulmonary blastomas*, which usually occur in the periphery of the lung, are thought to arise from mesoderm. Treatment is by surgical resection, but the prognosis is poor.

Primary sarcomas of the lung, which are very rare, include fibrosarcomas, leiomyosarcomas, hemangiopericytomas, and osteosarcomas. Treatment is by surgical resection. More recently, Kaposi's sarcoma has been recognized as a cause of pulmonary disease in patients with the acquired immunodeficiency syndrome (AIDS). It may be difficult to distinguish from infection. The diagnosis requires lung biopsy.

Olnibene FP, Steis RG, Macher AM, et al.: Kaposi's sarcoma causing pulmonary infiltrates and respiratory failure in the acquired immunodeficiency syndrome. Ann Intern Med 102:471, 1985. *Description of 66 patients with acquired immunodeficiency syndrome and 30 episodes of pulmonary Kaposi's sarcoma.*

Tumors Metastatic to the Lung

The lung may be involved from both hematogenous and lymphatic spread of carcinomas and sarcomas. Patients are often asymptomatic; however, metastatic lesions may cause dyspnea, cough, and chest pain. Diffuse hematogenous tumor spread may cause vascular obstruction manifested by corpulmonale with hilar enlargement and clear lung parenchyma.

The radiographic appearance of pulmonary metastases may give some clue to the primary tumor. Solitary nodules are usually associated with cancers from breast, colon, kidney, rectum, cervix, and melanoma. These tumors may also diffusely involve the lung, leading to multiple large nodules or micronodules. In addition, a micronodular pattern is also seen with tumors from the thyroid, trophoblastic tissue, or bone sarcomas. Large, well-defined pulmonary nodules, sometimes with associated hilar enlargement, occur with testicular germinal cell tumors.

Tumors that spread lymphatically include carcinomas from the stomach, pancreas, thyroid, larynx, and lung. These tumors may spread to lung lymphatics through hilar lymph nodes or from involvement of parenchymal lymphatics due to hematogenous metastases. Enlargement of lung lymphatics is radiographically visible as linear shadows similar to Kerley's lines.

Pleural involvement may appear as a pleural-based mass or as pleural effusion. Metastatic lesions, particularly synovial cell tumors and other bone tumors, may lead to pneumothorax. Certain metastatic lesions may cavitate: metastatic sarcomas, carcinomas of the colon, and epidermoid carcinomas of the head, neck, and the female reproductive system. Osteogenic sarcomas or chondrosarcomas display calcification in metastatic lesions.

The diagnosis of metastatic lesion is confirmed by histologic examination of tissue obtained by sputum cytology, fiberoptic bronchoscopy, or occasionally thoracotomy. Cytologic findings are positive in as many as 50 per cent of patients. Bronchoscopy and needle biopsy have similar success rates. Decisions on aggressiveness in seeking confirmation by tissue study of suspected metastatic lesions must be made thoughtfully. The risk to the patient must be weighed against the question of how the confirmation of metastasis will alter the management of the patient.

Treatment will usually be based upon management of the primary neoplasm. Certain metastatic lesions should be considered for surgical resection, especially those arising from osteogenic sarcomas. On occasion, resection of a solitary metastasis from other primary sources has been reported to be associated with increased survival, but usually without any controlled study. In considering surgical resection of a metastasis, the following criteria should be met: (1) absence of other metastatic lesions within the lung on CT, (2) no evidence of metastasis involving other organs, and (3) sufficient physiologic reserve to tolerate a more extensive resection if simple wedge resection is deemed inadequate. In general, this means that criteria used for determining tolerance of surgical resection of primary lung cancer should be applied when contemplating resection of metastatic lesions.

In summary, surgical resection of pulmonary metastasis should be considered when the primary tumor is under control, the patient is a good surgical risk, other approaches to treatment are unsatisfactory, and all of the tumor can be resected.

Beattie EJ: Surgical treatment of pulmonary metastases. Cancer 54:2729, 1984. *Brief review of metastatic lesions to the lung that may be appropriate for multiple surgical resections.*

Mountain CF, McMurtrey MJ, Hermes KE: Surgery for pulmonary metastasis: A 20-year experience. Ann Thorac Surg 38:323, 1984. *Report of results of the M.D. Anderson Hospital and Tumor Institute with surgical resection in 443 patients with various tumors metastatic to the lung.*

BENIGN NEOPLASMS OF THE LUNG

Benign neoplasms of the lung are uncommon. They may occur as solitary nodules within lung parenchyma or as endobronchial lesions. Symptoms are nonspecific and include cough, dyspnea, chest pain, and pneumonia.

HAMARTOMAS. Hamartomas, the most common benign tumors of the lung, are usually diagnosed in adults. The tumors consist of unorganized elements such as fat, fibrous tissue, epithelial tissue, cartilage, and calcification. Calcification leads to the "popcorn" radiographic appearance of the tumor. The majority of hamartomas occur as solitary nodules within lung parenchyma, but about 10 per cent are endobronchial. Hamartomas should be removed because of the potential complications of hemorrhage and bronchial obstruction resulting in atelectasis and pneumonia.

PAPILLOMAS. Papillomas, which arise form the trachea and bronchi, are most commonly found in children. They may be diffuse, leading to repeated pneumonias, bronchiectasis, atelectasis, and chronic infection. Because of diffuse involvement, management may be difficult and may require repeated bronchoscopy for attempt at removal of these tumors. Malignant changes may also occur.

Uncommon benign tumors of the lung include granular cell myoblastomas, lipomas, fibromas, leiomyomas, chondromas, and hemangiomas. They usually first appear as masses radiographically. Complications are similar to those of other benign neoplasms. Surgical removal is the usual treatment.

Arrignoni MG, Woolner LB, Bernatz PE, et al.: Benign tumors of the lung: A ten-year surgical experience. J Thorac Cardiovasc Surg 60:589, 1970. *Excellent review of 130 patients with benign tumors of the lung. Includes clinical, radiographic, and pathologic features.*

SOLITARY PULMONARY NODULE

A solitary pulmonary nodule is a single lesion, regardless of size, surrounded by lung parenchyma on at least two thirds of its circumference, not touching the hilum or mediastinum, and without associated atelectasis or pleural effusion. Important etiologies of solitary pulmonary nodules include neoplasia, infection, and collagen vascular disease. Because of wide varieties of cause and differing treatments, determining the etiology is very important (Table 70–6).

Etiology

Both benign and malignant tumors may manifest as a solitary pulmonary nodule. Approximately 40 per cent of solitary pulmonary nodules are malignant, and of these 85 to 90 per cent are bronchogenic carcinoma. Bronchogenic carcinomas that are detected as solitary nodules have a much more favorable prognosis (24 per cent five-year survival) than those with more complicated presentations (5 to 8 per cent

TABLE 70–6. ETIOLOGIES OF SOLITARY PULMONARY NODULES

1. Primary lung malignancies
2. Metastatic malignancies to the lung
3. Benign tumors or tumor-like conditions
   Hamartoma — Pseudolymphoma
   Herniation of omentum — Herniation of liver
   Hemangioma
4. Pulmonary infections
   Fungal — Mycobacterial
   Bacterial — Hydatid cyst
5. Foreign body pneumonitis
   Lipid pneumonia — Amyloidosis
   Pneumoconiosis — Aspiration pneumonia
   Talc granulomas
6. Pulmonary vascular disorders
   Pulmonary infarct — Pulmonary hemosiderosis
   Pulmonary hemorrhage

five-year survival). Patients detected with solitary nodules at stage I of bronchogenic carcinoma have been reported to have almost a 50 per cent five-year survival. Most benign hamartomas appear as solitary pulmonary nodules. Three to 10 per cent of solitary pulmonary nodules are due to malignancies metastatic to the lung from other organs, especially from renal cell carcinoma, Wilm's tumor, Ewing's sarcoma, choriocarcinoma, bladder carcinoma, rhabdomyosarcoma, osteosarcoma, melanoma, and carcinomas of the breast, colon, testis, head, and neck.

The most common infection that presents as solitary nodules is that caused by *Coccidioides immitis.* Echinococcal cysts also may appear as a single nodule, as may the lesions of *Histoplasma capsulatum* and *Blastomyces dermatitidis.* Tuberculosis rarely manifests as a solitary pulmonary nodule.

Certain collagen vascular disorders may present as pulmonary nodules, especially rheumatoid arthritis and Wegener's granulomatosis. Although usually multiple lesions occur, occasionally only a single nodule may be seen. Unusual causes of solitary nodules are pulmonary infarcts and vascular malformations.

Evaluation

The sequence of the approach to a patient with a solitary pulmonary nodule is outlined in Figure 70–1. Evaluation of patients with solitary pulmonary nodules begins with a thorough history and physical examination. Travel to an area endemic for fungal disease such as coccidioidomycosis suggests, but does not prove, this etiology. Weight loss and other constitutional symptoms are consistent with malignancy, although early stages may be asymptomatic. Joint changes may suggest rheumatoid nodules. Age is also an important consideration. Primary lung cancer is uncommon in patients who have never smoked and who are below the age of 30 years. Patients over the age of 50 years with new solitary nodules, particularly if they have smoked, have an increased incidence of malignancy. Geography is also important. Fungal disease is a more common etiology in persons who reside or have recently visited the American Southwest, whereas malignancy is a more common cause of solitary nodules in individuals living in areas nonendemic for fungal infections such as coccidioidomycosis.

An important step in the evaluation of a solitary pulmonary nodule is a comparison of its radiographic appearance with that of a previous film. A lesion that has not enlarged in two or more years suggests a benign etiology. On the other hand, if the nodule is new or if there has been progressive enlargement, malignancy or infection is much more likely. Most malignant solitary nodules have a volume doubling time of 60 to 150 days with a mean of 120 days. In spherical lesions, an increase in diameter of 26 per cent equates to one doubling in volume. Calcification within the node is usually a sign of a benign lesion. Patterns of calcification seen with benign lesions are a dense central nidus of calcium, a concentric or laminated pattern, a diffuse pattern, or a clustered or "popcorn" pattern. Small amounts of calcium may be seen within

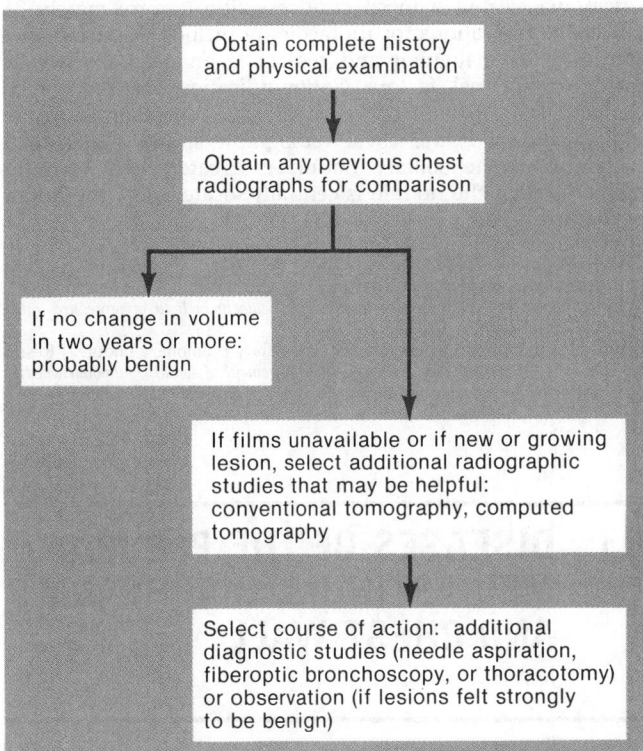

FIGURE 70–1. Approach to the patient with a solitary pulmonary nodule.

1 to 3 per cent of bronchogenic carcinomas or osteosarcomas metastatic to the lung. Computerized tomography has two important roles in evaluating solitary pulmonary nodules. First, imaging and densitometry can be helpful in detecting calcification. Tomograms of the lung may also serve this purpose. Second, other nodules not seen with standard anteroposterior and lateral chest radiographs may be detected on CT. The use of CT densitometry to identify malignancy by low density numbers remains experimental.

If a previous radiograph is not available, or if an enlarging lesion is suspected, the ultimate determination of etiology of a solitary nodule is dependent upon either culture confirmation of infection or histologic examination. A lesion can be considered benign only if a specific diagnosis is obtained. Sputum for tuberculosis should be obtained only if tuberculosis is highly suspected. Cytologic findings in sputum are positive in only 10 per cent or less of patients with endobronchially invisible bronchogenic carcinomas and 20 per cent of patients with malignancies metastatic to the lungs.

Once the etiology of a solitary nodule is ascertained, treatment will depend upon cause. When a lesion is not obviously benign, percutaneous transthoracic needle aspiration, fiberoptic bronchoscopy, or thoracotomy is indicated. Needle aspiration biopsy yields a specific diagnosis in 85 to 90 per cent of cases. It is helpful to establish a diagnosis of malignancy in patients in whom surgery is not contemplated but in whom a specific diagnosis will help guide management. Fiberoptic bronchoscopy with transbronchial biopsy and bronchial brushing has the advantage over needle aspiration because it is useful in staging lung cancer and has a lower complication rate. Success in obtaining a diagnosis is dependent upon the size of the nodule. Solitary pulmonary nodules less than 2 cm in size or within 2 cm of the hilum are difficult to diagnose with bronchoscopy. Thoracotomy is the most direct means of establishing a diagnosis. It also offers the best chance for cure of lung cancer. The possibility of small cell lung cancer is not necessarily a reason for avoiding thoracotomy. Surgical resection of small cell lung cancer presenting as a solitary pulmonary nodule may have a five-year survival comparable to that with other forms of nodular bronchogenic carcinoma treated with surgical resection (approximately 24 per cent). Indications for thoracotomy include suspicion that the lesion is malignant and resectable and the absence of major surgical risk factors. Contraindications are severe underlying lung disease or heart disease. Mediastinoscopy is indicated only if the chest radiograph shows mediastinal widening, if the solitary nodule is greater than 3 cm in diameter, or if the nodule is centrally located near the hilum of the lung.

Khouri, NF, Melziane MA, Zerhouni EA, et al.: The solitary pulmonary nodule: Assessment, diagnosis and management. Chest 91:128, 1987. *Practical review of clinical approach to solitary nodules, particularly in light of procedures other than thoracotomy.*

Stauffer JL: What to do when you detect a solitary pulmonary nodule. J Respir Dis 7:17, 1986. *Excellent summary of management of solitary pulmonary nodule based upon etiologic considerations and the yield of particular diagnostic approaches. Practical and rational.*

71 DISEASES OF THE PLEURA, MEDIASTINUM, DIAPHRAGM, AND CHEST WALL

Jerome S. Brody

THE PLEURA

ANATOMY AND PHYSIOLOGY. The pleura is composed of a single layer of mesothelial cells supported by a sparse network of connective tissue, vessels, and lymphatics. The parietal pleura covers the surface of the chest wall, diaphragm, and mediastinum, from which it separates with ease. It receives its blood supply from the systemic circulation and contains sensory nerve endings. The visceral pleura covers and adheres to the entire surface of both lungs. It receives its blood supply from the low-pressure pulmonary circulation and contains no sensory nerve fibers. Either pleural surface can be the site of a primary disease process; pleural disease, however, is most often an extension of, or a reflection of, disease that arises elsewhere.

The visceral and parietal pleural surfaces are separated by a potential space that is filled with 10 to 30 ml of fluid, which spreads out in a layer several angstroms thick. This serous fluid has a protein concentration of less than 2 grams per deciliter and a pH and glucose concentration similar to those of blood. The fluid in the pleural space turns over at a rate of 35 to 75 per cent per hour in a fashion dependent in part on Starling forces similar to those governing interstitial fluid exchange. Hydrostatic pressures are systemic in the parietal pleura (30 cm H_2O), pulmonary in the visceral pleura (10 cm H_2O), and subatmospheric in the pleural space itself (–5 cm H_2O at end expiration in normals). Colloid oncotic pressure results in pressure gradients of 25 cm H_2O from pleural space to each pleural surface. The net result of these forces is an inflow pressure gradient of 5 to 10 cm H_2O from parietal pleura to pleural space and an outflow pressure gradient of 5 to 10 cm H_2O from pleural space to visceral pleura. Augmenting this outflow pressure gradient are factors other than Starling forces such as pulmonary lymphatic flow, the relatively greater vascular bed in the visceral pleura, and the increased number of microvilli on visceral pleura mesothelial cells, all of which favor movement of fluid out of the pleural space.

The major forces involved in pleural fluid movement can help explain why fluid may accumulate in the pleural space. Excess hydrostatic forces or decreased oncotic pressures produce filtrates across intact capillary walls and result in protein-poor transudates. Breakdown of the normal formation-resorp-

tion mechanism because of damage to pleural capillaries (e.g., produced by inflammation) or blocking of lymphatics results in protein-rich exudates.

DIAGNOSTIC PROCEDURES. *History and Physical Examination.* Pleural pain and dyspnea are the symptoms most frequently associated with pleural disease, although considerable pleural disease can occur in the absence of symptoms. Pleural pain is usually unilateral, arising from irritation or inflammation of the parietal rather than visceral pleura. Because nerve fibers of the parietal pleura are derived from intercostal nerves, the pain may be referred to the abdomen, neck, or shoulder. Pleuritic pain is usually unilateral, sharp, and accentuated by deep breathing, coughing, or movement of the chest cage. The patient may find relief by splinting the area of involvement. Pleural pain often disappears once pleural effusion develops.

A collection of pleural fluid may produce respiratory dysfunction by compressing normal lung tissue and creating ventilation-perfusion mismatches, or by flattening the diaphragm and placing it at a mechanical disadvantage. These effects produce dyspnea in patients with otherwise normal lung function but may precipitate respiratory failure in patients with underlying lung disease.

The physical examination in pleural disease varies considerably, depending on the nature of the accompanying lung or systemic disease. Patients usually have rapid, shallow respirations, impaired chest wall motion (splinting), intercostal tenderness, and decreased breath sounds over the affected area. A pleural friction rub is the characteristic physical sign, but it is often entirely absent or audible for only 24 to 48 hours after the onset of the pain. Impaired percussion note, absent tactile fremitus, decreased or absent breath sounds, and E to A change of the spoken voice (egobronchophony) at the upper border of the fluid are frequent signs of pleural effusion.

Radiologic Examination. Up to 300 ml of pleural fluid may fail to be seen on the posteroanterior chest film. However, as little as 150 ml can be seen in a lateral decubitus film. Early signs of fluid accumulation include blunting and medial displacement of the normally sharp costophrenic angle and widening of the shadow between the gas-containing stomach and lower margin of the left lung. Larger volumes of fluid track up the pleural space, outlining the pleural fissures and producing a concave shadow with its highest margin along the pleural surface. Large amounts of pleural fluid may accumulate in the area between the lung base and diaphragm (subpulmonic effusion), producing the radiologic appearance of an elevated hemidiaphragm. In patients with small or subpulmonic effusions, bilateral decubitus roentgenograms will often reveal the presence of free pleural fluid and allow visualization of underlying lung tissue. Collections of pleural air and fluid (hydro-, pyo-, or hemopneumothorax) usually produce horizontal rather than concave areas of fluid. Loculated pockets of pleural fluid, pleural-based tumors, and parenchymal disease are often difficult to localize and define anatomically. Ultrasonic studies and computed tomography have provided more precise anatomic definition of pleural and contiguous parenchymal abnormalities.

Thoracentesis. Removal of pleural fluid serves both diagnostic and therapeutic functions. Diagnostic thoracentesis should be performed when the cause of the effusion is uncertain. Therapeutic thoracentesis should be performed when the effusion is producing symptoms or when infection is present within the pleural space. The patient is usually placed in a sitting position; the area of fluid is defined by physical examination; and, using sterile techniques, the fluid is removed. Diagnostic thoracentesis requires relatively small amounts of material, which may be obtained through a small-gauge needle. Therapeutic thoracentesis usually involves removing large amounts of fluid. However, no more than 1000 to 1500 ml of fluid should be removed at one time, since re-expansion pulmonary edema may occur as the fluid compressing the underlying lung is removed. Although pleural fluid can be classified as either transudative or exudative, the difference between transudate and exudate is relative and serves only to suggest likely categories of disease.

Transudates (Table 71–1) are defined by (1) a total protein content less than 3.0 grams per deciliter (or with a pleural fluid to serum protein ratio of less than 0.5) and (2) a lactic dehydrogenase (LDH) level of less than 200 units per milliliter (or a pleural to serum LDH level of less than 0.6). Such fluids usually have white blood cell counts less than 1000 per cubic millimeter. Transudates are usually seen in congestive heart failure or hypoalbuminemia, or with movement of peritoneal fluid into the pleural space.

Exudates (Table 71–2) exist if any one of the above criteria does not hold. They are most frequently produced by infection or malignancy. As there is overlap in these categories, white cell counts and differentials, acid-fast and Gram's stains, aerobic and anaerobic cultures, and cytologic analysis of fluid should be included in all studies of pleural fluid. A predominance of polymorphonuclear leukocytes is most compatible with bacterial infection, while a predominance of lymphocytes, particularly with a paucity of mesothelial cells, suggests tuberculosis. Lymphomas and lymphatic leukemias producing pleural disease also produce lymphocytic effusions. Pleural fluid eosinophilia is a nonspecific finding usually associated with effusions of long duration. Blood-tinged (serosanguineous) fluid may be produced by as few as 5000 red blood cells per cubic millimeter. Malignancy, trauma, and pulmonary infarction are the most frequent causes of bloody pleural effusion, although congestive heart failure and infection can produce serosanguineous effusions. Substantial amounts of pleural fluid with a high hematocrit (>10 per cent) nearly always indicate trauma, a neoplasm that has bled into the pleural space, or a vascular abnormality. A variety of special diagnostic studies can be performed on pleural fluid, and these studies will be mentioned under discussion of specific disease entities.

Pleural Biopsy. Needle biopsy of the pleura with a hook type needle (Cope or Abrams needle) is indicated in exudative effusions when the diagnosis is uncertain. Pleural biopsy provides a specific tissue diagnosis most frequently in tuberculosis and malignancy. Histologic examination with acid-fast stains and culture of pleural tissue add significantly to the diagnostic evaluation of tuberculous effusions. In each instance, pleural implants may be patchy so that diagnostic yield increases with repeat biopsies. Biopsy is usually reserved for those patients who have sufficient pleural fluid to separate safely visceral and parietal pleura. In patients with small or loculated effusions, localization of the fluid with ultrasound can increase the yield and safety of pleural biopsy.

Exploration of the Pleura. In 5 to 10 per cent of cases, a diagnosis cannot be established on the initial evaluation. In most instances, if one waits, either the effusion will not recur or its cause will become evident. The alternative approach, surgical exploration of the pleura, will usually provide the diagnosis. However, even in some of these patients the diagnosis will not be established. In most of these cases the effusion will not recur, although in 25 per cent the cause will prove to be a malignancy. An alternative to surgery is exploration of the pleura through a thoracoscope inserted percutaneously under general anesthesia. Experience with this approach has been limited in this country.

PLEURAL INFLAMMATION AND EFFUSION. *Pleural Transudates (Simple Hydrothorax).* The most common cause of pleural transudates is congestive heart failure. Left ventricular failure increases hydrostatic pressure in visceral pleural vessels, thereby diminishing reabsorption. Right ventricular failure increases parietal pleural and central venous pressures, thereby increasing transudation and decreasing lymphatic reabsorption. Pleural effusions are often a manifestation of biventricular failure. Pleural effusion resulting from cardiac disease is most often bilateral and usually larger on the right side. If unilateral, right-sided effusions are most frequent. On rare occasions, effusions are localized within fissures, simulating lung masses that vanish as congestive heart failure regresses (phantom tumors). Chronic effusions from cardiac causes may increase their protein concentration such that the fluid may appear exudative. Hypoalbuminemia of any cause may produce transudative pleural effusions; these are usually bilateral and associated with fluid accumulation elsewhere in the body. Intra-abdominal disease may also produce large transudative hydrothoraces. Pleural effusions occur in 5 to 10 per cent of patients with cirrhosis of the liver. In these patients, ascites is usually evident, but massive effusions may appear with little or no demonstrable ascites. In this setting, peritoneal fluid appears to traverse the diaphragm either through lymphatics or through minor channels between muscle fibers in the diaphragm. The effusions are usually right sided but may be bilateral or left sided. A similar mechanism is thought to be responsible for all the pleural fluid that appears following peritoneal dialysis.

Tuberculosis. Localized tuberculosis of the pleura occurs in most patients with pulmonary tuberculosis but is usually clinically inapparent. Pleural tuberculosis may be the first manifestation of primary infection, producing a febrile illness with serous fluid and often no evidence of parenchymal disease. The effusion in this setting results from hypersensitivity to tubercular protein in pleural tubercles. The acute illness usually subsides, even if untreated, although a few such patients develop progressive primary tuberculosis. The purified protein derivative is usually positive, but skin test conversion may not yet have occurred. Patients with pleural manifestations of primary infection have a high risk of future disease, as two thirds develop clinically apparent tuberculosis within the succeeding five years. A second form of pleural tuberculosis occurs when parenchymal disease, usually reinfection tuberculosis, extends into the pleural space, producing a tuberculous empyema. Diagnosis in this case is relatively simple, since the patient will have a positive tuberculin skin test, evidence of parenchymal disease, and often positive sputum smears. Pleural fluid is exudative and usually reveals lymphocytosis; occasionally a predominance of polymorphonuclear leukocytes may be found initially. Acid-fast bacilli are

TABLE 71–2. EVALUATION OF PLEURAL FLUID EXUDATES

Test	Disease(s)
pH (<7.20)	Infection, malignancy, rheumatoid arthritis, esophageal rupture
Glucose (<60 mg/dl)	Infection, malignancy, rheumatoid arthritis
Amylase (>200 units/dl)	Pancreatic disease, malignancy, esophageal rupture
Rheumatoid factor, ANA,* LE* cells	Collagen vascular disease
Complement (decreased)	Lupus erythematosus, rheumatoid arthritis
Biopsy (+)	Malignancy, tuberculosis
RBC* (>5000/μl)	Pulmonary embolus, malignancy, trauma
Chylous effusion (triglycerides >110 mg/dl)	Trauma, malignancy

*ANA = Antinuclear antibodies; LE = lupus erythematosus; RBC = red blood cells.

TABLE 71–1. CHARACTERISTICS OF PLEURAL FLUID TRANSUDATES

	Absolute Value	Pleural Fluid: Serum Ratio
Protein	<3.0 grams/dl	<0.5
Glucose	>60 mg/dl	1.0
WBC*	<1000	—
LDH*	<200 IU/liter	<0.6

*WBC = White blood cells; LDH = lactic dehydrogenase.

rarely seen in pleural fluid, but histologic examination for granulomas and culture of material obtained at biopsy, together with culture of pleural fluid, yield the diagnosis in 80 to 90 per cent of cases. When uncertain, the pleural biopsy and purified protein derivative skin test should be repeated and the patient treated for tuberculosis until culture results are available. Treatment of all types of pleural tuberculosis is with standard antibiotic regimens (see Ch. 302), although tube drainage of tuberculous empyema may be necessary.

Pleural Effusions with Pneumonia. Inflammation of adjacent pleura occurs in most patients with pneumonia whatever the cause. The extent of pleural inflammation in bacterial pneumonia varies widely. There may be minor inflammation producing pleural pain with no clinically detectable fluid, exudative effusions containing inflammatory cells but no bacteria (parapneumonic or sympathetic effusion), or large collections of purulent fluid containing numerous bacteria (empyema). Antibiotics are usually sufficient for treating parapneumonic effusions, with thoracentesis being reserved for diagnosis or for relieving dyspnea.

Empyema tends to occur in bacterial diseases associated with tissue necrosis, e.g., infections with anaerobes, staphylococci, and gram-negative organisms. Gram's stains and aerobic and anaerobic cultures of pleural fluid are mandatory, although Gram's stains of sputum and the clinical picture are often the best initial means of identifying the infecting organism. Empyema fluid should be completely removed either by one to three thoracenteses, using a large-bore venous catheter, or by closed tube drainage. Appropriate systemic antibiotics are also required. Since bacteria are not always seen on Gram's stain, thick purulent fluid with more than 100,000 cells per cubic millimeter or fluid with pH values less than or equal to 7.20 should be treated as a presumptive empyema with drainage. In some instances, placement of the tube or catheter will require ultrasound or computed tomography to locate loculated effusions. Occasionally an empyema will be associated with air in the pleural space resulting from tissue necrosis, infection with a gas-forming organism, or communication of the bronchial tree with the pleural space (bronchopleural fistula). Tube drainage and adequate antibiotic coverage will result in closure of most such fistulas. Untreated, however, they can communicate with skin (bronchopleurocutaneous fistula) and require surgical therapy (open drainage with rib resection, decortication, myoplasty involving insertion of flaps of skin or intercostal muscles into the empyema space, or occasionally thoracoplasty). Surgery, however, should be postponed until prolonged drainage and antibiotic therapy have failed.

Pleural involvement by nonbacterial, nontuberculous infections is uncommon. Viral and mycoplasmal pneumonias rarely produce pleural symptoms. Fungal disease is also not characterized by pleural disease except in coccidioidomycosis, in which a hypersensitivity pleuritis over frank empyema can occur.

Pulmonary Embolus and Infarction. Pulmonary embolus frequently produces pleural disease, with more than half of patients having detectable effusions. These effusions are usually exudates, which often contain blood, although occasionally transudates may be found. Unless repeated embolization occurs, the effusion disappears with time and requires no treatment. Pulmonary embolus is discussed in detail in Ch. 67.

Hemothorax. Frank blood in the pleural space (pleural fluid hematocrit greater than 25 per cent of peripheral blood hematocrit) may be associated with either blunt or penetrating chest trauma, but may also result from spontaneous pneumothorax, hematologic disorders, and pleural malignancies. Left-sided hemothorax, particularly when associated with a widened superior mediastinum, may indicate dissection or rupture of the aorta. Pleural blood often does not clot and can be removed by thoracentesis. Small amounts of blood are readily

reabsorbed via the lymphatics, but large collections should be removed by tube drainage. Persistent pleural bleeding requires surgical intervention.

Chylothorax. The leakage of thoracic duct lymph or chyle into the pleural space is most frequently due to *trauma* but may be due to *granulomatous disease* or to invasion of the thoracic duct by *tumor.* Lymphomas are most commonly implicated, although mediastinal involvement from any carcinoma can produce a chylothorax. The symptoms of chylothorax are those of the underlying lesion unless the chylothorax is large enough to produce pulmonary symptoms. Since chyle collects within the posterior mediastinum following trauma, the chylothorax does not appear until the mediastinal pleura ruptures, often days after the trauma. The chylous fluid is a milky exudate and, if allowed to stand, a creamy layer forms on top. The lipid content of the fluid is high, as manifested microscopically by sudanophilic fat droplets and a high concentration of neutral fat and fatty acids. Cholesterol content is low, and the fluid contains few cells. Initial therapy is conservative with repeated thoracenteses or tube drainage. Most cases involving trauma require surgical intervention and ligation of the thoracic duct at the site of the rupture. Radiation therapy may be of benefit in some cases when chylothorax is due to malignancy. *Pseudochylothorax* or cholesterol effusion, a milky effusion with high cholesterol and low neutral lipid and fatty acid content, is seen in patients who have longstanding pleural effusions and is often associated with large numbers of degenerating leukocytes and the presence of cholesterol crystals. Treatment is usually not required, but occasionally pleural decortication may be indicated.

Miscellaneous Disorders. Systemic lupus erythematosus (SLE) and *rheumatoid arthritis* are frequently associated with pleuritis and pleural effusion. Pleural abnormalities may be the first manifestation of each of these diseases, but most often pleural changes occur after the diagnosis has been established.

SLE may have pleural involvement in over 70 per cent of patients. Sometimes transient episodes of pleuritic pain are the only manifestation, but pleural effusions are seen in up to 50 per cent of cases. They may be the only radiographic abnormality, or there may be associated nonspecific parenchymal infiltrates. The effusions are usually exudates containing varying numbers of leukocytes. Lower than normal concentrations of hemolytic complement and its C3 and C4 components are present, and classic LE cells may be found in the fluid.

Rheumatoid arthritis may result in pleural effusions in approximately 5 per cent of patients. The effusion may be associated with rheumatoid lung disease, but most often it occurs in the absence of other pulmonary changes. The effusions are exudates, often with a predominance of lymphocytes, often have a low pH, and usually contain extremely low concentrations of glucose (less than 15 mg per deciliter and in some cases less than 5 mg per deciliter). Rheumatoid factor may be present, but this is a nonspecific finding. Pleural biopsy may reveal typical rheumatoid nodules, and occasionally palisades of histiocytes, similar to those in rheumatoid nodules, appear in the fluid. In contrast to SLE effusions, rheumatoid pleural effusions may persist for weeks or months and may require repeated thoracenteses.

Subdiaphragmatic abscess resulting from hepatic disease, gastrointestinal perforations, or prior surgery may be associated with pleuritic chest pain, fever, and abdominal findings. Elevation of a hemidiaphragm on the affected side and impaired diaphragmatic motion are characteristic. Exudative pleural effusions, occasionally containing bacteria, and basilar pneumonias are frequent. Treatment includes surgical drainage of the abscess and antibiotics.

Pancreatitis or *pancreatic pseudocysts* may be associated with pleural effusions, most often on the left side, although a significant number are bilateral. Effusions usually are not large. They are exudates, may be blood tinged, and contain levels of amylase that exceed those in serum. Effusions may be due to irritation and inflammation of the diaphragmatic pleura, extension of fluid through diaphragmatic lymphatics, or actual communication of a pseudocyst with the pleural space. The effusion will subside with treatment of the pancreatic problem. Acute pancreatitis may also be a cause of the adult respiratory distress syndrome (ARDS).

Meigs' syndrome is the association of ascites, benign fibroma or other ovarian tumors, and frequently massive and recurrent pleural effusions. The effusion is usually a transudate but may be exudative or serosanguineous. Removal of the tumor relieves the ascites and effusion. The mechanism for the formation of pleural and peritoneal fluid has not been completely explained. The diagnosis should be considered in women with pleural effusion of obscure origin, especially if there is evidence of concurrent ascites and pelvic disease.

Uremia is associated with a polyserositis, which may include the pleural space. The effusions are exudates and often contain varying amounts of blood. At least half the effusions are asymptomatic. Effusions resolve with treatment of the uremia, but repeated thoracenteses may be necessary to control symptoms.

Asbestosis is frequently associated with pleural disease (see Ch. 536). Asbestos is the main cause of pleural plaques, which often appear along diaphragmatic and pericardial pleura. These plaques often calcify 20 to 40 years after exposure and bear no direct relation to amount of asbestos exposure. They cause no functional impairment and do not lead to mesotheliomas. Pleural fibrosis is seen in 10 to 20 per cent of asbestos workers. It is usually bilateral, is not associated with interstitial fibrosis, and may in rare instances lead to functional impairment. Pleural effusion from asbestos is often bilateral, may be recurrent, is an exudate, and is often serosanguineous. There is no direct relation between duration or intensity of exposure and pleural effusions. In contrast to other complications of asbestosis, the latency for pleural effusions is less than 20 years from the initial exposure. Other rare causes of pleural effusions are sarcoidosis, myxedema, hypersensitivity reactions, hepatitis, and amebiasis.

NEOPLASMS OF THE PLEURA. *Metastatic Tumors.* Involvement of pleura by malignancies arising elsewhere is common. In middle and older age groups, metastatic disease (through either pleural implants or mediastinal lymphatic obstruction) accounts for 30 to 40 per cent of pleural effusions. Carcinomas of the lung and breast are the neoplasms that most commonly involve the pleura, although virtually any neoplasm may be implicated. Involvement of pleura is considered a sign of inoperability in bronchogenic carcinomas other than superior sulcus tumors. Malignant pleural fluid is usually exudative and may contain blood. Pleural fluid cytology is positive in 20 to 25 per cent of cases, and pleural biopsy provides a diagnosis of malignancy in an additional 25 to 40 per cent of cases. The course of malignant pleural effusions usually involves reaccumulation of fluid despite repeated thoracenteses. Under such circumstances, treatment is aimed at obliterating the pleural space with tube drainage or with one of a number of irritating substances. Intrapleural tetracycline is the present drug of choice, since it produces pleural symphysis in the majority of cases with no systemic and few local side effects. For best results, 1000 mg of the drug is introduced through a chest tube, is left in the pleural space for 24 hours, and then is drained as the pleural surfaces are approximated by suction applied to the tube.

Mesothelioma. Mesothelioma, the main primary pleural tumor, may be benign or malignant. Benign mesotheliomas are rare, have the histologic appearance of a fibroma, and generally present as localized tumor masses. They usually arise from visceral pleura and may reach a rather large size, compressing normal lung and thereby causing symptoms. Parietal pleural lesions may be pedunculated. In either case,

benign mesotheliomas appear on roentgenogram as smooth lobulated masses along the pleural surface. Hypertrophic pulmonary osteoarthropathy and clubbing are particularly common in patients with benign mesothelioma. Treatment involves surgical removal. Malignant mesotheliomas are related to asbestos exposure in 80 to 90 per cent of cases, although the dose relationship is a weak one. Smoking is not a factor. These tumors are diffuse and infiltrate the pleura widely, often completely encasing the lung. Symptoms of cough, chest pain, and dyspnea are frequent late in the disease, as are bloody pleural effusions. Although the diagnosis of a malignancy is made readily by the demonstration of malignant cells either in pleural fluid or from a pleural biopsy, distinguishing mesothelioma pathologically from metastatic disease on small tissue samples can be difficult. Prognosis is poor, with median survivals on the order of one year. Surgery is not possible, and radiation and chemotherapy have been largely unsuccessful to date.

Pneumothorax. A pneumothorax is an accumulation of gas within the pleural space. Gas may appear in the pleural space as a result of (1) perforation of the visceral pleura and entry of gas from the lung; (2) penetration of the chest wall, diaphragm, mediastinum, or esophagus; or (3) gas generated by microorganisms in an empyema. Spontaneous rupture of pleura and entry of air from the lung may occur in the absence of known disease (simple pneumothorax) or may occur as a result of parenchymal lung disease (secondary pneumothorax).

Simple spontaneous pneumothorax occurs most commonly in previously healthy men 20 to 40 years of age and is due to rupture of subpleural blebs that appear at the apex of the lung. The cause of these blebs and their predominance in men is not known. The right side is more frequently involved than the left, and recurrence is frequent (30 per cent on the same side, 10 per cent on the opposite side). The clinical presentation involves sudden onset of chest pain with dyspnea appearing in proportion to the size of the pneumothorax. The precipitating event is usually not clear, although some occur during vigorous effort, particularly with rapid large swings in intrathoracic pressure. The pneumothorax may vary in size from minor, being visible only on an expiratory film, to 100 per cent of the hemithorax being filled with air producing collapse of the lung. Small amounts of pleural fluid are present in 25 per cent of simple pneumothoraces. Tension pneumothorax (produced by increasing positive pressures in the hemithorax through a "ball-valve" air leak) is rare but can shift the mediastinum and compromise circulation. Treatment of a simple pneumothorax depends on its size. Small pneumothoraces occupying less than 25 per cent of the hemithorax in asymptomatic individuals can be treated on an outpatient basis without removing the air, since they will reabsorb over a period of seven to ten days. Larger pneumothoraces may be treated by removing air through a small catheter, and pneumothoraces of over 50 per cent or those associated with lung collapse should be treated with a chest tube initially connected to suction and, once the lung is expanded, placed under water seal drainage. The tube should be left in place for two to four days. For recurrent simple pneumothoraces, surgical obliteration of the apical pleural space (scarification, abrasion, or even decortication in certain circumstances) should be undertaken at the time of the second or third episode. Tension pneumothorax requires immediate decompression of the involved side with insertion of a large-bore needle through an intercostal space.

Secondary or *complicated pneumothorax* occurs as a result of trauma or as a result of some other pulmonary disease. Widespread emphysema is the most common pulmonary process producing secondary pneumothorax. Pneumothorax may complicate pulmonary infection by rupture of infected material into the pleural space (pyopneumothorax). Less common pulmonary diseases associated with pneumothorax are bronchial asthma, staphylococcal pneumatoceles, and advanced pulmonary fibrosis. Eosinophilic granuloma is an interstitial disease that is characteristically associated with spontaneous pneumothorax. Pneumothorax may also appear as a complication of mechanical ventilation when high intrathoracic pressures are utilized. In contrast to simple or primary pneumothorax, in which dyspnea and evidence of ventilatory compromise are unusual unless the pneumothorax is large, relatively small pneumothoraces may produce severe respiratory symptoms when superimposed on pre-existing pulmonary disease. Thus, treatment of patients with secondary pneumothorax is more aggressive, with thoracotomy tube drainage being employed more frequently. Persistent pleural leaks (bronchopleural fistulas) and tension pneumothorax are also more frequent with secondary pneumothorax, particularly in those patients who develop a pneumothorax while on mechanical ventilation.

Adams VI, Unni KK, Muhm, JR, et al.: Diffuse malignant mesothelioma of pleura. Diagnosis and survival in 92 cases. Cancer 58:1540, 1986. *A complete clinical, radiologic, and pathologic review of pleural mesotheliomas. Correlation of clinical findings and prognosis.*

Black LF: The pleural space and pleural fluid. Mayo Clin Proc 47:493, 1972. *An excellent discussion of the physiology of normal and abnormal pleural fluid formation. Not much has been added since this article was published.*

Epler GR, McLoud TC, Gaensler EA: Prevalence and incidence of benign asbestos pleural effusion in a working population. JAMA 247:617, 1982. *Puts asbestos pleural effusion in perspective. Reviews diagnostic criteria and epidemiology and emphasizes early onset of pleural effusion as a complication of asbestos exposure.*

Health and Public Policy Committee, American College of Physicians: Diagnostic thoracentesis and pleural biopsy in pleural effusions. Ann Intern Med 103:799, 1985. *A consensus about efficacy and cost effectiveness of various tests used in the evaluation of pleural effusions.*

Light RW, MacGregor MI, Luchsinger PC, et al.: Pleural effusions: The diagnostic separation of transudates and exudates. Ann Intern Med 77:507, 1972. *The "classic" paper that separates transudates and exudates on the basis of pleural fluid to serum ratios of protein and LDH.*

Malden LT, Tattersall MH: Malignant effusions. Q J Med 58:221, 1986. *An extensive review of the pathophysiology, diagnostic considerations, and treatment options for patients with malignant pleural effusions.*

Ryan CJ, Rodgers RF, Unni KK, et al.: The outcome of patients with pleural effusion of indeterminate cause at thoracotomy. Mayo Clin Proc 56:145, 1981. *An interesting study of the natural history of pleural effusions that could not be diagnosed at thoracotomy.*

THE MEDIASTINUM

ANATOMY. The mediastinum is the anatomic space that lies in the mid-thorax. It separates the two pleural cavities and is defined by the diaphragm below and the suprasternal thoracic outlet above. The mediastinum contains several vital structures contiguous to one another in a relatively small space. Thus, abnormalities within the mediastinum, regardless of their cause, can produce a number of serious symptoms. It is convenient for clinical purposes to divide the mediastinum into *anterior*, *middle*, and *posterior* areas. The anterior mediastinal compartment is bounded posteriorly by the pericardium, ascending aorta, and brachial cephalic vessels and anteriorly by the sternum. This compartment contains the thymus gland, substernal extensions of the thyroid and parathyroid glands, blood vessels, pericardium, and lymph nodes. The middle mediastinal compartment extends from the posterior limit of the anterior compartment to the anterior border of the vertebral bodies. The middle mediastinum contains the heart, great vessels, trachea, main bronchi, esophagus, and phrenic and vagus nerves. The posterior mediastinum extends from the anterior surface of the vertebral bodies to the dorsal chest wall. This compartment contains the vertebral bodies, the descending thoracic aorta, the esophagus, the thoracic duct, the azygous and the hemiazygous veins, the lower portion of the vagus nerve plus the sympathetic chains, and a posterior group of mediastinal nodes.

SIGNS AND SYMPTOMS. *Chest pain, cough, hoarseness,* and *dyspnea* are the most common complaints. Less common symptoms are *stridor, dysphagia,* and *Horner's syndrome*. However, most patients with mediastinal masses are asymptomatic. Occasionally, specific syndromes are associated with primary lesions of the mediastinum. Nearly half of all thymomas are associated with myasthenia gravis (see Ch. 518). Mesotheliomas, fibrosarcomas, and occasional teratomas have been associated with hypoglycemia. Parathyroid tumors may present with hypercalcemia. Neurogenic tumors may result in pressure against the spinal cord, causing a variety of symptoms. Because of the crowding within the normal mediastinum of a large number of structures, more than one organ is likely to be affected by a given disorder. Signs and symptoms of mediastinal disorders are thus nonspecific. The physical findings of mediastinal air or inflammation are specific and discussed below. Physical findings in a patient with a mediastinal mass, however, are unusual unless the mass is large or impinges on a vital structure. Rarely, the mass may be so large that the pleural cavity is obliterated, leading to findings consistent with pleural effusion. Occasionally, a mediastinal tumor may produce superior vena caval obstruction with typical signs of facial edema, dilated neck veins over the thorax, and edema of the upper extremities. A mass can also erode into the trachea, esophagus, or great vessels with life-threatening sequelae.

DIAGNOSIS. Radiographic studies are the most helpful procedures in evaluating patients with mediastinal disorders. A large percentage of such lesions are first detected on routine chest roentgenograms (Fig. 71–1A). Computed tomography (CT) has dramatically improved visualization and definition of mediastinal structures and will replace routine tomography in time (Fig. 71–1B). The angiographic definition of great vessels and barium esophagograms are often of considerable value in defining mediastinal lesions.

In those patients in whom specific diagnoses cannot be established by radiographic methods, surgical approaches to obtaining tissue for histologic diagnosis are necessary. Anterior and some middle mediastinal lesions can be approached through mediastinoscopy or mediastinotomy. Both procedures provide lymph nodes for histologic and cultural examination without the need for major surgery. Thoracotomy is necessary when tissue from middle and posterior mediastinal lesions is required. Thoracotomy not only provides the opportunity for tissue diagnosis but also allows drainage or definitive resection of specific lesions.

SPECIFIC DISEASES. *Infections.* Acute mediastinitis is rare and most often results from endoscopy, surgery, or trauma to the esophagus. Fever, chest pain, widening of the mediastinal shadow by x-ray, and a history of trauma or manipulation of the esophagus suggest the diagnosis. X-ray studies with contrast material may demonstrate esophageal perforation. Complicating pleural effusions are occasionally observed and, if untreated, often develop into an empyema. Repair of the esophageal perforation, surgical drainage of mediastinal abscesses, and antibiotic therapy should be employed. Chronic fibrosing mediastinitis caused by extension of granulomatous disease (especially histoplasmosis) from mediastinal lymph nodes is rare but may cause severe irreversible mediastinal fibrosis with superior vena caval obstruction.

Pneumomediastinum. Air may enter the mediastinum either as a result of a tear in the esophagus or tracheobronchial tree or because of the dissection of air from ruptured alveoli along the peribronchovascular sheath. Rupture of the esophagus usually is associated with instrumentation or trauma. Pneumomediastinum from alveolar rupture may occur spontaneously in individuals with no underlying lung disease or may be a complication of severe diffuse disease or artificial ventilation. In many cases of pneumomediastinum, air will rupture through the mediastinal pleura producing an associated pneumothorax, which may be bilateral. The air may dissect into the subcutaneous tissues of the neck and produce generalized subcutaneous emphysema. In children, the air

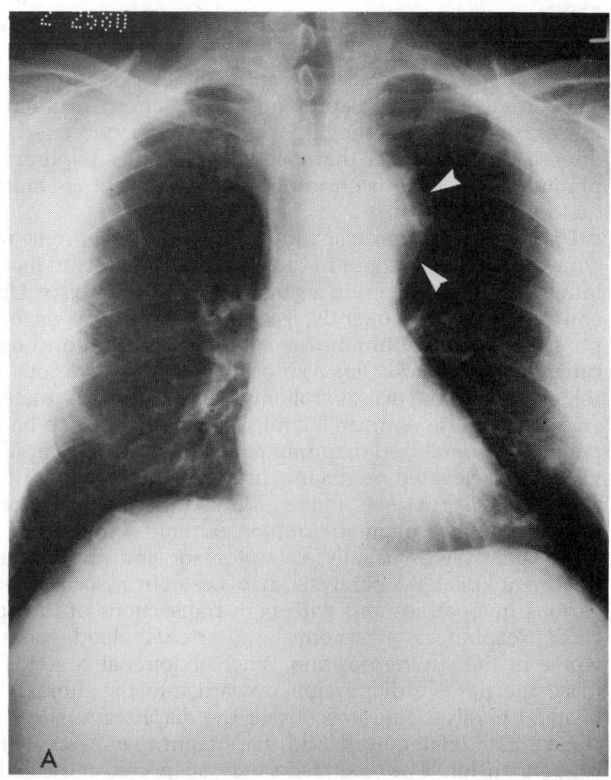

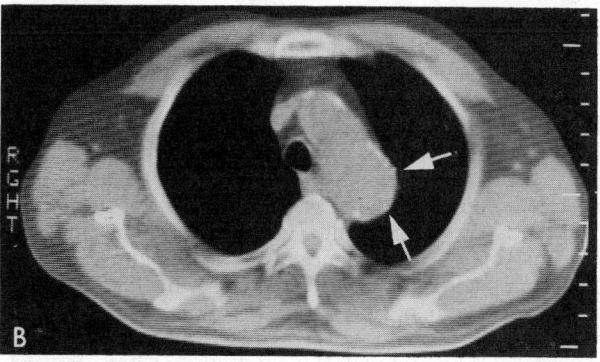

FIGURE 71–1. *A,* Posteroanterior chest roentgenogram of a 61-year-old man with mass noted adjacent to aortic arch *(arrows)*. On lateral film the mass projected posteriorly. There was a history of an automobile accident 17 years previously. *B,* CT scan shows large mass projecting from the aorta *(arrows)*. Dense calcium can be seen in the wall of this post-traumatic aortic aneurysm, which enhanced with injection of a small bolus of contrast medium (film not shown).

may collect within the mediastinum, compressing the great vessels. Patients with pneumomediastinum may be asymptomatic or at times may develop substernal chest pain indistinguishable from that of myocardial infarction. Physical examination may reveal subcutaneous emphysema in the neck, and auscultation often reveals a mediastinal crunch, a crackling sound synchronous with cardiac systole, best heard over the left sternal border when the patient is upright *(Hamman's sign).* A lateral chest roentgenogram is most effective in demonstrating air in the mediastinum. A simple, spontaneous pneumomediastinum usually subsides without treatment. When pneumomediastinum is severe, complicates airway or esophageal rupture, or involves compression of great vessels, surgical drainage and vigorous treatment of the underlying disease are required.

Tumors. Tumors of the mediastinum are the most common major disorder of this region. In young adults they are often

primary in the mediastinum and benign; in older adults they are often malignant and metastatic. Figure 71–2 lists the usual position of common mediastinal tumors. Of primary mediastinal tumors, approximately 20 per cent represent cysts, 20 per cent are neurogenic, 20 per cent are thymomas, 10 per cent are lymphomas, 10 per cent are teratomas, and the remainder are of miscellaneous origin. As noted above, most mediastinal tumors are asymptomatic, but when symptoms do arise they are the result of compression of vital structures within the mediastinum and usually represent malignant lesions. Surgical removal is the treatment of choice of most benign mediastinal tumors, even if asymptomatic, to prevent obstructive symptoms and potential malignant changes. Most malignant tumors are inoperable, although some, such as small cell carcinoma or lymphoma, may respond to radiation therapy or chemotherapy.

Benjamin SP, McCormack LJ, Effler DB, et al.: Primary tumors of the mediastinum. Chest 62:297, 1972. *A review of nonvascular mediastinal tumors. Many patients were asymptomatic, with masses being discovered on routine roentgenograms.*

Brown LR, Muhn JR: Computed tomography of the thorax: Current perspectives. Chest 83:806, 1983. *An excellent state-of-the-art review of the role that CT scanning plays in diagnosis of mediastinal and other thoracic diseases.*

Pugatch RD, Faling LJ, Robbins AH, et al.: CT diagnosis of benign mediastinal abnormalities. Am J Roentgenol 134:685, 1980. *Makes case for computed axial tomography as the initial procedure and most productive tool for evaluation of mediastinal abnormalities detected on plain chest roentgenogram. Excellent pictures and definition of mediastinal anatomy.*

THE DIAPHRAGM

The diaphragm is an airtight sheet of muscle and tendon lined by parietal pleura on one side and peritoneal membrane on the other. Its muscle fibers arise from the lower ribs and thoracic vertebrae and converge and insert into the margins of the crescentic central tendon. There is a hiatus for each of the principal structures that pass from thorax to abdomen. Motor and sensory fibers reach the diaphragm via the phrenic nerves, with separate innervation to the right and left halves. The diaphragm is the principal muscle of respiration. Diaphragmatic contraction tends to displace abdominal contents downward and to raise the ribs upward and outward, thus creating the negative intrapleural pressure of inspiration.

FIGURE 71–2. Locations of mediastinal tumors.

DIAPHRAGMATIC HERNIAS. Herniation of abdominal or retroperitoneal structures may occur through congenitally weak or incompletely fused areas of the diaphragm, may result from traumatic rupture, or may occur through the esophageal hiatus. The latter accounts for over three fourths of all diaphragmatic hernias and is considered in Ch. 98.

Hernias posteriorly through the foramina of Bochdalek are the most common form of hernia in infancy, occurring more often on the left than the right. The hernial opening may be large because of a virtual absence of the diaphragm owing to failure of its posterolateral portion to close. In this instance, abdominal viscera may extend freely into the left pleural space, producing respiratory distress and requiring immediate surgical repair. When the defect is small, the peritoneum and pleura usually fuse, producing a sac that contains the herniated contents. In adults, the defect is usually small and is discovered on routine chest roentgenogram. The defect is usually posterolateral, and the hernial contents usually contain retroperitoneal fat or the upper pole of the kidney or, rarely, the spleen.

Hernias anteriorly through the foramina of Morgagni are rare and tend to occur in the obese or in patients who have increased intra-abdominal pressure. The hernia commonly presents as an anterior, rounded density in the region of the right cardiophrenic angle. It usually contains omentum, but occasionally stomach, bowel, or liver may appear when hernias are large. Auscultation of borborygmi over the chest, radioisotope scans of the liver, routine gastrointestinal contrast films, and induction of a pneumoperitoneum followed by an upright film of the abdomen may all be useful diagnostic procedures. Therapy of both types of hernias may not be needed, especially when old films demonstrate that the abnormality has been present for a long time. Occasionally surgery is necessary for diagnosis or to relieve strangulation of hernia sac contents.

Traumatic hernias of the diaphragm may result from direct injury to the diaphragm or indirectly from severe abdominal compression. Signs and symptoms may occur immediately owing to extension of abdominal contents into the pleural space with resultant strangulation. More often, a latent period, which may extend for several years, intervenes before either respiratory or abdominal symptoms develop. Diagnosis is accomplished roentgenographically, and treatment is surgical.

DISORDERS OF DIAPHRAGMATIC MOTION. A variety of structural and functional abnormalities interfere with the ability of the diaphragm to develop inspiratory muscle strength. The resulting impairment of diaphragmatic function may be involved in many forms of respiratory failure.

Hiccup. Hiccup, or singultus, is a common disturbance produced by spasm of the diaphragm followed by sudden closure of the glottis during an inspiratory effort. A characteristic sound is produced as the glottis closes, and discomfort may be experienced as thoracic pressure is lowered by continued contraction of the diaphragm. Hiccup is usually of short duration but may persist for days or weeks. Hiccup is most often of unknown cause, presumably resulting from functional gastrointestinal disturbances. Occasionally, hiccups are a sign of serious disease, such as central nervous system disorders (encephalitis, brain stem strokes, tumor), uremia, herpes zoster, and pleural or abdominal processes that invade or irritate the diaphragm. Prolonged hiccups are sometimes thought to be psychogenic in origin. Hiccups usually subside spontaneously or when the initiating disease has been successfully treated. In persistent, debilitating hiccups, local anesthesia or actual crushing of one of the phrenic nerves may be required (crushing theoretically produces paralysis of only several months, but permanent paralysis is frequent).

Diaphragmatic Flutter. This is a rare disorder in which rapid rhythmic contractions of the diaphragm occur at a rate of 1 to 8 per second, lasting for seconds or as long as weeks or months. The contractions produce a cogwheel type of respiration and, when frequent, may hamper gas exchange. They are not accompanied by an inspiratory sound, and one or both halves of the diaphragm may be affected. Etiology is unclear, although psychogenic causes, central nervous system disease, and diseases that might irritate the diaphragm or phrenic nerve have been implicated. Treatment is similar to that for hiccup.

Diaphragmatic Paralysis. Interruption of the phrenic nerve anywhere from its origin in the C3–C5 nerve roots to its entry into the diaphragm produces diaphragmatic paralysis. Unilateral paralysis is frequently associated with invasion of the phrenic nerve by tumor (usually metastatic bronchogenic carcinoma). Paralysis has also been reported in various neurologic disorders such as poliomyelitis and herpes zoster. In an occasional patient, unilateral paralysis appears to be idiopathic. The paralyzed diaphragmatic leaf is not only nonfunctional but elevated, reducing lung volume on the side of paralysis. Diagnosis is made fluoroscopically by observing paradoxical diaphragmatic motion on sniff and cough. Unilateral paralysis is usually asymptomatic and rarely requires treatment. Bilateral paralysis may occur in association with various myopathies and with high transections of the spinal cord. Respiratory symptoms and arterial blood gases are worse in the supine position, since abdominal contents displace the passive diaphragm upward into the thorax. With bilateral paralysis, fluoroscopy of the diaphragm is less conclusive as a bilaterally flaccid diaphragm may drop with rib cage expansion. The diagnosis can be suspected at the bedside by observing inward, instead of outward, motion of the abdomen on inspiration. The diagnosis can be confirmed by recording muscle action potentials or by measuring esophageal and gastric (transdiaphragmatic) pressures on inspiration. Electrical stimulation of the phrenic nerve with measurement of conduction time may be helpful in diagnosing peripheral neuropathy. The hypoventilation of bilateral paralysis often produces respiratory failure. The hypoventilation of bilateral phrenic nerve paralysis can be treated by ventilating the patient on an intermittent or continuous schedule or by implanting and pacing phrenic nerve electrodes.

Eventration. Diaphragm eventration is a localized elevation of the diaphragm resulting from impaired muscle development or local muscle weakness. The diaphragm muscle is either absent or atrophic in the area of eventration. The elevation is usually on the right side of the anteromedial portion of the diaphragm. It most often appears in middle-aged, obese patients. The condition is usually asymptomatic, being recognized on routine chest roentgenograms. It must be differentiated from neoplasms, paralysis, and hernias and rarely requires surgical treatment.

Celli BR: Respiratory muscle function. Clin Chest Med 7:567, 1986. *A comprehensive up-to-date review covering clinical aspects of respiratory muscles clearly and concisely.*

Loh L, Goldman M, Davis JN: The assessment of the diaphragm function. Medicine 56:165, 1977. *A clear and easy-to-read review of diaphragm function and its importance clinically. Reference is made (Q J Med 45:87, 1976) to the role of diaphragm function in respiratory failure.*

THE CHEST WALL

The chest bellows serves to move air in and out of the lungs and is made up of the bony thoracic cage and the various muscles of respiration.

The neuromuscular–chest cage system is a major determinant of ventilatory patterns and of static and dynamic lung volumes. Disease of this system may influence total alveolar ventilation and ventilation-perfusion relationships and thus be responsible for hypoxemia or hypercapnia. Disorders of chest bellows function may be classified into two broad categories according to whether they result from impairment of the neuromuscular apparatus or from impairment of mechanical properties of the chest wall. The former are discussed as individual diseases in Part XXII. Only the latter group will be discussed here.

KYPHOSCOLIOSIS. This deformity of the chest wall is due to a combination of posterior angulation (kyphosis) and lateral angulation and rotation (scoliosis) of the spine. Scoliosis is categorized as to the right or left according to the direction of the convexity of the primary curvature. Idiopathic scoliosis is more frequently to the right in the thorax with a compensatory left curvature in the lumbar region.

The severity of scoliosis may be quantified by measuring the angle between upper and lower portions of spinal curve on a roentgenogram. Greater angles signify more severe deformity and imply greater respiratory impairment. In thoracic kyphoscoliosis the rib cage is distorted so that on the convex side of the spine the ribs are widely separated and rotation of the spine angulates them posteriorly, producing the kyphotic hump. On the concave side, the ribs are crowded and displaced anteriorly. Because of the kyphosis and loss of thoracic height, the lower anterior chest wall tends to bulge forward. Although mild degrees of kyphoscoliosis are common, severe distortion of the chest cage is unusual. Kyphoscoliosis usually begins in childhood but becomes more prominent during the rapid growth years of adolescence. In most cases (80 per cent) there is no discernible etiology; neurologic disorders that influence chest wall muscles and congenital abnormalities account for a small percentage of cases.

Patients are usually asymptomatic in early life. When kyphoscoliosis is severe (angle greater than 90 degrees) or when patients develop pulmonary infections (as a result of locally impaired bronchial clearance mechanisms), dyspnea appears. In these instances, gradual progression, respiratory failure, and cor pulmonale occur with death in the fourth through sixth decades. Patients with mild or moderate kyphoscoliosis (angle less than 50 degrees) who remain free of respiratory infections may have normal life expectancy.

Depending upon the degree of kyphoscoliosis, static lung volumes are reduced with preservation of residual volume; chest wall compliance is reduced, with lung compliance being slightly reduced or normal. Airflow rates are usually reduced only in proportion to the reduction of vital capacity. Studies of regional lung function tend to show variable shifts of ventilation and perfusion owing to the chest wall deformity. Arterial blood gases are also variable. Many patients have mild hypoxemia, secondary to ventilation-perfusion mismatch, but severe hypoxemia and hypercapnia occur only late in the disease and are most commonly associated with superimposed infection.

A variety of methods have been used to restore normal curvature or prevent progressive curvature of the spine. These include surgery, plaster casts, and various types of traction. With most, the cosmetic effect is greater than the physiologic effect, although they may prevent progression of curvature, particularly in those patients with idiopathic kyphoscoliosis. Efforts should be made to prevent airways disease; the patient should discontinue smoking, and respiratory infections should be treated early and vigorously. In patients with severe disease, episodic use of intermittent positive pressure breathing has been found to increase transiently functional residual capacity and total thoracic compliance and may be of value in ambulatory management. Episodes of acute respiratory failure, usually associated with respiratory infections, may require intubation and assisted ventilation. In some patients with chronic respiratory failure, night time ventilatory assistance may be effective in controlling symptoms and respiratory failure. Home oxygen should be used in those patients with severe hypoxemia.

PECTUS EXCAVATUM. This is a congenital deformity of the lower portion of the sternum with symmetric bowing of the anterior ribs. The defect, which is often familial, is thought to be due to a short central tendon of the diaphragm. When the deformity is severe, the heart and mediastinal structures are displaced laterally, but significant functional impairment is rare. Surgical correction is not necessary and is done only for cosmetic purposes.

ANKYLOSING SPONDYLITIS. This disease is characterized by fusion of costotransverse and vertebral joints and may also involve sternomanubrial and clavicular joints (see Ch. 434). The chest cage tends to be fixed in an inspiratory position, with the result that vital capacity is decreased while residual volume and functional residual capacity are increased. Although a small number of patients develop idiopathic upper lobe fibrosis, in most patients gas exchange is normal and respiratory disease is unusual.

FLAIL CHEST. Trauma to the chest that produces multiple anterior rib fractures may lead to instability of a large area of the anterior chest wall. This occurs most commonly in motor vehicle accidents or following cardiopulmonary resuscitation. Paradoxical motion occurs during respiration, with the injured area moving in an opposite direction from the remainder of the chest wall. Hypoxemia is common in flail chest, although alveolar hypoventilation with hypercapnia is rare. Hypoxemia is most often the result either of lung contusion with subsequent ventilation-perfusion mismatch or of breathing at low lung volumes and atelectasis. Artificial ventilation with volume ventilators is not necessary in many cases. Aggressive supportive care with attention to maintaining adequate oxygenation and clearance of airway secretions is the best approach to therapy.

Bergofsky EH: Respiratory failure in disorders of the thoracic cage. Am Rev Respir Dis 119:643, 1979. *A detailed clinical and physiologic review of the chest cage and its disorders. Contains an extensive list of references. Easy reading and "state of the art" for this topic.*

Hoeppner VH, Cockcroft DW, Dosman JH, et al.: Nighttime ventilation improves respiratory failure in secondary kyphoscoliosis. Am Rev Respir Dis 129:240, 1984. *Demonstrates effectiveness of now well-accepted approach to treatment of respiratory failure in patients with chest wall or diaphragmatic paralysis and other mechanical problems.*

Sharkford SR, Smith DE, Zarins CK, et al.: The management of flail chest. Am J Surg 132:759, 1976. *A retrospective review of personal cases and of the literature, establishing that not all patients with flail chest need to be intubated and ventilated.*

72 RESPIRATORY FAILURE

John F. Murray

INTRODUCTION

Adequate respiration consists of the uptake of sufficient amounts of O_2 and the elimination of sufficient amounts of CO_2 to maintain Po_2 and Pco_2 in arterial blood at their respective normal values. It follows that *respiratory failure* is associated with disturbances in the exchange of O_2 and CO_2 between gas in alveoli and blood in pulmonary capillaries and that these abnormalities must be reflected by changes in the Po_2 and Pco_2 in arterial blood. Thus respiratory failure is defined as a condition in which arterial Po_2 is below the normal range (excluding hypoxemia from intracardiac right-to-left shunting of blood) or arterial Pco_2 is above the normal range (excluding respiratory compensation for metabolic alkalosis). This definition, which is physiologically precise as well as clinically applicable, implies that the diagnosis of respiratory failure depends chiefly on laboratory analysis of arterial blood and not on clinical findings.

Respiratory failure is not a disease but a disorder of function that can be caused by a variety of conditions that affect the lungs; in some instances, the lungs are completely normal (e.g., overdose of sedative drugs). Respiratory failure is analogous to heart failure and renal failure, both of which represent the consequences of impaired normal function resulting from numerous disparate diseases.

Respiratory failure is traditionally divided into acute and

chronic varieties, depending on the time it takes for the abnormalities in gas exchange to occur. This arbitrary classification does not take into account the common clinical occurrence of an acute worsening of arterial P_{O_2} and P_{CO_2} in a patient who already has chronic respiratory failure as a result of some underlying disorder. However, the distinction between acute and chronic respiratory failure has important etiologic and therapeutic implications and will be referred to frequently.

PATHOPHYSIOLOGY OF RESPIRATORY FAILURE

In human beings, respiration has been subdivided into four functional processes: *ventilation, diffusion, perfusion,* and *control of breathing.* Each of these contributes uniquely to the maintenance of normal values of P_{O_2} and P_{CO_2} in arterial blood. Therefore, abnormalities in any one of the four processes, if sufficiently severe, will cause respiratory failure; furthermore, in many common respiratory disorders, multiple abnormalities coexist.

Normal Gas Exchange

The physiology of normal gas exchange is described in Ch. 59 and will not be reviewed here. However, understanding what is meant by normal is important, because arterial P_{O_2} varies with age, and both arterial P_{O_2} and P_{CO_2} vary according to the altitude (i.e., the prevailing barometric pressure) at which the person happens to be when the blood specimen is obtained and to the extent of acclimatization. The normal range includes the biologic variabilities among individuals and the analytic variations inherent in the measurements. Because the diagnosis of respiratory failure should be made in the laboratory and not at the bedside, the physician's ability to establish the diagnosis depends on the accuracy of the laboratory tests used to measure P_{O_2} and P_{CO_2}. Normal mean arterial P_{O_2} (Pa_{O_2}) values in subjects 20 years of age or older can be calculated from the regression equation $Pa_{O_2} = 100.1 - 0.323$ (age in years). The normal range of variation is ± 5 mm Hg from the mean value. Arterial P_{CO_2} does not vary with age and is normally within the range of 40 ± 5 mm Hg in healthy persons at sea level. Values of P_{O_2} *below* or P_{CO_2} *above* normal limits indicate the presence of respiratory failure.

Abnormal Gas Exchange

The pathophysiology of abnormal gas exchange is also discussed in Ch. 59. Hypoventilation, impaired diffusion, ventilation-perfusion mismatching, right-to-left shunting of blood, and breathing air with a low P_{O_2} all cause arterial hypoxia (a decrease below normal of P_{O_2}); in contrast, for practical purposes, only hypoventilation causes arterial hypercapnia (an increase above normal of P_{CO_2}). In view of the therapeutic importance of recognizing the abnormal mechanism(s) leading to a patient's respiratory failure, each will be reviewed briefly.

HYPOVENTILATION. Alveolar hypoventilation is present when the arterial P_{CO_2} is increased. Furthermore, as arterial P_{CO_2} increases, P_{O_2} decreases *except* when the patient is breathing gas with an enriched concentration of O_2. Because arterial P_{O_2} and P_{CO_2} change in opposite directions by nearly the same amount during hypoventilation, the contribution of hypoventilation to the patient's arterial hypoxia can be readily assessed. (In a 60-year-old person, for example, if $P_{O_2} = 50$ mm Hg and $P_{CO_2} = 70$ mm Hg, both have changed from their normal values by the same amount [30 mm Hg] and "pure" hypoventilation is present; in contrast, if $P_{O_2} = 30$ mm Hg and $P_{CO_2} = 70$ mm Hg, the change from normal of P_{CO_2} does not account for the entire change in P_{O_2}; therefore, some other cause in addition to hypoxia from hypoventilation must be present.) Arterial hypoxia from alveolar hypoventilation is not associated with an increased alveolar-arterial P_{O_2} difference and is "corrected" by breathing 100 per cent O_2.

IMPAIRED DIFFUSION. Abnormalities of diffusion do not cause arterial hypoxia in persons at rest unless they are extremely severe. Although these occur in occasional patients with respiratory failure, for practical purposes the possible contributions of an abnormality of diffusion to a given patient's arterial hypoxia can be ignored except during exercise or at high altitude. This practice is permissible because diffusion disturbances, even when marked, cause only relatively small increases in the patient's alveolar-arterial P_{O_2} difference, and this abnormality, if it exists, is readily corrected by adding small amounts of O_2 to the inspired air.

VENTILATION-PERFUSION IMBALANCE. When gas exchange units receive more blood flow than ventilation, arterial hypoxia results. Mismatching of ventilation-perfusion is by far the most common cause of arterial hypoxia and can be recognized by giving the patient 100 per cent O_2 to breathe; this causes the alveolar-arterial P_{O_2} difference from pure mismatching that is present while the patient breathes room air to decrease and arterial P_{O_2} to increase to normal values (>550 mm Hg). The importance of breathing 100 per cent O_2 is shown in Figure 72–1; in the presence of a severe ventilation-perfusion disturbance ($\sigma = 2.0$ in the figure), even an $F_{I_{O_2}}$ of 0.8 fails to raise P_{O_2} to normal values but 1.0 does. Although a "pure" ventilation-perfusion inequality can lead to CO_2 retention, this is an uncommon cause of hypercapnia because as arterial P_{CO_2} tends to increase, it stimulates peripheral and central chemoreceptors and increases ventilation; this, in turn, reduces P_{CO_2} back to normal values but, owing to the shape of the oxyhemoglobin dissociation curve, does not correct the hypoxia.

RIGHT-TO-LEFT SHUNTS. Shunts of blood from right to left may occur through abnormal anatomic communications in the lung (e.g., pulmonary arteriovenous fistula) but much more frequently by perfusion of lung units that are completely unventilated because they are either collapsed (atelectasis) or filled with fluid (pulmonary edema, pneumonia, intra-alveolar hemorrhage). Regardless of the cause, an alveolar-arterial P_{O_2} difference results that increases when the patient breathes 100 per cent O_2 compared with the value obtained while

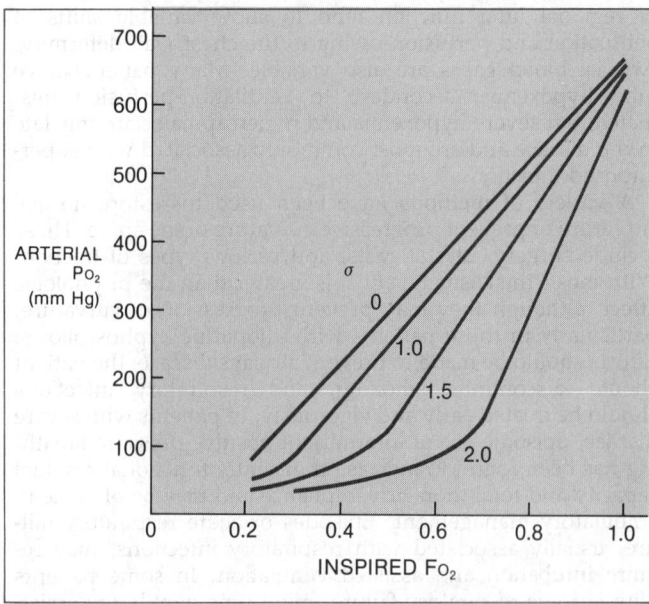

FIGURE 72–1. Graph showing the effects of changing inspired O_2 concentration (F_{O_2}) on arterial P_{O_2} in the presence of varying amounts of ventilation-perfusion inequality. When ventilation and perfusion are evenly matched ($\sigma = 0$), the relationship between inspired F_{O_2} and arterial P_{O_2} is linear. As ventilation-perfusion inequalities worsen ($\sigma = 1.0$ to 2.0), the effect of breathing a given F_{O_2} is progressively less. (Modified from West JB, Wagner PD: Bioengineering Aspects of the Lung. New York, Marcel Dekker, Inc., 1977. Reprinted with permission of the authors and publisher.)

breathing room air. For reasons similar to those occurring in patients with ventilation-perfusion imbalances, CO_2 retention seldom occurs in patients with right-to-left shunts.

DECREASED INSPIRED PO_2. Expected values of arterial PO_2 are corrected for the influence of decreasing barometric pressure; strictly speaking, therefore, the effects of altitude on inspired PO_2 and the resulting decreased arterial PO_2 are not an abnormal cause of hypoxia, even though the hypoxia may be severe and dangerous. Occasionally, pathologic hypoxia occurs when ambient PO_2 is reduced because of combustion of O_2 or because of dilution by some other gas. However, this phenomenon is not of importance when interpreting the results of analysis of arterial blood specimens obtained in the hospital or clinic.

HYPERCAPNIA. In contrast to arterial hypoxia, which may result from five different pathophysiologic derangements, arterial hypercapnia can always be interpreted as signifying alveolar hypoventilation. This is true because arterial PCO_2 (Pa_{CO_2}) is governed by the relationship between CO_2 production ($\dot{V}CO_2$) and alveolar ventilation ($\dot{V}A$): $Pa_{CO_2} = k\dot{V}CO_2/\dot{V}A$. Normally, however, even when CO_2 production increases markedly, alveolar ventilation increases proportionately and arterial PCO_2 is maintained within narrow limits. Thus an increase in arterial PCO_2 can always be viewed as respiratory failure in the sense that alveolar ventilation is inadequate to eliminate all the CO_2 being produced at that time. Severe ventilation-perfusion imbalances and right-to-left shunts can produce CO_2 retention, but this is uncommon because, as already emphasized, alveolar ventilation usually increases and corrects the disturbance.

An increase or decrease in PCO_2 in the blood has a direct effect on the amount of carbonic acid in the blood and a reciprocal effect on pH. Acute changes in PCO_2 have a more profound effect on pH than chronic changes owing to differences in plasma bicarbonate. With acute increases or decreases in PCO_2, there is little change in bicarbonate level and a considerable change in pH; after three to five days of sustained changes in PCO_2, renal compensation has increased plasma bicarbonate in hypercapnia and decreased it in hypocapnia, both tending to restore pH toward normal. Many patients with respiratory failure have mixed respiratory and nonrespiratory acid-base disturbances. Knowledge of the time course of a patient's problem as well as the magnitude of changes in plasma bicarbonate is extremely useful in providing the necessary understanding for appropriate treatment of all components of the disorder.

Right Heart Failure

Acute respiratory failure can cause acute right heart failure (acute cor pulmonale). The normal right ventricle is not a good pressure generator and cannot sustain sudden pressure loads over 40 to 50 mm Hg. Thus acute right heart failure may develop in any condition in which pulmonary vascular resistance increases abruptly; this happens most commonly in patients with multiple pulmonary emboli with obstruction of much of the pulmonary vascular bed (usually >60 per cent). At times, acute cor pulmonale complicates the course of patients with severe bronchial asthma or other forms of marked airways obstruction.

Acute right heart failure may also occur in patients with chronic lung disease during an episode of acute respiratory failure. Most of these patients have right ventricular hypertrophy (chronic cor pulmonale) to begin with, and a subclinical or stable condition is aggravated by the added effects of the superimposed acute lung disease (usually bronchitis or pneumonia). In these patients, right ventricular function is worsened for several reasons: (1) Alveolar hypoxia and acidemia cause pulmonary arterial vasoconstriction; (2) certain lung diseases reduce the cross-sectional area available for perfusion; (3) hyperinflation of the lung increases pulmonary vas-

cular resistance; and (4) arterial hypoxia may depress myocardial contractility. These factors are important to recognize because they are reversible and usually respond well to appropriate treatment of the intercurrent acute disorder.

CAUSES OF RESPIRATORY FAILURE

Because respiratory failure is defined as the presence of arterial hypoxia with or without hypercapnia, it is obvious that a large variety of disorders are capable of producing these abnormalities. For convenience, the multiple causes of respiratory failure can be classified, depending on which component of the respiratory system is involved. Because most of these disorders characteristically cause either acute or chronic respiratory failure, they can be subdivided further into these categories.

Diseases Causing Airways Obstruction

ACUTE. Obstruction may result from acute diseases that involve any portion of the upper and lower airways. The presence of respiratory failure depends on the magnitude and extent of the narrowing. Obstruction of the *extra*thoracic airway (nasopharynx, larynx, extrathoracic portion of the trachea) usually causes stridor, a characteristic alteration of breathing that is associated with harsh, high-pitched respiratory noises that are louder and more pronounced during inspiration than expiration. In contrast, obstruction of the *intra*thoracic airways causes wheezing, an abnormality of breathing in which expiration is louder and longer than inspiration.

Obstruction of the upper airways can result from (1) inflammation-induced swelling of the mucosa secondary to infections, allergic reactions, and, less commonly, thermal or mechanical injuries and (2) impaction of foreign bodies or, occasionally, tumors. Acute obstruction of the upper airways is particularly likely to develop in infants and young children who have smaller and hence more vulnerable upper passages than older children and adults.

Acute obstruction of the lower airways is usually caused by swelling of the mucosa, secretions in the lumen, or bronchospasm. Accordingly, bronchial asthma, infections, bronchiolitis, and the inhalation of chemicals (such as nitrogen dioxide in silo-filler's disease) are important causes of acute respiratory failure.

CHRONIC. Diffuse obstruction may result from disorders originating in large bronchi (bronchiectasis), small bronchi (bronchitis), or the lung parenchyma (emphysema). These abnormalities characteristically progress gradually and lead to chronic respiratory failure. Of considerable importance are the intercurrent episodes of acute disease, usually pneumonia or bronchitis, that complicate the underlying disorder and often worsen the severity of existing respiratory failure.

Diseases Causing Parenchymal Infiltration

ACUTE. The most common cause of acute infiltration of the parenchyma is pneumonia, which usually has an infectious origin but occasionally is caused by inhalation or aspiration of a toxic chemical. Whether acute respiratory failure develops depends on the extent and severity of the disease. Immunologic reactions from drugs, migrating parasites, or leukoagglutinins are uncommon causes of acute respiratory failure but are important because of their special therapeutic requirements.

CHRONIC. There are over 100 different conditions that can cause chronic diffuse parenchymal infiltration. When severe, any of these can cause chronic respiratory failure. As in patients with chronic airways obstruction, patients with chronic infiltrative diseases may have intercurrent episodes of bronchopulmonary infection that cause acute worsening of their underlying respiratory status.

TABLE 72–1. PARTIAL LIST OF CONDITIONS THAT HAVE BEEN ASSOCIATED WITH THE ADULT RESPIRATORY DISTRESS SYNDROME

Shock of any etiology	Inhaled toxins
Infections	O₂ (high concentrations)
Gram-negative sepsis	Smoke
Viral pneumonia	Corrosive chemicals (NO₂, Cl₂,
Bacterial pneumonia	NH₃, phosgene, cadmium)
Trauma	Hematologic disorders
Fat emboli	Intravascular coagulation
Lung contusion	Massive blood transfusion
Nonthoracic trauma (including	Metabolic disorders
head injury)	Pancreatitis
Liquid aspiration	Uremia
Gastric juice	Paraquat ingestion
Fresh and salt water (drowning)	Miscellaneous
Hydrocarbon fluids	Increased intracranial pressure
Drug overdose	(including seizures)
Heroin	Eclampsia
Methadone	Postcardioversion
Propoxyphene	Radiation pneumonitis
Barbiturates	Postcardiopulmonary bypass
Colchicine	

Diseases Causing Pulmonary Edema

CARDIOGENIC. Pulmonary edema in patients with heart disease may be acute or chronic in onset; both varieties are caused by an increase in the hydrostatic pressure within pulmonary capillaries. Pulmonary edema may follow an acute myocardial infarction or acute left ventricular failure of any cause (hypertensive crises, arrhythmias), or it may be precipitated in patients with valvular or other forms of chronic heart disease by sudden changes in their cardiorespiratory status (from arrhythmias, hypoxemia, or increased systemic blood pressure). Chronic pulmonary edema is found in patients with chronic, usually refractory, heart failure, but even in these patients the amount of edema increases and decreases according to changing hemodynamics and therapy.

INCREASED PERMEABILITY. Acute pulmonary edema can accompany certain conditions that do not involve the heart. The basic pathophysiologic abnormality in most of these disorders appears to be an increased permeability of the pulmonary capillary endothelium. Pulmonary edema resulting from increased permeability is an important and apparently steadily increasing cause of acute respiratory failure, especially in patients who are hospitalized with serious medical or surgical illnesses that initially do not involve the lungs. After a latent period of 6 to 24 hours, these patients develop progressive arterial hypoxia, decreased compliance, and extensive roentgenographic infiltrations; in fatal cases, the lungs are found to be nearly airless, intensely congested, and filled with a proteinaceous edema fluid that also contains large numbers of red blood cells; occasionally, hyaline membranes are found. This constellation of clinical, physiologic, and radiologic findings is known as the *adult respiratory distress syndrome* and has been reported as a complication of many apparently unrelated conditions (Table 72–1). The feature common to all these disorders is the presence of diffuse injury to the alveolar-capillary membrane. Once damage has occurred, probably by many different pathways, and the permeability of the membrane is increased, pulmonary edema follows; thus the clinical, physiologic, and radiologic manifestations are similar, regardless of the cause of the injury. The adult respiratory distress syndrome is described at greater length in Ch. 73.

Pulmonary Vascular Diseases

ACUTE. Pulmonary embolism is usually accompanied by a decreased arterial Po₂ and Pco₂, the former from ventilation-perfusion mismatching and the latter reflecting the hyperventilation that nearly always occurs. Pulmonary embolism is also an important cause of worsening respiratory failure in patients with underlying chronic lung disease. Fat emboli and emboli from platelet-fibrin aggregates can cause marked hypoxia by increasing the permeability of the alveolar-capillary membrane and producing severe pulmonary edema.

CHRONIC. Pulmonary vasculitis and recurrent thromboembolism are not common conditions and, when present, usually do not cause respiratory failure until the late stages of the disease. Recurrent thromboembolism occurs in intravenous drug abusers and in patients with chronic peripheral venous thrombi, sickle cell anemia, and schistosomiasis. Pulmonary vasculitis occurs in patients with scleroderma, other collagen diseases, and primary pulmonary hypertension.

Diseases of the Chest Wall and Pleura

ACUTE. The most important cause of sudden respiratory failure from acute disorders involving the thoracic cage is injury to the chest wall. Segmental fractures of several ribs or fractures of ribs on both sides of the sternum can result in a flail chest. Besides the impairment of ventilatory function that results from the unstable chest wall, gas exchange abnormalities are often compounded by contusion of the lung underneath the site of injury. Spontaneous or traumatic pneumothorax is an important cause of acute respiratory failure, which may be severe and which often afflicts otherwise healthy persons.

CHRONIC. Severe idiopathic or acquired kyphoscoliosis can cause chronic respiratory failure, which is often associated with cor pulmonale. Patients with massive pleural effusion(s) or with thickened, constrictive pleural layer(s) may also have chronic respiratory failure.

Disorders of the Neuromuscular System

Disorders of the neuromuscular system are classified according to which part of the effector system is involved, i.e., the brain, neuronal pathways, or muscles of respiration, rather than into acute and chronic varieties. Patients with these disorders often have normal lungs; respiratory failure occurs from inability to ventilate normally.

BRAIN DISORDERS. Probably the most common cause of respiratory failure from impaired function of the central nervous system is the use of sedative drugs or anesthetic agents. Suppression of ventilatory drive from opiates, barbiturates, psychic depressants, alcohol, and a variety of sedative drugs results in hypoxia and hypercapnia that may be life threatening. Ventilatory stimuli can also be depressed by many diseases of the central nervous system, including vascular diseases, tumors, and infections.

SPINAL CORD AND PERIPHERAL NERVE DISORDERS. Injuries to the cervical or high thoracic spinal cord may produce immediate respiratory failure from paralysis of the muscles of respiration. Loss of anterior horn cell function in patients with poliomyelitis was an important cause of acute and chronic respiratory failure but is seldom encountered now because of the widespread use of vaccination. Polyneuritis, whether postinfectious (Guillain-Barré syndrome) or toxic, is an uncommon but important cause of respiratory failure in view of its inherent reversibility.

MUSCULAR DISORDERS. The final effectors in the system that controls breathing are the skeletal muscles of respiration. When these muscles are involved by generalized myopathies, such as muscular dystrophy or myasthenia gravis, respiratory failure results. Respiratory failure in patients with myasthenia gravis occurs during myasthenic or cholinergic crises. In contrast, respiratory failure in patients with muscular dystrophy is nearly always chronic and related to an advanced stage in the progression of the disease.

SLEEP APNEA. Brief periods of apnea occur in normal persons during deep sleep. Much more prolonged episodes associated with severe hypoxia have been documented in patients with massive obesity, chronic mountain sickness, enlarged tonsils, and many other disorders. Apnea results from either failure of ventilatory drive or obstruction of the upper airway. Severe sleep apnea can cause chronic respiratory failure, cor pulmonale, psychosis, and pathologic daytime sleepiness, a condition sometimes called the pickwickian syndrome, with somewhat dubious literary authenticity. Sleep apnea is discussed at greater length in Ch. 457.

CLINICAL MANIFESTATIONS

Given the great variety of disorders that can cause respiratory failure, it is obvious that the clinical manifestations in a given patient depend in large part on which underlying disease he or she has; these are dealt with elsewhere in this book. When respiratory failure ensues and if the blood gas disturbances are sufficiently severe, the signs and symptoms of hypoxia, and possible hypercapnia, become superimposed upon the signs and symptoms of the underlying disease. The clinical manifestations of hypoxia and hypercapnia are nonspecific and usually occur late in the evolution of the clinical problem. This statement underscores the earlier axiom that the diagnosis of respiratory failure is made in the laboratory and not at the bedside.

Hypoxia

The signs and symptoms of acute hypoxia are chiefly caused by abnormalities in central nervous system and cardiovascular function. Characteristic features are impaired judgment and motor instability, a clinical picture closely resembling acute alcoholism. As hypoxia worsens, the brainstem is affected and death results from depression of the medullary respiratory centers. The initial cardiovascular effects of acute hypoxia are tachycardia and increased blood pressure; when hypoxia is very severe, bradycardia, myocardial depression, and shock ensue. Recognizable cyanosis of the lips, mucous membranes, and nail beds usually occurs when the concentration of reduced hemoglobin in the capillaries is >5 grams per deciliter. Accordingly, cyanosis can result from decreases in either arterial P_{O_2} or blood flow. In patients with lung disease, cyanosis cannot be detected by most physicians until arterial P_{O_2} is <50 mm Hg; some observers cannot recognize cyanosis unless arterial P_{O_2} is <40 mm Hg!

In patients with chronic hypoxia, the central nervous system manifestations are drowsiness, inattentiveness, apathy, fatigue, and delayed reaction time. The chronic cardiovascular effects are often minimal, but pulmonary hypertension or even cor pulmonale with signs of right heart failure may be detected on clinical examination. One of the hallmarks of chronic hypoxia is erythrocytosis, which may cause noticeable plethora and changes in the hemoglobin concentration, hematocrit ratio, or red blood cell count. However, the increase in red blood cell mass in many patients with chronic hypoxia is masked by an almost proportionate increase in plasma volume; in these patients, the usual peripheral blood indices of the red blood cell production (hemoglobin, hematocrit) do not reveal the full extent of the erythropoietic response.

Hypercapnia

The physiologic consequences of hypercapnia depend not only on the amount of excess CO_2 in the body but also on the rate at which retention develops. Increases in P_{CO_2} from acute respiratory failure lead to a constellation of progressive disturbances of central nervous system function: apprehension, confusion, drowsiness, coma, and death. The vascular responses represent a mixture of vasoconstriction, from generalized sympathetic activity, and vasodilation, from local accumulation of CO_2; thus the cardiovascular abnormalities are variable and depend on whether vasoconstrictor or vasodilator influences predominate. There are usually tachycardia and sweating, but blood pressure may be high, low, or normal.

In contrast, if P_{CO_2} increases slowly, compensation takes place and the clinical consequences may be minimal at values of arterial P_{CO_2} that would cause death if reached suddenly.

There are numerous patients with arterial P_{CO_2} values over 100 mm Hg who are ambulatory and at times living active lives, although most breathe supplementary O_2 to prevent life-threatening hypoxia. Patients with hypercapnia from chronic respiratory failure frequently complain of headaches and drowsiness; these symptoms are probably attributable to the potent cerebral vasodilating effect of excess CO_2. In addition, patients with chronic hypercapnia may have papilledema, muscular twitching, coarse myoclonic jerky motions, and asterixis. At times, the neurologic findings simulate those of a brain tumor.

TREATMENT OF ACUTE RESPIRATORY FAILURE

The time course of worsening abnormalities varies in patients with acute respiratory failure from almost instantaneous (flail chest, pulmonary embolism) to a gradual crescendo during a period of several hours or even days (respiratory tract infections, bronchial asthma). The demands for treatment and the speed with which it must be provided obviously differ from one patient to another. It is difficult to generalize about such an extremely variable clinical condition, but the principles of treatment of acute respiratory failure are as follows: *first,* establish an airway, administer O_2, and maintain adequate alveolar ventilation; *second,* identify and treat the underlying condition and monitor the patient's progress carefully.

Establish an Airway

The upper airway tends to be occluded in unconscious patients because of relaxation of the oropharyngeal muscles and tongue and the presence of saliva, vomitus, and other secretions. When respiratory arrest occurs away from medical facilities, clear all material from the oropharynx and place the victim on his or her back with the head tilted backward as far as possible and extend the jaw forward. Sometimes these simple maneuvers are all that is required to enable breathing to resume spontaneously. If it does not, start mouth-to-mouth breathing; after three or four quick full breaths without allowing time for deflation to occur, maintain deep breaths once every five seconds until the emergency is over.

An airway can be established by three different methods: an oropharyngeal tube, an endotracheal tube passed via the nose or mouth, and a tracheostomy. Selection of the procedure depends on available facilities and personnel and on the site and severity of the obstruction.

OROPHARYNGEAL AIRWAY. An oropharyngeal airway is valuable in unconscious patients who are breathing spontaneously (e.g., during recovery from general anesthesia, after a cerebrovascular accident). An oropharyngeal airway is also useful in patients who are apneic during emergency resuscitation but who are receiving some form of assisted ventilation (mouth-to-mouth respiration, bag-mask system). Although an oropharyngeal tube is commonly used in these clinical circumstances, its role must be viewed as temporary, either while the patient is waking up or until an endotracheal tube can be inserted.

ENDOTRACHEAL TUBE. The preferred method of establishing an airway in most emergencies is with an endotracheal tube. Once inserted, the tube is used to remove secretions and to provide ventilation. Endotracheal tubes can usually be passed quickly through the nose or, at times, through the mouth into the trachea by an experienced person; the airway is then sealed by inflating a balloon near the tip of the tube. Endotracheal tubes should be used in nearly all patients with acute respiratory failure severe enough to require control of their airways.

TRACHEOSTOMY. Emergency tracheostomy was formerly the only way of quickly establishing an airway in patients with acute respiratory failure. Now, emergency tracheostomy is contraindicated except in one clinical situation: acute obstruction of upper airways (e.g., from foreign bodies, trauma, or inflammation). Otherwise, intubation with an endotracheal tube is the treatment of choice for acute respiratory failure. Tracheostomy, if needed, can be performed electively at a later time in the operating room under ideal conditions. There is virtually no mortality and very little morbidity with an elective tracheostomy, in contrast to the high incidence of complications associated with emergency tracheostomy performed at the bedside.

The decision to convert a satisfactory endotracheal intubation to a tracheostomy is not an easy one and must be individualized in each case. The availability of tubes of inert plastic with low pressure cuffs permits endotracheal tubes to be used for weeks rather than days without prohibitive injury; the main mechanical difference between endotracheal and tracheostomy tubes is the trauma to the vocal cords from the former and problems related to the stoma in the latter. The usual reasons for performing a tracheostomy in a patient with a satisfactory endotracheal tube are (1) failure to control secretions (sometimes it is difficult to suction the lungs adequately, especially the left side, through a long endotracheal tube) and (2) the need for prolonged (i.e., several weeks) intubation for assisted ventilation and/or removal of secretions (these circumstances are uncommon but occur particularly in patients with neuromuscular disease and chest wall injuries).

The presence of a tube and its cuff in the airways can cause necrosis of the mucosa of the trachea; at times the entire airway wall may be eroded with penetration of the esophagus (tracheoesophageal fistula) or a neighboring blood vessel (innominate artery), causing severe hemorrhage. Delayed complications after extubation are caused by damage to the trachea or larynx from the tube or cuff; injury to the vocal cords merely impairs phonation, but serious and life-threatening obstruction to airflow can result from stenosis or malacia of the tracheal wall. These complications should be considered and evaluated in any patient who complains of persisting hoarseness or who develops breathlessness or stridor at any time after endotracheal intubation.

HUMIDIFICATION. Insertion of an endotracheal or tracheostomy tube bypasses the normal source of humidification of the inspired air. When this occurs and unhumidified air or gas mixture is breathed, the result is drying of the mucosa and impairment of mucociliary clearance. Thus as long as the upper airway is bypassed, patients must receive air or a mixture of O_2 that is fully saturated with water vapor at their body temperature. This is easily accomplished if the patient is being ventilated with most commercial ventilators that have heated humidifiers in the circuit. If the patient is breathing spontaneously, humidified gas can be delivered through a T-piece connected to the endotracheal or tracheostomy tube. When proper humidification is carried out, remember that there is *no* insensible water loss through the respiratory tract when evaluating the patient's daily fluid balance.

Administer Oxygen

Acute respiratory failure, by definition, includes decreased arterial P_{O_2}. When respiratory failure is severe, death results from the central nervous system or cardiovascular consequences of hypoxia. During emergencies, supplementary O_2 is given without worrying about the concentration being used; in general, the higher the concentration of O_2, the better. After the patient's emergency condition has stabilized, attention is directed to administering O_2 in the lowest possible concentration required to correct the hypoxia. Any more O_2 than required to raise arterial P_{O_2} to a safe level exposes the patient to the direct toxicity of O_2 on the lung parenchyma and other undesirable effects: suppression of alveolar macrophage function and mucociliary clearance. In patients with chronic obstructive pulmonary disease, especially those with chronic hypercapnia, the administration of O_2 is likely to worsen the CO_2 retention. The further increase in P_{CO_2} can be explained in part by suppression of pre-existing hypoxic

ventilatory drive; the remaining increase can be accounted for through the effects of O_2 on tidal volume and the timing of inspiration. In general, the higher the inspired O_2 concentration, the greater the CO_2 retention; this observation underlies the use of "low-flow" O_2 for these patients as described below under Treatment of Chronic Respiratory Failure.

The usual goal of O_2 therapy in acute respiratory failure is to raise arterial P_{O_2} to between 60 and 80 mm Hg. Because these values lie on the flat portion of the oxyhemoglobin dissociation curve, most of the available hemoglobin is saturated with O_2; raising arterial P_{O_2} values even higher adds very little additional O_2 to the blood and may require increases in alveolar P_{O_2} concentrations to toxic levels. At times, especially when the mechanism of arterial hypoxia is right-to-left shunting of blood, arterial P_{O_2} may be considerably less than 60 mm Hg even with the patient breathing 100 per cent O_2. When this occurs, other maneuvers such as addition of end-expiratory pressure are required to raise arterial P_{O_2} and to allow a reduction in inspired O_2 concentration.

There are several ways of giving supplementary O_2 to a patient. Which method is chosen depends on the cause and severity of the arterial hypoxia and convenience to the patient. It is important to emphasize that no method can be relied upon to produce a certain increase in arterial P_{O_2}; the response depends on which physiologic mechanism(s) is responsible for the hypoxia. Thus it is always advisable to monitor the effects of O_2 administration by serial analyses of arterial blood.

NASAL CANNULAS OR PRONGS. The concentration of O_2 in the inspired air can be enriched by nasal cannulas, catheters, or prongs. These devices work well even when patients breathe through their mouths. However, because of the drying effects of unhumidified O_2 on the nasal mucous membranes, if >3 to 5 liters per minute is needed to achieve satisfactory arterial oxygenation, other methods of administration are advisable.

VENTURI MASKS. These masks work on the principle of entrainment of a fixed proportion of air that mixes with the O_2 being supplied and results in a constant inspired concentration: 24, 28, 35, or 40 per cent O_2. Although a properly used Venturi mask ensures that the inspired O_2 concentration is constant, the effects on arterial P_{O_2} vary considerably from one patient to another. The mask is somewhat uncomfortable and must be removed for eating and drinking. Because of these disadvantages and high cost, other simpler and cheaper methods usually suffice to deliver relatively low (21 to 41 per cent) concentrations of O_2.

RESERVOIR MASKS. When high concentrations of O_2 (40 to 80 per cent) are needed in patients who are not intubated, reservoir masks are used. To ensure optimal efficiency of operation, the masks must be tight fitting to avoid leaks; because this often causes discomfort, it is difficult to deliver high concentrations of O_2 by reservoir masks for long periods.

OTHER METHODS. Most of the recently developed mechanical ventilators have regulators that can be set to deliver an inspired O_2 concentration that ranges from 21 to 100 per cent. One of the best ways of ensuring that patients actually receive high concentrations of O_2 (60 to 100 per cent) is to use a mechanical ventilator connected to an endotracheal or tracheostomy tube.

Maintain Alveolar Ventilation

Emergency resuscitation after respiratory arrest requires ventilation by mouth-to-mouth respiration or a bag and mask device. As soon as possible thereafter, if the patient does not resume spontaneous breathing, intubation and ventilation by a mechanical ventilator are indicated. Similar considerations apply to patients with acute respiratory failure whose breathing is insufficient to maintain adequate gas exchange. The main indications for mechanical ventilation are ventilatory failure, shown by an elevated or rising P_{CO_2}, or severe refractory hypoxia, shown by a low P_{O_2} that cannot be corrected without high concentrations of O_2 and often end-expiratory pressure. Special indications include the need to produce alkalosis, as in head injuries and certain drug overdoses, to stabilize the thorax, as in traumatic injuries that result in flail chest, or to aspirate secretions, as in bronchopulmonary infections and failure to cough.

MECHANICAL VENTILATION. Two types of mechanical ventilators can be used to provide assisted ventilation: pressure ventilators, in which a certain (adjustable) airway pressure is reached by the machine during each breathing cycle, or volume ventilators, in which a constant (adjustable) tidal volume is delivered to the patient with each breath. Most commercially available ventilators of both types can be set either to cycle automatically or to assist breathing once it is initiated by the patient. Most instruments also provide means of controlling inspiratory and expiratory flow rates. Pressure ventilators were widely used for many years, but almost all hospitals now use volume ventilators, which are more versatile and more reliable.

END-EXPIRATORY PRESSURE. Mechanical ventilators ordinarily raise airway pressure during inspiration and allow it to fall to zero (atmospheric) pressure during expiration; this pattern of assisted ventilation is known as intermittent positive pressure ventilation, or IPPV. At times, it is desirable to add positive pressure to the airway during expiration as well as inspiration to hold the lung at a higher end-expiratory lung volume (functional residual capacity) than it would reach at zero end-expiratory pressure; this pattern of assisted ventilation is known as continuous positive pressure ventilation, or CPPV. Keeping the lung at a high end-expiratory lung volume prevents closure of alveoli and airways during expiration, redistributes pulmonary edema fluid out of alveoli, and often improves arterial Po_2 considerably. Positive end-expiratory pressure (or PEEP) is most useful in patients with the conditions that cause the adult respiratory distress syndrome (Table 72–1).

Although end-expiratory pressure usually results in an improvement in arterial Po_2 and O_2 content, it may also decrease cardiac output by impairing venous return. Accordingly, the actual delivery of O_2 to the tissues of the body may decrease. Thus it is important to monitor both the respiratory and circulatory responses to end-expiratory pressure to determine the optimal amount of pressure and the need for additional therapeutic interventions. Another common and serious hazard of end-expiratory pressure is its tendency to cause spontaneous pneumothorax and pneumomediastinum.

Identify and Treat the Underlying Condition

Acute respiratory failure always has a precipitating cause. Consequently, the cause of the condition should be identified as soon as possible after emergency measures have been started and the patient's condition has stabilized. Usually, the diagnosis can be established easily by a thorough history and physical examination, analysis of the blood and urine, and chest roentgenogram. Helpful auxiliary tests include those that evaluate central nervous system or cardiac function, those that determine the presence of drugs or poisons in the body, and bacteriologic study of secretions and blood.

Treatment obviously depends on the underlying cause, and the reader is referred to the appropriate chapters of this book for information about the therapy of specific pulmonary and other disorders that lead to acute respiratory failure. In all patients with acute respiratory failure, careful attention should be paid to fluid balance. Overhydration is a frequent and serious complication that can usually be avoided by careful attention to fluid replacement and, when needed, monitoring of pulmonary capillary (wedge) pressure.

Many patients cared for in intensive care units are nutritionally depleted at the time of admission or become so soon afterward. Because morbidity and mortality are closely linked to nutritional status, it is important that this be assessed and, when necessary, treated by appropriate enteral or parenteral supplementation.

Monitor the Patient's Progress

The need for monitoring varies from patient to patient according to the response to initial treatment. If the disorder is readily reversible (e.g., bronchial asthma), the patient may respond sufficiently to go home shortly after being seen and treated. Other less rapidly responding conditions causing acute respiratory failure often require hospital care, and seriously ill patients are best treated in special acute care facilities (intensive care units) when available. Intensive care units provide an institutional focus of trained personnel and special equipment for the care of critically ill patients.

All seriously ill patients should have frequent measurements of blood pressure, constant monitoring of heart rate, careful recording of fluid intake and output, and determination of weight daily. Arterial blood gas analysis should be performed as often as needed but usually at least once daily. Special studies include measurement of cardiac output and placement of a Swan-Ganz catheter in the pulmonary artery for determination of pulmonary arterial and wedge pressures and sampling of mixed venous blood; this information is very helpful in guiding fluid replacement and ventilator adjustments, including levels of end-expiratory pressure. In general, wedge pressure values should be maintained in the normal range (5 to 10 mm Hg) and not allowed to increase above 15 mm Hg, especially in patients with the adult respiratory distress syndrome. Less reliance is being placed now, compared with previous years, on values of mixed venous Po_2 as a guide to O_2 delivery, especially in disorders such as sepsis and the adult respiratory distress syndrome. Attention is currently directed at improving O_2 delivery by increasing cardiac output through pharmacologic means or by increasing O_2 content through transfusions of packed red blood cells.

TREATMENT OF CHRONIC RESPIRATORY FAILURE

Patients with chronic lung disease often have sufficient alterations in their arterial Po_2 and Pco_2 values that they are said to be in chronic respiratory failure. Therapeutic regimens for these patients, whose disease is relatively stable, are delivered mainly on an outpatient basis and are designed to meet two objectives: (1) preventing or minimizing the number and severity of the intercurrent complications that would otherwise occur and (2) treating maximally all reversible elements of the underlying disorder. Many of the specific remedies are used for both purposes, and the approaches to preventive and maintenance therapy for patients with the most common chronic lung diseases, asthma, bronchitis, and emphysema, are discussed in Ch. 60 and 61.

Despite emphasis on preventing intercurrent complications, these attacks continue to plague the lives of patients with chronic lung disease. Acute episodes of bronchopulmonary infection, pneumothorax, pulmonary embolism, surgical procedures, and misuse of sedatives all add their effects to those of the underlying lung disease and frequently produce serious disturbances of blood gases. These episodes are potentially life threatening, are usually associated with prolonged morbidity, and frequently require hospitalization. The principles of therapy are to maintain oxygenation while treating all new, presumably reversible, elements of the disease in an effort to restore the patient to his or her former state of health.

Oxygen

Patients with chronic obstructive lung disease and superimposed episodes of acute respiratory failure nearly always have severe hypoxia from a combination of hypoventilation and ventilation-perfusion mismatching. Typical arterial blood values are Po_2 of approximately 30 mm Hg, Pco_2 of 70 mm Hg, and pH of 7.30. Neither the hypercapnia nor the acidemia is life threatening, but the hypoxia is potentially fatal. Thus treatment is directed mainly at alleviating the disturbance in oxygenation; the changes in Pco_2 and pH will return to the ordinary values for that patient as the acute condition improves. In view of the possibility that O_2 therapy may depress ventilation further by withdrawing the hypoxic stimulus to breathe and affecting the pattern of breathing, O_2 is given initially in low concentrations (1 to 3 liters per minute). The goal is to raise Po_2 to satisfactory levels (50 to 60 mm Hg) without depressing ventilation to the extent that unacceptable increases in Pco_2 and decreases in pH (particularly) occur.

The O_2 is usually started at 2 liters per minute, and an arterial blood specimen is analyzed 15 to 30 minutes later to determine the patient's response. Depending on the Po_2 value, the flow of O_2 can be adjusted. If hypoventilation and acidemia result from too much O_2 (e.g., Po_2 80 mm Hg, Pco_2 80 mm Hg, and pH 7.25), the supplementary O_2 should *not* be discontinued but the flow rate should be decreased. This is necessary because the Po_2 decreases much faster than the stimulus to breathe returns, and cardiac arrest or other serious complications of hypoxia may result.

Intubation-Assisted Ventilation

Low-flow O_2 given in the manner described provides satisfactory relief of hypoxia in nearly all instances. Although the goal of low-flow O_2 is an arterial Po_2 of 50 to 60 mm Hg, at times one has to be satisfied with 40 to 50 mm Hg. When oxygenation cannot be achieved without intolerable hypercapnia and acidemia, the decision whether to intubate and ventilate the patient must be made. Experience with intubation and mechanical ventilation in this group of patients has been extremely unrewarding, particularly because of the prolonged need for assisted ventilation once intubation is performed and the poor prognosis for lengthy survival and return to useful life after recovery from the acute episode. Although each case must be considered individually, in general, patients with chronic obstructive pulmonary disease who develop superimposed acute respiratory failure should not be intubated. The major exception to this axiom is the need for ventilator support during the postoperative period. Doxapram (see Respiratory Stimulants, below) often allows administration of "extra" O_2 without depressing ventilatory drive.

Bronchodilators

Most intercurrent episodes of acute respiratory failure in patients with chronic obstructive pulmonary disease are associated with increased airways resistance from the presence of secretions, edema of the mucosa, and bronchospasm. Because it is impossible to discriminate among these, bronchodilator drugs are always included in the treatment regimen to take advantage of the reversibility of whatever element of bronchospasm is present.

When patients seek medical attention for intercurrent attacks, they frequently have already tried—and failed to respond to—oral and aerosolized bronchodilators. In this circumstance, intravenous aminophylline is a useful drug. Aminophylline can be injected slowly in 250-mg or 500-mg boluses, or, if the patient has been hospitalized and prolonged treatment is envisioned, by a loading dose (5.6 mg per kilogram of body weight) and constant sustaining infusion (0.9 mg per kilogram of body weight per hour). These dosages should be reduced in patients who have been receiving aminophylline, who are elderly, or, especially, who have liver disease or heart failure. It is advisable to determine the aminophylline plasma level at the outset in those who have been taking the drug and 24 to 36 hours after the constant infusion regimen has been started to ensure that values are in the therapeutic range (10 to 20 μg per milliliter) and to avoid toxicity.

Selective $beta_2$ sympathomimetic drugs, usually administered by aerosol, are another mainstay of treatment. Because

aerosolized drugs fail to penetrate effectively throughout the tracheobronchial system in the presence of airways secretions and severe narrowing, they are given more frequently than is customary, usually at 1- or 2-hour intervals for the first 12 to 24 hours.

The indications for and dosage of corticosteroids in this clinical setting are controversial, although there is an increasing tendency to use these drugs in virtually all patients with asthma or chronic obstructive lung disease whose exacerbation is severe enough to warrant hospitalization. Either methylprednisolone, 60 mg, or hydrocortisone, 100 mg, intravenously every six hours is indicated. Much higher doses of corticosteroids (e.g., methylprednisolone, 15 mg per kilogram of body weight per day in divided doses) have been recommended, but there is no evidence to suggest that these are more efficacious in this clinical setting than the lower doses recommended above.

Antimicrobials

Infections are the most frequent and important cause of acute respiratory failure in patients with chronic underlying lung disease. Intercurrent attacks usually begin as a typical cold, with rhinitis, pharyngitis, and headaches. Shortly afterward, lower respiratory involvement appears with increasing cough, sputum production, purulence, wheezing, and breathlessness. These episodes occur several times a year in most patients with chronic obstructive pulmonary disease. (It should be noted that fever, leukocytosis, and new roentgenographic infiltrations are uncommon in this syndrome.) When airway infection is present, the sputum is not only purulent but usually contains numerous microorganisms detectable by Gram's stain of the secretions. Sputum cultures, however, often fail to reveal pathogenic bacteria, although at times *Streptococcus pneumoniae* and/or *Hemophilus influenzae* may be grown. Regardless of the presence or absence of identifiable pathogens, oral treatment with ampicillin (250 to 500 mg every six hours), a combined preparation of trimethoprim-sulfamethoxazole (160 mg and 800 mg, respectively, every 12 hours), or tetracycline (250 to 500 mg every six hours) frequently results in decreased volume of sputum, thinning of the secretions, change in sputum appearance from purulent to mucoid, and improvement in blood gases.

When pneumonia is present, signified by the presence of new infiltration(s) on the chest roentgenogram, Gram's stain of the sputum is likely to show one bacterial species predominating, and the initial selection of antimicrobials should cover this organism. Therapy can be revised, if necessary, when the results of the sputum cultures are available.

Control of Secretions

Many patients complain of thick tenacious sputum that is troublesome to clear. Although it seems desirable to attempt to alter the character of these secretions to facilitate their removal, there is no clear evidence that it is possible to do so by pharmacologic means. Iodides, enzymes, detergents, and acetylcysteine, administered orally or by aerosol, have been tried extensively, but none has been shown convincingly to be effective. Moreover, each has potential toxic side effects. Similarly, mist tents and ultrasonic nebulizers, once widely used, are seldom employed today. The best way to control secretions is to control infection with antimicrobials and to ensure adequate (but not excessive) hydration by the administration of intravenous fluids.

Patients with troublesome sputum retention may require intermittent nasotracheal suction to control the volume of secretions. Manual or mechanical percussion serves to loosen secretions and enhances their removal in patients who have retained sputum in their airways. Respiratory physical therapy, especially when carried out by a skilled therapist, may result in an increase in arterial Po_2 related to the improvement in the distribution of ventilation from clearance of sputum.

Treatment of Heart Failure

Cor pulmonale is an inevitable complication of severe chronic lung disease. Right ventricular hypertrophy followed by heart failure occurs secondary to the increased work load imposed on the ventricle by the changes in the pulmonary circulation from the effects of lung disease. Resistance to blood flow through the lungs increases when pulmonary blood vessels are destroyed (as in emphysema), obstructed (as in pulmonary thromboembolism), narrowed (from vasoconstriction), or compressed (breathing at high lung volumes), or when the blood is unusually viscous (polycythemia). Patients whose cor pulmonale is well compensated or even inapparent while their chronic lung disease is stable often develop acute right heart failure during intercurrent attacks of acute respiratory failure. Peripheral edema, increased venous pressure, and an enlarged, painful liver are important clues to the presence of acute cardiac decompensation.

Most patients with right heart failure from cor pulmonale, even if severe, have a satisfactory diuresis when put to bed, given O_2 and treated appropriately for their underlying lung disease. Diuretics may make patients feel more comfortable by diminishing peripheral edema and hepatic and gastrointestinal congestion faster than spontaneous diuresis; but if used, the drugs should be administered orally in low doses. Intravenous ethacrynic acid or furosemide can cause excessive renal loss of Cl^- that worsens existing acid-base disturbances and depletes intravascular volume sufficiently to decrease cardiac output and blood pressure. A particularly dangerous situation occurs in patients who already have coexisting nonrespiratory (metabolic) alkalosis often from Cl^--losing diuretics, in addition to their hypercapnia from chronic respiratory failure; when the measures designed to improve ventilation lower arterial P_{CO_2}, the metabolic alkalosis becomes "unmasked" and arterial pH becomes markedly alkaline. When this occurs, the patients can develop cardiac arrhythmias, become comatose, or manifest convulsive seizures or other focal neurologic abnormalities.

If an element of pulmonary edema or pulmonary vascular congestion is present from left heart failure, this may also respond to diuretics. Whether left heart failure can occur secondary to purely right-sided disease is controversial. Of greater importance are coexisting causes of left-sided involvement (e.g., valvular disease, coronary atherosclerosis); furthermore, chronic hypoxia and severe polycythemia may impair left ventricular as well as right ventricular function.

Present evidence indicates that digitalis preparations are not beneficial in patients with cor pulmonale. Also, the use of digitalis is hazardous in patients with chronic respiratory failure owing to the sudden shifts in acid-base balance and electrolyte concentrations that may occur in these patients. Therefore digitalis drugs should be used only in patients with digitalis-responsive arrhythmias or coexisting left heart failure.

Respiratory Stimulants

With few exceptions, respiratory stimulants are obsolete. Nikethamide, picrotoxin, and ethamivan have been replaced by other less hazardous and more efficient methods of maintaining ventilation. Doxapram, a drug that works by stimulating carotid chemoreceptors rather than neurons in the brain, appears to be much safer than centrally acting stimulants. The chief use of doxapram is to minimize or prevent the depression of ventilation, with consequent increase in P_{CO_2} and decrease in pH, that occurs in some hypoxic patients with hypercapnia who are given O_2 to breathe. Almitrine, another drug that stimulates the carotid chemoreceptors but that can be administered orally, is widely used in Europe to improve arterial P_{O_2} in outpatients with chronic respiratory failure. This drug has not been approved by the Food and Drug Administration at the time of publication.

Sedation

All sedative drugs should be avoided in patients with chronic lung disease and intercurrent acute respiratory failure, including diazepam (Valium) and chlordiazepoxide (Librium), which can suppress ventilation. Exceptions to this cardinal rule are made from time to time, but usually only when the patient is being mechanically ventilated and sedation is required to enable breathing synchronous with the machine.

Postoperative Complications

Patients with chronic respiratory failure are high-risk operative candidates. Moreover, the closer the surgical incision to the thorax, the higher the incidence of postoperative complications. Despite this caveat, it is safe to say that virtually *all* patients who have respiratory failure can safely undergo *nonthoracic* surgery or *nonresectional* thoracic surgery. Postoperative complications can be anticipated and often prevented by attention to the general principles of care outlined in this chapter. Close observation and monitoring are usually required, and these can best be carried out in an intensive care unit.

Askanazi J (ed.): Nutrition and respiratory disease. Clin Chest Med 7:1, 1986. *Entire issue devoted to contribution of nutritional depletion to respiratory failure and how to prevent and treat it.*

Bone RC (ed.): Respiratory failure. Med Clin North Am 67:549, 1983. *Symposium of 13 articles that cover the most important topics related to respiratory failure.*

Brandstetter RD: The adult respiratory distress syndrome. Heart Lung 15:155, 1986. *Up-to-date review with 94 references.*

Robin ED: The cult of the Swan-Ganz catheter: Overuse and abuse of pulmonary flow catheters. Ann Intern Med 103:445, 1985. *Appropriate cautionary message that applies to all kinds of invasive monitoring devices.*

Zapol WM, Falke KJ (eds.): Acute Respiratory Failure. New York, Marcel Dekker, Inc., 1985. *Collection of comprehensive and authoritative articles with emphasis on respiratory failure following acute lung injury.*

PART VIII

CRITICAL CARE MEDICINE

73 CRITICAL CARE MEDICINE

Philip C. Hopewell

The practice of critical care medicine involves virtually all areas in general internal medicine. Severe illness represents one end of a spectrum of pathophysiologic derangement that shades into less severe illness related to the same organ systems. The same basic diagnostic and therapeutic principles therefore apply. A wide variety of clinical problems are commonly encountered in critical care units, many of which are discussed in other chapters. This section will focus on areas in critical care medicine that are not extensively described elsewhere in this text and on the aspects of medical care that are unique to critical care units.

In the critically ill patient, the interdependence of organ systems must remain in sharp focus. Limited attention to one component of the illness, even if that component is predominant, frequently will yield a therapeutic approach that is detrimental to the patient as a whole. Commonly, management of the critically ill patient presents extremely difficult dilemmas. For example, treatment directed toward reducing the pulmonary capillary wedge pressure in patients with the adult respiratory distress syndrome may adversely affect renal and central nervous system perfusion. Conversely, increasing the pulmonary artery wedge pressure to optimize cardiac output in a patient with ischemic heart disease may result in noncardiogenic pulmonary edema if there has been a pre-existing acute diffuse lung injury. Bronchodilating agents may increase cardiac irritability and therefore cause significant arrhythmias, particularly in the presence of hypoxemia or acid-base disturbances or both. Nephrotoxic antimicrobial agents may be essential in the treatment of sepsis in a patient with pre-existing or acute renal disease. The physician who is primarily responsible for the care of a gravely ill patient often must synthesize an overall diagnostic and treatment strategy that incorporates the views of various consultants with a more narrow focus and reconcile the conflicting effects of their recommendations.

ATTRIBUTES OF A CRITICAL CARE UNIT

A critical care unit is defined by its ability to provide the environment, facilities, and personnel for the care of severely ill patients. The important features required of such a unit are listed in Table 73–1.

TABLE 73–1. UNIQUE FEATURES OF CRITICAL CARE UNITS

1. High nurse-to-patient ratio
2. Ready accessibility of physicians
3. Ability to provide invasive hemodynamic monitoring
4. Availability of respiratory support techniques
5. Ability to provide supervised continuous intravenous infusions of pharmacologic agents

Critical care units may have a general orientation, treating all types of severely ill patients, or be more specialized, accepting only specific categories of patients as defined by the type of illness (for example, burn units), organ system involved (coronary and acute neurologic care units), specialty service designation (medical and surgical units), or patient age (neonatal intensive care units). In addition to the basic attributes listed in Table 73–1, specialized units provide medical personnel specifically skilled in the area of care provided by the unit and have available particular forms of technology with applications generally limited to the category of patients accepted by the unit.

Critical care units usually need administrative policies and procedures that differ from those of standard hospital units. Because of the gravity of illness of their patients, critical care units require clear delineation of administrative and medical lines of authority and responsibility. Likewise, there must be at least general guidelines for admission and discharge of patients, specifically described nursing roles, standing orders, and a program of continuing staff education. The existence of such policies reduces the apparent ambiguity often inherent in the difficult environment of a critical care unit and enables prompt decision making by both physicians and nurses.

Greenbaum DM: Standards for critical care medicine. *In* Shoemaker WC, Thompson WL, Holbrook PR (eds.): Textbook of Critical Care. Philadelphia, W. B. Saunders Company, 1984, pp 1004–1005. *Provides a summary description of facilities, personnel, and services available in critical care units in the United States.*
National Institutes of Health. Consensus development of conference on critical care medicine. Crit Care Med 11:466, 1983. *This report summarizes the discussions of a large consensus development group that addressed issues of critical care unit utilization, organization, training of personnel, and research needs.*

GENERAL PRINCIPLES OF ASSESSMENT OF SEVERE RESPIRATORY DYSFUNCTION

The discussion in this section will focus on the techniques of assessment generally applicable to severely ill patients in whom it usually is neither possible nor desirable to perform elaborate comprehensive assessments of pulmonary function. Patients often cannot cooperate, and measurements made under non–steady-state conditions are generally inaccurate. The basic components of normal respiratory function are discussed in Ch. 59 and the characteristic abnormalities of various types of lung disorders in other chapters of Part VII.

Nonspecific Indicators of Severity

Respiratory rate is perhaps the simplest measurement that can be made. Although influenced by many factors, the respiratory rate provides a general indication of cardiorespiratory function and may be the first clue to impending or early respiratory failure. In addition, periodic counting of respiratory rate serves as a simple monitoring technique.

The degree of pulsus paradoxus correlates with the forced expiratory volume in 1 second (FEV_1) in patients with acute airways obstruction and therefore may indicate the severity of airways narrowing. Similarly, the presence of suprasternal, supraclavicular, and intercostal space retractions also correlates roughly with the degree of airways obstruction.

The mental status of the patient is an important, albeit even more nonspecific, indicator of the status of cardiorespiratory function. Behavioral alterations may reflect changes in the partial pressure of oxygen (Pa_{O_2}) and carbon dioxide (Pa_{CO_2}) in arterial blood.

Measurements of Lung Function

The lung function studies applicable in severely ill patients are rather limited. Depending on the type and severity of illness and the patient's ability to cooperate, one may measure vital capacity (VC), maximal inspiratory pressure (MIP), timed forced expiratory volume, and peak expiratory flow rate (PEFR).

The vital capacity is the maximal volume of air that can be slowly exhaled after maximal inspiration and as such provides an indication of the patient's ventilatory capability (Fig. 59–2). The VC is influenced by the respiratory neuromuscular system, the chest wall, the elastic properties of the lung, and the caliber of the airways. It cannot therefore be used to identify specific abnormalities. Nevertheless, it is particularly helpful in assessing and following patients with neuromuscular illnesses and in evaluating patients being mechanically ventilated to determine if it is feasible to consider weaning from the ventilator. A minimal acceptable VC is 10 to 15 ml per kilogram of body weight.

The maximal inspiratory pressure is somewhat analogous to the VC in the information that it provides and the factors by which it is influenced. However, the ability to generate an acceptable inspiratory pressure, less (more negative) than -20 cm H_2O, does not necessarily imply that the VC will be adequate.

The timed forced expiratory volume, which is usually expressed as the forced expiratory volume in 1 second (FEV_1) over the forced vital capacity (FVC), measures the severity of airways obstruction in patients with asthma or chronic airways obstruction. The measurement may not be possible in patients with severe airways obstruction who have marked tachypnea. However, it does provide the best objective indicator of the degree of airways obstruction and, when measured serially, the response to therapy. Absolute FEV_1 values of less than 0.75 liter or less than 25 per cent of the predicted value are commonly associated with increased Pa_{CO_2} values and hence are indicative of severe obstruction.

Peak expiratory flow rate provides information similar to the FEV_1 in patients with airways obstruction. It has the distinct advantage of not requiring a full inhalation followed by a full forced exhalation, a maneuver that may actually worsen airways obstruction. The PEFR is measured by having the patient slowly inhale and then blow a short forced puff through the flowmeter, a maneuver similar to a cough. Values below 60 liters per minute are indicative of severe obstruction.

Arterial Blood Gas and pH Measurements

The *Pa_{O_2}, Pa_{CO_2}, and arterial pH* provide the most informative indication of integrated cardiorespiratory function. These values are not particularly sensitive to early cardiorespiratory abnormalities and are not specific for the kind of abnormality present, but they provide crucial information in patients with severe dysfunction. The mechanisms of normal gas exchange and its abnormalities are discussed in Ch. 59. This section will focus on the interpretation of arterial blood gas and pH values in the assessment of severely ill patients and how these interpretations can be used to ascertain the pathophysiology and indicate the proper approach to treatment.

HYPOXEMIA. Clinically significant reductions in Pa_{O_2} can result from *hypoventilation, mismatching of ventilation to perfusion,* and *shunting.* It is important to determine which of these mechanisms is operative in a given patient.

Hypoventilation as the cause of hypoxemia implies that the lung itself is normal and that the only necessary therapeutic

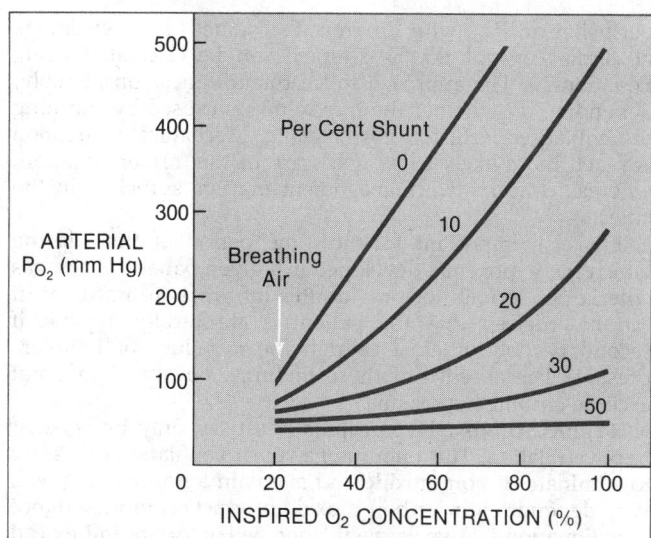

FIGURE 73–1. The relationship of Pa_{O_2} to Fi_{O_2} with increasing amounts of shunt. Note that with 30 per cent of the cardiac output being shunted there is only a slight increase in Pa_{O_2} with increasing Fi_{O_2} and with 50 per cent shunting, there is no increase in Pa_{O_2}. (From West JR: Pulmonary Pathophysiology: The Essentials. Copyright 1977, Baltimore, The Williams and Wilkins Company.)

goal is improved ventilation. This type of hypoxemia is characterized by a normal alveolar-to-arterial Po_2 difference $(P(A-a)_{O_2})$. The $P(A-a)_{O_2}$ can be determined by using the alveolar gas equation (Equation 5) to calculate Pa_{O_2} and by measuring Pa_{O_2}. In patients breathing room air, the difference should not be greater than 10 mm Hg, and with an increased fractional concentration of oxygen in inspired gas (Fi_{O_2}) sufficient to cause a Pa_{O_2} of 200 mm Hg or greater, the $P(A-a)_{O_2}$ should not be greater than 40 mm Hg.

Ventilation-perfusion mismatching and *shunting* can be distinguished by measuring the response to administration of 100 per cent oxygen. The Pa_{O_2} will increase normally to values of nearly 600 mm Hg if the hypoxemia is due purely to mismatching, whereas with a shunt the increase may be markedly reduced, depending on the magnitude of the shunt flow. Figure 73–1 shows the relationship between Pa_{O_2} and Fi_{O_2} with different shunt fractions, and Figure 73–2 demonstrates the effect of increasing amounts of mismatching of ventilation to

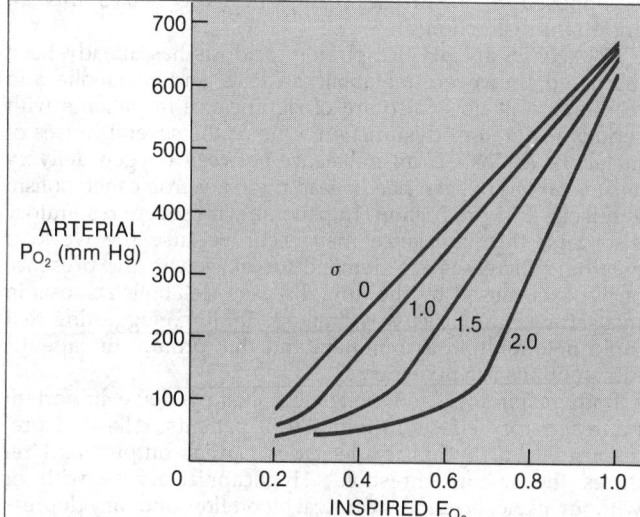

FIGURE 73–2. The relationship of Pa_{O_2} to Fi_{O_2} with increasing amounts of ventilation to perfusion mismatching (σ = standard deviation of log normal distribution of ventilation and perfusion). Note that even with marked mismatching the Pa_{O_2} increases to nearly normal values with very high Fi_{O_2}. (From West JR: Pulmonary Pathophysiology: The Essentials. Copyright 1977, Baltimore, The Williams and Wilkins Company.)

perfusion on Pa_{O_2} with different $F_{I_{O_2}}$ values. The percentage of cardiac output that is shunted can be calculated using Equation 10. The approach to treatment varies considerably, depending on whether the hypoxemia is caused by shunting or ventilation-perfusion mismatching. Mechanical ventilation is much more likely to be necessary in the former situation, whereas conservative management may be sufficient in the latter.

It is also important to know the period of time during which the hypoxemia developed in a given patient. Blood gas criteria per se will not provide this information; however, it can be inferred that the patient is chronically hypoxic if secondary polycythemia or right heart failure or both are present. The absence of these findings, however, does not exclude chronic hypoxemia.

HYPERCAPNIA. Hypercapnia is caused only by alveolar hypoventilation. The amount of alveolar ventilation necessary to eliminate carbon dioxide and maintain a normal Pa_{CO_2} will vary depending on carbon dioxide production in accordance with Equation 1. Alveolar ventilation will in turn be influenced by the amount of wasted ventilation as shown in Equation 4. Thus, increases in Pa_{CO_2} can occur because of increased production of carbon dioxide or increased wasted ventilation or both.

The relationship between Pa_{CO_2} and blood bicarbonate concentration determines the arterial pH, as indicated by the Henderson-Hasselbalch equation (Equation 13). The relationship between Pa_{CO_2} and arterial pH varies, however, depending on the time during which the Pa_{CO_2} has been increased and its rate of increase. Thus, by examining the relationships among Pa_{CO_2}, arterial pH, and $[HCO_3^-]$, the acuteness or chronicity of the carbon dioxide elevation can be inferred. Acute increases in Pa_{CO_2} are accompanied by only small increases in $[HCO_3^-]$ and arterial pH changes in a nearly linear fashion with Pa_{CO_2}. There is approximately a 0.0075 pH unit change in the opposite direction for every 1-mm Hg change in Pa_{CO_2}. Thus, an acute rise in Pa_{CO_2} from 40 mm Hg to 60 mm Hg would be expected to cause a decrease in arterial pH to 7.25. Over a period of one to three days, however, renal bicarbonate retention causes the $[HCO_3^-]$ to increase and buffer the arterial pH change. Thus, for a given change in Pa_{CO_2} the change in arterial pH is much less than when the change occurs acutely. These relationships are shown in Figure 73–3. Obviously the therapeutic implication of an acute as opposed to a chronic change in Pa_{CO_2} makes this an important distinction.

CHANGES IN pH. Respiratory acidosis has already been discussed; however, metabolic acidosis and metabolic and respiratory alkalosis also are of significance in patients with serious respiratory dysfunction. One of the several causes of metabolic acidosis is an imbalance between oxygen delivery and metabolic oxygen needs, leading to anaerobic metabolism and lactic acid production. In patients with severe respiratory disorders, this imbalance may occur because the work of breathing increases the demand for oxygen in the presence of hypoxia caused by the lung disease. Metabolic acidosis in this setting is a particularly ominous finding, suggesting that rapid deterioration is imminent and that prompt therapeutic interventions are necessary.

Both respiratory and metabolic alkalosis have important nonrespiratory effects in critically ill patients. Alkalosis predisposes to arrhythmias, decreases cardiac output, and reduces the seizure threshold. Hypocapnia per se with or without alkalosis reduces cerebral blood flow and may depress the level of consciousness. For these reasons alkalosis should be recognized as an important acid-base disturbance and corrective measures should be taken.

Calculations of Respiratory Variables

A number of equations and calculations are helpful in the assessment of respiratory function. Only brief descriptions of

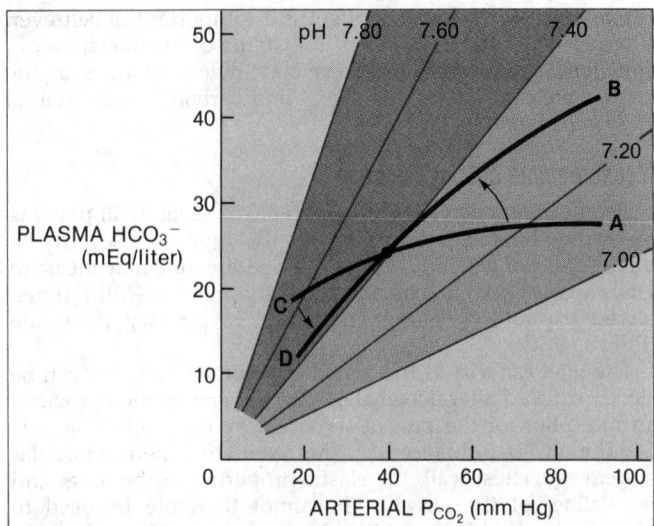

FIGURE 73–3. Effects of acute and chronic variations in Pa_{CO_2} on plasma HCO_3^- and pH. The line connecting points A and C represents the effects of an acute change in Pa_{CO_2} to a value above or below 40 mm Hg. Renal compensation over time results in a shift of the relationship to that represented by the line connecting points B and D as is indicated by the arrows. (From Murray JF: The Normal Lung. 2nd ed. Philadelphia, W. B. Saunders Company, 1986.)

the physiologic principles involved with the equations will be presented in this section.

Representative normal values for selected cardiorespiratory variables are listed in Table 73–2.

EQUATIONS RELATED TO VENTILATION. Arterial P_{CO_2} is related directly to carbon dioxide production ($\dot{V}_{CO_2}$ in milliliters per minute) and inversely to alveolar ventilation ($\dot{V}_A$ in liters per minute) as follows:

$$Pa_{CO_2} = K\frac{\dot{V}_{CO_2}}{\dot{V}_A} \tag{1}$$

where K is a constant.

The $\dot{V}_A$ is the difference between the tidal volume (V_T in liters) and the wasted or dead space ventilation (V_D) multiplied by the respiratory rate (F in breaths per minute).

$$\dot{V}_A = (V_T - V_D) \times F \tag{2}$$

Total minute ventilation ($\dot{V}_E$ in liters per minute) is the product of V_T and F.

$$\dot{V}_E = V_T \times F \tag{3}$$

TABLE 73–2. REPRESENTATIVE NORMAL VALUES FOR SELECTED RESPIRATORY AND HEMODYNAMIC VARIABLES

	Normal
Pa_{O_2}	95 mm Hg
Pa_{CO_2}	40 mm Hg
pH (arterial)	7.40
$P(A-a)_{O_2}$	<10 mm Hg
O_2 saturation	98%
Ca_{O_2}	19.8 ml/100 ml
$P\bar{v}_{O_2}$	40 mm Hg
$\dot{V}_{O_2}$	240 ml/min
$\dot{V}_{CO_2}$	192 ml/min
R	0.8
Respiratory rate	12
$\dot{V}_E$	6 L/min
V_D	150 ml
V_T	450 ml
V_D/V_T	.33
$\dot{Q}_T$	5 L/min
$\dot{Q}_S/\dot{Q}_T$	<7%
PVR	50–150 dyne sec/cm⁵
SVR	800–1200 dyne sec/cm⁵
$C\bar{v}_{O_2}$	14.6 ml/100 ml

From these three equations it can be seen that the factors determining the Pa_{CO_2} are V_T, V_D, F, and $\dot{V}_{CO_2}$.

The volume of wasted ventilation can be calculated from a modification of the Bohr equation:

$$V_D = \frac{(Pa_{CO_2} - Pe_{CO_2})}{Pa_{CO_2}} \times V_T \qquad (4)$$

where Pe_{CO_2} = the partial pressure of carbon dioxide in expired air. The V_D so derived is commonly expressed as a ratio of V_T. Normal values are from 0.30 to 0.35.

EQUATIONS RELATED TO OXYGENATION. The partial pressure of oxygen in the alveolus (PA_{O_2}) can be calculated from the *alveolar gas equation* as follows:

$$PA_{O_2} = FI_{O_2} (PB - 47) - Pa_{CO_2}/R \qquad (5)$$

where R = the respiratory exchange ratio ($\dot{V}_{CO_2}/\dot{V}_{O_2}$), PB = barometric pressure, and 47 = the partial pressure of water vapor in mm Hg in fully saturated air at body temperature. The value for R is usually assumed to be 0.8. Having calculated the PA_{O_2}, the $P(A-a)_{O_2}$ can then be determined, enabling a more precise quantitation of the degree of hypoxemia and mechanisms responsible for it.

Oxygen consumption ($\dot{V}_{O_2}$ in liters per minute) can be estimated fairly accurately from the relationship

$$\dot{V}_{O_2} = (FI_{O_2} - FE_{O_2}) \times \dot{V}_E \qquad (6)$$

where FE_{O_2} = the fractional concentration of oxygen in expired air.

Oxygen delivery to the tissues depends not only on Pa_{O_2} but also on arterial oxygen content (Ca_{O_2}) and cardiac output. The Ca_{O_2} (milliliters of oxygen per 100 milliliters of blood) is calculated as follows:

$$Ca_{O_2} = 1.34 \times [Hb] \times \left(\frac{per\ cent\ saturation}{100}\right) + (0.003 \times Pa_{O_2}) \qquad (7)$$

where 1.34 is the milliliters of oxygen carried by each gram of hemoglobin, [Hb] = the hemoglobin concentration in grams per 100 milliliters of blood, and per cent saturation = the saturation of hemoglobin with oxygen in arterial blood. The saturation can be measured directly or calculated from the oxyhemoglobin dissociation curve (Fig. 73–4). The constant 0.003 is the amount of dissolved (unbound) oxygen in blood in milliliters per mm Hg Pa_{O_2}.

Systemic oxygen transport (SO_2T) in milliliters per minute is calculated as follows:

$$SO_2T = Ca_{O_2} \times \dot{Q}T \qquad (8)$$

where $\dot{Q}T$ = cardiac output in liters per minute.

Thus, it can be seen that oxygen delivery to the tissues depends not only on Pa_{O_2} but on [Hb] and $\dot{Q}T$ as well. In evaluating and managing patients with severe respiratory dysfunction, all of these factors need to be taken into account.

The balance between oxygen supply and systemic oxygen demands can be evaluated by calculating the difference between Ca_{O_2} and the content of oxygen in mixed venous blood ($C\bar{v}_{O_2}$). The $C\bar{v}_{O_2}$ is calculated in the same manner as the Ca_{O_2} (Equation 7) but using the oxyhemoglobin saturation value in mixed venous (pulmonary artery) blood.

Using the $\dot{V}_{O_2}$ and the $C(a-\bar{v})_{O_2}$, the cardiac output can be calculated according to the Fick Principle:

$$\dot{Q}T = \frac{\dot{V}_{O_2}}{C(a-\bar{v})_{O_2}} \qquad (9)$$

The contribution of right-to-left shunting of blood to hypoxemia can be quantitated in patients receiving an FI_{O_2} of 1.0 using the following shunt equation:

$$\frac{\dot{Q}S}{\dot{Q}T} = \frac{Cc'_{O_2} - Ca_{O_2}}{Cc'_{O_2} - C\bar{v}_{O_2}} \qquad (10)$$

where $\dot{Q}S$ = the volume of shunted blood, Cc'_{O_2} = an approximation of end capillary blood oxygen content, assuming the Pc'_{O_2} to be the same as PA_{O_2} and calculating the Cc'_{O_2} on the basis of this assumption.

The effect of the per cent shunt on Pa_{O_2} as calculated from this equation is shown in Figure 73–1. This figure illustrates the lack of responsiveness of Pa_{O_2} to increases in FI_{O_2} (PA_{O_2}) once the $\dot{Q}S/\dot{Q}T$ exceeds 30 per cent.

ACID-BASE RELATIONSHIPS. The essential relationships among the factors controlling arterial blood pH are described in the Henderson-Hasselbalch equation:

$$pH = pK + \log \frac{[HCO_3^-]}{[H_2CO_3]} \qquad (11)$$

where pK, the dissociation constant, = 6.1 for plasma at 37° C. Because

$$[H_2CO_3] = Pa_{CO_2} \times 0.0301 \qquad (12)$$

where 0.0301 is the solubility constant of carbon dioxide in plasma at 37°, Equation 11 can be substituted as follows:

$$pH = 6.1 + \log \frac{[HCO_3^-]}{Pa_{CO_2} \times 0.0301} \qquad (13)$$

The relationships among these variables under acute and chronic conditions are shown in Figure 73–3.

LUNG MECHANICS. The stiffness of the lung and chest wall—that is, their resistance to inflation—is termed the *compliance of the respiratory system* (CRS). In patients being mechanically ventilated it is expressed by the following formula:

$$CRS = V_T/Pplateau - PEE \qquad (14)$$

where V_T is the tidal volume delivered by the ventilator, Pplateau is the inspiratory plateau pressure (see Fig. 73–5), and PEE is the end-expiratory pressure read from the manometer of the ventilator. The effect of airways resistance can be included in the measurement by using the peak inspiratory pressure (Ppeak) rather than Pplateau. This is termed the *effective compliance* (Ceff) or *dynamic compliance*.

$$Ceff = V_T/Ppeak - PEE \qquad (15)$$

Assuming that the compliance of the chest wall is stable, changes in CRS reflect changes in lung mechanical properties,

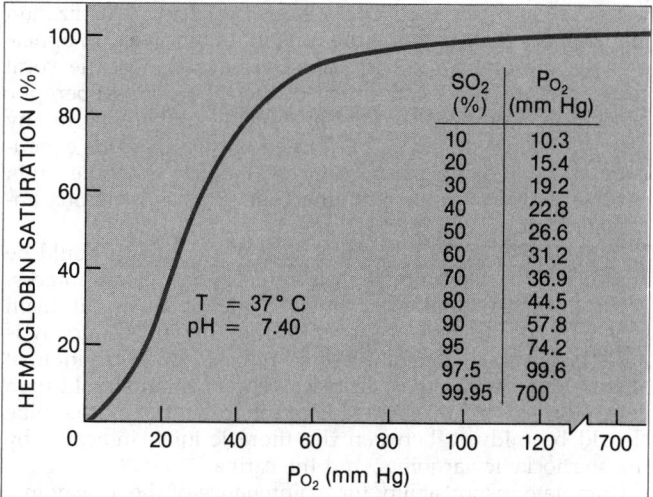

	SO_2 (%)	P_{O_2} (mm Hg)
	10	10.3
	20	15.4
	30	19.2
	40	22.8
	50	26.6
	60	31.2
	70	36.9
	80	44.5
	90	57.8
	95	74.2
	97.5	99.6
	99.95	700

FIGURE 73–4. Relationship of per cent hemoglobin saturation to Pa_{O_2} in man at 37° C and pH 7.40. Note that there is very little increase in hemoglobin saturation for increases in Pa_{O_2} above 60 mm Hg. (From Murray JF: The Normal Lung. 2nd ed. Philadelphia, W. B. Saunders Company, 1986.)

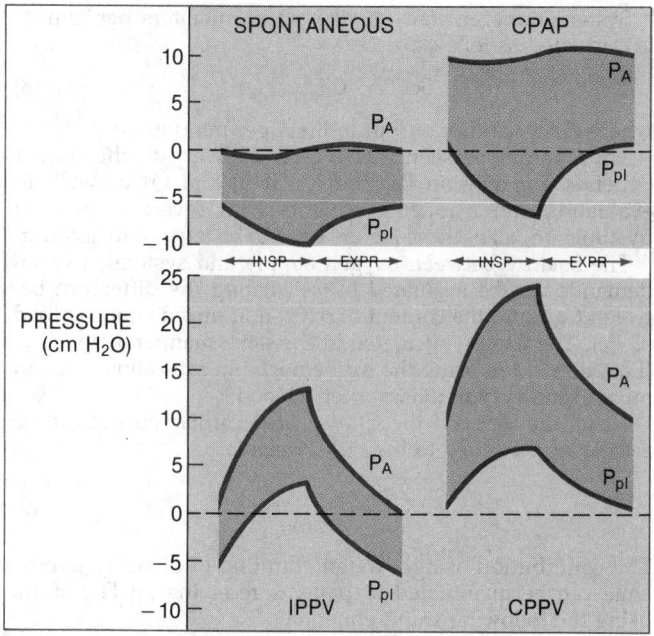

FIGURE 73–5. Schematic representations of airway (P_A) and pleural pressures (P_{pl}) with spontaneous respiration, spontaneous respiration with continuous positive airway pressure (CPAP), intermittent positive pressure ventilation (IPPV), and continuous positive pressure ventilation (CPPV). Note that with CPAP and CPPV, the pressure gradient between the airway and the pleural space is increased compared with spontaneous respiration and IPPV, respectively. (From Hinshaw HC, Murray JF (eds): Diseases of the Chest. Philadelphia, W. B. Saunders Company, 1980.)

whereas changes in Ceff may indicate changes in airways resistance (if inspiratory flow is unchanged) as well as lung compliance.

Murray JF: The Normal Lung. 2nd ed. Philadelphia, W. B. Saunders Company, 1986. *A concise review of normal lung function that provides the basis for an understanding of pulmonary pathophysiology.*

Lemaire F, Harf A, Teisseire BP: Oxygen exchange across the acutely injured lung. In Zapol WM, Falke KJ (eds.): Acute Respiratory Failure. New York, Marcel Dekker, 1985, pp 521–553. *An extensively referenced discussion of the abnormalities in oxygenation that occur in the adult respiratory distress syndrome.*

TECHNIQUES OF RESPIRATORY SUPPORT
External Devices for Administering Oxygen

Supplemental oxygen must frequently be administered by external devices in patients with any cardiorespiratory disorder that results in hypoxemia. The decision to use an external device as opposed to an endotracheal tube depends on the amount of oxygen needed and the potential consequences of failure to provide oxygen should the external device come off. Generally speaking, it is not prudent to rely on external devices for patients with hypoxemia severe enough to require an Fi_{O_2} of 0.5 and who could be expected to suffer major consequences should the device not be positioned properly.

A variety of types of delivery systems can be used to provide supplemental oxygen. The choice of a particular method depends on four factors: (1) the amount of oxygen needed, (2) the need for precise control of Fi_{O_2}, (3) the need for humidification, and (4) the patient's comfort. *Nasal prongs* are the simplest and most comfortable delivery device. However, the Fi_{O_2} provided cannot be quantitated reliably and humidification is poor. *Open face masks or face tents* provide a high flow of well-humidified, premixed air and oxygen with a moderately reliable Fi_{O_2} usually set by a Venturi device in a humidifier/mixer. *Tight-fitting face masks* provide higher but generally imprecise concentrations of oxygen. As with nasal prongs, humidification is minimal. The same sort of tight mask fitted with a nonrebreathing valve and a reservoir bag

can be used to provide even higher concentrations of oxygen but it is generally uncomfortable and the oxygen is poorly humidified. Positive end-expiratory pressure can also be supplied using a tight mask with an appropriate system of valves. The Fi_{O_2} is controlled much more precisely by the Venturi mask, which uses a calibrated Venturi device in the delivery line to provide high flows of gas containing 24, 28, 35, or 40 per cent oxygen. This sort of mask is used for patients with chronic airways obstruction and hypoventilation in whom there is concern that uncontrolled high oxygen concentrations will cause further hypoventilation by reducing ventilatory drive.

Ventilatory Assist Devices

A wide variety of devices can be used to provide ventilatory assistance without resorting to an endotracheal airway and mechanical ventilation. Generally, these devices are of limited usefulness; however, under proper circumstances, some may be quite helpful. Simple ventilators provide intermittent positive pressure ventilation via a mouthpiece but only transiently increase alveolar ventilation and, at least for this purpose, are of little value. External negative-pressure devices such as the cuirass ventilator, which fits over the chest wall and augments ventilation by lowering the pressure around the chest, causing it to expand, may be of value in patients with chronic neuromuscular diseases. Other ventilatory assist devices, including the rocking bed and surgically implanted phrenic nerve pacemakers, are of little general applicability.

Artificial Airways and Airway Management

When it is necessary, mechanical ventilation is best provided, at least initially, through an endotracheal tube passed through the mouth or nose. The oral route has the advantage of being more easily utilized under emergency circumstances, whereas the nasal route is better suited for long-term needs. Tracheostomy should be reserved for patients who will need long-term mechanical ventilation or who cannot tolerate either a nasal or an oral tube. The endotracheal tube should be fitted with a bonded high-volume, low-pressure cuff that will occlude the trachea around the tube, enabling positive pressure mechanical ventilation and preventing aspiration of oropharyngeal contents. Care should be taken to avoid overinflation of the cuff, which predisposes to pressure necrosis of the adjacent tracheal mucosa and to the development of a tracheoesophageal fistula or subsequent tracheal stenosis.

Semielective tube placement in a spontaneously ventilating patient may be accomplished via the nose without direct visualization of the vocal cords; however, direct visualization may be necessary to guide the tube into the larynx. In apneic patients the oral route with direct visualization of the vocal cords must be used. Placement of the tube over a fiberoptic bronchoscope may be helpful in difficult intubations. In any case intubation should be performed only by persons experienced with the procedure who are familiar with the often necessary pharmacologic adjuncts, such as intravenous anesthetics and muscle-relaxing agents.

Immediately after the tube is placed, the lungs should be auscultated to determine if air is entering both hemithoraces. Because of the relatively obtuse angle of the right main bronchus, positioning of the tip of the tube in this airway is quite common. If the tube seems to be in good position, it should be taped securely in place. The position should then be confirmed by a chest radiograph. The tip of the tube should be midway between the thoracic inlet, indicated by the sternoclavicular joints, and the carina.

Complete responsibility for maintenance of the airway in a patient with an endotracheal or tracheostomy tube rests with the persons caring for the patient. The patient can no longer humidify inspired air, cough effectively, or defend the lower airways against airborne microorganisms. Perhaps more important, the patient cannot call for help or unblock the tube should it become obstructed. For all of these reasons, in addition to the gravity of the illness for which the tube was placed, patients with artificial airways should nearly always be managed in a critical care unit.

Nasal or, in occasional circumstances, oral endotracheal tubes can be left in place with no absolute time limit in patients who continue to require mechanical ventilation or airway protection. Tracheostomy may be necessary, however, because of complications, such as infection or soft tissue necrosis in the upper air passages, including the nose. Occasionally, tracheostomy is more effective in facilitating removal of secretions than is an endotracheal tube. In addition, patients may find a tracheostomy more comfortable and may be able to eat and talk with a tracheostomy tube in place.

Endotracheal and tracheostomy tubes bypass the normal humidifying mechanisms in the upper airway; all inspired gas must therefore be fully humidified. Removal of pulmonary secretions using a suction catheter with sterile technique should be performed at regular intervals as determined by the volume of secretions present. All gas delivery circuits in direct communication with the airway should be sterile when connected and changed at least at 48-hour intervals.

Definitive indications for endotracheal intubation that apply to all situations are difficult to determine. Nevertheless, the criteria listed in Table 73–3 seem generally applicable. The decision to perform endotracheal intubation is often based on more subjective criteria and/or observation of the patient's course during a period of time. In each of the listed situations, the potential reversibility of the patient's underlying disorder must be taken into account in determining if intubation is indicated.

Mechanical Ventilation

INDICATIONS. As with endotracheal intubation, the indications for mechanical ventilation are not always easily definable. In general terms, however, mechanical ventilation is clearly necessary in the following situations: (1) progressive hypoxemia that is unresponsive to treatment of its underlying causes and in which external devices cannot provide a sufficiently high $F_{I_{O_2}}$ and (2) progressive hypoventilation with respiratory acidosis that is unresponsive to treatment of the underlying disorder. Less clear indications include: (1) "prophylactic" mechanical ventilation in patients in whom respiratory failure is anticipated, such as after thoracic or upper abdominal surgery and (2) patients who are barely maintaining adequate gas exchange at the expense of expending energy on the considerable work of breathing. Finally, mechanical ventilation is occasionally necessary in patients who require general anesthesia or heavy sedation to allow diagnostic or therapeutic intervention.

TYPES OF MECHANICAL VENTILATORS. The most important variable used to categorize mechanical ventilators is the mechanism determining the point at which the change-over from the inspiratory phase to the expiratory phase takes place (Fig. 73–5). This point may be determined by the volume of gas delivered (*volume-cycled*), the airway pressure achieved (*pressure-cycled*), or the elapsed time of inspiration (*time-cycled*). Both time-cycled and pressure-cycled ventilators have the

TABLE 73–3. INDICATIONS FOR ENDOTRACHEAL INTUBATION

1. Need for an $F_{I_{O_2}} > 0.5$ for more than a short time to maintain adequate oxygenation
2. Progressive hypoventilation with respiratory acidosis not responding to conservative management
3. Apnea
4. Loss of airway protective mechanisms
5. Inability to clear secretions
6. Need for heavy sedation or paralysis to control patient for diagnostic or therapeutic interventions

disadvantage of not necessarily delivering a constant tidal volume. For this reason volume-cycled ventilators are used most commonly. Many ventilators, however, have options that allow the device to be pressure- or time-cycled in addition to a volume-cycling mode.

FEATURES OF MECHANICAL VENTILATORS. Mechanical ventilators must have certain essential features in order to provide adequate ventilatory support in different patients with different types of respiratory disorders. Chief among these is the ability to deliver a wide range of tidal volumes (100 to 2000 ml), with an adjustable respiratory frequency (5 to 60) and an accurate adjustable $F_{I_{O_2}}$ (0.21 to 1.0). Additional important features include controls for adjusting the inspiration-expiration ratio (or the inspiratory flow rate) and the inspiratory pressure limit. The device should be capable of operating in an assist (patient-triggered) mode, a controlled (machine-triggered) mode, and an assist-control combination mode. The ventilator must be equipped with devices that monitor exhaled tidal volume, inspiratory pressure, the temperature of the inspiratory gas, and $F_{I_{O_2}}$ and have battery-operated alarms that signal loss of exhaled tidal volume, excessive inspiratory pressure, and reduction in $F_{I_{O_2}}$.

Preferably, ventilators should also have built-in controls for adjusting positive end-expiratory pressure (PEEP), for allowing intermittent mandatory ventilation (IMV), and for providing continuous positive airway pressure (CPAP) in spontaneously breathing patients.

PATTERNS OF VENTILATORY SUPPORT. Two basic patterns of ventilatory support may be employed in the management of patients with respiratory failure: (1) *intermittent positive pressure ventilation* (IPPV) and *intermittent mandatory ventilation* (IMV). The fluctuations in airway pressure that characterize spontaneous and mechanical ventilation are shown in Figure 73–5. The difference between IPPV and IMV is that there is no allowance for spontaneous ventilation with IPPV, whereas with IMV a portion of the patient's ventilation is spontaneous. The use of one or the other of these two patterns is often a matter of the physician's personal preference; however, some guidelines can be provided.

IPPV is clearly indicated in patients who have no spontaneous ventilation, who have severe pain with respiration and/or an unstable chest wall, or in whom the work of breathing represents a significant energy drain.

IMV offers the advantage of maintaining the condition of the respiratory muscles, and for this reason may be useful in patients who do not have chronic processes with pre-existing deconditioned muscles. In addition, patients may find IMV more comfortable than IPPV. Intermittent mandatory ventilation is also useful for patients who have significant reductions of cardiac output with mechanical ventilation, especially with PEEP, in that it may allow greater amounts of PEEP to be used. In patients who are not capable of synchronizing their inspiratory efforts with the ventilator and have a chaotic ventilatory pattern, IMV may allow adequate ventilation without the need for sedation or muscle-relaxing agents. It may also be a useful weaning technique in some situations.

POSITIVE END-EXPIRATORY PRESSURE (PEEP). As illustrated in Figure 73–5, PEEP increases the mean distending pressure across the walls of the airways and alveoli and thereby increases the volume of gas in the lung. This effect is beneficial in disorders characterized by pulmonary edema (usually noncardiogenic in origin) with consequent loss of functioning gas exchange units because of fluid filling or atelectasis. PEEP tends to re-expand collapsed units and to enable gas exchange to take place, thereby reducing intrapulmonary shunting of blood and improving Pa_{O_2}. PEEP can be added to IPPV to produce continuous positive pressure ventilation (CPPV) or to IMV. In addition, it can be used in spontaneously ventilating patients to produce CPAP or expiratory positive airway pressure (EPAP).

Positive end-expiratory pressure is not as clearly beneficial

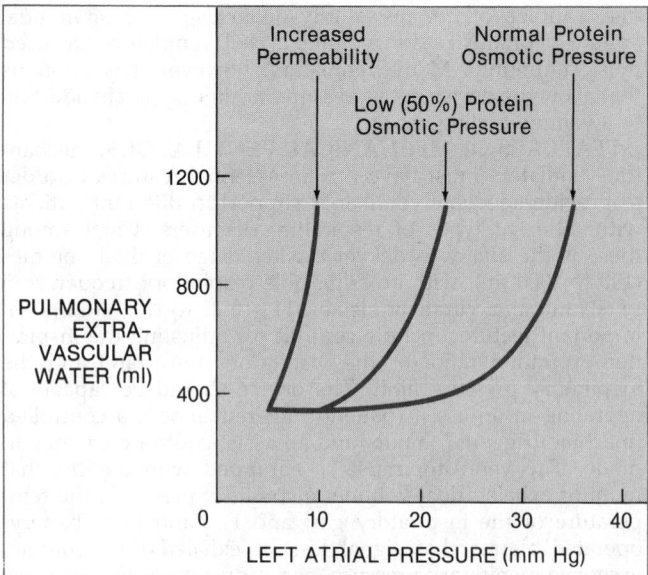

FIGURE 73–6. Schematic representation of the relationship of pulmonary extravascular water volume and left atrial or pulmonary artery wedge pressure. Curve at right represents the relationships when both capillary permeability and plasma protein osmotic pressures are normal; middle curve represents normal permeability but a reduction in plasma protein osmotic pressure of 50 per cent; left curve shows relationship when permeability of the capillaries is increased. (From Hopewell PC, Murray JF: Adult respiratory distress syndrome. In Moser KM, Spragg RG (eds.): Respiratory Emergencies. 2nd ed. St. Louis, The C. V. Mosby Company, 1982.)

and in fact may be harmful in patients with other types of respiratory failure, especially those failures caused by airways obstruction wherein the lung is already overinflated. In such cases further increases in lung volume may be hazardous. This dictum applies not only to CPPV but also to IMV with PEEP and to CPAP. PEEP may also decrease Pa_{O_2} in patients with focal infiltrative processes by increasing blood flow through the abnormal areas.

The conventional levels of PEEP range from 3 cm H_2O to 20 cm H_2O. Higher levels are occasionally used with IMV, but the indications for and the value of high levels of PEEP are not clearly defined.

CONSIDERATIONS IN INITIATING MECHANICAL VENTILATION. Once it is decided to initiate mechanical ventilation, a series of nearly equally important decisions should be made (Table 73–4). Much of the decision making is influenced by the pathophysiology of the underlying disorder for which mechanical ventilation is necessary. This is discussed in subsequent sections of this chapter.

VENTILATOR EMERGENCIES. Patients who are being mechanically ventilated are subject to a variety of potentially disastrous events that can occur suddenly and may be related either to the underlying disorder that made mechanical ventilation necessary or to malfunction of the ventilator or artificial airway. Such occurrences may rapidly be fatal. It is important that persons caring for critically ill patients develop a routine for assessment and management of these situations. The first indication that a problem is developing is usually

TABLE 73–4. DECISIONS IN INITIATING MECHANICAL VENTILATION

Type of ventilator
Pattern of ventilation (IPPV vs. IMV)
Mode (assist, control, or assist/control)
Tidal volume
Frequency
Fi_{O_2}
Inspiration:expiration ratio
End-expiratory pressure (PEEP vs. no PEEP)

that the patient is no longer being adequately ventilated, as manifested by patient distress, by activation of the high-pressure or low-VT alarm, or by sudden hemodynamic changes in the patient.

When the high-pressure limit is exceeded, problems that should be suspected include obstruction of the endotracheal or tracheostomy tube, obstruction in the patient's airways, or pneumothorax. Occasionally, migration of the tip of the tube into a mainstem bronchus (usually the right) will cause the high-pressure limit to be exceeded, but this is usually not so dramatic an occurrence. Less commonly, obstruction of the artificial airway may result from overinflation of the cuff with subsequent tube compression or herniation of the cuff over the tip of the tube.

When the high-pressure limit is exceeded and ventilation is ineffective, the first step is to disconnect the patient from the ventilator and begin hand ventilation with an anesthesia bag using an Fi_{O_2} of 1.0. At nearly the same time as bagging begins, the artificial airway should be checked for position and for evidence of external obstruction, such as kinking between the ventilator tubing connection and the nose or mouth or in the hypopharynx. If there is no external obstruction, the tube position seems correct, and compression of the bag is still difficult, the next step is to pass a suction catheter through the airway to check its patency and to remove mucous plugs or blood clots that may be causing the obstruction. If the obstruction is not removed, the tube cuff should be deflated to determine if it is causing the problem.

Assuming that the suction catheter can be passed, failure of these maneuvers to relieve the apparent obstruction indicates that the problem is within the patient and may be caused by major airway obstruction that was not removed by suctioning, sudden severe and more peripheral airways obstruction, or pneumothorax. The problem can usually be ascertained by a rapid physical examination of the chest. Tracheal obstruction is manifested by the finding of no or markedly reduced entry of air into the lungs. Mainstem bronchial obstruction is indicated by the absence of entry of air into the lung distal to the obstruction, causing a rocking motion of the chest with the affected side not expanding with inspiration and the unobstructed side being overinflated. Peripheral airways obstruction may be suspected from the patient's history and is usually indicated by wheezing, although with severe bronchoconstriction there may be little air movement and thus little or no wheezing. Pneumothorax in a patient being mechanically ventilated usually becomes a tension pneumothorax, characterized by difficulty with ventilation, reduction in arterial blood pressure, and an increase in central venous pressure. Examination of the chest shows no entry of air on the affected side, but, in contrast to the findings of mainstem bronchial obstruction, the affected side is hyperinflated and hyper-resonant to percussion. If the clinical situation allows, a chest roentgenogram can aid in a definitive diagnosis; however, a chest film showing a large tension pneumothorax may be viewed as being analogous to a 12-lead electrocardiogram in a patient with asystole.

Management of each of these situations is obviously different. Vigorous chest physical therapy and suctioning of the airway usually will remove obstructing mucous plugs or clots. Occasionally emergency fiberoptic bronchoscopy may be necessary. Tension pneumothorax requires prompt intervention to reduce the intrathoracic pressure. In an emergency situation a 14-gauge needle can be placed in the second anterior intercostal space. This will serve to relieve the tension with prompt restoration of the hemodynamic status and ability to ventilate the patient. After the needle is inserted, a chest tube should always be placed. Even if the diagnosis of pneumothorax was mistaken, a chest tube must be placed because of the high probability of lung puncture with the needle.

When the patient is suddenly not receiving adequate ventilation, but the high-pressure limit is not being exceeded, the problems that should be considered are leaks in the ventilator tubing or around the cuff of the artificial airway, ventilator malfunction, or a tracheoesophageal fistula. Again, the first step is to disconnect the ventilator and begin manual ventilation with an $F_{I_{O_2}}$ of 1.0. At the same time, the position of the tube and the inflation of the cuff of the endotracheal or tracheostomy tube should be checked. If the external pilot balloon is deflated, more air should be added. Leaks around the cuff may be caused by breaks in the cuff itself or in the external pilot balloon, or by enlargement of the trachea at the site of the cuff because of pressure on the tracheal wall. Occasionally, an endotracheal tube may be positioned too high in the airway with the cuff at the level of the vocal cords or higher, causing air to leak around the cuff. If the cuff itself is leaking, the tube must be replaced. With some kinds of tubes, the outer pilot balloon may be replaced, if defective, without changing the tube. If the leak is occurring because of tracheal enlargement, the problem may be solved by adding air to the cuff or by changing the level of the cuff within the trachea. If air is added, care should be taken not to exceed a measured intracuff pressure of 20 mm Hg.

Tracheal dilatation is often the precursor of a much more serious problem, formation of a tracheoesophageal fistula. This usually can be prevented by maintaining intracuff pressures of less than 20 mm Hg. When a fistula does develop, however, it is usually catastrophic. Patients with fistulas can sometimes be managed temporarily by placing the tube at a lower level in the trachea with the cuff below the fistula. Definitive management is surgical correction of the fistula.

WEANING FROM MECHANICAL VENTILATION. Patients being mechanically ventilated should be evaluated frequently to determine if their lung function has improved sufficiently to allow weaning from the ventilator and subsequent removal of the endotracheal tube. Factors other than the condition of the lungs play an important role in determining if the patient is ready to be weaned and in the outcome of the weaning process (Table 73–5).

The techniques and the rapidity of weaning vary considerably depending on the nature of the underlying disorders that caused the need for mechanical ventilation. There are some basic criteria that are generally applicable in determining if it is feasible to initiate weaning. First, the patient should be awake and fairly alert. Lung function should be adequate as indicated by the ability of the patient to generate a VC of greater than 10 ml per kilogram of body weight. This ability may also be inferred by the generation of a maximum inspiratory pressure of less (more negative) than -20 cm H_2O. In addition, the patient should not require an $F_{I_{O_2}}$ of greater than 0.5. Additional criteria that may be useful include a resting minute ventilation of less than 10 liters, the ability to double this volume voluntarily, a $P(A-a)_{O_2}$ less than 350 mm Hg at $F_{I_{O_2}} = 1$, and a V_D/V_T of less than 0.55.

In patients who meet these criteria, weaning can commence. The techniques used include progressive lengthening of periods of spontaneous ventilation with the endotracheal tube attached to a "T-piece," a similar arrangement but with CPAP, and IMV with a progressive reduction in the number of breaths delivered by the ventilator. Patients whose lungs were previously normal and who have required only a short period of mechanical ventilation usually can be weaned and extubated quickly. The weaning process is often much longer

TABLE 73–5. NONPULMONARY FACTORS THAT AFFECT WEANING FROM MECHANICAL VENTILATION

Cardiac function
Nutritional status
Electrolyte balance
Fluid balance
Pain
Mental status

in patients with chronic airways obstruction who have required a long period of ventilatory support.

Hudson LD: Diagnosis and management of acute respiratory distress in patients on mechanical ventilators. In Moser KM, Spragg RG: Respiratory Emergencies. St. Louis, C. V. Mosby Company, 1982, pp 202–213. *Describes the differential diagnosis of respiratory distress in patients who are being ventilated mechanically and discusses the steps to be undertaken in evaluation and management.*

Lanken PM: Weaning from mechanical ventilation. In Fishman AP (ed.): Update: Pulmonary Diseases and Disorders. New York, McGraw-Hill Book Company, 1982, pp 366–386. *Presents a comprehensive, well-referenced discussion of weaning. Reviews the basic pathophysiology of respiratory failure, criteria for weaning, and weaning techniques.*

Luce JM, Pierson DJ, Hudson LD: Intermittent mandatory ventilation. Chest 76:678, 1981. *A synthesis of information concerning the physiology and uses of IMV.*

Mushin WW, Rendell-Baker L, Thompson PW, et al.: Automatic Ventilation of the Lungs. 3rd ed. Oxford, Blackwell Scientific Publications, 1980. *The most comprehensive single-source reference on mechanical ventilation and ventilators that exists. Provides detailed technical information on nearly every commercially available positive pressure mechanical ventilator.*

Rizk NW, Murray JF: PEEP in pulmonary edema. Am J Med 72:381, 1982. *A concise updating of thinking concerning the effects of PEEP on lung fluid balance.*

Snider GL, Rinaldo JE: Oxygen therapy in medical patients hospitalized outside the intensive care unit. Am Rev Respir Dis 122(2):29, 1980. *A good description of the indications for and effects of supplemental oxygen with a discussion of the pros and cons of different techniques.*

Welch GW, Rippe JM: Airway Management and Endotracheal Intubation. In Rippe JM, Irwin RS, Alpert JS, et al. (eds.): Intensive Care Medicine. Boston, Little, Brown and Company, 1985, pp 3–16. *A comprehensive description of acute airway management, the indications for and techniques of endotracheal intubation, and complications resulting from intubation.*

PATHOPHYSIOLOGY, ASSESSMENT, AND CRITICAL CARE MANAGEMENT OF SPECIFIC FORMS OF RESPIRATORY FAILURE

The causes of respiratory failure may be categorized by the component of the respiratory system primarily involved and by the time course of the process. Life threatening or fatal respiratory failure may occur as the result of processes involving the respiratory neuromuscular system, the chest wall, the extrathoracic and intrathoracic airways, the lung parenchyma, and the pulmonary vasculature. Each of these produces respiratory failure by a different basic pathophysiologic mechanism and entails different approaches to treatment. In many instances, however, there is a mixture of the mechanisms that are causing respiratory failure. For example, fatigue of the respiratory muscles may be the final event precipitating fullblown respiratory failure in patients with other primary lung disorders. Thus, although the basic approach to management is determined by the major underlying pathophysiologic mechanism, a variety of secondary approaches may be called for as well.

Central Nervous System, Peripheral Nervous System, and Muscular Causes of Respiratory Failure

Processes such as sedative hypnotic drug overdose and brain injuries and infections can reduce or abolish central respiratory drive, resulting in respiratory failure that is characterized predominantly by hypoventilation. The airways and lung parenchyma are unaffected except by atelectasis, which may occur because of a lack of periodic hyperinflations (sighs). Once ventilation is provided, gas exchange is normal unless atelectasis has occurred. The same pathophysiologic pattern can result from high cervical spinal cord injuries, peripheral nervous system disorders such as Guillain-Barré syndrome, or muscular disorders such as myasthenia gravis.

Use of critical care in these instances is dictated by the requirement for careful observation and/or for ventilatory support. Generally ventilatory support is indicated for patients in this category who have hypoventilation that does not respond to initial conservative management.

Measurements of Pa_{CO_2}, Pa_{O_2}, and arterial pH in comatose or sedated patients provide a direct indication of alveolar ventilation and also inferential information on the status of the lung parenchyma. In patients with spinal cord injury or neuromuscular disease, measurements of arterial blood gas tensions and pH are similarly useful, but gas exchange may be well preserved until there is a marked reduction in ventilatory capability. Serial measurements of VC and maximal inspiratory pressure are therefore of value in predicting the likelihood of hypoventilation and the need for ventilatory support. In persons with normal ventilatory control mechanisms, hypoventilation does not occur with a VC of greater than 1 liter. Once the ventilatory capability is reduced to this degree, however, any further decrease is likely to be associated with a sudden increase in Pa_{CO_2}. Similarly, decreases in maximal inspiratory force to less than 20 cm H_2O are indicative of a critical reduction in ventilatory capability and the imminent possibility of hypoventilation. Apart from the direct respiratory consequences of these processes, critical care may be required to provide adequate airway protection and, in the case of drug overdose, to treat other toxic effects such as hemodynamic instability.

The pathophysiologic manifestations in this group of disorders are nearly identical, so that the approach to respiratory support of existing or imminent hypoventilation is the same. An oral or nasal endotracheal tube should be used to provide mechanical ventilation, preferably with a volume-limited ventilator. An initial tidal volume of 10 ml per kilogram of body weight is used in the control mode for apneic patients or in the assist/control mode for patients capable of initiating breaths. The ventilator frequency should be 8 to 10 breaths per minute with an inspiration-expiration ratio of 1:3. The appropriateness of this level of alveolar ventilation must be checked by measuring Pa_{CO_2}, Pa_{O_2}, and arterial pH approximately 10 minutes after initiating mechanical ventilation.

If the gas exchange abnormality is purely hypoventilation, use of supplemental oxygen should not be necessary. However, this is rarely the case. It is good practice to initiate mechanical ventilation using an FI_{O_2} of 1.0; after the initial measurement of Pa_{O_2}, FI_{O_2} should be adjusted downward. PEEP is generally not necessary in this category of illness but may be beneficial in preventing collapse or in re-expanding existing atelectatic areas of the lungs, complications not infrequent in patients with neurologic or muscular disorders.

Weaning from mechanical ventilation and the decision to remove the endotracheal tube should be made in accordance with the guidelines discussed previously. Generally, the weaning and extubation of drug-overdosed patients who do not have complications proceed quite rapidly once they are awake. Patients with chronic neuromuscular disorders present much more of a problem and may require long-term ventilatory support.

Respiratory Failure Caused by Chest Wall Abnormalities

The most frequently encountered cause of this type of respiratory failure is traumatic injury to the chest wall with consequent rib fractures. This is associated with pain that inhibits full lung inflation, with atelectasis, and occasionally with hypoventilation. Multiple ribs fractured in multiple places, in addition to causing pain, can interfere with lung inflation because of the loss of chest wall rigidity and subsequent paradoxic motion of the involved area, so-called *flail chest*. Atelectasis, hypoxemia, and hypoventilation in severe cases characterize the pathophysiologic picture. In addition, the underlying lung is frequently contused, which adds to the abnormalities of gas exchange. Chronic deformities of the chest wall or marked pleural disease also can result in respiratory failure, although in these situations the pathophysiologic alterations are more complex than in injuries to the chest wall and often involve parenchymal and vascular abnormalities as well.

The primary mode of assessment is measurement of arterial blood gas tensions. The basic indications for placement of an endotracheal tube are an inability to maintain adequate oxygenation with external oxygen delivery devices and significant increases in Pa_{CO_2}. The need for ventilatory support may be anticipated in patients who require large doses of narcotic agents to control their pain.

The pattern of mechanical ventilation utilized in patients with chest wall injuries is much the same as that described for patients with neuromuscular disorders. However, because of the greater likelihood of involvement of the lung parenchyma with atelectasis and hemorrhage, a higher V_T (12 to 15 ml per kilogram) and PEEP may be beneficial. The use of PEEP also helps to correct or prevent atelectasis and to stabilize the injured chest wall.

Weaning from mechanical ventilation does not necessarily have to await full stabilization of the chest wall, which can take weeks. Standard criteria can be used as the basis for making decisions concerning weaning and removal of the endotracheal tube.

Respiratory Failure Caused by Airways Obstruction

Impediments in the proximal portion of the airways (e.g., hypopharynx, larynx, and trachea) or generalized narrowing of the peripheral airways can severely obstruct airflow. With proximal obstruction hypoventilation is the major pathophysiologic abnormality. Gas exchange is normal once the obstruction is removed or bypassed. Similarly, hypoventilation is the hallmark of respiratory failure associated with diffuse airways obstruction (i.e., asthma, chronic bronchitis, and emphysema); however, the hypoventilation is invariably associated with hypoxemia due largely to ventilation-perfusion mismatching.

In this latter group of disorders, the primary abnormality is an increased resistance to airflow resulting from intrinsic narrowing of the airways or loss of airway tethering forces, or both. Regardless of the mechanism, the results are hypoxemia caused by mismatching of ventilation and perfusion and hypoventilation resulting from the airways obstruction itself plus fatigue of the respiratory muscles.

Measurements of airflow rates (FEV_1, PEFR) and arterial blood gas tensions are helpful in evaluating the severity of obstruction of airflow, and serial measurements describe the course of the episode and enable quantitation of response to treatment. The interpretation of a given set of arterial blood gas values varies considerably, depending on the time over which the abnormalities develop and their rate of change.

In patients with asthma or chronic airways obstruction, Pa_{CO_2} begins to increase when the FEV_1 is reduced to approximately 750 ml or less, or 25 per cent of its predicted value. With further reductions, Pa_{CO_2} tends to increase rapidly. Increased Pa_{CO_2} values occurring in association with FEV_1's of greater than 750 to 1000 ml may be the result of reduced ventilatory drive or increased production of carbon dioxide in a patient with a limited ability to increase the alveolar ventilation. As previously described, the distinction between acute and chronic hypoventilation can be determined by analyzing the relationships among Pa_{CO_2}, arterial pH, and $[HCO_3^-]$. Acute hypoventilation obviously dictates a more prompt response than chronic partially compensated respiratory acidosis.

The presence of metabolic acidosis is a more ominous finding than pure respiratory acidosis in the setting of airways obstruction. It implies a failure of the oxygen delivery system to provide sufficient amounts of oxygen to meet the demands imposed by the increased work of breathing. Such a situation cannot exist in steady state, and unless these patients rapidly improve, their condition will rapidly deteriorate.

Although hypoxemia invariably is present in patients with severe airways obstruction, the degree of reduction in Pa_{O_2} is generally in itself not sufficient to require respiratory support other than supplemental oxygen via external devices.

One cannot definitively state criteria for placement of an endotracheal tube and use of mechanical ventilation in patients with severe airways obstruction. Arterial blood gas and pH values at a single point in time showing marked acute respiratory acidosis or respiratory plus metabolic acidosis may be sufficient information on which to base the decision to provide mechanical ventilation. More commonly, however, it is necessary to evaluate the patient during a period of time while maximal conservative therapy is being administered and to evaluate the response to therapy. If the blood gas values are worsening or not improving in spite of maximal treatment, mechanical ventilation is the next logical step. In addition to the objective evaluation provided by arterial blood gas and pH measurements, subjective assessments are also of value. Patients who are confused, somnolent, or uncooperative may require ventilatory support because their mental status may indicate an end-organ effect of the blood gas abnormalities and because the patients cannot cooperate with conservative management.

Severe airways obstruction presents a difficult situation in which to apply mechanical ventilation. There is the need to allow adequate exhalation time in the presence of marked expiratory airflow slowing, but also slow inspiratory flows are desirable to optimize the distribution of ventilation and to minimize the airways pressure required to deliver the set V_T. To accomplish these goals, at least early in the course of mechanical ventilation, it is often necessary to sedate the patient to effect a slow respiratory frequency, which results in an appropriate inspiration-expiration ratio. The V_T should be approximately 10 ml per kilogram and the $F_{I_{O_2}}$ adjusted to provide an adequate Pa_{O_2}. As the airways obstruction improves, the need for sedation will decrease. In initiating mechanical ventilation in patients with chronic hypoventilation, it is important not to reduce the Pa_{CO_2} rapidly because it will result in uncompensated metabolic alkalosis. The minute ventilation should be set to reduce the Pa_{CO_2} gradually, allowing the arterial pH to go no higher than 7.50. In general, PEEP should not be used in patients with airways obstruction because it will further distend the already overinflated lungs.

Weaning patients with airways obstruction from mechanical ventilation also may present a difficult problem. Patients with asthma may be weaned and extubated quickly. However, patients with chronic airways obstruction may at best have marginal lung function with persistent retention of carbon dioxide. Generally speaking, the arterial blood gas pattern that is estimated to exist when the patient is "well" should be approximated while mechanical ventilation is still being used. Ideally, weaning can then proceed using previously described indicators. In many instances, however, patients with chronic airways obstruction never meet the objective criteria for weaning and extubation. When this occurs, the decisions in weaning and extubation are based on subjective criteria, such as level of alertness, patient cooperation, and prognosis. These factors obviously cannot be quantitated. Once the patient has demonstrated the ability to ventilate spontaneously for 30 to 60 minutes, the endotracheal tube should be removed.

It is important to try to determine which patients with chronic airways obstruction have a component of reversible respiratory dysfunction and which patients have simply reached the end stage of their disease. Although chronic mechanical ventilation is occasionally used to maintain life in a patient with end-stage chronic airways obstruction, the decision to pursue this course should be carefully considered by the patient, the family, and the physician, preferably before mechanical ventilation is begun.

Disorders of the Lung Parenchyma Causing Respiratory Failure

Disorders of the lung parenchyma can be divided into those that predominantly involve the interstitium and those that predominantly involve the alveolar airspaces. Accumulations of fluid in alveoli can be caused by cardiogenic pulmonary edema (left ventricular failure or mitral stenosis) or diffuse injury to the lung causing noncardiogenic pulmonary edema (adult respiratory distress syndrome [ARDS]). A list of the conditions that have been associated with ARDS is provided in Ch. 72.

Both cardiogenic and noncardiogenic pulmonary edema may cause respiratory failure that is characterized by hypoxemia caused by right-to-left intrapulmonary shunting of blood and ventilation-perfusion mismatching. In severe cases retention of carbon dioxide can occur. Although mechanical ventilation may be required in both forms of pulmonary edema, other therapeutic interventions and response to treatment are quite different. This section will focus on pulmonary edema resulting from an increase in the permeability of the alveolar-capillary membrane. Cardiogenic pulmonary edema is discussed in Ch. 43.

ADULT RESPIRATORY DISTRESS SYNDROME (ARDS). A constellation of clinical, radiographic, and pathophysiologic findings that result from diffuse injury to the lung parenchyma defines ARDS. The characteristics of the syndrome are (1) hypoxemia due to intrapulmonary shunting of blood, (2) increased lung stiffness (or decreased compliance), and (3) presence of diffuse infiltration on the chest roentgenogram. The common abnormality that accounts for these features is an increase in the permeability of the endothelium of the pulmonary capillary and the epithelium of the alveolar wall. This allows fluid to leak from the capillary into the alveolus even though the hydrostatic pressure within the capillary is normal; hence, noncardiogenic pulmonary edema results.

The injury to the lung that results in ARDS may be delivered via the airways or via the circulation. In many instances (e.g., aspiration of gastric juice or diffuse pneumonia), the mechanism by which the injury occurs is easily understood. However, in others (e.g., sepsis or pancreatitis), the mechanism is obscure.

Regardless of the type or mechanism of injury, both the pathophysiologic and the pathologic abnormalities are uniform. Grossly, the lung is edematous and hemorrhagic. Microscopic examination reveals intra-alveolar collections of proteinaceous fluid, red blood cells, and often inflammatory cells. Microthrombi or white blood cell aggregates may occasionally be seen in small vessels. After 24 to 48 hours, hyaline membranes line the inner aspects of alveoli and alveolar ducts. These membranes are formed by fibrin that has escaped through the leaking capillaries. Subsequently, as repair of the injury occurs, fibrosis may ensue although this is not an invariable consequence.

The pathophysiologic alterations affect lung volume, mechanical properties of the lung, and gas exchange. Reductions in VC and functional residual capacity (FRC) are characteristic of ARDS and are caused in part by fluid replacing alveolar air. As previously noted, one of the hallmarks of ARDS is the increased stiffness of the lung. This results not only from fluid in the alveoli but probably also from interaction between extravasated protein and surfactant, which increase surface forces at the air-liquid interface. The work of breathing considerably increases because of these effects on lung volume and lung compliance. The major and most frequent gas exchange abnormality is *hypoxemia*. This again is related predominantly to alveolar filling with fluid, causing these units to be the sites of shunting. In other less involved portions of the lung, ventilation-perfusion mismatching occurs and contributes to the hypoxemia.

In severe forms of ARDS, as the process evolves from injury to repair, the gas exchange abnormalities also evolve. Lung fibrosis may result in obliteration of capillaries and coalescence of airspaces to produce an increased V_D/V_T with overall alveolar hypoventilation, as indicated by an increased Pa_{CO_2}.

Definite abnormalities of gas exchange are seen only when the process has advanced to the stage of alveolar flooding.

Thus, such measurements of blood gas tensions are relatively insensitive in assessing the lung injury. Nevertheless, patients who either have or are at risk of developing ARDS should be carefully observed, and Pa_{O_2}, Pa_{CO_2}, and arterial pH should be measured frequently. Early in the course, the critical variable is the Pa_{O_2}. Because patients frequently hyperventilate at this stage, the $P(A-a)_{O_2}$ should be calculated to provide an accurate index of the course of the process. The occurrence of either respiratory or metabolic acidosis in this setting is an ominous finding. In addition to blood gas tensions, it is often necessary to measure the pulmonary artery wedge pressure both to determine if there is a contribution of cardiogenic pulmonary edema to the process and to serve as a guide for fluid management.

Patients who have fully developed ARDS invariably require mechanical ventilation. The determination of when to intervene with ventilatory support in patients who are at risk of developing ARDS or who have minor abnormalities of pulmonary function that suggest early ARDS may be quite difficult. The occurrence of edema and consequent loss of lung volume tends to be a self-perpetuating cycle, so that it is generally better to provide mechanical ventilation earlier rather than later.

When mechanical ventilation is undertaken, VT of 12 to 15 ml per kilogram of body weight should be used. Volumes of this magnitude are more effective in preventing or reversing atelectasis. In addition, use of PEEP has a well-documented role in the management of patients with ARDS. The beneficial effect of this pattern of ventilation is mainly attributable to the increase in FRC that it produces. By maintaining a continuously positive distending pressure across the walls of alveoli and airways, PEEP re-establishes their patency allowing gas exchange to resume in these units. Thus, shunting is decreased and Pa_{O_2} is improved.

Use of PEEP is not without hazards: (1) The increase in intrathoracic pressure caused by PEEP may reduce cardiac output. This appears to occur predominantly because of a reduction in venous inflow to the right side of the heart. It is therefore important to assess carefully the effects of PEEP not only on Pa_{O_2} but also on systemic oxygen transport by measuring cardiac output after PEEP is applied and after changes in PEEP. (2) The second potential complication of PEEP is the occurrence of pneumothorax. This seems more likely to occur later in the course of ARDS as architectural rearrangements take place in the lung that weaken its structure.

The application of PEEP may decrease Pa_{O_2} in situations in which there is considerable regional variation in the distribution of lung pathology. This results from shifting blood flow away from the more normal portions of the lung to the more abnormal portions and thereby increasing shunting.

Appropriate use of intravenous fluids is an important component of the management of ARDS. Pulmonary capillary permeability is increased and the regulatory mechanisms that normally tend to protect the lung from fluid overload are impaired. The prevailing capillary hydrostatic pressure therefore assumes an enhanced importance. Thus, administration of fluid, which increases the capillary hydrostatic pressure, tends to increase the amount of water in the lung. The relationship between capillary hydrostatic pressure and lung water content is shown schematically in Figure 73–6.

On the other hand, adequate pulmonary and systemic perfusion may also be important in preventing lung damage, and systemic perfusion is clearly important in maintaining renal, cardiac, and central nervous system functions. Thus, the effects of fluid administration should be carefully monitored with clear endpoints in mind. Rather than using systemic arterial pressure or central venous pressure alone to guide treatment, indexes of end-organ perfusion, such as urine output or mental functioning, should also be monitored. Frequently, at least early in the course of the process, a Swan-Ganz pulmonary artery catheter may be extremely helpful.

Sufficient fluid should be administered to maintain perfusion of critical organs with as little effect as possible on the pulmonary artery wedge pressure.

Crystalloid solutions are probably preferable to colloid solutions, at least early in the course of the process when the increase in capillary permeability is most marked. At present there are not sufficient clinical data to support the use of corticosteroids in the treatment of patients who either have or are at risk of developing ARDS.

Pulmonary Vascular Diseases

The major effects of pulmonary vascular obstruction are circulatory rather than respiratory. Nevertheless, both acute pulmonary embolism and chronic pulmonary vasculitis are commonly associated with hypoxemia. In the former it is thought to be caused by microatelectasis producing right-to-left shunting. In the latter, the gas exchange abnormalities probably relate to pulmonary parenchymal abnormalities adjacent to vascular inflammation and result from a mixture of shunting and ventilation-perfusion mismatching.

Both the assessment and the management of the respiratory abnormalities caused by pulmonary vascular disease are directed toward the vascular process itself. Rarely is mechanical ventilation necessary solely because of gas exchange abnormalities caused by pulmonary vascular disease. However, small and occasionally large pulmonary emboli may occur in patients with other respiratory illnesses, thus compounding their cardiorespiratory abnormalities.

Bell RC, Coalson JJ, Smith JD, et al.: Multiple organ system failure and infection in adult respiratory distress syndrome. Ann Intern Med 99:293, 1983. *A prospective study evaluating the role of multiple organ system failure and infection in patients with ARDS. The overall survival rate was 26.2 per cent and was significantly worse in patients who developed central nervous system, gastrointestinal, renal, endocrine, or coagulation disorders and in patients who had infections.*

Cherniack RM: Management of acute respiratory failure in chronic obstructive pulmonary disease. Semin Respir Med 8:158, 1986. *A detailed review of the pathophysiology and management of respiratory failure caused by chronic airways obstruction.*

Hopewell PC, Miller WT: Respiratory failure in status asthmaticus. Clin Chest Med 5:623, 1984. *Presents a review of the pathophysiology, assessment, and management of severe asthma.*

Hopewell PC, Murray JF: Adult respiratory distress syndrome. In Moser KM, Spragg RG (eds.): Respiratory Emergencies. 2nd ed. St. Louis, C. V. Mosby Company, 1982. *A comprehensive review of pathogenesis, pathophysiology, pathology, and management of ARDS.*

Hyers TM: Markers of acute lung injury in humans. Semin Respir Med 8(Suppl):65, 1986. *Describes the current status of our understanding of mediators and markers of acute lung injury.*

Montgomery AB, Stager MA, Carico CJ, et al.: Causes of mortality in patients with the adult respiratory distress syndrome. Am Rev Respir Dis 132:485, 1985. *An analysis of factors causing and contributing to death in patients with ARDS pointing out the importance of sepsis in causing and complicating the syndrome.*

Prewitt RM, Matthay MA, Ghignone M: Hemodynamic management in the adult respiratory distress syndrome. Clin Chest Med 4:251, 1983. *Discusses the important cardiopulmonary interactions in ARDS and optimal management strategies.*

Rinaldo JE, Rogers RM: Adult respiratory distress syndrome: Changing concepts of lung injury and repair. N Engl J Med 306:900, 1982. *An excellent review of ARDS emphasizing the mechanisms by which the lung injury might occur.*

CRITICAL CARE MONITORING

A critical care unit is unique in its ability to provide continuous and often invasive measurements of respiratory and hemodynamic status in severely ill patients. Such monitoring enables early detection of changes in the patient's condition and provides information that both directs therapy and assists in evaluating the response to treatment. The complexity of monitoring systems varies considerably, ranging from simple electrocardiographic monitoring with only a real-time screen display to automated "closed loop" systems wherein the monitored data, through a computer program, serve to regulate intravenous infusions of fluids and drugs. Usually, the kind of system employed relates to the kinds of patients being cared for in the unit.

Respiratory Monitoring

As a minimum, respiratory monitoring should consist of measurement of respiratory rate and periodic measurement of Pa_{O_2}, Pa_{CO_2}, and arterial pH. Respiratory rate can be measured and recorded automatically in nonintubated patients using impedance devices to which alarms can be attached. Both respiratory rate and V_T can be monitored in intubated, spontaneously breathing patients using a spirometer and appropriate alarms.

In patients who are being mechanically ventilated, monitoring of respiratory rate, exhaled V_T, and airway pressure is essential. Additional monitoring techniques are available but do not yet have a demonstrated role. These include breath by breath measurements of respiratory system compliance and volume-pressure and volume-flow relationships. In addition, multiplexed mass spectrometer-based systems are available for measurement of FI_{O_2} and exhaled carbon dioxide and oxygen. These systems may provide early indications of changes in Pa_{CO_2}, but their usefulness and general applicability remain to be determined.

The transcutaneous P_{O_2} and P_{CO_2} that are indirect reflections of Pa_{O_2} and Pa_{CO_2} can be measured continuously using heated skin electrodes. Measurement of transcutaneous P_{O_2} in infants has proved to be a helpful monitoring technique, but the value of this measurement in adults is uncertain.

Pulse oximeters are noninvasive monitoring devices that measure and record oxyhemoglobin saturation. This technique has proved to be useful in a variety of clinical situations, including weaning from mechanical ventilation and evaluating oxygenation during sleep and during procedures such as bronchoscopy.

Indwelling catheter electrodes for continuous intra-arterial measurement of Pa_{O_2}, Pa_{CO_2}, and arterial pH have been used but still have important technical limitations. More recently, a fiberoptic pulmonary artery catheter for continuous measurement of oxyhemoglobin saturation in mixed venous blood has been developed but does not have a defined role as yet.

Hemodynamic Monitoring

Most critical care units have the basic capacity to monitor and record heart rate and rhythm (usually with a built-in memory and recall capability), venous pressure, pulmonary arterial pressure, and systemic arterial pressure. In addition, many units have the instruments necessary for measurement of cardiac output.

Electrocardiographic monitoring is clearly of value in patients with specific cardiac disorders such as acute myocardial infarction or cardiac arrhythmia. This form of assessment is also essential in patients with any illness severe enough to require critical care. Abnormalities in heart rate or rhythm may signal the worsening of a respiratory condition, electrolyte abnormalities, or a variety of other noncardiac problems. Ideally, the system should have a built-in memory and should be able to display frequency and kinds of arrhythmias occurring in a given period of time. Both high-rate and low-rate alarms are necessary to complete the system.

Continuous *systemic arterial pressure monitoring* is of obvious value, assuming it is performed accurately. Changes in blood pressure can be detected immediately and therefore enable beat by beat assessment of the effects of such maneuvers as changes in ventilatory pattern or infusion of vasoactive drugs. Continuous measurement of the blood pressure decreases the amount of time necessary for staff members to spend with the patient. Finally, an arterial catheter provides ready access to arterial blood for measurement of blood gases.

Each of these advantages has a corollary disadvantage, however. If the equipment is not properly calibrated, an inaccurate reading may be obtained that may result in inappropriate decisions. Beat to beat variations in blood pressure may not warrant specific intervention. In many instances it is better for the nurse to be at the patient's bedside rather than watching a monitor screen. Finally, the presence of an arterial catheter may encourage withdrawal of more blood than is necessary for measurement of blood gases.

The advantages and disadvantages of arterial pressure monitoring must be taken into account in deciding when arterial catheter placement is indicated. In addition to the problems just listed, there are specific complications of arterial catheterization, which are discussed below (see Complications of Hemodynamic Monitoring, Systemic Arterial Pressure).

Given these considerations, the basic indication for monitoring arterial blood pressure is the presence or anticipation of hemodynamic instability as a result of either the disease process or the therapeutic intervention. In patients who require frequent measurement of arterial blood gases, insertion of an arterial catheter may be indicated to provide access to arterial blood.

The usual technique of monitoring systemic arterial pressure is to insert percutaneously a Teflon catheter into an accessible artery. The radial artery of the nondominant hand is usually the vessel of choice. The Allen test should be performed to determine the patency of the palmar arterial arch before insertion of the catheter. The femoral artery is the second choice for placement. The brachial artery, ulnar artery, and dorsalis pedis artery can also be used.

The catheter is connected via a stopcock to a rigid connecting tube that in turn is attached to a transducer. Commonly, a device that continuously flushes the catheter with a small volume of heparinized solution is also connected to the catheter.

Central venous pressure monitoring by a continuous technique is useful in quantitating and following the course of right ventricular failure, right ventricular infarction, tricuspid regurgitation, and cardiac tamponade. In addition, it is useful in evaluating the intravascular volume status of patients who have no pulmonary or cardiac disease.

Under normal circumstances, central venous pressure (CVP) is equivalent to right atrial and right ventricular diastolic pressures and bears a more or less constant relationship to the pulmonary wedge pressure (pulmonary artery wedge pressure [P_{PAW}] = CVP + 6 mm Hg). However, if cardiac or pulmonary disease is present, the CVP does not reflect the left atrial filling pressure (pulmonary artery wedge pressure). In fact, the CVP may provide misleading information leading to erroneous therapeutic decisions.

To monitor CVP a catheter is inserted percutaneously into either the subclavian or the external or internal jugular vein. An antecubital vein may also be used for catheter insertion either percutaneously or via a cutdown. Care should be taken to avoid passing the catheter into the right ventricle where it can cause ventricular arrhythmias. A chest roentgenogram should be obtained immediately after insertion of the catheter to determine its position and to check for pneumothorax or pneumomediastinum (with subclavian and internal jugular sites of catheter insertion).

The instrumentation for measurement of CVP is the same as that described for arterial pressure. The CVP measurements should be interpreted cautiously. In patients who have significant hemodynamic instability, the CVP should not be relied on as an accurate indicator of volume status, especially in the presence of cardiac or pulmonary disease.

In *pulmonary arterial pressure monitoring*, development of the balloon-tipped flotation catheter by Swan and Ganz increased both the ease and safety of catheter placement and, in addition, enabled bedside measurement of the wedge pressure. This catheter, in addition to having a central lumen with a distal opening to measure P_{PA}, has a balloon bonded to the catheter just proximal to the tip and a separate lumen for inflating the balloon. With the catheter properly positioned, inflation of the balloon occludes the vessel in which the tip resides, stopping blood flow and allowing measurement of

TABLE 73–6. INDICATIONS FOR PULMONARY ARTERIAL PRESSURE MONITORING

1. To help distinguish cardiogenic from noncardiogenic pulmonary edema.
2. To provide information in the differential diagnosis of hypotension.
3. To assist in determining the cause of hypoxemia.
4. To characterize the patterns of abnormal cardiac function after myocardial infarction.
5. To monitor the effects of various therapeutic interventions such as vasoactive agents, intravenous fluids, diuretics, digitalis, and CPPV.

the pulmonary artery wedge pressure. In addition to the basic single lumen No. 5 F catheter, there are a variety of modifications. The most versatile version is a No. 7 F size that has, in addition to the distal lumen, a proximal lumen for measurement of CVP and a thermistor near the tip that allows measurement of cardiac output using the thermal dilution technique.

Thus, the Swan-Ganz pulmonary artery catheter provides measurement of PPA, PPAW, CVP, and cardiac output. In addition, blood can be sampled from the pulmonary artery for measurement of oxygen content. The indications for monitoring PPA are listed in Table 73–6.

It is important to recognize the limitations of monitoring PPA. First, because of the effects of oscillations in pleural pressure on the measured intravascular pressure, the values are extremely difficult to determine in persons who are breathing rapidly. Second, the values are altered by PEEP; an accurate absolute value cannot be obtained in a patient in whom PEEP is being used. The measurement has a relative value, however, that can be used comparatively to evaluate a therapeutic maneuver unless the catheter is positioned in a portion of the lung in which alveolar pressure is greater than pulmonary venous pressure alone or PPA and pulmonary venous pressure (an unlikely occurrence). If this occurs, the reading of pulmonary artery wedge pressure will reflect alveolar pressure rather than left atrial pressure. Finally, pulmonary artery wedge pressure will not reflect the left ventricular filling pressure in the presence of mitral stenosis or pulmonary venous obstruction.

To obtain the maximal amount of information from the procedure, a recording of the wave form and pressures should be made as the catheter passes from the superior vena cava to the right atrium, right ventricle, and pulmonary artery. Figure 73–7 shows the normal wave forms encountered during passage of the catheter. Specific abnormal patterns may be seen in patients with tricuspid regurgitation or cardiac tamponade and constriction.

Insertion of the catheter is via the same choice of routes described for insertion of the catheter for measuring CVP. The instrumentation is also the same. The procedure must be performed with continuous electrocardiographic monitoring to allow identification of ventricular arrhythmias induced by

the catheter passing through the right ventricle. Because of the possibility of ventricular arrhythmias, lidocaine for immediate intravenous administration must be available. The catheter should be positioned so that a pulmonary artery wedge pressure tracing is seen with 1 ml of air in the balloon (for a No. 7 F catheter with a 1.5-ml capacity balloon). The catheter should then be secured in that position and a chest roentgenogram taken to confirm and record the position and to check for pneumothorax. The PPA tracing should be monitored continuously to detect distal migration and permanent wedging of the catheter, which may cause pulmonary infarction.

Measurements of cardiac output can be obtained easily and routinely using the thermistor-equipped Swan-Ganz catheter. Such measurements complement the pressure measurements described earlier and enable nearly complete characterization of the hemodynamic status of the severely ill patient.

The instrumentation required to perform thermal dilution determinations includes, in addition to the Swan-Ganz catheter, a cardiac output computer that processes the indicator-dilution measurements and calculates cardiac output. Such measurements are not without error, but, using standard techniques, the results are of acceptable accuracy.

Patterns of hemodynamic abnormalities are often of diagnostic value. Using the systemic and pulmonary arterial pressure, CVP, and cardiac output, the resistance across the pulmonary and systemic vascular beds can be calculated as follows:

$$PVR = \frac{\overline{PPA} - \overline{PPAW} \times 80}{\dot{Q}_T}$$

$$SVR = \frac{\overline{PSA} - \overline{PRA} \times 80}{\dot{Q}_T}$$

where PVR = pulmonary vascular resistance, SVR = systemic vascular resistance, $\overline{PPAW}$ = mean pulmonary artery wedge pressure, $\overline{PSA}$ = mean systemic arterial pressure, $\overline{PRA}$ = mean right atrial pressure. Normal values are 50 to 150 dyne-sec per centimeter^5 for PVR and 800 to 1200 dyne-sec per centimeter^5 for SVR.

Using these calculated variables plus the measured vascular pressures and cardiac output, patterns of hemodynamic abnormalities can be determined. Table 73–7 shows the hemodynamic patterns characteristic of the problems most frequently encountered in a critical care unit.

Liebowitz RS, Rippe JM: Arterial line placement and care. In Rippe JM, Irwin RS, Alpert JS, et al. (eds.): Intensive Care Medicine. Boston, Little, Brown and Company, 1985, pp 33–42. *A detailed description of indications, techniques, and complications of systemic arterial catheterization.*

Matthay MA: Invasive hemodynamic monitoring in critically ill patients. Clin Chest Med 4:233, 1983. *An excellent comprehensive review of indications, techniques, interpretation, and pitfalls of hemodynamic monitoring in critical care units.*

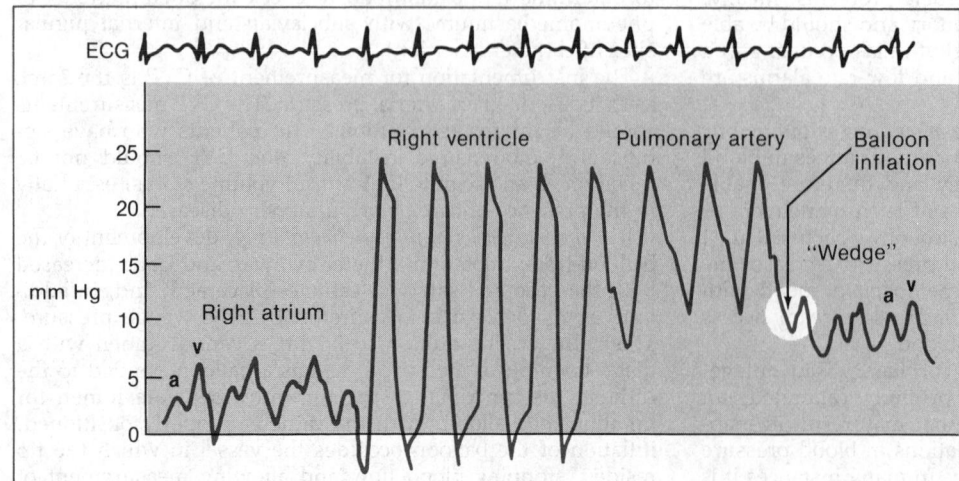

FIGURE 73–7. Tracing of pressures during passage of a Swan-Ganz catheter from the internal jugular vein into the pulmonary artery. Pressures and wave form are normal. (From Matthay MA: Invasive hemodynamic monitoring in critically ill patients. Clin Chest Med 4:233, 1983.)

TABLE 73–7. PATTERNS OF HEMODYNAMIC ABNORMALITIES IN SEVERELY ILL PATIENTS

Situation	$\bar{P}_{SA}$	$\bar{P}_{RA}$	$\bar{P}_{PA}$	$\bar{P}_{PAW}$	$C(a-\bar{v})_{O_2}$	$\dot{Q}_T$	PVR	SVR	$\bar{P}_{\bar{v}_{O_2}}$
Hypovolemic Shock	↓	↓	↓	↓	↑	↓	↑	↑	↓
Septic Shock	↓	↓	↓	↓	↓	↑	↑	↓	↓
Cardiogenic Shock	↓	↑	↑	↑	↑	↓	↑	↑	↓
Pulmonary Embolism	↓	↑	↑	→↓	↑	↓	↑	↑	↓
Airways Obstruction	→	→↑	↑	→	↑	↓	↑	→	→
Right Ventricular Infarct	↓	↑	→	↔↑	↑	↓	→	→↑	→↓
Cardiac Tamponade	↓	↑	↑	↑	↑	↓	→	↑	↓
End Stage Liver Disease	↓	→↓	→↓	→↓	↓	↑	→	↓	↑

P̄SA–mean systemic arterial pressure
P̄RA–mean right atrial or central venous pressure
P̄PA–mean pulmonary arterial pressure
P̄PAW–mean pulmonary arterial wedge pressure
C(a − v̄)O₂–arteriovenous O₂ content difference

Q̇T–cardiac output
PVR–pulmonary vascular resistance
SVR–systemic vascular resistance
P̄v̄O₂–mixed venous PO₂

Sheneff MG, Rippe JM: Central venous catheters. In Rippe JM, Irwin RS, Alpert JS, et al. (eds.): Intensive Care Medicine. Boston, Little, Brown and Company, 1985, pp. 16–33. *An excellent description of the indications, techniques, and complications of central venous catheterization.*
Sprung CL: The Pulmonary Artery Catheter. Baltimore, University Park Press, 1983. *A thorough review of indications, techniques, complications, and clinical applications of pulmonary artery pressure measurements.*
Tooker J, Huseby J, Butler J: The effect of Swan-Ganz catheter height on the wedge pressure–left atrial pressure relationship in edema during positive pressure ventilation. Am Rev Respir Dis 117:721, 1978. *An experimental study that demonstrated that positioning of the catheter tip in the upper lung zones resulted in wedge pressure measurements that were artifactually high.*

COMPLICATIONS OF CRITICAL CARE

The complications of critical care are often difficult to detect and separate from the complications of the illnesses that necessitated the care. Iatrogenic diseases uniquely associated with the technology that constitutes critical care clearly cause significant morbidity and occasionally death, however.

Some complications are straightforward and clearly related to an intervention taking place in a critical care unit, such as ventricular tachycardia occurring during the passage of a Swan-Ganz catheter through the right ventricle. The cause of other untoward events is less easy to discover. For example, cardiac arrhythmias and gastrointestinal hemorrhage are common in patients in critical care units but are not necessarily caused by the sort of care rendered in the unit. Confounding the issue further are errors in management that, because they occur in severely ill patients, may have much graver consequences than the same error would have in a less sick patient on a medical ward.

In addition to patient-related complications, the critical care environment takes its toll on the personnel who work there. The psychologic effects of working under what often are high-pressure conditions can result in nurse or physician "burnout." Moreover, personnel in the unit may be at greater risk for certain organic diseases.

The kinds of complications to which patients are prone relate to the kind of illness they have and to the diagnostic and therapeutic interventions carried out. Respiratory support has its unique complications as does hemodynamic support and monitoring.

Complications of Respiratory Support

Oxygen therapy administered by external devices may be associated with the following adverse effects: (1) discomfort related to the device or to administration of dry gas, (2) fires, and (3) hypoventilation because of uncontrolled administration of oxygen in patients who need a precisely controlled $F_{I_{O_2}}$. The first of these is not of great consequence and usually is easily managed by changing the device or improving the humidification. Fires related to oxygen delivery equipment may be catastrophic for the patient but fortunately are uncommon and generally preventable by prohibiting smoking where oxygen is being used. The last complication may be related to the wrong choice of an oxygen delivery device or to using too high a concentration of oxygen. It may also be unavoidable because of the pathophysiology underlying the disease. In any case, severe hypoventilation may be prevented by close observation of such patients and measurement of arterial blood gas tensions early in the course of oxygen administration.

Artificial airways may be associated with a number of complications. The placement of an endotracheal tube may cause immediate injury to the structures through which the tube passes—nose, hypopharynx, larynx, or trachea. The tube may be improperly positioned either at the time of placement or as a result of subsequent migration. This can result in the tube being either too low, usually in the right mainstem bronchus, or too high, with the cuff being at the level of the larynx or higher, causing an air leak around the cuff with inadequate ventilation. These problems may be minimized by the use of a tube that is easily visible on a roentgenogram and by taking a chest film immediately after placement or adjustment of the tube. In addition, daily chest roentgenograms should be obtained in patients with endotracheal tubes in place and the position of the tube noted.

Long-term problems from endotracheal tubes include necrosis of the nasal alae or internal nasal structures, sinus infection, retropharyngeal abscess formation, vocal cord damage, and tracheal injury. The tracheal injury may take the form of a tracheoesophageal fistula, which usually develops at the site of the cuff, or subsequent tracheal stenosis, also at the cuff site, that may not become apparent for several months after the tube is removed. Vocal cord or laryngeal injury may be apparent immediately after the tube is removed or may slowly progress over a period of several months.

The proper use of tubes with high compliance and low-pressure cuffs has greatly reduced the risk of injury at the cuff site. To reduce the risk still further, the pressures in the cuff should be checked periodically and kept below 20 mm Hg. The probability of injury at the other sites may be minimized by careful taping and stabilization of the tube, use of an appropriate-sized tube, and careful intubation technique. The tape holding the tube should be changed daily and the nose (if a nasal tube is used) inspected for areas of skin breakdown or necrosis.

Tracheostomy, because it bypasses the upper airway, avoids the problems associated with a tube passing through the aforementioned structures. However, tracheostomy itself has its own unique complications that more than offset its advantages. Early problems include hemorrhage, mediastinal and subcutaneous emphysema, and malpositioning of the tube. Subsequently, soft tissue infection, late hemorrhage, and tracheal stenosis may occur either at the site where the tube cuff impinged on the tracheal wall or, more commonly, at the site of the opening into the trachea. The overall frequency of complications, particularly the occurrence of tracheal stenosis, appears to be greater with tracheostomy than with endotracheal tubes. The frequency of tracheostomy complications can be reduced by careful operative techniques, use of tubes with low-pressure cuffs, effective stabilization of the tube, and meticulous wound care.

Obstruction of either endotracheal or tracheostomy tubes may occur as a result of inspissated secretions or blood clots. This problem may be prevented by adequate humidification of the inspired gas mixture and by frequent suctioning through the tube.

Both endotracheal and tracheostomy tubes are associated with an increased risk of *pulmonary infection.* The presence of the tube considerably compromises the normal mechanisms by which the airways rid themselves of potentially infecting agents. In addition, hospitalized patients, particularly those in critical care units, are much more likely to have colonization of the airways with organisms that are more pathogenic than those usually present. Both aerobic gram-negative organisms and staphylococci tend to replace the normal oropharyngeal flora in critically ill patients. The distinction between airway colonization with these organisms and true pulmonary infection may be quite difficult. Patients with endotracheal or tracheostomy tubes in place should have daily Gram's stains (not cultures) of aspirated sputum. Infection is often heralded by an increasing number of organisms and polymorphonuclear leukocytes present in the sputum with a subsequent increase in abnormalities on the chest roentgenogram and the appearance of or increase in fever. The finding of organisms in the sputum should not in itself be interpreted as indicating infection.

Mechanical ventilation may be associated with complications apart from the artificial airway, for example, *overventilation* and *underventilation, reduction in cardiac output,* and *pneumothorax* and/or *pneumomediastinum.* Use of the guidelines for mechanical ventilation discussed previously in this chapter will minimize the likelihood of either overventilation or underventilation. Nevertheless, Pa_{O_2}, Pa_{CO_2}, and arterial pH must be determined shortly after mechanical ventilation is initiated and after changes in either ventilator settings or the patient's condition.

The mechanisms by which mechanical ventilation and particularly CPPV reduce cardiac output are probably multifactorial, but the major effect seems to be a reduction of right ventricular inflow caused by decreased transmural right ventricular filling pressure. This effect is particularly evident in patients who are hypovolemic and may be offset by volume replacement. High levels of PEEP usually reduce cardiac output in normovolemic as well as hypovolemic patients. When cardiac output is reduced by PEEP, its beneficial effects must be weighed against the potential deleterious effects of further administration of intravenous fluids. In evaluating the usefulness of PEEP in a given patient, the overall effect on systemic oxygen transport should be measured and PEEP adjusted to yield the optimal balance between Pa_{O_2} and cardiac output.

Lung rupture with subsequent pneumothorax or pneumomediastinum probably relates to the increased transmural distending pressure in airways and alveoli. This pressure results in less distention of abnormal alveoli and relative overdistention of the more normal alveoli that can predispose them to rupture. For this reason, as well as to minimize the effects of pressure on cardiac output, the minimal amount of PEEP that is consistent with optimal oxygen transport should

be used. Peak airway pressure can be lowered by using inspiratory flows that are as slow as possible while still maintaining an appropriate inspiration-expiration ratio.

Oxygen toxicity is not a complication of mechanical ventilation per se but usually occurs in patients who are being mechanically ventilated with gas mixtures containing high concentrations of oxygen (see Ch. 537). Although it is not clearly determined, the threshold for clinically significant oxygen toxicity seems to be approximately 0.6 atmospheres, the important variable being Pi_{O_2} rather than Fi_{O_2}. Histologic changes in the lung that are compatible with oxygen toxicity have been noted in persons receiving lower concentrations of oxygen for long periods of time, but the clinical significance of these observations appears to be minimal.

The clinical syndromes produced by hyperoxia include tracheobronchitis, ARDS, and bronchopulmonary dysplasia. *Tracheobronchitis* is usually acute, manifested by substernal chest pain and nonproductive cough occurring after 12 to 24 hours of breathing oxygen at 1 atmosphere. The time course of *ARDS caused by oxygen* is not well defined and probably varies, being influenced by other factors in addition to the Fi_{O_2}. *Bronchopulmonary dysplasia* probably does not occur in adults but is common in neonates given high concentrations of oxygen.

The diagnosis of oxygen toxicity is extremely difficult to establish. Patients who require high oxygen concentrations already have sufficient clinical, physiologic, radiographic, and histologic abnormalities to obscure any additional changes caused by oxygen. Thus, at present the diagnosis is usually presumptive.

The prevention of oxygen toxicity rests with the general principle of using as low an inspired oxygen concentration as possible that provides the patient with adequate systemic oxygen transport. From the oxyhemoglobin dissociation curve (Fig. 73–4) it is apparent that at a Pa_{O_2} of 60 mm Hg, hemoglobin is nearly fully saturated. Further increases in Pa_{O_2} add little to oxygen transport. Thus, a Pa_{O_2} of 60 mm Hg, in general, should be regarded as satisfactory. In patients with ARDS the use of PEEP as previously described will often allow reduction of the Fi_{O_2}. At present, there are no proved biochemical approaches to the prevention of oxygen toxicity, although several theoretically attractive possibilities exist.

Complications of Hemodynamic Monitoring

There are primarily three types of problems associated with hemodynamic monitoring: local complications associated with vascular access, passage and final positioning of the catheter, and inappropriate decision making based on inaccurate data or misinterpretation of information from the monitoring device. The last complications can best be prevented by proper maintenance of equipment and accurate and frequent calibration checks. As a general rule, monitoring data that are not consistent with the clinical situation or on which crucial therapeutic decisions hinge should not be accepted until the system has been thoroughly checked, zeroed, and calibrated.

SYSTEMIC ARTERIAL PRESSURE. The most frequent complication of systemic arterial blood pressure monitoring is formation of a hematoma at the site of the arterial puncture. This may be prevented or minimized by careful insertion technique, manual application of pressure immediately after insertion, and use of a pressure dressing, with care taken not to compromise distal circulation. Actual laceration of the vessel may require surgical repair.

Peripheral nerve damage may result from direct injury at the time of insertion or from a hematoma. Prevention involves careful insertion technique and measures to reduce the likelihood of formation of a hematoma.

Ischemia distal to the site of catheter insertion may result from arterial obstruction by the catheter itself, because of a clot forming around the catheter or because of embolization from clots on the tip of the catheter. Use of the appropriate-sized catheter will reduce the likelihood of obstruction of flow. Newer materials such as polyamine resins and Teflon are minimally thrombogenic and decrease the risk of a clot forming around the catheter. Also, continuous flush devices that deliver a small constant volume of heparinized solution greatly decrease clotting at the catheter tip or in the lumen.

Local infection at the site of insertion of a percutaneous arterial catheter or in the vessel itself is less common than with venous catheters but nevertheless may be a problem. This risk can be minimized by careful asepsis at the time of catheter insertion, sterile dressings changed daily, and prompt removal of the catheter when it is no longer needed or serving its intended purpose.

CENTRAL VENOUS PRESSURE. The complications of central venous pressure monitoring include problems related to venous access, air embolism, infection, and venous thrombosis. When the subclavian or internal jugular vein is used for venous access, important complications include pneumothorax, hydrothorax, hemothorax, mediastinal hematoma, and subclavian or carotid artery puncture. If the left internal jugular or subclavian vein is used, the thoracic duct may be damaged, resulting in lymph fistula or chylothorax. Brachial nerve injury also may result from attempted subclavian vein catheterization. When an antecubital cutdown is used for central venous catheter placement, the brachial artery or median nerve may be injured. With each of these approaches local or intravascular infection or both and venous thrombosis may occur. If insertion is via a needle, withdrawal of the catheter through the needle may shear the catheter and create embolism of a foreign body.

Prevention of all of these complications is best approached through the use of meticulous insertion technique and maintenance of asepsis. Catheters placed and maintained with strict aseptic technique may be kept in place for long periods of time. However, under standard conditions in severely ill patients, they should not be left in place for more than 48 to 72 hours. A chest roentgenogram should be obtained promptly after catheter placement to look for evidence of pneumothorax or pleural fluid and to check the catheter position. Catheters that have entered the right ventricle should be withdrawn into the superior vena cava.

PULMONARY ARTERY PRESSURE. All of the complications attendant to central venous pressure monitoring may also occur with a pulmonary artery catheter. In addition, problems occur that are unique to this form of hemodynamic monitoring. The most common complication is a disturbance of cardiac rhythm or conduction or both. Premature ventricular contractions occur quite commonly as the catheter passes through the right ventricle. These generally are self-limited, at least with prompt catheter passage, but may occasionally require intravenous administration of 50 to 75 mg of lidocaine. Sustained ventricular tachycardia and ventricular fibrillation may also occur.

The frequency of ventricular arrhythmias can be minimized by inflating the balloon fully during catheter insertion and attempting rapid passage through the right ventricle. Guide wires and central venous catheters should not be advanced into the ventricle. Electrocardiographic monitoring with a visual display and audible signal should always be used during insertion. If ventricular arrhythmias occur, the catheter should promptly be withdrawn from the ventricle. Finally, intravenous lidocaine, a defibrillator, and resuscitation equipment should be immediately available.

During catheter insertion and occasionally after placement, right bundle branch block can develop. This usually does not present a problem unless there was a pre-existing left bundle branch block. In patients with left bundle branch block who need a pulmonary artery catheter passed, it may be advisable first to place a temporary transvenous pacemaker.

Intrapulmonary complications of Swan-Ganz catheters include pulmonary infarction and pulmonary artery rupture.

Pulmonary infarction occurs because the tip of the catheter has migrated into and obstructed a peripheral vessel or because of clot propagation at the catheter tip. These can be avoided by continuously monitoring the pulmonary artery pressure to look for a "permanent wedge" pressure tracing. If this is noted, the catheter should be withdrawn to a point where the pulmonary artery wedge pressure appears only after the balloon is inflated with 1 ml of air. Clot propagation is minimized by using the continuous flow device described previously. The likelihood of rupture of the pulmonary artery is also decreased by ensuring that the catheter is positioned properly in a more proximal vessel.

Psychologic Consequences of Critical Care

CONSEQUENCES FOR THE PATIENT. The patient-related psychologic consequences of critical care are difficult to define and quantitate. In many instances what might appear as disordered behavior in a critically ill patient in fact represents an appropriate response to a genuinely threatening situation. In others the behavior is an organic effect of the illness itself; for example, patients with chronic airways obstruction and hypoxemia have been found to have well-defined behavioral alterations. It is only logical to assume, however, that an environment so foreign and so frightening as a critical care unit that operates totally independent of and without concern for any biologic rhythm could in and of itself produce significant psychologic disturbances, especially when superimposed on the effects of critical illness. Pain and discomfort, sensory deprivation—often with beeps, hisses, and buzzes as the major input—erratic and interrupted sleep patterns, immobilization, and total dependence on others are certainly capable of contributing to clouding of consciousness, perceptual distortion, behavioral confusion, and delusional experiences.

Because of the difficulty in identifying and quantitating the psychologic consequences of critical care, specific preventive measures are not so clearly definable as with other complications. However, standard approaches in critical care management of patients should be geared to providing a milieu that is least likely to generate the factors previously cited as contributing to psychiatric syndromes. Patients should be treated as cognizant, intelligent human beings by all staff. Every attempt should be made to incorporate the patient into discussions regarding care. A patient, even one who appears to be comatose, should not be treated as an inanimate object around which an esoteric discussion is held. Monitoring equipment should not be used as a substitute for interpersonal contact. The equipment used and procedures performed should be carefully explained to the patient. Insofar as possible, the day-night sleep cycle should be maintained. Providing the patient with a calendar serves to create or maintain a correct time orientation. A television set in the room may provide more "normal" sensory input serving to over-ride the barrage of alarms and noises from ventilators and other sources. A liberal visiting policy allows needed "outside world" contact and helps to maintain contact with a familiar frame of reference. Sedative drugs and narcotics should be used only for specific indications such as for adequate pain relief. Benzodiazepines (such as diazepam or midazolam) and occasionally haloperidol (Haldol) can be extremely helpful in managing the psychiatric syndromes that do not respond to supportive treatment. Perhaps more important than all of these is the establishment of a pattern of behavior and interaction on the part of the critical care staff that fosters patient trust and confidence.

CONSEQUENCES FOR THE STAFF. Critical care staff members are also subject to the psychologic effects associated with providing care to severely ill patients. A variety of factors have been identified as contributing to the stress on critical care personnel, especially the nursing staff. First, the work is physically demanding and tiring. Second, patients, families, and physicians are emotionally demanding; emotional fatigue becomes superimposed on physical fatigue. The responsibilities are great and the performance expectations high while quite commonly the level of responsibility is not matched by decision-making authority. Such authority is vested in physicians who may have considerably less experience and expertise in critical care than the nurses. Nurses see what they may consider to be errors being made or patients getting worse and they are powerless to intervene in a meaningful way. These sorts of conflicts compound the already heightened emotional tension almost invariably present in critical care units. In addition, there are the genuine sorrow, distress, and sometimes guilt that accompany deaths occurring in the unit.

The important consequences of these factors are that patient care may be compromised and that the turnover of unit personnel is high. Prevention of these sorts of situations is not easy. Many of the problems are inherent in the job. However, provision of clearly defined administrative guidelines describing the lines of authority and responsibility may minimize the conflicts. Likewise, having standard policies that are developed and agreed upon by the nursing and physician staff members provides support for independent nursing action. Nursing administrative policies also have considerable influence on the emotional well-being of the staff. Staffing ratios, hours worked per shift, and work breaks all are important factors that can be manipulated to reduce stress among the critical care staff. Finally, it is important that there be a single physician in charge of the unit through whom "official" communication between the nursing and medical staff takes place and to whom members of each group can present their problems and complaints. This physician, working in concert with the head nurse, can develop mechanisms for dealing with the various stressful situations either as they arise or preferably before they occur.

Fisher AB: Oxygen therapy: Side effects and toxicity. Am Rev Respir Dis. 122:61, 1980. *A concise review of what is known about oxygen toxicity. Discusses approaches to prevention.*

Kieley WF, Procci WR: Psychiatric aspects of critical care. In Zschoche DA (ed.): Comprehensive Review of Critical Care. St. Louis, C. V. Mosby Company, 1981, pp 107–114. *A review of the kinds of psychiatric disorders commonly seen in critically ill patients with a discussion of specific approaches to management.*

Liebowitz RS, Rippe JM: Arterial line placement and care. In Rippe JM, Irwin RS, Alpert JS, et al. (eds.): Intensive Care Medicine. Boston, Little, Brown and Company, 1985, pp 33–42. *A detailed description of indications, techniques, and complications of systemic arterial catheterization.*

Robin ED: The cult of the Swan-Ganz catheter: Overuse and misuse of pulmonary flow catheters. Ann Intern Med 103:445, 1985. *Presents the view that pulmonary artery catheters are vastly overused relative to their proven benefits and complications.*

Seneff MG, Rippe JM: Central venous catheters. In Rippe JM, Irwin RS, Alpert JS, et al. (eds.): Intensive Care Medicine. Boston, Little, Brown and Company, 1985, pp 16–33. *An excellent description of the indications, techniques, and complications of central venous catheterization.*

Spring CL: Complications of pulmonary artery catheterization. In Spring CL (ed.): The Pulmonary Artery Catheter. Baltimore, University Park Press, 1983, pp 73–101. *An extensively referenced discussion of the complications occurring with Swan-Ganz pulmonary artery catheters. Presents the mechanisms by which the complications occur and the means for their prevention.*

Stauffer JL, Olson DE, Petty TL: Complications and consequences of endotracheal intubation and tracheostomy. Am J Med 70:65, 1981. *A prospective study of 150 patients requiring either endotracheal intubation or tracheostomy because of critical illness. Points out that, although the frequency of complications was similar with the two artificial airways, the complications of tracheostomy were much more likely to be severe than those associated with endotracheal tubes.*

SOCIAL AND ETHICAL ISSUES IN CRITICAL CARE
Indications for and Value of Critical Care

Although defining the value of critical care and its indications would not seem to pertain to a discussion of social and ethical issues, this is, in fact, the topic area in which such considerations are most appropriate. The kinds of technology used and techniques involved in critical care are rather easily described in a straightforward scientific manner. The ends achieved by these interventions are not so clearly defined. If the relationship was strictly one between science and health

or between medical practice and the patient's well-being, the discussion would be simple. Unfortunately, medical practice and the patient's well-being are not clearly and directly related when the connection is through the medium of a critical care unit. Critical care expensively consumes public resources, and its indications and values are poorly defined. The uses of critical care have therefore become a matter involving serious ethical and public policy considerations.

Critical care units have been utilized more or less in their present form for approximately 25 years, yet their contribution to health has not been quantitated. Studies of patients suspected of having a myocardial infarction have suggested that if there are no early (initial 2 hours in one study and 24 hours in the second) indications of complications, management in a coronary care unit does not offer any advantage over management in a general ward or at home. Unfortunately, no such studies exist for the usual category of patients admitted to a general critical care unit. The available data generally describe features of patients admitted to general critical care units and construct evaluative indexes that can be correlated with prognosis. In theory, patients for whom the index indicates a poor prognosis should not be admitted to a critical care unit because it is highly unlikely that all of the interventions available will produce a favorable result. In practice, most physicians caring for a gravely ill patient want the patient to have every opportunity to survive and will request that critical care be provided almost regardless of ultimate prognosis. This is a dilemma that to date has not been solved.

Some categories of patients such as those with end-stage malignancies or those who are very old should clearly not be treated in critical care units. Mentally competent adults who do not wish to undergo the potential rigors of critical care and so inform their physicians should not be admitted to such a unit. On the other hand, patients with significant cardiac arrhythmias, drug-overdosed patients, patients with reversible neuromuscular diseases, those with severe asthma, and victims of multiple trauma, in general, definitely benefit from critical care.

Death rates in critical care units vary considerably depending on the type of unit and the severity of illness of patients admitted. The apparent overall mortality ranges from approximately 10 per cent to 30 per cent. The mortality is higher if patients have a chronic disease. Patients who require mechanical ventilation do much less well than the group as a whole. In one study the need for mechanical ventilation for 48 hours, independent of the reasons for ventilation, was associated with an in-hospital mortality rate of 64 per cent, a one-year mortality rate of 70 per cent, and a three-year mortality rate of 72 per cent. In another study of patients with acute respiratory failure the mortality rate for those who required mechanical ventilation with an Fi_{O_2} of 0.5 or greater for more than 24 hours was 66 per cent; patients who required an Fi_{O_2} of 1.0 with a PEEP of 5 cm H_2O or more for 2 hours or an Fi_{O_2} of 0.6 and a PEEP of 5 cm H_2O for 12 hours or more had a mortality rate of 92 per cent.

Unfortunately, with the data available, physicians are not able to predict reliably who will benefit from critical care and who will not. For this reason much of the decision making regarding who should be admitted to a critical care unit will in the future probably be conditioned by social (i.e., public policy) and ethical considerations rather than by scientific analyses.

Specific Ethical Issues

The basic precepts of medical ethics are discussed in Ch. 5. In this section specific concerns that arise in critical care are addressed.

THE INFLUENCE OF PATIENT WISHES ON THE CARE GIVEN. The autonomy of a mentally competent patient must be respected. If the patient indicates that a specific intervention such as endotracheal intubation, mechanical ventilation, or cardiopulmonary resuscitation is not to be used, it should not be used. The concern with the patient's competence, however, often clouds the issue and makes the decision less than clear-cut. The physician charged with the care of the patient must thoroughly review the process by which the decision was made with the patient and, when appropriate, with the patient's family. If there is a question in the physician's mind as to the competence of the patient, consultation should be sought.

"DO NOT RESUSCITATE" ORDERS. Orders not to initiate cardiopulmonary resuscitation (CPR) may be written at the request of patients as just discussed or may be initiated by physicians caring for patients when to the best of the physician's knowledge CPR is an intervention that will not be successful in the broad sense of restoring meaningful life. In most instances, such decisions should be discussed with the patient and, when appropriate, with the family. The order should then be written in standard fashion in the order sheet, and a note describing the basis for the order and the discussions that took place with the patient and family should be included in the chart. These orders should be reviewed at least daily because circumstances may change. Such orders clarify the ambiguity that surrounds the decisions concerning critical care for a patient with an irreversible illness and relieve the nurse or uninvolved physicians from the responsibility of deciding not to initiate CPR in such a patient.

So-called "no code" patients may still benefit from critical care. Treating airways obstruction, heart failure, metabolic abnormalities, or arrhythmias may at least temporarily improve the patient's condition, making the existence of "do not resuscitate" orders a moot point.

TERMINATION OF LIFE SUPPORT SYSTEMS. Supportive measures may be discontinued when there is no hope for recovery. Continuation of such measures serves only to prolong the process of dying. Defining the hopeless situation, however, may be difficult. The most straightforward instance is that of brain death. Brain death has been defined by several sets of unambiguous medical criteria (see Ch. 457). The American Bar Association and a number of states have adopted the broader concept that "for all legal purposes a human body with irreversible cessation of brain function, according to usual and customary standards of medical practice, shall be considered dead."

Various prognostic indicators have been developed to allow prediction of the likelihood of recovery after severe brain insults. These provide guidance in instances in which all criteria for brain death are not present.

Black PMcL: Brain death. N Engl J Med 299:338 and 393, 1978. *An extensive review of all aspects of brain death, including legal considerations.*

Chassin MR: Costs and outcome of medical intensive care. Med Care 20:165, 1982. *In addition to discussing costs and outcomes in critical care, this report describes the growth of critical care units in the United States.*

Hill JD, Hampton JR, Mitchell JRA: A randomized trial of home-versus-hospital management for patients with suspected myocardial infarction. Lancet 1:837, 1978. *A report of the only well-designed prospective randomized study of the value of critical care (in this case, coronary care). Demonstrated that if the myocardial infarction was not complicated, hospital care offered no clear advantage over home care.*

Knaus WA, Droper EA, Wayne DP, et al.: Prognosis in acute organ-system failure. Ann Surg 202:685, 1985. *Presents the results of a prospective study relating acute organ-system failure to prognosis in patients admitted to critical care units.*

Lee MA, Cassèl CK: The ethical and legal framework for the order not to resuscitate. West J Med 140:117, 1984. *Describes the ethical consideration to be taken into account in determining a patient's resuscitation status and reviews the legal underpinnings of such decisions. Step by step guidelines in implementing the decision process.*

Levy DE, Bates D, Caronna JJ, et al.: Prognosis in nontraumatic coma. Ann Intern Med 94:293, 1981. *Presents the results of a prospective study of 500 patients with nontraumatic coma. Identifies factors that allow early identification of patients in whom recovery is very unlikely.*

Robin ED: A critical look at critical care. Crit Care Med 11:144, 1983. *A provocative discussion of the role of critical care in modern medical care. Presents a plea for objective evaluation of the indications and value of critical care.*

Schmidt CD, Elliott CG, Carmelli D, et al.: Prolonged mechanical ventilation for respiratory failure: A cost benefit analysis. Crit Care Med 11:407, 1983.

Defines the cost and benefits associated with prolonged (48 hours or more) mechanical ventilation primarily in medical patients.

Waner SH, Adelstein SJ, Cranford RE, et al.: The physician's responsibility toward hopelessly ill patients. N Engl J Med 310:955, 1984. *The report, written by a multidisciplinary group, discusses the role of patients and physicians in determining appropriate levels of care for patients who are hopelessly ill.*

CARDIOPULMONARY RESUSCITATION

Cardiopulmonary resuscitation is the supportive and sometimes definitive treatment applied to persons in whom, for whatever reason, effective cardiac and ventilatory activity has stopped. The situations in which this catastrophic event may occur unexpectedly include primary cardiac arrhythmias, arrhythmias associated with myocardial infarction, drowning, electrocution, acute upper airways obstruction, drug intoxication, and accidental trauma. In addition, cardiorespiratory arrest may result from a variety of underlying disease processes that reduce myocardial oxygen delivery or are associated with marked electrolyte or acid-base disturbances.

There are no data on the annual number of cardiorespiratory arrests occurring in this country. It is estimated, however, that more than 1 million persons have myocardial infarctions each year and that 540,000 persons die annually of coronary artery disease (Ch. 51). The majority of these deaths take place out of the hospital, usually within two hours of the onset of symptoms. These data have suggested that for CPR to be truly effective it should be applied in the community at large rather than being limited to an in-hospital technique. For this reason, a standard program for training lay persons in basic life support was developed and implemented throughout the country. By 1980 over 12 million persons in the United States had received training in basic life support.

In some communities more than 40 per cent of patients with documented ventricular fibrillation occurring out of the hospital have been resuscitated and in some subgroups survival has been as high as 60 to 80 per cent. These rates of success are generally attributed to the intervention of trained bystanders in initiating CPR and maintaining support until paramedical personnel arrive. The rate of survival following in-hospital cardiac arrest is much lower, ranging from 5 to 20 per cent. Different subgroups have markedly different rates, however. In one series patients with evidence of cardiac failure prior to the arrest had only a 2 per cent likelihood of survival and renal failure was associated with 3 per cent survival rate. Only 4 per cent of patients who were home-bound before hospitalization in which the cardiac arrest occurred survived. On the other hand 27 per cent of patients who were active before entering the hospital survived.

Pathophysiology of Cardiorespiratory Arrest

SYSTEMIC EFFECTS. Cardiorespiratory arrest results in the cessation of effective delivery of oxygen to body tissues. The immediate effects are the same as those described in the discussion of shock (Ch. 44). Catecholamine release results in peripheral vasoconstriction in an attempt to preserve blood flow to the brain and heart at the expense of cutaneous, muscle, and renal blood flow. Without oxygen, tissue metabolic processes become anaerobic with production of lactic acid, a by-product of anaerobic glycolysis, resulting in systemic metabolic acidosis. The amount of acidosis is determined largely by the balance between oxygen supply and oxygen demand. Thus, hypothermic patients, such as near-drowning victims, because of reduced oxygen needs have less lactate production and less tissue damage. Because there is no circulation or the circulation is much reduced, the lactic acid is not cleared from the tissues. As the hydrogen ion concentration increases, the effectiveness of catecholamines rapidly decreases, resulting in full vasodilation that abolishes the major mechanisms by which the blood volume is preferentially distributed to the brain and the heart. Irreversible damage to these critical organs ensues.

The critical determinants of the outcome of a cardiorespiratory arrest and resuscitation attempts are: (1) the reversibility of the abnormality leading to the cessation of effective cardiac output and (2) the success of the CPR in providing sufficient oxygen to the brain to prevent permanent damage.

CEREBRAL EFFECTS. Oxygen consumption by the brain ranges from 3 to 5 ml per minute per 100 grams of tissue during normal consciousness and cerebral blood flow (CBF) averages 50 to 60 ml per minute per 100 grams of tissue. Aerobic metabolism can be supported by as little as 0.21 ml of oxygen per minute per 100 grams of tissue. Experimentally, CBF carrying a normal amount of oxygen can be reduced to 16 to 18 ml per minute per 100 grams of tissue before electroencephalographic evidence of injury is seen. The determinants of CBF are the mean systemic arterial pressure ($\overline{PSA}$), the cerebrovascular resistance (CVR), and the intracranial pressure (ICP), which determines cerebral venous pressure. Thus,

$$CBF = \frac{\overline{PSA} - ICP}{CVR}$$

Under normal circumstances, CBF increases with increases in Pa_{CO_2} and with hypoxemia (below Pa_{O_2} 50 mm Hg) because of decreases in CVR.

Sudden cessation of blood flow to the brain, as occurs with cardiorespiratory arrest, results in unconsciousness within 10 seconds. Cerebral glycolysis is stimulated seven-fold, but endogenous stores of glucose are inadequate to maintain cellular viability for more than a few minutes. When brain adenosine triphosphate is reduced to 20 per cent of basal levels, which occurs within five minutes of cessation of effective CBF, lactate production ceases and irreversible neuronal damage results. Because oxygen utilization is nonuniform within the brain, some areas such as the frontal and temporal cortexes are more susceptible to ischemia than areas of lower metabolic activity. Restoration of cerebral perfusion after a period of no flow may result in transient increases in ICP, perhaps causing focal hypoperfusion and further ischemic injury.

CARDIAC EFFECTS. Myocardial oxygen consumption ranges from 8 to 10 ml of oxygen per minute per 100 grams of tissue for basal needs in the normally beating, nonischemic heart and 4 to 5 ml of oxygen per minute per 100 grams of tissue during ventricular fibrillation. Assuming normal Ca_{O_2} and an extraction of oxygen of 75 per cent, a myocardial blood flow of approximately 60 ml per minute per 100 grams of tissue would be required to meet oxygen needs in normal sinus rhythm. In ventricular fibrillation this figure would be 25 ml per minute per 100 grams of tissue. Myocardial blood flow (MBF) is determined by the $\overline{PSA}$, the coronary venous sinus pressure approximated by the mean right atrial pressure ($\overline{PRA}$), and the coronary vascular resistance CVR, as follows:

$$MBF = \frac{\overline{PSA} - \overline{PRA}}{CVR}$$

Coronary flow normally occurs during diastole when the aortic valve is closed. Thus, maintenance of coronary perfusion during CPR requires that the aortic valve close normally, that $\overline{PSA}$ remain elevated above $\overline{PRA}$, and that time for coronary filling be allowed. Coronary vascular resistance is likely to be minimal during ventricular fibrillation or asystole; however, in the presence of coronary artery disease, resistance and therefore flow will be nonuniform and probably cause regional ischemia and perhaps infarction. Fortunately, myocardial oxygen needs should also be low.

EFFECTS ON RESPIRATORY MUSCLES. Under normal circumstances the oxygen consumption of the respiratory muscles, primarily the diaphragm, is less than 5 per cent of total body oxygen consumption. However, as the work of breathing increases because of cardiac or pulmonary disorders or metabolic acidosis the oxygen needs of the respiratory muscles increase. In cardiogenic shock the respiratory muscles may become the most metabolically active tissues in the body. Because the oxygen need is increasing at a time when supply is decreasing, the ability of these muscles to maintain their work level may be impaired and hypoventilation may ensue.

Fatigue of the diaphragm may play an important role in augmenting the factors that lead to cardiorespiratory arrest. This suggests also that restoration of respiratory muscle function is an important goal in CPR. Restoration of function depends on improvement in muscle blood flow, which is determined by $\overline{PSA}$, $\overline{PRA}$, and muscle vascular resistance (MVR):

$$MBF = \frac{\overline{PSA} - \overline{PRA}}{MVR}$$

Furthermore, the oxygen needs of the respiratory muscles can be greatly reduced by effective mechanical ventilation.

RENAL EFFECTS. Renal blood flow suffers from the preferential redistribution of cardiac output to the brain and heart when hypotension occurs. Under baseline conditions, renal blood flow is approximately 25 per cent of the normal resting cardiac output and oxygen consumption is 9 to 10 ml of oxygen per minute per 100 grams of tissue. Although autoregulation of renal perfusion tends to maintain blood flow over a wide range of perfusion pressures, in shock the flow is markedly reduced. This may result in cellular injury and acute renal failure even if circulation is properly restored.

Administering Cardiopulmonary Resuscitation

IMMEDIATE INTERVENTIONS. The immediate sequence of events that should be undertaken by the person who first encounters a victim of a cardiorespiratory arrest is listed in Table 73–8. The mechanisms for providing the necessary support will, of course, vary depending on the training of the person or persons on the scene and whether or not the arrest occurs within a hospital.

Artificial Ventilation. An important determinant of success in CPR is the provision of adequate ventilation. The first step is to open the airway and assure its patency. The most common cause of obstruction is the tongue. This may be corrected simply by tilting the head backward and lifting the chin or lower jaw forward. Mouth-to-mouth ventilation can then be applied unless there is a foreign body obstructing the airway. A breath sufficient to make the chest wall rise should be given in 1 to 1.5 seconds.

A resuscitator's exhaled air may provide an FI_{O_2} of approximately 0.17 during mouth-to-mouth ventilation and carbon dioxide will be eliminated because of passive lung deflation. Commonly, however, gas exchange within the lungs is not normal and significant hypoxemia develops. For this reason supplemental oxygen should be administered as soon as it is available. Both oxygen administration and ventilation can be accomplished via a tight-fitting face mask and ventilation bag, preferably one capable of delivering an FI_{O_2} of 1.0. Endotracheal intubation provides the most reliable closed system of oxygen administration and also protects the airway against the aspiration of gastric contents.

Closed Chest Compression. Closed chest compression should be administered to patients who do not have a palpable pulse. The patient should be supine and on a firm surface. Sufficient pressure should be applied to the lower half of the

TABLE 73–8. IMMEDIATE SEQUENCE OF EVENTS IN CPR

Establish unresponsiveness
Call for help
Position victim
Open airway
Check for foreign body in airway
Institute mouth-to-mouth breathing
Check for pulse
Initiate closed chest compression

sternum to depress it 4 to 5 cm in most adults and 2 cm in children. The pressure should be relaxed after each compression, allowing the sternum to return to its relaxed position. The recommended compression-to-relaxation ratio is 1:1, and the rate of compressions should be a minimum of 80 per minute and 100 per minute if possible. The adequacy of closed chest compression should be determined by attempting to palpate a carotid or femoral pulse produced by the compression.

The mechanism by which closed chest compression causes blood to circulate is not clear. The original "cardiac pump" theory was that by compressing the chest the heart was squeezed between the sternum and the vertebral column, producing a mechanical systole in which right and left ventricular pressures exceed pulmonary artery and aortic pressures, respectively, causing forward blood flow. Release of the pressure caused diastolic filling of the ventricles due to the gradient between the peripheral venous system and the intrathoracic structures.

More recent data suggest that it is the total intrathoracic pressure that causes forward blood flow rather than cardiac compression ("thoracic pump" theory). For example, cough in itself has sustained cardiac output and consciousness in patients with ventricular fibrillation. A variety of experimental studies are consistent with this contention.

INTERMEDIATE INTERVENTIONS. The arrival of persons with more advanced training and equipment marks the second or intermediate phase of CPR. Electrocardiographic monitoring enables proper application of direct current countershock for defibrillation or conversion of ventricular tachycardia. A current of 200 to 360 joules should be used for ventricular fibrillation and 25 to 50 joules for ventricular tachycardias. The current given should be increased if there is no response to the initial shock. In patients with ventricular fibrillation, epinephrine should be administered routinely either intravenously (preferably by a central venous catheter) or via an endotracheal tube before countershock is applied. Epinephrine enhances myocardial contractility, constricts peripheral vasculature, and lowers the defibrillation threshold. This combination of effects operates to improve cerebral and cardiac perfusion and to increase the likelihood of defibrillation occurring. Standard doses are 0.5 to 1.0 mg or 5 to 10 ml of a 1:10,000 dilution. The dose can be repeated at approximately five-minute intervals. Although previous recommendations indicated that calcium chloride was useful in improving myocardial contractility, recent data have not demonstrated its usefulness, and because of theoretic adverse effects, calcium is not recommended for routine administration.

Lidocaine is the initial drug of choice to suppress ventricular ectopy in the setting of cardiorespiratory arrest. The usual dose is approximately 1 mg per kilogram (50 to 75 mg) given intravenously as a bolus injection. Additional boluses of 0.5 mg per kilogram may be given at 10-minute intervals to a total of 3 mg per kilogram. This is then followed by a continuous intravenous infusion of 1 to 4 mg per minute. Other agents that may be useful for ventricular arrhythmias not responsive to lidocaine include bretylium tosylate, procainamide, and verapamil. The doses and uses of these drugs are discussed in Ch. 45.

Atropine sulfate is useful in treating sinus bradycardia or complete heart block because it increases the rate of discharge of the sinus node and improves atrioventricular conduction. The usual dose of atropine sulfate is 0.5 mg administered intravenously and repeated at 5-minute intervals until the desired rate is achieved or a total dose of 2 mg is given.

Isoproterenol may also be used to treat hemodynamically significant bradycardia resulting from heart block that is refractory to atropine. Caution should be exercised in the use of both of these agents in that myocardial oxygen requirements increase with increases in heart rate. Thus, ischemia may be worsened by increasing heart rate above that necessary to provide an adequate cardiac output.

Contrary to previous recommendations, administration of bicarbonate is no longer thought to be beneficial and is not recommended for routine use.

INTERVENTIONS AFTER INITIAL RECOVERY. All patients who have been resuscitated successfully should be transferred as quickly as possible to a critical care unit. As a minimum, electrocardiographic monitoring should be provided. The need for invasive hemodynamic monitoring depends on the causes and consequences of the cardiorespiratory arrest. Often, at least transiently, it is necessary to provide mechanical ventilation. This allows rest and functional recovery of the respiratory muscles and minimizes total oxygen needs. The major determinant of return of brain function is the adequacy of cerebral perfusion during the period of cardiac arrest. Subsequently, after recovery of cardiac function, all factors that influence oxygen delivery to the brain should be evaluated and made normal where possible. Measures to prevent elevation in intracranial pressure (ICP), such as keeping the patient's head elevated, controlling arterial pH and Pa_{CO_2}, and treating seizures and agitation, should be undertaken. The effectiveness of measures designed to minimize brain damage, including the use of barbiturates, calcium channel–blocking agents, and systemic hypothermia, remains to be proven.

REASONS FOR FAILURE. Obviously, not all persons who sustain cardiac arrest can or should be resuscitated. Often the process leading to the arrest is irreversible or the resulting cardiac injury is so severe that it precludes successful resuscitation. In some instances, however, reversible factors may play a major role in the failure of CPR to restore an adequate cardiac output. These factors include severe electrolyte and acid-base disturbances, inadequate oxygenation or ventilation because of faulty technique, hypovolemia, pneumothorax (especially tension pneumothorax), and cardiac tamponade. Abnormalities of electrolyte and acid-base balance as well as inadequate oxygenation and/or ventilation usually manifest themselves as an inability to restore an adequate cardiac rate and rhythm. Hypovolemia, tension pneumothorax, and cardiac tamponade usually cause electromechanical dissociation in which the rate and rhythm of the heart are satisfactory but the cardiac output is inadequate. When electromechanical dissociation is detected, the initial response should be to administer epinephrine. Failure of epinephrine to increase cardiac output should prompt an immediate evaluation for mechanical factors that may be preventing adequate blood flow. If such factors are detected, pericardiocentesis, chest tube placement, or volume replacement may be lifesaving.

American Medical Association: Standards and guidelines for cardiopulmonary resuscitation (CPR) and emergency cardiac care (ECC). JAMA 255:2905, 1986. *This is the basic reference source describing CPR.*

Bedell SE, Delbanco TL, Cook EF, et al.: Survival after cardiopulmonary resuscitation in the hospital. N Engl J Med 309:569, 1983. *Reviews the results of in-hospital CPR and describes factors associated with prognosis.*

Cummins RO, Eisenberg MS: Prehospital cardiopulmonary resuscitation. Is it effective? JAMA 253:2408, 1985. *Presents a summary of the results of bystander-initiated resuscitation and concludes that it leads to improved survival.*

Luce JM, Ross BK, O'Quin RJ, et al.: Regional blood flow during cardiopulmonary resuscitation in dogs using simultaneous and nonsimultaneous compression and ventilation. Circulation 67:258, 1983. *An experimental study of the factors influencing organ blood flow in two forms of CPR.*

PART IX
RENAL DISEASES

74 APPROACH TO THE PATIENT WITH RENAL DISEASE

Thomas E. Andreoli

This chapter provides an overview of the cardinal manifestations of diseases of the kidney or urinary tract, together with a relatively simple classification of these disorders. There are five sections. The first section contains a brief consideration of the cardinal functions of the kidney. A more detailed analysis of renal physiology is presented in Ch. 75. Subsequently the cardinal urinary abnormalities of renal disease are described. The third section enumerates briefly the primary findings in the more common syndromes involving the kidneys and urinary tract, and the fourth section describes the consequences of complete or nearly complete failure of renal function, that is, the uremic syndrome. Finally, the last section considers the relationship between the adaptive response to a reduction in nephron mass and the potential contribution of one of these adaptive responses, renal hyperfiltration, to the pathogenesis of progressive renal disease.

CARDINAL ELEMENTS OF RENAL FUNCTION

URINE FORMATION. The kidneys maintain constancy of the volume and composition of body fluids by forming urine whose composition is ultimately determined by the dietary intake of solute and water and by the rate and kind of metabolic transformation of endogenous and exogenous carbohydrates, proteins, lipids, and nucleic acids. The kidneys also serve as the major route for the excretion of a large number of drugs. The formation of urine serves two purposes: a *regulatory* function, that is, the maintenance of a constant volume and composition for body fluids; and an *excretory* function, that is, elimination of endogenous and exogenous metabolic end-products.

Urine is formed by a sequence of five events:

1. The glomerulus filters approximately 180 liters of extracellular fluid daily across glomerular capillaries and the visceral epithelium of Bowman's capsule, using as a driving force the mean arterial pressure. The glomerular capillary endothelium and basement membrane and the visceral epithelium of Bowman's capsule are freely permeable to water and solutes of relatively low molecular weight (that is, under 6,000 to 8,000 daltons), moderately permeable to large molecular weight species such as myoglobin (molecular weight, approximately 16,000 daltons), and virtually impermeable to macromolecules such as albumin. Filtration is also influenced by molecular charge as well as size. The result is an isotonic, virtually protein-free filtrate whose daily volume is more than ten-fold greater than the volume of extracellular fluid (ECF).

2. The proximal tubule isotonically reabsorbs approximately two thirds of the glomerular filtrate. In the process certain alterations in the composition of tubular fluid are produced by specialized transport mechanisms: the preferential absorption of sodium with bicarbonate rather than chloride; the virtually complete absorption of organic solutes such as glucose and amino acids; and the absorption of organic acids such as uric acid and other nonamino acids in early segments of the proximal nephron, followed by secretion of these acids into tubular fluid in the late proximal nephron. Thus the volume of tubular fluid delivered to the loop of Henle is approximately one third of the volume of glomerular filtrate, has a sodium concentration equal to that of plasma and a bicarbonate concentration about 10 per cent of that in plasma, and contains little or no glucose or amino acids.

3. The loop of Henle dissociates the absorption of sodium and water. The descending limb of Henle passively abstracts water into the hypertonic medullary interstitium, concentrating the tubular fluid. Conversely, the water-impermeable thick ascending limb of Henle actively absorbs approximately 25 per cent of filtered sodium chloride but little water. As a result, about 18 liters of tubular fluid enter the distal convoluted tubule daily. This fluid, which is approximately 10 per cent of the initial glomerular filtrate, is also maximally dilute, having an osmolality of approximately 50 mOsm per kilogram of H_2O.

4. The distal convoluted tubule primarily absorbs sodium under the influence of aldosterone and secretes protons, ammonia, and potassium. Aldosterone regulates sodium absorption in this nephron segment.

5. The collecting duct system regulates the osmolality of urine. When antidiuretic hormone (ADH) is present, water is absorbed across the collecting duct and tubular fluid equilibrates osmotically with the hypertonic medullary interstitium; when ADH is absent, the water permeability of collecting ducts is at a minimum and a dilute urine is excreted.

THE KIDNEY AS AN ENDOCRINE RECEPTOR. Among many hormones that regulate renal function, three are of particular importance: parathyroid hormone (PTH), aldosterone, and antidiuretic hormone (ADH). PTH enhances the absorption of calcium and magnesium and inhibits the absorption of phosphate and bicarbonate in the proximal tubule by increasing intracellular cyclic 3',5'-adenosine monophosphate (cAMP). PTH also stimulates the renal conversion of 25-hydroxycholecalciferol, the major metabolite of vitamin D_3, to 1,25-dihydroxycholecalciferol, which is the major biologically active form of vitamin D_3 (Ch. 245).

Aldosterone and other mineralocorticoids stimulate the rate of sodium absorption in the distal nephron. Aldosterone also increases the rate of net potassium secretion and net proton secretion (and consequently, the rate of bicarbonate regeneration) by the distal nephron.

ADH promotes the formation of a hypertonic urine both by increasing the rate of salt absorption in the thick ascending limb of Henle and by increasing the water permeability of the collecting duct system. Both actions are mediated by ADH-dependent increases in cytosolic cAMP in those renal tubular segments.

THE KIDNEY AS AN ENDOCRINE ORGAN. The kidney plays a major role in prostaglandin production, in the operation of the kallikrein-kinin system, and in the degradation of low molecular weight proteins. The kidney is also the major site for the synthesis of erythropoietin and of renin. Erythropoietin is a glycoprotein produced by renal enzymatic action on a circulating precursor of hepatic origin. The principal action of erythropoietin is to stimulate the rate of red blood cell production by the bone marrow.

Renin is secreted by the granular cells of the juxtaglomerular apparatus in response to reductions in renal perfusion pressure or in effective circulating volume. Renin increases the rate of conversion of angiotensinogen to angiotensin I, which in turn is a precursor of angiotensin II. In turn, angiotensin II is a potent vasoconstrictor agent and a strong stimulus to thirst and to aldosterone production. Thus, the kidney, by way of renin production, plays a central role in the volume repletion reaction.

URINARY MANIFESTATIONS OF RENAL DISEASE (Ch. 76)

HEMATURIA. Hematuria indicates an abnormality in the kidneys or urinary tract, but not the particular form of renal disease. Hematuria of itself is not painful, but the passage of blood clots along the ureter or urethra may produce renal colic or dysuria, respectively. In general, hematuria occurs in the following disorders: (1) systemic disorders such as the hemoglobinopathies, coagulation disorders, sepsis, and, rarely, severe congestive heart failure; hematuria may also occur following severe exercise; (2) inflammatory and necrotizing glomerular diseases; hematuria also occurs in certain types of interstitial nephritis, particularly those that are acute, and in renal infarction; (3) diseases characterized by disruption of the normal structure of the kidneys or urinary tract, as in neoplasms, urolithiasis, trauma, or cystic disease of the kidney; and (4) irritative or inflammatory disorders of the kidneys, ureter, or lower urinary tract, as in pyelonephritis or lower urinary tract infection.

The presence of red blood cell casts indicates that the hematuria is of renal parenchymal origin. Proteinuria in combination with hematuria is a classic indicator of parenchymal renal disease; massive proteinuria (in excess of 3.0 grams per 24 hours) in combination with hematuria is typically, but not exclusively, a characteristic of glomerular disease.

Isolated, painless hematuria in the absence of associated urinary abnormalities such as red cell casts or proteinuria or of systemic disease or obvious entities such as urolithiasis or urinary tract infection generally requires more detailed studies such as renal ultrasonography, CT scanning, arteriography, or renal biopsy. The intent of such studies is the detection either of occult glomerular or interstitial disease or of renal tumors or cysts.

Isolated hematuria may occur in association with entirely normal renal imaging studies, a normal renal biopsy, and negligible proteinuria. This condition, which occurs most frequently in children and is often termed *benign recurrent hematuria of childhood*, is characterized by recurrent bouts of microscopic and gross hematuria. To date, there is no evidence that this disorder, when accompanied by normal glomerular architecture and negative glomerular immunofluorescence, leads to progressive renal disease.

PROTEINURIA. The normal daily rate of urinary protein excretion averages less than 150 mg per 24 hours. In certain instances, notably fever, severe congestive heart failure, and severe exercise, the rate of urinary protein excretion may be increased transiently in the absence of intrinsic renal disease. Furthermore, in young individuals, so-called "postural" proteinuria, defined as transient or consistent proteinuria in the upright but not recumbent position, may occur in the absence of histologically detectable lesions on renal biopsy.

Persistent proteinuria, occurring in both the recumbent and the upright positions and exceeding 750 mg per 24 hours, is a specific indicator of parenchymal renal disease. Proteinuria of less than 2.0 grams per 24 hours occurs commonly either in interstitial or in glomerular disease, but when in excess of 3.0 to 3.5 grams per 24 hours usually indicates glomerular disease and, more specifically, the nephrotic syndrome. However, massive proteinuria may also occur in severe congestive heart failure, in accelerated hypertension, and rarely in acute allergic interstitial nephritis.

URINARY LEUKOCYTES, CASTS, AND BACTERIA. *Pyuria* occurs when more than five to ten white blood cells per high-power field are found in centrifuged samples of the urinary sediment and indicates an inflammatory process within the kidneys or urinary tract. When leukocyte casts are also found, renal parenchymal inflammation is usually present.

Cylindruria, the presence of tubular urinary casts, is traditionally regarded as evidence of renal parenchymal injury. The matrix of most urinary casts is composed mainly of Tamm-Horsfall glycoprotein derived from the renal tubular epithelium. No single type of cast is explicitly diagnostic of any specific disease entity. In general, red cell casts are most often indicative of glomerular injury, white cell casts are suggestive of parenchymal inflammation, and so-called "broad" casts are formed within the region of the collecting duct or dilated nephron segments. The specific significance of granular, epithelial, hyaline, or fatty casts is not always clear.

Significant *bacteriuria* indicates bacterial colonization of urine. The presence of bacteria in freshly collected, clean-voided urine specimens generally correlates closely with bacterial colony counts in excess of 100,000 organisms per milliliter of urine, and a Gram's stain of the urinary sediment of a similarly collected specimen is generally helpful in identifying whether the offending organism is gram-positive or gram-negative.

MISCELLANEOUS URINARY FINDINGS. An evaluation of urinary *cytology*, done conveniently by a Wright's stain of the urinary sediment, is a useful diagnostic test for transitional cell tumors of the renal pelvis or ureter. Similarly, cytologic examination of bladder washings may be helpful in the diagnosis of bladder neoplasia (Ch. 93).

Pneumaturia, the passage of urine mixed with air, can occur in the presence of fistula tracts from either the bowel or the vagina into the bladder. These tracts may follow surgical procedures, pelvic infections, or inflammatory bowel disease. A plain film of the abdomen may also indicate the presence of air in the urinary bladder.

THE MAJOR RENAL SYNDROMES

Renal disorders are often nonspecific in their manifestations, as hematuria, azotemia, hypertension, or metabolic acidosis, for example. The interpretation of a group of findings obtained by history, physical examination, and routine laboratory studies, however, may be used to describe some of the more common syndromes and disorders affecting the kidneys and urinary tract, which are briefly described below.

THE PRERENAL SYNDROMES. The major classes of prerenal disorders are (1) renal hypoperfusion secondary to a reduction in effective circulating volume, and (2) renal ischemia because of occlusive disease in one or both renal arteries. Both sets of disorders are associated with hyperreninemia, but the clinical manifestations of the two diseases differ significantly (Table 74–1).

Renal hypoperfusion secondary to a *reduction in effective circulating volume* may occur in association with true volume contraction; an increase in vascular capacitance, as in sepsis; sequestration of fluid in interstitial compartments, as in ascites and the hepatorenal syndrome; or an inability to transfer fluid from the venous to the arterial limbs of the circulation, as in severe congestive heart failure, constrictive pericarditis, or pericardial tamponade. When the effective circulating volume is sufficiently reduced, the kidneys are hypoperfused, the glomerular filtration rate is reduced, and renin is released.

TABLE 74–1. THE PRERENAL (HYPOPERFUSION) SYNDROMES

Class of Disorder	Major Findings
Reduced Effective Circulating Volume	Oliguria Azotemia Reduced fractional sodium excretion Elevated plasma renin Normotension
Occlusive Renal Artery Disease	Hypertension Elevated plasma renin Azotemia: with severe, bilateral disease or an affected solitary kidney

This results in oliguria, an elevation in serum blood urea nitrogen (BUN) and creatinine concentrations, and a reduced fractional excretion rate for sodium (that is, generally less than 1 per cent). Although plasma renin levels are elevated, the patients are ordinarily normotensive, presumably because the effective circulating volume is decreased.

Renal ischemia produced by *occlusive disease* of the renal arteries results in renin release from the ischemic kidney without a reduction in effective circulating volume and consequently is manifested primarily as hypertension, since pressor activity is elevated while filling of the arterial tree is normal or only slightly reduced. If the renal arterial occlusive disease is limited to one kidney and the contralateral kidney retains normal function, azotemia is absent. However, if the hypertension results in injury to the unaffected kidney, azotemia may ensue. When both renal arteries are involved, azotemia occurs when renal ischemia is sufficiently severe that renal autoregulatory mechanisms are inadequate to maintain an adequate glomerular filtration rate.

THE RENAL PARENCHYMAL SYNDROMES. *Acute Glomerular Disorders*. GLOMERULONEPHRITIS AND THE NEPHROTIC SYNDROME (Ch. 81). Two major types of disorders affect the glomerulus: (1) the *acute nephritic syndrome*, characterized mainly by inflammatory and/or necrotizing lesions within glomeruli, and (2) the *nephrotic syndrome*, a predominantly noninflammatory derangement of the glomeruli characterized by an abnormal "leakiness" of the glomeruli to albumin and other macromolecules.

The etiologic, histologic, and clinical characteristics of the glomerulonephritic and nephrotic syndromes overlap to a considerable degree: (1) A given disease process—for example, systemic lupus erythematosus—may produce a mild, focal glomerulonephritis with hematuria, mild proteinuria, but no azotemia; a diffuse proliferative glomerulonephritis with hematuria, proteinuria and severe renal failure; or membranous nephropathy characterized by a relatively pure nephrotic syndrome. (2) Glomerular lesions may evolve; for example, Goodpasture's syndrome can begin as a mild, focal nephritis and progress to a diffuse, necrotic glomerulonephritis. (3) The extent of glomerular injury, as viewed on renal biopsy, correlates generally but inexactly with the severity of the clinical picture. (4) A given pathogenic mechanism—for example, immune complex disease—may in some instances result in acute glomerulonephritis and in other cases in a pure nephrotic syndrome. (5) In certain disorders such as membranoproliferative nephritis, both a nephritic picture and a nephrotic picture may coexist simultaneously.

These diverse glomerular disorders can be somewhat arbitrarily classified by four major patterns that may be defined by the initial presentation of the patient (Table 74–2). Table 74–3, in turn, lists the most common diseases that present as nephritic, nephrotic, and mixed syndromes.

THE MILD ACUTE GLOMERULONEPHRITIS SYNDROMES. In this class of glomerular inflammation, glomerular blood flow is sufficient to maintain the glomerular filtration at a normal or near normal rate. Mild acute glomerulonephritis is characterized by hematuria, red cell casts, modest proteinuria, minimal azotemia, and mild or no edema. Because renal perfusion is not severely compromised, hypertension or salt retention or both are generally absent.

THE DIFFUSE ACUTE GLOMERULONEPHRITIS SYNDROMES. These glomerulonephritic syndromes are usually characterized by diffuse glomerular inflammation and/or necrosis sufficiently severe that hematuria and proteinuria are accompanied by a reduction in filtation rate and, consequently, azotemia of varying degrees. Simultaneously, for reasons that are not well understood, sodium acquisitiveness in acute glomerulonephritis is considerably greater than that expected solely from the reduction in glomerular filtration rate. Plasma albumin is generally normal, so that a significant fraction of retained sodium remains in the vascular compartment and may result in hypertension, plasma volume dilution, circulatory overload, congestive heart failure, and a suppression of plasma renin activity.

NEPHROTIC SYNDROME. In the pure nephrotic syndrome the glomerular filtration barrier is abnormally permeable to macromolecules, so that massive proteinuria occurs even though the filtration rate may be normal. This large urinary loss of protein contributes to the characteristic hypoalbuminemia in such patients. Hypercholesterolemia also occurs and correlates closely with the degree of hypoalbuminemia.

Nephrotic patients are usually salt acquisitive and edematous. In the nephrotic syndromes the reduced plasma oncotic pressure leads to translocation of fluid to the interstitium, a reduced effective circulating volume, and a secondary sodium acquisitiveness and edema. Patients with the pure nephrotic syndrome often are normotensive, rarely develop circulatory overload, and frequently have elevated plasma renin activities. As further evidence for a reduced effective circulating volume, severely nephrotic patients may have postural hypotension even in the presence of anasarca and may have hemoconcentration and renal hypoperfusion with attendant azotemia following excessive diuretic use.

The Interstitial Nephritis Syndromes (Ch. 82). In the interstitial nephritis syndromes, the primary abnormality is damage to the tubulointerstitial system of the kidney with secondary glomerular damage. Thus renal tubular function tends to be deranged disproportionately to reductions in glomerular filtration rate.

Generalized tubulointerstitial disorders often damage the juxtaglomerular apparatus and therefore tend to impair renin production. As a consequence of hyporeninemia, aldosterone production is curtailed. This combination generally results in hyporeninemia, hypoaldosteronism, modest degrees of salt

TABLE 74–2. CLASSIFICATION OF MAJOR GLOMERULAR SYNDROMES

Class of Disorder	Major Derangement	Major Findings
1. Mild Acute Glomerulonephritis	Mild glomerular inflammation	Hematuria, proteinuria Absent or mild azotemia Absent or mild edema
2. Severe Acute Glomerulonephritis	Extensive glomerular inflammation Renal ischemia Primary tubular sodium acquisitiveness	Hematuria, proteinuria Azotemia Plasma volume expansion Hypertension Edema Circulatory overload (if severe)
3. Pure Nephrotic Syndrome	Glomerular protein leak	Massive proteinuria Reduced plasma oncotic pressure Anasarca Normotensive Sensitive to diuretics
4. Mixed Disorders	1 plus 3 or 2 plus 3	Hematuria Massive proteinuria Azotemia (variable) Hypertension (variable) Edema

wasting, hyperkalemia, and hyperchloremic metabolic acidosis. These abnormalities occur even when the glomerular filtration rate is only modestly reduced.

Urinary abnormalities such as hematuria and proteinuria are usually, but not always, relatively modest in patients with tubulointerstitial disease. Three general classes of tubulointerstitial diseases can be defined:

1. *Chronic tubulointerstitial disease* may occur as a consequence of any of a large number of diseases that produce chronic damage to the renal interstitium: chronic hypertension, with progressive ischemia to the renal interstitium; diabetes mellitus, in which microvascular disease within the kidney effects the same end result; occlusive disease of smaller renal vessels, as in sickle cell disease; chronic pyelonephritis; gout; and exogenous toxins, notably illicit alcohol containing lead, and analgesic abuse, particularly the combination of phenacetin and aspirin. Chronic interstitial disease is generally detected in individuals who have modest degrees of sodium wasting, hyperkalemia, metabolic acidosis, and an acid urine. These abnormalities may occur even when only mild degrees of azotemia exist. The plasma renin activity is generally reduced, as are rates of aldosterone secretion. Hematuria and massive proteinuria are not common in chronic interstitial disease.

2. *Acute allergic interstitial disease* occurs when patients are treated with antibiotics, notably penicillin and related drugs, or with nonsteroidal anti-inflammatory agents. In addition to producing electrolyte abnormalities similar to those described above for chronic interstitial nephritis, acute allergic interstitial nephritis may severely reduce glomerular filtration and be associated with marked hematuria and proteinuria and with oliguria.

Oliguria and azotemia associated with acute allergic interstitial nephritis may be difficult to differentiate from that of acute tubular necrosis. In this setting an electrolyte pattern of hyperkalemic, hyperchloremic metabolic acidosis, a reduced plasma renin activity and rates of aldosterone secretion, an elevated fractional excretion rate for sodium, eosinophilia, and the presence of eosinophils in the urine would strongly suggest acute allergic interstitial nephritis.

3. *Acute pyelonephritis*, a form of acute interstitial nephritis due to bacterial invasion of the kidney, usually produces a septic picture with fever, flank pain, leukocytosis, and dysuria (Ch. 86). Factors that predispose to acute pyelonephritis are often present, such as diabetes mellitus, obstructive uropathy, prior instrumentation of the urinary tract, or bacterial endocarditis with septic renal emboli. The most useful clues to the presence of acute pyelonephritis include findings of sepsis, costovertebral angle tenderness, pyuria, leukocyte casts, the presence of bacteria in unspun samples of urine, and positive urine cultures.

Isolated Tubular Defects (Ch. 84). In addition to tubular derangements secondary to diffuse tubulointerstitial disease, there are a number of specific defects of tubular function.

PROXIMAL TUBULAR DEFECTS. *Renal glycosuria* occurs when the glucose threshold of the proximal nephron is reduced. *Renal phosphate wasting* results when the rate of proximal absorption of phosphate is reduced. Similarly, *aminoaciduria* may result from tubular defects that are either generalized or specific. Finally, the rate of bicarbonate absorption by the proximal nephron may be reduced, resulting in profound bicarbonate wasting, a syndrome entitled *proximal renal tubular acidosis* (Ch. 84).

Renal phosphate wasting, renal glycosuria, renal aminoaciduria, and proximal renal tubular acidosis occurring simultaneously constitute Fanconi's syndrome (Ch. 84). These proximal tubular defects may be congenital or may be found in association with heavy metal poisoning of the proximal nephron, notably by copper in Wilson's disease, following

exposure to toxic agents such as maleic acid, and in the gammopathies.

POSSIBLE LOOP OF HENLE DEFECT. The pathogenesis of *Bartter's syndrome* has not been elucidated (Ch. 84). Yet it appears that many of the findings of Bartter's syndrome, including profound salt wasting, potassium wasting, and compensatory hypertrophy of the juxtaglomerular apparatus with hyperreninemia, may be the result of a salt-absorptive defect in the thick ascending limb. Most commonly, a clinical syndrome resembling Bartter's syndrome occurs because of surreptitious ingestion of furosemide or furosemide-like diuretics.

DISTAL TUBULAR DEFECTS. *Distal, gradient-limited renal tubular acidosis* represents a specific defect of the distal nephron (Ch. 84). In this disorder the distal nephron is abnormally permeable to protons and cannot therefore maintain an adequately acid urine. In contrast to patients who have tubulointerstitial disease, the classic electrolyte abnormalities in distal, gradient-limited renal tubular acidosis include a tendency to salt wasting, hyperchloremic metabolic acidosis, a urine that is relatively alkaline with respect to arterial pH, and profound hypokalemia. The hypokalemia of distal, gradient-limited renal tubular acidosis is probably a consequence of aldosterone release in response to salt depletion. In contrast to proximal renal tubular acidosis or to the hyperkalemic, hyperchloremic renal tubular acidosis of diffuse tubulointerstitial disease, gradient-limited distal renal tubular acidosis is frequently associated with severe nephrocalcinosis, renal calculi, renal infection, and progressive destruction of renal mass.

Distal, gradient-limited renal tubular acidosis may occur congenitally. The disorder may also occur as a consequence of exposure to exogenous agents, notably amphotericin B and lithium, and in association with the gammopathies.

COLLECTING DUCT DEFECTS. The unique tubular defect of the collecting duct is nephrogenic diabetes insipidus (NDI), in which the collecting duct is refractory to the action of ADH (Ch. 227). Patients with NDI are consistently polyuric, even when large amounts of ADH are administered. The disorder may occur congenitally; in association with certain systemic disorders, such as Sjögren's syndrome and sarcoidosis; and as a result of lithium intoxication or exposure to the antibiotic demethylchlortetracycline.

The Renal Calculus Syndrome. The origin and composition of renal calculi are described in Ch. 90; most renal calculi contain magnesium-ammonium-phosphate, calcium oxalate, uric acid, a combination of calcium oxalate and uric acid, or cystine as their main crystalloids. Of these, all but uric acid stones are radiopaque.

Renal calculi may be asymptomatic and detected only on routine radiographic examination of the kidney, especially isolated calculi that do not move down the urinary tract and staghorn calculi lodged within the renal pelvis. Calculi may obstruct urine flow and consequently lead to pyelonephritis. Therefore, in any patient in whom pyelonephritis is suspected, a careful radiographic and urologic examination for renal calculi is mandatory. *Renal colic* refers to the passage of a renal calculus from the renal pelvis into the ureter characterized by exquisite pain, generally beginning in the flank and radiating into the groin. Patients almost always describe renal colic as the worst pain they have ever experienced. Renal colic is almost invariably accompanied by hematuria, unless the calculus is lodged within a ureter and produces complete unilateral obstruction to urine flow. Under these circumstances, the urine voided by the patient represents red cell–free urine from the unaffected kidney.

Kidney stones are among the more common renal disorders. It is generally prudent, particularly in patients with multiple renal calculi or with a family history of renal calculi, to evaluate the patient for potential underlying causes for stone formation (for example, gout, absorptive hypercalciuria, cystinuria, distal, gradient-limited renal tubular acidosis, or primary hyperparathyroidism). The presence of nephrocalcinosis should alert the physician to the possibility of distal, gradient-limited renal tubular acidosis or to primary hyperparathyroidism.

The patient with renal colic also warrants an evaluation for obstructive uropathy on the affected side and for urinary tract infection. These approaches generally involve culture of the urine, plain films of the abdomen, and, when indicated, ultrasonography of the kidneys, excretory urography, evaluation of parathyroid function, and evaluation for an absorptive hypercalciuric state.

Renal Cystic Disease (Ch. 91). There are three major forms of renal cystic disease: single or multiple cysts, polycystic kidney disease, and microcystic disease of the renal medulla. The clinical characteristics, significance, and clinical presentations of these three kinds of renal cysts vary significantly. There is no evidence that true simple cysts, multiple simple cysts, or polycystic kidney disease progresses to renal neoplasia.

Isolated simple cysts, either single or multiple, form sporadically for unknown reasons within the renal parenchyma, generally within the renal cortex. Single cysts in particular usually cause no symptoms; they are generally detected in one of two circumstances: episodes of renal trauma that provoke cyst rupture and hematuria, or on routine excretory urography. The true single, simple cyst (in contrast to the cystic neoplasm, see below) is innocuous and needs no therapy. *Multiple simple cysts* probably represent an extension of the process described above and are also similarly innocuous unless they encroach on renal parenchyma. Multiple simple cysts should be distinguished from polycystic kidney disease, a disorder with a more ominous prognosis. These two forms of multicystic disease can be distinguished by excretory urography; in individuals with multiple simple cysts, the overall size of the kidney is normal and the calyceal system is not elongated and only minimally distorted.

Adult polycystic kidney disease is a form of nephropathy that is generally inherited by autosomal dominance with incomplete penetrance. If a parent has polycystic kidney disease, approximately one half of the progeny will ultimately develop the disorder, although the time at which polycystic kidney disease becomes manifest is highly variable.

Polycystic kidney disease may present with recurrent bouts of hematuria, renal colic, hypertension, or urinary tract infection because of intrarenal obstruction due to cysts. Many patients with polycystic kidney disease develop renal failure, although the rate and extent of development of renal failure depend on the degree of penetrance of the autosomal dominant trait.

Three factors distingish between patients with polycystic kidney disease and those with multiple simple cysts: (1) a positive family history consistent with an autosomal dominant trait; (2) enlargement of the kidneys, generally detected as a pole-to-pole diameter in excess of 15 to 17 cm and a cortical thickness in excess of 3 cm; and (3) elongation and deformation of the calyceal structure from the progressive enlargement of the parenchymal cysts.

Microcystic kidney disease of the renal medulla, a disorder of children generally inherited as a recessive trait, is characterized by progressive disruption and destruction of the renal medullary architecture by multiple cysts. The disease is generally detected when young children complain of fatigue and are noted to have mild degrees of proteinuria, anemia, and mild azotemia. The clinical course is characterized by an inordinately high requirement for salt intake in order to maintain blood pressure and an adequate filtration rate and by stunted growth due to chronic illness, to uremia, and to excessive urinary calcium losses. Nephrons are gradually destroyed, usually with progression to end-stage renal disease before the age of 30.

Renal Neoplasia (Ch. 93). Two major classes of renal tumors

occur in adults: *renal cell carcinomas* (sometimes called hypernephromas), which originate in the renal cortex, and *transitional cell tumors* of the renal pelvis. Hypernephromas are versatile tumors and are often difficult to diagnose. Many patients present simply with painless hematuria. However, hypernephromas also produce a number of unusual syndromes, including polycythemia, presumably due to excessive erythropoietin production; hypertension, presumably because the neoplasm acts as the equivalent of an arteriovenous fistula and results in renin release by the affected kidney; fever of unknown origin; and hypercalcemia (see Table 93–3).

Transitional cell tumors of the renal pelvis commonly present as hematuria, which may be painless or accompanied by renal colic from the clots that are passed. The systemic manifestations described for hypernephroma are uncommonly found in transitional cell tumors. Examination of urine cytology by a Wright's stain of the urinary sediment may provide a useful diagnostic clue to the presence of these tumors.

Acute Renal Failure (Ch. 78). Acute renal failure refers either to the sudden cessation of urine flow or to sudden oliguria. Acute renal failure caused by acute glomerular disorders is generally evident from the findings described above for the acute glomerulonephritic syndromes. The general approach to the differential diagnosis of individuals with acute renal failure, particularly in hospitalized patients, involves the distinction among three major classes of disorders: (1) the prerenal hypoperfusion syndromes indicated in Table 74–1; (2) intrarenal syndromes, especially acute tubular necrosis and acute allergic interstitial nephritis; and (3) postrenal syndromes, that is, oligoanuria resulting from urinary tract obstruction.

The general approach to these patients involves the following cardinal maneuvers: (1) an assessment of circulatory dynamics; (2) a careful history to assess possible antecedent hypotension or exposure to nephrotoxic agents, coupled with a measurement of the fractional excretion of sodium; and (3) renal ultrasonography to exclude the possibility of obstruction of both kidneys, or obstruction of a solitary kidney, as in an individual with renal agenesis or with renal transplantation. These maneuvers are generally helpful in distinguishing between prerenal, intrarenal, and postrenal causes of oliguria. Invasive hemodynamic monitoring, coupled with a fluid challenge, may still be required to exclude rigorously the possibility of oliguria due to a reduced effective circulating volume. A percutaneous renal biopsy may be needed to distinguish between acute tubular necrosis and acute allergic interstitial nephritis. Renal ultrasonography has reduced strikingly the need for retrograde ureteral catheterization as a means for excluding obstructive uropathy.

TABLE 74–3. MAJOR GLOMERULAR SYNDROMES

Common Presentation	Major Disorders
Acute Nephritic Syndrome	Post-infectious glomerulonephritis Vasculitides: SLE 　　　　　　Polyarteritis nodosa 　　　　　　Wegener's granulomatosis 　　　　　　Henoch-Schönlein purpura Rapidly progressive glomerulonephritis Goodpasture's syndrome Hemolytic-uremic syndrome
Nephrotic Syndrome	Minimal change disease (nil lesion) Membranous nephropathy Focal glomerulosclerosis Amyloidosis Essential cryoglobulinemia
Nephritic-Nephrotic Syndrome	Membranoproliferative glomerulonephritis 　　Type I 　　Type II (dense deposit disease) Mesangioproliferative glomerulonephritis 　　(IgG/IgA nephropathy) Diabetic glomerulosclerosis 　　(Kimmelstiel-Wilson lesion)

THE POSTRENAL SYNDROMES (Ch. 83). The postrenal syndromes result from obstruction of urine flow at various loci in the urinary tract from the renal papillae to the urethral meatus. Azotemia and oliguria occur in urinary tract obstruction only when the urinary tract is obstructed bilaterally or when obstruction exists in a sole functioning kidney. The degree of azotemia depends upon the extent of the obstruction; partial obstruction may produce only moderate degrees of azotemia, while complete obstruction of the urinary tract obviously produces anuria. Obstruction of urine flow can irreversibly damage the kidneys. If the obstruction is partial or nearly complete, renal function may be preserved for as long as four to five weeks following the onset of obstruction. Obstructive uropathy also carries with it the possible complication of urinary tract infection.

Bilateral ureteral obstruction most frequently occurs at three major sites: (1) the *ureteropelvic junction*, where the obstruction is generally due to scar formation or, less commonly, to renal vessels crossing the ureter; (2) the site where the ureters cross the *pelvic brim*—neoplasms are the primary cause of such obstruction, particularly extensive carcinoma of the cervix; and (3) the *ureterovesical junction*, because of either neoplasm or scar formation. Less commonly, other disorders such as *retroperitoneal fibrosis* or disseminated retroperitoneal lymphoma may cause bilateral ureteral obstruction between the ureterovesical junction and where the ureters cross the pelvic brim. The probability of renal calculi causing bilateral ureteral obstruction is small unless one kidney is already nonfunctional and a stone obstructs the outflow of urine from the other kidney. Prostatic enlargement is a common cause of partial or complete obstruction to urine outflow. In contrast to patients with ureteral obstruction, the urinary bladder distends and often results in overflow urinary incontinence. The patient may therefore present with azotemia secondary to a profound reduction in glomerular filtration and yet have significant volumes of urine flow.

Urinary tract obstruction represents a potentially remediable cause of renal failure; every attempt should be made to exclude obstructive uropathy in individuals who are oliguric or anuric. Renal ultrasonography has simplified this task greatly, since it noninvasively detects whether or not the renal calyces are dilated and the ureters narrowed, as occurs in ureteropelvic junction obstruction; or whether the ureters and renal calyces are both dilated, as occurs in ureterovesical obstruction or urethral obstruction.

RENAL FAILURE: THE UREMIC SYNDROME

The uremic syndrome (Ch. 79) occurs when the functional renal mass is reduced sufficiently that the kidney is no longer able to carry out excretory functions, functions relating to the regulation of the volume and composition of body fluids, functions as an endocrine receptor, and functions as an endocrine organ. The manifestations of *acute* uremia may differ from those of *chronic* uremia, but these differences relate more to the rate of development of renal failure than to fundamental differences in pathophysiology.

Uremia is in part a syndrome of "autointoxication." While the chemical agents responsible for this autointoxication have not been clearly identified, uremic syndromes may be ameliorated by dialysis (which generally removes molecules having molecular weights less than 1,000 to 2,000 daltons), and severe protein restriction may minimize the rate of development of the uremic symptoms. Thus it is plausible to presume that the retention of the end-products of protein metabolism, reflected primarily by the BUN and serum creatinine levels as well as by other factors such as acidosis, are responsible for many of the manifestations of the uremic syndrome.

Uremic symptoms that relate primarily to a reduction in glomerular filtration rate begin to occur when the GFR is reduced below 5 to 10 per cent of normal. The primary findings include central nervous system symptoms ranging

from lethargy and confusion to coma and seizures; a bleeding tendency, due at least in part to interference with adequate platelet function; peripheral neuropathy, which is most evident in individuals with long-standing rather than acute uremia; intense pruritus; and asthenia.

In uremia the major electrolyte alterations include hypocalcemia, presumably due to the inability to form 1,25-dihydroxycholecalciferol as renal mass is reduced and to hyperphosphatemia; hyperphosphatemia resulting from a reduction in glomerular filtration rate; and metabolic acidosis, which results from a reduction in the renal excretion of "fixed" acids (that is, incompletely combusted organic acids; and sulfate and phosphate, which represent the end-products of protein and nucleic acid metabolism, respectively).

The occurrence of hyperkalemia among uremic individuals is variable and depends on a number of factors, including the rate of potassium intake, the rate of tissue catabolism, and the rate at which renal failure has evolved. In general, patients in whom the uremic syndrome evolves acutely do not develop adaptive mechanisms (both renal and extrarenal) for potassium elimination and are therefore more prone to develop hyperkalemia. In contrast, individuals who approach end-stage renal disease gradually may often be normokalemic even when the glomerular filtration rate is less than 5 per cent of normal. Two factors may account for this phenomenon: (1) The development of renal disease is accompanied by asthenia and anorexia so that dietary intake of potassium may be minimized; and (2) both renal and extrarenal mechanisms for more efficient potassium excretion are gradually developed.

Uremia, whether acute or chronic, is a catabolic disorder. In individuals with acute renal failure, even extensive hyperalimentation fails to prevent the loss of approximately 0.5 to 1.0 pound daily. In individuals with chronic renal failure, weight loss is more gradual and less easily perceived by patients. But in both acute and chronic renal failure, asthenia and loss of lean body mass are inevitable sequelae.

As the functional renal mass is diminished, erythropoietin production is also reduced. Thus within two to three weeks of the onset of acute renal failure, the combination of diminished erythrocyte production and an accelerated rate of red cell destruction invariably reduces the hematocrit level to the range of 20 to 25 per cent. Similar hematocrits are found in patients with chronic renal failure, particularly prior to dialysis therapy. Polycystic kidney disease represents an exception in that profound reductions of glomerular filtration rate may occur coincident with the maintenance of an hematocrit well in excess of 30 per cent. Presumably, the large renal mass of polycystic kidney disease produces sufficient erythropoietin to maintain an adequate hematocrit.

Two symptoms of uremia are seen commonly in individuals with chronic renal failure but are rare in acute uremia: *peripheral neuropathy* and *renal osteodystrophy*. Peripheral neuropathy almost never develops in individuals with acute renal failure but is common in individuals with long-standing uremia who have not been treated with dialysis. Individuals with acute renal failure do not develop significant bone disease. In contrast, individuals with chronic, severe reductions in glomerular filtration rate and in functional renal mass often have significant bone disease, termed renal osteodystrophy (Ch. 249). At least four factors may contribute to the complex bone disorders in uremia: (1) The synthesis of 1,25-hydroxycholecalciferol in the kidney is reduced with consequent diminished calcium absorption from the gut. (2) The calcium malabsorption leads to secondary hyperparathyroidism, which mobilizes calcium from bone in an attempt to maintain a normal level of serum ionized calcium and in the process produces osteitis fibrosa (Ch. 247). (3) Bone calcium is exchanged for retained protons in buffering the metabolic acidosis of chronic renal failure with partial maintenance of acid-base homeostasis, but at the expense of progressive dissolution of bone. (4) The uremic state impairs protein synthesis in bone and with this the formation of osteoid.

In short, the uremic syndrome results from varying impairment in the ability of the kidney to meet all of its normal metabolic and physiologic obligations: to regulate the volume and composition of body fluids, to excrete the end-products of metabolism, to serve as an endocrine receptor, and to serve as an endocrine organ. Within that framework the particular manifestations of uremia in any given patient will depend largely on the rate at which kidney failure has occurred, the severity of the renal failure (that is, the extent to which residual nephron mass is able to maintain homeostasis), and the homeostatic stresses to which the individual is subjected.

ADAPTATION TO RENAL INJURY AND THE PATHOGENESIS OF PROGRESSIVE RENAL FAILURE

There are two added characteristics of nearly all forms of chronic renal disease that warrant particular consideration. First, nephron loss may be accompanied by *adaptive functional changes* in residual nephrons, which tend to minimize the effects of reducing the functional nephron mass on the chemical composition of blood. This argument, generally termed the *intact nephron hypothesis*, considers that, in chronic renal disease, the function of residual nephrons may be normal or supranormal. Among the cardinal adaptive characteristics described by the intact nephron hypothesis have been an increased glomerular filtration rate per nephron with elevated serum BUN concentrations or increased rates of protein feeding, and an increase in the rate of phosphate excretion per nephron mediated through secondary hyperparathyroidism, such that, in chronic renal failure, serum phosphate levels do not rise until the glomerular filtration rate is reduced to about 30 per cent of normal.

Second, these adaptive responses may ultimately be harmful to the kidney: For example, the maintenance of relatively normal serum calcium and phosphate concentrations in a setting of modest reductions in glomerular filtration rate (that is, to 30 to 40 per cent of normal) by secondary hyperparathyroidism is achieved at the expense of bone dissolution. Likewise, recent observations have provided evidence that increases in protein intake lead to glomerular hyperperfusion and that the elevated glomerular filtration rate produced by this hyperperfusion can result in progressive glomerular sclerosis. Thus, in principle, glomerular hyperperfusion produced by a protein intake that is large in relation to the residual nephron mass could contribute to the progression of chronic renal disease. A corollary to this hypothesis is the possibility that dietary protein restriction early in the course of chronic renal failure might slow the rate of progression of renal disease.

Brenner BM: Nephron adaptation to renal injury or ablation. Physiol 249:F324, 1985. *A detailed analysis of the relation between glomerular hyperfiltration and progressive renal damage.*

Coe FL, Favus MJ: Disorders of stone formation. In Brenner B, Rector F (eds.): The Kidney. 3rd ed. Philadelphia, W. B. Saunders Company, 1986. *A thorough review of the approach to patients with stone disease.*

Huh MP, Kelleher SP: Proteinuria and the nephrotic syndrome. In Schrier RW (ed.): Renal and Electrolyte Disorders. Boston, Little, Brown and Company, 1986. *A thorough review of the pathogenesis and clinical manifestations of proteinuria.*

Swartz RD: Fluid, electrolyte and acid base changes during renal failure. In Kokko JP, Tannen RL (eds.): Fluids and Electrolytes. Philadelphia, W. B. Saunders Company, 1986. *A comprehensive review of the laboratory derangements in renal failure.*

75 STRUCTURE AND FUNCTION OF THE KIDNEYS

Saulo Klahr

This chapter reviews the structure and function of the normal mammalian kidney as a framework for understanding the derangements that occur with kidney disease.

Renal Structure

The kidneys are located retroperitoneally with their upper and lower poles opposite the twelfth thoracic and third lumbar vertebrae, respectively. Because of the presence of the liver, the right kidney is generally inferior to the left. Each adult kidney weighs 130 to 170 grams and measures about 12 by 6 by 3 cm. Through the hilus of the kidney pass a renal artery and vein, lymphatics, a nerve plexus, and the *renal pelvis*, which subdivides into the *three major calices* and subsequently into eight or more *minor calices*. A coronal section of the kidney reveals two distinct regions: the medulla and the cortex. The *renal medulla* is composed generally of 12 to 18 conical masses, the *pyramids*. The base of each pyramid is located on the corticomedullary boundary, and the apex extends toward the renal pelvis, forming the *papilla*, which projects into the minor calix. Each papilla is perforated by the distal end of 15 or more *terminal collecting ducts* (of Bellini). The *renal cortex*, about 1 cm in thickness, covers the base of the pyramids and extends medially between the individual pyramids to form the renal columns (of Bertin).

BLOOD SUPPLY

Generally, each kidney is supplied by a single artery originating from the aorta at the level of the first lumbar vertebra. This artery generally divides into two branches (anterior and posterior) before entering the renal sinus. The anterior branch gives rise to upper, middle, and lower branches (*lobar arteries*). As these arteries enter the renal parenchyma they form the *interlobar arteries* that course toward the cortex along the lateral borders of the medullary pyramids. The interlobar arteries then run across the base of the renal medulla, forming the *arcuate arteries*. The *interlobular arteries*, branching at right angles from the arcuate vessels, course through the cortex to the periphery. They give rise to *afferent arterioles*, each of which ends in a fine capillary bed known as a glomerulus. Thus, the glomerulus is supplied by a single afferent arteriole and drained, in turn, by an *efferent arteriole*, which emerges at the glomerular vascular pole and immediately ramifies into numerous peritubular capillaries that surround the tubular segments of the cortex. The *vasa recta*, which extend medially into the medulla, are the capillaries that originate from efferent arterioles of juxtamedullary glomeruli.

The venous system follows the same pattern as the arterial system, with the capillaries forming venules that unite into interlobular, arcuate, lobular, and ultimately renal veins. Each renal vein drains into the inferior vena cava.

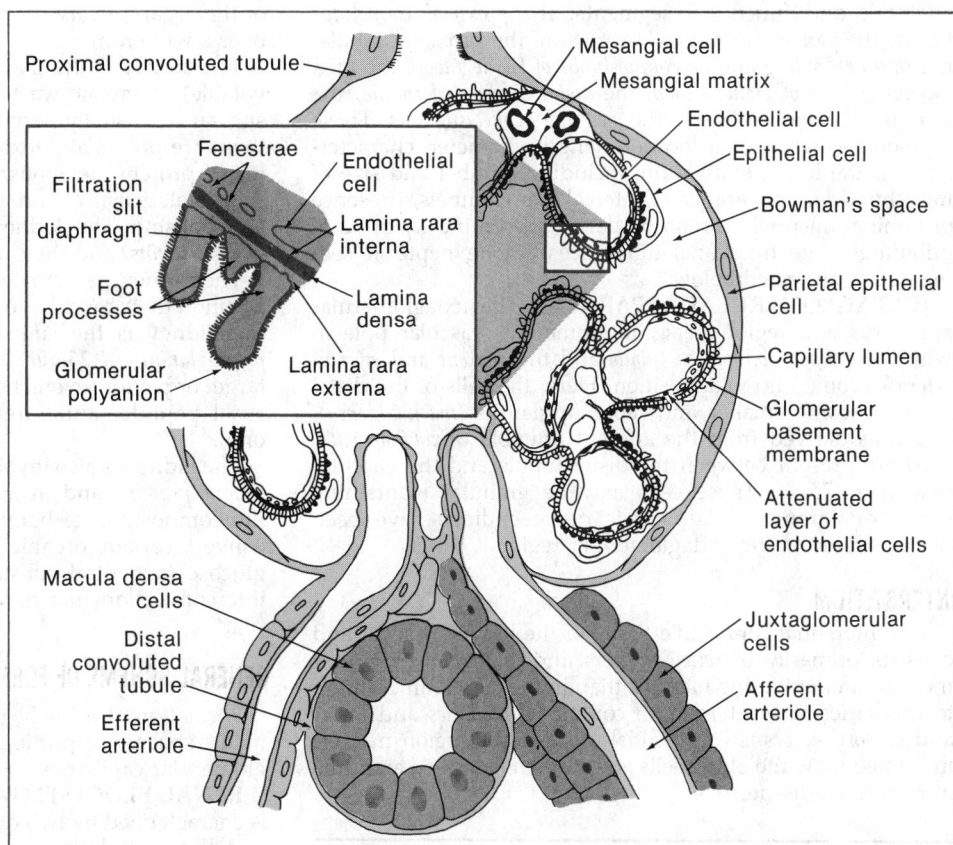

FIGURE 75–1. Schematic representation of the glomerulus, illustrating the three major types of cells (endothelial, epithelial, and mesangial) and the close relationship of the distal convoluted tubule to afferent and efferent arterioles ("juxtaglomerular apparatus"). Notice that there is no basement membrane interposed between the mesangium and the lumen of the capillaries. The inset shows a magnified view of the capillary wall, illustrating the gaps between the endothelial cells (fenestrae), the three layers of the basement membrane, and the foot processes of the epithelial cells. For more details see text.

THE NEPHRON

The nephron is the functional unit of the kidney. There are approximately 1,200,000 nephrons in each human kidney. Each is composed of a malpighian corpuscle (the *glomerulus* and *Bowman's capsule*) and its attached *tubule*. The tubule contains several distinct anatomic and functional segments: proximal tubule, loop of Henle, distal convoluted tubule, and cortical collecting tubule. The junction of cortical collecting tubules form the collecting ducts, which traverse the medulla and terminate at the tip of the papilla. There are two distinct populations of nephrons in the human kidney: those with glomeruli located in the outer cortex *(superficial nephrons)* and those with glomeruli situated near the corticomedullary junction *(juxtamedullary nephrons)*. The superficial nephrons, which constitute about 85 per cent of the total nephron population, have short loops of Henle that frequently do not penetrate the medulla. The juxtamedullary nephrons have long loops of Henle that extend into the inner medulla and are in close apposition to the vasa recta.

GLOMERULUS. The glomerulus (Fig. 75–1) is a network of capillaries originating from the afferent arteriole. After dividing into four to eight lobules to form the glomerular tuft, the capillaries rejoin to form the efferent arteriole, which leaves the glomerulus at the vascular pole. The glomerular tuft is surrounded by *Bowman's capsule,* which is an extension of the basement membrane and connective tissue of the proximal tubule. The *urinary* or *Bowman's space* separates the capsule from the glomerular tuft. Bowman's capsule contains a single layer of squamous cells *(parietal epithelial cells),* which undergo an abrupt transition to taller columnar cells typical of the proximal tubule at the urinary pole of the glomerulus. In the glomerular tuft there are three distinct cell types (endothelial, mesangial, and epithelial), a capillary wall (basement membrane), and an interstitial or supporting region (mesangium).

Capillary Wall. The capillary wall contains endothelial cells, a basement membrane, and epithelial cells (see Fig. 75–1).

The *endothelial cells* line the capillary lumen. Fenestrae or pores (approximate diameter of 700 Å) covered by thin diaphragms are present in the attenuated endothelium. The *basement membrane,* a structure with an average thickness in the adult of 3200 Å, contains three distinct areas: a central electron-dense *lamina densa* and, on either side, a *lamina rara externa* and *lamina rara interna* (see Fig. 75–1). The major constituents of the basement membrane are collagen and glycoprotein. Thickening of this structure is seen in a number of glomerular diseases. The *visceral epithelial cells,* or *podocytes,* are the largest of the glomerular cells. Extending from the body of the podocyte are primary processes, from which individual *foot processes,* or *pedicels,* project to come into contact with the lamina rara externa of the basement membrane. Between the foot processes is a space *(filtration slit* or *slit pore)* 250 to 400 Å wide, which is covered by a thin membrane, the *filtration slit diaphragm,* which is located approximately 600 Å from the basement membrane. This slit diaphragm is a zipper-like structure composed of rectangular pores (40 to 140 Å in a cross-section). The estimated total area of these pores is approximately 3 per cent of the total surface area of the glomerular capillaries. In renal diseases characterized by proteinuria the pedicels of the podocytes are replaced by a continuous band of cytoplasm adjacent to the lamina rara externa (fusion of foot processes).

The Mesangium. The mesangium, the interstitial portion of the glomerular lobules, is composed of *mesangial cells* (axial or intercapillary) and *mesangial matrix.* The latter is a homogeneous fibrillary material containing mucopolysaccharides and glycoprotein. The mesangial cells, which have phagocytic properties, resemble smooth muscle cells, contain myosin, and usually do not communicate directly with the vascular space. The mesangium is unique in that entry of a substance into the space does not require passage through a capillary basement membrane. In human glomerulonephritis, immune deposits are found in the mesangium, often exclusively.

THE TUBULE. The renal tubule is composed of distinct

anatomic and functional segments: the *proximal convoluted tubule*, the *pars recta* or *straight portion* of the proximal tubule, the *thin descending* and *ascending limbs of Henle's loop*, the *thick ascending limb of Henle's loop*, the *distal convoluted tubule*, the *cortical collecting tubule*, and the *medullary collecting duct*. These segments differ in their location, length, diameter, characteristics of the lining epithelium, including number and size of mitochondria, appearance of intercellular channels, presence of luminal microvilli (brush border), and complexity of basal infoldings. The functional differences among nephron segments are described below.

JUXTAGLOMERULAR APPARATUS. The juxtaglomerular apparatus is a region near the glomerular vascular pole in which the *distal convoluted tubule* and the *afferent* and *efferent* arterioles come into juxtaposition. Here, the cells of the distal tubule become smaller and more numerous (*macula densa*), and cells derived from the afferent arteriole (*juxtaglomerular cells*) are present between the distal tubule and the vascular pole (Fig. 75–1). These cells may be granular (containing renin) or agranular. Adrenergic nerve endings have been demonstrated in the juxtaglomerular region.

INTERSTITIUM

The interstitial connective tissue of the kidney is scant and consists primarily of *reticular fibers* and *interstitial cells*. It is more prominent in the medulla than in the cortex. In addition to capillaries, the interstitium contains *lymphatics* and *motor* and *sensory nerves*. In interstitial disease this region may be infiltrated by white blood cells and contain increased amounts of connective tissue.

Normal Renal Function

The principal functions of the kidney are summarized in Table 75–1. The kidneys have a central role in the *maintenance of volume and ionic composition of body fluids* (homeostasis). This function is accomplished by regulation of the rate of excretion of water and/or ions. Regulation entails feedback mechanisms that involve participation of the nervous system, the endocrine system, or both. Some of the homeostatic functions of the kidney are concerned with the balance of water, sodium, chloride, potassium, magnesium, phosphate, and hydrogen ions. The large changes in urine volume and composition, which occur in response to alterations in the diet, reflect the adaptability of the kidney to the requirements of homeostasis. There is no fixed normal volume or composition of the urine. Normal homeostatic renal function is defined by the capacity

TABLE 75–1. PRINCIPAL FUNCTIONS OF THE KIDNEY

1. Maintenance of volume and ionic composition of body fluids (homeostasis)

2. Excretion of metabolic waste products—e.g., urea, uric acid, creatinine

3. Detoxification and elimination of toxins, drugs, and their metabolites

4. Endocrine regulation of extracellular fluid volume and blood pressure
   a. Renin-angiotensin system
   b. Renal prostaglandins
   c. Renal kallikrein-kinin system

5. Control of red blood cell mass: erythropoietin

6. Endocrine control of mineral metabolism: formation of 1,25-dihydroxycholecalciferol and 24,25-dihydroxycholecalciferol

7. Degradation and catabolism of peptide hormones: insulin, glucagon, parathyroid hormone, calcitonin, growth hormone, etc.

8. Catabolism of low molecular weight proteins: light chains, beta$_2$-microglobulin

9. Metabolic interconversions: gluconeogenesis, lipid metabolism

of the organ to vary the volume and composition of the urine over a wide range.

The kidney is the main route of elimination of fixed (nonvolatile) metabolic waste products (*excretory function*). These substances usually serve no biologic function, and some of them are potentially toxic. Examples include urea (end-product of protein metabolism), uric acid (end-product of nucleic acid metabolism), and creatinine (end-product of creatine metabolism). The kidney also *eliminates exogenous chemicals* (*drugs, toxins*) and their metabolites.

The kidney participates in endocrine functions as well. In addition to its capacity to *metabolize and excrete certain hormones*, the kidney is the site of *production* of *renin, erythropoietin, prostaglandins, 1,25-dihydroxycholecalciferol*, and *kinins*. It is the target organ for several hormones (e.g., parathyroid hormone, atrial peptide, antidiuretic hormone, angiotensin, aldosterone).

The kidney is also involved in the *catabolism of small molecular weight proteins* and in *metabolic interconversions* that regulate the composition of body fluids. The ability of the kidney to convert certain organic acids (lactic, alpha-ketoglutaric) to glucose (a neutral substance) is an example of a metabolic interconversion that minimizes potential changes in plasma pH.

GENERAL SCHEME OF FORMATION OF URINE

Formation of urine begins with the ultrafiltration into Bowman's space of a portion of the plasma flowing through the glomerular capillaries.

RENAL BLOOD FLOW. Functionally, the renal circulation is characterized by two capillary beds in series: the glomerular and the peritubular capillaries. The glomerulus has a high intracapillary hydrostatic pressure because it is interposed between two arterioles, i.e., resistive vessels. Therefore, filtration is favored. The second capillary system (peritubular capillaries in the cortex, vasa recta in the medulla) is a high-flow, low-pressure system that acts as a reservoir for tubular reabsorption and secretion.

The kidneys receive 20 to 25 per cent of the cardiac output, or approximately 1.1 liters of blood per minute. In subjects with a physiologic hematocrit of 45 per cent, total renal plasma flow is about 600 ml per minute. Cortical blood flow is about 75 per cent and medullary blood flow 25 per cent of total renal blood flow. Only 1 per cent of the renal blood flow reaches the papilla. As blood flows through the glomerular capillaries, hydrostatic forces translocate about 20 per cent of the plasma volume (120 ml per minute) across the capillary wall into Bowman's space (glomerular filtration). The ratio of glomerular filtration rate (GFR) to renal plasma flow is called the *filtration fraction*.

Renal blood flow is maintained relatively constant (*autoregulation*) even in the face of wide variations (80 to 180 mm Hg) in perfusion pressure (i.e., mean pressure in the renal artery). This is achieved by changes in renal vascular resistance proportional to changes in perfusion pressure. Since the afferent and efferent arterioles determine renal vascular resistance, changes in arteriolar resistance will alter renal blood flow. When blood pressure falls below 80 or rises above 180 mm Hg, autoregulation is no longer operative and renal blood flow changes in proportion to pressure. In autoregulation, it appears that the afferent arteriole can sense transmural pressure and adjust wall tension to keep resistance proportional to pressure. Autoregulation of renal blood flow maintains a constant GFR despite altered perfusion pressure. Although the kidneys are innervated by adrenergic nerve fibers, renal sympathetic tone probably does not play a significant role in regulating renal blood flow under basal conditions. Thus, denervation or alpha- or beta-adrenergic blockers do not alter renal blood flow. However, augmented sympathetic activity (e.g., fright, pain, exercise, norepinephrine, congestive heart failure) increases renal vascular resistance and reduces renal blood flow. Both afferent and efferent arterioles contract, but GFR falls less than renal blood flow, suggesting that catecholamines exert their major effect at the efferent arteriole. Renal blood flow is increased by substances inducing fever (pyrogenic reaction).

GLOMERULAR FILTRATION RATE. The initial step in the formation of urine (ultrafiltration) occurs across the glomerular wall and separates the plasma water and its nonprotein constituents (crystalloids), which enter Bowman's space, from the blood cells and protein (colloids), which remain in the capillary lumen. The rate of glomerular ultrafiltration (GFR) is governed by the differences between transcapillary hydrostatic (ΔP) and colloid osmotic pressures ($\Delta \Pi$). GFR is influenced also by the filtration coefficient (K_f), which is a function of both total capillary surface area and the permeability per unit of surface area. Thus:

$$\text{GFR} = K_f (\Delta P - \Delta \Pi) \text{ or GFR} = K_f [(P_{GC} - P_{BS}) - \Pi_{GC}]$$

The difference in hydrostatic pressure (ΔP) between glomerular capillaries (P_{GC}) and Bowman's space (P_{BS}) favors filtration, whereas the colloid osmotic pressure inside the capillaries (Π_{GC}) opposes it. (The colloid osmotic pressure in Bowman's space is normally negligible and can be disregarded.) Hydrostatic pressure (P_{GC}) remains relatively constant along glomerular capillaries; however, the colloid osmotic pressure (Π_{GC}) undergoes a large progressive increase because filtration of "protein-free fluid" results in an increase of protein concentration along the capillary lumen. Hence, the mean effective pressure for ultrafiltration ($\Delta P - \Delta \Pi$) decreases along the glomerular capillary as $\Delta \Pi$ increases. In rats with surface glomeruli, the rise in glomerular capillary Π, as a function of length, is such that effective ultrafiltration pressure becomes zero before the end of the capillary. In other words, *filtration pressure equilibrium* ($P_{GC} = \Pi_{GC} + P_{BS}$) occurs, and filtration ceases before the end of the glomerular capillary. This fact makes GFR highly dependent on the flow rate of plasma entering the glomerulus, because at high flow rates, a slower rise in colloid osmotic pressure (Π_{GC}) occurs. Thus, glomerular filtration takes place across a greater length of the capillary. Hence, increased plasma flow tends to elevate GFR, whereas decreased plasma flow may cause a fall in GFR. As noted previously, renal blood flow and GFR are autoregulated within a wide range of renal arterial pressure. When perfusion pressure falls, the resistance of the afferent arteriole decreases. Thus, glomerular plasma flow and GFR are maintained. Below 80 to 90 mm Hg, renal plasma flow and GFR vary directly with arterial pressure, and the GFR ceases when the pressure falls below 50 mm Hg.

At a physiologic GFR of 120 ml per minute, the filtration rate per nephron (assuming 2,400,000 nephrons in both kidneys) would be 50 nanoliters per minute. However, just as superficial and juxtamedullary nephrons differ anatomically, they also appear to differ functionally. The larger juxtamedullary glomeruli have filtration rates that are about twice as high as the superficial ones. Single-nephron GFR probably is progressively lower in successively more superficial glomeruli. The physiologic implications of this extensive heterogeneity are not clear, although it has been suggested that redistribution of intrarenal blood flow toward deeper nephrons is associated with salt retention, and may contribute to edema in hepatic disease and congestive heart failure.

Alterations by disease states of any of the primary determinants discussed above may modify GFR. Thus, GFR can fall as a result of (1) decreased hydrostatic pressure in glomerular capillaries (marked hypotension); (2) increased hydrostatic pressure in Bowman's space (intratubular or urinary tract obstruction); (3) elevated glomerular plasma oncotic pressure as a consequence of increased concentration of proteins in the systemic circulation (dehydration: vomiting, diarrhea); (4) decreased renal blood flow (glomerular plasma flow), which may lead to filtration equilibrium at a more proximal region along the glomerular capillary, and hence may decrease the total surface area of capillary available for filtration (e.g., congestive heart failure, hepatic disease); or (5) a decrease in the filtration coefficient (K_f) due to a fall in permeability or to a reduction in total surface area available for filtration (intrinsic renal disease: certain nephrotoxins, acute or chronic glomerulonephritis).

Permselectivity of the Glomerular Capillary Wall. The glomerular capillary wall is highly permeable to small solutes and water. Molecules the size of inulin (molecular weight 5200) or smaller are present in the glomerular filtrate at the same concentration as in plasma water. Constituents with increasing *molecular size* exhibit progressively decreasing concentration in the filtrate. For example, albumin (molecular weight 69,000) is filtered to a very limited degree. However, plasma proteins with molecular sizes smaller than albumin are filtered at least to some degree.

In addition to molecular size, *molecular configuration, deformability,* and *net electrical charge* influence the filtration of macromolecules across the glomerular capillary wall. Negatively charged dextrans, of comparable size to albumin (a polyanion), have a clearance similar to that of albumin (less than 1 per cent that of inulin). In contrast, uncharged (neutral) dextran molecules of the same size as albumin are filtered at a much greater rate (20 per cent the rate of inulin), and filtration of cationic (positively charged) dextrans is even greater. Therefore, at constant molecular size, negative charge of the solute restricts and positive charge accelerates its filtration, suggesting that, phenomenologically, glomerular filtration occurs through pores with negative charges. A negatively charged glycoprotein ("*glomerular polyanion*"), predominantly found lining the foot processes of the epithelial cells, has been identified. Loss of these negative charges, in certain glomerular diseases, may lead to increased filtration of albumin.

HOMEOSTATIC AND EXCRETORY FUNCTIONS OF THE KIDNEY

The formation of urine begins with the elaboration of a protein-free plasma ultrafiltrate across the glomerular capillaries (*glomerular filtration*). As this ultrafiltrate flows through the renal tubule, solutes and water are reabsorbed from lumen to blood (*reabsorption*). Other solutes are secreted into the tubular lumen from the blood (*secretion*). In some cases, both processes (reabsorption and secretion) affect a given substance, permitting flexible regulation of its excretion. Quantitatively, about 170 liters of fluid is ultrafiltered daily, of which less than 1 liter to more than 10 liters may be excreted as urine, depending on the water balance of the individual. Large amounts of filtered sodium, chloride, calcium, magnesium, and phosphate are reabsorbed, with the quantity remaining in the final urine varying according to the dietary intake of each one of these solutes. Substances such as glucose, amino acids, and bicarbonate are almost completely reabsorbed and, under physiologic conditions, do not appear in the urine. The contribution of tubular transport to homeostasis is discussed in more detail below.

TUBULAR TRANSPORT. The renal tubule can be divided functionally into three major segments: (1) the proximal tubule, (2) the loop of Henle, and (3) the distal nephron. Although there are physiologic and morphologic subdivisions of these segments, it is possible to ascribe a general function to each. The proximal tubule reabsorbs, rather nonselectively, a large fraction (two thirds) of the glomerular filtrate. The loop of Henle has unique water and solute transport properties and serves to establish a hyperosmolar medullary interstitium that influences the ultimate concentration or dilution of the urine. The distal nephron is the site of fine regulation of water and electrolyte excretion and appears to be the main target of hormones that control these processes. Since the tubule segments are arranged in series, the function of any segment depends not only on its own intrinsic transport characteristics but also on the volume and composition of the fluid delivered to it from the previous segment.

Proximal Tubule. The proximal tubule reabsorbs sodium, several other solutes, and water at a high rate. Active sodium reabsorption and hydrogen ion secretion are the essential processes to which transport of chloride, several organic solutes, and water is coupled by a variety of mechanisms. Fluid transport is isosmotic, so that concentration gradients of solute across the wall are small. Functionally, the proximal tubule can be divided into three segments:

INITIAL PORTION OF THE CONVOLUTED SEGMENT. Sodium reabsorption in this portion occurs through cells and intercellular spaces. Transcellular reabsorption of sodium is active, generating a small transtubular electrical potential (1 to 5 mV, lumen negative) (Fig. 75–2). It requires entry of sodium across luminal (brush border) membranes and extrusion of sodium across basolateral membranes. Entry of sodium across luminal membranes is passive and occurs (1) by diffusion, (2) coupled to the transport of other solutes (e.g., glucose, amino acids, phosphate), and (3) in exchange with H^+ secreted from cell to lumen. Sodium extrusion from cells into the intercellular spaces and across the basolateral membrane is an active (energy-requiring) process that is accomplished by the sodium-potassium pump (Na^+, K^+-ATPase). Transport of sodium into the intercellular channels increases the concentration of solute in these spaces and creates an osmotic pressure gradient favoring the flow of water from lumen to intercellular spaces across the tight junctions that connect, toward the lumen, the lateral boundaries of the epithelial cells. The osmotic flow of water carries salt with it (solvent drag) and leads to bulk reabsorption of sodium.

Preferential reabsorption of bicarbonate resulting from H^+ secretion occurs in this segment, with bicarbonate concentration falling and chloride concentration increasing to an equivalent degree as the fluid flows along this segment of the tubule. The reabsorption of glucose and amino acids is active, is coupled to sodium transport, and is essentially complete in this segment. Some permeant solutes, such as urea, are partially reabsorbed by a passive mechanism because of the increase in their luminal concentration as water is absorbed.

DISTAL TWO THIRDS OF THE CONVOLUTED SEGMENT. The luminal fluid of the last two thirds of the convoluted tubule is characterized by a low concentration of bicarbonate and by the absence of glucose and amino acids. The tubular fluid remains isosmotic with plasma and has the same concentration of sodium as does the filtrate. The concentration of chloride in the lumen, however, exceeds the concentration of chloride in the peritubular capillary. This concentration gradient for chloride favors its diffusion out of the lumen generating a lumen-positive potential (which is on the order of 1 to 3 mV). In experiments in vitro in which luminal and peritubular fluids have identical compositions, active sodium transport occurs. Therefore, sodium reabsorption in this segment occurs by (1) active transport, (2) passive flow (because of the positive luminal potential), and (3) solvent drag.

STRAIGHT SEGMENT (PARS RECTA). This segment is the main site of secretion of organic acids (penicillin, uric acid). Its rate of sodium and fluid transport is slower, and its capacity for glucose and amino acid reabsorption is minimal when compared with that of the convoluted segments. The potential of the lumen is positive, and sodium and chloride are transported by the same mechanisms as in the last two thirds of the proximal convoluted tubule.

Modulation of Reabsorption by the Proximal Tubule. Proximal reabsorption conserves most of the filtered fluid and all of a number of essential solutes. Several factors modulate the transport rate at the proximal tubule and therefore influence the performance of subsequent segments by altering their load.

TRANSTUBULAR PHYSICAL FACTORS. The hydrostatic pressure (P) in the peritubular capillaries is markedly decreased compared with that in the glomerular capillaries. The colloid osmotic pressure (II) is increased owing to filtration of a "protein-free fluid" at the glomeruli. These "Starling forces" thus favor the uptake of fluid (from the interstitium) by the peritubular capillaries. When II falls or P rises, the uptake of fluid by peritubular capillaries decreases. This leads to fluid accumulation in the interstitium, increased hydrostatic pres-

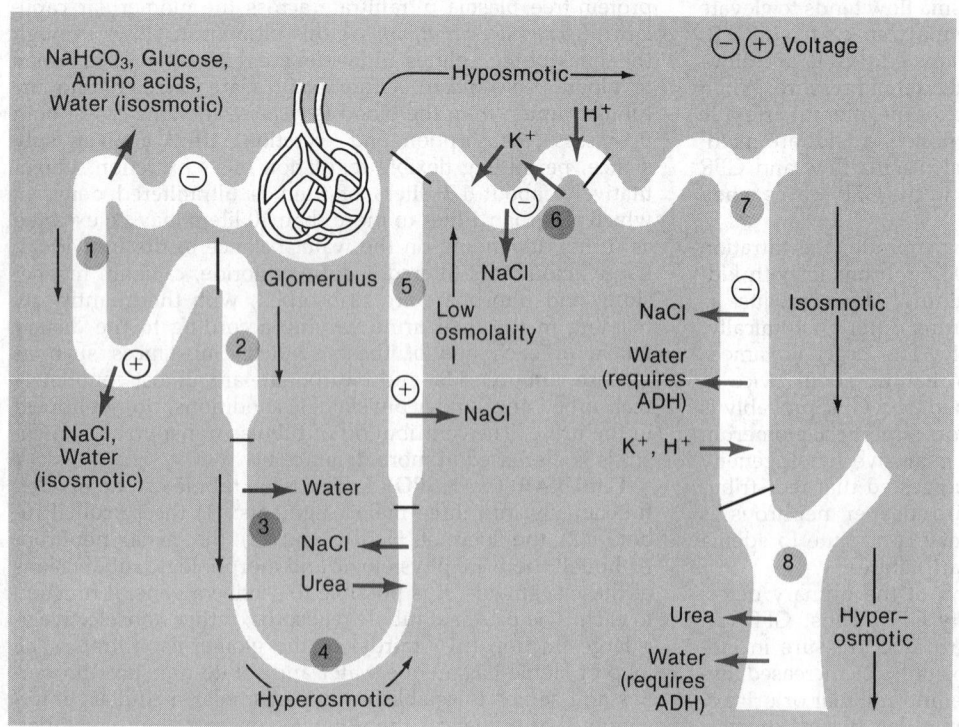

FIGURE 75–2. Schematic representation of the principal processes of transport in the nephron. In the convoluted portion of the proximal tubule (1) salt and water are reabsorbed at high rates, in isotonic proportions. Bulk reabsorption of most of the filtrate (65 to 70 per cent) and virtually complete reabsorption of glucose, amino acids, and bicarbonate take place in this segment. In the pars recta (2) organic acids are secreted and continuous reabsorption of sodium chloride takes place. The loop of Henle comprises three segments; the thin descending (3) and ascending (4) limbs and the thick ascending limb (5). The fluid becomes hyperosmotic, because of water abstraction, as it flows toward the bend of the loop and hyposmotic, because of sodium chloride reabsorption, as it flows toward the distal convoluted tubule (6). Active sodium reabsorption occurs in the distal convoluted tubule and in the cortical collecting tubule (7). This latter segment is water impermeable in the absence of ADH, and the reabsorption of sodium in this segment is increased by aldosterone.

The collecting duct (8) allows equilibration of water with the hyperosmotic interstitium when ADH is present. For further details see text. (Adapted from figure by A Iselin, from Burg MB: Hosp Pract 13:99, 1978. Reproduced with permission.)

sure in this space, and a delay in the egress of fluid from the lateral intercellular channels. The limiting junctions of these channels become more permeable, and backflux of fluid (from intercellular spaces to tubular lumen) occurs, thus diminishing net fluid reabsorption. When P falls or Π rises in the peritubular capillaries, as in dehydration, reabsorption of fluid increases.

Glomerular tubular balance refers to a direct relationship between GFR and the prevailing rates of proximal tubular reabsorption and has been ascribed to changes in Π in the peritubular circulation that result from changes in GFR (increases in GFR and hence in filtration fraction lead to a greater protein concentration and increases in Π in the efferent arterioles and peritubular capillaries; a decrease in GFR has the opposite effect). Thus, when GFR increases, a greater amount of fluid is delivered to the proximal tubule; however, the resulting rise in peritubular Π leads to a proportional increase in the reabsorption of fluid in this segment so that the percentage of the filtrate reabsorbed in the proximal tubule remains constant. An alternative mechanism accounting for glomerular tubular balance is a link between fluid reabsorption in the proximal tubule and flow rates of tubular fluid. Increases in GFR, and hence in proximal tubular flow, augment reabsorption; decreases in GFR and in flow decrease reabsorption.

EFFECTS OF HORMONES ON SODIUM REABSORPTION BY THE PROXIMAL TUBULE. Parathyroid hormone reduces sodium and fluid reabsorption in the proximal tubule; catecholamines may stimulate fluid reabsorption in this segment. However, the physiologic significance of these observations has not been established.

Loop of Henle. The loop of Henle, which is interposed between the proximal and distal tubules, is a hairpin-shaped structure extending into the renal medulla (Fig. 75–2). Under physiologic conditions it reabsorbs about 25 per cent of the filtered sodium and chloride and 15 per cent of the filtered water. In consequence, the isotonic fluid entering Henle's loop becomes hypotonic to plasma before entering the distal tubule.

The maintenance of water balance requires the excretion of urine of varied tonicity. The formation of a dilute (hypotonic to plasma) or concentrated (hypertonic to plasma) urine takes place by means of a *countercurrent system* that involves not only the loops of Henle but also the distal tubule, the collecting ducts, and the blood vessels supplying these segments. The excretion of a hypertonic urine involves two basic steps: (1) creation of a hypertonic medullary interstitium and (2) osmotic equilibration of the fluid that enters the medullary collecting duct with the hypertonic interstitium. Antidiuretic hormone (ADH) is required in this latter process. Hypotonic urine is excreted when the fluid that enters the medullary collecting duct does not equilibrate with the hypertonic interstitium owing to low levels or absence of ADH. Only the juxtamedullary nephrons contribute significantly to the production of medullary hypertonicity. However, the fluid from both superficial and deep nephrons drains into the collecting ducts and reaches osmotic equilibrium with the interstitium in the presence of ADH.

In normal human subjects the maximal osmolality of urine that can be achieved is around 1200 mOsm per kilogram. Since the tubular fluid reaches this osmolality by equilibration with the medullary interstitium, it follows that the interstitium must have a similar osmolality. *Countercurrent multiplication* is the process by which the interstitial osmolality is increased from 285 mOsm per kilogram in the cortex (the same osmolality as plasma) to 1200 mOsm per kilogram in the papillary tip. The thin descending and ascending limbs of juxtamedullary nephrons lie in close proximity to each other in the medulla. Flow through them is countercurrent. Fluid obtained from thin ascending limbs has a lower osmolality than fluid obtained from thin descending limbs at comparable levels in

the papilla. This is due to functional differences. Whereas the descending limb is highly permeable to water, slightly permeable to urea, and highly impermeable to sodium, the ascending limb is highly permeable to sodium, moderately permeable to urea, and impermeable to water. In normal mammals, the medullary interstitium is hyperosmotic owing to the accumulation of high concentrations of both urea and sodium chloride (see below). This composition and the properties of the two segments of the loop result in quite specific transport processes. The isotonic fluid delivered from the proximal tubule becomes progressively hypertonic as it traverses the thin descending limb owing to net water flow from lumen to interstitium. The highest osmolality of the luminal fluid is achieved at the tip of the loop. This hyperosmolar fluid becomes diluted progressively as it flows up the thin ascending limb, owing to the movement of sodium without water from the lumen to the interstitium. Urea present in the interstitium diffuses inward. However, since the permeability of this segment to sodium chloride is greater than to urea, the net effect is a greater exit of sodium chloride than urea entry, resulting in net addition of solute to the interstitial fluid. In addition, since the thin ascending limb is impermeable to water, the fluid is diluted (hypotonic) with respect to the interstitial fluid at the same level. The thick ascending limb of the loop reabsorbs sodium chloride actively. This segment is essentially impermeable to water, even when ADH is present; therefore, salt transport from lumen to interstitial fluid decreases the osmolality of the luminal fluid and increases the osmolality of the interstitium. This increased osmolality of the outer medullary interstitium promotes the exit of water from the thin descending limb. The function of the thick ascending limb accounts for the countercurrent multiplication that occurs in the renal medulla. Although analysis of the electrochemical gradient (Fig. 75–2) might suggest active chloride transport, there is strong evidence that sodium transport is primary and active and that chloride is moved across the luminal membrane in cotransport with sodium as neutral sodium chloride. The amount of urea present in the fluid of the thick ascending limb is higher than in the fluid entering the thin descending limb. This is due to water abstraction, in excess of urea, out of the latter segment and net urea entry (recycled from the collecting duct) into the thin ascending and descending limbs of Henle's loop.

Urea and sodium chloride contribute most of the 1200 mOsm per kilogram of solute present at the papillary tip during antidiuresis. Antidiuretic hormone plays a critical role in this high interstitial urea concentration. In the cortical collecting duct ADH increases water but not urea permeability. This results, as water is lost from the tubular fluid, in a rise in concentration of urea in the tubular lumen. In the medullary collecting duct, ADH enhances the permeabilities of both water and urea. As water leaves the collecting duct, urea concentration increases further and urea enters the interstitium; it then enters the thin descending (very little) and ascending limbs, increasing the amount of urea in the tubular fluid (see above). The net result is that both urinary and medullary urea concentrations are maintained at high levels in the presence of ADH (antidiuresis).

The fluid emerging from the loop of Henle is virtually always hyposmotic (about 150 mOsm per kilogram) compared with plasma, regardless of the final urine osmolality. With low or absent ADH the luminal fluid in the cortical collecting duct does not equilibrate with the isosmotic cortical interstitium or in the medullary collecting duct with the hypertonic medulla. Hence, the volume of fluid delivered to the tip of the collecting duct is increased and its osmolality decreased compared with plasma. The osmolality of this fluid can be further decreased to as low as 30 mOsm per kilogram by the reabsorption of solute in excess of water in distal tubule and cortical and medullary collecting ducts (see below).

Since the maximal urine osmolality cannot exceed that in

the interstitium, the ability to conserve water by excreting a highly concentrated urine is reduced when the hypertonicity of the medullary interstitium is decreased. This may be due to reduced papillary urea accumulation such as occurs in protein malnutrition, as a consequence of decreased urea production, or due to reduced interstitial sodium chloride accumulation (use of loop diuretics, hypercalcemia). Reduced levels or absence of ADH (diabetes insipidus) or unresponsiveness of the collecting duct to the action of ADH (nephrogenic diabetes insipidus) may prevent equilibration of the fluid in the collecting duct with the hypertonic interstitium, leading to an impairment in water conservation.

Distal Nephron (Distal Convoluted Tubule, Cortical Collecting Tubule, and Medullary Collecting Duct). The distal nephron accomplishes the final and delicate adjustments in the reabsorption of water, sodium, chloride, phosphate, and calcium in response to aldosterone, ADH, and parathyroid hormone.

The *distal convoluted tubule* is defined anatomically as the segment that extends from the macula densa to the site of transition from homogeneous cells to a mixture of dark and light cells (typical of the collecting duct). The distal convoluted tubule is essentially impermeable to water and unresponsive to ADH. Sodium chloride is reabsorbed at a slower rate than in the proximal tubule or in the loop, but against large concentration gradients. The rate of reabsorption is proportional to the load. The transtubular electrical potential, lumen negative, is related to the reabsorption of sodium and varies from -10 in the initial portion to -45 mV in the distal portion. Most of the reabsorption of sodium chloride occurs transcellularly. Potassium is secreted in this segment from peritubular capillary into the lumen (see below). Acidification of the luminal fluid in the distal tubule has been attributed to an active H^+ transport mechanism located at the luminal membrane.

The *cortical collecting tubule* extends from the end of the distal tubule to the corticomedullary junction. Under basal conditions, water permeability is negligible in this segment. It is increased markedly by ADH. Sodium chloride is actively reabsorbed at this level; therefore, in the absence of ADH the luminal fluid osmolality falls further. When ADH is present the luminal fluid equilibrates with the cortical interstitial fluid and becomes isosmotic with plasma; at the same time, luminal urea concentrations rise (see above). The transtubular electrical potential is about 35 mV, lumen negative; it is related to active reabsorption of sodium and is highly dependent on the levels of mineralocorticoids, which increase sodium reabsorption. Potassium and hydrogen are secreted in this segment. Aldosterone increases sodium reabsorption as well as potassium and H^+ secretion in this portion of the nephron (Fig. 75–2).

The *medullary collecting duct* starts at the corticomedullary junction and ends on the surface of the papilla. Water and urea permeabilities are low in the absence of ADH. Continuous sodium chloride reabsorption at this level, in the absence of ADH, results in a further drop in urine osmolality. ADH increases water and urea permeability and allows the equilibration of the luminal osmolality with that of the hypertonic interstitium.

To recapitulate, in the proximal tubule salt and water are transported at high rates, in isotonic proportions. Bulk reabsorption of most of the filtrate (65 to 70 per cent) and virtually complete reabsorption of "metabolically useful" solutes (glucose, amino acids, bicarbonate) take place in this segment. The *loop of Henle* comprises three segments with strikingly different properties of active transport and permeability of water and solute. Because of these properties, the medullary interstitium is made hyperosmolar and acts as the driving force for final water reabsorption. The loop reabsorbs additional sodium chloride (about 25 per cent of that filtered) and water (about 15 per cent of the filtrate) and leaves about 10

per cent of the sodium and 15 per cent of the water to be reabsorbed in the last segments of the tubule.

The distal convoluted tubule and the collecting tubule can establish large sodium gradients between fluid in the lumen and in the peritubular capillary. The collecting ducts, water impermeable in the absence of ADH, become permeable to water in response to the hormone. It is in these segments that the final volume and osmolality of the urine are determined. Salt transport occurs at a slower rate than in the preceding segments but against large concentration gradients. The final regulation of salt excretion takes place in these segments, under the influence of aldosterone. Potassium and H^+ excretion are regulated also in these segments.

ROLE OF THE KIDNEY IN SODIUM CHLORIDE HOMEOSTASIS. Normally the kidney regulates sodium balance (and hence extracellular fluid volume) in a very efficient manner. The daily intake of sodium varies considerably. In the Western world the average diet contains about 170 mEq per 24 hours. About 98 per cent of this amount is excreted in the urine. However, even when the normal daily excretion of sodium is 165 to 170 mEq per day, i.e., sufficient to maintain sodium balance on a relatively high sodium intake, less than 1 per cent of the amount of sodium filtered (140 mEq per liter $\times$ 170 liters = 23,800 mEq per day) is excreted in the urine. Thus, maintenance of sodium homeostasis is primarily a function of the renal tubule and reabsorption of filtered sodium; changes in GFR appear to be quantitatively less important. Thus, (1) sizable increases in GFR, not accompanied by extracellular fluid (ECF) volume expansion, do not result in a marked natriuresis because of glomerular tubular balance (see above), and (2) the natriuresis of ECF volume expansion occurs under experimental conditions in which GFR is maintained constant or even decreased experimentally. When a normal subject increases the intake of salt, urine sodium excretion increases progressively, reaching, in three to four days, a steady-state level equal to and offsetting intake. During the interval of adjustment, positive sodium balance occurs, with an accompanying retention of water and consequent gain in body weight. When salt intake is suddenly reduced, the opposite effects are observed. Sodium excretion decreases, reaching a level equal to intake within three to five days with a reduction in total body water and body weight.

Several physiologic mechanisms ordinarily control sodium reabsorption by the kidney to maintain the sodium content of ECF. Changes in sodium mass are not sensed as such, but secondarily as changes in ECF volume. Total ECF volume changes are sensed through their effects on circulatory dynamics ("effective arterial blood volume"). The determinants of effective arterial blood volume are (1) the degree of filling of the arterial tree, which depends in large part on cardiac output, and (2) peripheral vascular resistance, which depends on the compliance of the peripheral vessels and the magnitude of the arterial runoff. Decreases in effective volume (dehydration, hemorrhage, venodilation, venous pooling) lead to renal retention of salt. Increases in effective volume (saline administration, excessive salt intake) lead to a rise in salt excretion by the kidney.

Factors That Influence the Tubular Reabsorption of Sodium. Alterations in effective arterial volume affect handling of sodium by the kidney through the renin-angiotensin-aldosterone system, the sympathetic nervous system, and other less well-defined factors. The last category probably includes changes in intrarenal hydrostatic and oncotic pressures (socalled physical factors), a natriuretic (or salt-losing) hormone, and possibly the distribution of blood flow within the kidneys (Fig. 75–3).

ROLE OF PHYSICAL FACTORS IN THE REABSORPTION OF SODIUM. A fall in effective arterial blood volume (dehydration, hemorrhage) and the consequent decline in blood pressure decrease renal perfusion. In response to reductions in renal perfusion pressure, glomerular plasma flow decreases more

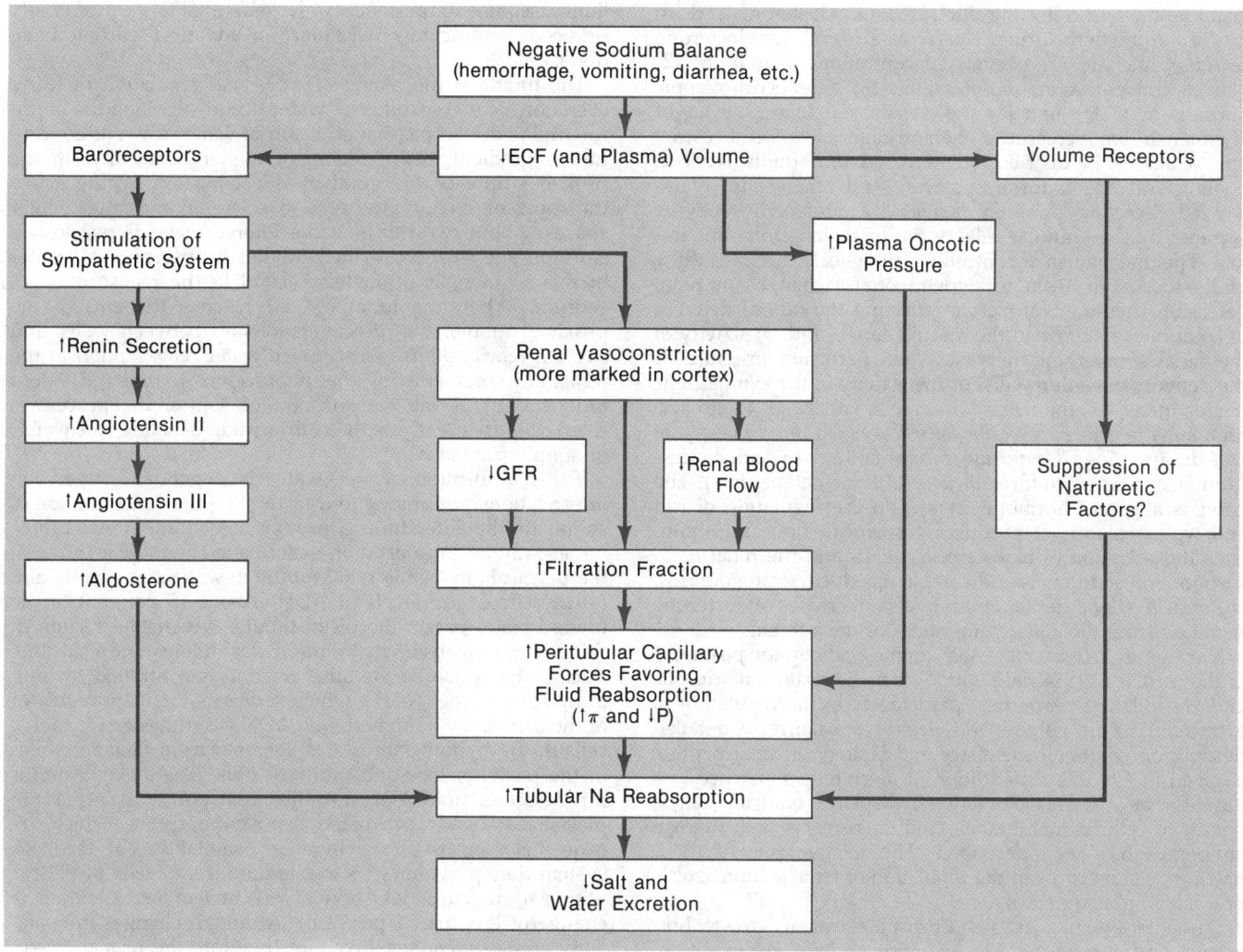

FIGURE 75–3. Mechanisms responsible for increased sodium reabsorption in the renal tubule in response to a negative sodium balance. These mechanisms and the accompanying stimulation of thirst and antidiuretic hormone secretion tend to restore the extracellular fluid (ECF) volume. The arrows indicate a decrease (↓) or an increase (↑). Oncotic pressure and hydrostatic pressure in peritubular capillaries are indicated by π and P, respectively.

than does glomerular capillary hydrostatic pressure, resulting in a fall in GFR that is proportionally less than the decline in renal plasma flow. This disparity is due to a greater vasoconstriction of efferent compared with afferent arterioles in response to increased levels of catecholamines and angiotensin II in the circulation. The lesser fall in GFR compared with renal plasma flow increases filtration fraction and hence the concentration of protein in the efferent arterioles and peritubular capillaries. In addition, vasoconstriction of the efferent arteriole results in a fall in hydrostatic pressure (P) in the peritubular capillaries. The increase in II and the decrease in P in the peritubular capillaries augment sodium and water reabsorption along the proximal segments of the nephron. Thus, in response to contraction of effective arterial volume, the glomerular and peritubular microcirculations act in concert to minimize fluid losses by both lowering GFR and augmenting salt and water reabsorption by the tubules (Fig. 75–3).

Expansion of the ECF volume elicits opposite effects. The increase in renal perfusion pressure leads to not only a rise in GFR but also a proportionally greater rise in renal plasma flow; consequently filtration fraction falls. The net effect is a decrease in peritubular protein concentration and hence in II, with a decrease in reabsorption of fluid by peritubular capillaries. The importance of such physical factors in the normal control of sodium and water reabsorption is not exactly clear. Since alterations in II and P in the peritubular capillaries influence fluid reabsorption mainly, if not exclusively, in the proximal tubule, it is likely that changes in physical factors are important only when fluid balance deficits or gains are very large (as, for example, with severe hemorrhage or marked expansion of the ECF volume). Whether significant changes in proximal reabsorption occur in response to more modest alterations in fluid balance (as might result, for example, in response to a diet very low or very high in sodium chloride) remains uncertain.

REDISTRIBUTION OF BLOOD FLOW. Another mechanism potentially altering sodium excretion is redistribution of blood flow. It has been suggested that certain nephrons, those with superficially placed glomeruli, have less capacity to reabsorb sodium than others. If so, at any given total GFR, the relative amounts of fluid filtered by the two different nephron populations would be an important determinant of sodium excretion. Redistribution of GFR toward the "high reabsorption nephrons" (juxtamedullary nephrons) would be associated with decreased sodium excretion because of the greater capacity of these nephrons to reabsorb sodium. Despite the attractiveness of this theory, evidence favoring it is scanty.

RENIN-ANGIOTENSIN-ALDOSTERONE. Sodium balance is controlled also by *mineralocorticoid hormones, mainly aldosterone.* Only a small but significant fraction (some 2 per cent) of the filtered sodium is under hormonal control. Yet loss or gain of an amount of sodium equivalent to 2 per cent of the filtered load (about 500 mEq per day) has profound effects on sodium balance. Aldosterone increases sodium reabsorption in the distal tubule and collecting duct. Lack of aldosterone leads to loss of sodium in the urine. The factors controlling aldosterone secretion include (1) plasma concentration of sodium, (2) plasma concentration of potassium, (3) adrenocorticotropic hormone (ACTH), and (4) angiotensin. Circulating levels of angiotensin are increased by hemorrhage, dietary salt restriction, changes in distribution of blood and fluids (venous pooling and edema-forming states), and other states of increased secretion of renin. *Renin* is a proteolytic enzyme secreted by the granular cells of the juxtaglomerular apparatus. The mechanisms controlling its release are not fully understood, but seem to depend on (1) changes in renal perfusion pressure, (2) factors reflecting the rate of delivery of sodium or chloride to the macula densa, and (3) activity of the renal sympathetic nerves. When perfusion pressure or the delivery of sodium falls, or the activity of the sympathetic nerves increases, the release of renin is enhanced. Renin acts on a substrate in plasma, *angiotensinogen*, to form *angiotensin I* (a decapeptide). *Converting enzyme* splits two amino acids from angiotensin I to form *angiotensin II* (an octapeptide). The latter is a potent hormone, central to the regulation of salt and water balance. It produces vasoconstriction and stimulates the secretion of aldosterone, thirst, and the renal reabsorption of sodium. Another split product of angiotensin, *angiotensin III* (a heptapeptide), also increases aldosterone secretion from the zona glomerulosa of the adrenal.

NATRIURETIC HORMONES. A 28–amino acid peptide produced in the cardiac atria (atrial peptide), which has both natriuretic and vasodilating properties, participates in the regulation of extracellular fluid volume and electrolyte balance. A detailed description of the biochemistry and biology of atrial peptide is given in Ch. 224. In addition, a natriuretic substance that inhibits Na^+, K^+-ATPase activity, displaces ouabain that is bound to cellular membranes, and cross-reacts with digoxin antibodies has been described. The relative role of these natriuretic substances in the regulation of renal sodium excretion has not been determined.

OTHER HORMONAL AGENTS. Cortisol, estrogen, growth hormone, and insulin all can enhance sodium reabsorption. Glucagon, progesterone, and parathyroid hormone can decrease it. It is almost certain that when circulating levels of these hormones are elevated (as, for example, estrogen during pregnancy), significant influences occur on sodium reabsorption and thereby excretion. However, there is no evidence that any of them, unlike the factors described previously, are controlled specifically as part of the homeostatic regulation of sodium balance. Of great interest is the possible role played by intrarenally produced substances such as *prostaglandins* and *kinins*. These agents are potent vasodilators and may reduce sodium reabsorption, by altering regional intrarenal vascular resistance or by direct actions on the tubular cells. Their levels change with alterations of sodium balance, but it is not yet clear how extensively they participate in the renal regulation of sodium excretion.

RENAL NERVES. The renal sympathetic nerves play a prominent role in sodium homeostasis by modulating (1) secretion of aldosterone via the renin-angiotensin system, (2) intrarenal physical factors, (3) the reabsorptive activity of the tubular cells themselves, and (4) GFR. Yet, because of the many other known (and potential) factors involved, a transplanted and, therefore, denervated kidney maintains sodium homeostasis quite well.

RENAL REGULATION OF WATER EXCRETION. The capacity to regulate renal excretion of water, independent of solute excretion, maintains the osmolality of body fluids within narrow limits despite wide variations in intake of water. Roughly 170 liters of water is filtered daily. Of this amount, less than 2 liters, or about 1 per cent of the amount filtered, is excreted. Except for setting an upper limit for the amount of water that can be excreted per unit time, GFR is not involved in the regulation of water excretion. This upper limit assumes importance only when GFR is profoundly reduced as in acute renal failure or advanced chronic renal disease.

The tubule is the major site for renal regulation of water excretion. Net absorption of water occurs all along the nephron and is due to passive diffusion of water down its concentration gradient into a region of higher osmolality. In the proximal tubule, this gradient is established by the active transport of sodium into the basolateral and intercellular spaces. About two thirds of the filtered water is reabsorbed isosmotically in the proximal tubule. Reabsorption of water in this segment is intimately related to the reabsorption of sodium. When the luminal fluid reaches the end of the proximal tubule, the direct relationship between water and sodium reabsorption is lost. Since water reabsorption in the remaining segments of the nephron is to a large extent independent of the reabsorption of solute, the process is referred to frequently as the reabsorption of solute-free water, or simply *free water*.

The reabsorption of free water is dependent largely on interrelationships among four factors: (1) the concentration of solute in the interstitium through which the renal tubule passes, (2) the concentration of solute in the tubular fluid, (3) the permeability of the renal tubule to water and solute, and (4) the circulating levels of ADH. About 15 per cent of the filtered water enters the distal tubule. A variable fraction of this water is reabsorbed by the distal tubules and collecting ducts. Absorption of this final fraction is controlled by antidiuretic hormone (ADH), which serves as the main regulator of the osmolality of body fluids. ADH is synthesized by nerve cells in the hypothalamus and liberated from their terminals in the posterior lobe and pituitary stalk. The major stimulus for the secretion of ADH into the circulation is an increase in plasma osmolality, mediated by osmoreceptors, which are exquisitely sensitive to changes in osmolality. The feedback system they provide helps to maintain the tonicity of plasma within a standard deviation of ± 2 mOsm per kilogram (a change of less than 1 per cent). Although changes in osmolality are the most sensitive and therefore the primary regulators of ADH release, alterations in ECF volume can modulate and sometimes override the effects of tonicity. However, secretion of ADH is not increased unless volume loss is greater than 10 per cent. Baroreceptor stimulation appears to mediate the increase in ADH secretion resulting from volume contraction. This effect is potentiated by elevated levels of circulating catecholamines, which act directly on these receptors. Angiotensin II, prostaglandins, and nicotine may also affect ADH release through activation of arterial baroreceptors. When a surfeit of body water develops, ADH release is inhibited and a dilute urine is excreted; when a water deficit is present, free water is reabsorbed and the urine becomes concentrated by mechanisms discussed previously.

The human kidney can dilute urine tenfold with respect to plasma (to about 30 mOsm per kilogram) but can concentrate it to a maximum of only fourfold with respect to plasma (to about 1200 mOsm per kilogram). The daily volume of urine depends on the intake of fluid and can be varied from 600 ml to over 24 liters. When a large load of water is ingested, the following events occur: (1) The osmolar concentration (osmolality) of plasma falls; (2) over the next 15 to 20 minutes ADH levels fall, and as a consequence the flow rate of urine increases, reaching a maximum in 45 to 60 minutes. The maximal increase in urine flow occurs when free water excretion is about 15 per cent of GFR.

ROLE OF THE KIDNEY IN THE PRESERVATION OF POTASSIUM BALANCE. The reader is referred to Ch. 77 for a detailed discussion of potassium balance and potassium distribution in body fluids.

The daily intake of potassium ranges from 50 to 150 mEq. Most of the potassium ingested is absorbed (less than 10 mEq is excreted in the stool); thus, maintenance of balance requires the daily renal excretion of an amount of potassium identical to that absorbed from the gut. Under physiologic conditions, approximately 70 per cent of the potassium filtered is reabsorbed in the proximal tubule. The loop of Henle reabsorbs the remaining 20 to 30 per cent. Distal segments of the nephron can both reabsorb and secrete potassium. The balance between distal reabsorption and secretion determines the net urinary excretion of this cation. On a normal diet (100 mEq per day) the kidneys excrete approximately 90 mEq of potassium per day. The potassium that appears in the urine is secreted in the distal tubule and collecting duct. The secretion of potassium is influenced by the potassium concentration in renal tubular cells and by the magnitude of the electrochemical gradient between cell interior and tubular lumen (see below). The factors that regulate potassium excretion in the urine are summarized in Table 75–2. If potassium intake is increased acutely, renal excretion of potassium can rise more than tenfold. About 50 per cent of the amount administered appears in the urine within 12 hours. The renal response to potassium deprivation is sluggish. Excretion falls to levels of 10 to 15 mEq per 24 hours only after 7 to 14 days of a potassium-free diet. During this interval a deficit of as much as 200 mEq of potassium may be incurred. In adults with increased catabolism (infections, surgery), the renal excretion of potassium may exceed the amount ingested.

Urinary excretion of potassium (Table 75–2) depends on its rate of secretion by the distal tubule. Increased net secretory rates of potassium in this segment could be due to (1) increased active uptake by the peritubular membrane leading to increased cell potassium concentration and increased passive leak across the luminal membrane, (2) increased permeability of the luminal membrane to potassium, (3) decreased active reabsorption of potassium by the luminal membrane, or (4) decreased electrical potential difference across the luminal membrane.

A high concentration of potassium in distal tubular cells is maintained through the action of a Na$^+$, K$^+$ exchange pump located in the peritubular membrane. Potassium uptake via this pump is stimulated by high plasma levels of potassium, alkalosis, aldosterone, and increased sodium reabsorption. All factors that raise cell potassium (increased peritubular pump activity, dehydration) favor its diffusion into the lumen. If the cellular potassium concentration falls (potassium deprivation, acidosis, dilution of body fluids), the rate of potassium translocation into the lumen falls and may be less than the potassium uptake across the luminal membrane. Under these conditions, net reabsorption of potassium may replace net potassium secretion.

TABLE 75–2. FACTORS THAT REGULATE POTASSIUM EXCRETION IN THE URINE

Condition		Effect on K$^+$ Excretion
Dietary K$^+$	High	Increase
	Low	Decrease
Serum levels of K$^+$	High	Increase
	Low	Decrease
Levels of mineralo- or glucocorticoid hormones	High	Increase
	Low	Decrease
Tubular fluid or urine flow rate	Fast	Increase
	Slow	Decrease
Sodium excretion in the urine	High	Increase
	Low	Decrease
Most diuretics		Increase
K$^+$-sparing diuretics (spironolactone, triamterene)		Decrease
Metabolic alkalosis		Increase
Metabolic acidosis		Decrease
Augmented urine excretion of impermeant anions (sulfate, carbenicillin)		Increase

The difference in electrical potential across the entire distal tubular cell is established by the active reabsorption of sodium and is about 50 mV (lumen negative to peritubular fluid). The cell interior is negative (–70 mV) in relation to the peritubular capillary. Thus, the luminal membrane potential difference is about 20 mV (cell negative to lumen). This electrical profile favors a greater leak of potassium across the luminal membrane than across the peritubular membrane. Thus, potassium is pumped into distal tubular cells and then leaks across the luminal membrane into the tubular lumen. Such passive translocation of potassium from the cell into the lumen depends not only on the electrical potential difference across the luminal membrane but also on the chemical concentration gradient. A decrease in luminal membrane potential difference (increased lumen electronegativity) or factors that increase cellular potassium or lower luminal potassium have been shown to augment potassium secretion.

Augmented sodium reabsorption in the distal tubule increases lumen electronegativity, which favors potassium secretion from the cell interior into the tubular fluid. Hence, increased distal sodium reabsorption will favor potassium excretion. For example, diuretic administration increases sodium delivery distally, which, in turn, increases potassium excretion, particularly in patients with secondary aldosteronism. Hyperkalemia increases potassium excretion by two mechanisms: It stimulates aldosterone secretion directly, and it also enhances renal secretion, presumably via increased cell content of potassium. Alkalosis enhances and acidosis depresses potassium secretion, probably by inducing corresponding changes in renal cell potassium. The rates of *distal tubular flow* also influence potassium excretion, presumably because of the rapid dissipation of the concentration of potassium in the tubular lumen at higher flow rates.

ROLE OF THE KIDNEY IN ACID-BASE BALANCE. The reader should consult the section on "Disturbances of Acid-Base Balance" in Ch. 77 for a detailed discussion of acid-base balance. The kidney maintains plasma pH in a physiologic range by regulating the concentration of plasma bicarbonate. This is accomplished by the excretion in the urine of 50 to 100 mEq of H$^+$ in the form of ammonium (NH$_4^+$) and titratable acid (the amount of alkali required to titrate the urine to the pH of plasma). Disodium phosphate (Na$_2$HPO$_4$) present in the filtrate is converted to NaH$_2$PO$_4$, which accounts for most of the titratable acid excreted in the urine. Net excretion of acid (titratable acid + ammonium excretion − bicarbonate excretion) equals the daily production of nonvolatile acids under physiologic conditions. Both the *reclamation* of filtered bicarbonate and the *regeneration* of bicarbonate depend on the secretion of H$^+$ from the tubular cells into the lumen. The secreted H$^+$ is generated within the tubular cells by the *carbonic anhydrase*–catalyzed hydration of CO$_2$ to H$_2$CO$_3$, which immediately dissociates into H$^+$ and HCO$_3^-$. The H$^+$ is secreted into the tubular fluid, and the bicarbonate, concomitantly produced intracellularly, enters the peritubular capillary. Thus, H$^+$ secretion results in addition of bicarbonate to plasma. When the H$^+$ secreted into the lumen combines with filtered bicarbonate, it forms H$_2$CO$_3$, which quickly dissociates to CO$_2$ and H$_2$O. As a consequence, a bicarbonate disappears from the lumen, and the net effect is bicarbonate reabsorption (reclamation).

At a physiologic GFR of 170 liters per day and a plasma bicarbonate level of 24 mEq per liter, the reabsorption of over 4000 mEq of bicarbonate requires the secretion of an equivalent amount of H$^+$, whereas the excretion of net acid requires the secretion of 50 to 100 mEq of H$^+$ daily (Table 75–3). The process of bicarbonate reclamation operates to reabsorb all the filtered bicarbonate below a critical serum concentration, the *bicarbonate threshold concentration*, which in adult humans is normally about 24 mEq per liter, essentially identical to the concentration of bicarbonate in plasma. When plasma bicarbonate concentration rises above this threshold, renal recla-

TABLE 75–3. ROLE OF THE KIDNEY IN ACID-BASE BALANCE

Function	mEq/24 hr
1. Reabsorption of filtered bicarbonate ("reclamation")	≅ 4000
2. Generation of new bicarbonate (net excretion of acid)	50–100
a. Ammonium excretion	35–65
b. Titratable acid excretion	15–35

mation is incomplete and the excess bicarbonate escapes into the urine, enabling the plasma bicarbonate concentration to return to the threshold level. Under physiologic conditions the virtually complete reabsorption of bicarbonate serves to preserve bicarbonate stores but does not replace the bicarbonate consumed in the buffering of nonvolatile acids. If the secreted H^+ combines with buffers, such as HPO_4^- or NH_3, a new bicarbonate ion (de novo synthesis) is added to the peritubular capillary blood. This results in replacement of the bicarbonate consumed in buffering the daily acid load (Table 75–3).

In the steady state, the net amount of H^+ excreted is equal to the H^+ load, about 50 to 100 mEq per day. At times, net acid excretion is absent or has a negative value. This occurs after ingestion of an alkaline load (bicarbonate or substances that can be metabolized to bicarbonate). Ammonium excretion accounts for two thirds and titratable acid for one third of the urinary excretion of acid. When the daily H^+ load increases (e.g., increased catabolism, infection), the rise in acid excretion by the kidney is usually due to increased ammonium excretion. Ammonia (NH_3), produced within the renal tubular cells from glutamine, diffuses into the peritubular capillary or lumen down its concentration gradient. In the lumen it combines with H^+ to form NH_4^+. As noted, each mole of NH_4^+ excreted will result in the de novo generation of 1 mole of bicarbonate. Thus, when metabolic acidosis develops and the need for regenerating bicarbonate increases, synthesis of ammonia and NH_4^+ excretion usually increase.

Hydrogen secretion occurs in both proximal and distal segments of the nephron. As the concentration of bicarbonate in the lumen decreases, the concentration of H^+ increases, and as a result a limitation is imposed on the net rate of H^+ secretion. The maximal H^+ gradient achievable between cell and collecting duct lumen is about 800:1 (luminal fluid pH of 4.5).

Factors That Regulate the Renal Secretion of Hydrogen Ions. The major factors that influence the renal secretion of H^+ are (1) *effective circulating volume*, (2) *arterial pH and P_{CO_2}*, (3) *plasma concentration of potassium*, and (4) *mineralocorticoids (aldosterone)*.

EFFECTIVE CIRCULATING VOLUME. Hydrogen ion secretion is increased by volume depletion (increased sodium reabsorption) and diminished by ECF volume expansion. Hydrogen secretion is stimulated also when significant amounts of nonreabsorbable anions, i.e., sulfate ions, are present in the distal nephron and when sodium reabsorption is enhanced by any mechanism. Thus, the effective circulating volume of the ECF and the amounts of nonreabsorbable anion accompanying sodium through the distal nephron are important determinants of renal H^+ secretion.

ARTERIAL pH AND P_{CO_2}. Net acid excretion is increased with acidosis and decreased with alkalosis. Acidosis, resulting from a decrease in the plasma concentration of bicarbonate (metabolic acidosis) or induced by an elevation in P_{CO_2} (respiratory acidosis), augments H^+ excretion and increases the renal synthesis of bicarbonate. Metabolic alkalosis (increased plasma bicarbonate) or respiratory alkalosis (decreased P_{CO_2}) has the opposite effects. The effects of arterial pH on net acid excretion are most likely mediated by changes in renal tubular cell pH. Elevations in arterial P_{CO_2} increase bicarbonate reabsorption, and a fall in arterial P_{CO_2} reduces bicarbonate reabsorption.

PLASMA POTASSIUM CONCENTRATION. Hypokalemia increases and hyperkalemia decreases bicarbonate reabsorption. These effects are due to changes in intracellular H^+ concentration induced by cation shifts between the ICF and the ECF. In hypokalemia, potassium leaves the cell and is replaced by H^+ and sodium. The increase in intracellular H^+ concentration (intracellular acidosis) leads to the enhanced H^+ secretion and bicarbonate reabsorption associated with potassium depletion. The opposite occurs with hyperkalemia.

ALDOSTERONE. Aldosterone stimulates secretion of both potassium and hydrogen in the distal nephron. Excess of aldosterone may cause metabolic alkalosis, and its deficiency may lead to metabolic acidosis by decreasing H^+ excretion.

ROLE OF THE KIDNEY IN MINERAL HOMEOSTASIS. The kidney regulates the homeostasis of minerals not only by modifying the excretion of phosphate, calcium, and magnesium (see below) but also by influencing the metabolism of vitamin D. Vitamin D_3 (cholecalciferol) is metabolized to 25(OH) cholecalciferol in the liver and subsequently to $1,25(OH)_2D_3$ and $24,25(OH)_2D_3$ in the kidney. The $1,25(OH)_2D_3$ is the calcemic hormone produced in the renal cortex in response to hypophosphatemia or elevated levels of parathyroid hormone (when hypocalcemia occurs), and $24,25(OH)_2D_3$ is produced preferentially when the balance of minerals is normal. The $1,25(OH)_2D_3$ increases absorption of calcium and phosphate from the gut as well as mineral mobilization from bone. The role of $24,25(OH)_2D_3$ is less well defined; it seems to promote bone mineralization and suppress parathyroid hormone release.

REGULATION OF PHOSPHORUS METABOLISM. The kidneys play a major role in maintaining the serum phosphorus concentration within narrow limits, about 3.0 to 4.5 mg per deciliter in adults. On an average diet, 1 gram of phosphorus is ingested daily, of which 700 mg is absorbed and the rest is excreted in the stool. The kidneys filter about 7 grams of phosphorus daily, of which 6.3 grams (90 per cent) is reabsorbed and 700 mg is excreted in the urine. As serum phosphorus and filtered load of phosphorus rise, the capacity to reabsorb phosphorus increases until a transport maximum (Tm) for phosphorus reabsorption is reached when serum phosphorus concentrations are between 6 and 9 mg per deciliter. Under physiologic conditions, about 70 per cent of the filtered phosphorus is reabsorbed in the proximal tubule and 10 to 15 per cent in the distal tubule and collecting ducts; thus, 5 to 20 per cent of the filtered phosphorus is excreted in the urine. In other words, the tubular reabsorption of phosphate (TRP) ranges normally from 80 to 95 per cent.

Numerous factors (the major ones being dietary phosphorus load and the serum levels of parathyroid hormone) affect the reabsorption of phosphorus. Phosphorus reabsorption approaches 100 per cent in patients fed a very low-phosphorus diet. In contrast, patients ingesting 2 to 3 grams of phosphorus daily can excrete 60 to 70 per cent of this amount in the urine. Changes in phosphorus intake affect phosphorus excretion directly and also by altering the levels of ionized calcium that modify the release of parathyroid hormone. Parathyroid hormone decreases phosphorus reabsorption in both proximal and distal segments of the nephron. An excess of parathyroid hormone may increase fractional excretion of phosphorus from a basal value of 10 per cent to 30 per cent or more. In the absence of parathyroid hormone the tubular capacity to reabsorb phosphorus is increased. Additional factors affect phosphorus reabsorption by the kidney. Volume expansion of the ECF, calcitonin, glucocorticoids, metabolic acidosis or alkalosis, and glycosuria increase urinary phosphorus excretion. On the other hand, administration of growth hormone and respiratory acidosis decrease phosphorus excretion. Vitamin D and its metabolites increase phosphorus reabsorption by the kidney.

RENAL REGULATION OF CALCIUM METABOLISM. Serum calcium concentrations in humans are maintained between 9 and 10 mg per deciliter despite wide variations in dietary calcium intake. Total serum calcium consists of ultrafilterable calcium (approximately 60 per cent of the total) and calcium bound to protein, primarily albumin. The ultrafilterable fraction includes both the ionized calcium (50 per cent of the total) and calcium complexed to citrate, bicarbonate, and phosphate, which represents 10 per cent of total serum calcium. Serum calcium levels are maintained relatively constant through modification of calcium absorption from the gastrointestinal tract, changes in renal calcium excretion, and mobilization of calcium from bone.

Approximately 1000 mg of calcium is ingested daily in the diet. About 800 mg appears in the stool (from unabsorbed dietary calcium and intestinal secretion) and 200 mg in the urine. The percentage of dietary calcium absorbed from the intestine increases when calcium intake is low and decreases when it is high. Parathyroid hormone and vitamin D participate in these adaptations. Thus, in patients fed a low-calcium diet, the development of mild and transient hypocalcemia increases the release of parathyroid hormone, which augments the renal conversion of $25(OH)D_3$ to $1,25(OH)_2D_3$. This latter compound increases intestinal calcium absorption and mobilizes calcium from bone, synergistically with parathyroid hormone. Thus, serum calcium returns toward normal. On the other hand, in patients fed a high-calcium diet, the mild hypercalcemia that may occur suppresses the release of parathyroid hormone, leading to decreased activity of the renal 1-hydroxylase enzyme and the preferential production of $24,25(OH)_2D_3$. This metabolite is less efficient than $1,25(OH)_2D_3$ in promoting calcium absorption from the intestine and in mobilizing calcium from the skeleton.

The kidneys filter approximately 10 grams of calcium per day, but usually less than 200 mg appears in the urine. Thus over 98 per cent of the filtered load is reabsorbed. Approximately 55 per cent of the filtered calcium is reabsorbed in the proximal tubule, 20 to 30 per cent in the loop of Henle, 10 to 15 per cent in the distal tubule, and 2 to 8 per cent in the terminal nephron, including the collecting duct. Most maneuvers that decrease sodium and fluid reabsorption in the proximal tubule (infusion of saline, administration of acetazolamide, or mild-to-moderate hypercalcemia) decrease calcium reabsorption in this segment as well. The reabsorption of calcium in the loop of Henle also parallels sodium reabsorption. It is only distal to the loop of Henle that calcium and sodium are influenced separately and independently.

Parathyroid hormone stimulates the renal absorption of calcium and decreases urinary calcium excretion. Acute parathyroidectomy increases calcium excretion despite a fall in total serum calcium and hence in the filtered load of calcium. However, the degree of calciuria declines when the plasma concentration of calcium falls below 7 mg per deciliter. Pharmacologic doses of vitamin D usually increase intestinal absorption of calcium and bone resorption, leading to increases in serum calcium, the filtered load of calcium, and urinary calcium excretion. Metabolic acidosis or phosphate depletion produces hypercalciuria. Both furosemide and ethacrynic acid inhibit sodium and calcium transport in the thick ascending limb of Henle's loop and increase calcium excretion. Chronic administration of thiazides results in natriuresis and hypocalciuria. This effect may be due to contraction of ECF volume and increased calcium reabsorption in the proximal segments. In addition, thiazides may potentiate the effect of parathyroid hormone on calcium reabsorption in the distal segment.

RENAL REGULATION OF MAGNESIUM METABOLISM. Total body magnesium is approximately 2000 mEq (or 25 grams). About 60 per cent of total body magnesium is found in bone. Another 20 per cent is present in muscle. Only a small fraction (about 1 per cent) is present in the ECF. The normal plasma concentration of magnesium in humans is 1.7 to 2.2 mg per deciliter, of which 80 per cent is ultrafilterable and the remainder protein bound. Most of the ultra-

filterable magnesium is ionized. Roughly 300 mg or 25 mEq of magnesium is ingested daily in the diet. About two thirds of this amount appears in the stool and one third is eliminated in the urine. The kidney filters about 2 grams of magnesium daily, and approximately 100 mg (5 per cent) appears in the urine; thus, 95 per cent of the filtered magnesium is reabsorbed. Renal excretion of magnesium can be reduced to less than 0.5 per cent of the filtered load during magnesium deprivation. On the other hand, during infusion of magnesium or among patients with advanced chronic renal insufficiency the kidney can excrete 40 to 70 per cent of the filtered magnesium. The proximal tubules reabsorb about 20 to 30 per cent of the filtered magnesium, with 50 to 60 per cent being reabsorbed in the loop of Henle. Expansion of the ECF volume, produced by infusion of saline or chronic administration of mineralocorticoids, reduces the reabsorption of magnesium. A diet deficient in magnesium or the administration of parathyroid hormone enhances the reabsorption of magnesium in the thick ascending limb of Henle's loop. Infusions of calcium, ingestion of alcohol, administration of glucose, diets containing large amounts of magnesium, and diuretics such as furosemide or ethacrynic acid increase the urinary excretion of magnesium.

OTHER NONEXCRETORY FUNCTIONS OF THE KIDNEY

In addition to its role in the secretion of renin and the metabolism of vitamin D already discussed, the kidney has several other nonexcretory functions.

REGULATION OF THE RED BLOOD CELL MASS. *Erythropoietin* promotes the differentiation, proliferation, and maturation of red blood cell precursors in the bone marrow. The site of synthesis of this glycoprotein within the kidney has not been clearly defined, but the juxtaglomerular cells have been implicated. The stimulus to increased erythropoietin production by the kidney appears to be decreased renal oxygen tension or decreased renal perfusion (anemia, hypoxia, renal ischemia) or circulatory alterations induced by vasoconstrictors such as norepinephrine, angiotensin, or vasopressin. Increased erythropoietin levels may be seen in association with renal artery stenosis, renal cysts, renal cell carcinoma, and hydronephrosis and after renal transplantation. Production of erythropoietin decreases with hyperoxia or an excess red blood cell volume.

RENAL METABOLISM OF PLASMA PROTEINS AND PEPTIDE HORMONES. The kidney is an important catabolic site for low molecular weight proteins (less than 50,000) but not for proteins with a molecular weight exceeding 68,000 (e.g., albumin, immunoglobulins).

Low molecular weight proteins are filterable. In the absence of tubular reabsorption they would be excreted quantitatively in the urine. Reabsorption of proteins or their catabolic products by the kidney prevents their loss in the urine, thereby conserving nutritionally important components. The proteins catabolized by the kidney are broken down to amino acids or polypeptides prior to return into the renal venous blood. The kidney, therefore, contributes to the regulation of their concentrations in plasma and precludes extensive loss of protein components in the urine.

In some patients with abnormalities of renal tubular function, low molecular weight proteins may appear in the urine in the absence of albumin owing to decreased tubular reabsorption. Conversely, in patients with reduced GFR the fractional catabolic rate of low molecular weight proteins (lysozyme, ribonuclease, beta$_2$-microglobulins, insulin, proinsulin, gastrin, glucagon, parathyroid hormone, Bence Jones protein, retinol binding protein, and growth hormone) is decreased and their levels in plasma are elevated.

Insulin, parathyroid hormone, and glucagon are catabolized by the kidney by filtration and subsequent tubular reabsorption as well as by peritubular uptake.

The catabolism of albumin, immunoglobulins, and larger

plasma proteins is relatively low, with the kidney accounting for less than 5 per cent of their fractional catabolic rate, unless the nephrotic syndrome is present, in which case albumin catabolism could be significantly increased owing to both urinary losses and increased tubular degradation.

THE KALLIKREIN-KININ SYSTEM. Kallikrein is a peptidase produced in various tissues, including the kidney, which acts on a specific substrate (kininogen) to split off a peptide, kinin. The kinin is destroyed by plasma and tissue peptidases (kininases). Kinins are potent vasodilators. The renal kallikrein-kinin system may constitute a local hormonal mechanism involved in the regulation of renal blood flow and sodium excretion. Renal kallikrein is probably produced by the cortex and excreted into the urine. It acts on a kininogen substrate to produce the potent vasodilator decapeptide (kallidin). Kallikrein excretion is augmented by reduced sodium intake. In contrast, high sodium intake decreases it. Administration of mineralocorticoids increases the excretion of kallikrein, and the increased kallikrein excretion of a low-salt diet is blocked by aldosterone antagonists (spironolactones). However, the role of the renal kallikrein system in sodium homeostasis is not yet established.

RENAL PROSTAGLANDINS. The prostaglandins are 20-carbon unsaturated fatty acids. Both vasodilator prostaglandins (PGE_2, prostacyclin, or PGI_2) and vasoconstrictor substances (thromboxanes) are synthesized in renal cortex (by arteries and glomeruli) and medulla (by interstitial and collecting duct cells) from free arachidonic acid, released from phospholipids. Renal prostaglandins may play a role in control of blood flow and GFR and in sodium and water excretion. They affect renin secretion as well. Prostaglandins may also modulate phosphorus transport and regulate renal ammonia synthesis. Their synthesis is stimulated by bradykinin, angiotensin II, ADH, and catecholamines. The last substances are vasoconstrictors that tend to diminish renal plasma flow. Therefore when constrictor stimuli are operative, renal prostaglandin production may increase, resulting in maintenance of renal blood flow.

Two other pathways of arachidonic acid metabolism have been described recently in the kidney: (1) an NADPH-dependent mono-oxygenase pathway that leads to the formation of 19- and 20-hydroxyeicosatetranoic acid (19-HETE and 20-HETE), 19-ketoarachidonic acid, and 1,20-dicarboxylic acid; and (2) a calcium-dependent lipoxygenase pathway with synthesis of 15-HETE, 12-HETE, and leukotrienes. The physiologic or pathophysiologic importance of these pathways is unknown, but it should be remembered that the HETE's are potent chemotactic compounds and, therefore, may play a role in inflammatory glomerular disease. Leukotrienes are known to contract vascular and nonvascular smooth muscle and enhance vascular permeability. Thus, they may play a role in the control of renal blood flow and GFR.

Brenner BM, Dworkin LK, Ichikawa I: Glomerular ultrafiltration. In Brenner BM, Rector JC (eds.): The Kidney. 3rd ed. Philadelphia, W. B. Saunders Company, 1986, pp 124–144. *A lucid chapter written by investigators who have made important contributions to our understanding of glomerular physiology.*

Dunn MJ: Renal prostaglandins. In Klahr S, Massry SG (eds.): Contemporary Nephrology. Vol III. New York, Plenum Publishing Company, 1985, pp 143–190. *A clear review of the role of arachidonic acid metabolites in health and disease.*

Jackson EK, Branch RA, Margolius HS, et al.: Physiological functions of the renal prostaglandins, renin and kallikrein systems. In Seldin DW, Giebisch G (eds.): The Kidney: Physiology and Pathophysiology. New York, Raven Press, 1985, pp 613–644. *An excellent chapter on intrarenal hormones and their mechanisms of action.*

Klahr S, Hruska KA: Effects of parathyroid hormone on the renal reabsorption of phosphorus and divalent cations. In Peck WB (ed.): Bone and Mineral Research. Vol 2. Amsterdam, Elsevier, 1983, pp 65–124. *A detailed view of phosphorus and calcium reabsorption in the kidney and its control by hormones and other factors.*

Lang F, Messner G, Rehwald W: Electrophysiology of sodium-coupled transport in proximal renal tubules. Am J Physiol 250 (Renal Fluid Electrol Physiol 19):F953, 1986. *A recent editorial review with up-to-date references on the coupling of sodium transport to that of other solutes.*

Tisher CC, Madsen KM: Anatomy of the kidney. In Brenner BM, Rector JC (eds.): The Kidney. 3rd ed. Philadelphia, W. B. Saunders Company, 1986, pp 3–60. *An authoritative and clearly written review of kidney structure.*

Valtin H: Renal Function: Mechanisms Preserving Fluid and Solute Balance in Health. 2nd ed. Boston, Little, Brown and Company, 1983. *This book presents the essential elements in renal fluid and electrolyte physiology, which every medical student should master.*

76 INVESTIGATIONS OF RENAL FUNCTION
Vincent W. Dennis

Methods are available to assess the functional integrity of the glomerular ultrafiltration barrier; the presence of urogenital inflammation; the overall rate of glomerular filtration; the ability to dilute, concentrate, or acidify urine; and the ability to conserve or to excrete specific solutes. Measurements of certain values in blood and urine detect abnormalities in renal function and may occasionally point to specific etiologies, but a final diagnosis usually requires direct or indirect visualization of the kidneys and urogenital system or morphologic examination of renal tissue.

PROTEINURIA. Increased urinary excretion of protein is one of the most common and most easily detected signs of renal disease. The normal excretion rate of urinary protein is less than 150 mg per 24 hours for adults, but values as high as 300 mg per 24 hours may occur in apparently healthy adolescents. The normal composition of urinary protein includes about 40 per cent albumin, 40 per cent tissue proteins originating from renal and other urogenital tissues, 15 per cent immunoglobulins and their fragments, and 5 per cent other plasma proteins. Abnormalities may occur in both the quantity and the composition of urinary proteins.

Urinary protein is usually detected by a colorimetric test ("dipstick test"), which depends on the ability of proteins, especially albumin, to alter the color reaction of a pH-sensitive dye. Such qualitative tests may detect protein concentrations as low as 15 mg per deciliter and result in a positive test if a normal amount of protein is present in a concentrated volume of urine. Conversely, abnormal rates of protein excretion may remain undetected in large volumes of dilute urine. It is therefore important to have some estimate of the degree of urine concentration when considering the significance of a positive qualitative test for protein. A positive qualitative test for urinary protein usually warrants quantification of the absolute protein excretion rate per 24 hours. Alternatively, the protein-creatinine ratio of a random daytime urine sample correlates well with values from 24-hour collections. The protein-creatinine method is quicker but less precise (Fig. 76–1). Proteinuria usually results from (1) elevated plasma concentration of normal or abnormal proteins, (2) increased glomerular permeability, (3) decreased tubular reabsorption of normally filtered proteins, and (4) alterations in renal hemodynamics (Table 76–1).

Overflow Proteinuria. Changes in plasma protein concentrations may alter the rates of protein excretion by both the normal and the abnormal kidney. This type of proteinuria may occur from the presence in plasma of increased concentrations of proteins not normally present in significant amounts. Examples include light-chain immunoglobulin fragments such as Bence Jones protein associated with plasma cell disorders (see Ch. 163) or myoglobin associated with rhabdomyolysis. The presence of increased concentrations of abnormal proteins in either plasma or urine may be confirmed by electrophoresis. Changes in the concentration of normal plasma proteins may also influence passage across the *abnormal* glomerular capillary wall. For example, increases or de-

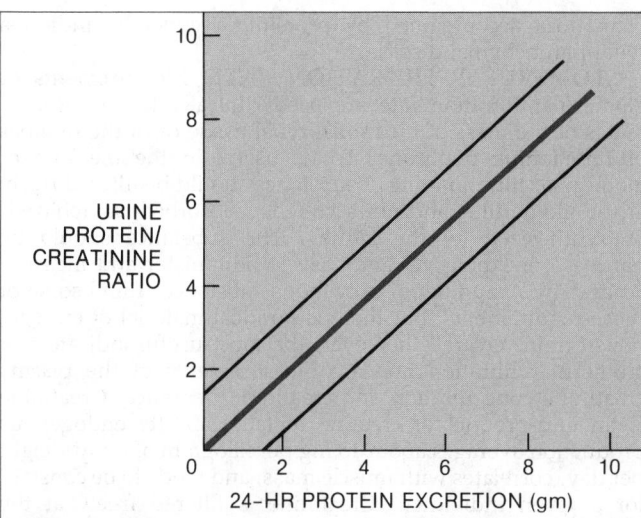

FIGURE 76–1. The lines and bands represent the 95 per cent confidence levels for the relationship between the protein-to-creatinine ratio in a random daytime urine sample to the amount of protein excreted in 24 hours.

creases in the plasma concentration of albumin may increase or decrease its rate of urinary excretion without necessarily indicating improvement or worsening of the renal conditions that led to proteinuria.

Increased Glomerular Permeability. The glomerular capillary wall consists of capillary endothelium, basement membrane, visceral epithelium, and mesangium. Each of these four anatomic components contributes directly or indirectly to the formation and maintenance of the functional ultrafiltration barrier that limits the passage of proteins into the urinary space. The glomerular capillary wall restricts the passage of plasma proteins according to their size (steric hindrance) and surface charge (electrostatic hindrance). At any given molecular size, negative charges on the glomerular capillary basement membrane hinder the passage of negatively charged molecules more than positively charged molecules.

A number of systemic and primary renal diseases may affect one or more glomerular structures and thereby increase the effective permeability of the glomerular capillary wall to proteins. The degree of proteinuria may range from 0.2 to greater than 20 grams per 24 hours. Proteinuria that exceeds about 3 to 5 grams of normal plasma protein per 24 hours provides direct evidence of increased effective permeability of the glomerular capillary wall, since these amounts exceed those that may be filtered by the normal glomerulus and reabsorbed by the renal tubules. Such massive losses of plasma proteins may be responsible for changes in plasma oncotic pressure and thereby set in motion the events that are manifest clinically as the nephrotic syndrome (see Ch. 81).

Because of its low molecular weight and its dominance among plasma proteins, albumin is typically the major urinary protein in this type of proteinuria. However, the relative proportion of albumin in the urine, even if corrected for changes in its proportion in plasma, is lower in some forms of renal diseases than in others. *Selective proteinuria* refers to the ability of the glomerulus to retain higher molecular weight proteins despite increased filtration of low molecular weight proteins. A highly selective proteinuria therefore consists almost exclusively of increased excretion of albumin, whereas a poorly selective proteinuria contains proportionately greater amounts of higher molecular weight proteins and is generally associated with severe disruption of the glomerular capillary wall. This selectivity may be attributed to the glomerulus only if the composition of urinary proteins is not affected significantly by downstream events such as tubular reabsorption. This requirement is presumably met with levels of proteinuria that exceed 3 to 5 grams per 24 hours, but the selectivity pattern of lesser amounts of proteinuria may be significantly influenced by tubular reabsorption. To define glomerular selectivity requires measurements of the relative clearances of specific proteins with increasing molecular weights such as albumin (69,000), transferrin (90,000), gamma globulin (150,000), and alpha$_2$-glycoprotein (820,000). Although attractive in theory and potentially useful as an index of the severity of glomerular damage, the techniques required to characterize the selectivity of proteinuria are generally too laborious and too imprecise to have achieved widespread clinical applicability. Nevertheless, heavy proteinuria characterized by the dominance of albumin and the absence of higher molecular weight globulins is typical of minimal change or nil lesion (see Ch. 81), whereas the detection of a nonselective pattern is highly suggestive of the presence of some other form of otherwise undefined glomerular disease.

Microalbuminuria refers to increases in albumin excretion that are detectable by sensitive immunoassay but not by current standard clinical techniques. The presence of microalbuminuria in diabetics may predict the development of diabetic nephropathy, whereas its absence may forecast a more favorable prognosis.

Tubular Proteinuria. Many polypeptides and low molecular weight proteins normally present in plasma are filtered freely at the glomerulus and are reabsorbed by the tubules. Examples include polypeptide hormones such as insulin, glucagon, and parathyroid hormone and plasma proteins smaller than 20,000 daltons. Once filtered, these proteins are absorbed by specific endocytic processes that bind and engulf the filtered proteins. The presence of tubular disorders, especially injuries that result from various antibiotics or heavy metals (see Ch. 82), may be associated with increased urinary excretion of low molecular weight proteins and relatively slight increases in the excretion of albumin (*tubular proteinuria*). This pattern is in marked contrast to the predominance of albumin in the urine of patients with glomerular disorders. Patients characterized clinically as having tubulointerstitial rather than glomerular diseases have increased urine protein excretion (generally less than 2 grams per 24 hours) and increased renal clearance of beta$_2$-microglobulin, especially relative to albumin. Beta$_2$-microglobulinuria is less likely to occur in those disease processes such as diabetes mellitus that cause proteinuria via effects on glomerular permeability. The clinical significance of tubular proteinuria is unclear at this time because

TABLE 76–1. TYPES OF PROTEINURIA*

Type	Mechanism	Quantity	Molecular Weight	Examples
Overflow	Increased filtration of abnormal plasma proteins across normal glomeruli	Variable (0.2 to >10g)	Low (<40,000)	Bence Jones proteinuria, myoglobinuria
Glomerular	Defective glomerular retention of normal plasma proteins	>3–5 grams	High (>68,000)	Glomerulonephritis, nephrotic syndrome
Tubular	Defective reabsorption of normally filtered plasma proteins	<2 grams	Low (<40,000)	Interstitial nephritis, antibiotic injury, heavy metals
Hemodynamic	Increased filtration and possibly decreased reabsorption	<2 grams	Variable (20,000–68,000)	Transient proteinuria, congestive heart failure, fever, seizures, exercise

*Values >150 mg per 24 hours.

there is still insufficient documentation of correlations between tubular proteinuria and detailed functional, biochemical, and morphologic descriptions of the underlying diseases in which it has been observed.

Proteinuria from Altered Renal Hemodynamics. Changes in protein excretion rate may also occur in response to changes in renal hemodynamics. Exercise, major motor seizures, change to the standing position, fever, and vasoactive agents such as renin, angiotensin, and norepinephrine increase urine protein excretion by mechanisms that seem related to reductions in renal blood flow. Changes in renal blood flow may also alter urine protein excretion in normal subjects as well as in those with abnormal rates of protein excretion. Possible mechanisms include local increases in protein concentration within the glomerular capillary, increased effective permeability of the glomerular capillary wall, increased transglomerular hydrostatic pressure, and increased effective filtration area. Hemodynamic increases in urine protein excretion are generally transient or additive to other causes of proteinuria.

LEUKOCYTURIA. The urinary leukocyte excretion rate in apparently healthy individuals ranges between 0 and 300,000 leukocytes per hour; rates greater than 400,000 per hour are generally regarded as abnormal. If appropriate cleansing precautions are used, there is no difference in leukocyte excretion rates between apparently healthy males and females or between urine samples obtained from suprapubic puncture and midstream urine.

In practice, leukocyte excretion rates are estimated indirectly by microscopic examination of urinary sediment resuspended after centrifugation of approximately 10 ml of urine. Abnormal leukocyturia probably exists when more than 5 white blood cells occur per high-power field. However, about 20 per cent of urine specimens from patients excreting more than 400,000 white blood cells per hour may demonstrate fewer than 5 leukocytes per high-power field. The indirect method thus underestimates the prevalence of abnormal leukocyturia, although increased numbers of white blood cells per high-power field appear to correspond well to increased rates of leukocyte excretion. Leukocyturia results frequently from urinary tract infection (see Ch. 86) but may also indicate other causes of inflammation, such as tubulointerstitial diseases (see Ch. 82).

HEMATURIA. The detection of hematuria is aided by the widespread use of the multifunctional "dipstick," which includes a section impregnated with orthotolidine. The test is sufficiently sensitive to detect the equivalent of greater than 10,000 red blood cells per milliliter of urine but is negative in normal individuals despite the wide range of red blood cell excretion rates. A positive orthotolidine test may also occur in the presence of free hemoglobin or myoglobin in urine. Free hemoglobin in the urine generally results from the lysis of red blood cells in the urine, but may also reflect free hemoglobin in the plasma. When indicated, this question can be resolved by direct measurements of plasma hemoglobin and haptoglobin concentrations. Myoglobin in the urine is detected by the differential precipitation of hemoglobin with ammonium sulfate, by spectrophotometry of the ferricyanide derivatives of hemoglobin and myoglobin, by the co-migration on paper electrophoresis of myoglobin with hemoglobin C, or, preferably, by direct immunoassay of myoglobin in plasma or urine. Myoglobinuria is usually accompanied by marked increases in plasma concentrations of creatine phosphokinase (CPK).

As with leukocytes, the presence of red blood cells in urine is quantified in terms of red blood cells per high-power field and is normally 0 to 1 in males but may be slightly higher in females. The persistent presence in males or females of even small numbers of red blood cells in urine is cause for concern and may indicate the presence of a coagulopathy, hemoglobinopathy, renal parenchymal disease, tumor, trauma, or inflammation anywhere along the renal and urinary tract.

Hematuria accompanied by proteinuria generally indicates renal parenchymal disease.

GLOMERULAR FILTRATION RATE. Measurements of glomerular filtration rate are used clinically largely as estimates of the mass of functional renal tissue or of the number of functioning nephrons. To be useful in the measure of glomerular filtration rate, a substance should be filtered freely at the glomerulus and not secreted, reabsorbed, catabolized, or synthesized by the kidney. The substance should be harmless, inexpensive, and easy to administer and measure accurately. A number of exogenous substances fulfill some of these requirements, but there is no ideal material of endogenous origin. Overall, however, the most useful indicators of glomerular filtration rate are measurements of the plasma creatinine concentration and creatinine clearance. Creatinine is an end-product of creatine metabolism. Its endogenous production averages about 15 mg per kilogram of body weight per day, correlates with muscle mass, and tends to be constant for a given individual. Creatinine is filtered freely at the glomerulus and is secreted by the proximal tubule to an extent that may increase with elevated plasma concentration. The excretion rate of creatinine thus reflects the combined effects of filtration and secretion, and normally the clearance of creatinine exceeds the glomerular filtration rate. The secretion of creatinine is inhibited by certain drugs such as cimetidine and trimethoprim, which may increase the plasma creatinine concentration without affecting glomerular filtration rate. Ketonemia may cause spurious increases in measurements of plasma creatinine because acetoacetate interferes with certain automated analytic techniques (Table 76–2).

Figure 76–2 shows the theoretic relationship between plasma creatinine concentration and creatinine clearance and the relationship between creatinine clearance and other measures of glomerular filtration rate, such as inulin clearance. The relationship between plasma creatinine and creatinine clearance is described by a rectangular hyperbola. This reflects the mathematical reality that values on the horizontal axis are determined by the reciprocals of values on the vertical axis, since the formula for creatinine clearance includes the serum creatinine concentration in the denominator. To the extent that creatinine clearance and glomerular filtration rate are equivalent, the same ideal relationship should apply between observed glomerular filtration rate and plasma creatinine concentration, but deviations from this ideal occur.

In the normal range, measurements of plasma creatinine concentration include a significant and variable component of noncreatinine chromogen that is not excreted in the urine. This overestimate offsets in part the error introduced by the renal secretion of creatinine, so that in this range creatinine clearances correlate well with other measures of glomerular filtration rate.

In the presence of renal failure, plasma creatinine concentration rises much more so than that of noncreatinine chromogens, and thus measurements of plasma creatinine concentration approach the true creatinine concentration. Moreover, in the presence of moderate degrees of renal failure, the secretory component of creatinine excretion may increase until the glomerular filtration rate falls below about 10 ml per minute. For these reasons, in the presence of moderate renal failure the clearance of creatinine tends to overestimate the glomerular filtration rate. In advanced renal

TABLE 76–2. FACTORS THAT AFFECT PLASMA CREATININE CONCENTRATION WITHOUT CHANGES IN GLOMERULAR FILTRATION RATE

Increase	
Ketonemia	Spurious increase in automated measurements by acetoacetate
Cimetidine, trimethoprim	Inhibition of tubular secretion
Decrease	
Muscle wasting	Reduced creatinine production

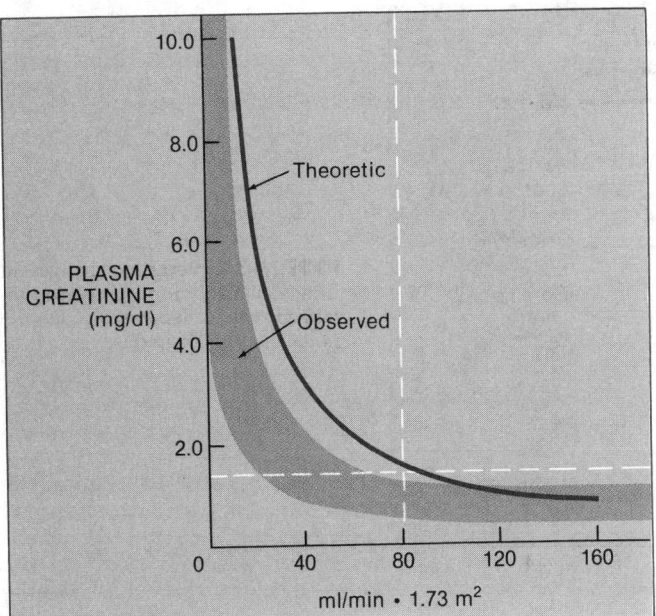

FIGURE 76–2. Relationship between plasma creatinine concentrations and various measures of glomerular filtration rate. The solid line depicts the theoretical relationship between plasma creatinine concentration and creatinine clearance. The color screened area represents the relationship between plasma creatinine and independent measures of glomerular filtration rate. The dashed lines denote the limits of normal values. Note the extent to which normal plasma creatinine values may occur in spite of reduced filtration rates.

failure (glomerular filtration rate less than 10 ml per minute), creatinine clearance again approximates the glomerular filtration rate (Fig. 76–2). Despite these shortcomings, measurements of plasma creatinine concentration and clearance of endogenous creatinine are useful indices of filtration rate largely because of the ease with which repeated observations may be made in individual patients along the course of their disease.

The most accurate measures of glomerular filtration rate in humans are obtained with the use of a number of exogenous substances such as inulin or a variety of radioisotopically labeled compounds such as ^{125}I-iothalamate. Standard clearance techniques for these measurements require injection of the compound to a steady-state plasma concentration and then the timed collection of urine.

The blood urea nitrogen (BUN) concentration is an imperfect quantitative indicator of renal filtration despite its frequent use for this purpose. Urea is synthesized by the liver from ammonia derived from the catabolism of proteins and amino acids. Urea production is therefore variable and is influenced by hepatic as well as dietary conditions. At the kidneys, urea is filtered, reabsorbed, and secreted. Reabsorption dominates, but the rate of reabsorption varies with the degree of hydration. Those conditions, such as dehydration, that tend to increase the renal reabsorption of volume also increase the reabsorption of urea. Accordingly, blood urea nitrogen concentration may increase without any abnormality in renal function. Conversely, in the presence of renal excretory failure and reduced filtration rate, the blood urea nitrogen concentration may be influenced significantly by the degree of dietary protein intake. For these reasons, measurement of plasma creatinine concentration provides a more reliable index of renal filtration rate than the BUN. The BUN is used mainly to quantify the balance between the accumulation and excretion of nitrogenous metabolites (i.e., the degree of uremia), especially in the presence of more than moderate reductions in glomerular filtration rate.

RENAL CONCENTRATING AND DILUTING ABILITY. The total solute concentration of urine is generally assessed clinically by measurement of urinary specific gravity, which relates the weight of a unit volume of urine to an equal volume of water. Because of its simplicity, this technique has persisted despite well-recognized deficiencies. Errors of technique relate primarily to poor calibration of the hygrometer, but even in the absence of faulty technique the specific gravity of urine provides only a rough indication of urine osmolality. For example, urines that contain high concentrations of urea have lower specific gravities than expected for their osmolality, and urines that contain higher density solutes, such as glucose, iodinated contrast material, or protein, have higher specific gravities relative to their osmolalities. Within these limitations, however, there is a useful correlation between the specific gravity and osmolality of urine such that urinary osmolality in milliosmoles per kilogram of water may be estimated as 40 times the increase in specific gravity of urine above the value of water, which is 1.000. Thus, urine with a specific gravity of 1.007 would have an estimated osmolality of 280 mOsm, similar to that of plasma, and urine with a specific gravity of 1.020 would be distinctly concentrated, with an estimated osmolality of 800 mOsm. Nonetheless, measurements of urine specific gravity represent only crude estimates of osmolality, and, when indicated, accurate measures of urine osmolality may be made easily by measurement of freezing-point depression in a cryoscopic osmometer.

Maximal urine concentrating ability is measured by restricting fluid intake until the patient loses a minimum of 3 per cent or a maximum of 5 per cent body weight, or until three consecutive urine specimens show no further increase in osmolality. These results are usually achieved within 16 hours of fluid restriction but may occur much earlier in patients with severe inability to conserve water. Once either one of these end-points is achieved, additional information may be obtained by the subcutaneous administration of 5 units of aqueous vasopressin to determine if any further increase in urine osmolality can be achieved. Normal subjects achieve maximal urine osmolality of 1000 ± 200 (SD) mOsm without further change after vasopressin. Patients who have complete or incomplete defects in antidiuretic hormone secretion, nephrogenic diabetes insipidus, or psychogenic polydipsia will have abnormal and distinctive patterns of response (Fig. 76–3).

Maximum diluting capacity of the kidney is assessed by the rapid administration of 1200 ml of water by mouth to a fasting subject. The osmolality of three hourly urine specimens is measured and should achieve values lower than 80 mOsm or specific gravity of 1.002. Measurements of the rate or extent of excretion of the administered water are quite variable and are not generally useful. Both maximal diluting and maximal concentrating ability of the kidney may be impaired by diuretics, especially potent loop diuretics such as furosemide and ethacrynic acid, and by diuretic states such as glucosuria.

ACIDIFICATION CAPACITY. The urine is normally more acidic than body fluids because of the endogenous production and renal excretion of nonvolatile acids derived primarily from sulfate and phosphate contained in dietary protein. Even at low pH, however, the amount of acid excreted as free hydrogen ion is negligible, and most hydrogen ion is excreted in the form of ammonium or titratable acids. For these reasons, the pH of a random specimen of urine provides only limited information about renal function and essentially no reliable information about the systemic acid-base status.

Assessment of the renal acidification capacity is accomplished by the *ammonium chloride tolerance test*. The basis of this test is to induce mild metabolic acidosis by the administration of ammonium chloride by mouth and to measure the maximal depression in urinary pH, maximal excretion rate of ammonium and titratable acid, and the percentage of excretion of the administered hydrogen ion equivalent. Because the purpose of the ammonium chloride is to induce metabolic acidosis, its administration is not necessary if acidosis is

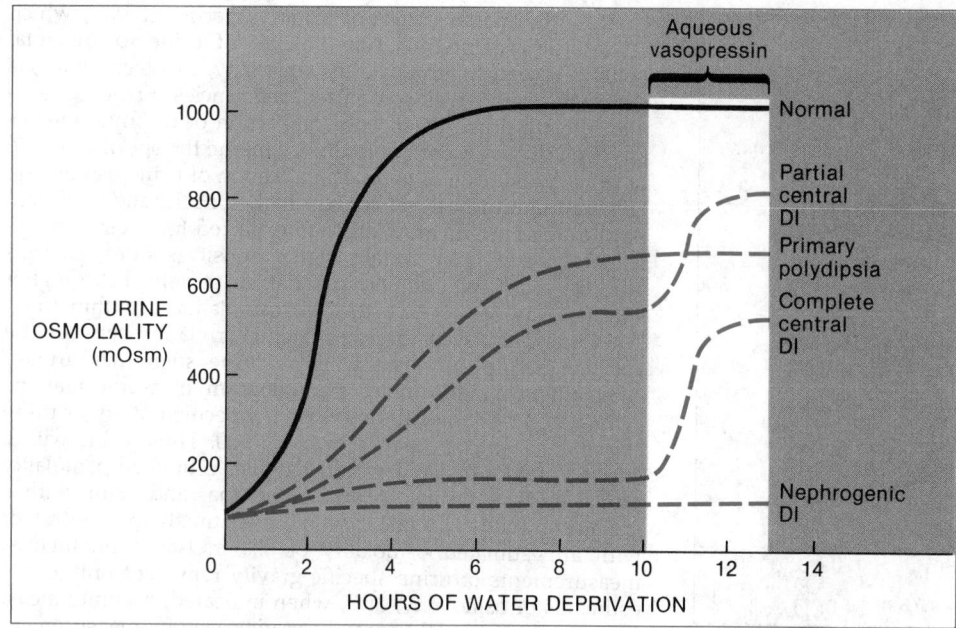

FIGURE 76–3. Patterns of changes in urine osmolality in response to prolonged water deprivation. DI denotes diabetes insipidus.

present spontaneously. Indications for the ammonium chloride test are generally restricted to those conditions, usually suspected abnormalities in distal tubular function, that are associated with only mild reductions in glomerular filtration rate. Ammonium chloride, 0.1 gram per kilogram, is administered by mouth, and urine is collected hourly for six to eight hours. A normal response is to achieve a urinary pH of 5.4 or less and to excrete at least 30 per cent of the administered hydrogen ion equivalent. An abnormal response consists of failure to acidify the urine below pH 5.4 despite a measured reduction in arterial pH. This indicates a defect in maximal acidification capacity. The ammonium chloride tolerance test is not generally performed in patients with renal insufficiency, but, if performed, these patients usually achieve reduction in the urinary pH below 5.4, although there is reduced excretion of ammonium and titratable acid.

URINARY ELECTROLYTES. Measurements of urinary sodium, potassium, and chloride may provide important information but only in a limited set of clinical circumstances. Two types of measurements are made. The absolute daily excretion of sodium, potassium, or chloride (milliequivalents per day) is derived from the electrolyte concentration of a 24-hour collection of urine. Such measurements provide quantification of the daily intake of these electrolytes provided that two requirements are met. First, total body weight must be constant to indicate balance between intake and output. Second, electrolyte excretion must be limited to the urine, and losses via the gastrointestinal tract or skin must be negligible. Under these conditions, the daily excretion of sodium, potassium, or chloride will reflect the dietary intake, but this information has only limited clinical value.

Measurement of the *concentration* of sodium, potassium, or chloride in a random urine sample may provide information of importance in certain circumstances such as the evaluation of hyponatremia, acute oliguria, volume depletion, hypokalemia, and metabolic alkalosis. In the evaluation of hyponatremia, a urinary sodium concentration less than 10 mEq per liter indicates the presence of reduced effective extracellular volume with an appropriate increase in mineralocorticoid and antidiuretic hormone (ADH) activity that leads to the renal retention of sodium and solute-free water. Higher urinary sodium concentrations indicate significant renal losses of sodium such as might occur from diuretics or, less commonly, from mineralocorticoid or glucocorticoid insufficiency or with volume expansion from the inappropriate secretion of ADH.

Similarly, in the evaluation of patients with reduced extracellular volume, urinary sodium concentrations greater than 10 to 20 mEq per liter indicate that the kidney is participating in the loss of sodium and volume, perhaps because of renal or adrenal insufficiency, whereas urinary sodium concentrations less than 5 to 10 mEq per liter indicate that losses of sodium and volume are occurring via extrarenal routes.

In the setting of acute oliguria, urine sodium concentration greater than 20 to 40 mEq per liter occurs frequently with acute renal failure or incomplete obstruction, whereas urine sodium concentrations are generally less than 20 mEq per liter in the presence of severe volume depletion (prerenal azotemia), acute glomerulonephritis, congestive heart failure, coexistent liver disease, or acute renal failure from radiocontrast material or acute rejection (Ch. 78). As is often the case, however, these values may be modified by many factors, including the administration of diuretics, and urine sodium concentrations are not generally regarded as sufficiently discriminatory to be useful in the differential diagnosis of acute oliguria.

The urine potassium concentration may be useful in the evaluation of unexplained hypokalemia. In the presence of hypokalemia, urine potassium concentrations greater than 20 mEq per liter indicate significant renal losses such as might occur from diuretics, increased mineralocorticoid activity, or magnesium deficiency. Urine potassium concentrations less than 10 mEq per liter indicate that the hypokalemia may be related to gastrointestinal losses such as may occur from the surreptitious use of laxatives or may indicate changes in plasma potassium concentration without potassium deficits such as may occur with hypokalemic periodic paralysis (see Ch. 516).

Urine chloride concentrations provide important information in the evaluation of metabolic alkalosis. Persistent metabolic alkalosis results most often from the depletion of chloride via the gastrointestinal tract or urine. In the presence of metabolic alkalosis, urine chloride concentrations greater than 10 mEq per liter suggest the presence of diuretic-induced increases in chloride excretion, severe depletion of potassium, Bartter's syndrome, or increased adrenocortical hormone activity. On the other hand, urine chloride concentrations less than 10 mEq per liter point to losses of chloride via extrarenal routes, usually vomiting, and indicate further that the metabolic alkalosis is likely to respond to replacement of volume and chloride.

IMAGING OF THE KIDNEYS AND UROGENITAL TRACT

Imaging techniques of importance in the evaluation of renal abnormalities include roentgenography, ultrasonography, radionuclide studies, and magnetic resonance imaging. These techniques are used (1) to visualize the number, size, and location of the kidneys; (2) to identify the presence and site of obstruction; (3) to detect and to characterize mass lesions; (4) to visualize renal arteries and veins; and (5) to guide percutaneous diagnostic and therapeutic interventions such as biopsy and nephrostomy. The choice of a technique is based on its relative simplicity, its safety, its potential to yield results that for a particular suspected disorder are neither falsely positive (lack of specificity) nor falsely negative (lack of sensitivity), and its potential to provide additional information not already available from previous studies.

ROENTGENOGRAPHIC STUDIES. The most simple radiologic study of the kidneys and urogenital system is the plain roentgenogram of the kidneys, ureter, and bladder (KUB), which will often reveal abnormal calcifications and may reveal renal size if not obscured by overlying bowel. If indicated, tomography may be necessary to determine the renal outlines.

Excretory Urogram. The excretory urogram, also known as the intravenous pyelogram, or IVP, is the standard radiologic method to detect anatomic abnormalities of the kidneys and ureters and to evaluate patients with renal abnormalities. The basic excretory urogram is performed by the intravenous injection of iodinated contrast material, which is filtered at the glomerulus and concentrated within the tubular lumina and collecting system by the renal reabsorption of volume. Visualization of the contrast material within the renal parenchyma yields a *nephrogram*, and visualization within the major collecting system yields a *pyelogram*. Each of these phases is dependent on the amount of radiocontrast material that is delivered to the kidneys and filtered and also on the degree of extraction of volume that concentrates the dye within the parenchyma and collecting system. Modern radiocontrast materials are not secreted. In view of these mechanisms, it is useful to limit hydration prior to an excretory urogram in an effort to increase the intrarenal concentration of the contrast material. In some patients, however, especially those with renal insufficiency, restriction of fluid intake prior to an excretory urogram appears to increase the rate of adverse reaction and is now deemed more harmful than beneficial.

A nephrogram normally appears within one to three minutes after injection of the contrast material. The nephrogram provides an opportunity to determine the number of kidneys, their size and configuration, and the possible presence of inhomogeneous areas or filling defects. In addition, the symmetric and timely appearance of nephrograms bilaterally provides qualitative information on the relative blood flow and filtration rate of each kidney. The pyelogram phase occurs within five minutes after the injection of dye as the nephrogram fades. This phase allows visualization of the caliceal system, ureters, and bladder and provides opportunities to detect abnormalities in shape, size, or drainage that might result from intrinsic defects or from extrinsic compression. Vascular or outflow obstructions may result in marked delays in the onset of both the nephrogram and the pyelogram phases.

Retrograde Pyelography. Retrograde pyelography is the direct injection of radiocontrast material into the ureter and upper urinary tract. The approach to this area is achieved via insertion of a ureteral catheter under direct visualization through cystoscopy. Some form of anesthesia may be required. Although retrograde pyelography was used frequently to assess renal size and to evaluate the possibility of ureteral obstruction in patients who presented with advanced renal failure, these questions are now resolved more readily with ultrasonography. Retrograde pyelography does provide more direct and improved visualization of the ureters and calices, and this visualization is useful in the localization and diagnosis of tumors and obstructions.

Antegrade Pyelography. Direct injection of radiocontrast material into a distended upper urinary tract or cyst may be achieved without the need for general anesthesia by the percutaneous injection of dye. This is performed under fluoroscopy or ultrasonography and requires the presence of a fluid-filled target such as a radiolucent or sonolucent mass. Antegrade pyelography may be useful to distinguish cysts from hydronephrosis.

Interventional Percutaneous Pyeloureteral Techniques. The combination of visualizing techniques such as roentgenographic fluoroscopy or ultrasonography and the availability of percutaneous catheters allows placement of a catheter in the renal pelvis, calices, or perirenal space if these spaces are distended by abnormal collections of fluid. Percutaneous catheter placement allows drainage and irrigation of pyonephrosis, abscesses, and obstructions, and placement of temporary nephrostomy catheters.

Renal Arteriography and Venography. The renal vasculature is visualized with radiocontrast material injected via a catheter introduced usually through the femoral vessels. Renal arteriography is performed most often to evaluate possible renal arterial stenosis as a cause or aggravating factor in systemic hypertension and to evaluate renal mass lesions. In general, cystic mass lesions are devoid of vasculature and may stretch and distort normal renal vessels and calices. Solid tumors are frequently vascular with irregular and erratic vessels that fill early as a blush of contrast material.

Renal venography is limited largely to searches for renal vein thrombosis and venous extension of renal cell carcinoma. Because renal venography requires the injection of dye against usually heavy renal venous outflow, turbulence may on occasion distort the distribution of dye and give the appearance of an intravascular filling defect. For this reason, renal venography is sometimes performed with intra-arterial infusion of epinephrine to reduce renal blood flow.

Digital Subtraction Angiography. Digital subtraction angiography uses high-quality image intensifiers and video camera recordings to visualize major arterial vessels following the rapid intravenous injection of radiocontrast material. Standard x-ray sources are used to produce sequential images at rates of about one per second beginning at the time of injection of radiocontrast material into a central or peripheral artery or vein. Images are intensified electronically, displayed on a video camera, digitized, and stored on magnetic tape in a memory system. Images obtained prior to the arrival of radiocontrast material at a particular vascular region are subtracted electronically from the subsequent images to enhance the contrast between vessels and other tissues. With regard to the detection of renal vascular diseases, digital subtraction venous angiography has an overall accuracy of about 70 to 80 per cent compared with conventional arteriography. Technically successful studies are generally sensitive enough to detect significant renal vascular lesions, but false-positive results may be as frequent as 20 to 30 per cent. Because venous angiography does not require an arteriotomy, it can be performed without hospitalization at considerably less cost than direct arteriography.

Computed Tomography. Computed tomography represents a sophisticated extension of roentgenography and may be performed with or without contrast material. Its usefulness in the evaluation of renal abnormalities consists primarily in its application as a tertiary mode after excretory urograms and ultrasonography to detect and localize mass lesions. Computed tomography may detect cystic masses as small as 0.5 cm in diameter, but the sensitivity is less for noncalcific solid masses (Fig. 76–4). Computed tomography is also useful to detect and evaluate obstruction and dilatation of the major collecting system in patients allergic to iodinated contrast

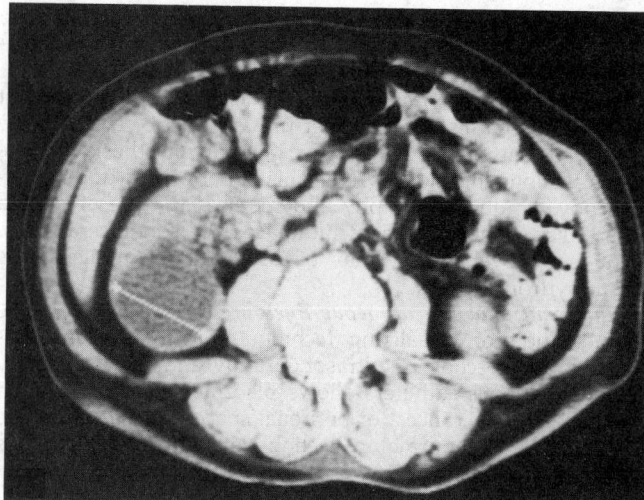

FIGURE 76–4. Computed tomography of the abdomen. The orientation is looking upward from toes to head. The right kidney is visualized at this level, but only a small portion of the left kidney is shown. There is a large, well-demarcated, homogeneous mass (white diagonal) in the right kidney which has the density of water rather than tissue. This is characteristic of a renal cyst.

material or for whom ultrasonography is inconclusive for technical reasons such as interference by bone, calcifications, or gas.

Adverse Effects of Urography. Two types of adverse effects should be considered in relation to the performance of excretory urograms, angiograms, or computed tomography with intravenous contrast material. First, any exposure to radiation is associated with a finite, statistical risk of permanent alteration in DNA. Depending on the question being asked, alternative modes of visualization such as ultrasonography might be considered in certain circumstances, especially those that involve pregnancy or repeated examinations over time.

The second type of adverse effect of excretory urography relates to toxic reactions to the iodinated contrast material. The overall incidence of adverse reactions to intravenous contrast is about 5 per cent for the general population and about 10 per cent for those with any allergies. The most common reactions involve nausea or urticaria; about 10 per cent of reactions will involve life-threatening events such as hypotension, laryngeal edema, or cardiac arrhythmias.

Excretory urography is a remarkably safe procedure, especially when performed in essentially healthy individuals. Not unexpectedly, excretory urography is less safe in individuals who are less healthy. Patients with diabetes mellitus and associated renal abnormalities are at increased risk to develop additional renal injury from excretory urography. Renal function may also deteriorate more frequently following excretory urography in patients with advanced age, marked dehydra-

tion, hyperuricemia, proteinuria, and pre-existing azotemia. Perhaps based on one or more of these factors, patients with multiple myeloma are at increased risk to develop adverse reactions to radiocontrast material. Appropriate precautions are indicated: consideration of alternative modes of visualization, attention to optimal hydration, and use of the minimal amount of contrast material consistent with an adequate examination.

ULTRASONOGRAPHY. Ultrasonography represents a major advance in the noninvasive visualization of the kidneys and genitourinary system. The acoustic impedance of a tissue to ultrasonic waves is the product of its density and the velocity of sound in that tissue. Significant differences in acoustic impedance occur among tissues that differ in their content of water, fat, collagen, minerals, and other solids, and interfaces between these tissues will reflect portions of the sound energy back to the transmitting transducer. These reflections are recorded as electrical signals and may be visualized by various display modes. The brightness modulation or B-mode displays echoes as bright dots plotted along the vertical and horizontal axes of an oscilloscope at positions corresponding to their point of origin in the area being scanned and, through so-called gray-scale processing, in degrees of brightness that correspond to their amplitude. So-called "real-time" imaging, or sonofluoroscopy, produces repetitive scans that give the impression of a continuous image.

Sonography can usually allow delineation of the renal outlines and measurement of the longitudinal and transverse dimensions (Fig. 76–5). Difficulties may arise from overlying ribs that may obscure the upper poles or from similarities in the acoustic impedance of perirenal fat and renal cortex such that the renal margins are poorly defined. The structures within the renal parenchyma are sufficiently similar that few intrarenal echoes are produced except by the vascular and caliceal structures of the renal pelvis. Advanced gray-scale examination of the kidney may permit identification of the cortex, medulla, arcuate vessels, and renal pyramids. The ureters are not normally visualized unless distended.

The primary applications of ultrasonography to the evaluation of renal abnormalities include assessment of renal size, especially in the presence of severe renal failure, evaluation of mass lesions detected by excretory urography, examination of the perinephric area, and detection and grading of hydronephrosis. Renal ultrasonography may serve as the primary imaging procedure for patients with unexplained acute renal failure, for diabetics and other individuals at higher risk for adverse reactions to contrast material, in the presence of pregnancy, and to diagnose suspected polycystic kidney disease.

Evaluation of Renal Mass Lesions. Ultrasonography is used widely and effectively in the evaluation of renal mass lesions detected by excretory urography. Fluid-filled cysts as small as 1 to 2 cm in diameter may be detected, but reliable detection

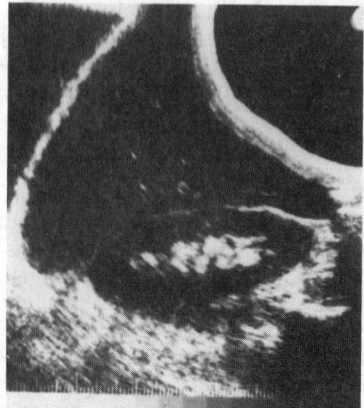

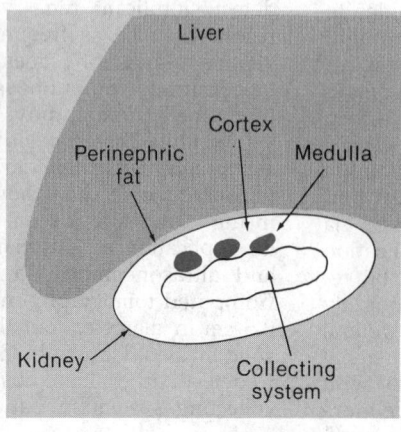

FIGURE 76–5. Ultrasonography and schematic of a normal right kidney. This was obtained anteriorly by transmission through the liver.

and evaluation of consistency generally require lesions greater than 2.5 to 3.0 cm. The primary application of ultrasonography is to describe the ultrasonographic characteristics of mass lesions according to three patterns: cystic, solid, or complex. Cystic lesions are free of internal echoes, have smooth, sharply defined margins, and cause accentuation of echoes from their far wall. Solid lesions have less distinct margins because of attenuation of the signal by solid tissue and also demonstrate internal echoes related to vessels, connective tissue, or hemorrhage. Complex lesions represent features of both patterns. Because of the inherent limitations of the technique, ultrasonographically defined lesions should be described simply as having the *characteristics* of cysts or solids. Physically solid lesions that may appear on ultrasonography as cysts include melanomas, lymphomas, and certain metastases. Localized areas of hydronephrosis may also appear as cysts.

Renal ultrasonography is most nearly diagnostic in adult polycystic kidney disease and severe hydronephrosis. In other instances, ultrasonography should be regarded as informative rather than diagnostic. In the evaluation of renal mass lesions, combinations of ultrasonography, computed tomography (Fig. 76–4), and arteriography may distinguish between benign cysts and potentially malignant solid tumors with remarkable accuracy. Clinical judgment will still be needed to decide whether even a 90 to 95 per cent level of accuracy is sufficient in an individual instance or whether surgery is indicated to obtain a definite diagnosis.

RADIONUCLIDE SCINTILLATION IMAGING. Radionuclide imaging has not achieved a major role in the evaluation of the kidneys and urinary tract. Two advantages of these techniques, however, make them useful in special circumstances. First, radionuclide imaging does not require the injection of radiocontrast material. Second, radionuclide studies are relatively simple and rapid and may be performed repeatedly at intervals of 24 to 48 hours. For these reasons, radionuclide imaging has perhaps its greatest application in the evaluation of patients at high risk for adverse reaction to radiocontrast material and in the evaluation of patients in the period immediately after renal transplantation. Otherwise, these techniques have few advantages over more direct radiologic and ultrasonographic methods.

With regard to the kidneys, radionuclide imaging techniques involve the intravenous injection of an agent labeled with a radionuclide that emits gamma radiation. Use of a scintillation camera allows the performance of dynamic studies that monitor the passage of a radiopharmaceutical agent through the vascular, renal parenchymal, and urinary tract compartments. Static studies examine the local accumulation of radionuclide activity. At present, radiopharmaceuticals of value in studies of the kidney contain either ^{131}I or ^{99m}Tc (technetium).

Static Imaging. Static imaging of the kidney consists of the administration of a radiopharmaceutical agent, usually ^{99m}Tc-glucoheptonate, that accumulates within the renal parenchyma and persists for several hours. Static imaging provides information on the location, size, and contour of functional renal tissue and may reveal areas of inhomogeneity or filling defects.

Dynamic Imaging. Dynamic scintillation imaging consists of the intravenous injection of a radiopharmaceutical agent and the visualization of its course through the vascular, renal parenchymal, and urinary collecting system by external monitoring of regional radioactivity with a scintillation camera. The time course of the appearance and disappearance of radioactivity is recorded in intervals as brief as one second. The radiopharmaceuticals used most frequently include ^{131}I-orthoiodohippurate, which is excreted by secretion with only a small component of filtration, and ^{99m}Tc-diethylenetriamine pentacetic acid (DTPA), which is excreted by filtration only. The time-activity data observed for the passage of either

radionuclide generally delineate three discrete phases. The vascular phase is the first 15 to 60 seconds after injection and consists of a rapid increase in radioactivity in the region viewed by the scintillation camera. The second phase occurs over the next three to five minutes and consists of slower accumulation of regional radioactivity. The third, or excretory, phase refers to the decrease in activity that occurs as the radionuclide is excreted from the region of interest. Unilateral or bilateral disturbances in renal blood flow, renal filtration, renal tubular function, or excretion cause disturbances in the various phases of this renogram. Although some efforts have been made to provide quantification of the various phases, interpretation of renograms still depends for the most part on the recognition of patterns in the scintillation displays. Dynamic imaging is especially useful for comparing excretory function between the right and left kidneys when renal dysfunction is asymmetric, such as may occur with congenital, vascular, or urologic disorders.

MAGNETIC RESONANCE IMAGING. Magnetic resonance imaging (MRI) represents a new and emerging diagnostic technology that uses high magnetic fields and radiofrequencies to construct images. The method avoids the use of ionizing radiation or the administration of contrast material. Imaging depends instead on the water content and the chemical behavior of hydrogen compounds in the tissues themselves. MRI provides images in a tomographic format similar to computed tomography (Fig. 76–6). The technique is very sensitive to blood flow and represents an excellent method for evaluating major vascular structures for patency or tumor involvement.

RENAL BIOPSY

Biopsy of the renal parenchyma by either the percutaneous or the open technique is useful (1) to define the morphologic expression of primary renal diseases, (2) to determine the type and extent of renal involvement by systemic diseases, and (3) to diagnose systemic diseases. The performance of renal biopsy is seldom necessary to *diagnose* systemic diseases. Diseases such as systemic lupus erythematosus, multiple myeloma, and diabetes mellitus, which may have typical but seldom diagnostic morphologic patterns, are diagnosed more

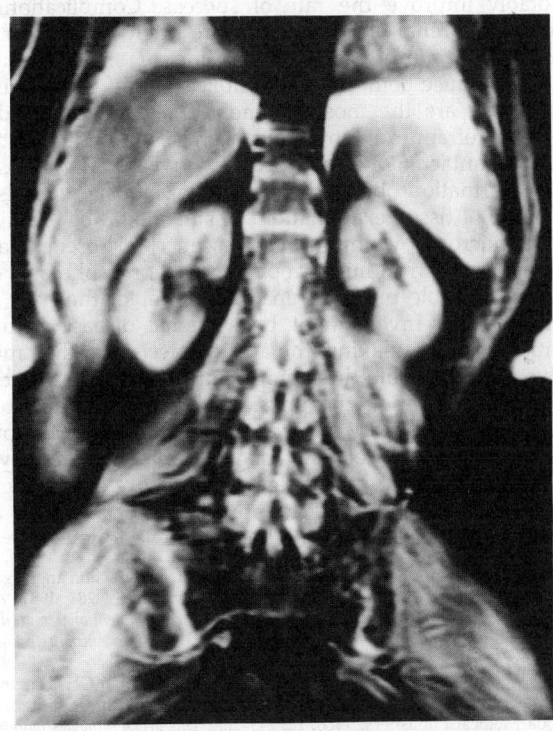

FIGURE 76–6. Magnetic resonance image of two normal kidneys in an elderly woman.

TABLE 76–3. INDICATIONS FOR RENAL BIOPSY

Presumptive presence of glomerular disease
    Heavy proteinuria (> 3 to 5 grams per 24 hours)
    Nephrotic syndrome
    Acute nephritic syndrome
Proteinuria with hematuria
Renal involvement by systemic disease
    Connective tissue disease
    Vasculitis
    Amyloidosis
    Suspected Goodpasture's disease
Unexplained acute renal failure
Persistent acute renal failure (beyond two to four weeks)
Renal transplantation
    Acute rejection
    Chronic rejection
    Recurrence of original disease

readily by other means. Systemic lupus erythematosus, diabetes mellitus, thrombotic thrombocytopenic purpura, Wegener's granulomatosis, and amyloidosis may on occasion display pathognomonic features on renal biopsy, but of these diseases only amyloidosis is likely to require renal biopsy for diagnosis.

Renal biopsy is performed most frequently via the percutaneous technique. The indications for percutaneous biopsy are listed in Table 76–3; the contraindications are the presence of a single kidney, bleeding disorders, and uncontrolled hypertension. In experienced hands, percutaneous renal biopsy is a safe and effective technique that should provide sufficient tissue in more than 90 per cent of the attempts. Complications occur in 5 to 10 per cent of the attempts, and the most frequent complication is gross hematuria that usually resolves uneventfully in 24 to 48 hours. The formation of a perirenal hematoma may on occasion require surgical evacuation. Microscopic hematuria occurs very frequently and is not generally considered as a complication. Complications that occur less frequently include persistent bleeding, formation of arteriovenous fistula, aggravation of hypertension, and inadvertent biopsy of nonrenal tissue such as muscle, liver, pancreas, spleen, or small bowel. Although fluoroscopy and ultrasonography may on occasion be useful or even necessary to localize the kidney for biopsy, it is not clear that these added maneuvers diminish the occurrence of complications or notably improve the rate of success. Complications of percutaneous renal biopsy occur more often in younger patients and in those with hypertension or small, diseased kidneys. Because hemorrhagic complications of percutaneous renal biopsy are the most common, the patient should be advised to refrain from strenuous exercises, especially lifting, and from contact sports for at least two weeks after biopsy.

The information obtained from a renal biopsy depends on the quality of tissue examination. Tissue should be examined by light microscopy, immunofluorescence microscopy, and, on occasion, electron microscopy. Accurate morphologic definition of possible primary renal disease or of the type and extent of renal involvement by systemic disease is often essential prior to making therapeutic decisions that might involve the use of life-threatening immunosuppressive therapy and to informing the physician and patient about the expected natural history of any renal abnormality. Moreover, for those renal disorders that may be treated ultimately by renal transplantation, knowledge of the nature of the original renal disease is important to predictions of whether that disease is likely to recur in the transplanted kidney.

Buonocore E, Meaney TF, Borkowski GP, et al.: Digital subtraction angiography of the abdominal aorta and renal arteries. Radiology 139:281, 1981. *Along with some early results from a comparison between conventional and digital subtraction angiography, there are some useful insights into relevant technology and procedures.*

Dennis VW, Robinson RR: Clinical proteinuria. In Stollerman GH, Harrington WJ, Lamont JT, et al. (eds.): Advances in Internal Medicine. Chicago, Year Book Medical Publishers, 1986, pp 243–263. *This article provides more detail on the mechanisms and clinical classifications of proteinuria isolated from other renal abnormalities.*

Kokko JP, Tannen RL: Fluids and Electrolytes. Philadelphia, W. B. Saunders Company, 1986. *This monograph is the finest and most thorough exposition of the laboratory evaluation of abnormalities in renal function and electrolyte metabolism. The chapter on clinical interpretation of laboratory values is especially relevant and well referenced.*

Mogensen CE: Microalbuminuria predicts clinical proteinuria and early mortality in maturity-onset diabetes. N Engl J Med 310:356, 1984. *This article advances the concept of microalbuminuria as a predictor of poor renal prognosis in patients with diabetes mellitus. It also refers to the theories and observations upon which the concept is based.*

Shemesh O, Golbetz H, Kriss JP, et al.: Limitations of creatinine as a filtration marker in glomerulopathic patients. Kidney Int 28:830, 1985. *Data provided in this article represent the modern basis upon which we interpret plasma creatinine values.*

77 DISORDERS OF FLUID VOLUME, ELECTROLYTE, AND ACID-BASE BALANCE

Thomas E. Andreoli

INTRODUCTION

Electrolyte abnormalities often occur as manifestations of underlying illnesses. In turn, fluid and electrolyte abnormalities, of themselves, produce systemic derangements. This chapter considers four major derangements of fluid and electrolyte balance, namely, volume disturbances, osmolality derangements, abnormalities of potassium balance, and acid-base disorders.

In health, the functional capacities of the mechanisms regulating water and electrolyte balance are so large that one can vary the intake of solutes and water over a wide range without developing perceptible metabolic disturbances. But when these mechanisms are impaired, the limits between which solute and water intake can be varied become narrower.

This concept is illustrated schematically in Figure 77–1. The safe range, or the range over which homeostasis is maintained, is bounded at the lower level by the minimal physiologic requirement and at the upper level by the maximal physiologic tolerance. These limits become progressively narrowed in disease. As the degree of functional impairment

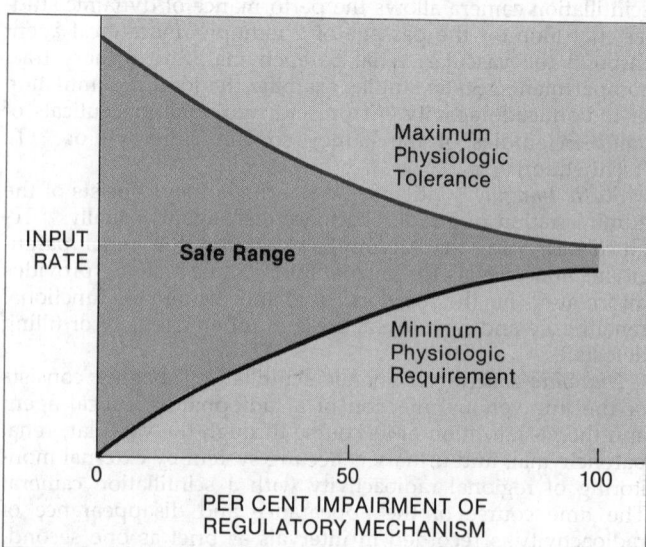

FIGURE 77–1. Upper and lower limits of intake. The safe range, or the range over which homeostasis is maintained, is bounded at the upper level by the maximum physiologic tolerance and at the lower level by the minimum physiologic requirement. Impairment of the regulating mechanism by disease narrows the safe range.

progresses, minimal requirements tend to increase while maximal tolerances tend to decrease. For example, salt intake in normal individuals can vary from approximately 10 mEq per day to several hundred milliequivalents per day without affecting volume homeostasis. In the presence of chronic renal disease, the minimal requirement rises and the maximal tolerance decreases, so that dietary salt intake must be kept within a much narrower range if volume depletion or volume overload is to be avoided.

Volume Disorders

PHYSIOLOGIC CONSIDERATIONS

Protection of extracellular fluid volume is the most fundamental characteristic of fluid and electrolyte homeostasis. It is helpful to use the term *effective circulating volume (ECV)*. The latter cannot be defined in an absolute sense. In operational terms, effective circulating volume may be viewed as adequate filling of the arterial tree, that is, an arterial flow rate sufficient to maintain adequate perfusion of body tissues. The mechanisms regulating volume balance respond primarily to changes in the effective circulating volume.

The Body Fluid Compartments

In healthy adults, body water comprises approximately 60 per cent of body weight and exists in two compartments: The intracellular compartment (ICF) contains two thirds of body water, or 40 per cent of body weight; the extracellular compartment (ECF) contains the remaining one third of total body water; and total blood volume, that is, plasma plus formed elements, constitutes one third of the total ECF volume. This "rule of thirds" for the body fluid compartments is useful in the assessment of most clinically encountered fluid and electrolyte disorders. Thus in a healthy 70-kg man, total body water comprises about 40 liters, of which 25 liters is intracellular. The functional extracellular fluid volume is 15 liters, 5 liters of which is blood; and since the normal hematocrit is 40 to 45 per cent, total plasma volume is approximately 2.75 to 3.0 liters.

More than 95 per cent of total body sodium is extracellular, and sodium and its associated anions, primarily chloride and bicarbonate, constitute the principal solutes of the ECF. Albumin and other macromolecules present in plasma are restricted to the vascular bed and constitute 5 per cent of plasma volume, so that plasma is about 95 per cent water. Since capillaries are freely permeable to water and small solutes, interstitial fluid is a protein-poor, but not entirely protein-free, ultrafiltrate of plasma.

Potassium is the principal cation of intracellular fluid, and nearly 98 per cent of total body potassium is intracellular. The principal anions of intracellular fluid vary among different cells. In muscle cells, they include phosphate, sulfate, and negatively charged macromolecules; and in red blood cells, they are the last-named anions, together with chloride and bicarbonate.

Regulation of Fluid Transfer Among Compartments

The transfer of fluid between vascular and interstitial compartments occurs at the capillary level and is governed by the balance between hydrostatic pressure gradients and plasma oncotic pressure gradients. This relation may be stated by the familiar Starling equation:

$$J_v = K_f (\Delta P - \Delta \pi)$$

where J_v is rate of fluid transfer between vascular and interstitial compartments, K_f is the water permeability of the capillary bed, ΔP is the hydrostatic pressure difference between capillary and interstitium, and $\Delta \pi$ is the oncotic pressure difference between capillary and interstitial fluids. Under normal circumstances, interstitial tissue pressure is low and the ΔP term in the Starling equation represents the integrated hydrostatic pressure gradient from arteriolar to venular ends of a capillary. Since interstitial fluid is protein poor, the $\Delta \pi$ term in the Starling equation represents the oncotic pressure of plasma proteins, principally albumin; 5 grams of albumin per deciliter of plasma exerts an oncotic pressure of about 15 mm of mercury.

Protection of Fluid Balance

As noted earlier, protection of the effective circulating volume is the single most fundamental characteristic of body fluid homeostasis. This primacy is underscored by the fact that, in circumstances in which multiple physiologic variables are threatened simultaneously, the homeostatic response invariably protects ECF volume even at the expense of aggravating another electrolyte disorder. For example, a volume-contracted patient who is replenished with water, and not sodium, will retain water and become hyponatremic in an attempt to avoid circulatory collapse. Likewise, the maintenance of metabolic alkalosis in patients who have vomited and are not repleted with salt depends, in part, on an elevated renal absorptive capacity for sodium bicarbonate. The latter maintains fluid balance at the expense of pH homeostasis.

Two cardinal mechanisms protect extracellular fluid volume: alterations in systemic hemodynamic variables and alterations in external sodium and water balance. Both mechanisms maintain filling of the arterial tree and consequently are activated by external fluid losses; by inability to transfer fluid from the interstitium to the venous system, for example, in ascites; or by impaired fluid transfer from venous to arterial systems, for example, in congestive heart failure, pericardial tamponade, or constrictive pericarditis.

The combination of alterations in systemic hemodynamic variables and alterations in external water and solute balance can be termed the integrated volume response (Table 77–1). Significantly, both limbs of the response, that is, systemic hemodynamics and external salt and water balance, are modulated by the same positive effectors and negative inactivators.

There are differences in the two response systems. Tachycardia, peripheral arteriolar vasoconstriction, and peripheral venoconstriction occur within minutes of external fluid losses, whereas renal salt and water conservation lag behind by 12 to 24 hours. The sensitivities of the two limbs also differ. For example, a 2 to 3 per cent decrease in extracellular fluid volume, which amounts to the loss of 40 to 60 mEq of sodium, results in virtual elimination of sodium from the urine but produces negligible changes in systemic hemodynamic factors such as heart rate, blood pressure, or systemic vascular resistance. Since there is 2500 to 3000 mEq of exchangeable sodium in the ECF, the system for conserving renal sodium is remarkably sensitive.

Renal Volume Regulation

Figure 77–2 provides a schematic summary of the renal factors regulating volume homeostasis. In general, the system

TABLE 77–1. THE INTEGRATED VOLUME RESPONSE

	Systemic Hemodynamic Changes	External Salt and Water Balance
Response	Tachycardia ↑ Peripheral resistance ↓ Venous capacitance	Thirst Renal Na⁺, water retention
Onset	Minutes	Hours
Major activators	Catecholamines Angiotensin II ADH	Catecholamines Aldosterone ADH
Major inactivators	Prostaglandins Atriopeptin	Prostaglandins Atriopeptin

ADH = Antidiuretic hormone.

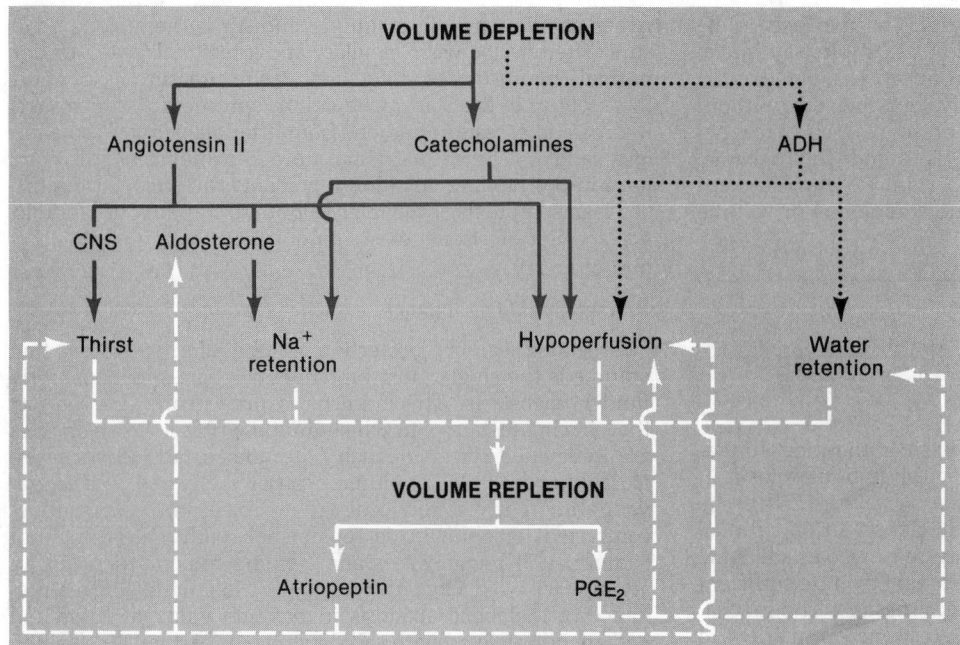

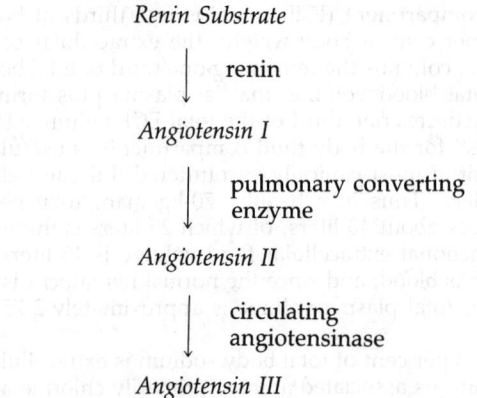

FIGURE 77–2. The volume repletion reaction. The solid arrows indicate positive mechanisms activated when volume depletion is modest; the dotted arrows indicate positive mechanisms activated with severe volume depletion. The dashed lines indicate negative feedback mechanisms.

is characterized by a positive limb, activated by volume contraction, and by negative feedback activated by volume repletion. In Figure 77–2 the solid lines and dotted lines represent volume conservation mechanisms activated by small and severe degrees of volume contraction, respectively; the dashed lines indicate negative feedback mechanisms activated by volume repletion. The separate details of this mechanism are as follows.

SENSING AND EFFECTOR ELEMENTS. Changes in effective ECF volume that exceed acceptable physiologic limits are sensed by baroreceptors located in both the high- and the low-pressure regions of the circulation. The low-pressure baroreceptors are located primarily in the left atrium and in major thoracic veins, whereas the arterial high-pressure baroreceptors are located in the sinus body and aortic arch. Both sets of baroreceptors respond to pressure and stretch stimuli associated with changes in effective circulating volume. Activation of these extrarenal baroreceptors by relatively slight reductions in effective circulating volume results in increased sympathetic nerve activity and in rises in plasma catecholamine activity.

This catecholamine response raises blood pressure by increasing arteriolar resistance and heart rate, while simultaneously decreasing venous capacitance. Increases in arteriolar resistance also reduce capillary hydrostatic pressure and therefore promote fluid transfer from interstitial fluid to the vascular compartment. Within the kidney this increase in arteriolar resistance results in renal hypoperfusion. Moreover, adrenergic nerve terminals are in direct contact with proximal renal tubular epithelial cells, and direct stimulation of renal sympathetic nerves increases proximal tubular sodium absorption.

A second effector mechanism activated by stimulation of extrarenal baroreceptors is release of antidiuretic hormone (ADH). When blood volume is isotonically contracted by more than 8 to 10 per cent, afferent stimuli carried by the ninth and tenth cranial nerves result in nonosmotic ADH release by the neurohypophysis. In turn, ADH enhances renal water conservation and, because the hormone also has potent vasoconstrictor activity, reduces renal perfusion.

In addition to these extrarenal baroreceptors the renal juxtaglomerular apparatus serves as an intrarenal baroreceptor system. Sympathetic nerve stimulation, reductions in afferent arteriolar blood pressure, or reductions in the rates of distal tubular sodium delivery enhance renin release by the juxta-

glomerular apparatus. Renal renin release into plasma accelerates the formation of angiotensin II according to the following general scheme:

$$
\begin{array}{c}
\textit{Renin Substrate} \\
\downarrow \text{renin} \\
\textit{Angiotensin I} \\
\downarrow \text{pulmonary converting enzyme} \\
\textit{Angiotensin II} \\
\downarrow \text{circulating angiotensinase} \\
\textit{Angiotensin III}
\end{array}
$$

The octapeptide angiotensin II has three major effects on volume conservation: (1) It is a potent pressor agent; on a molar basis, angiotensin II is a more potent vasoconstrictor than norepinephrine. (2) Angiotensin II is the major stimulus to aldosterone secretion and consequently is a key factor modulating renal sodium conservation. (3) The angiotensin II formed in the central nervous system is a potent stimulus to thirst. The heptapeptide angiotensin III is also a potent vasoconstrictor but is not as potent a stimulator of aldosterone secretion as is angiotensin II; angiotensin III also stimulates thirst.

RENAL ELEMENTS. The kidneys respond to slight reductions in effective circulating volume by increasing the rate of proximal tubular sodium absorption without disturbing either glomerular filtration rate or osmoregulatory mechanisms. In normal circumstances, approximately 70 per cent of filtered sodium is absorbed by the proximal nephron. So long as euvolemia persists, the fractional rate of proximal sodium absorption remains constant when the glomerular filtration rate is varied; this constant relation is referred to as *glomerulotubular balance.*

A number of factors modulate glomerulotubular balance in association with changes in effective circulating volume. In empiric terms, this modulation includes a down-setting of glomerulotubular balance in volume-expanded states and an increase in the rate of fractional proximal sodium absorption when filling of the arterial tree is impaired. Among these factors, the hemodynamic regulation of oncotic pressure in peritubular capillaries seems to have a dominant role. At relatively low concentrations, angiotensin II has a vasoconstricting effect on efferent, but not afferent, glomerular arterioles. Therefore this agent, by increasing glomerular filtration fraction, can increase peritubular capillary oncotic pressure and thereby enhance proximal tubular rates of sodium absorption. At high concentrations, angiotensin II, like norepinephrine, produces afferent glomerular arteriolar constriction, which results in reductions in glomerular filtration rate and in renal ischemia.

The kidney responds to modest sodium depletion by increasing the rate of tubular sodium absorption without altering glomerular filtration rate. Glomerulotubular balance is reset upward, so that a greater fraction of glomerular filtrate is absorbed in the proximal nephron; both direct stimulation of renal nerves and the effect of angiotensin II on efferent glomerular arterioles contribute in part to this resetting of glomerulotubular balance. Angiotensin II also provides a second mechanism for renal sodium conservation by increasing the rate of aldosterone secretion, which enhances sodium absorption in the terminal regions of the distal tubule. Finally, increased sodium absorption by more terminal portions of the collecting duct may also be part of the volume repletion reaction. When volume contraction becomes severe, the vasoconstrictive effects of high levels of norepinephrine and angiotensin II tend to reduce both the glomerular filtration rate and the rate of renal sodium excretion.

NEGATIVE FEEDBACK. As indicated in Figure 77–2, atriopeptin and E series prostaglandins (PGE) constitute the principal negative feedback elements of the renal volume regulatory response. The major features of these negative feedback mechanisms are as follows.

Prostaglandins, particularly of the E series, are potent vasodilators. Within the kidney, two cardinal loci of PGE_2 production include renal glomeruli, where angiotensin II activates eicosanoid production and release, and renal medullary interstitial cells, which produce and release PGE_2 in response to increases in medullary osmolality.

As indicated in Figure 77–2, E series prostaglandins suppress renal volume conservation by at least three effects: (1) These agents are natriuretic, although it is not yet established whether the natriuretic effect of prostaglandins is due to changes in renal hemodynamics or to a direct inhibition of tubular sodium absorption. (2) Prostaglandins are potent renal vasodilators and consequently play a major role in protecting the kidneys from ischemia in circumstances such as volume depletion, when levels of the vasoconstrictor agents, angiotensin II and norepinephrine, are increased. (3) PGE_2 is a direct antagonist of the renal tubular effects of ADH and thus impairs renal water conservation.

An important therapeutic principle follows from a consideration of the renal vasodilatory effects of prostaglandins. Specifically, the use of aspirin and other nonsteroidal anti-inflammatory agents should be avoided in circumstances characterized by a high degree of sodium avidity, that is, by a reduction in effective circulating volume. These agents inhibit prostaglandin synthesis and thus reduce the rate of prostaglandin production. Consequently, in sodium-avid states, the use of aspirin or other nonsteroidal anti-inflammatory agents will increase the rate of development of renal ischemia and hence azotemia.

Atriopeptin, or atrial natriuretic peptide, is the second negative feedback element in the renal volume regulatory response. This hormone is released from cardiac atrial storage granules in response to atrial distention; immunoreactive atriopeptin has also been identified within the central nervous system. Atriopeptin is discussed in detail in Ch. 224. In the present context, three actions of atriopeptin have particular pertinence: (1) Centrally released atriopeptin suppresses pituitary ADH release and angiotensin II–mediated thirst. (2) Atriopeptin of cardiac origin inhibits aldosterone secretion and hence renal Na^+ conservation; atriopeptin may also block terminal nephron Na^+ absorption directly. (3) Atriopeptin is a potent vasodilator that increases renal blood flow strikingly. The last-named effect also accounts in part for the natriuretic effects of this peptide.

SUMMARY. When considered in an overall context, two features of the volume repletion reaction illustrated in Figure 77–2 are noteworthy. First, redundant mechanisms protect effective circulating volume. Thus, angiotensin II release, catecholamine release, and ADH release all produce overlapping results.

Second, the magnitude of the volume repletion reaction varies depending on the degree of volume contraction. In modestly volume-contracted states, peripheral vasoconstriction and renal sodium conservation occur, but renal blood flow, glomerular filtration rate, and osmoregulation are unaffected. When volume contraction becomes advanced, nonosmotic ADH release, angiotensin II–mediated thirst, and reductions in the rate of salt delivery to the loop of Henle act in concert to produce hyponatremia. Finally, when catecholamine release and angiotensin II release become sufficiently great that renal blood flow is compromised beyond autoregulatory limits, prerenal azotemia ensues.

VOLUME DEPLETION

DEFINITION. A true hypovolemic state is one in which there is a reduction in total body water, functional ECF volume, and ICF volume; it occurs when the rate of salt and water intake is less than the combined rates of renal plus extrarenal volume losses. In chronic volume-contracted states, input and output may be equal.

ETIOLOGY AND PATHOGENESIS. Three major groups of diseases, occurring individually or in combination, account for most clinically encountered states of true volume contraction. Table 77–2 summarizes these three sets of disorders and the more common specific diseases in each group.

Hormone Deficit. Volume contraction can occur whenever there is loss of ADH or aldosterone. Untreated *diabetes insipidus*, either pituitary or nephrogenic, produces profound volume contraction and hypertonic encephalopathy in patients denied free access to water. Approximately 10 per cent of the glomerular filtrate, or about 18 liters daily, reaches the early distal convoluted tubule. Under normal circumstances, this fluid is hypotonic and, so long as ADH is present, is concentrated by osmotic equilibration with the hypertonic renal medullary interstitium. In diabetes insipidus, a large fraction

TABLE 77–2. MAJOR CAUSES OF VOLUME DEPLETION

Renal Losses	Extrarenal Losses
Hormonal Deficit	**Hemorrhage**
Pituitary diabetes insipidus	**Cutaneous Losses**
Aldosterone insufficiency	Sweating
Addison's disease	Burns
Hyporeninemic hypoaldosteronism	
Interstitial nephritis	
Renal Deficits	**Gastrointestinal Losses**
Specific Tubular Nephropathies:	Vomiting
Renal tubular acidosis	Diarrheal disorders
Proximal	Gastrointestinal fistulas
Distal, gradient-limited	Tube drainage
Bartter's syndrome	
Nephrogenic diabetes insipidus	
Diuretic abuse	
Postobstructive diuresis	
Excessive Filtration of Nonelectrolytes:	
Osmotic diuresis	
Generalized Renal Disease:	
Chronic renal failure	

of hypotonic tubular fluid may escape reabsorption and appear in the urine. Thus the obligatory loss of solute-free water in diabetes insipidus may be as high as 10 to 18 liters daily. Both forms of diabetes insipidus are discussed in Ch. 227.

Addison's disease may impair aldosterone production and hence lead to renal sodium wasting. A second major cause of aldosterone lack occurs in *hyporeninemic hypoaldosteronism*, which may accompany interstitial renal disease. Disorders that damage the renal interstitium, such as hypertension, diabetes mellitus, gout, sickle cell disease, chronic ingestion of lead-containing illicit alcohol, and analgesic abuse, can suppress the ability of the juxtaglomerular apparatus to produce renin. In turn, the low rate of renin secretion results in low rates of aldosterone secretion. Thus hyporeninemic hypoaldosteronism represents a disorder in which impaired aldosterone production results in renal salt wasting, hyperkalemia, and metabolic acidosis. It is not yet known why hyperkalemia, which is a potent stimulus to aldosterone secretion, fails to enhance rates of aldosterone secretion in patients with hyporeninemic hypoaldosteronism.

Renal Deficits. A number of disorders impairing renal tubular sodium or water conservation can lead to volume contraction. For convenience, these derangements may be grouped into three classes.

First, various tubular nephropathies are characterized by specific deficits in salt or water absorption. As mentioned above, nephrogenic diabetes insipidus and interstitial renal disease may produce water or sodium wasting, respectively. Because interstitial renal disease often results in hyperchloremic, hyperkalemic metabolic acidosis, the term "renal tubular acidosis, type IV" is often applied to this disorder. However, the general term "renal tubular acidosis" also includes other sodium-wasting disorders accompanied by hyperchloremic acidosis, such as proximal tubular acidosis, a specific proximal defect in bicarbonate reabsorption, and gradient-limited distal renal tubular acidosis, a specific defect in distal tubular sodium bicarbonate regeneration (Ch. 84).

Alternatively, Bartter's syndrome is a specific tubular nephropathy that results in failure of sodium chloride absorption by distal regions of the nephron; the disorder is accompanied by excessive production of prostaglandins by the renal medullary interstitium and is characterized by sodium chloride wasting, juxtaglomerular hyperplasia, high renin levels, and secondary hyperaldosteronism; the last-named results in hypokalemic metabolic alkalosis.

Inhibition of tubular sodium absorptive processes due to *chronic diuretic abuse* may also lead to salt wasting, volume contraction, and specific metabolic acid-base abnormalities. These abnormalities are discussed below in connection with Table 77–5 (see below). Diuretics such as furosemide and thiazides produce serum electrolyte changes indistinguishable from those of Bartter's syndrome.

Profound but reversible defects in tubular salt and water absorption may occur during *postobstructive diuresis*, that is, shortly after relief of partial or complete urinary tract obstruction. Salt and water losses may also occur in the *diuretic phase* of acute tubular necrosis. However, profound salt and water losses associated with the diuretic phase of acute tubular necrosis are seen uncommonly if extracellular fluid volume is carefully controlled during oliguric acute tubular necrosis.

Third, glomerular filtration of large amounts of nonelectrolytes may produce volume deficits by overwhelming renal tubular reabsorptive capacity for salt and water; in this instance, water losses predominate so that hypernatremia generally occurs. This phenomenon, termed *osmotic diuresis* or *solute diuresis*, occurs in diabetic ketoacidosis, hyperglycemic hyperosmolar coma, or hyperalimentation with large glucose loads in chronically debilitated patients; in patients with burns, in whom there are abnormally high rates of urea production; and during mannitol or glycerol administration

to patients with central nervous system disorders requiring reductions of intracranial pressure.

Finally, in *chronic renal failure* of any cause, there is an obligatory loss of sodium. As indicated in Figure 77–1, chronic renal failure of any cause is associated with a significant increase in the minimal physiologic requirement for maintaining sodium balance. The extent of obligatory sodium loss in chronic renal failure is most pronounced in cystic renal diseases, notably medullary cystic disease and polycystic kidney disease (Ch. 91).

Extrarenal Losses. In addition to hemorrhage, two other classes of extrarenal losses account for volume contraction. Simple dehydration may result from increased insensible water loss in *excessive sweating* due to high ambient temperatures or to fever. Because sweat usually contains less than 50 mEq per liter of sodium, the ICF and the ECF share the water loss, and body water osmolality rises while ECF volume loss is modest. *Burns* allow the loss of large amounts of plasma and interstitial fluid through affected areas and therefore can lead rapidly to profound ECF losses.

Finally, gastrointestinal volume losses occur when portions of the 8 to 10 liters of normal gastrointestinal secretions are lost, particularly in secretory diarrheas. Volume depletion is most commonly the consequence of vomiting, gastric drainage, or diarrhea but may occur with any type of bowel fistula. Loss of hydrochloric acid from the stomach may produce metabolic alkalosis, whereas loss of sodium bicarbonate from pancreatic secretions lost through the lower gastrointestinal tract, as in diarrhea, may produce metabolic acidosis.

CLINICAL MANIFESTATIONS. The clinical findings in states of true volume contraction are due both to underfilling of the arterial tree and to the renal and hemodynamic responses to this underfilling. In mild or partially compensated volume contraction, particularly when the latter has occurred gradually, the patient may exhibit nothing more than mild postural giddiness, postural tachycardia, and weakness. In more advanced stages of volume depletion, particularly those occurring acutely, there may be recumbent hypotension, tachycardia, and a reduced urine volume. Finally, when volume contraction is severe, the combination of profound fluid loss and increased sympathetic activity produces circulatory collapse characterized by oliguria, a nondetectable blood pressure (except by Doppler studies), recumbent tachycardia, and cold extremities. In short, mild-to-severe volume contraction may range from minimal symptoms to life-threatening circulatory collapse.

The lack of physical findings does not exclude the presence of mild-to-moderate volume contraction in a given patient. In postoperative patients, 7 to 10 per cent blood volume losses are often accompanied by normal vital signs and by only slight decreases in the central venous pressure or the pulmonary capillary wedge pressure.

Skin turgor and the moistness of mucous membranes are valuable indices to the volume of body water in infants but are unreliable in adults. In young adults, reductions in skin turgor do not occur unless profound volume contraction is present; and normal loss of skin elasticity makes skin turgor difficult to assess in older patients. Likewise, mouth breathing and other factors affect the oral mucosa independently of external volume balances.

The signs and symptoms of volume contraction, regardless of cause, are referable to a reduction in effective circulating volume. Consequently, the clinical findings in volume contraction depend primarily on the interplay among four major factors: the magnitude of the volume loss; the rate of volume loss; the nature of the fluid loss, that is, whether the fluid loss is primarily water, a combined sodium plus water loss, or a blood loss; and finally, the responsiveness of the vasculature to volume reduction. Some simple considerations illustrate these relations.

The clinical manifestations of volume contraction are obviously related intimately to the volume and rate of fluid loss. For example, an acute gastrointestinal hemorrhage of 1 liter of blood can easily result in oliguria, coupled with the signs and symptoms of circulatory collapse, while the hematocrit remains constant. In other words, the hemorrhage is sufficiently acute that fluid flux from the interstitial to the vascular bed makes a negligible contribution to expanding the vascular bed. However, the same amount of gastrointestinal blood loss occurring more slowly—for example, over a one-day period—permits a partial transfer of fluid from the interstitium to the vascular bed and consequently produces a fall in hematocrit; but since the effective circulating volume is at least partially restored by this fluid shift, the volume of urine flow and the hemodynamic response to volume contraction may be minimally affected.

Second, the kind of fluid loss significantly affects the clinical findings in volume contraction. Consider, for example, a 1-liter loss of different kinds of body fluids in a 70-kg man having a total body water of 40 liters and a hematocrit of 45 per cent. The acute loss of 1 liter of predominantly solute-free water, as in diabetes insipidus, produces a 2.5 per cent reduction in blood volume; urine flow and systemic hemodynamics are minimally affected. The acute loss of 1 liter of predominantly extracellular fluid produces a 6.6 per cent reduction in blood volume, since sodium is confined to the ECF; in this circumstance, modest oliguria and recumbent tachycardia ensue. Lastly, the acute loss of 1 liter of blood by hemorrhage reduces blood volume by 20 per cent, thus resulting in profound oliguria and near circulatory collapse.

Finally, peripheral vasoconstriction and tachycardia represent important physiologic responses to volume losses. Consequently, the signs and symptoms of volume contraction, even of modest degree, are amplified appreciably in patients with diminished myocardial reserve or reduced sympathetic nervous system function. The former occurs commonly in cardiomyopathies of any cause or in pericardial tamponade or pericardial constriction. The latter occurs commonly in patients subjected to prolonged bed rest, in diabetic patients with autonomic neuropathy, and as a consequence of therapy with certain antihypertensive drugs.

DIAGNOSIS. The pulse, blood pressure, and changes of these variables with position, together with a clinical estimate of the venous pressure and skin temperature, provide an initial assessment of circulatory dynamics. Because these findings may be inconclusive in moderate degrees of volume contraction, invasive hemodynamic monitoring may be required in critically ill patients who are hemodynamically unstable. In such patients, the central venous pressure may correlate poorly with cardiac output and with pulmonary vascular volume. Measurement of the pulmonary capillary wedge pressure with a Swan-Ganz (flow-directed) catheter may therefore be required.

However, even the pulmonary capillary wedge pressure may remain within normal limits when blood volume has been reduced by 5 to 10 per cent. Consequently, a fluid challenge is useful in the evaluation of critically ill patients in whom a volume deficit is thought to be a contributory factor to a reduced cardiac output. A convenient way of achieving this goal is to administer 500 ml of normal saline over 1 to 3 hours and to measure the change in the pulmonary capillary wedge pressure or the cardiac output, as estimated by thermal dilution.

The cardinal laboratory findings associated with volume contraction follow directly from the volume repletion mechanism summarized in Figure 77–2. The kidney initially responds to a decrease in effective circulating blood volume by reducing urine volume and sodium excretion. Severe degrees of volume contraction also reduce filtration rate and result in prerenal azotemia.

The urinary sodium concentration and the fraction of filtered sodium excreted in the urine, denoted as FE_{Na}, are clinically useful indices of renal sodium avidity. The FE_{Na} is calculated as the urine to plasma sodium concentration ratio divided by the urine to plasma creatinine concentration ratio. In the volume-contracted state, the urinary sodium concentration is generally less than 10 mEq per liter and the FE_{Na} is less than 1 per cent, whereas in acute tubular necrosis, the urinary sodium concentration is greater than 40 mEq per liter and the FE_{Na} is greater than 1 per cent. These indices are useful in the differential diagnosis between acute oliguric tubular necrosis and volume contraction associated with prerenal azotemia, with certain notable exceptions.

The urinary sodium indices are not reliable determinants of volume contraction when there is obligatory renal sodium wasting, as in interstitial nephritis. When volume contraction is due to the renal losses listed in Table 77–2 (except for diabetes insipidus), the urinary sodium concentration and the FE_{Na} may both be elevated even when volume losses are large enough to produce azotemia. The urinary sodium excretion may also be elevated in volume contraction due to upper gastrointestinal losses associated with vomiting or gastric drainage. This occurs during early metabolic alkalosis if the filtered load of bicarbonate exceeds the renal tubular reabsorptive capacity for bicarbonate. During this interval, the urinary chloride concentration is a more reliable index of renal salt avidity. Finally antecedent diuretic therapy may invalidate FE_{Na} measurements.

TREATMENT. The major goal of the treatment of volume contraction is to expand the effective circulating volume by replacing fluid deficits. The type of fluid, the route and rate of fluid administration, and the total amount of fluid to be given will vary with the particular circumstance. For example, a mild, nonpersisting upper gastrointestinal hemorrhage may be treated appropriately by infusion of normal saline, whereas a major, persisting upper gastrointestinal hemorrhage will generally require replacement with whole blood.

The degree to which a given volume of crystalloid solution expands the effective circulating volume depends on solution composition. If glucose metabolism is normal, the infusion of 5 per cent dextrose in water (D_5W) is equivalent to administering solute-free water, which distributes uniformly in total body water. Since less than 10 per cent of total body water is in the intravascular compartment, infusion of 1 liter of 5 per cent dextrose in water expands the intravascular volume by 75 to 100 ml, that is, by about 2 per cent.

Solutions containing sodium as the principal solute preferentially expand the extracellular fluid volume. Infusion of 1 liter of a normal saline solution increases blood volume by about 300 ml, or about 6 per cent; the remaining portion is distributed in the interstitial compartment. Hypotonic sodium-containing salt solutions expand intravascular volume in a manner intermediate between that of 5 per cent dextrose in water and normal saline.

Colloid-containing solutions, such as iso-oncotic albumin solutions and plasma, preferentially expand the intravascular compartment, since large molecules like albumin are mainly restricted to the intravascular space. Finally, blood, which contains formed elements, is the most potent expander of the intravascular space. A unit of packed red blood cells will remain entirely in the vascular bed. A unit of whole blood having a hematocrit of 45 per cent will retain all formed elements in the vascular bed; of the remaining 55 per cent volume of that unit, more than 40 per cent of the plasma will also remain in the vascular bed because of the oncotic effect of plasma proteins.

Three other factors concerning fluid replacement therapy warrant consideration: (1) When large volumes of glucose-containing solutions are given rapidly, an increase in plasma glucose concentration that results in glycosuria produces an obligate renal loss of sodium and water that aggravates volume losses. (2) Iso-oncotic albumin solutions expand intravascular volume rapidly. The half-life of infused albumin in critically ill patients is only four to six hours, however, and the cost of an iso-oncotic albumin solution is approximately 90 times greater than that of an equal volume of normal saline. For these reasons, the use of iso-oncotic albumin solutions should be limited to hemodynamically unstable patients in whom rapid intravascular expansion is critical. (3) Because volume contraction is associated with vasoconstriction, both in the venous and arterial circuits, transient changes in the pulmonary capillary wedge pressure may not reflect accurately the volume status of the patient. During volume expansion, the wedge pressure rises and subsequently falls. The initial pressure elevation is due to fluid infusion into a vasoconstricted, low-capacity vascular bed and should not be misinterpreted to indicate adequacy of volume repletion. The subsequent reduction in wedge pressure coincides with decreases in arterial resistance coupled to increases in venous capacitance.

CIRCULATORY COMPROMISE WITHOUT TRUE VOLUME CONTRACTION

DEFINITION. In the previous section, we considered those disorders characterized by inadequate filling of the arterial tree that occurred because of fluid losses between the patient and the external environment. Clearly, the cardinal signs and symptoms of these disorders are referable to responses accompanying the integrated volume repletion reaction (Fig. 77–2). There are also disorders in which inadequate arterial filling occurs in the absence of external fluid losses. The signs and symptoms of these disorders mimic closely those that characterize true volume contraction.

ETIOLOGY AND PATHOGENESIS. Table 77–3 lists three commonly encountered classes of derangements that may present clinically with tachycardia, acute hypotension, oliguria, azotemia, and a reduced Fe_{Na}. These disorders can be termed "non–volume-contracted circulatory compromise," with the understanding that the term "non–volume-contracted" refers to the absence of body fluid losses between the patient and the external world.

Impaired Cardiac Output. A profound collapse of cardiac output, due to acute myocardial infarction with pump failure (cardiogenic shock) or to acute pericardial tamponade, may clearly result in circulatory collapse. In this instance, failure to fill the arterial tree and to maintain an effective circulatory volume occurs because the heart fails to translocate blood adequately from venous to arterial beds.

Increased Vascular Capacitance. Circulatory collapse and its attendant signs and symptoms will occur when there is a sudden increase in the capacitance of the vascular bed, most notably in the venous part of the circulation. This kind of increase in ratio of vascular capacitance to vascular volume occurs most commonly in sepsis but may also be seen in circumstances in which peripheral vasodilators, particularly those having a postarteriolar locus of action, are administered injudiciously.

TABLE 77–3. CIRCULATORY COMPROMISE WITHOUT EXTERNAL FLUID LOSSES

I. **Impaired cardiac output**
   Acute myocardial infarction
   Pericardial tamponade
II. **Increased Vascular Capacitance**
   Septic shock
III. **Vascular → Interstitial Fluid Shifts**
   Acute pancreatitis
   Bowel infarction
   Rhabdomyolysis
   Noncardiogenic pulmonary edema

Vascular-Interstitial Fluid Shifts. Profound hypotension, tachycardia, progressive oliguria, and azotemia are also encountered when there is a rapid translocation of fluid from vascular to interstitial compartments, presumably because of a sudden, profound increase in the permeability characteristics of peripheral capillaries. Some common derangements of this type include infarction of the small or large intestine, extensive tissue trauma, acute pancreatitis, and rhabdomyolysis. An analogous mechanism, namely, a marked increase in the permeability of pulmonary capillaries, is also presumed to account for the formation of noncardiogenic pulmonary edema in the adult respiratory distress syndrome.

DIAGNOSIS AND THERAPY. The diagnosis and therapy of acute myocardial infarction with circulatory collapse and of acute pericardial tamponade are considered in detail in Section IV of this book. It is, however, worth citing certain factors particularly germane to the management of fluid therapy in such patients. In individuals affected either by right ventricular infarction or by pericardial tamponade, maintenance of adequate filling of the systemic arterial tree depends critically on providing a relatively high venous preload to the right side of the heart. Attempts at volume contraction in patients with right ventricular infarcts or pericardial tamponade may exacerbate systemic hypotension. Thus treatment of these disorders generally requires concomitant hemodynamic monitoring with a flow-directed Swan-Ganz catheter to avoid excessive preload to the left side of the heart.

In patients with left ventricular infarction and systemic hypotension, particular attention should be directed to excluding the possibility that antecedent true volume depletion—for example, with prolonged diuretic therapy and salt restriction prior to the myocardial infarction—may be a significant contributor to what otherwise might be mistaken for true cardiogenic shock. The combined findings of acute left ventricular infarction, systemic arterial hypotension, a reduced pulmonary capillary wedge pressure, and an antecedent history of prolonged diuretic therapy, when taken together, indicate that improved systemic hemodynamics may be achieved by cautious attempts at volume expansion carried out in combination with serial measurements of the cardiac output and the pulmonary capillary wedge pressure.

The distinction between hypotension as being due either to true volume contraction or to an increase in the capacitance/volume ratio of the vascular bed, as occurs in sepsis, is often difficult. This distinction is particularly difficult in individuals who have been in intensive care units for prolonged periods of time and in those at high risk for developing sepsis, such as cancer patients treated with potent chemotherapeutic agents. A useful clue to the presence of septic circulatory collapse is the occurrence of warm extremities coupled with hypotension and oliguria, since true hypovolemia, particularly when advanced, is ordinarily accompanied by profound peripheral vasoconstriction and hence cool and often cyanotic extremities.

True hypovolemia and sepsis may also coexist. In such a circumstance, invasive hemodynamic monitoring may be helpful. Both in true hypovolemia and in sepsis, the pulmonary capillary wedge pressure is reduced; but in septic circulatory collapse, the calculated systemic vascular resistance falls, because of peripheral vasodilation, whereas in true hypovolemia, peripheral vasoconstriction ordinarily raises the systemic vascular resistance. The diagnosis of disorders producing rapid transfer of fluids from the vascular bed to the interstitium, such as trauma, acute pancreatitis, or rhabdomyolysis, is generally evident from clinical appraisal.

The treatment of patients with sepsis and an increased vascular capacitance/volume ratio, as well as those individuals with rapid vascular to interstitial fluid shifts, has as a mainstay the administration of sufficient sodium-containing fluids, generally isotonic saline, to permit adequate filling of the arterial tree. This therapy necessarily expands total body water, particularly in the vascular and interstitial compartments. Consequently, during recovery from the underlying disorder, care must be taken to avoid unnecessary expansion of the vascular bed and consequently the risk of volume-mediated cardiac decompensation.

VOLUME EXCESS

DEFINITION. Volume-expanded states are characterized by an increase in total body water, which is accompanied, in most but not all circumstances, by an increase in total body sodium. Total body salt and water may be increased while the effective circulating volume is decreased. In other words, certain volume-expanded states are characterized by dissociation between total body salt and water and the effective circulating volume.

ETIOLOGY AND PATHOGENESIS. Volume expansion occurs whenever the rate of salt or water intake exceeds the rate of renal plus extrarenal losses; in chronic volume expansion, the external salt and water balance may be normal. A convenient way of considering volume-expanded states is to view them in the context of three different classes of physiologic explanations (Table 77–4).

Disturbances in Starling Forces. The most common diseases encountered in which both volume expansion and edema occur are those in which derangements in the Starling forces regulating fluid transfer between capillaries and interstitium tend to promote expansion of the interstitial compartment at the expense of the effective circulating volume. Consequently, renal sodium retention and edema occur. By definition, this group of disorders is characterized by increases in capillary hydrostatic pressure, by decreases in capillary oncotic pressure, or by a combination of these two factors.

Four groups include most edematous states characterized by abnormal Starling forces (Table 77–4). First, the systemic venous pressure may be increased because of primary cardiac disorders, such as right heart failure or constrictive pericarditis. Second, there may occur local elevations in pulmonary or systemic venous pressure, as in left heart failure, vena caval obstruction, or portal vein obstruction. Third, a reduction in plasma oncotic pressure, and consequently a net increase in the tendency for fluid transudation from capillaries to interstitium, accounts plausibly for edema formation in the nephrotic syndrome. Finally, a combination of these factors may be responsible for edema formation. For example, both hypoalbuminemia and portal hypertension are major contributory factors to the development of ascites in hepatic cirrhosis.

Plasma renin activity and aldosterone concentrations in these disorders tend to be elevated, although the results also tend to be variable. In advanced cases of disorders characterized by increases in local or systemic venous pressure, most notably in severe congestive heart failure and in cirrhosis, hyponatremia may occur; this finding represents an ominous prognostic sign. Finally, edema formation due to such derangements of Starling forces may result in the "third space" phenomenon, namely, the sequestration of large volumes of interstitial fluid in regions such as the pleural or peritoneal cavities.

Primary Hormonal Excess. These disorders include those disturbances in which there is unregulated production of mineralocorticoids or ADH. The volume expansion that occurs in states of mineralocorticoid excess, such as primary hyperaldosteronism, is due to sodium retention and is accompanied by a primary, preferential expansion of the ECF and consequently by hypertension. The serum sodium level is generally normal. In the syndrome of inappropriate ADH production (SIADH), primary water retention occurs. Consequently, the volume expansion involves both the ICF and ECF; dilutional hyponatremia is the hallmark of SIADH, whereas hypertension is uncommon. Edema is not characteristic in either of these two disorders. Instead, patients with primary aldosteronism or SIADH reach a volume-expanded steady state in which output equals input.

Primary Renal Sodium Retention. The kidneys may also retain sodium abnormally when the effective circulating volume is normal and there is no effector excess. For example, in acute glomerulonephritis unidentified renal mechanisms are primarily responsible for edema formation. Patients with acute glomerulonephritis retain salt and water and become hypertensive without reductions in glomerular filtration rate or in effective circulating volume. Furthermore, sodium retention and edema develop when plasma renin activity and aldosterone concentration are normal or reduced and when the serum albumin concentration is normal. Thus, the renal tubule may be abnormally avid for sodium in acute glomerulonephritis. Congestive heart failure may occur as a secondary consequence of the volume expansion.

DIAGNOSIS AND TREATMENT. The recognition and management of volume-expanded states depend on proper identification and treatment of the underlying disorder. Clearly, the cornerstones of therapy in volume-expanded states characterized by sodium excess include salt restriction and diuretics. Table 77–5 provides a summary of some of the major diuretics used commonly and certain of their properties. For convenience, these drugs have been classified according to their sites of action in the nephron.

Proximal Diuretics. The cardinal example of a proximal tubular diuretic is acetazolamide, a carbonic anhydrase inhibitor that blocks proximal reabsorption of sodium bicarbonate. Consequently, prolonged use of acetazolamide may lead to hyperchloremic acidosis, in contrast to all other diuretics, which act at loci prior to the late distal nephron. Metolazone, a congener of the thiazide class of diuretics, blocks sodium chloride absorption in two nephron sites by unknown mechanisms. Specifically, in addition to an action on the early distal tubule, metolazone also inhibits proximal tubular sodium chloride absorption. Since the major locus for phosphate absorption is in the proximal nephron, the phosphaturia accompanying metolazone administration exceeds considerably that observed with other thiazide class diuretics.

Loop Diuretics. Loop diuretics, such as ethacrynic acid and furosemide, produce diuresis by inhibiting the coupled entry on Na^+, Cl^-, and K^+ across apical plasma membranes in the thick ascending limb of Henle. The latter is responsible for the reabsorption of approximately 25 per cent of filtered sodium. The natriuretic dose-response characteristics of these diuretic agents are considerably more linear than those of all other currently used diuretics. Consequently, the loop diuretics are, for practical purposes, the most potent diuretics currently available; therefore these drugs are commonly referred to as "high-ceiling" diuretics.

Early Distal Tubule Diuretics. Early distal tubule diuretics, such as thiazide and metolazone, interfere primarily with sodium chloride absorption in the earliest segments of the distal convoluted tubule. The thiazide diuretics appear to exert their effect by blocking sodium entry from tubular fluid across apical plasma membranes into distal tubular cells.

TABLE 77–4. DISORDERS OF VOLUME EXCESS

I. Disturbed Starling Forces
(Reduced effective circulating volume; edema formation)
Systemic Venous Pressure Increases
  Right heart failure
  Constrictive pericarditis
Local Venous Pressure Increases
  Left heart failure
  Vena cava obstruction
  Portal vein obstruction
Reduced Oncotic Pressure
  Nephrotic syndrome
Combined Disorders
  Cirrhosis

II. Primary Hormone Excess
(Increased effective circulating volume)
Primary aldosteronism
Cushing's syndrome
SIADH

III. Primary Renal Sodium Retention
(Increased effective circulating volume)
Acute glomerulonephritis

SIADH = Syndrome of inappropriate antidiuretic hormone production.

TABLE 77–5. CHARACTERISTICS OF COMMONLY USED DIURETICS

Diuretic	Primary Effect	Secondary Effect	Complications
I. Proximal Diuretics			
Acetazolamide	↓ Na$^+$/H$^+$ exchange	↑ K$^+$ loss, ↑ HCO$_3^-$ loss	Hypokalemic, hyperchloremic acidosis
Metolazone	↓ Na$^+$ absorption	↑ K$^+$ loss, ↑ Cl$^-$ loss	Hypokalemic alkalosis
II. Loop Diuretics			
Furosemide	} ↓ Na$^+$:K$^+$:2Cl$^-$ absorption	↑ K$^+$ loss, ↑ H$^+$ secretion	Hypokalemic alkalosis
Ethacrynic acid			
III. Early Distal Diuretics			
Thiazide	} ↓ Na$^+$ absorption	↑ K$^+$ loss, ↑ H$^+$ secretion	Hypokalemic alkalosis
Metolazone			
IV. Late Distal Diuretics			
Aldosterone Antagonists			
Spironolactone			
Nonaldosterone Antagonists	} ↓ Na$^+$ absorption	↓ K$^+$ loss, ↓ H$^+$ secretion	Hyperkalemic acidosis
Triamterene			
Amiloride			

With the exception of acetazolamide (which impairs bicarbonate absorption), hypokalemia and metabolic alkalosis may complicate the administration of proximal diuretics, loop diuretics, and early distal tubular diuretics. This occurs because the rate of sodium delivery to terminal distal tubular regions, where a significant fraction of potassium and proton secretion occurs, is a major factor promoting these two processes. Consequently, an increased delivery of salt to the late distal nephron, occasioned by inhibition of sodium reabsorption in the proximal tubule, the ascending limb of Henle, or the early distal tubule, leads to accelerated rates of proton and potassium secretion and consequently to hypokalemia and metabolic alkalosis.

Late Distal Nephron Diuretics. Finally, a group of agents inhibit sodium absorption in terminal regions of the distal tubule and concomitantly suppress indirectly potassium secretion and proton secretion. Spironolactone competes with aldosterone; the primary use of this agent is restricted to conditions of aldosterone excess, either primary or secondary. Alternatively, both triamterene and amiloride operate independently of aldosterone. These agents directly block sodium uptake by late distal tubular cells and concomitantly suppress indirectly both potassium and proton secretion. Accordingly, hyperkalemic, hyperchloremic metabolic acidosis may complicate the injudicious use of spironolactone, triamterene, or amiloride.

One factor common to the treatment of disorders with reduced effective circulating volumes and expanded ECF volumes merits particular consideration. A major factor in edema formation is an increase in the Starling forces promoting fluid translocation from the vascular to interstitial spaces. When potent diuretics are administered to patients with portal hypertension or with hypoalbuminemia, urinary sodium excretion may exceed the rate at which salt and water are transferred from the interstitium to the vascular bed. As a result, vigorous diuretic therapy may result in volume contraction, reduced salt delivery to diluting segments, nonosmotic ADH release, and consequently hyponatremia. In advanced cases of diuretic abuse, hypotension, hemoconcentration, and azotemia also occur.

A like effect occurs in volume-expanded patients, particularly those exhibiting a third space effect and having significant hypoalbuminemia, if relatively large volumes of ascitic fluid are removed by paracentesis. In this circumstance, the transudation of fluid from the vascular space to the interstitial space may result in circulatory collapse.

Campbell WB, Currie MG, Needleman P: Inhibition of aldosterone biosynthesis by atriopeptins in rat adrenal cells. Circ Res 57:113, 1985. *The role of atriopeptin in negative feedback of aldosterone synthesis is discussed.*

Laragh JH: Atrial natriuretic hormone, the renin-aldosterone axis and blood pressure–electrolyte homeostasis. N Engl J Med 313:1330, 1985. *A general discussion of atriopeptin.*

Laski ME: Diuretics—mechanism of action and therapy. Semin Nephrol 6:210, 1986. *A topical summary of diuretic action.*

Lifschitz MD, Stein JH: Hormonal regulation of renal salt excretion. Semin Nephrol 3:196, 1986. *A good review of sodium excretion and its modulation by hormones.*

Needleman P, Greenwald JE: Atriopeptin: A cardiac hormone intimately involved in fluid, electrolyte and blood-pressure homeostasis. N Engl J Med 314:828, 1986. *The role of atriopeptin in negative feedback of volume control is described.*

Reid IA: The renin-angiotensin system and body function. Arch Intern Med 145:1475, 1985. *The role of renin and angiotensin in volume regulation.*

Osmolality Disturbances

PHYSIOLOGIC CONSIDERATIONS

In normal individuals, the serum osmolality is virtually constant from day to day and the serum sodium concentration is an accurate index to body water osmolality. In fact, the normal ranges for serum sodium concentrations or for serum osmolalities in populations of healthy individuals depend on small differences in body water osmolality among individuals, rather than on variations in body water osmolality in a given individual.

It is useful to define "effective ECF osmolality," since the osmoregulatory mechanisms that adjust water balance in normal individuals are determined primarily by changes in cell volume that result from variations in effective ECF osmolality. In dilutional states, the measured and effective ECF osmolalities are approximately equal, since ECF dilution also produces ICF dilution and, at least acutely, cell swelling. Osmoregulatory mechanisms are activated when ECF hypertonicity is due to a solute that is excluded from cells and therefore produces, at least acutely, cell shrinkage; in this case, the measured and effective ECF osmolalities are approximately equal. If the ECF osmolality is increased by solutes such as urea, which penetrate cell membranes readily, acute cell shrinkage does not occur and osmoregulatory mechanisms are not activated. In this case, the measured ECF osmolality is greater than the effective ECF osmolality.

The serum osmolality can be approximated from the following formula:

$$\text{Osmolality} = 2[\text{Na}^+] + \frac{[\text{glucose}]}{18} + \frac{[\text{BUN}]}{2.8}$$

where the glucose and blood urea nitrogen (BUN) concentrations are expressed as milligrams per deciliter and the serum sodium concentration is expressed as milliequivalents per liter. In normal circumstances, glucose contributes 5.5 mOsm per kilogram of H$_2$O and urea contributes 2 to 6 mOsm per kilogram of H$_2$O to the serum osmolality. When hyperglycemia occurs, the effective ECF osmolality rises because glucose entry into cells is limited. When azotemia occurs, the effective ECF osmolality does not rise because urea enters cells readily.

Cell Volume Regulation

Starling forces regulate fluid transfer between the ICF and the ECF. Because plasma membranes cannot tolerate even small hydrostatic gradients, the operational Starling forces between ICF and ECF are almost entirely osmotic. Significant changes in cell volume, particularly in the central nervous system, are by themselves potentially lethal. Thus the goals of fluid transport between the ECF and ICF are to maintain constancy of cell volume and to maintain a negligible hydrostatic pressure gradient between cells and the ECF. Since cell membranes are freely permeable to water, these two goals are achieved when the ECF osmolality is normal and intracellular and extracellular osmolalities are identical.

Since cell membranes are partially permeable to sodium and potassium, there is a tendency for sodium to leak into cells and for potassium to leak out of cells. Because impermeant macromolecules account for a large fraction of intracellular anions, passive sodium and potassium movements tend toward a Donnan distribution, in which total intracellular cations would exceed total interstitial cations, in precise analogy to the way in which total plasma water cations exceed total interstitial cations. If these passive cation movements across cell membranes were unopposed, osmotic water movement into cells would tend to produce cell lysis. Consequently, active transport mechanisms are required to balance intracellular and interstitial cation concentrations.

Specifically, both sodium leakage from the ECF into cells and potassium leakage out of cells into the ECF are counterbalanced exactly by active outward sodium transport coupled to active inward potassium transport. These active transport events maintain the intracellular cation (and therefore osmolar) content equal to that of extracellular fluid and also maintain the predominant extracellular and intracellular distributions of sodium and potassium, respectively. Thus because cellular cation pumps balance cellular cation leaks, cells are *operationally* impermeable to sodium and to potassium. Active sodium efflux coupled to active potassium influx is mediated by membrane-bound $(Na^+ + K^+)$–adenosine triphosphatase (ATPase), and the activity of these cellular cation pumps accounts for more than 50 per cent of the basal caloric consumption.

Cation transport mediated by $(Na^+ + K^+)$-ATPase is the major factor regulating cell volume when the effective ECF osmolality is normal. When the effective ECF osmolality is increased or decreased, additional processes are required to maintain the constancy of cell volume. These auxiliary mechanisms are of particular importance in minimizing potentially lethal changes in brain volume because of osmotic water shifts into or out of brain cells.

In chronic hypotonic disorders, cell swelling is offset by the loss of potassium chloride from cells. This potassium chloride efflux mechanism appears to be activated by small increases in cell volume produced by ECF dilution. In chronic hypernatremia, brain shrinkage is minimized by the accumulation of additional solutes within brain cells. These latter solutes, often called "idiogenic osmoles," include amino acids and other unidentified solutes. As will be discussed in the section on Treatment, these auxiliary transport processes affect significantly the therapeutic approach to patients with osmoregulatory failure.

Water Balance

The key elements regulating water balance are summarized in Figure 77–3. The solid lines indicate osmoregulatory mechanisms, which, as indicated above, maintain constancy of cell volume. When the effective circulating volume is reduced by more than 10 per cent, volume-mediated stimuli participate in the regulation of water balance. These pathways, indicated by the dotted lines in Figure 77–3, are the same as those shown in Figure 77–3 for extreme volume contraction. Finally,

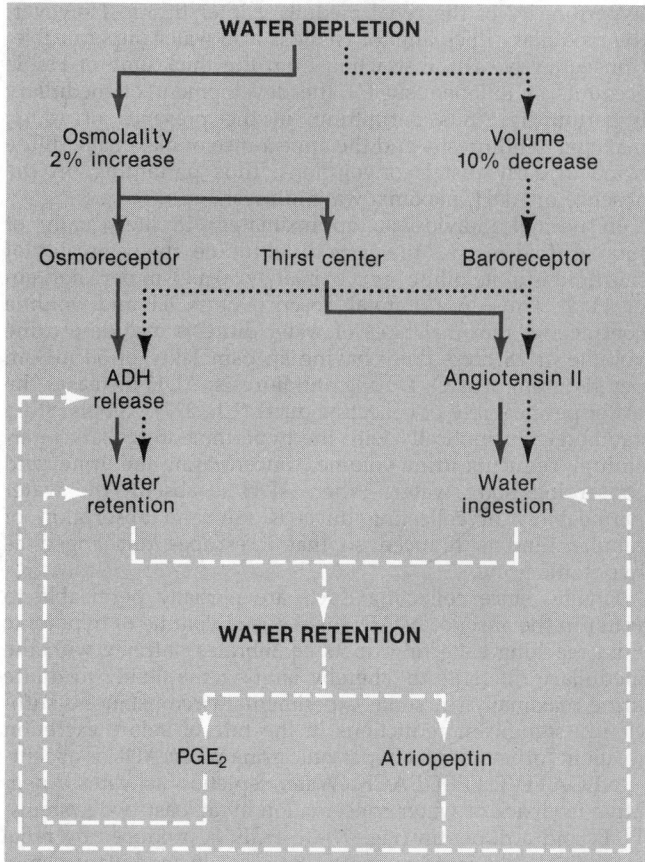

FIGURE 77–3. The water repletion reaction. The solid arrows are positive water conservation processes activated by osmolality increases; the dotted lines indicate volume-activated water conservation. The dashed lines show negative feedback.

the dashed lines in Figure 77–3 indicate the negative feedback limbs activated by water conservation.

SENSORS AND EFFECTORS. Three kinds of *sensor* elements adjust water balance. Two of these, osmoreceptors and the thirst center, respond to small changes in effective ECF osmolality, whereas baroreceptors respond to changes in effective circulating volume. The osmoreceptors are situated in the supraoptic and paraventricular nuclei of the hypothalamus, whereas the thirst center is in the organum vasculosum of the anterior hypothalamus. As little as a 2 per cent increase in effective ECF osmolality produced by solutes such as sodium chloride, but not urea, causes shrinkage of osmoreceptor cells and thirst center cells. The osmoreceptors stimulate the release of the *effector* hormone ADH from storage sites in the posterior pituitary gland. The stimulation of thirst by the thirst centers depends on centrally produced angiotensin II.

When the effective circulating volume is reduced by more than 10 per cent, volume-dependent mechanisms stimulate ADH release. Activation of extrarenal baroreceptors by blood volume depletion produces afferent signals, carried by the ninth and tenth cranial nerves, which result in nonosmotic ADH release. Volume contraction also acts as a potent stimulus to thirst via angiotensin II.

THE ANTIDIURETIC RESPONSE. The cardinal characteristics of the antidiuretic response depend primarily on the integrated activity of two regions of the nephron: the medullary thick ascending limb of Henle, referred to as the diluting segment; and the collecting duct, which may be termed the concentrating segment.

The medullary thick ascending limb absorbs a large amount, possibly as much as 25 per cent, of the filtered load of sodium. Some of this reabsorbed sodium is trapped in the renal medullary interstitium, thus accounting in large part for the hypertonicity of the renal medullary interstitium. However, the medullary thick limb of Henle is also water impermeable. Consequently, salt abstraction from the thick limb of Henle accounts simultaneously for the development of medullary hypertonicity, thus permitting, in the presence of ADH, maximal antidiuresis, and the appearance of maximally dilute urine in early distal convolutions, thus permitting, in the absence of ADH, maximal water diuresis.

In normal individuals, approximately 18 liters daily of tubular fluid reaches the early distal tubule; the osmolality of this fluid is quite dilute, approximately 50 mOsm per kilogram of H_2O. Thus in the total absence of ADH and volume contraction, maximal rates of water diuresis include a urine volume of 18 liters daily having an osmolality of 50 mOsm per kilogram of H_2O. During antidiuresis, ADH increases the water permeability of collecting ducts (Ch. 227). Tubular fluid equilibrates osmotically with the hypertonic medullary interstitium, reducing urine volume, concentrating the urine, and conserving body water. When ADH is absent, the water permeability of collecting ducts is low and absorption of tubular fluid is reduced so that it escapes unchanged as hypotonic urine.

Finally, since collecting ducts are partially permeable to water in the absence of ADH, a reduced volume of hypotonic fluid reaching collecting ducts equilibrates partially with the medullary interstitium, thereby limiting the ability to dilute urine maximally. In some experimental circumstances, sufficiently significant reductions in the rate of solute excretion result in formation of a hypertonic urine when ADH is absent.

NEGATIVE FEEDBACK. Water repletion activates a negative feedback of water conservation by at least two systems, PGE_2 and atriopeptin (Fig. 77–3). PGE_2 is produced by renal interstitial cells in response to increases in medullary osmolality. In turn, PGE_2 impairs water conservation by inhibiting the actions of ADH on nephron segments involved in the antidiuretic response, namely, the medullary thick ascending limb and the collecting duct.

Immunoreactive atriopeptin is elaborated within the central nervous system as well as by secretory granules in cardiac atria. This centrally released atriopeptin is capable of suppressing both ADH release and angiotensin II–stimulated thirst (Ch. 224).

HYPOTONIC DISORDERS

DEFINITION. A hypotonic disorder is one in which the ratio of solutes to water in body fluids is reduced, and the serum osmolality and serum sodium are both reduced in parallel. True hypotonicity must be distinguished from disorders in which the *measured* serum sodium is low while the measured serum osmolality is either normal or increased.

The distinction among these disorders is listed in Table 77–6. The measured serum sodium can be reduced either because there is an increased concentration of small, nonsodium solutes restricted to the ECF or because of a laboratory

TABLE 77–6. DISTINCTION BETWEEN APPARENT AND REAL HYPOTONICITY

Condition	Measured Serum [Na]	Measured Serum Osmolality
True hypotonicity	↓	↓
Increased nonsodium ECF solutes		
Hyperglycemia	↓	↑
Mannitol administration	↓	↑
Increased nonsodium ECF and ICF solutes		
Ethanol	normal	↑
Ethylene glycol	normal	↑
Methanol	normal	↑
Isopropyl alcohol	normal	↑
Laboratory artifact		
Hyperlipemia	↓	normal
Hyperproteinemia	↓	normal

TABLE 77–7. HYPONATREMIA REFERABLE TO IMPAIRED RENAL EXCRETION OF WATER

I. Reduced Sodium Delivery to the Diluting Segment
  Starvation
  Beer potomania
  ? Myxedema
II. Primary Excess of ADH
  SIADH
  Drug-induced ADH production
  Drug potentiation of ADH action
  Trauma
  Potassium depletion
  ? Myxedema
  ? Acute intermittent porphyria
	III. Mixed Disorders
	  Volume contraction (Addison's disease)
	  Edema with deranged Starling forces (congestive heart failure, constrictive pericarditis, and cirrhosis)

artifact. In hyperglycemia or excessive mannitol administration these solutes, which are restricted to the ECF, draw water from the cellular compartment. The serum sodium level is therefore reduced even though the serum osmolality may be increased. When a small, nonsodium solute is distributed in total body water, as in ethanol intoxication or in azotemia, the serum osmolality rises but the serum sodium concentration remains normal, resulting in an "osmolar gap."

In hyperlipemic or hyperproteinemic states, the volume of water in a given sample of serum sent for laboratory analysis is reduced. The flame photometer measures the total amount of sodium in a correspondingly reduced volume of water per unit volume of serum; therefore the serum sodium level appears low. However, the measured serum osmolality, which is a colligative property of aqueous solutions, is measured as normal, since the actual concentration of sodium per unit volume of water is normal. These instances of spurious hyponatremia are becoming less common as more laboratories adopt the use of ion-selective electrodes to measure the serum sodium concentration.

ETIOLOGY AND PATHOGENESIS. Hyponatremia and simultaneous body water hypotonicity develop whenever water intake exceeds the sum of renal plus extrarenal water losses; in chronic hyponatremia, the net water intake and net water output may be equal. Thus hyponatremia and body fluid hypotonicity occur when there is a primary increase in water ingestion, when the ability of the kidney to dilute urine maximally is limited, or when a combination of these factors is operative.

Dilutional hyponatremia may be the consequence of an absolute increase in water intake that exceeds the ability of a normal kidney to excrete free water, as in *primary polydipsia*, often referred to as psychogenic polydipsia. Patients with this disorder ingest unusually large volumes of water, often in excess of 10 to 15 liters daily, and generally develop mild, clinically asymptomatic hyponatremia. Profound hyponatremia is rare in these patients because the ability of the kidney to excrete large volumes of maximally dilute urine is not impaired.

More commonly, hyponatremia occurs because the ability of the kidney to excrete a maximally dilute urine is reduced. This inability to dilute urine maximally occurs because of (1) reductions in the rate of salt absorption by the diluting segment, that is, the thick ascending limb of Henle; (2) sustained nonosmotic release of ADH; or (3) a combination of these factors. Table 77–7 summarizes these disorders.

Reduced Sodium Delivery to Diluting Segments. These disorders occur when a reduced sodium intake, without significant sodium depletion or ECF volume contraction, decreases the rate of sodium delivery to the diluting segment and consequently impairs the maximal rate of dilute urine formation, the minimal urine osmolality, or both. Beer potomania, although an uncommon disorder, illustrates this mechanism for hyponatremia nicely.

Patients with beer potomania derive a substantial part of their caloric intake from the ingestion of large volumes of beer, which contains little salt or protein. Because sodium and urea are the major urinary solutes, dietary restriction of these solutes, particularly sodium, increases the fractional rate of proximal sodium absorption, diminishes the rate of salt delivery to diluting segments, and in turn limits the daily rate of formation of dilute urine. For example, the minimal urinary osmolality is approximately 50 mOsm per kilogram of H_2O; consequently, the excretion of 15 liters of highly dilute urine requires the excretion of 750 mOsm of solute. If the daily urinary solute excretion falls, the maximal amount of dilute urine formed daily is also reduced. Moreover, partial equilibration of reduced volumes of collecting duct fluid with the renal medullary interstitium impairs even further the daily excretion of dilute urine.

Hyponatremia due to reduced solute intake is not restricted to individuals with beer potomania but may occur during starvation, when intake may be dramatically reduced without parallel reductions in water intake. This form of hyponatremia occurs with increasing frequency in elderly patients in nursing homes who are inadequately supervised.

Patients with beer potomania or starvation are to be distinguished from individuals in whom a reduced effective circulating volume accompanied by an increase in total body water or by a reduction in glomerular filtration rate reduces the rate of salt delivery to diluting segments and collecting ducts (see below). In short, beer potomania and starvation are classic examples in which a reduced rate of delivery to the diluting segment, in the absence of ADH release, blunts significantly urinary diluting power in the absence of profound gains or excesses in total body water.

Primary Effector ADH Excess. THE SYNDROME OF INAPPROPRIATE ADH PRODUCTION (SIADH). In SIADH hyponatremia occurs as a result of sustained endogenous production and release of ADH or ADH-like substances; the effective circulating volume is normal or increased, and there are no other physiologic or pharmacologic stimuli to ADH release. Table 77–8 lists the major causes of SIADH. A similar process may account in part for the hyponatremia seen in myxedema.

Antidiuretic hormone, or a peptide having comparable biologic activity, is produced by tumors. Increased ADH levels, estimated by either bioassay or radioimmunoassay, have also been noted in patients with cranial disorders such

TABLE 77–8. MAJOR CAUSES OF SIADH

Malignant Neoplasia
  Carcinoma: bronchogenic, pancreatic, ureteral, prostatic, bladder
  Lymphoma and leukemia
  Thymoma and mesothelioma
Central Nervous System (CNS) Disorders
  Trauma
  Infection
  Tumors
  Porphyria
Pulmonary Disorders
  Tuberculosis
  Pneumonia
  Ventilators with positive pressure

as skull fractures, subdural hematomas, subarachnoid hemorrhage, and brain tumors; in acute intermittent porphyria; and possibly in myxedema. Four different patterns of plasma ADH concentrations have been described in patients with SIADH. Figure 77–4 illustrates three of these patterns; the shaded area in Figure 77–4 illustrates the normal relation between plasma ADH levels and serum osmolality. The pattern denoted as "erratic ADH release" in Figure 77–4 accounts for about 37 per cent of patients with SIADH; the hormone is released completely independently of osmotic control. About one third of patients with SIADH have a "reset osmostat"; there is an abnormally low threshold for ADH secretion, but if sufficiently hyponatremic, these patients with SIADH can produce a maximally dilute urine. About 16 per cent of patients with SIADH exhibit the "ADH leak" pattern, namely, sustained ADH production below the osmotic threshold, and normal increases in serum ADH levels with osmotic challenge (Fig. 77–4). Finally, about 14 per cent of patients with SIADH have no detectable abnormality in ADH levels; they fail, for reasons not yet understood, to dilute urine maximally.

The typical features of SIADH are listed in Table 77–9. The cardinal results of the sustained water conservation in SIADH are twofold: hyponatremia and volume expansion. In fact, patients with SIADH who are allowed free access to water generally gain about 3 kg in water weight, or, in other words, nearly 10 per cent of body water. In that respect, patients with SIADH differ from those with hyponatremia secondary to salt depletion, Addison's disease, or diuretic excess, since patients with the latter disorders are volume contracted. However, patients with SIADH, although volume expanded, do not develop edema and thus differ in that respect from patients with congestive heart failure or cirrhosis.

When total body water is expanded by about 10 per cent by water conservation in SIADH, a natriuresis occurs even in the face of hyponatremia. Thus the patient with SIADH reaches a steady state in which body water is expanded by water retention and in which natriuresis, even in the face of hyponatremia, prevents edema formation.

The causes for the natriuresis that is characteristic of SIADH are multiple. Volume expansion will result in enhanced release of atriopeptin, which enhances urinary sodium wasting both by enhancing glomerular filtration and probably by suppressing tubular sodium absorption. Second, the volume expansion of SIADH also reduces the rate of proximal tubular sodium absorption, as well as the rate of proximal uric acid absorption.

In short, SIADH is a disorder in which hormone-stimulated water conservation results in hyponatremia, volume expansion, and consequently an increased glomerular filtration rate, tubular sodium wasting, and reduced net tubular absorption of creatinine and uric acid, but no edema formation. These

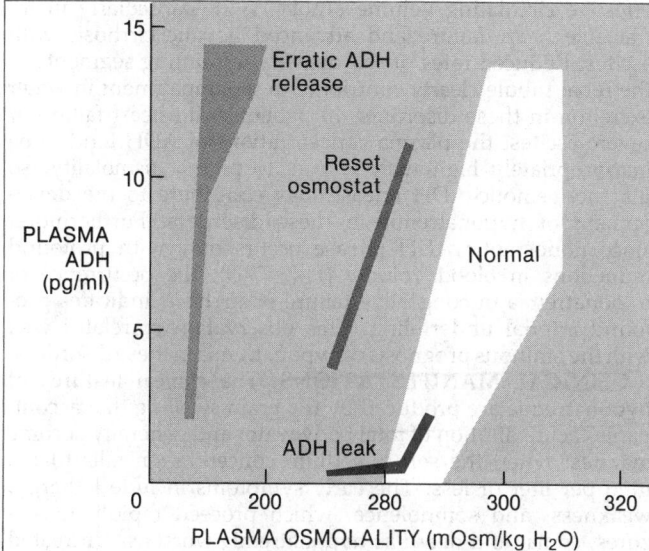

FIGURE 77–4. The patterns of serum ADH abnormalities in SIADH. The shaded areas indicate the normal relation between increases in effective ECF osmolality and ADH levels; the normal osmotic threshold is lower than the normal serum osmolality. The three shaded areas indicate ADH patterns in SIADH. (Adapted from Zerbe R, Strope L, Robertson G: Vasopressin function in the syndrome of inappropriate diuresis. Ann Rev Med 31:315, 1980.)

TABLE 77–9. MAJOR CHARACTERISTICS OF SIADH

Hyponatremia
Volume expansion without edema
Natriuresis
Hypouricemia
Normal or reduced serum creatinine level
Normal thyroid and adrenal function

characteristics are summarized in Table 77–9. Finally, as indicated in connection with Figure 77–4, the urine osmolality in patients with SIADH may be either inappropriately high for the level of serum osmolality or maximally dilute.

OTHER CAUSES OF EXCESSIVE ADH PRODUCTION AND/OR RELEASE. Table 77–7 lists other circumstances in which an increased level of ADH is the primary factor responsible for hyponatremia. A number of commonly used drugs stimulate ADH release: vincristine, cyclophosphamide, carbamazepine, phenothiazines, morphine, barbiturates, chlorpropamide, amitriptyline, thiothixene, and clofibrate. Chlorpropamide also potentiates the effect of ADH on the water permeability of collecting ducts. The posterior pituitary peptide oxytocin (Pitocin) also has an antidiuretic action, although oxytocin is a much less potent antidiuretic agent than vasopressin. Thus the administration of intravenous hypotonic solutions containing oxytocin for the purpose of inducing labor may result in profound hyponatremia. Trauma or surgical stress also stimulates ADH release.

Ordinarily, diuretic-induced hyponatremia is related to volume contraction; this kind of body fluid dilution will be discussed below. Chronic severe potassium depletion induced by diuretics also can result in ADH release, although the mechanisms by which potassium depletion stimulates ADH release are unknown.

Mixed Disorders. Hyponatremia occurs commonly in true volume contraction and in edematous states in which filling of the arterial tree is impaired. The former disorders include patients in whom both ECF and total body water are reduced; the latter group comprises those patients with deranged Starling forces, notably local or systemic increases in venous pressure, which result in inadequate filling of the arterial tree. In both sets of disorders, two factors contribute, individually or in unison, to the pathogenesis of hyponatremia: nonosmotic, volume-mediated ADH release and reductions in the rate of sodium delivery to the diluting segment.

Volume contraction is a potent nonosmotic stimulus to ADH release. Figure 77–5 shows the relations between osmotic and nonosmotic, volume-mediated stimuli and plasma ADH levels in experimental animals; entirely comparable responses occur in humans. Increases in plasma osmolality are related linearly to increases in plasma ADH levels. The relation between blood volume depletion and plasma ADH levels is nonlinear. However, with depletion of more than 7 to 10 per cent blood volume, plasma ADH levels rise sharply and produce an antidiuretic effect even when the plasma osmolality is reduced below normal. In other words, volume-mediated, nonosmotic ADH release occurs primarily when circulatory dynamics are moderately to severely advanced; in that circumstance, volume-mediated stimuli over-ride osmotically mediated ADH release, and hyponatremia ensues.

A second factor that accounts for hyponatremia in volume-contracted states is an inability to dilute urine maximally because the rate of sodium delivery to diluting segments in the thick ascending limb is reduced. This occurs because increased rates of proximal tubular sodium absorption are stimulated by reduced sodium intake or by inadequate filling of the arterial tree in conditions with combined ECF volume expansion and reduced arterial tree filling. The significance of volume contraction as a pathogenic factor in this type of hyponatremia can be gauged by noting that hyponatremia occurs during volume contraction in experimental animals with pituitary diabetes insipidus.

Hyponatremia is a common feature of untreated Addison's disease and occurs because of a combination of circumstances. In mineralocorticoid deficiency, ECF volume contraction, glomerular filtration reduction, enhanced proximal tubular salt absorption, and volume-mediated, nonosmotic ADH release appear to be the major factors responsible for an inability to handle water loads. Glucocorticoid deficiency also impairs the ability to handle water loads. One of the factors responsible

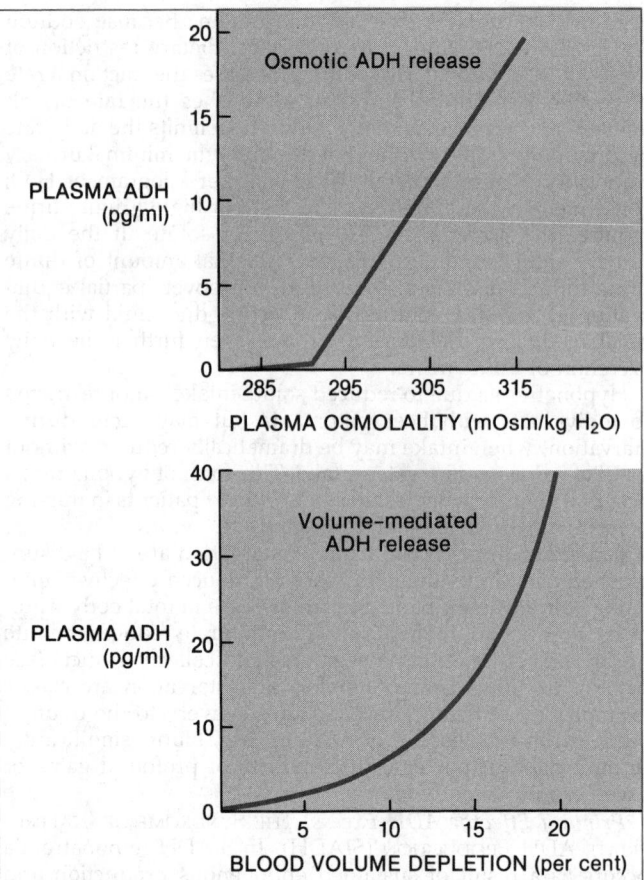

FIGURE 77–5. Relation between plasma ADH concentrations and either effective ECF osmolality (upper plot) or the per cent of blood volume depletion (lower plot). (Adapted from Dunn FL, Brennan TJ, Nelson AE, et al.: The role of blood osmolality and volume in regulating vasopressin secretion in the rat. J Clin Invest 52:3212, 1973.)

for water retention in Addison's disease is nonosmotic ADH release, which results from impaired cardiac function.

Hyponatremia occurs commonly in advanced stages of disorders characterized by edema formation and a reduced effective circulating volume (Table 77–7), particularly in intractable heart failure and advanced hepatic cirrhosis with ascites. Reduced rates of salt delivery to diluting segments of the renal tubule clearly contribute to the impairment in water excretion in these disorders. In patients with heart failure or severe ascites, the plasma concentrations of ADH tend to be inappropriately high with respect to plasma osmolality, so that nonosmotic ADH release may contribute to the development of hyponatremia in these disorders. Furthermore, since nonosmotic ADH release occurs only with profound reductions in blood volume (Fig. 77–5), the occurrence of hyponatremia in congestive failure or cirrhosis indicates profound arterial underfilling. This observation correlates well with the ominous prognosis of hyponatremia in these disorders.

CLINICAL MANIFESTATIONS. The clinical features of hyponatremia are produced by the brain swelling that accompanies acute dilution of total body water and generally become manifest when the serum sodium concentration falls to 120 mEq per liter or less. The early symptoms include lethargy, weakness, and somnolence, which proceed rapidly to seizures, coma, and death as hyponatremia worsens. Untreated acute water intoxication is nearly uniformly fatal and represents a medical emergency. In chronic hyponatremia, central nervous system manifestations are far less common, even when the serum sodium concentration is as low as 100 mEq per liter, because the loss of brain solutes, principally potassium chloride, minimizes brain cell swelling for a given reduction in body water osmolality.

DIAGNOSIS. Hyponatremia should be considered whenever there is a sudden deterioration in central nervous system function, particularly in circumstances such as intractable heart failure, hepatic cirrhosis with ascites, or the administration of large volumes of intravenous fluids. The hyponatremic patient should be evaluated to determine the underlying condition that produced body fluid dilution. This evaluation should include a careful history and physical examination; measurement of the serum creatinine, BUN, and electrolytes; measurement of the urinary sodium concentration, or the FE_{Na}; measurement of serum and urine osmolalities; and, when appropriate, evaluation of thyroid and adrenal function.

The history and physical examination are generally adequate for recognizing disorders such as beer potomania or compulsive water ingestion or for noting the ingestion of drugs that stimulate ADH release or enhance ADH action. The presence of edema is characteristic of individuals in whom hyponatremia occurs because of a reduced effective circulating volume coupled to ECF volume expansion. In myxedema or Addison's disease, the typical clinical or laboratory findings of these disorders are generally present (Ch. 229 and 230).

The most difficult differential diagnosis among hyponatremic disorders involves the distinction between patients who are modestly volume contracted and those who have SIADH. In both circumstances, the serum sodium and the serum osmolality are reduced, whereas the urine osmolality is inappropriately high with respect to the reduced serum osmolality. Nonosmotic water conservation in SIADH and in volume contraction is recognized by the presence of a urine osmolality greater than 120 to 150 mOsm per kilogram of H_2O in association with a reduced serum osmolality. The distinction between the two disorders therefore depends on a clinical and laboratory assessment of effective circulating volume.

Patients who are volume contracted may provide a history of volume losses or of diuretic ingestion and may exhibit the signs of ECF volume contraction discussed previously in the section on Volume Depletion. When the volume losses are due to extrarenal causes, the urinary sodium concentration is less than 10 to 15 mEq per liter and the FE_{Na} is generally less than 1 per cent. The presence of hyperuricemia may also be a useful index to the possibility of ECF volume contraction. Prerenal azotemia may occur if the volume contraction is severe. Patients with SIADH are generally normovolemic or slightly volume expanded and therefore exhibit none of the signs of volume contraction. The serum BUN and creatinine levels are normal, and the serum uric acid level is generally reduced. The urinary sodium concentration usually exceeds 30 mEq per liter, and the FE_{Na} is greater than 1 per cent. Tests of adrenal function yield normal results.

The above studies usually discriminate between SIADH and extrarenal volume contraction. When ECF volume contraction is due to renal salt wasting, urinary sodium losses generally persist unless volume contraction is profound. Moreover, as noted previously (see Volume Depletion), the blood pressure and pulse may be normal in states of modest volume contraction. A useful diagnostic and therapeutic maneuver in this situation is to observe the results of water restriction. When water intake is restricted to 600 to 800 ml daily, patients with SIADH exhibit a highly characteristic response: A 2- to 3-kg weight loss is accompanied by correction of hyponatremia and cessation of salt wasting, usually over a period of two to three days. If weight loss fails to correct both hyponatremia and urinary sodium wasting simultaneously, the diagnosis of SIADH is doubtful. Rather, renal sodium wasting with ECF volume contraction, due to Addison's disease or the other renal salt-losing disorders listed in Table 77–2, is the more probable diagnosis.

TREATMENT. The goal of treatment in hyponatremia is to correct body water osmolality and therefore restore cell volume to normal by raising the ratio of sodium to water in extracellular fluid. The increase in ECF osmolality draws water from cells and therefore reduces their volume. The choice of therapeutic approach, and whether or not net sodium and water balance is adjusted to be positive or negative during therapy, depends on the serum sodium concentration, the rate at which hyponatremia has developed, the clinical status of the patient, and the underlying disorder.

Acute Hyponatremia. Acute hyponatremia associated with a serum sodium concentration below 120 mEq per liter and with central nervous system manifestations requires immediate therapy. In volume-contracted states, the treatment of choice is to raise the serum sodium level to 125 mEq per liter over a six-hour interval by administering hypertonic 3 to 5 per cent saline. Since the desired effect is to correct body water osmolality, the amount of sodium administered must be sufficient to raise total body water osmolality to approximately 250 mOsm per kilogram of H_2O, that is, to approximately twice the desired serum sodium concentration. A convenient formula for calculating this sodium requirement is as follows:

$$[125 - \text{measured serum Na}^+] \times 0.6 \text{ body weight} = \text{required mEq of Na}^+$$

The serum sodium level is in milliequivalents per liter, and the body weight is in kilograms. Since 60 per cent of body weight is water, the formula allows an estimate of the amount of sodium required to raise body water osmolality to 250 mOsm per kilogram of H_2O.

The administration of hypertonic saline solutions is hazardous in volume-expanded, salt-retaining states such as congestive heart failure. Furthermore, in SIADH associated with volume expansion and sodium wasting, hypertonic saline alone is ineffective in correcting hyponatremia because the administered salt is excreted promptly in a relatively concentrated urine.

A preferable alternative is to use normal saline in combination with furosemide administration. The diuretic induces urinary salt loss and therefore reduces the risk of ECF volume expansion. Moreover, the diuresis induced by furosemide is characterized by the excretion of urine having a sodium concentration that is appreciably lower than that in plasma. Consequently, the combination of intravenously administered normal saline with a furosemide-induced diuresis of urine that is dilute with respect to plasma provides an effective way of raising the serum sodium level in SIADH or other volume-expanded states. By adjusting the rates of salt administration to be less than urinary salt losses, reductions in ECF volume can be produced simultaneously.

Rapid elevation of serum sodium concentrations to levels greater than 125 mEq per liter is hazardous. Since loss of brain solute represents one of the compensatory mechanisms for preserving brain cell volume in dilutional states, a serum sodium level of 140 mEq per liter may be relatively hypertonic to brain cells that have become partially depleted of solute as a result of hyponatremia. Consequently, raising the serum sodium rapidly to levels greater than 120 to 125 mEq per liter can result in central nervous system damage.

Chronic Hyponatremia. Mild, asymptomatic chronic hyponatremia is generally managed by correction of the underlying disorder, when the hyponatremia occurs in volume contraction or in salt-retaining states such as congestive heart failure or hepatic cirrhosis with ascites. Chronic hyponatremia in SIADH may be easily corrected by restricting water intake to 800 to 1000 ml daily, provided that patients can adhere to the program of water restriction. An alternative approach involves the use of agents such as lithium or demethylchlortetracycline, which interfere with the renal tubular effects of ADH. However, both agents have other adverse effects. As another alternative, some workers have recommended reducing renal ability for urinary concentration by administering large oral loads of urea, thereby producing a modest osmotic diuresis.

HYPERTONIC DISORDERS

DEFINITION. A hypertonic disorder is one in which the ratio of solutes to water in total body water is increased. All hypernatremic states are hypertonic. In some hypertonic disorders, the increase in effective ECF osmolality is due to nonsodium solutes, for example, uncontrolled hyperglycemia.

ETIOLOGY AND PATHOGENESIS. Hypernatremia develops whenever water intake is less than the sum of renal and extrarenal water losses; in chronic hypertonic states, net water balance may be zero. The most common causes for clinically significant hypernatremia occur as a consequence of three pathogenic mechanisms: impaired thirst; solute or osmotic diuresis; excessive losses of water, either via the kidneys or extrarenally; and combinations of these derangements. These disorders are grouped in Table 77–10 according to the primary pathogenic mechanism. There is also a group of miscellaneous disorders, such as hypokalemia, hypercalcemia, and interstitial renal disease, and chronic renal failure, which either impair partially renal urinary concentrating ability or blunt partially the responsiveness of collecting ducts to ADH. These disorders rarely cause significant hypernatremia and will not be discussed further.

Inadequate Intake of Water. This problem occurs in patients who are comatose or who are otherwise unable to communicate thirst. Because of the exquisite sensitivity of thirst mechanisms to changes in effective body water osmolality, hypernatremia due to inadequate water intake is rare in conscious patients allowed free access to water. Rarely, patients will have a primary thirst deficiency. Patients with Cushing's syndrome or primary hyperaldosteronism commonly have slight elevations in the serum sodium level for unknown reasons.

Finally, "essential hypernatremia" is characterized by a slightly elevated serum sodium level that occurs in the conscious state. The defect in patients with essential hypernatremia appears to be an insensitivity of thirst centers and osmoreceptors to osmotic stimuli. However, both thirst and antidiuresis occur when these patients are volume contracted. Consequently, it has been inferred that volume-mediated stimuli to thirst and ADH release are intact in patients with essential hypernatremia. This disorder may be either congenital or acquired, sometimes in association with histiocytic infiltration of the central nervous system.

Osmotic Diuresis. This is another mechanism for producing renal water losses in excess of sodium losses and therefore hypertonicity. Osmotic diuresis occurs commonly in uncontrolled glycosuria and may occur during mannitol administration for the treatment of increased intracranial pressure. Since these solutes are restricted to the ECF, the serum sodium level is generally reduced in the early stages of osmotic diuresis, and the effective ECF osmolality is increased primarily by the impermeant nonsodium solute. In prolonged osmotic diuresis, net water losses may be sufficiently great that hypernatremia develops. In this circumstance, the increase in effective ECF osmolality is due to the combined effects of hypernatremia and the nonsodium solute. Hyper-

natremia due to an osmotic urea diuresis can occur if large amounts of protein and amino acids are administered by nasogastric tube, or if tissue catabolism is great, as in burns. In this circumstance, hypernatremia is entirely responsible for the increased effective ECF osmolality.

Hypernatremia may also occur when large amounts of hypertonic sodium solutions are administered, particularly in patients whose renal function is compromised. Two common examples of this condition include the rapid intravenous administration of multiple ampules of sodium bicarbonate during cardiopulmonary resuscitation and the administration of large amounts of sodium bicarbonate to patients with lactic acidosis.

Excessive Water Losses. Impairment of ADH production, release, or action, as in pituitary or nephrogenic diabetes insipidus, respectively, can lead to profound water deficits and to hypernatremia. In such circumstances, the urine volumes are large, the urine osmolality is low, and the net rate of solute excretion is low, in contrast to individuals undergoing osmotic diuresis, in whom rates of urinary solute excretion are elevated.

Striking water losses may also occur with excessive sweating, particularly during rigorous physical activity by untrained individuals exercising in high humidity. This phenomenon plays a major role in the evolution of heat stroke.

Combined Disorders. Finally, hypertonic dehydration may occur as a combination of these events. A common example in modern clinical practice involves the injudicious administration of large amounts of carbohydrate or amino acids by nasogastric tube, coupled with limited amounts of water, to stroke patients unable to communicate thirst.

CLINICAL MANIFESTATIONS AND DIAGNOSIS. Since two thirds of body water is intracellular, primary water losses tend to have modest effects on circulating volume unless fluid losses are profound. Rather, the clinical manifestations are produced by brain shrinkage that results from increases in effective ECF osmolality. Thus the symptoms of hypertonicity produced either by hypernatremia or by impermeant nonsodium solutes such as glucose are referable to the central nervous system and range from somnolence and confusion to coma, respiratory paralysis, and death. The degree of symptomatology varies with the degree of hypertonicity and with the rate at which hypertonicity develops. In acute hypertonicity, symptoms generally appear when the effective ECF osmolality exceeds 320 to 330 mOsm per kilogram of H_2O, and coma and respiratory arrest may occur when the ECF osmolality exceeds 360 to 380 mOsm per kilogram of H_2O. Chronic hypertonicity generally produces fewer central nervous system manifestations, because brain cells accumulate idiogenic osmoles, which minimize the tendency for brain shrinkage.

TREATMENT. The treatment of acute hypernatremia requires the administration of isotonic dilute saline solutions, generally by an intravenous route. The following factors should be borne in mind when treating acute hypernatremia.

In the severely volume-contracted patient with severe hypernatremia, the administration of isotonic saline solutions has two advantages. It provides fluid resuscitation in impending cardiovascular collapse. Moreover, the isotonic salt solution, which is hypotonic with respect to the hypertonic patient, avoids an unnecessary rapid fall in the serum sodium level.

Rapid correction of hypertonicity to a normal serum osmolality is hazardous. Since accumulation of idiogenic osmoles by brain cells is a compensatory mechanism for preserving brain volume in hypertonic disorders, a normal serum osmolality may be relatively hypotonic to brain cells that have accumulated idiogenic solutes. Hence if the serum osmolality is reduced rapidly, central nervous system damage due to brain swelling may occur. A useful guide to circumventing this difficulty is to reduce the serum sodium level by no more

---

TABLE 77–10. MAJOR CAUSES OF HYPERNATREMIA

I. **Impaired Thirst**
    Coma
    Essential hypernatremia
II. **Solute Diuresis**
    Osmotic diuresis: diabetic ketoacidosis, nonketotic hyperosmolar coma, mannitol administration
III. **Excessive Water Losses**
    Renal
        Pituitary diabetes insipidus
        Nephrogenic diabetes insipidus
    Extrarenal
        Sweating
IV. **Combined Disorders**
    Coma plus hypertonic nasogastric feeding

than 1 mEq per liter during every two hours of the first two days of treatment.

Finally, if solutions of 5 per cent dextrose in water are administered at a rapid rate, hyperglycemia and osmotic diuresis may occur and hence aggravate the hypertonic state. In this circumstance, the use of a 2.5 per cent dextrose solution in one-quarter normal saline is advisable. This solution has been particularly useful in treating hypernatremia associated with volume contraction in children with pituitary or nephrogenic diabetes insipidus.

Anderson RJ, Chung H-M, Kluge R, et al.: Hyponatremia. A prospective analysis of its epidemiology and the pathogenetic role of vasopressin. Ann Intern Med 102:164, 1985. *A study of the frequency and causes of hyponatremia in hospitalized patients.*

Arieff AI: Hyponatremia, convulsions, respiratory arrest, and permanent brain damage after elective surgery in healthy women. N Engl J Med 314:1529, 1986. *A detailed analysis of the central nervous system complications of acute hyponatremia.*

Ayus JC, Krothapalli RK, Arieff AI: Changing concepts in treatment of severe symptomatic hyponatremia. Am J Med 78:897, 1985. *A review of the controversy surrounding the treatment of hyponatremia and its relation to central pontine myelinolysis.*

Buckalew VM Jr: Hyponatremia: Pathogenesis and management. Hosp Pract 21:49, 1986. *An excellent description of the treatment of hyponatremia.*

Gennari FJ: Serum osmolality—uses and limitations. N Engl J Med 310:102, 1984. *An introduction to the concepts of osmolality and tonicity with guides to the appropriate laboratory evaluation of osmolality disorders.*

Hebert SC, Culpepper RM, Andreoli TE: The posterior pituitary and water metabolism. In Wilson JD, Foster DW (eds.): Williams Textbook of Endocrinology. Philadelphia, W. B. Saunders Company, 1985, pp 614–652. *A complete discussion of the physiology of water metabolism, hypernatremia, and hyponatremia.*

Manning PT, Schwartz D, Katsube NC, et al.: Vasopressin-stimulated release of atriopeptin: Endocrine antagonists in fluid homeostasis. Science 229:395, 1985. *The role of atriopeptin in the negative feedback of water balance.*

Miller M, Dalakos T, Moses AM, et al.: Recognition of partial defects in antidiuretic hormone secretion. Ann Intern Med 73:721, 1970. *A concise guide to testing procedures for states of ADH insufficiency and a rational scheme for interpreting the test results.*

Narins RG, Jones ER, Stom MC, et al.: Diagnostic strategies in disorders of fluid, electrolyte and acid-base homeostasis. Am J Med 72:496, 1982. *A good clinical approach to osmolality disturbances.*

Thompson CS, Andreoli TE: Hyponatremia and hypernatremia. In Callaham ML (ed.): Current Therapy in Emergency Medicine. Philadelphia, B. C. Decker, 1987, pp 739–744. *A practical guide to the diagnosis and treatment of hyponatremia and hypernatremia.*

Zerbe R, Strope L, Robertson G: Vasopressin function in the syndrome of inappropriate diuresis. Ann Rev Med 31:315, 1980. *The patterns of ADH response in SIADH.*

Disturbances in Potassium Balance

PHYSIOLOGIC CONSIDERATIONS

The body contains approximately 3500 mEq of potassium, of which only 60 mEq, or about 2 per cent, is extracellular. In normal circumstances external potassium balance depends mainly on dietary potassium intake and renal potassium excretion; fecal potassium losses are only about 10 mEq per day unless diarrhea is present. Since 98 per cent of potassium is located intracellularly, primarily in skeletal muscle, regulation of the serum potassium concentration depends not only on external potassium balance but also on potassium exchanges between the intracellular and extracellular compartments.

Transfer Between ICF and ECF

The intracellular compartment acts as a large potassium reservoir in series with the small ECF potassium pool. In potassium-depleted states a 1 mEq per liter fall in the serum potassium level requires the loss of about 100 to 200 mEq of potassium; hence the bulk of external potassium loss comes from the cellular compartment. Conversely, if large amounts of potassium are administered acutely, the rise in serum potassium level is less than would be expected if the administered potassium were distributed solely in the ECF. In this situation, cellular uptake of potassium obviously occurs and prevents greater increases in the serum potassium concentration. This ability of cells to accumulate potassium can be enhanced strikingly by chronic administration of high-potassium diets.

A number of *effector* mechanisms regulate the partition of potassium between the ICF and ECF. These include active and passive ionic transcellular transport processes.

ACTIVE TRANSPORT PROCESSES. The cardinal transport process regulating K^+ distribution between ICF and ECF is cell membrane–bound $(Na^+ + K^+)$-ATPase, which actively transports potassium into cells and therefore counterbalances the passive leak of potassium from cells into interstitial fluid. Insulin is a second effector that promotes potassium transfer from ECF to ICF; this hormone promotes cellular uptake of potassium independently of cellular glucose uptake by increasing $(Na^+ + K^+)$-ATPase activity. Furthermore, hyperkalemia augments insulin release. Thus hyperkalemia may be the sensor that stimulates release of insulin, which then serves as an effector for potassium entry into cells. Finally, beta-adrenergic agents such as epinephrine and isoproterenol promote cellular uptake of potassium.

PASSIVE TRANSPORT PROCESSES. A number of passive effector mechanisms also regulate the partition of potassium between the ICF and the ECF. Alterations in the pH of ECF reproducibly shift potassium between the ICF and the ECF: Systemic acidosis, whether metabolic or respiratory, promotes potassium efflux from cells, whereas systemic alkalosis, either metabolic or respiratory, promotes cellular potassium uptake. As a general rule, a reduction in plasma pH of 0.1 unit raises the serum potassium level by 0.6 mEq per liter, whereas a plasma pH increase of 0.1 unit produces a similar reduction in serum potassium. The mechanisms for these pH-induced potassium shifts between ICF and ECF are not understood.

Second, cellular shrinkage produced by increases in effective ECF osmolality raises the intracellular potassium concentration and thereby increases the driving force for passive potassium leakage from the ICF to the ECF. This leakage may result in hyperkalemia when large glucose loads are administered to insulin-deficient diabetic patients who also have hyporeninemic hypoaldosteronism; the insulin lack limits cellular re-entry of potassium, and the aldosterone deficiency limits renal potassium excretion. Increases in cell potassium concentrations produced by cellular shrinkage also contribute significantly to the hyperkalemia of diabetic ketoacidosis, because hyperglycemia raises cell potassium levels by cell shrinkage and insulin lack prevents accelerated potassium re-entry into cells.

Finally, brain cells and renal tubular cells lose potassium when exposed to chronic ECF hypotonicity. However, muscle cells, which are the largest component of ICF potassium, do not appear to participate in this process. Consequently, hypotonic disorders, by themselves, have little effect on the serum potassium level or on external potassium balance.

Renal Handling of Potassium

The kidneys process potassium strikingly differently from the way in which they process sodium. Sodium excretion involves filtration, partial tubular absorption, and appearance of nonabsorbed sodium as urinary sodium excretion. When dietary sodium intake is varied, there is a prompt adjustment in urinary sodium excretion, either in the upward direction, when sodium intake is increased, or in the downward direction, when sodium intake is curtailed.

In contrast, virtually all dietary potassium, ordinarily about 50 to 200 mEq per day, appears in the urine because of tubular secretion of potassium by terminal nephron segments. These regions of the nephron can increase rates of potassium secretion significantly if dietary potassium intake is augmented; and they carry out net absorption of potassium in kaliopenic states. In other words, these terminal nephron segments

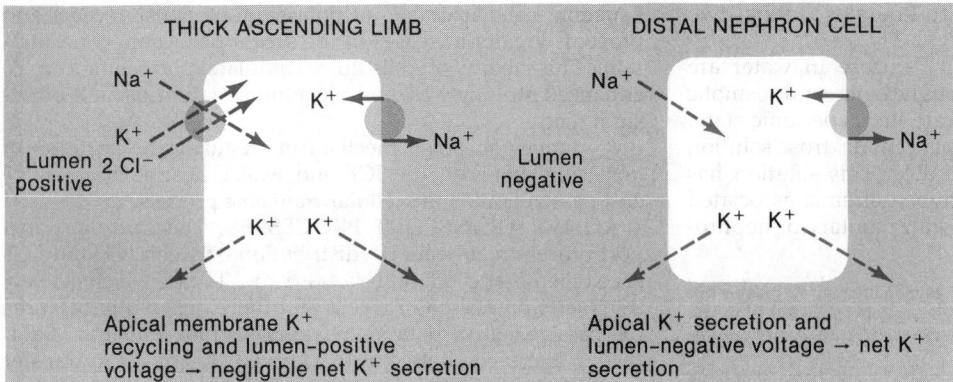

THICK ASCENDING LIMB

Na⁺
K⁺
Lumen 2 Cl⁻
positive
K⁺
Na⁺
K⁺   K⁺

Apical membrane K⁺
recycling and lumen–positive
voltage → negligible net K⁺ secretion

DISTAL NEPHRON CELL

Na⁺
Lumen
negative
K⁺
Na⁺
K⁺   K⁺

Apical K⁺ secretion and
lumen–negative voltage → net K⁺
secretion

FIGURE 77–6. Handling of potassium in late nephron segments, including the thick ascending limb and the distal nephron. The dashed arrows represent passive transport processes and the solid arrows represent active transport processes. In the thick ascending limb, K⁺ recycling into cells by Na⁺:K⁺:2 Cl⁻ cotransport and the lumen-positive voltage reduce the rate of net K⁺ secretion. Most urinary K⁺ comes from net K⁺ secretion by terminal nephron segments.

regulate external potassium balance by adjusting *renal output* to balance *intake*.

A convenient way of considering distal nephron handling of potassium, and the ways in which effector mechanisms modulate this process, is shown in Figure 77–6. The dashed lines indicate passive processes, and the solid lines denote active transport processes. Basolateral membranes of all terminal nephron segments, including the thick limb of Henle, the distal tubule, and the collecting duct, share two common characteristics: a passive leakage pathway for K⁺ efflux and an active (Na⁺ + K⁺)-ATPase for cellular K⁺ uptake. The apical membranes of these nephron segments also contain passive potassium leakage pathways, which can be blocked by barium. In the thick ascending limb of Henle, apical membranes contain a furosemide-sensitive coupled entry step that involves electroneutral Na⁺:K⁺:2Cl⁻ cotransport, driven by the electrochemical sodium gradient between lumen and cells. In distal tubular and collecting ducts, Na⁺ entry into cells involves sodium-specific channels that are blocked by amiloride. Thus in the ascending limb, coupled electroneutral sodium entry into cells does not result in luminal electronegativity (in fact, the lumen in the thick ascending limb is electropositive), whereas in the distal tubule and collecting duct, amiloride-sensitive ionic sodium entry produces luminal electronegativity.

The majority of net K⁺ secretion occurs in these latter two segments and is driven indirectly by the rate of sodium entry into cells, which increases luminal electronegativity and increases the activity of basolateral (Na⁺ + K⁺)-ATPase, thus raising cell potassium concentrations. In the loop of Henle, little net potassium secretion occurs, because the lumen is electropositive and because coupled Na⁺:K⁺:2Cl⁻ transport from lumen to cells recycles secreted potassium back into cells.

The major elements of the *effector systems* that regulate distal nephron potassium excretion include the rate of distal tubular sodium delivery; dietary potassium intake; plasma pH; aldosterone; impermeant anions; and tubular flow rates. When distal sodium delivery rates are increased, increased sodium entry into cells across apical membranes is accompanied by increased activity of pump (Na⁺ + K⁺)-ATPase, which tends to raise intracellular potassium concentrations. Second, either an increase in dietary potassium intake or an increase in plasma pH tends, as indicated above, to raise cellular potassium content. Third, urinary excretion of impermeant anions such as sulfate, carbenicillin, or penicillin produces greater luminal electronegativity. Fourth, aldosterone and mineralocorticoids, whose kaliuretic effects may be dissociated from their sodium-sparing effects, increase the permeability of luminal membranes to potassium. These hormones may also augment distal tubular (Na⁺ + K⁺)-ATPase activity. Among these factors, the rate of aldosterone secretion and the rate of distal salt delivery to terminal nephron segments are the cardinal variables.

Each of the above factors modulates one or another portion

of a generalized mechanism, namely, an electrochemical gradient favorable to the passive movement of potassium from tubular cells to urine and consequently for net potassium secretion. Conversely, reductions in sodium delivery, potassium restriction, reductions in plasma pH, and mineralocorticoid lack all reduce the magnitude of passive potassium movement from cells to tubular fluid and therefore tend to decrease net potassium secretion. Finally, increases in tubular flow rates, as in osmotic diuresis, also promote potassium secretion, whereas reductions in tubular flow rates decrease potassium secretion. The mechanism responsible for this effect is unknown.

The net rate of urinary potassium excretion in any given circumstance therefore depends on the interplay of these multiple factors in modulating the common effector mechanism for potassium secretion. For example, mineralocorticoid excess in primary aldosteronism commonly leads to severe potassium wasting. This kaliuresis can be curtailed by dietary sodium restriction and accentuated by dietary sodium loading. Conversely, in hyporeninemic hypoaldosteronism, hyperkalemia may be prevented by insuring a liberal intake of sodium.

The renal adaptation to excess potassium loads occurs over a 24- to 36-hour period. Consequently, hyperkalemia from the ingestion of large oral potassium loads is uncommon in normal individuals. But the renal response to dietary potassium restriction is more sluggish and requires seven to ten days for full development. Even under the latter circumstances, urinary potassium losses are rarely less than 20 mEq daily.

Excitable Tissues and the ICF/ECF Potassium Ratio

The clinical consequences of hypokalemia and hyperkalemia are generally due to changes in the excitable characteristics of heart, skeletal muscle, and smooth muscle. Excitable tissues, such as nerve, heart, and skeletal muscle, share certain common properties. At rest excitable tissues are far more permeable to potassium than to sodium. The cell interior is electronegative with respect to extracellular fluid, and this voltage is largely determined by the logarithm of the ratio of intracellular (K_i) to extracellular (K_o) potassium concentrations. When excitable tissues are suddenly depolarized to their threshold voltage, sodium permeability increases profoundly with an accompanying increase in the sodium to potassium permeability ratio. This sodium entry into the cells of excitable tissues occurs through sodium-specific channels having electronegative sites that are activated by sudden depolarization. During depolarization, rapid sodium entry produces the initial spike of the action potential, and the cell interior becomes electropositive.

This voltage-dependent increase in sodium permeability during depolarization to threshold is the most fundamental characteristic of excitable tissues (except in tissues such as the atrioventricular node, where Ca⁺⁺ influx into cells is responsible for the action potential). If an excitable cell is partially depolarized in the resting state, the rate of rise of action potentials is reduced; the prolonged resting depolarization, by undefined mechanisms, reduces the increase in sodium permeability that accompanies the action potential. This effect of resting depolarization on reducing sodium permeability during action potentials is referred to as inactivation.

Repolarization of excitable cells occurs more slowly than depolarization. During repolarization, potassium permeability rises with respect to sodium permeability, and there is passive potassium efflux from the cell to the ECF. This potassium efflux restores the electronegativity of the cell interior. In nerve and skeletal muscle potassium efflux occurs almost immediately after the initial spike of the action potential. In cardiac muscle potassium efflux follows the absolute refractory period and coincides with the relative refractory period (phase 3) of the cardiac action potential.

Hyperkalemia reduces the K_i/K_o ratio and consequently partially depolarizes electrical tissues at rest. Hyperkalemia also increases the potassium permeability of excitable cells. The results of these changes on cardiac excitation are illustrated in the left hand panel of Figure 77–7. Because partial resting depolarization decreases the rate of sodium entry into cells during excitation, the rate of phase zero depolarization is slower and the peak of phase zero depolarization is markedly reduced. The increased potassium permeability accelerates repolarization and shortens the plateau phase. The net effect of progressive hyperkalemia is therefore to make the heart progressively refractory to excitation.

The effects of hypokalemia on excitable tissues are more complex. Because the K_i/K_o ratio rises in hypokalemia, excitable cells at rest should be hyperpolarized. This occurs initially, but resting depolarization eventually follows, because the high K_i/K_o ratio, by itself, reduces the potassium permeability of excitable cells. The effects of hypokalemia on cardiac muscle fibers are shown in the right hand panel of Figure 77–7. At rest the cell is partially depolarized because the reduced potassium permeability allows the high extracellular to intracellular sodium ratio to make the cell interior less negative. The initial spike of the action potential is less affected than in hyperkalemia because the reduced potassium permeability offsets the reduced sodium permeability during phase zero depolarization. Since potassium efflux determines the rate of repolarization, the reduced potassium permeability prolongs the relative refractory period. The net effect of these changes in cardiac tissue is to increase the likelihood of sinus bradycardia, and, because of a prolonged relative refractory period, the risk of arrhythmia formation. In skeletal muscle the reduction in membrane permeability to potassium produced by hypokalemia leads, in severe hypokalemia, to generalized paralysis.

HYPOKALEMIA AND POTASSIUM DEPLETION

DEFINITION. Chronic hypokalemia generally reflects a reduction in total body potassium. A 1-mEq reduction in serum potassium level generally implies the net loss of 100 to 200 mEq of potassium from the body. In extreme body potassium depletion the serum potassium level may be as low as 1.5 to 2.0 mEq per liter. Acute reductions in serum potassium level without parallel reductions in total body potassium occur when potassium is shifted from extracellular to intracellular compartments.

ETIOLOGY AND PATHOGENESIS. Hypokalemia and simultaneous potassium depletion occur whenever renal plus extrarenal potassium losses exceed potassium intake. In advanced body potassium depletion, intake and output of potassium may be equal. The four major causes for hypokalemia are given in Table 77–11.

Inadequate Intake. Reduced potassium intake may result in potassium depletion and hypokalemia because maximal renal conservation of potassium requires, as indicated above, seven to ten days. During this interval, the net renal potassium loss may be as much as 150 to 200 mEq.

Excessive Renal Losses. Many of the causes for renal potassium wasting can be analyzed in terms of factors that modulate the common effector system for potassium secretion. *Mineralocorticoid excess* accelerates distal tubular potassium secretion (Fig. 77–6). Consequently, hypokalemia occurs regularly in primary hyperaldosteronism, in Cushing's syndrome, and in secondary hyperaldosteronism. *Chronic licorice ingestion* produces a syndrome that mimics primary hyperaldosteronism, because glycyrrhizinic acid, a component of licorice extract, has physiologic properties similar to those of aldosterone.

In *Bartter's syndrome* sodium chloride wasting and secondary aldosteronism may contribute to potassium depletion (Ch. 84). However, potassium depletion in Bartter's syndrome may also occur either when aldosterone secretion rates are normal or following bilateral adrenalectomy. Consequently, it is believed that a tubular defect in potassium handling also contributes to the hypokalemia of Bartter's syndrome.

Most diuretics having a locus of action prior to the late distal tubule (Table 77–5) increase urinary potassium losses. Enhanced sodium delivery to distal nephron segments is the major factor responsible for the kaliuresis produced by these diuretics, and sodium restriction or volume depletion tends to minimize diuretic-induced potassium losses. Carbonic anhydrase inhibitors such as acetazolamide inhibit proximal bicarbonate absorption and thereby accentuate potassium losses. Distal tubular segments are relatively impermeable to

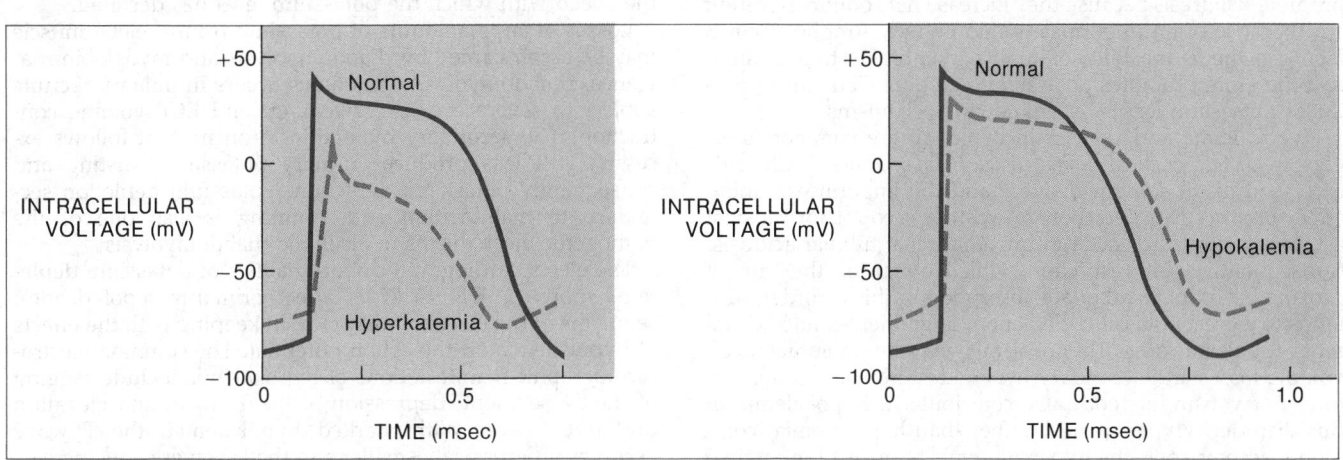

FIGURE 77–7. The effect of increases or decreases in serum potassium on the cardiac action potential. The solid lines represent the normal cardiac action potential; the dashed lines represent the cardiac action potential with either hyperkalemia (*left*) or hypokalemia (*right*).

TABLE 77—11. MAJOR CAUSES OF HYPOKALEMIA

I. Inadequate Intake	III. Gastrointestinal Losses
II. Excess Renal Loss	Vomiting
Mineralocorticoid excess	Diarrhea, particularly
Bartter's syndrome	secretory diarrheas
Diuresis	Villous adenoma
Diuretics with a pre–late	IV. ECF → ICF Shifts
distal locus	Acute alkalosis
Osmotic diuresis	Hypokalemic periodic
Chronic metabolic alkalosis	paralysis
Antibiotics	Barium ingestion
Carbenicillin	Insulin therapy
Gentamicin	Vitamin B_{12} therapy
Amphotericin B	Thyrotoxicosis (rarely)
Renal tubular acidosis	
Distal-gradient limited	
Proximal	
Liddle's syndrome	
Acute leukemia	
Ureterosigmoidostomy	

bicarbonate; consequently, increased delivery of bicarbonate to distal nephron regions has an impermeant anion effect that increases luminal electronegativity in these nephron regions.

Osmotic diuresis is commonly associated with increased renal potassium losses, because increased tubular flow rates enhance net potassium secretion. In diabetic ketoacidosis renal potassium losses are common. Yet patients with diabetic ketoacidosis and a reduced total body potassium commonly present with hyperkalemia, because metabolic acidosis tends to promote potassium shifts from the ICF to the ECF. Consequently, profound hypokalemia may develop if body potassium is not replenished concomitantly with insulin therapy and ECF volume expansion (Ch. 231).

Potassium depletion is seen frequently in *chronic metabolic alkalosis*. When the alkalosis is associated with volume contraction, secondary hyperaldosteronism results in renal potassium losses. Potassium depletion in chronic metabolic alkalosis is also enhanced if bicarbonaturia is present, because of the impermeant anion effect produced by bicarbonate delivery to terminal nephron segments. In fact, the hypokalemia associated with upper gastrointestinal fluid losses, as in vomiting or nasogastric suction, is primarily the result of the renal potassium losses produced by secondary hyperaldosteronism or bicarbonaturia or both. The potassium losses from the upper gastrointestinal tract are small, since upper gastrointestinal tract fluid contains only about 10 mEq of potassium per liter.

Hypokalemia may develop during therapy with certain *antibiotics*. Carbenicillin or other penicillin-like antibiotics exist as sodium or potassium salts of impermeant anions and promote kaliuresis because they increase net sodium excretion and because of an impermeant anion effect. Amphotericin B increases the permeability of luminal membranes to potassium and therefore promotes potassium secretion. Gentamicin produces potassium losses by unknown mechanisms.

Hypokalemia and potassium depletion are common findings in *distal, gradient-limited renal tubular acidosis* (Ch. 84). Increased distal sodium delivery and the impermeant anion effect produced by bicarbonate wasting account for most of the potassium losses seen in proximal renal tubular acidosis. Consequently, salt restriction, which enhances the rate of proximal sodium bicarbonate absorption in this disorder, also tends to correct potassium depletion. In gradient-limited distal renal tubular acidosis, hypokalemia may be accentuated by volume losses and secondary hyperaldosteronism. Other factors, not yet understood, also contribute to hypokalemia in this disorder. Hyperkalemia, rather than hypokalemia, commonly accompanies the hyperchloremic acidosis of interstitial disease (type IV acidosis).

Liddle's syndrome is a rare tubular disorder characterized by hypokalemia, metabolic alkalosis, hypertension, and normal aldosterone secretion rates. Therapy with triamterene, but not with aldosterone antagonists such as spironolactone, ameliorates the disorder. These findings suggest that terminal nephron sodium avidity and potassium secretion independent of aldosterone are major factors in the pathogenesis of Liddle's syndrome. Thus in operational terms, Liddle's syndrome may be described as distal nephron hyperfunction, in regard to Na^+ absorption and H^+ and K^+ secretion.

Gastrointestinal Losses. These provide the major route for potassium depletion, other than the kidney. As indicated above, potassium depletion associated with vomiting is referable primarily to renal potassium losses. Diarrhea produces significant potassium losses, since diarrheal fluid contains 30 mEq per liter of potassium. The most striking diarrheal potassium losses occur in secretory diarrheas, such as with non–beta islet cell tumors of the pancreas, which produce vasoactive intestinal polypeptide, and in laxative abuse. In both secretory diarrheas and chronic laxative abuse, hypokalemia is probably caused by increased rates of K^+ secretion through apical membrane K^+ channels. Villous adenomas of the colon produce potassium depletion because of excessive colonic K^+ secretion from the adenoma. Hypokalemia is uncommonly seen in inflammatory bowel disease.

ECF-ICF Shifts. Acute hypokalemia with a normal total body potassium may occur because of *potassium shifts* from the ECF to the ICF. In *hypokalemic periodic paralysis*, acute shifts of potassium from the ECF to the ICF produce limb and trunk paralysis. The periodic attacks are often precipitated by high-carbohydrate meals. Patients with the disorder can often abort attacks by exercising affected muscles. The chronic use of acetazolamide can prevent attacks. A condition resembling hypokalemic periodic paralysis occurs with the ingestion of *barium salts* and is endemic in China, where the disorder is referred to as "Pa-Ping." Barium appears to produce hypokalemia by blocking K^+ channels in skeletal muscle and thus blocking efflux of potassium from the ICF to the ECF. *Insulin* therapy and *vitamin B_{12}* therapy also promote potassium shifts from the ECF to the ICF. Hypokalemia can also result rarely from thyrotoxicosis, especially in Asian males, for reasons that are unclear.

CLINICAL MANIFESTATIONS. The clinical effects of potassium deficiency are manifest in one or more organ systems, including skeletal muscle, heart, kidneys, and the gastrointestinal tract. The most serious disturbances are those affecting the neuromuscular system. At serum potassium concentrations in the range of 2 to 2.5 mEq per liter, muscular weakness is likely to occur; with more severe hypokalemia, the patient may develop areflexic paralysis, in which case respiratory insufficiency is an immediate threat to survival. The severity of the neuromuscular disturbance tends to be proportional to the speed with which the potassium level has declined.

Losses of large amounts of potassium from skeletal muscle may be accompanied by rhabdomyolysis and myoglobinuria. Hence, rhabdomyolysis sometimes occurs in military recruits subject to severe exercise, sweating, and ECF volume contraction. The secondary hyperaldosteronism that follows excessive salt loss produces urinary potassium wasting and consequently potassium depletion. Potassium depletion secondary to malnutrition and vomiting is also one of the pathogenic mechanisms in alcoholic rhabdomyolysis.

The electrocardiographic abnormalities of potassium depletion, shown in Figure 77–8, affect primarily repolarization segments of the electrocardiogram, in keeping with the effects of hypokalemia on the action potential. The common electrocardiographic manifestations of hypokalemia include sagging of the ST segment, depression of the T wave, and elevation of the U wave. With marked hypokalemia, the T wave becomes progressively smaller and the U waves show increasing amplitude. In some cases the merging of a flat or positive T wave with a positive U wave may erroneously be interpreted as a prolonged QT interval. Ordinarily, there are no serious clinical consequences from the abnormalities in cardiac exci-

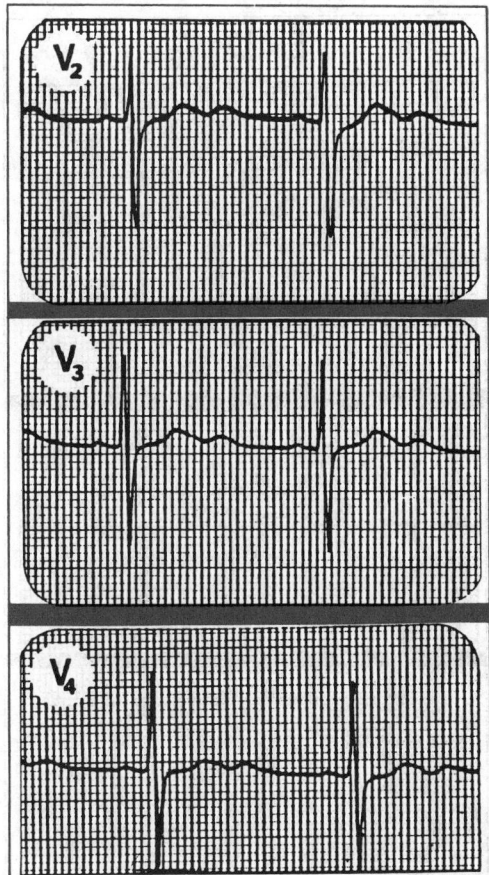

FIGURE 77-8. The electrocardiographic manifestations of hypokalemia. The serum potassium was 2.2 mEq/L. Note that the ST segment is prolonged, primarily because of a U wave following the T wave, and that the T wave is flattened.

tation. In patients treated with digitalis hypokalemia may precipitate serious arrhythmias.

Longstanding potassium depletion may produce renal tubular damage, referred to as hypokalemic nephropathy. Potassium deficiency also affects smooth muscle of the gastrointestinal tract and can result in paralytic ileus.

TREATMENT. The treatment of hypokalemia involves replacement therapy with potassium salts and attempts to correct the underlying disorder. Since diuretic abuse is probably the most common cause for hypokalemia in routine clinical practice, every attempt should be made to identify diuretic ingestion.

Except in extreme circumstances, oral rather than parenteral potassium replacement is prudent. However, when gastrointestinal function is impaired, or when neuromuscular manifestations of hypokalemia are present, parenteral therapy with potassium may be advisable. Since potassium deficits involve both the ICF and the ECF, their correction requires the transfer of administered potassium from the ECF into the ICF. The major problem in parenteral therapy is to avoid intravenous administration of potassium at rates sufficiently great to produce hyperkalemia. A prudent protocol to follow is to add potassium chloride to intravenous solutions at a final concentration of 40 to 60 mEq per liter and to administer no more than 10 to 20 mEq of potassium per hour. Except in unusual circumstances, the total amount of potassium administered daily should not exceed 200 mEq. The serum potassium level should be monitored at appropriate intervals; the frequency of monitoring should be determined by the patient's clinical condition, by the initial serum potassium, by the rate at which the serum potassium changes in a given patient, and by the patient's renal function. Because the electrocardiographic

manifestations of hypokalemia are subtle, the electrocardiogram should not be used as a guide to replacement therapy.

Although potassium chloride is the salt of choice for intravenous potassium replacement, oral potassium chloride solutions are not well tolerated because of gastrointestinal irritation. Enteric-coated potassium chloride tablets are to be avoided, because they produce small bowel ulcerations. Oral potassium is administered most conveniently in the form of organic salts such as gluconate or citrate. This form of therapy is, however, not effective in hypokalemic metabolic alkalosis with hypochloremia. In this circumstance, chloride supplementation is required together with potassium replacement and is most easily achieved by administering sodium chloride supplementation.

HYPERKALEMIA AND POTASSIUM EXCESS

DEFINITION. Chronic hyperkalemia can occur with little or no increase in total body potassium. However, acute increases in serum potassium concentrations, produced by potassium shifts from the ICF to the ECF, can occur even when total body potassium is normal or reduced.

ETIOLOGY AND PATHOGENESIS. Hyperkalemia develops whenever the rate of potassium intake or the rate of potassium efflux from cellular to extracellular fluids exceeds the sum of renal plus extrarenal potassium losses. The renal mechanisms for potassium excretion adapt efficiently to increases in the rate of potassium influx to extracellular fluid, particularly from dietary sources. Hence acute or chronic hyperkalemia due to exogenous potassium intake is uncommon, unless renal mechanisms for potassium excretion are compromised. In the latter setting injudicious potassium administration may result in hyperkalemia. This occurs most commonly when intravenous potassium chloride is administered too rapidly; when potassium salts of antibiotics such as penicillin are administered; when transfusions are given with blood that has been stored for long periods of time; or when salt substitutes containing potassium are used. The occurrence of hyperkalemia in these settings usually requires that renal potassium excretion be impaired.

Acute or chronic hyperkalemia occurs most commonly either because of diminished *renal excretion* or because there is a sudden *transcellular shift* of potassium from the ICF to the ECF. The major causes for hyperkalemia listed in Table 77–12 follow this format.

Diminished Renal Excretion. Hyperkalemia may occur in *acute oliguric renal failure* of any cause. In *chronic renal failure* hyperkalemia generally does not occur until the glomerular filtration rate has reached markedly low levels. Hyperkalemia may be precipitated in chronic renal failure, however, either by the development of acidosis or, as indicated above, by the injudicious administration of potassium salts. Hyperkalemia also occurs with little or modest reduction in the glomerular filtration rate, if there is impairment of potassium secretion by terminal nephron regions. This occurs in *Addison's disease*, in *hyporeninemic hypoaldosteronism*, and with the injudicious

TABLE 77–12. MAJOR CAUSES OF HYPERKALEMIA

I. Diminished Renal Excretion	II. Transcellular Shifts
Reduced GFR	Acidosis
Acute oliguric renal failure	Cell destruction
Chronic renal failure	Trauma, burns
Reduced tubular secretion	Rhabdomyolysis
Addison's disease	Hemolysis
Hyporeninemic hypoaldosteronism	Tumor lysis
	Hyperkalemic periodic paralysis
Potassium-sparing diuretics	Diabetic hyperglycemia
	Insulin dependence plus aldosterone lack
	Depolarizing muscle paralysis
	Succinylcholine

GFR = Glomerular filtration rate

administration of *potassium-sparing diuretics* such as triamterene or spironolactone. The tendency toward hyperkalemia in these circumstances can be aggravated by ECF volume contraction, which reduces sodium delivery to terminal nephron segments, or by acidosis, which promotes cellular potassium efflux.

Transcellular Shifts. The second class of disorders causing acute hyperkalemia includes situations in which there is an abrupt shift of potassium from the ICF to the ECF. This occurs in acidosis or in circumstances that result in *cell destruction;* the latter occurs commonly with tissue trauma, burns, rhabdomyolysis, or hemolysis, and with lysis of large masses of tumor cells. As indicated previously, hypokalemia predisposes to rhabdomyolysis. Thus the sudden occurrence of hyperkalemia in potassium-depleted patients is a diagnostic clue to the development of rhabdomyolysis.

Hyperkalemic periodic paralysis is an autosomal dominant disorder in which sudden increases in serum potassium level result in muscle paralysis. The hyperkalemia is often provoked by dietary potassium intake or by exercise. Myotonia occurs commonly in the disorder and appears either between attacks or immediately preceding attacks. The pathogenesis of the disorder is not understood. The acute paralytic attack can be treated by intravenous administration of calcium gluconate or glucose and insulin. Chronic treatment with diuretics such as acetazolamide minimizes the frequency of attacks.

Paradoxical hyperkalemia occurs when *sudden hyperglycemia* develops in insulin-dependent diabetics who also have interstitial renal disease and associated hyporeninemic hypoaldosteronism. The sudden increase in ECF osmolality draws water from cells, raises intracellular potassium concentrations, and therefore promotes passive potassium efflux from cells. The insulin lack minimizes cellular re-entry of potassium, and the aldosterone deficiency blunts renal potassium excretion. Insulin therapy promptly corrects the hyperkalemia. Finally, anesthetic agents or other drugs that cause a *depolarizing muscle paralysis*, such as succinylcholine, promote potassium efflux from muscle cells. The loss of cell electronegativity in this situation increases passive potassium efflux from muscle cells.

Pseudohyperkalemia may occur in thrombocytosis or leukocytosis, because clotting of blood promotes potassium release from these cells and may be identified by noting that the *serum* potassium level is elevated while the *plasma* potassium level is normal. This kind of artifact occurs most commonly in patients with myeloproliferative disorders.

CLINICAL MANIFESTATIONS. The most important clinical manifestations of hyperkalemia relate to alterations in cardiac excitability. For this reason the electrocardiogram is the single most important guide in appraising the threat posed by hyperkalemia and in determining how aggressive a therapeutic approach is necessary.

The electrocardiographic manifestations of hyperkalemia, shown in Figure 77–9, follow directly from the effects of hyperkalemia on cardiac action potentials (Fig. 77–7). The earliest manifestation of hyperkalemia is the development of peaked T waves, which become evident when the serum potassium level exceeds 6.5 mEq per liter. This peaking of the T waves is a manifestation of the accelerated repolarization of the cardiac action potential produced by hyperkalemia. When the potassium concentration exceeds 7 to 8 mEq per liter, diminished cardiac excitability results in prolongation of the PR interval followed by a loss of P waves and widening of the QRS complex. These changes indicate progressive inexcitability of cardiac muscle and are referable to hyperkalemia-induced inactivation of sodium permeability during the initial spike of the action potential. When the serum potassium level exceeds 8 to 10 mEq per liter, the electrocardiogram may develop a sine wave pattern and cardiac standstill can occur.

The correlation between serum potassium concentrations and electrocardiographic abnormalities is approximate at best;

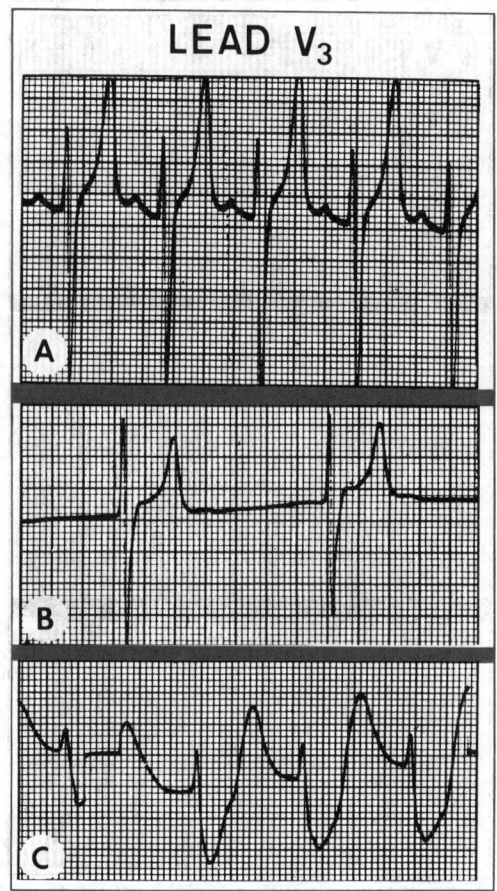

FIGURE 77–9. The effects of progressive hyperkalemia on the electrocardiogram. All of the illustrations are from lead V_3. *A*, Serum K^+ = 6.8 mEq/L; note the peaked T waves together with normal sinus rhythm. *B*, Serum K^+ = 7.7 mEq/L; note the peaked T waves and absent P waves. *C*, Serum K^+ = 8.9 mEq/L; note the absent P waves, marked prolongation of the QRS complex, and peaked T waves.

in a given patient, progression from peaked T waves to a sine wave pattern may occur rapidly, particularly if the serum potassium concentration rises rapidly. Therefore the development of peaked T waves in conjunction with hyperkalemia should be viewed as a serious disorder; more advanced electrocardiographic manifestations of hyperkalemia should be treated as life-threatening medical emergencies.

TREATMENT. Three kinds of maneuvers are used in the treatment of hyperkalemia: agents such as glucose plus insulin or sodium bicarbonate, which promote the transfer of potassium from the ECF to the ICF; maneuvers that enhance potassium elimination from the body, such as diuretics, exchange resins, or dialysis; and the use of calcium, which does not alter serum potassium concentrations but counteracts the effects of hyperkalemia on cardiac excitability.

Both insulin and sodium bicarbonate promote potassium entry into cells. The administration of 25 grams of glucose, together with 10 units of regular insulin, is an effective way of reducing the serum potassium level rapidly. The glucose may be administered over 30 minutes as a 20 per cent solution, or it may be given as a 50 per cent glucose solution. Insulin promotes potassium entry into cells, and glucose is administered to prevent hypoglycemia. In insulin-dependent diabetic patients in whom sudden hyperglycemia has precipitated the hyperkalemia, insulin administration alone suffices to reduce the serum potassium concentration.

The administration of 40 to 150 mEq of sodium bicarbonate intravenously over a 30- to 60-minute interval also promotes potassium entry into cells, particularly if acidosis is also present. This maneuver should be used with caution in patients with compromised renal function because of the risks of hypernatremia and of ECF volume overload.

None of the maneuvers described above removes potassium from the body. Gastrointestinal potassium losses may be produced by the use of cation exchange resins in the sodium cycle, such as sodium polystyrene sulfonate (Kayexalate). Each gram of the resin contains approximately 1 mEq of sodium and exchanges for about 1 mEq of potassium. This stoichiometry is not precise, since the sodium form of the resin also exchanges for other cations in gastrointestinal secretions, including calcium. In chronic hyperkalemia, 20 grams of Kayexalate may be given three or four times a day in a 70 per cent solution of sorbitol. The sorbitol creates an osmotic diarrhea and enhances resin passage through the gastrointestinal tract. In acute circumstances, Kayexalate may also be administered by enema, generally as 100 grams of resin suspended in 200 ml of 20 per cent sorbitol. The use of chronic Kayexalate therapy in patients with chronic renal failure carries with it the risk of sodium overload.

In settings of extreme hyperkalemic cardiotoxicity, when P waves are absent and the QRS complexes are widened, the administration of calcium gluconate, 10 to 30 ml of a 10 per cent solution over a 10- to 20-minute interval, may be life saving. This approach should be undertaken with constant electrocardiographic monitoring and should be used with extreme caution in patients who have received digitalis. In the latter circumstance, calcium administration may unmask digitalis intoxication, especially if other agents are used simultaneously to reduce the serum potassium level. Calcium salts should not be added to bottles of intravenous fluids containing bicarbonate, because water-insoluble calcium salts will form.

The influence of calcium salts in minimizing the cardiotoxic effects of hyperkalemia may be understood by noting, as described in the section on Physiologic Considerations, that depolarization of excitable tissues by elevating serum K^+ concentrations inactivates sodium channels and that the extracellular sides of these sodium channels are electronegative. Divalent cations such as calcium provide a remarkably effective way of screening these electronegative sites. Thus calcium salts raise the voltage gradient across sodium channels by screening electronegative surface charges of these channels on their extracellular fluid sides and consequently restoring the voltage-dependent excitability of these channels.

Finally, acute hemodialysis or peritoneal dialysis provides another mechanism for potassium removal from the body. This approach is particularly advantageous in acute renal failure; when patients are volume expanded and sodium administration may produce congestive heart failure; or when there is a continued efflux of large amounts of potassium from the ICF to the ECF, as in burns or rhabdomyolysis.

Brown RS: Extrarenal potassium homeostasis. Kidney Int 30:116, 1986. *A summary of cellular uptake processes for potassium.*

Field MJ, Giebisch GH: Hormonal control of renal potassium excretion. Kidney Int 27:379, 1985. *A thorough account of renal potassium handling.*

Ponce SP, Jennings AE, Madias NE, et al.: Drug induced hyperkalemia. Medicine 64:357, 1985. *A summary of drugs that provoke hyperkalemia.*

Tannen RL: Potassium disorders. In Kokko JP, Tannen RL (eds.): Fluids and Electrolytes. Philadelphia, W. B. Saunders Company, 1986. *A complete discussion of hypokalemia and hyperkalemia.*

Tsien RW, Hess P: Excitable tissue—the heart. In Andreoli TE, Hoffman JF, Fanestil DD, et al. (eds.): Physiology of Membrane Disorders. New York, Plenum, 1986, pp 469–490. *A meticulous description of the ionic basis for the cardiac action potential.*

Disturbances in Acid-Base Balance

PHYSIOLOGIC CONSIDERATIONS

The pH of arterial blood and interstitial fluid normally ranges between 7.38 and 7.42 despite wide variations in dietary intake of acids or alkali. The arterial pH range over which cardiac function, metabolic activity, and central nervous system function can be maintained is narrow; the widest range of pH values compatible with life is from 6.8 to 7.8, or an interval of one pH unit.

The major buffer system in extracellular fluid is the bicarbonate–carbonic acid pair. The relation between pH, bicarbonate, and carbonic acid concentrations in ECF may be expressed according to the familiar Henderson-Hasselbalch equation:

$$pH = pK + \log \frac{HCO_3^-}{H_2CO_3}$$

where pK is the carbonic acid dissociation constant, HCO_3^- is the plasma bicarbonate concentration, and H_2CO_3 is the plasma carbonic acid concentration. The H_2CO_3 concentration is given by $\alpha PaCO_2$, where α is the CO_2 solubility constant, and has a value of 0.03, and $PaCO_2$ is the arterial carbon dioxide tension. Therefore, with a $PaCO_2$ of 40 mm Hg, the Henderson-Hasselbalch equation becomes the following:

$$7.4 = 6.1 + \log \frac{24 \text{ mM/L}}{1.2 \text{ mM/L}}$$

The arterial pH provides a qualitative, but not quantitative, index to total body water acid-base status because, at any given time, about two thirds of an acid or alkali load is buffered by proton shifts into or out of the ICF, respectively. For this reason, some prefer to use the term "acidemia" for acidosis and "alkalemia" for alkalosis to connote that plasma pH measurements provide quantitative information about the pH status of plasma and interstitial fluid and only qualitative information about total body acid-base balance.

A convenient way to consider the total body buffering capacity is as follows. Bicarbonate is predominantly an extracellular anion, and the total ECF bicarbonate content in a 70-kg man having 15 liters of ECF is (24 mEq/liter × 15 liters), or 360 mEq HCO_3^-. However, about two thirds of a given acid or alkali load is buffered within cells. Consequently, the total body buffering capacity, often referred to as the "bicarbonate space," is calculated as:

$$(\text{Arterial } HCO_3^- \times 0.6 \text{ body weight})$$

that is, using total body water as an index to total buffering capacity. The bicarbonate space is also an index to net acid excess or net base excess. If the arterial HCO_3^- concentration in a 70-kg man is reduced to 15 mEq per liter while the $PaCO_2$ remains constant, the net acid excess (or net base deficit) is (24 − 15) mEq/liter × 42 liters = 378 mEq. Conversely, if the arterial HCO_3^- concentration rises to 33 mEq per liter while the $PaCO_2$ remains constant, the net base excess (or acid deficit) is 378 mEq.

Proton shifts between the ECF and ICF stabilize the plasma pH against acute fluctuations. But the ultimate maintenance of pH balance requires that input of acid or base into the body be matched by output of acid or base, so that the HCO_3^-/H_2CO_3 ratio and the total bicarbonate content in the ECF remain constant. The cardinal systems involved in these external processes are the kidneys, for bicarbonate balance, and the lungs, for carbon dioxide balance.

Carbon Dioxide Production and Elimination

VOLATILE ACID INPUT. The largest source of endogenous acid production is from combustion of glucose and fatty acids to carbon dioxide and water or, in other words, to a volatile acid. During aerobic glycolysis, that is, cellular respiration, glucose oxidation involves oxygen utilization and carbon dioxide production according to the following reaction:

$$C_6H_{12}O_6 + 6O_2 \rightarrow 6CO_2 + 6H_2O$$

Since red blood cells contain carbonic anhydrase (c.a.), carbon dioxide hydration in erythrocytes yields the following:

$$CO_2 + H_2O \overset{c.a.}{\rightleftharpoons} H_2CO_3 \rightleftharpoons H^+ + HCO_3^-$$

The protons formed from carbonic acid dissociation are buffered by hemoglobin, whereas bicarbonate leaves red blood cells in exchange for chloride (the familiar chloride shift). In other words, carbon dioxide generation is equivalent to carbonic acid formation, and the bulk of hydrogen ion formed is buffered intracellularly.

A simple way of calculating the daily rate of nonvolatile acid production is to note, from the above reactions, that the production of 1 mole of metabolic water and 1 mole of carbon dioxide represents, through dissociation of carbonic acid, the formation of 1 mole of hydrogen ions.

Since the molecular weight of water is 18, 1 liter of water contains about 55 moles of water. Consequently, the average rate of metabolic water production, about 400 ml daily, yields 22,000 mmol of water and an equal number of carbon dioxide molecules. Thus the rate of volatile acid production amounts to about 22,000 mEq of hydrogen ion daily. The cellular combustion of carbohydrates and fatty acids to carbon dioxide and water is remarkably efficient. Under normal circumstances, organic anions such as lactate and ketoacids, which derive from incomplete combustion of carbohydrates and fatty acids, have plasma concentrations of approximately 5 mEq per liter.

VOLATILE ACID OUTPUT. Pulmonary ventilation excretes the carbon dioxide formed by cellular respiration. During blood transit through the lungs, bicarbonate re-enters red blood cells and combines with protons to form carbonic acid, which dissociates to carbon dioxide and water. The carbon dioxide so formed diffuses freely through red blood cells and alveolar epithelium, so that the rate of carbon dioxide excretion is governed primarily by the rate of minute ventilation.

MODULATION OF RESPIRATION. The prime factors normally regulating alterations in the rate of minute ventilation are subtle changes in cerebrospinal fluid (CSF) pH or arterial pH. Sensor chemoreceptors in central medullary centers or in the carotid body are activated by small reductions in CSF pH or arterial pH, respectively; the pH reduction can result either from carbon dioxide accumulation or from nonvolatile acid accumulation, which reduces the plasma bicarbonate concentration. In most circumstances, central medullary chemoreceptors provide the major impetus to altering ventilatory response, and the carotid body chemoreceptors serve as relatively minor stimuli to ventilation. The medullary respiratory centers therefore serve as the major *effector* mechanism for regulating carbon dioxide output by increasing ventilation rate.

The ventilatory response for carbon dioxide removal involves an increase in both tidal volume and respiratory rate. On an average, for every 1 mEq per liter reduction in plasma bicarbonate produced by metabolic acidosis, increased minute ventilation will produce a 1.2 mm Hg fall in the $PaCO_2$. In most circumstances, the maximum reduction in $PaCO_2$ produced by the hyperventilatory response to severe metabolic acidosis is to a $PaCO_2$ of 12 to 15 mm Hg; hyperventilation to $PaCO_2$ values less than 10 mm Hg in metabolic acidosis almost never occurs. Conversely, an increase in arterial pH reduces the rate of minute ventilation and therefore results in carbon dioxide retention. For increases in plasma bicarbonate concentrations to 35 mEq per liter, the $PaCO_2$ usually remains less than 50 mm Hg. When profound metabolic alkalosis occurs, the $PaCO_2$ may rise further but virtually never exceeds 65 mm Hg.

Renal Bicarbonate Processing

In addition to volatile acid production due to carbon dioxide formation, cellular metabolism also results in the formation of a number of nonvolatile acids. The major source for nonvolatile acid production is the metabolism of sulfur-containing amino acids such as cysteine and methionine, which results in sulfuric acid formation. Consequently, the daily rate of nonvolatile acid production is closely related to dietary protein intake and to the rate of endogenous protein catabolism. Nonvolatile acids also derive from oxidation of phosphoproteins and phospholipids, which results in phosphoric acid formation; nucleoprotein degradation, which yields uric acid; and incomplete combustion of carbohydrates and fatty acids, which produces lactic acid and the ketoacids.

The daily rate of nonvolatile acid production under normal conditions is about 1 mEq per kilogram of body weight. Thus daily nonvolatile acid production would consume the total body fluid buffering capacity in about two weeks, were it not for the fact that the kidneys excrete nonvolatile acids and, in so doing, regenerate bicarbonate. Since the minimal urine pH ordinarily attainable is 5.0 and the amount of nonvolatile acid to be excreted is about 70 mEq daily, renal hydrogen ion excretion, which is equivalent to renal bicarbonate regeneration, occurs mainly as protons trapped in an undissociated form by urinary buffers.

The kidneys also filter large quantities of bicarbonate daily: For a normal plasma bicarbonate concentration of 24 mEq per liter and a glomerular filtration of 180 liters daily, the net amount of bicarbonate filtered daily is approximately 4300 mEq, or about four times the total body buffering capacity. Thus in addition to generating new bicarbonate, the renal tubules must also absorb filtered bicarbonate.

BICARBONATE REABSORPTION. Virtually all filtered bicarbonate is absorbed, together with sodium, by the proximal tubule. Consequently, the rate of proximal bicarbonate reabsorption is modulated by the same *effectors* that regulate proximal sodium absorption. Among these, the effective circulating volume exerts a central effect. Volume expansion, which resets glomerulotubular balance downward, reduces the fractional rate of proximal bicarbonate reabsorption. Conversely, volume contraction raises the bicarbonate threshold by increasing the fractional rate of proximal tubular sodium bicarbonate reabsorption.

Two other *effectors* regulate, in operational terms, the rate of bicarbonate reabsorption. One of these is the arterial $PaCO_2$: High $PaCO_2$ values raise the apparent bicarbonate threshold, whereas low $PaCO_2$ values reduce the rate of bicarbonate reabsorption. This factor accounts for the compensatory increase in plasma bicarbonate concentrations in respiratory acidosis. Second, hypokalemia also increases the rate of bicarbonate reabsorption, presumably by raising the intracellular hydrogen ion concentration. This factor accounts for the fact that, in hypokalemic, hypochloremic metabolic alkalosis associated with volume contraction, alkalosis can persist after volume deficits are restored. In this circumstance, correction of potassium deficits is required for correction of the alkalosis.

BICARBONATE REGENERATION. The excretion of nonvolatile acids and the simultaneous renal regeneration of bicarbonate occur principally in distal nephron segments. Distal renal tubular cells hydrate carbon dioxide to carbonic acid, which dissociates to protons, which are secreted into urine, and bicarbonate anions, which are absorbed into blood. The secreted protons titrate urinary buffers, principally phosphate, while sodium is absorbed. Thus the overall reaction is as follows:

$$\underset{\text{(filtered)}}{Na_2HPO_4} + H^+ + HCO_3^- \longrightarrow \underset{\text{(excreted)}}{NaH_2PO_4} + \underset{\text{(absorbed)}}{NaHCO_3}$$

Titratable acid formation normally accounts for about one third of renal acid excretion. The remaining two thirds of acid excretion is accounted for by ammonia (NH_3) secretion by the following sequence:

$$\underset{\text{(filtered)}}{NaR} + NH_3 + H^+ + HCO_3^- \longrightarrow \underset{\text{(reabsorbed)}}{NaHCO_3} + \underset{\text{(excreted)}}{NH_4R}$$

where NaR is the filtered sodium salt of a nonvolatile acid, NH_3 is ammonia produced by renal tubular cells, and the protons and bicarbonate come from carbon dioxide hydration by tubular cells.

Distal acid excretion and bicarbonate absorption are accompanied by sodium absorption. Consequently, *effector* systems that enhance distal sodium absorption, such as aldosterone or increased rates of sodium delivery to terminal nephron segments, also promote terminal nephron hydrogen ion excretion. Three other *effector* mechanisms also increase the rate of hydrogen ion excretion: (1) Delivery of sodium to terminal nephron segments in association with impermeant anions such as sulfate favors proton movement from tubular cells to lumen. (2) Hypokalemia enhances hydrogen ion excretion, particularly in sodium-acquisitive states, presumably because hypokalemia is accompanied by a fall in intracellular pH. (3) Acidosis stimulates ammoniagenesis by renal tubular cells; consequently, in metabolic acidosis, increases in the rate of renal acid excretion are referable primarily to increased rates of ammonium excretion. In other words, these last-named three effector systems enhance renal acid excretion by creating a favorable situation for proton transfer from tubular cells to urine. Conversely, aldosterone deficiency, alkalosis, or reduced rates of salt delivery to terminal nephron segments reduce renal capacity for acid excretion.

pH Disequilibria Between Plasma and CSF

Central rather than arterial chemoreceptors are the prime sensors for pH-mediated changes in respiration. The ventilatory responses to pH changes mediated by respiratory processes or by metabolic processes therefore differ. The blood-brain barrier is freely permeable to carbon dioxide. Consequently, pH changes produced exclusively by hyperventilation or hypoventilation occur almost simultaneously in arterial plasma and in the CSF, and the respiratory response to primary increases or decreases in $PaCO_2$ occurs almost instantaneously. The blood-brain barrier imposes a lag, however, in the rate at which arterial bicarbonate equilibrates with the CSF. Thus in metabolic acidosis, the arterial pH and bicarbonate concentration fall more rapidly than they do in the CSF; and in metabolic alkalosis, the CSF pH and bicarbonate concentration rise more slowly than they do in arterial plasma. Consequently, in the early stages of acute metabolic acidosis, there may be a one- to three-hour delay in the development of a maximal hyperventilatory response. Conversely, when metabolic acidosis is corrected rapidly, hyperventilation may persist for a few hours because of a delay in the rise of cerebrospinal fluid pH.

An unusual situation relating to this effect occurs in diabetic ketoacidosis and in certain other metabolic acidoses associated with impaired central nervous system function. In these situations, carotid body chemoreceptors, rather than central medullary chemoreceptors, provide the major stimulus to respiration driven by a reduced arterial pH. The rapid correction of ECF acidosis by bicarbonate administration reduces the rate at which carotid body chemoreceptors drive ventilation. When this occurs, $PaCO_2$ levels in plasma and in the CSF rise almost simultaneously; but because of a lag in the rate of bicarbonate entry into the CSF, the CSF bicarbonate/carbonic acid ratio tends to fall. In severe diabetic ketoacidosis, this situation can result in an actual fall in CSF pH simultaneously with a rise in arterial pH produced by intravenous bicarbonate administration.

DEFINITION OF ACID-BASE ABNORMALITIES

The arterial pH is determined by the ratio of the bicarbonate/carbonic acid buffer system, as expressed in the Henderson-Hasselbalch equation. These data also provide an index to total body acid-base balance, because, as indicated in the preceding section, the majority of body buffering occurs within cells. Acid-base disturbances can therefore occur either by altering the serum bicarbonate concentration, referred to as a "metabolic" disorder, or by altering arterial carbon dioxide tension, referred to as a "respiratory" disorder. A convenient way for considering these disturbances is illustrated in Figure 77-10, which illustrates pH isobars (for pH 7.0, 7.4, and 7.8) calculated according to the Henderson-Hasselbalch equation for the bicarbonate concentrations and $PaCO_2$ values listed on the ordinate and abscissa, respectively.

TYPES OF ACID-BASE ABNORMALITIES. The left hand panel in Figure 77-10 shows the directional changes in $PaCO_2$ and bicarbonate concentrations that *initiate* the four basic types of acid-base abnormalities. *Respiratory acidosis* results from hypoventilation and reduces pH by raising the $PaCO_2$. *Respiratory alkalosis* results from hyperventilation and raises pH by reducing the $PaCO_2$. *Metabolic alkalosis* occurs when increases in the plasma bicarbonate concentration raise pH, and *metabolic acidosis* occurs when reductions in plasma bicarbonate decrease pH.

Any of these initial acid-base disturbances activates *compensatory responses*, illustrated in the right hand panel of Figure 77-10, that tend to minimize the pH changes produced by the initial acid-base abnormality. By comparing the directional arrows in the left and right hand panels of Figure 77-10, it becomes evident that the initial disturbance in any of these four acid-base abnormalities tends to displace the arterial pH away from the pH 7.4 isobar and that the compensatory response partially restores arterial pH values toward the pH 7.4 isobar. The arterial pH, $PaCO_2$, and plasma bicarbonate concentrations illustrated in the right hand panel of Figure 77-10 are the values usually observed clinically in the four primary acid-base disturbances.

In respiratory acidosis increased renal bicarbonate reabsorption raises plasma bicarbonate concentrations to offset increases in $PaCO_2$ values. Since the renal response to an increased $PaCO_2$ requires 24 to 28 hours, a given increase in $PaCO_2$ will result in a more severe acidosis acutely rather than chronically. In respiratory alkalosis, renal bicarbonate excretion minimizes the tendency to an increased arterial pH but generally is inadequate to prevent arterial pH increases, particularly in acute hyperventilatory states.

In metabolic acidosis, compensatory hyperventilation can reduce the arterial $PaCO_2$ to 12 to 15 mm Hg, but in severe metabolic acidosis it is never adequate to restore the arterial pH to normal. In metabolic alkalosis, plasma bicarbonate concentrations in excess of 35 mEq per liter result in a compensatory hypoventilation that can raise the $PaCO_2$ to 50 mm Hg. In severe metabolic alkalosis, $PaCO_2$ values as high as 60 to 65 mm Hg may occur, particularly in azotemic patients.

THE ANION GAP. Sodium is the principal cation in extracellular fluids. The sum of plasma chloride plus bicarbonate concentrations is less than the serum sodium concentration; the remaining anions required for electroneutrality, generally not reported with routine serum electrolyte measurements, are referred to as unmeasured anions, or as the anion gap. A convenient formula for calculating the anion gap is the following:

$$\text{Anion gap} = Na^+ - (Cl^- + HCO_3^-)$$

where Na^+, Cl^-, and HCO_3^- are the serum sodium, chloride, and bicarbonate concentrations, respectively. The anion gap includes primarily phosphates and sulfates derived from tissue metabolism; lactate and ketoacids arising from incomplete combustion of carbohydrates and fatty acids; and negatively charged protein molecules, principally albumin. The normal value for unmeasured anions, or the anion gap, is 10 to 12 mEq per liter; albumin and other proteins normally account for about half of the anion gap.

An *increased* anion gap generally indicates the presence of

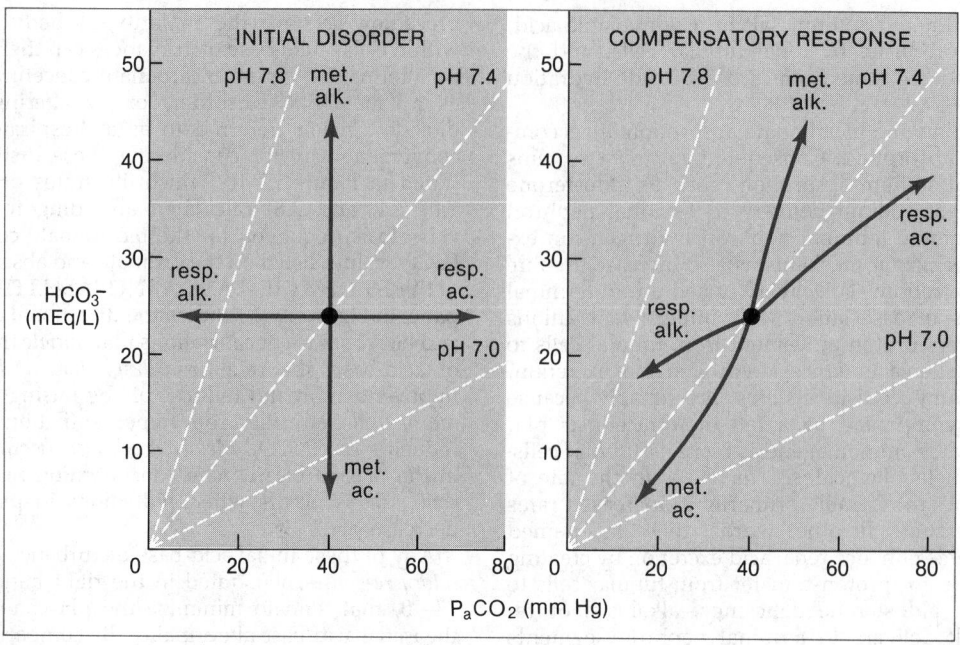

FIGURE 77–10. Schematic frame of reference for considering acid-base disturbances. The dotted lines are the pH isobars for pH values of 7.8, 7.4, and 7.0 computed from the Henderson-Hasselbalch equation for given combinations of arterial bicarbonate values (vertical axes) and arterial carbon dioxide tensions (horizontal axes). The graph on the left shows the initial derangement in HCO_3^- concentrations in metabolic acidosis and metabolic alkalosis and the initial P_aCO_2 derangement in respiratory acidosis and respiratory alkalosis. Note that each of the four changes in either HCO_3^- or P_aCO_2 tends to displace the arterial pH from the pH 7.4 isobar. The graph on the right, labelled compensatory response, indicates the general trend of pH, HCO_3^- and P_aCO_2 changes actually observed in the four primary acid-base disturbances: respiratory acidosis, respiratory alkalosis, metabolic acidosis, and metabolic alkalosis. Respiratory acidosis and alkalosis are accompanied by compensatory renal bicarbonate retention and loss, respectively. Metabolic acidosis and alkalosis are accompanied by compensatory hyperventilation and hypoventilation, respectively. Note that the compensatory response in each of the four acid-base disorders tends to restore arterial pH values toward the pH 7.4 isobar.

metabolic acidosis. The factors responsible for this kind of metabolic acidosis are discussed in the next section.

A *reduced* anion gap provides an index to certain other disorders. The anion gap will be reduced if the sodium concentration falls while the chloride plus bicarbonate concentrations are unchanged or, in other words, when the concentration of another cation in serum is increased while the serum osmolality remains normal. This may occur in multiple myeloma of the immunoglobulin G (IgG) variety, if the myeloma proteins are cationic at pH 7.4. Hyperviscosity syndromes may also result in a reduced anion gap because of a laboratory artifact: When serum is excessively viscous, automatic pumps deliver decreased volumes of serum to a flame photometer, producing artifactual reductions in sodium concentrations. Rarely, lithium intoxication, hypermagnesemia, and hypercalcemia raise nonsodium cation concentrations sufficiently high to reduce the anion gap.

The anion gap will also be decreased if the serum sodium concentration remains normal while the serum chloride plus bicarbonate concentrations are increased. This occurs most commonly in hypoalbuminemia. A low anion gap also occurs in bromide intoxication, since colorimetric techniques for serum chloride determinations give spuriously high values for chloride plus bromide when bromide is present in relatively high concentrations in serum.

METABOLIC ACIDOSIS

ETIOLOGY AND PATHOGENESIS. A convenient way to consider the metabolic acidoses is to divide them into two groups, normal anion gap and increased anion gap metabolic acidoses (Table 77–13). The pathogeneses of these two groups differ appreciably.

NORMAL ANION GAP METABOLIC ACIDOSIS. The metabolic acidoses having a *normal anion gap* result whenever there are abnormally high net bicarbonate losses. This may

occur because the kidneys fail to reabsorb or regenerate bicarbonate; because there are extrarenal losses of bicarbonate; or because excessive amounts of substances yielding hydrochloric acid have been administered.

Bicarbonate Losses. Bicarbonate losses occur either when the proximal tubule fails to absorb virtually all filtered bicarbonate, that is, when the apparent bicarbonate threshold is reduced, or when there are losses of bicarbonate from the gastrointestinal tract.

Renal bicarbonate wasting occurs in *proximal renal tubular acidosis*, either alone or as part of Fanconi's syndrome (Ch. 84). The apparent threshold for bicarbonate in this disorder is set below the normal value of 26 mEq of bicarbonate per deciliter of glomerular filtrate and may be as low as 15 to 20

TABLE 77–13. MAJOR CAUSES OF METABOLIC ACIDOSIS

Normal Anion Gap	Increased Anion Gap
I. Bicarbonate Loss	**I. Reduced Excretion of**
Proximal renal tubular acidosis	**Inorganic Acids**
Dilutional acidosis	Renal failure
Carbonic anhydrase inhibitors	**II. Accumulation of Organic Acids**
Primary hyperparathyroidism	Lactic acidosis
Diarrheal states	Ketoacidosis: alcoholic
Small bowel drainage	diabetic
Ureterosigmoidostomy	starvation
II. Failure of Bicarbonate	Ingestion: salicylates
Regeneration	paraldehyde
Distal, gradient-limited renal	methanol
tubular acidosis	ethylene glycol
Hyporeninemic	
hypoaldosteronism	
Diuretics: triamterene,	
spironolactone	
III. Acidifying Salts	
Ammonium chloride	
Lysine hydrochloride	
Arginine hydrochloride	
Parenteral hyperalimentation	

mEq of bicarbonate per deciliter of glomerular filtrate. Consequently, bicarbonate wasting occurs whenever the plasma bicarbonate level is raised above the apparent renal threshold for bicarbonate.

Attempts to correct the acidosis of proximal renal tubular acidosis by bicarbonate administration are generally unrewarding, because increases in the plasma bicarbonate level produced by administering bicarbonate salts are accompanied by corresponding increases in bicarbonaturia. A promising approach to this disorder involves reducing the effective circulating volume by sodium restriction. This maneuver exploits the fact that ECF contraction resets glomerulotubular balance upward and consequently increases the fractional rate of sodium, and hence bicarbonate, reabsorption by the proximal tubule.

A converse of this situation is sometimes referred to as *dilutional acidosis.* Individuals who are volume expanded reduce the fractional rate of sodium bicarbonate absorption by the proximal tubule and consequently develop mild reductions in plasma bicarbonate concentrations. *Carbonic anhydrase inhibitors* such as acetazolamide inhibit proximal sodium bicarbonate absorption, resulting in metabolic acidosis. *Primary hyperparathyroidism* also reduces the apparent bicarbonate threshold in the proximal tubule; mild degrees of hyperchloremic acidosis are commonly noted in patients with this disorder.

Gastrointestinal bicarbonate wasting can occur in several circumstances. Both pancreatic and small bowel secretions are rich in bicarbonate; pancreatic fluid, for example, has a pH of approximately 8.0. Hence *diarrheal states* and *ileal drainage* can result in significant bicarbonate losses. *Ureterosigmoidostomy* results in metabolic acidosis because the colon can secrete bicarbonate in exchange for chloride. Thus in patients with this surgical procedure, urine reaching the colon is alkalinized by bicarbonate exchange for chloride, thereby producing a net bicarbonate loss.

Failure of Bicarbonate Regeneration. The second major group of disorders producing hyperchloremic acidosis includes those disorders in which the ability of the distal nephron to regenerate bicarbonate is impaired. *Distal, gradient-limited renal tubular acidosis* and chronic interstitial renal disease with *hyporeninemic hypoaldosteronism* are prototypes of this kind of metabolic acidosis (Ch. 84). The nature of these two disorders is, however, different. In gradient-limited distal renal tubular acidosis, proton secretion may be normal, but because the distal tubule is unable to maintain a steep urine to blood proton concentration gradient, secreted protons are recycled back to blood. The administration of large quantities of phosphate salts permits the excretion of large amounts of titratable acid in this disorder, because the pH of the phosphate buffer system is 6.8, that is, relatively high. Potassium wasting and hypokalemia are common in distal gradient-limited renal tubular acidosis, owing at least in part to secondary hyperaldosteronism stimulated by sodium wasting.

In hyporeninemic hypoaldosteronism, which generally occurs in association with interstitial disease, the distal tubular derangements include diminished rates of sodium absorption and diminished rates of proton and potassium secretion. Consequently, sodium wasting and hyperkalemic, hyperchloremic acidosis are the hallmarks of this disorder. Diuretics such as *triamterene, spironolactone, and amiloride*, which interfere with distal tubular sodium absorption, proton secretion, and potassium secretion, also result in hyperkalemic, hyperchloremic metabolic acidosis (Table 77–5).

Acidifying Salts. The third major group of conditions producing hyperchloremic acidosis includes the administration of *acidifying salts* such as ammonium hydrochloride, lysine hydrochloride, or arginine hydrochloride. In each instance, metabolism of the ammonium or of the amino acids leads to hydrochloric acid formation. *Parenteral hyperalimentation* without the administration of adequate amounts of bicarbonate or

bicarbonate-yielding solutes (such as lactate or acetate) can also produce hyperchloremic metabolic acidosis. The acidosis occurs because the synthetic amino acids used in hyperalimentation mixtures contain positively charged amino acids such as arginine, lysine, and histidine, which yield proton equivalents when metabolized.

INCREASED ANION GAP METABOLIC ACIDOSIS. Metabolic acidoses characterized by an increased anion gap occur either because the kidneys fail to excrete inorganic acids, such as phosphate or sulfate, or because there is net accumulation of organic acids.

Reduced Acid Excretion. Renal failure, either acute or chronic, results in metabolic acidosis with an increased anion gap due to retention of sulfates and phosphates. In chronic renal failure metabolic acidosis occurs because the net amount of ammonium excreted daily falls as functional renal mass diminishes. The plasma bicarbonate concentration in most patients with chronic renal failure ranges between 16 and 20 mEq per liter. Although this degree of acidosis appears relatively modest, the daily acid load is buffered by bone salts; this buffering may contribute to the osteopenia of chronic renal failure (Ch. 249). In acute tubular necrosis, acidosis occurs because of generalized tubular dysfunction, including impaired net acid excretion. The plasma bicarbonate level generally remains above 16 mEq per liter unless sepsis, profound hypoxia, or extensive tissue necrosis complicates the disorder.

Organic Acid Accumulation. Accumulation of organic acids represents the second major cause for metabolic acidosis with an increased anion gap and is the most common cause for acute metabolic acidosis. Normally, the complete combustion of carbohydrates and fatty acids to carbon dioxide and water is highly efficient and results in the production of approximately 22,000 mEq of hydrogen ion per day. Thus the lungs eliminate, as expired carbon dioxide, more than 300 times as much acid as the 70 mEq of fixed acid excreted daily by the kidneys as titratable acid plus ammonia. Processes that impair cellular respiration, and therefore result in nonvolatile rather than volatile acid production, lead to profound metabolic acidosis. In these circumstances, the interplay of three cardinal factors determines the magnitude of the anion gap acidosis.

One of these is the rate of lipolysis, regulated by insulin, and the rate of glycolysis. Diabetic ketoacidosis is the prototype of such an anion gap acidosis. The second variable is the rate of cellular respiration, which in practical terms is determined by the rate of tissue perfusion with oxygen and the functional state of mitochondria. Lactic acidosis due to hypoperfusion or phenformin thereby is an anion gap acidosis caused by impaired cellular respiration.

The last factor determining the magnitude of the anion gap for such conditions is the extent of renal perfusion, which in turn regulates the proximal renal tubular threshold for organic acid excretion. Thus in diabetic ketoacidosis, volume expansion with normal saline can convert a large anion gap acidosis to a normal anion gap acidosis, not by correcting the underlying metabolic derangement, which requires insulin, but simply by increasing the rate of renal organic acid excretion.

The syndrome of *lactic acidosis* results from impaired cellular respiration. Lactic acid is produced in muscle, red blood cells, and other tissues as a consequence of anaerobic glycolysis. Lactic acid oxidation involves reduction of nicotine adenine dinucleotide (NAD) by lactic acid dehydrogenase (*LDH*) according to the following reaction:

$$\text{Lactate} + \text{NAD} \overset{LDH}{\rightleftharpoons} \text{pyruvate} + \text{NADH}$$

Cellular respiration involves mitochondrial oxidation of pyruvate and NADH to carbon dioxide and water. When lactic acidosis occurs because of impaired cellular respiration, the lactate to pyruvate ratio (L/P) rises, as does the NADH/NAD ratio. Thus glycolysis in a setting of impaired cellular respiration results in increased production of nonvolatile lactic acid. Lactic acidosis should not be confused with states in which serum lactate levels are elevated with normal L/P and NADH/NAD ratios, as, for example, in vigorous exercise. Lactic acidosis is also characterized by negative serum nitroprusside (Acetest) reactions, since Acetest tablets react with acetoacetic acid and acetone, but not with lactic acid or beta-hydroxybutyric acid. In lactic acidosis the beta-hydroxybutyric acid/acetoacetic acid ratio is elevated in parallel with the increased NADH/NAD ratio.

Lactic acidosis occurs most commonly in disorders characterized by inadequate oxygen delivery to tissues, such as shock, septicemia, and profound hypoxemia. Drug-induced lactic acidosis may occur with phenformin therapy and isoniazid toxicity; in both circumstances, oxygen utilization by tissues is thought to be impaired. Lactic acidosis also occurs in association with leukemia and diabetes mellitus. A negative serum Acetest reaction in patients with diabetes acidosis is a valuable clue to the coexistence of diabetic ketoacidosis and lactic acidosis. There is also a spontaneous, idiopathic form of lactic acidosis in debilitated patients, which is almost uniformly fatal.

A second group of disorders characterized by an anion gap metabolic acidosis includes those disorders in which cellular respiration may not be impaired, but accelerated rates of organic acid production, particularly from lipolysis, result in an increased anion gap. *Alcoholic ketoacidosis* occurs in patients with chronic alcoholism and a recent history of binge drinking, little or no food intake, and recurrent vomiting. Hypoglycemia may be present. The major pathogenic mechanism for alcoholic ketoacidosis is accelerated lipolysis and beta-hydroxybutyric acid production because of reduced insulin secretion. The Acetest reaction is variably positive, and the beta-hydroxybutyrate/acetoacetate ratio is elevated. Lactate utilization is diminished in this disorder. Patients with alcoholic ketoacidosis have beta-hydroxybutyric acid, rather than lactic acid, as the principal nonvolatile acid. *Diabetic ketoacidosis* is the most common cause for metabolic acidosis with an increased anion gap and occurs because of increased rates of ketogenesis due to insulin lack and inadequate carbohydrate combustion. *Starvation* produces metabolic acidosis by essentially the same mechanism: increased hepatic ketogenesis with reduced caloric intake. Thus in a general sense, alcoholic ketoacidosis, diabetic ketoacidosis, and starvation share at least one common feature: accelerated lipolysis and ketogenesis due to insulin lack.

Finally, a number of ingested substances result in severe metabolic acidosis with a large anion gap. *Salicylism* produces a complex set of acid-base abnormalities. Salicylates stimulate ventilation through central mechanisms; the decrease in $PaCO_2$ then results in reductions in plasma bicarbonate concentrations. Since salicylate is a relatively strong acid, the ingestion of large quantities of salicylate can, by itself, contribute to metabolic acidosis and an increased anion gap. Salicylates also interfere with mitochondrial function. As a consequence, a number of as yet unidentified organic acids accumulate in serum and are the major factors responsible for the anion gap acidosis of salicylism.

A number of other agents, including *paraldehyde, methanol,* and *ethylene glycol,* also produce severe metabolic acidosis with organic acid accumulation. In methanol poisoning, formic acid (an end-product of methanol metabolism) accounts in large part for the reduction in serum bicarbonate concentration. In ethylene glycol intoxication, glycolic and lactic acid accumulation accounts for the majority of the reduction in plasma bicarbonate level; however, oxalate deposition in tissues is clearly a major factor in ethylene glycol toxicity. The organic acids responsible for an increased anion gap in paraldehyde intoxication have not been identified.

DIAGNOSIS AND TREATMENT. The diagnosis of metabolic acidosis requires analysis of serum electrolytes and, when indicated, measurement of arterial pH and $PaCO_2$. A cardinal clinical manifestation of metabolic acidosis is hyperventilation, which, when severe, is manifest as Kussmaul's respiration. In patients with chronic metabolic acidosis, however, hyperventilation may be difficult to detect clinically.

Severe metabolic acidosis exerts a negative inotropic effect on the heart, which depends, at least in part, on the fact that acidosis diminishes tissue responsiveness to catecholamines. Thus in lactic acidosis, negative inotropy sets the stage for a potentially lethal chain of events: poor tissue perfusion → lactic acidosis → decreased cardiac function → further reduction in tissue perfusion.

Acidosis also affects the delivery of oxygen to tissues. In acidosis, the Bohr effect shifts the oxyhemoglobin dissociation curve to the right. This compensatory mechanism permits the delivery of oxygen to inadequately perfused tissues. However, the protective characteristics of the Bohr effect may be offset by the effect of pH variation on red blood cell 2,3-diphosphoglycerate (2,3-DPG). Increases in red cell 2,3-DPG also shift the oxyhemoglobin dissociation curve to the right. However, acidosis tends to reduce red blood cell 2,3-DPG; this may offset partially the compensatory Bohr effect and therefore aggravate inadequate tissue oxygenation in acidosis.

Since metabolic acidosis is a manifestation of a variety of different diseases, the treatment of metabolic acidosis varies depending on the underlying process and on the acuteness and severity of the acidosis. Certain general principles serve as useful guidelines for therapy. Those disorders characterized by *failure of bicarbonate regeneration* or *reduced excretion of inorganic acids* represent acidoses in which the kidneys fail to excrete a normal load of nonvolatile acid or, in other words, fail to regenerate approximately 70 mEq of bicarbonate daily. Thus the treatment of these metabolic acidoses requires removal of the offending agent, if patients are receiving triamterene or spironolactone, and the administration of relatively modest amounts of bicarbonate. In chronic renal failure, alkali therapy is generally not required unless the plasma bicarbonate level falls below 16 to 18 mEq per liter. If the acidosis is more severe, bicarbonate supplementation in the form of Shohl's solution (see below) may be instituted. Caution should be exercised to avoid sodium overload or the appearance of tetany, if overalkalinization occurs.

In distal, gradient-limited renal tubular acidosis, the administration of 30 to 60 mEq of bicarbonate daily usually corrects the acidosis. This can be given conveniently in the form of Shohl's solution, which is a mixture of sodium citrate and citric acid; 1 ml of Shohl's solution yields the equivalent of 1 mmol of sodium bicarbonate. Potassium supplementation is also required in the disorder. In children with distal renal tubular acidosis, greater quantities of bicarbonate, in the range of 5 to 14 mEq of alkali per kilogram daily, are usually required to avoid growth retardation.

The therapy of patients with metabolic acidosis due to *external bicarbonate loss* varies with the nature of the disorder. As indicated above, sodium restriction, and an attendant rise in the apparent bicarbonate threshold, may be helpful in treating proximal renal tubular acidosis. In acute metabolic acidosis due to gastrointestinal losses, the net bicarbonate deficit may be roughly calculated, as indicated previously, from the reduction in "bicarbonate space," or total body buffering capacity, as follows:

$$(24 \text{ mEq/L} - \text{measured plasma HCO}_3^-) \times 0.6 \text{ body weight (kg)}$$

Bicarbonate therapy should be instituted when the arterial pH falls below 7.1. It is prudent to administer sufficient sodium bicarbonate intravenously to raise the plasma bicarbonate concentration to 16 mEq per liter over a 12- to 24-hour interval, rather than to repair the entire bicarbonate deficit. Calculation of the bicarbonate deficit in this manner is valid only if there are no further bicarbonate losses. If the latter persist, as in cholera or other types of secretory diarrhea, the daily amount of bicarbonate given to maintain the plasma bicarbonate concentration in the range of 16 mEq per liter may actually exceed the calculated bicarbonate space.

The treatment of acidoses due to *accumulation of organic acids* varies with the disorder. In *lactic acidosis* therapy should be directed toward improving tissue perfusion. Because the disorder results from a failure of conversion of lactic acid and other organic acids to carbon dioxide and water, large amounts of sodium bicarbonate, sometimes in excess of 1000 mEq per 24-hour period, have been used in attempts to avoid lethal acidosis.

The treatment is complicated by the fact that the response to alkali therapy is not predictable. In experimental lactic acidosis, dichloroacetate can raise arterial pH by suppressing endogenous lactic acid production, but bicarbonate therapy worsens the disorder by increasing the rate of splanchnic bed lactate production. Moreover, large amounts of sodium bicarbonate (in the form of ampules containing 44.5 mmol of sodium bicarbonate per 50 ml) can produce cellular shrinkage due to hypertonicity and circulatory overload due to ECF volume expansion.

The treatment of *alcoholic ketoacidosis* generally requires only the administration of saline solutions and glucose. Alkali therapy should not be used unless the metabolic acidosis is in the lethal range. The same considerations apply to starvation ketosis. The insulin release provoked by glucose administration suppresses lipolysis and consequently the overproduction of ketoacids.

In *diabetic ketoacidosis*, insulin therapy promotes glucose utilization and consequently complete oxidation of ketoacids; simultaneously, ketogenesis is reduced. Therefore alkali therapy is ordinarily not required in the disorder. Furthermore, because the hyperventilatory response to acidosis in some diabetic patients is governed by arterial rather than central medullary chemoreceptors, intravenous sodium bicarbonate administration may result in arterial alkalinization, a reduction in the rate of minute ventilation, and a potentially lethal fall in CSF pH. Sodium bicarbonate therapy in diabetic ketoacidosis should therefore be reserved for initial therapy of the disorder when the arterial pH is below 7.0 to 7.1 and cardiac contractility is impaired. Finally, because *salicylates, methanol,* and ethylene glycol are by themselves tissue toxins, appropriate therapy for these disorders includes not only alkalinization but also hemodialysis for removal of the offending agent. Ethanol can be administered to slow the rate of metabolism of methanol to formic acid.

METABOLIC ALKALOSIS

ETIOLOGY AND PATHOGENESIS. The maintenance of the plasma bicarbonate concentration depends on renal bicarbonate reabsorption and renal bicarbonate regeneration (that is, net acid excretion). Consequently, although metabolic alkalosis may be *initiated* by the loss of hydrogen ion from the body—for example, during gastric drainage—the *maintenance* of a sustained metabolic alkalosis requires that the net rate of renal bicarbonate reabsorption or renal bicarbonate generation, or both, be greater than normal. In other words, a steady-state elevation of plasma bicarbonate concentrations to levels greater than 24 mEq per liter requires increased activity of one or more of the effector mechanisms regulating bicarbonate handling by renal tubules. In normal individuals it is therefore difficult to produce metabolic alkalosis by simple alkali loading.

Table 77–14 lists the major clinical causes of metabolic alkalosis. The table includes two disorders in which the apparent threshold for proximal bicarbonate reabsorption is increased, namely, volume contraction and potassium depletion, and disorders that increase net bicarbonate regeneration, including increased rates of distal salt delivery and mineralocorticoid excess, either primary or as a consequence of volume contraction. Table 77–14 also lists Liddle's syndrome, in which the pathogenesis of alkalosis is obscure.

TABLE 77–14. MAJOR MECHANISMS FOR METABOLIC ALKALOSIS

ECF volume contraction
Potassium depletion
Increased distal salt delivery
Mineralocorticoid excess
Liddle's syndrome
Bicarbonate loading (post-hypercapneic alkalosis)
Delayed conversion of administered organic acids

Volume contraction can sustain metabolic alkalosis because of an increase in the apparent rate of bicarbonate reabsorption by the proximal tubule. The most common cause for initiating this kind of alkalosis is hydrochloric acid loss because of vomiting or gastric suction. In the early stages of gastric fluid losses there is a modest sodium bicarbonate diuresis, but urinary sodium chloride excretion is reduced. As volume contraction becomes increasingly severe, sodium conservation occurs and potassium bicarbonate is excreted in an attempt to maintain pH homeostasis. Finally, when potassium depletion becomes severe, urinary sodium plus potassium excretion is sharply reduced and paradoxical aciduria occurs: The urine is acid while the plasma bicarbonate level and pH are both elevated. *Contraction alkalosis* is a frequently misunderstood term; the designation should be reserved for those patients in whom metabolic alkalosis has developed and volume contraction maintains the alkalosis by increasing the apparent proximal tubular threshold for bicarbonate reabsorption. Thus contraction alkalosis is a mirror image of the dilutional acidosis listed in Table 77–13.

Potassium depletion from any cause, when sufficiently severe, can sustain metabolic alkalosis initiated by acid loss, for example, during gastric drainage. Presumably, potassium loss from cells is accompanied by increased hydrogen ion concentrations within cells, including renal tubular cells. Thus potassium depletion, when sufficiently severe, can raise the rate of renal tubular bicarbonate reabsorption and hence maintain a metabolic alkalosis. Consequently, when serum potassium concentrations are reduced to about 2 mEq per liter, metabolic alkalosis due to gastric fluid loss becomes saline resistant but responsive to potassium chloride administration.

Situations in which there occurs *enhanced delivery of sodium chloride* to terminal nephron segments enhance renal acid excretion and therefore lead to metabolic alkalosis by increasing the rate of renal bicarbonate generation. This effect occurs with loop diuretics (Table 77–5), such as furosemide or ethacrynic acid, and with the proximal tubular diuretic metolazone. These diuretics also contribute to the maintenance of metabolic alkalosis by contracting ECF volume and by promoting potassium depletion. Salt wasting is common in *Bartter's syndrome*; metabolic alkalosis due to renal bicarbonate generation is therefore a common feature of the disorder. The administration of large amounts of *impermeant anions* such as carbenicillin also favors distal hydrogen ion secretion. Thus carbenicillin therapy is one of the few circumstances in which an increased anion gap and metabolic alkalosis can be produced simultaneously by the same agent.

Mineralocorticoid excess, either primary or secondary, can also result in metabolic alkalosis because of renal bicarbonate generation. The disorder can occur in volume-expanded patients, for example, in primary hyperaldosteronism, in which the alkalosis is unresponsive to sodium chloride loading; and in patients with a reduced effective circulating volume and secondary hyperaldosteronism. The alkalosis of mineralocorticoid excess occurs primarily because of increased generation of bicarbonate by terminal nephron segments (or, in other words, by increased renal acid excretion) and is clearly accentuated by potassium depletion. *Liddle's syndrome* is a disorder of unknown cause in which metabolic alkalosis, hypokalemia, and hypertension occur because of an increase in sodium avidity by terminal nephron segments, which can be blocked by triamterene therapy.

When viewed in this context, the disorders listed in Table 77–14, with the exception of posthypercapneic alkalosis, result in metabolic alkalosis by two general kinds of mechanisms. First, metabolic alkalosis may be initiated by a loss of acid from nonrenal sources, for example, gastric fluid loss; and the kidney maintains the metabolic alkalosis by raising the rate of proximal tubular bicarbonate reabsorption. This is the primary mechanism responsible for the alkalosis associated with ECF volume contraction or potassium depletion. Second, the generation of metabolic alkalosis may occur intrarenally, because of increased rates of renal bicarbonate generation (or net acid excretion). This appears to be the major factor responsible for the alkalosis accompanying increased rates of salt delivery to the terminal nephron, mineralocorticoid excess, and Liddle's syndrome. Obviously, there may be considerable degrees of overlap. For example, loop diuretics increase rates of salt delivery to terminal nephron segments and therefore enhance bicarbonate generation. However, these agents also produce hypokalemia and ECF volume contraction and as a consequence raise the apparent threshold for bicarbonate reabsorption. Likewise, in primary aldosteronism, increased distal nephron bicarbonate generation as a cause for alkalosis is accentuated by the effects of hypokalemia on bicarbonate reabsorption.

In normal circumstances it is nearly impossible to produce metabolic alkalosis by increasing dietary alkali intake. In certain situations, however, *bicarbonate loading* can produce either a transient or a steady-state alkalosis. One such circumstance is *posthypercapneic alkalosis*. Patients with chronic hypercapnia develop compensatory increases in plasma bicarbonate concentrations: On an average, chronic hypoventilation results in a 0.3 mEq per liter rise in serum bicarbonate level for each 1.2 mm Hg increase in excess of $PaCO_2$ of 40 mm Hg. If ventilatory status is improved acutely, the $PaCO_2$ will fall quickly but the plasma bicarbonate level will remain elevated, particularly if the patient is salt acquisitive because of congestive heart failure or ECF volume contraction. A common way to accentuate posthypercapneic alkalosis is to maintain patients on ventilators having high positive end-expiratory pressures (PEEP), which causes a central-tourniquet effect that reduces cardiac output.

Delayed conversion of *accumulated organic acids* is a second mechanism for producing transient metabolic alkalosis. This may occur after insulin therapy for diabetic ketoacidosis, during the recovery phase of lactic acidosis, and following high-efficiency hemodialysis. In the last-named circumstance, acetate in the dialysis bath is taken up rapidly during dialysis. The accumulated acetate, which represents "potential bicarbonate," is then converted to bicarbonate after dialysis has been completed. Prolonged metabolic alkalosis because of alkali loading is a common feature of the *milk-alkali syndrome*. The alkalosis occurs because of prolonged ingestion of absorbable alkali in patients with impaired renal function due to hypercalcemic nephropathy. Frequent vomiting and attendant ECF volume contraction may also contribute to alkalosis in this disorder.

CLINICAL FEATURES AND DIAGNOSIS. There are no specific signs or symptoms of metabolic alkalosis. Relatively severe metabolic alkalosis can result in cardiac arrhythmias. Severe metabolic alkalosis can also result in severe hypoventilation, especially in patients with reduced renal function. Tetany and increased neuromuscular irritability, which are quite common in acute respiratory alkalosis, are very rare in chronic metabolic alkalosis. Rather, since hypokalemia generally accompanies metabolic alkalosis, muscular weakness and hyporeflexia are often seen in chronic metabolic alkalosis.

The diagnosis is inferred in most cases by routine measurements of serum electrolytes and can be confirmed by arterial blood gas analysis. Hypokalemia is generally present. The finding of an unexplained hypokalemic metabolic alkalosis is

suggestive of the presence of Cushing's syndrome due to an extrarenal neoplasm.

The urinary chloride concentration is a useful index for distinguishing metabolic alkalosis due to volume contraction from that due to primary mineralocorticoid excess. In volume-contracted states, the urinary chloride concentration is generally less than 10 mEq per liter. Volume-contracted patients with Bartter's syndrome, or volume-contracted patients taking diuretics, generally have elevated urinary chloride concentrations. The combination of postural hypotension, hypokalemic metabolic alkalosis, and a urinary chloride concentration greater than 20 mEq per liter is therefore suggestive of diuretic abuse or Bartter's syndrome.

TREATMENT. In metabolic alkalosis associated with hypokalemia and volume contraction, appropriate therapy consists of volume expansion with saline solutions and of potassium replacement (see section on Disturbances in Potassium Balance). If the metabolic alkalosis is sufficiently severe that significant hypoventilation is present ($PaCO_2 > 60$ mm Hg), the administration of dilute hydrochloric acid or other acidifying salts, such as lysine hydrochloride or arginine hydrochloride, may be required. The use of these amino acid salts carries with it the risk of hyperkalemia that is in excess of that expected simply from the change in arterial pH, presumably because these agents promote potassium efflux from cells. Neither ammonium chloride, lysine hydrochloride, nor arginine hydrochloride should be used in patients with significant liver disease.

If diuretic abuse can be identified, use of these agents should be discontinued. Indomethacin may correct partially the abnormalities of Bartter's syndrome, although potassium supplementation is almost invariably required. Triamterene is effective in preventing potassium wasting in Liddle's syndrome.

Hypokalemia and metabolic alkalosis due to primary hyperaldosteronism are best treated by potassium chloride supplementation, which tends to correct the metabolic alkalosis partially. Dietary sodium restriction in this disorder also tends to reduce renal potassium wasting. Of course, neither of these maneuvers provides definitive therapy for primary hyperaldosteronism.

MIXED METABOLIC DISORDERS

Mixed metabolic derangements occur commonly. Consequently, the evaluation of metabolic acid-base abnormalities depends on a simultaneous assessment of the anion gap as well as the serum bicarbonate level. Electroneutrality requires that the sum of the principal anions in serum ($Cl^- + HCO_3^- +$ anion gap) equal the serum sodium level. Thus unless the serum sodium level changes, a change in the serum concentration of one or more of these principal anions necessitates a reciprocal change in the remaining anions.

Table 77–15 indicates the pattern of serum anion concentra-

TABLE 77–15. ANION PATTERNS IN METABOLIC ACID-BASE DISORDERS

Condition	Serum Anion Concentrations		
	HCO_3^-	Cl^-	Anion Gap
Simple Disorders			
Hyperchloremic acidosis	↓	↑	nl
Anion gap acidosis	↓	nl	↑
Metabolic alkalosis	↑	↓	nl
Mixed Disorders			
Metabolic alkalosis + anion gap acidosis	nl, ↑ or ↓	↓	↑
Anion gap acidosis + hyperchloremic acidosis	↓	↑	↑
Metabolic alkalosis + hyperchloremic acidosis	nl	nl	nl

nl = normal

tions in single and mixed acid-base disorders. In the single acid-base disturbances, the change in the concentration of one anion is usually balanced by a reciprocal change in one other anion. For example, in hyperchloremic acidosis, the increase in chloride concentration equals the decrease in bicarbonate concentration.

In mixed disorders, the anion patterns are more complex. In a mixed metabolic alkalosis combined with an anion gap acidosis (e.g., diabetic ketoacidosis complicated by vomiting), the identifying pattern is an increased anion gap offset partially or entirely by a reduction in chloride; the serum bicarbonate level is variable. In an anion gap plus hyperchloremic acidosis, the reduction in bicarbonate is offset by increases in both chloride and the anion gap. Finally, in metabolic alkalosis combined with hyperchloremic acidosis (e.g., vomiting combined with interstitial nephritis), offsetting changes in serum bicarbonate and chloride concentrations may result in normal anion concentrations.

RESPIRATORY ACIDOSIS

ETIOLOGY AND PATHOGENESIS. Respiratory acidosis occurs whenever there is impairment in the rate of alveolar ventilation. Carbon dioxide elimination involves the following sequence: transfer of carbon dioxide from tissues to the lungs in the form of venous bicarbonate; formation of carbon dioxide within red blood cells by a reversal of the chloride shift, described previously in connection with tissue buffering mechanisms; perfusion of the lungs with systemic venous blood; diffusion of carbon dioxide from pulmonary capillaries to alveoli; and alveolar ventilation. Under normal circumstances, the rate of carbon dioxide hydration within red blood cells and the rate of carbon dioxide diffusion from pulmonary capillaries into alveoli are sufficiently rapid that carbon dioxide accumulation is virtually synonymous with hypoventilation.

Acute respiratory acidosis occurs when there is a sudden depression of the medullary respiratory center, as in narcotic overdose or anesthesia; when there is paralysis of the respiratory muscles, as in profound hypokalemia, neuromuscular disorders (myasthenia gravis), or the administration of agents that impair neuromuscular transmission (aminoglycoside antibiotics); when there is airway obstruction, as in foreign body aspiration or profound bronchospasm; when trauma, such as flail chest, impedes ventilation; and when an acute insult is imposed on a chronic hypercapneic state.

Chronic respiratory acidosis generally occurs in individuals with chronic bronchitis, emphysema, and bullous lung disease; in patients with extreme kyphoscoliosis; and in individuals with extreme obesity (pickwickian syndrome).

The arterial pH and plasma bicarbonate concentrations differ in acute and chronic respiratory acidosis. The compensatory response to carbon dioxide retention is to increase the apparent renal threshold for bicarbonate reabsorption. In general, the plasma bicarbonate concentration rises by approximately 0.3 mEq per liter for every millimeter of Hg increase in the $PaCO_2$ over 40 mm Hg, until the $PaCO_2$ reaches 80 mm Hg. This compensatory increase in plasma bicarbonate concentration requires two to three days for complete expression. Conversely, when chronic hypercapnia is relieved suddenly, there is a two- to three-day lag in renal bicarbonate excretion, resulting in posthypercapneic alkalosis.

These concepts are also useful in evaluating the possibility of mixed acid-base disorders occurring in association with respiratory acidosis. For example, since the rate of compensatory bicarbonate retention is delayed in acute respiratory acidosis, the presence of an elevated plasma bicarbonate concentration in a setting of acute carbon dioxide retention should be an index to the simultaneous occurrence of acute respiratory acidosis and metabolic alkalosis. Likewise, because renal bicarbonate reabsorption is an effective compensatory mechanism for chronic carbon dioxide retention, plasma bicarbonate concentrations below 28 to 30 mEq per liter in patients having chronic $PaCO_2$ values in excess of 50 mm Hg should alert one to the possible coexistence of acute metabolic acidosis and chronic respiratory acidosis.

Since hypercapnia is synonymous with alveolar hypoventilation, patients with carbon dioxide retention are invariably hypoxemic. A compensatory polycythemia occurs commonly in chronic hypercapneic states.

CLINICAL MANIFESTATIONS. The clinical manifestations of respiratory acidosis vary depending on the severity of the disorder and on the rate at which carbon dioxide retention has occurred. Acute increases in $PaCO_2$ values result in somnolence, in confusion, and ultimately in *carbon dioxide narcosis*. Asterixis may also be present. Because carbon dioxide is a cerebral vasodilator, the blood vessels in the optic fundi are often dilated, engorged, and tortuous; in severe hypercapneic states, frank papilledema may occur.

TREATMENT. The only practical treatment for acute respiratory acidosis involves treatment of the underlying disorder and ventilatory support. The possibility of drug abuse should always be considered in otherwise healthy patients who suddenly develop acute respiratory depression; consequently, naloxone (Narcan) therapy should be considered in all comatose patients seen in the emergency room in whom no apparent cause for respiratory depression can be identified.

In patients with chronic hypercapnia who develop sudden increases in $PaCO_2$ values, attention should be directed toward identifying factors such as pneumonia or pulmonary embolism, which may have aggravated the underlying disorder. It should be emphasized again that oxygen therapy in patients with chronic hypercapnia should be instituted with extreme caution, since hypoxemia may be the primary stimulus to respiration in this setting. Consequently, in such patients, sudden increases in the arterial $PaCO_2$ produced by oxygen administration may result in cessation of respiration. The administration of alkalinizing salts has no place in the management of chronic respiratory acidosis.

RESPIRATORY ALKALOSIS

ETIOLOGY AND PATHOGENESIS. Respiratory alkalosis occurs when hyperventilation reduces the arterial $PaCO_2$ and consequently increases arterial pH. Acute respiratory alkalosis is most commonly the result of the hyperventilation syndrome in anxiety. Acute hyperventilation may also occur because of damage to the respiratory centers; in acute salicylism; in fever and septic states; and in association with pneumonia, pulmonary emboli, or congestive heart failure. The disorder may also be produced iatrogenically by injudicious mechanical ventilatory support. Chronic hyperventilation occurs in the acclimation response to exposure to high altitudes (a low ambient oxygen tension), in advanced hepatic insufficiency, and in pregnancy.

During acute hyperventilation, plasma bicarbonate concentrations fall by approximately 3 mEq per liter when the $PaCO_2$ falls to about 25 mm Hg. This fall in plasma bicarbonate level is due largely to proton shifts from the ICF to the ECF and tends to minimize acute changes in arterial pH. In chronic hyperventilation, renal bicarbonate loss provides the compensatory response to the reduction in $PaCO_2$. In experimental studies with dogs, approximately two to four days are required for a maximal renal compensatory response, which involves approximately a 0.4 mEq per liter reduction in plasma bicarbonate concentrations for every millimeter of Hg fall in $PaCO_2$.

Hyperventilation and respiratory alkalosis may also occur, as mentioned previously, following the correction of metabolic acidosis and particularly in diabetic ketoacidosis. In all likelihood, hyperventilation persists in this setting because of the lag in the rate at which plasma bicarbonate concentrations rise with respect to ECF bicarbonate concentrations during correction of metabolic acidosis.

CLINICAL MANIFESTATIONS AND TREATMENT.
Chronic hyperventilation may be asymptomatic. The acute hyperventilation syndrome is characterized by light-headedness, paresthesias, circumoral numbness, and tingling of the extremities. Tetany occurs in severe cases. Both the acute metabolic alkalosis and the reduction in ionized calcium contribute to the increased neuromuscular excitability.

The treatment of acute respiratory alkalosis involves correction of the underlying disorder. When severe anxiety provokes the hyperventilation syndrome, air rebreathing with a paper bag generally terminates the acute attack. If this maneuver fails, sedation may also be required.

Gabow PA: Disorders associated with an altered anion gap. Kidney Int 27:472, 1985. *A good summary of anion gap acidoses.*

Gabow PA, Clay K, Sullivan JB, et al.: Organic acids in ethylene glycol intoxication. Ann Intern Med 105:16, 1986. *An analysis of the plasma organic acids in ethylene glycol intoxication, showing significant accumulation of glycolic and lactic acids.*

Graf H: Effects of dichloroacetate in the treatment of hypoxic lactic acidosis in dogs. J Clin Invest 76:919, 1985. *Experimental observations on the beneficial effects of dicholoroacetate therapy in experimental lactic acidosis.*

Halperin ML, Hammeke M, Josse RG, et al.: Metabolic acidosis in the alcoholic: A pathophysiologic approach. Metabolism 32:308, 1983. *An analysis of acidosis in alcoholic patients.*

Hamm L, Jacobson HR: Mixed acid-base disorders. In Kokko JP, Tannen RL (eds.): Fluids and Electrolytes. Philadelphia, W. B. Saunders Company, 1986. *A thorough account of acid-base disturbances.*

Madias NE: Lactic acidosis. Kidney Int 29:752, 1986. *A superb discussion of lactic acidosis.*

Narins RG, Emmett M: Simple and mixed acid-base disorders: A practical approach. Medicine 59:161, 1980. *A good clinical summary of acid-base disturbances.*

Oster JR, Epstein M: Acid-base aspects of ketoacidosis. Am J Nephrol 4:137, 1984. *An account of ketosis and its relation to acidosis.*

Steinmetz PR, Palmisano J: Disorders of proton secretion by the kidney. In Andreoli TE, Hoffman JF, Fanestil DD, et al. (eds.): Physiology of Membrane Disorders. New York, Plenum, 1986. *A complete discussion of renal acidification and renal acidosis.*

78 ACUTE RENAL FAILURE
Jared J. Grantham

DEFINITION

Acute renal failure is a syndrome characterized by a relatively rapid decline in renal function that leads to the accumulation of water, crystalloid solutes, and nitrogenous metabolites in the body. Clinically significant acute renal failure is usually associated with a daily increase in the serum creatinine and urea nitrogen levels (azotemia) greater than 0.5 and 10 mg per deciliter, respectively. *Oliguria*, a rate of urine flow less than 400 ml per day, is commonly observed, but in some cases the urine output may exceed this limit (*nonoliguric* acute renal failure). Complete cessation of urine flow, *anuria*, is relatively uncommon.

ETIOLOGY

Acute renal failure may be seen in a wide variety of clinical settings (Table 78–1). A systematic approach to the causes of acute renal failure facilitates diagnosis in the individual patient. It is important to remember that acute renal failure is a bilateral process, except in patients with only one functioning kidney.

Prerenal

Prerenal causes lead to renal failure by decreasing the effective perfusion of kidney parenchyma. An absolute decrease in blood volume (hypovolemia), the most common prerenal disorder, may be caused by skin, gastrointestinal, and renal losses of water and electrolytes, hemorrhage, and sequestration of fluids in body cavities. In some conditions the kidneys respond as though the blood volume were de-

TABLE 78–1. CAUSES OF ACUTE RENAL FAILURE SYNDROME

Location of Primary Disorder	Clinical Examples
Prenal	
Absolute decrease in effective blood volume	Hemorrhage, skin losses (burns, sweating), GI losses (diarrhea, vomiting), renal losses (diuretics, glycosuria), fluid pooling (peritonitis, burns)
Relative decrease in blood volume (ineffective arterial volume)	Congestive heart failure, dysrhythmias, sepsis, anaphylaxis, liver failure
Arterial occlusion	Bilateral thromboembolism, thromboembolism of solitary kidney, aortic or renal artery aneurysm
Postrenal	
Ureteral obstruction	Bilateral or solitary kidney (calculi, neoplasm, clot, retroperitoneal fibrosis, iatrogenic)
Venous occlusion	Bilateral or solitary kidney (renal vein thrombosis, neoplasm, iatrogenic)
Intrarenal	
Vascular	Vasculitis, malignant hypertension, vasopressors, eclampsia, microangiopathy, hyperviscosity states, nonsteroidal anti-inflammatory drugs, hypercalcemia, iodinated radiocontrast agents
Glomerulus	Acute glomerulonephritis
Tubular injury	
Ischemia	Profound hypotension, postrenal transplant, vasopressors, microvascular constriction
Intratubular pigments	Hemoglobinuria, myoglobinuria
Intratubular proteins	Myeloma
Intratubular crystals	Uric acid, oxalate, sulfonamides, pyridium
Tubulointerstitial	Interstitial nephritis due to drugs, infection, radiation
Nephrotoxins	Antibiotics (gentamicin, kanamycin, neomycin, amikacin, tobramycin, streptomycin, cephaloridine, amphotericin B); metals (mercury, bismuth, uranium, arsenic, silver, cadmium, iron, antimony); solvents (carbon tetrachloride, glycol, tetrachlorethylene); iodinated contrast agents; streptozotocin, cisplatin

creased, when in fact the measured volume is normal or even increased. These oliguric states include congestive heart failure (which may be precipitated by myocardial infarction or dysrhythmia), sepsis, anaphylaxis, and liver failure. Bilateral renal artery occlusion can occur spontaneously owing to emboli from the heart or from an atheromatous aorta. Embolism of atheroma occurs commonly in the course of difficult surgical procedures involving the abdominal aorta.

Postrenal

Although quite rare, *bilateral ureteral obstruction* may be due to calculi, shed papillae in analgesic nephropathy, thrombus, neoplasms, and iatrogenic causes. Commonly in bilateral obstruction one kidney is blocked for several days or weeks before obstruction of the contralateral kidney causes acute renal failure. Acute ureteral obstruction of a solitary kidney is seen occasionally. Acute renal failure can be caused by *urethral obstruction* due to prostatic hypertrophy, prostatitis, bladder and prostate tumors, bladder rupture, calculi, and iatrogenic causes. In hospitalized patients with indwelling urinary catheters, the patency and correct placement of the catheter should always be checked in the evaluation of acute renal failure.

Bilateral renal venous occlusion is rare but may be seen in hypercoagulable states, with intra-abdominal neoplasms, or secondary to surgical procedures.

Intrarenal

The renal arterial and arteriolar *blood vessels* may be involved in vasculitis, malignant hypertension, eclampsia, and microangiopathies. Pronounced vasospasm leading to acute renal failure may be seen in scleroderma, during systemic infusions of norepinephrine, secondary to the use of nonsteroidal anti-inflammatory compounds, iodinated radiocontrast agents, or diet pills, or in hypercalcemic states.

Glomerular inflammation (acute glomerulonephritis, Ch. 81) may cause acute renal failure by sharply reducing renal blood flow. *Renal tubules* are susceptible to a number of insults. *Ischemic* injury, sometimes progressing to frank necrosis, may be seen secondary to profound hypotension, especially in elderly persons. Rarely, ischemia may be severe enough to cause irreversible necrosis of renal parenchyma. About one half of kidneys transplanted from cadaver sources undergo oliguric renal failure. The intravenous administration of powerful vasoconstrictors, such as norepinephrine, may cause acute ischemic tubular injury in certain susceptible patients. Renal tubules are susceptible to injury by high levels of urinary pigments (hemoglobinuria, myoglobinuria), especially in the setting of renal hypoperfusion and ischemia. Several serum proteins are potentially nephrotoxic, including kappa and lambda light chains, which may be abundantly excreted in patients with multiple myeloma. Renal tubules may be occluded by uric acid, oxalate, sulfonamide, or pyridium crystals, leading to acute renal failure.

A wide variety of chemicals are potential tubular toxins. Antibiotics of the aminoglycoside class (one of the most common iatrogenic nephrotoxins), streptomycin, cephaloridine, and amphotericin all injure renal tubules when given in excessive doses. These agents are apparently nephrotoxic even at low therapeutic doses in patients who are oliguric or hypotensive or who have underlying renal disorders. The combined effects of aminoglycosides and certain cephalothin drugs appear to be additive in causing acute renal failure. Heavy metal poisoning is seen rarely but may cause acute tubular necrosis and renal failure. Iodinated radiocontrast agents may directly injure renal tubules in patients with underlying disorders such as diabetes mellitus, systemic lupus erythematosus, and chronic renal insufficiency from nearly any cause. Chemotherapeutic agents such as streptozotocin and cisplatin almost routinely cause acute renal injury that may progress to acute renal failure. Phencyclidine, a psychotropic agent, has caused acute renal failure in a few patients.

INCIDENCE

Acute renal failure is a relatively common syndrome. The incidence in the general outpatient population is not known; in one study about 5 per cent of patients on medical and surgical units in a general hospital experienced an episode of acute renal failure. Approximately 60 per cent of cases are related to surgery or trauma; the remainder have medical or obstetric causes. Overall, about one half of cases of acute renal failure in hospitalized patients may be iatrogenic.

PATHOGENESIS

Ischemia and nephrotoxins are the most common causes of acute renal failure listed in Table 78–1. There are at least three important phases in the acute renal failure syndrome due to ischemia or nephrotoxins. In the first, or *initiation* phase, the kidneys are subjected to an insult that produces parenchymal injury (e.g., temporary cessation of renal blood flow; nephrotoxins or pigments; see Table 78–1 and Fig. 78–1). In some patients who are hypovolemic, the initiation phase can be overridden by plasma volume expansion and the acute renal failure syndrome aborted. More commonly, however, the initiation phase causes profound renal vasoconstriction and an initial decrease in renal blood flow. The initiation phase is followed by the *maintenance* phase, during which renal vasoconstriction may persist, thereby decreasing the formation of glomerular filtrate. The hydraulic permeability of the glomeruli is usually decreased, diminishing further the ability of glomeruli to form filtrate. In addition to factors operating within the glomeruli, injury to renal tubules causes the cells to slough from the basement membranes to form casts that can obstruct urine flow. Moreover, the damaged epithelium of the tubules allows the small amount of glomerular filtrate that is formed to leak back into the peritubular capillaries. These four factors, vasoconstriction, decreased glomerular permeability, intratubular obstruction, and tubular back leak of filtrate (Figs. 78–1 and 78–2), operate in concert to depress the effective glomerular filtration rate in the ischemic and nephrotoxic types of acute renal failure listed in Table 78–1.

In some cases the renal blood flow may return to relatively normal levels 24 to 48 hours after the initiation phase. Despite this, the glomerular filtration rate (GFR) remains very low owing to the decreased glomerular hydraulic permeability, tubular obstruction, or tubular back leak of filtrate.

The third stage in the pathogenetic sequence is the *recovery* phase. Provided that the initiating causes remit, healing of renal parenchyma and recovery of function may be expected in most types of acute renal failure.

CLINICAL MANIFESTATIONS

The onset of acute renal failure usually follows the initiating event by an interval varying from a few hours to as long as several days. Patients and physicians usually first notice a reduction in urine volume in the oliguric types of acute renal failure. Facial edema, tight fitting rings, and weight gain reflect the retention of water. Rarely pulmonary edema may be an initial manifestation. Renal pain is uncommon except in association with acute infection, urolithiasis, and tumors. Hematuria is seen in nephritic syndromes and vascular occlusive states but is uncommon in nephrotoxic and transient ischemic states.

The serum creatinine and urea levels rise steadily. In severely oliguric persons of average size the serum creatinine level rises about 1.5 to 2 mg per deciliter per day. When the measured increase in serum creatinine exceeds this range, one should consider hypercatabolic factors; when the measured increase is less, renal clearance of creatinine may be greater than the rate of urine volume flow would suggest. The serum urea nitrogen level usually rises in concert with

FIGURE 78–1. Pathogenesis of acute renal failure.

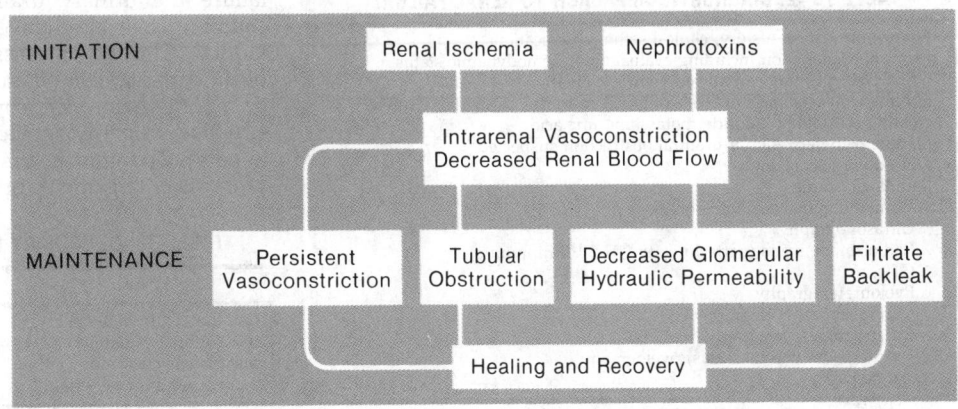

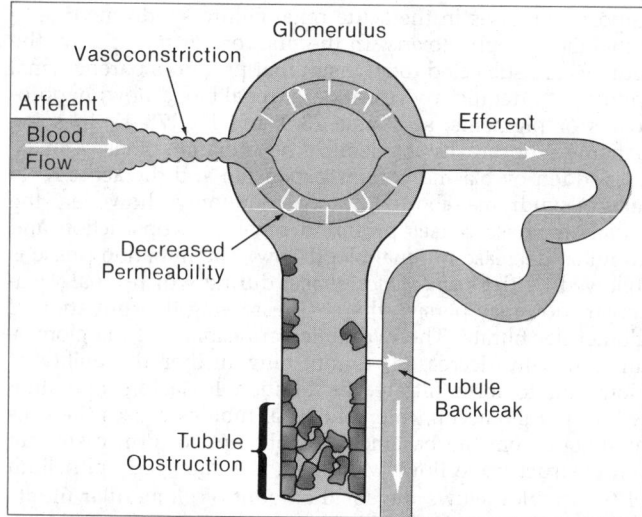

FIGURE 78–2. Possible mechanisms contributing to oliguria in acute renal failure.

the creatinine level. However, urea production is altered by food intake, by tissue catabolism, and by blood within the intestines; consequently, the urea levels do not reflect the performance of the kidneys as well as do creatinine levels.

Hyperkalemia due to inadequate renal excretion of potassium may be life threatening early in the course of acute renal failure. Metabolic acidosis due to inadequate renal excretion of hydrogen ions is seen later on. Hyponatremia may be seen in patients who drink unlimited amounts of water or other fluids. Hypocalcemia, hyperphosphatemia, hyperuricemia, and anemia usually develop after several days unless there are mitigating factors such as rhabdomyolysis and hemolysis. Serum amylase levels may be twice normal in the absence of pancreatitis.

The uremic syndrome develops gradually and, in addition to the features mentioned above, is characterized by the progressive development of anorexia, nausea, vomiting, nervous irritability, hyperreflexia, asterixis, seizures, and coma. Hemorrhagic signs include ecchymoses, gastric and colonic hemorrhage, and pericarditis.

DIAGNOSIS

When renal failure is recognized it is important to determine the probable cause and remediable factors underlying kidney dysfunction. Table 78–2 lists several key components in the diagnostic approach to renal failure.

The initial objective is to determine if the renal failure is acute or chronic. The diagnostic evaluation starts at the patient's bedside. With conversant ambulatory patients the onset of renal dysfunction can usually be determined based

TABLE 78–2. DIAGNOSTIC APPROACH TO RENAL FAILURE

1. Review of medical history, clinical setting, medications
2. Physical examination including evaluation of hemodynamic status
3. Urinalysis including careful sediment examination
4. Simultaneous chemical analysis of blood and urine. Osmolality, urea, creatinine, sodium, chloride, potassium, uric acid
5. Bladder catheterization if urethral obstruction suspected
6. Fluid-diuretic challenge
7. Radiologic studies
   Plain abdominal roentgenogram
   Ultrasonography
   Radioisotope scans (pertechnetate ^{99m}Tc, ^{131}I-hippurate)
   CT scan
   Pyeloureterography
     Intravenous pyelography
     Retrograde pyelography
     Antegrade (percutaneous) pyelography
8. Renal biopsy

on historical changes in urine output (oliguria, polyuria, nocturia), abnormal urine color, and changes in body weight. Chronic renal failure is further indicated by anemia, osteodystrophy, lipiduria, bilaterally small kidneys, neuropathy, and a modestly elevated serum level of uric acid.

In the differential diagnosis of acute renal failure it is important to distinguish among *prerenal*, *postrenal*, and *intrarenal* factors.

Prerenal Failure

Prerenal failure is suggested by a history of rapid weight loss, flu-like illness, lack of fluid ingestion, bleeding, nasogastric aspiration, diuretic therapy, or orthostatic dizziness. In prerenal failure due to *extracellular fluid volume contraction* the physical examination may reveal orthostatic hypotension and tachycardia, poor venous filling and a "thready" pulse, and peripheral vasoconstriction with cool extremities and dry mucous membranes. When prerenal failure occurs in *euvolemic* or *hypervolemic* patients, one usually finds signs of congestive heart failure or liver failure, including distended veins, a third heart sound, pulmonary rales and wheezes, ascites, jaundice, and peripheral edema.

Urinary indices (Table 78–3) show concentrated urine (relatively high specific gravity and osmolality), low fractional excretions of sodium and chloride, and a high urine to plasma creatinine ratio. Diuretics can diminish the diagnostic usefulness of urinary indices and should not be used prior to collecting urine for analysis. Urinalysis and urine sediment examination are usually unremarkable except for hyaline casts.

When the physical and chemical findings point to prerenal acute azotemia due to a *decrease in extracellular fluid volume*, a fluid challenge of 500 to 1000 ml of isotonic saline may stimulate urine formation in the average adult. In the author's opinion, mannitol and diuretics are contraindicated in volume-depleted patients with prerenal azotemia. In prerenal azotemia associated with an *expanded extracellular fluid volume*, diuretics may be indicated as part of the general plan to improve cardiac function.

Prerenal azotemia due to occlusion of renal arteries is revealed by radioisotope screening tests and arteriography. Urine output generally is scanty. Urinalysis may show hematuria and proteinuria, and urinary indices show an inability to concentrate urinary solutes (Table 78–3).

Postrenal Failure

Obstruction to the flow of urine may be acute or chronic (see Ch. 83). In most cases of acute obstruction of the *upper tract* the patient notices pain in the flank or lower abdominal regions and fluctuating urine output. *Urethral* obstruction usually causes urinary frequency, dribbling, and lower abdominal fullness. In urinary tract obstruction infected urine is commonly observed.

The onset of renal failure due to obstruction of the urinary drainage system can be difficult to determine. To cause renal failure the urinary drainage from both kidneys must be compromised; alternatively the patient may have only one kidney. Chronic progressive processes, such as retroperitoneal neoplasia, can obstruct the drainage of one ureter weeks or months before the contralateral ureter is obstructed. Obstructive uropathy should be suspected in patients with adenopathy, abdominal scars, palpable bladder, flank tenderness, prostatic enlargement, or pelvic masses with induration.

TABLE 78–3. URINARY INDICES IN ACUTE RENAL FAILURE

Index	Prerenal	Acute Tubular Injury
Urine osmolality mOsm/kg H_2O	> 500	< 350
Urine sodium mEq/liter	< 20	> 40
Urine/plasma creatinine	> 40	< 20
Fractional sodium excretion	< 1	> 1

Urinary findings are nonspecific. The sediment contains leukocytes and erythrocytes in infected patients. The urinary indices are variable. In acute obstruction the indices are identical to those seen in prerenal failure; in obstructions more than two days in duration the indices are similar to those seen in intrarenal tubular injury (Tables 78–2 and 78–3).

When urethral obstruction is suspected bladder catheterization may be diagnostic. With upper tract obstruction ultrasonography in the hands of an experienced radiologist is the most useful diagnostic test. Rarely, acute obstruction of the urinary tract may occur without dilation of the renal pelvis and cannot be detected by sonography. The ^{131}I-hippurate scan is a noninvasive test that is useful for determining the potential for return of renal function in obstructive uropathy. Bilateral upper tract obstruction is usually nonsynchronous. In such cases the hippurate scan shows asymmetric accumulation of the isotope. The kidney showing the most intense uptake of hippurate is the best candidate for return of function after relief of obstruction. Intravenous pyelography is useful to localize the site of obstruction, but adequate renal function is needed to concentrate the contrast material in the urinary tract. Retrograde pyelography should be reserved for those cases in which the noninvasive methods are not available or those in which equivocal results have been obtained. In some cases the CT scan may provide anatomic confirmation of obstruction.

Occlusion of the renal veins is suggested by a history of a hypercoagulable state, pulmonary emboli, hematuria, or proteinuria. Urinary indices are not diagnostic. Radioisotope studies of renal perfusion may be suggestive, but definitive diagnosis depends on renal arteriography or venography.

Intrarenal Failure

Renal failure due to intrinsic dysfunction is suggested by a history of multisystem disease (e.g., SLE, vasculitis), fever, malaise, skin rash, hypertension, gross hematuria, hypotensive episode, or exposure to nephrotoxins.

The urinalysis is an invaluable guide in the diagnosis of intrarenal failure. Acute glomerulonephritis is characterized by hematuria, proteinuria, erythrocyte casts, and granular casts. Lipid bodies and broad waxy casts suggest a chronic process. Pus casts indicate acute or chronic interstitial inflammation. Urinary eosinophils are seen in allergic interstitial nephritis. Crystalluria is observed in urate and oxalate disorders. Physicians should be able to recognize these formed elements in the urine and should personally examine a freshly prepared urine sediment. Acute inflammation of the preglomerular arterioles may or may not be associated with alterations in glomerular capillaries. In the absence of glomerular capillary inflammation the urinalysis reflects ischemic tubular injury due to reduced renal blood flow. Acute tubular injury does not give specific urinary sediment findings, but cellururia, epithelial cell casts, and coarse granular casts should raise the index of suspicion.

Urinary indices (Table 78–3) are very helpful in differentiating between conditions that cause injury to preglomerular arterioles and glomeruli and those that cause acute tubular injury. In the former the indices show a prerenal pattern, whereas in acute tubular injury the fractional excretion of sodium is increased and the urinary osmolality approaches that of plasma. The conditions that may exhibit low or normal fractional sodium excretion at some point in the course of the acute renal failure syndrome are listed in Table 78–4.

Radiologic tests are relatively nonspecific in the evaluation of intrarenal failure. The ^{131}I-hippurate scan shows accumulation of isotope in both kidneys if some renal perfusion is preserved and viable tubules remain. Renal arteriography may show microaneurysm formation in polyarteritis nodosa. Renal biopsy is usually indicated in the evaluation of glomerulonephritis, vasculitis, or interstitial nephritis but is not

TABLE 78–4. CONDITIONS ASSOCIATED WITH FRACTIONAL SODIUM EXCRETION (FE$_{Na}$) LESS THAN 1 PER CENT IN ACUTE RENAL FAILURE SYNDROME

Intense Intrarenal Vasoconstriction
1. Iodinated radiocontrast
2. Acute bilateral ureteral obstruction
3. Severe burns
4. Sepsis
5. Pigment excretion (myoglobin, hemoglobin)
6. Nonsteroidal anti-inflammatory drugs
7. Amphotericin B
8. Norepinephrine, dopamine
9. Liver disease
10. Cardiopulmonary bypass

Vascular Inflammation
1. Acute glomerulonephritis
2. Acute vasculitis
3. Renal transplant rejection

commonly used when pyelonephritis or acute tubular injury is suspected.

TREATMENT

There are at least four major objectives in the treatment of acute renal failure: (a) correct the reversible causes, (b) prevent additional injury, (c) convert oliguric to nonoliguric renal failure, and (d) provide general metabolic support during the maintenance and recovery phases of the syndrome.

Correct Reversible Causes

Prerenal and postrenal factors contributing to renal function should be corrected insofar as is possible. Drugs that interfere with renal perfusion or that are directly nephrotoxic should be stopped. In hypotensive patients the blood pressure should be restored by discontinuing antihypertensive drugs and administering isotonic volume-expanding solutions. In elderly patients with longstanding hypertension, a "normal" blood pressure of 110/70 may in fact be inadequate to generate glomerular filtrate. If there is doubt about the status of the plasma volume, an intravenous challenge of isotonic saline (500 to 1000 ml) is warranted. In the states listed in Table 78–4 associated with a low fractional sodium excretion due to intrarenal vasoconstriction, a volume challenge combined with 40 to 80 mg of intravenous furosemide may reverse the oliguric state, and in some cases prevent the maintenance phase of acute renal failure.

Prevention of Additional Injury

Radiocontrast agents are potentially harmful to patients in the maintenance phase of acute renal failure, and alternative diagnostic methods should be used whenever possible. CT scans are often done with contrast enhancement, and physicians are not always aware of this "hidden" source of iodinated radiocontrast material. Nonsteroidal anti-inflammatory drugs and nephrotoxic antibiotics should be avoided if possible. Drug dosages should be adjusted according to guidelines for renal failure, and plasma drug levels should be monitored when possible.

Convert Oliguria to Nonoliguria

Oliguria in and of itself is not harmful, and a normal urine flow rate does not accelerate the healing process in the acute renal failure syndrome. Nonetheless, experience shows that the management of patients with acute renal failure is simplified and the survival rate may be improved by converting oliguria to nonoliguria with diuretics and fluid administration. A trial of furosemide (2 to 10 mg per kilogram intravenous) is warranted. If urine output exceeding 40 ml per hour is achieved, additional doses of diuretic may be given periodically.

General Support

Conservative management without dialysis may be adequate in many cases. Indwelling urinary catheters should be avoided in uncomplicated cases. Intermittent catheterization using careful sterile technique is usually sufficient in oliguric obtunded patients. In all patients careful attention to fluid status is crucial to successful management. Daily weight measured by a competent assistant or physician is essential in the evaluation of changes in fluid balance. Catabolic patients may be expected to lose about 0.5 kg per day. As a rule of thumb, patients can be allowed to drink a volume of fluid (water, tea, coffee) equal to 500 ml plus the amount of the preceding 24-hour urine output. In febrile patients this fluid limit can be increased. In anorectic patients the fluids are given intravenously.

Sodium, potassium, and chloride are not given to patients in the maintenance phase of acute renal failure, except inadvertently in the food they eat. This may amount to about 1 mEq per kilogram of Na, K, and Cl daily. Protein intake is restricted to 0.7 to 1 gram per kilogram of body weight per day and is principally composed of foods high in essential amino acid content. Carbohydrates and fats are given to insure an adequate caloric intake. In patients who cannot eat, intravenous infusion of essential amino acids and glucose may be necessary, but this regimen contributes a considerable fluid load.

In addition to measurements of daily weight, fluid intake and fluid output, serial determinations of blood pressure (supine and upright), serum electrolytes, creatinine, urea nitrogen, and blood hematocrit are essential for patient management. Hyperkalemia exceeding 6 mEq per liter is a potentially serious complication that can be handled temporarily by ingestion of polystyrene sulfonate exchange resin (25 to 50 grams) in a solution containing sorbitol. Electrocardiographic changes showing widened QRS complexes or AV dissociation demand immediate treatment with intravenous sodium bicarbonate (88 mmol), glucose and insulin (25 units regular insulin per liter of 10 per cent glucose), and calcium gluconate (10 per cent solution, 10 to 30 ml). These measures will generally control the serum potassium level until dialysis can be initiated. (See Ch. 77 for a discussion of hyperkalemia.)

Dialysis may be necessary in certain patients in the maintenance phase of acute renal failure. The indications for dialysis include severe hyperkalemia (serum $K^+ > 6.5$ mEq per liter after treatment), severe metabolic acidosis (serum bicarbonate < 10 mEq per liter after bicarbonate therapy), pulmonary edema due to fluid overload, progressive azotemia (urea nitrogen > 100, creatinine > 10 mg per deciliter), encephalopathy, seizures, bleeding diathesis, pericarditis, and uremic enteropathy.

In uncomplicated cases, peritoneal dialysis may be the most suitable method of treatment. This procedure avoids the wide shifts in blood volume and blood solute composition encountered in hemodialysis, and anticoagulants are not used. Peritoneal dialysis can be used for prolonged treatment if recovery of renal function is slow.

In many cases, one must remove solutes and water from the blood faster than can be achieved by peritoneal dialysis. Also, patients with acute renal failure frequently have pre-existing abdominal injuries. In such cases hemodialysis is the preferred dialytic method. One has rapid access to the circulation by percutaneous catheterization of femoral or subclavian veins. Alternatively, external plastic shunts can be placed in adjacent arteries and veins in the lower or upper extremities. In hemorrhagic states, systemic heparinization is not feasible, and regional anticoagulation with citrate or prostacyclin may be necessary.

PROGNOSIS

The prognosis for patient recovery must be viewed from at least two perspectives: (1) patient survival, and (2) recovery of renal function.

Patient Survival

With the advent of modern dialysis techniques few if any patients with the acute renal failure syndrome die of uremia. Death is usually a consequence of the underlying disease that caused the acute renal failure or secondary to trauma and/or sepsis. The mortality rate in traumatized septic patients with acute renal failure is disturbingly high (40 to 80 per cent).

Recovery of Renal Function

The prognosis for recovery of renal function depends on the nature of the underlying disorder that initiated the renal dysfunction. All acute renal failure due to prerenal causes is potentially reversible. In postrenal failure, renal function may be expected to stabilize or improve significantly if the obstruction is relieved.

Acute renal failure due to intrarenal causes has a variable outcome. Glomerulonephritis and vasculitis may respond to immunosuppressive therapy, with complete recovery of renal function. Acute renal failure due to renal tubular injury is usually reversible provided that the cause of ischemia is removed or nephrotoxins are avoided. Recovery of renal function to near normal levels is more likely in nonoliguric than in oliguric patients, and in subjects who have strong images by the ^{131}I-hippurate renal scan. The duration of the period of poor renal function is highly variable. Recovery of renal function takes longer in elderly patients than in young persons. Recovery is also prolonged in patients who develop acute renal failure in addition to a chronic renal disorder that compromises baseline function.

The major improvements in renal function usually appear in the first and second weeks after the beginning of the recovery phase. Some mild defects in renal function may persist for months or years after a bout of acute tubular injury.

PREVENTION

The opportunity for major prevention of acute renal failure is in the hands of physicians and surgeons. As noted, hospital-acquired acute renal failure was seen in nearly 5 per cent of all patients admitted to one general hospital; nearly one half of these cases were iatrogenic.

A few simple measures will diminish the incidence of acute renal failure acquired in the hospital: (1) Patients should be adequately hydrated before receiving iodinated radiocontrast material. (2) Adequate hydration is necessary before certain surgical procedures, specifically repair of abdominal aortic aneurysm and renal transplantation. (3) Adequate hydration is essential before and during chemotherapy using cisplatin and streptozotocin. (4) Pretreatment with allopurinol before chemotherapy of massive tumors will diminish uric acid excretion. (5) Nonsteroidal anti-inflammatory drugs should be avoided in patients with renal diseases. (6) Nephrotoxic antibiotics should be avoided or carefully monitored. (7) Antibiotic combinations that synergistically potentiate acute tubular injury should be avoided (gentamicin and cephalothin, for example).

Bennett WM, Muther RS, Parker RA, et al.: Drug therapy in renal failure: Dosing guidelines for adults. Ann Intern Med 93:62, 286, 1980. *A handy, well-referenced guide to drug dosages in acute renal failure.*

Brezis M, Rosen S, Epstein FH: Acute renal failure. In Brenner BM, Rector FC Jr (eds.): The Kidney. 3rd ed. Philadelphia, W. B. Saunders Company, 1986, pp 735–799. *This is an exhaustive up-to-date compendium with 1003 references.*

Harwood TH, Hiesterman DR, Robinson RG, et al.: Prognosis for recovery of function in acute renal failure. Arch Intern Med 136:916, 1976. *A simple noninvasive radioisotope test (^{131}I-hippurate) is shown to be useful in judging the prognosis for recovery of renal function.*

Hou SH, Bushinsky DA, Wish JB, et al.: Hospital-acquired renal insufficiency: A prospective study. Am J Med 74:243, 1983. *A disturbing study that establishes in one hospital the risk for developing acute renal failure.*

Myers BD, Morna SM: Hemodynamically mediated acute renal failure. N Engl J Med 314:97, 1986. *The clinical patterns of acute renal failure are examined systematically in this excellent paper.*

Porter GA: Nephrotoxic Mechanisms of Drugs and Environmental Toxins. New York, Plenum Press, 1982. *A comprehensive collection of essays by an excellent group of authorities who deal with topics of increasing clinical interest.*

79 CHRONIC RENAL FAILURE

Juha Kokko

INTRODUCTION

Chronic renal failure (CRF) is a functional diagnosis characterized by a progressive and generally irreversible decline in glomerular filtration rate (GFR). It is caused by a large number of diseases. Figure 79–1 summarizes the causes of chronic renal failure in North American patients on chronic maintenance dialysis according to 1978 figures from the National Dialysis Registry. In some geographic locations diabetes and hypertension are more common disease processes leading to dialysis than the National Dialysis Registry indicates for the entire country. In this classification "glomerulonephritis" is not a specific disease but reflects a heterogeneous group of glomerular disorders in which the common expression is renal failure. This chapter considers the pathophysiology and clinical manifestations of CRF, an approach to the patient with CRF, and principles of management.

PATHOPHYSIOLOGY AND CLINICAL MANIFESTATIONS

The clinical constellation of signs and symptoms of end-stage renal failure is known as the "uremic syndrome" (Table 79–1). In the initial phases of advancing renal failure most organ functions remain normal so that the patient often seeks medical attention only when his or her disease has progressed to the uremic stage. Normally, the adult patient is unaware of advancing renal failure until the GFR has decreased to 20 ml per minute. At this phase adherence to strict therapeutic principles is of utmost importance to prevent the complications of CRF. When conservative medical management is no longer adequate, alternative approaches such as dialysis or transplantation (see Ch. 80) must be considered.

The uremic syndrome results from derangements of function of many systems of the body, although the prominence of specific symptoms may vary from patient to patient (Table 79–1). No organ system is spared. The pathophysiology and clinical manifestations of uremia will be discussed by com-

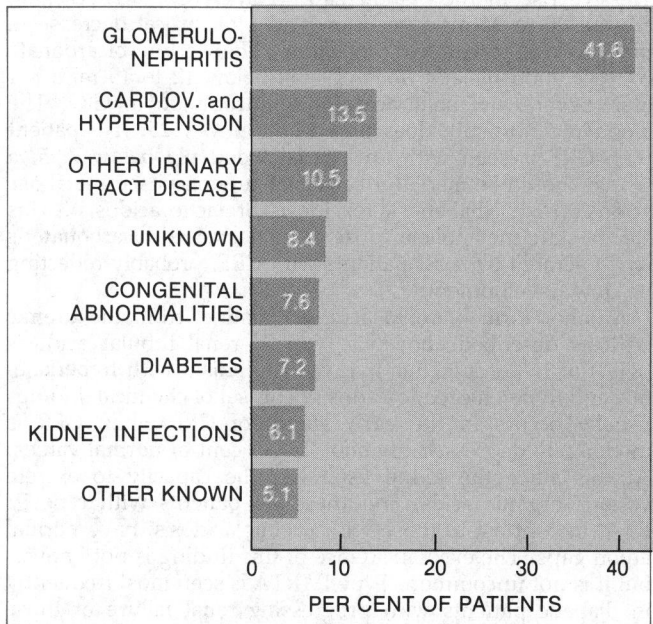

FIGURE 79–1. Histogram of primary renal diseases leading to dialysis. (Data based on National Registry data as represented by Wernman in Dialysis Transplantation 7:1034, 1978.)

TABLE 79–1. THE UREMIC SYNDROME OF CHRONIC RENAL FAILURE*

1. Electrolyte disorders
   a. Potassium: hyperkalemia, total body depletion
   b. Sodium: salt-losing nephropathy, sodium retention
   c. Acidosis: metabolic acidosis with high "anion gap," type IV renal tubular acidosis (hyporeninemic hypoaldosteronism)
   d. Calcium (see Table 249–1): tendency toward hypocalcemia—complicated mix of phosphate retention, second-degree hyperparathyroidism, calcitriol ↓
   e. Magnesium: mild hypermagnesemia
   f. Phosphate: hyperphosphatemia contributes to acidosis and to disorders of calcium metabolism

2. Cardiovascular abnormalities
   a. Accelerated atherosclerosis
   b. Hypertension
   c. Pericarditis

3. Hematologic abnormalities
   a. Anemia: erythropoietin ↓, Fe deficiency
   b. Leukocyte dysfunction
   c. Hemorrhagic diathesis: defective platelet function

4. Increased susceptibility for infections
   a. Impaired cellular immunity
   b. Leukocyte dysfunction

5. Gastrointestinal disorders
   a. Anorexia, nausea, vomiting
   b. GI bleeding

6. Renal osteodystrophy (see Table 249–1)
   a. Osteomalacia
   b. Osteitis fibrosa (secondary hyperparathyroidism)
   c. Osteosclerosis
   d. Osteoporosis

7. Neurologic abnormalities
   a. Central nervous system: insomnia, fatigue, psychologic symptoms
   b. Peripheral neuropathy

8. Myopathy: especially of proximal muscles

9. Impaired carbohydrate tolerance: peripheral resistance to insulin

10. Hyperuricemia: clinical gout is rare

11. Pruritus

*These manifestations occur to differing degrees in individual patients, depending on the severity and duration of renal failure, its cause, and unknown variables in the host.

ponents even though this is arbitrary and not all of them may be present in the same patient. This clinical description will be followed by a short summary of the retained "toxins" that have been considered of importance in the development of the uremic syndrome.

Components of the Uremic Syndrome

WATER, ELECTROLYTE, AND ACID-BASE METABOLISM IN UREMIA. Renal and extrarenal compensatory mechanisms maintain electrolyte and water metabolism near normal until the late stages of renal failure. However, characteristic changes can occur at that time.

Potassium. The normal human dietary intake of potassium is 1 to 1.5 mEq per kilogram of body weight per day, more than 90 per cent of which is excreted by the kidneys. Essentially all the filtered potassium is normally reabsorbed so that only a small fraction is delivered to the early distal nephron. The potassium excreted in the urine has been largely secreted by nephron segments beyond the macula densa, chiefly by passive diffusion down an electrochemical gradient, and to a lesser extent by active transport processes. In each case intracellular concentration of potassium is important in net potassium secretion. The accumulation of potassium in the distal tubular cells is related to the activity of Na-K-ATPase in the basolateral region of the cell. The greater the activity of this pump, the higher the rise in intracellular potassium and the greater the secretory rate of potassium. The activity of Na-K-ATPase is controlled by diet and mineralocorticoid status (both high-potassium diet and mineralocorticoids lead to high renal Na-K-ATPase). Both normal and uremic subjects adapt to high-potassium diets by increasing potassium excretion per nephron. In addition, the gut increases its ability to secrete potassium in response to a rise in intracellular potassium concentration.

In spite of these adaptive processes, potassium homeostasis in CRF patients is not normal. In advanced CRF the serum potassium concentration tends to be higher than normal even though body stores of potassium are often reduced. Hyperkalemia can be accentuated by trauma, surgery, anesthesia, blood transfusion, increased acidosis, or sudden changes of dietary intake. It can produce the usual spectrum of cardiac abnormalities, but many patients are asymptomatic until cardiac arrest occurs. Occasional patients complain of muscle weakness or paresthesias. The major warning signs are those detected by electrocardiography.

Total body potassium content may be low in CRF: (1) Many patients with CRF have anorexia and reduced dietary intake of potassium. (2) There is greater than normal loss of intracellular potassium to extracellular compartments with subsequent loss from the body. Of special importance is the low intracellular content of potassium in muscle. The low intracellular potassium concentration may reflect a decrease in Na-K-ATPase activity, as well as displacement of intracellular potassium by hydrogen ion. Patients with chronic renal failure tolerate acute increases in serum potassium concentration with less cardiotoxicity than do patients without kidney disease. Vigorous dialysis can restore the intracellular concentration of potassium to normal, suggesting the removal of circulating inhibitor of potassium transport.

Sodium. The kidney has a remarkable capacity to maintain total body sodium content within normal limits until the very end stages of functional deterioration. To accomplish this the remaining nephrons of the CRF patient must excrete a proportionately greater quantity of dietary sodium to maintain total body sodium balance within normal limits. This observation has led to a search for a humoral factor(s) that might be responsible for the increased natriuresis per nephron of the failing kidney.

Sodium excretion can be varied only over a restricted range in renal failure, and this narrows as GFR declines. Nevertheless, most patients remain in sodium balance until their GFR is below 5 ml per minute. Rarely, patients exhibit inappropriate natriuresis; more commonly patients have a tendency toward sodium retention and volume expansion because their dietary intake exceeds the blunted ability of the diseased kidney to excrete the usual sodium load.

SODIUM WASTING. Those patients who have CRF and *salt-losing nephropathy* may lose sodium to the point of extracellular volume contraction and hypotension. These patients will require sufficient dietary salt to prevent their hypotensive symptoms. A wide variety of renal diseases may be associated with salt wasting, but the most common are pyelonephritis, medullary cystic disease, hydronephrosis, interstitial nephritis secondary to analgesic abuse, and milk-alkali syndrome. Presumably in these conditions the collecting ducts are incapable of reabsorbing sufficient quantities of delivered sodium.

SODIUM RETENTION. Some patients are unable to increase sodium excretion to appropriate levels with increases in sodium intake. Most of these patients come to a new steady state with total body weight a few pounds higher than their euvolemic weight. When these patients then receive an extra sodium load they usually excrete it promptly, thus maintaining their new state of volume expansion. They behave as if they have reset their feedback control system for sodium reabsorption. This situation is more common in patients with glomerular than with tubulointerstitial disease. These patients often have the physical findings of expanded extracellular fluid volume: hypertension, peripheral edema, pulmonary congestive state, enlarged heart, and functional flow murmur.

The clinical picture is often interpreted as heart failure, and valvular heart disease is suspected erroneously. A small percentage of patients with normal cardiac output become relentless sodium retainers and require hemodialysis for volume control. These patients tend to be diabetic. Surreptitious intake of salt may play a role, but other unknown factors may also be of etiologic significance.

Acid-Base Balance. The kidney normally regulates blood pH within narrow limits by reabsorption (proximal tubule) and regeneration (distal tubule) of bicarbonate or by secretion of hydrogen (distal convoluted tubule and collecting duct segments). When diets high in alkali content are ingested, the kidney excretes less acid; whereas with acid ash diets and endogenous acid production, the kidney reabsorbs and regenerates bicarbonate and secretes hydrogen ion in amounts sufficient to maintain normal pH. A maximally acid urine in the human has a pH of 4.5 to 5.0. However, the total quantity of acid that can be excreted is a function of the amount of buffer that can be excreted. The excreted buffers may be filtered or generated. Quantitatively the most important filtered buffer is phosphate; the most important newly generated buffer is ammonium.

In chronic renal disease with progressively fewer functioning nephrons there is progressively less ammonia produced for the titration of secreted acid. Thus in CRF the urine pH may be maximally acid, but the total amount of hydrogen ion is low. In disease processes that disproportionately affect the medulla, the ability to form maximally acid urine is lost early. Metabolic acidosis, which may be partially compensated by respiratory mechanisms, develops when exogenous intake and endogenous production of acid exceed renal excretory capacity. In metabolic acidosis there is recruitment of extrarenal buffering mechanisms. Either the excess hydrogen ions are buffered by bone salts and other extracellular mechanisms or they enter the cells to be buffered by intracellular mechanisms. These buffering mechanisms allow for maintenance of relatively stable, albeit lower than normal, blood bicarbonate concentrations when the urinary excretion rate cannot keep up with endogenous production of acid. Tissue stores of buffer are partly consumed over long periods of time. Loss of bone salts contributes to the development of osteomalacia and renal osteodystrophy (Ch. 249). With recruitment of the various buffer mechanisms and with a decreased ability of the kidney to excrete various organic acids, there is a progressive rise in the "anion gap" [$Na - (Cl + HCO_3)$], to around 20 to 24 mEq per liter, and a reciprocal decrease in plasma bicarbonate concentration. The serum bicarbonate concentration usually does not fall below 12 to 15 mEq per liter. Severe metabolic acidosis is uncommon in CRF. The blood pH normally does not drop below 7.25. If a patient with CRF is seen with an arterial blood pH below 7.25, a search should be made for causes of superimposed metabolic acidosis (e.g., diabetic ketoacidosis or lactic acidosis). This steady-state metabolic acidosis with decreased bicarbonate is well tolerated by most patients with CRF, probably reflecting its slow development.

Another form of renal acidosis, distinct from the uremic acidosis described above, is type IV renal tubular acidosis (RTA) or hyporeninemic hypoaldosteronism with hyperkalemia and hyperchloremic acidosis. This set of chemical findings usually occurs in the early stages of CRF when GFR is moderately depressed to about 25 per cent of normal values. At this stage the kidney still has the capacity to excrete various organic acids, and therefore patients with type IV RTA, in contrast to those with uremic acidosis, have normal anion gaps. The exact incidence of this finding is not known, but it is not uncommon. Type IV RTA is seen most frequently in diabetic patients with progressing renal failure or those with predominantly tubulointerstitial disease. It is described further and compared with other types of RTA in Ch. 84.

Chloride. Patients with CRF are unable to regulate chloride excretion. For example, CRF patients excrete greater amounts of sodium when they are given an excess of sodium bicarbonate than following administration of an equivalent amount of sodium chloride. With increased intake of NaCl there is retention of salt and fluid and weight gain. Many CRF patients are in a stable volume-expanded state. The preferential retention of chloride in CRF patients does not usually lead to a reciprocal decrease in bicarbonate concentration, and thus CRF patients tend to be proportionately hyperchloremic with respect to sodium concentration.

Calcium. The total serum calcium concentration in CRF patients is significantly lower than normal, although usually above 7.5 mg per deciliter. Great variability exists, and occasionally the calcium level is very low. CRF patients tolerate the hypocalcemia quite well, and rarely is a patient symptomatic from the decreased calcium concentration. Tetany is surprisingly uncommon. It is occasionally precipitated by the infusion of sodium bicarbonate, but the usual muscle twitching and cramping of CRF are unrelated to hypocalcemia.

CRF patients have decreased intestinal absorption of calcium, and in consequence fecal calcium loss exceeds that of normal subjects. Jejunal and ileal malabsorption of calcium in CRF can be corrected by oral administration of active vitamin D analogues with increases in serum calcium concentrations.

In addition, patients with either acute or chronic renal failure are resistant to the normal calcemic action of parathyroid hormone (PTH). The mechanism of resistance may be secondary to a decreased permissive effect of $1,25(OH)_2D_3$ on bone action of PTH. Renal osteodystrophy is discussed in Ch. 249.

A subgroup of CRF patients develops hypercalcemia after some months on hemodialysis. Most often the hypercalcemia is due to persistent secretion of PTH from glands that have previously undergone hyperplasia. Occasionally these patients become symptomatic with bone pain or exhibit signs of metastatic calcification. Parathyroidectomy may be indicated if other causes of hypercalcemia can be ruled out.

Magnesium. Patients with CRF tend to have modest elevations in serum magnesium concentration when GFR has fallen below 20 per cent of normal. Urinary excretion of magnesium is diminished, but often intestinal magnesium absorption continues normally. Most CRF patients with hypermagnesemia have no associated symptoms or findings. Nevertheless, it is prudent to discontinue magnesium-containing antacids and cathartics in patients with GFR below 20 ml per minute.

Phosphate. The most important determinant of serum phosphate level is the relationship between net reabsorption of phosphate from the gut and excretion of phosphate by the kidney. The serum phosphate concentration is significantly higher than normal in patients with GFR below 20 ml per minute.

The major reason for hyperphosphatemia is decreased excretion of phosphate with advancing renal disease. The retained phosphate is of major pathogenetic importance in the development of the secondary hyperparathyroidism of CRF. It is postulated that in the evolution of CRF there are periodic decreases in phosphate excretion as nephrons progressively drop out. The resultant increases in plasma phosphate concentration lead to reciprocal decreases in serum calcium concentration, increased secretion of PTH, and increased tubular rejection of phosphate. This adaptive mechanism will maintain a normal serum phosphate concentration until GFR has fallen to approximately 20 per cent of normal. However, if usual dietary phosphorus intake continues in patients with far advanced renal disease, these adaptive mechanisms cannot compensate fully and hyperphosphatemia ensues. If dietary phosphorus is decreased in proportion to the decrease in GFR, hyperphosphatemia can be prevented and the expected rise in serum parathyroid hormone blunted. In addition, intestinal absorption of phosphate can be reduced by use of compounds that bind phosphate in the gut in nonabsorbable form.

CARDIOVASCULAR ABNORMALITIES. Cardiovascular complications are common in patients with CRF and can be classified into three main categories: atherosclerosis and hyperlipidemia, hypertension, and pericarditis.

Atherosclerosis. Accelerated atherosclerosis is one of the major factors limiting the longevity of patients with chronic renal failure. Although the plasma lipid pattern may be normal in CRF, the most characteristic abnormality is elevated triglyceride concentrations with normal or slightly elevated plasma cholesterol levels (type IV). A smaller percentage of patients has type IIa or IIb hyperlipoproteinemia. The incidence of elevated triglyceride concentrations is increased in patients maintained on chronic hemodialysis as compared with nondialyzed patients. Cardiovascular death is particularly common after the fifth year of dialysis. There appears to be a positive relationship between the elevation of plasma triglycerides and the increased incidence of occlusive coronary disease. The cause of hypertriglyceridemia in CRF is unknown, but current evidence favors a defect in triglyceride removal rather than an increase in triglyceride production. The most probable cause of the decreased removal rate of very low density lipoproteins is a defect in hepatic lipoprotein lipase activity.

Hypertension. Hypertension is common in chronic renal disease, being present in the majority of patients at the onset of maintenance dialysis. At least two factors contribute to its high incidence in CRF: (1) The tendency toward sodium retention and volume expansion is perhaps the most important. Expansion of the extracellular volume is accompanied by an initial rise of cardiac output, which may persist, followed by a rise in peripheral resistance. Patients with volume-sensitive hypertension may have increasing problems with blood pressure control as they progress into renal failure. (2) Alterations of the renin-angiotensin axis are also important contributors to the pathogenesis of hypertension. Although the absolute plasma values for renin and angiotensin are variable in CRF, plasma renin activity is inappropriately high for the degree of sodium retention in most patients. This view is supported by the efficiency of angiotensin-converting enzyme inhibitors in controlling hypertension and by those few patients whose hypertension can be controlled only by bilateral nephrectomy.

Pericarditis. "Uremic pericarditis" is a term that refers to pericarditis of unknown etiology occurring in association with uremia. Conventionally, pericarditis is not classified as "uremic" if an infectious etiology can be documented. Some authorities have attempted to divide pericarditis in renal failure into two subsets: "uremic" and "dialysis-associated." The former is said to occur in a uremic patient prior to initiation of dialysis, whereas the latter occurs in a uremic patient who is undergoing chronic hemodialysis. However, since the pathologic pericardial characteristics are similar in these two clinical settings and since the etiology has not been identified, the division of pericarditis in renal failure into two distinct subtypes appears arbitrary, and therefore the continued use of the term "uremic pericarditis" seems justified. In the older literature, uremic pericarditis was more commonly seen in nondialyzed patients, whereas currently it is most common in patients who are not dialyzed adequately. It is most likely caused by some unknown biochemical substance. Characteristically, the pericardial fluid is hemorrhagic. The onset of pericarditis is usually signaled by pain, often on the left side of the chest with respiratory accentuation. Pain is often severe and frequently associated with a friction rub. The friction rub can be loud, generalized, and even palpable. Tamponade can occur with signs of falling blood and pulse pressures, raised jugular venous pressure, and poorly perfused extremities. The hemorrhage is thought to originate from sheared pericardial capillaries that have developed in response to uremic inflammation of the pericardium. It is recognized that in previously nondialyzed patients, uremic pericarditis responds to dialysis more rapidly than in patients who develop pericarditis during dialysis. However, the pericarditis in this latter group usually responds to intensification of hemodialysis.

HEMATOLOGIC ABNORMALITIES. Hematologic abnormalities are among the most consistent manifestations of uremia. These abnormalities include anemia, bleeding, and granulocyte and platelet dysfunction.

Anemia. Many patients with CRF have severely reduced hematocrits. Hematocrits in the 20 to 25 per cent range are not uncommon. The manifestations of anemia include pallor, tachycardia, a wide pulse pressure with accentuation by exercise, a systolic ejection murmur best heard over the pulmonary area, and the precipitation of angina pectoris in patients with underlying coronary artery disease.

The primary cause of anemia in CRF is a deficiency of erythropoietin, which is a glycoprotein normally produced in the kidney in response to anoxia. It is responsible for normal red blood cell differentiation from stem cells. The decreased erythropoietin may be the result of destruction of renal parenchyma, the presence of circulating inhibitors, or protein deprivation that in turn decreases erythropoietin production. The result is normochromic, normocytic anemia.

Other factors may contribute to anemia. Many patients on maintenance hemodialysis programs are iron deficient. Iron absorption from the gut may be decreased in CRF patients and restored to normal following hemodialysis. Furthermore, iron deficiency may develop in dialyzed patients because of frequent blood sampling, loss of blood in hemodialysis tubing and coils, and periodic accidental losses from hemodialysis access sites. Red blood cell survival is shortened in uremia, probably due to some extrinsic factor: (1) Red blood cells isolated from uremic patients and infused into nonuremic individuals have a normal life span. (2) Aggressive hemodialysis increases the red blood cell survival to or toward normal. In addition, many patients with CRF have added intrinsic erythrocytic factors contributing to anemia, which include decreased Na-K-ATPase activity, pentose phosphate dysfunction, microangiopathic hemolytic component as a result of hypersplenism, and folate deficiency due to its dialyzability in chronic hemodialysis patients.

Leukocyte Dysfunction. In addition to anemia, there are other hematologic abnormalities in CRF. Although the granulocyte count is usually normal, some patients have a tendency toward granulocytopenia. Moreover, the chemotactic response of granulocytes is subnormal.

Hemorrhagic Diathesis. A hemorrhagic tendency, manifested by epistaxis, menorrhagia, or excessive bleeding or bruising after trauma, is common in late renal failure but seldom life threatening. Whole blood clotting time and prothrombin time are usually normal. Bleeding time may be prolonged, perhaps related to the associated abnormalities of platelet function. Platelets are often decreased in number owing to increased peripheral destruction. In addition, there are functional defects such as decreased adhesiveness and aggregation. These abnormalities are often corrected by hemodialysis and may be secondary to a dialyzable uremic toxin. The hemorrhagic diathesis of uremia is discussed further in Ch. 166 and 167.

INFECTIONS. Most patients with CRF develop serious infections during the course of their disease. Theoretically, this assumed susceptibility to infection could be due to deranged or deficient humoral or cellular immunity, impaired inflammatory reaction, or increased exposure to pathogenic bacteria and viruses. Humoral immunity is, in general, intact. Although exceptions exist, most patients have a normal humoral response to vaccines. Cellular defense mechanisms are often deficient. Skin tests may show impairment of delayed hypersensitivity. Patients with CRF may have low lymphocyte counts, and their lymphocytes do not respond normally to mitogenic stimulation. Abnormal lymphocyte function may be due to some dialyzable factor, since it is nearly normal after vigorous dialysis or after suspension of lymphocytes harvested from uremic patients in nonuremic sera. The neutrophil count is usually normal in chronic renal failure, and it rises appropriately in response to infection. However, a transient decrease may occur following hemodialysis owing to sequestration of leukocytes in pulmonary capillaries. In addition, leukocytes of uremic subjects have a decreased ability to phagocytize bacteria. The chemotactic response of polymorphonuclear leukocytes is also depressed; this function improves with hemodialysis. Additionally, patients on hemodialysis are frequently exposed to bacterial and viral infections. Staphylococcal sepsis is not uncommon. The presumed portal of entry is cutaneous contamination through the arteriovenous hemodialysis access. Gram-negative sepsis also occurs with increased frequency. Often an infected urinary tract can be implicated as the cause. Superinfection with *Candida albicans* is very common, mainly affecting the buccal mucosa. There is a significant increase in frequency of hepatitis in dialysis patients owing to multiple transfusions and increased exposure, secondary to either hepatitis B virus or non-A non-B viruses. The disease is usually asymptomatic, but it can be severe. A significant fraction of CRF patients who contract hepatitis become chronic carriers.

GASTROINTESTINAL DISORDERS. Gastrointestinal symptoms are common in patients with uremia. Their symptoms have varying presentations and may be quite distressing. The most common early symptom is loss of appetite. Many uremic patients then progress to develop nausea and vomiting, sometimes severe enough to cause loss of salt and water leading to volume depletion and negative caloric balance causing weight loss. The specific cause of these symptoms has not been identified.

Gastrointestinal bleeding is also common in uremic patients. Often it is of minor magnitude detected by positive stool guaiacs, but it also can be severe. The gastrointestinal bleeding may be the result of scattered petechiae, ulceration, or other specific lesions. Undoubtedly the platelet defects contribute to the increased frequency of gastrointestinal bleeding characteristic of uremic patients.

OSTEODYSTROPHY. The term "renal osteodystrophy" is an all-inclusive term for the skeletal changes in uremia, which include, in decreasing order of frequency, osteitis fibrosa, osteomalacia, osteoporosis, and osteosclerosis. Osteitis fibrosa is almost universal in terminal renal failure; it may be found in as many as 90 per cent of patients starting regular dialysis, the exceptions being those with rapidly progressive disease and a short experience of uremia. A substantial minority will exhibit abnormal radiographs, but very few will complain of bone tenderness or muscle weakness. Few patients survive more than a year or two on dialysis without evidence of bone disease. The pathogenesis and clinical features of renal osteodystrophy are discussed in greater detail in Ch. 249.

NEUROPATHY. Many patients with CRF have abnormalities in central and peripheral nervous system function. Tiredness, insomnia, and psychologic symptoms, including agitation, irritability, depression, regression, and rebellion, are common. Patients tend to have fewer such symptoms if they are eating a nutritious diet and are well dialyzed. Patients with secondary hyperparathyroidism caused by uremia have abnormal electroencephalograms (EEG) characterized by increased frequency of slow wave activity. Patients with secondary hyperparathyroidism caused by CRF may show improvement in their EEG and psychologic symptoms after parathyroidectomy. The mechanism by which PTH exerts these effects is not known, but in the uremic dog PTH increases brain calcium content and abnormal EEG changes of uremia require elevated levels of PTH. Brain calcium content is higher in patients with CRF than in patients who die without renal failure.

Peripheral neuropathy is also common in CRF. Clinical manifestations include painful paresthesias of extremities, twitchings, "restless leg syndrome," loss of deep tendon reflexes, muscular weakness, and occasional sensory deficits. Lower extremities are involved much more frequently than upper extremities. Diminished deep tendon reflexes and vibratory sense may be found, but the most reliable objective measurement of peripheral neuropathy in CRF is slowing of nerve conduction velocities. Peripheral neuropathy can be drug induced, but its pathophysiology in most patients is unknown. However, symptoms of neuropathy can be improved by prolonging the period of dialysis and by use of membrane dialyzers with larger membrane surface areas. Also, patients on chronic peritoneal dialysis have been said to have fewer symptoms than patients on extracorporeal hemodialysis. These findings suggest that the development of peripheral neuropathy is related to dialyzable uremic toxins of the "middle molecule" range.

MYOPATHY. Muscular weakness develops slowly, but it is common in patients with end-stage renal failure. Proximal muscles are affected more than distal muscles. It is not uncommon to see some wasting of the limb and cervical muscles. There are no distinct histologic features of uremic myopathy. The resting transmembrane potential difference of skeletal muscle cells is abnormally low, and the average mean duration of the action potential is significantly shortened in uremic individuals. In inadequately dialyzed uremic patients intracellular sodium and chloride contents are elevated, whereas potassium content is reduced. These findings are consistent with either increased permeability of the muscle membrane to these ions or a decrease in active efflux of sodium. However, it is doubtful that these are primary muscle membrane abnormalities, since all the abnormalities can be corrected by dialysis. Indeed, resting skeletal muscle membrane responses have been used as an index of adequacy of hemodialysis. Although a number of hormones and factors have been proposed as causal of uremic myopathy, the identity of such a factor(s) remains conjectural.

CARBOHYDRATE METABOLISM. Carbohydrate metabolism is often abnormal in patients with chronic renal failure. Glucose tolerance is reduced as shown by a rapid rise and delayed return to normal of the blood glucose concentration after an oral or intravenous glucose load. Fasting blood glucose values are normal or slightly elevated. This state of impaired glucose tolerance is often termed *uremic pseudodiabetes mellitus*. Severe hyperglycemia does not occur unless the patient receives a large load of glucose, e.g., during peritoneal dialysis with hypertonic glucose solutions. Nevertheless, the requirement for exogenous insulin decreases in insulin-dependent diabetics as renal failure progresses. At least two different mechanisms are responsible for the simultaneous coexistence of abnormal glucose tolerance and a decreased requirement for exogenous insulin: (1) enhanced peripheral resistance to insulin, and (2) a decreased renal clearance of insulin.

Increased peripheral resistance to insulin in uremia is manifested by a diminished forearm uptake of glucose in response to insulin and by elevated concentrations of circulating insulin as compared with normal subjects. A number of possibilities exist to explain the insulin resistance. First, some uremic substances may interfere with the action of insulin, since aggressive hemodialysis decreases exogenous requirements for insulin. Second, potassium deficiency may alter the nature of insulin released from the pancreas. Indeed, proinsulin to insulin ratios rise in nonuremic patients who are potassium deficient. Third, there is decreased binding of insulin to

peripheral receptors in CRF. Whatever the reason(s), patients with CRF clearly have some degree of peripheral resistance to insulin.

Insulin is filtered and metabolized by the kidney. With progressing CRF the urinary clearance of insulin approaches GFR, presumably reflecting a decreased uptake of filtered insulin by the proximal convoluted tubule. Nevertheless, blood insulin concentrations rise owing to decreased extraction of insulin by renal tubular epithelial cells. These observations explain the decrease in insulin requirements of diabetics with progressing CRF, but it is also necessary to postulate a degree of peripheral resistance to insulin to explain the carbohydrate intolerance ("uremic pseudodiabetes") of nondiabetic subjects with CRF.

URIC ACID. Approximately two thirds of the total uric acid excretory load is normally removed each day by the kidney. With progression of CRF hyperuricemia is a consistent finding once GFR has decreased to 20 per cent of normal. However, the correlation between the rise of serum uric acid and the severity of chronic renal failure is poor. Only rarely does the serum uric acid concentration rise above 10 mg per deciliter unless dehydration is superimposed. Whether or not the elevated serum uric acid levels hasten the development of end-stage renal disease is not known.

PRURITUS. Generalized pruritus is a frequent symptom of CRF and is occasionally severe and intractable. Usually there are no dermatologic findings. To date no single causative factor has been identified. Implicated factors include some dialyzable product of uremia, high calcium-phosphorus product in extracellular fluid with deposition of calcium salts in the dermal structures, and abnormalities in nerve end-plates. Symptomatic relief has been reported with more frequent dialysis, parathyroidectomy, dietary protein restriction, and exposure to sunburn spectrum of ultraviolet light.

Role of Retained Toxins

The kidney has a remarkable capacity to regulate the excretion of a variety of substances to maintain their blood concentrations at optimal levels. During the evolution of renal insufficiency until GFR is severely compromised this capacity is maintained by adaptive mechanisms whereby the remaining nephrons either metabolize or excrete greater than normal quantities of the substance in question. Adaptive mechanisms do not exist for substances that are freely filtered and neither reabsorbed nor secreted. Urea and creatinine are the classic examples of this group of compounds. Their clearance rates are close approximations of the glomerular filtration rate. However, most substances are not only filtered but also reabsorbed, secreted, or metabolized. In general, the blood concentrations of the latter group of substances do not rise until the later stages of renal disease. Many of the putative uremic toxins belong in this latter group.

The symptoms of uremia are, in part, caused by dialyzable substances that accumulate from failure of their renal excretion. Azotemic patients improve symptomatically after initiation of hemodialysis. No single substance has evolved as the cause of uremic symptoms. Multiple compounds no doubt contribute. The list of the suggested "uremic toxins" is long (e.g., guanidines, amines, phenols, indoles) and beyond the scope of this chapter. Urea and "middle molecules" (presumed polypeptides with molecular weights between 1000 and 1500) have received the most attention and will be discussed here.

UREA. Since blood urea nitrogen rises rapidly with decreasing GFR, and since intravenous injections of urea to animals produced neurologic symptoms, it was only natural to suspect that high urea concentrations produced uremic symptoms. However, this view is no longer held. For example, in studies in which patients were dialyzed for prolonged periods of time against a dialysate with a high concentration of urea, only minimal symptoms of headache, lethargy, emesis, or tremor were noted with postdialysis blood urea concentrations as high as 200 mg per deciliter. This is strong presumptive evidence that the clinical manifestations of chronic renal failure are not secondary to urea itself. In addition some patients have uremic symptoms at serum urea concentrations as low as 60 mg per deciliter. Therefore other factors in end-stage renal disease are of importance in producing uremic symptoms.

"MIDDLE MOLECULAR WEIGHT" TOXINS. The origin of the "middle molecular weight" toxin concept came from the clinical observation that patients who were peritoneally dialyzed had fewer uremic symptoms than patients who were hemodialyzed to the same blood urea concentration with small surface area dialyzers. It was argued that the peritoneum was more permeable to substances in the molecular weight range of 500 to 5000 than were the small pore hemodialyzers. Significant effort has been spent to identify specific compounds in this molecular range that might be toxic. Although a great number of compounds have been identified, there have been few correlative studies to establish "cause and effect" relationships. However, toxic effects of "middle molecules" isolated from uremic serum include inhibitions of hemoglobin synthesis, glucose utilization, lymphoblast transformation, leukocyte phagocytic activity, and nerve conductivity. Although the "middle molecular weight" toxin theory has not been established with certainty, clinical observations are consistent with the view that there are compounds in this molecular weight range that may play a role in the pathogenesis of the uremic syndrome.

APPROACH TO THE PATIENT WITH UREMIA

The principles of approach to the uremic patient are the same as those toward any patient who comes to the attention of the physician. A detailed clinical history is imperative, with special emphasis on urinary tract symptoms such as nocturia, hematuria, dysuria, polydipsia, and polyuria. Also of special importance is a complete history of systemic diseases, of exposure to toxins and infections, and of renal diseases in the family. The medical history will often be of diagnostic significance. The physical examination should emphasize the blood pressure, retina, cardiovascular system, renal examination with auscultation for bruits and palpation of size, rectal examination for size of prostate in males, gynecologic examination for pelvic masses in females, extremity examination for edema and nail bed findings, and neuroskeletal examination for evidence of myopathy, neuropathy, and osteodystrophy. Laboratory tests should include a complete blood count and urinalysis.

Additional studies should be designed to elucidate whether a patient has acute reversible renal failure, acute worsening of CRF resulting from aggravating factors, or a chronic progressive disease. Again, the history is important. It is unlikely that a patient with acute renal disease is asymptomatic with elevations of serum creatinine and blood urea nitrogen above 10 and 100 mg per deciliter, respectively. On the other hand, patients, especially if young, with slowly progressing CRF are often asymptomatic with much higher elevations of serum creatinine and blood urea nitrogen. Thus, if in the absence of other diseases, a patient complains of nausea, vomiting, anorexia, and weakness and the creatinine and blood urea nitrogen are below 10 and 100 mg per deciliter, respectively, the chances are that the patient is suffering from an acute process. Unfortunately exceptions to this rule exist. Also, in chronic renal failure the hematocrit tends to be lower, phosphate concentration higher, uric acid concentration lower, and urine sediment more benign. However, none of these tests is specific enough to differentiate with certainty between acute and chronic renal failure.

X-ray determination of the kidney size can be helpful in determining the chronicity of renal disease. The x-rays can be in the form of plain abdominal films, tomograms, or intravenous urograms (if the blood urea nitrogen is less than 100 mg per deciliter). Of these the plain abdominal film is least expensive, free from complications, and often informative. Renal sonograms can be used to estimate renal size and identify hydronephrosis or cystic masses. If the kidneys are significantly reduced in size, this almost always indicates chronicity and irreversibility. Normal kidney size tends to favor an acute process, although exceptions exist. Chronic renal processes in which kidney size may be normal or larger than normal include polycystic renal disease, amyloidosis, scleroderma, and diabetes mellitus. Thus normal renal size does not rule out a chronic process.

It is also important to differentiate between renal versus extrarenal causes of azotemia. Extrarenal causes of progressive uremia may be either pre- or postrenal. Prerenal causes are those disease processes that decrease the blood flow to the kidneys. This may be due to true extracellular fluid (ECF) volume depletion or to effective volume depletion as seen with cardiac and liver failure. This is discussed in more detail in the management section under "Aggravating Factors." Also, it is imperative to rule out postrenal causes of azotemia, namely, lower or upper urinary tract obstruction. Lower urinary tract obstruction may be diagnosed by having the patient void completely and then measuring the residual urine volume in the bladder via catheterization. The presence of residual urine indicates lower urinary tract obstruction. Occasionally sufficient time has elapsed between voluntary voiding and insertion of the catheter so that "new" urine is formed. When the physician is unsure of the significance of 5 to 10 ml of residual urine, he or she may elect to instill 20 to 40 ml of air into the bladder. If this air is passed (which the patient experiences as a "whistling" sound) during the next voiding, then the bladder can empty completely and lower urinary tract obstruction is ruled out. In males by far the most common cause is an enlarged prostate. Any time a uremic patient is seen with anuria, it is imperative that lower urinary tract obstruction be ruled out, especially if accompanied by symptoms such as hesitancy in initiating the urinary stream, slow urinary stream, and incontinence. Upper urinary tract obstruction can be established by ruling out residual urine in the bladder and demonstrating dilated renal calices, pelvis, and ureter(s) above the obstruction. This can be established by intravenous and retrograde pyelography or by renal sonograms. In addition to the dilated urinary tract systems, delayed visualization and delayed clearance of the dye on intravenous urograms characteristically exist. The most common causes of upper urinary tract obstruction include renal stones, congenital obstruction, and bladder cancer.

Once it has been determined that uremia is secondary to renal parenchymal disease and not due to pre- or postrenal causes, the physician must determine if a treatable form of parenchymal disease is present. The most common forms of treatable renal disease are listed in Table 79–2. The following additional tests may be helpful and are often considered: renal arteriography and renal biopsy. In general, although renal arteriography produces excellent visualization of the kidney,

TABLE 79–2. TREATABLE* TYPES OF PARENCHYMAL RENAL DISEASE

Acute hypertensive nephropathy
Analgesic nephropathy
Hemolytic-uremic syndrome
Hypercalcemic nephropathy
Lupus nephritis
Multiple myeloma
Oxalate nephropathy
Pyelonephritis
Renal vein thrombosis
Wegener's granulomatosis

*The mode of therapy and results in these disease processes are variable. All these processes may present with such severe end-stage renal disease that no form of conservative management is effective.

it is of limited diagnostic value in patients with uremia. It may be helpful in patients suspected of having polyarteritis nodosa, tumors (although uremia is an uncommon association), and renal disease secondary to severe hypertension.

Renal biopsy may give a definitive histologic diagnosis provided it is performed before the disease has progressed to such a degree that the only possible morphologic interpretation is "end-stage kidney disease." Renal biopsy can be performed by a percutaneous route with local anesthesia or as an open biopsy under general anesthesia, but it should be carried out only by those who are trained in its use. The associated morbidity and mortality are low, but the possibility of complications nevertheless exists. For these reasons renal biopsy is probably indicated in only a small number of patients with uremia. While a consensus does not exist among nephrologists, biopsy should not be done unless the physician has strong feelings that the information to be gained will influence management. Contraindications to renal biopsy include uncorrectable bleeding tendencies, severe hypertension, bacteriuria, suspicion of perinephric abscess, hydronephrosis, and extreme obesity. Biopsy is often useful in patients with normal sized kidneys and progressive renal disease if they have (or are suspected to have) nephrotic syndrome, collagen vascular disease (especially systemic lupus erythematosus), tubulointerstitial disease, or rapidly progressive glomerular disease.

MANAGEMENT

The management of CRF patients can be divided conveniently into three separate categories: treatment of aggravating factors, treatment of specific complications of uremia, and consideration of optimal diet and general principles in the long-term follow-up of patients with CRF. We will consider those principles of management that are common to all forms of CRF regardless of etiology.

Aggravating Factors

Patients with CRF are highly susceptible to factors that may cause a deterioration of renal function. These must be sought meticulously and treated immediately so that the underlying renal failure will not be worsened permanently. Table 79–3 lists factors that may rapidly increase the serum creatinine concentration in a patient with previously stable CRF. The relative incidence of these factors causing acute deterioration of renal function is dependent on the demographics of the patient population. Thus, generalized frequency distribution cannot be formulated; however, it is important for the physician to consider each of these general categories as a differential diagnostic possibility when evaluating a patient with progressive renal disease.

TABLE 79–3. AGGRAVATING FACTORS FOR PROGRESSION OF RENAL DISEASE

1. Vascular volume depletion
   a. Absolute: aggressive use of diuretics, gastrointestinal fluid losses, dehydration, etc.
   b. Effective: low cardiac output, renal hypoperfusion with atheroembolic disease, ascites with liver disease, nephrotic syndrome, etc.

2. Drugs: aminoglycosides, prostaglandin synthesis inhibitors in a setting of renal hypoperfusion, diuretics in dosage to cause volume depletion, etc.

3. Obstruction
   a. Tubular: uric acid, Bence Jones protein, etc.
   b. Post-tubular: prostatic hypertrophy, necrotic papillae, ureteral stones, etc.

4. Infections: sepsis with hypotension, urinary tract infections, etc.

5. Toxins: radiographic contrast materials, etc.

6. Hypertensive crises

7. Metabolic: hypercalcemia, hyperphosphatemia, etc.

Volume Depletion. One of the most common causes of rapidly rising serum creatinine concentration in a CRF patient is vascular volume depletion. Vascular volume depletion can be the result of either absolute volume depletion or contraction of the effective arterial blood volume. A common cause of absolute volume depletion is the combination of aggressive use of diuretics coupled with restricted intake of salt and fluids. Another common cause of absolute volume depletion of CRF patients is gastrointestinal loss of fluid from either vomiting or diarrhea. Vascular volume depletion can also be "effective." Effective arterial blood volume (EABV) is a dynamic concept that refers to blood volume that perfuses various volume receptors. Under circumstances of decreased EABV, the renal blood flow decreases. The kidneys of CRF patients are especially sensitive to decreases in renal blood flow. Therefore, aggravating factors that cause decreases in EABV can produce rapid rises in serum creatinine concentrations (Table 79–3). Physical signs of volume depletion should thus be sought. In addition, urinary electrolyte measurements will often suggest volume depletion. Although CRF patients normally have an elevated fractional urinary excretion of sodium and chloride (the degree being dependent on the severity of the decrease in GFR), these patients are able to decrease their fractional excretion of sodium and chloride in response to volume depletion. A decrease in previously determined high fractional excretion of sodium and chloride of 2 per cent (or a decrease in fractional excretion to less than 1 per cent) is highly suggestive of either true or effective volume depletion. Patients with CRF may rapidly and irreversibly decrease their GFR with volume depletion, so it is imperative for treatment, either oral or intravenous fluid replacement, to be started as soon as feasible. Patients with CRF who are not on chronic dialysis should be hospitalized if there is any doubt that adequate volume repletion can be carried out on an outpatient basis.

Drugs. Patients with CRF are often treated with various types of drugs, a number of which are nephrotoxic. Table 79–3 lists the nephrotoxic drugs. Of these, the aminoglycoside antibiotics are a common cause of worsening renal failure. In addition, prostaglandin synthesis inhibitors can decrease the creatinine clearance in CRF patients, especially in a setting of decreased EABV. It is beyond the scope of this chapter to review different drug-related nephrotoxins, but it is prudent to obtain a detailed drug ingestion history whenever a CRF patient with an accelerating rate of renal failure is seen.

Obstruction. Acute (less than a day) or subacute (less than a few weeks) obstruction of the urinary tract can occur from multiple causes in CRF patients. Urinary tract obstruction is conveniently divided into tubular and post-tubular causes. The more common etiologies for tubular obstruction include uric acid crystal deposition (as observed with malignancies) and Bence Jones protein deposition (in association with multiple myeloma). More common causes of post-tubular obstruction include prostatic hypertrophy and/or prostatism; necrotic papillae, especially in patients with diabetes; and ureteral stones. When the clinical symptoms suggest urinary tract obstruction, it is important that prompt diagnostic and therapeutic measures are undertaken. Rapid in-and-out catheterization will rule out bladder obstruction, whereas ultrasonography is useful in ruling out ureteral obstruction. These measures are simple and safe and often will prevent progression of azotemia.

Infection. Urinary tract infections are significantly increased when obstruction is present. The rate of infection rises especially after repeated catheterization. Although infection limited to the urinary tract rarely causes progression of renal failure, nevertheless, specific attention should be directed toward evaluating the degrees of proteinuria, pyuria, and bacteriuria and any changes from baseline abnormalities. Increased proteinuria and exaggerated pyuria suggest urinary tract infection. A culture of clean-voided urine should be done under these circumstances. If infection is documented, specific antibiotics are indicated. Care must be exercised to adjust the drug dosage for the degree of renal failure. A number of antibiotics are nephrotoxic, and the susceptibility to neprotoxicity increases with advancing renal failure. Uremic patients are also more prone to other infections such as pneumonia and sepsis on a de novo basis. These systemic infections, if present, in turn may compromise renal blood flow and result in worsening uremia. The index of suspicion should be high for sepsis in hypotensive CRF patients with urinary tract infection in whom the serum creatinine level is rising.

Toxins. The list of potential nephrotoxins is long. Therefore, it is important to obtain a good history in CRF patients with a rising serum creatinine level. In a hospitalized CRF patient, when the serum creatinine starts to rise rapidly, one must consider exposure to radiocontrast materials. Volume-depleted CRF patients, especially diabetics and patients with multiple myeloma, are susceptible for development of worsening renal disease. Fortunately, the prognosis is quite good if the patients are adequately hydrated.

Hypertensive Crisis. A good percentage of patients with CRF are hypertensive. Indeed, hypertension is one of the significant risk factors that may accelerate the rate of progression of renal disease. Thus strict attention must be paid to adequate control of blood pressure in CRF patients. Occasionally, patients with CRF will develop malignant hypertension with rapidly deteriorating renal function. It is imperative that the blood pressure is controlled rapidly in these patients.

Metabolic. Of the metabolic abnormalities that worsen the progression of renal disease, the rises in calcium-phosphorus products are among the most common. The rise in $Ca \times P$ product may not only cause soft tissue calcification but also be a precipitating factor in progression of renal disease. This is especially true in patients with multiple myeloma. An increased $Ca \times P$ product may become more frequent with the recent increase in the use of oral $CaCO_3$ to control hyperphosphatemia.

Complications of Uremia

WATER AND ELECTROLYTE ABNORMALITIES. Treatment of altered states of calcium, phosphorus, and bicarbonate balance is discussed in Ch. 249, "Renal Osteodystrophy."

Hyperkalemia. The mean serum potassium is higher than normal, whereas the total body potassium content is lower than normal in CRF. Serum potassium concentrations up to 6 mEq per liter are well tolerated in CRF patients. However, patients with CRF have difficulty in excreting a sudden increase in potassium load. Therefore potassium concentrations above 6 mEq per liter should be treated. One should initially determine whether the hyperkalemia is a result of some aggravating factor such as volume depletion, tissue breakdown, transient worsening of acidosis, action of drugs such as spironolactone or triamterene, fever, or high intake of potassium; or whether hyperkalemia is a consequence of steady metabolic events. If hyperkalemia is of modest degree and due to some aggravating factor, the therapy should be directed toward correcting the source of hyperkalemia. However, if hyperkalemia is severe, paralysis of skeletal muscles and electrocardiographic changes may be present. This represents a medical emergency and requires immediate transfer of potassium intracellularly and rapid excretion of potassium from the body. The treatment of hyperkalemia is described in detail in Ch. 77.

Abnormalities of Sodium Balance. Total body sodium content dictates total extracellular fluid volume. Although fractional excretion of sodium per nephron increases as renal disease progresses, patients with CRF are nevertheless susceptible to both volume contraction and volume expansion. Since even mild volume depletion may affect renal function

adversely in CRF patients, it is prudent to maintain these patients in a somewhat expanded state (on the "wet side"). Volume-sensitive hypertension and pulmonary edema will be limiting factors, but it is even more hazardous to keep a patient completely edema free. If a patient should develop orthostatic hypotensive symptoms, salt intake should be liberalized. Ideally, dietary salt intake should be decreased in proportion to the decrease in GFR. Some of the sodium should be given as sodium bicarbonate as described for renal osteodystrophy, below. If the patient is poorly compliant and becomes volume expanded, the use of diuretics such as furosemide or bumetanide is indicated, assuming that underlying kidney function is sufficient to permit a satisfactory clinical response to these drugs. If volume expansion causes severe symptoms and does not respond to conventional techniques, acute peritoneal or hemodialysis is indicated. Hypo- and hypernatremia are treated with the same general principles of water restriction or free water administration as in any other patient. Neurologically symptomatic, life-threatening hyponatremia may require the administration of hypertonic sodium chloride, but this risks potential volume expansion. One should be prepared for the possibility of acute dialysis to remove extra volume.

CARDIOVASCULAR ABNORMALITIES. It is important to control the cardiovascular complications of CRF to realize the potential longevity of chronic hemodialysis. Hypertriglyceridemia and hypertension are the primary risk factors leading to accelerated atherosclerosis and high cardiovascular mortality. It is not clear whether the course of atherosclerotic vascular disease in CRF patients can be altered. Even patients who have undergone successful renal transplantation seem to have an increased incidence of cardiovascular deaths. Nevertheless, it seems advisable to adhere to the same dietary principles in patients with hypertriglyceridemia and CRF as in patients without CRF (see Ch. 50). If clofibrate is used, its dosage level should be decreased proportionately to the degree of renal failure to prevent its adverse side effects.

Hypertension is the result of numerous interrelated factors in CRF patients. It is most commonly volume dependent and volume sensitive. Thus one of the primary objectives is to decrease intravascular volume, an approach that will be sufficient to control hypertension in many patients. If the patient has an adequate urine volume, the judicious use of diuretics together with a decrease in the dietary intake of salt and water is indicated. Of the available diuretics, furosemide and bumetanide are preferred because of their low renal toxicity. Volume can be removed in patients on dialysis by ultrafiltration during the procedure. If volume contraction is not sufficient, then the same general principles apply to the treatment of hypertension as in any other patient (see Ch. 47). Additional drugs such as methyldopa, hydralazine, and beta blockers such as propranolol and metoprolol may be required. Captopril, an oral inhibitor of angiotensin-converting enzyme, has been shown to be particularly useful in some patients. Minoxidil, a direct smooth muscle vasodilator, has also been advocated in a small group of patients with otherwise refractory hypertension. There still exists an extremely small number of patients with malignant hypertension that cannot be controlled by any medical regimen. These patients may respond to bilateral nephrectomy.

The diagnosis of uremic pericarditis requires hospitalization and treatment for fear of impending cardiac tamponade. The best initial therapy is daily dialysis for approximately a week. Indomethacin is not effective in uremic pericarditis. If pericarditis remains refractory to increased frequency of dialysis, intrapericardial injection of nonabsorbable steroids may prove therapeutic. Some patients will require partial pericardiectomy if they develop circulatory impairment that does not respond to medical management.

HEMATOLOGIC ABNORMALITIES. Anemia of CRF

often improves with maintenance hemodialysis. The rise in hematocrit is not due to stimulation of erythropoietin production but rather to the removal of some circulating factor that inhibits the normal response to erythropoietin.

Besides achieving the best possible metabolic status of the patient with either hemodialysis or transplantation, there exist two general considerations for treatment of anemia: long-term medical treatment and transfusion. The general aim of medical treatment is to increase the hematocrit to values as high as possible without secondary side effects. Because patients with CRF, especially those on maintenance hemodialysis, are iron deficient, supplemental iron should be given. Iron can be given daily as a ferrous salt or on a periodic basis as intravenous iron dextran. Oral iron supplementation is inexpensive and is associated with very few side effects. Unfortunately, not all patients rebuild their iron stores to normal even if given 900 mg of ferrous sulfate per day. These patients probably do not absorb iron normally in spite of hemodialysis. They require periodic intravenous iron dextran. There is no consensus on frequency or dosage, and there is the potential of iron overload with hemosiderosis and occasional anaphylactoid reaction. While some patients have a gratifying hematologic response to periodic intramuscular injections of androgens, many patients do not respond at all (especially anephric patients) and many have untoward side effects to androgens. Most CRF patients do not have folate deficiency unless they are receiving maintenance dialysis treatment. Folic acid is dialyzable, and therefore it is standard practice to order small daily doses of folate (1 mg per day orally) in the hope of increasing erythropoiesis.

Clinical trials have been recently carried out with recombinant human erythropoietin for the treatment of uncomplicated anemia in patients with end-stage renal disease. Gratifying and dose-dependent rises in hematocrits occurred in response to intravenous erythropoietin administration when given three times weekly after dialysis. If the results of this study are confirmed, they represent a major breakthrough in treatment of anemia of end-stage renal disease.

The above findings with erythropoietin may change the indications for transfusions. Many CRF patients tolerate extraordinarily low hematocrits surprisingly well. This may be due to increased release of oxygen from hemoglobin during chronic anemia. Nevertheless, before erythropoietin becomes available to all centers, some patients do require periodic transfusions. If patients are unduly tired and unable to do routine tasks, packed red blood cell transfusions can be given in amounts sufficient to abate the symptoms. If such symptoms improve, this provides strong presumptive evidence that the weakness was due to anemia and not to uremia per se. It is rare that transfusions are necessary in CRF patients if the hematocrit is above 20 per cent. However, notable exceptions are provided by patients with angina pectoris. In these patients the physician may be forced to transfuse the patient even at hematocrit values in the low 30's. This situation may become more common as the mean age of dialysis patients increases.

INFECTIONS. Infections are more common in uremic than nonuremic patients. The general approach to the use of antibiotics should be the same in both groups of patients. Ideally, the antibiotic dose should be adjusted by monitoring the serum concentration of the antibiotic. However, this often is not feasible and therefore after an initial normal loading dose, dosage levels must be adjusted for the degree of renal failure if the antibiotic is excreted by the kidney (Table 79–4). Some antibiotics are more nephrotoxic than others, and nephrotoxicity is potentiated by CRF. If drug sensitivities allow a choice in treatment of a given infection, the physician should choose the least nephrotoxic antibiotic that is therapeutic.

RENAL OSTEODYSTROPHY. Hyperparathyroidism, decreased amounts of active vitamin D metabolites, and chronic metabolic acidosis all contribute to the development of renal osteodystrophy as noted above. The goals of treatment are to normalize these abnormalities to the extent possible. Renal osteodystrophy is described in detail in Ch. 249.

NEUROPATHY. No specific treatment exists for either central or peripheral neuropathy. However, both objective and subjective improvement may occur by prolonging the periods of dialysis and by use of larger surface area dialyzers. Also, gratifying improvement of peripheral neuropathy has been noted following successful renal transplantation.

MYOPATHY. No specific therapy exists for myopathy. Patients may improve dramatically with adequate dialysis. Some patients have shown improvement of myopathy following treatment with active vitamin D analogues.

CARBOHYDRATE METABOLISM. Abnormalities of carbohydrate metabolism in the nondiabetic patient are of no or minimal clinical significance. In the diabetic patient, insulin dosages must be adjusted to maintain serum glucose values at normal levels. Often smaller insulin doses will be adequate as CRF progresses.

URIC ACID. Although uric acid levels are consistently elevated in CRF, they are rarely much above 10 mg per deciliter. However, even if the uric acid levels are significantly higher there is little or no evidence to suggest that asymptomatic hyperuricemia should be treated. It is our practice to treat elevated uric acid levels in uremic patients only when there are tophaceous deposits or symptomatic gout. If treatment is elected, allopurinol is the drug of choice, since patients with CRF do not respond to uricosuric agents. The allopurinol dose should be decreased to 100 mg per day in chronic uremic patients due to potential toxic side effects.

PRURITUS. No specific therapy has withstood the test of time in the treatment of pruritus. A few patients get relief following topical application of emulsified oils or the use of oral antihistamine agents. Some patients have benefited from lowering the serum phosphate concentration by phosphate binders. There are reports of beneficial effects of ultraviolet light. Parathyroidectomy has sometimes relieved intractable pruritus.

Diet

An appropriate diet can be critically important in the management of patients in chronic renal failure, for it may provide symptomatic improvement and also may slow the rate of loss of residual renal function. Although nutritional and caloric intake should be individualized for obese and malnourished patients, some general principles are applicable to all patients. In general, the higher the amount of protein in the diet, the higher will be the serum urea concentration. This occurs because amino acids are metabolized to form urea in addition to all other nitrogenous waste products that have been implicated as factors causing the uremic syndrome. Reducing the amount of protein in the diet will lower the blood urea concentration and reduce symptoms. Moreover, the difficulties in controlling serum phosphorus and acidosis will be ameliorated, since a high-protein intake is always associated with a high intake of phosphates as well as other inorganic ions. However, if dietary protein is too low, protein malnutrition will occur with loss of strength, body weight, and muscle mass. This can be avoided if the protein requirements are met by providing 0.6 gram of protein per kilogram of body weight per day, of which at least 60 per cent contains proteins rich in essential amino acids, e.g., eggs, lean meat, and milk. Although a high-calorie intake can improve nitrogen utilization at very low nitrogen intakes, it is not necessary to force large numbers of calories on these patients as long as minimum protein requirements are being met. Providing about 3 kilocalories per day generally suffices, although this may be lowered for obese patients or raised for patients weighing less than their ideal body weight. Accumulated waste produces can be reduced even further by lowering the daily protein intake to approximately 20 grams of protein per

TABLE 79–4. ANTIBIOTIC DOSAGE IN CRF

Major Reduction in Dosage	Moderate Reduction in Dosage	Minor or No Reduction in Dosage	Agents That Should Not Be Used
Flucytosine	Ampicillin	Amphotericin B	Bacitracin
Gentamicin	Carbenicillin	Cefotaxime	Chlortetracycline
Kanamycin	Cefazolin	Cefoperazone	Nitrofurantoin
Oxytetracycline*	Cephaloridine	Chloramphenicol	
Streptomycin	Cephalothin	Clindamycin	
Tetracycline*	Cloxacillin	Doxycycline	
Tobramycin	Co-trimoxazole	Erythromycin	
Vancomycin	(trimethoprim-	Isoniazid	
	sulfamethoxazole)	Lincomycin	
	Methicillin	Nafcillin	
	Moxalactam		
	Oxacillin		
	Penicillin G		
	Ticarcillin		

*Although tetracyclines are not significantly nephrotoxic per se, their dosage should be reduced in CRF because of their hepatotoxicity with increased blood levels (especially with chlortetracycline) and because their antianabolic actions cause an increase in blood urea nitrogen disproportionate to the degree of renal failure. If tetracyclines are indicated in renal failure, doxycycline is the drug of choice because it is cleared by hepatic routes.

day, but only if the diet is supplemented with essential amino acids or a mixture of essential amino acids and their alpha-ketoanalogues. Such a regimen will maintain adequate protein nutrition for prolonged periods of time in patients with advanced renal failure. Alpha-ketoanalogues of essential amino acids are aminated in the body to form essential amino acids and hence body protein. Nitrogen, which otherwise would have accumulated as waste products, is therefore used to build body proteins. Low-protein diets in which daily minimum requirements are met and the very-low-protein diet supplemented with mixtures of amino acids and alpha-ketoanalogues may slow the rate of loss of residual renal function and possibly postpone the time when therapy with chronic hemodialysis becomes necessary. Diets should be supplemented with the water-soluble B vitamins plus vitamin C and folic acid; there is no need to supply additional vitamin A or E. Vitamin D should be reserved for treatment of severe renal osteodystrophy. In general, there is no need to place a severe restriction on dietary sodium unless there is hypertension or edema. Most patients with chronic renal failure can readily excrete sodium until renal function is markedly impaired (creatinine clearances less than 10 ml per minute), but they cannot rapidly stop excreting salt when dietary sodium is markedly restricted. For most patients, the diet should contain at least 1.5 to 2 grams of sodium per day. As long as the amount of urine excreted is greater than 1 liter per day, it is unusual to have to restrict potassium in the diet. Using these guidelines, uremic symptoms and the consequences of renal insufficiency can be controlled for most patients. Once

chronic hemodialysis becomes necessary, the diet should be altered to meet the added requirements related to dialysis therapy.

General Principles of Follow-up

Patients with CRF should be seen at regular intervals to monitor the progress of their disease. The frequency of these visits will depend upon the presence of other diseases, e.g., hypertension and heart failure, and on how rapidly residual renal function is being lost. All patients should be seen at least every three months, at which time a medical history is taken and a physical examination is performed. In addition, laboratory values including hematocrit, white blood cell count, serum urea nitrogen and creatinine concentrations, and electrolyte values should be obtained. Monitoring the progress of renal insufficiency is generally accomplished by measuring the serum creatinine concentration as an indirect index of GFR. Alternatively, 24-hour urine collections can be obtained to measure creatinine and urea clearances, since the average of these two values gives a close approximation of GFR. For most patients, the loss of residual renal function proceeds at a constant rate; this rate is different for each patient, although generally patients with polycystic renal disease have a slower rate of loss of renal function than those with diabetic nephropathy. To monitor the progress of the disease, the reciprocal of the serum creatinine concentration can be plotted against time for an individual patient, as shown in Figure 79–2. For most patients, this relationship is remarkably linear and can be used to estimate when a patient will become a candidate for maintenance hemodialysis. When the reciprocal of serum creatinine concentration reaches 0.1 or less (a creatinine concentration of 10 mg per deciliter), the patient is close to the time when dialysis becomes necessary. Moreover, a sudden change in the slope of this line can indicate that some other factor, such as obstruction, infection, or uncontrolled hypertension, is accelerating the rate of loss of residual renal function.

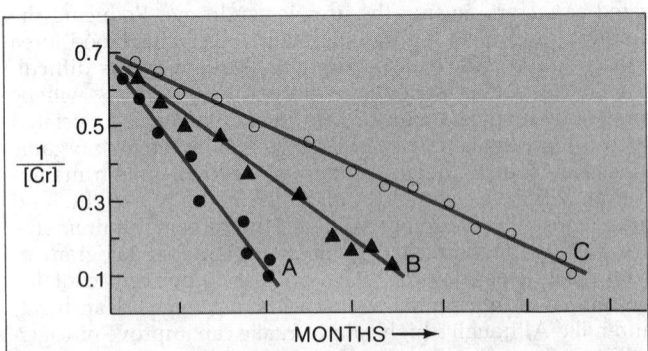

FIGURE 79–2. Plot of reciprocal of serum creatine concentration (vertical axis) against time (horizontal axis) in three hypothetical patients. This is a useful way to determine the rate of predetermined slope reflecting the underlying cause of CRF. For example, patient A reflects rapidly progressing renal failure such as seen with diabetes mellitus, patient B might represent nephrosclerosis secondary to essential hypertension, and patient C might reflect the slower rate of progression of polycystic disease.

Anderson S, Brenner BM: Effects of aging on the renal glomerulus (review). Am J Med 80:435, 1986. *This article reviews nicely the consequences of aging on renal function. It reminds us that the reduction in creatinine clearance with aging is accompanied by a reduction in daily production of creatinine. Thus, the serum creatinine level in the elderly patient does not reflect the same high creatinine clearance as in the younger patient. This becomes of importance in the management of elderly patients receiving nephrotoxic drugs. The article also proposes a provocative hypothesis based on animal studies that limitation of dietary protein intake may delay the age-related loss in renal function.*

Bricker NS: Sodium homeostasis in chronic renal disease. Kidney Int 21:886, 1982. *This article is an examination of factors regulating sodium homeostasis in normal and chronic renal failure patients.*

Chan MK, Varghese Z, Moorhead JF: Lipid abnormalities in uremia, dialysis and transplantation. Kidney Int 19:625, 1981. *An excellent overview editorial that discusses clearly the complex lipid abnormalities in uremic and dialysis patients.*

DeLuca HF: The vitamin D hormonal system: Implications for bone diseases. Hosp Pract April 1980, pp 57–63. *Dr. DeLuca reviews clearly the factors important in the pathophysiology of renal osteodystrophy, with special emphasis on the central role of vitamin D.*

Eschbach JW, Adamson JW: Anemia of end-stage renal disease. Kidney Int 28:1, 1985. *An excellent editorial review that discusses the mechanisms that contribute to the anemia and treatments that have been proposed for anemia of end-stage renal disease.*

Eschbach JW, Egrie JC, Downing MR, et al.: Correction of the anemia of end-stage renal disease with recombinant human erythropoietin. N Engl J Med 316:73, 1987. *This is an important report of results from phase I and II clinical trials using recombinant human erythropoietin to treat uncomplicated anemia in end-stage renal failure patients undergoing hemodialysis. The authors demonstrate a remarkable dose-dependent rise in hematocrit in response to intravenous erythropoietin given three times weekly after dialysis.*

Giordana C (ed.): Fourth Capri Conference on Uremia. Kidney Int 28(Suppl. 17):S1–S193, 1985. *This supplement represents contributions from 48 leading interdisciplinary specialists on various aspects of uremia. Clinical symptoms, pathogenesis, and treatment of uremia and its complications are discussed in great detail.*

Oldrizzi L, Rugin C, Valvo E, et al.: Progression of renal failure in patients with renal disease of diverse etiology on protein-restricted diet. Kidney Int 27:553, 1985. *This is a long-term study on more than 200 patients with renal disease of diverse etiology in which the authors demonstrate that the administration of protein-restricted diet delays the progression of functional renal deterioration.*

Wineman RJ: End-stage renal disease: 1978. Dialysis Transplantation 7:1034, 1978. *A review of demographic characteristics of end-stage renal disease as derived from the National Dialysis Registry.*

80 TREATMENT OF IRREVERSIBLE RENAL FAILURE

80.1 Dialysis

Robert G. Luke

Each year approximately 1 in 10,000 of the United States population develops end-stage renal disease (ESRD) and requires one of the various forms of renal replacement therapy: chronic hemodialysis in a center or at home; intermittent peritoneal dialysis—usually at home; continuous ambulatory peritoneal dialysis; or transplantation from a live-related or cadaveric donor. Most of the costs of such treatment are covered for almost all of the United States population by the Renal Medicare Program, and by the late 1980's approximately 100,000 patients are expected to participate. The most common causes of end-stage renal disease are chronic glomerulonephritis, nephrosclerosis, chronic pyelonephritis (reflux nephropathy), diabetic glomerulosclerosis, and polycystic kidney disease. The overall incidence of end-stage renal disease is 4.5 times greater in blacks than in Caucasians; hypertensive nephrosclerosis accounts for 33 per cent of the cases in blacks but only 8 per cent in whites.

Choices of renal replacement therapy is dictated by the availability of a live-related donor (best results), the age of the patient (transplantation is less frequently performed over the age of 55 years), and the presence of important systemic extrarenal disease (which may preclude surgery or immunosuppression). Preliminary hemodialysis is usually necessary before transplantation. Home hemodialysis or intermittent peritoneal dialysis requires the support of a partner, an adequate home, self-motivation by the patient, and reasonably stable medical circumstances. Such patients have better rehabilitation and survival rates than those on in-center hemodialysis, but this may relate to patient selection factors. The cost of home dialysis is less than in-center dialysis. In general, patients are best served when all modalities of treatment for end-stage renal disease are readily available and well integrated.

TECHNICAL ASPECTS

As renal excretory function becomes progressively impaired, solutes accumulate in the body and eventually contribute to the uremic syndrome (see Ch. 79) and, ultimately, to death. These solutes, especially those of low molecular weight such as urea, can be removed efficiently from the blood by the process of diffusion across a semipermeable membrane down a chemical concentration gradient (dialysis). Substances higher in concentration in the dialysate than in the plasma, such as bicarbonate, will diffuse into the plasma (Fig. 80–1). The membrane must be nontoxic and compatible with red blood cells, white blood cells, platelets, and plasma proteins. Either a synthetic membrane in the process of extracorporeal hemodialysis or, in peritoneal dialysis, the lining membrane of the peritoneal cavity is used.

Hemodialysis

Membranes of varying hydraulic conductivity and solute permeability can be used in dialyzers of varying surface area and extracorporeal blood volume (100 to 250 ml in adults) to accommodate patients of different sizes, including infants. To remove accumulated sodium chloride and water, ultrafiltration across artificial membranes is induced by a transmembrane hydrostatic pressure, either positive on the blood side or negative on the dialysate side (Fig. 80–1). The removal of over 1 liter of fluid per hour is feasible and predictable based on the ultrafiltration coefficient of the dialyzer. The essential components of a dialysate delivery and monitoring system of an artificial kidney apparatus are shown in Figure 80–2. Blood flow rates of 200 to 300 ml per minute are usual. Heparin is given intermittently or infused continuously (1000 to 10,000 units in total) to prevent clotting of blood in the dialyzer during the usually three- to six-hour procedure; dosage is controlled by the whole blood or activated clotting time.

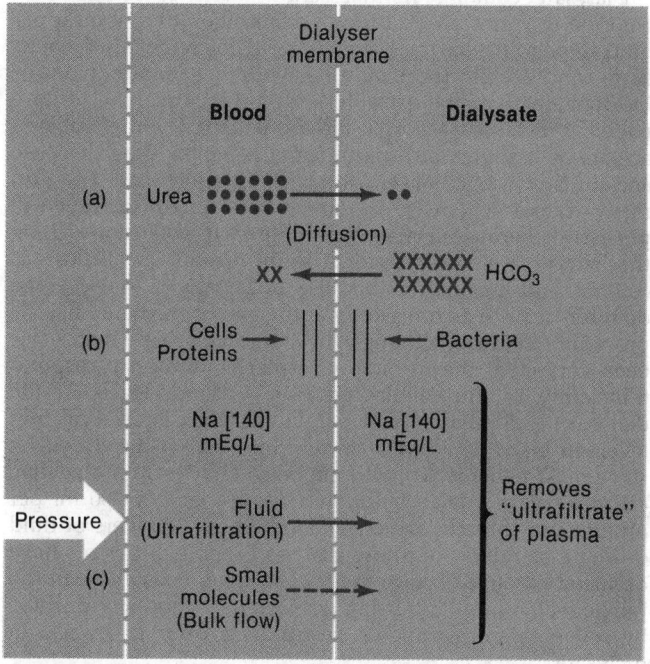

FIGURE 80–1. Mechanisms of removal of solute and fluid during dialysis. (*a*) Diffusion of urea from high concentration in blood into dialysate and of bicarbonate from higher concentration dialysate into lower concentration in the blood of patient with renal failure. (*b*) The dialysis membrane is impermeable to red blood cells and plasma proteins and to bacteria in the dialysate (but not to endotoxins). (*c*) The dialysate sodium is freely diffusible and determines the plasma sodium; fluid is removed by application of a transmembrane pressure (in peritoneal dialysis by increased glucose and hence osmotic pressure in the dialysate). The fluid is accompanied by small molecules such as sodium and chloride by convection (solvent drag).

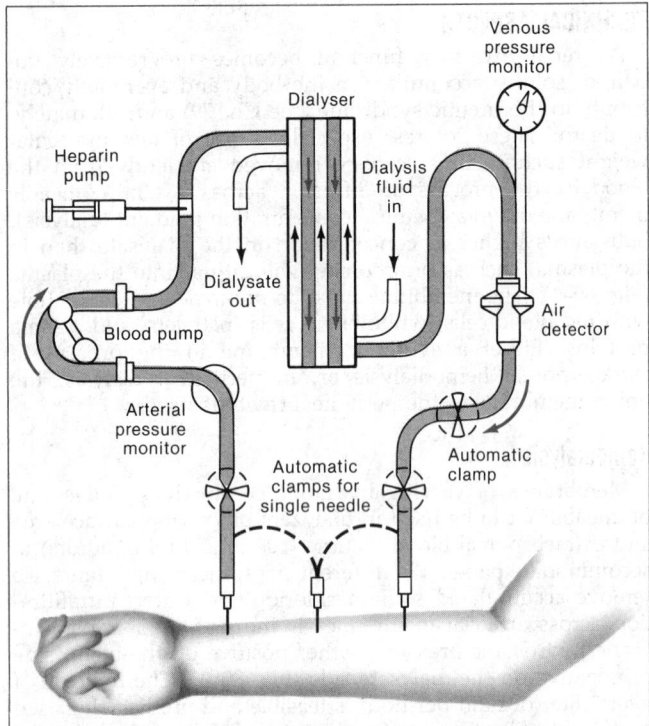

FIGURE 80—2. Essential components of a dialysis delivery system which, together with the dialyzer, makes up an "artificial kidney." In isolated ultrafiltration no dialysis fluid is used (bypass mode). Also shown is the apparatus for using a single needle for inflow and outflow of blood from the patient. (From Keshaviah PR, Shaldon S: In Drukker W, Parsons FM, Maher JF (eds.): Replacement of Renal Function by Dialysis. 2nd ed. Boston, Martinus Nijhoff Publishers, 1983, p. 224.)

Dialysate contains normal serum levels of sodium and chloride, a variable potassium concentration (0 to 4 mEq per liter) depending on the patient's need for removal of potassium, and acetate (normally metabolized to bicarbonate) or bicarbonate (35 mEq per liter) to correct the renal failure patient's metabolic acidosis. Bicarbonate may be preferable to acetate as a source of base in some patients, either because acetate is not metabolized normally (in which case the normally transient increase in "anion gap" in the plasma will persist) or because it may contribute to hypotension during the hemodialysis procedure. A slight respiratory alkalosis is common during dialysis because of loss of CO_2 across the dialyzer. It persists transiently at the end of the hemodialysis procedure because, although the extracellular base deficit has been corrected, the respiratory center continues to respond transiently to intracellular acidosis. Calcium levels in the dialysate—3.5 mEq per liter—are higher than ionized calcium levels in blood to allow a calcium influx from the dialysate, since most patients with chronic renal failure are in negative calcium balance. Dialysate flow rates are usually 500 ml per minute and thus the patient's blood "sees" 120 liters of fluid during a standard four-hour dialysis. Various problems have occurred because of trace metals and other substances in the public water supply, but tap water is now routinely purified by reverse osmosis and/or deionization prior to its use in dialysate.

Peritoneal Dialysis

In peritoneal dialysis clearances of low molecular weight substances are less than for hemodialysis (for example, a urea clearance of 20 to 25 ml per minute versus 150 ml per minute for hemodialysis), but clearance of some larger, perhaps also toxic, substances is greater because of the greater permeability of the peritoneal membrane to these larger molecules and the longer duration of treatment. When required, fluid removal is carried out by means of osmotic movement of water using high concentrations of glucose (1500 to 4500 mg per deciliter) in the dialysate. Exchange volumes during peritoneal dialysis are commonly 1 to 3 liters each hour. Several types of automated machines are available that make dialysate from concentrate, deliver set volumes of fluid into the abdomen, and then allow drainage after a set "dwell" time. The commonest type now in use is the cycler, which is relatively simple, uses commercially prepared dialysate in bottles, and automatically cycles up to a total of 16 liters of dialysate in and out of the abdomen for a period of 8 hours (often overnight). Because peritoneal dialysis is less efficient than hemodialysis, dialysis times are much longer (Table 80–1). Therefore chronic intermittent peritoneal dialysis is practical only for use at home.

Continuous Ambulatory Peritoneal Dialysis (CAPD)

This technique makes use of the fact that small molecular weight solutes reach complete equilibration with peritoneal fluid in four to six hours. Thus the patient exchanges 1.5 to 3.0 liters of sterile dialysate containing hypertonic glucose (1.5, 2.5, or 4.25 per cent) and physiologic electrolytes three to five times a day through a Tenckhoff peritoneal dialysis catheter and is able to maintain adequate removal of solutes and water. Since insulin-dependent diabetics have more complications of vascular access because of their vasculopathy and since regular insulin can be given in the dialysate with excellent control of the blood sugar, CAPD offers advantages to patients with diabetic glomerulosclerosis. In infants and children the higher peritoneal surface area relative to body size also facilitates CAPD. In contrast to poorer dialysis of small molecular weight solutes compared with hemodialysis, dialysis of larger molcules (>500 daltons) is increased (see Table 80–1). Larger "middle molecules" may accumulate in chronic hemodialysis patients and contribute to complications such as pericarditis. Many patients have been managed successfully by CAPD for several years, but technique failure rates remain higher than for chronic hemodialysis, mainly because of problems with the peritoneal catheter or recurrent peritonitis.

CLINICAL USE

During hemodialysis, the major limiting factor for clearance of small molecular weight substances such as urea is the "unstirred layer" barrier to diffusion at the blood-membrane interface. Clearance does not increase significantly beyond blood flow rates of 250 ml and dialysate flow rates of 500 ml per minute. Surface areas of 1.0 to 1.3 square meters are usually adequate to reduce blood urea by about 50 per cent during a three- to four-hour hemodialysis. In contrast, the limitation to clearance of a larger molecular weight substance such as inulin is the permeability of the membrane, and inulin clearance for most commonly used hemodialysis membranes is quite small (Table 80–1). The permeability of the peritoneal membrane (the effective surface area of which is estimated to be between 0.5 and 1 square meter in adults) for larger molecular weight substances is much greater than the artificial membranes, but dialysate flow rates in intermittent peritoneal

TABLE 80–1. TIME-AVERAGED CLEARANCE (ml/min)*

Technique	Weekly Duration	Urea Clearance	B₁₂ Clearance	Inulin Clearance
		(60)†	(1350)†	(5200)†
Hemodialysis	3 × 4 = 12 hr	11 (160)‡	2.5 (30)	0.3 (4)
Intermittent PD	4 × 10 = 40 hr	6 (25)	1.5 (7)	1.2 (5)
CAPD	Continuous	7	5	3
Normal kidney	Continuous	60	120	120

*Does not include residual renal function.
†Molecular weight (daltons).
‡Figures in parenthesis are actual clearances during procedure.
PD, peritoneal dialysis; CAPD, chronic ambulatory peritoneal dialysis.

TABLE 80–2. CONTINUOUS AMBULATORY PERITONEAL DIALYSIS (CAPD)

Advantages	Disadvantages
Requires no machine	Peritonitis due to contamination during bag changes*
Maintains constant plasma solutes	
Less restricted dietary intake	Patient time: 4 exchanges at 30 to 40 minutes/7 days per week
Less expensive (?)	
No dependence on helpers or nurses	Loss of protein in dialysate (8 to 12 grams/day)—requires increased protein intake
Enhanced mobility	
Better control of blood pressure (?)	
Good control of blood glucose by intraperitoneal insulin in diabetic patients	Hyperlipidemia and obesity (glucose in PD fluid)
Less cardiovascular stress	Long-term adequacy of peritoneal membrane as dialyzer (?)

*Majority of cases can, however, be treated on an outpatient basis with intraperitoneal antibiotics.

dialysis are much less (35 ml per minute). Thus urea clearance for peritoneal dialysis is much less than for hemodialysis, and inulin clearance is relatively greater (Table 80–1). Peritoneal blood flow has been estimated at 50 to 100 ml per minute and is clearly a factor that may critically limit clearance in states of markedly reduced cardiac output. Unfortunately, the causes of toxicity in the uremic syndrome are poorly understood, so that the ideal dialysis regimen or membrane cannot be defined. Techniques that remove small molecular weight end-products of protein metabolism, such as urea, are quite successful and compatible with prolonged survival and reasonable well-being, however.

Permanent vascular access is usually obtained by creation of an end-to-side arteriovenous fistula in the forearm or insertion of a prosthetic arteriovenous graft when the vessels themselves are inadequate. A permanent indwelling peritoneal catheter is made of radiopaque Silastic 25 cm long and includes an intra-abdominal (located in the pelvis), subcutaneous (with a Dacron felt cuff barrier to bacteria at each end), and external segment. Most ESRD patients continue to be managed, however, by chronic in-center hemodialysis, and only about 20 per cent of all dialysis patients are on some form of home dialysis, including chronic ambulatory peritoneal dialysis. The advantages and disadvantages of the latter technique are outlined in Table 80–2.

Initiation of Dialysis

Before initiating chronic dialysis careful discussion with the patient and family should address the issue of whether such treatment is in the patient's best interest. For example, if there is extensive irremediable extrarenal disease, such as severe cerebrovascular disease or a painful malignancy, it may be wiser to continue conservative treatment only.

Initiation of dialysis should occur when conservative management of chronic renal failure is beginning to be inadequate but before the development of uremic symptoms. In general, dialysis becomes necessary at a creatinine clearance of 4 to 8 ml per minute or a serum creatinine of about 10 mg per deciliter. However the patient's general clinical state is more important than the level of blood urea nitrogen or creatinine. It is especially important to institute therapy before the onset of pericarditis, peripheral neuropathy, or an impaired nutritional state secondary to anorexia or other uremic gastrointestinal symptoms, as subsequent recovery is then quite prolonged and mortality rate increased. Vascular access should be placed, if feasible, a few months before dialysis to allow it to mature adequately. Of the permanent types of access, only the Scribner shunt (a Teflon external connector between the radial artery and a forearm vein) is available for use immediately. If uremia develops abruptly, acute vascular access can be maintained for up to several weeks by an indwelling subclavian vein catheter or intermittently via the femoral vein. Permanent peritoneal access is placed one to two weeks prior to use to prevent fluid leaks, which predispose to peritoneal and subcutaneous infections.

In *diabetic nephropathy* renal failure may accelerate microangiopathic complications—especially retinopathy, gastropathy, and peripheral neuropathy—and many nephrologists therefore prefer to initiate replacement therapy earlier in such patients, perhaps when serum creatinine approximates 5 to 8 mg per deciliter. The progression of diabetic glomerulosclerosis to ESRD at that stage also tends to be quite rapid.

Hypertension is an important complication in most patients who reach end-stage renal disease. Antihypertensive medications can usually be tapered after initiation of dialysis, and blood pressure can be controlled by adjustment of plasma and extracellular fluid volume by ultrafiltration during dialysis and by dietary salt and water restriction. Sympatholytic drugs or drugs that cause postural hypotension are best avoided, since they interfere with the ability to remove fluid adequately by ultrafiltration. A reduction in urinary volume commonly accompanies the onset of dialysis because of lessening of solute osmotic diuresis. The concept of "dry weight" is a clinically important one in a chronic dialysis patient, regardless of modality of therapy. This is the postdialysis weight at which the patient has an acceptable blood pressure and a plasma volume adequate for avoiding symptoms of diminished cardiac output or of pulmonary congestion. Short-term changes in weight are always due to salt and water deficits or excesses, but careful supervision is required to detect changes in body mass in either direction over longer periods. Interdialytic weight gains should not exceed 2 to 3 kg but unfortunately often do so in patients who are not compliant with dietary salt and fluid restrictions.

Most dialysis patients thus have "volume-dependent" hypertension and require antihypertensive medications only if they are noncompliant with salt and water intake. In perhaps 10 per cent of patients, however, blood pressure is "renin dependent," and progressive ultrafiltration is accompanied by persistent rebound hypertension after hemodialysis due to rising circulating levels of angiotensin II. Previously bilateral nephrectomy was sometimes employed to control blood pressure in such patients, but the advent of such potent drugs as captopril and minoxidil has virtually eliminated the need for this procedure. Furthermore, it is especially important to avoid bilateral nephrectomy when some recovery of renal function may occur in time, as after an episode of primary or secondary malignant hypertension or after rapidly progressive glomerulonephritis. Indeed, anephric patients fare less well overall during chronic dialysis because of absence of erythropoietin production and, possibly, of $1,25(OH)_2$ cholecalciferol, and because of loss of residual renal clearance of larger molecular weight substances.

Dialysis disequilibrium describes a syndrome in which confusion, headache, and focal neurologic signs develop owing to more rapid dialysis of solutes from the plasma than from the intracellular compartment, especially from the brain. Thus an osmotic gradient can be set up between brain cells and extracellular fluid and lead to cerebral edema. This complication usually occurs in patients with acute or chronic renal failure and uremic symptomatology and/or a very high blood urea nitrogen (BUN). Short dialysis with a low blood flow usually prevents this problem, which does not occur in maintained chronic dialysis patients and is extremely rare during initiation of any of the forms of peritoneal dialysis because of their lesser efficiency.

Hepatitis B (Hb_sAg) is carried in the plasma of some patients with chronic renal failure, who therefore constitute a serious risk to dialysis staff and other patients, since there is repeated exposure to the patient's blood. Separate dialysis facilities and staff are needed for such patients if home dialysis or transplantation is not feasible. Routine monitoring for Hb_sAg is now performed in patients initially testing negative for the antigen, and active immunization is available and indicated for patients and staff. Non-A, non-B hepatitis also remains an epidemiologic problem.

**TABLE 80–3. RELATIVE INDICATIONS FOR
PERITONEAL (PD) OR HEMODIALYSIS (HD)
FOR MANAGEMENT OF ACUTE RENAL FAILURE**

Clinical Circumstance	Comment
1. Recent cerebral surgery, vascular accident or trauma	PD preferred; risk of hemorrhage with heparin and of fluid shifts in brain during HD
2. Hypercatabolic states (e.g., multiple injuries)	HD preferred; PD may not provide adequate clearance of urea, etc.
3. Recent cardiac surgery or myocardial infarction	PD preferred; increased risks of hypotension and arrhythmias with HD
4. Recent abdominal surgery	HD preferred; loss of fluid via incisions during PD; ileus requires surgical placement of PD catheter
5. Acute hemorrhage or severe coagulopathy	PD preferred; but in certain circumstances HD without heparin feasible
6. Complicating severe lung disease	HD preferred; PD may cause atelectasis and impair vital capacity by interfering with movement of diaphragm

Hemodialysis and acute intermittent peritoneal dialysis are also employed in the treatment of acute renal failure, the most frequent cause of which is acute tubular necrosis (see Ch. 78). These patients are often quite ill, and survival is aided by frequent "prophylactic" dialysis to maintain a blood urea nitrogen (BUN) of less than 100 mg per deciliter. The relative merits of hemodialysis and peritoneal dialysis for acute renal failure are outlined in Table 80–3.

Continuous Arteriovenous Hemofiltration

The technique of continuous arteriovenous hemofiltration can be uniquely valuable, especially in patients with acute cardiorenal failure and a low cardiac output. This procedure employs a membrane with a very high ultrafiltration coefficient, which allows fluid and solute removal at low blood perfusion pressures and flow rates. No blood pump or complex monitoring devices are required, and the procedure can be readily performed in an intensive care setting with femoral artery and vein cannulation in very ill, often fluid-overloaded patients in whom hemodialysis or peritoneal dialysis would be very difficult or impossible. Intravenous administration of electrolyte replacement solutions may be necessary with intravenous nutrition if indicated. Heparin is needed.

ROUTINE MANAGEMENT

Patients on chronic hemodialysis usually require a slightly reduced protein intake (0.8 to 1.0 gram per kilogram), but a more stringent control of salt and potassium intake, to maintain satisfactory levels of blood urea nitrogen, potassium, and blood pressure. Hyperkalemia remains a significant cause of death in chronic dialysis patients, usually due to dietary indiscretion. Monitoring of adequacy of dialysis requires assessment both of clinical well-being, including nutritional state, and of BUN and serum electrolytes, including calcium and phosphorus. The BUN reflects urea production rates and is dependent on protein intake and endogenous protein catabolism as well as on adequacy of urea removal by dialysis. Provided nutrition and protein intake are adequate, a BUN less than 90 to 100 mg per deciliter immediately prior to dialysis is usually acceptable. Plasma chemistries are checked monthly, or less often in stable home patients, in the absence of clinical problems. Adequate clearances can usually be achieved by a total of 12 (9 to 15) hours of hemodialysis per week on a thrice-weekly schedule. In most patients supplemental oral base (sodium bicarbonate) is not required; serum HCO_3 should be kept above 20 mEq per liter in the predialysis blood. Dialysis is almost always inadequate to maintain serum phosphorus in an acceptable range (3.5 to 5.0 mg per deciliter) and, as in the conservative management of renal failure, oral

aluminum-containing phosphate binders are necessary. Constipation is a frequent result and needs treatment by, for example, the use of an osmotic cathartic such as 70 per cent sorbitol. In some patients, aluminum-containing binders contribute to aluminum-related bone disease; calcium or magnesium carbonate may be used to substitute partially as phosphate binders. Because of loss of water-soluble vitamins, including folic acid, from the blood during dialysis, routine administration of supplements of these substances is necessary. Oral iron is also given because there is a chronic small loss of blood that cannot be returned to the patient at the end of each dialysis. Anabolic steroids such as nandrolone decanoate can improve the red blood cell production in dialysis patients and hence are commonly administered. Recently human erythropoietin, produced by recombinant DNA technology, has been shown to be capable of returning the hematocrit to normal in patients on chronic hemodialysis. This observation has obvious therapeutic implications for the future.

COMPLICATIONS OF CHRONIC DIALYSIS

The major clinical complications experienced by patients on chronic dialysis are renal osteodystrophy, anemia, vascular access infections and thromboses, pericarditis, and ascites (Table 80–4). The major cause of death remains cardiovascular disease, but the high incidence of coronary atherosclerosis probably reflects the risk factors of hypertension and hyperlipidemia (and perhaps of a high calcium-phosphate product) rather than any specific effects of chronic dialysis per se. Dialysis does cause some cardiovascular stress during the procedure owing to ultrafiltration and reduction of plasma volume and to a modest reduction in arterial oxygen levels (by 10 to 20 mm Hg). This latter is due either to hypocarbia secondary to loss of CO_2 across the dialyzer and/or to sequestration of blood leukocytes in alveolar capillaries after the activation of complement by the dialyzer membrane; a transient leukopenia is usual during the first hour of dialysis. Episodes of hypotension and hypoxia secondary to those dialysis effects frequently provoke angina in patients with coronary vascular disease.

Renal osteodystrophy is discussed elsewhere from the standpoint of both pathogenesis and treatment (see Ch. 249). Normal serum levels of calcium, phosphate, bicarbonate, and parathormone should be maintained. Calcium supplements, phosphate binders, and $1,25(OH)_2$ cholecalciferol may be needed. Rarely soft tissue calcification, hypercalcemia, and progressive osteitis fibrosa cystica may necessitate subtotal parathyroidectomy. Osteomalacia usually responds to $1,25(OH)_2$ cholecalciferol, but one resistant type, in which an excess of aluminum is found on bone biopsy, appears to respond only to diminishing bone aluminum by chelating agents such as desoxyferamine.

Anemia is a constant finding. The hematocrit in a well-dialyzed, well-nourished dialysis patient is usually in the range of 25 to 35 per cent. However, in anephric patients it

**TABLE 80–4. COMPLICATIONS IN
PATIENTS ON CHRONIC DIALYSIS**

Accelerated cardiovascular disease	Hepatitis B (Hb_sAg) carrier state
Hypertension	During dialysis
Renal osteodystrophy	Hypotension
Anemia	Cramps
Serositis	Bleeding
Pericarditis	Leukopenia with pulmonary
"Dialysis ascites"	sequestration of WBC's
Pleural effusion	Hypoxia
Access infections and thrombosis	Electrolyte disturbances
Dialysis dementia	Dialysis disequilibrium
Pseudogout, tenosynovitis	CAPD
Pruritus	Exacerbation of symptoms of
Poor nutrition	abdominal hernia or back pain

WBC's, white blood cells.

is usually 12 to 20 per cent. Transfusion is not indicated unless anemia is contributing to symptoms, heart failure, or angina. The major cause of the anemia appears to be lack of erythropoietin together with depression of erythropoiesis by azotemia. As noted above, synthetic human erythropoietin is likely to be available soon for use in man. Iron deficiency anemia is not uncommon and may be indicated by a lowered serum ferritin level. Eosinophilia is quite common in chronic dialysis patients and appears to be of little clinical importance.

Serositis, as manifested by pleural effusion, ascites, or pericarditis, may complicate chronic dialysis. The pathogenesis is not established, although onset often accompanies periods of infection, stress, or protein catabolism. The diagnosis in each case is dependent on elimination of other causes. In general, the abnormal fluid has the characteristics of an exudate and, especially in the case of the pericardial sac, may be hemorrhagic. Patients with pericardial effusion may develop pericardial tamponade, especially during dialysis, when intravascular volume and pressure in the right side of the heart are being reduced. Atrial arrhythmias are also common. If pericardial effusion occurs, dialysis should be carried out daily with very careful control of anticoagulation. If hemodynamic, radiologic, or ultrasonic assessment shows no improvement, surgical treatment by pericardial stripping or medical treatment by pericardiocentesis and insertion of a locally long-acting steroid such as triamcinolone is indicated. "Dialysis ascites" can be an intractable management problem. Poor nutrition and fluid overload often contribute, and insertion of a LeVeen shunt (one-way valve with bacterial filter between peritoneum and vena cava) may be necessary. Tuberculosis is an important differential cause of these complications, and diagnosis is dependent on histologic findings and culture, since anergy is common. Pleural effusion is less common and less troublesome than pericarditis and ascites.

Access infections are commonly due to *Staphylococcus aureus* infection, may be associated with bacteremia or septicemia, or even bacterial endocarditis, and may require excision of the graft. Access problems are the most frequent cause of admission to hospital in the dialysis population. These include thrombosis, aneurysms, and infection of the graft. Arteriovenous fistulas last, on the average, longer than synthetic grafts, but each may function for several, even many, years. Steal syndromes may develop with pain in the hand during dialysis, especially in patients with diabetic vascular disease. Very high blood flows through fistulas may contribute to congestive heart failure, but this is quite unusual.

Dialysis dementia is a progressive fatal disease of the central nervous system associated with speech and motor defects, dementia, and seizures. It is now much less frequent, probably because of improved procedures for preparation of dialysate water and reduction in its aluminum content. Motor paralysis due to peripheral neuropathy is also now rare in well-dialyzed patients.

Pseudogout and *tenosynovitis* occur quite frequently in dialysis patients and respond well to drugs such as indomethacin. *Pruritus* is a troublesome symptom and is sometimes attributable to a high blood calcium-phosphate solubility product or to hyperparathyroidism. In some cases pruritus, despite correction of the above factors, remains resistant to treatment.

The dialysis procedure itself may be complicated by hypotension and muscle cramps; both are related to rates of ultrafiltration and usually respond to injections of small amounts of hypertonic fluids such as 0.3 M NaCl or 20 per cent mannitol. Contributory causes of hypotension are autonomic insufficiency, diminished cardiac function, and hypotensive drugs. In patients who are prone to ventricular ectopy it is important to avoid hypoxia by use of supplemental oxygen and rapid changes in serum potassium by modifying dialysate potassium concentration. This is especially true in patients on cardiac glycosides. Other complications of the dialysis procedure are air embolism, bleeding secondary to heparin, loss of blood due to clotting of the dialyzer, and electrolyte disturbances due to errors in the dialysate. Fortunately these are all now quite unusual. Indeed, death or serious morbidity due to complications of the hemodialysis procedure itself in properly trained or supervised patients is now exceedingly rare.

LIMITATIONS OF DIALYSIS

For chronic dialysis, hemodialysis remains the "gold" standard, and many patients continue to do well after over ten years on this form of treatment. The three-year survival rate for American patients aged 20 to 25 years is 85 to 90 per cent; for those 60 to 65 years, 60 per cent; and for those with diabetic renal disease, 40 per cent. This form of treatment is inherently limited, however, not only because of low clearances (see Table 80–1) but also because the endocrine and regulatory functions of the native kidney are not replaced by the "artificial kidney." Indeed, life saving as it is, the latter term is a misnomer; the patient with an endogenous creatinine clearance of even 15 ml per minute is usually better off than one on maintenance chronic dialysis or CAPD.

Drukker W, Parsons FM, Maher JF: Replacement of Renal Function by Dialysis. Edition 2. Boston, Martinus Nijhoff Publishers, 1983. *This is a complete reference work for all technical and clinical aspects of dialysis.*
Eschbach JW, Egrie JC, Downing MR, et al.: Correction of the anemia of end-stage renal disease with recombinant human erythropoietin: Results of a combined phase I and II chemical trial. N Engl J Med 316:73, 1987. *This is an important new development that may become standard therapy in the future.*
Golper TA: Continuous arteriovenous hemofiltration in acute renal failure. Am J Kidney Dis 6:373, 1985. *This extensive review describes the clinical indications and advantages and disadvantages for continuous arteriovenous hemofiltration (CAVH) and compares it with traditional dialysis therapies for renal failure.*

80.2 Renal Transplantation
William J. C. Amend, Jr.

HISTORICAL PERSPECTIVE. Clinical renal transplantation had its successful beginnings at the Peter Bent Brigham Hospital in 1954 with the successful implantation of a kidney from a healthy identical twin donor into a young patient with chronic renal failure. This predated by some years the technique of chronic, repetitive hemodialysis and offered hope to patients with chronic renal failure. Unfortunately, most patients do not have an identical twin donor. Success in extending this transplantation technique to patients who were genetically dissimilar to their organ donor (the donor being a relative, nonrelative, or cadaver, or even a subhuman primate) had to await the discovery and use of various immunosuppressant techniques.

More recently, advances in organ preservation, knowledge of histocompatibility, tests in vitro involving pretransplant immunologic responses, immunosuppression, and other aspects of patient management have greatly improved the likelihood of transplant functional success. A greater utilization of both dialysis and transplantation has occurred from (1) technical and scientific improvements, (2) physician and patient awareness of treatment availability, and (3) economic support for its clinical applications (through legislative appropriation). At present, approximately 8000 patients per year receive a renal transplant, and approximately 85,000 patients per year receive some form of chronic dialytic support in the United States.

DONOR ASPECTS. Organ transplants can be generally divided into two types: (1) those from a living donor (related or nonrelated) and (2) those from a cadaver donor.

Living Donor. A prospective donor should have no significant medical history and be of an acceptable age (18 to 60 years). High motivation and normal emotional responses are necessary. Preliminary tissue-typing tests are performed, including ABO typing, HLA serotyping (human leukocyte antigen typing), and a direct lymphocyte crossmatch between donor lymphocytes and recipient sera. Biologic relatives are preferred, since there is an increased chance of tissue-typing compatibility. The post-transplant clinical response can be roughly predicted after this histocompatibility testing and with other immune tests performed in vitro (see "Immunologic Aspects," below, and Ch. 425). Finally, the donor undergoes intensive medical testing, culminating in pyelography and renal arteriography. If these medical tests are completely normal, the person can serve as a low-risk donor with the probability of near normalization of renal function following a half-year period of compensatory renal hypertrophy in the remaining kidney. Renal donors have shown little functional deterioration, proteinuria, or hypertension for a subsequent 2 to 20 years.

Cadaver Donor. Cadaver donations come after death from brain trauma, subarachnoid bleeding, or some other sudden, terminal event that occurs in a previously healthy individual. After brain death has been determined, the next of kin is contacted for permission for organ donation. When permission is given, a transplant team or regional organ bank is contacted for organ procurement. Often a cadaver donor serves for multiple organ purposes (i.e., kidney, lung, heart, pancreas, liver). The kidneys are removed and maintained at cold temperatures (4 to 6° C) with either a saline flush solution (cold preservation) or pulsatile perfusion (Belzer technique). While the kidneys are stored, the donor-recipient matching is performed at a histocompatibility laboratory, utilizing lymphocytes from donor lymph nodes obtained during the procurement procedure. These tests must be carried out rapidly (within 6 to 24 hours) in order to utilize the cadaver kidney before irreversible, storage-induced damage occurs. Computer-assisted analysis allows for the selection of recipients from a cadaver-transplant waiting list. This necessary speed of matching is in marked contrast to the methodical pretransplant immune testing (sometimes taking weeks) in live-related donor renal transplants.

RECIPIENT CHARACTERISTICS. The transplant recipient may have end-stage renal failure from a variety of causes. The most common are glomerulonephritis, diabetes mellitus, nephrosclerosis, and polycystic disease. Dialysis patients with severe chronic pulmonary disease, with severe obesity, with known cancer within three years of surgery, or with known active infection are considered unsuitable transplant candidates. Psychologic or compliance problems may be relative contraindications.

Recurrent urinary tract infections, persistently high antiglomerular basement membrane antibody levels, or resistant forms of renin-dependent hypertension often indicate the need for pretransplant bilateral nephrectomy. Also, if ureteral reflux is demonstrated with or without positive urine cultures, preliminary bilateral nephrectomy is performed. Recipients with certain forms of renal disease must be carefully informed regarding the absolute and relative risks of recurrent disease possibilities.

IMMUNOLOGIC ASPECTS. *Histocompatibility.* Increasing degrees of genetic similarity between donor and recipient confer upon organ transplants increasing chances for successful transplant function. When the transplant is between identical twins (isografts), there is no genetic disparity and hence no likelihood of rejection. The transplant success in these instances relates to nonrejection factors such as technical problems or the possibility of recurrent disease. More commonly, organ transplants are performed between two genetically dissimilar members of the same species (allografts or homografts).

Histocompatibility is defined as the degree to which the tissues of two individuals are alike. Cell surface antigens (phenotypes appearing on white cells and endothelial cells) are determined by histocompatibility genes, known as the HLA system (Ch. 425). Each genetic locus expresses its phenotypic information independently on human lymphocytes (T and/or B cells). A combination of five genetic loci on the sixth human chromosome is known as the major histocompatibility locus (MHL) and encompasses genotypes for both Class I and Class II antigens.

The antigens of the serologically defined loci (such as A, B, C, and DR) can be determined over six hours, whereas the antigens of the lymphocyte-defined loci (D) are determined by lymphocyte blastogenesis occurring in vitro over three to five days. A haplotype is that genetic information (from adjoining gene loci) that would be carried on any one chromosome. All individuals have leukocyte phenotypes that are made up of two haplotypes for the various HLA antigens.

Prior to a transplant, a patient with kidney failure undergoes tissue typing to assess his or her histocompatibility and to compare this with potential donors. By noting the various A, B, and DR leukocyte phenotypes (and their distribution) in a family, such as in Figure 80–3, it is possible to construct haplotypes involving these three histocompatibility antigens. In the example shown, the patient is a two-haplotype match to one sister, one-haplotype match to two siblings and both parents, and a zero-haplotype match to one sister. The last sibling could be of the same match grade as a randomly obtained, live-unrelated, or cadaver donor. In addition, ABO compatibility is currently felt to be necessary, so that donor selection includes both red-cell and white-cell tissue antigen systems. If there are no compatible relatives who might be a donor, the potential histocompatibility match from a nonrelative (living or cadaver donor) is shown in Figure 80–3.

As noted in Figure 80–4, functional survival of the transplant is excellent when two full haplotypes (HLA-identical) are shared and is less when only one haplotype is shared. Many centers employ pretransplant donor-specific blood transfusions, DST (see below under "Immune Responses"), for one-haplotype as well as zero-haplotype transplants (the latter being completely mismatched, such as a wife-husband match). Thus far, these are as successful as the pairs with the best HLA-match grades. Cadaver kidney transplant results are also depicted in Figure 80–4. HLA A and B locus matching does not improve cadaver-donated graft success rates in most centers in the United States. On the other hand, pretransplant blood transfusions have an important beneficial effect on graft survival. Recently, matching for the DR locus has improved cadaver graft success in some, but not all, regions of the United States. Most importantly, newer immunosuppressive agents, such as cyclosporine, have markedly improved two-year cadaver graft survivals.

Immune Responses. Organ transplants evoke a variety of responses in the recipient. If there has been previous sensitization (from blood transfusions, previous transplants, or pregnancy) a *hyperacute rejection* can immediately occur. This is based on a recipient antibody–donor endothelial cell reaction and resembles a Shwartzman's phenomenon. The result is cortical necrosis with no treatment possible. This is avoided with carefully performed pretransplant donor-recipient lymphocyte crossmatching. This crossmatching must particularly involve a T cell–type crossmatch. Interestingly, despite a positive T cell crossmatch with historic sera (sera from the patient more than one year before transplant), the transplant can be successfully performed as long as more recent sera are negative with the T cell crossmatch.

If a weaker degree of sensitization, perhaps to a minor histocompatibility locus, has occurred, a slightly delayed secondary humoral response can occur. This is termed an *acute-accelerated rejection*, which is pathologically similar to the hyperacute rejection. This likewise is irreversible, but it occurs in a delayed manner two to six days post-transplant.

In the more usual circumstances, the allograft is initially invaded by recipient macrophage and monocyte cells. If antigenic differences to the allograft are noted, these cells will process the antigen with a T lymphocyte and activate this T

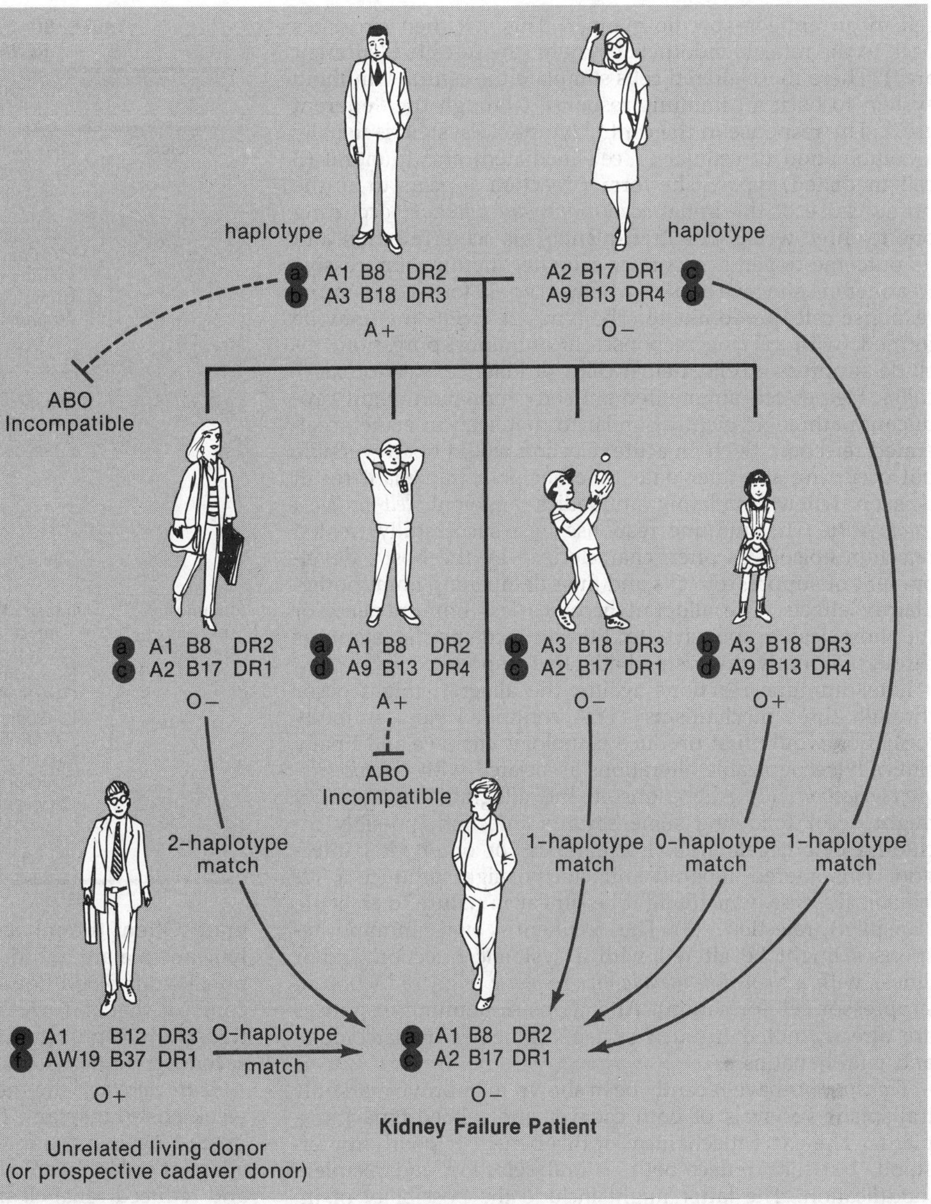

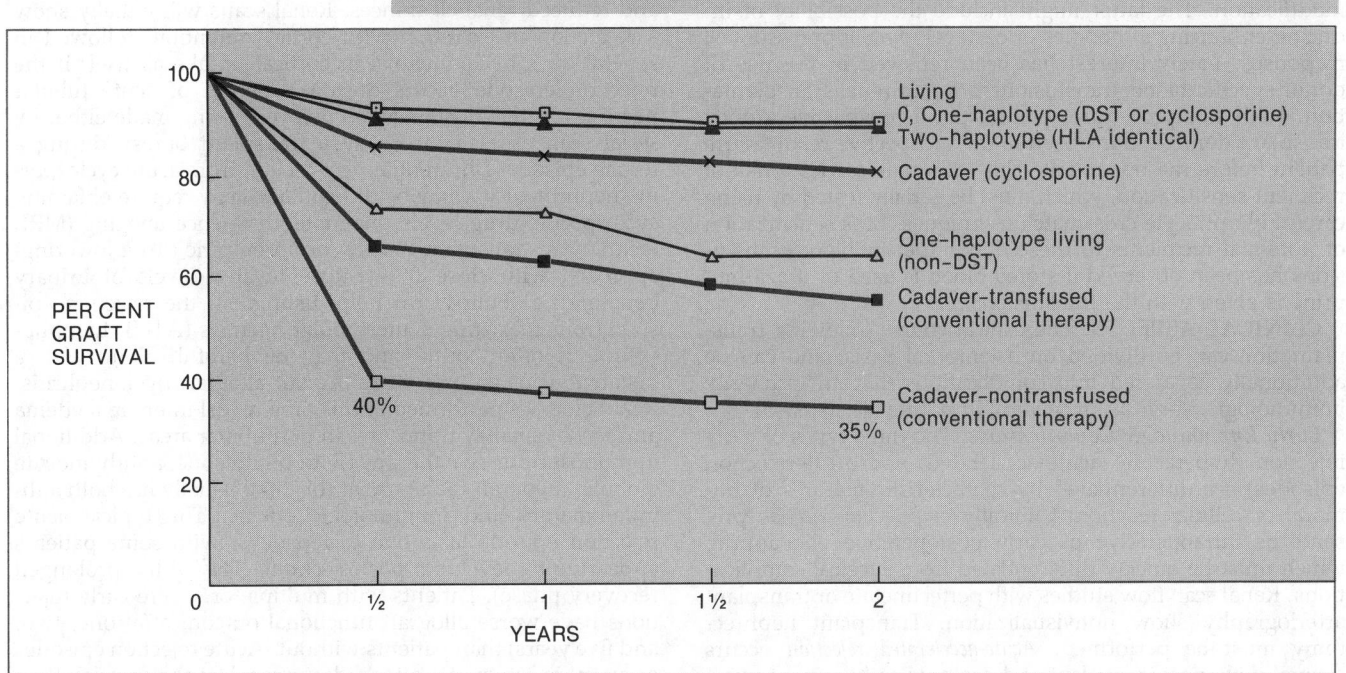

FIGURE 80–3. Family tree of HL-A genotypes and unrelated HL-A genotype.

FIGURE 80–4. Two-year renal transplant graft survivals utilizing various transplant strategies.

cell in an antigen-specific manner. This cell then circulates back to the reticuloendothelial system (the so-called "afferent arc"). There these altered cells stimulate the central lymphoid system to elicit an immune response (through the "efferent arc"). The response in the central lymphoid system is usually a combination of cellular (T cell–mediated) and humoral (B cell–mediated) types. The former reaction appears to be the prime cause of the initial *acute transplant rejection*, occurring one to three weeks post-transplant. This acute rejection and its outcome depend in part on whether immunosuppressive treatment is effective and on whether certain forms of immune response cells predominate. The types of T cells that may be formed (with varying responses to immunosuppression) include suppressor cells, helper cells, or killer cells (cytotoxic T cells). Helper cell–augmented antibody formation might produce a pathologic picture similar to that seen in acute accelerated rejection. Such an acute rejection would be irreversible but occurring at a later date. Another poor transplant result is seen when circulating antibodies augment *cell-mediated cytotoxicity*. The immune response in a successfully treated rejection episode is often characterized by the host's development of suppressor cells and their dampening immunoregulatory effects. The allograft becomes less immunogenic or the host less responsive to this antigen-specific stimulus through a poorly understood adaptive response.

Later immune reactions against the allograft might occur through three mechanisms: (1) A continued slow antibody formation would first produce pathologic changes and finally clinically recognizable alterations associated with *chronic allograft rejection*. (2) Alterations in the allograft's antigenicity might occur following some sorts of infection, possibly including cytomegalovirus, Epstein-Barr, or other viral infection. This altered allograft antigenicity might produce a *late immune response*, which might be similar in nature to an acute transplant rejection. (3) The recipient's own immune responses might be altered with a systemic infection and/or illness with a *change in the adaptive response* (e.g., reduction in suppressor cell formation). Alterations in immune responses are already noted in such systemic illnesses as sarcoidosis and viral hepatitis.

Transfusions have recently been shown to improve markedly transplant survivals of both cadaver and related-type transplants. The exact mechanism of this benefit is poorly understood, but may reflect both natural selection and recipient modification. The latter might include the possibility of inducing enhancing antibodies or of developing suppressor cell responses. Lately interest has been renewed in the use of donor-specific blood transfusions prior to renal transplantation. With this procedure, blood from a prospective kidney transplant donor is transfused to the prospective renal failure patient before the transplant. This technique carries a risk of recipient sensitization, which must be serially tested by using careful lymphocyte crossmatch techniques. Less sensitization of potential recipients to these donor-specific blood transfusions has been observed if stored blood is used or if azathioprine is given with the transfusions.

CLINICAL ASPECTS. The clinical course following transplantation can be divided on a temporal basis, and can be additionally separated into complications that are primarily immunologic, surgical, or medical in nature (Table 80–5).

Early Immunologic Complications. The three types of early rejection (hyperacute, acute-accelerated, and acute-rejection episodes) are differentiated by characteristic features of humoral or cellular reaction. Clinically, *hyperacute rejection* presents as intraoperative or early postoperative oligoanuria, which must be quickly differentiated from surgical complications. Renal scan flow studies with pertechnetate or transplant arteriography show nonvisualization. Transplant nephrectomy must be performed. *Acute-accelerated rejection* occurs several days post-transplant and presents as fulminant rejections with fever, oliguria, tenderness, and enlargement of the

TABLE 80–5. COMPLICATIONS FOLLOWING RENAL TRANSPLANTATION

	Early Complications (< 2 months)	Late Complications (> 2 months)
Immunologic	Hyperacute rejection Acute accelerated rejection Acute rejection	Acute rejection Chronic rejection
Surgical	Procurement/perfusion injury Urinary leak Obstruction	Lymphocele Reflux Obstruction—stone, cicatrization Renal artery stenosis
Medical	Renal failure—acute tubular necrosis, acute rejection	Progressive renal failure or nephrotic syndrome—chronic rejection, recurrent disease Transplant pyelonephritis Hypertension Atherosclerotic events Erythrocytosis
Immunosuppression-related	Impaired host defense—infections Moon facies, obesity Poor wound healing Gastrointestinal bleeding Leukopenia, thrombocytopenia Steroid psychosis Cyclosporine nephrotoxicity Cyclosporine hepatotoxicity	Impaired host defense—infections Moon facies, obesity, hirsutism Aseptic necrosis, osteoporosis Steroid myopathy Hypophosphatemia Cataracts Steroid hyperglycemia Neoplasia Hepatitis, pancreatitis Cyclosporine nephrotoxicity

graft. Often, thrombocytopenia and microangiopathic hemolytic anemia are found. Again, renal scans will reveal little or no allograft blood flow, consistent with cortical necrosis. The course is that of irreversible renal failure, which again requires transplant nephrectomy. This form of rejection represents a secondary humoral or cell-mediated response.

Acute rejection, the most common type, occurs after the first week post-transplant. It is felt to be a primary, cell-mediated process against the foreign donor cells. It is characterized by allograft enlargement, fever, malaise, oliguria, hypertension, and reduced renal clearances. Renal scans will initially show a reduction in excretion with cortical retention, followed in several days by reductions in cortical uptake as well. If the rejection episode occurs during a period of acute tubular necrosis, its diagnosis may be delayed, being made either by serial scan assessment or by a transplant biopsy during a febrile episode. Differentiating rejection from acute cyclosporine nephrotoxicity may be difficult and may require obtaining cyclosporine drug levels, magnetic resonance imaging (MRI) techniques, transplant biopsy, or an empiric (drug-lowering) approach with close follow-up. Elevated levels of urinary beta$_2$-microglobulins also help distinguish the rejection episode from coexisting acute tubular necrosis (ATN). Lymphocyturia is often found and may be helpful, along with a negative urine culture, in ruling out allograft pyelonephritis. Renal biopsies performed at this time reveal interstitial edema and foci of small lymphocytes in peritubular areas. Additional immunosuppressive therapy (with prednisone, antithymocyte globulin, allograft radiation) at this time usually has both anti-inflammatory and immunologic effects. The typical acute rejection episode lasts five to ten days, with some patients appearing to develop a postrejection ATN (with a prolonged recovery phase). Patients with multiple or severe early rejections have worse allograft functional outcomes (at one, two, and five years) than patients without. Acute rejection episodes occur more commonly after cadaver renal transplantation than after live-donor transplantation.

Early Surgical Complications. After cavader transplantation, there may be initial ATN on the basis of donor-agonal changes, warm ischemia (in excess of 30 minutes), or excessive donor-sympathetic responses at or near the time of the cadaver organ procurement. ATN per se does not affect the eventual transplant outcome. The patient will, however, require post-transplant dialysis. Rarely, storage or perfusion injury can occur. In either case, a technically poor result will occur with suboptimal renal function. In addition, the use of cyclosporine superimposed on this injury may be disadvantageous. These problems are usually not seen with live-donor transplants, since there can be careful preoperative management of the donor's hydration status and a marked reduction in warm ischemic injury. Attentive surgical technique lowers the possibilities of vesicoureteral reflux, of urinary leak from the neocystostomy site, and of lymphocele formation.

Early Medical Complications. Medical problems initially noted post-transplant include continuing renal failure (from ATN or rejection), during which the patient requires dialysis. As noted above, cyclosporine may induce varying degrees of drug-related acute nephrotoxicity. Hypophosphatemia can be seen after normal renal function is regained. Persisting secondary hyperparathyroidism causes exaggerated phosphaturia. This parathyroid hyperplasia usually regresses during the first half-year following successful transplantation. Correction of the patient's anemia or an increase in a diabetic patient's daily insulin requirement gives a favorable transplant prognosis, since the transplanted kidney has already begun normal renal endocrine function.

Immunosuppression commonly used following renal transplantation may include one or a combination of glucocorticosteroids, azathioprine or cyclophosphamide, antithymocyte globulin (either polyclonal or monoclonal antibodies against T cells or T cell subsets), cyclosporine or some other lymphocyte depletion technique such as thoracic duct drainage or, more recently, total lymph node irradiation. All these therapies confer what is termed "nonspecific immunosuppression." Despite different mechanisms of action, generalized impairments of cell- or humoral-mediated immune responses are produced.

Hypercortisolism accounts for many of the undesired side effects and morbidity in renal transplant patients. In the early post-transplant period, poor wound healing, reduced host defenses, psychologic changes, and steroid-induced hyperglycemia are particularly common. Growth may be retarded in children receiving daily glucocorticosteroids. In an attempt to reduce these problems, many transplant patients are shifted to once-daily or alternate-day dose regimens (see Ch. 30). Other immunosuppressive agents also reduce host defenses in a nonspecific fashion. The patient becomes more susceptible to viral, protozoal, fungal, or bacterial infection. Infections, particularly pulmonary, must be aggressively diagnosed and specific treatment rapidly begun. The patient's immunosuppression should be reduced if infection is suspected, even at the potential risk of transplant rejection loss. Bone marrow suppression, liver abnormalities, or hemorrhagic cystitis can also occur from one or more of these antimetabolites. The type and dosage of the drugs must be adjusted with monitoring of these signs and/or with drug blood levels (cyclosporine).

Late Immunologic Complications. Occasionally, an acute rejection process occurs more than two to three months after a transplant. This may occur either spontaneously or more frequently following an abrupt change in immunosuppressant therapy. Usually, rejection processes are more of a chronic, vascular type in the months to years following the transplant. Chronic rejections are clinically asymptomatic and are detected by renal functional abnormalities (progressive azotemia, proteinuria) and often have associated hypertension.

Late Surgical Complications. Late problems are primarily of a urologic type. Vesicoureteral reflux is not seen if the reflux-correcting "tunnel" procedure is employed at the time of transplantation. Lymphoceles may not be detected until years after the transplant and can be associated with partial obstruction, infection, or hypertension. Since allografts are denervated, stone passage is painless and is usually associated only with (temporary) renal impairment, hematuria, or signs of an associated urinary tract infection.

Late Medical Complications. Atherosclerotic disease, already a noteworthy complication of dialysis, is frequently present. Predisposing risk factors include smoking and significant hypertension and lipid abnormalities seen during uremia and dialysis. Opportunistic infectious problems still can occur in long-term situations. Careful evaluation for any post-transplant patient with a febrile illness is necessary. Fungal, protozoal, or viral infections are particularly serious and require rapid diagnosis and supportive therapy. Immunosuppression should be diminished if host resistance is compromised. Aseptic necrosis or osteonecrosis, particularly of weight-bearing joints, is an unfortunate complication seen in 15 per cent of these patients. It principally affects hip, knee, and shoulder joints and is related to pre-existing secondary hyperparathyroidism, in addition to the transplant corticosteroid therapy. Excellent rehabilitation therapy, however, can be provided with arthroplastic surgery. Hypertension frequently occurs after transplantation and may be related to rejection (either acute or chronic), residual kidney or renal pressor mechanisms (from the native kidneys), glucocorticoid or mineralocorticoid effects (cyclosporine per se), urologic abnormalities (lymphoceles or obstruction), or transplant renal artery stenosis. Evaluation of severe hypertension necessitates a urologic and renovascular workup, with the need for selective venous renin measurements from three kidney sites. Infusions of angiotensin-converting enzyme inhibitors might also be important in detecting renin-dependent, angiotensinogenic hypertension.

Certain forms of neoplasms are particularly noted in transplant patients. Cervical dysplasia and carcinoma may be related to herpes type 2 involvement. Excessive cases of immunoblastic lymphoma, leukemia, and cutaneous malignancies have also been noted. However, a generalized increase of malignancies (solid tumors as well as other forms of lymphoproliferative disorders) has not been demonstrated. It is not known whether the immunosuppression lowers tumor surveillance in these patients or whether the allograft alters the patient's own immune response (from a chronic antigen exposure). Rarely, a patient will develop post-transplant erythrocytosis. Such patients should be evaluated to establish the primary nature of this disorder. Often, recurrent phlebotomies are necessary for one to two years. It is felt that the erythropoietin source comes from the native kidneys (nonsuppressed in a nonuremic milieu).

The transplant kidney may develop the nephrotic syndrome with or without clearance deterioration. Usually, particularly if the primary renal disease was nonimmunologic, this is secondary to chronic rejection. By pathologic examination, chronic rejection has elements either of a predominantly arteriolar lesion with an intimal reaction or of a glomerular lesion with generalized basement membrane thickening and mesangial proliferation. Clinically, progressive hypertension and proteinuria are hallmark features of early phases of chronic rejection, with the eventual development of intractable renal failure. On the other hand, patients with certain forms of renal disease (Table 80–6) may be predisposed to recurrence of the original disease in their allografts. This was first noted in a high frequency with identical twin transplants, but must be suspected in all patients with these primary renal diseases. Renal biopsy or immunologic tests must be performed for diagnosis. Treatment of such conditions in the allograft is the same as that of primary disease. Transplant pyelonephritis is characterized by pain and swelling over the transplant and by usual accompanying renal functional dete-

TABLE 80–6. RECURRENT DISEASES OF RENAL ALLOGRAFTS

Primary Disease	Comments
Membranous glomerulonephritis	Same immunologic pattern; appearance is similar to that of chronic rejection
Rapidly progressive glomerulonephritis	Fulminant course in isografts; "crescents" on pathology; graft failure
Anti-GBM* glomerulonephritis	With and without preliminary bilateral nephrectomy; graft failure
Juxtamedullary focal glomerulosclerosis	With and without graft failure
IgA nephropathy	Immunofluorescence with and without graft failure
Membranoproliferative disease	
Type 1	With and without graft failure
Type 2 ("dense deposit")	Graft failure often
Oxalosis	Deposits and graft failure
Cystinosis	Deposits without graft failure
Henoch-Schönlein syndrome	
Hemolytic uremic syndrome	
Diabetes mellitus	Glomerular lesions nodular and diffuse; no graft failure (yet)

*GBM, glomerular basement membrane

rioration. Potential urologic problems should be tested for in this circumstance.

Patients who are positive for hepatitis B surface antigen (before or after the transplant) have a serious probability of developing chronic active hepatitis, cirrhosis, and/or hepatomas. Caution must be taken in recommending transplantation in such patients at the present time.

Transplant patients often regain fertility, and contraceptive advice is indicated. Despite theoretic risks of genetic malformation and a higher incidence of miscarriage and spermatozoal malformation, no severe congenital malformations have been described, and many successful pregnancies have occurred.

Psychologically, much anxiety and depression can occur with transplant- or immunosuppressive-related problems. The glucocorticoids directly affect the emotions of such patients, making the reactive nature of their emotional responses even more labile during such stresses. Despite an otherwise excellent physical status, some patients remain overly concerned that the transplant may "fail." Most patients with well-functioning renal transplants attain a degree of rehabilitation similar to their premorbid status.

Over a period of time, the patient seems to adapt immunologically to the transplant in a poorly understood manner. Even after an initial success of two years or more, there continues to be a relationship between the degree of histocompatibility and the long-range functional prognosis. There is a greater chance of late transplant failure in cadaver renal transplants than in forms of related renal transplants. Also, one-haplotype transplants do less well than fully matched sibling pairs. After an initial two years of transplant success, the T½, or half-life, probabilities for two-haplotype transplants are 34 years, for one-haplotype transplants 10 years, and for cadaver transplants 7.5 years. This analysis is practically important when discussing the long-range prognosis with a transplant recipient. The prognosis of certain patient populations, those with diabetes, for instance, is worsened because of systemic complications in these groups.

When a patient rejects a first renal transplant within the first year, transplant nephrectomy is usually necessary. Rejected foreign tissue left in situ will produce a symptom constellation of fever, allograft tenderness, generalized malaise, cachexia, and weight loss. Transplants that undergo chronic rejection, if well tolerated, may be left in place.

Retransplantation (a second or third time) can be attempted if the first transplant fails. An effort is made to avoid similar histocompatibility antigens in subsequent transplants or at least to assess whether specifically shared lymphocytotoxic antibodies have developed subsequent to the first transplant.

A similar clinical course (regarding rejection probabilities) can be anticipated in later transplants, suggesting that the recipients' own immune regulation is an important factor in transplant success. Choosing a different immunosuppressive agent for a second transplant might be important to attain better transplant success.

Prognosis. Three to 5 per cent of patients receiving a cadaver renal transplant are at risk of dying each year. Related-donor transplants have improved the likelihood of patient survival. The risk of death in certain patient groups (transplant recipients with diabetes or other systemic disease) is higher than in those patients who are otherwise healthy. A successful transplant permits the best opportunity for complete rehabilitation of a patient with chronic renal failure.

Calne RY: Organ transplantation: From laboratory to clinic. Br Med J 291:1751, 1985. *An informational recounting of the development of organ transplantation.*

Hunsicker LG: Impact of cyclosporine on cadaveric renal transplantation: A summary. Am J Kidney Dis 5:335, 1985. *A nice review of cyclosporine's beneficial results and toxicity problems. Summarizes many institutions' results.*

Opelz G: Correlation of HLA matching with kidney graft survival in patients with or without cyclosporine treatment. Transplantation 40:240, 1985. *Large collaborative study that emphasizes the role of donor-recipient histocompatibility.*

Strom TB: The improving utility of renal transplantation in the management of end-stage renal disease. Am J Med 73:105, 1982. *A thorough review of the subject, particularly good with the discussion of immunosuppression.*

81 GLOMERULAR DISORDERS
William G. Couser

About 80,000 patients in the United States require hemodialysis or transplantation for chronic renal failure at an annual cost in excess of 2 billion dollars. Two thirds of these have some glomerular disease. First described in the writings of Richard Bright in the early nineteenth century, these diseases have subsequently intrigued many clinician-investigators who have attempted to separate and classify them solely on the basis of clinical manifestations and histopathology. Inconsistent terminology and confusing classification systems proliferated, sufficient to befuddle generations of medical students.

The past two decades have witnessed a marked improvement in this situation: (1) Experimental models of glomerular diseases have been produced by immunizing animals with either renal antigens or various foreign proteins, thus confirming a long-held suspicion that most such diseases have an immunologic basis. (2) The histologic and functional abnormalities in these models were found to be associated with the development of immune deposits in glomeruli, demonstrated by immunofluorescence (IF) and electron microscopy (EM). The widespread application of percutaneous renal biopsy as a routine clinical diagnostic tool has allowed experimental observations to be applied to understanding the pathogenesis of glomerular lesions in humans. In this chapter, glomerular diseases are classified on a clinical basis into three groups: (1) primary renal diseases that usually present with the abrupt onset of hematuria, red cell casts, proteinuria, and decreased glomerular filtration rate (acute nephritic syndrome or glomerulonephritis [GN]); (2) primary renal diseases that usually present with the insidious onset of heavy proteinuria and relatively normal glomerular filtration rate (nephrotic syndrome); and (3) secondary glomerular diseases resulting from renal involvement by a variety of systemic illnesses, which may be either nephritic or nephrotic. This approach has the virtue of simplicity, but it is useful only if its limitations are fully appreciated. Separation between primary and secondary renal diseases is sometimes difficult and arbitrary. For example, IgA nephropathy is recognized as a primary renal disease and Henoch-Schönlein purpura is classified as a secondary one, although they probably represent only differing clinical manifestations of the same process and often overlap. Most of the diseases that present as acute GN may cause the nephrotic syndrome, although they do so uncommonly, and some nephrotic glomerular diseases may occasionally exhibit nephritic features.

IMMUNE MECHANISMS AND THE GLOMERULAR RESPONSE TO INJURY

Two immunologic mechanisms of glomerular disease are generally accepted: (1) Rare patients develop glomerulonephritis due to deposition of antibody to glomerular basement membrane (GBM) antigens, which results in a typical uninterrupted linear staining pattern along all glomerular capillary walls by immunofluorescence microscopy, (see Fig. 81–7). (2) Much more commonly, glomerulonephritis is associated with discontinuous, or granular, deposits of immunoglobulin and complement (see Figs. 81–2B, 81–3B, and 81–8). These deposits may occur at three sites: (1) within the glomerular mesangium, as in IgA nephropathy, Henoch-Schönlein purpura, and early lupus nephritis; (2) along the subendothelial surface of the capillary wall between endothelial cells and GBM, as seen in more severe forms of lupus nephritis and type I membranoproliferative glomerulonephritis (MPGN); and (3) on the outer, subepithelial surface of the capillary wall, as in membranous nephropathy and the so-called subepithelial "humps" in post-streptococcal glomerulonephritis. Granular, or immune complex, deposits at mesangial and subendothelial sites either can result from the passive glomerular trapping of preformed immune complexes from the circulation or may form in situ owing to initial glomerular localization of free antigens followed by antibody binding to them. Subepithelial immune complex deposits appear to form only on a local basis. Figure 81–1 illustrates schematically how immune deposits at each of these sites are related to normal glomerular structures and some of the morphologic lesions that result.

Several glomerular diseases that are believed to be immunologically mediated do not have immune deposit formation in glomeruli. For example, minimal change nephrotic syndrome (MCNS) exhibits a marked increase in capillary wall permeability without immune deposits or histologic changes; and idiopathic rapidly progressive glomerulonephritis (RPGN) is characterized by severe glomerular inflammatory changes with crescent formation without detectable immune deposits.

The type and severity of histologic and functional glomerular disease induced by immune deposits in glomeruli depend on many factors, including the quantity, composition, and site of the deposits. Most glomerular antibody deposits contain predominantly IgG, which activates complement via the classic complement pathway. When deposits are in mesangial and subendothelial sites they are accessible to circulating inflammatory cells. Chemotactic and immune adherence mechanisms recruit participation of neutrophils and macrophages, and these effector cells cause direct damage to glomeruli by release of proteolytic enzymes and toxic oxygen metabolites. An inflammatory glomerular lesion results, with clinical manifestations that include hematuria, proteinuria, and loss of renal function. IgA deposits activate complement less well and predominantly by the alternate complement pathway. When immune deposits form at a subepithelial site, as in membranous nephropathy, they are not accessible to circulating cells and the resulting lesion is a noninflammatory one, with the nephrotic syndrome apparently induced by a direct effect of the C5b-9, or membrane attack complex, portion of complement on capillary wall permeability. Thus, glomerular immune complex deposits may induce a spectrum of both clinical and histologic manifestations. The clinical consequences range from the acute nephritic syndrome with acute renal failure, as seen in some cases of post-streptococcal glomerulonephritis, to idiopathic nephrotic syndrome with

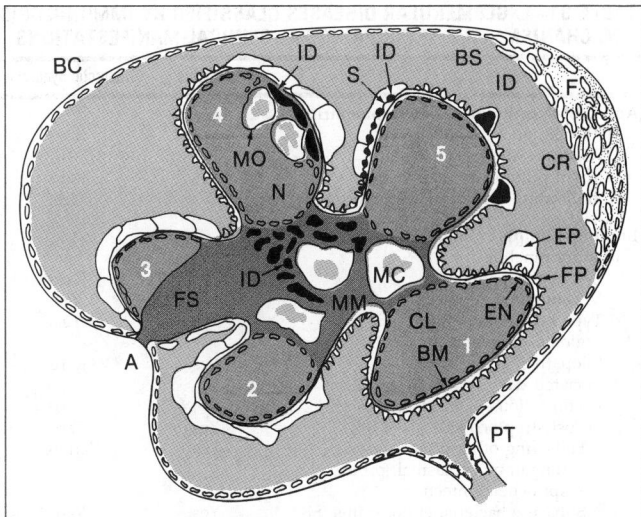

FIGURE 81–1. A highly schematized illustration of a cross-section of a single glomerulus showing normal glomerular architecture and some of the characteristic changes seen in glomerular diseases. One lobule with five capillary loops is illustrated within Bowman's capsule (BC). The capillary loops are supported by the intercapillary mesangium, containing mesangial cells (MC) and mesangial matrix (MM). Note that the normal glomerular capillary wall (loop 1) is composed of three layers: Endothelial cells (EN), basement membrane (BM), and epithelial cells (EP) with epithelial cell foot processes (FP).

Loop 2 illustrates minimal change nephrotic syndrome with only diffuse effacement, or "fusion," of epithelial cell foot processes. Foot process effacement is also seen in other areas where increased capillary permeability with proteinuria would occur. In loop 3 a focal sclerotic lesion (FS) is seen with collapse of the capillary loop and adhesion (A) to Bowman's capsule. Immune complex deposits (ID) are shown in black at three sites: within the mesangial matrix (loop 4); as subendothelial deposits between endothelial cells and basement membrane as seen in class IV SLE and type I MPGN (loop 4); and as the diffuse, finely granular subepithelial deposits of membranous nephropathy (left, loop 5) with intervening "spikes" (S) of basement membrane, or the larger, more widely spaced subepithelial humps (right, loop 5) seen in post-streptococcal glomerulonephritis. Mesangial and subendothelial deposits usually elicit an infiltrate of neutrophils (N) and monocytes (MO) that may displace endothelial cells and directly injure basement membrane, as shown in loop 4. With severe injury, fibrin (F) leakage into Bowman's space (BS) may induce formation of a cellular crescent (CR) composed of proliferating parietal epithelial cells and circulating mononuclear cells as shown from 1 to 3 o'clock. CL = Capillary lumen; PT = proximal tubule.

normal renal function, as in membranous nephropathy. Table 81–1 lists the glomerular diseases, classified by the mechanisms that produce them and with their major clinical presentations noted.

ACUTE GLOMERULONEPHRITIS
Pathophysiology of the Acute Nephritic Syndrome

The terms *acute GN* and *acute nephritic syndrome*, which are synonymous, refer to the abrupt onset of hematuria and proteinuria, usually associated with some impairment in renal function and often with retention of salt and water, leading to hypertension and edema. Virtually all of these abnormalities are present in patients with post-streptococcal GN (PSGN) but are less frequently found in other causes of the acute nephritic syndrome. The most common primary renal diseases that produce the acute nephritic syndrome are summarized in Table 81–2, where their major distinguishing clinical and pathologic features are compared. The syndrome may also result from membranoproliferative glomerulonephritis (MPGN), which is discussed under diseases that cause the nephrotic syndrome, and from glomerular involvement in several of the systemic diseases to be discussed subsequently.

HEMATURIA. Hematuria is the hallmark of the acute

TABLE 81–1. GLOMERULAR DISEASES CLASSIFIED BY IMMUNOLOGIC MECHANISMS AND THEIR PRINCIPAL CLINICAL MANIFESTATIONS

	Nephritis	Nephrotic Syndrome
Anti-GBM Antibody Glomerulonephritis		
With pulmonary involvement (Goodpasture's syndrome)	Yes	Rare
Without pulmonary involvement	Yes	Rare
Complicating membranous nephropathy	Yes	Yes
Immune Complex Glomerulonephritis		
Primary renal diseases		
IgA nephropathy	Yes	Rare
Membranous nephropathy	No	Yes
Type I membranoproliferative glomerulonephritis (MPGN)	Yes	Yes
Idiopathic	Yes	Rare
Associated with systemic diseases		
Postinfectious glomerulonephritis		
Post-streptococcal	Yes	Rare
Following other bacterial, viral, fungal, mycoplasmal, protozoal, spirochetal infections	Yes	Variable
Subacute bacterial endocarditis (SBE)	Yes	Rare
"Shunt nephritis"	Yes	Yes
Visceral abscesses	Yes	No
Collagen vascular diseases		
Systemic lupus erythematosus (SLE)	Yes	Yes
Henoch-Schönlein purpura (HSP)	Yes	Yes
Essential mixed cryoglobulinemia (EMC)	Yes	Yes
Diseases of Undefined but Probably Immune Pathogenesis		
Minimal change–focal sclerosis group	No	Yes
Idiopathic rapidly progressive glomerulonephritis (RPGN)	Yes	Rare
Type II MPGN (dense deposit disease)	Yes	Yes
Vasculitides: Polyarteritis nodosa (PAN)	Yes	Rare
Hypersensitivity vasculitis	Yes	No
Wegener's granulomatosis	Yes	Rare
Hemolytic uremic syndrome (HUS) and thrombotic thrombocytopenic purpura (TTP)	Rare	No

nephritic syndrome. When hematuria is associated with proteinuria (> 500 mg per day) and red blood cell (RBC) casts, it usually reflects an acute glomerular inflammatory process that may have the potential for rapid loss of renal function. RBC's probably reach the urine through breaks or "gaps" in the capillary wall and form casts as they become embedded in concentrated tubular fluid with an increased protein concentration. Hematuria and RBC casts may occasionally be seen in other diseases in which capillary wall disruption occurs, such as malignant hypertension and hereditary nephritis.

PROTEINURIA. In acute GN, proteinuria invariably accompanies hematuria but rarely exceeds 3.5 grams per day and is therefore in the "non-nephrotic" range. Proteinuria in acute GN reflects an increased urinary content of serum proteins due to some combination of three factors: (1) a generalized increase in the permeability characteristics of the glomerular capillary wall itself, (2) altered glomerular hemodynamics, and (3) mechanical disruptions in capillary wall structure. Thus proteinuria in acute GN is "nonselective" and contains serum globulins as well as albumin. The pathophysiology of glomerular protein excretion is discussed in more detail below under "Nephrotic Syndrome."

IMPAIRED RENAL FUNCTION. When glomerular inflammation severe enough to cause hematuria and proteinuria is present, the glomerular filtration rate (GFR) is usually reduced. This may range from a minimal reduction in GFR with normal serum creatinine values to oliguria or anuria requiring dialysis. Multiple factors account for the reduced GFR, including the effects of acute immune injury on glomerular pathophysiology and the development of glomerular intracapillary thromboses, acute tubular necrosis secondary to glomerular ischemia, tubular obstruction by casts, and compression of the glomerular tuft by proliferating epithelial cells forming crescents. The return of renal function to normal depends not only on cessation of the process that initiated the injury but also on the extent of irreversible structural changes that have occurred, such as necrosis, sclerosis, and fibrosis.

HYPERTENSION. Hypertension is a common manifestation of the acute nephritic syndrome in PSGN and may be a presenting sign in older patients. It is largely volume dependent, reflecting impaired renal excretion of sodium and water with reduced levels of plasma renin and aldosterone. Hypertension can generally be controlled by strict adherence to sodium restriction.

EDEMA. Edema in the acute nephritic syndrome, like hypertension, reflects extracellular fluid volume expansion due to renal retention of salt and water. The mechanisms of renal sodium retention in acute GN are poorly understood but include a reduced filtered sodium load as well as enhanced

TABLE 81–2. SUMMARY OF PRIMARY RENAL DISEASES THAT PRESENT AS ACUTE GLOMERULONEPHRITIS

Diseases	Post-streptococcal Glomerulonephritis (PSGN)	IgA Nephropathy	Goodpasture's Syndrome	Idiopathic Rapidly Progressive Glomerulonephritis (RPGN)
Clinical Manifestations				
Age and sex	All ages, mean 7, 2:1 male	15–35, 2:1 male	15–30, 6:1 male	Mean 58, 2:1 male
Acute nephritic syndrome	90%	50%	90%	90%
Asymptomatic hematuria	Occasionally	50%	Rare	Rare
Nephrotic syndrome	10–20%	Rare	Rare	10–20%
Hypertension	70%	30–50%	Rare	25%
Acute renal failure	50% (transient)	Very rare	50%	60%
Other	1–3 week latent period	Follows viral syndromes	Pulmonary hemorrhage; iron deficiency anemia	None
Laboratory Findings	↑ ASO titers (70%) Positive streptozyme (95%) ↓ C3–C9 Normal C1, C4	↑ Serum IgA (50%) IgA in dermal capillaries	Positive anti-GBM antibody	None
Immunogenetics	HLA-B12, D "EN" (9)*	HLA-Bw 35, DR4 (4)*	HLA-DR2 (16)*	None established
Renal Pathology				
Light microscopy	Diffuse proliferation	Focal proliferation	Focal→diffuse proliferation with crescents	Crescentic GN
Immunofluorescence	Granular IgG, C3	Diffuse mesangial IgA	Linear IgG, C3	No immune deposits
Electron microscopy	Subepithelial humps	Mesangial deposits	No deposits	No deposits
Prognosis	95% resolve spontaneously 5% RPGN or slowly progressive	Slow progression in 25–50%	75% stabilize or improve if treated early	75% stabilize or improve if treated early
Treatment	Supportive	None established	Plasma exchange, steroids, cyclophosphamide	Steroid pulse therapy

*Relative risk

sodium reabsorption in either the distal nephron or deep juxtamedullary nephrons. Edema and fluid retention are seen in over 90 per cent of patients with acute PSGN but are less common in other diseases causing the acute nephritic syndrome. Unlike nephrotic edema, edema in the nephritic syndrome is often present in nondependent areas such as eyelids, face, and hands. The key to management is effective sodium restriction, since diuretics may not be effective in the acute stage of GN.

Couser WG: Mechanisms of glomerular injury in immune-complex disease. Kidney Int 28:569, 1985. *A current, in-depth review of the pathogenetic mechanisms that underlie immune glomerular diseases.*
Madaio MP, Harrington JT: Medical intelligence. Current concepts: The diagnosis of acute glomerulonephritis. N Engl J Med 309:1299, 1983. *This short review provides a useful outline of the diagnosis and classification of acute glomerulonephritis, emphasizing the distinctive clinical and laboratory features of each of the diseases that cause the acute nephritic syndrome.*
Whitley K, Keane WF, Vernier RL: Acute glomerulonephritis: A clinical overview. Med Clin North Am 68:259, 1984. *This article reviews the pathogenetic mechanisms, clinical presentations, laboratory features, and renal biopsy findings in each of the major disease entities that cause acute glomerulonephritis.*

Isolated Hematuria

The presence of persistent abnormal hematuria (more than five RBC's per high-power field in more than one fresh-voided urine specimen), without systemic disease, RBC casts, significant proteinuria, or impaired renal function, is a common medical problem that may or may not reflect renal parenchymal disease. It is more common in children and adolescents than in adults. A careful medical and urologic evaluation must be performed with appropriate laboratory, radiologic, and urologic procedures to exclude nonglomerular lesions of the urinary tract such as infection, prostatism, papillary necrosis, polycystic and medullary sponge kidney, renal or urinary tract tumors, arteriovenous malformations, renal stones, blood dyscrasias, and hemoglobinopathies. The "loin pain-hematuria syndrome" is a disorder usually seen in young women taking oral contraceptives who develop recurrent episodes of gross hematuria accompanied by loin pain and mild hypertension in the absence of proteinuria or reduced renal function. The condition appears to be benign and is reversible when oral contraceptives are discontinued.

If no cause of hematuria can be found and no evidence of systemic or renal disease is present, isolated hematuria appears to be a benign entity, and only careful follow-up is indicated. Renal biopsy would be performed in such patients only if evidence of progressive renal disease developed or if the patient required further evaluation for other purposes such as insurance or employment. When such patients do undergo renal biopsy, the results usually reveal a mild, nonprogressive form of glomerular disease, often focal GN with or without mesangial IgA deposits. Only about 20 per cent of such patients will have normal renal biopsies.

Copley JB: Isolated asymptomatic hematuria in the adult. Am J Med Sci 29:101, 1986. *An excellent review of the causes of hematuria and the approach to diagnosis with a useful algorithm for evaluating patients who have only hematuria without proteinuria or renal dysfunction.*
Trachtman H, Weiss RA, Bennett B, et al.: Isolated hematuria in children: Indications for a renal biopsy. Kidney Int 25:94, 1984. *This paper reviews the findings in 76 children and adolescents biopsied for isolated hematuria and identifies a family history of hematuria and episodes of gross hematuria as the best predictors of significant renal pathology.*

Isolated Proteinuria

A more detailed discussion of proteinuria is given in Ch. 76. Like isolated hematuria, non-nephrotic range proteinuria *without* hematuria or decreased renal function may indicate a significant glomerular disease, but usually does not. When increased urinary protein excretion is suggested by qualitative analyses such as the dipstick, it must be confirmed by an accurate measurement of 24-hour protein excretion. Values in excess of 150 mg per day in adults, and 140 mg per square meter per day in children, are regarded as abnormal if an accurate 24-hour urine collection has been obtained. Abnormal protein excretion may be intermittent or persistent (fixed).

INTERMITTENT PROTEINURIA. The most common causes of intermittent proteinuria are *exercise*, assumption of the *upright position* (postural proteinuria), and *fever*. Up to 10 per cent of routine medical admissions may exhibit transient proteinuria. The basis for proteinuria in most of these conditions is probably hemodynamic (see above), although subtle alterations in glomerular architecture have not been excluded. Total protein excretion is usually less than 2.0 grams per day, renal function is normal, and 20-year follow-up studies have shown resolution of the proteinuria in a majority of cases with no evidence of progressive renal disease.

PERSISTENT PROTEINURIA. Persistent or fixed proteinuria can also occur without glomerular disease. *"Overflow" proteinuria* occurs when excess production of filterable, low molecular weight proteins exceeds the tubular reabsorptive capacity, as occurs with the production of lysozyme (molecular weight 14,000) in myelomonocytic leukemia or L-chains in plasma cell dyscrasias such as multiple myeloma. In some cases up to 5.0 grams of L-chains may be excreted daily. Another nonglomerular cause of proteinuria is renal tubular disease in which normal quantities of proteins such as lysozyme or beta$_2$-microglobulin are filtered but not reabsorbed. This can result in urinary excretion of up to 2.0 grams of such proteins daily in a variety of interstitial nephropathies and disorders of tubular function.

Isolated, fixed, non-nephrotic proteinuria of glomerular origin is associated with an increased incidence of hypertension and a somewhat decreased life expectancy in long-term follow-up studies, but progressive renal disease is rare. Renal biopsy in such patients usually reveals some glomerular abnormality. The spectrum of lesions in isolated proteinuria is wide and similar to that discussed above in isolated hematuria. In patients with fixed proteinuria of less than 2.0 grams per day without hematuria, systemic disease, or impaired renal function, renal biopsy is usually not performed unless a change in clinical status occurs or the patient requests a biopsy for other purposes.

Abuelo JG: Proteinuria: Diagnostic principles and procedures. Ann Intern Med 98:186, 1983. *A well-written summary of the different types of proteinuria, their causes and prognosis, with emphasis on the approach to evaluation of patients with mild proteinuria and normal renal function.*

SPECIFIC RENAL DISEASES THAT PRESENT AS ACUTE GLOMERULONEPHRITIS (GN) (see Table 81–2)

The prototype of acute postinfectious GN is post-streptococcal GN (PSGN), but glomerular disease may follow infection with a variety of other bacterial and nonbacterial agents: both gram-positive and gram-negative bacteria, viruses, mycoplasma, fungi, protozoa, helminths, and spirochetes. Many of these associations have been noted only in patients with endocarditis or infected ventriculoatrial shunts. It is important to distinguish between specific postinfectious glomerular diseases such as PSGN and the nonspecific role of many infections, particularly viral illnesses, in producing "exacerbations" of underlying glomerular disease. These exacerbations are usually evidenced by a transient increase in proteinuria and hematuria associated with the infection, usually without an intervening latent period.

Post-Streptococcal Glomerulonephritis (PSGN)

Etiology, Incidence, and Epidemiology. GN occurs only following infection with a group A (beta-hemolytic) streptococcus of nephritogenic M type, usually type 12 in the United States. Streptococcal pharyngitis is the most common antecedent event in the North, and PSGN occurs with a frequency of less than 5 per cent after a latent period of 6 to 20 days (average 10). The disease is often sporadic, occurs in the winter and spring, is more common in males, and is accompanied by serologic evidence of recent streptococcal infection in over 80 per cent of cases. In the South streptococcal pyoderma or impetigo is more common, the attack rate is higher (25 to 50 per cent), the latent period is longer (14 to 21 days, average 20), and the disease affects males and females equally, often occurring in epidemic form in more temperate climates in the summer and fall.

Pathogenesis. Granular immune complex deposits in glomeruli cause the clinical and histologic features of PSGN. The presence of these deposits, hypocomplementemia, and the latent period between infection and the onset of GN suggest that the disease is similar to experimental acute serum sickness, in which acute GN is mediated by formation of glomerular deposits containing antigen and antibody to it eight to ten days following a single injection of antigen. The deposits are thought to reflect glomerular trapping of circulating immune complexes, but they may also form on a local basis. Streptococcal antigens have been identified in glomerular deposits early in PSGN in some patients. The presence of C3 in the deposits and the prominent infiltrate of neutrophils and mononuclear cells in the acute stage suggest a lesion that is mediated by complement, neutrophils, and macrophages.

Pathology. Figure 81–2 illustrates the typical findings in acute PSGN by light microscopy, IF, and EM. The histologic lesion in PSGN is a diffuse (all glomeruli involved) proliferative GN with a marked hypercellularity involving glomerular endothelial and mesangial cells, as well as neutrophils and mononuclear cells with narrowing or occlusion of capillary loops (Fig. 81–2A). Proliferation of epithelial cells in Bowman's space results in formation of glomerular "crescents" in severe disease. Extensive crescent formation is seen in about 5 per cent of patients and correlates with a more severe initial disease and reduced likelihood of complete recovery. Coarsely granular deposits of IgG and C3 occur along the glomerular capillary walls and in the mesangium (Fig. 81–2B). By EM there are discrete electron-dense subepithelial nodules or "humps" (Fig. 81–2C) that persist for about eight weeks. Subepithelial humps are a highly characteristic feature of PSGN, although they may occasionally be seen in other types of bacterial postinfectious GN and type I MPGN.

Clinical Findings. PSGN is the prototype of the acute nephritic syndrome and causes all of the findings discussed above under "Pathophysiology of the Acute Nephritic Syndrome." The disease is most common in children between 3 and 12 years of age, with a mean age of about 7, and is rare in infancy and in adults over 50. The typical presentation of

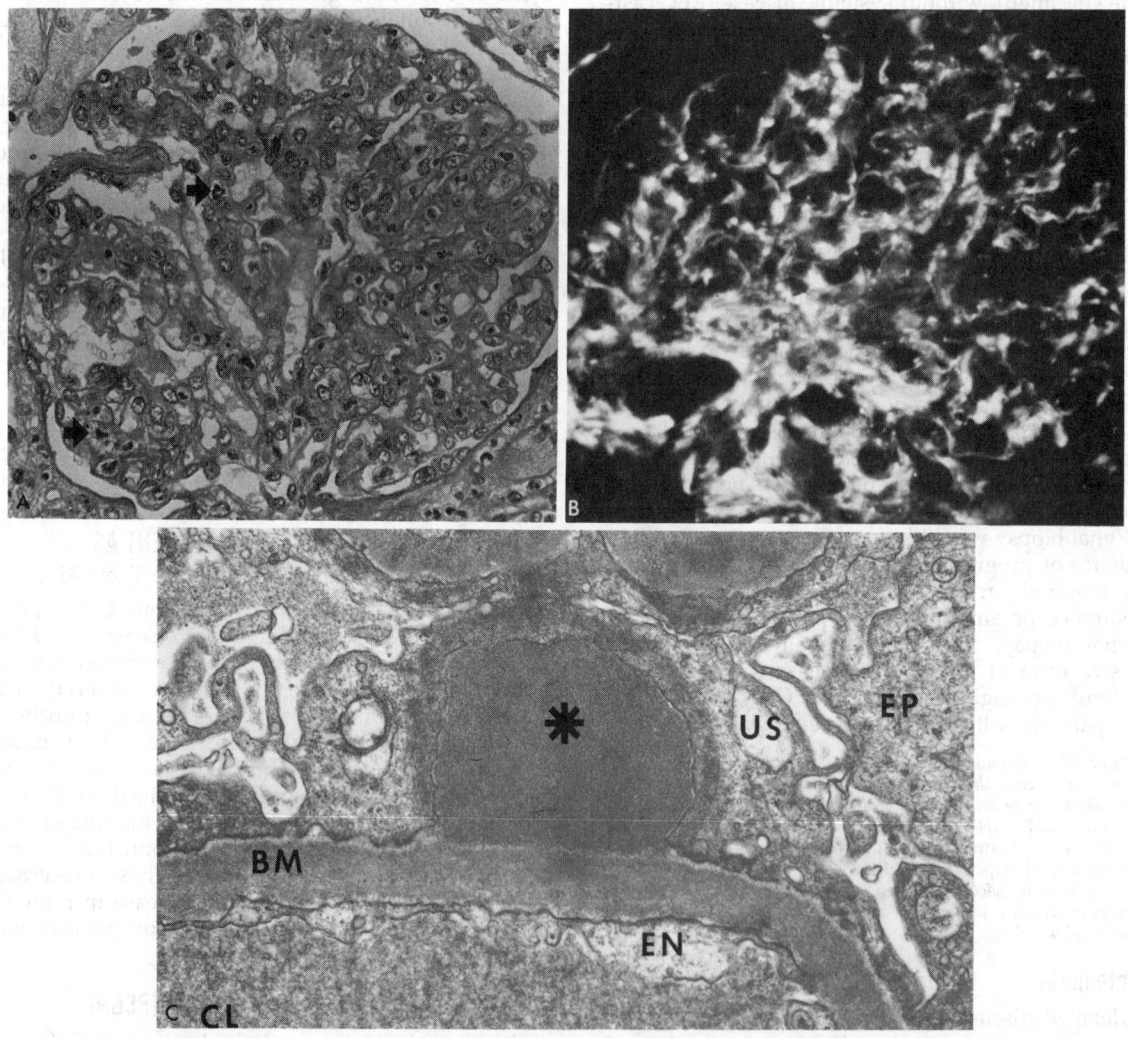

FIGURE 81–2. The renal lesion of post-streptococcal glomerulonephritis (PSGN). *A,* Light microscopic section of a renal biopsy from a patient with acute PSGN showing a marked increase in glomerular cells and infiltration by polymorphonuclear leukocytes (*arrows*) (periodic acid–Schiff stain; × 300). *B,* Immunofluorescent staining for IgG from the same biopsy reveals a coarse granular pattern of deposits on the capillary walls and in the mesangium (× 350). *C,* Electron microscopy in acute PSGN reveals a characteristic electron-dense "hump" on the subepithelial surface (*) with effacement of epithelial foot processes around the deposit. BM = Basement membrane; CL = capillary lumen; EN = endothelial cell; EP = epithelial cell; US = urinary space (× 14,400). (Reproduced with permission from Couser WG, Salant DJ, Stilmant MM. In Flamenbaum W, Hamburger RJ (eds.): Nephrology. Philadelphia, JB Lippincott Company, 1982, pp 265–301.)

PSGN is the abrupt onset of hematuria (90 per cent), which is usually evident as dark or *"smoky" urine*, accompanied by *malaise* and sometimes gastrointestinal symptoms such as abdominal pain, nausea, and vomiting. Central nervous system manifestations may include headaches and occasionally seizures. *Edema* is an early and frequent sign, often in a periorbital distribution most evident on arising and sometimes progressing to peripheral edema and anasarca. *Hypertension* is present in 60 to 70 per cent of patients and reflects renal retention of salt and water with volume overload. Proteinuria is usually present as well. About 20 per cent of hospitalized patients develop nephrotic range proteinuria, usually transiently and during the recovery phase. Renal function is impaired in about 50 per cent of patients.

Prognosis. Three clinical courses can be defined in PSGN: complete recovery, no recovery, or partial recovery with progressive disease. In over 90 per cent of cases complete recovery occurs with spontaneous diuresis in an average of four to seven days. Even patients who require dialysis during the acute phase usually recover spontaneously without specific therapy. Abnormal hematuria and proteinuria may persist for up to two years. Progressive renal disease is a very uncommon consequence of PSGN, however, if renal function returns to normal and proteinuria is less than 500 mg per day.

Fewer than 5 per cent of patients with PSGN have oliguria lasting more than nine days; the prognosis in these patients is worse. Although spontaneous complete recovery has been reported with oliguria or anuria for up to 25 days, this is unusual. Many patients with prolonged oliguria will have a crescentic glomerular lesion. About half of these will still recover spontaneously. In the remainder, the disease behaves like rapidly progressive glomerulonephritis (RPGN) with no recovery at all or with only partial recovery of renal function, which may be followed by persistent proteinuria and progressive renal disease leading to renal failure in months to years. Patients with PSGN who have oliguric renal failure lasting over one week, particularly adults, should undergo a renal biopsy. If extensive crescent formation is found they should be considered for therapy as outlined below under "Treatment."

Laboratory Features. Laboratory findings consist of an abnormal urinalysis, elevated antibodies against streptococcal exoenzymes, and reduced serum complement levels. The urinalysis usually reveals signs of glomerular inflammation with proteinuria, RBC's, white blood cells (WBC's), and casts. RBC casts are present in 60 to 85 per cent of cases when a freshly voided urine is examined. The urine is often concentrated and exhibits biochemical characteristics of prerenal azotemia, including a low urine sodium, indicating severe glomerular disease with good preservation of tubular function.

Beta-hemolytic streptococci are detected by culture in only 25 per cent of untreated patients, but serologic tests generally confirm recent streptococcal infection. The anti–streptolysin O (ASO) titer exceeds 200 Todd units within one to three weeks and may remain elevated for months. An increase in ASO titer may not be seen if penicillin therapy is initiated early or if the antecedent infection was in the skin. Antibodies to other streptococcal enzymes are usually elevated as well. The streptozyme test utilizes five of these antigens in a single assay and is quite sensitive and specific. Over 90 per cent of patients with PSGN have a reduced level of total hemolytic complement or C3 during the first two weeks of illness, with most returning to normal within eight weeks. The pattern of complement component depression suggests alternate pathway activation, with levels of C1q and C4 usually normal.

Diagnosis. The differential diagnosis of acute GN with hypocomplementemia includes other forms of postinfectious GN such as subacute bacterial endocarditis (SBE) or shunt nephritis, systemic lupus erythematosus (SLE), and type I membranoproliferative glomerulonephritis (MPGN). Only MPGN is difficult to exclude by clinical and laboratory criteria. A similar pattern of alternate complement pathway activation is seen in MPGN, a disease that also may occasionally follow streptococcal infection (see p. 597), and MPGN must be considered when nephrotic range proteinuria and hypocomplementemia persist for longer than two months. The diagnosis of PSGN can usually be made by the presence of typical clinical features of the acute nephritic syndrome following a streptococcal infection by an appropriate latent period, and by hypocomplementemia and serologic evidence of recent streptococcal infection. Because patients with PSGN usually recover spontaneously and no specific therapy is indicated, the diagnosis is often made clinically without a renal biopsy. Biopsy is indicated, however, if atypical features are present, such as prolonged oliguria, anuria, persistent hypocomplementemia, the nephrotic syndrome, or clinical or serologic evidence of systemic disease.

Treatment. In most patients with PSGN there is no need for specific therapy, since spontaneous recovery can be anticipated. Antibiotics should be given if cultures are positive for group A streptococci, but penicillin therapy does not alter the incidence or severity of PSGN. Manifestations of sodium retention such as hypertension, edema, and congestive heart failure can usually be managed with careful sodium restriction, but diuretics and antihypertensive agents may be employed if necessary. Dialysis may be required temporarily in some patients, most of whom will still recover normal renal function spontaneously.

There are no data on which to base a recommendation for therapy in patients with prolonged oliguria and a crescentic glomerular lesion on biopsy. Although up to 50 per cent of such patients may recover spontaneously, the prognosis is sufficiently guarded to warrant considering therapy with pulse steroids or plasma exchange as outlined below under RPGN.

Nissenson AR, moderator: Post-streptococcal acute glomerulonephritis: Fact and controversy. Ann Intern Med 91:76, 1979. *An excellent overview of the microbiology, epidemiology, clinical manifestations, laboratory features, pathogenesis, and sequelae of PSGN, with 128 references.*
Rodriguez-Iturbe B: Epidemic poststreptococcal glomerulonephritis. Kidney Int 25:129, 1984. *An excellent review of the pathogenesis, laboratory findings, clinical features, and long-term prognosis in acute post-streptococcal nephritis, with 65 references.*

Glomerulonephritis in Subacute Bacterial Endocarditis (SBE)

Glomerular disease in SBE ranges in severity from the proteinuria and hematuria seen in 70 per cent of patients, usually with normal renal function, to occasional cases of crescentic GN with acute renal failure. It is more common in chronic cases with right-sided cardiac involvement and negative blood cultures, as may occur in patients who abuse drugs. A wide variety of organisms have been implicated, most commonly *Staphylococcus aureus* and *Streptococcus viridans*. A similar syndrome may be seen in patients with infected ventriculoatrial shunts for hydrocephalus (shunt nephritis), often due to *Staphylococcus albus*. Serologic abnormalities are often present, including hypocomplementemia with activation of both the classic and the alternate complement pathways, cryoglobulinemia, and positive rheumatoid factor. Renal biopsy usually demonstrates a focal proliferative GN, often with necrosis and intra-capillary thrombi. Granular deposits of IgG, IgM, and C3 occur in mesangial and subendothelial areas, implicating an immune complex rather than an embolic mechanism in the pathogenesis of the lesion. Renal function usually returns to normal following appropriate antibiotic therapy and eradication of the infection. However, recovery may be slow if the lesion is severe or crescents are present.

Feinstein EI, Eknoyan G, Lister BJ, et al.: Renal complications of bacterial endocarditis. Am J Nephrol 5:457, 1985. *This discussion, with 69 references, of endocarditis and glomerulonephritis in a patient who is an intravenous drug abuser presents a comprehensive review of glomerular disease associated with both endocarditis and drug abuse.*

Neugarten J, Gallo GR, Baldwin DS: Glomerulonephritis in bacterial endocarditis. Am J Kidney Dis 3:371, 1984. *This paper reviews 107 patients with endocarditis and notes that 22 per cent had glomerulonephritis with a spectrum of renal lesions and that Staphylococcus aureus was the predominant organism. The relationship among renal lesion, therapy, and prognosis is discussed.*

Glomerulonephritis with Visceral Abscesses

The abrupt onset of acute renal failure associated with proteinuria, hematuria, and red cell casts may occur in patients with a pyogenic visceral abscess. Abscesses are most frequently located in the respiratory tract but have been reported at numerous other sites, including the abdomen and uterus. Endocarditis may be present but usually is not, and blood cultures are commonly negative. In contrast to PSGN, SBE, and shunt nephritis, serologic studies, including complement levels, are usually normal. A variety of bacteria have been implicated. The glomerular lesion is usually a proliferative GN with crescents, and monocytes may be prominent in glomeruli. IF and EM studies usually do not reveal immune deposits, so that the pathogenesis of this lesion is unclear. Recovery of renal function has occurred in about half of the patients reported with acute renal failure who were successfully treated to eradicate the infection, but the overall mortality is quite high.

Beaufils M: Glomerular disease complicating abdominal sepsis. Kidney Int 19:609, 1981. *A detailed review of nonstreptococcal postinfectious glomerulonephritis, including SBE- as well as abscess-related lesions. The frequency with which renal biopsies reveal glomerular disease as a cause of acute renal failure in patients with sepsis is striking, since most such patients would not be as extensively studied in the United States.*

Glomerular Disease in Acquired Immunodeficiency Syndrome (AIDS)

Up to 50 per cent of patients with AIDS have abnormal proteinuria and 10 per cent develop nephrotic syndrome. A variety of glomerular, tubular, and interstitial lesions have been noted, presumably induced by infections, drug exposure, and other factors. However, a majority of patients with nephrotic syndrome have focal glomerular sclerosis (see p. 594). A rapid loss of renal function may occur in this subset of patients.

Rao TKS, Filippone EJ, Nicastri AD, et al.: Associated focal and segmental glomerulosclerosis in the acquired immunodeficiency syndrome. N Engl J Med 310:669, 1984. *This paper documents the significant incidence of proteinuria and nephrotic syndrome in patients with AIDS associated with a lesion of focal segmental glomerulosclerosis usually accompanied by rapid deterioration of renal function.*

IgA Nephropathy (Berger's Disease)

Overview and Incidence. In 1968 Jean Berger reviewed 55 biopsies of children with so-called benign hematuria, idiopathic hematuria, or recurrent hematuria of childhood and noted a high frequency of mesangial IgA deposits and a variety of glomerular lesions, most commonly focal GN. IgA nephropathy is the commonest cause of primary glomerular disease in Europe, Australia, and probably the United States. The disease is now regarded as a monosymptomatic form of *Henoch-Schönlein purpura* (HSP), but clinical manifestations are milder than in HSP and are usually confined to the kidney. HSP is discussed later in this chapter and also in Ch. 166.

Pathogenesis. The pathogenesis of the renal lesion in IgA nephropathy and HSP is not known. It appears to be a consequence of mesangial formation of immune deposits composed predominantly of IgA (see Fig. 81–3B). The IgA probably represents the antibody component of an immune complex containing a nonrenal antigen. A similar glomerular lesion may develop in liver disease associated with elevated portal pressure. The glomerular IgA deposits appear to be predominantly polymeric and of mucosal origin, which may reflect the association of disease activity with viral infections of the upper respiratory and gastrointestinal tracts.

Pathology. The typical lesion of IgA nephropathy has a focal distribution, meaning that some glomeruli are involved while others are spared, and is also segmental, with lesions in some glomerular tufts but not others (Fig. 81–3A). Mesangial expansion and hypercellularity are common, but the characteristic lesion is a focal and segmental proliferative GN. When crescents are present they are usually small and rarely involve more than 30 per cent of glomeruli. Immune deposits are present diffusely in the mesangium of all glomeruli and contain IgA as the predominant immunoglobulin, accompanied by C3 in 60 per cent and IgG in 30 per cent of cases (Fig. 81–3B). C1q and C4 are usually absent, suggesting alternate complement pathway activation. Some patients have deposits along the subendothelial aspect of the capillary wall

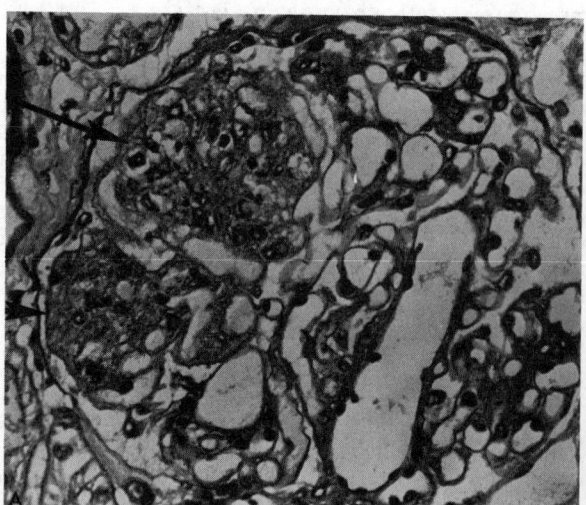
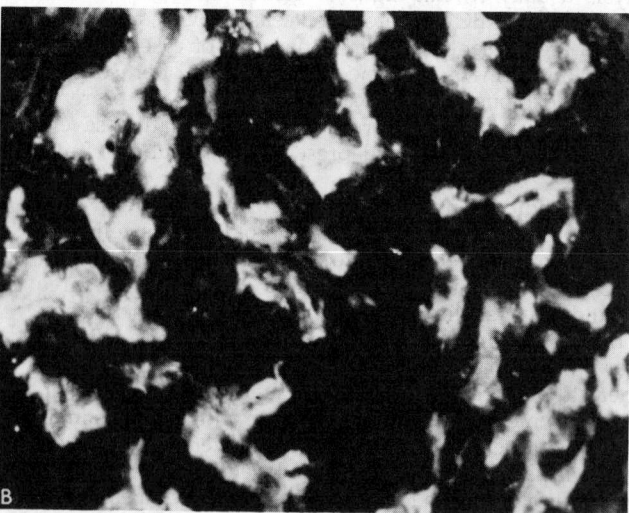

FIGURE 81–3. The renal lesion of IgA nephropathy. *A,* Light microscopic section from a patient with gross hematuria and focal glomerulonephritis due to IgA nephropathy. There is segmental involvement of the glomerulus, which shows mesangial matrix increase and hypercellularity in two lobules (*arrows*). Adjacent lobules are essentially normal (periodic acid–Schiff stain, × 350). *B,* Immunofluorescence microscopy on the same biopsy reveals bright, diffuse staining for IgA in all mesangial areas. No significant capillary wall staining is present. IgG and C3 may be found in a similar pattern but with less intensity (× 450). (Reproduced from Couser WG, Salant DJ, Stilmant MM. In Flamenbaum W, Hamburger RJ (eds.): Nephrology. Philadelphia, JB Lippincott Company, 1982, pp 265–301.)

or in the subepithelial space and generally have more severe disease and more proteinuria.

Clinical and Laboratory Findings and Diagnosis. IgA nephropathy is two to three times more common in males than in females, and most patients present before the age of 35. The classic presentation is with *gross hematuria* that occurs coincident with, or immediately following (24 to 48 hours), a viral upper respiratory infection (50 per cent), flu-like illness (15 per cent), a gastrointestinal syndrome (10 per cent), or other infectious prodrome. Associated findings often include mild fever, malaise, myalgias, dysuria, and loin pain. The remainder of cases are identified during medical evaluation for persistent, asymptomatic hematuria or proteinuria. The absence of a latent period, as well as normal levels of complement and anti-streptococcal antibodies, distinguishes this disease clinically from PSGN. Moreover, other features of the acute nephritic syndrome, including edema and hypertension, are seen in fewer than half of the patients. Only about 25 per cent of patients have impaired renal function during active disease, and the serum creatinine rarely exceeds 3 mg per deciliter. Proteinuria is usually less than 1 gram per day.

Gross hematuria usually lasts only two to six days, but microscopic hematuria often persists between attacks. Fifty per cent of patients will have only a single episode of gross hematuria. The remainder have recurring episodes for many years, usually "triggered" by viral infections.

There are no laboratory findings diagnostic of IgA nephropathy. About half of all patients have elevated serum levels of IgA that do not correlate with disease activity. Circulating immune complexes containing IgA are present intermittently, and deposits of IgA, C3, and fibrin may be present in the dermal capillaries of normal skin. The incidence of this disease is greater in persons with HLA-Bw 35 and HLA-DR4 phenotypes.

Course and Prognosis. Progression to renal failure occurs in 15 to 20 per cent of patients within 6 months, and a 50 per cent death or dialysis rate is projected over 20 years. While there are no clinical or pathologic features that permit accurate prediction of progression, patients who tend to do worse are male, have a prolonged clinical course, develop hypertension or proteinuria exceeding 3 grams per day, or have extensive glomerular sclerosis present on biopsy.

Treatment. No specific form of therapy has been shown to alter the long-term clinical course of this disease. Rigorous control of hypertension is important. Mesangial deposits of IgA occur with a high frequency in renal allografts but rarely compromise graft function.

Boyce NW, Holdsworth SR, Thomson NM, et al.: Clinicopathological associations in mesangial IgA nephropathy. Am J Nephrol 6:246, 1986. *Data are presented on the clinical features and histopathology of 112 patients, emphasizing presenting manifestations and features predictive of long-term course.*
Rodicio JL: Idiopathic IgA nephropathy. Kidney Int 25:717, 1984. *An in-depth review of the differential diagnosis, clinical features, pathology, diagnosis, course, and therapy of IgA nephropathy, with an appended commentary on pathogenesis by Michael P. Madaio, M.D.*

Rapidly Progressive Glomerulonephritis (RPGN)

Overview. The term RPGN is applied to any glomerular disease in which rapid loss of renal function occurs in association with extensive crescent formation in many glomeruli, usually over 50 per cent (Fig. 81–4). Volhard and Fahr first noted the association between crescents and a poor prognosis in 1914, and the term RPGN was first applied by Ellis in 1942.

RPGN may occur in severe cases of a wide variety of glomerular diseases, which are listed in Table 81–3, or it may occur alone as a primary renal disease. The classification system used here is based on pathogenetic mechanisms. Accurate prognosis and selection of appropriate therapy require that the underlying mechanisms be defined. About 20 per cent of cases of RPGN are mediated by anti-GBM antibody deposition and 40 per cent by glomerular immune complex formation (usually in association with some systemic disease

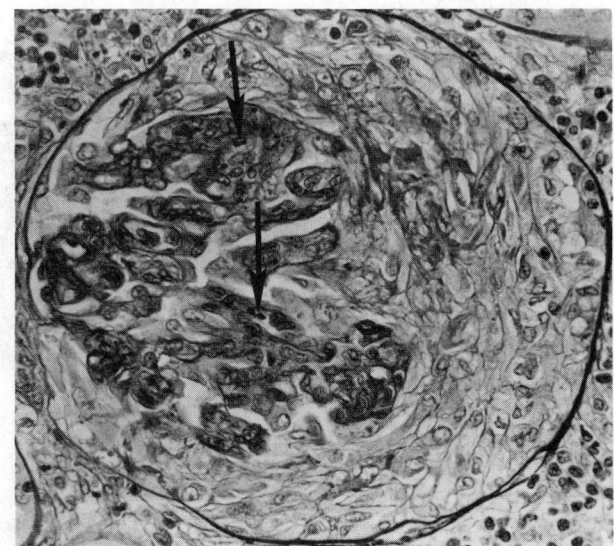

FIGURE 81–4. Light microscopy from a patient with idiopathic RPGN reveals the presence of a large cellular crescent in Bowman's space surrounding and compressing the glomerular capillary. A few polymorphonuclear leukocytes are seen in the glomerulus (*arrows*) (periodic acid–Schiff stain, × 275). (Reproduced from Couser WG, Salant DJ, Stilmant MM. In Flamenbaum W, Hamburger RJ (eds.): Nephrology. Philadelphia, JB Lippincott Company, 1982, pp 265–301.)

process such as PSGN or SLE), and 40 per cent are primary renal lesions with no significant glomerular immune deposits, which are classified here as idiopathic RPGN (Table 81–3).

RPGN DUE TO ANTI-GBM ANTIBODY. Although much is known of the mediation of immune glomerular injury from studies of experimental anti-GBM nephritis, this mechanism accounts for fewer than 5 per cent of cases of GN seen clinically. Anti-GBM GN is characterized by the abrupt onset of a proliferative GN, usually with crescents, and a characteristic linear deposition of IgG along the GBM by IF (Fig. 81–5). In about two thirds of cases, pulmonary hemorrhage accompanies GN, and the disease is termed Goodpasture's syndrome. The remaining one third of patients have anti-GBM nephritis without pulmonary involvement.

Goodpasture's Syndrome. PATHOGENESIS. The events that initiate anti-GBM antibody production are not known. Anti-

TABLE 81–3. CLASSIFICATION OF RAPIDLY PROGRESSIVE (CRESCENTIC) GLOMERULONEPHRITIS

Type of RPGN	Frequency
Anti-GBM Antibody–Mediated RPGN	20%
Goodpasture's syndrome	
Idiopathic anti-GBM nephritis	
Membranous nephropathy with crescents	
RPGN Associated with Granular Immune Deposits	40%
Postinfectious	
Post-streptococcal glomerulonephritis	
Bacterial endocarditis	
"Shunt" nephritis	
Visceral abscesses, other nonstreptococcal infections	
Noninfectious	
Systemic lupus erythematosus	
Henoch-Schönlein syndrome	
Mixed cryoglobulinemia	
Solid tumors	
Primary Renal Disease	
Membranoproliferative glomerulonephritis	
IgA nephropathy	
Idiopathic "immune complex" nephritis	
RPGN Without Glomerular Immune Deposits	40%
Vasculitis	
Polyarteritis	
Hypersensitivity vasculitis	
Wegener's granulomatosis	
Idiopathic RPGN	

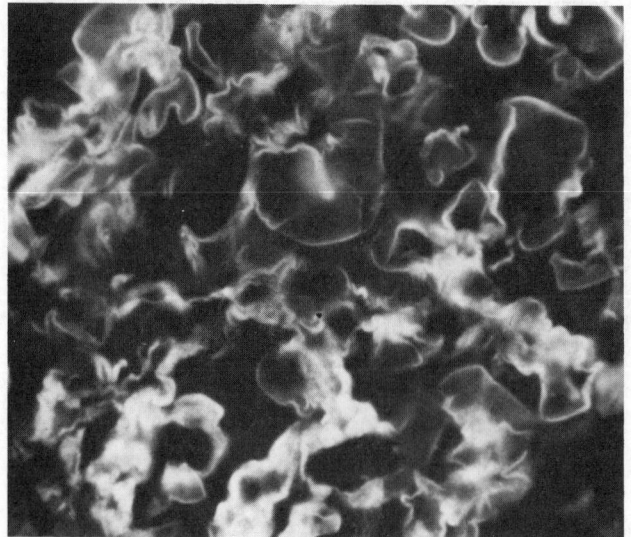

FIGURE 81–5. Immunofluorescence microscopy on a renal biopsy from a patient with Goodpasture's syndrome reveals continuous, uninterrupted, linear deposition of IgG along all capillary walls. This pattern is characteristic of anti-GBM disease (× 450). (Reproduced from Couser WG, Salant DJ, Stilmant MM. In Flamenbaum W, Hamburger RJ (eds.): Nephrology. Philadelphia, JB Lippincott Company, 1982, pp 265–301.)

body reactive with GBM and alveolar basement membrane mediates the glomerular disease in anti-GBM nephritis with and without pulmonary hemorrhage. The development of lung hemorrhage appears to require the presence of prior lung damage to allow antibody deposition. Genetic factors are clearly important in this disease. There is a strong association with HLA-DRw2 (relative risk 15 to 34 times normal). Anti-GBM antibody production is a self-limited event usually lasting several months. Exacerbations of disease associated with increased antibody levels may be triggered by infectious complications. Antibody binding to GBM mediates glomerular injury by mechanisms that involve complement activation and participation of both neutrophils and macrophages. Fibrin deposition in Bowman's space is believed to initiate glomerular crescent formation.

PATHOLOGY. The early histologic lesion in Goodpasture's syndrome is a focal proliferative and necrotizing GN that progresses to diffuse involvement with crescent formation. Extensive interstitial infiltrates may also be present, perhaps due to antibody deposition on tubular basement membranes. There is a characteristic, continuous, linear pattern of IgG deposition along the capillary wall, accompanied by C3 in about 70 per cent of cases (Fig. 81–5). Tubular basement membrane deposits may also occur. EM is not diagnostic.

CLINICAL FEATURES. Goodpasture's syndrome is a disease of young males (6:1 male-to-female ratio) characterized by a triad of *pulmonary hemorrhage, GN,* and *anti-GBM antibody production.* It usually begins with pulmonary hemorrhage manifest as hemoptysis, pulmonary alveolar infiltrates by x-ray, dyspnea, and iron deficiency anemia. The pulmonary symptoms are followed within days to weeks by development of hematuria, proteinuria, and rapid loss of renal function. Over half of patients with Goodpasture's syndrome are azotemic when first seen. Hypertension and fluid retention are uncommon. Preceding flu-like illness or exposure to other pulmonary toxins such as volatile hydrocarbon solvents and cigarettes is common. Until recently, 80 per cent of cases required treatment for end-stage renal disease within one year, although some patients with mild disease recover spontaneously. Up to 30 per cent of patients may die as a consequence of the pulmonary hemorrhage.

LABORATORY FINDINGS AND DIAGNOSIS. The only laboratory finding specific for anti-GBM nephritis is the demonstration

of antibody to GBM in the serum or as linear deposits of IgG in glomeruli. The antibody can be detected quickly in serum by indirect IF using normal human kidney substrate in a test that is similar to the fluorescent antinuclear antibody test. The indirect IF assay is positive in 80 to 90 per cent of patients with Goodpasture's syndrome. A more sensitive radioimmunoassay is also commercially available and is positive in over 95 per cent of patients. It is urgent to make a diagnosis and to initiate therapy early in RPGN of all types. An anti-GBM assay, as well as a renal biopsy, should therefore be obtained as soon as possible after the diagnosis of RPGN is suspected. The demonstration of anti-GBM antibody is critical, since a variety of other diseases may result in similar pulmonary and renal manifestations, including SLE, polyarteritis nodosa, Wegener's granulomatosis, and other forms of systemic necrotizing vasculitis.

TREATMENT. As in all forms of RPGN, the success of treatment is critically dependent upon how quickly it is initiated. The overall survival rate in Goodpasture's syndrome has risen from less than 10 per cent 15 years ago to over 50 per cent today owing to earlier diagnosis and detection of milder cases, better general medical care, and probably some improvements in specific therapy for the disease. There is little evidence that oral steroids or immunosuppressive agents alone significantly alter the course of the renal lesion. The pulmonary hemorrhage commonly responds either to high-dose oral prednisone therapy or to intravenous "pulse" methylprednisolone (see treatment of idiopathic RPGN below). However, steroid pulse therapy does not appear to benefit the renal lesion. Most centers now treat anti-GBM disease with vigorous plasma exchange therapy combined with prednisone, 1 mg per kilogram per day, and cyclophosphamide, 2 to 3 mg per kilogram per day. Plasma exchanges of up to 4 liters per day are performed on a daily or alternate-day basis until anti-GBM antibody is no longer detectable in the circulation and disease progression has halted. Therapy may require several weeks. Replacement is with albumin, or, when pulmonary hemorrhage is active, with fresh frozen plasma. Overall survival in anti-GBM nephritis appears to be improved by plasma exchange therapy. However, the response rate in patients who are oliguric on presentation or who have serum creatinines exceeding 6 mg per deciliter is very low, again emphasizing the need for early diagnosis. In patients with end-stage renal disease due to anti-GBM nephritis, renal transplantation appears to be safe if delayed until anti-GBM antibody is no longer detectable in the serum.

Anti-GBM Glomerulonephritis Without Pulmonary Hemorrhage. Some patients have the same anti-GBM antibody–mediated renal disease as seen in Goodpasture's syndrome, but antibody localization does not occur in lungs and pulmonary hemorrhage is therefore absent. The patients are generally older than those with Goodpasture's syndrome (mean age about 50), and males and females are equally affected. In all other respects, the clinical and pathologic findings, course, and treatment are the same as those discussed above for Goodpasture's syndrome. Because such patients present with an idiopathic form of acute RPGN without pulmonary hemorrhage and may respond to plasma exchange therapy, it is important that the possibility of anti-GBM nephritis be considered in all patients who present in this fashion and that circulating anti-GBM antibody studies and renal biopsy be performed early.

Savage COS, Pusey CD, Bowman C, et al.: Antiglomerular basement membrane antibody mediated disease in the British Isles 1980–4. Br Med J 292:301, 1986. *Experience with 71 patients in a single center is reviewed, disclosing two patterns of disease: young women in their twenties with Goodpasture's syndrome and women in their sixties with glomerulonephritis alone. The poor response to plasma exchange in patients with serum creatinine levels exceeding 6 mg per deciliter or in those requiring dialysis is emphasized.*

Walker RG, Scheinkestel C, Becker GJ, et al.: Clinical and morphological aspects of the management of crescentic anti–glomerular basement membrane antibody (anti-GBM) nephritis/Goodpasture's syndrome. Q J Med 543:75,

1985. This review of 22 patients with anti-GBM nephritis details the clinical features of this disease. Anuria and greater than 80 per cent crescents are identified as poor prognostic signs, and a beneficial effect of plasma exchange is suggested.

RPGN DUE TO GLOMERULAR IMMUNE COMPLEX FORMATION. Patients with RPGN associated with granular deposits of immunoglobulin and complement in glomeruli account for about 40 per cent of all patients seen with crescentic GN. In most cases the glomerular disease is a manifestation of some well-defined systemic illness such as SLE, Henoch-Schönlein purpura, or other forms of vasculitis, or of another well-defined primary renal disease such as PSGN, MPGN, or, rarely, IGA nephropathy. In all of these disorders the correct diagnosis can usually be made from the associated clinical, laboratory, and pathologic findings. Prognosis depends considerably on the underlying disease. For example, about 50 per cent of patients with RPGN secondary to streptococcal infection will recover spontaneously without specific therapy, while in RPGN due to SLE spontaneous recovery virtually never occurs. Therapy for the glomerular disease per se is the same as that outlined below under treatment for idiopathic RPGN and includes the use of methylprednisolone pulse therapy and/or plasma exchange.

IDIOPATHIC RPGN. *Pathogenesis.* RPGN as a primary renal disease is usually not associated with significant glomerular deposits of anti-GBM or immune complexes. The disease mechanism in such patients is undefined but probably immune in nature. Whatever the mechanism leading to capillary wall damage, leakage of fibrin into Bowman's space apparently initiates epithelial cell proliferation and crescent formation. Some of the vague prodromal clinical manifestations, as well as the presence of crescentic GN without immune deposits, are quite similar to findings in several of the vasculitides. This disease may be a form of vasculitis and may share a common pathogenetic mechanism, although inflammatory changes are confined primarily to the glomerular capillaries.

Pathology. There is extensive glomerular crescent formation with circumferential cellular crescents usually involving 50 to 100 per cent of glomeruli (see Fig. 81–4). Earlier cases may show fewer or smaller crescents and later ones reveal more fibrosis of crescents and glomerular obsolescence. There is a rough correlation between the percentage of glomeruli with crescents, the severity of clinical disease, and the prognosis. Changes in the glomerular tuft itself may be minimal. Prominent proliferative changes suggest a postinfectious etiology and a better prognosis. Interstitial changes are frequently prominent, and vasculitis is absent. Fibrinogen and fibrin polymers are present in the crescents. The glomeruli at most show only focal granular deposits of IgM and C3, which are nonspecific. EM may show "gaps" or rupture of the capillary wall but usually does not show immune deposits.

Clinical Manifestations and Diagnosis. Idiopathic RPGN is a disease of older patients (mean age 58). There is a slight male predominance. The disease tends to present in clusters. Many patients have a prodrome that resembles a viral illness with myalgias; arthralgias; loin, back, and abdominal pain; fever; and malaise. Minor hemoptysis is common, and fleeting pulmonary infiltrates may be seen by x-ray. No specific inciting events have been identified. RPGN presents as an acute nephritic syndrome, including *hematuria, proteinuria,* and *rapidly decreasing renal function,* often without hypertension or edema. As in anti-GBM nephritis, the progression of renal disease is usually very rapid, with up to 50 per cent of patients oliguric at the time of presentation and half of these sufficiently uremic to require immediate dialysis. The remaining patients may require dialysis within one to three weeks. At the time of presentation the disease is often relatively acute and potentially reversible.

The laboratory features of idiopathic RPGN are entirely nonspecific. ASO titers, antinuclear and anti-GBM antibodies, circulating immune complexes, and complement levels are normal or negative. The diagnosis is made by renal biopsy in a patient with deteriorating renal function, evidence of glomerular disease in the urine sediment, absence of anti-GBM antibody, and lack of clinical or serologic evidence of other systemic diseases such as SLE.

Treatment and Prognosis. Treatment with oral steroids and/or cytotoxic agents has been of little apparent benefit, and a death or dialysis rate of about 75 per cent in two years is reported. Favorable prognostic factors include a young age at the time of onset, a history of a preceding infectious episode, absence of oliguria and hypertension, serum creatinine below 6 mg per deciliter at presentation, and fewer than 50 per cent crescents in the renal biopsy. Success rates approaching 75 per cent have been reported in patients treated with either methylprednisolone pulse therapy or plasma exchange. Methylprednisolone, 30 mg per kilogram to a maximum of 3 grams, is given intravenously over 20 minutes on a daily or alternate-day basis three times, followed by oral prednisone, 2 mg per kilogram, which is tapered over several months. About 75 per cent of patients, including some who were oliguric and on dialysis, have shown a dramatic response, with a return of renal function to normal or nearly normal levels. Responses have generally been evident within five to ten days and have continued over four to six weeks. However, long-term follow-up data in such patients are limited, and some will progress to renal failure later despite an impressive initial response. Very similar results have been reported in patients treated with intensive plasma exchange (plus prednisone and cyclophosphamide). This treatment is extremely expensive and, compared with pulse therapy, probably has a higher incidence of complications, primarily bleeding and infection. Neither form of therapy has yet been shown in a prospective, controlled study to improve long-term patient or kidney survival over what might be achieved with more conservative measures. Until such data are available, the author's feeling is that both pulse therapy and plasma exchange probably do represent significant advances in the treatment of idiopathic RPGN. Steroid pulse therapy is safer and cheaper and appears to be as effective as plasma exchange. There are no data on the efficacy of cytotoxic drugs in this disease. However, if there is evidence of segmental necrotizing glomerular lesions or systemic manifestations consistent with vasculitis, cyclophosphamide should probably be given concurrently with steroids.

Idiopathic RPGN appears to recur rarely in allografted kidneys.

Couser WG: Idiopathic rapidly progressive glomerulonephritis. Am J Nephrol 2:57, 1982. *This review discusses the classification, clinical features, pathology, pathogenesis, and treatment of idiopathic RPGN in considerable detail, with 159 references.*

Glassock RJ: Natural history and treatment of primary proliferative glomerulonephritis: A review. Kidney Int 28:S136, 1985. *In this review of treatment of several forms of glomerulonephritis, the section on crescentic glomerulonephritis provides a thoughtful and comprehensive review of the literature on treatment of RPGN, with useful guidelines and recommendations.*

Hind CRK, Paraskevakou H, Lockwood CM, et al.: Prognosis after immunosuppression of patients with crescentic nephritis requiring dialysis. Lancet 1:263, 1983. *This paper reviews the experience with plasma exchange and immunosuppression in 48 patients with all forms of RPGN and acute renal failure requiring dialysis. No patients with acute anti-GBM disease responded, while about two thirds of patients with other forms of RPGN, including idiopathic, vasculitic, and Wegener's, showed a sustained improvement in renal function. The urgency of early diagnosis is emphasized.*

NEPHROTIC SYNDROME

The nephrotic syndrome is not a disease; it is a group of signs and symptoms commonly seen in patients with glomerular diseases that are characterized by a marked increase in capillary wall permeability to serum proteins rather than (or sometimes in addition to) glomerular inflammatory changes. The primary abnormality in nephrotic syndrome is the excretion of large amounts (greater than 3.5 grams per day) of protein in the urine. Other manifestations that may occur

TABLE 81–4. SUMMARY OF PRIMARY RENAL DISEASES THAT PRESENT AS IDIOPATHIC NEPHROTIC SYNDROME

	Minimal Change Nephrotic Syndrome (MCNS)	Focal Glomerular Sclerosis (FGS)	Membranous Nephropathy	Membranoproliferative Glomerulonephritis (MPGN)	
				Type I	*Type II*
Frequency*					
Children	75%	10%	<5%	10%	
Adults	15%	15%	50%	10%	
Clinical Manifestations					
Age	2–6, some adults	2–6, some adults	40–50	5–15	
Sex	2:1 male	1.3:1 male	2:1 male	male-female	
Nephrotic syndrome	100%	90%	80%	60%	
Asymptomatic proteinuria	0	10%	20%	40%	
Hematuria	20%	60–80%	60%	80%	
Hypertension	10%	20% early	Infrequent	35%	
Rate of progression	Does not progress	10 years	50% in 10–20 years	10–20 years	5–15 years
Associated conditions	Allergy, Hodgkin's disease	None	Renal vein thrombosis, cancer, SLE	None	Partial lipodystrophy
Laboratory Findings	Manifestations of nephrotic syndrome	Manifestations of nephrotic syndrome	Manifestations of nephrotic syndrome	Low C1, C4, C3–C9	Normal C1, C4, low C3–C9 C3 nephritic factor
Immunogenetics	HLA-B8, B12 (3.5)†	Not established	HLA-DRW3 (12–32)†	Not established	
Renal Pathology					
Light microscopy	Normal	Focal sclerotic lesions	Thickened GBM, spikes	Thickened GBM, proliferation, lobulation	
Immunofluorescence	Negative	IgM, C3 in lesions	Fine granular IgG, C3	Granular IgG, C3	C3 only
Electron microscopy	Foot process fusion	Foot process fusion	Subepithelial deposits	Mesangial and subendothelial deposits	Dense deposits
Response to Steroids	90%	15–20%	May slow progression	Not established	

*Approximate frequency as a cause of idiopathic nephrotic syndrome. About 10 per cent of adult nephrotic syndrome is due to various diseases that usually present with acute glomerulonephritis (Table 81–2).
†Relative risk.

secondary to *proteinuria* include *hypoalbuminemia, edema, hyperlipidemia*, and *lipiduria*. In contrast to the acute nephritic syndrome, the onset of the nephrotic syndrome is usually insidious, gross hematuria and red cell casts are infrequent, and renal function is often normal at the time of presentation.

The list of diseases that may cause the nephrotic syndrome is extensive and includes virtually every disorder that may affect the glomerulus. About one third of adults and 10 per cent of children have the nephrotic syndrome as a manifestation of some systemic disease, usually diabetes, SLE, or amyloidosis. In two thirds of adults, and most children, the nephrotic syndrome is idiopathic and a manifestation of one of three types of primary glomerular disease: minimal change nephrotic syndrome (MCNS) or its variants, membranous nephropathy, or membranoproliferative glomerulonephritis (MPGN). The relative frequencies of these diseases and their identifying characteristics are presented for comparison in Table 81–4. It is important to note that the occurrence of the nephrotic syndrome in patients over 45 may be associated with occult malignancy. The association of Hodgkin's disease with MCNS and of solid tumors of the lung, breast, and GI tract with membranous nephropathy is discussed below. All of the diseases discussed in the section on acute GN can also cause the nephrotic syndrome, although they do not commonly do so.

Pathophysiology of the Nephrotic Syndrome

PROTEINURIA. Glomeruli are normally perfused with plasma containing over 60,000 grams of protein per day, but less than 150 mg of protein is excreted in the final urine. The filtration barrier, which includes the endothelial cells, basement membrane, epithelial cells, and slit diaphragms, restricts the transcapillary passage of proteins on the basis of their size, shape, and electrical charge. The size barrier is primarily at the level of the endothelial cells and GBM. It restricts filtration of molecules between about 18 and 42 Å and effectively prevents filtration of neutral molecules larger than 42 Å. Circulating proteins such as albumin (36 Å) are further

restricted from crossing the capillary wall by an electrical charge barrier conferred by the polyanionic sialoprotein coating on endothelial and epithelial cells and heparan sulfate–proteoglycans in the lamina rara externa and interna. Thus, molecules with a net negative charge (anionic) are less freely filtered, or encounter smaller "pores" in the capillary wall, than positively charged (cationic) molecules of the same size. Most serum proteins are anionic at physiologic pH and may be filtered in increased amounts if the charge barrier is reduced, as it is in some glomerular diseases.

Glomerular hemodynamic factors also alter protein filtration. Thus, in situations of reduced renal perfusion, renal blood flow (RBF) may be reduced while GFR is maintained by adaptive changes in other determinants of GFR such as intracapillary hydraulic pressure. Under these circumstances the filtration fraction (GFR/RBF) is increased, resulting in a higher than normal protein concentration at the efferent end of the glomerular capillary. This may produce an increased diffusion of protein across the capillary wall, resulting in proteinuria in the absence of glomerular disease in conditions such as congestive heart failure and other states of reduced renal perfusion (see isolated proteinuria above).

Proteinuria, the hallmark of the nephrotic syndrome, exceeds 3.5 grams per day in adults or 40 mg per square meter per hour in children. Fixed nephrotic range proteinuria with the nephrotic syndrome generally occurs only in the presence of diffuse glomerular disease. The immune mechanisms that may cause an increase in the permselective properties of the glomerular capillary wall may induce a loss of net negative charge on the capillary wall, as appears to occur in MCNS, leading to a marked increase in urinary albumin excretion without significant change in the excretion of other serum proteins (*selective proteinuria*). Other diseases with extensive capillary wall immune deposits, such as membranous nephropathy, or disorders of basement membrane biochemistry or structure, such as those found in diabetes or hereditary nephritis, are associated with apparent structural defects and increased filtration of all serum proteins (*nonselective proteinuria*). Over 40 grams of protein may be excreted in the urine each day in some patients. It is this loss of protein that leads to the other clinical and biochemical manifestations of the nephrotic syndrome.

HYPOALBUMINEMIA. Serum albumin concentration decreases to less than 3.0 grams per deciliter when the rate of urinary protein loss and renal catabolism of filtered albumin (which may exceed 10 grams per day in the nephrotic syndrome) exceeds the rate of hepatic synthesis. Hepatic albumin synthesis is normally 12 to 14 grams per day in adults and may increase in the nephrotic syndrome but can be limited by various factors, including age, poor nutritional status, and liver disease. Thus, some patients may exhibit significant hypoalbuminemia with proteinuria of less than 10 grams per day, while others excreting larger amounts of protein are better able to maintain serum albumin levels.

EDEMA. Edema in the nephrotic syndrome results in part from a reduction in plasma oncotic pressure such that capillary hydraulic pressure exceeds oncotic pressure in peripheral capillaries and fluid leaves the capillaries. Although the reduction in effective circulating volume that occurs may result in increased renal retention of salt and water through normal compensatory mechanisms, over 50 per cent of patients with the nephrotic syndrome have normal or increased plasma volume and normal or low levels of plasma renin during sodium retention, suggesting a primary renal contribution to salt retention in the nephrotic syndrome through mechanisms that remain poorly defined.

HYPERLIPIDEMIA. Hyperlipidemia is common in the nephrotic syndrome and is inversely proportional to the serum albumin concentration. Hypercholesterolemia and elevated phospholipids are the most constant abnormalities observed, but increased levels of low and very low density lipoproteins, triglycerides, and chylomicrons are also seen. The primary mechanism appears to be increased hepatic synthesis of cholesterol, triglycerides, and lipoproteins, but reduced catabolism of these compounds has also been demonstrated.

LIPIDURIA. In a nephrotic urine sediment lipids are seen as free fat, oval fat bodies (degenerated renal tubular epithelial cells containing cholesterol esters), and fatty casts, all of which exhibit a Maltese cross pattern under polarizing light. Lipiduria parallels the level of urine protein excretion rather than the serum lipid levels.

Complications of the Nephrotic Syndrome

The most clinically important metabolic complications of the nephrotic syndrome are severe protein malnutrition, which may require appropriate nutritional supplementation, hypercoagulability with a tendency to form thrombi in both renal and peripheral veins leading to thromboembolic complications, and acute renal failure.

Hypercoagulability is thought to be a consequence of altered clotting factor levels in the nephrotic syndrome, including reduced levels of factors IX, XI, and XII; elevated levels of factors V and VIII, fibrinogen, beta-thromboglobulin, and platelets; a reduction in levels of antithrombin III and antiplasmin; and increased susceptibility of platelets to aggregation. There is a high incidence (10 to 40 per cent) of thrombus formation in renal, pulmonary, and peripheral veins, and occasionally in arteries, with frequent thromboembolic phenomena. The incidence of renal vein thrombosis appears to be particularly high in patients with the nephrotic syndrome due to membranous nephropathy. Routine anticoagulation is not indicated unless emboli occur.

Acute renal failure in the nephrotic syndrome very rarely occurs owing to rapid progression of the underlying renal disease, since most diseases that cause the nephrotic syndrome progress very slowly. However, acute renal failure does occur as a consequence of several potentially treatable disorders superimposed on nephrotic glomerular disease. These include (1) reduced renal perfusion due to low plasma volume, which can result in acute tubular necrosis, particu-

larly following a surgical procedure or biopsy; (2) interstitial renal edema in patients with MCNS and significant peripheral edema, who may develop intrarenal swelling sufficient to produce increased intrarenal pressure, cessation of filtration, and acute renal failure (this may be reversible with diuretic therapy); (3) drug-induced allergic interstitial nephritis, particularly in patients receiving diuretic therapy; (4) bilateral acute renal vein thrombosis; and (5) reduced glomerular perfusion due to nonsteroidal anti-inflammatory drugs, which inhibit synthesis of vasodilatory prostaglandins and reduce glomerular plasma flows in states of volume contraction or diffuse glomerular disease. Nonsteroidal anti-inflammatory agents may also cause acute allergic interstitial nephritis, which may be accompanied by a reversible nephrotic syndrome with a glomerular lesion like that in MCNS.

Other complications that may also be associated with the nephrotic syndrome include reduced levels of IgG (which may dispose to bacterial infection), proximal tubular dysfunction with signs of Fanconi's syndrome, deficiencies of trace metals such as iron, copper, and zinc, and loss of vitamin D with development of osteomalacia and secondary hyperparathyroidism. Measurements of thyroid function such as T_4 radioimmunoassay and T_3 resin uptake may falsely suggest reduced function, but free T_4 and TSH levels are generally normal.

Coggins CH: Management of nephrotic syndrome. In Brenner BM, Stein JH (eds.): Contemporary Issues in Nephrology. Vol 9. New York, Churchill Livingstone, 1982, p 283. *A clear review of the approach to clinical management of each of the systemic manifestations of nephrotic syndrome independent of the glomerular disease that causes them.*

Kaysen GA, Myers BD, Couser WG, et al.: Biology of disease: Mechanisms and consequences of proteinuria. Lab Invest 54:479, 1986. *An in-depth review that correlates the pathophysiology of glomerular protein filtration with observations in patients with nephrotic syndrome and discusses the mechanisms and the consequences of massive urinary protein loss.*

Reineck HJ: Mechanisms of edema formation in the nephrotic syndrome. In Brenner BM, Stein JH (eds.): Contemporary Issues in Nephrology. Vol 9. New York, Churchill Livingstone, 1982, p 31. *A clear and comprehensive analysis of this controversial topic, with suggestions on management.*

Primary Renal Diseases That Present as the Nephrotic Syndrome

Minimal Change Nephrotic Syndrome (MCNS)

As indicated in Table 81–4, MCNS accounts for about 75 per cent of cases of idiopathic nephrotic syndrome in children and up to 20 per cent of adults. Synonyms include minimal change disease, nephropathy or glomerulopathy, lipoid nephrosis, and nil disease.

Pathogenesis. The pathogenesis of MCNS is not known. The disease is characterized by a loss of net negative charge on the capillary wall and can recur promptly in the transplanted kidney, suggesting the presence of a circulating factor that neutralizes or destroys glomerular polyanion, resulting in loss of the charge barrier and a selective type of proteinuria. The association of MCNS with Hodgkin's disease, its responsiveness to steroids and alkylating agents, and the tendency for remission to follow some viral infections, particularly measles, have focused attention on the possibility of an abnormality in T lymphocytes, perhaps involving production of a lymphokine with properties that induce increased glomerular capillary permeability. However, attempts to demonstrate such a substance have not been successful thus far.

Pathology. By definition, the diagnosis of MCNS requires the absence of abnormalities by light microscopy and of immune deposits by IF. Diffuse epithelial cell foot process effacement, or "fusion," is the abnormality usually seen by EM, but some morphologic abnormalities may occur in MCNS, including mild-to-moderate focal or diffuse proliferation of mesangial cells; mesangial deposits of IgM, IgA, or C3 by IF; and the presence of focal glomerular sclerosis (FGS) by light microscopy. In the presence of FGS, response to steroids is poor, and progressive loss of renal function is commonly seen. This has led several authors to consider FGS as a separate disease (see below). However, in some patients the FGS lesion appears to develop late in the course of MCNS and may simply be a histologic marker of a more severe and less responsive form of MCNS mediated by a similar mechanism.

Mesangial proliferation and mesangial IgM deposits may occur together or separately and usually predict a poor (or delayed) response to steroids and an increased possibility of progression. As with FGS, there have been attempts to classify such patients into separate disease categories (mesangial-proliferative GN, IgM nephropathy). When progression occurs in patients with MCNS and mesangial proliferation and/or IgM deposits, glomeruli develop changes typical of FGS.

Clinical Features. The peak incidence of MCNS is in children two to six years of age, in whom it virtually always presents as a full-blown nephrotic syndrome. In childhood, males are affected twice as commonly as females. One third of patients will have a preceding upper respiratory tract infection or other identifiable antecedent event. In the absence of volume contraction, renal function and blood pressure are normal, but up to one third of patients may have a reduced GFR when first seen due to hypovolemia and reduced renal perfusion. Urine protein excretion may exceed 40 grams per day in severe cases, and serum albumin is less than 2.0 grams per deciliter in over 90 per cent of children. The complications of this disease are discussed above under complications of the nephrotic syndrome in general. In addition, there is an association between MCNS and Hodgkin's disease in which the nephrotic syndrome may be the presenting sign of an occult lymphoma. Allergic reactions to nonsteroidal anti-inflammatory agents may produce nephrotic syndrome and MCNS on biopsy, usually associated with interstitial nephritis and reduced renal function.

Laboratory Findings. The laboratory findings in MCNS are those of the nephrotic syndrome of any etiology. Proteinuria is "selective" (greater than 90 per cent albumin) in about 85 per cent of cases. Complement levels are usually normal. A consistent finding is a marked reduction in ASO titers (less than 100 Todd units).

Course and Treatment. Before steroids and modern antibiotics were available the spontaneous remission rate in MCNS was estimated at 25 to 40 per cent. During that era, the mortality rate in children exceeded 50 per cent in five years owing to infections or thromboembolic complications. The mortality rate now is about 7 to 12 per cent in nephrotic children and less than 2 per cent in those who respond to steroids. Some of this improvement reflects the development of effective antibiotics and better general medical care. Steroid therapy has never been shown in a controlled study to improve survival in patients with MCNS. However, the usual dramatic resolution of the nephrotic syndrome following steroid administration, as well as the fact that survival has improved since the presteroid era, has led to the widespread belief that such treatment is beneficial.

Conventional doses of oral prednisone are 60 mg per square meter per day in children and 2 mg per kilogram per day in adults, given daily for four weeks, followed by alternate-day therapy for four more weeks and then a tapering course over four to six months. Within four weeks, 90 per cent of children will have responded, and 90 per cent of adults will respond within about eight weeks. There is little value in continuing steroid therapy beyond eight weeks if abnormal levels of proteinuria persist. The 10 per cent of patients who fail to respond generally have FGS (see below).

Of the steroid responders, roughly 50 per cent will remain free of proteinuria or develop infrequent relapses that respond to steroids, eventually entering permanent remission. The remainder will either become "frequent relapsers" (more than twice a year) or steroid dependent, often with a high incidence of steroid side effects. Some can be managed conservatively with salt restriction, diuretics, and a high-protein diet. In children, the clinical manifestations of the nephrotic syndrome are usually more severe, and steroid toxicity may require the use of an additional drug. Both cyclophosphamide, 2 to 3 mg per kilogram per day (75 mg per square meter per day in children), and chlorambucil, 0.2 to 0.3 mg per kilogram per day, given for 8 to 12 weeks, have been shown to increase the frequency and duration of remission in steroid-sensitive MCNS. However, because of their gonadal toxicity, teratogenic potential, and other side effects, these agents should be used only when both the nephrotic syndrome and steroid side effects are severe. About half of such patients treated with a second drug are reported to be in remission four years later, suggesting that complete remission can be achieved with drug therapy in almost 90 per cent of patients with MCNS.

Hoyer JR: Idiopathic nephrotic syndrome with minimal glomerular changes. In Brenner BM, Stein JH (eds): Contemporary Issues in Nephrology. Vol 9. New York, Churchill Livingstone, 1982, p 145. *This is an excellent and current review of all aspects of MCNS, including the clinical features, pathogenesis, pathology, and treatment.*

Nolasco F, Cameron JS, Heywood EF, et al.: Adult-onset minimal change nephrotic syndrome: A long-term follow-up. Kidney Int 29:1215, 1986. *This paper reviews the clinical course and response to therapy in 89 adults with MCNS and documents a higher incidence of complications and slower response to therapy compared with children with this disease.*

Focal Glomerular Sclerosis (FGS)

Overview. FGS is a histologic lesion found in some patients with otherwise typical MCNS, and it correlates well with steroid resistance and progressive renal failure. Controversy exists regarding whether it should be classified as a separate glomerular disease or should be viewed as one end of a spectrum that ranges from pure steroid-responsive MCNS with no morphologic abnormalities to typical FGS. This spectrum includes patients who have either mesangial proliferation by light microscopy and/or mesangial IgM deposits with or without evidence of FGS. The author favors the views that mesangial proliferation, mesangial IgM deposits, and FGS are part of the MCNS spectrum. However, the clinical features of patients with idiopathic nephrotic syndrome and FGS in early biopsies are sufficiently different from those who do not have these lesions to warrant separate consideration.

Pathogenesis. The etiology and pathogenesis of the lesion of FGS are unknown. Presumably, the basic mechanism underlying the generalized increase in capillary wall permeability may be the same as that in MCNS, and the structural lesion may be the consequence of either the greater severity of this process in such patients or the presence of some additional, as-yet-unidentified factor(s). Experimentally, a marked increase in mesangial trafficking and deposition of circulating macromolecules occurs in association with altered glomerular permeability. Mesangial dysfunction, with loss of contractile properties and regulation of local capillary loop hemodynamics, may precede the development of FGS. This could result in persistent glomerular vasodilatation, hypertension, and hyperfiltration, with consequent structural damage to the capillary wall.

Pathology. The diagnosis of FGS is made by renal biopsy in which sclerotic lesions are seen only in some glomeruli (focal) and within an affected glomerulus are present only in some capillary loops (segmental). The presence of sclerosis involving occasional entire glomeruli (global sclerosis) is a common finding that increases with age in all patients and does not have prognostic significance. The FGS lesion itself is an expansion of the mesangial matrix with wrinkling and collapse of adjacent capillary loops, development of PAS-positive intracapillary hyaline deposits, adhesions to Bowman's capsule, and often foamy cells and focal epithelial cell proliferation (Fig. 81–6). Glomeruli that do not contain the lesion of FGS exhibit changes identical to those of MCNS, indicating that the increase in capillary permeability is a

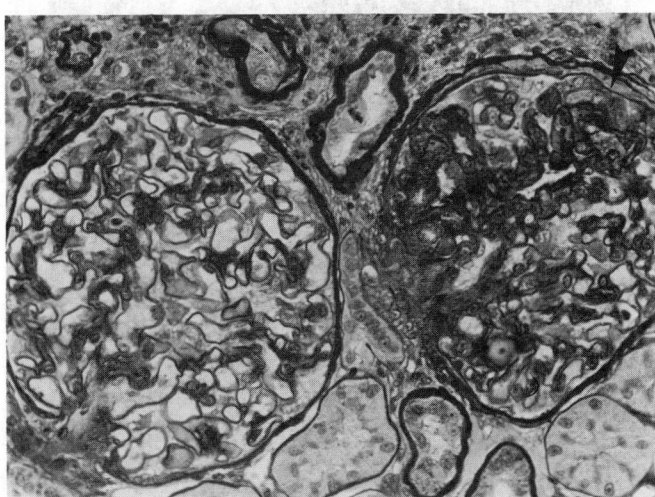

FIGURE 81–6. Renal biopsy from a patient with nephrotic syndrome, FGS, and decreased renal function. By light microscopy the glomerulus on the left appears almost normal with only slight mesangial matrix increase, while the glomerulus on the right is partially sclerotic with an adhesion to Bowman's capsule at one o'clock (*arrowhead*). Two atrophic tubules with thickened basement membranes in the upper part of the field are surrounded by fibrosis and mononuclear cells. (Periodic acid–Schiff stain, × 350.) (Reproduced from Couser WG, Salant DJ, Adler S, et al. In Brenner BM, Lazarus JM (eds.): Acute Renal Failure, Philadelphia, WB Saunders Company, 1983, p 403.)

diffuse one not confined to the areas of sclerotic lesions. Interstitial infiltrates and tubular atrophy usually accompany lesions of FGS. IgM and C3 are frequently deposited nonspecifically in sclerotic lesions and may occasionally be seen more diffusely in the mesangium.

Clinical Features. FGS is present in 5 to 15 per cent of patients with idiopathic nephrotic syndrome and is associated with a higher frequency of hematuria (65 per cent), hypertension (10 per cent), and renal insufficiency (10 per cent) than is seen in MCNS (Table 81–4). Sterile pyuria is also common. Proteinuria is nonselective, presumably reflecting the focal areas of structural damage to the capillary wall associated with lesions of FGS. While most patients have the nephrotic syndrome, a significant minority are detected with asymptomatic proteinuria, a finding that is rarely seen in MCNS. When all of these features accompany the finding of FGS in an early biopsy, only about 20 per cent of such patients will respond to steroid therapy and many of these do not remain steroid responsive. The presence of the nephrotic syndrome, hematuria, hypertension, decreased renal function, and mesangial hypercellularity on biopsy tends to indicate a poor prognosis.

A smaller group of patients appears to have clinically typical MCNS without hematuria or hypertension but shows early lesions of FGS on biopsy. Often such biopsies are obtained later in the course of the disease after several episodes of steroid-responsive nephrotic syndrome, and such patients may remain steroid responsive for many years and progress very slowly or not at all. When all patients with FGS on initial biopsy are studied, only about 40 per cent are in renal failure at the end of ten years.

Laboratory Features. There are no distinctive laboratory abnormalities, except for the increased incidence of hematuria and presence of nonselective proteinuria, that differentiate patients with FGS from those with pure MCNS.

Course and Treatment. Patients with FGS on initial biopsy, especially if hematuria, hypertension, and nephrotic syndrome are present, rarely respond to steroids and progress to renal failure in an average of about ten years. The level of proteinuria is clearly related to prognosis, and 80 per cent of all patients with non-nephrotic proteinuria retain normal renal

function for over ten years. About 15 to 20 per cent of all patients with FGS and the nephrotic syndrome will show a response to steroids, sometimes months to years after therapy, a phenomenon that justifies a trial of steroid therapy as outlined above for MCNS in such patients. If steroid responsiveness is present, the prognosis is considerably better, and such patients may behave like those with MCNS. Alkylating agents such as cyclophosphamide and chlorambucil have been shown to increase the frequency and duration of steroid-induced remission in FGS as they have in MCNS. Immunosuppressive drugs may occasionally be effective in steroid-resistant patients.

Patients with FGS who progress to renal failure have a high incidence of recurrent disease in renal transplants. Factors that have been correlated with recurrence include mesangial hypercellularity, a rapidly progressive course (less than three years), and receipt of a well-matched living-related donor transplant. In four antigen matches, the recurrence rate may be as high as 80 per cent, although it is less than 50 per cent for all patients with end-stage renal disease due to FGS. With recurrence, patients develop the nephrotic syndrome within a few hours to one week, accompanied by lesions of FGS in the transplant and usually a shortened graft survival. This phenomenon is important both in emphasizing the necessity for accurate diagnosis of renal disease in patients prior to transplantation and in selecting and counseling potential kidney donors.

Korbet SM, Schwartz MM, Lewis EJ: The prognosis of focal segmental glomerulosclerosis of adulthood. Medicine 66:304, 1986. *This detailed analysis of 46 patients with idiopathic nephrotic syndrome and focal glomerulosclerosis emphasizes clinical features, prognosis, and therapy.*

Southwest Pediatric Nephrology Study Group: Focal segmental glomerulosclerosis in children with idiopathic nephrotic syndrome: A report of the Southwest Pediatric Nephrology Study Group. Kidney Int 27:442, 1985. *This report reviews the clinical features, pathology, response to treatment, and clinicopathologic correlations in 75 children with FGS. The overlap with MCNS and the relatively poor prognosis are emphasized.*

HEROIN NEPHROPATHY. In some centers up to 25 per cent of new cases of FGS and 10 per cent of all cases of end-stage renal disease occur in young adults with a history of parenteral drug abuse, usually including heroin. Other renal lesions such as GN secondary to bacterial endocarditis, hepatitis B–associated membranous nephropathy, large vessel vasculitis, amyloidosis, and interstitial nephritis related to embolized foreign material are also seen in addicts. However, the entity of nephrotic syndrome with FGS, hypertension, and rapidly progressive renal disease appears to be the most common drug-related lesion. A similar lesion may cause nephrotic syndrome in patients with AIDS (see above). Discontinuation of drug use has resulted in stabilization or improvement in renal function in some patients, but no other form of therapy has proved beneficial. The role of the injected drugs or other foreign substances in the pathogenesis of this lesion is not known.

Dubrow A, Mittman N, Ghali V, et al.: The changing spectrum of heroin-associated nephropathy. Am J Kidney Dis 5:36, 1985. *This study of 35 heroin abusers with nephrotic syndrome confirms the presence of FGS as a common underlying lesion but emphasizes the increasing frequency with which amyloid is seen as the cause of nephrotic syndrome.*

Membranous Nephropathy

Overview. Membranous nephropathy is an uncommon disease in childhood but is the commonest cause of idiopathic nephrotic syndrome in adults, in whom it accounts for about 50 per cent of all cases (Table 81–4). As with all other causes of idiopathic nephrotic syndrome, the diagnosis can be made only by renal biopsy.

Pathogenesis. Experimentally, subepithelial immune deposits may result from antibody binding to an epithelial cell membrane antigen or to exogenous antigens that become localized at this site, usually on the basis of charge-charge interactions with glomerular anionic structures. It has not been established which of these mechanisms is the predominant one in humans, but the idiopathic form of membranous nephropathy may be an autoimmune disease. Subepithelial immune deposits appear to induce proteinuria by a mechanism that probably involves the C5b–9, or membrane attack, portion of the complement system.

The role played by inciting agents such as drugs or hepatitis virus in initiating this process is unknown. A strong association exists between idiopathic membranous nephropathy and HLA-DRw3 (relative risk about four), an association also noted in patients who develop membranous nephropathy while taking drugs. Although most cases are idiopathic, some develop in association with a variety of other conditions, including *drugs* (penicillamine, gold, captopril), *infectious agents* (hepatitis B, various parasitic infestations), *SLE*, and *malignancy*, particularly solid tumors of the lung, breast, and gastrointestinal tract. The nephrotic syndrome may be the presenting sign of an otherwise occult neoplasm, and older patients with idiopathic membranous nephropathy should be carefully evaluated for malignancy. An identical lesion occurs in about 15 per cent of patients with SLE and may be the presenting sign of this disease when other systemic and serologic manifestations are absent. Young females who present with what appears to be idiopathic membranous nephropathy must be carefully followed for later development of SLE. Other associations such as those with Sjögren's syndrome, mixed connective tissue disease, diabetes, thyroiditis, syphilis, sarcoidosis, and sickle cell disease are documented but rare.

Pathology. By light microscopy glomeruli may appear entirely normal early, but as the disease progresses, a diffuse thickening of capillary walls occurs without any increase in glomerular cellularity (Fig. 81–7). A silver methenamine stain will usually demonstrate the spike-like extensions of basement membrane between areas of subepithelial deposits, and the subepithelial deposits themselves may be seen with a PAS stain. A diffuse, very finely granular pattern of immune deposits of IgG and C3 is found along the subepithelial surface of all capillary loops (Fig. 81–8). EM demonstrates electron-

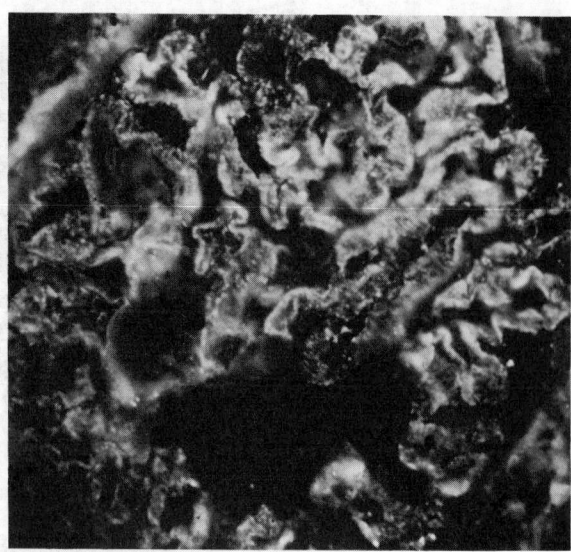

FIGURE 81–8. Immunofluorescence microscopy in membranous nephropathy demonstrates diffuse, finely granular staining of IgG (and C3) on all capillary walls, usually without mesangial deposits (× 400). (Reproduced from Couser WG, Salant DJ, Stilmant MM. In Flamenbaum W, Hamburger RJ (eds.): Nephrology. Philadelphia, JB Lippincott Company; 1982, pp 265–301.)

dense deposits in an exclusively subepithelial distribution with effacement of overlying foot processes (Fig. 81–9).

Clinical Manifestations. The mean age of onset of idiopathic membranous nephropathy in the United States is 40 to 50, and males predominate about 2 to 1. However, the disease has been reported in patients as young as 2 and over 70. Over 80 per cent of patients present with the nephrotic syndrome, but 20 per cent may be seen first with asymptomatic proteinuria. Microscopic hematuria is present in about 60 per cent of cases in adults, but red cell casts are rare. Hypertension is uncommon and renal function is usually normal at the time of presentation. The association of membranous nephropathy with other disease processes has been discussed above under "Pathogenesis."

Two complications of this disease are important: (1) Several patients have been reported to develop a *superimposed anti-*

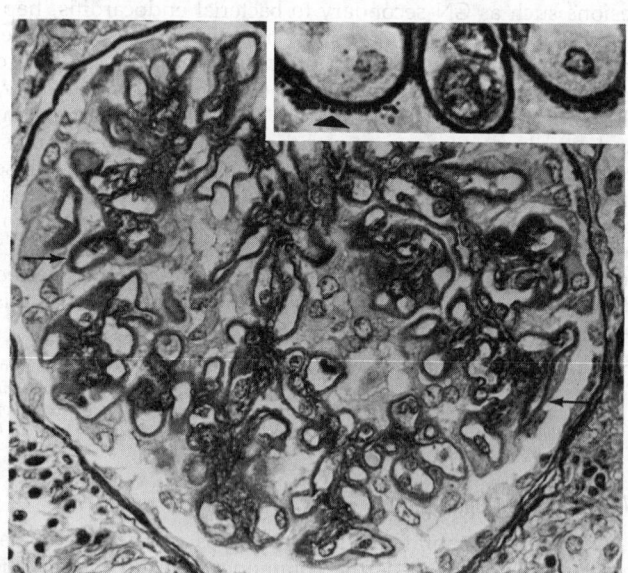

FIGURE 81–7. Light microscopy in early membranous nephropathy shows minimal thickening of the glomerular capillary walls (*arrows*) without any increase in cells or mesangial matrix. In the inset, three capillary loops stained with silver methenamine demonstrate the "spike" of basement membrane between deposits (*arrowheads*) (periodic acid–Schiff stain, × 350; inset: silver methenamine stain, × 900). (Reproduced from Couser WG, Salant DJ, Stilmant MM. In Flamenbaum W, Hamburger RJ (eds.): Nephrology. Philadelphia, JB Lippincott Company, 1982, pp 265–301.)

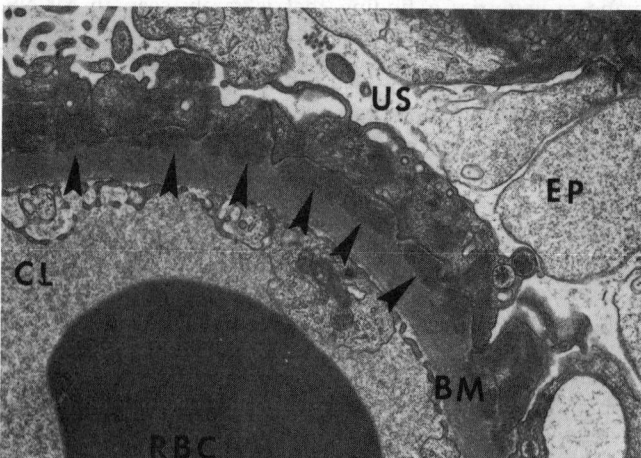

FIGURE 81–9. Electron micrograph of a glomerulus in membranous nephropathy showing many electron-dense subepithelial deposits (*arrowheads*) between the basement membrane and effaced epithelial cell foot processes. A red blood cell is present in the capillary lumen (× 15,000). BM = Basement membrane; CL = capillary lumen; EP = epithelial cell; RBC = red blood cell. (Reproduced with permission from Couser WG, Salant DJ, Adler S, et al. In Brenner BM, Lazarus JM (eds): Acute Renal Failure. Philadelphia, WB Saunders Company, 1983, p. 406).

GBM nephritis with crescent formation and a clinical course similar to that of RPGN. This possibility must be considered in otherwise stable patients who experience a rapid deterioration in renal function accompanied by a nephritic urine sediment. (2) An incidence of *renal vein thrombosis* as high as 50 per cent has been reported in membranous nephropathy. Any patient in whom a thromboembolism is suspected should be studied for renal vein thrombosis and treated with long-term anticoagulation to reduce thromboembolic complications if a venous thrombosis is demonstrated.

Laboratory Studies. There are no laboratory abnormalities specific for idiopathic membranous nephropathy. Because of the frequency of various associated conditions, the laboratory workup should include determinations of antinuclear and anti-DNA antibody, serum complement levels, rheumatoid factor, cryoglobulins, hepatitis B antigen, VDRL, and tests to exclude diabetes. In older patients, a careful clinical and radiologic search for occult malignancy is justified. If the patient has unusual flank pain, hematuria, or a reason to suspect pulmonary emboli, the renal veins should be studied by venography.

Course and Treatment. The disease has a widely variable clinical course with substantial fluctuations in proteinuria and an uncertain prognosis. The spontaneous remission rate is about 25 per cent in adults. Another 25 per cent of patients will have persistent nephrotic range proteinuria for many years but will retain normal renal function. The remaining 50 per cent of adults, and 10 to 15 per cent of children, experience a slowly progressive deterioration of renal function that results in end-stage renal disease in an average of about 15 years, although more rapid progression may be seen. No clinical or pathologic criteria have been identified that will predict the future clinical course in an individual patient.

The variable clinical course in idiopathic membranous nephropathy makes any assessment of benefits from therapy difficult, since large numbers of patients must be followed in a prospective controlled fashion to obtain meaningful data. One such study in adults with idiopathic membranous nephropathy and normal renal function compared treatment with 100 to 150 mg of prednisone every other day for two months with a placebo and demonstrated a slower rate of deterioration in renal function in patients treated with prednisone. Several retrospective studies have reached similar conclusions. Concomitant administration of cytotoxic drugs may further improve these results. Since fewer than 50 per cent of patients will develop progressive disease, the author recommends cytotoxic drugs only in patients with evidence of progressive loss of renal function.

Recurrent membranous nephropathy in a renal transplant is rare but has been reported in several patients who have progressed to end-stage renal disease in a period of four years or less. Recurrence usually has not adversely affected graft survival. Significantly more cases of de novo membranous nephropathy have been reported in renal allografts than cases of recurrence, and the disease is a relatively common cause of the nephrotic syndrome in transplant patients.

Cameron JS: Pathogenesis and treatment of membranous nephropathy (Nephrology Forum). Kidney Int 15:88, 1979. *A very complete and thoughtful discussion of membranous nephropathy by an experienced clinical investigator. It includes a review and discussion of the data on steroid treatment in this disease with Dr. Cecil Coggins.*

Ponticelli C: Prognosis and treatment of membranous nephropathy. Kidney Int 29:927, 1986. *This excellent summary reviews the causes of membranous nephropathy, the factors that influence prognosis, and the data on benefits of therapy. The results of a prospective study by the author suggesting a beneficial effect of treatment with a cytotoxic drug as well as steroids are reviewed and discussed in detail.*

Membranoproliferative Glomerulonephritis (MPGN)

Overview. The term membranoproliferative glomerulonephritis (MPGN) refers to a clinicopathologic entity found primarily in young adults and characterized by idiopathic nephrotic syndrome, hypocomplementemia, and a histologic lesion having the lobular appearance of glomeruli with both thickening of the basement membrane and cellular proliferation. This entity has also been called lobular GN, chronic hypocomplementemic GN, and mesangiocapillary GN. These histologic and clinical features are probably common to at least two separate and perhaps unrelated diseases, which are now referred to as type I MPGN (that with subendothelial immune deposits) and type II MPGN (dense deposit disease). Type I MPGN is about twice as common as type II, and the two diseases cause about 10 per cent of cases of idiopathic nephrotic syndrome in both children and adults (Table 81–4). However, unlike the other glomerular diseases that cause idiopathic nephrotic syndrome, about 20 per cent of patients present with an acute nephritic syndrome, and nephritic features are common in both of these diseases.

Pathogenesis. TYPE I MPGN. Several features of type I MPGN suggest that it is a chronic immune complex GN: (1) the granular deposits of IgG and C3 in a subendothelial and mesangial distribution, (2) the activation of the classic complement pathway, (3) the frequent presence of cryoglobulins and circulating immune complexes, (4) the presence of similar lesions in patients with some forms of postinfectious GN, including shunt nephritis and nephritis associated with chronic hepatitis B antigenemia, and (5) the production of similar lesions in animals immunized chronically with a foreign serum protein. However, the etiology of the disease, the nature of the antigen(s) involved, and the reasons for the chronicity of the process remain unknown.

TYPE II MPGN. This disease does not appear to be an immune deposit disease, and the nature of the dense deposits remains unclear. Despite much study of the unique abnormalities in complement metabolism associated with this disease, and the identification of C3 nephritic factor in the serum, the role of the complement abnormalities, if any, in the pathogenesis of the disease remains undefined. There is no animal model of dense deposit disease, and similar lesions have not been described in other renal diseases.

Pathology. TYPE I MPGN. Light microscopy reveals a diffuse proliferative GN with thickening of the glomerular capillary walls, increase in mesangial cells and matrix, and a lobulated appearance of the glomerulus (Fig. 81–10). The thickened capillary walls are due to subendothelial immune deposits and interposition of mesangial matrix between GBM and endothelium, resulting in a double contour, splitting, or "tram

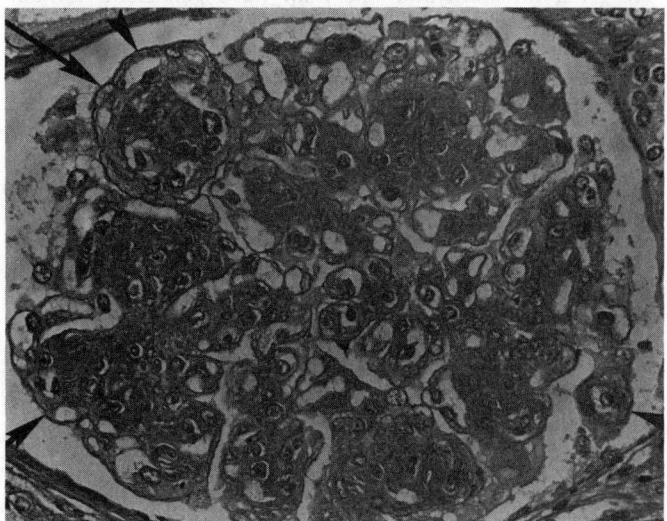

FIGURE 81–10. Light microscopy in membranoproliferative glomerulonephritis shows glomerular hypercellularity, segmental thickening of the basement membrane (*arrowheads*), and lobulation of glomerulus (*arrows*). (Periodic acid–Schiff, × 350.) (Reproduced from Couser WG, Salant DJ, Stilmant MM. In Flamenbaum W, Hamburger RJ (eds.): Nephrology. Philadelphia, JB Lippincott Company, 1982, pp 265–301.)

track" appearance of the capillary walls on silver stain. Crescents are present in less than 10 per cent of cases. Coarsely granular deposits of C3, and often of IgG, IgM, C4, properdin, and fibrin, occur in the mesangium and in peripheral capillary loops in a pattern much like that seen in diffuse proliferative, or class IV, SLE. By EM there are dense subendothelial and mesangial deposits present as well as mesangial matrix interposition with capillary wall thickening and narrowing of the capillary lumen.

TYPE II MPGN. The histologic findings in type II MPGN are very similar to those in type I disease except that crescents are present in up to 30 per cent of patients and correlate with a worse prognosis. The dense deposits may be seen as PAS-positive, ribbon-like deposits within the capillary wall as well as along Bowman's capsule and tubular basement membrane. C3 is present along the margins of these deposits, resulting in a double linear pattern on the capillary walls as well as surrounding deposits of similar material in the mesangium (mesangial rings). Granular immune deposits of IgG are much less common than in type I disease. EM reveals extensive replacement of the lamina densa with homogenous, dark-staining material that may also be seen in the mesangium, Bowman's capsule, and tubular basement membrane.

Clinical Features. There are only minor differences in the clinical manifestations of types I and II MPGN. What follows is a description of patients with the more common type I disease. The differences observed in type II disease are commented on below. MPGN is a disease of children and young adults, rarely seen before age 5 and relatively uncommon after age 30. Males and females are affected approximately equally. The nephrotic syndrome is the presenting sign in about 50 per cent of patients and develops during the course of the disease in over 80 per cent. Up to 20 per cent may present with an acute nephritic syndrome (which is more common in type II), and the remainder are detected with asymptomatic hematuria or proteinuria or both. Preceding upper respiratory tract infections have occurred in about half of patients with type I MPGN and may have been streptococcal. Hematuria is a common feature of the disease. Hypertension is present in one third, and 25 per cent have a reduced GRF on initial presentation.

The clinical course is quite variable. One third of patients develop end-stage renal disease within 6 to 10 years, one third have persistent nephrotic syndrome with relatively stable renal function, and one third have persistent non-nephrotic proteinuria or hematuria. Fewer than 5 per cent experience spontaneous remissions. In the long term at least 50 per cent of patients with type I will reach end-stage renal disease in 15 to 20 years, while type II progresses somewhat more rapidly (6 to 10 years). Poor prognostic signs in individual patients include a reduced GFR at onset, the presence of the nephrotic syndrome, early hypertension, gross hematuria, and the presence of either crescents or sclerosis on a renal biopsy.

Type I MPGN recurs in about 25 per cent of patients who receive renal transplants but rarely interferes with graft function.

The clinical features of type II disease that differ from those of type I include a higher frequency of both the nephrotic syndrome and acute nephritic episodes, a lower frequency of asymptomatic hematuria and proteinuria, more rapid progression to renal failure (probably due to the greater frequency of nephritic episodes), more frequent and persistent hypocomplementemia (see below), and a higher frequency of recurrence in transplants. Type II disease is also associated with partial lipodystrophy in some patients.

Laboratory Abnormalities. Type I MPGN is characterized by fluctuating levels of complement with depression of both classic (C1q, C4) and alternate pathway components at some time in most patients. In type II disease, hypocomplementemia is more frequent and persistent, and only alternate

pathway activation is usually seen with a reduction in C3 and other alternate pathway proteins such as properdin and factor B, while classic pathway components are usually normal. Most type II patients have a circulating IgG autoantibody (C3 nephritic factor, or C3 Nef) directed against the C3 convertase of the alternate complement pathway. The definitive diagnosis of either type I or type II MPGN can be made only by renal biopsy with complete IF and EM studies.

Treatment. Improvement or stabilization in renal function in MPGN has been reported with two-year courses of alternate day steroid therapy and with a "cocktail" of drugs including steroids, cytotoxic agents, anticoagulants, and antiplatelet agents. However, side effects of such treatments are significant. Administration of the platelet inhibitor dipyridamole, 225 mg per day, and aspirin, 975 mg per day, significantly reduces the rate of loss of renal function in type I MPGN with minimal side effects. This regimen is the one of most demonstrable benefit and least toxicity at present. Too few patients with type II MPGN have been studied prospectively to be certain that similar results are achieved with that lesion.

Cameron JS, Turner DR, Heaton J, et al.: Idiopathic mesangiocapillary glomerulonephritis. Comparison of types I and II in children and adults and long-term prognosis. Am J Med 74:175, 1983. *An excellent clinical review of 104 well-studied patients that discusses the clinical and laboratory findings in types I and II MPGN, the differences between children and adults, and the long-term prognosis and prognostic features.*

Donadio JV, Anderson CF, Mitchell JC III, et al.: Membranoproliferative glomerulonephritis: A prospective clinical trial of platelet-inhibitor therapy. N Engl J Med 310:1421, 1984. *In a prospective, randomized, double-blind, controlled trial of dipyridamole and aspirin versus placebo in 40 patients, most with type I MPGN, the author demonstrates better maintenance of renal function in the treated group without significant complications*

West CD: Childhood membranoproliferative glomerulonephritis: An approach to management. Kidney Int 29:1077, 1986. *This review by the investigator who first described this disease in 1965 discusses the clinical characteristics of 51 patients and reviews data on therapy, concluding that long-term steroid therapy is beneficial in altering the natural history.*

GLOMERULAR INVOLVEMENT IN SYSTEMIC DISEASES

The most common systemic diseases resulting in glomerular involvement are the various forms of vasculitis. With the group of diseases referred to as systemic necrotizing vasculitis, a distinction is made between necrotizing vasculitis involving medium-sized and larger vessels (the polyarteritis nodosa group including classic PAN, allergic granulomatosis, and "overlap" syndromes), and necrotizing vasculitis involving small vessels and capillaries (hypersensitivity vasculitis or microscopic PAN plus several well-defined clinical syndromes, including SLE, HSP, and mixed essential cryoglobulinemia). The only other common vasculitic syndrome with significant renal involvement is Wegener's granulomatosis.

Polyarteritis Nodosa (PAN)

Classic PAN, a disease of older adults sometimes associated with drug abuse (particularly amphetamines) and heptitis B antigenemia, is described in detail in Ch. 440. Renal involvement, which occurs in 90 per cent of cases, is usually manifest first as hematuria with an active urine sediment and mild proteinuria. In 70 per cent of cases, the renal lesion is primarily an ischemic one caused by vasculitic involvement of arcuate and interlobular arteries. This is best demonstrated by abdominal angiography and is generally not seen on renal biopsy. Aneurysmal dilatation is present in renal, hepatic, and mesenteric vessels. In 30 per cent of patients, a focal necrotizing GN with crescents may be seen. Both types of glomerular involvement may sometimes occur in the same patient. Immune deposits are generally not found in the glomerulus, and the pathogenesis of the renal disease is uncertain. Renal failure is a major cause of death and either may be a slowly progressive process or develop acutely in association with accelerated hypertension. In patients with PAN who develop hypertension and acute renal failure, renal cortical necrosis is common, and there is little reversibility. More often, the disease is a slowly progressive one in which vigorous control of hypertension, use of oral steroids, and addition of cytotoxic agents such as cyclophosphamide have achieved five-year survivals of over 80 per cent of patients in uncontrolled studies.

Milder renal lesions may occur in the other two subgroups of this category. In allergic granulomatosis, allergic symptoms, asthma, pulmonary involvement, and eosinophilia are prominent features of the disease. In the overlap syndromes, both allergic manifestations and small vessel involvement may occur in the presence of the classic large vessel involvement seen in PAN.

Balow JE: Renal vasculitis. Kidney Int 27:954, 1985. *A comprehensive review of the classification, pathogenesis, and clinical features of the various forms of systemic necrotizing vasculitis involving the kidney. The utility of angiography in the diagnosis of PAN and the indications for cytotoxic drug therapy are stressed.*

Wegener's Granulomatosis

Wegener's granulomatosis is a granulomatous and necrotizing vasculitis but also involves large vessels, usually of the upper and lower respiratory tract and kidney (see Ch. 441). The disease presents most frequently in the fourth or fifth decade of life and affects more males than females. Presenting signs usually are respiratory and include purulent rhinorrhea, painful sinusitis, otitis, keratoconjunctivitis, oral ulcerations, and multiple bilateral nodular pulmonary infiltrates. Renal involvement eventually develops in over 80 per cent of patients and untreated may result in the death of up to 30 per cent. Early renal involvement is manifest by hematuria, proteinuria, and mild renal impairment with a focal and necrotizing proliferative GN, usually without immune deposits. However, severe diffuse necrotizing and crescentic GN may develop rapidly. Necrotizing granulomatous vasculitis may be seen in biopsies of the respiratory tract but is often not evident in renal biopsies. The presence of granulomas may be the only pathologic finding that distinguishes Wegener's granulomatosis from PAN. Spontaneous improvements in renal disease have not been reported. There are no characteristic laboratory abnormalities in Wegener's granulomatosis. Although the diagnosis can usually be made on clinical grounds, a renal biopsy is generally performed early in the disease to identify potentially severe renal involvement that may be clinically silent and to distinguish Wegener's granulomatosis from other diseases with pulmonary and renal manifestations, such as Goodpasture's syndrome, which would be treated differently. Prognosis and therapy are discussed in Ch. 441.

Fauci AS, Haynes BF, Katz P, et al.: Wegener's granulomatosis: Prospective clinical and therapeutic experience with 85 patients for 21 years. Ann Intern Med 98:76, 1982. *This paper from the NIH describes in detail the clinical manifestations of 85 patients with Wegener's granulomatosis and the treatment protocol now used to induce remissions in over 90 per cent of patients.*

Hypersensitivity Vasculitis (Microscopic PAN, Allergic Vasculitis, Leukocytoclastic Angiitis)

This disease is a form of systemic necrotizing vasculitis of small vessels in which the clinical manifestations do not fall into a well-recognized syndrome such as SLE, HSP, or essen-

tial mixed cryoglobulinemia (see Ch. 439). The disease is believed to be a manifestation of immune complex formation in small vessels and frequently follows exposure to some offending antigen such as an infectious agent, drug, or foreign protein by about a seven- to ten-day latent period. However, about half of patients will not have an identifiable antecedent event. The skin is most commonly involved, with palpable purpura. Other frequent manifestations include microangiopathic hemolytic anemia and pulmonary infiltrates with hemoptysis.

Clinical renal involvement is present in about 50 per cent of cases and is usually manifest initially as asymptomatic proteinuria associated with a segmental necrotizing GN or biopsy. Impairment in renal function is present in 20 to 40 per cent of cases, and up to 10 per cent may develop acute oliguric renal failure. On biopsy, these patients generally have extensive necrotizing glomerular lesions with abundant crescent formation and negative IF studies. Treatment considerations are similar to those outlined above for idiopathic RPGN, including high-dose steroid pulse therapy and possibly plasma exchange. There is more evidence to support the use of additional cytotoxic agents, such as cyclophosphamide, in the treatment of RPGN due to vasculitis than is present in idiopathic RPGN.

Serra A, Cameron JS, Turner DR, et al.: Vasculitis affecting the kidney: Presentation, histopathology, and long-term outcome. Q J Med 210:181, 1984. *Fifty-three patients with vasculitis involving the kidney are reviewed. The finding of a segmental necrotizing glomerular lesion accompanied by systemic symptoms such as fever, malaise, or weight loss was considered diagnostic of a small vessel vasculitis. Clinical features in such patients were identical to those who had histologic evidence outside the kidney. The paper is an excellent review of the wide spectrum of clinical manifestations of vasculitis and the frequency of crescentic glomerulonephritis in such patients as well as the relatively poor prognosis.*

Systemic Lupus Erythematosus (SLE)

The current diagnostic criteria and clinical manifestations of SLE are considered in more detail in Ch. 436. This section will discuss only the renal involvement. About 70 per cent of patients will have clinical manifestations of renal disease ranging from microscopic hematuria and proteinuria to an acute nephritic syndrome with acute renal failure and typical nephrotic syndrome. Renal biopsies reveal some abnormalities in most patients.

CLASSIFICATION. The most common classification system used for renal involvement in SLE is the World Health Organization (WHO) classification based on histopathologic criteria (Table 81–5).

Class I (Normal Kidneys). Only very rarely do patients with diagnostic criteria for SLE have entirely normal kidneys by light microscopy, IF, and EM, and they do not have clinical manifestations of glomerular disease.

Class II (Minimal or Mesangial Lupus Nephritis). This is the earliest and mildest form of renal involvement in SLE and is characterized by mesangial deposits of immunoglobulin and C3 with (Class IIB) or without (Class IIA) focal proliferative changes by light microscopy. Clinical manifestations of proteinuria and hematuria are present in most patients, but the nephrotic syndrome and renal insufficiency are very

TABLE 81–5. HISTOLOGIC CLASS, CLINICAL PRESENTATION, AND PROGNOSIS IN SLE NEPHRITIS

Histologic Type	WHO Class	Frequency (%)*	Proteinuria (%)	Nephrotic Syndrome† (%)	Azotemia‡ (%)	Death (%)	Uremic Death (%)
Normal	I	<5					
Mesangial	II	15	68	0	12	18	0
Focal proliferative	III	20	100	15	18	30	11
Diffuse proliferative	IV	50	100	87	75	58	36
Membranous	V	15	100	88	20	38	6

*Per cent of patients biopsied with SLE who show this lesion.
†Proteinuria exceeding 3.0 grams per 24 hours.
‡Serum creatinine exceeding 1.2 mg per deciliter or BUN exceeding 25 mg per deciliter.

uncommon and do not develop unless progression to a more severe lesion occurs, as happens in about 20 per cent of patients. Five-year survival is over 90 per cent, and no specific therapy is indicated for the renal lesion.

Class III (Focal Proliferative Lupus Nephritis). This is a stage in a continuum between mesangial lesions alone and diffuse proliferative lupus nephritis. Focal proliferative changes are present in fewer than 50 per cent of glomeruli, but all glomeruli contain immune deposits of IgG, IgA, C3, and usually IgM and fibrin-related antigens. Deposits are predominantly mesangial, but occasional subendothelial deposits may be seen. All patients have proteinuria, but the nephrotic syndrome and renal insufficiency occur in fewer than 20 per cent and may remit following steroid therapy. Serologic abnormalities including hypocomplementemia are more severe than in Class II disease. Long-term prognosis with this lesion is also good (90 per cent five-year survival). However, there is a relatively high incidence of transformation to Class IV disease, resulting in a reduction in five-year survival to about 70 per cent, with almost half of the deaths occurring from renal failure. The most reliable predictor of progression is probably the presence of subendothelial deposits by EM.

Class IV (Diffuse Proliferative Lupus Nephritis). This is the severest of the glomerular lesions in lupus, with proliferation seen in over 50 per cent of glomeruli, frequently with crescent formation and necrosis. Extensive mesangial and subendothelial deposits contain all immunoglobulins, C3, and fibrin. Mesangial and subendothelial deposits are present by EM, often with subepithelial deposits as well. Proteinuria is seen in all patients, and nephrotic range proteinuria is present in 50 per cent at onset and 90 per cent some time during the course of the disease. Renal function is decreased in 75 per cent at the time of presentation, and serologic evidence of disease activity, including hypocomplementemia, elevated levels of anti-DNA antibody, and circulating immune complexes, is present in most patients. The long-term prognosis for this lesion has improved considerably over the years, with most centers now achieving survival rates of about 75 per cent at five years. The best prognosis is in those patients in whom a remission of the nephrotic syndrome and normalization of serologic parameters are achieved within one year of starting therapy.

Class V (Membranous Lupus Nephritis). About 15 per cent of patients with SLE will develop a glomerular lesion that may be indistinguishable from idiopathic membranous nephropathy with extensive subepithelial deposits of all immunoglobulins and C3. The nephrotic syndrome and a slowly progressive renal disease are common (see Table 81–4). Patients may have undetectable levels of antinuclear antibody at the time of presentation. The incidence of systemic manifestations of SLE and serologic abnormalities in general is also lower in patients with a membranous lesion. The long-term prognosis for patients with this lesion does not differ significantly from those with Class II disease. As in idiopathic membranous nephropathy, there appears to be an increased incidence of renal vein thrombosis. Steroid therapy as discussed under idiopathic membraneous nephropathy is usually recommended.

TREATMENT OF LUPUS NEPHRITIS. In patients with active renal disease and a class III or IV lesion, steroids have a beneficial effect in lupus nephritis. High-dose steroid therapy is given for a period of four to six weeks and subsequently tapered and adjusted according to responses in renal function, serologic parameters, and extrarenal disease. In the presence of crescents and deteriorating renal function, steroid pulse therapy, as discussed above under idiopathic RPGN, may result in more rapid return to maximal renal function. The addition of a cytotoxic agent such as cyclophosphamide to oral steroid therapy may result in better preservation of renal function in a subset of patients with evidence of active Class III or IV disease and mild chronic changes by biopsy. Thus a renal biopsy appears to be useful as a basis for selecting therapy in patients with active lupus nephritis. Administration of cyclophosphamide as a monthly intravenous pulse may provide a therapeutic effect equivalent to a daily oral dose with fewer side effects.

With development of renal failure, disease activity in SLE usually subsides. Renal transplantation has been carried out in a large number of patients without significant problems.

Austin HA, Muenz LR, Joyce KM, et al.: Prognostic factors in lupus nephritis: Contribution of renal histologic data. Am J Med 75:382, 1983. *Newer histologic parameters have been shown to be useful in selecting patients with lupus nephritis who may benefit from administration of a cytotoxic drug in addition to steroids. This paper establishes the value of age, sex, and initial level of renal functions, as well as the chronicity index determined from the renal biopsy, as important prognostic factors in lupus nephritis.*

Austin HA III, Klippel JH, Balow JE, et al.: Therapy of lupus nephritis: Controlled trial of prednisone and cytotoxic drugs. N Engl J Med 314:614, 1986. *This prospective study of 106 patients with active lupus nephritis suggests a beneficial effect of intravenous cyclophosphamide in reducing the risk of end-stage renal disease only in the subset of high-risk patients identified by the presence of chronic histologic changes. The data support the claim that monthly intravenously administered cyclophosphamide is less toxic than a daily dose. This is the best study currently available on the efficacy of cytotoxic drug therapy in lupus nephritis.*

Ballow JE, moderator: Lupus nephritis. Ann Intern Med 106:79, 1987. *This review from a group with extensive experience in the classification and treatment of lupus nephritis summarizes current understanding of the pathogenesis and treatment of renal disease in SLE.*

Henoch-Schönlein Purpura (HSP)

Henoch-Schönlein syndrome, or anaphylactoid purpura, is another systemic necrotizing vasculitis of small vessels in which systemic manifestations include palpable purpura (100 per cent) on the lower extremities and buttocks due to a leukocytoclastic vasculitis of dermal vessels, arthralgias of large joints, usually the knees and ankles (70 per cent), gastrointestinal involvement with colic and bleeding (25 per cent), and renal involvement (see Ch. 167). About 30 per cent of patients have clinical evidence of renal disease in the form of hematuria or acute nephritic syndrome. Except for the systemic manifestations, the disease is very similar in its morphologic and clinical characteristics to IgA nephropathy but is of somewhat greater severity. Typically the disease presents with an acute nephritic syndrome, usually without edema or hypertension, developing within three months of the onset of other systemic manifestations of HSP. Many patients have an infectious episode prior to the onset of renal disease. Up to 25 per cent of adults may develop a severe crescentic lesion with RPGN. The nephrotic syndrome has been reported to develop in over 50 per cent, and progressive renal failure occurs in at least 25 per cent of patients. The renal involvement is much less severe in children. Predictors of progressive disease include presentation with an acute nephritic syndrome, nephrotic syndrome, crescents, and subepithelial deposits or subendothelial "lead-shot" lesions by EM. Most patients have self-limited episodes of renal involvement, usually lasting one week or less. However, recurrences are common.

Laboratory features are not distinctive and do not differ from those described for IgA nephropathy. Renal biopsy may reveal a spectrum of lesions ranging fom focal mesangial proliferation to diffuse crescentic GN, but the most characteristic lesion is a focal necrotizing GN in which necrosis and fibrin deposition are more common than in IgA nephropathy. IF and EM findings do not differ from those in IgA nephropathy with diffuse mesangial deposits of IgA and lesser amounts of IgG and complement. IgA deposits are also present in dermal capillaries of involved or uninvolved skin.

The pathogenesis of HSP is unknown but is presumed to be immunologic and similar to that of IgA nephropathy. Similar immunogenetic associations in the two diseases, as well as the clinical, histologic, and immunopathologic similarities, strongly suggest that a common underlying disease mechanism is involved.

No treatment has been shown to be of benefit in the nephritis of HSP. Short courses of steroids may be useful in controlling systemic manifestations but do not appear to benefit the renal lesion. Patients who develop crescents and a clinical picture of RPGN should be considered for treatment as outlined above under idiopathic RPGN.

Lee HS, Koh HI, Kim MJ, et al.: Henoch-Schönlein nephritis in adults: A clinical and morphological study. Clin Nephrol 26:125, 1986. *This paper provides a detailed analysis of the clinical and morphologic features as well as prognostic variables in 17 adult patients with Henoch-Schönlein nephritis.*

Meadow AR, Glasgow EF, White RHR, et al.: Schönlein-Henoch nephritis. Q J Med 41:241, 1972. *This older article provides an excellent review of the clinical features in a large series of adult patients with HSP.*

Essential Mixed Cryoglobulinemia (EMC)

Low concentrations of mixed cryoglobulins, usually type III with polyclonal IgG and IgM with rheumatoid factor activity, are seen in a variety of immune glomerular disorders, autoimmune diseases, vasculitides, and neoplastic syndromes, in which they rarely produce symptoms (Ch. 439). Type II mixed cryoglobulins, composed of monoclonal IgM rheumatoid factor and polyclonal IgG, are characteristic of a disorder called essential mixed cryoglobulinemia (EMC), in which dependent vascular purpura, Raynaud's phenomenon, arthralgias, weakness, and GN are the principal clinical manifestations. Cryoprecipitates from these patients often contain hepatitis B antigen. The disease is one of middle age and affects females somewhat more often than males.

Renal involvement is present in about 40 per cent of cases and is usually preceded by purpura and arthralgias. The severity of renal disease ranges from microscopic hematuria and proteinuria to an acute nephritic syndrome with acute renal failure. In contrast to most of the other vasculitic syndromes, the nephrotic syndrome is a rather frequent occurrence, and severe hypertension is common. Laboratory abnormalities include a markedly elevated sedimentation rate, cryoglobulins, rheumatoid factor activity, and sometimes an artifactual decrease in levels of early complement components, with C3 and later components often normal. The glomerular lesion is a diffuse proliferative and exudative GN, sometimes accompanied by vasculitis, with large PAS-positive proteinaceous deposits present in many capillaries. The subendothelial capillary deposits are composed predominantly of IgG and IgM, with lesser amounts of C3 and fibrin. In patients with acute nephritic syndrome and renal failure the prognosis is poor. However, in all patients with renal disease, over 50 per cent may recover with or without therapy, and the survival rate at ten years is about 75 per cent. Although steroids and cytotoxic agents alone have not been shown to be of consistent benefit in the renal lesion, plasma exchange therapy may improve the prognosis in patients with severe renal disease.

Tarantino A, DeVecchi A, Montagnino G, et al.: Renal diseases in essential mixed cryoglobulinaemia. Q J Med 197:1, 1981. *A detailed review of the renal manifestations, biopsy findings, and long-term course in 44 patients with EMC and renal disease, emphasizing the spectrum of disease and prognosis.*

Thrombotic Microangiopathy (Hemolytic Uremic Syndrome and Thrombotic Thrombocytopenia Purpura)

Hemolytic uremic syndrome (HUS) and thrombotic thrombocytopenic purpura (TTP) are referred to collectively by some authors as thrombotic microangiopathy. The two disorders can be clinically indistinguishable, probably have a common, although poorly understood, pathogenesis, and respond to similar therapy.

HEMOLYTIC UREMIC SYNDROME (HUS). HUS is a syndrome of microangiopathic hemolyic anemia, thrombocytopenia, and renal impairment, which usually occurs abruptly in children about three to ten days following episodes of gastroenteritis or viral upper respiratory tract infection. Gastroenteritis is often associated with verotoxin producing *Escherichia coli* infections. A similar syndrome occurs less commonly in adults, often associated with complications of pregnancy or during the postpartum period (postpartum acute renal failure) or associated with the use of oral contraceptives. HUS also occurs in adults following treatment with a variety of antineoplastic agents. Acute renal failure develops in up to 60 per cent of children but usually resolves spontaneously within about two weeks with only supportive therapy. Chronic renal failure occurs in only 10 per cent of patients, usually those who suffer loss of renal function in a gradual, progressive manner, who have oliguria lasting longer than two weeks, or who have total anuria. Laboratory features of the disease include microangiopathic hemolytic anemia, thrombocytopenia, increased numbers of reticulocytes, elevated bilirubin levels, reduced haptoglobin levels, and elevated levels of fibrin split products, usually with only minimal laboratory evidence of disseminated intravascular coagulation. In TTP (see below) levels of fibrin split products are less commonly elevated. The glomerular lesion is one of intimal hyperplasia of arterioles and intracapillary fibrin thrombi, sometimes with areas of focal necrosis. The anemia and thrombocytopenia are presumably due to trapping of platelets and destruction of red cells in the areas of capillary thrombosis. The pathogenesis of the syndrome is unknown but probably involves glomerular endothelial cell injury by some as yet unidentified circulating factor, with subsequent fibrin deposition and thrombosis. Decreased endothelial cell production of prostacyclin, a vasodilator and inhibitor of platelet aggregation, has been reported but may be a secondary event.

In typical HUS in children, only supportive therapy, including early dialysis, is required, since the rate of spontaneous recovery is very high. In adults, the prognosis is considerably worse because renal involvement is more severe and development of bilateral cortical necrosis more common. This is particularly true in cases associated with pregnancy and oral contraceptives. No form of therapy has been determined to be effective in HUS, although aspirin, antiplatelet agents, heparin, fresh frozen plasma infusions, and plasma exchange have all been advocated by some authors. In adults with severe disease, treatment with plasma exchange as described below for TTP, in addition to steroids, antiplatelet agents, and aspirin, is probably indicated.

THROMBOTIC THROMBOCYTOPENIC PURPURA (TTP). TTP is clinically and pathologically very similar to HUS (see Ch. 167). The differences that distinguish this end of the spectrum of thrombotic microangiopathy are (1) a more common occurrence in young adults, (2) fever as a frequent manifestation of the disease, (3) neurologic abnormalities that tend to predominate and cause death, and (4) a lesser degree of renal involvement with acute renal failure in only about 10 per cent of cases. Hematuria is the most common manifestation of renal disease. Proteinuria, generally less than 5 grams per day, and a serum creatinine in excess of 2 mg per deciliter occur in about 50 per cent of cases. Histologically the renal lesion is the same as that in HUS. TTP has a considerably worse prognosis than HUS, with about a 75 per cent mortality within three months, and spontaneous recovery is rare.

A wide variety of therapeutic regimens have been employed in TTP, including all of those listed above for HUS as well as intravenous infusion of prostacyclin and vigorous plasma exchange. The most promising results have been obtained with plasma exchange, often in combination with fresh plasma, antiplatelet agents, and steroids, a regimen that has produced rather dramatic clinical remissions in several patients with apparently severe and advanced disease. In refractory cases, splenectomy may confer an additional benefit.

Hakim RM Schulman G, Churchill WH Jr, et al.: Successful management of thrombocytopenia, microangiopathic anemia, and acute renal failure by plasmapheresis. Am J Kidney Dis 5:170, 1985. *This report describes successful treatment of six consecutive adult patients with thrombocytopenic, microangiopathic anemia and renal failure with plasmapheresis as well as fresh plasma and steroids. This approach is the treatment of choice for severe cases of thrombotic microangiopathy.*

Ridolfi R, Bell WR: Thrombotic thrombocytopenic purpura. Report of 25 cases and review of the literature. Medicine 60:413, 1981. *This is a comprehensive review article covering clinical features, renal involvement, pathology, and pathogenesis of TTP, with a detailed approach to therapy and over 200 references.*

CHRONIC GLOMERULONEPHRITIS

Chronic GN is not a separate disease. It represents the progressive stage of any of the primary or secondary glomerular diseases discussed in this chapter prior to development of end-stage renal disease. Thus, PSGN, IgA nephropathy, RPGN, focal glomerular sclerosis, membranoproliferative glomerulonephritis, membranous nephropathy, and SLE, as well as diseases such as hereditary nephritis, may result in chronic GN with progressive loss of renal function, proteinuria, abnormal urine sediments, and diminishing renal size. About 60 per cent of all cases of end-stage renal disease result from some form of chronic GN. In the early stages these lesions can be accurately diagnosed by renal biopsy and sometimes successfully treated. However, in patients with chronic disease, small kidneys, and creatinine clearances below 15 ml per minute, the changes on renal biopsy are rarely diagnostic, and there is little reversible component to the renal damage.

The clinical features of chronic GN are noteworthy only for the frequency with which progressive renal disease is asymptomatic. About 50 per cent of patients will present with advanced renal insufficiency without a clear past history of renal disease. In most patients with chronic renal failure and creatinine clearances below 25 ml per minute, progression to renal failure is inexorable. The rate of progression can be quite accurately predicted from plots of the reciprocal of serum creatinine concentration versus time and is quite consistent for individual patients although not for specific diseases. The clinical manifestations of chronic renal failure are discussed in more detail in Ch. 79.

In end-stage glomerular disease the renal cortex is thin, and glomeruli are acellular, sclerotic, and often replaced by collagenous material. Tubular atrophy, interstitial fibrosis, and cellular infiltrates are widespread. The mechanisms by which acute renal injury leads to progressive loss of renal function have not been well defined. In some acute inflammatory diseases such as RPGN, immune injury may be so severe that glomeruli are irreversibly destroyed by ischemia, necrosis, and thrombosis, resulting in acute renal failure and end-stage renal disease without a chronic or progressive phase. However, in most diseases progression is a much slower process that appears to continue long after the initial disease process has resolved.

The primary mechanisms of progression in glomerular disease may be hemodynamic. Loss of functioning nephron mass from an acute injury results in an adaptive increase in glomerular capillary plasma flow rates and transcapillary hydraulic pressure gradient (*glomerular hyperfiltration*) to maximize the GFR. Increased intraglomerular pressure appears to result in increased capillary permeability to protein and structural glomerular damage when sustained above a certain level over time. The histologic manifestation of this form of glomerular injury is focal glomerular sclerosis—a process that characterizes virtually all progressive renal diseases and results in gradual loss of filtering surface areas. Glomerular hyperfiltration induced experimentally can be substantially modified by restricting dietary protein intake or by treatment with angiotensin-converting enzyme inhibitors, which reduce efferent arteriolar constriction and thereby lower intraglomerular pressure. Thus, changes in dietary protein or specific drug therapy may be beneficial in slowing or halting progression in a variety of chronic renal diseases. The role of these treatments in chronic renal disease has not yet been defined but is the subject of intensive ongoing investigation.

Dunn BR, Anderson S, Brenner M: The hemodynamic basis of progressive renal disease. Semin Nephrol 6:122, 1986. *This paper reviews the experimental basis for postulating that progressive renal disease is hemodynamically mediated.*

and reviews the data suggesting that protein restriction therapy or angiotensin-converting enzyme inhibitors may prevent the loss of renal function in a wide variety of glomerular diseases.

Glassock RJ, Adler SG, Ward HJ, et al.: Primary glomerular diseases. In Brenner BM, Rector FC Jr (eds.): The Kidney. Philadelphia, W. B. Saunders Company, 1986, p 946. *This chapter presents a detailed discussion of the clinical and pathologic features, course, and therapy of chronic GN and is extensively referenced.*

Oldrizzi L, Rugiu C, Valvo E, et al.: Progression of renal failure in patients with renal disease of diverse etiology on protein-restricted diet. Kidney Int 27:553, 1985. *The study of 78 patients with chronic glomerulonephritis, polycystic kidney disease, and chronic interstitial nephritis documents a significantly reduced rate of loss of renal function in patients treated with protein and phosphorus restriction compared with controls. The results suggest that the beneficial effects of such treatment demonstrated experimentally in animal models probably apply to humans as well.*

82 TUBULOINTERSTITIAL DISEASES AND TOXIC NEPHROPATHIES

T. Dwight McKinney

COMMON FEATURES OF TUBULOINTERSTITIAL DISEASES

Tubulointerstitial disease (tubulointerstitial nephritis or nephropathy, interstitial nephritis) refers to a diverse group of acute and chronic disorders that primarily affect the renal tubules and interstitium. In contrast, in other primary renal diseases, most notably glomerulonephritis, the tubules and interstitium are only secondarily involved. Approximately 30 per cent of all cases of chronic renal insufficiency in the United States result from tubulointerstitial diseases. Usually the cause of tubulointerstitial disease can be identified. Renal function may improve or stabilize with appropriate therapy.

Clinical Manifestations

In tubulointerstitial diseases, functional renal tubular defects, which are present to some degree in advanced renal insufficiency of any cause, are frequently out of proportion to the degree of renal insufficiency as measured by reduction in glomerular filtration rate (GFR). In fact, the finding of such a disproportional loss of tubular compared with glomerular function should lead one to suspect the diagnosis of tubulointerstitial disease (Table 82–1). Urinary concentration in response to water deprivation or exogenous antidiuretic hormone may be reduced, particularly in chronic interstitial nephritis. This may result in decreased maximal urinary osmolarity, polyuria (generally <3 liters per day), and nocturia. Concentration defects, an acquired form of nephrogenic

TABLE 82–1. MANIFESTATIONS OF RENAL TUBULOINTERSTITIAL DISEASES

1. Tubular dysfunction disproportionate to reduction in GFR
2. Tubular abnormalities
   a. Reduced maximal urinary concentrating ability (polyuria, nocturia)
   b. Renal tubular acidosis (hyperchloremic metabolic acidosis)
   c. Partial or complete Fanconi's syndrome

Phosphaturia	Uricosuria
Bicarbonaturia	Glycosuria
Aminoaciduria	

   d. Sodium wasting
   e. Hyperkalemia
3. Renal endocrine deficiencies
   a. Hyporeninemic hypoaldosteronism (hyperkalemia, metabolic acidosis)
   b. Calcitriol deficiency (renal osteodystrophy)
   c. Erythropoietin deficiency (anemia)
4. Urinalysis
   a. May be normal but usually contains cellular elements
   b. Proteinuria is usually modest (<3.5 grams per day) and consists largely of low molecular weight "tubular" proteins such as lysozyme and beta$_2$-microglobulin

diabetes insipidus, may result from interference with the action of antidiuretic hormone on the collecting ducts or anatomic damage or disruption of the medullary structures involved in the urinary concentrating mechanism (Ch. 227). Damage to the proximal tubules may result in excessive urinary excretion of substances normally reabsorbed in this location. Bicarbonaturia (proximal renal tubular acidosis), phosphaturia, aminoaciduria, uricosuria, glycosuria, kaliuresis, and low molecular weight proteinuria may be seen. These losses may cause low plasma levels of some of these substances, particularly phosphate, bicarbonate, and urate. The presence of multiple proximal tubular defects is referred to as Fanconi's syndrome (Ch. 84). In addition to proximal renal tubular acidosis, failure of the distal nephron to acidify the tubular fluid maximally results in classic distal renal tubular acidosis. Hyperkalemic (type 4) distal renal tubular acidosis may also occur. All of these cause a hyperchloremic (normal anion gap) metabolic acidosis (Ch. 77). Hyperkalemia may result from a primary failure of potassium secretion by the distal nephron but more commonly results from decreased renal production of renin and subsequent secondary hypoaldosteronism. Patients with tubulointerstitial disease may also fail to conserve sodium normally. In some, this is due to the hyporeninemic hypoaldosteronism noted above. Renal sodium wasting may result in signs of extracellular fluid volume depletion when sodium intake is restricted and may cause worsening of renal function. With acute and, to a lesser extent, chronic interstitial nephritis, these tubular defects may be accompanied or, indeed, overshadowed by other signs, symptoms, and laboratory abnormalities of renal failure (Ch. 78 and 79).

Diagnosis

A specific diagnosis of tubulointerstitial renal disease can often be made or inferred from historical information, physical examination, or laboratory tests. Renal biopsy is the most definitive method of diagnosis, but this is not always necessary. Pathologic features are discussed below. Radiographic, ultrasonographic, and radionuclide examinations generally show only evidence of acute or chronic renal insufficiency but may provide a specific diagnosis such as urinary tract obstruction or polycystic kidney disease.

Prognosis and Treatment

The prognosis usually depends on the specific cause of tubulointerstitial renal disease as discussed below. General supportive therapy, e.g., treatment of electrolyte disorders, and management of acute and chronic renal failure are discussed in Ch. 78 and 79.

COMMON FEATURES OF TOXIC NEPHROPATHIES

The term toxic nephropathy refers to those renal disorders resulting directly or indirectly from exposure of the kidneys to exogenous chemicals and physical factors, including both drugs and environmental agents, and abnormal concentrations of substances normally present in the body fluids, such as calcium and uric acid. Drug-related renal disease is the most important cause of toxic nephropathy. Toxic nephropathy often results in tubulointerstitial disease, but it is not synonymous with it.

Several factors predispose the kidneys to toxic injury: (1) The kidneys receive approximately 20 per cent of the resting cardiac output and, therefore, are exposed to more blood-borne materials than any other organ except the lungs. (2) The high metabolic rate of the renal tubules required for active transport processes makes them particularly vulnerable to toxic insults. (3) The large glomerular capillary surface area is an available site for trapping immune complexes or for in situ antigen-antibody reactions. (4) Some substances (e.g., aminoglycosides) are selectively concentrated in the renal cortex because of specific transport processes located in the proximal tubules, whereas others (e.g., phenacetin) are concentrated in the medulla owing to the renal countercurrent system. This selective concentration accounts, in part, for the anatomic distribution of damage by some nephrotoxins. (5) Certain substances are converted to less soluble forms with resultant precipitation (e.g., urate to uric acid) consequent to acidification of tubular fluid in the distal nephron. This may lead to tubular obstruction.

Nephrotoxins injure the kidneys in a variety of ways, both direct and indirect (Fig. 82-1). Indirect injury, for example, may result from immunologic reactions or from secondary effects such as drug-induced hypotension or hemolysis. These mechanisms, alone or in concert, may cause an array of renal disorders ranging from isolated functional tubular defects to reversible acute renal failure to progressive end-stage renal disease.

ACUTE INTERSTITIAL NEPHRITIS

Pathology and Pathogenesis

Characteristically, in acute interstitial nephritis (AISN) mononuclear cells infiltrate the interstitium, particularly in the cortex. Eosinophils, especially in cases of drug-related AISN, and occasionally small numbers of polymorphonuclear leukocytes may also be present. Inflammatory cells may invade the tubule walls and, in severe cases, may be associated with areas of tubular necrosis. The infiltrate may be diffuse or patchy; the extent of the infiltrate corresponds in general to the degree of renal functional impairment. In addition to the cellular infiltrate, the renal tubules are separated by interstitial edema, but no fibrosis is present. With prolonged AISN, interstitial fibrosis may develop and the pathologic picture may merge into that of chronic interstitial nephritis. In primary AISN the glomeruli are generally normal, although there may be some mesangial prominence. The predominant mononuclear inflammatory cells in infiltrates are T cells. Both helper/inducer and suppressor/cytotoxic T cells are present, although their relative numbers may vary depending on the specific disease. These observations suggest that both T cell–mediated delayed hypersensitivity reactions and cytotoxic T cell injury may be involved in AISN. In some cases immunoglobulins and complement components are demonstrable in the interstitium and/or tubular basement membrane by immunofluorescence. Rarely, electron microscopy may reveal electron-dense deposits in these areas suggestive of immune complexes. Finally, in occasional cases there may be linear deposition of immunoglobulins and complement in the tubular basement membrane indicative of anti–tubular basement membrane antibodies. There is, therefore, considerable evidence for immune injury mediated by cellular and humoral mechanisms as the cause of AISN. Usually, however, the immunopathogenetic mechanisms involved in a given case of AISN remain unknown.

Etiology

Acute interstitial nephritis may result from a variety of causes (Table 82-2). Drug-related AISN is becoming more frequently recognized as an important cause of acute renal insufficiency, probably because of (1) the more widespread use of renal biopsy, (2) the increasing number of drugs being used, and (3) the characteristic clinical presentation.

DRUG-INDUCED ACUTE INTERSTITIAL NEPHRITIS. The list of drugs that have been implicated as etiologic in AISN continues to expand (Table 82-3). AISN is a rare complication of drug therapy, but because of the frequency with which these agents are used, drugs account for a substantial portion of all cases of acute renal failure.

Penicillins. A number of penicillin congeners may cause AISN, including amoxicillin, ampicillin, carbenicillin, methicillin, mezlocillin, nafcillin, oxacillin, and penicillin G. Meth-

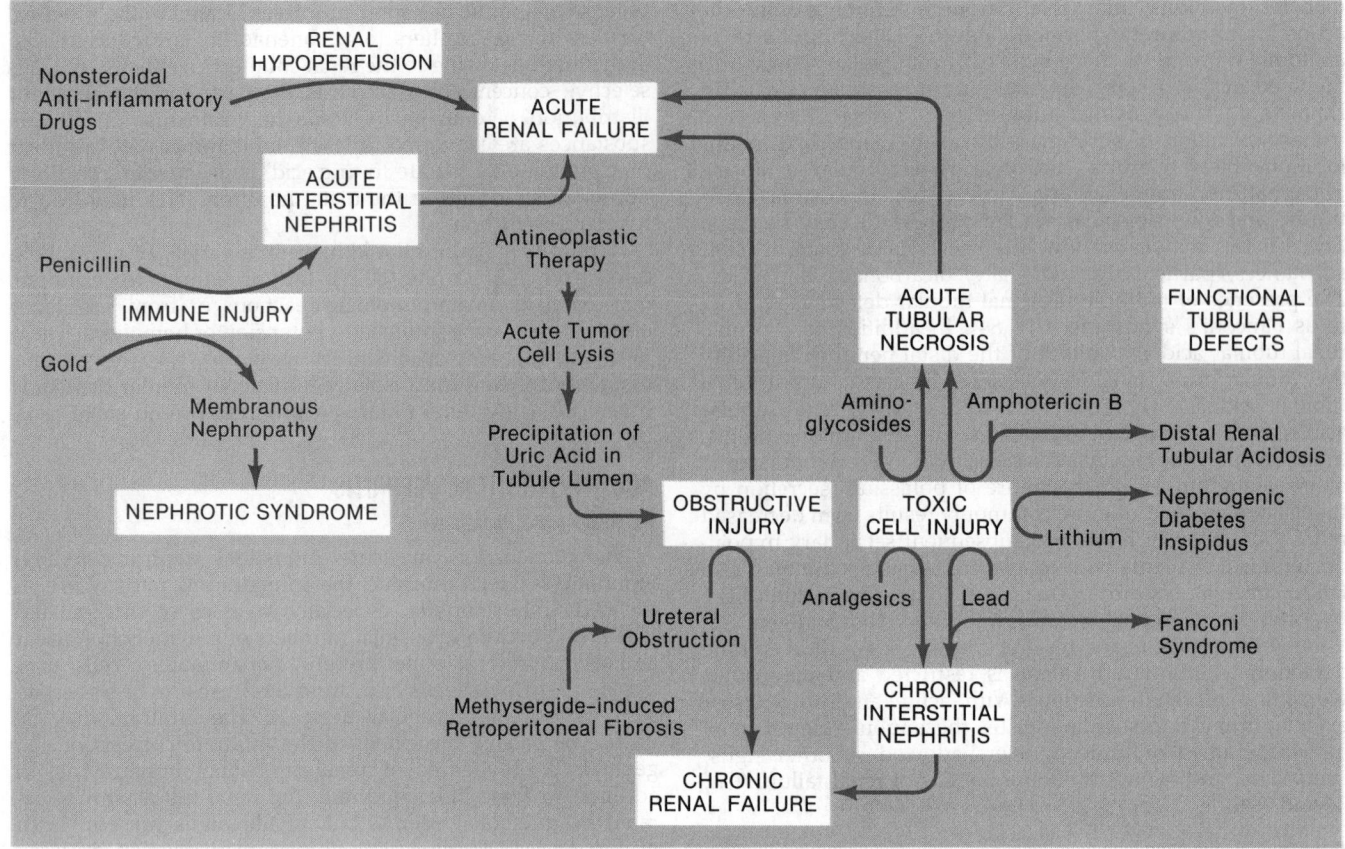

FIGURE 82–1. Types of toxin-induced renal disease.

icillin has been responsible for most reported cases, but the clinical syndrome is similar for the other penicillins. It is reasonable to presume that AISN may occur with any penicillin. Typically, penicillins have been taken for about two weeks prior to the onset of signs and symptoms of AISN, but this time interval has varied from two days to several weeks. The disorder appears to be more frequent in men and children. There is no correlation between the dosage of the drug administered and subsequent development of AISN. In one review of methicillin nephritis, the most frequent manifestations were as follows: hematuria, 97 per cent (this may be gross and associated rarely with red cell casts in the urinary sediment); proteinuria, 94 per cent (usually less than nephrotic range); pyuria, 93 per cent (eosinophiluria is frequently present and strongly suggests the diagnosis of AISN); fever, 87 per cent; eosinophilia, 79 per cent (this may be evanescent);

azotemia, 61 per cent in adults and 16 per cent in children (often associated with oliguria); and skin rash, 24 per cent. Serum IgE levels may be elevated. Renal sodium wasting and hyperchloremic metabolic acidosis with hyperkalemia (hyperkalemic distal renal tubular acidosis) may also occur. The pathogenesis of the disorder is uncertain. Binding of penicillin haptens to renal tubule basement membranes may result in formation of anti–tubular basement membrane antibodies, but evidence for this mechanism is not convincing in most patients.

For treatment, the offending drug must be discontinued and another appropriate drug for the underlying infection should be substituted. In the majority of cases this will result in restoration of renal function. Recovery may require several weeks, with some patients needing interval dialysis. A short course of high-dose corticosteroids (60 mg per day of pred-

TABLE 82–2. CAUSES OF ACUTE INTERSTITIAL NEPHRITIS

1. Drug-related (Table 82–3)
2. Systemic infections
   Brucellosis   Mycoplasmal pneumonia
   Cytomegalovirus   Polyomavirus
   Diphtheria   Rocky Mountain spotted fever
   Infectious mononucleosis   Streptococcal infections
   Legionnaires' disease   Syphilis
   Leptospirosis   Toxoplasmosis
3. Primary renal infections
   Bacterial pyelonephritis (Ch. 86)
   Renal tuberculosis
   Fungal nephritis
4. Immune disorders
   Acute glomerulonephritis associated with anti-tubular basement membrane antibodies and/or secondary interstitial nephritis (Ch. 81)
   Systemic lupus erythematosus
   Acute rejection of a renal transplant (Ch. 80.2)
   Necrotizing vasculitis
5. Other conditions
6. Idiopathic

TABLE 82–3. DRUGS ASSOCIATED WITH ACUTE INTERSTITIAL NEPHRITIS

Antimicrobial Drugs

Cephalosporins	Para-aminosalicylic acid
Chloramphenicol	Penicillins*
Colistin	Polymyxin B
Erythromycin	Rifampin*
Ethambutol	Sulfonamides*
Isoniazid	Tetracyclines
	Vancomycin

Nonsteroidal Anti-inflammatory Drugs (Table 82–6)

Miscellaneous

Allopurinol*	Methyldopa
Antipyrene	Phenindione*
Azathioprine	Phenylpropanolamine
Bismuth	Phenytoin
Captopril	Probenecid
Cimetidine	Sulfinpyrazone
Clofibrate	Sulfonamide diuretics*
Gold	Triamterene

*Most frequent or clinically important.

nisone for one to two weeks) may possibly accelerate the recovery process, but the added risk in patients with underlying infections must be weighed against possible benefits.

Sulfonamides. Both antimicrobial sulfonamides and sulfonamide diuretics (thiazides, furosemide, chlorthalidone, acetazolamide) have been implicated in AISN. Although frequently these are prescribed in combination with other drugs (e.g., sulfamethoxazole plus trimethoprim as antimicrobials and hydrochlorothiazide plus triamterene as diuretics), it is most likely that the sulfonamide moiety of these combinations is responsible for AISN. Typically, evidence for AISN develops several days after therapy is begun, but rechallenge of a patient with a previous past history of sulfonamide-induced AISN may result in signs and symptoms within hours of exposure. The clinical presentation is in many ways similar to that described for the penicillins. Pyuria, hematuria, eosinophilia, and azotemia are frequent. A skin rash is present in a minority of patients. Renal failure may be severe and may require temporary dialysis, but recovery is the rule when the offending drug is discontinued. A brief course of corticosteroids may hasten recovery if no contraindication to their use is present.

Drug-induced AISN should be particularly considered in patients with underlying renal disease, such as nephrotic syndrome, who are treated with sulfonamide diuretics and who experience a more rapid decline in renal function than expected or other manifestations, such as eosinophilia, that suggest an allergic reaction. If diuretic therapy is required in a patient in whom a diagnosis of AISN is made by renal biopsy or presumed to be present based on characteristic clinical findings, a nonsulfonamide diuretic such as ethacrynic acid should be prescribed.

Antituberculous Drugs. A number of patients have developed AISN while receiving chemotherapy for tuberculosis, usually while being treated with more than one agent. Although rifampin, isoniazid, ethambutol, and para-aminosalicylic acid have all been incriminated as causing AISN, the evidence is most compelling for rifampin. AISN appears to occur more often and to be more severe with intermittent therapy with rifampin or after reinstitution of therapy following a drug-free interval than during continuous therapy. Fever, chills, flank pain, and anuria may develop after readministration of a single dose of rifampin. In contrast to other types of acute renal failure, transient hypercalcemia of unknown cause has been reported in several patients developing AISN during therapy for tuberculosis. Discontinuing the offending drugs is generally followed by recovery of renal function, although sometimes rather slowly. Corticosteroids do not appear to be beneficial in hastening recovery of renal function.

Allopurinol. Allopurinol-associated AISN generally develops after several days of treatment (mean interval of three weeks). Most patients have an exfoliative maculopapular skin rash, fever, eosinophilia, and decreased renal function. In addition, most have evidence of acute hepatic injury. Elevations of serum glutamic-oxaloacetic transaminase, sometimes to values in excess of 1000 U per liter, are present in about two thirds of patients. This form of allopurinol toxicity is severe and carries a mortality of approximately 20 per cent. Deaths result from severe systemic reactions, sepsis, gastrointestinal bleeding, or acute hepatic or renal failure. The cause of allopurinol toxicity is uncertain. Clinical and laboratory manifestations suggest a severe systemic hypersensitivity reaction. Most reported patients have been treated with conventional doses of the drug (200 to 400 mg per day), but most have had underlying renal insufficiency prior to development of allopurinol toxicity. Serum concentrations of the major metabolite of allopurinol, oxipurinol, are elevated in renal insufficiency. It may be that hypersensitivity to this or another metabolite may be responsible for the syndrome. In addition, about one half of the reported patients were receiving con-

comitant diuretic therapy. Whether this represents a causal relationship or merely coincidence is uncertain, as allopurinol is commonly prescribed to treat hyperuricemia that develops with diuretic therapy. Treatment of allopurinol toxicity consists of discontinuing the drug and instituting supportive measures, including dialysis, when indicated. Although corticosteroids have been given to many patients, it is uncertain whether they are efficacious. The incidence of allopurinol toxicity can be reduced by prescribing the drug only for clearly documented indications such as recurrent gouty arthritis or uric acid nephrolithiasis and not for asymptomatic hyperuricemia *per se* (including diuretic-induced hyperuricemia). The dose should be reduced in patients with underlying renal insufficiency.

Other Drugs Associated with AISN. Of the numerous other drugs reported to cause AISN, perhaps the most important are the anticoagulant phenindione and the nonsteroidal antiinflammatory drugs. For the remainder of the agents listed in Table 82–3, AISN appears to be a very rare complication. Nevertheless, when manifestations characteristic of AISN occur in patients receiving these drugs (or other drugs not listed), the diagnosis of AISN should be entertained. In this setting it may be simplest to discontinue the suspect drug and replace it with an alternative agent. On the other hand, in patients for whom no suitable alternative exists, it may be necessary to confirm or exclude the diagnosis of AISN by renal biopsy.

AISN ASSOCIATED WITH INFECTION. Systemic bacterial, viral, rickettsial, mycoplasmal, and parasitic infections have been associated with AISN. Infections with group A beta-hemolytic streptococci are, perhaps, the most frequent, especially in children. The pathogenesis of AISN related to systemic infection is uncertain. Possibly, renal deposition of antigens related to the infectious agent elicits humoral and cell-mediated immune reactions that result in renal injury as discussed earlier. Many patients with AISN associated with systemic infections have received antibiotic therapy and may have drug-induced AISN (see above). Therapy of AISN due to systemic infections consists of treatment of the underlying infection and supportive therapy. The prognosis for recovery of renal function is usually quite favorable.

Acute bacterial pyelonephritis is a common cause of AISN. The clinical presentation with fever, chills, flank pain, and bacteria is characteristic (Ch. 86). Similarly, renal parenchymal fungal and mycobacterial infections may cause acute renal interstitial inflammation. All of these can result in renal scarring but only rarely cause acute renal failure.

AISN ASSOCIATED WITH IMMUNE DISORDERS. Varying degrees of acute and chronic interstitial nephritis may accompany numerous renal or systemic diseases of presumed immune origin. Several types of glomerulonephritis are associated with interstitial inflammation that may be out of proportion to the degree of glomerular injury (Ch. 81). In some, there may be antibodies to the tubular basement membranes. Although glomerulonephritis is generally the primary renal lesion in systemic lupus erythematosus, interstitial nephritis is the predominant finding in some patients (Ch. 81 and 436). Acute and chronic interstitial inflammation is the hallmark of renal transplant rejection (Ch. 80.2). Renal involvement with necrotizing vasculitis is generally manifest as a focal segmental glomerulonephritis, but in some patients, particularly those with Wegener's granulomatosis, there may be prominent interstitial involvement.

OTHER CONDITIONS ASSOCIATED WITH AISN. Sarcoidosis (Ch. 69), may involve the kidneys in a number of ways, including acute (granulomatous) interstitial nephritis, chronic interstitial nephritis (often associated with hypercalcemia and hypercalciuria), and primary glomerulonephritis. Rarely, AISN may cause acute renal failure in sarcoidosis. There have been isolated case reports of AISN following therapy with recombinant leukocyte interferon.

IDIOPATHIC AISN. In a number of patients with AISN, a specific cause cannot be identified. Some of these have evidence, such as eosinophilia, suggesting a hypersensitivity reaction to an unknown antigen. In addition to acute interstitial inflammation, renal biopsies sometimes demonstrate evidence for anti–tubular basement membrane antibodies. Others have granulomatous interstitial nephritis in the absence of an obvious etiology. The course of idiopathic AISN is variable; with some patients recovering spontaneously or in response to corticosteroid therapy and others progressing to renal insufficiency.

CLINICAL MANIFESTATIONS

In AISN the GFR may decline abruptly, often accompanied by oliguria. The urinary sediment typically contains numerous leukocytes. In cases of drug-induced AISN, eosinophils are often present as well. Hematuria is ordinarily present, and red blood cell casts, although rare, may be observed. Proteinuria is usually present but modest (<3.5 grams per day), except in AISN due to nonsteroidal anti-inflammatory drugs (see below). The fractional excretion of sodium tends to be high, as it is in most cases of acute tubular necrosis (see Ch. 78). A spectrum of renal tubular defects may be present (Table 82–1). In cases of drug-induced AISN (see above), other manifestations of drug allergy, such as fever, skin rash, and eosinophilia, are frequent. In AISN occurring as part of a systemic process, such as systemic lupus erythematosus, clinical and laboratory manifestations of the primary disease may dominate the clinical presentation. The diagnosis of AISN is established by examination of renal tissue obtained by biopsy (or autopsy). In drug-induced AISN, the diagnosis is often inferred from characteristic clinical and laboratory findings. The outcome of AISN depends on the underlying disease process. In drug-induced disease, renal function generally improves once the offending drug is stopped. Corticosteroid therapy may be beneficial, as discussed above. With prolonged and severe AISN, variable degrees of chronic renal insufficiency may result.

CHRONIC INTERSTITIAL NEPHRITIS

Pathology

Chronic interstitial nephritis (CISN) is characterized pathologically by interstitial fibrosis with atrophy and loss of renal tubules. The glomeruli may be normal but frequently are contracted. There is generally a patchy interstitial infiltrate of chronic inflammatory cells. The renal vasculature may show evidence of associated hypertension. In addition to these general findings, there may be others that suggest a specific disease, such as casts typical of multiple myeloma.

Etiology (Table 82–4)

CISN may result from persistence or progression of many of the acute forms of interstitial nephritis (Table 82–2) or may evolve without an obvious preceding phase of acute injury. Many of the specific causes of CISN are discussed subsequently; some of the remainder are commented on briefly below.

Urinary tract obstruction (including vesicoureteral reflux), the single most important cause of CISN, is discussed in Ch. 83. Perhaps the second most important group of disorders comprises those caused by nephrotoxins, most of which are discussed later as toxic nephropathies. In addition to exogenous toxins, certain endogenous chemical abnormalities may result in CISN. The major renal complication of *chronic hypokalemia* and potassium depletion is nephrogenic (vasopressin-resistant) diabetes insipidus, which results in mild polyuria, but chronic interstitial nephritis with modest renal insufficiency may also rarely occur. *Hypercalcemia* also produces mild polyuria due to nephrogenic diabetes insipidus. Acute hypercalcemia also acts on the glomeruli and renal vasculature to

TABLE 82–4. CAUSES OF CHRONIC INTERSTITIAL NEPHRITIS

1. Persistence or progression of acute interstitial nephritis (Table 82–2)
2. Chronic urinary tract obstruction (Ch. 83)
3. Nephrotoxins
   Drugs: analgesics, nitrosoureas
   Endogenous substances: hypercalcemia, hypokalemia, oxalate, uric acid
   Metals: cisplatin, copper, lead, lithium, mercury
   Radiation
4. Chronic bacterial pyelonephritis (Ch. 86) or renal tuberculosis (Ch. 302)
5. Immune disorders
   Chronic glomerulonephritis with interstitial nephritis (Ch. 81)
   Chronic rejection of a renal transplant (Ch. 80.2)
   Systemic lupus erythematosus (Ch. 436)
   Sjögren's syndrome (Ch. 438)
6. Associated with neoplasia or paraproteinemias
   Leukemia | Waldenström's macroglobulinemia (Ch. 163)
   Lymphoma | Cryoglobulinemia (Ch. 81)
   Amyloidosis (Ch. 210) | Multiple myeloma (Ch. 163)
7. Cystic diseases
   Medullary cystic disease
   Polycystic kidney disease (Ch. 91)
8. Miscellaneous
   Diabetes mellitus | Advanced renal failure
   Sickle cell hemoglobinopathies | Idiopathic
   Vascular diseases

reduce GRF in a manner largely reversible with correction of hypercalcemia. Chronic hypercalcemia results in nephrocalcinosis and chronic interstitial nephritis with reduced glomerular filtration rate that may be only slowly and incompletely reversible. In addition, nephrocalcinosis may cause distal renal tubular acidosis (Ch. 84). In the absence of urinary tract obstruction, *chronic bacterial pyelonephritis* rarely causes severe renal failure. Renal *tuberculosis* can result in acute and chronic tubulointerstitial disease. Tuberculous ureteral strictures may cause hydronephrosis.

A variety of *immune disorders* may be associated with both acute and chronic interstitial nephritis, including several types of glomerulonephritis (Ch. 81), chronic renal transplant rejection (Ch. 80.2), and systemic lupus erythematosus (Ch. 436). Renal involvement in *Sjögren's syndrome* is usually in the form of CISN. The most common functional abnormalities are distal renal tubular acidosis and urinary concentrating defects (Ch. 438).

Neoplastic and *paraproteinemic* disorders may be associated with CISN. In patients with lymphomas and leukemias, particularly acute lymphoblastic leukemia, neoplastic cells may infiltrate the renal interstitium and cause renal enlargement. Adjacent renal tubules may be compressed and destroyed, but renal function is rarely compromised. Renal disease in patients with *amyloidosis* (Ch. 210), *Waldenström's macroglobulinemia* (Ch. 163), and *mixed cryoglobulinemia* (Ch. 81) usually involves the glomeruli, but, rarely, there may be prominent tubulointerstitial involvement. Renal failure is a common cause of death in patients with *multiple myeloma*, especially in patients with Bence Jones proteinuria (monoclonal immunoglobulin light chain paraproteins). CISN, often associated with cast nephropathy, is the most important cause of renal failure in multiple myeloma. Large, dense eosinophilic casts occur within the tubule lumina, surrounded by a chronic interstitial infiltrate. Renal failure appears to result both from obstruction of the renal tubules by these casts and/or from direct toxic effects of the Bence Jones proteins. In addition to renal insufficiency, multiple myeloma may cause proximal and distal renal tubular acidosis, Fanconi's syndrome, urinary concentrating defects, and the nephrotic syndrome. The last is usually associated with renal amyloidosis. Recovery from renal failure due to CISN with cast nephropathy is rare in contrast to that occurring from other abnormalities in these individuals, particularly hypercalcemia.

Miscellaneous Factors

In *diabetes mellitus* and *sickle cell hemoglobinopathies*, CISN may be accompanied by papillary necrosis. Hyperkalemia and hyperkalemic distal renal tubular acidosis may occur in both. In diabetic patients this is generally due to hyporeninemic hypoaldosteronism. Urinary concentrating defects are particularly common in sickling disorders. Chronic reduction in renal blood flow from a variety of *renal vascular disorders* causes atrophy of both the renal tubules and the glomeruli, along with interstitial fibrosis. *Advanced renal disease* of any etiology results in interstitial fibrosis with mild interstitial inflammation, tubular atrophy, and glomerular sclerosis characteristic of the "end-stage" kidney. Cysts of varying size may also be present. In many cases these changes are so severe that it is not possible to determine whether the underlying cause of renal failure was tubulointerstitial, glomerular, or vascular in origin. In occasional cases of *CISN*, sometimes accompanied by granulomas, no recognized cause can be identified.

Clinical and Laboratory Manifestations

The clinical manifestations may be primarily those of renal tubular functional defects (Table 82–1) or may primarily reflect those of advanced renal failure. Sterile pyuria may be seen, but, in contrast to AISN, eosinophilia and eosinophiluria are not. Historical and laboratory findings may suggest a specific diagnosis, e.g., flank pain and radiographic or ultrasonographic evidence of hydronephrosis suggesting obstructive nephropathy. Clinical presentations unique to certain entities are discussed elsewhere.

TOXIC NEPHROPATHIES (Table 82–5)

Drug-induced acute interstitial nephritis, an important type of nephrotoxic renal injury, is discussed in the preceding section with other causes of acute interstitial nephritis. Other important toxic nephropathies are discussed below.

Analgesic Nephropathy

Chronic interstitial nephritis leading to chronic renal failure may result from excessive consumption of certain analgesic agents. In the United States 2 to 10 per cent of all cases of end-stage renal disease are thought to be due to analgesic nephropathy (AN). In other countries, AN is an even more important cause of chronic renal failure. For example, about 20 per cent of all cases of end-stage renal disease in Australia result from AN. The drugs most commonly associated with AN are phenacetin or acetaminophen (phenacetin is largely converted to acetaminophen soon after ingestion), usually in combination with aspirin. Generally, the offending agents are taken in the form of proprietary drugs, but sometimes they are obtained by prescriptions from physicians. In many countries the availability of phenacetin in proprietary drugs is now greatly restricted.

Pathogenesis and Pathology

Although phenacetin, acetaminophen, and aspirin may be nephrotoxic when consumed in large quantities over extended periods of time, there is some debate about which of these may be the most noxious to the kidney. The combination of acetaminophen or phenacetin with aspirin appears to be more nephrotoxic than either drug alone. Prospective epidemiologic studies show a convincing correlation between the amount of analgesics consumed and the development of renal disease. The generally accepted requirement for the presumptive diagnosis of AN is a cumulative ingestion of 3 kg or more of the above drugs or daily consumption of 1 gram per day for three or more years. In most reported cases of AN, consumption has far exceeded these amounts and has usually consisted of mixtures of phenacetin or acetaminophen and aspirin.

The pathogenesis of AN is still uncertain. Both aspirin and acetaminophen are concentrated within the kidney, and for acetaminophen, and perhaps aspirin, a concentration gradient exists within the kidney from the renal cortex to the medulla. Phenacetin and acetaminophen are metabolized to reactive species that covalently bind to proteins and result in oxidative tissue damage by depleting reducing equivalents such as glutathione. Aspirin may exacerbate this toxicity by inhibition of the hexose monophosphate shunt, which is a major metabolic pathway for maintaining glutathione stores. In addition, aspirin is a potent inhibitor of prostaglandin synthesis. This latter action may lead to a reduction in renal medullary blood flow and result in ischemic damage. In addition to aspirin, other nonsteroidal anti-inflammatory drugs that also inhibit prostaglandin synthesis (e.g., phenylbutazone, ibuprofen, and indomethacin) have been associated with papillary necrosis in humans and in experimental animals. The ultimate importance of these other drugs as a cause of chronic interstitial nephritis will require long-term observations, as many of them have been only recently used on a wide scale.

In the initial stages of AN, there is patchy necrosis of interstitial cells, loops of Henle, and capillaries in the inner medulla, with calcium deposition and lipid accumulation in the involved areas. With continued exposure to these drugs, the process progressively involves the outer medulla and often results in total papillary necrosis. In advanced stages, the renal cortex is thin and the renal tubules are atrophic. There is interstitial fibrosis accompanied by a round-cell infiltrate. The glomeruli are initially spared, but later they and the arterioles become sclerotic. If AN is complicated by bacterial infection, focal collections of acute inflammatory cells are evident. The necrotic papillae may remain in situ, often with cavities in them, or they may totally detach from the medulla and slough into the renal pelvis.

Clinical and Laboratory Manifestations

AN is usually associated with a characteristic group of signs, symptoms, and laboratory findings. The diagnosis of AN is often overlooked because patients frequently do not admit to taking analgesics or, if they do, will not provide a true estimate of the amount consumed. When the diagnosis is suspected, therefore, the possibility of AN should be vigorously pursued by discussions with family members and physicians who have cared for the patient previously. AN occurs more frequently in women (usually middle age) with a female to male ratio of 3:1 to 6:1. Although patients may consume analgesics for a variety of complaints, especially headaches, more often than not there is no disease that warrants taking large amounts of analgesics. In many patients there is a large psychologic component to their clinical presentation. In some patients there is a family history of heavy analgesic use. Anemia is present in most patients and is frequently more severe than can be attributed to their degree of renal insufficiency. In addition to renal insufficiency, anemia may result from hemolysis or gastrointestinal blood loss due to peptic ulcer disease or gastritis, which also occur commonly. Hypertension is present in about one half of patients, but generally appears after renal disease is obvious. Malignant hypertension occasionally develops.

TABLE 82–5. PROMINENT OR COMMON NEPHROTOXINS

Anticonvulsants: paramethadione, phenytoin, trimethadione
Antihypertensive drugs: captopril, methyldopa
Antimicrobials: aminoglycosides, amphotericin B, cephalosporins, ethambutol, isoniazid, para-aminosalicylic acid, penicillins, rifampin, sulfonamides, tetracyclines
Antineoplastic agents: cisplatin, methotrexate, mitomycin-C, nitrosoureas, radiation
Sulfonamide diuretics: acetazolamide, chlorthalidone, furosemide, thiazides
Endogenous compounds: Bence Jones proteins, calcium, hemoglobin, myoglobin, oxalate, uric acid
Halogenated alkanes, hydrocarbons, and solvents: carbon tetrachloride, ethylene glycol, paraquat, toluene
Iodinated radiographic contrast media
Metals: arsenic, bismuth, cadmium, copper, gold, lead, lithium, mercury
Nonsteroidal anti-inflammatory drugs (Table 82–6)
Miscellaneous compounds: acetaminophen, allopurinol, amphetamines, azathioprine, cimetidine, cyclosporine, heroin, methoxyflurane, methysergide, D-penicillamine, phenacetin, phenindione, silicon

Urinalysis frequently reveals pyuria. Urinary tract infections are present in approximately one half of patients at some point and may be associated with leukocyte casts in the urinary sediment. Sloughing of a necrotic papilla into the urinary tract may be associated with gross hematuria, flank pain (ureteral colic), and passage of tissue in the urine. Proteinuria is generally modest (<2 grams per day), but as the disease progresses, occasional patients develop focal sclerosing glomerulopathy with heavy proteinuria. Generally, progression to end-stage renal failure occurs over a period of several years. An abrupt decline in renal function may accompany ureteral obstruction from sloughed papillae. Renal tubular abnormalities may be reflected by hyperchloremic metabolic acidosis due to decreased renal acidification, mild polyuria with an inability to concentrate the urine above the osmolality of blood due to nephrogenic diabetes insipidus, and an inability to reduce appropriately urinary sodium excretion with sodium deprivation (renal salt wasting).

Early in the course of the disease, the kidneys may be of normal size and contour when evaluated radiographically or by ultrasonography. In the late stages, the kidneys are small with a thin cortex and an irregular surface. A variety of findings on intravenous urography or retrograde pyelography—including caliceal clubbing, papillary cavities, and caliceal filling defects due to the presence of a sloughed papilla (ring sign)—may suggest papillary necrosis. Demonstration of papillary necrosis in the absence of its more common causes (e.g., diabetes mellitus, urinary tract obstruction, often with infection, or sickle cell disease) should suggest AN. Finally, patients with AN are at increased risk for development of transitional cell carcinoma of the urinary tract, particularly of the renal pelvis. The appearance of hematuria should lead to prompt evaluation to exclude a uroepithelial neoplasm. This evaluation should generally include examination of the urine for neoplastic cells, cystoscopy, and retrograde pyelograms.

Prevention and Therapy

Obviously, avoidance of drugs implicated as causes of AN will prevent the disorder. Public education about the dangers of excessive analgesic consumption is important. In Canada removal of phenacetin from proprietary analgesic mixtures has been associated with a decline in the incidence of AN. This has not been the case in Australia, however.

The most important factor in treatment of established AN is cessation of analgesic use. For individuals who habitually abuse analgesics, this requires a great deal of education and encouragement. Often psychologic counseling is needed. For patients with diseases requiring analgesics—e.g., rheumatoid arthritis—alternative forms of therapy are indicated. With cessation of analgesic use renal function will generally stabilize or improve. If renal disease is clearly established and drug use continues, renal function inexorably declines, often to the point of end-stage renal disease, over a period of several years. Urinary tract infections, ureteral obstruction from sloughed papillae, hypertension, and dehydration are conditions that may cause a more rapid decline in renal function, and all should be treated promptly.

Nonsteroidal Anti-inflammatory Drugs

During the last decade, a large number of drugs that inhibit production of the various prostaglandins have been marketed. These agents are referred to collectively as nonsteroidal anti-inflammatory drugs (NSAID'S) (Table 82–6). With more widespread use of these drugs, several renal and electrolyte complications have been recognized.

The functions of renal prostaglandins have yet to be completely elucidated. Nevertheless, vasodilator prostaglandins (PGE_2, PGI_2) appear to be important in maintaining renal blood flow in states of sodium depletion or when "effective" arterial blood volume is low. These states are generally asso-

TABLE 82–6. NONSTEROIDAL ANTI-INFLAMMATORY DRUGS

Aclofenac	Meclofenamate
Diclofenac	Mefenamate
Fenclofenac	Naproxen
Fenoprofen	Phenylbutazone
Galfenine	Piroxicam
Ibuprofen	Salicylates
Indomethacin	Sulindac
Ketoprofen	Tolmetin

ciated with elevated levels of circulating angiotensin II and catecholamines. By causing renal vasodilation, prostaglandins preserve renal blood flow while allowing angiotensin II and catecholamines to maintain systemic blood pressure by increasing systemic vascular resistance. Prostaglandins may also cause a natriuresis, stimulate renin release, and antagonize the effect of antidiuretic hormone. Many of the renal and electrolyte complications of prostaglandin inhibition by NSAID's (Table 82–7) are predictable, based on these recognized functions of the prostaglandins.

HEMODYNAMICALLY MEDIATED ACUTE RENAL FAILURE. This has been reported in several patients receiving NSAID's, most notably indomethacin. This type of renal failure appears to result from renal hypoperfusion and occurs shortly after drug therapy is instituted. Patients at risk are those with sodium depletion (e.g., from diuretic therapy) or low "effective" arterial blood volumes (e.g., nephrotic syndrome, congestive heart failure, and hepatic cirrhosis with ascites), older individuals, and patients with underlying renal disease. Individuals receiving triamterene may be especially at risk. This type of acute renal failure is usually associated with oliguria and low fractional excretion of sodium (see Ch. 78). The urinary sediment is generally unremarkable. Renal biopsies have shown evidence of acute tubular necrosis. Azotemia generally resolves promptly after discontinuation of the offending drug. Occasional patients, however, require temporary dialysis.

ACUTE INTERSTITIAL NEPHRITIS (AISN). AISN resulting in acute renal failure has been described in several patients in association with NSAID's, particularly fenoprofen. Heavy proteinuria, often in the nephrotic range, is peculiar to this form of drug-induced AISN. In addition to copious proteinuria, there are other features of AISN due to NSAID's that differ from those associated with other drugs. For example, eosinophilia, eosinophiluria, and skin rashes are uncommon. As with other types of drug-induced AISN, however, urinalysis frequently reveals microscopic hematuria and pyuria. In addition to histopathologic changes of AISN (described earlier), electron microscopy of the glomeruli reveals fusion of podocyte foot processes. Unlike hemodynamically mediated acute renal failure, AISN usually appears only after the offending drug has been administered for several days to several months. The disorder usually resolves with discontinuation of the drug, but recovery may not occur until several months later, and interval dialysis may be required. Corticosteroid therapy is believed by many to hasten recovery, and, in the absence of contraindications, it is reasonable to prescribe a short course of high-dose corticosteroids (1 mg per kilogram per day of prednisone) if renal failure is severe and

TABLE 82–7. RENAL AND ELECTROLYTE COMPLICATIONS OF NONSTEROIDAL ANTI-INFLAMMATORY DRUGS

1. Renal failure
   a. Hemodynamic (major risk factors are sodium depletion and low "effective" arterial blood volume)
   b. Acute interstitial nephritis with or without the nephrotic syndrome
   c. Glomerulonephritis associated with diffuse vasculitis
   d. Papillary necrosis with chronic interstitial nephritis
2. Sodium and fluid retention
3. Hyperkalemia, metabolic acidosis (occurs more often in patients with renal insufficiency, sodium depletion, or other factors predisposing to hyperkalemia)

spontaneous recovery does not occur within several days of stopping the drug.

OTHER RENAL COMPLICATIONS OF NSAID's. In addition to the above causes of acute renal insufficiency, *systemic vasculitis* with *glomerulitis* and *papillary necrosis* with chronic interstitial nephritis may occur rarely in association with NSAID's.

RETENTION OF SODIUM (AND FLUID). This is perhaps the most common renal side effect of NSAID's. Although this retention may not present a problem in persons with normal cardiovascular and renal function, it may result in worsening of pre-existing congestive heart failure or hypertension. Finally, inhibition of prostaglandin synthesis may result in *hyperkalemia* and *metabolic acidosis* due to inhibition of renin secretion and secondary hypoaldosteronism. Underlying renal insufficiency, sodium depletion, or concomitant administration of other drugs that predispose to hyperkalemia (e.g., potassium-sparing diuretics) increases the risk for developing the latter electrolyte abnormalities.

Antimicrobial Drugs

Renal damage from penicillin, sulfonamide, and antituberculous antimicrobials usually results from AISN, described earlier. Additional antibiotics may cause renal disease manifested in other ways.

AMINOGLYCOSIDES. The aminoglycosides, excreted primarily by glomerular filtration, accumulate in the renal cortex to levels higher than those in serum. They may cause several renal tubular functional abnormalities, the most clinically relevant of which are potassium and magnesium wasting, which may result in hypokalemia and hypomagnesemia. The most important manifestation of aminoglycoside renal toxicity, however, is acute renal failure. Evidently, this results from both a direct effect of these drugs on glomerular filtration and tubular toxicity causing acute tubular necrosis. Up to 10 per cent of patients receiving aminoglycosides develop some degree of acute renal failure, accounting for 10 to 15 per cent of all cases of this disorder in the United States. Generally, this failure is manifested by a rise in the serum creatinine level after several days of therapy with one of the aminoglycosides. At times, renal failure may become evident only after the drug has been discontinued. Acute renal failure is usually mild and of the nonoliguric variety. However, oliguria and severe renal failure requiring dialysis may be seen.

The most nephrotoxic aminoglycoside is neomycin, which is, therefore, not administered parenterally. It may rarely cause acute renal failure when given orally or by enema to decrease the bowel flora. The least nephrotoxic is streptomycin. Tobramycin and netilmicin are, perhaps, less nephrotoxic than gentamicin and amikacin. Risk factors for development of aminoglycoside toxicity include the dose of drug administered; the length of therapy; simultaneous administration of other potential nephrotoxins, particularly cephalosporins; renal insufficiency; advanced age; extracellular fluid volume depletion; and, possibly, potassium depletion. In older individuals the GFR is normally lower, although this is unaccompanied by an elevated serum creatinine level. Failure to consider this variable when calculating the dose of aminoglycosides is a major (and preventable) factor in production of acute renal failure.

Management of acute renal failure following aminoglycoside administration consists of discontinuing the drug and substituting another appropriate antibiotic, if continued treatment is necessary. Supportive measures are similar to those indicated with acute renal failure of other causes (Ch. 78). The prognosis for recovery of renal function after several days is excellent.

CEPHALOSPORINS. Acute renal failure due to acute tubular necrosis was an important complication of cephaloridine, the first cephalosporin widely used in clinical medicine.

Renal failure due to acute tubular necrosis and acute interstitial nephritis may rarely accompany treatment with the newer cephalosporins also. The combination of a cephalosporin and an aminoglycoside carries a risk higher than for either drug alone, requiring close monitoring of renal function when this combination of drugs is used.

TETRACYCLINES. Tetracyclines inhibit protein synthesis and, therefore, shunt amino acids into urea. The enhanced synthesis of urea elevates the blood urea nitrogen (BUN) without a concomitant elevation of serum creatinine or a reduction in GFR. In normal individuals this is of little consequence. In patients with underlying insufficiency, however, the increase in azotemia may be dramatic. With the exception of doxycycline and minocycline, which do not accumulate in renal failure and which require only minor dosage adjustments, tetracyclines should be avoided in individuals with significant renal insufficiency. Demeclocycline causes a dose-related nephrogenic diabetes insipidus. This property has been used to treat some hyponatremic patients, particularly those with the syndrome of inappropriate secretion of antidiuretic hormone. Demeclocycline has been reported to cause acute renal failure, however, when used to treat hyponatremic patients with hepatic cirrhosis. Although the renal failure is reversible, demeclocycline (and other tetracyclines) should be avoided in these patients. Outdated tetracyclines can cause Fanconi's syndrome.

AMPHOTERICIN B. Most patients receiving more than 2 grams of this antifungal agent develop one or more renal abnormalities. Defects in distal nephron function are the first to appear: distal renal tubular acidosis, nephrogenic diabetes insipidus, and renal potassium wasting. These alterations may occur without a reduction in GFR and are generally reversible with discontinuation of the drug. Metabolic acidosis and hypokalemia should be treated with supplemental alkali and potassium salts. Acute renal insufficiency, which may be progressive and incompletely reversible, is a major side effect of amphotericin B. This is dose related and appears to result both from direct renal tubular toxicity and from ischemia due to renal vasoconstriction. Acute renal failure is more likely to occur in patients who are sodium depleted from whatever cause: diuretics, vomiting, and so on. Sodium repletion may protect against amphotericin B nephrotoxicity. Once moderate azotemia is present (BUN > 50 mg per deciliter), consideration should be given to prescribing the drug on alternate days or to temporarily discontinuing therapy until renal function improves. The risk of renal insufficiency has to be weighed, of course, against the severity of the underlying infection and whether alternative antifungal therapy is available.

Radiographic Contrast Agents

Acute renal failure resulting from acute tubular necrosis is an uncommon, but important, complication of iodinated radiographic contrast agents used, for example, in intravenous urography, arteriography, or contrast-enhanced computed tomography. The incidence of acute renal failure associated with these agents has varied in large series from 0 to 13 per cent but is much higher in certain groups of patients. Risk factors include underlying renal insufficiency, diabetes mellitus, older age, dehydration, history of prior acute renal failure following use of contrast agents, multiple contrast procedures in a short period of time, concomitant exposure to other nephrotoxins, and, perhaps, multiple myeloma. In addition, acute renal failure is more likely after administration of larger doses of these agents. Clearly, individuals at highest risk are diabetic patients with renal insufficiency. The incidence of acute renal failure following exposure to these agents in this population of patients may be as high as 75 per cent. In the absence of other risk factors, diabetes *per se* does not appear to pose a major risk. The same is true for multiple myeloma.

The pathogenesis of radiocontrast-induced acute renal failure is uncertain. Several possible mechanisms have been suggested, including ischemia resulting from renal arteriolar vasoconstriction due to the hypertonicity of these agents, tubular obstruction due to precipitation of proteins, and direct tubular toxicity. In addition, as with any drug, anaphylaxis with hypotension is a rare cause of acute renal failure. Patients who develop acute renal failure generally become oliguric within 24 hours of exposure to radiocontrast agents. This usually persists for two to four days, and the peak in serum creatinine elevation typically occurs within seven days. Renal insufficiency is usually moderate and resolves in a few days, but it may be severe and necessitate temporary dialysis. With advanced underlying renal disease, the acute insufficiency may be irreversible. In patients at risk, the serum creatinine concentration should be measured the day after exposure to these agents to determine if nephrotoxicity has occurred. A persistent nephrogram at this time also suggests renal injury.

Prevention of renal failure in patients at high risk includes avoidance of dehydration, minimizing the amount of contrast administered (no more than 0.88 mg of iodine per kilogram of body weight), and using alternative diagnostic methods such as ultrasonography, if possible. Hypertonic mannitol (25 to 50 grams given over one hour) immediately following exposure to radiographic contrast agents may reduce the incidence of acute renal failure in high-risk patients. Treatment of acute renal failure due to contrast agents is similar to that resulting from other etiologies (Ch. 78).

Nephropathies Resulting from Anti-neoplastic Therapy

Several drugs used in the treatment of neoplasia may produce renal toxicity. Some of these may cause isolated abnormalities in renal tubular function, whereas others may produce acute or chronic renal insufficiency. For some of these compounds, renal damage represents the dose-limiting toxicity.

CISPLATIN. Cisplatin and its metabolites are eliminated primarily by urinary excretion. Acute tubular necrosis, which may occur after intravenous administration of the drug, is dose related, being uncommon with single doses less than 50 mg per square meter but occurring in most patients with doses above 100 mg per square meter. The cause of cisplatin toxicity is uncertain, but it appears similar to that produced by other heavy metals (see below). Concomitant administration of cisplatin and other nephrotoxins, such as aminoglycosides, increases the risk of acute renal failure. Generally, azotemia appears a few days after administration of the drug and is usually reversible over a period of two to four weeks. With severe acute renal failure and/or repeated administration of cisplatin, chronic renal insufficiency due to chronic interstitial nephritis may develop. The incidence of acute renal failure due to cisplatin can be reduced by ensuring adequate hydration and establishing a saline diuresis prior to and during administration of the drug and by continuously infusing the drug slowly over several hours or a few days. Hypomagnesemia due to renal magnesium wasting may occur in as many as 50 per cent of patients treated with cisplatin. Hypomagnesemia may be severe, may develop in the absence of renal insufficiency, and may persist for several weeks following cisplatin therapy. Other renal tubular abnormalities, such as potassium wasting, decreased urinary concentrating ability, and low molecular weight proteinuria may also be observed but are generally of little clinical importance.

METHOTREXATE. This folic acid antagonist is eliminated principally by urinary excretion. Nephrotoxicity is rare with low doses (5 to 60 mg per square meter). With high-dose therapy (500 to 7500 mg per square meter), the drug precipitates in the renal tubule lumina and causes acute renal failure from tubular obstruction. Direct tubular toxicity may also play a role. Nephrotoxicity may be reduced by vigorous (intravenous) hydration to maintain a urine flow of greater than 100 ml per hour for several days following high-dose therapy. In

addition, the urine pH should be kept above 7 by alkali administration, since methotrexate is more soluble in alkaline solutions. Development of renal insufficiency prolongs the half-life of methotrexate and increases the likelihood of systemic toxicity.

NITROSOUREAS. A number of nitrosoureas used in cancer chemotherapy, including streptozocin, BCNU, CCNU, and methyl CCNU, may produce several types of renal toxicity. Streptozocin may cause proteinuria, sometimes resulting in nephrotic syndrome, due to glomerular injury; acute tubular necrosis leading to acute renal failure; and a variety of renal tubular abnormalities, including proximal renal tubular acidosis, glycosuria, phosphaturia, and aminoaciduria. Proteinuria is generally the first manifestation of renal toxicity. Should this occur, therapy should be withheld and only cautiously restarted if this resolves. Azotemia developing after streptozocin should lead to permanent discontinuation of the drug. The other nitrosoureas given in multiple courses over several weeks have been associated with a very high incidence of chronic renal insufficiency. In one series the majority of patients receiving at least six courses of therapy developed insidious chronic renal insufficiency, sometimes resulting in uremia, without an antecedent episode of acute renal failure and without abnormalities in the urinary sediment. The principal pathologic findings are chronic interstitial nephritis and glomerular sclerosis. Any nitrosoureas should generally be discontinued at the first sign of an otherwise unexplained decrease in renal function.

MITOMYCIN-C. There is a 5 to 40 per cent incidence of nephrotoxicity following mitomycin-C therapy. Toxicity is dose related and generally appears after repeated courses and/or a cumulative dose of 60 mg per square meter. Renal injury is manifested by proteinuria (usually mild) and azotemia. Renal insufficiency may develop gradually or abruptly. In the latter instance, the clinical features are similar to those of the hemolytic uremic syndrome (Ch. 81) and include thrombocytopenia, microangiopathic hemolytic anemia, and acute renal failure. Renal pathologic findings consist of glomerular alterations (mesangial fragmentation, capillary thrombi, and hemorrhage) and thrombosis and fibrinoid necrosis of the arterioles. There is no established therapy except for supportive measures for renal failure developing after administration of mitomycin-C. Renal function should be monitored closely in patients receiving this drug, and therapy should probably be discontinued if otherwise unexplained azotemia occurs.

MISCELLANEOUS ANTINEOPLASTIC AGENTS. Nephrotoxicity has occasionally been reported with other cancer chemotherapeutic agents, including 5-azacytidine, daunorubicin, doxorubicin, mithramycin, dacarbazine, and recombinant leukocyte A interferon. Finally, therapy resulting in massive acute killing of neoplastic cells may cause the tumor lysis syndrome (see below).

RADIATION NEPHRITIS (Also see Ch. 539). Exposure of the kidneys during abdominal irradiation for cancer may subsequently result in damage of varying degree. Manifestations range from mild proteinuria, urinary concentrating defects, and benign hypertension with a reduced GFR to malignant hypertension with end-stage renal failure. Evidence for renal damage occurs several months to years after renal irradiation, and the severity bears a general relationship to the amount of irradiation received. Clinically evident renal injury is uncommon with less than 1000 to 2000 rads but develops in approximately 50 per cent of patients receiving doses higher than this. In the early stage of radiation nephritis, there is tubular necrosis, medial and intimal thickening of the small renal arteries, and damage to the glomerular endothelium. Later, glomerular sclerosis, collagenous thickening of the small renal arteries, and interstitial fibrosis are prominent. It is unclear whether the primary injury is to the renal tubular epithelium or to the vascular endothelium, both tissues being equally sensitive to radiation damage in experimental situations. The incidence of radiation nephritis can be minimized by limiting the total dose of abdominal irradiation in a single course to 2000 rads over two weeks and by shielding the kidneys as much as possible. Malignant hypertension resulting from unilateral radiation nephritis can be cured by nephrectomy.

URIC ACID AND THE TUMOR LYSIS SYNDROME. Patients with certain hematologic malignancies, particularly acute lymphoblastic leukemia and poorly differentiated lymphomas, may rarely develop spontaneous acute renal failure from obstruction of the renal tubules by uric acid. More frequently, this complication occurs following chemotherapy or radiation therapy, which kills cells and releases massive amounts of purine uric acid precursors. The resulting hyperuricemia greatly increases the filtered load of uric acid. Its solubility is exceeded, and precipitation occurs in the renal tubules, often resulting in acute obstructive renal failure. A ratio of urinary uric acid/creatinine concentrations greater than 1:1 suggests the diagnosis of acute uric acid nephropathy. During massive cell lysis, phosphate is also released in large amounts, and hyperphosphaturia with intrarenal precipitation of calcium phosphate may contribute to the renal failure. Hyperkalemia due to release of intracellular potassium may also be observed. Prevention of acute renal failure secondary to massive tumor cell killing includes establishing a urine output of 3 or more liters per 24 hours and treatment with high-dose allopurinol (300 to 400 mg per square meter per day) prior to institution of cytotoxic therapy. The role of urinary alkalinization is uncertain. Although this will increase the solubility of uric acid, a high urine pH will favor precipitation of phosphate salts in the renal tubules. If renal failure occurs despite the foregoing precautions, hemodialysis is indicated for supportive therapy and for removing uric acid. This allows renal function to recover, generally in a few days. Chronic interstitial nephritis (gouty nephropathy), a rare complication of chronic hyperuricemia and gout, is discussed in Ch. 195.

Metal Nephropathies

The diagnosis and treatment of intoxication with trace metals are discussed in detail in Ch. 542. Only certain aspects of this subject related to the kidney are discussed below. Acute intoxication with some metals may cause both acute renal injury with a reduction in GFR and renal tubular dysfunction. With chronic intoxication, the most common form of injury is chronic interstitial nephritis manifested by renal tubular abnormalities with or without reduction in GFR. In certain instances glomerular injury may also occur. Metal intoxication is often treated by chelation therapy. Unfortunately, some of the drugs used for this purpose, e.g., penicillamine, may also be nephrotoxic, as discussed below.

LITHIUM. Lithium carbonate, used in the treatment of affective disorders, causes a variety of renal abnormalities. The most frequent is a form of vasopressin-resistant nephrogenic diabetes insipidus, probably due to decreased production of cyclic adenosine monophosphate (AMP) by collecting ducts in response to the hormone. This is of little consequence in most patients. Polyuria (urine volumes > 3000 ml per day) may result but usually abates when lithium therapy is stopped. The diuretic amiloride may significantly reduce the polyuria associated with lithium. Incomplete distal renal tubular acidosis and mild renal sodium wasting may also result from lithium therapy. Chronic interstitial nephritis is more common in individuals with psychiatric disorders than in the general population. The risk of this nephritis occurring in lithium-treated patients seems to be only minimally higher than in similar but untreated patients. In patients taking lithium, a history of acute lithium intoxication, however, appears to predispose to development of chronic renal insufficiency.

LEAD. Lead poisoning may result from acute exposure, e.g., from ingestion of lead-containing paint, but more often from chronic exposure, e.g., in foundry and battery workers or from consumption of illicit alcoholic beverages or "moonshine"). Acute intoxication, more common in children, is manifested primarily by abdominal colic, hemolytic anemia, and encephalopathy. Acute interstitial nephritis with eosinophilic inclusions in the proximal tubular cells, tubular necrosis with a reduction in GFR, and Fanconi's syndrome may also occur. Whether acute lead intoxication without further exposure results in chronic renal disease in later years is unclear. Chronic lead intoxication causes interstitial nephritis with variable reductions in GFR and renal tubular dysfunction. Some patients develop gout and hypertension as a result of chronic lead intoxication ("saturnine gout"). Some patients with "essential" hypertension and renal failure have excess body burdens of lead. Therefore, chronic lead intoxication should be considered in individuals with the triad of gout, hypertension, and chronic renal insufficiency. A history of exposure to lead should be sought and a CaNa$_2$-EDTA infusion carried out to evaluate lead stores (Ch. 542). Treatment of acute lead intoxication consists of preventing further exposure to the metal, supportive care, and chelation with dimercaptopropanol (BAL) or CaNa$_2$-EDTA. Chronic renal insufficiency resulting from lead may sometimes improve during chelation therapy but may also progress despite this therapy.

MERCURY. Acute intoxication with mercurial salts may cause tubular necrosis and severe renal failure. The strong affinity of mercury for sulfhydryl groups, along with the hypotension that frequently accompanies acute intoxication, probably accounts for the acute renal injury. Acute exposure may occur rarely in industrial settings or with intentional ingestion of mercurial salts. Treatment of acute mercury poisoning with mercurial salts consists of chelation therapy with dimercaptopropanol or penicillamine and supportive care (Ch. 542). Chronic exposure to organomercurials may result in subtle renal damage manifested by increased urinary excretion of low molecular weight proteins and renal tubular enzymes (tubular proteinuria). Chelation therapy is ineffective in removing organomercurials. Chronic exposure to mercurial compounds may also cause the nephrotic syndrome as a result of glomerular damage, most commonly from membranous nephropathy. The pathogenesis of this disorder is uncertain, as mercury is not demonstrable in the glomeruli.

GOLD. Proteinuria may complicate the treatment of rheumatoid arthritis with gold salts, more frequently with parenteral than with oral administration. Proteinuria may develop at any time, but usually after several months of therapy. Rarely, it may be severe enough to result in the nephrotic syndrome associated with membranous nephropathy. It is unlikely that gold *per se* is directly responsible for the glomerular injury, since the metal can be demonstrated in the renal tubules, but not in the glomeruli. Gold may in some way modify an intrinsic protein such that it becomes antigenic and elicits the immune reactions that produce membranous nephropathy. Membranous nephropathy may also occur in patients with rheumatoid arthritis who have not been treated with gold. The appearance of proteinuria in a patient receiving gold should prompt discontinuation of the drug. This will generally result in disappearance of the proteinuria, but this may occur only several months later.

ARSENIC. Arsenic is used in a number of industrial applications and is present in several commercial products such as insecticides. In addition, illicit alcohol may be contaminated with the metal. Gastrointestinal symptoms and peripheral neuropathy are the most prominent manifestations of acute arsenic poisoning, but acute tubular necrosis may also occur. Like mercury, arsenic has a high affinity for sulfhydryl groups of proteins. Cellular damage resulting from this interaction and from hypotension are the most likely causes of acute renal damage. Treatment of arsenic poisoning includes supportive measures and chelation therapy with dimercaptopropanol. Arsine gas may cause acute renal failure secondary to hemoglobinuria from acute hemolysis and from hypotension.

CADMIUM. With chronic low-level exposure—for example, in alkaline battery workers—cadmium accumulates in the renal cortex. This may result in mild proteinuria, of both glomerular and tubular origin, and in early renal insufficiency. The incidence of proteinuria increases with the length of exposure.

MISCELLANEOUS METALS. *Bismuth* has been reported to cause both acute tubular necrosis and the nephrotic syndrome. Acute *copper* poisoning may result in acute tubular necrosis, most likely resulting from hemolysis with hemoglobinuria and from hypotension. Chronic copper accumulation in Wilson's disease (Ch. 205) may be associated with proximal renal tubular acidosis and other components of Fanconi's syndrome and mild renal insufficiency. In rare instances, renal injury has been reported with *antimony*, *thallium*, and *uranium* intoxication. *Platinum* nephrotoxicity is discussed under cisplatin.

Oxalate

End-stage renal failure from chronic interstitial nephritis and from recurrent nephrolithiasis is the major complication of primary hyperoxaluria and may rarely occur in enteric hyperoxaluria as well (Ch. 182).

Acute intoxication with ethylene glycol is the major cause of acute renal failure due to oxalate. Ethylene glycol is the major component of antifreeze and is usually ingested by desperate alcoholics, by children accidently, or in a suicide attempt. Ethylene glycol is metabolized to several toxic substances, one of which is oxalic acid. Intoxication with ethylene glycol causes acute renal failure, profound metabolic acidosis of the anion gap variety (Ch. 77), and acute central nervous system and pulmonary dysfunction. Renal failure results from massive deposition of oxalate within the renal tubules. This is usually accompanied by large numbers of calcium oxalate crystals in the urinary sediment. Ethylene glycol intoxication is managed by (1) administration of ethyl alcohol to slow the metabolism of ethylene glycol by competing for alcohol dehydrogenase; (2) hemodialysis to remove the parent compound, to allow treatment with sodium bicarbonate therapy, which may be required in amounts that would otherwise result in pulmonary edema and hypernatremia, and to treat acute renal failure; and (3) administration of pyridoxine and thiamine to help shunt ethylene glycol into other metabolic pathways that result in less toxic metabolites. If patients survive acute intoxication, chances for recovery of renal function are good, but many will require temporary dialysis for several days prior to functional renal recovery.

As noted below, acute renal failure accompanying methoxyflurane anesthesia may result, in part, from oxalate.

Captopril

This angiotensin-converting enzyme inhibitor used in the treatment of hypertension and congestive heart failure has been associated with both acute renal failure and the nephrotic syndrome. Acute renal failure has been reported in patients with bilateral renal artery stenosis or stenosis of the renal artery supplying a solitary kidney. Usually captopril-associated acute renal failure is thought to be hemodynamic in origin, resulting from loss of autoregulation of renal blood flow and glomerular filtration rate. Sometimes, however, acute renal failure has been accompanied by skin rash, eosinophilia and eosinophiluria, a constellation of findings strongly suggesting allergic interstitial nephritis. Acute renal failure in both the above settings generally resolves with discontinuation of captopril but may recur upon rechallenge with the

drug. Membranous nephropathy with the nephrotic syndrome may also occur in association with captopril therapy. This complication may resolve slowly after discontinuation of the drug. Membranous nephropathy occurring during therapy with captopril and penicillamine (see below) may possibly be related to the active sulfhydryl group that they contain.

D-Penicillamine

Therapy with this drug for metal chelation, rheumatoid arthritis, scleroderma, or cystinuria is complicated by proteinuria in 4 to 7 per cent of patients, often sufficiently severe to result in the nephrotic syndrome. Proteinuria, which may be associated with mild azotemia, usually results from membranous nephropathy (Ch. 81). Rarely, rapidly progressive glomerulonephritis accompanied by pulmonary hemorrhage occurs. Proteinuria generally resolves or decreases when therapy with D-penicillamine is discontinued, but usually only after several months.

Methoxyflurane

This fluorinated anesthetic agent may cause a dose-related postoperative nephrogenic diabetes insipidus and acute renal failure. Similar complications have rarely been reported with enflurane. The initial polyuric acute renal failure may progress to oliguria in severe cases. Renal function may recover after several days, but persistent renal failure, which has required long-term dialysis, may develop. The pathogenesis of methoxyflurane-induced acute renal failure is uncertain. The drug is metabolized to fluoride and oxalate. Although oxalate is nephrotoxic (see above), it is believed that the major toxic product is fluoride, since nephrotoxicity correlates with blood levels of this ion and fluoride produces nephrotoxicity in experimental animals. Volume depletion due to the urinary concentrating defect may also contribute to acute renal failure.

Miscellaneous Nephrotoxins

Exposure to *hydrocarbons*, frequently in the form of paint or glue sniffing, has been associated with a variety of (generally) reversible abnormalities, including azotemia, renal tubular acidosis, Fanconi's syndrome, proteinuria, hematuria, and pyuria. Similar findings may result from exposure to halogenated alkane solvents such as *carbon tetrachloride* and insecticides such as *paraquat*. *Silicon* exposure—for example, in sandblasters—has been implicated in a connective tissue–like disease with multiple serologic abnormalities and progressive renal failure associated with both glomerular and renal tubular pathologic changes that appear to be immune mediated.

Heroin abuse is associated with a variety of glomerular lesions, including amyloidosis, and glomerulonephritis due to bacterial endocarditis or hepatitis B infection. In a number of patients, however, these etiologies cannot be implicated as the cause of the heroin-associated glomerular disease. Most commonly, focal sclerosing glomerulopathy is found, often resulting in the nephrotic syndrome. Heroin-associated nephropathy generally results in progressive renal failure unless abuse of the drug is stopped.

The nephrotic syndrome may occur as a rare complication of *trimethadione* and *methimazole*. *Sulfonamides* and intravenous *amphetamines* may cause systemic vasculitis that results in renal damage from segmental renal infarction or glomerulonephritis (Ch. 81 and 439). Acute renal insufficiency is a major complication of cyclosporine therapy of organ transplantation (Ch. 80.2). *Nifedipine*, like many other drugs, may cause prerenal azotemia because of hypotension but, in addition, may also rarely cause reversible acute renal failure in the absence of a fall in blood pressure and without abnormalities in the urinary sediment.

Retroperitoneal fibrosis as a complication of long-term treatment of migraine headaches with *methysergide* may obstruct the ureters. *Anticoagulant therapy* may cause ureteral obstruction from intraluminal blood clots or from ureteral compression by a retroperitoneal hematoma.

ACUTE AND CHRONIC INTERSTITIAL NEPHRITIS

Adler SG, Cohen AH, Border WA: Hypersensitivity phenomena and the kidney: Role of drugs and environmental agents. Am J Kidney Dis 5:75, 1985. *An excellent review of the various types of immune-mediated renal injury that may result from numerous pharmacologic agents.*

Boucher A, Droz D, Adafer E, et al.: Characterization of mononuclear cell subsets in renal cellular interstitial infiltrates. Kidney 29:1043, 1986. *Using monoclonal antibodies, the authors found that the predominant mononuclear cells in interstitial cellular infiltrates of 33 renal biopsies, including 11 with acute or chronic interstitial nephritis, were T cells. However, the relative proportions of the different T cells subsets varied among the biopsies.*

Cotran RS, Rubin RH, Tolkoff-Rubin NE: Tubulo-interstitial diseases. In Brenner BM, Rector FC Jr (eds.): The Kidney. Edition 3. Philadelphia, W. B. Saunders Company, 1986. *An excellent review of this topic (353 references).*

Lins LE: Reversible renal failure caused by hypercalcemia. Acta Med Scand 203:309, 1978. *In 13 patients with hypercalcemia of differing etiology, there was a direct correlation between serum concentrations of calcium and creatinine before and after treatment of their hypercalcemia.*

McCluskey RT: Immunologically mediated tubulo-interstitial nephritis. In Cotran RS (guest ed.), Brenner BM, Stein JH (eds.): Tubulointerstitial Nephropathy, Vol. 10 of Contemporary Issues in Nephrology. New York, Churchill-Livingstone, 1982, p 121. *A comprehensive review of this subject utilizing both clinical and experimental observations.*

Riemenschneider T, Bohle A: Morphologic aspects of low-potassium and low-sodium nephropathy. Clin Nephrol 19:271, 1983. *This report describes the renal histopathology and clinical findings in 40 patients with chronic hypokalemia of varying etiologies.*

Stone WJ: Renal complications of neoplastic paraproteinemias. In McKinney TD (ed.): Renal Complications of Neoplasia. New York, Praeger, 1986. *A recent review of this subject with emphasis on clinical manifestations and management.*

DRUG-INDUCED ACUTE INTERSTITIAL NEPHRITIS

Ditlove J, Weidmann P, Bernstein M, et al.: Methicillin nephritis. Medicine 56:483, 1977. *In this report the authors describe 4 of their patients with methicillin nephritis and review 68 others previously reported in the literature.*

Galpin JE, Shinaberger JH, Stanley JH, et al.: Acute interstitial nephritis due to methicillin. Am J Med 65:756, 1978. *This report describes 14 cases of methicillin nephritis, 8 of whom were treated with prednisone.*

Hande KR, Noone RM, Stone WJ: Severe allopurinol toxicity. Am J Med 76:47, 1984. *This report describes 7 patients with allopurinol toxicity treated by the authors and reviews another 78 cases from the literature. Dosage guidelines for allopurinol for patients with varying degrees of renal insufficiency are proposed.*

Magil AB, Ballon HS, Cameron EC, et al.: Acute interstitial nephritis associated with thiazide diuretics. Am J Med 69:939, 1980. *This report describes the clinical characteristics and renal biopsy findings in three patients who developed AISN while being treated with a combination of hydrochlorothiazide and triamterene.*

Nessi R, Bonoldi GL, Redaelli B, et al.: Acute renal failure after rifampicin: A case report and survey of the literature. Nephron 16:148, 1976. *One case of acute renal failure that developed after rifampin administration is presented, along with a review of 36 previously reported cases.*

Pusey CD, Saltissi D, Bloodworth L, et al.: Drug associated acute interstitial nephritis: Clinical and pathological features and response to high dose steroid therapy. QJ Med 52:194, 1983. *In this report nine cases of drug-related AISN are described, four of which were associated with sulfonamides. Seven episodes were treated with high-dose methylprednisolone with rapid improvement in renal function.*

TOXIC NEPHROPATHY (GENERAL REFERENCES)

Heptinstall RH: Renal complications of therapeutic and diagnostic agents, analgesic abuse and addiction to narcotics. In Heptinstall RH (ed.): Pathology of the Kidney. Edition 3. Boston, Little, Brown and Company, 1983. *This chapter provides a thorough discussion and representative photographs of the renal histopathology of these toxic compounds.*

Humes HD, Weinberg JM: Toxic nephropathies. In Brenner BM, Rector FC Jr (eds.): The Kidney. Edition 3. Philadelphia, W. B. Saunders Company, 1986. *A recent, extensive, and well-written review with 579 references.*

Roxe DM: Toxic nephropathy from diagnostic and therapeutic agents. Am J Med 69:759, 1980. *A brief summary of this topic with 141 references.*

ANALGESIC NEPHROPATHY

Blohme I, Johansson S: Renal pelvic neoplasms and atypical urothelium in patients with end-stage analgesic nephropathy. Kidney Int 20:671, 1981. *This paper describes 4 cases of renal pelvic carcinoma among 84 patients with end-stage analgesic nephropathy. In addition, urothelial atypia was found in the renal pelvis of 27 of 56 patients whose kidneys were removed immediately prior to or after renal transplantation. No atypia was found in other types of renal disease.*

Buckalew VM Jr, Schey HM: Renal disease from habitual antipyretic analgesic consumption: An assessment of the epidemiologic evidence. Medicine 65:291, 1986. *This paper reviews the worldwide evidence which indicates that habitual analgesic use is an important cause of renal diseases (74 references).*

Eknoyan G, Qunibi WY, Grissom RT, et al.: Renal papillary necrosis: An update. Medicine 61:55, 1982. *A comprehensive review of the various causes of papillary necrosis, including analgesic nephropathy.*

Kincaid-Smith P (ed.): Analgesic nephropathy. Kidney Int 13:1, 1978. *This entire issue is devoted to virtually every aspect of clinical and experimental analgesic nephropathy.*

NONSTEROIDAL ANTI-INFLAMMATORY DRUGS

Carmichael J, Shankel SW: Effects of nonsteroidal anti-inflammatory drugs on prostaglandins and renal function. Am J Med 78:992, 1985. *This paper summarizes in tabular form many cases of the various renal syndromes that have been reported with the NSAID's in current use (146 references).*

Clive DM, Stoff JS: Renal syndromes associated with nonsteroidal anti-inflammatory drugs. N Engl J Med 310:563, 1984. *An excellent review of this topic with 157 references.*

Dunn MJ, Patrono C (eds.): Renal effects of nonsteroidal anti-inflammatory drugs. Am J Med 81(Suppl 2B):1, 1986. *The several papers from the proceedings of this recent symposium deal with most aspects of this topic (1068 references).*

ANTIMICROBIAL DRUGS

Appel GB, Neu HC: The nephrotoxicity of antimicrobial agents. N Engl J Med 296:663, 722, 784, 1977. *This three-part series provides an extensive review of this topic (272 references).*

Heidemann HT, Gerkins JF, Spickard WA, et al.: Amphotericin B nephrotoxicity in humans decreased by salt repletion. Am J Med 75:476, 1983. *This report describes five patients, four of whom were sodium depleted, who developed renal insufficiency with amphotericin B therapy. Sodium repletion was associated with improved renal function, which allowed completion of therapy.*

Humes HD, Weinberg JM, Knauss TC: Clinical and pathophysiologic aspects of aminoglycoside nephrotoxicity. Am J Kidney Dis 2:5, 1982. *This in-depth review discusses both clinical and experimental features of aminoglycoside nephrotoxicity (215 references).*

Perez-Ayuso RM, Arroyo V, Camps J, et al.: Effect of demeclocycline on renal function and urinary prostaglandin E_2 and kallikrein in hyponatremic cirrhotics. Nephron 36:30, 1984. *In this report, five of eight hyponatremic cirrhotic patients given demeclocycline developed acute reversible renal insufficiency with a reduction in GFR from an average of 72 to 31 ml per minute.*

RADIOGRAPHIC CONTRAST–INDUCED NEPHROTOXICITY

Anto HR, Chou SY, Porush JG, et al.: Infusion intravenous pyelography and renal function. Arch Intern Med 141:1652, 1981. *In this report there was a 22 per cent incidence of worsening renal function in 37 patients with underlying renal insufficiency (mean serum creatinine 4.1 ml per deciliter) given 50 grams of mannitol immediately following intravenous urography. This compares with a 70 per cent incidence in a similar group of patients not receiving mannitol previously reported by the same authors.*

Berkseth RO, Kjellstrand CM: Radiologic contrast-induced nephropathy. Med Clin N Am 68:1, 1984. *A comprehensive review of this topic (101 references).*

NEPHROTOXICITY ASSOCIATED WITH ANTINEOPLASTIC THERAPY

Chiuten D, Vogl S, Kaplan B, et al.: Is there cumulative or delayed toxicity from cis-platinum? Cancer 52:211, 1983. *This study of 95 patients receiving repeated courses of cisplatin in doses of 50 to 75 mg per square meter suggests that cumulative nephrotoxicity is low (around 4 per cent) if adequate hydration and diuresis are established prior to and during administration of the drug.*

Giroux L, Bettez P, Giroux L: Mithramycin-C nephrotoxicity: A clinicopathologic study in 17 cases. Am J Kidney Dis 6:28, 1985. *This is a good description of clinical and pathological findings in this disorder.*

Goldberg ID, Garnick MB, Bloomer WD: Urinary tract toxic effects of cancer therapy. J Urol 132:1, 1984. *This brief review provides a concise discussion of the genitourinary complications of radiation therapy, cisplatin, methotrexate, and nitrosoureas.*

Hainsworth JD, Johnson DH, Porter LL: Nephrotoxicity associated with antineoplastic therapy. In McKinney TD (ed.): Renal Complications of Neoplasia. New York, Praeger, 1986. *A recent review of this topic with a particularly extensive discussion of cisplatin nephrotoxicity.*

Hande KR: Hyperuricemia, uric acid nephropathy and the tumor lysis syndrome. In McKinney TD (ed.): Renal Complications of Neoplasia. New York, Praeger, 1986. *A recent comprehensive review of this topic.*

METAL NEPHROPATHIES

Craswell PW, Price J, Boyle PD, et al.: Chronic renal failure with gout: A marker of chronic lead poisoning. Kidney Int 26:319, 1984. *This is one of several recent papers that confirms the association of renal failure, gout, and chronic lead intoxication.*

Cullen MR, Robins JM, Eskenazi B: Adult inorganic lead intoxication: Presentation of 31 new cases and a review of recent advances in the literature. Medicine 62:221, 1983. *This article describes clinical characteristics in 31 patients with lead intoxication resulting from industrial exposure, along with a review of the topic (207 references).*

Falck FY Jr, Keren DF, Fine LJ, et al.: Protein excretion patterns in cadmium exposed individuals. High resolution electrophoresis. Arch Environ Health

39:69, 1984. *In this study, 7 of 39 men chronically exposed to industrial sources of cadmium had mild proteinuria, and 5 had mild elevations of serum creatinine concentrations.*

Gerhardt RE, Crecelius EA, Hudson JB: Moonshine-related arsenic poisoning. Arch Intern Med 140:211, 1980. *This paper reviews 12 cases of arsenic poisoning, 50 per cent of which resulted from "moonshine" ingestion. Five patients with acute or semiacute poisoning had renal damage.*

Johanson GFS, Hunt GE, Duggin GG, et al.: Renal function and lithium treatment: Initial and follow-up tests in manic depressive patients. J Affective Disord 6:249, 1984. *In this study, several renal function tests were serially examined in 61 patients receiving long-term lithium therapy. Twelve per cent of them had a low GFR, which correlated with previous episodes of acute lithium intoxication.*

Katz WA, Blodgett RC Jr, Pietrusko RG: Proteinuria in gold-treated rheumatoid arthritis. Ann Intern Med 101:176, 1984. *In this report 41 of 1283 (3 per cent) patients receiving oral gold treatments for rheumatoid arthritis developed proteinuria. In 9 this was in the nephrotic range. The results suggest that oral gold is less nephrotoxic than parenteral gold therapy.*

Tubbs RR, Gephardt GN, McMahon JT, et al.: Membranous glomerulonephritis associated with industrial mercury exposure. Am J Clin Pathol 77:409, 1982. *This report describes two patients with industrial exposure to mercury who developed biopsy-proven membranous nephropathy with heavy proteinuria. In one case proteinuria resolved after cessation of exposure to mercury, and this correlated with a decline in urinary mercury excretion from high to normal values.*

Wedeen RP: Occupational renal disease. Am J Kidney Dis 3:241, 1984. *This review discusses numerous important aspects of intoxication with several metals and other industrial toxins.*

MISCELLANEOUS NEPHROTOXINS

Bolton WK, Suratt PM, Sturgill BC: Rapidly progressive silicon nephropathy. Am J Med 71:823, 1981. *The clinical and pathologic features of four cases of this syndrome are described.*

Diamond JC, Cheung JY, Fang LST: Nifedipine-induced renal dysfunction. Am J Med 77:905, 1984. *This paper describes four patients with underlying renal insufficiency who had reversible acute declines in renal function during nifedipine therapy in the absence of hypotension.*

Gabow PA, Clay K, Sullivan JB, et al.: Organic acids in ethylene glycol intoxication. Ann Intern Med 105:16, 1986. *This paper describes three patients with ethylene glycol intoxication, acute renal failure, and metabolic acidosis successfully treated by a combination of ethanol infusion and hemodialysis.*

Hricik DE, Browning PJ, Kopelman R: Captopril-induced functional renal insufficiency in patients with bilateral renal artery stenosis or renal artery stenosis in a solitary kidney. N Engl J Med 308:373, 1983. *Eleven patients are described who developed reversible renal insufficiency four days to two months after institution of therapy with captopril.*

Llach F, Descoeudres C, Massry SG: Heroin-associated nephropathy: Clinical and histologic studies in 19 patients. Clin Nephrol 11:7, 1979. *A variety of glomerular lesions were present in these patients, the majority of which resulted in the nephrotic syndrome.*

Ntoso KA, Tomaszewski JE, Jimenez SA, et al.: Penicillamine-induced rapidly progressive glomerulonephritis in patients with progressive systemic sclerosis: Successful treatment of two patients and a review of the literature. Am J Kidney Dis 8:159, 1986.

Streicher HZ, Gabow PA, Moss AH, et al.: Syndromes of toluene sniffing in adults. Ann Intern Med 94:758, 1981. *Clinical features of 25 cases of toluene sniffing are reported. The most prominent renal-electrolyte manifestation was hyperchloremic metabolic acidosis.*

83 OBSTRUCTIVE NEPHROPATHY

Floyd C. Rector, Jr.

Obstruction of the urinary tract may produce profound structural and functional changes in the kidneys and, if uncorrected, may result in complete, irreversible loss of renal function. Early diagnosis and appropriate correction, therefore, are essential for preserving or restoring renal function and preventing the progression to end-stage renal failure. The obstructing lesions may occur at any site in the urinary tract from the renal tubules to the terminal urethra. The clinical presentation is variable, depending on the site of obstruction and whether the obstruction is acute or chronic, complete or partial, unilateral or bilateral, or complicated by urinary tract infection.

INCIDENCE AND ETIOLOGY. In a large series of autopsies the prevalence of hydronephrosis has varied from 3.5 to 3.8 per cent. Clinically significant urinary tract obstruction occurs less frequently than noted at postmortem examination;

TABLE 83–1. CAUSES OF OBSTRUCTIVE UROPATHY

Intraluminal
Stone
Bladder tumor
Papillary necrosis
Clot
Ureteral tumor
Bence Jones proteinuria
Acute urate nephropathy

Intramural
Congenital
  Ureteropelvic dysfunction (10 per cent bilateral)
  Ureterovesical stricture (simple or ureterocele)
  Bladder neck obstruction
  Pinpoint meatus
Acquired
  Urethral stricture
  Ureteral stricture (tuberculosis, etc.)
  Neurogenic bladder dysfunction

Extramural
Prostatic obstruction
Ureteropelvic juncture—vessels, bands, etc.
Aortic aneurysm
Periureteral fibrosis
Retroperitoneal tumor or nodes
  Extraurinary growth (carcinoma of colon, diverticulitis)
Pelvic tumor
Inadvertent ligature

nevertheless it is a rather common disease in all age groups. Hydronephrosis is a contributing factor to destruction of renal function in 15 to 25 per cent of uremic patients.

Obstructive uropathy can result from three general types of obstruction (Table 83–1): (1) mechanical obstruction of the lumen of the urinary tract; (2) functional or anatomic abnormalities of the ureter, bladder, or urethra; or (3) compression from masses or processes extrinsic to the urinary tract. The prevalence of the various causes of obstruction varies with age and sex. The most common causes are congenital abnormalities of the urinary tract (e.g., urethral valves, vesicoureteral reflux, cystocele) in children, pregnancy and pelvic malignancy in women, renal stones in young men, and prostatic hypertrophy in elderly men. Acute ureteral obstruction from calculi results in the hospitalization of 1 out of 1000 Americans each year. Benign prostatic enlargement occurs in 80 per cent of men over 60 years, and 10 per cent of these require surgery for the correction of obstruction. Vesicoureteral reflux is most common in young girls, but also occurs to some extent in approximately 5 per cent of adults. Neurogenic bladder dysfunction is a serious medical problem frequently complicated by incontinence, recurrent urinary tract infection, bladder stones, and hydronephrosis; this disorder can occur secondary to traumatic injuries of the spinal cord or to metabolic and neurologic diseases (diabetes mellitus, multiple sclerosis, myelodysplasia, senile dementia, and vascular disease).

PATHOLOGY AND PATHOPHYSIOLOGY. Obstruction of the lower urinary tract produces profound structural and functional changes in the kidney and, if complete, can irreversibly destroy renal function within four to six weeks. This is the consequence of combined mechanical and hormonal factors (Table 83–2). Superimposition of urinary tract infection or renal immunologic injury (antibody formation secondary to the release of renal antigens into the circulation) will accelerate and intensify this destruction of renal function.

Immediately following obstruction of one ureter, pressures in the pelvis and tubules increase, causing the pelvis and tubules to dilate and the renal papillae to become flattened. Secondary to the increased tubular pressure and dilatation there is a marked decrease in glomerular filtration rate, disruption of the junctional complexes between tubular cells permitting backleak of solutes from tubule lumen to blood, and inhibition of sodium reabsorption and potassium and hydrogen secretion in the distal nephron.

Concomitant with these mechanical changes there is stimulation of prostaglandin production within the kidney. Increased levels of PGI_2 (prostacyclin) stimulate the release of renin (sufficient to cause acute hypertension) and produce

TABLE 83–2. EFFECTS OF OBSTRUCTION ON RENAL FUNCTION

I. Mechanical
  A. Increased tubular pressure
    1. Disruption of junctional complexes—increased tubule permeability
    2. Decreased collecting duct Na transport; decreased H^+ and K^+ secretion
    3. Decreased GFR
  B. Increased renal interstitial pressure
    1. Altered proximal reabsorption
    2. Impaired countercurrent function

II. Hormonal
  A. Increased PGI_2 synthesis
    1. Stimulated renin release
    2. Cortical vasodilation
  B. Increased PGE_2 synthesis
    1. Medullary vasodilation
    2. Inhibition of vasopressin action
    3. Inhibition of aldosterone action
    4. Inhibition of Cl^- transport in thick ascending limb
  C. Increased thromboxane A_2 synthesis
    1. Cortical vasoconstriction
    2. Decreased number of functioning nephrons
  D. Retained natriuretic factors in blood

III. Other
  A. Decreased glomerular permeability
  B. Decreased mesangial clearance of immune complexes

vasodilation in the renal cortex. Increased levels of PGE_2 produce vasodilation in the renal medulla, block the action of vasopressin, and further inhibit salt transport in the loop of Henle and distal nephron. As a consequence of these hormonal changes there is an initial rise in renal blood flow, lasting four to six hours. Thereafter, renal blood flow progressively falls to levels of 10 to 15 per cent of normal despite continued increased production of PGI_2 and PGE_2. This fall in blood flow is the result of intense renal vasoconstriction produced by increased levels of the prostaglandin derivative thromboxane A_2, one of the most potent vasoconstrictors known. Associated with these mechanical and hormonal changes the kidney becomes severely ischemic, with many nephrons ceasing to function. The residual nephrons have reduced filtration rates and impaired ability to conserve sodium, secrete potassium, and acidify and concentrate the urine. The tubules progressively atrophy, the medulla is destroyed, and by four to six weeks the cortex consists of only a thin shell of connective tissue with few remaining glomeruli.

If the obstruction is corrected prior to this stage of irreversible renal damage, there may be significant recovery of renal function. Experimental studies in dogs have shown 45 to 50 per cent recovery after two weeks of complete obstruction, 15 to 30 per cent recovery after three to four weeks of obstruction, but no recovery after six weeks of complete obstruction.

In contrast to the changes observed with complete obstruction, with partial obstruction, particularly if bilateral, the renal pelvis may become tremendously dilated, holding 2 to 3 liters of urine, and yet structure and function of the renal cortex may be relatively well preserved. Functionally, filtration rate and blood flow may be only slightly (or moderately) reduced, and the major abnormality may be the inability to concentrate the urine and/or secrete potassium and hydrogen ions.

CLINICAL MANIFESTATIONS OF URINARY TRACT OBSTRUCTION.

The clinical manifestations of urinary tract obstruction depend on the site of obstruction and on whether it is acute or chronic. Patients with obstruction below the bladder (prostate, urethra) may have decreased force and caliber of the urinary stream, intermittency, postvoid dribbling, hesitancy, and nocturia. Neurogenic dysfunction of the bladder with incomplete emptying may cause urgency, frequent urination, and urinary incontinence (overflow incontinence). These symptoms, however, do not occur with obstruction at higher levels in the urinary tract. Urinary tract obstruction may also present as asymptomatic hydronephrosis, as renal colic, as either acute or chronic renal failure, or occasionally as a specific renal tubular disorder (Table 83–3).

Pain. The pain associated with urinary tract obstruction is produced by distention of the renal capsule, and the intensity of the pain is related to the rate of distention. With chronic, low-grade obstruction the renal collecting system can be tremendously dilated without producing pain. This form of obstruction will be discovered either accidentally or during the workup for urinary tract infection, renal failure, or renal tubular abnormalities. Occasionally, in patients with chronic asymptomatic hydronephrosis the urinary tract may become acutely and painfully distended during a diuresis induced by large fluid intake (e.g., water, beer). Therefore, intermittent flank pain induced by fluid intake should suggest the presence of urinary tract obstruction. Pain induced by urination should suggest vesicoureteral reflux. Acute obstruction of a ureter with a stone may produce one of the most severe forms of pain encountered in clinical medicine. Usually the pain is located in the lower abdomen or flank, radiating into the groin on the obstructed side.

Renal Failure. Chronic obstruction of one kidney will result in unilateral hydronephrosis if the obstruction is partial, and in a nonfunctioning kidney if the obstruction is complete. Unilateral obstruction will not produce renal failure if the opposite kidney is functional. However, obstruction of a single functioning kidney or bilateral obstruction can give rise to either acute or chronic renal failure.

Acute renal failure secondary to obstruction is usually associated with severe oliguria or anuria, although it may occasionally present as "high output" acute renal failure. Variable output from day to day should suggest the presence of lower urinary tract obstruction. Acute renal failure can arise from sudden occlusion of the lower urinary tract or from widespread intratubular obstruction secondary to precipitation of Bence Jones protein in patients with multiple myeloma or of uric acid in patients with myeloproliferative disorders treated with chemotherapy.

TABLE 83–3. CLINICAL MANIFESTATIONS OF URINARY TRACT OBSTRUCTION

1. Lower tract symptoms: urgency, hesitancy, incontinence, nocturia

2. Chronic hydronephrosis
  a. Asymptomatic
  b. Intermittent pain

3. Renal colic

4. Renal failure
  a. Acute
    (1) Intratubular
    (2) Lower tract
  b. Chronic
    (1) Hydronephrosis
    (2) Infection ± lithiasis
    (3) Interstitial nephritis
    (4) Reflux nephropathy
    (5) Papillary necrosis

5. Recurrent urinary tract infection

6. Renal tubule dysfunction
  a. Concentration defect
    (1) Nocturia, polyuria
    (2) Nephrogenic diabetes insipidus
  b. Distal renal tubular acidosis
  c. Potassium secretory defect

7. Hypertension
  a. Acute—renin dependent
  b. Chronic—volume dependent

8. Polycythemia

9. Postobstructive diuresis

Urinary tract obstruction is an important pathogenetic factor in 15 to 25 per cent of patients with end-stage renal failure and uremia. This progression to chronic renal failure can occur as a consequence of progressive hydronephrosis or by the destructive effects of recurrent urinary tract infections. In fact, it is unusual for chronic, recurrent pyelonephritis to occur in the absence of mechanical problems in the lower urinary tract. Urinary tract obstruction may also produce chronic interstitial nephritis unrelated to infection. Recently, several patients with chronic vesicoureteral reflux have been found to have severe chronic glomerulonephritis. The mechanism is not known.

Infection. Recurrent urinary tract infection may be superimposed on urinary tract obstruction and present with the typical symptoms of fever, flank tenderness, and dysuria. The incidence of urinary tract infection ranges from 8 to 15 per cent in patients with urinary tract obstruction who have not been previously instrumented. Instrumentation (bladder catheters, cystoscopy), neurogenic bladder dysfunction, and bladder stones all increase the incidence of chronic infection. Once infection is established in the obstructed urinary tract, it is extremely difficult to eradicate and may contribute significantly to morbidity and the rate of destruction of renal function.

Tubular Dysfunction. A small percentage of patients may present with renal tubular abnormalities as the principal manifestation of their urinary tract obstruction. The most frequent of these abnormalities is inability to concentrate the urine. Usually, this is characterized by isosthenuria, nocturia, and modest polyuria, but occasionally may express itself as vasopressin-resistant nephrogenic diabetes insipidus with the excretion of large volumes (greater than 4000 ml per day) of dilute urine. The factors contributing to the defect in concentrating ability are destruction of the renal medulla and the antagonistic effects of PGE_2 against the renal action of vasopressin. Occasionally, patients with obstruction may present with renal tubular acidosis of the distal type, characterized by hyperchloremic acidosis with an inability to lower urine pH below 6.0 in response to acid loading. Less commonly, patients with obstruction may present with hyperkalemia secondary to a renal tubular defect in potassium secretion. When hyperkalemia occurs it is invariably associated with hyperchloremic acidosis.

Hypertension. Hypertension occurs in approximately 30 per cent of patients with acute unilateral obstruction. The hypertension tends to be mild and transient (rarely lasting longer than one week) and is caused by increased renin secretion. In general, hypertension is not a feature of chronic unilateral obstruction, although there have been a few cases of high-renin hypertension reported, which were corrected by removal of the obstructed kidney. In contrast, a high percentage of patients with chronic bilateral hydronephrosis have hypertension. These patients do not have elevated renin levels, and the hypertension appears to be the consequence of retained salt and water.

Polycythemia. A rare manifestation of obstructive nephropathy is polycythemia. In the small number of patients in whom this disorder has been observed, the erythrocytosis rapidly resolves following nephrectomy and is thought to be due to abnormal production of erythropoietin by the obstructed kidney.

Postobstructive Diuresis. Following the surgical correction of lower urinary tract obstruction the patient may undergo a marked diuresis ("postobstructive diuresis"). Both clinically and experimentally, postobstructive diuresis is associated with bilateral, but not with unilateral, obstruction. In most instances the diuresis is transient and does not result in significant contraction of extracellular volume. In these cases the diuresis is the consequence of the excretion of salt, urea, other solutes, and water retained during the period of obstruction, and continues until the volume and composition of the extracellular fluid return to normal. In a few instances, however, the diuresis represents a true salt and water wastage, with depletion of extracellular volume and its associated findings (e.g., postural hypotension, tachycardia). A natriuretic factor, normally excreted into the urine, may be retained during periods of bilateral obstruction and causes salt wasting when the obstruction is released. There also appears to be a vasopressin-resistant component to the diuresis, possibly caused by high levels of renal prostaglandins.

DIAGNOSIS AND EVALUATION. Urinary tract obstruction should be suspected in patients who have lower urinary tract symptoms (diminished stream, urgency, hesitancy, incontinence); recurrent urinary tract infections; pain in the flank, groin, or lower abdomen; abdominal masses; or unexplained uremia or oliguric acute renal failure. The patient's history should be evaluated for previous stone disease, drug ingestion, diabetes mellitus, or neurologic disorders. The physical examination should evaluate the abdomen and flanks for pain or masses, the external genitalia, the prostate in men, and the pelvic structures in women. In selected circumstances, postvoiding urine volume measured by bladder catheterization may provide the key to diagnosis. This test, however, must be performed with great care to avoid inducing infection.

In patients presenting with acute oliguric renal failure, other causes of oliguria-anuria must be excluded. These include (1) extracellular volume depletion, (2) renal arterial or venous occlusion, (3) acute glomerular disease or vasculitis, (4) cortical necrosis, (5) acute tubular necrosis, and (6) urinary tract obstruction. Workup of these patients should include history of drug exposure (antibiotics, radiopaque dyes, analgesics, chemotherapy), evidence for multiple myeloma or uric acid nephropathy, and status of extracellular fluid volume. The urine should be carefully examined for red cell casts, renal tubular cell casts (renal failure casts), urate crystals, and red cells. Urine sodium concentration is helpful in that it should be low (less than 10 mEq per liter) in prerenal azotemia, acute glomerular disease, or renal vasculitis, but will be relatively high in acute tubular necrosis and urinary tract obstruction.

The key to the diagnosis of urinary tract obstruction is the demonstration of a dilated urinary collecting system. One of the most useful techniques for identifying dilation of the renal pelvis, particularly in acutely oliguric patients, is ultrasonography. This technique is rapid and noninvasive and avoids the potential hazards of radiocontrast dyes. The intravenous urogram with nephrotomography is also a useful procedure in patients in whom radiocontrast agents are not contraindicated. In the presence of renal failure it is necessary to use a higher dose of dye. In most patients, even those with severe reduction of glomerular filtration rate (GFR), there should be adequate visualization to determine kidney size, whether there are one or two kidneys, and whether the renal pelvis is dilated. If the obstruction is acute, the nephrogram will be delayed but quite dense, whereas if the obstruction is more chronic, the nephrogram will be faint. Delayed films, 24 to 36 hours after dye injection, may be necessary to visualize the renal pelvis and collecting system sufficiently to identify the site of obstruction. More recently, computed tomography has proved useful in identifying urinary tract obstruction and its cause. In performing these tests it must be remembered that the renal pelvis may not be dilated at the time of study if the obstruction is partial and/or intermittent or if the patient is severely volume depleted. In evaluating patients with intermittent flank pain, it is important, therefore, to perform the study at a time when the patient is having pain or after induction of osmotic or water diuresis. In severely ill patients, it is important to correct any deficits of extracellular volume prior to the test.

Once the presence of urinary tract obstruction is established, more complex urologic procedures such as retrograde pyelography, percutaneous antegrade pyelography, cystoscopy, and voiding cystograms may be needed to identify the site of obstruction, the presence of vesicoureteral reflux, and the functional status of the bladder. Renal radionuclide scans are helpful in determining the relative function of the two kidneys and are particularly useful in determining the residual function of a unilaterally obstructed kidney.

TREATMENT. The general aims of therapy are (1) relief from the symptoms of obstruction, (2) prevention or eradication of infection, and (3) preservation of renal function. Obstruction complicated by infection and sepsis is a potentially lethal disease requiring relief of obstruction as soon as possible. Complete obstruction, uncomplicated by infection, is not a medical emergency, but should be evaluated and corrected promptly for optimal preservation of renal function. In this situation uremia, if present, should first be treated by dialysis before proceeding with surgical correction of the obstruction. Elective repair of urinary tract obstruction is indicated in patients with recurrent urinary infections, persistent pain, urinary retention, recurrent bleeding, or progressive renal damage. Simple uncomplicated postvoid residual urine, vesicoureteral reflux, and dilation of the collecting system are not indications for surgery.

The specific method used for relief of obstruction depends on the general status of the patient, whether the situation requires an emergency or elective procedure, the location of the obstruction, whether the obstructing lesion is benign or malignant, whether the obstruction is mechanical or neurogenic, and the functional status of the obstructed kidney.

In the septic patient requiring an emergency procedure, the obstruction can be relieved either by urethral or ureteral catheters or by percutaneous placement of a nephrostomy tube into the dilated renal pelvis. These bypass procedures can also be used electively in the presence of complete obstruction to gain time for diagnostic studies and the evaluation of residual renal function. Occasionally, one may elect to leave these diversion tubes in place permanently. Despite the inevitable urinary infection associated with the presence of these tubes, the patients may survive for years with little or no further loss of renal function. However, whenever possible, the tubes should be removed and a more definitive procedure performed. If the obstructed kidney is nonfunctional and has no chance of recovering function (chronic obstruction or complete acute obstruction for more than three to four months), then nephrectomy may be the most judicious procedure. A discussion of surgical procedures is beyond the scope of this chapter.

Acute obstruction of a ureter with a renal stone is usually transient and will correct spontaneously in 85 to 90 per cent of the cases. If the stone is greater than 5 mm, it may become impacted in the ureter and require surgical removal within a few days. If a stone lodged in the ureter does not produce complete obstruction, one can delay for two to four weeks to see if spontaneous passage will occur. If the stone is not passed, it should then be surgically removed. Manipulation or removal of ureteral stones by a basket catheter is sometimes successful, but this procedure runs the risk of ureteral injury with subsequent stricture.

Functional obstruction secondary to neurogenic bladder is a complicated and difficult management problem. Helpful maneuvers are frequent voiding, double voiding, suprapubic pressure on the bladder during voiding, and the use of cholinergic drugs. Intermittent catheterization may also be used, with the addition of anticholinergic or sympathomimetic drugs to prevent incontinence between catheterizations. More severe cases may require a permanent indwelling catheter or, preferably, surgical reimplantation of the ureters into an ileal conduit.

Klahr S (guest ed.): Obstructive uropathy. In Kurtzman N (ed.): Seminars in Nephrology, Vol II, No 1, March, 1982. *A superb multiauthored review of the physiologic, biochemical, and hormonal changes in the obstructed kidney.*

Klahr S, Buerkert J, Morrison A: Urinary tract obstruction. In Brenner BM, Rector FC (eds.): The Kidney. 3rd ed. Philadelphia, W. B. Saunders Company, 1986, pp 1443–1490. *An extensive review of the pathophysiology of obstructive uropathy written for nephrologists; with 379 references.*

Okegawa T, Jonas PE, DeSchryver K, et al.: Metabolic and cellular alterations underlying the exaggerated renal prostaglandin and thromboxane synthesis in ureter obstruction in rabbits. J Clin Invest 71:81, 1983. *Acute unilateral ureteral obstruction produces an inflammatory reaction in the obstructed kidney with an interstitial infiltrate of monocytes and fibroblasts. These inflammatory cells account for the increased cyclo-oxygenase activity and the exaggerated production of PGE_2 and thromboxane A_2.*

84 SPECIFIC RENAL TUBULAR DISORDERS

Martin G. Cogan

INTRODUCTION

The diverse reabsorptive functions of the kidney are generally segregated such that specific nephron segments are responsible for specific transport functions. As described in Ch. 75, the proximal nephron is responsible for the reabsorption of most of the filtered bicarbonate, glucose, amino acids, uric acid, phosphate, and low molecular weight proteins. The loop of Henle reabsorbs over half the filtered sodium chloride as well as divalent cations. The distal nephron (including the cortical and medullary collecting ducts), under the influence of aldosterone, reabsorbs the final quantity of sodium, secretes hydrogen ions to lower the pH of the urine and titrate buffers, and secretes potassium ions. The terminal collecting ducts can be induced by antidiuretic hormone to permit water reabsorption and thereby cause urinary concentration.

Genetic and acquired conditions exist that can affect one or more of the reabsorptive or secretory transport processes within each of these nephron segments, as illustrated in Table 84–1. Depending on the transport sites affected, these diseases therefore lead to abnormal wastage or retention of specific solutes. For instance, within a given nephron segment, there may be a selective transport defect for a single solute (e.g., bicarbonate in proximal renal tubular acidosis or glucose in renal glycosuria) or for a class of solutes (e.g., dibasic amino acids in cystinuria). Alternatively, those solutes modulated by a specific hormone may be affected by a hormone-deficient or -resistant state (e.g., in hypoaldosteronism or diabetes insipidus). Finally, there are diseases that affect all solutes normally transported by a given nephron segment (e.g., all proximal transported solutes in Fanconi's syndrome). Luminal, cellular, or peritubular components of the overall transport process can be responsible for each of these situations. The following sections, and other chapters (195, 196, 227, 230, 246, and 247) as identified in Table 84–1, describe some of the more common transport defects of the individual nephron segments.

DISORDERS OF PROXIMAL NEPHRON FUNCTION

The proximal nephron is responsible for reabsorbing 80 to 99 per cent of several filtered solutes, including glucose, amino acids, and bicarbonate. Appearance of one or more of these solutes in the urine at normal filtered loads implies a disorder of proximal transport.

Renal Glycosurias

The renal glycosurias are caused by inherited or acquired defects in proximal tubule glucose reabsorption such that glycosuria occurs in the absence of hyperglycemia.

PATHOPHYSIOLOGY. Glucose is reabsorbed across the luminal membrane of the proximal tubule by a stereospecific carrier that requires sodium. The amount of glucose reabsorbed changes in proportion to filtered glucose load until a

TABLE 84–1. CLINICAL SYNDROMES DUE TO NEPHRON TRANSPORT DEFECTS

Proximal Nephron

I. *Selective transport defects*
  A. Renal glycosurias
    1. Primary
    2. Combined:
      a. Glucose/galactose malabsorption
      b. Glucoglycinuria
  B. Renal aminoacidurias
    1. Basic aminoacidurias
      a. General: cystinuria (cystine, lysine, arginine, ornithine)
      b. Specific: hypercystinuria, dibasic aminoaciduria (lysine, arginine, ornithine), lysinuria
    2. Neutral aminoacidurias
      a. General: Hartnup disease
      b. Specific: methioninuria, tryptophanuria, histidinuria
    3. Iminoglycinuria
      a. General (proline, hydroxyproline, glycine)
      b. Specific: glycinuria
    4. Dicarboxylic aminoaciduria
      a. General (glutamic, aspartic acids)
  C. Proximal renal tubular acidosis
    1. Primary: idiopathic or genetic
    2. Transient (infants)
    3. Carbonic anhydrase deficiency, inhibition, alteration
      a. Drugs: acetazolamide, sulfanilamide, mafenide acetate
      b. Idiopathic?
  D. Renal uric acid disorders (see Ch. 195, 196)
  E. Phosphate and calcium disorders (see Ch. 246, 247)
II. *Nonselective transport defects: Fanconi's syndrome*
  A. Primary: idiopathic or genetic
  B. Genetically transmitted systemic diseases
    1. Cystinosis
    2. Lowe's syndrome
    3. Wilson's disease
    4. Tyrosinemia
    5. Hereditary fructose intolerance
    6. Pyruvate carboxylase deficiency
  C. Dysproteinemic states
    1. Multiple myeloma
    2. Monoclonal gammopathy
  D. Secondary hyperparathyroidism with chronic hypocalcemia
    1. Vitamin D deficiency or resistance
    2. Vitamin D dependency
  E. Drugs and toxins
    1. Outdated tetracycline
    2. Methyl-3-chromone
    3. Streptozotocin
    4. Glue
    5. Gentamicin
  F. Heavy metals
    1. Lead
    2. Cadmium
    3. Mercury
  G. Tubulointerstitial diseases
    1. Sjögren's syndrome
    2. Medullary cystic disease
    3. Renal transplantation
  H. Other diseases
    1. Nephrotic syndrome
    2. Amyloidosis
    3. Osteopetrosis
    4. Paroxysmal nocturnal hemoglobinuria

Loop of Henle

I. *Bartter's syndrome*
II. *Drugs*
  A. Furosemide
  B. Bumetanide
  C. Ethacrynic acid

Distal Nephron

I. *Selective transport defects*
  A. Classic distal RTA
    1. Primary: genetic or idiopathic
    2. Genetically transmitted systemic diseases
      a. Ehlers-Danlos syndrome
      b. Hematologic disorders: hereditary elliptocytosis, sickle cell anemia, carbonic anhydrase I deficiency or alteration
      c. Medullary cystic disease
      d. With nerve deafness
      e. Glycogenosis type III
    3. Autoimmune diseases
      a. Hypergammaglobulinemia: hyperglobulinemic purpura, cryoglobulinemia, familial
      b. Sjögren's syndrome
      c. Thyroiditis
      d. Pulmonary fibrosis
      e. Chronic active hepatitis
      f. Primary biliary cirrhosis
      g. Systemic lupus erythematosus
    4. Diseases associated with nephrocalcinosis
      a. Primary hyperparathyroidism
      b. Vitamin D intoxication
      c. Hyperthyroidism
      d. Hypercalciuria: idiopathic or genetic
      e. Hereditary fructose intolerance
      f. Medullary sponge kidney
      g. Fabry's disease
      h. Wilson's disease
    5. Drug or toxic nephropathies
      a. Amphotericin B
      b. Toluene
      c. Glue
      d. Analgesics
      e. Cyclamate
    6. Tubulointerstitial diseases
      a. Chronic pyelonephritis secondary to urolithiasis
      b. Obstructive uropathy
      c. Renal transplantation
      d. Leprosy
      e. Hyperoxaluria
    7. Miscellaneous
  B. RTA of glomerular insufficiency
  C. Hypermineralocorticoid and other potassium secretory disorders (see Ch. 230)
II. *Nonselective transport defects: generalized distal RTA, hyperkalemia, and renal salt wasting*
  A. Primary mineralocorticoid deficiency (see Ch. 230)
  B. Hyporeninemic hypoaldosteronism
    1. Diabetic nephropathy
    2. Tubulointerstitial nephropathies
    3. Nephrosclerosis
    4. Nonsteroidal anti-inflammatory agents
  C. Mineralocorticoid-resistant hyperkalemia
    1. Without salt wasting: genetic
    2. With salt wasting
      a. Childhood forms
      b. Tubulointerstitial nephropathies: methicillin, obstructive nephropathy, transplantation, sickle cell disease
      c. Drugs: spironolactone, amiloride, triamterene

Loop and Medullary Collecting Ducts

I. *Diabetes insipidus* (see Ch. 227)
II. *SIADH* (see Ch. 227)
III. *Other concentrating and diluting disorders*

---

maximal reabsorptive capacity or "Tm" is reached, as shown in Figure 84–1. Somewhat before saturation is attained, glucose reabsorption is incomplete, representing the "splay" in the response. The initial point of the splay represents that filtered glucose concentration or load, called the "threshold," at which reabsorption no longer equals filtration and glucose appears in the urine. The normal threshold concentration is 200 to 240 mg per deciliter, well above the normal plasma glucose concentration, so little glucose (< 125 mg per day) appears in the urine of a normal individual. The kinetics of glucose reabsorption have been analogized to an enzyme system: The Tm is equivalent to the $\dot{V}max$, whereas the Km

is related to the degree of splay. In the two major types of renal glycosurias, either the capacity (type A, Vmax or Tm mutation) or the affinity (type B, Km, or degree of splay mutation) of glucose reabsorption is altered (Fig. 84–1). In either case, the threshold is reduced so glucose is spilled into the urine at a normal plasma glucose concentration. The glycosuria is markedly exaggerated when filtered glucose concentration is elevated by intravenous hypertonic glucose infusion.

SYMPTOMS AND ETIOLOGIES. Renal glycosurias (Table 84–1) are relatively unusual, with an incidence (depending on the stringency of diagnostic criteria) of about 0.2 to 0.6 per

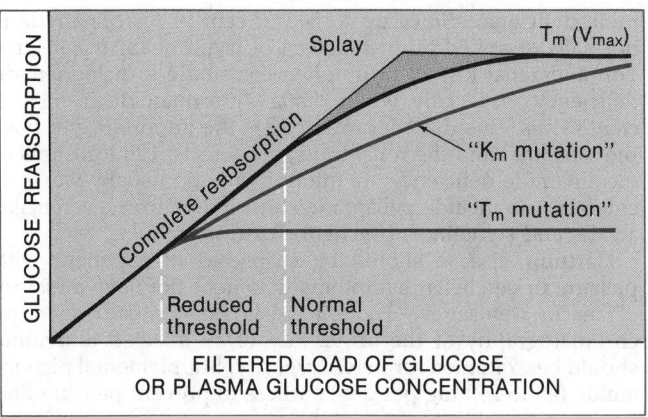

FIGURE 84–1. Kinetics of renal glucose reabsorption and the two variants of renal glycosuria. (Modified from Cogan MG: Disorders of proximal nephron function. Am J Med 72:278, 1982.)

cent. They are usually inherited in an autosomal recessive manner. Homozygotes have more severe glycosuria than heterozygotes. Usually, but not invariably, Vmax and Km variants of the syndrome are inherited separately. On renal biopsy, there are no consistent pathologic distinguishing features. Unlike the aminoacidurias, there is no coexisting intestinal transport defect for glucose. Renal glycosuria is completely asymptomatic (i.e., affected individuals do not have polydipsia or polyuria).

Intermittent glycosuria is not infrequent during pregnancy (second and third trimesters) and during the terminal phases of chronic renal insufficiency. In both cases, an increase in tubular flow rate, due to an increase in total or just single nephron glomerular filtration rate (GFR), is probably the primary cause of the functional alteration in glucose transport kinetics. In a rare syndrome in children, malabsorption of two sugars, glucose and galactose, in both the jejunum and the kidney causes diarrhea and mellituria.

DIAGNOSIS AND TREATMENT. Diagnosis should be based on finding a urinary glucose excretion of greater than 500 mg per 24 hours (on a diet containing 30 kilocalories per kilogram, of which 50 per cent is carbohydrate) in the absence of hyperglycemia (plasma glucose < 140 mg per deciliter). The glucose oxidase method should be used to confirm that the excreted sugar is glucose in order to exclude other mellituric conditions (pentosuria, fructosuria, sucrosuria, maltosuria, galactosuria, and lactosuria). Appropriate tests to rule out coexistent tubular transport defects (of amino acids, bicarbonate, phosphate, and uric acid) typical of the Fanconi syndrome should be performed, and diabetes mellitus must be excluded, using standard clinical and laboratory evidence. If desired, differentiation of the Vmax or Km variants can be accomplished by glucose loading.

The condition is completely benign with respect to symptoms and to renal functional deterioration. Treatment is unnecessary. Prolonged fasting should be avoided to prevent the unusual complication of hypoglycemia and ketosis.

Cystinuria and Other Renal Aminoacidurias

The renal aminoacidurias are inherited disorders in which one or a group of amino acids are excreted by the kidney (in the absence of hyperaminoacidemia) and are usually also malabsorbed by the intestine (Table 84–1).

GENERAL CONSIDERATIONS. Amino acids are avidly reabsorbed in the proximal nephron so that only about 2 per cent of the filtered amino acid load is excreted in the urine (except for glycine, 5 per cent, and histidine, 8 per cent). In general, most amino acids are transported by a stereospecific carrier across the luminal membrane of the proximal nephron accompanied by sodium and driven by the lumen-to-cell

sodium gradient. Under some circumstances, amino acids can also be secreted. Reabsorptive kinetics are similar to those of glucose (Fig. 84–1). Five major luminal membrane carriers for reabsorption exist, each of which transports a specific group of amino acids: basic amino acids (cystine, lysine, arginine, and ornithine); acidic amino acids (glutamic and aspartic acids); neutral amino acids (alanine, serine, threonine, valine, leucine, isoleucine, phenylalanine, tyrosine, tryptophan, and histidine); iminoglycine amino acids (proline, hydroxyproline, and glycine); and beta-amino acids (beta-aminoisobutyric acid, beta-alanine, and taurine). Inherited dysfunction of a carrier results in urinary loss of the entire amino acid group: cystinuria (basic aminoaciduria); dicarboxylic aminoaciduria; Hartnup disease (neutral aminoaciduria); and iminoglycinuria. There is no clinical disorder yet described of beta-amino acid transport. There are also other carriers (> 25 are estimated to exist) that selectively transport only one or several members of a given amino acid group. Disorders of these carriers cause even more selective aminoaciduria: hypercystinuria, histidinuria, and lysinuria.

Many of the amino acid carriers in the proximal nephron are also expressed on the luminal membrane of gastrointestinal epithelial cells. Defective gastrointestinal absorption therefore occurs conjointly with increased renal excretion of the amino acid or acids in question. Amino acid dimers can be normally absorbed by the gut, however, so that nutritional problems arising from amino acid malabsorption are unusual. Furthermore, gut absorption is not so constrained by time as that in the renal tubule, i.e., does not require such rapid efficiency.

For diagnosis of a renal aminoaciduria, a high plasma level of the amino acid must first be excluded. Excessive filtration of an amino acid can overwhelm the tubular transport carrier for it and other members of its amino acid family and result in one or more aminoacidurias. These "overflow" aminoacidurias are discussed in Ch. 187–193. In contrast, the renal aminoacidurias are associated with low or normal levels of plasma amino acid concentrations because the aminoaciduria is due to defective proximal tubular transport.

CYSTINURIA. One of the most common aminoacidurias is *cystinuria* (basic aminoaciduria), an autosomal recessive disease estimated to affect about 1:7000 individuals (between 1:1000 and 1:20,000, depending on the population studied). Urinary spillage of lysine, arginine, and ornithine is asymptomatic. Cystine, however, is the least soluble of naturally occurring amino acids, and it therefore tends to precipitate to form cystine urolithiasis. Cystinuria accounts for about 1 to 2 per cent of all urinary calculi. Stone formation usually becomes manifest during the second and third decades of life, though presentation may occur from infancy to the ninth decade, and males are more severely affected. Cystine stones are yellow-brown and have a granular appearance. Such stones are radiopaque, can create staghorn calculi, and frequently form a nidus for calcium oxalate stone formation. Symptoms include renal colic, which may be associated with obstruction or infection or both. Evidence associating cystinuria with central nervous system disorders has been tenuous. A more general discussion of nephrolithiasis is found in Ch. 90.

The diagnosis of cystinuria should be entertained in any patient with a renal calculus, even if the stone is composed primarily of calcium oxalate (since cystine might have been the formation nidus). The typical hexagonal crystals may be recognized on urinalysis, especially in a concentrated, acidic, early morning specimen. A useful screening test is the cyanide-nitroprusside test, which will detect a cystine excretion rate of about 75 to 125 mg per gram of creatinine. Because of false-positive results, a definitive diagnosis requires thin-layer or ion-exchange chromatography or high-voltage electrophoresis. Excretion rates in an adult of greater than 18 mg of cystine per gram of creatinine confirm the diagnosis. The dibasic amino acids will also be increased in excretion per gram of creatinine: lysine > 130 mg; arginine > 16 mg; and ornithine > 22 mg. Persons with homozygous cystinuria routinely excrete more than 250 mg of cystine per gram of creatinine, usually about 0.5 to 1.0 gram per day. Cystinuria has three allelic variants, classified according to whether coexisting intestinal and renal basic amino acid transport is completely absent (types I and II) or variably reduced (type III) and whether heterozygotes have normal (type I) or supernormal (types II and III) urinary cystine and basic aminoaciduria.

Medical therapy of cystinuria is aimed at decreasing the urinary concentration below the solubility limit of 300 mg of cystine per liter. The most practical approach is to increase fluid intake to about 3 to 4 liters per day. The polyuria must be maintained at all times, including nighttime, when the urine otherwise tends to become concentrated and acidic. Cystine solubility also can be increased by alkalinizing urine pH, but a urine pH of greater than 7.5 is necessary to achieve a salutary effect. Avoidance of excessive intake of methionine, the metabolic precursor of cystine, is a reasonable adjunctive therapy but is ineffective as a sole therapy. When conservative measures fail, D-penicillamine is recommended, usually in a dose of 1 to 2 grams per day. This drug forms a mixed disulfide of penicillamine-cysteine, which is much more soluble than cystine alone. Free cystine excretion then falls to an acceptable level. Unfortunately, penicillamine causes fever and a rash in as many as 50 per cent of patients, and sometimes arthralgias. More severe hypersensitivity reactions also occur, including membranous nephropathy and nephrotic syndrome, pancytopenia or thrombocytosis, epidermolysis, hypogeusia, and a Goodpasture-like syndrome. In some cases the drug can be readministered at a lower dose following an adverse reaction. Pyridoxine should be given as a supplement, since penicillamine can deplete this cofactor. Other investigational agents, such as N-acetyl-D-penicillamine and mercaptopropionylglycine, have been reported to be efficacious. There have been conflicting reports regarding the utility of glutamine administration. Chlordiazepoxide has also been found to reduce cystine excretion.

HARTNUP DISEASE. Hartnup disease, a neutral aminoaciduria, is a rare autosomal recessive disorder (1:16,000 births) in which the clinical presentation is dominated by nicotinamide deficiency. Since up to 50 per cent of nicotinamide is normally supplied by metabolism of tryptophan, malabsorption and renal loss of tryptophan contribute to nicotinamide deficiency, especially when dietary nicotinamide is insufficient. Thus, this disorder exemplifies the importance of both the intestinal and the renal transport defects. Clinical signs of nicotinamide deficiency are intermittent and usually worse in children and include pellagra in sun-exposed areas, cerebellar ataxia, and sometimes psychiatric disturbance.

Hartnup disease should be suspected in a patient with pellagra or cerebellar symptoms who does not have a history of niacin deficiency. The diagnosis can be confirmed by chromatography of the urine. Sibs of an affected individual should be examined for heterozygosity. Supplemental nicotinamide (40 to 250 mg per day) suffices to prevent pellagra and neurologic problems.

OTHER AMINOACIDURIAS. Less common aminoacidurias lacking clinical manifestations include iminoglycinuria, isolated hypercystinuria (without hyperexcretion of other basic amino acids), isolated glycinuria, and dicarboxylic aminoaciduria. Mental retardation predominates in the rare disorders of hyperdibasic aminoaciduria, isolated lysinuria, histidinuria, and methioninuria.

Proximal Renal Tubular Acidosis (RTA)

Proximal (type II) RTA is a hyperchloremic, hypokalemic metabolic acidosis due to a selective defect in proximal acidification, which is characterized by a normally acidic urine during acidosis but marked bicarbonate wasting when plasma bicarbonate concentration is normalized.

PATHOPHYSIOLOGY. The proximal nephron reabsorbs 85 to 90 per cent of the filtered bicarbonate, predominantly by Na^+/H^+ exchange and the enzymatic degradation of H_2CO_3 to CO_2 and H_2O by carbonic anhydrase (Fig. 84–2). Interference with the normal operation of Na^+/H^+ exchange or of carbonic anhydrase activity will therefore result in excess delivery of bicarbonate to the distal nephron and, because of the limited distal bicarbonate reabsorption capacity, into the urine. Thus, the urinary wastage of 15 per cent or more of the filtered bicarbonate load at a normal blood bicarbonate concentration is pathognomonic of proximal RTA. The excess delivery of the relatively impermeant bicarbonate to the distal

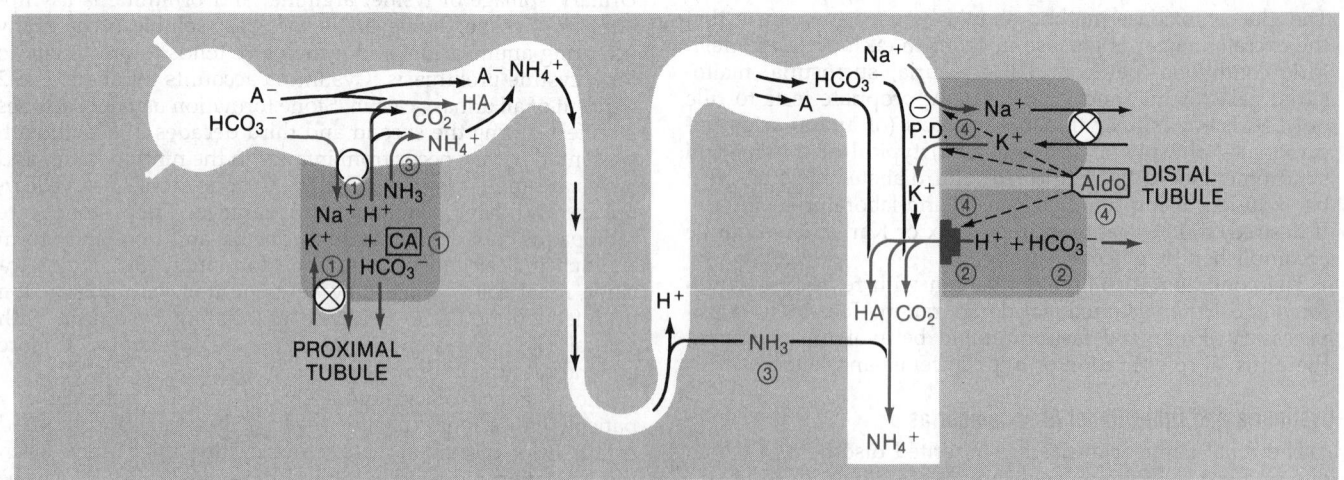

FIGURE 84–2. Sites of impaired renal acidification (RTA). The proximal tubule reabsorbs most of the filtered bicarbonate by hydrogen ion secretion. Proximal acidification is sodium- and carbonic anhydrase–dependent and is energetically driven by the lumen-to-cell sodium gradient. Disorders of proximal acidification, proximal RTA, may result from defects (labelled 1) in the Na^+/H^+ exchanger, carbonic anhydrase activity, or the activity of the basolateral Na^+-K^+ ATPase. The distal nephron is regulated by aldosterone to reabsorb sodium and secrete hydrogen ions. Distal acidification is responsible for titrating both remaining filtered buffer (labelled A^-) to form titratable acids (HA) and proximally produced ammonia (NH_3) to form ammonium (NH_4^+). Disorders of distal acidification include defects of the proton pump or basolateral bicarbonate exit step (labelled 2) in classic distal RTA, of ammonia production or delivery (labelled 3) in the RTA of glomerular insufficiency, or in aldosterone levels or target sites (labelled 4) in generalized distal RTA.

TABLE 84–2. RENAL TUBULAR ACIDOSES

Type	Renal Defect	Plasma [K+]	Proximal Acidification HCO_3^- Reabsorption (During HCO_3^- Loading)	Distal Acidification $U_{pH_{min}}$ (During Acidosis)	$(U_{NH_4^+}\cdot V) + (U_{TA}\cdot V)$ (During Acidosis)
Proximal (type II)	↓ Proximal acidification	↓	↓	< 5.5	N
Classic distal (type I)	↓ Distal pH gradient	↓	N	> 5.5	↓
Glomerular insufficiency	↓ NH_3 production	N	N	< 5.5	↓
Generalized distal (type IV)	↓ Aldosterone action	↑	N	< 5.5	↓

Abbreviations: $U_{pH_{min}}$ = minimal urinary pH; $(U_{NH_4^+}\cdot V) + (U_{TA}\cdot V)$ = urinary ammonium plus titratable acid excretion; N = normal.

nephron also results in accelerated potassium secretion and hypokalemia. As the plasma bicarbonate concentration and filtered load fall owing to defective proximal bicarbonate reabsorption and subsequent urinary bicarbonate wastage, absolute bicarbonate delivery to the distal nephron progressively decreases. At a certain point, usually when the plasma bicarbonate concentration is 15 to 18 mM, the distal nephron can cope with the delivery out of the proximal tubule. At this stage, bicarbonaturia disappears, urinary pH can be lowered normally, and net acid excretion equivalent to endogenous acid production resumes. Acid-base homeostasis is reestablished at the expense of metabolic acidosis.

SYMPTOMS AND ETIOLOGIES. Manifestations of proximal RTA are attributable to acidemia (growth retardation, anorexia and malnutrition, volume depletion), potassium depletion (muscular weakness, polyuria, nocturia, polydipsia), and disordered calcium/phosphate/parathormone/vitamin D metabolism (osteomalacia and other bone diseases). Proximal RTA is a rare disorder, usually found when carbonic anhydrase is defective or is inhibited or in conjunction with the full Fanconi syndrome (Table 84–1).

DIAGNOSIS AND TREATMENT. Laboratory findings of proximal RTA are those of a hyperchloremic, hypokalemic metabolic acidosis. When the patient is acidemic, the urine is acidic and net acid excretion equals endogenous acid load (Table 84–2). When bicarbonate is infused to normalize the plasma bicarbonate concentration, massive bicarbonaturia results (≥ 15 per cent of the filtered load). Proximal RTA is usually not isolated but rather associated with the full Fanconi syndrome.

Therapy of the underlying disease should be undertaken if possible (e.g., multiple myeloma) or offending drugs or toxins discontinued (e.g., heavy metals). When this is not possible, proximal RTA is treated with large amounts of sodium and potassium bicarbonate. As the plasma bicarbonate concentration rises with treatment, distal bicarbonate delivery increases, causing more potassium wasting and the need for further potassium supplementation. Because of the inability to correct the disorder fully with bicarbonate alone, volume contraction utilizing diuretics is also used to stimulate fractional proximal bicarbonate reabsorption. Therapy with vitamin D is indicated when signs of vitamin D deficiency exist.

Nonselective Proximal Nephron Dysfunction: Fanconi's Syndrome

In the Fanconi syndrome, the entire array of proximal transport functions is impaired, resulting in glycosuria, generalized aminoaciduria, proximal RTA, phosphaturia, and uricaciduria.

PATHOPHYSIOLOGY. The lumen-to-cell sodium gradient provides the driving force in the proximal tubule for the absorption of glucose, amino acids, phosphate, and organic acids and for secretion of hydrogen ions needed to reabsorb bicarbonate. Disruption of this common driving force serves as an attractive hypothesis to explain the global functional impairment of reabsorption of solutes in the proximal tubule observed in the Fanconi syndrome. Collapse of the sodium gradient could arise by several mechanisms: a primary disturbance of the Na^+-K^+ adenosinetriphosphatase (ATPase); in-

creased permeability of the cell to sodium; or reduced metabolic energy due to an abnormality in the redox potential or in intracellular phosphate supply.

In addition to the solutes described above, there is disordered reabsorption, and sometimes depressed serum concentrations, of calcium, magnesium, citrate, and low molecular weight proteins. Enhanced sodium delivery to the distal nephron causes kaliuresis and hypokalemia. Since the proximal nephron is the principal site of conversion of 25-OH vitamin D to 1,25-$(OH)_2$ vitamin D, the circulating level of this latter hormone is also diminished.

SYMPTOMS AND ETIOLOGIES. As a result of the complex disorders of mineral and vitamin D metabolism, the most prominent clinical finding of the Fanconi syndrome is metabolic bone disease, either rickets in children or osteomalacia in adults (see also Ch. 246). Nausea, episodic vomiting, anorexia, and growth retardation in children are frequent. Other clinical findings include symptoms of hypokalemia, such as polyuria and muscle weakness.

Causes of the Fanconi syndrome are listed in Table 84–1. The most common inherited disorder is *cystinosis*, in which cystine accumulates in cells, specifically in lysosomes, of the kidney, liver, gut, lymphoid tissues, conjunctiva, and cornea and in bone marrow–derived cells and fibroblasts. Cystinosis should be distinguished from cystinuria, described above. Cystinosis may present as the Fanconi syndrome, followed by renal failure, in the first two years of life (infantile nephropathic form) or in the adolescent years. It is usually relatively benign if it first appears in adulthood, causing only asymptomatic cystine deposits in the conjunctiva, cornea, and bone marrow. An interesting inducible form of the Fanconi syndrome is *hereditary fructose intolerance* (HFI) caused by a deficiency of aldolase B activity. Ingestion of fructose in affected individuals causes acute symptoms, including nausea, vomiting, abdominal pain, and neurologic dysfunction. Chronic fructose ingestion can cause symptoms associated with the Fanconi syndrome and with liver dysfunction.

In adults, acquired Fanconi's syndrome is most often due to dysproteinemias, heavy metal (especially chronic cadmium or acute lead) exposure, or immunologic diseases (Table 84–1). An older adult presenting with the Fanconi syndrome should be assumed to have multiple myeloma until proven otherwise.

DIAGNOSIS AND TREATMENT. Diagnosis of the Fanconi syndrome is established by finding consequences of the full array of proximal nephron dysfunction: glycosuria, generalized aminoaciduria, proximal RTA, phosphaturia, hypouricemia, hypovitaminosis D, and secondary hypokalemia. Underlying causes of the Fanconi syndrome (Table 84–1) should be sought. Serum and urine electrophoresis should be obtained to rule out multiple myeloma in adults.

Treatment of the Fanconi syndrome itself requires attempts to normalize the electrolyte and vitamin imbalance. Supplements of bicarbonate (up to 15 to 20 mEq per kilogram of body weight daily), potassium, phosphate, magnesium, and vitamin D are necessary. Treatment of the underlying disease, of course, varies widely. Effective results have been reported in the treatment of cystinosis with cysteamine, of Wilson's disease with penicillamine, of hereditary fructose intolerance with fructose restriction, and of heavy metal intoxication with removal from metal exposure or chelation (for lead).

DISORDERS OF FUNCTION OF THE ASCENDING LIMB OF THE LOOP OF HENLE

The thick ascending limb of Henle reabsorbs sodium chloride by means of a luminal Na-K-2Cl system. A lumen-positive potential difference and parallel transport systems effect potassium, calcium, and magnesium reabsorption. Defective reabsorption by the thick ascending limb of Henle occurs during diuretic treatment or in Bartter's syndrome.

Bartter's Syndrome

Bartter's syndrome consists of a constellation of findings including hypokalemia and metabolic alkalosis with hyperreninemic hyperaldosteronism. Hypertension and edema are absent.

PATHOPHYSIOLOGY. Evidence that dysfunction of the thick ascending limb of Henle is the proximate cause of Bartter's syndrome comes primarily from free-water clearance studies. The pathophysiologic consequences of diminished loop sodium chloride reabsorption is illustrated in Figure 84–3. Mild extracellular volume depletion causes hyper-reninemic hyperaldosteronism and the juxtaglomerular hyperplasia found on renal biopsy. Enhanced sodium chloride delivery to the collecting duct stimulates potassium secretion (exacerbated by concurrent hyperaldosteronism) leading to hypokalemia, as well as hydrogen ion secretion resulting in metabolic alkalosis. Accelerated kinin and prostaglandin (especially PGE_2 and prostacyclin) production occurs and may account for the vascular unresponsiveness to pressors and various other phenomena known to occur in Bartter's syndrome.

SYMPTOMS AND ETIOLOGY. Symptoms of Bartter's syndrome are usually manifested in childhood. Inheritance is autosomal recessive, with a higher penetrance in males. Adult cases have also been reported. Presenting features relate primarily to the hypokalemia, including muscle weakness and a vasopressin-unresponsive urinary concentrating defect, characterized by polyuria, nocturia, and enuresis. Divalent cation wasting and metabolic alkalosis may conspire to cause symptoms characteristic of hypocalcemia, including Trousseau's and Chvostek's signs. The electrolyte abnormalities can also present acutely as intestinal ileus or chronically as growth retardation in children. Affected patients are normotensive and nonedematous, have a normal GFR, and can usually conserve sodium chloride when dietary salt is restricted, though at the expense of signs of moderate extracellular volume compromise.

DIAGNOSIS AND TREATMENT. Other conditions associated with hypokalemia, metabolic alkalosis, and secondary hyper-reninemic hyperaldosteronism must be excluded before making a diagnosis of Bartter's syndrome. Surreptitious vomiting, chronic diarrheal states, or surreptitious diuretic or laxative administration can cause symptoms indistinguishable from those of Bartter's syndrome. These disorders are associated with extracellular volume depletion, and therefore the urinary chloride level is less than 20 mEq per liter, unless diuretics are being actively consumed. Thus, diagnosis of Bartter's syndrome must be preceded by confirmation that urinary chloride concentration is more than 20 mEq per liter and by negative screens for diuretics in the urine and for laxatives in the stool (phenolphthalein test). States of primary hyper-reninism or hypermineralocorticoidism can be readily excluded, since they are usually associated with hypertension.

Therapy of Bartter's syndrome is primarily aimed at ameliorating the hypokalemia by disrupting the renin-angiotensin-aldosterone and kinin-prostaglandin axes. Potassium supplementation, magnesium repletion, propranolol, spironolactone, prostaglandin inhibition, and captopril have all been used, but each has usually been met with incomplete success.

DISORDERS OF DISTAL NEPHRON FUNCTION

The distal nephron, including the distal convoluted tubule and the collecting ducts, is responsible for reabsorbing the final quantity of sodium in the tubule fluid and for secreting potassium and hydrogen ions. Inherited and acquired defects exist for selective or combined disorders of sodium, potassium, and acid-base regulation.

Classic Distal Renal Tubular Acidosis (RTA)

Classic distal (type I) RTA is a hypokalemic, hyperchloremic metabolic acidosis due to a selective defect in distal acidification and is characterized by inability to lower the urine pH normally and therefore by subnormal urinary net acid excretion.

PATHOPHYSIOLOGY. The distal nephron (especially the cortical and medullary collecting ducts) is normally capable of lowering the urine pH fully 2 to 3 pH units below that of blood to titrate filtered buffers (principally phosphate) to form

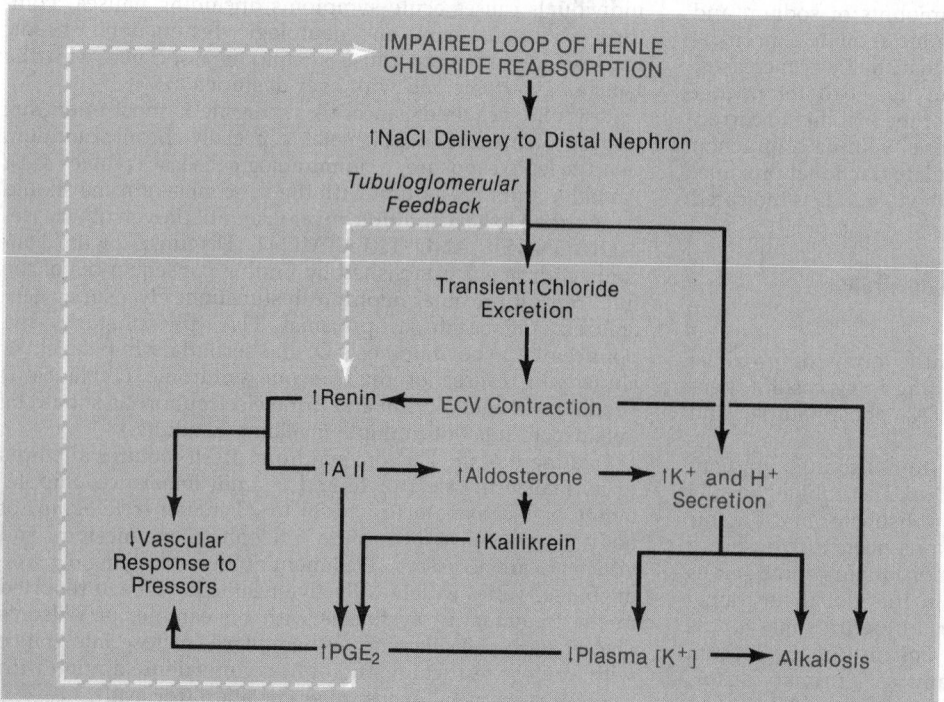

FIGURE 84–3. Pathophysiology of Bartter's syndrome. The primary sodium chloride reabsorptive defect is presumed to reside in the thick ascending limb of the loop of Henle. (From Cogan MG, Rector FC Jr: Acid-base disorders. In Brenner BM, Rector FC Jr [eds.]: The Kidney. 3rd ed. Philadelphia, W. B. Saunders Company, 1986, pp 457–518.)

titratable acids and endogenously produced ammonia to form ammonium (Fig. 84–2). If the distal nephron is incapable of lowering the luminal pH below 5.5 when challenged by metabolic acidosis, a classic distal RTA is present. Because of the inappropriately high urine pH, net acid excretion (titratable acid plus ammonium minus bicarbonate) is subnormal, less than acid production by the body. Accelerated potassium secretion occurs, presumably because there is reduced competition by proton secretion for the electrochemical driving forces in the distal nephron. The acidification defect may result from an insufficient number of proton-secreting pumps in the distal nephron. Alternatively, there may be backleak of acid across the luminal membrane, so that establishment of a pH gradient is prevented even when proton secretion is normal.

SYMPTOMS AND ETIOLOGIES. Distal RTA is found both in infants and children and in adults. Symptoms may be of acidosis or hypokalemia, as described above. Nephrocalcinosis and nephrolithiasis are common, either as a cause or as a result of classic distal RTA. However, bone disease is not as frequent as in proximal RTA. Classic distal RTA may also be genetic (most frequently autosomal dominant) or due to autoimmune diseases, drugs and toxins, and various tubulointerstitial diseases (Table 84–1.)

DIAGNOSIS AND TREATMENT. The findings of hyperchloremic, hypokalemic metabolic acidosis with an inappropriately high urine pH (> 5.5) and diminished net acid excretion confirm the diagnosis (Table 84–2). In individuals with a normal plasma bicarbonate concentration, the failure to lower urine pH to less than 5.5 following an acute acid challenge with NH_4Cl defines the syndrome of incomplete classic distal RTA (see Ch. 77 for details of the NH_4Cl test). Proximal bicarbonate reabsorption as tested by bicarbonate loading is normal. Treatment with alkali is generally very effective. The daily dose of alkali in adults is 1 to 3 mEq per kilogram, to compensate for the normal acid production by the body plus a small amount of urinary bicarbonate wastage. In contrast to proximal RTA, urinary potassium wasting is ameliorated with alkali therapy. Children require more alkali, about 5 to 14 mEq per kilogram per day. Prognosis with respect to stabilization of glomerular filtration rate in adults or growth in children is excellent with provision of adequate alkali therapy.

RTA of Glomerular Insufficiency

This disorder is a normokalemic, hyperchloremic metabolic acidosis associated with moderate renal insufficiency (glomerular filtration rate of 20 to 30 ml per minute), due to deficient ammonia delivery, and is characterized by an appropriately low urine pH but subnormal urinary net acid (ammonium) excretion.

PATHOPHYSIOLOGY. When the GFR falls to about 20 to 30 ml per minute owing to any intrinsic glomerular or tubulointerstitial disease, a normokalemic metabolic acidosis is frequently found. The cause of this acidosis is thought to be either deficient ammonia production or impairment in the urinary trapping of ammonia as ammonium (Fig. 84–2). In either case, proximal bicarbonate reclamation and the ability to lower the urine pH to less than 5.5 are intact, but the failure to generate sufficient acid excretion to equal intake results in systemic acidosis.

SYMPTOMS AND ETIOLOGY. The degree of metabolic acidosis is generally mild, and plasma bicarbonate concentration is usually greater than 15 mEq per liter. The acidemia has been suggested by some investigators to exacerbate the osteodystrophy of progressive renal disease. Although tubulointerstitial diseases are thought to produce this form of RTA more commonly than glomerular diseases, this distinction has been difficult to verify. This hyperchloremic metabolic acidosis should be distinguished from the high anion gap (normochloremic) metabolic acidosis due to retained organic acids that usually occurs when glomerular insufficiency is more severe (GRF < 20 ml per minute). The two acidoses may coexist.

DIAGNOSIS AND TREATMENT. A hyperchloremic, normokalemic metabolic acidosis that occurs when GFR falls to about 20 to 30 ml per minute is typical of the RTA of glomerular insufficiency. Although net acid, specifically ammonium, excretion is subnormal, the urine pH is appropriately acidic (Table 84–2). Mineralocorticoid levels are not diminished. An elevated anion gap (uremic acidosis) is generally seen only when GFR is less than 20 ml per minute. Treatment consists of 1 to 3 mEq per kilogram per day of alkali therapy to compensate for daily acid ingestion and production.

Nonselective Distal Nephron Dysfunction: Generalized Distal RTA, Hyperkalemia, and Renal Salt Wasting

These disorders arise from global dysfunction of the distal nephron due to aldosterone deficiency or antagonism and are characterized by hyperkalemic, hyperchloremic (type IV) metabolic acidosis due to subnormal net acid excretion and frequently by renal salt wasting.

PATHOPHYSIOLOGY. When sodium is reabsorbed in the distal nephron under the influence of aldosterone, luminal sodium concentration can be reduced to very low levels, less than 10 mEq per liter (sometimes ≤1 mEq per liter). Sodium reabsorption creates a lumen-negative potential difference, favoring secretion of potassium and hydrogen ions (Fig. 84–2). Disruption of sodium reabsorption and of potassium and hydrogen secretion may therefore be ascribable to a defect in the integrity of the distal nephron cell, deficient aldosterone production or action, diminished sodium reabsorption, or blunting of the lumen-negative potential by enhanced chloride reabsorption. Any of these processes will lead to diminished total hydrogen ion and potassium excretion and therefore metabolic acidosis with hyperkalemia. The hyperkalemia will also serve to depress renal ammoniagenesis independently, which exacerbates the defect in renal acidification. The ability to reabsorb bicarbonate (a proximal nephron function) and to lower the urinary pH normally (a qualitative distal nephron function at low buffer strength) remains intact (Table 84–2).

SYMPTOMS AND ETIOLOGIES. The symptoms of generalized distal RTA in children or adults usually relate to the acidosis itself or occasionally to the neuromuscular consequences of hyperkalemia. Renal salt wasting can cause extracellular volume depletion and hypotension when sodium chloride intake is reduced. The most common forms of generalized distal RTA are due to reduction in aldosterone level or prevention of its action (Table 84–1). The adrenal synthesis of aldosterone may be directly impaired, as in Addison's disease or in inherited enzymatic defects, such as 18- or 21-hydroxylase deficiencies. More commonly, primary hyporeninemia due to diabetic nephropathy, hypertensive nephrosclerosis, or tubulointerstitial diseases can also reduce aldosterone levels. Finally, end-organ unresponsiveness to mineralocorticoid with high circulating levels of aldosterone can be found in various tubulointerstitial diseases, especially those that have a predilection for the medulla and papilla of the kidney (e.g., analgesic abuse, sickle cell disease, and obstructive nephropathies).

DIAGNOSIS AND TREATMENT: HYPERKALEMIC, GENERALIZED DISTAL RTA. Generalized distal RTA is unique among the hyperchloremic metabolic acidoses in being a hyperkalemic disorder (Table 84–2). Glomerular filtration rate is invariably reduced in the forms associated with hyporeninemia or tubulointerstitial nephropathy but may be at levels (≥ 30 ml per minute) above that typically found in the RTA of glomerular insufficiency.

Treatment of the hyperkalemia and generalized distal RTA is effected with mineralocorticoid (9-α-fludrocortisone 0.1 mg per day) when deficient. When hyporeninemia is the cause, high doses of the synthetic mineralocorticoid are required (up to 0.5 mg per day) because of associated mineralocorticoid resistance. Hypertension can be precipitated with this treatment. Alternatively, providing modest amounts of alkali to compensate for daily acid generation (1 to 3 mEq per kilogram per day) can be used. Treatment of the hyperkalemia by dietary potassium restriction, potassium-wasting diuretics, or cation-exchange resins can also ameliorate or even correct the acid-base disorder.

DIAGNOSIS AND TREATMENT: RENAL SALT WASTING. Renal salt wasting becomes apparent when dietary sodium chloride intake becomes less than the minimal threshold for sodium chloride excretion. In normal persons, abrupt dietary sodium restriction to 10 mEq per day causes urinary sodium excretion to fall to a comparable level (10 mEq per day) within three to five days. Only a transient period occurs in which urinary sodium excretion exceeds intake and slight weight loss occurs ($\leq$ 1 kg). Renal salt wasting is diagnosed when, in response to acute reduction of sodium intake (10 mEq per day), urinary sodium excretion remains inappropriately elevated, typically greater than 50 mEq per day and weight loss is significant (> 3 kg). Progressively severe extracellular volume depletion occurs with development of hypotension and renal insufficiency. This diagnostic maneuver is not without hazard, since symptomatic hypovolemia or hyperkalemia can be precipitated, and should be performed under close supervision.

Therapy for renal salt wasting due to aldosterone deficiency or partial resistance requires physiologic or supraphysiologic mineralocorticoid replacement, as described above. In all other cases, sodium chloride supplementation is indicated to prevent volume depletion in the event sodium intake is curtailed. The dose of sodium chloride prescribed, in the diet plus salt tablets, should exceed that amount of sodium chloride spilled into the urine by the patient when dietary salt was restricted.

GENERAL

Cogan MG: Disorders of proximal nephron function. Am J Med 72:275, 1982. *This paper presents an overview of the physiology, pathophysiologic mechanisms, and clinical disorders of proximal nephron function.*

Sebastian A, Hulter HN, Kurtz I, et al.: Disorders of distal nephron function. Am J Med 72:289, 1982. *This article is a thoughtful, pathophysiologically oriented overview of the various clinical dysfunctions of potassium and hydrogen ion secretion.*

RENAL GLYCOSURIAS

Wen S-F: Glycosurias. In Gonick HC, Buckalew VM Jr. (eds.): Renal Tubular Disorders. New York, Marcel Dekker, Inc., 1985, pp 159–199. *This chapter presents an excellent discussion of the physiology of glucose transport and the pathophysiology and clinical spectrum of the renal glycosurias.*

RENAL AMINOACIDURIAS

Foreman JW, Segal S: Aminoacidurias. In Gonick HC, Buckalew VM Jr. (eds.): Renal Tubular Disorders. New York, Marcel Dekker, Inc., 1985, pp 131–157. *This chapter presents an excellent overview of the physiology of amino acid transport and the clinical spectra of the aminoacidurias.*

Segal S, Thier SO: Cystinuria. In Stanbury JB, Wyngaarden JB, Fredrickson DS, et al. (eds.): The Metabolic Basis of Inherited Disease. 5th ed. New York, McGraw-Hill Book Company, 1983, pp 1774–1791. *This is an authoritative review of the most common of the aminoacidurias.*

FANCONI'S SYNDROME

Brewer ED: The Fanconi syndrome: Clinical disorders. In Gonick HC, Buckalew VM Jr. (eds.): Renal Tubular Disorders. New York, Marcel Dekker, Inc., 1985, pp 475–544. *This is a superb, exhaustive review of the pathophysiology, clinical presentations, and principles of treatment of the multiple causes of the Fanconi syndrome.*

Roth KS, Foreman JW, Segal S: The Fanconi syndrome and mechanisms of tubular transport dysfunction. Kidney Int 20:705, 1981. *An excellent review of the pathogenetic mechanisms of this syndrome.*

BARTTER'S SYNDROME

Gill JR, Bartter FC: Evidence for a prostaglandin-independent defect in chloride reabsorption in the loop of Henle as a proximal cause of Bartter's syndrome. Am J Med 65:766, 1978. *This paper describes in vivo studies pinpointing the tubular site of the reabsorptive defect in Bartter's syndrome.*

Stein JH: The pathogenetic spectrum of Bartter's syndrome. Kidney Int 28:85, 1985. *This article reviews the variety of clinical presentations and current concepts of pathogenesis of this heterogeneous syndrome.*

RENAL TUBULAR ACIDOSIS

Arruda JAL, Kurtzman NA: Mechanisms and classification of deranged distal urinary acidification. Am J Physiol 239:F515, 1980. *This paper provides a critical and insightful examination of the causes of classic and generalized distal RTA.*

Cogan MG, Arieff AI: Sodium wasting, acidosis and hyperkalemia induced by methicillin interstitial nephritis. Evidence for selective distal tubular dysfunction. Am J Med 64:500, 1978. *This article describes the standard evaluation and treatment of a patient with marked renal salt wasting.*

Cogan MG, Rector FC Jr.: Acid-base disorders. In Brenner BM, Rector FC Jr. (eds.): The Kidney. 3rd ed. Philadelphia, W. B. Saunders Company, 1986, pp 457–518. *This chapter is a comprehensive review of acid-base homeostasis including the RTA's.*

Harrington JT, Cohen JJ: Metabolic acidosis. In Cohen JJ, Kassirer JP (eds.): Acid-Base. Boston, Little, Brown & Company, 1982, pp 121–226. *This chapter describes the pathophysiology and clinical manifestations of metabolic acidoses.*

Rector FC Jr., Cogan MG: The renal acidoses. Hosp Pract 15:99, 1980. *This article provides an introduction to the diagnosis and pathophysiology of the hyperchloremic metabolic acidoses.*

Schambelan M, Sebastian A, Biglieri EG: Prevalence, pathogenesis and functional significance of aldosterone deficiency in hyperkalemic patients with chronic renal insufficiency. Kidney Int 17:89, 1980. *This paper provides one of the most comprehensive reviews of the heterogeneous causes of generalized distal (Type IV) RTA.*

85 DIABETES AND THE KIDNEY
Bryan D. Myers

INCIDENCE AND PREVALENCE

Among the 15,000 patients entering chronic dialysis and kidney transplantation programs in the United States each year, the development of end-stage renal failure can be attributed to diabetes mellitus in approximately 25 per cent. Diabetic glomerulopathy, a complex disorder associated with a diffuse expansion of collagenous components of the glomerulus, is the predominant cause of the renal failure. The diabetic patient is also prone to other renal diseases such as pyelonephritis, papillary necrosis, and obstructive nephropathy that occasionally cause or exacerbate renal failure (Ch. 83 and 86). Diabetic patients with glomerulopathy are more susceptible to these associated renal disorders than are those who do not have glomerulopathy. Most victims of end-stage diabetic renal disease have longstanding type I diabetes, defined here as juvenile-onset and insulin-dependent diabetes (see Ch. 231). Patients with type II diabetes, characterized by a more advanced age of onset and not requiring insulin for control of hyperglycemia, are not spared from diabetic glomerulopathy and comprise a substantial minority among diabetic patients in end-stage renal failure programs.

CLINICAL AND LABORATORY FEATURES OF DIABETIC GLOMERULOPATHY

The natural history of diabetic glomerulopathy has been best documented in type I patients. Early abnormalities of glomerular function and structure appear to be invariable in all type I diabetics, but only 30 to 50 per cent will develop a progressive, proteinuric form of diabetic glomerulopathy. The evolution of the glomerulopathy in this subset of type I diabetics may be thought of as a continuum of glomerular injury divisible into three stages (Fig. 85–1). The first stage of occult glomerulopathy cannot be diagnosed by conventional laboratory techniques and lasts for approximately ten years. It is followed by two clinically evident stages of increasingly severe glomerular injury. Both are identified by the presence of proteinuria, while the milder, intermediate second stage

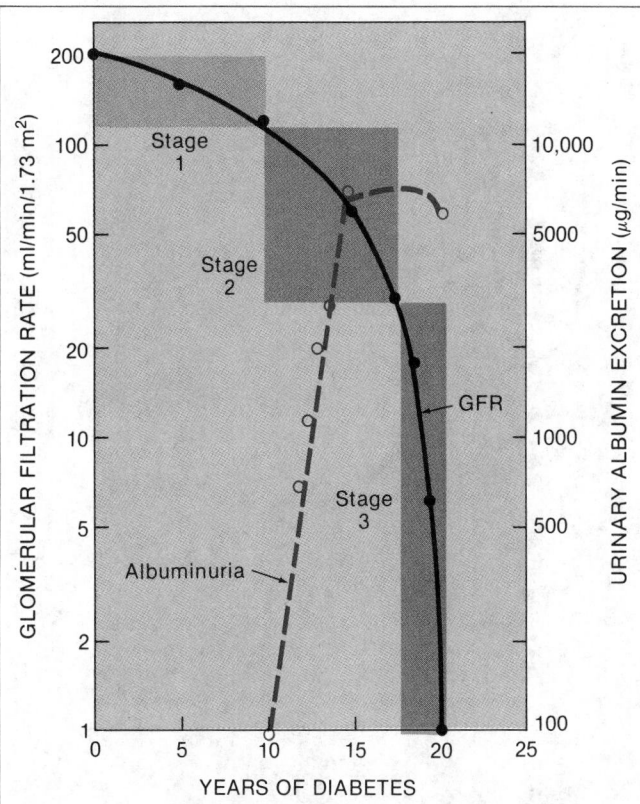

FIGURE 85–1. The glomerular filtration rate (●—●) and albumin excretion rate (○—○) have been plotted against time to chart a hypothetical course typical of diabetic glomerulopathy. The course of the disease has been divided into three stages, which are described in the text.

merges with the advanced third stage with the development of azotemia. The clinical and laboratory features of this prolonged and progressive glomerular disease will be reviewed by each stage separately.

Stage 1—Occult Diabetic Glomerulopathy

During this stage, the type I diabetic patient is devoid of clinical symptoms and signs of glomerulopathy. The most striking laboratory finding is a 20 to 40 per cent *elevation of the glomerular filtration rate* (GFR) above that found in age-matched normal controls. Although ultrastructural alterations can be demonstrated in the glomerular capillary wall and mesangium in the early stages of the disease, they do not appear to account for the observed glomerular hyperfiltration. Striking elevations of GFR in poorly controlled diabetic patients can be lowered within a matter of hours following restoration of normoglycemia. A parallel *increase in renal plasma flow*, measured by the clearance of *p*-aminohippurate, and also reversible by lowering blood glucose levels, points to a hemodynamic basis for the hyperfiltration. Notwithstanding the responsiveness of vasomotor regulation in the kidney to alterations in the metabolic milieu, GFR tends to remain elevated even with good metabolic control of the diabetic state. Not until proteinuria ushers in the intermediate second stage of the glomerulopathy does the GFR fall into the normal range.

The stage 1 glomerular hyperfiltration is accompanied by a subtle increase in the urinary albumin excretion rate that is not measurable by conventional techniques. Healthy adolescents and young adults excrete albumin in their urine at rates of up to 15 μg per minute. Many patients with type I diabetes of short duration excrete albumin at rates in excess of 15 μg per minute but less than the 100 μg per minute, which is roughly the threshold detectable by conventional techniques. This "microalbuminuria" is inferred to represent an increase in the transglomerular filtration of albumin rather than a de-

crease in tubular reabsorption of a normal, filtered albumin load. Microalbuminuria tends to be associated with the most striking degrees of hyperfiltration observed among type I diabetics, suggesting that it may also have a hemodynamic basis. It is exaggerated by exercise, which causes an increase in the intraluminal hydraulic pressure of the glomerular capillaries, and is blunted, although not abolished, by restoration of normoglycemia.

Early in the course of type I diabetes there is a consistent *increase in kidney size*. Hyperfiltration, renal hyperemia and enlargement, and microalbuminuria are all characteristic of this early occult stage, but hypertension, an important complication of diabetic glomerulopathy, is not prevalent. The incidence of hypertension in large diabetic populations without proteinuria is no different from that in nondiabetic populations.

Stage 2—Intermediate Diabetic Glomerulopathy

This stage is heralded by the development of persistent, easily measurable proteinuria. Once proteinuria has become manifest its magnitude tends to reflect the rate of deterioration of glomerular capillary wall function that typifies the second stage of diabetic glomerulopathy. As indicated in Figure 85–1, proteinuria tends to increase exponentially with time and to be related inversely to GFR.

After several years of proteinuria, urinary losses reach nephrotic proportions (> 3.5 grams per 24 hours) and the patient will frequently become edematous. The proteinuria is also paralleled by an increasing prevalence of hypertension. Thus stage 2, intermediate diabetic glomerulopathy, is characterized by *increasing proteinuria, declining GFR*, and the development of *hypertension* and *edema*.

The proteinuria of stage 2 diabetic glomerulopathy has no pathognomonic characteristics, but several features distinguish it from other glomerular diseases: (1) From the onset of the second stage, immunoglobulins and other large plasma proteins are excreted in the urine in large quantities along with albumin, signifying an early loss of barrier size-selectivity in this disorder. (2) Persistent and ultimately massive urinary losses of plasma proteins in stage 2 diabetic glomerulopathy are rarely accompanied by hypoproteinemia. Inasmuch as the conventional definition of the nephrotic syndrome requires hypoproteinemia in addition to massive proteinuria and edema, stage 2 diabetic glomerulopathy does not truly exemplify the nephrotic syndrome. An important role in edema formation is ascribed to reduction of plasma oncotic pressure in patients with the nephrotic syndrome as classically defined; the absence of hypoproteinemia, and hence the maintenance of normal plasma oncotic pressure, in stage 2 diabetic glomerulopathy implicates alternate mechanisms of edema formation. (3) Neither can edema formation, or, for that matter, hypertension, be related to a stimulated renin-angiotensin-aldosterone system. To the contrary, diabetic glomerulopathy is usually associated with an inability to cleave the inactive precursor of renin, with the result that concentrations of active renin in plasma are low and angiotensin production is depressed. Plasma concentration and urinary excretion rate of aldosterone tend also to be depressed, despite the presence of edema. In fact, proteinuric diabetic glomerulopathy probably constitutes the commonest example of hyporeninemic hypoaldosteronism, and such patients not infrequently exhibit the syndrome of generalized distal type IV renal tubular acidosis (see Ch. 84). Thus, both the mechanism by which edema is formed and the basis for the widespread prevalence of hypertension in stage 2 diabetic glomerulopathy remain obscure.

Stage 3—Advanced Diabetic Glomerulopathy

The third, advanced stage represents the terminal 2 or 3 years of what is typically a 20- to 25-year process. Its onset is delineated by the development of *azotemia*. Retention of urea, creatinine, and other nitrogenous compounds will generally become apparent once the GFR has declined to less than one third of normal levels. As with the intermediate stage that precedes it, GFR in the third and terminal stage of diabetic glomerulopathy has been observed to decline at rates approaching 1 ml per minute per month. Thus in the prototypical case illustrated in Figure 85–1, GFR is predicted to decline from a normal value approximating 120 ml per minute at the onset of stage 2 to zero at the end of stage 3 over a period of 10 years. Not only does GFR decline irrevocably, resulting in progressive azotemia but *edema* and *hypertension* tend to worsen in the third and final stage of the disease. Similarly, *proteinuria* continues to be massive and *hypoproteinemia* finally results. Although reduced plasma protein concentration and the lowered GFR serve to lower the filtered protein load, urinary protein excretion rate is maintained at massive levels, reflecting increasing leakiness of the glomerular capillary wall to large plasma proteins.

By the time the third, advanced stage of diabetic glomerulopathy is reached, *widespread microangiopathy* involving the retinae and peripheral nerves is invariable. Although its extent varies among patients, retinopathy is frequently associated with visual impairment sufficient to result in functional blindness. The effects of peripheral and more particularly of autonomic neuropathy may be equally devastating. This is particularly true when autonomic neuropathy results in partial paresis of the bladder. Progressive urinary retention may exacerbate renal insufficiency in stage 3 glomerulopathy by resulting in a superimposed obstructive nephropathy. Obstructive nephropathy in turn may predispose the already vulnerable patient to ascending pyelonephritis and/or ischemic papillary necrosis, thereby compromising renal function even further. (For more detailed discussion of obstructive nephropathy, see Ch. 83.)

Given the prolonged duration of diabetes mellitus, by the time stage 3 glomerulopathy is reached many patients will be 40 years of age or more, an age group in which atherosclerosis, accelerated in part by the presence of longstanding hypertension, will adversely affect several organ systems. Coronary artery disease, cerebrovascular disease and stroke, and peripheral vascular disease are all common in the third stage of diabetic glomerulopathy, and account collectively for the majority of fatalities. The eventual need for substitution therapy in end-stage renal failure programs occurs in a setting, therefore, in which serious extrarenal complications are prevalent and impair the effectiveness of rehabilitation generally achieved by such therapy.

DIAGNOSIS

Proteinuria due to diabetic glomerulopathy is accompanied by typical changes of glomerular histopathology. These include a striking accumulation of matrix components of the mesangium and a widening of the glomerular capillary wall due to a thickened glomerular basement membrane. The former change results in an acellular expansion of the mesangium, which is most commonly diffuse in nature and hence termed diffuse intercapillary glomerulosclerosis. Not infrequently mesangial matrix accumulation occurs in a segmental fashion, resulting in the formation of acellular spherical nodules at the center of single or multiple peripheral glomerular lobules (Fig. 85–2), referred to as nodular glomerulosclerosis. A nodular accumulation of mesangial matrix material, indistinguishable from that observed in diabetic subjects, has been associated with dysproteinemia, notably that associated with a monoclonal proliferation of B lymphocytes or plasma cells. Provided that the latter entity is excluded, however, the finding of diffuse or nodular glomerulosclerosis in a proteinuric diabetic subject is diagnostic of diabetic glomerulopathy.

A diagnosis of diabetic glomerulopathy can be made with a high degree of certainty in a proteinuric diabetic patient, without resort to biopsy, which carries a finite risk for the

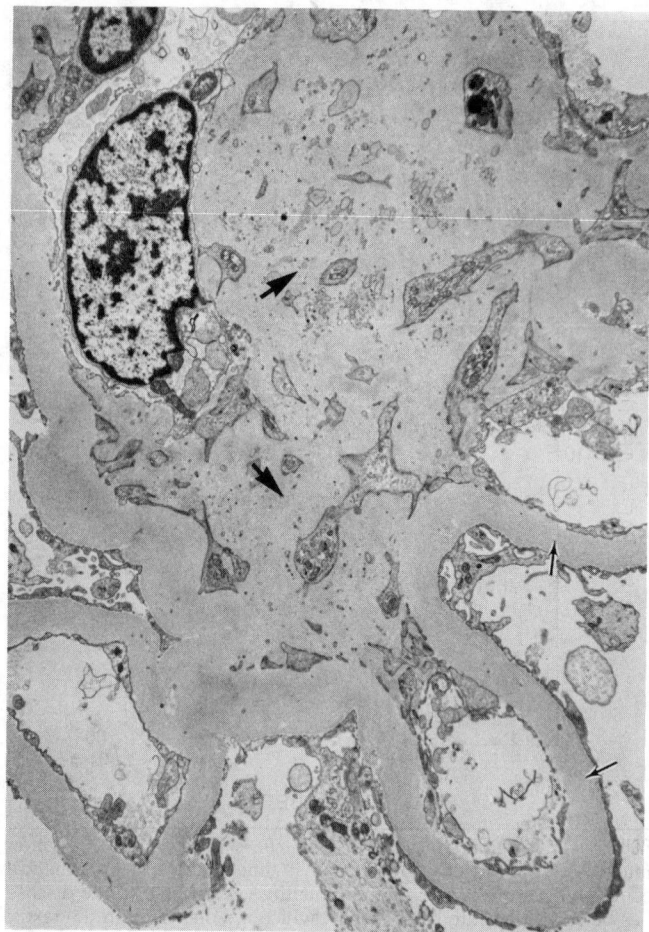

FIGURE 85–2. Electron photomicrograph of a portion of a glomerulus from a patient with proteinuric, diabetic glomerulopathy (magnification × 5000). A striking increase in collagenous components has resulted in (1) widening of the basement membrane of peripheral capillary loops (*small arrows*), and (2) expansion of the matrix of the glomerular mesangium (*large arrows*). The latter alteration is responsible for compressing and ultimately obliterating the glomerular capillary network.

patient. Background and proliferative retinopathy, for example, are correlated strongly with the presence of diffuse or nodular glomerulosclerosis in a proteinuric diabetic. The diagnostic probability can be further strengthened by using noninvasive imaging techniques, such as ultrasonography or nephrotomography, to demonstrate kidney enlargement. Nephrotoxic acute renal failure caused by contrast agents occurs more commonly in patients with diabetic glomerulopathy than in any other patient category. For this reason nephrotomography (or other radiologic procedures) should be performed without the use of contrast agents whenever possible. The coexistence of retinopathy and nephromegaly in diabetic patients with proteinuria is so constant that the performance of a diagnostic renal biopsy need be considered only when these factors are absent, particularly when the duration of diabetes is less than 10 years. In these circumstances, a renal biopsy has frequently revealed other, and presumably unrelated, primary glomerulopathies such as minimal change nephropathy, membranous glomerulopathy, and proliferative glomerulonephritis (Ch. 81).

PATHOGENESIS AND PATHOPHYSIOLOGY

The diabetic state per se is the presumed forerunner of glomerulopathy. Glomerular basement membrane widening and increased mesangial matrix, the earliest ultrastructural markers of glomerulopathy, are absent at the onset and can be detected only after some years of type I diabetes. An identical sequence has been observed in experimental diabetes induced in a variety of mammalian species with the use of pancreatic beta cell toxins or pancreatectomy.

As in humans, GFR is substantially elevated in the rat with experimental diabetes of short duration. The early hyperfiltration is a consequence of altered vasomotion in the major resistance vessels of the renal cortex. Dilatation of the efferent and especially the afferent glomerular arterioles results in an elevation of glomerular capillary perfusion rate and pressure. By contrast, those determinants of GFR that are intrinsic to the glomerular capillary wall, namely hydraulic conductivity and the surface area available for filtration, are unaltered. Thus hyperfiltration early in the course of diabetes appears to have a purely hemodynamic basis. It remains to be determined which factor or factors associated with the diabetic state are responsible for the deranged renal vasoregulation. Hyperglycemia per se, or elevated levels of vasodilator glucoregulatory hormones such as glucagon and growth hormone, may be implicated. Abnormalities of other hormonal regulators of glomerular perfusion rate and pressure have also been identified. Thus diminished production and activity of angiotensin II, but increased production of vasodilator prostaglandins, by glomerular cells isolated from diabetic rats point to an imbalance in favor of local vasodilatation of renal cortical microvessels. Experimental maneuvers that further increase glomerular overperfusion in the diabetic rat, including surgical reduction of renal mass or feeding a high-protein diet, are followed by heavier proteinuria and more severe glomerulosclerosis than observed in diabetic rats with a normal complement of nephrons and fed conventional rat chow. Conversely, measures that prevent glomerular hyperemia and hypertension—such as partial constriction of the renal artery with a clip, the administration of angiotensin-converting enzyme inhibitor, or dietary protein restriction—largely prevent the development of proteinuria as well as the histopathologic damage observed in diabetic rats not so protected. These findings are taken to indicate that hemodynamic factors serve as a stimulus for an ensuing accumulation of mesangial matrix components and, hence, subsequent glomerulosclerosis.

Whether or not glomerular capillary hypertension and hyperperfusion are unique causes of an accumulation of mesangial matrix components, there seems little doubt that this lesion is responsible for the progressive reduction of GFR that typifies the second and third stages of clinical diabetic glomerulopathy. As shown in Figure 85–2, expansion of the mesangial matrix occurs at the expense of the surrounding glomerular capillary loops, with progressive reduction of the surface area available for filtration. By the time the end of the third stage of diabetic glomerulopathy has been reached, the mesangium will have encroached upon most glomerular capillary loops to the point that they have become almost totally obliterated.

The process by which the glomerular basement membrane becomes widened has been presumed to be responsible for the alteration in the glomerular capillary wall, causing it to become permeable to large plasma proteins. Surprisingly, however, there is no correlation whatsoever between glomerular basement membrane width and proteinuria. While the structural basis of proteinuria remains obscure, the functional nature of the disturbance in glomerular permselectivity has been elucidated by the use of in vivo physiologic techniques in which the clearance of probe filtration markers of graded size has been used to define the size-selective properties of the glomerular filter. One such study has revealed that proteinuria in diabetic glomerulopathy can be accounted for by the development within the glomerular capillary wall of a subpopulation of enlarged, protein-permeable pores. In contradistinction to the diffuse widening of the basement membrane seen by electron microscopy (Fig. 85–2), the enlarged pores can be estimated to be few in number and to behave as isolated defects in the glomerular capillary wall.

PROGNOSIS AND TREATMENT

The profound loss of filtering surface area and the disruption of glomerular membrane pore structure that underlie stage 2 and 3 glomerulopathy in diabetics are unlikely to be reversible. Attempts to maintain blood glucose in such patients in a normal range have failed to prevent or attenuate the progression of renal insufficiency. Meticulous control of hypertension, however, may slow the rate of decline of GFR. Together with antihypertensive therapy, attention to and correction of coexistent cardiac failure, obstructive nephropathy, pyelonephritis, and other events that may lower GFR independently of the glomerulopathy represent the mainstay of therapy of proteinuric glomerulopathy.

On the basis of our current understanding of the pathophysiology and pathogenesis of diabetic glomerulopathy, a strong case can be made for trying to prevent the advent of progressive stage 2 disease by correcting glomerular overperfusion during the first decade of diabetes. The subset of patients most likely to benefit from early, protective therapy is that with microalbuminuria (50 to 200 μg per minute) and an elevated GFR, particularly when associated with ophthalmoscopic evidence of diabetic retinopathy. Measures that are likely to lower glomerular perfusion rate and pressure include restoration of euglycemia by custom-tailored insulin replacement regimens and dietary protein restriction. The rationale for protective therapy is based on purely theoretic considerations, however. Prolonged and carefully controlled trials have yet to be conducted to confirm the efficacy and safety of such measures.

Once end-stage renal failure has supervened, the diabetic patient should be referred for treatment to a dialysis and/or transplantation center (Ch. 79 and 80). Many diabetic patients respond favorably to and enjoy a good quality of life with these modalities of treatment. With special attention to the unique problems of the diabetic patient with renal failure, the survival rates achieved with chronic hemodialysis or with chronic ambulatory peritoneal dialysis, or following renal transplantation, are today approaching those achieved for nondiabetic patients.

Hostetter TH, Rennke HG, Brenner BM: The case for intrarenal hypertension in the initiation and progression of diabetic and other glomerulopathies. Am J Med 72:375, 1982. *A lucid review of the pathophysiology of diabetic glomerulopathy citing virtually every important reference to this subject.*

Hostetter TH, Troy JL, Brenner BM: Glomerular hemodynamics in experimental diabetes mellitus. Kidney Int 19:410, 1981. *An elegant micropuncture study demonstrating the hemodynamic basis for glomerular hyperfiltration in early experimental rat diabetes.*

Luetscher JA, Kraemer FB, Wilson DM: Increased plasma inactive renin in diabetes mellitus. N Engl J Med 312:1412, 1985. *The abnormalities in the renin-angiotensin system in diabetic glomerulopathy are clearly delineated.*

Mauer SM, Steffes MW, Ellis EN, et al.: Structural-functional relationships in diabetic nephropathy. J Clin Invest 74:1143, 1984. *A review of the authors' use of electron microscopy and elegant morphometric techniques to chart the evolution and progression of diabetic glomerulopathy.*

Myers BD, Winetz JA, Chui F, et al.: Mechanisms of proteinuria in diabetic nephropathy: A study of glomerular barrier function. Kidney Int 21:96, 1982. *Modern physiologic techniques and mathematical modeling are used to describe the glomerular capillary wall as an ultrafiltration membrane; the defect in the glomerular filter of proteinuric diabetics is elucidated.*

Omachi R: The pathogenesis and prevention of diabetic nephropathy. West J Med 145:222, 1986. *This summary of a recent medical grand rounds offers a review of the topic with 57 references.*

Viberti GC, Bilous RW, Mackintosh D, et al.: Monitoring glomerular function in diabetic nephropathy. Am J Med 74:256, 1983. *A careful prospective study of the effects of metabolic control on proteinuric glomerulopathy. Its message is pessimistic.*

Zatz R, Meyer TW, Rennke HG, et al.: Predominance of hemodynamic rather than metabolic factors in the pathogenesis of diabetic glomerulopathy. Proc Natl Acad Sci USA 82:5963, 1985. *The protective effect of lowering glomerular pressures and flows on sclerosing diabetic glomerulopathy is well documented.*

86 URINARY TRACT INFECTIONS AND PYELONEPHRITIS

Vincent T. Andriole

DEFINITION

Urinary tract infection refers to both microbial colonization of the urine and tissue invasion of any structure of the urinary tract. Bacteria are most commonly responsible, although yeast, fungi, and viruses may produce urinary infection. Urinary tract infections may be relatively mild, such as the "honeymoon cystitis" syndrome, or catastrophic, such as a perinephric abscess in a diabetic. Urinary tract infections are often categorized by the site of infection, which is convenient for the purpose of discussion. However, it is often not possible to diagnose the various types of infections on clinical grounds alone.

Significant bacteriuria refers to sufficient numbers of bacteria in the urine to denote active infection rather than contamination. A bacteria count over 100,000 organisms per milliliter in a fresh "clean-catch" midstream specimen is a reliable indicator of active urinary tract infection but does not indicate whether the infection is cystitis or pyelonephritis. In addition, women with acute cystitis may have $>10^3$ but $<10^5$ bacteria per milliliter in midstream urine cultures.

Asymptomatic bacteriuria refers to large numbers of bacteria in the urine without producing symptoms. Dysuria and frequency in the absence of significant bacteriuria are common problems among young women. This entity has been called the *acute urethral syndrome* and is often caused by *Chlamydia trachomatis*.

Cystitis and *acute pyelonephritis* are symptomatic infections of the bladder and kidney, respectively. *Perinephric and renal abscesses*, uncommon complications of urinary infections, usually occur in (1) urinary tract obstruction, (2) bacteremia, particularly staphylococcal or candidal bacteremia, and (3) immunocompromised individuals, particularly diabetics.

Complicated infections refer to bacteriuria in association with structural or neurologic defects in the voiding mechanism (vesicoureteral reflux, neurogenic bladder), foreign bodies (stones or indwelling catheter), or intrinsic renal disease (diabetic nephropathy or polycystic renal disease).

Chronic pyelonephritis refers to the pathologic and radiologic findings of chronic cortical scarring, tubulointerstitial damage, and deformity of the underlying calix. Chronic bacterial pyelonephritis can be *active*, which occurs in patients with persistent *complicated* infection, or *inactive*, which consists of focal sterile scars of a past infection. Recurrent infection can result in multiple scars combined with active foci of infection. In the absence of obstruction, reflux, foreign bodies, or an immunocompromised host (notably the diabetic patient), urinary tract infections rarely cause the shrunken, scarred kidneys of end-stage chronic pyelonephritis.

Other disease states can produce renal lesions that mimic "chronic pyelonephritis." Identical characteristics can be observed, in the absence of infection, in patients who suffered from severe vesicoureteral reflux in childhood. This entity, *reflux nephropathy*, refers to the radiographic triad of intrarenal reflux and vesicoureteral reflux, scarring, and loss of parenchymal mass in the absence of other obstructive lesions and can ultimately lead to end-stage renal failure with scarred, shrunken kidneys. "Reflux nephropathy" may result from "autoimmune" renal damage rather than bacterial infection of the kidney. Nevertheless, the combination of recurrent infection and reflux nephropathy can also result in chronic pyelonephritis. *Analgesic nephropathy* may produce papillary necrosis and may also mimic bacterial pyelonephritis on radiography.

PATHOGENESIS

The normal urinary tract is free of bacteria except for some organisms normally present near the external meatus and some staphylococci and diphtheroids normally found in the distal urethra. Urine, as a culture medium, generally supports bacterial multiplication. However, high concentrations of urea and hyperosmolality (which are present in the renal medulla), an acid pH, and urinary organic acid are generally unfavorable to bacterial growth. In addition, the dynamics of the urinary flow (washout) and antibacterial properties of the lining membrane of the urinary tract and of the vaginal and periurethral epithelial cells appear to be important defense mechanisms.

Urinary tract infections result most commonly from ascending transurethral invasion of the bladder by pathogenic gramnegative aerobic bacilli normally present in the large bowel and perineum, particularly of women. Sequentially, bacteria migrate from the anus to the periurethral area and along the urethra into the bladder, where infections occur if the organisms become established. This pathogenic mechanism helps explain the higher rate of urinary tract infection in women, whose urethras are shorter than those of men, and the marked frequency of the urinary infection associated with instrumentation of the urethra and the bladder.

Other pathways from the large bowel to the urinary passages and kidneys include the hematogenous and lymphatic routes. The hematogenous route, a less common mechanism for renal infection, generally, but not always, requires antecedent structural damage to the kidney. Staphylococcal bacteremia can produce multiple microabscesses in the kidney (*renal carbuncle*). Disseminated *Candida albicans* infections in the immunocompromised host can involve the kidney. Finally, septic emboli, particularly in the setting of bacterial endocarditis, represent a classic mode for hematogenously disseminated infection of the kidney.

The renal medulla, because of its unique hypertonicity, is much more susceptible to infection than the cortex. In experimental pyelonephritis, as few as 10 to 100 *Escherichia coli* may produce infection in the medulla, whereas 100,000 are required to infect the cortex. The increased susceptibility of the medulla is thought to be due to impaired leukocyte mobilization and phagocytosis in the hypertonic environment.

Microbial virulence factors are also important in the pathogenesis of symptomatic urinary infections. *E. coli* strains isolated from patients with pyelonephritis are more likely to (1) possess large amounts of K (capsular) antigen, (2) adhere in larger numbers to human urinary epithelial cells, and (3) possess surface pili, than are strains found in asymptomatic bacteriuria. The virulence of *Proteus* species may be related to their urease content and ammonia production.

CLINICAL MANIFESTATIONS

The symptoms of acute urinary tract infections are varied and include frequency, dysuria, burning pain on urination, suprapubic discomfort, passage of cloudy and occasionally blood-tinged urine, fever, costovertebral angle tenderness or flank pain, and rigors. Urinary tract symptoms, particularly dysuria, occur in 20 per cent of women each year, although only half seek medical attention. Approximately equal numbers of these women will have either the acute urethral syndrome (urethritis), bladder bacteriuria (cystitis), or renal infection.

In general, clinical grounds form an uncertain basis for separating patients with the acute urethral syndrome from those with either bladder or renal bacteriuria because frequency, burning, and suprapubic pain are found approximately equally in all three groups of patients. Costovertebral angle tenderness and fever may be present as frequently in patients with the acute urethral syndrome as in those with renal bacteriuria. Rigors occur almost equally (15 per cent) in patients with the acute urethral syndrome and those with cystitis. Similarly, tenderness in the region of one or both kidneys occurs not infrequently in lower urinary tract infections. However, sudden fever to 38.9° to 40.6°C, shaking chills, aching costovertebral or flank pain, and symptoms of sepsis are more characteristic of acute pyelonephritis than of cystitis or urethritis.

Laboratory tests show a polymorphonuclear leukocytosis in both cystitis and pyelonephritis. Pyuria is seen in urethritis, cystitis, and pyelonephritis, but white blood cell casts are more typical of pyelonephritis. Stain of the sediment and urine cultures reveal numerous bacteria, usually gram-negative bacilli. Cultures of blood may also be positive in some cases of pyelonephritis. A simple but convenient way of identifying infection of the urinary tract is by examining the urine (see below): The microscopic presence of bacteria in the urine generally indicates more than 100,000 colonies per milliliter of urine. However, the microscopic absence of bacteria does not exclude the diagnosis of urinary infection.

Impaired renal function or acute hypertension is rarely seen in acute pyelonephritis, but renal concentrating ability may be impaired. Also, subclinical forms of acute pyelonephritis may occur because tests that differentiate "upper" (kidney) from "lower" (bladder) infection may indicate the presence of renal infection in the absence of flank pain or fever. However, the only reliable tests, ureteral catheterization and bladder washout, are considered to be research maneuvers. Search for antibody-coated bacteria in the urine as a marker of renal bacteriuria may be performed, but the sensitivity and specificity of this test are not optimal. Pyelonephritis at times presents with symptoms that do not point to the urinary tract. Some patients may have only backache without demonstrable renal tenderness. Others have upper or lower abdominal pain together with symptoms of disturbed gastrointestinal function. Some complain only of general fatigue.

In the absence of obstructive lesions of the urinary tract or host immunocompromise, as in diabetics, upper or lower urinary tract infections are generally self-limited, lasting 10 to 14 days. When obstruction or host immunocompromise is present, pyelonephritis may be complicated by papillary necrosis, perinephric abscess, or renal carbuncle. These complications should be suspected when persistent flank pain, fever, and leukocytosis are unresponsive to otherwise adequate chemotherapy (see below).

Acute urinary tract infection complicated by pyelonephritis may occur in patients subjected to urethral instrumentation, particularly long-term indwelling catheters. Sepsis from pyelonephritis is a major cause of death in individuals having neurologic disorders requiring long-term indwelling catheters.

DIAGNOSIS
Microscopic Methods

Rapid diagnostic methods are available either (1) by preparation of a Gram's stain of either centrifuged or uncentrifuged urine and examination with an oil immersion lens or (2) by study of either centrifuged or uncentrifuged urine, employing the high-dry objective under reduced light, with or without methylene blue stain. The presence of any bacteria on Gram's stain of centrifuged urine correlates best (97 per cent) with quantitative culture (100,000 bacteria per milliliter of urine). Examination of the unstained sediment for the presence of any bacteria is also very helpful and can be done during routine examination for formed elements. Pyuria, arbitrarily defined as ten or more leukocytes per high-power field in the centrifuged specimen, can also be detected by the leukocyte esterase dipstick test. The presence of pyuria in a midstream urine sample suggests the likelihood of a urinary tract infection. Some erythrocytes may be seen in the urine, and gross hematuria may occur when inflammation in the bladder is intense. Proteinuria is not common in urinary infections, but

in fulminant pyelonephritis, as in other severe acute interstitial nephritides, significant degrees of proteinuria may occur transiently.

Significant Bacteriuria

The concept of "significant bacteriuria" was introduced to distinguish between those bacteria that actually multiply in the urine and bacteria that are contaminants. This distinction can be made by knowledge of the site and manner in which the urine is collected from the patient and by enumeration of the number of organisms present in the sample. The criterion of 100,000 or more organisms per milliliter of urine for the diagnosis of significant bacteriuria is an excellent operational definition when the clear-voided method is used, in both males and females, to collect specimens that are processed promptly. However, bacterial counts lower than 100,000 colonies per milliliter may occur in patients with true bacteriuria. Specifically, some women with acute bacterial cystitis, who present with dysuria and frequency (the acute urethral syndrome), may have as few as 100 bacteria per milliliter of urine. Isolation of multiple species from the urine usually indicates contamination, especially in the asymptomatic person.

Urine collected by suprapubic aspiration or bladder catheterization is less likely to be contaminated. In this instance, bacterial counts of fewer than 100,000 organisms per milliliter are likely to be significant.

Bacteriologic Findings

The species of bacteria most likely to be recovered from individuals with bacteriuria depends upon prior history of infection, prior antimicrobial therapy, hospitalization, and instrumentation of the urinary tract. Enterobacteriaceae are the most common organisms identified. *E. coli* accounts for more than 80 per cent of all species recovered in uncomplicated cases, whereas *Proteus, Klebsiella, Enterobacter, Pseudomonas*, enterococci, and staphylococci are more often found in patients who have had previous infection or instrumentation. Occasionally, *Serratia marcescens, Acinetobacter, Candida albicans*, and *Cryptococcus neoformans* may produce infection of the urinary tract in diabetics and in immunosuppressed or corticosteroid-treated patients. Coliforms are also the most common organisms responsible for the acute urethral syndrome in women who have fewer than 10^5 bacteria per milliliter of urine, although *Staphylococcus saprophyticus* and *Chlamydia trachomatis* are responsible for some cases. Patients with the acute urethral syndrome caused by *Chlamydia trachomatis* have pyuria but sterile bladder urine when cultured with standard bacteriologic media.

Anaerobes are commonly present in the distal urethra and the vagina and are abundant in the gut, but they rarely produce urinary tract infection. Suprapubic aspiration of urine or examination of tissues is needed to prove anaerobic infections. When responsible, anaerobes are usually associated with complicated, longstanding infections.

Radiology

Radiographic evaluation of the urinary tract is undertaken to detect correctable lesions that may contribute to the severity or recurrence of urinary tract infections. Evaluation is indicated in men with any type of urinary tract infection or in instances of documented bacteremia. In women, urography is not indicated unless a complication, such as papillary necrosis, perinephric abscess, renal carbuncle, or tumor, is suspected because the patient is unresponsive to otherwise adequate chemotherapy.

EPIDEMIOLOGY AND NATURAL HISTORY

Bacteriuria in the newborn population has been difficult to study because of problems inherent in urine collection. Cultures of urine obtained by bladder puncture suggest an incidence of 1 to 2 per cent. Infection of the urinary tract in this age group may be part of a generalized, life-threatening gram-negative sepsis and is more common in boys than girls. Symptomatic urinary infections are more prevalent among girls in preschool years and are often associated with obstructive or neurogenic lesions. Urologic investigation is valuable in this age group. *Urologic evaluation is mandatory in males of any age because of the high frequency of structural abnormalities found* (valves, malformation, and obstructive and neurogenic lesions).

The incidence of bacteriuria among school girls is 1 to 2 per cent; it is only 0.03 per cent in boys of the same age. The incidence of bacteriuria in females rises about 1 per cent per decade.

Urinary infection is common after marriage. The pathogenesis of the "honeymoon cystitis" syndrome remains unclear. Physical factors associated with sexual activity in previously sexually nonactive women may play a prominent role. Many patients with "honeymoon cystitis" (up to 50 per cent) will have dysuria due to local irritation rather than infection, and this should be clearly differentiated by culture.

Bacteriuria of pregnancy varies from 2 to 6 per cent, depending upon age, parity, and socioeconomic group. Acute symptomatic pyelonephritis will develop later in pregnancy in approximately 20 per cent of these women. However, there is no evidence that isolated episodes of pyelonephritis in pregnant women lead to chronic urinary tract infections after these women cease childbearing activities. Early detection and treatment of bacteriuria in pregnancy will prevent the emergence of symptomatic infection.

Elderly women may have frequencies of bacteriuria as high as 10 per cent; this rate may increase in hospitalized patients, particularly diabetics. Bacteriuria in the male begins to appear in "prostate years" and is often initiated by instrumentation.

Role of Instrumentation

Bacteriuria persists in 1 to 2 per cent of relatively healthy individuals following a single catheterization; the risk is higher in the debilitated patient and in males with prostatic obstruction. With open indwelling catheter drainage, bacterial colonization exceeds 90 per cent within three to four days. This may lead to life-threatening pyelonephritis and gram-negative sepsis. Fortunately, it is largely preventable by (1) careful criteria for catheterization and (2) use of aseptic closed drainage. The catheter should be removed as soon as it is no longer needed.

Intermittent self-catheterization coupled with abdominal pressure may be of benefit in patients with neurogenic bladders and may result in minimal urinary tract infections.

TREATMENT

The goal of treatment is to eradicate bacteria from the urinary tract in order to relieve symptoms, prevent renal damage, and diminish the likelihood of spread of infections to other sites. Prophylaxis is used to prevent recurrent symptomatic infection. Suppression, although rarely effective, is used to diminish the number of bacteria in the urine or tissue. Indications for therapy depend on the potential of infection to give rise to symptoms or damage to the urinary tract and the likelihood that treatment will be effective (Fig. 86–1).

Asymptomatic Bacteriuria

Asymptomatic bacteriuria should probably not be treated except in those patients who are at high risk of developing symptomatic infections. Thus, treatment of asymptomatic bacteriuria is indicated in pregnant patients to prevent symptomatic illness in the third trimester; in patients who may have major predisposing factors to renal disease, such as diabetic or polycystic kidneys, or who have anatomic or neurologic abnormalities; and in patients who are immunocompromised or who will undergo urologic manipulation. If the treatment fails to eradicate asymptomatic infections in such individuals, further treatment should be reserved for acute symptomatic episodes. In contrast, asymptomatic bacteriuria in females should not be treated in the absence of underlying structural or neurologic lesions, since the likelihood that renal damage will occur is slight. Furthermore, short courses of therapy, when effective, are commonly followed by reinfection. In addition, asymptomatic bacteriuria in patients with indwelling catheter and in the very elderly or nonambulatory patients should not be treated, because the toxicity and expense of therapy may outweigh the risk of disease.

Symptomatic Urinary Tract Infection

Acute uncomplicated episodes of symptomatic bacteriuria localized to the lower urinary tract (bladder or urethra) can be treated effectively with oral single-dose therapy, either amoxicillin, 3 grams, or co-trimoxazole (trimethoprim, 0.32 gram, plus sulfamethoxazole, 1.6 grams), two double-strength tablets. Single-dose therapy will usually fail to eradicate either renal bacteriuria or complicated infections. In addition, single-dose therapy is more effective in suburban compared with inner-city women with cystitis and in women less than 25 years of age compared with women over 40 years of age. Higher cure rates may be achieved in inner-city or older women with trimethoprim, 0.16 gram, plus sulfamethoxazole, 0.8 gram, twice daily for three days. Symptomatic urethritis caused by *Chlamydia trachomatis* should respond to oral doxycycline (100 mg twice daily) or tetracycline (500 mg four times daily) for seven days.

Pyelonephritis requires a 7- to 14-day or longer course of therapy. Complicated infections in which obstruction or a foreign body is not removed may not respond to such a course. Hematogenous pyelonephritis requires specific therapy directed at the invading organism.

The choice of an oral or parenteral agent depends upon the severity of the infection and the patient's ability to take the oral agent. Drugs are selected on the basis of cost, side effects, and antibacterial spectrum. Antimicrobial susceptibility tests should be used to guide therapy of recurrent episodes. Effective oral agents include sulfonamides, tetracyclines, ampicillin, amoxicillin, cinoxacin, cephalosporins, co-trimoxazole, trimethoprim, and nitrofurantoin. The last three drugs are useful in recurrent infections, because emergence of resistant strains occurs infrequently.

The initial attack of urinary tract infection is usually due to *E. coli*, which is sensitive to most antimicrobial agents and therefore may be treated "blindly" with the agents described above with equal success. However, the widespread use of these agents for other infections has decreased their previous reliability. For example, approximately 40 per cent of *E. coli*, including those that are community acquired, are now resistant to ampicillin.

Microscopic examination of urine and urine cultures have been the mainstay for accurate diagnosis of urinary tract infections. Pretreatment urine cultures are probably not essential, however, and are not cost effective in selected young women with acute dysuria and pyuria, in whom the probability of uncomplicated bacterial cystitis is high. These patients respond to short-course empiric therapy. Urine cultures can be reserved for those in whom therapy has failed. In contrast, pretreatment urine cultures should be obtained in symptomatic infants, children, men, and the elderly; patients with suspected pyelonephritis or complicated infection; patients with relapsing infections; those with *symptomatic* catheter- or instrument-associated nosocomial infection; and pregnant women to detect covert bacteriuria of pregnancy.

When therapy is successful, bacteriuria should disappear within 24 hours even if pyuria and symptoms continue. A

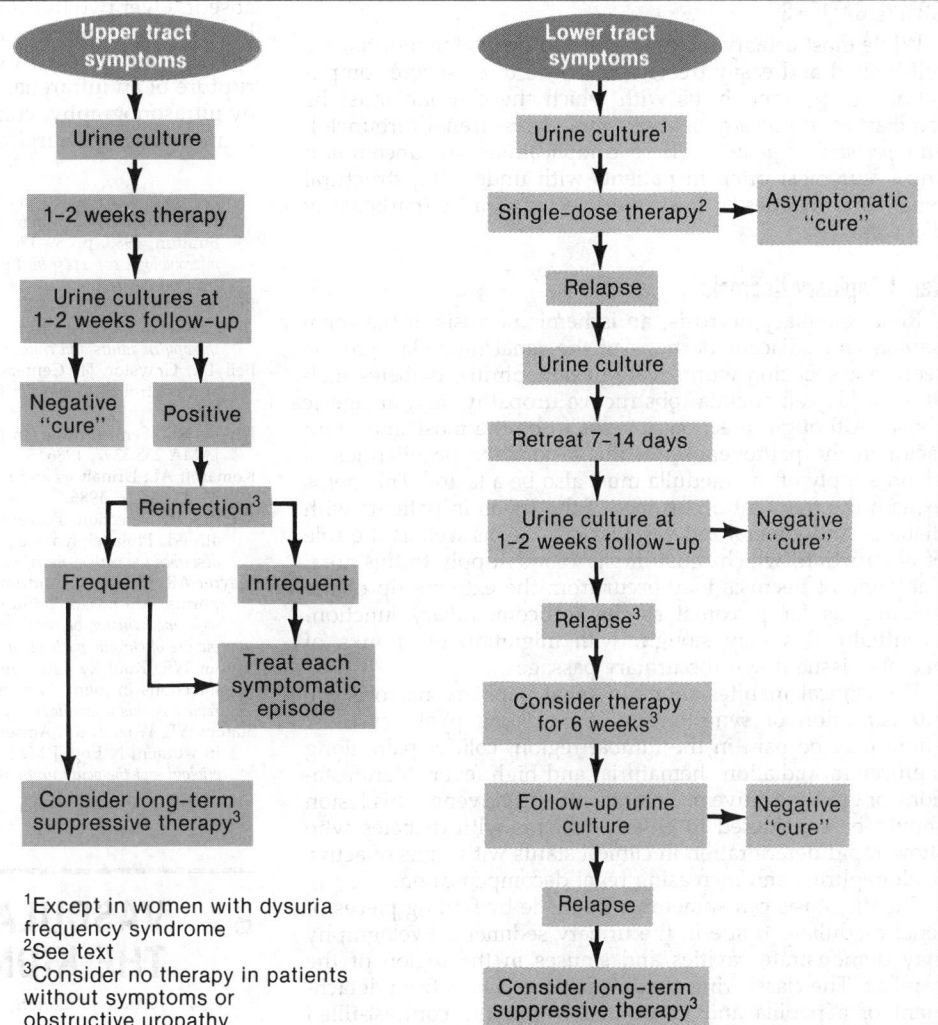

FIGURE 86—1. Management of urinary infections.

Flowchart (left side):

Upper tract symptoms → Urine culture → 1–2 weeks therapy → Urine cultures at 1–2 weeks follow-up → Negative "cure" / Positive → Reinfection[3] → Frequent / Infrequent → Treat each symptomatic episode / Consider long-term suppressive therapy[3]

Flowchart (right side):

Lower tract symptoms → Urine culture[1] → Single-dose therapy[2] → Asymptomatic "cure" / Relapse → Urine culture → Retreat 7–14 days → Urine culture at 1–2 weeks follow-up → Negative "cure" / Relapse[3] → Consider therapy for 6 weeks[3] → Follow-up urine culture → Negative "cure" / Relapse → Consider long-term suppressive therapy[3]

[1]Except in women with dysuria frequency syndrome
[2]See text
[3]Consider no therapy in patients without symptoms or obstructive uropathy

repeat urine culture should be obtained after 72 hours of treatment in those patients who have had a pretreatment culture. A positive culture at this time denotes treatment failure. It is important to recognize bacteriologic failure early and to change to another drug. Parenteral agents, such as ampicillin, a cephalosporin, or an aminoglycoside, may be required in some instances or when the patient is too ill to receive an oral agent. A follow-up culture one week after the completion of antimicrobial therapy is recommended to document a cure.

Some authors recommend routine follow-up cultures several times over the ensuing year to detect recurrent bacteriuria, but this practice is prohibitively expensive and difficult to justify on medical grounds in asymptomatic patients.

Recurrent Infections

Recurrence of infection in the few weeks after treatment is usually due to persistence of the same focus, whereas later recurrence, particularly in females, is more often a result of reinfection. Frequent recurrent infections may be managed either by close follow-up and treatment of each episode or by prophylaxis with nitrofurantoin, trimethoprim, or co-trimoxazole as a single bedtime dose.

Urinary antiseptics such as methenamine mandelate or hippurate require an acid urine, preferably at pH 5.5, and are of little value unless their use is accompanied by agents that consistently lower urinary pH, such as high-dose ascorbic acid (1000 mg daily). Methenamine, however, is an effective "suppressant" agent and is best used after infection is eradicated by a more effective drug.

Prophylaxis when given for three to six months is effective for recurrent infections of the reinfection type in women. Cessation of prophylaxis, however, results in a significant incidence of recurrence in individuals having structural abnormalities of the urinary tract or intrinsic renal structural defects. In those circumstances prophylaxis should be reinstituted. Generally, the therapeutic agent should be changed if bacteriuria persists during treatment. This latter circumstance usually means an organism resistant to the agent is now colonizing the urine. Prophylaxis is ineffective in patients with indwelling catheters and will only lead to emergence of resistant bacteria.

The patient should be instructed to drink fluids generously and void frequently. Double voiding in patients with vesicoureteral reflux is recommended. Voiding after sexual intercourse is felt by some to decrease the chance of recurrent infection, but postcoital use of prophylactic agents is probably more effective.

Complicated Infections

Complex urinary infections, i.e., those in the presence of obstructive uropathy, neurogenic bladders, or catheters, are exceedingly difficult to eradicate. They are often best left untreated except for management of acute episodes. Suppressive therapy should be considered ineffective if bacterial populations in the urine are not reduced to less than 1000 per milliliter. The key to management is relief of obstruction or the removal of foreign bodies. Intermittent catheterization has benefited some patients with neurogenic bladders.

COMPLICATIONS

While most urinary infections, including pyelonephritis, are self-limited and easily treated, there are three severe complications of pyelonephritis with which the clinician must be familiar: *renal papillary necrosis, renal abscess* (renal carbuncle), and *perinephric abscess*. These complications are uncommon and occur most often in patients with underlying structural renal abnormalities or host immunocompromise (particularly diabetes).

Renal Papillary Necrosis

Renal papillary necrosis, an ischemic necrosis of the renal papilla and adjacent portions of the renal medulla, may be seen in association with severe pyelonephritis, diabetes mellitus, sickle cell anemia, obstructive uropathy, and analgesic abuse. Although infection appears to be the most important factor in the pathogenesis of this lesion, the peculiarities of blood supply of the medulla must also be a factor. This helps explain the frequent occurrence of the lesion in patients with diabetes and generalized vascular disease, as well as the role of obstruction, which must impair blood supply to this area. The zone of necrosis may occur from the extreme tip of the pyramid as far proximal as the corticomedullary junction. Eventually this may slough, with migration of chunks of necrotic tissue down the urinary passages.

The clinical manifestations of renal papillary necrosis are intensification of symptoms of pre-existing pyelonephritis. There may be pain in the lumbar region, colicky pain along the ureteral radiation, hematuria, and high fever. Manifestations of gram-negative bacteremia may supervene. This lesion should be considered in elderly patients with diabetes who show rapid deterioration in clinical status with signs of active pyelonephritis and increasing renal decompensation.

The diagnosis can sometimes be made by finding pieces of renal medullary tissue in the urinary sediment. Pyelography may demonstrate cavities and sinuses in the region of the papillae. The classic ring-shadow pattern results from detachment of a papilla and its outline within the contrast-filled cavity.

Therapy should be directed toward control of infection and measures employed to improve the status of patients who have diabetes mellitus or who are habitual abusers of analgesic agents.

Renal Abscess

Renal abscesses usually occur as a result of extension of a pyelonephritis process. Up to one half of the cases, however, arise from hematogenous spread, by virulent organisms such as *S. aureus*, from a distant focus.

A renal abscess may be identified by intravenous pyelography, ultrasonography, computed tomography, or magnetic resonance imaging. It should be suspected whenever a urinary tract infection fails to respond to an adequate course of appropriate antibiotics. Blood and urine cultures may be negative, so empiric antibiotic regimens may be needed to cover gram-negative rods and staphylococci. Surgical drainage is usually required in addition to parenteral antibiotics, although early diagnosis may eliminate the need for surgery in some patients.

Perinephric Abscess

Perinephric abscesses are notoriously difficult to diagnose. They have an insidious onset, with symptoms usually present for over two weeks at the time of presentation. Fever and unilateral flank pain are common presenting symptoms. The diagnosis should be considered in the evaluation of any patient with a fever of unknown origin. A recent history of urinary tract infection should alert one to the possibility of a perinephric abscess, although this piece of history is often absent. Over two thirds of patients with perinephric abscesses have either diabetes or kidney stone disease.

Perinephric abscesses occur almost exclusively from the rupture of an intrarenal abscess. Diagnosis can be established by ultrasonography, computed tomography, or magnetic resonance imaging. Surgical drainage is mandatory.

Andriole VT: Current concepts of urinary tract infections. In Weinstein L, Fields BN (eds.): Seminars in Infectious Disease, Vol III. New York, Thieme-Stratton, 1980, pp 89–130. *The author's review of practical diagnostic methods, microbiologic concepts, host defenses, clinical syndromes, and treatment of urinary tract infections.*
Bailey RR (ed.): Single Dose Therapy of Urinary Tract Infection. Sydney, Australia, ADIS Health Science Press, 1983. *A multiauthor text on single-dose therapy in adults and children.*
Bell TA, Grayston JT: Centers for Disease Control guidelines for prevention and control of *Chlamydia trachomatis* infections. Ann Intern Med 104:524, 1986.
Jenkins RD, Fenn JP, Matsen JM: Review of urine microscopy for bacteriuria. JAMA 255:3397, 1986.
Komaroff AL: Urinalysis and urine culture in women with dysuria. Ann Intern Med 104:212, 1986.
Kunin CM: Detection, Prevention and Treatment of Urinary Tract Infections. 4th ed. Philadelphia, Lea & Febiger, 1986 (in press). *An excellent text that describes the pathogenesis, management, and prevention of urinary infections.*
Mayrer AR, Miniter P, Andriole VT: Immunopathogenesis of chronic pyelonephritis. Am J Med 75 (Suppl 1B):59, 1983. *Recent studies describing immunologic mechanisms of renal injury and scarring, which produce a histopathologic picture of chronic pyelonephritis.*
Stamm WE, Koutsky LA, Benedetti JK, et al.: *Chlamydia trachomatis* urethral infections in men. Ann Intern Med 100:47, 1984. *An excellent and concise review of this underdiagnosed type of infection.*
Stamm WE, Wagner KF, Amsel R, et al.: Causes of the acute urethral syndrome in women. N Engl J Med 303:409, 1980. *A detailed description of the various etiologies of the acute urethral syndrome in women.*

87 VASCULAR DISORDERS OF THE KIDNEY
Jordan J. Cohen

RENAL ARTERY OCCLUSION

Partial occlusion (stenosis) of the main renal artery, or one or more of its branches, is common and typically results in hypertension. The clinical features of renovascular hypertension are discussed in Ch. 47. This section considers total or nearly total occlusion of the arterial supply to all or a portion of the kidney.

CAUSES (see Table 87–1). Thrombosis in situ rarely occurs in the absence of a severely diseased or damaged vessel. Macroemboli of the renal circulation are far more common as a cause of complete occlusion than are in situ thrombi. (Atheroemboli are considered in the following section.) Approximately 90 per cent of renal artery emboli originate in the heart. Of these, most arise from the left atrium and are a consequence of atrial fibrillation due to arteriosclerotic heart disease. Although 20 per cent of the cardiac output normally goes to the kidney, only 2 to 3 per cent of the systemic emboli derived from the heart lodge in the renal circulation. The number, the size, and the consistency of individual embolic particles vary with the nature of the underlying process and determine the extent of renal involvement. Large emboli can occlude the main renal artery, but, more frequently, embolic material reaches primary or secondary branches of the vessel. Thus, total infarction of the kidney is much less common than is ischemia or segmental infarction. The presence of one or more accessory renal arteries in 20 to 30 per cent of people and of a generally rich capsular circulation also reduces the likelihood of extensive infarction. In most instances, the embolic event involves only one kidney; bilateral emboli and

TABLE 87–1. CAUSES OF RENAL ARTERY OCCLUSION

Thrombosis, in situ
    Progressive atherosclerosis
    Blunt trauma
    Inflammation (e.g., polyarteritis, thromboangiitis
      obliterans)
    Aortic or renal artery aneurysm
    Aortic or renal artery dissection
    Angiographic catheter
    No obvious cause ("spontaneous")

Macroemboli
    Atrial fibrillation
    Mitral stenosis
    Mural thrombus
    Atrial myxoma
    Infective endocarditis
    Prosthetic valve
    Paradoxical emboli (patent foramen ovale)

Atheroemboli
    Abdominal aorta surgery
    Blunt trauma
    Angiographic catheters
    Anticoagulation (?)
    No obvious cause ("spontaneous")

emboli to a solitary kidney do occur and are associated with greater morbidity.

CLINICAL MANIFESTATIONS. Sudden occlusion of a renal artery, whether from embolus or thrombosis, results in a wide spectrum of clinical manifestations in accordance with the caliber of the vessel or vessels involved and with the pre-existing status of the renal circulation. Occlusion of a primary or secondary branch of the renal artery in a patient with well-established collateral circulation due to chronic, high-grade stenosis may produce little or no infarction and, hence, few or no signs or symptoms; conversely, occlusion of the main renal artery in an otherwise normal kidney may result in immediate infarction of most of the organ and in a dramatic clinical presentation. Renal infarction typically results in the acute onset of vague, nonspecific flank pain that is described as dull and aching in character. The pain may, however, resemble that due to renal colic, cholecystitis, or pancreatitis. Nausea and vomiting are frequent; gross hematuria is *not* common. The symptoms usually subside within three to four days.

Fever is an infrequent finding at onset but often appears within one to two days. Blood pressure does not usually rise above baseline values. The white blood cell count is usually elevated, and a leftward shift in the differential count is characteristic. Microscopic hematuria is common but may be absent. Striking elevations of serum lactate dehydrogenase (LDH) levels and lesser evaluations of serum glutamic-oxalo-acetic transaminase (SGOT) are characteristic. The blood urea nitrogen (BUN) and creatinine levels typically rise transiently in unilateral infarction; more severe and protracted degrees of renal functional impairment, including acute oliguric renal failure, may follow bilateral renal infarction or infarction of a solitary kidney.

DIAGNOSIS. The diagnosis of renal artery occlusion and infarction is often difficult because the clinical findings are frequently meager and nonspecific. As a result less than 1 per cent of autopsy-proven cases may be diagnosed ante mortem. The intravenous pyelogram typically reveals reduced or absent function in the involved kidney or kidneys; retrograde pyelography usually reveals no abnormality. Indeed, a normal retrograde study in a kidney that makes no urine and fails to visualize on intravenous pyelography is virtually diagnostic of arterial occlusion. Radionuclide scanning of the kidney may show segmental perfusion defects or complete absence of perfusion. Definitive diagnosis of renal artery occlusion, however, requires renal angiography. In addition, angiography can often distinguish between embolic and thrombotic occlusion. Angiography should be reserved for those patients in whom the diagnostic information is crucial for making management decisions because the risk of the procedure in this setting is appreciable.

TREATMENT. The choice of therapy of renal artery occlusion varies widely with individual circumstances (Table 87–2). As a rule, unilateral renal artery occlusion should be treated conservatively, especially if a branch vessel or vessels are involved; observation alone or coupled with anticoagulation often results in recanalization and avoids the high risk of surgery. Patients with bilateral occlusion or occlusion in a solitary kidney generally fare better with operative intervention. Although early intervention maximizes recovery of renal function, sufficient time should be taken for stabilizing the patient's underlying medical condition to reduce the operative risk; mortality rates as high as 35 per cent have been reported in patients undergoing acute revascularization procedures. Fibrinolytic therapy followed by anticoagulation can be considered as an alternative to surgery in selected cases. Recovery of renal function is a complex function of the duration and magnitude of the occlusion, the extent of collaterals, the degree of associated cardiovascular disease, and the skill and experience of the operative team. Hemodialysis can be used as a temporizing maneuver if the degree of renal functional impairment warrants. Recovery of renal function has been reported to occur after as long as one month of oliguric renal failure due to renal artery occlusion. Given that irreversible renal damage occurs within 60 minutes of total renal ischemia induced experimentally, such occurrences of recovery after lengthy delay underscore the important role of renal collaterals.

Percutaneous transluminal angioplasty has proved successful as an alternative to surgery for stenotic lesions of the renal artery and shows promise for occlusive lesions as well. Nephrectomy should not be considered unless unequivocal evidence of total infarction is present.

RENAL ARTERY ATHEROEMBOLI

CAUSES. Renal artery atheroembolization is a complication of severe erosive (ulcerative) atheromatosis of the abdominal aorta. Atheroemboli may occur with great frequency in patients with this condition, but, fortunately, in only a small fraction does the process culminate in significant clinical abnormalities. Common events that can trigger the release of cholesterol-laden embolic material from ulcerative plaques are listed in Table 87–1.

CLINICAL MANIFESTATIONS. Atheroemboli characteristically lodge in vessels smaller than the interlobular arteries. As a consequence, macroscopic renal infarction does not usually occur, and the clinical picture is usually bland. The insidious development of renal insufficiency is the mode of presentation in most instances of severe atheroemboli. Hypertension is frequently present and may be severe. Distal embolization in the lower extremities, occasionally associated with livedo reticularis, is frequent. Acute pancreatitis and gastrointestinal bleeding can occur and indicate more widespread embolization. Laboratory findings are nonspecific and give evidence of steady or episodic decline in renal function over a period of days, weeks, or even months. Eosinophilia is common, but its cause is unknown. Urinalysis reveals nothing characteristic and is frequently normal. Kidney size is usually normal or only slightly reduced.

DIAGNOSIS. Diagnosis is made by renal biopsy. Choles-

TABLE 87–2. TREATMENT OPTIONS FOR RENAL ARTERY OCCLUSION

Observation
Anticoagulation
Thrombolytic therapy followed by anticoagulation
Percutaneous transluminal angioplasty
Surgical embolectomy or endarterectomy
Partial or total nephrectomy

TABLE 87-3. CAUSES OF RENAL VEIN THROMBOSIS

Reduced renal blood flow (especially in infants)
Nephrotic syndrome (especially in membranous glomerulopathy)
Renal cell carcinoma
Inferior vena caval thrombosis
External compression (e.g., retroperitoneal fibrosis, tumor)

terol crystals contained in the embolic material are dissolved during routine preparation of the histologic sections, leaving pathognomonic biconvex, cleftlike structures in the occluded vessels.

TREATMENT. No effective therapy is available for this condition. Anticoagulants are *not* helpful and may in fact foster atheroemboli by delaying healing of the atheromatous ulcers in the aorta. Unfortunately, once renal manifestations are evident, the process often progresses unrelentingly to renal failure.

RENAL VEIN THROMBOSIS

CAUSES (see Table 87-3). Renal vein thrombosis in infants is typically an acute catastrophic event triggered by a volume-depleting illness such as profuse diarrhea. The consequences are sudden cessation of renal function, engorgement and enlargement of the kidneys, and ultimate renal infarction and atrophy if venous obstruction is not relieved. Fortunately, acute renal vein thrombosis of such magnitude is rare in older children and adults.

Renal vein thrombosis in adults is typically of insidious onset and is almost always superimposed on an established disease. It occurs most frequently in association with idiopathic nephrotic syndrome, especially that due to membranous glomerulopathy. Predisposing factors may include reduced antithrombin III levels, reduced intravascular blood volume (often aggravated by diuretic therapy), thrombocytosis, and elevated liver-derived clotting factors. Patients with renal cell carcinoma often develop renal vein thrombosis consequent to tumor invasion of the renal vein.

CLINICAL MANIFESTATIONS. In the typical circumstance in which gradual occlusion of the renal vein occurs, the process may progress without any outward sign. Mild abdominal or back pain may be present, but severe pain is uncommon. Pulmonary emboli occur during the course of approximately half of all patients with chronic renal vein thrombosis and are frequently the initial manifestation of the condition. Renal vein thrombosis can also cause unexplained deterioration in renal function in patients with the nephrotic syndrome. Chronic renal vein thrombosis itself results in no characteristic findings on physical examination or laboratory testing. Heavy proteinuria occurs frequently in patients with this condition but reflects the presence of pre-existing nephrotic syndrome; it is not the result of renal vein thrombosis itself.

DIAGNOSIS. The index of suspicion may be heightened greatly by the clinical setting (e.g., recurrent pulmonary emboli in a patient with neophrotic syndrome) or by findings on intravenous pyelography (e.g., large kidneys with splayed calices due to interstitial edema, notching of the upper ureters due to collaterals). Definitive diagnosis, however, requires visualization of the renal vein. Adequate visualization of the main vein can often be obtained with ultrasound, computerized tomography, or magnetic resonance imaging. Selective renal venography may be required for unequivocal visualization of the vessel and its branches.

TREATMENT. Long-term anticoagulation remains the treatment of choice in chronic, subtotal renal vein thrombosis. Fibrinolytic therapy for a few days prior to instituting anticoagulation should be considered in patients with more serious manifestations of renal vein thrombosis (e.g., acute flank pain coupled with a rising serum creatinine level, rapidly recurring pulmonary emboli).

Harrington JT, Kassirer JP: Renal vein thrombosis. Ann Rev Med 33:255, 1982. *An excellent, clinically relevant review.*

Keating MA, Althausen AF: The clinical spectrum of renal vein thrombosis. J Urol 133:938, 1985. *A well-referenced review of historical and modern concepts of the etiology and management of renal vein thrombosis.*

Lessman RK, Johnson SF, Coburn JW, et al.: Renal artery embolism: Clinical features and long-term follow-up of 17 cases. Ann Intern Med 89:477, 1978. *An excellent detailed review and follow-up of one of the larger series of patients with renal artery embolism; emphasizes the nonoperative management.*

Sniderman KW, Sos TA: Percutaneous transluminal recanalization and dilation of totally occluded renal arteries. Radiology 142:607, 1982. *A report of seven patients treated by this technique.*

Stanley JC, Whithouse WMJ: Occlusive and aneurysmal disease of the renal arterial circulation. DM 30:7, 1984. *A readable review emphasizing the diagnosis and therapy of common afflictions of the renal arteries.*

Wagoner RD, Stanson AW, Holley KE, et al.: Renal vein thrombosis in idiopathic membranous glomerulopathy: Incidence and significance. Kidney Int 23:368, 1983. *A well-referenced study of a moderately large series of cases.*

88 RENAL DISEASE IN PREGNANCY

John P. Hayslett

The detection and clinical management of renal disease in the gravid woman is complicated by concern for fetal development and survival, as well as for the health of the patient. In addition, clinical evaluation must account for physiologic changes in volume status and renal function that accompany pregnancy.

RENAL FUNCTION IN PREGNANCY. Pregnancy is characterized by a gradual, cumulative retention of 500 to 900 mEq of sodium and 6 to 8 liters of water, which are distributed between maternal extracellular fluid and the fetus. Despite an expansion in plasma volume of 30 to 45 per cent, mean blood pressure falls approximately 15 per cent owing to a reduction in peripheral vascular resistance. The glomerular filtration rate increases by 30 to 50 per cent by the twelfth week of gestation; the elevation is sustained until term and is position dependent (Fig. 88-1). An evaluation of glomerular filtration rate should take into account expected levels during gestation and should not compare measured values with reported normal values obtained in the nonpregnant individual. Because of the marked position dependence, a convenient way of measuring filtration rate in later pregnancy is with a timed (e.g., four hours) water-loaded creatinine clearance with the woman positioned in the lateral recumbent position.

Owing to the increase in glomerular filtration rate and expanded plasma volume, the levels of creatinine and blood urea nitrogen fall to approximately 0.5 mg per deciliter and 9 mg per deciliter, respectively. Plasma concentrations above 0.8 mg per deciliter of creatinine and 13 mg per deciliter of urea nitrogen should alert the physician to the possibility of renal insufficiency. Plasma osmolality falls from approximately 280 mOsm · kg H_2O^{-1} to 270 owing to a resetting of the osmostat; plasma uric acid falls to 3 to 4 mg per deciliter and plasma bicarbonate to approximately 20 mEq per liter (owing to mild respiratory alkalosis). Glucosuria and aminoaciduria may occur during pregnancy as a result of a transient reduction in the renal threshold of absorption. The ureters dilate during pregnancy and for as long as 12 weeks post partum with no implication of outflow obstruction.

TOXEMIA OF PREGNANCY

DEFINITION. Toxemia, unique to human pregnancy, is characterized by hypertension, edema, and proteinuria. Clinically the syndrome is divided into the stages of preeclampsia and eclampsia, the latter when convulsions have occurred. Onset is usually insidious after the thirty-second week of pregnancy, but it may occur as early as the twenty-fourth

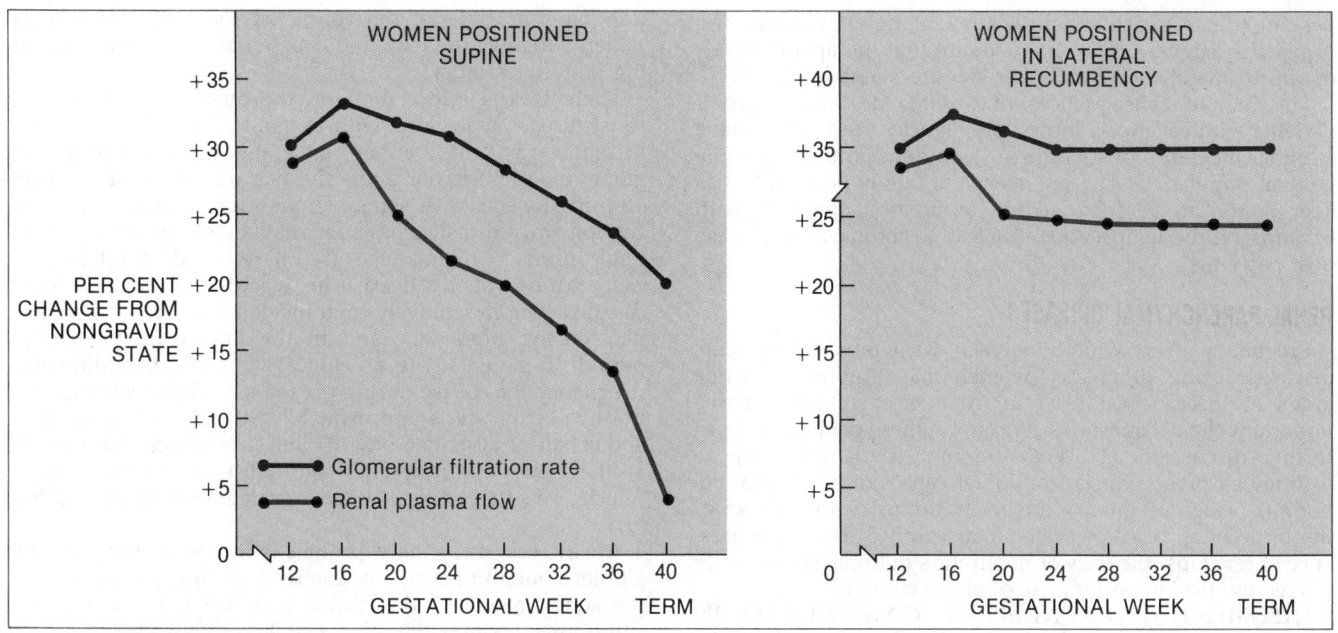

FIGURE 88–1. The early increment of glomerular filtration rate and effective renal plasma flow is position dependent and is sustained if subjects are studied in lateral recumbency. (Adapted from Pippig L: Clinical aspects of renal disease during pregnancy. Med Hyg 27:181, 1969. In Lindheimer MD, Katz AI: Kidney Function and Disease in Pregnancy. Philadelphia, Lea and Febiger, 1977.)

week. In women with a hydatidiform mole, toxemia has been reported to occur in the first trimester. The usual sequence is edema and hypertension, followed by proteinuria, although proteinuria may occasionally precede hypertension. Signs of toxemia spontaneously subside after delivery. Clinical criteria for diagnosis vary depending on changes of blood pressure considered to be abnormal in pregnancy. In general, hypertension in the third trimester is defined by a blood pressure measurement of 140/85 mm Hg or greater if sustained for four to six hours, or an increase of 30 mm Hg or more in systolic blood pressure and 15 mm Hg or more in diastolic pressure above values measured during the early stages of pregnancy. The major differential diagnosis involves a distinction among toxemia, essential hypertension, and primary renal disease, although toxemia can be superimposed on the other two clinical entities.

INCIDENCE. Toxemia of pregnancy occurs worldwide with an incidence that varies between 2 per cent and 25 per cent in different populations. In the United States the quoted incidence is 6 to 7 per cent. Individuals with a poor socioeconomic status are at higher risk for developing the syndrome; the incidence is reduced after introduction of adequate prenatal care with special attention to weight gain and monitoring of blood pressure. The syndrome occurs predominantly in primigravidas and in multiparous women over 35 years of age.

CLINICAL MANIFESTATIONS. Clinical symptoms may include headache, visual disturbances, and apprehension. While diastolic hypertension may be prominent, systolic blood pressure seldom exceeds 160 mm Hg except when associated with underlying hypertension. Funduscopic examination may reveal segmental arteriolar narrowing and a generalized glistening fundus indicative of retinal edema. The ocular changes reflect vasoconstriction. Signs of central nervous system hyperexcitability are regarded as ominous, since they often precede convulsions with a high maternal and fetal death rate. Laboratory findings include a rate of protein excretion usually less than 2 grams per day, but higher levels in the range seen in the nephrotic syndrome may occur. There is a reduction in glomerular filtration rate and renal plasma flow to about 60 per cent of that in pregnancy control subjects. Owing to elevated levels of glomerular filtration rate in normal

pregnancy, however, blood urea and serum creatinine levels may not appear to be elevated in toxemic patients, especially if compared with nonpregnant control values. Plasma uric acid levels rise in toxemia to about 5.0 mg per deciliter in mild toxemia and to over 7.0 mg per deciliter in severe states, owing to a fall in its renal clearance. It is suggested that uric acid levels provide a guide for estimating severity of toxemia.

PATHOGENESIS AND PATHOLOGY. The cause of toxemia is not understood. Plasma levels of aldosterone and renin are lower in toxemic women than in normal pregnant individuals but still may be inappropriately high in relation to salt intake and volume status. Many primigravidas who eventually develop toxemia exhibit increased sensitivity to the pressure effects of infused angiotensin many weeks before they become hypertensive. In addition, although a reduction in placental blood flow is found in toxemia, it is not known whether this is a primary change or is secondary to systemic hypertension.

The histopathologic renal changes in toxemia, primarily confined to the glomerulus, are termed *glomerular capillary endotheliosis*. The glomeruli are large and swollen, with encroachment on capillary lumina by swollen and vacuolated endothelial and mesangial cells. Occasionally, small subendothelial deposits and fibrin deposits may be seen, but immunofluorescence studies are negative for deposition of immunoglobulins. The characteristic lesion of endotheliosis seems to be invariably present in toxemia, even in patients with mild clinical preeclampsia, but resolves during an interval of a few weeks or months after delivery.

TREATMENT AND PROGNOSIS. All patients suspected of having preeclampsia should be hospitalized. The majority of patients with mild preeclampsia respond to bed rest and sedation. If they do not, antihypertensive agents are administered, usually in the form of vasodilators and alpha methyldopa. In general there are strong arguments for avoiding diuretic agents in the treatment of hypertension in pregnancy because of risks of reducing placental blood flow. The definitive treatment for toxemia is delivery, which is indicated as soon as fetal maturity is achieved. The occurrence of hyperreflexia or convulsions requires immediate efforts to reduce the level of hypertension and depress central nervous system hyperexcitability. Most obstetric units employ parenteral magnesium sulfate to achieve these aims, along with monitoring of plasma magnesium levels to assure that therapeutic levels of approximately 6 to 8 mEq per liter are maintained.

The remote consequences of toxemia are controversial. Patients with eclampsia in first pregnancies seem not to have a higher incidence of subsequent hypertension than does the general population. The prevalence of late hypertension has been found to be increased in multiparous patients with eclampsia. Preeclampsia does not lead to chronic renal disease post partum.

RENAL PARENCHYMAL DISEASES

Pregnancy may occur in women with pre-existing renal disease; during pregnancy women may acquire the same kinds of disease that exist in the nongravid state. Three important clinical questions concerning these patients warrant further discussion: (1) What are the criteria that help to distinguish preeclampsia from other causes of renal dysfunction? (2) Does pregnancy adversely influence the course of the underlying renal or systemic disease? (3) Does the presence of renal insufficiency or nephrotic syndrome significantly reduce the likelihood for a successful fetal outcome?

DIFFERENTIAL DIAGNOSIS OF RENAL DISEASE IN PREGNANCY. Since the clinical hallmarks of preeclampsia, e.g., hypertension, proteinuria, and edema, are also manifested by most other types of renal parenchymal disease, a diagnostic evaluation cannot be based on these clinical features alone. Preeclampsia does not occur before the twenty-fourth week of gestation, except in hydatidiform mole or multiple gestation pregnancies. The differential diagnosis is therefore simplified if clinical signs of renal disease are known to exist prior to conception or in the early stages of pregnancy. In patients who are not observed until the last trimester of pregnancy, however, identification of the cause of renal dysfunction is often difficult. Multisystem involvement resulting in abnormal liver function tests and coagulation studies suggests preeclampsia. The renal biopsy finding of the pathognomonic changes of preeclampsia provides the only absolute method of confirming the diagnosis of toxemia. When it is necessary to establish the diagnosis, renal biopsy should be performed during the week immediately following delivery. During pregnancy, therefore, management in most cases must rely on a presumed clinical diagnosis. Since the clinical manifestations of preeclampsia usually resolve spontaneously within four to six weeks post partum, persistence of hypertension, proteinuria, or renal insufficiency strongly suggests a primary renal disease.

Information on the relative incidence of the various causes of hypertension and proteinuria during gestation has been reported in a large series of patients in whom the diagnosis was confirmed by renal biopsy performed within six days of delivery. In most of these patients a presumed diagnosis of preeclampsia was made during pregnancy. Among primigravidas the incidence of preeclampsia, primary renal disease, and hypertensive glomerulosclerosis was 83 per cent, 12 per cent, and 5 per cent, respectively. In multiparous patients, in contrast, preeclampsia occurred in only 38 per cent of patients, while renal disease accounted for 26 per cent of cases, and hypertensive renal disease for 24 per cent.

INFLUENCE OF PREGNANCY ON UNDERLYING RENAL DISEASE. Pregnancy does not significantly alter the course of pre-existing primary renal disease due to either glomerular or tubulointerstitial injury in patients with normal or nearly normal renal function. The effect of pregnancy on underlying disease, when renal insufficiency is more severe, (serum creatinine >2.0 mg per deciliter) is less certain because of insufficient data. Although increased proteinuria, often to nephrotic levels, occurs in nearly one half of patients with a glomerulonephropathy, there is no constant relationship between pregnancy and long-term changes in glomerular filtra-

tion rate. In general, the course of renal disease in these patients follows the expected course defined by the underlying pattern of injury.

There is less information on the effect of pregnancy on renal disease associated with systemic disorders. Pregnancy in diabetic patients neither accelerates the onset of diabetic glomerulosclerosis nor alters the natural course of renal disease in subjects with signs of renal dysfunction before conception. In contrast, pregnancy may adversely influence systemic lupus erythematosus (SLE), reflected in relapse and exacerbations of this disease in patients with an established diagnosis and a relatively high incidence of de novo onset of SLE during pregnancy and in the immediate postpartum period. In patients with no clinical signs of active SLE before pregnancy the course during pregnancy is relatively mild and the live birth rate is approximately 90 per cent. In contrast, about half of all patients with clinical evidence of active SLE at the time of conception have subsequent exacerbations, which are often severe and associated with increased fetal loss.

An increase in urinary protein excretion in subjects with glomerulonephropathies is common during pregnancy and frequently results in the clinical manifestations of nephrotic syndrome. Sodium retention usually tends to become more severe in the last trimester. In most cases the level of proteinuria spontaneously returns to pregestational levels after delivery. Low birth weight has been reported by some to correlate directly with low serum albumin levels, but this finding has not been seen in all patient series. An increase in the rate of edema formation should be anticipated during the later stages of pregnancy in patients with moderate or severe proteinuria and can be blunted by the introduction of a diet with low sodium content. The use of diuretics in pregnancy is controversial because of the possible induction of reduced placental blood flow. Conservative measures including dietary measures and bed rest are preferred. The judicious use of natriuretic agents may be useful in patients who fail to respond to conservative measures and has not been shown to increase fetal death.

INFLUENCE OF RENAL DISEASE ON FETAL OUTCOME. In the absence of hypertension and severe renal insufficiency, e.g., serum creatinine greater than 2.0 mg per deciliter, the live birth rate is greater than 90 per cent in most patients with primary renal disease. Pregnancies associated with mild to moderate renal insufficiency, however, result in an increased rate of preterm delivery and small-for-gestational-age births. Severe renal insufficiency reduces the incidence of live births to 20 to 50 per cent. Since there is no evidence that pregnancy alters the natural course of primary renal diseases or most types of renal disease due to systemic disease, early termination of pregnancy is not indicated on medical grounds. Clinical management should include control of hypertension and careful monitoring of fetal growth to maximize the likelihood of fetal maturity at birth.

ACUTE RENAL FAILURE IN PREGNANCY

Acute renal failure during pregnancy results from severe injury to tubular epithelial cells due to renal ischemia or to the action of nephrotoxic agents (Ch. 78). The cell injury may be reversible, with an eventual complete restoration of renal function; it may be irreversible and lead to renal cortical necrosis. Renal cortical necrosis is characterized by the development of fibrosis within the cortex in a diffuse or patchy pattern, with relative sparing of the medullary portions of the kidney. Although cortical necrosis is uncommon in nonpregnant individuals, it is a frequent complication of obstetric conditions, especially in subjects beyond the age of 30 years and in association with abruptio placentae. It has been suggested that increased reactivity of the renal vasculature to vasoactive amines in pregnancy and local activation of coagulation may play an important role in the induction of tissue injury leading to cell death.

In addition to the usual causes of acute renal failure, some types of renal insults are unique to pregnancy. Septic abortion and hyperemesis gravidarum may cause renal failure in early pregnancy, while severe preeclampsia, placenta previa, and abruptio placentae are causative factors in the later stages of pregnancy. Clinical management of acute renal failure in pregnancy is comparable to that in nonpregnant patients (Ch. 78). Because of the reported high rate of fetal death, delivery should be performed as soon as the maternal condition has been stabilized and fetal maturity is ascertained. There is inadequate experience with dialysis treatment in gravid patients with acute renal failure to assess its possible usefulness.

Hayslett JP: Pregnancy does not exacerbate primary glomerular disease. Am J Kidney Dis 6:273, 1985. *An analysis of the literature concerning the effect of pregnancy on the underlying renal disease.*

Katz AI, Davison JM, Hayslett JP, et al.: Pregnancy in women with kidney disease. Kidney Int 18:192, 1980. *An analysis of a large series of pregnancies associated with primary renal disease. An excellent source for references.*

Pritchard JA: Management of preeclampsia and eclampsia. Kidney Int 18:259, 1980. *A clear and concise description of the regimen used to treat toxemic women in obstetric units.*

89 HEREDITARY CHRONIC NEPHROPATHIES

Wadi N. Suki

Several genetically transmitted renal disorders of unknown pathogenesis may fall under this heading. This chapter will discuss two of these disorders, Alport's syndrome and the nail-patella syndrome. Some hereditary disorders of renal tubular function are described in Ch. 84. Other genetic disorders that may be associated with renal disease are listed in Table 89–1.

ALPORT'S SYNDROME

DEFINITION. Also known as "chronic hereditary nephritis," this syndrome is characterized by the familial occurrence in successive generations of a progressive nephritis, more severe in males, manifested invariably by hematuria and frequently associated with a sensorineural hearing deficit.

GENETICS. The mode of transmission in most kindreds is consistent with autosomal dominant inheritance with discrepant penetrance in the two sexes, males being affected earlier and more severely than females. Male and female offspring of an affected female are at equal risk (1 in 2) for inheriting this disorder, whereas male offspring of an affected male are at a greatly reduced risk (1 in 8) compared with the female (1 in 2). Autosomal recessive and sex-linked dominant inheritances also have been described in certain kindreds, suggesting that this disorder may be genetically heterogeneous.

INCIDENCE AND PREVALENCE. Several hundred kindreds of all races and geographic origins have been described. Alport's syndrome accounts for nearly 5 per cent of patients with end-stage renal disease.

PATHOLOGY AND PATHOGENESIS. Early in the disease the kidneys may be normal or large in size, but they shrink with progression of the disease. Under light microscopy the glomeruli may be normal or show some hypertrophy of epithelial cells and increase in mesangial matrix. Later changes consist of mesangial cell proliferation, thickening and splitting of glomerular and tubular basement membranes, thickening of Bowman's capsule, tubular cell atrophy, interstitial fibrosis, and the presence of foam cells. Electron microscopy characteristically reveals both thinning and irregular thickening of

TABLE 89–1. INHERITED RENAL DISEASES*

Disorders of Tubular Function
 Proximal tubule
  Cerebro-oculorenal syndrome of Lowe
  Cystinosis (Fanconi's syndrome)
  Cystinuria
  Galactosemia
  Glycogen storage (von Gierke's) disease
  Glycinuria
  Hartnup disease
  Hepatolenticular degeneration (Wilson's disease)
  Hereditary fructose intolerance
  Hypophosphatemic vitamin D–resistant rickets
  Iminoaciduria
  Proximal renal tubular acidosis
  Pseudohypoparathyroidism
  Renal glucosuria
 Distal/collecting tubule
  Distal renal tubular acidosis
  Nephrogenic diabetes insipidus
Disorders of Renal Structure
 Agenesis
 Cystic disorders
  Hepatocerebrorenal syndrome of Zellweger
  Medullary sponge kidney
  Medullary cystic disease
  Polycystic kidney disease, adult type
  Polycystic kidney disease, infantile type
  Renal retinal dysplasia
 Duplication
 Renal malformations with extrarenal anomalies
Biochemical Disorders
 Alkaptonuria
 Cystinosis
 Diabetes mellitus
 Glycosphingolipidosis (Fabry's disease)
 Hepatolenticular degeneration (Wilson's disease)
 Hyperuricemia
 Primary hyperoxaluria (oxalosis)
 Xanthine oxidase deficiency
Systemic Disorders
 Amyloidosis
 Asphyxiating thoracic dystrophy (Jeune's disease)
 Charcot-Marie-Tooth disease
 Laurence-Moon-Biedl syndrome
 Osteo-onychodysplasia (nail-patella syndrome)
Hereditary Chronic Nephropathies
 Benign recurrent hematuria
 Hereditary chronic nephritis
 Hereditary chronic nephritis with hyperprolinemia
 Hereditary chronic nephritis with thrombocytopathy
 Hereditary immune nephritis
 Infantile nephrosis

*Includes diseases that affect the kidney secondarily.

the glomerular and tubular basement membranes, with splitting of the lamina densa into several lamellae separated by lucent zones containing electron-dense round granulations.

The etiology and pathogenesis of Alport's syndrome are unknown. It has been speculated that an inherited deficiency of a collagenous or noncollagenous component of basement membrane may be responsible for thinning and rupture followed by repair and focal thickening.

CLINICAL MANIFESTATIONS. The disease is discovered in 70 per cent of patients by the age of six years, the rest of the cases being discovered at any age thereafter up to and well into adulthood. Persistent or intermittent microscopic hematuria is universally present. Gross hematuria, especially after exercise or respiratory infections, may occur in 60 per cent of affected children but rarely in adults. Proteinuria is present in 70 per cent of patients. It is usually mild but reaches the nephrotic range in 30 to 40 per cent of patients. Sensorineural hearing loss in the high-frequency (4000 to 8000 Hz) range is observed in 40 to 60 per cent of patients, predominantly males. Its detection may require audiometric testing, but it may progress to clinical deafness. Ocular disorders, especially anterior and posterior lenticonus and spherophakia, are seen in 15 per cent of patients. The renal disease may be mild and nonprogressive, especially in women, or may progress with the development of azotemia and hypertension culminating in chronic renal failure and uremia. Progression occurs predominantly in males, with a predilection to those with massive proteinuria, deafness, and lenticonus. Renal failure may occur in childhood or in adulthood, and in affected males usually before age 40 years. Affected females may experience decline of renal function during pregnancy.

In several kindreds patients with classic Alport's syndrome have been reported to have thrombocytopenia with giant platelets manifested clinically by bruising, epistaxis, and gastrointestinal bleeding, and in the laboratory by prolonged bleeding time. A few cases have also been associated with hyperprolinemia (Ch. 191).

DIAGNOSIS. The presence of progressive renal disease in one family member younger than age 50, other than the proband, and the presence of neural hearing loss in the patient or a relative form the basis for the diagnosis of Alport's syndrome in a patient with hematuria with or without proteinuria, azotemia, or hypertension. Differential diagnosis includes benign familial hematuria, a nonprogressive disorder characterized by a uniformly thin glomerular capillary basement membrane; and IgA nephropathy (Berger's disease), a glomerulonephritis with distinctive findings on light, electron, and especially immunofluorescent microscopic examination of the renal glomerulus. The audiometric findings, ocular manifestations, and family history, coupled with the changes in the glomerular and tubular basement membranes, usually should distinguish Alport's syndrome from other renal disorders.

TREATMENT. There is no specific treatment for Alport's syndrome, and no therapy is known to alter its course. Only conventional management of progressive renal disease is available. Peritoneal dialysis or hemodialysis and related or cadaveric donor kidney transplantation have been utilized with degrees of success at least matching those in other renal disorders. In fact, improvement of hearing deficit has been reported after renal transplantation. Recurrence of the renal lesion has not been observed following transplantation, but several patients have developed Goodpasture's syndrome.

NAIL-PATELLA SYNDROME

An autosomal dominant trait also known as osteo-onychodysplasia, this disorder of mesenchymal tissue is characterized by atrophic or absent fingernails, hypoplasia or aplasia of the patella, accessory conical iliac horns, thickening of the scapula, and subluxation of the radial heads at the elbow. In 40 per cent of patients the kidneys may be involved, as manifested by mild proteinuria and rarely hematuria. Occasionally the nephrotic syndrome and progression to renal failure (27 per cent) may be observed. Light microscopy shows glomerular cellular proliferation, mesangial sclerosis, and basement membrane thickening. Electron microscopy reveals areas of rarefaction in the lamina densa of the glomerular basement membrane filled with bundles of curvilinear fibrils having the typical periodicity of collagen. No specific therapy exists for this disorder. Renal transplantation has been carried out without evidence of recurrence of the disease in the transplanted organ.

Bennett WM, Musgrave ME, Campbell RA, et al.: The nephropathy of the nail-patella syndrome. Am J Med 54:304, 1973. *A good description of the renal disorder in the nail-patella syndrome.*

Gubler C, Levy M, Broyer M, et al.: Alport's syndrome. A report of 58 cases and a review of the literature. Am J Med 70:493, 1981. *An excellent review of the clinical and histologic features of Alport's syndrome in children.*

90 RENAL CALCULI

Charles Y.C. Pak

DEFINITION

Renal calculi (kidney stones, nephrolithiasis) are abnormal concretions occurring in the kidneys, consisting of crystalline components and an organic matrix. They are typically located within the calices or pelvis and may become lodged in the ureter or bladder as they are passed. Nephrolithiasis should be differentiated from nephrocalcinosis, which is calcification of renal parenchyma. Stones originating in the bladder (bladder stones) are rare in industrialized countries, although they were common in antiquity and are still frequent in certain countries in Southeast Asia.

Nephrolithiasis affects 1 to 5 per cent of the population, with a recurrence rate in afflicted individuals of 50 to 80 per cent and an annual incidence rate of 0.1 to 0.3 per cent. Calcareous (calcium-containing) renal stones account for 80 to 95 per cent of stones and are principally composed of calcium oxalate and calcium phosphate, usually occurring as mixtures. The remaining stones are composed of uric acid, cystine, magnesium ammonium phosphate (struvite), and, rarely, xanthine (Table 90–1).

ETIOLOGY AND PATHOGENESIS

Renal stones form by an initial crystallization of a nidus (termed nucleation) from a supersaturated urine with subsequent crystal growth and aggregation of the nidus into a macroscopic stone. Kidney stones are not simply masses of crystals. They usually have an organic matrix that gives form, cohesiveness, and sometimes a remarkably regular structure to the stone. At the present time, abnormalities in the amount or composition of stone matrix have not been demonstrated to be important in stone pathogenesis. It is impossible to dissolve the amounts of calcium, oxalate, and phosphate present in normal urine in 1 or 2 liters of distilled water. Obviously, therefore, there are substances present in normal urine that impede crystallization and sustain supersaturation. These normal inhibitors are not fully characterized but seem to include pyrophosphate, citrate, magnesium, and certain organic macromolecules (such as glycosaminoglycans and glycoproteins).

All patients with stones are presumed to have some physiologic derangements that make them susceptible to stone formation, although no cause can be demonstrated by current

TABLE 90–1. COMPOSITION OF RENAL STONES*

Type	Percentage
Calcium oxalate	70
Calcium phosphate	10
Hydroxyapatite	
Brushite	
Tricalcium phosphate	
Carbonate apatite	
Magnesium ammonium phosphate	5–10
Uric acid	< 5
Cystine	1
Xanthine	< 1

*Some stones occur as mixtures. Percentages are calculated for the predominant stone types.

TABLE 90–2. PATHOGENESIS OF NEPHROLITHIASIS

Cause	Percentage of Patients with Stones	Sex Predominance	Stone Composition
Hypercalciuria			
Absorptive hypercalciuria	35–50	Male	Ca oxalate, Ca phosphate
Renal hypercalciuria	5–15	Equivalent	Ca oxalate, Ca phosphate
Fasting hypercalciuria with normal PTH*	5–25	Male	Ca oxalate, Ca phosphate
Primary hyperparathyroidism	4–10	Female	Ca phosphate, Ca oxalate
Hyperoxaluria			
Primary	Rare	Equivalent	Ca oxalate
Enteric	2	Equivalent	Ca oxalate
Hyperuricosuric calcium nephrolithiasis	10 (pure) 30–50 (mixed)	Male	Ca oxalate, Ca phosphate
Hypocitraturic calcium nephrolithiasis			
Renal tubular acidosis	1–10	Equivalent	Ca phosphate, Ca oxalate
Other	10 (pure) 10–50 (mixed)	Male	Ca oxalate, Ca phosphate
Uric acid stone diathesis	3–10	Male	Uric acid, Ca oxalate, Ca phosphate
Cystinuria	1–3	Equivalent	Cystine
Infection lithiasis	< 10	Female	Struvite, carbonate apatite
Low urine volume	< 5 (pure) 10–50 (mixed)	Female	Ca oxalate
No physiologic disturbance	< 5	Female	Ca oxalate

*PTH = parathyroid hormone.

techniques in 3 per cent of patients. These derangements alter urinary concentration of stone-forming constituents and of inhibitors to cause supersaturation and facilitate crystallization (Table 90–2).

Supersaturation of crystalloids can result from (1) too little urine output (a concentrated urine), (2) an absolute increase in the amount of a stone constituent excreted over a period of time, such as calcium, oxalate, or uric acid, or (3) an alteration in urine pH. Low urinary pH (< 5.5) increases urinary saturation of uric acid, whereas high urinary pH raises that of calcium phosphate and magnesium ammonium phosphate.

Reduction in the concentration of inhibitors of crystallization in the urine may be of great importance in stone pathogenesis. Some inhibitors (such as citrate) may be directly measured in urine, providing diagnostic utility. Other inhibitors (such as glycoproteins) that are difficult to analyze can sometimes be assessed indirectly from the overall inhibitor activity against crystallization of stone-forming salts.

Other factors may be important in stone formation. (1) *Stasis*: Most embryonic stones are probably harmlessly washed out in the urine. Stasis allows time for nascent stone to grow. (2) *Heterogeneous nucleation*: Crystallization may begin in a supersaturated solution that is seeded with a crystal of a different (heterogeneous) composition but one that has an analogous surface topography. This process of one crystal growing on the surface of another is known as epitaxy. Many stones are mixed in composition and perhaps represent epitaxial growth. Of greatest practical importance, however, is the fact that calcium oxalate crystals can be nucleated by uric acid or sodium hydrogen urate crystals. This is the presumed cause of the calcium oxalate stone diathesis associated with hyperuricosuria (see below).

HYPERCALCIURIA. As noted, calcium is a constituent of 80 to 95 per cent of kidney stones. Hypercalciuria is the single most frequent abnormality found in patients with stone diathesis. Hypercalciuria is often statistically defined and varies with body size and diet. In general, the normal upper limit for urinary calcium is 300 mg per day on a diet containing 1000 mg of calcium per day (some authorities use a figure of 4 mg per kilogram per day) and 200 mg per day on a diet with a daily composition of 400 mg of calcium and 100 mEq of sodium (urinary calcium tends to parallel urinary sodium so that dietary sodium should ideally be controlled). Hypercalciuria can result from (1) enhanced absorption from dietary

sources, (2) primary renal wastage with secondary enhanced absorption, (3) excessive resorption from storage in bone, or (4) a combination of the above (Fig. 90–1). These different forms will be discussed briefly.

Absorptive hypercalciuria, the most common abnormality, is encountered in 35 to 50 per cent of patients with kidney stones. Increased absorption of dietary calcium may rarely occur from excessive ingestion of milk and other dairy products, from vitamin D excess (Ch. 245), or from the altered vitamin D metabolism associated with sarcoidosis (Ch. 69). Absorptive hypercalciuria usually refers, however, to a primary idiopathic increase in intestinal absorption of calcium. The consequent rise in serum calcium concentration tends to suppress parathyroid function (PTH ↓). Hypercalciuria ensues from the increased renal filtered load of calcium and the reduced renal tubular reabsorption of calcium associated with

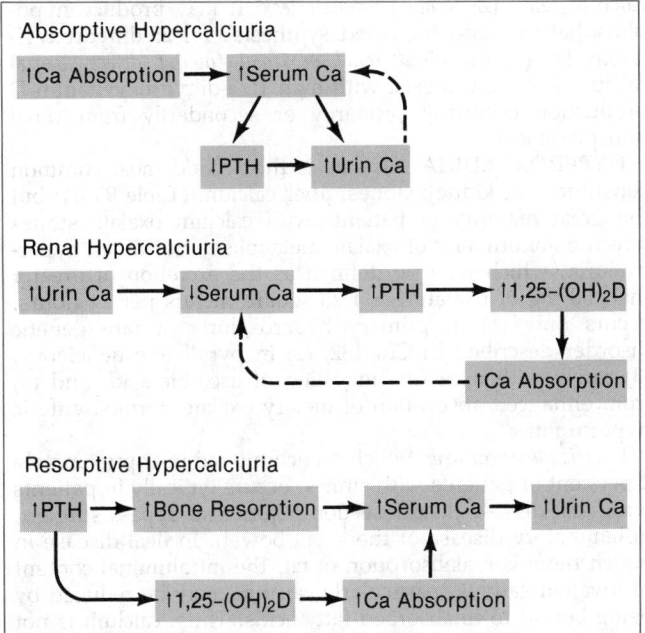

FIGURE 90–1. Pathophysiologic schemes for hypercalciuria. (After Pak CYC: Kidney stones. In Foster DW, Wilson JE [eds.]: Williams Textbook of Endocrinology. Philadelphia, W. B. Saunders Company, 1985, pp 1256–1273.

suppression of the secretion of parathyroid hormone (PTH). Serum calcium is typically maintained within the normal range because of compensatory hypercalciuria. In its usual presentation, the disorder tends to be familial and is believed to occur independently of hypophosphatemia or altered vitamin D metabolism. There is some evidence that it represents a jejunal disease characterized by a selective intestinal hyperabsorption of calcium in this intestinal segment.

Renal hypercalciuria, as a form of "idiopathic hypercalciuria," occurs less commonly than absorptive hypercalciuria and originates from an impaired renal tubular reabsorption (renal leak) of calcium. The ensuing decline in serum calcium causes secondary hyperparathyroidism, which in turn stimulates the renal synthesis of 1,25-dihydroxyvitamin D (Fig. 90–1). Thus, the skeletal mobilization and intestinal absorption of calcium may be secondarily increased, effects that restore serum calcium concentration to normal and further contribute to the hypercalciuria. The possibility that there may be a more generalized disturbance in proximal tubular function is shown by an exaggerated natriuretic response to thiazide and calciuric response to a carbohydrate load.

Resorptive hypercalciuria results from excessive bone resorption, most commonly from the hypersecretion of PTH. Four to 10 per cent of all kidney stones are caused by primary hyperparathyroidism (Table 90–2); conversely, 10 to 40 per cent of patients with primary hyperparathyroidism present with renal stones. The hypercalcemia of hyperparathyroidism causes hypercalciuria by augmenting the renal filtered load of calcium. The intestinal calcium absorption may also be increased secondarily, consequent to parathyroid hormone–dependent stimulation of the synthesis of 1,25-dihydroxyvitamin D; this increased calcium absorption further contributes to the hypercalciuria. Hypercalciuria secondary to net bone resorption is also seen in thyrotoxicosis, multiple myeloma, pseudohyperparathyroidism of malignancy, metastatic disease of bone, and immobilization (acute osteoporosis) and with spontaneous or iatrogenic Cushing's syndrome.

Fasting hypercalciuria with normal levels of serum PTH is neither absorptive hypercalciuria (because of the presence of apparent renal calcium leak) nor renal hypercalciuria (since parathyroid stimulation is lacking). This picture may result from several disturbances. (1) *Enhanced 1,25-dihydroxyvitamin D synthesis*: It may cause parathyroid suppression and an acquired renal calcium leak. (2) *Renal phosphate leak*: It may produce hypophosphatemia and increased synthesis of 1,25-dihydroxyvitamin D. (3) *Combined renal proximal tubular defect*: Renal calcium leak may coexist with high 1,25-dihydroxyvitamin D production occurring primarily or secondarily from renal phosphate leak.

HYPEROXALURIA. Oxalate is the second most common constituent of kidney stones, after calcium (Table 90–1), but the great majority of patients with calcium oxalate stones have no abnormality of oxalate metabolism. Sustained hyperoxaluria, which may be defined as the excretion of greater than 60 mg of oxalate per 1.73 square meters per 24 hours, occurs only (1) in primary hyperoxaluria, a rare genetic disorder described in Ch. 182, (2) in pyridoxine deficiency, (3) rarely with excessive ingestion of ascorbic acid, and (4) from enhanced absorption of dietary oxalate, termed enteric hyperoxaluria.

Enteric hyperoxaluria, which is encountered in approximately 2 per cent of patients with stones, occurs typically in patients with ileal disease (ileal resection, jejunoileal bypass surgery, inflammatory disease of the small bowel). In ileal disease in which there is malabsorption of fat, the intraluminal content of divalent cations, particularly calcium, may be reduced by being bound to unabsorbed fatty acids. Thus, calcium is not normally available to bind and limit oxalate absorption. The resulting enlarged free intestinal oxalate pool increases absorption and renal excretion of oxalate. Oxalate absorption may be stimulated primarily as well, especially in the colon,

since patients with ileostomies do not have hyperoxaluria. Low urine volume (from an excessive intestinal loss of fluid) and defective urinary inhibitor activity (from an impaired renal excretion of citrate and magnesium) probably contribute to calcium stone formation in ileal disease.

In hypercalciuria associated with increased calcium absorption (e.g., absorptive hypercalciuria), a mild increase in oxalate excretion to the higher ranges of normal may be found (up to 50 mg per day). The total amount of oxalate absorbed from the gut may be high because more calcium is absorbed and less calcium is available intraluminally to bind oxalate.

HYPERURICOSURIC CALCIUM OXALATE STONE DIATHESIS. Hyperuricosuria may be the only discernible biochemical abnormality associated with calcium oxalate stones (10 per cent), although it often coexists with hypercalciuria (30 to 50 per cent). Most patients with hyperuricosuric calcium oxalate nephrolithiasis do not suffer from clinical gout. The hyperuricosuria is usually dietary in origin, since a history of high purine intake may often be disclosed and normal urinary uric acid excretion values may be restored by purine restriction. Less commonly, hyperuricosuria results from a primary overproduction of uric acid. The urinary pH typically exceeds 5.5, so that dissociated urate rather than uric acid predominates. It is believed that urates facilitate crystallization of calcium oxalate, either directly by inducing heterogeneous nucleation or indirectly by removing macromolecular inhibitors through adsorption.

HYPOCITRATURIA. Citrate reduces urinary saturation of calcium salts by complexing calcium, as well as inhibits the crystallization of these salts. Thus, hypocitraturia would be expected to increase the tendency toward the formation of calcium-containing kidney stones. Hypocitraturia is encountered in any acidotic condition, such as renal tubular acidosis, chronic diarrheal states, thiazide-induced hypokalemia (which causes intracellular acidosis), and ingestion of excessive animal protein (which has a high acid-ash content). Distal (type I) renal tubular acidosis, often in an incomplete form, may first manifest with nephrolithiasis. The cause for stone formation is multifactorial and probably includes hypercalciuria (from induced renal leak of calcium by acidosis), enhanced dissociation of phosphate, an increased saturation of calcium phosphate (from high urinary pH), as well as an impaired inhibitor activity (from defective excretion of citrates). Renal tubular acidosis is described in greater detail in Ch. 84. Hypocitraturia of excessive intestinal alkali loss has been found not only in ileal disease (enteric hyperoxaluria) but also in postgastrectomy states and ulcerative colitis. Hypocitraturia should be suspected in patients with hypercalciuric nephrolithiasis who continue to form stones while on thiazide therapy. Another cause of hypocitraturia is urinary tract infection (probably from bacterial degradation of citrate). The cause for hypocitraturia often remains unknown. Hypocitraturia may occur as a sole abnormality (5 per cent) but is usually associated with other causes of nephrolithiasis (10 to 50 per cent).

URIC ACID STONES. Approximately two thirds to three fourths of the uric acid synthesized in the body is excreted in the urine. The rest is excreted in the intestine and largely destroyed by bacterial degradation. Uric acid excretion varies widely with diet. Urinary values greater than 600 mg per 1.73 square meters per 24 hours after three days of a diet moderately restricted in purine probably represent endogenous overproduction. In the study of patients with kidney stones, it is more important to measure uric acid excretion on the patient's usual diet. In this case, an excretion of more than 750 mg for women and more than 800 mg for men would be considered abnormally high.

Uric acid stones usually form in urines with a pH of less than the dissociation constant for uric acid (5.5), especially when there are absolute increases in uric acid (hyperuricosuria). Thus, the amount of urinary free uric acid is increased. Uric acid stones often occur in primary gout, which may be accompanied by low urinary pH and hyperuricosuria (Ch. 195), or in secondary causes of purine overproduction, such as myeloproliferative states, glycogen storage disease, and malignancy. Chronic diarrheal syndromes (ulcerative colitis, regional enteritis, jejunoileal bypass surgery) may cause uric acid stones by inducing net alkali deficit (thereby reducing urinary pH) and lowering urine volume (thereby augmenting urinary concentration of uric acid). Most patients with uric acid stones do not have clinical gout. Some patients with uric acid stones may also form calcium-containing stones.

CYSTINURIA. A cystine kidney stone forms only in a patient with the genetic disorder cystinuria (Ch. 84). Other forms of aminoaciduria are not associated with the excretion of enough cystine to form stones. Cystinuria is characterized by a disturbance in renal and intestinal handling of lysine, arginine, ornithine, and cystine. Stone formation, occurring in a minority of patients with cystinuria, is the result of an excessive renal excretion of cystine and its low solubility in urine. Cystine solubility is pH dependent; at pH 5, 170 to 300 mg of cystine may be dissolved in each liter of urine, whereas at pH 7.5, 220 to 500 mg of cystine may go into the solution. Many patients with homozygous cystinuria who are prone to cystine stone formation excrete more than 250 mg of cystine per day.

INFECTION. Urinary tract infections with urea-splitting organisms may be associated with renal stones of struvite (magnesium ammonium phosphate) and varying amounts of calcium phosphate. Ammonia formed by enzymatic degradation of urea by bacterial urease undergoes hydration to form ammonium and hydroxyl ions. The resulting alkalinity of urine augments dissociation of phosphate to form more triphosphate ions and reduces the solubility of struvite. Thus, the urinary environment becomes supersaturated with respect to struvite. Although struvite stones may form de novo from infection alone, they may sometimes occur as a complication of other causes of renal calculi, such as hypercalciuria. The presence of a struvite stone is presumptive evidence for concurrent or previous urinary tract infection.

MISCELLANEOUS. A minority of patients (less than 5 per cent) present with low urine volume (< 1 liter per day) without any of the previously mentioned causes. Habitual decreased drinking of fluids may have contributed to stone formation. It has been reported that oxalate exchange in peripheral red blood cells is significantly increased in patients with "idiopathic" calcium oxalate nephrolithiasis and that this disturbance may be corrected by treatment with thiazide or amiloride. The significance of this finding is uncertain, since intestinal absorption and renal excretion of oxalate (given without calcium) are normal, and urinary oxalate is not affected by thiazide in patients with absorptive or renal hypercalciuria.

RENAL STRUCTURAL ABNORMALITIES. Nephrolithiasis may also be found in association with *renal structural abnormalities*, such as ectopic kidney, polycystic kidney, and horseshoe kidney. In this situation, it is generally believed that stones, usually composed of struvite or calcium phosphate, form secondarily to urinary tract infection. Medullary sponge disease is often associated with calcareous renal calculi. There is no convincing evidence that the structural abnormality causes stone formation, since metabolic abnormalities (such as the three forms of hypercalciuria) are usually found in medullary sponge disease, in similar distribution to that of patients without this disease.

IDIOPATHIC STONE DIATHESIS. In less than 5 per cent of patients, no physiologic abnormality can be discerned. The cause for stone formation remains unknown.

CLINICAL MANIFESTATIONS

Patients with renal stones may be asymptomatic; may pass small, sandlike concretions with relatively little pain; or may experience severe symptoms from ureteral obstruction, localized trauma, or infection. Renal colic is the manifestation of ureteral spasm produced by the irritation of a stone and accompanying obstruction. Microscopic hematuria is almost invariably present; gross hematuria, even clots, may sometimes accompany renal colic. Pain may begin in the costovertebral angle or the flank and may migrate toward the groin; sometimes pain moves into, and may be most severe in, the testis or penis in the male. Pain may subside after the stone or clot has passed, but the process may take several hours, even days, if the stone is impacted or if ureteral swelling impedes migration. Women frequently report that the pain of renal colic is more severe than that of labor. Infection arising from stones may lead to fever, flank tenderness, dysuria, and frequency of urination.

DIAGNOSIS

INITIAL SCREEN. The first step in the diagnosis of the cause of a kidney stone is to secure the stone for analysis, if at all possible. The analysis should preferably be carried out by a crystallographic technique, which can sometimes reveal the sequence of stone formation from the central nidus to the periphery.

All patients with renal stones should have a carefully taken history, abdominal roentgenographic examination, urinalysis and culture, and a routine blood screen.

A positive family history of renal calculi suggests absorptive hypercalciuria or, more rarely, cystinuria, primary hyperoxaluria, or type I renal tubular acidosis. Absorptive hypercalciuria should be suspected in middle-aged white men who have a history of recurrent calcium-containing stones and a family history of renal stones. Renal hypercalciuria may be present in patients with a history of recurrent urinary tract infection, especially if the infection preceded the onset of the stone disease. A high-calcium diet may aggravate the stone disease in those with an intestinal hyperabsorption of calcium. Patients with gout may form stones of either uric acid or calcium oxalate. A history of chronic diarrhea, ileal disease, or intestinal surgery should arouse the suspicion of uric acid or calcium oxalate stones (enteric hyperoxaluria or hypocitraturic calcium nephrolithiasis). A high purine intake may cause hyperuricosuria and contribute to stone formation in hyperuricosuric calcium oxalate nephrolithiasis. Acetazolamide may impair renal acidification and cause formation of calcium phosphate stones. Excessive ingestion of vitamin D and of oxalate-rich foods (such as spinach and brewed tea) may increase oxalate excretion.

Calcium-containing stones, struvite stones, and cystine stones are radiopaque. Uric acid stones and the rarely encountered xanthine and 2,8-dihydroxyadenine stones are radiolucent (see Ch. 196). A staghorn calculus suggests a cystine or struvite stone. Positive urine culture for *Proteus, Pseudomonas, Klebsiella,* or *Staphylococcus* in association with an alkaline urine indicates that the stone is probably struvite. On a routine blood screen, primary hyperparathyroidism is suggested by hypercalcemia and hypophosphatemia (Ch. 247); gouty diathesis by hyperuricemia; and defective acidification by the electrolyte picture of hyperchloremic metabolic acidosis.

IN-DEPTH EVALUATION. The objective of in-depth evaluation, applicable particularly to those with recurrent calculi, is to discern the specific metabolic cause for the nephrolithiasis. Ideally, it should include a measure of parathyroid function (serum immunoreactive PTH); 24-hour urinary calcium (on defined diets with respect to calcium and sodium intake); 24-hour urinary calcium, oxalate, uric acid, citrate, total volume, and pH (on random diets); and a measure of renal tubular reabsorption and intestinal absorption of calcium (from urinary calcium levels during fasting and following excessive oral ingestion of calcium). Hypercalciuria should be defined with respect to the particular diet during which urinary calcium is determined as noted above. If the stone is not known to contain calcium, a qualitative test for urine cystine is indicated.

The nature of parathyroid function distinguishes the three forms of *hypercalciuria*. Primary hyperparathyroidism is suggested by parathyroid stimulation in the setting of hypercalcemia, absorptive hypercalciuria by normal or suppressed parathyroid function with normocalcemia and hypercalciuria, and renal hypercalciuria by parathyroid stimulation with normocalcemia and hypercalciuria. The fasting urinary calcium level is invariably increased in renal hypercalciuria and is frequently elevated in primary hyperparathyroidism, whereas it is typically normal in absorptive hypercalciuria. Intestinal calcium absorption is always increased in absorptive hypercalciuria and is often high in renal and resorptive hypercalciurias. Fasting hypercalciuria with normal parathyroid function is suggested by high fasting urinary calcium levels in the setting of normal levels of serum calcium and PTH.

In *enteric hyperoxaluria*, the urinary calcium level is typically low (< 100 mg per day) and the urinary oxalate level is high (often > 100 mg per day). Serum calcium and magnesium levels may be low, parathyroid function may be stimulated, metabolic acidosis may be present, and the urinary citrate level is low (< 320 mg per day). Hypocitraturia is also found in hypocitraturic calcium nephrolithiasis.

Urinary uric acid consistently exceeds 600 mg per day (and often > 750 to 800 mg per day), and pH is greater than 5.5 in *hyperuricosuric calcium oxalate nephrolithiasis*. Urinary pH is usually low (< 5.5) *in uric acid lithiasis* and high (> 7.5) in *struvite lithiasis*. Urine pH is high (> 6.9) in complete type I *renal tubular acidosis* and high normal or high (> 6) in the incomplete form.

TREATMENT

Kidney stones are heterogeneous in pathogenesis and not infrequently are manifestations of a generalized multisystem disorder. By and large, kidney stones cannot be treated medically in the sense of causing their dissolution. The goal of treatment is to stop growth or new formation of stones by correcting the specific underlying physicochemical and physiologic derangements. Stone prophylaxis often entails a prolonged program. It is particularly important, therefore, to ensure patient compliance, few complications, and reasonable costs.

GENERAL TREATMENT. The initial treatment program, applicable to all patients with renal calculi, consists of a high fluid intake to ensure a minimum urine volume of 2 liters per day. At least 3 liters of fluids should be drunk each day, distributed throughout the day. In general, any fluid (with the exception of milk and oxalate-rich tea in certain disorders to be enumerated) may be consumed. In patients with intestinal hyperabsorption of calcium, dairy products and certain calcium-rich foods should be avoided. Oxalate intake should be restricted in patients with calcium oxalate stones. An excessive dietary intake of sodium should be discouraged, since this may enhance calcium excretion. Urinary tract infection should be vigorously treated.

Activity of Stone Diathesis. As noted, as many as 5 per cent of the population may have a kidney stone at some time. Some patients, usually men, have a single calcium oxalate stone in middle life and are not subsequently affected. Clearly, it would not be wise to begin a lifetime program of pharmacologic intervention without some knowledge of the prognosis of the stone diathesis in the individual patient. In the absence of remediable disorders, such as primary hyperparathyroidism, it is often wise following a first stone episode to institute the general measures noted above and then to follow patients carefully with sequential radiographs to document whether new stones are forming or old stones are enlarging before more vigorous measures are instituted.

SPECIFIC MEDICAL TREATMENT. Specific programs may be required when the aforementioned conservative measures are ineffective in controlling stone formation and there is continued activity of stone diathesis.

Treatment of Hypercalciuria. The surgical removal of abnormal parathyroid tissue is clearly the treatment of choice for kidney stones secondary to the hypercalciuria of primary hyperparathyroidism. Following parathyroidectomy, serum 1,25-dihydroxyvitamin D levels, intestinal calcium absorption, and urinary calcium levels decline toward normal. Parathyroidectomy may also ameliorate the extrarenal manifestations of primary hyperparathyroidism, such as bone disease and peptic ulcer disease (Ch. 100). Similarly, the hypercalciuria of vitamin D excess, sarcoidosis, thyrotoxicosis, multiple myeloma, and malignancies may respond to specific therapies directed toward those systemic entities. The main problem is in the management of remaining forms of hypercalciuria. Several agents that have proved to be useful will be individually discussed.

Thiazides (and related compounds such as chlorthalidone) are unique among diuretics in their ability to augment the renal tubular reabsorption of calcium and therefore to reduce urinary calcium. At a dosage of hydrochlorothiazide of 50 mg once or twice a day, or an equivalent amount of related drugs, thiazides represent the treatment of choice for renal hypercalciuria. Thiazides correct the renal leak of calcium and thereby reverse the sequence of parathyroid hyperactivity, increased synthesis of 1,25-dihydroxyvitamin D, and enhanced absorption of intestinal calcium. The urinary saturations of calcium oxalate and calcium phosphate are reduced. Thiazides may be equally effective in the control of absorptive hypercalciuria, at least during the first two years of therapy. However, some patients may show an attenuation of the hypocalciuric response with chronic treatment. Moreover, thiazide therapy may cause hypokalemia and hypocitraturia. To overcome these problems, urinary calcium levels should be monitored, and potassium supplement (preferably as potassium citrate) should be provided.

Sodium cellulose phosphate (Calcibind) should be used only in patients with normophosphatemic absorptive hypercalciuria without bone disease in whom hypercalciuria cannot be controlled by dietary calcium restriction. When given orally, it forms a nonabsorbable complex with calcium that is then excreted in the feces. About 2.5 to 5 grams of this resin with each meal is sufficient to limit the amount of luminal calcium available for absorption and to restore normal urinary calcium levels. This reduces urinary saturation of calcium salts, particularly that of calcium phosphate, without overly stimulating parathyroid function or causing bone disease. Urinary oxalate may increase, because less calcium may be available intraluminally to complex oxalate, so that a moderate dietary restriction of oxalate is recommended. Oral magnesium supplementation should be provided, since this drug also binds magnesium. Sodium cellulose phosphate is contraindicated in primary hyperparathyroidism, in other states of excessive skeletal calcium mobilization, in renal hypercalciuria, and in states of normal intestinal calcium absorption because it tends to stimulate parathyroid function and thereby produces or aggravates bone disease.

Orthophosphates, as neutral or alkaline soluble salts of sodium or potassium or both, are potentially absorbable from the intestinal tract, unlike sodium cellulose phosphate. When given orally (at a dosage of 1.5 to 2.0 grams of phosphorus per day in divided doses), they decrease urinary calcium and increase urinary phosphate levels. They reduce urinary saturation of calcium oxalate, although they may increase that of calcium phosphate. Moreover, urinary inhibitor activity may be increased, probably consequent to the increased renal excretion of inhibitors, such as pyrophosphate and citrate.

Orthophosphates are optimally indicated in the management of renal phosphate leak because of the possibility that they may restore normal levels of serum 1,25-dihydroxyvitamin D and calcium absorption. Orthophosphates are contraindicated in moderate or severe hypercalcemia and in renal failure because of the danger of metastatic calcification and in urinary tract infection because of the danger of struvite or calcium phosphate stone formation.

Treatment of Enteric Hyperoxaluria. Oral administration of large amounts of calcium or magnesium has been recommended for the control of nephrolithiasis of enteric hyperoxaluria. Although urinary oxalate levels may decrease, the concurrent rise in urinary calcium may obviate the beneficial effect of this therapy in some patients. Cholestyramine does not generally cause a sustained reduction in oxalate excretion. A limitation of dietary oxalate intake and potassium citrate therapy (to be discussed) may be helpful in lowering oxalate and increasing citrate levels in urine, respectively. A high fluid intake is essential to overcome intestinal fluid loss.

Treatment of Hyperuricosuric Calcium Nephrolithiasis. This form of hyperuricosuria usually results from a diet high in purine precursors of uric acid. It should therefore be subject to effective dietary therapy. Unfortunately, many patients cannot or do not choose to maintain this dietary restraint. Allopurinol, 300 mg per day orally, will produce normal or subnormal levels of urinary uric acid and thereby may inhibit urate-induced crystallization of calcium oxalate.

Treatment of Hypocitraturic Calcium Nephrolithiasis. In renal tubular acidosis (distal), sodium citrate or potassium citrate (60 to 120 mEq per day in divided doses) may augment citrate excretion (see Ch. 84 for details). In the absence of renal insufficiency, potassium citrate is preferable because it could reduce urinary calcium and correct potassium deficiency. In *chronic diarrheal states,* potassium citrate in a liquid form is recommended to allow for rapid absorption (60 to 120 mEq per day). Hypocitraturia is sometimes very severe and recalcitrant to alkali therapy. In *thiazide-induced hypocitraturia,* potassium citrate (30 to 60 mEq per day in two divided doses in a slow-release tablet form) is generally sufficient to correct both hypokalemia and hypocitraturia. In other causes of hypocitraturia, a sufficient dose of potassium citrate may be provided to restore normal urinary citrate levels. The efficacy of potassium citrate is shown in Figure 90–2.

Treatment of Uric Acid Stones. In uric acid diathesis, administration of potassium citrate may increase urinary pH and create an environment in which uric acid is more soluble. Moderate amounts of alkali (40 to 60 mEq of potassium citrate per day in divided doses), sufficient to raise urinary pH to a range of 6 to 6.5, are recommended. Alkali therapy, especially at high dosages, may be complicated by the formation of calcium stones. The potassium salt rather than sodium salt of bicarbonate or citrate may be preferable in preventing this complication. If hydration and alkali therapy are ineffective, allopurinol should be used to decrease uric acid stone formation. See the discussion in Ch. 195 on gout for more details.

Treatment of Cystinuria (see Ch. 84). If a high fluid intake and alkali therapy are ineffective in reducing cystine concentration below saturation of cystine, D-*penicillamine* (2 grams per day in divided doses) may be required. This compound reduces urinary cystine content by forming a more soluble mixed disulfide with cysteine. Unfortunately, penicillamine treatment may be complicated by serious side effects, including nephrotic syndrome, dermatitis, and pancytopenia. An investigational drug, alpha-mercaptopropionylglycine, may exert similar action on cystine excretion, with apparent reduced toxicity.

Treatment of Struvite (Magnesium Ammonium Phosphate) Stones. If a longstanding effective control of infection with urea-splitting organisms can be achieved, there is some evidence that new struvite stone formation can be averted or some dissolution of existing stones may be achieved. Unfortunately, such a control is difficult to obtain with antibiotic therapy alone. It is difficult to eliminate the infection com-

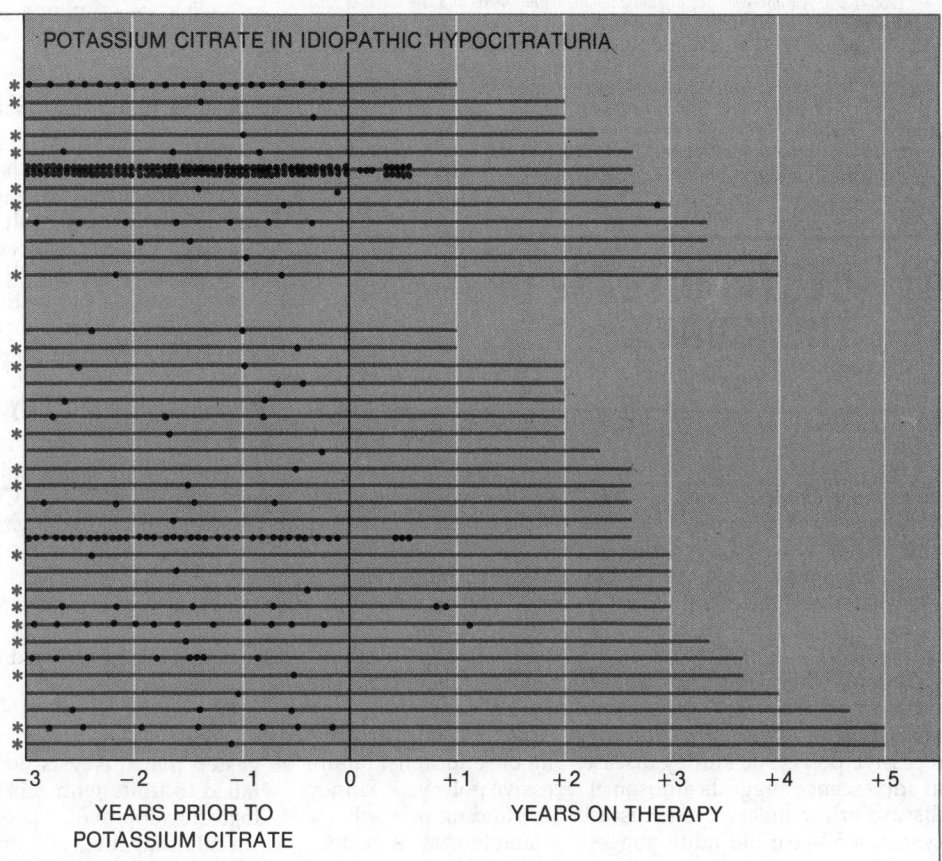

FIGURE 90–2. Effect of potassium citrate therapy on new stone formation. Each line represents one patient. An asterisk before the line indicates the presence of pre-existing stone(s). Each point shows new stone formation.

pletely from an existing struvite stone because the stone often harbors the organisms within its interstices. Even if sterilization of urine is achieved by antibiotic therapy, reinfection often occurs from harbored organisms. Addition of acetohydroxamic acid, a urease inhibitor, at a dosage of 250 mg three times per day, may be more effective in controlling struvite stone formation. If not, surgical removal of stones should be considered.

Surgical Treatment

Removal of stones may become mandatory when nephrolithiasis is complicated by obstruction, infection, gross hematuria, or intractable pain. Dramatic progress has been made in techniques for stone removal. Certain stones may now be removed less invasively via percutaneous nephroscopy and by extracorporeal shock wave lithotripsy. The latter procedure, now widely introduced in the United States, utilizes focused, electrically generated shock waves to fragment stones within a human kidney without incision. Single stones of moderate size ($\leq$ 1 cm in diameter) located in the renal pelvis are particularly amenable to this treatment. The risk of obstruction, pain, and retained fragments is higher for multiple stones and larger stones. Not all stones are amenable to shock wave lithotripsy alone (e.g., staghorn calculi and stones in lower ureter). The criteria for the choice of different methods are undergoing rapid refinement as further experience is gained with new approaches.

Coe FL: Nephrolithiasis: Pathogenesis and Treatment. Chicago, Year Book Medical Publishers, 1979. *A detailed review of current concepts of cause and treatment of calcareous as well as noncalcareous stones.*

Drach GW, Dretler S, Fair W, et al.: Report of the United States cooperative study of extracorporeal shock wave lithotripsy. J Urol 135:1127, 1986. *A review of results of extracorporeal shock wave lithotripsy among 2501 patients undergoing this procedure in the United States.*

Millman S, Strauss AL, Parks JH, et al.: Pathogenesis and clinical course of mixed calcium oxalate and uric acid nephrolithiasis. Kidney Int 22:366, 1982. *A useful review of the intriguing and important interactions of uric acid and oxalate in stone pathogenesis.*

Pak CYC: Kidney stones. In Foster DW, Wilson JD (eds.): Williams Textbook of Endocrinology. Philadelphia, W. B. Saunders Company, 1985. pp 1256–1273. *A comprehensive discussion of the pathogenesis and treatment of renal calculi.*

Pak CYC, Britton F, Peterson R, et al.: Ambulatory evaluation of nephrolithiasis: Classification, clinical presentation and diagnostic criteria. Am J Med 69:19, 1980. *A detailed description of the outpatient protocol that provides diagnostic criteria for different causes of nephrolithiasis.*

Pak CYC, Fuller C, Sakhaee K, et al.: Long term treatment of calcium nephrolithiasis with potassium citrate. J Urol 134:11, 1985. *A detailed study describing mechanism of action and utility of potassium citrate in calcium nephrolithiasis.*

91 CYSTIC DISEASE OF THE KIDNEY

Patricia A. Gabow

Renal cystic diseases are disorders characterized by the presence in the kidneys of epithelium-lined cavities filled with fluid or semisolid debris. The cysts may be single or multiple, inherited or acquired, occurring in infancy or old age, clinically silent or symptomatic, producing renal insufficiency. This discussion will focus on simple cysts, polycystic kidney disease, acquired cystic disease, and medullary cystic disorders (Table 91–1).

Certain clinical settings suggest various disorders. The presence of abdominal masses in a neonate or infant should raise the consideration of autosomal dominant or autosomal recessive polycystic kidney disease. The onset of renal failure in adolescence suggests autosomal recessive polycystic kidney disease or medullary cystic disease. The finding of a solitary cyst in a 50-year-old adult suggests a simple cyst. A history of renal disease in a family raises the possibility of autosomal dominant polycystic kidney disease or medullary cystic disease. Recurrent renal stones can occur in autosomal dominant polycystic kidney disease or with medullary sponge kidneys. The onset of gross hematuria in a patient undergoing chronic hemodialysis raises the possibility of acquired cystic disease.

SIMPLE CYSTS

Simple renal cysts, the most common and clinically least significant of all the cystic disorders, increase in frequency with age (from 0.1 to 4 per cent in children to 50 per cent in the population over 50 years of age). Often the cysts are asymptomatic and are discovered during abdominal imaging studies performed for other reasons. Occasionally patients with simple cysts present with hematuria or flank pain, thereby raising the question of malignancy within the cyst. Evaluation should begin with renal ultrasonography, which in a simple cyst will demonstrate smooth walls, good sound transmission, and no intracystic debris. If the ultrasonographic pattern differs from these characteristics, but the lesion is clearly cystic rather than solid, patients should undergo cyst puncture with ultrasonographic guidance. In this manner, cyst fluid can be obtained for cytology and for measurement of lactic dehydrogenase (LDH) and lipids, and contrast material can be injected to delineate the cyst wall architecture. This approach differentiates simple cysts from malignancy with 96 per cent or greater accuracy (Table 91–2). If the functional and structural characteristics of a cyst suggest malignancy, obviously surgery should be considered. For another discussion of renal masses, see also Ch. 93.

Kleist H, Jonsson O, Lundstam S: Quantitative lipid analysis in the differential diagnosis of cystic renal lesions. Br J Urol 54:441, 1982. *Cyst fluid analysis is discussed.*

Lang E, Johnson B, Chance HL, et al.: Assessment of avascular renal mass lesions: The use of nephrotomography, arteriography, cyst puncture, double contrast study and histochemical and histopathologic examination of the aspirate. South Med J 65:1, 1972.

Mir S, Rapola J, Koskimies O: Renal cysts in pediatric autopsy material. Nephron 33:189, 1983. *Data from autopsy material in 6521 children are presented.*

Zeman RK, Cronan JJ, Rosenfield AT, et al.: Imaging approach to suspected renal mass. Radiol Clin North Am 23:503, 1985. *A comprehensive review of the subject.*

POLYCYSTIC KIDNEY DISEASE

Polycystic kidney disease includes autosomal dominant polycystic kidney disease (ADPKD) and autosomal recessive polycystic kidney disease (ARPKD). These disorders were previously labeled adult polycystic kidney disease and infantile or childhood polycystic kidney disease, respectively. It is now clear, however, that pattern of inheritance rather than age of onset is the distinguishing characteristic. ADPKD not uncommonly is manifested in childhood and even occasionally in infancy or in utero.

Autosomal Dominant Polycystic Kidney Disease (ADPKD)

ADPKD, inherited in an autosomal dominant pattern, is primarily characterized by cyst development and growth of cysts in the kidneys. Cyst formation or outpouchings may also occur in other organs, particularly in the liver, but also in the pancreas, ovaries, gastrointestinal tract, and vascular tree. ADPKD has a worldwide occurrence with 1/200 to 1/1000 people affected. A gene for ADPKD is carried on chromosome 16, but the gene product is not known. Complete penetrance of the gene is estimated to occur by the time the individual is 90 years of age.

PATHOGENESIS AND PATHOLOGY. The pathogenesis of ADPKD has not been established. An early theory suggested that the cysts were "dead ends" of renal tubules that failed to unite with other nephron segments during embryologic development. Microdissection of renal tubules, however, reveals that the cysts are outpouchings occurring at various

TABLE 91–1. CHARACTERISTICS OF RENAL CYSTIC DISORDERS

Feature	Simple Cysts	ADPKD	ARPKD	ACKD	MCD	MSK
Inheritance pattern	None	Autosomal dominant	Autosomal recessive	None	Often present, variable pattern	None
Prevalence	Common, increasing with age	1/400 to 1/1000	Rare	40% in dialysis patients	Rare	Common
Age of Onset	Adult	Usually adults	Neonates, children	Older adults	Adolescents, young adults	Adults
Presenting symptom	Incidental finding: hematuria	Pain, hematuria, infection, family screening	Abdominal mass, renal failure, failure to thrive	Hematuria	Polyuria, polydipsia, enuresis, renal failure, failure to thrive	Incidental, urinary tract infections, hematuria, renal calculi
Hematuria	Occurs	Common	Occurs	Occurs	Rare	Common
Recurrent infections	Rare	Common	Occurs	No	Rare	Common
Renal calculi	No	Common	No	No	No	Common
Hypertension	Rare	Common	Common	Present from underlying disease	Rare	No
Method of diagnosis	Ultrasound	Ultrasound	Ultrasound	CT scan	None reliable	Excretory urogram
Renal size	Normal	Normal to very large	Large initially	Small to normal, occasionally large	Small	Normal

ADPKD = Autosomal dominant polycystic kidney disease; ARPKD = autosomal recessive polycystic kidney disease; ACKD = acquired cystic kidney disease; MCD = medullary cystic disease; MSK = medullary sponge kidney.

points along intact nephrons. Cyst puncture and cyst fluid analysis demonstrate transport characteristics compatible with various nephron segments. For example, some cysts have sodium concentrations similar to that of plasma, whereas others have low sodium concentrations, suggesting that the cysts are of proximal and distal tubular origin, respectively. Exposure to an environmental toxin or bacterial product in a susceptible individual has been postulated with no direct evidence. By electron microscopy polypoid lesions have been noted throughout the cyst walls in both experimental cystic disease and human ADPKD. These polyps have been envisioned as obstructing tubules with retrograde tubular bulging or cyst formation, but this theory fails to explain the extrarenal cysts. In addition, obstructive uropathy does not produce cystic renal changes. The observation of polyp formation suggests that ADPKD is a disorder of altered cell growth. Cell proliferation must occur to provide for the epithelial lining of the renal cysts. The basement membrane has been noted to be abnormally split in ADPKD, suggesting that it is intrinsically abnormal. The concept that ADPKD is a disorder of extracellular matrix formation, i.e., basement membrane and other collagen types, offers the best current pathogenetic explanation for the extrarenal manifestations. The genetic defect may result in both altered cell growth and abnormal matrix formation because of the close inter-relationship of cell growth and cell supporting structure. In fact, cell cultures from cysts of patients with ADPKD demonstrate both altered cell growth and abnormal basement membrane structure.

Kidneys in ADPKD can be normal in size with few cysts, particularly early in the course of the disorder. Ultimately, the kidneys enlarge and may attain the size of a football, weighing as much as 8 kg. The end-stage kidney appears to be virtually replaced by cysts (Fig. 91–1). The cysts can contain clear fluid, purulent-appearing fluid, or blood. The cut surface

TABLE 91–2. DIFFERENTIATING CHARACTERISTICS OF BENIGN AND MALIGNANT CYSTS

Feature	Benign	Malignant
Color of fluid	Straw color	Turbid or reddish
Cytology of fluid	Normal	Atypical or malignant cells
LDH of fluid	Low	High
Mean total lipid of fluid (mmol/liter)	0.3	13.2
Mean cholesterol of fluid (mmol/liter)	0.18	8.5
Cyst wall	Smooth	Irregular

LDH = Lactate dehydrogenase.

of the kidney reveals cysts throughout the renal parenchyma (Fig. 91–2).

CLINICAL MANIFESTATIONS. Individuals usually present for screening either because of a family history of the disease or because of symptoms. *Pain* and *hematuria* are the most common clinical manifestations. Flank pain and back pain are more common than abdominal pain. The pain can be constant or intermittent, mild or severe and disabling. Both microscopic and gross hematuria occur. One third of patients will have microscopic hematuria on a random urinalysis. Episodes of hematuria occur in about 30 per cent of patients and are often precipitated by trauma or strenuous exercise. Headaches, gastrointestinal complaints, nocturia, frequency, and polyuria are other presenting symptoms. Some patients also present with renal complications of ADPKD, such as urinary tract infections, renal calculi, or retroperitoneal bleeding.

The extrarenal manifestations of ADPKD are summarized in Table 91–3. The most common extrarenal involvement in ADPKD is that of hepatic cysts, which occur in 40 per cent to 60 per cent of patients. As with renal cysts, hepatic cysts appear to increase in number or size, or both, over time and can eventuate in massive hepatomegaly, but they rarely produce functional impairment. However, hepatic cysts can become infected. Colonic diverticulosis, often resulting in perforation and intra-abdominal abscess formation, has been reported in 83 per cent of patients with ADPKD undergoing chronic hemodialysis treatment, compared with a prevalence of 32 per cent in dialysis patients with other renal disease. Both hiatal and inguinal hernias may be more frequent in

TABLE 91–3. SYSTEMIC INVOLVEMENT IN AUTOSOMAL DOMINANT POLYCYSTIC KIDNEY DISEASE (ADPKD)

I. Genitourinary
    Polycystic kidney
    Hypernephroma
    Renal calculi
    Ovarian cyst (?)
II. Gastrointestinal
    Hepatic cysts
    Pancreatic cysts
    Diverticuli
III. Cardiovascular
    Hypertension
    Cardiac valvular abnormalities
    Berry aneurysms
    Thoracic aortic aneurysms
IV. Hematopoietic
    Erythrocytosis

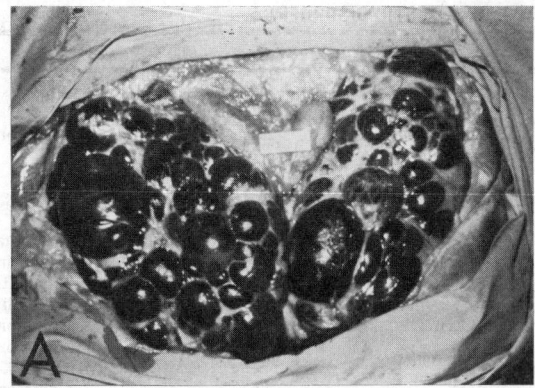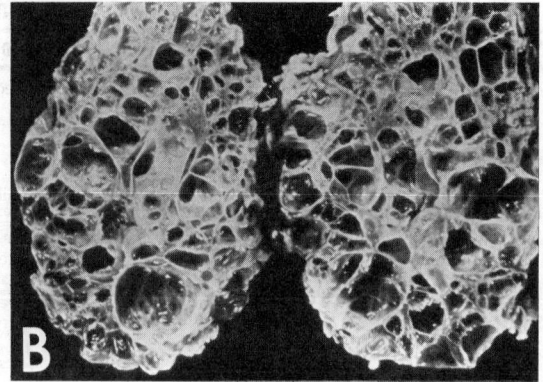

FIGURE 91–1. Autosomal dominant polycystic kidney disease (ADPKD) in situ (*A*) and on cut section (*B*). Note diffuse, bilateral distribution of cysts. (Courtesy of F. E. Cuppage, Kansas City, KS.)

patients with ADPKD. An occasional patient will also demonstrate pancreatic cysts.

Hypertension, the most common cardiovascular manifestation of ADPKD, occurs in 60 per cent of patients before the onset of renal insufficiency. The hypertension does not appear to be related to the renin-angiotensin system. *Berry aneurysms* occur in 10 per cent to 40 per cent of patients with ADPKD; it is not clear what percentage of these actually rupture. No known clinical factors predict which patients with ADPKD are at high risk for rupture. Rarely a subarachnoid hemorrhage is the presenting manifestation of ADPKD. Thoracic aortic aneurysms and cardiac valvular abnormalities (especially aortic and mitral valve involvement, occasionally with myxomatous degeneration) also seem to be increased in prevalence.

Ovarian cysts occur in ADPKD, but the relationship of this common abnormality to the genetic defect is not known. Occasionally patients with ADPKD demonstrate erythrocytosis. This is presumed to reflect increased erythropoietin production by the cystic kidney.

The incidence of bilateral renal malignancy appears to be higher in patients with ADPKD than in the general population. A person with this malignancy may present with asymmetric renal enlargment, increasing frequency or amount of hematuria, and weight loss, but the presence of these symptoms in the absence of malignancy, and the underlying structural abnormalities in the kidney, often make the diagnosis of renal malignancy difficult.

The natural history of renal functional impairment with ADPKD is variable. Renal failure may occur as early as the first decade of life in children with early symptomatic disease, or renal function may be well maintained into the eighth decade. End-stage renal disease rarely occurs before 40 years of age. Approximately 50 per cent of patients have well-preserved renal function at 70 years of age. Renal function is less well maintained in ADPKD patients with hypertension. Other factors that influence long-term prognosis are less well defined.

DIAGNOSIS. The diagnosis of ADPKD depends upon the demonstration of the characteristic bilateral renal cystic involvement, now best established by renal ultrasonography. Not infrequently, screening studies of families will demonstrate only a few unilateral cysts or only one or two cysts in each kidney. This situation requires differentiation of ADPKD from multiple simple cysts (Table 91–4). The patient's age and the presence of extrarenal involvement are most helpful in this instance (Fig. 91–3). Since simple cysts are uncommon in

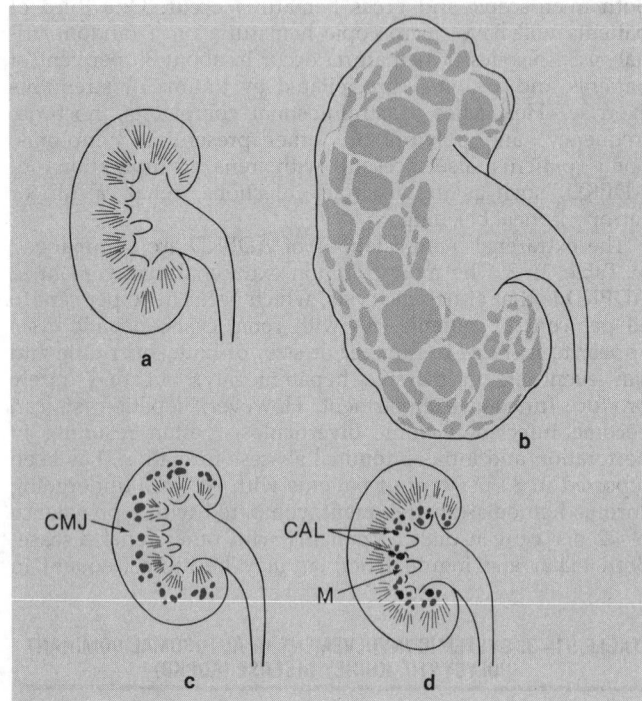

FIGURE 91–2. Schematic drawings of a cut section of (*a*) a normal kidney, measuring 12 cm with normal papilla, cortex, medulla, and corticomedullary junction and (*b*) a kidney from a patient with ADPKD. The kidney is large, measuring 29 cm, and contains cysts throughout the cortex and medulla which vary in size from 1 mm to 5 cm. *c*, A kidney from a patient with medullary cystic disease. The kidney is small, measuring 8 cm, with a scarred surface. The cysts are at the corticomedullary junction (CMJ) and are small, measuring 1 to 5 mm across. *d*, A kidney from a patient with medullary sponge kidney. There are multiple ductal dilatations measuring 1 to 5 mm in diameter, giving the medulla (M) a porous appearance. Some dilatations contain calculi (CAL). (*c* and *d* adapted from Spence HM, Singleton R: What is sponge kidney disease and where does it fit in the spectrum of cystic disorders? J Urol 107:176, 1972.)

TABLE 91–4. COMPARISON OF MULTIPLE SIMPLE CYSTS AND EARLY ADPKD

Feature	Multiple Simple Cysts	ADPKD
Family history	No	≈ 60%
Ultrasonographically demonstrable cysts in other family member(s)	No	≈ 90%
Sex distribution	M > F	M = F
Renal size	Normal	Normal to mildly enlarged
Kidneys involved	Usually unilateral, may be bilateral	Usually bilateral, may be unilateral early
Cyst distribution	Cortical	Cortical and medullary
Cyst size	Usually < 2 cm, occasionally larger	< 2 cm early
Blood in cysts	Rare	Common
Hepatic cysts	No	40–60%; likelihood increases with age
Berry aneurysm	No	10–40%
Hypertension	Rare	60%

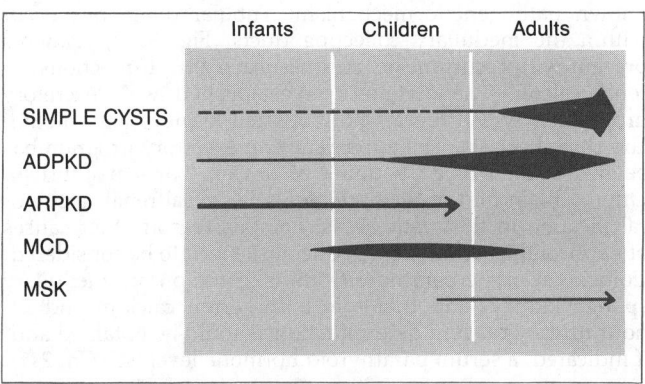

FIGURE 91–3. Ages of renal cystic disease.

children, the finding of any cysts in a child in a family with ADPKD strongly suggests the disorder. In an individual over age 50 with similar ultrasonographic findings, however, the diagnosis is much less certain. The presence of extrarenal involvement, particularly hepatic cysts, lends support to the diagnosis of ADPKD. In the absence of extrarenal involvement, which is often absent early in the course of the disease, the best method of establishing a diagnosis in a patient with only unilateral cysts or very few cysts is follow-up abdominal ultrasonography in two to three years. If renal cystic involvement increases or if extrarenal involvement occurs, the diagnosis of ADPKD can be made. If there is a need for more immediate definitive diagnosis, computerized axial tomography will occasionally reveal more diffuse cystic involvement than is apparent by ultrasonography. The role of magnetic resonance imaging remains to be defined. The finding of a gene linkage with a gene for ADPKD on chromosome 16 opens the possibility in the near future for definitive diagnosis of the gene carrier state prior to the development of gross structural abnormalities.

It is not important to establish the presence of extrarenal involvement in all patients with ADPKD. Currently, routine total abdominal ultrasonography for diagnosis of hepatic, pancreatic, or ovarian cysts is not recommended. Moreover, routine carotid angiography or computerized axial tomography of the head in search of a berry aneurysm is not recommended in asymptomatic patients with ADPKD. Echocardiography need not be performed routinely to assess valvular disease.

TREATMENT. The treatment for patients with ADPKD is generally aimed at preventing complications of the disease and at preserving renal function. First, patients and family members should be educated about the inheritance and manifestations of the disease. Patients with large kidneys should be cautioned about risks of contact sports, since significant renal trauma seems to occur more frequently in structurally abnormal kidneys. Episodes of gross hematuria should be managed conservatively with bed rest, analgesics, and hydration. Urinary tract instrumentation, including Foley catheter placement, should be avoided because of the increased risk of serious urinary tract and renal cyst infections in patients after such instrumentation. Patients suspected of having a urinary tract infection should have urine and blood cultures obtained. Selection of appropriate antibiotic therapy depends on the presumed site of infection. Bladder and renal parenchymal infections can be treated as they are treated in other patients. Failure to respond to appropriate antibiotic treatment suggests cyst infections. In this instance the antibiotic chosen must be one that has been shown to enter cyst fluid. These include chloramphenicol and trimethoprim-sulfamethoxazole.

Hypertension should be aggressively treated. The roles for restriction of phosphorus or protein, or both, or for cyst puncture in the preservation of renal function have not yet been established in ADPKD. Patients should have their blood pressures monitored. A serum creatinine level should be obtained yearly prior to the development of renal insufficiency and at least every six months thereafter. Repeat imaging studies need not be performed unless new clinical symptoms occur. Computerized axial tomography is the method of choice for establishing the diagnosis of complications such as intracystic or retroperitoneal hemorrhage, renal calculi, or renal malignancy. A more general discussion of the treatment of renal failure is found in Ch. 80.

Bach JF, Crosnier J, Funck-Brentano JL, et al.: Liver changes and complications in adult polycystic kidney disease. In Grunfeld (ed.): Advances in Nephrology, Vol. 14. Chicago, Year Book Medical Publishers, 1985, pp 1–20.

Gabow PA, Ikle DW, Holmes JH: Polycystic kidney disease: Prospective analysis of nonazotemic patients and family members. Ann Intern Med 101:238, 1984. *A comprehensive presentation of symptoms, signs, and ultrasonography in a large, young, nonazotemic patient population.*

Grantham JJ, Gardner KD Jr (eds): Polycystic Kidney Disease. Proceedings of the First International Symposium on ADPKD. Kansas City, MO, PKR Foundation, 1985. *Contains many interesting discussions on all aspects of ADPKD.*

Schwab SJ, Bander SJ, Klahr S: Renal infection in autosomal dominant polycystic kidney disease. Am J Med 82:714, 1987.

Welling LW, Grantham JJ: Cystic and developmental diseases of the kidney. In Brenner BM, Rector FC Jr. (eds.): The Kidney. 3rd ed. Philadelphia, W. B. Saunders Company, 1986, pp 1341–1376. *An admirable summary of all cystic disorders in the kidney, with 279 references.*

Wilson PD, Schrier RW, Breckon RD, et al.: A new method for studying human polycystic kidney disease epithelia in culture. Kidney Int 30:371, 1986.

Autosomal Recessive Polycystic Kidney Disease (ARPKD)

Autosomal recessive polycystic kidney disease (ARPKD) is a rare disorder that has been classified into perinatal, neonatal, infantile, or juvenile types based on age of onset. The presenting manifestations include abdominal masses, failure to thrive, and urinary tract infections. The pathogenetic mechanism is not understood. The kidneys are large early in life and may diminish in size with time. The cut surface of the kidney reveals radially oriented fusiform cysts. As in ADPKD, ultrasonography is the diagnostic method of choice. Examination of the parents and, in some instances, liver biopsy of the affected child are necessary to distinguish ARPKD from the childhood presentation of ADPKD. Normal findings on renal ultrasonography in the parents strongly suggest ARPKD. In addition, children with ARPKD, particularly the juvenile form, often have hepatic involvement with hepatic fibrosis, frequently resulting in portal hypertension. Children with ARPKD usually progress to end-stage chronic renal failure before adolescence; in the perinatal form, this occurs within the first few weeks of life. Treatment of the chronic renal failure of ARPKD is similar to that of other childhood renal insufficiency.

Blyth H, Ockenden BG: Polycystic disease of kidneys and liver presenting in childhood. J Med Genet 8:257, 1971. *A discussion of classification of this disorder.*

ACQUIRED CYSTIC KIDNEY DISEASE (ACKD)

Acquired cystic disease refers to the development of cysts in previously noncystic kidneys in patients with end-stage renal disease, almost exclusively in those undergoing dialysis. Forty per cent of patients undergoing chronic dialysis appear to develop this disorder. Most patients have no symptoms attributable to this complication, but some patients develop hematuria, and about 16 per cent of ACKD patients develop renal tumors. Unlike ADPKD or ARPKD, computerized axial tomography is the diagnostic method of choice in ACKD because the kidneys are often small and prone to malignancy. Episodes of hematuria can be treated as in ADPKD. Severe, recurrent hematuria can be treated with renal arterial embolization, as it is not critical to preserve renal parenchyma in dialysis patients. Renal tumors less than 3 cm can be followed with yearly computerized axial tomography; larger tumors require surgery because of their greater propensity for malignancy.

Gehrig JJ Jr, Gottheiner TI, Swenson RS: Acquired cystic disease of end-stage kidney. Am J Med 79:609, 1985. *Excellent review of clinical and pathologic data.*

Levine E, Grantham JJ, Slusher SL, et al.: CT of acquired cystic kidney disease and renal tumors in long-term dialysis patients. Am J Roentgenol 142:125, 1984. *Role of computerized tomography (CT) in assessing ACKD is fully discussed and documented.*

MEDULLARY CYSTIC DISORDERS

Medullary cystic disease and medullary sponge kidney are the most common of the medullary cystic disorders. Medullary cystic disease has also been labeled nephronophthisis, cystic medullary complex, and renal-retinal dysplasia (because of the coincidence of retinitis pigmentosa in some families). Medullary cystic disease is uncommon; only about 300 cases have been reported. A familial pattern appears to be present in a majority of cases. Both autosomal recessive and autosomal dominant patterns of inheritance have been reported. Recessive transmission may occur more often in the childhood presentation of the disease and dominant inheritance more commonly in the adult presentation of the disorder.

PATHOGENESIS AND PATHOLOGY. No pathogenetic theory has been proposed for this disorder. The kidneys are small and generally display some cysts at the corticomedullary junction and in the medulla (Fig. 91–2). An acystic form of the disorder appears to occur. The glomeruli are hyalinized, and the tubules vary in appearance, some being atrophic and others being tortuous. The tubular basement membrane is often irregular with areas that are thickened and others that are thinned and split. The interstitium reveals fibrosis and mononuclear cell infiltrate. This interstitial involvement suggests some as yet undefined relationship with other immune and nonimmune tubulointerstitial disease. It has been postulated that medullary cystic disease may be the end-stage form of other tubulointerstitial disease.

CLINICAL MANIFESTATIONS. A majority of patients present in childhood or early adolescence with polydipsia, polyuria, and enuresis. Often the children demonstrate growth retardation and anemia. The polyuria and enuresis with secondary polydipsia are presumed to reflect a defect in urinary concentrating ability, which apparently occurs early in the disease.

Renal salt wasting has also been suggested to occur in the disorder to a degree in excess of the impaired sodium conservation that accompanies any end-stage renal disease. Certainly the possibility of salt wasting should be considered in a patient with this disorder prior to sodium restriction.

DIAGNOSIS. Diagnosis of the disorder is often difficult. The urinalysis is often unremarkable, and proteinuria is generally minimal. Imaging studies reveal only small end-stage kidneys. Some patients are simply labeled as having "chronic renal failure" or "chronic pyelonephritis." The disorder should be considered in children or young adults who present with renal insufficiency, small kidneys, and a family history of renal disease. No specific treatment exists. Management is the same as that appropriate for any child with renal insufficiency, with attention to growth, bone disease, and, in particular, sodium balance. The possibility of retinal abnormality must also be considered in initial evaluation.

Avasthi PS, Erickson DG, Gardner KD: Hereditary renal-retinal dysplasia and the medullary cystic disease–nephronophthisis complex. Ann Intern Med 84:157, 1976. *The association is described, and the inheritance of medullary cystic disease is described.*

Chamberlin BC, Hagge WW, Stickler GB: Juvenile nephronophthisis and medullary cystic disease. Mayo Clin Proc 52:485, 1977. *Six cases are presented, and literature is reviewed.*

Helczynski L, Landing BH: Tubulointerstitial renal diseases of children: Pathologic features and pathogenetic mechanisms in Fanconi's familial nephronophthisis, antitubular basement membrane antibody disease, and medullary cyst disease. Pediatr Pathol 2:1, 1984.

Steele BT, Lirenman DS, Beattie CU: Nephronophthisis. Am J Med 68:531, 1980. *The clinical data and follow-up information on 21 patients are presented.*

MEDULLARY SPONGE KIDNEY

Medullary sponge kidney is a relatively common disorder affecting between 1/5000 and 1/20,000 individuals. There is no known pathogenetic mechanism. Tubular dilatations occur within the medullary collecting ducts (Fig. 91–2). Patients present with recurrent hematuria, urinary tract infections, or renal calculi. The diagnosis is established with excretory urography, which reveals normal-sized kidneys with medullary ductal ectasia. The appearance on excretory urogram has been described as a "bouquet of flowers" or a paintbrush. Often a plain film of the abdomen will reveal renal calculi or calcification in the cystic areas. For this reason other causes of nephrolithiasis and nephrocalcinosis need to be considered. Coincident hyperparathyroidism is common in medullary sponge kidney, and therefore both serum calcium and 24-hour urinary calcium determinations should be obtained and, if indicated, a serum parathyroid hormone level (see Ch. 247). Conversely, as many as 20 per cent of patients presenting with nephrolithiasis may have medullary sponge kidney. Other clinical manifestations of medullary sponge kidney reflect the structural alterations in the renal papillae that occur in the disease and include a decreased renal concentrating ability, an inability to acidify the urine maximally with an incomplete renal tubular acidosis and an impairment in renal potassium excretion in response to acute potassium loading. However, despite these defects, serum electrolyte concentrations are almost always normal. Treatment includes appropriate management of renal infections and of renal calculous disease (Ch. 86 and 90). Urinary tract obstruction must be considered during acute episodes of renal colic. In the absence of obstruction, renal function remains normal.

Green J, Szylman P, Sznajder II, et al.: Renal tubular handling of potassium in patients with medullary sponge kidney. Arch Intern Med 144:2201, 1984. *Presentation of renal tubular defects in medullary sponge kidney.*

Morris RC, Yamaughi H, Palubinskas AJ, et al.: Medullary sponge kidney. Am J Med 38:883, 1965. *Twenty patients with medullary sponge kidney and some related abnormalities are discussed.*

Parks JH, Coe FL, Strauss AL: Calcium nephrolithiasis and medullary sponge kidney in women. N Engl J Med 306:1088, 1982.

Zawada ET Jr, Sica DA: Differential diagnosis of medullary sponge kidney. South Med J 77:686, 1984. *Differential diagnosis—a case report with excretory urography.*

92 ANOMALIES OF THE URINARY TRACT

Richard D. Williams

Congenital aberrations of the urinary tract occur in over 10 per cent of the population. They vary in severity from lesions incompatible with life to those that are insignificant and detected only incidentally during studies prompted by unrelated causes. Often the anomalies, although not intrinsically detrimental, predispose to infection, lithiasis, and chronic renal failure, which lead to their recognition.

KIDNEY

ANOMALIES OF NUMBER. *Bilateral renal agenesis* is rare (1 in 4800 births), more frequent in males (3 to 1 ratio), and typically accompanied by oligohydramnios, Potter's facies, and pulmonary hypoplasia; this complex results in death within a few days of birth. *Unilateral renal agenesis* is more common (1 in 1100 births), generally involves the left kidney, and is seen more often in males (ratio 1.8 to 1). Renal absence is considered secondary to lack of a ureteral bud. Occasionally, a presumptive diagnosis of unilateral renal absence may be made in males when an ipsilateral vas deferens is absent on palpation. In only 10 per cent of renal agenesis cases is the adrenal absent. Extrarenal tissue or *supernumerary kidneys* are extremely rare (only 60 cases have been described); they are distinct from ureteral and caliceal duplication to be described later.

ANOMALIES OF POSITION (ECTOPIA). These are due to abnormal renal ascent: They include lumbar and pelvic and the less common thoracic or crossed ectopic varieties (Fig. 92–1). As a group they occur in 1 in 900 cases and reach clinical significance only when they are mistaken for tumor during exploratory surgery or because of associated genital anomalies. Anomalies of fusion fall into this same category, since the abnormality leads to lack of ascent; *fused pelvic kidneys* or *horseshoe kidneys* (typically fused at their lower poles) are prevented from normal ascent by the inferior mesenteric artery (Fig. 92–2). These latter two anomalies are associated with recurrent infection and calculi in 10 to 20 per cent of patients and with a high incidence of ureteropelvic junction obstruction. *Nephroptosis* is the descent toward the pelvis of a normally ascended kidney when the upright posture is assumed; it is seen in adults and is perhaps due to poor renal fixation in the retroperitoneum. This condition, which is not an anomaly per se, is usually asymptomatic and rarely, if ever, needs surgical correction. Anomalies of rotation, commonly termed *malrotation,* are due to incomplete ventromedial rotation during ascent and are rarely related to any functional abnormality.

ANOMALIES OF THE RENAL PARENCHYMA. There is a heterogeneous group of cystic and dysplastic lesions of the kidney. The most important group of disorders comprises those that produce cystic abnormalities, described in detail in Ch. 91. *Renal dysplasia* occurs in several forms: (1) *Multicystic kidneys* are malformed, nonfunctioning, generally unilateral, and invariably associated with ipsilateral ureteral atresia. When both kidneys are involved the manifestations and prognosis are similar to those in patients with bilateral renal agenesis. (2) *Segmental dysplasia* or *hypoplasia* is rare; it is not usually associated with significant renal complications, except in the bilateral and generalized form. (3) *Total renal dysplasia* is associated with lower urinary tract obstruction such as *posterior urethral valves* or functional bladder outlet obstruction, as in the "prune-belly" syndrome.

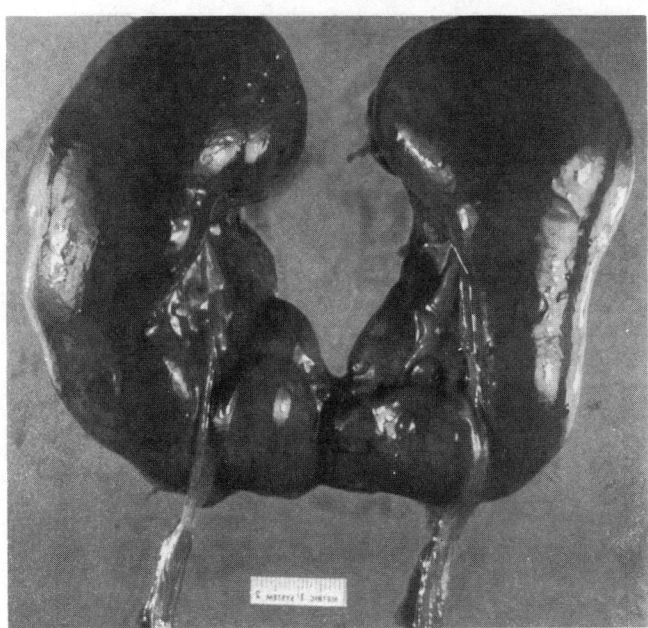

FIGURE 92–2. Gross pathologic specimen of horseshoe kidneys.

RENAL VASCULATURE

Multiple renal arteries occur in 15 to 20 per cent of the population. They are of little significance, except when they are inadvertently injured during an operation or (rarely) when they cause caliceal infundibular obstruction or (more often) *ureteropelvic junction obstruction. Congenital renal artery aneurysms* are infrequent; they are differentiated from acquired lesions by their location at the bifurcation of the main renal artery or at a distal branch point. The lesions require surgical treatment only if resulting hypertension is uncontrolled or if they are calcified and/or have a diameter of more than 2.5 cm. *Congenital arteriovenous fistulas* are rare but may result in hematuria, hypertension, and/or cardiac failure (if large), necessitating surgical intervention.

COLLECTING STRUCTURES AND URETER

Caliceal anomalies include *diverticuli, hydrocalycosis, megacalycosis,* and *infundibular stenosis.* They are clinically important only when urinary stasis results in recurrent infection and/or stone formation. *Ureteropelvic junction obstruction* is one of the more frequent causes of hydronephrosis in childhood (Fig. 92–3). Bilaterality is not unusual and the condition is often asymptomatic; however, flank pain (particularly following diuresis), urinary infection, and gross hematuria (following minor trauma) are frequent findings on presentation. Relief of symptoms as a rule follows surgical repair (pyeloplasty), although normalization of the radiologic abnormality is infrequent.

Ureteral duplication is the most common ureteral anomaly; it may be incomplete, with the duplicated ureters combining to form only one entrance per side into the bladder, or complete, with two or more ureters coursing toward the bladder on one or both sides. Most often all completely duplicated ureters enter the bladder. The ureter from the upper pole is always placed inferior in the bladder to that of the lower pole and often drains in an ectopic site, such as the bladder neck, prostate, or seminal vesicle in the male or midurethra in the female. The ureter from the lower pole often obtains poor implantation within the bladder, which may result in vesicoureteral reflux and possibly recurrent infection and hydroureteronephrosis. Ureteral ectopia can also occur in the absence of duplication but results in similar sequelae.

Ureteral reflux may be unrelated to duplication but due to an abnormal implantation of the ureter into the bladder with a resulting poorly developed trigone and deficient lower

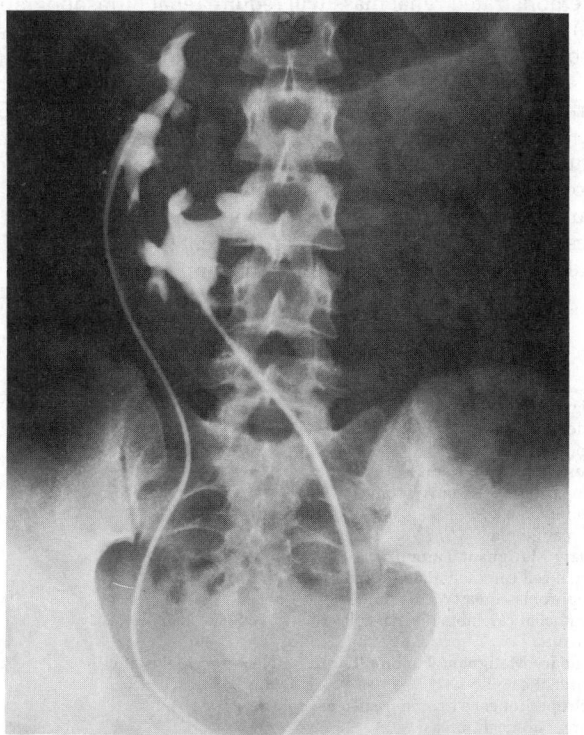

FIGURE 92–1. Bilateral retrograde ureteropyelogram of crossed renal ectopia.

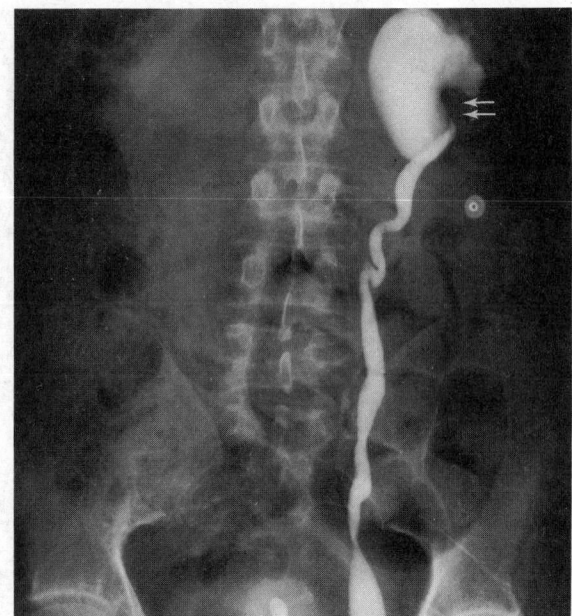

FIGURE 92–3. Retrograde ureteropyelogram showing ureteropelvic junction obstruction due to an aberrant lower pole renal artery (*arrows*).

ureteral muscle. This condition can cause recurrent urinary infection in children; however, surgical reimplantation is necessary only in severe cases. Other ureteral anomalies include *ureterocele*, a congenital distal ureteral meatal stenosis; *megaloureter*, an abnormality of the ureteral musculature allowing massive ureteral dilatation, often without caliceal distortion; *ureteral valves*; *ureteral diverticuli*; and *retrocaval ureter*, an anomaly of the formation of the vena cava causing the ureter to course behind the cava.

BLADDER

Anomalies of the bladder are very infrequent and include (1) *complete absence* (agenesis), which results in a persistent cloaca; (2) *duplication*, which may be complete with separate ureteral openings drained by separate urethras, or incomplete with a septum or hour-glass deformity; (3) *urachal* anomalies, which may appear as a patent connection to the umbilicus, a *diverticulum* at the dome of the bladder, or a *urachal cyst* along the course of the partially obliterated urachus; and (4) *exstrophy*, which is the most common severe anomaly of the bladder. Exstrophy represents a midline defect in closure of the bladder wall, lower abdominal muscles, pubic bones, and anterior urethra (*epispadias*). The "prune-belly" syndrome is a complex anomaly in which absence of the abdominal muscles is associated with bilateral cryptorchidism, ureteral dilatation and reflux, and an irregular capacious bladder with a dilated proximal urethra.

URETHRA

Hypospadias is the most common urethral anomaly in males (1 in 300 live births). The lesion results from failure of ventral fusion of the urogenital folds. It may present as a ventrally displaced meatus on the distal penile shaft or, in more severe forms, with the meatus opening more proximal on the shaft or in the perineum. These latter forms are often associated with a ventral penile chordee. Isolated *epispadias* (failure of dorsal closure of the urethra) occurs in males or females and is usually associated with incontinence. Congenital *urethral strictures* are infrequent. Although *meatal stenosis* is common, it is thought to be acquired, inasmuch as it generally is seen only in circumcised boys. Congenital *urethral diverticuli* are not rare, yet they generally are small and of no consequence. Finally, *megalourethra*, a markedly dilated anterior urethra,

often associated with poor development of the erectile corpora, is rarely seen.

Arey LB: Developmental Anatomy. 7th ed. Philadelphia, W.B. Saunders Company, 1974. *The most complete text describing the derivation of congenital anomalies.*

Perlmutter AD, Retik AA, Bauer SB: Anomalies of the upper urinary tract. In Harrison et al.: Campbell's Urology. 5th ed. Philadelphia, W.B. Saunders Company, 1986, p 1665. *A complete and well-referenced treatise of the subject.*

93 TUMORS OF THE KIDNEY, URETER, AND BLADDER
Richard D. Williams

Benign and malignant renal tumors are either primary in the kidney and its surrounding connective tissue or collecting structures, or secondary (involving the kidney from adjacent organs or distant sites of origin). By definition, any mass within the kidney is a "renal tumor," but only solid masses are considered in this chapter. Cystic lesions of the kidney are discussed in Ch. 91. A classification of renal tumors is presented in Table 93–1.

APPROACH TO THE PATIENT WITH A RENAL MASS

In the past, most renal masses were detected on excretory urograms (IVP) during an evaluation prompted by signs or symptoms of disease (Table 93–2). Surgical exploration was often necessary for definitive diagnosis and treatment. Today, there are multiple new modalities for the accurate diagnostic study of renal masses, and because of their sensitivity an increasing number of incidental renal masses are being identified in asymptomatic patients. A systematic algorithmic approach should result in less than 10 per cent of renal masses being indeterminate prior to surgery (Fig. 93–1). Its use will often obviate the requirement for surgical definition.

The IVP with nephrotomography is still the study of first choice and can accurately define 75 per cent of renal masses. A demonstrated renal mass will require renal ultrasonography (US) to determine more accurately whether the mass is cystic or solid. If the mass fulfills all US criteria for a simple cyst (65 per cent of renal masses) there is little need for further workup, inasmuch as US is over 95 per cent accurate (Ch. 91). In the symptomatic patient, however, further workup, including needle aspiration cytology or computed tomographic (CT) scan or both, may be appropriate. When a mass is suspected on IVP but not confirmed on US (15 per cent of cases), either an isotopic scan of the renal cortex (DMSA) or renal CT is required, particularly in symptomatic patients.

TABLE 93–1. CLASSIFICATION OF RENAL TUMORS

Benign Tumors
  Adenoma
  Oncocytoma
  Mesoblastic nephroma
  Hamartoma-angiomyolipoma
  Leiomyoma
  Hemangioma
Primary Malignant Tumors
  Renal cell carcinoma (adenocarcinoma)
  Nephroblastoma (Wilms' tumor)
  Urothelial carcinoma (renal collecting system and pelvis)
  Sarcoma
Secondary Malignant Tumors (Direct Extension or Metastatic)
  Adrenal carcinoma
  Retroperitoneal sarcoma, pancreas, colon
  Lung, stomach, breast
  Reticuloendothelial—lymphoma and Hodgkin's disease, and hematologic—leukemia and multiple myeloma

TABLE 93–2. PRESENTING SYMPTOMS, LABORATORY FEATURES, OR PHYSICAL FINDINGS IN PATIENTS WITH RENAL CELL CARCINOMA

Finding	Occurrence (%)
Hematuria	50–60
Elevated erythrocyte sedimentation rate (ESR)	50–60
Abdominal mass	24–45
Anemia	21–41
Flank pain	35–40
Hypertension	22–38
Weight loss	28–36
Pyrexia	7–17
Hepatic dysfunction	10–15
Classic triad (gross hematuria, flank pain, and palpable abdominal mass)	7–10
Hypercalcemia	3–6
Erythrocytosis	3–4
Acute varicocele	2–3

Data from Skinner DG, et al.: Diagnosis and management of renal cell cancer. Cancer 28:1165, 1971; Chisholm GD: Nephrogenic ridge tumors and their syndromes. Ann NY Acad Sci 230:402, 1974; Fallon B: Renal parenchymal tumors. *In* Culp DA, Loening SA (eds.): Genitourinary Oncology. Philadelphia, Lea & Febiger, p 202, 1985.

If the mass on US is solid or complex (20 per cent of cases), a renal CT scan (both with and without intravenous injection of iodine contrast) has replaced renal arteriography as the next diagnostic step. CT is as accurate as, and obviates the potential morbidity of, angiography in defining renal masses. Contrast enhancement of the usually highly vascular renal cancer on a CT study leaves little doubt as to the nature of a solid mass. In addition, CT can give sufficient local staging information to allow definitive surgical management. When contrast enhancement is coupled with areas of a negative CT number (relative tissue density in Hounsfield units) typical of fat, a diagnosis of angiomyolipoma is appropriate and no further workup or immediate treatment will be required. In indeterminate cases, arteriography or needle aspiration cytology or both may be needed to define the diagnosis further; however, in these unusual cases, final definition will likely require surgery.

In general, the nature of primary renal parenchymal masses in adults will be readily defined via this algorithm. Another advance that might further shape the algorithm suggested above is magnetic resonance imaging (MRI). MRI is nearly equal to CT in diagnosing renal masses but is better in local tumor staging (defining perirenal fat, para-aortic nodal and adjacent organ extension, and intravascular tumor thrombi). With the advent of paramagnetic agents capable of contrast-like enhancement, MRI may permit differentiation between tumor types.

Cronan JJ, Zeman RK: Renal mass imaging: The internist's role. Am J Med 81:1026, 1986. *A succinct discussion of the imaging modalities available for renal mass evaluation, including cost and efficacy considerations.*

Cronan JJ, Zeman RK, Rosenfeld AT: Comparison of computerized tomography, ultrasound and angiography in staging renal cell cancer. J Urol 127:712, 1982. *A definitive study showing CT to be the most accurate modality for staging renal cell carcinoma (RCC).*

Hricak H, Demas BE, Williams RD, et al.: MRI in the diagnosis and staging of renal and perirenal neoplasms. Radiology 154:709, 1985. *The initial report correlating pathologic data and MRI findings in renal cancer.*

Richie JP, Garnick MD, Seltzer D, et al.: CT scan for diagnosis and staging of renal cell cancer. J Urol 129:1114, 1983. *A substantial series of patients studied by CT with surgical correlation results.*

BENIGN RENAL TUMORS

Renal adenoma is the most common benign solid parenchymal lesion. Those under 3 cm in size have been designated as "benign," yet they tend to occur in circumstances similar to lesions larger than 3 cm (which are considered cancerous), i.e., in patients above 40 years of age, with a male to female ratio of 2 or 3 to 1. Small "renal adenomas" (< 3 cm) are virtually indistinguishable histologically from renal adenocarcinomas and a few have in fact metastasized. Since the biology

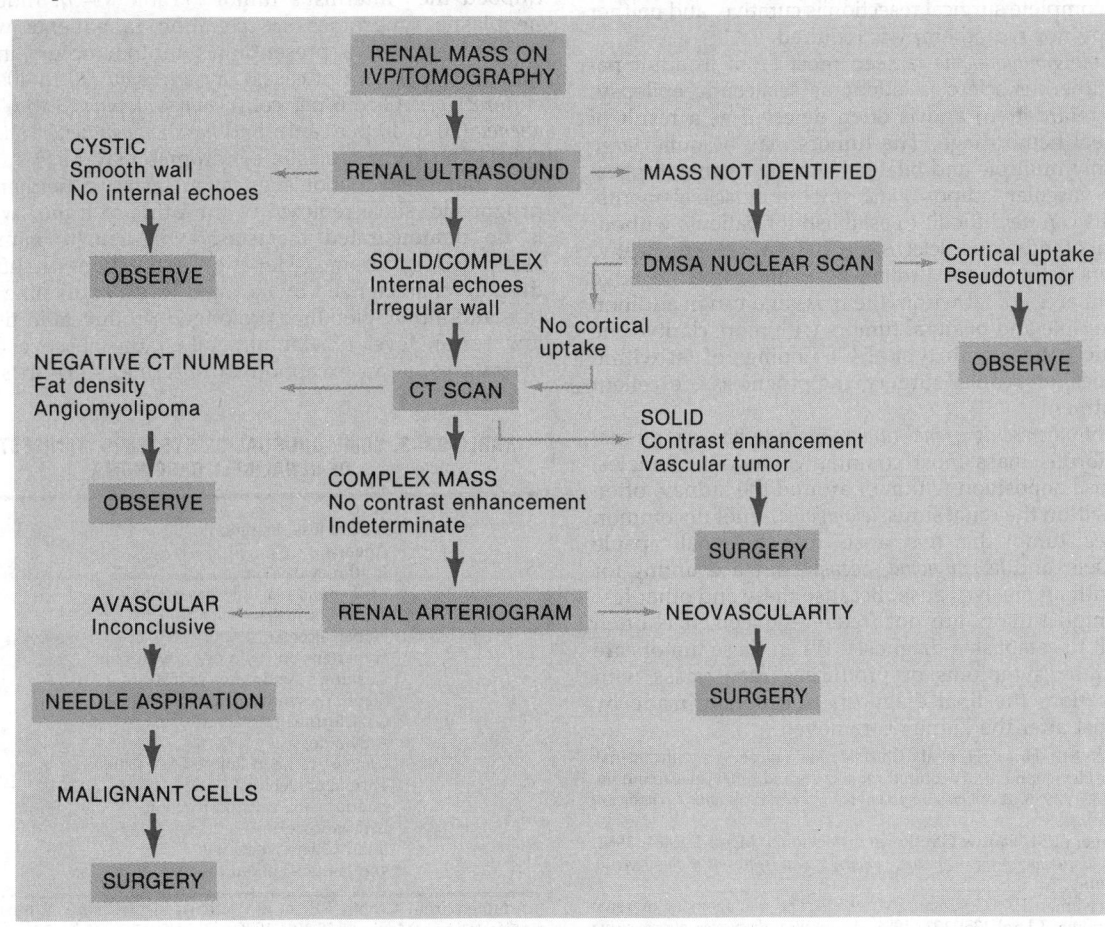

FIGURE 93–1. Algorithm for the work-up of a renal mass.

of these small tumors cannot be predicted preoperatively, most urologic oncologists consider them to be malignant and recommend radical nephrectomy. Trials of a subtotal nephrectomy in highly selected lesions are appropriate, however, since there are surprisingly good survival rates following partial nephrectomy for renal cancer in solitary kidneys and after subtotal nephrectomy in bilateral disease, and since the frequency of diagnosis of small, asymptomatic renal tumors is increasing because of the liberal use of CT scanning.

Renal oncocytoma, a subtype of adenoma accounting for 5 to 7 per cent of renal tumors, has a characteristic pale brown gross appearance and contains cells with an acidophilic cytoplasm. These tumors, although sometimes several centimeters in size, are generally asymptomatic. The typical spoke-wheel pattern on angiography is not sufficiently specific to exclude a malignant lesion preoperatively, and therefore treatment continues to be radical nephrectomy.

Acquired renal cystic disease is a new entity described in up to 45 per cent of patients with end-stage renal disease after three years of chronic hemodialysis. Approximately 10 per cent of these patients develop renal tumors that vary histologically from benign adenomas and oncocytomas to renal cell carcinomas. The tumors tend to be multiple and bilateral. The metastatic rate of these tumors is only about 6 per cent. The etiology is thought to be due to a poorly excreted, nondialyzable metabolite, since the entity has been described in patients with renal failure but who are not yet on dialysis. These tumors tend to present with gross hematuria. It is recommended that all patients be screened by annual renal ultrasonography after three years of chronic dialysis.

Mesoblastic nephroma, a benign congenital renal tumor of early childhood, must be distinguished from the highly malignant nephroblastoma, or Wilms' tumor. Unlike the latter, however, the mesoblastic nephroma is commonly diagnosed at birth or within the first few months of life. The prognosis is excellent; complete surgical resection is curative, and neither chemotherapy nor radiotherapy is required.

Hamartoma-angiomyolipoma is seen most often in adult patients with tuberous sclerosis (adenoma sebaceum, epilepsy, and mental retardation) and is often detected as a result of retroperitoneal hemorrhage. The tumors may be quite large and commonly multiple and bilateral. As their name implies, they contain vascular, adipose, and smooth muscle elements. The diagnosis can be difficult to establish for patients without the stigmata of tuberous sclerosis. Computed tomography, however, can define these tumors by exhibiting a negative CT number in areas of fat within the mass and can in addition delineate multiple and bilateral tumors with more clarity. The asymptomatic patient with typical CT findings of fat within the tumor does not require surgery; the prognosis is excellent without treatment.

A variety of *other benign renal tumors* include *fibroma*, a renal medullary fibrous mass most commonly found in females; *lipoma*, adipose deposition within or around the kidney, often perihilar or within the renal sinus; *leiomyoma*, a not uncommon retroperitoneal tumor that may arise from the renal capsule or renal vessels; and *hemangioma*, occasionally accounting for hematuria with an elusive cause. Because these and other less common benign tumors are not frequently seen, it is often quite difficult to establish a diagnosis. When these tumors are accompanied by symptoms or produce a renal mass with caliceal distortion, the final diagnosis is generally made by the pathologist after the kidney is removed.

Bretan PN, Busch MP, Hricak H, et al.: Chronic renal failure: A significant risk factor in the development of acquired renal cysts and renal cell carcinoma. Cancer 57:1871, 1986. *A complete review of the reported cases with discussion of the probable causes.*

Lieber MM, Tomera KM, Farrow GM: Renal oncocytoma. J Urol 125:481, 1982. *An excellent discussion of the diagnosis, pathology, and treatment of this recently recognized entity.*

Oesterling JE, Fishman EK, Goldman SM, et al.: The management of renal angiomyolipoma. J Urol 135:1121, 1986. *An excellent discussion of presenting findings and conditions for conservative management.*

PRIMARY MALIGNANT TUMORS

RENAL CELL CARCINOMA. Renal cell carcinoma is the most common renal malignancy in adults, accounting for 6 per cent of all malignancies and approximately 7500 deaths per year in the United States. The tumor is also called renal adenocarcinoma, Grawitz' tumor, hypernephroma, and nephrocarcinoma, although renal cell carcinoma (RCC) has become a universally accepted designation. RCC appears to arise from cells of the proximal convoluted tubule. Risk factors include pipe and cigar smoking and maleness (ratio of 2 or 3 to 1). Persons with HLA antigen types BW44 and DR8 may be more prone to develop renal cancer, and evidence suggests that oncogenes localized to the short arm of chromosome 3 may have etiologic implications. RCC is occasionally familial and is more common in patients with von Hippel-Lindau disease, horseshoe kidneys, adult polycystic kidney disease, and acquired renal cystic disease from renal failure. Histologically, RCC is of three varieties: the classic "clear cell" type characterized by uniformly large, cholesterol-laden cells with small nuclei and rare mitoses; a granular cell type exhibiting a darker staining cytoplasm containing numerous mitochondria, and more numerous mitoses; and an uncommon spindle cell (sarcomatoid) variety that has fusiform cells and variability in cell size.

Clinical Manifestations. The classic presenting triad of *hematuria, flank pain,* and a *palpable abdominal mass* is seen in less than 10 per cent of patients and among those only with far advanced local tumors (Table 93–2). Gross or microscopic hematuria alone, however, is present in approximately 60 per cent of patients with RCC. The detection of renal tumors in asymptomatic patients has increased, but 30 per cent of patients continue to have local extension or metastatic disease at the time of diagnosis. Because of its protean manifestations and propensity for curious metastatic sites, RCC has been dubbed the "internist's tumor" (Table 93–3). Indeed, paraneoplastic syndromes are common in patients with RCC: *pyrexia* (fever as a presenting symptom occurs in approximately 15 per cent of cases), *hypertension* (20 to 40 per cent), *erythrocytosis* (3 to 6 per cent), *hypercalcemia* (3 to 6 per cent), *anemia* (20 to 40 per cent), and *hepatic dysfunction* (10 to 15 per cent). The paraneoplastic syndromes may raise suspicion of RCC but they do not suggest metastases; neither are they prognostic, since removal of the primary tumor when there is no demonstrated metastasis will usually eliminate the associated syndrome. Hepatic dysfunction (Stauffer's syndrome), characterized by elevated levels of alkaline phosphatase and alpha$_2$-globulin, prolonged prothrombin time, and a low serum level of albumin, all in the absence of hepatic metastases, is an exception to this rule, since in such cases

TABLE 93–3. SOME UNUSUAL OR SYSTEMIC MANIFESTATIONS OF RENAL CELL CARCINOMA

Fever
Weight loss, inanition
Anemia
Erythrocytosis
Leukemoid reaction, eosinophilia
Thrombocytosis
Hypercalcemia
Hypertension (with or without renin ↑)
Cushing's syndrome (ACTH)
Stauffer's syndrome (hepatopathy)
Galactorrhea (prolactin)
Amyloidosis
Congestive heart failure (A-V fistula)
Thrombophlebitis
Inferior vena cava obstruction
Left varicocele
Budd-Chiari syndrome
von Hippel–Lindau disease

Adapted from Cronin RE, et al.: Renal cell carcinoma: Unusual systemic manifestations. Medicine 55:191, 1976.
ACTH = adrenocorticotropic hormone; A-V = arteriovenous.

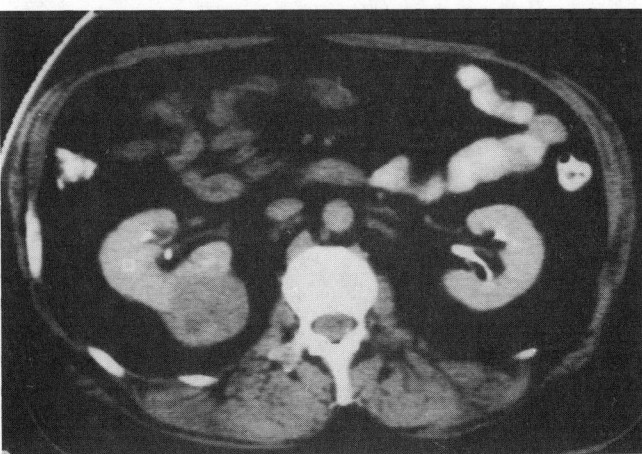

FIGURE 93–2. Contrast-enhanced abdominal CT scan showing renal cell cancer in the right kidney.

there is an unexplained high recurrence rate after definitive treatment of localized disease.

Diagnosis. There is no specific diagnostic laboratory test for RCC. The physician must often suspect RCC in patients with unexplained constitutional symptoms. The diagnostic evaluation relies on the algorithm previously described for investigation of renal mass (Fig. 93–1). A mass suspected on IVP with nephrotomograms should be confirmed by ultrasonography. If it is solid on US, an abdominal CT scan will, in approximately 95 per cent of cases, be sufficient to establish the diagnosis (Fig. 93–2). MRI can also establish the diagnosis and be useful for staging (Fig. 93–3). A renal vein or caval thrombus is common and may change the surgical approach to treatment, so the presence of a thrombus should be determined by ultrasonography, CT scanning, or MRI. In equivocal cases a venacavogram may be necessary for definition and/or determination of the cephalad extent of the thrombus before operation. The CT scan may be capable of determining local extension and/or local lymph node involvement, although it has not been found to be specific enough in most cases to obviate exploratory surgery for confirmation.

Staging and Treatment. It is important to determine the presence of metastases before determining therapy. No ben-

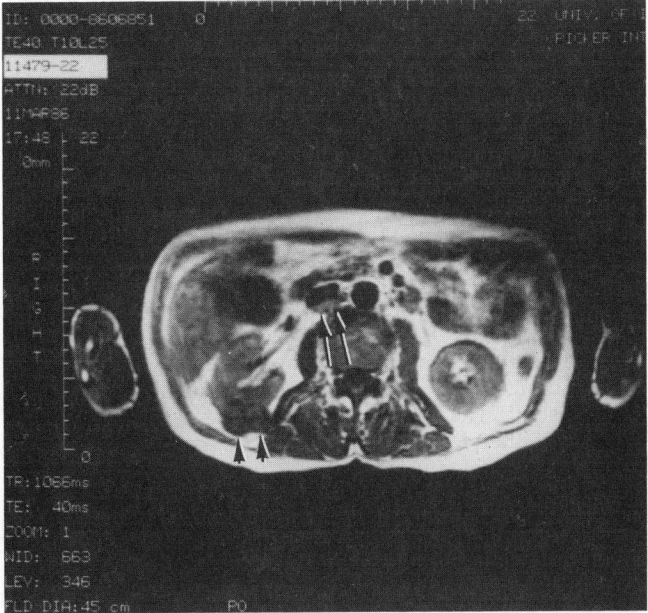

FIGURE 93–3. Transaxial MRI showing a renal cancer in the right kidney (*short arrows*) and a tumorous retroperitoneal lymph node (*long arrows*).

TABLE 93–4. STAGING SYSTEM FOR RENAL CARCINOMA

Stage I	Tumor confined to the renal parenchyma
Stage II	Tumor involving the perinephric fat or adrenal but confined within Gerota's fascia
Stage III A.	Tumor thrombus in renal vein or vena cava
B.	Tumor involving regional nodes
C.	Tumor involving lymph nodes and renal vein or vena cava
Stage IV	Tumor extending into adjacent organs (liver, colon, pancreas, duodenum) or distant metastases

efit has been ascribed to removal of the primary tumor in patients with known metastases unless the patient is symptomatic, the metastasis is solitary and amenable to resection, or a promising medical therapeutic protocol is planned (see below). Spontaneous regression of metastases following surgical removal of the primary tumor is calculated at 0.5 per cent, whereas the surgical mortality is nearly 2 per cent. The primary metastatic sites beyond the ipsilateral adrenal and local lymph nodes are lung and long bones. A chest roentgenogram and CT and a radionuclide bone scan are routine staging modalities. Lymphangiography has not been helpful in staging RCC patients.

Therapy of RCC depends entirely on the staging system summarized in Table 93–4. In patients with Stages I, II, and III A, treatment consists of a radical nephrectomy, which includes removal of the kidney and ipsilateral adrenal intact within its surrounding fascia, as well as removal of a possible intracaval thrombus. The local hilar lymph nodes will be included, but a formal para-aortic node dissection is not warranted. The prognosis for patients so treated approximates a 50 to 70 per cent five-year survival. Patients with lymph node involvement (Stage III A, C) have a 15 to 35 per cent five-year survival, and those with distant metastases (Stage IV) generally have less than a 5 per cent five-year survival.

Treatment of metastatic disease has included radiotherapy, chemotherapy, and immunotherapy, with none of these modalities emerging as clearly beneficial in effecting long-term survival. Hormonal therapy with medroxyprogesterone has less than a 5 per cent response rate. A variety of other hormonal agents, including testosterone, tamoxifen, nafoxidine, and estramustine, have similarly shown few responses. Approximately 20 per cent of patients with metastatic RCC were reported to respond to vinblastine. Immunotherapy with bacille Calmette-Guérin (BCG), *Corynebacterium parvum*, and xenogeneic immune ribonucleic acid (RNA) has been tried with limited success. Recent trials of recombinant alpha-interferon are reported to show up to a 30 per cent response rate with an occasional complete remission. An additional form of immunotherapy entails production of augmented autologous lymphocytes (LAK cells) by incubation with interleukin-2 in vitro. LAK cells are then reinfused into the patient. Early results show greater than 80 per cent response rate in patients with pulmonary metastases, but the toxicity of the treatment is great, and the durability of remissions is unknown. Although radiation therapy is not important in primary treatment, it can provide short-term control of symptomatic bone metastases.

Cronin RE, Kaehny WD, Miller PD, et al.: Renal cell carcinoma: Unusual systemic manifestations. Medicine 55:291, 1976. *This article presents eight cases with unusual aspects of RCC and contains a comprehensive review of the literature.*

DeKernion JB: Treatment of advanced renal cell cancer—traditional methods and innovative approaches. J Urol 130:2, 1983. *A superb and inclusive review of the treatment of disseminated RCC.*

Garnick MB, Richie JP: Renal neoplasia. In Brenner BM Rector FC, Jr (eds.): The Kidney. 3rd ed. Philadelphia, W. B. Saunders Company, 1986, pp 1533–1550. *An excellent general review of renal cell carcinoma, sarcomas of renal origin, and Wilms' tumor, with 141 references.*

Holland JM: Cancer of the kidney—natural history and staging. Cancer 32:1030, 1973. *The classic article on RCC containing a complete description of the staging system.*

Niedhart JA: Interferon therapy for the treatment of renal cancer. Cancer 57 (suppl):1696, 1986. *Complete review of the interferon treatment studies for RCC.*

Richie JP, Garnick MD: Primary renal and ureteral cancer. In Rieselbach RE, Garnick MB (eds.): Cancer and the Kidney. Philadelphia, Lea & Febiger,

1982, pp 662–706. *An excellent general review in a book devoted to the interrelationships of neoplastic diseases and renal disease; 185 references.*

Rosenberg SA: The adoptive immunotherapy of cancer using the transfer of activated lymphocytic cells and interleukin-2. Semin Oncol 13:200, 1986. *The initial report of the LAK cell therapy of human malignancies.*

NEPHROBLASTOMA. Nephroblastoma (Wilms' tumor) is the most common malignant neoplasm of the urinary tract in childhood. It is diagnosed in one third of cases when the child is under the age of two and in two thirds of cases when the child is under the age of four.

Clinical Manifestations and Diagnosis. The tumor is palpable in as many as 80 per cent of cases, often noted by a parent. Pain is initially present in 50 per cent of cases, hematuria (usually microscopic) in 10 to 20 per cent, and hypertension in approximately 60 per cent. The diagnosis is established first by IVP, which commonly shows caliceal distortion. Calcification within the mass occurs in 10 to 15 per cent of cases. Abdominal ultrasonography or CT scans are useful to determine tumor extension and the possibility of bilaterality (this occurs in approximately 10 per cent of patients). Arteriography is rarely utilized.

If there still is doubt about the differential diagnosis (after the studies just described are done), measurement of urine vanillylmandelic acid should help rule out neuroblastoma. The metastatic workup should be directed to the lungs, liver, and opposite kidney. A chest roentgenogram and CT and an abdominal CT are sufficient. Nephroblastoma, as is the case with RCC, often produces a tumor thrombus in the inferior vena cava, which may have to be delineated by venacavography. Abdominal ultrasonography is also a reasonable alternative to establish this possibility.

Treatment. The development of successful treatment of nephroblastoma (Wilms' tumor) is rightfully heralded as one of the most significant advances in cancer therapy of the past few years. The prognosis has improved from a 25 per cent survival in the 1960s to a current rate of over 85 per cent disease-free survival, if there is no distant dissemination or unfavorable histology.

The initial treatment of nephroblastoma is complete surgical removal of the primary tumor and kidney, even when there are metastases. A transabdominal approach will allow the safest access and the necessary visibility of the liver, para-aortic nodes, and contralateral kidney for complete staging. Occasionally radiotherapy or chemotherapy may be required preoperatively to decrease the bulk of massive tumors. Combined therapy is indicated postoperatively in all patients but is dependent upon accurate staging, completeness of surgical extirpation, and tumor histology. A tumor confined to the kidney in children under two years of age requires only postoperative administration of actinomycin D and vincristine, whereas for all others the best results are obtained with radiation therapy to the tumor bed plus administration of actinomycin D and vincristine. Doxorubicin is also an active agent in the treatment of this disease. Additional areas of current investigation are (1) radiation therapy and the addition of doxorubicin to vincristine and actinomycin D for patients with extensive local disease and favorable histology, and (2) radiation therapy with triple drug versus quadruple drug (addition of cyclophosphamide) for cases with unfavorable histology (anaplasia or sarcomatous elements). Wilms' tumor may occasionally be seen in adults; similarly, RCC occurs but rarely in children.

D'Angio GJ, Evans A, Breslow N, et al.: The treatment of Wilms' tumor: Results of the second National Wilms' Tumor Study. Cancer 47:2302, 1981. *A follow-up of the first NWTS report establishing improved results with complete staging and chemotherapy only in younger patients.*

UROTHELIAL TUMORS. Malignant tumors of the urothelial lining of the urinary tract include those involving the collecting structures of the kidney (renal pelvis and calices), ureter, and bladder. These tumors are transitional cell cancers (TCC) in over 90 per cent of cases, with an occasional

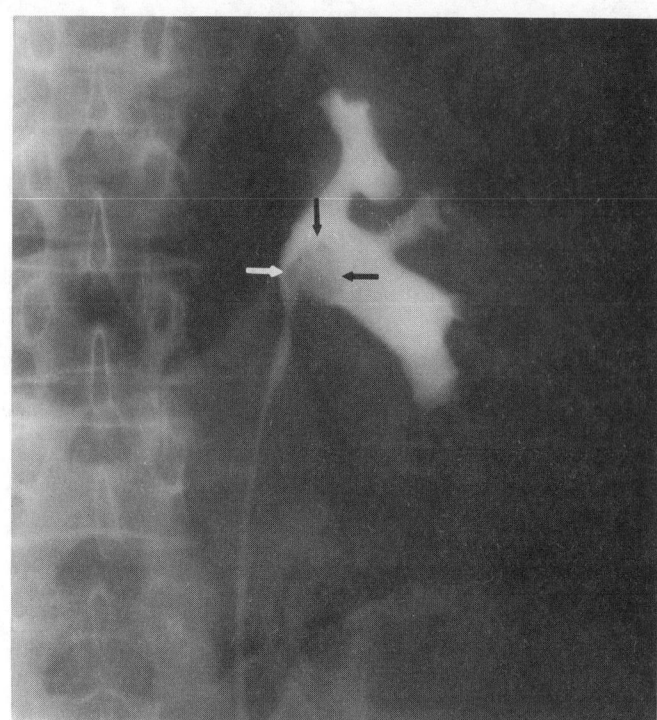

FIGURE 93–4. Retrograde pyelogram showing a transitional cell cancer in the pelvis of the right kidney (*arrows*). (Reproduced with permission from Williams RD: Renal, perirenal, and ureteral neoplasms. In Gillenwater JY, Grayhack JT, Howards SS, et al.: Adult and Pediatric Urology. Chicago, Year Book Medical Publishers, 1987.)

squamous cell carcinoma (often in association with chronic inflammation due to stone formation in the upper tracts and with *Schistosoma haematobium* infestation in the bladder) and rarely adenocarcinoma (commonly associated with embryologic hindgut remnants such as a persistent urachus in the dome of the bladder). TCC tends to be multifocal, occurring bilaterally in the upper tracts in a few cases but with an increasing frequency of simultaneous occurrence or recurrences in the ureter and particularly in the bladder. In each location there is a strong association of TCC with cigarette smoking, exposure to certain industrial chemicals (particularly aromatic amines), and chronic abuse of phenacetin-containing analgesics.

TCC of the Renal Pelvis and Calices. CLINICAL MANIFESTATIONS AND DIAGNOSIS. The presenting finding is gross or microscopic hematuria in more than 60 per cent of cases. In contrast to RCC, constitutional symptoms and paraneoplastic syndromes are few. Generally the diagnosis is made by the finding of a filling defect in a calix, infundibulum, or renal pelvis on IVP (Fig. 93–4). Ultrasonography can be utilized to eliminate the possibility of a nonopaque calculus. Examination of the urine by an experienced cytologist can be diagnostic of TCC, although the site will be undetermined. Cystoscopy with retrograde pyelography, including ureteral wash or brush cytology, may be required to establish the diagnosis. Ureteroscopy may be useful in equivocal cases. CT scanning may be useful in determining local extent of tumor but is usually unnecessary. Arteriography is generally not diagnostically useful. The tumors tend to metastasize to lung and bone, and therefore a chest roentgenogram and CT and a bone scan are often indicated. Since these tumors tend to be multifocal, careful preoperative scrutiny of the opposite side of the urinary tract (on IVP) and of the bladder and urethra by direct cystourethroscopy is recommended.

TREATMENT AND PROGNOSIS. Treatment of renal urothelial cancer is radical nephroureterectomy, with removal of the entire ureter. Because 40 to 50 per cent of patients will have or develop similar tumors within the bladder, direct cystourethroscopy is a necessary postoperative routine, usually done quarterly the first year, twice the second year, and then annually.

Most of these tumors are low grade and noninvasive, and the five-year tumor-free survival rate after complete removal of the ipsilateral upper tract is more than 90 per cent. Patients with high-grade and/or invasive lesions, however, have a poor prognosis (<15 per cent five-year survival). Chemotherapeutic combinations, which have begun to show activity in TCC of the bladder, are also efficacious in metastatic TCC of the upper tracts (see below).

TCC of the Ureter. CLINICAL MANIFESTATIONS AND DIAGNOSIS. These tumors are most often detected secondary to gross or microscopic hematuria, but occasionally present with renal colic due to obstructing blood clots. Diagnosis is commonly made by the finding of a ureteral filling defect on IVP. If the ureter is totally obstructed with a resultant lack of contrast excretion, cystoscopy with retrograde ureterography or ureteroscopy is required to demonstrate the lesion. As in renal pelvis TCC, ureteral urine or brush cytology can be diagnostic. Abdominal CT scans can aid in local staging, as can chest roentgenograms, and CT and bone scanning assist in detecting distant metastases.

TREATMENT AND PROGNOSIS. Prognosis is determined by the histologic grade of the lesion and the depth of invasion. Selected low-grade lesions may be successfully treated by segmental resection, particularly in patients with renal insufficiency or a solitary kidney, but the definitive approach remains nephroureterectomy, as in renal pelvis TCC. Prognosis of low-grade noninvasive lesions is greater than 70 to 80 per cent five-year survival, but for the higher grade, usually invasive lesions the prognosis is dismal. Treatment of metastatic disease is rarely successful; however, as with TCC of the renal pelvis, the newer combinations of chemotherapy are promising (see below).

TCC of the Bladder. Bladder cancer affects over 20,000 people and accounts for nearly 10,000 deaths annually in the United States. Men are affected at least twice as often as women.

CLINICAL MANIFESTATIONS AND DIAGNOSIS. Hematuria occurs at presentation in 68 per cent of patients and classically is total (throughout the stream) whether microscopic (as tested by a three-glass test) or gross. The degree of hematuria does not parallel the size of the lesion. Bladder irritability (frequency and dysuria) in the absence of infection is also a common (25 per cent) presenting complaint, particularly in males.

Intravenous pyelography is not sufficiently sensitive to detect small bladder tumors, but it is helpful in detecting upper tract TCC in the 10 per cent of patients with simultaneous lesions and in predicting bladder wall invasion in patients with concomitant unilateral ureteral obstruction. Urine cytology may establish the diagnosis of TCC but not the site. Definitive diagnosis requires cystoscopy and transurethral bladder biopsy under anesthesia, at which time a bimanual examination can predict whether the tumor has extended beyond the bladder wall. Metastases are local into adjacent pelvic structures and lymph nodes and distant to lungs and bones, and therefore staging of deeply invasive tumors is by chest roentgenograms, CT of the chest and abdomen, and bone scanning.

TREATMENT AND PROGNOSIS. Nearly 80 per cent of bladder TCC's are low grade and noninvasive (stage 0) or invade only into the lamina propria (stage A). Patients with such lesions have an 85 per cent five-year survival rate when treated by complete transurethral resection of the tumor(s). The lesions tend toward multiple recurrences in more than 50 per cent of patients and therefore cystoscopic surveillance is a mandatory postoperative routine. Intravesical chemotherapy with thiotepa, doxorubicin, mitomycin-C, or more recently BCG has been used successfully for prophylaxis in patients with multiple or recurrent superficial low-grade tumors, resulting in an approximate 50 per cent reduction in recurrences. Importantly, only about 20 per cent of patients presenting with superficial bladder TCC will subsequently develop high-grade and/or invasive disease.

Unfortunately, 80 per cent of patients with invasive bladder TCC are found so at initial presentation. In patients with deeply invasive disease, stage B_1 refers to superficial muscle invasion, stage B_2 to deep muscle invasion, and stage C to full-thickness bladder wall invasion. In the absence of metastases current best efforts at cure of invasive disease require pelvic lymphadenectomy and radical cystectomy (complete removal of the bladder and prostate in males and the bladder, urethra, and uterus in females). This approach affords a 50 to 60 per cent five-year survival rate in patients with stage B_1, B_2, or C disease. Patients with pelvic lymph node (stage D_1) or distant metastases (stage D_2) have less than a 15 per cent five-year survival rate.

Metastatic disease is difficult to treat, but combination chemotherapy with vinblastine, methotrexate, and cisplatin with or without doxorubicin is showing a durable 30 per cent complete remission rate. This significant advance, if consistent, may alter the surgical approach to bladder TCC in the future.

SARCOMAS. Renal sarcomas are rare; they include rhabdomyosarcoma, liposarcoma, fibrosarcoma, osteogenic sarcoma, and, most commonly, leiomyosarcoma (60 per cent). In general, sarcomas are quite malignant and usually detected at a late stage, and thus have a poor prognosis. The diagnosis approach is similar to that for RCC. Treatment is surgical with wide local excision; however, local recurrence and subsequent distant metastases are the rule.

Droller MJ: Transitional cell cancer: Upper tracts and bladder. In Walsh PC, Gittes RF, Perlmutter AD, (eds).: Campbell's Urology. Philadelphia, W. B. Saunders Company, 1986, pp 1343–1440. *A detailed and complete discussion of uroepithelial cancer diagnosis and treatment.*

McCarreen JP, Mullis D, Vaughn ED: Tumors of the renal pelvis and ureter: Current concepts and management. Semin Urol 1:75, 1983. *A definitive review of upper tract urothelial cancer.*

Myers F, Palmer J, Harrigan J: Chemotherapy of disseminated TCC. In Williams RD (ed.): Advances in Urologic Oncology. New York, Macmillan, 1987. *A discussion of cisplatin/methotrexate/vinblastine chemotherapy showing a 40 to 50 per cent overall complete remission/partial remission rate.*

SECONDARY MALIGNANT TUMORS

Tumors of the lung, stomach, and breast most commonly metastasize to the kidney, but the metastases are usually clinically silent except for microscopic hematuria. More than 50 per cent of patients with primary lung cancer have renal metastases at autopsy. Routine use of staging abdominal CT in a variety of primary malignancies is expected to increase the premorbid diagnosis of secondary renal tumors. Adjacent tumors of the adrenal, colon, and pancreas, and sarcomas may spread contiguously into the kidney. Reticuloendothelial tumors, such as lymphoma and Hodgkin's disease, and hematologic malignancies, such as leukemia and multiple myeloma, may infiltrate the kidney, but this type of renal involvement is almost never primary or symptomatic. Other forms of renal involvement in multiple myeloma are described in Ch. 163.

PART X
GASTROINTESTINAL DISEASES

94 INTRODUCTION

Marvin H. Sleisenger

Digestive diseases in the United States account for a large part of the economic burden of illness, of total days of illness among adults, of all admissions to general hospitals, and of all major surgical operations. The prompt recognition of digestive disease and its treatment are thus plainly important. In order best to discharge this responsibility, knowledge of the pathophysiologic basis for signs and symptoms of gastrointestinal disease is most helpful. This introduction to the chapters on gastrointestinal diseases will be concerned with this broad subject.

APPROACH TO THE PATIENT WITH GASTROINTESTINAL DISEASE. In the approach to a patient with gastrointestinal disease the physician must obtain an accurate history of illness, correctly interpret the principal symptoms of digestive disease, conduct a thorough physical examination in which findings often characteristic of specific gastrointestinal diseases and syndromes are assiduously sought, and make intelligent use of laboratory tests and other diagnostic aids. An accurate history of digestive disease requires attention to details that mark the duration of the disability, establishing relationships between the waxing and waning of symptoms and external factors such as stress, eating, or fasting. Understanding the pathophysiologic basis of symptoms and signs helps greatly to establish the location, nature, and urgency of the problem.

The majority of patients with digestive disease have had their illness for years. The common diseases are chronic: *acid-peptic disease* affecting the esophagus, stomach, or duodenum; *alcoholic disease* of the *liver* and *pancreas; calculous biliary tract disease; inflammatory bowel disease; postprandial dyspepsia; irritable bowel;* and *cancer* of the stomach, intestines, pancreas, or liver. To be sure, some gastrointestinal diseases may be acute and even catastrophic; the *acute abdomen* is a general phrase of importance in both medical and surgical practice.

THE VALUE OF A THOROUGH HISTORY. The duration of symptoms in patients with digestive diseases ranges from moments to decades. In an emergency room a physician may be called to see a previously healthy person suffering the symptoms and displaying the signs of an acute intra-abdominal disorder requiring a rapid decision about whether surgery is indicated. The next patient seeking care may be an elderly person with a problem of four or more decades' duration. This patient is also ill but does not appear to be. Differences exist in the incidences of digestive problems in patients' families, in their reactions to stress, in their dietary habits, in the degree of involvement of other organ systems, and in the degree to which their illnesses affect general health and activity.

The natural history of many gastrointestinal diseases is marked by characteristic patterns of symptoms. Complaints often have a particular intensity, a periodicity (time of day, month, or season), and a relationship to fatigue, stress, eating, or drinking alcohol. For example, patients with irritable bowel tend to have low-grade, nagging, cramplike lower abdominal distress for decades. The distress may be aggravated by certain foods and may wax and wane with the appearance and disappearance of stress. Although the discomfort may be intense at times, its intensity contrasts with the acute, sudden, and excruciating pain of the patient with an acutely obstructed small intestine, ureter, or common bile duct; a perforated duodenal ulcer; a dissecting aneurysm; or an acutely ischemic small intestine. Pain of gastrointestinal disease may be intermediate between acute and chronic, and between severe and mild, e.g., the epigastric distress of duodenal ulcer. It rarely incapacitates and is usually relieved quickly with appropriate therapy. However, a change in these characteristics, i.e., increased duration and less relief with antacids, may signal a possible penetration and deserves special attention. Complications are common in the natural history of many other gastrointestinal diseases. The patient with longstanding irritable bowel may also have diverticulosis and suddenly rupture a diverticulum. Knowledge of the natural history of digestive diseases is essential to understanding changes in patterns of symptoms, particularly pain.

The *locus* and *timing* of the distress are important in determining which organ of the digestive tract is affected. Upper abdominal discomfort related to meals usually means that the stomach, duodenum, gallbladder, or pancreas is the site of the problem. Periumbilical pain one-half hour or so postprandially may indicate that the small intestine is involved. When the discomfort is in the lower abdomen and is associated with an abnormal bowel habit or rectal bleeding or is relieved by bowel movement or flatus, the colon is likely to be at fault. The *nature* of the pain is also important. Aching pain is characteristic of ulcer disease, boring pain of pancreatic disease, and cramping pain of both small and large intestines.

The presence of associated symptoms is important in evaluating gastrointestinal disease. Fever, arthritis, conjunctivitis, uveitis, and erythema nodosum may all be associated with the diarrhea of chronic inflammatory bowel disease. Continuing weight loss and evidence of malnutrition with vitamin deficiencies usually reflect a serious organic disease; however, such malnutrition may result from anorexia, early satiety, or forced vomiting often associated with laxative abuse in order to lose weight (*bulimia*), all related to neuropsychiatric problems (Ch. 13). Type and location of pain, presence of diarrhea, a relationship of symptoms to diet and alcohol, and history of prior surgery all help the clinician better to define the disease underlying the malnutrition and possible malabsorption. The historical facts associated with *weight loss* due to digestive disease are crucial for correct diagnosis. Is anorexia due to depression or physical illness? If the appetite is normal, is decreased intake due to *dysphagia, nausea, early satiety,* or *fear* of postprandial symptoms? Some individuals lose weight, despite good appetite and adequate food intake, because of *malabsorption* or *occult intra-abdominal malignancy.* The chronic alcoholic may get enough calories from ethanol to supply energy needs and may not lose weight; however, his or her diet lacks important ingredients such as essential amino acids and fatty acids, vitamins, minerals, and electrolytes.

EMOTION AND STRESS. *Emotion* and *stress* play a large role in many gastrointestinal disorders. Patients who are massively obese or who have *anorexia nervosa* or *bulimia* are emotionally disturbed, and their eating habits are expressions of the disturbance extended over prolonged periods of time. These aberrant eating habits may represent bizarre conscious or unconscious attempts to lose weight or somehow to resolve personal or family conflicts. No clear association among personality, stress, and the pathogenesis of duodenal ulcer has been established. Nevertheless, it is clear that recurrence of symptoms can often be correlated with emotional tension.

It has long been held that emotion plays a role in the pathogenesis of ulcerative colitis, but patients with this disease have not been shown to have an abnormal prevalence of psychiatric illness or an abnormal number of "critical life incidents." There is a higher incidence of both psychoneurotic behavior and critical life incidents in patients with irritable bowel than in those with ulcerative colitis.

A personality disorder often underlies the habitual abuse of alcohol, found in many patients with diseases of the digestive system. No amount of effort in treating the esophagus (reflux esophagitis), stomach (erosive gastritis), pancreas (acute and chronic pancreatitis), or liver (acute alcoholic hepatitis, cirrhosis) will favorably affect the clinical course of these patients without attention to the basic problem.

THE PHYSICAL EXAMINATION: COMMON SIGNS OF GASTROINTESTINAL DISEASE. Certain signs of serious illness must be sought on physical examination of patients with complaints of digestive disease. The abdominal findings in patients with acute abdominal problems that require immediate surgery are discussed in Ch. 115.

Evidences of Malnutrition. Malnutrition is common in serious gastrointestinal diseases. It is characterized principally by signs of weight loss, mainly disappearance of fat depots and decreased muscle mass. Malnutrition is often associated with signs of *vitamin* and *mineral deficiencies*. Erythroderma, glossitis, cheilosis, muscle tenderness, angular stomatitis, bronzing of exposed skin, nasolabial seborrhea, dementia, and peripheral neuropathy all reflect deficiency of B soluble vitamins. Glossitis, peripheral neuropathy, and lemon-tinted pallor may reflect vitamin B_{12} deficiency. Rough skin may be due to hyperkeratosis follicularis (vitamin A deficit?) or perifolliculitis of vitamin C deficiency. Petechiae, ecchymoses, or other evidences of easy bruising may reflect vitamin K deficiency. Pallor and glossitis may be due to folate deficiency while pallor, lingual atrophy, koilonychia, and splenomegaly point to iron deficiency. Petechiae and ecchymoses may reflect vitamin K deficiency; failure to grow, kyphosis, and skeletal deformities are evidences of vitamin D lack. Xerophthalmia results from insufficient vitamin A. Deficiencies of trace metals may be suspected on physical examination. Copper and zinc deficiencies are associated with loss of taste acuity, and zinc deficiency with severe dermatitis, hyperpigmentation, as well as alopecia and evidence of dementia. Central nervous system damage, due principally to deficiency of vitamin B_1 and ranging from recent ophthalmoplegia and confusion to dementia and cerebellar ataxia, may be noted, particularly in alcoholics.

Patients with *protein deficiency* not only lose subcutaneous fat and muscle mass but also may have edema; decreased turgor and dyspigmentation of skin; dryness, brittleness, and lightening of hair; hepatomegaly; and mental dullness. Inadequate protein intake slows growth of children and impairs bone integrity in adults. Protein malnutrition caused by gastrointestinal disease is usually not selective, being coupled with subnormal caloric intake, and this is called *protein-calorie malnutrition*. Lack of essential fatty acids leads to skin eczema.

Other Important Signs. Physical signs pointing to disease in a particular organ system are also important. Thus, jaundice, hepatomegaly, splenomegaly, ascites, and spider angiomas all indicate chronic and severe liver disease. Palpable abdominal masses may be found in patients with *pancreatic pseudocyst, malignancies* of the gastrointestinal tract, *Crohn's disease,* intraperitoneal *abscesses, lymphoma, dissecting aortic aneurysms,* malignant extrahepatic biliary tract obstruction (*enlarged gallbladder*), or *lacerated* or *infarcted spleens.* Abdominal distention with evidence of gas-filled loops of bowel is often noted in patients with malabsorption resulting from diffuse proximal small bowel disease or from conditions associated with bacterial overgrowth.

Fever may be present during periods of inflammatory activity in patients with acute and chronic inflammatory disease of the gut, pancreatitis, cholecystitis, cholangitis, lymphoma, abscesses (intra-abdominal, hepatic, retroperitoneal, and perirectal), and acute progressive infarction of the bowel. The duration of fever varies and reflects the nature of the underlying disease. For example, fever is present for hours in acute suppurative cholangitis or acute small bowel infarction, and for days or even weeks in alcoholic hepatitis, Crohn's disease, pancreatitis with extensive necrosis or sepsis, abscesses (including liver), or lymphoma.

PATHOPHYSIOLOGIC BASIS FOR COMMON SYMPTOMS OF GASTROINTESTINAL DISEASE. An understanding of the pathophysiologic basis of the important symptoms of digestive disease will help in their correct interpretation and thus in arriving at an effective plan for diagnosis and treatment.

Anorexia. Disturbances of appetite, such as *anorexia* and *early satiety*, are common in digestive disease. *Hunger* is the desire for food accompanied by unpleasant epigastric sensations. *Appetite* is the desire for food after hunger ceases. *Satiety* is the loss of the desire to eat after ingesting food. The control of both hunger and satiety is complex, involving neurotransmitters, including neuropeptides, which regulate hypothalamic centers that control hunger and satiety. Cholecystokinin (CCK) peptides, released after feeding, elicit satiety, whereas opioids (endorphins, enkephalins), norepinephrine (alpha$_2$) pancreatic polypeptides, growth hormone–releasing factor, as well as other gut-brain peptides, stimulate eating.

Gastric distention and delayed gastric emptying inhibit feeding, probably via the actions of CCK, glucagon, and somatostatin. In turn, hormonal action depends upon intact vagal afferent innervation of the stomach. The factors that initiate hunger and affect appetite and satiety and are related to release of neuropeptides in gut and brain are not clearly defined but may include arteriovenous (A-V) glucose gradients, sugar intake, physical activity, and behavior.

The causes of anorexia are both physical and psychologic. *Anorexia nervosa* is a psychologic disorder in which appetite virtually does not exist and hunger is greatly reduced. Anorexia, of course, is associated with many organic diseases, intestinal and extraintestinal. In many patients anorexia is clearly associated with continuing intra-abdominal pain or fever; in others, with chronic or recurrent nausea. In those with cancer of the stomach or pancreas but without pain, its basis is not known.

Hyperphagia. The complex factors underlying excessive feeding include (1) inability to regulate energy intake according to nutritive value for the food, (2) cultural influences, (3) possible failure of normal response to feeding, i.e., failure of release of peptides that delay gastric emptying or defective receptor mechanism for them, and (4) a hypothalamic lesion, although this has not as yet been demonstrated in humans. Another group, usually young females, will alternate cramming of food and induced vomiting (*bulimia*) with periods of anorexia.

Abdominal Pain. The most frequent symptom that brings a patient with digestive disease to the physician is pain, most commonly abdominal, but not infrequently located in the chest or back. Pain warns the patient of possible imminent tissue damage and is usually caused by anoxia, inflammation, or stretching of smooth muscle or organ capsules. Pain from the viscera and peritoneum is mediated by the sympathetic nervous system. The afferent endings are located in the smooth muscle of hollow organs, in the peritoneum, and in organ capsules. These afferents are identified with dermatomes, which correspond with segments of the spinal cord. They travel with afferents from the periphery. This association is the basis of *referred pain* to extra-abdominal structures.

Pain originating from hollow viscera is called *visceral*; it is midline, dull, and often associated with nausea. The location depends upon the organ involved. Pain from the esophagus is usually felt over the site but occasionally in the suprasternal notch. Pain from the stomach and duodenum is epigastric or to the right of the midline in the epigastrium. Jejunal and ileal pain is often periumbilical, although distal ileal pain may be perceived in the right lower quadrant. Colonic pain is lower abdominal in location, often poorly localized. Pain from the gallbladder and common bile duct is in the right upper quadrant or epigastrium; when severe, it is often felt in the midline of the upper back. Pancreatic pain is midline or to the left of the epigastrium and often radiates through to the midline of the upper back.

Pain may be felt at a site distant from the organ involved, either by referral or by involvement of neighboring structures. Thus, an abscess in the lower abdomen over the psoas may refer its pain to the hip or groin; spasm of the esophagus may lead to pain felt down the inner aspect of the left upper arm, as in the pain of myocardial ischemia. The pain in the trapezius ridge areas of the shoulders may be associated with irritation of the diaphragmatic pleura by an inflammatory process such as a subdiaphragmatic abscess. The physician must be familiar with the common areas of pain reference and with the influence on pain patterns of involvement by contiguity.

Intra-abdominal pain is often due to *inflammation* or *ischemia*. Edema and spasm narrow the involved segment; smooth muscle proximal to the narrowed gut stretches, causing pain. In addition, ischemia and inflammation lower the pain threshold by releasing local bradykinin, serotonin, histamine, prostaglandins, and lactic acid. Pain is due in part also to the stretching of smooth muscle in blood vessels. Sensory nerve fibers may be directly involved by a tumor (e.g., paraspinal sensory nerve roots may be entrapped by cancer of the pancreas, other retroperitoneal malignancies).

Initially *visceral* pain is felt in the midline and is dull in character regardless of the organ involved. As inflammation or ischemia progresses, the pain will shift gradually to the site of the organ affected. Thus, in a matter of hours the pain of acute appendicitis shifts from the midline to the right lower quadrant, and that of cholecystitis from the midline to the right upper quadrant.

The patient's behavior during the pain is important in correct interpretation. Pain caused by stretching of smooth muscle of the gut, ureter, or common bile duct is colicky. The patient tends to be restless, and the pain is not aggravated by movement. The patient with peritoneal irritation, on the other hand, prefers to lie quietly, since jarring or movement exacerbates the pain.

FACTORS AFFECTING INTENSITY AND PERCEPTION OF PAIN. The patient's description of pain is influenced by neural, psychologic, and cultural factors. Perception is reduced by environmental stress, as in battle, probably owing to release of enkephalins. Likewise, depression blunts perception. The neural influences reside within the spinal cord, particularly the dorsal horns, which integrate central and peripheral impulses with those of pain, altering them before they reach the brain. Perception is also affected by cultural influences, ranging from demonstrativeness to stoicism. Finally, age affects pain perception. Patients in the eighth decade and

beyond often have a significant rise of pain threshold. Degree of discomfort is often disproportionately low even with sepsis, perforation, and infarction in this group.

Vomiting. Vomiting is the rapid evacuation of gastric contents in retrograde fashion from stomach through mouth. It must be distinguished from *rumination*, the asymptomatic regurgitation of food, rechewing, and reswallowing. It is immediately due to a forceful contraction of the abdominal muscle with the cardia and mouth open. It is most often the final stage of a three-part act. The first is *nausea*, a most unpleasant feeling, difficult to define but universally recognizable. Gastric motor activity is diminished, and duodenal pressure increases with reflux of duodenal contents into the stomach. Nausea is followed by *retching*, which comprises spasmodic respiratory movements opposed by expiratory contractions of the abdominal muscles and raises the cardia of the stomach, an important preparatory maneuver to evacuation, which is the third stage. Paraphenomena of vomiting include hypersalivation, some reverse peristalsis of the small intestine, evidences of abnormal vagal stimulation (principally bradycardia), and the urge to defecate. Vomiting is controlled by bilateral vomiting centers in the dorsal portions of the lateral reticular formation of the medulla, activated by so-called chemoreceptor trigger zones (CTZs) located near the postrema.

Drugs and ionizing radiation cause nausea and vomiting by stimulating the chemoreceptor trigger zones; this pathway also mediates the nausea and vomiting of motion sickness, uremia, diabetic ketoacidosis, and use of general anesthetics. Vagal afferents may also stimulate the vomiting centers, bypassing the chemoreceptor trigger zones. Examples include distention of the smooth muscle of the gut, particularly when sudden; substances noxious to the mucosa of the stomach such as copper sulfate or mustard; and irritation and inflammation of the peritoneum. Thus, a large number of diseases and disorders that affect the intestine, bile ducts, ureters, and peritoneum are associated with nausea and vomiting. The symptom complex is often nonspecific and not helpful in differential diagnosis of intra-abdominal disorders. Additional pathways to the vomiting center are stimulated by noxious smells and tastes, but the location of the involved supramedullary receptors is not known. Apparently, many different pathways in the brain stem as well as different neurotransmitters are involved in the multiple stimuli that cause nausea and vomiting.

TYPES OF VOMITING. Important features of vomiting that may characterize a particular category of underlying disease are its amount, duration, content, and relationship to meals.

When a patient vomits during or immediately after a meal, it is most likely to be psychogenic, although such vomiting, particularly after a heavy meal, may be due to edema and spasm of the pylorus associated with a pyloric canal ulcer. (However, in these latter cases, the patient often has pain that is relieved by emesis, in contrast to failure of pain relief by vomiting in patients with cancer of the pancreas or biliary tract disease, for example.) Vomiting an hour or more after a meal is more compatible with gastric outlet obstruction, acute pancreatitis, or motility disorder of the stomach (diabetic neuropathy, postvagotomy). Vomiting of material eaten many hours previously also fits in the category of organic obstruction. Often patients with chronic outlet obstruction will have large, dilated stomachs and on examination will be noted to have a succussion splash. This sign is important in distinguishing psychogenic from organic obstruction in chronic vomiting. Alcoholics, pregnant women, and uremic persons have nausea and vomiting early in the morning on arising. Some patients with increased intracranial pressure may have vomiting unassociated with meals or nausea; classically, it has been described as projectile or forceful, although this is by no means always the case.

Large amounts of vomitus, food and secretions, usually

TABLE 94–1. COMMON DISEASES AND DISORDERS ASSOCIATED WITH NAUSEA AND VOMITING

Psychogenic
Drug-induced
Intra-abdominal problem:
    Colic, sepsis, perforated viscus
Inflammation: ischemia
Toxins and poisons (ingested, inhaled, injected)
Metabolic disorders and diseases
Gastric outlet obstruction
Duodenal and high small bowel obstruction
Intracranial diseases
Viral gastroenteritis
Cyclic vomiting, childhood
Pregnancy
Due to pain, intra-abdominal or extra-abdominal

indicate nearly complete or complete obstruction. This may also result, however, from severe gastric atony and dilatation, or, in rare instances, from hypersecretion of gastric juice in the Zollinger-Ellison syndrome without outlet obstruction.

QUALITY OF VOMITUS. *Content* of the vomitus is important in the determination of the underlying disorder. Undigested food indicates a gastric outlet obstruction. If there is blood in the vomitus, an inflammatory or malignant disease of the stomach should be suspected. Vomitus without bile indicates that the problem is prepyloric, whereas consistent appearance of bile suggests that the problem is postpyloric. The presence of bile may signify only that the increase in pressure in the duodenum was sufficiently great that, with a relaxed pylorus, duodenal contents entered the stomach preceding evacuation. Large-volume vomitus of high acidity (pH 1.5 or less) suggests gastrinoma, although outlet obstruction with an active duodenal ulcer may have a similar output and pH.

Odor may also be helpful. A fecal smell to vomitus suggests lower intestinal obstruction, a fistula between the stomach and colon or between the upper small intestine and colon, or bacterial overgrowth of the stomach or small intestine (long-standing obstruction).

Nausea and vomiting that follow the recent onset of a persisting abdominal pain provide a clue to a likely important event within the abdomen, an event that often requires hospitalization and, in some cases, surgery.

CLASSIFICATION OF DISEASES AND DISORDERS ASSOCIATED WITH VOMITING. The major categories of disorders associated with vomiting are summarized in Table 94–1.

Psychogenic vomiting, a chronic and complex disturbance, takes place immediately after eating or during the meal. It is often self-induced and, although chronic, is compatible with good health over many years. It is frequently associated with anorexia nervosa or follows the binge eating of bulimia.

The clinical entities associated with nausea and vomiting that command immediate attention are *intra-abdominal*, *intracranial*, and *metabolic diseases*. In the abdomen they include gastric outlet obstruction; intestinal obstruction; gastrointestinal inflammation; perforation of a viscus; peritonitis; pancreatitis; abscess; acute distention of smooth muscle in bile ducts, the ureter, and the small intestine; and acute ischemia. In general, nausea and vomiting often follow severe pain, extra-abdominal as well as intra-abdominal. In addition, ileus of the intestine and stomach, and acute gastric dilatation with atony, no matter what the cause, are often associated with nausea and vomiting. In these instances, organic outlet obstruction or intestinal obstruction cannot be demonstrated.

Intracranial disease causing increased intracranial pressure (tumor, hematoma), many *toxic* and *metabolic encephalopathies* (including infection), migraine headache, and *gastric neuropathies* are examples of neurologic diseases associated with vomiting.

In medical practice nausea and vomiting are most commonly *drug induced.* The list of offending drugs is lengthy; most drugs are capable of causing nausea and vomiting in susceptible individuals. Whether the afferent stimuli originate from the action of drugs on the gastrointestinal tract or from the direct effect of drugs on the chemoreceptor zone is not clear in most instances. Anticholinergic agents, however, may cause vomiting by inhibiting motor activity in patients with partial outlet obstruction. The most common causes of gastric outlet obstruction are chronic ulcer disease of the pylorus or duodenum and antral carcinoma.

COMPLICATIONS OF VOMITING (Fig. 94–1). The major consequences of prolonged vomiting include *dehydration, hypokalemia,* and *alkalosis.* Dehydration is due to fluid loss. Hypokalemia results from exchange of sodium for potassium in the renal tubule in an effort to conserve sodium lost in vomitus, from diminished potassium intake, and from loss of potassium in the vomitus. Alkalosis follows loss of hydrogen ions in the vomitus and is exacerbated by a contraction of extracellular fluid, with noncommensurate loss of bicarbonate and shift of hydrogen into cells resulting from potassium deficiency. So-

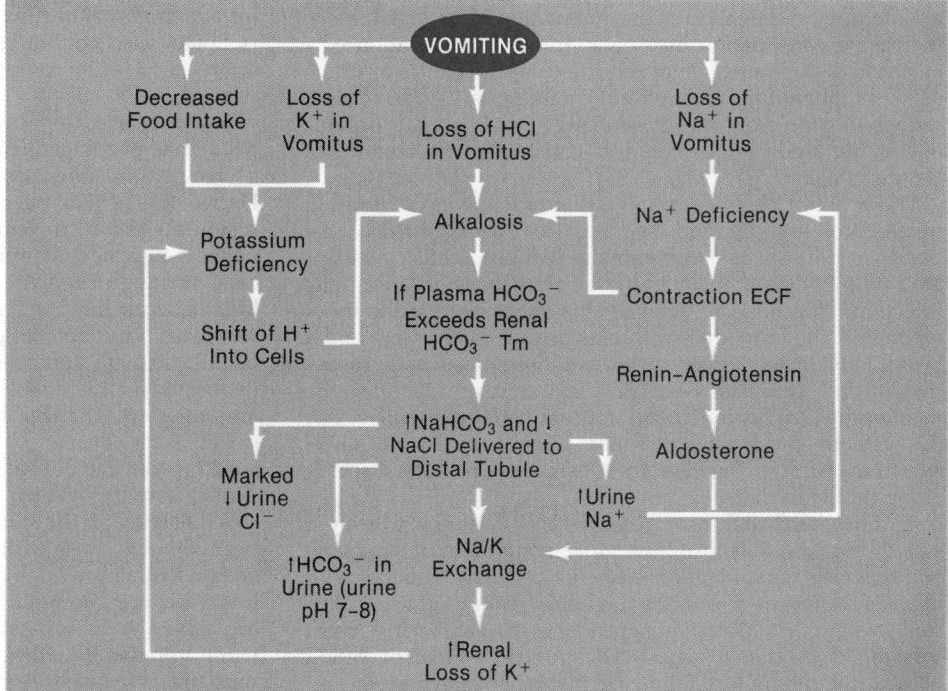

FIGURE 94–1. Metabolic consequences of vomiting. (From Feldman M: In Sleisenger MH, Fordtran JS [eds.]: Gastrointestinal Diseases. 3rd ed. Philadelphia, W. B. Saunders Company, 1983.)

dium depletion results from loss of sodium in the vomitus and, in some instances, renal loss of sodium. Urine is concentrated; a variable amount of bicarbonate is lost, depending upon whether or not the renal transport maximum (Tm) for bicarbonate is exceeded. The urinary excretion of sodium, potassium, and chloride is low if the Tm for bicarbonate is not exceeded. On the other hand, if the Tm for bicarbonate is exceeded, sodium, potassium, and bicarbonate will be high in the urine, and urine chloride will be low.

Signs and symptoms that result from the metabolic consequences of vomiting include muscle weakness, polydipsia, impaired urinary concentration, and abdominal distention (caused by hypokalemia); muscle cramps, weakness, somnolence, and even stupor (caused by hyponatremia and marked dehydration); and hypotension and low urinary output (caused by dehydration and intravascular volume contraction).

Change in Bowel Habit: Constipation and Diarrhea. Normal bowel habit ranges from one bowel movement per one to three days to three to four stools per day. Generally patients readily discern significant changes in their own pattern. Some persons may have only one stool per week or longer for many years. Severe constipation may be lifelong, as in congenital aganglionosis of the colon (Hirschsprung's disease). The definition of diarrhea is also difficult. It is not based entirely on numbers of bowel movements, although patients with diarrhea most frequently have more than three bowel movements per day. The definition most often used is based on volume—a daily stool bulk that exceeds 150 ml. A patient may have three or more small bowel movements a day but not be considered to have diarrhea. The physician who is consulted for long-standing constipation or diarrhea is obliged to investigate the complaint. Hitherto undiagnosed chronic treatable disease may be found.

Change in bowel habit must always be taken seriously even if it has occurred gradually over many months or even years. The recent onset of constipation or diarrhea may represent a reaction to stress, a change in diet, an enteric infection, malignancy of the colon, or a result of a metabolic disease. The majority of patients with nonorganic causes of constipation (bowel movement frequency of less than two per week) will increase the number of movements to three or more if placed on a high-fiber diet. A few patients will complain of lifelong inability to have bowel movements without vigorous catharsis or enemas. Such patients may also have megacolon and require investigation of the innervation of the distal colon. Increasing constipation may be a chronic manifestation of a systemic disease such as myxedema or of the effects of drugs such as phenothiazines or anticholinergics. A decreasing caliber of stool, on the other hand, may connote organic obstruction and may be due to a constricting malignancy of the distal colon.

The onset of diarrhea of more than a few weeks' duration necessitates investigation (see Ch. 103). Its significance depends in part on its accompanying features. Thus, if associated with bleeding and fever in a recent traveler, an enteric infection (shigellosis or amebiasis) is suggested. At the other extreme is the individual with diarrhea for many years and a bowel habit characterized by several loose, nonbloody movements after breakfast each day and occasionally after the evening meal. This individual appears healthy, is active, has no systemic symptoms, and most likely has irritable bowel syndrome (IBS). In between these extremes are many diseases associated with diarrhea.

Chronic diarrhea may or may not be associated with weight loss. If the patient is losing weight, the question of *malabsorption syndrome* must be addressed (see Ch. 104). Patients with this syndrome have abnormal stools—bulky, light in color, foul smelling, and greasy in appearance and character. Weight loss might be due to associated anorexia or fear of eating because of discomfort following meals, both symptoms resulting possibly from an inflammatory or malignant disease of the intestine, liver, or pancreas. Does the diarrhea persist despite the patient's abstaining from eating? If so, a secretory tumor of the pancreas, thyroid, or enterochromaffin tissue may be responsible. On the other hand, if the diarrhea is ameliorated by restricting food and fluid and if the stool water prior to such restriction has contained lower than normal concentrations of sodium and potassium, a disorder causing so-called osmotic diarrhea must be suspected. It results from the intraluminal generation of osmotically active material from unabsorbed disaccharides, hexoses, fatty acids, and amino acids. The bacterial metabolites of these substances are osmotically active, drawing fluid into the lumen of the intestine. The amount and rate of transit are such that the colon cannot reabsorb most of the water and electrolyte presented to it. A more extensive discussion of the pathophysiology of diarrhea and its differential diagnosis is presented in Ch. 103.

Gastrointestinal Bleeding. Gastrointestinal bleeding may be gross or occult. Gross bleeding may be caused by a variety of disorders, including erosions of the stomach; tears and varices of the lower esophagus; peptic ulcer of the lower esophagus, stomach, duodenum, or jejunum; angiodysplasia or other vascular anomalies (telangiectasia, blue rubber nevi, and so on); tumors of the stomach and small intestine (particularly leiomyomas); sudden, severe ischemia of the small or large intestine; diverticula of the colon; or rupture of arterial aneurysms or of bypass aortic grafts into the gut lumen. The bleeding may be dramatic clinically, particularly if bright red blood has been vomited or passed in large quantities from the rectum. Many patients, particularly those with bleeding from the upper tract (stomach, duodenum, and proximal jejunum), note only black tarry stools (melena). Regardless of the character of the bleeding, the patient's condition is determined by the amount and rapidity of loss. Most often such persons require hospitalization, emergent study, and appropriate treatment, including emergency surgery (see Ch. 114).

CARDIOVASCULAR RESPONSES TO ACUTE GASTROINTESTINAL HEMORRHAGE. Tachycardia is the earliest response to loss of blood volume in otherwise healthy persons, and it is accentuated by change in position from lying to standing. With continuing hemorrhage diastolic hypotension appears. At first it is evident only when the patient assumes an upright or standing posture; later it is present without change in position. A fall in diastolic blood pressure is not ordinarily noted until the patient has lost in excess of 20 to 25 per cent of intravascular volume within a few hours. Systolic hypotension is noted with continuing hemorrhage and also will not be appreciated early unless the patient assumes an upright posture.

The decreased cardiac output of significant acute gastrointestinal hemorrhage is manifested in the skin as coolness and a clammy moisture, occasionally with peripheral cyanosis. Decreasing cardiac output and cerebral ischemia cause confusion, agitation, or obtundation. With the upright posture, patients may note symptoms of blurred vision, roaring in the ears, vertigo, or a dizzy sensation; in severe cases or in later life, patients may suffer syncope. The aging brain is very sensitive to hypoperfusion and, hence, anoxia. In the elderly and those with compromised cerebral circulation, hypoperfusion may initiate cerebral thromboses. Even in those who are still alert, changes in the electroencephalogram may be noted.

Fall in cardiac output is often accompanied by changes in cardiac function. Thus, patients with significant arteriosclerotic disease of the coronary arteries may develop angina pectoris, and even without pain ischemic changes on the electrocardiogram such as ST segment depression or T wave inversion are common. On occasion the patient suffers an acute myocardial infarction. Oliguria is a common manifestation in patients with severe blood loss from the gastrointestinal tract. At onset of bleeding, urinary osmolality and specific gravity are increased and sodium concentrations are usually less than 20 mEq per liter. With severe shock and marked renal hypoperfusion, acute cortical or tubular necrosis may supervene. The gastrointestinal tract itself is not immune from the manifestations of a severe decrease in cardiac output brought about by hypovolemia. The liver is not severely injured unless hypotension is severe and prolonged. However, the tubular gastrointestinal tract (particularly the small bowel beyond the ligament of Treitz, cecum, transverse colon, and descending colon, may suffer the effects of ischemia (see Ch. 106). Nonocclusive ischemia of these areas of the tubular gastrointestinal tract can be associated with a rapid deterioration of the patient.

With occult bleeding, patients may or may not have other symptoms indicative of disturbance in a particular part of the gastrointestinal tract. Many elderly persons complain of the effects of a progressive anemia. Unexplained iron deficiency with stools containing occult blood in such patients often reflects carcinoma of the cecum and right colon. Between these extremes are patients who intermittently pass small amounts of blood by rectum. These are patients who must be suspected of having malignancy, ischemia, or inflammatory disease of the distal colon. Chronic occult bleeding in elderly persons, particularly those with aortic valve disease, may be due to angiodysplastic lesions of the gut, particularly of the cecum and right colon.

Intestinal Gas. Patients are frequently bothered by symptoms caused by intestinal gas. These are *eructation*, the distress of *bloating* with borborygmi, and *excessive flatus*.

The major intraluminal gases are nitrogen (N_2), carbon dioxide (CO_2), and methane (CH_4); all these gases but N_2 are produced in the bowel lumen. About 600 ml of gas is passed per rectum per day, of which over 400 ml is produced enterically. The amount of hydrogen and CO_2 depends to a significant degree upon the diet. Unabsorbed carbohydrate and protein, particularly greens and vegetables, are broken down by colonic bacteria to yield hydrogen and carbon dioxide. CH_4 is produced by only about one third of the adult population.

Although complaints referable to intestinal gas have classically been attributed to excessive air swallowing, it is clear that this habit is not responsible for a major contribution either to the amount of intestinal gas or to the symptoms. Normally, swallowed air is quickly expelled. It may cause distress in only a very limited number of persons who do not normally expel it.

ERUCTATION (BELCHING). Air that is expelled by belching is usually that recently swallowed into the esophagus. Repeated belching may on occasion be associated with serious organic disease, particularly with gastric outlet obstruction or gastric dilatation. The vast majority of patients who belch frequently in order to relieve distress are overanxious (constantly swallowing air, thus the word "aerophagia").

ABDOMINAL DISTRESS OF DISTENTION (BLOATING). Bloating and "gas pains" have classically and erroneously been thought to be due to excessive gas. In fact, abnormal intestinal motor activity usually accounts for these symptoms. Usually, the intestinal contents move along in an orderly fashion, stimulated particularly by eating. Disorders of motility both in the small bowel and in the colon may move gas faster than normal. However, there may be areas of resistance to rapid passage owing to organic disease or, more commonly, to motor dysfunction associated with spasm, noted particularly in the irritable bowel syndrome. Bowel proximal to a narrowed area dilates, whether narrowing is a stricture or spasm, stretching the smooth muscle and eliciting pain of a cramping nature. Organic causes of disturbed motility may also underlie these symptoms, e.g., progressive intestinal obstruction caused by a stricture or tumor. Recent onset of these complaints always warrants thorough investigation.

The *irritable bowel syndrome* is associated with a motor disturbance and often with abdominal bloating. The discomfort of these patients may indeed be due to gas, albeit in normal amounts. It may be alleviated by dietary exclusion of gas-forming foods, including lactose, thus relieving complaints of many years to decades.

EXCESSIVE FLATUS (GAS PER RECTUM). Excessive flatus results from ingesting foods notorious as substrates for gas formation, from an overgrowth of gas-producing bacteria in the gastrointestinal tract, or from malabsorption of carbohydrates (e.g., lactase deficiency). Patients have excessive gas resulting from bacterial action on unabsorbed carbohydrate in the colon (or in the small gut if there is bacterial overgrowth), with release of hydrogen as the most important gas but also of CO_2. Only about one third of normal individuals produce intestinal methane, but a larger number (80 per cent) of patients with cancer of the colon do so. Methane production presumably reflects a special bacterial colonization of the colon. Some patients have normal amounts of flatus per day but complain of increased frequency of flatus following a meal. This complaint is most likely due to a hyperactive gastrocolic reflex, which characterizes many patients with irritable bowel syndrome.

Patients who pass more than a normal amount of gas may complain of bloating and pain. Analysis of flatus demonstrates unusually high percentages of hydrogen and carbon dioxide. Whether it is due to a particular disease of the small intestine, pancreatic insufficiency, bacterial overgrowth of the small intestine, or lactase deficiency requires definition. Excessive colonic production of gas also may be caused by the ingestion of abnormal amounts of fruit and vegetables which contain nonabsorbable carbohydrates, and may respond to dietary restriction of lactose, legumes, and wheat.

Jaundice. Jaundice is due to elevated levels of either conjugated or unconjugated bilirubin in plasma and extracellular fluid. It is a common and important sign of disease of the liver or biliary tract, or of hemolysis. Hyperbilirubinemia may result from excessive production of bilirubin (hemolysis), reduced excretion of bilirubin into the bile (liver disease), or obstruction of the flow of bile into the intestine (biliary tract disease). Rarely jaundice is caused by hereditary diseases producing defects in the hepatic uptake of bilirubin or its glucuronidation. Impaired capacity to secrete conjugated bilirubin into the bile may also be due to inherited metabolic defects. The pathophysiology of bilirubin metabolism is discussed in greater detail in Ch. 118.

Jaundice is not usually detectable in natural light below plasma bilirubin levels of 2 to 2.5 mg per deciliter. Jaundice caused by conjugated bilirubin is associated with dark urine, since conjugated bilirubin is water soluble and therefore excreted in the urine. On the other hand, nonconjugated bilirubin is lipid soluble and protein bound so that it is not excreted in the urine.

The most common cause of jaundice is injury to the hepatocyte by virus, toxin, or drug. The clinical significance of jaundice in a patient therefore depends to a large extent on its duration, intensity, and relationship to possible infection or drug use, and on the presence or absence of factors that may cause obstruction (cholelithiasis). Gradual obstruction of the extrahepatic ductal system with progressive jaundice in an elderly person not taking hepatotoxic drugs and with no evidence of viral infection most frequently indicates *choledocholithiasis*, malignancy of the bile ducts (*cholangiocarcinomas*), or a *periampullary malignancy*. In jaundice due to choledocholithiasis, serum bilirubin rarely exceeds 12.0 mg per deciliter but is commonly much higher with periampullary or bile duct malignancies. *Pruritus* is common in many patients with jaundice; it may be due to severe intrahepatic cholestasis, extrahepatic obstruction, recurrent jaundice of pregnancy, or primary biliary cirrhosis.

Low-grade fever (100° to 101°F) usually accompanies viral or alcoholic hepatitis and, occasionally occurs in so-called *sclerosing cholangitis,* but is dramatically high (102° to 104°F) in cholangitis due to choledocholithiasis. Careful search on physical examination for evidences of liver disease is crucial in evaluating patients with jaundice. The presence of masses, particularly of a palpable gallbladder, indicating long-standing progressive common bile duct obstruction by cancer (*Courvoisier's sign*), is a most important finding. In many instances, the routine laboratory examinations, including liver function tests, are of great help but must be interpreted with caution. The differential diagnosis of jaundice may require use of the specialized diagnostic techniques discussed in Ch. 95 and 96.

Most patients with gastrointestinal disease complain of one (or more) of the symptoms and demonstrate some of the signs that have been discussed. The significance attached to these signs and symptoms determines which road to diagnosis and treatment will be taken. This approach to patients ensures intelligent reference to detailed descriptions of the clinical possibilities and leads to wise choices of tests and procedures. In the chapters that follow, symptoms and signs will be more fully described in terms of specific diseases of the various organs constituting the digestive system, and a wide range of diagnostic tests and procedures will be included. In this way the science of medicine and gastroenterology is brought to bear on good patient care.

Baile CA, McLaughlin CL, Della-Fera MA: Role of cholecystokinin and opioid peptides in control of food intake. Physiol Rev 66:172, 1986. *A comprehensive review of the complex regulation of food intake with emphasis upon the role of neuropeptides that act upon hypothalamic centers.*

Sleisenger MH, Fordtran JS: Gastrointestinal Disease. 4th ed. Philadelphia, W. B. Saunders Company, 1988. Chapters 1, 9, 10, 14, 15, 17, 20, 22, 25, and 28.

95 DIAGNOSTIC IMAGING PROCEDURES IN GASTROENTEROLOGY

Susan D. Wall

With the development of increasingly complex diagnostic imaging procedures in gastroenterology, the importance of direct communication with the consulting radiologist has increased. Clinical information regarding each diagnostic question is essential to tailoring the studies; none are "routine." In addition to conventional plain films of the abdomen and barium examination of the gastrointestinal tract, radiographic procedures of interest to the gastroenterologist include computed tomography, ultrasonography, endoscopic retrograde cholangiopancreatography, percutaneous transhepatic cholangiography, enteroclysis, radionuclide scanning, and magnetic resonance imaging.

COMPUTED TOMOGRAPHY

The faster scan time (two to three seconds) and higher spatial resolution available with current computed tomography (CT) have improved greatly the images of the alimentary tract as well as of the pancreas (Fig. 95–1), liver, and gallbladder. Computed tomography continues to be an important modality for the investigation of possible hepatic tumor, pancreatic carcinoma, and retroperitoneal adenopathy. Less well known is its contribution to the evaluation of the acute abdomen. When the diagnosis is unclear, CT is helpful in diagnosing possible pancreatitis (Fig. 95–2), perforated viscus, and subdiaphragmatic abscess and in assessing the extent of Crohn's disease or bowel ischemia. It can detect extraluminal abscess associated with appendicitis and diverticulitis (Fig. 95–3) and can sometimes help in the decision regarding

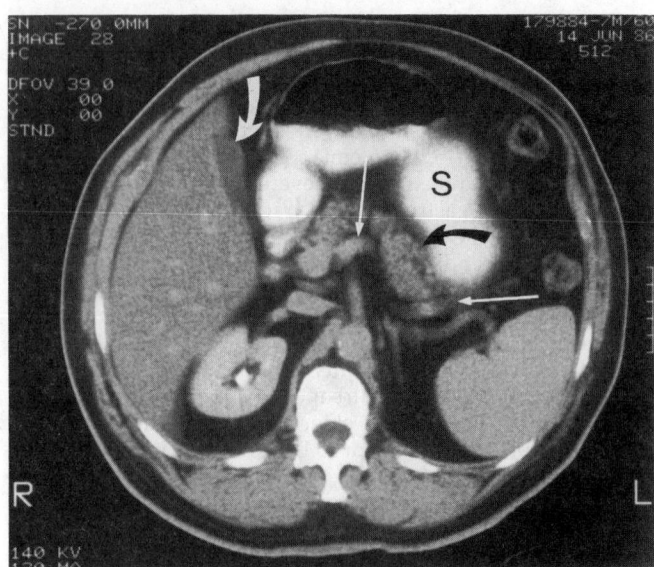

FIGURE 95–1. Normal computed tomogram. One cm thick transverse image (supine, patient's right to reader's left) is at the level of the pancreas (*black arrow*), which is behind the contrast filled stomach (S). The splenic artery is posterior to the splenic vein (*straight white arrows*), which abuts the posterior margin of the tail and neck of the pancreas. The density of the right kidney is enhanced because of intravenous contrast material. *Curved white arow* points to gallbladder.

surgical versus nonsurgical management. Computed tomography also can detect free intra- (Fig. 95–4) or retroperitoneal air and small amounts of contrast material that have extravasated from the gastrointestinal tract (Fig. 95–3); it provides excellent visualization of the mesentery. It is the modality of choice for evaluation of suspected complications of pancreatitis, such as abscess, pseudocyst, and colonic or mesenteric inflammation.

Percutaneous fine needle aspiration (PFNA) with CT guidance can diagnose pancreatic carcinoma, primary and metastatic tumor of the liver, and sometimes tumor involvement of enlarged lymph nodes. False-negative results occur, but this procedure often obviates the need for diagnostic laparotomy. Furthermore, PFNA can diagnose suspected abscess (Fig. 95–3), which can be variable and nonspecific in its radiographic appearance. Percutaneous drainage of intra-abdominal or pelvic abscess with CT guidance is a nonsurgical treatment option for selected patients; it can palliate others until surgery is performed.

Computed tomography sometimes replaces barium contrast examination as the initial study of the gastrointestinal tract. Barium examination, which provides mucosal detail and delineation of the intraluminal contour, cannot demonstrate thickening of the wall and causes severe artifact on CT images, precluding the possibility of a diagnostic study. Moreover, even unsuspected disease in the gastrointestinal tract, both primary and secondary, often is detected initially with CT. Assessment of thickening of the esophageal, gastric, and bowel wall is possible with current CT, and surrounding organs may also be evaluated, especially regarding inflammatory processes such as diverticulitis, appendicitis, Crohn's disease, pancreatitis, and possible perforated ulcer. Computed tomography has limited value in the regional staging of gastrointestinal malignancies because of its limited accuracy in determining tumor invasion into adjacent tissues. Indications for preoperative evaluation of patients with rectosigmoid colon carcinoma, for example, include suspected extensive disease or complications such as perforation. Computed tomography is more helpful in determining recurrence postoperatively. A baseline study is performed two to four months after resection, with follow-up comparison studies every six months for two years. New or enlarging masses in the pelvis

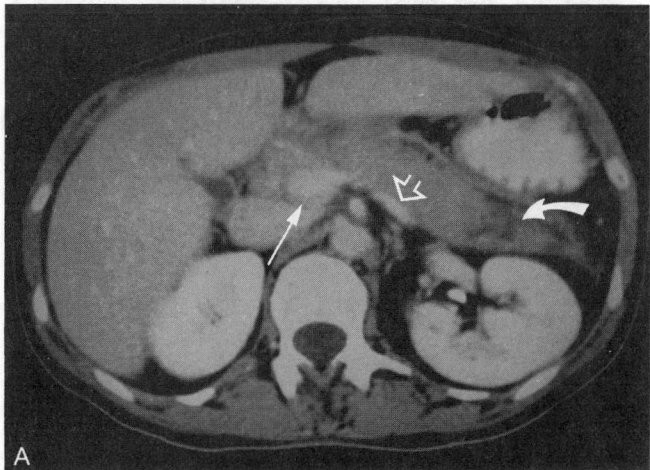

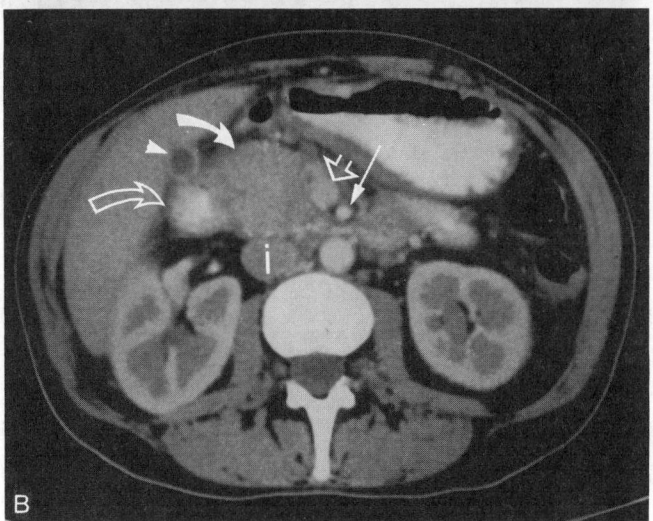

FIGURE 95–2. Computed tomography of pancreatitis. *A,* The body and tail of the pancreas are enlarged. Ill-defined area of low density (*curved arrow*) in the pancreatic parenchyma represents early finding of developing pseudocyst. The enhanced splenic vein (*open arrowhead*) and splenoportal confluence (*straight arrow*) delineate the posterior margin of the pancreas. *B,* The head of the pancreas (*closed curved arrow*), which is swollen, is surrounded by the contrast-filled duodenum (*open curved arrow*) laterally and the inferior vena cava (i) posteriorly. The gallbladder (*closed arrowhead*), superior mesenteric vein (*open arrow*), and superior mesenteric artery (*straight arrow*) are seen. Early intravenous bolus enhancement of the kidneys provides cortical-medullary differentiation.

suggest recurrent tumor; CT-guided biopsy can be performed for tissue diagnosis.

Bret PM, Fond A, Casola G, et al.: Abdominal lesions: A prospective study of clinical efficacy of percutaneous fine-needle biopsy. Radiology 159:345, 1986. *An excellent prospective study and discussion of the influence of percutaneous fine needle biopsy on diagnostic workup, therapeutic choice, and cost benefit.*

Quint LE, Glazer GM, Orringer MB, et al.: Esophageal carcinoma: CT findings. Radiology 155:171, 1985. *A review of the literature and report of their findings; the latter indicates low accuracy of staging CT.*

Thompson WM, Halvorsen RA, Foster WL Jr, et al.: Preoperative and postoperative CT staging rectosigmoid carcinoma. Am J Roentgenol 146:703, 1986. *An excellent review of the literature and of their experience.*

ULTRASONOGRAPHY

Abdominal ultrasonography (US) is noninvasive, requires no ionizing radiation, and can be performed with a portable unit. In experienced hands it has excellent results; operator dependence is decreasing as equipment improves. Ultrasonography is superior to other modalities in differentiating cystic from solid lesions and is highly sensitive in detecting ascites. Because of the superb ability to demonstrate gallstones (Fig. 95–5), US has replaced oral cholecystography for the diagnosis

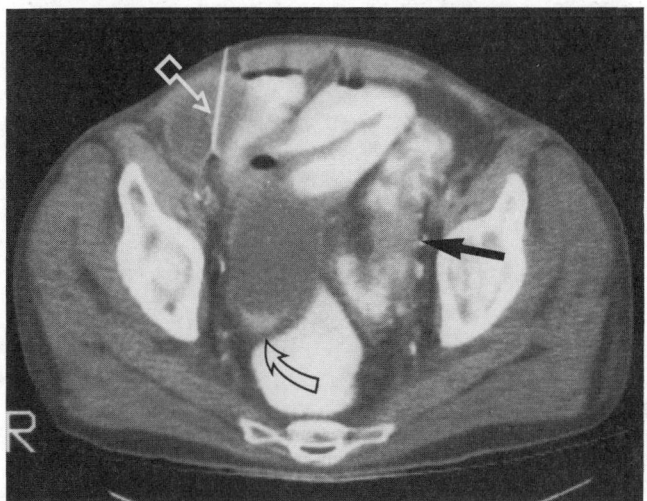

FIGURE 95–3. Computed tomography of diverticular abscess. Percutaneous fine-needle aspiration (*boxed white arrow*) of pelvic fluid collection diagnosed abscess in this patient with thickening of the wall of the sigmoid colon (*straight black arrow*) and diverticulitis. Note second fluid collection with small amount of contrast material (*curved black arrow*) extravasated from the diseased colon. Abscesses were drained percutaneously until the patient was well enough for surgery.

of cholelithiasis. It is an effective and efficient first examination for suspected liver tumors. Ultrasonography is the primary screening examination for hepatobiliary disease and often is the only study needed. Dilatation of the intra-and extrahepatic biliary system can be detected (Fig. 95–6), but the distal common bile duct often is not seen adequately with US. Similarly, the tail or body of the pancreas or both are well visualized less often than the head, principally because of interference by the overlying gas-filled bowel. Ultrasonography, which plays a complementary role with CT in many diseases, often is the preferred modality when follow-up examination is needed, as in pancreatic pseudocyst, abdominal aortic aneurysm, and drained fluid collections. Percutaneous fine needle aspiration and drainage procedures can be performed with ultrasonographic guidance, sometimes with greater ease and less cost compared with CT.

Recent advances in ultrasound involve the application of a transducer to an exposed organ at surgery or through an

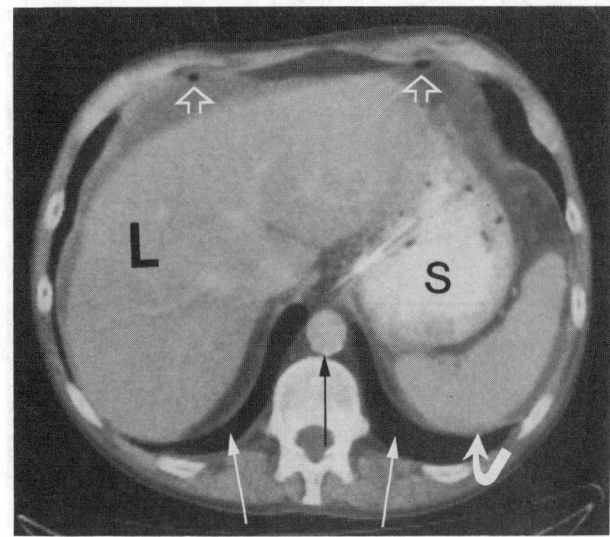

FIGURE 95–4. Computed tomography of pneumoperitoneum. Two small collections of free intraperitoneal air (*open arrows*) are seen in the nondependent areas of the upper abdomen in this patient with colon perforation. Note the air-filled lungs (*straight white arrows*), spleen (*curved arrow*), stomach (S), and liver (L). The aorta (*black arrow*) is anterior to the spine.

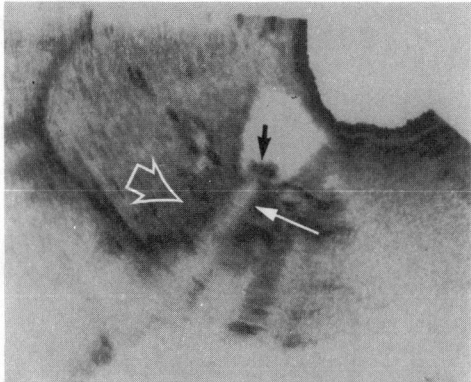

FIGURE 95–5. Ultrasound of cholelithiasis. Sagittal image (patient's head to reader's left) demonstrates a single gallstone (*black arrow*). The sound waves easily pass through the fluid (bile) in the gallbladder—hence the "posterior acoustical enhancement" (*open arrow*) characteristic of a cystic structure. The echogenic stone impedes the sound waves—hence the "posterior shadowing" (*straight white arrow*) characteristic of a gallstone. This "static" ultrasound image produces black echoes on white background.

endoscope. Ultrasonography has facilitated the intraoperative search for pancreatic islet cell tumor and occasionally finds unsuspected multiple tumors. Endosonography requires an end-viewing fiberoptic gastroscope, which is modified to incorporate a transducer. Although still in the developmental stage, this new imaging procedure has been shown to demonstrate the thickness of the esophagus, stomach, and duodenum and to identify both diffuse and focal intramural lesions. It may also be valuable for diagnosis of early pancreatic lesions.

Cummings S, Papadakis M, Melnick J, et al.: The predictive value of physical examination of ascites. West J Med 142:633, 1985. *Excellent comparison of ultrasonography and physical examination in detecting ascites with a useful list of references.*
Gordon SJ, Rifkin MD, Goldberg BB: Endosonographic evaluation of mural abnormalities of the upper gastrointestinal tract. Gastrointest Endosc 32:193, 1986. *A good presentation of some of the early work with this procedure.*
Jeffrey RB Jr, Laing FC, Wing VW: Extrapancreatic spread of acute pancreatitis: New observations with real-time US. Radiology 159:707, 1986. *A succinct comparison of US and CT in acute pancreatitis with state of the art equipment by experts in the field.*

ENDOSCOPIC RETROGRADE CHOLANGIOPANCREATOGRAPHY

Endoscopic retrograde cholangiopancreatography (ERCP) is performed with the fluoroscopic guidance of the radiologist.

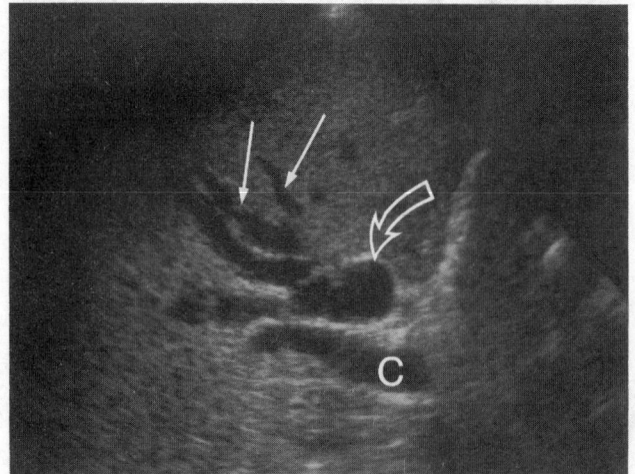

FIGURE 95–6. Ultrasound of dilated bile ducts. Dilatation of the intrahepatic (*straight arrows*) and extrahepatic (*curved arrow*) bile ducts is well demonstrated on the sagittal ultrasound image of a patient with distal biliary obstruction. (C indicates the inferior vena cava.) This real-time ultrasound image produces white echoes on black background.

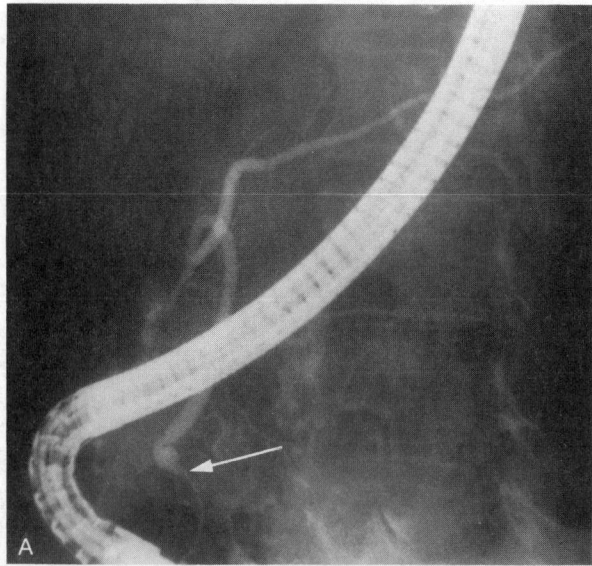

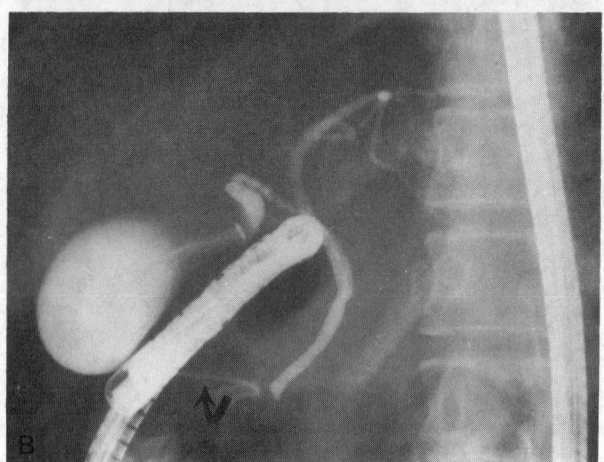

FIGURE 95–7. Normal endoscopic retrograde cholangiopancreatogram. *A,* Normal pancreatogram. The cannula (*arrow*) at the tip of the fiberoptic endoscope has been inserted into the papilla of Vater under direct visualization and the pancreatic duct opacified. *B,* Normal cholangiogram. The gallbladder, cystic duct, common hepatic duct, and common bile duct are visible. *Arrow* indicates cannula in the papilla of Vater.

The papilla of Vater is visualized through a fiberoptic endoscope, and the common bile duct or the pancreatic duct or both are cannulated. Water-soluble iodinated contrast material is injected, and images are taken of the opacified biliary tree or pancreatic duct (Fig. 95–7). ERCP is performed specifically to evaluate the pancreatic duct or follows US or CT demonstrating distal biliary obstruction. When a constricting or obstructing lesion is seen in the distal common bile duct, biopsy or papillotomy can be performed. A further discussion of ERCP is contained in Ch. 76.

TRANSHEPATIC CHOLANGIOGRAPHY

Percutaneous transhepatic cholangiography is used to visualize the intra- and extrahepatic biliary tree following CT, US, or ERCP that has demonstrated proximal obstruction of the common hepatic or common bile duct. It is performed by injecting water-soluble iodinated contrast material through a flexible 23-gauge needle introduced percutaneously into the intrahepatic biliary tree under fluoroscopic guidance. After the biliary tree is opacified, multiple radiographs are taken in order to characterize the suspected site of blockage or narrowing (Fig. 95–8). This study provides the surgeon with the best demonstration of possible anastomotic sites of the biliary tree in the porta hepatis. Serious complications such as bile peri-

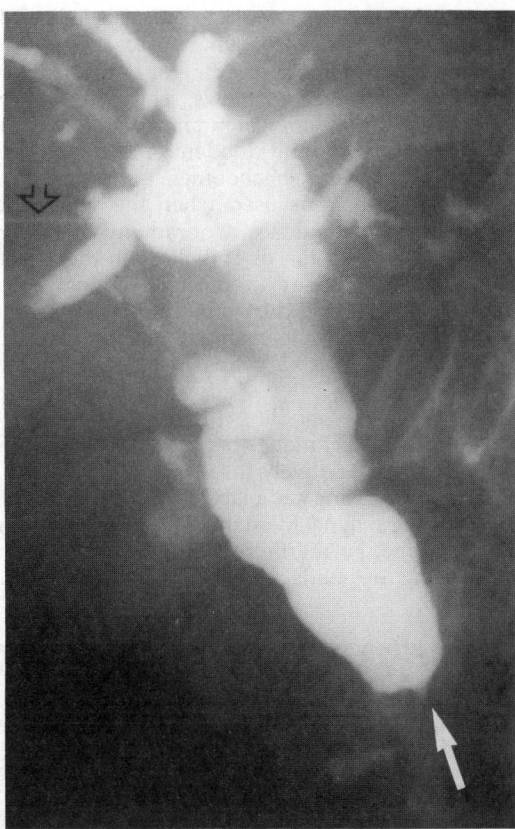

FIGURE 95–8. Percutaneous transhepatic cholangiogram. Dilatation of the biliary tree is demonstrated after percutaneous puncture and opacification of a dilated intrahepatic duct with a long 23-gauge needle (*open black arrow*). The distal common bile duct is abruptly narrowed and obstructed (*white arrow*) owing to cholangiocarcinoma.

tonitis or intraperitoneal hemorrhage occur in less than 2 per cent of cases. Biliary obstruction can be treated in patients who are poor surgical risks by several interventional procedures, including percutaneous stricture dilatation, percutaneous drainage, or insertion of a biliary endoprosthesis. The last procedure can be performed percutaneously or via an ERCP in conjunction with a percutaneous transhepatic technique.

Lammer J, Neumayer K: Biliary drainage endoprostheses: Experience with 201 placements. Radiology 159:625, 1986. *An excellent discussion of procedure, complications, and patient tolerance.*

ENTEROCLYSIS

Procedures used to study the small bowel include the "dedicated" small bowel follow-through, single- and double-contrast enteroclysis, and the peroral pneumocolon. Examination of the small bowel should not accompany most studies of the esophagus, stomach, and/or duodenum because the high-density barium used for the latter interferes with visualization of detail of the small bowel, especially the jejunum. Consequently, lesions that are present may be seen poorly or may be missed, and often it is nearly impossible to exclude abnormality. Hence, the traditional "upper gastrointestinal series with small bowel follow-through" is no longer the optimal examination for small intestinal disease. An exception to this is the patient in whom the terminal ileum is the only suspected site of involvement. In this case, the peroral pneumocolon may be the most precise approach. It is performed with introduction of insufflated air per rectum when orally administered thin barium has reached the cecum. With reflux of air across the ileocecal valve, double-contrast images of the terminal ileum are obtained.

Enteroclysis, also known as small bowel enema, refers to the direct introduction of contrast material after intubation of the first loop of jejunum or, less optimally, the distal duodenum. It allows for a controlled rate of delivery of contrast material independent of gastric emptying and thus optimizes luminal distention. The double-contrast method uses air or methylcellulose to provide fine detail to the folds of the small bowel. Enteroclysis has been advocated as the most accurate method for the detection of focal lesions in the small bowel. However, it is comparable to a dedicated (tubeless) small bowel study for the detection of lesions due to Crohn's disease and tumor and is only slightly more sensitive for adhesions. A dedicated small bowel study does not immediately follow examination of the esophagus, stomach, or duodenum; it is performed with frequent, intermittent spot films by the radiologist. Enteroclysis, which is more lengthy and requires more expertise by the radiologist, is tolerated less well by the patient and, most importantly, involves a much greater radiation exposure.

Ott DJ, Chen YM, Gelfand DW, et al.: Detailed per-oral small bowel examination vs. enteroclysis. Part I: Expenditures and radiation exposure, and Part II: Radiographic accuracy. Radiology 155:29, 1985. *An excellent comparison study of these two modalities; the enteroclysis technique was single contrast.*

Wolf KJ, Goldberg HI, Wall SD, et al.: Peroral pneumocolon: The usefulness in evaluating the normal and abnormal ileocecal region. *A study of 170 patients; demonstrates its value in detecting ulcerations, edematous mucosa, and cobblestone patterns.*

RADIONUCLIDE IMAGING

Acute cholecystitis is usually due to obstruction of the cystic duct by a calculus. Scanning with technetium-labeled iminodiacetic acid (^{99m}TcHIDA), which is excreted by the hepatobiliary system, is valuable when such a diagnosis is in question. Visualization of the liver, bile ducts, gallbladder, and bowel occurs within 60 minutes of injection in normal, fasting patients (Fig. 95–9). Visualization of the gallbladder excludes the diagnosis of obstruction of the cystic duct. Nonvisualization of the gallbladder with normal visualization of the common bile duct and bowel indicates cystic duct obstruction (Fig. 95–10). Nonvisualization of both the gallbladder and the bowel can occur in conditions involving cholestasis without cystic duct obstruction, such as hepatocellular disease, total parenteral nutrition, and obstruction of the distal common bile duct. Ultrasonography is more sensitive regarding the detection of gallstone but is less accurate in the diagnosis of acute cholecystitis.

Gastric mucosa secretes ^{99m}Tc pertechnetate. It can be used to detect ectopic gastric mucosa, especially in Meckel's diverticulum and sometimes in Barrett's esophagus. Ectopic gastric mucosa is present in most symptomatic Meckel's diverticula and in nearly all that bleed, but only half of the bleeding Meckel's diverticula in adults are detected by this study. False-positive results are common. This method of detecting Meckel's diverticulum is far more useful in children.

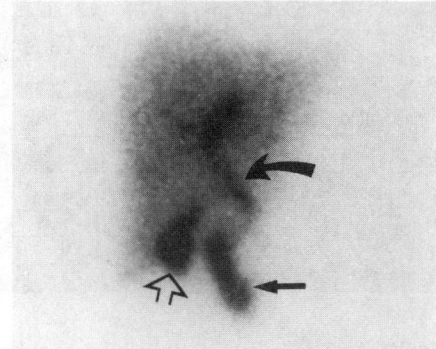

FIGURE 95–9. Normal Tc HIDA scan. Technetium-99m labeled iminodiacetic acid (HIDA) has been excreted by the liver in this normal, fasting patient. Within 60 minutes of intravenous injection, there is visualization of the common bile duct (*curved arrow*), gallbladder (*open arrow*), and duodenum (*straight arrow*).

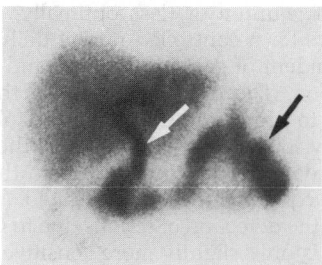

FIGURE 95–10. Tc HIDA of acute cholecystitis. Visualization of the common bile duct (*white arrow*) and small bowel (*black arrow*) without visualization of the gallbladder indicated obstruction of the cystic duct in this fasting patient with acute cholecystitis.

There are two nuclear medicine procedures available for the detection of acute and chronic gastrointestinal bleeding sites, both of which rely upon the extravasation of the radionuclide into the intestinal lumen. Injected ⁹⁹ᵐTc sulfur colloid remains in the circulation only briefly, and therefore its use requires active bleeding (approximately 2 ml per minute) at the time of the study. This disadvantage, which is shared with angiography, does not apply to ⁹⁹ᵐTc-labeled autologous erythrocytes because they remain in circulation. With the latter procedure, intermittent bleeding of 10 to 20 ml per hour may be detected on delayed views. The reliability of both procedures is greater for the colon and small bowel than for the esophagus, stomach, and duodenum because of overlapping structures in the upper abdomen. *Angiography* for gastrointestinal hemorrhage is used when the site of bleeding cannot be identified by endoscopy or radionuclide imaging or when transcatheter infusion or embolization therapy is indicated. Visceral angiography of most abdominal pathologic conditions has been replaced by other diagnostic procedures, but it is indicated still in the evaluation of vascular occlusive disease, in polysystemic vasculitis, and preoperatively for hepatic tumors.

Disorders of gastric motility are not well evaluated by barium radiographic techniques because these techniques are not quantitative, are relatively insensitive, and are not physiologic. Procedures using radiolabeled food with continuous gastric monitoring may yield quantitative data such as gastric half-emptying time. Furthermore, with radionuclide imaging, gastric emptying of solids versus liquids can be assessed simultaneously.

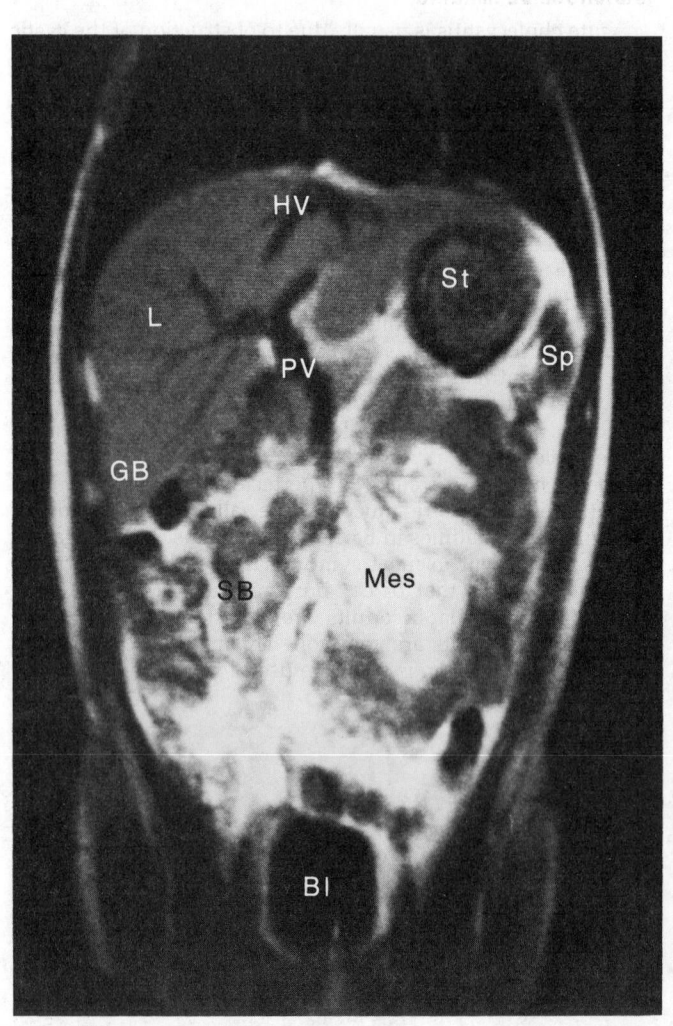

A

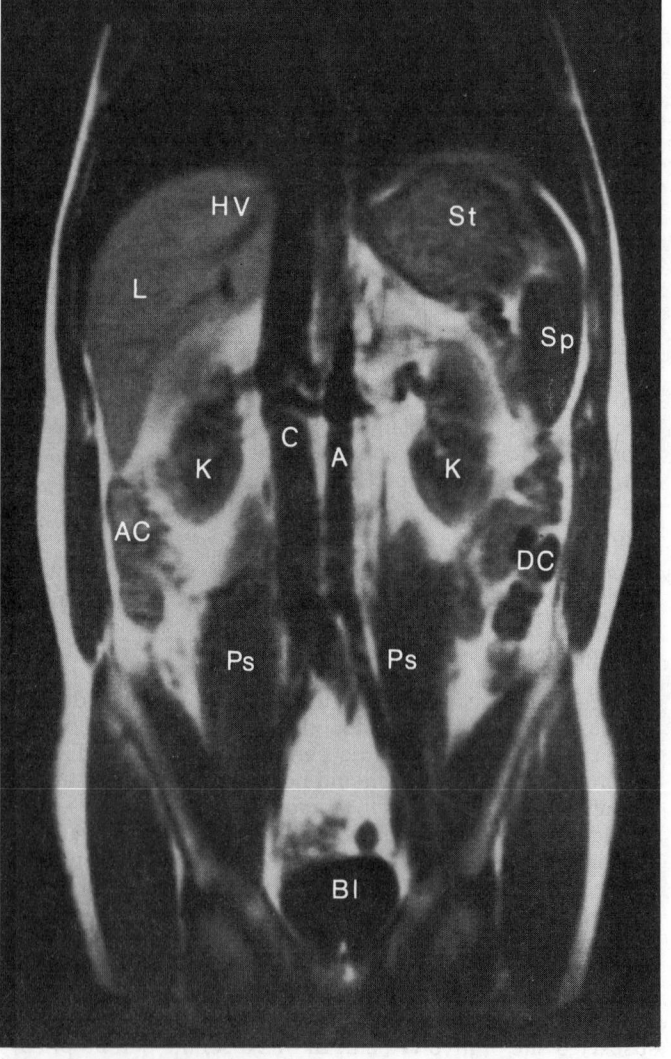

B

FIGURE 95–11. Normal abdominal magnetic resonance. *A*, T1 weighted coronal image of the anterior abdomen demonstrates the liver (L), spleen (Sp), stomach (St), gallbladder (GB), hepatic veins (HV), portal vein (PV), small bowel (SB), mesentery (Mes), and urinary bladder (B1). *B*, T1 weighted coronal image of the posterior abdomen demonstrates the inferior vena cava (C), aorta (A), kidneys (K), ascending colon (AC), descending colon (DC), and psoas muscles (Ps) in addition to the structures noted in the anterior abdomen in *A*. (Courtesy of General Electric Company, Milwaukee, WI.)

Intravenous injection of indium 111–labeled leukocytes is sometimes indicated in the febrile patient, especially if symptomatic less than two weeks with an acute inflammatory process of uncertain origin. This technique has a sensitivity of 85 to 90 per cent and a specificity of 90 to 95 per cent. Importantly, for the detection of abscess, it can be performed with a portable unit for the patient too ill to go to the radiology department for other imaging procedures.

Liver scanning with ^{99m}Tc-sulfur colloid is used for the assessment of size, shape, and position; identification of space-occupying lesions such as tumor, abscess, or hematoma; and evaluation of hepatocellular disease. Sensitivity for the detection of primary and metastatic tumor is comparable to that of CT (which is slightly more accurate) and that of US (which is slightly less sensitive). The newer technique of liver scanning with SPECT (single photon emission computed tomography) imaging produces three-dimensional cross-sectional tomographic images and eliminates the overlapping influences of the surrounding radioactivity. Thus, the sensitivity for small (2 cm) space-occupying lesions is increased.

Arnstein NB, Shapiro B, Eckhauser FI, et al.: Morbid obesity treated by gastroplasty: Radionuclide gastric emptying studies. Radiology 156:501, 1985. *A study of 50 postgastroplasty patients by experts in radionuclide imaging.*

Kudo M, Hirasa M, Takakuwa H, et al.: Small hepatocellular carcinomas in chronic liver disease: Detection with SPECT. Radiology 159:697, 1986. *Comparison with US, CT, angiography, and alpha-fetoprotein.*

Schwartz MJ, Lewis JH: Meckel's diverticulum: Pitfalls in scintigraphic detection in the adult. Am J Gastroenterol 79:611, 1984. *A review of 37 Meckel scan studies in addition to their own experience; emphasis on adults.*

MAGNETIC RESONANCE IMAGING

A very brief and simplified summary of the physics of magnetic resonance (MR) imaging is presented here as a background. Hydrogen nuclei (protons) have a dipole moment and therefore behave as would a magnetic compass. In MR scanning, the protons align with the strong magnetic field but are easily perturbed by a brief radiofrequency (RF) pulse of very low energy and then are altered in their alignment. As the protons return to their orientation with the magnetic field, they release energy of a radiofrequency that is strongly influenced by the biochemical environment. T1 and T2 relaxation times are a description of the released energy, which is detected, mathematically analyzed, and displayed as a two-dimensional proton-density map according to the "signal intensity" of each tissue. Because the water molecule contains two hydrogen nuclei, changes in distribution of water in tissue, as well as its overall concentration, strongly influence the "intensity" of the MR signal. Hence, MR can provide superior contrast differentiation of tissues with varying amounts of water compared with conventional radiographic modalities, which depend only upon the attenuation of the roentgenographic beam. In addition, fat emits a strong signal because of the abundance of lipid protons. Other advantages of MR include its noninvasiveness, lack of ionizing radiation, and ability to image directly in transaxial, sagittal, coronal (Fig. 95–11), and nonorthogonal planes. Its disadvantages include cost, limited availability, slow scanning time, and problems associated with the powerful magnetic field. The last-named precludes imaging patients with a cardiac pacemaker or metallic clips on intracranial blood vessels. Moreover, critically ill patients cannot easily be monitored because of limited access to the patient during the study and because the strong magnetic field prohibits the presence of resuscitative equipment made of metal.

Physiologic motion limits the diagnostic capability of MR in

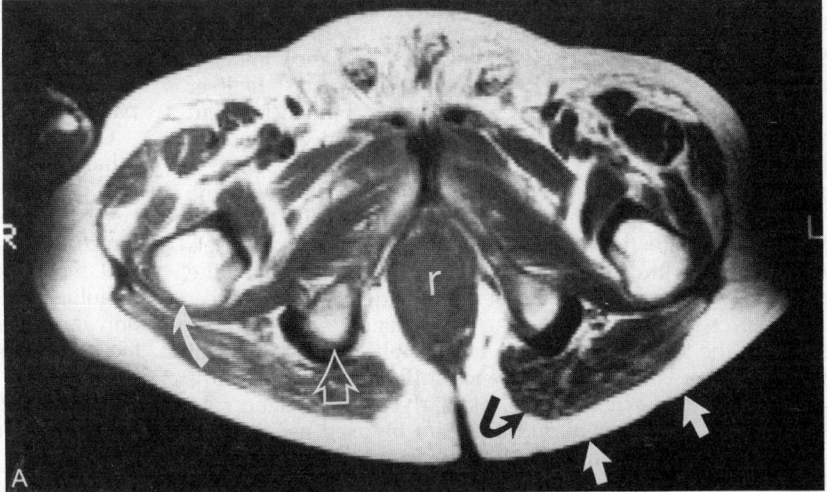
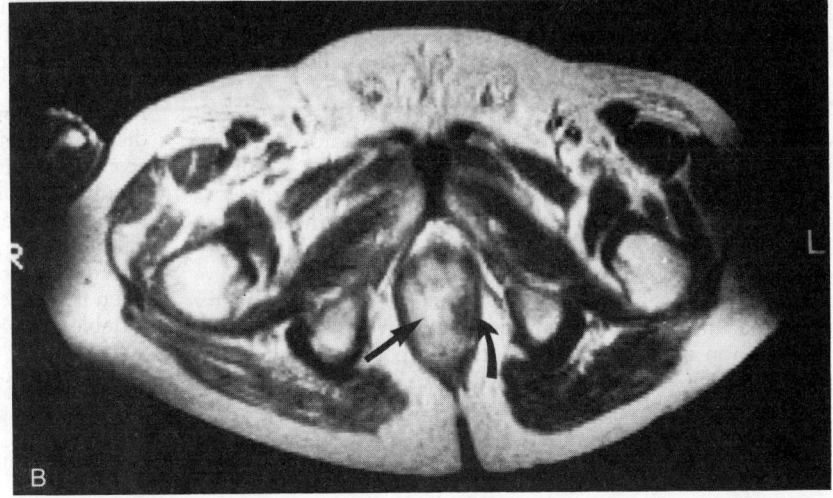

FIGURE 95–12. Magnetic resonance of rectal tumor. *A,* Transverse T1 weighted image (TR = 0.5 sec, TE = 30 msec) demonstrates thickening of the rectum (r) due to cloacogenic carcinoma, which is isointense with the surrounding uninvolved muscle. Normal structures demonstrated include the gluteus muscle (*curved black arrow*), which is emitting a low-intensity signal, subcutaneous fat (*white arrows*), which is emitting a high-intensity signal, the right ischium (*open arrow*) and the right femoral head (*curved white arrow*). *B,* T2 weighted image of the same area demonstrates a relative increase in the signal intensity of the tumor (*straight arrow*) because of prolongation of its T2 relaxation time. It now can be differentiated from the adjacent, noninvolved muscle (*curved arrow*), which has retained a normal low-intensity signal. (Courtesy of Diasonics, San Francisco, CA.)

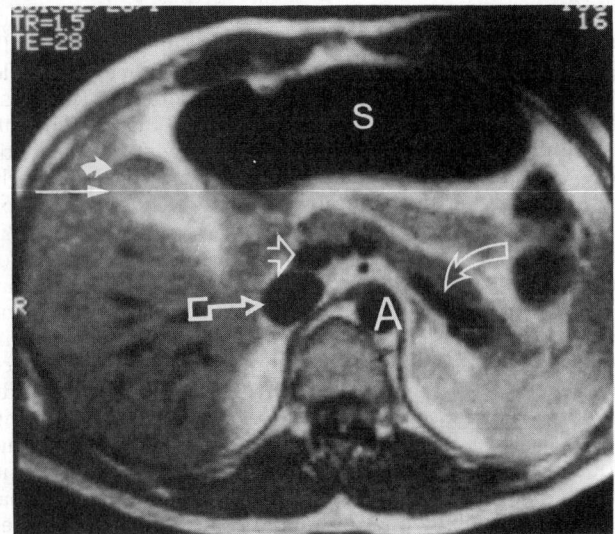

FIGURE 95–13. Magnetic resonance of normal gallbladder. Transverse MR image (TR = 1.5 sec, TE = 628 msec) demonstrates layering of nonconcentrated bile (*closed curved arrow*) (low signal intensity) upon concentrated bile (*straight arrow*) (high signal intensity) within the gallbladder. Note the absence of signal from the air-distended stomach (S) and the patent blood vessels including the splenic vein (*open curved arrow*), portal vein (*open arrow*), aorta (A), and inferior vena cava (*boxed arrow*). (Courtesy of Diasonics, San Francisco, CA.)

the abdomen. With current imaging times of minutes (as opposed to a few seconds for CT), respiration and peristalsis cause blurring and artifact, especially of pancreatic and bowel images. New techniques are being developed to decrease the scan time to seconds. Thereafter, MR imaging may become valuable for the mesenteric alimentary tract. Currently, it images well only the fixed portions, as in the rectum (Fig. 95–12) and distal esophagus. Magnetic resonance imaging may have a greater sensitivity to primary and metastatic liver tumors compared with CT, US, and nuclear medicine; but whether it has greater specificity has not been established. Magnetic resonance can sometimes differentiate hepatic neoplasia from fatty infiltration, either diffuse or focal, with the use of chemical shift imaging, a specifically modified imaging technique. Magnetic resonance can also image blood vessels noninvasively and as such may be useful to evaluate the patency of surgical shunts for portal hypertension. The effect of the presence of a paramagnetic substance, such as ferric iron, on the T1 and T2 relaxation times alters the MR signal intensity of involved tissue. Hence, MR can detect hemosiderosis and hemochromatosis. Similarly, paramagnetic substances such as gadolinium-DTPA can be used as contrast-enhancing agents. Magnetic resonance can image the gallbladder, detect cholelithiasis, and differentiate concentrated from nonconcentrated bile (Fig. 95–13). With further development, it may become the procedure of choice for assessing not only morphology but also function of the gallbladder and for diagnosing acute cholecystitis.

Magnetic resonance spectroscopy (MRS) of tissue specifically localized by imaging techniques is a new procedure that is still in the research stage of development. It has not yet achieved clinical applicability in the abdomen, but early work indicates some promise of diagnostic value in the study of high-energy phosphate metabolism (^{31}P) and in imaging sodium (^{23}Na), fluorine (^{19}F), and carbon (^{13}C). Such a procedure, which would facilitate the in vivo study of the biochemistry of normal and diseased organs, is technically more demanding than proton imaging. Because of great potential clinical impact, research is progressing rapidly.

Bernardino ME, Steinberg HV, Pearson TC, et al.: Shunts for portal hypertension: MR and angiography for determination of patency. Radiology 158:57, 1986. *Demonstrates MRI to be an accurate, noninvasive method of determining shunt patency and presence of collateral vessels.*

Evens RG, Jost RG, Evens RG Jr: Economic and utilization analysis of magnetic resonance imaging units in the United States in 1985. Am J Roentgenol 145:393, 1985. *A study of the utilization, costs, and revenue for users of MRI in 1985.*

Lee JKT, Heiken JP, Dixon WT: Hepatic metastases studied with MR and CT. Radiology 156:423, 1985. *Good discussion of a comparative study with up-to-date references; results suggest MRI indicated for clarification of equivocal or negative CT findings.*

Pykett IL: NMR imaging in medicine. Sci Am 246:78, 1982. *An excellent, understandable review of the physical principles of MRI.*

von Schulthess GK, Higgins CB: Blood flow imaging with MR: Spin-phase phenomena. Radiology 157:687, 1985. *A concise examination and analysis of the current concepts regarding MRI flow imaging.*

ACKNOWLEDGMENT: I wish to express my appreciation to Michael P. Federle, M.D., for helpful review of this manuscript. S.D.W.

96 GASTROINTESTINAL ENDOSCOPY

Jack A. Vennes

Remarkable progress in optical engineering and in fiberoptics during the past two decades has revolutionized the management of many gastrointestinal disorders. Fiberoptic techniques were initially used primarily for diagnosis, but increasingly they have been used for therapy. Excellent optical resolution and tip control permit direct visualization of mucosal abnormalities, with photographic record as desired. End-viewing instruments are adapted to visualize all mucosal surfaces of the esophagus, stomach, and duodenum or, alternatively, the entire colon. An internal channel permits routine aspiration, air insufflation, mucosal biopsy, or cytologic examination. Various therapeutic devices can also be precisely directed. Side-viewing instruments are used for visualizing the ampulla of Vater and for cannulation of the biliary and pancreatic ductal systems for contrast visualization.

Coincident with the development of fiberoptic techniques, other new diagnostic and often therapeutic modalities have also been developed using radiographic, ultrasound, or nuclear scanning. The problem is often to decide, therefore, which of these diagnostic and therapeutic alternatives is best and most cost effective for patients. Proper sequencing of radiologic, ultrasonic, nuclear, and endoscopic techniques is only gradually becoming clear and is often determined by factors of cost, morbidity and locally available skill and experience.

The diagnostic accuracy and therapeutic success of most procedures are dependent on operator skill and experience. Inexperience not infrequently results in increased complications—including the complication of an erroneous diagnosis. Endoscopic training programs are generally available, integrated with the disciplines of gastroenterology or colorectal or general surgery.

Endoscopy is contraindicated if there is severe cardiac or respiratory failure or a probable perforated viscus or if the diagnostic results are unlikely to affect management. Endoscopic procedures should be carefully discussed with patients in advance for reassurance. Procedures done by trained personnel are generally well tolerated after light parenteral sedation and analgesia. Topical pharyngeal anesthesia usually improves acceptance of upper tract endoscopy and indeed is often the only medication required for safe, minimally uncomfortable examinations with modern small-caliber endoscopes.

ESOPHAGOGASTRODUODENOSCOPY

Endoscopic examination of the entire esophagus, stomach, and duodenum (EGD) is accomplished with routine examination to the deep descending duodenum. All mucosal sur-

TABLE 96–1. INDICATIONS FOR ESOPHAGOGASTRODUODENOSCOPY (EGD)

A. Upper abdominal distress that persists despite an appropriate trial of therapy
B. Upper abdominal distress associated with signs suggesting serious organic disease (e.g., anorexia and weight loss)
C. Dysphagia or odynophagia
D. Esophageal reflux symptoms that are persistent or progressive despite appropriate therapy
E. Persistent vomiting of unknown cause
F. Other system disease in which the presence of upper gastrointestinal pathologic conditions might modify other planned management; examples include patients with a history of gastrointestinal bleeding who are scheduled for renal transplantation, long-term anticoagulation, and chronic nonsteroidal therapy for arthritis
G. Radiographic findings of:
   1. A neoplastic lesion, for confirmation and specific histologic diagnosis
   2. Gastric or esophageal ulcer
   3. Evidence of upper tract stricture or obstruction
   4. Mass
H. Gastrointestinal bleeding:
   1. As the first procedure in most actively bleeding patients
   2. When surgical therapy is contemplated
   3. When rebleeding occurs after acute, self-limited blood loss
   4. When portal hypertension or aortoenteric fistula is suspected
   5. For endoscopic therapy of upper gastrointestinal bleeding
   6. For presumed chronic blood loss and iron deficiency anemia when colonoscopy findings are negative

From Appropriate Use of Gastrointestinal Endoscopy. American Society for Gastrointestinal Endoscopy, 1986.

faces are visualized, and photographic records are often made of visually recognized abnormalities. Histologic and cytologic diagnosis can be made as indicated.

COMPLICATIONS. Complications from EGD are rare with modern small-caliber, flexible instruments but do occur. A morbidity of 0.13 per cent and a mortality of 0.0004 per cent have been reported. During or following endoscopic examination, perforation has occurred in the upper esophagus near the cricopharyngeus, through Zenker's diverticula, and through areas of tumor. Use of sedative or analgesic drugs may transiently suppress respiration, especially in elderly patients or those with severe obstructive pulmonary disease. Aspiration during endoscopy is very unlikely unless there is vomiting due to massive bleeding or gastric outlet obstruction. Cardiovascular complications, sepsis, prolonged bleeding, or thrombophlebitis from intravenous medications occur rarely.

INDICATIONS. Indications for diagnostic EGD are listed in Table 96–1. Esophagogastroduodenoscopy is most often indicated in the evaluation or discovery of possible acid-peptic disease, malignancy, or gastrointestinal bleeding. Endoscopy used "just in case" disease is found leads to overutilization, but blind management of a presumed disease without diagnostic confirmation often turns out to be underutilization. Both extremes are frequently cost *in*effective. Therapeutic use of endoscopic techniques will be briefly discussed with each procedure in this chapter.

Patients frequently seek medical help for upper abdominal discomfort and associated dyspeptic symptoms of relatively recent onset. If other findings indicative of serious disease are absent, a trial of therapy may be indicated as a first diagnostic test. Much less than 1 per cent of such patients have a malignancy as the cause of their dyspepsia. Most will respond to a trial of therapy directed toward their presumed acid-peptic problem. Esophagogastroduodenoscopy is therefore indicated for the perhaps 30 per cent of patients with dyspeptic symptoms that continue despite therapy for 14 days.

Irritable bowel syndrome does not usually require endoscopy, but there are occasional exceptions. Other problems that usually do not require endoscopy include intermittent dyspepsia, heartburn responding to medical therapy, and asymptomatic or uncomplicated hiatus hernia. Uncomplicated duodenal bulb ulcer seen on radiograph that responds to therapy does not usually require endoscopy unless symptoms recur quickly.

Acid-Peptic Disease

Acid-peptic disease, i.e., reflux esophagitis, gastric ulcer, duodenal ulcer, and duodenitis, can be strongly suspected on the basis of the history, but one cannot confidently predict the specific site or pathologic condition. Symptoms of reflux esophagitis are quite specific, but other gastroduodenal lesions frequently coexist (Ch. 98). The presence of esophageal reflux symptoms correlates well with the presence of endoscopic findings and less well with histologic findings. Local symptoms in the mid or lower esophagus are usually predictive of disease location, whereas high substernal symptoms may be due to disease anywhere in the esophagus. Gastric or duodenal ulcers are usually symptomatic, but in patients with previous gastric or duodenal ulcer, asymptomatic recurrences are discovered in 5 per cent or more of patients who have had endoscopy in long-term studies.

Esophagogastroduodenoscopy is more sensitive and specific than radiographic studies of the upper gastrointestinal tract, although neither is infallible. Radiographic studies are least sensitive in evaluating lesions without apparent depth, such as flat stomal postgastrectomy ulcers, giant duodenal ulcers involving an entire wall of the duodenal bulb, or erosive esophagitis.

Cancer

Malignant lesions of the upper gastrointestinal tract are generally evident as exophytic masses protruding into the lumen (Ch. 101). Flat, infiltrative lesions do occur occasionally, however. In the esophagus, such lesions may resemble a benign stricture, and in the stomach (linitis plastica), the primary features are stiffness and poor distensibility. Malignancy may occasionally present as ulceration, accurate evaluation of all esophageal and gastric ulcers is therefore mandatory and challenging. At least 75 per cent of malignant ulcers are correctly identified, by endoscopic visual criteria, as asymmetric folds or nodules that randomly form the crater rim and extend irregularly into surrounding mucosa. Malignant tissue is often seen as multihued. Benign ulcers are typically smoother with more crater depth and with more symmetry and less randomness, and a zone of erythema is present at the junction of the crater and rim.

Histologic and cytologic data should be added to the evaluation of all suspicious lesions and most gastric ulcers. This results in a sensitivity (positive when disease is present) and specificity (negative when disease is absent) of 95 per cent. Brush or lavage cytology is a particularly important adjunct in evaluating the smooth, infiltrative esophageal stricture or the linitis plastica gastric lesion or the occasional superficial, spreading, flat gastric cancer. Primary gastric lymphoma may present as an ulcer, ulcerated mass, or large, asymmetric folds. Specific histologic features are frequently present only in submucosal tissue.

Mucosal polyps are rare in the stomach and rarer still in the duodenum and esophagus. Submucosal or intramucosal polypoid defects overlain with normal mucosa are usually pancreatic rests or leiomyomas and can be left in place. Adenomatous polyps have premalignant potential, which increases with size. All polypoid lesions should be endoscopically visualized, with biopsy or removal with snare cautery. Multiple small, hyperplastic polyps are not premalignant and need not all be removed, and no surveillance is indicated. Adenomas should be excised endoscopically when feasible. Very large lesions may require surgical removal. Surveillance is indicated after removal of gastric adenomatous polyps.

Other upper gastrointestinal malignancies originating in the pancreas or biliary tree do not usually extend into gastric or duodenal mucosa, and they require other diagnostic studies (see below). Ampullary carcinoma is usually visible *if* the papilla of Vater is adequately seen via a conventional end-viewing endoscope or a side-viewing instrument (see below).

Upper Gastrointestinal Bleeding (see Ch. 114)

Esophagogastroduodenoscopy is the most informative procedure when further information is indicated for management of the acutely bleeding patient, particularly if it is done within 12 hours of admission. Information obtained includes (1) location and identity of the bleeding source; (2) whether bleeding is continuing; (3) whether bleeding is arterial; (4) which of multiple lesions is bleeding; and (5) whether a visible vessel is present in an ulcer base. These endoscopic observations are available in 85 per cent of patients with acute bleeding and influence prognosis and management decisions. There is no evidence that endoscopy initiates further bleeding. A precise diagnosis of the source of gastrointestinal bleeding would seem to be the logical basis for an improved outcome; however, controlled clinical studies have not shown this to be true. Endoscopic methods for controlling active bleeding are proving effective in current controlled trials. When indications for these techniques become clearer, more early endoscopy of acute bleeding will likely be indicated.

The source of chronic gastrointestinal blood loss or iron deficiency anemia in men is usually discovered in the colon. Esophagogastroduodenoscopy may be indicated by history suggesting upper tract sources or after negative findings on colonoscopy.

Therapeutic Applications of Esophagogastroduodenoscopy

Therapeutic endoscopic procedures commonly carried out in the upper gastrointestinal tract include removal of foreign bodies, dilation of benign or malignant esophageal strictures, sclerotherapy of bleeding esophageal varices, and electrocoagulation of focal bleeding lesions. Foreign bodies in the esophagus or stomach can usually be removed by techniques that employ snares, forceps, and protective overtubes to prevent soft tissue injury or aspiration. Impaction of food may occur because of an underlying esophageal abnormality, and careful esophagoscopy after removal of food may reveal a benign or malignant stricture or may suggest a motility disorder.

Esophageal strictures found to be benign on careful evaluation can be successfully dilated. If the course of the esophagus is tortuous, if the stricture is tight and does not admit the endoscope, or if epiphrenic diverticula are present, dilation is safely done over a guide wire passed under fluoroscopic control. Tapered bougies, metal olives, or inflatable balloons of progressively increasing diameter may be passed over the wire. Following this, endoscopy and biopsy are done to assess whether there is a malignant lesion. Less complex strictures that only partially occlude the lumen may, after endoscopy, be safely dilated with tapered bougies without wire guidance and without further endoscopy. A maintenance dilation schedule with individualized intervals and techniques is important.

Management of malignant esophageal strictures is directed to the goal of allowing the patient to swallow food, liquids, and oral secretions. The options available include surgery, radiation therapy, or such endoscopic procedures as repeated esophageal dilation, dilation and endoscopic placement of a stent across the malignant narrowing (or across a tracheoesophageal fistula), or use of laser energy to restore the lumen by tumor destruction. All of these latter procedures have quite good reported results; all require skill for success and safety; and all can be done without prolonged hospitalization. Local skills are often valid determinants. Quality survival time is usually brief, but 85 to 90 per cent of patients can be helped.

Several endoscopic measures have proved effective in controlling upper gastrointestinal bleeding. Endoscopic variceal sclerosis by intravariceal and perivariceal injection of various sclerosants controls the acute variceal hemorrhage of portal hypertension in 90 per cent of patients. Prophylactic sclerosis may also prevent future hemorrhage. The effect of either acute or prophylactic sclerotherapy on long-term survival is currently undergoing prospective controlled testing.

Focal nonvariceal bleeding can often be controlled using electrocoagulation with monopolar or bipolar current delivery or combined electrocoagulation and thermal heater probe techniques or laser photocoagulation. Argon or neodymium yttrium aluminum garnet (YAG) laser energy is carried through the endoscope via a flexible wave guide and converted to thermal energy when precisely directed to an absorptive (bleeding) area. Bleeding is controlled in up to 90 per cent of lesions, including those with brisk arterial bleeding, but rebleeding rates are significant with all methods. Laser equipment is expensive and not portable. Perforation, though of low risk, is a definite hazard with all techniques. Eighty-five per cent or more of upper gastrointestinal bleeding stops spontaneously; how then shall we select those patients who need endoscopic control of bleeding? A visible vessel in the ulcer base, a fresh adherent clot, or continuing active bleeding are all observable risk factors for further bleeding (and risk of death) and are indications for endoscopic therapy, most frequently with electrocoagulation or heater probe techniques. Surgical management will continue to be required for some whose bleeding is excessive.

Percutaneous endoscopic gastrostomy (PEG) is a useful method for providing selected patients with long-term enteral feeding. Candidates are those with a functioning gut and chronically inadequate oral intake. Some may have recurrent aspiration secondary to upper esophageal dysfunction. Specific indications include neurologic disorders that affect the swallowing mechanism or that result in diminished food intake secondary to a decreased sensorium or cancer of the pharynx or upper esophagus that does not totally obstruct (so that an endoscope can be passed). Percutaneous endoscopic gastrostomy is not indicated in postgastrectomy patients or in those with midline abdominal scar, severe, uncorrectable coagulopathy, or respirator dependency. The decision to initiate chronic enteral feeding can be a difficult one, involving the wishes of patient and family and the gravity of the underlying disease. Once the decision is made, however, PEG is a simple and safe method.

COLONOSCOPY AND FLEXIBLE SIGMOIDOSCOPY

The entire colon is now routinely accessible to high-resolution viewing with biopsy, brush cytology, polypectomy, and photography of observed lesions. Much has been learned of the polyp-cancer progression, and significant control of colon cancer is within cost-effective reach of the trained endoscopist.

COMPLICATIONS. Diagnostic colonoscopy has a complication rate of 0.5 per cent, which rises to 1 per cent when polypectomy is added, with hemorrhage and perforation being the principal complications.

INDICATIONS. The indications for colonoscopy are listed in Table 96–2. As with EGD, colonoscopic examination is primarily used to evaluate possible cancer, inflammation, and bleeding. The procedure is contraindicated in the presence of fulminant colitis; acute, severe diverticulitis; or probable perforated viscus. Colonoscopy is generally not indicated for stable irritable bowel syndrome, acute diarrhea, upper gastrointestinal bleeding, or rectal bleeding with an anorectal source on anoscopy or sigmoidoscopy. Other nonindications include routine follow-up of inflammatory bowel disease (except as noted in Table 96–2) and routine preoperative examination of patients undergoing elective abdominal surgery for noncolonic disease.

Flexible sigmoidoscopy (FFS) is usually carried out with 60-cm instrumentation, although a 35-cm endoscope is available. Training requirements are less rigorous than those for colonoscopy. Indications for flexible sigmoidoscopy are listed in Table 96–3. At least 60 per cent of colon cancers and potential

TABLE 96–2. INDICATIONS FOR COLONOSCOPY

A. Evaluation of an abnormality on barium enema that is likely to be clinically significant, such as a filling defect or stricture
B. For discovery and excision of colonic polyps:
    1. When polyps are seen on barium enema radiograph
    2. When neoplastic polyps are detected by proctosigmoidoscopy
C. Evaluation of unexplained gastrointestinal bleeding:
    1. Clinically significant hematochezia
    2. Melena with a negative upper gastrointestinal workup
    3. Presence of unexplained fecal occult blood
D. Unexplained iron deficiency anemia
E. Surveillance for colonic neoplasia
    1. Examination to "clear" entire colon of synchronous cancer or neoplastic polyps in a patient with a treatable cancer or neoplastic polyp
    2. Follow-up examination at two- to three-year intervals after resection of a colorectal cancer or neoplastic polyp and an adequate initial "clearing" colonoscopy
    3. Patients with a strongly positive family history of colonic cancer
    4. In patients with chronic ulcerative colitis: colonoscopy every one to two years with multiple biopsies for detection of cancer and dysplasia in patients with:
        a. Pancolitis of greater than seven years duration
        b. Left-sided colitis of over 15 years duration (no surveillance needed for disease limited to rectosigmoid)
F. Chronic inflammatory bowel disease of the colon if more precise diagnosis or determination of the extent of activity of disease will influence immediate management
G. Therapeutic colonoscopy, as control of bleeding or colonic decompression

From Appropriate Use of Gastrointestinal Endoscopy. American Society for Gastrointestinal Endoscopy, 1986.

colon cancers (neoplastic polyps) are located in the rectosigmoid and lower descending colon and thus are in reach of the "screening" FFS. Flexible sigmoidoscopy has the same contraindications as colonoscopy and is generally not indicated when colonoscopy is indicated (see Table 96–3). Flexible sigmoidoscopy is specifically not indicated for polypectomy because colonoscopy is needed, and full colonic preparation is necessary to prevent possible explosions during electrocautery. Preparation for FFS is simple, using two enemas, whereas preparation for colonoscopy requires a two-day liquid diet preparation or total gut lavage with large volumes of an isotonic solution. The place for FFS is assured as a more comfortable, more productive replacement for rigid proctosigmoidoscopy at nearly equivalent cost.

Polyps and Cancer of the Colon (see Ch. 107)

Colonoscopy to evaluate the possibility of colon cancer or its precursor polyps is usually indicated after an abnormality is detected by barium enema or proctosigmoidoscopy or if there is unexplained lower gastrointestinal bleeding. If occult blood is detected in the interior of a passed stool, colonoscopy will identify an age-related 20 to 30 per cent incidence of adenomatous polyps and 8 to 15 per cent incidence of cancers. During active bleeding, colonoscopy may encounter technical difficulties in accurately locating the bleeding source. Repeat colonoscopy may be necessary after cessation of bleeding for accurate colonic assessment.

After endoscopic removal of neoplastic polyps or after resection of colon cancer, continued surveillance is indicated, since the patient is now identified as being at risk for later colon cancer. A "clearing" examination may be optionally done within 12 months to be certain no polyps or cancers were missed at the first examination. Thereafter, follow-up examination every three years will detect new lesions before they become infiltrating carcinomas, since the process from polyp inception to infiltrating cancer appears to take up to

TABLE 96–3. INDICATIONS FOR FLEXIBLE FIBEROPTIC SIGMOIDOSCOPY (FFS)

A. Screening of asymptomatic patients at risk for colonic neoplasia
B. Evaluation of suspected distal colonic disease when there is no indication for colonoscopy
C. Evaluation of the entire colon in conjunction with barium enema radiographs

From Appropriate Use of Gastrointestinal Endoscopy. American Society for Gastrointestinal Endoscopy, 1986.

seven years. The only way to rule out cancer within a polyp is to remove it completely for histologic examination. Other conditions associated with increased risk for cancer also require surveillance (Table 96–2).

Most colonic polyps are hyperplastic and are not premalignant. In neoplastic polyps, cancer risk increases with increasing dysplasia and villoglandular transformation and also with size. Pedunculated polyps with an uninvolved stalk and with cancer confined to the mucosa can be cured by snare cautery removal. Most colonoscopists remove all polyps greater than 5 mm in diameter. Polyps less than 5 mm may be neoplastic; coagulation or a coagulation biopsy technique during colonoscopy is used to remove them.

Inflammatory Bowel Disease (see Ch. 105)

Most patients with inflammatory bowel disease do not require colonoscopy for diagnosis. At times, however, colonoscopy may provide unique and important information. Differentiation between granulomatous colitis (Crohn's disease) and ulcerative colitis is usually possible with colonoscopy and multiple biopsies. The anatomic extent of disease can be determined. The presence or absence of inflammatory bowel disease can be determined more accurately when clinically suspected despite absence of radiographic or sigmoidoscopic findings.

Diagnostic colonoscopy in ulcerative colitis is at times necessary to evaluate a stricture or a mass seen on barium enema. Occasionally, strictures are malignant with submucosal tumor spread. Pseudopolyps are not premalignant and need not be histologically examined. Polyps may be neoplastic or malignant, however, and those that are larger than 1 cm in diameter and are friable and irregular in color or configuration should be biopsied. In surveillance examinations of patients with ulcerative colitis, multiple biopsies are obtained throughout the involved colon. When moderate-to-severe dysplasia is consistently found, colectomy is usually recommended.

Polypectomy is the main therapeutic use of colonoscopy. Endoscopic control of bleeding is not usually feasible. Electrocautery of angiodysplastic lesions in the cecum and ascending colon has been successful, but new lesions may appear within months. Dilation of anastomotic strictures by balloons passed over a guide wire or through the endoscope is occasionally useful.

ENDOSCOPIC RETROGRADE CHOLANGIOPANCREATOGRAPHY (ERCP)

The side-viewing endoscope and the technique for identifying and cannulating the ampulla of Vater allow for radiographic study of both the common bile duct and the pancreatic duct in 80 to 90 per cent of attempts (Figs. 96–1 and 96–2). Failure may result from anatomic distortions due to prior surgery, tumor infiltration, or the duodenal edema of acute pancreatitis.

COMPLICATIONS. In 1 per cent of patients, acute pancreatitis follows ERCP, usually beginning within two hours of the procedure as a clinically mild complication. Biliary sepsis occurs less commonly but is more serious and even life threatening. Introduction of even a few bacteria into a semiclosed space—bile duct, gallbladder, pancreatic pseudocyst—may occasionally have serious septic consequences. Organisms may be introduced from the unsterile gastrointestinal tract or from instruments. Stringent cleaning and disinfection techniques are mandatory, including periodic cultures of equipment. Sepsis is prevented by prompt surgical, endoscopic, or transhepatic decompression within 24 hours of ERCP, plus judicious use of appropriate parenteral antibiotics.

INDICATIONS. Indications for ERCP are listed in Table 96–4. Endoscopic retrograde cholangiopancreatography is generally not helpful in evaluating abdominal pain of obscure origin in the absence of objective findings suggesting pan-

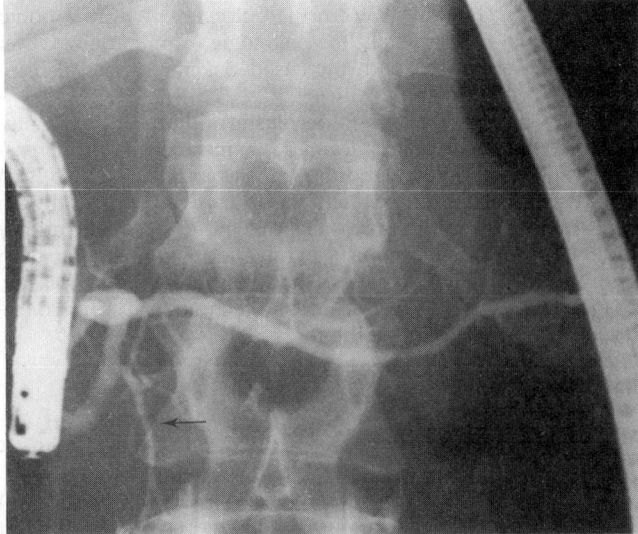

FIGURE 96—1. Normal pancreatogram, endoscopic retrograde cholangiopancreatography. The main pancreatic duct tapers normally from the tail near the hilum of the spleen to the papillary orifice (obscured by the tip of the endoscope). Lateral branches, partially filled with contrast, are of fine caliber and straight, draining the main gland and the uncinate process (*arrow*).

creatic or biliary disease. Known or suspected gallbladder disease is not an indication for ERCP in the absence of evidence for bile duct involvement. Study of patients with acute pancreatitis is usually deferred until a second episode has established its recurrent nature, unless there is evidence to suggest gallstone disease. Pancreatic malignancy clearly demonstrated on CT or ultrasound need not be further evaluated with ERCP except for stent placement.

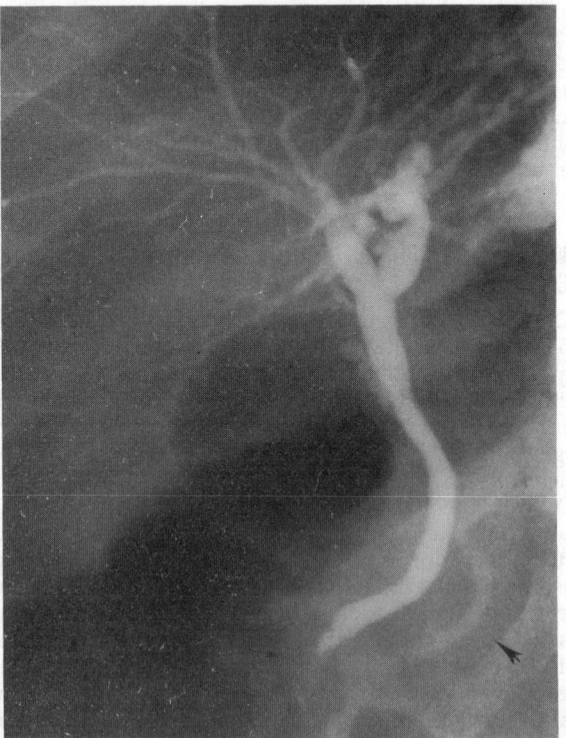

FIGURE 96—2. Normal cholangiogram. The normal-caliber, smoothly tapering intrahepatic ducts are well outlined with contrast, draining into right and left hepatic ducts. The cystic duct stump, remnant of previous cholecystectomy, divides the common hepatic duct above from the common bile duct below as they course medially around the black air-filled duodenum. The intramural duct is faintly visible (*small arrow*), terminating at the papilla. The main pancreatic duct is faintly visible medially (*large arrow*).

TABLE 96—4. INDICATIONS FOR ENDOSCOPIC RETROGRADE CHOLANGIOPANCREATOGRAPHY (ERCP)

A. Evaluation of the jaundiced patient suspected of having treatable biliary obstruction
B. Evaluation of the patient without jaundice (with or without prior cholecystectomy) whose clinical presentation suggests bile duct disease
C. Therapeutic pancreatic or biliary endoscopy, e.g., endoscopic sphincterotomy, balloon dilatation of strictures, stent placement across strictures; these procedures frequently require follow-up endoscopy
D. Evaluation of signs or symptoms suggesting pancreatic malignancy when results of ultrasound (US) and/or computed tomography (CT) are equivocal or normal
E. Evaluation of recurrent or persistent pancreatitis of unknown etiology
F. Preoperative evaluation of the patient with chronic pancreatitis
G. Evaluation of possible pancreatic pseudocyst undetected by CT or US and for known pseudocyst prior to planned surgical therapy

From Appropriate Use of Gastrointestinal Endoscopy. American Society for Gastrointestinal Endoscopy, 1986.

Other tests besides ERCP provide diagnostic evidence of pancreatic and biliary disease: percutaneous transhepatic cholangiography (PTC), computed tomography (CT), and ultrasound (US). Transabdominal fine-needle aspiration cytology with CT, US, or ERCP guidance is also helpful, as malignant cells are found by this means in 85 per cent of patients with pancreatic cancer.

In evaluating suspected biliary obstruction, a cholangiogram is usually obtained prior to therapy (Fig. 96–3). When the patient has fever, pain, and icterus, choledocholithiasis is suspected with high clinical accuracy. One may then proceed directly to cholangiography by PTC or preferably by ERCP if endoscopic sphincterotomy is planned. Ultrasound is usually obtained to assess ductal dilatation, but this is of limited value, as calculi often reside in undilated ducts.

When the presence of extrahepatic obstruction and its etiology are less certain, US as the initial study provides useful information at reasonable cost. For example, a normal gallbladder without calculi makes choledocholithiasis unlikely. Masses in the pancreas, bile duct, or porta hepatis, diffuse pancreatic enlargement, or grossly dilated bile ducts direct an appropriate specific disease evaluation.

Ultrasound and CT have improved greatly in their ability to detect pancreatic malignancy (Ch. 109). Equivocal results at times require confirmation by ERCP. Cut-off or stenosis of pancreatic duct and often of bile duct (double duct sign) is a

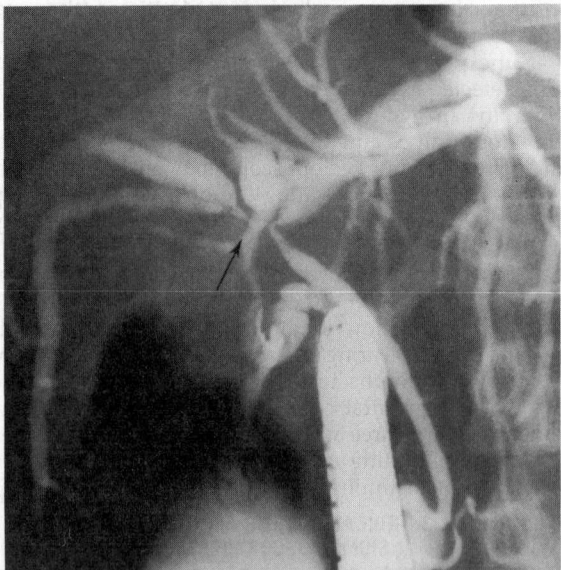

FIGURE 96—3. Retrograde cholangiogram: bile duct cancer. Multiple strictures at the bifurcation of the common hepatic duct (*arrow*) are due to a primary bile duct cancer (Klatskin tumor). Intrahepatic ducts are dilated and partially obstructed. The extrahepatic ductal system distal to the tumor is of normal caliber, here seen coursing medial to the endoscope.

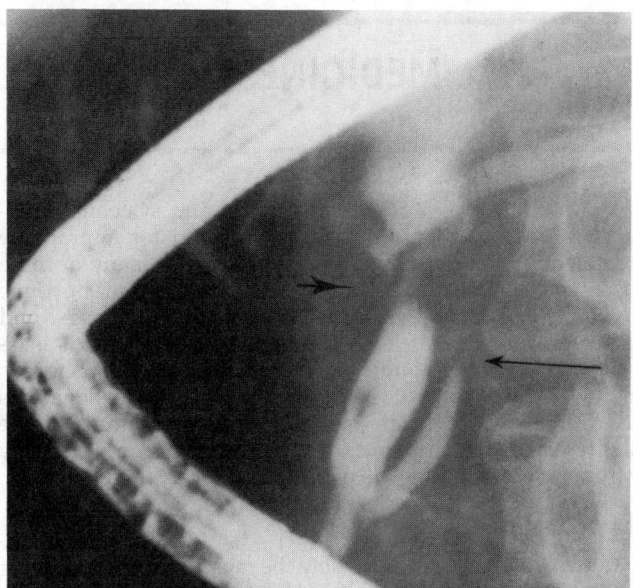

FIGURE 96–4. Pancreatogram and cholangiogram: pancreatic cancer. Both ducts are outlined by retrograde instillation of contrast at the bottom of the picture. Both the common bile duct (*large arrow*) and the pancreatic duct (*small arrow*) are strictured in the classic "double duct sign" of pancreatic cancer.

reliable ERCP finding suggestive of carcinoma (Fig. 96–4). Patients with chronic pain and suspected chronic pancreatitis who are surgical candidates should have preoperative pancreatography and cholangiography to assess patency of the main pancreatic duct and to assess possible stricture of the intrapancreatic bile duct. Differentiating chronic pancreatitis from pancreatic cancer may be difficult, as the pancreatic duct is often dilated and tortuous with dilated, stubby lateral branches (Fig. 96–5). Downstream stricturing in the pancreatic head is the hallmark of malignancy, however.

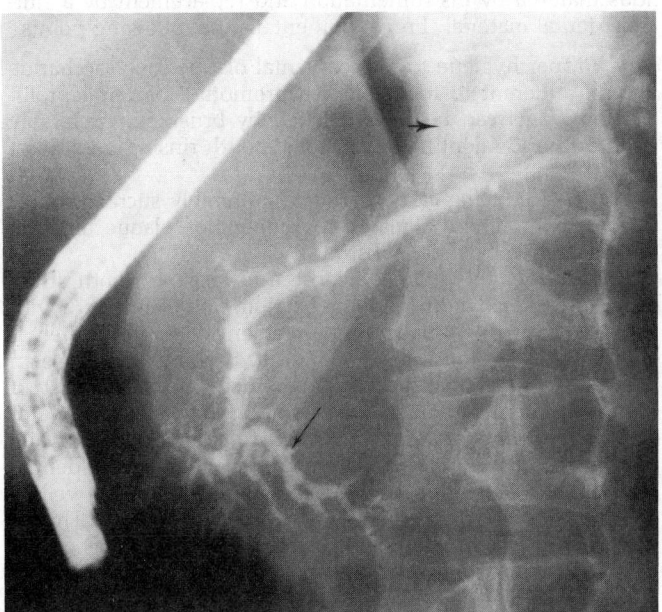

FIGURE 96–5. Pancreatogram: chronic pancreatitis. The main pancreatic duct is moderately dilated and unobstructed. The lateral branches are dilated, tortuous, and stubby. The duct from the uncinate process is prominent (*small arrow*). A small pseudocyst (*large arrow*) is barely visible overlying the spine in this oblique view. Filling defects in the main pancreatic duct may be calculi or air bubble artifact. With progression of the disease the main pancreatic duct may become more tortuous and dilated.

Therapeutic Applications of Endoscopic Retrograde Cholangiopancreatography

By endoscopic retrograde sphincterotomy (ERS), soft tissues and sphincter fibers of the papilla and intraduodenal portion of the common bile duct are divided with electrocautery to relieve ductal obstruction due to common duct stones or papillary stenosis. Endoscopic retrograde sphincterotomy has assumed a major role in the management of choledocholithiasis and offers a relatively safe and simple alternative to surgical management.

Biliary obstruction is relieved by ERS in 85 to 90 per cent of attempts. Complications of hemorrhage, pancreatitis, perforation, and cholangitis occur in 3 to 8 per cent of cases with a mortality rate of 0.4 per cent. Late complications of restenosis or re-formed stones occur in 1 to 8 per cent of patients.

Endoscopic retrograde sphincterotomy is now widely considered the therapy of choice for patients with symptomatic stones in the common bile duct. The procedure is often carried out immediately following ERCP as soon as the presence of stones in the duct is confirmed. It is clearly safer and cheaper than surgery in these generally elderly patients and more successful than percutaneous transhepatic extraction. Cholangitis and gallstone pancreatitis usually respond dramatically to decompression. About 40 per cent of patients with symptomatic choledocholithiasis have never had cholecystitis, and therefore their gallbladders are intact. Almost all contain calculi. After removing duct calculi with ERS, should the gallbladder be electively removed to preclude further cholecystitis or migration of stones into the now open biliary tree? Or may the gallbladder be left in place and removed only as future symptoms dictate? Experience with patients at high surgical risk suggests the safety and success of waiting, as the probability of cholecystitis does not exceed 5 to 10 per cent per year in these generally elderly patients.

Papillary stenosis is a poorly defined disorder or group of disorders in which recurrent biliary colic or occasionally pancreatitis are thought to result from fibrosis or sphincter dysfunction. Diagnostic criteria include a dilated bile duct, slow ductal drainage, cholestasis following painful episodes, and elevated basal sphincter of Oddi pressure during manometry. The problem arises most commonly in women who have had a cholecystectomy either for cholelithiasis or for biliary colic–like pain without stones. Endoscopic retrograde sphincterotomy is often curative for carefully selected patients with papillary stenosis.

Placement of plastic stents across biliary strictures is the second major therapeutic extension of ERCP. Most strictures are caused by inoperable pancreatic or bile duct carcinoma, and other treatment options are surgical or transhepatic decompression. A catheter containing a guide wire is introduced through the stricture, and a stent is passed over the catheter. The proximal end is left in the duodenum, bile drainage is restored, and barbed flaps prevent dislodgment of the stent. The procedure is successful in 90 per cent of attempts. Present-day stents remain patent for five months or more and can be rather easily replaced.

LAPAROSCOPY

Laparoscopy permits direct inspection of much of the anterior abdominal space. A pneumoperitoneum is created and a (usually) rigid or flexible laparoscope is introduced through a puncture in the abdominal wall, with the patient under local anesthesia and mild sedation. The procedure is well tolerated; complications of bleeding or bowel perforation occur in only 0.1 to 0.2 per cent. When it is clinically important to assess focal or diffuse liver disease, laparoscopy, by combining assessment of gross appearance and guided biopsy, is 90 per cent accurate, substantially better than percutaneous blind liver biopsy. This is true whether the disease is diffuse (cirrhosis) or focal (metastatic nodules). More than two thirds of the liver and variable parts of the gallbladder, spleen, peritoneum, and diaphragm can usually be visualized. The colon and small bowel are variably open to inspection.

The major indications for laparoscopy are (1) inspection and guided biopsy of the liver in suspected diffuse or focal disease, when the information will affect therapy and (2) evaluation of exudative ascites (malignancy versus inflammation). Determination of the presence or absence of abdominal metastases may be important in assessing operability. The procedure is contraindicated in the presence of acute peritonitis, intestinal obstruction, severe coagulopathy, infection of the abdominal wall, or severe ascites in patients with portal hypertension.

FUTURE OF ENDOSCOPY

Endoscopic instrumentation is approaching optimal size and optical resolution, in both conventional and emerging electronic video endoscopy equipment. The number of skilled endoscopists has increased so that precise diagnostic studies are generally available to most patients.

Fiberoptics are contributing enormously to management of gastrointestinal disease and will continue to do so. A clearer understanding of the colonic polyp-cancer progression will likely be available in the next few years. Colonoscopic polypectomy will play a key role in altering the course of this major malignancy. It is likely that nearly all cases of common duct stones will be treated endoscopically, until such time as extracorporeal lithotripsy for bile stones becomes generally available and successful. Measures for successful control of gastrointestinal bleeding are greatly improving. Their influence on mortality should soon become clear.

Optimal management of patients with benign or malignant biliary obstruction is not clearly dependent on a single technique. Endoscopists, radiologists, and surgeons working together will likely evolve an integrated approach with indications for each of several options.

Cello JP, Grendell JH, Crass RA, et al.: Endoscopic sclerotherapy versus portacaval shunt in patients with severe cirrhosis and variceal hemorrhage. N Engl J Med 311:1589, 1984. *The effect of sclerotherapy on short- and long-term outcome is not clear at present.*

Decker W, Tytgat GN: Diagnostic accuracy of fiberendoscopy in detection of upper intestinal malignancy: A follow-up analysis. Gastroenterology 73:710, 1977. *Review of fiberendoscopic studies in 1005 patients revealed an overall correct endoscopic interpretation in 92.7 per cent of 135 patients with gastric malignancy. Diagnosis was correct in 98.8 per cent, owing largely to the number of biopsies (GTR >10) in gastric ulcer patients.*

Dolley CP, Larson AW, Nigel HS, et al.: Double contrast barium meal and upper gastrointestinal endoscopy. Ann Intern Med 101:538, 1984. *In the best controlled study to date comparing endoscopy and barium meal radiographs, endoscopy was more sensitive (92 per cent versus 54 per cent) and specific (100 per cent versus 92 per cent).*

Ferrucci JT, Mueller PR: Interventional radiology of the biliary tract. Gastroenterology 82:974, 1982. *Relief of biliary obstruction is best handled with a team approach involving interventional radiologist, endoscopist, surgeon, and ultrasonographer. Radiologic techniques are discussed.*

Gilbert DA, Silverstein FE, Tedesco FJ, et al.: The national ASGE survey on upper gastrointestinal bleeding. Gastrointest Endosc 27:94, 1981. *A comprehensive, valuable review of collated experience with 2225 patients.*

Kahn K, Greenfield S: Endoscopy in the evaluation of dyspepsia. Ann Intern Med 102:266, 1985. *A clear and important statement of the Clinical Efficacy Assessment Project of the American College of Physicians concerning the diagnostic use of a trial of therapy.*

Proceedings of the NIH Consensus Workshop on Upper Gastrointestinal Bleeding. Dig Dis Sci (suppl):1, 1981. *Papers on the value of endoscopy in upper gastrointestinal bleeding that were used as background for the consensus workshop outlining the role of endoscopy in this condition.*

Scharschmidt BF, Goldberg H, Schmid R: Approach to the patient with cholestatic jaundice. N Engl J Med 308:1515, 1983. *A reasoned approach to this problem, which currently has several contending "solutions."*

Utilization Committee: Appropriate Use of Gastrointestinal Endoscopy. Manchester, MA, American Society for Gastrointestinal Endoscopy, 1986. *The source of the tables used in this chapter and a clear consensus statement on the current status of gastrointestinal endoscopy.*

Vennes JA: Management of calculi in the common duct. Semin Liver Dis 3:162, 1983. *Discussion of present-day evaluation of choledocholithiasis and management with endoscopic sphincterotomy.*

97 ORAL MEDICINE

Sol Silverman, Jr.

Many oral diseases representing local and systemic conditions must be recognized by the physician for appropriate treatment or referral. Signs and symptoms of many of these diseases, as well as effective management, can be quite variable. Fortunately, most oral diseases are benign and noncontagious. Many of the conditions are progressive, making correct diagnosis and early treatment important factors in minimizing morbidity. Precancerous lesions and malignancies occur frequently enough to be of constant concern in the differential diagnosis. Some of the most common and clinically important oral diseases will be reviewed briefly in this chapter.

DENTAL CARIES

Caries (tooth decay) is possibly the most widespread human disease and the greatest cause of loss of teeth prior to the age of 35.

ETIOLOGY. Bacteria, substrate, and a susceptible tooth are required for the carious lesion. Although a variety of microorganisms can be responsible for dental decay, the most important appear to be certain streptococcal strains. Substrate for bacterial growth is a critical factor, primarily carbohydrates in the form of sucrose have been shown to be most harmful in promoting dental plaque, bacterial growth, and the carious lesion. Most natural teeth are susceptible to decay unless preventive measures are instituted.

SIGNS AND SYMPTOMS. Early decay can be detected by careful clinical examination and x-ray evaluation. When the lesion becomes moderately advanced, missing tooth structure, surface softness, discoloration, and sensitivity become apparent.

MANAGEMENT. Treatment requires removal of the carious material by instrumentation and replacement by a suitable dental material. Prevention entails the following points.

1. Proper hygiene to reduce dental plaque (polysaccharide matrix adherent to tooth surface promoting bacterial proliferation). This can be accomplished by brushing, preferably with a fluoride dentifrice, vigorous mouth rinsing, and flossing.

2. Diet (reducing carbohydrates, preferably sucrose-source foods) to minimize a major component of plaque and the most effective bacterial substrate.

3. Fluoride, to produce a more acid-resistant tooth structure, to enhance tooth remineralization, and to interfere with bacterial growth. A fluoride supplement of approximately 1 mg daily during tooth development has been shown to be an effective means of reducing dental decay. The amount of fluoride depends upon that occurring in the communal water supply and the amount of water consumed daily. Daily fluoride mouth rinses and topical applications by the dentist also are very effective supplements for children, as well as for adults who continue to have caries problems. This is particularly true in adults with reduced saliva (e.g., as occurs with Sjögren's syndrome, irradiation effects, drug-induced xerostomia). Fluoride ingestion does not increase the risk for development of cancer.

Newbrun E: Sugar and dental caries: A review of human studies. Science 217:418, 1982. *Studies reviewed indicate that frequent or high intake of sugary foods predisposes to dental decay.*

DENTAL ABSCESS

If the carious process (bacterial infection with tooth decalcification) progresses to the dental pulp, pulpitis (inflammation of the dental pulp) ensues. Spontaneous sensitivity and reactions to temperature changes are often the first signs. The pulpitis may be reversible if the carious process is removed; however, if it continues, abscess formation takes place. The abscessed tooth is manifested by pain that may be spontaneous, in response to temperature changes or to pressure. Dental abscesses can sometimes be caused by deep fillings or trauma, which initiates the pulpal inflammatory process.

DIAGNOSIS. The abscessed tooth is classically diagnosed by its tenderness to slight percussion, reactivity to heat, and a periapical radiolucency visualized in dental x-rays. Progression of the abscess can lead to severe pain, swelling, lymphadenopathy, and fever. The discomfort may be continuous or intermittent, and cannot always be localized to the offending tooth.

Occasionally abscess formation is not accompanied by symptoms and is detected by routine x-ray examination. In these cases the dental abscess or granuloma often converts into a cyst or may develop a fistular tract, establishing chronic low-grade drainage ("gumboil" or parulis).

Ludwig's angina can be a rare complication if appropriate drainage, removal of the infectious source, or effective antibiotics are not instituted.

MANAGEMENT. Emergency care involves drainage, antibiotics (preferably penicillin, with erythromycin being used in penicillin-sensitive individuals), and analgesic drugs. Definitive treatment is by endodontic therapy (root canal filling) or extraction.

PERIODONTAL DISEASE

This condition is the most common cause for the loss of teeth beyond the age of 35. Periodontal disease is manifested by the loss of dental bone support (alveolar process of mandible and maxilla), which creates dental pockets (gingival and bony crevices around the teeth). This further promotes accumulation of bacteria and debris, calculus formation, worsening of the inflammatory process, further acceleration of bone loss, and loosening of the teeth. This process may be accompanied by gingivitis, purulent exudates, swelling, and pain.

ETIOLOGY. Although the most common cause of periodontal disease is poor hygiene (formation of plaque and calculus), in some individuals causative factors remain unknown. Bacterial toxins and inflammation are the common denominators, and immunologic mechanisms have been implicated. Inheritance does not play an important role. In addition to staining tooth structure, tobacco usage has been shown to increase the risk for gingivitis, periodontal disease, and earlier loss of teeth. Diabetes also encourages periodontal disease by suppressing local cell systems that control bacterial proliferation and inflammation. Associations between periodontal disease and other metabolic diseases, gastroenteropathies, and nutritional deficiencies have not been established. The loss of bone through the aging process is a common denominator, and periodontal disease in younger persons is extremely rare, even with poor hygiene.

DIAGNOSIS. Early periodontal disease may go unrecognized, since it is often asymptomatic and without clinically obvious signs. As periodontal disease continues, however, it usually can be detected by gingival erythema and swelling, tooth mobility, and a gingival exudate associated with discomfort or pain. Periodontal disease is confirmed by examination for dental pockets and more accurately assessed by loss of bone seen in x-rays. Certain conditions, such as histiocytosis, hypophosphatasia, and the Papillon-Lefèvre syndrome, can simulate precocious periodontal disease when the jaw bones are affected and teeth are lost prematurely.

PREVENTION AND TREATMENT. Optimal home care (brushing, rinsing, and flossing) and periodic dental office prophylaxes (curettage and polishing) are extremely important factors in removing the causative dental plaque (similar but not identical to plaque causing dental caries). For advanced periodontal disease, surgical alterations of gingiva and alveolar bone, as well as splinting teeth together, may be helpful in slowing or preventing further deterioration. In acute flares, hydrogen peroxide mouth rinses (3 per cent H_2O_2 with equal parts warm water) and antibiotics (preferably penicillin) are usually effective. Although a nutritious diet is important, this will not prevent periodontal disease. Effective human vaccines are not yet available.

Joseph CE, Farnoush A: Current concepts of periodontitis. J Calif Dent Assoc 12:43, 1984. *Assessment of causative factors, pathogenesis, and control of periodontal disease.*

ACUTE GINGIVITIS

This condition, often referred to as acute necrotizing ulcerative gingivitis (ANUG) and Vincent's infection, does not follow any epidemiologic patterns, and there is no evidence that it is contagious. With proper microbiologic testing methods, it does seem to be often associated with fusiform and spirochete organisms. Poor oral hygiene and suboptimal nutrition are frequently found. ANUG can mimic gingival changes occasionally seen in individuals with blood dyscrasias or viral infections.

DIAGNOSIS. The condition is usually characterized by its acute nature associated with pain, fetid oral odor, and gingival ulcerations (Fig. 97–1). There may be associated tendency toward bleeding. Most often there is no associated fever or lymphadenopathy, but malaise may be present.

The diagnosis is established by ruling out other, more serious systemic disease and by response to treatment. This condition differs from chronic gingivitis, which may be asymptomatic and due to poor home care, irritating fillings, or pocket formation (incipient periodontal disease).

TREATMENT. The most conservative approach is by improving oral hygiene, hydrogen peroxide mouth rinses (3 per cent H_2O_2 mixed with equal parts warm water), and dental prophylaxis. Adequate nutrition is important, and antibiotics are useful in cases of fever, lymphadenopathy, or severe oral signs and symptoms. Penicillin is the drug of choice (1000 to 1500 mg daily), with erythromycin in similar dosages an alternative. If good home care is continued, recurrence is unlikely.

When ANUG does not respond to treatment, other diseases must be considered, requiring more extensive laboratory tests. Diseases such as erythema multiforme, lichen planus, pemphigoid, and pemphigus may mimic a chronic or subacute gingivitis. In these instances a biopsy will assist the diagnosis and corticosteroids will control signs and symptoms.

APHTHOUS ULCERS

Aphthous ulcers (canker sore, ulcerative stomatitis) occur in up to 40 per cent of the population. There appears to be a

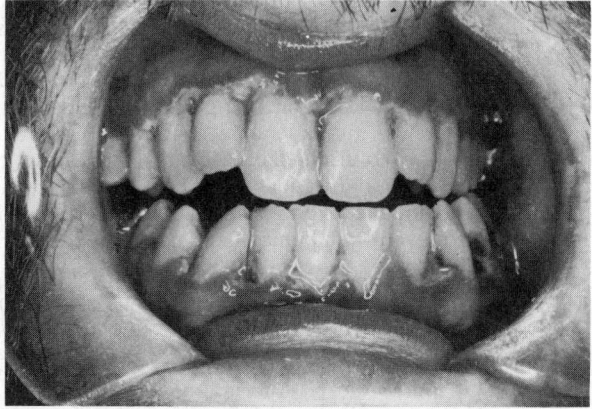

FIGURE 97–1. Acute necrotizing ulcerative gingivitis. Note typical necrosis of marginal gingiva. These signs, associated with pain and fetid odor, were present for one week.

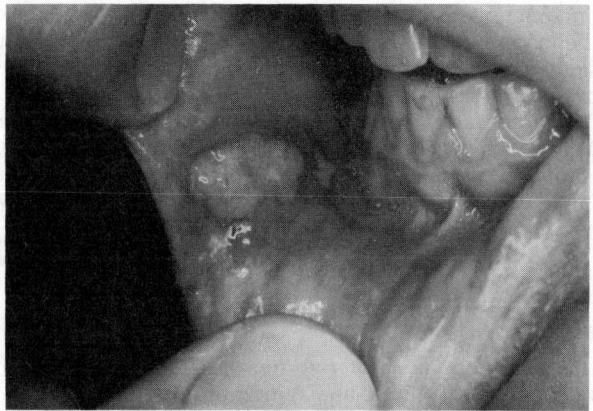

FIGURE 97–2. Aphthous ulcers. These idiopathic ulcerations usually do not exceed 5 to 6 mm in size and heal in 10 to 14 days. This large (major) aphthous ulcer had been present for one month and did not heal for two months.

genetic tendency, since offspring of parents with aphthous ulcers have a greater risk for developing them. Aphthae usually appear by age 20 and without sex preference. There is a tendency to have fewer and less severe attacks as time progresses. Viral, bacterial, or other causative agents have never been proved; immunologic factors are being implicated. Certain foods, fever, and stress may bring on attacks in predisposed persons.

DIAGNOSIS. The diagnosis of aphthae is made by clinical appearance and history. Most commonly they appear as shallow, pseudomembrane-covered ulcerations with a surrounding erythematous halo. They are often tender and heal spontaneously in one to two weeks. Aphthae may occur as multiple small ulcers, or sometimes they appear as single large ulcerations (major aphthae), which usually incur more pain and a longer healing period (Fig. 97–2). This implies a difference in the host and not the disease. Some patients will never be free of ulcers; as one ulcer heals, others occur.

Blood examination or smears are not helpful. Biopsies show nonspecific inflammation and ulceration; the initial inflammatory cell is the lymphocyte. The larger lesions can mimic more serious diseases, since the inflammatory process involves underlying musculature, causing more induration and pain.

Aphthous ulcers may be associated with inflammatory bowel disease and Behcet's syndrome. In the differential diagnosis care must be taken not to confuse aphthae with the oral manifestations of erythema multiforme, erosive lichen planus, primary herpetic stomatitis, pemphigoid, pemphigus, drug reactions, and mucosal manifestations of blood dyscrasias.

TREATMENT. Frequently, special treatment is unnecessary. Empirical approaches, using bland mouth rinses, topical preparations, vitamins, and mild sedatives and analgesics, may be helpful in some persons. The most effective management is by administering short courses of corticosteroids systemically. Frequently less than 40 mg prednisone daily for two to three days will give adequate control of signs and symptoms (this also confirms the inflammatory nature of aphthae). The dosage and duration of corticoid treatment may vary with individual patients and their characteristic patterns of disease. Vaccines and antibiotics have not proved beneficial.

Olson JA, Greenspan JS, Silverman S Jr: Recurrent aphthous ulcerations. J Calif Dent Assoc 10:53, 1982. *Comprehensive review of clinical features, pathogenesis, and management.*

Silverman S Jr, Lozada-Nur F, Migliorati C: Clinical efficacy of prednisone in the treatment of patients with oral inflammatory ulcerative diseases: A study of fifty-five patients. Oral Surg 59:360, 1985. *Benefits of prednisone treatment were shown by comparing time-dosage schedules, reduction of signs and symptoms, and drug side effects.*

ORAL HERPETIC INFECTIONS

Herpes simplex virus (HSV) infects the mouth in a variety of ways. Diagnostic techniques are usually impractical, and treatment is supportive. Evidence for a contagious nature is lacking. A history of these lesions has not been associated with an increased risk for cancer.

COLD SORE (HERPES LABIALIS). The most common bothersome lesion is the cold sore. In the prone individual the latent virus is activated by an external irritant (cold, fever, trauma) and yields the characteristic vesicle or vesicles that subsequently scab and usually take one to three weeks to heal. The lesion is not associated with any rise in HSV antibody titer, and no effective preventive or therapeutic agents (vaccines, vitamins, ointments, and antivirals) are available. Therefore, an empirical approach with which any patient gets the best result is still indicated (see Ch. 533). In more severe attacks, acyclovir, 1200 to 2000 mg daily, may be helpful.

RECURRENT INTRAORAL HSV. Intraoral recurrent herpetic lesions should not be confused with recurrent aphthous ulcers. Recurrent herpetic infections are rare and only occur on the gingiva or hard palate. They are usually characterized by shallow, small, irregular erosive lesions on an erythematous mucosa. Pain is usually no more than moderate, and the lesions are usually self-limiting in seven to ten days.

PRIMARY HERPETIC GINGIVOSTOMATITIS. Primary herpetic gingivostomatitis is the most acute form of oral herpetic infection. Usually 90 per cent of the population is infected before puberty, but most persons do not develop noticeable lesions or complaints. Signs and symptoms can include ulcerations on an erythematous and edematous mucosa (Fig. 97–3). This is often accompanied by lymphadenopathy, fever, and malaise, which can be confused with more serious illnesses. The condition is self-limiting; signs and symptoms usually become progressively severe for one week and disappear by the end of the second week. Treatment is supportive with antipyretic-analgesic agents, rest, and nutritional supplements.

During the course of disease, HSV antibody titer rises at least four-fold and confers lifelong immunity. Blood tests usually show only a slight lymphocytosis. Cytologic smears show pseudogiant cells (squamous) typical of the herpetic infection.

Approximately 10 per cent of adults, as shown by seroepidemiologic study, either did not become infected in childhood or have not developed adequate antibodies. Therefore, this infection is not limited to children. Adult infections of primary herpetic gingivostomatitis are usually more severe than the childhood form. Both forms can be mistaken for more severe diseases such as erythema multiforme, infectious mononucleosis, blood dyscrasias, and pemphigus. Persons who are

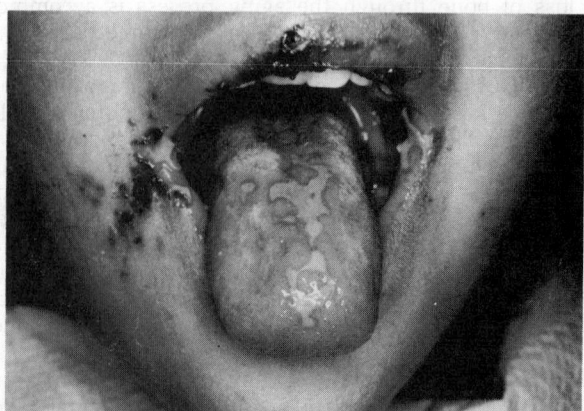

FIGURE 97–3. Primary herpetic gingivostomatitis in a five-year-old youngster. These acute attacks render lifelong immunity.

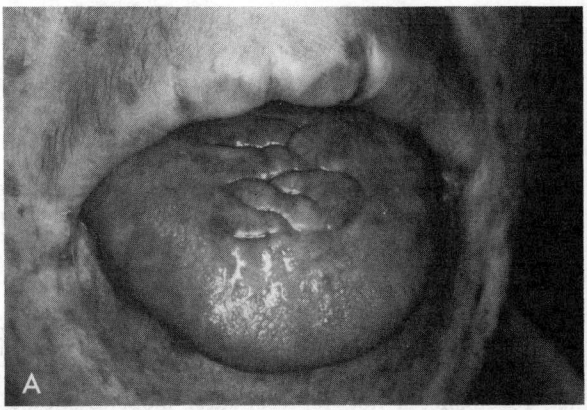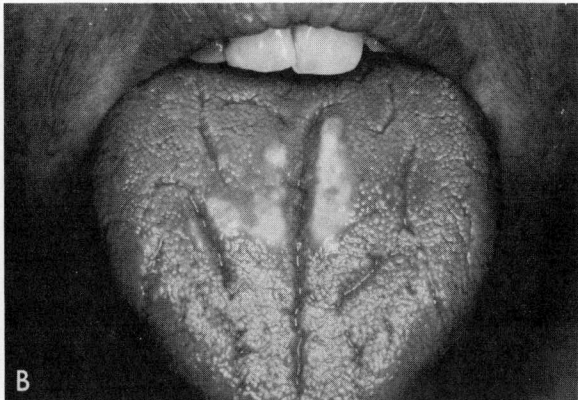

FIGURE 97–4. Candidiasis of tongue. *A,* Note depapillation and angular cheilitis. This patient had an idiopathic iron deficiency anemia. *B,* Note painful white surface colonies. This attack followed a course of antibiotics.

immunosuppressed, e.g., cancer and kidney transplant patients, have an increased risk for developing a primary herpetic stomatitis. Acyclovir (1200 mg daily per os or intravenously) has proved effective in controlling these conditions.

Hirsch MS, Schooley RT: Treatment of herpesvirus infections. N Engl J Med 309:963, 1983. *Reviews HSV infections and management.*

CANDIDIASIS (Moniliasis, Thrush)

Candida albicans (see Ch. 375) is a normal oral flora resident in about 30 to 40 per cent of the population. For unclear reasons, the fungi can become overpopulated and produce clinical signs and symptoms. Most frequently oral candidal infections are associated with antibiotic use (suppressing oral bacterial flora and making more carbohydrate substrate available), diabetes mellitus, xerostomia, immunosuppression, and the wearing of dentures (poor hygiene).

DIAGNOSIS. Oral candidiasis is often recognized by complaints of generalized mouth discomfort. It may be acute or chronic. While examination frequently reveals the typical surface creamy white fungal colonies, often the manifestation is that of irregular or widespread erythema (Fig. 97–4). Occasionally there will be erosive changes. Angular cheilitis is a common finding.

Since the clinical appearance is often only suggestive, smears or cultures (to observe pseudomycelia and spores) may be required to confirm the diagnosis. If biopsies are obtained, special staining with the periodic acid–Schiff (PAS) method may show the fungus, which grows in the most superficial epithelial stratum.

TREATMENT. The first step in treatment is to rule cut underlying factors, such as hyperglycemia, xerostomia, and anemia. Hydrogen peroxide–saline mouth rinses (3 per cent H₂O₂ diluted with equal parts warm saline) are helpful. Specific treatment includes orally dissolving nystatin vaginal troches (100,000 units three or four times daily). Nystatin suspension is not as effective, since the contact time with the oral mucosa is much less. Clotrimazole tablets (10 mg dissolved orally five times daily) appear to be equally or more effective than the nystatin. Ketoconazole (200 mg per os daily with food) offers an effective alternative to oral dissolution, which some individuals find objectionable. The angular cheilitis is most effectively treated with Mycolog II cream (nystatin-triamcinolone). Oral candidiasis does not appear to be contagious or related to infections at other sites. Unless the underlying cause is identified and corrected, oral infections can recur.

Mackowiak PA: The normal microbial flora. N Engl J Med 307:83, 1982. *Reviews microbial florae and their interrelationships in health and disease.*

Renner RP, Lee M, Andors L, et al.: The role of *C. albicans* in denture stomatitis. Oral Surg 47:323, 1979. *Reviews biology of oral* Candida, *techniques for measurement and differential diagnosis of clinical appearance. Increased fungal infections were shown in denture wearers.*

ORAL FINDINGS IN ACQUIRED IMMUNODEFICIENCY SYNDROME (AIDS)

Oral signs and/or symptoms of the acquired immunodeficiency syndrome (AIDS) or the AIDS-related complex (ARC) may be the first evidence or complaint indicating the possibility of AIDS virus (HIV) infection. The most common oral infection is chronic candidiasis. This is suspected when there is no other explanation (e.g., dentures, diabetes, leukemia, medicines) other than the possibility of HIV infection and immunosuppression in high-risk individuals (see Ch. 346). A unique white lesion, termed hairy leukoplakia, which occurs almost exclusively on the lateral borders of the tongue in homosexual and bisexual males, is a sign of HIV infection and indicates a high risk for developing AIDS (Fig. 97–5). The Epstein-Barr virus has been isolated from the lesion. Oral Kaposi's sarcoma (KS), often asymptomatic, has been found in over half of the patients with skin KS and sometimes as the sole lesion of KS. It can occur on any oral mucosal surface (predominantly on the palate) as a flat or raised lesion (Fig. 97–6). Other oral findings that should arouse suspicion of HIV infection include progressive periodontal disease (loss of gingival tissue and alveolar bone) for which there is no other obvious explanation; unusually frequent or extensive oral aphthae and herpes simplex lip lesions (cold sores); unilateral mucosal or facial skin vesicles of varicella zoster; cytomegalovirus-induced xerostomia; increased number of allergies usually manifested by mucosal or skin rashes; and condyloma acuminatum (venereal warts), which may occur on any mucosal surface and appear as papillomas.

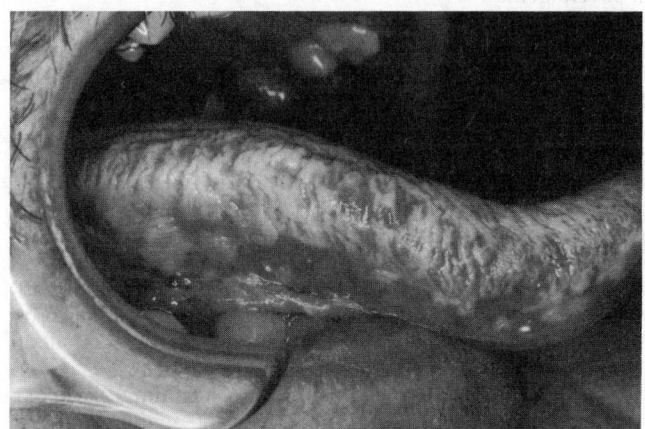

FIGURE 97–5. Hairy leukoplakia in a 31-year-old homosexual male. This unique tongue lesion almost always indicates AIDS virus infection and a high risk for developing AIDS. This patient was diagnosed as having pneumocystic pneumonia four months later.

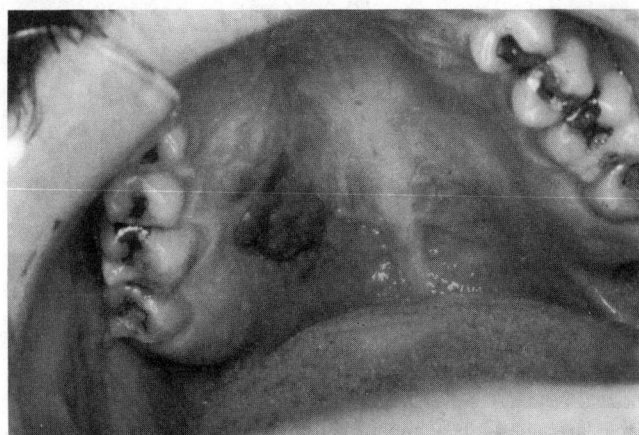

FIGURE 97–6. This exophytic vascular-appearing growth on the palate is a biopsy-proved Kaposi's sarcoma in a 29-year-old homosexual male.

Silverman S Jr, Migliorati CA, Lozada-Nur F, et al.: Oral findings in people with or at high risk for AIDS: A study of 375 homosexual males. J Am Dent Assoc 112:187, 1986. *A study of 375 homosexual-bisexual males, describing and illustrating oral signs and symptoms of ARC and AIDS and discussing risks and control measures.*

GLOSSITIS

Inflammatory conditions of the tongue are moderately common and quite variable. Asymptomatic glossitis may be due to the aging process (atrophy of the filiform papillae) or due to such idiopathic conditions as geographic tongue (glossitis migrans) and median rhomboid glossitis (central papillary atrophy). Occasionally glossitis may reflect a blood dyscrasia or a variety of debilitating diseases involving malnutrition. By careful clinical examination, history, and ruling out other diseases, the asymptomatic atrophic tongue can usually be classified.

Complex clinical problems may be associated with patients having symptomatic glossitis (glossopyrosis, glossodynia). Frequently examination of the tongue will not reveal any specific lesions or depapillation. The symptoms are often a manifestation of anxiety or depression. Occasionally the glossitis may be due to a drug reaction. Xerostomia or dehydration may be causative factors, and candidiasis must be ruled out. Rarely, anemia or hyperglycemia may induce these changes. Glossitis is not caused by poor oral hygiene, dentures, or other tooth-related problems. Tobacco use may contribute to the discomfort, as may certain foods. In many cases the etiology remains unknown, and by default they are classified as psychogenic.

MANAGEMENT. Approach to the patient with a symptomatic tongue usually involves a careful history and consideration of discontinuing or altering drugs. Tobacco must be discontinued, at least temporarily. Blood dyscrasias and hyperglycemia should be ruled out with the appropriate tests. Inspection for any obvious dental or oral pathologic condition is in order, and these should be corrected even though it is unlikely that they may play a role. Occasionally a malignancy of the tongue may create these symptoms, therefore, a careful examination must be performed. Reassuring a patient that there is no sign of malignancy is sometimes an important part of management. Candidiasis should be eliminated by appropriate cultures or smears or by instituting a short trial of antifungal agents.

A systematic pharmacologic approach, including placebos, vitamins, tranquilizers, and antidepressant agents, may be utilized after the other diagnostic approaches are exhausted. Occasionally sialogogues (pilocarpine or bethanechol) or anti-inflammatory agents (corticoids) are helpful. If all these approaches fail and a diagnosis cannot be established, then any acceptable supportive therapy may be attempted, e.g.,

hypnosis, biofeedback, or even periodic recall visits for reassurance.

Dreizen S: The telltale tongue. Postgrad Med 75:150, 1984. *Reviews diseases of the tongue with reference to cause, appearance, and management.*

LEUKOPLAKIA–ERYTHROPLAKIA

These terms designate white and red patches that may occur on any oral mucosal surface (Fig. 97–7). There may be associated discomfort, and an etiologic factor is not always apparent.

MANAGEMENT AND DIAGNOSIS. The first practical approach is to remove all irritants, such as tobacco use, ill-fitting dentures, poor hygiene, spicy or hot foods, and any other potentially injurious habits, in order to see if the lesions are reversible. If not, representative biopsies should be obtained. Most often leukoplakia will be a manifestation of benign hyperkeratosis and erythroplakia a reflection of epithelial atrophy and inflammation. If a lesion cannot be classified as any specific disease entity, then at the very least it should be followed closely because of the risk for malignant transformation (thus the term precancerous lesion). If the biopsy indicates dysplasia, then a more aggressive attempt should be made to remove these lesions surgically. A red component also increases the risk for malignant transformation. Carbon dioxide laser resection or evaporation has been an effective surgical modality. Removal does not guarantee permanent control or cancer prevention.

DIFFERENTIAL DIAGNOSIS. Occasionally a white-and/or red-appearing oral lesion may already be squamous carcinoma. Alternatively, it may represent a classifiable benign lesion such as lichen planus, erythema multiforme, or pemphigoid. In these latter conditions, topical or systemic corticosteroids will help confirm the diagnosis by at least partial control of the lesion. For leukoplakia and erythroplakia, corticosteroids, keratinolytic agents, vitamin A, and other approaches have not been uniformly effective.

Silverman S Jr, Gorsky M, Lozada F: Oral leukoplakia and malignant transformation. A follow-up study of 257 patients. Cancer 53:563, 1984. *Describes profiles and establishes risk factors in patients with precancerous oral lesions.*

ORAL CANCER

Cancer of the mouth accounts for about 4 per cent of all cancers. The tongue is the most common site, although it may occur in any mouth site. More than 90 per cent are squamous carcinomas, commencing in the oral epithelial lining. The average age of onset approximates 60 years, and there is a 2 to 1 male to female prevalence. Oral cancer occurs in all ethnic groups.

ETIOLOGY. The increased risk and cause-effect relationship among tobacco use, alcohol consumption, and mouth

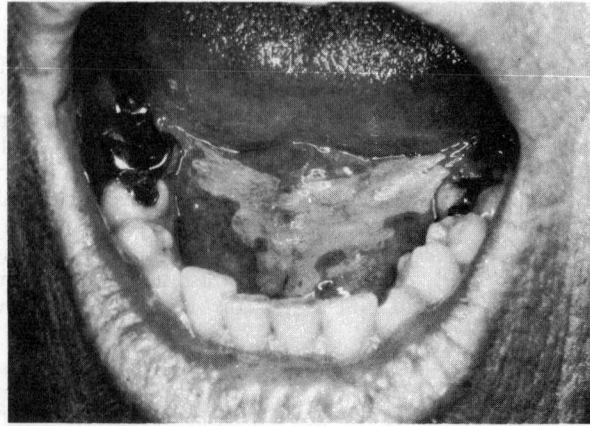

FIGURE 97–7. Leukoplakia of floor of mouth. This lesion, which was asymptomatic, had been present for four years. The cause was related to cigarette smoking.

cancer have been well documented. Abstinence is significant in preventive measures. Since patients with one oral cancer have an extremely high risk for developing second head and neck malignancies (about 20 per cent), discontinuation of tobacco and alcohol is critical. Although various forms of oral irritation, food carcinogens, and herpesvirus have been implicated, studies have not confirmed an associated risk factor.

DIAGNOSIS. There are no reliable signs or symptoms associated with mouth cancer. This causes delay by the patient in seeking professional advice, and conversely the varied features often delay diagnostic procedures. The most common finding is that of a painful ulceration associated with induration. Early malignant changes often can appear as essentially asymptomatic white and/or red surface patches. Patients often describe these changes as lumps or irritations.

Biopsy is the only acceptable method of diagnosis. Exfoliative cytology and vital staining with toluidine blue (1 per cent aqueous toluidine blue, decolorized with 1 per cent acetic acid) are useful adjuncts to clinical opinion when biopsy is delayed or extent of disease is being determined.

TREATMENT. The survival rate for oral cancer is relatively poor, in most studies averaging less than 50 per cent. This is usually due to late detection, promoting lesions that are locally extensive with diffuse margins, large tumor volume, and spread to the neck (cervical lymphadenopathy). While spread to neck nodes is rather common, approximating 50 per cent, involvement of other organ systems occurs in less than 15 per cent of advanced cases.

Curative therapy utilizes radiation and surgery. Often these modalities are used in combination, which seems to increase cure rates slightly, although also increasing morbidity. In advanced cases chemotherapy is also used (most effective drugs include methotrexate, bleomycin, and cisplatin); the sequences, dosages, and combinations vary.

REHABILITATION. Rehabilitation is essential, since treatment often compromises appearance, function, and attitude. For surgical defects maxillofacial prosthetic appliances are very effective. Paraprofessionals are useful in improving speech and swallowing defects. Radiation, which is frequently used, alters saliva and taste, interfering with oral comfort and nutrition. Dietary consultation can often assist food acceptance. Xerostomia usually can be improved by the administration of pilocarpine, 5 mg four times a day, or bethanechol, 50 mg three times a day, if more conservative methods (sugarless gum or candy drops) are unsuccessful. Supplements of elemental zinc (up to 100 mg daily) have improved taste perception in some patients. Jaw bone and mucosal necrosis is also increased with radiation, and special care must be taken regarding dental procedures, extractions, and other forms of dental trauma. The risk is proportional to the radiation dosage, becoming most critical above 6500 rads. Antibiotics and time will often control the necrosis; however, surgery is sometimes required.

Silverman S Jr, Greenspan D: Early detection and diagnosis of oral cancer. J Calif Dent Assoc 13:29, 1985. *Comprehensive review of epidemiology, survival, and early detection and diagnosis; tables and photos.*

98 DISEASES OF THE ESOPHAGUS

Charles E. Pope II

CLINICAL SYMPTOMATOLOGY

The esophagus would seem to be a relatively simple portion of the gastrointestinal tract. Its duty, the transport of solids, liquids, and gas, usually is performed unobtrusively. The structure of the esophagus is not complex. Yet malfunction can lead to such trivial complaints as heartburn or overwhelming clinical problems such as aspiration, obstruction, and hemorrhage. A good clinical history will often be the most valuable diagnostic test. The laboratory diagnosis of esophageal malfunction often exceeds our therapeutic capabilities.

Esophageal disorders can be expressed by a group of symptoms that are unique to this organ. The esophagus also shares other symptoms with the rest of the gastrointestinal tract. The clinician should concentrate on the unique symptoms, as further investigations will usually uncover an esophageal cause.

DYSPHAGIA. Consciousness of bolus arrest during swallowing, even if transient, indicates esophageal dysfunction. The patient will usually use the term "sticks," "hesitates," "pauses," or "hangs up" and will often indicate the site of arrest with a finger.

Bolus arrest closely associated with the act of swallowing is dysphagia. The sensation of a substernal lump present one-half hour after eating is not dysphagia. Most patients consider mild dysphagia a normal phenomenon. "I just swallowed something that was too big." Thus, often they will not spontaneously mention the presence of dysphagia unless questioned closely.

A specialized type of dysphagia occurs when the bolus cannot be propelled from the mouth or hypopharynx into the esophagus, so-called "transfer dysphagia." This type of dysphagia is most commonly related to neurologic disease or to pharyngeal muscle weakness.

The sensation of dysphagia is localized to the suprasternal notch or substernally. The exact location of the sensation is of little use in pinpointing the site of bolus arrest. Dysphagia for a liquid bolus usually indicates an esophageal motor disorder. Dysphagia for solids can be seen either with an organic obstruction (stricture or cancer) or secondary to esophageal motor disorders.

The patient's response to dysphagia can also provide useful information about the cause of dysphagia. If the bolus must be regurgitated, and if an attempt to force the bolus down with water is met by a sudden return of the fluid, then an organic obstruction should be suspected. If the patient is able to force the bolus down by posturing, by performing a Valsalva's maneuver, by repeated swallowing, or by ingesting fluid, then a motor disorder is more likely. Inexorable progression of dysphagia over months usually signals the presence of organic narrowing, either a lumen-obliterating carcinoma or a stricture caused by active peptic esophagitis.

Dysphagia is never an expression of a pure psychiatric disorder; it is not a manifestation of hysteria. Some patients with well-established esophageal disease such as achalasia will report that their dysphagia is often worse at a time of severe emotional tension. Such observations have led many patients (and unfortunately some physicians) to believe that dysphagia is a matter for the psychiatrist rather than the gastroenterologist. Such an opinion can lead to subsequent embarrassment or tragedy, especially if an esophageal carcinoma is overlooked.

ODYNOPHAGIA. Pain upon swallowing, odynophagia, is another cardinal symptom of esophageal disease. Bolus arrest producing dysphagia can sometimes progress to a sensation of pain as esophageal obstruction continues. However, odynophagia usually occurs during the transit of the bolus and disappears once the swallowed material has left the esophagus. It may be mild in intensity so that the patient is merely aware of the location of the swallowed bolus. This is most commonly seen in patients with reflux disease. It can be of such intensity that the patient will refuse to swallow any solids or liquids and will expectorate saliva. Odynophagia can be seen after involvement of the mucosa by *reflux*, by *radiation*, or by *viral* or *fungal infections*. Odynophagia can be an uncommon manifestation of carcinoma or of a localized ulcer caused by a lodged tablet. Odynophagia thus localizes a process to the esophagus but gives no clue to pathogenesis.

HEARTBURN (PYROSIS). Heartburn or pyrosis is the most common manifestation of esophageal disease, so much so that it is difficult to recruit "normal" subjects, if strict histories are taken to eliminate any who have ever had heartburn. The term "burning" rather than "pain" is usually used, although heartburn can increase in intensity until it is perceived as pain. Patients commonly illustrate heartburn with a movement of the open hand up and down the sternum. This is in contrast to the stationary tightly clenched fist of angina pectoris. Heartburn is usually relieved, even if only temporarily, by taking antacids. A constant burning, unrelieved by antacids, may well be of esophageal origin, but it does not represent heartburn. Heartburn is often worse after recumbency or lifting; and may follow overeating or alcoholic indiscretion.

REGURGITATION. Regurgitation of fluid contents into the mouth often accompanies heartburn. Sometimes such regurgitation is associated with eructation; often it accompanies bending over, lifting, or lying down at night. The bitter regurgitated fluid is often described as yellow-brown or green. Regurgitation at night may lead to stridor or to wheezing, a hoarse voice, and other respiratory symptoms from unrecognized reflux. Less commonly, regurgitated fluid is not from the stomach or duodenum, but from fluid retained in an *achalasic esophagus* or in a large *pharyngeal diverticulum*. An uncommon but fascinating process that can be confused with regurgitation is *rumination*. In this condition, recently eaten food is propelled back into the mouth from the stomach by a strong contraction of the abdominal wall musculature. The food commonly is rechewed, reswallowed, and again returned to the mouth (Ch. 215).

ESOPHAGEAL COLIC. In addition to the discomfort from severe reflux, which can advance from heartburn into pain, abnormal motor activity of the esophageal muscle can cause severe pain clinically indistinguishable from angina pectoris in terms of intensity, radiation, relationship to exercise, and even response to nitroglycerin. Chest pain of esophageal origin can radiate directly through to the back and is often found in patients who also notice dysphagia. Esophageal colic can last from five to ten seconds to hours.

HEMATEMESIS. Although vomiting blood is less specific for esophageal disease than are many of the symptoms listed above, hematemesis can signal the presence of esophageal varices, of mucosal ulceration resulting from esophageal reflux, of a rent of the mucosa of the lower esophagus, or, uncommonly, of an ulcerating carcinoma or leiomyoma of the esophagus. Although bleeding from the esophagus may be life threatening, more often it is a slow ooze, usually caused by esophageal reflux disease, which presents clinically as an iron deficiency anemia.

Berk JE (ed.): Bockus' Gastroenterology. 4th ed. Philadelphia, W. B. Saunders Company, 1985, pp 666–850. *Reference textbook chapters on esophagus. Good source for recent references.*

Pope CE II: Chapters on the esophagus. In Sleisenger MH, Fordtran JS (eds.): Gastrointestinal Disease. 4th ed. Philadelphia, W. B. Saunders Company, (in press). *Reference textbook on esophageal disease.*

GASTROESOPHAGEAL REFLUX DISEASE

DEFINITION. Gastroesophageal reflux disease (GERD) refers to the varied clinical manifestations of reflux of stomach and duodenal contents into the esophagus. It is preferable to the term "reflux esophagitis" because the latter expression tends to mean different things to the clinician, the endoscopist, and the pathologist. Although it may be associated with a sliding hiatus hernia, "symptomatic hiatus hernia" is a term that tends to put the emphasis on the wrong anatomic entity and pathophysiology. Gastroesophageal reflux disease can be characterized by any combination of symptoms and radiologic, endoscopic, or pathologic changes. In its milder manifestations, it is a common disease; its most florid state is uncommon but may be life threatening.

PATHOGENESIS. Several factors must work in concert to produce clinical effects of esophageal reflux. All persons will demonstrate short bursts of reflux if monitored with an intraesophageal pH probe over 24 hours. This reflux is seen postprandially and usually in the upright position. Those in whom reflux has produced symptoms or pathologic changes will demonstrate more prolonged episodes of reflux, which tend to occur at night. The factor or factors that cause this difference are not known. However, important differences between persons with and without reflux might help explain these findings.

The *lower esophageal sphincter* (LES) is a specialized bundle of circular muscle at the lower end of the esophagus with different physical and pharmacologic characteristics when compared with the circular muscle above and below it. There is a tendency for mean LES pressure to be significantly lower in subjects with GERD compared with normal persons, but LES pressures are not very useful in predicting whether reflux is present in an individual patient unless the pressure is very low. The most common event associated with reflux appears to be an *inappropriate relaxation of the lower esophageal sphincter*, i.e., LES relaxation unassociated with either swallowing or the distention of the esophageal body by refluxed fluid. Thus, two abnormalities of LES may be associated with reflux: a sphincter with very low tone, as measured by lower esophageal sphincter pressure, or inappropriate relaxation of a normally competent sphincter.

Several factors are important in removing refluxed material. The upright position facilitates esophageal emptying by gravity. Peristaltic waves initiated by swallowing or by esophageal distention help remove the refluxed material. Acid placed within the esophagus is cleared less well by patients with GERD than by normal subjects, even though the manometric tracings seen in both groups seem identical. Clearing occurs in two phases. The bulk of the fluid is returned to the stomach by a peristaltic contraction; the remainder of the acid film clinging to the esophageal wall is neutralized by swallowed saliva.

The composition and perhaps the quantity of the refluxed material also play a role in the production of GERD. Gastric acid and pepsin seem clearly important in the pathogenesis of GERD. Bile salts and possibly pancreatic enzymes may be responsible in those patients in whom acid is absent. The combination of bile salts plus acid is more injurious to the esophagus than either agent alone. Other less well-studied factors such as altered or abnormal esophageal mucus, swallowed saliva of high bicarbonate content, and diminished resistance of the esophageal mucosa to digestion may be important in determining the amount of mucosal damage in GERD.

Esophageal squamous epithelium reacts to reflux by an increase in the basal cell or germinative layer. The dermal pegs are increased in height and may become more vascular. If the process becomes more severe, the epithelial layer is destroyed, with the appearance of microulcers and classic signs of inflammation in the lamina propria, such as infiltration with polymorphonuclear leukocytes and edema. Even deeper lesions cause first submucosal, then muscular inflammation and fibrosis, resulting in an esophageal stricture. Why reflux is so common, yet inflammation and stricture formation so relatively uncommon, is not known.

Other conditions can be associated with the pathogenesis of reflux. Reflux during pregnancy, once thought to be due to the increased abdominal pressure from the fetus, may be due mainly to diminished LES strength caused by extra estrogen and progesterone. Weight gain also tends to aggravate reflux through an unknown mechanism. As expected, resection of the lower esophageal area for cancer or myotomy for achalasia can lead to severe postoperative reflux (see below).

ROLE OF HIATUS HERNIA. The presence of a hiatus

hernia is now considered to be much less of a factor in GERD than previously thought. Some radiologists find hiatus hernias in a large percentage of patients, no matter what the reason for the examination. Others rarely demonstrate a hiatus hernia. It is not appropriate to spend a great deal of time trying to define whether a hiatus hernia is present or absent in dealing with most patients with GERD. The important entity to investigate is reflux, not hiatus hernia.

SYMPTOMS OF GASTROESOPHAGEAL REFLUX DISEASE. *Heartburn* is the most common manifestation of GERD. It can vary from an occasional mild burning after overeating to an ever-present, severe discomfort that severely limits a patient's lifestyle. It may be accompanied by *regurgitation* of gastric contents either into the mouth or into the respiratory tree. This latter group of patients may complain of nocturnal wheezing, hoarseness, a need to clear the throat repeatedly, and a sensation of deep pressure at the base of the neck. This group of symptoms may be the primary clinical presentation and more prominent than the classic symptoms of GERD.

Dysphagia is often present in those with significant GERD. Although dysphagia may be severe and even mark the onset of stricture formation, it usually is mild and must be carefully sought. Dysphagia of GERD is for solids, and the dysphagia is usually overcome by swallowing repeatedly or by washing down the bolus with some water. Dysphagia without anatomic strictures has been noted in about three fourths of patients scheduled for antireflux surgery. Many patients with GERD will not complain of bolus arrest, but rather of being aware of the location of each solid morsel as it travels down the esophagus.

Blood loss may result from esophageal erosion and shallow ulcers. Rarely producing life-threatening hemorrhage, the erosions are much more likely to weep quietly over a prolonged period of time, producing iron deficiency anemia. Some of these patients have very few other clinical manifestations of GERD, and the condition is discovered by endoscopy during an evaluation of occult gastrointestinal bleeding. Patients who vigorously and repeatedly abuse alcohol seem prone to develop severe erosive esophagitis with bleeding; this lesion heals with abstinence from alcohol without other major antireflux therapy.

DIAGNOSIS. The history and clinical manifestations of GERD are the most important diagnostic aids in the establishment of the diagnosis; objective testing is used to quantify the extent and severity of the process. In the evaluation of an individual, questions to be answered dictate the appropriate test.

Does reflux exist and, if so, to what degree? This question might arise either if another condition such as pulmonary disease is present and a causal relationship is being sought, or if some idea of the frequency and extent of reflux is important. Reflux during a barium swallow in adults is uncommon unless vigorous provocative maneuvers are employed. When spontaneous reflux of barium is seen, it usually denotes free reflux. Children reflux barium more easily than do adults. The pH probe can be used either for short-term studies of 15 to 30 minutes or for more prolonged periods (24 hours). If repeated bursts of reflux are demonstrated during a 15-minute period, then severe reflux is present. At the same time, the ability of the esophagus to clear itself of refluxed acid can be evaluated. Usually a manometric catheter is attached to the pH probe in order to locate it in the esophagus; this catheter can also estimate the LES pressure. Only very low values of LES pressure such as 1 to 2 mm Hg (normal, about 20 mm Hg) are of prognostic value.

Twenty-four-hour pH monitoring can be performed with a portable unit, which allows the patient to follow an almost normal lifestyle. During the prolonged monitoring period, the relationship between symptoms (heartburn, pain, wheezing) and episodes of reflux can be ascertained, and calculations can be made of the number of episodes of reflux and the amount of time the esophagus is acidified.

Reflux can be measured noninvasively by scanning of the esophageal area with a gamma camera after placing a solution of ^{99m}Tc sulfur colloid in the stomach. An abdominal binder is used to stress the gastroesophageal junction if free reflux is not seen. This technique seems to be of most value in infants and children, who tolerate esophageal tubes very poorly.

Could reflux be responsible for the patient's symptoms? This question might be asked if pain is the predominant symptom rather than more classic heartburn. This question can be answered with the same catheter assembly used to measure LES pressure and acid reflux. After a five-minute period of dripping normal saline through one of the pressure catheters whose opening has been localized to the upper esophagus, this infusion is changed to 0.1 N hydrochloric acid without the patient's knowledge. Reproduction of the symptoms within 30 minutes of acid infusion (usually four to five minutes into the infusion) and rapid disappearance of the symptom with a switch back to saline infusion suggests an esophageal cause of the discomfort.

As another approach, the patient is asked to signal the time of discomfort during prolonged pH monitoring of the esophagus. If the patient signals discomfort at the same time that reflux is demonstrated by the pH probe, then a causal relationship is made more likely. Prolonged pH monitoring is not used widely clinically because of the expense of hospitalization. The development of portable pH monitors has made this approach more feasible.

What has reflux done to the esophageal mucosa? A barium swallow will detect gross changes such as stricture formation or a deep esophageal ulcer but will miss the much more common shallow ulcerations and erosions. These will be detected by direct inspection with the endoscope. Only discrete lesions such as erosions and ulcerations should be taken as proof of esophageal damage; such endoscopic findings as erythema, edema, or friability are subject to wide interobserver variation. If the mucosa appears absolutely normal, as it is in approximately one third of patients with moderate-to-severe symptoms of GERD, a suction biopsy can demonstrate the changes of reflux.

A logic tree of how these tests might be used is shown in Table 98–1. A patient whose symptoms are severe enough to seek medical attention might be screened with a barium swallow. Uncommonly, reflux will be demonstrated, a stricture found, or a deep ulcer seen. This might lead to immediate endoscopy for more complete evaluation. If a patient presents with hematemesis and reflux symptoms, endoscopy might appropriately be used as the first step. After first evaluation, it is appropriate to begin therapy (see Treatment, below). Only if there is a poor response to therapy should an acid perfusion test be used to confirm the diagnosis. At the same time, the presence of reflux can be checked, an estimate of LES pressure and acid clearance obtained, and the presence or absence of peristaltic waves determined.

More intensive therapy should be instituted at this point. If it fails and the patient is still symptomatic, endoscopy can be employed to see if gross disease is still present in the face of maximal therapy. If the appearance of the mucosa is normal grossly in the presence of overwhelming symptoms, suction biopsies can be obtained to search for objective evidence of reflux damage. This scheme will restrict extensive testing to those who have failed medical therapy and who are presumably candidates for surgical treatment. This algorithm can be modified if the patient has blood loss or severe dysphagia. Endoscopy should follow a screening barium radiographic examination of such patients.

COMPLICATIONS OF GASTROESOPHAGEAL REFLUX DISEASE. *Esophageal Stricture.* Of the many who complain of symptoms of GERD, only a few will develop esophageal

TABLE 98–1. DIAGNOSIS OF REFLUX

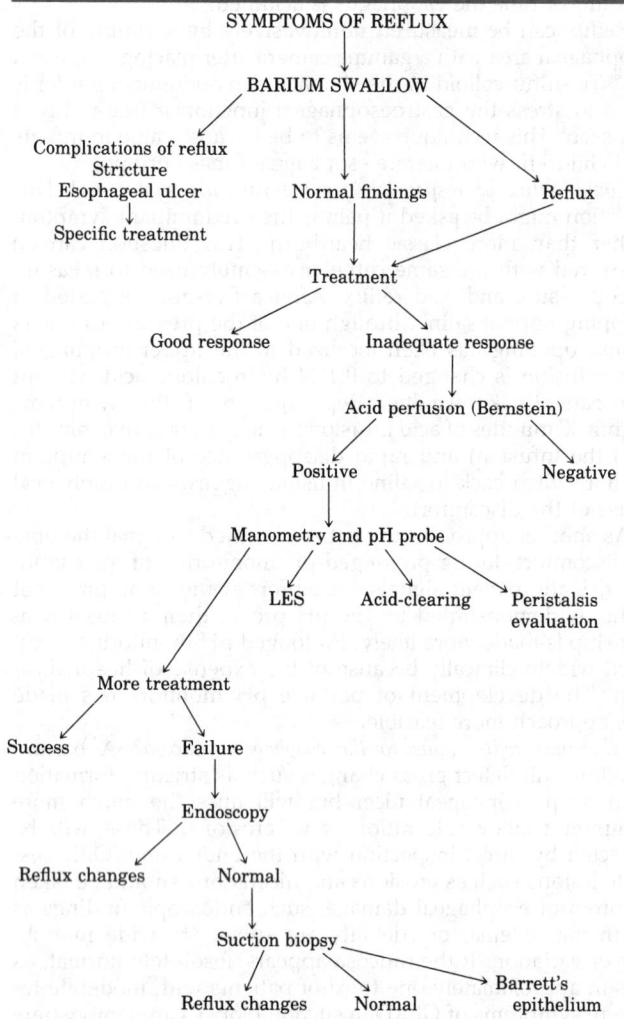

SYMPTOMS OF REFLUX

BARIUM SWALLOW

Complications of reflux
Stricture
Esophageal ulcer → Specific treatment

Normal findings

Reflux

Treatment

Good response

Inadequate response

Acid perfusion (Bernstein)

Positive

Negative

Manometry and pH probe

LES

Acid-clearing

Peristalsis evaluation

More treatment

Success

Failure

Endoscopy

Reflux changes

Normal

Suction biopsy

Reflux changes

Normal

Barrett's epithelium

TABLE 98–2. CLINICAL FEATURES OF PULMONARY ASPIRATION

1. Onset of "asthma" in patients over 30 years without a family history of asthma or industrial exposure
2. Nocturnal or early morning cough
3. Nocturnal wheezing
4. Hoarseness, especially on arising
5. The need to clear the throat repeatedly
6. A feeling of constant pressure deep in the neck

through to the back. Brisk hemorrhage is another manifestation, from erosion either through to an esophageal artery or, more catastrophically, into the nearby aorta. The presence of an ulcer can be suspected on a barium swallow and confirmed endoscopically. The ulcer is usually found to reside in columnar (Barrett's) epithelium.

Columnar Epithelium. In some patients who have suffered severe esophageal ulceration as a result of GERD, the healing epithelium is replaced not with squamous epithelium but with a specialized columnar epithelium. The junctional zone between squamous and columnar epithelium can progress orad over years. Columnar epithelium is found at and below midesophageal strictures and around deep esophageal ulcers, although it can be found on routine biopsy of patients with severe GERD. Its major clinical importance is not only as a marker of severe reflux but also as a precursor for adenocarcinoma of the esophagus (see under Esophageal Tumors).

Pulmonary Aspiration. If refluxed material breaches the upper esophageal sphincter, it may easily spill into the larynx and tracheobronchial tree. Some patients react to such a spill with intense respiratory stridor. Others seem to tolerate the presence of refluxed contents in the larynx and tracheobronchial tree with milder laryngeal or respiratory symptoms. It is even possible that the gastric contents do not have to reach the larynx, instillation of acid in the esophagus of susceptible individuals while they are in the upright posture can be shown to cause closing of small bronchial airways, presumably by a vagal reflex.

None of the clinical features of pulmonary aspiration (Table 98–2) is pathognomonic. Taken together they point toward reflux and aspiration as a possible etiology. Diagnostic proof of the relationship is difficult with current techniques. Radioisotopes placed in the stomach have been demonstrated the next morning to be in the lungs by gamma camera scanning, but this cannot be demonstrated in the majority of patients. Only correction of reflux with subsequent disappearance of pulmonary symptoms can prove the relationship.

TREATMENT OF GASTROESOPHAGEAL REFLUX DISEASE AND ITS COMPLICATIONS. *Medical Management.* Most mildly symptomatic patients with reflux and some moderately afflicted individuals can be helped by manipulations designed to alter the frequency or type of esophageal reflux. Many patients respond to the simple measures outlined in Table 98–3. Elevation of the head of the bed by 6 to 8 inches is the simplest and most effective form of therapy. Twenty-four–hour pH monitoring has shown that this simple measure decreases the frequency and length of reflux epi-

TABLE 98–3. TREATMENT OF GASTROESOPHAGEAL REFLUX DISEASE

Simple Measures
1. Elevation of head of the bed
2. Avoidance of food and fluid intake before bedtime
3. Reduction of fat in diet
4. Liquid antacid (aluminum hydroxide, magnesium hydroxide) one and three hours after meals and at bedtime
5. Avoidance of cigarettes and alcohol
6. Weight loss

Measures for Resistant Cases
1. Alginic acid–antacid (Gaviscon), 15 ml four times a day
2. Bethanechol (Urecholine),* 10 or 25 mg four times a day
3. Metoclopramide (Reglan),* 10 mg three times a day
4. Cimetidine,* 300 mg four times a day
5. Ranitidine,* 150 mg twice a day

*This use is not listed in the manufacturer's directive.

strictures. Usually beginning at the lower end of the esophagus, strictures may migrate over years to the midesophagus or higher. Columnar epithelium will be found below the stricture. Presumably those who develop strictures have had deep circumferential ulceration of the esophageal mucosa due to reflux damage. Instead of healing with only minimal submucosal and muscular fibrosis, these patients develop esophageal obstruction with a narrowed esophageal lumen. If reflux can be controlled, these strictures will disappear.

Dysphagia is the clinical hallmark of esophageal stricture formation. Unlike the relatively mild dysphagia seen in uncomplicated GERD, the dysphagia in patients with strictures tends to be constant and slowly progressive, causing the patient to alter the type of food taken. If a bolus becomes arrested in the stricture, it is usually necessary for the bolus to be regurgitated back into the mouth before further intake of food or fluids is possible.

Strictures are most easily evaluated by barium swallow. Sometimes the extent of the strictured area is overestimated unless the esophagus below the stricture can be fully distended by barium. For mild strictures, the ingestion of a bread or marshmallow bolus can draw attention to slight luminal narrowing when the bolus impacts there. Once demonstrated, endoscopy with biopsy and/or brush cytology is in order to make certain that the stricture is benign.

Esophageal Ulcer. In addition to the more common shallow ulcerations, deep esophageal ulcers may complicate severe GERD. These ulcers, which retain barium and usually project outside the wall of the esophagus, characteristically produce severe and unrelenting pain, often with radiation of the pain sodes. The use of pillows to elevate the thorax does not work well, as patients tend to roll off the pillows during the night. A foam rubber wedge can be used if the bed frame cannot be moved. Avoiding food and fluid for at least three hours before retiring decreases the amount of material available for reflux at night. Avoidance of food that the patient finds distressing, such as fatty foods, chocolate, and onions, makes sense but has never been subjected to clinical trial.

Neutralization of acid is approached by taking 30 ml of aluminum hydroxide–magnesium hydroxide antacid one and three hours after meals and at bedtime. In recalcitrant cases, hourly antacids may be tried, with substitution of pure aluminum hydroxide gel to control diarrhea produced by the magnesium ion. Most patients will not tolerate such a regimen for long.

An attempt should be made to have the patient stop smoking, drinking alcohol, and overeating. Most patients, however, apparently prefer to suffer with reflux symptoms rather than to give up these mainstays of life.

If these simple measures are not effective, more vigorous treatment is indicated. Alginic acid–antacid, 15 ml after each meal and at bedtime, is more effective than placebo and as effective as antacids. It is worth trying, but often will not control symptoms of severe reflux. Bethanechol* is a parasympathomimetic agent that can be used in doses of 10 or 25 mg four times a day. Metoclopramide,* 10 mg three times a day, can be helpful, but central nervous system side effects can limit its usefulness. Cimetidine,* 300 mg four times a day, or ranitidine,* 150 mg twice a day, although not approved for therapy of heartburn, improves symptoms significantly when compared with placebo.

Surgical Management. In a patient in whom adequate trial of medical management as outlined above has not brought good results in a six-month period, and in whom there is good objective evidence of reflux, surgical correction of reflux should be considered. Current surgical therapy, regardless of exact techniques, attempts to restore sphincter competence by surrounding the lower end of the esophagus with a cuff of gastric fundal muscle. This is done either completely, as in the Nissen fundoplication, or partially (Hill repair, Belsey repair).

It is difficult to choose one operation or method over another, as most published surgical reports do not carefully define the exact indications for the operation, the length and type of preoperative medical management, or the use of objective tests pre- and postoperatively. Follow-up tends to be short and incomplete; the postoperative assessments are usually made by those responsible for choosing or operating upon the patients. Therefore, no firm statement can be made about the true efficacy of surgery in the correction of reflux.

A surgeon experienced in the techniques of antireflux surgery is necessary for good postoperative results. Technique is all important. Although some individual surgeons have enviable postoperative results, antireflux surgery has a relatively poor reputation in many medical communities. Currently, a conservative approach toward antireflux surgery seems indicated.

Treatment of Complications. Esophageal strictures, if only mildly symptomatic, can be handled by careful attention to dietary intake, improvement of dentition, and institution of medical therapy. Techniques of dilation have proliferated in recent years, but they still require an experienced operator. Short, simple strictures can be dilated with weighted rubber or Teflon dilators (Hurst, Maloney). Tortuous or angulated strictures are more easily approached over a previously placed guide wire. This, in turn, can be passed through an endoscope or under radiographic control. Graded steel olives (Eder-Peustow), a dilator with graded increases of size (Celestin), or a balloon with a fixed maximal diameter (Cooke) can be

passed over the previously placed wire. Alternatively, a balloon of fixed maximal diameter can be passed through the large channel of an endoscope during diagnostic endoscopy, and dilation can be done under direct vision. Once the lumen is restored to a diameter of 13 to 15 mm, most patients swallow without difficulty. If the stricture is stable and requires dilation only every four to six months, nothing else is necessary.

Some patients will not tolerate dilation or require vigorous dilation every three to four weeks. This is an indication for definitive antireflux operation, following which the stricture may regress. Unfortunately, many strictures persist after attempts at antireflux surgery. Esophageal replacement by colon, jejunum, or stomach is a surgical maneuver of last resort; such procedures have relatively high morbidity and mortality. Those afflicted by strictures often have significant lung and cardiovascular disease that makes them unsuitable operative candidates.

If a patient has a peptic stricture that does not respond to dilation and if surgery is deemed too risky because of the patient's age or condition, irradiation of the stomach may be tried. Fifteen hundred rads to the stomach is usually well tolerated and produces anacidity for weeks to months after therapy is completed. Acid production usually returns at a later date, but often at a lower level. This procedure sometimes facilitates dilation of the stricture.

Esophageal ulcers also represent a major therapeutic problem. Although cimetidine therapy may heal an ulcer, antireflux surgery, if tolerated, is a more reliable mode of treatment. If not, gastric radiation can be employed as in esophageal stricture.

Columnar epithelium may be premalignant. There is no way short of esophageal resection to make certain that the epithelium can be removed. Adequate antireflux therapy will cause regression of columnar epithelium in a rare patient, but further study is necessary before antireflux surgery can be recommended as a treatment for columnar epithelium. The effect of long-term cimetidine therapy on recurrence of either esophagitis or the columnar epithelium is not known.

Treatment of the pulmonary complications of reflux depends on the age of the patient. Infants who present with recurrent bronchitis can be treated by postural methods and by thickening the formula. In adults, attention to posture at night is most important (see above). Since diagnostic methods that establish a direct causal relationship between reflux and lung disease are lacking, caution is advised in offering surgery to those who present with primary pulmonary problems and in whom reflux is demonstrated.

Castell DO, Wu WC, Ott DS: Gastroesophageal Reflux Disease. Mt. Kisco, NY, Futura Publishing Company, 1985, pp 1–324. *Monograph with good literature review.*
Spechler SJ, Goyal RK: Barrett's esophagus. N Engl J Med 315:362, 1986. *Up-to-date review of columnar epithelium.*

MOTOR DISORDERS OF THE ESOPHAGUS

DEFINITION AND PATHOGENESIS. The muscular tube of the esophagus is guarded at both ends by specialized bundles of muscle, the upper and lower esophageal sphincters (UES, LES). Material from the oropharynx is injected at a high velocity (in the case of liquids), and precise coordination is required to link the muscles of the oropharynx, UES, body of the esophagus, and LES into a functional unit. Failure of any or all of these components will result in an esophageal motor disorder.

Failure of the oropharyngeal and UES units can be caused either by primary muscle disease such as *myotonia dystrophica* or *dermatomyositis* or by neurologic lesions involving the innervation of these muscle groups. *Brain stem infarcts, multiple sclerosis,* and *amyotrophic lateral sclerosis* serve as examples for the latter process.

The pathogenesis of motor abnormality of the esophageal

---

*This use is not listed in the manufacturer's directive.

body is less well understood. The striated muscle that constitutes the upper one quarter to one third of the body can be affected by primary muscle disease, such as *myotonia dystrophica*, or by metabolic disease affecting muscle function, such as *hypothyroidism*. The smooth muscle seems more resistant to muscular disease, but the intrinsic nervous network can be involved in *Chagas disease* and *achalasia*. In the latter disease, there is infiltration of Auerbach's plexus with lymphocytes or actual disappearance of the neuron cell bodies in the plexus.

The motor disorders of the body of the esophagus have historically been classified as *achalasia* or *diffuse spasm*. In achalasia, dysphagia and esophageal retention predominate; the radiograph shows a dilated esophagus with a distal beak, and manometry reveals a high pressure in the LES with no or incomplete relaxation as well as only simultaneous low-amplitude contractions in response to a swallow. Diffuse spasm has been characterized as a clinical syndrome of esophageal colic or dysphagia or both; segmental contractions seen by radiograph; and a manometric picture of some peristaltic waves interspersed with periods of slight simultaneous elevation of the baseline pressure in several leads surmounted by simultaneous contractions. Another common manometric abnormality is high-amplitude, long-duration waves that are peristaltic and can be associated with either esophageal colic or dysphagia or both (nutcracker esophagus). There are many variations of these "classic" diseases, and progression from diffuse spasm to achalasia has been documented in the same individual. Many nonspecific motor disorders of the esophagus do not fit these syndromes. The pathophysiology of these nonspecific disorders has not been described. It seems best at the present state of knowledge to be descriptive of the features of a motor disorder without being too precise about an actual name of the disorder.

SYMPTOMS. The type of symptom produced is a function of the level and extent of the problem. *Weakness of the oropharyngeal musculature* may cause *transfer dysphagia*—the inability to propel a solid or liquid bolus from the pharynx to the esophagus. Patients are aware usually that they cannot begin the act of deglutition. Solids are usually more trouble than liquids. Palatal weakness may lead to *nasal regurgitation* of fluids or to *laryngeal aspiration* because of muscular failure to seal off the larynx. Such weakness may be signaled by a nasal quality of the voice.

Incoordination of UES relaxation has been suggested as a cause of transfer dysphagia and for the production of Zenker's diverticulum, but current high-fidelity methods fail to show such incoordination. Transfer dysphagia accompanied by a prominent cricopharyngeal impression on a barium swallow ("cricopharyngeal achalasia") similarly shows no defect in relaxing or in timing when studied by modern manometric methods.

Motor disorders in the body of the esophagus produce either *dysphagia* or *pain*, or both. The dysphagia may be intermittent or continuous. It may be manifest both for solids and for liquids. It is rare for the arrested material to be regurgitated; often posturing (throwing the shoulders back and extending the neck) or a Valsalva maneuver will help the material pass into the stomach.

Pain or esophageal colic is the other major clinical presentation of motor disorders. The pain is usually substernal, described as a feeling of pressure or aching, radiating to the back as well as to the neck, jaw, and arms. It can range in intensity from a transient discomfort to an overwhelming, agonizing pain similar to that of a major myocardial infarction or dissecting aortic aneurysm. The pain may last for only five to ten seconds or may be present for hours. The differentiation between angina pectoris and esophageal colic may be impossible on clinical grounds; both may be related to exercise, have the same intensity and distribution, and respond to sublingual nitroglycerin.

Failure of the lower esophageal sphincter may present with two separate symptom complexes. If the sphincter fails to relax on deglutition (as occurs in achalasia), there will be dysphagia and retention of contents in the body of the esophagus. This failure, coupled with loss of peristalsis (achalasia), leads to marked esophageal retention, regurgitation, and overflow of esophageal contents into the tracheobronchial tree. If there is primary muscle failure of the sphincter, as occurs in *scleroderma*, massive reflux and the consequences of GERD will follow.

DIAGNOSIS. A careful history is essential in choosing the correct diagnostic tools for evaluating esophageal motor disorders. If the difficulty is thought to be in the oropharynx and upper esophageal sphincter, a cineradiograph would offer the most information. The cine film allows for frame-by-frame analysis of this rapidly moving portion of the gastrointestinal tract. Incoordination of tongue and palate, unilateral pharyngeal weakness, and aspiration of small amounts of barium into the trachea on swallowing can be shown. Air double-contrast examinations of the pharynx can elucidate an unsuspected hypopharyngeal carcinoma. A diverticulum or prominence of the cricopharyngeal muscle can also be seen. Manometric examination of the hypopharynx and upper esophageal sphincter has not been helpful.

Radiology offers the best chance of diagnosis when the motor disorders have relatively static changes. In achalasia the body of the esophagus commonly dilates with retention of food, secretions, and barium (Fig. 98–1). Special attention can be paid to the terminal end of the esophagus. In achalasia, there is a smooth, tapering beak. Any irregularity of this beak should lead to a vigorous search for an infiltrating neoplasm of the cardia, which can exactly mimic achalasia clinically and radiologically.

If the esophageal muscle is atonic, as is seen in far-advanced scleroderma, barium and even air will be retained for long periods of time in the supine position. Assumption of the upright position will rapidly clear the barium from the esoph-

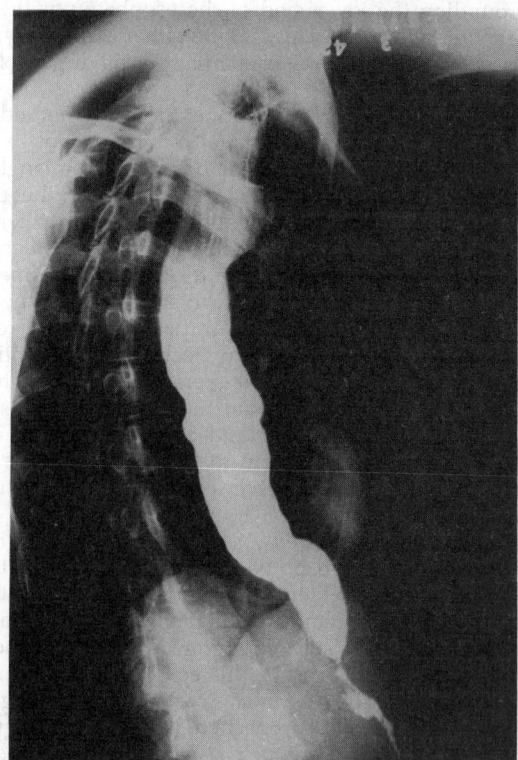

FIGURE 98–1. Radiologic appearance of achalasia. The esophageal body is dilated and terminates in a narrowed segment. (Courtesy of Dr. FE Templeton. From Pope CE II: In Sleisenger MH, Fordtran JS [eds.]: Gastrointestinal Disease. 3rd ed. Philadelphia, W. B. Saunders Company, 1983.)

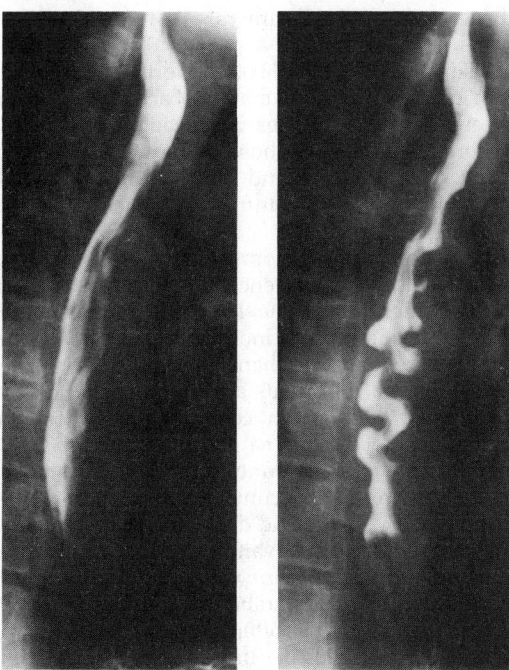

FIGURE 98–2. Radiologic appearance of diffuse spasm. Two spot films were taken within 10 seconds of each other. A fairly normal appearance on the left changes rapidly to an appearance of numerous contractions. (Courtesy of Dr. CA Rohrmann. From Pope CE II: In Sleisenger MH, Fordtran JS [eds.]: Gastrointestinal Disease. 3rd ed. Philadelphia, W. B. Saunders Company, 1983.)

agus and leave a double-contrast view of a dilated esophagus.

The radiologist has more difficulty when the motor abnormality is more intermittent (Fig. 98–2). Such a radiologic appearance is not always evidence for a clinically important motor disorder; elderly patients will often show similar radiologic findings and yet be totally asymptomatic.

Manometric examination allows more prolonged evaluation of esophageal motor function and is the only method that allows lower esophageal sphincter function to be directly determined. Normally, a swallow causes a peristaltic wave to be detected sequentially by pressure detectors spaced along the esophagus. Aperistalsis (no response to a swallow), simultaneous single or multiple contractions, prolonged contractions of high amplitude and low velocity, and spontaneous activity not related to swallowing can be recorded. Some of the "classic" patterns associated with diseases are shown in Figure 98–3. Many subjects present with dysphagia and/or chest pain in different patterns. It is best to describe the radiologic and manometric findings in the individual patient and then try to relate them to the classic syndrome most closely resembled. Also, one syndrome (diffuse spasm) may progress over time to another (achalasia).

Manometric examination can be of special benefit in the evaluation of chest pain if the patient happens to have an attack of chest pain during the examination. If the chest pain is accompanied by motor activity that allows the manometrist to predict onset, intensity, and disappearance of the chest pain by watching the manometric tracing, the diagnosis of an esophageal origin of chest pain is firmly established. Similarly, if pH is being simultaneously monitored and the episodes of chest pain correlate closely with drops in intraesophageal pH, an esophageal origin of pain is likely. Conversely, if typical chest pain occurs but there is no change in motor activity or pH over control values, an esophageal cause of pain is unlikely. Unfortunately, such definitive statements can be made only in about 20 per cent of the patients examined.

Pharmacologic stimulation of the esophagus has been employed for diagnostic purposes using such agents as mecholyl, pentagastrin, bethanechol, and ergonovine, but no universally successful stimulus has yet been found. The possibility of serious coronary ischemia or cardiac arrhythmia with ergonovine limits the usefulness of this agent.

Endoscopy has little usefulness in the evaluation of most motor disorders except for inspection of the cardia with a retroflexed view from the stomach to rule out an infiltrating carcinoma. Possibly transport of radionuclides as measured by a gamma camera will aid in the detection and evaluation of motor disorders.

FIGURE 98–3. Idealized manometric patterns. *A,* The normal swallow consists of a progressive wave with a wave of short duration and rapid rise time in the striated upper esophagus. The lower esophageal sphincter shows a fall in pressure coincident with swallowing. *B,* In achalasia the striated muscle sometimes but not always produces a typical wave. The smooth muscle portion of the esophagus has a simultaneous low-amplitude contraction that follows the striated muscle contraction. The elevated pressure in the LES shows either incomplete or no relaxation. *C,* Diffuse spasm shows an elevation of the baseline after swallowing, on top of which are superimposed repetitive simultaneous contractions. LES pressure may be high and relaxation may terminate prematurely. *D,* High-amplitude, long-duration waves (nutcracker esophagus). The wave is peristaltic but of high amplitude. Duration is increased and velocity of propagation may be decreased. *E,* Scleroderma. Striated muscle contraction is normal, but the amplitude of contraction in the smooth muscle is reduced or may be absent. Sphincter pressure is low.

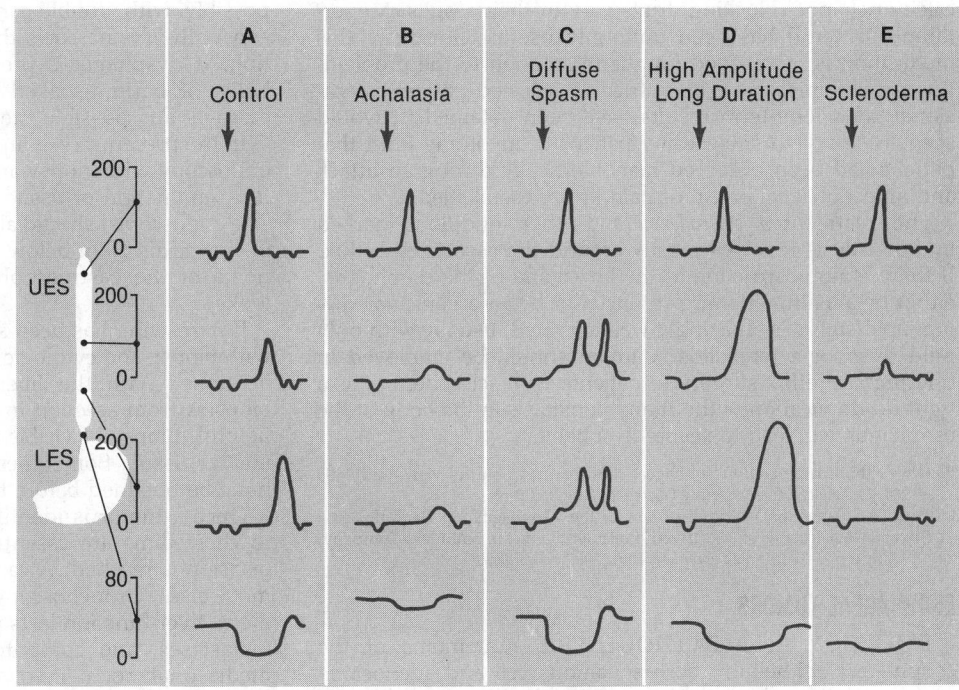

TREATMENT. Of the various motor disorders of the esophagus, only *achalasia* seems amenable to relief. Since the problem in achalasia is one of obstruction of the lower end of the esophagus by a sphincter that will not relax, all forms of therapy are directed at relief of this obstruction. Short-term improvement in clinical symptoms and in scintigraphic esophageal emptying may occur with isosorbide dinitrate, a long-acting nitrate, or with nifedipine, a calcium channel blocker. The place of long-term pharmacologic management of achalasia has not been established. Dilation with a large Hurst bougie may give temporary relief; a few patients have been maintained for long periods of time with weekly self-dilations. Much more effective is brisk dilation with a pneumatic bag under radiographic control. This should be performed by an expert, since the rate of perforation even in good hands is about 5 to 15 per cent. Bag dilation is preferable initially for all patients.

Surgery is reserved for those in whom bag dilation fails or those who do not wish to be exposed to the risk of perforation. Direct section of the lower esophageal sphincter muscle (myotomy) is carried out, sparing some gastric muscle fibers to prevent postoperative reflux (Heller procedure). Amazingly, after both bag dilation and myotomy, manometry reveals return of normal peristalsis in 20 per cent of those with achalasia. This observation is difficult to explain in view of the degeneration of Auerbach's plexus in the intramural nervous network, thought to explain the pathogenesis of this disease.

Treatment of most other motor disorders is much more difficult. Patients with diffuse spasm can be given nitroglycerin or anticholinergics, but the results are disappointing. Balloon dilation has also been suggested to be of benefit in diffuse spasm, but it is difficult to understand how stretching of the lower esophageal sphincter segment would benefit a process that involves the entire esophageal body. Division of all the circular muscle with a long myotomy has been tried, but the long-term results of this procedure are not always favorable.

Treatment of other nonspecific motor disorders associated with chest pain can be equally frustrating. Prescribing sublingual nitroglycerin is justifiable. If it is ineffective, long-acting nitrate therapy will probably not work. Anticholinergic drugs will benefit only a few. Preliminary reports on the use of calcium channel blocking drugs vary in their results. Meperidine (Demerol) has been uniformly useful. Obviously this medication is not a good long-term solution to the problem. Long myotomies have been tried in selected patients; occasional good long-term results have been obtained. It would seem wise not to subject any patient to myotomy until that patient had been observed manometrically during an attack and an esophageal origin of pain firmly established.

The treatment of *scleroderma* and other conditions marked by aperistalsis revolves mostly around the associated reflux. If there is no obstruction at the lower end of the esophagus, either by a malfunctioning sphincter or by an organic narrowing, aperistalsis is amazingly well tolerated, usually with only mild dysphagia for solids. Caution should be employed in offering antireflux surgery to patients with scleroderma, as a tight fundoplication without any peristalsis in the body of the esophagus will lead to severe dysphagia.

Blackwell JN, Castell DO: Oesophageal chest pain: A point of view. Gut 25:1, 1984. *Review of the esophagus as a source of anginal pain.*

Ouyang A, Cohen S: Motor disorders of the esophagus. In Berk JE (ed.): Bockus' Gastroenterology. 4th ed. Philadelphia, W. B. Saunders Company, 1985, pp 690–704. *Good current review of motor disorders.*

ESOPHAGEAL TUMORS

ETIOLOGY AND PATHOGENESIS. Carcinoma of the esophageal epithelium, both squamous cell and adenocarcinoma, is by far the most common and important tumor of the esophagus. Benign neoplasms (leiomyoma, papilloma, and fibrovascular polyps) are rarer by far. Squamous cell cancer has an incidence of 4 per 100,000 in males (United States), rising to 130 per 100,000 in North China. It is associated with both alcohol intake and tobacco smoking in countries where these substances are used. Esophageal cancer occurs more commonly in those who have developed squamous cancers of the head and neck, in those with lye strictures, and in patients with untreated or inadequately treated achalasia.

Adenocarcinoma of the esophagus arises in columnar (Barrett's) epithelium. The sequence of dysplasia, adenoma formation, and adenocarcinoma has been demonstrated. The actual incidence of adenocarcinoma in a patient with columnar epithelium is probably less than the original estimate of 10 to 15 per cent but still represents a significant problem.

SYMPTOMS. In Western countries, the most common clinical symptom of carcinoma is *progressive dysphagia* over a six- to eight-month period until only liquids can be taken. The obstruction reflects circumferential involvement of the esophageal wall by tumor and does not occur until the cancer is biologically rather far advanced. The dysphagia may be accompanied by a *steady, boring pain*, which signals mediastinal involvement and inoperability. In the Orient but not in the United States, pain is often a relatively early sign of a localized and thus resectable tumor. Unexplained persistent chest pain should always be investigated by a careful double-contrast radiographic view of the esophagus or by endoscopy.

More advanced lesions manifest themselves with *halitosis, weight loss,* and *coughing after drinking fluid.* The last-named symptom is caused either by near-complete esophageal lumen obstruction with overspill into the larynx or by the development of a tracheoesophageal fistula. Hoarseness from involvement of the recurrent laryngeal nerve by tumor and hematemesis are unusual symptoms. Nail bed clubbing can be seen with both benign and malignant tumors.

Since dysphagia is the most common presenting symptom of neoplasm of the esophagus, the physician is responsible for making absolutely certain that cancer is not the cause of dysphagia. Early diagnosis affords the only chance for cure. Early diagnosis allows the patient, family, and physician to plan better all aspects of the patient's future.

DIAGNOSIS. The clinical suspicion of a cancer of the esophagus should lead immediately to an esophagogram, possibly with double-contrast techniques. Any irregularity, especially if it narrows the lumen, mandates further evaluation. If dysphagia is present, the radiologist should give a bolus of barium-soaked bread or a large marshmallow to discover any possible sites of arrest.

In the presence of symptoms but a normal barium swallow, endoscopy with biopsy and brushing of any suspicious lesion for examination of tissue and of exfoliated cells is indicated. The endoscopist should always obtain a good retroflexed view of the cardia from below to make certain that an adenocarcinoma of the gastroesophageal junction has not been overlooked.

If narrowing has been seen by barium swallow, endoscopy with biopsy and cytologic brushings of the involved area must be done. With the fiberoptic endoscope, numerous blind biopsies from as deep in the lesion as possible will be most helpful. Biopsy of visible tissue will often reveal only inflammatory tissue. Sometimes as many as eight or nine biopsies must be obtained before tumor is recovered.

Once a tumor is identified, certain procedures in addition to chest films are essential for staging before a therapeutic decision is reached. A careful physical examination for nodal metastases, bronchoscopy for evidence of tracheal involvement, liver function tests plus ultrasound for evidence of liver metastases, and computed tomographic (CT) scanning for mediastinal nodal involvement, esophageal wall thickness, and liver metastases are necessary before the final therapeutic plan is decided upon. A chest roentgenogram is mandatory.

TREATMENT. The ideal form of treating cancer of the esophagus, either for cure or for palliation, has not yet been developed. No series exists in which patients were carefully staged with the best noninvasive methods available and then randomized to different treatment modalities.

Surgical resection of squamous cell carcinoma and adenocarcinoma of the lower one third of the esophagus is preferred in most centers if the patient does not have widespread metastases. Surgery offers the benefit of rapidly restoring esophagogastric continuity. Perhaps only one quarter of all patients presenting to a medical-surgical center will have a resectable tumor; of these patients 20 per cent will not survive the operative period, and five-year survival will be only 5 to 10 per cent, even with extensive resections. Long-term survival cannot be predicted in the individual case by the operative findings. There is growing enthusiasm for palliative resection with restoration of gastrointestinal continuity with stomach or colon. Surgical results in China and Japan, with hospital deaths of 5 per cent and five-year survivals of 20 to 30 per cent, are better than those quoted for the United States. Whether this represents better technical skill, a different type of patient, or earlier diagnosis is not certain.

Radiotherapy is employed in lesions of the upper one third of the esophagus and often in middle third tumors as well. This form of therapy has little hospital mortality, although it carries some short-term and long-term morbidity. With ideal home situations, radiotherapy can be carried out on an outpatient basis. Approximately 40 per cent of tumors cannot be destroyed with conventional 6000-rad therapy. Combination of pre- and postoperative radiation with resective therapy has been employed, but there is no good evidence that such combined therapy is better. Adenocarcinomas occasionally respond to radiotherapy but are not as radiosensitive as squamous cell carcinomas.

When obvious extraesophageal spread is present, palliation with bougienage to restore and maintain an adequate esophageal lumen may be done. If performed with a guide wire under fluoroscopic guidance, such therapy is not hazardous in skilled hands. If dilation does not offer lasting relief, then a Silastic tube can be placed perorally for relief of esophageal obstruction. Such tubes are also of great benefit in the treatment of a malignant tracheoesophageal fistula. Another promising approach is the destruction of intraluminal tumor and restoration of an adequate lumen by laser therapy or an intraluminal heat-coagulating probe.

Choice of therapy will depend on the location and size of the lesion, presence or absence of spread, cell type, and the skills of the medical community. Until an adequate randomized trial after adequate staging is carried out, choice of treatment modality will continue to be a matter of preference.

Earlam R, Cunha-Melo JR: Oesophageal squamous cell carcinoma. Br J Surg 67:381, 457, 1980. *Two articles present exhaustive literature reviews of surgical and radiotherapy of esophageal carcinoma.*

Livstone EM: General considerations of tumors of the esophagus. In Berk JE (ed.): Bockus' Gastroenterology. 4th ed. Philadelphia, W. B. Saunders Company, 1985, pp 818–840. *Review of diagnostic and therapeutic considerations in esophageal carcinoma.*

OTHER CONDITIONS

RINGS AND WEBS. During early development, the lumen of the esophagus becomes completely obliterated and then is recanalized to form the adult hollow viscus. A failure of this process leads to atresia or a residual web. Such webs usually occur in the upper esophagus, often with eccentric openings; occasionally they are multiple. A much more common web or ring is located in the terminal esophagus, has a symmetric opening, and is usually at the junction between squamous and the normal transitional or columnar epithelium of the stomach (Fig. 98–4). This latter ring (Schatzki's ring) can be demonstrated in many individuals if cine studies of the lower esophageal zone are used. It produces symptoms infrequently

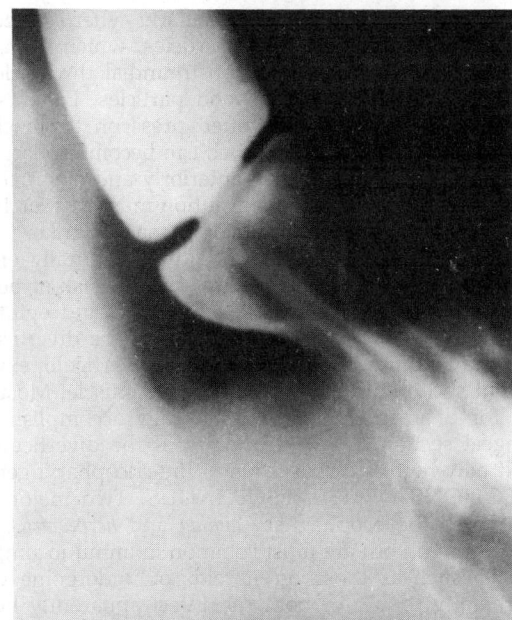

FIGURE 98–4. Lower esophageal ring (Schatzki's ring). This ring consists of a symmetric thin web located in the terminal esophagus. (From Pope CE II: In Sleisinger MH, Fordtran JS [eds.]: Gastrointestinal Disease. 3rd ed. Philadelphia, W. B. Saunders Company, 1983.)

but in a characteristic manner. An acquired web located in the postcricoid area is sometimes associated with iron deficiency anemia.

All these types of webs or rings cause dysphagia for solids, and the impacted bolus usually has to be regurgitated. The lower esophageal ring (Schatzki's ring) has a characteristic clinical presentation that allows the diagnosis to be made by history. Every three to four months, after a bolus of meat or bread, the patient will complain of dysphagia and total inability to swallow solids or liquids. The bolus will be regurgitated, and then the patient can continue to eat normally. If the patient comes to the emergency room with an impacted bolus of meat, nothing will be seen after the impacted bolus is removed with the operating endoscope, and the disorder will be labeled as "hysterical dysphagia." The lower esophageal ring is not well seen with the rigid endoscope, as the lower portion of the esophagus cannot be distended enough to force the ring into prominence.

Treatment of all webs involves mechanical disruption either with a dilator or with the endoscope. Treatment of iron deficiency anemia is said to cause the postcricoid webs to disappear. Only very rarely will a surgical approach to a web or ring be necessary.

DIVERTICULA OF THE ESOPHAGUS. Zenker's diverticulum of the pharynx is not anatomically an esophageal diverticulum, as its neck is above the upper esophageal sphincter muscle, but custom has dictated its inclusion in description of esophageal diverticula. An epiphrenic diverticulum usually occurs on the right side of the esophagus just above the lower esophageal sphincter. Other diverticula are at the level of the carina and are known as traction diverticula, although traction by scar tissue is rarely demonstrated. Scleroderma is occasionally associated with numerous wide-mouthed diverticula scattered along the length of the esophagus. Large-amplitude motor waves have been associated with midbody diverticula and either achalasia or motor incoordination with epiphrenic diverticula.

Symptoms vary widely; many diverticula are found by accident during barium examination of the esophagus. If a patient with dysphagia is found to have a diverticulum, it is difficult to tell whether the diverticulum or the associated motor disorder is the cause. Zenker's diverticulum often has a classic symptom complex, particularly when it becomes large. It retains saliva and food particles, which may either be aspirated or cause repeated postprandial throat clearing with production of liquid and food particles. Patients with this type of diverticulum can often press on the neck and empty the diverticulum. The pouch can become so large that it can compress the esophagus anteriorly and obstruct it. In the presence of diverticula great caution must be exercised in passing tubes into the esophagus or stomach. Zenker's diverticulum is a special problem, since tubes naturally enter it rather than the esophageal opening, and the risk of perforation into the mediastinum is great. Traction and epiphrenic diverticula do not require treatment. Zenker's diverticulum, if large, may require diverticulectomy or diverticulopexy with coincident section of the cricopharyngeus muscle. Most techniques for diverticulectomy automatically accomplish cricopharyngeal section at the same time. If the diverticulum is small, it may regress after section of the cricopharyngeus.

INFECTIONS OF THE ESOPHAGUS. Two major infections involve the esophagus: *Candida* and *herpesvirus* infections. Although both are most common in immunocompromised hosts such as those on steroids or undergoing cancer chemotherapy, either or both can infect apparently healthy hosts. Both can be found incidentally at autopsy or during endoscopy for other indications. Most commonly, infection of the mucosa leads to odynophagia of rather marked degree. Dysphagia for both solids and liquids usually accompanies the odynophagia and can be of such intensity that weight loss is rapid.

Although the radiograph occasionally reveals a shaggy mucosa in the case of monilial involvement, and occasionally even a stricture, endoscopy is the best method of detecting and confirming infectious involvement. *Candida* can present as isolated white plaques, which can be confused with glycogenic acanthosis, or progress to form confluent ulcerations with an overlying membrane. Herpesvirus tends to produce isolated ulcers, but extensive involvement can produce confluent ulcerations. Biopsy of the ulcerated area usually shows either invasive hyphae of *Candida* or characteristic nuclear changes of the squamous cells when herpesvirus is present. Cytologic washings occasionally demonstrate the same change.

Treatment depends on correct identification of the etiologic agent. For *Candida* infection, an assessment of the degree of severity is needed. For mild disease, topical therapy with 250,000 units of nystatin (Mycostatin) every two hours will suffice. For more serious infections, low-dose intravenous amphotericin therapy has been successful, the dose being individualized on the basis of weight and renal status. Treatment with miconazole and ketoconazole appears promising. For severe esophageal infections, ketoconazole should be given in doses of 200 mg to 400 mg per day for eight to ten days. Herpesvirus infection is treated symptomatically with viscous lidocaine.

ESOPHAGEAL INJURIES. *Caustic Ingestion.* Caustic burns of the esophagus occur in children by accident; adults usually suffer such burns because of suicide attempts. Lye crystals, and especially liquid lye preparations for drain cleaning, are the most common cause. The speed of lye injury is so great that attempts to neutralize the caustic are futile. Detergents and Clorox also find their way into the esophageal lumens of both children and adults. The history is all important, but the degree of esophageal injury still must be assessed endoscopically as an emergency. Significant esophageal damage has been seen even without oral burns; conversely, oral burns do not necessarily mean that the material has reached the esophagus. If there is no esophageal reaction after apparent caustic ingestion, further care directed toward the esophagus will not be necessary.

The accepted therapy of a definite lye or caustic burn remains unsupported by clinical trials. For burns with solid lye or other solid agents, steroids have been recommended, at an initial dose of 80 mg per day, tapering to 20 mg per day until esophageal healing. Most clinicians also use broad-spectrum antibiotics such as ampicillin, 500 mg four times a day. If liquid lye has been the damaging agent, serious consideration of emergency esophagogastrectomy is in order, as lesser measures have met with unacceptably high mortality.

Damage by Medication. A new form of iatrogenic illness of the esophagus has recently become evident. Ingested pills tend to lodge in the esophagus and damage the mucosa in a localized area. Tetracycline, doxycycline, ascorbic acid, and quinidine have all been indicted, and the list will undoubtedly grow. Normal individuals can retain small capsules in the esophagus, even when swallowing in the upright position. The clinical syndrome consists of steady burning or chest pain, accompanied by local odynophagia, all occurring four to six hours after ingestion of one of the offending capsules or tablets. Endoscopy (not clinically necessary) usually shows a localized mucosal ulcer, which heals without a scar within a week. Symptomatic therapy is adequate, but prophylaxis seems to be a more practical idea. Pills of the offending class should be taken in the upright position with several swallows of water.

Esophageal Trauma. The esophagus is well protected by the thoracic cage, but can be involved either by blunt trauma (automobile accidents) or by penetrating missiles (gunshots, knives). Often the surgeon's attention is directed toward more life-threatening damage to heart, lungs, or major blood vessels, and it is understandable that a rent in the esophagus may thus be overlooked. This unfortunate oversight, however, will be followed by mediastinitis, which may worsen an already grave situation. Iatrogenic perforation with endoscope, dilator, or, very rarely, nasogastric tube leads to a similar complication.

Vomiting itself can cause esophageal injury, either mucosal (*Mallory-Weiss*) or through-and-through rupture (*Boerhaave's syndrome*). The mucosal lesion first described by Mallory and Weiss has been recognized much more frequently since the advent of rapid emergency endoscopy with fiberoptic endoscopes. Classically, the patient has repeated attacks of retching, productive at first of gastric contents, and later of bright red blood. One quarter of patients shown to have a Mallory-Weiss tear have no prior history of vomiting. The tear is usually in the gastric mucosa just below the gastroesophageal junction, although it can extend through the junction and up into the esophageal mucosa. Diagnosis of this condition is almost always made at endoscopy; the rent is usually seen as the endoscope is being withdrawn from the stomach into the esophagus. The majority of such lesions heal with conservative therapy. Angiographic or surgical therapy is necessary in less than 5 per cent.

Vomiting can also cause a complete tear in the esophageal wall. Unlike the Mallory-Weiss lesion, the tear in Boerhaave's syndrome is located above the gastroesophageal junction on the left side. It usually follows vomiting, but other marked increases in intra-abdominal pressure such as lifting a heavy weight or straining at stool have been associated with a tear. The clinical diagnosis can be extremely difficult; often patients with esophageal rupture are thought to have a myocardial infarct, pneumothorax, a perforated viscus, or pancreatitis. Air in the mediastinum or the rapid appearance of a hydrothorax on the left usually leads to the correct diagnosis.

The diagnosis of esophageal perforation can usually be established by a cautious radiographic examination with water-soluble material. Barium may be used only if a rent is not demonstrated by the water-soluble agent. Immediate surgical repair is the accepted method of treatment of esophageal perforation. In those too ill for surgery, treatment consists of nasogastric suction, antibiotics, and subsequent mediastinal drainage if necessary.

Pope CE II, McDonald GB: Rings and webs; Diverticula; Involvement of the esophagus by infections, systemic illnesses, and physical agents. In Sleisenger MH, Fordtran JS (eds.): Gastrointestinal Disease. 4th ed. Philadelphia, W. B. Saunders Company (in press). *Textbook review of these various conditions.*

99 GASTRITIS

Charles T. Richardson

DEFINITION. Inflammation of the stomach mucosa may be diffuse and involve all parts of the stomach or localized to the fundus and body or antrum (see Fig. 100–1). Even within a specific area (e.g., the antrum), inflammation may be diffuse or localized. Gastritis is classified as acute or chronic primarily on the basis of histologic and/or endoscopic findings and long-term clinical follow-up. Acute gastritis is believed to be a self-limited disease, whereas chronic gastritis by definition persists for long periods of time.

ACUTE GASTRITIS

ETIOLOGY. Nonsteroidal anti-inflammatory drugs (such as aspirin), ethanol, bile salts, and pancreatic enzymes damage the gastric mucosa and are believed to cause both acute and chronic gastritis (see Chronic Gastritis, below). How these chemical agents cause gastritis is not known. They are thought to disrupt the so-called "gastric mucosal barrier" (the ability of gastric mucosa to restrict movement of hydrogen ions from lumen to mucosa), thereby allowing back-diffusion of acid and pepsin, and in this manner to contribute to the development of gastritis. Inhibition of prostaglandin synthesis by nonsteroidal anti-inflammatory drugs also may be a factor in the pathogenesis of acute gastritis in patients who are treated with these drugs.

Acute gastritis also occurs in the setting of severe medical or surgical illnesses such as respiratory failure, sepsis, renal failure, hypotension, or trauma. This form of acute gastritis is called "stress"-induced gastritis and may produce "stress" bleeding. Mucosal ischemia is believed to be an important factor in the pathogenesis of "stress"-related gastritis. Gastric acid is also likely to be involved, since in experimental models mucosal damage does not occur in the absence of acid. Bile and pancreatic juices also may be contributing factors.

Infectious agents cause some forms of acute gastritis. An example is a rare but fulminant and often fatal form of acute bacterial gastritis called acute phlegmonous gastritis. Streptococci are most commonly the cause, although staphylococci, *Escherichia coli*, and *Proteus* have been cultured from stomachs of patients with acute phlegmonous gastritis.

Gastric *Campylobacter*-like organisms (GCLO) are found in some patients with either acute or chronic gastritis. Although evidence suggests that these organisms cause gastritis, a cause-and-effect relationship has not been firmly established, since these same bacteria have been found also in gastric mucosa of normal humans.

An epidemic form of acute gastritis has been reported to be associated with decreased gastric acid secretion (hypochlorhydria). Since gastritis occurred in a number of different persons who were in contact with each other over a relatively brief period of time, an infectious etiology was suspected. In fact, some investigators have postulated that this acute gastritis with hypochlorhydria was due to GCLO.

Additional causes of acute gastritis include roentgen irra-

diation, ingestion of corrosive substances, and ingestion of staphylococcal exotoxin.

CLINICAL MANIFESTATIONS. Patients with acute gastritis secondary to aspirin, other nonsteroidal anti-inflammatory drugs, or "stress" may have hematemesis and/or melena and pain, nausea, and vomiting. This form of acute gastritis is called acute hemorrhagic or erosive gastritis. At times, bleeding can be so severe that patients develop hypotension or shock. In contrast, other patients with acute gastritis secondary to nonsteroidal anti-inflammatory drugs may have minimal gastrointestinal bleeding detected only by testing stools for occult blood.

Finding acute gastritis on biopsy does not necessarily mean that a patient has clinically important disease, since as many as 30 per cent of otherwise healthy, asymptomatic persons can have acute gastritis on biopsy. Also, some forms of acute gastritis with known cause, such as acute irradiation gastritis, are not associated with symptoms. However, patients with other causes of gastritis may have symptoms. For example, some patients with epidemic gastritis with hypochlorhydria have epigastric pain, nausea, and vomiting.

The physical examination in patients with acute gastritis is usually normal unless bleeding or other illnesses such as liver disease or arthritis are present. If bleeding occurs, the patient may have a reduced hematocrit, increased blood urea nitrogen, and a positive nasogastric aspirate or stool guaiac test for blood. Unless there are concomitant diseases, other laboratory studies are usually normal (see Ch. 114).

DIAGNOSIS. Most clinically significant forms of acute gastritis are associated with mucosal abnormalities that can be visualized at endoscopy (Table 99–1). For example, in acute gastritis secondary to aspirin or "stress," the gastric mucosa often appears congested, and petechial hemorrhages, erosions, and superficial ulcerations cover the mucosal surface. These changes may be diffuse, although the fundus and body are most severely affected.

In the strictest sense, the diagnosis of acute gastritis is made by the pathologist from the histologic findings of the biopsy specimen. Inflammatory cells (usually neutrophils and mononuclear cells) infiltrate the lamina propria, whereas the glandular areas are distorted by edema and hemorrhage. Exudate often fills the gastric pits and/or glands (pit and/or gland abscesses). In severe forms of gastritis (e.g., aspirin- or "stress"-induced), focal sloughing of surface epithelial cells can occur, producing superficial erosions and ulcerations.

NATURAL HISTORY. The major feature differentiating acute from chronic gastritis is the tendency for mucosal changes in acute gastritis to revert to normal. The time over which this occurs depends on the type of acute gastritis and on the method used to detect the endpoint. For example, in acute hemorrhagic gastritis the endoscopic appearance of the gastric mucosa may revert to normal within 24 to 48 hours after bleeding has stopped. Histologic reversion to normal may require a longer period of time.

Some patients with epidemic gastritis with hypochlorhydria have had moderate-to-severe gastritis on biopsy from 2 to 5 months after initial diagnosis and moderate gastritis even up to 12 months. Acute gastritis is a reversible lesion, but histologic abnormalities may persist for months in some forms. Whether acute gastritis progresses to chronic gastritis in some patients is not known.

TREATMENT. Most patients with acute gastritis do not require treatment. For example, acute gastritis found on biopsy in asymptomatic, healthy persons need not be treated. Treatment with antacids may be warranted in symptomatic patients who have a histologic diagnosis of acute gastritis and in whom other causes of symptoms have been excluded. Since there have been no controlled clinical trials evaluating antacids in the treatment of acute gastritis, the effectiveness and dosage are not known. Bismuth-containing compounds

TABLE 99–1. TYPES OF GASTRITIS, METHOD OF DIAGNOSIS, AND ENDOSCOPIC, BARIUM X-RAY, AND/OR HISTOLOGIC FINDINGS

Types of Gastritis	Method of Diagnosis*	Endoscopic, Barium X-ray, and/or Histologic Findings
Acute		
Drug-induced (salicylates or other nonsteroidal anti-inflammatory drugs or alcohol)	Endoscopy	Congested mucosa with petechial hemorrhages and erosions.
	Histology	Neutrophils and mononuclear cells infiltrate the lamina propria; edema and hemorrhage distort the glands; inflammatory cells fill the pits and glands, forming small abscesses.
Stress-induced (secondary to severe medical or surgical diseases or trauma)	Endoscopy	Erythema, petechial hemorrhages, and erosions cover most of the mucosa.
	Histology	Inflammatory cells (primarily neutrophils) infiltrate the lamina propria; edema and hemorrhage distort the glands; pit and gland abscesses and focal sloughing of surface cells can be seen.
Chronic		
Superficial	Histology	Inflammatory cells (neutrophils, lymphocytes, plasma cells, and a few eosinophils) are limited to the gastric pits and upper lamina propria.
Atrophic	Histology	Inflammatory cells are located superficially but also invade deeper into the lamina propria; thinning of the mucosa with loss of glandular elements and intestinal metaplasia may occur.
Gastric atrophy	Histology	More severe form of atrophic gastritis; a marked reduction in mucosal thickness with loss of parietal and chief cells occurs; only a few inflammatory cells are present.
Special Types		
Giant hypertrophic	Endoscopy or barium x-ray	Large folds are usually confined to the fundus and body but may involve the antrum.
	Histology	Hyperplasia of mucus, parietal, and chief cells; large cystic spaces containing mucus are often seen.
Eosinophilic	Endoscopy or barium x-ray	Rigid, nondistensible antrum and/or thickened mucosal folds are usually seen.
	Histology	Eosinophils infiltrate the lamina propria, submucosa, and muscular layers.
Granulomatous	Endoscopy or barium x-ray	Involved portions of the stomach are narrowed and rigid.
	Histology	Granulomas are found in the mucosa and submucosa and occasionally can be found in the muscular layer and serosa.

*Some clinicians and investigators believe that gastritis is always a histologic diagnosis and that the findings on endoscopy and barium radiography only suggest what the pathologist might find on the histologic stain.

are believed to eradicate GCLO from gastric mucosa. Therefore, some investigators have advocated using Pepto-Bismol to treat patients suspected of having GCLO-induced gastritis.

Patients with acute hemorrhagic gastritis present special therapeutic problems. Many of these patients experience severe upper gastrointestinal bleeding that requires treatment, including fluid and blood replacement and nasogastric lavage. Since acid and pepsin probably play a role in the pathogenesis, it seems reasonable to reduce gastric acidity and concomitantly peptic activity with antacids and/or cimetidine or ranitidine. Recent results suggest that sucralfate also may be useful in preventing "stress"-induced ulceration and bleeding. Surgical therapy is to be avoided if at all possible because of its inordinately high morbidity and mortality.

Initially, an antacid (usually 30 ml of a liquid aluminum-magnesium preparation) is prescribed every hour during the day and night; higher doses or more frequent administration may be needed in some patients. A combination of antacid plus cimetidine or ranitidine has been recommended by some physicians. Measurement of intragastric pH every hour and administration of medications in doses to keep intragastric pH above 3.5 have been suggested. Such a regimen prevents "stress"-induced ulcerations and bleeding in a large percentage of critically ill patients and is recommended in treating such patients; however, there is no evidence that maintaining pH above 3.5 controls bleeding or assists in healing acute hemorrhagic gastritis once it occurs.

CHRONIC GASTRITIS

CLASSIFICATION. Chronic gastritis is usually classified on the basis of mucosal histology and/or the anatomic portion of the stomach involved. Although endoscopic and radiologic criteria for classifying chronic gastritis have been reported, gastric mucosal biopsy is the most reliable means of diagnosis. Biopsies should be obtained from several different areas, since chronic gastritis may be a localized disease.

HISTOLOGY. Chronic gastritis is divided into superficial gastritis, atrophic gastritis, and gastric atrophy (Table 99–1). When inflammatory cells are limited to the gastric pits and upper lamina propria, gastritis is classified as superficial. In atrophic gastritis inflammatory cells invade deeper into the lamina propria and glandular epithelium. Lymphoid follicles may also be seen. As the disease progresses, thinning of the mucosa occurs with loss of glandular elements. In some patients intestinal metaplasia develops with loss of parietal and chief cells and development of goblet cells, absorptive cells, and intestinal villi. Finally, in patients with gastric atrophy, parietal and chief cells are absent, mucosal thickness is reduced markedly, and only a small number of inflammatory cells are present.

LOCATION. Chronic atrophic gastritis has been divided into Type A and Type B, based primarily on the anatomic portion of the stomach involved and the presence or absence of parietal cell antibodies. In Type A gastritis the fundus and body of the stomach are involved, whereas the antrum is relatively normal. Parietal cell antibodies are found in a large percentage of patients, and pernicious anemia may develop. On the other hand, in Type B gastritis the antrum is involved primarily, although inflammation is found frequently in the fundus and body. Parietal cell antibodies do not occur. Immunologic, functional, and clinical differences between these two types of gastritis will be discussed below.

ETIOLOGY. The causes of chronic gastritis are unknown. Radiation injury, nutritional deficiencies, endocrine disorders, and infectious diseases have been postulated but not proved to cause chronic gastritis. Gastric *Campylobacter*-like organisms (GCLO) have been found in association with histologic evidence of chronic gastritis, but a cause-and-effect relationship has not been established (see Acute Gastritis, above). Repeated insults to the gastric mucosa by mechanical, thermal, or chemical agents have also been thought to cause chronic musocal changes. Long-term alcohol or aspirin ingestion may lead to chronic gastritis, although this has not been clearly established.

Reflux of duodenal juice into the stomach is believed to irritate gastric mucosa and perhaps lead to chronic gastritis. Lysolecithin, which is formed when phospholipase A from pancreatic juice reacts with lecithin from bile, appears to be the most damaging constituent of refluxed duodenal juice. Lysolecithin, bile, and pancreatic juice are postulated to initiate the process leading to gastritis by removing the mucus layer from the epithelial surface. This leads to damage of the "mucosal barrier," allowing diffusion of gastric acid and pepsin into the mucosa. This, in turn, leads to further mucosal damage.

Immunologic injury may play a role in the pathogenesis of chronic gastritis in some patients. Patients with atrophic gastritis of the fundus and body (Type A gastritis) usually have antibodies against parietal cells, and some, but not all, of these patients develop pernicious anemia. Approximately 90 per cent of patients with pernicious anemia have parietal cell antibodies. Many also have antibodies to intrinsic factor, which may be of two types: (1) a blocking antibody, which reacts with the vitamin B_{12}–intrinsic factor binding site and blocks the binding of vitamin B_{12} and intrinsic factor; or (2) a binding antibody, which can react either with intrinsic factor alone or with intrinsic factor–vitamin B_{12} complex.

Antibody to gastrin-producing cells occurs in a few but not all patients with gastritis primarily involving the antrum (Type B gastritis). This finding adds further support for the role of immunologic abnormalities in the development of chronic gastritis. These patients do not have parietal cell or intrinsic factor antibodies and do not develop pernicious anemia.

Whether parietal cell and other cellular antibodies lead to mucosal destruction or whether they are markers of mucosal damage caused by other mechanisms is not known. Repeated injection of cellular antibodies can lead to gastric atrophy and decreased acid secretion in laboratory animals, suggesting that development of antibodies may be the initiating event. Serum of some patients with pernicious anemia has been found to contain an autoantibody that is cytotoxic to canine gastric mucosal cells. On the other hand, patients with adult-onset hypogammaglobulinemia can develop gastric atrophy and pernicious anemia even though they do not have antibodies to parietal cells or intrinsic factor.

Genetic influences also have been implicated in the development of chronic gastritis. Family members of patients with pernicious anemia have a higher incidence of atrophic gastritis, achlorhydria, vitamin B_{12} malabsorption, and parietal cell and intrinsic factor antibodies than does the general population. The role of genetics in patients with chronic gastritis who do not have pernicious anemia has not been adequately explored.

Theoretically, gastric atrophy could also develop from the absence of a mucosal trophic factor such as gastrin, urogastrone, or epidermal growth factor, or from end-organ resistance to one of these factors. So far, there are no studies evaluating these possibilities.

CLINICAL MANIFESTATIONS. As with acute gastritis, many patients with chronic gastritis and no other underlying disease are asymptomatic and have a normal physical examination. For example, it is rare for patients with pernicious anemia to have symptoms related to gastritis or gastric atrophy. Symptoms such as nausea, vomiting, and epigastric pain can occur in patients with chronic gastritis; however, studies have shown a poor correlation between presence or absence of symptoms and histologic evidence of gastritis. Thus a biopsy diagnosis of chronic gastritis should not be used as the sole explanation for upper gastrointestinal symptoms, and other causes such as peptic ulcer disease, gastric cancer, or cholelithiasis should be excluded.

Other clinical findings in patients with chronic gastritis relate to abnormalities in laboratory studies. Gastric acid secretion usually is lower than normal and is especially low or absent in patients with atrophic gastritis or gastric atrophy. Decreased secretion of pepsin also occurs. Patients with gastritis involving the fundus and body but sparing the antrum (Type A gastritis) usually are hypo- or achlorhydric and have elevated serum gastrin concentrations presumably secondary to an alkaline antral pH (sometimes as high as in patients with Zollinger-Ellison syndrome). When gastritis involves the antrum primarily (Type B gastritis), acid secretion is usually diminished but serum gastrin concentration is in the normal range.

In patients with pernicious anemia, the vitamin B_{12} absorption test (Schilling test) is abnormal when performed in the absence of exogenous intrinsic factor, and in untreated patients signs and symptoms of vitamin B_{12} deficiency may develop. Some patients with pernicious anemia have clinical and laboratory evidence of other diseases such as Hashimoto's thyroiditis, hypothyroidism, hyperthyroidism, insulin-dependent diabetes mellitus, or vitiligo.

NATURAL HISTORY. Chronic gastritis is a longstanding disease that increases in frequency with advancing age. The process in an individual patient is thought to progress over time from superficial gastritis to chronic atrophic gastritis to gastric atrophy, but this has not been established. It is also not known whether all patients who later in life are found to have gastric atrophy initially had superficial gastritis. In one study, patients with chronic superficial gastritis were followed for 10 to 20 years. Superficial gastritis persisted, relatively unchanged, in half of the patients, whereas progression to atrophic gastritis occurred in most of the remainder. Reversion to normal was also noted in a few patients.

Associations have been reported between chronic gastritis and gastric polyps, benign gastric ulcer, and gastric cancer. Although benign gastric ulcers usually occur in an area of chronic superficial or atrophic gastritis, it is not known whether gastritis precedes and perhaps leads to gastric ulcer formation or whether gastritis develops in response to ulceration. Gastric cancer may occur more frequently in patients with both Types A and B gastritis; however, numerically the incidence is higher in Type B.

TREATMENT. Most patients with chronic gastritis do not require treatment for the following reasons: (1) the pathogenesis of chronic gastritis is poorly understood; thus, it is difficult to design rational therapy; (2) most patients with chronic gastritis are asymptomatic; and (3) there is no evidence that therapy prevents sequelae such as gastric atrophy, pernicious anemia, or cancer.

Although pernicious anemia cannot be prevented, it seems reasonable to follow patients with known gastric atrophy for development of either signs or symptoms of pernicious anemia or low serum B_{12} levels. Glucocorticoid therapy can partially reverse the gastric mucosal changes in patients with pernicious anemia, but chronic therapy with steroids is impractical and dangerous.

Patients with pernicious anemia should be evaluated for other diseases such as thyroid disease or diabetes mellitus, and their relatives should be screened for pernicious anemia. Whether or not patients with pernicious anemia and/or gastric atrophy should be screened periodically for gastric cancer is controversial.

SPECIAL TYPES OF GASTRITIS

GIANT HYPERTROPHIC GASTRITIS. Several relatively uncommon clinical syndromes are characterized by gastric mucosal hypertrophy. These syndromes are usually included under the heading of giant hypertrophic gastritis, although inflammatory cells are not always present. The most commonly recognized syndrome is *Menetrier's disease*, which is characterized by gastric mucosal hypertrophy, hyposecretion of gastric acid, increased loss of protein from the stomach, edema, weight loss, and occasionally pain, nausea, and vomiting. Another syndrome, *hypertrophic hypersecretory gastropathy*, is similar but is associated with hypersecretion of acid. These syndromes are more commonly found in men than in women and usually occur between the ages of 30 and 50, although a childhood variety has been described. Gastric atrophy and parietal cell antibodies have been reported as late developments in a few patients.

Diagnosis is based on clinical findings, appearances of large mucosal folds on upper gastrointestinal x-ray series or endoscopy, and histologic appearance of mucosal biopsies (Table 99–1). Large mucosal folds are usually limited to the fundus and body of the stomach, although the antrum may be involved. Mucosal biopsy reveals hyperplasia of all three glandular elements—parietal, chief, and mucus-secreting cells. Because of the enlarged folds, other diseases such as Zollinger-Ellison syndrome, infiltrating carcinoma, lymphoma, or amyloid must be excluded.

In some patients medical therapy with anticholinergic drugs has led to reduced gastric secretion, decreased protein loss, and clinical improvement. Cimetidine also has been reported to decrease protein loss, although the mechanism is unknown. One or both of these therapies should be tried prior to surgical intervention. Some patients have been treated successfully with vagotomy and pyloroplasty. In a few patients, persistent, severe protein loss or recurrent gastrointestinal hemorrhage may necessitate total gastrectomy.

EOSINOPHILIC GASTRITIS (GASTROENTERITIS). Eosinophilic infiltration of the gastrointestinal tract can involve the stomach and/or small intestine. Peripheral eosinophilia also commonly occurs. The pathogenesis is poorly understood, although allergic or immunologic factors are thought to be involved. Both IgE-mediated and IgE-independent mechanisms have been implicated.

Gastric involvement is usually limited to the antrum. On biopsy eosinophils infiltrate the mucosa and the muscular layer (Table 99–1). This leads to antral rigidity and thickening of mucosal folds. Delayed gastric emptying and/or gastric outlet obstruction may occur. On x-ray it is often difficult to differentiate eosinophilic gastritis from granulomatous disease or neoplasm. Clinically, patients usually present with pain, nausea, and vomiting. Occasionally, eosinophils may invade the serosa, leading to ascites.

Eosinophilic gastritis is often a self-limited disease, but in some patients symptoms persist or recur. Corticosteroid therapy has been useful in alleviating obstructive signs and symptoms as well as ascites.

GRANULOMATOUS GASTRITIS. Granulomas can be found in the stomach as part of generalized diseases such as tuberculosis, histoplasmosis, sarcoidosis, syphilis, or Crohn's disease, or may be limited to the stomach and unassociated with other diseases. Two examples of the latter are eosinophilic granuloma (a separate disease from eosinophilic gastritis) and isolated (idiopathic) granulomatous gastritis.

On upper gastrointestinal x-ray the involved portions of the stomach appear rigid and narrowed and the x-ray appearance is often similar to that of malignancy (Table 99–1). The antrum is most often involved, although granulomas can be found also in the mucosa of the body and fundus. Mucosal biopsies reveal granulomas in the mucosa and submucosa, and in surgical specimens granulomas have been found in the muscular layer and serosa. Ulcerations may also occur. Because of the malignant appearance on x-ray, cancer must be ruled out in all patients by multiple biopsies and/or cytology.

Because of problems with differentiating granulomatous gastritis from malignancy, the condition in most patients is diagnosed at the time of surgery. If the diagnosis of granulomatous gastritis is made preoperatively, a search should be made for a primary disease and therapy should be tailored to the specific disease (e.g., tuberculosis). If an etiology cannot be found and malignancy has been excluded, the patient should be observed for several weeks, since spontaneous resolution of isolated granulomatous gastritis has been reported. If resolution does not occur, surgical therapy is indicated.

GASTRITIS FOLLOWING GASTRIC SURGERY. Gastritis is a common histologic and endoscopic finding after either a subtotal gastrectomy or antrectomy has been performed for peptic ulcer disease. This form of gastritis is often referred to as bile reflux or alkaline gastritis, reflecting the theory that it is caused by the reflux of bile or pancreatic juice or both into the gastric remnant. Features believed to be compatible with the diagnosis include (1) epigastric pain, heartburn, nausea, and vomiting (often vomiting of bile-containing material) and/or weight loss; (2) presence of bile in the gastric remnant; (3) endoscopic evidence of gastritis; and (4) histologic evidence of gastritis. None of these features, however, are specific for the diagnosis. For example, such symptoms frequently occur following ulcer surgery with or without histologic or endoscopic evidence of gastritis. Furthermore, histologic or endoscopic changes can occur in postoperative patients who are asymptomatic. The presence of bile in the gastric remnant also does not mean necessarily that patients have bile-induced gastritis, because it is very easy for bile and other duodenal contents to reflux into the gastric remnant. Thus, caution should be exercised in making the diagnosis of bile reflux gastritis.

Cholestyramine or aluminum hydroxide antacids, as bile acid–binding agents, have been given to patients with postgastrectomy gastritis but usually do not alleviate symptoms or reverse the histologic appearance of gastritis. As noted, bile acids alone may not be responsible for symptoms associated with "bile reflux gastritis"; other substances such as pancreatic secretions may be needed. Corrective surgery has consisted of procedures designed to divert duodenal contents away from the gastric remnant. The most commonly used operation is called a Roux-en-Y diversion. Some, but not all, studies have shown this procedure to be successful in relieving symptoms in some patients. Thus, surgery should be reserved for patients with incapacitating symptoms.

Meyer JH: Reflections on reflux gastritis (editorial.) Gastroenterology 77:1143, 1979.

Miller TA: Stress erosive gastritis. In Moody FG, Carey LC, Jones RS, et al. (eds.): Surgical Treatment of Digestive Disease. Chicago, Year Book Medical Publishers, 1986, pp 203–215. *A review of the pathophysiology, methods of prophylaxis, and the medical and surgical treatment of stress erosive gastritis.*

Peura DA, Johnson LF: Cimetidine for prevention and treatment of gastroduodenal mucosal lesions in patients in an intensive care unit. Ann Intern Med 103:173, 1985. *Results of this study demonstrate that cimetidine is better than placebo at treating mucosal abnormalities already present in the stomach or duodenum and is better than placebo in preventing mucosal disease from occurring in patients who are critically ill and who are in an intensive care unit.*

Priebe HJ, Skillman JJ, Bushnell LS, et al.: Antacid versus cimetidine in preventing acute gastrointestinal bleeding: A randomized trial in 75 critically ill patients. N Engl J Med 302:426, 1980. *Antacid was better than cimetidine for protecting seriously ill patients from developing acute upper gastrointestinal tract bleeding.*

Sauerbruch T, Schreiber MA, Schussler P, et al.: Endoscopy in the diagnosis of gastritis: Diagnostic value of endoscopic criteria in relation to histological diagnosis. Endoscopy 16:101, 1984. *Histologic examination of biopsy specimens obtained from the stomach is a better method for diagnosing gastritis than endoscopic appearance.*

Weinstein WM: Gastritis. In Sleisenger MH, Fordtran JS (eds.): Gastrointestinal Disease. 4th ed. Philadelphia, W. B. Saunders Company, 1987.

100 PEPTIC ULCER

100.1 Pathogenesis
Charles T. Richardson

DEFINITION

Ulcers are defects in the gastrointestinal mucosa that penetrate the muscularis mucosa. This distinguishes them from superficial erosions that do not extend through the muscularis mucosa. Peptic ulcers usually occur in the stomach, pylorus, or duodenal bulb but also can develop in the esophagus and the postbulbar duodenum. In patients with markedly increased acid secretion (as in Zollinger-Ellison syndrome) ulcers sometimes develop in the distal duodenum and jejunum.

Peptic ulcers occasionally occur in the ileum in or near Meckel's diverticula.

Originally, all ulcers in the upper gastrointestinal tract were believed to be caused by the aggressive action of hydrochloric acid and pepsin on the mucosa. Thus they became known as "peptic ulcers." Although acid and pepsin are secreted by most patients with benign ulcers, they are not the only causes of ulcers. Ulcers probably result from several different pathogenetic mechanisms. In general, ulcers occur when luminal aggressive factors overcome opposing mucosal defenses. Mechanisms believed important in the pathogenesis of ulcer disease are discussed in greater detail below.

NORMAL PHYSIOLOGY

STRUCTURE. The stomach is divided into four anatomic regions: the cardia, fundus, body, and antrum (Fig. 100–1). *Parietal cells*, which secrete acid, and *chief cells*, which secrete pepsinogen, are located primarily in the fundus and body, although a few are found in the antrum. *Gastrin (G) cells* are located in the antrum.

Gastric mucosa is made up of a series of pits and glands (Fig. 100–2). The pits contain surface epithelial cells, whereas the glands contain mucous, parietal, endocrine, and chief cells. Normal gastric juice is a mixture of parietal secretion (acid and intrinsic factor) and nonparietal secretions (mucus, bicarbonate, sodium, potassium, and pepsinogen).

CONTROL OF GASTRIC SECRETION. Three endogenous chemicals (acetylcholine, gastrin, and histamine) stimulate acid secretion (Fig. 100–3): (1) *Acetylcholine*, believed to be a neural transmitter, is released by vagal efferent neurons. Vagal stimulation of acid secretion occurs when humans see, smell, taste, chew, or think about appetizing food. Local neurons within the wall of the stomach also release acetylcholine and are activated when the stomach is distended. (2) *Gastrin* is a hormone responsible for acid secretion. Protein in food is the most potent stimulant of gastrin release, but vagal stimulation, calcium, other cations such as magnesium and aluminum, and alkalinization of the antrum also release gastrin. Gastrin release is inhibited by acid within the lumen of the antrum. (3) *Histamine* stimulates acid secretion via a paracrine mechanism. Mastlike cells that contain histamine are located in the lamina propria of the stomach in close proximity to parietal cells. When histamine is liberated from mast cells, it diffuses through intercellular spaces to reach parietal cells. Gastrin or acetylcholine or both may release histamine from mast cells. Acetylcholine, gastrin, and histamine are believed to act on receptors on parietal cell membranes to cause acid secretion (see Ch. 100.3, on medical therapy of peptic ulcer disease).

Mechanisms within parietal cells that lead to acid secretion

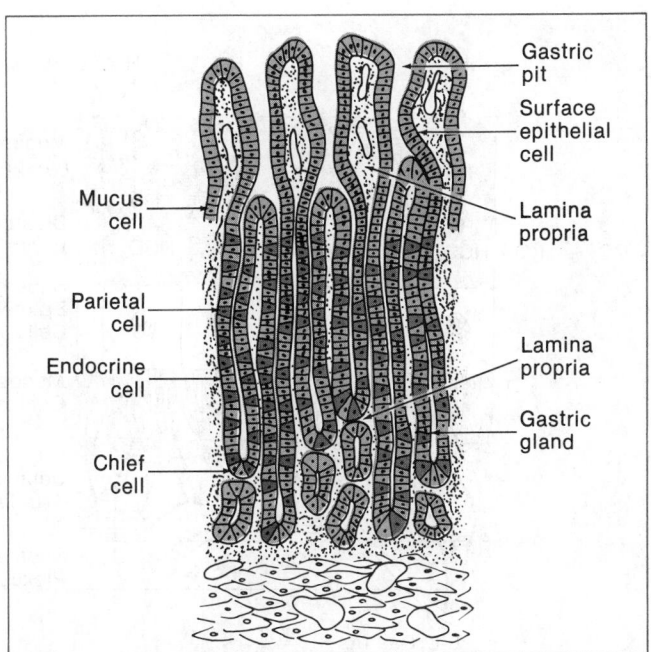

FIGURE 100–2. Diagram demonstrating the cell types lining the pits and glands of the gastric mucosa.

are not well defined. It is believed that cyclic adenosine monophosphate (AMP) is important in the mediation of histamine-stimulated acid secretion, while calcium entry into parietal cells is believed to play a role in acetylcholine-stimulated secretion. A hydrogen/potassium adenosine triphosphatase (ATPase) enzyme is located on the luminal surface of parietal cells (Ch. 100.3). This enzyme serves as a proton pump, which is the final step in secretion of hydrogen ions.

PRODUCTS OF GASTRIC SECRETION. In the pathogenesis of peptic ulcer the two most important products of gastric secretion are hydrochloric acid and pepsin.

Secretion of Acid. Basal acid output (BAO) is the amount of acid secreted under fasting or unstimulated conditions. Peak acid output (PAO) or maximum acid output (MAO) is acid secreted in response to an injection of either pentagastrin or histamine, the maximal amount of acid that a normal subject or patient with ulcer disease can secrete. MAO reflects the number of parietal cells in an individual, and the ratio of BAO to MAO represents the fraction of parietal cell mass functional under basal conditions. Thus, if a patient has an increased amount of gastrin, acetylcholine, or histamine near

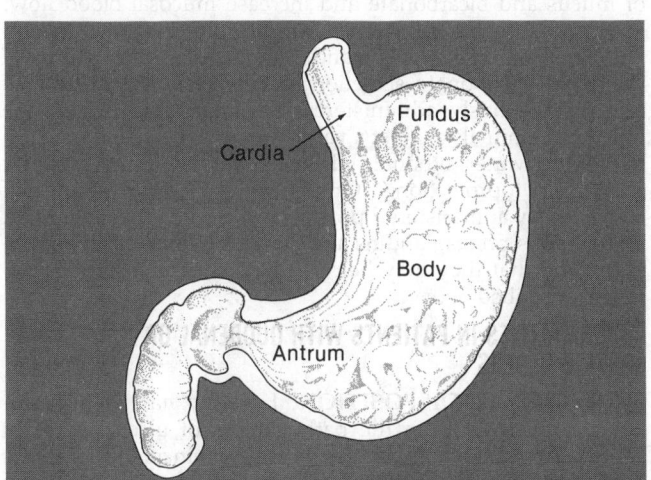

FIGURE 100–1. Anatomic divisions of the stomach.

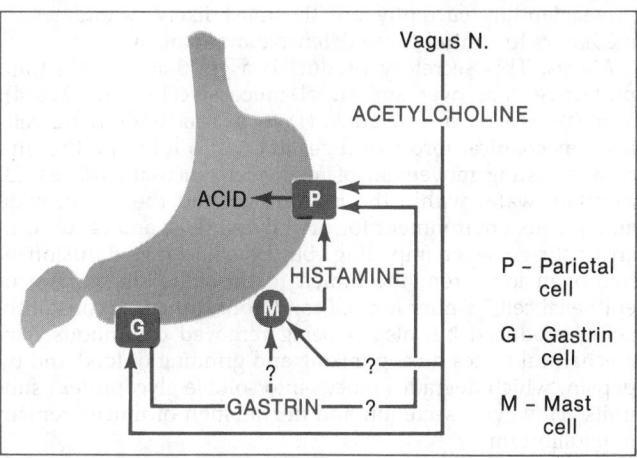

FIGURE 100–3. Model illustrating the chemical stimulants of acid secretion. Acetylcholine originates in the vagus nerves; gastrin is released from gastrin cells in the antrum; and histamine is liberated from mast cells in the lamina propria of the gastric mucosa.

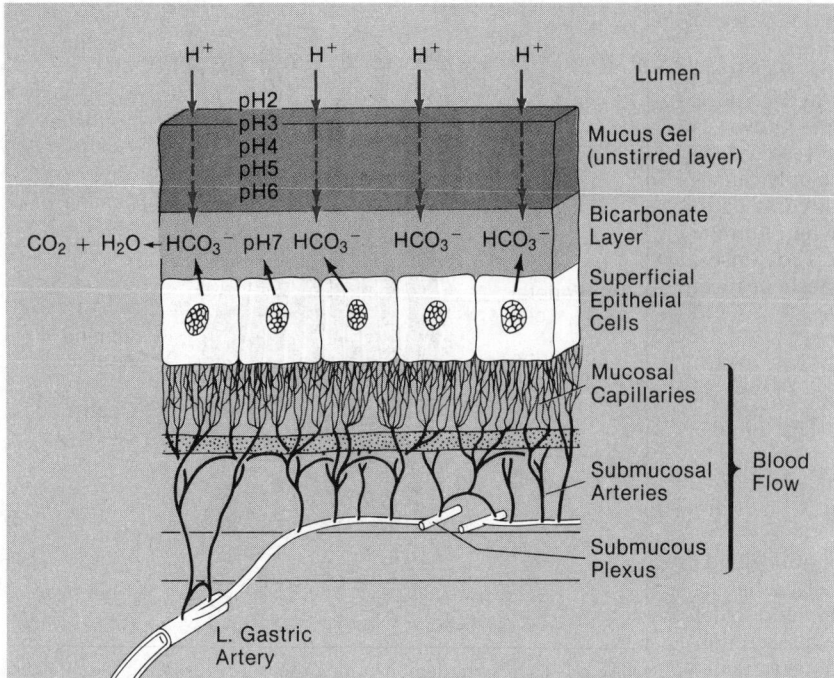

FIGURE 100–4. Model illustrating mechanisms maintaining mucosal integrity. Superficial epithelial cells secrete mucus and bicarbonate, which aid in maintaining a pH gradient between lumen and mucosa and protect the underlying epithelial cells from damage by acid and pepsin. Epithelial cell renewal and mucosal blood flow also are believed to be important mechanisms in maintaining mucosal integrity.

parietal cells or if there is increased sensitivity of parietal cells to normal amounts of these stimulants, BAO will be increased, as will the BAO/MAO ratio. Such a patient is said to have a basal acid hypersecretory state (see below).

Upper and lower limits of normal acid secretion are shown in Table 100–1. Men secrete more acid than women. This can be explained, in part, by differences in body size, but men secrete more acid than women even when corrections are made for weight and lean body mass.

Secretion of Pepsin. Pepsin is secreted into the lumen as an inactive precursor, pepsinogen. Pepsinogen secretion usually accompanies acid secretion. Although mechanisms controlling pepsinogen secretion are less well understood, cholinergic stimulation is believed to be a major mediator. Once pepsinogen is secreted into the gastric lumen, it is converted by acid to pepsin, the active enzyme. The optimal pH for conversion of pepsinogen to pepsin ranges between 1.8 and 3.5.

MAINTENANCE OF NORMAL MUCOSAL INTEGRITY. Several mechanisms are believed important in protecting gastric and duodenal mucosa from damage by acid, pepsin, bile, pancreatic enzymes, and other possible aggressive factors. These defensive mechanisms include mucus, bicarbonate, mucosal blood flow, and cell renewal. Endogenous prostaglandins currently are the most likely candidates as mediators to control these defensive mechanisms.

Mucus. This secretory product is a gel that forms a thin, protective coat over superficial mucosal cells (Fig. 100–4). Mucus has several functions: (1) to protect underlying cells from mechanical forces of digestion; (2) to lubricate the mucosa, assisting movement of food over mucosal surfaces; (3) to retain water within the mucous gel and thereby provide an aqueous environment for underlying cells; and (4) to form an unstirred layer impeding, but not blocking, diffusion of hydrogen ions from the lumen to the apical membrane of epithelial cells. Under normal conditions, mucus is constantly being produced but also is being removed continuously by mechanical forces during mixing and grinding of food and by pepsin, which degrades mucus into soluble glycoprotein subunits. However, secretion and degradation of mucus remain in equilibrium.

Bicarbonate. A bicarbonate-rich fluid is secreted by surface epithelial cells in the stomach and duodenum and also by Brunner's glands in the duodenum. Although some bicarbonate reaches the lumen, much of the secreted bicarbonate

remains below or within the mucous layer (Fig. 100–4). Thus, the mucosal surface is in contact with fluid that contains a high pH relative to the lumen of the stomach. Under normal conditions, hydrogen ions are neutralized by bicarbonate (producing carbon dioxide and water) as they diffuse through the mucous gel layer. A pH gradient is thus established between the lumen and surface epithelial cells.

Mucosal Blood Flow. The rich blood supply of the stomach and duodenum is important in maintaining normal mucosal integrity. Gastric and duodenal mucosae are supplied by arborizing mucosal capillaries that traverse the glandular area of the stomach and duodenum. Beneath the muscularis mucosa, an extensive system of submucosal arteries and a submucous plexus of arteries and veins regulate the blood supply to surface epithelial cells (Fig. 100–4).

Cell Renewal. Normal cell renewal is also an important factor in maintaining mucosal integrity. Cells are constantly dying and are being replaced by new cells. In order for this system to function normally, there must be a balance between cell loss and cell renewal. Disruption of this steady state may lead to mucosal damage.

Endogenous Prostaglandins. Prostaglandins of the E, F, and I types are found in the gastric and duodenal mucosa. When administered exogenously, prostaglandins stimulate secretion of mucus and bicarbonate and increase mucosal blood flow. Prostaglandins also may have a trophic effect on the mucosa. Duodenal mucosal prostaglandins appear to stimulate basal duodenal bicarbonate secretion and its response to luminal acid. Exogenously administered prostaglandins protect the mucosa of animals against a variety of noxious agents, including boiling water, ethanol, bile acids, and aspirin, a property termed "cytoprotection." On the basis of such studies of exogenously administered prostaglandins, it is presumed that endogenous prostaglandins also possess cytoprotective properties and that they may help regulate the defensive mechanisms described above.

ABNORMALITIES IN PATIENTS WITH DUODENAL OR GASTRIC ULCERS

GENETIC PREDISPOSITION. Heredity has been postulated to play a role in the pathogenesis of ulcer disease in some patients. Several families with a high incidence of ulcers have been described. The mechanism or mechanisms whereby genetic factors contribute to ulceration in these families is unclear. Originally, it was believed that familial aggregations of ulcer disease represented polygenic inheritance because the genetics of peptic ulcer could not be explained by a single autosomal, sex-linked, dominant, or recessive defect. Polygenic or multifactorial disorders are believed to be caused by the interaction of several genes with environmental factors. Thus, the hereditary component in ulcer disease was believed to reflect the combined contribution of many different genes in an individual patient. More recently, polygenic inheritance has seemed less likely than genetic heterogeneity. In this form of inheritance a number of genetically determined abnormalities share a common clinical manifestation—in this case, the ulcer crater. A number of rare genetic syndromes are associated with peptic ulcer disease. Multiple endocrine neoplasia I syndrome is the most common example (Ch. 241). Additionally, several pathophysiologic abnormalities believed to be associated with increased acid and pepsin secretion or increased gastric emptying have been discovered and several of these have been found in "ulcer families." For example, in several families an increased level of serum pepsinogen I was inherited as an autosomal dominant trait. Since serum pepsinogen I concentrations reflect chief cell mass and correlate with maximum acid output, members of these families may have developed ulcers because of either increased pepsin or acid secretion or increased secretion of both. Other abnormalities, such as those leading to diminished mucosal defense, may be inherited also. The true importance, if any, of hereditary factors in the pathogenesis of peptic ulcer disease in most patients has not been established.

ABNORMALITIES IN SECRETION OF ACID AND PEPSIN. Approximately 30 to 40 per cent of patients with duodenal ulcer disease have acid secretion rates above the upper limits of normal shown in Table 100–1. The remainder have values within the normal range. Since pepsinogen secretion usually accompanies acid secretion, approximately the same percentage of ulcer patients will have increased or normal pepsinogen secretion.

Most patients with gastric ulcers have either normal or lower than normal acid secretion rates. Only a minority of patients with gastric ulcer disease (for example, a few patients with Zollinger-Ellison syndrome) have secretion rates above the normal range. The fact that most gastric ulcer patients have normal or lower than normal acid secretory rates does not exclude acid and pepsin as the cause of gastric ulcer disease in an individual patient but suggests that other factors may be involved (see below). This same concept applies to patients with duodenal ulcers who have normal rates of acid secretion. In fact, the exact role acid or pepsin or both play in the pathogenesis of either gastric or duodenal ulcers is not known. It is assumed that acid is involved in the pathogenesis of ulcer disease in patients with higher than normal rates of acid secretion (see below).

There are three known mechanisms for increased basal acid secretion: (1) increased stimulation by *gastrin* (Zollinger-Elli-

son syndrome, retained antrum syndrome, and antral gastrin [G] cell hyperplasia or hyperfunction); (2) increased stimulation by *acetylcholine* (vagal hyperfunction); and (3) increased *histamine* stimulation (systemic mastocytosis or basophilic leukemia). Other causes of basal hypersecretion may exist, but so far they have not been described. Ulcers presumably occur in patients with these disorders because of increased levels of acid and pepsin. All of the currently recognized syndromes causing increased basal acid secretion are rare. Of the group Zollinger-Ellison syndrome is the most common and will be discussed separately (see Ch. 100.6).

REFLUX OF BILE AND PANCREATIC JUICE. Bile acids, lysolecithin, and pancreatic enzymes are believed to be aggressive factors that lead to ulceration in some patients, especially some of those with gastric ulcers. It has been postulated that duodenal contents reflux into the stomach causing gastritis that, in turn, predisposes to gastric ulceration. Some patients with gastric ulcers may have an incompetent pyloric sphincter that allows reflux of bile or pancreatic enzymes or both into the stomach.

Two mechanisms have been proposed whereby bile and pancreatic juice may damage gastric mucosa: first, alteration of mucus overlying surface epithelial cells, reducing its protective effect; and second, damage to the so-called gastric mucosal barrier (the ability of the stomach to maintain electrical and hydrogen ion concentration gradients between lumen and blood). When these protective mechanisms are disrupted, the mucosa becomes more permeable to the damaging effects of acid and pepsin. Although bile and pancreatic juice have been postulated as the cause of ulcers in some patients, a cause-and-effect relationship has not been clearly established.

ABNORMALITIES OF MUCOSAL DEFENSE. Little is known at the present time about how disruptions in mucosal integrity may lead to ulceration, although there are several theoretic ways in which this might occur. For example, some patients may secrete *reduced amounts of mucus* or *structurally abnormal mucus*. Both could lead to a weaker mucous gel layer.

Diminished blood flow may lead to cell injury and ulceration in some patients. Gastric mucosal ischemia is believed to be a factor in the pathogenesis of acute mucosal injury, as occurs in patients with severe medical or surgical illnesses (stress ulceration). Whether similar reductions in blood flow contribute to the development of chronic gastric or duodenal ulcers is not known. There are fewer collateral blood vessels on the lesser curvature of the stomach compared with the greater curvature. Whether this anatomic difference in blood supply leads to reduced blood flow to the lesser curvature with subsequent ulceration in some patients is not known, but most gastric ulcers do occur on the lesser curvature.

Decreased bicarbonate secretion is a theoretic possibility as a cause for diminished mucosal defense. Gastric bicarbonate secretion has been measured in patients with duodenal ulcer disease and found not to be significantly different from that in normal subjects. However, results of a recent study suggest that bicarbonate secretion from the duodenum may be decreased in duodenal ulcer patients. Reduced pancreatic bicarbonate secretion into the lumen of the duodenum could lead to increased acidity in the duodenal bulb with subsequent duodenal ulceration. There is no evidence, however, that patients with pancreatic insufficiency have a higher incidence of duodenal ulcers. The role of possible *abnormalities in cell renewal* in the pathogenesis of peptic ulcer is entirely speculative at the present time.

Prostaglandin content in gastric or duodenal mucosa might be diminished, leading to abnormalities of mucosal defense (see above). The preliminary studies have led to conflicting reports, however, so that it is impossible at this time to evaluate adequately the possible role of endogenous prostaglandins in the pathogenesis of gastric or duodenal ulcers.

EMOTIONAL STRESS. The mechanism or mechanisms by

TABLE 100–1. UPPER (ULN) AND LOWER (LLN) LIMITS OF NORMAL ACID SECRETION IN HEALTHY MEN AND WOMEN

	Acid Output (mmol/hr)*			
	Basal	*Peak*	*Maximum*	*Basal/Maximum*
Men (N = 172)				
ULN	10.5	60.6	47.7	0.31
LLN	0	11.6	9.3	0
Women (N = 76)				
ULN	5.6	40.1	31.2	0.29
LLN	0	8.0	5.6	0

*Acid output (volume of gastric juice times concentration of acid) is measured in 15-minute intervals and is expressed in mmol/hr. Basal acid output is the sum of acid secreted during four 15-minute periods. Peak acid output is the sum of the highest two 15-minute periods after pentagastrin or histamine stimulation multiplied by two. Maximum acid output is the sum of four 15-minute intervals after pentagastrin or histamine stimulation.

which emotional stress might contribute to ulcer disease in some patients are unclear. Certain emotions such as hostility, resentment, guilt, and frustration are associated with increased gastric acidity. Furthermore, basal acid secretion has been reported to increase during stressful interviews and prior to surgery in ulcer patients or before difficult school examinations in healthy subjects. Patients have been described who developed acid hypersecretion and gastric ulcer disease during periods of severe emotional stress. With alleviation of stress, acid secretion diminished and symptoms and ulcerations disappeared. Thus, it appears that certain emotions can cause increased acid secretion that in turn may lead to ulceration in certain patients. Emotional stress may alter factors that maintain mucosal integrity and thereby result in ulcers because of decreased mucosal defense. Although emotional stress is likely to be a factor in the pathogenesis of ulcer disease in some patients, its exact role is uncertain.

DELAYED GASTRIC EMPTYING. For a number of years delayed gastric emptying was believed to be a major factor in the pathogenesis of gastric ulcer disease. It was postulated that delayed gastric emptying caused retention of food in the stomach; in turn, this retention led to increased gastrin release, higher rates of acid secretion, and gastric ulceration. Prolonged gastric emptying, perhaps due to antral hypomotility, was also believed to cause stasis and delayed clearing of duodenal contents (bile and pancreatic enzymes) that had refluxed into the stomach. This in turn could damage gastric mucosa, cause gastritis, and lead to ulceration. Neither of these proposed pathogenetic mechanisms was ever established. Currently delayed emptying is believed to be related to ulceration in only a minority of patients.

EXOGENOUS FACTORS. The most important exogenous factors that have been associated with peptic ulcer disease are cigarette smoking and the use of nonsteroidal anti-inflammatory drugs. The possible association with adrenocorticosteroid therapy, infectious agents, alcohol or caffeine is more tenuous.

Cigarette Smoking. Whether cigarette smoking is related to the pathogenesis of ulcer disease is unclear, although epidemiologic data suggest an association between the two: (1) Smoking is more common among patients with ulcers than among control subjects. (2) There is a positive correlation between the quantity of cigarettes smoked and the prevalence of ulcer disease. (3) Death due to peptic ulcer disease is more likely among patients who smoke than among those who do not. (4) Duodenal ulcers are less likely to heal in cigarette smokers than in nonsmokers. (5) Duodenal ulcers recur more frequently in smokers than in nonsmokers. Whether this applies also to patients with gastric ulcers is not known.

Two mechanisms have been postulated whereby smoking may lead to ulceration: reduction of pyloric sphincter pressure and decreased pancreatic bicarbonate secretion. Smoking has been shown to reduce pyloric sphincter pressure in some patients with gastric ulcers. This, in turn, may lead to increased duodenogastric reflux of bile and pancreatic enzymes into the stomach with subsequent damage to the gastric mucosa. Nicotine reduces pancreatic bicarbonate secretion and may thereby lead to duodenal ulcers by impairing neutralization of acid by bicarbonate in the duodenal bulb. There is no proof, however, that either of these mechanisms actually causes ulceration.

Nonsteroidal Anti-inflammatory Drugs. These medications inhibit prostaglandin synthesis and cause decreased mucus and bicarbonate secretion, diminished mucosal blood flow, and perhaps reduced cell renewal. Aspirin and other nonsteroidal anti-inflammatory drugs cause superficial mucosal erosions in the stomach, presumably by reducing the factors believed important in maintaining mucosal integrity. It is unclear, however, whether these drugs also cause chronic gastric or duodenal ulcers. Chronic gastric ulcers seem to occur more frequently in patients taking large doses of aspirin

than in control populations, but a definite relationship between the intake of aspirin and other nonsteroidal anti-inflammatory drugs and the development of chronic ulcers has never been established. These drugs may play a role in the pathogenesis of chronic gastric ulcers in some patients. Their role in the development of duodenal ulcers seems less likely.

Adrenocorticosteroid Therapy. An association between treatment with glucocorticoids (especially prednisone) and peptic ulcer disease has been both supported and denied in conflicting studies. Any relationship between steroid therapy and ulcer disease remains controversial, therefore.

Infectious Agents. Cytomegalovirus (CMV) has been isolated from gastric ulcers in a few patients receiving immunosuppressive drugs and in patients with post-transfusion CMV mononucleosis. *Candida albicans* also has been found in gastric ulcers in several patients. Whether these organisms caused the ulcers or whether the organisms were there secondarily is not known. Herpesviruses have never been isolated from gastric or duodenal ulcers, but one study indicated that antibodies to Herpesvirus type I occurred more frequently and in higher titers in patients with duodenal ulcers than in control subjects.

Gastric *Campylobacter*-like organisms (GCLO) have been associated with acute and chronic gastritis (see Ch. 99). Some postulate that these organisms may be related to the pathogenesis of gastric or duodenal ulcers, but such a relationship remains to be established.

Alcohol or Caffeine-Containing Beverages. Even though both of these substances stimulate acid secretion, there is no evidence that either causes gastric or duodenal ulcers.

Grossman MI (ed.): Peptic Ulcer. A Guide for the Practicing Physician. Chicago, Year Book Medical Publishers, 1981. *This book is an objective review of information relative to the pathogenesis of peptic ulcer disease, including the role of environmental and hereditary factors.*

Miller TA: Protective effects of prostaglandins against gastric mucosal damage: Current knowledge and proposed mechanisms. Am J Physiol 245:G601, 1983. *An excellent review of mechanisms that maintain normal mucosal integrity, the regulation of these mechanisms, and some of the ways in which alterations in these mechanisms may lead to mucosal diseases.*

Richardson CT: Gastric ulcer. In Sleisenger MH, Fordtran JS (eds.): Gastrointestinal Disease. 4th ed. Philadelphia, W. B. Saunders Company, 1987. *The factors involved in the pathogenesis of gastric ulcer are discussed.*

Soll AH: Duodenal ulcer diseases. In Sleisenger MH, Fordtran JS (eds.): Gastrointestinal Disease. 4th ed. Philadelphia, W. B. Saunders Company, 1987. *The pathophysiologic abnormalities found in various groups of duodenal ulcer patients are discussed.*

100.2 Epidemiology, Clinical Manifestations, and Diagnosis

Lawrence R. Schiller

EPIDEMIOLOGY

Peptic ulcer disease is a common disorder; 5 to 10 per cent of all individuals develop peptic ulcer in their lifetime. Although ulcer disease is a common cause of morbidity, it is a relatively rare cause of death. The annual prevalence of symptomatic peptic ulcer disease in the United States is approximately 18 per 1000 adults, but the current mortality rate is only 2.5 per 100,000. Approximately 350,000 new cases of ulcer present each year in the United States.

Ulcer incidence varies by site, sex, and age. Symptomatic duodenal ulcer is more common than symptomatic gastric ulcer in both men (5.5 to 1) and women (2.8 to 1). Men are twice as likely as women to develop a duodenal ulcer but equally likely to develop a gastric ulcer; sex differences may be narrowing, however. Duodenal ulcer usually first produces symptoms between the ages of 25 and 55 years (peak occurrence at age 40) and gastric ulcer most commonly between 40 and 70 years of age (peak occurrence at age 50).

Hospitalization and mortality rates for peptic ulcer disease seem to be declining in the United States, suggesting that the prevalence of peptic ulcer may be declining. It is unclear whether this reflects an actual change in the prevalence of peptic ulcers, a change in the criteria for hospitalization, or a change in the way mortality data are recorded. Studies from other countries suggest that morbidity and mortality from ulcer disease vary widely with geography and may not be declining with time. Before 1900 duodenal ulcer was a rarity and gastric ulcer was a disorder diagnosed mainly in young women. The reasons for reported changes in prevalence and sex incidence with time and for geographic differences are not known.

SYMPTOMS

DYSPEPSIA. Peptic ulcer usually presents as a painful upper abdominal disorder with the constellation of symptoms known as *dyspepsia*. Dyspepsia is poorly defined by both patients and physicians and often includes such symptoms as nausea, vomiting, anorexia, and fullness and bloating in addition to pain or discomfort. Most patients thought to have ulcers because of "typical dyspepsia" are not found to have peptic ulcer by radiography or endoscopy but instead have other diseases or are classified as having "non-ulcer" (functional) dyspepsia.

A list of clinical features and their frequency in gastric ulcer, duodenal ulcer, and "non-ulcer" dyspepsia is provided in Table 100–2. It is impossible to differentiate these conditions from each other or from other diseases producing upper abdominal symptoms, such as cholelithiasis, by any one clinical feature. In practice physicians make the correct diagnosis on the basis of history in patients with dyspepsia less than 50 per cent of the time. In contrast, the use of structured questionnaires and computer-generated multivariate analysis of clinical findings has been remarkably successful in predicting diagnoses in patients with upper abdominal symptoms (80 to 90 per cent correct). This suggests that information leading to a correct diagnosis is contained within the history, but that physicians may be obtaining or analyzing the data incorrectly.

PAIN. The clinical diagnosis of ulcer disease has usually been based on the location of pain, its character, and the factors aggravating or alleviating it. For example, ulcer pain is classically described as being located in the epigastrium and as burning or gnawing in character. Pain in this location also occurs in a majority of patients with "non-ulcer" dyspepsia, however, and pain of this character actually occurs in a minority of patients with either gastric or duodenal ulcer (Table 100–2). Some patients describe ulcer pain as a cramping sensation not unlike hunger pangs, but descriptions of the character of pain are often hard to obtain in an unbiased way and are difficult to assess. Typical ulcer pain is said to be relieved by ingestion of food or antacids, but this is also quite variable. A better predictor of the presence of peptic ulcer (especially duodenal ulcer) is an episodic pattern of pain. Individual episodes of pain usually are short lived, lasting for minutes rather than hours. Episodes of pain usually occur in clusters lasting from days to weeks, interspersed with long symptom-free periods. Some patients with ulcer report annual recurrences of pain during particular seasons such as spring or fall.

The cause of ulcer pain remains unknown. Ulcer pain is usually attributed to increased acidity at the ulcer site and the relief of pain to a decrease in luminal acidity. This theory is consistent with the typical onset of pain several hours after a meal, when gastric emptying has reduced the buffering capacity of gastric contents and intraluminal acidity rises. Attempts to induce pain by perfusing the ulcer site with acid have not uniformly produced pain, however. In several studies ingestion of placebo with no buffering capacity was as effective as ingestion of active antacid in relieving ulcer pain. In addition, ingestion of food sometimes worsens pain. Alternative mechanisms for the production of ulcer pain have been proposed, such as abnormal gastric or duodenal motor function, but are similarly unproved.

COMPLICATIONS. Peptic ulcers frequently fail to produce dyspepsia or pain and therefore may present de novo as a complication, such as bleeding, obstruction, or perforation. These are discussed in Ch. 100.5.

PHYSICAL EXAMINATION

The physical examination is usually not helpful in uncomplicated peptic ulcer disease. Epigastric tenderness is an insensitive and nonspecific finding and correlates poorly with the presence of an active ulcer crater. When ulcer disease is complicated by obstruction, perforation, penetration, or bleeding, important physical findings may be present (see Ch. 100.5).

Rarely, peptic ulcer is associated with multisystem syndromes that may produce physical findings. For instance, systemic mastocytosis, stiff skin syndrome, pachydermoperiostosis, and multiple lentigenes–ulcer syndrome may have cutaneous findings. Ulcer-tremor-nystagmus syndrome and amyloidosis may produce both peptic ulcer and neurologic findings.

DIAGNOSTIC VISUALIZATION

The initial diagnosis of ulcer depends on visualizing the ulcer crater by radiography or endoscopy. Radiography is well tolerated (even in patients in fragile condition), readily available, and comparatively inexpensive, making it an excellent screening test. However, radiography may miss as many as 20 per cent of peptic ulcers. Endoscopy is more accurate and allows directed biopsy and cytologic study of suspicious lesions but cannot always be done safely in uncooperative patients or those whose condition is unstable. In the United States, where endoscopy currently costs from three to five times as much as radiography, upper gastrointestinal radiographs, preferably with both single-contrast and double-contrast techniques, are often the initial diagnostic test. In symptomatic patients with no radiographic abnormalities or with equivocal evidence of ulcer, endoscopy can establish or exclude the diagnosis of active ulcer disease. In situations in

TABLE 100–2. CLINICAL FEATURES OF GASTRIC ULCER, DUODENAL ULCER, AND "NON-ULCER" DYSPEPSIA*

Clinical Feature	Gastric Ulcer (%)	Duodenal Ulcer (%)	"Non-ulcer" Dyspepsia (%)
Features of pain:			
Primary pain location			
Epigastric	67	61–86	52–73
Right hypochondrium	6	7–17	4
Left hypochondrium	6	3–5	5
Radiation to back	34	20–31	24–28
Frequently severe	68	53	37
Gnawing pain	13	16	6
Clusters (episodic)	16	56	35
Occurs at night	32–43	50–88	24–32
Within 30 min of food	20	5	32
Increased by food	24	10–40	45
Food relief	2–48	20–63	4–32
Not related to food or variable	22–53	21–49	22–65
Relief by alkali	36–87	39–86	26–75
Anorexia	46–57	25–36	26–36
Weight loss	24–61	19–45	18–32
Nausea	54–70	49–59	43–60
Vomiting	38–73	25–57	26–34
Heartburn	19	27–59	28
Fatty food intolerance	—	14–72	53
Bloating	55	49	52
Belching	48	59	60

*From Soll AH, Isenberg JI: Duodenal ulcer disease. In Sleisenger MH, Fordtran JS (eds.): Gastrointestinal Disease. 3rd ed. Philadelphia, W.B. Saunders Company, 1983, pp 625–672.

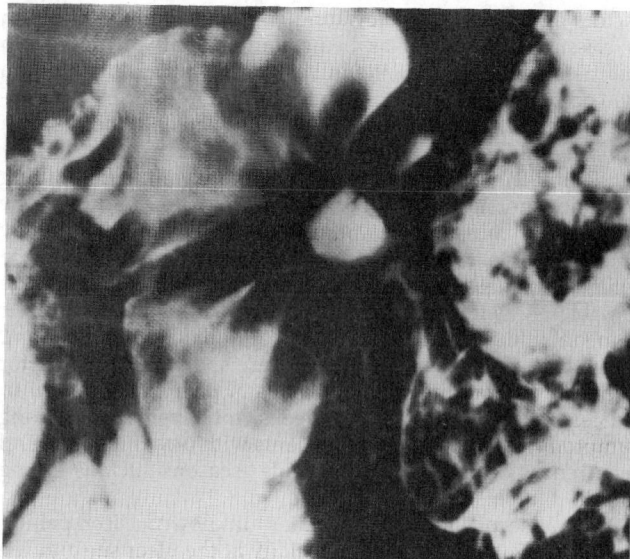

FIGURE 100–5. Duodenal ulcers are recognized when barium is retained within an ulcer niche. In this example barium has collected in an ulcer at the base of the duodenal bulb along the posterior wall. Folds radiate to the margin of this ulcer. (From Goldberg HI: In Sleisenger MH, Fordtran JS [eds.]: Gastrointestinal Disease. 2nd ed. Philadelphia, W. B. Saunders Company, 1978.)

which there is little difference in cost between endoscopy and radiography, endoscopy is preferable in the investigation of patients with dyspepsia because of its greater sensitivity in diagnosis.

DUODENAL ULCER. If a duodenal ulcer is demonstrated radiographically (Fig. 100–5), no further diagnostic evaluation is necessary and treatment can be started. Since duodenal ulcers are rarely malignant, endoscopic biopsy is not necessary. Follow-up examinations to assess healing of a duodenal ulcer need not be done routinely. However, if symptoms fail to subside with therapy, endoscopy should be done to prove the diagnosis of ulcer before considering surgery (see Ch. 100.4)

GASTRIC ULCER. If a gastric ulcer is found on the radiograph (Fig. 100–6), malignancy should be rigorously excluded, particularly if there is any suspicion by the radiologist that the ulcer may be malignant. Malignancy should be suspected if (1) the ulcer is located completely within the gastric wall or in an intraluminal mass, (2) there is nodularity of the ulcer base or of adjacent gastric mucosa, (3) there are no folds radiating to the ulcer margin, or (4) the ulcer is large. Malignancy can best be excluded by direct endoscopic visualization of the gastric ulcer to obtain brush cytologic specimens and to obtain a minimum of six to eight punch biopsy specimens for careful pathologic examination. This approach will lead to an accurate diagnosis in more than 95 per cent of cases. Some investigators recommend that patients with radiographically benign-appearing gastric ulcers not have endoscopy initially but that malignancy be excluded by repeating a radiographic study or by endoscopy after a period of therapy to prove that the ulcer has healed completely. Whether initially endoscoped and found benign or not, all gastric ulcers should be followed to healing. This can be done best by endoscopy after treatment for 8 to 12 weeks to allow healing to occur. Surgery may be needed to exclude malignancy in nonhealing gastric ulcer even if multiple endoscopic biopsies yield negative results (Ch. 100.4).

LABORATORY STUDIES

SERUM GASTRIN LEVELS. Radioimmunoassay of gastrin is useful in screening patients with known ulcer disease for Zollinger-Ellison syndrome and other rare hypersecretory states. The reasons for identifying these patients are (1) they

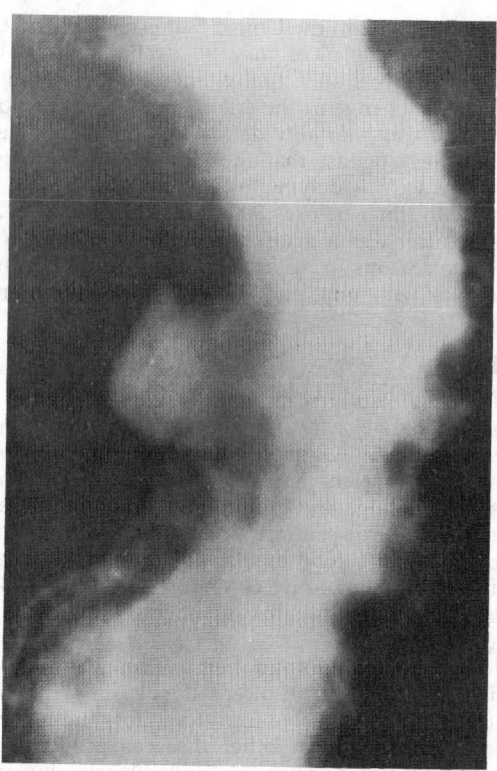

FIGURE 100–6. This ulcer of the lesser curve of the stomach demonstrates several features typical of benign gastric ulcers: The ulcer crater projects beyond the contour of the gastric wall, the margin of the ulcer crater is sharply defined and smooth, the ulcer is surrounded by a broad lucent band—an ulcer collar—resulting from edema at the ulcer orifice, and mucosal folds radiate from the ulcer collar. (From Goldberg HI: In Sleisenger MH, Fordtran JS [eds.]: Gastrointestinal Disease. 2nd ed. Philadelphia, W. B. Saunders Company, 1978.)

may have a more severe course marked by excessive complications such as bleeding, obstruction, or perforation; (2) therapy is different, particularly surgical therapy (see Ch. 100.4); (3) associated but undiagnosed diseases of other organs, such as multiple endocrine neoplasia type I, may cause morbidity; and (4) gastrinomas associated with Zollinger-Ellison syndrome may be malignant and cause death from metastasis. Early recognition of Zollinger-Ellison syndrome makes possible effective control of symptoms and sometimes allows resection of tumor and cure of the disease (Ch. 100.6).

Measurement of serum gastrin concentrations in all patients with peptic ulcer disease is not cost effective because the incidence of Zollinger-Ellison syndrome is low (less than 1 per cent of patients with peptic ulcer disease). Table 100–3 lists the selective clinical situations in which obtaining a fasting serum gastrin level may be useful, although even with this selectivity the likelihood of identifying a patient as having Zollinger-Ellison syndrome is low.

If fasting serum gastrin concentrations are elevated (> 200 pg per milliliter) in patients not taking medications that alter intragastric pH, gastric acid secretion should be measured in

TABLE 100–3. CLINICAL SITUATIONS IN WHICH MEASUREMENT OF SERUM GASTRIN LEVELS IS INDICATED

Family history of peptic ulcer
Ulcer associated with hypercalcemia or other manifestations
   of multiple endocrine neoplasia type I
Multifocal peptic ulcer
Peptic ulceration of postbulbar duodenum or jejunum
Peptic ulceration associated with diarrhea*
Chronic unexplained diarrhea*
Enlarged gastric folds on upper GI x-ray
Before surgery for "intractable" ulcer
Recurrent ulcer after ulcer surgery

*Not due to antacid ingestion.
GI = Gastrointestinal.

order to prove that gastrin levels are not elevated in response to hypochlorhydria or achlorhydria, such as that due to pernicious anemia, atrophic gastritis, gastric cancer, or vagotomy. A finding of high serum gastrin levels and increased basal acid output limits the differential diagnosis to only a few entities (Table 100-4). If both fasting gastrin levels and basal acid secretion are very high (> 1000 pg per milliliter and > 15 mmol per hour, respectively), a diagnosis of Zollinger-Ellison syndrome is likely.

When fasting gastrin levels or basal acid outputs or both are less markedly elevated and the diagnosis of Zollinger-Ellison syndrome is unclear, the response of serum gastrin concentration to an intravenous injection of secretin may be helpful. In individuals with Zollinger-Ellison syndrome, intravenous injection of pure Secretin-Kabi, 2 U per kilogram of body weight, results in a prompt and pathognomonic rise of gastrin of > 200 pg per milliliter within two to ten minutes. Patients with other hypergastrinemic conditions (Table 100-4) and normal individuals do not show this elevation. Gastrin secretion rises with calcium infusion also, but this rise is less reliable diagnostically than that following injection of secretin.

Differentiation of other rare hypergastrinemic syndromes (Table 100-4) can be made on the basis of (1) history of ulcer surgery (retained antrum syndrome, discussed in Ch. 100.4) or small bowel resection, (2) demonstration of gastric outlet obstruction by radiography or endoscopy, (3) laboratory evidence of renal failure, or (4) response of serum gastrin levels to a meal. Patients with antral G cell hyperplasia or hyperfunction more than double their already elevated fasting gastrin levels after ingestion of a protein meal. Patients with Zollinger-Ellison syndrome do not usually have this exuberant response to a meal.

ACID SECRETORY TESTING. Gastric acid secretion is measured by placing a vented nasogastric tube in the gastric antrum under fluoroscopic guidance and aspirating gastric juice with a suction pump. By measuring the volume and acid concentration (determined either by titration to pH 7.0 or indirectly from pH measurements), the quantity of acid secreted by the stomach can be calculated. Basal acid output (BAO) is defined as the amount of acid produced during four consecutive 15-minute periods. Vmax for acid secretion is estimated by injecting a maximally effective dose of gastric secretagogue. Pentagastrin (6 μg per kilogram), the biologically active carboxyl-terminal fragment of gastrin, is preferred for this purpose. Histamine or betazole (Histalog) can also be used. Stimulated secretion is expressed as peak acid output (PAO, the sum of the two highest consecutive 15-minute periods after injection multiplied by 2) or as maximal acid output (MAO, the sum of four consecutive 15-minute periods after injection). Values for acid secretion in healthy subjects and ulcer patients are shown in Table 100-1. In the absence of hypergastrinemia, measurement of gastric acid secretion is usually unnecessary in patients with peptic ulcer. Basal and peak acid output are increased in duodenal ulcer patients as a group (see Ch. 100.1), but knowledge of the level of acid secretion has no therapeutic implications for the individual patient at present. Measurement of acid secretion rates is sometimes useful preoperatively so that postoperative values can be compared and the effect of the operation on acid secretion can be assessed (see Ch. 100.4). When ulcer disease occurs in the presence of achlorhydria, malignancy should be suspected.

TABLE 100-4. CAUSES OF INCREASED FASTING SERUM GASTRIN CONCENTRATIONS AND INCREASED BASAL ACID OUTPUT

Zollinger-Ellison syndrome
Retained antrum syndrome
Massive small bowel resection (?)
Chronic gastric outlet obstruction (?)
Renal failure
Antral G cell hyperplasia or hyperfunction

TABLE 100-5. COMMON DISEASES THAT MAY PRODUCE EPIGASTRIC PAIN SIMULATING PEPTIC ULCER

Myocardial infarction
Pleurisy
Pericarditis
Esophagitis
Cholecystitis
Pancreatitis
Irritable bowel syndrome

DIFFERENTIAL DIAGNOSIS

Peptic ulcer can usually be distinguished from painful intestinal disorders that customarily produce discomfort in the periumbilical or lower quadrants of the abdomen (e.g., appendicitis or diverticulitis). Disorders affecting the viscera of the upper abdomen or chest are more difficult to differentiate from peptic ulcer disease (Table 100.5). Differentiation of these disorders can often be made by considering the acuteness of pain, lack of response to eating or antacids, changes of pain with changes in position, radiation of pain, and the presence of physical findings such as rebound tenderness, all of which are atypical in uncomplicated peptic ulcer disease. Because ulcer disease is common and ulcer symptoms are often variable, however, peptic ulcer must be considered as a possible cause of abdominal symptoms even in patients with atypical symptoms.

FUNCTIONAL DYSPEPSIA. *Functional dyspepsia* ("nonulcer" dyspepsia) is diagnosed when a symptomatic individual is not found to have an ulcer or other structural disease, such as cholelithiasis. Women in their twenties are especially likely to have this condition. The causes of this syndrome are unknown. It is likely that several different problems can lead to dyspepsia. It has been estimated that 20 to 30 per cent of patients with this diagnosis eventually develop peptic ulcer; therefore, some of these patients may really have evanescent ulcers that evade diagnosis. Some of these patients have a disruption of normal gastric motor function. Gastrokinetic agents such as metoclopramide or domperidone have been found to reverse both symptoms and motor dysfunction in some of these patients. Longer clinical trials are needed before such therapy can be generally recommended for patients with functional dyspepsia.

GASTRIC CANCER. Many patients with gastric cancer present with dyspepsia (Ch. 101). This diagnosis should be considered in particular when dyspepsia is associated with weight loss or evidence of occult gastrointestinal blood loss in an elderly individual or when radiographic or endoscopic appearances of gastric ulcer are suspicious for malignancy. However, a diagnosis of cancer should also be considered in any individual with a benign-appearing gastric ulcer, since roughly 2 to 5 per cent of such ulcers contain foci of gastric carcinoma.

MISCELLANEOUS DISORDERS. A variety of other diseases can produce dyspepsia that may mimic that of peptic ulcer. These conditions include *infiltrative diseases* of the stomach such as hypertrophic gastritis, tuberculosis, syphilis, Crohn's disease, and other granulomatous gastritides (see Ch. 99); *duodenal obstruction* by polyps, webs, or an annular pancreas; and *intestinal parasitosis* by Giardia or Strongyloides. More common diseases causing dyspeptic symptoms include *biliary tract disease* and *pancreatitis*. These can often be differentiated from ulcer disease by history, but tests such as sonography, cholecystography, and serum amylase determinations are usually necessary to confirm their diagnosis.

Bonnevie O: Changing demographics of peptic ulcer disease. Dig Dis Sci 30(Suppl. Nov. 1985):8S, 1985. *Well-referenced review of changing trends in ulcer disease from a European perspective.*

Cotton PB, Shorvon PJ: Analysis of endoscopy and radiography in the diagnosis, follow-up and treatment of peptic ulcer disease. Clin Gastroenterol 13:383, 1984. *Thoughtful and detailed analysis of the role of radiography and endoscopy in ulcer patients.*

de Dombal FT: Analysis of foregut symptoms. In Baron JH, Moody FG (eds.): Butterworth's International Medical Reviews, Gastroenterology 1, Foregut. London, Butterworth & Co, Ltd, 1981, pp 49–66. *Excellent review of new approaches to foregut symptoms, including multivariate analysis.*

Kurata JH, Haile BM: Epidemiology of peptic ulcer disease. Clin Gastroenterol 13:289, 1984. *Precise analysis of current statistics with discussion of epidemiologic problems.*

Lagarde SP, Spiro HM: Non-ulcer dyspepsia. Clin Gastroenterol 13:437, 1984. *Wide-ranging review of this diffuse syndrome.*

Thompson WM, Kelvin FM, Gedgaudas RD, et al.: Radiologic investigation of peptic ulcer disease. Radiol Clin North Am 20:701, 1982. *Review of state of the art for radiology of peptic ulcer with many excellent examples.*

100.3 Medical Therapy

Walter L. Peterson

In the healthy human stomach and duodenum there is an effective balance between the potential of gastric acid and pepsin to damage mucosal cells and the ability of these cells to protect themselves from injury. Disruption of this balance leads to peptic ulcers. In some patients the imbalance occurs primarily because of acid (and pepsin) hypersecretion, in others primarily because of some abnormality in mucosal defense, and in still others because of both mechanisms. However, once an ulcer has formed, healing may be promoted by manipulating either factor, regardless of which was primarily responsible for the ulcer. For example, although aspirin is believed to produce a gastric ulcer by disrupting mucosal defense in some way, the ulcer may be treated by a drug that reduces gastric acidity, such as cimetidine.

Therapeutic agents for peptic ulcer disease can be classified as those that act primarily by reducing levels of acid and pepsin in the gastric lumen and those that act primarily by enhancing mucosal defense. Since pepsin's activity is pH dependent, reduction of acidity reduces peptic activity simultaneously.

DRUGS THAT REDUCE GASTRIC ACIDITY

Gastric acidity may be reduced either by inhibiting secretion of acid from parietal cells or by neutralizing acid that has been secreted.

INHIBITION OF ACID SECRETION. Secretion may be reduced either by blocking the interaction of histamine or acetylcholine with their receptors on parietal cells (histamine H_2-receptor antagonists or antimuscarinic drugs) or by interfering with the intracellular machinery of the parietal cell (prostaglandins or substituted benzimidazoles) (Fig. 100–7).

H_2-RECEPTOR ANTAGONISTS. The effects of histamine are mediated through H_1 and H_2 receptors. H_1 receptors are located in the smooth muscle of the bronchus and small bowel, and H_2 receptors are located on parietal cells and the uterus. H_1 receptors are blocked by classic antihistamines such as diphenhydramine (Benadryl), while H_2 receptors are blocked by specific H_2-receptor antagonists. All such drugs effectively lower both fasting and food-stimulated gastric acid secretion.

The first commercially available H_2-receptor antagonist was *cimetidine* (Tagamet), whose structure, like histamine, contains an imidazole ring. Side effects with cimetidine, which are uncommon and almost always reversible, include mental confusion (especially in elderly patients with hepatic or renal insufficiency), gynecomastia, impotence, and interaction with other commonly prescribed drugs. Cimetidine competitively antagonizes the metabolism (via the cytochrome P-450 system) of warfarin, theophylline, propranolol, phenytoin, chlordiazepoxide, and diazepam. Although blood levels of these drugs rise when given concomitantly with cimetidine, the clinical importance of such rises is unsettled. *Ranitidine* (Zantac), which possesses a furan ring, is the second H_2-receptor antagonist to gain widespread human use. Its putative advantages over cimetidine include a five- to tenfold increase in potency, and to date fewer reported side effects. It does not cross the blood-brain barrier well and therefore may not cause mental confusion. Although it has less of an effect on the cytochrome P-450 system, it may also interfere with the metabolism of drugs. *Famotidine* (Pepcid), containing a thiazole ring, is yet another H_2-receptor antagonist that is now available.

ANTIMUSCARINIC DRUGS. The classic antimuscarinic drugs reduce fasting and food-stimulated acid secretion by about 50 per cent and 30 per cent, respectively. However, these drugs also block other muscarinic receptors and produce unwanted side effects such as drowsiness, blurred vision, and urinary hesitancy. The centrally active tricyclic antidepressant drugs trimipramine and doxepin also possess antimuscarinic properties. Pirenzipine is a tricyclic antimuscarinic compound that does not cross the blood-brain barrier and therefore has no antidepressant activity or central nervous system side effects. Pirenzipine (not available in the United States) is believed to block certain types of muscarinic receptors (e.g., those controlling acid secretion) at doses that do not block other muscarinic receptors (e.g., those controlling heart rate and smooth muscle contraction). Thus, acid secretion can be controlled by doses of drug too small to produce side effects such as tachycardia and bladder atony.

PROSTAGLANDINS. Several methylated analogues of prostaglandins E_1 and E_2 have been shown to reduce gastric acid secretion, probably by interfering with generation of cyclic adenosine monophosphate (cAMP) in the parietal cell. Diarrhea occurs in about 10 per cent of patients treated with these agents, although it is usually mild and self-limited. Concern has also been voiced that prostaglandins may induce abortions. At the time of writing, none of the prostaglandin analogues has been approved for use in the United States.

SUBSTITUTED BENZIMIDAZOLES. Drugs of this class, the prototype of which is omeprazole,* are extremely potent inhibitors of gastric acid secretion. These drugs inhibit H^+/K^+ adenosine triphosphatase (ATPase), an enzyme found at the acid secretory surface of parietal cells that mediates final transport of hydrogen ions (via exchange with potassium ions) into the gastric lumen (Fig. 100–7). There is a prolonged duration of action, even when blood levels of drug are undetectable. Studies are underway to determine clinical efficacy and safety profiles in humans. In animals given high doses of omeprazole, gastric carcinoid tumors have developed. These tumors are likely a result of the profound hypergastrinemia that results from the prolonged achlorhydria induced by omeprazole.

NEUTRALIZATION OF GASTRIC ACID. Antacids react with hydrochloric acid to form a salt and water, thereby

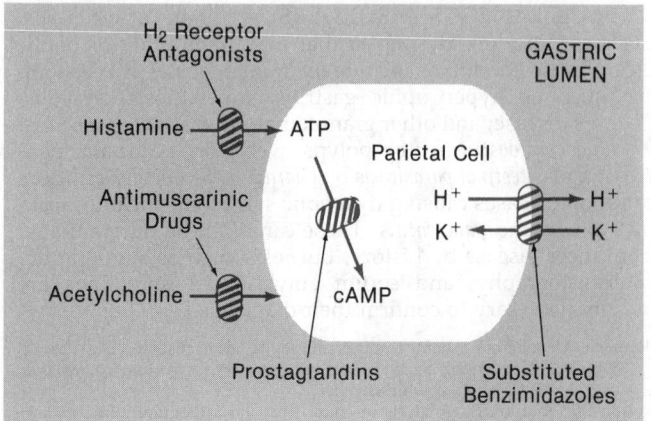

FIGURE 100–7. Sites of action of four drugs employed to inhibit acid secretion.

---

*Investigational drug.

reducing gastric acidity. Sodium bicarbonate, a classic antacid, is not recommended for long-term use because of its short duration of action and its propensity to produce alkalosis and sodium retention. Neither is calcium carbonate suggested for therapy of peptic ulcer because it may cause acid rebound (sustained hypersecretion of gastric acid after antacid has emptied from the stomach) and may cause the milk-alkali syndrome. Antacids most widely recommended are those containing varying proportions of magnesium and aluminum hydroxide. Serious side effects with these two compounds are uncommon. However, antacids containing proportionately larger amounts of magnesium hydroxide often produce diarrhea, whereas those with large amounts of aluminum hydroxide may produce constipation. All antacids can result in "taste fatigue" for individual patients. Most antacids used today are relatively low in sodium content.

Beyond individual preferences for antacid flavors, patients with ulcer may choose any of the commercially available magnesium and aluminum hydroxide antacids as long as neutralizing capacity is considered. Most clinical studies with antacids specify doses in terms of in vitro neutralizing capacity (for example, 140 mmol seven times per day), and antacids vary in potency. Table 100–6 lists several commonly prescribed antacids with the volume required to neutralize 70 to 140 mmol of hydrochloric acid in vitro.

DRUGS THAT ENHANCE MUCOSAL DEFENSE

Mucosal protection is more of a conceptual term than one with a firm definition because it is not known exactly what constitutes "mucosal defense." Mucus, bicarbonate secretion, and blood flow may all play roles, and some of the drugs that "enhance mucosal defense" may indeed affect these variables. However, a more general description of these drugs is that they exert a beneficial effect on an ulcer *without affecting luminal gastric acidity*. Since they do not belong in the first group, they fall by default into the second group.

SUCRALFATE. Sucralfate (Carafate) is the aluminum hydroxide salt of a sulfated disaccharide, sucrose octasulfate. The exact mechanisms of action are not understood. It has been suggested that sucralfate (1) forms a viscous shield over an ulcer crater, preventing acid from reaching regenerating ulcer tissue, (2) adsorbs bile acids or pepsin or both in the lumen, or (3) stimulates the generation of local prostaglandins. The drug should not be taken at the same time as food, antacids, or other medications. Binding with food or antacids may limit the effectiveness of the drug, and binding by sucralfate of the other medications may limit their absorption.

PROSTAGLANDINS. Prostaglandins play a poorly defined role in mucosal integrity, but their absence may permit development of ulcers of the stomach and duodenum. However, when given exogenously in doses that do not affect acid secretion, prostaglandin analogues do not promote ulcer healing. It may well be that the properties of prostaglandins that maintain "mucosal integrity" have little to do with ulcer healing.

TABLE 100–6. VOLUMES (IN ML) OF SEVERAL COMMONLY PRESCRIBED LIQUID ANTACIDS REQUIRED TO NEUTRALIZE 70 OR 140 MMOL OF HYDROCHLORIC ACID

	70 mmol	140 mmol
Maalox Therapeutic Concentrate Mylanta II	15	30
Gelusil II	20	40
Maalox Mylanta Gelusil Riopan Alternagel*	30	60
Amphojel*	50	100

*Aluminum hydroxide antacids.

BISMUTH. Tripotassium dicitrato-bismuthate (DeNol), a complex bismuth salt, chelates with protein (e.g., necrotic ulcer tissue) at acidic pH levels. Its mechanism of action is unknown, although recent evidence suggests it is bactericidal for Campylobacter pyloridis, an organism that may play a role in some patients with peptic ulcer disease. Side effects are minor. The drug in liquid form has an unpleasant odor and, like all bismuth compounds, it will darken stools. DeNol is unavailable in the United States at the time of writing.

LICORICE EXTRACTS. Carbenoxolone is a synthetic derivative of glycyrrhetic acid, a substance found in licorice. It appears to promote ulcer healing by several mechanisms. The drug produces thick mucus, inhibits peptic activity (independent of pH), and may actually increase the longevity of mucosal cells. Because carbenoxolone possesses licorice's aldosterone-like side effects (salt retention, hypertension, hypokalemia), it is not the preferred drug for peptic ulcer therapy; it is unavailable in the United States.

TREATMENT OF PATIENTS WITH PEPTIC ULCER

At this writing, five drugs are available in the United States as first-line therapy for patients with peptic ulcers: cimetidine, ranitidine, famotidine, antacids, and sucralfate. One or more of the prostaglandin analogues may soon be available. Because of their side effects, currently available antimuscarinic drugs should be used as adjunctive therapy only. While selecting one of the first-line drugs, a physician should also be aware of several factors that at one time or another have been considered important in ulcer therapy.

COMPLEMENTARY FACTORS IN PEPTIC ULCER THERAPY. Factors to consider in this category include diet, smoking, alcohol or analgesic use, sedatives, and the need for hospitalization.

Diet. Diet therapy was once the standard in the treatment of peptic ulcer disease. Now, it is clear that no specific diet is of proven benefit in ulcer therapy. Patients should avoid whatever foods cause them discomfort but otherwise eat whatever they like. Because food, especially milk, stimulates acid secretion, between meal or bedtime snacks should be taken in moderation.

Smoking. There are many important reasons (other than the presence of a peptic ulcer) to encourage patients to stop smoking. However, data are very persuasive that patients who do not smoke heal ulcers more often and more rapidly than those who smoke. The mechanism of this adverse effect on peptic ulcers is not known, although components of cigarettes may reduce endogenous generation of prostaglandins.

Alcohol. There is no evidence that alcohol ingestion retards ulcer healing. Nevertheless, because alcohol damages gastric mucosa, patients with ulcers who choose to drink should be advised to drink in moderation.

Analgesics. Drugs that inhibit prostaglandin synthesis (aspirin, nonsteroidal anti-inflammatory drugs) can produce gastric ulcers and therefore patients with this disorder should stop the drugs if possible. Although the evidence that these drugs cause duodenal ulcer is unconvincing, patients with refractory or bleeding duodenal ulcer should be advised not to take them.

Sedatives. Although emotional stress may play a role in the pathogenesis of peptic ulcers in some patients, routine use of sedative drugs is of no proven benefit in ulcer therapy.

Hospitalization. Hospitalization should be reserved for patients with complications of ulcer disease (bleeding, perforation, penetration, obstruction) (see Ch. 100.5) or patients with ulcer pain refractory to routine medical management. In other situations, hospitalization is not warranted and has not been shown to lead to more rapid healing.

TREATMENT OF PATIENTS WITH UNCOMPLICATED DUODENAL ULCER. In selecting a drug with which to treat a patient with duodenal ulcer (or gastric ulcer, see below), four factors must be considered: effectiveness, safety, convenience, and cost (Table 100–7).

Effectiveness. All available drugs are equally effective in hastening healing of duodenal ulcer when compared with placebo, with approximately 70 per cent of patients experiencing ulcer healing by four weeks and 90 per cent by six weeks. Each also promptly relieves ulcer pain, although often not significantly better than placebo.

Safety. Although side effects do occur with these drugs, they are uncommon and usually not serious. As examples, one can anticipate diarrhea occurring with large doses of magnesium hydroxide antacid or one may need to monitor serum levels of some drugs (e.g., theophylline or phenytoin) when taken in conjunction with cimetidine. Sucralfate is theoretically the safest, since it is not absorbed.

Convenience. Antacids have been proved effective in United States studies only when large doses of a liquid antacid are taken seven times daily, an inconvenience for many patients. Sucralfate must be taken four times daily on an empty stomach. The H_2-receptor antagonists with their once-a-day dosing are clearly the most convenient.

Cost. Cost varies according to the regimen and the locale where the drug is purchased. As shown in Table 100–7, antacid in large doses is the most expensive regimen in Dallas, followed by ranitidine, famotidine, sucralfate, and cimetidine.

Recommendation. Patients should initially be treated with adequate doses of a single drug. Cimetidine, ranitidine, and famotidine are the first-line drugs of choice, primarily because of convenience. Sucralfate and antacids are just as effective as H_2-receptor antagonists but are somewhat less convenient. Prostaglandins may offer yet another option. Treatment should continue for four to six weeks, and if the patient is symptom free, the medication is stopped. Documentation of ulcer healing by radiography or endoscopy is unnecessary in the patient with routine duodenal ulcer.

APPROACH TO PATIENTS WITH DUODENAL ULCER IN WHOM FIRST-LINE THERAPY FAILS. Failure of first-line therapy for duodenal ulcer is defined as the development of a complication (bleeding, perforation, penetration) while the patient is on therapy or persistence of ulcer symptoms after several weeks of therapy. For patients who do not require surgery, there are several alternatives for continued medical therapy. These options include changing to a different drug, increasing drug dosage, combining two drugs, or any combination of these. There are no adequate data to support any of these particular approaches.

If symptoms persist after one or more changes in medical therapy, surgery should be considered (see Ch. 100.4). However, before it is performed, the patient should undergo endoscopy to verify the existence of an unhealed ulcer, compliance with the medication regimen should be established, and the Zollinger-Ellison syndrome should be excluded. A period of medical therapy in a hospital may benefit some patients with peptic ulcer disease of this severity.

TREATMENT OF PATIENTS WITH GASTRIC ULCER. Cimetidine, ranitidine, and famotidine will each lead to complete healing in 85 per cent of benign gastric ulcers by eight weeks (Table 100–7). Liquid antacids in doses of 70 mmol (15 to 50 ml) seven times daily produce results comparable to those with cimetidine, although once again the inconvenience of such a regimen may be a disadvantage. Results of sucralfate therapy are currently being evaluated.

Because 2 to 3 per cent of benign-appearing gastric ulcers harbor a malignancy (not a problem with duodenal ulcer), special efforts are taken to make sure that the ulcer is benign and that it heals completely. Assuming that endoscopic biopsies were taken at the time of initial diagnosis and showed no evidence of malignancy, proof of healing can be obtained by either radiography or endoscopy. Unless the ulcer was very large initially, it will usually heal in eight weeks. If the ulcer is unhealed at this time, repeat endoscopic biopsies should be taken to confirm the benignity of the ulcer and if no evidence of tumor is found, medical therapy should be continued for another four to eight weeks. Since very few ulcers that have not healed after eight weeks of therapy will ultimately heal if the same dose of medication is continued, either the dose of drug should be increased or antacids should be added. A specific duration for continued therapy should be specified (e.g., another four or eight weeks), after which the patient should be operated upon if the ulcer has not healed.

TABLE 100–7. COMPARISON OF DRUGS TO TREAT DUODENAL (DU) AND GASTRIC (GU) ULCERS

Drugs	Dose	Regimen	Effective for Healing of DU	GU	Approximate Cost to Patient for 30-Day Course‡
1. *H_2-Receptor Antagonists*					
Cimetidine	300 mg	q.i.d.	Yes	Yes	$49
	400 mg	b.i.d.	Yes	Yes*	$48
	800 mg	h.s.	Yes	Yes*	$51
Ranitidine	150 mg	b.i.d.	Yes	Yes	$54
	300 mg	h.s.	Yes	Yes*	$59
Famotidine	40 mg	h.s.	Yes	Yes*†	$57
2. *Antacids*§					
Liquid	35 mmol	1 and 3 h p.c.	Yes†	NT	$15
	70 mmol	1 and 3 h p.c. and h.s.	NT	Yes	$36
	140 mmol	1 and 3 h p.c. and h.s.	Yes	NT	$72
Tablet	30 mmol	1 h p.c. and h.s.	Yes†	Yes†	$6
3. *Sucralfate*	1 gram	q.i.d.	Yes	Probably*	$49
	2 gram	b.i.d.	Yes*†	NT	$49
4. *Prostaglandins*					
Arbaprostil**	100 µg	q.i.d.	Yes*	NT	
Enprostil**	35µg	b.i.d.	Yes*	Yes*	Not yet available
Misoprostol**	50 µg	q.i.d.	No	No	
	100 µg	q.i.d.	Yes*	Probably*	
	200µg	q.i.d.	Yes*	Yes*†	
	400 µg	b.i.d.	Yes*	NT	

*Not approved by United States Food and Drug Administration at time of writing.
†Not studied in United States.
‡Mean of four drugstores in Dallas, Texas (in July 1986; famotidine, February, 1987).
§Maalox Therapeutic Concentrate (Rorer, Inc.): 35 mmol per 7.5 ml liquid; 30 mmol per one tablet.
**Investigational drug.
No antacid has been approved by the United States Food and Drug Administration for treatment of peptic ulcer.
NT = Not tested; h.s. = hora somni; p.c. = post cibum.

LONG-TERM MAINTENANCE THERAPY. Once an ulcer has healed with full-course therapy, long-term treatment with any of the H$_2$-receptor antagonists, antacids, or sucralfate will significantly reduce the high incidence of recurrent ulcer (as high as 70 to 80 per cent in one year). However, not every patient requires such therapy. Patients who have bled from an ulcer should receive maintenance therapy in the hope that rebleeding will not occur and that surgery will not be necessary. Maintenance therapy is also given to those patients with frequent or especially severe recurrences for whom surgery might otherwise be considered. Unless a patient is a poor operative candidate, surgery is recommended if the ulcer recurs during maintenance therapy.

TREATMENT OF PATIENTS WITH ZOLLINGER-ELLISON SYNDROME. Patients with Zollinger-Ellison syndrome (ZES) pose a special problem. Because of constant gastrin-induced hypersecretion of acid, they are always at risk of ulceration and ulcer complications. The treatment is discussed in Ch. 100.6.

Berstad A, Weberg R: Antacids in the treatment of gastroduodenal ulcer. Scand J Gastroenterol 21:385, 1986. *Up-to-date review of studies using various doses of antacids to treat peptic ulcer.*

Feldman M: Inhibition of gastric acid secretion by selective and nonselective anticholinergics. Gastroenterology 86:361, 1984. *Scholarly discussion of pharmacology of anticholinergic drugs.*

Hawkey CJ, Rampton DS: Prostaglandins and the gastrointestinal mucosa: Are they important in its function, disease, or treatment? Gastroenterology 89:1162, 1985. *Extensive review of all aspects of prostaglandins as they relate to gastroduodenal disease.*

Lauritsen K, Rune SJ, Bytzer P, et al.: Effect of omeprazole and cimetidine on duodenal ulcer. N Engl J Med 312:958, 1985. *Illustrates the results achievable in treatment of duodenal ulcer when acid secretion is profoundly suppressed.*

Pounder RE: Duodenal ulcers that will not heal. Gut 25:697, 1984. *Complete, practical approach to the ulcer that does not heal with first-line therapy.*

Richardson CT: Gastric ulcer. In Sleisenger MH, Fordtran JS (eds.): Gastrointestinal Disease. 4th ed. Philadelphia, W. B. Saunders Company (in press). *Includes a detailed discussion of clinical results with therapeutic agents for gastric ulcer.*

Soll AH: Duodenal ulcer. In Sleisenger MH, Fordtran JS (eds.): Gastrointestinal Disease. 4th ed. Philadelphia, W. B. Saunders Company (in press). *Presents for duodenal ulcer what the preceding reference does for gastric ulcer.*

Strum WB: Prevention of duodenal ulcer recurrence. Ann Intern Med 105:757, 1986.

100.4 Surgical Therapy

Richard C. Thirlby

INDICATIONS

Peptic ulcers can be managed medically in most patients. However, surgery may be required to treat patients with complications of ulcers (hemorrhage, perforation, or obstruction) or patients with intractable ulcer disease. The decision to operate for intractability is difficult and is made primarily on subjective criteria. The physician and the patient must decide when pain and multiple ulcer recurrences become intolerable or intractable. Patients should be considered candidates for surgery when medical therapy has failed. Failure of medical therapy occurs when an ulcer does not heal on medication, when ulcers recur during maintenance medical treatment, or after multiple ulcer recurrences. Pain, interruption of livelihood or lifestyle, and history of major complica-

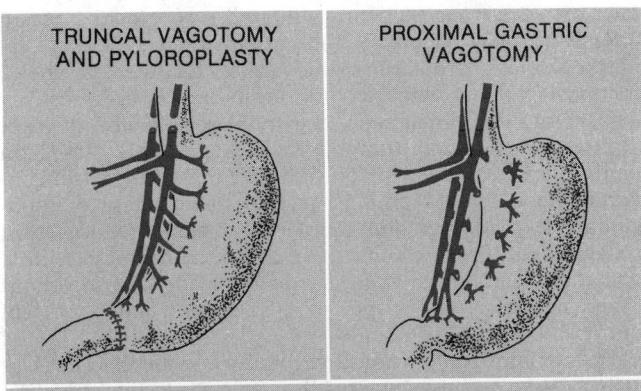
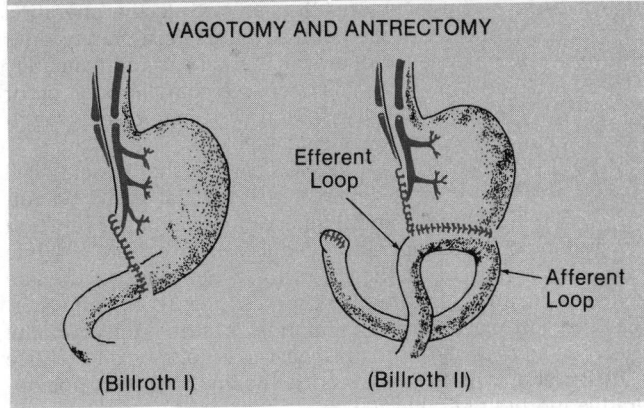

FIGURE 100–8. Model illustrating surgical procedures for peptic ulcer disease.

tions all influence the decision to refer patients for surgery. Pain per se is not an indication. Endoscopy should be performed before surgery to document the presence of an active ulcer in a patient with intractable pain, because the pain may arise from another cause.

SURGICAL PROCEDURES

SUBTOTAL GASTRECTOMY. Subtotal gastrectomy (65 to 75 per cent gastrectomy) was the standard operation for duodenal ulcer disease for many years. This procedure was effective in preventing ulcer recurrence in 90 to 95 per cent of cases, but the incidence of long-term postoperative complications was excessive (Table 100–8). This procedure is no longer recommended for treating patients with duodenal ulcers but is occasionally necessary in treating patients with gastric ulcers (see below).

TRUNCAL VAGOTOMY AND PYLOROPLASTY. Vagotomy eliminates cephalic (vagal) stimulation of acid secretion and reduces basal acid output by 80 to 90 per cent and maximal (peak) acid output by 50 to 60 per cent. Truncal vagotomy also denervates the antral pump mechanism, leading to delayed gastric emptying. This can be overcome by adding a drainage (gastric emptying) procedure to vagotomy either as a pyloroplasty (Fig. 100–8) or a gastrojejunostomy.

Operative mortality with vagotomy and pyloroplasty is less than 1 per cent (Table 100–8). Even when this procedure is performed as an emergency, operative mortality is relatively

TABLE 100–8. SURGICAL PROCEDURES FOR TREATMENT OF PEPTIC ULCER DISEASE

| | Operative Mortality | | Late Postoperative Complications | | | | | |
| | | | Dumping | | Diarrhea | | | |
	Elective	Emergency	Mild*	Severe	Mild*	Severe	Weight Loss	Incidence of Recurrent Ulcers
Subtotal gastrectomy	1%	10%	60%	5%	15%	0%	50%	5–10%
Truncal vagotomy and pyloroplasty	<1%	<7%	20%	2%	20%	2%	5–39%	7–10%
Truncal vagotomy and antrectomy	1%	9–15%	30%	2–5%	20–30%	2%	10–42%	1%
Proximal gastric vagotomy	0.1%	1%	0.5%	0%	1–2%	0%	0–5%	10%

*Nearly all patients have some change in bowel habits. Numbers are averages of many series and reflect clinically important symptoms.

low in contrast to an operative mortality of 9 to 15 per cent after emergency vagotomy and antrectomy (see below). Vagotomy and pyloroplasty is the surgical treatment of choice for most patients with bleeding ulcers and is also used by some surgeons to treat patients with intractable ulcer disease.

TRUNCAL VAGOTOMY AND ANTRECTOMY. Resection of the gastric antrum, or antrectomy, removes gastrin-containing mucosa and diminishes the gastric phase of food-stimulated acid secretion. Antrectomy alone reduces acid secretion, and the combination of an antrectomy with a vagotomy leads to an even greater reduction of acid output (reducing basal acid output by 90 per cent and peak acid output by 70 to 80 per cent).

The combination of truncal vagotomy and antrectomy (Fig. 100–8) is frequently considered the standard elective operation for duodenal ulcer disease because ulcers recur rarely after this procedure. However, operative mortality is approximately 1 per cent, and long-term postoperative complications occur frequently (Table 100–8). Therefore, proximal gastric vagotomy is gaining favor in some centers.

PROXIMAL GASTRIC VAGOTOMY. The parietal cell mass can be selectively denervated (proximal gastric vagotomy) (Fig. 100–8) while antral innervation and motor function remain intact. This operation reduces acid secretion while maintaining normal gastric emptying. Since many of the late sequelae of other acid-reducing procedures (e.g., dumping, diarrhea) are secondary to abnormal gastric emptying, the theoretic advantage of proximal gastric vagotomy is to reduce acid secretion with minimal mortality and long-term postoperative morbidity (Table 100–8).

Proximal gastric vagotomy is probably not indicated in patients with gastric outlet obstruction, active pyloric channel ulcers, prepyloric ulcers, or actively bleeding ulcers. Complicated peptic ulcer disease (history of bleeding or perforation) or high acid outputs do not contraindicate this procedure. Proximal gastric vagotomy is becoming the operation of choice in many hospitals for patients undergoing elective operations for duodenal ulcers.

SPECIAL CONSIDERATIONS IN PATIENTS WITH GASTRIC ULCERS

The indications for operation and the surgical management of gastric ulcers are the same as for duodenal ulcers except that gastric cancer is a concern in patients with nonhealing gastric ulcers. If endoscopy with multiple biopsies and brush cytology specimens indicates that a gastric ulcer is benign, cancer is excluded with 95 to 98 per cent certainty (see Ch. 101). However, if an ulcer has not healed after 12 weeks of medical management (15 weeks in patients with initial ulcers > 2.5 cm in diameter), surgery is usually indicated to exclude the possibility of cancer.

While proximal gastric vagotomy is currently the procedure of choice for most patients with duodenal ulcers, antrectomy alone with resection of the ulcer is indicated in most patients with gastric ulcers (Fig. 100–8). Sometimes a subtotal gastrectomy is necessary to remove all of the gastric ulcer–prone epithelium. Vagotomy may not be necessary, because many patients with gastric ulcers have normal or low acid secretion rates. Some patients, on the other hand, also have duodenal ulcers or prepyloric gastric ulcers and require vagotomy in addition to an antrectomy.

LATE POSTOPERATIVE COMPLICATIONS

POSTPRANDIAL DUMPING. This can occur whenever the pyloric mechanism is disrupted by pyloroplasty, gastroduodenostomy (Billroth I) (Fig. 100–8), or gastrojejunostomy (Billroth II). The dumping syndrome rarely develops after proximal gastric vagotomy (Table 100–8). The syndrome is transient in most patients and can usually be managed by dietary manipulations (see below).

TABLE 100–9. DIETARY TREATMENT OF DUMPING SYNDROMES AND POSTVAGOTOMY DIARRHEA

1. Follow low-carbohydrate, high-protein, high-fat diet.
2. Avoid refined carbohydrates and concentrated carbohydrates such as sugar, jelly, cake, pie, pudding, candy; substitute complex carbohydrates such as starch.
3. Eat six small meals a day.
4. Drink fluids between meals rather than immediately before or during meals.
5. Eat slowly.

Postprandial dumping syndrome is divided into early and late symptoms. *Early* symptoms occur immediately after a meal and are both intestinal (nausea, vomiting, epigastric pain, diarrhea, and dyspepsia) and vasomotor (flushing, dizziness, tachycardia, and diaphoresis). The initiating event is believed to be rapid gastric emptying, and symptoms may be caused by several pathophysiologic events: (1) duodenal or jejunal distention produced by the food bolus, (2) contraction of circulating blood volume due to displacement of fluid into the hyperosmolar solution in the gut (especially after consumption of refined carbohydrates), and (3) release of vasoactive hormones (serotonin, bradykinin, vasoactive intestinal peptide).

Late postprandial dumping symptoms occur one to three hours after a meal and are believed to result from hypoglycemia. The mechanism is presumed to be a rapid rise in blood glucose after ingestion of a large carbohydrate meal. This leads to an exaggerated insulin response followed by reactive hypoglycemia.

Treatment of the dumping syndrome is largely dietary (Table 100–9). Medications such as serotonin antagonists or antimuscarinic drugs are ineffective in most patients. Reconstructive surgery aimed at slowing the transit of food through the small intestine using reversed intestinal segments or Roux-en-Y jejunal interposition may be indicated in the 2 to 5 per cent of patients who are severely disabled (Fig. 100–9).

POSTVAGOTOMY DIARRHEA. Diarrhea is common following gastric surgery, especially when vagotomy is included. In 20 to 30 per cent of patients, diarrhea is clinically important and in 2 per cent it is incapacitating (see Table 100–8). The pathogenesis is unclear, and diagnosis of postvagotomy diarrhea should not be made without excluding *inflammatory bowel disease, lactose deficiency, celiac sprue,* or other causes of diarrhea, because gastric surgery may unmask previously silent diseases.

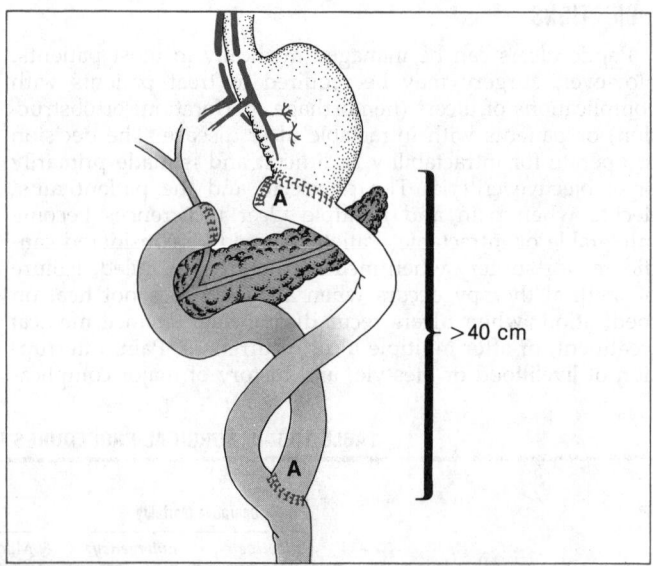

FIGURE 100–9. Model illustrating truncal vagotomy, antrectomy, and Roux-en-Y gastrojejunostomy (see text). Jejunum is divided at A-A' with distal end (A) anastomosed to stomach. Pancreaticobiliary secretions are thus diverted from the stomach by at least 40 cm of interposed intestine (pancreaticobiliary secretions shown in red).

Treatment of postvagotomy diarrhea is largely dietary (Table 100–9). Medications (antidiarrheal agents, opiates, cholestyramine, and aluminum hydroxide–containing antacids) may be helpful in some patients. Approximately 2 per cent of patients will require reoperation (using reversed intestinal segments) to control disabling diarrhea.

WEIGHT LOSS. Weight loss occurs frequently after antrectomy (see Table 100–8). In general, it develops in proportion to the extent of gastric resection and occurs most commonly after a Billroth II gastrojejunostomy (see Fig. 100–8). Weight loss after gastric surgery most commonly results from inadequate caloric intake. Early satiety resulting from a small gastric remnant may cause patients to limit meal size. Fear of eating because of postprandial symptoms or diarrhea may also prevent patients from consuming adequate calories. Other causes of weight loss include bacterial overgrowth that can occur in the afferent limb (blind loop) of a Billroth II anastomosis (see Fig. 100–8), relative pancreatic insufficiency, and in rare cases celiac sprue. Bacterial overgrowth leads to hydrolysis of conjugated bile salts and also damage to small intestinal absorptive cells. In turn, this causes malabsorption of fat, fat-soluble vitamins, and other nutrients. Bacteria also utilize vitamin B_{12}; this may lead to B_{12} deficiency.

Antibiotics or surgical conversion of a Billroth II to a Billroth I anastomosis will reduce bacterial overgrowth and may restore vitamin B_{12}, fat, and fat-soluble vitamin absorption toward normal. Converting a Billroth II to a Billroth I anastomosis also may increase absorption by better mixing of food with pancreatic secretions, which further reduces malabsorption. Weight loss and malabsorption may be helped also by dietary manipulations (Table 100–9), antidiarrheal drugs, pancreatic enzymes, or a gluten-free diet in patients with celiac sprue.

ANEMIA. Anemia after surgery for ulcer disease can be caused by deficiency of iron, vitamin B_{12}, or folate. Iron deficiency is frequent after gastric resection. Malabsorption of iron and bleeding from recurrent ulcers or peristomal gastritis contribute to iron deficiency. Vitamin B_{12} deficiency may occur either because of atrophic gastritis (loss of parietal cells that secrete intrinsic factor) or because of bacterial overgrowth in the afferent loop of a Billroth II anastomosis (see Fig. 100–8). Folate deficiency is uncommon and presumably is caused by malabsorption of folate from food and by decreased ingestion of dietary folate.

Evaluation of anemic patients after surgery for peptic ulcer requires measurements of serum iron, B_{12}, and folate and assessment of stool for occult blood. Parenteral administration of vitamin B_{12} (1000 µg per month intramuscularly) and oral or intravenous iron (Imferon) may be required if deficiencies are documented. If bacterial overgrowth is suspected in patients with a Billroth II anastomosis, antibiotics (e.g., tetracycline, 250 mg four times daily) may be helpful.

ALKALINE REFLUX GASTRITIS AND ESOPHAGITIS. Reflux of duodenal contents, particularly bile, into the gastric remnant is believed to cause gastritis and esophagitis (see Ch. 99). Symptoms include continuous, burning abdominal pain, nausea, and vomiting of bile-containing material. Establishing reflux and inflammation as the cause of symptoms is difficult, since many asymptomatic postgastrectomy patients have similar endoscopic or histologic findings. No test definitively confirms that the symptoms are caused by reflux.

Results of medical treatment with drugs that bind bile salts (cholestyramine or aluminum hydroxide–containing antacids) are poor. Roux-en-Y jejunal interposition prevents reflux of duodenal contents into the gastric remnant and esophagus and may relieve symptoms in some patients (Fig. 100–9). However, it is difficult to select patients who may benefit from this operation, because the diagnosis is often in doubt.

AFFERENT LOOP SYNDROME. This can occur in patients who have a Billroth II–type gastroenterostomy (Fig. 100–8). Symptoms occur when pancreatic and biliary secretions collect in a partially obstructed afferent loop, causing distention and pain. Eventually, the fluid bypasses the partial obstruction, rushes into the stomach, and provokes vomiting. Thus, the symptom complex is characterized by postprandial cramping epigastric pain followed by projectile vomiting. Pain is relieved after vomiting. The vomitus is voluminous, contains bile, and does not contain food because food has left the stomach and passed through the efferent loop. Management of severe symptoms requires operative revision of the gastrojejunal anastomosis.

POSTOPERATIVE RECURRENT PEPTIC ULCER

Postoperative ulcers can develop in the stomach, the duodenum, or the jejunum in patients with a Billroth II gastrojejunostomy (marginal ulcer) (Fig. 100–8). The incidence varies for the different operations (Table 100–8). The clinical presentation is characterized by pain in only one half of patients, and complications, especially bleeding, are frequent. Diagnosis of postoperative recurrent ulcer is best made by endoscopy because upper gastrointestinal barium studies are poor at identifying postoperative ulcers, particularly after a Billroth II gastrojejunostomy.

Incomplete vagotomy is responsible for postoperative recurrent ulcers in the majority of patients. Other uncommon causes include *Zollinger-Ellison syndrome, retained antrum syndrome, ulcerogenic drugs* (aspirin or other nonsteroidal antiinflammatory drugs), *silk surgical sutures* at the anastomosis, or *antral G cell hyperplasia*. Serum gastrin concentrations should be measured in all patients with recurrent ulcers to rule out Zollinger-Ellison syndrome (see Ch. 100.6) or retained antrum syndrome.

Sham feeding is the best test for diagnosis of incomplete vagotomy (see Ch. 100.1). An appetizing meal is presented to a patient, and the meal is chewed but not swallowed. Acid output is measured during the test by aspirating gastric secretions through a nasogastric tube. Acid output induced by sham feeding greater than 10 per cent of pentagastrin-stimulated peak acid output implies intact vagal innervation of the stomach. The insulin test, or Hollander test, of vagal function is no longer recommended because it is dangerous; hypoglycemic seizures, strokes, myocardial infarction, and deaths have been reported. It is also less reliable and less specific than the sham feeding test.

Until recently, the treatment of postoperative recurrent ulcers caused by incomplete vagotomy was surgical. The advent of histamine H_2-receptor antagonists has made medical management the first choice. Postoperative recurrent ulcers will heal with standard doses of histamine H_2-receptor antagonists in 60 to 90 per cent of patients, and reoperation may not be necessary. Lifetime maintenance therapy (cimetidine, 400 to 800 mg, or ranitidine, 150 mg, at bedtime) is required in most patients to prevent further recurrence and complications. The indications for reoperation in patients with recurrent ulcer secondary to incomplete vagotomy are (1) failure to heal with cimetidine or ranitidine, (2) recurrence on maintenance therapy with H_2-receptor antagonists, (3) a complication (bleeding, obstruction, or perforation) associated with recurrent ulcer, or (4) noncompliance with long-term medical therapy. The choice of reoperation should be individualized. If sham feeding confirms incomplete vagotomy, transthoracic revagotomy usually should be performed if the patient has had an emptying procedure such as pyloroplasty or a type of gastroenterostomy such as Billroth I or II at the initial operation. Antrectomy may be indicated in some patients who have had only a vagotomy as their initial procedure.

Herrington JL, Davidson J, Shumway SJ: Proximal gastric vagotomy: Follow-up of 109 patients for 6–13 years. Ann Surg 204:108, 1986. *Long-term follow-up on 109 patients after proximal gastric vagotomy. The incidence of side effects was very low, and the recurrent ulcer rate was 9.2 per cent.*

Herrington JL, Scott HW, Sawyers JL: Experience with vagotomy-antrectomy and Roux-en-Y gastrojejunostomy in surgical treatment of duodenal, gastric and stomal ulcers. Ann Surg 199:590, 1984. *Report of a large experience with Roux-en-Y gastrojejunostomy in the treatment of patients with postoperative recurrent ulcer, postgastrectomy syndromes, and complicated duodenal ulcer.*

Jordan PH Jr: Operations for peptic ulcer disease and their early postoperative complications. In Sleisenger MH, Fordtran JS (eds.): Gastrointestinal Disease. 4th ed. Philadelphia, W. B. Saunders Company (in press). *A general review of the surgical treatment of peptic ulcer disease, including indications for surgery and a description of the operations.*

Knight CD, VanHeerden JA, Kelly KA: Proximal gastric vagotomy: Update. Ann Surg 197:22, 1983. *Seven-year experience with proximal gastric vagotomy in 298 patients evaluated and treated in the Mayo Clinic.*

100.5 Complications
Mark Feldman

Approximately one of three patients with peptic ulcer disease experiences *bleeding, perforation,* or *obstruction* at some point in the course of his or her disease. A complication may be the first manifestation, or it may occur later. Patients with a peptic ulcer in the pyloric channel or postbulbar duodenum, with combined duodenal and gastric ulcer, and with Zollinger-Ellison syndrome are especially likely to experience complications.

BLEEDING

Bleeding is the most common complication of peptic ulcer disease, occurring in 15 to 20 per cent of patients with duodenal ulcer and 10 to 15 per cent of patients with gastric ulcer. Risk of bleeding is unrelated to duration of ulcer disease; one of four patients will have no history of ulcer disease when he or she presents with bleeding. The mortality rate for a single bleeding episode (5 to 10 per cent) has not changed in the past several decades.

Hemorrhage results from erosion of the ulcer into a blood vessel. The most common sign of acute bleeding is melena, with or without hematemesis. Although these symptoms usually indicate major blood loss (> 1000 ml), melena may occur with loss of as little as 50 to 75 ml of blood. In some patients with major hemorrhage, gastrointestinal transit of blood may be so rapid that the stool is bright red or maroon. Moreover, a nasogastric aspirate may not contain blood if active bleeding from a duodenal ulcer does not reflux into the stomach. Thus, the combination of hematochezia and a bloodless nasogastric aspirate can occur in patients with bleeding peptic ulcer. The hemoglobin and hematocrit on admission may not reflect the severity of bleeding if sufficient time has not elapsed to allow for compensatory hemodilution. Therefore, the severity of acute bleeding is better assessed by the blood pressure and pulse rate. A systolic blood pressure of less than 100 mm Hg and a pulse rate of more than 100 beats per minute, both taken with the patient supine, suggest major blood loss, as do a fall in blood pressure of greater than 10 mm Hg and an increase in pulse of more than 20 beats per minute after the patient assumes an upright position.

Peptic ulcer is the commonest source of acute upper gastrointestinal bleeding (accounting for 40 to 50 per cent of cases). The differential diagnosis, however, includes esophagogastric varices, erosive and hemorrhagic gastritis, and Mallory-Weiss laceration. Less common causes include benign and malignant gastric neoplasm, esophagitis, duodenitis, vascular anomaly (e.g., angiodysplasia and arteriovenous malformation), and aortoenteric fistula, usually in patients with a prosthetic aortic graft. Peptic ulcers may also cause chronic or intermittent bleeding, resulting in iron deficiency anemia. In such instances, it is mandatory to exclude other causes of chronic blood loss, such as colonic cancer, before attributing the bleeding to a peptic ulcer.

Certain factors may, if present, adversely affect clinical outcome in patients with bleeding peptic ulcers: (1) severe, continuing hemorrhage (arbitrarily defined as the need for three or more units of blood in the first 24 hours or six or more units in the first 48 hours after pre-existing losses have been replaced); (2) early rebleeding, usually occurring within 3 to 5 days of initial stabilization; (3) age greater than 60 years; (4) associated diseases, especially involving the cardiovascular system, lungs, and liver (particularly active alcoholic liver disease); (5) history of ingestion of nonsteroidal anti-inflammatory drugs; and (6) endoscopic visualization of a blood vessel or clot in the base of the ulcer.

Various therapeutic measures have been employed in patients with bleeding ulcers, including nasogastric suction, antacid therapy, and inhibition of gastric acid-pepsin secretion with intravenous or oral histamine H_2-receptor antagonist drugs. None of these measures, alone or in combination, has been proved to stop active bleeding, to prevent rebleeding, to decrease need for surgery, or to reduce mortality. As an exception H_2-receptor antagonists may be modestly effective in patients with bleeding gastric ulcers.

Ulcers that are actively bleeding or that have endoscopic stigmata of recent bleeding are sometimes treated endoscopically using electrodes (monopolar, bipolar, heater probes) or laser (argon, neodymium: yttrium aluminum garnet). Unfortunately, the efficacy of these modalities has not yet been adequately documented by controlled clinical trials. Endoscopic therapy of actively bleeding ulcers may someday replace surgical therapy in many patients.

Continuous bleeding from an ulcer or major bleeding that recurs in the hospital commonly is an indication for surgery. Urgent surgery is required in approximately 15 per cent of patients with bleeding peptic ulcers, carrying with it a mortality rate two- to threefold higher than that of elective surgery. Emergency surgical therapy for bleeding duodenal ulcer consists of suture ligation of the bleeding vessel, along with either (1) truncal vagotomy and pyloroplasty or (2) truncal vagotomy and antrectomy. The procedure of emergency vagotomy and pyloroplasty has a higher in-hospital rebleeding rate than truncal vagotomy and antrectomy but a lower operative mortality rate. For bleeding gastric ulcer, the distal stomach, including the ulcer, is usually resected. If the ulcer is quite proximal in the stomach, the ulcer is usually biopsied and oversewn, followed by distal gastrectomy. Emergency surgery stops bleeding in 90 to 95 per cent of cases. In poor surgical candidates, angiography with arterial embolization using Gelfoam or autologous clot may stop bleeding.

Following discharge from the hospital, a patient has a 30 to 50 per cent chance of bleeding again from an ulcer, a twofold or greater risk than for the overall population of patients with peptic ulcers. This enhanced risk remains approximately the same after a second or third bleeding episode. The severity of the initial bleeding event is not correlated with the severity of subsequent bleeding. Chronic medical therapy or surgery does not clearly reduce the subsequent risk of rebleeding.

PERFORATION

An ulcer may penetrate the wall of the duodenum or stomach, resulting in (1) *free perforation*—rupture into the peritoneal cavity with spillage of duodenal or gastric contents; (2) *penetration*—erosion into and confinement by a solid organ, such as pancreas, liver, or spleen; or (3) *fistula formation*—extension into a hollow viscus, such as the common bile duct, pancreatic duct, gallbladder, or intestine.

Free perforation occurs in 6 to 11 per cent of patients with duodenal ulcer and in 2 to 5 per cent of patients with gastric ulcer, usually during the course of known peptic ulcer disease. Free perforation occurs more commonly in men, in elderly patients, and in patients who ingest nonsteroidal anti-inflammatory agents. Duodenal ulcers that bleed are more often posterior; duodenal ulcers that perforate are usually anterior. A duodenal ulcer may occasionally perforate posteriorly into the lesser sac and cause back pain rather than signs of generalized peritonitis. Most perforated gastric ulcers arise from the lesser curvature. In approximately 10 per cent of cases, peptic ulcer perforation is complicated by significant bleeding.

Free perforation characteristically causes sudden, severe, constant abdominal pain that reaches maximal intensity rapidly. The pain is initially present in the upper abdomen but quickly becomes generalized. Movement exacerbates the pain so that the patient prefers to lie on his or her back without moving. Marked abdominal tenderness to palpation and diffuse, boardlike rigidity of the abdominal wall musculature are present. Hypotension and tachycardia usually occur owing to intraperitoneal fluid losses. Hemoconcentration and leukocytosis are usually present, whereas fever often is absent. The serum amylase level is mildly elevated in one of six patients. Upright abdominal or chest radiographs show free air (pneumoperitoneum) in approximately 75 per cent of cases. If pneumoperitoneum is not evident and there is clinical suspicion of perforation, it may be helpful to insufflate 400 to 500 ml of air into the stomach through a nasogastric tube and then to obtain upright radiographs of the chest and abdomen (pneumogastrography) or to administer a contrast agent such as meglumine diatrizoate (Gastrografin) through the tube or by mouth. A definite diagnosis of perforated peptic ulcer often is not established until surgery is performed. The differential diagnosis of perforated ulcer is discussed in Ch. 100.2.

The presentation of free perforation may be atypical: (1) A perforation may close rapidly with only minimal contamination of the peritoneal cavity and with rapid, spontaneous clinical improvement. (2) Abdominal pain and physical findings may be less impressive in elderly patients and in patients with neurologic or psychiatric problems or both. Such patients may present with unexplained shock. (3) Fluid may leak into the peritoneal cavity slowly and collect in the right paracolic gutter, resulting in a clinical presentation simulating that of acute appendicitis.

Treatment of free perforation is usually surgical. In most cases, surgery is carried out to establish the diagnosis and to patch the perforation with a piece of omentum (Graham's closure). Whether definitive ulcer surgery should be carried out also at the time of patching a perforation is controversial. Many physicians will perform parietal cell vagotomy, truncal vagotomy and pyloroplasty, or truncal vagotomy and antrectomy for perforated duodenal ulcer (or distal gastrectomy for perforated gastric ulcer) if there has been a long history of ulcer disease or previous ulcer complications. If perforation occurred more than 8 to 12 hours earlier, definitive surgery is usually not performed because of extensive peritoneal soiling. If a perforated gastric ulcer is not resected, the ulcer should be biopsied because 10 per cent of perforated gastric ulcers are malignant. Medical therapy of free perforation, usually reserved for high-risk patients, consists of nasogastric suction, intravenous fluids, and systemic broad-spectrum antibiotics. Some patients whose perforation appears to have become sealed off and who are improving rapidly can also be treated medically.

Mortality from free perforation is approximately 5 to 15 per cent for duodenal ulcer and somewhat higher for gastric ulcer, especially if the gastric ulcer is near the cardia. The most important factors associated with a poor outcome in perforated duodenal ulcer are longstanding (> 48 hours) perforation prior to surgery; preoperative shock; serious concurrent illnesses; and, possibly, old age.

Penetration into solid organs such as the pancreas occurs with unknown frequency, since penetration can be diagnosed with certainty only at surgery or autopsy. These patients almost always have a long history of ulcer disease and usually present with intractable ulcer pain. Serum amylase and lipase levels may be elevated with posterior penetrating ulcers.

A *fistula*, an uncommon form of perforation, from a duo-denal ulcer usually extends into the common bile duct; one from a gastric ulcer usually extends into the colon or duodenum. Patients with duodenocholedochal fistula may be asymptomatic but have air in the biliary tree, or they may present with cholangitis and abnormal liver function tests. The fistula is usually demonstrated by an upper gastrointestinal series, in which case barium refluxes from the duodenal bulb into the biliary tree. The fistula may close during medical treatment, although surgery may be required in some cases. Gastrocolic or gastrojejunocolic fistula caused by perforated gastric ulcer is often associated with ingestion of nonsteroidal anti-inflammatory drugs. These patients may present with diarrhea and malabsorption. The usual treatment is surgical. A gastric ulcer in the antrum may also perforate into the duodenal bulb, resulting in two or even three channels from the stomach to the duodenum.

OBSTRUCTION

Gastric outlet obstruction occurs in approximately 5 per cent of patients with duodenal or gastric ulcer and is especially common if the ulcer is located in the pyloric channel. Obstruction is caused by edema, smooth muscle spasm, fibrosis, or a combination of these processes. Obstruction usually occurs after ulcer disease of many years duration but may occasionally occur as the initial manifestation. Mortality rates from obstruction in peptic ulcer disease are 7 to 26 per cent, depending on the age of the patient and the presence or absence of associated diseases.

Obstruction delays gastric emptying and commonly causes nausea, vomiting, epigastric fullness or bloating, anorexia, early satiety, and a fear of eating (sitophobia). Significant weight loss may result. Epigastric pain is frequent and may be relieved temporarily by vomiting. Symptoms have usually been present for weeks or months. Vomiting, which may be delayed an hour or more after eating, is often copious and may contain undigested food but usually no bile. Physical examination may reveal volume depletion (hypotension, tachycardia, and dry skin and mucous membranes), visible peristalsis in the epigastrium, or a succussion splash over the stomach.

Any of the following objective measurements support the diagnosis of gastric retention: (1) aspiration of more than 300 ml of gastric fluid four or more hours after a meal (a large-bore tube may be necessary for measuring this), (2) aspiration of more than 200 ml of gastric fluid the morning after an overnight fast, or (3) removal of more than 400 ml of gastric fluid 30 minutes after instilling 750 ml of isotonic saline into the empty stomach (*saline load test*). Gastric retention may be appreciated on a plain abdominal radiograph (large, dilated stomach containing solid debris) and documented by an upper gastrointestinal series or radionuclide scintigraphy. Gastric retention is not always caused by gastric outlet obstruction. It may result from gastric atony, as in diabetic gastroparesis, from vagotomy, or as a side effect of medications. Gastric outlet obstruction, which is caused by peptic ulcer disease in 80 to 90 per cent of cases, can usually best be established by endoscopy. The other common cause is carcinoma of the antrum. Less common causes include gastric lymphoma, pancreatic carcinoma, pancreatitis, hypertrophic pyloric stenosis, eosinophilic gastritis, Crohn's disease, antral caustic stricture, antral polyp, and annular pancreas.

Laboratory studies usually reflect intravascular volume depletion (hemoconcentration, prerenal azotemia) and a hypokalemic, hypochloremic metabolic alkalosis due to vomiting. If extensive weight loss has occurred, hypoalbuminemia, cutaneous anergy, and a low serum transferrin concentration may be present. The urine is usually concentrated and contains less than 10 mEq of chloride per liter, but the urinary sodium concentration and pH are variable, depending on the renal tubular threshold for bicarbonate reabsorption.

Therapy of gastric outlet obstruction has three goals: gastric decompression and resolution of obstruction; replacement of fluids and electrolytes; and nutritional support. Gastric decompression is accomplished by continuous nasogastric suction for at least 72 hours. With prolonged obstruction, gradual gastric dilation occurs, and this interferes with the contractile function of gastric smooth muscle. Electrolyte disturbances such as hypokalemia can also contribute to gastric motor dysfunction. Saline load tests, performed serially, may have prognostic value. For example, a return of more than 300 ml after 24 hours of nasogastric suction suggests that obstruction will not resolve and that surgery may be required. After 72 hours, a return of less than 200 ml is a favorable sign and usually indicates that the tube can be removed and the patient can be fed liquids. Intravenous fluids and electrolytes are given to replace pre-existing and current losses. Isotonic saline containing 10 to 20 mEq of potassium chloride per liter is satisfactory in most cases. Losses of gastric acid from continuous gastric aspiration can be curtailed by administering H_2-receptor antagonists (cimetidine or ranitidine) intravenously. If suction is carried out for only a few days, 5 per cent dextrose solution administered intravenously, along with soluble vitamins, may suffice. If prolonged suction proves necessary, parenteral intravenous hyperalimentation should be instituted. This is especially valuable if the patient has lost significant lean body mass.

Approximately 50 per cent of patients with obstruction respond acutely to medical management. This response is related to the relative degrees of edema, spasm, and fibrosis, because edema and spasm may resolve. Obstruction relieved by medical therapy not infrequently occurs again within the next several years, requiring surgery at that time. Medical therapy may be effective for many years, however, so that it may be prudent to attempt it initially rather that to proceed directly to surgery in all patients. If obstruction does not resolve in three to seven days, surgery is usually necessary. There is controversy over which operation is best: truncal vagotomy and antrectomy, truncal vagotomy and drainage (pyloroplasty or gastrojejunostomy), or subtotal gastrectomy. Some surgeons are reluctant to perform truncal vagotomy for fear of postoperative gastric atony, although this complication is uncommon. Gastrojejunostomy (without gastric resection or truncal vagotomy) is associated with a high rate (30 to 40 per cent) of recurrences of ulcer. Nonsurgical dilation of the obstructed pylorus using balloons passed through an endoscope is a newly introduced therapy, the long-term efficacy of which remains to be established.

Collier D St J, Pain JA: Non-steroidal antiinflammatory drugs and peptic ulcer perforation. Gut 26:359, 1985. *Demonstrates an association between ingestion of these drugs and perforation in patients older than 65.*

Collins R, Langman M: Treatment with histamine H_2 antagonists in acute upper gastrointestinal hemorrhage. Implications of randomized trials. N Engl J Med 313:660, 1985. *Reviews data from 27 randomized trials, emphasizing end points of rebleeding, need for operation, and death.*

Fleischer D: Endoscopic therapy of upper gastrointestinal bleeding in humans. Gastroenterology 90:217, 1986. *Comprehensive and critical review of current modalities for endoscopic therapy of upper gastrointestinal bleeding, including bleeding ulcers.*

Graham D: Complications of peptic ulcer disease and indications for surgery. In Sleisenger MH, Fordtran JS (eds.): Gastrointestinal Disease. 4th ed. Philadelphia, W. B. Saunders Company (in press). *Comprehensive review with extensive references.*

Hogan RB, Hamilton JK, Polter DE: Preliminary experience with hydrostatic balloon dilation of gastric outlet obstruction. Gastrointest Endosc 32:71, 1986. *Uncontrolled study suggests that endoscopic dilation can delay or prevent surgery in most patients with gastric outlet obstruction, although long-term follow-up was short (4 to 14 months).*

Koo J, Lam SK, Boey J, et al.: Gastric acid secretion and its predictive value after vagotomy for perforated duodenal ulcer. Scand J Gastroenterol 18:929, 1983. *Controlled study of 101 patients with perforated duodenal ulcer found an ulcer recurrence rate of 3 per cent after proximal gastric vagotomy, 6 per cent after truncal vagotomy and pyloroplasty, and 43 per cent after simple closure without vagotomy.*

Lieberman DA, Keller FS, Katon, RM, et al.: Arterial embolization for massive upper gastrointestinal tract bleeding in poor surgical candidates. Gastroenterology 86:876, 1984. *Reviews embolization techniques in treating high-risk patients with bleeding ulcers.*

Peoples JB: Peptic ulcer disease and the nonsteroidal anti-inflammatory drugs. Am Surg 51:358, 1985. *Retrospective study suggests that patients with bleeding ulcers require surgery and die more often if they have been receiving these drugs prior to admission.*

100.6 Zollinger-Ellison Syndrome

Charles T. Richardson

DEFINITION

The Zollinger-Ellison syndrome is defined by both chemical and clinical criteria: (1) an increased serum gastrin concentration, (2) an increased basal acid output, (3) an increased ratio of basal to peak (pentagastrin-stimulated) acid output, and (4) the presence of peptic ulcer disease or diarrhea or both. Not all patients with an elevated serum gastrin concentration and hypersecretion of acid have tumors that can be identified at surgery. Presumably, such patients have tumors that are too small to be found at exploratory laparotomy, or they have hyperplasia of the islets of Langerhans, a condition known as microadenomatosis.

CLINICAL MANIFESTATIONS

Zollinger-Ellison syndrome can develop at any age; it occurs most frequently, however, between ages 35 and 65 years and more commonly in men than in women.

Abdominal pain resulting from an ulcer is the most common clinical finding. Ulcers usually occur in the duodenal bulb but also may develop in the postbulbar duodenum, jejunum, stomach, or esophagus. Complications of ulcer disease, such as bleeding or perforation, occur in 40 to 50 per cent of patients at some time during their course and may be the presenting manifestation. *Diarrhea* is a frequent complaint and may precede ulceration in some patients or occur without ulcers in others (5 to 10 per cent). *Fat malabsorption* (steatorrhea) is occasionally noted.

About 20 to 30 per cent of patients with Zollinger-Ellison syndrome have multiple endocrine neoplasia (MEN I) syndrome and thus have a hereditary form of peptic ulcer disease (Ch. 241). These patients may have parathyroid or pituitary tumors and clinical findings such as hypercalcemia, renal stones, or increased prolactin levels. It is unlikely that peptic ulcer disease occurs with increased frequency in association with parathyroid adenomas except in patients who also have MEN I syndrome.

In some patients, Cushing's syndrome can develop as a result of either pituitary disease or ectopic adrenocorticotropic hormone (ACTH) production by gastrinomas. Patients with ectopic ACTH production frequently have metastatic gastrinoma, for example, in the liver.

PATHOPHYSIOLOGY

Peptic ulcers in patients with Zollinger-Ellison syndrome presumably result from increased secretion of acid and pepsin driven by excessive amounts of circulating gastrin. Gastrin also has a trophic effect on parietal (acid-secreting) cells that leads to an increased parietal cell mass. Since parietal cell mass correlates with maximum acid output, some patients with Zollinger-Ellison syndrome also have increased maximum (peak) acid outputs.

Diarrhea results almost exclusively from the large volumes of fluid secreted by the stomach and is relieved in most patients by aspirating gastric juice via a nasogastric tube or more conveniently by treating patients with histamine$_2$ (H_2)-receptor antagonists (see below). Independent of stimulating acid secretion, gastrin may also play a role in the development of diarrhea by reducing intestinal absorption of water and electrolytes.

Steatorrhea may occur for several reasons. First, acid damages small bowel epithelial cells. This, in turn, causes a mucosal defect that limits transport of fat and perhaps other nutrients across the mucosa. Second, pancreatic lipase is inactivated by acid. This leads to decreased breakdown of triglycerides and contributes to fat malabsorption. Third, acid may decrease the amount of conjugated bile acids in the duodenum and upper jejunum. This results in inadequate formation of micelles, this, in turn, may lead to fat malabsorption.

DIAGNOSIS

Zollinger-Ellison syndrome should be suspected in patients who have (1) ulcers in unusual locations, such as the post-bulbar duodenum or jejunum, (2) ulcers that persist despite medical treatment, (3) ulcers and diarrhea, (4) abnormally large gastric folds or thickened duodenal and/or jejunal folds, (5) ulcers and manifestations of other endocrine tumors such as renal stones, (6) a family history of ulcer disease, and (7) recurrent ulcers after ulcer surgery.

These criteria call for measurement of the serum gastrin concentration (Table 100–3). If the level is abnormally high, a gastric analysis should be performed. Zollinger-Ellison syndrome is a likely diagnosis if the serum gastrin level is elevated, basal acid output is increased (>10.6 mmol per hour in men and 5.6 mmol per hour in women), and the ratio of basal to peak acid output (pentagastrin stimulated) is greater than 0.40:1.0. The diagnosis can be confirmed by performing a secretin stimulation test (see Ch. 100.2). This test is especially helpful in patients with serum gastrin concentrations or basal acid outputs that are only slightly increased. A positive secretin test, along with an increased serum gastrin concentration and basal acid output, establishes the diagnosis of Zollinger-Ellison syndrome in over 95 per cent of patients.

Tumors are found at surgery in 40 to 70 per cent of patients with Zollinger-Ellison syndrome and are usually located in the pancreas. Tumors have also been found in the duodenum, stomach, greater omentum, transverse mesocolon, and other areas of the peritoneal cavity. Computerized axial tomography (CT) is useful in detecting gastrinomas and therefore should be performed in patients suspected of having the Zollinger-Ellison syndrome. A positive CT scan is almost always correct, whereas a negative CT scan is less reliable. Angiography is a helpful adjunct to CT if a laparotomy is planned but is not indicated in every patient with the Zollinger-Ellison syndrome. Since some gastrinomas have been found in the stomach or duodenum, upper endoscopy also should be performed to look for tumors. Techniques such as intraoperative sonography or transhepatic venous sampling to measure gastrin from tributaries draining the pancreas or duodenum have been helpful in some centers in localizing tumors, but these tests are not available in most hospitals.

THERAPY

For many years total gastrectomy was the treatment of choice for patients with Zollinger-Ellison syndrome and in some hospitals remains the treatment of choice. All of the acid-secreting mucosa as well as the antrum is removed, with subsequent cure of peptic ulcers and diarrhea. However, many of the late postoperative complications that occur in patients with ordinary peptic ulcer disease develop after total gastrectomy (see Ch. 100.4). Furthermore, in some centers mortality is higher with total gastrectomy than with other surgical procedures for ulcer disease.

With the advent of H₂-receptor antagonists, it has become possible to treat patients medically. Antagonism of the H₂-receptor with either cimetidine, ranitidine, or famotidine effectively reduces acid secretion in most patients and decreases symptoms related to the disease. However, larger than normally prescribed doses, as well as more frequent administration, are often required. For example, 600 mg of cimetidine every four hours or 300 mg of ranitidine every eight hours may be necessary to reduce acid secretion adequately.* A few patients have required even larger and more frequent doses of cimetidine or ranitidine. For example, a few patients have required as much as 5 to 10 grams of cimetidine daily. The dose of cimetidine or ranitidine may be reduced by treating patients concomitantly with an antimuscarinic drug such as glycopyrrolate or isopropamide (see Fig. 100–7), since antimuscarinic drugs have been shown to enhance the inhibitory effect on acid secretion of H₂-receptor antagonists. A new drug, omeprazole, is currently being tested for treating patients with Zollinger-Ellison syndrome. This compound is a potent inhibitor of acid secretion, and in many patients, acid secretion can be inhibited by taking the drug once daily (see Ch. 100.3).

Medical treatment with H₂-receptor antagonists is not ideal for two reasons: First, complications of ulcer disease have occurred in some patients, and second, medical therapy does not provide an opportunity to search for resectable tumors, more than half of which are believed to be malignant. Because of this, a reasonable approach to treating patients with Zollinger-Ellison syndrome is laparotomy to search for resectable tumors present in about 20 to 30 per cent of patients, followed by medical therapy with H₂-receptor antagonists.

Vagotomy may be combined with H₂-receptor antagonists in some patients to reduce acid secretion and to add to the inhibitory effect of cimetidine or ranitidine. Treatment with H₂-receptor antagonists is still necessary, although the dose of medication can sometimes be reduced. Regardless of the therapy used (tumor search followed by medical therapy alone or medical therapy combined with vagotomy), close follow-up to ensure compliance with the regimen is mandatory.

---

*May exceed maximum recommended daily dose.

Jensen RT, Doppman JL, Gardner JD: Gastrinoma. In Brooks, F, Dimagno E, Gardner JD, et al.: The Exocrine Pancreas: Biology, Pathology and Disease. New York, Raven Press, 1986, pp 727–745. *An excellent review of the clinical manifestations, diagnosis, and treatment of patients with Zollinger-Ellison syndrome.*

Jensen RT, Gardner JD, Raufman J-P, et al.: Zollinger-Ellison syndrome: Current concepts and management. Ann Intern Med 98:59, 1983. *A review of the literature relative to diagnosis and treatment of Zollinger-Ellison syndrome, including the experience with patients treated at the National Institutes of Health.*

McGuigan JE: The Zollinger-Ellison Syndrome. In Sleisenger MH, Fordtran JS (eds.): Gastrointestinal Disease. 4th ed. Philadelphia, W. B. Saunders Company (in press). *A review of the pathophysiology, diagnosis, and treatment of Zollinger-Ellison syndrome.*

---

101 NEOPLASMS OF THE STOMACH†

Sidney J. Winawer

The majority of gastric neoplasms are malignant, in contrast to the colon, where the reverse is true. Although gastric carcinoma is steadily decreasing in the United States, it still represents a major public health problem throughout the world. In some countries it is the most frequent cancer and the leading cause of death from cancer. In the United States gastric carcinoma is responsible for 90 to 95 per cent of malignant disease of the stomach. Approximately 5 per cent of all primary gastric malignancy is Hodgkin's disease (HD) and non-Hodgkin's lymphoma, particularly the latter, since HD rarely involves the stomach as a primary site. The sarcomas, including leiomyosarcoma, liposarcoma, neurogenic sarcoma and fibrosarcoma, are all relatively rare malignant tumors that may involve the stomach. Leiomyosarcoma of the stomach represents about 1 per cent of gastric cancers.

---

†This revised chapter was originally written by Paul Sherlock, to whom this is dedicated.

CARCINOMA OF THE STOMACH

EPIDEMIOLOGY. The incidence of gastric cancer varies markedly in different areas of the world. It is extremely common in Japan, Latin America west of the Andes, some parts of the Caribbean, and Eastern Europe; moderately common in Finland, Austria, and Czechoslovakia; and uncommon in the United States, Australia, New Zealand, and other Anglo-Saxon countries. Colorectal cancer tends to be rare where gastric cancer is common and vice versa. The low incidence in the United States is a recent development, since gastric cancer was the most common known cancer in the United States 40 to 50 years ago. Other countries that previously had a high incidence have also begun to show a decrease. The reasons for this are unknown. Environmental factors are considered important in the etiology of gastric cancer, as evidenced by populations migrating to areas of either low or high risk and taking on the risk of the area of migration. Japanese moving to Hawaii have a decreased incidence of gastric cancer in subsequent generations, and there is a further reduction with migration to the mainland. The incidence of colonic cancer increases with this migration.

ETIOLOGY. *Dietary influences* are thought to be important, but without direct proof. Consumption of barbecued meals, smoked or pickled fish and sauces, and alcohol and deficiencies of magnesium and vitamin A have all been postulated but unproved as causes of gastric cancer (Table 101–1).

Nitrosamines are powerful carcinogens for animals. They can be formed easily from common, secondary, tertiary, and quaternary amines by combining these with nitrite (the nitrosation reaction). This reaction can take place under varying conditions of pH and temperature, so that nitrosamines may be formed in the soil, under conditions of food storage, during food preparation such as frying bacon, or in the body. Bacteria may play a role by catalyzing the amine nitrite union or by reducing nitrate to nitrite. Thus the achlorhydric stomach is considered a favorable site for nitrosamine synthesis. The necessary amines can be found in many foods and medications, whereas nitrate and nitrites are found naturally in food and water and are present in food preservatives. Ascorbic acid (vitamin C) blocks the nitrosation reaction in the test tube. The increased intake of vitamin C and refrigeration have been postulated to be responsible for the decrease in gastric cancer in this country over the last few decades, but the nitrite hypothesis itself remains to be validated.

Blood group A is associated with a higher incidence of gastric cancer even in areas of the world where gastric cancer is rare. This fact and the aggregation of gastric cancer in certain families have raised the possibility of a genetic component.

Pernicious anemia had been considered a premalignant condition. However, the prior high incidence of gastric cancer seen in this disease is no longer seen. This may be a reflection of the progressively decreasing incidence of gastric cancer being observed worldwide. Although atrophic gastritis is usually seen in association with gastric cancer, this disorder is extremely common, and the vast majority of such patients never develop cancer.

Adenomatous polyps of the stomach, especially those larger than 2 cm, may occasionally give rise to carcinoma. Most stomach polyps are hyperplastic and do not become malignant.

Subtotal resection for benign disease results in chronic atrophic gastritis from either bile reflux or removal of the gastrin trophic factor. This has been shown to produce gastric cancer in animals. It has also been shown to result in gastric cancer after a ten-year interval in persons living in countries at increased risk for gastric cancer, especially in men, who are at higher risk than women.

Immunologic deficiencies, particularly the common variable type, may cause a predisposition to gastric cancer.

Gastric ulcer does not transform into cancer. Cancer foci may be present in association with an ulcer, however. All gastric ulcers must be suspected of having small areas of malignancy even when the ulcer appears benign by radiograph or endoscopy. Biopsy and cytologic examination will reveal the true nature of the lesion.

INCIDENCE AND PREVALENCE. It is estimated that there were 23,000 new cases of gastric cancer and 14,000 deaths from gastric cancer in the United States in 1986. Although this is a substantial number, a dramatic decline in the incidence of stomach cancer has occurred here and in many other countries. The magnitude of the decline varies. In the United States the age-adjusted mortality rate for males dropped from 28 per 100,000 in 1930 to 9.7 per 100,000 in 1967. The rate of decline has been the steepest among United States whites and in the older age group of all race-sex categories. Carcinoma of the stomach occurs most frequently between the ages of 50 and 70 years and is rare in patients younger than 30 years. The incidence and mortality rise steeply with age. Rates are higher in males than females by 2 to 1. The incidence of gastric cancer is higher for United States blacks than whites, but the marked difference noted earlier in the century is diminishing. Risk of gastric cancer is greatest among those of low socioeconomic status.

PATHOLOGY. Carcinoma of the stomach is adenocarcinoma that usually is manifested pathologically in one of four ways (Fig. 101–1): (1) Most often it appears as a bulky mass with deep central ulceration projecting into the lumen and invading the wall. (2) The tumor may infiltrate and narrow a portion of the lumen, most often in the antrum. Less commonly, the infiltration extends throughout the entire stomach,

TABLE 101–1. DIETARY FINDINGS FROM CASE CONTROL STUDIES OF GASTRIC CANCER*

Positive Association	Negative Association
Salted fish	Vegetables
Pickled vegetables	Fruit
Salty foods	Milk
Smoked fish	Meat
Starchy foods	Squash
Cabbage, potatoes	Eggplant
Cooked cereals	Lettuce
Bacon	Celery
	Animal fat

*United States (including Hawaii), Japan, Norway, England, and Israel.

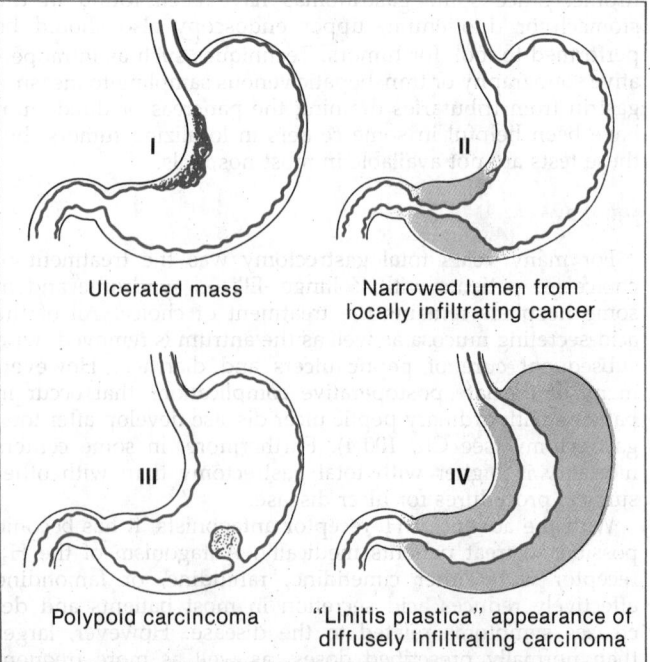

FIGURE 101–1. Diagrammatic representation of various presentations of gastric carcinoma.

I — Ulcerated mass

II — Narrowed lumen from locally infiltrating cancer

III — Polypoid carcincoma

IV — "Linitis plastica" appearance of diffusely infiltrating carcinoma resulting in *linitis plastica*—a fixed, nondistensible stomach with absence of normal folds and a narrowed lumen. (3) Polypoid or exophytic carcinoma with or without a stalk may occur and be difficult to distinguish from a benign polyp on radiograph. (4) More rarely, carcinoma of the stomach may occur as a superficially spreading tumor involving only the mucosal surface and producing a granular appearance. This is unlike linitis plastica, which extends through the entire thickness of the wall.

Gastric carcinomas may be well-differentiated adenocarcinomas or may be so anaplastic as to resemble diffuse histiocytic lymphoma or sarcoma. A true carcinoma in situ is rarely found and is confined entirely to the glands. This is more commonly seen at the surface of large adenomatous polyps of the stomach.

In about 75 per cent of patients with carcinoma of the stomach the tumors are found in the distal third. The lymphatic flow from such tumors is in the direction of the subpyloric nodes and porta hepatis and along both curvatures. The tumor very rarely spreads to the pancreaticolineal nodes, in contrast to proximal and midstomach lesions. Celiac and pancreatic nodal involvement occurs from lesions in all areas. In addition to invasion of lymph nodes, gastric carcinoma invades local structures: the lower end of the esophagus by submucosal spread, the pancreas, the transverse colon, the peritoneum, and, rarely, the duodenum. Hematogenous spread results in pulmonary, pleural, liver, brain, and bone metastases.

CLINICAL MANIFESTATIONS (Table 101–2). Early carcinoma of the stomach is frequently asymptomatic. *Anorexia* and *weight loss* are nonspecific symptoms and not well correlated with the size of the tumor. *Early satiety*, particularly with linitis plastica; *bloating; dysphagia; epigastric distress;* or more severe epigastric boring pain may be later symptoms. *Vomiting* is commonly a later symptom that may be caused by pyloric obstruction but may occur with other levels of obstruction. Vomiting also occurs without obstruction and may be secondary to the motility disturbance that a fixed mass in the wall produces. The pain is similar to that of peptic ulcer in about one fourth of patients, particularly when the tumor has ulcerated. In most patients, however, the pain usually occurs after eating and is not relieved by foods or antacids. Boring pain radiating to the back may indicate penetration of the tumor into the pancreas.

Dysphagia may occur with more proximal lesions, particularly when they have invaded the area around the cardioesophageal junction or spread submucosally to the esophagus, which is common in fundal lesions. Weakness and fatigue from *anemia* caused by chronic occult blood loss are common, although massive bleeding and hematemesis are unusual. Angina pectoris, congestive heart failure, and cerebral ischemia may occur because of the anemia. Perforation occurs in a small percentage of patients and can simulate peptic ulcer. When the tumor metastasizes, symptoms will depend upon organ involvement and may include jaundice, diarrhea, bone pain, cough, fever, hiccups, central nervous system disturbances, and abdominal bloating from ascites.

Physical examination during the early stages of gastric carcinoma may be completely unremarkable. Later there may be signs of weight loss and anemia. When the tumor has disseminated, hepatomegaly from metastases, jaundice, or ascites from peritoneal implants may be present. Splenomegaly may occur if the portal or splenic vein is invaded. A palpable *epigastric mass* is present in less than one half of patients and usually, but not always, indicates extensive involvement. Left supraclavicular adenopathy (Virchow's node), a nodular perirectal wall (Blumer's shelf), or umbilical nodules give evidence of metastatic spread.

Several extragastric signs may precede the detection of an underlying malignancy. These include recurrent thrombophlebitis (Trousseau's syndrome); acanthosis nigricans, a verrucous, hyperpigmented, elevated skin lesion involving primarily the flexor spaces of the body; neuromyopathy characterized by localized sensory and/or motor disturbances; and profound central nervous system involvement with abrupt onset of confusion, memory defects, hostility, or ataxia. More detailed descriptions of the paraneoplastic syndromes are contained in specific chapters in Part XIII.

Laboratory studies usually disclose iron deficiency or megaloblastic anemia if the tumor is associated with untreated pernicious anemia. *Occult blood in the stool*, even with a single determination, is present in about one half of the patients. Most patients have gastric acid present but in reduced amounts. A few have achlorhydria after maximal stimulation with pentagastrin. A few have hypersecretion, especially with antral tumors. Therefore the presence of acid does not ensure that carcinoma is not present. Abnormalities in liver function, particularly a markedly elevated alkaline phosphatase and 5'nucleotidase level, suggest liver metastases. Microangiopathic hemolytic anemia has been reported in several patients with gastric cancer. Rarely, protein-losing enteropathy occurs with ulcerated carcinomas of the stomach.

DIAGNOSIS. *Roentgenologic Diagnosis.* Most gastric cancers will be suspected on roentgenologic examination. The standard upper gastrointestinal series has been refined to include barium contrast studies capable of detecting very small lesions. With the gastric mucosa covered by a thin layer of barium and distended with air or gas, multiple projections are taken, which outline almost the entire stomach surface. Refinement of technique can be accomplished by using high-density barium, CO_2, simethicone for gas dispersion, and glucagon to induce gastroparesis. With such methods films showing fine detail may be produced and small mucosal lesions visualized.

The radiologist is usually able to define the characteristics of a benign versus malignant lesion and is on occasion even able to suggest a histologic diagnosis. For example, lymphoma of the stomach may be suspected by the extensive involvement, multiple shallow ulcerations, and giant rugal hypertrophy caused by infiltrative disease, and by the fact that the duodenum may be involved in the neoplastic process. A gastric ulcer often gives difficulty, but radiologic accuracy is in the range of 80 per cent. Characteristic radiographic signs that suggest a malignant lesion are the presence of an ulcer in a mass, irregular folds stopping short of the ulcer crater, and an irregular ulcer base. It is essential to determine the nature of the ulcer by endoscopy with biopsy and cytology when any doubt exists. Generally the location of an ulcer is not too important in determining malignancy. Ulcers on the greater and lesser curvatures have about equal frequency of malignancy. Rigidity, loss of distensibility, unchanging contour, and irregular peristalsis are characteristic of a malignant lesion; when extensive infiltration from linitis plastica is present, a "leather bottle" appearance may result.

Endoscopy with Biopsy and Cytology. Fiberoptic endoscopy has increased the diagnostic yield over radiology alone. When combined with biopsy and brush cytology, the diagnostic accuracy is in the range of 95 to 99 per cent in various series. About one half of early gastric cancers present as small ulcerations; some have slight elevation or depression of the

TABLE 101–2. ADENOCARCINOMA OF THE STOMACH

Associated With	Clinical Manifestations
Environment—geographical differences	Anorexia, early satiety, weight loss
Diet—? nitrosamines	Dysphagia, vomiting, weakness
Blood group A—genetic	Epigastric distress to severe, boring pain
Atrophic gastritis	Anemia, occult blood in stools
Adenomatous polyps (>2 cm)	Epigastric mass, signs of metastases
Subtotal resection for benign ulcer disease in high-risk countries	Rare—Virchow's node, Blumer's shelf, Trousseau's syndrome, acanthosis nigricans

adjacent mucosa. The next most common type is a small polyp. Appearance at endoscopy may be misleading. Directed tissue sampling techniques, such as biopsy or brush cytology, should be used on any suspicious area, whether it is raised, depressed, or ulcerated. With more advanced carcinoma a specific tissue diagnosis can also be achieved with high accuracy by directed biopsy and cytology. The use of endoscopy to diagnose malignancies of the stomach is described in greater detail in Ch. 96.

Other Techniques. Maximal gastrin-stimulated gastric acid determination defines achlorhydria. This is less important now with fiberoptic endoscopy, biopsy, and cytology.

Elevation of carcinoembryonic antigen (CEA) is a late finding in gastric carcinoma but can define metastatic disease before it is clinically evident. The immunologic detection of fetal sulfoglycoprotein antigen (FSA) in the gastric juice of patients with cancer has been noted. The sulfoglycoprotein of carcinomatous gastric juice often has blood group A glycoprotein, which has been associated with gastric cancer.

TREATMENT. At present *surgery* provides the only satisfactory curative treatment for gastric cancer. The high frequency of regional node metastases plays a major role in the choice of the surgical procedure and the results of various therapeutic efforts. When the tumor is localized in the distal portion of the stomach, the omentum as well as nodes in the region of the porta hepatis and the pancreatic head are dissected, and a generous subtotal gastrectomy is performed. For tumors in the pars media and the proximal stomach, total gastrectomy may be indicated to obtain an adequate margin and for dissection of the predictable lymphatic spread in all directions. Distal pancreatectomy and splenectomy are usually necessary. There is little doubt that operative mortality is greater after total gastrectomy than after subtotal resection, and the procedure should be avoided whenever possible.

With extensive bleeding or obstruction, a palliative limited subtotal gastric resection can be done even in the presence of residual cancer. Palliative total gastrectomy should almost never be done. Resection of recurrent cancer in the gastric remnant may be of palliative value even when a cure is not obtained.

Chemotherapy is often suggested for unresectable gastric adenocarcinoma in an effort to decrease symptoms and prolong survival. The most widely used drug has been 5-fluorouracil (5FU), with an overall partial response rate of 15 to 20 per cent. Other agents such as mitomycin-C, doxorubicin (Adriamycin), and the various nitrosoureas have also been used as single agents with varying response. Combined use of several agents has not proved to be more effective than single agents so far.

Adjuvant chemotherapy following apparently curative surgery is an attractive concept for gastric carcinoma because of its high recurrence rate. Micrometastases are undoubtedly frequently present after surgery, and it has been postulated that chemotherapy might be most effective against such minimal disease. However, multiple trials with single agents have not been successful. Several trials using adjuvant chemotherapy with combinations of agents are in progress and may provide an answer to this very important question, although to date no effective adjuvant program has been demonstrated.

Radiation therapy is generally unsatisfactory, since gastric carcinomas are usually radioresistant. Occasionally palliation may be obtained for persistent bleeding, obstruction, or pain. An occasional patient with inoperable gastric carcinoma has had prolonged survival with radiation therapy. A controlled study combining 5FU with radiation therapy for inoperable metastatic disease resulted in a synergistic effect in both response rate and survival. Further studies are needed utilizing this combination modality.

Patients with gastrointestinal cancer frequently have complications associated with their disease or its treatment that require vigorous supportive treatment. Many aspects of the patients' general condition require consideration and treatment, including the management of infection; anemia; gastrointestinal bleeding; fluid and electrolyte loss secondary to vomiting, diarrhea, or fistula formation; disabling ascites; pain; and poor nutrition. Endoscopic LASER treatment is also being evaluated as a palliative approach to keeping the lumen open in unoperated upon or recurrent cancer in order to maintain nutrition. Total parenteral nutrition is being utilized more frequently to supply the daily caloric requirement of patients with gastric cancer. Preoperative and postoperative use of this modality enables patients to withstand the rigors of surgery and to tolerate more effectively the postoperative period, including the use of chemotherapy.

PROGNOSIS. The five-year survival rate depends upon whether or not adjacent lymph nodes contain cancer. The presence of perigastric lymph node metastases indicates a less than 15 per cent chance for survival. Early diagnosis plays a role in prognosis because a long period of time between the onset of cancer and its diagnosis favors lymphatic spread. In the Japanese studies, resection of gastric cancer limited to the mucosa and submucosa had a more than 80 per cent cure rate; when disease was limited to the mucosa, cure rate was 90 to 95 per cent. Linitis plastica and infiltrating lesions have a very poor prognosis compared with polypoid or exophytic disease.

PREVENTION. Until we learn more of the etiologic factors in gastric carcinoma we cannot practice primary prevention. We can only practice a limited degree of secondary prevention, i.e., detect the disease at an earlier stage in minimally symptomatic people in order to prevent its devastating consequences. The mass survey approach utilized in Japan is not practical in the United States because of the relatively low incidence of gastric cancer.

LYMPHOMA OF THE STOMACH (Ch. 158 and 160)

Primary lymphoma represents about 5 per cent of all primary malignant tumors of the stomach, and non-Hodgkin's lymphoma accounts for most of these. It is extremely rare for Hodgkin's disease (HD) to involve the stomach as a primary lesion. Patients with lymphoma are generally about a decade younger than those with carcinoma of the stomach, and males are affected most frequently. Pain is the most frequent symptom, and mild anemia is common, owing to gastrointestinal bleeding (which on occasion can be massive). A palpable mass is the most common presenting physical finding. Studies of maximal stimulation of gastric acid secretion have not been done in a large group of patients, but achlorhydria seems to be unusual. Secondary lymphoma involving the stomach is common in the course of disseminated lymphoma but is difficult to diagnose.

Lymphoma of the stomach frequently presents radiographically as a bulky mass and less frequently as a diffusely infiltrating tumor—the most common form of secondary lymphoma—giving the appearance of large folds on upper gastrointestinal series, frequently associated with multiple nodular defects and ulcerations. Lymphoma of the stomach often resembles superficially spreading carcinoma, linitis plastica, or solitary adenocarcinoma. Gastroscopy with directed biopsy and brush cytology gives a higher yield than was previously appreciated. Exophytic lesions provide a diagnosis in about 88 per cent of cases; the infiltrative type does not yield as high an accuracy.

Pseudolymphoma is a gastric lesion that may be confusing. This diffuse or discrete lesion is an atypical inflammatory response in the region of benign gastric ulcers. It is frequently difficult for the pathologist to differentiate pseudolymphoma from a true lymphoma.

In patients with lymphoma of the stomach there is a significant incidence of nontumorous lesions such as stress ulcer, hemorrhagic gastritis, and monilial gastritis. Therefore in such patients with upper gastrointestinal bleeding or other symptoms referable to the stomach, it is important that a careful diagnostic approach be undertaken to determine the possible nontumor cause of the sign or symptom.

Treatment of primary lymphoma of the stomach is usually surgical resection followed by 3600 to 4000 rads of radiotherapy, particularly if lymph nodes are involved. Some have advocated radiotherapy alone because of the marked sensitivity of lymphoma to radiation. If lymphoma involves the stomach secondarily, radiotherapy or chemotherapy or both are indicated. The five-year survival following surgery for primary lymphoma of the stomach is in the range of 50 per cent for non-Hodgkin's lymphoma and less for HD, suggesting that HD is already disseminated when initially found in the stomach. The best prognosis for primary tumors occurs with small lesions confined to the stomach, differentiated into tumor follicles without lymph node involvement and with only superficial infiltration of the wall.

OTHER MALIGNANT TUMORS OF THE STOMACH

Leiomyosarcoma of the stomach represents about 1 per cent of gastric cancers and may present with a large intramural mass with central ulceration. Systemic symptoms are minimal, but massive bleeding or a palpable mass of which the patient is aware may be the presenting complaints. The tumor may be slow growing; five-year survival following resection is in the range of 50 per cent. Metastases to the liver and nodes are common, but these patients have a better prognosis than those with other metastatic tumors. Liposarcoma, fibrosarcoma, myxosarcoma, and neurogenic sarcoma are extremely rare and present with symptoms similar to those of leiomyosarcoma. Neurogenic sarcoma can be associated with von Recklinghausen's disease.

Metastatic disease to the stomach from other sites is not common but may simulate primary gastric cancer. Malignant melanoma and breast and lung carcinomas are the most frequent offenders. In breast cancer the metastatic lesions may be ulcerative, of linitis plastica type, or polypoid.

LEIOMYOMAS AND BENIGN TUMORS

Leiomyomas are commonly found at postmortem examination but are rarely of clinical significance. They occur equally in men and women, and are usually found in the midportion and antrum of the stomach. They may grow toward the mucosa, encroach on the lumen, and cause mucosal effacement and secondary ulceration. They may grow in the direction of the serosa, producing a mass that is predominantly extrinsic. Simultaneous inward and outward growth results in a dumbbell shape. These features are also characteristic of leiomyosarcomas, and differentiation on radiography or gastroscopy is difficult. Bleeding is common and epigastric pain may simulate peptic ulcer disease. On roentgen examination the findings are usually an intramural filling defect with or without secondary ulceration. Gastroscopic examination reveals effaced but normal mucosa overlying the mass. Central ulceration may be seen.

Asymptomatic leiomyomas need not be removed while symptomatic lesions are excised locally.

Neurofibroma occasionally associated with von Recklinghausen's disease, neuroma, lymphangioma, ganglioneuroma, lipoma, carcinoid, and hamartoma associated with Peutz-Jeghers syndrome all may involve the stomach. About 10 per cent of hamartomas of the stomach and duodenum in Peutz-Jeghers syndrome become malignant.

ADENOMAS

Adenomas of the stomach are relatively rare lesions. Most polyps of the stomach are hyperplastic, not neoplastic, and do not become malignant. Adenomatous polyps are the usual neoplastic type of polyp. These are more frequent in men than in women and are generally seen in patients over 50.

Bleeding, dyspepsia, and nausea are the most common symptoms, but most patients are asymptomatic. The diagnosis may be strongly suspected when a rounded smooth defect in the stomach on upper gastrointestinal series or a mass covered by mucosa with or without a stalk is detected by radiograph or endoscopy.

The size of polyps strongly influences management. It is rare for a polyp under 2 cm to show malignant change. In view of their potential for malignancy (present and future), polyps larger than 2 cm or polyps of any size causing significant symptoms should be removed. Pedunculated polyps can now be safely removed by cautery-snare technique via the fiberoptic endoscope. For sessile polyps more than 2 cm in diameter, a segmental gastric resection may be necessary to rule out carcinoma. If carcinoma is diagnosed histologically at the time of surgery, subtotal gastric resection should be done. Multiple gastric polyps are usually hyperplastic and of no significance.

TUMORS OF THE DUODENUM

Adenocarcinoma of the duodenum is rare but is more common than lymphoma, which, in turn, arises more commonly in the jejunum and ileum. The second and third portions of the duodenum are the usual sites of adenocarcinoma except when associated with Crohn's disease, in which it is in the ileum. Cancer in the duodenal bulb is exceedingly rare. Adenocarcinoma of the duodenum more frequently affects men and develops at a younger age than carcinoma of the stomach or colon. The tumor tends to grow into the lumen or to invade the wall of the duodenum. Cramping abdominal pain, anorexia, weight loss, vomiting, and melena are common. Jaundice or fever may result from obstruction of the ampulla of Vater or the common bile duct when the carcinoma involves the second portion of the duodenum. The tumor may simulate benign postbulbar ulceration. The diagnosis is usually made by radiologic examination and confirmed by endoscopy. Pancreaticoduodenectomy is necessary. Five-year survival ranges between 4 and 15 per cent.

Lymphoma, leiomyosarcoma, carcinoid, metastatic cancer, and benign tumors may involve the duodenum, and these are discussed in more detail in Ch. 107. In general, these lesions are manifested as an intramural and submucosal mass with the exception of lymphoma and metastatic cancer, which frequently are exophytic and ulcerate. Any tumor, benign or malignant, may occur in a diverticulum at the descending portion of the duodenum. Aberrant pancreatic tissue may produce a submucosal filling defect in the duodenum, which may resemble a neoplastic lesion. Also, hyperplasia or adenoma of Brunner's glands may produce multiple polypoid defects in the duodenal bulb and is frequently associated with hypersecretion, duodenal ulcer and, rarely, Zollinger-Ellison syndrome. A prominent ampulla of Vater may resemble a neoplastic lesion radiographically. Endoscopy may be necessary to clarify the situation.

Brooks JJ, Enterline HT: Primary gastric lymphomas. A clinicopathologic study of 58 cases with long-term follow-up and literature review. Cancer 51:701, 1983. *A large series of primary gastric lymphomas with long-term follow-up (average 12.8 years). Five- and ten-year survival rates were 57 and 46 per cent, respectively. Statistically significant prognostic variables were smaller tumor size, superficial mural invasion (submucosal only), and pathologic stage I disease.*

Correa P: Clinical implications of recent developments in gastric cancer pathology and epidemiology. Semin Oncol 12:2, 1985. *A comprehensive review of etiologic factors in gastric cancer. Worldwide epidemiology, risk factors, mucosal abnormalities, and genetics are discussed.*

Douglass HO, Nava HR: Gastric adenocarcinoma—management of the primary disease. Semin Oncol 12:32, 1985. *Excellent review of the overall management of patients with gastric cancer, including surgery and postoperative supportive care. Pathology and preoperative staging are also discussed.*

Kurtz RC, Lightdale CJ, Winawer SJ, et al: Endoscopy and gastrointestinal neoplasm: Diagnosis and management. Curr Probl Cancer 5:4, 1980. *This monograph describes the techniques and applications of endoscopy in patients with cancer of the gastrointestinal tract, including the stomach. Great technical progress has been made in recent years.*

Le Chevalier T, Smith FP, Harter WK, et al.: Chemotherapy and combined modality therapy for locally advanced and metastatic gastric carcinoma. Semin Oncol 12:46, 1985. *An overview of recent results. Response rates are still disappointing, and combination protocols have not as yet been dramatically better.*

Ming SC: Gastric carcinoma. A pathological classification. Cancer 39:2475, 1977. *The classification described provides a simple basis for evaluation of various aspects of gastric cancer.*

O'Brien MJ, Burakoff R, Robbins EA, et al.: Early gastric cancer, clinicopathologic study. Am J Med 78:195, 1985. *Early gastric cancer as seen in United States patients is discussed. The disease is not seen often in the United States because of late diagnosis but is the same disease as early gastric cancer seen in Japan.*

Phillips JC, Lindsay JW, Kendall JA: Gastric leiomyosarcoma: Roentgenologic and clinical findings. Am J Dig Dis 15:239, 1970. *The typical clinical and roentgenologic findings are reviewed in 11 patients. The tumors were predominantly exogastric lesions. Ulcerations were present in five cases. Hemorrhage, fever, abdominal pain, and a palpable abdominal mass are helpful clinical points.*

Schafer LW, Larson DE, Melton LJ, et al.: Risk of development of gastric carcinoma in patients with pernicious anemia: A population-based study in Rochester, Minnesota. Mayo Clin Proc 60:444, 1985. *This study demonstrates the present lack of significant risk of gastric cancer in patients with pernicious anemia. The prior association was probably related to the higher incidence of gastric cancer worldwide. The risk for gastric cancer is no longer being expressed in this population.*

Shiu MH, Papacristou DN, Kurloff C, et al.: Selection of operative procedure for adenocarcinoma of the midstomach. Ann Surg 192:730, 1980. *This paper demonstrates the varying survival following different types of surgery for gastric cancer. Early-stage cancers seemed to benefit from an elective, more radical procedure.*

Sonenberg A: Endoscopic screening for gastric stump cancer—would it be beneficial? Gastroenterology 87:489, 1984. *This paper provides a current perspective as well as a review of recent literature. Gastric stump cancer is a real entity but is expressed primarily in individuals living in countries at high risk for gastric cancer.*

Winawer SJ, Posner G, Lightdale CJ, et al.: Endoscopic diagnosis of advanced gastric cancer. Factors influencing yield. Gastroenterology 69:1183, 1975. *Diagnostic yield was higher for exophytic lesions than for infiltrative tumor, and directed brush cytology alone was more productive than directed biopsy alone. Combination of infiltrative character and location in antrum or cardia often resulted in nondiagnostic biopsy and cytology specimens.*

102 DISORDERS OF GASTROINTESTINAL MOTILITY

Sidney Phillips

Normal Motility of Stomach, Small Intestine, and Colon

MOTILITY AND OVERALL FUNCTIONS OF THE BOWEL. Motility embraces all movements of the gastrointestinal tract and its contents. As such, the subject encompasses contractions of smooth muscle, the intraluminal pressures thereby developed, and the transit of contents that results from gradients of pressure. Movements of chyme along the bowel are modified by the actions of specialized segments of intestine and the sphincters, and the whole is integrated by neural and humoral levels of control. Motility is best understood teleologically, i.e., as a process that facilitates the nutritive functions of the gut.

After solid food is chewed and moistened by saliva, it moves rapidly, in small boluses, into the stomach. Acting as a simple conduit, the esophagus is well served by strong bands of smooth muscle, integrated toward propulsive peristaltic motility, that push solid food to the stomach, even against the forces of gravity. Moreover, the lower and upper esophageal sphincters prevent acid-peptic reflux from corroding the esophageal mucosa and entering the bronchial tree. (Ch. 98 covers esophageal function and disease in detail.)

The stomach has three major functions: (1) accommodating meals of variable volumes, (2) grinding of solid food into small particles, and (3) the finely tuned process of gastric emptying. This last function is an important control of the load of chyme presented to the small bowel for digestion and absorption. Thus, the gastric fundus exhibits "receptive relaxation," a decrease in basal tone that is mediated by vagal reflexes and that reduces pressure in the body and fundus during a meal. Receptive relaxation provides accommodation for that meal, and food remains in the stomach for acid-peptic digestion to proceed. Later in the postcibal period basal tone returns; this increase in intraluminal pressure facilitates emptying of the liquid phase of mixed meals. Meanwhile, the antrum has developed strong, rhythmic peristaltic contractions that propel food to the prepyloric antrum. Solids are ground against the terminal antrum, triturated, and retropelled to the proximal antrum for another cycle of grinding. The pylorus allows only small solids (<1 mm) to pass through with the meal; larger solids are retained and emptied between meals. By a combination of these forces and the integrated action of duodenal musculature, pressure gradients are developed whereby gastric emptying is controlled very precisely. Sensitive receptors in the duodenal mucosa respond to intraluminal fat and hydrogen ions or hypertonicity of the contents, setting in motion a feedback mechanism that brakes emptying. In this way, contents entering the duodenum are prepared for their subsequent contact with pancreaticobiliary secretions. These controls are disturbed most dramatically when the pylorus is destroyed surgically; dumping syndromes or gastric stasis may be unfortunate, and all too common, sequelae.

Transit through the small bowel is steady but slow, a series of gentle to-and-fro movements of chyme, well suited to the mixing of food with digestive enzymes. Further, exposure of digestive products to the absorptive cells is maximized. Moreover, a normal pattern of motility is important in maintaining relative sterility of the small bowel. Disordered motility leads to bacterial overgrowth ("blind loop syndrome") and a malabsorption syndrome (see Ch. 104).

The colon can be thought of as two functional entities. The proximal half dehydrates its contents, removing salt and water very effectively. In addition, it stores feces, which undergo bacterial biotransformation by the fecal flora. Some components of dietary fiber can be digested only in this way. The motor activity of this segment subserves these functions of storing and mixing via its back-and-forth movements and mixing waves (haustra). The distal colon and rectum store formed stools until evacuation is convenient. The necessary propulsion and excretion are achieved by coordination of peristaltic contractions and voluntary elevations of intra-abdominal pressure. The anal sphincters relax in concert with these propulsive forces.

GASTROINTESTINAL SPHINCTERS. In physiologic terms, a sphincter is an area of high intraluminal pressure within the bowel. Sphincters separate areas of lower pressure and thus are able to modify the flow of intestinal contents. Sphincters respond to distention or changes of pressure within the adjacent bowel by either tightening or relaxing. Sphincters may be recognized anatomically by the presence of specialized bands of muscle (upper esophageal sphincter) or may be associated with no clearly defined or unique tissue (lower esophageal sphincter) (see Ch. 98). The pylorus has a concentrated bundle of circular muscle characteristic of a sphincter, but it contracts and relaxes in concert with adjacent bowel. Functionally, the pylorus is not clearly distinct from the antrum or duodenum and can be considered as having only certain characteristics of a "sphincter." The ileocecal junction has the appearance of a valve but can function like a sphincter. One of its important roles is to prevent reflux of fecal flora into the small intestine. The anal sphincters are well developed anatomically and function as true sphincters.

ELECTRICAL AND MECHANICAL CORRELATES OF MOTILITY.

Contractions of smooth muscle cells are determined by the state of polarization-depolarization of the cell membranes, contraction occurring only when action potentials ("spikes") are superimposed on an appropriate background level of depolarization. Throughout the stomach and intestines a baseline fluctuation of basal electrical activity is present in the muscularis, as measured by extracellular electrodes embedded in the muscle layers. This omnipresent "basic electrical rhythm" (BER, slow wave or pacesetter potential) originates at specific sites ("pacemakers") located in the proximal stomach, proximal duodenum, and midcolon. The potentials so generated, at 3 per minute in stomach, 12 per minute in duodenum, and 3 to 12 per minute in the colon, spread distally along muscle bundles, thus establishing a maximal frequency at which the smooth muscle can contract. In other words, antral pacesetters of 3 per minute establish this as the maximal rate of antral contractions. The corresponding rate in the proximal duodenum is 12 per minute, but this rate slows progressively, in a caudad direction along the bowel, so that the terminal ileal rate is 8 to 9 per minute. When spike discharges are present on any slow wave complex, adjacent smooth muscle contracts (Fig. 102–1). At each level, not all pacesetter potentials have action potentials; in other words, the smooth muscle may contract at its maximal rate, not contract at all, or exhibit any intermediate level of activity. The state of fasting or feeding is a major determinant of the degree of muscular activity that actually occurs. The colonic pacemaker is probably located in the transverse colon, and pacesetter potentials spread distally and proximally. Such a system may well provide the basis for to-and-fro movement in the colon, allowing storage, desiccation, and fermentation in the cecum.

FASTING AND POSTCIBAL MOTILITY.

The fasting bowel is not quiescent; it exhibits cycles of contractility that are interrupted by food. With a periodicity of approximately two hours, an intense burst of motor activity begins in the stomach, in which every pacesetter potential has an action potential associated with it. This wave of activity passes caudally through duodenum, jejunum, and ileum. The velocity of this "front" is such that on reaching the ileum another "front" (or migrating motor complex) originates in the stomach. At any single locus, a cycle of activity lasts approximately 2 hours during fasting, each intense burst of motility lasting 5 to 15 minutes. The remainder of the 2-hour cycle is taken up with quiescence (lasting about 1 hour—"phase I"), intermittent contractile activity (about 45 minutes—"phase II"),

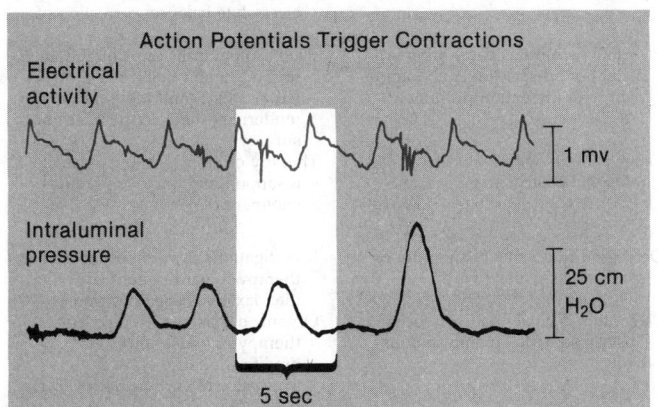

FIGURE 102–1. Simultaneous electrical and mechanical activity in the canine jejunum. The electrical signal was recorded from an extracellular electrode in the tunica muscularis; it shows a regular cycle of depolarization-repolarization at 12 to 14 cycles per minute. Superimposed on some of these cycles (basic electrical rhythm, slow wave, or pace-setter potential) are more rapid oscillations (fast waves, spikes). When spiking occurs, the smooth muscle contracts, causing intraluminal pressure to rise (lower tracing).

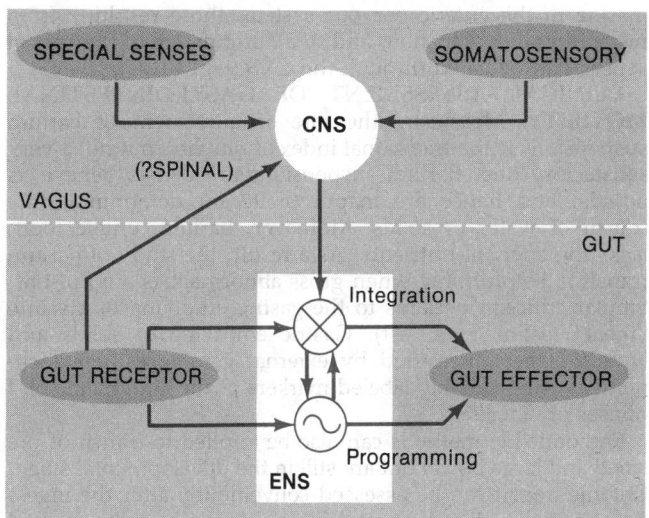

FIGURE 102–2. Scheme for the control of intestinal motility. Possible stimuli for gut receptors include wall tension, serosal inflammation, and luminal chemoreceptors. The signals are integrated and programmed by the enteric nervous system within the bowel and then act on effector tissues (smooth muscle, absorptive, or secretory cells). The vagus nerves are 80 to 90 per cent afferent and other, less well-defined, pathways go via abdominal ganglia and the spinal cord to the CNS. Input from the special senses is best demonstrated by the cephalic phase of gut function. The somatosensory input is illustrated by altered intestinal motility in response to cold or pain stress. (From Wingate DL: Viewpoints on Digestive Diseases, Vol 17, No 5, November, 1985. Reproduced with permission of the publishers, American Gastroenterological Association.)

and then the migrating complex ("phase III"). The migrating complex has been described by Code as the "interdigestive housekeeper." The function proposed is one of sweeping secretions, desquamated cells, and food residue distally in preparation for another meal. Food interrupts the cycle, replacing it with the "fed pattern" of intermittent contractions (similar to phase II) that last for 4 to 10 hours. Whereas transit is rapid in phase III of fasting, it is slower after a meal.

CONTROL OF GASTROINTESTINAL MOTILITY.

The cholinergic system has important control of the proximal gut. Vagal denervation impairs receptive relaxation of the stomach and, by reducing gastric accommodation to large volumes, speeds the emptying of liquids. Vagal denervation also diminishes the important duodenal "brake" on gastric emptying. Antral contractions are also weakened by vagotomy, and hence the grinding and emptying of solids are reduced. The sympathetic nervous system becomes more important in the distal bowel, particularly in the coordination of rectal contractions and relaxation of the anal sphincters. A third system ("noncholinergic-nonadrenergic") also exists, although the exact neurotransmitters responsible for it are as yet unclear. Among the candidates are adenosine triphosphate (ATP) ("purinergic"), dopamine-like compounds, and neuropeptides. A number of peptides can alter gastrointestinal motility, but whether they have physiologic roles is unclear. Cholecystokinin-pancreozymin contracts the gallbladder and intestinal smooth muscle. Other stimulating hormones include gastrin and motilin, and inhibitory hormones include secretin, glucagon, vasoactive intestinal polypeptide, and gastric inhibitory polypeptide.

Neurohumoral control of gut motility is coordinated ultimately by interactions between the enteric nervous system (nerve cells and axons of the intramural plexuses), the intra-abdominal ganglia, and the central nervous system. An important new concept is the autonomy of the enteric nervous system ("mini-brain" in the gut), which is, in turn, modulated by the central nervous system (CNS) (Fig. 102–2). Recognition of these different levels of control gives a basis for a general separation of intestinal dysmotility into those conditions originating in the enteric nervous system, those resulting from more central dysfunction, and those originating in the special senses but mediated through the CNS (Fig. 102–2).

CLINICAL ASSESSMENT OF GASTROINTESTINAL MOTILITY. Measuring the rate of movement of barium suspensions is the traditional index of motility, but not a very satisfactory one. Barium suspensions are dense, behave as liquids, and hence are inappropriate for determining the transit of water or solids. Moreover, barium, unlike food, lacks the effect of nutrients. As a result, the study of barium transit is helpful only when gross abnormalities are present. Similar criticism pertains to the gastric emptying of a saline "meal" (saline load test). Gastric emptying of solids and liquids is best measured by external gamma camera techniques, using suitably labeled markers of the liquid and solid phases of "meals."

Radionuclide methods can also be applied to transit of the small and large bowel but are still in the developmental stage. Colonic transit can be assessed conveniently after the ingestion of small radiopaque markers; stools can be radiographed to determine mouth-to-anus transit times, or abdominal radiographs may be used to quantify transit through different segments of the colon. The arrival time of a bolus of fermentable carbohydrate in the cecum can be identified by the excretion of hydrogen in the breath. Hydrogen is generated in the body only by bacterial fermentation of carbohydrate. In this way, mouth-to-cecum transit times can be measured noninvasively. The measurement of intraluminal pressures by transducers or water-filled catheters is used extensively in the diagnosis of esophageal and anorectal disease. Application of these techniques to the stomach, small intestine, and colon is restricted largely to research studies.

Christensen J: Motility of the colon. In Johnson LR (ed.): Physiology of the Gastrointestinal Tract. 2nd ed. New York, Raven Press, 1987. *Complete review with reference to basic mechanisms; includes some material on pathophysiology of disease.*

Meyer JH: Motility of the stomach and gastroduodenal junction. In Johnson LR (ed.): Physiology of the Gastrointestinal Tract. 2nd ed. New York, Raven Press, 1987. *Comprehensive review of the physiology of the region; contains all major references to basic mechanisms.*

Sarna SK: Cyclic motor activity; migrating motor complex: 1985. Gastroenterology 89:894, 1985. *Extensive review of intestinal motility, with emphasis particularly on the basic mechanisms and control of fasting patterns. Contains all important references.*

Wingate DL: Backwards and forwards with the migrating complex. Dig Dis Sci 26:641, 1981. *Complete historical and scientific review of small intestinal motility with emphasis on the normal physiology. Referenced extensively.*

Disorders of Gastroduodenal Motility

PYLORIC STENOSIS: GASTRIC OUTLET OBSTRUCTION

ETIOLOGY AND PATHOGENESIS. A transient syndrome occurs when acute peptic ulcers involve the pyloric canal. A chronic, cicatricial condition often complicates recurrent ulceration in the pyloroduodenal region, and vomiting may be severe. Carcinoma is also a cause of gastric outlet obstruction.

TABLE 102–1. COMMON DISORDERS OF GASTROINTESTINAL MOTILITY

Disorder	Suggested Mechanisms	Clinical Features	Treatment and Comments*
Stomach			
Congenital			
Hypertrophic pyloric stenosis	Hypertrophied, nonpropulsive muscle, neuronal agenesis	First-born males; vomiting without bile	Ramstedt's operation is curative
Postoperative			
Gastroparesis	Poor mechanical drainage; vagotomy	Early: excessive gastric aspirations; late: easy satiety, bezoars	Radiology and endoscopy to rule out mechanical obstruction; soft diet; cholinergic drugs; metoclopramide, 10 mg q.i.d.†
Dumping syndrome	Rapid gastric emptying; hypovolemia; hypoglycemia; inappropriate release of gastrointestinal peptides	Early: weakness, dizziness, palpitations, diarrhea; late: features of hypoglycemia	Dry diet; reduced sugar intake; rest after meals; surgery may be required
Others			
Gastroparesis (idiopathic or diabetic)	Diminished motor fronts; ? pylorospasm	Fullness; nausea; vomiting; bezoars	Juvenile diabetics; soft diet; drug treatment with metoclopramide or cholinergic drugs
Small Bowel			
Adynamic ileus	Postoperative; electrolyte disturbances; peritonitis	Vomiting; abdominal distention	Intestinal decompression; maintenance of fluid and electrolyte balance; correction of cause
Mechanical obstruction	Bands; hernias; tumors, etc.	Proximal: vomiting, pain, minimal distention; distal: lower abdominal pain with distention prominent	Plain radiographic films of abdomen; fever, feculent vomiting, leukocytosis, and rebound tenderness indicate the need for surgery
Pseudo-obstruction	(See Table 102–2 for causes)	Older patients with features of intestinal obstruction	Therapy of idiopathic form usually disappointing; metoclopramide, cholinergics[2]
Large Bowel			
Constipation	(See Table 102–3 for causes)	Decreased frequency or quantity of stool; stools usually hard	Investigations toward specific cause; therapy toward patient education, diet; laxatives used judiciously
Irritable bowel syndrome	Disorder of small bowel and large bowel motility	Pain; altered bowel habit; associated "psychosomatic" manifestations likely	Organic disease to be ruled out; therapy is reassurance, modification of diet, and avoidance of chronic use of drugs
Megacolon			
Congenital	Absence of intramural nerve plexuses ("aganglionosis")	Obstipation, meconium ileus from birth; rectum empty; narrow segment on barium radiograph	Diagnosis by manometry and rectal biopsy; corrected by surgery
Acquired	Secondary to constipation	History of constipation; older age groups; rectum full	Disimpaction of feces; treatment of constipation

*It is essential in all suspected disorders of gastrointestinal motility to rule out mechanical obstruction or organic disease as a cause for symptoms.
†Two new "prokinetic" drugs (Domperidone, Cisapride) are unavailable in the United States at the time of writing. Both show promise as alternative therapies of gastroparesis and pseudo-obstruction.

In infants, hypertrophy of pyloric muscle may occur, leading to severe degrees of obstruction. Hypertrophic pyloric stenosis occurs rarely in adults, although in later life it is difficult to distinguish a specific "hypertrophic syndrome" from the multiple, variable manifestations of chronic peptic ulcer disease.

Congenital Hypertrophic Pyloric Stenosis

INCIDENCE. This lesion occurs in two to four infants per 1000 live births, is more common in firstborn children, and is four to five times more frequent in males. A familial incidence is reported, as is an increased incidence in twins. Some degree of muscle spasm is present, since partial relaxation may occur during anesthesia or with the use of anticholinergic drugs. The morphology of the affected muscle may be similar to that of Hirschsprung's disease (see later); neurons are sparse or absent, but nerve fibers are present.

CLINICAL MANIFESTATIONS. The infant usually seems normal at birth, but regurgitation is noted at one to three weeks post partum and rapidly progresses to projectile vomiting, dehydration, and weight loss but without anorexia. The vomitus contains no bile. Gastric peristalsis may be visible, and the hypertrophied pylorus may be palpable in the epigastrium.

DIAGNOSIS. The radiologic appearances are characteristic: an elongated, narrow pylorus surrounded by the hypertrophied muscle, which may be seen as a soft tissue shadow. In adults, the pyloric region may protrude proximally into the antrum, resembling a uterine cervix at endoscopy.

TREATMENT. After correction of acid-base and electrolyte imbalance, a trial of anticholinergics and small feedings is justified in milder examples, but surgical correction will usually be necessary. Pyloromyotomy in the fashion of Ramstedt is performed; a simple longitudinal incision of the circular muscle suffices, with an excellent prognosis. In adults, resection of the pylorus and distal antrum with vagotomy is usually advisable.

POSTOPERATIVE DISORDERS

Surgical therapies for peptic ulcer disease often result in profound alterations of the finely tuned process of gastric emptying (see also Ch. 100). The most radical surgical procedures for peptic ulceration resect the antrum and pylorus, thus removing the physical effect of the distal stomach in the grinding of solid food, as well as removing the pyloric sieve. The lesser procedure of total gastric vagotomy is usually combined with pyloroplasty or gastroenterostomy ("drainage"), since reduced antral grinding in the vagotomized stomach leads to retention of solids. If the "drainage" maneuver is less than adequate, stagnation of solids may occur, although, at the same time, gastric emptying of liquids may be excessively rapid. This "dumping" of liquids is readily explicable by impairment of vagally innervated receptive relaxation of the proximal stomach, a process that permits storage of volume without undue elevation of intragastric pressure. Thus, after gastric surgery many disorders of gastric emptying are encountered, including rapid emptying of liquids (dumping syndrome), reduced emptying of solids (gastroparesis), or a combination of both. Certain mechanical complications of gastroenterostomy are also recognized, including obstruction of afferent jejunal loops and intussusception of jejunal limbs into the gastric remnant. The least traumatic surgical procedure, proximal gastric vagotomy, reduces gastric hypersecretion by denervation of the parietal cells alone. Innervation of the antrum and pylorus being preserved, gastric emptying is minimally affected.

Diagnostic steps for the patient with postoperative problems include a careful history, which must determine the exact temporal relationship of symptoms to meals, degree of nausea, nature of vomitus, and ability to handle liquid or solid diet. Barium meal examination is often unhelpful, testing as it does only the emptying of a dense liquid without nutrient content. However, failure to empty some barium by 30 minutes or retention of most barium at six hours signals a severe abnormality. Endoscopy may reveal fasting retention of foods or solid masses (bezoars) in the stomach and is useful to exclude mechanical obstruction. This common and confusing syndrome can be better evaluated by the use of gamma-labeled mixed meals monitored by external gamma cameras, thus allowing selective evaluation of emptying patterns for labeled liquids and solids.

Dumping Syndrome

DEFINITION, CLINICAL FEATURES, AND INCIDENCE. This symptom complex of sweating, weakness with orthostatic features, tachycardia, and sometimes diarrhea following meals occurs transiently in one third or more of patients after gastric surgery. Although most common and severe after gastric resection and gastroenterostomy (Billroth II), it may complicate any operation for peptic ulceration. Symptoms appear as soon after surgery as patients begin a regular diet. Although usually subsiding by 3 to 12 months after surgery, symptoms may persist and be debilitating. Liquid meals, especially those containing large amounts of carbohydrate, are most likely to evoke symptoms. Patients learn that recumbency minimizes symptoms and often discover that avoidance of sugars and desserts helps.

ETIOLOGY AND PATHOGENESIS. No other syndrome in gastroenterology has received more scrutiny and yet yielded so little uniform information as to its cause and rational treatment. Hypovolemia caused by pooling of interstitial fluid in the gut (as a result of uncontrolled entry of hyperosmolar fluids into the small bowel), hypoglycemia, and hormonal imbalance have received most attention. Among the humoral agents incriminated are serotonin and neurotensin. The symptoms can be mimicked in some patients by depletion of extracellular volumes (and corrected by volume expansion), by hypoglycemia, and by distention of a balloon in the small intestine.

DIAGNOSIS. The diagnosis is established by the characteristic history and the exclusion of other diseases likely to produce similar symptoms. Radiology and endoscopy of the upper gastrointestinal tract are required to rule out organic or mechanical problems.

TREATMENT. Reassurance that the symptoms will subside with time will often be sufficient treatment. Patients should be advised to eat small meals, separating fluids from the more solid components of major meals. Lying down after large meals may help, as will avoidance of sweetened drinks and desserts. The prognosis is good with regard to major incapacitation, although minor symptoms may continue indefinitely if certain combinations of diet and activity are pursued.

Gastroparesis and Bezoars

DEFINITION AND PATHOPHYSIOLOGY. Many patients demonstrate mild degrees of gastric retention of solids after gastric surgery, although few (<10 per cent) have major problems. Motility studies reveal diminished phase III activity ("motor fronts") in the stomach but normal cyclic activity in the small bowel.

CLINICAL MANIFESTATIONS. Postprandial fullness, nausea, and vomiting are the major features. Occasionally, solid material may completely obstruct the stoma or the esophagus. The most important consequence, however, is superficial ulceration of the stomach, which often bleeds.

DIAGNOSIS. Bezoars are detected by barium meal examination or endoscopy. The latter procedure has additional therapeutic potential, since boluses can be broken up mechanically and washed into the small intestine or removed by gastric lavage. Barium studies reveal intraluminal filling defects, often of massive dimensions.

TREATMENT. Physical disruption of bezoars by endoscopy, repeated gastric lavage, or both will be helpful. Chemical disruption by papain or cellulase has been successful also. Patients should then be advised to chew their food well and avoid large amounts of raw fruit and vegetables. Metoclopramide can accelerate the delayed emptying of solids after gastric surgery, although most studies report only short-term benefits. Metoclopramide (10 mg) or bethanechol (5 mg) has been shown experimentally to stimulate gastric contractions and to speed emptying of solids.

PROGNOSIS. In general, dietary measures and gradual recovery of gastric contractile function can be expected to alleviate symptoms. In some patients, however, a permanent change in eating patterns is required.

Intussusception

Jejunal intussusception into the stomach may occur after Billroth II gastric resection or, less often, after gastroenterostomy. Although it is sometimes asymptomatic, pain and gastric outlet obstruction may result. The radiologic picture of a "coiled spring" filling defect and the endoscopic appearances are characteristic. When intussusception is severe, surgical correction is required.

GASTROPARESIS DIABETICORUM

DEFINITION AND INCIDENCE. Severely impaired gastric emptying without evidence of mechanical obstruction is a well-recognized complication of diabetes mellitus. It is unknown whether lesser degrees of gastric stasis are responsible for milder symptoms and the variable control of blood sugar so common in diabetics with longstanding disease.

PATHOGENESIS AND CLINICAL FEATURES. The cause is unknown, but autonomic denervation of the proximal gut seems likely. Patients may be of any age and either sex and are usually "juvenile-onset" diabetics whose disease is of more than ten years' duration. Retinopathy, nephropathy, and other complications are common. The pathophysiologic features are an absence of phase III activity "fronts" in the distal stomach and increased tone across the pylorus, with the motor pattern of the small bowel being normal. Nausea, vomiting, poor and variable control of blood sugar levels, and weight loss are the major presenting symptoms. Esophageal reflux, esophagitis, and even repeated episodes of Mallory-Weiss syndrome from vigorous vomiting may be seen.

DIAGNOSIS. The clinical picture is characteristic, but mechanical obstruction must be excluded by radiology and upper gastrointestinal endoscopy. Fluoroscopy may suggest reduced antral contractions or display retained food and secretions.

TREATMENT AND PROGNOSIS. Dietary management with soft foods well cooked and chewed should be instituted, since pharmacologic maneuvers provide little long-term benefit. Metoclopramide is certainly the best agent available at this time. Unfortunately, drug resistance is common, and long-term benefit is less common. Cholinergic agents (bethanechol 5 to 10 mg) are worthy of trial but are not often effective. Surgical treatment (e.g., gastroenterostomy) may be attempted, but only temporary benefit should be anticipated.

IDIOPATHIC GASTROPARESIS

DEFINITION AND INCIDENCE. Otherwise healthy persons may develop symptoms suggestive of gastroparesis, sometimes acutely in association with a flulike illness. Vomiting in nonbacterial gastroenteritis (e.g., those caused by parvoviruses or Norwalk and Hawaii agents) is accompanied by slow gastric emptying. Some patients diagnosed as having psychogenic vomiting actually have impaired motility and gastric emptying.

PATHOGENESIS AND CLINICAL FEATURES. Abnormalities of the gastric pacemaker potential have been reported in some persons with delayed emptying. Electrogastrography

can be performed, using intraluminal or external electrodes, "tachygastria" and other arrhythmias have been noted. The abnormal electrical potentials in turn lead to a failure to develop "spikes" and adequate contractions of smooth muscle. Gastric retention, more often for solids than liquids, causes bloating, nausea, and vomiting.

DIAGNOSIS. Mechanical obstruction and peptic ulceration must be excluded carefully, but it is still uncertain how often those pathophysiologic disturbances are present in patients with "nonulcer dyspepsia."

PROGNOSIS AND TREATMENT. Most examples are transient, perhaps in association with a viral illness. Occasionally, when the problem is chronic, surgery has been required. Some evidence suggests that prostanoids are implicated in "tachygastria" and trial of a nonsteroidal anti-inflammatory drug should be considered.

MISCELLANEOUS CONDITIONS

Gastric diverticula are uncommon, single, and asymptomatic. True diverticula are always located in the upper quarter of the stomach, usually on the posterior wall. Their only significance is in their diagnostic confusion with peptic ulcers or ulcerating neoplasms. Endoscopy may be required for this differentiation. Pseudodiverticula are scarred areas of dilatation, usually in the prepyloric antrum, in association with peptic ulcer disease.

Gastric volvulus is torsion of the stomach along its long axis, the esophagogastric junction and pylorus remaining fixed. Large hiatal hernias or diaphragmatic defects may be predisposing factors. An acute volvulus is often an abdominal emergency, particularly if the gastric blood supply is compromised. The chronic form is more common, bloating, regurgitation, dysphagia, and pain may occur and the diagnosis is made radiologically. Surgical treatment is required for acute volvulus and for severe symptomatic chronic volvulus.

Acute dilatation of the stomach is best considered as a localized form of paralytic ileus (see below); it is seen after abdominal operations or immobilization in body casts, during diabetic ketoacidosis, or as an acute side effect of anticholinergics. Distention of the stomach may become massive if nasogastric suction is not instituted, and mucosal bleeding may lead to "coffee-ground" emesis.

Aerophagia is a normal accompaniment of swallowing but may be exaggerated in anxious persons, leading to epigastric bloating. Bloating often induces patients to attempt repeated belches, each of which perpetuates the swallowing of gas. Organic disease must be excluded, and the chewing of gum and ingestion of carbonated beverages should be avoided.

Malagelada J-R, Camilleri M, Stanghellini V: Manometric Diagnosis of Gastrointestinal Motility Disorders. New York, Thieme-Stratton, 1986. *A monograph on the diagnosis of motility disorders but dealing also with normal physiology and the pathophysiology of the common and uncommon disorders of motility. The bibliography is extensive and will guide the reader into any area.*

Meyer JH: Chronic morbidity after ulcer surgery. In Sleisenger MH, Fordtran JS (eds.): Gastrointestinal Disease. 4th ed. Philadelphia, W. B. Saunders Company, 1988. *Comprehensive review of all the major problems encountered after gastric surgery. Includes pathophysiology, clinical features, and treatment.*

Disorders of Small Bowel Motility

INTRODUCTION

Normally, progression of food through the small intestine is slow and steady. Although the "head" of a barium meal may reach the terminal ileum in one to two hours, mean transit time (for 50 per cent of a meal) is slower and the "tail" is even more delayed. The only documented examples of intestinal hurry are in patients with "short bowel syndrome," seen after extensive resection of the small bowel, and the malabsorption that accompanies jejunoileal bypass. In these conditions, the major defect is inadequate contact between chyme and the digestive-absorptive surface (see Ch. 104).

The chronic stasis of delayed transit through the small intestine, from any cause, is often accompanied by an overgrowth of intestinal flora, since normal motility helps maintain the relative sterility of the small bowel. The *"blind loop syndrome"* can be produced experimentally by ganglionic blocking drugs (nonobstructive or adynamic ileus) and by partial mechanical obstruction. The blind loop syndrome occurs clinically (1) in conditions causing stasis (chronic obstruction, giant jejunal diverticula, and surgical blind pouches), (2) when a fistula is present between the colon and the upper bowel, and (3) with disturbances of the interdigestive motor complex (see Ch. 104).

ILEUS: ADYNAMIC AND MECHANICAL

DEFINITION AND ETIOLOGY. Ileus signifies impairment of caudad transit of intestinal contents. It can be subdivided into two broad categories: (1) adynamic or paralytic and (2) mechanical. The difference between these categories is important clinically: Mechanical causes are usually treated surgically, whereas adynamic ileus requires medical management. Adynamic ileus occurs in association with abdominal surgery or external trauma, when the peritoneum is exposed to irritants (bacterial toxins, bile, blood, pancreatic enzymes, or intestinal contents), in severe electrolyte imbalance, and after intra-abdominal vascular accidents. The etiopathogenesis is unknown, although disordered sympathetic tone is presumed. Ileus can also be induced by ganglionic blocking drugs.

Mechanical obstruction may occur at any level of the small bowel or colon; it can be separated pathogenetically into lesions lying outside the bowel (e.g., adhesive bands, obstructed hernias), those within the wall (e.g., intramural tumors, hematomas, strictures), and those within the lumen (e.g., epithelial tumors, foreign bodies, intussusception).

PATHOPHYSIOLOGIC CONSEQUENCES. The proximal bowel distends, and its function becomes compromised. In experimental obstruction of the canine small intestine, absorption from distended bowel segments diminishes after 6 to 12 hours and is replaced by secretion of sodium and water. Increased intraluminal pressure, elevation of portal venous and lymphatic pressures, ischemia, and the toxic effects of rapid bacterial multiplication in the involved segment are among the mechanisms proposed to account for these changes.

Once obstruction is established, edema, petechial hemorrhages, and finally necrosis and gangrene develop in the bowel wall. These changes are most pronounced when occlusion or strangulation of the vasculature occurs, as in closed-loop obstruction, which produces exceedingly high intraluminal pressure. Excessive permeability of the damaged intestinal mucosa allows proteins to leak from blood into the intestinal lumen; conversely, bacteria and their toxins enter the damaged and permeable mucosa. Peritonitis, therefore, frequently complicates untreated obstruction. Additional injury to ischemic mucosa may be caused by compounds in the intestinal lumen, including pancreatic enzymes, bile acids, and bacterial enterotoxins. The sequence whereby untreated obstruction leads to irreversible shock and death is uncertain. Extracellular fluid volume depletion, free perforation of the bowel, bacterial toxins, gram-negative septicemia, and splanchnic vasoconstriction all have been implicated. The general role of bacteria is well established experimentally, since mortality from obstruction is reduced in newborn or germ-free animals, or when broad-spectrum antibiotics have been given previously.

Hypovolemia, hyponatremia, and hypochloremia are the major abnormalities observed. During the course of ileus, several liters of extracellular fluid may become sequestered in the intestine. Experimental obstruction of the distal small bowel results in leakage of as much as 50 per cent of the plasma volume into this "third space." Additional fluid may accumulate in the peritoneal cavity. Plasma concentrations of electrolytes are initially normal, since the fluid lost is isotonic, but the patient usually drinks sodium-poor fluid, so that hyponatremia develops. Severe vomiting depletes chloride, and alkalosis may be prominent in obstruction of the upper intestine. Impairment of renal function secondary to hypovolemia and starvation, with consequent ketosis, may combine to produce mild acidosis.

CLINICAL MANIFESTATIONS. The symptoms and signs depend on the level of obstruction, its duration, and whether the cause is obstructive or adynamic. Paralytic ileus may cause little pain and be manifested only by abdominal distention and vomiting. Increased volumes of aspirate obtained from nasogastric suction and oliguria may be early manifestations of paralytic ileus in the patient already under close observation, e.g., postoperatively. The symptoms of mechanical obstruction are vomiting, cramping abdominal pain, distention, and obstipation. When obstruction is episodic, relief may be heralded by watery, voluminous stools. When proximal, obstruction produces earlier vomiting, epigastric or midabdominal pain, and minimal distention. Distal obstructive lesions are associated with less vomiting, lower abdominal pain, and more prominent abdominal distention with obstipation. Physical signs are those of the metabolic disorder, particularly extracellular dehydration and hypovolemia, abdominal distention with variable tenderness, and a mass that might indicate the underlying lesion. Bowel sounds are high pitched, frequent, and rushing in mechanical obstruction. Adynamic ileus has lesser physical signs; distention is prominent, but tenderness is less pronounced unless the ileus is associated with peritonitis. Bowel sounds are infrequent to absent early in ileus in contrast to mechanical obstruction. Bowel sounds may disappear later in the course of mechanical obstruction.

DIAGNOSIS. Plain abdominal radiographic films are vital for diagnosis, to determine the level of obstruction, and to distinguish mechanical from adynamic ileus. Air-fluid levels in obstructed bowel will be seen in upright or lateral decubitus films. Mechanical obstruction often also demonstrates a sharp demarcation between dilated bowel above and collapsed bowel below the point of obstruction. Such a transition is not seen in ileus, in which dilatation is uniform throughout small and large intestines.

Colonic gas shadows are recognized by the presence of haustra, which are asymmetric and do not extend across the entire diameter of the bowel. Valvulae conniventes of the small bowel are regular, symmetric shadows across the entire diameter. Contrast material will pool above an obstruction and should not be given by mouth. Proctosigmoidoscopy and a barium enema, without preparation, can be performed cautiously when the obstruction is thought to be in the colon. Other diagnostic measures to determine a cause of ileus should then be considered. Overall metabolic evaluation will include measurements of serum electrolytes and the status of acid-base balance, blood urea, hematocrit, and serum protein levels, as well as careful monitoring of urine volume.

TREATMENT. The primary goals of therapy for ileus or obstruction are (1) intestinal decompression, (2) restoration or maintenance of fluid and electrolyte balance, and (3) treatment of the cause. Most instances of adynamic ileus are transient, and a medical approach can achieve all three goals. However, when the obstruction is mechanical, initial decompression is achieved by intubation, but definitive decompression and removal of the obstruction usually require surgery.

Nasogastric aspiration is usually sufficient for decompression, because this removes air before it reaches the intestine. Fluid replacement is aimed at replacing the lost water, sodium, chloride, and potassium. Alkalosis or acidosis should be corrected. Central venous pressure should be monitored to assure adequate replacement as well as to avoid fluid overload, particularly in patients with compromised cardiovascular reserve. Repeated observations are made of serum electrolytes as well as blood pressure, urinary output, and hematocrit. When fever, leukocytosis, or signs of peritonitis suggest perforation or strangulation, appropriate antimicrobials are administered to suppress growth of intestinal bacteria. Strangulation with impending gangrene demands surgery within six hours.

Jones RS: Intestinal obstruction, pseudo-obstruction, and ileus. In Sleisenger MH, Fordtran JS (eds.): Gastrointestinal Disease. 4th ed. Philadelphia, W. B. Saunders Company, 1988. *A more detailed description of the causative lesions, clinical features, and practical management of obstruction of the small and large intestines.*

INTESTINAL PSEUDO-OBSTRUCTION

DEFINITION. Pseudo-obstruction implies a syndrome with clinical features akin to mechanical obstruction but for which there is no obstructive lesion. When the episode is single and transient, pseudo-obstruction is more appropriately included among examples of adynamic ileus. Thus, the term should be applied to chronic or recurrent episodes of obstruction. The underlying causes are either unknown or untreatable diseases, and pseudo-obstruction has a poor prognosis.

ETIOLOGY. So-called "primary idiopathic pseudo-obstruction" has no known cause. It affects families, and the defect appears to be transmitted as an autosomal dominant trait. Relatives of patients with the syndrome may have only radiologic and manometric evidence of abnormal intestinal motility or the full-blown disease. Primary pseudo-obstruction can be subdivided into (1) hollow visceral myopathy and (2) autonomic neuropathies. Pseudo-obstruction also occurs as a manifestation of other diseases (Table 102–2), termed secondary intestinal pseudo-obstruction.

PATHOGENESIS. The pathophysiology of both primary and secondary forms is unknown, but the mechanisms are probably diverse. Category 1 of Table 101–2 includes diseases in which the smooth muscle itself is directly replaced by infiltrates, fibrous tissue, or other noncontractile elements. Category 2 lists diseases in which intramural nervous tissue is involved, either destroyed (Chagas' disease) or histologically intact but functionally disturbed ("ganglioneuromato-

TABLE 102–2. CAUSES OF SECONDARY INTESTINAL PSEUDO-OBSTRUCTION*

1. **Diseases involving intestinal smooth muscle ("intestinal myopathies")**
   Collagen vascular diseases
     Scleroderma
     Dermatomyositis
     Polymyositis
     Systemic lupus erythematosus
   Amyloidosis
   Primary muscular diseases
     Myotonic dystrophy
     Progressive muscular dystrophy
2. **Neurologic diseases ("intestinal neuropathies")**
   Chagas' disease
   Hirschsprung's disease
   Familial autonomic dysfunction
   Parkinson's disease
3. **Endocrine diseases**
   Hypothyroidism
   Diabetes mellitus
   Hypoparathyroidism
   Pheochromocytoma
4. **Drug effects**
   Phenothiazines, tricyclic antidepressants, antiparkinsonian drugs, ganglion blockers, clonidine
5. **Miscellaneous associations**
   Ceroid deposits in bowel
   Nontropical sprue
   Jejunal diverticulosis
   Paraneoplastic neuropathy

*Modified, with permission of the authors, from Faulk DL, Anuras S, Christensen J: Gastroenterology 74:922, 1978.

sis"). Category 2 also includes diseases with extensive denervation, as when there is other evidence of autonomic dysfunction with involvement of the urinary bladder (diabetes mellitus and other neuropathies). Disturbances of hormonal regulation of intestinal function may also occur as a paraneoplastic syndrome. Certain drugs as listed in Table 102–2 may occasionally be associated with pseudo-obstruction.

CLINICAL MANIFESTATIONS. Patients with pseudo-obstruction may be of any age but, as anticipated from the nature of the underlying causes, are more often middle aged or older. The clinical presentation may vary from one of persistent symptoms of moderate severity to more acute episodes of pain, distention, and vomiting, closely mimicking the more common circumstance of mechanical obstruction. The symptoms and signs are those of retarded transit and stagnation of intestinal contents, a variable spectrum of dysphagia, regurgitation, vomiting, distention, obstipation, diarrhea, and malabsorption. Abdominal pain is quite variable also and, when prominent, makes differentiation from mechanical obstruction quite difficult. Manifestation of neuromuscular incoordination of other systems, notably the urinary bladder, may be present, as may the features of any underlying disease. Severe and chronic pseudo-obstruction may produce malnutrition and inanition.

DIAGNOSIS. The diagnosis of pseudo-obstruction requires the painstaking exclusion of mechanical obstruction. Free flow of contrast must be demonstrated after a barium meal with small bowel follow-through and with a barium enema. Failure to recognize a correctable mechanical obstruction may have grave consequences. The differentiation of pseudo-obstruction from slowly progressive distal obstruction (as, for example, with carcinoid tumors, radiation enteritis, and other fibrosing lesions) can also be quite difficult. Adjunctive evidence of a generalized disorder of muscle function can be obtained from motility studies of the esophagus, from cystometric studies, and from clinical evidence of underlying disease. When malabsorption is present, other causes of steatorrhea must be excluded. In some instances, exploratory laparotomy cannot be avoided, and full-thickness biopsy of involved intestine can be helpful.

TREATMENT. Pharmacologic treatment of pseudo-obstruction, although rational, has generally been unrewarding. Cholinergic agents and metoclopramide have the most appeal but are usually ineffective; hormones such as cholecystokinin-pancreozymin and a related peptide, cerulein, have also been tried with poor results. Corticosteroids have not augmented motility or reduced steatorrhea. Elevated serum levels of prostaglandins have been reported, as has partial relief with indomethacin. However, in an uncommon disease with an unpredictable natural history, any therapeutic information is largely anecdotal. Acute episodes require nasogastric suction and parenteral fluids, sometimes leading to parenteral alimentation. When a "blind loop syndrome" is present, antibiotics can be helpful. Surgical resection of more severely affected segments can help very occasionally but should not be entertained lightly; each laparotomy merely increases the likelihood of adhesive obstruction, further confusing an already complex problem. The prognosis is poor, and some patients have required total (home) parenteral nutrition.

Anuras S, Mitros FA, Sofer RT, et al.: Chronic intestinal pseudo-obstruction in young children. Gastroenterology 91:62, 1986. *Report of eight children with symptoms beginning between the ages of a few weeks to five years. All had marked dilatation of the entire intestine and megacystis. The disease was variable among individual examples, but, in most, the smooth muscle appeared normal.*

Schuffler MD, Baird HW, Fleming CR, et al.: Intestinal pseudo-obstruction as the presenting manifestation of small-cell carcinoma of the lung. Ann Intern Med 98:1983. *A carefully studied and well-documented example of a paraneoplastic neuropathy of the gastrointestinal tract. Though a rare syndrome, it exemplifies one of the multiple mechanisms of motor control that can be disturbed by disease.*

Snape WJ Jr: Pseudo-obstruction and other obstructive disorders. Clin Gastroenterol 11:3, 1982. *Succinct review of pathophysiology and clinical features of the syndrome. Contains all major original references.*

DIVERTICULA OF THE SMALL INTESTINE

Duodenal diverticula are common and only rarely of any significance. Although a few examples of ulceration and bleeding have been documented, duodenal diverticula are of little diagnostic significance in upper gastrointestinal hemorrhage. Jejunal diverticula are important when stasis and bacterial overgrowth occur, resulting in the "blind loop syndrome" (see Ch. 104).

Meckel's diverticulum is the most common congenital abnormality of the gut, occurring in 2 per cent of the population. Meckel's diverticula are situated 30 to 90 cm proximal to the ileocecal sphincter on the antimesenteric wall of the ileum. Although usually 5 to 7 cm in length, they can be much longer. Gastric mucosa is present within the lumen in about one third of these diverticula. They are usually asymptomatic, but occasionally bleed, perforate, become inflamed, or obstruct the ileum. The presence of gastric mucosa and the capacity of this tissue to take up selectively radioisotopes of technetium form the basis of a diagnostic test using external gamma-camera scintillography. The diverticulum "lights up" and can be occasionally identified in this way.

Disorders of Colonic Motility

INTRODUCTION

The colon's multiple functions—desiccation of feces, bacterial metabolism of unabsorbed materials, storage of stools, and voluntary defecation—are served by a complex pattern of motility. The walls of the cecum and ascending and transverse colons show radiologic indentations ("haustra") that correspond to low-pressure mixing waves, as recorded by intraluminal pressure transducers. These waves are thought to provide a "back-and-forth" mixing that facilitates reabsorption of salt and water. This motor pattern probably also increases the digestive potential for bacterial enzymes on dietary fiber. Transit through the descending colon is more rapid, although feces are stored in the sigmoid region. Entry of stools into the rectum triggers a coordinated sequence of rectal events, voluntary elevations of intra-abdominal pressure, and relaxation of the anal sphincters whereby controlled and voluntary defecation is possible.

Dietary fiber, components that are resistant to digestion by mammalian enzymes, may modify colonic motor function. Modern analytic techniques have now identified the important components of fruits, vegetables, and the outer shells of cereals that constitute fiber. The major components of fiber are celluloses (large, unbranched polymers of glucose), hemicelluloses (highly branched polymers of five-carbon sugars), pectins (gel-forming carbohydrates), and lignins (noncarbohydrate polymers of phenylpropanes). The differing chemical compositions within each of these classes and wide variations among the natural sources of fiber in foods contribute to the variable clinical effects of different fibers. In most instances, fiber decreases transit time through the colon and increases fecal bulk while undergoing some degree of digestion by the fecal flora. Gases (hydrogen, carbon dioxide, and, in one third of adults, methane) and organic anions (butyrate, propionate, acetate) are generated. Undigested components of fiber have physical effects on feces by entrapping ions and water within their complex matrices. Fiber deficiency has been incriminated in several colonic diseases, including simple constipation, diverticulosis, hemorrhoids, and carcinoma of the colon.

Vahovny GV, Kritchevsky D: Dietary Fiber in Health and Disease. New York, Plenum Press, 1982. *A simple but comprehensive monograph that contains much that will be useful for clinicians wishing to know more about modern views on fiber. Excellent chapters on "what is fiber," physical properties of fiber in the bowel, and effects of fiber on colonic function.*

SIMPLE CONSTIPATION: LAXATIVES AND THEIR ABUSE

DEFINITION. Most normal adults experience brief episodes of constipation when their living habits change abruptly. Normal frequency of stools is approximately three or more per week; moreover, defecation should be painless, not require undue straining, and be satisfyingly complete. Patients may complain of constipation if any of these criteria is not fulfilled. In order to determine whether a patient has constipation, stool frequency and fecal weight should be measured over a period of two weeks during which the intake of fiber in the diet is adequate and no constipating drugs are being taken. On such a schedule a stool should be passed with ease at least every other day.

ETIOLOGY. Constipation is a symptom and not a disease. The major causes are listed in Table 102–3. In many instances a combination of factors will be present, e.g., diets that contain little fiber, complicated by drugs that constipate, being ingested by an individual who is debilitated, with poor muscular tone, and who has a poor habit for defecation. Clearly, the list of underlying causes in Table 102–3 dictates that constipation that continues despite the program outlined above must be evaluated carefully.

PATHOGENESIS. The major abnormality is slow transit of feces through the colon, an abnormality that can be documented best by observing the time required for small radiopaque pellets to be excreted. There is no evidence that fluid absorption by the colon is excessive, except to the degree that augmented absorption can be explained by slower transit. In some persons, stools are held up at the rectal outlet, since the muscles of the pelvic floor and anal sphincter fail to relax during defecatory efforts. In most instances of secondary constipation, a pathogenic mechanism cannot be specified.

CLINICAL MANIFESTATIONS AND DIAGNOSIS. Many symptoms are falsely attributed to constipation; these include halitosis, distention, belching, rectal gas, abdominal discomfort, headache, and even temper tantrums. However, severe fecal impaction can cause intestinal obstruction with spurious ("overflow") diarrhea, stercoral ulceration with bleeding, and even acute abdominal crises. Features of underlying disease may be present by history or on physical examination. Other

TABLE 102–3. MAJOR CAUSES OF CONSTIPATION

1. **"Functional causes"**
   Fiber-deficient diets
   Inadequate evacuatory habits
   Variants of "irritable bowel syndrome"
   Psychoses and mental deficiency
   Debilitation and extreme old age
2. **Colonic diseases**
   Chronic obstructive lesions (e.g., tumors, strictures)
   Ulcerative proctitis
   Collagen vascular diseases with muscular abnormalities
3. **Rectal diseases**
   Stricture (e.g., ulcerative colitis, postsurgical)
   Painful conditions (fissure, abscess)
   Prolapsed rectal mucosa
   Rectocele
4. **Neurologic diseases**
   Hirschsprung's disease
   Ganglioneuromatosis
   Chagas' disease
   Intestinal pseudo-obstruction
   Spinal cord injuries and disease
   Parkinson's disease
   Cerebral tumors and cerebrovascular disease
5. **Metabolic diseases**
   Porphyria
   Hypothyroidism
   Hypercalcemia
   Pheochromocytoma
   Uremia
6. **Drugs**
   Analgesics, antacids (calcium and aluminum compounds), anticholinergics, anticonvulsants, antidepressants, bismuth salts, ganglion blockers, heavy metal poisonings, drugs for parkinsonism and psychotherapy

physical findings may include tenderness of the colon to abdominal palpation and sigmoidoscopic visualization of melanosis coli, a superficial, brown pigmentation of the rectal mucosa that is seen in persons who use anthraquinone laxatives habitually. Abuse of laxatives can have other serious sequelae (see below).

TREATMENT. When treatable diseases are excluded, it is important to educate the patient about the colon's functions. Establishment of a daily ritual, aided by an increase in dietary fiber through use of fruit and vegetables or the addition of psyllium hydrophilic colloids (Metamucil), should be the major approach. Patients need to be told that such agents are not cathartics and that a prompt evacuation will not follow their use. The patient should gradually increase a regular (three times daily) dosage of psyllium hydrophilic colloids until an effect is achieved and then continue that dosage. One teaspoonful (7 grams) of powder three times a day may suffice, as an example. Chronic use of more potent laxatives should be avoided. In fecal impaction, enemas may soften and dislodge hard feces; suppositories and "wetting agents" may also help. When all else fails, manual removal, under appropriate sedation, may be necessary.

Laxatives are classified conventionally into several classes: (1) Osmotic agents are poorly absorbed molecules that retain water in the bowel lumen through osmotic pressure. Sulfates, phosphates, and magnesium salts are in this category. (2) Stool softeners, such as dioctyl sodium sulfosuccinate, are thought to be "wetting agents," although they also stimulate fluid secretion in a way similar to the next class. (3) "Stimulant laxatives," which vary in potency from the relatively mild to the powerful purgatives, include phenolphthalein, senna, the biguanides, and castor oil. All these drugs stimulate intestinal secretion of fluid and also augment propulsive motor activity. (4) Bulking agents are derivatives of plant fiber. For regular use, only this last class can be considered totally harmless. The major stimulants can destroy intramural nerve plexuses in the large bowel, causing "cathartic colon." This serious sequel of lifelong laxative abuse features a radiologic appearance similar to that of ulcerative colitis, a "pipestem" colon lacking haustra and with abnormal propulsive activity. Laxative abuse can also cause major electrolyte imbalance, mild steatorrhea, and a protein-losing enteropathy.

Binder HJ: Pharmacology of laxatives. Ann Rev Pharmacol Toxicol 17:355, 1977. *Succinct review of classification of laxatives, including sections on influence of laxative on fluid absorption and secretion, intestinal motility, and side effects of laxative abuse.*

Devroede GJ: Constipation: Mechanisms and management. In Sleisenger MH, Fordtran JS (eds.): Gastrointestinal Disease. 4th ed. Philadelphia, W. B. Saunders Company, 1988. *This is the most complete scientific evaluation of constipation. By focusing on the important underlying diseases, the author develops a strong approach that will not always be needed for simpler examples. But valuable understanding of this common and variable symptom will arise from careful review, and the clinician wishing to understand this common symptom will gain much from such review.*

IRRITABLE BOWEL SYNDROME

DEFINITION AND INCIDENCE. The key features of the irritable bowel syndrome are abdominal discomfort, alterations of bowel habit, and no demonstrable organic cause. It is the most common gastrointestinal disorder in Western societies, constituting up to 50 per cent of all referrals for subspecialty opinion. It is more common in women than men and occurs in the middle years of life. Numerous terms are applied to the syndrome, but several are inappropriate and even harmful. The entity is not an inflammation, and thus "mucous" or "spastic" *colitis* is incorrect. Functional diarrhea is sometimes considered as a separate entity, although irritable bowel syndrome may be characterized by episodes of diarrhea, often alternating with constipation.

ETIOLOGY AND PATHOGENESIS. Although causative mechanisms are unknown, it is likely that the syndrome includes a number of entities for which specific causes will eventually be uncovered. For example, the definition of lactase deficiency has allowed some patients who earlier would have been designated as having irritable bowel to receive a specific diagnosis and therapy. Psychologic and social stresses are often present in patients with irritable bowel syndrome and may be related in a temporal sense to exacerbations of symptoms. They are thought to be at least aggravating factors but may be causative.

Investigations of the pathophysiology have centered on motility studies of the colon. The colonic neuromusculature is abnormally sensitive to stress in the irritable bowel syndrome. Thus, although basal contractions are not very different from normal, meals, emotional stresses, mechanical distention, and pharmacologic stimuli elicit greater numbers of more powerful contractions. In the sigmoid colon, higher intraluminal pressures have been incriminated as a mechanism for pain and the development of diverticula and muscular hypertrophy. Studies of colonic myoelectrical activity reveal an increased incidence of waves at a rate of three per minute and fewer at six per minute, when compared with control subjects. More sensitive methods have uncovered abnormalities of muscle function in the esophagus and small intestine. Thus, it seems likely that the pathophysiology may involve an "irritability" of the entire gut in some persons.

CLINICAL FEATURES. Particular traits of personality have been attributed to patients with irritable bowel syndrome. They are often rigid, methodical persons who are conscientious, with obsessive-compulsive tendencies. Depression and hysteria are the most common psychiatric illnesses.

Abdominal pain is the most common complaint. This pain may be of any type or severity but characteristically is not severe enough to interfere with sleep. Pain is often related to meals, sometimes suggesting peptic ulcer disease, and possibly triggered in the colon by the "gastrocolic reflex." Pain may be relieved by passing flatus, which is often thought by the patient to be excessive in amount. Variants of irritable bowel syndrome include the "splenic flexure syndrome," in which colonic gas appears to be localized to that region. In fact, volumes of intestinal gas are not increased in the irritable bowel syndrome, rather, the patient is overly sensitive to normal volumes of gas or to intestinal distention by balloons. Some disturbance of bowel habit is always present as diarrhea, constipation, or a variable pattern. Stools are described as marbles, pellets, and "rabbity" mucus and undigested food are described but are of no significance. Bleeding is not a feature unless hemorrhoids are also present, and weight loss does not occur unless depression is a major feature. Associated features—emotional lability, lethargy, headaches, and benign cardiovascular symptoms—are likely psychosomatic manifestations. The program of investigation, which includes stool analysis, clinical laboratory surveys, proctosigmoidoscopy, and barium enema, is designated to eliminate underlying organic disease.

TREATMENT AND PROGNOSIS. Sympathetic explanation of the nature of the disorder and a careful exclusion of other diseases of the colon with subsequent reassurance are keys to successful management of these patients. A positive approach can be taken, irritable bowel syndrome is *not* a "wastebasket" but a disorder of intestinal function with an as yet unknown pathogenesis. Drug therapy should be avoided if at all possible. Psychoneuroses may require treatment, and severe pain may require a non-narcotic analgesic. Anticholinergic spasmolytics may also be helpful, and episodes of diarrhea may require treatment with antimotility agents. Constipation should be explained and treated with hydrophilic colloids and diet (see above). Patients should eliminate foods from the diet *only* when a specific food predictably increases symptoms and when exclusion of that food has been shown to help. The rigid use of a "low-residue" diet has no place and may well aggravate many features of the syndrome. The disorder is chronic, and it is unlikely to be modified greatly by any single measure. The aim should be to reduce symptoms to a tolerable level that interferes minimally with the patient's normal activities.

Connell AM: Motility and its disturbances. Clin Gastroenterol 11:3, 1982. *Excellent monograph with chapters covering irritable bowel syndrome, emotions and the gastrointestinal tract, and diverticular disease.*
Thompson WG: The Irritable Bowel. Gut 25:305, 1984. *An extensive review with 112 references. It summarizes well current views on the prevalence, pathophysiology, diagnosis, and treatment of this very common disorder.*

DIVERTICULOSIS COLI

DEFINITION AND INCIDENCE. Colonic diverticula are outpouchings of mucosa through the muscular layers and therefore contain no smooth muscle in their walls. They occur in close proximity to the teniae coli, where the muscular coats of the colon are perforated by an arteriole. The prevalence of colonic diverticula increases with age above 30 to 40 years, and they are present in over 50 per cent of octagenarians in the United States. Since most patients remain asymptomatic, simple diverticulosis is more an anatomic abnormality than it is a disease. However, the term "diverticular disease" is often applied to a spectrum that extends from uncomplicated diverticula, which are thought by some to be variants of the irritable bowel syndrome, to the serious complications of diverticula: bleeding, perforation, and diverticulitis (see Ch. 115).

PATHOGENESIS. Diverticula with muscle hypertrophy seem to be related to spasm of colonic muscle with raised luminal pressures and muscular hypertrophy in the sigmoid colon. "Simple" diverticula have no associated hypertrophy of muscle or evidence for high intraluminal pressures. The former or "spastic" type has been related both to irritable bowel syndrome and to a deficiency of fiber in the Western diet. Fiber is thought to protect by increasing fecal bulk, which, in turn, increases the diameter of the colon. By Laplace's law, the smaller the radius of a cylinder, the greater the pressure generated at a given tension. It is proposed that heightened pressure herniates mucosa and submucosa through the wall of the colon at points of intrinsic weakness. The fiber theory rests to a large extent on the increased incidence of spastic diverticulosis in Western society when compared with societies in which more fiber is ingested. This theory is supported by the increased incidence of diverticulosis in the past century, associated with increasing refinement of the Western diet. The pathogenesis of "simple" diverticula is unknown.

CLINICAL FEATURES. Most patients with diverticula are asymptomatic. When diverticula are present in patients with irritable bowel syndrome, it is virtually impossible to determine their role in the cramping left lower quadrant pain, constipation, or alternating constipation and diarrhea of which these individuals complain. Episodes of more severe distress, lasting for hours or a few days, are classified clinically as *acute diverticulitis*. Although tenderness and a sausage-shaped mass may be noted in the left lower quadrant, fever and leukocytosis characteristic of diverticulitis are absent in bouts of "diverticular disease." On occasions, however, there will be clinical overlap between the symptoms of "diverticular disease" and those of diverticulitis. Bleeding of two types can be seen with diverticula, those with or without diverticulitis. Minimal or occult bleeding may complicate either form of the disease. Significant gross bleeding is seen most often in asymptomatic patients and is less common in those with diverticulitis.

DIAGNOSIS. The diagnosis of diverticula in the colon is by barium enema examination. The diverticula are seen as outpouchings, particularly in the sigmoid colon. Muscular spasm and hypertrophy may be present, giving a "sawtooth," asymmetric pattern to the barium column. In appropriate cases evidence of diverticulitis should be sought—i.e., extraintestinal flow of barium, indicating chronic perforation of the

bowel. The differential diagnosis from carcinoma can be difficult, or impossible in some instances. Proctosigmoidoscopy may be painful but may reveal diverticula, luminal spasm, and fixed angulation of the sigmoid from prior disease.

TREATMENT. The only plausible program for treating diverticula of the colon is designed to increase stool bulk; the aim is to prevent constipation and the development of high pressures within the lumen of the colon. Bran, hydrophilic colloids, and dietary supplements of vegetables and fruits should be used. However, the clinical success of these programs is still uncertain. Spasmolytic anticholinergics and nonopiate analgesics may be needed. Narcotics increase intraluminal pressure and should be avoided. During follow-up visits an assessment must be made as to whether the episodes of pain represent diverticulitis, since this diagnosis raises the question of surgical treatment if recurrences are frequent. (For a discussion of treatment of diverticulitis see Ch. 98.)

Almy TP, Howell DA: Diverticular disease of the colon. N Engl J Med 302:324, 1980. *This medical progress article gives an excellent summary of current knowledge concerning the pathogenesis, clinical picture, and treatment of colonic diverticula. It also supplies 119 pertinent references.*

MEGACOLON: CONGENITAL (HIRSCHSPRUNG'S DISEASE) AND ACQUIRED

DEFINITION. Hirschsprung's disease is colonic dilatation resulting from a functional obstruction of the rectum, where there is a congenital absence of intramural neural plexuses ("aganglionosis") and a "narrow segment." Acquired megacolon may be secondary to any of the causes of constipation discussed under that heading and may be assumed if colonic dilatation was not present at an earlier examination.

INCIDENCE. Congenital aganglionosis occurs in one of each 5000 live births, is five to ten times more common in boys, and is more common in sibs of probands and in children with Down's syndrome or other congenital abnormalities. Acquired megacolon occurs in the young, the very old, and the infirm.

PATHOGENESIS. Aganglionosis is due to arrest of the caudad migration of cells from the neural crest, cells that are destined to develop as intramural plexuses; thus, the aganglionic segment always extends from the internal anal sphincter a variable distance proximally. In most instances, the aganglionic segment is within the rectum and sigmoid colon; involvement of very short segments, only in the region of the anal sphincters, has also been described. The aganglionic segment is permanently contracted, causing dilatation proximal to it. Pressure studies of the anorectal segment demonstrate an absence of normal relaxation of the internal sphincter in response to rectal distention. This abnormality is absent in acquired megacolon, which has no specific pathogenesis but is merely the extreme end-result of severe constipation of many possible causes.

CLINICAL MANIFESTATIONS AND DIFFERENTIAL DIAGNOSIS. Children with congenital megacolon have obstipation, intestinal obstruction, and meconium ileus in the first days of life. Later in life the presentation is less dramatic. It does not then mimic acute intestinal obstruction, but is characterized by severe constipation and recurrent fecal impactions. Although most children have difficulty before the second month of life, very short segment aganglionosis may not cause severe symptoms until after infancy.

Congenital megacolon must be differentiated from other causes of neonatal intestinal obstruction, particularly intestinal atresia and imperforate anus. The differential diagnosis from acquired megacolon is also important. Fecal incontinence is common in acquired megacolon but does not occur in Hirschsprung's disease. Other underlying causes of severe constipation (Table 102–3) should also be sought. Digital examination of the rectum shows the rectum to be empty in congenital megacolon; barium enema usually confirms the absence of stool from the rectal ampulla and will demonstrate the narrowed distal segment in three fourths of patients. In acquired megacolon, dilatation of the bowel extends as far distal as the anal sphincter. Definitive diagnosis of Hirschsprung's disease is made by the absence of ganglion cells from Meissner's and Auerbach's plexuses, as seen in a full-thickness biopsy of the rectum. Hirschsprung's disease can be excluded when ganglion cells are seen within Meissner's submucosal plexus in more superficial biopsies; however, failure to see ganglion cells may be due to faulty technique, and their absence from punch or suction biopsies is not diagnostic of congenital megacolon.

TREATMENT. When a diagnosis of congenital megacolon is established, the treatment of choice is definitive surgery, although preliminary decompression by a colostomy may be necessary to relieve acute obstruction. In other instances, decompression can be achieved by a regular program of enemas. A number of surgical approaches are well established, and the procedure of choice should be left to the surgeon.

Treatment of acquired megacolon is medical. It involves disimpaction of feces by laxatives and enemas, a retraining of bowel habits, and behavioral modifications.

Phillips SF: Megacolon: Congenital and acquired. In Sleisenger MH, Fordtran JS (eds.): Gastrointestinal Disease. 4th ed. Philadelphia, W. B. Saunders Company, 1988. *A description of congenital and acquired megacolon in children, including clinical features, diagnosis, and treatment.*

MOTOR DYSFUNCTION IN SPINAL CORD TRANSECTION

DEFINITION. Whether due to trauma or intrinsic neurologic disease, cord transection causes a predictable disturbance of gastrointestinal motility, the recognition and management of which is key to adequate acute and long-term management of these patients.

PATHOGENESIS. The exact level of denervation and the rapidity of onset, instantaneous in many traumatic transections but slower with some intrinsic diseases, will modify the clinical picture. However, three clinical stages can be generally recognized.

CLINICAL FEATURES AND TREATMENT. In the acute stage of spinal shock, motility, transit, and evacuation are markedly depressed. Although most emphasis has been placed upon the symptoms of obstipation and abdominal distention, acute gastric dilatation and paralysis of the small intestine can also be serious complications. This phase, which lasts usually only a few days, may require nasogastric suction, rectal decompression, and the use of stimulants (e.g., neostigmine [Prostigmin*], 0.3 to 0.5 mg). During a second stage, automatic reflex activity of the bowel is established. By this time, the functions of the upper gut are usually nearly normal, but emptying of the colon may require suppositories or digital removal to reinforce reflex defecation. In the chronic stage of "reconditioning," bulking agents, stool softeners, and a program featuring planned attempts at defecating will be required. Postprandial timing and a sitting posture will be helpful at this point. The anal sphincteric reflexes are retained in most paraplegics.

Guttmann L: Spinal Cord Injuries: Comprehensive Management and Research. 2nd ed. Oxford, Blackwell Scientific, 1976. *The most comprehensive discussion of pathophysiology, clinical features and practical therapy of this problem; written by the pioneer of systematic care for spinal injuries.*

*This use is not listed in the manufacturer's directive.

Drugs That Modify Intestinal Motility

Whether or not diarrhea should be equated with rapid movement of contents through the bowel and constipation with slow transit, drugs that are used to treat these conditions are often assumed to alter motility and, hence, to modify absorption. Few reliable data are available, however, to support the concept that rapid transit impairs absorption, or the reverse. Indeed, dual effects seem more likely; thus, antidiarrheals of proven efficacy, such as the opiates, slow transit and may also have primary effects on epithelial function to enhance absorption. Some newer drugs that modify intestinal motility and transit have been introduced recently, but some are still under investigation and are not freely available in the United States at the time of writing.

AGENTS THAT REDUCE MOTILITY AND/OR TRANSIT

1. **Muscarinic blockers of the belladonna-atropine class** ("anticholinergics") have been used traditionally to reduce gastric secretion and intestinal motility. They reduce antral propulsion, delay gastric emptying, and block contractions in the small and large intestines. Some synthetic compounds (e.g., dicyclomine) are suggested to have more specific effects on "spastic" smooth muscle. Most of these drugs have generalized side effects (e.g., ophthalmologic, or on the urinary tract) that limit their usefulness.

2. **Opiates** are effective antidiarrheals, but they actually increase contractile activity in the small intestine. They stimulate propulsive activity initially and briefly, but transit is slowed later. Decreased propulsion despite increased numbers of contractions presumably reflects the stimulation of nonpropulsive, segmenting patterns of motility. Newer antidiarrheals, such as loperamide and diphenoxylate, are thought to act mainly peripherally when given by mouth, without much central opiate effect. Central effects are seen when they are administered parenterally or in large doses.

3. **Alpha-2 adrenergic agonists,** such as clonidine and lidamidine, have antidiarrheal potential. They modify the balance between absorption and secretion of fluids but also reduce motility and slow transit. Their pharmacologic actions include considerable potential for cardiovascular side effects (postural hypotension), especially if the agent (e.g., clonidine) crosses the blood-brain barrier.

4. **Neuropeptides.** Glucagon relaxes and inhibits intestinal smooth muscle and is used often in diagnostic procedures such as intestinal endoscopy and radiology. A brief action and the need for parenteral administration limit its therapeutic utility. Somatostatin inhibits the release of other gastrointestinal peptides, reduces intestinal secretion, and slows transit. It has been used successfully to control the symptoms of the carcinoid syndrome (Ch. 243).

5. **Calcium channel blockers** act at the level of the smooth muscle cell and are being tested for the treatment of "spastic" conditions such as diffuse esophageal spasm and the pain of irritable bowel syndrome.

AGENTS THAT ENHANCE MOTILITY AND/OR TRANSIT

1. **Traditional agents** include those that increase acetylcholine-like activity at the level of the smooth muscle cell, either by anticholinesterase (neostigmine) or choline-like (bethanechol) activity. Durations of action are brief; generalized effects on multiple systems must be anticipated; and they have limited clinical utility, although bethanechol has been used to correct slow gastric emptying.

2. For the treatment of slow transit, including constipatiuon, a novel class of drugs ("prokinetics") has emerged. They appear to act peripherally, possibly through enhancing the release of acetylcholine, although the precise mechanisms are still unclear. **Metaclopramide** normalizes slowed gastric emptying and has proved useful in the treatment of diabetic gastroparesis. Drug resistance has limited its long-term utility, and it has little action on the distal small bowel or colon. **Domperidine**, which has antidopaminergic properties, has effects that are also confined largely to the stomach and duodenum. **Cisapride** has been tested extensively in Europe

and appears more likely to provide broader stimulation of the small and large bowels.

3. The traditional "stimulant laxatives" promote propulsive motility, especially in the colon. The mechanisms of action are unclear, and long-term use may lead to permanent changes in the enteric nervous system and colonic atony.

Burks TF: Actions of drugs on gastrointestinal motility. In Johnson LR (ed.): Physiology of the Gastrointestinal Tract. New York, Raven Press, 1981. *Classic pharmacologic treatment of the subject, extensively referenced for background and basic sciences.*

First International Cisapride Investigators' Meeting. Digestion 34:137, 1986. *A group of 50 preliminary reports on the use of this novel stimulant of intestinal motility, which appears to act from esophagus to colon.*

103   DIARRHEA

Guenter J. Krejs

Diarrhea is defined as the presence of stool liquidity (instead of formed or soft stool) and an increase in daily stool weight, the upper normal limit of which is 200 grams in industrialized societies. Diarrhea is usually associated with increased stool frequency (more than three bowel movements per day) and is often accompanied by urgency, perianal discomfort, and incontinence. Some patients may have increased frequency and liquidity of stools, however, when their daily stool weights are less than 200 grams. Since diarrhea results from a disturbance in the normal flow and transport of gut fluids, the normal physiology of absorption in the digestive tract will first be considered.

NORMAL PHYSIOLOGY

DELIVERY, FLOW, AND ABSORPTION RATES. During fasting, the intestine contains very little fluid, but when three normal meals per day are eaten, about 9 liters of fluid are delivered to the proximal duodenum. Approximately 2 liters of this fluid are from ingested food and liquids, the rest being digestive secretions.

The volume of chyme that passes through different segments of the small bowel depends on the type of food that has been eaten. For example, meals containing high concentrations of sugar are hypertonic, and when such meals are ingested, the volume of material passing through the jejunum is even greater than the volume that enters the proximal duodenum. On the other hand, after isotonic or hypotonic meals (such as a meal of steak, potatoes, and tea), the volume of fluid traversing the jejunum is much less than that which was delivered to the duodenum. (These considerations are especially important in patients who have had gastric surgery or intestinal resection.) In either case, the osmolality of chyme is adjusted toward that of plasma as fluid travels through the duodenum and upper jejunum, and by the time chyme reaches the ileum, most of the dietary sugars, amino acids, and fats have been absorbed. Fluid arriving at the ileum is mainly an isotonic salt solution and therefore similar in its ionic composition to plasma. The ileum absorbs much, but not all, of this salt solution. About 1 liter per day of this isotonic unabsorbed ileal fluid enters the colon. Although ileal fluid resembles plasma with regard to its sodium and potassium concentrations, the concentrations of chloride and bicarbonate are quite different, being approximately 70 and 60 mEq per liter, respectively.

The colon can absorb 2 to 4 liters of isotonic salt solution per day (even more in patients with secondary hyperaldosteronism associated with salt depletion). The presence of nonabsorbable and osmotically active solutes from the diet and from bacterial action, a relatively slow rate of absorption

from the rectosigmoid, and timely bowel movements prevent complete fluid absorption and desiccation of the fecal mass. About 100 ml of fluid is excreted in the feces; its sodium and chloride concentrations are about 50 mEq per liter, while the potassium concentration is about 90 mEq per liter. This fluid also contains a high concentration of volatile fatty acids (from bacterial action on nondigestible carbohydrates), which dissipate most of the unabsorbed or secreted bicarbonate ions and which often cause stool fluid to be hypertonic to plasma. Since the gastrointestinal tract does not have a diluting mechanism, the osmolality of fecal fluid is never less than the osmolality of plasma.

To summarize, daily volumes of fluid traversing the duodenum are 9 liters, traversing the ileocecal valve area are 1 liter, and traversing the anal sphincter are 0.1 liter. Stated in another way, the small bowel absorbs 8 liters of fluid per day and empties 1 liter into the colon, and the colon absorbs 0.9 liter. Theoretically 2 to 4 liters of fluid would have to be delivered to the colon per day before diarrhea would ensue, provided that delivery rates were steady, the fluid contained no abnormal solutes, and colon function was normal. Unfortunately, the latter qualifications do not apply in many gastrointestinal diseases.

TRANSPORT PHYSIOLOGY. The mechanisms responsible for fluid absorption differ in different regions of the gut and in different species. According to the model for the ileum shown in Figure 103–1, the brush border membrane contains a carrier that facilitates the simultaneous entry of Na^+ and glucose into the cells; Na^+ cannot enter without glucose. A separate pair of exchange carriers works together to facilitate the simultaneous and electrically neutral entry of Na^+ and Cl^-. Na^+ enters in exchange for H^+, and Cl^- enters in exchange for HCO_3^-. If these two exchange carriers operate at the same rate, Na^+ and Cl^- are absorbed in equal amounts, and H^+ and HCO_3^- are secreted in equal amounts and react in the lumen to form CO_2 and water. However, the anion carrier usually operates more rapidly than the cation carrier, and there is a net secretion of HCO_3^-. (This accounts for the high concentration of HCO_3^- and the low concentration of Cl^- in fluid that the ileum delivers to the colon.) Once inside the cell (via either the Na^+/H^+ exchange or the Na^+-glucose carrier), Na^+ is pumped out of the cell across the basolateral membrane by a pump that is probably an Na^+-K^+ adenosine triphosphatase (ATPase). Chloride and glucose exit the basolateral membrane by facilitated or passive diffusion.

Sodium pumping at the basolateral membrane causes a potential difference (PD) across the mucosa (serosal side positive). However, the tight junctions between small bowel mucosal cells (the "shunt pathway") are "leaky," and passive diffusion of anions (in the absorptive direction from lumen to plasma) or cations (in the secretory direction) readily dissipates the PD. Therefore, the residual PD across small bowel mucosa is only 2 to 4 mV.

Colonic cells and colonic transport are somewhat different. The brush border membrane apparently has a carrier for Na^+ that is not influenced by glucose or other actively absorbed nonelectrolytes (glucose is not absorbed in the colon). There is no convincing evidence for Na^+-H^+ exchange, but the brush border membrane appears to have an anion exchange carrier that facilitates chloride absorption and bicarbonate secretion. The tight junctions are "tight," so the electrical gradient generated by the basolateral membrane pump is sustained. The PD is, therefore, about 30 mV (serosal side positive).

Potassium movement in all regions of the gut is passive, in response to electrochemical gradients. Thus, passive potassium absorption in the colon is retarded (owing to the high lumen negative PD), and the potassium concentration in fecal fluid is much higher than in plasma (up to 100 mEq per liter). Water movement throughout the gut is passive, secondary to osmotic pressure gradients generated by active solute transport.

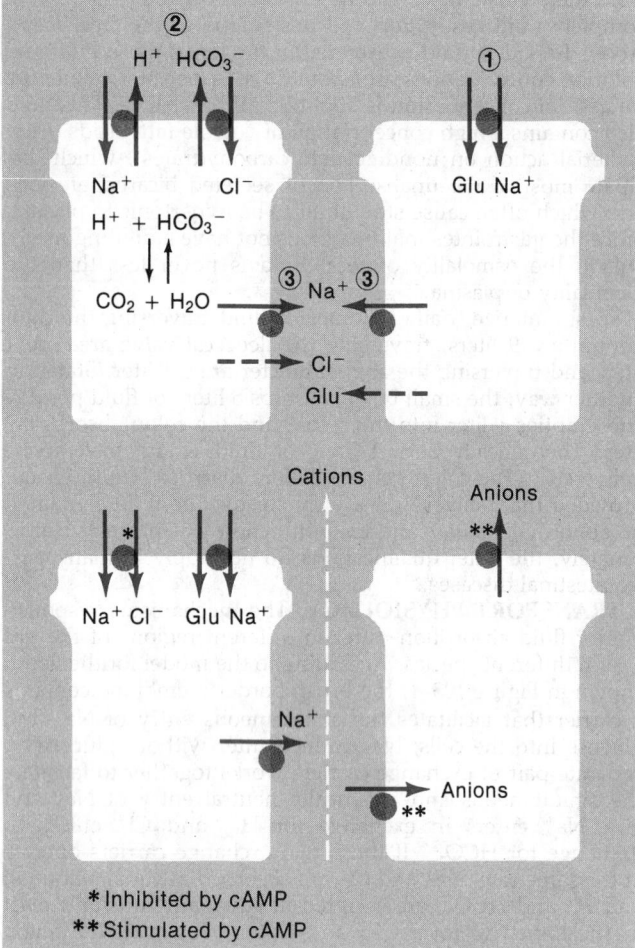

*Inhibited by cAMP
**Stimulated by cAMP

FIGURE 103–1. *Top,* Active transport mechanisms in the human ileum. *1,* Brush border glucose-sodium carrier. *2,* Double exchange carriers for neutral NaCl entry. *3,* Basolateral membrane sodium pump. *Bottom,* Model of cyclic AMP–mediated change in intestinal transport. Active anion secretion is stimulated (**), and there is inhibition of neutral NaCl entry across the brush border membrane (*). The glucose-sodium entry carrier and the basolateral membrane sodium pump are intact. Cations are secreted passively via the tight junction pathway.

NORMAL SMALL BOWEL SECRETION. Small intestinal cells normally secrete as well as absorb electrolytes and water, with the secretory rate normally being of less magnitude than the absorptive rate, so that the net effect of small bowel transport processes is absorption of fluid. (Although it is possible that the same cell might both absorb and secrete, the putative small bowel secretion probably originates in crypt cells, whereas absorption takes place from villous cells.) This is an extremely important concept, because it means that a hormone or toxin might reduce net absorption rate in either of two ways: (1) by stimulating secretion, and (2) by inhibiting absorption. In either case, the observed effect is reduced absorption. Similarly, a hormone or a toxin might cause small bowel secretion by stimulating active secretion, so that it overwhelms the normal absorptive process; or a hormone or a toxin could cause secretion by inhibiting absorption, so that the normal small bowel secretion is unmasked. In fact, many toxins and hormones appear capable of both stimulating secretion and inhibiting normal absorption (see below). In patients with diarrhea caused by toxins or hormones, it is difficult to ascertain which of these factors is predominant.

In the colon, absorption takes place from the surface epithelial cells. There is no evidence for or against a normal colonic secretion.

PATHOPHYSIOLOGY OF DIARRHEA

Diarrhea may result from one or more of the following four mechanisms. There is, in addition, a miscellaneous group for which a single mechanism cannot currently be identified:

1. Poorly absorbable, osmotically active solutes in the intestinal lumen.
2. Active ion secretion.
3. Deranged intestinal motility.
4. Altered mucosal morphology or loss of absorptive surface.
5. Miscellaneous (several mechanisms or pathophysiology not clearly understood).

Osmotic Diarrhea

Osmotic diarrhea is caused by the accumulation of nonabsorbed solutes in the gut lumen. There are three main subtypes: (1) ingestion of poorly absorbable solutes, such as saline purgatives; (2) maldigestion of ingested food, such as in lactase deficiency; and (3) failure of a mucosal transport mechanism, such as in glucose-galactose malabsorption (Table 103–1). Being osmotically active, these solutes cause water and salts to be retained within the intestinal lumen, resulting in diarrhea.

Osmotic diarrhea stops when the patient fasts (or stops ingesting the poorly absorbable solute). Furthermore, the fecal fluid has a large solute gap, i.e., normal electrolytes do not account for much of the fecal fluid osmolality (fecal solute gap = [osmolality] − 2[(Na$^+$) + (K$^+$)]; the factor of 2 is to account for anions in stool water). An exception is congenital chloridorrhea, in which unabsorbed chloride prevents water absorption. In chloridorrhea the chloride concentration in fecal fluids exceeds the sum of the concentration of sodium and potassium. Such fecal fluid analysis is performed on supernatant stool water following centrifugation of a stool sample in a test tube (30 minutes at 2000 g). In most instances, electrolytes and osmolality will provide meaningful information only if the stools are liquid enough that at the end of centrifugation the supernatant stool water constitutes at least one third of the total sample. In osmotic diarrhea resulting from carbohydrate malabsorption, the concentration in stool of short-chain fatty acids is high, and thus the pH is low (pH 4.0 to 6.0). In some instances it is necessary to measure magnesium (normal less than 12 mM), sulfate (normal less than 5 mM), and phosphate (normal less than 12 mM) in stool water to identify the cause of osmotic diarrhea, especially in surreptitious laxative abuse.

Normal fecal fluid, which can be isolated from stool by dialysis methods, often has a modest solute gap (mainly because of unabsorbed carbohydrates and their bacterial products). Therefore, the presence of a solute gap is suggestive of osmotic diarrhea only if stool volume losses are substantially higher than normal. For example, a modest osmotic gap with

TABLE 103–1. CAUSES OF OSMOTIC DIARRHEA

1. *Ingestion of poorly absorbable solutes*
   Magnesium sulfate, sodium sulfate, citrate-containing laxatives
   Some antacids—Mg(OH)$_2$
   Mannitol, sorbitol (chewing gum, diet candy)
2. *Maldigestion*
   Disaccharidase deficiencies (lactose, sucrose-isomaltose, trehalose intolerance)
   Gastrocolic fistula, jejunoileal bypass, short bowel syndrome
   Postgastrectomy, postvagotomy state
   Chronic intestinal ischemia
   Lactulose therapy
3. *Mucosal transport defects*
   Glucose-galactose malabsorption
   Chloridorrhea
   Congenital sodium diarrhea
   General malabsorption in diffuse disease of small bowel mucosa

a stool weight of only 200 grams per 24 hours would not by itself be suggestive of osmotic diarrhea.

Secretory Diarrhea

The net effect of a secretory stimulus on intestinal mucosa can be either inhibition of absorption or a net luminal gain (secretion) of water and electrolytes. This sequence of net movement changes may follow a dose-response curve, with a low secretagogue dose (e.g., circulating vasoactive intestinal polypeptide concentration) inhibiting intestinal water and ion absorption and a high dose causing net secretion. On a cellular level, both processes can occur at the same time, with inhibition of villus absorption and enhancement of crypt secretion in the small bowel.

Secretory diarrhea is recognized clinically by certain features: Stools are large in volume and watery (more than 1 liter per day), and diarrhea persists with fasting. The stool osmolality can be totally accounted for by normal ionic constituents: $([Na^+] + [K^+]) \times 2$ equals stool osmolality, which is close to the osmolality of plasma. Table 103–2 gives the major causes of secretory diarrhea. A few examples are discussed in detail.

ENTEROTOXIN-INDUCED SECRETION. The classic disease in this category is Asiatic cholera (Ch. 287). Intestinal secretion is caused by cholera toxin; the morphologic appearance of intestinal mucosa, however, remains normal. An increase in intracellular cyclic adenosine monophosphate (cAMP) in cholera mediates active ion secretion by the enterocytes (Fig. 103–1B). Patients may lose 10 to 20 liters of watery stool per day. Mortality was high prior to the introduction of oral rehydration solutions. This therapy is successful because glucose-stimulated sodium absorption remains normal despite ongoing secretion.

Enterotoxigenic *Escherichia coli* strains can produce one or more of at least three types of toxins (one heat-labile and two heat-stable toxins). Intestinal secretion caused by these toxins is responsible for many episodes of acute diarrhea, including traveler's diarrhea (Ch. 289). Enterotoxin is produced by a large number of other bacteria, some of which are also capable of tissue invasion (*Campylobacter jejuni*, *Yersinia enterocolitica*, *Salmonella*, *Shigella*, *Clostridium difficile*, *Staphylococcus aureus*, *Klebsiella pneumoniae*, *Aeromonas*, *Plesiomonas*).

PANCREATIC CHOLERA SYNDROME (Ch. 233). High circulating levels of VIP (vasoactive intestinal polypeptide) cause intestinal water and electrolyte secretion that results in large-volume diarrhea. In adults, VIP production usually comes from tumors originating in pancreatic islet cells, whereas in children these tumors are often ganglioneuromas or ganglioneuroblastomas. The disease can be mimicked by prolonged intravenous VIP infusion in healthy subjects. This syndrome is also known as Verner-Morrison syndrome, VIP-oma syndrome, or watery diarrhea-hypokalemia-hypochlorhydria (WDHH) syndrome. Diarrhea disappears when plasma VIP levels return to normal following tumor resection. Fifty per cent of patients have metastatic disease at diagnosis, however, so that resection is not possible.

In one study of patients with pancreatic cholera, mean daily stool weights averaged 4224 grams during a regular diet and 1817 grams during fasting. Hypokalemia and metabolic acidosis due to large fecal potassium and bicarbonate losses are prominent features, whereas hypochlorhydria is variable. Cosecretion of calcitonin, pancreatic polypeptide, PHM (peptide histidine methionine), or helodermin by these tumors has been found in a number of patients.

IDIOPATHIC SECRETORY DIARRHEA. Patients with this syndrome present with the large-volume secretory diarrhea and other clinical features of pancreatic cholera, but no evidence of tumor or of an abnormally elevated concentration of a circulating secretagogue can be found. These patients undergo extensive negative investigations that often include exploratory laparotomy. Autopsy examination may also be unrevealing, and the etiology remains unknown. Both the severity of this syndrome and the prognosis vary widely. Spontaneous resolution of the diarrhea may occur after several months. A few patients respond to opiates.

CARCINOID SYNDROME (Ch. 243). Diarrhea is a common manifestation of the carcinoid syndrome, occurring in about 70 to 80 per cent of patients. In most patients, intestinal secretion can be demonstrated. Serotonin and substance P elicit intestinal water and ion secretion in experimental animals, and these agents are often elevated in the plasma of patients with the carcinoid syndrome. In other patients, the diarrhea appears episodic and possibly associated with the hypermotility that can be demonstrated when serotonin is given intravenously to normal volunteers. In addition, other contributing causes for diarrhea may be (1) bile salt catharsis if ileal resection was required for tumor removal, (2) lymphatic obstruction due to tumor mass, or (3) subacute intestinal obstruction as a consequence of bowel wall fibrosis induced by the tumor.

MEDULLARY CARCINOMA OF THE THYROID (Ch. 229). Diarrhea occurs in 30 per cent of patients with medullary carcinoma of the thyroid and may precede the presence of a palpable thyroid mass. Circulating calcitonin is the major mediator of intestinal secretion in this syndrome. Since this tumor may be part of multiple endocrine neoplasia syndromes (Ch. 241), first-degree relatives need to be investigated by measuring basal and postprovocation (intravenous pentagastrin) plasma calcitonin concentrations. Other than in medullary carcinoma of the thyroid, calcitonin is also found in high concentrations in the plasma and tumor tissue of a number of patients with endocrine pancreatic tumors (VIPoma, somatostatinoma), but usually it is not the predominant peptide.

ZOLLINGER-ELLISON SYNDROME (Ch. 100). The secretory diarrhea that occurs in gastrinoma (Zollinger-Ellison syndrome) has a unique pathophysiology. Due to the gastric hypersecretion caused by high concentrations of circulating gastrin, an excessive load of acidic fluid enters the small bowel and overwhelms the intestinal absorptive capacity. In such patients, daily delivery of up to 24 liters of acidic fluid to the jejunum can occur in the fasting state. Although the percentage of decrease in luminal flow rates in the intestine is similar to that in healthy subjects, the remaining fecal volume is often still in excess of 1 liter per day. Other factors that may play a role in causing diarrhea in gastrinoma are the functional

TABLE 103–2. INTESTINAL SECRETION: DIARRHEAL SYNDROMES AND CORRESPONDING SECRETORY STIMULI

Diarrheal Syndromes	Secretory Stimulus
Traveler's diarrhea, Asiatic cholera	Enterotoxins (*Escherichia coli*, *Vibrio cholerae*)
Laxative abuse	Laxatives (phenolphthalein, senna, bisacodyl)
Pancreatic cholera syndrome	Vasoactive intestinal polypeptide
Medullary carcinoma of the thyroid	Calcitonin
Carcinoid syndrome	Serotonin, substance P
Zollinger-Ellison syndrome	Gastrin
Secreting villous adenoma of the rectum	Prostaglandins
Small intestinal obstruction	Intestinal distention
Diarrhea in patients with portal hypertension plus severe hypoalbuminemia	Increased hydrostatic vascular pressure and tissue pressure
Congenital chloridorrhea (intestinal secretion in some instances); lethal familial protracted diarrhea	Congenital mucosal ion transport defects
Giardiasis, strongyloidosis, amebiasis	Unknown mechanism activated by protozoa
Idiopathic chronic secretory diarrhea (pseudopancreatic cholera syndrome)	Unknown
Collagen vascular diseases (scleroderma, systemic lupus erythematosus, mixed connective tissue disease)	Unknown
Intestinal lymphoma	Unknown

or morphologic impairment of the mucosal brush border by the abnormal acid milieu, the direct effect of excessive gastrin on the small bowel mucosa (reducing absorption), and inactivation of pancreatic lipase by the acidic fluid, causing a mild degree of steatorrhea. Low intraluminal pH may also cause some of the primary bile acids to become insoluble, leading to a reduction of micelle formation and a mild degree of steatorrhea.

BILE ACID DIARRHEA. Watery diarrhea in cholerrheic enteropathy results from the secretory effect of malabsorbed bile acids on colonic mucosa. Interruption of the normal enterohepatic circulation of bile acids can be caused by three types of bile acid malabsorption. Type I is due to ileal disease or resection. Type II, which is less common, consists of a selective ileal transport defect for bile acids. Type III is bile acid malabsorption in the postcholecystectomy and postvagotomy state. Cholestyramine is the treatment of choice for Type I and Type II bile acid diarrhea. Patients with Type III are rarely found to have secretory concentrations of fecal bile acids and rarely respond to cholestyramine.

Deranged Intestinal Motility

On a priori grounds, three major derangements might cause diarrhea: (1) Abnormally reduced peristalsis may allow bacterial overgrowth in the small bowel. (2) "Intestinal hurry" may reduce contact time between the small bowel mucosa and its contents and thus result in delivery of abnormally large and qualitatively abnormal fluid loads to the colon. This occurs in spite of the fact that absorption in the small bowel is normal per unit of time. (3) Premature emptying of the colon caused by an abnormality of its contents, or by intrinsic colonic "irritability" or inflammation, results in a reduced contact between luminal contents and colonic mucosa and therefore increased volume and liquidity of the stools.

Some diarrheal diseases due, at least in part, to deranged motility are irritable bowel syndrome, malignant carcinoid syndrome, postvagotomy diarrhea, diarrhea resulting from diabetic neuropathy, diarrhea resulting from thyrotoxicosis, and the diarrhea associated with postgastrectomy dumping syndrome. Abnormal motility may also contribute to acute diarrhea caused by infections. Stool analysis in diarrhea due to a motility disturbance may be consistent with that in osmotic diarrhea if nutrient absorption is impaired in the small bowel or may resemble that in secretory diarrhea, if, following nutrient absorption, the ileocecal transit volume remains largely unabsorbed. Alternatively, a mixed pattern can exist, with electrolytes accounting for an osmolality equal to that of plasma and an additional component making stool water hyperosmolar, owing mainly to bacterial metabolism of malabsorbed carbohydrates in the collection unit following passage of the stool. Irritable bowel syndrome and fecal incontinence will be discussed in more detail.

IRRITABLE BOWEL SYNDROME. In the United States, up to 50 per cent of all patients seen by primary care physicians for digestive tract problems have irritable bowel syndrome. Diarrhea is usually referred to as functional diarrhea, since no obvious cause can be found on extensive routine clinical testing. On special investigations, altered myoelectric activity in the large bowel and a significant acceleration in small bowel transit have been demonstrated in patients with irritable bowel syndrome and diarrhea. At the present time, however, it is unclear what clinical relevance these findings may have in the diagnostic and therapeutic management of such patients.

Although functional diarrhea as part of the irritable bowel syndrome is generally considered a diagnosis by exclusion, this does not mean that extensive testing is necessary when one is initially confronted with such a patient. Rather, a positive diagnosis can often be made at the first interview. This is based mainly on a typical history: abdominal pain of long duration (often for several years), discomfort and pain in different areas of the abdomen, bloating associated with various so-called food intolerances, and alternating diarrhea and constipation. Functional diarrhea may show a temporal relation to meal intake, and nocturnal diarrhea is typically absent. Furthermore, signs of systemic disease, such as weight loss, are usually absent. Classically, patients are female and in their 20's and 30's, and a history of emotional conflict, stress, or anxiety is common.

In functional diarrhea, stool weight rarely exceeds 500 grams per day (normal less than 200 grams). In a patient who complains of an increased frequency of defecation, a normal or nearly normal 24-hour stool weight may be the first clue to fecal incontinence, a diagnosis often confused with functional diarrhea.

INCONTINENCE. Most patients whose major disability is due to fecal incontinence present to their physician with "diarrhea." Either they are embarrassed to mention the incontinence, or they interpret it as a manifestation of severe diarrhea. If patients do mention incontinence, the physician also usually attributes it to voluminous diarrhea. In most instances, however, these patients are suffering primarily from a defect in the continence mechanisms rather than from severe diarrhea. As a matter of fact, quantitative stool collections usually reveal rather small fecal volumes, even though stools are soft to liquid in consistency. In any case, the major problem in most such patients is in the anal continence mechanisms. The most frequent causes for sphincter dysfunction are previous anal surgery for fissures, fistulas, or hemorrhoids; episiotomy or tear during childbirth; anal Crohn's disease; and diabetic neuropathy.

Anal sphincter training may improve sphincter function and reduce the frequency of incontinent episodes. It is also important to establish the cause of diarrhea if possible, since effective therapy of the diarrhea will usually prevent further incontinence. Symptomatic therapy with opiate drugs is helpful in some patients. There is recent interest in surgical treatment for incontinence, but no good prospective studies have been done. No therapy for incontinence in patients with diarrhea, whether involving drugs, biofeedback, or surgery, has included objective data that convincingly establish its benefit.

Morphologic Alterations

Efficient intestinal absorption requires that the intestinal mucosa be intact with a well-functioning blood supply and intact neural connections. A large number of diseases can cause diarrhea by disrupting the normal anatomy of the intestine (Table 103–3).

VIRAL GASTROENTERITIS. It is estimated that every year 5 million children less than two years of age will die in

TABLE 103–3. DIARRHEA DUE TO DISRUPTION OF STRUCTURAL INTEGRITY OF THE INTESTINE

Viral gastroenteritis
Bacterial infection with tissue invasion
Sprue (tropical, nontropical, collagenous)
Whipple's disease
Radiation enteritis
Drugs (e.g., chemotherapeutic agents)
Amyloidosis
Collagen vascular diseases (systemic lupus erythematosus, scleroderma, mixed connective tissue disease)
Inflammatory bowel disease (Crohn's disease, ulcerative colitis, microscopic and collagenous colitis)
Eosinophilic gastroenteritis
Intestinal lymphoma
Ileocecal tuberculosis
Intestinal ischemia, mesenteric vasculitis
Diverticulitis
Pelvic inflammatory disease
Acquired immunodeficiency syndrome (AIDS)

developing countries as a consequence of acute diarrhea. Rotavirus is responsible for at least 50 per cent of these infections. The pathogenesis of viral diarrhea is thought to be as follows. The virus enters the absorptive epithelial cells on the tip of the villus, and these cells are sloughed off. Crypt cells then move quickly to replace the lost enterocytes. These cells, however, are immature and cannot absorb effectively. Their sucrase and lactase activities are low, whereas adenylate cyclase activity and cAMP content are normal (in contrast to cholera, in which sucrase and lactase activities are normal and adenylate cyclase activity and cAMP content are increased). There is no enhanced water and electrolyte secretion in viral gastroenteritis; however, sodium-stimulated glucose absorption is markedly diminished. Malabsorption of water, electrolytes, and nutrients results until the infection subsides and mature enterocytes again coat the surface of the villus.

SPRUE (Ch. 104). The changes associated with sprue involve villous atrophy and a marked diminution in the effective absorptive surface of the bowel. When studied with intestinal perfusion techniques, such patients demonstrate jejunal secretion. This can be expected from the observation that the mucosa in total villous atrophy consists only of crypts, and crypts normally secrete fluid and electrolytes. Diarrhea is a result of fat and carbohydrate malabsorption. Typically, there is no diarrhea when these patients fast, suggesting that the colon reabsorbs the small bowel secretions. In rare cases patients with sprue have severe secretory diarrhea; a stool output as high as 5 liters a day has been observed.

RADIATION ENTERITIS. Acute radiation enteritis usually occurs within the initial weeks of radiation exposure and is characterized by abdominal cramping, diarrhea, nausea, and vomiting. With the passage of time, symptoms abate, and a quiescent period ensues. The average onset of further symptoms is one year, but symptoms may occur at any time. Malabsorption of varying degree for bile acids, fat, carbohydrate, and vitamin B_{12} is observed. Interference with absorption occurs owing to infiltration of the mucosa by inflammatory cells and luminal narrowing of the submucosal arterioles with fibrin plugs. Disturbances in motility due to the effects of radiation on the muscularis propria can also contribute to the diarrhea. Late-appearing structural changes with intermittent obstruction, mucosal ulceration, and fistula formation may also lead to diarrhea. Medical therapy with antidiarrheal agents, broad-spectrum antibiotics for bacterial overgrowth, and prednisone rarely provides total control of symptoms. Ultimately, 15 per cent of patients will require surgical intervention, such as segmental resection or fistula closure.

LOSS OF ABSORPTIVE SURFACE. The diarrhea that results from intestinal resection may be on the basis of the region removed (e.g., ileum, with its special transport sites for active bile acid absorption) or of the length of bowel resected. At least 50 per cent of the small bowel is required in order to avoid diarrhea and malnutrition associated with the short bowel syndrome.

AIDS (ACQUIRED IMMUNODEFICIENCY SYNDROME) (Ch. 346). Small intestinal morphologic alterations and consequent malabsorption and diarrhea are common among patients with the acquired immunodeficiency syndrome. Infectious agents (*Giardia, Salmonella, Cryptosporidium,* and *Stronglyoides*) and Kaposi's sarcoma can cause gastrointestinal disturbancs in AIDS. There remains a group of patients, however, who do not have identifiable infectious or parasitic agents or Kaposi's sarcoma but who still manifest diarrhea, malabsorption, and weight loss. Such patients have abnormal D-xylose and fat absorption. Duodenal biopsies reveal blunting of the villi and an inflammatory infiltrate in the lamina propria. This condition is referred to as AIDS enteropathy. Other patients with AIDS may demonstrate a histiocytic infiltrate (pseudo-Whipple's disease) containing numerous acid-fast organisms. *Mycobacterium avium intracellulare* has been isolated in these patients.

TABLE 103–4. MISCELLANEOUS CAUSES OF DIARRHEA

Drugs
    Diuretics, cardiac glycosides, propranolol, quinidine, colchicine, antibiotics, methotrexate, 6-mercaptopurine, 5-fluorouracil, guanethidine, ethanol
Endocrine disorders
    Addison's disease, hypoparathyroidism
Neurologic diseases
    Tabes dorsalis, multiple sclerosis, myelitis, encephalitis, heat stroke, Charcot-Marie-Tooth disease, myotonia dystrophica, orthostatic hypotension
Toxicologic disorders
    Lead poisoning
Immunoglobulin deficiency
Allergy
Systemic mastocytosis

MICROSCOPIC COLITIS. Some patients with chronic diarrhea demonstrate inflammation of colonic mucosa despite a normal appearance of the colon on barium enema and colonoscopy. The histologic changes consist of excess neutrophils and round cells in the lamina propria, cryptitis, and reactive changes of surface epithelial cells. When colonic absorption is measured in these patients by perfusion techniques, water and electrolyte absorption is either abolished or abnormally low. Thus, the normal ileocecal transit volume (1 liter per day) remains largely unabsorbed, and stool weights are typically in the range of 400 to 800 grams per day.

Miscellaneous Causes of Diarrhea

Table 103–4 gives a list of diseases in which several of the discussed mechanisms may cause diarrhea or in which the pathophysiology is not clearly understood.

DIAGNOSIS

Although the cause of diarrhea is obvious in many clinical situations, in many others it is not. Here we are concerned with a diagnostic approach to the patient with diarrhea in whom the cause is unknown.

History and Physical Examination

When the stools are consistently large in volume, the underlying cause of diarrhea is likely to be located in the small bowel or in the proximal colon. By contrast, in small-volume diarrhea, in which the patient has frequent urges to defecate but passes only small amounts of feces or mucus, the disorder is usually in the left portion of the colon and rectum. Passage of blood mixed in with the diarrheal stool usually indicates inflammation of the mucosa, less often a neoplasm. Passage of nonbloody mucus suggests irritable bowel syndrome, as does a history of small-volume diarrhea alternating with constipation. Frothy stools and excessive flatus suggest fermentation of unabsorbed carbohydrates. Excessively foul stools suggest putrefaction of unabsorbed amino acids. Visible oil or fat indicates severe steatorrhea. Fecal soiling (incontinence) suggests an anal sphincter defect. Diarrhea in a patient with features of anorexia nervosa suggests laxative abuse.

There are, of course, many other pertinent facts obtainable from the history, including previous surgery, drug intake (Table 103–4), symptoms of systemic illness, travel, and related illnesses in family members. In chronic and recurrent diarrhea, an association of exacerbation of diarrhea with emotional stress should be sought, an association that may suggest irritable bowel syndrome. The patient's sexual history should be discussed, as male homosexuals have a high incidence of shigellosis, giardiasis, other intestinal infections, and the usually recognized venereal diseases. Diarrhea may be the presenting manifestation of AIDS.

The physical examination may provide clues to the cause of diarrhea. Some physical findings, as well as other clinical associations that may assist in the diagnosis of diarrhea, are listed in Table 103–5.

TABLE 103–5. CLUES TO DIAGNOSIS OF DIARRHEA FROM OTHER SYMPTOMS, SIGNS, AND LABORATORY TESTS

Symptom or Sign Associated with Diarrhea	Diagnoses To Be Considered
Arthritis	Ulcerative colitis, Crohn's disease, Whipple's disease
Liver disease	Ulcerative colitis, Crohn's disease, bowel malignancy with metastasis to liver
Fever	Ulcerative colitis, Crohn's disease, amebiasis, lymphoma, tuberculosis
Marked weight loss	Malabsorption, inflammatory bowel disease, cancer, thyrotoxicosis
Eosinophilia	Eosinophilic gastroenteritis, parasitic disease
Lymphadenopathy	Lymphoma, Whipple's disease, AIDS
Neuropathy	Diabetic diarrhea, amyloidosis
Postural hypotension	Diabetic diarrhea, Addison's disease, idiopathic orthostatic hypotension
Flushing, large liver	Malignant carcinoid syndrome
Proteinuria	Amyloidosis
Perianal disease or right lower quadrant abdominal mass	Crohn's disease
Purpura	Celiac disease
Peptic ulcer	Zollinger-Ellison syndrome, antacid therapy, gastrocolic fistula
Following cholecystectomy	Bile acid malabsorption
Frequent infections	Immunoglobulin deficiency, AIDS
Immunodeficiency	Giardiasis, nodular lymphoid hyperplasia, celiac sprue
Hyperpigmentation	Whipple's disease, celiac disease, Addison's disease
Good response to corticosteroids	Ulcerative colitis, Crohn's disease, Whipple's disease, Addison's disease, pancreatic cholera, eosinophilic enteritis
Good response to antibiotics	Bacterial overgrowth in small intestine, tropical sprue, Whipple's disease, celiac disease

Diagnostic Tests

ROUTINE EXAMINATION OF STOOL. Unless the diagnosis is readily apparent from the history and physical examination, certain relatively simple studies on the stool should routinely be performed. Regardless of the clinical classification, the information obtained will usually narrow the diagnostic possibilities.

Stain for Pus. The presence or absence of intestinal inflammation can often be ascertained by examination of a stained stool specimen. Wright's or methylene blue stains are satisfactory. The presence of large numbers of white blood cells is diagnostic of inflammation. The presence of rare, scattered white cells is within normal limits.

In patients with acute or traveler's diarrhea, pus in the stool suggests invasion of the mucosa by *Shigella, E. coli, Entamoeba histolytica, Salmonella, Campylobacter*, gonococci, or other invasive organisms. In general, shigellosis and invasive *E. coli* infections cause more pus than *Salmonella* and *E. histolytica* infections. Antibiotic-related colitis may or may not be associated with pus. Diarrhea caused by noninvasive organisms that produce enterotoxins (toxigenic *E. coli*, for example), viruses, and *Giardia* is not associated with pus in the stool.

In patients with chronic and recurrent diarrhea or diarrhea of unknown etiology, pus suggests colitis of some type—idiopathic ulcerative colitis, Crohn's colitis, antibiotic-associated colitis, amebic colitis, ischemic colitis, or tuberculous colitis. Pus is especially abundant in idiopathic ulcerative colitis and tends to be less so in amebic colitis. It is usually absent in microscopic colitis. Absence of pus on a single examination does not, of course, absolutely rule out any of these entities. Radiation-induced disease of the large or small bowel and Crohn's disease limited to the small intestine may or may not be associated with pus in the stool. Pus is not present in the stools of patients with irritable bowel syndrome, most causes of malabsorption syndrome, laxative abuse, viral gastroenteritis, and giardiasis.

Occult Blood. Occult (or gross) blood in association with diarrhea usually indicates inflammation and therefore usually has the same significance as pus in the stools (see above). When blood is present in diarrheal stools that do not contain pus, one should consider neoplasms of the colon, heavy metal poisoning, and acute ischemic damage to the gut.

Sudan Stain for Fat. If excess fat is evident on Sudan stain, steatorrhea is probably present, and the various causes of malabsorption syndromes should be considered (see Ch. 104). Most such patients will have chronic and recurrent diarrhea; steatorrhea in a patient with acute or traveler's diarrhea suggests giardiasis.

Alkalinization. A pink color following alkalinization of a stool or urine sample indicates phenolphthalein ingestion as the cause of diarrhea. The test is so easily and quickly done, and the significance of a positive result is so great, that it should be carried out routinely in female patients with chronic diarrhea. Surreptitious laxative ingestion is rarely seen in males.

OTHER TESTS. Evidence of systemic illness will have obvious implications in the etiology of diarrhea (Table 103–5). For instance, a history of flushing and diarrhea will lead to determination of urinary 5-hydroxyindole acetic acid (Ch. 243). The order in which tests are carried out, assuming that further tests are necessary, will vary according to the physician's intuition regarding a particular patient. Certain of the diagnostic tests deserve brief discussion here.

Search for Infectious and Parasitic Organisms. It is important to complete the examination for parasites and to have adequate bacterial cultures in progress prior to examination of the patient with radiologic contrast media because barium interferes with successful demonstration of pathogens. Failure to find *Giardia* in stool samples is not strong evidence against giardiasis; sometimes it is necessary to examine duodenal fluid in order to demonstrate this organism. *Cryptosporidium* can be revealed by acid-fast stain of feces subjected to a flotation technique for concentration. Special culture methods are required if the presence of infection by *Gonococcus, Campylobacter*, or *Yersinia* is to be established. A microimmunofluorescent test with monoclonal antibodies can be used on a rectal mucosal smear to assess for chlamydial proctitis. Serologic tests for amebae and lymphogranuloma venereum may assist in the diagnosis in some patients. Finally, tests for clostridial toxin in fecal fluid will help in the diagnosis of pseudomembranous colitis.

Proctosigmoidoscopy. Proctosigmoidoscopy is helpful in establishing the presence or absence of mucosal inflammation. In antibiotic-associated diarrhea, it may reveal pseudomembranes. Proctosigmoidoscopy is often essential in patients with chronic and recurrent diarrhea and in patients with diarrhea of unknown etiology. The findings are especially apt to be abnormal in those whose stools contain pus or blood or both; they are usually normal in patients with diarrhea caused by the various malabsorption syndromes.

Proctosigmoidoscopy to investigate diarrhea should be done without enemas, laxatives, or suppositories. Such preparation may wash away exudate, distort the mucosa, induce trauma, and possibly obscure evidence of disease or create the false impression of disease. In almost all instances, fecal matter can easily be aspirated or pushed aside, and since most abnormalities are diffuse, fecal matter does not interfere greatly with a satisfactory examination. The presence of solid stool in the rectum of a patient who supposedly has diarrhea is also revealing, suggesting that an acute diarrhea is subsiding, that the patient may have irritable bowel syndrome, that the diarrhea is an illusion, or that the diarrhea is secondary to fecal impaction.

Since proctitis may not be evident grossly, even to the experienced eye, mucosal smears should always be obtained and stained for pus. The mucosa should be carefully examined for melanosis coli, although melanosis may be present microscopically even if it is not present grossly.

Rectal Biopsy. Biopsy can often be helpful in the evaluation of patients with diarrhea. The main disorders that might be detected by biopsy, but not by smears and stool examination, are amyloidosis, Whipple's disease, microscopic colitis, granulomatous inflammation, melanosis coli, intestinal spirochetosis (other than that caused by *Treponema pallidum*), and schistosomiasis. Biopsy is indicated in patients with diarrhea of unknown origin, especially in a search for melanosis coli and unsuspected colitis that may not have been evident grossly. It is the opinion of this author that irritable bowel syndrome should not be diagnosed until after a rectal mucosal smear has shown that pus is not present and a rectal biopsy is found to reveal no abnormality. The biopsy should be taken from the posterior wall of the rectum on a valve. Although the risk is uncertain, some clinicians believe that a rectal biopsy with large forceps predisposes to a colonic perforation if a barium enema is done within ten days of the biopsy.

Quantitative Fecal Fat. Collected stools (usually for 72 hours) should be quantitatively analyzed for fat content (1) when malabsorption is suggested by the history and physical examination, (2) when the qualitative test for fecal fat is positive, or (3) routinely in patients with diarrhea of unknown origin. If steatorrhea is present, the differential diagnosis of malabsorption syndrome can be pursued (see Ch. 104). Of course, the results of this test must be interpreted with knowledge of the approximate intake of dietary fat. Stool weight in grams (which is equivalent to stool volume in milliliters) should also be noted and recorded (see below).

Twenty-four-hour Stool Volume. For reasons indicated under History and Physical Examination above, knowledge of stool volume helps localize the region of the intestine that is most likely responsible for diarrhea, and in several instances specific information on stool volume is of great diagnostic help. For example, stool volumes greater than 500 ml per day are rarely seen in patients with irritable bowel syndrome, and stool volumes of less than 1000 ml per day provide evidence against pancreatic cholera syndrome. In addition, very large measured stool volumes will alert the physician to the need for vigorous fluid replacement therapy.

Collection of 24-hour stool specimens is easy to do in the initial phases of a diarrhea workup, prior to barium radiographs, enemas, or other preparations. With a little effort, it can be accurately done on an outpatient basis. If a record of stool frequency is kept, the average volume of each stool can be calculated, and the results may give useful insight.

In special instances, e.g., in diarrhea of unknown origin, it is useful to measure stool electrolytes and osmolality and to determine whether or not the diarrhea persists during a 48-hour fast (while the patient is given glucose and salt solutions intravenously). These results will help establish whether the diarrhea is secretory or osmotic in type (see Pathophysiology, above). If the osmolality of stool water is less than 250 mOsm per kilogram, water has been added to the stool to simulate diarrhea. A sodium concentration in fecal water that is higher than that of plasma indicates contamination by urine.

Vasoactive Intestinal Polypeptide (VIP) and Other Circulating Agents. The pancreatic cholera syndrome should be considered if diarrhea of unknown origin has lasted longer than four weeks, is secretory in type, and is severe (more than 1 liter per day and/or associated with hypokalemia and salt and water depletion), and if surreptitious laxative abuse and organic disease of the gastrointestinal tract have been excluded. The incidence of this syndrome is 1 in 10 million population per year. Only in this rare subgroup of patients is serum assay for VIP, PHM, and calcitonin likely to be helpful. Other gastrointestinal hormones such as pancreatic polypeptide (PP) may be elevated in plasma and serve as markers of endocrine pancreatic malignancy. In the United States, Dr. O'Dorisio's laboratory (Columbus, Ohio) and, in England, Dr. Bloom's laboratory (London) offer a gastrointestinal hormone profile that can be obtained from a single plasma sample. Blood needs to be drawn in iced tubes containing ethylenediamine tetra-acetic acid (EDTA) with aprotinin added to inhibit serum peptidases (aprotinin [Trasylol], 0.5 ml [5000 Kallikrein Inactivator Units] per 10 ml of blood). After immediate centrifugation in a refrigerated centrifuge, plasma is stored at $-25°C$ or lower until sent in a frozen state on dry ice to the appropriate laboratory.

Therapeutic Trials. In some instances therapeutic trials are indicated as diagnostic tests. (Obviously, in most instances, the results must be considered suggestive rather than conclusive.) These trials may include pancreatic enzymes, antibiotics (also as part of the Schilling test), metronidazole or quinacrine (for giardiasis), cholestyramine (for bile acid malabsorption), indomethacin (for prostaglandin synthetase inhibition), and various diets (lactose free, carbohydrate free, low fat, and avoidance of any specific food to evaluate the unlikely possibility of food allergy).

THERAPY

The most satisfactory therapy is to cure the underlying disease. When this is not possible, certain drugs may ameliorate the disease and thus reduce the severity of diarrhea (prednisone for inflammatory bowel disease is an example). In a few instances, the disease cannot be ameliorated, but there is fairly specific therapy for the diarrhea, such as cholestyramine for bile acid malabsorption.

At present, unfortunately, in many patients the disease process responsible for diarrhea cannot be satisfactorily suppressed, and specific therapy is lacking. Supportive and symptomatic therapy is required in such instances.

Fluid Replacement

The most important aspect of therapy in acute and traveler's diarrhea, and in some patients with chronic diarrhea, is prevention or correction of salt and water depletion. This can be done by oral ingestion of liquids and salty foods, oral glucose-saline solutions, or intravenous fluid therapy, as dictated by the clinical situation. Two points deserve emphasis. First, soft drinks, tea, and citrus juices contain little, if any, sodium chloride (even Gatorade contains only 23 mEq per liter of sodium chloride). Second, oral glucose-saline solutions or liquids plus salty foods will actually worsen the diarrhea (in terms of stool volume) as they help correct fluid depletion. The oral rehydration solution recommended by the World Health Organization contains the following in millimoles (grams) per liter; glucose, 111 (20); NaCl, 60 (4); KCl, 20 (2); NaHCO_3, 30 (2); and osmolality is 331 mOsm per kilogram. In some patients, particularly those with short bowel syndrome, a high sodium concentration is needed in the oral rehydration solution to achieve a positive sodium and fluid balance. To prevent hypertonicity of such a solution, glucose is best given as a polymer. Glucose polymer consists of linear chains of mostly five to nine glucose units and is obtained from hydrolysis of starch. Glucose polymer is available as Polycose (Ross Laboratories, Columbus, Ohio) or Moducal (Mead Johnson, Evansville, Indiana) and in England as Caloreen (Roussel Ltd., Wembly Park, England). Glucose polymer is readily hydrolyzed in the gut lumen, providing glucose to the sodium-glucose carrier in the brush border. The solution contains the following in millimoles (grams) per liter: glucose polymer, 20 (20); NaCl, 120 (7); KCl, 10 (1); and osmolality is 280 mOsm per kilogram. Various flavoring substances can be added to this solution (e.g., Kool Aid).

Avoidance or Treatment of Perianal Discomfort

Helpful therapy consists of the following: (1) avoidance of soap, toilet paper, washcloths, and towels; (2) gentle washing with warm water on absorbent cotton after each bowel movement, followed by gentle, thorough drying with absorbent cotton; (3) if seepage is present, absorbent cotton retained next to the anal orifice and held in place by snug underwear; (4) sitz baths for 10 minutes two or three times a day; and (5) hydrocortisone creams (1 per cent). In addition to these measures, patients may obtain relief by additional gentle cleaning with soft pads containing witch hazel (Tucks). Locally applied anesthetic ointments may be transiently helpful, but ointments restrict perspiration and anesthetics may irritate the perianal skin, so these agents should be used only for short periods of time. It is important to recognize specific treatable conditions, such as perianal moniliasis.

Opiates

Codeine, diphenoxylate with atropine (Lomotil), and loperamide reduce urgency, bowel movement frequency, and stool volume in a wide variety of acute or chronic diarrheal illnesses. This is not to say that they have a beneficial effect in every patient; but they do in most, so that when groups of patients are studied, both stool frequency and stool volume are reduced to a statistically significant extent. Of the three drugs, loperamide and codeine are usually somewhat superior to diphenoxylate; loperamide may have less tendency than codeine to cause addiction. Codeine, however, is much less expensive. In chronic diarrhea, the drugs may be given once a day in a maximally tolerated dose or several times daily in smaller doses.

Opiate drugs are generally thought to reduce diarrhea through reducing the propulsive activity of the gut and thereby reducing stool frequency. This mechanism might also enhance contact time between intestinal mucosa and luminal contents. Assuming that at least part of the gut mucosa is in an absorbing and not a secretory state, this would allow greater absorption of fluid and thereby reduce stool volume. In vitro opiates have also been reported to stimulate sodium chloride absorption and to have antisecretory action against several secretagogues. These effects cannot be demonstrated in clinical situations using therapeutic doses of opiate drugs.

Opiates should not be used in patients with severe ulcerative colitis with impending toxic megacolon, and there is evidence suggesting that they may prolong the diarrhea in shigellosis and perhaps in diarrheal diseases caused by other invasive bacteria and in antibiotic-associated diarrhea. These reservations notwithstanding, opiates are often of benefit in the symptomatic relief of diarrhea in patients with less severe ulcerative colitis and with many acute infectious diarrheal illnesses. Obviously, they should be prescribed only when diarrhea is causing significant disability.

There are rare case reports suggesting that opiate drugs can be a cause of paradoxical diarrhea.

Bismuth Subsalicylate

Bismuth subsalicylate may prevent infection with enterotoxin-producing E. coli organisms. In addition, this agent will bring mild symptomatic relief in patients with acute infectious diarrhea, whether bacterial or viral in origin. The mechanism of the effect is unknown. The dose is 30 to 60 ml every 30 minutes for eight doses. Patients should be warned that this medication may turn their stools black. If the patient is on other medications, possible drug interaction should be considered.

Antibiotics in Acute and Traveler's Disease (Ch. 289)

For at least two reasons, antibiotics should not usually be used. First, in most patients they will not shorten the duration of illness. Second, their use risks the development of antibiotic-associated diarrhea or colitis, superimposed on whatever was causing the diarrhea initially. This greatly confuses the problem if the diarrhea becomes chronic.

In mild disease (small-volume diarrhea, no chills or fever, no blood or pus in the stool), antibiotics should not be prescribed unless a specific indication emerges from the bacteriology and parasitology laboratory. In patients who are severely ill, especially if they have blood or pus in the stool, antibiotic therapy aimed at shigellosis is reasonable, pending the result of stool culture.

Antisecretory Drugs

A specific and potent inhibitor of intestinal secretion is not available. On the basis of in vitro observations and individual case reports, a number of agents can be tried on an empiric basis. Phenothiazines inhibit secretion caused by cholera toxin and E. coli enterotoxins; aspirin, indomethacin, and other nonsteroidal anti-inflammatory agents reduce secretion mediated by prostaglandins (inhibition of prostaglandin synthesis); glucocorticoids decrease mucosal inflammation and enhance NaCl absorption (increase in Na-K-ATPase activity); nicotinic acid, clonidine, lidamidine,* and lithium carbonate may increase intestinal NaCl absorption (inhibition of adenylate cyclase), and cromoglycate may inhibit release of mediators of allergic reaction in the intestine. When diarrhea is due to circulating agents (VIPoma, carcinoid), a somatostatin analogue given subcutaneously may abolish diarrhea by decreasing secretagogue release from tumor tissue.

Bo-Linn GW, Vendrell DD, Lee E, et al.: An evaluation of the significance of microscopic colitis in patients with chronic diarrhea. J Clin Invest 75:1559, 1986. *First description of microscopic colitis as a separate disease entity. Patients reveal abolished water and electrolyte absorption during colonic perfusion studies.*

Field M, Fordtran JS, Schultz SG (eds.): Secretory Diarrhea. Bethesda, Md., American Physiological Society, 1980. *Sixteen chapters by different experts on various aspects of the pathophysiology of secretory diarrhea. The emphasis is on basic research, although there is a highly original chapter on the pharmacology of antidiarrheal drugs.*

Krejs GJ (ed.): Diarrhoea. Clin Gastroenterol 15, No 3, 1986. *Thirteen chapters on the pathophysiology and clinical investigation of diarrhea. Contains re-evaluation of criteria for defining secretory diarrhea and extensive description of diarrhée motrice (diarrhea due to motility derangement).*

Krejs GJ: VIPoma syndrome. Am J Med (in print). *An extensive description of pancreatic cholera syndrome, the most prominent example of secretory diarrhea caused by a circulating agent.*

Krejs GJ, Fordtran JS: Diarrhea. In Sleisenger MH, Fordtran JS (eds.): Gastrointestinal Disease. 3rd ed. Philadelphia, W. B. Saunders Company, 1983, pp 257–279. *A detailed description of the physiology of the human intestinal tract with regard to water and electrolyte movement and the pathophysiology of chronic diarrhea.*

Lambert HP (ed.): Infections of the GI tract. Clin Gastroenterol 8, No 3, 1979. *Twelve excellent chapters by different experts dealing with the pathophysiology of diarrhea, viral infections, pathogenic mechanisms in bacterial diarrhea, E. coli, Shigella, food poisoning, typhoid and paratyphoid fever, Campylobacter enteritis, traveler's diarrhea, antibiotic-associated colitis, antibiotic resistance, and antimicrobial agents. The book contains much practical and clinically useful information.*

Read NW, Krejs GJ, Read MG, et al.: Chronic diarrhea of unknown origin. Gastroenterology 78:264, 1980. *A detailed account of the clinical problems encountered in patients with intractable and difficult-to-diagnose chronic diarrhea.*

Santangelo WC, Krejs GJ: Gastrointestinal manifestations of the acquired immunodeficiency syndrome. Am J Med Sci 292:328, 1986. *Complete review of enteric infections, parasitic infestations, enteropathy, gastrointestinal bleeding, and neoplasms in patients with AIDS.*

*Investigational agent.

104 MALABSORPTION

Phillip P. Toskes

The malabsorption syndrome refers to a clinical condition in which a number of nutrients and minerals are not normally absorbed; almost always, however, lipids fail to be normally absorbed. At times the absorption of a single nutrient may be selectively impaired. A sound knowledge of normal absorptive processes allows the physician to pursue a logical approach to the diagnosis and treatment of the patient with malabsorption.

NORMAL ABSORPTION OF NUTRIENTS

Absorption is the integration of those processes whereby the products of digestion pass from the lumen of the intestine through the small intestinal enterocyte to appear in the general circulation via the lymphatics or the portal vein. Although the digestive process is initiated by acid and pepsin within the stomach, the exocrine pancreas has the major role in digesting fat, carbohydrate, and protein by its secretion of lipase, amylase, and proteases. Fat is eventually broken down to monoglycerides and fatty acids; carbohydrate, to disaccharides and monosaccharides; and proteins, to peptides and amino acids. These forms of nutrients are absorbed through the intestinal enterocyte. The villi and microvilli of the small intestine provide an enormous area for absorption. The motility of the intestine and the contraction of the microvilli allow molecules to pass through an "unstirred layer" adjacent to the microvilli.

Nutrients pass through the enterocyte by several processes: active transport, passive diffusion, facilitated diffusion, and endocytosis. Active transport and passive diffusion are the main mechanisms whereby nutrients pass through membranes. *Active transport* moves nutrients against a chemical or electrical gradient, requires energy, is carrier mediated, and is subject to competitive inhibition. *Passive diffusion* does not require energy and allows nutrients to pass through a membrane according to chemical concentration and electrical gradients. Passive diffusion, best typified by water absorption, is not carrier mediated and does not demonstrate competitive inhibition. *Facilitated diffusion* is similar to passive diffusion but may be carrier mediated and may be subject to competitive inhibition. *Endocytosis* is a process whereby nutrients are engulfed by parts of the cell membrane. Although endocytosis may be most important in the neonatal period, this absorptive mechanism may also occur to some extent in the adult and may be involved in the absorption of antigens.

Absorption of nutrients may be regionalized (Table 104–1). Although many nutrients can be absorbed throughout the small intestine, each nutrient has a major site of absorption. When areas of the intestine are damaged or resected, the remaining intestine usually adapts effectively to absorb the nutrients that would normally have been absorbed by those areas. Two noteworthy exceptions to this adaptation process are cobalamin (vitamin B_{12}) and bile salts. If the distal ileum has been resected, the subject can *never* actively absorb these two nutrients again. This has important clinical implications, especially for cobalamin. Patients who have had their distal ileum resected must receive monthly parenteral cobalamin or they will develop macrocytic anemia and neuropathy secondary to cobalamin deficiency (Ch. 136).

TABLE 104–1. REGIONALIZATION OF NUTRIENT ABSORPTION

Nutrient	Major Site of Absorption
Fat	Proximal small intestine
Protein	Mid small intestine
Carbohydrate	Proximal and mid small intestine
Iron	Proximal small intestine
Calcium	Proximal small intestine
Folic acid	Proximal and mid small intestine
Cobalamin (vitamin B_{12})	Distal small intestine (ileum)
Other water-soluble vitamins	Proximal and mid small intestine
Bile salts	Distal small intestine (ileum)
Water and electrolytes	Small intestine and colon (especially cecum)

Fat Absorption

Dietary fat is ingested largely as long-chain triglycerides, the absorption of which is a complex process involving the pancreas, liver, small intestine, and lymphatics (Fig. 104–1). Nevertheless, the process is very efficient; the coefficient of fat absorption is greater than 93 per cent, i.e., less than 7 per cent of ingested fat escapes absorption and appears in the stool per day. A breakdown in any one of these steps (Fig. 104–1) leads to malabsorption of fat (steatorrhea). A thorough knowledge of this physiologic process allows a logical approach to be pursued in the evaluation of the patient with steatorrhea.

Some triglyceride digestion begins in the stomach by lingual and gastric lipases. Triglyceride is emulsified in the stomach, and fat is slowly emptied into the duodenum, where its entry and that of acid release cholecystokinin-pancreozymin and secretin. As a result, the pancreas secretes enzymes and bicarbonate, and the gallbladder contracts to release bile salts. Bicarbonate maintains the pH of the intestinal lumen above 4, allowing pancreatic lipase to be effective in hydrolysis of triglycerides to yield free fatty acids and monoglycerides. Another pancreatic protein, colipase, facilitates the interaction between lipase and triglyceride for effective lipolysis. Fatty acids and monoglyceride interact with conjugated bile salts to form molecular aggregates or micelles (Fig. 104–1). A critical concentration of bile salts for micelle formation (5 to 15 μmol per milliliter) is maintained by a very efficient enterohepatic circulation of bile salts. Although the total bile salt pool is only 2 to 4 grams, 95 per cent of bile salts is actively absorbed in the ileum and returned to the liver by the portal venous system. Each day 20 to 30 grams of bile salts recirculate in this enterohepatic circulation. Only about 200 to 600 mg of bile salts is excreted in the feces per day and must be replaced by hepatic biosynthesis from cholesterol.

Micellar fat passes through the "unstirred" water layer covering the surface of the enterocyte. Because of their solu-

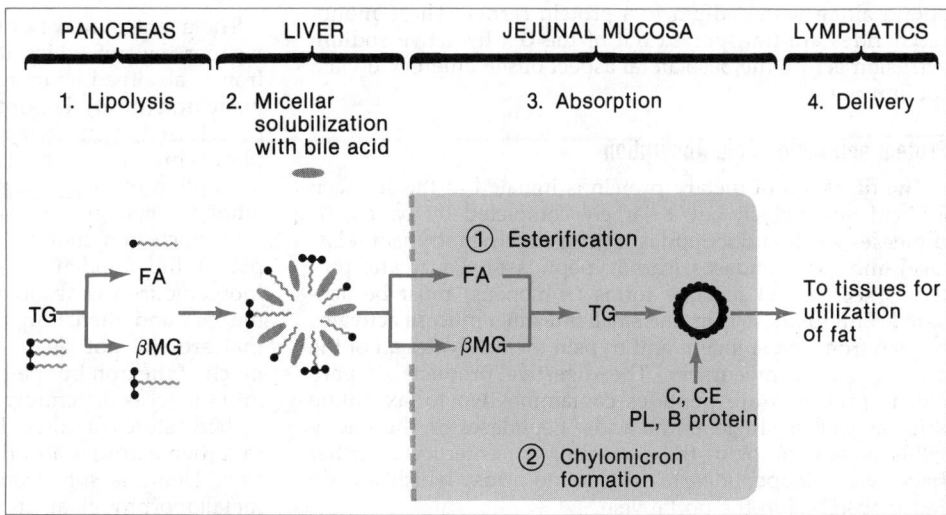

FIGURE 104–1. Schematic of intestinal absorption, showing the participation of the pancreas, liver, and intestinal mucosal cell in fat absorption. (From Wilson FA, Dietschy JM: Gastroenterology 61:911, 1971. Copyright 1971, The Williams & Wilkins Company, Baltimore.)

bility in the lipid-rich surface membrane, the fatty acids and monoglycerides are released and diffuse into the enterocyte. Fatty acid–binding protein (low molecular weight cytosolic protein) avidly binds long-chain fatty acids in the enterocyte and transports them to the smooth endoplasmic reticulum, where they are re-esterified with monoglyceride to form triglyceride. Absorbed cholesterol is also largely esterified with fatty acids for optimal transport. The intestine must also synthesize phospholipids and specific proteins (apoproteins) in order to incorporate these nonpolar lipids into lipoproteins, the major transport vehicles for fat transport in lymph and plasma (Ch. 183). These polar components are added to the surface of the lipid droplet, producing lipoproteins called chylomicrons. Chylomicrons are concentrated in the Golgi apparatus and then discharged through the lateral basal portion of the cell to the interstitium and mesenteric lymph to be delivered via the thoracic duct to the vena cava.

Medium-chain triglycerides (C-6 to C-12 fatty acids) are absorbed quite differently and more effectively than are long-chain triglycerides (C-16 to C-18 fatty acids) described above. Medium-chain triglycerides (MCT) (1) are more completely hydrolyzed by pancreatic lipase, (2) do not require bile salts for absorption, (3) can be directly taken up into the enterocyte and hydrolyzed by a mucosal lipase to fatty acids, (4) do not need to be re-esterified, (5) are not incorporated into lipoproteins, and (6) can pass directly into the portal venous system, transported as fatty acids bound to albumin. These characteristics of MCT allow its therapeutic use to improve fat absorption in a number of diseases in which dietary triglyceride absorption is impaired.

Fat-soluble vitamins (A, D, E, K) are absorbed after micellar solubilization and are transported into lymph with chylomicrons. In the case of vitamin A, the free vitamin is esterified within the enterocyte with palmitic acid, transported via chylomicrons in the lymph and stored as retinol palmitate in the liver. Vitamin metabolism is described more fully in Ch. 217.

Carbohydrate Absorption

Carbohydrate is ingested in the form of starch, sucrose, and lactose. Salivary and pancreatic amylases hydrolyze starch to oligosaccharides and disaccharides. All carbohydrate must be digested to a final monosaccharide product before it can be absorbed. Disaccharides are split by membrane-bound disaccharidases located on the microvilli of the enterocyte. Lactose is digested by lactase to glucose and galactose; sucrose, by sucrase to glucose and fructose, and maltose by maltase to two molecules of glucose. These monosaccharides are then transported through the enterocyte to the portal blood. Glucose and galactose are absorbed by active transport requiring sodium. Fructose is transported by facilitated diffusion. Glucose is transported into the enterocyte, probably bound along with sodium to a protein carrier. These monosaccharides are transported out of the cell by active sodium extrusion across the basolateral aspect of the enterocyte via a sodium pump.

Protein and Amino Acid Absorption

The digestion of dietary protein is initiated in the stomach by acid and pepsin but is largely completed by pancreatic proteases, both endopeptidases (trypsin, chymotrypsin, elastase) and exopeptidases (carboxypeptidase). Pancreatic proteases secreted in inactive forms (zymogens) must be activated. Enterokinase from the small intestinal mucosa activates trypsin from trypsinogen, and trypsin then activates all of the other protease precursors. The digestive products of pancreatic proteases are peptides containing two to six amino acids as well as single amino acids. Peptidases on the microvillus membrane or in the cytosol of the enterocyte further hydrolyze oligopeptides to free amino acids, which are directly absorbed in the portal vein.

The L forms of amino acids are actively transported in the enterocyte by specific energy-requiring, sodium-dependent processes. There are several specific transport systems for amino acids: (1) the dibasic amino acid system, which is often abnormal in cystinuria, (2) the neutral amino acid system, which is abnormal in Hartnup disease; (3) the iminoglycine system, and (4) the dicarboxylic acid system. Intact di- and tripeptides are also actively transported across the enterocyte membrane without hydrolysis by peptidases on the microvillus membrane. These peptides are hydrolyzed in the cytosol of the enterocyte to amino acids, which are then released into the circulation.

Water and Electrolyte Absorption

Over 7 liters of water (both ingested and reabsorbed from intestinal secretion) is absorbed by the small intestine per day through the process of passive diffusion. Absorption of water often follows that of glucose and electrolytes in order to maintain isotonicity of intraluminal contents.

Sodium is actively transported linked to an exchange with H^+ in the jejunum and ileum and with Cl^- and HCO_3^- in the ileum. Na^+ transport is enhanced by glucose absorption in the jejunum (via the glucose-Na^+ carrier on the microvillus membrane) and by solvent (water) drag. Some Na^+ also moves down a gradient across the mucosa, i.e., by passive diffusion. Changes in the concentration of sodium in the lumen depend on relative rates of exchange of both sodium and water between blood and lumen. Potassium passively diffuses from the lumen of the proximal small intestine and into the lumen of the distal small intestine.

Calcium Absorption

Calcium is actively absorbed in the duodenum largely regulated by the active form of vitamin D_3—1,25-dihydroxycholecalciferol (calcitriol). Vitamin D_3 from the diet is metabolized first by the liver (25-hydroxylation) and then by the kidney (1-hydroxylation) to form 1,25-dihydroxycholecalciferol ($1,25[OH]_2D_3$) (Ch. 245). This process is influenced by parathyroid hormone levels, which are regulated by plasma levels of ionized calcium. Calcitriol stimulates the synthesis of calcium-binding protein, alkaline phosphatase, and a calcium-activated ATPase—all involved in active calcium transport. Absorption of vitamin D, a fat-soluble vitamin, is often impaired in the malabsorptive syndromes such that calcium absorption is diminished. Fatty acids within the lumen of the intestine may also directly impair absorption by binding calcium. In turn, the unavailability of ionized calcium in the lumen leads to excessive absorption of oxalate and a resulting propensity to form calcium oxalate kidney stones.

Iron Absorption (Ch. 135)

The average intake of iron from dietary sources is 15 to 25 mg per day, of which 0.5 to 2.0 mg is normally absorbed. Iron is absorbed as inorganic iron (cereals, vegetables) or as heme iron (meat). For optimal absorption, inorganic iron must be released from dietary components to soluble iron complexes in the intestinal lumen. Gastric acid enhances the absorption of inorganic iron (both Fe^{+++} and Fe^{++}) by facilitating its chelation with sugars, amino acids, bile, and ascorbic acid. Such iron complexes remain in solution at the alkaline pH of the duodenum—the major site of iron absorption. Inorganic iron is absorbed from the intestinal lumen by the mucosa and then transported to the blood by mechanisms that are still not clear. A mucosal regulatory system keeps much of the iron trapped within the enterocyte, to be excreted into the feces depending on the need for iron, as determined by body stores of iron or by the rate of erythropoiesis. Organic iron (heme iron) is absorbed more efficiently than is inorganic iron. Heme is split from globin and absorbed as an intact metalloporphyrin at an alkaline pH. Iron is released from heme by heme oxygenase intracellularly. In plasma, iron is transported bound to transferrin, a specific globulin, to various tissues for use or storage.

Iron absorption is increased in iron deficiency, pregnancy, idiopathic hemochromatosis, and any conditions in which there is active erythropoiesis. Absorption is decreased in chronic infection and after the ingestion of large amounts of iron. Diffuse disease of the duodenum such as nontropical sprue may impair iron absorption and lead to iron deficiency.

Folic Acid Absorption

Dietary folic acid is conjugated with glutamyl peptides, prior to its absorption, these polyglutamates must be deconjugated to monoglutamates by folic deconjugase, an enzyme found on the microvillus membrane. Folate monoglutamates are absorbed by active transport at low concentrations of folate and by passive diffusion at high concentrations of folate. Folic acid undergoes an enterohepatic circulation. Since its body stores are limited, the major cause of folate deficiency is poor dietary intake of fresh fruits and vegetables. Folic acid deficiency may also occur if there is extensive damage to the proximal small intestine (e.g., nontropical sprue) or secondary to the use of a number of medications (sulfasalazine, phenytoin, trimethoprim) that inhibit its absorption. Other causes of folate deficiency are listed in Table 136–1.

Cobalamin (Vitamin B₁₂) Absorption (Ch. 136)

The current concept of cobalamin absorption and transport is depicted in Figure 104–2. Cobalamin, found in animal protein, is released from protein in the stomach by the synergistic action of both acid and pepsin. Cobalamin initially binds to a cobalamin-binding protein (R binder or cobalophilin), also secreted by the stomach. The cobalophilin-cobal-

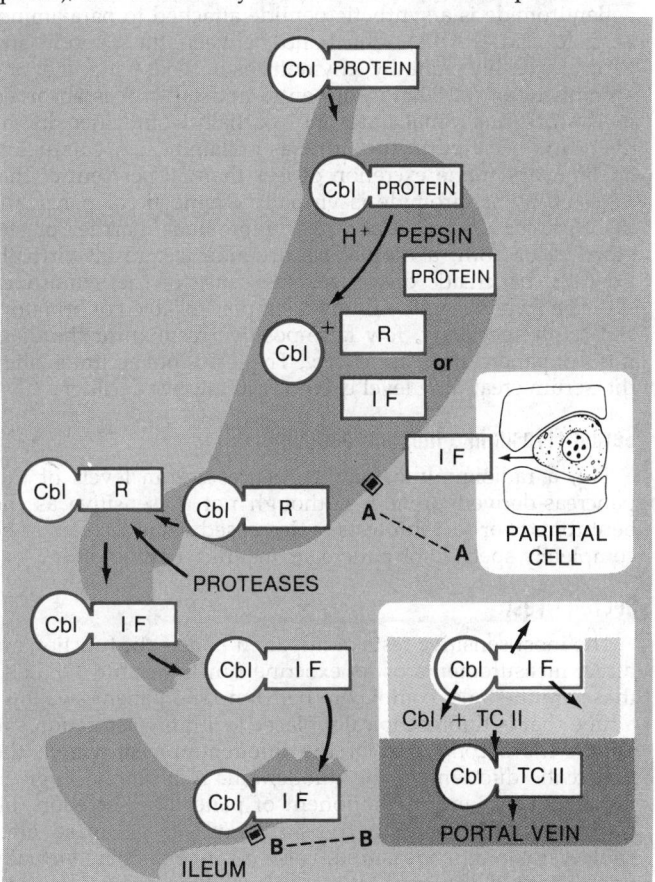

FIGURE 104–2. Cobalamin absorption and transport. Cbl = Cobalamin, R = R-protein or cobalophilin, IF = intrinsic factor, TC II = transcobalamin II. (From Toskes PP: J Clin Gastroenterol 2:287, 1980.)

amin complex is degraded by pancreatic proteases within the duodenal lumen, with release of cobalamin to bind with gastric intrinsic factor (a glycoprotein secreted by the parietal cells). After intrinsic factor binds cobalamin, the intrinsic factor–cobalamin complex passes down the small intestine until it reaches the distal 60 cm of the ileum, where it binds to a specific receptor of the brush border. In the absence of the terminal ileum, intrinsic factor–mediated cobalamin absorption ceases, although large doses of cobalamin (milligram in contrast to microgram amounts) may lead to adequate absorption by passive diffusion throughout the gastrointestinal tract.

Intrinsic factor does not enter the ileal cell and is not absorbed. Transcobalamin II (TCII), the most important transport protein for cobalamin, picks up cobalamin in the ileal mucosa and promotes its uptake by tissues throughout the body. The TCII-cobalamin complex enters tissues via endocytosis, with cobalamin being released by lysosomal proteolysis.

At equilibrium, the majority of circulating cobalamin is attached to cobalophilin, which is also found in saliva, gastric secretions, intestinal secretions, semen, and tears. It also moves continuously in an enterohepatic circulation. The function of the ubiquitous cobalophilins is unclear, but they may prevent or retard the absorption and dissemination of a variety of cobalamin analogues, either produced by bacteria or even found within multivitamin supplements.

CLASSIFICATION AND CLINICAL MANIFESTATIONS OF MALABSORPTION

Causes of Malabsorption

Table 104–2 divides the causes of the malabsorption syndrome into nine categories, based upon its pathophysiology (Fig. 104–1). Some conditions have multiple reasons for malabsorption but are arbitrarily classified under one major category. The differential features and management of important types of this syndrome are detailed later in the chapter.

Clinical Manifestations

Patients with the malabsorption syndrome usually present with diarrhea, weight loss, and malnutrition. These patients often complain that their stools are bulky, greasy, and excessively malodorous and that they float and are difficult to flush down the toilet. Steatorrheal stools float not because of their fat content but because of their high gas content. Patients with severe malabsorption, as exemplified by that secondary to pancreatic insufficiency, may complain of oil seeping out of the rectum. The symptoms and signs of malabsorption are varied and involve a number of organ systems. Patients may demonstrate one or more of these manifestations depending on the severity of their malabsorption. The different symptoms and signs that such patients may show and the causes of these symptoms and signs are detailed in Table 104–3. These aspects of the history and physical examination are crucial in evaluating a patient with malabsorption.

DIAGNOSIS OF MALABSORPTION

Although there may be selective malabsorption of nutrients, most patients with clinically relevant malabsorption have steatorrhea. Consequently, documentation of steatorrhea is important and is the cornerstone of the diagnostic evaluation of patients with malabsorption. The only truly reliable means to document the presence of steatorrhea is the quantitative chemical analysis of fat in a 72-hour stool collection while the patient is ingesting a high-fat diet (at least 100 grams per day). On such a diet normal subjects excrete less than 7 grams of fat per day (coefficient of absorption of >93 per cent). Unfortunately, the quantitative fecal fat determination is cumbersome to perform and difficult to obtain in most hospitals.

TABLE 104–2. CLASSIFICATION OF THE MALABSORPTION SYNDROME

1. Impaired digestion
   a. Primary pancreatic exocrine insufficiency
   b. Gastric surgery (Billroth I and II, vagotomy, and pyloroplasty)*
   c. Gastrinoma*
2. Reduced bile salt concentration
   a. Liver disease
   b. Small intestine bacterial overgrowth (scleroderma, diabetes mellitus, primary motility disturbances, postgastrectomy, achlorhydria)*
   c. Ileal disease or resection*
3. Abnormalities of intestinal mucosa
   a. Disaccharidase deficiency
   b. Impaired monosaccharide transport
   c. Folate or cobalamin deficiency
   d. Nontropical sprue
   e. Nongranulomatous ileojejunitis
   f. Amyloidosis
   g. Crohn's disease*
   h. Eosinophilic enteritis
   i. Radiation enteritis*
   j. Abetalipoproteinemia
   k. Cystinuria
   l. Hartnup disease
4. Inadequate absorptive surface
   a. Short bowel syndrome
   b. Jejunoileal bypass*
5. Infection
   a. Tropical sprue
   b. Whipple's disease*
   c. Acute infectious enteritis
   d. Parasitic infections
6. Lymphatic obstruction
   a. Lymphoma*
   b. Tuberculosis
   c. Lymphangiectasia
7. Cardiovascular disorders
   a. Congestive heart failure
   b. Constrictive pericarditis
   c. Mesenteric vascular insufficiency
8. Drug-induced
   a. Cholestyramine
   b. Neomycin
   c. Colchicine
   d. Phenindione
   e. Irritant laxatives
9. Unexplained
   a. Carcinoid syndrome
   b. Diabetes mellitus*
   c. Adrenal insufficiency
   d. Hyper- and hypothyroidism
   e. Mastocytosis
   f. Hypogammaglobulinemia

* = Multiple reasons for malabsorption.

Furthermore, the documentation of steatorrhea only indicates that the patient has the malabsorption syndrome—it does not indicate the pathophysiology or confer a specific diagnosis.

Table 104–4 details some alternative tests (other than the quantitative fecal fat determination) that can be employed to detect the presence and the cause of malabsorption in a given patient. The tests are categorized into screening tests and those that are more specific in localizing the site of the malabsorption. It is usually necessary to utilize a number of malabsorptive tests to establish the cause of the malabsorption.

Qualitative Stool Fat

The microscopic examination of stool for the presence of fat is a helpful test if performed properly and if the patient is ingesting a high-fat diet. Two specimens of stool are placed on two slides. To the first slide, two drops of water and two drops of 95 per cent ethyl alcohol are added, followed by two drops of a fat stain (e.g., Sudan III). The specimen is microscopically examined for orange neutral fat (triglyceride) globules. The globules should be larger than a red cell and should be numerous per high-power field. To the second slide, several drops of 36 per cent acetic acid are added, then several drops of Sudan III. The slide is heated until it begins to boil.

Microscopically, the presence of large orange globules or spicules represents free fatty acids. Part 1 is positive in patients with pancreatic insufficiency, detecting undigested triglyceride; part 2, in patients with small bowel disease, detecting free fatty acids. Figure 104–3 demonstrates a positive part 1 test in a patient with pancreatic insufficiency. There is a 25 per cent false-negative rate when steatorrhea is mild, i.e., <10 grams per 24 hours. The false-positive rate is about 15 per cent. This test is simple to perform and inexpensive.

Urinary D-Xylose Test

The urinary xylose excretion test distinguishes between malabsorption due to small intestinal disease and that due to pancreatic exocrine insufficiency. A five-hour urinary excretion of 5 grams or greater is normal following the oral administration of 25 grams of D-xylose to a well-hydrated subject. Decreased xylose absorption and excretion are found in patients with damage to the proximal small intestine and in bacterial overgrowth in the small intestine (the bacteria catabolize the xylose). Patients with pancreatic steatorrhea usually have normal xylose absorption. As with any urinary excretion test, decreased renal function or incomplete collection of the urine may invalidate the test. Impaired renal function is most important when evaluating an elderly patient who may not have obvious renal disease, but whose creatinine clearance may be low. Decreased urinary xylose values may also be seen in patients with ascites. Although a blood level of 30 mg per deciliter or greater one hour after ingestion of xylose may indicate normal absorption, there appears to be a great deal of overlap between control subjects and those with malabsorption.

Bentiromide Urinary Excretion Test

Bentiromide is a synthetic peptide attached to para-amino-benzoic acid (PABA) The bond between the peptide and PABA is easily split by chymotrypsin. Following the oral administration of 500 mg of bentiromide, PABA is absorbed in the proximal small intestine, partially conjugated in the liver, and excreted in the urine as arylamines. A cumulative six-hour arylamine excretion of less than 50 per cent of that ingested as bentiromide is virtually diagnostic of pancreatic insufficiency. In a patient with symptomatic diarrhea or steatorrhea or both, a normal bentiromide test result virtually excludes pancreatic disease as the cause of the symptoms. The use of bentiromide offers a simple, reliable confirmatory test (high specificity, few false-positive results) for the diagnosis of pancreatic insufficiency. The test is not accurate when the serum creatinine level exceeds 2.0 mg per deciliter.

Serum Trypsin-like Immunoreactivity (TLI)

TLI, a radioimmunoassay, measures serum levels of this pancreas-derived protein. Although not as sensitive as the bentiromide or secretin tests, a decreased value appears to be completely specific for pancreatic insufficiency.

Secretin Test

The most sensitive tests of impaired pancreatic function are direct measurements of its exocrine function; unfortunately, these are the most complex to perform. The patient swallows a tube that is fluoroscopically placed, with the aspiration site within the second part of the duodenum near where the pancreatic duct enters the duodenum. A hormone is given intravenously, and a component of pancreatic secretion (bicarbonate after secretin; trypsin, amylase, or lipase after cholecystokinin) is measured. False-positive tests are virtually nonexistent if the tube has been properly positioned, and false-negative tests are not relevant because the secretin test will invariably be abnormal if the steatorrhea is secondary to pancreatic insufficiency.

TABLE 104—3. SYMPTOMS AND SIGNS OF MALABSORPTION

History	Pathophysiology	Physical Examination	Pathophysiology
Diarrhea	Increased secretion and impaired absorption of water and electrolytes, unabsorbed dihydroxy bile acids, unabsorbed fatty acids	Pallor	Anemia secondary to iron, folate, or cobalamin deficiency
		Glossitis, stomatitis, cheilosis	Iron, folate, cobalamin, and other vitamin deficiencies
Greasy, bulky, malodorous stools that are difficult to flush	Increased fat in stool		
Oil seeping from rectum	Unabsorbed triglyceride (pancreatic insufficiency)	Ecchymosis, purpura	Vitamin K malabsorption
		Acrodermatitis	Zinc and fatty acid deficiency
Weight loss despite good appetite	Loss of calories from malabsorption	Dehydration, hypotension	Water and electrolyte malabsorption
Excessive flatus	Fermentation of unabsorbed carbohydrates by colonic bacteria	Edema	Protein malabsorption (decreased serum albumin)
Diffuse abdominal pain	Inflammation or infiltration of tissue (pancreatic insufficiency, Crohn's disease, lymphoma)	Peripheral neuropathy	Cobalamin deficiency
Postprandial (30 minutes after eating) midabdominal pain	Intestinal ischemia		
Abnormal bruisability	Vitamin K malabsorption		
Weakness and fatigue	Protein, electrolyte, fat, iron, folate, cobalamin malabsorption		
Milk intolerance	Lactase deficiency		
Bone pain	Calcium and protein malabsorption		
Tetany, paresthesias	Calcium and magnesium malabsorption, cobalamin deficiency (paresthesias only)		
Night blindness	Vitamin A malabsorption		
Nocturia	Delayed absorption of water, hypokalemia		
Amenorrhea	Protein malabsorption		

TABLE 104—4. TESTS FOR MALABSORPTION

Test	Normal Values	Comments Relevant to Patients with Malabsorption
Screening Tests		
1. Serum carotene	>0.06 mg/dl	Decreased; very good test if poor oral intake has been excluded
2. Serum calcium	9.0 to 10.5 mg/dl	Decreased, not very sensitive
3. Serum cholesterol	150 to 250 mg/dl	Decreased, not very sensitive
4. Serum albumin	4.0 to 5.2 mg/dl	Decreased, not very sensitive
5. Serum magnesium	1.7 to 2.0 mEq/liter	Decreased, not very sensitive
6. Prothrombin time	Control value	Increased, not very sensitive
7. Qualitative stool fat	No fat globules per hpf*	Numerous fat globules per hpf; part 1 for neutral fats, part 2 for split fats (see text)
Specific Tests		
1. Serum iron	80–150 μg/dl	Malabsorbed in proximal small bowel disease
2. Serum folate	5–21 ng/ml	Decreased in proximal small bowel disease, may be increased in bacterial overgrowth
3. Serum cobalamin (vitamin B_{12})	200–900 pg/ml	Malabsorbed in distal small bowel disease, pernicious anemia, bacterial overgrowth, chronic pancreatitis
4. Urinary D-xylose	>5 grams/5 hr	Decreased in small bowel disease and bacterial overgrowth, normal in pancreatic disease
5. Bentiromide test	Arylamine excretion >57% in 6 hr	A value of <50 per cent is diagnostic of pancreatic insufficiency
6. Serum trypsin–like immunoreactivity (TLI)	29–80 ng/ml	A value of <20 ng/ml is specific for pancreatic insufficiency
7. Secretin test	HCO_3^- conc >80 mEq/liter Vol >1.8 ml/kg/hr	Most sensitive test of pancreatic function
8. ^{57}Cyanocobalamin urinary excretion test	>8% 24 hr	Decreased in pernicious anemia, chronic pancreatitis, bacterial overgrowth, ileal disease
9. Urine 5-HIAA	1.7–8.0 mg/24 hr	Markedly elevated in carcinoid syndrome, minimally elevated in any kind of malabsorption
10. Breath tests		
a. ^{14}C-xylose	<0.0013% of administered dose as breath $^{14}CO_2$ at 30 min	Elevated in bacterial overgrowth
b. cholyl-1-^{14}C-glycine	<1% of administered dose as breath $^{14}CO_2$ at any interval over 4 hr	Elevated in bacterial overgrowth or bile acid malabsorption
c. Lactulose H_2	<10 ppm rise in breath H_2 over baseline at any interval for 120 min	Elevated in bacterial overgrowth; increase in fasting breath H_2 suggests bacterial overgrowth; up to 27% of subjects may not have flora that produces H_2
d. Lactose-H_2	<20 ppm rise in breath H_2 over baseline at any interval for 180 min	Elevated in lactase deficiency
11. Small intestinal culture	≤10^5 organisms per ml jejunal secretions	>10^5 organisms per ml jejunal secretions indicates bacterial overgrowth
12. Small intestinal biopsy	See Figure 104–4	See Table 104–7

*hpf = High-power field, 5-HIAA = 5-hydroxyindoleacetic acid.

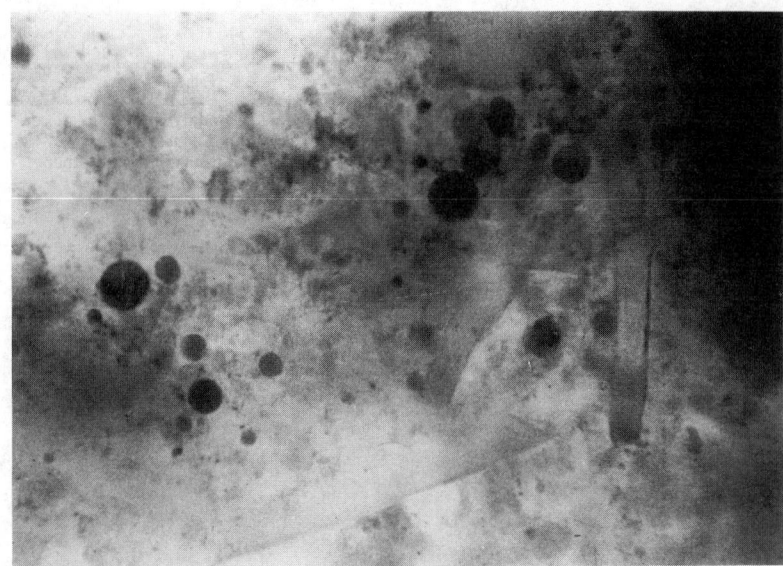

FIGURE 104–3. Positive fecal fat stain. Note the many globules of undigested triglycerides.

Tests for Cobalamin (Vitamin B₁₂) Absorption (Ch. 136)

In the Schilling test, 1.0 μg of ^{57}Co-cyanocobalamin is administered orally, followed by 1000 μg of nonlabeled cobalamin given intramuscularly to help "wash out" that fraction of the isotope that has been absorbed. If the subsequent 24-hour urinary excretion of the radioactivity is less than 8 per cent of that administered, cobalamin malabsorption is present. There are four common clinical causes of cobalamin malabsorption, which can be sorted out by a differential Schilling test (Table 104–5). If an abnormal test result improves with the concomitant administration of hog intrinsic factor or pancreatic extract (six to eight conventional tablets or three enteric-coated microsphere capsules), the cobalamin malabsorption is secondary to pernicious anemia or exocrine pancreatic insufficiency, respectively. If cobalamin malabsorption still persists, the tests should be repeated after four days of antimicrobial therapy (metronidazole, 250 mg three times daily). If the malabsorption of labeled cobalamin is corrected by this therapy, bacterial overgrowth was the etiology. Metronidazole is the antimicrobial agent of choice because anaerobes such as *Bacteroides* are usually responsible for the cobalamin malabsorption. If the malabsorption still persists, damage to the ileal receptor (Crohn's disease, ileal resection, lymphoma, Imerslund's syndrome) is probably present and the patient must always receive a monthly injection of cobalamin (100 μg). In the face of renal impairment, 4 ml of plasma may be obtained eight hours after the administration of labeled cobalamin. A value greater than 0.6 per cent of the orally administered dose is considered normal.

There are two caveats concerning the Schilling test: (1) Severe cobalamin deficiency itself may damage the ileum such that the ileal receptors may not bind the intrinsic factor–cobalamin complex. This may confuse interpretation of the Schilling test. Thus, it is advisable to wait until one week of cobalamin therapy (100 μg per day intramuscularly) has been completed before performing the differential Schilling test. (2) Two other clinical conditions are associated with cobalamin deficiency—cobalamin deficiency secondary to lack of intake (as in complete vegetarians) and the failure to absorb food-bound cobalamin because of decreased acid secretion—that are not associated with an abnormal Schilling test (Table 104–5). The patient's history is the key to the former, and a test of protein-bound cobalamin absorption will detect the latter.

Breath Tests

Two breath tests are reliable enough to receive routine clinical use—the lactose-H₂ breath test for detecting lactase

TABLE 104–5. THE DIFFERENTIAL SCHILLING (^{57}CO-CYANOCOBALAMIN) TEST

	Stage 1: Free Cobalamin	Stage 2: Free Cobalamin and Intrinsic Factor	Stage 3: Free Cobalamin and Pancreatic Extract	Stage 4: Free Cobalamin and Antibiotics	Comment
Pernicious anemia	Abnormal	Normal	Abnormal	Abnormal	In face of severe cobalamin deficiency, test should be performed only after a week of cobalamin therapy
Chronic pancreatitis	Abnormal	Abnormal	Normal	Abnormal	Although cobalamin malabsorption is common, cobalamin deficiency is rare
Bacterial overgrowth	Abnormal	Abnormal	Abnormal	Normal	Anaerobicidal antibiotic is needed
Ileal disease	Abnormal	Abnormal	Abnormal	Abnormal	Once receptor is permanently damaged, cobalamin malabsorption is permanent
Complete vegetarian* (vegan)	Normal	Normal	Normal	Normal	Cobalamin deficiency secondary to poor intake, absorption normal
Hypo- or achlorhydria*	Normal	Normal	Normal	Normal	Absorption of cyanocobalamin (free B₁₂) does not depend on acid; food B₁₂ (protein-bound) does; must employ protein-bound cobalamin absorption test

*Cobalamin deficiency with normal Schilling test.

TABLE 104–6. BREATH TESTS FOR BACTERIAL OVERGROWTH

Procedure	Simplicity	Sensitivity	Specificity	Safety
^{14}C-xylose	Excellent	Excellent	Excellent	Good
Cholyl-1-^{14}C-glycine	Excellent	Fair	Poor	Good
Lactulose-H_2	Excellent	Fair–good	Fair	Excellent

Modified from King CE, Toskes PP: The use of breath tests in the study of malabsorption. Clin Gastroenterol 12:591, 1983.

deficiency and the ^{14}C-xylose breath test for the diagnosis of small intestine bacterial overgrowth.

The *lactose-H_2 breath test* has replaced the lactose intolerance test because of superior sensitivity and specificity. Lactose (1 gram per kilogram) is administered orally, and an increase in breath H_2 of more than 20 ppm over basal breath H_2 indicates lactose malabsorption. This test depends upon the release of H_2 from unabsorbed lactose by bacterial metabolism.

The ^{14}C-xylose breath test is a sensitive and specific test for bacterial overgrowth. Following the oral administration of xylose (1 gram, 5 to 10 μCi), breath $^{14}CO_2$ concentration is monitored at 30 and 60 minutes, with an increase of $^{14}CO_2$ at 30 minutes being the most reliable assessment. Neither false-negative nor false-positive results appear to be a clinically significant problem. Xylose is catabolized by gram-negative aerobes, which are always part of the overgrowth flora, whereas other breath tests often utilize substrates that are catabolized by gram-negative anaerobes, which may or may not be present in the overgrowth of bacteria. The small dose of xylose (1 gram) is either catabolized by the overgrowth flora or absorbed in the proximal bowel, leaving very little xylose to "dump" into the colon, causing a possible false-positive result. An abnormal xylose breath test indicates, similar to a culture, the presence of increased numbers of bacteria within the lumen of the proximal small intestine. Whether or not the abnormal test indicates that therapy is necessary is a decision the clinician must make. Table 104–6 lists two other breath tests used to diagnose bacterial overgrowth, both of which suffer from inadequate sensitivity and specificity.

A ^{14}C-triolein breath test has received some use as a test of fat absorption, but it does not appear to separate control subjects from those with malabsorption very reliably, especially if the steatorrhea is not severe.

Culture of the Small Intestine

The proximal small intestine of normal subjects has less than 10^5 organisms per milliliter of jejunal fluid—usually less than 10^3, largely streptococci and staphylococci, and only an occasional coliform or *Bacteroides*. The ileocecal area is a transition zone with both a qualitative and a quantitative change toward the pattern that is found in the colon. In the colon, there is a marked increase in both aerobes (>10^7 organisms per milligram of stool) and anaerobes (>10^{10} organisms per milligram of stool). The qualitative change is also remarkable, with a preponderance of anaerobes (*Bacteroides, Clostridium*, enterococci) and coliforms (*Escherichia coli, Klebsiella*). In small intestine bacterial overgrowth, the small intestine becomes populated with a colon-like flora. Cultures should be considered suspicious if more than 10^3 organisms per milliliter are present (especially when anaerobes are identified) and clearly abnormal when more than 10^5 organisms per milliliter are present.

Biopsy of the Small Intestine

Biopsy of the small intestine is an important test in the evaluation of malabsorption presumed to be secondary to disease of the small intestine itself. Most instruments (Rubin's tube, Crosby's capsule, Carey's capsule) utilize a blind suction biopsy technique, but biopsies can be obtained endoscopically as well. Figure 104–4 illustrates the findings of a normal biopsy. Note the long, frondlike villi. The lining columnar epithelium is regular with basal orientation of the nuclei. There is not much cellular infiltration of lamina propria. The villus/crypt ratio favors the villus, with villus height normally being three to four times the height of the crypts.

For contrast, note Figure 104–5, which represents a biopsy from a patient with nontropical sprue (adult celiac disease). There is total villus atrophy, elongated crypts, and a dense infiltration of chronic inflammatory cells in the lamina propria, and at higher magnification the surface epithelial cells are cuboidal, not columnar. Total villus atrophy, as shown in Figure 104–5, is almost always nontropical sprue (adult celiac disease), but it is not a specific lesion, since it may occasionally be observed in other diseases such as lymphoma, Whipple's disease, tropical sprue, ileojejunitis, or bacterial overgrowth. Table 104–7 lists disorders associated with abnormalities in the biopsy of the small intestine and points out that there are very few disorders in which multiple biopsies are consistently abnormal and diagnostic, i.e., a diagnostic diffuse lesion.

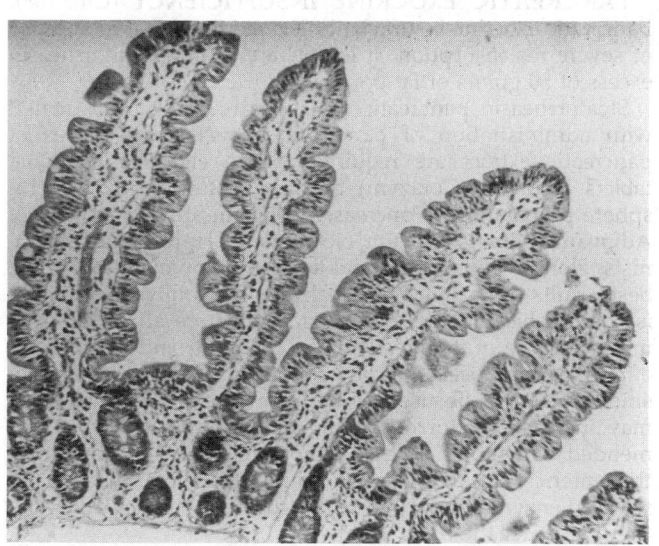

FIGURE 104–4. Appearance of normal small intestine on biopsy.

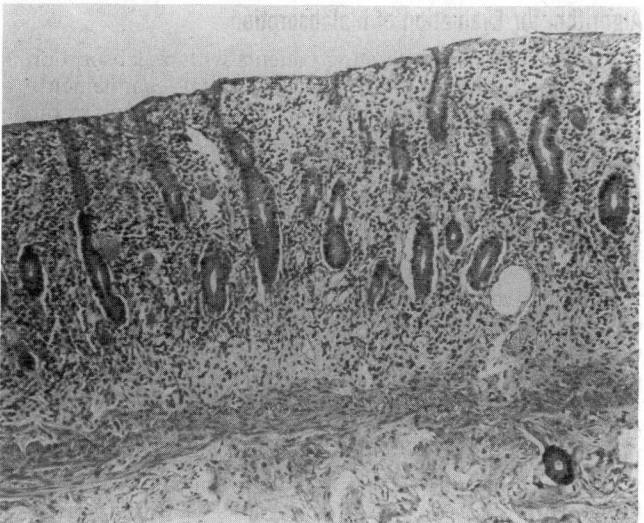

FIGURE 104–5. Small intestinal biopsy from a patient with nontropical sprue showing total villus atrophy.

TABLE 104–7. VALUE OF SMALL INTESTINAL BIOPSY

I. **Conditions in which the biopsy is consistently abnormal and diagnostic:**
   Abetalipoproteinemia
   Immunodeficiency syndrome
   Whipple's disease

II. **Conditions in which the biopsy is diagnostic but the lesion is often patchy:**
   Amyloidosis
   Capillariasis
   Coccidiosis
   Crohn's disease
   Cryptosporidiosis
   Eosinophilic enteritis
   Giardiasis
   Lymphangiectasia
   Lymphoma
   Mastocytosis
   Strongyloidiasis

III. **Conditions in which the biopsy is often abnormal but not diagnostic:**
   Bacterial overgrowth
   Cobalamin (vitamin B_{12}) deficiency
   Celiac sprue (nontropical)
   Drug enteritis
   Folate deficiency
   Infectious gastroenteritis
   Protein-calorie malnutrition
   Radiation enteritis
   Tropical sprue
   Unclassified sprue
   Zollinger-Ellison syndrome

IV. **Conditions in which the biopsy is invariably normal:**
   Functional bowel disease
   Liver disease
   Pancreatic disease
   Primary disaccharidase deficiency
   Ulcerative colitis

Gastrointestinal Radiology

With the possible exception of pancreatic calcification on plain film of the abdomen, radiographs of the intestinal tract do not play a primary role in the diagnostic evaluation of malabsorption. Function tests as described previously are more sensitive and more specific and afford the patient little, if any, radiation exposure. The radiation exposure received from a small bowel series may be considerable. The traditional signs of malabsorption on small bowel radiographs—segmentation or clumping of the barium (moulage sign)—were noted when thick barium was used in contrast to the thin barium commonly employed now. Small bowel radiographs are most frequently used now to determine why bacterial overgrowth has occurred (e.g., the presence of diverticula or dilation of the small intestine in scleroderma) or to confirm a clinical diagnosis of Crohn's disease.

Algorithm for Evaluation of Malabsorption

An algorithm for evaluating patients with malabsorption is presented in Table 104–8. The algorithm complements a thorough history and physical examination. A serum carotene determination and a microscopic fat stain of the stool are the best screening tests and together will detect the presence of steatorrhea about 85 per cent of the time, especially if the patient is excreting more than 15 grams of fat per day. Once steatorrhea has been confirmed, the clinician should ask whether the steatorrhea is secondary to pancreatic disease or to small bowel disease. The urinary xylose test helps differentiate between these two categories. If xylose absorption is normal, tests of pancreatic function should be pursued. If diffuse calcification of the pancreas is present on a plain film of the abdomen, there is likely to be approximately 80 per cent damage to the exocrine pancreas. The bentiromide test has about the same sensitivity as plain film calcification and will be abnormal 80 to 90 per cent of the time if the steatorrhea has a pancreatic cause. A serum trypsin level will complement the bentiromide test, adding specificity to the evaluation. If these simple tubeless tests of pancreatic function are not

TABLE 104–8. ALGORITHM FOR EVALUATION OF MALABSORPTION

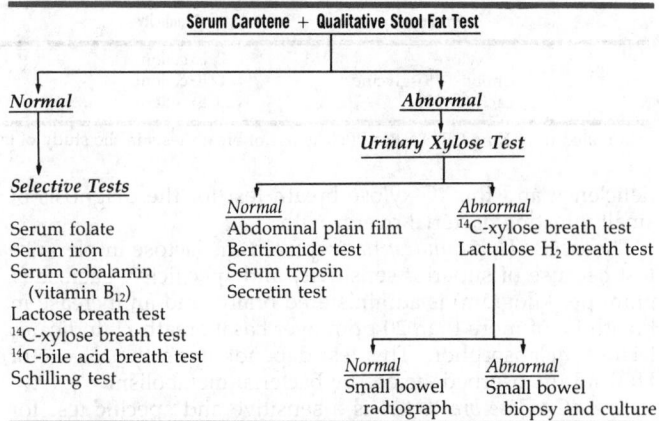

diagnostic, a direct tube test like the secretin test should be performed.

If the xylose test is abnormal, small bowel tests should be performed. A breath test (^{14}C-xylose, lactulose H_2) will detect bacterial overgrowth. If normal, a small bowel radiograph, culture, and biopsy should be done, with the radiograph suggesting the site to be biopsied. If steatorrhea is not present, tests designed to detect selective malabsorption of single nutrients can be pursued (lactose H_2 breath test, the Schilling test, and so on).

The algorithm is logical and cost effective, emphasizing inexpensive, noninvasive, outpatient evaluation. A specific diagnosis can often be made for less than $300 with minimal or no discomfort to the patient. If more complicated tests are needed, such as the secretin test or small bowel biopsy, the expense and discomfort to the patient will increase. The algorithm also emphasizes initial testing for the more common causes of malabsorption (pancreatic insufficiency, bacterial overgrowth) and delayed testing for less common disorders (nontropical sprue, Whipple's disease, and so on).

DIFFERENTIAL FEATURES AND TREATMENT OF INDIVIDUAL FORMS OF THE MALABSORPTION SYNDROME

Numerous disorders can be associated with malabsorption (Table 104–2). Although there may be specific therapy for individual disorders (gluten-free diet for nontropical sprue, pancreatic enzymes for pancreatic insufficiency), there are many nonspecific therapies for malabsorption (Table 104–9).

Impaired Digestion

PANCREATIC EXOCRINE INSUFFICIENCY (Ch. 108). Pancreatic exocrine insufficiency is a relatively common cause of severe malabsorption. It is not rare to note steatorrhea in excess of 50 grams of fat per day.

Steatorrhea in pancreatic disease is relatively well treated with administration of pancreatic extract. Large doses of pancreatic extract are required: six to eight conventional tablets (Viokase, Cotazym) or three enteric-coated, microsphere preparations (Pancrease, Cotazym-S) with each meal. Adjuvant therapy (sodium bicarbonate, H_2-receptor antagonists) along with conventional tablet therapy may lead to the best results by raising duodenal pH. The adjuvant of choice is sodium bicarbonate (650-mg tablet before and after each meal) because of its effectiveness, low cost, and lack of side effects at this dose. Antacids containing calcium or magnesium are not to be used as adjuvant therapy because they may increase steatorrhea. Adjuvant therapy is not recommended with enteric-coated preparations, for it may cause the enteric coat to open up within the stomach and the released enzymes may then be destroyed by gastric acid before they can enter the duodenum.

POSTGASTRECTOMY STATES (Ch. 100.4). The pathogenesis of the malabsorption noted in patients with gastric surgery (Billroth I, Billroth II, vagotomy and antrectomy, vagotomy and pyloroplasty) is multifactorial: (1) loss of reservoir function with rapid emptying and dispersion of food through the small intestine, thereby diluting the normal

TABLE 104–9. AGENTS USED IN THE TREATMENT OF MALABSORPTION

1. **Calcium**
   Oral: Requires 1200 mg elemental calcium daily as
   a. Calcium gluconate (91 mg Ca^{++}/gm), 5–10 gm 3 times per day *or*
   b. Calcium carbonate (500 mg Ca^{++}/tablet)1–2 gm per day in divided doses *or*
   c. Calcium carbonate, 2 tablets supplied as Caltrate or 2½ tablets as Os-Cal 500
   Intravenous: Calcium gluconate injection (10% solution, 9.1 mg Ca^{++}/ml), 10–30 ml administered slowly)

2. **Magnesium**
   Oral: Magnesium gluconate, 500-mg tablets (20 mg Mg^{++}/tablet), 1–4 gm daily in divided doses
   Intramuscular: (20% sol.) 10 ml 2–3 times daily
   Intravenous: Magnesium sulfate, 0.5 per cent sol., up to 1000 ml at a rate not faster than 1.0 mEq/min

3. **Iron**
   Oral: Ferrous sulfate, 325 mg (65 mg elemental iron) 3 times daily
   Intramuscular: Imferon must be calculated according to severity of anemia; detailed instructions accompany preparation

4. **Cyanocobalamin** (vitamin B$_{12}$)
   Intramuscular: 100 µg daily for 2 weeks, then 100 µg monthly

5. **Folic acid**
   Oral: 5 mg daily for 1 month; maintenance 1 mg daily

6. **Vitamin B complex**
   Any multivitamin preparation that contains US RDA amounts; use 2 tablets daily; intramuscular preparations are available for severe deficiencies

7. **Fat-soluble vitamins**
   a. Vitamin A
      Vitamin A capsules (25,000 units per capsule), 100,000–200,000 units daily in severe deficiencies; maintenance, 25,000–50,000 units daily.
      Caution: Vitamin A toxicity can occur with recommended doses if hypertriglyceridemia is present
   b. Vitamin D
      Vitamin D (as vitamin D$_2$ or D$_3$), 30,000 units daily; dosage varies considerably depending on response as determined by level of serum calcium and urinary calcium
   c. Vitamin K
      Oral: Menadione, 4–12 mg daily; vitamin K tablets (Mephyton), 5–10 mg daily
      Intravenous: Acute bleeding episodes: vitamin K (Mephyton), 50-mg ampule administered slowly over 10-min period; repeat in 8–12 hr if prothrombin time has not returned to normal

8. **Cholestyramine**
   4-gm pk, 1–2 pk before breakfast and lunch

9. **Medium-chain triglyceride** (MCT oil)
   Administer 60% of fat intake as MCT oil, 40% as dietary long-chain triglyceride

10. **Human albumin, salt poor** (0.25 gm/ml)
    Intravenous administration of 50–100 gm daily for 3–7 days to elevate a severely depressed serum albumin level

11. **Immune serum globulin** (0.165 gm/ml)
    Intramuscular injection of 0.05 ml/kg each 3–4 wk in patients with hypogammaglobulinemia and recurrent infection

12. **Adrenocorticosteroids**
    Prednisone, 40–60 mg daily for 2 wk, then decrease by 5 mg each week to maintenance of 5–15 mg daily

13. **Antidiarrheal agents**
    Oral: Diphenoxylate hydrochloride (Lomotil), 5.0 mg (2 tablets) initially and after each loose bowel movement, not to exceed 8 tablets daily; loperamide hydrochloride (Imodium), 2-mg capsules, 2 capsules initially and then 2 capsules after each loose bowel movement, not to exceed 8 capsules daily

14. **Drugs for parasites**
    Oral: Metronidazole (Flagyl), 250-mg tablet 3 times daily for 1 wk, or quinacrine hydrochloride (Atabrine), 100-mg tablet 3 times daily for 1 wk for *Giardia lamblia.* Thiabendazole (25 mg/kg/day): strongyloidiasis, 2–3 days; *Capillaria phillipinensis,* 30 days; *A. duodenale, N. americanus,* 25 mg/kg/day twice daily for 2 days.

output of pancreatic enzymes; (2) postcibal asynchrony, i.e., in a patient who has undergone a Billroth II procedure, food may get to the jejunum before bile salts and pancreatic enzymes do; and (3) occurrence of stasis, leading to bacterial overgrowth of the small intestine. Postgastrectomy steatorrhea is usually mild (<10 grams of fat per day) but occasionally may be marked. Severe steatorrhea in this setting is usually the result of bacterial overgrowth or rarely is secondary to pancreatic insufficiency. Because the duodenum (the major site for calcium and iron absorption) is bypassed when a Billroth II procedure is performed, clinically significant problems related to calcium and iron malabsorption may result.

GASTRINOMA (Ch. 100.6). Multiple mechanisms contribute to the malabsorption observed in patients with a gastrinoma (Zollinger-Ellison syndrome). The extreme hypersecretion of acid irreversibly inactivates lipase, causing a secondary pancreatic insufficiency. In addition, this acid environment precipitates bile salts and may cause abnormal small bowel histologic findings. All of these abnormalities have been shown to revert to normal after effective therapy with large doses of H$_2$-receptor antagonists (cimetidine or ranitidine).

Reduced Concentration of Bile Salts

LIVER DISEASE. Steatorrhea (usually mild) may occur in acute or chronic liver disease, presumably owing to impaired synthesis and excretion of conjugated bile salts. Patients with liver disease who manifest clinically significant steatorrhea should have their pancreatic function evaluated, since these patients will often have pancreatic exocrine insufficiency responsive to pancreatic extract therapy. Metabolic bone disease (bone pain, spontaneous pathologic fractures) resulting from malabsorption of calcium and vitamin D may occur, particularly in those with biliary cirrhosis (Ch. 246).

BACTERIAL OVERGROWTH. Overgrowth of bacteria within the small intestine accompanied by nutrient malabsorption is called the stasis, stagnant loop, or blind loop syndrome. The normal subject usually has sparse bacterial growth in the proximal small intestine (see section on Diagnosis—Culture of the Small Intestine). In the stasis syndrome, the proximal small intestinal flora resembles that of the colon and the overgrowth flora competes with the human host for ingested nutrients. The resultant malabsorption is due to a disturbed intraluminal environment (catabolism of carbohydrate by gram-negative aerobes, deconjugation of bile salts by anaerobes, binding of cobalamin by anaerobes) and patchy damage to the small intestinal enterocyte, perhaps secondary to toxins secreted by the overgrowth flora.

In healthy persons, bacteria within the small intestine are controlled by the cleansing motion of the small intestine, gastric acid secretion, and luminal immunoglobulins. Any alteration of these protective factors may lead to bacterial overgrowth (Table 104–10). In the past, bacterial overgrowth was thought to be related largely to blind loops and other structural abnormalities. Now the emphasis is on motor disturbances, often with no structural abnormality, and on states of decreased acid secretion. Indeed, bacterial overgrowth is one of the major, if not the major, cause of clinically significant malabsorption in the elderly, who often have both decreased acid secretion and a motility disturbance of the small intestine.

The diagnosis has become much more practical with the development of noninvasive breath tests (see section on Diagnosis—Breath Tests, Tables 104–4 and 104–6). This has greatly increased the awareness of this syndrome. Intestinal cultures have been expensive, awkward to perform, and usually not utilized extensively in clinical practice.

In the past, treatment was often empiric, not based on a firm diagnosis but dictated by a clinical impression. Broad-spectrum antibiotics (tetracycline) were prescribed for 7 to 10 days and the clinical response monitored. Up to 60 per cent of the anaerobes (*Bacteroides*) now may be resistant to tetra-

TABLE 104–10. CLINICAL CONDITIONS ASSOCIATED WITH BACTERIAL OVERGROWTH

I. **Gastric proliferation of bacteria**
Hypo- or achlorhydria, especially when combined with motor or anatomic distrubances
II. **Small intestinal stagnation**
Anatomic
Afferent loop of Billroth II partial gastrectomy
Duodenal or jejunal diverticulosis
Surgical blind loop (end-to-side anastomosis)
Surgical recirculating loop (side-to-side anastomosis)
Obstruction (stricture, adhesion, inflammation, cancer)
Motor
Scleroderma
Idiopathic intestinal pseudo-obstruction
Derangements of interdigestive motor complex
Diabetic autonomic neuropathy
III. **Abnormal communication between proximal and distal gastrointestinal tract**
Gastrocolic or jejunocolic fistula
Resection of ileocecal valve
IV. **Miscellaneous**
Hypogammaglobulinemia
Chronic pancreatitis

Modified from King CE, Toskes PP: Small intestine bacterial overgrowth. Gastroenterology 76:1035, 1979.

cycline. It behooves the physician to establish the diagnosis firmly, for the antibiotics needed may have serious side effects.

The mainstays of therapy are antimicrobial therapy and nutritional support. If there is a surgically correctable cause of the overgrowth, surgery should be performed if possible. Most patients with overgrowth do not have a surgically correctable cause (e.g., they have scleroderma, diverticulosis, or diabetes) and must receive lifelong antimicrobial and nutritional therapy.

A ten-day course of a cephalosporin (Keflex), 250 mg four times a day, and metronidazole (Flagyl), 250 mg three times a day, is very effective in suppressing the flora and correcting malabsorption. Tetracycline is an alternative, but the resistance problem must be appreciated. If these fail, chloramphenicol (50 mg per kilogram per day in four divided doses) is also very effective. Anaerobicidal agents by themselves (metronidazole, clindamycin) do not seem to be as effective as the combination of an aerobicidal and an anaerobicidal agent.

Three therapeutic patterns occur. Usually a ten-day course of an effective antimicrobial program will correct the malabsorption for months; some patients may need cyclic therapy (one week out of every six); rarely a patient may need continuous therapy for several months. Antibiotic sensitivity assays of the overgrowth flora are not recommended because of the multitude of organisms present.

Nutritional therapy (especially with medium-chain triglyceride oil) is very important but often ignored. Medium-chain triglyceride administration is ideal therapy for this condition, since this form of fat does not need bile salts for absorption. Other agents such as cobalamin, vitamin D, and calcium are given in doses detailed in Table 104–9.

ILEAL DISEASE OR RESECTION. Disease of the distal ileum leads to an interruption of the enterohepatic circulation of conjugated bile acids, resulting in a diminished bile acid pool and steatorrhea. The degree of steatorrhea is proportional to the amount of diseased or resected intestine. When less than 100 cm of intestine is damaged or resected, proximal to the ileocecal valve, the steatorrhea is mild and choleretic diarrhea tends to be the most frequent problem. The malabsorbed bile acids dump into the colon and impair water and electrolyte absorption. When more than 100 cm of small intestine is resected, the steatorrhea is large owing to a number of factors, including a diminished bile acid pool, loss of the absorptive function of the ileum, and bacterial overgrowth (loss of the ileocecal valve). Choleretic diarrhea can usually be managed with cholestyramine (Table 104–9).

Abnormalities of the Intestinal Mucosa

DISACCHARIDASE DEFICIENCY AND MONOSACCHARIDE MALABSORPTION. The most common disaccharide deficiency is lactose deficiency, which may be primary or secondary. Primary lactase deficiency is common throughout the world, with 60 to 90 per cent of American Indians, black Americans, and Asians being deficient with varying degrees of lactose intolerance. Only 5 to 15 per cent of Caucasians are lactase deficient. Any disease that damages the enterocyte may lead to secondary lactase deficiency.

Lactase-deficient subjects are intolerant to milk, experiencing bloating, abdominal cramps, and diarrhea. The lactose within milk cannot be hydrolyzed to glucose and galactose. It remains in the intestinal lumen, where it is fermented by bacteria, producing organic acids, which increase the osmotic load, inducing shifts of water into the intestinal tract. The end result is distention of the intestine and diarrhea.

Primary lactase deficiency may not manifest itself until adulthood, yet the reason for this delayed appearance is not clear. Subtotal gastrectomy or pyloroplasty and vagotomy may unmask the condition by increasing the load of ingested lactose on the jejunal mucosa. Although the diagnosis is often made by taking a history, the lactose-H_2 breath test is the best way to document lactose intolerance (see Diagnosis section and Table 104–4). Treatment of primary lactase deficiency is through avoidance of milk products or through the ingestion of one to two capsules of Lactrase when dairy products are ingested. Lactrase, derived from *Aspergillus oryzae*, is commercially available.

Sucrase deficiency is quite rare. In afflicted patients, diarrhea occurs after ingesting sucrose. Elimination of sucrose, dextrins, and starches from the diet is effective.

Monosaccharide (glucose-galactose) malabsorption is a rare disorder present from birth. All sugars metabolized to glucose or galactose cannot be tolerated. Therapy consists of utilizing fructose as a source of sugar.

NONTROPICAL SPRUE (ADULT CELIAC DISEASE, CELIAC SPRUE, GLUTEN-SENSITIVE ENTEROPATHY). Nontropical sprue is a disease of unknown etiology characterized by malabsorption resulting from gluten-induced damage to the differentiated villus epithelial cells of the small intestine. Gluten is a high molecular weight protein found in wheat, rye, oats, and barley. The mechanism for this toxic effect is not known, but the most accepted theory at present is that metabolites of gluten initiate an immunologic reaction in the enterocyte. The enterocyte is often strikingly damaged, and biopsy of the small intestine demonstrates characteristic changes (see Fig. 104–5 and discussion of small bowel biopsy in Diagnosis section). Malabsorption is secondary to the impaired transport of nutrients through the damaged enterocyte. In addition, a net secretory state for water and electrolytes has been noted in the jejunum, and pancreatic exocrine function may be secondarily diminished owing to a decreased release of secretin and cholecystokinin from the damaged small bowel mucosa.

Genetic factors appear important in this disease. Nontropical sprue is closely linked to two histocompatibility antigens, HLA-B8 and HLA-DW3. These antigens are present in 60 to 90 per cent of patients with this disease and in only 20 to 30 per cent of the general population. An additional antigen has been found on the surface of B lymphocytes in 70 to 80 per cent of patients with nontropical sprue and in 15 per cent of normal controls. The same antigen is present in 100 per cent of the patients' parents. Perhaps these antigens evoke antibodies to gluten, which result in the binding of gluten to the enterocyte with subsequent mucosal damage.

Patients with nontropical sprue usually have severe malabsorption—steatorrhea, diarrhea, weight loss, and many of the other symptoms and signs detailed in Table 104–3. Symptoms typically begin in infancy, disappear in late childhood, and reappear in the third to sixth decade of life. The proximal small intestine is usually the most severely damaged, and the symptoms, signs, and laboratory evaluation reflect this (Tables 104–3 and 104–4). At times, the clinical presentation may be quite subtle, e.g., anemia secondary to iron deficiency or bone pain from osteomalacia without obvious diarrhea or steatorrhea. Small bowel biopsy is essential in this disease, for a diagnosis of nontropical sprue commits the patient to a very restricted diet indefinitely.

The cornerstone of therapy is the withdrawal of all gluten from the diet, i.e., all grains must be eliminated except rice and corn. Most patients will respond to dietary restriction with a remarkable decrease in symptoms and signs within a few days to a week. In some patients, however, it may take months before a significant improvement is noted. Function tests such as urinary xylose excretion return to normal within a few weeks of gluten withdrawal. Post-treatment biopsies demonstrate marked improvement in most patients and completely normal histologic findings in many. The patient with the characteristic syndrome and biopsy findings who does not respond to gluten withdrawal is usually not adhering to the diet. Some patients may have the characteristic clinical picture and flat biopsy and in reality are not responding because they have another disease such as Whipple's disease, nongranulomatous ileojejunitis, giardiasis, lymphoma, or collagenous sprue. Collagenous sprue, a variant of nontropical sprue, demonstrates not only the characteristic changes in the small intestinal biopsy but also masses of eosinophilic hyaline material in the lamina propria. Such patients have a poor prognosis. Corticosteroid therapy (Table 104–9) or parenteral hyperalimentation may be needed in some patients.

Small bowel lymphoma and carcinoma in general seem to be increased in patients with nontropical sprue. The appearance of abdominal pain in a patient with sprue should suggest lymphoma. Whether or not these complications are fewer in those who adhere strictly to a gluten-free diet is controversial.

Two other associated abnormalities in patients with sprue are (1) ulcers of the jejunum and ileum with abdominal pain, bleeding, and perforation, which are unresponsive to therapy, and (2) dermatitis herpetiformis. Some patients with this skin lesion may have latent sprue. The dermatitis is pruritic, vesicular, and papular and responds to sulfone treatment. Sulfone does not improve the intestinal lesion, but some of these lesions may respond to gluten withdrawal.

NONGRANULOMATOUS ILEOJEJUNITIS. This disease has features of both Crohn's disease and nontropical sprue, even a flat small intestinal biopsy. There is an abrupt onset with fever, abdominal pain, at times splenomegaly, and elevated white count—all suggesting lymphoma. Malabsorption may be profound, resulting in a therapeutic trial of steroids and a gluten-free diet—often to no avail.

CROHN'S DISEASE (Ch. 105.2). Malabsorption in Crohn's disease results from several problems: (1) decreased absorptive surface from active disease or surgical resection, (2) bile salt depletion from ileal disease, and (3) bacterial overgrowth secondary to dilatation of the bowel and resection of the ileocecal valve.

EOSINOPHILIC ENTERITIS. Peripheral blood eosinophilia and infiltration of the gastrointestinal tract by eosinophils characterize this disease. Three patterns of involvement are seen: (1) involvement of the muscle layers of the stomach and small intestine causing obstruction, (2) involvement of the mucosa of the small intestine causing malabsorption, and (3) involvement of the subserosa causing ascites. Most patients have no evidence of allergy or food sensitivity. Corticosteroids and occasionally surgery are employed successfully.

RADIATION ENTERITIS (Ch. 115 and 539). Radiation injury to the intestine may lead to malabsorption from (1) extensive mucosal damage, (2) lymphangiectasia from lymphatic obstruction, and (3) bacterial overgrowth. Malabsorption may occur shortly after exposure to radiation or years

later. Most patients with clinically significant malabsorption appear to respond to therapy for bacterial overgrowth.

ABETALIPOPROTEINEMIA (Ch. 183). This rare disease represents a defect in chylomicron formation. The intestinal cells are lacking apoprotein B, and therefore fat absorption cannot occur normally. Biopsy of the small intestine shows the epithelial cells to be engorged with fat even after an overnight fast. The clinical manifestations are steatorrhea, neurologic disease (ataxia, retinitis pigmentosa), very low serum cholesterol and triglyceride levels, and "spiny red cells" (acanthocytes). Therapy consists of substitution of dietary fat with medium-chain triglyceride and administration of fat-soluble vitamins, especially vitamin E.

Inadequate Absorptive Surface

SHORT BOWEL SYNDROME. Extensive resection of the small intestine is usually performed for Crohn's disease, intestinal infarction, or trauma. Acute hyperalimentation in these patients has been life-saving, and the ability of the remaining gut to adapt for increased nutrient absorption by hypertrophy of residual small intestinal villi is remarkable. Patients do rather well despite extensive resection if approximately 90 to 100 cm of duodenum and jejunum and the terminal ileum (intact ileocecal valve) remain.

Treatment consists of parenteral hyperalimentation for weeks to months until evidence exists that the remaining gut is functional. Gradual introduction of oral feedings, high in protein content, vitamins, and minerals, as well as medium-chain triglyceride (MCT), forms the basis for maintenance therapy. Antidiarrheal agents and cholestyramine may help (Table 104–9). Occasionally, pancreatic extract therapy and H₂-receptor antagonists are necessary to treat the transient acid hypersecretion and secondary pancreatic insufficiency that may occur. Steroids may increase water absorption. Finally, some patients must receive hyperalimentation at home indefinitely.

JEJUNOILEAL BYPASS. Some patients with morbid obesity have had a surgical procedure performed (14 inches of proximal jejunum is anastomosed to 4 inches of terminal ileum) that induces malabsorption. In addition to many of the problems detailed above in the short bowel syndrome, other serious complications occur, such as oxalate kidney stones, intestinal pseudo-obstruction, cirrhosis, and arthritis. Because of these complications, the operation has been abandoned.

Infection

TROPICAL SPRUE. The pathogenesis of this malabsorptive disorder occurring in tropical regions (Far East, India, Caribbean) is poorly understood. An overgrowth of coliforms within the jejunum has been demonstrated in these patients. Such organisms have been shown to elaborate an enterotoxin that induces fluid secretion. Tropical sprue is not a true bacterial overgrowth, since anaerobes (particularly *Bacteroides*) are conspicuously absent. Malabsorption of many nutrients occurs, especially folic acid, cobalamin, and fat. The intestinal biopsy does not demonstrate total villus atrophy, but rather nonspecific changes in the villi (shortening, thickening) and cellular infiltration of the lamina propria. Successful therapy has been achieved with cobalamin, folic acid, or antibiotics. A two-month course of a broad-spectrum antibiotic (e.g., tetracycline, 250 mg orally four times daily) and folic acid, 5.0 mg daily, is most effective. In those patients with cobalamin deficiency, 1000 μg of cobalamin should be given intramuscularly for two consecutive days. Improvement of malabsorption following therapy with folic acid or cobalamin alone casts doubt upon infection as the sole etiology.

WHIPPLE'S DISEASE. Patients (usually male) who present with Whipple's disease manifest steatorrhea, weight loss, abdominal pain, nondeforming arthritis, fever, peripheral lymphadenopathy, and neurologic abnormalities (nystagmus, ophthalmoplegia, cranial nerve defects). Protein-losing enteropathy may be present because of lymphatic obstruction.

Small bowel biopsy is diagnostic, demonstrating heavy infiltration of the mucosa and lymph nodes by macrophages that stain positive with periodic acid–Schiff reagent (PAS). Biopsy of the small intestine also shows blunting of villi and dilated lymphatics. The macrophages are filled with rod-shaped bacilli, which disappear after antibiotic therapy and reappear prior to an exacerbation of the disease. Although these rodlike structures resemble bacilli, no bacteria have been consistently cultured from patients with this disease—hence the bacterial etiology of Whipple's disease has not been proved.

Untreated, this is a fatal disease. These patients should be treated for at least a year and probably indefinitely. The antibiotic of choice appears to be trimethoprim-sulfamethoxazole, 500 mg given orally four times daily.

Lymphatic Obstruction

LYMPHOMA (INTESTINAL). Malabsorption occurs in patients with intestinal lymphoma from (1) mucosal invasion, (2) lymphatic obstruction, and (3) bacterial overgrowth secondary to dilatation of the bowel with stasis. Antibiotic therapy will often completely correct the clinical manifestations of malabsorption (diarrhea, steatorrhea), suggesting that bacterial overgrowth is an important cause of malabsorption in these patients. Abdominal pain, fever, and steatorrhea are principal complaints; lymphadenopathy and hepatosplenomegaly are uncommon. The small bowel biopsy may mimic nontropical sprue but not respond to a gluten-free diet. The diagnosis is usually made by the finding of malignant lymphoid cells in the mucosa or submucosa via small bowel biopsy or by full-thickness biopsy at surgery. As many as 10 per cent of patients with nontropical sprue may develop lymphoma.

LYMPHANGIECTASIA. Primary or congenital lymphangiectasia is characterized by diarrhea, mild steatorrhea, edema, enteric loss of protein (protein-losing enteropathy), and abnormal dilated lymphatic channels on small intestinal biopsy (Fig. 104–6). The main clinical feature of this disorder, which affects primarily children and young adults, is asymmetric edema secondary to the hypoplastic peripheral lymphatics and chylous effusions. Lymphocytopenia and depressed serum protein levels are a result of the protein-losing enteropathy. The hypoplastic lymphatics lead to an obstruction in lymph flow, increased pressure within lymphatics, dilated lymphatic channels in the intestine, and finally rupture of the lymphatic channels, discharging lymph into the bowel lumen. Therapy is directed to decreasing lymph flow via a low-fat diet and substitution of dietary fat with medium-chain triglycerides (MCT), which are transported by the portal venous system rather than the lymphatic system.

Although protein-losing enteropathy is a hallmark of intestinal lymphangiectasia, many other disorders can also cause enteric protein loss. The mechanisms are multifactorial: (1) exudation of protein through inflamed or engorged mucosa (gastric cancer, hypertrophy of gastric mucosa, ulcerative colitis), (2) loss of protein because of abnormal enterocytes (nontropical sprue, scleroderma), and (3) passage of proteins into the intestine secondary to increased pressure within lymphatics (lymphangiectasia, constrictive pericarditis, lymphoma).

Enteric protein loss can be detected by intravenously administering various labeled macromolecules and measuring the radioactivity in the feces. These tests are cumbersome to perform and not readily available. Recently, alpha$_1$-antitrypsin has been used as a marker for this disorder. Alpha$_1$-antitrypsin (similar size as albumin) can be measured in the feces by immunodiffusion.

Cardiovascular Disorders

Any disorder causing poor perfusion of the intestine may lead to steatorrhea. Atherosclerosis and vasculitis may both affect the mesenteric blood supply.

Drug-Induced Malabsorption

This entity is not very common and usually produces clinically insignificant malabsorption. Steatorrhea secondary to therapy with cholestyramine and neomycin is thought to be a result of precipitation of bile salts. The mechanism or mechanisms of most drug-induced malabsorption is not well understood.

Unexplained Malabsorption

Other than that in diabetes and perhaps in the carcinoid syndrome, the malabsorption occasionally observed in endocrine disorders (adrenal insufficiency, thyroid disease) is not at all understood. In diabetes, malabsorption may result from neuropathic changes (diarrhea) or bacterial overgrowth (steatorrhea). In systemic mast cell disease, there may be massive infiltration of the small intestine with mast cells, blunting of intestinal villi, and marked acid hypersecretion (Ch. 427). Malabsorption, however, does not appear to correlate well with any of these abnormalities. Hypogammaglobulinemia is at times associated with severe malabsorption. Although the pathogenesis is not well defined, such patients may have giardiasis, bacterial overgrowth, and histologic abnormalities of the small intestine (patchy villus atrophy, nodular lymphoid hyperplasia). Plasma cells are absent within the intestine.

Malabsorption in the Elderly

Elderly patients may develop malabsorption from any of the disorders listed in Table 104–2, but bacterial overgrowth appears to be the most common cause of clinically significant steatorrhea in this population. The elderly often have decreased gastric acid secretion and abnormalities in intestinal motility that predispose them to malabsorption from bacterial overgrowth. The hypo- or achlorhydria may lead to cobalamin (vitamin B$_{12}$) deficiency from malabsorption of food-bound

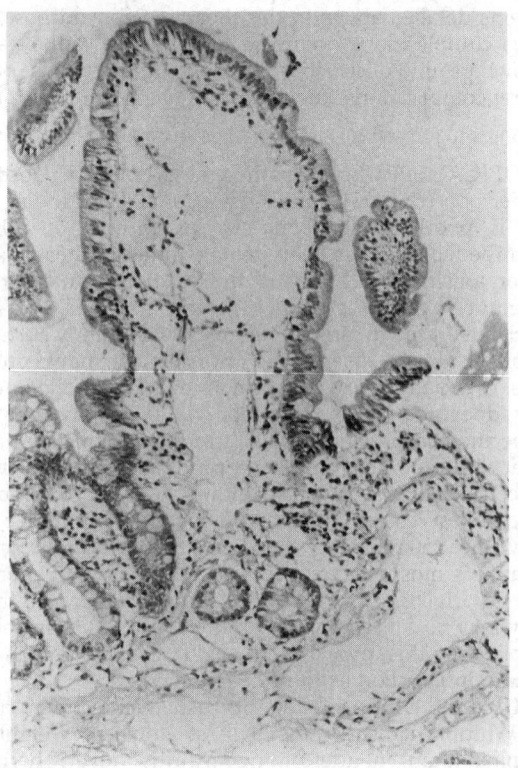

FIGURE 104–6. Small intestinal biopsy from a patient with intestinal lymphangiectasia. Note the dilated lymph channels (clear spaces).

cobalamin (Table 104–5). Such patients may be treated effectively just with tablets of cyanocobalamin (unbound B_{12}), since they have intrinsic factor in adequate amounts. Recognition of this problem may avoid parenteral administration of cobalamin.

Malabsorption in the Acquired Immunodeficiency Syndrome (AIDS) (Ch. 346)

Patients with AIDS often have diarrhea, malabsorption, and weight loss. Although these patients often have enteric infections and intestinal involvement with Kaposi's sarcoma, there are significant numbers of patients with AIDS who have malabsorption without these two abnormalities. In some patients with AIDS, biopsy of the small intestine demonstrates large numbers of histiocytes within the lamina propria. Although such findings on biopsy may be confused with Whipple's disease, in patients with AIDS these histiocytes contain acid-fast bacilli, representing *Mycobacterium avium-intracellulare*. Still other patients with AIDS have malabsorption with the only abnormality found being that of a nonspecific mild-to-moderate chronic inflammatory response in the small bowel biopsy. The malabsorption in this last group of patients may be due to bacterial overgrowth or other unidentified enteric infections.

Cole SG, Kagnoff MF: Celiac disease. Ann Rev Nutr 5:241, 1985.

Florent C, L'Hirondel C, Desmazures C, et al: Intestinal clearance of α_1-antitrypsin: A sensitive method for the detection of protein-losing enteropathy. Gastroenterology 81:777, 1981. *New method of documenting protein-losing enteropathy.*

Gaskin KJ, Durie PR, Hill RE: Colipase and maximally activated pancreatic lipase in normal subjects and patients with steatorrhea. J Clin Invest 69:427, 1982. *Points out the importance of colipase.*

Gillin JS, Shike M, Alcock N, et al: Malabsorption and mucosal abnormalities of the small intestine in the acquired immunodeficiency syndrome. Ann Intern Med 102:619, 1985. *Good discussion of causes of malabsorption in patients with AIDS.*

Keinath RD, Merrell DE, Vlietstra R, et al: Antibiotic treatment and relapse in Whipple's disease. Long-term follow-up of 88 patients. Gastroenterology 88:1867, 1985. *Current discussion of therapy in this disease.*

King CE, Toskes PP: Comparison of the 1-gram ^{14}C-xylose, 10-gram lactulose-H_2, and 80-gram glucose-H_2 breath tests in patients with small intestine bacterial overgrowth. Gastroenterology 91:1447, 1986.

King CE, Toskes PP: Small intestine bacterial overgrowth. Gastroenterology 76:1035, 1979. *Comprehensive review of the subject.*

King CE, Toskes PP: The use of breath tests in the study of malabsorption. Clin Gastroenterol 12:591, 1983. *Thorough overall review of clinical usefulness of these tests.*

Montgomery RD, Haboubi NY, Mike NH, et al.: Causes of malabsorption in the elderly. Age Ageing 15:235, 1986.

Simon CL, Gorbach SL: The human intestinal microflora. Dig Dis Sci (Suppl) 31:147, 1986.

Sleisenger MH, Fordtran JS (eds.): Gastrointestinal Disease. 4th ed. Philadelphia, W. B. Saunders Company, 1988, Ch. 18, 19, 57, 61, 66–68. *Normal absorption and malabsorption in well-referenced text of gastroenterology.*

Toskes PP: The bentiromide test for pancreatic exocrine insufficiency. Pharmacotherapy 4:74, 1984. *Review of worldwide experience with this noninvasive test of pancreatic function.*

Weser E, Fletcher JT, Urban E: Short bowel syndrome. Gastroenterology 77:572, 1979. *Excellent review of this important problem.*

Westergaard H: The sprue syndromes. Am J Med Sci 290:249, 1985.

105 INFLAMMATORY BOWEL DISEASE

105.1 Introduction

Irwin H. Rosenberg

The term *inflammatory bowel disease* is broadly used to refer to idiopathic chronic inflammatory diseases of the intestine, principally *ulcerative colitis* and *Crohn's disease*. Ulcerative colitis, as the name implies, is an inflammatory, ulcerating process of the colon; Crohn's disease is a transmural granulomatous enteritis that may involve any part of the intestine, but primarily the distal small intestine and colon. These two conditions of unknown etiology share a number of clinical, epidemiologic, immunologic, and genetic features, including extraintestinal complications and response to treatment. Therefore, they are often considered together despite distinguishing clinical and pathologic features. These diseases may represent different pathologic responses to a common cause, or they may turn out to be unrelated in etiology and pathogenesis. These two major forms of inflammatory bowel disease will be discussed separately for convenience, but it will prove useful to compare and contrast them throughout.

105.2 Crohn's Disease

Irwin H. Rosenberg

DEFINITION. *Crohn's disease* is a subacute and chronic inflammatory process of unknown cause that may involve any part of the intestinal tract, especially the distal ileum, colon, and anorectal region. Although earlier reports are suggestive, Crohn's disease was first clearly described as an inflammatory condition of the terminal ileum by Burrill Crohn and his colleagues in 1932 and called *regional ileitis*. Shortly thereafter reports of similar transmural granulomatous inflammation of portions of the small and large bowel made the term "regional enteritis" more appropriate. A similar granulomatous inflammation of the colon, distinguishable from ulcerative colitis, was subsequently described and termed "Crohn's disease of the large intestine." The pattern in over 50 per cent of patients with Crohn's disease is *ileocolitis*, which involves the distal small bowel with variable, segmental involvement of the colon. *Ileitis* is a common designation for Crohn's disease confined to the ileum. *Crohn's colitis* refers to predominant involvement of the colon.

EPIDEMIOLOGY. Like ulcerative colitis, Crohn's disease is more common in northern Europe and the United States, less frequent in central Europe and the Middle East, and infrequent in Asia and Africa. Crohn's disease has a prevalence roughly half that of ulcerative colitis. The incidence and prevalence of Crohn's disease rose gradually through the 1960's and 1970's. The incidence has stabilized in most European and North American countries. In the United States this disease affects 50,000 to 100,000 patients at any time, with 5000 to 10,000 new cases diagnosed each year. The incidence of Crohn's disease is approximately equal in males and females. The age of onset profile of Crohn's disease is shown in Figure 105–1. Crohn's disease is uncommon before age ten; the peak incidence occurs in the next two decades and declines thereafter. A later peak of incidence has been reported at 55 to 60 years, but whether this represents a true secondary peak or the effect of hospitalization for other disorders (e.g., ischemic bowel) remains uncertain.

American blacks and American Indians are at less than one fifth the risk of the white population for inflammatory bowel disease. There is growing evidence that the incidence of inflammatory bowel disease in blacks is rising. In Japan the incidence of inflammatory bowel disease has been relatively low, but now is rising steadily. The prevalence of Crohn's disease is six times higher for Jewish men and three times higher for Jewish women. The incidence of inflammatory bowel disease among Jews in Israel is lower than that of Jews in the United States or in northern Europe. Israeli Jews of European (Ashkenazic) ancestry are at considerably greater risk than are Jews of Mediterranean or Middle Eastern (Sephardic) ancestry. Inflammatory bowel disease occurs with equal frequency in urban and rural populations. Some of these demographic features are summarized in Table 105–1.

FAMILIAL-GENETIC PATTERN. There are definite famil-

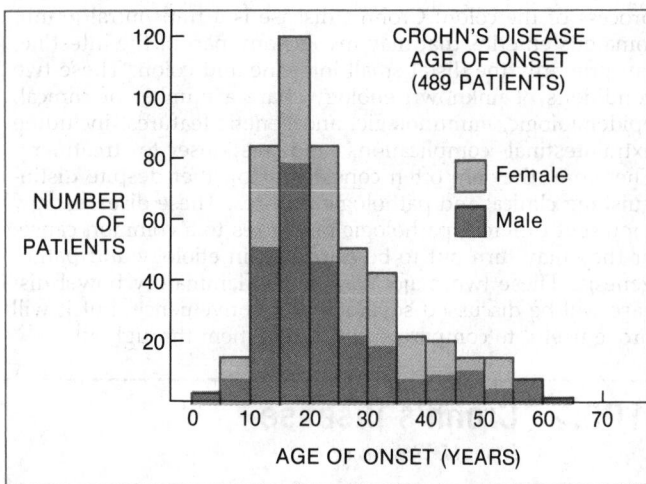

FIGURE 105–1. Age of onset of 489 patients with Crohn's disease. (From Rogers BHG, Clark LM, Kirsner JB: J Chron Dis 24:743, 1971.)

ial clusters of patients with both ulcerative colitis and Crohn's disease. In one large series, 17.5 per cent of patients had a positive family history for a similar disorder. As many as five members in a single family with inflammatory bowel disease have been reported. Three fourths of family clusters involve either ulcerative colitis or Crohn's disease, but in one fourth of such families both ulcerative colitis and Crohn's disease are found in the same pedigree. Disease concordance has occurred in some, but not all, monozygotic twins.

ETIOLOGY AND PATHOGENESIS. Both Crohn's disease and ulcerative colitis are diseases of unknown etiology. The patterns of prevalence described above suggest both host and environmental factors. Individual susceptibility factors are suggested by the specific ethnic patterns of occurrence and the phenomenon of family clustering. Familial occurrence might also represent exposure of the patient and family members to common environmental factors. Parallel trends in disease incidence with increasing technologic development in Asia as well as Europe and the United States also suggest environmental factors. Some of the many and disparate theories of the etiology of Crohn's disease will be reviewed briefly.

Psychogenic Factors. Significant emotional events have often seemed to be temporally related to the onset or exacerbation of inflammatory bowel disease, leading to the hypothesis that psychogenic factors are important in its etiology or pathogenesis. The nervous system may profoundly influence the motor, secretory, vascular, and metabolic functions of the digestive system, but it is difficult to postulate that these variables would lead to the type of segmental involvement or transmural inflammation often seen in Crohn's disease. Psychogenic factors are probably important in their contribution to symptomatic exacerbations.

Infectious Origin. From the time of the first descriptions of this condition, etiologic interest has emphasized possible bacterial or other microbiologic causes. The similarity of the inflammatory response to that with mycobacterial infection, the fever and toxemia in some patients, and the response of some to antimicrobial therapy have been recurrent clinical

TABLE 105–1. DEMOGRAPHIC FEATURES OF CROHN'S DISEASE

Worldwide distribution
More common in whites than nonwhites
Increased frequency among European stock
More common among Jews (especially Ashkenazic) than
  non-Jews (3 to 6 times)
Most frequent age of onset: 15 to 30 years
Aggregation in families

Modified from Donaldson RM Jr: In Sleisenger MH, Fordtran JS (eds.): Gastrointestinal Disease. 3rd ed. Philadelphia, W. B. Saunders Company, 1983.

observations. Sporadically, microbial isolates have been made from tissues of patients with Crohn's disease, most recently cell wall–deficient mycobacteria and ribonucleic acid (RNA) viruses. However, evidence for an etiologic role for any of these agents has been lacking. Earlier reports of transmission of an infectious agent or agents in animal models or of viral isolations have not been confirmed by multicenter trials using standardized methods and interlaboratory exchanges of tissue homogenates. *Yersinia enterocolitica* infection can produce an acute ileitis, and *Campylobacter* and *Clostridium difficile* have been reported in association with exacerbations of Crohn's disease, but these agents are not implicated in the etiology. Nevertheless, the search for microbiologic agents represents one current approach to understanding the etiology of the inflammatory bowel diseases.

Immunologic Factors. Whether or not microorganisms are directly implicated in the etiology of these diseases, they may be involved in their pathogenesis in concert with altered immune mechanisms. Some of the extraintestinal manifestations of inflammatory bowel disease suggest the presence of antigen-antibody complexes in these sites. Serum concentrations of the major immunoglobulin classes follow no predictable pattern among patients with ulcerative colitis or Crohn's disease and fail to show a consistent relationship to the state of activity or severity of the diseases. Circulating lymphocytes from patients with inflammatory bowel disease may be cytotoxic to cultures of human fetal or adult colonic epithelial cells. Responses of circulating lymphocytes to nonspecific mitogens are generally intact, especially in patients with ulcerative colitis. Some abnormalities of proportions or numbers of circulating B and T lymphocytes, particularly T-suppressor cells, have been reported. None of these immunologic changes has been clearly shown to be implicated in the etiology or pathogenesis of inflammatory bowel disease. Lymphocytes and macrophages isolated from the intestinal tissue itself tend to show "inappropriate" immune responses, perhaps genetically determined, which are thought to result in a persistent, and thus pathologic, local mucosal response to unidentified antigens. Whether these abnormalities in the behavior of macrophages and regulatory T lymphocytes are central or peripheral to the etiopathogenesis of Crohn's disease remains the challenging question.

MEDIATORS OF INFLAMMATION. Endogenous mediators, such as prostaglandins and leukotrienes, participate in the inflammatory/metabolic responses in Crohn's disease. Increased amounts of these highly active agents have been measured in the involved tissues of patients, thereby providing a rationale for the use of drugs that might blunt the action of known mediators of inflammation or of fat-modified diets to limit availability of their fatty acid precursors.

PATHOLOGY. Crohn's disease may involve any segment of the alimentary canal or any combination of segments. There are, however, pathologic changes that characterize the inflammatory process in any segment of involved bowel. The involved portion of the bowel, usually the distal ileum and adjacent right colon, is thickened and hyperemic with some serosal fibrin deposition and adhesions between adjacent loops of bowel (Fig. 105–2). The adjacent mesentery is commonly thickened with migration or "creeping" of mesenteric fat onto the serosal surface of the bowel. Mesenteric lymphatics are engorged, and mesenteric lymph nodes are commonly enlarged and matted.

Diseased segments of bowel wall are thickened. The mucosa may be nearly normal or only mildly hyperemic, or there may be elongated linear ulcerations, usually in the long axis of the bowel. In more advanced cases the mucosal architecture is destroyed by multiple ulcerations, with only small islands of mucosa remaining. Numerous aphthoid ulcers may be present in the mucosa. Deep ulcers or clefts may extend into the thickened and edematous submucosa and sometimes through to the serosal surface.

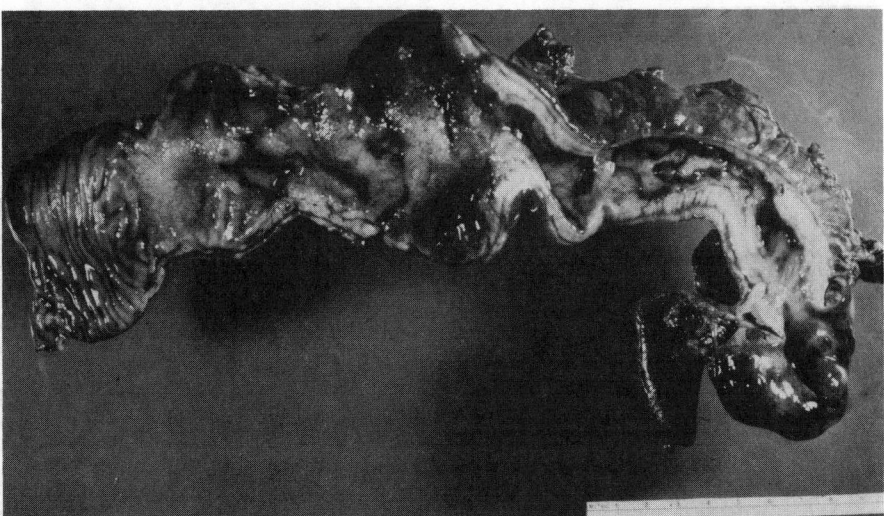

FIGURE 105–2. Resected specimen of ileum showing thickening of the wall, loss of normal mucosa, scarring, and stricture in Crohn's disease. "Creeping fat" is visible on the serosal surface.

Fistulas form readily in this setting of a transmural inflammation when deep ulcerations and fissures combine with obstruction and stenosis to form a penetrating, pressure-relieving pathway to adjacent and adherent loops of bowel or other viscera, and sometimes to the abdominal wall. Ileoileal, ileosigmoid, and ileocecal communications are most common, but communication with other parts of the gastrointestinal tract, including the stomach, duodenum, and gallbladder, has been reported. Fistulas may also occur from the intestine to the urinary bladder, the renal collecting system, and the female genital tract, most often the vagina.

The inflammatory process involves all layers of the bowel and consists of infiltration of lymphocytes, histiocytes, and plasma cells with characteristic aggregation to form noncaseating granulomas. Focal granulomas are found in about half of the cases; in the remainder, well-defined lymphoid aggregates are found.

These pathologic changes and their progression correlate with many of the important clinical manifestations of Crohn's disease. Abdominal pain and cramps reflect the narrowed lumen and partial obstruction that result from thickening of the bowel wall. Diarrhea may represent disordered mucosal absorptive-secretory function or abnormal motility of either small or large bowel. The transmural inflammation increases adherence of loops of bowel, producing signs of peritoneal irritation and the formation of abdominal masses.

CLINICAL PRESENTATION. When Crohn's disease affects primarily the distal small intestine (*Crohn's ileitis* or *regional enteritis*), the most characteristic clinical pattern emerges. A young person, usually in the second or third decade, will present with a period of episodic abdominal pain, largely postprandial and often periumbilical, occasionally with low-grade fever and mild diarrhea. Such episodes often remit spontaneously but recur with increasing frequency and severity, with pain eventually localizing to the right lower quadrant.

The *abdominal pain* often has the characteristics of partial intestinal obstruction, made worse by eating and improved by rest, local heat, and fasting. The effect of early ileitis on bowel habits may be variable. *Diarrhea* is rarely more severe than four or five stools daily, and rectal bleeding is uncommon. *Weight loss* is frequent. In children growth retardation and delayed sexual maturation may be the presenting clinical features in Crohn's disease. The patient may be aware of *tenderness in the right lower quadrant* and even of a palpable mass in that region. The similarity of this presentation to that of acute appendicitis commonly results in an abdominal exploration, and diagnosis is then made surgically. When the involvement of the small intestine is more diffuse in the syndrome of jejunoileitis, the presentation may include more diffuse abdominal pain and more prominent weight loss, growth retardation, and sometimes peripheral edema.

In Crohn's colitis or ileocolitis the presentation is characterized by lower abdominal, crampy pain worsened by eating, by diarrhea, and by fever. Crohn's colitis tends to be more subtle in onset than ulcerative colitis and thus may not be diagnosed until anemia or other systemic complications predominate.

One third of all patients with Crohn's disease and one half with Crohn's colitis develop perirectal or perianal fistulas with pain, mass, purulent drainage, and often fever. Perianal complications may represent communication of a fistulous tract from the small bowel along the presacral gutter to the perirectal area but more commonly are a complication of deep, penetrating ulceration in Crohn's colitis of the lower colon. When drainage is impaired, local abscess formation occurs.

Extraintestinal manifestations such as arthritis, ankylosing spondylitis, and erythema nodosum may precede or strongly influence the presenting syndrome. These extraintestinal manifestations of Crohn's disease will be discussed subsequently.

DIAGNOSIS. The diagnosis of Crohn's disease may be delayed for months or even years in patients whose symptoms are subtle and insidious and in those in whom extraintestinal manifestations focus attention away from the bowel. Crohn's disease should be suspected in patients of any age, but particularly in those in the younger age groups, when there is a history of recurrent episodes of abdominal pain worsened by eating, and a change in bowel habits with intermittent or persisting diarrhea. The presence of pain, tenderness, and a mass in the right lower quadrant should strongly heighten the suspicion of this diagnosis. A history of weight loss is common. In addition, unexplained arthritis, perianal disease, recurrent fevers, or, in children, cessation of normal growth should raise the question of Crohn's disease even if gastrointestinal symptoms are minimal.

Physical Examination. A moderately ill patient may be pale, underweight, and febrile (temperature seldom greater than 38°C). An abdominal examination often demonstrates tenderness or a mass in the right lower abdominal quadrant. The bowel sounds may be hyperactive. Examination of the extremities may reveal signs of large joint arthritis or, rarely, clubbing. Uveitis, iritis, and skin manifestations (see below) may occasionally be present. Peripheral edema may reflect protein depletion. Examination of the rectum and perianal area may identify perianal fistulas, fissures, or an abscess. A purulent vaginal discharge in a woman with Crohn's disease is strongly suggestive of enterovaginal fistula.

Radiographic Examination. The diagnosis of Crohn's dis-

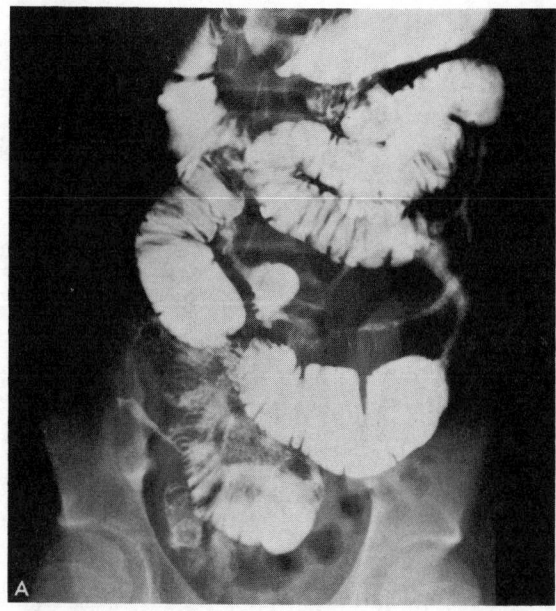

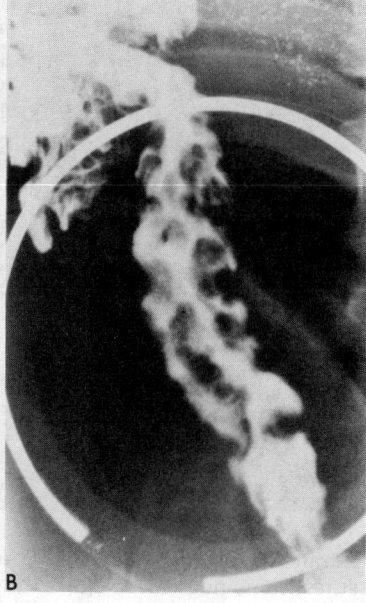

FIGURE 105–3. *A,* Small bowel radiograph in Crohn's disease demonstrating extensive jejunoileitis with areas of narrowing and mucosal damage alternating with "skip areas" of more normal bowel. *B,* Cobblestone appearance of the terminal ileum in Crohn's disease.

ease depends in considerable measure on the presence of characteristic radiographic findings in the bowel. The abdominal plain film may demonstrate dilated loops of small bowel in the presence of partial obstruction. The diagnosis depends, however, upon upper and lower intestinal barium contrast studies (Figs. 105–3 and 105–4). Characteristic changes on the small bowel roentgenogram include segmental narrowing, obliteration of the normal mucosal pattern with or without evidence of ulceration, enteroenteric fistula formation, or the classic "string sign" of the contrast medium shown on segmental films of the terminal ileum, particularly when changes are localized to the most distal small bowel and the adjacent right colon (Fig. 105–3).

Most radiologists prefer air contrast radiography of the colon to delineate the presence or extent of disease in the large bowel (Fig. 105–4). In 85 per cent of patients with Crohn's disease of the large bowel, there will also be involvement of the distal small bowel, which is best demonstrated by antegrade barium studies as described above. It is important to distinguish between "backwash ileitis" associated with

ulcerative colitis and true mucosal involvement of ileal Crohn's disease. In Crohn's colitis there is a characteristic asymmetric and segmental pattern with areas of disease separated by areas of apparently normal colonic tissue.

The most subtle changes in the small bowel are thickening and edema of the valvulae conniventes. Earliest changes in the large bowel are the appearance of small aphthous ulcers on air-contrast examinations. Loss of haustral markings may be a subtle early finding. Mucosal ulcers are likely to be longitudinal. When severe ulcerative disease is present, the alternation of ulcers with regenerating mucosa produces the "cobblestone" appearance (Fig. 105–3*B*). As the disease progresses, there is increasing scar formation with total loss of mucosal pattern and narrowing of the segments of involved bowel. The presence of fistulous tracts from one loop of bowel to another can often be demonstrated. The presence of distinctly narrowed segments of bowel need not be taken as clear evidence of cicatricial and irreversible obstruction. These findings are often manifestations of severe edema and thickening of the bowel and may improve substantially following treatment. The newer technique of enteroclysis—instillation of barium directly into the small bowel by tube—may add precision to small intestinal studies.

Laboratory Diagnosis. No laboratory test is diagnostic for Crohn's disease. Anemia may result from blood loss or iron or folate deficiency. Sedimentation rate and other acute phase reactants, including serum orosomucoid, may be elevated. Examination of the stool may reveal the presence of occult blood and increased fat. Fecal leukocytes call attention to inflammatory processes as a basis for the diarrhea. A low serum albumin reflects malnutrition and increased enteric protein loss. Low serum calcium or magnesium may be seen in patients with severe diarrhea and steatorrhea. An abnormal Schilling test of vitamin B_{12} absorption reflects extensive disease or resection of the ileum. Other tests of intestinal absorption, including the quantitative fecal fat, xylose absorption test, and lactose absorption test, are helpful in assessing the extent and severity of disease. Analyses of the circulating levels of iron, folate, vitamin B_{12}, 25-hydroxy vitamin D, and plasma zinc may demonstrate evidence of micronutrient depletion.

Proctosigmoidoscopy. In contrast to ulcerative colitis, the rectum is uninvolved in more than half of the patients with Crohn's disease. Proctosigmoidoscopy may simply show mild erythema associated nonspecifically with diarrhea. Rarely, a biopsy of the normal-appearing rectum will reveal inflammatory changes and even granuloma, but such biopsies are not a necessary part of the diagnostic evaluation.

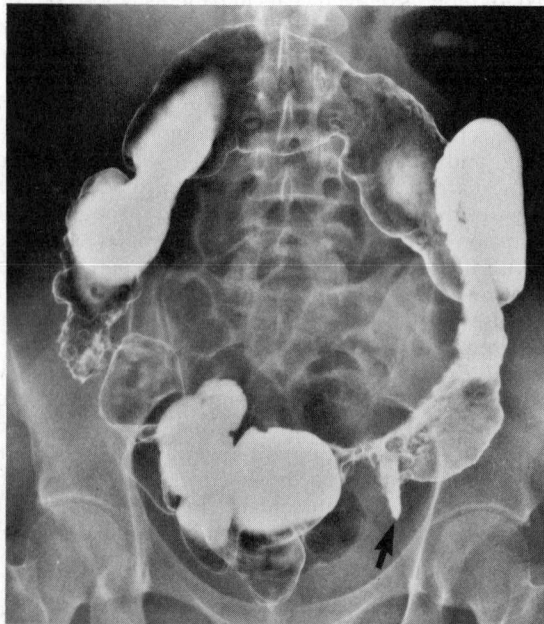

FIGURE 105–4. Typical Crohn's colitis demonstrated by air-contrast exam. Note asymmetric involvement, loss of normal haustral markings, and early fistula in the sigmoid region (*arrow*).

Colonoscopy. Colonoscopy may be valuable in determining the extent and severity of colonic involvement and in evaluating strictures or polypoid masses. Colonoscopic biopsies are helpful for verification of the diagnosis in difficult cases.

LOCAL COMPLICATIONS. Chronic, transmural inflammation of the bowel with progressive scarring leads to a number of local complications. Hemorrhage is uncommon, but *chronic blood loss* leading to iron deficiency often occurs. Local scarring and narrowing of the bowel lead to *intestinal obstruction* of varying severity. Free *intestinal perforation* occurs rarely; more often there is fistulous communication between loops of bowel or into matted mesentery, which presents as a tender, inflammatory mass with fever. Fistulas can occur to any abdominal viscus, as previously noted.

Perianal fistulas and related fissures and abscesses affect nearly half of all patients with Crohn's disease. Indurated, nonhealing rectal fissures, draining perianal fistulas, or local abscesses may cause local pain, fever, and progressive perineal distortion. Abscesses must be drained, with special attention to the integrity of the anal sphincter muscles and the threat of fecal incontinence. A judicious and persistent combination of bowel rest and dietary, drug, and surgical therapy is required (see Treatment).

MALABSORPTION AND NUTRIENT-LOSING ENTEROPATHY. Predictably, malabsorption is found largely in those patients with extensive inflammatory involvement or following partial resection of the small intestine. The ileum is the major site of absorption of both vitamin B_{12} and bile salts. Ileitis may therefore result in malabsorption of this vitamin as well as steatorrhea on the basis of the interrupted enterohepatic circulation of bile salts. Malabsorption of fat-soluble vitamins, including vitamin D, and of water-soluble vitamins, such as folate, has been reported in Crohn's disease. There is a tendency, especially in those who have had resection of the ileocecal valve, to develop bacterial overgrowth, which further contributes to malabsorption. Enteric protein loss through the damaged epithelium may be an important contributor to protein and associated trace metal depletion. The reader is referred to Ch. 103 for a more extensive discussion of malabsorption.

SYSTEMIC AND EXTRAINTESTINAL COMPLICATIONS (see Table 105–2). *Nutritional Complications.* Nutritional complications are common in inflammatory bowel disease. The majority of patients admitted to the hospital will exhibit some degree of nutritional depletion. Assessment of the nutritional status should be part of the initial evaluation of the patient in order to recognize and treat nutritional complications early. Deficiencies of protein, calories, minerals, vitamins, and trace metals are well documented in both Crohn's disease and ulcerative colitis. These deficiencies may result from inadequate dietary intake, malabsorption, or intestinal loss of protein, as noted above. In addition, increased nutritional requirement relating to the chronic inflammatory response and faster cell turnover in the diseased gut is probable but less well documented.

Growth Retardation. Retarded skeletal growth, often with a delay in sexual maturation, is frequently observed in children whose onset of Crohn's disease occurs before puberty. In some patients a slowing or arrest of linear growth occurs years before the diagnosis of Crohn's disease is made and may be the condition that brings the patient to medical attention. The pathogenesis of growth retardation is complex. No hormonal deficiencies have been demonstrated in these patients. Corticosteroids administered daily in high doses for colitis or Crohn's disease may suppress growth in some patients. Lower doses or alternate-day steroid therapy may allow restoration of normal growth by suppressing the activity of the disease. Abnormalities of intestinal absorption have not been prominent in those patients carefully studied. Caloric insufficiency is of central etiologic importance and usually results from a dietary intake that is limited by the young

TABLE 105–2. EXTRAINTESTINAL MANIFESTATIONS OF THE INFLAMMATORY BOWEL DISEASES

Nutritional and metabolic abnormalities
 Weight loss, growth retardation in children
 Hypoalbuminemia—nutritional, protein-losing enteropathy
 Vitamin deficiencies
 Deficiencies of calcium, magnesium, or zinc
Hematologic abnormalities
 Anemia—bleeding, Fe deficiency, folate deficiency
 Leukocytosis, thrombocytosis
Skin and mucous membrane
 Pyoderma gangrenosum
 Erythema nodosum
 Stomatitis with multiple aphthous ulcers
Musculoskeletal
 Ankylosing spondylitis, sacroiliitis (HLA-B27 associated)
 Peripheral arthritis of large joints
 Osteoporosis, osteomalacia
Hepatic and biliary manifestations
 Fatty liver
 Pericholangitis
 Sclerosing cholangitis
 Cirrhosis
 Gallstones
 Carcinoma of the bile ducts
Renal complications
 Kidney stones—uric acid, calcium oxalate
 Obstructive uropathy
 Fistulas to urinary tract
 Amyloidosis (rare)
Eye complications
 Conjunctivitis, episcleritis, uveitis
 Iritis

patient in response to abdominal pain and diarrhea. Protein, vitamin, and mineral deficiencies are less regular.

Hepatobiliary Complications. Hepatobiliary complications of Crohn's disease (and of ulcerative colitis) include a spectrum from clinically inapparent histologic abnormalities through progressive and sometimes life-threatening liver disease. The possibility that chronic or intermittent portal bacteremia or the return from the gut to the liver of toxic metabolic products, such as lithocholic acid, may be responsible for hepatic injury has been suggested but not proved. Neither viral hepatitis after blood transfusion nor drug toxicity can account for a significant proportion of liver disease in these patients. *Fatty infiltration* of the liver is found in virtually all biopsy or autopsy specimens of patients with inflammatory bowel disease. Abnormalities other than fatty infiltration are found in the majority of liver specimens obtained by needle biopsies in patients with inflammatory bowel disease: *pericholangitis* (50 to 70 per cent), *chronic active hepatitis, cirrhosis,* extrahepatic obstruction associated with *primary sclerosing cholangitis,* and, most rarely, *carcinoma of the bile ducts.* Fewer than 25 per cent of such patients will have increased alkaline phosphatase activity; jaundice is even less common. However, when serious or progressive liver disease is present histologically, liver function tests are usually abnormal.

Pericholangitis refers to a lymphocytic inflammatory response in the entire portal triad, not only periductal as the name implies. Most patients with pericholangitis demonstrated by biopsy are asymptomatic, and the majority have normal liver function tests. Some may have recurring episodes of cholestasis, jaundice, and pruritus with increased serum alkaline phosphatase. In a few patients the full picture of ascending cholangitis, shaking chills, fever, and jaundice will occur. Recurrent right upper quadrant pain may cause diagnostic confusion with gallstone disease, which is also more common in patients with Crohn's disease. Occasionally, pericholangitis will progress to cirrhosis. Those patients with pericholangitis found incidentally on liver biopsy at the time of surgery without a history of cholangitis or hepatic function abnormalities are likely to have a benign course without progressive hepatic deterioration.

Sclerosing cholangitis is an uncommon inflammatory and sclerosing lesion of extra- and intrahepatic bile ducts causing biliary obstruction and recurrent cholangitis. Its relationship to pericholangitis is uncertain. In some patients inflammation extends from the portal triads to the intra- and extrahepatic ducts. The extent of anatomic abnormality is best determined by endoscopic retrograde cholangiography. Corticosteroids are often used to suppress inflammation, and antibiotics are used to treat episodes of cholangitis. Promising results have recently been reported with low-dose methotrexate therapy. In some patients adequate bile drainage may have to be established surgically. Carcinoma of the bile ducts, although extremely rare in Crohn's disease, is sometimes seen in the setting of sclerosing cholangitis.

Gallstones develop with increased frequency in patients with Crohn's disease whether or not bile duct abnormalities exist. This tendency is often attributed to bile salt malabsorption in the diseased ileum, leading to a diminished bile salt pool and a relative increase in the ratio of cholesterol to bile salts in bile.

Renal Complications. Renal complications in Crohn's disease include *obstructive uropathy, nephrolithiasis, fistulas* to the renal collecting system, and rarely, *amyloidosis.* Fistulas from the bowel to the renal excretory system may present as the passage of gas or fecal material in the urine. The diagnostic changes may be more subtle and simply involve recurrent episodes of pyuria or infection. Right-sided hydronephrosis resulting from cicatricial and inflammatory obstruction of the right ureter may be asymptomatic, and some advocate the regular use of ultrasonography in the full evaluation of the patient with Crohn's disease. Corrective surgery by unsheathing of the right ureter may prevent progressive destruction of the right kidney.

The most common renal complication is *nephrolithiasis.* There is an increased incidence of uric acid stones in both Crohn's disease and ulcerative colitis, probably related to increased cell turnover and the excretion of a concentrated urine of increased acidity. The most frequent type of kidney stone in patients with Crohn's disease, however, is composed of calcium oxalate as its main crystalloid. Patients with extensive disease of the distal small intestine, particularly those who have had resections of the distal small bowel, have excessive absorption of dietary oxalate and low urinary excretion of citrate and are therefore at increased risk for the formation of calcium oxalate stones (see Ch. 90 for more details).

Miscellaneous Complications. Both *peripheral arthritis* and *spondylitis* occur in Crohn's disease as in ulcerative colitis, affecting approximately 10 to 20 per cent of patients. Osteoporosis, especially in patients who receive high doses of corticosteroids, is common even though usually asymptomatic. Osteomalacia usually reflects subclinical vitamin D deficiency. *Erythema nodosum* is seen in approximately 9 per cent of patients with Crohn's disease, but *pyoderma gangrenosum* and *erythema multiforme* are rare. Ocular complications include *episcleritis, uveitis,* and *iritis* in 3 to 4 per cent of patients.

DIFFERENTIAL DIAGNOSIS. The classic presentation of Crohn's disease with a characteristic history, a palpable right lower abdominal mass, and typical radiographs offers little diagnostic challenge. The presentation, however, may be highly variable. With an acute onset, Crohn's disease may be mistaken for appendicitis, particularly in a young person with right lower quadrant rebound tenderness and leukocytosis. Diarrhea, however, is uncommon in appendicitis. If progression of symptoms and signs is rapid and the opportunity to diagnose Crohn's disease by the typical radiographic findings is not feasible, exploration may be necessary. An *appendiceal abscess* is particularly difficult to distinguish from a mass associated with Crohn's disease by radiography.

Infection by *Yersinia enterocolitica* causes an acute or subacute mesenteric adenitis and may produce diarrhea, abdominal pain, and fever. Infection by *Campylobacter fetus* may resemble acute or subacute colitis. Successful diagnosis requires attention to the specific requirements for culturing these organisms. Distinction of Crohn's disease from *ileocecal tuberculosis* or from fungal infections involving the bowel is usually possible on epidemiologic grounds. Intestinal tuberculosis is rare in the United States and western Europe and is usually seen in native-born Americans only in the presence of extensive pulmonary tuberculosis. Persons raised in areas where milk-borne tuberculosis is common often have ileocecal tuberculosis without pulmonary disease.

Benign lymphoid hyperplasia of Peyer's patches in the ileum is seen on barium radiographs in children and young adults in a setting of infection or fever. This benign condition is distinguishable from Crohn's disease on radiographic grounds, since no mucosal abnormality or luminal narrowing occurs.

Patients with a more chronic course present a more extensive differential diagnosis. *Nongranulomatous ulcerative jejunoileitis,* another inflammatory condition of the small bowel of unknown etiology, has more prominent malabsorption, nutrient-losing enteropathy, and nonspecific shallow small bowel ulcers on intestinal biopsy. This distinction in rare cases, however, requires exploration and surgical biopsies.

Lymphoma or *lymphosarcoma* of the small bowel may produce a picture similar to that of Crohn's disease. Once initiated, the symptoms of this malignant process are usually more persistent and more rapidly progressive than those of Crohn's disease. Palpable abdominal masses tend to be firmer. A diffuse nodularity of the bowel without segmental narrowing characteristic of Crohn's disease on small bowel series suggests abdominal lymphoma. Occasionally *carcinoid* of the ileum or other malignancies will be extensive and invasive enough to be mistaken for Crohn's disease by radiography.

Radiation enteritis involving the distal ileum and colon after pelvic irradiation for carcinoma is distinguished from Crohn's disease mainly by history.

Eosinophilic gastroenteritis may present with diarrhea, malabsorption, and protein-losing enteropathy, but the pattern of the intestinal involvement demonstrated by radiographic or endoscopic techniques, peripheral blood eosinophilia, and positive findings on intestinal biopsy are distinguishing features.

When Crohn's disease involves the duodenum or stomach, it may be mistaken for duodenal ulcer disease, or even the Zollinger-Ellison syndrome when there are multiple ulcerating lesions. The pain pattern tends to be different in these conditions. Crohn's disease causes more persistent or postprandial abdominal pain and symptoms of obstruction. Endoscopy and biopsy in addition to radiographic findings may be helpful in distinguishing these conditions from Crohn's disease.

For distinction between Crohn's ileitis and backwash ileitis associated with ulcerative colitis and for the differentiation of Crohn's colitis and ulcerative colitis, the reader is referred to Table 105–3.

TREATMENT. There is no known cure for Crohn's disease. Treatment is empiric and is directed at alleviating the symptoms and manifestations of the disease. Symptomatic remissions may occur during therapy, or even in its absence, but the disease is lifelong, and surveillance by the physician must be a continuing process. In addition to medical and sometimes surgical management, general support is very important, including attention to the psychologic stresses imposed by the disease on the patient and the family. In addition, the physician must anticipate, identify, and, when possible, prevent the common nutritional and metabolic complications described above.

Medical Management. Medical management of Crohn's disease requires a comprehensive assessment of the clinical status of the patient. It is particularly important to determine the extent and severity of the disease, largely by radiologic and

TABLE 105-3. A COMPARISON OF THE CLINICAL AND PATHOLOGIC FEATURES OF CROHN'S COLITIS AND ULCERATIVE COLITIS

Feature	Crohn's Colitis	Ulcerative Colitis
Intestinal		
Malaise, fever	Common	Uncommon
Rectal bleeding	Sometimes	Common
Abdominal tenderness	Very common	May be present
Abdominal mass	Very common (especially with ileocolitis)	Not present
Abdominal pain	Very common	Unusual
Fistulas	Very common	Very uncommon
Endoscopic		
Rectal disease	Occasionally	Very common
Diffuse, continuous, symmetric involvement	Uncommon	Very common
Aphthous or linear ulcers	Common	Very unusual
Cobblestoning	Common	Very unusual
Friability	Unusual	Very common
Radiologic		
Continuous disease	Uncommon	Very common
Ileal involvement	Very common	"Backwash ileitis"
Asymmetry	Very common	Uncommon
Strictures	Common	Uncommon
Fistulas	Very common	Uncommon
Pathologic		
Discontinuity	Common	Uncommon
Rectal involvement	Uncommon	Common
Intense vascularity	Uncommon	Common
Ileal involvement	Common	Nonexistent
Aphthous ulcers	Common	Very uncommon
Transmural involvement	Common	Very uncommon
Lymphoid aggregates	Common	Uncommon
Crypt abscesses	Uncommon	Very common
Granulomas	Common	Uncommon
Linear clefts	Common	Uncommon

proctoscopic methods, and to assess the presence or absence of the complications. Only on the basis of this complete information, and a knowledge of the patient as an individual, can a full program of nutritional, drug, and supportive therapy be rationally planned. The physician-patient relationship is challenging and critical.

Nutritional Treatment. Nutritional assessment is based on a careful diet history to determine the extent of calorie insufficiency, to document weight loss, and to analyze nutritional status on the basis of body measurements and laboratory tests. In prepubertal patients assessment of growth pattern is a critical part of the evaluation.

For ambulatory patients dietary goals should be set that are adequate for the nutritional needs of the patient, but that minimize stress on the inflamed and often narrowed segments of bowel. Evidence of lactose intolerance should be sought by history and, when possible, confirmed by *blood* or *breath test analysis* (see Ch. 104). Removal of lactose-rich foods, such as milk and ice cream, in the lactase-deficient patient may have a prompt symptomatic benefit. In many patients with cramping and diarrhea, decreasing the intake of fiber-containing foods may be beneficial, and in those with steatorrhea a decrease of fat intake to 70 to 80 grams per day may substantially improve diarrhea. Attention to restoration of an adequate diet must always accompany these deletions.

The hospitalized patient presents a different management problem. More than half of such patients suffer from deficiencies of calories, protein, certain vitamins, and minerals. Most such patients take an inadequate diet limited by the worsening of intestinal symptoms after eating. One approach in such patients is to put the inflamed and narrowed bowel "at rest" by removing the stimulus of food intake on intestinal secretion and motility. Many patients derive symptomatic benefit from partial rather than total bowel rest with the delivery of nutrients enterally in the form of low residue–defined formula diets. Rarely can adequate nutritional maintenance be achieved by the oral intake of these formula diets alone owing to limitations of palatability. The use of small-caliber nasogastric tubes for continuous or intermittent drip provides a well-

tolerated alternative means of delivery that is often associated with a marked decrease in bacterial flora, stool frequency, and symptoms. In more severely ill patients, and in those who cannot tolerate enteral feeding or who lack adequate intestine for absorption, total parenteral nutritional support is used increasingly.

For the severely malnourished patient, total parenteral nutrition can be used to achieve nutritional repletion during the diagnostic investigation, to prepare the nutritionally depleted patient for surgery, and, when required, to maintain the patient through the postoperative period. For the patient with a short bowel disability following major intestinal resections, total parenteral nutrition can be used in the immediate postoperative period or even for prolonged nutritional support at home until the adaptive responses permit oral nutritional maintenance. In patients with fistulas total parenteral nutrition and bowel rest may lead to closure of the fistulas with sustained remission in 20 to 50 per cent of patients. The combination of nutritional support therapy and corticosteroids appears more effective than either modality alone.

Specific attention to vitamin and mineral depletion will help in the management of anemia and bone disease and should aid the healing process and the overall sense of well-being. Calcium and magnesium losses may be particularly high in the presence of poor intake, severe diarrhea, and steatorrhea. Vitamin D deficiency may lead to metabolic bone disease in Crohn's disease patients, particularly after intestinal resection. This deficiency can usually be corrected with adequate amounts of oral vitamin D, approximately 4000 IU daily. Vitamins can usually be replaced by a therapeutic multivitamin preparation containing three to five times the normal daily requirement. Zinc deficiency should be considered, especially in patients with prolonged and severe diarrhea who may require replacement therapy. In patients on parenteral nutrition, addition of trace metals to parenteral fluids is mandatory.

Therapy in Growth-Retarded Patients. The young patient whose growth is retarded presents a special challenge. In some patients the institution of a medical regimen, including sulfasalazine or corticosteroids, preferably on an alternate-day regimen, will suppress symptoms and disease activity sufficiently to improve dietary intake and restore growth. Restoring normal nutrition is crucial to success of medical therapy. Nutrition may be restored by total parenteral nutrition, including episodic administration at home, or by administering a defined, minimal-residue formula diet by enteral tube. Surgery, timed to permit a maximal growth spurt during puberty, is recommended by some for intractable disease in ulcerative colitis or Crohn's ileocolitis unresponsive to medical management. In such instances the possibility of a period of relative freedom from symptoms and potential growth restitution must be balanced against the strong likelihood of recurrence of Crohn's disease and the need for repeated resections later.

Sulfasalazine. Containing a sulfonamide, sulfapyridine, and salicylate in azo linkage, sulfasalazine is the most commonly used drug in inflammatory bowel disease. Sulfasalazine in the usual dose of 3 grams a day orally has been established by means of a national cooperative study as effective treatment for the management of exacerbations of Crohn's disease, particularly of Crohn's disease of the colon. Sulfasalazine in combination with prednisone was not better than prednisone alone in treatment of an acute exacerbation of Crohn's disease. The effectiveness of sulfasalazine in Crohn's disease limited to the small intestine remains in question. No drug regimen has been proved to reduce recurrences of Crohn's disease after clinical remission, whether spontaneous, induced by drugs, or after resective surgery. Still, in many centers sulfasalazine therapy, once instituted, is maintained. Side effects of sulfasalazine treatment are discussed in Ch. 105.3.

Newer Drugs Containing 5-Aminosalicylate (5-ASA). Increasingly, 5-ASA is recognized as the active moiety of sulfasalazine. Topical 5-ASA is equivalent to sulfasalazine in resolving rectal inflammation. Oral preparations of 5-ASA designed to deliver the drug to the lower bowel by slow-release tablets or by azo linkage to other compounds have yielded encouraging initial results and are used increasingly, especially in sulfasalazine-sensitive patients. Major trials are in progress in America and Europe.

Antimicrobial Therapy. Despite the fact that no specific microbiologic agent has been implicated in the etiology or pathogenesis of Crohn's disease (see above), antibiotics are often used empirically in this inflammatory disorder. Parenteral antibiotics are commonly used in the acutely ill patient with fever and signs of peritoneal irritation and sometimes as an adjunct in programs for bowel rest or with corticosteroid therapy. The use of antibiotics, including tetracycline and trimethoprim-sulfamethoxazole, in ambulatory patients with Crohn's disease has yielded some promising results, but these observations require confirmation in controlled trials.

Metronidazole has a broad spectrum of activity against anaerobic bacteria that predominate in the gastrointestinal tract and are present in markedly increased numbers in inflammatory bowel diseases. Metronidazole has been used as an adjunct in the management of perianal fistula in Crohn's disease with reported success. A recent controlled trial has demonstrated the efficacy of metronidazole, 10 mg per kilogram per day in divided doses, in the management of acute exacerbations of Crohn's disease.

Corticosteroid Therapy. Corticosteroids are used to suppress inflammation in the bowel and the coincident systemic manifestations of inflammation. The decision to use corticosteroids in Crohn's disease is one that should be made with care. Prednisone in doses of 0.25 to 0.75 mg per kilogram for four months is usually effective in the treatment of an exacerbation of Crohn's disease, but prolonged corticosteroid use does not seem to prevent exacerbations of the disease. Therefore, the usual practice is to treat the acute exacerbation with 40 to 60 mg of prednisone per day for two to four weeks followed by tapering doses as symptoms permit. Some patients, unable to be tapered off prednisone, may continue to take low doses for protracted periods. In prepubertal patients it is particularly important to give corticosteroids on an alternate-day regimen, if at all possible, to reduce growth retardation. Such an alternate-day regimen should be used when possible even in adult patients. Novel corticosteroid preparations for topical use with better therapeutic to toxicity ratios are largely of interest in the treatment of ulcerative colitis.

Immunosuppressive Therapy. Azathioprine* and 6-mercaptopurine* have been used with encouraging results in the management of patients with Crohn's disease. In Crohn's disease, as well as in ulcerative colitis, the use of daily doses of 1.0 to 1.5 mg per kilogram has permitted the lowering of corticosteroid doses without symptomatic exacerbation in controlled trials. As a single agent, however, azathioprine demonstrated no superiority over a placebo in a four-month trial. When 6-mercaptopurine is used for longer periods, it may be effective in the management of some patients with Crohn's disease if sufficient time is allowed for the immunosuppressive effects to be accomplished. Toxic side effects may limit the use of these agents, especially in women of childbearing age (see Ch. 176).

Antidiarrheal Drugs. Patients may be symptomatically improved by drugs given to diminish intestinal motility and diarrhea. Loperamide, diphenoxylate, tincture of opium, or paregoric can be used to reduce diarrhea in Crohn's disease. Anticholinergic drugs are helpful in some patients in diminishing stool frequency. All these antimotility drugs should be used carefully, with special attention to narcotic dependence in the case of codeine, paregoric, and opium. Symptoms of obstruction may be exacerbated with all of these drugs.

Surgery for Ileitis or Ileocolitis. Surgical resection of bowel involved in Crohn's disease is occasionally required but is undertaken with reluctance because of the high rate of recurrence of the disease. In one study recurrence after resection of the involved distal small bowel or ileum and adjacent colon was 50 per cent in 5 years, 75 per cent in 10, and 91 per cent in 15. Still there is a prominent place for surgery in the management of many patients with Crohn's disease. Surgery is clearly indicated for high-grade intestinal *obstruction* unresponsive to medical therapy, for *perforation*, and for *fistulas* to other abdominal organs such as the bladder. Patients lacking these clear indications may undergo resective surgery for *intractable disease* with the knowledge that recurrence is likely but still seeking temporary symptomatic relief. Surgery in the adolescent with growth retardation has been discussed earlier. The most common operation is resection of the involved portions of the terminal ileum with an ileocolonic anastomosis. Such an anastomosis should retain as much of the right colon as possible, since the right colon may be critical in determining the extent of debility from postiliectomy diarrhea.

Surgery for Crohn's Colitis. Indications for surgery in Crohn's colitis are similar to those for ulcerative colitis (see Ch. 105.3). Uncontrolled bleeding, perforation, and toxic dilatation are rarer than in ulcerative colitis but may occasionally demand acute surgical intervention. Most commonly surgery is performed for clinical intractability of the disease despite full medical management. Intractability usually means inability to work or function socially despite therapy, inadequate growth and development in children, unresolved perianal complications, or unremitting systemic complications such as iritis or liver disease. The surgical approach may be that of total proctocolectomy and resection of involved terminal ileum with ileostomy, or a subtotal colectomy with ileosigmoid, ileorectal, or ileoanal anastomosis. For any resection with internal anastomosis, recurrence rate is in excess of 75 per cent in ten years. In many patients a period of several years of relative freedom from symptoms without ileostomy makes ileorectal or ileosigmoid anastomosis the surgical approach of choice. For patients with extensive involvement of colon, including the rectum, total proctocolectomy with ileostomy is usually performed. The need for surgical revision of the ileostomy, usually caused by complications resulting from recurrent inflammatory disease, may be as high as 40 per cent in five years. The actual rate of recurrence of Crohn's disease after ileostomy is uncertain but is probably less than 15 per cent in five years. Thus Crohn's colitis, in contrast to ulcerative colitis, is not cured by total proctocolectomy.

PROGNOSIS. Crohn's disease exacts a very substantial cost in altered patient lifestyle and in regular, often intensive medical care. A pattern of remissions and exacerbations is usual. Although disease-free intervals may extend for years and, rarely, for decades, the most characteristic and discouraging feature of Crohn's disease is its almost relentless tendency to recur despite intensive medical treatment or after surgery. The benefits of some years free of symptoms after surgical resection are substantial in many patients. About 50 per cent of patients require surgical treatment eventually. Surgery is rarely if ever curative, however, so every effort should be made to manage all aspects of the patient's illness. Overall mortality attributed to Crohn's disease or its complications ranges from 5 to 18 per cent in various reports. It is lower in patients with disease limited to the small intestine.

The outlook for patients with Crohn's disease has improved steadily with advances in general and supportive treatment. Further progress may be expected as our understanding of the etiology of Crohn's disease increases.

---

*This use is not listed in the manufacturer's directive.

Donaldson RM Jr: Crohn's disease. In Sleisenger MH, Fordtran JS (eds.): Gastrointestinal Disease. 4th ed. Philadelphia, W.B. Saunders Company,

1988. *Excellent, balanced review of all phases of Crohn's disease, supplemented by illustrative radiographs and 129 references.*

Gitnick G: Evidence for infectious agents in IBD. In Gitnick G (ed.): Current Gastroenterology, Vol 7. Chicago, Year Book Medical Publishers, 1987.

Greenstein AJ, Janowitz HD, Sachar DB: The extraintestinal complications of Crohn's disease and ulcerative colitis: A study of 700 patients. Medicine 55:401, 1976.

Hanauer S: New Drug Therapies for inflammatory bowel disease. In Gitnick G: Current Gastroenterology. Vol 7. Chicago, Year Book Medical Publishers, 1987.

Kirsner JB, Shorter RG: Recent developments in "nonspecific" inflammatory bowel disease. N Engl J Med 306:775, 837, 1982. *An authoritative review with emphasis on concepts of etiopathogenesis.*

Mendeloff AL: The epidemiology of inflammatory bowel disease. Clin Gastroenterol 9:259, 1980. *A comprehensive review and critique comparing the behavior of Crohn's disease and ulcerative colitis in a volume devoted to inflammatory bowel disease.*

The National Cooperative Crohn's Disease Study. Gastroenterology 77:825, 1980. *Twelve articles summarizing the results of a cooperative study, clinical characteristics, drug therapy, diagnostic studies, complications, and adverse reactions.*

105.3 Ulcerative Colitis
Bernard Levin

DEFINITIONS. Ulcerative colitis is a chronic disease of unknown etiology characterized by inflammation of the mucosa and submucosa of the large intestine. The inflammation usually involves the rectum down to the anal margin and extends proximally in the colon for a variable distance. Terms in common usage refer to the anatomic extent of the disease: *pancolitis* for involvement of the entire colon; *ulcerative proctitis* or *proctosigmoiditis* for diseases limited to the rectum or rectosigmoid; and *left-sided colitis* for disease of the descending colon.

Ulcerative colitis has an estimated incidence of 2 to 7 cases per 100,000 and a prevalence of 40 to 100 cases per 100,000 population in the United States. For ulcerative proctitis both the incidence and prevalence are roughly comparable to those for colitis. Although both Crohn's disease and ulcerative colitis are being increasingly recognized, there is no evidence that the incidence of ulcerative colitis is actually increasing. In the United States between 200,000 and 400,000 persons suffer from inflammatory bowel diseases, with about 30,000 new cases diagnosed each year. Ulcerative colitis affects women more frequently than men and exhibits a bimodal age distribution, with a first peak of incidence between the ages of 15 and 20 years and a secondary small peak at ages 55 to 60 (Fig. 105–5). The incidence of ulcerative colitis in blacks may be as low as one third that in whites, and its incidence among Jews is about three to five times greater than among non-Jews.

FAMILIAL AND GENETIC FEATURES. There is an increased familial incidence of inflammatory bowel disease, both for ulcerative colitis and for Crohn's disease, but without a clear-cut pattern of inheritance. In one study about 4 per cent of a control population had a family history of inflammatory bowel disease, whereas 11 per cent of those with chronic inflammatory bowel disease had a family history of these disorders. The onset of disease in patients from affected families occurred at a lower age than in those without family histories.

Patients with inflammatory bowel disease and ankylosing spondylitis have a likelihood of 50 to 90 per cent of possessing the histocompatibility antigen HLA-B27, whereas the antigen is found in 6 to 9 per cent of the control population. The antigen is present in even higher prevalence in patients with spondylitis without inflammatory bowel disease (see Ch. 434). An increased incidence of ankylosing spondylitis has been reported in relatives of patients with ulcerative colitis or Crohn's disease. These findings continue to arouse interest in genetic factors in the pathogenesis of chronic inflammatory bowel disease.

ETIOLOGY AND PATHOGENESIS. The etiology of chronic ulcerative colitis is unknown. Furthermore, no satisfactory animal model of the human disorder has been discovered.

Psychogenic Factors. Considerable debate has occurred about the role of psychosomatic factors in the initiation and further development of ulcerative colitis. Once the illness has become manifest, it is often impossible to distinguish its influences on behavior from the patient's premorbid personality. Any illness characterized by severe diarrhea, rectal bleeding, and a variety of constitutional symptoms, especially when occurring in a young, previously healthy person, constitutes a stressful situation and can destroy a patient's self-confidence. Regressive behavior may result. Hospitalized children with colitis are often compulsively neat, demanding, and immature for their age. Adults may exhibit exaggeration of dependency needs during periods of active disease. Conflicting data exist about the occurrence of significant life-stress crises at the time of onset of the disease.

Infectious Agents. Ulcerative colitis is characterized by an inflammatory reaction in the bowel resembling that caused by known microbiologic pathogens such as *Shigella*. However, no organism has been reproducibly demonstrated to be responsible for the condition. Nevertheless, microbial infection remains a possible cause because of the recent recognition of bacterial causes of enteritis and colitis (*Yersinia enterocolitica* and *Campylobacter fetus jejuni*). The possible role of viral agents in the etiology of inflammatory bowel disease is discussed in more detail in relation to Crohn's disease (see Ch. 105.2).

Immunologic Factors. An immunologically mediated pathogenic mechanism is suggested by the frequent presence of personal and family histories of atopic diseases in patients with ulcerative colitis and the concomitant presence of conditions such as erythema nodosum, arthritis, uveitis, and vasculitis. Circulating anticolon antibodies have been described in ulcerative colitis, but these remain of unknown significance. The beneficial effects of corticosteroid therapy for ulcerative colitis are consistent with its immunosuppressive as well as its anti-inflammatory effects.

Some of the extraintestinal manifestations of ulcerative colitis such as skin rashes, arthritis, and vasculitis suggest immune complex deposition. Activation of the alternative complement pathway in ulcerative colitis is suggested by the observations of normal or elevated levels of C3PA and markedly reduced levels of properdin convertase in sera from patients with extraintestinal complications of the disease.

Antilymphocyte antibodies have been found in up to 40 per cent of patients with ulcerative colitis and in up to 50 per

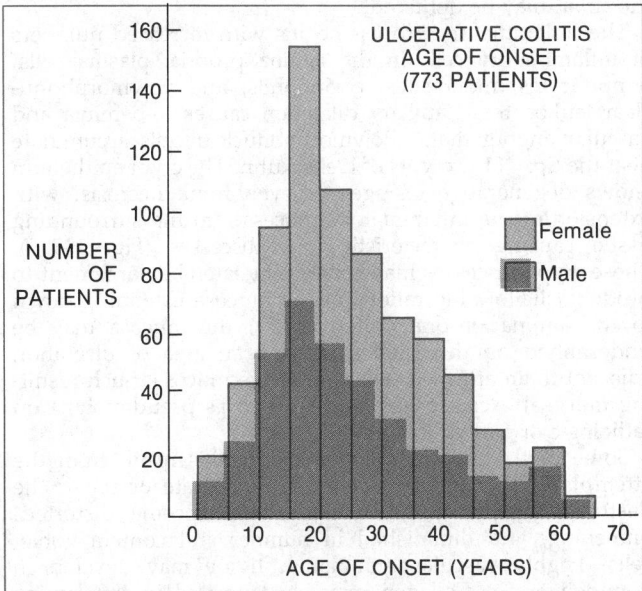

FIGURE 105–5. Age of onset in 773 patients with ulcerative colitis. (From Rogers BHG, Clark LM, Kirsner JB: J Chron Dis 24:743, 1971.)

cent of family members and unrelated household contacts of patients with inflammatory bowel disease. In contrast, these antibodies were found in only 4 per cent of control family members. Lymphocytotoxic antibodies have been found in sera from patients with inflammatory bowel disease and from their unaffected spouses more frequently than sera from age-matched controls and their spouses. Such data suggest exposure to a common environmental agent, but genetic factors must also be implicated, since there is an increased prevalence of lymphocytotoxic antibody in sera from consanguineous relatives without household contact as well.

The T lymphocytes of patients with inflammatory bowel disease do not proliferate normally when stimulated with autologous non–T cells, and suppressor T cell generation is also impaired in these patients. Such failure of suppression may create a "permissive environment," allowing abnormal responses to antigens.

Observations of immunologic events at the intestinal mucosal level have suggested decreased spontaneous antibody secretion in intestinal mononuclear cells compared with peripheral blood mononuclear cells, which showed increased synthesis and secretion of IgG, IgM, and IgA. This suggests the possibility that a primary mucosal immunodeficiency in the bowel of patients with inflammatory bowel disease weakens the mucosal barrier, thereby facilitating both a local inflammation and a heightened systemic immune response.

PATHOLOGY. Pathologic changes in the colon in ulcerative colitis readily predict the clinical features of the disease. In 75 per cent of patients disease involves only the left side of the colon. In the remainder, the entire colon is involved (pancolitis). Extensive vascular engorgement and mucosal ulceration result in bleeding. The damaged mucosa is less able to absorb sodium and water, and watery diarrhea results. Iron deficiency anemia results from blood loss, and hypoalbuminemia may reflect transmucosal loss of protein. The histologic changes in ulcerative colitis are nonspecific, but the chronicity and distribution pattern are characteristic.

Ulcerative colitis involves primarily the mucosa of the colon. Unlike the segmental lesions of Crohn's disease, the mucosa is inflamed continuously, occasionally terminating at some point in the colon where the abnormality gradually changes to a normal appearance over a distance of a few centimeters. The involved mucosa is red and granular and bleeds diffusely. The macroscopic lesions may progress from small, petechial ulcerations to deeper, linear ulcers separated by islands of inflamed but intact mucosa. In severe cases, large areas of the colon may be denuded.

The inflammatory process begins with increased numbers of inflammatory cells in the lamina propria: plasma cells, lymphocytes, monocytes, eosinophils, and polymorphonuclear leukocytes. Capillary dilatation causes hyperemia and vascular engorgement. Polymorphonuclear cells accumulate near the tips of the crypts of Lieberkühn. The crypt epithelium shows degenerative changes or even frank necrosis, with extension of the inflammatory process into the surrounding tissue causing characteristic microabscesses (Fig. 105–6). These crypt abscesses may coalesce by lateral enlargement to produce shallow ulcerations of the mucosa extending down to the lamina propria. Alternatively, the mucosa may be undermined on three sides, leaving an area of ulceration adjacent to an attached fragment of the mucosa. Such resulting mucosal excrescences may be seen as pseudopolyps on radiologic or endoscopic examination.

Some of the features of ulcerative colitis result from the attempts of the inflamed colon to regenerate or repair the destroyed crypts. Regenerating crypts become distorted, branching, and diminished in number and contain goblet cells. Highly vascular granulation tissue may develop in denuded areas. Collagen may be deposited in the lamina propria, and the muscularis mucosae may hypertrophy.

The alternating processes of superficial ulceration and gran-

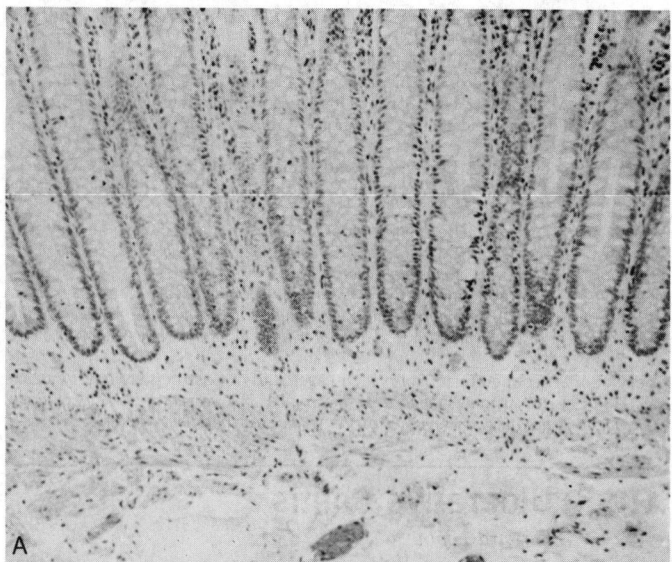

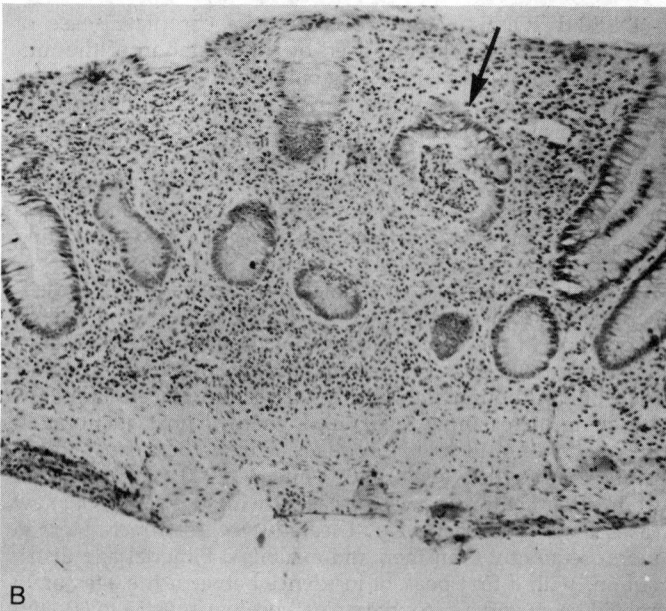

FIGURE 105–6. Rectal biopsies from (A) a normal patient and (B) a patient with ulcerative colitis. In B, note mucosal atrophy, branching of a gland, cellular infiltration, and crypt abscess (*arrow*). × 100. (From Cello JP: In Sleisenger MH, Fordtran JS [eds.]: Gastrointestinal Disease. 3rd ed. Philadelphia, W. B. Saunders Company, 1983.)

ulation followed by re-epithelialization can lead to the development of polypoid excrescences. These are inflammatory polyps (pseudopolyps) that are not neoplastic. Longstanding disease gives rise to hyperplasia of the muscularis mucosae, and this change, accompanied by postinflammatory fibrosis, causes shortening of the colon. The haustrations are lost, and the large bowel has the appearance of a smooth tube. Strictures may be caused by the localized fibromuscular hyperplasia; a distinction must be made between these and malignant strictures.

In the most severe cases, the inflammation can involve the submucosa and even the serosa and lead to perforation. In toxic dilatation of the colon, a particularly severe and acute form of this disease, the diameter of the lumen of the colon is greatly increased and the bowel wall is thinned, with a serious risk of spontaneous perforation.

CLINICAL MANIFESTATIONS AND COURSE. The five most common symptoms of ulcerative colitis are *rectal bleeding, diarrhea, abdominal pain, weight loss,* and *fever*. The patient is usually in the second, third, or fourth decade of life at the onset of symptoms. Ulcerative colitis may begin in a subtle manner or with catastrophic suddenness. Patients may relate the acute onset of symptoms to a recent emotional upset, to an upper respiratory infection, or occasionally to oral antibiotic therapy.

When signs and symptoms of colonic inflammation (including malaise, lower abdominal discomfort, and an increased number of bowel movements with rectal bleeding) are not marked, the designation *mild ulcerative colitis* is often used. This form of the disease, which accounts for roughly half of all patients with ulcerative colitis, is less likely to be recognized and may not be diagnosed for months or even years. The mortality is negligible, and the long-term prognosis for these patients does not differ from that of a control population. The development of colonic cancer in mild ulcerative colitis is about one seventh of that occurring in the more severe forms of the disease.

Moderate ulcerative colitis describes a more abrupt onset of the disorder, typically associated with four to five loose and bloody bowel movements per day. In this form of the disease, which accounts for about 30 per cent of ulcerative colitis, abdominal cramps may be severe and may awaken the patient at night. Low-grade fever, fatigue, and malaise may be prominent symptoms, as may some of the extracolonic manifestations (see below). The patient may have anorexia and weight loss. Some patients with moderate colitis may become progressively worse, with increasingly severe diarrhea, bleeding, and fever. The immediate mortality in patients with moderate colitis is low because of the efficacy of corticosteroid therapy, but the long-term prognosis for avoiding colectomy is guarded. Exacerbations of the disease often occur and may require intensive medical management over extended periods. The risk of developing cancer of the colon is increased and probably affects this group most significantly.

Severe or fulminant ulcerative colitis presents usually in a dramatic fashion with *profuse diarrhea, rectal bleeding,* and *fever,* which may be as high as 39°C. This form of the disease occurs in about 15 per cent of patients with ulcerative colitis. Abdominal cramps, rectal urgency, and profound weakness are common presenting symptoms. Intermittent nausea, anorexia, and weight loss are also present. Occasionally patients with initially less severe disease may worsen and present a picture of fulminant colitis. Physical examination reveals an acutely ill, pale, weak, and febrile patient. Tachycardia, hypotension, and even shock may be present. Examination of the abdomen reveals generalized tenderness; localized tenderness, especially with "rebound," signals the onset of peritoneal irritation. This suggests that the inflammatory process has extended beyond the mucosa. Absence of bowel sounds should suggest the diagnosis of toxic dilatation, and this serious complication must be carefully excluded.

TOXIC DILATATION OF THE COLON (TOXIC MEGA-COLON). In severe ulcerative colitis, the patient may become gravely ill with signs and symptoms of a general toxic state associated with abdominal pain, distention, rebound tenderness, and dilatation of the diameter of the colon on plain abdominal roentgenograms to 6 cm or greater (Fig. 105–7). In a patient with severe active colitis, toxic megacolon may be precipitated by a barium enema examination (and its antecedent preparation), potassium depletion, or anticholinergic or narcotic medication. The complication may also develop spontaneously. Medications that may decrease colonic motility should be avoided in these patients. Severe inflammation disrupts the neural and muscular elements that maintain normal tone. This allows the intraluminal pressure to expand the colon well beyond its normal width. Bacteria overgrow and are thought to produce toxins that intensify the complication and contribute to the hazard of peritonitis. Diffusion of these toxic products into the systemic circulation contributes to the toxic state.

Clinical signs include fever, tachycardia, dehydration, and abdominal tenderness and distention. The loss of bowel

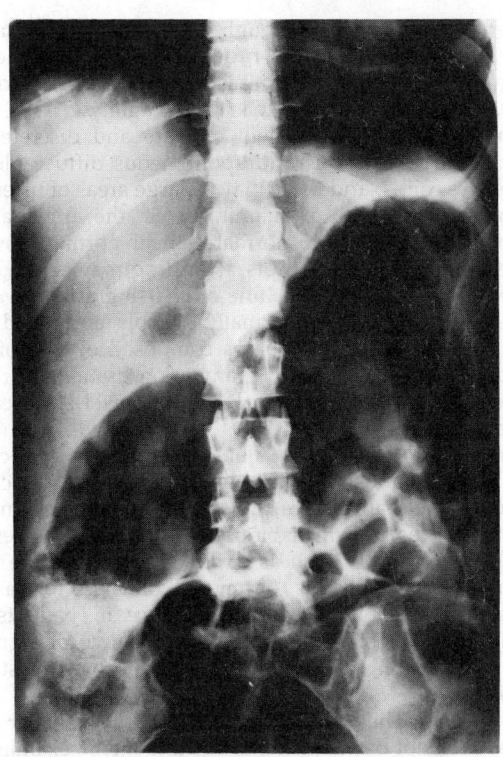

FIGURE 105–7. Plain film of the abdomen from a patient with ulcerative colitis and toxic megacolon. Note that the air in the colon silhouettes an irregular colonic mucosa. (From Cello JP: In Sleisenger MH, Fordtran JS [eds.]: Gastrointestinal Disease. 3rd ed. Philadelphia, W. B. Saunders Company, 1983.)

sounds is a significant finding. The colon is found to be dilated with severe mucosal disease demonstrated by a plain film of the abdomen (Fig. 105–7). Marked leukocytosis, hypokalemia, anemia, and hypoalbuminemia are frequently present. The mortality rate in toxic dilatation of the colon may be as high as 20 to 30 per cent. Intensive medical therapy with early colectomy can decrease mortality (see Treatment).

DIAGNOSIS. The diagnosis of ulcerative colitis is usually made on the basis of its clinical features, the demonstration of inflammation of the rectal and sigmoidal mucosa on proctosigmoidoscopy, and the exclusion of specific infections by appropriate stool culture and examination for parasites. The diagnosis may be supported by radiologic examination, fiberoptic colonoscopy, and rectal biopsy.

Proctosigmoidoscopy. This is the most reliable diagnostic study in ulcerative colitis because the observer may inspect the mucosa directly. This examination is indicated in every patient with rectal bleeding. At the same time, fresh stool samples may be obtained for culture and microscopy to determine the presence of fecal leukocytes or trophozoites. The mucopurulent exudate should be aspirated, mixed with a drop of warm saline, and examined microscopically for motile, hematophagous trophozoites of *Entamoeba histolytica.* It is important to exclude the diagnosis of amebiasis before beginning corticosteroid therapy.

The gross appearance of the rectal mucosa is nonspecific in acute colitis. Specific causes such as shigellosis and *Campylobacter* infections should be excluded by cultures obtained at the time of proctosigmoidoscopy. Particularly, but not exclusively, in patients with prior antibiotic therapy acute colitis may be caused by the enterotoxin of *Clostridium difficile.* Such patients may have endoscopic features of pseudomembranous colitis (see Ch. 279). It is preferable to avoid enemas prior to proctosigmoidoscopy in a patient suspected of having ulcerative colitis because they may confuse by irritating normal rectal mucosa and by aggravating mild abnormalities. Despite its name, in the early phases ulcerative colitis does not produce visible ulcers, but rather the red, diffusely bleeding, granular mucosa looks as though it has been gently sandpapered. Edema and erythema produce a markedly reddened, swollen mucosa with a diminished vascular pattern, the changes of hyperemia, petechiae, and fragility.

In moderate colitis, purulent exudate and discrete small ulcers appear. Gross pus and spontaneous diffuse bleeding mark severe colitis, and there may be large areas of ulceration. After appropriate therapy in mild cases, the appearance of the rectum may return to normal or near normal; however, repeated attacks with attempts at healing may cause loss of the normal vascular pattern, fine or coarse granularity of the mucosa, blunting of the normally sharply angulated rectal valves, and inflammatory polyps composed of tags of damaged mucosa and heaped-up granulation tissue. After many cycles of inflammation and healing, the bowel may scar and become stenosed.

Rectal Biopsy (Fig. 105–6). A biopsy usually is not necessary to make the diagnosis of ulcerative colitis if the clinical and sigmoidoscopic features are typical. However, there may be certain instances in which biopsy is helpful: (1) to exclude other forms of colitis such as Crohn's disease of the colon, pseudomembranous colitis, or amebic colitis; (2) to search for mucosal dysplasia in cancer surveillance in patients with longstanding colitis; or (3) to confirm equivocal sigmoidoscopic findings in a patient with a history suggestive of ulcerative colitis.

Radiography. The patient who is ill with moderate or severe colitis should not be subjected to barium enema examination. In such patients radiologic examination is unnecessary for diagnosing ulcerative colitis and may be dangerous. Preparation of the patient by use of cathartics and enemas will worsen the condition significantly.

In the acutely ill patient the plain abdominal film should be employed in the initial evaluation. The extent of disease can be predicted by observing the patterns of fecal residue in the colon as well as the mucosal outline and haustral patterns. Failure to recognize early a grave complication such as toxic megacolon increases the risk of morbidity and mortality. The diagnosis of toxic dilatation is made on both clinical and radiographic grounds. Patients suspected of having toxic megacolon (fever, abdominal tenderness and distention, decreased or absent bowel sounds) may be seen on plain film to have dilatation of the midtransverse colon to a diameter of 6 cm or more (Fig. 105–7).

Barium enema examination may provide the following important information: (1) When sigmoidoscopy confirms the diagnosis of colitis, and after specific infectious causes have been excluded, it helps to determine the extent and severity of the mucosal lesions. If the sigmoidoscopy is negative in a patient with rectal bleeding and diarrhea, barium examination will be helpful in making the diagnosis of another cause such as neoplasm, Crohn's disease of the colon, or ischemic colitis. (2) In patients with equivocal findings at sigmoidoscopy or on a rectal biopsy, it may demonstrate features of ulcerative colitis more proximally. (3) The barium enema may detect complications such as colonic cancer in patients with longstanding colitis.

The postevacuation film of a single-contrast barium enema also provides information about mucosal detail. Unless the double-contrast (barium and air) technique is used, however, fine mucosal abnormalities may be overlooked and the extent of the involvement underestimated.

In the acute stage of ulcerative colitis, fine granularity reflects mucosal edema and hyperemia. As the disease progresses, superficial erosions develop and adherent barium produces a stippled appearance. Tiny ulcerations may be seen as these enlarge, and "collar-button"–like projections appear that involve the colon circumferentially. As the disease progresses, the normal colonic mucosal surface is lost; however, it may regenerate with healing. Inflammatory polyps may appear as rare or numerous intraluminal filling defects (Fig.

105–8). The inflammatory process also may affect the muscular layers of the colon, producing a smooth, foreshortened colon without haustra. After recovery from a first attack, haustral markings may reappear. After longstanding mucosal and submucosal thickening in some patients with ulcerative proctitis or colitis, the presacral space may enlarge. This is seen best on a lateral view of the barium-filled rectum.

A small bowel follow-through radiographic study should be performed after acute symptoms are controlled to help exclude the diagnosis of Crohn's disease. In ulcerative colitis involving the entire colon, the ileocecal valve may be dilated and incompetent. The terminal ileum may be dilated, but discrete ulceration is seen only when Crohn's disease is present.

Colonoscopy. Colonoscopy has little place in the diagnosis of acute ulcerative colitis and may be hazardous because of the risks of perforation and hemorrhage. Since the entire colon may be examined by colonoscopy, it is extremely useful in the patient who does not have acute and severe symptoms when the diagnosis and extent of inflammatory bowel disease are uncertain. Colonoscopy is most commonly used in obtaining multiple biopsies in patients with longstanding colitis in a search for neoplastic changes.

DIFFERENTIAL DIAGNOSIS. Numerous other causes of diarrhea must be considered in the differential diagnosis of ulcerative colitis, but the clinical presentation, sigmoidoscopic findings, and radiologic features are used to make a definite diagnosis. The differential diagnosis of rectal bleeding includes hemorrhoids, colonic adenomas and carcinomas, angiodysplastic lesions, bleeding disorders, and diverticular disease. The differential diagnosis of gastrointestinal bleeding is discussed in greater detail in Ch. 114.

Viral infections, bacillary dysentery, and toxigenic strains of *Escherichia coli* may cause acute colitis and occasionally simulate ulcerative colitis. Diarrhea is a prominent symptom of these diseases, but rectal bleeding is uncommon except in *shigellosis*, which rarely lasts more than a few days. *Campylobacter* infections may closely mimic nonspecific ulcerative colitis. Their diagnosis is particularly important, since these infections respond well to appropriate antibiotic therapy. *Salmonella* infections may present as an acute or subacute diarrheal disorder. *Yersinia enterocolitica* produces an acute

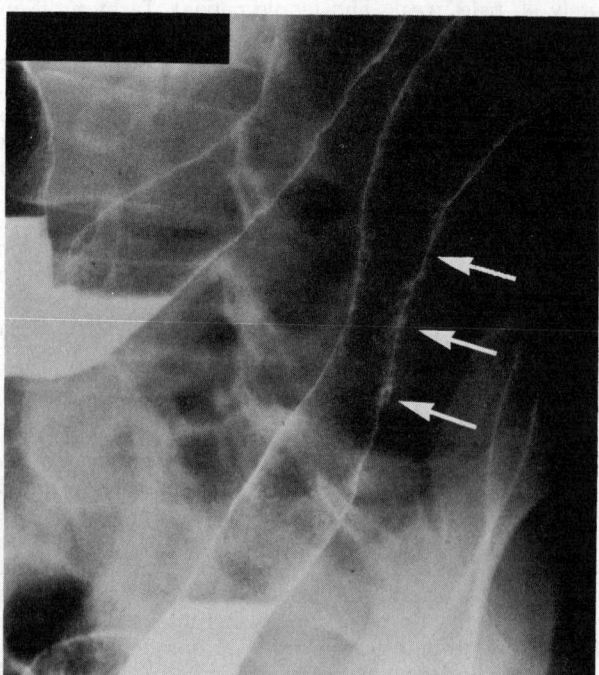

FIGURE 105–8. Double-contrast enema in patient with active ulcerative colitis with discrete collar button ulcers (*arrows*) in an anhaustral and diffusely granular colon.

bacterial ileitis and mesenteric adenitis, which more closely resemble an acute attack of Crohn's disease.

Ischemic colitis is more common in elderly individuals and often causes a segmental form of colitis. Typically, roentgenographic features of "thumbprinting" caused by intramural hemorrhage are observed. Infarction of the colon, affecting primarily the right side of the colon, may be seen in young women taking oral contraceptives. This clinical picture of acute lower abdominal pain, fever, and rectal bleeding may resemble acute ulcerative colitis, but the course will help distinguish this entity.

Amebiasis may occasionally be difficult to distinguish from ulcerative colitis in its early phases. A history of foreign travel may be elicited but is not essential. Mild, diffuse hyperemia on sigmoidoscopic examination is not uncommon. Later, distinctive features include discrete large ulcers with overhanging edges. Fresh preparations of mucopus must be examined for the presence of trophozoites (see Ch. 390).

Gonococcal proctitis may present with rectal burning and diarrhea, a mucopurulent discharge, or bleeding. On sigmoidoscopic examination, generalized redness and edema of the rectal mucosa may be indistinguishable from ulcerative proctitis. The rectal discharge should be cultured for gonococci.

Pseudomembranous colitis is usually associated with a preexisting history of antibiotic use. This condition is generally related to the growth of *Clostridium difficile*, which produces a toxin that can be identified in stools. In patients with pseudomembranous colitis, proctoscopic examination reveals raised, initially small, yellowish plaques on intensely red and later ulcerated mucosa. The plaques may be covered by mucus, which must be swabbed off before the plaque can be seen. The mucosa bleeds when the membrane is stripped.

The following diseases also may cause rectal inflammation: *histoplasmosis, leukemic* and *lymphomatous infiltration, solitary ulcer syndrome, malakoplakia,* and *lymphogranuloma venereum*. The last-named disorder presents with the passage of blood, mucus, and pus from the rectum, but patients also may have perianal fistulas and inguinal adenopathy. Patients with *radiation proctitis* will have a history of radiation therapy for cancer of the cervix, prostate, or testis, but the proctoscopic appearance is indistinguishable from that of nonspecific ulcerative colitis. It is important to recognize that the workup of homosexual patients with proctitis or colitis should include a search for common and uncommon viral, bacterial, and parasitic pathogens.

The most difficult differential diagnosis is that between ulcerative colitis and Crohn's disease of the colon. *Crohn's colitis* presents with diarrhea but usually not with rectal bleeding. Crohn's colitis also is frequently associated with perianal lesions. Characteristic features of these two diseases are compared in Table 105–3. Clinical data, endoscopic examinations, and barium enemas can differentiate Crohn's disease of the colon from ulcerative colitis in 80 to 85 per cent of patients with inflammatory bowel disease. In approximately 15 to 20 per cent of patients differentiation is not possible, and the type of colitis remains undetermined. The differentiation is useful in that it affects the approach to treatment and the assessment of prognosis.

LOCAL COMPLICATIONS. Local complications include hemorrhoids, anal fissures, perianal or ischiorectal suppuration, rectovaginal fistulas, and rectal prolapse. These complications appear most frequently when diarrhea is severe. Anal fissures improve with control of the colitis. Perirectal abscesses and rectal fistulas heal with incision and drainage of abscesses and unroofing of fistulous tracts.

More significant complications include massive hemorrhage, colonic strictures, inflammatory polyps, adenomatous polyps, adenocarcinoma, and toxic dilatation. *Massive hemorrhage* occurs in about 5 per cent of patients. Prompt replacement of circulating blood volume, correction of hypoprothrombinemia, and early colectomy if bleeding is uncontrollable are the principles of management of this condition.

Colonic strictures are seen in some patients on barium examination or during colonoscopy. Occasionally these apparent strictures may be due to spasm and will disappear after the intravenous administration of glucagon. It is essential to ensure that strictures are benign by colonoscopic biopsy and brushing cytology. Nevertheless it is not always possible to exclude a deeply infiltrating carcinoma by these means, and colectomy should be considered if any doubt exists about the diagnosis. *Inflammatory polyps* do not require removal except in cases in which it is impossible to distinguish them grossly from true adenomas. *Adenomatous polyps*, when identified, should be removed at the time of colonoscopy. Their association with carcinoma of the colon is of particular significance in the patient with longstanding colitis, and the patient's colon warrants careful evaluation for the presence of other adenomas or carcinoma (see Ch. 107).

Carcinoma of the large bowel occurring as a complication of ulcerative colitis is correlated with the extent of disease and its duration. The overall prevalence of cancer in all patients with ulcerative colitis is between 3 and 5 per cent. For those with pancolitis and a duration of disease greater than ten years, the risk is 10 to 20 times greater than that of the general population (see Fig. 107–4). In children ulcerative colitis usually involves the entire colon; more adults have disease limited to the distal colon. The risk of developing cancer is similar in both children and adults with universal disease, viz. 13 per cent after 15 years, 23 per cent after 20 years, and 42 per cent after 25 years of the disease. Some authorities have suggested that the risk of complicating cancer is much lower and that most published studies are from referral centers with a markedly biased patient composition.

The patients who develop colonic cancer are often in a quiescent stage of their illness, and diagnosis often is delayed because the symptoms of bleeding or diarrhea may be attributed initially to a recurrence of the colitis. The tumors in colitis may be flat and small and not detectable even by expert colonoscopic and radiologic techniques. The prognosis of carcinoma of the colon in ulcerative colitis tends to be worse than that developing in the absence of colitis, because the diagnosis is often made late and the lesions are often multifocal and display a high grade of malignancy.

Some physicians advocate elective proctocolectomy after 10 to 12 years of the active ulcerative colitis to avoid progression to colonic cancer. The patient, however, may be very reluctant to undergo this procedure, particularly if the colitis or the side effects of medication are minimal. In biopsies obtained at proctoscopy or colonoscopy, the presence of epithelial dysplasia (neoplastic change) in the mucosa may provide an early indication of increased vulnerability to colonic cancer. Multiple biopsies are required and interpretation by an experienced pathologist is essential. These issues are discussed in detail in Ch. 107.

EXTRAINTESTINAL COMPLICATIONS (see Table 105–2). Two characteristic skin lesions occur in ulcerative colitis: *pyoderma gangrenosum* and *erythema nodosum. Erythema nodosum* is characterized by the appearance of dull, red, raised, painful nodules usually on the skin of the legs. This lesion, which is more common in women than in men, is roughly correlated with the activity of the mucosal disease and is likely to develop when arthritis also accompanies the attack of colitis. It is seen in both ulcerative colitis and Crohn's disease. *Pyoderma gangrenosum* is seen in 5 per cent of patients with ulcerative colitis and is characteristic of that disease. The lesion starts with the appearance of a furuncle on the skin and later appears as a painful, indurated area surrounded by violaceous, undermined skin. Topical and systemic corticosteroids have been used to suppress the colonic inflammation with a parallel improvement of the lesions of pyoderma gangrenosum. Favorable responses to dapsone (Avlosulfon) therapy also have been reported.

There are two separate types of *joint involvement* in ulcerative colitis and Crohn's disease: (1) sacroiliitis with or without ankylosing spondylitis and (2) a specific form of peripheral arthritis. The prevalence of *ankylosing spondylitis* in chronic ulcerative colitis and Crohn's disease varies from 1.6 to 12.6 per cent, at least 30 times more common than in the general population. The symptoms of ankylosing spondylitis are pain and stiffness in the spine with loss of normal lumbar lordosis. *Sacroiliitis* may be symptomatic or associated only with mild pain in the region of the sacroiliac joints. On routine radiologic examination, changes compatible with sacroiliitis were identified in approximately 20 per cent of patients with ulcerative colitis and Crohn's disease. When spondylitis occurs unassociated with ulcerative colitis, the histocompatibility antigen HLA-B27 is found in roughly 90 per cent of patients. Seventy-five per cent of patients with ankylosing spondylitis who have simultaneous inflammatory bowel disease have this antigen. The *peripheral arthritis* associated with both Crohn's disease and ulcerative colitis occurs in about 10 to 12 per cent of patients with both conditions. The arthritis is a transient, acute, painful swelling that usually affects one or more large joints and is accompanied by a sterile serous joint effusion. The knees are commonly affected, but any joint may be involved. Arthritis rarely precedes the onset of the inflammatory bowel disease but may begin at any time during its course. It is more common in patients with extensive bowel involvement and at times of a flare-up of intestinal symptoms. Peripheral arthritis is more common in patients with perianal disease.

There appears to be a *hypercoagulable state* in ulcerative colitis, with reported increases in the platelet count and in the plasma levels of factor V, factor VIII, and fibrinogen. This may account for the enhanced susceptibility to thromboembolic phenomena exhibited by these patients.

Conjunctivitis, iritis, and/or episcleritis occur as complications in 3 to 10 per cent of patients with ulcerative colitis or Crohn's colitis (and a smaller percentage of those with regional enteritis). Iritis is the most important because of its threat to vision. There is a high incidence of iritis in patients with both spondylitis and colitis. Iritis presents as a red, painful eye with discomfort increased in the dark owing to pupillary dilatation. *Stomatitis* with multiple aphthous ulcers may occasionally be severe.

The incidence of *kidney stones*, particularly urate stones, in patients with ulcerative colitis is approximately twice that in the normal population. Following colectomy and ileostomy, the incidence of urate stones may be as high as 20 times normal. Prevention is best achieved by ensuring adequate hydration and reducing urine acidity but may on occasion require the use of allopurinol (see Ch. 90).

Hepatobiliary complications of both ulcerative colitis and Crohn's disease range from asymptomatic *pericholangitis* to *sclerosing cholangitis, chronic active hepatitis* and *cirrhosis*, and *bile duct carcinoma*. The *nutritional abnormalities* commonly seen in patients with ulcerative colitis are usually not as severe as those seen with Crohn's disease, but growth retardation is not unusual (see Ch. 105.2).

TREATMENT. Management of the patient with ulcerative colitis requires a comprehensive review of the patient's medical, nutritional, and psychologic needs. Ulcerative colitis tends to follow an acute relapsing course with quiescent intervals in some patients, during which the rectal mucosa may appear normal. No method other than colectomy is known to cure ulcerative colitis. During remission treatment is designed to prevent relapse. In patients with chronic active inflammation, therapy is intended to suppress inflammation.

General Therapy. Dietary and nutritional decisions are important in the management of ulcerative colitis and of Crohn's disease (see Nutritional Treatment in Ch. 105.2). The fiber content of the diet should be reduced during periods of diarrhea. In lactose-intolerant patients restriction of lactose intake (avoidance of dairy products) may ameliorate the diarrhea. Alternatively, bacterial lactase is commercially available and may be used to reduce the lactose content of milk to well tolerated levels. Nutritionally balanced, minimal-residue liquid nutritional formulas are available and are acceptable as supplements to most patients. In the severely ill, catabolic patient, parenteral alimentation may be employed to put the bowel at rest, largely to prepare patients for colectomy or for the postoperative recovery period.

The causes of anemia may be multiple and may include the anemia of chronic illness (see Ch. 135), blood loss with resulting iron deficiency, or folate deficiency. Oral iron may be poorly tolerated, necessitating the use of parenteral iron. Folate deficiency is associated with sulfasalazine therapy as well as with inadequate dietary intake owing to reduction in folate-containing foods such as fresh fruits and leafy vegetables.

In the patient with mild or moderate colitis, agents to reduce diarrhea may be useful. These include diphenoxylate with atropine (2.5 to 5 mg), codeine (15 to 30 mg), deodorized tincture of opium (6 to 10 drops), paregoric (4 to 8 ml), or loperamide (2 to 4 mg) before meals and at bedtime. Tincture of belladonna (10 drops) four times a day and other anticholinergics may be used to decrease abdominal cramps. Extreme care must be exercised in the use of these medications in the moderately ill patient because of the risk of precipitating toxic dilatation.

Nonspecific measures include attention to psychologic stresses in the patient's life, often involving interactions with close relatives. Patients should be encouraged to have adequate amounts of rest and sleep. As with any other chronic illness, patient education is important in enabling the patient and family to understand the nature of the disease and its effects on the individual. Formal psychiatric counseling is reserved for a minority of patients, although most benefit from a sympathetic, supportive relationship with their physicians, which may involve modest amounts of psychotherapy.

Therapy for Severe Acute Colitis. Early diagnosis and recognition of this condition are important in reducing mortality. An early decision between intensive medical treatment and immediate surgery may be necessary, particularly if there is evidence of perforation or of peritonitis, or if there is uncontrollable hemorrhage. Toxic dilatation is perhaps the most threatening type of acute severe ulcerative colitis. Failure of toxic dilatation to respond to medical management within 24 to 36 hours is ominous, since the mortality of such patients is very high unless colectomy is performed. Adequate replacement of circulating plasma volume with crystalloid, plasma, and blood is essential. Broad-spectrum antibiotics (cefoxitin or imipenem-cilastin) and intravenous corticosteroids are used. Hydrocortisone, 300 mg intravenously daily, is effective but may cause sodium and water retention. Alternatives include intravenous prednisolone, 60 mg daily, or methylprednisolone, 48 mg daily, in four divided doses.

Successful treatment depends on prompt recognition, early surgical consultation, and intensive resuscitative, antibacterial, and anti-inflammatory therapy. Important measures include intravenous fluids, plasma, blood, nasogastric suction, antibiotics, and intravenous corticosteroids. It is essential that the patient be re-evaluated every four to six hours by the physician and surgeon, and that plain abdominal films be obtained twice daily. Failure to respond to maximal therapy within 24 to 36 hours makes prompt surgical intervention essential. Usually the surgeon will choose to perform an abdominal colectomy with ileostomy, leaving the rectum in place for a subsequent operation when the patient has recovered from this severe episode. Early surgical intervention has resulted in decreased mortality in the acute phase. Overall mortality (in both medically and surgically treated patients) is high, between 12 and 30 per cent. About one fifth of patients with toxic dilatation require surgery after failure to respond to medical treatment. Patients who do not undergo surgical therapy during the attack of toxic dilatation often require elective surgery within 6 to 12 months because of subsequent failure of medical therapy.

If the patient with severe ulcerative colitis does not respond to full treatment within five to ten days, many clinicians advise colectomy (even in the absence of toxic megacolon) as soon as the patient's general condition has been stabilized. Postoperative mortality can be reduced by earlier operation, by correction of malnutrition, and by appropriate antibiotic therapy.

If the patient's general condition responds to maximal therapy and there is improvement in the sigmoidoscopic appearance of the rectal mucosa, oral feeding can commence along with the use of oral corticosteroids. If liquids are tolerated well, solid foods are added gradually as tolerated. Sulfasalazine, 2 to 4 grams orally daily, is usually then added. The oral corticosteroid dose should initially be about 40 mg of prednisone a day. If the clinical response continues to be satisfactory, this dose can be reduced by 5 mg daily every week to a dose of 20 mg of prednisone daily. This dose should be administered for a period of six to eight weeks before it is slowly tapered. Slow reductions in dosage sometimes help individual patients to withdraw eventually from this medication. Repeated brief courses of steroids for treatment of recurrences do not cause as many disabling side effects as does continuous use. Alternate-day dosage is associated with fewer side effects, but this regimen may have diminished symptomatic benefit in some patients. An alternate-day regimen may be of particular value in prepubertal children to avoid the growth suppression of large daily doses of corticosteroids.

Moderate-to-Mild Acute Colitis. For mild or moderate attacks of colitis, hospitalization is usually not required. In addition to the general measures already described, sulfasalazine is used with or without corticosteroids, depending on the severity of diarrhea and systemic symptoms. For mildly symptomatic colitis with predominantly left-sided disease, oral sulfasalazine and topical corticosteroid therapy are often satisfactory.

Corticosteroid can be applied locally to the rectal and colonic mucosa as hydrocortisone (100 mg) administered in 100 ml of saline either by enema or by slow rectal infusion. This volume of fluid always reaches the sigmoid colon, but the proximal spread is variable. Approximately one third is absorbed systemically. Suppositories and foam can be used for disease confined to the rectum. Newer nonabsorbed topical corticosteroid preparations diminish systemic side effects.

Sulfasalazine is largely unabsorbed and is metabolized by colonic bacteria to sulfapyridine and 5-aminosalicylic acid. The 5-aminosalicylic acid may exert a therapeutic effect by interfering with prostaglandin synthesis, a mediator of inflammation. Synthesis of prostaglandin E_2 by cultured rectal mucosa from patients with colitis and prostaglandin synthetase activity of the rectal mucosa are increased in active colitis. Adverse reactions to sulfasalazine, including headaches, arthralgias, nausea, skin rashes, and mild hemolysis, occur in up to 15 to 20 per cent of patients. More severe blood dyscrasias, high fever, leukopenia, and agranulocytosis are rare. A reversible loss of fertility may occur in some patients. Many of these side effects occur in patients taking 4 grams or more of sulfasalazine per day; reduction to a dose of 2 to 3 grams is often effective. Sulfapyridine is acetylated in the liver after absorption before being excreted in the urine. Many of the patients with adverse effects are genetic slow acetylators. Sulfasalazine is effective in treating moderate colitis, and continued treatment lessens the frequency of recurrent attacks. Newer compounds, such as sustained-release 5-aminosalicylic acid, have been devised to transport this compound into the colon without sulfapyridine.

Active Chronic Colitis. For patients with chronic symptoms resulting from persistent inflammation, topical corticosteroids in addition to sulfasalazine and antidiarrheal preparations are used. Azathioprine* may be of benefit in the rare patient who is dependent on corticosteroids and for whom surgical management is inappropriate. In general, there is a reluctance to use azathioprine in children or in adults who have not completed their families in view of the mutagenic potential of the drug. The aim in quiescent colitis is to prolong remission. Sulfasalazine (2 to 3 grams per day orally) has been demonstrated to be effective. The newer 5-aminosalicylic acid formulations may also be useful in such patients.

Surgical Therapy. Proctocolectomy with construction of an ileostomy cures ulcerative colitis and leads to a remission or improvement in many of the peripheral manifestations. Absolute indications for subtotal or total colectomy are (1) *perforation*, with or without abscess formation; (2) *colonic carcinoma*, for which total proctocolectomy and lymph node dissection are required; and (3) *massive hemorrhage*. Relative indications are as follows: (1) Severe acute colitis with or without toxic dilatation of the colon (toxic megacolon), with failure to respond to maximal therapy. The current trend is toward earlier surgical intervention in this group of patients after restoration of plasma volume, administration of antibiotics, corticosteroids, and total parenteral nutrition for as long as possible preoperatively. In the absence of toxic dilatation many clinicians are willing to wait for seven to ten days before advising surgery. It is indefensible to extend medical therapy in a patient who continues to bleed and who has high fever, tachycardia, severe diarrhea, depleted intravascular and extravascular volumes, hypoalbuminemia, and electrolyte depletion. (2) Failure of medical management. The patient with chronic symptoms or frequent relapses over a period of five years or longer, particularly in the face of corticosteroid-induced complications, has the promise of improved quality of life after proctocolectomy and ileostomy. Although this decision is particularly difficult in children, it should not be delayed, since the risk of growth retardation in children is great (see Growth Retardation, Ch. 105.2). (3) Suspicion of cancer. In a patient with extensive colitis of long duration the presence of dysplastic changes or a mass lesion with overlying dysplasia may be used as a basis for recommending proctocolectomy. Other considerations may include chronic symptoms or the presence of a highly suspicious persisting stricture even after endoscopic biopsy and cytology have failed to reveal malignancy.

The internist, surgeon, and stoma therapist all play an important role in the pre- and postoperative education and management of the patient with proctocolectomy and ileostomy. The mortality of elective proctocolectomy is approximately 1 to 3 per cent. Over two thirds of patients have no postoperative complications such as hemorrhage, intra-abdominal sepsis, or intestinal obstruction. Between 10 and 15 per cent of patients with a standard ileostomy (Brooke) following proctocolectomy will require some form of surgical revision of the stoma. The reoperation rate for the continent ileostomy (Kock) is as high as 20 to 30 per cent in some series, and postoperative complications and dysfunction not requiring operation are common. The continent ileostomy is contraindicated in Crohn's disease, in fulminating ulcerative colitis, in cases of diagnostic uncertainty, in emotionally unstable patients, and when experienced surgeons are unavailable. Other, rare complications include impotence (less than 2 per cent, in contrast to a universal incidence after an abdominoperineal resection for carcinoma of the rectum) and damage to the ureters. Healing of the perineal wound may be delayed for up to six months. Patients who are about to undergo or have undergone proctocolectomy with ileostomy will benefit from referral to groups such as the Ileostomy

---

*This use is not listed in the manufacturer's directive.

Association or Ileoptomists. Ingenious procedures have been developed with the goal of preserving rectal muscle and anal sphincter function. These include ileoanal anastomosis after construction of an ileal reservoir in the pelvis. Particularly in the young, intelligent patient, such procedures may be useful alternatives to the conventional ileostomy.

ULCERATIVE COLITIS AND PREGNANCY. About one third of patients with inactive ulcerative colitis have exacerbation and about two thirds with active disease have worsening of their condition either during pregnancy or in the early postpartum period. For those with continuing active colitis the worsening is likely to occur in the first trimester. When the first attack of ulcerative colitis occurs during pregnancy or the postpartum period, symptoms are often severe. About 10 per cent of pregnancies in women with ulcerative colitis will terminate in spontaneous abortions.

The general diagnostic and therapeutic measures previously described apply to pregnant patients. Radiographic studies should be minimized and proctoscopy performed only when necessary, especially during the first trimester. The usual indications for corticosteroid therapy apply. Sulfasalazine therapy during pregnancy has not been reported to have adverse effects on the fetus. Azathioprine is not used during pregnancy, although no adverse effects upon the fetus have been reported. Therapeutic abortion has little place in the management of pregnant patients with ulcerative colitis except for the rare instances of women in the first trimester who are desperately ill and are likely to lose the child. Women with quiescent ulcerative colitis should not be discouraged from pregnancy. In the presence of active colitis, pregnancy should be postponed until control of the colitis has been achieved for at least one year.

ULCERATIVE PROCTITIS. Ulcerative proctitis probably represents ulcerative colitis limited to the rectum. Typically the patient presents with mild or moderate rectal bleeding, rectal tenesmus, and an increased number of bowel movements. Symptomatic episodes recur periodically several times a year.

The macroscopic and microscopic features are similar to those described previously for ulcerative colitis, although only the distal 3 to 10 cm of the rectum may be involved. On sigmoidoscopy there is usually a sharp line of demarcation between the distal inflammatory process and normal proximal rectal or lower sigmoid mucosa.

Therapy includes the general measures described for ulcerative colitis, with the use of sulfasalazine, 2 to 3 grams per day by mouth, and topical corticosteroids. Commonly used preparations include enemas containing 100 mg of hydrocortisone or 40 mg of methylprednisone, administered once daily. Steroid suppositories (25 mg of hydrocortisone) or steroid foam (90 mg of hydrocortisone per dose) may be inserted into the rectum once or twice daily. Newer forms of therapy include topical 5-aminosalicylic acid and nonabsorbable corticosteroids. Response to treatment is usually very satisfactory, although occasional patients may remain symptomatic despite intensive therapy.

PROGNOSIS OF ULCERATIVE COLITIS. The outlook for recovery from a first attack of ulcerative colitis is very good. Mortality, which is about 5 per cent, occurs almost exclusively in those who have a severe form of the disease involving the entire colon. The mortality is higher in patients over 60 years, approximately 17 per cent, compared with 2 per cent in patients between ages 20 and 59. Toxic megacolon has a mortality rate of about 20 per cent. Death generally results from the complications of massive hemorrhage, systemic infections, pulmonary embolism, or associated cardiac disorders. Better medical therapy and earlier colectomy for patients who do not respond to medical therapy have improved the overall acute prognosis.

After the first attack about 10 per cent of patients will have a remission lasting up to 15 years or more. An additional 10

per cent will experience continuously active colitis. The remainder (80 per cent) experience remissions and exacerbations of their disease over the ensuing years irrespective of the severity of the initial attack. About one fifth of patients with ulcerative colitis require proctocolectomy at some stage in their illness. After the first postoperative year, the long-term prognosis for patients with colectomy for ulcerative colitis is similar to that of the general population. With continuous improvements in medical and surgical management, the outlook for both survival and quality of life continues to improve.

Allan RN, Keighley MRB, Alexander-Williams J, et al. (eds.): Inflammatory Bowel Disease. Edinburgh, Churchill-Livingstone, 1983. *A multiauthored, well-referenced book covering all aspects, with representation from North America and Britain.*

Cello JP: Ulcerative colitis. In Sleisenger MH, Fordtran JS (eds.): Gastrointestinal Disease. 4th ed. Philadelphia, W. B. Saunders Company, 1988. *An excellent general review with an extensive bibliography.*

Dozois RR (ed.): Alternatives to continent ileostomy. Chicago, Year Book Medical Publishers, 1985. *A detailed consideration of newer surgical alternatives in the management of ulcerative colitis.*

Faintuch JS, Levin B, Kirsner JB: Inflammatory bowel disease and malignancy. CRC Crit Rev Oncol Hematol 2:323, 1985. *An extensive review of the association of neoplasia with ulcerative colitis and Crohn's disease.*

Hanauer SB, Kirsner JB (eds.): Inflammatory Bowel Disease: A Guide for Patients and Their Families. New York, Raven Press, 1985. *A useful text for the education of patients and family members with helpful, common-sense advice.*

Kirsner JB, Shorter RG (eds.): Inflammatory Bowel Disease. Philadelphia, Lea & Febiger, 1987. *An in-depth monograph with chapters by leading authorities on incidence trends, pathology, etiology, and medical and surgical therapy.*

Riddell RH, Goldman H, Ransohoff DF, et al.: Dysplasia in inflammatory bowel disease: Standardized classification with provisional clinical applications. Hum Pathol 14:931, 1983. *A definitive description of colonic dysplasia, including an illustrative atlas.*

106 VASCULAR DISEASES OF THE INTESTINE

James H. Grendell

ANATOMY, PHYSIOLOGY, AND PATHOPHYSIOLOGY OF THE MESENTERIC CIRCULATION

The intra-abdominal portions of the digestive tract receive their blood supply almost entirely from three relatively large arteries arising from the aorta. The anatomy of these vessels, including their anastomotic interrelationships and potential for collateral formation, determines the consequences of acute or chronic vascular occlusion.

The celiac axis, the most cephalad of the three major arteries, usually originates at a level between the twelfth thoracic and the first lumbar vertebrae, passing next to the median arcuate ligament of the diaphragm (Fig. 106–1). Its branches supply the liver and biliary structures (hepatic artery), spleen (splenic artery), and the stomach (left gastric and gastroepiploic, short gastrics, and branches of the gastroduodenal, including the right gastroepiploic). The gastroduodenal artery gives rise to the superior pancreaticoduodenal arteries, which not only provide part of the blood supply to the pancreas and duodenum but also form anastomoses with the inferior pancreaticoduodenal arteries, which are derived from the superior mesenteric artery. These interconnections, the pancreaticoduodenal arcades, are an important potential route for collateral blood flow between the celiac and the superior mesenteric arteries.

The superior mesenteric artery originates behind the pancreas at the level of the first lumbar vertebra, just caudal to the celiac axis (Fig. 106–2). In addition to the inferior pancreaticoduodenal arteries, the superior mesenteric artery gives rise to branches supplying the small and large intestines from the distal duodenum to the distal transverse colon. These intestinal branches form a series of three or four arcades before entering the wall of the intestine as arteriae rectae. Although

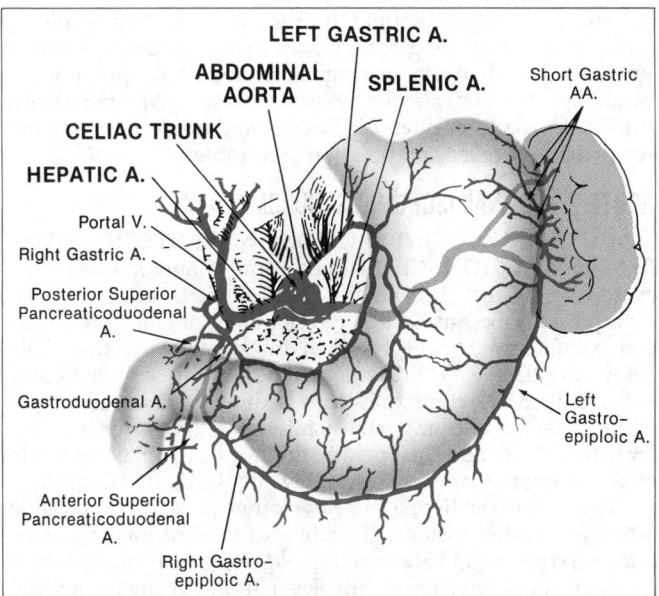

FIGURE 106–1. Arterial supply to the stomach and duodenum, showing major branches of the celiac axis and the superior portion of the pancreaticoduodenal arcades. (From Grendell JH, Ockner RK: In Sleisenger MH, Fordtran JS [eds.]: Gastrointestinal Disease. 3rd ed. Philadelphia, W. B. Saunders Company, 1983.)

there is considerable potential for collateral flow within the primary and secondary arcades, the arteriae rectae appear to represent end-arteries, and few, if any, important anastomotic connections are present within the bowel wall itself. Accordingly, selective occlusion of these more distal vessels, as may occur in vasculitis, may lead to segmental infarction.

The inferior mesenteric artery, the smallest of the three major arteries, supplies the distal transverse colon, the descending and sigmoid colon, and the proximal portions of the rectum.

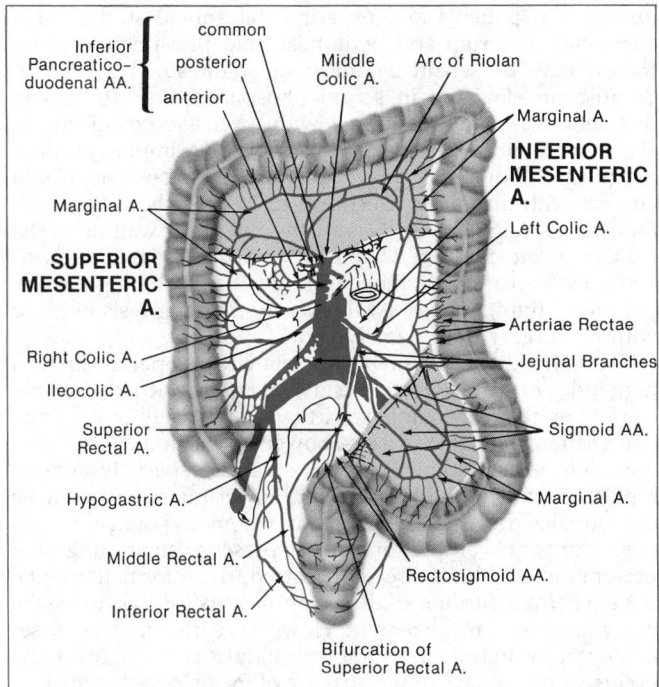

FIGURE 106–2. Arterial supply to the small and large intestines, showing the inferior portion of the pancreaticoduodenal arcades and the anastomoses between superior and inferior mesenteric arteries (arc of Riolan or "meandering mesenteric," and the marginal artery). (From Grendell JH, Ockner RK. In Sleisenger MH, Fordtran JS [eds.]: Gastrointestinal Disease. 3rd ed. Philadelphia, W. B. Saunders Company, 1983.)

Its branches form a series of arcades ending in arteriae rectae similar to what is found in the superior mesenteric artery's distribution. Branches of the inferior mesenteric artery connect with those of the superior mesenteric artery via the arc of Riolan ("meandering mesenteric artery") and the marginal artery (Fig. 106–2), and with the inferior and middle rectal branches of the hypogastric (internal iliac) arteries.

In general, veins parallel arteries in the smaller branches and for portions of the main mesenteric trunks. However, rather than entering the vena cava directly, the superior mesenteric and splenic veins join to form the portal vein, which enters the liver after receiving additional blood from the gastric circulation via the coronary vein. The inferior mesenteric vein usually drains into the splenic vein.

The blood supply to the intra-abdominal portion of the gastrointestinal tract is richly endowed with anastomotic interconnections that help protect against the consequences of occlusive vascular disease. If the occlusive process is chronically progressive, these interconnections usually permit sufficient collateral flow to maintain intestinal viability. In fact it is possible for *all* of the intra-abdominal digestive tract to be adequately supplied by only one of its three primary arterial sources. Conversely, the collateral supply may be only marginally adequate or nonexistent in certain areas, such as the arteriae rectae and intramural arteries. Also potentially vulnerable are the "watershed" areas in the distal transverse colon and splenic flexure and at the junction of the superior and middle portions of the rectum, where branches of the inferior mesenteric artery anastomose with branches of the superior mesenteric and hypogastric arteries, respectively. This may, in part, explain why segmental infarction of the colon occurs most commonly in the region of the splenic flexure and rectosigmoid.

The mesenteric circulation is regulated by three different means: (1) *Intrinsic regulation* or local modulation of blood flow occurs in response to changes in arteriolar transmural pressure or to alterations in tissue oxygenation in order to maintain adequate blood flow and oxygen delivery. Examples of this include the vasodilatation observed after brief periods of arterial occlusion (reactive hyperemia) and during digestion of a meal (functional hyperemia). Functional hyperemia may also, in part, be due to the effects of regulatory gastrointestinal peptides. (2) *Extrinsic neurologic regulation* of intestinal blood flow is mediated by sympathetic postganglionic fibers originating from the splanchnic nerves, which cause constriction of arteries and arterioles and a reduction in intestinal blood flow. Continued stimulation of these nerves, however, leads to a partial or in some cases complete recovery of flow (autoregulatory escape). (3) *Circulating endogenous and exogenous agents* may affect mesenteric blood flow. Increased arteriolar resistance is caused by α-adrenergic agonists, vasopressin, angiotensin II, prostaglandin F_2, and digitalis glycosides. Vasodilatation and increased blood flow result from the actions of β-adrenergic agonists, prostaglandin E_2, and the gut hormones cholecystokinin, gastrin, and glucagon.

The microcirculation of the intra-abdominal digestive organs is controlled by (1) the arteriole that, as the major site of resistance, is the most important local determinant of overall mesenteric blood flow, and (2) the precapillary sphincter, which determines capillary perfusion.

Several factors are important in determining the extent, severity, or possible reversibility of ischemic processes or events. The first of these is the abruptness of a vascular occlusion; more gradually occlusive processes may permit development of collaterals. A second factor is size and configuration of a vessel; emboli most commonly enter the large, obliquely situated superior mesenteric artery. A third factor is the level of involvement of a localized occlusive process. Vasculitis involving arteriae rectae or intramural arteries does not allow for development of collateral blood flow and may result in ischemia of a limited segment of intestine.

Intestinal ischemia may occur in hypoxic or low cardiac output states in the absence of an anatomic obstruction to blood flow (nonocclusive intestinal infarction). It is postulated that this may result from (1) the formation of toxic superoxide anions, (2) loss of the protective function of small intestinal brush border glycoproteins against the deleterious effects of luminal pancreatic proteases and bacterial toxins, or (3) shunting of oxygen from the villus tip caused by a countercurrent exhange resulting from the arrangement of blood vessels in the villus.

CHRONIC INTESTINAL ISCHEMIC SYNDROMES

ABDOMINAL ANGINA. This uncommon syndrome is due to severe atherosclerosis involving at least two of the three major arterial supplies to the intestine. There is usually a history of intermittent dull or cramping midabdominal pain characteristically beginning 15 to 30 minutes after eating and lasting for 1 to 2 hours. This is the period of increased intestinal blood flow and oxygen consumption required for digestion and absorption. Patients may also have lost a substantial amount of weight owing mainly to a decrease in food consumption resulting from fear of the pain associated with eating. Mild-to-moderate malabsorption may also be present. Physical examination usually uncovers evidence of atherosclerotic disease involving other vessels. The presence or absence of an abdominal bruit is not of diagnostic value. A presumptive diagnosis may be made on the basis of a strongly suggestive history and the angiographic demonstration of significant (> 50 per cent) narrowing of at least two of the three major arteries. Often there is evidence of collateral flow. Many patients who are asymptomatic, however, may show similar angiographic findings. Surgical treatment has included bypass, endarterectomy, and reimplantation procedures with significant relief of symptoms in most patients. Percutaneous transluminal angioplasty has also been employed successfully and offers the possibility that nonoperative approaches may also prove useful in some patients. As many as 50 per cent of patients with acute mesenteric arterial occlusion (see below) give a history suggestive of previous abdominal angina. Successful treatment of chronic intestinal ischemia may prevent such a catastrophic outcome.

CELIAC COMPRESSION SYNDROME. Recurrent abdominal pain in some individuals has been found to be associated with narrowing of the celiac axis alone. These patients, generally younger women in otherwise good health, complain of epigastric pain of variable frequency and duration. The pain may or may not be related to meals and is infrequently accompanied by nausea and vomiting. An epigastric bruit that does not radiate to the lower abdomen is the only physical finding that has been frequently described. Lateral views of the celiac axis during angiography demonstrate narrowing near its origin. At surgery this has usually been ascribed to compression by the median arcuate ligament of the diaphragm. In some cases, however, the stenosis has been reported to be due to neurofibrous tissue of the celiac ganglion or to intimal narrowing of the vessel itself. Surgical therapy has involved either division of the obstructing structure or bypass grafting, usually with relief of symptoms. The symptoms have recurred with time in some patients. The validity of this syndrome is a matter of considerable controversy for several reasons: (1) similar degrees of celiac axis narrowing have been found incidentally at angiography or autopsy in a substantial number of patients without symptoms of this syndrome, and (2) stenosis of the celiac axis alone would not be expected to result in symptomatic intestinal ischemia because of mesenteric collateral vessels. Some investigators believe that the pain is not truly ischemic but may arise in the celiac ganglion, which is removed or disrupted by most surgical treatments for this syndrome. Resolution of this controversy will require more precise clinical and pathophysiologic definition of the syndrome, including detailed follow-up studies. Surgery should be reserved for those patients with preoperative angiographic evidence of celiac stenosis who would otherwise undergo exploratory laparotomy for disabling and unexplained abdominal pain. At operation a thorough search for other disorders should precede treatment for presumed celiac compression syndrome.

ACUTE INTESTINAL ISCHEMIC SYNDROMES

ACUTE BOWEL INFARCTION: MESENTERIC ARTERIAL OCCLUSION. Gradual occlusion of one or sometimes even two of the three major mesenteric arteries may be asymptomatic because of the development of adequate collateral circulation. However, when intestinal blood flow falls below a critical level, ischemic necrosis of the supplied areas will result. Most commonly this is due to advanced *atherosclerotic disease* affecting at least two of the major visceral branches of the aorta. Generally the most proximal segments of these arteries are most severely involved. In addition to *embolism*, which is discussed below, other causes of mesenteric arterial occlusion include dissecting *aortic aneurysm, fibromuscular hyperplasia,* and *systemic vasculitides,* which may involve the mesenteric arteries at any level from the major arterial trunks to the intramural arteries. An association has also been reported with the use of *oral contraceptives*.

Diagnosis. The early diagnosis of acute intestinal infarction is often difficult. The history usually is not very helpful, but evidence of "abdominal angina" (see above) or other conditions predisposing to thrombosis may aid in the evaluation. Patients frequently have *severe abdominal pain* that initially may be colicky in nature and periumbilical in location. Bowel sounds not only may be present but may even be hyperactive. At this stage the patient's complaint of pain often appears out of proportion to physical findings or laboratory studies. As ischemia progresses, pain becomes constant and poorly localized. Systemic manifestations become prominent and severe, including *tachycardia, hypotension, fever, leukocytosis, acidosis,* and the presence of *blood* in nasogastric aspirate, vomitus, or stool. It has been suggested, on the basis of small numbers of patients and experimental animal studies, that elevations in serum and peritoneal fluid phosphate concentration may be sensitive indicators of intestinal infarction. Because an elevation in serum phosphate concentration in this setting is often associated with extensive bowel injury, acute renal insufficiency, and acidosis, it implies a poor prognosis. Abdominal radiographs usually show evidence of an *ileus* with distended, thick-walled loops of bowel and air-fluid levels (Fig. 106–3). Gas in the intestinal wall or portal vein is a late finding. Ultimately, when ischemic necrosis becomes transmural, signs of *peritonitis,* including bloody peritoneal fluid, appear. At this point, the prognosis (with or without surgery) is extremely poor.

The early diagnosis of bowel infarction depends upon a high index of suspicion and exclusion of other intra-abdominal conditions that can manifest virtually identically (e.g., acute pancreatitis, perforated viscus, bowel obstruction). A decision regarding extensive radiographic studies, especially angiography, in patients with suspected bowel infarction must be individualized. For the patient in whom hypotension, acidosis, or signs of peritonitis are present, suggesting that perforation may have already occurred, the information to be obtained from further studies may not justify the necessary delay in surgical management. However, earlier in the course, angiography may help define the nature and extent of the occlusive process or, in the absence of major vessel occlusion, suggest the diagnosis of nonocclusive infarction. Interpretation, however, is often difficult and clinical judgment is based only in part on angiographic findings. Computed tomography shows promise of becoming a rapid, noninvasive means of confirming the diagnosis of acute bowel infarction by identifying characteristic changes in the appearance of the bowel wall and mesentery.

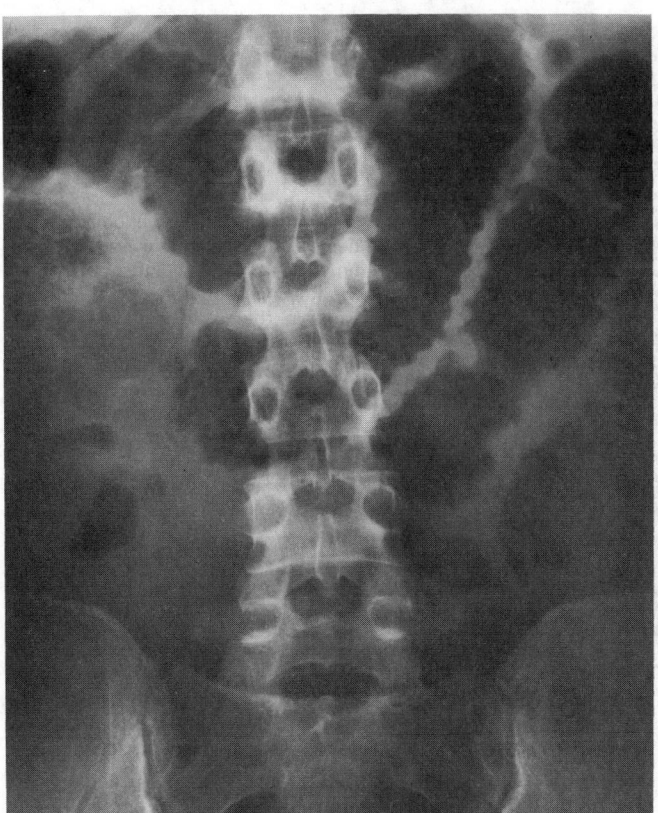

FIGURE 106–3. A supine abdominal x-ray in a patient with acute infarction of the small intestine showing dilated loops of small bowel with irregular thickening of the bowel wall.

Treatment. Initial supportive therapy, aimed at stabilization of the patient's condition prior to surgery, includes nasogastric suction, replacement of fluid and electrolyte deficits, administration of broad-spectrum antibiotics after blood cultures have been obtained, and cardiopulmonary support, if needed. As soon as the patient's condition is adequately stabilized and the diagnosis strongly suspected, prompt surgical exploration should be performed. At surgery, resection of necrotic bowel is the primary objective. An attempt may be made to revascularize the remaining viable intestine by bypass graft or endarterectomy if the patient's condition is sufficiently stable to perform the additional surgery.

At the time of operation it is important but sometimes difficult to define the limits of viable bowel in order to resect completely irreversibly diseased intestine while at the same time avoiding unnecessary development of the short bowel syndrome. It is often necessary to perform a "second-look" operation 12 to 36 hours after the initial exploration to identify and resect any additional bowel that in the interim proves to be nonviable. Infarction of large segments of intestine carries essentially a 100 per cent mortality rate without surgery. Even with surgery the mortality rate is > 50 per cent in most series because of delay in diagnosis or because of other complicating factors such as advanced age or atherosclerotic disease involving other vital organs.

Mesenteric vasculitis (e.g., as may occur in lupus erythematosus, polyarteritis nodosa, dermatomyositis, rheumatoid vasculitis, and Henoch-Schönlein purpura) may cause segmental intestinal infarction not conforming to the distribution of the major arteries. Vascular occlusion may not be demonstrable angiographically if only intramural arteries and arterioles are involved. Although some patients may require emergency surgery for intestinal necrosis and perforation, these complications are less common than with occlusions of the major arteries or their principal branches. In some cases the acute episode may resolve spontaneously, which may leave the patient with a segmental stricture demonstrable by barium contrast studies.

MESENTERIC ARTERY EMBOLISM. Emboli to the mesenteric circulation most commonly involve the superior mesenteric artery because of its size and the oblique angle of its origin from the aorta. These emboli usually arise from mural thrombi in the heart in patients with atherosclerotic or valvular heart disease but may also arise from vegetations of bacterial endocarditis, atrial myxomas, valvular prostheses, or atherosclerotic plaques in the thoracic or upper abdominal aorta, either spontaneously or during angiography. Patients may have a history of previous embolic episodes or exhibit evidence of simultaneous peripheral embolization (e.g., to the brain or extremities). Typically patients described the *abrupt onset of severe midabdominal cramping pain,* accompanied by vomiting or diarrhea. Although patients may feel and appear severely ill, early in the course objective physical findings are sparse. If the diagnosis is not made promptly and appropriate treatment undertaken, a mesenteric embolus will lead to bowel infarction. Angiography may demonstrate mesenteric artery occlusion in the absence of collateral circulation, indicating the acute nature of the process. Computed tomography may also strongly suggest the diagnosis early in the course of the disease in a patient with acute onset of abdominal pain of unknown source. Following supportive measures as needed to stabilize the patient's condition, immediate exploration with embolectomy and resection of any infarcted bowel is indicated. A "second-look" procedure will sometimes be necessary. The characteristic setting in which mesenteric embolism occurs, as well as its abrupt onset, offers a greater opportunity for early diagnosis and treatment. For this reason, and because the patients generally are younger, the prognosis is more favorable than for most nonembolic causes of bowel infarction. Some patients who are successfully treated by embolectomy without need for bowel resection may develop a transient malabsorption syndrome persisting for several months.

NONOCCLUSIVE INTESTINAL INFARCTION. In some patients clinical findings suggestive of mesenteric arterial occlusive disease or embolism occur without a demonstrable obstruction to arterial flow. This syndrome, now recognized with increasing frequency, usually occurs in the setting of severe congestive heart failure, shock, hypoxia, or a recent myocardial infarction. In addition, it has been reported following cocaine ingestion, possibly related to α-adrenergic stimulation due to the drug. The clinical course often evolves more slowly than is seen with occlusive processes. Occasionally a precipitating event is not identifiable. The use of α-adrenergic vasoconstrictors (and possibly digitalis glycosides) may also contribute to the development of this process. Because of its high degree of metabolic activity, the mucosa has the greatest requirement for intestinal blood flow of the various layers of the bowel wall. Thus it will show the earliest evidence of ischemic injury. At times, it may be the only portion to undergo hemorrhagic infarction. However, infarction may ultimately become transmural and occur in a patchy and irregular distribution, not conforming to the area supplied by a major vessel. Early angiography is useful to exclude a major vessel occlusion, which would usually require vascular surgery. In at least 50 per cent of such patients angiography reveals irregular narrowing of the major arterial branches and arcades (due to spasm) and impaired filling of the intramural vessels. Therapy consists of supportive measures and surgical exploration to resect infarcted bowel if the patient's situation suggests the need for this. Selective infusion of vasodilators into the mesenteric circulation has been suggested, but its therapeutic efficacy remains to be established. This syndrome generally carries a very poor prognosis, primarily because it is usually associated with shock or severe cardiopulmonary disease.

ISCHEMIC COLITIS. Ischemic injury to the colon may be

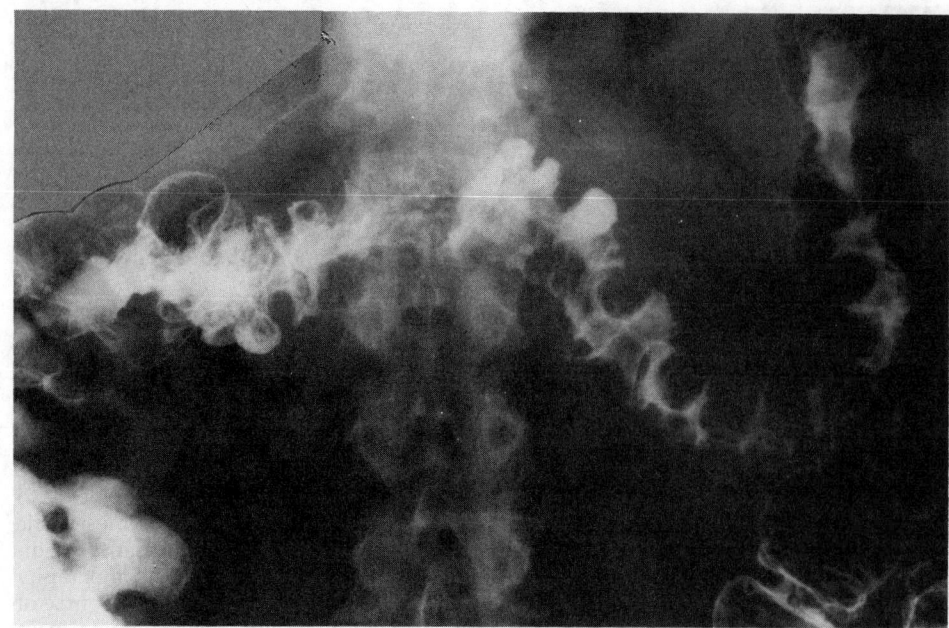

FIGURE 106–4. A barium enema in a patient with ischemic colitis showing narrowing and "thumbprinting" (nodular indentations of the bowel wall) in the distal transverse colon. This is one of the "watershed" areas of the colon between two adjacent arterial supplies (superior and inferior mesenteric arteries) where ischemia is more likely to develop.

caused by advanced atherosclerosis or interruption of the colonic blood supply during surgery (e.g., abdominal aortic aneurysmectomy, aortoiliac reconstruction, abdominoperineal resection) or may occur in association with "hypercoagulable" states, amyloidosis, vasculitis, ruptured aortic aneurysm, colorectal cancer, or the use of oral contraceptive agents. In addition, nonocclusive colonic ischemia may occur in states of low cardiac output or hypoxia. Nonocclusive colonic ischemia may be mediated primarily by the renin-angiotensin system, to which the colonic vasculature appears to be remarkably sensitive. The syndrome of ischemic colitis may be quite variable in its extent, severity, and prognosis. However, extensive infarction and perforation appear to be infrequent. Localized or segmental ischemia is more common, particularly affecting those areas of the colon that lie on the "watershed" between two adjacent arterial supplies, i.e., the splenic flexure (superior and inferior mesenteric arteries) and the rectosigmoid (inferior mesenteric and internal iliac arteries). Characteristically, patients over the age of 50 are most often affected with *abrupt onset of lower abdominal cramping pain, rectal bleeding,* and, to variable degrees, *vomiting* and *fever.* Some patients give a history of similar symptoms occurring intermittently for weeks to months before presentation. Left-sided abdominal tenderness and peritoneal signs may be present, as well as evidence of generalized atherosclerotic disease. Sigmoidoscopy may be normal; may show evidence of mild, nonspecific proctitis; or may reveal a spectrum of findings, including multiple discrete ulcers, blue-black hemorrhagic submucosal blebs, or an adherent pseudomembrane. Angiography generally has not proved useful in the diagnosis of patients in this setting. The differentiation of ischemic colitis from infections of the colon, diverticulitis, and idiopathic inflammatory bowel disease (ulcerative colitis, Crohn's disease of the colon) may be very difficult. Initial management consists of general supportive measures, including antibiotics. In those patients in whom perforation or infarction of the colon appears likely, early surgical exploration is indicated; however, many patients will improve without surgery. Subsequent barium enema will often show a characteristic picture of intramural hemorrhage and edema, including "thumbprinting," tubular narrowing, and "sawtooth" irregularity (Fig. 106–4). Some patients will proceed to complete resolution of the clinical process and radiographic abnormalities. Others will develop a residual stricture that eventually may require surgical resection.

MESENTERIC VENOUS THROMBOSIS. This condition, which accounts for about 5 to 15 per cent of patients with intestinal ischemia, almost always involves the superior mesenteric vein. It is associated with a variety of conditions: stasis in the mesenteric venous bed (portal hypertension, congestive heart failure), abdominal neoplasms, intra-abdominal inflammation (peritonitis, abscess, inflammatory bowel disease), abdominal surgery and trauma, a variety of presumed hypercoagulable states (antithrombin III deficiency, polycythemia vera), and use of oral contraceptives. Occasionally a predisposing condition is absent. Patients may have abrupt onset of a clinical picture indicative of acute bowel infarction; however, many others have a more gradual course with development of progressive abdominal discomfort over a period of weeks. Physical findings are nonspecific. The presence of a small amount of bloody peritoneal fluid is typical and may be an important clue to the diagnosis in patients with a subacute clinical course. Selective superior mesenteric angiography shows intense spasm of the arteries to the involved segment of bowel and absence of venous drainage.

Following initial supportive care to stabilize the patient's condition, an operation should be performed to resect infarcted or severely ischemic bowel. Reconstructive venous surgery is not generally possible. Because there is about a 25 per cent rate of recurrent thrombosis within the first several weeks postoperatively, anticoagulation is recommended except in patients who have underlying disease processes that would make this too hazardous. A "second-look" operation to search for recurrent thrombosis may also be required if there is unexplained clinical deterioration following initial surgery. In general, the prognosis is more favorable than for patients with mesenteric arterial disease, with reported mortality as low as 20 per cent.

MISCELLANEOUS DISORDERS

INTRAMURAL INTESTINAL HEMORRHAGE. This may follow abdominal trauma or may occur in the setting of ischemic bowel injury, vasculitis, or bleeding diatheses. Some patients have a picture suggesting a perforated viscus (severe abdominal pain, tenderness, leukocytosis), but most have cramping abdominal pain and vomiting suggestive of partial or complete bowel obstruction. Hematemesis or melena and fever may be present. Occasionally a palpable abdominal mass caused by the presence of a hematoma may be noted. Barium studies of the small intestine typically show a "stacked coins" or "thumbprint" appearance. Usually intramural intestinal hemorrhage can be managed conservatively with nasogastric suction, intravenous hydration and electrolytes, and correction of an underlying coagulopathy, when possible. In those patients with high-grade or unremitting intestinal obstruction, or in whom signs of peritonitis develop (suggesting perforation), surgery is necessary.

PARAPROSTHETIC-ENTERIC AND AORTOENTERIC FISTULAS. Following aortic aneurysmectomy and other procedures in which vascular prostheses are placed in the abdomen or retroperitoneum, fistulas may form between the graft and adjacent bowel. This may occur as early as several weeks postoperatively but in most cases is delayed by at least two years. This complication usually results from local infection or damage to the intestine or its blood supply at surgery, with subsequent erosion of the bowel wall by the graft. Patients may present with massive upper or lower gastrointestinal bleeding or both that may be rapidly fatal without emergency surgery. In a number of patients, however, bleeding may be initially intermittent, resembling that from a number of more common lesions. In these patients, early consideration of this diagnosis with urgent evaluation by upper endoscopy, radiolabeled red blood cell studies, computed tomography, and/or angiography may be required to establish the diagnosis and need for surgical intervention.

Unoperated upon abdominal aortic aneurysms and aneurysmal dilatations of other major abdominal arteries may erode into the gastrointestinal tract, causing upper or lower gastrointestinal bleeding or both of various degrees of severity.

SUPERIOR MESENTERIC ARTERY SYNDROME. This uncommon syndrome of postprandial epigastric pain, distention, and vomiting has been attributed to compression of the third portion of the duodenum between the superior mesenteric artery anteriorly and the fixed retroperitoneal structures posteriorly. This has been described as occurring most commonly in individuals who have lost a substantial amount of weight or are of "asthenic habitus," and in children with rapid growth in the absence of corresponding weight gain or who have been fixed in a position of hyperextension by a cast following spinal injury or surgery. Barium contrast studies show distention of the proximal duodenum, and lateral aortograms or abdominal sonograms have shown a narrowing of the angle between the aorta and the superior mesenteric artery. The differential diagnosis includes generalized disorders of gastrointestinal motility, such as scleroderma, and anorexia nervosa. Recommended treatment has included the use of small feedings and elemental diets with the patient lying prone or on the left side in the knee-chest position after eating. In refractory cases duodenal mobilization or duodenal-jejunal bypass has reportedly been effective in relieving symptoms. Since apparent compression of the duodenum by the superior mesenteric artery does not prove clinically significant obstruction, the diagnosis of this syndrome must be made only after other possible causes of duodenal stasis have been excluded. This entity is frequently overdiagnosed unless strict diagnostic criteria are employed.

VASCULAR MALFORMATIONS INCLUDING ANGIODYSPLASIA. Hemangiomas of the small intestine are very uncommon vascular tumors found throughout the bowel, particularly the jejunum. They represent one of the causes of gastrointestinal bleeding that may be very difficult to locate. These lesions are most reliably diagnosed by abdominal angiography.

Vascular malformations can occur in the gastrointestinal tract in association with diseases involving the skin, such as the *hereditary hemorrhagic telangiectasia (Osler-Weber-Rendu) syndrome, blue rubber bleb nevus syndrome,* and the *CREST syndrome* (calcinosis, Raynaud's phenomenon, esophageal hypomotility, sclerodactyly, and telangiectasia). In addition, vascular malformations may occur as a primary process (*angiodysplasia,*

vascular ectasia) chiefly involving the colon but also occurring in the stomach or small intestine. This latter process is being increasingly recognized as a frequent cause of lower intestinal bleeding, especially in patients over the age of 60. An association of angiodysplasia with aortic stenosis has also been reported but not fully established. Angiodysplastic lesions of the stomach and small intestine may be the most common source of upper gastrointestinal bleeding in patients with chronic renal failure.

Angiodysplastic lesions consist of ectatic, tortuous submucosal veins and groups of ectatic mucosal vessels lying just under the gastric, intestinal, or colonic epithelium or at times on the luminal surface unprotected by any intestinal epithelium. The etiology of these lesions remains uncertain. One theory suggests that they develop as a result of chronic low-grade obstruction of the submucosal veins as they penetrate the muscularis propria; another theory proposes that these lesions develop because of chronic mucosal ischemia.

Larger vascular malformations, including some primary angiodysplastic lesions, may be visualized by selective mesenteric arteriography. Many of these lesions are small and are best demonstrated by endoscopy. Such lesions are present in a large number of older individuals without apparent gastrointestinal blood loss. For those patients who have chronic or recurrent gastrointestinal blood loss without other apparent cause, surgery has been recommended if vascular malformations could be identified and localized (e.g., right colectomy for lesions in the cecum). This approach is often unsatisfactory, and bleeding may recur either because some lesions in other parts of the gastrointestinal tract may not have been appreciated at the initial evaluation or because new lesions may subsequently develop. For these reasons, nonoperative endoscopic approaches have been developed to obliterate vascular malformations by such techniques as laser photocoagulation, electrocoagulation, or thermal coagulation (heater probe).

Baur CM, Millay DJ, Taylor CM, et al.: Treatment of chronic visceral ischemia. Am J Surg 148:138, 1984. *Illustrates the efficacy of surgical treatment for abdominal angina in properly selected patients.*

Cello JP, Grendell JH: Endoscopic laser treatment for gastrointestinal vascular ectasias. Ann Intern Med 104:352, 1986. *Demonstrates the effective use of nonoperative therapy for this disorder.*

Cooke M, Sande MA: Diagnosis and outcome of bowel infarction on an acute medical service. Am J Med 75:984, 1983. *Highlights the difficulty of differentiating bowel infarction from other intra-abdominal catastrophes.*

Croft RJ, Menon GP, Marston A: Does "intestinal angina" exist? A critical study of obstructed visceral arteries. Br J Surg 68:316, 1981. *A provocative report demonstrating the difficulty in relating gastrointestinal symptoms to angiographic findings.*

Federle MP, Chun G, Jeffrey RB, et al.: Computed tomographic findings in bowel infarction. Am J Roentgenol 142:91, 1984. *This report demonstrates the potential value of computed tomography in the diagnosis of vascular diseases of the intestine.*

Grendell JH, Ockner RK: Vascular diseases of the bowel. In Sleisenger MH, Fordtran JS (eds.): Gastrointestinal Disease. 4th ed. Philadelphia, W.B. Saunders Company, 1988. *A comprehensive survey including pathophysiology, diagnosis, and management.*

Hines JR, Gore RM, Ballantyne GH: Superior mesenteric artery syndrome: Diagnostic criteria and therapeutic approaches. Am J Surg 148:630, 1984. *Emphasizes the importance of strict diagnostic criteria to avoid overdiagnosis of this entity.*

Kiernan PD, Pairolero PC, Hubert JP Jr, et al.: Aortic graft–enteric fistula. Mayo Clin Proc 55:731, 1980. *A detailed review of clinical features, management, and prognosis.*

Rogers DM, Thompson JE, Garret WV, et al.: Mesenteric vascular problems: A 26-year experience. Ann Surg 195:554, 1982. *This article describes an extensive surgical experience with a variety of vascular diseases of the intestine.*

Zuckerman GR, Cornette GL, Clouse RE, et al.: Upper gastrointestinal bleeding in patients with chronic renal failure. Ann Intern Med 102:588, 1985. *Demonstrates the importance of angiodysplastic lesions as a source of upper gastrointestinal bleeding in patients with chronic renal failure.*

107 NEOPLASMS OF THE LARGE AND SMALL INTESTINE

Sidney J. Winawer

NEOPLASMS OF THE LARGE INTESTINE

Adenocarcinoma of the large intestine is a worldwide health problem of major importance, especially in western countries. The incidence of this cancer in the United States is more than 145,000 per year; more than half of those affected will die of their disease within five years of the time of diagnosis. With the exception of skin cancer, cancer of the colon, along with lung cancer and breast cancer, is one of the three leading malignancies in this country in terms of annual new cases. New concepts and new technologies for diagnosis and treatment of this cancer have evolved over the past few years, providing opportunities for earlier detection and improved survival.

The colon is the site of a variety of other malignant tumors. Its second most common primary malignant tumor is the epidermoid or squamous cell carcinoma of the anal canal and rectum. Other primary malignant tumors that can involve the colon include lymphomas, leiomyosarcomas, and malignant carcinoid tumors as well as direct invasion by tumors from adjacent sites such as stomach, uterus, ovary, and prostate. Rarely tumors from such sites as breast and lung metastasize to the colon.

The most frequent tumors that involve the large intestine are adenomas, which are present in as many as 30 to 40 per cent of asymptomatic patients over the age of 40. A variety of other benign tumors, including lipomas, leiomyomas, and benign carcinoid tumors, occur in the colon. Of these all are rare except for lipomas of the ileocecal valve. Adenomas of the large intestine will be discussed first because of their frequency and their association with cancer of the colon.

Polyps of the Colon

A polyp in a generic sense is any lesion that arises from the surface of the gastrointestinal tract and protrudes into the lumen (Fig. 107–1). Polyps are usually defined pathologically as overgrowths of epithelial tissue that may be either hyperplastic or neoplastic, benign or malignant, and of various histopathologic subtypes. They are noted clinically in the large bowel as negative shadows in the lumen demonstrated by barium enema or by direct visualization during proctosigmoidoscopy or colonoscopy. They may be single or multiple, pedunculated (on a stalk) or sessile (flat and without a stalk), and sporadic in occurrence or part of a dominantly transmitted familial polyposis syndrome. Their importance lies in their frequency, their occasional production of symptoms (bleeding), and most of all their potential for malignant transformation. They are to be distinguished from pseudopolyps, which have an inflammatory mass in association with normal epithelium.

PATHOLOGY. In addition to carcinoma of the large intestine, which may present as a polypoid mass, four distinct types of benign polyps arise from colonic epithelium: (1) hyperplastic (metaplastic), (2) tubular adenomas, (3) villous adenomas, and (4) mixed type. *Hyperplastic polyps*, which account for about 25 per cent of all polyps and for most of the polyps of the rectum, tend to be small and asymptomatic, and are not considered to be neoplastic, based on the histologic criteria of normal cellular differentiation and a sharp line of demarcation between the polyp and the normal mucosa. *Neoplastic polyps* or adenomas have the same distribution in the colon as do cancers of the colon and account for most of the polyps above the area of the rectum. They are usually less than 1 cm in diameter (75 per cent), may be sessile or pedunculated, and represent localized neoplastic tumors of colonic epithelium. Histologically they have abnormal cellular differentiation and exhibit predominantly tubular structure. *Villous adenomas* typically are spongy, exophytic, and larger than adenomatous polyps (60 per cent > 2 cm). They exhibit a predominantly glandular pattern representing overgrowth of poorly differentiated cells from the base of the crypts of Lieberkühn. They have a high association with malignant transformation. *Mixed type adenomas* contain both tubular and villous components, and the villous component tends to increase with the size of the polyp.

RELATIONSHIP OF COLONIC ADENOMAS TO CANCER. The evidence that links benign adenomas (the neoplastic polyps classified as adenomas, mixed or villous) to adenocarcinoma of the colon is compelling: (1) the epidemiology of adenocarcinomas and adenomas of the colon is similar wherever studied in the world; (2) adenocarcinomas of the colon occur in the same anatomic distribution as adenomas of the colon; (3) the risk for colorectal cancer is high in patients with a prior history of adenomas, but is lower if adenomas are removed; (4) as adenomas grow in size, the frequency of finding cancer in the adenoma increases; (5) residual adenomatous tissue can sometimes be found in colorectal cancers on pathologic examination; and (6) the association of cancer and adenomas is particularly strong in the inherited colorectal cancer syndromes, with adenocarcinomas having been documented to have arisen from the underlying adenomas. In brief, there is now very little doubt that colorectal cancer arises from an antecedent premalignant tumor of the colon, the benign adenoma.

The premalignant nature of adenomas is related to size and

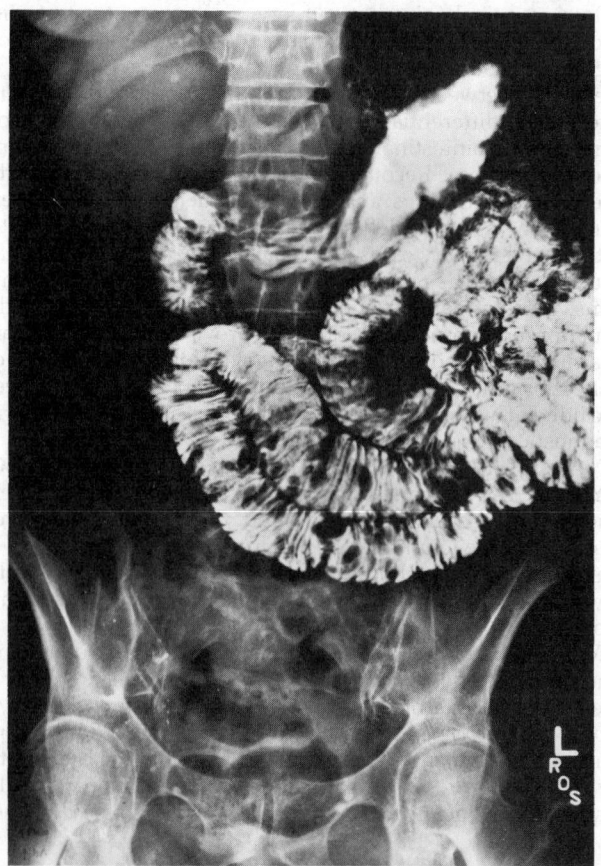

FIGURE 107–1. Barium study of the upper gastrointestinal tract showing multiple polyps of the small bowel in a patient with Peutz-Jeghers syndrome.

histology. The frequency of cancer in adenomas is 1 per cent in adenomas less than 1 cm in size; 10 per cent in adenomas between 1 and 2 cm in size; and 30 per cent in adenomas greater than 2 cm in size. The relationship of cancer to adenomas is much greater in adenomas with villous components than in adenomas without villous components. Cancer in adenomas is usually well differentiated and occurs most commonly in the tip of the adenoma without invasion of the muscularis mucosae. These are called in situ or focal cancers and are not immediately dangerous. Less commonly, cancers in adenomas invade the muscularis mucosae, and therefore have the potential to grow down the stalk, invade lymphatics, involve adjacent lymph nodes, and metastasize.

The occurrence of adenomas signifies an important transformation of the colonic mucosa to a premalignant state. Thus, it is understandable that additional adenomas often concurrently exist (synchronous adenomas) and others will appear subsequently (metachronous adenomas). The synchronous rate for adenomas is 50 per cent, and the metachronous rate is 30 to 40 per cent. Synchronous and metachronous rates for colorectal cancers are 1.5 to 5 per cent and 5 to 10 per cent, respectively. Multiple adenomas appear to be associated with a higher frequency of metachronous adenomas and metachronous cancers.

CLINICAL MANIFESTATIONS. Most polyps are asymptomatic. When symptoms do occur, they most frequently result from *bleeding* (hematochezia or iron deficiency anemia, depending on the location of the polyp and the rate of blood loss). When polyps are very large they may rarely cause *abdominal pain* from partial intestinal obstruction or from induced intussusception. Villous adenomas may rarely result in *watery diarrhea* with severe potassium depletion or in excessive secretion of mucus with loss of sufficient protein to produce hypoalbuminemia (an unusual form of "protein-losing enteropathy").

TREATMENT AND FOLLOW-UP. Because of the association of polyps with cancer of the colon, it is recommended that they be removed when identified.

Colonoscopic Polypectomy. Pedunculated polyps of any size can be removed by cautery snare through the colonoscope (see Fig. 96–3). Sessile polyps smaller than 2 cm can generally also be removed by cautery snare through the colonoscope. Controversy exists as to whether sessile polyps larger than 2 cm should be removed by colonoscopy or by surgery. Although large sessile polyps can be excised segmentally via the colonoscope, this approach is challenged because many of them already are cancerous, the risk of complications during removal is significantly increased, and the completeness of removal is uncertain. Since there is also risk involved in surgery, each case must be individualized. Suspicion that a polyp may be a polypoid adenocarcinoma warrants a biopsy and brushing for cytology. If the diagnosis of carcinoma is confirmed, surgery is indicated. Benign-appearing polyps are totally excised, not biopsied, and the entire polyp is submitted for pathologic examination. Polyps up to 7 or 8 mm in size can be removed by a combination of biopsy and fulguration. This is a particularly rapid and effective means for treating these small lesions.

After endoscopic polypectomy the patient must be followed periodically. Usually a repeat colonoscopy is performed one year later to search for missed synchronous lesions, and then approximately every three years thereafter to search for metachronous lesions. If the patient has multiple adenomas, colonoscopy is often done annually for several years.

Focal cancer in an adenoma demands special consideration. If the cancer is in the tip of the polyp and has not penetrated the muscularis mucosae, no further surgery need be done. If the cancer has penetrated the muscularis mucosae and lymphatic invasion has been demonstrated, if the cancer is poorly differentiated, or if it has extended down to the line of cautery, then follow-up laparotomy and segmental resection are indicated. In such circumstances there will be approximately a 5 per cent frequency of regional lymph node metastases.

Inherited Polyposis Syndromes of the Large and Small Intestines

There are a number of heritable syndromes characterized by polyposis of the intestine with or without additional extraintestinal manifestations. Some of these syndromes have a greatly increased frequency of cancer, and some have a slightly increased frequency of cancer.

Familial polyposis of the colon, an autosomal dominant trait, is characterized by multiple adenomas of the large intestine and rarely of the ileum as well (Fig. 107–2). In this disorder, which occurs approximately once each 8000 births, hundreds and sometimes thousands of polyps develop throughout the entire colon, beginning in childhood. Virtually all patients with familial polyposis develop carcinoma of the colon by age 40, so subtotal colectomy should be carried out early in adult life in affected persons. An intensive survey of other family members must be conducted because of the inheritance pattern; some cases occur without a family history and probably represent spontaneous mutations.

Gardner's syndrome is a dominantly transmitted disorder characterized by the triad of adenomas of the colon, bone tumors (osteomas), and soft tissue tumors (lipomas, sebaceous cysts, fibromas, fibrosarcomas) (Fig. 107–3A). Other associated features include retroperitoneal fibrosis, pigmented ocular fundus lesions, supernumerary teeth, and a tendency toward the development of carcinomas of the thyroid, adrenal, and duodenum in the region of the ampulla of Vater. There may be osteosclerosis of the skull in addition to the osteomas of the mandible and maxillary regions. The colonic polyps resemble those of familial polyposis and have the same potential for malignancy. The treatment is therefore subtotal colectomy and a careful survey for other affected members of the family.

Turcot's syndrome represents the rare association of adenomas of the colon with a variety of tumors of the central nervous system. The polyps have a high frequency of malignant transformation. The central nervous system lesions have included medulloblastoma, ependymoma, and glioblastoma. The mode of transmission is thought to be autosomal recessive, although this is unclear.

Peutz-Jeghers syndrome is a rare familial disorder, with autosomal dominant transmission, characterized by multiple intestinal polyposis and mucocutaneous pigmentation (Fig. 107–3B). The polyps, which occur in the small intestine, large intestine, and stomach, are mostly hamartomas rather than true adenomas and as such have a low potential for malignant transformation. It is estimated that 2 to 3 per cent of patients with this syndrome develop adenocarcinoma of the intestinal tract, with the small intestine being more frequently involved than the colon. Pigmentation is particularly marked in the buccal mucosa, in the hard and soft palate, on the lips, on the soles of the feet, on the dorsum of the hands, and around the mouth and nostrils. More rarely exostoses, ovarian tumors, and polyps of the bladder and nose have been described. Surgical removal of gastric and small bowel polyps is reserved only for complications such as bleeding or intestinal obstruction. True adenomas can occur in the colon in this disorder. These can usually be removed endoscopically.

Generalized juvenile polyposis refers to a familial syndrome with autosomal dominant transmission characterized by hamartomatous polyps in the colon and rectum and to a lesser extent in the small intestine and stomach. Symptoms usually begin in the first decade of life with bleeding, diarrhea, and abdominal pain. There are no extraintestinal manifestations. There seems to be an increased incidence of carcinoma of the intestine in the families with generalized juvenile polyposis, probably from true adenomas that occur with higher frequency in these families.

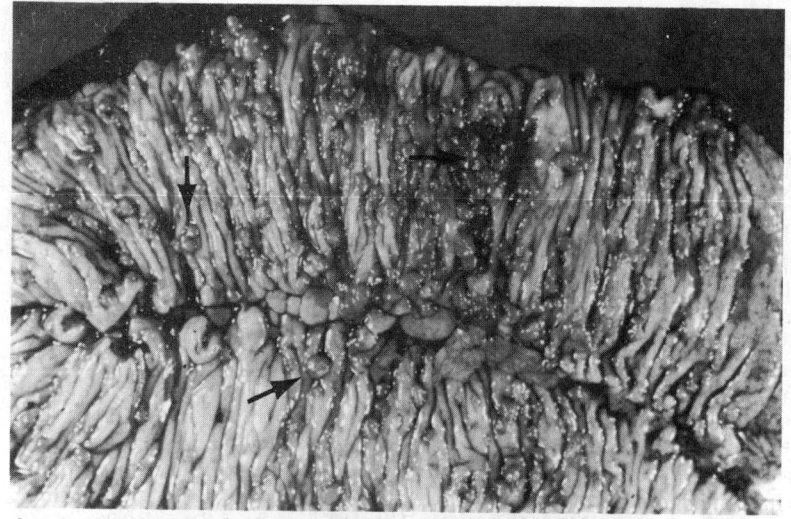

A

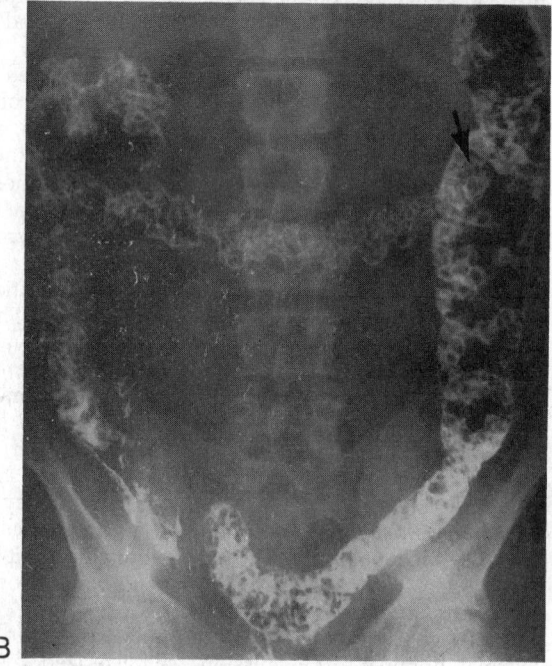

B

FIGURE 107–2. *A*, Patients with familial polyposis have multiple adenomatous polyps carpeting the colon, as demonstrated in this gross specimen. Note that the colon is diffusely studded with sessile and occasional pedunculated adenomatous polyps (*arrows*). Many of the larger polyps contain villous elements, and occasionally villous adenomas are found. Although no carcinoma was seen in this patient, nearly all patients will eventually develop colorectal carcinoma if surgery is not performed. *B*, This barium enema examination of a patient with familial polyposis represents diffuse studding of the large bowel with adenomatous polyps. Note the marked variation in size of these polyps. Although this patient did not have osteomas or soft tissue tumors, the barium enema is similar to that seen in Gardner's syndrome. (From Boland CR, Kim YS: In Sleisenger MH, Fordtran JS [eds.]: Gastrointestinal Disease. 3rd ed. Philadelphia, W. B. Saunders Company, 1983.)

Cronkhite-Canada syndrome refers to the rare association of generalized intestinal polyposis, dystrophy of the fingernails, alopecia, and cutaneous hyperpigmentation. The polyps are hamartomas; no familial association has been clearly established.

Adenocarcinoma of the Colon

EPIDEMIOLOGY. Colorectal cancer is more prevalent in the developed countries, suggesting a relationship to economic development. Its incidence is high in North America, New Zealand, and Europe and low in South America, Africa, and Asia. The United States has one of the highest rates of colorectal cancer in the world. Migrants to a particular geographic area assume the colonic cancer risk of that area. This is well illustrated by the higher incidence of the disease among blacks in America compared with those in Africa, in Puerto Ricans who have migrated to the mainland compared with those in Puerto Rico, and in first- and second-generation Japanese immigrants to Hawaii and the mainland United States compared with Japanese in Japan. In the United States the incidence of colorectal cancer is higher in the north than in the south, in urban areas compared with rural areas, and in whites compared with blacks. There is a slightly increased risk among certain occupations such as factory wood-workers.

ETIOLOGY. Migrant studies strongly suggest that *environmental factors*, particularly *diet*, are important in the etiology of colorectal cancer. There is a low incidence of appendicitis, adenomas, diverticulosis, ulcerative colitis, and colorectal cancer in the South African Bantu and other African populations in which diets contain more fiber and less animal fat than is the case with diets in more developed areas. High-fiber diets produce rapid intestinal transit so that any potential carcinogen is in contact with the mucosa for a shorter period of time. The various components of fiber may bind carcinogens or cocarcinogens or increase intraluminal bulk, and thereby dilute carcinogens. A direct association between *increased fat and animal protein* intake (particularly beef) in the western diet and the rising incidence of colonic cancer has been suggested. In Japan, the intake of fat (mostly unsaturated) provides only 12 per cent of the total caloric intake; in the United States fat intake represents 40 to 44 per cent of the total caloric intake. It has been postulated that the western diet with its high beef and fat content favors the establishment of bacterial flora capable of producing enzymes such as beta-glucuronidase and azoreductase, resulting in increased metabolism of acid and neutral sterols to carcinogens and cocarcinogens. Studies are in progress concerning putative mutagens in feces, including nitrosamide, which has been demonstrated in the feces of persons on high-beef diets. Reduction in mutagenicity

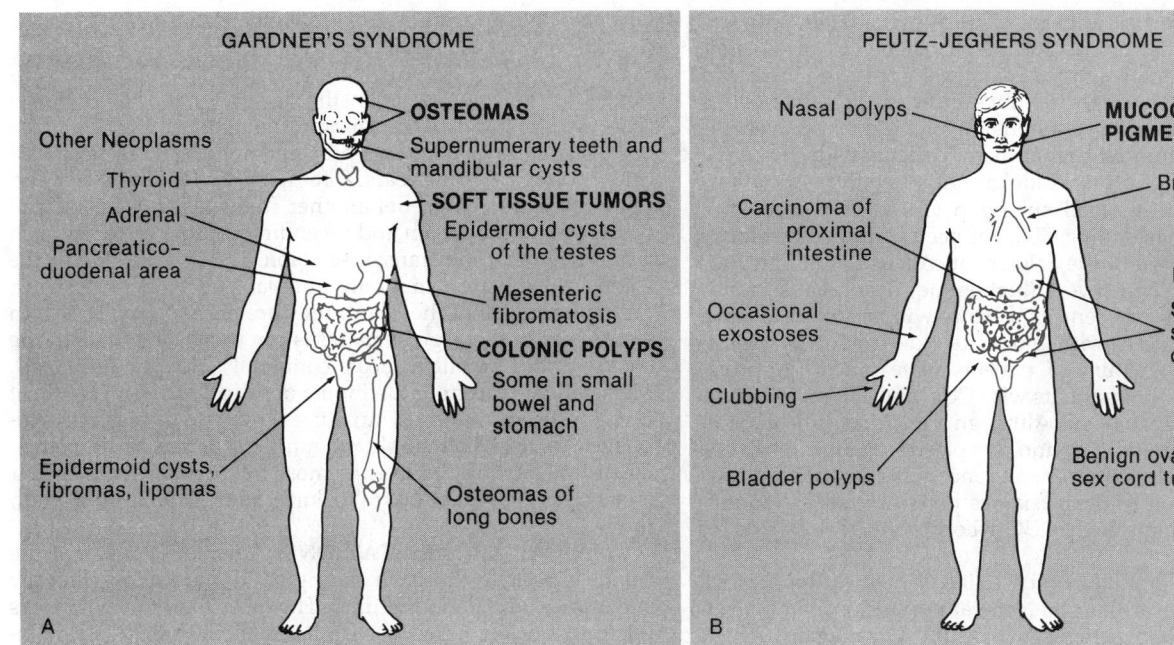

FIGURE 107–3. *A,* Schematic representation of Gardner's syndrome. The triad of colonic polyposis, bone tumors, and soft tissue tumors (heavy print) are the primary features; other features are indicated in lighter print. *B,* Schematic presentation of the Peutz-Jeghers syndrome. Mucocutaneous pigmentation and benign gastrointestinal polyposis (heavy print) are the primary features of this syndrome. Lighter print shows the secondary features. (From Boland CR, Kim YS: In Sleisenger MH, Fordtran JS [eds.]: Gastrointestinal Disease. 3rd ed. Philadelphia, W. B. Saunders Company, 1983.)

and in levels of nitrosamide in the stool has been noted in patients on high doses of ascorbic acid and alpha-tocopherol. Dietary calcium has recently been shown possibly to offer protection against colorectal cancer. The mechanism of this protection either may be a direct effect on the mucosal cells or may be the result of the combination of calcium with fatty acids and bile acids, thereby eliminating their toxic effect on the mucosa. Obviously much remains to be learned about the proposed relationship of diet to colorectal cancer, concerning both the validity of the association and the chemical link between diet and the induction of neoplastic transformation.

SUSCEPTIBILITY. In addition to general risk factors that influence susceptibility on a broad basis (Table 107–1), there are a number of specific factors that affect risk in the individual (see accompanying table). One of these factors is age. The risk for colorectal cancers begins to increase slightly at age 40 and more sharply at age 50, doubling with each decade and reaching a maximum at age 75. Additional risk factors include a prior history of colorectal cancer or adenoma, a prior history of female genital cancer, underlying ulcerative colitis of long standing, and a family history of one of the inherited colon cancer syndromes (see below).

Prior Colonic Cancer or Adenoma. Patients who have had one colorectal cancer are at increased risk for a subsequent colorectal cancer (metachronous lesion) occurring at a future time from the initial or index lesion. A prior adenoma of the

colon also increases risk for subsequent colorectal cancer. The association of adenomas and cancer of the colon has been previously discussed in detail.

Ulcerative Colitis. One third of deaths related to chronic ulcerative colitis (CUC) are due to colorectal cancer, which occurs in an overall incidence 7 to 11 times greater in patients with CUC than in the general population. The risk of cancer in ulcerative colitis can be related to two recognized variables: (1) the duration of active colitis, and (2) the anatomic extent of colonic involvement by the pathologic process.

The relationship between duration of ulcerative colitis and the cumulative risk of colorectal cancer for both adults and children is shown in Figure 107–4. In adults the risk begins to rise after seven years, and 20 per cent of patients with cancer and CUC develop their malignancies between seven and ten years from the onset of colitis. Extent of colonic involvement by CUC also affects risk for cancer. Pancolitis carries a greater risk than colitis confined to the left side of

TABLE 107–1. COLORECTAL CANCER RISK FACTORS*

Standard Risk:	Age over 40, men and women
High Risk:	Inflammatory bowel disease
	History of female genital or breast cancer
	History of colonic cancer or adenoma
	Peutz-Jeghers syndrome
	Familial polyposis syndromes
	Family cancer syndromes
	Hereditary site-specific colonic cancer
	History of juvenile polyps
	Immunodeficiency disease

*From Stearns MW Jr (ed.): Neoplasms of the Colon, Rectum, and Anus. New York, John Wiley & Sons, 1980, pp 9–22. Reprinted with the kind permission of the publisher.

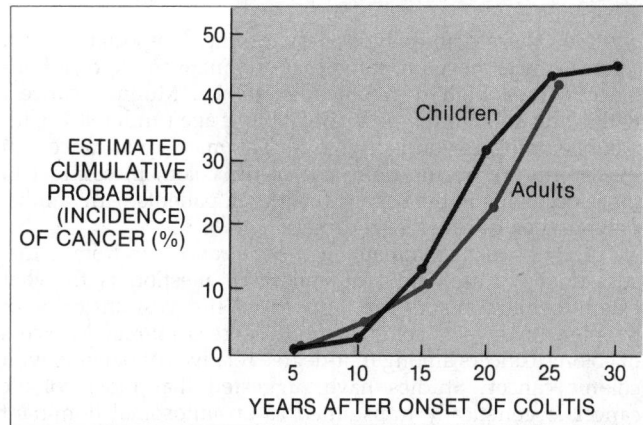

FIGURE 107–4. Estimated cumulative incidence with time of cancer complicating ulcerative colitis in adults and children with panproctocolitis. (From Stauffer JQ: In Sleisenger MH, Fordtran JS [eds.]: Gastrointestinal Disease. 2nd ed. Philadelphia, W. B. Saunders Company, 1978.)

the colon, where risk appears later, approximately 15 years after onset. Colitis confined to the rectosigmoid carries minimal risk, and ulcerative proctitis appears to have no increased risk for cancer. The high risk for cancer in ulcerative colitis has been considered by some investigators to be an overestimate resulting from referral of many patients with ulcerative colitis and cancer to centers that have reported the association.

In recent years a small subgroup (10 to 15 per cent) of patients with longstanding CUC has been identified by biopsy as having dysplasia of the colonic mucosa as an indicator for risk of cancer. When severe (high-grade) dysplasia is found, approximately 50 per cent of patients will be found to have simultaneous cancer; with moderate (low-grade) dysplasia, approximately one third of patients have cancer. Approximately 80 per cent of patients with CUC and colorectal cancer have dysplasia on biopsy. Although there are difficulties in histologic interpretations and dysplastic changes may be patchy, nevertheless the general concept is an important one; the demonstration of dysplasia has potential value in identifying those patients with CUC who are at greatest risk for colorectal cancer.

Patients with granulomatous colitis are also at higher risk for colorectal cancer than the general population, but considerably less so than patients with CUC. Once again, risk is related to the duration of disease.

Heredity and Colonic Cancer. Inherited predisposition to colonic cancer can be divided into two major categories: the polyposis type (familial polyposis, Gardner's syndrome, juvenile polyposis, Peutz-Jeghers syndrome, and Turcot's syndrome) and the nonpolyposis types (site-specific colonic cancer, the familial cancer syndromes, and Muir's [Torre's] syndrome). The familial polyposis syndromes have been discussed previously.

When it is stated that certain patients with a heritable predisposition to colonic cancer belong to a "nonpolyposis group," it is meant only that the colon is not carpeted by a myriad of small polyps. There is increasing evidence, however, that even in this group colorectal cancer develops from adenomas as in the familial polyposis syndromes. These adenomas are either single or multiple but if multiple are only in small numbers. Three major patterns are seen in this group: (1) Cancer confined to the colon and rectum (site-specific). In site-specific colonic cancer the transmission from generation to generation is only for colorectal cancer. (2) Multifocal cancer involving other sites in the gastrointestinal tract or the female sex organs (ovary, uterus, and breast) as well as the colon and rectum. This is sometimes called the "family cancer syndrome." (3) Muir's (Torre's) syndrome, a rare disorder resulting in multiple adenocarcinomas and epidermoid carcinomas in many organs in association with a large number of sebaceous cysts.

All of these "nonpolyposis syndromes" associated with colonic cancer have an autosomal dominant mode of inheritance with a high degree of penetrance. Multiple cancers within the colon often occur at a young age (under 40), with risk beginning as young as age 20. The majority of cancers in this group are on the right side of the colon, in contrast to those occurring in the usual patient or in patients with familial polyposis or Gardner's syndrome.

The autosomal dominant high-penetrance syndromes discussed above are rare. An important question is to what extent genetic factors are present in the vast majority of people who develop colonic cancer. There is a threefold excess of colonic cancers among first-degree relatives of patients with colonic cancer. Studies have suggested that most colonic cancer is genetically transmitted as an autosomal dominant low-penetrance disease. Environmental factors, especially diet, then modulate the expression of the disease in genetically susceptible individuals. This susceptibility or predisposition is first manifest as abnormalities in mucosal phenotypic expression of cell proliferation and cell differentiation,

later by the appearance of adenoma, and finally by the development of adenocarcinoma.

PATHOLOGY. Approximately 50 per cent of adenocarcinomas of the colon occur in the distal 25 cm of large bowel (Figs. 107–5 and 107–6). This percentage was higher in the past, but there has been a "proximal migration" of neoplasia in the colon in recent years. The distal descending colon and upper sigmoid represents another frequent site of colorectal cancer, as do the cecum and ascending colon. Cancer is much less frequent in the transverse colon. On the left side of the colon, cancers are commonly annular and tend to obstruct; on the right side of the colon, they are primarily polypoid. In fact, either of these gross patterns can occur anywhere in the colon, and all colonic cancers commonly ulcerate and bleed. Metastatic spread from carcinoma of the colon occurs by direct invasion of surrounding structures, by way of regional lymphatics, or less commonly by multiple peritoneal implants. Of distant organs the liver is most frequently involved, but metastases may also occur to lung, and to bone and brain rarely.

CLINICAL MANIFESTATIONS. Adenocarcinomas of the colon, especially those on the right side, are often clinically silent for a long period of time. The most common symptoms relate to *bleeding* (anemia with its manifestations or hematochezia) and *obstruction* (change in bowel habits, sometimes pain). When the lesion is in the right colon, the bleeding is often occult, since the blood tends to be well mixed with stool and therefore escapes notice. Tumors of the cecum and ascending colon rarely obstruct, at least early in their course, so that a change in bowel habits or pain is less useful as an early symptom. Polypoid lesions of the left side of the colon may be associated with frequent and sometimes loose stools. With obstructing left-sided lesions, changes in bowel habits are usually those of gradual but progressive constipation, tenesmus, or a reduction in stool caliber, and hematochezia is much more frequent. Because of the frequency of tumor ulceration and bleeding, testing chemically for occult blood is an excellent survey technique and leads to an earlier diagnosis with a greater chance for cure. The general symptoms of malignancy—weakness, malaise, anorexia, weight loss—are frequent but nonspecific. Adenocarcinoma of the colon may present with a localized perforation, which becomes sealed off, or with signs of peritonitis (fever, generalized discomfort, rebound tenderness) when the perforation enters freely into the abdominal cavity. An abdominal mass or the signs and

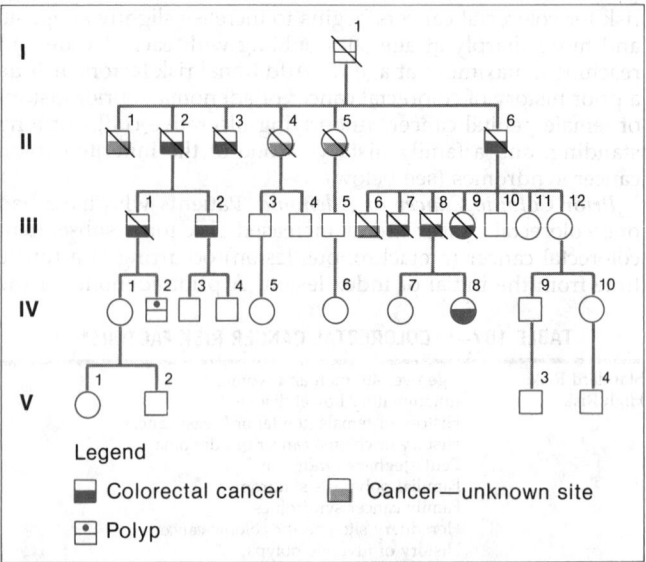

FIGURE 107–5. Pedigree of family with high prevalence of colorectal cancer. (From Kussin SZ, et al.: Am J Gastroenterol 72:448, 1979. Reprinted with permission of the publishers of the American Journal of Gastroenterology.)

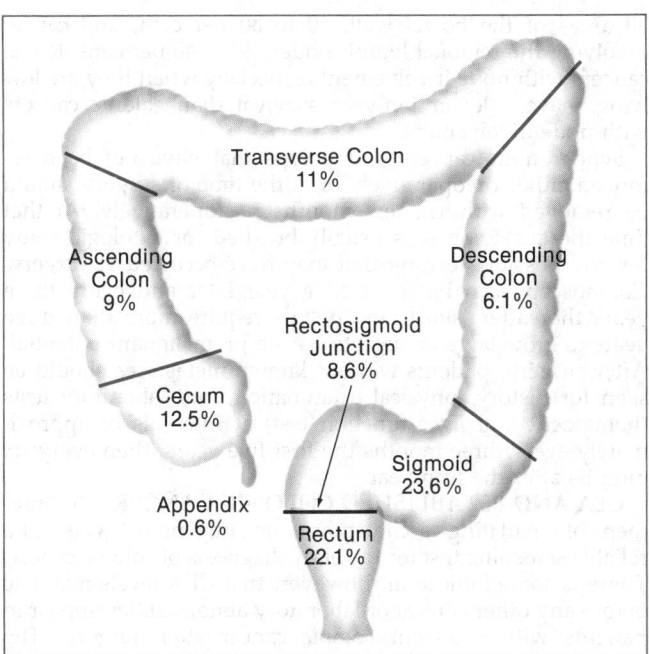

FIGURE 107–6. Distribution of large bowel cancer by anatomic segment according to the third national cancer survery (segment unspecified). (From Shottenfeld D, Fraumeni J Jr [eds.]: Cancer Epidemiology and Prevention. Philadelphia, W. B. Saunders Company, 1982, pp 703–727.)

symptoms of metastasis to the liver may be the earliest complaints.

Cancers at the mucocutaneous junction or in the anal canal or rectum may present with rectal bleeding, change in bowel habits, mass, or perineal pain. These can also present with symptoms referable to invasion of adjacent organs, including hematuria, urinary frequency, and vaginal fistulas.

DIAGNOSIS. *Differential Diagnosis.* The diagnosis of colorectal cancer must be considered when patients present with a change in bowel habits, a recent decrease in caliber of the stool, rectal bleeding, unexplained abdominal pain, or iron deficiency anemia. Overall the most common causes for bright red rectal bleeding are non-neoplastic, but the frequency of neoplastic lesions as the cause for bleeding increases progressively over age 40 and is especially high in those with a family history of colonic cancer. Bright red rectal bleeding can also be caused by angiodysplasia of the colon, diverticulosis, and a variety of other benign and malignant tumors of the colon (see Ch. 114).

A change of bowel habits can be produced by many other neoplastic lesions as well as by several benign disorders. Change in the character of the stool to a pellet type with more difficulty in passage is as common in progressive diverticular disease and muscle hypertrophy of the colon as in colonic malignancy (see Ch. 102). Diarrhea and incontinence can be a manifestation of many colonic and small intestinal diseases in addition to colorectal cancer. A recent change in bowel habits in one who has always had regular bowel habits, particularly if the person is at risk for colorectal cancer, clearly raises the possibility of a colonic neoplasm. The character of rectal bleeding cannot distinguish benign from neoplastic disorders. Blood appearing only on the toilet paper is indeed most commonly from hemorrhoids or a fissure, but it can also be from rectal cancer. Although a profuse bleeding episode is more likely to be the result of angiodysplasia, diverticulosis, ulcerative colitis, or ischemic colitis, it may be due to a large ulcerating neoplasm of the right colon.

Metastatic Colonic Cancer. Metastases of colonic cancer may be present before resection or may occur after it, producing different patterns of symptoms. Metastases to liver with progressive hepatomegaly may produce pain from dis-

tention of the liver capsule. Spread within the pelvis can result in pressure on the urinary bladder, obstruction of the rectosigmoid, sciatic nerve pain, and sometimes small bowel obstruction. Metastases to lung and bone are usually silent until very advanced. Intra-abdominal metastases may produce multiple areas of small and large bowel obstruction. Implants on the peritoneum sometimes cause ascites. Metastatic lesions can also occur in the skin, within the subcutaneous tissues, in suture lines, and within the bowel lumen. Intraluminal recurrences of colorectal cancer are unusual and follow surgery performed under adverse circumstances such as obstruction, or a low anterior resection for rectal cancer that leaves only a very narrow distal margin free of tumor. When tumor recurs within the colon, it more commonly is an intra-abdominal growth from the serosa into the lumen.

Diagnostic Approach. The history, physical examination, and common laboratory tests are essential for early diagnosis of colonic cancer. The history should combine the patient's symptoms with important clues such as the prior removal of an adenoma or even of a colorectal cancer, a history suggesting ulcerative colitis, or a family history suggesting one of the inherited colonic cancer syndromes. Physical examination may reveal evidence for Peutz-Jeghers syndrome, soft tissue tumors suggesting Gardner's syndrome, or the possibility of Muir's syndrome, and will provide clues as to any possible spread of the tumor to the liver, peripheral nodes, or skin. The digital rectal examination is important to determine the presence of a low-lying tumor or of perianal or pelvic disease. Laboratory testing might reveal iron deficiency anemia, occult blood in the stool, or an abnormality of liver function. Evaluation of the patient would also include a chest roentgenogram to search for pulmonary metastases.

When patients have symptoms or signs of colorectal cancer, the digital rectal examination should be followed by either proctoscopy and barium enema or colonoscopy. Proctoscopy may be performed with a rigid instrument, but this has had poor patient acceptance and physician application. Flexible sigmoidoscopes are more comfortable for the patient and have produced a much higher diagnostic yield because of the more complete insertion (see Ch. 96). A double-contrast barium enema is more revealing of mucosal lesions than the single-column study. In a well-prepared patient the majority of colorectal cancers can be detected by the combination of these two techniques. A barium enema should not be ordered without a prior proctoscopy, since there may be a distal lesion that could be obstructive and result in a perforation during the examination if the radiologist is not alerted to its presence. In addition, the patient may not have a neoplastic lesion but may have another disease, such as ulcerative colitis, which can readily be diagnosed by proctoscopy. If this disease is very active, a barium enema may in fact be undesirable.

Colonoscopy will be successful in uncovering lesions not detected by the barium enema, especially polyps but also cancers. Colonoscopy is also desirable in patients who have had an abnormality detected by barium enema. If the lesion detected radiologically appears to be cancer, it should be located endoscopically and confirmed by biopsy. In addition, a search for synchronous lesions and polyps should be carried out. If the lesion seen on radiographs is clearly an obstructing cancer of the left side, then colonoscopy is not necessary and may actually be hazardous. When the barium enema has uncovered only a polyp, colonoscopy can be utilized to remove the polyp, to search for other polyps, and to rule out an associated malignancy.

During colonoscopy, tissue sampling would include not only biopsies but also brushings for cytology, which increases the sensitivity of tissue diagnosis. In longstanding ulcerative colitis, biopsies are useful to look for dysplasia as an indication of premalignancy. These are obtained from the cecum to the rectum.

TREATMENT. *Surgery.* The goal of treatment for primary

malignant neoplasms of the colon is to remove them as completely as possible. The best hope for cure is surgical removal of the segment of colon harboring the neoplasm, including omentum with lymph nodes. Cancers of the right and left colons are treated by hemicolectomies; cancer of the sigmoid and upper rectum above 5 cm from the anal verge is resected anteriorly with removal of a wide margin of normal colon above and below the tumor. In low anterior resections, the surgeon wishes to leave 2 to 3 cm of tumor-free margin distal to the tumor. Lesions within 4 cm of the anal verge are usually treated by a combined abdominal-perineal resection (APR). It is desirable to do a lower anterior resection rather than an APR if at all possible, since APR is not associated with increased survival and leaves the patient with a permanent colostomy. The availability of staplers allows the surgeon to do a low anterior resection of tumors closer to the anal verge than previously possible.

Epidermoid cancers in the anal canal may be treated by local excision if superficial. If deeper, an APR is required. A period of preoperative radiation and chemotherapy in these cases will usually shrink the tumor and improve the likelihood of successful resection.

Patients may require surgery for palliation as well as for cure. Obstruction usually requires a colostomy, followed at a later time by closure of the colostomy. In most patients with obstruction, however, a primary resection and colostomy can usually be accomplished in one stage. Carcinoma that has perforated also is usually treated by primary resection and colostomy with later closure of the colostomy. Patients with obvious metastatic disease may require surgery for their tumor if it bleeds or obstructs significantly. Palliative treatment with radiation and/or chemotherapy of the metastases may then proceed.

Radiation Therapy. Radiation may be used preoperatively and in patients who have evidence of recurrent disease, especially in the pelvis, or localized recurrences intra-abdominally. Adjuvant use of radiation and chemotherapy in rectal cancer has been associated with a longer tumor-free interval after surgery.

Chemotherapy. Chemotherapy of colorectal cancer is used primarily for metastatic disease. Unfortunately, chemotherapeutic agents are usually unsuccessful in the treatment of adenocarcinoma of the colon. 5-Fluorouracil (5-FU) has been disappointing because of its poor efficacy. Most combination agent trials have not been very encouraging for adenocarcinoma of the colon. For epidermoid cancers of the anal canal, the combination of mitomycin C and 5-FU in sequence with radiation has been effective in producing tumor regression preoperatively. Chemotherapy is most effective for liver metastases and is not as effective as radiation for pelvic recurrence or an isolated single mass. Current trials suggest that there may be some benefit for adjuvant chemotherapy in patients with rectal cancer judged histologically to be at high risk of recurrence, but as yet no benefit has been demonstrated for patients with colonic cancer. There has also been interest in direct infusion of the liver with floxuridine (FUDR) and other agents through a surgically placed catheter connected to a pump implanted subcutaneously. The efficacy of this method compared with systemic chemotherapy has not been demonstrated conclusively.

Most other primary malignancies of the colon are treated by resection. Metastatic disease to the colon may require surgery for obstruction or bleeding. Disseminated cancers involving the colon, such as lymphoma, melanoma, or breast cancer, usually require systemic treatment for the primary tumor.

PROGNOSIS AND FOLLOW-UP. The overall ten-year survival for patients after surgery for colorectal cancer is approximately 42 per cent. The survival correlates directly with the stage of the disease: cancer confined to the mucosa, 80 to 90 per cent ten-year survival; cancer extending through all areas of the bowel wall, 60 to 80 per cent; and cancer involving the regional lymph nodes, 30 to 40 per cent. Rectal cancers with node involvement, especially when they are low lying, have a lower ten-year survival than colonic cancers with node involvement.

Synchronous cancers and polyps that have not been removed either preoperatively or at the time of surgery should be removed within a few months postoperatively. At that time the anastomosis is usually brushed for cytologic study for any possible seeding that may have occurred at surgery. Colonoscopy can be repeated a year later and every three years thereafter, since new polyps require more than three years to grow large enough to have a premalignant potential. After surgery, patients without known metastases should be seen for history, physical examination, and laboratory tests (hematocrit and liver function test) at intervals of approximately every three months the first five years, then every six months after the fifth year.

CEA AND ESTABLISHED COLONIC CANCER. Measurement of circulating carcinoembryonic antigens (CEA) is not a reliable screening test for the early diagnosis of colonic cancer. There is some indication, however, that CEA levels may rise before any other clinical or laboratory abnormalities appear in patients with recurrent colonic cancer after surgery. The common cause for such an increase in the CEA is widespread metastatic disease, particularly involving the liver. In a few patients, however, rising CEA may reflect a small, localized, potentially resectable intra-abdominal metastasis. Although still investigational, it has been suggested that the CEA measurement be performed every three months. If a significant rise in the CEA is detected, the patient should undergo an intensive investigation, including liver function tests, computed tomographic scan, colonoscopy, and chest radiographs; if all are negative, a "second-look" exploration could be considered to search for a localized, potentially resectable intra-abdominal metastasis. In patients who have a rising CEA with negative workup there is an 80 per cent chance of finding recurrent tumors, 30 per cent of which are resectable. However, this approach has, as yet, not been of demonstrated effectiveness and must be viewed as controversial and investigational. Re-exploration and resection of recurrences have not been shown to prolong survival.

PREVENTION OF COLORECTAL CANCER. Prevention may be defined as (1) primary, the identification and eradication of agents in the environment that produce colorectal cancer, and attempted control of genetic factors; and (2) secondary, the identification and eradication of premalignant lesions, and the detection and resection of cancer while it is still curable. No effective primary preventive measures are yet available. Despite the previously cited evidence that diet may be related in some way to the evolution of colorectal cancer, there is no current proof that proscription of any diet in favor of a low-fat and high-fiber regimen would be effective.

Secondary prevention as defined above has been more rewarding with the introduction of better methods of screening for early cancer or premalignant adenomas. Effective screening requires the application of relatively simple and inexpensive tests to a large number of people in order to identify those who are likely to have disease. There are several critical questions to consider in any screening program: (1) What are the expected benefits in terms of survival of those patients whose disease is discovered by screening tests and treated, and in terms of the possible mortality reduction from colorectal cancer in the entire screened population? (2) Can high-risk subgroups be identified? (3) Are effective screening tests available? (4) Are community health resources adequate for the diagnostic workup and treatment of persons with positive screening tests? (5) What are the costs, patient compliance, and risks of screening?

It is justifiable to consider screening for colorectal cancer in the United States, since it is a high-risk country by worldwide epidemiologic standards. It is assumed that earlier diagnosis would lead to longer survival. In general, screening programs that have been in progress for colorectal cancer have demonstrated earlier staging and better survival of patients with cancer detected through screening but have not had sufficient time to prove that the screened group has a lower mortality from colorectal cancer. Screening for rectosigmoid cancer with periodic sigmoidoscopy may lead to earlier detection and improved long-term survival and even to a less than expected incidence of cancer at this anatomic site, probably because of identification and eradication of polyps. Screening for colorectal cancer can be classified in two ways: general screening of patients at average risk, and screening of patients in high-risk subgroups.

Average-Risk Patients. In average-risk groups (all of those not in one of the defined high-risk groups), suggested screening includes testing stool specimens for occult blood annually with impregnated guaiac slides and by sigmoidoscopy every three to five years. Guaiac solutions, Hematest, and benzidine have been discarded because of too many false-negative and false-positive results. Testing with six slides over a period of three days, with the patient making smears from two different parts of the same stool each day while on a high-fiber, meat-free diet, has resulted in detection of early colorectal cancer. Current trials using this approach have been promising but need further time for long-term results. This test is useful only in totally asymptomatic patients and should not be used as a substitute for clinical judgment in patients who have symptoms of neoplastic disease or who have already reported a history of rectal bleeding. The effective utilization of this test requires follow-up studies of patients who have positive tests, positive being defined as one or more positive slides. Diagnostic workup must include colonoscopy to search for lesions that are missed by the barium enema and an upper gastrointestinal series if no colonic neoplasm is detected. Approximately 30 per cent of patients with positive tests will have neoplastic lesions, mostly adenomas but also colorectal cancers. The stool blood test in its present form will detect 70 to 80 per cent of colorectal cancers present. More specific sensitive fecal occult blood tests using immunologic methods and quantitative assays for human hemoglobin are being evaluated. The fecal occult blood test is not very sensitive for rectosigmoid tumors and therefore is complemented by sigmoidoscopy. Rigid sigmoidoscopes have been used; however, flexible scopes of 30 to 60 cm in length have been tested and appear to increase the yield of polyps and cancers and provide a more comfortable examination.

High-Risk Groups. GENETIC. Familial polyposis requires early surgery. Patients with a family history of polyposis or Gardner's syndrome should have sigmoidoscopy at least annually beginning at puberty. Female patients with a history of genital or breast cancer should have periodic fecal occult blood testing and sigmoidoscopy, beginning as soon as they are identified. Patients with site-specific colonic cancer or the family cancer syndrome must be examined with barium enema and/or colonoscopy beginning at age 20, since one cannot comfortably rely only on fecal occult blood testing in these very high-risk patients. A reasonable screening approach would be a fecal occult blood test annually and colonoscopy every three to five years. The search would be primarily for adenomas, for which the colonoscope is much more sensitive than radiography. The number of patients with nonpolyposis inherited colonic cancer syndromes is not known. It has been estimated that these patients account for 1000 to 5000 cases of colorectal cancer annually.

PRIOR ADENOMA OR COLONIC CANCER. Patients with a prior history of adenoma or colonic cancer should be examined periodically by colonoscopy. Once the colon has been cleared of all synchronous lesions, screening every three years is sufficient, since excisable metachronous lesions usually do not develop sooner and often require years to evolve.

ULCERATIVE COLITIS. No well-established data exist on the optimal detection of cancer early in ulcerative colitis or granulomatous colitis, or at what intervals screening should be conducted. One suggestion is that multiple biopsies be obtained by colonoscopy once a year or once every other year after the patient has had universal colitis for 7 years or left-sided colitis for 15 years. If moderate or severe dysplasia is seen on these biopsies and confirmed in several specimens at several examinations, total colectomy should be considered. Patients with granulomatous colitis should be evaluated endoscopically if they have a change in their symptoms or develop a stricture (which may harbor a tumor).

NEOPLASMS OF THE SMALL INTESTINE

EPIDEMIOLOGY. Cancer is rare in the small intestine; only about 2000 cases occur in the United States each year. Small bowel cancer, like cancer of the large intestine, is more common in developed Western countries than in underdeveloped countries. With rare exceptions, the incidence for males is higher than that for females.

ETIOLOGY AND RISK FACTORS. Some cancers originating in the small intestine are related to pre-existing premalignant states, such as Crohn's disease of the small intestine or gluten-sensitive enteropathy. Small intestinal cancer may rarely develop from polyps of the Peutz-Jeghers syndrome or from polyps in patients with familial polyposis or Gardner's syndrome. The incidence of small bowel malignancy, especially lymphoma, is also increased in patients with various hereditary syndromes involving decreased humoral or cellular immunity. Lymphoma is by far the most common malignancy complicating celiac disease. A particular type of small intestinal lymphoma, called Mediterranean lymphoma, is endemic in the Middle East, affecting Sephardic Jews, Arabs, Armenians, and Iranians; environmental factors in the area have not been adequately studied.

Several hypotheses have been suggested to explain this striking rarity of small intestinal malignancies, especially adenocarcinomas, compared with adenocarcinomas of the colon. The bacterial population of the colon, quantitatively much greater than that of the small intestine, may convert bile acids or other products to carcinogens. Ingested carcinogens may be diluted in the small intestine by the large volume of liquid present there. Also, the transit time through the small bowel is much faster than through the colon, limiting the exposure of the small intestinal epithelium to carcinogens. The rapid cell proliferation of the small intestinal mucosa may also be important in preventing malignancy.

PATHOLOGY. Four types of neoplasms, adenocarcinomas, carcinoids, lymphomas, and leiomyosarcomas, account for over 95 per cent of malignant small bowel tumors. The most common tumor of the small intestine is asymptomatic benign carcinoid, most often found at postmortem examination. The most common tumor detected clinically in the small intestine is metastatic malignancy (lymphoma, melanoma, and carcinoma of the breast, kidney, ovary, and testicle). Adenocarcinomas are most common in the proximal small intestine, and carcinoids and lymphomas are most common in the distal small intestine.

CLINICAL MANIFESTATIONS. Small carcinoid tumors are asymptomatic, but larger carcinoid tumors can obstruct or bleed. The vast majority of symptomatic carcinoid tumors produce features of the carcinoid syndrome; the primary tumor of the small intestine is asymptomatic (see Ch. 243). Leiomyosarcomas often cause bleeding, and lymphomas present with a spectrum of clinical manifestations, including intestinal obstruction, bleeding, fever and malabsorption. Adenocarcinomas have characteristic clinical presentations, depending on their location: in the postbulbar area they may simulate peptic ulcer disease; in the periampullary area they can obstruct the common bile duct, causing jaundice; and beyond the periampullary area they can obstruct the bowel.

Adenocarcinomas of the distal small bowel usually develop as a complication of Crohn's disease and are most often found at surgery in patients operated on for longstanding Crohn's disease and obstruction. The clinical manifestation of benign polyps of the small intestine is usually bleeding. Most, however, are silent.

DIFFERENTIAL DIAGNOSIS. Tumors of the small intestine that present with bleeding or obstruction of the small bowel must be differentiated from many other causes of these symptoms. Bleeding can be secondary to Meckel's diverticulum, vascular anomaly, or duodenal ulcer, among other diagnoses. Obstruction can be due to adhesions, internal hernias, volvulus, or strictures. Obstructive jaundice can be due to tumors in the area of the ampulla as well as to carcinoma of the pancreas, bile duct cancer, impacted common duct stone, acute pancreatitis, and many other causes. Investigation of a patient with suspected small bowel tumor depends on the location and the clinical presentation. Patients presenting with atypical duodenal ulcer disease usually require upper gastrointestinal radiographs. Patients presenting with obstructive jaundice usually require sonography and either percutaneous transhepatic cholangiography or endoscopic retrograde cholangiopancreatography (ERCP). Those with small intestine obstruction require a period of decompression followed by radiologic study of the small bowel. Where tumors are accessible to direct visualization, such as the terminal ileum by colonoscopy and ileoscopy, or the upper duodenal area by upper gastrointestinal endoscopy, the procedures should be performed to confirm the presence of tumor and to obtain a tissue diagnosis.

THERAPY. Treatment is primarily surgical for adenocarcinomas, leiomyosarcomas, and malignant carcinoids. Primary lymphoma of the small intestine is usually treated surgically, although in poor-risk patients radiation therapy may provide the same benefit. Radiation therapy may be used postoperatively if there is evidence of spread beyond the bowel wall. If the lymphoma of the small intestine is part of a disseminated process, then chemotherapy is usually the treatment of choice (see Ch. 158).

PROGNOSIS AND PREVENTION. The prognosis of small intestinal adenocarcinomas is generally poor, with survival extremely low for the majority of patients. The prognosis for leiomyosarcoma and primary lymphomas of the small bowel is good if the lesion can be entirely removed by surgical resection, but this is rarely possible. Patients with malignant carcinoid tumors may survive for long periods, even after extensive metastases (see Ch. 243).

So little is known of the etiology of carcinoid tumors and leiomyosarcomas of the small bowel that no speculation regarding their prevention can be made. Primary small intestinal lymphomas could possibly be decreased in the Middle East by public health measures that decrease the high incidence of chronic bowel inflammation and parasitic infestation in this area. Diagnosis and treatment of celiac disease may reduce the frequency of superimposed malignancies. Surgical resection, rather than bypass, for Crohn's disease may decrease the incidence of adenocarcinoma in this high-risk group. In Peutz-Jeghers and multiple polyposis syndromes, adenomas in the duodenum could be monitored and potentially removed endoscopically.

GENERAL REVIEW

Bresalier R, Kim YS: Malignant neoplasms of the small and large intestine. In Sleisenger MH, Fordthan JS (eds.): Gastrointestinal Disease. 4th ed. Philadelphia, W. B. Saunders Company, 1988.
Winawer SJ, Enker WE, Lightdale CJ: Malignant tumors of the colon and rectum. In Berk JE (ed.): Bockus Gastroenterology. 4th ed. Philadelphia, W. B. Saunders Company, 1985, pp 2531–2574.

EPIDEMIOLOGY

Schottenfeld D, Winawer SJ: Large intestine. In Schottenfeld D, Fraumeni J Jr (eds.): Cancer Epidemiology and Prevention. Philadelphia, W. B. Saunders Company, 1982, pp 703–727. *A critical overview of the present concepts in the worldwide epidemiology of large bowel cancer.*

ETIOLOGY

Weisburger JH, Reddy BS, Spingarn NE, et al.: Current views on the mechanism involved in the etiology of colorectal cancer. Burkitt DP: Fibre in the aetiology of colorectal cancer. Goldin B: The role of diet and the intestinal flora in the etiology of large bowel cancer. In Winawer SJ, Schottenfeld D, Sherlock P (eds.): Colorectal Cancer: Prevention, Epidemiology, and Screening. Progress in Cancer Research. Vol. 13. New York, Raven Press, 1980, pp 19–41. *This series of papers reviews the evidence for the three major factors (fat, fiber, and bacterial flora) currently felt to be important in the etiology of colorectal cancer.*

RISK

Burt RW, Bishop DT, Cannon LA, et al.: Dominant inheritance of adenomatous colonic polyps and colorectal cancer. N Engl J Med 312:1540, 1985.
Devroede G: Risk of cancer in inflammatory bowel disease. In Winawer SJ, Schottenfeld D, Sherlock P (eds.): Colorectal Cancer: Prevention, Epidemiology, and Screening. Progress in Cancer Research. Vol. 13. New York, Raven Press, 1980, pp 325–334. *This paper carefully examines the relative risk among the subgroups of patients with inflammatory bowel disease.*
Kussin SZ, Lipkin M, Winawer SJ: Inherited colon cancer: Clinical implications. Am J Gastroenterol (State of the Art) 72:448, 1979. *A review of the literature of inherited colonic cancer with a focus on the possible link of genetic factors to sporadic cancer.*

DIAGNOSIS

Hunt RH, Waye JD (eds.): Colonoscopy. Techniques, Clinical Practice and Colour Atlas. England, Chapman and Hall, 1981. *A comprehensive treatise by various authors on technique and practical application.*

TREATMENT

DeCosse JJ (ed.): Clinical Surgical International. Large Bowel Cancer. Vol 1. New York, Churchill-Livingstone, 1981. *The subject of treatment is extensively covered in this book.*

CARCINOEMBRYONIC ANTIGEN (CEA)

Zamcheck N: Current status of CEA. In Winawer SJ, Schottenfeld D, Sherlock P (eds.): Colorectal Cancer: Prevention, Epidemiology, and Screening. Progress in Cancer Research. Vol. 13. New York, Raven Press, 1980, pp 219–234. *The current status of CEA in the follow-up of patients after surgery is discussed in detail in this paper by one of the senior investigators in the field.*

PREVENTION

Gilbertsen VA, Nelms JM: The prevention of invasive cancer of the rectum. Cancer 41:1137, 1978. *Unique long-term study demonstrating the impact of proctosigmoidoscopy on the natural history of rectosigmoid cancer.*
Lipkin M, Newmark H: Effect of added dietary calcium on colonic epithelial–cell proliferation in subjects at high risk for familial colonic cancer. N Engl J Med 313:1381, 1985.
Rozen P, Winawer SJ: Secondary prevention of colorectal cancer: An international perspective. Basel, Karger, 1986. *A compendium of papers from worldwide programs, including screening.*
Sherlock P, Lipkin M, Winawer SJ: The prevention of colon cancer. A combined clinical and basic science seminar. Am J Med 68:917, 1980. *Screening is examined from the viewpoint of the spectrum of risk, with heavy emphasis on markers being investigated in high-risk groups.*
Simon JB: Occult blood screening for colorectal carcinoma: A clinical review. Gastroenterology 88:820–837, 1985. *An update of screening issues and screening program results.*
Winawer SJ, Fleisher M, Baldwin M, et al.: Current status of fecal occult blood testing in screening for colorectal cancer. Cancer 32:100, 1982. *A comprehensive review of the background and status of fecal occult blood testing.*

SMALL INTESTINE

Lightdale CJ, Koepsell TD, Sherlock P: Small intestine. In Schottenfeld D, Fraumeni JF Jr (eds.): Cancer Epidemiology and Prevention. Philadelphia, W. B. Saunders Company, 1982, pp 692–702. *An excellent review of various epidemiologic and etiologic aspects of small intestinal tumors.*

108 PANCREATITIS

Michael D. Levitt

The pathogenesis of pancreatitis remains obscure and treatment is therefore supportive rather than specific. Only in the area of diagnostic procedures have there been major recent advances. The physician can now diagnose acute and chronic pancreatitis accurately, but the ability to influence the course of the disease has progressed little during the past ten years.

NORMAL ANATOMY AND PHYSIOLOGY OF EXOCRINE PANCREAS. The exocrine pancreas consists of acinar cells that synthesize digestive enzymes. These enzymes reside in zymogen granules within the cells and are deposited into the central ductule of the acinus. The ductules coalesce to form larger ducts, finally draining into the main pancreatic duct (Wirsung), which empties into the duodenum at the ampulla of Vater. Pancreatic secretion is stimulated by two hormones produced in the duodenum: (1) *secretin*, which is released in response to acid in the duodenum, stimulates a pancreatic juice high in volume and [HCO_3^-]; (2) *cholecystokinin-pancreozymin* (CCK-PZ), which is released in response to fatty acids and amino acids in the duodenum and results in a secretion rich in enzymes.

The enzymes secreted by the pancreas are grouped into those that digest starch (amylase), fat (lipases), and protein (trypsin and other proteolytic enzymes). The proteolytic enzymes are secreted in an inactive form, thus preventing autodigestion of the pancreas. Trypsinogen is activated to trypsin in the duodenal lumen, and trypsin then activates the other proteolytic enzymes. Protease inhibitors in the pancreas and pancreatic juice provide additional protection against autodigestion.

CLASSIFICATION OF PANCREATITIS. Pancreatitis is classified as acute or chronic by clinical pathologic criteria. Clinically, an attack of pancreatitis is defined as *acute* if the patient becomes asymptomatic following recovery, whereas in *chronic* pancreatitis the patient has persistent pain or insufficient exocrine or endocrine pancreatic secretion. The term *relapsing* denotes recurrent attacks that may occur in either acute or chronic pancreatitis. The pathologic findings in acute pancreatitis range from mild interstitial edema (which may not warrant the designation of pancreatitis), to acute inflammatory infiltrate, to necrosis and hemorrhage with virtually complete destruction of the gland. Since laparotomy is contraindicated in acute pancreatitis, pancreatic pathology is seldom documented by examination of tissue. Chronic pancreatitis is characterized by the disappearance of acinar tissue and the presence of fibrosis, calcification, and cyst formation. Pancreatitis will occur in roughly 0.5 per cent of the population and accounts for about 1 death annually per 100,000 population.

ACUTE PANCREATITIS

PATHOGENESIS. The final common pathway of acute pancreatitis is thought to be autodigestion by activated enzymes. The exact mechanism that provokes this process of autodigestion remains speculative. There is an association between pancreatitis and the clinical conditions listed in Table 108–1. Familiarity with these conditions is useful clinically, since the diagnosis of pancreatitis is often suggested by the coexistence of one of these states, and the prevention of recurrent pancreatitis usually hinges on the elimination of the

TABLE 108–1. ETIOLOGIC FACTORS IN PANCREATITIS

Alcoholism
Biliary tract disease
Trauma—postoperative, abdominal injuries, post-ERCP
Infections—mumps, coxsackievirus and echovirus, mycoplasma, parasitosis
Metabolic—hyperlipidemia, hyperparathyroidism, pregnancy, uremia, postrenal transplant
Drugs
  Multiple reports
    Immunosuppressive—corticosteroids, azathioprine, L-asparaginase
    Diuretics—thiazides, furosemide, ethacrynic acid
    Miscellaneous—phenformin, oral contraceptives, tetracycline
  Rare or questionable reports
    Acetaminophen, isoniazid, rifampin, propoxyphene
Vascular—shock, lupus erythematosus, periarteritis, atheromatous embolism
Mechanical—pancreas divisum, ampullary stenosis, ampulla of Vater tumor, duodenal diverticula, duodenal Crohn's disease, duodenal surgery
Penetrating duodenal ulcer
Familial

predisposing condition. No cause of acute pancreatitis is uncovered in about 15 per cent of cases. In the United States, the majority of patients with acute pancreatitis have *alcoholism* or *gallstones* as an etiologic factor.

Alcoholic pancreatitis develops in susceptible persons after heavy ethanol ingestion for many years. Chronic alcoholism may produce proteinaceous plugs in the small pancreatic ducts, causing atrophy of the acini drained by the obstructed duct. These chronic, irreversible pathologic changes antedate the first attack of acute pancreatitis, and 10 per cent of alcoholics develop pancreatic insufficiency without a recognized acute attack. The factors triggering the superimposition of an acute attack on this chronic process are not understood.

Gallstone pancreatitis is virtually always associated with fecal excretion of gallstones, whereas a much lower frequency of fecal stones is found in patients with gallstones who do not have pancreatitis. Thus, passage of a gallstone through the ampulla of Vater creates conditions favorable to the development of pancreatitis. This condition is not simply obstruction, since ligation of the ampulla does not cause pancreatitis. Rather, some factor such as reflux of biliary or duodenal contents or stimulation of pancreatic secretion appears necessary to produce pancreatitis. This "large duct" form of pancreatitis differs from the "small duct" type observed in alcoholics, in that the former seldom leads to chronic pancreatitis or pancreatic calcifications and is cured by cholecystectomy.

Postoperative pancreatitis, the third most commonly identified cause of acute pancreatitis, may follow any type of abdominal surgery. Biliary tract procedures and retroperitoneal node dissections have the highest incidence of this complication.

Hypertriglyceridemia, often with lactescent serum, occurs in about 15 per cent of patients with acute pancreatitis. Many of these patients are alcoholics who have an underlying abnormality of lipid metabolism, which is particularly pronounced during the acute attack. The apparent decrease in frequency of attacks of pancreatitis following dietary therapy for hypertriglyceridemia suggests that hyperlipidemia is a cause of pancreatitis.

Vascular insufficiency of the pancreas is a more common cause of pancreatitis than is generally recognized. Pancreatitis (usually asymptomatic) was observed in postmortem examination of 10 per cent of patients who died with hemorrhagic shock. Pancreatitis is a well-recognized complication of ischemia resulting from vasculitis or cholesterol emboli.

Pancreas divisum is a common (5 per cent) anatomic variant in which the portion of the pancreas (tail, body, and part of head) derived from the embryologic dorsal pancreas is drained through the duct of Santorini and the minor papilla rather than via the duct of Wirsung and the ampulla of Vater. Pancreas divisum occurs in 20 to 25 per cent of patients with otherwise unexplained pancreatitis. Presumably, this variant drainage is sometimes inadequate, although sphincterotomy of the minor ampulla has yielded only equivocal benefit in the prevention of pancreatitis.

Drugs have been linked to the development of pancreatitis (Table 108–1). This linkage is generally rather weak with the exception of antimetabolites such as L-asparaginase, which is associated with a 10 per cent frequency of pancreatitis. Frequently it is difficult to exclude the possibility that pancreatitis is a complication of the disease for which the drug was prescribed. For example, the high frequency of pancreatitis reported in patients taking diuretics may reflect the increased incidence of pancreatitis in patients with various forms of vascular disease.

Pancreatitis may be inherited as an autosomal dominant trait, which often begins in childhood. This type of pancreatitis has an increased incidence of late-developing pancreatic carcinoma.

CLINICAL PRESENTATION. The hallmark of acute pancreatitis is *abdominal pain.* This diagnosis should be considered in every patient presenting with abdominal discomfort. The time from onset to peak intensity of the pain ranges from seconds to hours. The pain, which tends to be steady rather than colicky, varies in intensity from minor to agonizing. At the onset of the attack, the pain is often localized to the epigastrium and left upper quadrant but as the attack progresses, it becomes diffuse and radiates to the back. The back pain results from retroperitoneal irritation and is partially relieved by flexing the trunk. Acute pancreatitis may be relatively painless, and massive hemorrhagic necrosis of the gland, frequently in postoperative patients, may be an unexpected postmortem finding. *Vomiting* occurs in 70 to 90 per cent of the cases, but often brings about only minimal relief of the abdominal discomfort. The past medical history is important, since pancreatitis is usually associated with one of the underlying conditions listed in Table 108–1, and there frequently is *a previous history* of similar attacks of pain.

Nonspecific physical findings include fever, tachycardia, and hypotension. *Abdominal tenderness* is virtually always present; however, abdominal guarding and rigidity may be surprisingly slight, given the apparent distress of the patient. Although rarely palpable on initial examination, an abdominal mass subsequently develops in 10 to 20 per cent of patients. Occasionally, in hemorrhagic pancreatitis, retroperitoneal blood dissects into the flanks or around the umbilicus, producing Grey Turner's or Cullen's sign, respectively.

History and physical examination are seldom diagnostic of acute pancreatitis, and the differential diagnosis includes all causes of abdominal pain. Features favoring the existence of pancreatitis include a left upper quadrant component of the pain (as opposed to the right-sided nature of gallbladder pain), steady pain (as opposed to the colic of bowel disease), vomiting that does not relieve pain (the discomfort of gastritis and bowel obstruction are transiently relieved by vomiting), and abdominal rigidity less than that expected for pain (perforated peptic ulcer has marked rigidity). The absence of a condition associated with pancreatitis (Table 108–1) reduces the possibility of pancreatitis, whereas a previous history of documented pancreatitis is the single most reliable indicator that the present attack is also due to pancreatitis.

LABORATORY TEST. *Amylase.* In few disease states does the diagnosis rely so heavily on a single laboratory determination as is the case with acute pancreatitis and the measurement of serum amylase. The patient with abdominal pain and an elevated serum or urine amylase level is usually considered to have pancreatitis, whereas a patient with identical symptoms and physical findings but normal amylase levels seldom is diagnosed as having pancreatitis. The sensitivity and specificity of the amylase measurements cannot be evaluated, since the actual presence or absence of pancreatitis is seldom verified by some independent, more reliable technique.

Amylase is produced in large quantity by the pancreas, salivary glands, and certain malignant tumors, and in lesser quantity by the fallopian tubes and lungs. Normally, most of the amylase secreted by the pancreas and salivary glands enters and is confined to the gut. A small fraction enters the plasma, accounting for the normal serum amylase activity, of which about two thirds is salivary isoamylase and one third pancreatic isoamylase.

In pancreatitis, increased quantities of pancreatic amylase escape into the lymph and blood flow of the pancreas. An increase in pressure in the pancreatic duct owing to obstruction or injection of contrast material during endoscopic retrograde cholangiopancreatography (ERCP) causes amylase to regurgitate into the plasma usually with little or no accompanying inflammation.

Amylase is cleared from the plasma with a half-life of about two hours, about 20 per cent being excreted in the urine. Two thirds of the amylase filtered by the glomerulus is normally reabsorbed or catabolized by the renal tubule.

A variety of conditions other than pancreatitis may cause an elevated serum amylase level. Inflammation or trauma to the salivary glands causes excessive release of salivary amylase into the serum. Chronic, unexplained elevations of serum amylase activity are almost always due to increases in salivary-type isoamylase, although there is usually no clinical evidence of salivary gland disease. In mesenteric infarction and perforated peptic ulcer, amylase from the intestinal lumen may leak into the circulation. These conditions must always be differentiated from pancreatitis in patients with abdominal pain and hyperamylasemia. Ruptured ectopic pregnancy, ovarian cysts, and various forms of pulmonary disease have also been reported to be associated with elevations of serum amylase. A chronic, very high serum amylase level may result from the production of amylase by metastatic tumors originating in the lung, reproductive tract, or pancreas. Serum amylase levels may also be elevated because of slow clearance from the blood. Uncomplicated renal failure is commonly associated with serum amylase values up to two times normal; higher levels suggest associated pancreatitis. Macroamylasemia is an asymptomatic state in which amylase is bound to serum proteins, thus forming a complex that is slowly cleared from the serum. Confusion results when the macroamylasemic patient has associated abdominal pain.

The rate of excretion of amylase in the urine is increased out of proportion to the serum amylase level in pancreatitis and may be elevated when the serum amylase is normal. This disproportionate elevation apparently results from the inhibition of tubular reabsorption of amylase in acute pancreatitis; thus, a greater portion of the filtered amylase appears in the urine. Although a more sensitive indicator of pancreatitis than is the serum level, the urinary amylase may be falsely normal when renal failure complicates pancreatitis. Spuriously elevated values occur in virtually all the nonpancreatitic conditions that cause hyperamylasemia (except macroamylasemia and renal disease) and in a variety of conditions with proximal renal tubular malfunction, including thermal burns, diabetic acidosis, and postoperative states.

Serum amylase originates from a variety of organs in addition to the pancreas, but serum lipase, trypsin, or pancreatic isoamylase is derived almost entirely from the pancreas. These enzymes, although technically more difficult to measure than amylase, may therefore provide in the future a more specific and sensitive indicator of pancreatitis.

The appropriate interpretation of amylase measurements may be summarized as follows. The patient with an acute attack of abdominal pain and an elevated serum amylase activity in all likelihood has acute pancreatitis, provided that perforated ulcer and bowel infarction are excluded. An elevated urinary amylase with a normal serum amylase is suggestive, but less diagnostic, of pancreatitis. The height of the amylase elevation does not correlate with the severity of the pancreatitis. For example, extremely high values, which return to normal over one to two days, are often associated with the passage of common duct stone and minimal, if any, inflammation of the pancreas. Elevation of amylase activity beyond 7 days is usually associated with relatively severe pancreatitis, and a protracted clinical course and elevation for more than 14 days suggest the possibility of a pseudocyst or pancreatic ascites. Chronic elevations of serum amylase activity associated with mild or no abdominal symptoms are seldom due to pancreatic disease but rather to renal failure, macroamylasemia, salivary hyperamylasemia, or tumor hyperamylasemia. Serum isoamylase assay can readily distinguish pancreatic from salivary hyperamylasemia. Serum lipase levels can also be used to distinguish pancreatic from salivary hyperamylasemia, since lipase is not produced by the salivary gland.

Other Laboratory Tests. The leukocyte count is usually elevated. Early in the course of acute pancreatitis, the hematocrit often rises to supranormal levels owing to *hemoconcentration* resulting from the massive loss of serum into the peritoneal and retroperitoneal spaces. *Hyperglycemia* often occurs, possibly resulting from increased glucagon and/or decreased insulin release. The serum in pancreatitis is frequently lactescent, and for unknown reasons the serum amylase level is frequently normal in this situation. *Hypocalcemia* is indicative of severe pancreatitis and is postulated to result from sequestration of calcium in soaps in areas of fat necrosis. In addition, there is a probable failure of the usual mechanisms that regulate calcium homeostasis. The presence of any of these nonspecific findings—elevated hematocrit, hyperglycemia, hypocalcemia, or hyperlipemia—in a patient with abdominal pain should always arouse suspicion of acute pancreatitis. Methemalbuminemia results from the extravascular destruction of hemoglobin and is the only laboratory finding that directly indicates that the pancreatitis is hemorrhagic. Evidence of cholestasis (elevated serum bilirubin and alkaline phosphatase) occurs in as many as 25 per cent of patients with acute pancreatitis, owing to compression of the common bile duct as it passes through the edematous pancreas. The cholestasis usually clears spontaneously in seven to ten days.

Roentgenograms. Roentgenograms of the abdomen should be obtained to rule out the presence of free air, signifying a perforation. In pancreatitis nonspecific ileus is usually observed. Somewhat more specific for pancreatitis, but not diagnostic, are localized gas collections in loops of bowel overlying the pancreas.

Imaging Techniques. Until recently, the pancreas could be only indirectly visualized radiographically via its impression of other viscera. The development of techniques to visualize the pancreas directly by means of ultrasound, computed tomography (CT), and ERCP has marked a great advance.

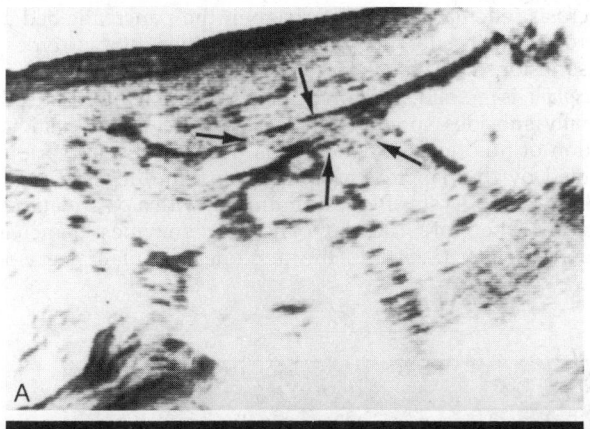

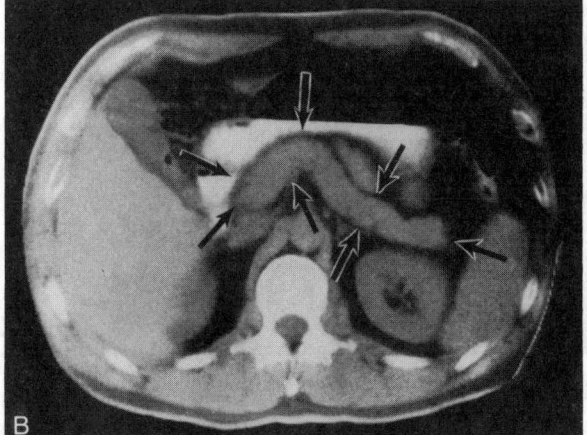

FIGURE 108–1. Normal pancreas demonstrated by ultrasound (*A*) and computed tomography (*B*). (Courtesy of Dr. Eugene P. DiMagno, Mayo Medical School, Rochester, Minnesota.)

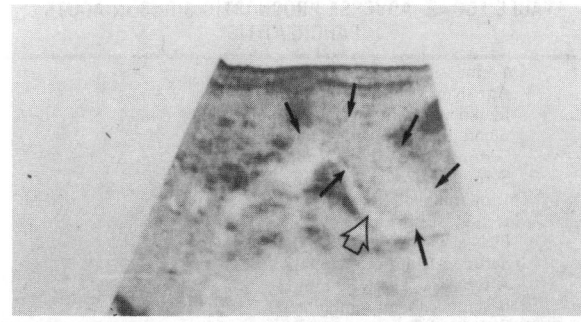

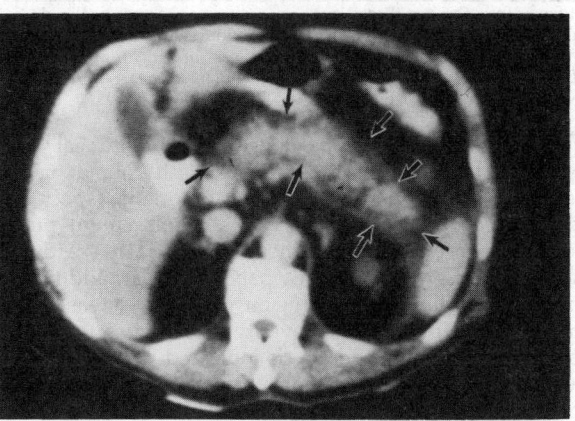

FIGURE 108–2. Diffusely enlarged pancreas of acute pancreatitis demonstrated by ultrasound (*above*) and computed tomography (*below*). The large arrow on the sonogram points to the splenic vein. (Courtesy of Dr. Henry I. Goldberg, Department of Radiology, University of California at San Francisco.)

Computed tomographic scanning demonstrates a diffusely enlarged pancreas in over 90 per cent of patients during an acute attack of pancreatitis, whereas ultrasound is less sensitive owing to problems with overlying gas (Figs. 108–1 and 108–2). Computed tomography is not required for the diagnosis of pancreatitis in most patients and should be reserved for very ill patients in whom the diagnosis is in doubt. This procedure is particularly valuable in the deteriorating patient who might have a gut perforation or infarction, since the pancreas appears normal in such patients, in contrast to the distinctly abnormal scan in severe acute pancreatitis. Endoscopic retrograde cholangiopancreatography exacerbates acute pancreatitis and is contraindicated during an acute attack.

TREATMENT. About 50 per cent of patients with acute pancreatitis have relatively mild and self-limited disease and probably would recover without benefit of medical therapy; 40 per cent are quite ill but survive their attack; and 10 per cent succumb despite the best of therapy. Virtually all deaths occur during the first or second attack of acute pancreatitis, recurrent attacks having a very low mortality rate. It is frequently difficult to judge the severity of the attack during the initial stages; therefore most patients with acute pancreatitis should be hospitalized, with a possible exception being the patient having recurrent attacks of chronic pancreatitis.

A number of objective measurements (Table 108–2) have been found to correlate with a poor prognosis.

Surgical intervention during the acute, symptomatic stage of pancreatitis is associated with a greater morbidity and mortality than is medical therapy, so the initial treatment of acute pancreatitis should be medical rather than surgical. Medical therapy is largely symptomatic and supportive, and there is little evidence that the acute inflammation of the pancreas is altered by this therapy. Meperidine should be used for pain relief because of the theoretic problem of spasm of the sphincter of Oddi with morphine. In severe pancreatitis, as much as 6 to 10 liters of plasma and blood may be

TABLE 108–2. ADVERSE PROGNOSTIC SIGNS IN ACUTE PANCREATITIS*

On admission:
    Age over 55
    Leukocyte count over 16,000/mm³
    Blood glucose over 200 mg/dl
    Serum LDH over 350 IU/liter
    Serum GOT over 250 sigma Frankel U/dl
During initial 48 hours:
    Hematocrit decrease over 10%
    BUN rise over 5 mg/dl
    Serum calcium below 8 mg/dl
    Arterial PO_2 below 60 mm Hg
    Base deficit over 4 mEq/liter
    Estimated fluid sequestration over 6 liters

*If fewer than three of these signs are present, mortality is negligible (<1 per cent) and few are seriously ill. If more than four signs are present, mortality may be 25 per cent and an additional 50 per cent of patients are seriously ill.
LDH = lactate dehydrogenase; GOT = glutamic-oxaloacetic transaminase, BUN = blood urea nitrogen.

sequestered in the retroperitoneal and peritoneal spaces. Prompt replacement of these losses with colloid or whole blood is probably the single most important aspect of the initial medical therapy. Such volume replacement probably accounts for recent sharp declines in the frequency with which acute renal failure complicates pancreatitis. In addition, this therapy helps maintain perfusion of the pancreas, a factor that seems to diminish the severity of experimental pancreatitis. Cautious insulin therapy is indicated for marked hyperglycemia, and intravenous calcium may be required for hypocalcemia.

For years, the major objective of therapy for acute pancreatitis was to "put the pancreas at rest" by reducing the humoral stimuli to pancreatic secretion. To this end, the patient received no oral alimentation, and gastric suction was carried out to prevent gastric HCl from entering the duodenum, thus minimizing secretin release. This therapy was based on limited evidence of benefit in experimental pancreatitis and on the clinical observation that the abdominal pain of pancreatitis appeared to subside more rapidly following the initiation of nasogastric suction. Two controlled studies in mild to moderately severe pancreatitis failed to demonstrate any significant benefit from nasogastric suction, and in such patients this form of therapy is optional. The value of suction in severe hemorrhagic pancreatitis has not been confirmed; however, the associated ileus that invariably complicates severe pancreatitis provides a strong indication for nasogastric suction.

TABLE 108–3. COMPLICATIONS OF ACUTE PANCREATITIS

Pancreatic—phlegmon, pseudocyst, abscess, ascites, hemorrhage
Contiguous organs—portal venous thrombosis, bowel necrosis, intraperitoneal bleeding, obstruction of common duct
Systemic
  Cardiovascular—hypotension, nonspecific ST-T changes, pericardial effusion
  Pulmonary—pleural effusion, shock lung, atelectasis
  Renal—acute renal failure
  Gastrointestinal—gastritis
  Hematologic—disseminated intravascular coagulation
  Metabolic—hypocalcemia, hyperglycemia, hypertriglyceridemia
  Fat necrosis—subcutaneous, bone
  Central nervous system—psychosis

The use of peritoneal dialysis to remove toxins in the peritoneal cavity should be considered when the patient's condition deteriorates despite standard medical therapy. A randomized trial of peritoneal dialysis showed striking short-term benefit in severe pancreatitis; however, late deaths due to sepsis resulted in similar overall mortalities for the dialyzed and control groups.

A number of therapies have been shown to be ineffective in controlled studies: proteolytic enzyme inhibitors such as aprotinin (Trasylol), glucagon to reduce pancreatic secretion, anticholinergics to reduce gastric and pancreatic secretion, and prophylactic antibiotics to prevent infection in the pancreatic bed.

COMPLICATIONS. The most important complications associated with acute pancreatitis are listed in Table 108–3. In the absence of these complications, recovery usually occurs in one to two weeks. A frequent cause of death during the first few weeks of the illness is the development of the *adult respiratory distress syndrome* (ARDS) secondary to increased alveolar capillary permeability. Prompt recognition and treatment with O_2 and positive end-expiratory pressure (PEEP) breathing appear to be lifesaving in some of these patients. Necrosis, edema, and hemorrhage in the pancreatic bed and surrounding tissues may lead to formation of two types of mass lesions, which can be differentiated by sonography. A *phlegmon* is a solid, inflamed mass of pancreatic tissue that usually subsides spontaneously. A *pseudocyst* is a cystic collection of fluid and necrotic debris whose walls are variously formed by the pancreas and other surrounding organs (Fig. 108–3). Pseudocysts often communicate with a pancreatic duct and are, therefore, rich in pancreatic enzymes. Pancreatic secretions may track into the peritoneal or pleural cavities,

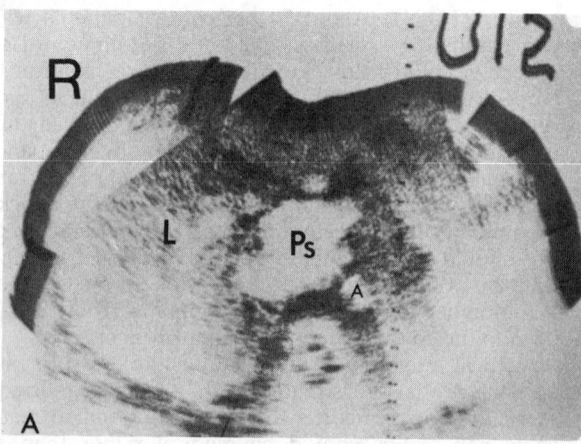 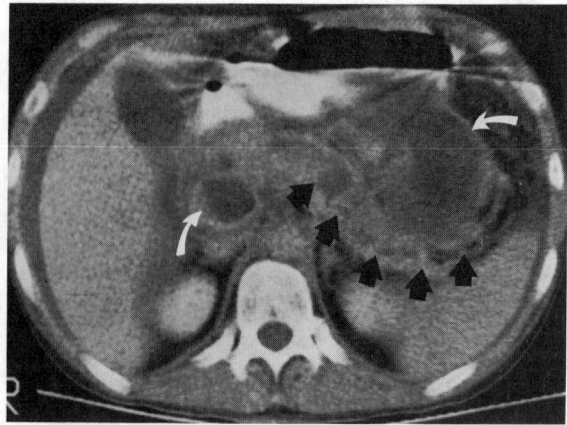

FIGURE 108–3. *A*, A pseudocyst demonstrated by ultrasound. Ps = pseudocyst; A = aorta; L = liver; R = right of patient. (Courtesy of Dr. Dennis A. Sarti, Dept. of Radiological Sciences, University of California at Los Angeles, and Radiology 125:789, 1977.) *B*, A CT scan through the region of the tail, body, and head of the pancreas demonstrates the presence of two pancreatic pseudocysts (*curved white arrows*). The larger of the two extends from the tail of the pancreas anteriorly to compress a portion of the greater curvature of the stomach, here denoted by contrast material in the dependent portion and an air/fluid level. The smaller of the two is well circumscribed and located in the head of the pancreas. Both pseudocysts are of low CT density and well-described margins. In addition, the pancreatic duct (*black arrows*) is dilated and irregular in contour, a finding typical of a chronic pancreatitis. (Courtesy of Dr. Henry Goldberg, University of California at San Francisco.)

resulting in pancreatic ascites or a pleural effusion. The pancreatic origin of these fluids is established by the finding of a fluid amylase concentration many-fold higher than that of serum. A serious complication of either phlegmons or pseudocysts is the development of an *abscess*, which is usually heralded by increasing pain, hectic fever, and leukocytosis. Immediate surgical drainage of the lesion is indicated, since nonoperative therapy carries a mortality of nearly 100 per cent.

Large pseudocysts are usually palpable, but smaller cysts are detected only by sonography or CT scanning. Many pseudocysts (particularly the smaller ones) are relatively asymptomatic and resolve spontaneously; some pseudocysts (usually the larger ones) cause marked discomfort and have the potentially lethal complications of hemorrhage or perforation. It is usually safe to follow smaller, asymptomatic pseudocysts or larger, uncomplicated cysts that are diminishing in size. The cyst that is expanding or causing appreciable discomfort should be drained, either surgically via anastomosis of the cyst to the gut or percutaneously via a needle. The indications for the traditional surgical as opposed to the newer percutaneous procedures remain to be determined. Complications of abscess, hemorrhage, or rupture require immediate surgical intervention.

It is very important to prevent the recurrence of acute pancreatitis by the treatment of conditions listed in Table 108–1. Abstinence from ethanol frequently does not prevent the progression of alcoholic pancreatitis but may reduce the frequency and severity of attacks. Studies to rule out the presence of gallstones are mandatory, since cholecystectomy in such patients nearly always prevents subsequent attacks. Cholecystectomy usually should be carried out after the subsidence of symptoms but during the initial hospitalization. Treatment of hypertriglyceridemia with a low-calorie, low-fat diet, as well as abstinence from alcohol, seems to prevent some subsequent attacks of hyperlipemic pancreatitis. Hypercalcemia as the cause of pancreatitis may be obscured during the acute attack and should be excluded by a serum calcium determination following recovery. Endoscopic retrograde cholangiopancreatography should be performed in patients who have had more than one attack of otherwise unexplained pancreatitis. Lesions, potentially correctable by surgery, that may be detected by ERCP include small gallstones missed by sonography, an isolated stricture in the main pancreatic duct, an undetected pseudocyst, pancreas divisum, or ampullary stenosis.

CHRONIC PANCREATITIS

ETIOLOGY. Chronic pancreatitis may be associated with most of the conditions listed in Table 108–1, with the exception of gallstone disease, which produces only recurrent acute attacks. Alcoholism is by far the most common cause of chronic pancreatitis in the United States; in some parts of the world, protein-calorie malnutrition is the major cause.

PATHOPHYSIOLOGY. In chronic alcoholism (with or without superimposed acute pancreatitis), proteinaceous plugs in the pancreatic ducts apparently lead to atrophy of the acinar tissue, fibrous tissue replacement, and dilatation of the ductular system. Calcification of these ductular plugs accounts for the diffuse, stippled calcification of the pancreas observed in about 30 per cent of patients. Pseudocysts are also a frequent finding. The normal secretion of pancreatic enzymes far exceeds that required for digestion, and malabsorption occurs only when enzyme secretion falls to less than 10 per cent of normal. Clinically significant malabsorption of fat-soluble vitamins is relatively rare in pancreatic insufficiency (as compared with small bowel mucosal disease), since normal lipolysis is relatively unimportant for the absorption of the fat-soluble vitamins. The pathophysiology of pancreatic malabsorption is discussed in detail in Ch. 104. Impaired

glucose tolerance is common, but diabetic ketosis and coma are rare. The vascular, neurologic, and renal complications of diabetes mellitus are seldom seen in the hyperglycemia of chronic pancreatitis. Cobalamin malabsorption occurs in about 50 per cent of patients with chronic alcoholic pancreatitis, because of failure to digest cobalamin-binding proteins, but pernicious anemia is relatively uncommon.

CLINICAL MANIFESTATIONS. *Pain* is the predominant symptom in about 90 per cent of patients. It may take the form of recurrent acute attacks often superimposed on a background of low-grade abdominal pain or relatively constant pain usually aggravated by food ingestion. The discomfort is most often epigastric and in the left upper quadrant with radiation to the back and is characteristically relieved by forward flexion of the trunk. Physical examination of the abdomen usually reveals less abdominal tenderness than expected in view of the often disabling pain of which the patient complains.

As the disease progresses, insufficient pancreatic secretion results in *malabsorption* manifested by the passage of bulky, foul-smelling stools. The failure to digest triglycerides may result in the passage of fat droplets that float as a visible scum on the toilet water, a finding that indicates that the steatorrhea is due to pancreatic insufficiency rather than small bowel mucosal disease. The combination of malabsorption and poor oral intake often leads to appreciable weight loss. Malabsorption is described more extensively in Ch. 104.

Less common clinical manifestations of chronic pancreatitis include cholestasis caused by compression of the common duct as it passes through the head of the pancreas; subcutaneous fat necrosis presenting as erythematous, tender nodules, usually on the lower extremities; and intramedullary fat necrosis, causing bone pain. The complications of chronic pancreatitis are listed in Table 108–4.

DIAGNOSIS. The diagnosis of chronic pancreatitis usually requires no additional laboratory confirmation in the alcoholic patient with a past history of acute pancreatitis who subsequently develops chronic abdominal pain and steatorrhea. When the patient presents with chronic abdominal pain and steatorrhea without previous history of acute pancreatitis, the usual diagnostic problem is to distinguish chronic pancreatitis from carcinoma of the pancreas. Diffuse, stippled pancreatic calcification is observed radiographically in about 30 per cent of patients with chronic pancreatitis and is virtually diagnostic. Sonography or CT scanning should be the next step to rule out the presence of a solid, localized pancreatic mass suggesting carcinoma and to demonstrate calcifications not seen with a survey abdominal film. Pancreatic exocrine insufficiency is most readily documented by the bentiromide test. Bentiromide is a peptide linked to para-aminobenzoic acid (PABA) via a bond that is split by chymotrypsin. Free PABA is absorbed from the gut and excreted in urine. If diarrhea or steatorrhea is due to pancreatic insufficiency, PABA is not liberated from ingested bentiromide, and hence urinary excretion of PABA is subnormal. If the existence of chronic pancreatitis remains in doubt, it may be useful to measure pancreatic secretory function by collecting duodenal aspirate during secretin stimulation. Pancreatic secretion in chronic pancreatitis usually has decreased $[HCO_3^-]$ and low output of enzymes; however, similar results may be observed in

TABLE 108–4. COMPLICATIONS OF CHRONIC PANCREATITIS

Pseudocyst formation
Pancreatic abscess
Obstruction of the common bile duct
Diabetes mellitus
Drug addiction
Exocrine insufficiency
Peptic ulcer
Fat necrosis—bone pain, subcutaneous
    tender nodules

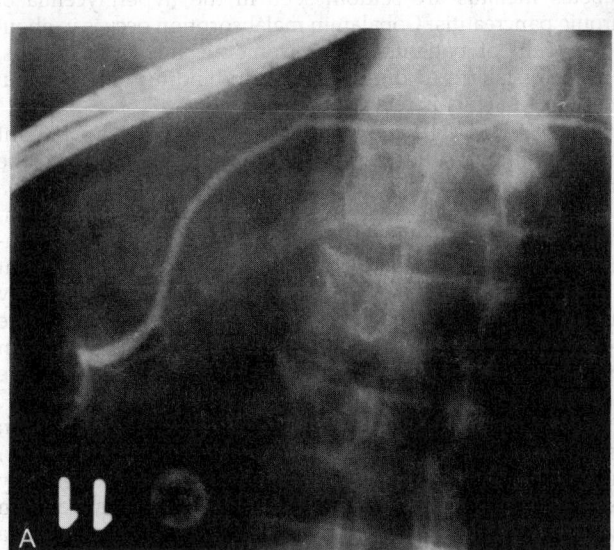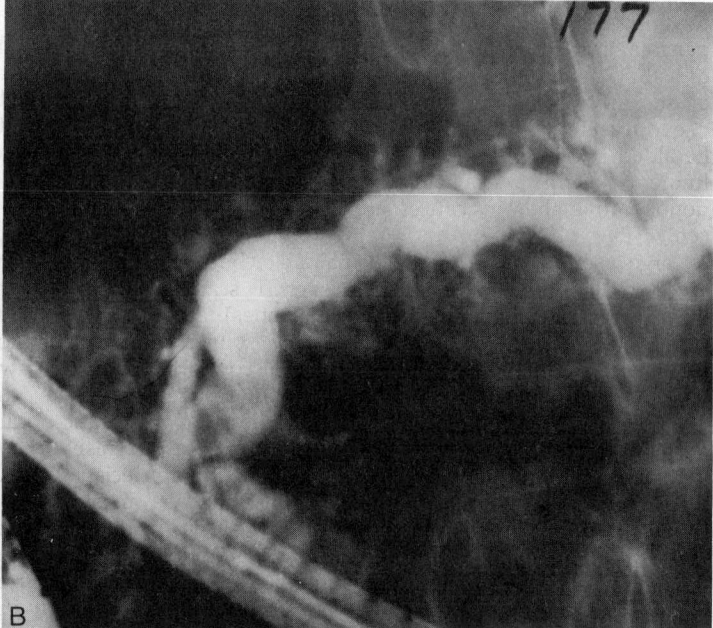

FIGURE 108–4. Normal pancreatic ductogram as demonstrated by ERCP (*A*), contrasted with dilatation of ductal system in chronic pancreatitis (*B*). (Courtesy of Dr. Stephen E. Silvis, Chief, Specialized Diagnostic and Treatment Unit, Medical Service, Veterans Administration Medical Center, Minneapolis, MN.)

carcinoma of the pancreas. Endoscopic retrograde cholangio-pancreatography is almost always diagnostic in chronic pancreatitis. The main pancreatic duct is found to be irregularly strictured and dilated ("chain of lakes"), and the major branches have a "beaded" appearance owing to dilatation (Fig. 108–4). In pancreatic carcinoma a localized stricture of the main duct is observed, with dilatation distal to the stricture.

TREATMENT. Chronic symptomatic pancreatitis denotes irreversible pathologic damage to the pancreas. Although the course of the disease may not be modified, the conditions that predispose to pancreatitis (particularly alcoholism) should be eliminated if possible.

Pain. Pain is the predominant problem of most patients with chronic pancreatitis. In fact, there are few benign diseases associated with such persistent, disabling pain for which current medical or surgical therapy is so unsatisfactory. The cause of the pain is unclear, although its frequent relation to food ingestion suggests that pancreatic secretion plays a role. Large doses of pancreatic supplements appear to reduce the pain of some patients, presumably via a negative feedback on pancreatic secretion. Efforts should be to treat with nonaddicting analgesics, such as salicylates or acetaminophen. Unfortunately, most patients with chronic pancreatitis sooner or later become addicted to narcotics and the withdrawal of the narcotics is difficult to achieve. Dietary regimens or other forms of medical manipulation are rarely useful in the management of the pain. Fortunately, as the pancreatitis "burns out" the pain often gradually disappears, leaving exocrine and endocrine deficiency as the major clinical problems.

Because of the inadequacy of medical therapy, a variety of surgical procedures have been employed for the treatment of the pain of chronic pancreatitis. If the patient has a localized stricture of the main pancreatic duct or a pseudocyst, resection of the pancreas distal to the stricture or drainage of the cyst may produce remarkable improvement. However, most patients do not have such surgically treatable lesions. Although widely employed in the past, sphincterotomy and various procedures designed to interrupt the pain fibers from the pancreas appear to be of limited value. The Puestow procedure is designed to allow free drainage of the entire pancreatic duct into the small bowel. The main pancreatic duct is "filleted" along its entire linear extent, and a loop of jejunum

is then anastomosed longitudinally over the opened duct. There is disagreement as to the benefit derived from the Puestow procedure. At best, not more than two thirds of patients obtain some pain relief, and most studies have not taken into account the decreasing pain that is part of the natural history of chronic pancreatitis.

Exocrine Deficiency. A second problem associated with chronic pancreatitis is malabsorption and diarrhea caused by deficient secretion of pancreatic enzymes. This problem can be controlled, although absorption is frequently not normalized, by the administration of 4 to 8 capsules of a pancreatic enzyme preparation with each meal. A low pH in the stomach irreversibly denatures the pancreatic enzyme. Therefore if malabsorption does not respond to pancreatic supplements, the additional administration of antacids or cimetidine to raise the pH of the stomach will enhance delivery of active enzyme into the duodenum and improve absorption. The treatment of pancreatic exocrine deficiency is described in greater detail as part of the general approach to patients with malabsorption (see Ch. 104).

PROGNOSIS. Few patients die of chronic pancreatitis per se. The incidence of carcinoma of the pancreas is, at most, only slightly increased above normal, except in the familial form of pancreatitis. Thus, the prognosis is largely a function of the associated alcoholism or of other diseases that may be associated with chronic pancreatitis.

Arvanitakis C, Cooke AR: Diagnostic tests of exocrine pancreatic function and disease. Gastroenterology 74:932, 1978. *Extensive review and bibliography of exocrine pancreatic function tests.*

Ettien JT, Webster PD III: The management of acute pancreatitis. Adv Intern Med 25:169, 1980. *Excellent review and bibliography of treatment of acute pancreatitis.*

Field BE, Hepner GW, Shabot MM, et al.: Nasogastric suction in alcoholic pancreatitis. Dig Dis Sci 24:339, 1979. *Controlled study showing no benefit from nasogastric suction in acute pancreatitis.*

Husband JC, Meire HG, Kreel L: Comparison of ultrasound and computer-assisted tomography in pancreatic diagnosis. Br J Radiol 50:855, 1977. *Compares the images of the ultrasound and computed tomography in acute and chronic pancreatitis.*

Isaksson G, Ihse I: Pain reduction by an oral pancreatic enzyme preparation in chronic pancreatitis. Dig Dis Sci 28:97, 1983. *Provides data on controlled trial of pancreatic supplements for control of pain of chronic pancreatitis.*

Ranson JH: The surgical treatment of acute pancreatitis. NY Acad Med Bull 58:601, 1982. *Review of surgical intervention in acute pancreatitis.*

Ranson JHC, Rifkind KM, Turner JW: Prognostic signs and nonoperative peritoneal lavage in acute pancreatitis. Surg Gynecol Obstet 143:209, 1976.

Evaluates the prognostic significance of various clinical and laboratory findings in acute pancreatitis.

Sarles H: Chronic calcifying pancreatitis—chronic alcoholic pancreatitis. Gastroenterology 66:604, 1974. *Review of pathogenesis of chronic, alcoholic pancreatitis.*

Soergal KH: Acute pancreatitis. Grendell JH, Cello JP: Chronic pancreatitis. In Sleisenger MR, Fordtran JS (eds.): Gastrointestinal Disease. 4th ed. Philadelphia, W. B. Saunders Company, 1988. *Excellent review of acute and chronic pancreatitis.*

Winship D, et al.: Pancreatitis: Pancreatic pseudocysts and their complications. Gastroenterology 73:593, 1977. *Review of etiology, diagnosis, course and treatment of pseudocysts.*

109 CARCINOMA OF THE PANCREAS

John P. Cello

DEFINITION. Carcinoma of the pancreas is an insidiously developing, relentlessly progressive, and nearly universally fatal malignancy arising in the epigastric retroperitoneum. Over 90 per cent of carcinomas of the pancreas are adenocarcinomas, derived from the simple cuboidal epithelium of the pancreatic duct. Five per cent of adenocarcinomas of the pancreas are of islet cell origin, often manifested early by the secretion of hormones. These islet cell malignancies are discussed in Ch. 233. Even rarer forms of pancreatic malignancy include acinar cell, epidermoid, adenocanthomas, sarcomas, and cystadenocarcinomas.

INCIDENCE AND EPIDEMIOLOGY. Carcinoma of the pancreas is responsible for over 24,000 new cases of cancer and 20,000 cancer-related deaths annually in the United States. This accounts for 5 per cent of all cancer-related deaths among both men and women. It is the second most common tumor of the digestive system (after colonic cancer) and the fourth most common cause of cancer deaths (after lung, breast, and colonic cancer). Men are more frequently afflicted than women (2:1 in most clinical studies). Although carcinoma of the pancreas may be seen in patients at any age, the mean age of onset is the seventh and eighth decades of life.

For unknown reasons, the age-adjusted mortality rate from carcinoma of the pancreas has been increasing in Western society over the past half century, whereas carcinoma of the stomach has decreased sharply in incidence. Pancreatic cancer is higher than expected among New Zealand Maoris, native Hawaiians, blacks, diabetics, and urban dwellers in higher latitudes.

Cigarette smoking is the strongest environmental factor associated with an increased risk for pancreatic cancer. The odds ratios for male and female smokers developing pancreatic cancer are 3:1 and 2:1, respectively, when compared with nonsmokers. Other environmental factors reported to increase the risk of pancreatic cancer include meat consumption; high fat intake; exposure to oil refining, gasoline, and paper manufacturing; and possibly asbestos in drinking water. A negative correlation has been suggested between pancreatic cancer and increased consumption of raw fruits and vegetables. There is little to suggest an association with either alcohol abuse or coffee consumption.

PATHOPHYSIOLOGY AND CLINICAL MANIFESTATIONS (see Table 109–1). Ductal adenocarcinoma of the pancreas is characterized pathologically by a dense fibrotic or desmoplastic reaction producing a compact, hard mass of tissue. The pancreas lacks a mesentery. It lies adjacent to the bile duct and other vital porta hepatis structures and is surrounded by duodenum, stomach, and colon; the most common clinical manifestations of pancreatic cancer are those related to the encroachment of these adjacent structures. There are few characteristic signs or symptoms that immediately point to a diagnosis of pancreatic cancer. At the time of

TABLE 109–1. SYMPTOMS AND ROUTINE LABORATORY TESTS IN CARCINOMA OF THE PANCREAS

Symptoms*	Percentage	Laboratory Test†	Percentage Abnormal
Abdominal pain	74	Alkaline phosphatase	82
Jaundice	65	5'-Nucleotidase	71
Weight loss	60	LDH	69
Diarrhea	27	SGOT	64
Weakness	21	Albumin	60
Constipation	8	Bilirubin	55
Hematemesis/melena	7	Amylase	17
Vomiting	6		
Abdominal mass	1		

*Modified from Anderson A, Bergdahl L: Am Surg 42:173, 1976.
†Modified from Fitzgerald PJ, Fortner JG, Watson RC, et al.: Cancer 41:868, 1978.
LDH = lactate dehydrogenase; SGOT = serum glutamic-oxaloacetic transaminase.

diagnosis more than half of the patients complain of constant, dull *epigastric abdominal pain* occasionally going to the back. This usually implies invasion of adjacent retroperitoneal organs or splanchnic nerves. *Insidious weight loss* with anorexia and occasionally with a curious aversion for meats, accompanied by a metallic taste in the mouth, diarrhea, weakness, and vomiting, may also be seen. *Vomiting* may indicate gastric or duodenal invasion or extensive peritoneal metastases. *Hematemesis* and *melena* are occasionally noted by patients with duodenal or gastric involvement as the tumor erodes into these richly vascularized adjacent structures. *Jaundice* is noted in over 50 per cent of patients, the vast majority of whom have large tumor masses arising from the head of the pancreas encasing the distal common bile duct. On rare occasions, however, a small focal mass in the head of the pancreas will obstruct the distal common bile duct and produce early jaundice. About one quarter of the patients with pancreatic malignancy have a large, hard, palpable abdominal mass noted at the time of presentation. Occasionally, the jaundice and weight loss may be accompanied by a palpable, distended gallbladder *(Courvoisier's sign)*, which is suggestive of the obstructing periampullary lesion. Patients with carcinoma of the pancreas may also have *thrombophlebitis, psychiatric disturbances,* or *diabetes mellitus.*

DIAGNOSIS. The insidious development of pancreatic malignancy without characteristic signs or symptoms and its low five-year survival rate have given rise to the search for newer, more sensitive and specific diagnostic tests. More patients with pancreatic cancer will have *anemia* resulting from nutritional deficiency, indolent blood loss into the bowel, or the anemia of "chronic disease." An *elevated erythrocyte sedimentation rate* is common, as is the presence of blood in the stools on chemical testing. On occasion, the obstructive jaundice together with blood loss into the duodenum may produce a characteristic *silver-colored stool.*

Serologic biochemical tests cannot definitively make or exclude the diagnosis of pancreatic malignancy (see Tables 109–1 and 109–2). On occasion, patients with pancreatic malignancy will have *elevated serum amylase* due to associated pancreatitis. *Elevation of serum alkaline phosphatase* (often greater than five to ten times the upper limits of normal values) occurs commonly in patients with pancreatic malignancy and is due either to distal common bile duct obstruction or to multiple hepatic metastases. In patients with bile duct obstruction, relentlessly progressive *hyperbilirubinemia* is noted, with the direct-reacting fraction predominant.

An array of serologic markers for the detection of pancreatic cancer has been reported with sensitivities ranging from 10 to 88 per cent. None of these markers can or should be used to make or exclude a diagnosis of pancreatic cancer. The most promising at present are carcinoembryonic antigen (CEA), galactosyltransferase isoenzyme II (GT-II), and antibody CA-19–9. An elevated serum level of CEA has been noted in over

TABLE 109–2. EVALUATION OF SENSITIVITY AND SPECIFICITY OF TESTS FOR PANCREATIC CANCER

	Ultrasound Positive in*	CT Positive in	ERCP Positive in	CEA Positive in	GT-II Positive in
Pancreatic cancer	64%	79%	93%	34%	67%
Other malignancies	13%	7%	0	26%	55%
Benign diseases	1%	4%	0	2%	2%

*"Positive in" refers to an imaging result suggestive of pancreatic cancer or an abnormally high serum level of CEA or GT-II. (Modified from Podolsky D, McPhee MS, Alpert E, et al.: N Engl J Med 304:1313, 1981.)

CT = computed tomography, ERCP = endoscopic retrograde cholangiopancreatography; CEA = carcinoembryonic antigen; GT-II = galactosyltransferase isoenzyme II.

70 per cent of patients with pancreatic malignancy. Elevation of CEA is not, however, specific for either pancreatic cancer or gastrointestinal tract malignancies in general (see Ch. 172). Elevated CEA levels are noted in patients with cirrhosis, chronic pancreatitis, renal failure, and some nongastrointestinal malignancies. Sixty-seven per cent of patients with pancreatic cancer had elevated GT-II levels in one study; however, 55 per cent of patients with other cancers and 2 per cent of patients with chronic pancreatitis also had elevated serum levels of this enzyme.

Nearly 90 per cent of patients with pancreatic cancer are reportedly positive for a serum mucin antigen detected by monoclonal antibody 19–9 (CA-19–9). A specificity of 95 per cent has been suggested, i.e., 95 per cent of patients *without* pancreatic cancer have negative results on the CA-19–9 antibody test. Other serologic and skin test markers for pancreatic cancer are promising, yet incompletely evaluated: pancreatic cancer–associated antigen (67 per cent sensitivity), oncofetal pancreatic antigen (88 per cent sensitivity), and skin test reactivity to Thomsen-Friedenreich antigen (88 per cent sensitivity).

The *upper gastrointestinal tract series* may demonstrate widening of the "C-loop" of the duodenum and mass indentation along the medial aspect of the descending duodenum in patients with cancer of the pancreatic head. Anterior displacement of the stomach and/or displacement of the ligament of Treitz from the greater curvature of the stomach may be noted radiographically in patients with carcinoma of the pancreatic body or tail. The upper gastrointestinal series is, however, a poor screening test in making an early diagnosis of pancreatic malignancy, especially in patients with carcinoma of the body and tail of the pancreas. Barium radiography will also interfere with computed tomographic (CT) scanning and thus should not be done initially in patients who are suspected of having pancreatic disease, either benign or malignant.

The abdominal imaging techniques of ultrasound and computed tomography (CT) (see Ch. 95) have markedly enhanced our ability to visualize the pancreas. Pancreatic malignancy is characteristically seen on *ultrasound* and *CT scanning* as either an asymmetrically or a uniformly enlarged and nonhomogeneous pancreas. In addition to the mass enlargement of the pancreas, marked dilation of the extrahepatic and intrahepatic bile ducts will be readily apparent in patients with bile duct obstruction (see Fig. 95–6). Metastases to the liver and peripancreatic lymph nodes may also be detected by either ultrasound or CT scanning. The sensitivity and specificity of both ultrasound and CT scanning in pancreatic cancer exceed 90 per cent. The larger mass lesions will almost certainly be demonstrated by both ultrasound and CT. However, the lower limits of resolution in both techniques are in the range of 1 to 2 cm; thus small, potentially resectable pancreatic cancers, especially those not altering the contour of the gland, may be overlooked. Nonetheless, these two tests are the most helpful in identifying patients with pancreatic disease and, when combined with cytologic studies, can establish the diagnosis of pancreatic cancer in the majority of instances (see below).

Many invasive diagnostic procedures are available for investigating tumors of the pancreas (see Ch. 95). *Angiography* will usually demonstrate displacement of the pancreatic arcades or tumor encasement of celiac, splenic, gastroduodenal,

or superior mesenteric arteries. Moreover, the venous phase of the angiogram may demonstrate occlusion of the splenic vein and portal vein. With *secretin or cholecystokinin (CCK) stimulation of the pancreas*, the volume of pancreatic juice that can be collected via a duodenal sump (Dreiling) tube is characteristically decreased, but the bicarbonate and trypsin concentrations remain normal. *Transhepatic cholangiography* (THC) in patients with pancreatic malignancy obstructing the common bile duct will usually demonstrate a long, irregular, tapered segment of the common bile duct as it passes through the pancreatic malignancy. The radiographic findings are similar to those shown for cholangiocarcinoma in Figure 95–8. Difficulty may be encountered, however, in differentiating malignant stricturing of the distal common bile duct caused by pancreatic malignancy from that produced by scarring in a patient with chronic pancreatitis.

Endoscopic retrograde cholangiopancreatography (ERCP) provides the only means of directly opacifying the pancreatic duct (see Ch. 96). Since most pancreatic cancer is ductal adenocarcinoma, even small mass lesions will occlude branches of the main pancreatic duct. The characteristic finding of an abrupt cutoff of the pancreatic duct or the stricturing of both pancreatic and common bile duct (so-called "double duct sign") is virtually diagnostic of pancreatic carcinoma (Fig. 109–1).

Intraoperative transduodenal biopsy was previously the only means of obtaining tissue for histologic demonstration of malignancy. *Cytologic study of fluid* collected during ERCP may demonstrate malignant cells in the majority of patients. *Guided*

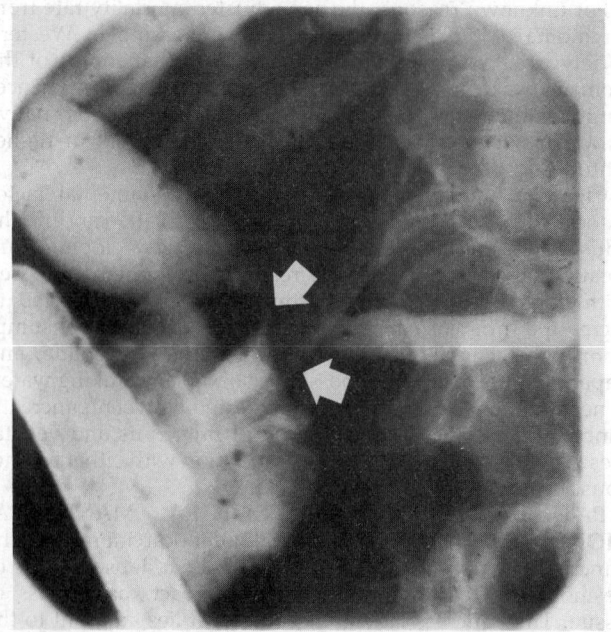

FIGURE 109–1. Endoscopic retrograde cholangiopancreatography (ERCP) in carcinoma of the head of the pancreas. A classic "double duct sign" is seen with stricturing of both the distal common bile duct and pancreatic duct (*arrows*). A markedly enlarged proximal common bile duct is filled with contrast material. A 2-cm pancreatic adenocarcinoma was successfully removed by Whipple's resection. However, death occurred within six months of recurrent disease.

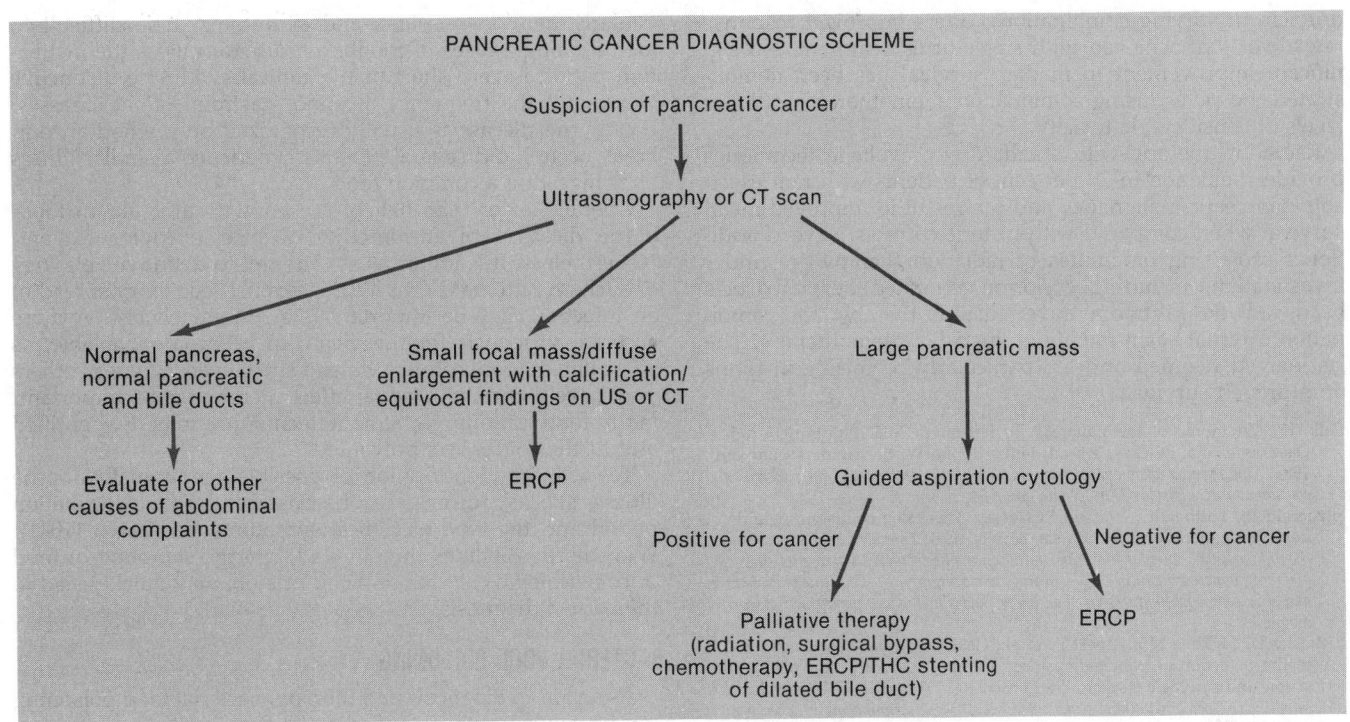

PANCREATIC CANCER DIAGNOSTIC SCHEME

Suspicion of pancreatic cancer

Ultrasonography or CT scan

Normal pancreas, normal pancreatic and bile ducts

Small focal mass/diffuse enlargement with calcification/ equivocal findings on US or CT

Large pancreatic mass

Evaluate for other causes of abdominal complaints

ERCP

Guided aspiration cytology

Positive for cancer

Negative for cancer

Palliative therapy (radiation, surgical bypass, chemotherapy, ERCP/THC stenting of dilated bile duct)

ERCP

FIGURE 109–2. Suggested approach to the patient with the suspicion of pancreatic cancer. The initial evaluation should include adequate noninvasive imaging by either ultrasonography or computed tomography.

fine-needle aspiration cytology of the pancreas is now possible using either ultrasound or CT guidance. In most series, 80 to 90 per cent sensitivity and 100 per cent specificity in the presence of pancreatic cancer have been demonstrated.

LOGICAL USE OF DIAGNOSTIC METHODS. A schematic approach to the diagnosis of pancreatic cancer is summarized in Figure 109–2. In the patient who is suspected of having pancreatic malignancy, ultrasound should be performed first. If the ultrasound scan is inadequate in visualizing the pancreas, a CT study should then be done. In those patients with an accessible pancreatic mass (the situation in most patients with pancreatic cancer), a guided aspiration biopsy or cytologic examination of the mass lesion should be performed, using either ultrasound or CT guidance. In those patients with histologic or cytologic confirmation of malignancy, appropriate therapy may be initiated. For those patients with large pancreatic mass lesions but negative cytologic studies, an ERCP should be performed to demonstrate ductal changes of either pancreatic cancer or chronic pancreatitis. In patients with small focal enlargement or pancreatic calcification, ERCP should be performed to differentiate focal pancreatic disease such as malignancy from either chronic pancreatitis or a normal gland. A normal ultrasound scan and/or CT with a normal ERCP (all of which can and should be done on an outpatient basis) virtually excludes pancreatic cancer.

DIFFERENTIAL DIAGNOSIS. There are no characteristic signs or symptoms of carcinoma of the pancreas, especially for a cancer arising in the body or tail of the gland. In patients *without* jaundice, the vague abdominal pains, anorexia, weight loss, and malaise are all nonspecific and may be difficult to distinguish from those in patients with gastric ulcer, gastric cancer, other intra-abdominal malignancies, chronic pancreatitis, and even severe depression. In a reliable elderly patient, however, these complaints should lead to a suspicion of pancreatic or other malignancy. Epigastric abdominal masses from pancreatic cancer should be distinguished from an enlarged left hepatic lobe, gastric or colonic masses, large omental metastases, and pancreatic pseudocyst or chronic pancreatitis.

Most patients with carcinoma of the pancreatic head have obstructive jaundice. Other periampullary malignancies such

as ampullary, duodenal, and cholangiocarcinomas and porta hepatis node metastases should be differentiated from pancreatic cancer, since they may have better prognoses than pancreatic cancer following radical surgery. Benign conditions causing obstructive jaundice, such as common bile duct gallstones, chronic pancreatitis, or bile duct strictures, must always be clearly differentiated from malignant obstruction of the bile duct. Intrahepatic cholestasis from drugs, toxins, hepatitis, abscess, cirrhosis, and even alcoholic hepatitis must be distinguished from extrahepatic cholestasis, usually by employing biochemical tests and noninvasive imaging techniques.

THERAPY. Despite the technical advances mentioned above, pancreatic cancer usually manifests clinically at a nonresectable stage of disease. Pancreatic cancer is usually treated by combinations of surgery, chemotherapy, and radiation therapy. Whipple's resection (pancreaticoduodenectomy) or subtotal or total pancreatectomy should be reserved for patients with small focal mass lesions without any evidence of involvement of adjacent vascular structures or distal metastases. The operative mortality of Whipple's procedure is 20 per cent, with a mean five-year survival of only 5 per cent. Mean survival in an unselected series of patients undergoing Whipple's resection is not significantly better than with the palliative biliary bypass alone. Total pancreatectomy, combining the en bloc resection of pancreas and spleen, may improve mean survival when compared with palliative bypass and Whipple's resection. In symptomatic patients with large, bulky tumor masses obstructing the common bile duct, palliative surgical bypass with a choledochojejunostomy or cholecystojejunostomy should be considered. Percutaneous transhepatic or endoscopic retrograde stenting of the common bile duct may likewise palliatively decompress the dilated biliary tree. These last two techniques, in experienced hands, should be employed, rather than laparotomy palliative duct decompression, in poor-risk surgical patients with large, bulky tumors.

Single-agent chemotherapy offers limited palliation but no improved survival in patients with nonresectable pancreatic cancer. Combination chemotherapy, employing agents such as 5-fluorouracil (5-FU), mitomycin C, streptozocin, and doxorubicin in varying combinations, offers improved response rates over that achieved with single-drug treatment. No significant improvement in median survival has been demonstrated, however, using combination chemotherapy, often at levels of considerable toxicity.

Radiation therapy with standard supravoltage techniques provides palliation in 70 per cent of patients with nonresectable pancreatic malignancy and can result in improved mean survival when compared with historic controls. Several additional promising modalities of radiation therapy are under investigation, including cyclotron-generated heavy particle beam radiation, intraoperative radiation therapy, and combination external beam radiation plus 5-FU chemotherapy. The last-named regimen appears particularly promising in terms of improved survival.

Cello JP: Carcinoma of the pancreas. In Sleisenger MH, Fordtran JS (eds.): Gastrointestinal Disease. 4th ed. Philadelphia, W. B. Saunders Company, 1988. *This recent review covers the general topic of carcinoma of the pancreas and contains an extensive and up-to-date list of 54 references.*

Fitzgerald PJ, Fortner JG, Watson RC, et al.: The value of diagnostic aids in detecting pancreas cancer. Cancer 41:868, 1978. *Thorough analysis is made of the diagnostic accuracy of invasive and noninvasive tests in 184 patients suspected of having pancreatic cancer. CT scanning, celiac angiography, alkaline phosphatase, and ^{75}Se-selenomethionine, in that order, had the highest percentage of correct diagnoses.*

Podolsky D, McPhee MS, Alpert E, et al.: Galactosyltransferase isoenzyme II in the detection of pancreatic cancer: Comparison with radiologic, endoscopic and serologic tests. N Engl J Med 304:1313, 1981. *GT-II was the most sensitive (67 per cent) and specific (98 per cent) for discriminating between benign and malignant pancreatic disease. As a single test, only ERCP was more sensitive than GT-II. When GT-II was combined with ultrasound or with CT, sensitivities of 92 and 88 per cent, respectively, were noted.*

Van Dyke JA, Stanley RJ, Berland LL: Pancreatic imaging. Ann Intern Med 102:212, 1985. *Review of the available imaging techniques of the pancreas. Computed tomography is the best for initial evaluation of the patient with suspected pancreatic disease. No single test will always provide all necessary diagnostic information.*

110 FOOD POISONING

David F. Altman

Food poisoning, which may be defined as clinical syndromes arising from the ingestion of food that either is contaminated or is itself toxic, may cause illness in three distinct ways: (1) by contamination of food with microorganisms or their products (most common); (2) by its contamination with poisonous chemicals; or (3) by ingestion of poisonous plants or animals.

As the gastrointestinal tract is the mode of entry for these various contaminants, most illnesses associated with food poisoning involve some form of gastroenteritis, with either upper or lower gastrointestinal manifestations predominating. Other syndromes are often identifiable by extraintestinal (par-

ticularly neurologic) signs and symptoms. It is difficult to identify single cases of foodborne disease unless the incubation period is very short or the clinical syndrome distinctive because of the frequency of minor gastrointestinal illnesses. Foodborne disease is usually recognized only when an outbreak occurs and several persons experience a similar illness after ingesting a common food.

Overall, fewer than half of the known outbreaks of foodborne disease are attributed to a specific etiologic agent. Nevertheless, it is important to attempt to define the etiology of such an outbreak. Prophylaxis against secondary spread of an infection may be important (e.g., in shigellosis). A more accurate prognosis for the victim may become available, as some illnesses are self-limited and short-lived, whereas others may have a chronic residual effect. Perhaps most important, faulty food handling or storage techniques may be identified and further outbreaks prevented.

To facilitate identification of possible agents in foodborne illness, such syndromes can be classified by their incubation period and the type of clinical symptoms (see Table 110–1). With the possibilities thus limited, specific sampling of food or bacteriologic cultures of blood or stool may quickly lead to the correct diagnosis.

BACTERIAL FOOD POISONING

As an aid to diagnosis and therapy, bacterial food poisoning can be conveniently classified as (1) that due to the ingestion of living microorganisms, (2) that due to the ingestion of a toxin produced by microorganisms in food prior to its ingestion, or (3) that due to enterotoxins produced in the gut by pathogens only after their ingestion.

The most important "infectious" types of food poisoning, requiring ingestion of living organisms, are *Salmonella* gastroenteritis and *Shigella* dysentery, which are dealt with in Ch. 284 and 285, respectively. Other organisms responsible in this way include *Campylobacter jejuni*, *Escherichia coli*, *Vibrio cholerae*, *Vibrio parahaemolyticus*, *Bacillus cereus*, and *Clostridium perfringens*. In addition, epidemics of listeriosis transmitted by food and a foodborne outbreak of streptococcal pharyngitis have both been reported.

The "toxin" type of food poisoning most often identified is due to *Staphylococcus aureus*. The syndrome of botulism caused by ingestion of the toxin produced by *Clostridium botulinum* is discussed in Ch. 280.

Staphylococcal Food Poisoning

ETIOLOGY. This form of food poisoning is caused by an enterotoxin produced by multiplying staphylococci before the contaminated food is ingested. Nearly all strains known to elaborate enterotoxins are coagulase-positive *Staphylococcus aureus*; however, some coagulase-negative strains have also been incriminated. The two major sources of contamination are human carriers (usually nasal or skin) and cows with mastitis, the former accounting for nearly 90 per cent of

TABLE 110–1. CLINICAL INDICATORS OF THE ETIOLOGY OF FOODBORNE ILLNESS

Predominant Symptomatology	Mean Incubation Period			
	< 2 Hours	2–7 Hours	8–14 Hours	> 14 hours
Upper intestinal	Heavy metals	S. aureus B. cereus		
Lower intestinal			C. perfringens B. cereus	V. cholera Enterotoxic or invasive E. coli Shigella spp. V. parahaemolyticus Salmonella
Both upper and lower gastrointestinal				V. parahaemolyticus
Extragastrointestinal, i.e., some gastrointestinal plus others, usually paresthesias or other abnormal sensory complaint	Scombrotoxin Shellfish toxin Mushroom toxin (early)	Ciguatoxin	Mushroom toxin (delayed)	C. botulinum

outbreaks. Staphylococcal food poisoning requires not only contamination of food with the microorganisms but also a period of some hours during which they may multiply, as may occur during slow cooling after cooking or if food is held at ambient temperature. Subsequent reheating may destroy the organism but not the remarkably heat-resistant toxin, and it is the latter that causes the clinical illness.

PATHOGENESIS, CLINICAL MANIFESTATIONS, AND TREATMENT. Little is known about the mode of action of the enterotoxins. In experimental animals they cause destruction of gastrointestinal mucosal cells and evoke an inflammatory response. Effects on other organ systems, including the emetic centers in the brain, also have been postulated. Symptoms usually begin two to four hours after ingestion of the toxin, heralded by salivation and followed rapidly by nausea, vomiting, abdominal cramping, and diarrhea. The illness usually is short, rarely lasting 24 hours, and often is subsiding by the time medical attention is sought. It may occasionally be life-threatening, especially in the elderly or in persons with other serious illness. Therapy is supportive and symptomatic, the primary goal being to restore extracellular fluid volume with parenteral fluids as necessary. Antibiotic therapy may worsen the course of the illness.

PREVENTION. Proper food handling is essential for the prevention of staphylococcal food poisoning. Sanitary measures and personal hygiene can prevent contamination of the food to some degree. More importantly, food handlers must recognize that enterotoxin is not produced at ordinary domestic refrigerator temperatures. Foods should not be left to cool slowly, especially in large containers, and should be taken from the refrigerator (and reheated, if required) immediately before serving.

Clostridial Food Poisoning

ETIOLOGY. *Clostridium perfringens* type A has been the third most common bacterial cause of food poisoning in the United States for the last several years. Clostridial poisoning typically occurs in fairly large outbreaks. The organism is ubiquitous, being found in most samples of raw meat, human and animal feces, flies, soil, and dirt from kitchens. Both heat-sensitive and heat-resistant strains have been known to cause outbreaks. The conditions necessary for an outbreak generally include the cooking of meat, poultry, or beans at a temperature (usually less than 100° C) high enough to kill vegetative forms but insufficient to destroy heat-resistant spores. Oxygen is driven out of the food, thereby lowering the oxidation-reduction potential of the medium. During slow cooling the spores germinate, encouraged by the relatively anaerobic environment and the rich supply of amino acids and other growth factors. If the food is not reheated to a temperature high enough to inactivate the recently multiplied organism, ingestion may result in illness.

PATHOGENESIS AND CLINICAL MANIFESTATIONS. Ingestion of living organisms is necessary for the production of clostridial food poisoning, but the pathogenesis of the clinical manifestations remains to be defined. Several toxins have been suggested, but none is clearly responsible for human disease. The incubation period is usually 8 to 12 hours after ingestion, but may be as long as 24 hours. The usual symptoms are abdominal cramps and diarrhea; vomiting is rare, as are headache, chills, and fever. The illness is self-limited, rarely lasting more than 24 hours. Treatment rarely is necessary and should always be confined to efforts at symptomatic relief. The few deaths recorded have been in elderly or debilitated patients.

PREVENTION. Food is best served immediately after cooking. If it is to be kept, it should be cooled rapidly. Cooked meat should always be kept either cold, below 5° C, or hot, over 60° C. This is especially true of food prepared in large batches.

Vibrio parahaemolyticus Food Poisoning

V. parahaemolyticus is a gram-negative facultative anaerobe found in marine water and fauna throughout the world. It lives in sediment of coastal and estuarian waters during cold winter months. As the temperature rises in spring and summer, the organism leaves the sediment and colonizes animal life, especially shellfish and crustaceans. Not all strains are pathogenic.

The pathogenesis of the illness is not clearly defined, and different serotypes may produce disease by different mechanisms. The presence of fecal leukocytes and occasionally bloody diarrhea implies bacterial invasion and damage of the gut mucosa.

Virtually all outbreaks of *V. parahaemolyticus* food poisoning have occurred during warm months of the year and have been associated with the ingestion of raw or improperly refrigerated seafood. Although originally described in Japan, cases have occurred in other parts of Asia and on the Atlantic, Gulf, and Pacific coasts of the United States. The incubation period is usually between 12 and 24 hours, but has been as long as 96 hours. Explosive watery diarrhea is present in more than 90 per cent of cases, with nausea, vomiting, and abdominal cramps as common accompaniments. Fever, headache, and chills occur less often. The diagnosis is suspected when a typical illness occurs after eating seafood, and is confirmed by recovery of the organism from stool. Treatment is rarely necessary, as the illness infrequently lasts more than two days. However, in protracted cases, antibiotic treatment with tetracycline or ampicillin may shorten the illness.

Prevention depends on the recognition both of the potential for contamination of seafood with *V. parahaemolyticus* during warm months and of the predisposition of organisms to multiply under conditions of inadequate refrigeration. Cooked seafood may also become cross-contaminated when stored under proper conditions with a raw source.

Bacillus cereus Food Poisoning

Bacillus cereus, an aerobic, motile, spore-forming, gram-positive rod, has been increasingly recognized as a cause of foodborne disease. There appear to be two separate clinical forms of the disease. An emetic form, clinically identical to staphylococcal food poisoning, is associated with contaminated fried rice. A diarrheal form has a longer incubation period and predominantly lower gastrointestinal symptoms, reminiscent of *Clostridium perfringens* food poisoning. Cell-free filtrates derived from *B. cereus* strains responsible for this latter form of illness stimulate the adenylate cyclase–cyclic adenosine monophosphate (cAMP) system in intestinal epithelial cells, and their activity is destroyed by heat, thus resembling cholera enterotoxin. The illnesses are usually mild and self-limited, and antibiotics are not indicated. No fatalities have been reported. As the organism commonly occurs in soil and in many dried or processed foods, careful food handling is most important in prevention of the disease. *B. cereus* may be found in uncooked rice, for example, and heat-resistant spores may survive boiling. If the rice is left unrefrigerated, the spores may then germinate and produce toxin. Flash frying or rewarming before serving is often not sufficient to destroy the preformed, heat-stable toxin. The disease thus can be prevented by prompt refrigeration of boiled rice.

Blake PA: Diseases of humans (other than cholera) caused by vibrios. Ann Rev Microbiol 34:341, 1980. *A comprehensive review of clinical and microbiologic aspects of Vibrio-caused disease.*

Centers for Disease Control: Foodborne disease outbreaks, annual summary, 1982. In CDC Surveillance Summaries, 35:7ss, 1986. *An annual compendium of reports of foodborne diseases in the United States, with analysis of vehicles of transmission and contributing factors to contamination for each type of infection identified.*

Holmberg SD, Blake PA: Staphylococcal food poisoning in the United States: New facts and old misconceptions. JAMA 251:487, 1984. *Information on the epidemiology and clinical characteristics of this entity.*

Horowitz MA: Specific diagnosis of foodborne disease. Gastroenterology 73:375, 1977. *A clinician's guide to the clinical and epidemiologic differential diagnosis of foodborne diseases.*

Schlech WF III, Lavigne PM, Bortolussi RA, et al.: Epidemic listeriosis—evidence for transmission by food. N Engl J Med 308:203, 1983. *This is a thorough account of a heretofore suspected but unproved type of food-related illness.*

Terranova W, Blake PA: *Bacillus cereus* food poisoning. N Engl J Med 298:143, 1978. *A brief but comprehensive review of the various forms of this illness.*

CHEMICAL FOOD POISONING

Food poisoning caused by chemicals may be related either to the accidental contamination of food prior to its preparation or during storage or to a food additive or preservative. Thus various forms of metallic poisoning, discussed in Ch. 542, can occur when food, particularly acid liquids, comes in contact with certain metals, especially cadmium, copper, tin, or zinc.

The so-called Chinese restaurant syndrome, in which individuals develop sensations of burning skin, facial pressure, chest pressure, and headaches 10 to 20 minutes after eating certain Chinese foods (especially won ton soup), has been attributed to the use of monosodium L-glutamate (MSG). The symptoms appear to be a pharmacologic effect of MSG, obeying a dose-effect relationship, but with a widely variable threshold for an oral dose.

Sodium nitrite, widely used as a preservative in smoked meats, has been blamed for the "hot dog headache" seen in some persons. In addition, because of its metabolism to nitrosamines it is suspected to be a potential carcinogen, although evidence for this is inconclusive.

Food additives such as aspartame and pesticides have been incriminated as a cause of foodborne disease. Although the former have not been conclusively identified as the source of illness, outbreaks of the latter have been documented. A recent episode of contamination of watermelons by aldicarb caused gastrointestinal and neurologic symptoms in over 1000 individuals.

Schaumburg HH, Byck R, Gerstil R, et al.: Monosodium L-glutamate: Its pharmacology and role in the Chinese restaurant syndrome. Science 163:826, 1969. *A careful analysis of MSG pharmacology and its dose-effect relationships.*

POISONOUS ANIMALS AND PLANTS

Fish and Shellfish Poisoning

Vertebrate fish may contain various toxins capable of causing human illness. Most commonly this is due to toxin contained in musculature (ichthyosarcotoxins), of which nine types have been described. The most common fish poisonings worldwide—ciguatera, scombroid, and puffer fish poisoning—are attributable to ichthyosarcotoxins.

Two forms of shellfish poisoning, paralytic and neurotoxic, have been described. These are caused by toxins derived from dinoflagellates contaminating the shellfish.

CIGUATERA FISH POISONING. Ciguatera fish poisoning is caused by ciguatoxin, a lipid-soluble, heat-stable substance for which chemical structure has not been determined. More than 400 fish species have been implicated, generally bottom-dwelling shore fish found in temperate and tropical zones.

The onset of the illness usually occurs one to six hours after, but may be as soon as a few minutes or as long as 30 hours after, ingestion of toxic fish. Gastrointestinal symptoms, including abdominal cramps, nausea, vomiting, and diarrhea, predominate at the outset, along with numbness, pruritus, and paresthesias of the lips, tongue, and throat. Paresthesias may later involve the extremities, and in severe cases there may be abnormal temperature sensations, cranial nerve palsies, hypotension, bradycardia, and even respiratory paralysis. Acute symptoms usually subside within a few days and require only symptomatic, supportive therapy. The return of pruritus with alcohol ingestion is thought to be almost pathognomonic of this syndrome. Weakness and sensory disturbances may persist for months or years.

SCOMBROID FISH POISONING. Scrombroid fish poisoning is the only form of ichthyosarcotoxism in which toxins are formed by the action of bacteria, in this case particularly *Proteus morgani*, on fish flesh. The chemical nature of the scombrotoxin is unknown, but it is thought to consist of histamine and related substances. Most fish that have caused outbreaks are members of the suborder *Scombroidea*, most commonly mahi-mahi, tuna, mackerel, and bonito. Symptoms begin within a few minutes of ingestion and resemble those of a histamine reaction: flushing, headache, dizziness, abdominal cramps, nausea, vomiting and diarrhea, and occasionally urticaria and generalized pruritus. The illness has a median duration of four hours in the reported outbreaks. Antihistamines have provided symptomatic relief, which has been reported to be rapid and complete with intravenous cimetidine. Production of the toxin is inhibited by proper refrigeration, perhaps reflecting the temperature optimum of 20 to 30° C for the enzymatic conversion of histidine to histamine. Improper refrigeration of fresh-caught fish has been observed in most outbreaks of this illness.

PUFFER FISH POISONING (TETRODOTOXIN POISONING). Many puffer fish found in the Pacific, Atlantic, and Indian Oceans are inherently toxic. The tetrodotoxin found in their viscera is a neurotoxin, and its effects are nearly identical to the saxitoxin that produces paralytic shellfish poisoning (see below).

PARALYTIC SHELLFISH POISONING. Paralytic shellfish poisoning is caused by the ingestion of bivalve mollusks contaminated with the neurotoxin of the dinoflagellates *Gonyaulax catanella* or *Go. tamarensis*. Although a "red tide," related to "blooming" of the dinoflagellates, has been associated with paralytic shellfish poisoning, not all red tides are toxic, and some outbreaks have occurred in the absence of a red tide. The toxin of *Go. catanella*, saxitoxin, appears to act by blocking the propagation of nerve and muscle action potentials.

The illness begins within 30 minutes of ingestion of a toxic mollusk and is characterized by paresthesias of the mouth, lips, face, and extremities and by nausea, vomiting, and diarrhea. In more severe cases, muscle weakness or paralysis and respiratory embarrassment may occur. Deaths, though rare, have occurred within the first 12 hours. Treatment consists of a cathartic or enema in severe cases to remove unabsorbed toxin. Gastric lavage may be used if vomiting has not occurred. Mechanical ventilatory assistance may be required.

NEUROTOXIC SHELLFISH POISONING. *Gymnodinium breve* is a toxic dinoflagellate that causes a red tide off both the Gulf and Atlantic coasts of Florida. Within three hours of the consumption of shellfish contaminated with this toxin, patients experience paresthesias, abnormal temperature sensations, ataxia, nausea, vomiting, and diarrhea. The disease is self-limited and milder than paralytic shellfish poisoning. No deaths have been reported.

MUSHROOM POISONING

Of the more than 2000 identified species of mushrooms, fewer than 50 are poisonous. However, even expert mycologists may have difficulty identifying poisonous species. Moreover, with the increased interest in "organic" foods and in the hallucinogenic substances found in certain species, poisoning from the ingestion of wild mushrooms has been increasing in frequency.

The principal toxin is amanitine, which contains cyclic octapeptides. Phalloidin, another putative toxin, appears to have some hepatocellular toxicity, but mushrooms with phalloidin but without amanitine have been consumed without ill effect. Amanitine selectively inhibits nuclear ribonucleic acid (RNA) polymerase II. Mushrooms containing these toxins belong to the genera *Amanita* and *Galerina*. *Amanita verna* (the "destroying angel"), *A. virosa,* and *A. phalloides* (the "death cap") are the species most often associated with mushroom poisoning in the United States, and *A. phalloides* accounts for more than 90 per cent of such deaths in Europe.

Symptoms of *A. phalloides*–type mushroom poisoning characteristically occur in three stages. The first is characterized by the abrupt onset of abdominal pain, nausea, vomiting, and diarrhea 6 to 24 hours after ingestion. This may be accompanied by severe fluid and electrolyte disturbances and fever. The second stage, occurring during the next 24 to 48 hours, involves worsening of hepatic and renal function despite resolution of the initial symptoms. Finally, during the third and fourth days after ingestion, hepatic and renal function deteriorates, accompanied occasionally by cardiomyopathy and coagulopathy, convulsions, coma, and death. The mortality rate is between 40 and 90 per cent.

The diagnosis of mushroom poisoning may be difficult. The delayed onset of symptoms may cause patients not to associate the illness with the ingestion of wild mushrooms. The mushroom toxins can be detected in gastric aspirate, vomitus, or stool by thin-layer chromatography in some laboratories. Treatment remains supportive, including renal dialysis when indicated. Thioctic acid has been used experimentally since 1968 as an antidote for *A. phalloides*–type mushroom poisoning, but this treatment now appears to be ineffective. There has been a report of a successful orthotopic liver transplantation in a child, but timing of surgery and availability of a suitable donor will continue to make this rarely possible.

Plant Alkaloids, Mycotoxins, and Other Poisonings

These various forms of food poisoning remind us of historic knowledge of the pharmacologic effect of plant alkaloids and other toxicants found naturally in foods. Although formerly used with therapeutic intent, plant alkaloids are now more often ingested accidentally and often in large doses. Reports now appear of digitalis intoxication from home-brewed teas made with foxglove or oleander, diarrhea from senna tea, which contains the stimulant cathartic anthraquinone, and liver failure from *Senecio longilobus,* which contains highly hepatotoxic pyrrolizidine alkaloids. Other highly toxic plants include *Atropa belladonna* (deadly nightshade) and *Datura stramonium* (thorn apple, jimson weed), whose berries and seeds can cause an atropine effect, *Conium maculatum* (hemlock), which contains several alkaloids with severe central nervous system depressant effects, and *Phytolacca americana* (pokeweed), whose leaves and berries have strong emetic properties.

Lathyrism, a slowly progressive spastic paraplegia, is associated with the ingestion of sweet peas of the species *Lathyrus sativus.* Large amounts of this may be ingested during famines in Africa and Asia. The toxic principle appears to be beta-aminoproprionitrile. Interestingly, this substance, when given to poultry and other experimental animals, causes degeneration of the aortic media, with resulting dissecting aortic aneurysms or aortic rupture. This effect is not seen in humans.

Mycotoxins may contaminate some moldy foods. Ergotism, characterized by intense vasospasm, is the most familiar syndrome caused by this ingestion. Other mycotoxins, including aflatoxin, have been identified. This product of *Aspergillus flavus* contaminates grains stored in warm, damp areas, and has been associated with the development of hepatocellular carcinoma. Small amounts of aflatoxin have been found in commercial peanut butter in the United States.

Hughes JM, Merson MH: Fish and shellfish poisoning. N Engl J Med 295:1117, 1976. *A thorough review of the pathophysiology and clinical manifestations of this group of illnesses.*

Olson KR, Pond SM, Seward J, et al.: *Amanita phalloides*–type mushroom poisoning. West J Med 137:282, 1982. *This is a comprehensive review of the clinical manifestations of mushroom poisoning, the various species involved, and a brief guide to their identification. Therapeutic options are presented.*

Poisoning associated with herbal teas. MMWR 26:257, 1977. *Case reports and discussions of several types of herbal poisonings.*

Wogan GN: Mycotoxins. Ann Rev Pharmacol 15:437, 1975. *A review of the current understanding of the pharmacology and health impact of mycotoxins.*

111 DISEASES OF THE RECTUM AND ANUS

David F. Altman

DISEASES OF THE RECTUM

INTRODUCTION. The rectum primarily serves a storage function by allowing convenient disposition of fecal waste. Most diseases of the rectum involve some inflammatory change that alters neuromuscular control over defecation and results in symptoms of constipation or diarrhea, tenesmus, and urgency.

The sigmoidoscope and forceps biopsy instruments are most useful to examine the rectum. In contrast, the barium enema gives poor resolution in the rectum and therefore is unreliable as a primary diagnostic tool. Sigmoidoscopy using flexible fiberoptic instruments permits more of the rectum and sigmoid to be examined with decreased patient discomfort.

PROCTITIS. Inflammatory disease of the rectum may be caused by radiation injury, trauma from a foreign body, ischemia or infection, or other processes. Chronic inflammatory disease of unknown etiology, perhaps related to more generalized inflammatory bowel diseases, is a frequent occurrence.

INFECTIOUS PROCTITIS. Inflammatory disease in the rectum may be caused by several infectious agents. The syndromes of bacillary dysentery and amebiasis are discussed in Ch. 285 and 390, respectively. Venereally transmitted diseases, especially gonorrhea, syphilis, lymphogranuloma venereum (LGV), and non–LGV chlamydial serotypes, may involve the rectum primarily (see Ch. 306, 307, and 310). These diseases have their greatest impact in the male homosexual population; e.g., asymptomatic rectal carriage of gonorrhea may be detected in up to two thirds of tested subjects, and frequent sexual contact permits rapid spread of the infection.

Diagnosis of anorectal gonorrhea is best made by obtaining culture material with a sterile cotton swab inserted approximately 2.5 cm into the anal canal, swept around a peripheral arc for ten seconds, and then inoculated immediately on selective growth medium. Rarely, disseminated gonococcal infection with bacteremia has been reported after anorectal gonorrhea. Treatment is the same as for other localized gonococcal infections (see Ch. 306).

Herpes simplex virus is known to cause an acute proctitis in homosexual men. Anorectal pain and discharge are the most common presenting complaints, and these are often accompanied by constipation, tenesmus, and hematochezia. Neurologic involvement, with urinary bladder dysfunction, paresthesias, erectile difficulties, and gluteal or thigh pain, is also seen. Proctoscopy will often show an acute distal proctitis with ulcerations. Rectal biopsy shows acute inflammation, and intranuclear inclusions, if seen, confirm the diagnosis. Treatment is supportive and symptoms resolve spontaneously, although there may be periodic recurrences.

NONSPECIFIC ULCERATIVE PROCTITIS. Nonspecific ulcerative proctitis most commonly produces symptoms of rectal bleeding, tenesmus, and often a mucosanguineous anal discharge. The bleeding seldom is severe, and patients with diarrhea often describe no increase in stool volume but rather frequent passage of small amounts of mucus or blood. Systemic symptoms, such as fever and weight loss, rarely occur. Indeed, the patient usually feels remarkably well in spite of the primary complaints noted above. Extraintestinal manifestations of inflammatory bowel disease, especially arthritis, uveitis, and dermatitis, also are rare. The diagnosis is made when (1) sigmoidoscopy reveals inflammation of the rectal mucosa with a clearly demarcated upper border above which the mucosa is normal, (2) the remainder of the colon and small intestine is found to be normal by barium radiograph and/or colonoscopy, and (3) a rectal biopsy demonstrates changes indistinguishable from those of chronic ulcerative colitis.

Differential diagnosis includes Crohn's ileocolitis, radiation proctitis, and infectious disease of the rectum, especially bacillary dysentery, amebiasis, lymphogranuloma venereum, and gonorrheal proctitis. A detailed history and physical examination, appropriate cultures of stool and rectal mucus, biopsy, and serologic studies for chlamydiae should suffice to distinguish among these possibilities.

Treatment is primarily that used for more generalized inflammatory bowel disease, with the exception that systemic corticosteroids are rarely or never used. Topical corticosteroids, administered once or twice daily either as suppositories or as enemas, often provide a satisfactory response. Sulfasalazine or other poorly absorbed sulfa preparations may also be used either orally or rectally. With treatment the disease usually runs a course with periodic exacerbations. Rectal strictures may occur, but carcinoma of the rectum seems to be only a small risk. However, biannual sigmoidoscopy is warranted to follow the course of the illness. Fewer than 15 per cent of patients with ulcerative proctitis develop diffuse ulcerative colitis.

FECAL IMPACTION AND STERCORAL ULCER. Incomplete evacuation of feces over an extended period of time may result in the formation of an obstructing mass of firm stool in the distal colon or rectum. *Fecal impaction* occurs most often in children with undiagnosed congenital megacolon or psychiatric disorders, in patients with painful anal diseases, and in elderly, debilitated, or sedentary persons. Patients may complain only of a sensation of fullness in the lower abdomen, anorexia, and malaise. Liquid stool above the fecal mass may distend the proximal colon and then pass around the obstruction. This may be misinterpreted as diarrhea, and inappropriate treatment may be instituted. The diagnosis is most easily made on digital rectal examination, but when the impaction is located more proximally in the sigmoid colon, only an abdominal mass may be felt.

A large fecal impaction usually requires both administration of enemas and mechanical disimpaction digitally. Treatment consisting of saline enemas and oral mineral oil is usually successful once the fecal mass has been broken up. More extraordinary enema solutions have included milk and molasses in equal volumes and water-soluble radiographic contrast material. Warm oil or soapsuds enemas rarely are necessary; in fact, they may be injurious to the rectal mucosa.

Fecal impactions may be associated with the development of intestinal obstruction, volvulus, megacolon, or rectal prolapse. Colonic perforation can occur spontaneously, usually during the attempted passage of the fecal mass. More often, perforation is iatrogenic and is signaled by the onset of fever, abdominal pain and distention, or shock shortly after disimpaction. Surgical treatment is required, and without early diagnosis mortality is high.

Stercoral ulcers in the rectum and colon probably result from pressure necrosis produced by the fecal mass. The ulcer is irregular and has a dark gray or purple outline. Biopsies reveal little inflammation. The ulcer heals rapidly after the mass is removed, but complications of bleeding or perforation have been reported.

Prevention of recurrent impaction is essential. In patients with illness predisposing to the development of impaction, prophylaxis may consist of the use of stool-wetting or bulk-forming agents. Mild laxatives may also be used when necessary.

SOLITARY RECTAL ULCER. Discrete, usually single ulcerations of unknown cause may develop in the rectum as well as in other areas of the colon. Solitary ulcer of the rectum is commonly a chronic condition in which the patient complains of painless passage of blood and/or mucus with stool and, less frequently, of dull rectal pain. In contrast, ulcers in the proximal colon usually cause acute abdominal pain. Although this condition has been called solitary ulcer, sigmoidoscopy reveals multiple lesions in 30 per cent of patients. Usually located 7 to 10 cm from the anal verge, the ulcers are shallow and occasionally have heaped-up or nodular borders. The ulcers may be round, linear, or irregular in outline and average 2 cm in diameter. They are chronic, lasting many years, and no treatment has been uniformly successful. Fortunately, complications are rare. The cause of solitary rectal ulcers has not been established. Trauma does not appear to be a major factor. Possibly the ulcer is related to the unusual entity *colitis cystica profunda,* with the ulcer resulting from rupture or cystic degeneration of heteroptic colonic mucosa. Solitary rectal ulcer must be distinguished from other diagnostic possibilities requiring more specific therapy, particularly carcinoma, Crohn's disease, and lymphogranuloma venereum. Biopsy of the rim of the ulcer is most helpful in diagnosis.

PROCTALGIA FUGAX. Proctalgia fugax is episodic severe rectal pain, probably related to spasm of the coccygeus and levator ani muscles. Anorectal infection, fracture of the coccyx, or chronic prostatitis may cause symptoms that mimic those of proctalgia fugax. Chronic trauma from poor sitting posture is said to be causative, but psychologic factors often are prominent. The pain is severe, lasting up to 45 minutes, and even may awaken the patient from sleep. The physical examination is generally normal except for muscle tenderness detected on digital rectal examination. Warm baths, muscle massage, and improvement of posture often constitute successful therapy. In most patients, the symptoms resolve spontaneously over a period of months to years.

Trauma to the coccyx can result in severe pain, termed *coccygodynia.* This may also be related to muscle spasm secondary to the trauma. The diagnosis is made by eliciting pain during movement of the coccyx, and treatment consists of administration of warm sitz baths, massage of the spastic muscles, tranquilizers such as diazepam, and local anesthetic injections.

Chronic ischemia of the rectum may also cause severe anorectal pain accompanied by fecal incontinence and rectal bleeding. This is most often seen in patients over age 50 and may follow anal surgery. Arteriography may show inferior mesenteric artery occlusion or a vascular steal.

Devroede G, Vobecky S, Masse S, et al.: Ischemic fecal incontinence and rectal angina. Gastroenterology 83:970, 1982. *A brief but comprehensive description of this entity, including histology, radiography, and rectal manometry.*

Goldberg M, Hoffman GC, Wombolt DG: Massive hemorrhage from rectal ulcers in chronic renal failure. Ann Intern Med 100:397, 1984. *Reports of the occurrence of solitary rectal ulcers in patients with chronic renal failure.*

Goodell SE, Quinn TC, Mkrtichian PA-C, et al.: Herpes simplex virus proctitis in homosexual men: Clinical, sigmoidoscopic and histopathological features. N Engl J Med 308:868, 1983. *This series of articles provides an overview of the etiology, diagnosis, and management of anorectal infections seen in homosexual men.*

McMillan A, Lee FD: Sigmoidoscopic and microscopic appearance of the rectal mucosa in homosexual men. Gut 22:1035, 1981. *In a study of 100 men who practiced anal intercourse, the authors demonstrated the presence of proctitis on both gross and histologic inspection, without microorganisms identified.*

Quinn TC, Goodell SE, Mkrtichian PA-C, et al.: Chlamydia trachomatis proctitis. N Engl J Med 305:195, 1981.

Rompalo AM, Stamm WE: Anorectal and enteric infections in homosexual men. West J Med 142:647, 1985. *A comprehensive review of the particular infectious problems of this population.*

Thompson WG: Proctalgia fugax in patients with the irritable bowel, peptic *ulcer, or inflammatory bowel disease. Am J Gastroenterol 79:450, 1984. A current review of the clinical presentation that also dispels the association with irritable bowel syndrome.*

DISEASES OF THE ANUS

By virtue of its strategic location and function, diseases of the anus occasion many complaints. Examination of the anal canal is best performed by external inspection, with the glutei spread and the patient bearing down, and with an anoscope. Most patients with common anal disorders can be well cared for without surgery or referral to a proctologist.

HEMORRHOIDS. Hemorrhoids are dilated vessels of the hemorrhoidal plexuses in the anal canal and lower rectum. By age 50, fully 50 per cent of people have hemorrhoids. *Internal hemorrhoids* arise from the superior (internal) hemorrhoidal venous plexus and are covered by rectal mucosa. *External hemorrhoids* are dilatations of the inferior (external) hemorrhoidal plexus and are covered with pain-sensitive anoderm and perianal skin. The pathogenesis of hemorrhoids remains controversial. They are not varicose veins of the rectum. The upright human posture may combine with downward pressure from defecation to cause enlargement of hemorrhoidal vessels. This effect may be enhanced when prolonged straining stretches the pelvic muscles and diminishes muscle tone, thereby causing a failure of retraction of the anal cushion after defecation. Manometric studies of the anal sphincters in patients with internal hemorrhoids often show elevated resting pressures and abnormal low-frequency pressure waves undulating at less than two cycles per minute. These changes are found in 40 per cent of patients with hemorrhoids but in only 5 per cent of people without hemorrhoids. It has been postulated that these pressure changes contribute to the development of the hemorrhoids.

Hemorrhoids are usually asymptomatic but may cause bleeding, prolapse, or a mucous anal discharge. Pain is not caused by hemorrhoids except when they thrombose. Chronic bleeding from internal hemorrhoids may be severe enough to cause iron deficiency. Prolapse of an internal hemorrhoid usually is mild, but eventually the hemorrhoid may become irreducible, leading to thrombosis. The differential diagnosis is not difficult; however, rectal bleeding should not be attributed to hemorrhoids until completion of the anorectal examination, including sigmoidoscopy.

Conservative therapy, consisting of warm sitz baths and stool softeners, usually suffices for hemorrhoids that cause only scant bleeding or minimal discomfort. Internal hemorrhoids that bleed persistently or prolapse are most successfully treated with sclerosis by the submucosal injection of a sclerosing agent (e.g., 5 per cent phenol in oil) into the tissue at the upper pole of the hemorrhoid (not into the hemorrhoid itself). Elastic band ligation has been widely used with success, but several cases of fatal sepsis after this procedure have raised concern. Photocoagulation of hemorrhoids is a new and very promising technique. These measures are not appropriate for the pain-sensitive external hemorrhoids. When these thrombose, the clot can be excised under local anesthesia. If pain is subsiding when the patient comes for treatment, simple therapy with analgesics, sitz baths, and stool softeners will usually suffice. Ointments and suppositories widely advertised for therapy of hemorrhoids have at best limited value.

ANORECTAL ABSCESS AND FISTULA. *Anorectal abscesses* are infections of the tissue spaces in and adjacent to the anorectum. Clinical features, dependent on the size and location of an abscess, usually include a throbbing, constant pain either in the perianal area or higher in the rectum. A large abscess may produce fever. The abscess is palpated externally near the anus or internally by digital rectal examination. These abscesses are classified according to their location in the anatomic spaces. The perianal abscess, just beneath the anal skin, is the most common. Other sites include the ischiorectal fossa, the intermuscular plane between the internal and external sphincters, the pelvirectal space above the levator ani and below the pelvic peritoneum, and the retrorectal space. Infection usually arises in an anal crypt. Patients with Crohn's disease, hematologic disorders, and other immune-deficient states are particularly susceptible to the development of anorectal abscesses. Prompt surgical drainage of the abscess is the treatment of choice.

Anorectal fistulas, hollow fibrous tracts lined by granulation tissue and connecting the anal canal or rectum with the perianal skin, may result from the rupture or surgical drainage of an anorectal abscess. Such fistulas may also develop from tuberculosis, Crohn's disease, carcinoma, radiation therapy, lymphogranuloma venereum, and anal fissures. Patients complain of the constant and irritating drainage of pus, blood, mucus, and occasionally stool. Treatment requires both control of the underlying disease and surgical fistulotomy.

ANAL FISSURE. An anal fissure is a longitudinal elliptical or rounded defect that occurs in the anoderm (usually in the posterior midline) and that extends into the anal canal as far as the pectinate line. The cause is most often anal trauma, usually the passage of a large, firm stool. The patient complains of severe tearing or burning anal pain and occasionally of the passage of a few drops of blood. In a patient with a chronic anal fissure, a swelling at the lower end of the fissure, the "sentinel pile," may be perceived as an anal mass. Chronic spasm and inflammation can lead to anal stenosis. Observation of fissures out of the midline or of multiple fissures should raise the question of inflammatory bowel disease, carcinoma, tuberculosis, syphilis, or other venereal disease. Most fissures heal spontaneously, and local anesthetics, sitz baths, and stool softeners give good results in most cases. Chronic fissures may require surgical excision or sphincterotomy.

PRURITUS ANI. Itching of the perianal skin is a symptom, not a diagnosis. The causes are many and varied. Principal categories of etiologies include anorectal diseases (e.g., fistulas, fissures, neoplasms); dermatologic diseases (psoriasis, eczema, lichen planus, seborrheic dermatitis); contact dermatitis (including reaction to agents commonly used to treat the pruritus); infections and parasites (especially pinworms, scabies, and pediculosis); inappropriate hygiene (either insufficient or excessive); and systemic diseases, especially diabetes mellitus and chronic liver disease. Also, many patients are thought to have pruritus on the basis of irritant stools. Normal feces are weakly acid, and diarrheal stools tend to be alkaline, which may be irritating to perianal skin. Specific therapy of one of the aforementioned conditions is the preferred approach; however, most patients require a general regimen, including avoidance of topical agents, laxatives, and tight underclothing, and careful hygiene after defecation with use of nonmedicated talcum powder if necessary. Occasionally, patients benefit from the sparing application of 1 per cent hydrocortisone to the skin, especially at night, when the symptoms seem to be worst. Anecdotal reports suggest benefit from the use of *Lactobacillus acidophilus* preparations or malt soup extract (Maltsupex) to produce a more acid colonic flora.

ANAL MALIGNANCY. Epidermoid carcinomas of the anus of various histologic types (e.g., squamous cell, basal cell, cloacogenic) constitute about 2 per cent of cancers of the large bowel. Homosexual men who practice anal-receptive intercourse may be at increased risk for this neoplasm. The lesions tend to spread widely both directly into the perianal structures and via lymphatic and hematogenous metastases. Bleeding, pain, and a mass are the usual presenting symptoms. Pruritus, mucoid drainage, and change in bowel habits may also occur. Surgical excision is necessary except in the anoderm well below the pectinate line, where small lesions may respond to irradiation. Overall five-year survival rates of 60 per cent have been reported for surgically treated patients.

Other malignancies more rarely seen in the anus include malignant melanoma, mucinous adenocarcinoma, and extramammary Paget's disease. Each of these may produce trivial symptoms and may have widely metastasized by the time of discovery. Wide surgical excisional biopsy must be performed for a suspected lesion. Abdominoperineal resection is still the treatment of choice, but its impact on survival in melanoma is unclear.

Kaposi's sarcoma of the perianal skin, anus, and rectum may occur, particularly as a manifestation of the acquired immune deficiency syndrome (AIDS). In fact this may be the earliest manifestation of the syndrome. Symptoms are rare, as is clinically significant bleeding. Local therapy of isolated lesions with radiation has been successful in selected cases, but this does not address the problem of the underlying immune defect.

FECAL INCONTINENCE. Anal sphincter dysfunction can be a most devastating result of perianal disease, anal surgery, or certain neurologic diseases. Various surgical reconstructive techniques have been employed with some success. Operant conditioning, using biofeedback techniques, has been highly successful in some individuals, and the long-term result has been good.

Bush RA, Owen WF Jr: Trauma and other noninfectious problems in homosexual men. Med Clin North Am 70:549, 1986. *A comprehensive review of these problems, their diagnosis, and treatment.*

Lieberman DA: Common anorectal disorders. Ann Intern Med 101:837, 1984. *An excellent review of pathogenesis, diagnosis, and treatment.*

112 DISEASES OF THE PERITONEUM

Michael D. Bender

ANATOMY AND PHYSIOLOGY. The peritoneum is a continuous mesothelial membrane that lines the abdominal cavity and its contained viscera. The peritoneal cavity is subdivided by peritoneal reflections and mesenteric attachments into several compartments or recesses, which are clinically important because they determine the location and spread of pathologic processes such as abscesses and metastases. The omentum, a double layer of fused peritoneum, plays an important role in peritoneal defense mechanisms by closing perforations, containing infection, and providing blood supply. The microvascular anatomy of the peritoneum consists of long, straight vessels arranged in two layers at right angles to each other, which helps account for the efficiency of the peritoneal membrane as an exchange interface.

The visceral peritoneum does not contain pain receptors; afferent stimuli are transmitted via the visceral autonomics. In contrast, the parietal peritoneum is supplied by spinal nerves that also innervate the abdominal wall. As a result, irritation of the parietal peritoneum produces well-localized somatic pain, whereas irritation of the visceral peritoneum produces a less well-defined discomfort that is poorly localized. The diaphragmatic portion of the peritoneum is supplied by the phrenic nerve centrally and by intercostal nerves peripherally. As a result, pain caused by diaphragmatic irritation may be referred either to the shoulder or to the thoracic and abdominal wall.

The peritoneal surface, a semipermeable membrane, allows for the passive diffusion of water and solutes between the abdominal cavity and the subperitoneal vascular (blood and lymphatic) channels. In general, water and solutes of molecular weight less than 2000 are absorbed from the peritoneal cavity via the blood vascular system; larger molecules and particulate substances enter the lymphatics. Movement of particles from the peritoneal cavity into the subdiaphragmatic lymphatics is facilitated by discontinuities that exist between the peritoneal mesothelial cells and the lymphatic endothelial cells. Basement membranes are scanty or absent so that particles of substantial size may move freely from the abdominal cavity into the subdiaphragmatic lymphatics, a process that may be facilitated by respiratory motion of the diaphragm itself. Water and electrolytes equilibrate rapidly (within two hours) between the blood vascular compartment and the free peritoneal cavity. *Net* fluid movement from the abdominal cavity into the plasma occurs at a maximal rate of approximately 30 to 35 ml per hour both in normal persons and in patients with portal hypertension and ascites. This rate cannot be exceeded despite vigorous diuresis; rather such diuresis only serves to remove fluid from other body compartments, and may cause hypovolemia. The importance of transperitoneal fluid exchange is also illustrated in peritonitis, in which fluid movement into the peritoneal cavity caused by increased vascular permeability can be rapid and massive and may lead to hypotension and shock.

The peritoneum heals readily after damage. Peritoneal injuries normally heal without the formation of adhesions, but in the presence of infection, ischemia, or foreign bodies, adhesions may result. In these situations, fibrinogen released into the peritoneal cavity is converted to fibrin, and then to fibrous adhesions.

DIAGNOSIS. The cardinal symptoms of peritoneal disease are *abdominal pain* and *ascites*. More variable in their occurrence are fever, distention, nausea and vomiting, and altered bowel habits. Direct tenderness, rebound tenderness, and involuntary spasm of the abdominal musculature are the major signs of peritoneal irritation. These signs and symptoms may be minimal or absent in the elderly or debilitated patient and will vary, depending on the location, cause, and acuteness of the underlying process. Because of this, peritoneal disease should be considered in any patient whose abdominal pain is difficult to diagnose.

Radiographically, ascites may be manifested by abdominal haziness, separation of bowel loops, or widening of the flank stripe on plain abdominal films. Otherwise, peritoneal disease reflects itself indirectly on barium contrast studies. Angulation, separation, or rigidity of bowel loops may indicate visceral peritoneal involvement. *Ultrasonography* and *computed tomography* may be useful in demonstrating relatively small amounts of peritoneal fluid, and especially in distinguishing free fluid from cystic masses. Computed tomography also has occasionally been successful in the demonstration of peritoneal implants and in the examination of the retroperitoneum.

If ascites is present, *abdominal paracentesis* is essential to establish its cause (see below). *Peritoneal biopsy*, particularly with the Cope needle, is a relatively simple and safe bedside technique that may yield a positive diagnosis of neoplastic or infectious causes in 50 to 60 per cent of cases. *Peritoneoscopy*, performed under the proper circumstances by a physician experienced in this technique, can be accomplished with little morbidity or mortality. A successful examination may obviate the need for exploratory surgery and may permit biopsy under direct vision of involved portions of the peritoneum or liver. If a diagnosis cannot be made in a patient with obvious peritoneal disease by means of the aforementioned procedures, *exploratory laparotomy* may be necessary.

ASCITES

CLINICAL FEATURES. The accumulation of fluid within the peritoneal cavity is a common clinical finding with a wide range of causes. Its pathophysiology varies with the cause; possible factors are outlined in Table 112–1. The pathophysiology of ascites associated with portal hypertension is considered in Chapter 127.

Small amounts of ascites may be asymptomatic, but as it

TABLE 112–1. FACTORS IN ASCITES FORMATION

Cirrhotic Ascites
Increased portal venous hydrostatic pressure
Decreased portal venous colloid osmotic pressure
Increased hepatic lymph formation
Decreased renal sodium excretion
Decreased renal free water excretion
Noncirrhotic Ascites
Increased subperitoneal capillary permeability
Decreased peritoneal lymphatic drainage
Leakage from disrupted abdominal viscera

increases the patient becomes aware of abdominal distention and a sense of fullness and discomfort. Larger amounts of ascites, especially if the abdomen is tensely distended, may cause respiratory distress, anorexia, nausea, early satiety, pyrosis, or frank pain. Body weight may vary, depending on the state of nutrition and the underlying disease process. On physical examination the flanks bulge, and a fluid wave may be demonstrable. Shifting dullness is somewhat more sensitive but may be nonspecific. Although it is difficult to detect less than 1.5 to 2 liters of fluid, placing the patient on his or her hands and knees and percussing flatness over the dependent abdomen (puddle sign) may demonstrate smaller amounts. Indirect evidence such as penile or scrotal edema, umbilical herniation, or pleural effusion may suggest the presence of ascites.

The diagnosis of ascites may be facilitated by plain abdominal films, ultrasonography, or computed tomography.

EVALUATION OF ASCITES FLUID. Once the diagnosis of ascites is made by examination, imaging techniques, or paracentesis, laboratory analysis of the fluid removed is essential to determine its cause. Evaluation of ascites fluid consists of routine studies to characterize the fluid and other studies that may be chosen depending on the clinical situation, as noted in Table 112–2.

Fluids with protein concentrations *exceeding 3 grams per 100 ml* are designated exudates, and below these values, transudates. Other characteristics that may help separate transudates from exudates include ascites-lactate dehydrogenase (LDH), and ascites-serum protein and LDH ratios. The *serum-ascites albumin gradient*, which reflects the oncotic pressure gradient between the vascular bed and the ascitic fluid, is elevated in association with increased portal pressure, whereas a low gradient occurs in conditions in which portal hypertension is not a factor in the genesis of ascites. Tests that help distinguish transudates from exudates, and their common causes, are listed in Table 112–3. Although this classification is useful, exceptions in both directions occur not infrequently. For this reason, ascitic fluid chemistries must be interpreted only in the context of all other clinical and laboratory findings.

A large number of red cells suggests the diagnosis of neoplasm, especially hepatocellular or ovarian carcinoma. Other causes of bloody ascites include tuberculosis, trauma, perforated viscus, and spontaneous bleeding associated with cirrhosis. An ascitic fluid leukocyte count of more than 500 per cubic millimeter is strongly suggestive of a peritoneal inflammatory process, such as infection or tumor infiltration. A predominance of polymorphonuclear leukocytes suggests acute bacterial infection, whereas lymphocytes and monocytes characterize chronic inflammatory disease, especially tuberculosis, but there are exceptions. Cytologic examination is essential if malignancy is suspected and may be expected to yield accurate results in more than half of cases. Samples of fluid should be cultured for bacteria, acid-fast bacilli, or fungi in the appropriate clinical setting, such as fever, undiagnosed pain, or deterioration in a patient with cirrhosis. Other chemical determinations that may be helpful in diagnosis are listed in Table 112–2.

TREATMENT: GENERAL CONSIDERATIONS. Although small or moderate amounts of ascites are often only esthetically displeasing, ascites frequently has a detrimental effect on the overall sense of well-being of the patient. Massive ascites may require urgent removal for severe abdominal discomfort, respiratory distress, cardiac dysfunction, or ulceration or impending rupture of an umbilical hernia. Paracentesis is the method of choice for rapid removal of fluid, as it rapidly reduces intra-abdominal pressure and improves cardiac performance. The risk to the patient of a single, large paracentesis of 2 to 5 liters is minimal and is not associated with a change in plasma volume in cirrhotic patients with edema. One should not hesitate to remove ascites in sufficient volume to treat the complications of tense ascites noted above, but repeated paracentesis to control ascites is rarely warranted.

In patients with intractable, disabling, massive ascites that does not respond to repeated paracentesis or diuretic therapy, peritoneovenous shunting has been successful. Because of numerous complications, careful consideration must be given before recommending peritoneovenous shunting (see Ch. 127). Details of nutritional and diuretic management of ascites are discussed in Chapter 127.

DIFFERENTIAL DIAGNOSIS OF ASCITES. More than 90

TABLE 112–2. LABORATORY ANALYSIS OF ASCITIC FLUID

Test	Abnormal Values	Clinical Situations
Red cell count	> 10,000/mm³	Routine
White cell count and differential	> 500/mm³	Routine
Total protein*	> 3 gm/dl	Routine
LDH*	> 200 IU/liter	Routine
Albumin†	< 1.1	Routine
Bacterial culture	+	Routine
Acid-fast, fungal culture	+	History or findings of Tbc; cirrhosis; immunosuppressed patient
Cytology	+	Neoplasm
Amylase‡	Ascites > serum	Pancreatitis, alcoholism, cirrhosis
Glucose‡	Ascites < serum	Tuberculosis, neoplasm, secondary bacterial peritonitis
Triglycerides‡	Ascites > serum	Chylous (milky) ascites
Starch granules (polarizing microscopy)	+	Postoperative abdominal pain
pH§	< 7.35	Spontaneous bacterial peritonitis
Lactate§	> 25 mg/dl	Spontaneous bacterial peritonitis
CEA	> 10 ng/ml	Adenocarcinoma
Hyaluronic acid¶	> 0.25 mg/ml	Mesothelioma

*Simultaneous blood value for ratio.
†Serum albumin − ascites albumin = gradient. See text.
‡Simultaneous blood value for comparison.
§Also abnormal in neoplastic, tuberculous, and pancreatic ascites.
¶Liquid chromatographic method.
LDH = lactate dehydrogenase; CEA = carcinoembryonic antigen, Tbc = tuberculosis.

TABLE 112–3. DIAGNOSIS OF TRANSUDATIVE VERSUS EXUDATIVE ASCITES

	Transudate	Exudate
Protein	< 3 gm/dl	> 3 gm/dl
LDH	< 200 IU/liter	> 200 IU/liter
Protein ascites/serum ratio	< 0.5	> 0.5
LDH ascites/serum ratio	< 0.6	> 0.6
Albumin gradient*	> 1.1	< 1.1
Common causes	Congestive heart failure	Neoplasm
	Constrictive pericarditis	Tuberculosis
	Inferior vena cava obstruction	Pancreatitis
		Myxedema
	Budd-Chiari syndrome	Vasculitis
	Cirrhosis	
	Nephrotic syndrome	
	Hypoalbuminemia	

*Serum albumin − ascites albumin.
LDH = lactate dehydrogenase.

TABLE 112–4. CAUSES OF ASCITES NOT ASSOCIATED WITH PERITONEAL DISEASE*

I. **Portal hypertension**
   A. Cirrhosis
   B. Hepatic congestion
      1. Congestive heart failure
      2. Constrictive pericarditis
      3. Inferior vena cava obstruction
      4. Hepatic vein obstruction (Budd-Chiari syndrome)
   C. Portal vein occlusion
II. **Hypoalbuminemia**
   A. Nephrotic syndrome
   B. Protein-losing enteropathy
   C. Malnutrition
III. **Miscellaneous**
   A. Myxedema
   B. Ovarian disease
      1. Meigs' syndrome
      2. Struma ovarii
      3. Ovarian overstimulation syndrome
   C. Pancreatic ascites
   D. Bile ascites
   E. Chylous ascites
   F. Urine ascites and nephrogenic ascites

*From Bender MD, Ockner RK: In Sleisenger MH, Fordtran JS (eds.): Gastrointestinal Disease. 3rd ed. Philadelphia, W. B. Saunders Company, 1983.

per cent of patients with ascites have *cirrhosis, neoplasm, congestive heart failure,* or *tuberculosis.* Causes of ascites may be divided into diseases not involving the peritoneum (Table 112–4) and diseases of the peritoneum (Table 112–5). Of those cases not associated with peritoneal disease, cirrhosis is by far the most common (Ch. 126). Portal hypertension caused by diseases of the heart and great veins accounts for a substantial number of patients with ascites of obscure origin. Included in this group are patients with congestive heart failure, constrictive pericarditis, and inferior vena cava and hepatic vein obstruction (Budd-Chiari syndrome). Clinically, patients with these conditions may not be readily distinguish-

TABLE 112–5. DISEASES OF THE PERITONEUM

I. **Infections**
   A. Bacterial peritonitis
   B. Tuberculous peritonitis
   C. Fungal diseases
      1. Candidiasis
      2. Histoplasmosis
      3. Coccidioidomycosis
      4. Cryptococcosis
   D. Parasitic diseases
      1. Schistosomiasis
      2. Enterobiasis
      3. Ascariasis
      4. Strongyloidiasis
      5. Amebiasis
II. **Neoplasms**
   A. Secondary malignancy
   B. Mesothelial hyperplasia and benign mesothelioma
   C. Primary malignant mesothelioma
   D. Pseudomyxoma peritonei
III. **Granulomatous peritonitis**
   A. Exogenous
   B. Endogenous
   C. Iatrogenic
IV. **Sclerosing peritonitis**
V. **Miscellaneous**
   A. Vasculitis
   B. Familial paroxysmal peritonitis (familial Mediterranean fever)
   C. Eosinophilic gastroenteritis
   D. Whipple's disease
   E. Gynecologic disease
      1. Endometriosis
      2. Deciduosis
      3. Gliomatosis
      4. Leiomyomatosis
      5. Dermoid cyst
      6. Melanosis
   F. Splenosis
   G. Peritoneal lymphangiectasia
   H. Peritoneal cysts
   I. Peritoneal encapsulation

*Modified from Bender MD, Ockner RK: In Sleisenger MH, Fordtran JS (eds.): Gastrointestinal Disease. 3rd ed. Philadelphia, W. B. Saunders Company, 1983.

able from those with hepatic cirrhosis; a high index of suspicion is necessary, and special procedures may be required in order to establish or exclude the diagnosis.

Hypoalbuminemia of any cause, including nephrotic syndrome and protein-losing enteropathy, may be associated with a classically transudative ascites.

Various endocrine conditions may be associated with ascites. These include *myxedema,* in which the fluid is typically protein rich, and diseases of the ovary, among them *Meigs' syndrome,* in which transudative ascites is associated with ovarian fibroma or cystadenoma, struma ovarii, ovarian edema, and "ovarian overstimulation syndrome."

Pancreatic ascites usually occurs in the presence of chronic pancreatitis or pseudocyst. The most common etiologic factors are alcohol and trauma. The ascites fluid amylase concentration is elevated, often to extremely high levels. Diagnosis of ductal disruption and pseudocyst leakage is usually possible with endoscopic retrograde pancreatography. Drainage of the pseudocyst and repair of duct injury often have been effective in managing this complication, particularly in traumatic cases. In the chronic alcoholic with pancreatic ascites, a trial of conservative management is indicated before surgery is undertaken. Leakage of bile may be associated with the development of *bile ascites,* a condition for which surgical repair of the biliary tract is usually necessary. This situation is not necessarily associated with the fulminant clinical picture of fever, leukocytosis, and peritonitis, i.e., *bile peritonitis,* which appears to result from superimposed infection.

Chylous ascites is due to the presence of lipoproteins and chylomicrons in the peritoneal cavity and is the result of lymphatic obstruction or leakage. These lipid-rich particles impart a turbidity to the fluid that facilitates its diagnosis. However, not all turbid abdominal fluids are "chylous." Establishment of the diagnosis requires direct evidence that the turbidity is indeed the result of neutral lipid, a determination best made by analysis of the fluid for triglyceride concentration. Other turbid abdominal fluids may be due to cellular debris and are designated *pseudochylous ascites,* a condition occasionally associated with abdominal neoplasm or infection. The differential diagnosis of true chylous ascites depends upon its chronicity and the age of the patient. *Chronic chylous ascites* in adults is caused in over 80 per cent of cases by abdominal neoplasm, usually lymphoma, with associated obstruction and disruption of the abdominal lymphatics resulting from extensive lymph node involvement. Inflammatory causes include tuberculosis, pancreatitis, cirrhosis, and adhesions. *Acute chylous ascites* ("chylous peritonitis") is associated with abrupt onset of abdominal pain. In some cases, this syndrome is due to trauma, intestinal obstruction, or rupture of a chylous cyst, but identifying a specific cause may not be possible even at laparotomy. In children, congenital malformations of the lymphatics, including intestinal lymphangiectasia, account for a higher proportion of the cases of chylous ascites. Treatment of chylous ascites depends on the underlying cause. General measures include (1) the use of low-fat diets with medium-chain triglyceride supplementation (these are transported by the portal vein rather than the lymphatics); (2) total parenteral nutrition, to achieve bowel rest and allow healing of damaged lymphatics; and occasionally (3) peritoneovenous shunting, if other measures are unsuccessful.

Urine ascites may result from trauma to the urinary tract, high-grade obstruction caused by posterior urethral valves in the neonate, or renal transplantation. Ascites also may occur in a few patients maintained on chronic hemodialysis. The cause appears to reflect a number of factors including prior peritoneal dialysis or infection, fluid overload, hypertension, poor nutrition, or hypoalbuminemia. Management may be difficult, but if aggressive dialysis does not help, renal transplantation seems to offer the best chance of relieving chronic ascites.

INFECTIONS OF THE PERITONEUM

ACUTE BACTERIAL PERITONITIS. Bacterial peritonitis most commonly results from perforation of an abdominal viscus caused by trauma, obstruction, infarction, neoplasm, foreign bodies, or primary inflammatory disease (Ch. 54). Peritonitis may also be associated with chronic indwelling catheters used for chronic ambulatory peritoneal dialysis, peritoneovenous shunting, and intraperitoneal chemotherapy. The peritoneum has several defense mechanisms in response to bacterial contamination: (1) Bacteria may be cleared from the peritoneum via the diaphragmatic lymphatics. (2) Opsonins, polymorphonuclear leukocytes, and macrophages enter the peritoneal cavity, where phagocytosis of bacteria can occur. (3) The peritoneum and omentum can contain localized infections and enclose small visceral perforations, in part by exudation of fibrin-containing fluid.

Regardless of etiology, abdominal pain, nausea, vomiting, tachycardia, and fever are usually present. The severity of these symptoms is related to the extent of contamination; in generalized peritonitis, shock is often present and may be profound, whereas signs and symptoms may be minimal if infection is localized. In severe cases, there may be exquisite, diffuse direct and rebound tenderness and rigidity of the abdomen; bowel sounds are usually diminished or absent, and distention may be present. Despite its dramatic presentation, recognition of acute peritonitis may be difficult in those patients in whom the clinical manifestations are masked or suppressed, such as the elderly patient or those receiving corticosteroids. In these patients, a high index of suspicion is necessary, since minor or isolated signs such as tachycardia or unexplained hypotension may herald peritonitis.

Laboratory findings are nonspecific and may include leukocytosis, hemoconcentration (from fluid loss into the peritoneum), and subdiaphragmatic air or distended intestinal loops on plain abdominal films. In debilitated or obtunded, elderly patients, *peritoneal lavage* may help establish or rule out the presence of peritonitis. One liter of fluid is instilled through a peritoneal dialysis catheter; a positive lavage fluid contains more than 500 white blood cells per cubic milliliter of fluid or more than 50,000 red blood cells per milliliter or, on Gram's stain, reveals bacteria.

The principal systemic complications of peritonitis are septicemia, shock, ileus, and widespread organ failure, including respiratory, renal, hepatic, and cardiac failure. Local complications include wound infection, abscess, anastomotic breakdown, and fistula formation.

The initial management of peritonitis includes restoration of fluid and electrolyte balance, institution of nasogastric suction to reduce distention and improve pulmonary function, oxygen, analgesics to control pain, and early antibiotic therapy. In advanced peritonitis, polymicrobial aerobic and anaerobic organisms are usually found, requiring broad-spectrum coverage. A frequently used regimen combines an aminoglycoside for aerobes with clindamycin or metronidazole for anaerobes. Cephalosporins are popular for their low toxicity and broad-spectrum coverage, especially the third-generation compounds such as cefoxitin and ceftazidime, which provide broad aerobic and anaerobic coverage (see Ch. 28). Total parenteral nutrition may be necessary in severe peritonitis with major catabolic losses.

In patients who are seen early after a recognized perforation of a viscus and who are good operative candidates, early surgery is usually indicated. In a few patients who are very poor operative risks, it may be desirable to attempt to control the process nonoperatively and to encourage its localization by antibiotic drugs and other conservative measures. Localized abscesses so formed may be drained later when circumstances are more favorable.

Despite the use of antibiotics, modern anesthesia, and intensive support systems, the mortality of generalized peritonitis remains at 50 per cent. Factors adversely affecting prognosis include older age, malnutrition, shock, and organ failure.

ABDOMINAL ABSCESSES. Intra-abdominal abscesses form from a collection of necrotic tissue, bacteria, and white blood cells contained in one of the spaces of the peritoneal cavity and walled off from the rest of the peritoneal cavity by inflammatory adhesions. The contamination is almost invariably derived from endogenous gut flora that escapes as a result of inflammatory perforation, ischemia, traumatic injury, or a surgical procedure. Abscesses within the abdomen localize in three distinct areas: the subphrenic spaces, the intermesenteric area (including the paracolic gutters and interloop areas), and the pelvis. The subphrenic and pelvic localizations reflect the dependent position of these spaces in the recumbent patient and the effect of diaphragmatic movement in drawing fluid up into the subphrenic spaces.

The diagnosis of intra-abdominal abscesses is often a difficult challenge, particularly in immunologically depressed patients with malignancy or malnutrition or patients receiving perioperative antibiotics; all of these may mask clinical signs of sepsis. Fever is the most reliable finding. Other signs and symptoms include malaise, pain, nausea, vomiting, anorexia, tachycardia, abdominal tenderness, and abdominal distention. A subphrenic localization is suggested by thoracic symptoms and signs, including dyspnea, chest pain, decreased breath sounds, dullness, and radiologic evidence of impaired diaphragmatic motion, pleural effusion, or atelectasis. Pelvic localization is suggested by urinary or rectal symptoms and careful vaginal or rectal examination. Leukocytosis with a left shift in the differential count, the usual finding, may be absent. Elevated bilirubin or hepatic enzymes may be a clue to the presence of intra-abdominal sepsis. In summary, a high degree of suspicion is important, and the possibility of an abdominal abscess should be suggested by otherwise unexplained fever, sepsis, leukocytosis, ileus, poor postoperative recovery, or organ dysfunction.

Diagnosis is facilitated by imaging procedures. Plain films may reveal nonmovable gas bubbles, often with air-fluid levels, and barium contrast studies may suggest a mass by displacement of normal structures. Ultrasonography, computed tomography, and gallium citrate 76 or indium 111 leukocyte labeling are newer modalities to diagnose and visualize abscesses. Of these, computed tomography is the most sensitive and specific. Occasionally the diagnosis is made only at the time of abdominal exploration.

Antimicrobial therapy usually suppresses the process and helps to contain it but may also obscure its recognition. Prior computed tomography–guided percutaneous aspiration, with Gram's stain and culture of the obtained fluid, may quickly confirm the presence or absence of an abscess and expedite selection of the proper antibiotic.

Appropriate drainage is indispensable for treatment of an intra-abdominal abscess. Computed tomography–guided percutaneous drainage has increasingly been utilized but may be less successful in abscesses associated with multiple cavities, viscous debris, or a source of continued contamination, such as a perforated viscus or fistula. If percutaneous drainage is inappropriate, surgical drainage should be undertaken.

PRIMARY (SPONTANEOUS) BACTERIAL PERITONITIS. Bacterial peritonitis may occur in the absence of an acute intra-abdominal precipitating factor. In this circumstance, the offending organism may not be enteric, and the syndrome is more likely to occur in patients who have pre-existing ascites, impaired immunologic defenses, or a cause for bacteremia such as localized infection elsewhere in the body or indwelling catheters. A widely recognized example of this circumstance is the child with nephrotic syndrome and ascites who develops primary peritonitis. The pathogenesis is probably hematogenous seeding of the peritoneum, particularly suggested by the frequent identification of extra-abdominal pathogens such as *Streptococcus pneumoniae*. The mortality rate associated with this entity has diminished considerably during recent decades because of the availability of antimicrobial drugs.

More common is spontaneous bacterial peritonitis in patients with advanced, decompensated cirrhosis and ascites. This syndrome is discussed in Chapter 127.

OTHER INFECTIONS. *Tuberculous peritonitis* is discussed in detail in Ch. 302. This disorder may present in a variety of ways, ranging from an acute abdomen to an insidiously developing, otherwise unexplained ascites resembling cirrhosis. Accordingly, its presence should be suspected in all patients with ascites, particularly in patients from endemic areas, in cirrhotic patients, and in immunosuppressed patients. Fewer than half of the patients have active disease elsewhere in the body, and tuberculosis skin testing and appropriate cultures of ascites fluid for tubercle bacilli should be regarded as routine in the evaluation of ascites. The diagnosis is strongly suggested by a high percentage of lymphocytes in the abdominal fluid and may be confirmed by means of a positive culture, peritoneal biopsy, laparoscopy, or, if necessary, exploratory laparotomy. The very satisfactory response of this condition to appropriate chemotherapy adds to the importance of early diagnosis.

Fungal and parasitic diseases may be associated with peritoneal involvement and occasionally with ascites. The most common fungal peritonitis is due to *candidiasis*, which may occur after contamination of the peritoneal cavity caused by perforated ulcer, trauma, surgery, or peritoneal dialysis. Other disorders, including histoplasmosis, coccidioidomycosis, cryptococcosis, ascariasis, amebiasis, and schistosomiasis, are quite uncommon, but deserve consideration in otherwise unexplained cases of peritoneal disease with or without ascites.

TUMORS OF THE PERITONEUM

SECONDARY CARCINOMATOSIS. Secondary malignancy is the most common form of neoplastic involvement of the peritoneum. More than 75 per cent of such tumors are classified as adenocarcinoma, mainly from ovary, pancreas, and colon, but peritoneal involvement by sarcoma, lymphoma, leukemia, carcinoid, and multiple myeloma has been described. Ascites formation in these patients appears to result from the combination of increased capillary permeability and obstruction of channels that drain the peritoneal cavity by way of the subdiaphragmatic lymphatics. The clinical picture is usually that associated with advancing malignancy, including weakness and weight loss, and variable complaints referable to the abdomen such as pain, distention, nausea, or vomiting. Radiographic findings may include angulation, fixation, or displacement of intestinal loops, or submucosal edema reflecting lymphatic obstruction. Ultrasonography or computed tomography may help confirm the presence of ascites and associated mass lesions. On abdominal paracentesis, the fluid obtained usually has a high LDH and protein content (more than 3.0 grams per deciliter); cellular composition is variable, and occasionally the fluid is grossly bloody (see Tables 112–2 and 112–3). The diagnosis is made by cytology in approximately 50 per cent of patients, and, if that is negative, by computed tomography–guided percutaneous biopsy or peritoneoscopy. Occasionally surgical exploration may be necessary.

Malignant ascites formation is a grave prognostic sign, with few patients surviving beyond six months after onset. Treatment of this condition involves the intraperitoneal administration of antitumor agents, including alkylators, antimetabolites, or radioactive isotopes. The standard intracavitary treatments use a small drug volume, but recent trials have used a large volume (2 liters) administered through a semipermanent indwelling catheter to allow for uniform drug distribution, high local drug levels, and repetitive treatments. Intra-abdominal quinicrine or other sclerosing agents have occasionally been successful in producing a fibrous serositis,

thereby obliterating the free peritoneal space and reducing further fluid exudation, but the usefulness of this approach is limited by the frequent occurrence of fever, nausea, vomiting, and abdominal pain.

Salt restriction and diuretics may be tried but are often unsuccessful. Paracentesis is useful, and removal of large volumes may be well tolerated; although it may reduce body protein stores, it is often indispensable for patient comfort. In selected patients, peritoneovenous shunting affords palliation in 75 per cent of cases.

PRIMARY MESOTHELIOMA. The mesothelium may undergo hyperplasia or metaplasia, and rare benign cystic and papillary mesotheliomas have been described, but most mesothelial neoplasms are malignant. Primary mesotheliomas are tumors arising from the epithelial and mesenchymal elements of the mesothelium. Approximately 25 per cent involve the peritoneum, often in association with the more frequent pleural localization. Exposure to asbestos is the most established etiologic factor (see Ch. 536), although it is unclear if asbestos fibers produce peritoneal disease by passage from the intestinal lumen, penetration of the diaphragm, or via retrograde lymphatic transport.

Mesothelioma is most common in males over the age of 50 and is associated with the gradual onset of abdominal pain and distention, anorexia, nausea, vomiting, weight loss, and ascites. Blood counts and chemistries are rarely helpful, and barium contrast films reveal nonspecific findings. Ultrasonography and computed tomography demonstrate ascites in sheetlike masses that may suggest the diagnosis. Paracentesis yields an exudate that may be hemorrhagic, and high fluid hyaluronic acid concentrations suggest the diagnosis. Peritoneoscopy reveals extensive studding of peritoneal surfaces with nodules and plaques. However, laparotomy is often necessary to provide adequate biopsies and rule out a primary neoplasm. Even with biopsy or cytologic specimens, the variable histologic characteristics of epithelial and mesenchymal elements may make it difficult to differentiate from other malignancies.

The prognosis of peritoneal mesothelioma is exceedingly poor, with a median survival of about one year after diagnosis. Death usually results from cachexia or obstruction rather than metastatic disease. Tumor response and increased survival have been reported after chemotherapy (especially doxorubicin) and/or radiotherapy. Intensive combination therapy with surgical debulking, whole abdominal radiotherapy, and intraperitoneal doxorubicin and cisplatin may provide substantial palliation in selected, early cases.

PSEUDOMYXOMA PERITONEI. Pseudomyxoma peritonei is a rare condition in which the peritoneal cavity becomes distended with a mucinous, semisolid, translucent material. The two major causes of this "mucinous ascites" are mucinous cystadenomas and cystadenocarcinomas of the ovary and appendix, although other tumors of the genitourinary and gastrointestinal tract have been associated with the process. Extensive pseudomyxoma is invariably associated with cystadenocarcinomas, although they may be low grade.

The condition usually presents as an increase in abdominal girth with little in the way of other clinical signs of disease. At surgery, the abdominal cavity is found to contain gelatinous material existing in a variety of states, including cystic masses, lying freely without apparent attachment or anchored to the peritoneal surface. If the tumor is indeed malignant, it appears to be low grade and rarely metastasizes. As a result, the course of the disease is prolonged and is characterized by recurrent episodes of intestinal obstruction and fistula formation. Surgical removal of the ovary, appendix, and as much mucin as possible and intraperitoneal instillation of an alkylating agent are usually indicated.

GRANULOMATOUS PERITONITIS. The peritoneum responds to a wide variety of stimuli with a granulomatous inflammatory reaction. *Exogenous* causes include mycobacteria, parasites, fungi, or organic material; *endogenous* causes are rare and include keratin in squamous tumors, meconium, sarcoidosis, and Crohn's disease. The most common etiology is *iatrogenic*, due to contamination at the time of surgery from starch, talc, cotton, or wood fibers used in surgical gloves, gowns, or drapes. *Starch granulomatous peritonitis* presents two to nine weeks postoperatively with pain, tenderness, fever, distention, nausea, and vomiting, and may suggest adhesions or abscesses. If it is considered, the diagnosis can be made by demonstrating starch granules in peritoneal fluid. Short-term indomethacin or corticosteroids often speeds recovery.

SCLEROSING PERITONITIS. This unusual form of peritonitis manifests with symptoms of intestinal obstruction caused by the encasement of the entire small bowel in a fibrotic membrane or "cocoon." It has been reported following peritoneovenous shunting, chronic ambulatory peritoneal dialysis, practolol (but not other beta blockers) administration, intraperitoneal chemotherapy and as an idiopathic form in young females. The etiology is unclear but may involve toxins or subacute infections that stimulate fibroblast proliferation.

MISCELLANEOUS DISEASES OF THE PERITONEUM. The peritoneal membrane may be affected by a wide variety of systemic diseases, including systemic lupus erythematosus (see Ch. 436) and other collagen vascular diseases, Whipple's disease (see Ch. 104), familial Mediterranean fever (see Ch. 209), and eosinophilic gastroenteritis. Rarely, unusual tissues deposit on the peritoneum, which may cause low grade peritoneal symptoms or be mistaken for metastatic carcinoma. Examples include endometrial, decidual, glial, and splenic tissue. Several other unusual conditions affecting the peritoneum have been described (Table 111–5).

Antman KH, Pomfret EA, Aisner J, et al.: Peritoneal mesothelioma: Natural history and response to chemotherapy. J Clin Oncol 1:386, 1983. *A concise report of 23 patients from two oncology centers with a large experience in mesothelioma.*
Bastani B, Sharietzadeh MR, Dehdashti F: Tuberculous peritonitis—report of 30 cases and review of the literature. Q J Med 56:549, 1985. *Presents clinical data from Iran, as well as a thorough review of clinical statistics from studies over the last 20 years.*
Bender MD, Ockner RK: Ascites. In Sleisenger MH, Fordtran JS (eds.): Gastrointestinal Disease. 4th ed. Philadelphia, W. B. Saunders Company, 1988.
Bender MD, Ockner RK: Diseases of the peritoneum, mesentery and diaphragm. In Sleisenger MH, Fordtran JS (eds.): Gastrointestinal Disease. 4th ed. Philadelphia, W. B. Saunders Company, 1988. *A broad review, extensively referenced.*
Hau T, Haaga JR, Aeder MI: Pathophysiology, diagnosis, and treatment of abdominal abscesses. Curr Probl Surg 21:1, 1984. *A comprehensive monograph covering all aspects of abdominal abscesses, including current perspectives on percutaneous drainage.*
Press OW, Press NO, Kaufman SD: Evaluation and management of chylous ascites. Ann Intern Med 96:358, 1982. *An analysis of 28 cases from one institution, seen over 20 years.*
Weaver DW, Walt AJ, Sugawa C, et al.: A continuing appraisal of pancreatic ascites. Surg Gynecol Obstet 154:845, 1982. *Reviews a series of 42 alcoholic patients with chronic pancreatitis. Preoperative endoscopic retrograde cholangiopancreatography (ERCP) is emphasized to plan the surgical approach.*

113 DISEASES OF THE MESENTERY AND OMENTUM

Michael D. Bender

GENERAL CLINICAL FEATURES. Patients with mesenteric disease usually have nonspecific symptoms such as abdominal pain, distention, or intestinal obstruction. The most frequent physical finding is a mass, which may be mobile. There are no specific laboratory findings, but mesenteric disease may be suspected if calcifications, displacement of bowel loops, or pressure deformities are observed radiographically. Ultrasonography and computed tomogra-

phy are useful in identifying mesenteric and omental masses. However, definitive diagnosis usually depends on direct inspection and biopsy, either surgically or by peritoneoscopy.

MESENTERIC INFLAMMATORY DISEASE. This syndrome includes a spectrum of conditions ranging from acute inflammation to a chronic fibrosing process associated with intestinal obstruction, ascites, and steatorrhea. Included are such conditions as "mesenteric panniculitis" and "retractile mesenteritis." The cause of this syndrome is not known, but it is believed to represent the sequel to some inciting event such as trauma, infection, or ischemia in the mesentery. Fat necrosis occurs, evoking an inflammatory reaction with subsequent scarring and granuloma formation.

The condition is most commonly seen in males and in late adulthood. The acute syndrome ("mesenteric panniculitis"), which constitutes the presentation of 60 per cent of cases, is characterized by recurring abdominal pain, weight loss, nausea, vomiting, and fever. In most patients, a tender abdominal mass is palpable; leukocytosis may or may not be present. The remaining 40 per cent of cases are identified by the discovery of a mass on examination or at surgery. Radiographic examination is nonspecific, showing the effects of an abdominal mass and variable scarring that includes displacement and separation of intestinal loops with angulation, stenosis, and extrinsic compression. In some patients the condition evolves into a more chronic process ("retractile mesenteritis"), characterized by continuing pain, fever, weight loss, and various signs of intestinal obstruction, ascites, and steatorrhea. At surgery, the small bowel mesentery is found to be the principal site of involvement; it is thickened and fibrotic, particularly at the root. Resection of the mass is often not possible, and generally should not be attempted. Microscopically in mesenteric panniculitis there is infiltration of adipose tissue by foamy macrophages and lymphocytes, with fat necrosis, fibrosis, and calcification. In retractile mesenteritis, the thickening and fibrosis are more pronounced, and there is less evidence of acute necrosis and inflammation. Infrequently, the mesocolon or parietal peritoneum may be involved, or the process may occur in association with retroperitoneal fibrosis.

Most patients seem to have prolonged survival and become asymptomatic after a period of months to years. A minority exhibits the more chronic symptoms noted earlier. The role of corticosteroids is uncertain; although they may be effective in the management of those patients in whom acute symptoms predominate, there is no evidence that they affect the long-term prognosis or progression of the disease. In 15 per cent of patients, malignant lymphomas develop; the basis for this apparent association is not known.

MESENTERIC AND OMENTAL CYSTS AND TUMORS. Mesenteric cysts usually develop as the result of anomalies in the mesenteric lymphatic system but may also be of mesothelial origin. They may spontaneously wax and wane in size; usually they do not cause symptoms in patients less than 10 years of age. Symptoms are related to the size and position of the cyst, which on physical examination is nontender, round, and mobile. Spontaneous rupture, hemorrhage, or infection may occur, but these complications are unusual. Treatment consists of surgical enucleation or excision.

Mesenteric tumors are rare and usually arise from the cellular elements normally present in the mesentery. They include fibromas, myxomas, lipomas, and other less common neoplasms of mesenchymal or neural origin. Most are well-differentiated, low-grade fibrosarcomas that produce symptoms such as pain, weight loss, abdominal mass, and compression of adjacent organs. They may be treated successfully by surgical excision. Others are more highly malignant and may metastasize distantly. *Mesenteric lymphoid tumors* also occur, and certain of these have been associated with unexplained abnormalities in iron metabolism with hypochromic microcytic anemia. *Metastatic tumors* of the mesentery are more common than primary tumors and are usually due to enlarged lymphomatous or carcinomatous lymph nodes.

Tumors of the omentum, unlike those of the mesentery, are chiefly muscular in origin (leiomyomas, leiomyosarcomas). About 40 per cent of these are malignant and cause symptoms by virtue of local invasion and development of an abdominal mass; distant metastasis is unusual.

MISCELLANEOUS DISEASES. *Torsion of the omentum* is an acute surgical condition that mimics acute appendicitis or cholecystitis. It usually occurs in patients over age 30 and causes right-sided abdominal pain with nausea, vomiting, fever, leukocytosis, and occasionally a mass. Omentectomy is indicated. *Idiopathic primary omental infarction* presents a similar clinical picture and is invariably diagnosed only at laparotomy. *Mesenteric fibromatosis* (desmoid tumor) is a benign, noninflammatory fibrous proliferation of the mesentery, which occurs mainly in patients with familial polyposis of the colon or Gardner's syndrome.

Bender MD, Ockner RK: Diseases of the peritoneum, mesentery and diaphragm. In Sleisenger MH, Fordtran JS (eds.): Gastrointestinal Disease. 4th ed. Philadelphia, W. B. Saunders Company, 1988. *A broad review, extensively referenced.*

Vanek VW, Phillips AK: Retroperitoneal, mesenteric and omental cysts. Arch Surg 119:838, 1984. *Surveys the literature and gives a complete overview of cystic lesions.*

114 GASTROINTESTINAL HEMORRHAGE

Walter L. Peterson

Gastrointestinal (GI) hemorrhage is a common clinical problem. Despite increased availability of intensive care units and improved methods of diagnosis, mortality from upper gastrointestinal hemorrhage is still approximately 10 per cent, which represents almost no decline over the past 30 years. The most likely reason for this observation is that the efficacy of available therapy is little better today than 30 years ago. This is especially true for the group of patients who account for the largest share of overall mortality, i.e., those with bleeding esophageal or gastric varices. This chapter describes general considerations in the management of the patient with gastrointestinal hemorrhage. The important goals in this regard are (1) hemodynamic stabilization of the patient, (2) cessation of bleeding by the least invasive technique possible, and (3) prevention of recurrent hemorrhage. The overall approach to the patient with GI hemorrhage is shown in Figure 114–1.

RECOGNITION OF GASTROINTESTINAL HEMORRHAGE

PRESENTING SIGNS AND SYMPTOMS. Patients with GI hemorrhage have either obvious efflux of blood from the GI tract or no external manifestation (i.e., occult bleeding). Efflux of blood is manifested as (1) *hematemesis*, in which bright red or "coffee-ground" material is vomited; (2) *melena*, which is black, tarry, sticky, odoriferous stool;* and (3) *hematochezia*, the passage of bright red or maroon stool. Occult bleeding may occur with (1) signs and symptoms of *hypovolemia*; (2) *anemia*, either symptomatic or detected only by routine laboratory screening; or (3) chemical evidence of *occult blood* in the stool.

OBJECTIVE CONFIRMATION. Objective evidence that blood has entered the GI tract may be obtained by examining the gastric aspirate or stool for blood. If blood is not grossly evident, a chemical test for occult blood—for example, Hem-

---

*Melena must not be confused with dark stools produced by iron or bismuth compounds.

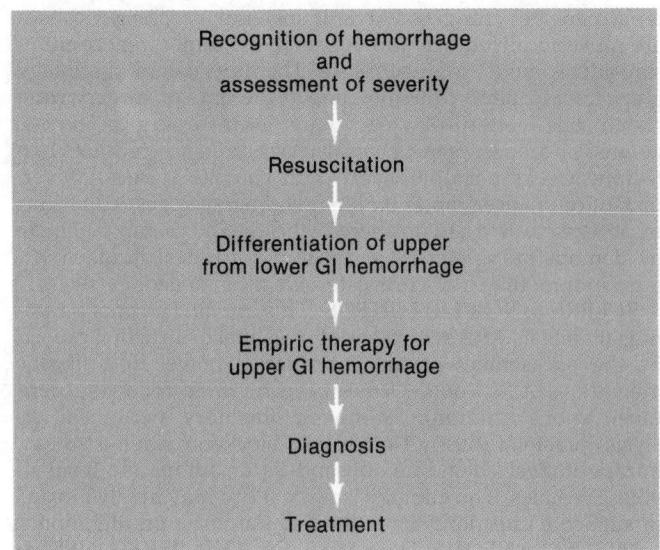

FIGURE 114–1. Approach to the patient with gastrointestinal hemorrhage.

occult—can be performed on a stool specimen. False-positive results occur 1 to 2 per cent of the time. Vitamin C may produce false-negative tests. The hematocrit should always be measured to substantiate blood loss from any source or site, although the hematocrit may be normal immediately after an acute bleeding episode (see below).

RAPIDITY AND MAGNITUDE OF HEMORRHAGE. After confirming that a patient is bleeding (or recently has bled), the physician must determine whether it is continuing, determine its rapidity and magnitude, and begin resuscitation. These are important steps that must precede any concern for the site of gastrointestinal hemorrhage, whether upper or lower.

The rapidity of hemorrhage is gauged initially by the manner in which bleeding is manifested. Hematochezia or repeated episodes of copious hematemesis suggest brisk hemorrhage, as does inability to clear the nasogastric aspirate of bright red blood with gastric lavage. The ultimate measure of rapidity of hemorrhage remains the amount and rapidity of blood transfusions required to restore and maintain the vascular volume.

The magnitude of hemorrhage can be estimated by the clinical presentation. Melena can be produced experimentally by as little as 100 to 200 ml of blood, although in clinical practice the presence of melena almost always indicates at least 500 ml of blood loss. Upper gastrointestinal (UGI) bleeding manifested by hematochezia suggests losses of 1000 ml or more. By contrast, as little as 25 ml blood loss will produce a guaiac-positive stool.

Acute blood losses greater than 1000 ml are more accurately estimated by evidence of hypovolemia manifested by tachycardia, hypotension, or a fall in blood pressure upon change of position (orthostatic hypotension). These signs must be evaluated with knowledge of the physiologic compensatory responses following an acute GI hemorrhage (see below). To interpret these signs too literally may lead to underestimation of the severity of the hemorrhage, a cardinal danger in the management of such patients.

PATHOPHYSIOLOGY OF ACUTE BLEEDING. The hematocrit and blood pressure measured initially in a bleeding patient reflect four basic factors: (1) pre-existing blood volume, (2) the volume of blood lost, (3) the rate at which it is lost, and (4) the extent of endogenous volume replacement. Following loss of 20 per cent of the circulating blood volume (1000 ml), there is an immediate fall in blood pressure, a rise in heart rate, and peripheral vasoconstriction. The hematocrit initially remains unchanged. Only as fluid enters the vascular space from extravascular compartments does the hematocrit fall and blood pressure rise. The heart rate may soon return to normal or actually fall below normal and may therefore be an unreliable sign of the severity of a hemorrhage. As noted, the level of the hematocrit depends on the rapidity and completeness of dilution of the remaining blood as well as the severity of the hemorrhage. An isolated hematocrit reading, unless low, is of little help.

The blood pressure is the most important sign of the state of blood volume and most accurately mirrors the severity of the situation. However, it is also affected by the patient's age, pre-existing blood pressure, and ability to mobilize fluid. For example, a dehydrated patient who bleeds acutely may be unable to restore volume. The resulting blood pressure will be low and the hematocrit may remain normal or high. A low hematocrit, low blood pressure, or rapid heart rate usually indicates a severe hemorrhage. A normal hematocrit, normal blood pressure, or normal heart rate must be interpreted with caution.

INITIAL THERAPY

RESUSCITATION. Initial therapy (resuscitation) is independent of the source of bleeding. Rather, it is dependent on the rapidity and magnitude of hemorrhage. Generally, patients should be placed in an intensive care unit unless it is clear that the bleeding is mild or chronic and the patient does not require resuscitation. It is also prudent to obtain surgical consultation to follow the patient through resuscitation, diagnosis, and therapy, so that rapid surgical assistance is available if needed. Resuscitation is directed toward supporting the vascular volume and providing adequate tissue oxygenation. Large intravenous catheters should be inserted, at times into a large central vein, and fluids begun. The physician must remember that the dilutional effect of exogenous fluids will lower the hematocrit. Nasal oxygen (2.0 to 3.0 liters per minute) may be necessary, particularly for elderly persons or those with cardiac or pulmonary disease. Urine output and systemic blood pressure should be closely monitored and, if necessary, central venous or pulmonary wedge pressures as well. Blood is sent for typing and crossmatching as well as for other laboratory data (especially determinations of clotting factors). An electrocardiogram and chest radiograph should be obtained and, to record the patient's progress, a flow sheet for fluids, vital signs, and other values is initiated.

The blood products administered depend upon the rapidity of hemorrhage and the resources of individual blood banks. Patients with active bleeding should receive whole blood if possible; but if packed red blood cells must be used to treat active bleeding, fresh frozen plasma should be given with every 4 to 6 units.

In patients whose plasma volume has been restored from extravascular compartments, packed red blood cells are sufficient. Packed cells are indicated especially in elderly patients with chronic bleeding who are in shock and in whom whole blood may produce vascular volume overload. Fresh frozen plasma should be given to patients whose bleeding has ceased only if there are demonstrated needs. For example, patients with cirrhosis may have special needs for clotting factors present in fresh frozen plasma.

When and how much blood is transfused varies from patient to patient and is dependent upon several factors. These include the volume of blood lost, the presence or absence of continuing hemorrhage, the chronicity of blood loss, and the patient's clinical response to blood loss. For example, a young patient may tolerate without transfusion a hematocrit of 25 per cent or less quite well, especially if bleeding has been chronic; on the other hand, an older patient, at the same hematocrit, may have postural hypotension, confusion, or angina pectoris and require transfusion. Patients with continuing hemorrhage usually require blood regardless of the absolute hematocrit level. A hematocrit of 30 per cent has proved to be a satisfactory level to achieve

with transfusions. Nevertheless, the requirements for numbers of units of blood must often be determined individually, based on the patient's clinical status.

DISTINGUISHING BETWEEN UPPER AND LOWER GASTROINTESTINAL HEMORRHAGE

As restorative therapy is begun, thought should be given to whether the source of bleeding is from the upper or lower gastrointestinal tract. Hematemesis connotes a source of bleeding above the ligament of Treitz. Melena results from the breakdown of blood during its transit through the intestinal tract. The longer blood remains in the GI tract, the more likely melena will occur. Therefore, melena occurs most often from upper GI bleeding lesions and only occasionally from bleeding sites as distal as the right colon. Hematochezia represents either a very rapid, massive (1000 ml) UGI hemorrhage or, more likely, a lower intestinal source. Hypovolemia, anemia, or occult stool blood may be manifestations of either upper or lower GI hemorrhage. To confirm or detect a UGI source, a nasogastric tube is placed. A bloody aspirate is diagnostic of UGI hemorrhage; a clear aspirate effectively rules out active bleeding from the esophagus and stomach. When the gastric aspirate is negative for blood, the source of bleeding is usually lower GI, but an actively bleeding postpyloric lesion (such as duodenal ulcer) may still be present. Obviously the nasogastric aspirate may be negative if bleeding has ceased.

Other findings in UGI bleeding include hyperactive bowel sounds, leukocytosis, low-grade fever, and elevation of the blood urea nitrogen (BUN). Elevation of the BUN in acute UGI bleeding probably represents a combination of (1) absorption of a high protein load (approximately 15 grams of globin plus plasma proteins per 100 ml of blood) with resulting increased synthesis of urea and (2) hypovolemia with reduced renal perfusion.

EMPIRIC THERAPY FOR UPPER GASTROINTESTINAL HEMORRHAGE

If the patient is suspected of having UGI hemorrhage, a nasogastric tube is placed to document that its source is esophageal, gastric, or (in many cases) immediately postpyloric and to gauge the rapidity of bleeding. If the aspirate is a flow of fresh blood, this tube is withdrawn and is replaced with a large-bore orogastric tube for gastric lavage. Large volumes (500 to 1000 ml) of iced saline or tap water are lavaged through the orogastric tube, although room temperature fluids may function as well. The fluid is removed from the stomach by gravity drainage, avoiding excess suction, which can damage the gastric mucosa. Gastric lavage serves several purposes: the rate of bleeding is gauged, blood clots are evacuated, and hemostasis may be promoted. Although cause and effect have not been proved, gastric lavage is associated with cessation of such bleeding in 85 to 90 per cent of patients. No therapeutic intervention, including cimetidine, has been shown to improve upon the results obtained with lavage alone. The amount of lavage fluid required varies from patient to patient. Gastric contents will clear in some with 1 to 2 liters of fluid, whereas in others 10 or more liters may be required.

If bleeding does not subside during lavage, levarterenol (Levophed, 8 mg in 100 ml of normal saline) may be instilled into the stomach through the nasogastric tube. Such local vasoconstrictor therapy may be effective as a stopgap measure, although no controlled evidence is available to prove its effectiveness.

If hemorrhage ceases during lavage, empiric therapy should be begun for the most common cause of UGI hemorrhage in the nonalcoholic—i.e., peptic ulcer. One such approach is to maintain gastric pH as close to neutrality as possible during the initial 24 to 72 hours when recurrent hemorrhage is most likely. This may be accomplished by blocking acid secretion with an H_2-receptor blocking agent and monitoring gastric pH hourly. Hourly doses of supplemental antacids (beginning with 30-ml aliquots of an aluminum-magnesium preparation) are then instilled through the nasogastric tube to maintain the pH near 7. When a particular dose of antacid is found that will reliably maintain the pH near 7, the nasogastric tube can be withdrawn and antacids given orally. After three days, therapy is continued with standard doses of ulcer medication (see Ch. 100).

DIAGNOSTIC APPROACH TO DETERMINE THE SPECIFIC CAUSE OF HEMORRHAGE

To this point in a patient's course, attention has been directed toward establishing that GI hemorrhage has occurred, determining its rapidity and magnitude, localizing the source as upper or lower GI, and initiating resuscitation. During this time, it is important to obtain a careful history and perform a thorough physical examination. Although the information obtained often provides only valuable clues, it may at times be diagnostic. The subsequent approach to treatment depends on whether or not bleeding continues or ceases with initial therapy.

UPPER GASTROINTESTINAL HEMORRHAGE. Helpful historic information includes prior episodes of bleeding, associated illnesses (e.g., cirrhosis), medications taken (especially analgesics and anticoagulants), or prior abdominal surgery (for peptic ulcer or for placement of aortic vascular prostheses). Has the patient experienced epistaxis or hemoptysis? Does the patient tell of dyspepsia, heartburn, or retching prior to hematemesis, which may indicate peptic ulcer, reflux esophagitis, or a Mallory-Weiss mucosal tear, respectively? On physical examination, the physician should look for cutaneous manifestations of underlying diseases such as Osler-Weber-Rendu syndrome, Ehlers-Danlos syndrome, pseudoxanthoma elasticum, and the blue rubber bleb nevus syndrome. Is there adenopathy to suggest malignancy? Or jaundice, palmar erythema, spider angiomas, or hepatosplenomegaly to suggest cirrhosis?

If Hemorrhage Continues Despite Initial Therapy. If bleeding continues even after vigorous gastric lavage, further therapy may be invasive and will differ depending upon the actual source of bleeding. Therefore, rapid, accurate diagnosis is required and is best achieved with panendoscopy. In the occasional situation in which bleeding is so brisk as to preclude visualization by endoscopy, and if time will allow, arteriography will often delineate an actively bleeding arterial site. If none is found, venous bleeding from varices is inferred. Arteriography offers the additional advantage of permitting infusion of vasoconstrictor drugs or embolization of a substance such as Gelfoam into the offending vessel as a means of treatment. Barium studies of the UGI tract are not appropriate in this setting, because only potential bleeding sites can be seen and because the contrast material may hinder further diagnostic procedures such as endoscopy or arteriography.

Rapid bleeding from fistulization of an aortofemoral bypass graft into the duodenum is a special situation. The nasogastric aspirate is often clear, but melena or marked hematochezia suggests a UGI site. In a patient with an aortofemoral graft, endoscopy of the esophagus, stomach, and proximal duodenum should be done immediately to exclude a bleeding site other than a graft-enteric fistula. The fistula itself, if present, is rarely seen at endoscopy. Arteriography may not reveal the bleeding from the graft and should not be done. Immediate surgery is indicated in patients with grafts if no other site of hemorrhage is visualized.

If Hemorrhage Ceases with Initial Therapy. In most patients (85 per cent or more), hemorrhage ceases with initial therapy or is not active at the time of admission and urgent diagnosis is not required. Most patients should undergo either a barium

UGI series or panendoscopy for diagnostic evaluation. The UGI series is a safe, inexpensive procedure that will detect most UGI malignancies and many peptic ulcers. This is especially true if a double-contrast radiographic examination is performed. Panendoscopy is more specific and sensitive, and hence a more accurate diagnostic tool (especially for superficial bleeding lesions). Clinical settings in which endoscopy is the preferable diagnostic test are shown in Table 114–1.

Angiography is rarely indicated in patients who cease bleeding, for it will detect only abnormal vascular patterns that are rare and may or may not be the actual source of bleeding. Nevertheless, in selected cases of UGI bleeding in which UGI radiographs and endoscopy are unrevealing, arteriography may be helpful (see The Diagnostic Dilemma, below).

LOWER GASTROINTESTINAL HEMORRHAGE. Remote and recent historical points that are important in assessing lower gastrointestinal hemorrhage include a prior history of rectal bleeding (hemorrhoids, diverticulosis, or polyps), a recent change in stool caliber (colonic cancer), acute abdominal pain with bleeding (ischemic colitis), or recurrent or bloody diarrhea (inflammatory bowel disease). A history of familial colonic polyposis or of an aortofemoral bypass graft would also be very important. On physical examination, one should palpate for abdominal masses, look for external hemorrhoids, and note any masses present on digital rectal examination. Inflammatory bowel disease or familial polyposis may have extracolonic manifestations involving skin, bones, or joints (see Ch. 105 and 107).

If Hemorrhage Continues Despite Initial Therapy. Anoscopy and proctosigmoidoscopy can detect lesions involving the lower 20 to 25 cm of the colon, such as hemorrhoids, polyps, inflammatory bowel diseases, ischemic colitis, or rectosigmoid cancer. On many occasions, however, all that can be seen is blood coming from somewhere above the level reached by the instruments. While an angiography team is being assembled, it is reasonable to perform a quick upper endoscopy to exclude a postpyloric bleeding site in the UGI tract. If endoscopy is negative, and if bleeding persists, angiography will sometimes localize the site of lower intestinal bleeding, although perhaps not the specific lesion (see above for the approach to possible bleeding from aortofemoral grafts). This is especially helpful in patients bleeding from diverticula or vascular anomalies. Intra-arterial infusions of vasopressin may even stop the bleeding before surgical intervention is required. Barium enema examination should not be performed, as it will preclude subsequent angiography. Colonoscopy is difficult in the face of continuing hemorrhage, but may be performed if bleeding slows to an ooze.

Detection of intestinal extravasation of a radioisotope such as technetium 99m (^{99}Tc)–labeled sulfur colloid is a noninvasive means to localize active bleeding. ^{99}Tc sulfur colloid is rapidly cleared from the blood by the liver and spleen, which means that bleeding may be detected only a short time. Attachment of ^{99}Tc to the patient's own red blood cells avoids this problem. While important therapeutic decisions should probably not be based solely on the results of radionuclide scanning until more experience has been gained, this technique may provide clues to the location of bleeding and may at the least be a helpful screening test prior to arteriography.

TABLE 114–1. CLINICAL SETTINGS FOR ENDOSCOPY IN PATIENTS WITH UGI BLEEDING*

1. Radiologic technique is inadequate
2. Patient has had gastric resection
3. Endoscopic or surgical therapy is planned
4. More than one lesion may be present (especially in patients with varices)
5. Vascular graft is in place

*These are settings in which endoscopy is preferable to a barium UGI series.

If Hemorrhage Ceases with Initial Therapy. Patients whose bleeding ceases spontaneously during resuscitation should in most instances undergo colonoscopy at the earliest convenient time. This is the quickest, most convenient, and most accurate means of making a diagnosis. If colonoscopy is not performed, the patient should undergo proctoscopy and then be observed for 48 hours before further diagnostic evaluation. A barium enema is not performed before this time for fear of being unable to utilize arteriography (because of residual barium) should hemorrhage recur. After 48 hours a barium enema may be obtained. In some patients, the results of the barium enema, when coupled with the clinical findings, may complete the evaluation. In others, colonoscopy may be performed (after cleansing the colon) to confirm or biopsy lesions detected by barium enema, to exclude other sources of bleeding in the large number of patients who may have diverticulosis as an incidental finding, and to detect mucosal lesions or small polyps missed by barium enema. Patients who experience recurrent hemorrhage during the first 48-hour period may require angiography or, if bleeding again ceases or slows, colonoscopy, if not yet performed. If evaluation of the patient with presumed lower GI bleeding is unrewarding, UGI sources should be excluded with an UGI series and possible endoscopy; lesions below the ligament of Treitz but above the terminal ileum may be sought with a small bowel series (see The Diagnostic Dilemma, below).

SPECIFIC CAUSES OF HEMORRHAGE AND THEIR TREATMENT

The causes of GI bleeding are shown in Table 114–2. The ligament of Treitz is generally considered the dividing point for upper and lower GI lesions. However, because jejunal and ileal lesions are so rarely the cause of GI bleeding, lower GI bleeding almost always comes from the colon.

UPPER GASTROINTESTINAL HEMORRHAGE. The three most common causes of serious upper gastrointestinal bleeding are peptic ulcer, acute mucosal lesions, and esophageal varices.

Peptic ulcer (gastric, duodenal, or postsurgical anastomotic ulcers) will in most cases require urgent surgery if bleeding does not cease. In some patients, surgery may be precluded, or at least delayed, by application of one of the available endoscopic modalities to coagulate the bleeding lesion thermally. Unfortunately, use of such techniques is not based on clear results from controlled clinical trials. Only laser therapy has been well studied, and results are conflicting. If bleeding ceases, therapy after the first three days (see above) is the same as for nonbleeding ulcers, i.e., antacids, sucralfate, or histamine H_2-receptor antagonists (see Ch. 100). Use of endoscopically delivered thermal therapy to prevent rebleeding in selected patients remains unsettled. *Acute mucosal lesions* (esophagitis, gastritis, or Mallory-Weiss tears) that continue

TABLE 114–2. CAUSES OF GI BLEEDING

Upper GI	Upper or Lower GI	Lower GI
Duodenal ulcer	Neoplasms	Hemorrhoids
Gastric ulcer	Carcinoma	Anal fissure
Anastomotic ulcer	Leiomyoma	Diverticulosis
Esophagitis	Sarcoma	Meckel's diverticulum
Gastritis	Hemangioma	Ischemic bowel disease
Mallory-Weiss tear	Lymphoma	Inflammatory bowel
Esophageal varices	Melanoma	disease
Hematobilia	Polyps	Solitary colonic ulcer
Menetrier's disease	Arterial-enteric fistulas	Intussusception
	Vascular anomalies	
	Osler-Weber-Rendu	
	Blue rubber bleb nevus	
	CREST syndrome	
	Arteriovenous malformations	
	Angiodysplasia (vascular ectasia)	
	Hematologic diseases	
	Elastic tissue disorders	
	Pseudoxanthoma elasticum	
	Ehlers-Danlos	
	Vasculitis syndromes	
	Amyloidosis	

bleeding often respond to intra-arterial infusions of vasoconstrictor drugs such as vasopressin, thereby precluding the need for surgery. Such treatment, of course, necessitates catheterization of visceral arteries, usually the celiac. In some centers embolic therapy with blood clot or Gelfoam is also used. If bleeding ceases, acute mucosal lesions are treated with measures to reduce gastric acidity, although Mallory-Weiss lesions usually require no specific therapy. If aspirin is believed to be the cause of acute gastric mucosal bleeding, other analgesics should be substituted. This should be done cautiously, since most other analgesics (with the exception of enteric-coated aspirin) also may cause mucosal bleeding. "Stress" gastritis can be prevented in patients predisposed to this lesion by the prophylactic administration of frequent, large doses of a potent antacid.

Continuing hemorrhage from *esophageal or gastric varices* is a condition for which no therapy has been convincingly shown to be satisfactory. A low-dose, constant intravenous infusion of vasopressin* (0.1 to 0.4 unit per minute) is often recommended. This therapy may be no better than placebo at stopping variceal bleeding. Use of vasopressin may also result in unwanted side effects of arterial vasoconstriction, including mesenteric ischemia and angina pectoris. Concomitant use of nitroglycerin may reduce the incidence of side effects. Balloon tamponade will often stop the bleeding but at a substantial risk of esophageal perforation or pulmonary aspiration. Because emergent or even urgent surgery for variceal hemorrhage carries with it an extremely high mortality in patients with cirrhosis of the liver, new techniques such as transhepatic obliteration of varices or endoscopic sclerotherapy have been developed. Because the transhepatic angiographic technique requires puncture of a diseased, easily bleeding liver, and because there are more endoscopists available than angiographers, endoscopic sclerotherapy has more or less been given pre-eminence. Although controlled data are scarce, it appears that urgent endoscopic sclerotherapy will stanch variceal bleeding most of the time. If hemorrhage has ceased, and depending upon the individual circumstances, consideration may be given to means of preventing future episodes of hemorrhage. Propranolol, a beta-blocking agent that lowers portal pressure, has been suggested as one form of long-term therapy to prevent recurrent variceal bleeding. However, reductions in portal pressure are often trivial, and controlled trials do not uniformly show efficacy. More reliable is portal vein decompressive surgery, which prevents recurrent bleeding in a large proportion of patients. Hepatic encephalopathy often occurs after portal vein decompression, however, so many experts recommend obliteration of the varices via repeated endoscopic injections of varices with a sclerosing solution. This technique reduces the incidence of recurrent esophageal (but not gastric) variceal bleeding without interrupting portal blood flow to the liver.

Malignant lesions producing UGI hemorrhage are usually treated surgically, while rare *vascular lesions* such as Osler-Weber-Rendu syndrome or angiodysplasia may respond either to experimental thermal obliteration with endoscopic electro- or laser coagulation or, if localized, to segmental surgical resection.

LOWER GASTROINTESTINAL HEMORRHAGE. *Hemorrhoids* are treated medically with sitz baths and lubricating suppositories, by banding, or surgically, depending on the severity and frequency of bleeding episodes (see Ch. 111). *Ischemic colitis, inflammatory bowel disease,* and *cancer* only rarely produce bleeding severe enough to necessitate immediate surgery and are managed as they would be if hemorrhage had not been the presenting symptom. Hemorrhage from *diverticulosis* that continues after initial therapy may respond to intra-arterial vasopressin therapy. If not, diagnostic arteriography may localize the bleeding site to permit segmental colonic resection rather than subtotal colectomy. *Vascular*

---

*This use is not listed in the manufacturer's directive.

anomalies located by arteriography may also respond to intra-arterial vasopressin. Indication for elective surgical resection of diverticula or vascular anomalies that cease bleeding either spontaneously or with vasopressin depends upon the severity and frequency of bleeding episodes.

THE DIAGNOSTIC DILEMMA

The diagnostic approach just described for patients with gastrointestinal hemorrhage will fail to disclose a diagnosis in many patients. Fortunately such failure is not detrimental to most, particularly during a period of observation. Nevertheless, failure to locate and define the source of bleeding jeopardizes patients with multiple episodes of hemorrhage that require repeated hospitalizations and blood transfusions, particularly high-risk elderly patients with a potentially curable lesion.

There are at least three reasons for failure to diagnose the bleeding lesion. First, it may be in a location that is relatively inaccessible to standard radiographic procedures and endoscopy. The best example is a lesion of the small bowel, i.e., a middle GI lesion. Second, there may be single or multiple lesions that are potential bleeding sites, and documentation of the one responsible may be virtually impossible. Third, the lesion responsible for the hemorrhage may be overlooked because of its subtle manifestation or because diagnosticians are unfamiliar with the lesion.

Lesions of the small bowel include tumors, vascular anomalies, and Meckel's diverticula. An infusion small bowel series, in which a tube is positioned in the third portion of the duodenum to allow a controlled, steady infusion of barium, permits the radiologist to follow the column of barium more closely than with the standard small bowel series. Tumors of the small bowel may be detected with this technique. If this procedure is unrewarding, visceral angiography may detect abnormal vascular patterns of tumors or vascular anomalies, although contrast material will not enter the lumen unless bleeding is active (at least 0.5 ml of blood loss per minute). Meckel's diverticula are sources of bleeding primarily in young patients and may at times be localized by using a technetium isotopic scan. This test is often difficult to interpret.

Confirmation that a lesion is actually the site of hemorrhage requires either endoscopy or arteriography performed while the patient is bleeding. In the UGI tract this may be of particular importance in patients with esophageal varices, whereas in the lower GI tract it is important in the patient with suspected bleeding from diverticulosis or angiodysplasia. For example, a patient may present with a lower GI hemorrhage that ceases spontaneously. Barium enema and/or colonoscopy disclose only diverticula. If the patient at a later time has another hemorrhage, arteriography may demonstrate that a diverticulum is bleeding in a particular area of the colon, or it may disclose a lesion such as angiodysplasia that was overlooked on colonoscopy. The role of radionuclide scanning in patients whose conditions present a diagnostic dilemma remains to be settled.

Vascular anomalies are subtle lesions with which many physicians may be unfamiliar. These range from the hereditary telangiectasias of Osler-Weber-Rendu to angiodysplasia, which may account for an important proportion of GI hemorrhage in elderly patients. This lesion is believed to be an acquired one that develops as part of the aging process. In theory, many years of low-grade obstructions of submucosal veins ultimately lead to small arteriovenous communications in the mucosa and submucosa. This lesion was originally recognized by arteriography as a cause of bleeding in the cecum and may be responsible for a substantial proportion of bleeding episodes previously ascribed to right-sided diverticula. Because many of these malformations are submucosal, they cannot alway be seen by colonoscopy or at surgery.

Angiodysplasias arising in the mucosa have been described endoscopically as bright red, flat, and fernlike. These vascular lesions have been found both in the cecum and in the UGI tract. As more endoscopists become familiar with this lesion, it will likely become a more frequently listed cause of both upper and lower gastrointestinal hemorrhage in the elderly.

Angiodysplasia localized to the cecum and ascending colon may be treated with right hemicolectomy. In fact, some investigators suggest resection after the first episode of hemorrhage. An alternative form of therapy is thermal coagulation, using electrocoagulation or laser. This technique would appear especially useful when there are multiple, widely scattered lesions or when they are present in the UGI tract and surgical resection would result in undesirable postoperative complications.

Fleischer D: Endoscopic therapy of upper gastrointestinal bleeding in humans. Gastroenterology 90:217, 1986. *An up-to-date review with extensive bibliography.*

Flesicher D: Etiology and prevalence of severe persistent upper gastrointestinal bleeding. Gastroenterology 84:538, 1983. *A nice evaluation of severe upper gastrointestinal bleeding.*

Graham DY, Smith JL: The course of patients after variceal hemorrhage. Gastroenterology 8:800, 1981. *Demonstrates the dismal prognosis for variceal bleeders.*

Larson DE, Farnell MB: Upper gastrointestinal hemorrhage. Mayo Clin Proc 58:371, 1983. *An in-depth review of all aspects of upper gastrointestinal bleeding with excellent reference list.*

Lieberman DA, Keller FS, Katon RM, et al.: Arterial embolization for massive upper gastrointestinal tract bleeding in poor surgical candidates. Gastroenterology 86:876, 1984. *One of the largest series of severe bleeders treated with arterial embolization.*

Peterson WL: Gastrointestinal bleeding. In Sleisenger MH, Fordtran JS (eds.): Gastrointestinal Disease. 4th ed. Philadelphia, W. B. Saunders Company, 1988. *A much expanded, fully referenced review of gastrointestinal bleeding.*

Rector WB: Drug therapy for portal hypertension. Ann Intern Med 105:96, 1986. *Scholarly review of pharmacologic agents used to treat variceal bleeding.*

Rutgeerts P, Van Gompel F, Geboes K, et al.: Long term results of treatment of vascular malformations of the gastrointestinal tract by Neodymium Yag laser photocoagulation. Gut 26:586, 1985. *One of the largest published experiences with laser treatment of vascular anomalies.*

Zinner MJ, Zuidema GD, Smith PL, et al.: The prevention of upper gastrointestinal tract bleeding in patients in an intensive care unit. Surg Gynecol Obstet 153:214, 1981. *The best study of prophylactic prevention of "stress" bleeding.*

115 MISCELLANEOUS INFLAMMATORY DISEASES OF THE INTESTINE

Marvin H. Sleisenger

Acute Appendicitis (Including the Acute Abdomen)

DEFINITION. Appendicitis is acute inflammation of the vermiform appendix. It is rare before the age of two and reaches a peak incidence in the second and third decades. The vast majority of patients are between the ages of 5 and 30. Although incidence of the disease declines after the age of 40, the annual incidence is about 1.5 per thousand for males and 1.9 per thousand for females between the ages of 17 and 64. The disease is important because it is common and curable; it therefore constitutes the most important entity in the differential diagnosis of the acute abdomen.

PATHOLOGY. Usually, the appendix is swollen, hyperemic, warm, and covered with exudate. However, in the early stages it may appear only slightly discolored and, in the late stages, gangrenous with perforation. Microscopically, the picture ranges from some acute inflammatory cells in the lumen and mucosa to acute inflammatory changes transmurally with superficial mucosal ulcerations; in advanced stages, one or more perforations may be noted, particularly in patients over the age of 60.

ETIOLOGY AND PATHOGENESIS. Although the vast majority of cases have no obvious cause for obstruction, identifiable etiologies include *calculi, Enterobius vermicularis, Kaposi's sarcoma, Burkitt's lymphoma, adenocarcinoma, schistosomiasis,* and *carcinoid tumors.* The initiating event in acute appendicitis appears to be obstruction, followed by increased intraluminal pressure, reduced venous drainage, thrombosis, hemorrhage, edema, and bacterial invasion of the wall. The appendiceal artery (an end-artery) becomes occluded and perforation results.

Calculi are thought to be the most common cause of the initial obstruction. A small percentage of inflamed appendices contain a radiologically demonstrable calculus, compared with 2.7 per cent of normal ones. Gangrene and perforation are more common in appendices with calculi. The calculi are composed of inspissated fecal material, calcium phosphate–rich mucus, and inorganic salts. Although fecaliths are more common in populations eating a low-fiber diet, the incidence of appendicitis is decreasing in the West, and 70 per cent of patients with acute appendicitis do not have calculi. Whether the increasing use of high-fiber diets underlies this reduction of incidence is not yet proved.

CLINICAL PICTURE AND DIAGNOSIS. The duration of appendicitis is usually 12 to 48 hours from onset to hospitalization. Over 95 per cent of patients complain of *pain* at onset, classically referred to the epigastric or periumbilical areas and later localizing in the right lower quadrant. This sequence, however, is not found in all patients and is notably absent in *retrocecal appendicitis.* Further, in a significant number of patients, particularly women in the late second or third trimester of pregnancy, the pain will not localize clearly to the right lower quadrant, being either diffuse or in the lower abdomen. In *pelvic appendicitis* the pain may be in the left lower quadrant. When retrocecal, the pain may be referred to the thigh or right testicle. Dysuria is present frequently in both types of appendicitis.

Pain referred to the midepigastrium is due to stretching of the organ during early inflammation. Initially it is vague and mild, but it gradually increases over about four hours and may be colicky. It tends to subside, and when the process has reached the serosa and the peritoneum, it localizes over the site of disease. In some patients distress appears to be alleviated at the time of perforation; after perforation, localization of pain will depend on whether or not the process is quickly walled off locally. Thus if the spreading infection is not contained, generalized abdominal discomfort of variable severity will result. *Anorexia* and *nausea* (with or without vomiting) are the second and third most frequent symptoms. In almost all instances, pain precedes the appearance of these other complaints, and its principal feature is *persistence.* About 10 per cent of patients will have constipation; diarrhea is uncommon. Temperature usually ranges between 38 and 38.6°C; higher levels usually indicate perforation.

PHYSICAL EXAMINATION. The findings on physical examination depend not only upon the stage of the inflammation but also upon the age of the patient. Tenderness to palpation is the most common (99 per cent), important, and reliable sign; indeed, without it, diagnosis is unlikely. It is usually confined to McBurney's point (one finger) in the right lower quadrant, corresponding to the usual location of the organ. However, although rectal tenderness is present in about one third of patients, it may be so severe as to indicate pelvic peritonitis and thus probable *pelvic appendicitis.* On initial examination in a minority of patients, a mass may be felt in the right lower quadrant or in the pelvis or transrectally. Localized rebound pain is found in 75 per cent. Generalized rebound tenderness indicates diffuse peritonitis. Bowel sounds may be present or absent; absence associated with

distention and generalized rebound tenderness is consistent with perforation and diffuse peritonitis. The patient with acute appendicitis often does not seem ill. The physician must not be deceived; the diagnosis rests upon persisting pain and localized tenderness.

On occasion, tenderness may be elicited in the case of retrocecal appendicitis by stretching the psoas by hip extension. Very rarely, because of the odd location of the appendix, tenderness may be in the right upper quadrant or even the left lower quadrant.

LABORATORY FINDINGS. Laboratory studies consistently show a leukocytosis with an increase in polymorphonuclear cells—over 10,000 per cubic millimeter and greater than 75 per cent, respectively. Urinalysis is usually normal; however, about 15 per cent of patients have either a slight amount of protein or mild pyuria or hematuria. Presence of a calcified fecalith in the right lower quadrant on flat film of the abdomen is helpful, but it is present in only a small percentage of patients. Other findings on flat film include possible obliteration of the right psoas shadow, right lower quadrant sentinel loop ileus, and a right lower quadrant soft tissue mass with or without gas bubbles. With perforation and generalized peritonitis, fluid in the peritoneal cavity and obliteration of the peritoneal lines may be noted.

DIFFERENTIAL DIAGNOSIS OF APPENDICITIS AND OF THE ACUTE ABDOMEN. Appendicitis is first on the list of conditions causing acute abdominal pain that require surgery or immediate consultation with a surgeon. Computerized tomography (CT) is now increasingly used in diagnosis, demonstrating swelling, perforation, and fecaliths in a high proportion of cases, and appears to be more helpful than a plain film early in the disease. About 15 per cent of patients operated upon for acute appendicitis will have a normal appendix; in view of the gravity of unoperated upon disease, this figure is entirely acceptable. Here a few principles regarding the acute surgical abdomen in the setting of the differential diagnosis of acute appendicitis will be reviewed.

Pain Characteristics. Conditions associated with pain of sudden onset include *perforated viscus,* more commonly a *peptic ulcer* or a *colonic diverticulum,* or, rarely, a *carcinoma of the colon* or *acute ischemia* (although acute ischemia does not always cause acute or severe pain in the elderly); the onset of pain in *acute small bowel obstruction, choledocholithiasis, ureteral obstruction, rupture of an abdominal aortic aneurysm,* and *dissection of the abdominal aorta* may also be abrupt. The more gradual onset of pain usually indicates an inflammatory lesion—*cholecystitis, acute pancreatitis, diverticulitis,* and *appendicitis.* However, the pain of diffuse *inflammatory bowel disease* is not localized as it is in appendicitis, except as a consequence of perforation or fistulization in Crohn's disease. The pain of pelvic inflammatory disease is usually associated with menstruation and has been present for 24 or more hours, whereas appendicitis pain is more often intermenstrual and rarely is suffered so long except with perforation.

The type and radiation of the pain also help in differential diagnosis. For example, evidence of irritation of the diaphragm may be found on the right in *acute cholecystitis* and on the left in *acute pancreatitis*; sudden, severe pain referred to the tips of the shoulders, associated with diffuse intra-abdominal pain and, later, distention, is more typical of perforated viscus, particularly *peptic ulcer. Ureteral obstruction* causes pain that is frequently referred to the genitalia or groin. Steady, continuous pain is more characteristic of inflammation, as in appendicitis; on the other hand, intermittent or crampy pain is more characteristic of *obstruction of a hollow viscus* such as the gallbladder or small bowel.

Pain precedes nausea and vomiting in *appendicitis*; on the other hand, vomiting may be an early symptom of *acute cholecystitis* or *acute pancreatitis.* Bile-stained vomitus associated with acute cramping upper abdominal pain suggests *small bowel obstruction*; blood in the vomitus points toward a mucosal lesion proximal to the third portion of the duodenum. Relief of pain by vomiting suggests *gastric outlet obstruction*. Vomiting, of course, may accompany any intra-abdominal conditions, particularly if the patient is in great pain and has ileus or generalized peritonitis.

Physical Findings. Physical examination of the patient with an acute abdomen is of great importance, and the range of findings expected in acute appendicitis has been discussed. Unlike many causes of acute and severe abdominal pain, *mesenteric ischemia* is not associated with notable abdominal tenderness for six or more hours after onset. Localized tenderness and temperature elevation associated with continuing pain over a period of hours reflect either *localized peritonitis*, with or without perforation, or *vascular necrosis* of an ischemic organ. In such instances, the temperature is approximately 38.5 to 39.5°C. Higher temperatures are more often associated with urinary tract infections or bacterial pneumonias. Marked epigastric tenderness in a patient with a steadily increasing boring type of epigastric pain for several hours, particularly if accompanied by falling blood pressure, suggests *acute pancreatitis*. A rapidly rising pulse rate strengthens this possibility but is present with *perforation of a viscus*, a *gangrenous bowel*, or *rupture of an aneurysm*, as well.

Diffuse peritonitis is reflected by resistance of movement and change in position because of accentuation of pain; on the other hand, colic caused by *obstruction* of bile ducts, ureter, or small bowel early in its course is associated with restless movement. Later, in biliary tract and small bowel obstruction, infection and compromise of the blood supply may ensue and will cause the appearance of signs of localized tissue necrosis and peritonitis. The abdomen should be carefully examined for scars of previous surgery that may now underlie an *intestinal obstruction* caused by adhesions; hernias must be sought. A succussion splash indicates marked *gastric outlet obstruction*. A large, pulsatile midabdominal mass points to *dissection of the abdominal aorta*. *Rupture of an aortic aneurysm* is usually very sudden; pain is brief, since shock quickly supervenes. Abdominal examination reveals distention.

In examining the patient with an acute abdomen, the physician should palpate in that quadrant that is farthest removed from the site of distress. The important findings that indicate a surgical condition include persistent, localized tenderness with unequivocal rebound, indicating localized peritonitis, and guarding. Guarding must be interpreted circumspectly, because it may be voluntary or involuntary. If it is the latter, underlying peritoneal irritation is likely. Generalized involuntary guarding is a classic finding for a perforated intra-abdominal viscus. The presence of an abdominal mass not previously noted, particularly when associated with other findings of inflammation, gangrene, or perforation, is very strong evidence for a surgical condition. Likewise, free air in the abdominal cavity, as evidenced by distention, absence of bowel sounds, and absence of liver dullness in the setting of acute abdominal pain, reflects a perforated viscus. Bowel sounds may be more active and high pitched in early obstruction or continuously active in diffuse acute inflammation (nonsurgical) of the small bowel. With increasing distention of small bowel loops, the sounds become less frequent and more high pitched. Bruits are an important finding, because they may reflect the presence of *arterial aneurysms*, the dissections of which may be the cause for the abdominal pain.

Rectal examination is crucial in differential diagnosis. Unequivocal tenderness indicates pelvic inflammation, and a mass usually reflects the presence of an abscess. As noted above, this examination often reveals positive findings in *acute appendicitis*. A glove specimen of stool must always be examined for occult blood. In females with acute abdominal pain, pelvic examination is essential to complement a careful gynecologic history.

Laboratory Aids in Diagnosis. The laboratory examination, consisting of urinalysis, complete blood count, serum electrolytes, blood urea nitrogen (BUN) and creatinine, serum amylase, radiographic examination of the abdomen and chest, and sonography of the abdomen, is essential in the differential diagnosis of the acute abdomen.

A *polymorphonuclear leukocytosis* strongly substantiates an acute intra-abdominal process with inflammation or necrosis; a low hematocrit reflects a disorder that is also capable of producing bleeding—*mucosal ulcerations*, *intestinal carcinoma*, *ischemia*, or *dissecting aneurysms*. An elevated hematocrit and BUN suggest dehydration, usually caused by vomiting and deficient fluid intake.

Urinalysis is vital in differential diagnosis, because the presence of pyuria, particularly white cell casts and bacteria on the smear of urinary sediment, is strong evidence for urinary tract infection and interdicts surgical exploration. Microscopic hematuria (numerous red cells) suggests stone or tumor of the genitourinary tract; red cell casts, on the other hand, suggest glomerulitis. A few scattered white and red cells may be seen in the sediment of about 20 per cent of patients with acute appendicitis. Examination of a *stool specimen* for blood and white blood cells is indicated in patients with right lower quadrant pain, fever, and *diarrhea*. *Salmonella* enterocolitis (and other bacterial infections) may be confused with acute appendicitis.

Important blood chemistries are *serum amylase*, elevation of which usually reflects acute pancreatitis; however, it may not be elevated in chronic relapsing pancreatitis, and it is elevated in other conditions such as *perforated peptic ulcer, strangulated obstruction* of the small bowel with perforation, *acute cholecystitis, cholangitis, acute renal failure*, and *ruptured tubal pregnancy*.

Visual Aids in Diagnosis. Roentgenologic examinations of importance include chest and flat films of the abdomen and CT scans, including contrast films with water-soluble, iodine (1 to 2 per cent)-containing substances. Radionuclide studies and ultrasonography are often useful as well. The flat and upright films of the abdomen may show free air in the peritoneal cavity, reflecting a perforation of a hollow viscus (80 per cent of cases are due to perforated ulcer, followed by perforated diverticulum and appendicitis). They also support the diagnosis of acute small bowel obstruction, indicate the likelihood of calculus disease of either gallbladder or urogenital tract, outline a large obstructed stomach, and reveal a variety of soft tissue masses that may reflect cysts or abscesses. Collections of extraintestinal gas often point to abscesses; occasionally, the biliary tree may be outlined by air, thus revealing a fistula to bowel. Diffuse calcification of the region of the pancreas indicates chronic pancreatitis. As noted, calculi in the right lower quadrant may rarely help in the diagnosis of acute appendicitis. Flat film of the abdomen also may yield findings characteristic of acute pancreatitis, including "sentinel" loops and a "cut-off" of the colon. A cross-table lateral view will outline an abdominal aortic aneurysm. A routine chest radiograph is essential in order to reveal free intraperitoneal air under the diaphragm, to demonstrate pneumonia, or to show an elevated diaphragm on the left with or without pleural effusion and partial atelectasis, as noted in acute pancreatitis, or on the right, reflecting subphrenic abscess.

Sonography is particularly helpful in demonstrating gallstones, obstruction of the extrahepatic biliary tract (dilated intrahepatic ducts), collections of fluid including abscesses, defects in the liver, and obstruction of the urinary tract. Ultrasonography may also indicate *colonic diverticulitis, Crohn's disease, intramural hemorrhage*, or *intussusception* by revealing a thickened bowel wall. It may also help in diagnosing "closed loop" obstruction.

Computerized tomographic scans are increasingly used in difficult cases, especially when flat films and sonograms are not helpful. Computerized tomography may detect choledocholithiasis, the swollen pancreas of acute pancreatitis; inflammatory pseudocyst of the pancreas; intra-abdominal abscess; enlarged lymph nodes; subcapsular hematomas of liver, spleen, or kidney; dissection of the aorta; colonic diverticulitis; and with contrast, perforated or thickened bowel of Crohn's disease or cancer.

Radionuclides given intravenously may help by visualizing the gallbladder (technetium 99m, labeled iminodiacetic acid or derivative compounds) or by localizing an intra-abdominal abscess (gallium citrate 67). Visualization of the gallbladder by technetium 99m scan renders the diagnosis of acute cholecystitis highly unlikely. Radiolabeled agents may also detect localized inflammation and abscess. Gallium 67 collects in granulocytes and mononuclear cells; indium 111–labeled white cells of the patient are given intravenously. These agents are most useful when CT scanning and ultrasonography yield negative findings in the search for an inflamed organ or mass.

Nonsurgical conditions that cause acute abdominal pain are important in the differential diagnosis of acute appendicitis. Chief among these are *pyelonephritis, pneumonia, pulmonary infarction, acute myocardial infarction,* and *pericarditis,* all of which may cause acute upper abdominal pain. Acute distention of the liver and its capsule resulting from *acute right heart failure* may simulate *acute cholecystitis; acute hepatitis,* viral or toxic (including alcohol), may closely simulate acute biliary tract disease. In these instances, however, an enlarged, tender liver will be felt. Further, serum glutamic-oxaloacetic transaminase (SGOT) determinations will be markedly elevated. (However, acute obstruction of the common duct with cholangitis may transiently raise SGOT to levels of 1000 units or more for 24 to 48 hours.)

Systemic diseases, such as *sickle cell disease, acute intermittent porphyria, tabes dorsalis, heavy metal poisoning,* and *diabetic neuropathy,* all may present pictures simulating an acute surgical abdomen.

Acute pancreatitis usually is characterized by pain of many hours' to days' duration, associated with a history suggestive of biliary tract disease or indicative of acute and chronic alcoholism, and in its early stages abdominal tenderness is usually localized to the epigastrium. Markedly elevated plasma amylase (within 48 hours of onset) will help establish the diagnosis. Elevation of serum bilirubin above 3.0 mg per deciliter and of alkaline phosphatase indicates obstruction of the common bile duct, and occasionally ultrasonography or CT scan, in addition to indicating obstruction, may help in establishing choledocholithiasis as the cause of the pancreatitis.

SPECIAL CONSIDERATIONS IN DIFFERENTIAL DIAGNOSIS OF ACUTE APPENDICITIS. Great care must be extended to establish the diagnosis of this condition in the very young and very old. Children with diffuse abdominal pain that is preceded by anorexia, nausea, and vomiting and is often associated with diarrhea are more likely to have *acute infectious gastroenteritis,* in some cases due to *Yersinia enterocolitica, Campylobacter,* or *Salmonella.* Acute enteric infection with *Salmonella* must always be suspected, particularly in young adults with right lower quadrant pain, fever, and diarrhea. *Acute mesenteric adenitis,* presumably caused by viral illnesses and often associated with diffuse abdominal pain, is frequently confused with acute appendicitis in children. The difficulty is in those patients in whom there is some right lower quadrant tenderness and slight elevation of the white count. In such instances a diagnosis must be established at operation, because it is far safer to undertake a negative exploration than to neglect removal of an acutely inflamed appendix. Clinical differentiation of acute appendicitis from *Meckel's diverticulitis* is impossible. The acute onset of *Crohn's disease* involving terminal ileum may be very difficult to distinguish from acute appendicitis, although such patients usually have cramping abdominal pain and diarrhea.

In young women diagnosis is confused by problems in the reproductive system, such as *ruptured graafian follicles, twisted ovarian cysts, ectopic pregnancy, dysmenorrhea, ruptured endometrioma,* and *acute pelvic inflammatory disease. Ruptured ectopic pregnancy* is usually of dramatic suddenness and is often associated with shock and massive blood loss; these findings in a pregnant woman make the diagnosis virtually certain. The *ruptured graafian follicle* is noted in midcycle; fever and leukocytosis are uncommon. Tenderness on moving of the cervix on vaginal examination points toward a *twisted ovarian cyst,* the pain of which is out of proportion to the general well-being of the patient. The pain of *gonococcal salpingitis* is more diffuse, and tenderness is not so well localized as in appendicitis. Localized pain and tenderness in a pregnant woman whose pregnancy remains normal and who is not bleeding indicate probable appendicitis.

The differential diagnosis of appendicitis in the elderly may also be difficult. The classic picture is seldom noted, the history may be inadequate or misleading because of infirmity or the effects of medication, and the appendix perforates early. Findings on physical examination are usually not as dramatic, and, despite complications, fever may be only slightly elevated. Accuracy in diagnosis of patients over 60 years of age is below 70 per cent, and the incidence of perforation without a localized or generalized peritonitis at surgery is nearly 70 per cent—more than twice as high as all other age groups combined.

In elderly patients the principal problems in differential diagnosis are *cholecystitis, diverticulitis, mesenteric thrombosis, intestinal obstruction, incarcerated hernia,* and *perforated ulcer.*

Right-sided acute diverticulitis may simulate acute appendicitis in every respect. In a few instances, *left-sided diverticulitis* may localize tenderness to the right lower quadrant, because the sigmoid is often more redundant in the elderly. The patient also may have an episode of diarrhea associated with cramping or steady lower abdominal pain, slight temperature elevation, and, later, evidence of moderate-to-complete large bowel obstruction. When differential diagnosis is difficult, a cautiously administered barium enema or a CT scan with contrast may help greatly in excluding acute diverticulitis as the cause of the problem.

In all instances, elderly patients must not be subjected to the risk of exploration falsely. Accordingly, all efforts should be extended to make certain that *acute myocardial* or *pulmonary infarction, pneumonia,* or other systemic disease or toxin, in addition to intra-abdominal conditions that do not require immediate surgery, are not responsible for acute abdominal pain simulating appendicitis.

TREATMENT. Unless strongly contraindicated, the only therapy for acute appendicitis is surgical removal of the appendix. Since mortality correlates with perforation and, except in elderly patients, perforation correlates with duration of symptoms, early diagnosis and appendectomy are essential for the lowest acceptable morbidity and mortality for the disease. To avoid the catastrophe of unoperated-upon acute appendicitis, normal appendices may have to be removed in 20 to 25 per cent of patients.

In patients in whom complications (*perforation, peritonitis,* and *abscess*) have already occurred or are suspected, dehydration must be corrected; continuous nasogastric suction should be started; and gentamicin, 1.0 to 1.5 mg per kilogram, clindamycin, 1.6 to 2.5 grams, and metronidazole, 2.0 grams, given parenterally per day in divided doses, should be administered prior to surgery.

Patients with obvious acute appendicitis for whom no surgeon is available may be treated with head-up position of the bed; intravenous fluids; gentamicin, 1.0 to 1.5 mg per kilogram, clindamycin, 1.6 to 2.4 grams, and ampicillin, 2.0 grams, intravenously in divided doses daily; and nasogastric suction. The chance for recovery in otherwise healthy individuals with this program is surprisingly good. However, these patients must be scheduled for appendectomy six weeks later, or appendicitis is likely to recur.

MORBIDITY AND MORTALITY OF SURGERY. Overall, about 15 per cent of patients with acute appendicitis develop complications postoperatively; this figure is about 35 per cent in those with perforation and localized peritonitis at the time of surgery and is 70 per cent in those with perforation and generalized peritonitis. The complications include *wound infection, intra-abdominal abscess,* mechanical *small bowel obstruction, fecal fistula,* and, much more rarely, *intraperitoneal hemorrhage. Pylephlebitis* is extremely rare (1 in 1000).

The overall mortality of acute appendicitis ranges from 0.18 to 1.6 per cent and is due principally to the inter-related factors of age and perforation. Indeed, mortality over the age of 60 ranges from 6.4 to 14 per cent. The cause of death in this group may be attributed equally to septic and nonseptic complications.

Alvarado A: A practical score for the early diagnosis of acute appendicitis. Ann Emerg Med 15:557, 1986. *Predictive factors for diagnosis in order of importance are localized tenderness in the right lower quadrant, leukocytosis, migration of pain, shift to the left in the neutrophils, temperature elevation, nausea, vomiting, anorexia, and direct rebound pain.*

Brender JD, Marcuse EK, Koepsell TD, et al.: Childhood appendicitis: Factors associated with perforation. Pediatrics 76:301, 1985. *Delay in treatment—the interval between first recognized symptoms of abdominal pain and surgery—was most predictive of perforation. A treatment delay of more than 36 hours was associated with a 65 per cent or greater incidence of perforation.*

Lau WY, Fan ST, Yiu TF, et al.: Acute appendicitis in the elderly. Surg Gynecol Obstet 161:157, 1985. *A prospective study of 104 patients more than 60 years old with appendicitis. Showed clinical features similar to those of the younger patient; however, the elderly patient may have little or no pain, and the incidence of appendiceal perforation is increased.*

Schrock TR: Acute appendicitis. *In* Sleisenger MH, Fordtran JS (eds.): Gastrointestinal Disease. 4th ed. Philadelphia, W. B. Saunders Company, 1988. *A concise yet comprehensive article on every aspect of the subject. A handy reference.*

Way LW: Abdominal pain and the acute abdomen. *In* Sleisenger MH, Fordtran JS (eds.): Gastrointestinal Disease. 4th ed. Philadelphia, W. B. Saunders Company, 1988. *An excellent chapter containing all important information on diagnosis of the acute abdomen, identifying the cause and the accepted approaches to management.*

Diverticulitis of the Colon

DEFINITION. *Diverticulitis* of the colon is a focal inflammation in the wall of the apex of a diverticulum, most commonly of the sigmoid, caused by inspissated feces. It is more common in those with multiple diverticula that have appeared at an early age. Peridiverticulitis results from necrosis with micro- or macroperforation. An abscess then forms, its size depending on the size of the rupture; small ones may subside with scarring, while larger abscesses involve pericolonic tissue and may even dissect along, or within, the bowel wall. Occasionally they rupture into contiguous organs (bladder, ureter, vagina, and small bowel).

CLINICAL PICTURE. The predominant clinical symptoms of diverticulitis are *pain* and *fever.* The pain is usually prominent and is frequently constant. Most commonly, it is localized in the left lower quadrant, because the sigmoid and descending colon are the sites of the largest number of diverticula. The patient may have a few loose stools or become constipated, and only rarely is rectal bleeding noted. Bleeding from diverticula is not associated with inflammation and perforation. It is usually bright red and may be copious. Bleeding colonic diverticula must be differentiated from ischemic colitis, acute amebic and *Shigella* dysenteries, *ulcerative colitis,* and *tumors of the colon* (see Ch. 114). When the perforation and sepsis are of sufficient magnitude, the patient may also have chills with fever as high as 39 to 39.5°C. Usually, however, the fever is low grade, between 38 and 39°C.

Although the pain may be somewhat intermittent and even colicky at onset, it usually becomes steady and is of the same quality as noted in acute appendicitis. Indeed, acute diverticulitis has often been referred to as "left-sided appendicitis." The patient may seek medical help after only a few hours or,

when the situation is not so severe, after a few days of lingering but nagging lower quadrant pain and low-grade fever. Rarely, a *diverticulum of the right colon* will perforate, causing right lower quadrant pain with fever, closely simulating appendicitis. Diagnosis is usually made at laparotomy.

Physical examination is extremely important in establishing the diagnosis. Since the process usually quickly involves the serosal surface and peritoneal cover, marked, localized tenderness will be found, both direct and rebound. Frequently, a tender mass may be discerned. When present for more than a few days, this mass may be astonishingly firm, even hard, and the distinction grossly from carcinoma is almost impossible. The abdomen is often slightly distended. Rectal examination also will be painful, because inflamed bowel is often within reach of the finger; also, a mass may be palpable if a sizable abscess has formed.

In some instances the patient will have complications of diverticulitis; *dysuria, pyuria, pneumaturia,* or *passing gas or feces through the vagina.* These symptoms are due to perforation of bladder or vagina by the diverticulitis (colovesical and colovaginal fistulas). The vast majority of these patients, usually elderly, do not relate these symptoms to a prior attack of severe pain. The presenting symptom may be septic fever, caused by pericolic, pelvic, or subdiaphragmatic abscess. The inflammatory process may penetrate other pelvic organs, but such fistulization is often clinically undramatic. Rarely, the diverticulum perforates freely. In this instance the signs of free perforation are evident—that is, distention of the abdomen, generalized rebound tenderness, and absent bowel sounds. It is unusual also for diverticulitis to cause persistent colonic obstruction (see below).

DIAGNOSIS. Diverticulitis should be suspected particularly in patients with known diverticula who develop fever, leukocytosis, and signs of pericolic and peritoneal inflammation in the left lower quadrant. The diagnosis is even more likely if a mass is palpable. Fever between 38.5 and 39°C is also compatible with the diagnosis; when the process is more extensive and with formation of a *pericolic abscess* and its complications, the temperature is usually over 39°C, and the white count is proportionately higher. Urinalysis will reflect varying degrees of involvement of the urinary tract by this septic process; that is, with mild ureteral irritation a few red and white cells may be seen in the urinary sediment, but with direct involvement of the ureter or invasion of the ureter or the bladder, the urine may be frankly septic and contain large numbers of red cells.

Some patients suffer much left flank pain owing to *hydronephrosis* resulting from obstruction of the ureter by a *pericolic abscess.* An intravenous pyelogram shows no function or an obstructed kidney on the left, and a sonogram or CT scan demonstrates unilateral hydronephrosis.

The use of radiographs is of crucial importance in the diagnosis, especially a flat film of the abdomen. Evidence of pericolic perforation and abscess formation may be suspected from collections of air and fluid in the left lower quadrant. Free air may be seen under the diaphragm in instances of free perforation. Sonography may reveal a localized thickening of the wall of the involved colon. Computerized tomographic scans are particularly helpful by showing inflamed pericolic fat in nearly all cases, the involved diverticula in 85 per cent, and thickening of the bowel wall in 75 per cent. Sonography, CT scan, or scintigraphy (gallium citrate 67) may localize an abscess. A fistula to the bladder or ureteral obstruction may be seen with ultrasonography or by CT scan.

Sigmoidoscopy should be carefully performed with minimal preparation. Air insufflation should not be used, and the importance of the examination is to exclude other conditions (see below). Usually with diverticulitis the instrument cannot be passed beyond the rectosigmoid junction, which is occluded by fixation, angulation, and spasm.

Clinicians debate the advisability of using a barium enema

in the diagnosis of diverticulitis, particularly in its acute phase. The concern is that the increased intraluminal pressure may cause perforation. The history, physical examination, laboratory information, flat film of the abdomen—and, in many cases, ultrasonography or CT scan—are sufficient to make the clinical diagnosis in most instances. Barium enema should await some subsidence of the acute phase of the illness. The exceptions to this dictum are those instances in which the *acute ischemic colitis* of the left colon and perforation of a left colonic carcinoma cannot otherwise be excluded. Colonoscopy or flexible sigmoidoscopy also is not indicated unless the diagnosis is not clear and the patient has gross rectal bleeding, since the techniques often do not reveal the perforated diverticulum.

The roentgenographic features characteristic of diverticulitis are the presence of barium outside a diverticulum, the delineation of a pericolic mass (Fig. 115–1), or the demonstration of a fistula originating in the colon. In some instances the distinction between diverticulitis and carcinoma or Crohn's disease may be difficult (see below). The presence of irregularity, thickening, or even a sawtooth appearance of the bowel is not sufficient to make the diagnosis of diverticulitis, because these are typical for diverticula without perforation.

After diagnosis of diverticulitis has been established, ultrasonography should be done to ascertain whether or not obstructive involvement of the urinary tract is present, particularly on the left side. In some instances, as noted above, urinary symptoms may be the predominant feature, and ultrasonography or radiographic examination of the urinary tract may have to be performed early.

DIFFERENTIAL DIAGNOSIS. For many years symptoms of *diverticulosis* have been attributed incorrectly to *diverticulitis*. *Diverticulosis* may periodically be associated with marked local tenderness, a palpable sigmoid loop, and some degree of large bowel obstruction, and thus the picture suggests diverticulitis. However, such patients do not have fever, the localized tenderness gradually recedes, the white count is not elevated, and there is no evidence of involvement of contiguous organs. Barium enema will reveal an irregular luminal contour with a narrowed sigmoid, possibly even a so-called "sawtooth" appearance of the mucosa. Barium must be noted outside the diverticulum, a fistula seen, or evidences of a pericolic or intramural mass detected before the diagnosis of diverticulitis is definitely made.

Carcinoma of the colon must be distinguished from diverticulitis because of similarity of age during which both diverticulitis and cancer of the colon appear. The differential diagnosis is especially difficult, because in about 25 per cent of patients with diverticulitis the lumen is narrowed, suggesting carcinoma. Differentiation from cancer is more difficult if diverticulitis has appeared insidiously. Chronic obstruction, more persistent rectal bleeding, and weight loss are more characteristic of *cancer*. However, the tumor may be obscured on barium enema in 50 per cent of patients with diverticula. Localized tenderness with rebound, leukocytosis, and fever support the diagnosis of diverticulitis. In some cases, however, it may be impossible to distinguish the two conditions, especially when the barium enema has features common to both—i.e., a mass, luminal irregularities, and partial obstruction. In such patients CT scan with contrast and colonoscopy may be very helpful in excluding cancer. Rapid disappearance of the obstruction strongly suggests diverticulitis. In some patients correct diagnosis can be made only at surgery, and, in a few, only from surgical biopsy or by the disappearance of the occlusion following colostomy.

Crohn's disease of the colon may be difficult to exclude in the face of marked luminal narrowing or multiloculated channels parallel to the bowel wall on radiograph. Clinically, although both may produce pain, partial obstruction and lower abdominal mass, some rectal bleeding, fever, and leukocytosis, the past history differs. The patient with Crohn's colitis usually will have had previous episodes of lower abdominal pain, fever, and diarrhea. Sigmoidoscopy may reveal the rectum to be involved with granulomatous disease. Also, evidence elsewhere in the bowel of granulomatous disease, such as cobblestoning, long intramucosal sinus tracts, and skip areas, will help in the differential diagnosis (see Ch. 105).

Ischemic colitis of the left colon in elderly patients may produce signs and symptoms of bowel necrosis and localized peritonitis that are difficult to distinguish from diverticulitis. In these instances, gross rectal bleeding is prominent, and a barium enema is of crucial importance, because so-called "thumbprinting" will be found in ischemic colitis, especially in the area of the splenic flexure and descending colon (see Ch. 106).

TREATMENT OF DIVERTICULITIS. Patients with low-grade fever and no evidence of mass, fistula, or obstruction may be treated with clear liquids by mouth and ampicillin (2.0 grams) or a cephalosporin (4.0 to 6.0 grams) per day in divided dosage intravenously. If the patient has fever of 39° C or more or has a tender mass or other evidence of greater extent of infection, gentamicin, 1.0 to 1.5 mg per kilogram, clindamycin, 1.6 to 2.4 grams, and metronidazole, 2.0 grams, are given parenterally in divided doses daily. In such patients nasogastric suction and intravenous fluids are given to maintain intravascular volume, urinary output, and electrolyte balance. About 50 per cent of complicated cases will require surgery. Surgical consultation must be obtained early in all cases in which a mass is palpable or when there is suspicion of peritonitis or involvement of a contiguous organ.

Most patients respond well to this type of therapy with abatement of the fever, tenderness, and evidence of partial obstruction. Long-term therapy becomes identical with that for diverticulosis (see Ch. 102).

COMPLICATIONS AND INDICATIONS FOR SURGERY. Surgical intervention is necessary for the complications of diverticulitis, such as an *enlarging mass* despite therapy, *generalized peritonitis, persisting intestinal obstruction,* or the development of a *fistula,* most commonly to the urinary bladder and rarely to other contiguous structures, such as the left hip, infecting joint or bone. In unusual cases, acute diverticulitis may bleed massively, requiring laparotomy. If possible, a one-stage procedure is carried out; if not, a temporary colostomy is established after resection of a fistula or drainage of a septic area. More definitive resection and reanastomoses are carried out later. Elective surgery is indicated for recurrent attacks of diverticulitis and for the inability to exclude a carcinoma as-

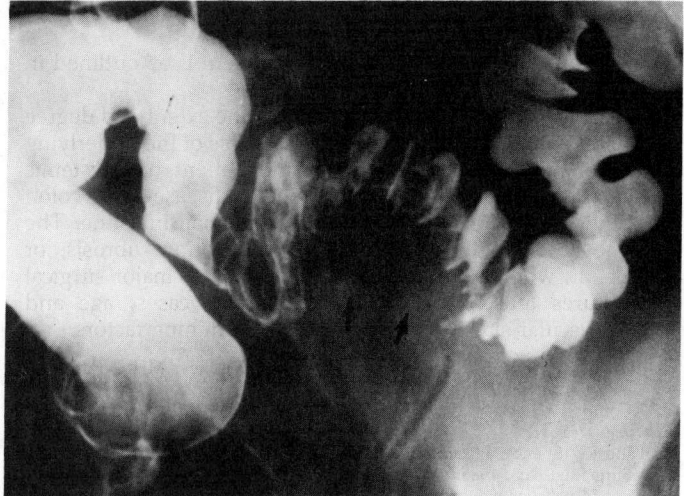

FIGURE 115–1. A paracolic mass that deforms and displaces the sigmoid lumen is delineated in a patient with diverticulitis and a palpable left lower quadrant mass. (From Almy TP, Naitove A: In Sleisenger MH, Fordtran JS [eds.]: Gastrointestinal Disease. 3rd ed. Philadelphia, W. B. Saunders Company, 1983.)

the cause for persisting deformity after recovery from the acute phase.

Almy TP, Howell DA: Diverticular disease of the colon. N Engl J Med 302:324, 1980. *A marvelously lucid update of every aspect of the subject.*

Almy TP, Naitove A: Diverticula of the colon. In Sleisenger MH, Fordtran JS (eds.): Gastrointestinal Disease. 4th ed. Philadelphia, W. B. Saunders Company, 1988. *A complete description of etiology, pathogenesis, and clinical pictures and complications of colonic diverticula, including diverticulitis.*

Hulnick DH, Megibow AJ, Balthazar EJ, et al.: Computerized tomography in evaluation of diverticulitis. Radiology 152:491, 1984. *CT scanning was very helpful in the diagnosis of 43 cases with demonstration of inflamed pericolic fat in 98 per cent of cases, of the involved diverticula in 84 per cent, and of a thickened wall in 70 per cent.*

Radiation Enterocolitis

Damage to the small intestine and colon may result from radiation therapy for abdominal and pelvic malignancy.

INCIDENCE. Incidence of severe radiation injury varies between 2.5 and 25 per cent of patients treated with radiotherapy for pelvic and intra-abdominal malignancy. Minor degrees of damage are common, as evidenced by impaired ileal absorption of conjugated bile acids in many women who are irradiated for pelvic cancer. It is noted most commonly after the total dosage exceeds 5000 rads. Transient histologic inflammatory change may, however, be found in the rectal mucosa of nearly 75 per cent of individuals receiving such therapeutic irradiation. The small intestine is more frequently affected than the rectum.

PATHOGENESIS AND PATHOLOGY. Damage results from interference with replication of radiosensitive epithelial cells, particularly of the crypt, leading to varying degrees of damage to the mucosal surface. Often it is reversible if dosage is not too great or treatment is not prolonged. Such damage may follow dosage of less than 5000 rads. Damage to the mesothelial cells of the small submucosal arterioles results in varying degrees of occlusion and mucosal transmural necrosis. Accordingly, hyperemia and ulceration of the mucosa are frequent. With extreme damage, diffuse edema is followed by extensive fibrosis with multiple strictures and irreversible damage. Such serious damage is more common in diabetics, in those with previous abdominal surgery, and in patients with serious vascular disease.

The pathologic changes range from diminution of crypt cell mitosis and shortening of villi of the small intestine to varying degrees of hyperemia, edema, and inflammatory cell infiltration of the mucosa. Mucosal thickness decreases. Progress of damage is marked by crypt abscesses, sloughing of epithelial cells, and, later, mucosal ulcerations, diffuse or localized, are found. Two to 12 months after radiotherapy, the damage to the blood vessels becomes prominent. In these instances, repair of acute damage does not ensue. The mucosa and submucosa become progressively ischemic and fibrotic. *Abscesses* and *fistulas* may form with sinus tracts between loops of intestine and between intestine and neighboring organs. A more general discussion of radiation injury is found in Ch. 539.

CLINICAL PICTURE. Symptoms may appear early, that is, during the first or second week of therapy, or late, that is, six months or more after completion of therapy. Early, diarrhea and mild rectal bleeding may appear, resembling ulcerative colitis. Sigmoidoscopy reveals an edematous mucosa that may be friable; in more extreme instances, the acute changes also reveal a patchy or diffusely necrotic mucosa.

Later, symptoms of radiation include gross rectal bleeding, decrease in stool caliber, and progressive difficulty in defecation with marked constipation, all indicating severe rectal involvement. Small intestinal symptoms result from either fibrosis and obstruction or fistulization and abscess formation. These serious complications are clinically apparent, on the

average, 20 to 24 months after the insult. Those with fistulas are more likely to have synchronous lesions; areas most severely affected are the mid and distal small intestine and the rectosigmoid. If the damage is especially diffuse, malabsorption may be noted, as described in Ch. 104.

DIAGNOSIS. Diagnosis of *radiation enteritis* is suspected with any of the aforementioned symptoms in patients who have received significant radiation. Sigmoidoscopy shows a picture that ranges from variable degrees of edema to a markedly inflamed and necrotic mucosa. Multiple telangiectases are common, as is rectal stricture. Since most cases are fairly clear cut, biopsy is usually not indicated.

Barium studies of the intestine are not specific and range from changes of diffuse edema and spasm to diffuse fibrosis with strictures, fistulas, and ulceration in more severe cases. Thus the picture may resemble localized malignancy in the colon or diffuse granulomatous disease in the small intestine. Long strictured areas may also be noted, however, in the colon.

Differential diagnostic usefulness of small vessel angiography of the intestine in radiation enteritis remains to be confirmed.

TREATMENT. Improving methods for monitoring radiotherapy and delivering rads in small increments will probably reduce the incidence of this complication; however, the increasing incidence of malignancy and of the efficacy of radiotherapy will probably increase the total number of such patients.

Symptoms caused by early reaction consist of mild diarrhea and perhaps some minimal bleeding that can be managed by reduction of dose by 10 per cent, with the judicious use of tranquilizers, anticholinergic drugs, local analgesics, agents that increase stool bulk, and warm sitz baths for those with rectal involvement. An elemental diet free of gluten, milk protein, and lactose may benefit patients with early radiation reaction. If watery diarrhea is a problem, treatment with cholestyramine (4 to 6 grams per day) to bind bile salts may help greatly. If rectal bleeding is prominent, treatment with steroid retention enemas should be initiated as in ulcerative colitis (see Ch. 105). If the bleeding is more significant, transfusions may be required and even, possibly, surgery. Rectal strictures may be dilated, provided that it is early in their course and they are not extensive. Lubricants and stool softeners are often helpful; however, the progress to symptomatic occlusion of the lumen may necessitate proximal colostomy. Fistulas should be resected and abscesses drained. Resection of bowel and anastomoses are hazardous in view of the impaired blood supply, and anastomoses should always be made to uninvolved intestine.

In patients with malabsorption, treatment is as outlined in Ch. 104.

PROGNOSIS. Prognosis depends on the extent and degree of damage, the age of the patient, the course of the underlying malignancy, and whether or not the patient has systemic vascular disease. Unfortunately extensive disease of the colon usually means significant disease in the small intestine. The prognosis is guarded in those with ulceration, fibrosis, or fistulas in whom repeated resections or other major surgical procedures must be carried out. In such cases, age and cardiovascular status are also crucial determining factors.

Earnest DH, Trier JS: Radiation enterocolitis. In Sleisenger MH, Fordtran JS (eds.): Gastrointestinal Disease. 4th ed. Philadelphia, W. B. Saunders Company, 1988. *A comprehensive discussion of the radiation damage to small and large gut.*

Galland RB, Spencer J: Radiation-induced gastrointestinal fistulae. Ann R Coll Surg Engl 68:5, 1986. *Of 70 patients with radiation enteritis, 10 (14 per cent) had 14 radiation-induced fistulas. The median latent period between radiotherapy and presentation of the fistula was 20 months. The fistulas were often multiple and/or associated with other radiation-induced lesions, patients presenting with fistulas being significantly more likely to have synchronous lesions compared with those who presented with strictures.*

Galland RB, Spencer J: Surgical management of radiation enteritis. Surgery 99:133, 1986. *This study of 70 patients with 63 strictures, 14 fistulas, 12 perforations, and 8 bleeds shows that use of nonirradiated bowel for at least one end of an anastomosis significantly improves the results of resection of irradiated bowel.*

Small Intestinal Ulceration: Isolated and Diffuse

ISOLATED NONSPECIFIC ULCERS

This inflammatory disease of unknown etiology is rare. About 75 per cent are ileal and 25 per cent jejunal. Often they are multiple. These ulcers may be caused by ingestion of enteric-coated potassium chloride. Such ulceration may also be associated with *vascular disease* (systemic lupus erythematosus, polyarteritis nodosa, rheumatoid arthritis), *hematologic disorders, granulomatous diseases, trauma, infections, Behçet's syndrome,* and *neoplasia.*

The clinical picture consists of periumbilical colicky pain and perhaps nausea and vomiting. Frequently, however, the patient presents with small bowel obstruction, bleeding, or perforation. Duration of illness is usually weeks to months but may be years. Accordingly, examination may show signs of obstructions, or peritonitis may be present.

Laboratory investigation is normal unless the patient has been bleeding or has had protracted vomiting; plain films of the abdomen are of great value if small bowel is obstructed or has perforated. Barium contrast studies in the uncomplicated cases are most often unrevealing, although in rare instances ulceration and narrowing may be noted. Upper endoscopy may reveal the ulcer or ulcers if located in the high jejunum.

Treatment for the disease is conservative if no complications have occurred. If the involved segment is bleeding, perforated, or stenotic, it should be resected.

Boydstun JS, Gaffey TA, Bartholomew LG: Clinico-pathological study of non specific ulcer of small intestine. Dig Dis Sci 26:911, 1981. *Comprehensive review of the Mayo Clinic's experience with 29 patients.*

Thomas WE, Williamson RC: Nonspecific small bowel ulceration. Postgrad Med J 61:587, 1985. *Good report of clinical and radiologic features of this entity.*

DIFFUSE ULCERATION OF JEJUNUM AND ILEUM

Diffuse ulceration of the small bowel may be found in *gluten-sensitive enteropathy (celiac sprue), lymphoma, idiopathic chronic ulcerative enteritis* (also known as *chronic ulcerative nongranulomatous jejunoileitis*). It may also be found after oral administration of flucytosine. Patients with *gluten-sensitive enteropathy* may develop diffuse ulceration of jejunum and ileum, usually signaling a rapid decline in their clinical course despite elimination of gluten from the diet, with increased diarrhea, malabsorption, and, in some patients, perforation or hemorrhage. In instances of mild degrees of ulceration, steroids may induce remission; however, the majority are refractory to medical therapy and require appropriate resection of involved gut. Mortality in this group is high. The condition in patients with lymphoma and diffuse ulceration also is often refractory to resection and radiotherapy.

Chronic ulcerative enteritis and *eosinophilic gastroenteritis* affect the small intestine, usually in patients under 50. They are characterized by diarrhea, weight loss, variable degrees of malabsorption, and protein-losing enteropathy. *Chronic ulcerative enteritis* is a much graver illness, often with fever, ascites and edema, a rapidly progressive course unresponsive to steroids, and a high mortality. The etiology is unknown. Biopsy, peroral or at laparotomy, reveals nonspecific diffuse inflammation and mucosal ulcers. Prednisolone, 60 to 100 mg intravenously daily over two to three weeks, may be associated with remission in about one half of these patients. Infection, intraperitoneal or systemic, is the common cause of death.

Eosinophilic gastroenteritis may be localized to stomach, small intestine, or colon—so-called *eosinophilic granuloma*. It consists of infiltration by sheets of eosinophils into the submucosal and muscle layers. It is associated with systemic illnesses or peripheral eosinophilia and appears in the fourth to sixth decades. Steroids are often effective, but surgery may be indicated. *Universal eosinophilic gastroenteritis,* on the other hand, is a disease of younger persons, is often associated with allergies, always has a peripheral eosinophilia (greater than 20 per cent), affects stomach and small intestine diffusely, and is associated with diarrhea, crampy pain, weight loss, hypoalbuminemia, and often occult bleeding. Rarely, it responds to elimination of certain foods, particularly fish or meat. Most patients, however, require treatment with steroids, usually short-term (ten days to two weeks), but some may require long-term administration of 10 mg of prednisolone daily.

Bayless TR: Small intestinal ulceration: Isolated and diffuse. In Sleisenger MH, Fordtran JS (eds.): Gastrointestinal Disease. 4th ed. Philadelphia, W. B. Saunders Company, 1988. *Excellent clarification and description of isolated and diffuse ulceration of the small gut.*

Heyman, IN: Allergic disorders of the intestine and eosinophilic gastroenteritis. In Sleisenger MH, Fordtran JS (eds.): Gastrointestinal Disease. 4th ed. Philadelphia, W. B. Saunders Company, 1988. *A concise review of eosinophilic disease of the gut.*

PART XI

DISEASES OF THE LIVER, GALLBLADDER, AND BILE DUCTS

116 CLINICAL APPROACH TO LIVER DISEASE

Robert K. Ockner

The liver plays a central and varied role in many essential physiologic processes. It is the sole source of albumin and many other plasma proteins, and of blood glucose in the postabsorptive state; it is the major site of lipid synthesis and source of plasma lipoproteins; and it is the principal organ in which a wide variety of endogenous and exogenous substances such as ammonia, steroid hormones, drugs, and toxins undergo biotransformation. To the extent that biotransformation "detoxifies" or inactivates a substance, the liver may be viewed as serving a regulatory or protective function for the whole organism; to the extent that such biotransformation results in the formation of toxic products, as in the case of certain drugs, the liver may bear the brunt of their adverse effects.

The clinical manifestations of liver diseases are also varied. Moreover, the clues by which the clinician may be first alerted to the existence of liver disease, even when advanced, may be subtle, consisting of seemingly trivial information gleaned during a careful history (e.g., increased fatigue, or the reversal of sleep pattern or personality change of early hepatic encephalopathy), physical examination (e.g., prominence of breast tissue and small testes in a man with cirrhosis, or excoriation reflecting pruritus), or routine laboratory screening tests (e.g., mild decreases in one or more of the formed elements of the blood because of portal hypertension–associated hypersplenism). Careful assessment is equally important in the patient with obvious liver disease, to address more complex questions. For example, does what seems to be acute hepatitis in fact represent relapse of previously subclinical chronic hepatitis, or delta-agent (hepatitis D) infection in a hepatitis B carrier? (See Ch. 121.) Or does the deteriorating course of a patient with known cirrhosis represent the natural progression of the disease, or a superimposed common bile duct stone, adverse drug reaction, or hepatocellular carcinoma?

HISTORY. Some very *nonspecific symptoms* may be important evidence of liver disease, including fatigue, malaise, fever, change in sleep pattern or behavior, diminished libido, anorexia, weight loss, nausea, and vomiting. *Pruritus* is an important symptom of *cholestasis* (impaired bile secretion), and may be present in the absence of jaundice. *Jaundice* is often first noted by family members or friends, and, especially in dark-skinned individuals, may appear first as a yellow discoloration of the conjunctivae (*"scleral icterus"*). Since jaun-

dice in most forms of liver and biliary disease reflects cholestasis (see below), such patients will often observe that stool color lightens while urine gets darker as the excretion of "bile pigments" is diverted from bile to urine. Right upper quadrant *abdominal discomfort* or *pain* may reflect a rapidly enlarging liver with distension of Glisson's capsule because of acute hepatic inflammation or congestion, an acutely inflamed gallbladder, common bile duct obstruction by an impacted gallstone, or abscess or tumor in the liver or adjacent areas.

The history may provide important clues to the presence of *complications of liver disease*, especially those reflecting *portal hypertension* and *portal-systemic shunting*. Early hepatic *encephalopathy* may cause subtle changes in affect or sleep pattern. More overt symptoms include episodic somnolence, confusion, combativeness, ataxia, incoordination, or obtundation. A history of *abdominal swelling* suggests ascites, and may be most easily recalled by the patient as a change in the fit of clothing, possibly associated with *edema*. Ascites may also occur in many other conditions, including hepatic vein or inferior vena cava occlusion, congestive cardiac failure and constrictive pericarditis, and a wide variety of neoplastic and inflammatory processes (see Ch. 112). A history of *gastrointestinal bleeding* in a patient with liver disease may suggest esophageal varices, but can also reflect other lesions such as *gastritis, Mallory-Weiss syndrome,* and *peptic ulcer.*

The history is of major importance in the identification of potentially significant *etiologic* or *predisposing factors*. Viral hepatitis is suggested by a history of contact with jaundiced persons, exposure to persons known to have hepatitis or to a common source of hepatitis, ingestion of uncooked or partially cooked shellfish, prior blood transfusion, work with subhuman primates, employment in certain health professions (especially in dialysis or transplantation units), accidental inoculation, sexual promiscuity (especially in the homosexual community), sharing of needles, travel to geographic areas with inadequate public health programs, and consumption of water or uncooked vegetables in such areas. Foreign travel may also suggest parasitic disease such as amebic liver abscess. Q fever hepatitis may occur in individuals in proximity to livestock. Exposure to drugs, ethanol, and other potential dietary, occupational, or environmental toxins must be reviewed in detail. The information obtained may require supplementation or corroboration by family members or other close associates, especially in regard to ethanol consumption. It is often possible to document previous liver function through recourse to *medical records*, and this is particularly useful in evaluating the chronicity of liver disease. A *family history* of jaundice, liver disease, or neonatal jaundice may suggest an inherited disorder such as Wilson's disease, alpha₁-antitrypsin deficiency, or hemochromatosis.

PHYSICAL EXAMINATION. Scleral *icterus* may be detected at a serum bilirubin concentration as low as 2.0 to 2.5 mg per deciliter. Although *spider telangiectasias*, most prominent around the shoulders and upper trunk, and *palmar erythema* are nonspecific and may be present to a limited extent in normal subjects (especially women in pregnancy), they are potentially important signs of liver disease, and usually imply chronicity. Excoriations reflect pruritus and suggest significant cholestasis, not necessarily accompanied by jaundice. *Xanthomas* and *xanthelasmas* are not specific for hepatobiliary disease, but may be a sign of prolonged cholestatic hypercholesterolemia. Changes in hair pattern, gynecomastia, and small or soft testes may reflect the *hormonal changes* that accompany cirrhosis in men. Prominence of cutaneous veins in the epigastrium or around the umbilicus may indicate a *portal-systemic collateral circulation* and, therefore, portal hypertension.

Examination of the heart and lungs may provide evidence of congestive cardiac failure, constrictive pericarditis, or diseases of the lungs or pleura that may be associated with liver dysfunction, cause pain referred to the abdomen, or reflect processes involving the subdiaphragmatic regions such as tumor or abscess.

Examination of the *liver* should include documentation of its *size*, and is best recorded both as the distance to which the lower edge extends below the costal margin, and its overall vertical span as determined by percussion. These dimensions should be related to a reproducible landmark such as the midclavicular line. The *form* and *consistency* of the liver should be noted: e.g., smooth, with a sharp edge; nodular and rockhard; firm with a rounded and irregular edge. A rapidly decreasing liver size during the course of severe acute hepatitis may be a sign of massive hepatic necrosis. An abdominal mass, tenderness, or muscular spasm may suggest secondary involvement of the liver or biliary passages by a neoplastic or inflammatory process. *Ascites*, most readily detected as dullness or bulging in the flanks, fluid wave, or shifting dullness, may be caused by advanced liver disease, or superimposed infectious or neoplastic processes.

A diffusely tender and enlarged liver suggests hepatitis or congestion, whereas tenderness in a relatively limited area at or below the lower margin in the region of the interlobar fissure may reflect acute cholecystitis. A visible or palpable gallbladder is abnormal and may be an important sign of primary gallbladder pathology, or of cystic or common bile duct obstruction, the latter usually neoplastic in jaundiced patients (Courvoisier's sign). Splenomegaly may be the first evidence of portal hypertension of any cause, or may reflect primary splenic pathology such as neoplasm or infection.

Neurologic evaluation is of particular importance with respect to signs of hepatic encephalopathy. These are discussed in detail in Ch. 128, but, as noted, these may be very subtle, consisting initially of a personality change, a mild confusional state, or lethargy. A *flapping tremor* (asterixis), characteristic of metabolic encephalopathy of any cause, is usually present in more obvious cases. In advanced hepatic encephalopathy almost any form of neurologic abnormality may be present, including seizures, lateralizing signs, and abnormal posturing. Despite this, it is essential in patients with liver disease to consider other causes of central nervous system pathology such as the effects of ethanol, sedatives or other toxins, hypoglycemia, trauma, hemorrhage, infection, and primary or secondary neoplasms.

Schiff L, Schiff E (eds.): Diseases of the Liver. Philadelphia, J. B. Lippincott Company, 1982.
Sherlock S: Diseases of the Liver and Biliary System. Oxford, Blackwell Scientific Publications, Ltd., 1985.
Wright R, Millward Sadler GH, Alberti KGMM, et al. (eds.): Liver and Biliary Disease. 2nd ed. London, W. B. Saunders Company, 1985.
Zakim D, Boyer T (eds.): Hepatology: A Textbook of Liver Disease. Philadelphia, W. B. Saunders Company, 1982.
Four current and comprehensive textbooks that serve to introduce the topic and provide literature references dealing with the broad field of hepatobiliary structure, function, and disease.

117 HEPATIC METABOLISM IN LIVER DISEASE
Robert K. Ockner

Intermediary metabolism may be profoundly disturbed in liver disease, and in some instances the resulting changes may overshadow the underlying disease process.

CARBOHYDRATE METABOLISM. Except during the absorption of dietary carbohydrate, maintenance of blood glucose levels depends entirely on the liver. Two distinct mechanisms are involved: *glycogenolysis* and *gluconeogenesis*. In glycogenolysis, glucose is released from hepatic glycogen by the enzyme phosphorylase, converted to its active form by the interaction of glucagon or epinephrine with specific liver cell surface receptors and subsequent activation of glycogen phosphorylase kinase via the calcium messenger system. Insulin, conversely, stimulates the incorporation of glucose into hepatic glycogen. Normal hepatic glycogen stores are sufficient to sustain blood glucose concentrations in the absence of exogenous carbohydrate for only about 24 hours; beyond that, maintenance of blood glucose in the fasting state depends entirely on hepatic gluconeogenesis. Gluconeogenesis, i.e., the de novo synthesis of glucose, largely from lactate, pyruvate, and amino acid precursors, is stimulated by glucagon and epinephrine and inhibited by insulin.

Thus, the normally functioning liver is responsive to a continually changing nutritional and hormonal milieu. During the fed state (relative glucose and insulin excess), glucose production (gluconeogenesis and glycogenolysis) is minimal; instead, dietary glucose either is stored as glycogen or is converted to fatty acids (*lipogenesis*), largely to be secreted from the liver in the form of triglyceride-rich lipoproteins and destined for storage in adipose tissue. In the fasting state, the process is reversed, and relative glucagon excess with respect to insulin favors energy consumption rather than energy storage. Thus, liver glycogen is mobilized, and gluconeogenesis is increased; glucose is no longer diverted to lipogenesis, but is exported into plasma. The decrease in fatty acid synthesis is associated with increased fatty acid oxidation, which becomes the principal energy source for the liver.

In liver disease, disturbances in glucose homeostasis usually produce *hypoglycemia* or *glucose intolerance*. Mild hypoglycemia (blood glucose concentrations between 45 and 60 mg per deciliter) occurs in about 50 per cent of patients with uncomplicated acute viral hepatitis. As a rule, these patients are not hyperinsulinemic; rather, hypoglycemia may reflect several hepatic abnormalities, including diminished glycogen stores, diminished glycogenolytic response to glucagon, diminished gluconeogenesis, and impaired repletion of hepatic glycogen during the fed state. In most cases, the hypoglycemia is not clinically significant, but in very severe acute liver injury of any cause, such as virus- or drug-induced massive hepatic necrosis or Reye's syndrome, hypoglycemia may be an important component of the syndrome of acute liver failure. Hepatic hypoglycemia may also occur in the absence of overt liver damage. For example, *alcoholic hypoglycemia* classically occurs in persons whose only important source of calories over a period of days is ethanol; hypoglycemia in this setting reflects both a depletion of hepatic glycogen stores and inhibition of gluconeogenesis by ethanol. Hypoglycemia should be considered in the differential diagnosis of altered mental status in any patient with significant acute liver disease or exposure to ethanol or other toxins.

Glucose intolerance, on the other hand, is more typically associated with chronic liver disease and cirrhosis. Plasma insulin concentrations tend to be high, suggesting a state of *insulin resistance*. Both insulin receptor number and binding affinity have been found to be diminished in peripheral blood monocytes, suggesting a more generalized receptor defect. In addition, insulin resistance may in part reflect increased plasma glucagon concentrations and in part a diminished insulin effect on the liver because the hormone is diverted to the peripheral circulation via portal-systemic shunts. Regardless of the mechanism, the glucose intolerance associated with chronic liver disease, per se, is rarely of clinical significance. Occasionally, patients with chronic liver disease may also have other disorders such as *hemochromatosis* and *chronic pancreatitis*, in which *diabetes mellitus* may contribute to glucose intolerance.

LIPID METABOLISM. The liver plays a central role in the metabolism of fatty acids and other lipids and lipoproteins. Of the total daily turnover of plasma nonesterified fatty acids (free fatty acids) derived from adipose tissue, about one third enter the liver, where they are esterified to triglycerides or other esters, or undergo oxidation, largely in the mitochondria. The balance between esterification and oxidation is closely regulated, as is the rate of de novo fatty acid synthesis. In the fasting state, fatty acid synthesis is inhibited, whereas fatty acid oxidation is increased at the expense of the esterification pathways. In the fed state, de novo fatty acid synthesis and esterification are favored, whereas oxidation is diminished. Exclusive of dietary sources and de novo synthesis, a total of approximately 60 to 70 grams of plasma nonesterified fatty acid (>200 mmol) is taken up by the liver each day in the average adult, and in the fasting state fatty acids are the major energy source for the liver. Interference with hepatic fatty acid metabolism may either cause or be caused by clinically significant abnormalities of hepatic structure and function.

Fatty liver usually reflects excess accumulation of triglyceride, which may be deposited as large vacuoles displacing the nucleus, or as small droplets, in which the nucleus remains central. It may be viewed as an imbalance between the rate of triglyceride biosynthesis on the one hand, and the rate of triglyceride disposition (primarily secretion into plasma in the form of very low density lipoproteins) on the other. This imbalance may result from many factors that can affect either or both sides of the equation. Conditions associated with large vacuolar fatty liver include obesity, protein-calorie malnutrition (e.g., kwashiorkor, jejunoileal bypass), diabetes mellitus, corticosteroid therapy, and ethanol ingestion (see Ch. 126). Small-droplet fat accumulation (see below) is characteristic of obstetric fatty liver (acute fatty liver of pregnancy), Reye's syndrome, Jamaican vomiting sickness, and tetracycline and valproic acid hepatotoxicity and, occasionally, is ethanol related. Accumulation of triglyceride in the liver cell is usually associated with hepatomegaly and reflects abnormal liver function, but does not *by itself* appear to cause severe, progressive, or lasting liver damage.

Conversely, interference with fatty acid oxidation at any of several stages may have profound consequences. For example, *alcoholic ketosis* is attributed to an ethanol- or acetaldehyde-mediated impairment of the tricarboxylic acid cycle, resulting in incomplete oxidation of the products derived from beta-oxidation of fatty acids. A far more profound derangement of hepatic function is caused by hypoglycin, a low molecular weight compound present in the unripened fruit of the ackee tree and the cause of *Jamaican vomiting sickness*. In this disorder, hypoglycin metabolites are converted to coenzyme A thioesters and to carnitine derivatives. Since these cannot be metabolized further, they effectively sequester the cellular carnitine pool. Fatty acid oxidation is inhibited, and there is a corresponding decrease in ATP production and gluconeogenesis. Continuing fatty acid esterification under these conditions leads to a form of fatty liver characterized by *small-droplet fat* deposition, associated in severe cases with

liver failure and hypoglycemia. Despite the histopathologic and clinical similarities among this entity and *Reye's syndrome*, *obstetric fatty liver*, and *tetracycline* and *valproic acid hepatotoxicity*, in none of these latter conditions has the pathogenesis been fully elucidated.

Another clinically important aspect of hepatic lipid metabolism concerns the synthesis of *cholesterol* and *bile acids* and the excretion of biliary lipids. The liver is the major source of endogenously synthesized cholesterol (approximately 0.5 gram per day). Together with cholesterol of dietary origin, this newly synthesized cholesterol enters a "metabolically active" hepatic cholesterol pool, from which is derived the cholesterol destined for secretion into bile or into plasma (in lipoproteins), for synthesis of liver cell membranes, and for conversion to bile acids. Bile acid synthesis accounts for the disposition of approximately half of the total daily turnover of cholesterol and, as such, is an important determinant of body cholesterol stores. Relative rates of secretion of bile acids, cholesterol, and phosphatidyl choline (lecithin) into bile are important factors in the pathogenesis of cholesterol gallstones, but the mechanism(s) by which the secretion of these substances is effected and controlled is incompletely understood.

AMINO ACID AND PROTEIN METABOLISM. Except for the immunoglobulins, most plasma proteins, including albumin, clotting factors, transferrin, alpha$_1$-antitrypsin, and the nonalimentary lipoproteins, are synthesized in the liver. The synthesis of each is controlled by specific regulatory mechanisms. In all cases, however, synthesis and secretion are dependent on the integrity of many aspects of cell function, including the transcriptional mechanisms in the nucleus, the translational mechanisms in the rough endoplasmic reticulum, and the secretory mechanisms in the Golgi apparatus. Despite these common features, individual proteins are affected differently in liver disease. This nonuniformity may result from several factors such as the availability of an essential *nutritional* component (e.g., the vitamin K–dependent clotting factors), *hormonal* influences (e.g., very low density lipoproteins), *genetic* determinants (e.g., ceruloplasmin or alpha$_1$-antitrypsin), the effects of drugs or toxins (e.g., the warfarin-like anticoagulants or ethanol), or the response of selected proteins such as fibrinogen (and other "acute phase reactants," including C-reactive proteins, ceruloplasmin, haptoglobin, and transferrin) to inflammatory processes. In addition, the *kinetics* of synthesis and turnover of a particular protein are major determinants of response of its plasma concentration to acute liver injury. In general, plasma concentrations of proteins of which the turnover is rapid (e.g., clotting factors, plasma half-time of hours to days) are more likely to be depressed by severe acute liver injury than are those of proteins that turn over more slowly (e.g., albumin, plasma half-time of 2½ to 3 weeks). Finally, *catabolism* of certain plasma proteins may be accelerated (e.g., clotting factors in *disseminated intravascular coagulation*, or albumin in *protein-losing enteropathy*). For these reasons, although liver disease generally tends to depress the plasma concentration of proteins of hepatic origin, plasma concentration of such proteins may not accurately reflect the severity of the liver disease in a given patient. Interpretation of the prothrombin time, partial thromboplastin time, and serum albumin concentrations in the evaluation of liver disease is discussed in Ch. 119.

Amino acids, in addition to their obvious importance in protein synthesis, also participate in other reactions in the liver. Of special significance is the role of certain amino acids as precursors for gluconeogenesis, as discussed above. Amino acids may undergo *transamination*, in which the alpha-amino group is transferred to an alpha-keto acid, as in the alanine transaminase (ALT)–mediated deamination of alanine to pyruvate; the resulting transfer of the amino group to alpha-ketoglutarate converts this acceptor to glutamate. Alternatively, amino acids may undergo *oxidative deamination*; in this case, an alpha-keto acid is formed as the amino group is converted to ammonium ion and, ultimately, to urea (see below).

BIOTRANSFORMATION AND DETOXIFICATION. The liver is the major site of chemical modification of a wide variety of exogenous drugs and toxins, as well as endogenous substances such as hormones. The reactions potentially involved are numerous and, in many instances, involve the cytochrome P-450–dependent microsomal mixed function oxidase system. The basic principles of drug disposition are discussed in Ch. 24, but several aspects warrant special emphasis in the context of liver function and disease. First, while biotransformation of an endogenous or exogenous substance may *inactivate* it or render it more suitable for urinary or biliary excretion, there are many examples of compounds upon which activity or toxicity is conferred by this process. A number of clinically significant hepatotoxins are *activated* in this way, and there is good evidence that some "idiosyncratic" hepatic drug reactions may reflect individual differences in drug metabolism rather than an immunologic response (see Ch. 122). Second, diseases of the liver may seriously impair the biotransformation of exogenous substances, thereby resulting in an *increased sensitivity* to certain drugs (e.g., sedatives and opiates), or may enhance the biologic effect of endogenous hormones (e.g., contributing to the feminizing effects of chronic liver disease) or toxins (e.g., diminished hepatic conversion of ammonia to urea in hepatic encephalopathy). Finally, one substance may significantly influence the hepatic biotransformation of another. Examples of this particular form of *drug-drug interaction* include the well-recognized induction of the microsomal drug-metabolizing system by prior administration of phenobarbital and its inhibition by various toxins.

A particularly important hepatic detoxification pathway converts *ammonium ion* to urea via the Krebs-Henseleit *urea cycle*, in which ornithine, citrulline, argininosuccinate, and arginine are intermediates and which involves both mitochondrial and cytosolic components (see Fig. 192–1). Glutamate, formed from NH_4^+ and alpha-ketoglutarate, is the principal NH_2 donor. Ammonium ion is produced in abundance in the intestinal tract, especially the colon, by the bacterial degradation of luminal proteins and amino acids and of endogenous urea, 25 per cent of the daily production of which diffuses into the intestinal lumen. The NH_4^+ so formed diffuses into the portal circulation and is transported to the liver, where it is converted to urea by the mechanism described above. As discussed in Ch. 128, *hepatic encephalopathy* in part reflects the failure of this important detoxification process (or of analogous pathways for other *enterogenous toxins*) because of extensive acute liver cell necrosis or direct entry of portal blood into the peripheral circulation via spontaneous or surgically created portal-systemic shunts.

Arias IM, Popper H, Schachter D, et al.: The Liver: Biology and Pathology. New York, Raven Press, 1982. *An in-depth and well-documented presentation of many more basic aspects of normal and abnormal hepatic structure and function.*

Popper H, Schaffner F (eds.): Progress in Liver Diseases. Vol. 8. Orlando, Grune & Stratton, 1986. *Authoritative reviews of several basic and clinical aspects of liver function in health and disease.*

Zakim D, Boyer T (eds.): Hepatology: A Textbook of Liver Disease. Philadelphia, W. B. Saunders Company, 1982.

118 BILIRUBIN METABOLISM AND HYPERBILIRUBINEMIA

Bruce F. Scharschmidt

BILIRUBIN METABOLISM (See Fig. 118–1)

BILIRUBIN CHEMISTRY. Bilirubin consists of four pyrrole rings linked by three carbon bridges. Unconjugated bilirubin is virtually water-insoluble at physiologic pH because its $-COOH$ and $-NH$ groups are involved in strong intramolecular hydrogen bonds and are therefore unable to interact with water. These intramolecular hydrogen bonds are disrupted by conjugation of the $-COOH$ groups with glucuronic acid as occurs in the liver cell, thus greatly enhancing the aqueous solubility of the molecule and altering its biologic properties. In contrast to the more polar water-soluble conjugates, relatively nonpolar unconjugated bilirubin diffuses across most biologic membranes such as the blood-brain barrier, placenta, and intestinal and gallbladder epithelium. It is excreted in bile in only trace amounts. Thus, hepatic conjugation confers upon bilirubin the properties that permit its elimination from the body and thereby prevents damage to the central nervous system. Exposure of bilirubin to light appears reversibly to convert unconjugated bilirubin to one of several isomers that are also unable to form intramolecular hydrogen bonds, and hence have increased water solubility. These photoisomers are excreted by the liver without conjugation; this may be the primary mechanism by which phototherapy lowers serum bilirubin concentration in neonatal hyperbilirubinemia.

BILIRUBIN FORMATION. Bilirubin is formed by selective cleavage of the heme ring at the alpha-methene bridge. Daily bilirubin production in adults averages about 4 mg per kilogram, of which about 70 per cent results from degradation of the heme moiety of hemoglobin in senescent erythrocytes. Most of the remainder results from the breakdown of nonhemoglobin hemoproteins in the liver, principally the cytochromes P-450. A minor fraction of bilirubin production results from premature destruction of newly formed erythrocytes in the bone marrow or circulation. In certain clinical disorders (e.g., megaloblastic anemia) destruction of young or developing erythroid cells is increased and may account for a substantial proportion of total bilirubin production. The most common cause of increased bilirubin production is increased breakdown of hemoglobin heme resulting from hemolysis.

Senescent erythrocytes are normally sequestered and degraded in the mononuclear phagocytic cells of the spleen, liver, or bone marrow. In contrast, the heme moiety of methemalbumin, methemoglobin, free hemoglobin, and haptoglobin-bound hemoglobin is taken up and catabolized by hepatic parenchymal cells. Microsomal heme oxygenase, the heme-cleaving enzyme, is most abundant in the liver, spleen, and bone marrow and exhibits substrate-mediated induction by heme or hemoglobin. The conversion of heme to biliverdin,

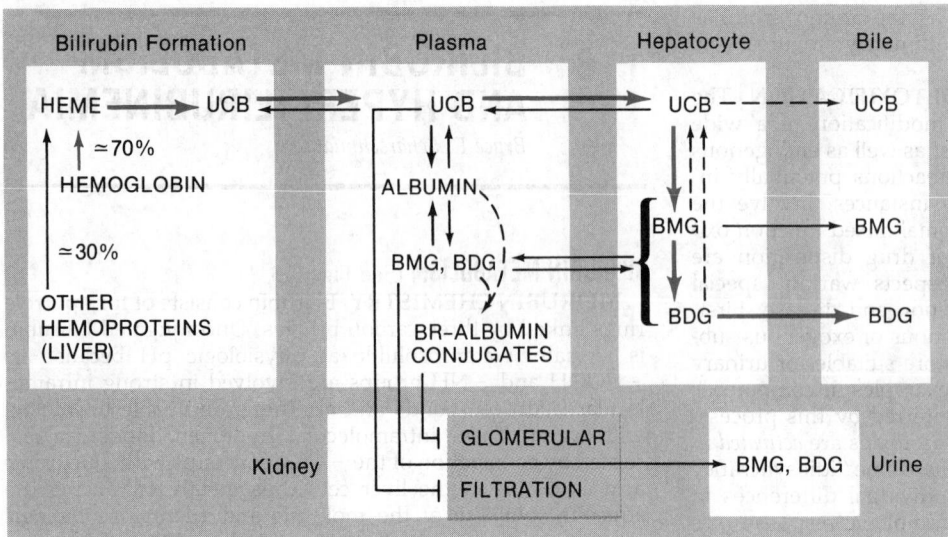

FIGURE 118–1. Overview of bilirubin metabolism. Unconjugated bilirubin (UCB) formed from the breakdown of hemoglobin heme and other hemoproteins is transported in plasma reversibly bound to albumin and is converted in the liver to bilirubin monoglucuronide (BMG) and diglucuronide (BDG), the latter being the predominant form secreted in bile. BMG and BDG together normally account for less then 5 per cent of serum bilirubin. In the presence of hepatobiliary disease, BMG and BDG accumulate in plasma and appear in urine. Bilirubin glucuronides in plasma also react nonenzymatically with albumin and possibly other serum proteins to form protein conjugates, which do not appear in urine and have a plasma half-life similar to that of albumin.

which is rate limiting for bilirubin formation, is followed by reduction of biliverdin to bilirubin by cytosolic biliverdin reductase. The reason mammals convert nontoxic, water-soluble biliverdin to water-insoluble bilirubin is unclear. Bilirubin, unlike biliverdin, is able to cross the placenta, however.

BILIRUBIN BINDING TO PLASMA PROTEINS. Unconjugated bilirubin is bound reversibly to albumin at a primary high affinity site (10^8 M^{-1}). At plasma concentrations exceeding its molar equivalence with albumin (about 35 mg per deciliter), bilirubin also binds to at least two low-affinity sites. A variety of compounds, including certain sulfonamides, penicillin derivatives, furosemide, and radiographic contrast media, may displace bilirubin from its albumin-binding sites and increase the risk of kernicterus in neonates. Presumably because of its tight albumin binding and low water solubility, unconjugated bilirubin is not excreted in urine. Conjugated bilirubin is somewhat less tightly bound to albumin than is bilirubin. It is filtered to a greater extent at the glomerulus, is incompletely reabsorbed by the renal tubules, and therefore does appear in the urine in small amounts in patients with conjugated hyperbilirubinemia.

In addition to the reversible binding to albumin just described, another bilirubin fraction binds very tightly, perhaps covalently, to albumin. This pigment fraction (called delta-bilirubin, biliprotein) has a serum half-life of about 17 days, similar to that of albumin. It has been detected only in patients with conjugated hyperbilirubinemia, in whom it may constitute a substantial proportion of direct-reacting fraction as measured by conventional assays (see below). The identification of this protein-bound fraction helps explain the occasionally slow resolution of hyperbilirubinemia in patients convalescing from hepatitis or in whom biliary obstruction has been relieved, as well as the disappearance of bilirubinuria in these patients prior to the resolution of jaundice.

HEPATIC BILIRUBIN TRANSPORT. Uptake of bilirubin and other substances tightly bound to protein is facilitated by large fenestration in the cells of the sinusoidal lining that permits plasma proteins to enter the space of Disse and directly contact the hepatocyte plasma membrane. Uptake of bilirubin and other organic anions such as sulfobromophthalein across the sinusoidal membrane of the hepatocyte displays several features characteristic of carrier-mediated transport, including saturability and competition. Uptake of albumin-bound bilirubin by the putative membrane carriers may indeed be facilitated by transient binding of the albumin-bilirubin complex to the cell surface. Once inside the liver cell, bilirubin and other organic anions appear to bind to cytoplasmic proteins such as ligandin. Ligandin, which con-

stitutes 2 per cent of cytoplasmic protein in human liver, may alter net uptake by reducing bilirubin efflux back into plasma. In addition to transport through the cytoplasm, bilirubin may be directly transferred from the plasma membrane to the membranes of the endoplasmic reticulum, where conjugation occurs.

In the process of conjugation, the carboxyl groups of one or both propionic acid side chains of bilirubin are esterified, usually with glucuronic acid. Glucose and xylose conjugates are formed in trace amounts only. Formation of bilirubin monoglucuronide and diglucuronide is catalyzed by microsomal UDP-glucuronyltransferase. Transport of conjugated bilirubin from the hepatocyte into bile, like the uptake step, seems to show saturability and competition and therefore is presumably carrier mediated. Excretion and/or conjugation, but not uptake, appears to be rate limiting for overall bilirubin transport from blood to bile. Bilirubin diglucuronide predominates in human bile (70 to 80 per cent), with the isomeric monoglucuronides present in small amounts.

ENTEROHEPATIC CIRCULATION. Absorption of conjugated bilirubin from the gallbladder and small intestine is negligible. In the terminal ileum and colon, bilirubin is converted by bacterial enzymes into colorless urobilinogens and related products, including urobilins. Most urobilinogen that is absorbed from the intestine is re-excreted in bile and ultimately in feces; a small fraction appears in urine. Urobilinogen is absent from the bile and urine of patients with complete biliary obstruction; however, fecal and urinary urobilinogen levels correlate poorly with bilirubin production rate and are of little clinical utility. In addition to urobilins, the normal brown color of stool may reflect the presence of nonbilirubin pigments, perhaps of plant origin, which are also excreted in bile and undergo enterohepatic circulation.

CONCENTRATION IN PLASMA. About 95 per cent of circulating bilirubin in healthy adults is unconjugated. In contrast, circulating bilirubin in patients with hepatocellular or biliary tract disease consists predominantly of monoconjugates and diconjugates. The conventional diazoassay, which is employed in most clinical laboratories, tends to overestimate total plasma bilirubin concentration in patients with hepatobiliary disease, perhaps because of the detection of protein-bound pigment, i.e., delta-bilirubin. Moreover, determination of conjugated bilirubin based on measurement of the direct-reacting fraction is frequently in error. Nonetheless, for practical clinical application, conventional laboratory techniques are generally adequate. Plasma bilirubin concentration, which ranges normally between 0.3 and 1.0 mg per deciliter, varies directly with bilirubin production and inversely with hepatic bilirubin clearance. Thus it is possible to interpret all forms of hyperbilirubinemia in terms of increased production and/or decreased clearance.

INHERITED DISORDERS OF BILIRUBIN METABOLISM

The hereditary disorders of hepatic bilirubin metabolism constitute a heterogeneous group of disorders characterized by impaired ability of the liver to transport or conjugate bilirubin (Table 118–1). The common and benign entity of *Gilbert's syndrome* and the exceedingly rare and almost uniformly lethal Type I *Crigler-Najjar syndrome* represent opposite ends of this spectrum. Routine tests of liver function are generally normal in all these disorders, but a variety of abnormalities in the hepatic handling of bilirubin and other cholephilic anions such as sulfobromophthalein have been described. Many of these disorders, including Gilbert's syndrome, the *Dubin-Johnson syndrome*, and *Rotor's syndrome*, may be mistaken for acquired hepatobiliary disease. They are all of interest because of the insight they provide into hepatic bilirubin transport and conjugation.

GILBERT'S SYNDROME. Because of its frequency (up to 7 per cent of the population), Gilbert's syndrome is the disorder most likely to be encountered by the clinician. Mild unconjugated hyperbilirubinemia is recognized most commonly during the second and third decades of life because of the presence of scleral icterus, often first noted with fasting or as an incidental laboratory finding. Although a variety of nonspecific symptoms have been described, it is unlikely that any significant symptoms are attributable to Gilbert's syndrome itself. Gilbert's syndrome results from a decrease in the hepatic clearance of unconjugated bilirubin, probably due to impaired conjugation. Up to one half of patients with Gilbert's syndrome have a very slight decrease in red cell survival detectable by ^{51}Cr labeling. The principal clinical importance of this disorder is that it may be confused with more serious acquired hepatobiliary disease. From a practical standpoint, the diagnosis of Gilbert's syndrome is made by demonstrating low-grade unconjugated hyperbilirubinemia in a patient with a normal physical examination and otherwise repeatedly normal laboratory tests of liver function. Normal concentrations of bile acids in serum are also helpful in excluding liver disease. Liver biopsy demonstrating normal histology is almost never necessary. An exaggerated hyperbilirubinemic response to fasting, lipid withdrawal, or nicotinic acid administration has been found to be helpful by some investigators, but these tests are neither sensitive nor specific enough to warrant routine use. In patients with overt hemolysis, direct measurement of hepatic bilirubin clearance may be necessary to establish the diagnosis. Gilbert's syndrome and the other inherited disorders of hepatic bilirubin metabolism are outlined in Table 118–1.

BENIGN RECURRENT CHOLESTASIS. In contrast to the inherited disorders in which hepatic bilirubin metabolism or excretion is selectively impaired, this entity is characterized by recurrent attacks of cholestasis manifested by pruritus, conjugated hyperbilirubinemia, and elevated serum levels of alkaline phosphatase and bile salts. Individual attacks may persist from weeks to months, do not result from biliary obstruction, and typically remit spontaneously. Attacks frequently begin in childhood, recur at highly variable intervals, and do not generally lead to cirrhosis or decreased longevity. The etiology of this disorder is unknown, but an inherited basis is postulated because of its early age of onset and familial nature.

There are also inherited forms of hemolytic anemia (e.g., hereditary spherocytosis), which may produce modest unconjugated hyperbilirubinemia due to increased bilirubin production. These disorders are discussed in detail in Ch. 138.

ACQUIRED HYPERBILIRUBINEMIA

HEMOLYSIS. Hemolysis increases bilirubin production and generally produces low-grade unconjugated, indirect-

TABLE 118–1. THE HEREDITARY DISORDERS OF HEPATIC BILIRUBIN METABOLISM

	Gilbert's Syndrome	Type I Crigler-Najjar Syndrome	Type II Crigler-Najjar Syndrome	Dubin-Johnson Syndrome	Rotor's Syndrome
Incidence	Up to 7% of population	Very rare	Uncommon	Uncommon	Rare
Inheritance	? Autosomal dominant	Autosomal recessive	? Autosomal dominant	Autosomal recessive	Autosomal recessive
Defect(s) in bilirubin metabolism	Decreased hepatic UDP-glucuronyl-transferase activity, (?) slow hepatic bilirubin uptake, associated mild hemolysis in up to 50% of patients	Absence of hepatic UDP-glucuronyltransferase activity	Markedly decreased or undetectable UDP-glucuronyltransferase activity	Impaired biliary excretion of conjugated bilirubin	Impaired biliary excretion of conjugated bilirubin
Plasma bilirubin concentration (mg/dl)	≤3 in absence of fasting or hemolysis, predominantly unconjugated	17–50, usually >20, all unconjugated	6–45, usually <20, all unconjugated	1–25, usually <7, about 60% conjugated	1–20, usually <7, about 60% conjugated
Clinical sequelae	None	Death in infancy from kernicterus in almost all cases	Usually none, rarely kernicterus	Probably none	Probably none
Plasma sulfobromophthalein disappearance rate	Mildly abnormal in some patients (45-min retention <15%)	Usually normal	Usually normal	Slow initial disappearance with frequent secondary rise (45-minute retention <20%)	Markedly slowed, no secondary rise (45-minute retention 30–50%)
Oral cholecystography	Normal	Normal	Normal	Faint or nonvisualization	Usually normal
Hepatic histology (light microscopy)	Normal, occasionally increased lipofusion	Normal	Normal	Coarse pigment in centrolobular cells	Normal
Reduction of plasma bilirubin concentration by phenobarbital	Yes	No	Yes	Minimal	Unknown
Diagnosis	Clinical and laboratory findings, response to fasting occasionally helpful, liver biopsy not usually necessary	Clinical and laboratory findings, lack of response to phenobarbital	Clinical and laboratory findings, response to phenobarbital	Clinical and laboratory findings, sulfobromophthalein disappearance, urinary coproporphyrin excretion	Clinical and laboratory findings, sulfobromophthalein disappearance
Treatment	None necessary	None uniformly effective	Phenobarbital if bilirubin concentration markedly elevated	None available, avoid estrogens (may worsen jaundice)	None available

reacting hyperbilirubinemia. Because of the enormous reserve of the hepatic bilirubin transport mechanism, hepatic bilirubin clearance remains constant, and plasma bilirubin concentration increases linearly with bilirubin production rate in most individuals. Since the bone marrow cannot increase erythrocyte production more than about eight-fold, ongoing *steady-state hemolysis* by itself cannot account for a sustained increase in plasma unconjugated bilirubin concentration above 4 to 5 mg per deciliter. Concentrations consistently exceeding this indicate hepatic dysfunction irrespective of the presence of hemolysis. In contrast, *acute hemolysis*, even in patients with normal hepatic function, may produce elevations in total plasma bilirubin concentration that greatly exceed 5 mg per deciliter.

INEFFECTIVE ERYTHROPOIESIS. Bilirubin production is increased and hence the plasma concentration of unconjugated, indirect-reading bilirubin may be elevated in a variety of disorders associated with ineffective erythropoiesis. Markedly increased ineffective erythropoiesis is the basis of the rare disorder known as *shunt hyperbilirubinemia* or *idiopathic dyserythropoietic jaundice*.

FASTING HYPERBILIRUBINEMIA. Fasting causes an increase in the plasma concentration of unconjugated, indirect-reacting bilirubin owing primarily to a decrease in hepatic bilirubin clearance. This effect may be particularly marked in patients with Gilbert's syndrome and the Type II Crigler-Najjar syndrome. Both dietary composition and total caloric intake are important, since a normocaloric but lipid-free diet produces a response similar to that observed with complete fasting, and the effect of complete fasting is reversed by feeding small amounts of lipid. The mechanism of the decrease in hepatic bilirubin clearance with fasting is unclear. A slight increase in bilirubin production contributes to fasting hyperbilirubinemia.

POSTOPERATIVE HYPERBILIRUBINEMIA. Postoperative hyperbilirubinemia (>2 mg per deciliter), also called postoperative intrahepatic cholestasis or postoperative jaundice, usually occurs in patients who have undergone major surgery. The incidence of postoperative hyperbilirubinemia is about 15 per cent following open heart surgery compared with about 1 per cent after elective abdominal surgery and may be increased in patients with pre-existing liver disease. Hyperbilirubinemia, usually predominantly conjugated, occurs from one to ten days after surgery, can become quite marked, and is typically accompanied by a two- to four-fold elevation of the alkaline phosphatase and 5'-nucleotidase with minimally abnormal transaminase levels and prothrombin time. The etiology of the hyperbilirubinemia is probably multifactorial, with both increased bilirubin production (from breakdown of transfused erythrocytes and resorption of hematomas) and impaired hepatic excretory function (from hypotension, hypoxemia, or bacteremia) being potentially important contributing factors. Postoperative hyperbilirubinemia is usually benign and resolves as the overall condition of the patient improves. It is important to distinguish it from postoperative jaundice caused by biliary obstruction or hepatocellular necrosis resulting from shock, anesthetic injury, or posttransfusion hepatitis. The latter is typically accompanied by markedly abnormal transaminase levels and prothrombin time.

DIFFUSE HEPATOCELLULAR INJURY. Hyperbilirubinemia associated with disorders such as viral hepatitis reflects one aspect of a global insult to hepatocellular function. The hyperbilirubinemia is of importance primarily as an index of the severity of hepatocellular injury. In unusual cases in which hyperbilirubinemia seems disproportionate to the hepatic injury, as reflected by serum transaminase levels and prothrombin time, a search for causes of increased bilirubin production (e.g., hemolysis) or decreased hepatic bilirubin clearance (e.g., infection) is worthwhile.

MISCELLANEOUS. Mild unconjugated hyperbilirubinemia is occasionally found in a variety of unrelated conditions. *Cyclic premenstrual unconjugated hyperbilirubinemia* appears related to serum progesterone levels. Administration of *chenodeoxycholic acid* and certain drugs such as *propranolol, rifampin,* and *probenecid* has been associated with apparently mild, reversible unconjugated hyperbilirubinemia in some instances due to reaction of the drug or a metabolite with the diazo reagent.

Fevery J, Blanckaert N: What can we learn from analysis of serum bilirubin? J Hepatol 2:113, 1986. *A brief synopsis of the interpretation of serum bilirubin measurements in relation to current concepts of bilirubin metabolism, the recent development of newer assays, and the recognition of the protein-bound bilirubin fraction.*

Ostrow JD (ed.): Bile Pigments and Jaundice: Molecular, Metabolic, and Medical Aspects. New York, Marcel Dekker, 1986. *A series of 24 exhaustively referenced monographs covering all aspects of bilirubin metabolism, which, collectively, represent the most comprehensive and authoritative treatment of this subject currently available.*

Weiss JS, Gautam A, Lauff JJ, et al.: The clinical importance of a protein-bound fraction of serum bilirubin in patients with hyperbilirubinemia. N Engl J Med 309:147, 1983. *A concise description of the protein-bound fraction—in whom it occurs and what it means.*

119 LABORATORY TESTS IN LIVER DISEASE

Robert K. Ockner

Unlike tests employed in the clinical evaluation of other organ systems (e.g., arterial blood gases, creatinine clearance, plasma hormone assays), "liver function" tests for the most part are highly empirical, and often do not indicate either the integrity of liver function or the severity of a disease process. Despite this, and provided that their limitations are recognized, they may be useful in screening for hepatobiliary diseases, diagnostic evaluation, and following the course of the disease. In this chapter, the generally available laboratory tests for the diagnosis of hepatobiliary disease are discussed with regard to physiology, pathophysiology, and clinical usefulness.

BILIRUBIN. The metabolism of bilirubin and its measurement are discussed in detail in Ch. 118.

TRANSAMINASES. *Transaminases (aminotransferases)* catalyze the transfer of amino groups from aspartate or alanine to alpha-ketoglutarate. The enzymes are named either by the products of the reaction (glutamic and oxalacetic, or glutamic and pyruvic transaminases, SGOT or SGPT, respectively) or, as is currently preferred, by the amino-group donor (aspartate or alanine transaminases, AST or ALT, respectively). Specific isozymes of AST are present in liver cell mitochondria and cytoplasm, whereas ALT is confined to the cytoplasm. Increased serum transaminase activity in liver disease is assumed to reflect leaking from injured cells. Transaminases are not present in appreciable concentrations in urine. Although they are present in bile, activity there does not reflect that in serum, and clearance of these enzymes from plasma does not depend on secretion into bile or urine. Since the mechanisms and determinants of transaminase entry into or clearance from plasma are not fully defined, interpretation of serum activity is necessarily empirical. Generally the height of the transaminase activity reflects the severity of hepatic necrosis, but there are important exceptions. In even the most severe forms of acute *alcoholic hepatitis*, for example, levels seldom exceed 200 to 300 IU per liter. In contrast, serum transaminase activities of 1000 IU or more are often present in mild uncomplicated acute *viral hepatitis* or sudden high-grade *biliary obstruction*, as may occur during passage of a gallstone. Conversely, initially elevated serum transaminase activities may fall as the clinical course of massive hepatic necrosis deteriorates, suggesting that the liver is so severely damaged that little enzyme activity remains.

Despite these caveats, the serum transaminase activities may be helpful in certain circumstances: First, they are useful as *screening tests* for liver disease. Although AST levels may be increased in diseases of other organs (e.g., myocardium and skeletal muscle), values more than ten times the upper limit of the normal range usually reflect hepatic or biliary pathology. Moreover, the ALT is relatively specific for hepatobiliary disease. In the context of other clinical and laboratory findings, identification of the source of increased serum transaminase activity is not usually difficult. Second, it is distinctly uncommon for the AST to exceed 15 times the upper limit of normal in bile duct obstruction, except when it occurs suddenly, or is associated with cholangitis. Third, in contrast to most other forms of parenchymal liver disease, in which the ALT activity usually equals or exceeds the AST, in *alcoholic hepatitis* this relationship is reversed, and this may be useful diagnostically. Finally, transaminase values are often useful in monitoring the course of acute or chronic parenchymal liver disease, although, as noted, they are potentially misleading in certain circumstances.

ALKALINE PHOSPHATASE. This group of enzymes is present in many tissues, including liver, bile ducts, intestine, bone, kidney, placenta, and leukocytes; hepatic alkaline phosphatase itself appears heterogeneous. The phosphatases catalyze the release of inorganic phosphate from a phosphate ester substrate, at alkaline pH. Their biologic function is unknown, except for an apparent relationship to bone deposition. Normally, serum alkaline phosphatase activity reflects mainly the liver and bone isozymes. In some persons, especially those of blood types O or A who are secretors of the ABO red cell antigens and are positive for the Lewis antigen, intestinal alkaline phosphatase may account for 20 to 60 per cent of total serum activity. In the later stages of pregnancy, the placental contribution may be substantial. A number of less common sources of alkaline phosphatase have been identified. These include a variant associated with hepatoma, and the so-called *Regan isozyme*. The latter is apparently identical to the placental enzyme, but originates in a variety of tumors, especially lung; it also may be detected rarely in the serum of normal subjects.

Serum alkaline phosphatase activity may be increased in many conditions not associated with hepatobiliary disease, including bone disorders, pregnancy, normal growth, and occasionally the presence of malignancy not involving either bone or liver (e.g., the Regan isozyme), and for this reason the organ or tissue of origin must be identified. In some cases, this is obvious because of other clinical and laboratory findings. When the source is less apparent, several methods have been used to differentiate hepatobiliary from other isozymes, such as heat stability or electrophoretic separation of isozymes. Most practical and available is the measurement of the serum *5'-nucleotidase, leucine aminopeptidase,* or *gamma-glutamyl transpeptidase* activities, which tend to parallel that of alkaline phosphatase in hepatobiliary disease, but do not usually increase in bone disease. However, the first two of these may increase during pregnancy (see below).

Serum hepatobiliary alkaline phosphatase activity is usually increased in bile duct obstruction, parenchymal disease, or infiltrative or mass lesions of the liver. This increased serum activity reflects increased enzyme synthesis rather than decreased biliary excretion or leakage from damaged cells. Although the highest levels usually occur with bile duct obstruction, very high values may also be associated with intrahepatic cholestasis or infiltrative or mass lesions. On the other hand, it is most unusual for the serum alkaline phosphatase activity to remain relatively normal in the presence of significant bile duct obstruction, especially in association with jaundice. Con-

versely, increased alkaline phosphatase may be the only clinically apparent abnormality in bile duct stricture or in lesions that produce obstruction of a single hepatic lobe or segment. As many as one third of patients with isolated elevations of serum hepatobiliary alkaline phosphatase activity may have no demonstrable underlying liver or biliary disease.

LEUCINE AMINOPEPTIDASE, 5'-NUCLEOTIDASE, AND GAMMA-GLUTAMYL TRANSPEPTIDASE. Leucine aminopeptidase (LAP) is a ubiquitous cellular peptidase, whereas 5'-nucleotidase (5'-NT) is a plasma membrane enzyme that cleaves the inorganic phosphate from adenosine 5'-phosphate or inosine 5'-phosphate. The serum activity of both enzymes usually increases in cholestasis, and their major clinical value is that they may be of help in identifying the source of elevated serum alkaline phosphatase activity.

Since these enzymes may be increased in late pregnancy, they are most useful in the nonpregnant patient. Although elevated serum activity of either of these enzymes suggests a hepatobiliary origin of increased alkaline phosphatase, the converse is not true, and liver alkaline phosphatase occasionally may be increased while the others remain normal.

Gamma-glutamyl transpeptidase (GGTP) is present in many tissues. It increases in serum not only in hepatobiliary disease but also after myocardial infarction, in neuromuscular diseases, in pancreatic disease in the absence of biliary obstruction, and during the ingestion of ethanol and other inducers of hepatic microsomal enzymes. The GGTP has been proposed as a sensitive screening test for hepatobiliary disease, and for the monitoring of abstinence from ethanol. This test may be used to identify the source of an alkaline phosphatase increase, but it offers no clear advantage over the other available tests.

ALBUMIN AND GLOBULIN. *Albumin* is synthesized exclusively in the liver at a rate of 100 to 200 mg per kilogram of body weight per day. The synthetic rate is influenced by systemic or liver disease and by nutritional state, thyroid hormone, glucocorticoids, plasma colloid osmotic pressure, and toxins such as ethanol and carbon tetrachloride. The mechanism of albumin degradation in health is not known; the rate is increased in exfoliative dermatitis, severe burns, nephrotic syndrome, and protein-losing enteropathy. Thus, albumin concentration, which reflects the balance between synthesis and degradation or loss, may be importantly influenced by factors other than the functional state of the liver, and therefore this test is not specific. On the other hand, if other factors can be excluded, hypoalbuminemia may be an important sign of liver disease, and serum albumin concentration may be a useful, albeit slowly responsive, indicator of changing hepatic function. Although hypoalbuminemia reflects diminished synthesis in some patients with cirrhosis and ascites, in others synthesis is normal and hypoalbuminemia is caused by a redistribution among the extracellular fluid compartments, including the peritoneal cavity.

Serum globulins are of limited diagnostic utility in hepatobiliary diseases. As a group, they are heterogeneous with respect to site and regulation of production, physical properties, and physiologic function. Their concentration, as measured by serum protein electrophoresis or salt fractionation, may be influenced by a wide variety of hepatic and extrahepatic factors and disease states. The mechanism for their increased serum concentration in liver disease is not fully understood, but probably is multifactorial, and may include stimulus to increased antibody production resulting from increased entry of bacterial antigens into the systemic circulation, or release of antigenic material from injured liver cells. An important exception to this generalization is the finding of a diminished concentration of the alpha$_1$-globulin fraction as demonstrated by serum protein electrophoresis. Since approximately 85 per cent of this fraction is accounted for by alpha$_1$-antitrypsin, a decrease in its concentration may be an important sign of an alpha₁-antitrypsin deficiency, an inherited disorder associated with neonatal hepatitis, cirrhosis, and pulmonary emphysema (see Ch. 125). Elevated IgM concentrations are common in primary biliary cirrhosis, but other clinical, laboratory, and imaging procedures are of greater diagnostic value. Diffuse increases in globulin concentrations are commonly seen in cirrhosis and may be especially pronounced in HbsAg-negative chronic active hepatitis (see Ch. 123).

PROTHROMBIN TIME. This test, usually performed by the one-stage (Quick) method, measures the rate at which prothrombin in citrated plasma is converted to thrombin in the presence of added calcium, tissue thromboplastin, and activated clotting factors. It depends on the plasma concentration not only of prothrombin but also of other clotting factors synthesized in the liver, including V, VII, X, and fibrinogen. Prothrombin time (or, expressed as a percentage of a standardized control sample, prothrombin content) may be abnormal if plasma concentrations of prothrombin itself or of the other important factors are reduced below a critical level. This may reflect an increased rate of degradation, as in disseminated intravascular coagulation, a decreased rate of synthesis, or both.

Synthesis of fibrinogen, prothrombin and of factors V, VII, IX, X, XI, XII, and XIII occurs in the liver. Synthesis of prothrombin and factors VII, IX, and X depends on an adequate supply of *vitamin K*, which activates preformed polypeptides in the liver by stimulating the synthesis of the calcium-binding residue, gamma-carboxyglutamic acid. Thus, an abnormal prothrombin time that reflects decreased production of these factors may be caused rarely by *inherited abnormalities* and much more commonly by *vitamin K deficiency, liver disease*, or both. Vitamin K is abundant in many foods, and a portion of the vitamin that is produced by intestinal bacteria may also be available to the host. Thus, deficiency of the vitamin is most often caused by one of the *malabsorption syndromes*, including biliary obstruction and other causes of cholestasis. Rarely, it may reflect antimicrobial suppression of intestinal bacteria. Any acute or chronic liver disease may cause an abnormal prothrombin time if the synthesis of essential clotting factors is impaired. In acute liver disease, hypoprothrombinemia often indicates an unfavorable prognosis.

An abnormal prothrombin time may be of diagnostic value in the evaluation of the jaundiced patient. In general, when it is prolonged on the basis of vitamin K deficiency alone, e.g., because of cholestasis-induced malabsorption, it will return to near normal levels within hours after parenteral administration of vitamin K. In contrast, when clotting factor synthesis is diminished because of parenchymal liver disease, response to vitamin K may be slight or absent. Unfortunately, for several reasons this simple and attractive diagnostic approach does not always reliably differentiate obstructive from parenchymal liver disease. First, hypoprothrombinemia may reflect more then one factor, e.g., biliary obstruction associated with parenchymal liver disease or disseminated intravascular coagulation. Second, vitamin K malabsorption and a prolonged but correctable prothrombin time may result from cholestasis of any cause, including parenchymal disease such as primary biliary cirrhosis, cholestatic hepatitis, and drug-induced cholestasis. Finally, a partial response to vitamin K administration may be misleading. Because of these shortcomings, the response to an abnormal prothrombin time to parenteral vitamin K administration must be interpreted in the context of other available information.

The *partial thromboplastin time* is used to assess the "intrinsic" clotting mechanism, and reflects the activity of all clotting factors except for platelet factor 3, factor XIII, and factor VII. For this reason, the test is complementary to the prothrombin time and may indicate deficiencies of other clotting factors or the presence of a circulating anticoagulant.

SERUM LIPIDS AND LIPOPROTEINS. Parenchymal liver disease and bile duct obstruction may be associated with significant abnormalities in serum lipids and lipoproteins. In acute parenchymal liver disease, there may be loss of the alpha₁-lipoprotein band normally present on serum lipoprotein electrophoresis, reflecting abnormal composition and physical properties of the high-density lipoproteins. There may also be a transient hypertriglyceridemia, reflecting the presence in serum of abnormal low-density lipoproteins rich in triglycerides. These changes appear attributable in part to deficient activity of plasma lecithin: cholesterol acyltransferase (LCAT), an enzyme of hepatic origin that esterifies plasma cholesterol. The changes are transient, and with resolution of the acute liver injury, plasma lipids and lipoproteins return to their previous state.

In cholestasis the serum concentrations of unesterified cholesterol and phospholipids are increased, and the development of xanthomas and xanthelasma is related to the severity and duration of this abnormality. Of the increased plasma unesterified cholesterol, a major fraction is accounted for by the presence of an abnormal low-density lipoprotein, designated *LPX*. LPX consists mainly of unesterified cholesterol and phosphatidyl choline (lecithin), in a 1:1 molar ratio, with a small amount of protein, largely a mixture of albumin and the C apolipoproteins. In negative-staining electron microscopy, LPX assumes the shape of a disc that may form rouleaux. The similarity of the lipid composition of LPX to that of bile (primarily free cholesterol and lecithin), together with other evidence, suggests that it represents the entry into plasma either of biliary lipid or of lipid from the hepatocyte normally destined for secretion into bile. LPX is not currently of value in the differential diagnosis of jaundice. Its concentrations are correlated with the far simpler determination of plasma-free cholesterol concentration, but not with other tests of liver function.

MITOCHONDRIAL ANTIBODY. In approximately 90 per cent of patients with primary biliary cirrhosis, serum contains antibodies directed against a lipoprotein component of the inner mitochondrial membrane. The antibodies are neither organ nor species specific, and are demonstrated by immunofluorescent techniques employing rat kidney, liver, and stomach and human thyroid, stomach, and kidney. They include the three main immunoglobulin classes and are complement fixing. In patients with primary biliary cirrhosis, the titer is not related to the increased level of serum IgM or the stage or severity of the disease.

Mitochondrial antibodies are also present in up to 25 per cent of patients with chronic active hepatitis and postnecrotic cirrhosis and in 7 to 8 per cent of asymptomatic relatives of patients with primary biliary cirrhosis. They are rarely present in extrahepatic biliary obstruction. A small percentage of patients with nonhepatic diseases may also exhibit positive tests; these include the collagen-vascular disorders, thyroiditis, myasthenia gravis, Addison's disease, autoimmune hemolytic anemia, and chronic biologic false-positive reactions for syphilis. Several types of mitochondrial antibodies have thus far been identified; M₂ is the type usually found in primary biliary cirrhosis. Mitochondrial antibodies are demonstrable in only 0.4 to 0.7 per cent of the general population.

In the differential diagnosis of jaundice the mitochondrial test is useful in two respects. First, a negative result renders the diagnosis of primary biliary cirrhosis unlikely but does not exclude it. Second, because of its rarity in extrahepatic biliary obstruction, a positive result tends to suggest parenchymal liver disease, but it does not exclude bile duct obstruction. Since the incidence of gallstones in patients with primary biliary cirrhosis is approximately 40 per cent, and is also increased in other forms of cirrhosis, the mitochondrial antibody test cannot be regarded as a reliable basis for distinguishing "medical" from "surgical" jaundice.

ANTINUCLEAR AND SMOOTH MUSCLE ANTIBODIES. Either or both of these tests may be positive in a variable percentage of patients with chronic active hepatitis, usually among those cases not associated with hepatitis B infection. They have also been demonstrated in a minority of patients with primary biliary cirrhosis. As is true of the mitochondrial antibody, these factors are neither organ nor species specific. They probably do not play a role in pathogenesis. The presence of these antibodies in serum may suggest but does not differentiate among chronic hepatitis, postnecrotic cirrhosis, or primary biliary cirrhosis, and clearly does not exclude a bile duct lesion.

TESTS FOR HEPATITIS VIRUS INFECTION. These tests and their clinical significance are discussed in Ch. 121.

URINE AND STOOL EXAMINATIONS. The presence of bilirubin in urine indicates that a significant fraction of plasma bilirubin is conjugated, and is strong evidence of hepatobiliary disease. Jaundice in the absence of bilirubinuria indicates an exclusively unconjugated hyperbilirubinemia, i.e., reflecting hemolysis, ineffective erythropoiesis, or an inherited disorder of bilirubin conjugation. For several reasons, urine and fecal *urobilinogen* determinations usually do not provide useful information in the evaluation of hepatobiliary disease (see Ch. 125). Testing of stool for occult blood is essential, and may provide the first evidence of an alimentary tract lesion related or unrelated to hepatobiliary disease, a bleeding diathesis, or an explanation for the appearance of hepatic encephalopathy. In selected cases, depending on the clinical circumstances, stool culture or examination for ova and parasites may provide information of importance in the diagnosis of liver disease.

HEMATOLOGIC TESTS IN LIVER DISEASE. Diseases of the liver may be associated with a wide variety of hematologic abnormalities, including qualitative and quantitative changes in the formed elements, and in clotting function. The abnormalities depend not only on the etiology of the liver disorder but also on whether it is acute or chronic, or associated with complications such as liver failure or portal hypertension.

In acute liver disease not associated with liver failure, major changes in the formed elements are uncommon and consist primarily of mild anemia, reflecting either low-grade hemolysis or marrow depression. Macrocytosis may be present. Slight leukopenia is not uncommon and often is associated with atypical lymphocytes.

Rarely, a severe aplastic anemia may complicate acute viral hepatitis, especially non-A, non-B. The pathogenesis is unknown, the prognosis is very poor, and treatment is largely ineffective. In other forms of acute liver disease, hematologic abnormalities, e.g., marrow suppression, may be caused by toxins such as ethanol or drugs. Zieve's syndrome also occurs in the alcoholic. It consists of hemolytic anemia and hypertriglyceridemia; the basis for this association is not understood. Coagulopathy may complicate massive hepatic necrosis, reflecting depressed hepatic synthesis of clotting factors or disseminated intravascular coagulation.

In chronic liver disease, a number of abnormalities of the erythrocytes may be present. Target cells, often associated with cholestasis, result from an expansion of the cell membrane, with relative preservation of the cholesterol-phospholipid ratio. Spur cells (acanthocytes) are most often found in advanced cirrhosis, usually alcoholic, and reflect a more profound relative and absolute increase in membrane-free cholesterol.

Red cells, white cells, and platelets may be decreased in patients with portal hypertension, primarily because of hypersplenism. A number of other abnormalities may be present, but to a large extent these are caused by associated nutritional, pathologic, or pharmacologic influences. Examples include iron deficiency, megaloblastic, and sideroblastic anemias.

LIVER BIOPSY. Performed by a blind technique or under direct vision during laparoscopy, this procedure is of value in the diagnosis of diffuse or localized parenchymal diseases (e.g., cirrhosis, chronic hepatitis, hemochromatosis) and hepatomegaly. Because bile duct obstruction is often associated with nonspecific parenchymal changes, biopsy is not ordinarily a preferred initial diagnostic procedure in the evaluation of the patient with cholestatic jaundice. Rather, imaging and cholangiographic methods are more rewarding in this setting. Liver biopsy requires the cooperation of the patient, except in infants, and normal clotting function. Relative or absolute contraindications include the presence of biliary sepsis, right pleural disease, ascites, coagulopathy, and high-grade bile duct obstruction.

IMAGING TECHNIQUES AND CHOLANGIOGRAPHY. These techniques are discussed in detail in Ch. 95. In the following chapter, their utility is considered briefly in the context of the diagnosis of jaundice.

Arias IM, Popper H, Schachter D, et al.: The Liver: Biology and Pathobiology. New York, Raven Press, 1982. *An in-depth and well-documented presentation of many more basic aspects of normal and abnormal hepatic structure and function.*

Popper H, Schaffner F (eds.): Progress in Liver Diseases. Vol. 8. Orlando, Grune & Stratton, 1986.

Wright R, Millward-Sadler GH, Alberti KGMM, et al. (eds.): Liver and Biliary Disease. 2nd ed. London, W. B. Saunders Company, 1985.

Zakim D, Boyer T (eds.): Hepatology: A Textbook of Liver Disease. Philadelphia, W. B. Saunders Company, 1982. *A comprehensive textbook. Provides references dealing with hepatobiliary structure, function, and disease.*

120 APPROACHES TO THE DIAGNOSIS OF JAUNDICE

Robert K. Ockner

Jaundice may be caused by a wide range of disorders (Ch. 118). Excluding hemolysis, ineffective erythropoiesis, and congenital errors of bilirubin metabolism (any of which may be present *in addition to other causes*), jaundice can be broadly classified as *intrahepatic* or *extrahepatic*. Included among the intrahepatic causes are (1) hepatocellular diseases such as viral or drug-induced acute or chronic liver disease, (2) various metabolic and infiltrative disorders such as anoxia, Wilson's disease, and metastatic tumor, and (3) disorders of the intrahepatic biliary system such as primary biliary cirrhosis, intrahepatic sclerosing cholangitis, and congenital disorders associated with cystic dilatation of the smaller bile ducts. Extrahepatic causes of jaundice, i.e., large bile duct obstruction, include choledocholithiasis, bile duct strictures, chronic pancreatitis with bile duct compression, and tumors affecting the bile duct itself or critically situated contiguous structures such as lymph nodes in the porta hepatis, the ampulla of Vater, or the head of the pancreas.

In view of the magnitude and diversity of the differential diagnosis, the clinical approach must be equally broad. A careful history and physical examination are of paramount importance, emphasizing a search for clues that might suggest a cause such as exposure to a jaundiced person or a potentially toxic drug (viral or drug-induced hepatitis), an antecedent history of pruritus and xanthelasma (chronic cholestasis such as primary biliary cirrhosis), recurrent abdominal pain and nausea (gallstone disease), chronic ulcerative colitis (sclerosing cholangitis), or epigastric pain, weight loss, and distended gallbladder (cancer of the head of the pancreas). Routinely available laboratory studies are also helpful (see Ch. 119). In general, serum aminotransferase activities do not exceed 10 to 15 times the upper limit of normal in patients with bile duct obstruction, unless there is superimposed bacterial cholangitis or the obstruction occurs suddenly, and is high grade. In the latter instance, usually associated with impaction of a gallstone in the common bile duct, the aminotransferase level, which may exceed 1000 IU, usually also falls quite rapidly (over a few days) toward normal. Alkaline phosphatase activities usually exceed two to three times normal, but very high values may be seen in both intrahepatic and extrahepatic processes. Elevation of serum cholesterol tends to suggest chronic cholestasis but is of little help in differential diagnosis. Amylase activity may be elevated because of pancreatitis induced by passage of a gallstone that also causes bile duct obstruction, or may reflect pancreatitis of some other cause that secondarily causes compression of the intrapancreatic portion of the distal common bile duct. Hepatitis serologies may help in diagnosis, but obstructive biliary disease may be superimposed on chronic parenchymal liver disease such as chronic hepatitis B or cirrhosis.

Despite the seemingly limitless number of diagnostic possibilities and of permutations and combinations of clinical and laboratory findings, the clinical evaluation (that based on history, physical examination, and routine laboratory tests) is quite accurate and serves to identify correctly the cause of jaundice in 80 to 85 per cent of cases. It is for confirmation of these clinical diagnoses (when needed) and for the elucidation of the clinically more obscure processes that other diagnostic procedures are available. The availability and accuracy of these procedures have increased dramatically in recent years, and the decision regarding their proper use has become a critically important part of the judgmental process involved in the management of these problems.

The diagnostic approach to the jaundiced patient does not lend itself readily to generalizations or inflexible algorithms. Rather, a host of highly individual factors must be taken into account. These include the evolving clinical course and current status of the patient; the differential diagnosis; the availability, reliability, and safety of diagnostic procedures in a given institution; and the experience and judgment of a consulting surgeon. Despite these reservations, some general guidelines are valid in many instances and may serve, with appropriate modification, as the basis for an approach to diagnosis.

First, as noted above, the diagnosis in most patients will be obvious or strongly suggested by routine clinical and laboratory findings. For example, if the patient appears to have viral or drug-induced acute hepatitis, if this presumptive diagnosis is supported by appropriate laboratory studies, and if the patient is doing well, more elaborate or invasive studies are usually unnecessary as continuing observation and follow-up studies will suffice.

Second, if more information is needed in a patient with unexplained cholestatic jaundice, liver biopsy is often not helpful, since in many cases of parenchymal cholestasis the histopathology is nonspecific. Moreover, parenchymal liver disease not only does not exclude biliary tract disease but may in fact predispose to it (e.g., the increased incidence of gallstones in cirrhosis). Thus, although biopsy can be performed with reasonable safety in the presence of bile duct obstruction, in most cases it will not be the initial diagnostic procedure of choice.

Of the available radiographic and imaging procedures, ultrasound scanning and computed tomography are attractive because they are noninvasive and provide accurate information concerning caliber of the bile ducts. Because of its lesser cost, the absence of radiation exposure, and its ability to detect stones in the gallbladder accurately, ultrasonography may be preferred. However, these two tests suffer from a finite, albeit small error rate (both false positives and false negatives) in the diagnosis of bile duct obstruction. This is not unexpected in view of the fact that these techniques provide information as to the caliber of the bile duct; the presence or absence of biliary obstruction can only be inferred. Clearly, the syndrome of biliary tract obstruction is so varied that the relationship between completeness and duration of the obstructive process on the one hand and the caliber of the ducts on the other must also vary. For these reasons, the noninvasive tests, although useful in initial assessment, may not be definitive.

Direct cholangiography is currently the most reliable approach to the nonoperative diagnosis of cholestatic jaundice. It may be accomplished either percutaneously, with the Chiba ("skinny") needle, or endoscopically. In most centers, the probability of duct visualization with the percutaneous transhepatic technique approaches 100 per cent in the presence of bile duct obstruction. The success rate with parenchymal jaundice is variable but generally lower. The procedure is rapid and simple, is readily performed in most institutions, and involves minimal cost and technical experience. For these reasons, percutaneous transhepatic cholangiography represents the best combination of accuracy, speed, low risk, and low cost, and therefore is suggested as the single most valuable of the currently available invasive techniques (see also Ch. 95).

Endoscopic retrograde cholangiography, although more demanding of patient and physician, more expensive, and more time consuming, nonetheless has a definite place. It can be safely performed in the patient with abnormal clotting function, whereas the percutaneous study cannot. It may demonstrate duct pathology when the percutaneous approach has failed, and may be especially suitable in those patients in whom the intrahepatic bile ducts are not dilated, or in whom there may be associated pancreatic disease. Finally, it may permit a direct therapeutic approach in certain cases, e.g., endoscopic sphincteroplasty and stone extraction for patients with retained impacted common bile duct stones or gallstone-associated pancreatitis. Each of these procedures carries with it certain risks, which are discussed in Ch. 96.

Niederau C, Sonnenberg A, Muelle J: Comparison of the extrahepatic bile duct size measured by ultrasound and by different radiographic methods. Gastroenterology 87:615, 1984. *An interesting comparison among commonly used techniques with evidence for some important differences.*

Scharschmidt BF, Goldberg HI, Schmid R: Approach to the patient with cholestatic jaundice. N Engl J Med 308:1515, 1983. *A concise summary, useful approach, and comprehensive bibliography.*

Vennes JA, Bond JH: Approach to the jaundiced patient. Gastroenterology 84:1615, 1983. *A balanced editorial addressing the clinical problem in general and two accompanying articles in particular.*

121 ACUTE VIRAL HEPATITIS

Robert K. Ockner

DEFINITION. Acute viral hepatitis is caused by any of several agents and presents as a spectrum of syndromes ranging from entirely subclinical and inapparent to rapidly progressive and fatal. In most cases, it is self-limited and uncomplicated, but, depending on the viral agent involved, there is a variable incidence of clinically significant extrahepatic manifestations or of progression to chronic liver disease. These diseases represent an infection by a viral agent with relative or absolute predilection for the hepatocyte. After a variable incubation period, viral replication in the liver cell approaches a maximum, followed by the appearance of viral components in body fluids and/or excreta, liver cell necrosis with an associated inflammatory response, changes in laboratory tests of liver function, and symptoms and signs of liver damage. The immunologic response of the host appears to play an important but not fully defined role in pathogenesis.

ETIOLOGY. Viral hepatitis is caused by three major agents and several minor ones. The vast majority of cases are accounted for by hepatitis viruses A and B, and the so-called non-A, non-B agents, of which there appear to be at least two. Selected characteristics of each are summarized in Table 121–1, and each is considered in greater detail below. The

TABLE 121-1. CHARACTERISTICS OF COMMON CAUSATIVE AGENTS OF ACUTE VIRAL HEPATITIS

	Hepatitis A	Hepatitis B	Hepatitis D	Hepatitis Non-A, Non-B (Two or More Agents)
Causative agent	27 nm RNA virus	42 nm DNA virus; core and surface components	36nm hybrid particle with HBsAg coat	Apparent similarities to hepatitis B virus
Transmission	Fecal-oral; H₂O-, food borne	Parenteral inoculation, or equivalent; direct contact	Similar to HBV	Same as for B; epidemic form attributed to HAV-like agent
Incubation period	2–6 weeks	4 weeks–6 months	Similar to HBV	2–20 weeks
Period of infectivity	2–3 weeks in late incubation and early clinical phases	During HBsAg positivity (occasionally only with anti-HBc positivity)	During HDV RNA or anti-HDV positivity	Unknown
Massive hepatic necrosis	Rare	Uncommon	Yes	Uncommon
Carrier state	No	Yes	Yes	Yes (? for epidemic form)
Chronic hepatitis	No	Yes	Yes	Yes (not for epidemic form)
Prophylaxis (see text)	Hygiene; immune serum globulin	Hygiene; hepatitis B immune globulin; vaccine	Hygiene; HBV vaccine	Hygiene; ? immune serum globulin; avoid commercial blood

delta (δ) agent (hepatitis D) may cause an acute or chronic hepatitis syndrome limited to those individuals with simultaneous or pre-existing hepatitis B virus infection (see below). Other viral agents that cause an acute hepatitis syndrome include the Epstein-Barr virus (infectious mononucleosis), cytomegalovirus, herpes simplex, yellow fever, and rubella; the clinical disorders caused by these agents are considered in greater detail elsewhere in the text.

PATHOLOGY. The lesion of ordinary acute hepatitis A, B, and non-A, non-B consists of focal necrosis of individual hepatocytes associated with a mononuclear inflammatory response, and expanded portal areas that are infiltrated predominantly by lymphocytes and in which bile ducts may be especially prominent (bile duct "proliferation"). There is often a variable, but usually minor, degree of necrosis of hepatocytes bordering the portal areas (so-called periportal hepatitis or piecemeal necrosis). Necrosis of an individual liver cell, whether periportal or within the lobule, is usually reflected in its replacement by a cluster of mononuclear cells, or it may be represented by balloon degeneration or by a shrunken cell with homogeneous eosinophilic cytoplasm and a condensed pyknotic nucleus ("acidophil body"). The regular pattern of the cords of hepatocytes is disrupted, mitotic figures and cholestasis are common, and Kupffer cells are prominent. Although these features are characteristic of typical acute viral hepatitis, they are not specific, individually or collectively. Thus, the same overall pattern of injury is seen in certain forms of drug-induced liver disease, and its individual components are seen in many processes of diverse etiology and duration. Mononuclear cell portal infiltrates, periportal hepatitis, and bridging or confluent necrosis may be especially prominent in chronic forms of hepatitis.

More severe variants of the acute necrotic process include "bridging" necrosis, "confluent" or "submassive" necrosis, and massive necrosis. In these, the necrotic process simultaneously involves contiguous groups of cells rather than single cells in isolation. As a result, there may be variable collapse or condensation of stroma. Bridging necrosis, so named because the continuous zones of necrosis may extend between (i.e., "bridge") adjacent portal and/or central areas, may be a necessary, if not sufficient, antecedent to evolution to a subacute form of hepatitis with progressive deterioration of liver function leading over several months to death in liver failure, or to chronic hepatitis or to cirrhosis. Such a predisposition is not conclusively established, however. Thus, bridging necrosis is compatible with complete clinical and histologic recovery and therefore does not per se constitute evidence of chronic or progressive liver disease.

Submassive and massive hepatic necrosis are reflected in a more severe clinical course and a less favorable prognosis. Massive necrosis, in which broad areas of hepatocytes are destroyed, with condensation of stromal elements and portal structures (bile ducts and vessels), is usually manifested clinically as fulminant hepatic failure (see Ch. 128). This syndrome is characterized by severely deranged liver function, hepatic encephalopathy, and a high case fatality rate. In survivors, however, despite the severity of the acute process, a chronic course is unusual, and liver histology typically returns nearly to normal.

In the recovery phase there is regeneration of hepatocytes and a largely complete restoration of normal lobular architecture. It is distinctly uncommon for the healing that follows a circumscribed acute hepatitis to be accompanied by fibrous scar formation or by nodular regeneration. In the latter, hepatocytes cluster in an abnormal configuration lacking a central vein and other components of the normal lobular architecture. These two manifestations of an *abnormal* healing process (fibrosis and nodular regeneration) are the essential components of cirrhosis, a form of chronic liver disease that almost always reflects ongoing injury and repair rather than a single acute event.

CLINICAL AND LABORATORY MANIFESTATIONS. The earliest symptoms of acute viral hepatitis typically are nonspecific, predominantly constitutional and gastrointestinal. They may include malaise, fatigue, anorexia, nausea, vomiting, and arthralgias, and may suggest a "flu" or upper respiratory syndrome to both patient and physician. Classically, the patient may describe a loss of taste for coffee or cigarettes. Fever, if present, is usually mild. Abdominal discomfort may reflect an enlarged tender liver. Arthritis occurs in 10 to 15 per cent of cases; in hepatitis B it appears to represent immune complex deposition, but it also occurs with similar frequency in hepatitis A, in which immune complexes have not been demonstrated. Urticaria may occur occasionally.

After a period of several days to a week or more, the prodromal phase may lead to an icteric phase. The earliest clinical manifestation of a rising serum concentration of direct-reacting bilirubin is bilirubinuria, followed by a lightening of stool color, scleral icterus, and, in light-skinned individuals, frank jaundice. Constitutional symptoms often abate during the icteric phase, especially in children, in whom the disease is characteristically less severe. In adults, the gastrointestinal components of the prodrome may persist or even increase for a time. If cholestasis worsens, pruritus may cause increasing discomfort.

Physical findings are variable and depend on the stage of the illness. The only objective finding during the prodrome, apart from mild fever, may be an enlarged and tender liver, associated in perhaps 20 per cent with splenomegaly. Jaundice may or may not appear; indeed, it is likely that the vast majority of cases remain anicteric. Excoriations reflect the intensity of pruritus. Spider nevi occasionally develop during an acute hepatitis, but since their appearance is unusual, it should suggest the possibility of a more chronic process.

Laboratory studies are highly variable, but almost by definition the clinical onset is accompanied by rising activities of serum transaminases; usually the ALT (SGPT) exceeds the AST (SGOT). An elevated serum bilirubin is predominantly direct reacting; very high concentrations, e.g., greater than 15 to 20 mg per deciliter, indicate a severe lesion or may reflect associated hemolysis. The alkaline phosphatase is usually moderately increased, whereas serum albumin concentration may decrease slightly. A diffuse hyperglobulinemia is common. Prothrombin time is prolonged in more severe cases, and a persisting or increasing prolongation is an unfavorable prognostic sign. Mild and clinically insignificant hypoglycemia occurs in perhaps 50 per cent of cases; more profound hypoglycemia may complicate fulminant hepatic failure. Hematologic tests are also quite variable. Usually the total leukocyte count is normal or slightly decreased and atypical lymphocytes may be present. In more severe cases, total leukocytes may be increased, with relative or absolute neutrophilia. Hemoglobin and hematocrit are usually relatively normal, but occasionally there may be a coincidental hemolytic process, and rarely the course is complicated by aplastic anemia. Urinalysis is usually nonspecific except for the presence of bilirubin.

An important aspect of the laboratory approach to acute viral hepatitis is the etiologic serodiagnosis. Although establishing a specific etiologic diagnosis will not usually influence management, it may have a bearing on prognosis, and is particularly useful epidemiologically and for the immunization of contacts. These tests are considered below, in the discussions of hepatitis A, hepatitis B, hepatitis D, and prevention.

After an icteric phase lasting usually from several days to several weeks, the patient enters a convalescent phase in which there is gradual improvement in symptoms and laboratory tests. The healing process may require several weeks, during which time residual weakness and malaise are common. Normalization of laboratory tests is usually complete within four months. Persistence of abnormalities beyond six months suggests that the process may have become chronic; in this circumstance, liver biopsy may be indicated if there is no evidence of continuing improvement.

COMPLICATIONS AND EXTRAHEPATIC MANIFESTATIONS. The two most important complications of acute viral hepatitis are massive hepatic necrosis (fulminant hepatitis) and progression to chronic hepatitis. Fortunately, these are uncommon, especially in hepatitis A, in which chronicity does not occur and massive necrosis is less common than in hepatitis B and non-A, non-B.

Massive hepatic necrosis with fulminant hepatic failure occurs in fewer than 1 per cent of cases of acute viral hepatitis and is usually signaled by deepening jaundice, increasing prothrombin time, and hepatic encephalopathy, which, in its earliest stages, may appear only as a subtle personality change. Serum transaminase levels may remain high, but in many cases will fall, often in association with a decrease in liver size. These changes are assumed to reflect extensive loss of parenchymal mass and, in the presence of other evidence of a deteriorating course, are unfavorable prognostic signs. The diagnosis and management of acute hepatic failure and encephalopathy are considered in greater detail in Ch. 128.

Evolution to chronic hepatitis is a more common complication of acute hepatitis B, D, and non-A, non-B. It is suggested by persistence of abnormal serum transaminases, with or without other laboratory abnormalities and clinical symptoms, beyond an arbitrarily selected endpoint. Authorities differ as to where that endpoint belongs; guidelines range from four to twelve months, but most would accept six months as reasonable. Clearly, however, judgments must be individualized as to when an acute process becomes chronic (or, more pragmatically, when investigations such as liver biopsy should be performed). For example, as long as the patient continues to show evidence of clinical and laboratory improvement, there is little to be gained from a more vigorous diagnostic or

therapeutic approach. Conversely, evidence suggestive of chronic liver disease (e.g., signs of portal hypertension or progressive deterioration of laboratory tests) appearing before six months may justify earlier diagnostic intervention. Since many of the histopathologic features associated with chronic hepatitis also may be components of an acute process, however, liver biopsies obtained too early in the course may be difficult to interpret and potentially misleading. Chronic hepatitis is also considered in the discussions of hepatitis B, D, and non-A, non-B, below, and in greater detail in Ch. 123.

The *cholestatic hepatitis syndrome* occurs occasionally as a complication of acute viral hepatitis. Patients may exhibit a relatively prolonged course dominated by cholestatic features, including pruritus, dark urine, light stools, direct-reacting hyperbilirubinemia, and elevation of alkaline phosphatase. Some of these cases are associated with hepatitis A virus infection. Almost without exception, however, the prognosis is favorable. The major problem in management posed by this variant is its occasionally difficult differentiation from biliary obstruction and the possible need to exclude disorders such as gallstones, stricture, and tumors by means of appropriate imaging and cholangiographic techniques. Brief corticosteroid therapy may be useful symptomatically and is well tolerated, but has no long-range impact.

Aplastic anemia may very rarely complicate the icteric or convalescent phase of acute viral hepatitis, especially non-A, non-B. Its pathogenesis is unknown, and its prognosis poor. Among the relatively few survivors, there is no clear evidence of a beneficial effect of glucocorticoids or anabolic steroid treatment. Other formed elements may also be depressed, and pancytopenia, agranulocytosis, and thrombocytopenia have been reported.

Extrahepatic manifestations of acute viral hepatitis also include *arthralgias* and *arthritis*, and *urticaria*. These are usually most prominent during the prodromal phase and, in hepatitis B, appear to reflect deposition of immune complexes. They also may occur in non-A, non-B hepatitis. Other manifestations of hepatitis B infection, such as *glomerulonephritis* and *vasculitis*, are also associated with immune complex deposition and are discussed in Ch. 81 and 63, respectively. A tentative association of *essential mixed cryoglobulinemia* with hepatitis B infection also has been reported. *Pancreatitis* is found in 12 to 40 per cent of cases of fatal acute viral hepatitis, and serum amylase activity may be elevated in up to 30 per cent of nonfatal cases; the true overall incidence and mechanism of pancreatitis in viral hepatitis are not known. Myocarditis, pneumonitis, and other extrahepatic manifestations are rare, and in their presence other systemic disorders should be considered.

SPECIFIC ETIOLOGIC CATEGORIES OF VIRAL HEPATITIS

HEPATITIS A. This form of hepatitis also has been referred to as infectious hepatitis, short-incubation hepatitis, or MS-I hepatitis. The causative agent (hepatitis A virus) is a 27-nm diameter RNA virus that is readily and almost exclusively transmitted via the fecal-oral route. In this important respect it differs significantly from hepatitis B, D, and most cases of non-A, non-B. Accordingly, when the etiology of water-borne, point-source, food-handler–related, and institutional hepatitis outbreaks has been defined, hepatitis A almost invariably has been implicated. An epidemic form of non-A, non-B hepatitis may also be spread by contaminated water supplies. In addition, hepatitis A occurs sporadically and is spread by direct person-to-person contact; there appears to be an increased incidence among promiscuous homosexuals. Spread of hepatitis A in day care centers may involve not only children but also the staff and the families of affected children. Although parenteral transmission is theoretically possible, it must occur rarely. The incidence of the disease appears to correlate in a general way with personal hygiene and the efficacy of public health measures, as suggested by the apparent influence of socioeconomic status on the incidence of

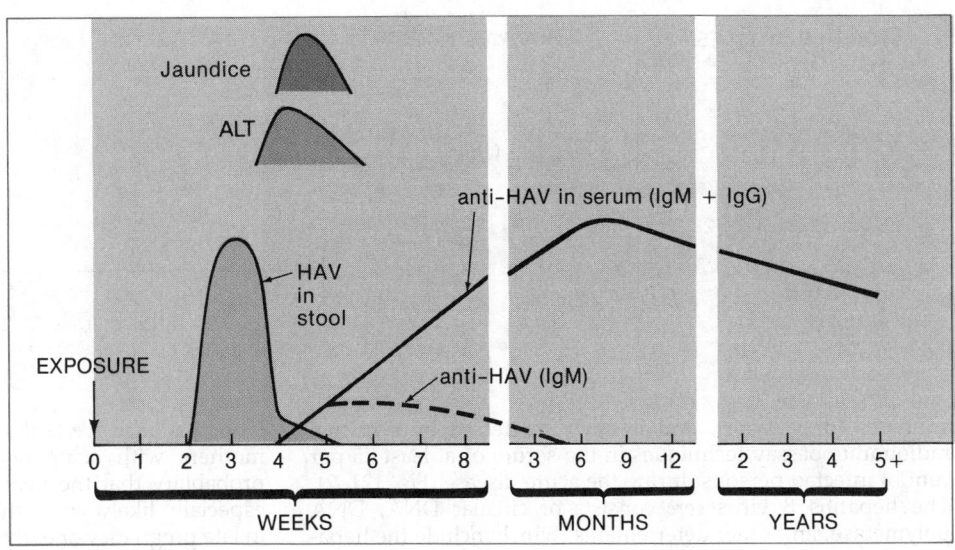

FIGURE 121–1. Sequence of clinical and laboratory findings in a patient with hepatitis A. Fecal shedding of virus is brief in duration, and ends with the appearance of anti-HAV in serum. IgM anti-HAV may persist in serum for a year or more after the acute illness. (From Krugman S, Gocke DJ: Viral Hepatitis. Philadelphia, W. B. Saunders Company, 1978.)

hepatitis A antibodies (anti-HAV), which averaged 45 per cent in one study of an urban population in the United States and approximated 90 per cent in residents of Costa Rica. There is no evidence for the existence of a chronic form of hepatitis A or a carrier state. The "reservoir" for the virus appears to consist of the large number of clinically inapparent acute cases, as well as those persons in the late incubation period of overt hepatitis A in whom shedding of virus occurred prior to the clinical onset.

Hepatitis A infection typically has an incubation period of two to six weeks. Fecal shedding of virus occurs during the final week of the incubation period and the prodromal phase, and declines as serum transaminases reach maximal levels (Fig. 121–1 and Table 121–1). Although there is a transient viremia during this interval, parenteral transmission of the disease is very rare. Viral shedding in stool declines as antibody (anti-HAV) appears in serum. Initially, antibody is predominantly of the IgM class, but an IgG antibody soon appears, and after several weeks to a few months the IgM antibody disappears. The IgG antibody perisists in serum for many years; its exclusive presence indicates prior experience with, and immunity to, the hepatitis A virus. The presence of the IgM antibody, on the other hand, almost always indicates current or very recent infection (Table 121–2), although occasionally this antibody may persist for up to one year or more. Shedding of virus is limited to a two- to three-week period. An IgA antibody to HAV appears in the feces of patients at about the time fecal shedding of virus ceases and persists for several weeks.

The acute illness itself is quite diverse in its clinical manifestations and course. The majority of cases probably are clinically inapparent, especially in children, or are perceived as a nonspecific "flu" syndrome. Jaundice, when it occurs, is usually mild. Symptoms usually subside, and serum transaminases return to normal within three to four months. Hepatitis A virus infection has been implicated in some cases of acute cholestatic hepatitis. Rarely, hepatitis A causes massive hepatic necrosis and fulminant hepatic failure, but this complication is much less common than in hepatitis B and non-A, non-B.

The ease with which hepatitis A is transmitted among contacts and via water and food, as well as the demonstrated efficacy of immune serum globulin in prevention or amelioration of the disease, underscores the value of individual and public health measures to control the spread of infection. The application of these to the management of the individual patient and his or her contacts is discussed below.

HEPATITIS B. In marked contrast to hepatitis A, hepatitis B virus infection may cause a wide variety of acute or chronic

hepatic and extrahepatic diseases, as well as a chronic carrier state. Its presentation as an acute hepatitis is typical of those cases that previously were designated serum hepatitis, homologous serum jaundice, long-incubation hepatitis, or MS-II hepatitis, although it is now apparent that many of these cases may also represent non-A, non-B hepatitis (see below). The hepatitis B virus (HBV) differs in almost every respect from hepatitis A (Tables 121–1 and 121–2; Fig. 121–2). The complete infective virion, or *Dane (HBV) particle*, is a DNA virus of 42 nm diameter, consisting of antigenically distinct surface and core components. The *surface coat* is largely lipid and protein, and may exist in serum or other body fluids either as a component of the Dane particle or as separate 20-nm diameter spheres or cylinders. Its major antigenic determinant (hepatitis B surface antigen, HBsAg) includes several

TABLE 121–2. SEROLOGIC TESTS IN VIRAL HEPATITIS

Agent	Terminology	Definition	Significance
Hepatitis A (HAV)	Anti-HAV IgM type	Antibody to HAV	Current or recent infection or convalescence
	IgG type		Current or previous infection; indicates immunity
Hepatitis B (HBV)	HBsAg	HBV surface antigen	Positive in most cases of acute or chronic infection
	HBeAg	e antigen; HBV core component	Transiently positive in acute hepatitis, and in some chronic cases; reflects Dane particle concentration and infectivity
	Anti-Hbc (IgM or IgG)	Antibody to HBV core antigen	Positive in all acute and chronic cases and in carriers; thus, marker of HBV infection; not protective; IgM anti-HBc reflects active virus replication
	Anti-HBe	Antibody to e antigen	Transiently positive during convalescence and in some chronic cases and carriers; not protective; reflects low infectivity and possible integration of HBV DNA into host genome
	Anti-HBs	Antibody to surface antigen	Becomes positive late in convalescence in most acute cases; protective
Hepatitis D (HDV)	Anti-HDV (IgM or IgG)	Antibody to HDV antigen	Similar to anti-HBc in indicating infection; not protective

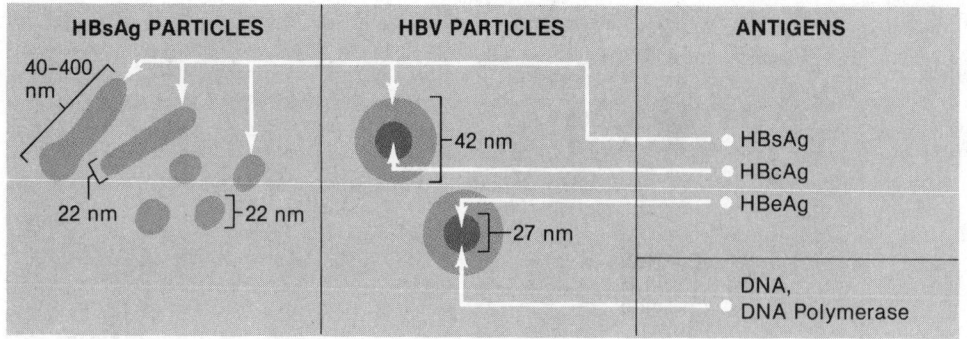

FIGURE 121-2. Forms of HBV in plasma, showing location of the various components and antigenic determinants. (From Koff RS: In Sanford JP, Luby JP [eds.]: The Science and Clinical Practice of Medicine. Infectious Diseases. Vol. 8. New York, Grune & Stratton, 1981, by permission.)

subtypes (d, y; w, r), and it can be detected by sensitive radioimmunoassay techniques in the serum of at least 75 per cent of infected persons during the acute disease (Fig. 121–2). The hepatitis B virus *core* consists of circular DNA, DNA polymerase, and other determinants, which include the hepatitis B core antigen (HBcAg) and two or three related e antigens (HBeAg). The biologic significance of HBcAg and HBeAg is not fully understood, but they are structurally related, and each elicits a humoral antibody response (anti-HBc and anti-HBe, respectively) during the course of the hepatitis B infection, which may be of diagnostic or prognostic significance. HBV-DNA can be detected in serum by molecular hybridization, is the most sensitive test for the presence of infective virus, and may be more widely employed in the near future.

In contrast to hepatitis A, *transmission* of hepatitis B by the fecal-oral route is relatively unimportant; infection may follow oral ingestion, but large doses appear necessary. Instead, the virus is present in virtually all body fluids and excreta, and transmission of this disease occurs primarily via parenteral routes. Therefore, it usually requires either overt inoculation (e.g., transfusion, or injection via a contaminated needle) or intimate personal contact (e.g., between sexual partners, patients and health professionals, and mother and newborn infant). The disease occurs with an increased frequency among sexual partners of acutely infected individuals, as well as among chronically exposed persons, including health professionals and patients exposed to blood and blood products (e.g., workers and patients in clinical laboratories, dialysis and oncology units), the sexually promiscuous (especially male homosexuals), drug users who share needles, and handlers of primates (which are susceptible to infection). In urban centers, hepatitis B may account for up to 50 per cent of sporadic cases of acute hepatitis, even in the absence of documented parenteral inoculation. This attests to the importance of person-to-person contact in the spread of this disease.

Unlike hepatitis A, hepatitis B infection may be chronic, either in association with demonstrable liver disease or in otherwise seemingly healthy carriers. Less than 1 per cent of the general population of the United States and Western Europe is HBsAg-positive. This low incidence contrasts with incidence of anti-HBs of about 10 per cent in the same population, providing additional evidence that in most patients with acute hepatitis B the infection is self-limited and followed by immunity, and only infrequently leads to chronic liver disease or a carrier state. The incidence of HBsAg positivity is much higher in less-developed areas (up to 15 per cent) and among certain subpopulations with increased exposure and/or impaired immunity, such as patients with Down's syndrome, leprosy, or lymphoproliferative disorders; addicts; and patients undergoing dialysis. In addition to acute cases, therefore, these chronically infected individuals constitute the "reservoir" that serves to perpetuate the virus. Historically, it is likely that transmission of the disease has occurred not so often via overt parenteral inoculation but rather via sexual contact or from mother to newborn. In the latter instance (*vertical transmission*), i.e., in infants born to mothers with acute or chronic infection, there is a high probability that the neonate will acquire the disease. This is especially likely when the mother develops acute hepatitis B in late pregnancy or early post partum or has chronic hepatitis. Transmission appears to correlate with the presence of HBeAg in maternal serum, reflecting the concentration of Dane particles. Characteristically, these infants remain chronically infected for many years, either as "carriers" or with a persisting low-grade and chronic hepatitis. They are probably at increased risk of developing hepatocellular carcinoma (see Ch. 129). Vertical transmission may be an important mechanism by which the reservoir of the virus is sustained from generation to generation.

The *incubation period* of acute hepatitis B, as defined by the appearance of clinical symptoms, varies between four weeks and six months, with an average of about 50 days. If the incubation period is defined instead in terms of the interval between exposure and the first *serologic* evidence of viremia, it may be as brief as two weeks, especially after exposure to large parenteral doses. Two weeks to two months prior to the clinical onset, HBsAg becomes detectable in serum (see Fig. 121–3 and Table 121–2). At about the time of the clinical onset and the rise in serum transaminase activities anti-HBc becomes detectable. Initially, an IgM anti-HBc is present in high titer and persists for several months to one year; thereafter IgG anti-HBc predominates. In chronic HBV infections, IgM anti-HBc is likely to be detectable during periods in which the virus is actively replicating. IgG anti-HBc persists for up to several years after acute hepatitis and is present in all chronic carriers. It appears to play no role in host defenses; rather, it serves as a reliable marker of hepatitis B infection currently or within the preceding few years. The Dane particle markers (HBeAg and DNA polymerase) usually become detectable in serum prior to the increase in transaminase. The duration of HBsAg positivity is highly variable. It may persist for a few days to two to three months; persistence beyond this time may indicate a chronic course. Characteristically, HBsAg becomes undetectable prior to the appearance of anti-HBs. This antibody can be demonstrated in 80 to 90 per cent of patients, usually late in convalescence, and indicates relative or absolute immunity. Its appearance generally suggests a successful response to the infection, but there are exceptions to this in certain patients with chronic hepatitis (see Ch. 123).

Several important qualifications should be noted in interpreting the results of hepatitis B serologic tests. First, in a significant number of patients with acute hepatitis B the serum is negative for HBsAg, presumably because the antigen is very low in titer or evanescent. For this reason, a single negative HBsAg test does not exclude the diagnosis. Anti-HBc is more sensitive in this regard and may be the only serologic indication of hepatitis B infection. A negative test for anti-HBc effectively excludes the diagnosis. On the other hand, a positive test for anti-HBc in an HBsAg-negative serum could merely reflect a prior episode of hepatitis B. These HBsAg-negative, anti-HBc–positive patients may be classifi-

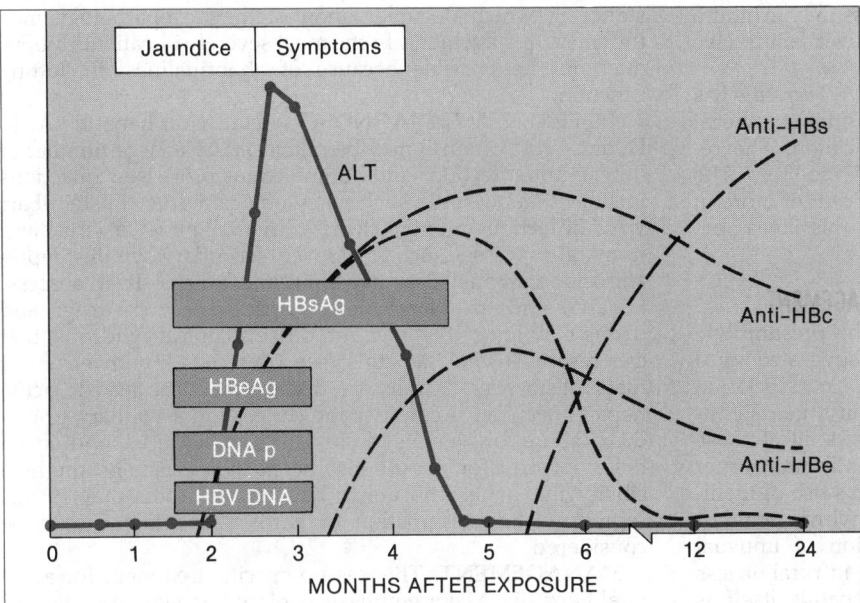

FIGURE 121–3. Sequence of clinical and laboratory findings in a patient with acute hepatitis B, followed by recovery. HBsAg-emia is the initial manifestation. "Dane particle markers" (HBeAg, DNA polymerase, and HBV DNA) precede the ALT rise and are transient. Anti-HBc (IgM, then IgG) appears during the acute illness; after the disappearance of anti-HBsAg and before the appearance of anti-HBs, anti-HBc may be the only marker of hepatitis B infection. (Adapted from Hoofnagle J, Schafer DF: Serologic markers of hepatitis B virus infection. Semin Liver Dis 6:4, 1986.)

able on the basis of the anti-HBs: if this test is positive early in the course of an acute hepatitis, it is evidence against the diagnosis of acute hepatitis B. Detection of IgM anti-HBc suggests recent acute or chronic HBV infection during a phase of active virus replication, as noted above. In those IgM-anti-HBc–negative subjects in whom HBV infection appears to have antedated the acute illness, the possibility of superimposed infection by hepatitis D (delta-agent), a non-A, non-B virus, or other causes of an acute hepatitis syndrome must be considered.

The *clinical course* of acute hepatitis B is more variable and usually more prolonged than that of hepatitis A. It is also more often associated with extrahepatic manifestations, including urticaria and other rashes, arthritis, and, much less commonly, glomerulonephritis and vasculitis. The immune complexes that appear to cause these extrahepatic manifestations consist of HBsAg, anti-HBs, and complement components. Glomerulonephritis and vasculitis are also associated with chronic hepatitis B infection and are not necessarily accompanied by apparent liver disease. Indeed, up to one third of all cases of polyarteritis nodosa may be caused or associated with hepatitis B virus infection.

Approximately 90 per cent of patients with acute hepatitis B recover completely and become HBsAg negative. Fewer than 1 per cent develop massive hepatic necrosis, but this complication is more common than in hepatitis A. Of the 10 per cent of patients who remain HBsAg positive beyond three or four months, in a significant number the antigen will clear over a period of six months to a year or more without evidence of chronic hepatitis developing. Many of those with prolonged HBsAg positivity, however, appear destined either to become chronic carriers or to develop chronic persistent or chronic active hepatitis (see Ch. 123).

HEPATITIS D (DELTA-AGENT). Infection with this unusual agent may be regarded as a complication of hepatitis B. The delta-agent is an incomplete RNA virus that requires antecedent or simultaneous HBV infection to infect the host cell. The agent exists in plasma in a coat of HBsAg and is present in the nuclei of infected hepatocytes. HDV infection is reflected by the presence of anti-HDV antibody (IgM acutely; IgG chronically) or HDV RNA in serum. Almost invariably the serum is positive for HBsAg and anti-HBc and, in most, anti-HBe. It is most commonly found among intravenous drug addicts and recipients of multiple transfusions. In subjects who are acutely and simultaneously infected with

HBV and HDV there is no apparent increase in the probability that chronic hepatitis will ensue. In individuals chronically infected with HBV, however, superimposed acute HDV infection usually also becomes chronic and is associated with the histopathologic findings of chronic active hepatitis. Acute HDV infection may cause fulminant hepatic failure.

HEPATITIS NON-A, NON-B. A large number of cases of acute viral hepatitis are caused by at least two other agents. Progress is being made in the identification of these agents, but it still is not possible to document the infection on a routine basis. Consequently, the designation non-A, non-B remains appropriate, since these forms of hepatitis are essentially diagnoses of exclusion.

Non-A, non-B hepatitis is the major cause of *post-transfusion hepatitis*. It occurs in approximately five to ten cases per 1000 transfusions and can be transmitted in whole blood, packed cells, platelets, plasma, and especially clotting factor concentrates. The incidence of post-transfusion hepatitis B has been greatly reduced by screening of donors for HBsAg. Non-A, non-B also is a common cause of hepatitis in needle users and accounts for 20 per cent or more of sporadic cases, i.e., those not associated with obvious contact or parenteral inoculation. A significant number of those cases of hepatitis previously referred to as serum hepatitis or homologous serum jaundice actually represented non-A, non-B hepatitis infections. Conversely, it is also now clear that some cases of "non-A, non-B" hepatitis actually represent HDV infection. Moreover, certain monoclonal antibodies may detect HBsAg in cases otherwise negative for this determinant and therefore are classified as non-A, non-B.

Hepatitis B and non-A, non-B also have many similar clinical manifestations. Thus, the incubation period of non-A, non-B hepatitis is longer than that of hepatitis A, ranging from two to twenty weeks, with an average of eight weeks. The acute illness is also quite variable. The incidence of massive hepatic necrosis appears comparable to that of hepatitis B, and together these two categories account for the great majority of cases.

Finally, post-transfusion and sporadic non-A, non-B hepatitis is associated with both an apparent carrier state (inferred from the fact that it may be transmitted by blood from apparently healthy donors) and chronic hepatitis. The incidence of chronic hepatitis after non-A, non-B transfusion hepatitis approaches 50 per cent. In some of these patients the disease is mild and may spontaneously subside or remit after a year of more, but in others the process may exhibit a progressive course and lead to cirrhosis and liver failure (see Ch. 123).

In recent years, an *epidemic form of non-A, non-B hepatitis* has been described, associated with outbreaks in India, Southeast Asia, Burma, North Africa, and the Soviet Union. The responsible agent appears morphologically similar to HAV. The illness is associated with a mortality of 10 per cent or more in pregnant women. There is no evidence that this illness becomes chronic.

GENERAL APPROACHES TO DIAGNOSIS AND MANAGEMENT

DIAGNOSIS. In its classic presentation, the presumptive diagnosis of acute viral hepatitis is readily suggested by a compatible history and physical examination, in association with laboratory evidence of hepatocellular injury, i.e., significantly increased serum transaminases. Because all of these features are nonspecific, however, it is essential that other possible etiologic factors be considered, such as use of medications or illicit drugs, alcohol, exposure to environmental or industrial toxins, and the possible acquisition of unusual infections as suggested by travel or residence in rural or less well developed areas. Exposure to viral hepatitis itself is suggested by contact with jaundiced persons or persons known to have developed hepatitis, sexual promiscuity (especially among male homosexuals), transfusion of blood or blood products, or the sharing of needles by drug users. Among health professionals, workers in dialysis and oncology units, surgeons, dentists, and clinical laboratory technicians are at increased risk, as is anyone in direct contact with blood blood products, or other body fluids. Despite the importance of a careful inquiry into these possible risk factors, many patients with acute viral hepatitis will report no significant exposures.

A careful and complete physical examination will help establish the diagnosis (tender hepatomegaly is the most common finding) and help exclude other processes that occasionally mimic acute viral hepatitis, such as acute hepatic congestion, disseminated sepsis or liver abscess, or biliary tract disease with or without cholangitis.

Serodiagnosis of viral hepatitis is now possible, with certain limitations (see above). A positive test for the IgM class of anti-HAV or a rising titer of total anti-HAV is strong evidence for acute hepatitis A. Conversely, if the test for anti-HAV is negative well into the convalescent phase, the diagnosis is excluded. A single positive test for anti-HAV is of little diagnostic value, since this could reflect a previous infection.

Although an acute hepatitis syndrome associated with HBsAg positivity has been taken as presumptive evidence for acute hepatitis B, none of the tests generally available at this time permits early and unequivocal diagnosis or exclusion of this entity. An important exception is that the presence of anti-HBs early in the course of acute hepatitis tends to exclude acute HBV infection. Since the classic pattern in which both HBsAg and anti-HBc are positive acutely may not be present in all cases (although anti-HBc itself is virtually always positive), a single negative test for HBsAg does not definitively exclude acute hepatitis B. Medical records, if available, may be of help by providing information about prior liver function tests, hepatitis serologies, or blood donation. Since donated blood has been screened routinely for HBsAg since 1972, such information may be quite helpful in the evaluation of hepatitis B serologies. As tests for the non-A, non-B agents become available, accurate serodiagnosis of hepatitis syndromes will be greatly facilitated.

If a *liver biopsy* is performed, it may demonstrate the pathologic features of acute viral hepatitis. However, these are nonspecific, and in the vast majority of cases biopsy is not indicated. Its use should be reserved for patients in whom the diagnosis is uncertain or in whom there is concern regarding chronicity or a deteriorating course, or any circum-

stance in which documentation of the histopathology may influence management. In the most severely ill patients biopsy may not be possible because of abnormalities of clotting function.

DIFFERENTIAL DIAGNOSIS. Acute viral hepatitis A, B, D, and non-A, non-B may be mimicked by a large number of other acute infections and noninfectious processes. Infections include other viruses such as cytomegalovirus, Epstein-Barr virus (infectious mononucleosis), and yellow fever virus; and nonviral processes such as Q fever, secondary syphilis, leptospirosis, salmonellosis, pyogenic and amebic liver abscess, malaria, and toxoplasmosis. A wide variety of drugs and toxins may injure the liver and cause a clinical syndrome that can resemble viral hepatitis (see Ch. 122). Inborn errors of metabolism such as Wilson's disease may also lead to acute hepatic necrosis. Acute hepatic congestion secondary to cardiac failure or venous occlusion, cholecystitis, and acute biliary obstruction should also be excluded. Finally, the possibility that what appears to be acute hepatitis may in fact represent the exacerbation of chronic hepatitis should be considered.

MANAGEMENT. There is no specific treatment for acute viral hepatitis. Major emphasis is placed on symptomatic and supportive care and on the prevention of transmission. Prevention is considered in detail below.

Most patients with acute viral hepatitis do not require hospitalization and are appropriately managed at home. Rest is advisable, but strict confinement to bed is not necessary beyond what is dictated by the patient's own sense of fatigue and malaise. No specific dietary measures are indicated, but most patients find a low-fat, high-carbohydrate diet more palatable. During the most severe phases of the illness, anorexia and nausea may be so extreme that oral intake of any kind is minimal. In such instances, attention to fluid balance is important, and it may be necessary to advise the intake of small amounts of clear fluids at frequent intervals. Although there is an appropriate reluctance to administer medication to the patient with liver disease, judicious use of small doses of antinausea agents such as hydroxyzine, trimethobenzamide, and even prochlorperazine is occasionally necessary and usually well tolerated. As the patient's symptoms decrease and appetite improves, intake can be liberalized, usually according to taste. Alcoholic beverages should be avoided throughout the course of the acute illness. Ambulation and activity may be increased as symptoms and laboratory tests improve; the most useful advice is that such activity should be limited so as to avoid causing fatigue. The decision to return to employment or school must take into consideration the patient's symptoms, the strenuousness of the work, and the potential for transmission of the disease; this, in turn, is a function of the viral etiology and the closeness of contact with others. In general, transmission is quite unlikely after two to three weeks in hepatitis A, whereas spread of hepatitis B or non-A, non-B ordinarily requires direct person-to-person contact.

Hospitalization is indicated for those patients in whom severe nausea and vomiting prevent maintenance of adequate fluid balance, in whom there is evidence of progressive deterioration, especially with encephalopathy or prolongation of prothrombin time, or in whom invasive diagnostic studies are indicated.

There is no convincing evidence to justify the use of corticosteroids in acute hepatitis, regardless of its severity. The management of fulminant hepatitis poses special problems in patient monitoring and support and is discussed in detail in Ch. 128.

PREVENTION. The entire area of hepatitis prophylaxis has been dramatically changed by the availability of an effective vaccine for hepatitis B. In this vaccine, the immunizing antigen is HBsAg, prepared from donor sera or, more recently, by recombinant DNA technology employing yeast; an appropriate immune response is reflected by the appearance of anti-HBs. Hepatitis A virus has been propagated in tissue culture, and a vaccine may also be available in the near future for this disease. Finally, continuing progress in the identification, isolation, and characterization of non-A, non-B viral hepatitis agents suggests the possibility of active immunization, although not for some time. Pending the advent of generally available and effective vaccines for all of the viral causes of acute hepatitis, prevention must depend mainly on personal hygiene and public health measures directed at minimizing the exposure of potentially susceptible individuals, and on the appropriate use of passive immunization.

The use of public health and hygienic measures rests on the premise that body fluids and excreta of infected individuals are potentially infective. Clearly there are certain exceptions, depending on the specific virus involved, the clinical stage of the infection, the amount of potentially infective material involved, and the nature of the exposure. For example, because of the ease with which hepatitis A is spread via the fecal-oral route, contact of such patients with others should be minimized, and their excreta and essentially all materials handled by them during their brief period of infectivity should be carefully disposed of. In contrast, hepatitis B and D are not commonly spread via the fecal-oral route. Although excreta are to be regarded as infective in these patients, the more important concern is transmission via puncture by contaminated needles (or equivalent exposure to infective material) or intimate personal (sexual) contact, especially during the period of HBsAg positivity. Non-A, non-B hepatitis in the United States more closely resembles hepatitis B in its transmissibility, but common-source outbreaks analogous to those caused by hepatitis A virus have recently been documented in India, Southeast Asia, Burma, North Africa, and the Soviet Union (see above). Because of these differences among the agents and differences in the approach to passive immunization, serologic diagnosis of the acute viral hepatitis case is useful, even though most patients with these disorders may be expected to do well regardless of etiology. In practice, however, rapid serodiagnosis is not always possible, and for this reason certain generalizations regarding the early management of the patient and his or her contacts are appropriate and are discussed below, along with measures for specific agents.

Hepatitis A. Since the infection is spread primarily via the fecal-oral route, including transmission by handling food, in drinking water, and potentially by fomites, strict attention to hygiene on the part of the patient and his or her attendants, whether in home or hospital, is of utmost importance during the period of viral shedding (Fig. 121–1). Direct body contact should be limited to that necessary for care; attendants should wear gloves, and careful handwashing is appropriate. Food, utensils, clothing, linen, needles, and excreta should be handled separately and carefully, also by gloved attendants. The virus is readily inactivated by boiling or by exposure to formalin, chlorine, or ultraviolet irradiation. In the hospital setting, strict isolation is not usually required for cooperative and informed patients with hepatitis A. In the home, similar measures should be implemented to the extent possible.

Close contacts of patients with hepatitis A should receive passive immunization with immune serum globulin as soon as possible, preferably within the first few days. The official recommended dose is 0.02 ml per kilogram up to a maximum of 2 ml, although up to 5 ml has been advocated. This would apply to immediate family members, sexual contacts, or others with whom the patient has been in close contact during the presumed period of infectivity. Casual contacts in the workplace or school probably do not require passive immunization unless there is reason to suspect mutual handling of food, beverages, or contaminated items. On the other hand, it is important to inquire about other possible cases among work or classroom associates. If there is reason to suspect a possible point-source outbreak, then all similarly exposed persons should receive immune serum globulin and appropriate epidemiologic information obtained.

The mode of transmission of hepatitis A also renders its prevention a matter of concern for those who intend to travel in areas where public health and sanitation measures may be suboptimal. In such circumstances, drinking water, fresh fruits and vegetables, and shellfish may be contaminated and should be avoided if possible. For these persons, administration of a standard dose (0.02 ml per kilogram) of immune serum globulin may be expected to afford protection for up to three months; for longer periods, a dose of 0.05 ml per kilogram is recommended and should be repeated at four- to six-month intervals.

Hepatitis B. Although this agent is less readily transmitted via the fecal-oral route, due consideration should be given to the general hygienic measures outlined for hepatitis A, in both home and hospital. Transmission ordinarily requires direct contact with the patient or the equivalent of a parenteral inoculation of infective material. Thus, in the home, children are far less likely than the spouse to acquire hepatitis B from an acutely infected adult. In the hospital, strict isolation may not be necessary if excreta, needles and other medical supplies, and personal utensils are identified, carefully handled, and discarded.

Passive immunization with immune serum globulin enriched in anti-HBs (hepatitis B immune globulin, or HBIG) is protective against hepatitis B infection in certain circumstances and when used in accordance with established guidelines. Because this material is expensive, it should not be used indiscriminately. At present, its use is officially recommended in the following specific situations:

1. Inoculation of material known to be contaminated with the hepatitis B virus, e.g., inadvertent puncture of a health professional by a needle from an HBsAG-positive patient, or accidental transfusion of HBsAg-positive blood or blood products.
2. Splash of HBsAg-positive material into the eye or on an open skin wound or eruption, as may occur in a laboratory accident or during a surgical or diagnostic procedure.
3. Ingestion of HBsAg-positive material, as may occur during a laboratory pipetting accident.
4. Sexual partners of patients with *acute* hepatitis B (partners of patients with chronic hepatitis B presumably have been previously exposed) within 14 days of contact.
5. Infants born to HBsAg-positive mothers, especially those who have had acute hepatitis B during the final trimester of pregnancy or first two months post partum, or who are positive for both HbsAg and HBeAg at the time of delivery.

The rational use of HBIG depends on two essential components. First, it must be documented that the material to which the person has been exposed contains HBsAg, and this requires identification of the source and appropriate serologic confirmation. For example, accidental puncture of the skin by one of several used needles in a disposal container effectively precludes meeting this requirement and, therefore, the use of HBIG. Second, the exposed person must actually be at risk. If, at the time of exposure, he or she is already positive for HBsAg (i.e., infected) or anti-HBs, (i.e., immune if the s/n value by radioimmunoassay exceeds 10), nothing will be gained from the administration of anti-HBs (HBIG). Ideally, therefore, the serologic status of both "donor" and "recipient" should be documented before the decision to administer HBIG is made. In practice, however, this is not usually possible within the few days' interval after exposure in which HBIG appears to be most effective. As a practical alternative to this dilemma, one possible approach is to immediately obtain serum from both the donor and the person at risk. Pending results of the HBsAg assays, the latter may be given 5 ml of ordinary immune serum globulin. HBIG may be administered later, if indicated by the test results. This approach represents a compromise between the need to institute early passive immunization on the one hand and to avoid indiscriminate use of HBIG on the other, and at a cost that is small relative to that of the HBIG itself. Other approaches are possible. In the family situation, the value of administering HBIG to the spouse remains controversial, but it is generally accepted that its use is not required for children, since they are at low risk.

Hepatitis B Vaccine. As noted, a safe and effective vaccine has been developed for the prevention of hepatitis B. It became generally available in the summer of 1982, after extensive field trials in the homosexual population, in which there is a high incidence of hepatitis B and a high and predictable rate of acquisition of the infection owing to frequent and promiscuous sexual contacts in certain segments of this population. The vaccine consists of highly purified and triple-inactivated HbsAg obtained from the serum of chronic carriers. More recently a recombinant vaccine utilizing HBsAg synthesized in yeast has become available. The vaccine is administered in three 20 μg-doses: initially and one month and six months later, and usually elicits production of anti-HBs in the recipient. Intramuscular injection is important, and is more likely effective with deltoid than with gluteal administration. (Smaller doses are used for children, and larger doses for dialysis and immunocompromised patients.) The vaccine is safe, but caution is recommended by the manufacturer for use in pregnant women. Although most subjects who have completed the three-dose immunization are protected against hepatitis B infection, there are important exceptions, especially among immunosuppressed subjects. The duration of this protection probably is of the order of five years, and is indicated by an anti-HBs titer of s/n >10 by radioimmunoassay.

The vaccine is recommended for use in high-risk groups and individuals. These include, but are not limited to, health professionals (especially those with high exposure risk such as surgeons, dentists, and dialysis workers), susceptible dialysis patients, and those subject to multiple transfusions (e.g., hemophiliacs), certain residents and staff of custodial care institutions, parenteral illicit drug users, heterosexual and household contacts of HBsAg carriers, Alaskan Eskimos, and sexually active and promiscuous male homosexuals. Available evidence suggests that it is also effective, when the first vaccine dose is combined with HBIG, in the passive-active immunization of health professionals after accidental needle stick, and in infants born to HBsAg-positive mothers. The cost-effectiveness of screening of potential vaccine recipients (e.g., anti-HBs determination) varies with the circumstance. In general, in those groups in which prevalence of hepatitis B is relatively low, screening is not cost effective, whereas it is useful in groups with a high prevalence (e.g., the homosexual community). For most health professionals, screening is marginally cost effective and depends on the prevalence of hepatitis B infection in the particular subgroup. In any case, it is established that administration of the vaccine to individuals already infected or immune is without harmful sequelae.

Hepatitis D. There is no established method for active or passive immunization. Since HDV infection requires simultaneous or antecedent HBV infection, prevention of HBV, e.g., by the vaccine, protects against HDV. Since previously infected HBV subjects are at risk for HDV infection, care should be taken to minimize exposure to HDV-containing materials, e.g., HBV-positive serum or secretions.

Hepatitis Non-A, Non-B. There is at present no generally available means of documenting exposure to, or infection by, this group of agents, but it appears to be transmitted in a manner that more closely resembles that of hepatitis B than hepatitis A. Thus close personal contact and parenteral inoculation appear necessary, suggesting that prophylactic measures suitable for hepatitis B are appropriate.

A problem largely confined to non-A, non-B hepatitis at present is that of post-transfusion hepatitis. The single most effective means of reducing the incidence of this disorder is the exclusion of blood obtained from commercial (paid donor) sources. There is a correlation between both elevated aminotransferase activity and anti-HBc positivity in donor unit plasma and the probability of post-transfusion hepatitis in a recipient, and exclusion of such units is desirable. The possible role of pre-exposure (i.e., pretransfusion) immune serum globulin in the prevention of the disorder remains unclear, and at present immune serum globulin is not officially recommended for its prevention.

Alter HJ (ed.): Hepatitis. Semin Liver Dis 6:1, 1986. *A minisymposium in which clinically relevant aspects of acute and chronic hepatitis are discussed by a group of recognized experts.*

Centers for Disease Control: Postexposure prophylaxis of hepatitis B. Ann Intern Med 101:351, 1984. *A summary of official recommendations.*

Dienstag JL: Non-A, non-B hepatitis. Gastroenterology 85:439, 743, 1983. *A thorough consideration of putative agents and summary of clinical, epidermiologic, and prophylactic aspects.*

Favero MS, Maynard JE, Leger RT, et al.: Guidelines for the care of patients hospitalized with viral hepatitis. Ann Intern Med 91:872, 1979. *Specific recommendations based on established concepts of epidemiology. A useful guide.*

Gregory P: Steroid therapy in severe viral hepatitis. N Engl J Med 294:681, 1976. *Convincing evidence that corticosteroids are not helpful, and potentially harmful in severe acute viral hepatitis.*

Health and Public Policy Committee, ACP: Hepatitis B vaccine. Ann Intern Med 100:149, 1984.

Jacobson IM, Dienstag JL: The delta hepatitis agent: Viral hepatitis, type D. Gastroenterology 86:1614, 1984. *Excellent and well-referenced editorial that summarizes concepts and progress toward the understanding of basic and clinical aspects of this newer facet of hepatitis B infection.*

Popper H, Schaffner F (eds.): Progress in Liver Diseases. Orlando, Grune & Stratton, 1986. *Several current and authoritative summaries of various aspects of acute hepatitis.*

Vyas GN, Dienstag JL, Hoofnagle JH (eds.): Viral Hepatitis and Liver Disease. Orlando, Grune & Stratton, 1984. *Proceedings of a March 1984 International Symposium. Progress and concepts in virtually all aspects of the field are presented, discussed, and referenced.*

122 TOXIC AND DRUG-INDUCED LIVER DISEASE

Robert K. Ockner

DEFINITION AND GENERAL PRINCIPLES OF DIAGNOSIS AND MANAGEMENT

Pharmacologic and chemical agents may produce a wide variety of acute or chronic liver diseases. At the one extreme they may take the form of asymptomatic and seemingly inconsequential abnormalities in liver function, whereas at the other they may include fatal acute massive hepatic necrosis or progressive chronic hepatitis, cirrhosis, and liver failure. This spectrum of histopathologic changes, clinical and laboratory features, and prognosis therefore is as broad as that of all other forms of liver disease. Several characteristics of these disorders create special problems for the clinician. First, the mere *association* of a given drug with disturbed liver function does not necessarily imply causality, either in an individual case or in general, and this problem accounts for much of the uncertainty in the field. Second, in a specific instance it may be unclear whether liver dysfunction is caused by a drug, by the underlying disorder for which the implicated drug is being used, by some other concurrent treatment, or by an independent process. Furthermore, in most forms of drug-induced liver injury, there exist important yet poorly understood differences in individual susceptibility. Although some of these differences may be immunologically mediated, this has not been established, and other factors such as differences in drug metabolism are probably of greater significance. Finally, not only may the histopathologic changes seen in drug-induced liver injury be very similar to those of other common entities such as viral hepatitis or biliary obstruction, but some drugs may produce more than one kind of lesion.

Since most forms of drug-induced liver injury are not associated with a specific histopathology, diagnosis must depend chiefly on the history of exposure, consistent clinical, laboratory, and (when appropriate) biopsy findings, and improvement subsequent to removal of the presumed toxin. For those agents that produce small-droplet lipid deposition, such as tetracycline or valproic acid, or those that produce prominent centrilobular necrosis, such as acetaminophen (especially when associated with significant blood levels of the drug), the diagnosis can be made with reasonable certainty on the basis of laboratory and biopsy findings. In most instances, however, unequivocal diagnosis cannot be made without demonstration of recurrent liver damage in response to rechallenge with the implicated drug. With rare exceptions, however, this maneuver is not justified; moreover, for those agents that cause a viral hepatitis–like reaction (e.g., halothane or isoniazid), there is the distinct possibility of a severe or even fatal outcome. Although assumption of such risks may be necessary on rare occasions, in most instances some degree of diagnostic uncertainty is acceptable as long as alternative drugs are available.

The appropriate management of drug-induced liver disease consists of discontinuation of the implicated drug(s) and supportive care for acute hepatitis or liver failure as needed. Only in acetaminophen hepatoxicity is there convincing evidence that specific pharmacologic intervention is beneficial (see below). There is no clear evidence that corticosteroids are of value in the treatment of drug-induced liver disease, although they may suppress systemic manifestations, especially when there is an associated serum sickness–like syndrome. Complications of hepatic adenomas, whether or not estrogen-associated, may require a surgical approach.

HISTOPATHOLOGIC CLASSIFICATION OF DRUG-INDUCED LIVER DISEASE

The classification shown in Table 122–1, although useful conceptually, should not obscure the fact that a given agent may cause more than one form of liver injury. For example, isoniazid may produce a nonspecific focal hepatitis, an acute viral hepatitis–like lesion, or chronic active hepatitis, whereas oral contraceptives may cause hepatocellular cholestasis or liver cell adenoma and have been implicated in hepatic vein thrombosis.

ZONAL NECROSIS. Zonal necrosis is most commonly produced by hepatotoxins that cause a predictable and dose-related injury that also can be produced in laboratory animals. Examples include the centrilobular necrosis associated with *carbon tetrachloride* and *acetaminophen* toxicity. For these and some other agents, toxicity depends on their conversion in the liver cell to a toxic derivative. Despite the predictability

TABLE 122–1. CLASSIFICATION OF DRUG-INDUCED LIVER DISEASE

Category	Examples
Predictable hepatotoxins with zonal necrosis	Acetaminophen, carbon tetrachloride
Nonspecific hepatitis	Aspirin, oxacillin
Viral hepatitis-like reactions	Halothane, isoniazid, phenytoin
Cholestasis	
Noninflammatory	Estrogens, 17α-substituted steroids
Inflammatory	Chlorpromazine, antithyroid agents
Fatty liver	
Large droplet	Ethanol, corticosteroids
Small droplet	Tetracycline, valproic acid
Granulomas	Phenylbutazone, allopurinol
Chronic hepatitis	Methyldopa, nitrofurantoin
Tumors	Estrogens, vinyl chloride
Vascular lesions	6-Thioguanine, anabolic steroids

and dose dependency that characterize this class of agents, there are significant differences in individual susceptibility, in part reflecting differences in rates of conversion to toxic products. The acute lesion either is fatal or is followed by essentially complete recovery. A similar lesion may result from chronic exposure, but it is not certain that this leads to progressive liver disease and cirrhosis.

NONSPECIFIC HEPATITIS. Nonspecific hepatitis consists of isolated foci of liver cell necrosis and inflammation, without the characteristic features of viral hepatitis. It also appears to exhibit a variable dose dependency. Neither the mechanism of the injury nor the basis for individual differences in susceptibility is known. Examples include *aspirin* and *oxacillin*.

VIRAL HEPATITIS–LIKE REACTIONS. These may mimic the broad spectrum of clinical, histopathologic, and prognostic variants of viral hepatitis, from an acute uncomplicated process, to bridging or submassive necrosis, to fatal massive necrosis. Examples include *halothane, isoniazid, ketoconazole, methyldopa, sulfonamides,* and *phenytoin*. There are marked differences in individual susceptibility to this form of injury, accounting for its sporadic occurrence and for the common belief that it represents a form of drug allergy. Although there appears to be a specific antibody to hepatocyte surface membranes in the serum of patients with severe halothane hepatitis, it is not certain whether this is important in pathogenesis or represents a secondary immune response to membrane antigens exposed during the halothane-induced injury. Furthermore, in the hepatitis associated with isoniazid and phenytoin, there is strong evidence that cell injury is mediated by a toxic drug metabolite. Thus, differences in individual susceptibility need not imply an immunologic mechanism, but may reflect the influence of genetic, dietary, environmental, or pharmacologic factors on drug metabolism.

CHOLESTASIS. Cholestasis is a very common manifestation of drug-induced liver injury and takes two distinct forms. In the first, caused principally by *natural and synthetic estrogens* and by *17 alpha-substituted androgenic and anabolic steroids*, there is usually little or no evidence of hepatocellular necrosis or a substantial inflammatory response. The injury is most simply viewed as the impaired secretion of bile by the liver cell, probably reflecting a direct steroid effect on the physical properties of cellular membranes or the activities of enzymes involved in this process. Although large doses may minimally impair bile secretion in most subjects, certain persons seem especially sensitive. These differences in individual susceptibility clearly are not allergic, and appear at least in part genetically determined. The lesion is completely and rapidly reversible.

In the second form of cholestatic injury, there is significant hepatocellular necrosis and portal and lobular inflammation; acidophil bodies and eosinophils are variably present. Systemic features, including fever, rash, and arthralgias, are not uncommon. This form of injury is produced by a broad group of agents, including the *phenothiazines, oral hypoglycemic* and *antithyroid* agents, and the *macrolide antibiotics* (e.g., erythromycin estolate). Its prognosis is generally favorable and complete recovery may be expected, except in very few individuals in whom chlorpromazine leads to a prolonged but ultimately resolving cholestatic course; rarely, the reaction may prove fatal. Marked differences in individual susceptibility associated with systemic features have suggested drug allergy as the basis for this form of injury. Chlorpromazine, however, is converted to a number of variably toxic metabolic products; this may account not only for the frequently abnormal liver function observed in patients receiving large doses for prolonged periods but also for the smaller number who develop the overt inflammatory and necrosing cholestatic lesion.

FATTY LIVER. Fatty liver usually represents the accumulation of triglyceride within the hepatocyte, and also may occur in two forms. In the most common, associated with *ethanol, corticosteroids, protein-calorie malnutrition, obesity, uncon-*

trolled diabetes mellitus, and after *jejunoileal bypass,* the fat accumulates in large droplets that displace the liver cell nucleus and confer upon it an adipocyte-like appearance. Despite this distortion, liver function may be well preserved.

A much less common pattern is seen in association with *tetracycline* or *valproic acid* hepatotoxicity, and occasionally with alcoholic liver disease, and superficially resembles that seen in *Reye's syndrome, obstetric fatty liver,* and *Jamaican vomiting sickness.* It consists of fat deposited in smaller droplets throughout the liver cell, the nucleus remaining central. This pattern is usually associated with significant, occasionally fatal, disturbances in liver function.

GRANULOMAS. Granulomas are found in the liver in certain forms of drug-induced liver injury, and may be associated with extrahepatic granulomas and prominent systemic features. Included among the agents responsible are *phenylbutazone, quinidine, allopurinol, phenytoin, halothane,* and *hydralazine.*

CHRONIC HEPATITIS. Chronic hepatitis has been associated with an increasing number of drugs, including *amiodarone, dantrolene, isoniazid, methyldopa, nitrofurantoin, oxyphenisatin, perhexilene maleate, phenytoin, propylthiouracil, sulfonamides, acetaminophen,* and *aspirin.* Although these agents more often cause acute liver injury, prolonged use may occasionally result in a chronic progressive process leading in some instances to cirrhosis. In many cases, the lesion is largely or completely reversible, but in severe cases this may require many months after the drug is discontinued. Rarely, progressive liver failure and death may ensue despite cessation of the drug. *Ethanol* abuse occasionally is associated with a lesion similar to that of chronic active hepatitis.

TUMORS. Tumors caused by drugs and other chemical agents may be of several types, including *hepatic adenoma (and possibly hepatocellular carcinoma)* associated with *oral contraceptive* use, and *angiosarcoma* caused by prolonged exposure to *vinyl chloride* monomer or Thorotrast. The mechanisms by which these tumors are produced are not known, but their clinical and laboratory features generally resemble those of similar tumors occurring "spontaneously." A possible exception is the apparently greater size, vascularity, and tendency to sudden hemorrhage of hepatic adenomas associated with oral contraceptive use (see Ch. 129).

VASCULAR LESIONS. Vascular lesions of several kinds occasionally are caused by drugs. Oral contraceptives have been implicated as a cause of hepatic vein thrombosis. Hepatic *veno-occlusive disease,* a process that affects the smaller tributaries of the hepatic vein, has been associated with the use of *antitumor agents,* including *6-thioguanine* and *cytarabine* as well as with ingestion of *pyrrolidizine alkaloids,* e.g., from plants of *Senecio* and *Crotalaria* species ("bush tea poisoning"). *Oral contraceptives* and *anabolic steroids* have been identified as causes of *peliosis hepatis,* a condition in which the liver lobule contains extrasinusoidal blood-filled spaces; this lesion is also seen in certain chronic wasting neoplastic and inflammatory diseases.

SELECTED EXAMPLES OF DRUG-INDUCED LIVER DISEASE

ACETAMINOPHEN. Hepatotoxicity caused by acetaminophen is a classic example of a predictable, dose-dependent form of zonal necrosis. This readily available agent has been used with increasing frequency in suicide attempts. It causes death in acute liver failure, often associated with renal failure, and usually with doses in excess of 10 to 15 grams. Within several hours patients develop nausea, vomiting, and hypotension. This initial phase may then subside and the patient may exhibit few symptoms, but over the next 24 to 48 hours there appears clinical and laboratory evidence of progressive deterioration of liver function.

The injury apparently is caused by toxic products of acetaminophen biotransformation; above threshold levels these toxic products overwhelm the capacity of detoxification mechanisms (e.g., conjugation with glutathione or other acceptors) and appear to react directly with critical cell constituents or lead to the formation of highly reactive free radicles. The rate of formation of these toxic products reflects not only drug dose but also the activity of the cytochrome P-450–dependent microsomal drug metabolizing system. When the activity of this pathway has been stimulated by inducers such as phenobarbital or ethanol, increased amounts of toxic product are formed. The activity of this pathway and the availability of endogenous acceptors such as glutathione are probably important determinants of individual differences in susceptibility to acetaminophen toxicity. In addition, glutathione is important in many and diverse aspects of cell function; thus, depletion of this critically important substance may have major adverse effects apart from its unavailability to combine with toxic drug metabolites.

Although acute toxicity usually requires a dose in excess of 10 to 15 grams, the clinical history is quite unreliable as the basis for assessing prognosis in a given case. Far more useful is the acetaminophen plasma level: When it exceeds 200 mg per liter at four hours, 100 mg per liter at eight hours, or 50 mg per liter at 12 hours after ingestion, severe liver damage may occur. Subsidence of the early gastrointestinal symptoms is not necessarily a favorable prognostic sign, and measurement of the plasma concentration is important both for prognosis and for treatment. Treatment of the higher-risk patients with *N*-acetylcysteine within the first ten hours after ingestion may significantly improve chances for survival. *N*-acetylcysteine has been thought to act by providing additional cysteine for glutathione synthesis, but other possible mechanisms are not excluded. The recommended dose of *N*-acetylcysteine (Mucomyst) is 140 mg per kilogram orally initially, followed by maintenance doses of 70 mg per kilogram every four hours for a total of 72 hours. (In Britain, an intravenous preparation is available and is administered as follows: 150 mg per kilogram initially over 15 minutes, 50 mg per kilogram over the next four hours and 100 mg per kilogram over the next 16 hours.) In all cases, supportive care is also indicated, and early gastric aspiration may permit recovery of a substantial portion of the ingested dose. In survivors, recovery is virtually complete; there is no evidence of chronic progressive liver disease, but in some cases serum bile acid concentrations may be increased, and there may be residual hepatic fibrosis.

In addition to the acute effects of a massive overdose, acetaminophen may also cause liver injury when taken for a long time at doses within the therapeutic range (3 to 8 grams per day). On liver biopsy, either centrilobular necrosis or a picture suggestive of chronic hepatitis may be found. This injury is fully reversible after the drug is discontinued.

ASPIRIN. Usually in doses in excess of 3.0 grams per day, aspirin may cause abnormalities in serum transaminases and other liver function tests, associated with a biopsy picture of either a nonspecific or chronic hepatitis. Not unexpectedly, these effects are seen most often in patients with diseases such as juvenile and adult rheumatoid arthritis and systemic lupus erythematosus, in which long-term high-dose salicylate therapy may be employed. The mechanism of the injury is not known, but its clear-cut dose dependency suggests a toxic effect of either aspirin or a product of its biotransformation.

The diagnosis of aspirin hepatotoxicity should be suspected in any subject with abnormal liver function on a regimen of high-dose salicylate therapy. Serum salicylate concentrations will usually be found to exceed 20 mg per deciliter. The injury is rapidly and completely reversible when salicylates are discontinued. A potential source of confusion may arise when liver functions are abnormal in a patient with features of "autoimmune" disease and a liver biopsy suggestive of chronic active hepatitis. If the patient is taking salicylates and the serum salicylate concentration is compatible, this constellation of findings should suggest salicylate hepatotoxicity and should be managed accordingly, before giving consideration to corticosteroid treatment for chronic active hepatitis.

There has been recent concern regarding aspirin treatment of viral syndromes in children and its possible etiologic or contributory role in the development of Reye's syndrome. While a causal relationship has not been established, currently available epidemiologic evidence is sufficiently convincing to justify avoidance of aspirin in these circumstances.

CHLORPROMAZINE. This agent characteristically produces a cholestatic reaction, associated with variable local and systemic symptoms, including fever, anorexia, nausea, abdominal discomfort, and, occasionally, rash. On biopsy, a hepatocellular and canalicular cholestasis is found, together with a significant but variable lobular and portal inflammatory infiltrate and liver cell necrosis. The sporadic occurrence of this reaction, and its systemic features and frequently associated eosinophilia, have suggested "drug allergy." However, chlorpromazine may cause a form of toxic liver injury. Thus, among those using this drug in high doses or for prolonged periods, there is a high incidence of abnormal liver function tests. Furthermore, in acute animal experiments, chlorpromazine at doses approximating those used clinically causes an acute dose-related impairment of bile secretion. Finally, certain chlorpromazine metabolites have been shown to affect adversely several factors necessary for the formation of bile. Individual differences in susceptibility to chlorpromazine cholestasis may reflect corresponding differences in the rate of formation of the more toxic metabolites.

The prognosis of chlorpromazine cholestasis is generally favorable. Rarely, patients may exhibit a prolonged course resembling primary biliary cirrhosis despite discontinuation of the agent, but in these cases eventual recovery, even after three to four years, also is the rule. Fatal hepatic necrosis is rare. Therapeutic intervention is not indicated, other than discontinuation of the drug and symptomatic support (e.g., cholestyramine or colestipol for puritus); if cholestasis is prolonged, replacement of fat-soluble vitamins may be necessary.

ERYTHROMYCIN ESTOLATE. The lauryl sulfate salt of propionyl erythromycin may cause a cholestatic reaction with components of inflammation and necrosis of liver cells. A similar reaction occasionally has been associated with erythromycin ethylsuccinate and erythromycin propionate. Erythromycin estolate hepatotoxicity often presents as an acute syndrome of a right upper-quadrant pain, fever, and variable cholestasis, and there are several well-documented cases in which such patients were subjected to major surgery for presumed cholecystitis or cholangitis. The prognosis for the hepatic lesion is uniformly excellent, but the reaction may be expected to recur if the drug is readministered. The mechanism of the injury is unknown.

HALOTHANE. This anesthetic agent is now generally accepted as a rare cause of a viral hepatitis-like reaction and, even more rarely, of fatal massive hepatic necrosis. The mechanism of the injury is unknown. An immunologic basis has been invoked because most clinically apparent cases occur in persons with a history of prior exposure to halothane or a related agent, and because antibodies to hepatocyte surface membranes can be demonstrated in patients' serum (see above). On the other hand, halothane is predictably hepatotoxic in animals when circumstances favor its metabolism via reductive pathways, and its incidence appears to be higher among individuals with genetically determined impairment of enzymatic mechanisms for detoxifying harmful drug metabolites. Halothane hepatitis usually becomes evident approximately seven to ten days after anesthesia, but with repeated exposures the interval between administration of halothane and the clinical onset decreases. The course is indistinguishable from that of viral hepatitis, and the hepatitis may terminate fatally within days, or the patient may progress

to rapid and complete recovery or exhibit a more prolonged course with eventual recovery. Despite earlier evidence to the contrary, single-exposure halothane hepatitis does not appear to lead to chronic hepatitis.

ISONIAZID (INH). The overall incidence of clinical hepatitis among persons taking *isoniazid* (INH) for single drug chemoprophylaxis against tuberculosis approximates 1 per cent, with a case fatality rate of about 10 per cent. Clinically and histologically, the disease resembles the wide spectrum of viral hepatitis, and may appear as a relatively mild acute process, a subacute or chronic hepatitis, or fatal massive necrosis. There is an important age effect on incidence, which may exceed 2 per cent among persons over the age of 50. Most cases become manifested within two to three months after the start of the drug, but the onset may be delayed for up to 12 months. Despite earlier reports to the contrary, there seems to be no apparent relationship between acetylator status (rapid as opposed to slow acetylators) and risk of hepatotoxicity.

In addition to the 1 per cent overall incidence of overt hepatitis, there is approximately a 10 to 20 per cent incidence of subclinical liver injury, manifested by mild to moderate increases in serum transaminase activity reflecting a focal nonspecific hepatitis. The laboratory abnormalities associated with this lesion appear nonprogressive and will subside in most patients despite continued administration of the drug.

The mechanism of neither of these two forms of expression of isoniazid hepatotoxicity is fully understood. However, there is evidence that a toxic metabolite may be involved. There is no evidence to suggest "drug allergy"; indeed, patients with isoniazid hepatitis usually lack clinical manifestations, such as skin rash and arthralgias, which might suggest drug allergy.

The clinical presentation of isoniazid hepatitis may be nonspecific, consisting initially of a "flu" syndrome or low-grade fever. For this reason, any patient receiving isoniazid should be followed at regular intervals and advised to report intercurrent symptoms. If these are found to be associated with clinical or laboratory evidence of disturbed liver function, the drug should be discontinued, pending further evaluation. A more difficult question concerns the appropriate management of the patient with an asymptomatic transaminase elevation early in the course of isoniazid treatment. Since there is at least a 90 per cent probability (especially in younger patients) that this finding reflects a transient and self-limited event rather than significant hepatitis, it is not generally recommended that liver function tests be routinely monitored in patients taking isoniazid. However, a several-fold elevation in transaminase levels in a patient over 35 years of age, even in the absence of symptoms, must be regarded as potentially serious and may be sufficient to justify discontinuation of the drug. As a general rule, the risk-benefit ratio for isoniazid chemoprophylaxis rises rapidly after age 35. In this group it is often best to err on the side of caution in deciding whether to employ chemoprophylaxis and by stopping the drug when in doubt regarding possible hepatotoxicity.

The management of suspected isoniazid hepatitis, apart from discontinuing the drug, is supportive. Fulminant hepatic failure should be treated as described in Ch. 128. There is no evidence that corticosteroids are of value in either acute or chronic forms of the disease.

RIFAMPIN. This antituberculous agent may cause liver injury. It reversibly impairs the hepatic uptake of bilirubin and sulfobromophthalein from plasma; it is also an inducer of the microsomal cytochrome P-450–dependent drug-metabolizing system. This latter effect has been cited as the mechanism by which rifampin may cause an unusually precipitous and severe form of isoniazid hepatitis when the two agents are administered together, but this possible drug interaction is not conclusively established. Rifampin itself has been implicated as a cause of acute hepatitis, but in most reported cases isoniazid was also being used; thus, the true incidence of rifampin hepatitis is unknown.

METHYLDOPA. This drug appears to be the only important antihypertensive agent with a significant incidence of hepatotoxicity. It is similar to isoniazid in that minor and apparently inconsequential abnormalities in liver function occur in perhaps 5 per cent of subjects, whereas overt acute or chronic hepatitis is much less common. There is a high incidence of serologic indicators of altered immunity in users of this drug, but hepatic injury does not correlate with Coombs' test positivity and may be mediated by a toxic drug metabolite. Most reported cases have resembled acute viral hepatitis, but this agent is also important among the growing list of drugs implicated as causes of chronic active hepatitis.

ORAL CONTRACEPTIVES. These hormonal agents have been associated with several adverse effects on the hepatobiliary system: (1) hepatocellular cholestasis, (2) hepatic vein thrombosis, (3) liver cell neoplasia, and (4) increased predisposition to cholesterol gallstone formation.

The *cholestatic effects* of oral contraceptives are largely attributable to the estrogenic component. Among oral contraceptive users, the majority exhibit subtle disturbances in bile secretory function (e.g., as demonstrated by measurement of the transport maximum for sulfobromophthalein), whereas only a few develop clinical cholestasis, with associated pruritus and jaundice. Histologically, there is usually little or no inflammation or hepatocellular necrosis. The syndrome is completely reversible, usually within two to three months, when the pill is discontinued. An entirely analogous situation may occur during the later stages of pregnancy, in which subclinical or mild cholestasis is common (e.g., mild pruritus), whereas clinically overt cholestasis ("recurrent intrahepatic cholestasis of pregnancy") is unusual and resolves rapidly after parturition. Cholestasis of pregnancy can be reproduced by subsequent administration of estrogens; it may be caused by a direct physical effect of the natural or synthetic estrogen on membrane components important in the bile secretory process. The obvious marked individual differences in susceptibility to this effect, although clearly not related to "drug allergy," are not well understood. The possible importance of genetic factors is suggested by the higher incidence of this problem among women with the Dubin-Johnson syndrome, the substantial differences in its incidence among descendants of certain Indian tribes in Chile, apparently unrelated to current location, diet, or other environmental factors, and the recent documentation of the familial occurrence of recurrent cholestasis of pregnancy.

Treatment of oral contraceptive-induced cholestasis consists of discontinuation of the drug, and symptomatic support (e.g., bile acid sequestrants for pruritus) as needed. Resolution should be rapid and complete; persistence of abnormalities beyond two or three months, or worsening at any time after the pill is discontinued, suggests the possibility that the agent may have simply unmasked some pre-existing clinically inapparent condition, and additional diagnostic evaluation may be indicated.

Farrell G, Prendergast D, Murray M: Halothane hepatitis. Detection of a constitutional susceptibility factor. N Engl J Med 313:1310, 1985. *Evidence for a genetically determined predisposition to halothane hepatitis based on impaired drug metabolism.*

Goldman IS, Winkler ML, Raper SE, et al.: Increased hepatic density and phospholipidosis due to amiodarone. AJR 144:541, 1985. *CT abnormalities in patients with histologically documented amiodarone hepatotoxicity.*

Kaplowitz N, Aw TY, Simon FR, et al.: Drug induced hepatotoxicity. Ann Intern Med 104:826, 1986. *A useful current review of mechanisms and clinical aspects of drug hepatotoxicity.*

Lewis JH, Zimmerman HJ, Benson GD, et al.: Hepatic injury associated with ketoconazole therapy. Analysis of 33 cases. Gastroenterology 86:503, 1984. *A summary and analysis of reported cases to date with histologic documentation and useful guidelines.*

McMaster KR, Hennigas GR: Drug-induced granulomatous hepatitis. Lab Invest 44:61, 1981. *A summary of implicated agents, with histopathologic documentation.*

Ockner RK: Drug-induced liver disease. In Zakim D, Boyer T (eds.): Hepatology.

Philadelphia, W. B. Saunders Company, 1982, pp 691–722. *A classification and summary of pharmacologic agents that may cause liver injury, including consideration of mechanisms and clinical aspects.*

Seeff LB, Cuccherini BA, Zimmerman HJ, et al: Acetaminophen hepatotoxicity in alcoholics. A therapeutic misadventure. Ann Intern Med 104:399, 1986. *This paper and an accompanying editorial by M. Black and J. Raucy provide and review evidence regarding the mechanism by which alcohol use increases susceptibility to acetaminophen hepatotoxicity.*

Zimmerman HJ (ed.): Drug-induced liver disease. Semin Liver Dis 1:89, 1981. *A useful, multiauthored summary of advances and perspectives.*

Zimmerman HJ: Hepatotoxicity. The Adverse Effects of Drugs and Other Chemicals on the Liver. New York, Appleton-Century-Crofts, 1980. *A comprehensive and authoritative source. Well organized, readable, and thoroughly referenced.*

Zimmerman HJ: Hepatotoxic effects of oncotherapeutic agents. In Popper H, Schaffner F (eds.): Progress in Liver Diseases. Orlando, Grune & Stratton, 1986, vol 8, pp 621–642. *A useful and current summary, thoroughly referenced.*

123 CHRONIC HEPATITIS
Robert K. Ockner

GENERAL CONSIDERATIONS

DEFINITION. Chronic hepatitis is a sustained inflammatory process in the liver lasting more than six months to one year. It encompasses a wide spectrum of syndromes of diverse etiology, pathogenesis, histopathology, and clinical manifestations. In most, there is a variable element of hepatocellular necrosis. In its more severe forms, this inflammatory and necrotic process may lead to collapse of stromal elements, distortion of the lobular architecture, and a reparative process consisting of fibrosis and nodular regeneration (i.e., cirrhosis). The cell necrosis is associated with an inflammatory response that may be predominantly portal, periportal, or lobular in its distribution.

ETIOLOGY. Chronic hepatitis (Table 123–1) can be caused by *hepatitis B* (with or without superimposed hepatitis D) and *non-A, non-B* virus infection, *drugs* and *toxins* (see below and Ch. 122), and *inborn errors of metabolism* such as *Wilson's disease* and *alpha₁-antitrypsin deficiency*. In addition, there are one or more poorly understood types of *unknown etiology* in which clinical and laboratory features suggest but do not prove an immunologically mediated process.

CLINICAL AND LABORATORY MANIFESTATIONS AND DIAGNOSIS. Patients with chronic hepatitis may be entirely asymptomatic and exhibit only minimal abnormalities in routine laboratory tests, or may be incapacitated by progressive liver failure and the complications of portal hypertension. At any given time, the clinical and laboratory features may not correlate well with histopathology or long-term prognosis. For this reason, and because concepts of the natural history and response to treatment are changing for some of these disorders, decisions regarding diagnosis, management, and prognosis are often difficult and uncertain.

TABLE 123–1. CAUSES OF CHRONIC HEPATITIS

Chronic viral infections	
Hepatitis B	
Hepatitis B with superimposed hepatitis D	
Hepatitis non-A, non-B	
Drugs and toxins, including	
Acetaminophen	Nitrofurantoin
Amiodarone	Oxyphenisatin
Aspirin	Perhexilene maleate
Dantrolene	Phenytoin
Ethanol	Propylthiouracil
Isoniazid	Sulfonamides
Methyldopa	
Wilson's disease	
Alpha₁-Antitrypsin deficiency	
Idiopathic (? "autoimmune")	

These aspects of the various chronic hepatitis syndromes are considered in greater detail in the balance of this chapter.

PATHOLOGY. In most forms of chronic hepatitis there is a prominent portal inflammatory reaction, consisting mainly of mononuclear cells, especially small lymphocytes and plasma cells. There is also variable necrosis and inflammation involving hepatocytes immediately adjacent to the portal area. In this *periportal hepatitis* (or *"piecemeal necrosis"*) the inflammatory process invades the peripheral portions of the hepatic lobule, so that individual liver cells or nests of cells are isolated within the inflammatory zone. Periportal hepatitis is not specific for chronic hepatitis, and often is present in uncomplicated acute hepatitis and several other processes. For this reason it does not necessarily reflect a chronic or progressive process, and its significance can be judged only in the context of associated pathologic and clinical findings.

The lobular architecture may be substantially disrupted, as indicated by extension of the portal inflammatory and necrotic process into the lobule to a depth sufficient to span adjacent portal and/or central areas, i.e., *"bridging necrosis."* Although bridging necrosis can occur as part of an otherwise uncomplicated and self-limited acute hepatitis, it reflects a more severe injury that has a greater propensity to lead to progressive deterioration over a period of weeks to months (*"subacute hepatic necrosis"*) or to chronic active hepatitis and cirrhosis. Thus, its presence, or the presence of submassive necrosis or significant fibrosis in a patient with liver disease lasting more than six months, suggests a chronic and progressive process. Paradoxically, among survivors of the most extreme forms of acute liver injury, i.e., massive hepatic necrosis, chronic progressive liver disease is uncommon. Although the classification of chronic hepatitis that follows is based on histopathology, overlap is common, and differentiation of one from the other may be difficult.

CHRONIC PERSISTENT HEPATITIS

DEFINITION AND PATHOLOGY. Chronic persistent hepatitis is a nonprogressive inflammatory process largely confined to the portal areas. There is little or no periportal or lobular hepatitis; significant fibrosis and cirrhosis are absent. Of the small number of patients with acute hepatitis B whose illness becomes chronic, most will be found to have this lesion, and it is the most common form of chronic hepatitis. By definition, the diagnosis of persistent hepatitis is not appropriate if there is significant stromal collapse, fibrosis, or nodular regeneration.

CLINICAL AND LABORATORY MANIFESTATIONS. Chronic persistent hepatitis may be entirely asymptomatic or associated with nonspecific symptoms, including fatigue, anorexia, abdominal discomfort, or right upper-quadrant pain. Extrahepatic manifestations such as arthritis, glomerulonephritis, and vasculitis are rare. Jaundice, if present, is usually very mild. Physical findings are usually limited to palmar erythema, a few spider telangiectasias, and mildly tender hepatomegaly; the spleen occasionally is slightly enlarged. By definition, complications of advanced liver disease and portal hypertension, such as evidence of a collateral circulation, ascites, and encephalopathy, are absent.

Laboratory abnormalities are also mild, and include moderate increases in serum transaminases, bilirubin, and globulins. Albumin concentration and prothrombin time are usually normal. The serum is positive for HBsAg in perhaps 20 to 30 per cent of patients; other serologic tests such as mitochondrial, smooth muscle, and antinuclear antibodies are usually negative.

DIAGNOSIS, PROGNOSIS, AND MANAGEMENT. In any patient with persisting abnormalities of liver function, ethanol or other potential hepatotoxins should be discontinued, at least temporarily, to determine their possible etiologic significance. Because its clinical and laboratory features are totally nonspecific, the diagnosis of persistent hepatitis cannot be made without liver biopsy, but even biopsy does not always make it possible to distinguish this syndrome with certainty from chronic active hepatitis. In particular, HBsAg-positive individuals are subject to worsening of their hepatitis during a "reactivation" in which active virus replication is spontaneous or induced by immunosuppressive agents.

The outlook for persistent hepatitis usually is favorable, in that progression to cirrhosis or liver failure does not occur. However, the syndrome may last for ten years or more, and may cause continuing or intermittent discomfort or disability. Because of the difficulties inherent in the biopsy diagnosis of this group of disorders, continuing observation is important. Evidence of significant clinical deterioration may indicate the presence of a more serious process such as chronic active hepatitis, cirrhosis, or hepatocellular carcinoma and would be reason to consider repeating the liver biopsy. No specific treatment is indicated or available for chronic persistent hepatitis. Symptomatic and nutritional support is appropriate, and exposure to potential hepatotoxins should be avoided. For patients in whom alcohol has been excluded etiologically, small amounts of alcoholic beverages are permissible if they do not cause worsening of symptoms or laboratory tests. A form of chronic persistent hepatitis may be found in those patients in whom corticosteroid treatment of idiopathic or "autoimmune" chronic active hepatitis has induced a remission. The prognosis of this variant is less favorable, since about 50 per cent of such patients may have relapse after steroid therapy is discontinued.

CHRONIC LOBULAR HEPATITIS

This is a less well defined variant of chronic hepatitis in which the predominant lesion is a scattered single-cell necrosis in the lobule, with a relatively minor portal inflammatory component. It is, in effect, a variant of chronic persistent hepatitis, appearing not to progress to cirrhosis or liver failure except in those subjects in whom the disease becomes more active. Aside from those few patients in whom hepatitis B infection is present (with or without hepatitis D), a specific etiology is not identifiable.

CHRONIC ACTIVE HEPATITIS

DEFINITION. This is the most serious form of chronic hepatitis because of its potential for progression to cirrhosis and liver failure. It has been designated by a number of other essentially synonymous terms, such as *lupoid hepatitis, autoimmune hepatitis, plasma cell hepatitis, chronic aggressive hepatitis,* and *chronic active liver disease.*

ETIOLOGY. Approximately 20 per cent of cases are associated with, and presumably caused by, *chronic hepatitis B infection,* with or without superimposed hepatitis D infection (see Ch. 121). Chronic active hepatitis may also follow non-A, non-B hepatitis. Drugs that can cause the syndrome include *amiodarone, dantrolene, isoniazid, methyldopa, nitrofurantoin, oxyphenisatin, perhexilene maleate, phenytoin, propylthiouracil,* and *sulfonamides.* Long-term use of *acetaminophen, aspirin,* and *ethanol* occasionally may cause similar changes, as may *Wilson's disease* and *alpha₁-antitrypsin deficiency.* In a large number of cases the etiology is unknown, although many of this group exhibit clinical features and serologic abnormalities suggestive of autoimmunity. Despite such suggestive evidence, however, a truly "autoimmune" basis for chronic hepatitis has not been conclusively established, and in many instances phenomena that might be considered to reflect such a mechanism are also found in that form of the disease associated with hepatitis B virus infection. With time, specific etiologies may be identified for additional subsets of chronic active hepatitis.

PATHOLOGY. The syndrome is characterized by expansion of portal areas, which are infiltrated by lymphocytes and plasma cells, by periportal hepatitis, and by a variable degree of bridging necrosis, collapse, and fibrosis. In one third or more of patients, macronodular cirrhosis is present at the time of diagnosis. Except for the characteristic features of alpha₁-antitrypsin deficiency, which can be demonstrated by histochemistry, the various causes of chronic active hepatitis cannot be differentiated from one another on the basis of pathology.

CLINICAL MANIFESTATIONS. The course of chronic active hepatitis may be highly variable. The onset is usually insidious, but in perhaps one third of cases may resemble an acute hepatitis. It may affect all age groups and both sexes. However, HBsAg-negative cases occur mainly in young adult females, often associated with a more severe course and autoimmune features, whereas HBsAg-positive cases are more common in males and are often minimally symptomatic. Patients may be asymptomatic or may exhibit a wide range of local or constitutional symptoms typical of liver disease, such as fatigue, malaise, fever, anorexia, jaundice, or ascites.

Extrahepatic manifestations are often quite prominent and at times may dominate the clinical picture, especially in young females. These include amenorrhea, various skin rashes, glomerulonephritis, polyserositis, thyroiditis, vasculitis, Sjogren's syndrome, pneumonitis, depression of the formed elements of the blood, and an apparently increased incidence of ulcerative colitis.

Physical findings may also be quite variable. Patients may exhibit only a few spider telangiectasias, possibly with mild enlargement of liver and/or spleen, and may or may not be jaundiced. In advanced cases with cirrhosis, patients may have ascites, evidence of collateral circulation, or encephalopathy. In young women, acne and hirsutism may reflect the hormonal effects of chronic liver disease. Evidence of other extrahepatic manifestations may also be prominent, as noted above.

LABORATORY FINDINGS. Transaminases are usually increased over a range from minimally abnormal to in excess of 1000 IU. Globulins usually are diffusely increased, and the albumin value often is low. The alkaline phosphatase is usually only slightly to moderately increased; major increases should suggest the possibility of biliary tract disease or infiltrative or mass lesions. Prothrombin time generally reflects the severity of the disease, but may also be influenced by vitamin K deficiency. Because of their variability, the laboratory tests often poorly reflect the pathologic process; for this reason they do not always provide a reliable basis for the assessment of natural history or response to treatment.

Chronic active hepatitis is often characterized by the presence of a number of unusual but nonspecific immunoglobulins in serum, especially in patients who are negative for HBsAg. These include smooth muscle antibodies (positive in about two thirds), antinuclear antibodies (about one half), and antimitochondrial antibodies (about one third). Antibodies to a liver plasma membrane protein also have been demonstrated; their significance is unknown.

DIAGNOSIS. Diagnosis of chronic active hepatitis requires liver biopsy. In addition to the pathology, it is essential to establish a specific etiology, if possible, e.g., chronic hepatitis B infection, drugs, ethanol, Wilson's disease, or alpha₁-antitrypsin deficiency. Exposure to drugs and toxins usually can be identified by means of a careful history, including, when appropriate, questioning of family members or friends.

A positive test for HBsAg suggests that hepatitis B virus infection is causative, but even in these persons drugs, toxins, or superimposed hepatitis D also should be considered. Conversely, some cases of chronic active hepatitis may be caused by hepatitis B virus despite HBsAg-negative serum (in these patients serum usually has been positive for anti-HBc, but it may not be possible to definitively establish or exclude the diagnosis except by demonstrating the presence of HBV DNA

in serum or liver by molecular hybridization). In some patients with chronic hepatitis B, a relapse—either spontaneous or following immunosuppressive therapy—may be followed by an apparent remission associated with seroconversion from HBe-positive to anti-HBe-positive and loss of other Dane particle markers from serum. This seroconversion is considered to represent a change from an actively replicative to a nonreplicative or integrated state of the HBV DNA. However, patients in this latter phase of the disease are still subject to reactivation of their disease, either spontaneous or resulting from immune suppression. Wilson's disease should be excluded in any patient with chronic hepatitis who is under the age of 40. Appropriate tests for this purpose include slit-lamp examination for Kayser-Fleischer rings, and measurement of serum ceruloplasmin and urinary copper excretion. If all tests are negative, additional studies are not necessary; when the suspicion persists, measurement of liver copper concentration or incorporation of radioactive copper into serum ceruloplasmin may be necessary (see Ch. 205). Alpha₁-antitrypsin deficiency can be excluded by protease-inhibitor phenotyping of serum and, in liver biopsy specimens, by the presence of PAS-positive material in hepatocytes after diastase treatment of the tissue section.

The *different diagnosis* includes *chronic persistent hepatitis, postnecrotic cirrhosis*, and some cases of *primary biliary cirrhosis* in which clinical and pathologic features may resemble those of chronic active hepatitis.

TREATMENT. Treatment of chronic active hepatitis not attributable to drugs, Wilson's disease, or alpha₁-antitrypsin deficiency has been studied in several large clinical trials. The great majority of patients included for study were symptomatic and had clinically obvious liver disease, and most were negative for HBsAg; however, criteria for inclusion, treatment programs, controls, and duration of follow-up differed substantially among the studies.

Generally, *corticosteroids*, with or without low-dose azathioprine, improve laboratory test results, reduce symptoms, suppress the inflammatory response seen on biopsy, and decrease short-term and long-term morbidity and mortality Thus, in the Mayo Clinic study, a favorable clinical, biochemical, and histologic response was seen initially in 56 per cent of patients, whereas spontaneous improvement occurred in only 20 per cent of placebo-treated controls; early mortality and progression to cirrhosis were also decreased. Similarly favorable results were observed in studies conducted at other institutions.

Despite this seemingly beneficial overall response, several factors that importantly influence the natural history and response to treatment must be considered in making the decision to institute a chronic treatment program with potentially significant adverse effects. First, corticosteroid therapy is not indicated for chronic hepatitis B (with or without hepatitis D), as these patients do not benefit and their status may even deteriorate as a result. Second, chronic hepatitis does not usually progress to cirrhosis or liver failure in the absence of bridging necrosis on liver biopsy; the absence of such changes would weigh significantly against the use of corticosteroids. Third, there is no evidence that corticosteroids are of benefit in asymptomatic chronic active hepatitis. Fourth, since the reported series contain an unknown number of patients with chronic non-A, non-B hepatitis, and since the natural history of this disorder is highly variable, it is difficult to assess the impact of corticosteroids in this group, although the presence or absence of "autoimmune" features seemed to be of little consequence in the Mayo Clinic series. Finally, since many patients with chronic active hepatitis would fail to meet the criteria for inclusion in some of the published series, any decision regarding their treatment is necessarily an extrapolation from a limited study population.

In view of this substantial uncertainty concerning the value of corticosteroids in certain subsets of chronic active hepatitis, it is very difficult to make broadly applicable recommendations as to their use. In general, however, an initially favorable response would most likely be expected in a young, HBsAg-negative female with progressive disease characterized by prominent symptoms and autoimmune features and no recent transfusion or other exposure to non-A, non-B hepatitis. Since there appear to be exceptions, such decisions must be individualized.

In the Mayo Clinic study, an initial daily dose of 60 mg of prednisone or of 30 mg of prednisone combined with 50 mg of azathioprine, tapering gradually over several weeks to months to a daily maintenance dose of 20 mg of prednisone or 10 mg of prednisone plus 50 mg of azathioprine, was found to be most effective. The azathioprine was of no value when given alone, but permitted use of the lower prednisone dose, thereby reducing the incidence of significant steroid-related complications, which otherwise approximated 60 per cent. Alternate-day treatment was less effective. If a favorable response is not observed within two to three months, treatment should be discontinued.

Patients being treated for chronic active hepatitis should be examined and have their liver function checked periodically. The possible side effects of drug treatment should be monitored and liver biopsies should be repeated at intervals of six months to one year, depending on the circumstances. Return of liver enzymes to a level less than twice the upper limit of normal, together with a liver biopsy showing subsidence of the inflammatory and necrotic process to a picture similar to that of persistent hepatitis, is considered a successful response and warrants an attempt gradually to discontinue treatment. In about 50 per cent of patients, this attempt will succeed and additional corticosteroid treatment will not be needed. In the remainder, evidence of relapse may suggest the need for reinstitution of therapy.

Unfortunately the disease may eventually progress to cirrhosis despite an apparently favorable clinical response, especially in those patients in whom repeated recurrences of activity require treatment over a period of three years or longer. Over these longer intervals the advisability of continued corticosteroid therapy must be judged not only on the basis of symptoms and laboratory and biopsy findings but also in recognition of the possibility of diminishing returns in the face of increasing risks. The possible effectiveness of other experimental approaches to the treatment of chronic active hepatitis, including the use of interferon and adenine arabinoside in chronic hepatitis B, remains to be determined.

SPECIAL CLINICAL PROBLEMS

Two circumstances are encountered in clinical practice with sufficient frequency that they deserve particular comment with reference to diagnostic approach and management.

UNEXPECTED INCREASE OF SERUM TRANSAMINASES. The advent and common use of multiphasic laboratory screening techniques have led to the identification of individuals in whom transaminase activities are abnormal but who lack clinical evidence of liver disease. If the abnormal finding is confirmed, and if it does not reflect muscle or other extrahepatic disease, it may have either of two possible implications: (1) It may reflect a subclinical acute process (e.g., acute viral hepatitis), or (2) it may reflect a chronic process (e.g., chronic toxic or viral hepatitis). If the patient is asymptomatic or nearly so, a period of observation is appropriate, and follow-up studies and hepatitis serologies should be obtained. Alcohol and potentially hepatotoxic drugs and toxins should be avoided. Improvement would presumably reflect resolution of a self-limited process or the response to removal of a toxin, e.g., ethanol. Worsening of the results may herald the clinical onset of a more overt syndrome, the

proper evaluation of which would depend on the circumstances. Persistence of the abnormality beyond six to twelve months may reflect a chronic hepatitis and may justify liver biopsy.

HEPATITIS B SURFACE ANTIGEN POSITIVITY. Approximately 0.1 to 0.2 per cent of the population of the United States is positive for HBsAg. At any given time, most of these persons exhibit no overt evidence of liver disease and are designated carriers. The meaning of the term *carrier* varies, however, and has been used to include all chronically positive individuals, or only those who have no apparent liver disease.

The practical question of significance concerns the management of the patient with a positive test. If the result is confirmed, it could indicate (1) a subclinical acute hepatitis B, (2) chronic hepatitis (persistent or active) or cirrhosis, or (3) a "healthy" carrier state. Although differentiation of these conditions may require liver biopsy, HBsAg-positive persons who have no clinical or laboratory evidence of liver disease usually have normal or nonspecific biopsy findings. For the few among this group of *asymptomatic persons with normal liver function tests* who may have chronic active hepatitis on biopsy, there is no evidence that corticosteroid treatment is indicated. Therefore, these individuals can be followed at intervals without first obtaining a liver biopsy. Those HBsAg-positive persons who do have clinical and/or laboratory signs of liver disease should be managed in accordance with the severity and duration of the process; persistence of the abnormalities beyond six months may suggest a chronic hepatitis and the need for liver biopsy.

Alter HJ (ed.): Hepatitis. Semin Liv Dis 6:1, 1986. *A minisymposium in which clinically relevant aspects of acute and chronic hepatitis are discussed by a group of recognized experts.*

Bonino F, Smedile A: Delta agent (type D) hepatitis. Semin Liv Dis 6:28, 1986. *A summary of this unusual agent prepared by workers in the unit where it was first identified.*

Czaja AJ: Natural history, clinical features and treatment of autoimmune hepatitis. Semin Liv Dis 4:1, 1984. *A summation of the Mayo Clinic experience.*

Czaja AJ, Davis GL, Ludwig J, et al.: Autoimmune features as determinants of prognosis in steroid-treated chronic active hepatitis of uncertain etiology. Gastroenterology 85:713, 1983. *Follow-up data in chronic non-B disease, indicating little difference between patients with and without "autoimmune" features.*

Czaja AJ, Ludwig J, Baggenstoss AH, et al.: Corticosteroid-treated chronic active hepatitis in remission. Uncertain prognosis of chronic persistent hepatitis. N Engl J Med 304:1, 1981.

Davis GL, Czaja AJ, Ludwig J: Development and prognosis of histologic cirrhosis in corticosteroid-treated hepatitis B surface antigen-negative chronic active hepatitis. Gastroenterology. 87:1222, 1984. *A useful observation, based on the Mayo Clinic experience, that histologic cirrhosis in these patients may not have major effects on prognosis.*

Davis GL, Hoofnagle JH, Waggoner JG: Spontaneous reactivation of chronic hepatitis B virus infection. Gastroenterology 86:230, 1984. *A series of cases in which clinically significant reactivation was not preceded by immunosuppressive therapy.*

Gregory P: Interferon in chronic hepatitis B. Gastroenterology 90:237, 1986.

Sherlock S, Thomas HC: Treatment of chronic hepatitis due to hepatitis B virus. Lancet 2:1343, 1985. *Two concise overviews of the current status of antiviral therapy.*

Hoofnagle JH, Dusheiko GM, Seeff LB, et al.: Seroconversion from hepatitis B e antigen to antibody in chronic type B hepatitis. Ann Intern Med 94:744, 1981. *Information on natural history and possible implications of spontaneous changes in the e-anti-e system with time.*

Liaw Y-F, Chu C-M, Chen T-J, et al.: Chronic lobular hepatitis: A clinicopathological and prognostic study. Hepatology 2:258, 1982. *A generally benign disorder warranting no specific treatment.*

Scott J, Gollan JL, Samourian S, et al.: Wilson's disease presenting as chronic active hepatitis. Gastroenterology 74:645, 1978. *A thorough clinical and pathologic description of 17 patients presenting with features of chronic active hepatitis. Emphasis is placed on the often difficult problem of different diagnosis.*

Scullard GH, Smith CI, Merigan TC, et al.: Effects of immunosuppressive therapy on viral markers in chronic active hepatitis B. Gastroenterology 81:987, 1981. *Evidence that viral replication may be potentiated.*

Sherman M, Shafritz DA: Hepatitis B virus and hepatocellular carcinoma: Molecular biology and mechanistic considerations. Sem Liv Dis 4:98, 1984. *A useful summary of the continually evolving concepts in this important area.*

Vyas GN, Deinstag JL, Hoofnagle JH (eds.): Viral Hepatitis and Liver Disease. Orlando, Grune & Stratton, 1984. *Proceedings of a March, 1984, international symposium. Concepts in virtually all aspects of the field are presented, discussed, and referenced.*

124 PARASITIC, BACTERIAL, FUNGAL, AND GRANULOMATOUS LIVER DISEASE

Bruce F. Scharschmidt

PARASITIC DISEASE OF THE LIVER AND BILIARY TRACT

The parasitic disorders of humans are discussed in detail in Part XIX. Those parasitic disorders that commonly involve the liver and biliary tract are outlined in Table 124–1. With respect to diagnosis, the most important first step is a carefully obtained history of travel or residence in an endemic area and potential exposure to the parasite. For example, prior travel or residence in Central Africa or the Middle East in a patient with hepatomegaly and portal hypertension suggests the diagnosis of *schistosomiasis*. In East Asia, prior ingestion of raw or undercooked freshwater fish in a patient with biliary disease should raise the possibility of *clonorchiasis* or *opisthorchiasis*. A history of cattle or sheep raising in a patient being investigated for hepatic mass should suggest *echinococcosis* and interdict the use of needle biopsy until the possibility of a cystic lesion has been excluded. Ingestion of uncooked freshwater plants (e.g., watercress) from cattle- or sheep-raising areas may be an important clue to the presence of *fascioliasis*, and a history of contact with pet cats and dogs, particularly puppies, is typically obtained from patients with *toxocariasis*.

Tender hepatomegaly and eosinophilia are commonly present during the invasive phase of many helminthic disorders, including *ascariasis, toxocariasis, strongyloidiasis, schistosomiasis,* and *fascioliasis*, yet the diagnosis may not be suspected until weeks, months, or even years later when complications resulting from the presence of eggs or the adult parasite appear. At this time, eosinophilia may no longer be present. Except in echinococcosis, serologic and skin tests are of limited value in the helminthic disorders, and the diagnosis generally requires demonstration of larvae or ova in feces or tissue.

Protozoan disorders also frequently involve the liver, and *malaria* is among the most common causes of hepatomegaly worldwide. However, hepatic involvement in malaria and in most protozoan infections represents a relatively minor component of the overall clinical disorder. The outstanding exception is *amebiasis*, of which hepatic amebic abscess is the most life-threatening manifestation (see Liver Abscess, below). In comparison to the helminthic disorders, protozoan infections are less frequently accompanied by eosinophilia and can more often be diagnosed by serologic tests.

Treatment of the helminthic disorders is discussed in Ch. 392 to 413. In addition to eradication of the parasite, biliary tract surgery may be necessary in patients with ascariasis, clonorchiasis, opisthorchiasis, or fascioliasis who develop complications such as biliary obstruction, infection, or stone formation. Patients with schistosomiasis and recurrent life-threatening hemorrhage caused by esophageal varices may be candidates for portacaval anastomosis. However, all adult worms should be eradicated prior to such surgery to prevent systemic dissemination of ova. The treatment of amebic liver abscess is discussed later in this chapter. Treatment of other protozoan disorders involving the liver is discussed in Ch. 381 to 391.

MYCOTIC LIVER DISEASE

Hepatic involvement is frequently absent or constitutes a minor component of mycotic disease in man, but virtually all fungal infections, when disseminated, can involve the liver. These include histoplasmosis, cryptococcosis, mucormycosis, aspergillosis, coccidioidomycosis, North and South American blastomycosis, candidiasis, sporotrichosis, and actinomycosis. Hepatic pathologic changes may include granulomas, hepatocellular necrosis, and abscesses. The manifestations, diagnosis, and treatment of mycotic disease are discussed in detail in Ch. 368 to 379.

HEPATIC MANIFESTATIONS OF SYSTEMIC BACTERIAL INFECTION

Many systemic infections can be accompanied by minor abnormalities of standard liver function tests and, less commonly, jaundice. Since these changes typically occur in the absence of demonstrable invasion of the hepatic parenchyma by the infecting organism(s), they are generally attributed to the hepatic effects of various toxins. For example, bacterial endotoxin has been implicated in the cholestasis occasionally associated with gram-negative bacterial infections. Staphylococcal exotoxin(s) appears responsible for the cholestasis that sometimes accompanies the toxic shock syndrome. Fever and hypoxemia also adversely affect liver cell function. Infection by gram-positive cocci (particularly pneumococcus), gram-negative cocci (e.g., gonococcus), and gram-negative bacilli (particularly *Escherichia coli* infections in infants) may all be accompanied by jaundice. The jaundice and/or abnormal liver function tests in these patients resolve with successful treatment of the infection, and the importance of these abnormalities lies primarily in the fact that they may be mistaken for other disorders such as viral hepatitis or biliary tract obstruction.

In addition, certain organisms can affect the liver directly. Hepatic invasion by streptococci or salmonellae is a rare cause of liver dysfunction and a hepatitis-like illness. Gonococcal perihepatitis *(Fitz-Hugh-Curtis syndrome)* typically occurs in women with concomitant or recent pelvic inflammatory disease and causes an acute inflammatory reaction in the hepatic capsule accompanied by right upper quadrant pain and fever. "Violin-string" adhesions between the anterior abdominal wall and liver surface may result. *Treponema pallidum* may also invade the liver, and secondary syphilis is accompanied by a hepatitis-like illness in up to 10 per cent of cases. Hepatitis associated with secondary syphilis differs from most other forms of acute hepatic injury in that it is typically associated with markedly increased alkaline phosphatase activity in serum.

LIVER ABSCESS

Pyogenic Liver Abscess

DEFINITION. A pyogenic liver abscess is a macroscopic collection of pus within the hepatic parenchyma that results from bacterial infection.

ETIOLOGY. Enteric flora (particularly *Escherichia coli* and *Klebsiella*) and pyogenic gram-positive cocci (particularly *Staphylococcus aureus*) are common causes of pyogenic liver abscess. With appropriate culture techniques, anaerobic bacteria have been isolated from one half or more of pyogenic abscesses, and multiple bacterial species are present in up to two thirds of cases. While mycotic and mycobacterial infections are unusual causes of macroscopic hepatic abscesses in healthy individuals, systemic candidiasis with multiple hepatic abscesses has been recognized with increasing frequency in patients with leukemia and neutropenia. Failure to isolate any organism from a presumed pyogenic abscess occurs relatively frequently and may reflect inappropriate sample handling or culture technique or misdiagnosis of an amebic abscess.

INCIDENCE. Liver abscess is an uncommon disorder, accounting for less than 1 per cent of most necropsy series. This relative infrequency is somewhat surprising when one

TABLE 124–1. COMMON PARASITIC DISEASES OF THE LIVER AND BILIARY TRACT

Disorder (Organism)	Principal Endemic Areas	Nature of Hepatic Involvement		
		Pathophysiology	*Manifestations*	*Diagnosis*
Helminthic disorders				
Ascariasis (*Ascaris lumbricoides*)	Worldwide; most common in underdeveloped areas of Asia, Africa, and tropics	Initially larvae carried to liver by portal blood; later, adult worms may enter the biliary tree from the intestine and deposit eggs	Occasional hepatomegaly and fever during larval migration; later, granuloma formation, biliary obstruction, biliary colic, cholangitis, and stone formation	Identification of ova in feces
Toxocariasis (*Toxocara canis, T. cati*)	North and South America, Europe, India	Larval migration in hepatic parenchyma (visceral larva migrans)	Hepatomegaly, granuloma formation	Identification of larvae in tissue, serologic testing
Strongyloidiasis (*Strongyloides stercoralis*)	Tropics	Larval invasion of liver with hyperinfective syndrome (rare)	Granuloma formation	Identification of larvae in stool or duodenal juice, filarial complement fixation test
Echinococcosis (*Echinococcus granulosus, E. multilocularis*)	Worldwide	Growth of larval form (hydatid cyst) in liver	Signs and symptoms of a hepatic mass, cyst rupture, secondary infection, rarely portal hypertension with *E. multilocularis*	Serologic tests, including hemagglutination and complement fixation
Schistosomiasis (*Schistosoma mansoni, S. japonicum*)	East Asia, Central Africa, Middle East, and South America	Adult worms live in portal venous system, eggs carried to liver by portal blood	Granuloma formation, hepatomegaly, portal hypertension and its complications	Identification of eggs in feces or tissue (e.g., rectal mucosa, liver)
Clonorchiasis (*Clonorchis sinensis*)	East Asia	Worms grow and deposit eggs in bile ducts	Granuloma formation, biliary obstruction and infection, stone formation, cholangiocarcinoma	Identification of ova in stool
Opisthorchiasis (*Opisthorchis felineus, O. viverrini*)	Europe, Asia, and Thailand	Worms grow and deposit eggs in bile ducts	Similar to clonorchiasis	Identification of ova in stool
Fascioliasis (*Fasciola hepatica*)	Worldwide	Larvae migrate through hepatic parenchyma to the bile ducts	Hepatomegaly and fever during invasive phase; later, biliary obstruction and infection	Identification of ova in stool
Protozoan disorders				
Amebiasis (*Entamoeba histolytica*)	Worldwide	Invasion of hepatic parenchyma	Signs and symptoms of hepatic abscess, extension and rupture into adjacent structures	Serologic tests, including gel diffusion precipitin and indirect hemagglutination, for tissue invasion; sigmoidoscopy and stool examination for intestinal infection
Malaria (*Plasmodium falciparum, P. vivax, P. ovale, P. malariae*)	Africa, Asia, Central and South America	Pre-erythrocytic (all types) and exoerythrocytic stages (except *P. falciparum*) present in liver	Centrolobular necrosis with acute *P. falciparum* infection, hepatosplenomegaly with chronic malaria	Identification of plasmodia in blood smear
Visceral leishmaniasis (*Leishmania donovani*)	Mediterranean basin, Asia, Africa, South America	Infection of mononuclear phagocytic cells of liver and other organs	Hepatosplenomegaly, fever	Identification of parasite in tissue, serologic testing
Toxoplasmosis (*Toxoplasma gondii*)	Worldwide	Parasite multiplication in liver	Hepatosplenomegaly	Serologic tests, including indirect fluorescent antibody test and Sabin-Feldman dye test; isolation of organism from tissue or body fluid
Trypanosomiasis (*Trypanosoma brucei, T. gambiense, T. rhodesiense*) (*T. cruzi*)	Tropical Africa South and Central America	Hepatic involvement during acute systemic phase	Hepatosplenomegaly, hepatocellular necrosis and jaundice occasionally with *T. rhodesiense* infections	Identification of parasite in blood, tissue, or cerebrospinal fluid; serologic testing

considers the large blood flow to the liver and its strategic position between the portal and systemic circulations.

PATHOGENESIS. The most common predisposing cause for pyogenic hepatic abscess is currently biliary tract disease, including acute cholecystitis as well as disorders leading to obstruction of the ductal system. Infection in areas drained by the portal venous system (e.g., appendicitis, diverticulitis, Crohn's disease) may also result in pylephlebitis and pyogenic hepatic abscess, but this occurs less frequently now than in the preantibiotic era. Other causes include direct extension from adjacent structures other than the biliary tree (subphrenic or perinephric abscess), penetrating or blunt abdominal trauma, septicemia, and infection arising in necrotic primary or secondary tumor deposits. In many cases, no predisposing cause is apparent. Pyogenic liver abscesses may be single or multiple. Multiple small abscesses occur particularly frequently in association with pylephlebitis, biliary tract obstruction with cholangitis, and septicemia.

CLINICAL MANIFESTATIONS. The symptoms of hepatic abscess are usually those of a systemic febrile illness lasting from several days to weeks, although multiple small abscesses related to cholangitis or septicemia tend to appear dramatically and suddenly. No characteristics of the fever pattern reliably distinguish hepatic abscesses from abscesses elsewhere in the body. In addition to fever and symptoms of chronic illness, such as weight loss and anorexia, patients may complain of abdominal pain or distension. Jaundice is present in up to 20 per cent of cases and often indicates concomitant biliary tract disease with cholangitis. Extension or rupture into the pleural, pericardial, or peritoneal space occurs less commonly with pyogenic than with amebic abscesses.

The most common physical findings are hepatomegaly and

right upper quadrant tenderness. However, unlike the liver in acute hepatitis, a point of maximal tenderness may be demonstrable by palpation or percussion. Even without extension into the pleural space, basilar rales may be present, or the right hemidiaphragm may be elevated or fixed.

DIAGNOSIS. Routine laboratory studies are not particularly helpful. As with any abscess of comparable duration and severity, leukocytosis and anemia are frequently present. Alkaline phosphatase is elevated in most cases, and other liver function tests may be normal to mildly abnormal. Marked hyperbilirubinemia is uncommon.

Radiologic studies are frequently useful. Roentgenograms of the chest reveal abnormalities such as elevation of the right hemidiaphragm, basilar atelectasis, or pleural effusion in about half of cases. While radionuclide scanning detects most larger abscesses, ultrasonography is probably more sensitive in identifying smaller lesions and may help distinguish abscesses from simple cysts or tumors. Computed tomography is also capable of detecting even small lesions; however, the appearance of abscesses on computed tomography and ultrasonography is quite variable, and the distinction between abscess and tumor cannot always be made reliably by any imaging method.

Blood cultures have been positive in up to 60 per cent or more of reported cases and should be obtained routinely when a hepatic abscess is suspected. On the basis of clinical findings and chest roentgenograms, pyogenic liver abscesses are most commonly mistaken for pneumonia, hepatitis, cholecystitis, or cholangitis.

TREATMENT. When a hepatic abscess is strongly suspected on the basis of clinical, laboratory, and radiologic findings, blood cultures should be drawn and antibiotic therapy begun. Antibiotics should be chosen to include coverage for gram-negative enteric bacteria and anaerobic organisms as well as possibly for enterococci or *S. aureus*. If amebic abscess is a possibility, empiric therapy for this disorder (e.g., metronidazole) should be included.

Although surgical drainage of large solitary abscesses has long been the accepted approach to therapy and is still strongly recommended by many authorities, there are now several reported series of patients treated successfully without surgery. If such a nonoperative approach is chosen, accessible lesion(s) should be aspirated both to confirm the diagnosis and to obtain material for Gram's stain and culture. Aspiration is best performed under sonographic or computed tomographic guidance and should be performed after the beginning of antibiotic therapy and institution of appropriate supportive measures (Fig. 124–1). It is appropriate to drain as much of the abscess content as possible at the time of the diagnostic aspiration, and consideration should be given to leaving in a drainage catheter. Antibiotic therapy should be modified as necessary on the basis of the results of cultures of blood or abscess content. Antibiotics are generally administered parenterally for the first 10 to 14 days and continued for a total of four to six weeks. Even in patients successfully treated by this approach, abnormalities on radionuclide scanning or sonography may persist for months.

Surgical consultation is appropriate for all patients in whom hepatic abscess is strongly suspected, even if the nonoperative approach just outlined is elected, because emergency surgery may be necessary in patients who fail to respond to this treatment or in patients who suffer complications from percutaneous aspiration or drainage. For patients with multiple small abscesses not amenable to surgical drainage, antibiotic administration with attempted aspiration of the largest, most accessible lesions is the only therapy possible, and antibiotics must frequently be administered for several months in such cases. Conversely, surgical intervention is necessary for patients in whom the abscess(es) is due to a predisposing surgical disorder such as intra-abdominal sepsis or biliary tract obstruction. Percutaneous drainage of the biliary system

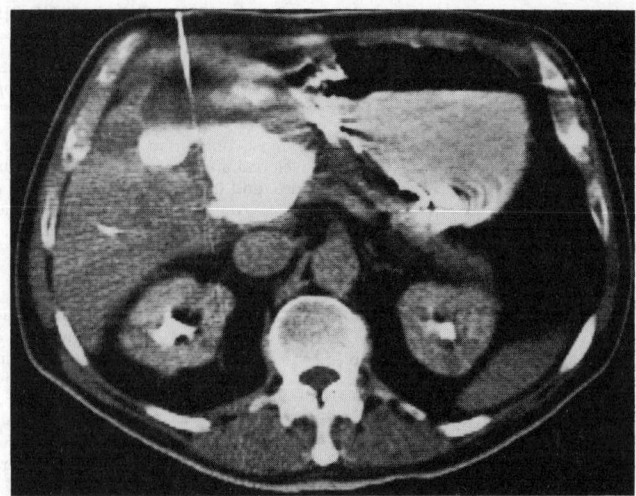

FIGURE 124–1. Computed tomogram showing CT-directed needle aspiration of a liver abscess. The needle is seen as the thin dense linear object entering the liver from the anterior abdominal wall. Contrast material has been introduced into the abscess cavity through the needle in order to outline the extent of the abscess.

may also be at least temporarily used in the latter group (see Ch. 130).

PROGNOSIS. The prognosis for patients with pyogenic hepatic abscesses has improved considerably since antibiotics have become available, but this remains a serious illness with reported mortality ranging from 10 to 60 per cent. The prognosis is adversely affected by the presence of multiple abscesses that cannot be surgically drained, advanced age, underlying malignant disease, or extension or rupture into the pleural, pulmonary, or pericardial cavities.

Amebic Liver Abscess

INCIDENCE. In developed countries, such as the United States, liver abscess is most commonly of bacterial origin. In contrast, amebic liver abscess predominates in areas of the world in which sanitation is poor and is a relatively common disorder in some countries. The factor(s) that predisposes to liver abscess in a patient with intestinal amebiasis is unknown. A more general discussion of amebiasis is found in Ch. 390.

CLINICAL MANIFESTATIONS. The clinical and laboratory features of amebic liver abscess are very similar to those of pyogenic liver abscess. Clues to the presence of an amebic as opposed to a pyogenic abscess include age less than 50 years, recent travel to an endemic area, and the absence of any evident intra-abdominal or biliary disease. Approximately 10 per cent of patients have symptoms of more than two weeks' duration, and occasionally symptoms have been present for months. While fever and leukocytosis are typical features of an amebic abscess, very high fever and a leukocyte count in excess of 20,000 per cubic millimeter may represent clues to secondary bacterial infection. Less than one half of patients have a history of recent diarrhea suggestive of intestinal amebiasis, and *Entamoeba histolytica* is identified in the stool of only one third of patients with an abscess. Extension of the abscess into the pleural space commonly causes cough, dyspnea, pleurisy, or even symptoms of a bronchohepatic fistula. Overall, extension or rupture into the pleural, pericardial, or peritoneal cavity occurs in up to 10 per cent of patients. Rupture into the pericardial or peritoneal cavity is particularly frequent with abscesses in the left lobe.

DIAGNOSIS. Routine laboratory studies, chest roentgenogram, radionuclide scan, ultrasound examination, and computed tomography reveal abnormalities very similar to those of pyogenic abscess. Although amebic abscesses are most commonly solitary and located in the right lobe, they may be multiple and can occur in other locations.

Serologic testing is extremely valuable in the diagnosis of amebic liver abscess. Indirect hemagglutination, the standard test performed by the Parasitology Division of the Centers for Disease Control in Atlanta, is positive in more than 90 per cent of patients with amebic liver abscess, and antibody titers remain elevated for many years. The gel diffusion precipitin test, which is available in most state laboratories and many local hospitals, is similarly positive in more than 90 per cent of cases, but reverts to negative in most patients within one year after successful treatment. This fact can be an advantage in distinguishing active disease from past infection.

TREATMENT. For patients with an amebic abscess, medical therapy alone is usually sufficient. Metronidazole (750 mg three times daily for ten days) is the drug of choice, and some authorities recommend that an intestinal amebicide such as diiodohydroxyquin (650 mg three times daily for 20 days) be given in addition. Chloroquine (500 mg daily for 10 weeks) is reportedly equally effective, but the long duration of treatment and lack of efficacy against intestinal amebae render it less desirable. A variety of alternative regimens also exist, including a single-day drug treatment regimen (see Ch. 390). Most patients report rapid symptomatic improvement after both forms of therapy and are afebrile by the end of the first week. However, since metronidazole is also effective against anaerobic bacteria present in pyogenic liver abscesses, a favorable therapeutic response to this agent cannot, by itself, be considered proof of an amebic versus a pyogenic abscess. Rare treatment failures have been reported, and it is particularly important in such cases to make sure that any concomitant intestinal infection has been eradicated. The role of needle aspiration in the treatment of amebic abscess is controversial. Some advocate it routinely and report excellent results; however, there are no controlled studies to support the therapeutic value of aspiration, and most patients recover with medical therapy alone. Aspiration should be undertaken only by skilled personnel, after appropriate medical therapy has been begun, and is probably most appropriate for patients with impending rupture as evidenced by increasing pleural or pericardial reaction or progressive hepatic enlargement, particularly with abscesses in the left lobe for patients in whom the diagnosis is uncertain and for patients who fail to respond to appropriate therapy within three to four days. Surgery is rarely necessary.

PROGNOSIS. The prognosis in uncomplicated amebic abscess is excellent with appropriate medical therapy, the mortality being as low as 1 per cent in some series. With extension or rupture into the pleural, pericardial, or peritoneal space, the mortality increases sharply. The presence of jaundice is associated with a higher incidence of complications and a higher mortality. Even after successful treatment, resolution of the radionuclide scan defect caused by an amebic abscess may require many months.

GRANULOMATOUS DISEASE OF THE LIVER

ETIOLOGY. The liver is one of the most frequent sites in the body for granuloma formation. By virtue of its large number of mononuclear phagocytic cells and strategic location, the liver clears the circulation of many substances, including microorganisms, antigens, and immune complexes. In addition, the liver is the major site of metabolism of many drugs and toxins. These factors help account for the 2 to 10 per cent incidence of granulomas found in liver biopsies.

Hepatic granulomas have been reported in association with a wide variety of infectious and other systemic illnesses, hepatobiliary disorders, and drugs or exogenous agents (Table 124–2). Since granulomas are not a rare finding in liver biopsy material, it is possible that some of the reported associations are spurious. The relative frequency with which various underlying disorders have been associated with hepatic granulomas varies with the patient population under study. Sarcoidosis, tuberculosis, and, more recently, drug reactions have

TABLE 124–2. HEPATIC GRANULOMAS (REPORTED ASSOCIATIONS)

Infections	Hepatobiliary disorders
Bacterial, mycobacterial, spirochetal	Primary biliary cirrhosis
Tuberculosis	Chronic active hepatitis
Atypical mycobacteria	Granulomatous hepatitis
Tularemia	Jejunoileal bypass
Brucellosis	**Systemic disorders**
Leprosy	Sarcoidosis
Typhoid fever	Wegener's granulomatosis
Granuloma inguinale	Vineyard sprayer's lung
Syphilis	Inflammatory bowel disease
Whipple's disease	Chronic granulomatous disease
Listeriosis	Allergic granulomatosis
Melioidosis	Granulomatous arteritis-
BCG immunotherapy	polymyalgia rheumatica
Cat-scratch disease	Melanoma
Viral	Hodgkin's disease
Infectious mononucleosis	Lymphoma
Cytomegalovirus	**Exogenous agents**
Chickenpox	Phenylbutazone
Influenza B	Alpha-methyldopa
Lymphogranuloma venereum	Sulfonamides
Rickettsial	Carbamazepine
Q fever	Hydralazine
Fungal	Procainamide
Coccidioidomycosis	Quinidine
Histoplasmosis	Allopurinol
Cryptococcosis	Phenytoin
Actinomycosis	Halothane
Blastomycosis	Penicillin
Aspergillosis	Nitrofurantoin
Nocardiosis	Chlorpromazine
Torulopsosis	Chlorpropamide
Candidiasis	Clofibrate
Parasitic	Oral contraceptives
Amebiasis	Beryllium
Giardiasis	Copper sulfate
Schistosomiasis	Parenteral foreign material
Clonorchiasis	(starch, talc, silicon, etc.)
Fascioliasis	
Toxocariasis	
Ascariasis	
Toxoplasmosis	
Strongyloidiasis	
Ancyclostomiasis	
Tongue worm (Pentastomida)	

accounted for the largest proportion of patients in the United States and Western Europe.

PATHOLOGY. Granulomas in the liver, as elsewhere, consist of a compact collection of mature mononuclear phagocytes. In well-developed granulomas, these phagocytic cells take the form of epithelioid cells. Giant cells and necrosis are frequent additional features, but their presence is not necessary for the pathologic diagnosis of granuloma. Although the morphologic features of the granuloma itself are seldom characteristic enough to permit a determination of etiology, this is occasionally possible (e.g., acid-fast bacilli in tuberculosis, ova in schistosomiasis, larvae in toxocariasis, fibrinoid ring plus central clear space in Q fever, birefringent granules in starch granuloma or in foreign substance injection as with parenteral drug abuse). The location of the granuloma or the presence of coexisting parenchymal liver disease may also be helpful, as in granulomatous arteritis and primary biliary cirrhosis.

CLINICAL MANIFESTATIONS. The predominant clinical manifestations are generally those of the underlying disorder. In many of the entities listed in Table 124–2, hepatic dysfunction either is not detectable or constitutes a minor component of the illness. Hepatomegaly is present in more than one half of all patients, whereas splenomegaly is less frequent. In the absence of a primary hepatobiliary disorder, peripheral stigmata (vascular spiders, palmar erythema) and complications (portal hypertension, ascites, encephalopathy) of chronic liver disease are uncommon. Serum alkaline phosphatase and transaminase levels are mildly to moderately elevated in up to two thirds of patients, and hyperbilirubinemia occurs in approximately one quarter of the cases. However, these generalizations do not apply to many individual cases. For example, portal hypertension is a frequent complication of schistosomiasis, and rare patients with sarcoidosis have striking cholestasis and jaundice.

DIAGNOSIS. Because hepatic granulomas are associated with a variety of disorders, many of which are infrequently encountered in clinical practice, the differential diagnosis of granulomatous disease of the liver is one of the most challenging problems in medicine. The histopathologic features and location of the granuloma(s) seldom indicate the etiology, and cultures of the biopsy specimen are usually negative. For example, acid-fast bacilli are demonstrable by appropriate stains in 10 to 25 per cent of biopsies from patients with extrapulmonary tuberculosis, and culture is also infrequently positive. In most cases, the finding of hepatic granulomas serves mainly to direct attention to the broad class of diseases known to cause a granulomatous response in the liver, and the specific diagnosis depends on cultures and/or biopsies from other sites, serologic tests, or skin tests. The generally low frequency with which liver biopsy yields a specific diagnosis, however, appears not to apply to patients with the acquired immune deficiency syndrome. Preliminary reports suggest that atypical mycobacteria and other organisms are detected by stain and culture in a high proportion of such patients with fever and abnormal biochemical studies.

The workup of the patient with hepatic granulomas should begin with a careful interview, probing previous illnesses, travel, occupational and environmental exposures, and drug use or abuse. Physical examination should include careful inspection of the skin and palpation of lymph nodes. A chest roentgenogram is valuable in detecting sarcoidosis and tuberculosis as well as certain fungal diseases. Serial thin sections of the biopsy material with special stains should be obtained to increase the likelihood of detecting acid-fast bacilli, fungi, ova, or foreign material. Bacterial, mycobacterial, and fungal cultures of the biopsy material as well as blood and possibly bone marrow should be obtained when the biopsy is performed as part of an investigation of fever. The appropriateness of additional tests, cultures, and biopsies depends upon the individual clinical circumstances. Despite a thorough search, a satisfactory cause for the granuloma(s) is not discovered in 20 per cent or more of cases. Such patients in whom no satisfactory explanation for the hepatic granulomas can be found and who have fever of unknown origin have been designated as having idiopathic *granulomatous hepatitis*. The existence of granulomatous hepatitis as an entity distinct from sarcoidosis has been disputed.

TREATMENT AND PROGNOSIS. The treatment is that of the underlying disorder. When the underlying disorder can be successfully treated or an offending drug or exposure terminated, clinical and biochemical evidence of liver dysfunction typically disappears. The granulomas themselves, however, may persist for a variable time, depending on the rapidity with which the inciting agent is removed. Patients with idiopathic granulomatous hepatitis have generally responded favorably to administration of corticosteroids. However, this approach should not be undertaken until a thorough search has failed to reveal a cause for the granulomas and generally after a trial of antituberculous therapy has failed.

Berger LA, Osborne DR: Treatment of pyogenic liver abscesses by percutaneous needle aspiration. Lancet 1:132, 1982. Herbert DA, Rothman J, Simmons F, et al.: Pyogenic liver abscesses: Successful nonsurgical therapy. Lancet 1:134, 1982. McCorkell, Niles NL. Pyogenic liver abscesses: Another look at medical management. Lancet 1:803, 1985. *These three articles summarize the results of nonoperative management.*

Conter RL, Pitt HA, Tompkins RK, et al.: Differentiation of pyogenic from amebic hepatic abscesses. Surg Gynecol Obstet 162:114, 1986. *A comprehensive review of 82 patients with emphasis on differential diagnosis and management.*

Drugs for parasitic infections. Med Letter 24:5, 1982. *A concise summary of this topic.*

Elliot DL, Tolle SW, Goldberg L, et al.: Pet-associated illness. N Engl J Med 313:985, 1985. *A succinct summary of a variety of parasitic, bacterial, rickettsial,*

and other infectious disorders (including many affecting the liver) with emphasis on clinical features and diagnosis.

Harrington PL, Gutierrez JJ, Ramirez-Rhondra CH, et al.: Granulomatous hepatitis. Rev Infect Dis 4:638, 1982. *An exhaustively referenced and thorough review of the disorders associated with hepatic granulomas.*

Katzenstein D, Rickerson V, Braude A: New concepts of amebic liver abscess derived from hepatic imaging, serodiagnosis, and hepatic enzymes in 67 consecutive cases in San Diego. Medicine 61:237, 1982. *A pertinent review that distinguishes acute from chronic cases.*

Orenstein MS, Tavitian A, Yonk B, et al.: Granulomatous involvement of the liver in patients with AIDS. Gut 26:1220, 1985. *Report of a small series of patients with AIDS in whom liver biopsy was found to be a high yield procedure for establishing the presence of mycobacterial infection.*

125 INHERITED, INFILTRATIVE, AND METABOLIC DISORDERS INVOLVING THE LIVER

Bruce F. Scharschmidt

The liver is involved in a variety of inherited, infiltrative, and metabolic disorders. Most of the disorders included in this chapter, e.g., Wilson's disease, hemochromatosis, the glycogen and lipid storage diseases, and amyloidosis, are discussed here only with respect to their hepatic involvement. A more comprehensive treatment of these entities can be found elsewhere in this textbook.

ALPHA₁-ANTITRYPSIN DEFICIENCY

Alpha$_1$-antitrypsin (A_1AT) deficiency is an inherited disorder associated with a decreased concentration of A_1AT in serum (see Ch. 61). This glycoprotein, which is found in other body fluids as well as in serum, inhibits a variety of proteolytic enzymes, including pancreatic trypsin, chymotrypsin, and elastase, as well as certain proteases produced by leukocytes and macrophages. It is normally present in a concentration of about 200 mg per deciliter in serum, where it accounts for 90 per cent of total antitrypsin activity and a major portion of the alpha-1-globulin fraction. A_1AT production is controlled by codominant alleles, and more than 25 different alleles have been identified by starch gel electrophoresis of serum. The most common allele at the P_i (protein inhibitor) locus is termed M (allele frequency 0.94 to 0.95 in the United States). The most important variant is Z, since P_iZZ accounts for virtually all patients with severe A_1AT deficiency. The liver plays a critical role in the pathophysiology of the disorder, as evidenced by the observation that A_1AT levels return to normal after liver transplantation and the P_i phenotype converts to that of the donor.

Severe A_1AT deficiency is associated with early-onset emphysema in some individuals, liver disease in others, and occasionally both liver and lung disease. The pathogenesis of the disorder is unclear; the deficiency state, by itself, is not sufficient to produce disease. About 10 per cent of individuals with P_iZZ phenotype develop overt liver disease in childhood and have signs and symptoms of cholestasis in the first few days to weeks of life. In a minority of infants, cholestasis persists or worsens and is associated with liver failure and death in a few years. Cholestasis typically remits by six months in the remaining patients, about half of whom nevertheless develop cirrhosis. The long-term prognosis for these children is uncertain. An as yet undefined proportion of infants with P_iZZ phenotype who do not develop neonatal cholestasis have also been shown to have elevated transaminase levels in serum and fibrosis or cirrhosis on liver biopsy. Severe deficiency, P_iZZ phenotype, is associated with a several-fold increase in the risk of developing both cirrhosis and hepatocellular carcinoma, particularly in males. Heterozygous A_1AT deficiency (phenotypes MZ and SZ) may also be associated with an increased incidence of liver disease and cancer, although the link is less clear than for severe deficiency.

The diagnosis of A_1AT deficiency can be suspected from serum protein electrophoresis and confirmed by measurement of A_1AT in serum either as trypsin inhibitory activity or by immunoassay. However, definitive diagnosis requires determination of protease inhibitor phenotype by starch gel electrophoresis or isoelectric focusing. This is particularly true of individuals with heterozygous A_1AT deficiency who may have serum levels of A_1AT in the low normal range. Patients with the Z allele, with or without liver disease, also exhibit characteristic rounded eosinophilic cytoplasmic inclusions in periportal hepatocytes. These inclusion bodies are immunologically related to A_1AT but differ in certain amino acids as well as in their content of sialic acid and other sugars. Importantly, such eosinophilic inclusions have been recently described as an apparently acquired defect in patients with alcoholic liver disease and are thus not diagnostic of inherited A_1AT deficiency. There is currently no specific therapy for this disorder; however, a number of patients have successfully undergone transplantation with favorable results (Ch. 128).

WILSON'S DISEASE

Wilson's disease is an autosomal recessive disorder with a prevalence worldwide of about 1 in 30,000 (see Ch. 205). Its clinical and pathologic manifestations result from excessive accumulation of copper in many tissues, including the brain, liver, cornea, and kidneys. Although the primary genetic defect remains undetermined, impaired biliary copper excretion rather than enhanced absorption is the cause of the copper accumulation. Unfortunately the diagnosis of this treatable disorder is often missed or delayed because of its rarity and diverse presentations. Hepatic disease is a common initial clinical manifestation in childhood and adolescence and may take the form of a self-limited illness resembling viral hepatitis, fulminant hepatic failure, or chronic active hepatitis; thus, biochemical screening for Wilson's disease is imperative in all patients under the age of 35 years who have liver disease of uncertain etiology. A majority of patients with fulminant hepatic failure die despite initiation of D-penicillamine therapy. Hemolysis represents an important clue to the presence of Wilson's disease and predisposes to the development of cholelithiasis. Neurologic manifestations typically appear between the ages of 12 and 30 years and are almost invariably accompanied by the presence of Kayser-Fleischer rings.

The diagnosis and treatment of Wilson's disease are discussed in detail in Ch. 205; however, certain points merit special emphasis here. First, while the combination of an abnormally low ceruloplasmin level in serum and Kayser-Fleischer rings establishes the diagnosis, about 15 per cent of patients having Wilson's disease presenting with hepatic manifestations have serum ceruloplasmin concentrations in the low normal range, and about one half of patients who seek medical help with chronic active hepatitis or fulminant hepatic failure have not yet developed Kayser-Fleischer rings. If the diagnosis of Wilson's disease is uncertain, a biopsy should be performed for quantitative copper determination. If coagulation abnormalities preclude a biopsy, measurement of incorporation of orally administered radiolabeled copper into ceruloplasmin or measurement of serum copper or urinary copper excretion may be useful.

HEMOCHROMATOSIS

Hemochromatosis is among the more common genetic disorders, with a calculated homozygous frequency of about 1 in 300 to 1 in 400 in certain high prevalence areas. The molecular basis of the underlying defect responsible for enhanced intestinal iron absorption remains undetermined. Males homozygous for the hemochromatosis allele, which is in close linkage with HLA-A3 on chromosome 6, show progressive accumulation of hepatic iron, and clinical evidence of disease usually develops in the fourth, fifth, or sixth decades of life. Most homozygous females do not develop clinical evidence of disease, presumably because of iron loss through menses and pregnancy. Heterozygotes may also show abnormal accumulation of hepatic iron, but the absolute amounts present are much less than in homozygotes, and clinical evidence of iron overload rarely develops.

Hepatic iron overload is most commonly manifested as moderate to marked hepatomegaly with initially well preserved liver function. Esophageal varices, ascites, and impaired hepatic synthetic function are present in more advanced cases. Other important clinical features include abnormal skin pigmentation, glucose intolerance, cardiac involvement, hypogonadism, and arthropathy. Hepatocellular carcinoma develops in up to one third of patients. These classic manifestations are present in only a minority of homozygotes. Indeed, there is considerable variability in the expression of the disorder, and it is possible that some homozygotes never develop overt disease. With appropriate phlebotomy therapy hepatic function frequently improves, and there are case reports that suggest regression of apparent cirrhosis.

Screening for hemochromatosis is probably best accomplished by measurement of transferrin saturation and serum ferritin. A saturation exceeding 50 per cent is present in nearly all homozygotes over 20 years of age, and a value less than 50 per cent largely precludes the diagnosis. However, the positive predictive value of a transferrin saturation exceeding 50 per cent is relatively low. In contrast, a transferrin saturation exceeding 80 per cent is a more reliable indicator of hemochromatosis, and a large study in Utah suggests that a transferrin saturation greater than 62 per cent most reliably separates homozygotes from heterozygotes and normal persons. Serum levels of ferritin are a generally accurate reflection of tissue iron stores and exceed 1000 ng per ml in most patients. However, occasional families with hemochromatosis and normal serum ferritin levels have been described and, conversely, serum ferritin is typically increased out of proportion to tissue iron stores in patients with hepatocellular necrosis. If either of these tests suggests iron overload, liver biopsy with quantitative iron determination and histochemical stains for iron should be performed. A variety of noninvasive methods for measurement of hepatic iron have been proposed for use in patients who cannot undergo a liver biopsy. Dual-energy computed tomography appears particularly promising, and nuclear magnetic resonance and magnetic susceptibility measurement are also undergoing evaluation. Hemochromatosis is discussed in detail in Ch. 206.

STORAGE DISEASES

The glycogen storage diseases may present as disorders of the liver as well as of the heart and musculoskeletal system. Hepatomegaly is a prominent feature of most of these disorders, whereas splenomegaly is found primarily in Type IV and less commonly in Type III. Patients with Type I and III glycogen storage disease frequently survive childhood and may be encountered by the physician treating adults. Patients with type I glycogen storage disease apparently have an increased incidence of hepatic adenoma as well as hepatocellular carcinoma. Portacaval anastomosis may improve growth and reverse certain metabolic abnormalities in selected Type I patients, although the mechanism for these beneficial effects is uncertain. The glycogen storage diseases are discussed in detail in Ch. 179. In addition to glycogen, the liver abnormally stores fatty acids, cholesterol, or complex lipids in the lipid storage disorders as well as various mucopolysaccharides and mucolipids. Although hepatomegaly is common to most of these disorders, the clinical consequences are attributable to involvement of the nervous and musculoskeletal systems.

PROTOPORPHYRIA

Protoporphyria is a disorder characterized by increased protoporphyrin content in erythrocytes, plasma, feces, and liver. It is inherited as an autosomal dominant trait and results from a deficiency of heme synthase (ferrochelatase), the enzyme that catalyzes the formation of heme from protoporphyrin and iron. It is most conveniently diagnosed by demonstrating an elevated level of erythrocyte protoporphyrin. Protoporphyria is usually a mild disorder manifested by mild photosensitivity and, rarely, hemolysis. Hepatobiliary complications include pigment gallstones and infrequent hepatic failure. About 18 cases of hepatic failure associated with protoporphyria have been reported. The hepatic failure, typically heralded by cholestasis, is associated with and presumably results from massive hepatic accumulation of birefringent crystals of protoporphyrin. Interruption of the enterohepatic circulation of protoporphyrin with cholestyramine or activated charcoal has been reported to deplete hepatic protoporphyrin deposits and restore liver function to normal in some patients with mild disease, but the value of such treatment in patients with severe cholestasis and established hepatic failure is unknown. Oral iron therapy has also been reported to decrease protoporphyrin production in a single patient. At present there is no way of identifying the small proportion of patients with protoporphyria who will develop significant hepatic disease.

CYSTIC FIBROSIS

In infants with cystic fibrosis, amorphous eosinophilic material in bile ducts and ductules, presumably representing inspissated secretions, may produce cholestasis (see Ch. 66). Later manifestations include cholangitis, fibrosis, and obstructive biliary cirrhosis. Up to 20 per cent of patients who survive to adolescence have cirrhosis with portal hypertension, and bleeding from esophageal varices represents a significant cause of morbidity in this older age group. Patients who have bled from varices and have good pulmonary function are candidates for shunt surgery. Since liver disease with portal hypertension has even been reported as a first manifestation of cystic fibrosis, the diagnosis should be considered in a young patient with otherwise unexplained liver disease.

AMYLOIDOSIS

Amyloid deposition in the liver is common in amyloidosis of all types (see Ch. 168). Hepatomegaly is present in approximately one half of patients with systemic amyloidosis; splenomegaly is present in about 10 per cent of patients; and mild elevation of the serum alkaline phosphatase is the most common biochemical abnormality. Cutaneous stigmata of chronic liver disease (e.g., spider angiomas, palmar erythema) and portal hypertension are unusual. Intrahepatic cholestasis with marked elevation of the serum bilirubin and alkaline phosphatase concentrations occurs in about 5 per cent of patients. The diagnosis of amyloidosis can usually be established without resorting to liver biopsy.

SARCOIDOSIS

Hepatic involvement in sarcoidosis represents a continuum from the presence of asymptomatic granulomas to cases in which hepatic involvement represents a prominent part of the overall clinical picture (see Ch. 69). Approximately two thirds to three quarters of patients with sarcoidosis have hepatic granulomas, making the liver one of the most commonly involved organs in this disease, and liver biopsy is often of value in establishing the diagnosis of sarcoidosis.

About 20 per cent of patients with sarcoidosis have hepatomegaly, and up to 40 per cent have abnormal liver function tests, most commonly a mild elevation of the level of alkaline phosphatase. Overt hepatic involvement is present in fewer than 20 per cent of patients. This may take several forms, including (1) hepatomegaly, generally with splenomegaly, and multiple abnormal liver function tests; (2) chronic cholestasis, which may closely mimic primary biliary cirrhosis; and (3) portal hypertension and its manifestations. The characteristic histologic feature of hepatic sarcoidosis is the presence of granulomas, frequently located in portal tracts. Chronic portal tract inflammation, hepatocyte poikilocytosis and anisocytosis, fibrosis, and even cirrhosis may be accompanying findings. Little information is available regarding the response of these hepatic lesions to corticosteroids, but a therapeutic trial is justified if significant symptoms are present and tuberculosis and other disorders producing hepatic granuloma have been excluded.

ENTERIC BYPASS

Hepatic disease related to enteric bypass surgery has typically been reported in patients who have had extensive bypass procedures for treatment of marked obesity. Jejunocolic bypass, an early operation, has now largely been abandoned because of a high incidence of complications, including cirrhosis and hepatic failure. Hepatic abnormalities are also common following jejunoileal bypass and may take several forms. Fatty change is present in up to two thirds of markedly obese patients prior to bypass surgery, and hepatic lipid content increases during the period of weight loss. Cirrhosis ensues in up to 5 per cent of patients, and death from liver failure accounts for a substantial proportion of the early postoperative mortality of 2 to 4 per cent. Histologic features may mimic those of alcoholic liver disease, including the presence of alcoholic hyalin. Longer-term follow-up studies suggest that hepatic abnormalities may not appear until several years after surgery in some patients.

The pathogenesis of these hepatic changes is unclear. Weight loss itself does not account for the progressive postoperative fat accumulation, since this does not occur in nonoperated obese patients who lose weight through dietary measures. However, hepatic disease resembling alcoholic hepatitis and even cirrhosis have been described in abstinent patients with obesity who have not undergone bypass surgery. Protein depletion, leading to a kwashiorkor-like state, may contribute to the fatty change. Increased production in the gut of potentially toxic substances may also play a role. For example, increased delivery of chenodeoxycholate to the colon results in increased production of the potentially hepatotoxic bile salt, lithocholate. The bypassed segment may also serve as a site for bacterial overgrowth and production of potentially toxic bacterial products.

Laboratory studies of hepatic function are frequently abnormal in the first few postoperative months following bypass surgery even in the absence of serious liver disease. Conversely, the absence of abnormal hepatic function tests or clinical evidence of liver disease during the first postoperative year does not preclude the possible later development of significant liver disease. Deterioration of synthetic or excretory function as evidenced by an abnormal prothrombin time that does not respond to vitamin K administration, hypoalbuminemia, or hyperbilirubinemia is an ominous sign. Biopsy is the only reliable way of assessing the severity of hepatic disease, and some advocate follow-up biopsies in all patients. Serious and persistent hepatic disease is an indication for reestablishing normal bowel continuity, which may be required in up to 25 per cent of patients. Currently, alternative procedures such as gastroplasty, which are associated with fewer hepatic and metabolic complications, are preferred in the morbidly obese patients.

INFLAMMATORY BOWEL DISEASE

Liver function tests may be transiently abnormal in up to one half of patients with chronic ulcerative colitis and less commonly in Crohn's disease, but significant and persistent biochemical abnormalities are present in fewer than 10 per cent of patients. A variety of histologic abnormalities have been described in these patients. *Pericholangitis* is defined as portal tract inflammation with or without periductular fibrosis in association with inflammatory bowel disease. Direct cholangiography has revealed sclerosing cholangitis in a substantial proportion of patients with pericholangitis. Moreover, the hepatic histologic changes in patients with radiologically documented sclerosing cholangitis are indistinguishable from those of pericholangitis in association with radiologically normal bile ducts (see Ch. 105). Thus, the term *small duct sclerosing cholangitis* has been suggested as preferable to pericholangitis to describe the heterogeneous collection of bile duct abnormalities seen in patients with inflammatory bowel disease and radiologically normal bile ducts. While portal bacteremia or other enteric toxins have been postulated to play a role in the pathogenesis of small- and large-duct sclerosing cholangitis associated with inflammatory bowel disease, such a cause-and-effect relationship between the bowel disease and these lesions does not account for the variable temporal relationship between the two and the often very mild bowel disease. A variable response of bile ducts and colon to some common factor better accounts for these clinical findings. Other hepatic abnormalities in patients with inflammatory bowel disease have included fatty change, chronic active hepatitis, cirrhosis, amyloidosis and granulomas.

No specific therapy is available for these hepatic abnormalities. Treatment should be directed at the underlying bowel disease, although this does not reliably produce improvement in the hepatic disorder. Progression of serious liver disease in ulcerative colitis is not consistently altered by colectomy, so this approach cannot be generally recommended.

TOTAL PARENTERAL NUTRITION

Total parenteral nutrition has been associated with a spectrum of hepatic abnormalities, including mild elevations in alkaline phosphatase and transaminase levels, cholestasis with jaundice, and, rarely, progressive hepatic disease resulting in death. Liver biopsy in these patients has frequently revealed fatty change, cholestasis, and mild periportal inflammation, with fibrosis or cirrhosis found in a minority. Some of these abnormalities have been due to the underlying disease or complicating infection, but total parenteral nutrition, by itself, can produce elevated serum bile salt levels and occasionally hyperbilirubinemia in both infants and adults. The degree of abnormality appears related to the duration and amount of parenteral alimentation. In infants, cholestasis associated with parenteral nutrition also increases in frequency with decreasing gestational age and birth weight, and adults with the short-bowel syndrome appear particularly at risk for severe liver disease. Hepatic function generally returns gradually to normal after total parenteral nutrition is discontinued. Modifying the infusate by lowering the caloric-nitrogen ratio or decreasing the total caloric intake has reportedly produced improvement in some patients, but this has not been systematically studied, and no one component of the parenteral formula has been clearly implicated as causative. Total parenteral nutrition also appears to predispose patients to the development of gallstones and cholecystitis, and these possibilities should be kept in mind when one is evaluating a patient receiving parenteral nutrition for hepatobiliary disease.

PREGNANCY

Liver size and liver histology remain normal during uncomplicated pregnancy. Serum levels of alkaline phosphatase and leucine aminopeptidase typically rise in the second and third trimesters and are of placental origin; aminotransferase and bilirubin levels are normal.

EFFECT OF PREGNANCY ON COEXISTING LIVER DISEASE. In the United States and Western Europe, pregnancy does not appear to alter the course of acute viral hepatitis. In underdeveloped countries, however, viral hepatitis in pregnancy, particularly during the third trimester, appears to run a more severe course and is associated with an unusually high incidence of fulminant hepatic failure with high fetal and maternal mortality. Pregnancy has not been shown to alter the course of chronic persistent or chronic active hepatitis, although maternal and fetal morbidity and mortality may be increased because of variceal bleeding and postpartum hemorrhage. Vertical transmission of hepatitis B virus infection occurs commonly when the mother contracts acute hepatitis B during the third trimester or is a chronic carrier (particularly if she also is HBeAg positive), and it is important that the infant receive appropriate passive and active prophylaxis at delivery (see Ch. 121).

LIVER DISEASES ASSOCIATED WITH PREGNANCY. *Hyperemesis gravidarum* of sufficient severity to require hospitalization may be accompanied by minor abnormalities in standard liver function tests. *Acute fatty liver of pregnancy* can be defined as a syndrome of acute hepatic dysfunction that develops in late pregnancy, is associated with microvesicular fat accumulation in hepatocytes, and resolves with delivery. It typically becomes apparent after the 30th week of gestation and is manifested initially by constitutional symptoms, often with abdominal pain, followed in many instances by overt evidence of hepatic failure, including encephalopathy and jaundice. In the past, intravenous tetracycline therapy was incriminated in some cases, but this is rarely true at present. The only known treatment is termination of the pregnancy. Early reports suggested that the disorder was associated with a very high mortality rate, but more recent reports suggest that there is a spectrum of disease severity and that milder cases without frank hepatic failure occur and have a favorable prognosis. It also appears that acute fatty liver may, at least in some instances, fall within the spectrum of hepatic dysfunction associated with *pre-eclampsia* or *eclampsia*, as these two disorders occasionally share certain features, including onset in late pregnancy, increased incidence in young primiparas, the presence of coagulopathy, hypertension, and proteinuria, and resolution upon delivery. Focal necrosis and, rarely, hepatic rupture may occur in women with *eclampsia*. *Cholestasis of pregnancy* generally occurs in the last four months of gestation (range 7 to 39 weeks). It is characterized by pruritus, sometimes followed by jaundice. It typically resolves within two weeks of delivery and frequently recurs in subsequent pregnancies or with administration of oral contraceptives. Serum alkaline phosphatase and bile salts are increased, and hyperbilirubinemia may be present. Serum transaminase is also frequently mildly increased. Although generally considered a benign condition, cholestasis of pregnancy has been associated with an increased incidence of premature labor and postpartum hemorrhage.

CIRCULATORY DISTURBANCE

Hepatic function and histology are commonly altered in patients with cardiovascular disease. Disorders associated with an elevation of systemic venous pressure typically produce hepatic venous congestion manifested by hepatomegaly, minor abnormalities of liver function tests, and centrolobular congestion without necrosis. Longstanding hepatic congestion may lead to cardiac cirrhosis with fibrous bands joining centrilobular areas (see Ch. 126). When hypotension is superimposed, even transiently, on hepatic congestion, severe centrilobular to midzonal necrosis, transaminase levels exceeding 1000 units, marked hyperbilirubinemia, and hypoprothrombinemia may result. Differentiating this disorder from viral hepatitis may be difficult, since the clinical features are similar and hepatic dysfunction often is not recognized until several days after the resolution of the circulatory failure. Unlike viral hepatitis, however, serum transaminase levels frequently fall very rapidly and may approach normal within days. If the circulatory insult is brief, patients usually recover from their hepatic injury uneventfully. Fatal fulminant hepatic failure has been reported, however. A similar form of acute hepatic injury is occasionally seen in persons without pre-existing cardiovascular disease who suffer severe or prolonged hypotension or in patients with severe isolated left-sided heart failure.

Alagille D: α-1-Antitrypsin deficiency. Hepatology, 4:11S, Jan-Feb Suppl. 1984. *A concise review of the clinical course of 45 children with neonatal cholestasis and A₁AT deficiency.*

Bassett ML, Halliday JW, Powell LW: Genetic hemachromatosis. Semin Liver Dis 4:217, 1984. *A concise, practically oriented, and well-referenced review.*

Eriksson S, Carlson J, Velez R: Risk of cirrhosis and primary liver cancer in alpha-1-antitrypsin deficiency. N Engl J Med 314:736, 1986. *Report of an autopsy study conducted in Sweden that provides the clearest evidence to date that this disorder predisposes to cirrhosis and liver cancer.*

Hocking MP, Duerson MC, O'Leary P, et al.: Jejunoileal bypass for morbid obesity. Late follow-up in 100 cases. N Engl J Med 308:995, 1983. *A summary of complications in patients with intact bypasses followed for more than five years.*

Kaplan MM: Acute fatty liver of pregnancy. N Engl J Med 313:367, 1985. *A short review focusing on practical clinical issues.*

McCullough AJ, Fleming CR, Thistle JL, et al.: Diagnosis of Wilson's disease presenting as fulminant hepatic failure. Gastroenterology 84:161, 1983. *This article summarizes the clinical features of this presentation of Wilson's disease and the value of various tests other than liver biopsy in making the diagnosis.*

O'Leary J: Hepatic complications of jejunoileal bypass. Semin Liver Dis 3:203, 1983. *A comprehensive review with pertinent references.*

Stanko R, Nathan G, Mendelow H, et al.: Development of hepatic cholestasis and fibrosis in patients with massive loss of intestine supported by prolonged parenteral nutrition. Gastroenterology 92:197, 1987. *Report of a small series of patients that suggests that the short-bowel syndrome predisposes to severe liver injury in patients undergoing parenteral alimentation.*

Wee A, Judwig J: Pericholangitis in chronic ulcerative colitis: Primary sclerosing cholangitis of the small bile ducts? Ann Intern Med 102:581, 1985. *A review of the spectrum of hepatobiliary disease seen in 107 patients with ulcerative colitis with emphasis on the relationship between histologic abnormalities noted on liver biopsy and sclerosing cholangitis.*

Zakin D, Boyer TD: Hepatology. Philadelphia, W. B. Saunders Company, 1982. *Consult chapters 12, 33, 42, 43, 44, and 48 for authoritative, and well-referenced reviews of the disorders discussed briefly in this chapter.*

126 CIRRHOSIS OF THE LIVER

Thomas D. Boyer

GENERAL CONSIDERATIONS. Cirrhosis is an irreversible alteration of the liver architecture, consisting of hepatic fibrosis and areas of nodular regeneration. When the nodules are small (less than 3 mm), uniform, and encompass one lobule, the term micronodular or unilobular cirrhosis is applied. In macronodular or multilobular cirrhosis the nodules exceed 3 mm, vary in size, and encompass more than one lobule. Frequently, features of both micronodular and macronodular cirrhosis are present in the same liver. Etiologic diagnosis may be impossible from the gross and microscopic appearance of the cirrhotic liver and must therefore be based on history, physical examination, biochemical and serologic tests, and histochemical stains. The causes of cirrhosis are listed in Table 126–1.

Patients with cirrhosis may have one of two general types of manifestations: (1) signs or symptoms related to hepatocellular necrosis, which are similar to those of acute hepatitis and include jaundice, nausea and vomiting, and tender hepatomegaly; or (2) signs or symptoms of the complications of cirrhosis, which are largely due to the rise in intrahepatic vascular resistance that leads to portal hypertension and its complications (ascites, formation of portal-systemic collaterals, encephalopathy, splenomegaly, and bleeding esophageal and

TABLE 126–1. CAUSES OF CIRRHOSIS

Drugs and toxins	*Metabolic*
Alcohol	Wilson's disease
Methyldopa	Hemochromatosis
Methotrexate	Erythropoietic protoporphyria
Isoniazid	Pediatric—alpha₁-antitrypsin
Perhexiline maleate	deficiency, galactosemia,
Amiodarone	hereditary fructose intolerance,
Oxyphenisatin	glycogen storage disease Type IV,
Infections	tyrosinosis
Hepatitis B and non-A non-B	*Cardiovascular*
Syphilis (tertiary)	Chronic right heart failure
Schistosoma japonicum	Budd-Chiari syndrome
Biliary Obstruction	Veno-occlusive disease
Carcinoma (pancreatic or bile duct)	*Miscellaneous*
Chronic pancreatitis	Chronic active hepatitis
Common duct stones	Primary biliary cirrhosis
Strictures	Sarcoidosis
Cystic fibrosis	Jejunoileal bypass
Biliary atresia	Neonatal hepatitis
Sclerosing cholangitis	*Cryptogenic*

gastric varices). Other, less specific manifestations of cirrhosis include gynecomastia, spider angiomas, parotid hypertrophy, and testicular atrophy. Patients frequently present a mixed picture with features of both hepatocellular necrosis and portal hypertension.

Agents that cause cirrhosis may have systemic effects as well. Extrahepatic features may dominate the clinical picture with little or no evidence of liver disease. For example, patients with alcoholic liver disease frequently have complaints referable to the central nervous system, peripheral nerves, heart, muscles, and gastrointestinal tract. Patients with disease such as primary biliary cirrhosis may have prominent eye and skin disorders. Patients with hemochromatosis may present with diabetes mellitus or arthritis, and patients with Wilson's disease, with central nervous system dysfunction, before liver disease becomes apparent. Thus, cirrhosis is frequently a subclinical illness, and a high index of suspicion may be necessary to establish a correct diagnosis.

ALCOHOLIC LIVER DISEASE

DEFINITION AND INCIDENCE. Alcoholic liver disease, a frequent and serious sequela of the chronic abuse of ethanol, occurs singly or intermingled in three forms: *fatty liver, alcoholic hepatitis,* and *cirrhosis.* Alcohol is the most common cause of liver disease in the Western world. Alcoholic cirrhosis is discovered in 1.6 to 9.9 per cent of all necropsies in the United States. The peak incidence is in patients 40 to 55 years of age; however, patients in their twenties may be seen with advanced alcoholic liver disease. The male to female ratio is 2:1.

ETIOLOGY AND PATHOGENESIS. *The relationship between alcohol abuse and cirrhosis* is well established. The incidence of cirrhosis and the per capita consumption of alcohol are directly related; countries with the greatest alcohol consumption also have the highest incidence of cirrhosis. Neither the pattern of drinking (spree versus daily) nor the type of alcoholic beverage consumed appears to be important in the genesis of liver disease. The single most important factor is the average daily consumption of ethanol. Levels of daily ethanol consumption exceeding 40 to 80 grams (36 to 72 oz of beer, 4.5 to 9 oz liquor, 15 to 30 oz of wine) for 10 to 15 years are associated with an increase in the incidence of cirrhosis. Women may be more susceptible to the toxic effects of ethanol than men, and a lower daily consumption of ethanol by women may lead to cirrhosis. As the daily level of alcohol consumed rises, the time required for the development of cirrhosis is reduced.

Ethanol is a hepatotoxin. Administration of alcohol to humans or animals leads to the development of fatty liver (hepatic steatosis). The mitochondria and endoplasmic reticulum of hepatocytes are altered morphologically and functionally. Ethanol also causes lactic acidemia, hyperuricemia, and hypoglycemia. Many of the effects of ethanol reflect its metabolism, which is catalyzed primarily by the cytosolic enzyme alcohol dehydrogenase as shown:

$$\underset{\text{Ethanol}}{CH_3CH_2OH} \xrightarrow[\underset{NAD^+ \longrightarrow NADH + H^+}{}]{\text{Alcohol dehydrogenase}} \underset{\text{Acetaldehyde}}{CH_3CHO}$$

(Other metabolic pathways via a microsomal ethanol oxidizing system or a catalase system appear to be of minor importance, except perhaps at high ethanol concentrations.) The acetaldehyde formed from ethanol is then oxidized to acetate by acetaldehyde dehydrogenase with NAD^+ as a cofactor. The lack of the active high affinity form of acetaldehyde dehydrogenase (50 per cent of Japanese) leads to high blood levels of acetaldehyde following ethanol ingestion. The high levels of acetaldehyde in these individuals are associated with flushing, vasodilatation, tachycardia, and aversion to ethanol. The limiting step in the rate of metabolism of ethanol is the availability of the cofactor NAD^+, which is converted to NADH during the aforementioned two reactions. This increased reducing potential in the cell favors the conversion of pyuvate to lactate. When blood levels of ethanol are high (more than 200 mg per deciliter), the resulting lactic acidemia decreases the clearance of urate by the kidneys and hyperuricemia develops. At lower levels of ethanol ingestion (blood level $\leq$ 150 mg per deciliter) increased production of urate is the cause of hyperuricemia. Inhibition of gluconeogenesis and fasting hypoglycemia may also follow ethanol abuse (Ch. 117). Fatty acid oxidation is impaired, and the esterification of fatty acids to triglycerides is increased. The latter effects, acting in concert with less well defined events, lead to the development of a fatty liver. The metabolism of ethanol may lead to increased levels of acetaldehyde in the blood and probably within the hepatocyte. Acetaldehyde is a reactive molecule and may interact with proteins and membrane lipids, causing alterations in their structure and function, which may lead to cell injury and death.

The metabolic effects of ethanol are relatively well understood, but the mechanism by which it causes chronic liver disease is not. There is evidence for impaired protein synthesis and secretion, mitochondrial injury, lipid peroxidation, cellular hypoxia, and cell-mediated and antibody-mediated cytotoxicity, but the relative importance of each of these in producing sustained cell injury is unknown.

Ethanol fed to animals receiving an otherwise balanced diet has not been shown to cause alcoholic hepatitis. In addition, only 10 to 20 per cent of alcoholics and about 50 per cent of ethanol-fed baboons develop cirrhosis despite similar levels of ethanol ingestion. Thus, *genetic, nutritional,* or *environmental* factors may act in concert with ethanol to cause liver disease.

Malnutrition is a common finding in alcoholics who have both poor diet and reduced intestinal absorption of dietary nutrients. Administration of ethanol to patients with active alcoholic liver disease does not appear to impair recovery if the patients also receive a balanced, high-calorie diet. Lesions identical to those of alcoholic hepatitis may develop following jejunoileal bypass for obesity, a condition in which protein malnutrition is common. Thus, malnutrition appears to potentiate the adverse effects of alcohol. Other factors, such as simultaneous exposure to other hepatotoxins, may also be important in the genesis of liver injury. Alcoholism and alcoholic liver disease are more common in certain populations, in twins, and within families, but there is no evidence of a genetically determined abnormality in the metabolism of ethanol that renders them more susceptible to liver injury.

DIAGNOSIS. The diagnosis of alcoholic liver disease should be considered in any patient who consumes more than 40 grams of ethanol daily. Tender hepatomegaly, fever, and jaundice are suggestive of alcoholic hepatitis, whereas ascites and venous collaterals suggest cirrhosis. Many patients, however, will lack any distinctive clinical features such that a firm diagnosis cannot be established without liver biopsy. In addition, up to 20 per cent of patients with clinical features of alcoholic liver disease are found on liver biopsy to have another type of hepatic disorder.

PATHOLOGY, CLINICAL PRESENTATION, AND THERAPY. Alcohol causes three major pathologic lesions and clinical illnesses: *fatty liver, alcoholic hepatitis, and cirrhosis.* Each of these may occur as an isolated event, or they may be present in any combination in a single patient. Therefore, although the three lesions will be described as single entities, many patients have all three and will have a mixed clinical picture. The histologic pattern is not specific for alcohol alone, but may also be found in the livers of patients who have undergone jejunoileal bypass for obesity, or as an unusual accompaniment of obesity or diabetes mellitus. Patients treated with the vasodilator perhexiline maleate or the antiarrhythmic drug amiodarone also may develop a lesion identical to alcoholic liver disease.

Fatty Liver. Fatty liver is the most common biopsy finding in alcoholics. The fat, either centrilobular or diffuse in location, is present in large droplets, which occupy most of the volume of the hepatocyte. Occasionally the fat is present in small droplets, resembling the lesion of Reye's syndrome or fatty liver of pregnancy. Patients with fatty liver are usually asymptomatic, but on occasion they may have abdominal pain, icterus, or vague gastrointestinal complaints. The liver is enlarged and may be tender, but is of normal consistency. Ascites, venous collaterals, and the stigmata of chronic liver disease, if present, are not attributable to the fatty liver per se, but reflect more serious lesions. The laboratory tests are only mildly abnormal in fatty liver. Jaundice, when present, is usually mild (bilirubin below 5 mg per deciliter), although intense cholestasis occasionally develops in patients with fatty liver. The AST, if elevated, is only modestly so (less than five times normal). The serum albumin and globulin are abnormal in about 25 per cent of patients. Patients with alcoholic fatty liver alone have an excellent prognosis. Withdrawal of the alcohol leads to a rapid resolution of the clinical illness and histologic lesion (fat disappears within three to six weeks). On rare occasions, these patients die suddenly from multiple fat emboli to the lungs.

Alcoholic Hepatitis. Alcoholic hepatitis (acute sclerosing hyaline necrosis) is a serious sequela of alcoholism because it may lead to hepatic failure or to cirrhosis. The pathologic lesion is most severe in central areas, and consists of hepatocellular necrosis and the triad of (1) *alcoholic hyalin,* (2) *infiltration by polymorphonuclear leukocytes,* and (3) *increased intralobular connective tissue* with or without occlusion of the hepatic venules and sclerosis of terminal hepatic (central) veins. Alcoholic hyalin (Mallory body) is an eosinophilic intracellular aggregate of proteinaceous material that is characteristically perinuclear in location. The origin of alcoholic hyaline is uncertain although it may be formed by intermediate filaments. It is present in only 30 per cent of liver biopsies in which the diagnosis of alcoholic hepatitis can be made on clinical and other histologic criteria. Alcoholic hyalin is not specific for alcoholic liver disease, since it has also been found in the livers of patients with Wilson's disease, primary biliary cirrhosis, hepatocellular carcinoma, and diabetes mellitus, as well as following jejunoileal bypass. Central vein sclerosis may be severe enough to cause a severe outflow block and portal hypertension in the absence of cirrhosis.

The clinical features of alcoholic hepatitis range from absence of symptoms to hepatic failure. Patients commonly complain of anorexia, nausea, vomiting, abdominal pain, and weight loss. Tender hepatomegaly is present in at least 80 per cent of patients. Ascites, jaundice, fever (temperature 37.2 to 39.4°C), splenomegaly, and encephalopathy are common but not invariable. Although fever is common, bacterial infection should be excluded since such patients are at an increased risk for developing pneumonia, urinary tract infections, sepsis, and bacterial peritonitis. The AST is frequently elevated; however, the degree of elevation is modest (less than 10 times normal) although on occasion it can exceed 15 times normal. The ALT may be normal and is almost always less than the AST. The AST/ALT ratio frequently exceeds two. This is in contrast to viral hepatitis, in which the AST frequently exceeds 15 to 25 times normal and the ALT is equal to or greater than the AST. Hyperbilirubinemia is common (60 to 90 per cent) in alcoholic hepatitis, and it may be marked (20 to 30 mg per deciliter). The alkaline phosphatase is usually elevated to less than three times normal, but an occasional patient has a cholestatic picture in which the alkaline phosphatase is unusually high. Prolongation of the prothrombin time, hypoalbuminemia, and hyperglobulinemia may be present. The white blood cell count frequently is elevated (>10,000) and may exceed 30,000 to 40,000 per cubic millimeter. Patients with alcoholic hepatitis may develop the hepatorenal syndrome, and a rising BUN and creatinine are poor prognostic signs.

Treatment for alcoholic hepatitis is nonspecific. Patients should receive a well-balanced diet, high in calories (2500 to 3000 kcal). Protein should be included in the diets unless encephalopathy is present. Anorexia is frequent, and tube or intravenous alimentation may be necessary. Improvement in the patient's nutritional state may be associated with more rapid resolution of the liver test abnormalities; however, the effect of nutritional support on survival is unclear. Prednisone has not been shown to decrease the morbidity or mortality in patients with mild to moderate disease. Use of steroids to treat patients with severe alcoholic hepatitis is controversial and cannot be recommended on the basis of available evidence. Propylthiouracil, penicillamine, anabolic steroids, and colchicine have also been used in the treatment of alcoholic hepatitis, but without documented success.

The *prognosis* for patients with alcoholic hepatitis is much worse than for those with fatty liver. Some patients who stop drinking may have complete resolution of the lesion. In most patients, however, alcoholic hepatitis persists (with clinical improvement), progresses to cirrhosis, or leads to hepatic failure and death. The hospital mortality for patients with severe disease (who cannot have biopsy or who have encephalopathy) exceeds 40 per cent, whereas for those with milder disease the expected death rate is 10 per cent or less.

Alcoholic Cirrhosis. *Alcoholic cirrhosis* usually consists of micronodules of regular size, but it can be macronodular or of a mixed type. Micronodular cirrhosis is not specific for alcoholic liver disease. Histologically, dense bands of connective tissue join portal and central areas. Scarring is most severe in the central regions, and collagen may deposit in the space of Disse. In addition, alcoholic hepatitis frequently coexists, as well as varying amounts of cholestasis, iron, and fat.

Clinically, cirrhosis is an asymptomatic disease in 10 to 20 per cent of patients. It is also commonly present in association with alcoholic hepatitis, and signs of acute liver injury may dominate the clinical picture. Patients may also have ascites, gastrointestinal bleeding, or encephalopathy. These major sequelae of cirrhosis are discussed in detail in the next chapter (Ch. 127). The liver may be large or small and usually has a firm consistency. Spider angiomas, palmar erythema, parotid enlargement, testicular atrophy and gynnecomastia (men), menstrual irregularities (women), and muscle wasting are frequently found; however, these findings are not specific for alcoholic cirrhosis. Upper abdominal pain associated with bloody ascitic fluid, right upper quadrant bruit, or a friction rub over the liver suggests hepatocellular carcinoma.

The *laboratory abnormalities* present in patients with cirrhosis may be similar to those of alcoholic hepatitis. The AST is normal to mildly elevated, and bilirubin is only slightly increased unless the picture is complicated by alcoholic hepatitis, hemolysis, sepsis, hepatic failure, or carcinoma. Anemia

is a common finding. The cause of the anemia is multifactorial, including blood loss, folate and pyridoxine deficiency, hemolysis, and the toxic effect of ethanol on the bone marrow. Hypersplenism or bone marrow suppression by ethanol may lead to thrombocytopenia or leukopenia. The serum sodium and potassium may be low in patients with ascites. Hypomagnesemia and hypophosphatemia are common, as is a mild respiratory alkalosis. The BUN and creatinine are increased in patients who have been treated with excessive diuretics or who are developing hepatorenal failure.

The *treatment* of alcoholic cirrhosis is also nonspecific. Deficiencies of vitamins (folate, thiamine, pyridoxine, vitamin K) and minerals (magnesium, phosphate) should be corrected. The sodium content of the diet need not be reduced unless there is sodium retention by the kidneys. Protein restriction is necessary only when there is clinical evidence of hepatic encephalopathy.

The *prognosis* for patients with alcoholic cirrhosis is dependent upon two features: presence of complications and continued abuse of alcohol. Patients without ascites, jaundice, or gastrointestinal bleeding have a better prognosis than those with these complications. Continued alcohol abuse reduces the expected five-year survival to only 40 per cent, whereas it is 60 per cent or greater in those who abstain.

Bosron WF, Li T-K: Genetic polymorphism of human liver alcohol and aldehyde dehydrogenases, and their relationship to alcohol metabolism and alcoholism. Hepatology 6:502, 1986. *A review of the genetics of these two enzymes and how studies of their polymorphism may help us to understand the inherited nature of alcoholism.*
D'Amico G, Morabito A, Pagliaro L, et al.: Survival and prognostic indicators in compensated and decompensated cirrhosis. Dig Dis Sci 31:468, 1986. *Analysis of variables associated with a poor prognosis in alcoholic and nonalcoholic cirrhosis.*
Galambos J: Cirrhosis. Philadelphia, W. B. Saunders Company, 1979. *An excellent monograph that reviews cirrhosis and its complications.*
Lieber C: Alcohol and the liver: 1984 update. Hepatology 4:1243, 1984. *A review of all of the factors that have been thought to play a role in the pathogenesis of alcoholic liver disease.*

PRIMARY BILIARY CIRRHOSIS

DEFINITION AND ETIOLOGY. Primary biliary cirrhosis, a cholestatic disorder, develops because of progressive destruction of small and intermediate-sized intrahepatic bile ducts. The extrahepatic biliary tree and larger intrahepatic bile ducts are patent. The cause of primary biliary cirrhosis is unknown. The injury to the bile ducts is thought to be on an immunologic basis, as there is a high frequency of serum autoantibodies, elevated levels of immunoglobulins (especially IgM), circulating immune complexes, and a reduced cell-mediated immune response in patients with this disease. In addition, the injured bile ducts are surrounded by lymphocytes and, on occasion, by granulomas. These findings, however, are nonspecific and do not establish the etiologic agent or agents responsible for the disease. Genetic factors may also be important, as the disease has been described in a mother and daughter, in siblings, and in twins. In addition, the incidence of positive tests for antimitochondrial antibodies in relatives of patients with primary biliary cirrhosis is increased. The high female preponderance suggests that estrogens or progesterone may be important in the pathogenesis of this disease.

PATHOLOGY. Primary biliary cirrhosis is characterized by progressive, nonsuppurative, destructive cholangitis, which occurs in four histopathologic stages: *ductal, ductular, scarring,* and *cirrhotic*. The lesions in the first two stages are distributed unevenly and may therefore be absent in needle biopsies of the liver. The characteristic lesion (ductal or Stage 1) consists of damaged interlobular and septal bile ducts surrounded by a dense infiltrate of lymphocytes and plasma cells. Well-formed granulomas are frequently seen near the injured bile ducts. In Stage 2 (ductular) of the disease, bile ductules proliferate and bile ducts are reduced in number. Portal fibrosis may be present or absent, and granulomata are found less often than in Stage 1. Later, as the inflammation subsides, scarring increases, most marked in portal areas with fibrous septa extending into the lobule (Stage 3). When cirrhotic (Stage 4), the liver may lose all of the characteristic lesions. Bile ducts are few in both Stages 3 and 4, and this paucity of bile ducts may be the only clue to the diagnosis of primary biliary cirrhosis. In one quarter of the cases, alcoholic hyalin is identifiable in the biopsy. Histologic features of chronic active hepatitis may also be present, leading to difficulties in diagnosis.

CLINICAL MANIFESTATIONS (Table 126–2). Ninety per cent of patients with primary biliary cirrhosis are female. The disease has been found in patients as young as 23 and as old as 72; however, the majority of patients are of ages 40 to 60. The onset is usually marked by *pruritus*, or by discovery of asymptomatic hepatomegaly. Sometimes the first abnormality is an elevated alkaline phosphatase noted on an automated screening panel. The itching may start during pregnancy or with the use of birth control pills. Following delivery or withdrawal of the medication, the itching usually continues; this is in contrast to *cholestasis of pregnancy*, in which pruritus resolves following parturition. Itching leads to excoriative dermatitis and thickening and darkening of the skin. Hepatomegaly and less frequently splenomegaly may be found at the time of diagnosis. *Jaundice* rarely precedes the onset of pruritus and may follow it by several years. *Portal hypertension* and *hepatic failure* are usually late events, and ascites or bleeding esophageal varices are uncommon presenting features. *Hypercholesterolemia*, secondary to the decreased biliary excretion of cholesterol, may be severe enough to produce xanthomas. *Osteomalacia* or more commonly *osteoporosis* may develop in these patients. The cause of the bone disease is incompletely understood; however, malabsorption of vitamin D and calcium are important pathogenic factors. Copper accumulates in the livers of patients with primary biliary cirrhosis because it cannot be efficiently secreted into the bile. The levels of hepatic copper may reach levels equal to those found in Wilson's disease, and rarely *Kayser-Fleischer rings* have been described.

ASSOCIATED DISEASES. Primarily biliary cirrhosis is associated with a variety of disorders. *Sjögren's syndrome* with dryness of the eyes and mouth is present in at least 70 per cent of patients when specific tests (Schirmer test, buccal biopsy, and others) are used (Ch. 438). These same patients may have hyposecretion by the pancreas. *Scleroderma* and the *CREST syndrome* (calcinosis, Reynaud's phenomenon, esophageal hypomotility, sclerodactyly, telangiectasia) are both increased in frequency in patients with primary biliary cirrhosis. The prevalence of *arthritis*, both seropositive and seronegative, is increased in these patients. *Thyroid autoantibodies* are found in about 25 per cent of patients, and in the antibody-positive patients thyroid dysfunction (primarily hypothyroidism) is common. *Renal tubular acidosis* also is present in patients with primary biliary cirrhosis. The pathogenesis of the renal tubular acidosis is unknown, but it may be secondary to deposition of copper in renal tubules.

LABORATORY FINDINGS. The *alkaline phosphatase* is elevated in almost all patients with primary biliary cirrhosis, although it may be normal in asymptomatic patients. The elevation is usually two to six times normal, but can be more than ten times normal. The serum bilirubin is usually normal or mildly elevated until the later stages of the disease are reached. Serum bile acids and cholesterol are increased frequently. Serum *immunoglobulin M* levels are increased in 75 per cent of patients with primary biliary cirrhosis. The finding, however, is not specific. Hypoprothrombinemia and hypocalcemia may be present and reflect deficiencies of vitamins K and D. The serum transaminases are normal to mildly elevated. Eighty-four to ninety-eight per cent of patients with primary biliary cirrhosis have *circulating antimitochondrial antibodies*. This antibody is directed toward an antigen in the inner mitochondrial membrane. The antibody is neither species nor organ specific. Antimitochondrial antibodies may be present in patients with HBsAg-negative chronic active hepatitis, cryptogenic cirrhosis, and collagen vascular diseases; however, test results are normal in patients with extrahepatic obstruction unless they also have primary biliary cirrhosis or chronic active hepatitis. A small percentage of patients (5 to 30 per cent) with primary biliary cirrhosis have antinuclear antibodies in their serum.

DIAGNOSIS. The diagnosis of primary biliary cirrhosis is established by finding a positive antimitochondrial antibody test and the characteristic pathology (Stage 1 or 2) on liver biopsy. It may be necessary to exclude extrahepatic obstruction in some patients in whom the diagnosis of primary biliary cirrhosis cannot be made with certainty, as *extrahepatic biliary obstruction* can clinically mimic primary biliary cirrhosis. Also, patients with primary biliary cirrhosis have an increased incidence of gallstones, which may cause biliary obstruction. Biliary tract disease may be excluded by either transhepatic or endoscopic retrograde cholangiography.

THERAPY AND PROGNOSIS. No specific therapy for primary biliary cirrhosis is available. Corticosteroids are not known to be effective in this disease and will aggravate the bone disease. D-Penicillamine, azathioprine, and colchicine have been used in the treatment of primary biliary cirrhosis. D-Penicillamine cannot be recommended because its use is associated with numerous complications without improvement in survival. Recently, treatment with colchicine has been shown to improve liver tests but not hepatic histology as compared to placebo-treated controls. Further experience is required in the use of colchicine before it can be recommended.

The treatment of primary biliary cirrhosis is directed toward its complications and includes correction of specific deficiency states and reduction in the pruritus. Dietary fat may be reduced to 40 grams daily to decrease steatorrhea and improve calcium absorption. Medium-chain triglycerides are absorbed directly into the portal vein without the presence of intraluminal bile salts, and these may be given as a dietary supplement. If the prothrombin time is prolonged, vitamin K (10 mg) is given intramuscularly every four weeks. The osteomalacia may be preventable through such measures as exposure to sunlight (10 to 20 minutes daily) and dietary supplementation with vitamin D and calcium. The serum 25(OH)D level should be measured, and, if low, it should be increased to the normal range with oral vitamin D. If the serum 25(OH)D levels fail to increase with vitamin D therapy, then oral 25(OH)D, 100 to 200 μg daily, may be given. Hepatic osteomalacia, but not osteoporosis, responds to treatment with metabolites of vitamin D. During the administration of vitamin D or its metabolites, the serum and urine calcium must be monitored closely to prevent development of hypercalcemia. See Ch. 246 and 250 for further discussion of osteomalacia and osteoporosis, respectively. Patients with thyroid antibodies should be tested for hypothyroidism.

The cause of the pruritus is unknown, but it may be secondary to increased tissue levels of bile salts. Cholestyra-

TABLE 126–2. CLINICAL FEATURES OF PRIMARY BILIARY CIRRHOSIS

Signs and Symptoms	Laboratory
Female preponderance (> 90%)	Antimitochondrial antibodies (> 90%)
Pruritus	
Jaundice	Elevated alkaline phosphatase, cholesterol, IgM, serum bile acids, and bilirubin
Skin hyperpigmentation	
Hepatosplenomegaly	
Xanthelasma/xanthoma	*Associated Diseases*
Bleeding diathesis (vitamin K deficiency)	Sjögren's syndrome
	Scleroderma/CREST syndrome
Bone pain (osteoporosis/ osteomalacia)	Arthritis
	Autoimmune thyroiditis
Ascites/variceal hemorrhage (late)	Renal tubular acidosis

mine and colestipol are anion exchange resins that bind bile salts in the intestines, preventing their reabsorption in the terminal ileum. Eight to twelve grams of cholestyramine is given daily in divided doses with breakfast and dinner. Fat-soluble vitamins should not be given at the same time as the resin. The hypercholesterolemia may also respond to cholestyramine therapy. Clofibrate should not be used in these patients, as there may be a paradoxical increase in the serum cholesterol.

Patients with primary biliary cirrhosis who are asymptomatic have a good prognosis, with a ten-year survival similar to age-matched controls. Patients who present with symptoms have, in contrast, an average life expectancy of 5.5 to 11 years. The development of jaundice, ascites, or cirrhosis is associated with a poor prognosis.

Kaplan M: Primary biliary cirrhosis. N Engl J Med 316:521, 1987. *A succinct Medical Progress article with an excellent bibliography of 124 references. A good place to start.*

Kaplan M, Alling DW, Zimmerman HJ, et al.: A prospective trial of colchicine for primary biliary cirrhosis. N Engl J Med 315:1448, 1986. *Sixty patients were treated for up to two years with either colchicine or a placebo. Treatment with colchicine led to an improvement in liver tests but did not affect symptoms or progression of the liver lesions.*

Roll J: A new treatment for primary biliary cirrhosis? Gastroenterology 89:1195, 1985. *An excellent discussion of the treatment and prognosis of patients with primary biliary cirrhosis.*

Roll J, Boyer J, Barry D, et al: The prognostic importance of clinical and histologic features in asymptomatic and symptomatic primary biliary cirrhosis. N Engl J Med 308:1, 1983. *Defines the clinical and pathologic features that predict survival.*

Warnes T: Treatment of primary biliary cirrhosis. Semin Liver Dis 5:228, 1985. *A review of the treatment of the disease and its complications.*

SECONDARY BILIARY CIRRHOSIS

DEFINITION, ETIOLOGY, AND PATHOLOGY. Secondary biliary cirrhosis is an uncommon sequela of longstanding obstruction of the biliary tree. Obstruction is usually present for more than one year (mean of about six years) before cirrhosis develops; however, intervals as short as four months from the onset of obstruction (jaundice) to the diagnosis of cirrhosis have been reported. Cirrhosis or fibrosis may also develop in the absence of jaundice in patients with prolonged partial biliary tract obstruction as may be seen in chronic pancreatitis. In adults, obstruction is due to gallstones, strictures, carcinoma, chronic pancreatitis, or sclerosing cholangitis. In children, biliary atresia and cystic fibrosis are common causes of secondary biliary cirrhosis.

The liver is usually enlarged and dark green. The surface is granular or occasionally nodular. The lobular pattern is usually preserved until the cirrhosis is advanced. The portal tracts are widened owing to fibrosis and proliferation of bile ducts. The hepatic parenchyma may contain bile plugs, infarcts, or lakes. There is focal hepatocellular necrosis. As the cirrhosis progresses, the fibrous septa extend into the hepatic parenchyma, forming pseudolobules. In advanced cirrhosis, there is nodular regeneration.

CLINICAL MANIFESTATIONS. *Jaundice* is common but not invariable, and the level of jaundice may fluctuate. Patients with strictures or stones may have suffered recurrent bouts of cholangitis or biliary colic. *Pruritus* is also a common complaint and may precede the onset of icterus. If the pruritus is severe, itching may lead to thickening and darkening of the skin. Xanthelasma and xanthomas may appear. *Steatorrhea* with diarrhea may be a major complaint, and *bone disease* may develop owing to malabsorption of vitamin D and calcium. Splenomegaly is common. Ascites and gastrointestinal bleeding develop later in the course of the disease and are uncommon presenting complaints.

LABORATORY TESTS. The serum bilirubin is usually moderately increased (3 to 15 mg per deciliter). The alkaline phosphatase is also almost always increased; however, in 25 to 30 per cent, the elevation is less than twice normal. The AST is usually elevated, but the elevations are moderate. The

prothrombin time may be prolonged and may improve with vitamin K administration. Hypoalbuminemia and hyperglobulinemia may also be present. Serum cholesterol and bile acids are frequently increased. *Lipoprotein X*, an abnormal lipoprotein, is found commonly in patients with extrahepatic obstruction (see Ch. 119). Lipoprotein X is also present in other forms of liver disease, and its absence does not exclude extrahepatic obstruction. Elevations of the white blood cell count in patients with extrahepatic obstruction suggest the presence of cholangitis or a hepatic abscess.

THERAPY AND PROGNOSIS. Relief of the biliary obstruction is the only specific form of treatment. In patients in whom the obstruction cannot be relieved, the correction of vitamin deficiencies and the use of cholestyramine to relieve itching, as outlined for the treatment of primary biliary cirrhosis, is warranted. In addition, there may be recurrent episodes of cholangitis requiring antibiotic treatment.

The prognosis for patients with carcinoma is poor, with most dying because of the malignancy and not because of the liver disease. The mortality for patients with benign obstructions (stone or stricture) depends on whether or not the obstruction can be relieved. When the obstruction cannot be relieved, mortality is high; however, survival may be prolonged (years) before the patient dies from hepatic failure or bleeding esophageal varices. Surgical relief of the biliary obstruction improves survival, although ascites and esophageal varices may develop later. The development of these complications, usually many years after apparently successful surgery, may be due to subclinical recurrence of partial biliary obstruction.

Littenberg G, Afroudakis A, Kaplowitz N: Common bile duct stenosis from chronic pancreatitis: Clinical and pathologic spectrum. Medicine 58:385, 1979. *Reviews the effects of the liver biliary obstruction secondary to chronic pancreatitis.*

CRYPTOGENIC CIRRHOSIS

DEFINITION AND ETIOLOGY. Cryptogenic (macronodular or postnecrotic) cirrhosis is any cirrhosis for which the etiology is unknown. The liver contains little or no necrosis or inflammation and has no diagnostic pathologic lesions (for example, alcoholic hepatitis). It lacks any specific lesions demonstrable by histochemical stains, e.g., alpha$_1$-antitrypsin or iron; and specific serologic tests, e.g., HBsAg, anti-HBc, AMA, and ceruloplasmin, are normal. It is assumed that most cases represent the end-stage of a previously active, chronic, or recurrent hepatitis, but alcoholic and other chronic liver diseases give rise to a very similar form of coarsely nodular cirrhosis. Cases previously called cryptogenic cirrhosis have been reported to be due to type B hepatitis despite the absence of detectable levels of HBsAg in the plasma. In these cases, HBV antigens or free or integrated HBV DNA was demonstrable in the liver cells. It is unclear, however, what role HBV infection played in the development of cirrhosis in this group of patients. Cryptogenic cirrhosis should become a less frequent diagnosis as our understanding of the causes of liver disease increases and we develop tests for agents such as non-A non-B hepatitis.

PATHOLOGY. The size of the liver is variable and its surface distorted by large regenerative nodules (macronodular), which may be several centimeters in diameter. The liver between the nodules appears to be collapsed and fibrotic. The microscopic appearance of the liver is one of regenerative nodules separated by connective tissue. The portal areas may be infiltrated by mononuclear cells, but the liver cells are well preserved, and active hepatocellular necrosis or hepatic steatosis is minimal or absent.

CLINICAL MANIFESTATIONS. Cryptogenic cirrhosis may remain clinically silent for many years and frequently is discovered unexpectedly, often during the evaluation of an unrelated condition. When the disease becomes "clinically manifest," its signs and symptoms are usually nonspecific (malaise, lethargy) or related to portal hypertension and include ascites, splenomegaly, hypersplenism, or bleeding esophageal varices. The liver frequently is of normal size or small. Splenomegaly is common; spider angiomas, ascites, and abdominal wall venous collaterals may also be present. Serum transaminases and bilirubin are usually normal to slightly increased. Hyperglobulinemia is common and may be the only laboratory abnormality.

DIAGNOSIS. Cryptogenic cirrhosis is a diagnosis of exclusion and is based on histologic and clinical evidence of cirrhosis in the absence of a definable etiology (see Table 126–1). Wilson's disease and hemochromatosis, although uncommon, are specifically treatable and should therefore be carefully excluded (see Ch. 205 and 206). A small number of patients with cryptogenic cirrhosis may have chronic hepatitis B infection despite the absence in the serum of detectable levels of HB_sAg. Measurement of anti-HB_c may be helpful in identifying these patients. Testing for antimitochondrial antibodies, ANA, and an LE preparation will help exclude primary biliary cirrhosis and chronic active hepatitis. Alpha$_1$-antitrypsin deficiency may be excluded by appropriate histochemical stains and serologic tests (see Ch. 125). Findings of hepatic congestion on biopsy may be indicative of occult cardiac disease or hepatic vein occlusion. A previous history of alcoholism may be the only evidence for alcohol as the cause of the cirrhosis.

TREATMENT AND PROGNOSIS. Specific therapy for this type of cirrhosis is lacking. Complications such as ascites, encephalopathy, and gastrointestinal bleeding should be managed as discussed in Ch. 114, 127, and 128. Patients who have asymptomatic cirrhosis may do quite well with a good five-year prognosis; however, the onset of ascites or bleeding esophageal varices is a poor prognostic sign.

CARDIAC CIRRHOSIS

ETIOLOGY. Cardiac cirrhosis is an uncommon complication of severe, prolonged, recurrent right heart failure of any cause, although it is usually due to rheumatic heart disease (mitral or aortic stenosis with tricuspid regurgitation), cardiomyopathy, or constrictive pericarditis.

PATHOLOGY. The gross appearance of the liver in acute hepatic failure is one of alternating red and pale areas (nutmeg liver). The red areas are congested central areas of the hepatic lobule, whereas the pale areas are the preserved hepatocytes. With recurrent bouts of heart failure, the centrilobular hepatocytes atrophy and fibrosis develops, and with time fibrous septa extend out into the rest of the lobule. Regenerative nodules develop later, and they arise from the periphery of the hepatic lobule.

CLINICAL MANIFESTATIONS, DIAGNOSIS, AND THERAPY. The clinical picture is usually dominated by the cardiac disease. Differentiation of patients with acute hepatic congestion from those with cardiac cirrhosis is difficult, as the clinical features are similar (see Ch. 125). The liver may be small or enlarged and firm. When tricuspid regurgitation is present, the absence of hepatic pulsation suggests cirrhosis. Ascites and splenomegaly are common. The bilirubin is usually only mildly increased, and either the unconjugated or conjugated pigment may predominate. The AST is often moderately elevated, but may be normal if the heart failure is controlled. The prothrombin time may be prolonged, and in the presence of significant liver disease Coumadin and related anticoagulants should be used with caution. The diagnosis of cardiac cirrhosis is established by performing a liver biopsy. However, in most situations, this is not warranted.

Reduction in the incidence of rheumatic fever and tuberculosis as well as advances in cardiovascular surgery in the Western world have made cardiac cirrhosis an uncommon disease. Its prognosis depends largely upon the course of the cardiac disease. If the latter can be successfully treated, hepatic function improves and liver disease stabilizes.

Dunn GD, Hayes P, Breen K, et al.: The liver in congestive heart failure: A review. Am J Med Sci 265:174, 1973. *Reviews both acute and chronic heart failure and their effects on the liver.*

127 MAJOR SEQUELAE OF CIRRHOSIS

Thomas D. Boyer

PORTAL HYPERTENSION

ANATOMY AND PHYSIOLOGY OF PORTAL VENOUS SYSTEM. The portal venous system begins in the capillaries of the intestines and terminates in the hepatic sinusoids. The portal vein is formed by the confluence of the superior and inferior mesenteric veins and splenic vein.

The liver receives about 1500 ml of blood each minute, two thirds of which is provided by the portal vein. The hepatic artery provides 40 to 60 per cent of the oxygen supply to the liver. The liver offers little resistance to the flow of blood, and the pressure within the sinusoids is low (less than 5 mm Hg above the pressure in the inferior vena cava). Since the veins in the portal system lack valves, increased resistance to flow at any point between the splanchnic venules and the heart will increase pressure in all vessels on the intestinal side of the obstruction.

DEFINITION AND PATHOGENESIS. Portal hypertension represents an increase in the hydrostatic pressure within the portal vein or its tributaries. This is manifested clinically by the development of *portal-systemic collaterals, splenomegaly,* and/ or *ascites.* Since portal hypertension may be present in the absence of clinical findings, it may be detectable only by measurement of pressures in the portal system. Pressures within the hepatic sinusoids may be measured by catheterizing the hepatic veins (wedged hepatic vein pressure) or the portal vein pressure may be measured directly by transhepatic or umbilical vein catheterization or at surgery. Portal hypertension is present when the wedged hepatic vein pressure is more than 5 mm Hg higher than the inferior vena cava pressure. Although generally considered to be a progressive disorder, portal hypertension may in fact decrease as the liver disease improves, i.e., alcoholic hepatitis. Portal hypertension also can be an acute and transient phenomenon, as may occur with acute right heart failure. Since the pressure in any vascular system is directly proportional not only to resistance but also to flow, portal hypertension may result from either increased blood flow in the portal vein or increased resistance to flow within the portal venous system.

Increased portal venous blood flow is an unusual cause of portal hypertension for two reasons: (1) Increases in portal vein flow cause a reflex decrease in hepatic artery blood flow, thereby tending to maintain relatively normal sinusoidal pressure. (2) The outflow resistance from the liver is so low that increases in portal vein flow must be very large to cause a significant increase in portal venous pressure.

Increased resistance to venous flow is the most common mechanism for the development of portal hypertension. Liver disease accounts for the majority of cases; however, occlusion of the portal or hepatic veins and cardiac disease also cause increased resistance to flow and increases in portal pressure. The diseases causing portal hypertension are listed in Table 127–1 and are discussed below.

CLINICAL MANIFESTATIONS. The clinical presentation

TABLE 127–1. CAUSES OF PORTAL HYPERTENSION

Increased hepatic blood flow
    Splenomegaly not due to liver disease
    Arteriovenous fistula
Diseases of cardiovascular system
    Portal vein occlusion
    Splenic vein occlusion
    Hepatic vein occlusion
    Veno-occlusive disease
    Web lesion or thrombosis of inferior vena cava
    Congestive heart failure–constrictive pericarditis
Liver diseases
    Cirrhosis—all causes
    Congenital hepatic fibrosis
    Schistosomiasis
    Idiopathic portal hypertension
    Sarcoidosis
    Alcoholic hepatitis
    Partial nodular transformation

of portal hypertension depends to a certain extent upon its cause. Essentially all forms may present with either *bleeding esophageal varices* or *splenomegaly* with or without *hypersplenism*. In portal vein thrombosis, as the liver is normal, ascites and jaundice are unusual. *Ascites* and other signs of hepatic disease (jaundice, spiders, encephalopathy) are common clinical features of cirrhosis. Occlusion of the hepatic veins almost always leads to development of ascites and varying degrees of hepatic dysfunction. Thus, the clinical findings may be important clues to the cause of the portal hypertension.

The development of portal-systemic collaterals is the major complication of portal hypertension. Several vessels may form collaterals. The veins that lie in the mucosa of the gastric fundus and esophagus are of greatest clinical interest because, when dilated, they form gastric and esophageal varices (Fig. 127–1). The remnant of the umbilical vein may also dilate. If

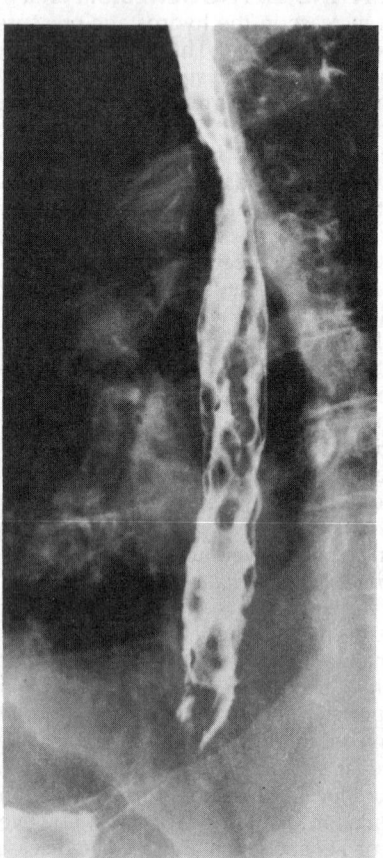

FIGURE 127–1. Barium esophagogram, demonstrating large varices involving the lower two thirds of the esophagus. (Courtesy of T. Munyer. From Zakim D, Boyer TD [eds.]: Hepatology: A Textbook of Liver Diseases. Philadelphia, W. B. Saunders Company, 1983.)

flow through this vessel becomes great enough, a loud venous hum may be audible over the path of the umbilical vein (Cruveilhier-Baumgarten syndrome). The umbilical vein enters the left portal vein, and therefore, if a venous hum is present, the cause of the portal hypertension must be intrahepatic or in the hepatic veins or inferior vena cava. Large collaterals also may form between the splenic and renal (chiefly left) veins. Dilated abdominal wall veins are common in patients with portal hypertension and are especially prominent when the patient stands. The hemorrhoidal veins may also act as collaterals. Varices may also form in unusual locations within the intestines (e.g., ileostomies, upper small bowel, and ascending, descending, and sigmoid colons), and these may bleed.

DISEASES CAUSING PORTAL HYPERTENSION (see Table 127–1). *Arteriovenous fistulas* may form between an artery and the portal vein or one of its tributaries as a consequence of abdominal trauma, liver biopsy, carcinoma (either intrahepatic or extrahepatic), or rupture of an arterial aneurysm (e.g., splenic). An upper abdominal bruit or a palpable thrill at surgery suggests this diagnosis in any patient with portal hypertension. The fistula can be localized by celiac angiography and is usually surgically correctable.

Splenomegaly resulting from hematologic diseases such as polycythemia rubra vera and myelofibrosis or an infiltrative process such as Gaucher's disease may, in rare instances, lead to portal hypertension. The enlarged spleen receives high blood flows from the splenic artery, leading to high flows within the splenic vein which are thought to cause the rise in portal pressure. These diseases also frequently involve the liver and the infiltrative process may increase intrahepatic resistance. However, the principal event in the genesis of the portal hypertension appears to be the high portal vein blood flow, since splenectomy usually cures the portal hypertension.

Splenic vein thrombosis may be caused by pancreatitis, abdominal trauma, or a locally invasive tumor. Pressure is increased only in areas drained by the splenic vein, whereas pressure in the portal vein is normal. The diagnosis should be suspected in a patient with gastric or esophageal varices but a normal liver biopsy, and is established by celiac angiography. Splenectomy is curative.

Portal vein thrombosis may develop following abdominal trauma or intra-abdominal sepsis, or in association with cirrhosis or hepatocellular carcinoma. In the majority of cases, however, the cause is unknown. This is primarily a disease of children, although adults may also develop portal vein thrombosis. The diagnosis is again suggested by the presence of portal hypertension in a patient with a normal liver biopsy. The diagnosis is established by angiography. Thrombi also may be identified using ultrasound or by CT scan. The surgical management of these patients may be difficult because of the absence of a patent vein to use for making a portal-systemic shunt.

Thrombosis of the hepatic veins (Budd-Chiari syndrome) may follow abdominal trauma or the use of birth control pills, or may occur in patients with diseases such as polycythemia rubra vera and paroxysmal nocturnal hemoglobinuria, which have an associated hypercoagulable state. Patients with hepatic vein thrombosis may develop an acute, subacute, or chronic illness in which abdominal pain and ascites are the major features. The liver is usually enlarged and tender. Elevations of the serum transaminases and bilirubin are usually mild, although they can be increased significantly in patients who have an acute illness. The initial clinical diagnosis is usually cirrhosis, and the correct diagnosis is not suspected until centrilobular congestion is seen on liver biopsy. Catheterization of the inferior vena cava and hepatic veins is a useful test in the evaluation of this condition. The presence of thrombi in the inferior vena cava can be established. The diagnosis of hepatic vein thrombosis is made by finding the characteristic pathology on liver biopsy, excluding cardiac disease that causes a similar histologic lesion, and inability to catheterize the hepatic veins. The outlook for patients with hepatic vein thrombosis is poor, with mortality of 50 to 90 per cent. The use of side-to-side portacaval shunts in these patients has been thought to prolong survival. Further experience is required before the proper role of this procedure can be evaluated. The use of anticoagulants has not been shown to affect survival.

Veno-occlusive disease (nonthrombotic occlusion of hepatic venules) also causes a Budd-Chiari–like syndrome. Veno-occlusive disease develops in patients who have ingested plants containing pyrrolidizine alkaloids, who have been treated for malignant disease with certain chemotherapeutic agents, or following bone marrow transplantation. It also is a common pathologic finding in patients with alcoholic hepatitis and cirrhosis. The disease is thought to be due to a toxic injury to the endothelium of the affected vessels. The occluded venules may be present in a liver biopsy, and an abnormal vascular pattern is found when contrast material is injected into the hepatic veins.

Thrombi, tumor, or a membrane in the inferior vena cava may obstruct the hepatic veins and give a clinical picture similar to that of hepatic vein thrombosis, with the additional features of peripheral edema and stasis dermatitis. Membranous obstruction near the terminus of the inferior vena cava has been described in all areas of the world but is most frequently observed in South Africa and the Orient. These patients also have a high incidence of hepatocellular carcinoma. The reasons for this latter association are unclear. Catheterization of the inferior vena cava will identify the obstructing lesion. Removal of the membrane surgically is sometimes possible and leads to resolution of the portal hypertension. Thrombectomy is usually not helpful.

Cirrhosis causes portal hypertension by increasing the intrahepatic vascular resistance. The increased resistance is thought to occur because of compression of vessels by regenerative nodules, distortion and reduction of the sinusoidal bed, and narrowing of portal vessels by the fibrous tissue. In alcoholic liver disease, serious portal hypertension may develop without cirrhosis. In some patients with acute alcoholic hepatitis, there is progressive obliteration of the central veins with resultant centrilobular fibrosis. These patients develop a severe outflow block, which leads to the formation of ascites or esophageal varices.

Portal hypertension due to noncirrhotic portal fibrosis may occur in four conditions. In *schistosomiasis*, the adult worm resides in the intestinal venules. The eggs are shed into these vessels and are swept into the portal vein and into the liver, where they lodge in and obstruct the portal venules. The host's immune response to the eggs leads to periportal fibrosis and the development of portal hypertension. (Schistosomiasis is discussed more fully in Ch. 400.) *Idiopathic portal hypertension* (Banti's syndrome) is a disease in which there is portal hypertension, no cirrhosis, and a patent portal vein. The liver biopsy may be normal, or there may be fibrosis in the periportal areas and in the space of Disse. The disease process is progressive, with the liver eventually becoming small and fibrotic. A similar clinical picture may be seen in patients exposed to arsenic, vinyl chloride, and copper salts. *Congenital hepatic fibrosis* also causes portal hypertension without cirrhosis. In the portal areas, there is marked hyperplasia of the bile ducts and stellate fibrosis. This condition may be present in association with cystic liver disease and Caroli's disease (intrahepatic ductal ectasia), with an associated polycystic renal lesion in many patients. The development of portal hypertension is the major consequence of this form of liver disease, as hepatic function is well maintained. Hepatic *sarcoidosis* may rarely lead to hepatic fibrosis and portal hypertension.

DIAGNOSTIC APPROACH TO PORTAL HYPERTENSION. Portal hypertension should be suspected in any patient with ascites or splenomegaly, and its presence is established when portal-systemic collaterals are found. One may find collaterals on physical examination (dilated abdominal wall or umbilical veins), or they may be identified in the esophagus or stomach by a gastrointestinal series or by endoscopy. It is important that the etiology of portal hypertension be identified, since some causes (splenic vein thrombosis) may be curable. A liver biopsy will provide useful information as to the presence of liver disease; central venous congestion suggests hepatic vein thrombosis or cardiac disease. If the biopsy is not diagnostic, then catheterization of the hepatic veins may be performed. Elevated pressure will establish the presence of liver disease. Also, inferior vena cava or hepatic vein thrombosis may be found during catheterization of the hepatic veins. If the wedge pressure is normal, then the cause of the portal hypertension is (1) occlusion of the portal vein or its tributaries, (2) liver disease that involves the periportal areas and portal venules (schistosomiasis or idiopathic portal hypertension) and therefore does not increase the wedge pressure, or (3) increased flow in the portal vein. Celiac angiography will usually differentiate among this group of patients. Ultrasonography or computed tomography may also be used to identify thrombi in the portal vein.

BLEEDING ESOPHAGEAL AND GASTRIC VARICES

PATHOGENESIS. Hemorrhage from esophageal varices is a major complication of portal hypertension. The mortality in adult patients with cirrhosis varies from 30 to 60 per cent for each bleeding episode. The varices form because of increased pressure in the portal vein. Bleeding from varices may occur when the portal pressure exceeds 11 to 12 mm Hg above inferior vena cava pressure. However, not all patients with pressures above these levels have bleeding varices. The tension on the vessel wall is greater in large as compared to small varices for a given level of pressure. Therefore, large varices are more likely to rupture and bleed than are smaller ones; reflux esophagitis and ascites do not appear to be important in the genesis of bleeding.

CLINICAL MANIFESTATIONS. The most common presentation is hematemesis. The bleeding may be massive with the rapid development of shock, or the bleeding may stop spontaneously only to recur later. On occasion, the patient may only complain of hematochezia or melena without an antecedent history of hematemesis. Features suggesting underlying liver disease such as hepatomegaly, ascites, or jaundice may be present or absent, depending on the etiology of the portal hypertension and the activity of the underlying hepatic disease.

DIAGNOSIS AND TREATMENT. The care of the patient with gastrointestinal bleeding is discussed in detail in Ch. 114. The restoration of the patient's blood volume takes precedence over all other therapy and diagnostic tests. The blood volume should be corrected rapidly but not excessively, since overexpansion may lead to the development of ascites or renewed bleeding. Proof that esophageal or gastric varices are the source of hemorrhage depends on endoscopy, since, even in those with known varices, 30 to 50 per cent will be bleeding from other lesions (especially gastritis).

The bleeding from varices in many patients stops without any specific therapy. The *medical management* of patients who continue to bleed includes *vasopressin, endoscopic sclerosis of varices,* and *balloon tamponade.* Long-term therapy with *propranolol* for the prevention of variceal hemorrhage is controversial and cannot be recommended.

Vasopressin, a potent vasoconstrictor, is believed to act by constricting the splanchnic arterioles, which results in a fall in portal flow and thus a drop in portal pressure. This drug should be given only to patients who can be carefully monitored, preferably in an intensive care unit. Vasopressin is infused into a peripheral vein at a rate of 0.2 to 0.4 unit per minute. This therapy will provide temporary control in about

60 per cent of patients. Unfortunately, about half of those initially controlled will have rebleeding, and the use of vasopressin has little effect on morbidity or mortality. The intravenous use of somatostatin or combined use of vasopressin and nitroglycerin may be as effective as vasopressin alone in controlling variceal hemorrhage, with fewer side effects. Further experience is required before these newer forms of therapy can be recommended. The gastric and esophageal varices lie in the mucosa of the gastric fundus and esophagus and are therefore susceptible to *balloon tamponade*. Tamponade is best accomplished by inserting a tube that has a gastric and an esophageal balloon (Sengstaken-Blakemore tube). Once placed in the stomach, the gastric balloon is inflated and pulled into the cardia of the stomach, tamponading the varices. If bleeding does not stop, then the esophageal balloon is inflated. This therapy is effective in controlling hemorrhage in 70 to 90 per cent of patients. There is a significant risk of aspiration during balloon tamponade, and 50 to 60 per cent of the patients will hemorrhage again. During endoscopy, the *direct injection of esophageal varices* with sclerosing agents has been described as a method for the control of acute bleeding and for the long-term management of these patients. Repeated injections over several weeks are required to obliterate the varices, and rebleeding during this period is common. Once they are obliterated the rate of rebleeding from the varices is reduced, and survival may be improved. Endoscopic sclerotherapy is associated with serious side effects and requires further clinical experience before its role in the management of bleeding varices is established.

In *surgical therapy* for portal hypertension the high pressure portal system is anastomosed to the low pressure systemic venous system to create a *portal-systemic shunt*. There are two basic types of shunts. One is *nonselective*, in that the entire portal-venous system is decompressed. The end-to-side and side-to-side portacaval and mesocaval shunts are nonselective. *Selective* shunts decompress only the varices. The pressure remains high in the portal vein, and portal flow into the liver is preserved. Thus the varices are decompressed with minimal disruption of the normal hepatic circulation. The distal splenorenal shunt is of this type. The selective shunt may cause less encephalopathy than the nonselective types of shunts without improving survival.

Portal-systemic shunts have been used in four clinical situations: (1) *Hypersplenism* is not an indication for a portal-systemic shunt, because the reduction in formed elements in the blood is usually not of clinical significance. (2) The *prophylactic shunt* is made in patients with cirrhosis and varices but who have never bled. Prophylactic shunts shorten survival compared to unoperated controls, with death from hepatic encephalopathy and liver failure. Thus prophylactic shunts should not be performed. (3) *Emergency shunts* may be used to control hemorrhage in actively bleeding patients. However, the operative mortality may exceed 50 per cent, so that emergency shunts should be used rarely and in a select group of patients. The indications for this operation are still controversial. (4) *Therapeutic portal-systemic shunts* are used in patients who have bled at least once from varices. Operations in these patients have been shown to effectively stop further bleeding from varices. Unfortunately, the patient's survival is not improved significantly because of an increased incidence of hepatic encephalopathy and liver failure when compared to unoperated controls. Possibly these results could be improved upon by better selection of patients for the operations. As might be expected, the majority of patients with poor hepatocellular function, i.e., those who are jaundiced with hypoalbuminemia, ascites, encephalopathy, and poor nutrition, tolerate a portal-systemic shunt less well than do patients without these complications of liver disease. Patients with more severe liver disease may well be better managed by sclerosis of their varices than by shunt operations. The choice of therapy (sclerosis or shunt) for bleeding varices in patients

with well-compensated cirrhosis is controversial. The morbidity and mortality from bleeding esophageal varices will remain high until current therapies are refined and new ones developed.

Benhamou J-P, Lebrec D: Portal hypertension. Clin Gastroenterol 14:1, 1985. *A multiple-authored review of portal hypertension and the treatment of bleeding varices.*

Boyer TD: Portal hypertension and its complications. In Zakim D, Boyer TD (eds.): Hepatology: A Textbook of Liver Disease. Philadelphia, W. B. Saunders Company, 1982, pp 464–499. *A current review of portal hypertension and its causes.*

Conn HO: Vasopressin and nitroglycerin in the treatment of bleeding varices: The bottom line. Hepatology 6:523, 1986. *An editorial that reviews the use of vasoconstrictors in the management of variceal hemorrhage.*

Groszmann R, Atterbury C: The pharmacological therapy of portal hypertension. Adv Intern Med 31:341, 1985. *An up-to-date review of the use of vasoconstrictors, vasodilators, or β-blockade for the treatment of bleeding varices.*

Mitchell MC, Boitnott JK, Kaufman S, et al.: Budd-Chiari syndrome: Etiology, diagnosis and management. Medicine 61:199, 1982. *An excellent review of hepatic vein thrombosis.*

Smith JL, Graham D: Variceal hemorrhage: A critical evaluation of survival analysis. Gastroenterology 82:968, 1983. *A careful evaluation of survival following an episode of hemorrhage from varices.*

The Copenhagen Esophageal Varices Sclerotherapy Project: Sclerotherapy after first variceal hemorrhage in cirrhosis: A randomized multicenter trial. N Engl J Med 311:1594, 1984. *A large trial that demonstrates a decrease in rebleeding and an improvement in survival in patients who survived long enough to have their varices obliterated.*

ASCITES

DEFINITION. Ascites is the presence of excess fluid in the peritoneal cavity. It is most frequently due to cirrhosis, but there are numerous other causes (see Ch. 112), and it cannot be assumed that the appearance of ascites is indicative of cirrhosis. For this reason, patients with a recent onset of ascites must be thoroughly evaluated to establish its cause.

PATHOGENESIS (Table 127–2). Ascites forms in patients with portal hypertension because of changes in the formation and reabsorption of hepatic and splanchnic lymph and because of alterations in the metabolism of salt and water by the kidneys.

Splanchnic Lymph Formation. Increases in portal venous pressure cause a rise in the pressure within the splanchnic capillaries, resulting in loss of fluid into the interstitial space. The capillaries of the intestine restrict the loss of protein to the interstitial space, and an oncotic gradient develops between the capillary and the extravascular space. This oncotic gradient returns the majority of the fluid to the capillary, and any fluid loss is usually removed by the intestinal lymphatics. For this reason, diseases that elevate the pressure only in the splanchnic bed, e.g., portal vein thrombosis, causes ascites uncommonly.

Hepatic Lymph Formation. In the noncirrhotic liver the endothelial lining of the hepatic sinusoids is discontinuous and does not effectively restrict plasma protein loss with even slight increases in sinusoidal pressure. Thus, in contrast to the intestines, the oncotic gradient between the sinusoids and extravascular space is small, and much of the fluid entering the interstitial space is not returned to the vascular space. These large amounts of fluid lost into the interstitial space must be returned to the vascular space via hepatic lymphatics. When the rate of formation of lymph exceeds the rate of removal, then fluid "weeps" out of the lymphatics and into

TABLE 127–2. FACTORS IN THE PATHOGENESIS OF CIRRHOTIC ASCITES

1. Increased hydrostatic pressure in hepatic sinusoids and splanchnic capillaries.
2. Overproduction of hepatic and splanchnic lymph secondary to (1), leading to a transudation of lymph into peritoneal space.
3. Limited or reduced reabsorption of water and protein by peritoneal lymphatics.
4. Sodium retention by the kidney secondary to hyperaldosteronism, increased sympathetic activity, alterations in metabolism of prostaglandins and kinins, and altered renal hemodynamics.
5. Impaired renal water excretion, in part caused by increased levels of ADH.

the peritoneal cavity. Diseases that cause marked elevations of the sinusoidal pressure, e.g., congestive heart failure and hepatic vein thrombosis, therefore commonly cause ascites with a high protein content. With cirrhosis the situation is more complex in that there is "capillarization" of the sinusoids such that an oncotic gradient forms between plasma and lymph. Large amounts of lymph are formed by the cirrhotic liver with overflow into the peritoneal space; however, the protein content of this fluid is low.

Peritoneal Reabsorption. The peritoneum plays an active role in the reabsorption of the ascitic fluid. Water and protein are reabsorbed by the lymphatics in the peritoneal membrane. The intra-abdominal pressure and character of the peritoneum are important factors in determining the rate of removal. The amount of fluid removed by the peritoneal lymphatics is variable but usually does not exceed 800 to 1000 ml every 24 hours.

Renal Function. An important factor in the genesis of ascites is the *retention of sodium* by the kidney. During the formation of ascites there is a positive sodium balance despite a total body sodium that is greater than normal. The pathogenesis of the sodium retention by the kidney is understood poorly; however, there is increased reabsorption of sodium by both proximal and distal tubules. The increased reabsorption of sodium may be mediated, in part, by increased plasma levels of aldosterone, increased sympathetic activity, and alterations in the renal production of prostaglandins and kinins. Reduced renal blood flow resulting from vasoconstriction also leads to enhanced sodium reabsorption.

CLINICAL MANIFESTATIONS AND DIAGNOSIS. Patients with ascites complain of increasing abdominal girth. The presence of ascites on physical examination is suggested by the findings of shifting dullness, a ballotable liver, or a fluid wave. Small amounts of ascites may be identified by abdominal ultrasound. Once the presence of ascites is suspected, diagnostic paracentesis should be performed. The character of the ascitic fluid in cirrhosis is variable; however, 80 to 90 per cent of patients have an ascitic fluid protein concentration of less than 2.5 grams per deciliter. The ascitic fluid lactic dehydrogenase and albumin concentrations are also low. The ascitic fluid white blood cell count is less than 500 per cubic millimeter in 90 per cent of patients with cirrhosis, and mononuclear cells predominate (>75 per cent).

MANAGEMENT. Resolution of the acute hepatic injury, following withdrawal of ethanol or a specific course of therapy, may reduce portal hypertension, and ascites may resolve spontaneously. In many patients, however, ascites is chronic and specific therapy is warranted. Accumulation of ascitic fluid occurs only in patients who are in positive sodium balance; therefore, *restricting sodium intake* will diminish or stop the accumulation of ascitic fluid. Diets containing 250 to 500 mg of sodium (10 to 20 mEq) are adequate to achieve sodium balance in most patients. The kidney is also unable to excrete a water load normally in some patients with ascites, in part because of high blood levels of antidiuretic hormone. *Fluid restriction* (1000 to 1500 ml daily) is sometimes necessary, therefore, to prevent hyponatremia. Many patients do not lose their ascites or edema with sodium restriction, and the use of *diuretics* becomes necessary. Spironolactone and triamterene act on the distal tubule and cause natriuresis with sparing of potassium. Spironolactone, 150 to 400 mg daily, causes diuresis in patients with mild to moderate sodium retention. Furosemide, thiazides, and ethacrynic acid are more potent diuretics and cause both natriuresis and potassium wasting. Furosemide, 40 to 80 mg daily, in combination with spironolactone or triamterene, causes diuresis in most patients with ascites. All diuretics cause a loss of fluid from the plasma. This fluid is then replaced by the reabsorption of ascitic or edema fluid. The rate of fluid lost should therefore not exceed the rate at which the ascites and edema fluids may be reabsorbed. The maximal rate of reabsorption of ascitic fluid

varies widely; however, fluid losses of 1 kg daily in patients with edema and ascites and 0.3 to 0.5 kg daily in those with only ascites are well tolerated. The BUN and electrolytes must be monitored for the development of azotemia and hypokalemia. The use of diets very low in sodium (250 to 500 mg) is possible in the hospital; however, this is rarely possible in an outpatient setting. Therefore, preceding discharge from the hospital, the patient's sodium intake should be increased (1 to 2 grams daily) and diuretics adjusted so that he or she is still in negative sodium balance.

A few patients with cirrhosis will not respond to diuretic therapy. Treatment in the hospital with increasing doses of diuretics leads to azotemia or hepatic encephalopathy. Other patients are controlled in the hospital but, upon discharge, rapidly reaccumulate their ascitic fluid. If these patients are incapacitated by the ascites, they may be candidates for other therapies. The *peritoneovenous (LeVeen) shunt* consists of a tube placed subcutaneously between the peritoneal cavity and the superior vena cava. There is a pressure-activated one-way valve that allows peritoneal fluid to enter the vascular space but prevents the backflow of blood into the tube. This shunt may be effective in controlling ascites; however, its use is associated with episodes of disseminated intravascular coagulation, sepsis, and frequent shunt thrombosis, thus limiting its application only to patients who have severe and incapacitating ascites. Even in this latter group of patients, its use is controversial. The shunt should not be used in patients whose condition can be managed by other therapies. Repeated *abdominal paracentesis* of 1 to 2 liters of ascitic fluid is a poor form of long-term therapy for resistant ascites. Patients presenting with massive ascites and difficulty in breathing, however, may be improved dramatically by the removal of 1 to 2 liters of fluid. Attempts to increase the venous oncotic pressure by infusions of albumin or plasma are not likely to cause sustained diuresis and are an expensive form of therapy.

SPONTANEOUS BACTERIAL PERITONITIS. Patients with cirrhosis and ascites may develop spontaneous bacterial peritonitis. There is no obvious cause for the peritonitis, i.e., perforation of the bowel, and it appears to occur because of bacterial seeding of the ascitic fluid via the lymph or blood or by bacteria traversing the bowel wall. The frequency of this complication in patients with ascites may be increasing, and its early recognition is essential (mortality exceeds 60 to 90 per cent even if treated). Patients with very low ascitic fluid protein levels (less than 1 gram per deciliter) appear to be at greater risk for developing peritonitis. The clues to the diagnosis are the presence of fever, abdominal pain or tenderness, or decreased bowel sounds in a patient with ascites. The diagnosis should also be suspected in patients with the sudden onset of hepatic encephalopathy or hypotension. Patients may be asymptomatic and the diagnosis suggested only by finding an elevated ascitic fluid white blood cell count, or by a positive ascitic fluid culture. The diagnosis is established by abdominal paracentesis, which should be performed in patients with onset of new ascites or in those with a change in their clinical course. The ascitic fluid white blood cell count is usually above 500 per cubic millimeter (93 per cent of cases), and more than 50 per cent of the cells are polymorphonuclear leukocytes. The ascitic fluid pH also is lower than the blood pH. Bacteria may be identified on Gram's stain. The ascitic fluid and blood should be cultured and treatment instituted before the results of culture are known, as delays in therapy may increase mortality. The organisms most frequently cultured are Enterobacteriaceae (mainly *E. coli*) and Group D streptococci, *Streptococcus pneumoniae*, and *Streptococcus viridans*. Other bacteria are cultured less frequently, and anaerobic bacteria are uncommon isolates. Initial antibiotic therapy should therefore include both an aminoglycoside and ampicillin or a newer cephalosporin antibiotic. The response to therapy is monitored by the fever pattern and by changes in the ascitic fluid white blood cell count. If therapy is effective, the ascitic fluid white blood cell count falls and the predominant cell again becomes mononuclear. Antibiotic therapy is continued for 10 to 14 days.

HEPATORENAL SYNDROME

DEFINITION AND PATHOGENESIS. The hepatorenal syndrome (functional renal failure) is a decrease in renal function that develops in a patient with serious liver disease in whom all other causes of renal dysfunction are excluded. The kidneys lack serious pathologic lesions. If the liver disease improves, normal renal function returns. The pathogenesis of the hepatorenal syndrome is unknown. There is intense intrarenal vasoconstriction and redistribution of blood flow. In addition, the plasma levels of renin and aldosterone are increased. These changes may be due to reduced "effective" plasma volume in some patients.

CLINICAL MANIFESTATIONS. Patients developing the hepatorenal syndrome frequently have severe hepatic disease and therefore are jaundiced and have other signs and symptoms of liver disease. Almost all of the patients with this syndrome have ascites. The illness is marked by oliguria. The urine is usually free of protein, and the urine sediment is normal. The urine sodium level is low (<10 mEq per liter), the urine-plasma creatinine ratio is high (>30:1), and the urine-plasma osmolality ratio is greater than 1.0. These urine findings are different from those of acute tubular necrosis, in which the urine sodium content is high (>30 mEq per liter), the urine-plasma creatinine ratio is low (<20:1), and the urine is isosmotic to plasma. The progression of the renal failure is variable, with some patients having a complete loss of renal function over several days, whereas in others the serum creatinine slowly increases over several weeks as the liver function gradually worsens.

DIFFERENTIAL DIAGNOSIS. Patients with liver disease may develop renal failure for a variety of reasons. These patients commonly receive diuretics and may develop prerenal azotemia. Renal function will improve with withdrawal of the medication. Acute tubular necrosis may occur following an episode of hypotension (bleeding or sepsis) or during fulminant hepatitis and can be distinguished from hepatorenal failure by the urine findings. Drugs (antibiotics, especially aminoglycosides, and nonsteroidal anti-inflammatory medications) may cause worsening of renal function in patients with cirrhosis. Acute pyelonephritis, with or without papillary necrosis, may also cause renal failure in patients with liver disease.

THERAPY AND PROGNOSIS. Specific causes of renal failure should be looked for and excluded. Any medications that are potential nephrotoxins should be withdrawn. A brief trial of plasma expansion with monitoring of urine output and serum creatinine may be attempted, to exclude hypovolemia as a cause of the renal failure. The volume of fluid infused should be limited (1000 ml), as overexpansion of the plasma volume may precipitate variceal hemorrhage. Infusions of vasodilators may transiently improve renal function; however, this does not improve survival. Uremia may be treated by dialysis; again, overall survival is not improved. The use of peritoneovenous shunts in these patients is being investigated, but their efficacy is as yet unproven. The prognosis for patients with the hepatorenal syndrome is poor, with over 90 per cent dying during hospitalization, usually from liver failure or complications of portal hypertension. Definitive therapies must await a better understanding of the pathogenesis of this syndrome.

Boyer T, Goldman I: Treatment of cirrhotic ascites. Adv Intern Med 31:359, 1985. *Discusses the overall management of cirrhotic ascites, including the role of the peritoneovenous shunt.*

Epstein M: Peritoneovenous shunt in the management of ascites and the hepatorenal syndrome. Gastroenterology 82:790, 1982. *An authoritative review of the good and bad effects of the peritoneovenous shunt.*

Epstein M (ed.): The Kidney in Liver Disease. 2nd ed. New York, Elsevier Biomedical, 1982. *A complete review of the renal functional alterations in liver disease. Multiple authors contributed to this work.*

Hoefs JC, Canawati HN, Sapico FL, et al.: Spontaneous bacterial peritonitis. Hepatology 2:399, 1982. *Describes the clinical features and hospital course of patients with spontaneous peritonitis.*

Reynolds T: Rapid presumptive diagnosis of spontaneous bacterial peritonitis. Gastroenterology 90:1294, 1986. *An expert's discussion of the value of the newer tests that have been proposed to be of value in the diagnosis of spontaneous bacterial peritonitis.*

128 ACUTE AND CHRONIC HEPATIC FAILURE AND HEPATIC TRANSPLANTATION
Bruce F. Scharschmidt

THE SYNDROME OF HEPATIC ENCEPHALOPATHY

DEFINITION AND SIGNIFICANCE. Hepatic encephalopathy (also called hepatic coma or portal-systemic encephalopathy) represents a constellation of neurologic signs and symptoms accompanying advanced, decompensated liver disease of all types and/or extensive portal-systemic shunting. Recognition of these signs and symptoms often represents an important clue to the presence of deteriorating liver function or superimposed complications. In addition, repeated neurologic evaluation of the encephalopathic patient provides valuable information regarding the patient's course and prognosis.

PATHOGENESIS. The pathogenesis of hepatic encephalopathy remains unclear. The encephalopathy is at least partially attributable to toxic materials that are derived from the metabolism of nitrogenous substrate in the gut and that bypass the liver through anatomic or functional shunts. This is the origin of the term *portal-systemic encephalopathy*, often used interchangeably with hepatic encephalopathy. *Ammonia* and *mercaptans* result from the degradation of urea or protein and sulfur-containing compounds, respectively, and both can produce coma when administered in large doses to animals. The presence of mercaptans in the breath of some encephalopathic patients probably accounts for the characteristic sweetish musty odor termed *fetor hepaticus*. Ammonia-induced changes in central nervous system metabolism include depletion of glutamic and aspartic acids and ATP. While often present in increased amounts in the blood or cerebrospinal fluid or both, the absolute concentration of ammonia, ammonia metabolites including glutamine, and mercaptans correlates only roughly with the presence or severity of encephalopathy. *Gamma-aminobutyric acid*, the principal inhibitory neurotransmitter in the mammalian brain, is also produced in the gut and is present in increased amounts in the blood of patients and animals with hepatic failure. A role for gamma-aminobutyric acid in hepatic encephalopathy is supported by the observation that visual evoked potentials in animals with hepatic failure mimic those of benzodiazepine-induced or barbiturate-induced coma, but differ from those of comatose states caused by administration of ether, ammonia, or mercaptans. A separate hypothesis holds that accelerated entry of *aromatic amino acids* into the central nervous system results in decreased synthesis of normal neurotransmitters such as norepinephrine and enhanced synthesis of *false neurotransmitters* such as octopamine. Other compounds such as short-chain *fatty acids* are also present in blood in increased amounts and have been proposed as potentially toxic. Finally, there is impaired integrity of the *blood-brain barrier* in animals with acute hepatic failure. It is possible that hepatic encephalopathy may represent the synergistic effects of a number of toxins acting on an unusually susceptible nervous system.

TABLE 128–1. STAGES OF HEPATIC ENCEPHALOPATHY

Stage 0	Subclinical encephalopathy associated with impaired psychomotor function
Stage I	Varied manifestations, often diagnosed in retrospect, including apathy, lack of awareness, anxiety, restlessness, slowed thinking, reversal of sleep rhythm
Stage II	Lethargy, drowsiness, disorientation, incontinence
Stage III	Deep somnolence (but patient can at least transiently be aroused), incoherent speech
Stage IV	Coma; patient may (Stage IVA) or may not (Stage IVB) respond to painful stimuli

NEUROLOGIC MANIFESTATIONS. The personality and mental changes of hepatic encephalopathy are frequently divided into stages (Table 128–1). Although this staging of encephalopathy is generally useful, marked individual variations occur, and many patients do not show an orderly progression of symptoms. Moreover, the clinical grading scale is relatively insensitive. Standardized testing has revealed psychomotor abnormalities in a high proportion of patients with cirrhosis in whom conventional neurologic examination is normal. Such *subclinical encephalopathy* is potentially important inasmuch as it may be associated with impaired functional capacity, including job performance and ability to drive an automobile. Patients with hepatic encephalopathy also display a characteristic spectrum of abnormal neurologic signs. Early signs may include asterixis, myoclonus, hyperactive muscle stretch reflexes, facial grimacing, and blinking, as well as primitive reflexes such as suck, snout, and grasp. As encephalopathy progresses, extensor toe responses, clonus, and decerebrate or decorticate posturing may be observed. Generalized flaccidity with absence of reflexes occurs preterminally.

In addition to the acute, reversible signs and symptoms already mentioned, rare patients with longstanding liver disease and portal-systemic shunting develop *irreversible neurologic dysfunction* characterized by tremor, rigidity, slurred speech, oral-facial dyskinesia, choreoathetosis, and ataxic gait. Spastic paraparesis is another rare manifestation of advanced chronic liver disease and portal-systemic shunting.

As with other types of metabolic encephalopathy, asymmetric neurologic findings are unusual, and brainstem reflexes such as the pupillary light response, oculovestibular response, and oculocephalic response are typically preserved until very late. Thus, asymmetric neurologic signs or abnormal brain stem reflexes may suggest a structural lesion of the central nervous system such as a subdural hematoma. Seizures are also uncommon in the absence of alcohol withdrawal and should alert the clinician to the possibility of a structural lesion or hypoglycemia. The disappearance of pupillary reactivity, of the oculocephalic or oculovestibular response, or of deep tendon reflexes is associated with a very poor prognosis in all types of metabolic encephalopathy, including hepatic encephalopathy (but excluding drug overdose). Electroencephalographic changes are sensitive indicators of hepatic encephalopathy but are not specific for this disorder. They include symmetric slowing observed initially over the frontal areas with later spreading laterally and posteriorly.

DIAGNOSIS. The diagnosis of hepatic encephalopathy is based upon the presence of compatible neurologic signs and symptoms in a patient with advanced liver disease and exclusion of other possible causes of the neurologic abnormalities. Routine laboratory studies, including electrolytes, calcium, blood urea nitrogen, creatinine, glucose, and standard liver function tests, are of help primarily in excluding other causes of metabolic encephalopathy and evaluating the presence and severity of hepatic disease. Toxicologic screening is also appropriate when ingestion of sedatives or toxins capable of altering neurologic function is suspected. Blood ammonia and cerebrospinal fluid levels of glutamine correlate only roughly with mental status and are therefore of limited value in most circumstances. Structural lesions such as a subdural hematoma are often a consideration and may require special radiologic studies. Other causes of encephalopathy such as the Wernicke-Korsakoff syndrome, sepsis, or menigitis must also be excluded, depending on the clinical circumstances.

TREATMENT. *Identification of Precipitating Factors.* The management of patients with hepatic encephalopathy is largely supportive. A thorough search should be made to detect and correct factors that may precipitate or aggravate encephalopathy (Table 128–2). All nonessential drugs should be stopped—particularly sedatives and potentially hepatotoxic agents. For the occasional patient who demonstrates manic disorientation as an early manifestation of encephalopathy, soft restraints are preferable to sedative hypnotic agents.

Decreasing Production and Absorption of Enteric Toxins. Therapy should also be directed at decreasing the production of putative toxins that result from enteric bacterial metabolism of nitrogenous substrates. The level of blood urea nitrogen should be lowered if possible since urea diffuses into the gut and is a substrate for ammonia production. Gut cleansing should be accomplished by enema, and oral administration of cathartics such as magnesium citrate is appropriate unless lactulose (see below) is administered. It is also generally appropriate to restrict dietary protein to about 40 grams per day in mildly encephalopathic patients and eliminate it in patients with more advanced or progressive encephalopathy. Several additional points regarding protein merit consideration. First, *vegetable protein* appears somewhat less likely to induce encephalopathy than animal protein and may be useful in the long-term management of patients with chronic or recurrent encephalopathy. Second, since protein-calorie malnutrition may play a role in the pathogenesis of alcoholic hepatitis, judicious administration of 40 to 80 grams of protein, with careful observation, may be appropriate for such patients even in the presence of encephalopathy. Finally, while oral or parenteral administration of *branched-chain amino acids* has been reported to be beneficial in the treatment of hepatic encephalopathy, controlled trials have not provided clear evidence of efficacy, and their use is not generally recommended.

In addition to these measures aimed at decreasing nitrogenous substrate, production of enteric toxins should be further inhibited by oral administration of a poorly absorbable antibiotic, such as neomycin in a dose of 1 to 2 grams every six hours, or by administration of lactulose. Lactulose is neither metabolized nor absorbed in the upper small bowel and is metabolized by ileal and colonic bacteria to organic acids. It is as effective as neomycin in lowering blood ammonia and reversing encephalopathy in patients with chronic liver disease. The mechanisms of action of lactulose may include increased bacterial assimilation of ammonia, decreased ammonia production, and possibly trapping of ammonia as NH_4^+ or ammonia precursors in the bowel lumen made more acidic by its metabolism. Lactulose therapy is commonly initiated by administering 50 ml of the syrup orally every two hours until diarrhea ensues. Thereafter, the dose is decreased to that amount necessary to produce two to four soft stools per day. Lactulose can also be given by retention enema. Concom-

TABLE 128–2. HEPATIC ENCEPHALOPATHY—COMMON PRECIPITATING FACTORS

Deterioration in hepatic function
Drugs (sedative or potentially hepatotoxic agents)
Gastrointestinal hemorrhage
Increased dietary protein
Azotemia
Hypokalemia
Infection
Constipation
Anesthesia and surgery
Hypoxia
Diuretics (hypokalemia, alkalosis, and hypovolemia)

itant administration of neomycin and lactulose may be useful in selected patients.

FULMINANT HEPATIC FAILURE

ETIOLOGY. Fulminant hepatic failure is defined as hepatic failure with Stage III or IV encephalopathy developing in less than eight weeks in a patient without pre-existing liver disease. It develops most commonly as a complication of viral hepatitis (usually B; B with superimposed delta; non-A, non-B; less commonly A), but may also result from exposure to a potentially hepatotoxic drug (e.g., acetaminophen) or anesthetic (halothane), exposure to a frank hepatotoxin (e.g., carbon tetrachloride), or from certain less common hepatic disorders (e.g., acute hepatic vein occlusion, acute fatty liver of pregnancy) and infections (herpes simplex virus). Reye's syndrome may present a similar clinical picture; however, it differs from most forms of fulminant hepatic failure in its presumed pathogenesis, its rarity beyond the second decade of life, and by the accumulation of microvesicular fat in hepatocytes. Wilson's disease may also present as acute hepatic failure and is particularly important to recognize because it is potentially treatable (see Ch. 205). Finally, a small group of patients exist in whom the duration of illness prior to the onset of encephalopathy may range from eight weeks to several months, but in whom, as in patients with fulminant hepatic failure, there is no evidence of previous liver disease. Serologic evidence of viral infection or toxic exposure is often lacking, and such *late-onset acute hepatic failure* (also called subacute hepatic necrosis or subacute hepatitis) is frequently attributed to non-A, non-B hepatitis. Apart from the somewhat slower tempo of their illness, these patients exhibit a clinical course and prognosis similar to patients who meet standard criteria for fulminant hepatic failure.

DIAGNOSIS. The diagnosis of fulminant hepatic failure requires the presence of Stage III or IV encephalopathy in a patient with severe, acute liver disease. Synthetic function of the liver as reflected by the prothrombin time is nearly always markedly abnormal. Serum bilirubin concentration is less helpful, since some patients may become very ill rapidly and progress to coma before the serum bilirubin is markedly elevated. Serum transaminase levels are usually elevated early in the illness but do not reliably distinguish between fulminant hepatic failure and acute hepatitis without encephalopathy.

TREATMENT. A thorough search should be made to detect and correct factors that may precipitate or aggravate encephalopathy (Table 128–2); however, encephalopathy in fulminant hepatic failure primarily reflects the severe nature of the underlying liver injury, and correcting potential precipitating factors is less likely to produce objective benefit than it is in patients with encephalopathy complicating chronic liver disease. Special attention must be directed to those complications that frequently occur in patients with fulminant hepatic failure. *Hypoglycemia* is common and results from impaired glycogenolysis and gluconeogenesis. Frequent monitoring of blood glucose is necessary, and administration of a 10 per cent dextrose solution is advisable. *Hyponatremia*, which is typically due to a combination of impaired renal clearance of free water and administration of excessive free water in the form of dextrose solutions, may require water restriction. *Hypokalemia*, which increases renal ammonia production, should be corrected. *Azotemia* frequently occurs and may result from hypovolemia, hepatorenal syndrome, or acute tubular necrosis. Hypovolemia should be corrected when present. Survival in patients with fulminant hepatic failure and either the hepatorenal syndrome or acute tubular necrosis does not appear to be improved by dialysis. In the patient with severe hypoprothrombinemia and serious *bleeding*, administration of fresh frozen plasma is appropriate in addition to measures directed more specifically at the source of

hemorrhage. The risk of gastrointestinal bleeding in patients with fulminant hepatic failure has been shown to be reduced by prophylactic administration of the H_2-receptor antagonist cimetidine. However, on the basis of studies in other critically ill patient groups, prophylactic administration of antacids is probably more effective and generally advisable. There is no evidence that heparin improves survival in patients with *disseminated intravascular coagulation* with hepatic failure. The risk of pulmonary, genitourinary, and other *infections* should be minimized by proper positioning of the patient to prevent aspiration and by judicious use of genitourinary and intravenous catheters. *Bacteremia* is a frequent complication of fulminant hepatic failure, with streptococci, *Staphylococcus aureus*, and *Escherichia coli* being the most commonly isolated organisms. *Hypoxemia* is commonly present even in the absence of obvious pulmonary pathology; it may result from both functional right-to-left shunting and ventilation perfusion imbalance and should be corrected by administration of oxygen. *Endotracheal intubation* should be performed for normal indications in fulminant hepatic failure and should be considered with onset of coma to prevent aspiration. *Pulmonary edema* may occur in the absence of left-sided heart failure and may require mechanical ventilation with positive end-expiratory pressure. *Hypotension* is common even in the absence of sepsis or bleeding and results from reduced systemic vascular resistance. However, pressors are often ineffective or only transiently effective. *Respiratory alkalosis* is a common early finding and requires no treatment. *Metabolic acidosis*, which occurs rarely and may be due to lactic acid accumulation, should be treated with bicarbonate. *Cerebral edema* is present in over half of patients dying of fulminant hepatic failure and may result in intracranial herniation. Moreover, in conjunction with systemic hypotension, it reduces cerebral perfusion and may cause brain death. Corticosteroids do not appear to be of benefit, but a single controlled study suggests that direct monitoring of intracranial pressure and treatment of intracranial hypertension with mannitol significantly improve survival. Treatment of clinically evident intracranial hypertension, manifested by unequal or abnormally reactive pupils, myoclonus, and/or decerebrate posturing, is certainly appropriate. Unfortunately, clinical signs may be an insensitive way of detecting intracranial hypertension. The decision regarding invasive intracranial pressure monitoring must thus be carefully individualized.

Experimental Measures. Because the mortality of fulminant hepatic failure is high even with optimal supportive care, a variety of other forms of therapy have been tried. Some of these—*corticosteroid administration, exchange transfusion*, and administration of L-*dopa* or *hepatitis B hyperimmune globulin* (for hepatitis B)—have been shown to be ineffective by controlled prospective clinical trials. Similar controlled observations for the remaining measures, which include *charcoal hemoperfusion, amino acid infusion, plasmapheresis, hemodialysis, total body washout, cross circulation* with a human volunteer or baboon, or *extracorporeal perfusion* through a human cadaver liver, pig liver, or baboon liver, are not available. However, the reported uncontrolled observations strongly suggest that these experimental forms of therapy offer *no advantage* over conventional supportive care.

PROGNOSIS. The short-term prognosis for patients with fulminant hepatic failure that progresses to coma is poor, the average reported survival being about 20 per cent. In contrast, the outlook for those patients who do survive an episode of fulminant hepatic failure with coma is quite good. Virtually all patients have returned to their previous state of health within two to three months, and follow-up liver biopsies have usually demonstrated no or minimal abnormalities. Patients with persistent biochemical or histologic abnormalities have frequently been found to have had pre-existing liver disease or to have continuing exposure to toxic or infectious agents, as for example through parenteral drug abuse.

CHRONIC LIVER DISEASE WITH ENCEPHALOPATHY

ETIOLOGY. Hepatic encephalopathy may also occur in patients with chronic liver disease, usually cirrhosis with portal-systemic shunting. Some patients with cirrhosis may be chronically encephalopathic. In most, however, encephalopathy tends to occur acutely and intermittently. In this latter group, the occurrence of encephalopathy reflects a worsening of hepatic function and/or the presence of one or more precipitating factors (Table 128–2).

DIAGNOSIS. As with fulminant hepatic failure, diagnosis requires the presence of signs and symptoms compatible with hepatic encephalopathy in a patient with underlying chronic liver disease. Routine tests of liver function are typically abnormal but are of little value in differential diagnosis. Unlike fulminant hepatic failure, encephalopathy in patients with chronic liver disease may be accompanied by only minimally abnormal liver function tests. A markedly elevated or rising prothrombin time in an encephalopathic patient with known chronic liver disease suggests superimposed acute hepatocellular necrosis. It is extremely important in patients with chronic alcoholic liver disease to exclude other causes of metabolic encephalopathy (e.g., hypoglycemia, alcohol intoxication, Wernicke-Korsakoff syndrome), meningitis, or structural lesions such as subdural hematoma.

TREATMENT. Unlike fulminant hepatic failure, encephalopathy in the patient with chronic liver disease is frequently not due to acute hepatocellular necrosis, but rather results from one or more potentially reversible precipitating factors. The essential first step in the management of these patients is to identify and, when possible, correct such factors as are outlined in Table 128–2. Additional general measures as outlined earlier for the treatment of hepatic encephalopathy should be undertaken. A small number of patients with chronic hepatic encephalopathy fail to respond to standard measures, and preliminary clinical studies suggest that administration of ornithine salts of branched-chain keto acids or bromocriptine may be helpful in this selected patient group.

The complications and additional supportive care required for these patients are similar to those described for fulminant hepatic failure. Overall, however, the severity and frequency of complications (e.g., hypoglycemia) are less than with fulminant hepatic failure. The various forms of experimental therapy that have been tried in fulminant hepatic failure also

TABLE 128–3. LIVER TRANSPLANTATION*

Hepatobiliary Disease	Per Cent of Total Patients	Per Cent One-Year Survival After 1983
Nonalcoholic cirrhosis	41	60
Hepatobiliary tumors	20	†
Biliary atresia	17	87
Metabolic disorders	7	66
Sclerosing cholangitis	6	78
Alcoholic cirrhosis	4	†
Hepatic vein occlusion	3	71
Fulminant hepatic failure and miscellaneous	2	†

*Based upon an analysis of 279 patients undergoing liver transplantation at several centers during 1983 and 1984.
†Too few patients for meaningful subgroup analysis

have no established role in the management of patients with chronic liver disease with encephalopathy.

PROGNOSIS. Because encephalopathy in patients with chronic liver disease is frequently precipitated by potentially reversible factors, the short-term prognosis is better than in fulminant hepatic failure. Most patients survive the acute episode, particularly if the encephalopathy is not attributable to a sudden deterioration of hepatic function. However, because the underlying chronic liver disease is commonly irreversible and slowly progressive, the long-term prognosis is guarded.

HEPATIC TRANSPLANTATION

Between 1963, when the first human liver transplantation was performed, and 1980, only about 300 such procedures were performed worldwide. Since 1980, more than 1000 liver transplantations have been performed, the number of liver transplant centers has increased from 3 to more than 30, and the results of transplantation have improved dramatically.

INDICATIONS AND RESULTS. Liver transplantation merits consideration in any patient with liver disease that is progressive, irreversible, not otherwise treatable, and sufficiently advanced that quality of life and lifespan are likely to be significantly improved. Table 128–3 summarizes the types of liver disease for which transplantation has most commonly been performed and the actuarial one-year survival in cohorts after 1983. Adults with nonalcoholic cirrhosis have repre-

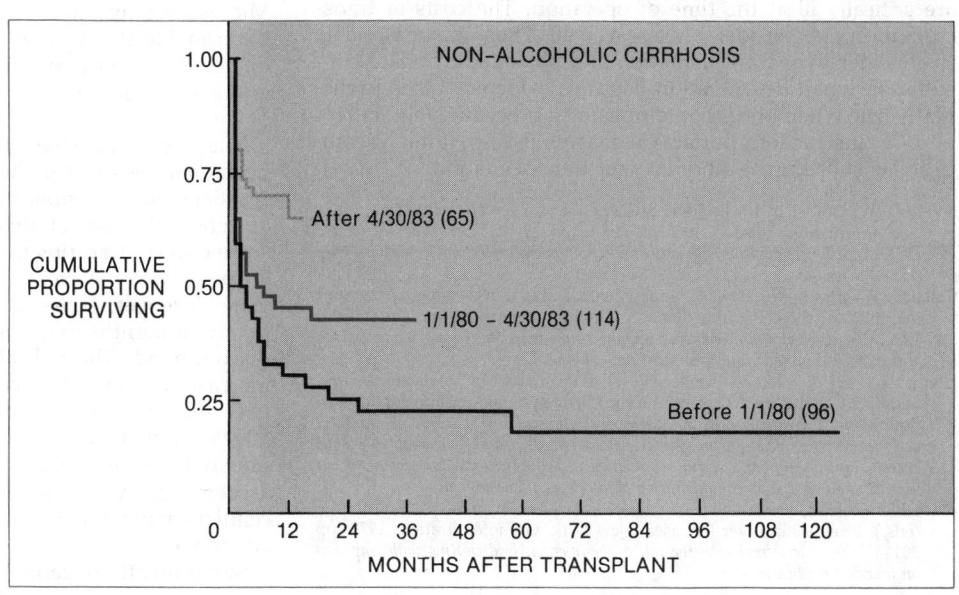

FIGURE 128–1. Actuarial survival of three consecutive cohorts of patients with non-alcoholic cirrhosis undergoing liver transplantation at several centers through August, 1984. The number of patients in each cohort is in parentheses.

sented the largest group of transplant recipients, and as with most other types of nonmalignant hepatobiliary disease, the results of transplantation have improved significantly. The recent improvement in survival likely reflects several factors, including the use of cyclosporin, newer surgical techniques, better supportive care, and the selection of patients with less advanced disease. These advances have greatly decreased postoperative mortality (Fig. 128–1). Most individuals (≥ 80 per cent) who survive the first three postoperative months live at least three years, and the quality of life for such individuals has been good, with about 80 per cent able to resume their former activities. Other diseases for which transplantation has yielded encouraging results have included biliary atresia, metabolic disorders (predominantly alpha$_1$-antitrypsin deficiency and Wilson's disease), sclerosing cholangitis, and hepatic vein occlusion. In contrast to nonmalignant disease, the results of transplantation for malignant hepatobiliary disease have been poor overall and have improved relatively little, with half or more of patients who survive the postoperative period dying of recurrent disease. The appropriateness of transplantation for most such patients thus remains controversial, as it does for patients with alcoholic liver disease. Relatively few patients with fulminant hepatic failure have undergone transplantation. However, preliminary reports of transplantation in this setting have been encouraging, particularly for patients whose disease is less fulminant and spans several weeks to months rather than days (see above.).

Contraindications to liver transplantation include the presence of extrahepatic malignant disease, serious and irreversible extrahepatic disease, active alcoholism, and portal vein thrombosis. Patients with hepatitis-B-virus–related liver disease and evidence of ongoing viral replication (see Ch. 123) have generally experienced recurrent disease in the donor liver and have therefore also been considered poor candidates.

Between 10 and 30 per cent of patients require a second or even third transplant because of failure of the first graft. Such graft failure is most commonly attributable to postoperative complications such as vascular thrombosis, primary graft nonfunction, or rejection; recurrence of the original disease accounts for few cases of graft failure.

TIMING OF TRANSPLANTATION. Tests for precisely measuring hepatic reserve are not available, and the prognosis for an individual patient is often hard to predict. Thus the timing of transplantation for an otherwise appropriate candidate is often difficult to judge. Survival of ambulatory patients undergoing transplantation is greater than that of those who are critically ill at the time of operation. The costs of transplantation are considerably less as well. Thus, it is reasonable to consider liver transplantation and obtain appropriate consultation when deterioration becomes evident. This is particularly true when one is contemplating a procedure (e.g. biliary tract reconstruction, portacaval anastomosis) that might compromise subsequent candidacy for transplantation.

Busuttil RW, Goldstein LI, Danovitch GM, et al.: Liver transplantation today. Ann Intern Med 104:377, 1986. *A well-referenced review that focuses on the UCLA experience and deals with patient selection, operative technique, postoperative care, and results.*

Canalese J, Gimson AE, Davis C, et al.: Controlled trial of dexamethasone and mannitol for the cerebral oedema of fulminant hepatic failure. Gut 23:625, 1982. *A controlled study reporting improved survival with aggressive monitoring of intracranial pressure and treatment with mannitol.*

Conn HO, Leevy CM, Vlahcevic ZR, et al.: Comparison of lactulose and neomycin in the treatment of chronic portal-systemic encephalopathy. A double-blind controlled trial. Gastroenterology 72:573, 1977. *A skillfully designed prospective study in patients with cirrhosis and chronic portal-systemic encephalopathy. Provides useful information regarding clinical assessment of encephalopathy as well as administration of lactulose and neomycin.*

Flute PT: Clotting abnormalities in liver disease. In Popper H, Schaffner F (eds.): Progress in Liver Diseases. New York, Grune & Stratton, 1979, pp 301–322. *A concise review of the role of the liver in blood clotting with emphasis on practical applications.*

Gimson AES, O'Grady J, Ede RJ, et al.: Late onset hepatic failure: Clinical, serological and histological features. Hepatology 6:288, 1986. *A complete characterization of patients without known prior liver disease in whom the total duration of illness exceeds eight weeks. Has a useful reference list.*

Jones EA, Schafer DF: Fulminant hepatic failure. In Zakim D, Boyer TD (eds.): Hepatology: A textbook of Liver Disease. Philadelphia, WB Saunders Company, 1982, pp 415–445. *An exhaustively referenced review of the pathogenesis and treatment of hepatic encephalopathy in the setting of rapidly deteriorating hepatic function. An excellent entry point into the literature.*

Plum F, Hindfelt B: The neurological complications of liver disease. In Vinken PJ, Bruyn GW (eds.): Handbook of Clinical Neurology. Amsterdam, North Holland Publishing Company, 1976, pp 349–377. *The clinical description of neurologic abnormalities is a particularly valuable part of this comprehensive review.*

Scharschmidt BF: Human Liver Transplantation: An analysis of 819 patients from eight centers. In Thomas HC, Jones EA (eds.): Recent Advances in Hepatology. New York, Churchill-Livingston, 1986, pp 175–189. *A comprehensive summary of the results of liver transplantation at several centers in the United States and Western Europe, with a brief consideration of costs and issues regarding patient selection.*

Summary of National Institutes of Health Consensus Development Conference on Liver Transplantation. Hepatology 4:1s–107s, 1984. *This conference, which had a major positive impact upon the field of liver transplantation, reviewed the indications for liver transplantation and results of the procedure in various patient groups.*

Uribe M, Marquez MA, Ramos GG, et al.: Treatment of portal-systemic encephalopathy with vegetable and animal protein diets: A control cross-over study. Dig Dis Sci 27:1109, 1982. *A controlled study of different protein sources with important practical details regarding diet.*

129 HEPATIC TUMORS

Bruce F. Scharschmidt

BENIGN HEPATIC TUMORS
Hepatocellular Adenoma

Hepatocellular adenomas occur almost exclusively in women. These tumors are most frequently detected during the childbearing years, particularly the third and fourth decades of life, but are occasionally found in postmenopausal women as well. Adenomas most commonly occur in the right lobe of the liver, are solitary in about one third of the cases, and are often quite large, with up to one half being 10 cm or more in diameter. Hepatocellular adenomas are usually well circumscribed, may be surrounded by a pseudocapsule, and often show areas of bile stasis, hemorrhage, and necrosis. Microscopically, these tumors consist of a monotonous array of normal to slightly atypical hepatocytes without portal tracts or bile ducts. Kupffer cells are markedly reduced in number or absent, and a few arteries and thin-walled veins are present.

The preponderance of this tumor in women suggests a hormonal role in its pathogenesis, and there is strong circumstantial evidence implicating oral contraceptives. The number of reported cases of this tumor has increased dramatically since oral contraceptives were introduced in 1960, and nearly 90 per cent of these are associated with oral contraceptive use. Moreover, some adenomas have clearly regressed in a period of months to years after use of oral contraceptives was discontinued. The risk of developing this tumor appears to increase steadily with increasing duration of oral contraceptive use, and the annual incidence is estimated to be 3 to 4 per 100,000 in women who have taken oral contraceptives continuously for several years. Although not generally regarded as a premalignant lesion, there are instances in which hepatocellular carcinoma appears to have arisen in an hepatocellular adenoma.

Symptomatic patients with hepatocellular adenomas present with signs and symptoms of an abdominal mass, tumor infarction, intratumor hemorrhage (pain, fever, leukocytosis), or, in about one third of cases, tumor rupture (pain, hemoperitoneum, circulatory collapse). The mortality in this last group is approximately 20 per cent. Because the true incidence of these tumors is unknown, the actual proportion that ruptures cannot be determined.

Because Kupffer cells are infrequent or absent, hepatocellular adenomas usually appear as a defect ("cold spot") on technetium 99m–sulfur colloid scans. The angiographic appearance is typically hypervascular, often with areas of hypovascularity. The management of hepatocellular adenomas is a matter of some debate. In patients taking oral contraceptives that can be discontinued, a several-month period of observation with repeated radionuclide scans is justifiable, particularly if the location, size, or number of tumors would make resection hazardous. Surgery is appropriate for most persistent resectable lesions.

Focal Nodular Hyperplasia

Focal nodular hyperplasia, which shows a female to male predominance of 2:1 to 7:1, has also been referred to as pseudotumor, focal cirrhosis, and hepatic hamartoma. Despite distinctive pathologic features, focal nodular hyperplasia and hepatocellular adenoma have often been confused in the medical literature. Unlike hepatocellular adenoma, a firm link between focal nodular hyperplasia and oral contraceptives has not been established. Focal nodular hyperplasia generally is a solitary tumor in the right lobe. It has a characteristic grossly lobulated appearance on cut section, which is produced by a central fibrous core with septa radiating in a stellate pattern. Hemorrhage and necrosis are rare. Microscopically, these fibrous septa contain bile ductules and inflammatory cells and are surrounded by normal or slightly atypical hepatocytes as well as Kupffer cells.

Unlike hepatocellular adenomas, focal nodular hyperplasia does not usually produce symptoms and is generally found incidentally at surgery or necropsy. In up to 20 per cent of the cases, it presents as an upper abdominal mass. Portal hypertension has been reported in association with multiple lesions, and rupture is rare. Because these tumors contain Kupffer cells, they frequently take up technetium 99m–sulfur colloid normally and may appear as voids, hot spots, or some combination of these on scan. Occasionally they exhibit uniform uptake of isotope equivalent to that of normal liver and are not visualized by technetium 99m–sulfur colloid scan. They are characteristically hypervascular on angiography with a visible capillary blush. Since focal nodular hyperplasia has no known malignant potential, asymptomatic lesions can be followed nonoperatively. If the lesion is encountered unexpectedly at surgery, simple wedge biopsy is appropriate if complete excision would be difficult.

Hemangioma

Cavernous hemangioma is probably the most common benign hepatic tumor, with a 0.4 to 7.3 per cent incidence in necropsy series and a predominance in females. The great majority of hemangiomas are asymptomatic and are found incidentally at surgery or necroscopy. These lesions can, however, present with signs and symptoms of an abdominal mass, infarction, rupture, or thrombocytopenia and hypofibrinogenemia.

Hemangiomas typically appear as a cold spot on conventional scans with technetium 99m–sulfur colloid; enhanced activity with blood pool scanning is frequently found and is highly specific. Their presence can occasionally be suspected on plain roentgenogram of the abdomen by the presence of calcified spicules radiating from the center of the lesion. The angiographic appearance of dense and persistent tumor stain-

ing is virtually diagnostic. Computed tomographic studies with rapid sequential imaging following the bolus injection of intravenous contrast material may also provide diagnostically useful information as may magnetic resonance imaging. Because of the accuracy of these imaging techniques in distinguishing hemangioma from a vascular carcinoma or angiosarcoma, resection is not usually necessary to establish a diagnosis, being necessary only for large symptomatic lesions. There are also case reports of regression following radiotherapy or hepatic artery ligation.

Other Benign Tumors

A variety of less common benign liver tumors may also occur in adults. They usually produce no symptoms unless very large. Included in this group are *bile duct adenomas, bile duct cystadenomas, fibromas, lipomas, leiomyomas, mesotheliomas, teratomas,* and *myxomas. Nodular regenerative hyperplasia* is a condition characterized by multiple nodules of varying size arising in a noncirrhotic liver. The nodules are composed of liver plates that are two cells thick. An association with rheumatoid arthritis, Felty's syndrome, CREST syndrome, oral contraceptives, and a variety of drugs is reported. The most common manifestation of nodular regenerative hyperplasia is portal hypertension.

MALIGNANT HEPATIC TUMORS
Hepatocellular Carcinoma

EPIDEMIOLOGY. In the United States and Western Europe, hepatocellular carcinoma (hepatoma) is increasing in incidence but remains relatively uncommon, accounting for less than 1 per cent of all causes of death at autopsy and 2.5 per cent or less of all malignant growths. In certain other areas of the world, including parts of sub-Saharan Africa, Southeast Asia, Japan, Oceania, and Greece, hepatocellular carcinoma is among the most frequent malignant tumor and is an important cause of overall mortality. Hepatocellular carcinoma is predominantly a disease of males and usually arises in a cirrhotic liver. The risk appears to be greatest in cirrhosis associated with hemochromatosis and hepatitis B virus infection, low in primary biliary cirrhosis and Wilson's disease, and intermediate in alcoholic and cryptogenic cirrhosis. Chronic hepatitis B virus infection may predispose to hepatocellular carcinoma: (1) The aforementioned areas of the world in which hepatocellular carcinoma is most prevalent are the same areas in which hepatitis B virus infection is most common. (2) Serologic evidence of hepatitis B virus infection is much more common in patients with hepatocellular carcinoma than in controls, an observation that has been made in all parts of the world, including the United States. (3) The incidence of hepatocellular carcinoma is about one hundredfold higher in individuals with hepatitis B virus infection than in noninfected controls. (4) Analysis of tumor tissue in patients with serologic evidence of hepatitis B virus infection has indicated the presence of hepatitis B virus integrated into the host genome. (5) Woodchucks and ducks infected with viruses that are related to the human hepatitis B virus also develop hepatocellular carcinoma.

Epidemiologic evidence has also suggested a link between hepatocellular carcinoma and ingestion of aflatoxins, mycotoxins produced by *Aspergillus flavus,* a mold that can grow in warm moist areas and contaminate peanuts and stored grains. Case reports have also suggested a link between hepatocellular carcinoma and alpha$_1$-antitrypsin deficiency and administration of androgenic steroids, Thorotrast, and possibly estrogenic steroids in the form of oral contraceptives (Table 129–1).

CLINICAL FEATURES. The most common presenting features of hepatocellular carcinoma are *abdominal pain,* the presence of an *abdominal mass,* and *weight loss.* Hepatocellular

TABLE 129–1. HEPATOCELLULAR CARCINOMA

Incidence
From 1–7 per 100,000 to > 100 per 100,000 in high-risk areas

Sex
4:1 to 8:1 male predominance, except fibrolamellar carcinoma

Associations
Cirrhosis
Hepatitis B virus infection (usually with cirrhosis)
Hemochromatosis (with cirrhosis)
Aflatoxin ingestion
Thorotrast
α_1-Antitrypsin deficiency (?)

Suggestive Clinical or Laboratory Findings
Hepatic bruit or friction rub
α-Fetoprotein ↑ (> 400 ng/ml)

Common Clinical Presentations
Abdominal pain
Abdominal mass
Weight loss
Deterioration of liver function

Unusual Manifestations
Bloody ascites
Tumor emboli to lung
Obstructive jaundice
Obstruction of hepatic or portal veins
Bloody ascites
Metabolic (erythrocytosis, hypercalcemia, hypercholesterolemia, carcinoid syndrome, sexual changes, hypoglycemia, acquired porphyria)

carcinoma may also present with rupture and hemoperitoneum, obstructive jaundice, unexplained deterioration in a patient with cirrhosis, or a variety of paraneoplastic syndromes, including erythrocytosis, persistent fever, hypercalcemia, and hypoglycemia. Hepatomegaly is present in about two thirds of patients. Other suggestive physical findings include the presence of a bruit, hepatic friction rub, or bloody ascites. Hepatocellular carcinoma may invade and obstruct the portal and hepatic veins and metastasizes most often to regional lymph nodes and the lungs. Alpha-fetoprotein levels in serum greater than 1000 ng per milliliter or progressively rising levels are highly suggestive of hepatocellular carcinoma. Unfortunately, only a minority of patients with hepatocellular carcinoma in most parts of the world, including the United States, have elevations of this magnitude, and low level elevations up to about 200 ng per milliliter are relatively nonspecific. For this reason, alpha-fetoprotein has proved disappointing in the screening of high-risk populations. Hepatocellular carcinomas typically fail to take up technetium 99m–sulfur colloid, but accumulate gallium 67 normally on radionuclide scan, and they generally appear as an irregular hypervascular mass with tumor "staining" and arterial displacement and/or encasement on angiography.

TREATMENT AND PROGNOSIS. The results of current treatment for hepatocellular carcinoma are discouraging. In the United States, median survival from the time of diagnosis is about six months. Because of the advanced stage of the disease at the time of diagnosis and the frequent coexistence of severe liver disease, only a small fraction of patients are candidates for hepatic resection. The presence of coexisting cirrhosis in a patient with well-preserved hepatic function does not altogether preclude surgery; however, such patients are unlikely to tolerate more than limited resection of a localized tumor. Prospective screening of high-risk patients in Japan has resulted in detection of earlier, smaller tumors and resulted in a higher proportion of tumors being resectable. While patients undergoing resection of such early tumors have shown remarkably high survival rates up to 3 years, the median period of asymptomatic growth of such tumors is about 3 years, and the utility of aggressive population screening and early surgery is as yet unclear. Adriamycin alone or in combination with other agents has produced objective tumor response in up to 50 per cent of patients, but has minimally affected survival. Radiation therapy has also yielded disappointing results. Hormonal therapy has been tried, but experience with this approach is too limited to judge its value. As discussed in Ch. 128, the results of liver transplantation for unresectable hepatocellular carcinoma have been disappointing, with a three-year survival of about 15 per cent.

A variant of typical hepatocellular carcinoma termed *fibrolamellar carcinoma* differs from the typical form of the disease in that it usually occurs in young adults without underlying cirrhosis, lacks the usual male predominance, is associated with a longer survival when untreated, and has been cured surgically in between 10 and 30 per cent of cases.

Other Primary Hepatic Malignancies

Cholangiocarcinoma occurs much less frequently than hepatocellular carcinoma and shows an association with clonorchiasis and opisthorchiasis in the Far East and with sclerosing cholangitis. It may present with obstructive jaundice when it involves major ducts in the area of the hepatic hilum. Truly mixed hepatocellular cholangiocarcinomas are rare. Angiosarcoma, an unusual tumor associated with vinyl chloride exposure as well as arsenic and Thorotrast administration, frequently causes thrombocytopenia and has a propensity to rupture, causing hemoperitoneum and circulatory collapse. Other unusual primary hepatic malignant tumors of adults include cystadenocarcinoma, squamous carcinoma, and hepatoblastoma.

As with hepatocellular carcinoma, treatment of these malignant hepatic tumors has been unsatisfactory. Resection is seldom possible. Of patients with cholangiocarcinoma who have undergone liver transplantation, the three-year survival has been about 7 per cent.

Tumors Metastatic to Liver

The liver and lung are the most frequent sites of metastatic cancer, and metastases constitute the largest group of hepatic tumors in adults. Necropsy studies have demonstrated hepatic metastases in more than half of patients with primary malignant tumors having portal venous drainage (e.g., stomach, colon, and pancreas). Other solid tumors that frequently metastasize to the liver include melanoma and tumors of the lung, oropharynx, and bladder. Next to the spleen, the liver is also the most common extranodal site of involvement by Hodgkin's disease, the non-Hodgkin's lymphomas, and malignant histiocytosis (histiocytic medullary reticulosis).

DIAGNOSTIC APPROACH TO THE PATIENT WITH A SUSPECTED HEPATIC NEOPLASM

Most hepatic neoplasms present as a right upper quadrant or epigastric mass. Additional clinical features that may provide clues regarding the specific type of tumor have been noted above and include pre-existing cirrhosis (hepatocellular carcinoma), portal or hepatic vein thrombosis (hepatocellular carcinoma), oral contraceptive use (hepatocellular adenoma), abdominal pain with hemoperitoneum and hypotension (hepatocellular adenoma; less commonly angiosarcoma, hepatocellular carcinoma, hemangioma), and unusual systemic manifestations (hepatocellular carcinoma). Cholangiocarcinoma and hepatocellular carcinoma can cause biliary obstruction, but this may potentially result from strategically located tumors of all types.

Physical examination most commonly reveals hepatomegaly or a discrete mass. The presence of a bruit or friction rub may suggest hepatocellular carcinoma but is not specific. Elevations of alkaline phosphatase and transaminase levels are the most common biochemical abnormalities. In general, however, liver function tests are not particularly helpful in diagnosis and may be entirely normal in some patients. Uncommon biochemical abnormalities in patients with hepatocellular carcinoma include the presence of a variant alkaline phosphatase, erythrocytosis, or hypercholesterolemia. A markedly elevated and/or progressively rising alpha-fetoprotein level is strongly suggestive of hepatocellular carcinoma.

Examination of tissue is ultimately required for the unequivocal diagnosis of hepatic tumors. In a patient with a known extrahepatic malignant tumor and clinical or biochemical evidence of hepatic metastases, radionuclide scanning or ultrasonography is a reasonable first step. The finding of single or multiple defects is consistent with metastatic disease, and a percutaneous biopsy can be expected to recover tumor in 50 to 75 per cent of such cases. Two biopsies performed through the same skin site and cytologic examination of the tissue core and aspirated fluid appear to enhance the yield without increasing the risk of bleeding. In patients with lymphoreticular malignant disease, percutaneous biopsy is less sensitive in demonstrating hepatic involvement than wedge biopsy obtained at laparotomy, and histologic evidence of hepatic involvement may be found even in the absence of clinical, biochemical, or radionuclide scan abnormalities.

The workup in suspected primary hepatic tumor must be individualized on the basis of the relative risks and benefits of establishing a diagnosis. Ultrasound examination or computed tomography, particularly following intravenous injection of iodinated contrast material, appears to be more sensitive than radionuclide scanning in the detection of small tumors and may be useful also in excluding a cyst. Angiography may occasionally permit a definite diagnosis, as with a hemangioma, and is helpful in assessing resectability. Because of the rapidly evolving capabilities of current imaging procedures, radiologic consultation is helpful in selecting the most appropriate method.

In a patient who is a candidate for operation and who has an apparently resectable lesion of uncertain or suspicious nature based on imaging studies, preoperative biopsy is usually not indicated. Two additional factors must be taken into account when assessing the appropriateness of a preoperative biopsy. First, needle biopsy of primary lesions such as hemangioma, angiosarcoma, and possibly hepatocellular adenoma is potentially dangerous owing to their propensity to hemorrhage, and biopsy of a possible echinococcal cyst is contraindicated. Second, definitive diagnosis of hepatocellular adenoma and focal nodular hyperplasia, which consist predominantly of normal or minimally abnormal hepatocytes, may be difficult from examination of a needle biopsy alone. In the patient who is not a candidate for surgery or in whom information regarding tumor type will importantly influence decisions regarding further evaluation and therapy, a diagnosis can often be established by needle biopsy. Compared with percutaneous biopsy, a laparoscopic approach facilitates directed biopsy of visible tumor deposits and may permit control of bleeding. Inspection of the liver at laparoscopy for evidence of cirrhosis or tumor deposits not evident from radiologic studies may also aid in determining the resectability of a lesion. A directed percutaneous aspiration biopsy has also yielded excellent results in certain centers. Non-neoplastic lesions that may mimic hepatic tumors include regenerative nodules, anomalous hepatic lobulation, cysts, and abscesses.

Kerlin P, Davis GL, McGill DB, et al.: Hepatic adenoma and focal nodular hyperplasia: Clinical, pathologic, and radiologic features. Gastroenterology 84:994, 1983. *A concise review comparing and contrasting these two common benign hepatic neoplasms.*

Kew MC: Hepatic tumors. Semin Liver Dis 4:89, 1984. *A concise and well-referenced review.*

Locker GY, Doroshow JH, Zwelling LA, et al.: The clinical features of hepatic angiosarcoma: A report of four cases and a review of the English literature. Medicine 58:48, 1979. *A review of information about this unusual tumor.*

Malt RA: Surgery for hepatic neoplasms. N Engl J Med 313:1591, 1985. *A brief and very practical summary of this topic.*

Nagasue N, Yukaya H, Ogawa Y, et al.: Hepatic resection in the treatment of hepatocellular carcinoma: Report of 60 cases. Br J Surg 72:292, 1985. *A particularly valuable summary of the results of surgery for early lesions in a generally cirrhotic patient population.*

Sheu J-C, Sung J-L, Chen D-S: Growth rate of asymptomatic hepatocellular carcinoma and its clinical implications. Gastroenterology 89:259, 1985. *A nearly unique report of sequential imaging of non-resected early tumors that has implications regarding screening programs for patients at high risk for hepatocellular carcinoma.*

Shinagawa T, Ohto M, Kimura K, et al.: Diagnosis and clinical features of small hepatocellular carcinoma with emphasis on the utility of real-time ultrasonography: A study in 51 patients. Gastroenterology 86:495, 1984. *A review of the clinical features, biochemical abnormalities, and utility of conventional imaging techniques in the diagnosis of hepatocellular carcinomas less than 5 cm in diameter.*

130 DISEASES OF THE GALLBLADDER AND BILE DUCTS

Peter F. Malet and Roger D. Soloway

Biliary tract disorders result from a variety of congenital, inflammatory, metabolic, infectious, and neoplastic conditions. These conditions often present in subtle ways and can pose challenging diagnostic problems. Ongoing improvements in diagnostic and therapeutic techniques have allowed the clinician to diagnose biliary tract disease more quickly and to treat patients more effectively.

NORMAL PHYSIOLOGY OF BILE FORMATION

Bile is an isotonic aqueous mixture consisting primarily of electrolytes, proteins, bile salts, cholesterol, phospholipids, and bilirubin. Secretion across the canalicular membrane of the hepatocyte accounts for about two thirds of total bile flow. Bile salt–dependent secretion comprises about one half of canalicular bile formation, while the other half is termed bile salt independent and consists mainly of electrolytes. The remaining one third of bile flow is an alkaline fraction generated by the epithelial cells lining the bile ducts; ductular secretion is stimulated by secretin, cholecystokinin, and gastrin. An as yet unquantitated contribution to canalicular bile flow consisting mainly of water and electrolytes occurs by way of the interhepatocytic space (paracellular pathway). The total volume of bile produced ranges from 500 to 800 ml per day.

Under basal (fasting) conditions, tonic contraction of the sphincter of Oddi diverts about half of the flow of hepatic bile into the gallbladder; the other half flows into the duodenum assisted by phasic peristalsis action of the sphincter. The gallbladder actively reabsorbs Na^+, Cl^-, and HCO_3^+ and passively resorbs H_2O. It is capable of concentrating bile tenfold within about four hours. The gallbladder mucosa secretes H^+ and mucin.

Cholecystokinin, released from the intestinal mucosa after meals by fat, amino acids, and H^+, simultaneously stimulates the gallbladder to contract and the sphincter of Oddi to relax, emptying bile into the duodenum.

Bile salts are synthesized by hepatocytes (Fig. 130–1) from cholesterol by a multistep process, the rate-limiting step of which is catalyzed by 7 alpha-hydroxylase, which is under inhibitory feedback control. Cholate and chenodeoxycholate, the two *primary* bile salts (that is, they are synthesized in the liver), are conjugated with either glycine or taurine before secretion to improve solubility. Bile salts are secreted by active transport across the biliary canalicular membrane. After entering the proximal small intestine, bile salts aid in fat absorption by forming *micelles* (Ch. 104) and then are largely reabsorbed in the mid and distal small intestine. Bile salts that reach the colon are partially deconjugated, which makes them more lipid soluble and facilitates their reabsorption. Cholate and chenodeoxycholate are also partially converted by bacterial 7 alpha-dehydroxylation to the *secondary* bile salts, deoxycholate and lithocholate, respectively. Deoxycholate is absorbed from the colon, reconjugated in the liver, and excreted in bile. Lithocholate is poorly reabsorbed; it is sulfated as well as reconjugated during hepatic transfer. Sulfation increases aqueous solubility and further reduces intestinal reabsorption. The average bile salt composition of bile is 35 per cent chenodeoxycholate, 35 per cent cholate, 25 per cent deoxycholate, 2 per cent ursodeoxycholate, and 2 per cent lithocholate. Each is conjugated with either glycine or taurine in a

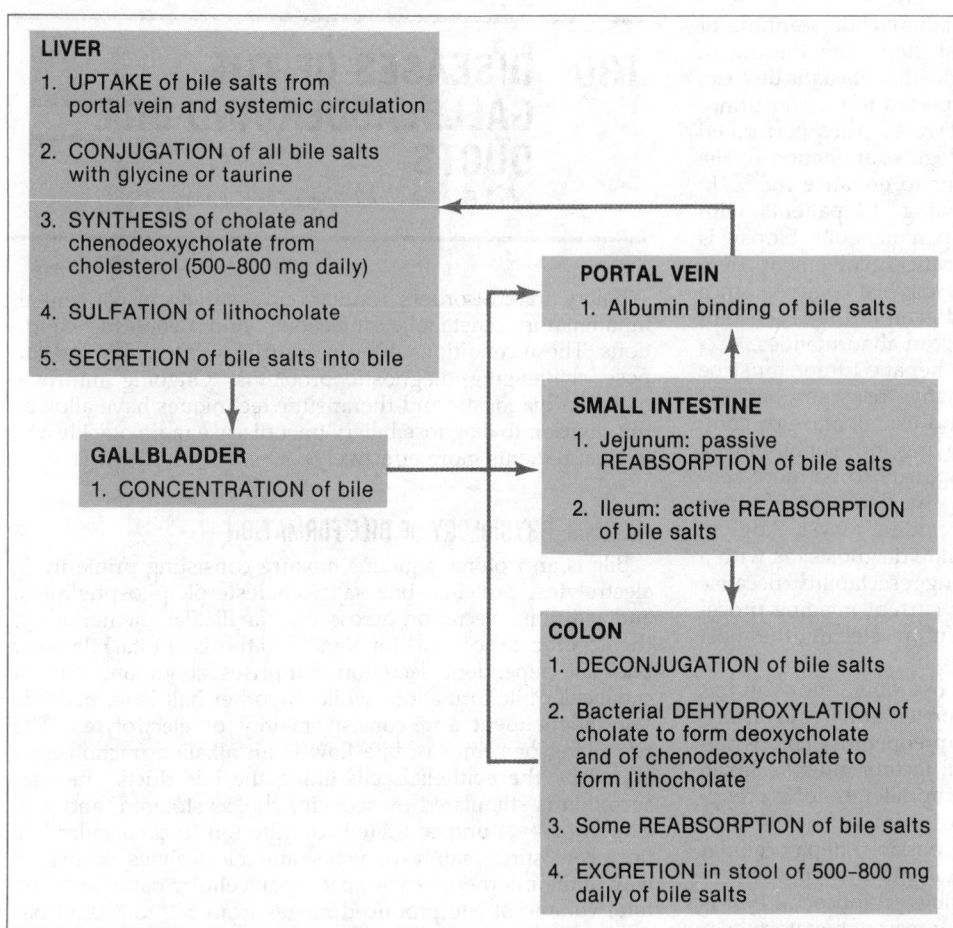

LIVER

1. UPTAKE of bile salts from portal vein and systemic circulation

2. CONJUGATION of all bile salts with glycine or taurine

3. SYNTHESIS of cholate and chenodeoxycholate from cholesterol (500–800 mg daily)

4. SULFATION of lithocholate

5. SECRETION of bile salts into bile

GALLBLADDER

1. CONCENTRATION of bile

PORTAL VEIN

1. Albumin binding of bile salts

SMALL INTESTINE

1. Jejunum: passive REABSORPTION of bile salts

2. Ileum: active REABSORPTION of bile salts

COLON

1. DECONJUGATION of bile salts

2. Bacterial DEHYDROXYLATION of cholate to form deoxycholate and of chenodeoxycholate to form lithocholate

3. Some REABSORPTION of bile salts

4. EXCRETION in stool of 500–800 mg daily of bile salts

FIGURE 130–1. The major steps in the enterohepatic circulation of bile salts. This cycle provides for conservation of bile salts by an effective reabsorption mechanism in the intestine.

ratio of 2 to 3:1. Bile salts are secreted in the form of micelles containing phospholipids (mainly lecithin), and cholesterol. These lipids account for 90 per cent of biliary solids.

Intestinal reabsorption of bile salts, which is about 95 per cent for a single passage, occurs by passive diffusion throughout the intestine and by active transport within the terminal ileum. The reabsorbed bile salts are largely bound to albumin in portal blood and are then almost completely removed by the hepatocytes in a single passage through the liver sinusoids. The bile salt pool, normally 1.8 to 3.0 grams, passes through the liver and intestine two or three times during each meal, producing six to nine cycles daily (i.e., each day about 20 to 25 grams of bile salts enter the duodenum); this cycling is termed the *enterohepatic circulation*. During an average day involving three meals, bile salts are in continuous motion with peaks of secretion during and following meals. At night, when the majority of the secreted hepatic bile eventually enters the gallbladder, and there is no stimulus for gallbladder contraction, the intestinal concentration of bile salts is much lower. Conservation of bile salts in this enterohepatic circulation is so efficient that only 15 to 25 per cent (500 to 600 mg) of the bile salt pool must be replaced by hepatic synthesis of new bile salts daily. If the efficiency of enterohepatic conservation is impaired by conditions such as biliary fistula, ileal Crohn's disease or ileal resection, hepatic synthesis of bile salts increases. The maximal synthetic rate (5 grams per day) will be insufficient to restore intraluminal concentrations to normal if external losses exceed this amount.

Bile salts are *amphophiles*, possessing water-soluble and fat-soluble sides. In an aqueous medium they are distributed randomly until a critical concentration (about 2 mM) is reached, at which point spontaneous aggregation forms multimolecular structures called micelles. In micelles the bile salt molecules line up with their hydrophilic portions facing the solvent (water) and their hydrophobic portions facing each other (Fig. 130–2). The hydrocarbon center of the micelle can

incorporate biliary lecithin and cholesterol, and the entire aggregate remains water soluble. The addition of lecithin expands micellar size and enhances the ability of bile salt micelles to incorporate other lipids. In addition, a variable amount of cholesterol is carried in lecithin-cholesterol vesicles. The ultimate cholesterol-carrying capacity of bile depends on the relative amounts of bile salts and lecithin as well as the total lipid concentration.

Besides electrolytes, other solutes in bile are bilirubin that has been conjugated in the liver with glucuronic acid (Ch. 118), proteins, and cations such as calcium, iron, copper, and zinc, and low concentrations of the end-products of drug and hormone metabolism.

PATHOPHYSIOLOGY OF GALLSTONE DISEASE

In Western cultures about 75 per cent of gallstones are composed principally of cholesterol (*cholesterol gallstones*) and 25 per cent of calcium bilirubinate and other calcium salts (*pigment gallstones*). Overall, about 15 per cent of gallstones are radiopaque, about two thirds of which are pigment and one third are cholesterol stones. The symptoms caused by gallstones are the same regardless of the chemical composition and to a large extent are independent of size. Stones can cause pain and jaundice by passage through the cystic and common bile ducts or can cause pain by intermittently becoming impacted in the neck of the gallbladder.

CHOLESTEROL GALLSTONES. Cholesterol stones are usually yellow green to tan and are round or faceted. They may be single or multiple; most range in size from 1 mm to 3 to 4 cm. Cholesterol accounts for 50 to 100 per cent of stone weight, the remainder consisting of mucin glycoproteins and less than 10 per cent calcium bilirubinate and/or other calcium salts. These stones occur three times as frequently in women as men, the difference beginning at puberty and declining after menopause. The incidence is higher with multiparity and with the use of birth control pills, which suggests an

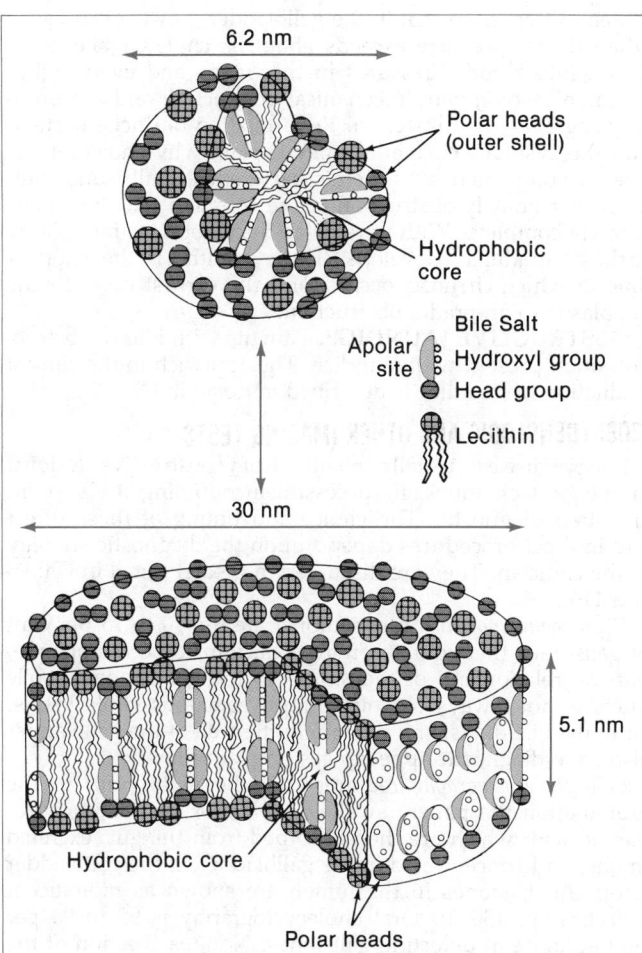

FIGURE 130–2. Dimorphic structure of a biliary mixed lipid micelle, which has been shown to exhibit a sphere → disc transition, depending upon whether the solution is bile salt–rich (sphere) or lecithin-rich (*disc*). The lecithin-rich micelle is larger and capable of dissolving and transporting a much larger amount of cholesterol. The transition depends upon the bile salt–lecithin molar ratio present in the micelle but may also be influenced by other constituents present in native bile. Bile salt molecules in both micellar forms are thought to form pairs (dimers) to avoid contact of the hydroxyl groups (*small clear circles*) with the nonpolar environment of the micellar core. (Adapted with permission from Muller K: Biochemistry 20:404, 1981. Copyright 1981 American Chemical Society.)

influence of female sex hormones. The incidence in blacks, whites, and American Indians increases in that order. About 75 per cent of American Indian women over the age of 25 years and 90 per cent of those over age 60 are affected. In the United States 20 per cent of 75-year-old men and 35 per cent of 75-year-old women have stones at autopsy. Environmental and dietary influences are important. For example, the incidence of gallstones in blacks in Africa is much lower than in blacks in the United States.

Cholesterol, which is insoluble in water, is normally carried in bile within bile salt-lecithin micelles. A completely clear micellar solution of bile is one in which cholesterol is completely solubilized. A prerequisite for cholesterol gallstone formation is an excess of cholesterol in relation to micellar carrying capacity, a condition that may result from decreased bile salt or increased cholesterol concentration in bile. When the cholesterol-solubilization capacity of micelles is exceeded, cholesterol forms either a *metastable* solution, which is clear initially but forms crystals and becomes cloudy after standing, or a *supersaturated* solution, which is visually turbid, containing either liquid or solid crystals of cholesterol.

Bile of patients with gallstones has relatively more choles-

terol than that of normal persons, although the overlap is great. In patients with gallstones, bile is supersaturated with cholesterol as it emerges from the liver, implicating the hepatocytes rather than the gallbladder as the cause of the abnormality. In some patients with gallstones the total bile salt pool is decreased in size, and the hepatocytes have decreased amounts of the enzyme 7 alpha-hydroxylase. These observations suggest that diminished bile salt secretion is a factor in the genesis of lithogenic bile in some patients. Another factor, particularly associated with obesity, is increased cholesterol secretion into hepatic bile.

The relationship between cholesterol and bile salt output is hyperbolic, so that when bile salt secretion declines, the cholesterol-bile salt ratio climbs and the bile becomes more lithogenic. During fasting, bile salts are sequestered in the gallbladder, hepatic secretion of bile salts declines, the rate of cholesterol secretion persists, and the bile becomes more lithogenic. Supersaturation of bile with cholesterol is therefore common after overnight or prolonged fasting. Normal human bile probably contains *solubilizing* or *antinucleating factors*, for example, apolipoprotein A-1, that prevent cholesterol crystallization.

Cholesterol saturation of bile appears to be a necessary but not a sufficient condition for cholesterol gallstone formation. Supersaturated bile from patients without gallstones does not form cholesterol crystals, even on prolonged incubation, while bile of identical lipid composition from patients with stones usually contains or forms such crystals. The gallbladder is considered to be important in gallstone formation, possibly by supplying a nidus (*nucleating factor*) for crystallization, such as mucin glycoproteins or other smaller proteins secreted by the epithelium, or by providing an area of stasis to facilitate precipitation. For example, stone formation occurs predominantly in the gallbladder, and cholesterol gallstones rarely recur after cholecystectomy.

PIGMENT GALLSTONES. Pigment stones are subdivided into two categories, black and brown stones, on the basis of differing compositional and clinical characteristics.

Black pigment stones are much more common in the West and are usually under 1 cm, irregular in shape, and featureless on cross-section. They form in the gallbladder and are composed of calcium bilirubinate, bilirubin polymers, calcium phosphate and carbonate, and mucin glycoproteins. There is no relationship between black stones and obesity, parity, saturation of bile with cholesterol, or bile salt pool size. Rather, old age and less than ideal weight are associated with black stone formation in the general population. The great majority of patients with black stones have no underlying disease, but patients with cirrhosis and hemolytic diseases are predisposed to develop these stones. There is no sexual predisposition; American Indians are rarely, and Scandinavians infrequently, affected. The concentration of unconjugated bilirubin is increased in the bile of some patients with these stones.

Brown pigment stones (calcium bilirubinate) have layers of calcium bilirubinate alternating with cholesterol and calcium salts of fatty acids. Bilirubin is thought to precipitate with calcium because beta-glucuronidase of bacterial, biliary epithelial, or hepatic origin deconjugates bilirubin diglucuronide to less soluble bilirubin monoglucuronide or unconjugated bilirubin. The fatty acids of biliary lecithin may be similarly precipitated as calcium salts because of hydrolysis by phospholipases. These stones are much more common in the Orient; the incidence decreases with the westernization of the culture and diet. They can form in the gallbladder and/or in intrahepatic or extrahepatic biliary ducts (Table 130–1). In Western nations they form primarily in the common bile duct years after cholecystectomy for cholesterol or black pigment stones. Unlike in the West, in the Orient stones frequently recur after removal and are associated with massive dilatation of the biliary tract and accompanying cholangiohepatitis (re-

TABLE 130–1. CONDITIONS ASSOCIATED WITH A PROPENSITY FOR GALLSTONE FORMATION

1. **Cholesterol**
   Obesity
   Ileal disease or resection
   Multiparity
   Drugs: clofibrate, estrogens
   Race: American Indian
   Cystic fibrosis
2. **Black pigment**
   Old age
   Cirrhosis
   Hemolysis
   Intravenous hyperalimentation
3. **Brown pigment**
   Oriental cholangiohepatitis
   Sclerosing cholangitis
   Caroli's disease
   Choledochal cysts
   Duodenal diverticula (perivaterian)

current pyogenic cholangitis), often resulting in secondary biliary cirrhosis and hepatic failure.

DISSOLUTION OF GALLSTONES. Attempts have been made to dissolve cholesterol gallstones by reversing some of the above pathogenetic mechanisms. Chenodeoxycholate (CDC), 12 to 15 mg per kilogram per day orally, will dissolve a substantial proportion of radiolucent cholesterol gallbladder stones within two years. CDC causes the bile to become unsaturated by mechanisms that are still unclear. Problems with CDC therapy include diarrhea and hepatoxicity. Ursodeoxycholate has a similar therapeutic effect, but is less hepatotoxic and diarrheogenic. These compounds are ineffective for dissolution of pigment stones, of radiopaque stones, of stones in gallbladders nonopacified by oral cholecystography, and of stones in obese patients. Candidates for dissolution treatment are mildly to moderately symptomatic patients who are bad risks for surgery because of other illnesses. Stones will usually dissolve in one or two years in 30 to 40 per cent of patients who receive CDC in a dose of 12 to 15 mg per kilogram daily. Ursodeoxycholate therapy achieves the same success rate in about half the time. Relative contraindications to therapy include chronic liver diseases, chronic diarrhea, and peptic ulcer disease. Women who may become pregnant should not be treated because of the potential (though not proven) for harmful effects of CDC on the fetus. When treatment is discontinued after initial dissolution, gallstones re-form in up to 50 per cent of patients within five years.

Current research into new methods of gallstone dissolution includes direct instillation of methyl-tert-butyl ether into the gallbladder lumen by percutaneous transhepatic catheter placement. This technique usually dissolves cholesterol gallstones within one to two days. Another technique undergoing study is extracorporeal shock-wave lithotripsy in which gallstones are fragmented into fine particles, using a technique that is similar to that already successfully used for renal stone fragmentation.

PATHOPHYSIOLOGY OF BILIARY OBSTRUCTION

Obstruction caused by a stone is the primary cause of all manifestations of gallstone disease. Obstruction of the cystic duct by gallbladder stones distends the gallbladder, producing biliary pain. If the obstruction persists, acute cholecystitis may ensue. The intermediary steps from obstruction to acute inflammation are discussed later. Whether complications such as empyema or perforation develop depends on whether secondary infection occurs. Cholecystectomy cures cholecystitis, but cholecystostomy, which only relieves the obstruction, will eliminate all the clinical manifestations of the disease.

Obstruction of the common duct may produce pain, jaundice, pruritus, infection, and biliary cirrhosis. Surgical procedures that decompress the duct upstream from the stone eliminate these manifestations. The situation in the ductal system differs from that in the gallbladder, however, because when ductal pressure exceeds about 25 cm/H_2O, bile is refluxed into blood. Pressures in this range and even higher commonly accompany mechanical obstruction and are probably aggravated by infection. Regurgitation of ductal bacteria into the systemic circulation may explain why cholangitis is often accompanied by systemic bacteremia, chills, and high fever. Fortunately obstruction of the common duct by stones is rarely complete. With unrelieved ductal obstruction, biliary cirrhosis gradually develops. Three months is the shortest time in which cirrhosis occurs, and the earliest cases follow neoplastic (high-grade) obstruction.

OBSTRUCTIVE JAUNDICE. Patients with biliary obstruction often present with jaundice. The approach to the clinical evaluation of jaundice is described in detail in Ch. 120.

ROENTGENOLOGIC AND OTHER IMAGING TESTS

Biliary disease usually results from obstructive lesions; radiologic techniques, if successful in outlining the system, are often diagnostic. The choice and timing of these direct and indirect procedures depend upon the diagnostic strategy of the clinician. They are discussed in greater detail in Ch. 95 and 116.

Plain roentgenograms can demonstrate the 10 to 15 per cent of gallstones that contain enough calcium to be radiopaque, but the relationship of the stones to the gallbladder or bile ducts is not always obvious. Emphysematous cholecystitis, air in the bile ducts, and calcium in the wall of the gallbladder also have diagnostic appearances on plain films.

Oral cholecystography requires that the night prior to the examination the patient swallow tablets of iopanoic or tyropanoic acid, which are then absorbed from the gut, excreted in bile, and concentrated in the gallbladder. If the gallbladder is opacified, stones in the lumen are shown as radiolucent defects (Fig. 130–3). Oral cholecystography is 90 to 95 per cent accurate in detecting gallstones. Nonopacification of the gallbladder occurs if the cystic duct is blocked or if the diseased gallbladder mucosa cannot concentrate the contrast material. The gallbladder may not be opacified for several reasons not related to gallbladder disease: if the patient has been vomiting, if the patient has been fasting for several days immediately before taking the tablets, or if absorption by the gut or excretion by the liver is faulty. If extrabiliary causes of a nonopacified gallbladder are excluded, nonopacification is 95 per cent reliable in indicating gallbladder disease.

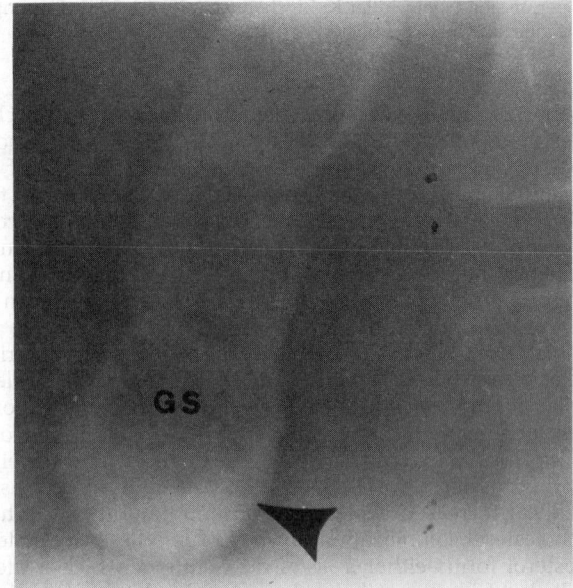

FIGURE 130–3. Oral cholecystogram showing a gallbladder (*arrowhead*) opacified by an orally administered contrast agent. The gallbladder is filled with four large round gallstones (GS).

Ultrasonography of the biliary tree may demonstrate gallstones or dilatation of the intrahepatic or extrahepatic ductal system (Fig. 130–4). It also has the advantage of being able to examine, if indicated, the liver and pancreas at the same time. Real-time ultrasonography is very reliable in detecting gallbladder stones (false positives are uncommon); it should be used as the first test for screening for gallstones. Unfortunately, less than one third of common duct stones are identified. Ductal dilatation is detected in about 90 per cent of cases of proven obstruction. Ductal dilatation usually indicates distal obstruction by neoplasm, stricture, or stone. The correlation between dilatation and obstruction is inexact because (1) the ducts may be dilated from previous disease or surgery although currently unobstructed, (2) cirrhosis or scarring from previous cholangitis may stiffen the ducts enough to prevent dilatation, and (3) lesions characterized by intermittent obstruction (e.g., common duct stones, stricture) may produce dilation followed by spontaneous decompression; ducts may appear undilated if the patient is examined after the duct has spontaneously decompressed.

Percutaneous transhepatic cholangiography (PTC) involves direct percutaneous puncture of an intrahepatic duct by a needle

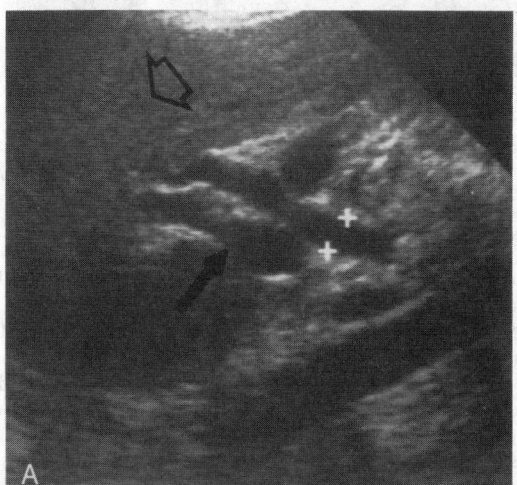

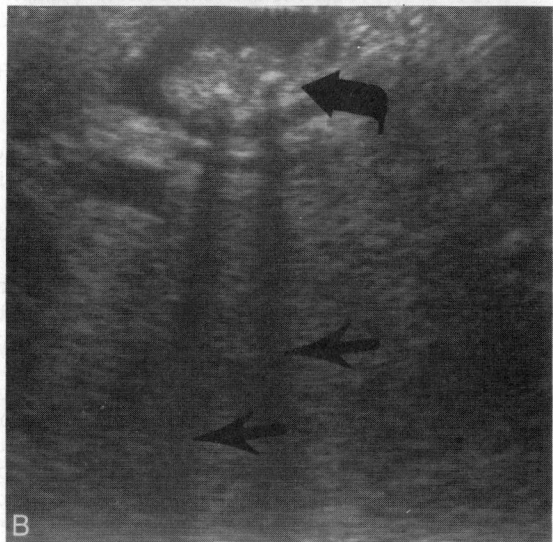

FIGURE 130–4. *A,* Real-time ultrasonography of the extrahepatic biliary tract showing a dilated common bile duct (the width of the duct measured between the two white crosses is 9 mm); the portal vein is seen as the anechoic area (*solid arrow*) directly beneath the common bile duct. The liver parenchyma is indicated by the arrowhead. *B,* Ultrasonography of a gallbladder containing gallstones and sludge (*curved arrow*) that appear as echogenic foci within the gallbladder lumen. The gallstones exhibit acoustic shadowing (*lower two arrows*), that is, paucity of echoes distal to the stones due to blockage of the echo waves by the solid stones. (Courtesy of Dr. Peter Arger.)

inserted through the eighth or ninth right intercostal space into the center of the liver. An abnormal clotting mechanism, significant ascites, and severe cholangitis are contraindications. PTC has proved particularly valuable in diagnosing gallstones within the intrahepatic biliary tract, biliary strictures, and neoplastic obstruction of the bile ducts (Fig. 130–5). A technically successful study can be obtained in nearly all patients with dilated ducts and in 70 per cent of patients with normal-sized ducts.

Endoscopic retrograde cholangiopancreatography (ERCP) involves cannulation of the common bile duct and pancreatic duct through the ampulla of Vater via the endoscope (see Fig. 95–7). With experience, a successful study of one or both ducts is possible in 80 to 90 per cent of attempts. ERCP is particularly useful in patients with normal-sized bile ducts or in whom pancreatic disease as a cause of bile duct obstruction is strongly suspected.

Both PTC and ERCP are usually contraindicated in active cholangitis unless a therapeutic maneuver is planned because as ductal pressure increases during injection of the contrast material, severe uncontrollable sepsis may be produced. Patients undergoing either of these procedures should usually receive premedication with antimicrobial agents regardless of whether there is a history of cholangitis.

Radionuclide imaging of the biliary tree may be accomplished by intravenous injection of a ^{99m}Tc-labeled derivative of iminodiacetic acid (e.g., HIDA, PIPIDA, or DISIDA). Normally, a high-quality image of the biliary tree appears within 30 minutes after administration of the radionuclide agent (see Fig. 95–9). This test is becoming the procedure of choice in verifying the diagnosis of acute cholecystitis. Filling of the ducts but not of the gallbladder supports the diagnosis of cholecystitis due to obstruction of the cystic duct by a stone. A false-negative study is rare; however, false-positive (nonfilling) studies are seen in patients with severe illnesses such as pancreatitis and cholestatic liver disease and in those receiving intravenous hyperalimentation. Ultrasonography is more useful in detecting common bile duct obstruction than is radionuclide imaging.

Computed tomography is usually performed after evidence of biliary ductal disease has been ascertained by ultrasonography or cholangiography. It is useful in defining pancreatic causes of biliary tract obstruction, in detecting paraductal lymph node enlargement, and in examining the liver for abscesses, intrahepatic ductal dilatation, and neoplasms.

CLINICAL CATEGORIES OF GALLBLADDER AND BILIARY TRACT DISEASES

Asymptomatic Gallstones

Approximately 60 to 80 per cent of patients in the United States with gallstones are asymptomatic, based on surveys using ultrasonography. In the past, patients with asymptomatic gallstones were advised to have a cholecystectomy. The trend now is to observe such patients and not to recommend surgery. Such asymptomatic patients may therefore be followed expectantly with prophylactic cholecystectomy reserved for the following two exceptions: (1) *diabetics,* because their mortality from acute cholecystitis is 10 to 15 per cent, mainly as a result of the coexisting diabetic complications, such as cardiovascular disease, and (2) patients with *calcified gallbladders,* often associated with carcinoma of the gallbladder. Asymptomatic patients with gallstones have approximately an 18 per cent chance of developing biliary pain in 20 years, and only 3 per cent will require cholecystectomy. Mortality from gallstone disease is low when a conservative plan is used of treating only those who present with typical biliary pain. Even with symptomatic patients, the decision to perform surgery is not always clear-cut. Patients with infrequent mild pain may prefer not to undergo cholecystectomy, or the physician may be hesitant to recommend surgery because of serious coexisting illnesses. Such patients may be

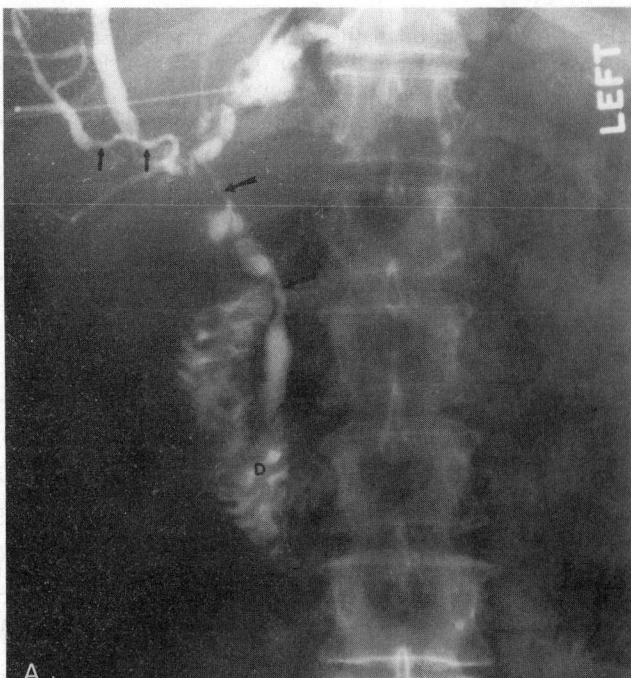 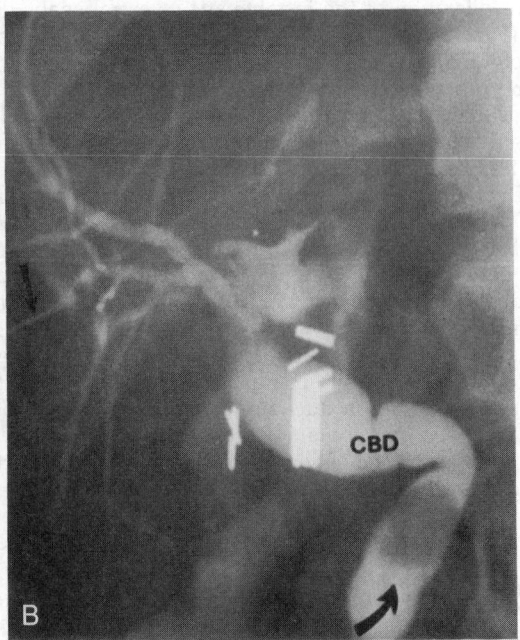

FIGURE 130–5. *A,* Percutaneous transhepatic cholangiogram demonstrating primary sclerosing cholangitis in a 54-year-old woman with a long history of Crohn's disease and biochemical evidence of cholestasis. There are strictures (*arrows*) scattered throughout her intra- and extrahepatic biliary tract; dye is seen to flow into the duodenum (D). *B,* Percutaneous transhepatic cholangiogram (skinny needle used for dye injection is indicated by arrow on left) showing a 1.5 × 2.0 cm gallstone (*curved arrow*) in the distal common bile duct (CBD) causing dilatation of the extrahepatic biliary tract. The metallic clips are from a prior cholecystectomy. The patient presented with a three-day history of RUQ pain and jaundice with a total bilirubin of 5.6 mg per deciliter. (Courtesy of Dr. Gordon McLean.)

suitable candidates for medical dissolution with chenodeoxycholate.

Symptomatic Gallstones

PATHOLOGY. The pathologic findings in the gallbladder wall and the clinical manifestations of gallstone disease often correlate poorly. In some patients the gallbladder is severely affected as the result of previous attacks of acute cholecystitis, with shrinking, scarring, and thickening of the wall, adhesions to adjacent viscera, and patchy replacement of the mucosa by granulation tissue or collagen. Nonopacification following oral cholecystography is frequent in such patients. At the other extreme the gallbladder may be grossly normal with only slight thinning of the mucosa, mild patchy scarring and inflammation, and a normally visualized oral cholecystogram. The term *chronic cholecystitis* is a descriptive pathologic term for such changes although it has been used to describe the clinical manifestations of chronically symptomatic gallstones.

CLINICAL MANIFESTATIONS. Symptomatic gallstones commonly produce a steady pain most often located in the epigastrium or right upper quadrant, thought to be caused by gallbladder distension arising from transient obstruction of the cystic duct by a gallstone. The onset of pain takes only a few minutes; it quickly reaches a plateau in intensity that may range from moderate to excruciating. After 30 minutes to several hours the pain subsides gradually. The pain usually does not wax and wane like intestinal colic; hence the preferred term is *biliary pain,* not biliary colic. Nausea and vomiting may accompany the attack, and only a vague residual ache or soreness may remain after the acute pain has dissipated. Tenderness, muscular guarding, a palpable mass, fever, and leukocytosis are absent, distinguishing this condition from acute cholecystitis. Many patients have simultaneous pain referred to the back near the scapula or to the right shoulder area. Attacks may occur daily or as seldom as once every few years. Dyspepsia, intolerance to fatty food, flatulence, heartburn, and belching may occur, but are not helpful

diagnostically because they often occur in persons with normal gallbladders.

Hydrops (mucocele) of the gallbladder refers to its distension with mucus (white bile) and gallstones; it may develop from cystic duct obstruction. Hydrops produces constant discomfort in the right upper quadrant and a palpable mass without the clinical findings of acute cholecystitis.

DIAGNOSIS. Real-time *ultrasonography* is the preferred test because it is 95 to 99 per cent sensitive in detecting gallbladder stones. It also has the advantage of allowing examination of the common bile duct, pancreas, and liver at the same time without radiation exposure. An oral cholecystogram after a double dose of contrast material (that is, taken on the two nights prior to the examination) will identify 90 to 95 per cent of gallstones. If nonopacification occurs and liver function and intestinal absorption are normal and other extrabiliary causes are excluded, gallbladder disease can be inferred with a high degree of certainty. In about 5 to 10 per cent of patients with gallstones, opacification of the gallbladder will be adequate during oral cholecystography, but calculi will not be demonstrated, either because the stones are too small to be seen or because they are of the same radiographic density as the contrast medium.

In patients with typical biliary pain in the absence of demonstrable gallstones by cholecystography or ultrasonography, examination of bile for crystals may prove helpful. A sample of bile is obtained from an orally placed duodenal tube and is examined microscopically for the presence of cholesterol crystals. If no crystals are seen initially the bile can be incubated at 37°C for 24 or 48 hours to look for crystal formation. The significance of calcium bilirubinate crystals is uncertain. In the presence of what seems to be biliary pain, a positive duodenal drainage test is highly suggestive that tiny stones are present or, in a few cases, that cholesterolosis is present.

The *differential diagnosis* includes other common causes of chronic abdominal symptoms such as peptic ulcer, reflux esophagitis, esophageal spasm, and pancreatitis, which may have manifestations similar to those of gallstones. Radicular pain from spinal lesions or rib pain from bone lesions may mimic biliary pain. Angina pectoris may cause pain thought to be abdominal, just as biliary pain may be felt in the precordial region. Postprandial pain or discomfort may result from the irritable bowel syndrome or intestinal tumors.

COMPLICATIONS. *Choledocholithiasis* is the most common complication, affecting about 15 per cent of patients with cholecystolithiasis. The incidence of common duct stones increases with advancing age. Patients with symptomatic gallstones often eventually develop an attack of *acute cholecystitis*. About two thirds of patients with acute cholecystitis have previously had symptomatic gallstones. Mirizzi's syndrome results from extrinsic compression of the common hepatic or common bile duct by a large stone passing through the cystic duct. Obstructive jaundice may develop. Calcification of the gallbladder (*porcelain gallbladder*) is an uncommon condition, but of special significance because of its frequent association with carcinoma of the gallbladder. The diagnosis is made from the radiographic demonstration of an eggshell-like rim of calcium in the gallbladder wall. Adenocarcinoma of the gallbladder is found mainly in elderly patients with cholelithiasis, most of whom have had biliary symptoms for many years.

TREATMENT. Dietary changes, anticholinergics, and antispasmodics have no effect on the course of the disease, but they sometimes provide temporary symptomatic relief. Analgesics should be used for relief of pain. *Cholecystectomy* is the treatment of choice. At operation the common bile duct is inspected, a cholangiogram is obtained, and the common duct is explored if there is evidence of choledocholithiasis.

Cholecystectomy relieves symptoms from gallstones; the postcholecystectomy syndrome is discussed later in this chapter. Loss of the gallbladder does not impair gastrointestinal function. The mortality in elective cholecystectomy is less than 0.5 per cent. In patients over 70 years of age, however, mortality rises to 2 to 3 per cent; most of the postoperative deaths are a result of pre-existing cardiopulmonary diseases.

Acute Cholecystitis

PATHOGENESIS. Acute cholecystitis is the result of cystic duct obstruction and chemical irritation rather than of bacterial infection. Filling the gallbladder of a dog with concentrated bile and obstructing the cystic duct produce acute inflammation. If the gallbladder is empty or distended with physiologic saline solution instead of bile, cystic duct obstruction is tolerated without inflammation. Obstruction is associated with the release of phospholipase from the gallbladder epithelium that can hydrolyze lecithin, releasing lysolecithin, an epithelial toxin. Simultaneously the epithelial barrier coating of mucin glycoproteins may be acutely disrupted, making the epithelium susceptible to injury by the detergent action of the concentrated bile salts.

Bacterial infection is secondary to biliary obstruction rather than being primary. Bacteria are not present in the gallbladders of asymptomatic or chronically symptomatic patients with cholesterol or black pigment gallstones. Early in acute cholecystitis, the gallbladder bile is sterile, but within a week after onset, bacteria may be present in bile in over 50 per cent of cases. Although infection is secondary, it may be ultimately responsible for the most serious sequelae of acute cholecystitis—empyema, gangrene, and perforation.

Acalculous cholecystitis, accounting for less than 5 per cent of cases, is more common in men and in patients with unrelated sepsis. Most cases have been associated with prolonged fasting after major trauma, e.g., war or automobile accident injuries, surgical operations, or severe burns. Rare cases are caused by *Salmonella typhosa*, polyarteritis nodosa, or ischemia of other causes. At operation the bile is viscous and full of sludge. Gangrene and perforation are more frequent, and the outcome is generally worse than in acute calculous cholecystitis.

PATHOLOGY. Early inflammation with subserosal edema, mucosal ulcerations, and submucosal hemorrhages progresses slowly to cellular infiltration of the wall after three to four days, which reaches its greatest intensity at the end of the first week. During the second week, patchy mural gangrene, small intramural abscesses, and collagen deposition appear. Resolution of the acute changes takes another week or more.

The term *empyema* describes the rare entity of a pus-filled gallbladder characterized clinically by a septic form of acute cholecystitis. Gangrene and perforation are most common in the fundus where the blood supply is meager or in the neck where stones become impacted. With perforation, gallbladder contents may spill into the free abdominal cavity (bile peritonitis) or, more often, are confined by adhesions (pericholecystic abscess). Sometimes an adherent viscus is penetrated, forming a cholecystenteric fistula through which the gallstones and pus may be discharged. Fistulization is most frequent with the duodenum, but jejunal and colonic fistulas have been described.

CLINICAL MANIFESTATIONS. An attack of acute cholecystitis begins with *abdominal pain* that increases gradually in severity. The pain is usually located in the right subcostal region from the start, but it sometimes begins in the epigastrium or left upper quadrant and then shifts to the region of the gallbladder as inflammation progresses. Two thirds or more of patients have had previous episodes of typical biliary pain. Early in the attack the patient may expect the symptoms to subside spontaneously as had happened before with similar pain, and medical aid is often not sought until 48 hours or more. Referred pain may be experienced in the back at the scapular level. Patients in their 70's and 80's may have few or no localizing symptoms.

Anorexia, nausea, and vomiting are often present, but vomiting is rarely severe enough to be confused with bowel obstruction and is generally less than in acute pancreatitis. In the absence of complications, chills are rare, and the temperature is about 38°C. Chills and high temperature suggest suppurative cholecystitis or associated cholangitis.

The right subcostal region is tender to palpation, and involuntary muscle spasm generally limits the examination. If the patient takes a deep breath while the subhepatic area is being palpated, heightened tenderness arrests inspiration (*Murphy's sign*).

In somewhat less than a quarter of the patients, a distended, tender gallbladder can be distinctly felt, an important finding that confirms the suspected diagnosis. The gallbladder cannot be felt in the rest of the patients because of obesity, rigidity of the abdominal wall, deep subhepatic location, or because it is small and shrunken from previous inflammation. Other related conditions characterized by a tender mass in the same area are pericholecystic abscess, acute cholecystitis complicating carcinoma of the gallbladder, torsion of the gallbladder, or gallbladder distension in obstructive cholangitis.

About 20 per cent of patients with acute cholecystitis have *mild jaundice* caused by edema of the nearby common duct or more likely by common duct stones. Rarely a tumor of the bile ducts is the underlying cause.

With treatment, improvement is usually noticeable within the first 12 to 24 hours, and the signs and symptoms gradually subside over three to seven days. Persistent severe pain, a rise in temperature or leukocyte count (> 10,000 per cubic millimeter), and appearance of shaking chills or of more severe local or generalized abdominal tenderness all indicate progression of the disease and suggest the need for surgery.

Empyema (suppurative cholecystitis) can produce systemic toxicity and mild increases in bilirubin, alkaline phosphatase, and the transaminases and may herald perforation. If this severe infection is controlled with antimicrobial drugs, a large tender gallbladder may remain palpable for several weeks, and return of well-being is similarly prolonged.

DIAGNOSIS. The diagnosis is strongly suggested by the clinical manifestations just described. Roentgenograms of the abdomen may show calcified gallstones or an enlarged gallbladder. Ultrasonography is probably the simplest and most reliable method of detecting gallbladder stones in these patients. Oral cholecystography is diagnostically unreliable because of unpredictable absorption and excretion of the contrast agent.

Radionuclide scanning following intravenous administration of 99mTc DISIDA or related compounds is the procedure of choice to verify a clinical impression of acute cholecystitis. If the gallbladder fills, the diagnosis of acute cholecystitis is quite unlikely. If the bile duct fills but the gallbladder does not, the diagnosis is strongly supported.

In the differential diagnosis, acute pancreatitis, acute appendicitis, and penetrated or perforated peptic ulcer are the conditions that most often cause major problems. Furthermore, acute cholecystitis and acute pancreatitis may coexist.

In women, *gonococcal perihepatitis* (Fitz-Hugh-Curtis syndrome), caused by intra-abdominal spread of the infection from the reproductive tract to the right upper quadrant, may be mistaken for acute cholecystitis, but adnexal tenderness is usually present on pelvic examination. A cervical smear usually reveals gonococci, and the patients are younger, often have higher temperature, and are in less distress than would be expected with cholecystitis. Shoulder pain and a friction rub over the liver, common in the Fitz-Hugh–Curtis syndrome, are not found in uncomplicated acute cholecystitis.

Acute hepatitis, either viral or alcoholic, sometimes produces marked right upper quadrant pain and tenderness. A history of recent binge drinking, high transaminase levels, and liver biopsy aid differentiation. Pneumonitis, pyelonephritis, and acute cardiac disease (particularly right-sided failure) all on occasion may cause acute pain suggestive of cholecystitis.

The use of 99mTc DISIDA will distinguish between the unusual location of pain in these disorders and acute cholecystitis.

TREATMENT. Most patients with acute cholecystitis will improve with either expectant treatment or cholecystectomy performed during the acute attack. In general, the decision regarding the kind of treatment should include the following considerations (Fig. 130–6): (1) whether the diagnosis is secure, (2) whether biliary complications have occurred or appear imminent, and (3) the overall condition of the patient (operative risk).

Upon the patient's admission to the hospital, nasogastric suction should be started if the patient has significant vomiting, and fluids should be given intravenously to correct dehydration. In many elderly patients the acute biliary condition may aggravate pre-existing cardiac, pulmonary, or renal disease and produce a more ominous prognosis if surgery is delayed or if adequate treatment is not given.

Antimicrobials are of principal value to prevent bacteremia and to treat suppurative complications. If the patient is seen shortly after symptoms begin, and if local signs and symptoms are mild, antimicrobial therapy need not be given. Otherwise, an antimicrobial regimen with coverage for gram-negative aerobes as well as enterococci is preferred. One that is often used is ampicillin plus gentamicin given parenterally. In seriously ill patients, such as those with empyema or perforation, it is wise to also add an antimicrobial with anaerobic coverage, such as clindamycin.

Cholecystectomy is generally considered the optimal therapy for acute cholecystitis, but only after the diagnosis is confirmed and the patient adequately prepared for operation. Many physicians still prefer to reserve surgery during the acute attack for those patients who develop complications and for those who become worse or fail to improve. Although this is still common practice, about 25 per cent of patients managed in this way require urgent operation for worsening disease. For patients who respond to nonoperative management, interval cholecystectomy is generally recommended. The timing of cholecystectomy in such patients has been debated, but the trend is to perform surgery later during the same hospitalization.

About 30 per cent of patients are good surgical risks; in these patients the diagnosis is obvious within 12 to 24 hours, and cholecystectomy can be scheduled promptly. Another 30 per cent are good surgical candidates, but the diagnosis is not quite firm. In this situation, a 99mTc DISIDA scan should be obtained to verify the clinical impression. Another 30 per cent of patients will have serious coexistent cardiac, respiratory, or other disease for which treatment takes precedence. The cholecystitis should be treated expectantly while the other problems are being corrected. Progression of local abdominal findings requires continued re-evaluation, balancing the risks of operation with the risks of continued delay.

About 10 per cent of patients require emergency surgery

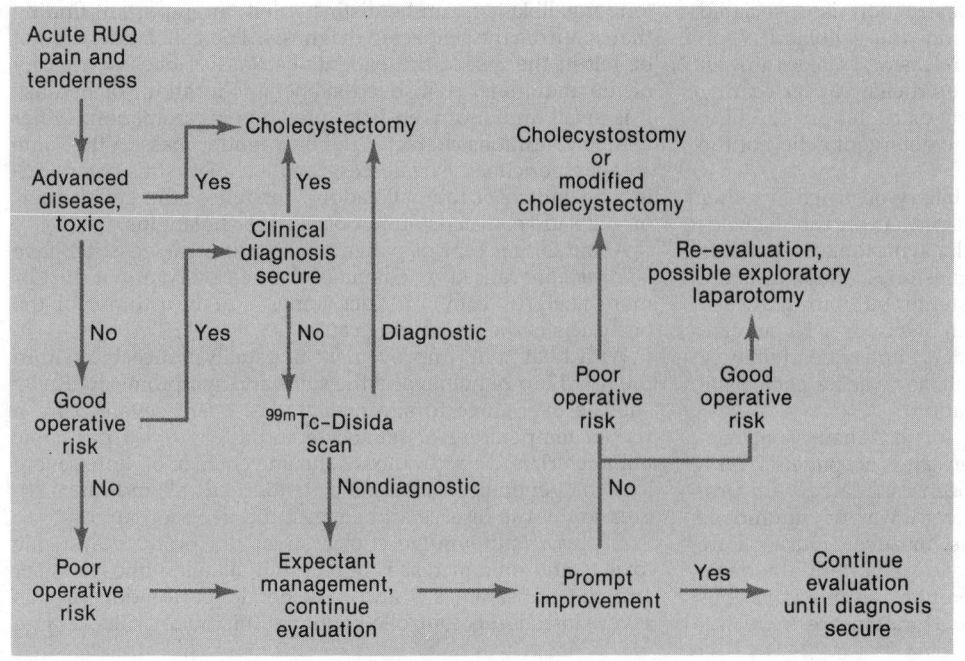

FIGURE 130–6. Schema for managing patients with right upper quadrant pain and tenderness who are thought possibly to have acute cholecystitis. This approach is based on a policy of early operation for appropriate patients and distinguishes between patients who are good versus poor operative risks.

for complications present on admission or that appear later during observation and medical management. When emergency operation becomes necessary, cholecystostomy may sometimes be preferable to cholecystectomy in the seriously ill patient. In this procedure the fundus is incised, stones and pus are removed from the lumen, and the organ is decompressed by catheter drainage, allowing the acute infection to resolve. Patients who recover should undergo cholecystectomy six to eight weeks later. Those who continue to be poor surgical risks may be followed expectantly if postoperative cholecystography shows that the gallbladder and common duct contain no residual stones. If stones are present, interventional radiologic techniques can be used to remove gallbladder stones through the cholecystomy tract after four to six weeks of tract maturation, and endoscopic sphincterotomy can be utilized to remove ductal stones. In seriously debilitated patients the cholecystostomy tube can be left in place indefinitely.

After the cholecystostomy tube is removed from a patient whose biliary system contains no calculi, within the first year about 50 per cent of patients develop new stones. Eventually 90 per cent of patients will again develop stones.

COMPLICATIONS. *Emphysematous Cholecystitis.* In emphysematous cholecystitis, a rare variant of acute cholecystitis, gas of bacterial origin can be seen in the gallbladder lumen and adjacent tissues. Clinically, emphysematous cholecystitis causes the same signs and symptoms as acute cholecystitis. Men are affected twice as frequently as women, about 30 per cent of patients have diabetes mellitus, and the gallbladder is acalculous in about half the cases. Gas does not develop until 24 to 48 hours after the attack begins, at which time a radiolucent halo outlines the lumen, and an air-fluid level may be seen on upright films. Subserosal and then pericholecystic emphysema appear with time. Differential diagnosis of the radiographic findings includes cholecystenteric fistula and appendiceal, perinephric, or subhepatic abscess. In about half the cases the gas-forming organisms are clostridia, and the rest are *Escherichia coli*, streptococci, and other bacteria of intestinal origin. Treatment is the same as for acute cholecystitis, but the somewhat more aggressive nature of emphysematous cholecystitis and the association with diabetes mellitus usually require prompt surgery.

Perforation. Perforation is usually manifested by greater sepsis and more marked abdominal signs. Perforation may take any of three forms: (1) free perforation into the abdominal cavity, (2) localized (contained) perforation with pericholecystic abscess, and (3) perforation into another viscus with fistula formation.

Free perforation, which has a 25 per cent mortality, is the least common type. It usually occurs early in the attack, often within the first three days, suggesting that when gangrene develops this quickly it cannot be walled off by adjacent viscera or the omentum. Clinically, free perforation classically causes toxicity with high temperatures (greater than 39°C), leukocytosis (over 15,000 per cubic millimeter), and diffuse abdominal tenderness and rigidity. In more than half the cases the correct diagnosis is unsuspected until laparotomy or autopsy, because a clear-cut history of preliminary right upper quadrant pain is often lacking. Treatment consists of intravenous antimicrobial therapy and emergency laparotomy with cholecystectomy.

Localized perforation most often appears in the second week of the attack at the peak of the inflammatory reaction. The diagnosis should be suspected with increasing local signs, especially when a mass suddenly appears. In most cases cholecystectomy can be performed, but in a severely ill patient cholecystostomy and drainage of the abscess may be wiser.

Fistula Formation. A fistula usually involves the nearby second portion of the duodenum or, less commonly, the colon, jejunum, stomach, or common bile duct. Rare fistulas have entered the renal pelvis or bronchus or extended through the abdominal wall (empyema necessitatis). After intestinal fistulization the contents of the gallbladder are discharged into the gut, often aborting the acute attack. Clinically, the fistula itself may not be suspected because it produces no unique findings; many are discovered incidentally later. In the absence of biliary obstruction a cholecystenteric fistula is not necessarily of pathophysiologic significance. Cholecystocolonic fistulas may cause malabsorption from diversion of bile or from bacterial overgrowth in the upper gut.

Gallstone Ileus. If a particularly large gallstone enters through the fistula, it may obstruct the intestine, a condition called gallstone ileus. The stone, passing through a cholecystenteric fistula, most often enters the gut in the duodenum, less commonly in the jejunum, ileum, colon, or stomach. It is often assumed that the initial event responsible for fistula formation is an attack of acute cholecystitis, but only 30 per cent of patients with gallstone ileus give a history of recent right upper quadrant pain. After entering the gut, the gallstone moves downsteam until it encounters an area of intestinal lumen too narrow to accommodate. Gallstones, usually more than 2.5 cm in diameter, most frequently obstruct the terminal ileum; they will block the colon only if its lumen has been narrowed by intrinsic disease.

On physical examination the findings are those of small-bowel obstruction. Infrequently the large stone can be felt as a mass on abdominal, vaginal, or rectal examination, but it is rarely correctly identified. Roentgenograms usually show air in the biliary tree if the films are carefully examined, and in some cases a radiopaque gallstone can be identified at the leading edge of the obstruction. Treatment consists of removing the obstructing gallstone through a small enterotomy. It is generally wise to leave the biliary disease undisturbed initially, because elderly patients tolerate long procedures poorly, and nothing much is gained by repairing the fistula primarily. Postoperatively, many patients remain asymptomatic, and the fistula may even close spontaneously; for them, expectant management is best. Some patients may require cholecystectomy later because of symptoms related to gallstones.

The mortality is 15 to 20 per cent because of delay in diagnosis and because of cardiopulmonary complications.

PROGNOSIS. The mortality in acute cholecystitis of 5 to 10 per cent is almost totally confined to patients over 60 years of age with serious associated disease. Suppurative complications are more common in the elderly, who can tolerate them least. In most instances, localized perforation can be managed satisfactorily at operation. Free perforation is considerably more ominous (25 per cent mortality), but is rare.

Choledocholithiasis and Cholangitis

In Western countries choledocholithiasis is usually the result of passage of gallstones formed in the gallbladder into the common duct. About 10 to 15 per cent of patients with asymptomatic cholecystolithiasis are thought to develop choledocholithiasis on this basis. Once in the common duct the stones may pass into the duodenum without causing symptoms. The frequency of this event is not known, but is probably greatly underestimated. Less commonly, stones form in a dilated duct behind a longstanding obstruction caused by a stricture or ampullary stenosis. About 5 per cent of patients with choledocholithiasis have no gallbladder stones; in such cases it is assumed that all the gallbladder stones escaped into the duct or, more rarely, that the stones formed primarily in the common duct. Stone type helps to determine site of origin: Cholesterol or black pigment stones more likely form in the gallbladder, while almost all brown pigment stones in patients in Western countries form in the bile ducts.

CLINICAL MANIFESTATIONS. The natural history of choledocholithiasis is incompletely known (Fig. 130–7). About 30 to 40 per cent of patients are asymptomatic at the time of

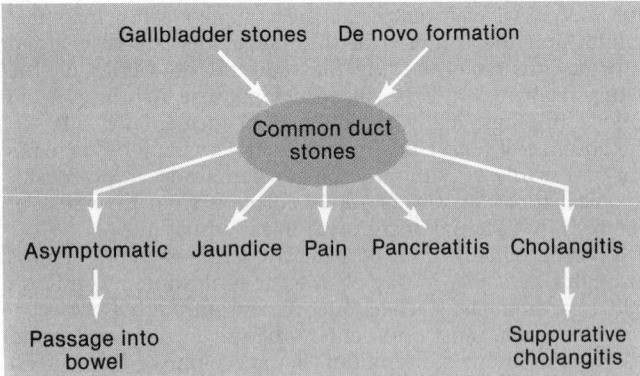

FIGURE 130–7. Natural history of choledocholithiasis. In most cases, common duct gallstones originate in the gallbladder. In some cases, particularly after the gallbladder has been surgically removed, stones may form in the common duct. The majority of stones in the common duct remain asymptomatic and may either remain in the duct without causing symptoms, pass into the bowel through the ampulla of Vater and be excreted in stool, or eventually result in symptoms, the most common of which are indicated. The exact frequency of each of these occurrences is not known.

diagnosis, implying a relatively benign course in many cases. How often asymptomatic stones remain undetected is, of course, unknown. Obstruction by stones of the biliary or pancreatic ducts may produce any of the following syndromes: biliary pain, jaundice or increased alkaline phosphatase alone (without pain), cholangitis, pancreatitis, or a combination of these. Secondary hepatic effects of persistent obstruction include biliary cirrhosis or hepatic abscesses.

Intermittent cholangitis, consisting of biliary pain, jaundice, and fever and chills (Charcot's triad), is the most common presenting symptom complex. In the absence of previous biliary surgery it is almost diagnostic of choledocholithiasis in Western countries. Intermittency of symptoms is quite characteristic, a manifestation of intermittent partial obstruction. Whenever pain, chills with fever, and jaundice fluctuate together over a span of a few days or a week, cholangitis from biliary obstruction is almost certainly the cause. In a typical attack, chills may precede the other symptoms, and bilirubinuria may follow. Epigastric or right upper quadrant pain, indistinguishable from biliary pain caused by gallbladder stones, is steady and very severe. Pain may be referred to the right infrascapular area, the upper back, the right shoulder, or even the precordium, suggesting coronary artery or esophageal disease.

The severity of fever and chills varies widely from the usual mild transient illness to overwhelming sepsis with shock (see Suppurative Cholangitis, below). In the average case, the temperature rises to 38.5 to 40°C, preceded by chills and positive blood cultures. Localized tenderness in the subcostal region may be associated with extreme guarding and rigidity, but more often the local findings are minimal or intermittent and are usually less severe than in acute cholecystitis.

In most cases of common duct obstruction caused by stones the gallbladder does not become distended, because it is scarred and inelastic, and the obstruction is recent, partial, or transient, the obverse of Courvoisier's law, i.e., a distended nontender gallbladder in a jaundiced patient signifies neoplastic obstruction of the bile duct.

DIAGNOSIS. In cholangitis the leukocyte count averages 15,000 per cubic millimeter, but may go much higher in severe cases. Bilirubin values are usually in the range of 2 to 4 mg per deciliter and are uncommonly higher than 10 mg per deciliter. Elevated serum alkaline phosphatase and 5'-nucleotidase levels are usually greater than three times the upper limit of normal. The AST generally remains below 200 units; however, transiently it may exceed 1000 units. In these instances the prompt drop of the AST level within 48 hours allows differentiation from viral hepatitis and suggests the diagnosis of obstruction.

The demonstration of gallbladder stones does not necessarily imply that stones in the bile ducts are responsible for the cholangitis. The same conditions considered for the patient with chronically symptomatic gallstones must be excluded for the patient with biliary pain caused by ductal calculi. In patients who have had cholecystectomy, differentiation between choledocholithiasis and biliary stricture as the cause of cholangitis usually depends on radiologic demonstration of the ducts. When the presenting syndrome is painless cholestatic jaundice, other causes, especially periampullary and biliary neoplasms, must be considered. With neoplastic obstruction, the bilirubin averages about 15 to 20 mg per deciliter and rarely fluctuates. Although jaundice from stones may be as intense, the level of bilirubin is characteristically less than 10 mg per deciliter, and it may rise and fall episodically. The diagnosis of intrahepatic cholestasis from causes such as drugs, viral hepatitis, or pregnancy should follow the schema outlined in Ch. 120. In such cases, opacification of normal bile ducts by PTC or ERCP may ultimately be required. Gallstone disease is common in cirrhosis, so choledocholithiasis and alcoholic liver disease may coexist.

Common duct stones may cause acute pancreatitis indistinguishable clinically from that resulting from alcohol or other causes and unaccompanied by specific signs of biliary disease (Ch. 108). Pancreatitis caused by biliary calculi, despite numerous attacks, rarely progresses to pancreatic calcification, chronic pain, and pancreatic insufficiency, as so often occurs in the alcoholic variety. Gallstone disease should be ruled out in every patient with acute pancreatitis, because further damage during such an episode and future attacks can be avoided if the gallstones are removed.

TREATMENT. The potential seriousness of cholangitis warrants hospitalization for diagnosis and treatment. After blood cultures are obtained, antimicrobial drugs effective against enteric organisms are given by the parenteral route. A regimen consisting of an aminoglycoside plus ampicillin for mild attacks with the addition of clindamycin in severe infection is usually successful. Failure to obtain a rapid response may mean that the organisms were not susceptible to the initial drugs, justifying the addition of another drug or a shift from the initial regimen on the basis of the result of cultures and drug susceptibility tests. The margin between mild and severe illness is small; antimicrobial therapy should be expected to control the acute attack within 48 to 72 hours, and if there is no improvement or worsening after this period, emergency surgery or endoscopic sphincterotomy must be considered seriously.

More than 90 per cent of patients respond satisfactorily to treatment, allowing an orderly attempt at diagnosis. Ultrasonography should be performed first to detect ductal dilatation. Direct opacification of the ducts can be attempted by PTC or ERCP. Both kinds of direct cholangiography are potentially hazardous in active cholangitis and should be postponed if possible until infection is well controlled; then one proceeds only under the protection of antimicrobial therapy. However, decompression of the bile duct using a percutaneous transhepatic catheter or by endoscopic sphincterotomy may provide the control needed when there is evidence of duct obstruction.

Deciding between endoscopic and surgical approaches to the management of choledocholithiasis should be on a case by case basis. If the gallbladder is present, cholecystectomy is performed and the common duct is opened and emptied of stones. A T tube is usually left in the duct to decompress biliary pressure in the postoperative period and to provide a route for subsequent cholangiography. With accurate diagnosis and treatment, choledocholithiasis is cured by cholecystectomy and choledocholithotomy. Recurrent ductal stone formation occurs infrequently except when the duct has become markedly dilated.

Selected patients with choledocholithiasis may be satisfactorily treated by endoscopic sphincterotomy. By means of the side-viewing duodenoscope, a wire (papillotome) is passed into the bile duct and the sphincter divided by electrocautery. Common duct stones 1.5 cm or smaller will usually pass into the duodenum. This technique may be unsuccessful with large stones or when the common duct is greatly dilated. Bleeding and pancreatitis are the principal complications, but are infrequent. Mortality in the procedure is less than 1 per cent in experienced hands. When endoscopic sphincterotomy is successfully used for cholangitis in patients with gallbladder stones, there is debate about whether to perform cholecystectomy at a later date. In our opinion this decision should be based on whether the patient subsequently develops symptoms referable to the gallbladder stones.

RETAINED COMMON DUCT STONES. The methods for detecting duct stones at operation are about 95 per cent reliable, which means, unfortunately, that a few are overlooked only to be discovered on postoperative T-tube cholangiograms. There are two approaches to remove residual stones without another laparotomy. Neither method should be tried until four to six weeks postoperatively to allow for maturation of the T-tube tract. One technique depends on the ability of mono-octanoin (glyceryl-1-mono-octanoate) to dissolve cholesterol gallstones. Mono-octanoin is infused into the duct at 5 ml per hour; care must be exercised to avoid producing pressures in the duct greater than 30 cm H_2O during infusion. The retained stones disappear in about one half of patients within a four- to eight-day treatment period. There is no solvent known to be effective against black pigment stones. Mono-octanoin has been partially successful for brown pigment stones.

Instrumental extraction is somewhat simpler and faster and is the treatment of choice. Under image-intensification fluoroscopy the T tube is pulled out, a Dormia ureteral basket is passed into the duct, and the stone is grasped and withdrawn. The best plan usually is to try instrumental extraction first and dissolution if it fails. If neither mechanical extraction nor chemical dissolution is successful, endoscopic sphincterotomy may allow the stone to pass into the duodenum. If that technique is unsuccessful, reoperation is necessary.

SUPPURATIVE CHOLANGITIS. The most severe form of cholangitis, suppurative cholangitis, involves the same causative factors as the "nonsuppurative" form, but differs in that obstruction is complete, ductal contents become purulent, and clinically the manifestations of sepsis overshadow those of cholestasis. Hypotension and mental changes such as lethargy or confusion appear in addition to right upper quadrant pain, chills, fever, and jaundice. Some elderly patients may be hypothermic and have minimal clinical signs. Because infection in the face of the high-grade obstruction progresses so rapidly the serum bilirubin does not reach very high levels before the patient becomes moribund from sepsis. Costly delays in diagnosis are frequent, a consequence of failure to recognize the significance of mild icterus and abdominal pain in a patient with sepsis. All but a few cases involve complications of choledocholithiasis, the others occurring with biliary stricture or neoplastic obstruction, usually from bile duct carcinoma with or without sclerosing cholangitis.

Laboratory tests reveal evidence of cholestasis with bilirubin values between 2 and 5 mg per deciliter and elevated serum levels of alkaline phosphatase, 5'-nucleotidase, and transaminases. The leukocyte count varies from subnormal to 40,000 per cubic millimeter. Hypoglycemia may sometimes be present.

Tenderness to palpation is present in the right upper quadrant, but rigidity is uncommon. In some cases secondary cholecystitis develops, and an enlarged tender gallbladder may be found on abdominal examination. Ultrasonography may show dilated bile ducts. Diagnosis rests on recognizing the evidence of biliary obstruction and its relationship to the sepsis and on verifying the initial impression by ultrasonography. After initial resuscitation—consisting of intravenous infusions, antimicrobial drugs (gentamicin or tobramycin plus ampicillin and clindamycin parenterally), and measures to restore cardiac, pulmonary, or renal function—decompression of the duct by emergency laparotomy, percutaneous transhepatic catheter placement, or endoscopic sphincterotomy offers the only hope of saving the patient. Biliary stents have been placed endoscopically to reduce obstruction and systemic sepsis.

At surgery when choledochotomy is performed, pus often squirts from the duct as a result of the high pressure. If the patient's condition permits, thorough exploration can be carried out to correct the obstruction by removing stones, repairing a stricture, or bypassing a tumor. Insertion of a T tube proximal to the obstruction is sufficient in patients who are unable to tolerate a longer operation, but sometime later it will be necessary to perform a second more definitive procedure before the T tube can be removed. The mortality is about 50 per cent, resulting from septic shock, renal or respiratory failure, acute hepatic insufficiency, or a combination of these complications.

Other Causes of Bile Duct Obstruction

Duodenal and pancreatic tumors are common causes of obstruction in the middle-aged or elderly. These important diseases are discussed in Ch. 107 and 109. Common bile duct obstruction may also be caused by a variety of uncommon disorders such as sclerosing cholangitis in patients with ulcerative colitis or by Oriental cholangiohepatitis in immigrants from Southeast Asia. Rare causes are compression by neoplastic paraductal lymph nodes or by duodenal Crohn's disease.

SCLEROSING CHOLANGITIS. Sclerosing cholangitis, a condition of unknown cause, consists of benign nonbacterial chronic inflammatory narrowing of the bile ducts. The entire ductal system is involved in most cases; less commonly the process may be confined to the extrahepatic or intrahepatic portion. The ratio of males to females is 3:2, and the peak incidence occurs in the third and fourth decades. More than half of the cases are associated with *ulcerative colitis* (Ch. 105) and, to a lesser extent, *regional enteritis*. The severity of sclerosing cholangitis does not parallel the activity of the colitis, and colectomy does not improve the cholangitis. Other much less commonly associated diseases are retroperitoneal fibrosis and Riedel's thyroiditis.

The initial complaint may be jaundice or pruritus, although more cases are being discovered at an asymptomatic stage. There may be mild upper abdominal pain and sometimes fever, but a clinical picture resembling bacterial cholangitis is uncommon in the absence of previous surgical exploration or instrumentation of the ducts. Hepatomegaly may be present in some cases; when secondary cirrhosis develops, ascites or splenomegaly may be found.

Jaundice may be constant or fluctuating, and bilirubin values are usually in the range of 2 to 10 mg per deciliter. The alkaline phosphatase is always increased, usually greater than three times the upper limit of normal, and remains increased despite variations in clinical manifestations. Transaminases are usually mildly increased. Antimitochondrial antibodies are normal.

Percutaneous transhepatic cholangiography or preferably endoscopic retrograde cholangiopancreatography is required to establish the diagnosis. The radiographs show diffuse or focal irregular ductal narrowing with intervening areas of normal caliber or dilatation; this "beaded" appearance is characteristic. Some patients develop gallstones behind the strictured areas as a result of stasis; these are usually brown pigment gallstones. Localized strictures may be difficult to distinguish from ductal carcinoma.

Treatment with corticosteroids or immunosuppressants has not been proved to be generally effective, but a few patients do respond. A trial of treatment is advocated by some experts. Cholestyramine is useful for pruritus. Antimicrobials are necessary if bacterial cholangitis develops.

In symptomatic patients the aim of therapy is to relieve biliary obstruction. If a segmental stricture is present, balloon dilatation can be attempted either percutaneously or, if the lesion is in the common bile duct, endoscopically. This involves the insertion into the bile duct of a balloon-tipped catheter; inflation of the balloon stretches the narrowed area and allows greater bile flow. Balloon dilatation may have to be repeated intermittently to provide sustained relief of obstruction; there is the risk of inducing bacterial cholangitis, particularly with the endoscopic approach. Percutaneous catheter drainage is another option, but often does not provide adequate drainage of all obstructed areas in diffuse disease. Surgical therapy is warranted in some cases to provide stenting in diffuse disease or to bypass severe distal common bile duct disease. Significant palliation follows surgery in most cases, but is not usually permanent. Most patients have episodic remissions and exacerbations, during which secondary biliary cirrhosis develops. Liver transplantation is now an option for those with advanced disease. Death may follow uncontrollable biliary sepsis with hepatic abscesses, liver failure, or bleeding from esophageal varices.

STRUCTURAL ABNORMALITIES. *Choledochal cysts* occasionally produce their initial clinical manifestations in young adults, presenting with jaundice, pain, or cholangitis. Diagnosis requires direct ductal visualization with PTC or ERCP; computed tomography or ultrasonography can provide information about surrounding structures. The most definitive surgical procedure is excision of the cyst, followed by Roux-en-Y choledochojejunostomy.

Caroli's disease, consisting of saccular intrahepatic bile duct dilations, most often becomes symptomatic in patients between the ages of 20 and 50 years, because of intrahepatic stone formation and cholangitis. Two forms are recognized: (1) disease of the ducts only and (2) ductal disease associated with hepatic fibrosis and medullary sponge kidney (more common). The latter patients often have complications of portal hypertension before cholangitis or obstructive jaundice appears. Antimicrobial therapy may control attacks of cholangitis, and surgical procedures to facilitate ductal emptying or to extract stones may help in some cases, but the intrahepatic anomaly cannot be definitively corrected unless lobectomy is possible for single lobe involvement.

PANCREATITIS. Pancreatitis can produce transient jaundice by obstruction of the distal common duct where it is surrounded by pancreatic tissue. Prolonged obstruction can result from pressure by an adjacent pseudocyst or entrapment of the distal common bile duct in severe pancreatic scarring from *chronic pancreatitis.* Diagnosis may be delayed in alcoholic patients in whom elevated alkaline phosphatase or bilirubin values are usually attributed to hepatocellular disease. Persistent elevation of the alkaline phosphatase value in an alcoholic should raise suspicion of the possibility of biliary obstruction, particularly if pancreatic calcification is present on plain abdominal radiographs. Jaundice resulting from chronic pancreatitis requires choledochoduodenostomy or Roux-en-Y anastomosis of jejunum to the common bile duct.

HEMOBILIA. Hemobilia classically presents with biliary pain, obstructive jaundice, and occult or gross intestinal bleeding. Most cases are caused by hepatic injury from external or operative trauma, with secondary bleeding into the ductal system. Other causes include biliary or hepatic neoplasms, ductal rupture of a hepatic artery aneurysm, hepatic abscess, and gallstones, or it may follow percutaneous needle biopsy of the liver or cholangiography. Hemobilia following

trauma is best treated by hepatic artery ligation, which is well tolerated except when there is advanced parenchymal disease; otherwise, direct management of the causative lesion is necessary.

PARASITIC DISEASE. An *echinococcal hepatic cyst* can rupture into the ducts and can give rise to biliary colic, jaundice, and cholangitis (Ch. 397). *Ascariasis* may produce biliary colic, jaundice, and cholangitis by worm invasion into the bile ducts from the duodenum (Ch. 406).

ORIENTAL CHOLANGIOHEPATITIS. Oriental cholangiohepatitis or *recurrent pyogenic cholangitis* is a common form of recurrent cholangitis in the Orient associated with brown pigment gallstone formation throughout the biliary tract. The cause is unclear, but the parasite *Clonorchis sinensis* is found in very few cases so does not seem to be a major causative factor. Most patients present with acute cholangitis; those with recurrent cholangitis may develop liver abscesses, biliary-enteric fistulas, or sepsis. In advanced cases, one (usually the left) or both lobar ducts may become honeycombed with scars or abscesses, producing atrophy of the hepatic parenchyma.

Direct cholangiography is necessary for a definitive diagnosis. Sphincteroplasty or choledochojejunostomy is usually performed to remove stones and sludge and provide adequate biliary drainage. Cholecystectomy or partial hepatic resection is required when the gallbladder or localized hepatic segments are involved.

BILIARY STRICTURE. Biliary stricture almost always results from *surgical injury* to the duct and usually follows cholecystectomy rather than procedures on the duct itself such as common duct exploration. Biliary stricture may also result from external trauma or scarring produced by choledocholithiasis.

The symptoms resemble those of cholangitis with choledocholithiasis. Differential diagnosis includes all the various causes of obstructive jaundice and cholangitis. Laboratory evidence consists of leukocytosis and elevated serum levels of bilirubin, alkaline phosphatase, and transaminases. The jaundice and cholangitis are generally mild and transient, and infection generally responds promptly to antimicrobial therapy. Diagnosis can be made with visualization of the biliary tract by either PTC or ERCP. With persistent obstruction over several years, secondary biliary cirrhosis or multiple intrahepatic abscesses may develop.

In almost all cases an attempt should be made to repair the stricture surgically by creating a new unobstructed conduit between normal duct on the hepatic side of the lesion and the proximal intestine rather than attempting direct end-to-end anastomosis of the duct after excision of the lesion. The overall success rate of these operations is about 75 per cent with an operative mortality of 10 per cent.

Balloon catheter dilatation of a short stricture at the time of either PTC or ERCP may be useful in some patients, particularly those who are poor operative risks.

Carcinoma of the Gallbladder

In the United States there are approximately 2500 deaths annually from carcinoma of the gallbladder, a number equal to the mortality from benign disease of the biliary tract. Gallbladder cancer accounts for 1 per cent of all cancer deaths and 3 per cent of gastrointestinal malignant disease. Women are affected more frequently than men by a ratio of 3 to 1, and the average age is 70 years. Because 70 to 80 per cent of cases occur in patients with gallstones, cholelithiasis is thought to be etiologically important, but the mechanism involved is unclear. Gallbladder cancer develops in fewer than 1 per cent of patients with cholelithiasis. The disease is five to ten times more frequent in American Indian populations.

Almost all gallbladder carcinomas are *adenocarcinomas;* the earliest spread is usually by metastasis to the hilar lymph nodes and adjacent hepatic parenchyma followed by direct extension to the liver and hilar structures. Distant metastases appear relatively late.

Patients have one of the following clinical pictures: (1) unremitting deep jaundice from common duct and hepatic involvement; (2) acute cholecystitis, usually with a palpable mass; (3) chronic intermittent right upper quadrant pain; and 4) advanced disseminated carcinoma. The diagnosis is not often considered preoperatively, but in some instances clinical clues are present. In about two thirds of patients a mass can be felt, and in one third there is local tenderness. In all but a few cases the gallbladder is not opacified during oral cholecystography, and even when it is, the tumor can rarely be demonstrated. The diagnosis can be suspected on ultrasound study if an intraluminal gallbladder mass is identified that does not change with position. The differential diagnosis is that of a cholesterol polyp or of a stone adherent to the gallbladder wall. Pathologic studies indicate that all apparent tumor would be removed in 25 per cent of cases by cholecystectomy, resection of a rim of adjacent liver, and dissection of the common duct lymph node chain. Even in this favorable group the five-year survival rate is 5 per cent. Most patients live for only a few months after the diagnosis.

Benign Tumors and Pseudotumors of the Gallbladder

Adenomyomatous hyperplasia, also called *adenomyomatosis*, is the most common of the benign tumors and pseudotumors of the gallbladder; there is hyperplasia of the mucosa with formation of intramural diverticula. The cause is unknown. Typically, neoplastic or inflammatory changes are absent. Adenomyomatosis is usually diagnosed by oral cholecystography as a diffuse, segmental, or focal sessile filling defect with a central umbilication and small peripheral opaque areas representing diverticula. Most often adenomyomatosis is asymptomatic. A few cases are associated with typical biliary pain that can be cured by cholecystectomy.

Cholesterolosis (strawberry gallbladder) is a condition of unknown cause characterized by an accumulation of cholesterol and other lipids in macrophages in the gallbladder mucosa. Unlike cholesterol gallstones, it does not appear to be necessarily related to biliary supersaturation with cholesterol. *Cholesterol polyps* are a focal form of cholesterolosis consisting of a core of macrophages filled with cholesterol covered with epithelium located at a villous tip. Generally, multiple polyps are present. The polyp is attached to the mucosa by a fragile stalk that can easily be broken. Cholesterol polyps appear on oral cholecystography or ultrasonography as a fixed filling defect on the gallbladder wall that does not change with position; in contrast to gallstones, no acoustic shadowing is seen on ultrasonography. Unless cholesterol polyps are present, cholesterolosis is difficult to detect by oral cholecystography. Most patients with cholesterolosis are asymptomatic. Some patients have concomitant gallstones and, if symptoms are present, they are attributed to the gallstones. Those few patients with cholesterolosis without gallstones who have typical biliary pain are often relieved by cholecystectomy.

Papillary and nonpapillary adenomas are benign neoplasms of the gallbladder. They are much less common than cholesterol polyps. Most adenomas are pedunculated; about two thirds are multiple. They appear as filling defects on oral cholecystography. Carcinoma in situ is found in about 5 per cent of adenomas, but the relationship between gallbladder adenomas and carcinoma is not clear.

Tumors of the Bile Duct

The main cause of early morbidity from tumors of the bile duct is biliary obstruction with gradual hepatocellular damage or secondary hepatobiliary infection. Tumors of the bile ducts are rarely benign. Papilloma, the most frequent, is often multifocal and therefore difficult to cure. Adenomas and granular cell tumors are localized, but are often difficult to treat surgically without radical excision. This section will be directed primarily to discussion of malignant tumors, but many of the same principles of pathophysiology and diagnosis will apply to the rare benign tumors.

Except for a rare squamous cell tumor, malignant bile duct tumors are adenocarcinomas with either a scirrhous or a papillary pattern. Grossly, three types of pathologic presentations occur: *focal stricture, diffuse thickening,* and *nodular mass.* The first two varieties can easily be mistaken for a benign process such as post-traumatic stricture or sclerosing cholangitis. In many cases, spread is confined to local lymph node metastases or hepatic invasion for months or years before there is more widespread abdominal or systemic involvement. The common hepatic duct or common bile duct is the site of origin in about two thirds of the cases. The eponym *Klatskin tumor* is often used to refer to adenocarcinoma at the bifurcation of the common hepatic duct. In contrast with carcinoma of the gallbladder, cholelithiasis is found in only one third of patients, and men slightly outnumber women. The average age at diagnosis is 70 years. A number of cases have been reported in younger patients with ulcerative colitis. Since some of these patients have previously undergone colectomy, it is thought that elimination of the diseased colon is not protective. Sclerosing cholangitis is a recognized complication in these same patients and may have identical clinical features, especially when it primarily affects the extrahepatic bile ducts. Caroli's disease and choledochal cysts are also associated with the development of carcinoma in a small percentage of cases. In the Orient, infestation with *Clonorchis sinensis* probably contributes to the higher incidence of bile duct carcinoma.

CLINICAL MANIFESTATIONS. The typical patient presents with unremitting severe jaundice, mild deep-seated upper abdominal pain, and weight loss. Pruritus is reported by many, usually but not always after the onset of jaundice. Pain, present in more than half the patients, is not colicky and tends to be steady; fever and chills are absent. Hepatomegaly without splenomegaly is found on abdominal examination. Tumors of the common duct sparing the cystic duct often produce in addition to jaundice a distended nontender palpable gallbladder (*Courvoisier's law*).

The serum bilirubin value exceeds 10 mg per deciliter in most cases, with a mean between 15 and 20 mg per deciliter. Complete obstruction of the ductal system results in a bilirubin value of 30 mg per deciliter or higher. The alkaline phosphatase is almost always increased, often more than ten-fold, and AST may be slightly elevated, although rarely higher than 200 units per liter. Obstruction of the right or left hepatic system alone causes a 10- to 30-fold increase in alkaline phosphatase with normal levels of bilirubin. Serum proteins are most often normal. The prothrombin time may be prolonged, but responds to parenteral vitamin K. Serum cholesterol is usually increased and averages about 400 mg per deciliter.

DIAGNOSIS. Ultrasonography or computed tomography shows dilatation of the intrahepatic bile ducts. Transhepatic or retrograde cholangiography demonstrates marked ductal dilatation and the site of the block.

The differential diagnosis includes primary biliary cirrhosis and drug-induced cholestatic jaundice. In neither of these conditions does the bilirubin generally reach levels over 12 to 15 mg per deciliter. Xanthelasma, found often with primary biliary cirrhosis, is only rarely seen with neoplastic obstruction. Antimitochondrial antibodies can be demonstrated in the serum of most patients with primary biliary cirrhosis. Sclerosing cholangitis, usually associated with chronic inflammatory bowel disease, is characterized by intermittent attacks of pain, jaundice, and fever. It also shows a characteristic pattern on transhepatic cholangiography or ERCP although it may be difficult to distinguish focal disease from carcinoma.

Choledocholithiasis and postoperative biliary stricture are less likely to present with deepening jaundice and weight loss. The jaundice fluctuates, is milder, and is usually associated with fever. PTC or ERCP will help to differentiate these diseases.

TREATMENT. Unfortunately, complete excision of the tumor is often impossible, because nonexpendable anatomic structures are involved early. Nevertheless, a few cures can be expected when radical surgery is judiciously employed, and palliation is often lengthy and of excellent quality.

Distal lesions require radical pancreaticoduodenectomy (Whipple's procedure) for complete removal. Because this operation has a 15 per cent mortality, it should be performed only if no gross tumor would be left behind. Tumors of the midportion of the common bile duct are sometimes amenable to complete resection. Localized tumors of the bifurcation of the hepatic duct can sometimes be treated by excision, even though microscopic deposits of tumor usually remain in the bed of the dissection. Reconstruction involves use of a Roux-en-Y hepaticojejunostomy. Radiotherapy with either external beam or intraluminal rods may provide some benefit.

For tumors with local or distant spread the goal is palliation. The treatment of choice is percutaneous or endoscopic stenting of the biliary tract with catheters having multiple portholes above and below the point of bile duct obstruction. Either type of tube can be changed periodically to prevent plugging. Distal tumors can be bypassed by cholecystojejunostomy or other types of biliary-enteric anastomoses.

PROGNOSIS. Cure is achieved in 5 to 10 per cent, and many patients survive in good condition for several years or more following palliative excision. If biliary drainage can be maintained with a tube, patients with unresectable lesions occasionally do well for a year of two. Death eventually results from hepatic replacement with tumor or intrahepatic sepsis from recurrent ductal obstruction.

Postcholecystectomy Syndrome

After cholecystectomy, 10 per cent of patients continue to have significant abdominal symptoms. In most patients the explanation for continued postoperative symptoms is that the gallstone disease was not the cause of their preoperative complaints. Patients with typical biliary pain are more often relieved by cholecystectomy than are those with the vague symptoms of fatty food intolerance, dyspepsia, or flatulence. Postcholecystectomy complaints can often be attributed to overlooked disease such as choledocholithiasis, pancreatitis, peptic ulcer, esophageal or small-bowel disease, or irritable bowel syndrome. These possibilities must be investigated by appropriate studies.

Stenosis of the sphincter of Oddi (ampullary stenosis), biliary dyskinesia, neuroma of the cystic duct stump, and other cystic duct remnant lesions are conditions that have returned to clinical favor as causes of the postcholecystectomy syndrome along with objective tests for detection such as ERCP with manometry.

Renewed interest in ampullary stenosis and biliary dyskinesia has followed the development of methods to perform endoscopic sphincterotomy. Early results suggest that a minority of patients with episodic typical biliary pain in the absence of stones have hypertension, dysmotility, and/or stenosis of the sphincter of Oddi. The appearance of a narrowed sphincter alone is insufficient to document either stenosis or dyskinesia. A provocative test has been used that involves injection of morphine (10 mg) and neostigmine methylsulfate (1 mg) intramuscularly. Pain and a rise in serum amylase levels are indications of ampullary stenosis. The results of this test, however, do not correlate with sphincter of Oddi pressures, and the test is sometimes positive in normal subjects. Clinicians should remain skeptical about a diagnosis of ampullary stenosis when the principal finding is abdominal pain. The diagnosis is more secure in patients with recurrent pancreatitis, increase of transaminases, cholangitis, and/or a dilated bile duct whose sphincter appears tight radiographically and will accept only a small probe. Treatment consists of division of the sphincter at operation or transendoscopically. Patients with recurrent pancreatitis should have an operative pancreatic septectomy in addition—division of that portion of the pancreas separating the distal common bile duct and pancreatic duct, thereby dividing that portion of the sphincter that extended onto the pancreatic duct.

Convincing evidence has been submitted to document the importance of each of the aforementioned conditions in specific cases. Dyskinesia of the sphincter without stenosis is very difficult to establish as a cause of the syndrome. Perhaps further data from manometric studies will elucidate a relationship between motor abnormalities and postoperative pain. In the management of such patients with chronic abdominal pain thought to be due to dyskinesia in the absence of objective findings, treatment can be tried with nitrates, anticholinergics, or calcium channel blockers. If this is unsuccessful, consideration can be given to endoscopic sphincterotomy, although its efficacy remains uncertain. Exploratory laparotomy has a low rate of success for diagnosis, and surgical correction of minor variations in the gut anatomy usually fails to cure.

Broughan TA, Sivak MV, Hermann RE: The management of retained and recurrent bile duct stones. Surgery 98:746, 1985. *Endoscopic sphincterotomy is preferable to surgery in a majority of cases.*

Brandy-Rauf PW, Pincus M, Adelson S: Cancer of the gallbladder. A review of 43 cases. Human Pathol 13:48, 1982. *A review of the clinicopathologic findings, epidemiology, and natural history of this virtually incurable disease.*

Chitwood WR Jr, Meyers WC, Heaston DK, et al.: Diagnosis and treatment of primary extrahepatic bile duct tumors. Am J Surg 143:99, 1982. *Covers the subject in detail.*

Cohen S, Soloway RD (eds.): Gallstones. New York, Churchill Livingstone, 1985. *A 341-page multiauthored book with 20 chapters covering virtually all aspects of gallstone disease. The first reference to use to get an authoritative perspective on a specific topic relating to stones.*

Delchier J-C, Benfredj P, Preaux A-M, et al.: The usefulness of microscopic bile examination in patients with suspected microlithiasis: A prospective evaluation. Hepatology 6:118, 1986. *Seeing cholesterol crystals in bile is highly correlated with the presence of small gallbladder stones that may be undetectable by radiologic techniques.*

Gracie WA, Ransohoff DF: The natural history of silent gallstones: The innocent gallstone is not a myth. N Engl J Med 307:798, 1982. *The best article to date describing a group of truly asymptomatic gallstones.*

Grundy SM: Mechanism of cholesterol gallstone formation. Sem Liv Dis 3:97, 1983. *A comprehensive review of the biochemistry leading to cholesterol stone formation, with 105 references.*

Jarvinen HJ, Hastbacka J: Early cholecystectomy for acute cholecystitis. A prospective randomized study. Ann Surg 191:501, 1980. *This controlled trial demonstrates the advantages of early surgery over expectant management for acute cholecystitis.*

Maton RN, Iser JH, Reuben A, et al.: Outcome of chenodeoxycholic acid (CDCA) treatment in 125 patients with radiolucent gallstones. Medicine 61:86, 1982. *Factors influencing efficacy, withdrawal, symptoms and side effects, and postdissolution recurrence.*

Sauerbruch T, Delius M, Baumgartner G, et al.: Fragmentation of gallstones by extracorporeal shock waves. N Engl J Med 314:818, 1986. *Whether or not this becomes the wave of the future awaits more studies.*

Scharschmidt BF, Goldberg HI, Schmid R: Current concepts in diagnosis: Approach to the patient with cholestatic jaundice. N Engl J Med 308:1515, 1983. *Excellent review of the most efficient approach to distinguishing intrahepatic from extrahepatic cholestasis.*

Silvis SE: What is the postcholecystectomy syndrome? Gastro Endoscopy 31:401, 1985. *A succinct editorial outlining what is and what is not known about this condition.*

Somjen GJ, Gilat T: Contribution of vesicular and micellar carriers to cholesterol transport in human bile. J Lipid Res 26:699, 1985. *Both the classically described micelles and the more recently described non–bile salt containing cholesterol vesicles are important in solubilizing cholesterol in bile.*

Trotman BW, Soloway RD: Pigment gallstone disease: Summary of the National Institutes of Health International Workshop. Hepatology 2:879, 1982. *Good starting point for understanding pigment stone disease, with 60 references.*

Wiesner RH, LaRusso NF: Clinicopathologic features of the syndrome of primary sclerosing cholangitis. Gastroenterology 79:200, 1980. *A review of 50 patients with sclerosing cholangitis.*

PART XII
HEMATOLOGIC DISEASES

131 INTRODUCTION
David G. Nathan

This introduction is primarily intended to provide a general background to diagnostic hematology and marrow function. The remaining chapters in Part XII emphasize fundamental physiologic principles and provide descriptions of relatively common hematologic disorders with the hope that the entire Part will influence the reader to consider such diseases broadly and systematically.

The nonmalignant disorders of erythrocytes, phagocytes, and platelets, including their precursors and progenitors, are initially discussed. Then follows a description of the acute and chronic proliferative disorders that involve the cells of the marrow and lymphoid systems, a series of chapters that ends with a discussion of bone marrow transplantation. The final chapters of Part XII are devoted to a review of the disorders of the fluid phase of blood coagulation and the vascular purpuras.

DIAGNOSTIC HEMATOLOGY. The circulating blood cells are the products of the terminal differentiation of recognizable precursors. In fetal life hematopoiesis occurs throughout the reticuloendothelial system. In the normal adult, the process of terminal differentiation of the recognizable precursors of erythrocytes, granulocytes, and platelets occurs exclusively in the marrow cavities of the axial skeleton with some extension into the proximal femoral and humeri, but the space is highly expandable when the demand for blood cell production is accelerated (Fig. 131–1).

Observations of differentiated blood cells by enumeration and relatively simple morphologic studies of properly prepared blood films provide the essential cornerstone of diagnostic hematology. Automated blood counts and cell sizing now provide both reproducibility and enhanced diagnostic capacity. For example, early red cell production failure may be heralded by unexpected macrocytosis. Peripheral blood cell morphology offers insight into the rate of effective hematopoiesis; the state of marrow nutrition with respect to vitamin B_{12}, folic acid, and iron; the presence of acquired and congenital disorders of the membrane; the energy metabolism or the hemoglobin of erythrocytes that leads to their accelerated destruction; the differential diagnosis of infections; the presence of allergic reactions; the acquired or congenital abnormalities of intracellular organelles; and the invasion of the marrow by malignant cells or infectious agents. The contributions of morphologic techniques to hematologic diagnosis depend entirely upon the adequacy of specimen preparation and the skill of the observer. Egregious errors are made when diagnostic pronouncements are based on inadequate material. The slavish enumeration of individual cells is rarely of aid without careful overall inspection and positive searches for diagnostic clues that are relevant to the case at hand. Morphology can be particularly misleading if the observer does not understand that many kinds of disorders induce similar changes in shape, particularly in the red cells.

Although circulating lymphocytes appear to be terminally differentiated cells, they are instead capable of rapid proliferative responses to appropriate stimuli during which they

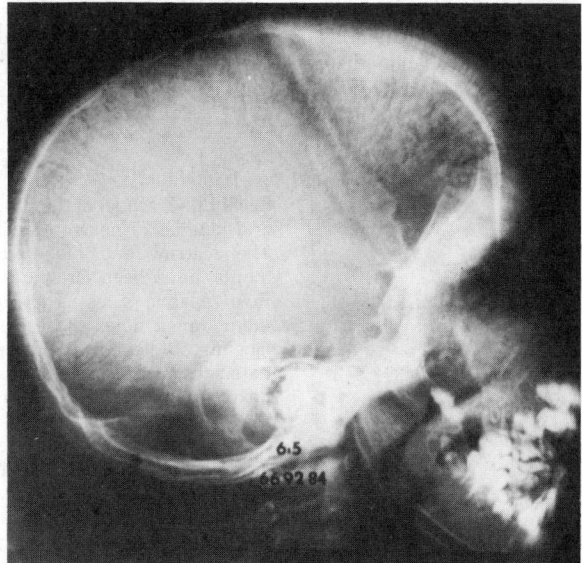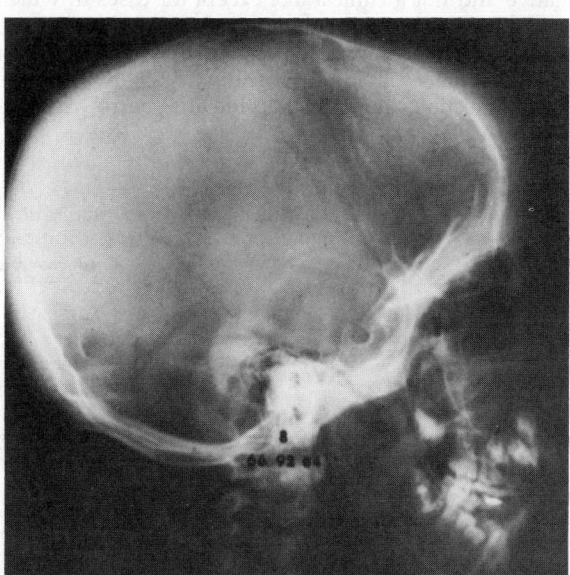

FIGURE 131–1. Roentgenograms of the skull of a patient with homozygous beta thalassemia at the age of 6½ years (*left*), before splenectomy and transfusion therapy, and at the age of eight years (*right*), after splenectomy and transfusion therapy to control anemia. Note the marked "hair-on-end" appearance in the left-hand radiograph, signifying expansion of the marrow space. (From Nathan DG: N Engl J Med 286:586, 1972.)

resume the appearance of relatively undifferentiated precursors. At this stage they are often called atypical, even though this blastic transformation is entirely appropriate. The functional subsets of lymphoid cells are not readily demonstrable by inspection, although "killer" lymphocyte function may be associated with larger cells that contain granules. Obtaining that important information requires studies of lymphocyte function and studies with specially prepared antibodies reactive with lymphocytes.

Well-prepared marrow films and biopsy specimens also contribute important information such as total marrow cellularity, the presence of invading malignant cells or infectious granulomas, the adequacy of the numbers of megakaryocytes, the ratio of myeloid to erythroid precursors, the state of marrow cell nutrition, the presence of abnormal storage cells, and even the deposition of abnormal crystals. In brief, the blood lends itself to biopsy and to structural, chemical, and functional studies far more readily than does any other human organ. Its cellular elements are diverse, bearing in common only a joint ancestral cell, origin in the marrow, and the property of being transported through vessels suspended in plasma.

PRECURSORS OF CIRCULATING BLOOD CELLS.

Erythrocytes. Much of the progress of differentiation of erythroid precursors can be appreciated morphologically, particularly the onset of hemoglobin synthesis and the maturation and extrusion of the nucleus. During this process each proerythroblast may give rise to approximately eight erythrocytes. The transit time from proerythroblast to emergence of reticulocytes is approximately five days. The transit time may decrease during anemic stress to as little as two days by means of skipped divisions. The red cells that emerge under conditions of stress are macrocytic and may contain as much as 25 per cent fetal hemoglobin (F cells). They may also bear additional fetal characteristics, particularly the presence of i antigen on their surfaces. More quantitative analyses of the transit of erythroid precursors during the process of maturation may be appreciated from the use of radioactive iron that, when injected intravenously, accumulates preferentially in the newly synthesized ferritin of proerythroblasts and ultimately emerges in peripheral blood incorporated into reticulocyte hemoglobin. The use of surface scanning following infusion of ^{59}Fe-labeled transferrin reveals the site as well as the rate of intramedullary erythropoiesis. This is largely an investigative and not a clinical tool except for cases in which the anatomic site of erythropoiesis needs to be determined, such as in myeloid metaplasia. A qualitative assessment of erythroid precursor activity throughout the body may be gained from injection of indium chloride and marrow scintigraphy. Indium-111 binds to transferrin and is incorporated into immature marrow erythroid precursors. Body scanning then reveals the distribution of marrow.

Granulocytes. The process of intramedullary granulocyte maturation involves changes in nuclear configuration and the accumulation of specific intracytoplasmic granules. A model that describes the production and kinetics of neutrophils is shown in Figure 131–2 (see also Ch. 148). It is highly compartmentalized. The relatively small peripheral blood pool is divided into two compartments in equilibrium, the circulating and the marginating pools. These pools provide entrance into the tissues. The level of peripheral cells is buffered by an immense marrow reserve of identifiable precursors, some of which are in the mitotic compartment and some in the maturing and storage compartment. The kinetics of proliferation of these recognizable precursors have been studied using labeled precursors of DNA. These so-called labeling indices, from which estimates of cell cycle times can be derived, have served as important approaches to the study of pharmacology and toxicity of chemotherapeutic agents.

Platelets. The differentiation of committed megakaryocytes, the precursors of platelets, involves a nuclear endoreduplication phenomenon which produces 16N and 32N megakaryoblasts. The endoreduplication ceases at the stage of the mature megakaryocyte. Platelet shedding from megakaryocytes is accomplished by the formation of multiple demarcation membranes within the cytoplasm of the cell, usually visible only by electron microscopy. Although the platelet appears at first to be a simple tissue fragment, its functions are diverse and hemostatically versatile. It must selectively adhere to abnormal surfaces and then sequentially secrete, aggregate, fuse, and retract to ensure a firm platelet-fibrin plug. In the process it assists in the coagulation cascade, synthesizes prostaglandins, and releases ADP and a variety of other substances of known and unknown function.

Lymphocytes. The geography of lymphocyte precursor maturation and differentiation is considerably more complex than that of the other hematopoietic cells. Primitive lymphoid precursors of B cell origin arise in the marrow, spleen, and lymph nodes where they continue their maturation and differentiation. Primitive T cell precursors arise in the marrow, travel to the thymus where they undergo further differentiation, and are finally exported to the spleen, lymph nodes, and marrow where they establish their final residence and perform many of their functions. Both T and B cells enter the peripheral blood circulation, which delivers them to tissue sites at which their functions may be required or their unbridled activity may cause disease (see Ch. 417). T cells previously "educated" in the thymus give rise to progeny that survive

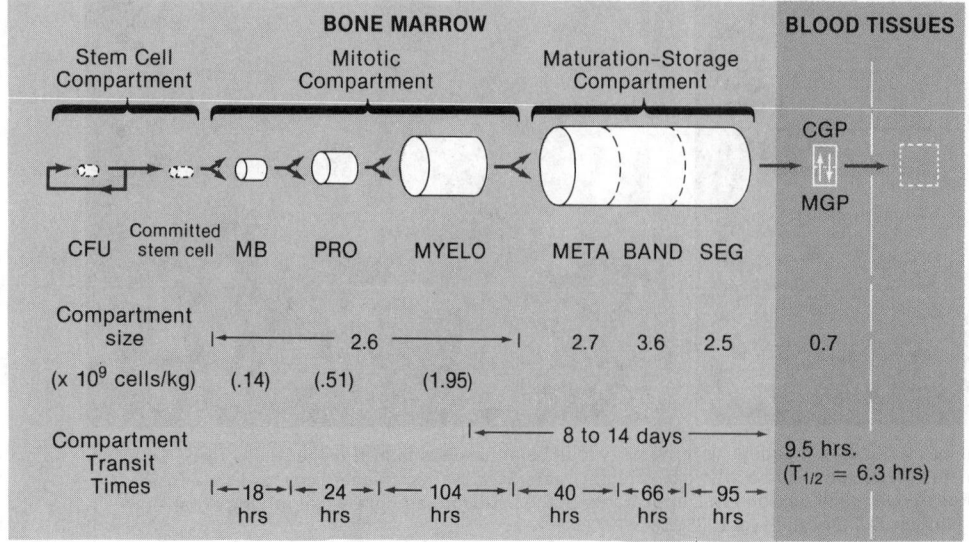

FIGURE 131–2. Model of the production and kinetics of neutrophils in man. The marrow and blood compartments have been drawn to show their relative sizes. The compartment transit times as derived from labeling studies with DF^{32}P and tritiated thymidine are shown on the next to last line and the last line. The less obvious symbols in the figure include CGP, the circulating granulocyte pool; MGP, the marginating granulocyte pool; CFU, the tripotential stem cell; MB, myeloblast; and PRO, promyelocyte. (From Wintrobe MM, Lee RG, et al.: Clinical Hematology. 7th ed. Philadelphia, Lea & Febiger, 1974, p 244.)

for the life of the individual. Circulating lymphocytes represent only a tiny fraction of the total lymphocyte pool. Analysis of these circulating cells may not reflect the nature of the total pool.

HEMATOPOIETIC PROGENITORS. The recognizable marrow precursors of the differentiated peripheral blood cells tend to occupy the attention of hematologists, but they are rarely primary causes of the hematopoietic cytopenias. It is true that various toxins or nutritional deficiencies can so seriously damage the orderly progression of precursor differentiation that effective production of fully differentiated blood cells is embarrassed. In general, however, deficient or excessive production of blood cells is due to abnormalities of *undifferentiated progenitor cells*. They must themselves undergo vital processes of maturation and amplification to give rise to the recognizable precursors of circulating differentiated blood cells.

Progenitor Maturation. Pluripotent stem cells are few in number, but the initial stages of their development lead to committed progenitors of the lymphoid and myeloid systems (Fig. 131–3). These committed progenitors are destined to produce the differentiated, recognizable precursors of the specific types of blood cells. Pluripotent stem cells are capable of slow but indefinite self-renewal, whereas the committed progenitor cells are not capable of indefinite self-renewal.

They "die by differentiation," and their numbers depend on influx from the pluripotent stem cell pool. The committed erythrocyte, phagocyte, and platelet progenitors and the precursors to which they give rise emerge as the result of the maturation of a tripotential progenitor usually called CFU-S for the spleen colony-forming unit described by Till and McCulloch in mice. They observed hematopoietic colonies in the spleens of lethally irradiated mice rescued with bone marrow cells of histoidentical donors. The spleen colonies contained megakaryocyte, granulocyte, and erythroid precursors. A small fraction of CFU-S is found to be replicating or in the act of DNA synthesis at any one time. As more committed progenitors are formed, the fraction of these cells undergoing DNA synthesis increases. These increasingly committed progenitors include CFU-M, the progenitors of megakaryoblasts; CFU-GM, progenitors of phagocytic precursors; and BFU-E, the erythroid burst-forming units that ultimately give rise to erythroid precursors. This last-named process of maturation ultimately leads to erythroid colony-forming units, CFU-E, the immediate progenitors of proerythroblasts. The process of maturation of erythroid progenitor cells is accompanied by the increasing size and increased sensitivity to erythropoietin, a hormone produced largely in the kidney in response to anemia or hypoxia, and in the liver, particularly in fetuses. Its deficiency contributes to the anemia

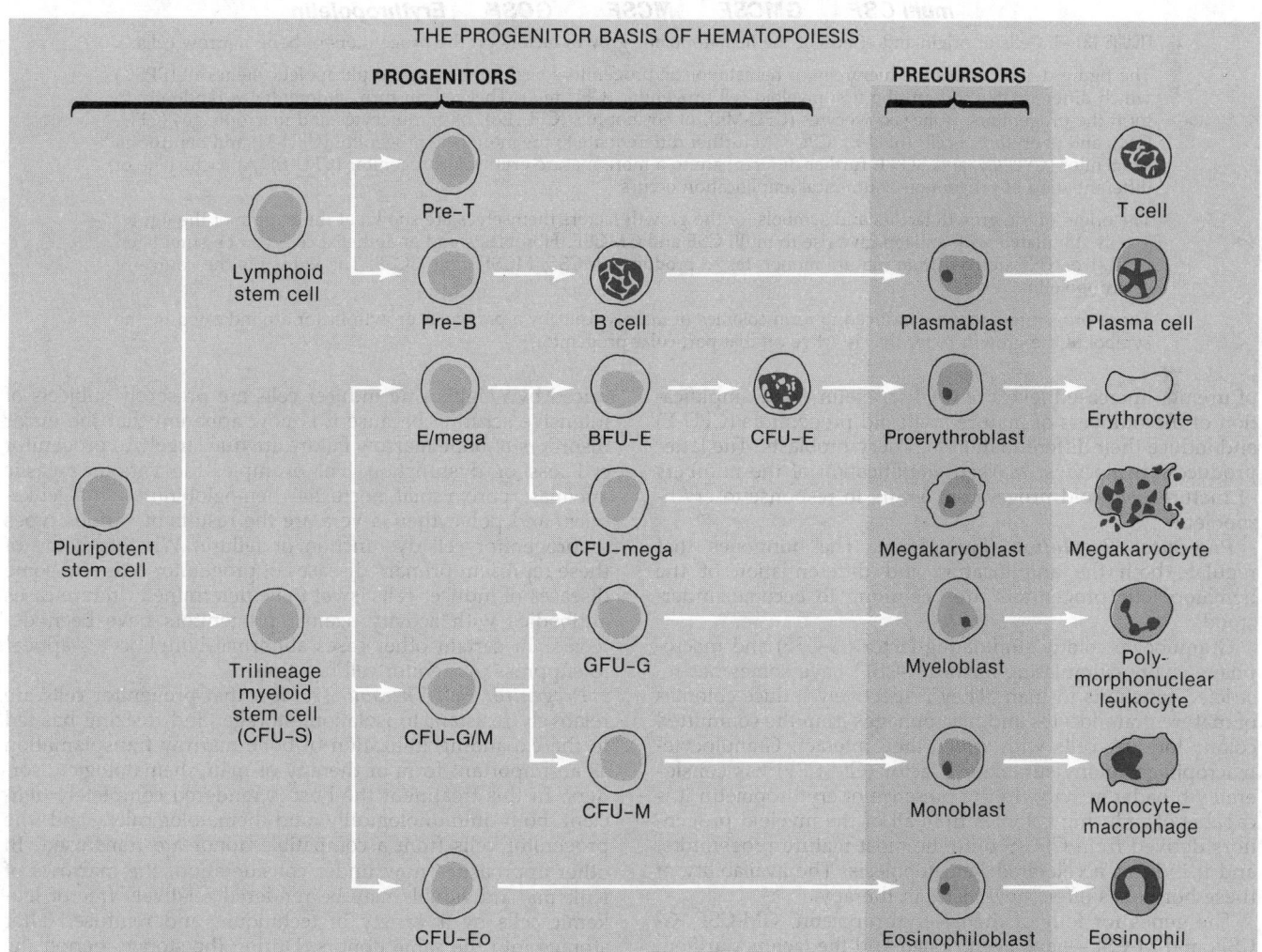

FIGURE 131–3. A schematic outline of the progenitor basis of hematopoiesis. Note the progressive restriction in the potential for terminal differentiation of the progenitors as they mature from left to right in the drawing. They finally form the recognizable marrow precursors from which the circulating blood cells, shown on the far right, are derived. Not shown in this outline is the process of self-renewal of fractions of the progenitor cell populations, particularly the immature progenitors. Also not shown is the progressive amplification of progenitors and precursors as they mature and differentiate. The bipotential erythroid-megakaryocyte progenitor shown in this drawing and referred to in the text has been demonstrated in the mouse, but not definitely in man.

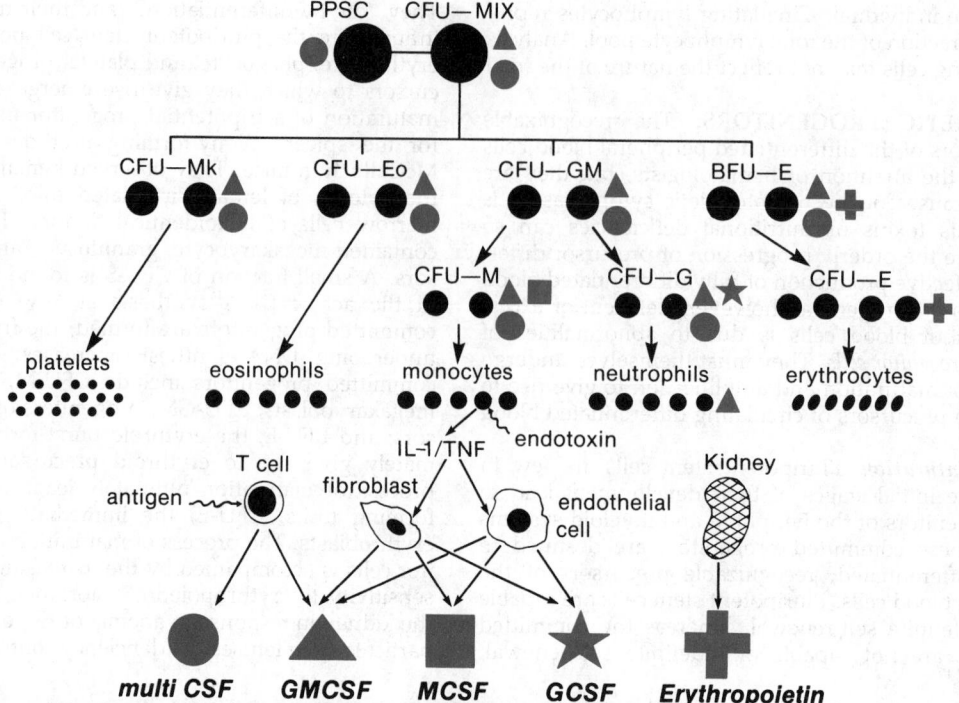

FIGURE 131–4. Cells of origin and effects of the hematopoietic growth factors on the progenitors of bone marrow cells.

The figure demonstrates the hierarchy of hematopoietic progenitors beginning with the pluripoietic stem cell (PPSC) which differentiates to form the first myeloid cell progenitor (CFU mix). This cell, in turn, differentiates randomly to form the progenitors of megakaryocytes (CFU-Mk), of eosinophils (CFU-Eo), of granulocytes and macrophages (CFU-GM), and of erythroid cells (BFU-E). CFU-GM further differentiate to the monocyte progenitor (CFU-M) and neutrophil progenitor (CFU-G), and BFU-E further differentiate to a more mature erythroid progenitor (CFU-E). At each stage of differentiation of progenitors, numerical amplification occurs.

The origin of the growth factors and symbols for the growth factors themselves are shown at the bottom of the figure. T cells stimulated with antigen give rise to multi CSF and GMCSF. Fibroblasts and endothelial cells can be stimulated by IL-1 or TNF derived from mature monocytes to produce GMCSF, MCSF, and GCSF. The kidney is the source of erythropoietin.

Those progenitors that are induced to form colonies of marrow cells by a particular growth factor are indicated by the symbol of the growth factor that is active on that particular progenitor.

of uremia. Increased levels of erythropoietin cause amplification of the numbers of mature erythroid progenitors (CFU-E) and induce their differentiation to proerythroblasts. The latter produce reticulocytes. Marked amplification of the numbers of mature erythroid progenitors occurs in response to erythropoietin.

Progenitor Regulation (Fig. 131–4). The hormones that regulate both the amplification and differentiation of the hematopoietic progenitors are beginning to become understood.

Granulocyte colony-stimulating factor (G-CSF) and macrophage colony-stimulating factor (M-CSF) have somewhat restricted functions in man. They respectively induce colonies of mature granulocytes and macrophages from the committed colony-forming cells with which they interact. Granulocyte-macrophage colony-stimulating factor (GM-CSF) has considerably broader activity. In the presence of erythropoietin it is capable of inducing colonies from all of the myeloid progenitors derived from CFU-S onto the most mature progenitors, and it induces accelerated hematopoiesis. The availability of these hormones offers new vistas in therapy.

The genes for four of them—erythropoietin, GM-CSF, G-CSF, and M-CSF—have been cloned and the factors purified. All are glycoproteins. The last three are produced by interleukin 1–stimulated fibroblasts and endothelial cells (the framework cells of marrow) and by activated T cells.

Progenitors and Marrow Failure. The hematopoietic progenitors can be detected in the null cell fraction of peripheral blood and in the mononuclear Ia+ cell fraction of marrow. Interactions of progenitor cells and the various factors pro-

duced by neighboring inducer cells are presently subjects of intensive scrutiny because it is now apparent that the major disorders of bone marrow failure are due largely to progenitor cell loss or dysfunction. For example, the various aplastic anemias, paroxysmal nocturnal hemoglobinuria, the leukemias, and polycythemia vera are the results of various types of progenitor cell dysfunction or failure. Whether some of these represent primary diseases of progenitor cells and some diseases of inducer cells is yet to be determined. In rare cases antibodies with activity against progenitors have been detected. In certain other cases abnormal lymphocytes appear to suppress progenitor cell function.

Progenitor Cell Therapy. The fact that progenitor cells are relatively resistant to isolation, storage, and freezing has led to the expanding utilization of bone marrow transplantation as an important form of therapy of many hematologic disorders. In this treatment the host is rendered completely deficient both immunologically and hematologically, and the progenitor cells from a compatible donor are transfused. In other approaches now under consideration, the marrows of leukemic individuals may be rendered relatively free of leukemic cells by a variety of techniques and reinfused after storage into the same donors. During the storage period the donors receive intensive ablative therapy. The frozen marrow cells are then infused to reconstitute hematopoietic function.

MARROW ANATOMY. Although most cases of bone marrow failure and malignancy are due to disorders of progenitors, the total microenvironment in which progenitors, inducer cells, and precursors interact to form mature differentiated peripheral blood cells is complex and subject to severe dys-

FIGURE 131–5. A schematic diagram of the factors that may be involved in controlling the release of marrow cells. The central relationship between the hematopoietic compartment and the marrow sinus is depicted. The drawing highlights the similarity of the egress process for the three major hematopoietic cells: reticulocytes in the top pathway, granulocytes and monocytes in the center pathway, and platelets in the lower pathway. Immature cells undergo biophysical changes under the influence of cytopoietins that favor egress. In the case of reticulocytes, enucleation precedes egress. This is shown by the solid black inclusion in the perisinal macrophage representing nucleophagocytosis antecedent to digestion of the erythroblast nucleus. The cytoplasmic protrusion of the megakaryocyte presumably detaches itself from the cell and will further fragment into platelets in the circulation. (From Lichtman MA, Chamberlain JK, Santillo PA: In Silber R, LoBue J, Gordon AS [eds.]: The Year in Hematology, 1978. New York, Plenum Medical Book Company, 1978, p 274.)

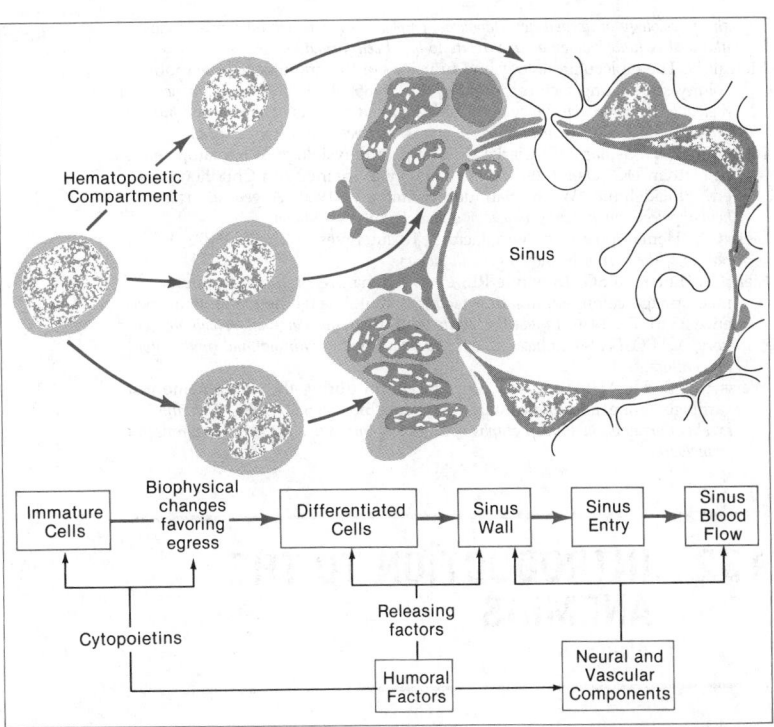

function. This is an obvious problem in myelofibrosis, or in infectious granulomatosis of the marrow. But certain other forms of bone marrow failure, such as aplastic anemia itself, may also be due to more subtle forms of microenvironmental failure. The marrow cavity is a vast network of vascular channels or sinusoids that separate groups of hematopoietic cells, including fat cells. The hematopoietic cells are found in the intrasinusoidal spaces. Clumps of megakaryocytes are found adjacent to marrow sinuses. They shed platelets, the fragments of their cytoplasm, directly into the lumen. This reduces the requirement for movement of bulky megakaryocytes, a mobility characteristic of the granuloid and erythroid differentiated precursors as they approach the point at which they egress from the marrow. The vascular and hematopoietic compartments are lined by reticular cells that form the adventitial surfaces of the vascular sinuses and extend cytoplasmic processes to create a lattice for the mesh of endothelial cells and fibronectin on which blood cells are found. The lattice is illustrated by reticulin stains of marrow sections and scanning electron photomicrographs. A schema of the egress of cells from marrow is shown in Figure 131–5.

KINETICS OF HEMATOPOIESIS. The marrow microenvironment supporting the progenitors and precursors must provide for the normal steady-state rates of renewal of the cellular elements of blood. Under homeostatic conditions, the production rates precisely equal destruction rates. The average life span of a human red cell is approximately 120 days. This means that approximately 5×10^4 red cells must be produced per day per microliter of blood in an adult. The average life span of platelets is seven to ten days for a daily production rate of 2×10^4 platelets per microliter of blood. The white blood cell compartment exhibits more complex kinetics. Granulocytes are rapidly turned over with an approximate intravascular life span of 6 to 12 hours in humans. To maintain a level of circulating granulocytes of 5×10^3 per microliter requires a daily production that is roughly comparable to that of red cell and platelet production, approximately 2×10^4 cells per microliter of blood. At the opposite extreme in terms of life span is the lymphocyte, which can exhibit lifetimes measured in months, or even years. This long life span of lymphocytes suggests that the daily renewal of certain lymphocyte progenitors occurs at a rate substantially lower than that of the progenitors of the other formed elements of blood.

The various symptoms of complete marrow failure are closely related to the life span and the turnover of the peripheral cells of the blood. Thus, patients with complete marrow failure initially lose granulocytes and therefore usually present with enhanced susceptibility to infection. Petechial bleeding caused by platelet deficiency rapidly follows, and finally pallor and symptoms of anemia occur. Loss of circulating lymphocytes and cellular immune function is an unusual event in such circumstances.

The turnover of red cells and platelets can be measured for diagnostic purposes, using $Na_2^{51}CrO_4$ as a labeling agent. Both the red cell and the platelet life spans can be estimated and the site of the red cell destruction determined. This can be a useful maneuver in decisions regarding splenectomy.

CONCLUSIONS. Modern cell biology and molecular genetics have revolutionized hematology, changing it from a largely descriptive field to a remarkable amalgamation of diagnostic and therapeutic ventures. The realization that differentiated marrow precursors arise from a population of lymphoid-appearing cells that have a fascinating developmental biology of their own has led to reclassification of the marrow failure syndrome and to new approaches to therapy, particularly with bone marrow transplantation. In addition, inquiries into the kinetics of progenitors and differentiated precursors have encouraged more rational approaches to the chemotherapy of malignant diseases. As approaches to the actual isolation of progenitors are developed, enumeration of these cells will soon be as commonplace as the evaluation of precursors and mature cells. This kind of enumeration will require specific antibodies and diagnostic instruments that are taking their places as standard aspects of the hematology of this era.

Burakoff SJ, Lipton JM, Nathan DG: Recapitulation of the immune response and hematopoietic system in bone marrow transplantation. In Nathan DG (ed.): Bone Marrow Transplantation. Clin Haematol 12:695, 1983. *A brief up-to-date review of regulation of hematopoiesis in two volumes devoted to basic and clinical aspects of marrow transplantations.*

Donahue, RE, Wang EA, Stone DK, et al.: Stimulation of hematopoiesis in primates by continuous infusion of recombinant human GM-CSF. Nature 321:872, 1986. *Purified recombinant human GM-CSF elicits dramatic leukocytosis and substantial reticulocytosis when infused into healthy monkeys and had a similar effect in one immunodeficient pancytopenic animal.*

Lipton JM, Nathan DG: The anatomy and physiology of hematopoiesis. In Nathan DG, Oski F (eds.): Hematology of Infancy and Childhood. 3rd ed. Philadelphia, W. B. Saunders Company, 1987. *A general review of the anatomy and physiology of normal hematopoiesis, emphasizing new developments in molecular and cellular biology as they relate to blood cell formation.*

Metcalf D: The molecular biology and functions of the granulocyte-macrophage colony-stimulating factors. Blood 67:257, 1986. *An up-to-date comprehensive review of the molecular biology and multiple in vitro effects of murine and human growth factors, their relationships, receptors, and possible role in leukemia.*

Nathan DG, Housman DE, Clarke BJ: The pathophysiology of hematopoiesis. In Nathan DG, Oski F (eds.): Hematology in Infancy and Childhood. 2nd ed. Philadelphia, W. B. Saunders Company, 1980. *A general review of hematopoiesis emphasizing physiology and clinical correlations.*

Sieff CA: Hematopoietic growth factors. J Clin Invest 79:1549, 1987. *A brief review of the currently known growth factors.*

Sieff CA, Emerson SG, Donahue RE, et al.: Human recombinant granulocyte-macrophage colony-stimulating factor: A multilineage hematopoietin. Science 230:1171, 1986. *In addition to its effect on granulocyte-macrophage progenitors, GM-CSF also induces colonies derived from erythroid and multipotent progenitors.*

Weiss RE, Reddi AH: Appearance of fibronectin during the differentation of cartilage, bone and bone marrow. J Cell Biol 88:630, 1981. *Contains an excellent array of photomicrographs of developing marrow cells within a fibronectin framework.*

132 INTRODUCTION TO THE ANEMIAS

Alan S. Keitt

Humans live in tenuous equilibrium with their life blood. Elaborate mechanisms have evolved to extract the nutrients for blood formation from available food stores and to conserve them by efficient recycling. The transition from hunter-gatherer to agricultural societies resulted in the replacement of most readily absorbable heme iron in the human diet by poorly absorbable iron in grains, thus rendering this balance precarious for a large part of the world's population. Other evolutionary strategies have concentrated genes for various red cell abnormalities that enhance survival in malarial areas but at the cost of producing anemia within a large minority of the population of these regions. Parasitic infestations and frequent pregnancies produce stress on iron balance in the same underdeveloped and populous areas. As a result of these combined nutritional, genetic, and parasitic factors, the global hematocrit is by no means optimal; anemia is perhaps the most frequent and significant worldwide health problem. Anemia does not have the same impact on the population of western societies, but it remains a cardinal indicator of disease and requires careful consideration and treatment.

Although defined by numbers, anemia is in reality a *process* that evolves within a clinical context. For the experienced hematologist, this clinical context is analogous to habitat for the ornithologist. A brief glance through the binoculars is often sufficient to identify the microspherocytes of autoimmune hemolytic anemia in a patient known to have systemic lupus erythematosus just as one instantly recognizes a wood duck in the woods because that is where it belongs. In the same vein, an unfamiliar stray may be noticed by the alert observer when it occurs outside of its usual clinical context. The importance of habitat in hematologic diagnosis cannot be overemphasized and is often neglected in the current proliferation of sequential algorithms for the diagnosis of anemia. Such constructions, which are based primarily on laboratory data, may fail to take into account changes occurring over time and often provide only a single point of entry to the process of anemia.

The great majority of anemias are diagnosed and treated by nonhematologists. Except for the primary blood dyscrasias, the diagnostic classification of the anemias is relatively simple and logical. The pathophysiologic classification, presented in Table 132–1, is most useful because it stresses the underlying mechanisms of the anemias and therefore helps one to predict some of the key diagnostic tests that are discussed below.

TABLE 132–1. PATHOPHYSIOLOGIC CLASSIFICATION OF ANEMIAS

I. **Hypoproliferative anemias**
  A. Marrow aplasias (Ch. 133)
  B. Myelophthisic anemia (Ch. 133)
  C. Anemia with blood dyscrasias
  D. Anemia of chronic disease (Ch. 134)
  E. Anemia with organ failure (Ch. 134)
    1. Renal failure
    2. Hepatic failure
    3. Hypothyroidism
    4. Hypopituitarism
II. **Maturation defects**
  A. Cytoplasmic
    1. Hypochromic anemias (Ch. 135)
  B. Nuclear
    1. Megaloblastic anemias (Ch. 136)
  C. Combined
    1. Myelodysplastic syndromes
III. **Hyperproliferative anemias**
  A. Hemorrhagic (Ch. 134)
    1. Acute blood loss
  B. Hemolytic (Ch. 137)
    1. Immune hemolysis (Ch. 139)
    2. Primary membrane defects (Ch. 138)
    3. Hemoglobinopathies (Ch. 143)
    4. Enzymopathies (Ch. 138)
    5. Toxic hemolysis—physical-chemical (Ch. 139)
    6. Traumatic or microangiopathic hemolysis (Ch. 139)
    7. Hypersplenism (Ch. 164)
    8. Parasitic infections (Ch. 139)
IV. **Dilutional anemias**
  A. Pregnancy
  B. Splenomegaly

DEFINITIONS OF ANEMIA

STATISTICAL CONSIDERATIONS. Anemia is defined as a reduction in either the volume of red blood cells (termed the hematocrit or packed cell volume [PCV]) or the concentration of hemoglobin in a sample of peripheral venous blood when compared with similar values obtained from a reference population. Normal values for red blood cell measurements are given in Table 132–2. By convention the normal range is defined to include 95 per cent of a reference population that is assumed to have a normal (gaussian) distribution. In this definition 2.5 per cent of "normal individuals" will fall below this arbitrary statistical limit and be classified as anemic. Some of these individuals in the general population will be truly anemic while others are *statistical outliers.* Unfortunately this statistical definition of anemia may fail to detect truly anemic patients whose hematocrits have decreased significantly without leaving the defined normal range. Here the only valid reference figure is a previous hematocrit in that individual.

RED CELL MASS. Anemia can be more rigorously defined as a reduction in red cell mass (a misnomer for the total volume of circulating erythroid cells in the body). Red cell mass can be accurately measured by isotope dilution using

TABLE 132–2. SELECTED HEMATOLOGIC VALUES IN NORMAL INDIVIDUALS OF VARIOUS AGES*

Age	Hemoglobin (gm/dl) mean (−2SD)	Hematocrit (%) mean (−2SD)	MCV (μ³) mean (−2SD)
1–3 days	18.5 (14.5)	56 (45)	108 (95)
0.5–2 yrs	12 (10.5)	36 (33)	78 (70)
12–18 yrs			
Male	14.5 (13)	43 (37)	88 (78)
Female	14.0 (12)	41 (36)	90 (78)
18–49 yrs			
Male	15.5 (13.5)	47 (41)	90 (80)
Female	14 (12.0)	41 (36)	90 (80)

*Values selected from Dallman PR: In Rudolph A (ed.): Pediatrics, 16th ed. New York, Appleton-Century-Crofts, Inc., 1977, p 1111. The values were derived by Coulter Counter. Values in parentheses represent two standard deviations below the mean, or the lower limit of normal assuming a normal distribution.

[51]Cr-labeled red cells, a procedure usually employed to establish increased red cell mass, i.e., erythrocytosis, rather than anemia. This measurement is occasionally useful for assessing anemia in patients with marked splenomegaly in whom the peripheral hematocrit underestimates the true red cell mass (see below).

EFFECTS OF AGE, SEX, AND ALTITUDE. Developmental changes in hematocrit are most evident during the first year of life (see Table 131–2). Adult levels of hematocrit are reached by late childhood in females. The higher hematocrit of males as compared with females begins at puberty as a result of stimulation of hematopoiesis by androgenic hormones.

Whether the hematocrit normally declines with aging is controversial. With age the cellularity of the bone marrow is progressively replaced by fat and in men over 60 the incidence of anemia increases progressively as well. Some studies show similar trends in women. Iron deficiency and chronic diseases are common in this age group but seem not to account entirely for the increased incidence of anemia. Mild anemia in the elderly, therefore, must still be considered as an indicator of potential ill health, but investigation of these patients frequently fails to indicate a precise etiology.

The hematocrit is increased in individuals living at high altitudes as an appropriate response to diminished oxygen content of the atmosphere and blood. This effect can be noticed above 4000 feet where significant desaturation of hemoglobin begins. The definition of anemia therefore requires adjustment to the altitude at which the individual lives.

COMPENSATION FOR ANEMIA

INCREASED PLASMA VOLUME. Initial symptoms of patients with anemia are related to efforts by the body to compensate for the diminished oxygen supply. Later symptoms of progressive anemia reflect failure of these compensatory mechanisms. The symptoms and signs differ markedly depending on the acuteness of onset of the anemia. The abrupt loss of 30 per cent of the circulating blood volume in a patient with gastrointestinal hemorrhage will result in marked postural hypotension, a fall in cardiac output, shunting of blood from skin to central organs, thirst, and air hunger (Ch. 114). In contrast, the gradual loss of 30 per cent of the circulating red cell mass in a patient with iron deficiency may occur without any symptoms at all. The major difference lies in the blood volume, which is maintained by a proportionate increase in plasma volume as a compensatory response in most chronic anemias but is compromised in acute hemorrhage. Because the central blood volume is maintained until very late in the course of a progressive chronic anemia, such *patients are susceptible to volume overload by transfusions.* The injudicious administration of whole blood and even packed red cells may precipitate acute congestive heart failure in a previously well compensated individual.

INCREASED CARDIAC OUTPUT. In chronic anemias cardiac output increases to circulate fewer red cells through the tissues more frequently. This process is abetted by the diminished viscosity of blood at low hematocrits but is ultimately limited by the capacity of the heart to respond to the increased work. An early sign of failing compensation in gradual-onset anemias is postural hypotension, which may be associated with palpitations, dizziness, throbbing headaches, and dyspnea on exertion.

REDUCED AFFINITY OF HEMOGLOBIN FOR OXYGEN. In anemia the oxyhemoglobin dissociation curve usually shifts in a manner to increase the quantity of oxygen released in tissues without appreciably altering the quantity of oxygen bound in the lungs (see Fig. 140–3). Red cell 2,3-diphosphoglycerate (2,3-DPG) regularly increases in anemic patients to mediate this effect. Maximum elevation of RBC 2,3-DPG increases oxygen delivery only about 30 per cent, but this is a highly efficient form of compensation requiring no significant expenditure of energy.

ASSESSMENT OF SYMPTOMS IN ANEMIA. Anemia is usually insidious in its onset and has no specific symptoms to alert the physician to its presence. Unusual fatigue is the earliest and most common complaint, but other more subtle changes such as loss of libido or alterations in mood or sleep patterns may be elicited prior to the awareness of the more typical cardiovascular symptoms mentioned above. The level of anemia at which symptoms occur is highly variable among individuals as would be expected from the widely differing degrees of physical activity, physical conditioning, circulatory adequacy, and sensitivity or stoicism of the population. In otherwise healthy individuals symptoms are usually present when the hemoglobin falls below 7 or 8 grams per deciliter.

Exceptions to this general rule are not infrequent. An occasional patient with a gradual-onset anemia may deny all symptoms despite a hemoglobin of 5 grams per deciliter. Conversely, and more commonly, patients with mild anemia of 9 or 10 grams of hemoglobin per deciliter may complain bitterly of fatigue and lassitude. A careful search for underlying systemic disease or depression is warranted in these patients. Finally, because oxygen transport is much more compromised by impaired circulation than by diminished oxygen-carrying capacity per se, patients with vascular or cardiac disease may become symptomatic with milder degrees of anemia. For example, angina, claudication, transient ischemic attacks, and cardiac failure can occur or be exacerbated with relatively mild anemia. In essence, each organ within each patient sets its own functional definition of anemia.

EVALUATION OF THE ANEMIC PATIENT

The remainder of this chapter outlines in considerable detail a systematic approach to the anemic patient. This involves the construction and interpretation of an initial data base derived from careful assessment of the clinical context, key physical findings, and certain basic laboratory tests. The confirmatory diagnostic procedures for specific types of anemia are detailed in the other chapters of this section and will be mentioned only briefly here. Good practice dictates that this initial data base be collected and analyzed prior to the random ordering of procedures or consultations, since it will provide definitive diagnoses in a surprisingly large number of patients and point toward efficient diagnostic approaches in most of the others.

How to Assess the Clinical Context

The answers to six basic questions provide the essential information with which to include or exclude the great majority of anemias.

1. Is the patient truly anemic?

The answer to this seemingly trivial but in fact crucial question requires an awareness of all of the aforementioned factors that can affect the normal hematocrit as well as appreciation of the insidious nature of mistakes in sampling and measurement of blood. An isolated low hematocrit in an otherwise completely normal clinical context bears repeating before an intensive investigation is undertaken.

Does the decreased hematocrit reflect a true decrease in red cell mass? Congestive heart failure and iatrogenic fluid overload commonly cause *dilutional anemia* that disappears once diuresis is obtained. In patients with *giant splenomegaly,* red cells may be concentrated in the enlarged spleen and diluted in an increased plasma volume that is in general proportional to their degree of splenomegaly. Both maldistribution and dilution contribute to the frequently observed reduction in peripheral venous hematocrit in such individuals who may have a normal red cell mass. This phenomenon should be distinguished from hypersplenism in which the red cells (or other elements) are destroyed by the spleen. In contrast, dehydrated or severely burned patients may have significant anemia that is masked by diminished plasma volume.

2. Is the anemia inherited or acquired?

Heritable forms of anemia are almost always intrinsic to the red cell or marrow while acquired anemias more often result from extrinsic factors. This distinction, often of fundamental aid in diagnosis, is by no means always simple because of the episodic nature and variable severity of many genetic disorders, particularly those involving red cells. An inherited susceptibility to hemolysis, for example, may require exposure to an oxidant drug or severe infection for anemia to occur (e.g., G6PD deficiency in blacks). Patients may be unaware of mild to moderate lifelong anemias until they have a routine blood test or develop symptoms during pregnancy or after a severe febrile infection.

A positive *family history* suggests an inherited red cell disorder. Because of the concentration of genes for certain hemoglobinopathies and enzyme defects in various African, Mediterranean, and Oriental populations, detailed information concerning *racial background* is pertinent. Clustering of involvement on one side of the family may give clues to autosomal dominant or sex-linked modes of transmission, while a history of consanguinity may accompany autosomal recessively transmitted diseases. The absence of family history by no means excludes a genetic mechanism of transmission, even in dominantly inherited disorders such as hereditary spherocytosis, which may arise by *spontaneous mutation* in a significant number of cases. The absence of congenital anemia can be implied in regular blood donors who will have been screened by the blood bank prior to each donation.

3. Is there evidence for blood loss?

Iron deficiency anemia is the most common anemia in the general population; in the developed western societies it almost always results from blood loss. Because of the frequency of iron deficiency a careful search for blood loss is mandatory in the initial evaluation of an anemic patient. Women of reproductive age are at particular risk because of the combined iron losses of menstruation (estimated at 20 to 30 mg per month) and pregnancy (estimated at 500 mg). Estimation of menstrual loss is difficult and requires specific questioning concerning the frequency of periods, the duration of heavy flow, the frequency of changing pads or tampons, and the appearance of clots.

Gastrointestinal bleeding caused by ulcers, cancers, anomalous vessels, and parasites is a frequent source of blood loss. The gastrointestinal route is virtually the only significant occult source of bleeding. Thus iron deficiency is a frequent presenting manifestation of otherwise unsuspected gastrointestinal pathology, which must be carefully sought once bleeding has been documented.

A number of causes of blood loss that are frequently forgotten are listed below:

Diagnostic phlebotomy. Hospitalized patients, especially children and patients receiving intensive care, may undergo extensive phlebotomy. Individuals with low iron stores (most menstruating females) are at risk for developing iron deficiency as a result, while patients with other marrow impairments will be slow to make up the loss.

Regular blood donation.

Soft tissue bleeding after trauma or surgery. Fractured hips in the elderly are notorious for copious tissue bleeding. Iron is not readily salvaged from such hematomas.

Urinary loss of hemosiderin in chronic intravascular hemolysis.

Pulmonary bleeding in idiopathic pulmonary hemosiderosis.

Bleeding in patients with *hemostatic defects* including hemophilias and hereditary hemorrhagic telangiectasia.

A useful ancillary question that may uncover the presence of iron deficiency relates to the frequent ingestion of starch, clay, or ice. Craving for non-nutritive material, or *pica*, is common in patients with iron deficiency. In black cultures, clay has been a favorite substance since antiquity, and starch seems to be a modern equivalent. Another favorite material is ice, crushed or in cubes, which is also used by whites. Not all individuals who use these materials are iron deficient: there is a cultural as well as a physiologic component. Curiously, the craving for such substances often disappears within 24 hours of treatment with medicinal iron. Iron deficiency is more extensively discussed in Ch. 136 and 206.

4. Is there evidence for hemolysis?

Hemolytic anemias are considerably less common than are the anemias of iron deficiency or chronic disease and may be more difficult to recognize. Inherited disorders of the red cell show a very wide spectrum of severity for reasons that are not entirely clear. The more severe cases, which are encountered in hospitals and hematology clinics, are easily recognized. In milder cases, however, the patient may be unaware of the disease.

The answers to several questions are important for the initial data base. First, the patient should be asked if he has ever had *jaundice*, or yellowing of skin or eyeballs, and if he has ever had hepatitis. The key to suspecting inherited hemolytic anemias is the presence of constant or episodic jaundice. While the hepatic conjugating mechanism can handle a considerable increase in bilirubin production consequent to the breakdown of hemoglobin, the exacerbation of hemolysis occurring during severe febrile infections often causes visible jaundice. This combination frequently leads to the misdiagnosis of recurrent hepatitis. However, not all patients with intrinsic red cell defects give this history—some are able to handle the bilirubin load without visible jaundice.

Second, the patient should be asked if he has ever noticed *darkening of the urine* resembling tea or cola. Bile is characteristically absent from the urine in patients with hemolysis because the predominant form of bilirubin in the plasma is unconjugated and is tightly bound to albumin (Ch. 118). However, during periods of increased hemolysis, alternate products of bilirubin degradation called *dipyrroles* sometimes appear in the urine, causing considerable darkening in its color. For most patients, dark urine means concentrated urine so that specific questioning concerning the color is essential in order to exclude simple dehydration. Other causes of dark urine include hemoglobinuria in patients with moderate to severe intravascular hemolysis and biliuria in patients with liver or biliary tract disease. A careful search for symptoms of *gallbladder disease* in the patient or the family is warranted because of the frequency with which patients with chronic hemolytic disorders develop pigment stones.

As *exceptions*, megaloblastic anemias and severe dyserythropoietic states, which show marked *ineffective erythropoiesis* (also termed intramedullary hemolysis) can also cause jaundice. Similarly, resorption of large *tissue hematomas* may suggest hemolysis because of the resulting anemia and jaundice.

5. Has the patient been exposed to medication or toxins that can result in anemia?

The frequency with which individuals ingest or inhale medications and recreational drugs and the ubiquitous nature of chemical toxins require that a careful search be made for such exposures in an anemic patient. Drug-induced anemias (lumping together both medications and chemical toxins) may be associated with marrow aplasia, maturational defects, and hemolysis by both direct or immune-mediated mechanisms. While it is frequently difficult to establish cause and effect between a given chemical and anemia, certain drugs are notoriously involved, and a history of their use should always be sought. *Alcohol* is probably the most common toxin associated with anemia. The various categories and some specific agents are listed in Table 132–3.

6. Is there a systemic illness or any nonhematologic organ dysfunction?

Assessment of the habitat within which an anemia arises

TABLE 132–3. DRUGS THAT MAY CAUSE ANEMIA

I. **Agents associated with marrow aplasia*** (see Table 133–3)
Antineoplastic drugs—antimetabolites, alkylating agents
Antimicrobials—chloramphenicol, quinacrine
Anticonvulsants—phenytoin, tridione
Insecticides
Solvents—benzene
Anti-inflammatory drugs—phenylbutazone, gold

II. **Agents associated with hemolytic anemia**
Oxidant drugs*
Antibiotics—sulfasalazine, sulfones, nitrofurantoins, nalidixic acid
Antimalarials—primaquine
Analgesics—acetanilid, pyridium
Miscellaneous compounds—methylene blue, naphthalene, phenylhydrazine, fava beans

Immune mediated
Penicillin, stibophen, alpha methyldopa, quinine, etc.

III. **Agents causing maturation defects**
Alcohol
Folate antagonists—trimethoprim, triamterene, methotrexate
Heme synthesis antagonists—INH, lead

IV. **Agents causing gastrointestinal blood loss**
Aspirin, nonsteroidal anti-inflammatory agents

*Hemolytic primarily in G6PD-deficient individuals.

TABLE 132–4. PHYSICAL FINDINGS IN VARIOUS ANEMIAS

Physical Finding	Associated Anemia
Skin	
Jaundice	Hemolysis, liver disease
Petechiae	Blood dyscrasia, autoimmune hemolysis with ITP
Telangiectasia	Iron deficiency
Spider angiomas	Liver disease
Facies	
Frontal bossing, maxillary prominence, hypertelorism	Severe congenital hemolysis
Eyes	
Scleral icterus	Hemolysis, liver disease
Retinal hemorrhages	Severe anemia of any cause
Retinal detachment	SC hemoglobinopathy
Mucous Membranes	
Glossitis	Vitamin B_{12}, folate, or iron deficiency
Angular cheilosis	Iron deficiency
Lymph Nodes	
Generalized adenopathy	Malignant lymphoma, blood dyscrasias
Cardiac	
Valvular murmurs	Traumatic hemolysis with iron deficiency, bacterial endocarditis with ACD
Abdominal	
Splenomegaly	Hypersplenism, chronic leukemias, hemolysis, etc.
Hepatomegaly	Liver disease
Pelvic and Rectal	
Hemorrhoids, masses	Blood loss, iron deficiency
Extremities	
Symmetric joint deformity	Rheumatoid arthritis, ACD, and iron deficiency
Congenital anomalies	Constitutional marrow aplasias
Leg ulcers	Chronic hemolysis, esp. sickle cell disease
Myopathy	Rare red cell enzymopathies (deficiency of phosphofructokinase)
Neurologic	
Diminished vibration, position sense, dementia	Vitamin B_{12} deficiency
Neuropathy	Lead poisoning
Mental retardation, spastic paresis	Rare red cell enzymopathies (deficiency of triosephosphate isomerase)

requires a careful search for systemic illness or organ dysfunction.

The Anemia of Chronic Disease (ACD). Most patients with *active inflammatory disease* or *advanced malignant disease* show a characteristic mild to moderate anemia. The severity of the anemia is in general related to the intensity of the inflammation or the extent of malignant spread, although occasionally relatively localized tumors may present with prominent systemic symptoms and anemia. Weight loss, fever, and night sweats may indicate underlying systemic inflammation. Chronic infections such as subacute bacterial endocarditis and active inflammatory processes such as *rheumatoid arthritis* and inflammatory bowel disease are almost always associated with ACD. The diagnosis of ACD and its differentiation from iron deficiency are discussed in Ch. 134.

Nonhematologic Organ Dysfunction. Patients with diminished renal, hepatic, or endocrine function are often anemic. The pathogenesis of these anemias is multifactorial, and there are relatively few constant distinguishing features. In each case, a significant degree of organ failure must be present to result in anemia. Therefore they are relatively easily excluded by simple measurement of renal, hepatic, thyroid, or pituitary function.

Anemia Associated with Immune Dyscrasias. Red blood cell production and destruction are intimately modulated by the immune system (Ch. 130). It is thus not surprising that immune dysfunction, due either to dysregulation or neoplasms or both, is commonly complicated by anemias. Autoimmune hemolytic anemia is classically associated with systemic lupus erythematosus or with B cell neoplasms, particularly chronic lymphocytic leukemia or diffuse large cell (histiocytic) lymphomas. The hallmark of this combination is a *positive Coombs test* (Ch. 137). Another B cell neoplasm, *multiple myeloma,* commonly presents with anemia due to marrow invasion or suppression or both. Thus the triad of skeletal symptoms (usually low back pain), renal dysfunction, and anemia should always prompt a search for myeloma (see Ch. 163).

The Physical Examination

As in the evaluation of any systemic disorder, a complete physical examination is essential in the patient who presents with anemia. However, particular attention should be paid to the presence of certain key findings that are of help in classifying the anemia (Table 132–4).

The Initial Laboratory Data Base

An essential minimum laboratory data base, most of which is obtained on every hospitalized patient, includes a complete blood count (or hemogram), an examination of the peripheral blood smear (usually performed as part of the leukocyte differential), examination of the stool for occult blood, and a reticulocyte count. These readily available procedures provide powerful and sometimes definitive diagnostic information.

THE HEMOGRAM. Modern automated cell counters provide a great deal of information to the physician for remarkably little effort by the laboratory. These instruments are designed to detect the passage of individual blood cells through either an electrically charged aperture or a laser beam. The resulting change in impedance or in light scatter as the cell passes is counted and quantitated. The size of the impedance change is proportional to the size of the cell causing it. Thus both the number and size distribution of cells are measured, which allows for derivation of the total volume of red cells (the hematocrit), as well as separation between cells of different sizes (red cells and platelets).

Red Cell Indices. The mean corpuscular volume (MCV) is the most useful of the red blood cell indices. Most hematologists consider the range of MCV's between 80 and 100 cubic microns as normal, although the actual range defined by statistical criteria is somewhat narrower.

The MCV provides a convenient basis for separating anemias into groups that are microcytic (less than 80 cubic microns), normocytic (80 to 100 cubic microns), and macrocytic (greater than 100 cubic microns). This classification is useful but limited by the fact that the great majority of anemic patients fall within the normocytic group and must be distinguished by other means.

MICROCYTOSIS. Microcytosis (see Table 132–5) almost always reflects *defective cytoplasmic maturation* due to impaired heme synthesis, as in iron deficiency, or defective globin synthesis, as in the thalassemias. Carriers of beta-thalassemia trait have MCV's that are almost always less than 80 and usually less than 70 cubic microns (Ch. 142). The alpha-thalassemia traits are often somewhat milder, with MCV's in the 70's. Moderate to severe iron deficiency is also associated with a decreased MCV. In patients with iron deficiency, the microcytosis is in rough proportion to the degree of anemia, whereas in carriers of thalassemias the microcytosis may be much greater with only mild or no anemia. Severe inflammatory disease can induce iron-deficient erythropoiesis in ACD. While the anemia is usually normocytic, occasionally in such patients the anemia is quite microcytic despite normal or increased iron stores. Other causes of reduced MCV include defects in heme synthesis such as occur in lead poisoning or inherited sideroblastic anemia (Table 132–5).

MACROCYTOSIS. Macrocytosis (see Table 132–5) usually reflects *aberrant nuclear maturation* or is a consequence of stressed erythropoiesis. Values for MCV of 130 cubic microns or more occur in severe megaloblastic anemias due to deficiency of vitamin B_{12} or folate (Ch. 136). Many moderate to severe hemolytic disorders are also macrocytic because of the presence of large prematurely released reticulocytes, which have been called shift cells (see next section).

Combinations of factors that cause macrocytosis and microcytosis, when they occur in the same patient, not infrequently create *exceptions* to these rules. For example, the rather common occurrence of alpha-thalassemia in blacks can mask the macrocytosis seen in pernicious anemia. Similarly, *combined nutritional deficiency* of iron and vitamin B_{12} or folic acid, such as often occurs during *pregnancy* or in *alcoholics*, can result in severe anemia with a normal MCV. Here the key to the diagnosis may rest in the accompanying leukocyte abnormalities of hypersegmentation.

Primary marrow diseases, especially aplastic anemias and refractory anemias associated with myelodysplastic syndromes, commonly have a moderately elevated MCV. Many moderate or severe hemolytic disorders are also macrocytic because of the presence of large prematurely released reticulocytes.

The mean corpuscular hemoglobin (MCH) and mean corpuscular hemoglobin concentration (MCHC), which are derived indices, provide ancillary information concerning cell size and hemoglobin content but are rarely as helpful as the MCV. The Coulter apparatus is relatively insensitive to elevation of the MCHC that is known to occur in spherocytic disorders.

TABLE 132–5. MICROCYTIC AND MACROCYTIC ANEMIAS

Microcytosis (MCV < 80μ³)	Macrocytosis (MCV > 100μ³)
Iron deficiency	Megaloblastic anemias
Thalassemias	Chemotherapy* (esp. hydroxyurea)
Anemia of chronic disease (usually normocytic)	Reticulocytosis*
	Aplastic anemias*
Sideroblastic anemias* Hereditary Lead poisoning	Hypothyroidism*
	Sideroblastic anemias* Acquired
Severe red cell fragmentation Burns* Hereditary pyropoikilocytosis	Myelodysplasias* Chromosome (5q−) deletion

*In many cases MCV may be borderline or within the normal range.

The Leukocyte and Platelet Count. Anemia should always be assessed in relation to total marrow function. Anemia with a diminished leukocyte and platelet count—*pancytopenia*—suggests primary marrow disease, megaloblastic anemia, or hypersplenism. A bone marrow study is frequently needed to establish the diagnosis of pancytopenia (see Table 133–3).

THE RETICULOCYTE COUNT. A reticulocyte is a young cell newly released from the bone marrow. Normal circulating reticulocytes in a nonanemic individual are morphologically indistinguishable from more mature red cells and must be counted after staining with new methylene blue. The percentage of cells showing bluish clumps or strands of RNA in 500 or 1000 total cells is referred to as the reticulocyte count. The normal reticulocyte circulates for approximately 24 hours before maturing and may spend a brief portion of that time in the spleen. Because normal red cells survive for an average of 120 days, the normal reticulocyte count is approximately 1 per cent (range 0.5 to 1.8 per cent). Anemia of any cause, by decreasing the denominator of the fraction by which the reticulocyte percentage is derived, will increase the count. For this reason the count is customarily corrected to a "normal" hematocrit of 45 per cent:

Corrected retic count = retic count × patient Hct/45

Additional corrections of the reticulocyte count have been proposed that take into consideration the increased time of maturation of the "shift" reticulocytes released prematurely from the marrow in severe anemia. These may circulate for considerably longer than 24 hours, but are also subject to a variable period of sequestration in the spleen. The uncertainty associated with estimating true reticulocyte maturation time in the circulation makes the interpretation of an elevated count a semiquantitative exercise.

While *reticulocytosis is a hallmark of hemolytic anemia*, it gives no information about longevity of red cells; rather it reflects entirely the ability of the marrow to respond. Reticulocytosis is most readily interpreted by several measurements over a significant time span. This allows one to assess whether the hematocrit is rising and the reticulocytosis is sustained. Persistent reticulocytosis of 5 per cent or greater (corrected) with a stable hematocrit over several weeks is highly suggestive of a continuing hemolytic process.

Young patients with congenital hemolytic anemias are at risk from transient suppression of marrow function by viral infection (see Ch. 133). They may have an *aplastic crisis* with a precipitous fall in hematocrit and a low reticulocyte count or absence of reticulocytes. Prompt diagnosis and treatment (by transfusions) of this life-threatening complication of chronic hemolysis depends on recognizing this *exception* to the general correlation between hemolysis and reticulocytosis.

Reticulocytosis with a rising hematocrit suggests either a transient hemolytic episode, such as might occur in G6PD deficiency with an exposure to an oxidant drug, or recovery from blood loss. Recovery of marrow function after reversible suppression, such as correction of vitamin B_{12} or folic acid deficiency, will also cause marked transient reticulocytosis with a rising hematocrit.

A markedly decreased corrected reticulocyte count of less than 0.5 per cent implies a primary suppression of the marrow rather than just inadequate response to anemic stress. The causes of marrow failure are discussed in Ch. 133. Severe reticulocytopenia (0.1 per cent or less) implies aplasia of the marrow, either aplastic anemia or its variant pure red cell aplasia. Reticulocyte counts are sometimes expressed as an absolute number, rather than as a percentage. A normal value represents 1 per cent of 5 million red cells or approximately 50,000 reticulocytes per cubic millimeter. Levels below 20,000 reticulocytes per cubic millimeter represent severe reduction in marrow output.

In the great majority of anemias that represent varying combinations of marrow inadequacy and peripheral loss or destruction of red cells, reticulocytes fall in an indeterminate range within the extreme values given above.

EXAMINATION OF THE PERIPHERAL BLOOD SMEAR. The diagnostic information to be gained from an educated appraisal of the blood morphology exceeds that of any other simple laboratory test. In addition to abnormalities in red cells, abnormal leukocytes or platelets can also contribute valuable diagnostic information. It would be misleading to claim that most anemias can be diagnosed from the peripheral smear alone. However, the large number of anemic processes that can be *excluded* by the smear as well as the frequency of definitive abnormalities make it highly useful.

When looking at a peripheral blood smear from a patient with anemia: (1) It is crucial to be aware of the treacherous effects of *artifact* on red blood cell morphology. Routine differential counts and platelet estimations are frequently performed on blood smears that are totally inadequate for evaluation of red cells. (2) One must seek not only the particular abnormal red cell that may give a clue to diagnosis, but also must *evaluate the background morphology* in which it arises. The frequency of poikilocytosis in anemia is such that one can find almost any cell one wishes by looking long enough. Thus several schistocytes found in association with numerous other abnormal shapes are insufficient evidence that traumatic hemolysis is a major cause of the anemia. Marked poikilocytosis usually represents either the effects of dyspoiesis due to nutritional or dysplastic disorders of the marrow or fragmenting accidents to red cells that occur in the circulation. The distinction between these alternatives is often difficult and may depend on ancillary data including marrow examination. In contrast, a particular abnormality such as spherocytosis when it occurs as a significant minority finding

TABLE 132-6. USEFUL FINDINGS FROM PERIPHERAL BLOOD MORPHOLOGY

Abnormalities in Red Cell Morphology	Associated Conditions
A. **Hypoproliferative group**	
Normal smear	Aplasias, ACD
Rouleaux	Myeloma
Burr cells	Renal failure
Blasts	Blood dyscrasias
Teardrops, nucleated RBC	Myelophthisic anemias
Extreme poikilocytosis	Myelodysplasias
B. **Maturation defect group**	
Hypochromia, microcytes	Iron deficiency
Targets (occasional)	Thalassemias
Elliptocytes (occasional)	
Oval macrocytes	
Hypersegmented neutrophils (>5% PMN's with 5 or more lobes)	Vitamin B_1- or folate deficiency
Prominent basophilic stippling	Lead poisoning, sideroblastic anemias
C. **Hyperproliferative group**	
Polychromasia ± nucleated RBC	Hemolysis, response to anemic or hypoxic stress
Sickle forms	Sickle cell disease or variants
Microspherocytes (smooth)	Hereditary spherocytosis, autoimmune hemolytic anemia
Microspherocytes (rough = echinocytes)	Glycolytic enzyme defects esp. postsplenectomy
"Bite" cells—Heinz bodies (special stain)	Oxidant hemolysis, G6PD deficiency
Schistocytes	Traumatic or microangiopathic hemolysis
Target cells (predominant)	HbC and E syndromes
Extreme microspherocytosis with budding	Burns, hereditary pyropoikilocytosis
D. **Changes not usually associated with anemia**	
Howell-Jolly bodies	Hyposplenism
Target cells	Obstructive jaundice
Elliptocytosis (predominant)	Hereditary elliptocytosis (may be hemolytic)

TABLE 132-7. INDICATIONS FOR BONE MARROW EXAMINATION IN ANEMIA

Presence of circulating nucleated red cells
Pancytopenias
Absence of reticulocytes
Presence of circulating blasts
Monoclonal gammopathies
Definitive estimation of marrow iron stores
Suspicion of sideroblastic anemia
Moderate to severe anemia of unknown cause
Combined nutritional deficiencies

in an otherwise relatively normal cell population assumes more significance. (3) It should be noted that *splenectomy* greatly enhances the range of morphologic diversity in almost any anemia.

A list of relatively specific aberrations in red cell morphology and their associated anemias is given in Table 132-6.

TESTING OF STOOLS FOR OCCULT BLOOD. Gastrointestinal bleeding is a frequent cause of iron deficiency anemia and, furthermore, it may indicate the presence of *carcinoma of the colon* or another malignant tumor. Examination of the stools for occult blood is therefore an essential part of the initial data base on every anemic patient. The most widely used procedure for occult fecal blood is the Hemoccult test, which depends on the presence of peroxidase activity of the heme in the sample. The test is sensitive enough to detect approximately 5 ml of blood in a 24-hour sample of stool, but difficulties arise if bleeding is *intermittent* or if the blood does not permeate the stool evenly (sampling error). Bleeding from the upper gastrointestinal tract and oral doses of vitamin C diminish the sensitivity of the test. Hydrating the stool smear with a drop of water before developing approximately doubles the sensitivity. Red meat and certain raw vegetables with high levels of endogenous peroxides, such as broccoli, may cause false positive tests.

A single negative glove or stool specimen is insufficient to exclude gastrointestinal bleeding as a cause of iron deficiency. At least three samples, and preferably six, should be tested on separate days, and one should never be satisfied with a negative result when there is no other explanation for iron deficiency.

Examination of the Bone Marrow in Evaluation of Anemias

The most common anemias—those associated with blood loss, chronic disease, hemolysis, or nutritional deficiency—do not normally require an examination of the marrow for definitive diagnosis. The available tests for assessing the sufficiency of iron, vitamin B_{12}, and folic acid in serum, when coupled with assessment of response to a therapeutic trial, are generally quite sufficient for simple deficiencies. Difficulties arise, however, in the complex case in which combined deficiencies or chronic disease is present. Since nutritional anemias, particularly in patients with alcoholism, are often multiple, marrow examination may be the only means to establish the adequacy of iron stores in this setting. Similar problems arise in iron deficiency when combined with chronic inflammatory disease such as active rheumatoid arthritis.

Virtually all of the other indications for marrow examination involve the suspicion of a *primary blood dyscrasia* or the invasion of the marrow space by an *extrinsic tumor or infection*. Exami-

TABLE 132-8. SOME USEFUL ANCILLARY TESTS WHEN THE INITIAL DATA BASE IS UNREVEALING

Coombs' test
Sedimentation rate
Creatinine
Liver function tests
Thyroid profile
Serum protein electrophoresis
Serum iron and transferrin

TABLE 132–9. LABORATORY APPROACH TO DIAGNOSIS OF CAUSE OF ANEMIA

Hematocrit	RBC Mass	Retics (corrected)	MCV	Smear	Other	Marrow	Diagnostic Group
	Clinical assessment; Exclude hemodilution	↑ → NL or ↑		Table 132–6 Group C	± Jaundice	Rarely indicated	Hyperproliferative Hemolytic
					Acute bleed	Not indicated	Hyperproliferative Hemorrhagic
			↑	Table 132–6 Group B	± Pancytopenia	Megaloblastic	Nuclear maturation defect—B₁-folate deficiency
Verify ↓ →	↓ →	NL or ↓ →	NL	Table 132–6 Group A	See Table 132–8	See Table 132–7	Hypoproliferative
			↓	Table 132–6 Group B	Iron studies NL or ↑	↑ Iron stores ± sideroblasts	Cytoplasmic maturation defect— thalassemias, etc.
					Chronic blood loss	↓ Iron stores	Cytoplasmic maturation defect—iron deficiency
	↓↓ — ↑			Normal	± Pancytopenia	Empty or loss of erythroid precursors	Hypoproliferative — aplasias

nation of aspirated smears in general gives superior cytologic information while the core biopsy provides crucial information concerning the overall cellularity, as well as the presence of fibrosis, tumor, or granulomas. Both procedures are complementary and are best performed together when the diagnosis is in doubt.

Firm indications for marrow examination in anemia are listed in Table 132–7.

USE OF LABORATORY DATA IN EVALUATION OF ANEMIAS. Careful assessment of the initial data base will almost always reveal diagnostic clues to follow. A list of useful ancillary procedures when no hints can be extracted from the data base are given in Table 132–8. In Table 132–9 a rational approach to the laboratory evaluation of anemias is summarized, with reference back to the previous tables in this chapter. The definitive diagnostic approaches to the various disorders are described in the accompanying chapters.

TREATMENT OF ANEMIAS

Therapies for the various causes of anemia are detailed in subsequent chapters. Some general therapeutic principles and common therapeutic errors are pertinent to this introduction. Therapy for anemia may be *specific,* as in the replacement of deficient iron, vitamin B₁₂, or folate; *diagnostic,* as in the therapeutic trial; or *symptomatic,* as in the administration of blood transfusions. It is a mark of good practice to carefully distinguish these differing therapeutic situations.

Specific therapy requires a definitive diagnosis, the absence of which converts it into a therapeutic trial. Therapeutic trials of iron or vitamin B₁₂ are consistent with good practice, provided that the response is documented quantitatively and the cause of any deficiency found is thoroughly investigated. Duration of treatment must be correlated with response and based on a thorough understanding of continuing requirements and body stores to avoid harm to patients. For example, patients may continue using iron supplements for years after a course of therapy and become at risk for iron overload. Conversely, the cessation of cobalamin therapy after a full response is obtained in pernicious anemia, a lifelong disease, will inevitably lead to a potentially damaging recurrence. Probably the most frequent error in the treatment of anemia

is the excessive use of specific remedies, e.g., iron or cobalamin, for questionable symptomatic indications.

Symptomatic treatment of anemia with blood transfusions must be undertaken within the same constraints as for any other medical disorder—that is, for *real symptoms* that outweigh the *real hazards* of therapy. Deviations from good practice most often involve (1) overestimation of the benefits of transfusion in a compensated patient, particularly when symptoms relate more to an underlying disease than to the anemia per se, and (2) underestimating the life-threatening risks of transfusion, both circulatory and infectious. Thus the sporadic use of small-volume transfusions for symptomatic indications is rarely consistent with good practice.

Blood volume. In Mollison PL: Blood Transfusion in Clinical Medicine. Oxford, Blackwell Scientific Publications. 7th ed. 1983, pp 65–92. *A gold mine of information concerning the many factors influencing blood volume in health and disease. Much of this material is not generally referenced in hematology texts.*
The approach to the patient with anemia. In Wintrobe MM: Clinical Hematology. Philadelphia, Lea and Febiger. 8th ed. 1981, pp 529–558. *A more leisurely approach to the subject with the usual comprehensive perspective and extensive historical references that have characterized this work throughout its many editions.*

133 ANEMIA DUE TO BONE MARROW FAILURE

Alan S. Keitt

The hematopoietic system consists of primitive migratory pluripotential stem cells, their progeny, and certain habitats to which these cells are attracted to undergo differentiation. The organization of these habitats is determined by specialized supporting cells that provide a framework in which the hematopoietic and lymphoid cells may operate. These organs are components of the reticuloendothelial system, named for the fibroblastic and endothelial cells that make up their supporting matrix. They share certain homologies in their vascular architecture, namely a system of cords and sinuses, which are lined by the supporting cells. In subprimates and during fetal life, all of the reticuloendothelial organs may harbor active hematopoietic tissue. In mature primates, however, the liver, spleen, and lymph nodes assume other specialized functions, and only the bone marrow continues to support effective hematopoiesis.

Marrow failure may arise by two basically distinct mechanisms: the aplastic and myelophthisic anemias. The *aplastic anemias* represent failure of the stem cell to undergo differentiation, either because of intrinsic damage, or interruption of its interactions with the particular cast of supporting cells that comprise its microenvironment. The *myelophthisic anemias* result from loss of essential habitat for hematopoiesis due to destruction of the macroenvironment of the bone marrow by neoplastic or inflammatory tissue. This latter group will be considered briefly in a separate section at the end of this chapter.

THE APLASTIC ANEMIAS
Definition

APLASTIC ANEMIA. This refers to a diverse group of potentially severe marrow disorders characterized by peripheral pancytopenia and a marrow that is largely devoid of hematopoietic cells but that retains the basic marrow architecture or stroma with replacement of hematopoietic cells by large amounts of fat. Aplastic anemia has been classified as *severe* when at least two of the following three criteria are present: (1) anemia with a corrected reticulocyte count <1 per cent, (2) neutrophils <500 per cubic millimeter, (3) platelets <20,000 per cubic millimeter. In addition, marrow hypocellularity must be present (estimated as <25 per cent of marrow space).

UNICELLULAR APLASIAS. Isolated deficiencies of each of the main hematopoietic cell lines, i.e., pure red cell aplasia (PRCA), occur somewhat less commonly than typical aplastic anemia. In some instances the unicellular aplasias may progress to frank aplastic anemia with pancytopenia, but a significant number of other cases will remain "pure." The unicellular aplasias exhibit relatively normal cellularity of the bone marrow with selective dropout of one set of precursors. These disorders presumably arise from failure of a "committed" rather than a pluripotential stem cell. There is no clear means at the present time of separating these disorders from those in which recognizable precursors of a given cell line occur in the marrow in the absence of mature forms. It is likely that these disorders are part of a spectrum of autoimmune cytopenias in which the target cells have differing degrees of maturation.

CONSTITUTIONAL APLASIAS. Inherited forms of the disease, both pancellular and unicellular, have been designated as constitutional aplasias. These frequently arise in combination with various congenital anomalies and probably involve fundamental intrinsic abnormalities of stem cells.

Etiology

The multiple causes and diverse associations of the various bone marrow failure syndromes are classified in Table 133–1. Approximately 50 per cent of cases arise de novo and are thus considered idiopathic. The remaining cases are associated with exposure to an extremely diverse array of chemicals or ionizing radiation or occur in the context of a neoplastic, autoimmune, or infectious disease. Such associations do not necessarily imply a causal relationship with the aplasia. There is little apparent clinical difference between the idiopathic and secondary forms of the disease.

DRUG-RELATED APLASIAS (Table 133–2). *Dose-Dependent Aplasias.* Chemotherapeutic agents used in the treatment of various neoplasms are virtually uniform in their cytotoxicity for hematopoietic stem cells. The resulting aplasia is usually reversible, and its severity depends on the amount of drug

TABLE 133–1. CLASSIFICATION OF THE ETIOLOGY OF APLASTIC ANEMIA AND RELATED DISORDERS

I. **Aplastic Anemias**
  A. *Acquired*

Idiopathic	Radiation
Autoimmune	Infections—hepatitis
Drugs (Table 133–2)	Pregnancy
Toxic chemicals	Paroxysmal nocturnal hemoglobinuria

  B. *Constitutional*
    Familial or congenital
    Fanconi's anemia
    Dyskeratosis congenita

II. **Unicellular Aplasias**
  A. *Pure red cell aplasia*
    1. Acquired

Thymoma	Autoimmune
Idiopathic	Drugs and toxins

    2. Constitutional
      Diamond-Blackfan
      anemia
  B. *Agranulocytosis/granulocytopenia*
    1. Acquired

Idiopathic	Felty's syndrome
Drugs and toxins	Thymoma

    2. Constitutional
      Congenital
      Familial-benign, severe, cyclic
  C. *Thrombocytopenia*
    1. Acquired
      Idiopathic
      Autoimmune-systemic lupus erythematosus
      Drugs and toxins
    2. Constitutional
      Amegakaryocytic thrombocytopenia (associated with congenital anomalies)
      Autosomal recessive thrombocytopenia

exposure. Agents that are cycle specific such as cytosine arabinoside and methotrexate act preferentially on the more mature stem cells, which are known to have a higher mitotic rate than the more primitive pluripotential stem cells. As a result, patients manifest pancytopenia prior to the depletion of the pluripotent stem cells on which ultimate marrow regeneration depends. Other agents such as busulfan and the nitrosoureas attack both cycling and noncycling stem cells and therefore can lead to prolonged or irreversible aplasia unless used with great caution. Certain other drugs that are not used for cancer chemotherapy show reversible, dose-related marrow suppression as an adverse side effect. These include phenytoin, phenothiazines, thiouracil, methicillin, and chloramphenicol.

Idiosyncratic Aplasias. Another large group of seemingly unrelated drugs, which may or may not show dose-related marrow suppression, is associated with the rare occurrence of disastrous aplasia in a small number of sensitive individuals. The prototype of this group is *chloramphenicol*, for many years the leading cause of idiosyncratic drug-related aplastic anemia. Chloramphenicol has restricted usage in developed countries, but it is still widely available and heavily used in Third World countries, where accurate assessment of fatalities is unavailable.

In contrast to the dose-dependent aplasias, idiosyncratic reactions may occur weeks or months after exposure to small amounts of chloramphenicol. The frequency of this reaction is estimated between 1:24,000 and 1:40,000 of the exposed population. Even the use of topical ophthalmic solutions has been associated with aplasia. A latent period does not always occur; the rapid development of severe aplasia during therapy is not uncommon.

Chloramphenicol also manifests reversible dose-related marrow suppression primarily affecting erythroid precursors probably as a result of its inhibition of mitochondrial protein and heme synthesis. This effect of chloramphenicol is associated with prominent vacuolization and sideroblastic changes in developing erythroblasts.

There is evidence from studies of identical twin concordance that some patients who develop severe idiosyncratic aplasia from chloramphenicol have an underlying genetic suscepti-bility. The nature and frequency of this putative sensitivity is unknown. The management and prognosis of chloramphen-icol-related aplasia does not differ from that of other idiosyn-cratic drug reactions or of the idiopathic form of the disease and will be discussed subsequently. Drugs that have been associated with the development of marrow aplasias are listed in Table 133–2.

ENVIRONMENTAL TOXINS (Table 133–2). Solvents and insecticides comprise the major group of toxins that have been linked to aplastic anemia. Of these, benzene is the most important and has received the most experimental attention. *Benzene* appears to have heterogeneous effects on marrow function and may induce various combinations of aplasia, myelofibrosis, or frank leukemia. The abnormalities in marrow function may arise during or years after exposure to benzene. Most recognized cases have resulted from rather heavy and prolonged industrial exposures. Aplastic anemia after glue sniffing probably relates to the presence of benzene deriva-tives in glues.

INFECTIONS. *Hepatitis.* Severe aplastic anemia may fol-low an episode of apparent viral hepatitis. The association seems to be with non-A, non-B hepatitis and is twice as common in males as in females, usually occurring in patients under 20 years of age. The hepatitis is not unusually severe, whereas the subsequent aplasia is often quite severe and has a high mortality.

Parvovirus. Selective transient loss of erythroid precursors in the marrow with reticulocytopenia is a well-recognized occurrence in patients with congenital hemolytic anemias and has been termed *aplastic crisis.* Although the suppression of erythropoiesis is self limited, the rapid fall of hematocrit that is a result of the short lifespan of the remaining red cells may induce severe life-threatening anemia. Human parvovirus infection has been linked to aplastic crisis in hereditary sphero-cytosis and sickle cell anemia, and the virus has been shown to selectively inhibit erythroid progenitors in cell cultures. The association with parvovirus appears quite specific. The apparent tropism of the virus for the erythroid stem cell has rekindled speculations concerning a viral etiology for aplastic anemia.

TABLE 133–2. CHEMICAL AND PHYSICAL AGENTS ASSOCIATED WITH THE DEVELOPMENT OF PANCYTOPENIA AND A HYPOPLASTIC MARROW*†

ANTINEOPLASTIC AGENTS: alkylating agents, antimetabolites, antimitotic agents, antibiotics, radiation

ANTIMICROBIAL AGENTS: *chloramphenicol, organic arsenicals, quinacrine,* streptomycin, penicillin, methicillin, oxytetracycline, chlortetracycline, sulfonamides, sulfisoxazole (Gantrisin), sulfamethoxypyridazine (Kynex), amphotericin B

ANTICONVULSANTS: mephenytoin (Mesantoin), *trimethadione (Tridione),* phenacemide (Phenurone), phenytoin, ethosuximide (Zarontin), carbamazepine (Tegretol)

ANTITHYROID DRUGS: carbethoxythiomethylglyoxaline (Carbimazole), methylmercaptoimidazole (Tapazole), potassium perchlorate, propylthiouracil

ANTIDIABETIC AGENTS: tolbutamide, chlorpropamide, carbutamide

ANTIHISTAMINES: tripelennamine (Pyribenzamine)

ANTIRHEUMATIC AGENTS: *phenylbutazone, gold compounds,* acetylsalicylic acid, indomethacin, penicillamine, colchicine

SEDATIVES AND TRANQUILIZERS: meprobamate, chlorpromazine, promazine, chlordiazepoxide (Librium), mepazine

MISCELLANEOUS: acetazolamide (Diamox)

TOXIC CHEMICALS: solvents (*benzene,* glue, toluene, carbon tetrachloride), insecticides (chlorophenothane [DDT], parathion, chlordane, pentachlorophenol), bismuth, mercury, arsenic, colloidal silver

*Adapted from Wintrobe MM: Clinical Hematology. 8th ed. Philadelphia, Lea & Febiger, 1981. Drugs associated with 20 or more reported cases are in italics.

†Additional drugs that are associated only with agranulocytosis are not listed here (see Ch. 150).

PRELEUKEMIA. Most forms of marrow aplasia, both ac-quired and congenital, have been associated with the occa-sional development of acute leukemia. One characteristic sequence of events occurs in children who present with typical aplastic anemia but respond rapidly to corticosteroid therapy. These patients ultimately relapse with typical acute lympho-cytic leukemia of childhood. Rarely, acute myeloid leukemias may arise after years of mild or moderate marrow aplasia, particularly in patients with exposure to benzene or radiation.

Pathogenesis

The pathogenesis of aplastic anemia remains elusive. The diversity of the clinical contexts in which it arises (Table 133–1) and the heterogeneity of responses to different thera-pies suggest that several or perhaps many different mecha-nisms are involved. Two dominant hypotheses have emerged: (1) a *primary stem cell failure,* i.e., an intrinsic defect of the hematopoietic stem cell that renders it unable to differentiate (such a lesion could arise by exposure of a susceptible indi-vidual to an environmental chemical, by viral infection of the stem cell, or by other unknown mechanisms); (2) an *immu-nologically mediated attack* either on the stem cell itself or on other components of the complex network of cells and factors that are necessary for normal hematopoiesis (reviewed in Ch. 131). It predicts that in some cases, continued suppression of the marrow would prevent simple replacement of stem cells by marrow transplantation.

EVIDENCE FOR DEFECTIVE STEM CELLS. Approxi-mately one half of patients with aplastic anemia who have received marrow transplants from an *identical twin* have had engraftment with rapid, complete, and sustained recovery of marrow function. The simplest interpretation of these dra-matic therapeutic results is that the donor marrow has re-placed absent or defective stem cells in the patient, since external factors, such as antibodies, would presumably attack the new cells as well. The data give no information about the nature of the original stem cell lesion, however.

EVIDENCE FOR IMMUNE-MEDIATED MARROW FAIL-URE. In the remainder of the attempted transplants between identical twins, the donated marrow is rejected by the aplastic recipient. In most of these patients, however, grafting can be subsequently carried out after a course of cyclophosphamide therapy, and they then show sustained and complete recovery of marrow function. What cyclophosphamide does in these patients is unclear: (1) It might eliminate a population of immune cells and interrupt an immune reaction against the donor stem cells, or (2) it might eliminate residual defective stem cells from preferred architectural "niches" that are es-sential for normal stem cell differentiation, allowing access of the donor stem cells to these particular microenvironmental sites.

Antilymphocyte Globulins. Antilymphocyte globulins (ALG) or antithymocyte globulins (ATG), complex hetero-antisera raised in animals against thymic lymphocytes, can significantly ameliorate the course of aplastic anemia in many patients. The clinical responses, which are obtained in 30 to 65 per cent of patients, are incomplete; they may occur after several months of therapy, and cytopenias may persist. How-ever, transfusion requirements are often abated, and the granulocyte and platelet counts may rise above the critical levels necessary to prevent infection or bleeding. These anti-sera are generally assumed to act by immunosuppression, but they also bind to many hematopoietic cells and may have other targets that are not presently defined. Unfortunately, different antisera vary considerably in efficacy, and there is no current method to assay the active components by means other than in vivo therapeutic trials in humans.

In Vitro Studies. Colony growth in normal marrow in vitro cultures is suppressed by various mononuclear cell fractions, usually containing T cells, derived from some patients with aplastic anemia. The interpretation of these results is complicated, however, by the presence of alloimmunization consequent to transfusion therapy of these patients. When alloimmunization is absent (no previous transfusion or in identical twin coculture experiments), inhibition is observed more rarely (10 to 15 per cent) than was initially supposed. As other evidence for the role of cellular immune suppression, erythroid and granulocytic colonies can be grown from marrows of some patients with aplastic anemia only after removal of T cells.

Unicellular Aplasias. Autoimmunity is clearly important in causing some of the unicellular aplasias, particularly in pure red cell aplasia (PRCA). This disease often arises in patients with other manifestations of immune dysfunction. Thymoma, hypogammaglobulinemia, monoclonal gammopathy, antinuclear antibodies, and Coombs-positive hemolysis have all been reported in association with PRCA. Serum inhibitors of erythropoiesis have been described using marrow culture techniques. Immunoglobulin fractions derived from affected patients have shown specific staining of erythroblast nuclei by immunofluorescence as well as complement-dependent cytolysis of erythroblasts. These patients also frequently respond to combinations of prednisone or Cytoxan; reduction in the post-treatment level of serum inhibitor has been demonstrated in some instances. *Transient erythroblastopenia of childhood*, a self-limited form of PRCA, is also associated with antibody-mediated marrow suppression.

SUMMARY. Marrow aplasia syndromes are associated with agents that are known to be both cytotoxic and leukemogenic (e.g., alkylating agents, benzene, and ionizing radiation) as well as with constitutional disorders that may also terminate in acute leukemia (e.g., Fanconi's anemia). This implies that intrinsic genetic damage to stem cells may occur that prevents normal differentiation. The degree to which the proliferative potential of these damaged stem cells is preserved may then determine whether aplasia or leukemia ensues. This apparent dichotomy is reminiscent of the effects of retroviral infections of immune cells that can induce either malignant transformation or selective aplasia of the same cell type. Marrow failure in other cases seems to be associated with inhibition of normal stem cell differentiation as a result of cellular or humoral autoimmunity. It is premature to invoke immune marrow suppression in most patients with aplastic anemia simply because they respond to ALG.

Incidence

Fortunately aplastic anemia is rare. The incidence of idiopathic aplastic anemia was 11 new cases per million population per year in Sweden from 1973 to 1977. This is about one-fourth the incidence of acute leukemia in the general population. There is a fivefold increase in the incidence of this disease after the age of 65 years. Aplastic anemia seems to be more common in the Orient, although this has not been firmly established.

Clinical Description

ONSET. The clinical features of the disease relate almost entirely to the effects of inadequate numbers of functional peripheral blood cells. The onset is usually insidious but may be dramatic, depending on the severity and rapidity with which the aplasia progresses. Bleeding manifestations may be the first indication of severe disease. These include gingival bleeding, epistaxis, and petechial hemorrhages, all of which are characteristic of severe thrombocytopenia. Fatigue and pallor are usually noted at presentation. Infections frequently begin with bacterial invasion of vulnerable areas of the gastrointestinal tract, namely, the oropharynx or the rectum. Opportunistic infections are unusual at presentation, but may occur in patients with very low lymphocyte counts and after immunosuppressive therapy. Systemic symptoms are not prominent unless there is extensive infection, and weight loss is unusual.

PHYSICAL EXAMINATION. Pallor is frequent; its absence in a patient with the acute onset of petechial hemorrhages is much more likely to be associated with immune thrombocytopenic purpura. Retinal hemorrhages are not uncommon and correlate with the severity of anemia rather than thrombocytopenia. The spleen is not enlarged; splenomegaly strongly suggests an underlying blood dyscrasia or hypersplenism rather than marrow aplasia. The constitutional forms of marrow aplasia (Fanconi's anemia, dyskeratosis congenita, Diamond-Blackfan anemia, and others) are frequently associated with congenital anomalies that should be carefully noted. The onset of marrow disease in some of the constitutional disorders may occur in the second or third decade so they must be considered in the differential diagnosis of aplasia in the young adult or adolescent.

Diagnosis

The diagnosis of aplastic anemia is usually straightforward. It is based on the combination of peripheral cytopenias with the characteristic empty marrow replaced with fat.

PERIPHERAL BLOOD FINDINGS. The basic structural framework of the marrow remains relatively intact, so the peripheral red cells do not show marked abnormalities except for a tendency toward macrocytosis. Nucleated red cells occur rarely in simple aplasia; their presence raises the possibility of a myeloproliferative or myelophthisic process instead. The total lymphocyte count may be normal, but is often very low in severe cases and after therapy with steroids or other immunosuppressive agents.

BONE MARROW FINDINGS (Fig. 133–1). The empty marrow replaced by fat is the key diagnostic feature. Residual foci of mainly erythropoietic tissue are often found, however, that can alter the impression of aspirated material. A large-needle biopsy (>1 cm) is an essential adjunct in evaluating the degree of aplasia. If a single biopsy and aspirate are equivocal, repeating is warranted.

Assessment of marrow cellularity is at best semiquantitative, and the degree of hypocellularity has not been shown to correlate well with prognosis. This probably results from unavoidable heterogeneity of sampling this large organ. Benign lymphoid nodules may be found; this finding must not be confused with involvement by malignant lymphoma. The unicellular aplasias arise in the setting of normal marrow cellularity with absence of a single cell line. In some cases of PRCA, as in agranulocytosis, immature precursors may be found in the absence of any mature forms.

ANCILLARY STUDIES. Because of the frequent association of paroxysmal nocturnal hemoglobinuria (PNH), the *Ham test* or *sucrose hemolysis test* is frequently performed in patients with marrow aplasia, especially if there is any degree of reticulocytosis (Ch. 137). Occasional patients have had hypogammaglobulinemia; therefore, measurement of serum immunoglobulins is warranted. A search for *thymoma* should be performed by computed tomography in patients with pure red cell aplasia. When there is a question of a constitutional aplasia, skeletal and renal radiographs are indicated to assess the presence of congenital anomalies.

DIFFERENTIAL DIAGNOSIS. A list of causes of peripheral pancytopenia is presented in Table 133–3. The most important distinction to be made in assessing aplastic anemia is to exclude the presence of leukemia, which may occasionally be characterized by marked marrow hypocellularity and pancytopenia. Splenomegaly, circulating immature cells, and increased marrow reticulin all suggest a primary blood dyscrasia or myelofibrosis rather than simple aplasia.

Management

INITIAL ASSESSMENT. A general approach to the initial assessment and subsequent management of patients with

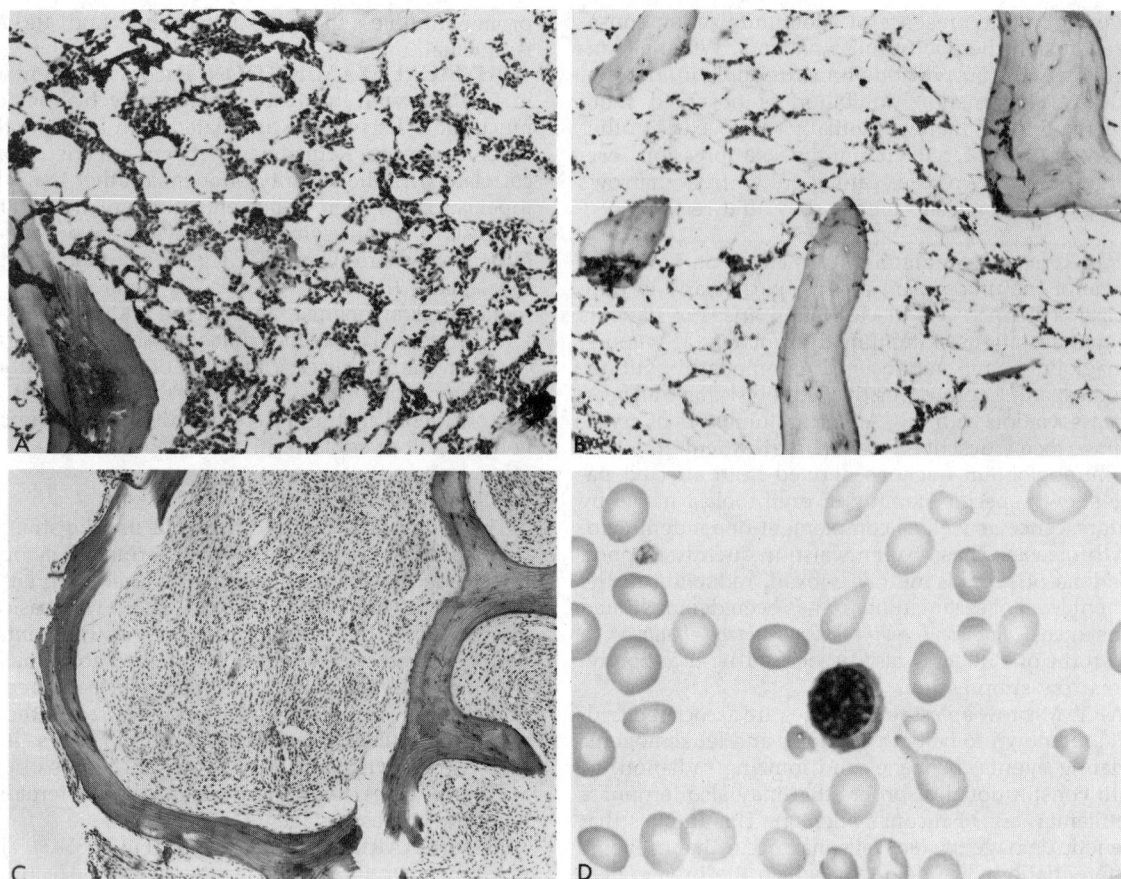

FIGURE 133–1. *A,* Normal bone marrow biopsy. Note even mixture of hematopoietic tissue and fat. *B,* Bone marrow biopsy from a patient with aplastic anemia. Note the increase in fat at the expense of normal hematopoietic tissue. *C,* Bone marrow biopsy from a woman with metastatic breast carcinoma. Note the dense fibrosis. *D,* Peripheral smear from a patient with idiopathic myelofibrosis. Note frequent teardrop forms and the nucleated red cell.

aplastic anemia is presented in Figure 133–2. The most important first task, once the diagnosis is firm, is to assess severity. When severe disease is present, or judged to be imminent when blood counts are falling, *rapid action is essential.* After the initial assessment it is usually best to refer the patient to a center that is experienced in handling the formidable problems associated with the evaluation and care of this disease. The disease is sufficiently rare that new patients are extremely valuable for the important clinical trials that will guide future therapy. Of course, any potentially toxic drugs should be discontinued, and the patient should be removed from any environmental source of marrow toxins during the assessment period.

THERAPY DIRECTED AT REVERSAL OF APLASIA.
Bone Marrow Transplantation. Indications for bone marrow transplantation are being redefined as experience grows with the use of ALG. Transplant candidates must have an HLA-compatible donor, usually a sibling, which markedly limits the use of the procedure. The results of transplantation are excellent in patients under the age of 20 years who have not previously received a transfusion; it is the preferred therapy for this group. The incidence of graft-versus-host disease with its attendant morbidity and mortality becomes unacceptable in patients over age 40. The details of the procedure and the results in aplastic anemia are reviewed in Ch. 165.

Antilymphocyte Globulin. ALG, administered as a single series of injections over a one- to two-week period, improves

TABLE 133–3. CAUSES OF PANCYTOPENIA

A. Aplastic anemias (Table 133–1)	D. Megaloblastic anemias
B. Myelophthisic anemias (Table 133–4)	E. Myelodysplastic syndromes
C. Hypersplenism	F. Overwhelming sepsis

survival in patients with severe aplastic anemia. The characteristics of the response have been described above (see Pathogenesis). Serum sickness is noted in all patients. Responses have been noted in idiopathic aplasia as well as in aplasia associated with drugs or hepatitis. Older patients respond at least as well as do younger ones.

These encouraging results seem to offer improved survival for the majority of patients with the disease who lack a compatible donor. Use of ALG is still experimental therapy, and the optimal preparation of the reagent, the appropriate use of adjunctive therapies, and the long-term effects on survival remain to be established.

Androgens. As the only available therapy in the era before marrow transplantation and ALG, androgens have been widely used. They have also been incorporated into a number of the ALG trials as adjunctive therapy. It is not clearly established that androgens induce remissions in severe aplastic anemia more frequently than they occur spontaneously. With less severe aplasia, however, androgens may improve the hematocrit and lessen transfusion requirements. In occasional patients who are androgen dependent relapse has occurred repeatedly when androgens are discontinued. Granulocyte and platelet responses are much less common than is a rise in hematocrit. Both the injectable forms of testosterone enanthate* (5 to 8 mg per kilogram once weekly) and synthetic oral agents, e.g., oxymetholone (2 to 4 mg per kilogram daily) have shown responses. Toxicity is significant; both groups of drugs cause masculinization with hirsutism, acne, fluid retention, and clitoral enlargement. The oral agents are associated with additional hepatic toxicity, including cholestatic jaundice and hepatocellular carcinoma.

---

*This use is not listed in the manufacturer's directive.

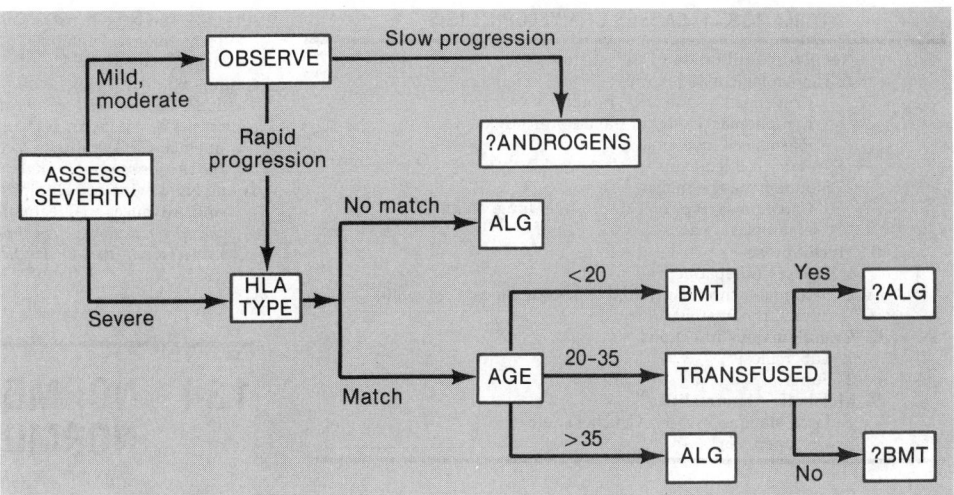

FIGURE 133–2. Schematic approach to the management of aplastic anemia. ALG = Antilymphocyte globulins ± androgens or high-dose steroids. BMT = Allogenic bone marrow transplantation. ? = Optimal therapy in doubt.

High-Dose Corticosteroids. Very high doses of methylprednisolone (100 mg per kilogram per day over a one- to two-week period) have been used in combination with ALG without a notable effect on the observed response rate. Methylprednisolone alone has given responses equivalent to those of ALG alone, including some complete remissions. Because of the marked immunosuppression of such doses and the risk of opportunistic infections in these already granulocytopenic patients, this treatment should be used with caution. It may prove to be a valuable form of therapy when access to transplantation and ALG is unavailable.

Pure Red Cell Aplasias. Immunosuppression has a more clearly defined role in the treatment of unicellular aplasias, especially in pure red cell aplasia. Combinations of cyclophosphamide and other cytotoxic agents and prednisone have induced excellent remissions in PRCA, but the disease eventually recurs in most individuals. About one third of patients with PRCA and thymoma have had remissions after thymectomy.

SUPPORTIVE CARE. Supportive care has assumed an increasingly important role in survival of aplastic anemia patients both before and after various therapeutic interventions.

Transfusions. Transplant candidates should have transfusion only when absolutely necessary because of the risk of sensitization and subsequent graft rejection. The number of donors should be restricted, and *family members must be avoided* until the question of transplantation is decided. Complete phenotyping of major and minor red cell antigens should be performed prior to transfusion. This will aid in the detection of red cell alloantibodies should they develop after repeated transfusions. The use of frozen red cells diminishes the development of leukocyte alloantibodies, but washed, leukocyte-poor packed cells are a more widely available and usually satisfactory substitute. Additional aspects of long-term transfusion therapy, including the use of iron chelators to reduce iron overload, are discussed in Ch. 141.

Platelet transfusions are of undoubted value to the bleeding patient, but their continued use is limited by the development of alloantibodies that render the patient refractory to random donor platelets. Such patients may benefit from platelets obtained by pheresis of an HLA-compatible donor. The onset of such refractoriness is highly variable, and nearly half of patients seem to tolerate random donor platelet support for long periods.

Aplastic patients frequently tolerate very low platelet counts with only cutaneous bleeding in the form of petechiae and traumatic ecchymoses. While conventional teaching has held that a count below 20,000 is the threshold value for a high risk of bleeding, it may in fact be much lower. Platelets should be reserved for actual bleeding episodes or when cerebral

hemorrhage is suspected. Patients with demonstrable increments after transfusions may reasonably be given prophylaxis as the count falls below 5000 or 10,000 per cubic millimeter. Platelets should be irradiated to avoid graft-versus-host disease if immunosuppressive therapy is given.

General Measures. Suppression of menstruation by appropriate hormonal manipulation is indicated for females with excessive blood loss. *Aspirin and all antiplatelet medications should be avoided.* Low doses of prednisone (10 to 15 mg) appear to decrease capillary bleeding in severely thrombocytopenic patients. Scrupulous attention to aseptic technique in administering intravenous infusions, avoidance of intramuscular injections, careful attention to handwashing by personnel, and isolation from obviously infected visitors are important. Rigid adherence to "reverse isolation" impedes proper nursing care without a corresponding benefit in reducing infections, which are largely acquired from endogenous or ubiquitous flora. Management of these infections in the compromised host is discussed in Ch. 258.

Prognosis

Patients with aplastic anemia appear to fall into two major subgroups: (1) a severely affected group as previously defined with a high mortality (perhaps as high as 96 per cent with no treatment) by six months, and (2) a mildly to moderately affected group with a considerably better outlook. Before the era of bone marrow transplantation and intensive supportive care the overall mortality in all patients was from 55 to 75 per cent. Survival in marrow transplant patients with severe aplasia who had a matched sibling donor ranges from 40 to 80 per cent and is adversely affected by increasing age and prior tranfusions. Graft-versus-host disease is the major factor in morbidity and mortality in these patients (Ch. 165). Long-term survival in ALG-treated patients is not established, but one- and two-year survival is approximately equivalent to that in the marrow transplant patients.

MYELOPHTHISIC ANEMIAS

Myelophthisis is an archaic term for any pathologic process that obliterates the normal marrow architecture. The microcirculatory anatomy of the marrow normally retains developing hematopoietic cells within extravascular spaces, called *cords*, until they are sufficiently mature to gain access to the general circulation by crossing the cordal-sinusoidal boundary. If this delicate network is disrupted, abortive attempts at hematopoiesis occur, which result in the release of immature blood cells into the peripheral blood. The presence of circulating nucleated red blood cells, myelocytes, or blasts and giant platelets is termed *leukoerythroblastosis*. This is a frequent although not invariable accompaniment of myelophthisis (Fig.

TABLE 133–4. CAUSES OF MYELOPHTHISIS

A. Neoplastic Infiltration of the Marrow
  1. Hematologic malignancies
    Leukemias—acute and chronic
    Lymphomas–Hodgkin's and non-Hodgkin's
    Plasma cell myeloma
    Hairy cell leukemia
  2. Nonhematologic malignancies
    Carcinomas–esp. breast, prostate, lung, stomach
    Neuroblastoma
B. Myelofibrosis
  1. Primary (idiopathic)
  2. Secondary–chronic myeloid leukemia, cancers, vasculitis
    (lupus, rheumatoid arthritis)
C. Granulomatous infections
  1. Tuberculosis
  2. Fungi
D. Metabolic Abnormalities
  1. Lipid storage diseases–Gaucher's, etc.
  2. Osteopetrosis

133–1). Transient leukoerythroblastosis may occur without myelophthisis under conditions of extreme erythropoietin-mediated marrow stress such as acute hemorrhage, abrupt hypoxemia, or severe chronic hemolysis.

The pathologic processes that cause myelophthisis can be usefully divided into four general categories (Table 133–4). *Metastatic carcinoma* has replaced tuberculosis as the most commonly associated condition. Many of these neoplastic marrow processes incite an intense fibrotic reaction that may obscure the malignant cells. The hematopoietic disorders that are most likely to cause myelofibrosis, idiopathic myelofibrosis, and chronic myelogenous leukemia are associated with marked megakaryocytic hyperplasia. Acute leukemias and well-differentiated lymphoid neoplasms, although they may totally replace the normal marrow, only rarely elicit a leukoerythroblastic response, for reasons that are not entirely clear.

The diagnosis of myelophthisis is frequently suggested by the presence of *nucleated red blood cells* or other immature forms on the peripheral smear. The total leukocyte and platelet count may be decreased if marrow replacement is extensive; however, there may be marked leukocytosis in idiopathic myelofibrosis or when a leukemoid reaction occurs. *Teardrop-shaped red cells* are commonly present along with other poikilocytes (Fig. 133–1). Occasionally the diagnosis is suggested by abnormal bone films showing focal lytic or blastic lesions, or a more widespread increase in bone density as in idiopathic myelofibrosis.

Definitive diagnosis of myelophthisis depends on adequate examination of the bone marrow (Fig. 133–1). *Because the aspirate is characteristically "dry," a needle or surgical biopsy is essential.* The marrow involvement is often patchy, and residual areas of normal or hyperplastic marrow may be found. Demonstration of increased reticulin fibers in the marrow biopsy with silver stains is a useful adjunct in myelofibrotic conditions. A careful search for malignant cells embedded within the fibrotic tissue should always be performed.

The therapy of myelophthisic anemias is entirely dependent on the recognition and appropriate treatment of the underlying pathologic process. Successful treatment of breast or prostatic carcinomas, either by cytotoxic or hormonal agents, can lead to complete resolution of the myelophthisis and recovery of normal marrow function. A dramatic example of the reversibility of the myelophthisic process has been demonstrated in the childhood disease osteopetrosis. This condition has been linked to an inherited defect in the mononuclear phagocytic system that is manifested by decreased osteoclast function. The resulting overgrowth of bony trabeculae that obliterates the marrow space can be completely reversed by bone marrow transplantation with restoration of normal hematopoiesis.

Alter BP: The bone marrow failure syndromes. In Nathan DG, Oski FA (eds.): Hematology of Infancy and Childhood. 3rd ed. Philadelphia, W.B. Saunders Company, 1987.

Ammus SS, Yunis AA: Acquired pure red cell aplasia. Am J Hematol 24:311, 1987. *Concise, well-referenced review.*

Gewirtz AM, Hoffman R: Current considerations of the etiology of aplastic anemia. CRC Crit Rev Oncol Hematol 4:1, 1985. *A current review emphasizing the various sources of data concerning the immune etiology of aplastic anemia.*

Young NS, Levine AS, Humphries RK (ed.): Aplastic Anemia; Stem Cell Biology and Advances in Treatment. New York, Alan R. Liss, Inc., 1984. *State-of-the-art reviews of current theories of pathogenesis and treatment by all of the most active investigators of aplastic anemia. The single most useful volume to date.*

134 NORMOCHROMIC NORMOCYTIC ANEMIAS

James P. Kushner

The normocytic normochromic anemias are those in which the average cell size (mean corpuscular volume; MCV) and the average cell hemoglobin concentration (mean corpuscular hemoglobin concentration; MCHC) are normal. These anemias occur in association with a large number of diseases, and the mechanisms responsible for the anemia are quite diverse. Frequently the anemia is only a minor manifestation of a systemic disease of much more serious consequence. The anemia, however, may be the first detected evidence of disease, and the finding of anemia may lead to studies resulting in correct diagnosis of an underlying disorder.

In spite of their highly variable causes, it is possible to approach normocytic normochromic anemias with a classification scheme that can direct the diagnostic investigation (Table 134–1). Central to this classification is the determination of whether the bone marrow is responding appropriately to a given degree of anemia. Normally functioning bone marrow can accelerate the rate of erythropoiesis up to eightfold. Accelerated erythropoiesis by normal bone marrow is reflected by an increase in the reticulocyte count. Reticulocytosis can be detected on routinely stained smears by the finding of a population of large polychromatophilic red cells. When reticulocytosis is pronounced the MCV may be moderately elevated because of the contribution of the large young erythrocytes to the measurement of the average cell size. Reticulocytosis is a manifestation of an appropriate marrow response to hemolytic anemia (see Ch. 137) and to acute posthemorrhagic anemia. These two conditions can generally be differentiated on clinical grounds.

When evidence of accelerated erythropoiesis in response to anemia is *not* found, it is likely that the underlying disorder

TABLE 134–1. CLASSIFICATION OF THE NORMOCYTIC NORMOCHROMIC ANEMIAS

I. **Anemia with appropriate marrow response**
  A. Acute posthemorrhagic anemia
  B. Hemolytic anemia (may be macrocytic when there is pronounced reticulocytosis) (Ch. 137–139)
II. **Anemia with impaired marrow response**
  A. Marrow hypoplasia
    1. Aplastic anemia (Ch. 133)
    2. Pure red cell aplasia (Ch. 133)
  B. Marrow infiltration
    1. Infiltration by malignant cells
    2. Myelofibrosis (Ch. 154)
    3. Inherited storage diseases
  C. Decreased erythropoietin production
    1. Kidney disease
    2. Liver disease
    3. Endocrine deficiencies
    4. Malnutrition
    5. Anemia of chronic disease (Ch. 135)

is directly or indirectly affecting the bone marrow. Intrinsic marrow disease should be strongly suspected when leukopenia and thrombocytopenia are also found, or when morphologic abnormalities are found on the blood smear. These morphologic abnormalities include nucleated red cells, teardrop-shaped poikilocytes, immature granulocytes, and large platelets or megakaryocyte fragments (dwarf megakaryocytes). Marrow aspiration and biopsy are nearly always indicated in the face of these findings.

When anemia is found in association with an impaired marrow response and no signs of intrinsic marrow disease are detected, it is likely that an underlying disease is producing an indirect effect on red cell production. Renal disease, liver disease, and a variety of endocrine disorders indirectly affect erythropoiesis in association with a reduction of erythropoietin production. The pathogenesis of the anemia of chronic disease may also involve this mechanism, in addition to the defect in the mobilization of reticuloendothelial iron stores (Ch. 135).

ACUTE POSTHEMORRHAGIC ANEMIA

DEFINITION. The anemia caused by loss of a large volume of blood may occur as a result of trauma or because of an underlying disease that affects blood vessels or the coagulation mechanism. Bleeding may be obvious when profuse hemorrhage occurs from a body orifice or from an external wound. If bleeding occurs within a body cavity, tissue space, or the gastrointestinal tract, the nature of the problem may not be immediately appreciated (Ch. 114). The manifestation of hemorrhage depends on the rate and magnitude of the bleeding and the time elapsed between the acute hemorrhage and the first clinical observations.

CLINICAL MANIFESTATIONS AND DIAGNOSIS. The characteristic sequence of events following a single acute hemorrhage can be divided into two phases. The first, lasting up to three days, reflects the volume of blood loss and is dominated by the manifestations of hypovolemia. Anemia may not be detected by measurement of the hematocrit or hemoglobin. The second phase occurs after the body has restored the blood volume to normal or near normal and is characterized by the findings of anemia and reticulocytosis.

As outlined in Table 134–2, a normal individual can rapidly lose up to 20 per cent of the blood volume without any signs or symptoms. Limited signs of cardiovascular distress appear with losses up to 30 per cent of the blood volume, but shock gradually appears only when the blood loss exceeds 30 to 40 per cent of the blood volume. As the plasma volume and red cell mass are reduced in proportional amounts, the hematocrit and hemoglobin fail to reflect the magnitude of blood lost.

TABLE 134–2. CLINICAL MANIFESTATIONS OF ACUTE BLOOD LOSS IN OTHERWISE HEALTHY INDIVIDUALS

Percentage of Blood Volume Lost	Amount Lost (ml)	Clinical Manifestations
10–20	500–1000	Usually none; vasovagal syncope may occur in 5%; tachycardia in response to exercise; mild postural hypotension may be noted
20–30	1000–1500	Few changes supine; light-headedness and hypotension commonly occur when upright; marked tachycardia in response to exertion
30–40	1500–2000	Blood pressure, cardiac output, central venous pressure, urine volume reduced even when supine; thirst, shortness of breath, clammy skin, sweating, clouding of consciousness and rapid, thready pulse may be noted
40–50	2000–2500	Severe shock, often resulting in death

Clinical signs and symptoms must be used initially to estimate the degree of blood volume depletion and in planning emergency treatment. When blood loss is more gradual, the plasma volume may be restored by endogenous mechanisms, and very large volumes of blood can be lost without clinical manifestations of shock.

Anemia is first detected following expansion of the plasma volume. In recumbent patients most of the plasma volume expansion has occurred by 24 hours; this expansion mainly is caused by movement of water and electrolytes into the intravascular space. In ambulatory patients plasma volume expansion occurs more slowly, mainly through the mobilization of albumin from extravascular sites. The hematocrit may not reach the minimum value until three or four days after the hemorrhagic episode. Erythropoietin secretion is stimulated shortly after the appearance of the anemia, and hyperplasia of marrow erythroid elements then begins.

Reticulocytosis is usually detected three to five days after the hemorrhagic episode, and maximal reticulocyte counts are reached at six to eleven days. The degree of reticulocytosis is related to the magnitude of hemorrhage but rarely exceeds 14 per cent. During the period of maximal reticulocytosis, polychromatophilia and macrocytosis can be detected on the peripheral blood smear, and the MCV may become transiently increased. If the initial evaluation is done during this state, the findings may be mistaken for those of hemolytic anemia. Differentiation from hemolytic anemia may be difficult if bleeding has occurred into a body cavity or tissue space, because resorption of blood from these areas often results in an increased production of unconjugated bilirubin and even mild jaundice. In contrast to the reticulocyte response both the platelet count and the leukocyte count may rise dramatically within hours of hemorrhage. Platelet counts as great as 1000×10^9 per liter may be detected within one to two hours, and leukocyte counts of 20 to 35×10^9 per liter may be reached by two to five hours. Elevated platelet and leukocyte counts generally return to normal within three to five days.

TREATMENT. During the hypovolemic phase therapy should be directed at stopping the hemorrhage, combating shock, and restoring the blood volume. Restoration of the blood volume may be achieved by intravenous infusion of crystalloid (electrolyte) solutions; colloid solutions of plasma protein, albumin, or dextran; or fresh whole blood. Complete reliance on fresh whole blood in the emergency situation is unwise for several reasons. First, large amounts of type O Rh-negative whole blood are required. If typing and crossmatching are done prior to transfusion, there may be a dangerous delay in therapy. Second, allergic transfusion reactions may restrict volume expansion or even produce plasma volume contraction. For the emergency situation crystalloid solutions are preferred.

A nonprotein crystalloid solution with a sodium concentration approximating that of plasma is the most widely used fluid therapy for hemorrhagic shock. Ringer's lactate, Ringer's acetate, or normal saline supplemented with 90 mmol of sodium bicarbonate (2 ampules) per liter may be used. Crystalloid solutions containing large amounts of glucose should be avoided, as they may induce osmotic diuresis, further depleting the vascular volume. An initial infusion of two to three times the volume of the estimated blood loss is administered. When larger volumes of crystalloid solutions are administered, peripheral edema often develops, as these solutions are rapidly distributed throughout the intravascular and extravascular compartments.

The use of protein-containing solutions (albumin or fresh frozen plasma) has been supported by some who claim that increasing the oncotic pressure within the vascular space is beneficial. There is little evidence to support this contention, as protein is extravasated into interstitial spaces throughout the body in patients in shock. Dextran solutions have been widely used in the treatment of hemorrhagic shock, but there is no convincing evidence to suggest they are superior to crystalloid solutions in acute emergencies. Acute renal failure has occurred in a few patients receiving dextran solutions. Dextran may cause difficulty in cross-matching and may interfere with platelet adhesiveness and the normal coagulation cascade.

The administration of 3 liters of a crystalloid solution over 15 to 20 minutes will generally resuscitate any patient in hemorrhagic shock if the hemorrhage has been arrested. Continued signs and symptoms of hypovolemia indicate continued bleeding and usually indicate the need for surgical intervention to control the hemorrhage.

Once the emergency has been dealt with, the bleeding lesion identified, and the bleeding stopped, attention can be directed to the anemia. The anemia itself rarely requires specific therapy and provision of a high-protein diet and oral iron supplementation will suffice in most cases. Blood transfusions may be reserved for those situations in which rapid correction of the anemia is required, as in preparation of the patient for surgery.

Billhardt RA, Rosenbush SW: Cardiogenic and hypovolemic shock. Med Clin North Am 70:853, 1986. *An up-to-date review of the crystalloid versus colloid controversy in the acute management of hypovolemic shock.*

Mollison PL: Blood Transfusion in Clinical Medicine. 7th ed. Oxford, Blackwell Scientific Publications, 1983. *The "bible" for detailed analysis of the measurement of blood volume and its restoration by transfusions.*

OTHER NORMOCYTIC NORMOCHROMIC ANEMIAS

ANEMIA OF CHRONIC RENAL INSUFFICIENCY. In contrast to the anemia found in association with most chronic diseases, the anemia associated with renal failure may be quite severe. Many factors may contribute to the anemia. Folate may be lost into the dialysate in patients receiving long-term dialysis therapy. Iron deficiency may develop because of blood loss from the genitourinary or gastrointestinal tracts or into the hemodialysis coil. Microangiopathic hemolytic anemia may occur in patients with renal failure because of malignant hypertension, or in the hemolytic-uremic syndrome. In the absence of any of these mechanisms the degree of anemia correlates roughly with the increase in the blood urea nitrogen and creatinine. Although red cell survival may be moderately shortened, the mechanism underlying the anemia is mainly reduced red cell production. Failure of the erythropoietin-secreting function of the kidney appears to be responsible for the impaired marrow response to the anemia.

Blood transfusions are infrequently required. The hematocrit rarely drops below 15 per cent, and most patients tolerate this degree of anemia remarkably well. Long-term dialysis therapy may result in a modest reduction in the degree of anemia, provided that folate or iron deficiency does not develop as a complicating factor. Androgens may be useful for patients who do not tolerate anemia well and require repeated transfusions. Weekly intramuscular injections of nandrolone decanoate (100 mg) or the oral administration of fluoxymesterone* (10 to 30 mg per day) have proved effective in reducing transfusion requirements. The administration of human erythropoietin derived from recombinant DNA has proved extremely effective in treating the anemia of chronic renal disease in early studies of patients maintained by hemodialysis. Following a successful renal homograft, normal and even supranormal hematocrit values may be achieved.

ANEMIA IN CIRRHOSIS AND OTHER LIVER DISEASE. Anemia is a frequent manifestation of liver disease; the pathogenetic mechanisms responsible may be more varied than those underlying the anemia of chronic disease. The anemia is generally normocytic and normochromic but occasionally it may be mildly macrocytic. It is unusual for the MCV to exceed 115 fl in the absence of advanced folate deficiency with frank megaloblastic changes in the marrow.

Etiologic factors implicated in the pathogenesis of the anemia associated with liver disease include chronic alcoholism and its effect on erythropoiesis; iron deficiency due to blood loss from gastritis, peptic ulcer, varices, and deficient coagulation factors; sequestration of erythrocytes and other formed elements of the blood by the enlarged spleen resulting from portal hypertension; exaggeration of the degree of anemia because of the increased plasma volume associated with cirrhosis; and alterations in the lipid composition of erythrocyte membranes.

ANEMIAS ASSOCIATED WITH ENDOCRINE DISORDERS. Anemia frequently accompanies disorders of the pituitary gland, the thyroid gland, the adrenal glands, and the gonads. In general the anemia is mild and by itself produces few symptoms. Reduced tissue oxygen requirements as a result of the endocrine disturbance may result in diminished renal production of erythropoietin. Loss of the stimulating effect of androgens on erythrocyte production may be a factor in some cases. Endocrine disorders tend to begin insidiously; the early symptoms are generally no more specific than fatigue and lassitude. When initial laboratory testing reveals anemia, the diagnostic studies may be directed to the hematopoietic system. Unless endocrine disease is included in the differential diagnosis of a normocytic normochromic anemia, the primary diagnosis may be overlooked.

Anagnostou A, Kurtzman NA: Hematological consequences of renal failure. In Brenner BM, Rector FC (eds.): The Kidney. 3rd ed. Philadelphia, W. B. Saunders Company, 1986. *A comprehensive treatise on the subject, with over 500 references.*

Eichner ER: The hematologic disorders of alcoholism. Am J Med 54:621, 1973. *A review of the hematologic effects of the pathogenetic agent responsible for most cases of advanced liver disease.*

Eschbach JW, Egrie JC, Downing MR, et al.: Correction of the anemia of end-stage renal disease with recombinant human erythropoietin: Results of a combined phase I and II clinical trial. N Engl J Med 316:73, 1987. *A clinical study demonstrating the efficacy of erythropoietin in the treatment of the anemia of end-stage renal disease.*

Williams WJ, Beutler E, Erslev AJ, et al. (eds.): Hematology. 3rd ed. New York, McGraw-Hill Book Company, 1983. *Extensive references to the anemias associated with renal and endocrine disorders.*

135 HYPOCHROMIC ANEMIAS

James P. Kushner

Anemias associated with a subnormal average cell hemoglobin concentration (mean corpuscular hemoglobin concentration; MCHC) are classified as hypochromic. When the average cell size (mean corpuscular volume; MCV) is also reduced the anemia is classified as hypochromic, microcytic. Hypochromia and microcytosis can be detected either by examination of the stained blood smear or by calculation of the erythrocyte indices (Table 135–1). The widespread use of electronic cell counting equipment makes available the erythrocyte indices at the same time that anemia is usually detected by the finding of subnormal values for the hemoglobin concentration and the volume of packed red cells (generally referred to as the hematocrit).

The developing erythrocyte requires iron, protoporphyrin, and globin for the biosynthesis of hemoglobin. Hypochromic

TABLE 135–1. RED CELL INDICES*
IN HYPOCHROMIC AND MICROCYTIC ANEMIAS

	MCV (fl)	MCHC (gm/dl)	MCH (pg)
Normal	83–96	32–36	28–34
Hypochromic	83–100	28–31	23–31
Microcytic	70–82	32–36	22–27
Hypochromic-microcytic	50–79	24–31	11–29

*Variations in the methods for measuring the red blood cell count, the volume of packed red cells, and the hemoglobin concentration could change the values slightly.

---

*This use is not listed in the manufacturer's directive.

TABLE 135–2. CLASSIFICATION OF ANEMIAS CHARACTERIZED BY DEFICIENT HEMOGLOBIN SYNTHESIS AND THE PRESENCE OF HYPOCHROMIC ERYTHROCYTES

I. **Disorders of iron metabolism**
   A. Iron deficiency anemia
   B. Anemia of chronic disease
   C. Hereditary atransferrinemia
   D. Congenital hypochromic-microcytic anemia with iron overload (Shahidi-Nathan-Diamond syndrome)
II. **Disorders of porphyrin and heme synthesis: sideroblastic anemias**
   A. Acquired sideroblastic anemias
      1. Idiopathic refractory sideroblastic anemia
      2. Complicating other diseases
      3. Associated with drugs or toxins—ethanol, INH, lead
   B. Hereditary sideroblastic anemias
      1. X chromosome–linked
      2. Autosomal recessive
III. **Disorders of globin synthesis**
   A. The thalassemias (Ch. 142)
   B. Hemoglobinopathies characterized by unstable hemoglobins (Ch. 144)

anemias, characterized by deficient hemoglobin synthesis, can be divided into three groups, depending on which of the three components required for hemoglobin biosynthesis is deficient (Table 135–2).

IRON DEFICIENCY ANEMIA

DEFINITIONS. Iron deficiency anemia occurs when body iron stores become inadequate for the needs of normal erythropoiesis. Body iron stores must be exhausted before red cell production is restricted; therefore, anemia occurs at a late stage of iron deficiency. In its fully developed form iron-deficient erythropoiesis is characterized by hypochromia and microcytosis of the circulating erythrocytes, low plasma iron and ferritin concentrations, and a transferrin saturation of about 15 per cent or less. Iron deficiency anemia is a sign of disease and is not in itself a complete diagnosis.

PREVALENCE. Iron deficiency is the most common cause of anemia throughout the world, although it is difficult to define precisely its prevalence. Published studies vary in the reported incidence of iron deficiency because of differences in the criteria used to identify iron deficiency as well as in the nature of the population sampled in terms of age, sex, economic status, and local environmental factors. In parts of Africa and India, where marginal dietary intake and excessive iron loss due to intestinal parasites are present together, over half the population may suffer from iron deficiency anemia.

In most developed countries about 3 per cent of men, 20 per cent of women, and over 50 per cent of pregnant women are deficient in iron as judged by plasma iron levels. As judged by serum ferritin levels, iron stores are greatly reduced in about 25 per cent of children, 30 per cent of adolescents, 30 per cent of menstruating women, 60 per cent of pregnant women, and 3 per cent of men.

IRON METABOLISM. The total iron content of a healthy human subject remains within relatively narrow limits. Loss of iron from the body is precisely matched by absorption of iron from food. Iron loss is not due to "excretion" in the usual sense but rather to loss of intact cells containing iron.

Epithelial cells from the gastrointestinal and urinary tracts, and from the skin, account for the normal daily iron loss in men of about 1 mg. In women, menstrual flow, childbearing, and lactation are additional routes of iron loss.

The body iron content in normal adult men is about 50 to 55 mg per kilogram of body weight and in women is about 35 to 40 mg per kilogram. This difference reflects the high incidence of iron deficiency in women and does not indicate any fundamental differences in iron metabolism between the sexes. Most of the body iron is found in hemoglobin, with smaller amounts in myoglobin and iron storage compounds (Table 135–3). Only a minute portion is found in plasma, where it is bound to transferrin.

The metabolism of iron is dominated by its role in hemoglobin synthesis. Iron incorporated into hemoglobin is utilized over and over again through an internal cycle, the *iron cycle* (Fig. 135–1). The plasma iron compartment, in which iron is bound to the transport protein transferrin, is central to this cycle. Iron moves from the plasma to erythroid precursor cells in the marrow. These cells synthesize hemoglobin and, with maturation, are released into the circulation. At the end of their 120-day lifespan the red cells are ingested by macrophages, principally in the splenic sinusoids, and the iron is extracted from the hemoglobin by the enzyme heme oxygenase. A small portion of this iron is stored in macrophages as ferritin or hemosiderin, but most is returned to the plasma where it becomes bound to transferrin, completing the cycle. In the normal adult male about 30 mg of iron completes the iron cycle daily. One to 2 mg of iron leaves the plasma daily and enters the liver and other tissues where it is utilized for the synthesis of other hemoproteins such as cytochromes and myoglobin.

ABSORPTION. The average intake of iron in the meat-containing diet in the United States is about 10 to 30 mg per day, but much greater variations occur in different parts of the world. Only 5 to 10 per cent of dietary iron (about 1 mg) is absorbed daily in order to balance precisely the amount lost. The amount of iron absorbed can increase up to fivefold if body iron stores are depleted or if erythropoiesis is accelerated. The amount absorbed decreases in states of iron overload or if there is erythroid hypoplasia. Total body iron balance is thus regulated at the absorptive step; the precise mechanism by which this control is accomplished has not been defined. Iron is absorbed chiefly in portions of the

TABLE 135–3. DISTRIBUTION OF IRON IN THE BODY

Compound	Iron Content (mg) Men (70 kg)	Iron Content (mg) Women (50 kg)	Per Cent of Total Body Iron Men	Per Cent of Total Body Iron Women
Hemoglobin	2670	1500	69.6	73.1
Myoglobin	350	220	9.1	10.7
Heme enzymes	8	7	0.2	0.3
Transferrin	6	5	0.2	0.2
Ferritin-hemosiderin	800	320	20.9	15.7
Total	3834	2052	100.0	100.0

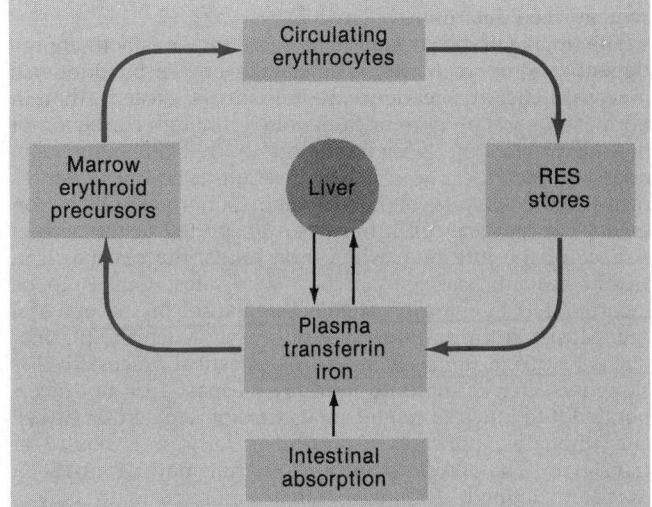

FIGURE 135–1. The internal iron cycle. In the plasma, iron bound to transferrin is transported to the marrow where it is transferred to developing red blood cells and incorporated into hemoglobin. The mature red blood cells are released into the circulation and after 120 days are ingested by macrophages in the reticuloendothelial system (RES). Here the iron is extracted from hemoglobin and returned to plasma, completing the cycle.

intestine proximal to the midjejunum, and very little is absorbed in more caudal intestinal segments.

Iron is absorbed by two distinct pathways in humans, one for iron in heme and the other for iron in ferrous and ferric iron salts. Heme iron is derived from the hemoglobin, myoglobin, and other heme proteins in foods of animal origin. Exposure to the acid and proteases of gastric juice liberates the heme from its apoprotein. Heme is rapidly taken up by gastrointestinal epithelial cells, and the iron is made available by enzymatic degradation of the porphyrin macrocycle. The absorption of heme iron is influenced very little by other dietary components.

The "bioavailability" of nonheme dietary iron, however, varies greatly. Availability is dependent on the oxidation state and solubility of the iron and the presence of chelating substances in the diet. Factors modifying the form in which iron is presented to the intestinal mucosal cell play an important role in the amount of iron that can be absorbed. At the acidic pH normally found in the stomach, both ferrous and ferric iron are soluble. Patients who have undergone gastrectomy, or who are achlorhydric for other reasons, demonstrate impaired absorption of iron. Cimetidine, a potent inhibitor of gastric acid secretion, may also impair the absorption of dietary iron. In the duodenum, as the pH rises, ferric iron is readily converted to insoluble ferric hydroxides. Agents such as ascorbic acid may promote iron absorption by reducing some ferric iron to ferrous iron, which remains soluble at neutral pH. Dietary constituents such as citrate may enhance the solubility of inorganic iron and hence enhance absorption. Phytates, neutral detergent fibers, and other substances present in cereals, grain, and corn impair iron absorption by binding iron as relatively insoluble complexes.

The clinical significance of the various luminal factors that influence iron absorption may be minimal in United States society, where the diet provides relatively large amounts of heme iron. In developing countries, however, diets are generally characterized by low meat content and high content of grains and vegetables. Such diets, with low heme iron content and high content of substances that impair nonheme iron absorption, may not meet the iron demands of many individuals. The manipulation of dietary iron content by large scale iron supplementation programs has been instituted in both developed and underdeveloped countries. The incidence of iron deficiency in the population is decreased by such programs, but the risks to individuals predisposed to iron loading remain to be determined (Ch. 206).

The uptake of iron from the intestinal lumen is both energy dependent and regulated. The uptake of ^{59}Fe by duodenal mucosal cells in iron-deficient individuals exceeds that in normal subjects by two- or three-fold. Although correction of the anemia in iron-deficient subjects by red cell transfusion does not decrease iron uptake, repletion of body iron stores restores the kinetics of iron uptake to normal. Once iron enters the mucosal cell it must be transported to the serosal surface of the intestine, where iron enters the plasma. Iron within the mucosal cell can have two fates. One is to be incorporated into ferritin within the cytosol of the mucosal cell. Most ferritin iron does not ultimately reach the plasma, but is lost from the body when the intestinal mucosal cell is sloughed after its three- to four-day lifespan. Iron not incorporated into mucosal cell ferritin is transported across the cell and ultimately appears in plasma as ferric iron bound to transferrin. The process of intracellular transport has not been precisely defined. Although transferrin appears to play a central role in iron absorption, other mechanisms must also be available, because the rare patients with congenital atransferrinemia show no evidence of deficient absorption.

TRANSPORT. Transferrin, the iron transport protein in plasma, is a glycoprotein with an approximate molecular weight of 80,000. The liver is the major source of transferrin synthesis and the protein is equally distributed in the intra-

vascular and extravascular spaces. Transferrin is capable of binding two iron atoms in the ferric state. In normal subjects the plasma concentration of transferrin is about 2.5 to 3.0 grams per liter. Plasma transferrin is usually quantified in terms of the amount of iron it will bind, a measure called the *total iron-binding capacity* (TIBC). In normal subjects only about one third of the available transferrin binding sites are occupied (TIBC = 33 per cent). Although there is a diurnal variation in plasma iron concentration, with the highest values in the morning and the lowest in the evening, no diurnal variation occurs in the TIBC. Although a number of genetically determined electrophoretic variants of transferrin have been demonstrated, all subtypes appear to function normally as iron transport proteins.

Transferrin has no known function other than as a transport protein and is reused for many cycles of iron transport. With the exception of very small amounts of iron in ferritin, all the iron in plasma is carried by transferrin. The affinity of transferrin for iron is sufficiently high that, theoretically, less than one free iron atom might be present in a liter of blood.

Significant physiochemical differences exist between the two iron-binding sites of transferrin when iron uptake and release are studied in vitro. In spite of these differences the two iron-binding sites function equivalently in the delivery of iron to cells in vivo. The two iron-binding sites are located on separate "halves" of the molecule but about 40 per cent of the amino acid sequence in the two halves is identical. This homology lends credence to the theory that transferrin arose from a duplication of a gene for an antecedent iron transport protein with a single iron-binding site. The evolutionary advantage of the doubled structure may be the reduction of losses in the glomerular filtrate.

CELLULAR UPTAKE. The initial event in the transfer of iron to cells is binding of diferric transferrin to specific, high-affinity receptors on the cell surface. When receptors are lost because of cell maturation (as occurs in developing erythrocytes in vivo) or artificial manipulations in vitro, the ability of the cell to take up iron from transferrin is lost. As cellular iron uptake is directly proportional to the number of transferrin cell surface receptors, it follows that cells with a high iron demand should have large numbers of receptors. The biosynthesis of hemoglobin by erythroid cells has a high iron requirement, and the human reticulocyte may have as many as 300,000 receptors per cell. Developing erythroid cells in the bone marrow may have even more.

In the process of iron uptake by cells the transferrin receptor–diferric transferrin complex is internalized into an acidic, nonlysosomal vesicle (Fig. 135–2). At the acidic pH of the vesicle, iron is readily dissociated from diferric transferrin, but the resulting apotransferrin remains bound to the receptor. The transferrin receptor–apotransferrin complex is transported back to the cell surface where, at neutral pH, the apotransferrin is liberated and becomes available for another cycle of iron binding and release.

Once iron enters the cell, two events occur. One is the delivery of iron to the mitochondria, where it is enzymatically incorporated into protoporphyrin to form heme. The other is the incorporation of iron into ferritin. Ferritin iron is a storage form of iron and is probably not utilized by the cell for heme synthesis. Ferritin iron may, however, be recycled for use by other cells.

STORAGE. Iron-free apoferritin is a spherical protein made up of 24 subunits that surround a central cavity. The central cavity of each apoferritin molecule can potentially store more than 4000 molecules of iron. When iron is present in the central cavity, the protein is termed ferritin. The importance of ferritin as an iron storage compound is emphasized by the wide distribution of structurally similar ferritins in both plant and animal tissues.

A number of isoferritins with differing isoelectric points have been demonstrated. Two different ferritin subunits exist,

FIGURE 135—2. Diagrammatic representation of heme biosynthesis within the erythroblast. The relationships between the iron pathway, the porphyrin biosynthetic pathway, the vitamin B_6 pathway, and the synthesis of transferrin receptors are illustrated. The biosynthesis of porphyrins is dependent upon the availability of pyridoxal phosphate as a cofactor at the rate limiting Δ-aminolevulinic acid synthase step. The biosynthesis of heme requires both protoporphyrin and iron. Iron uptake is dependent upon the interaction of diferric transferrin with high affinity cell surface receptors. Receptor synthesis is regulated by heme; when heme synthesis is impaired, more receptors are synthesized and the cell takes up more iron. T_f represents transferrin receptors for diferric T_f, I.V. the acidic, nonlysosomal intermediate vesicle, Fe^{+++} ferric iron, PP protoporphyrin, PBP porphyrin biosynthetic pathway, ALA Δ-aminolevulinic acid, ALA-s Δ-aminolevulinic acid synthase, PLP pyridoxal-5′-phosphate, and B_6 vitamin B_6.

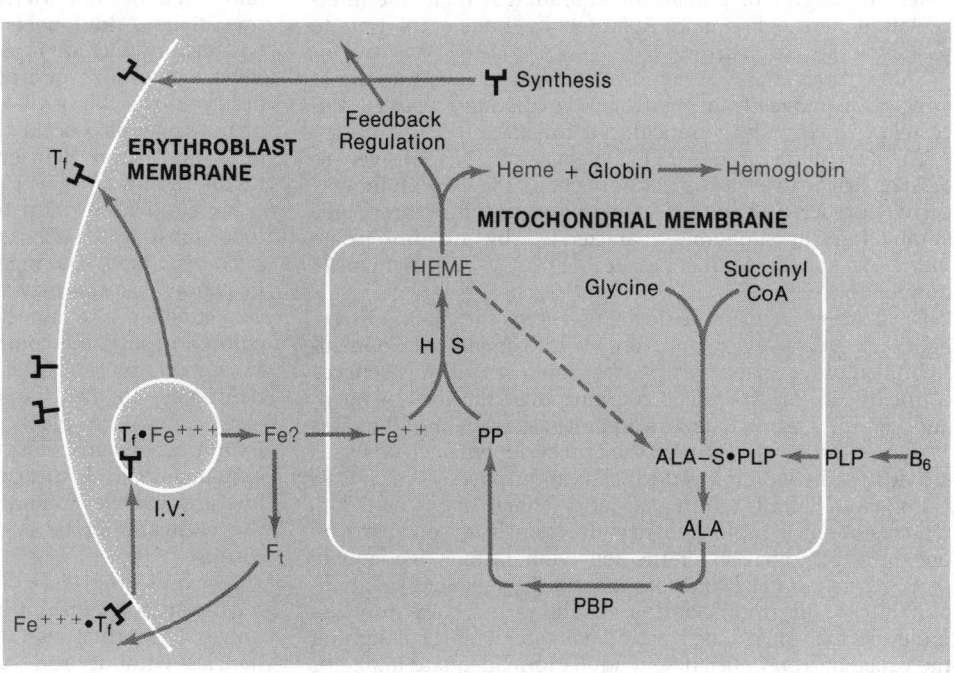

termed H (the major subunit of heart ferritin) and L (the major subunit of liver ferritin). These may be present in differing quantities within a given ferritin molecule, leading to heterogeneity. The H and L subunits are derived from different genetic loci.

Ferritin meets the requirement of cells for an efficient form of iron storage. It has a large capacity to store iron, maintains a reserve storage capacity (few ferritin molecules are iron replete), and can quickly both take up and release iron. Ferritin aggregates are visible by light microscopy in developing erythroid cells when bone marrow smears are stained with Prussian blue. These "siderotic granules" are found in the cytosol of normal developing erythroblasts and are absent in erythroblasts obtained from subjects with iron deficiency anemia.

Small amounts of iron-poor ferritin (mostly apoferritin) circulate in plasma and can be accurately measured by a widely available radioimmunoassay. Under most conditions the concentration of ferritin in the plasma correlates directly with body iron stores. Normal values range from 12 to 325 ng per milliliter with a mean of about 125 for men and 55 for women. The concentration of ferritin in iron-deficient individuals is less than 10 ng per milliliter, whereas in individuals with iron overload the concentration is proportional to the increase in tissue storage iron.

Hemosiderin is an insoluble iron aggregate with a ratio of iron to protein that is high. It is derived from ferritin; however, the reactions leading from ferritin to hemosiderin have not been resolved. Iron in hemosiderin disappears from tissues after repeated venesections, but the mechanism by which iron is mobilized is unknown.

THE MACROPHAGE. While net iron uptake occurs through the intestinal mucosa, most transferrin-bound iron (over 95 per cent) reflects iron recycled from damaged or aged red blood cells by macrophages in the spleen and other organs. Within the macrophage the membrane of ingested erythrocytes is disrupted and the iron in hemoglobin is oxidized to the trivalent state, forming methemoglobin. The heme and globin are dissociated and the iron liberated from hemin (ferric-protoporphyrin) by the microsomal enzyme heme oxygenase, yielding iron and biliverdin. In order to meet a variable demand for iron, macrophages maintain a

storage pool in ferritin and hemosiderin. Under normal conditions the amount of iron entering the macrophage approximates that leaving and there is little interchange between iron newly liberated from hemin and iron in the storage pool. Iron from recently destroyed erythrocytes passes quickly through the macrophage and appears in the plasma bound to transferrin.

When the red cell mass is expanding and erythrocytes are being produced more rapidly than they are being destroyed (e.g., following an acute hemorrhage), iron is mobilized from macrophages. The amount of iron leaving the macrophage under these conditions exceeds that entering. When red cell destruction exceeds production (e.g., in aplastic anemia), the amount of iron entering the macrophage exceeds that leaving and iron is deposited in stores. The control mechanism coupling the rate at which iron leaves the macrophage to the rate of erythrocyte production is unknown. Mobilization of iron from the storage pool is interfered with by infection, inflammation, and malignancy; such interference may be responsible for the anemia associated with chronic disease.

FERROKINETICS. Ferrokinetic studies, based on tracking ^{59}Fe as it moves from the plasma transferrin to the bone marrow and into circulating erythrocytes, make it possible to assess rates of both effective erythropoiesis and ineffective erythropoiesis. The term *ineffective erythropoiesis* refers to the production of defective erythrocytes that are destroyed before they leave the marrow (or very shortly thereafter). A small proportion of erythropoiesis is ineffective even in normal subjects, but in conditions such as megaloblastic anemia, thalassemia, and sideroblastic anemias, ineffective erythropoiesis becomes greatly exaggerated. The plasma ^{59}Fe disappearance, expressed as the half-life ($t\frac{1}{2}$), is normally between 60 and 120 minutes. More rapid disappearance (a shorter $t\frac{1}{2}$) is found in iron deficiency and conditions with accelerated erythropoiesis (such as polycythemia and hemolytic anemias). A long $t\frac{1}{2}$ indicates erythroid hypoplasia. The *plasma iron transport rate* (PIT) is a measure of the rate at which iron leaves the plasma. The PIT is a good index of total erythropoiesis, whether effective or ineffective. The PIT correlates well with the total nucleated red cell mass and the rate of red cell production. However, when erythropoiesis is reduced, or when the degree of transferrin saturation is high, the interpretation of the PIT is complicated by transfer of iron to tissues other than marrow.

The *erythrocyte iron turnover rate* (EIT) measures the rate at which iron moves from marrow to circulating red cells, and correlates well with the reticulocyte index.

The *marrow transit time* (MTT) evaluates the responsiveness of the marrow to erythropoietin. In general there is an inverse correlation between the MTT and the degree of erythropoietic stimulation. In situations characterized by an appropriate marrow response to anemia the MTT may be less than 24 hours.

Ferrokinetic measurements are useful for clinical and investigational purposes but are only approximations. Sophisticated computer analysis of plasma iron disappearance curves coupled with body surface counting over the liver, spleen, and sacrum may yield a more accurate assessment of the rates at which iron moves through the iron cycle, but such analyses are not routinely employed for clinical purposes.

PATHOGENESIS. Iron deficiency comes about as a late manifestation of prolonged negative iron balance caused by one or a combination of the following factors: inadequate dietary intake, malabsorption, blood loss, repeated pregnancies, and rapid growth during childhood. As daily iron loss under normal conditions is very small (about 1 mg), assigning the cause of iron deficiency in adults to inadequate intake or malabsorption implies chronicity measured in years. Iron losses that occur from the gastrointestinal tract or through excessive menstrual bleeding are far more important factors. Factors leading to negative iron balance can be divided into two broad categories: decreased iron uptake and increased iron loss (Table 135–4).

Decreased Iron Uptake. The daily dietary iron requirement for healthy adult men is about 5 to 10 mg. For premenopausal women the daily dietary requirement is higher, roughly 7 to 20 mg daily. In the United States the average diet contains about 6 mg per 1000 calories. The average man therefore consumes more iron than needed but many women subsist on a marginal iron uptake. Because of the adequacy of their diets and their larger iron stores, males in the United States rarely develop iron deficiency solely on the basis of an inadequate dietary intake of iron. Even in women some factor in addition to poor diet is usually necessary before overt anemia develops.

Gastric acid facilitates the absorption of ferric iron in the diet (although it has little effect on heme iron or ferrous iron),

TABLE 135–4. FACTORS PRODUCING NEGATIVE IRON BALANCE AND IRON DEFICIENCY

I. **Decreased iron uptake**
  A. Inadequate diet
  B. Impaired absorption
    1. Achlorhydria
    2. Gastric surgery
    3. Celiac disease
    4. Pica
II. **Increased iron loss**
  A. Gastrointestinal bleeding (Ch. 114)
    1. Neoplasm
    2. Duodenal and gastric ulcers
    3. Hiatal hernia
    4. Gastritis from salicylates, other drugs, or toxins
    5. Diverticulosis
    6. Ulcerative colitis and regional enteritis
    7. Hookworm
    8. Meckel's diverticulum
    9. Hemorrhoids
    10. Arteriovenous malformations
  B. Menometrorrhagia
  C. Repeated blood donations
  D. Repeated pregnancies
  E. Hemoglobinuria due to chronic intravascular hemolysis
  F. Hereditary hemorrhagic telangiectasia
  G. Idiopathic pulmonary hemosiderosis
  H. Disorders of hemostasis

and iron deficiency is a frequent complication following gastric operations. Additional factors that impair iron absorption after gastrectomy include rapid intestinal transit and bypass of the most active sites of iron absorption in the duodenum (as occurs in the Billroth II or Polya procedures). Malabsorption of iron may also occur in patients with adult celiac disease, and rarely iron deficiency anemia may be the dominant manifestation of celiac disease.

Impaired absorption of iron because of interactions with food substances such as phytates and vegetable fibers has been discussed. The ingestion of unusual substances, a practice known as *pica,* may also impair iron absorption. Although pica may be a manifestation of iron deficiency, in certain cultural groups the compulsive ingestion of substances such as clay (geophagia) or starch (amylophagia) may lead to iron deficiency. In the United States the practice appears to be most common in black women in the southern states. Clay interferes with iron absorption by acting in the gut as an ion exchange resin. Laundry starch is a carbohydrate with a very low iron content. When it is consumed in large quantities to the exclusion of other foods, a dietary deficiency of iron results.

Increased Iron Loss. Gastrointestinal bleeding is by far the most common cause of iron deficiency in men and is second only to menstrual loss as a cause in women. Repeated pregnancies without iron supplementation are a less common cause of iron deficiency in women.

Although any hemorrhagic lesion of the gastrointestinal tract may cause iron deficiency (Table 135–4), those most likely to do so are associated with chronic occult bleeding and the steady loss of small amounts of blood. To estimate the effect of blood loss on iron balance it is convenient to consider that 1.0 ml of blood contains about 0.4 mg iron. A steady blood loss of as little as 4 to 5 ml per day (1.6 to 2.0 mg iron) can result in negative iron balance and depletion of iron stores over several years. Failure to detect occult blood in the stool, even after repetitive testing, does not exclude gastrointestinal blood loss as the cause of iron deficiency. *Iron deficiency in men and in postmenopausal women must be considered to result from blood loss unless some other cause can be proven.* This is a critical dictum because iron deficiency anemia may be the first sign of a cancer of the gastrointestinal tract, and the anemia may lead to the diagnosis when the tumor is in an operable stage. Carcinoma of the cecum, for example, is often clinically silent until the symptoms of anemia appear.

Blood loss from erosive gastritis due to aspirin ingestion is becoming an increasingly frequent cause of iron deficiency. Chronic ingestion of as few as two aspirin tablets daily may lead to blood loss of up to 4.5 ml per day.

CLINICAL MANIFESTATIONS. Iron deficiency anemia is not a disease; it is a sign of disease. In some patients, iron deficiency anemia is discovered incidentally when the presenting signs and symptoms are those of the disease that led to the deficiency. In some patients signs and symptoms of both the underlying disease and the iron deficiency are found together. In others only the symptoms of iron deficiency are present and the disease leading to the deficiency is occult.

The onset of iron deficiency anemia is insidious and the progression of symptoms is gradual. Patients are often able to accommodate quite well to the anemia and may continue to perform strenuous work with few symptoms. Fatigue, irritability, palpitations, dizziness, breathlessness, and headache are all common complaints of symptomatic individuals with anemia of any type and do not in themselves suggest iron deficiency as the cause of the anemia. However, some clinical findings do specifically suggest the presence of iron deficiency.

Chlorosis, a peculiar greenish pallor of iron-deficient adolescent girls, was frequently described in the decades between 1890 and 1910, although now is rarely noted. Oral lesions associated with iron deficiency include angular stomatitis (ulcerations or fissures at the corners of the mouth), atrophy of the lingual papillae, and varying degrees of glossitis. *Ozena* (chronic atrophy of the nasal mucosa associated with a foul-smelling discharge) occurs in some patients with iron deficiency anemia, particularly in southeastern Europe. Thinning and flattening of nails and finally the development of spoon-shaped nails (koilonychia) have been described in patients with advanced iron deficiency.

The association of dysphagia, angular stomatitis, and lingual abnormalities with iron deficiency anemia (Plummer-Vinson or Paterson-Kelly syndrome) is rarely noted in the United States but is quite common in Great Britain and Scandinavia. The dysphagia is due to the development of a mucosal web at the juncture of the hypopharynx and esophagus. Multiple webs may develop, usually extending from the anterior wall of the esophagus into the lumen. Occasionally they may encircle the lumen, forming a cufflike structure. In other patients a stricture with or without a web may be found, drastically constricting the opening into the esophagus at the level of the cricoid cartilage. Relief of the dysphagia requires rupturing of the webs or dilatation of the stenosis, because repletion of the iron stores alone is not effective. Other gastrointestinal complaints such as anorexia, pyrosis, flatulence, nausea, belching, and constipation are common in association with advanced iron deficiency anemia.

Pica, as already mentioned, can be a cause of iron deficiency but it also may be a striking manifestation of iron deficiency. The ingestion of ice (pagophagia) is particularly common. Many patients compulsively eat one or other food items; oddly, the object of the unnatural dietary craving usually contains very little iron.

The spleen is slightly enlarged in about 10 per cent of patients with iron deficiency anemia. There are no specific pathologic changes in the organ and the splenomegaly recedes with correction of the iron deficiency. Neuralgic pains, numbness, and tingling without objective neurologic abnormalities are reported by 15 to 30 per cent of patients and rarely iron deficiency anemia may lead to increased intracranial pressure, papilledema, and the clinical picture of pseudotumor cerebri.

LABORATORY FINDINGS. The degree of anemia is variable and depends upon the duration of iron-limited erythropoiesis. Because of the hypochromia the hemoglobin concentration is usually reduced to a greater degree than the hematocrit. The mean corpuscular volume (MCV), mean corpuscular hemoglobin (MCH), and mean corpuscular hemoglobin concentration (MCHC) are all usually reduced. The degree of change in the red cell indices is related to both the duration and the severity of the anemia. Average values for patients with hemoglobin concentrations of 8 to 9 grams per deciliter are MCV of 74 fl, MCHC 28 grams per deciliter, and MCH of 20 pg.

A well-stained blood smear reveals an increase in the area of central pallor in the individual red corpuscles (hypochromia), microcytes, and marked variations in cell size (anisocytosis) and shape (poikilocytosis) (Fig. 135–3 and Color plate 2D). The plasma iron concentration is generally less than 50 μg per deciliter, and the total plasma iron-binding capacity (the transferrin concentration) is greater than 350 μg per deciliter. As a result the transferrin saturation is less than 15 per cent. The plasma ferritin concentration is generally less than 10 ng per milliliter. The last enzymatic reaction leading to the biosynthesis of heme (the ferrochelatase or heme synthase reaction) requires both iron and protoporphyrin as substrates. In iron deficiency excess protoporphyrin accumulates in the developing erythrocyte and is retained by the circulating erythrocytes. As a result the free erythrocyte protoporphyrin (FEP) is increased, generally about five times normal (normal range, 30 to 80 μg per deciliter of red cells).

Both the percentage and the absolute number of reticulocytes are usually normal. The osmotic fragility of the erythrocytes may be normal, but more often there is increased resistance to hemolysis in hypotonic salt solutions. Although the leukocyte count is usually normal, in very chronic iron deficiency a slight decrease in the absolute number of granulocytes may be seen. The platelet count is usually elevated to levels of about two to three times normal and returns to normal after therapy. Rarely, in severe, longstanding iron deficiency anemia, mild thrombocytopenia may be noted.

Examination of the bone marrow is generally not required to establish a diagnosis of iron deficiency anemia. An exception is the clinical situation when suspected iron deficiency coexists with a chronic disease. Although anemias associated with chronic disease may mimic iron deficiency (see below), they can be distinguished by examination of the marrow. In iron deficiency the marrow is usually normocellular and there is mild erythroid hyperplasia. Macrophage iron is absent or severely reduced. Fewer than 10 per cent of the marrow normoblasts contain siderotic granules visible with Prussian blue staining. In the anemia of chronic disease macrophage iron stores are normal or increased; however, as in iron deficiency, very few normoblasts contain siderotic granules.

The sequence of laboratory changes in slowly developing iron deficiency is fairly predictable. Initially, as iron stores are depleted, the serum ferritin concentration falls. At the earliest stage of iron deficiency the transferrin concentration rises, the plasma iron concentration falls, and the FEP increases. When

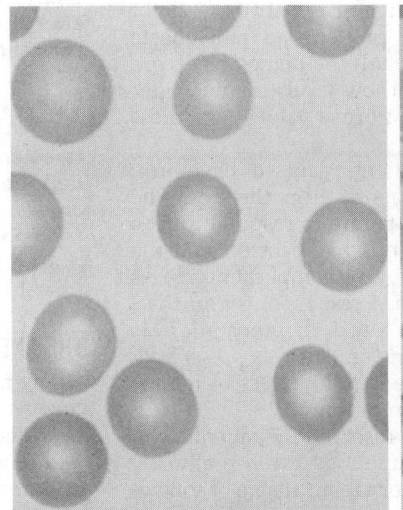
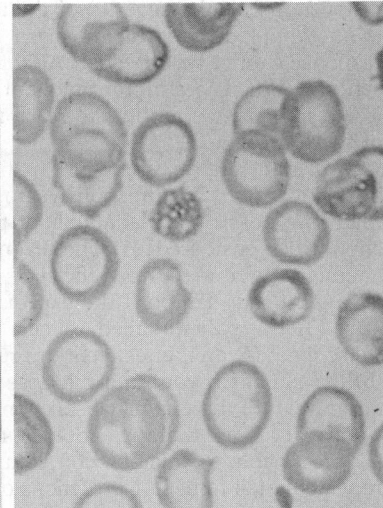

FIGURE 135–3. Blood smear from a patient with advanced iron deficiency anemia (*right*) and from a normal subject (*left*). The red cells from the iron-deficient subject are poorly hemoglobinized (hypochromic), smaller than normal (microcytic), and vary in size and shape (anisocytosis and poikilocytosis). (Wright's stain, × 1000.)

anemia first appears the morphology of the circulating erythrocytes and the erythrocyte indices are generally normal. As the anemia progresses the morphology becomes clearly hypochromic and microcytic and the indices reflect this.

TREATMENT. *Every effort must be made to recognize and if possible correct the underlying cause.* This should be possible in most patients. A simpler goal is correcting the anemia and replenishing body iron stores.

Iron is highly effective in treating iron deficiency but has no other legitimate therapeutic use. Iron exerts no beneficial effect on any of the anemias not caused by iron deficiency. A large number of preparations containing iron have been promoted for the oral treatment of iron deficiency, but none has any advantage over simple ferrous salts (ferrous sulfate, ferrous gluconate, and ferrous fumarate). Ferrous sulfate is the standard preparation for oral use. A daily dose of about 200 mg of elemental iron produces an optimal response. This dose is achieved with three ferrous sulfate tablets (each tablet contains 60 mg of elemental iron) given in divided doses with or just after a meal. Iron is best absorbed when the stomach is empty, but gastric irritation is extremely common when iron is taken this way. In spite of some reduction in absorption when iron is taken with meals, the gain in patient compliance is worth this slight disadvantage. Enteric-coated preparations, designed to reduce gastric irritation by retarding dissolution of the iron, cannot be recommended because with them the most actively absorbing regions of the intestine are bypassed and absorption is markedly reduced. Although large doses of ascorbic or succinic acid will increase iron absorption as much as 20 to 30 per cent, they add greatly to the expense of therapy.

Some patients given oral iron therapy complain of gastrointestinal symptoms (nausea, epigastric pain, cramps, diarrhea); however, it is rare that these symptoms are severe enough to require discontinuation of therapy. Gastric symptoms appear to be dose related and patients intolerant of full therapeutic doses may be able to take a dose of 120 mg per day. Gastric symptoms may be minimized by gradually increasing the dose during the first week of therapy. Regardless of the form of oral therapy used, it is important to continue treatment for 6 to 12 months after the anemia has been corrected. The prolonged therapy allows for repletion of iron stores.

When adequate doses of iron are given, there is often a rapid subjective improvement with a reduction of fatigue, lassitude, and other nonspecific symptoms. This response may occur within two or three days, before any evidence of a hematologic response can be detected. An increase in the number of reticulocytes is the first sign of hematologic response, and a maximal value of 5 to 10 per cent is usually achieved after about ten days of therapy. The height of the reticulocyte peak and the rate of hemoglobin regeneration are proportional to the severity of the anemia. With only slight to moderate degrees of anemia a pronounced reticulocyte response cannot be expected. Although the hemoglobin concentration increases more rapidly at low levels than at high, it takes about two months to reach normal values regardless of the starting level.

It is not rare to encounter patients said to have iron deficiency anemia unresponsive to oral iron therapy. The following possible explanations for failure to respond to iron should be considered: (1) The diagnosis is incorrect and the anemia is not due to iron deficiency; (2) a complicating illness is present that dampens the expected response to iron therapy; (3) the patient failed to take the iron preparation as prescribed; (4) an ineffective iron preparation was prescribed; (5) the patient is continuing to lose iron in excess of intake; and rarely (6) there is malabsorption of iron.

Parenteral iron therapy should be reserved for patients who (1) are unable to tolerate iron compounds given orally, (2) repeatedly fail to heed instructions or are incapable of following them, (3) are losing blood at a rate too rapid to be compensated by oral iron intake, (4) have a disorder such as ulcerative colitis or regional enteritis in which symptoms may be aggravated by oral iron therapy, or (5) are unable to absorb iron from the gastrointestinal tract.

Iron-dextran complex (Imferon) containing 50 mg of iron per milliliter is the preparation of choice for parenteral administration. The total dose required to correct the anemia and to replenish stores can be calculated by the following formula:

$$\text{Iron to be injected (mg)} = [15\text{-patient's Hb (gm/dl)}] \times \text{body weight (kg)} \times 3$$

Iron-dextran can be given intramuscularly or intravenously. Intravenous administration does not appear to have a higher incidence of adverse effects than the intramuscular route. Anaphylactic reactions are rare (0.1–0.6 per cent), but fever, arthralgia, myalgia, and regional adenopathy occur in about 5 per cent of patients. Intramuscular injections should be made into the upper outer quadrant of the buttock, and the skin displaced laterally prior to injection to prevent staining of the skin by reflux of the dark-brown iron solution along the injection path. A test dose of 0.5 ml should be given initially to test for hypersensitivity. Generally 2.5 ml is injected into each buttock (total 5 ml or 250 mg of iron) daily. Intravenous administration permits larger doses to be given in a single injection; thus the discomfort and inconvenience of repeated intramuscular injections can be avoided. After testing for hypersensitivity, 10 ml (500 mg of iron) of undiluted iron-dextran may be administered over about a five-minute period. In Great Britain and Europe it is usual to administer the entire dose calculated by the formula in a single intravenous infusion. A 1:20 dilution of iron-dextran in saline is prepared and administered at an initial flow rate of 20 drops per minute. After five minutes, if no side effects are observed, the rate is increased to 40 to 60 drops per minute. Dextrose solutions should not be used as a diluent because the incidence of superficial phlebitis may be as high as 25 per cent with this vehicle.

PROGNOSIS. The prognosis in iron deficiency relates only to the underlying disorder causing the anemia. Patients rarely if ever die of iron deficiency anemia itself, but may die of the underlying cause. Recurrence of iron deficiency anemia after treatment is common, emphasizing the importance of identifying and effectively treating the cause of the iron deficiency.

HYPOCHROMIC ANEMIAS NOT CAUSED BY IRON DEFICIENCY

Once iron deficiency has been excluded as the cause of a hypochromic anemia, a limited number of diagnostic possibilities remain. A presumptive diagnosis is generally possible after analysis of the history and physical examination and the basic hematologic parameters. If the diagnosis remains obscure, a useful approach is to segregate the diagnostic possibilities on the basis of an accurate determination of the serum iron. When the serum iron is reduced to levels at which the transferrin saturation is less than about 15 per cent, only iron deficiency and the anemia of chronic disease need be considered.

Hypochromic anemias due to defects in globin biosynthesis (the thalassemias and hemoglobinopathies characterized by unstable hemoglobins) are discussed in Ch. 142 and 144.

THE ANEMIA OF CHRONIC DISEASE

The anemia of chronic disease is not always hypochromic; however, because of its association with hypoferremia, it is best discussed under the heading of hypochromic anemias. Although the anemia of chronic disease is usually normocytic and normochromic, hypochromia and even microcytosis may be the dominant morphologic abormalities. When microcytosis is present it is usually not as marked as in iron deficiency. The MCV rarely falls below 72 fl.

DEFINITION. A mild-to-moderate anemia frequently accompanies chronic infections, inflammatory diseases such as rheumatoid arthritis, and cancers. Since these are so common, the anemia of chronic disease is frequently encountered and may be second only to iron deficiency anemia in overall incidence. The anemia of chronic disease is defined by the presence of a chronic disease, anemia, and hypoferremia despite abundant quantities of iron in macrophage stores.

ETIOLOGY AND PATHOGENESIS. Three factors seem to interact in the pathogenesis of the anemia: (1) impaired flow of iron from macrophages to plasma, (2) decreased erythrocyte lifespan, and (3) inadequate marrow response to the mild hemolysis.

Characteristically, the serum iron is decreased, total iron binding capacity is reduced (a point often useful in differentiating the anemia from iron deficiency anemia), and transferrin saturation is subnormal. Injection of ^{59}Fe-labeled red cells (or labeled hemoglobin) reveals rapid clearance by reticuloendothelial cells but defective reutilization of the iron for new hemoglobin synthesis. In bone marrow aspirates stained for iron there is an increase in hemosiderin and ferritin in the macrophages; however, the number of red cell precursors containing siderotic granules is reduced. A decrease in the amount of iron available for heme biosynthesis results in the production of hypochromic erythrocytes and, as in iron deficiency, an increase in free erythrocyte protoporphyrin (FEP) to levels of three to five times normal. In contrast to iron deficiency anemia the FEP increases slowly and does not become clearly abnormal until significant anemia has developed. A humoral factor has been implicated in the pathogenesis of the abnormal iron metabolism. This factor, termed *leukocyte endogenous mediator* (LEM), is released from neutrophils and macrophages during phagocytosis or after stimulation by bacterial toxins. LEM is a low molecular weight protein that, when injected into experimental animals, produces the abnormalities of iron metabolism that characterize the anemia of chronic disease.

The erythrocyte lifespan is about 80 days rather than the normal 120 days. When red cells from a patient with the anemia of chronic disease are transfused into normal subjects they survive normally. Conversely, normal red cells have a shortened survival when transfused into patients with anemia. This suggests that an extracorpuscular factor is involved in the pathogenesis of the hemolysis. However, no such factor has yet been identified. Normally the bone marrow should be able to compensate for such a modest reduction in erythrocyte survival. Failure of the marrow to do so implies that impaired production capacity is important in the pathogenesis of the anemia. The marrow response to anemia is under the control of erythropoietin. In patients with the anemia of chronic disorders erythropoietin levels are usually lower than expected for the degree of anemia. The marrow, however, is capable of responding appropriately to erythropoietin when the hormone is injected or when erythropoietin production is stimulated by hypoxia or cobalt administration. The precise mechanism causing failure of erythropoietin release in response to the slowly developing anemia is unknown.

The three basic abnormalities are interrelated in the pathogenesis of the anemia. For example, the response to erythropoietin suggests that the hormone directly or indirectly affects the block in iron metabolism. It appears that balance is eventually reached among the three factors, and thus the anemia is only mild to moderate and does not generally progress to the point at which transfusion therapy is required.

CLINICAL MANIFESTATIONS. Because this type of anemia occurs in association with so many diseases, the clinical manifestations vary widely. Although the signs and symptoms of the underlying disorder usually overshadow those of the anemia, in occasional patients the anemia is the first sign of the underlying disease.

DIAGNOSIS. The anemia develops during the first few months of the underlying illness and rarely progresses thereafter. The hematocrit generally remains constant in a range between 25 and 40 per cent. The red cell morphology is usually normal as is the reticulocyte count. The characteristic iron determinations are a transferrin saturation less than 15 per cent with a normal serum ferritin. In the marrow there is a decrease in the number of erythroid precursors containing cytoplasmic iron granules (sideroblasts), but reticuloendothelial cells contain normal or increased iron stores. Despite the hemolysis, the usual manifestations of increased blood destruction are absent. The serum bilirubin and the excretion of urobilinogen are generally normal.

TREATMENT. Correction of the anemia depends upon successful treatment of the underlying disease. Blood transfusions are not usually necessary because the anemia is generally mild to moderate and is not progressive. Therapy with cobalt, androgenic steroids, and corticosteroids offers more potential for harm than good. The block to iron flow cannot be bypassed and the administration of oral or parenteral iron is of no benefit. When bleeding causes superimposed iron deficiency, the administration of iron will restore hemoglobin levels to those of the underlying chronic disorder but not back to normal.

SIDEROBLASTIC ANEMIA

DEFINITION. When hypochromic anemia is associated with hyperferremia and increased transferrin saturation, a diagnosis of sideroblastic anemia is suggested. The sideroblastic anemias are a heterogeneous group of disorders associated with various defects in the porphyrin biosynthetic pathway. Porphyrin biosynthetic defects lead to diminished synthesis of heme, which in turn may be associated with an increase in cellular iron uptake (Fig. 135–2). The sideroblastic anemias are characterized by the association of anemia with the presence of an abnormal erythroid precursor in the marrow. The abnormal precursor, the ringed sideroblast, is a normoblast containing excessive deposits of iron within mitochondria. These iron-laden mitochondria, because of their perinuclear distribution, account for the Prussian blue–positive granules forming a full or partial ring around the nucleus of the ringed sideroblast (Color plate 2H). Normal sideroblasts contain one to four Prussian blue–positive ferritin aggregates in the cytoplasm and no visible iron in mitochondria.

PATHOGENESIS AND CLASSIFICATION. Mitochondrial iron excess appears to be a consequence of defective heme synthesis. A population of hypochromic erythrocytes, common to all the sideroblastic anemias, is morphologic evidence of the synthetic defect. Other common characteristics include abnormalities in porphyrin biosynthesis; an increase in total body iron stores; an increase in the serum iron concentration, often to the point of complete saturation of transferrin; and kinetic evidence of ineffective erythropoiesis. It is customary to divide the sideroblastic anemias into two groups, depending on whether the disorder appears to be acquired or inherited (Table 135–2).

Acquired Sideroblastic Anemias

IDIOPATHIC REFRACTORY SIDEROBLASTIC ANEMIA. This acquired disease of older adults has an unknown pathogenesis. The anemia develops insidiously and is often discovered during a routine examination. The anemia is usually slightly macrocytic. Examination of the peripheral blood smear reveals two populations of erythrocytes. One is entirely normal and the other is macrocytic and quite hypochromic with prominent basophilic stippling. Leukocyte and platelet counts are usually normal but leukopenia is occasionally noted and either moderate thrombocytopenia or thrombocytosis has been reported. FEP is increased, but the precise enzymatic defect(s) in porphyrin biosynthesis has not been defined. About 30 to 40 per cent of patients have a palpable spleen. Therapy with pyridoxine or folic acid is not successful and only rare patients respond to androgens. The median survival for patients with idiopathic refractory sideroblastic anemia is about ten years; most patients require no therapy. Transfusion therapy should be kept to a minimum because the chronic administration of erythrocytes has led to transfusional hemochromatosis. Therapy with daily subcutaneous infusions of deferoxamine may be of value to selected patients who require repeated transfusion. The condition in about 10 per cent of patients eventually shows evidence of transformation to acute leukemia. No reliable indicators predict the likelihood of leukemic transformation. The closest association between the development of leukemia and the presence of ringed sideroblasts is noted when sideroblastic anemia occurs following chemotherapy for a variety of malignant disorders. Alkylating drugs such as cyclophosphamide, nitrogen mustard, and melphalan are the most common offenders.

SIDEROBLASTIC ANEMIA COMPLICATING OTHER DISEASES. Acquired sideroblastic anemia associated with other diseases and with drugs or toxins is quite common; however, the anemia is usually only mild. Inflammatory diseases such as rheumatoid arthritis, neoplasms, and a variety of primary hematologic disorders have all been associated with a secondary sideroblastic anemia. The treatment, course, and prognosis are all related to the nature of the associated disease.

SIDEROBLASTIC ANEMIA ASSOCIATED WITH DRUGS OR TOXINS. Sideroblastic anemia is a common complication in hospitalized alcoholics. Withdrawal of alcohol results in a reticulocytosis and disappearance of the ringed sideroblasts within five to ten days. *Alcohol* may cause sideroblastic anemia by interfering with pyridoxine metabolism and thus indirectly affecting the activity of Δ-aminolevulinic acid synthetase, the rate-limiting enzyme in the porphyrin biosynthetic pathway. This mechanism likely also underlies the sideroblastic anemia occasionally seen in association with the administration of the antituberculous agent *isonicotinic acid hydrazide* (INH). The sideroblastic anemia that occurs in *lead poisoning* is caused by the inhibition by lead of the enzyme that converts Δ-aminolevulinic acid to porphobilinogen (Δ-aminolevulinic dehydratase) and the enzyme heme synthetase (ferrochelatase). As a result of these two enzymatic defects it is possible to screen for lead poisoning by detecting either increased urinary excretion of Δ-aminolevulinic acid or a markedly increased FEP.

Hereditary Sideroblastic Anemias

Hereditary sideroblastic anemia is almost always a disease of males and is most likely inherited as an X-linked recessive trait. Although the anemia is usually detected in the late teenage years, in rare cases the anemia is found first in either infancy or adult life. The anemia is severe (average blood hemoglobin 6.5 grams per deciliter) and the red cell indices indicate marked microcytosis and hypochromia. The inherited defect in some way involves the interaction between Δ-aminolevulinic acid synthetase and its cofactor pyridoxal phosphate. Individuals with hereditary sideroblastic anemia are not pyridoxine deficient; however, large amounts of vitamin B_6 produce partial correction of the anemia.

Beutler E, Fairbanks VF: The effects of iron deficiency. In Jacobs A, Worwood M (eds.): Iron in Biochemistry and Medicine II. New York, Academic Press, 1980, pp 394–428. *An extensive review of both the hematologic and nonhematologic manifestations of iron deficiency.*

Jacobs A (ed.): Disorders of iron metabolism. Clin Hematol 11:1, 1982. *A collection of review articles covering basic physiology, clinical diagnosis, and patient management of iron deficiency, sideroblastic anemias, and iron overload.*

Miescher PA, Jaffe ER, Finch CA (eds.): Semin Hematol vol. 19, no. 1, 1984. *An issue of a respected review journal devoted to the clinical aspects of iron deficiency and excess.*

Ward JH, Kushner JP, Kaplan J: Iron: Metabolism and clinical disorders. In Fairbanks VF (ed.): Current Hematology and Oncology. New York, John Wiley & Sons, 1984, vol 3, pp 1–50. *A review of basic iron metabolism with an extensive list of references.*

Williams WJ, Beutler E, Erslev AJ, et al. (eds.): Hematology. 3rd ed. New York, McGraw-Hill Book Company, 1983. *A comprehensive textbook of hematology with an excellent presentation of basic iron metabolism and its application to clinical medicine.*

Wintrobe MM, Lee GR, Boggs DR, et al. (eds.): Clinical Hematology. 8th ed. Philadelphia, Lea & Febiger, 1981. *The oldest standard textbook of hematology with an exhaustive description of the clinical manifestations of iron deficiency anemia.*

136 MEGALOBLASTIC ANEMIAS
William S. Beck

DEFINITION. Megaloblastic anemia (often a pancytopenia) is due to impaired DNA synthesis and is manifested by a readily recognized pattern of morphologic changes in bone marrow and blood cells that include giantism of these cells—and indeed of all proliferating cells in most cases—and various evidences of retarded cell division. The anemia is ordinarily macrocytic—i.e., the mean corpuscular volume (MCV) exceeds 100 cu μm—although not all macrocytic anemias are megaloblastic.

ETIOLOGY. Megaloblastic anemia is easily diagnosed in most cases. The differential diagnosis of the underlying disorder, however, may be more difficult because defective DNA synthesis can have many causes. It is convenient to divide the megaloblastic anemias into three major etiologic categories: (1) those that are associated with cobalamin (vitamin B_{12}) deficiency and respond to cobalamin therapy, (2) those that are associated with folate deficiency and respond to folic acid (pteroylmonoglutamate) therapy, and (3) those unresponsive to cobalamin or folic acid therapy. Deficiencies of cobalamin and folate may themselves have a great many specific causes. Pernicious anemia, for example, is but one cause of cobalamin deficiency. Accurate differential diagnosis is important because it guides the choice of therapy and usually discloses a significant underlying disorder.

The major etiologic categories and their underlying causes are summarized in Table 136–1. Cobalamin deficiency and folate deficiency are by far the most common categories. Together with iron deficiency anemia they constitute the bulk of the so-called nutritional anemias, which are among the most common of human ills. Both vitamin deficiencies lead to tissue coenzyme deficiencies that are usually corrected easily by repletion of the lacking vitamin. Hematopoiesis then reverts from megaloblastic to normoblastic. Other mechanisms obviously account for the megaloblastic anemias that are unresponsive to therapy with cobalamin and folic acid.

The approach to a patient suspected of megaloblastic anemia should proceed through several orderly steps. First, it is determined from the reticulocyte count and other tests whether a macrocytic anemia is due to bone marrow failure or erythrocyte loss or destruction. If marrow failure, the presence of megaloblastosis is established by demonstrating in blood and bone marrow the characteristic morphologic features to be described below. The broad etiologic category is then elucidated with serum vitamin assays and other procedures to be discussed. One then seeks a specific causal mechanism, administers specific treatment, and observes the response to treatment.

PATHOGENESIS AND PATHOLOGY OF MEGALOBLASTIC ANEMIA. The following discussion deals with the general features of megaloblastic anemia per se, irrespective of cause. The features of cobalamin and folate deficiency, irrespective of cause, and the major disorders responsible for these deficiencies will then be discussed.

TABLE 136–1. ETIOLOGIC CLASSIFICATION OF THE MEGALOBLASTIC ANEMIAS

Category	Etiologic Mechanisms
I. Cobalamin deficiency	
A. Decreased ingestion	Poor diet, lack of animal products, strict vegetarianism
B. Impaired absorption	1. Intrinsic factor deficiency
	Pernicious anemia
	Gastrectomy (total and partial)
	Destruction of gastric mucosa by caustics
	Anti-IF antibody in gastric juice
	Abnormal intrinsic factor molecule
	2. Intrinsic intestinal disease
	Familial selective malabsorption (Imerslund's syndrome)
	Ileal resection, ileitis
	Sprue, celiac disease
	Infiltrative intestinal disease (e.g., lymphoma, scleroderma)
	Drug-induced malabsorption
	3. Competitive parasites
	Fish tapeworm infestations (*Diphyllobothrium latum*)
	Bacteria in diverticula of bowel, blind loops
	4. Chronic pancreatic disease
C. Increased requirement	Pregnancy
	Neoplastic disease
	Hyperthyroidism
D. Impaired utilization	Enzyme deficiencies
	Abnormal serum cobalamin binding protein
	Lack of transcobalamin II
	Nitrous oxide administration
II. Folate deficiency	
A. Decreased ingestion	Poor diet, lack of vegetables
	Alcoholism
	Infancy
B. Impaired absorption	Intestinal short circuits
	Steatorrhea
	Sprue, celiac disease
	Intrinsic intestinal disease
	Anticonvulsants, oral contraceptives, other drugs
C. Increased requirement	Pregnancy, infancy
	Hyperthyroidism
	Hyperactive hematopoiesis
	Neoplastic disease, exfoliative skin disease
D. Impaired utilization	Folic acid antagonists: methotrexate, triamterene, trimethoprim
	Enzyme deficiencies
E. Increased loss	Hemodialysis
III. Unresponsive to cobalamin or folate therapy	
A. Metabolic inhibitors	Purine synthesis: 6-mercaptopurine, 6-thioguanine, azathioprine
	Pyrimidine synthesis: 6-azauridine
	Thymidylate synthesis: methotrexate, 5-fluorouracil
	Deoxyribonucleotide synthesis: hydroxyurea, cytosine arabinoside, severe iron deficiency
B. Inborn errors	Lesch-Nyhan syndrome
	Hereditary orotic aciduria
	Deficiency of formimino-transferase, methyltransferase, etc.
C. Unexplained disorders	Pyridoxine-responsive megaloblastic anemia
	Thiamine-responsive megaloblastic anemia
	Erythremic myelosis (Di Guglielmo's syndrome)

Mechanism of Megaloblastosis. Megaloblasts contain an increased amount of RNA and a normal or slightly increased amount of DNA per cell, the former presumably accounting for the cytoplasmic basophilia (blue color) in Wright's-stained smears. Thymidine is readily incorporated into their DNA. Hence, DNA synthesis can occur. There is, however, impairment of a critical step in the pathway of DNA synthesis—the synthesis of thymidylate (dTMP). In addition, there is a sharp increase in intracellular dUMP and dUTP levels and thus of the dUTP/dTTP ratio. As a result there is significant misincorporation of uracil into DNA. Much of this uracil is removed by an "editorial" enzyme system, but lack of available dTTP blocks final DNA repair. Hence, DNA is fragmented and DNA replication and cell division are blocked, while synthesis of RNA and protein proceed normally. Prolongation of this state results in permanent loss of the capacity for cell division and eventual cell death. In megaloblastic bone marrow the degree of impairment of DNA synthesis varies from cell to cell and from cell series to cell series. Usually, it is more severe among erythrocyte precursors than granulocyte precursors.

Morphology of Megaloblastic Cells (Color plate 2F). The features characteristic of the megaloblastic state are seen most vividly in the Wright's-stained smear of aspirated bone marrow. Among *erythrocyte precursors* megaloblastic changes occur at all stages of development. They are larger than corresponding cells of the normoblastic series and often have a higher than normal ratio of cytoplasmic area to nuclear area. Promegaloblasts, the most immature of the series and the most easily recognized, display brilliantly colored, deeply basophilic (blue), granule-free cytoplasm and lavender-tinted chromatin with a distinctive open and fine-grained texture that contrasts with strand-like pronormoblast chromatin. As the cell matures, the chromatin retains its odd texture and is slow to form coarse deeply basophilic clumps. Development of a dense pyknotic nucleus like that of an orthochromatic normoblast either fails to occur or is delayed. With the appearance of hemoglobin, the apparent maturity of the cytoplasm contrasts sharply with the apparent immaturity of the nucleus—a feature termed nuclear-cytoplasmic asynchronism. All of these changes are less well developed in mild or incipient megaloblastic anemias or in megaloblastic anemias associated with iron deficiency.

Granulocyte precursors may also display nuclear-cytoplasmic asynchronism and enlargement, most strikingly at the metamyelocyte stage. A "giant metamyelocyte" has ragged chromatin and a relatively large nucleus, sometimes of bizarre shape, that takes stain poorly and may be pinched off in several places, in anticipation perhaps of later hypersegmentation (Color plate 2E).

The *bone marrow* is extremely cellular, especially when anemia is severe. Megaloblastic changes may be seen in all cell lines, although major changes may be limited to the erythroid cells (Color plate 2F). Many mitotic figures (i.e., cells in metaphase) are found among them. The myeloid/erythroid ratio typically falls from 3 to about 1. Megaloblastic granulopoiesis is more evident in infection, in which increased granulocyte production has been stimulated. Unless iron deficiency is present, iron in reticulum cells is increased.

In the *blood*, erythrocytes usually display striking variations in size and shape and are normochromic (unless iron deficiency coexists) and macrocytic, with MCV's ranging from 100 to more than 140 cu μm. Macro-ovalocytes, large oval-shaped erythrocytes up to 14 μm in diameter, are usually present (Color plate 2E). The reticulocyte count is often lower than normal, both in absolute and relative (percentage) terms. Erythrocyte changes become more severe as the anemia worsens. When the hematocrit is low (<20 per cent), nucleated red cells may appear in the blood.

Many neutrophils have more than four segments; occasionally some have up to 16 segments. Hypersegmented neutrophils, or macropolycytes, may be quite large. This is a significant finding, because it is not masked by coexisting iron deficiency and in folate deficiency tends to occur before bone marrow cells are overtly megaloblastic. Hypersegmentation is probably due to abnormalities of nuclear division and chromatin.

Megaloblastosis actually occurs in all proliferating body cells, which share the underlying defect in DNA synthesis.

Thus epithelial cells of buccal mucosa, stomach, and vagina all display typical morphologic and biochemical abnormalities. These changes in many patients with cobalamin and folate deficiency account for such phenomena as glossitis (and mouth soreness), secondary gastric atrophy (and dyspepsia), and secondary malabsorption.

Pathophysiologic Features of the Megaloblastic State. Whatever its cause, megaloblastic anemia is associated with two pathophysiologic abnormalities: ineffective erythropoiesis and moderate hemolysis.

Ineffective erythropoiesis is indicated by (1) the marked increase in marrow erythroid precursors and the high ratio of erythroid precursors to released erythrocytes; (2) increase in plasma iron turnover to three to five times the normal level, despite the fact that iron uptake by individual erythroid precursors is normal; (3) decreased rate of reappearance of labeled plasma iron in blood erythrocytes; and (4) various signs of intramedullary destruction of megaloblasts. These include increased production of "early-labeled peak" bilirubin and endogenous carbon monoxide, phagocytosis of megaloblastic erythroid precursors by marrow reticulum cells, and high serum levels of lactic dehydrogenase (isozymes 1 and 2, which come from erythroid percursors) and muramidase (from leukocyte precursors). Other findings are slight to moderate increases in serum bilirubin, iron, and iron saturation, and decreases in haptoglobin (owing to ongoing hemolysis) and, in some patients, serum uric acid (owing to decreased DNA synthesis). Even when serum uric acid is not depressed, it usually rises sharply soon after the start of specific therapy.

Intramedullary hemolysis results from this ineffective erythropoiesis. A substantial degree of extramedullary hemolysis also occurs. Erythrocyte lifespan is moderately decreased (to one-half to one-third normal) when patient erythrocytes are infused into normal subjects, classic evidence of an intracorpuscular defect. Decreased survival of normal erythrocytes infused into untreated patients suggests the presence of an extracorpuscular defect as well.

Inadequate production of myeloid cells accounts for the neutropenia of megaloblastic anemia. Elevated serum muramidase levels reflect the increased rate of intramedullary myeloid cell destruction. Thus, the mechanism of leukopenia is ineffective granulopoiesis. Ineffective thrombopoiesis also occurs; its pathophysiology parallels that of ineffective erythropoiesis and granulopoiesis. A decreased rate of platelet production (despite the presence of megakaryocytes) accounts for the mild to moderate thrombocytopenia observed in many patients with megaloblastic anemia.

Unless iron deficiency is present, ineffective erythropoiesis is associated with features suggesting iron overload: increased plasma iron and iron saturation, increased plasma iron turnover, decreased incorporation of plasma iron into circulating hemoglobin, accumulation of iron in marrow reticulum cells, and increased iron stores in the liver (hepatic siderosis) and other tissues.

MEGALOBLASTIC ANEMIA OF COBALAMIN DEFICIENCY

Classic studies of pernicious anemia led directly or indirectly to much of our early knowledge of cobalamin. Until the demonstration by Minot and Murphy in 1926 of the successful treatment of pernicious anemia by feeding liver, the disease was often fatal. Potent liver extracts soon replaced oral liver, but difficulties plagued investigators attempting to purify the anti-pernicious anemia principle of liver. Cobalamin was finally discovered in 1948 when proportionality was found between the nutrient activity of liver extracts in cultures of *Lactobacillus lactis* Dorner and their therapeutic activity in pernicious anemia. The resulting microbiologic assay rapidly facilitated purification and identification of the vitamin.

Metabolic and Nutritional Aspects of Cobalamin. Cobalamin is synthesized only by certain microorganisms. Wherever it is found in nature, it can be traced to microorganisms growing in soil, sewage, intestine, or rumen. Animals thus depend ultimately upon microbial synthesis for their cobalamin supply. Foods in the human diet that contain cobalamin are essentially those of animal origin: meat, liver, fish, eggs, and milk. The average daily diet in Western countries contains 5 to 30 μg of cobalamin, of which only 1 to 5 μg (the minimal daily requirement) is absorbed. Total body content is 2 to 5 mg in an adult man; approximately 1 mg is in the liver. Hence, a deficiency state will not develop for several years after cessation of cobalamin absorption.

The cobalamin molecule (Fig. 136–1) includes a porphyrin-like moiety (termed *corrin*) and a central cobalt atom. The four cobalamins of importance in animal cell metabolism are *cyanocobalamin* (CN-Cbl) and its analogue *hydroxocobalamin* (OH-Cbl), and two coenzyme forms—*adenosylcobalamin* (AdoCbl) and *methylcobalamin* (MeCbl). In adenosylcobalamin, a 5'-deoxyadenosyl moiety is the ligand of cobalt. This compound, the main storage form of cobalamin in liver, is the coenzyme of *methylmalonyl CoA mutase*, an enzyme catalyzing the final step in the pathway of propionic acid metabolism, in which methylmalonyl CoA is converted to succinyl CoA. This is the major AdoCbl-dependent reaction in animal tissues. Methylcobalamin, which occurs in small amounts in liver but is the major cobalamin in serum, is the coenzyme for the conversion of homocysteine to methionine (Fig. 136–2). This methyltransferase enzyme serves primarily as a means for converting N^5-methyltetrahydrofolate (N^5-methyl FH_4) to tetrahydrofolate (FH_4).

Impairment of DNA synthesis in cobalamin deficiency has been attributed to slowing of the cobalamin-dependent pathway of methionine synthesis. This sequesters folate as N^5-methyl FH_4, a form that is unavailable to the critical thymidylate synthetase reaction. This theory, the so-called methylfolate trap theory, is supported by the occurrence in cobalamin deficiency of elevated serum folate (N^5-methyl FH_4) levels. Folate coenzymes in tissues are in the form of polyglutamates. The enzyme converting folate (folylmonoglutamate) to folylpolyglutamate is most active with FH_4 as substrate and is relatively inactive with N^5-methyl FH_4. When the latter form accumulates in cobalamin deficiency, it is unavailable for conversion to folylpolyglutamate, and thymidylate synthetase is further deprived of its essential cofactor. This situation accounts for depressed levels of folylpolyglutamates in cobalamin-deficient tissues.

Cobalamin in food is liberated by peptic enzymes and acid in gastric juice. The vitamin is then bound by one or more proteins in gastric juice. Electrophoresis reveals two binders or classes of binders in gastric juice, one with slow and one with rapid mobility, that have been designated *S-proteins* and *R-proteins*, respectively (Table 136–2). One of the binding proteins in gastric juice is intrinsic factor (IF), a glycoprotein of molecular weight 44,000 that binds a molecule of cobalamin with high affinity. Secretion of IF parallels HCl secretion by the parietal cells in man. R-cobalamin complexes may be

TABLE 136–2. MAJOR COBALAMIN-BINDING PROTEINS

Source	Protein(s)	Function	Class*
Gastric juice	Intrinsic factor (IF)	Promotes absorption of cobalamin in ileum	S
Gastric juice	"Haptocorrin(s)"	May be involved in formation of IF-cobalamin; binds cobalamin analogues	R
Plasma	Transcobalamin I (TC I)	May participate in plasma transport of cobalamin	R
Plasma	Transcobalamin II (TC II)	Promotes entry of cobalamin into cells	S
Plasma (and granulocytes)	Transcobalamin III (TC III)	Unknown	R

* R = rapid; S = slow. Based on electrophoretic mobility.

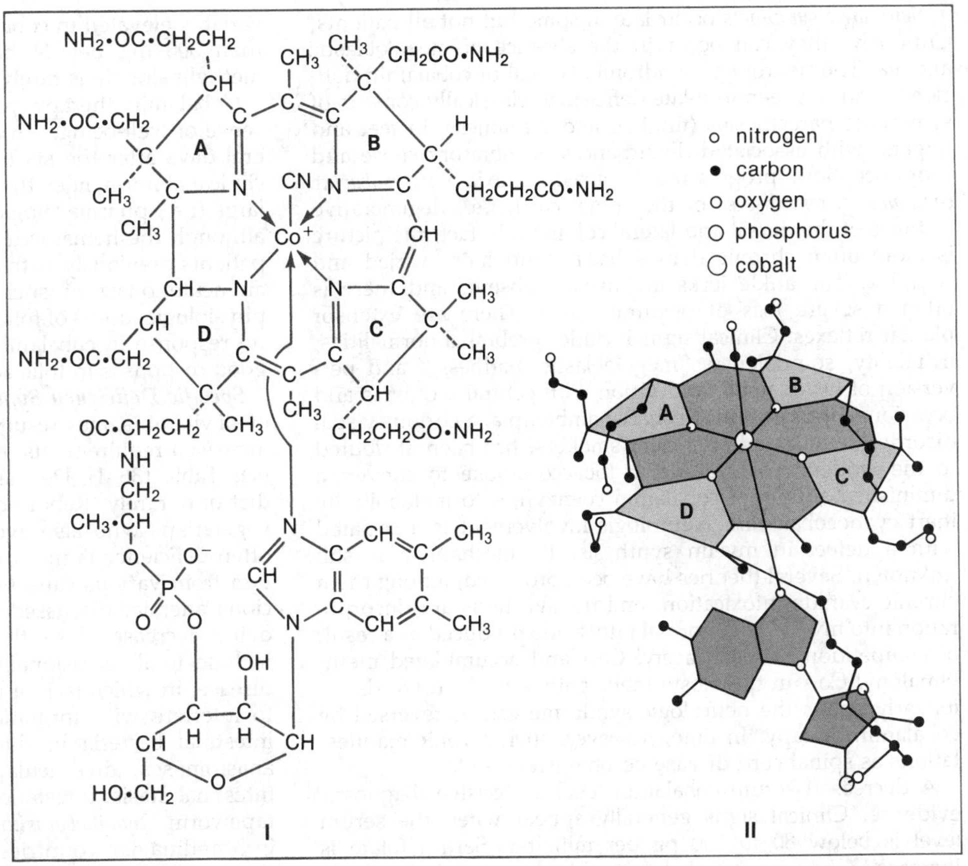

FIGURE 136–1. Chemical structure of cyanocobalamin. *Formula I*, Molecular structure. *Formula II*, Semidiagrammatic representation of three-dimensional structure showing relations of planar and nucleotide moieties. Hydrogen atoms and a number of oxygen atoms are omitted. (Adapted from Beck WS: N Engl J Med 266:708, 1962.)

o nitrogen
● carbon
o oxygen
O phosphorus
O cobalt

converted to IF-cobalamin with the participation of pancreatic proteases. The stable IF cobalamin complex encounters specific mucosal receptors in the microvilli of the ileum that bind to a specific site on the IF molecule. Attachment requires neutral pH, Ca^{++}, or other divalent cations, but no energy. Cobalamin is transferred into the ileal cell and ultimately transferred to portal vein blood. Thus, IF is essential for the intestinal absorption of ingested cobalamin.

Two types of anti-IF antibodies occur. "Blocking" antibodies prevent binding of cobalamin by IF and show little species specificity. "Binding" antibodies combine with IF-cobalamin and with free IF without impairing its ability to bind cobala-

min. Both types of antibodies occur in sera of some patients with pernicious anemia.

Binding proteins, which occur in serum, leukocytes, saliva, gastric juice, milk, and virtually all body cells, promote uptake of cobalamin by mitochondria and other organelles within cells.

Normal plasma contains 175 to 725 pg per milliliter of cobalamin (normal range varying with method and laboratory). All of it is protein-bound. The three major cobalamin-binding proteins of plasma are designated *transcobalamin I* (TC I), *transcobalamin II* (TC II), and *transcobalamin III* (TC III). They have only two known functions: TC II transports cobalamins through cell membranes, and all three prevent loss of cobalamins in urine, sweat, and other body secretions.

Serum cobalamin levels are most conveniently and accurately measured with a radioisotope dilution assay with IF as a binding agent. The results parallel those obtained using the microbiologic assays of the past. There are other cobalamin analogues in serum that will interfere with the assay if the less specific R proteins, rather than IF, are used as binders. The presence of these analogues raises many interesting questions. What is the source and fate of these analogues? Do they have pathophysiologic significance? Is it one of the roles of R-proteins, especially those of gastric juice, to bind these compounds (which may be of dietary origin) to minimize their absorption in the intestine?

Cobalamin Deficiency. The clinical picture of human deficiency includes the nonspecific manifestations of megaloblastic anemia and its sequelae—e.g., megaloblastosis, slowly progressing anemia, glossitis, increased serum lactic dehydrogenase—that occur as well in folic acid deficiency (and are described above), *plus* certain specific features that make possible the diagnosis of cobalamin deficiency, irrespective of the underlying cause. These include neurologic abnormalities, decreased serum cobalamin level, methylmalonic aciduria, and a characteristic response to cobalamin therapy and lack of response to therapy with physiologic doses of folic acid.

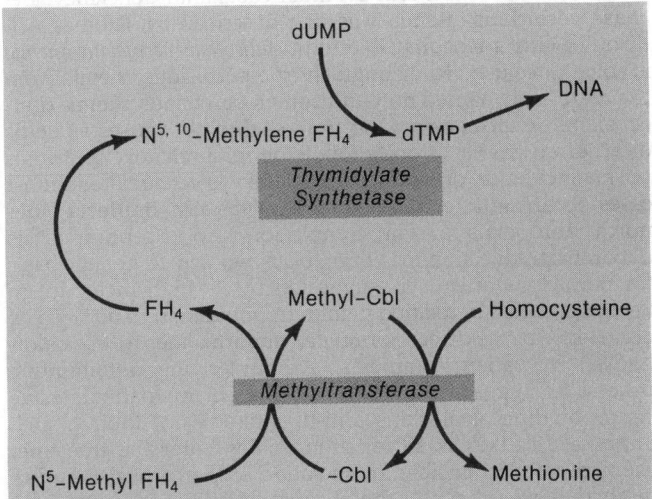

FIGURE 136–2. Diagram of relationship between N^5-methyl FH_4: homocysteine methyltransferase and thymidylate synthetase. In cobalamin deficiency, folate is sequestered as N^5-methyl FH_4. This ultimately deprives thymidylate synthetase of its folate coenzyme ($N^{5,\,10}$-methylene FH_4) and thereby impairs DNA synthesis.

Neurologic symptoms occur late in some but not all patients. Curiously, they can occur in the absence of megaloblastic anemia. The neurologic syndrome, typical of cobalamin deficiency and not seen in folate deficiency, classically consists of symmetric paresthesias (tingling and numbness) in feet and fingers, with associated disturbances of vibratory sense and proprioception, progressing to spastic ataxia with *subacute combined system disease* of the spinal cord, i.e., degenerative changes of the dorsal and lateral columns. In fact, the picture is more often chronic than subacute and more varied and complex. The ankle jerks are usually absent, and there is often a severe loss of postural sense. There are extensor plantar reflexes. Clinical signs include cerebral abnormalities, irritability, somnolence, "megaloblastic madness," and perversion of taste, smell, and vision with central scotomas and occasional optic atrophy. Tobacco amblyopia, a curious visual disorder in cobalamin-deficient smokers, has been attributed to the tendency of cyanide in tobacco smoke to convert a diminished supply of cobalamin coenzymes to metabolically inert cyanocobalamin. Neurologic involvement is associated with a defect in myelin synthesis. Its mechanism is still unknown. Several theories have been proposed, among them chronic cyanide intoxication, and the synthesis and incorporation into myelin of abnormal fatty acids produced as a result of competition between acetyl CoA and accumulated methylmalonyl CoA in the biosynthetic pathway of fatty acids. In its early stages the neurologic syndrome can be reversed by cobalamin therapy. In time, however, such chronic manifestations as spinal cord disease become irreversible.

A decreased serum cobalamin level is decisive diagnostic evidence. Clinical signs generally appear when the serum level is below 80 to 100 pg per milliliter. Serum folate is increased when serum cobalamin is depressed unless there is coexisting folate deficiency. Methylmalonic aciduria is also a sensitive index of cobalamin deficiency except in rare cases in which it is due to an inborn error of metabolism. It does not occur in folate deficiency. Normal subjects excrete only traces of methylmalonate, i.e., 0 to 3.5 mg per 24 hours. Levels are variably elevated in cobalamin deficiency, sometimes to more than 300 mg per 24 hours. In practice, assay of urinary methylmalonate is rarely necessary.

Cobalamin therapy produces within hours an improved sense of well-being. An abrupt reticulocyte crisis begins several days after the start of therapy (Fig. 136–3). Reversal of clinical abnormalities then ensues. A partial response follows large (i.e., pharmacologic) doses of folic acid (5 mg per day), although the hematocrit is not fully restored to normal, and patients previously without neurologic symptoms may suffer an acute onset of such symptoms. However, small (i.e., physiologic) doses of folic acid (200 to 400 μg per day) produce no response in cobalamin deficiency, whereas they produce good responses in folic acid deficiency.

Specific Deficiency Syndromes. Deficiency of cobalamin, as of all vitamins, may result from inadequate intake, abnormally increased requirements, or impaired utilization in the tissues (see Table 136–1). Deficiency of cobalamin results from poor diet only rarely. Reported instances have occurred mainly in vegetarians who also avoid dairy products and eggs. Most often deficiency is the result of diminished intestinal absorption from various causes. The most common cause is pernicious anemia, discussed below, in which a gastric mucosal defect decreases IF synthesis. Other and less common causes include total (occasionally subtotal) gastrectomy; pancreatic disease, in which lack of proteases in the duodenum appears to interfere with formation of IF-cobalamin; overgrowth of intestinal bacteria in the blind loop syndrome, strictures, anastomoses, diverticula, and other conditions producing intestinal stasis; infestation with the cobalamin-utilizing fish tapeworm *Diphyllobothrium latum* (once a common condition in Scandinavian countries); and organic disease of the ileum that interferes with cobalamin absorption despite the presence of adequate IF. Cobalamin deficiency resulting from increased requirements occurs mainly in pregnancy, presumably arising from the superimposition of fetal demands upon a background of poor nutrition. Impaired utilization of cobalamin occurs in various genetic defects, involving deletions or defects of methylmalonyl CoA mutase, TC II, and enzymes in the pathway of cobalamin adenosylation.

PERNICIOUS ANEMIA

Once a fatal disease and now the physician's favorite for its rich history, scientific importance, and cheerful prognosis, pernicious anemia is an atrophic gastropathy that leads to deficient IF secretion and eventual cobalamin deficiency. Because pernicious anemia was first described by Thomas Addison of Guy's Hospital, the term *addisonian pernicious anemia* is sometimes used to distinguish true pernicious anemia from the regrettably named non-addisonian pernicious anemia (i.e., cobalamin deficiency arising from such other causes as ileitis or acquired gastric atrophy following inflammatory gastritis).

The incidence of pernicious anemia is age related, most cases occurring after the age of 40. Typically, it affects older north Europeans of fair complexion. An exception is its apparent predilection for young black women. A genetic basis for pernicious anemia is suggested by its high incidence in Scandinavians, a relatively inbred population, and by the occurrence of the disease or related abnormalities (e.g., achlorhydria) in patients' families. An underlying autoimmune process is suggested by the fact that many patients have serum binding or blocking anti-IF antibodies. Although such antibodies can block IF function if they enter the intestine, they are not responsible for cessation of IF synthesis. Anti-IF antibodies also occur in the absence of pernicious anemia in the serum of patients with diabetes mellitus, thyroid disease, and other diseases. Serum from pernicious anemia may also contain antibodies against gastric parietal cell cytoplasm and thyroid acinar cell cytoplasm. Pernicious anemia occurs frequently in patients with thyrotoxicosis, Hashimoto's thyroid-

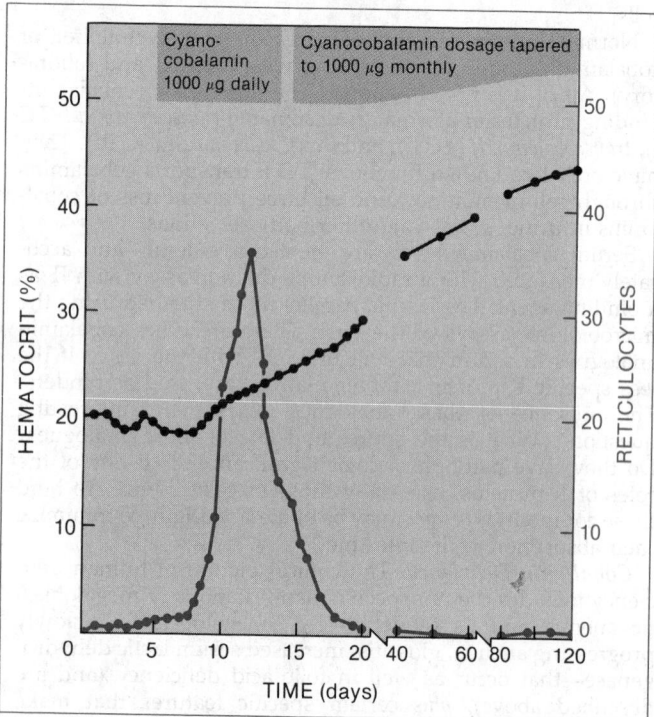

FIGURE 136–3. Time course of reticulocyte count and hematocrit level during treatment of pernicious anemia with cyanocobalamin. (Adapted from Beck WS, Goulian M: In DiPalma J [ed.]: Drill's Pharmacology in Medical Practice. 4th ed. New York, McGraw-Hill Book Company, 1971.)

itis, and several other diseases (hypogammaglobulinemia, vitiligo, rheumatoid arthritis, and gastric carcinoma). Most hematologists have the impression that the incidence of pernicious anemia is decreasing.

Clinically, there is a slow onset of megaloblastic anemia and laboratory signs of cobalamin deficiency. If untreated, the patient may eventually develop neurologic symptoms. Diagnostic features are achlorhydria after histamine stimulation and decreased levels of IF in gastric juice as revealed by direct assay in vitro (which is performed routinely in Europe but infrequently in the United States) or by decreased cobalamin absorption in an in vivo test of cobalamin absorption. In the absorption test known as the *Schilling test*, a fasting patient ingests 0.5 microcurie (0.5 to 2.0 μg) [⁵⁷Co]cyanocobalamin at time zero. A dose (1 mg) of unlabeled cyanocobalamin is injected at two hours, and radioactivity is measured in a 24-hour urine collection. If excretion of radioactivity is low, the test is repeated (in no less than five days) by the same procedure, except that 60 mg of hog IF is given orally with the radioactive cobalamin. If poor excretion and therefore presumably poor absorption was due to IF deficiency, the result with the addition of exogenous IF should be normal. If excretion is still low, ileal disease may be suspected. Renal disease with impaired glomerular filtration may delay excretion of radioactivity in the Schilling test. Since the Schilling test includes an injection of cobalamin it is a therapeutic commitment if therapy has not already been initiated.

Juvenile pernicious anemia includes four entities: (1) true pernicious anemia, which occurs infrequently between ages 2 and 14; (2) congenital IF lack, with no other abnormality of gastric secretion and no anti-IF antibody; (3) production of biologically inert IF (one case reported); and (4) familial selective malabsorption of cobalamin (Imerslund's syndrome) with normal absorption of other nutrients and normal gastric secretion of IF and HCl. The Schilling test reveals decreased cobalamin uncorrected for IF. Presumably, there is a defect of specific mucosal receptors for IF-cobalamin.

Therapy. Therapy consists in the parenteral administration of cobalamin (hydroxocobalamin or cyanocobalamin) in amounts that are ultimately sufficient to provide the 2 to 5 μg needed for the daily requirement and to replete liver stores and other reservoirs, which normally contain 2 to 5 mg of cobalamin. Because of its low cost and lack of toxicity, doses in excess of need are generally given. Parenterally administered cobalamin is bound to plasma proteins and cellular binding sites. If much more than 100 μg is given parenterally in a single dose, delay in encountering vacant binding sites promptly leads to renal excretion of unbound vitamin. Since hydroxocobalamin is bound more tightly by binding proteins than cyanocobalamin, it is less rapidly excreted by the kidney and more effective in achieving high serum cobalamin levels. Hypokalemia sometimes develops early in the course of treatment, especially in severely deficient patients, as a result of a sudden increase in the need for potassium in young red cells abruptly returning to normal hematopoiesis. The following treatment schedule is used in my clinic: (1) 500 to 1000 μg intramuscularly daily for two weeks; (2) the same dose twice weekly for an additional four weeks or until the hematocrit is normal; and (3) the same dose once monthly for the lifetime of the patient. A dosage schedule of 500 to 1000 μg every two weeks for six months is recommended for patients with neurologic manifestations. Neurologic symptoms persisting beyond 12 to 18 months are usually irreversible.

Oral cobalamin–IF preparations are not recommended, since the condition often becomes refractory to therapy. Oral therapy with cobalamin alone (500 to 1000 μg daily) should be reserved for the occasional patient who for some reason cannot receive parenteral therapy. This mode of therapy depends on intestinal absorption by passive diffusion, a process that is often unpredictable. Patients receiving oral medication who feel well may decide to stop their medication.

The patient with pernicious anemia should understand that he or she must be treated for life.

Since the response to cobalamin occurs within 48 to 72 hours, it is seldom necessary to subject the patient to the risks, discomfort, and expense of blood transfusion.

There is no need for iron therapy in pernicious anemia unless there is evidence of associated iron deficiency or reason to suspect that tissue iron reserves are deficient—as, for example, in women of early middle age who may have had heavy menstrual losses or several pregnancies. In such cases, hemoglobin and erythrocyte regeneration is delayed until iron is given. There is no need to administer folic acid or ascorbic acid in addition to the cobalamin, provided that the patient has an adequate diet. As long as cobalamin is given, folic acid therapy causes no harm. It is commonly elected to administer both cobalamin and folic acid to distressed patients with severe megaloblastic anemia without awaiting the diagnostic workup. In this situation, as in all cases of megaloblastic anemia, it is mandatory to obtain serum samples for vitamin assays before therapy starts.

With the exception of hereditary methylmalonic aciduria, cobalamin deficiency of whatever cause is the only valid indication for cobalamin therapy. It has been recommended, nevertheless, for many disorders in which there is no evidence of deficiency, especially for various types of neuropathy, liver disease, dermatologic disorders, and allergies, and as a "tonic" or appetite stimulant. The usefulness of cobalamin in these circumstances has not been proved, and its use for such purposes is not recommended.

MEGALOBLASTIC ANEMIA OF FOLATE DEFICIENCY

Converging lines of nutritional research led to the discovery of folic acid in the mid 1940's. In 1948 crystalline folic acid was obtained from liver and its structure confirmed by organic synthesis. Although experimental folic acid deficiency was known to produce megaloblastic anemia, it was not immediately recognized that folic acid is not the anti-pernicious anemia principle of liver, which was identified a year later. Confusion arose when folic acid therapy produced notable reticulocyte responses in pernicious anemia. Hemoglobin regeneration was incomplete, however, and relapses and neurologic complications occurred during treatment. Liver extracts active in pernicious anemia were then found by direct assay to contain little or no folic acid. Thus, it was recognized that cobalamin deficiency is the basis of the megaloblastic anemia of pernicious anemia and that folate deficiency is a distinctive cause of megaloblastic anemia.

Metabolic and Nutritional Aspects of Folic Acid. Folic acid is the trivial name for *pteroylmonoglutamic acid* (Fig. 136–4), parent compound of the large family of compounds known collectively as folate or folates. The molecule contains three moieties: a pteridine derivative, a *p*-aminobenzoic acid residue, and an L-glutamic acid residue. The first two combined constitute pteroic acid; hence folates are pteroylglutamates.

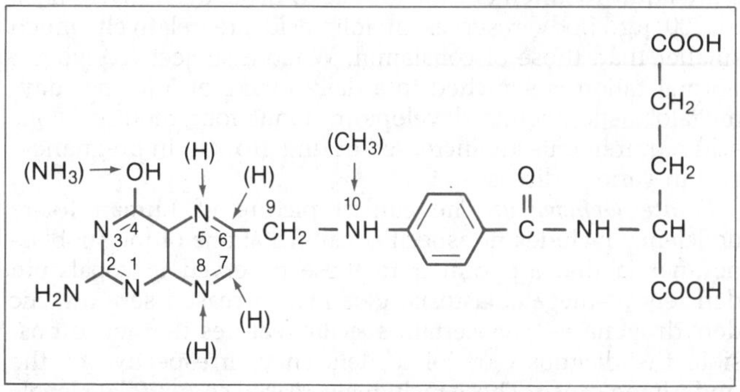

FIGURE 136–4. Chemical structure of folic acid (pteroylmonoglutamic acid). Substituents in parentheses are attached at the sites shown in the several folate derivatives described in the text. (From Beck WS [ed.]: Hematology. 4th ed. Cambridge, Mass., MIT Press, 1985.)

Folic acid occurs in nature largely in the form of folylpolyglutamates, in which multiple glutamic acid residues are attached by peptide linkages to the gamma-carboxyl group of the preceding glutamic acid residue. The synthetic folic acid used therapeutically is folylmonoglutamate. However, folylmonoglutamates are converted in cells to polyglutamates, which are apparently the true coenzymes of folate-dependent enzymes.

Folic acid occurs at three levels of oxidation: folic acid (F); 7,8-dihydrofolic acid (FH_2); and 5,6,7,8-tetrahydrofolic acid (FH_4). Reduction of F to FH_4 is a necessary prerequisite to the participation of folic acid in enzyme reactions. In this reduction, F is reduced to FH_2, which is then reduced to FH_4. In animal cells both reactions are catalyzed by a single NADPH-linked enzyme, *dihydrofolate reductase*, which is notably sensitive to inhibition by folate analogues containing a 4-amino group (Fig. 136–4) such as aminopterin and amethopterin, later renamed methotrexate (MTX).

The folate family consists largely of FH_4 derivatives bearing one of several "one-carbon" substituents on N^5 or N^{10} (or both). Specific enzymes interconvert many of these compounds. Folate derivatives differ in their ability to support various microorganisms. The major form of folate in human serum is N^5-methyl FH_4 (a monoglutamate), which is assayed with *Lactobacillus casei*. Satisfactory isotope dilution assay procedures are now available for the assay of serum folate.

In metabolism, FH_4 is a catalytic self-regenerating acceptor-donor of one-carbon units in anabolic and catabolic reactions involving one-carbon transfers. A number of metabolic systems in animal tissues are known to require folate coenzymes. Impairment of thymidylate synthesis is the key event in folate deficiency that produces major clinical manifestations (see Fig. 135–2). Methylation of deoxyuridylate to thymidylate, catalyzed by the enzyme thymidylate synthetase, is an essential step in the biosynthesis of DNA. Impairment of thymidylate synthesis in folate deficiency slows DNA synthesis with resulting megaloblastic transformation. Folate also participates in the breakdown of histidine and its catabolic product, formiminoglutamic acid (abbreviated FIGlu). Interference with this system in folate deficiency has no morbid effects, but it provides the basis for a diagnostic test for folate deficiency. When insufficient FH_4 is present to accept the formimino group, FIGlu accumulates in the urine, where it is easily detected.

Green vegetables are rich sources of folate, the richest being asparagus, broccoli, spinach, and lettuce, each of which contains more than 1 mg of folate per 100 grams dry weight. Folates are also found in liver, kidney, yeast, and mushrooms. An average daily American diet, prepared without special precautions, contains approximately 200 µg of folate by *Streptococcus faecalis* assay and an additional 400 to 500 µg of folate that is active only with *Lactobacillus casei*. Excessive cooking, particularly with large amounts of water, can remove or destroy a high percentage of the folate in foods. The minimal daily adult requirement for folic acid, or its derivatives, is 50 to 200 µg. Body reserves of folic acid are relatively much smaller than those of cobalamin. When a subject receiving a normal ration is switched to a daily intake of 5 µg per day, megaloblastic anemia develops in about four months. Folic acid requirements are increased during growth, in pregnancy, and in various diseases.

Folate Deficiency. The clinical picture of human folate deficiency includes nonspecific manifestations of megaloblastic anemia that are similar to those observed in cobalamin deficiency—megaloblastosis, glossitis, increased serum lactic dehydrogenase—*plus* certain specific features that make possible the diagnosis of folate deficiency, irrespective of the underlying cause. These include decreased serum folate levels (normal, 6 to 15 ng per milliliter), decreased red cell folate levels (normal, 150 to 600 ng per milliliter of cells), and full clinical response to therapy with physiologic doses of folic

acid. Features suggestive but not diagnostic of folate deficiency in a patient with megaloblastic anemia are lack of neurologic changes of the type seen in cobalamin deficiency, normal serum cobalamin and urine methylmalonic acid levels, and a history of circumstances almost certain to lead to folic acid deficiency, e.g., poor diet, malabsorption, or alcoholism.

Specific Deficiency Syndromes. As shown in Table 136–1, the major categories of folate deficiency are those due to decreased intake, increased requirements, and impaired utilization. Decreased intake is by far the most common. Because body folate reserves are small, deficiency develops rapidly in persons with an inadequate diet. As noted, excessive cooking may also promote deficiency, especially among peoples who live on finely divided foods such as rice. Megaloblastic anemia occuring in chronic liver disease is usually due to folate deficiency resulting from poor diet and impaired hepatic storage of folate. The macrocytic anemia accompanying liver disease is often normoblastic and unresponsive to folic acid therapy. Nutritional folate deficiency is often associated with multiple vitamin deficiencies. In such patients, a history of gross dietary inadequacy is usually easy to obtain. Folate is normally absorbed in the upper third of the small intestine and commonly malabsorbed in nontropical sprue (celiac disease) as described in Ch. 103. Tropical sprue is a malabsorptive disorder of unknown etiology that occurs frequently and endemically in the tropics—notably the West Indies, the Indian subcontinent, and Southeast Asia. It can be acquired by residents of temperate climates who go to the tropics, sometimes persisting long after return from the tropics. It may be due in part to deficiency of dietary folate, the malabsorption resulting from secondary gastrointestinal changes. Treatment with folic acid alone usually reverses all abnormalities, including defective folate absorption. Other causes of malabsorption are noted in Table 136–1. Low serum folate levels in patients receiving phenytoin (Dilantin) have been attributed to reversible drug-induced malabsorption of folylpolyglutamate. Oral contraceptives block deconjugation of folylpolyglutamate in certain women.

Pregnancy increases requirements for folate. Although true anemias of pregnancy are commonly due to iron deficiency or multiple nutritional deficiencies, two thirds of anemic pregnant women are folate deficient. Its frequency is attributable both to meager folate reserves and to the fact that pregnancy increases daily requirements for folate five- to tenfold, especially in the last trimester. The presence of multiple fetuses, poor diet (a frequent result of anorexia or nausea), infection, and lactation may further increase requirements. The capacity of the fetus to take up folic acid (and other nutrients) at the expense of the mother, even when the available supply is markedly reduced, is quite remarkable. Folic acid supplementation is desirable during pregnancy not only because requirements are increased but also because there is a suspected association between severe folate deficiency and such complications of pregnancy as abruptio placentae, embryopathology, spontaneous abortion, and bleeding. The folate requirement also rises sharply in hemolytic anemias associated with acute or chronic overactivity of the bone marrow and in most neoplastic diseases, especially metastatic cancer and the leukemias. The deficiency presumably reflects competitive utilization of the vitamin by tumor cells, a phenomenon that resembles the pre-emption of maternal nutrients by a fetus.

Impaired utilization of folate is caused by administration of 4-aminopteroylglutamates, aminopterin and methotrexate, powerful inhibitors of dihydrofolate reductase that can deplete folate coenzymes in tissues within hours. Citrovorum factor (leucovorin, folinic acid, N^5-formyl FH_4) effectively counteracts the actions of MTX by bypassing the inhibited reductase and is useful in the treatment of toxicity.

Therapy. Folic acid is usually administered orally in 1 mg tablets. Oral therapy is satisfactory for most needs. Even in the presence of intestinal malabsorption, the relatively large doses used ordinarily permit sufficient absorption to achieve repletion. The usual dose is 1 to 2 mg daily, although doses in excess of 1 mg are seldom necessary. Folic acid in these doses also partially corrects the hematopoietic and gastrointestinal manifestations of cobalamin deficiency. Neurologic abnormalities, however, may progress with disastrous results. This is the principal danger in the uncritical use of folic acid. Therapy for four to five weeks is usually adequate to replenish stores and correct anemia. Therapy is continued until diet or underlying problems are corrected. In some patients (e.g., those with malabsorption, chronic hemolysis, chronic exfoliative skin disease, or renal failure requiring hemodialysis), it must continue indefinitely.

A parenteral preparation containing 5 mg per milliliter of the sodium salt may be used in severely ill patients, in certain cases of malabsorption, or in patients incapable of taking oral medication. Citrovorum factor is available as a parenteral therapeutic preparation. Its main clinical indication is severe intoxication by folic acid antagonists that block folate reduction. In the absence of such inhibition, little is accomplished by treating folate deficiency with this compound instead of folic acid.

MEGALOBLASTIC ANEMIA UNRESPONSIVE TO COBALAMIN OR FOLIC ACID

Megaloblastic anemia is occasionally unaccompanied by cobalamin or folic acid deficiency and fails to respond to therapy with either vitamin. In some cases, folate or cobalamin deficiency coexists with megaloblastic anemia but is not responsible for it. Most of these occurrences arise in three situations (see Table 136–1): therapy with an antimetabolite drug that inteferes with DNA synthesis (common), inborn error of metabolism (rare), and refractory megaloblastic anemia of undetermined etiology, which is probably due to somatic mutation leading to loss of an enzyme in the pathway of DNA synthesis. Except for various dysplastic features, megaloblasts in the bone marrow of these patients generally resemble those in vitamin-deficiency megaloblastic anemia. The defect in all is probably an impaired capacity to duplicate DNA at a normal rate. Drug-induced megaloblastosis is potentially reversible. However, those cases caused by genetic error or acquired refractory megaloblastosis are irreversible and unfortunately difficult to treat with any but supportive measures.

Beck WS: Metabolic aspects of vitamins B₁₂ and folic acid. Erythrocyte disorders—anemias related to disturbance of DNA synthesis (megaloblastic anemias). In Williams WJ, Beutler E, Erslev AJ, et al. (eds.): Hematology, 3rd ed. New York, McGraw-Hill Book Company, 1983, pp 311–331, 434–465. *Sections of a standard hematology text that covers the megaloblastic anemias in detail. Extensive bibliographies.*

Castle WB: The conquest of pernicious anemia. In Wintrobe MM (ed.): Blood, Pure and Eloquent. A Story of Discovery, of People, and of Ideas. New York, McGraw-Hill Book Company, 1980, pp 283–318. *An engrossing historical essay by the one who in 1929 discovered intrinsic factor.*

Chanarin I, Deacon R, Lumb M, et al.: Cobalamin-folate interrelations: A critical review. Blood 66:479, 1985.

Shane B, Stokstad ELR: Vitamin B₁₂–folate interrelationships. Ann Rev Nutr 5:115, 1985. *These two reviews, published almost simultaneously reflect somewhat different views of a puzzling old problem: Why do cobalamin-deficient patients respond as they do to folate therapy? The answer is still not certain. Excellent bibliographies.*

Lindenbaum J: Status of laboratory testing in the diagnosis of megaloblastic anemia. Blood 61:624, 1983. *A brief guide to available methods. I agree with everything in it except the remarks on the deoxyuridine suppression test.*

Rosenberg LE: Disorders of propionate and methylmalonate metabolism. In Stanbury JB, Wyngaarden JB, Frederickson DS, et al. (eds.): The Metabolic Basis of Inherited Disease. 5th ed. New York, McGraw-Hill Book Company, 1983, p 474. *A thorough review of a group of inborn errors that may cause laboratory findings that could confuse an observer who is not alert to the possibilities. 191 references.*

137 HEMOLYTIC DISORDERS: INTRODUCTION

Manuel E. Kaplan

PATHOPHYSIOLOGY OF HEMOLYSIS. Human red blood cells normally survive for approximately 120 days after they are released from the bone marrow as reticulocytes, being destroyed only after they have become senescent. With advancing cell age the activities of various red cell enzymes decline, and the cells become denser and less deformable. Phagocytic cells of the spleen and liver are believed to recognize and destroy effete red cells, although splenectomy does not extend the red cell lifespan beyond 120 days.

A hemolytic disorder is defined as premature destruction of red cells, which may occur either because inherently defective red cells are produced or because noxious factors are present in the intravascular environment. Intrinsic abnormalities that predispose to hemolysis may occur in the red cell membrane or in its contained hemoglobin or enzymes. These are, for the most part, genetically determined. In contrast, the environmental abnormalities that prejudice red cell survival are almost all acquired. A classification of the causes of hemolytic anemia is given in Table 137–1.

To measure red cell survival, anticoagulated venous blood is incubated with radioactive chromium (^{51}Cr) to label intracellular hemoglobin and is then reinfused. Normally 50 per cent of the injected ^{51}Cr activity disappears from the blood (t½) in 29 ± 3 days rather than at 60 days, because ^{51}Cr is an imperfect label and slowly elutes from the red cells. Nevertheless, the results of such studies are clinically informative because rates of hemolysis are reliably quantified and the sites of red cell destruction can be identified by external scanning utilizing a collimated gamma scintillation counter.

CONSEQUENCES OF HEMOLYSIS. Accelerated destruction of red cells may occur intravascularly or, more commonly, after the cells have been culled from the circulation (sequestered).

Intravascular Hemolysis. Following intravascular hemolysis, hemoglobin is released into the plasma and is bound by haptoglobin, an alpha-globulin synthesized by the liver. The haptoglobin concentration of blood, normally about 100 mg per 100 ml, reflects the rate of haptoglobin synthesis and catabolism. Haptoglobin synthesis is usually diminished in

TABLE 137–1. CLASSIFICATION OF THE CAUSES OF HEMOLYTIC ANEMIA

I. Congenital hemolytic disorders (see Ch. 138)
   A. Membrane defects
   B. Enzyme defects
     1. Embden-Meyerhof pathway defects
     2. Hexose monophosphate shunt defects
   C. Hemoglobin defects
     1. Structural (hemoglobinopathies) (see Ch. 143)
     2. Synthetic (thalassemias) (see Ch. 142)
   D. Other
II. Acquired hemolytic disorders (see Ch. 139)
   A. Sequestrational hemolysis (hypersplenism)
   B. Immune hemolytic disorders
     1. Alloimmune
     2. Autoimmune
     3. Drug-induced
   C. Paroxysmal nocturnal hemoglobinuria
   D. Due to toxins and metabolic abnormalities
   E. Due to red cell parasites
   F. Due to red cell trauma

patients with parenchymal liver disease and may be increased in various inflammatory disorders, in which it acts as an acute phase protein. Free (uncomplexed) haptoglobin has a half-life of approximately four days. In contrast, hemoglobin-hapto-globin complexes are removed from the plasma within minutes, primarily by hepatic reticuloendothelial cells that catabolize both components of the complex. Haptoglobin catabolism usually exceeds haptoglobin synthesis in patients with significant intravascular hemolysis, and plasma haptoglobin levels fall, frequently to undetectable levels. If the quantity of hemoglobin entering the plasma exceeds the binding capacity of haptoglobin, hemoglobin appears in the glomerular filtrate, primarily as a 32,000 dalton alpha-beta dimer. The dimers are readily absorbed by cells of the proximal tubules that convert heme iron into ferritin and hemosiderin. After the tubular cells are sloughed, hemosiderin can be detected in the urinary sediment with a Prussian blue stain. Hemoglobinuria, which occurs only when the filtered load of alpha-beta dimer exceeds the absorptive capacity of the tubular cells, connotes rapid intravascular hemolysis. Persistent urinary loss of hemosiderin or hemoglobin or both may result in iron deficiency.

Hemoglobin in the plasma is unstable. Its heme prosthetic groups tend to dissociate and bind either to hemopexin, a beta-globulin, or to albumin, forming methemalbumin. Neither of these heme-protein complexes appears in the urine unless significant proteinuria is present. Because heme-hemopexin complexes are cleared rapidly from the blood, serum levels of hemopexin, like haptoglobin, are typically reduced or absent in the presence of significant intravascular hemolysis.

Erythrocytes contain high concentrations of the enzyme lactic dehydrogenase (LDH). Consequently, very high LDH levels are found in patients with intravascular hemolysis.

Extravascular Destruction. In most hemolytic disorders red cell destruction occurs extravascularly rather than intravascularly. Red cells are sequestered primarily within the spleen or liver or both and are phagocytized in situ. Although only a small fraction of the hemoglobin they contain escapes into the plasma, plasma haptoglobin levels characteristically fall, particularly when hemolysis is longstanding. However, plasma hemoglobin levels do not rise significantly, and no hemoglobinuria or hemosiderinuria occurs. Serum LDH levels are usually elevated, but not to the degree seen in intravascular hemolysis.

Hemoglobin derived from hemolyzed red cells is normally catabolized by reticuloendothelial cells to unconjugated, indirect-reacting bilirubin. As each heme tetrapyrrole ring is opened, one molecule of carbon monoxide is elaborated. The rate of formation of endogenously produced carbon monoxide has been used to quantify red cell destruction in vivo. However, this may not accurately reflect the rapidity of hemolysis since ineffective erythropoiesis (destruction of immature red cells in the bone marrow) also contributes to carbon monoxide formation. Unconjugated bilirubin produced by phagocytic cells is bound by albumin. The concentration of unconjugated bilirubin in the serum of a patient reflects the quantity of heme catabolized and the rate at which the liver is able to convert it into the direct-reacting, water-soluble product (Ch. 130). Serum levels of conjugated bilirubin are typically normal in patients with uncomplicated hemolytic disorders. Bilirubinuria does not occur unless the patient has concomitant hepatocellular or biliary disease.

Bone Marrow Response. The loss of circulating red cells results in an erythropoietic stimulus to the bone marrow proportional to the decline in the oxygen-carrying capacity of the blood. The normal bone marrow responds by increasing commensurately its erythropoietic activity. When examined morphologically, bone marrows of patients with hemolysis characteristically exhibit erythroid hyperplasia. Consequently, unless an underlying neoplastic disorder such as leukemia or lymphoma is suspected, diagnostic bone marrow studies are usually not indicated. The intensity of the marrow's erythropoietic response to hemolysis, which may reach a maximum of approximately eight times normal, is reflected by reticulocytosis in the peripheral blood. The reticulocyte percentage alone does not adequately reflect the degree of marrow compensation. This may be more reliably gauged by calculating the reticulocyte index (patient hematocrit times percentage reticulocytes/normal hematocrit). In some patients sustained reticulocytosis may compensate fully for the increased red cell destruction, and there is no anemia. More commonly, bone marrow compensation is incomplete so that anemia, of greater or lesser severity, supervenes. If bone marrow function is compromised by such factors as infection or folate deficiency the reticulocyte count will fall and the anemia will rapidly worsen because of the ongoing hemolytic process.

DIFFERENTIAL DIAGNOSIS OF HEMOLYTIC DISORDERS. *The Diagnosis of Hemolysis.* The presence of hemolysis as the cause of anemia is generally not difficult to establish. The clinical diagnosis is usually based on the presence of sustained reticulocytosis in a patient exhibiting no evidence of blood loss or of increasing hemoglobin concentration. Some or all of the following findings may occur:

1. *Evidence of enhanced marrow response:* polychromatophilia, reticulocytosis, marrow erythroid hyperplasia.
2. *Evidence for excessive release of red cell components:* (a) plasma—unconjugated bilirubin ↑, LDH ↑, haptoglobin ↓, hemopexin ↓, methemalbumin +, free hemoglobin ↑; (b) urine—hemosiderin +, hemoglobin +.
3. *Evidence of decreased red cell survival:* Decreased ^{51}Cr red cell t½.

The problem remains to determine the cause of the hemolytic process (see Table 137–1). Hemolysis is caused either by an abnormality of the red cell or an abnormality in its environment, the circulatory system in which the red cell resides. Red cell abnormalities associated with hemolysis may be congenital (genetically determined) or acquired. Congenital red cell defects resulting in hemolysis may involve the cell membrane, erythrocyte enzymes, or the contained hemoglobin. Acquired red cell defects that predispose to hemolysis may occur (1) under conditions of grossly abnormal (dysplastic) red cell maturation (such as marked deficiencies of iron, B_{12}, or folate) with bone marrow production and elaboration into the circulation of severely misshapen erythrocytes, and (2) in paroxysmal nocturnal hemoglobinuria (Ch. 139). More commonly, acquired hemolytic disorders are due to the presence in the circulation of such noxious factors as red cell antibodies, immune complexes containing activated complement components, chemical or metabolic "toxins," or parasites.

Clinical Findings. A patient with hemolysis may present with diverse complaints and physical findings that reflect the rapidity, underlying etiology, and pathophysiologic mechanism of red cell destruction. Patients with congenital hemolytic disorders are frequently anemic and intermittently jaundiced early in life. Usually a suggestive family history of anemia, jaundice, cholelithiasis, splenomegaly, and/or therapeutic splenectomy can be elicited. A significant proportion of patients with acquired hemolysis have an identifiable underlying disease such as systemic lupus erythematosus (SLE) or chronic lymphocytic leukemia (CLL). Patients with rapidly falling hemoglobin values resulting from hemolysis of any cause commonly complain of fatigue, palpitations, breathlessness, postural dizziness, and worsening of pre-existing angina. Physical examination typically discloses pallor, mild jaundice, and frequently splenomegaly. Other signs and symptoms referable to specific underlying disease may also be present: joint discomfort in SLE, painful acrocyanosis in cold agglutinin disease, lymphadenopathy in CLL.

Laboratory Findings. Patients with significant hemolysis

TABLE 137–2. MORPHOLOGIC ABNORMALITIES OF RED CELLS IN VARIOUS HEMOLYTIC DISORDERS

Abnormality	Hemolytic Disorder	
	Congenital	*Acquired*
Permanently sickled cells	Sickle cell anemia	—
Fragmented cells (schistocytes)	Unstable hemoglobins (Heinz body anemias)	Microangiopathic processes
		Prosthetic heart valves
Spur cells (acanthocytes)	Abetalipoproteinemia	Severe liver disease
Spherocytes	Hereditary spherocytosis	Immune, warm antibody type
		Liver disease
Target cells	Thalassemia	
	Hemoglobinopathies (Hb C)	
Agglutinated cells	—	Immune, cold agglutinin disease

typically exhibit reticulocytosis with polychromasia on peripheral smear, unconjugated hyperbilirubinemia, serum haptoglobin levels ranging from decreased to absent, erythroid hyperplasia of the bone marrow, and elevated serum LDH levels. In fact, as noted earlier, these findings form the basis of diagnosing an anemia as being hemolytic. Hemoglobinemia, hemoglobinuria, and hemosiderinuria occur only when rapid intravascular hemolysis is present. Significant intravascular red cell destruction occurs in relatively few situations, e.g., G6PD deficiency, certain infections (*Clostridium welchii*, falciparum malaria), paroxysmal nocturnal hemoglobinuria, paroxysmal cold hemoglobinuria, incompatible transfusions, and as a result of traumatic disruption of red cell membranes by excessive heat or mechanical stress.

The morphologic appearance of red cells is frequently abnormal in patients with hemolysis. Occasionally the abnormalities are so typical that they indicate the correct diagnosis (Table 137–2).

Further Studies. The overall clinical picture for which a patient with hemolysis seeks medical help is usually sufficiently informative to suggest a rational diagnostic approach. Frequently useful laboratory studies to elucidate the cause of a presumed congenital hemolytic process include osmotic fragility test, G6PD and pyruvate kinase screening tests, and hemoglobin electrophoresis. For a presumed acquired hemolytic disorder a direct antiglobulin (Coombs') test is invariably indicated and, less frequently, Ham's test for paroxysmal nocturnal hemoglobinuria.

TREATMENT OF HEMOLYTIC ANEMIA. Only general supportive measures will be discussed here since effective therapy usually requires definition of the cause and pathophysiologic mechanisms underlying the specific disease processes, as described in the subsequent two chapters.

Severely anemic patients should be placed at temporary bed rest to reduce cardiac output. Nasal oxygen may afford symptomatic relief. Transfusions with packed red cells should be utilized to correct hemodynamic abnormalities rather than to treat low hemoglobin or hematocrit values. To avoid iatrogenically induced hypervolemia, transfusions should be administered slowly. The physician must consider the potential dangers of transfusions, particularly in patients with autoimmune hemolytic disorders (see Ch. 139).

To maintain accelerated erythropoiesis patients with chronic hemolysis requires extra quantities of folic acid. Therefore, daily oral supplementation with folic acid, 1 to 2 mg per day, is recommended. The serum cobalamin concentration should be measured if concomitant cobalamin deficiency is suspected. When it is low, parenteral vitamin B_{12} should also be administered.

SPECIFIC HEMOLYTIC DISORDERS. The purpose of this brief introduction is merely to provide a background of the common pathophysiology of the hemolytic anemias as well as a general classification (Table 137–1). The anemias are discussed more extensively in Ch. 135 and 136. Specific

hemolytic diseases resulting from intracorpuscular abnormalities (usually caused by genetic abnormalities of the red cell membrane, of red cell enzymes, or of hemoglobin) are presented in the following chapter. Chapter 139 summarizes the acquired hemolytic disorders.

138 HEREDITARY DEFECTS IN THE MEMBRANE OR METABOLISM OF THE RED CELL

Samuel E. Lux

MEMBRANE DISORDERS
Normal Red Cell Membrane
Structure

Membrane Lipids. The red cell membrane, or *ghost*, is a mixture of phospholipids, unesterified cholesterol, and glycolipids, arranged in a bilayer, and traversed randomly by transmembrane protein channels and receptors. The phospholipids are asymmetrically arranged. Choline phospholipids (phosphatidyl choline and sphingomyelin) are found primarily in the outer half of the bilayer; amino phospholipids (phosphatidyl serine and phosphatidyl ethanolamine) and phosphatidyl inositols are confined to the inner half. The mechanism that maintains this arrangement is poorly understood, but there is evidence that the membrane skeleton (see below) is involved. It is probably important to sequester amino phospholipids, since their exposure triggers coagulation and causes red cells to adhere to phagocytes. The lipids are mobile in the plane of the membrane. This gives the membrane properties of a viscous two-dimensional fluid.

Membrane Proteins. The red cell membrane contains 10 to 15 major proteins and innumerable minor ones (Fig. 138–1). The proteins fall into two classes. (1) *Integral membrane proteins* traverse the bilayer, interact with the hydrophobic lipid core, and are tightly bound. They include functionally important transport proteins (e.g., protein 3) and glycoprotein surface antigens (e.g., glycophorin). (2) *Peripheral membrane proteins* are confined to the cytoplasmic membrane surface and include structural proteins, such as spectrin and actin, and some red cell enzymes (e.g., glyceraldehyde-3-phosphate dehydrogenase). These proteins bind to each other and to anchoring sites on integral proteins.

The major peripheral membrane proteins form a two-dimensional protein network that laminates the cytoplasmic membrane surface (Fig. 138–1). The principal components of this *membrane skeleton* are spectrin, actin, protein 4.1, and ankyrin. *Spectrin*, the major skeletal protein, contains two long, flexible chains that are aligned in parallel and twisted about each other. These dimers interact at their "head" end to form tetramers or higher-order oligomers (spectrin self-association) (Fig. 138–1). At the opposite ("tail") end, spectrin binds to *short filaments of actin*. This interaction is greatly strengthened by *protein 4.1*, which attaches to spectrin near the actin-binding site. Because multiple spectrins can bind to each actin filament, the spectrin-actin-4.1 complex is a molecular junction that allows spectrin filaments to branch and form a two-dimensional membrane skeleton. The skeleton is anchored to the overlying lipid bilayer by *ankyrin*, which binds to spectrin near the self-association site and links it to the cytoplasmic portion of protein 3 (Fig. 138–1). Interactions between protein 4.1 and some of the glycophorins and between various skeletal proteins and membrane lipids probably also occur, but are less well characterized.

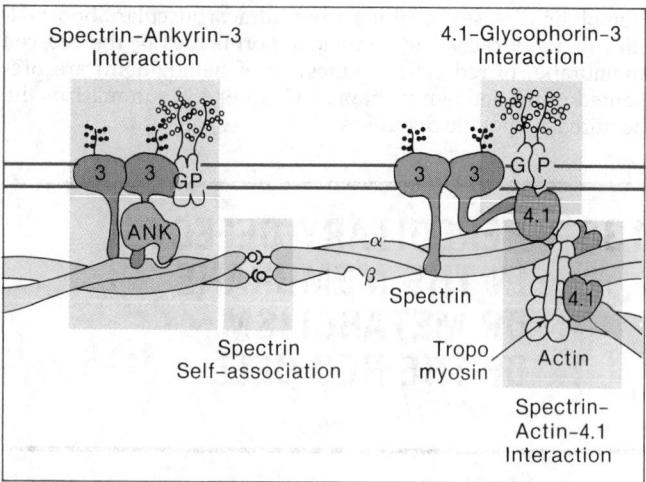

FIGURE 138–1. Schematic illustration of the organization of the major proteins of the red cell membrane and membrane skeleton.

Major Functions

Membrane Strength and Durability. In humans the red cell must be flexible enough to negotiate splenic and capillary channels less than half its diameter and still be strong and durable enough to survive the turbulent journey through the heart approximately 500,000 times during its 120-day lifespan. These properties are *determined by the membrane skeleton.* The membrane spontaneously vesiculates when spectrin and actin are selectively extracted or when spectrin is denatured (at 49°C). Mice with hereditary deficiencies of spectrin have extremely fragile red cells that rapidly fragment in the circulation, leading to marked spherocytosis and severe hemolysis.

Maintenance of Cell Volume. The red cell controls its volume and water content by regulating its intracellular concentration of Na^+ and K^+. This is possible because the membrane is relatively impermeable to cations. Normally, small passive cation leaks are balanced by the active transport of Na^+ outward and K^+ inward. These ion movements are powered by a pump that is fueled by the membrane enzyme $Na^+, K^+-ATPase$. Normally this system maintains intracellular Na^+ and K^+ at about 10 mEq per liter and 100 mEq per liter, respectively. The pump is regulated by the intracellular Na^+ concentration and has considerable ability to compensate for an increased leak of Na^+ into the cell. If this capacity is surpassed and the inward leak of Na^+ exceeds the K^+ leak out, red cells gain cations and water and swell. Unfortunately the pump does not compensate nearly as well to a decrease in intracellular K^+. Any increase in the outward leak of K^+ relative to Na^+ (normally $K^+[out]:Na^+[in] = 2:3$) leads to loss of total monovalent cations and water and results in cellular dehydration.

Calcium Homeostasis. Excessive intracellular Ca^{++} is very deleterious, and the red cell actively extrudes it with an efficient, calmodulin-regulated calcium pump that is driven by a $Ca^{++}-ATPase$. Intracellular Ca^{++} is normally almost undetectable (about 0.1 μM). If ATP levels fall below about 20 per cent of normal or if Ca^{++} leakage exceeds the capacity of the pump, Ca^{++} accumulates and changes the red cell from a biconcave disc to an echinocyte—a spiculated sphere with numerous short, regular projections. Elevated intracellular Ca^{++} also causes a selective loss of K^+ and water. The result is a crenated, dehydrated, almost indeformable cell that is highly susceptible to splenic sequestration and destruction.

Anion Exchange. Physiologically the red cell is a critical component of CO_2 transport. Red cells normally convert tissue CO_2 to HCO_3^- and carry the HCO_3^- to the lungs where they exchange it for Cl^-. The process is massive and requires a large number of transport channels (~1 million per red cell). These are formed by *protein 3* (Fig. 138–1).

Interactions Between Red Cells and the Spleen

Red cells that enter the spleen must squeeze their 7-μ wide bodies through narrow elliptical fenestrations that separate the splenic cords and sinuses to return to the circulation (Ch. 164). Normal red cells make this journey about 120 times per day and complete it in about 30 seconds, but abnormal cells may be detained for minutes to hours in the hypoxic, acidic, hypoglycemic environment of the splenic cords. This taxing metabolic stress is often fatal for old or defective erythrocytes.

Red cells are detained in the spleen if they are rigid or if they are coated with proteins such as IgG1, IgG3, or C3b that bind to receptors on splenic macrophages. Probably other, less well defined, changes in the red cell surface also attract phagocytes and lead to red cell death. Increased rigidity may result from (1) increased cytoplasmic viscosity (e.g., sickled cells and other dehydrated red cells); (2) intracellular rubbish (e.g., Heinz bodies); (3) membrane rigidity (e.g., secondary to oxidative cross-linking of the membrane skeleton); or (4) a decrease in the red cell surface-volume ratio.

Surface-Volume Ratio: Osmotic Fragility Test

Spherocytes are caused by a decrease in the surface-volume ratio of the red cell. Target cells form when this ratio is increased. Because the area of the red cell membrane is fixed (i.e., the membrane is not stretchable), the cell becomes progressively more rigid as its spheroidicity increases. Surface-volume ratio is assessed clinically by the *unincubated osmotic fragility test.* This test measures the ability of red cells to swell in a graded series of hypotonic solutions. Spherocytes are osmotically fragile; that is, they can tolerate less osmotic swelling than normal cells before they hemolyze. Target cells are osmotically resistant.

Hereditary Spherocytosis (HS)

Hereditary spherocytosis is an inherited hemolytic anemia characterized by osmotically fragile, partially spherical, spectrin-deficient red cells that are selectively trapped by the spleen. The disease occurs in all races, but is particularly common in northern Europeans, where the prevalence is about 1 in 5000. There are at least two patterns of inheritance: 75 per cent of the families show a classic autosomal dominant pattern. Most of the remainder have a nondominant (probably autosomal recessive) form.

Pathogenesis. Hereditary spherocytes transfused into normal subjects show impairment of survival, demonstrating clearly that they are intrinsically defective. The primary physiologic defect appears to be membrane instability. Red cell membranes from some HS patients fragment more easily than normal when stressed. This weakness suggests a defect of the membrane skeleton.

All HS red cells are spectrin deficient. Either quantitative or qualitative defects may occur in this major skeletal protein. The degree of spectrin deficiency correlates closely with the degree of spherocytosis, as measured by osmotic fragility, and with the severity of hemolysis and response to splenectomy. In general, patients with dominant HS have only mild deficiency (spectrin content 75 to 90 per cent of normal) and mild to moderate hemolysis. Patients with recessive HS often have a more severe deficit; sometimes so severe (30 to 50 per cent of normal) that it produces life-threatening, transfusion-dependent hemolysis.

In a subset of patients with dominant HS (perhaps 5 to 10 per cent) a qualitative defect in the beta chain of spectrin is also present. About 40 per cent of the spectrin molecules *lack the ability to bind protein 4.1.* (This is close to the expected proportion in the dominant form of HS, since only one of the two beta-spectrin genes will be abnormal.) The defective spectrin binds poorly to actin, weakening the skeleton. Red cells from these patients are also spectrin deficient, presumably because the mutant spectrin is catabolized more rapidly than normal. It is not yet known whether the decreased

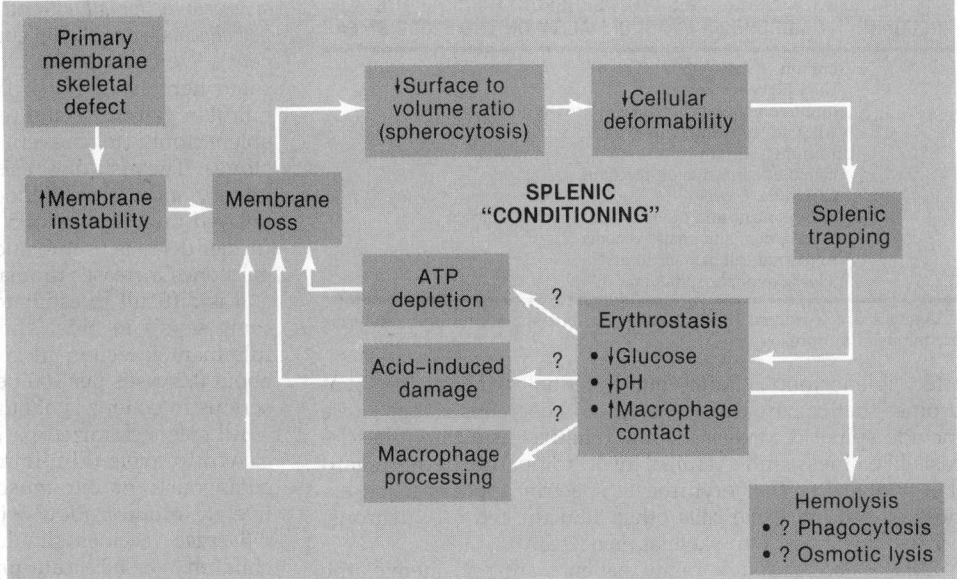

FIGURE 138–2. Currently favored model of the pathophysiology of hereditary spherocytosis.

spectrin observed in other HS patients is due to analogous, unidentified structural defects or whether it results from decreased synthesis of an otherwise normal protein.

It is speculated that HS red cells gradually lose the portions of lipid bilayer that overlie spectrin-deficient regions, and become progressively more spherocytic as they age in the circulation (Fig. 138–2). Eventually they are detained in the splenic cords where, for unknown reasons, their membrane loss is accentuated by the toxic cordal environment. This *"splenic conditioning"* can be mimicked in vitro by incubating red cells in the absence of glucose for 24 hours. Under these conditions hereditary spherocytes lose membrane fragments more rapidly than do normal red cells. This is the basis of the *incubated osmotic fragility test.* In vivo, conditioned spherocytes are prevalent in the splenic pulp, and some escape into the peripheral circulation as the characteristic HS hyperchromic microspherocytes. These impaired cells form the hyperspherical tail on osmotic fragility curves. Undoubtedly many HS red cells never escape the conditioning process. Those that do are especially susceptible to recapture and destruction by the spleen.

Clinical Features (Table 138–1). The hallmarks of HS are *anemia, jaundice,* and *splenomegaly.* The disease may present at any age. In neonates excessive jaundice is frequent (~50 per cent) and sometimes requires an exchange transfusion. After the neonatal period most patients develop partially compensated hemolysis with mild to moderate anemia (Hb = 9 to 11.5 grams per deciliter), intermittent mild jaundice (especially during viral infections), and splenomegaly. *Clinical severity can vary widely,* sometimes even within the same family. A small proportion of patients have life-threatening hemolysis and are transfusion dependent. A much larger proportion, roughly 25

per cent, have unusually mild disease. In these patients marrow erythropoiesis is sufficient to balance the modest rate of spherocyte destruction, and there is no anemia, little or no jaundice, and minimal splenomegaly. However, severe hemolysis and anemia may develop with illnesses that cause the spleen to hypertrophy, such as infectious mononucleosis. Hemolysis may also be exacerbated by long-term intensive physical activity, possibly because of increased splenic blood flow. Finally, in old age, when bone marrow function becomes sluggish, previously well compensated splenectomized patients may become dangerously anemic.

Complications. *Crises.* The clinical course is interrupted in most patients by periodic crises, characterized by worsening anemia. *Hemolytic crises* are the most frequent, but usually are mild and clinically insignificant. They are presumably secondary to the reticuloendothelial hyperplasia that accompanies many infections. *Aplastic crises* are less prevalent, but are often severe enough to threaten heart failure and require transfusion. They are frequently caused by a human parvovirus that invades hematopoietic stem cells and inhibits their growth. The infection typically presents in young children as a febrile illness or as fifth disease, a viral exantham; however, some older children and adults are also susceptible to the virus and aplastic crises. *Megaloblastic crises* occur when dietary intake of folic acid is inadequate for the increased needs of the erythroid HS bone marrow. This need is particularly acute during pregnancy. To prevent megaloblastic crises, all HS patients should receive daily supplements of folic acid (1 mg per day).

Gallstones. Untreated older children and adults with HS often develop bilirubinate gallstones secondary to increased bilirubin production. Only 5 per cent of children less than 10 years old are affected, but the prevalence rises to 40 to 50 per cent in the second to fifth decades and 55 to 75 per cent thereafter. The frequency after age 30 parallels the frequency in the general population, which suggests that gallstones in HS patients form primarily in the second and third decades. Ultrasonography is the most reliable method for detecting bilirubin stones. Only 50 per cent are radiopaque. Concern about cholecystitis and biliary obstruction is the major impetus for splenectomy in most patients. It is unfortunate, therefore, that there are no accurate data on the prevalence of these complications in patients with bilirubin stones to help assess the indications (risk-benefit ratio) for operation.

Other Complications. Occasional adult patients with HS develop gout, indolent ankle ulcers, or a chronic erythematous dermatitis on the legs. All of these complications disappear

TABLE 138–1. HEREDITARY SPHEROCYTOSIS

Clinical Manifestations	Laboratory Features
Anemia	Reticulocytosis
Splenomegaly	Spherocytosis
Intermittent jaundice	Elevated MCHC
From hemolysis	Increased osmotic fragility
From biliary obstruction	(especially incubated osmotic
Aplastic crises	fragility test)
Often dominant inheritance	Normal Coombs' test
Rare manifestations	Decreased red cell spectrin
Leg ulcers	
Spinal cord dysfunction	
Myocardiopathy	
Good response to splenectomy	

TABLE 138–2. DISEASES WITH SPHEROCYTOSIS AS THE PREDOMINANT MORPHOLOGIC ABNORMALITY ON THE BLOOD SMEAR

Common
  Hereditary spherocytosis
  Immunohemolytic anemias (warm antibody type)
  ABO incompatibility in neonates
Uncommon to rare
  Hemolytic transfusion reactions
  Clostridial sepsis
  Severe burns and other red cell thermal injuries
  Spider, bee, and snake venoms
  Acute red cell oxidant injury*
  Severe hypophosphatemia

*Acute red cell oxidant injury is common, but spherocytosis is rarely the predominant morphology.

after splenectomy. Rarer but potentially interesting syndromes that coexist with HS have also been described. These include spinal cord dysfunction, manifest as a multiple-sclerosis-like illness, and a familial myocardiopathy. In this regard it is tantalizing that erythrocyte spectrin appears to be expressed only in three cells other than the red cell: neurons, cardiac myocytes, and skeletal myocytes.

Diagnosis. Although many patients are not anemic, the *reticulocyte count is always increased* prior to splenectomy (except during an aplastic crisis). It is a much more dependable sign of hemolysis than is hyperbilirubinemia, since indirect bilirubin levels are elevated in only 50 to 60 per cent of patients. *Spherocytosis,* the hallmark of the disease, is the other most reliable finding (Color plate 2K). However, spherocytes are a frequent artifact in normal blood smears, so the physician must take care to examine only areas of the smear in which the red cells are well separated and some cells with central pallor are evident. Spherocytosis is also observed in a variety of other conditions (Table 138–2); however, with the exception of certain *immunohemolytic anemias* (which can be excluded with a Coombs test), most of these do not present any diagnostic difficulty.

In 20 to 25 per cent of patients, classic microspherocytes are sparse, and it may be difficult to recognize spherocytosis from the blood smear alone. In these patients the *unincubated* osmotic fragility (OF) test will sometimes be normal or only slightly increased, since it simply quantifies what is visible on the smear. The *incubated* OF, however, is almost always abnormal and is the most reliable available diagnostic test. HS red cells are somewhat dehydrated and therefore have an *increased mean corpuscular hemoglobin concentration (MCHC).* An MCHC level of 36 or greater is present in 50 per cent of HS patients and is useful confirmatory evidence of the disease. Since spectrin deficiency appears to be the primary defect, a direct assay of red cell spectrin content should be the most accurate test; however, at present this measurement is available in only a few research laboratories.

Once HS is diagnosed *a careful search for the disease should always be made in all close relatives.* It is tragic to see HS become symptomatic in elderly patients with a poor operative risk, whose condition could have been discovered earlier.

Treatment. *Splenectomy* dependably blunts both red cell conditioning and hemolysis in HS and is the recommended therapy. Following surgery, spherocytosis persists because the basic red cell defect is unchanged, but conditioned microspherocytes disappear and changes typical of the postsplenectomy state (Howell-Jolly bodies, target cells, siderocytes, and acanthocytes) become evident on the blood smear. During the operation the surgeon must be careful to search for accessory spleens, which occur in 20 to 30 per cent of patients. Recurrence of hemolysis due to regrowth of an accessory spleen is occasionally observed after years or even decades.

Splenectomy increases susceptibility to sepsis from pneumococci and certain other encapsulated bacteria. The major issues today are who should undergo splenectomy and how should they be treated postoperatively. It is impossible to answer either question absolutely. In general, *we recommend splenectomy for all HS patients with either anemia or significant hemolysis* (reticulocyte counts repeatedly greater than 5 per cent). We defer splenectomy in patients with mild compensated hemolysis, but if these patients subsequently develop bilirubin gallstones and require cholecystectomy, we advocate splenectomy to prevent the recurrence of common duct stones. The risk of sepsis after splenectomy is very high in infancy and early childhood; splenectomy should therefore be delayed until the age of 5 or 6 years. There is no evidence that further delay is useful, and it may be harmful, since the risk of gallstones increases dramatically after the age of 10 years.

It is difficult to estimate accurately the risk of postsplenectomy sepsis in older children and adults. The incidence of fulminant infection in splenectomized adults appears to be about 0.2 cases per 100 person-years, and the incidence of all serious infections is about 7 cases per 100 person-years.

All splenectomized patients should receive *polyvalent pneumococcal vaccine* (Pnu-Immune 23 or equivalent, 0.5 ml subcutaneously or intramuscularly), preferably given preoperatively. Immunization with meningococcal and *Hemophilus influenzae* vaccines should also be considered, especially in children. We advocate prophylactic antibiotics after splenectomy, with emphasis on protection against pneumococcal sepsis (i.e., Pen-Vee K or equivalent, 6 to 8 mg per kilogram twice daily), at least for the first two years after surgery when the incidence of infection is greatest. This is a controversial issue that depends on patient compliance, bacterial resistance in the local community, and a host of other factors.

All unsplenectomized patients with HS (and other hemolytic anemias) should receive *folic acid* (1 mg per day) to sustain erythropoiesis and prevent megaloblastic crises.

Hereditary Elliptocytosis (HE)

Hereditary elliptocytosis, usually inherited as an autosomal dominant trait, is relatively common (~1:2500), particularly in its nonhemolytic form. Clinically the disease is more heterogeneous than is HS (Table 138–3). All types of HE are due to defects in the membrane skeleton. A number of specific molecular defects have been defined, some of which are discussed in the following sections.

Common HE

This most prevalent form of HE (~90 per cent of cases) is usually caused either by defects in the head end of spectrin that interfere with spectrin self-association or by the partial

TABLE 138–3. HEREDITARY ELLIPTOCYTOSIS

Clinical Manifestations	Laboratory Features
Common HE	
Asymptomatic	Blood smear: elliptocytes, few or no poikilocytes
Dominant inheritance: one parent with HE	No anemia, little or no hemolysis (reticulocytes = 1 to 3%)
Variants:	Normal osmotic fragility
Some neonates with moderately severe hemolytic anemia and HPP-like smear. Converts to typical common HE by 1 to 2 years	Often defect in spectrin self-association or partial deficiency of protein 4.1
Some patients with mild chronic hemolysis	
Hereditary Pyropoikilocytosis	
Anemia	Blood smear: bizarre poikilocytes, fragments, spherocytes, ± elliptocytes
Splenomegaly	
Intermittent jaundice	
Aplastic crises	Reticulocytosis
Recessive inheritance: both parents normal or one or both parents with HE	Increased osmotic fragility
	Decreased red cell heat stability
	Marked defect in spectin self-association
Good response to splenectomy	
Spherocytic HE	
Anemia	Blood smear: rounded elliptocytes, ± spherocytes
Splenomegaly	
Intermittent jaundice	Reticulocytosis
Dominant inheritance pattern	Increased osmotic fragility
Good response to splenectomy	

absence of protein 4.1. Practically it is little more than a morphologic curiosity. Most patients have no anemia or splenomegaly and only mild hemolysis (reticulocyte counts of 1 to 3 per cent). The blood smear shows prominent elliptocytosis (usually >40 per cent; normal <15 per cent). Osmotic fragility is normal. A few cases (10 to 20 per cent) have moderate hemolysis and are classified as sporadic hemolytic variants. The reason for this variation is unknown.

In general, patients with common HE require no therapy; but they may develop significant hemolysis if the spleen hypertrophies in response to various stimuli (e.g., infectious mononucleosis, cirrhosis). In addition, the physician must be alert for *transient neonatal hemolysis*. Neonates in some HE families (particularly black families with a defect in spectrin self-association) have moderately severe hemolytic anemia with marked red cell budding, fragmentation, and poikilocytosis. The relative paucity of elliptocytes may create diagnostic confusion; however, the diagnosis is easily made from family studies, since one of the parents will have common HE. Hemolysis gradually declines in these infants during the first year or so of life, and the disorder evolves into typical common HE. This curious phenomenon is unexplained. Presumably it reflects a difference in the fetal red cell or the circulatory system of the newborn that augments the primary defect in spectrin self-association.

Hereditary Pyropoikilocytosis (HPP)

This rare autosomal recessive disorder is characterized by moderately severe hemolytic anemia, marked red cell fragmentation, and *bizarre poikilocytosis*. It is most common in blacks. When heated for short periods, HPP red cells fragment (and their isolated spectrin denatures) at 45 to 46°C instead of the normal 49°C. This *exceptional heat sensitivity* constitutes the primary test for the disease. Hemolysis decreases after splenectomy, the treatment of choice, but the bizarre red cell morphology and heat sensitivity are unchanged. HPP is related to common HE in that all HPP patients have a *defect in spectrin self-association* that is qualitatively identical to the defect in common HE, but more severe. In addition, patients with HPP often have first-degree relatives with HE. A current hypothesis is that HPP patients are either homozygous for common HE, homozygous for a related "silent" mutation, or doubly heterozygous for common HE and the putative silent gene defect.

Spherocytic HE

This variant (~10 per cent of cases) is clinically and pathophysiologically similar to hereditary spherocytosis. It is inherited in an autosomal dominant pattern. The primary molecular defect is unknown. Patients typically have moderate hemolysis, mild anemia, and splenomegaly. Elliptocytes are less prominent and are more rounded than in typical common HE. Spherocytes are often evident and occasionally may predominate; however, at least one family member will usually have clear-cut elliptocytosis. Patients with this form of HE, like those with HS, have osmotically fragile red cells and respond dramatically to splenectomy.

Hereditary Defects in Membrane Permeability

Hereditary Xerocytosis

In this rare, autosomal dominant disorder of red cell membrane permeability the ratio of K^+ loss to Na^+ gain exceeds the normal ratio of 2:3; as a result, total cation content and cell water decrease. This occurs as a secondary event in a variety of conditions (e.g., sickle cell disease and glycolytic enzyme deficiencies). Morphologically, dehydrated red cells are typically either targeted or contracted and spiculated. Because dehydration increases intracellular viscosity, these cells are relatively rigid and risk splenic sequestration and hemolysis.

Hereditary Hydrocytosis (Hereditary Stomatocytosis)

In this rare autosomal dominant disease, an inherited defect in Na^+ permeability causes massive Na^+ influx, which overwhelms the Na-K pump and leads to an increase in intracellular cations and water. In some families this results in severe hemolysis. In others, for unknown reasons, hemolysis is much milder. Patients with the severe variant respond well to splenectomy. The partially swollen red cells appear on blood smears as stomatocytes (i.e., red cells with a mouthlike band of pallor across the center of the stained cell). Stomatocytes are much more frequently seen as an acquired defect, without hydrocytosis, cation changes, or hemolysis, in patients with acute alcoholism or with various types of liver disease.

ENZYME DEFICIENCIES
Normal Red Cell Metabolism

Reticulocytes have no nuclei and lose their mitochondria and microsomes as they mature; consequently, mature red cells consume little oxygen and do not synthesize protein. Glucose, the main metabolic substrate of the cells, is metabolized via two major pathways: the *Embden-Meyerhof pathway* and the *hexosemonophosphate shunt* (Fig. 138–3).

The Embden-Meyerhof (EM) Pathway

Approximately 90 to 95 per cent of metabolized glucose is converted to lactate via the EM pathway. This is the *major pathway of ATP synthesis in mature red cells*. Only two moles of ATP are generated from glycolysis per mole of glucose consumed, very inefficient compared to cells that possess mitochondria and an active Krebs cycle (that generates 38 moles of ATP per mole of glucose). Nevertheless the meager amount of ATP produced permits renewal of 150 to 200 per cent of the total red cell ATP every hour. Red cell ATP is used to transport monovalent cations and calcium, to phosphorylate various proteins, to synthesize glutathione, to salvage nucleotides, and to produce the glucose phosphates needed to fuel glycolysis.

The EM pathway is also the major source of red cell NADH. This cofactor is essential for the maintenance of heme iron in the reduced state, an enzymatic process that is mediated by *NADH methemoglobin reductase*. Oxidation of heme iron to Fe^{+++} produces methemoglobin, which does not transport oxygen (Ch. 146).

Red cells have a uniquely high concentration of *2,3-diphosphoglycerate (2,3-DPG)*; only traces of this metabolic intermediate are present in other cells. This intermediate, formed by the Rapaport-Luebering shunt (Fig. 138–3), decreases the oxygen affinity of hemoglobin and increases oxygen delivery to peripheral tissues (Ch. 140).

Hexose Monophosphate (HMP) Shunt

Approximately 5 to 10 per cent of utilized glucose is normally directed through the HMP shunt. This pathway is the *major source of NADPH in human red cells*: Two moles of NADPH are produced for each mole of glucose metabolized. Under conditions in which the oxidation of NADPH is accelerated, diversion of glucose through the shunt can increase up to 10- or 20-fold.

The most important reactions associated with NADPH oxidation are those related to glutathione. Red cells contain relatively high concentrations (2 mM) of *reduced glutathione (GSH)*, a tripeptide (gamma-glutamylcysteinylglycine) that is synthesized by mature red cells (Fig. 138–3). GSH protects red cells from injury by oxidants such as superoxide anion (O_2^-), hydrogen peroxide (H_2O_2), and hydroxyl radical $(OH\cdot)$, which are produced continuously in normal red cells as byproducts of the oxidation of heme by its dangerous oxygen cargo. Large amounts of oxidants are generated by activated phagocytes (e.g., during infections) and by red cells in the

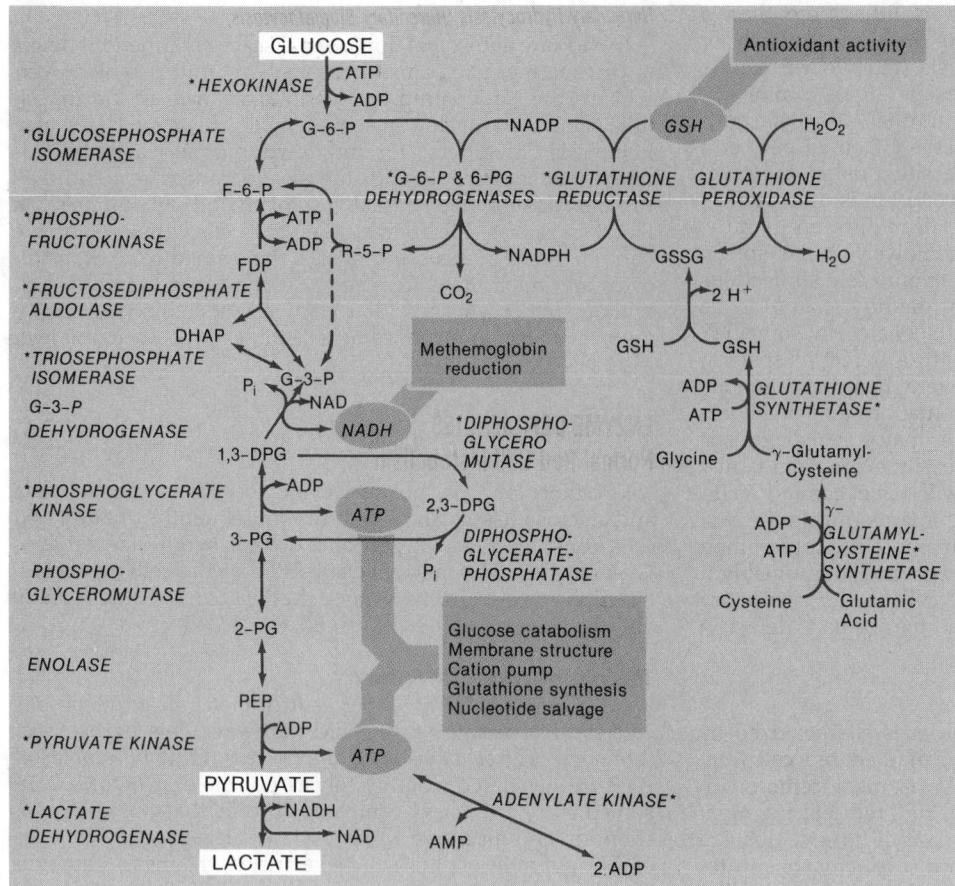

FIGURE 138–3. Glycolytic pathways and glutathione metabolism in the human erythrocyte. Asterisks indicate enzymes for which severe deficiency has been established. (From Valentine WN: Hemolytic anemia and inborn errors of metabolism. Blood 54:549, 1979. Reprinted by permission.)

presence of certain drugs. Injury to cell lipids and proteins occurs if these agents accumulate. Normally this is prevented by GSH. Detoxification of H_2O_2 can occur spontaneously, but it is enhanced by *glutathione peroxidase.* Catalase also degrades H_2O_2, but under physiologic conditions it is less important. In these reactions GSH is converted to *oxidized glutathione (GSSG)* and to mixed disulfides with protein thiols (Fig. 138–3). GSH levels are restored by *glutathione reductase.* In the process, NADPH is oxidized to NADP, which stimulates the HMP shunt, regenerating NADPH. This tight coupling of the HMP shunt with glutathione metabolism normally protects red cells from oxidant injury.

Defects in the HMP Shunt or Glutathione Metabolism

Almost all HMP shunt defects are due to *glucose-6-phosphate dehydrogenase* deficiency, the most common enzyme abnormality associated with hemolytic anemia. It affects millions of people throughout the world. In contrast, pyruvate kinase deficiency, the most common glycolytic defect, affects only hundreds to thousands of patients.

Glucose-6-Phosphate Dehydrogenase (G6PD) Deficiency

Pathophysiology. Defects in the HMP shunt or glutathione metabolic pathways impair the ability of red cells to defend themselves against oxidative assault. Oxidants produced by infections or oxidant drugs are normally detoxified by GSH, but GSH levels are not maintained in G6PD deficiency because of the diminished ability to generate NADPH. As a consequence the oxidants are free to damage vital cell constituents. Oxidation of hemoglobin produces the functionless *methemoglobin* and intracellular precipitates of denatured hemoglobin that are known as *Heinz bodies.* Heinz bodies are not visible in ordinary Wright's stained blood smears, but are revealed with supravital stains such as *methyl violet.* They attach to the membrane and damage it in poorly defined ways. In vitro, this causes increased membrane leakiness to cations, decreased osmotic fragility, and decreased deformability. In vivo, Heinz bodies are "pitted" from circulating red cells by the spleen and thus are more plentiful in splenectomized

patients. *"Bite cells,"* that is red cells with a localized invagination, possibly at the site of Heinz body removal, appear in the circulation during acute hemolytic episodes. Red cells with a submembranous hemoglobin-free area, *"blister cells,"* may also be seen. In addition to damage from Heinz bodies, G6PD-deficient red cells suffer oxidative cross-linking of spectrin and peroxidation of membrane lipids. Spectrin cross-linking decreases membrane flexibility and promotes splenic trapping. Lipid damage may be responsible for the intravascular hemolysis seen during acute hemolytic episodes.

More than 150 G6PD variants are now known, but only a few of these are common. The normal enzyme is termed G6PD[B] or Gd^B. It is present in about 70 per cent of American blacks and in more than 99 per cent of whites. Gd^{A+} is a normal variant found in about 20 per cent of American blacks. It has a greater electrophoretic mobility than Gd^B because of substitution of an asparagine for an aspartic acid in the amino acid sequence. Gd^{A-}, the most common variant associated with hemolysis, is found in about 10 per cent of American blacks and in many African black populations. It has the same electrophoretic mobility as Gd^{A+}, but its catalytic activity is decreased. Gd^{Med}, the second most common abnormal variant, is found in peoples of the Mediterranean area (Italians, Greeks, Sardinians, Sephardic Jews, Arabs, etc.), in India, and in southeastern Asia. Its electrophoretic mobility is normal, but its catalytic activity is markedly reduced. Gd^{Canton}, a relatively common variant in Oriental populations, produces a clinical syndrome similar to Gd^{A-}.

As normal red cells age in vivo, the activity of intracellular Gd^B decays slowly with a half-life of about 60 days (Fig. 138–4). Despite this loss of active enzyme, older normal red cells retain enough activity to produce NADPH and maintain GSH in the face of almost all oxidant stresses. The defect in Gd^{A-} results in a *labile enzyme* that disappears with a half-life of about 13 days. *Young red cells thus have normal enzyme activity, while older red cells are grossly deficient.* As a consequence of this heterogeneity, hemolysis is self-limited in individuals with Gd^{A-}.

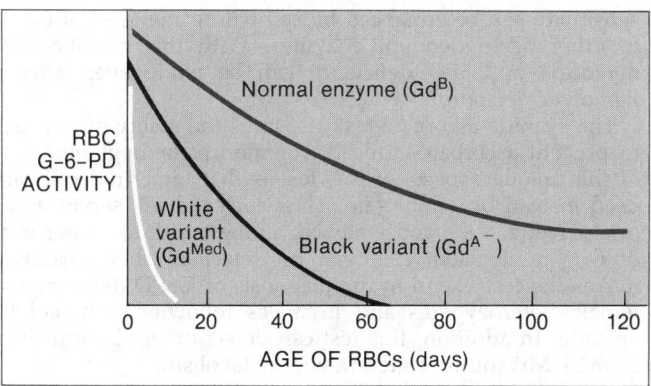

FIGURE 138–4. Intracellular decay of red cell G-6-PD as a function of cell age. The top curve shows the decay rate for Gd^B, the normal enzyme. The middle and lower curves show the greater than normal decay rates for the unstable Gd^A− and Gd^Med variants. Note that only the oldest Gd^A− red cells are markedly G-6-PD deficient and susceptible to hemolysis, whereas nearly all Gd^Med erythrocytes are vulnerable. Note also that after the most deficient Gd^A− red cells have been destroyed, the average G-6-PD level in the remaining cells will be near normal. This explains why G-6-PD assays after a hemolytic episode often fail to disclose the defect in Gd^A− males. (From Lux SE: Hemolytic anemias. Metabolic disorders. In Beck WS (ed.): Hematology. 4th ed. Cambridge, MA, The MIT Press, 1985, p 223. Reprinted with permission.)

This is shown graphically in Figure 138–5, which depicts the course of primaquine-induced hemolysis in an individual with Gd^A−. Acute hemolysis with hemoglobinuria and decreased ⁵¹Cr red cell survival develops when the drug is first administered, but this is followed by a recovery phase in which anemia and reticulocytosis abate and red cell survival improves despite continued administration of the drug. The reason is that once the oxidant-sensitive older red cells are destroyed, the remaining young cells are oxidant resistant. Since only about 50 per cent of the cells are oxidant sensitive to begin with in Gd^A−, the bone marrow can compensate by simply doubling its output. This apparent drug resistance persists as long as the offending drug is continuously administered. Note, however, that if the drug is stopped for two to three months, older red cells will survive and accumulate, and the patient will again become drug sensitive.

Gd^Med is considerably more unstable than Gd^A− (Fig. 138–4). Very little activity is present in mature red cells. Despite this, chronic hemolysis does not occur, which must indicate that endogenous oxidant stresses are normally very low. When

threatened by infections or oxidant drugs, however, these patients are at much greater risk because virtually their entire red cell population can be destroyed.

Clinical Features (Table 138–4). The most dramatic clinical presentation is acute intravascular hemolysis. These patients typically develop hemoglobinemia (pink to brown plasma), hemoglobinuria (red-brown to black urine), and jaundice acutely with an infection or within one to three days of exposure to an oxidant drug. In severe cases abdominal or back pain may be prominent. Symptoms of acute anemia (dizziness, headache, palpitations, dyspnea) may also develop. Heinz bodies and increased levels of methemoglobin appear in the red cells, and some bite cells and blister cells may be seen on the blood smear. In many cases, however, the red cell morphology is relatively normal. More often hemolysis is less dramatic, and a modest decline of hemoglobin (3 to 4 grams per deciliter) occurs, without hemoglobinuria or prominent symptoms. These episodes are easily overlooked unless the physician is alert.

The discovery of G6PD deficiency followed the observation that black soldiers developed explosive hemolysis after receiving primaquine for malaria. Subsequently, numerous other oxidant drugs were implicated as causative agents, some of which are listed in Table 138–5. The most common cause of hemolysis, however, is *infection*. Virtually every type of infection has been associated. One speculation is that oxidants generated by warring phagocytes trigger hemolysis by impinging on neighboring G6PD-deficient red cells. Hemolysis can also be precipitated by diabetic ketoacidosis and is exacerbated by uremia, because of an acquired inefficiency in the operation of the HMP shunt.

Severe hemolytic episodes occasionally follow exposure to *fava beans* (Italian broad beans) or their pollen, probably caused by divicine and isouramil, oxidant pyrimidine derivatives that are present in high concentrations in the beans. This rare phenomenon occurs mainly in individuals with Gd^Med; it is not seen in Gd^A−. This, and the fact that not all patients with Gd^Med are susceptible, indicates that other unknown factors must be involved.

In some patients with rare variants of G6PD, *chronic hemolysis* occurs in the absence of obvious oxidants. These cases are characterized by enzymes that are unable to maintain basal NADPH production. Variants generally have either a high K_m for NADP or a low K_i for NADPH.

Genetics. The gene for G6PD is located on the X chromosome, so its inheritance is sex linked. Males have one type of G6PD; females can have two types. For example, 70 per cent

FIGURE 138–5. Course of drug-induced hemolysis in an individual with Gd^A−. Note that hemolysis abates and apparent resistance to the drug develops after the initial hemolytic episode due to repopulation with young red cells. (Adapted from Alving AS: Bull World Health Organ 22:621, 1960. Reprinted with permission.)

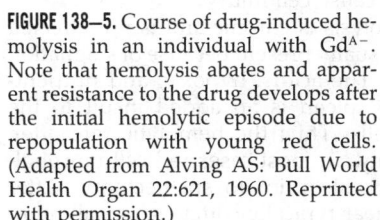

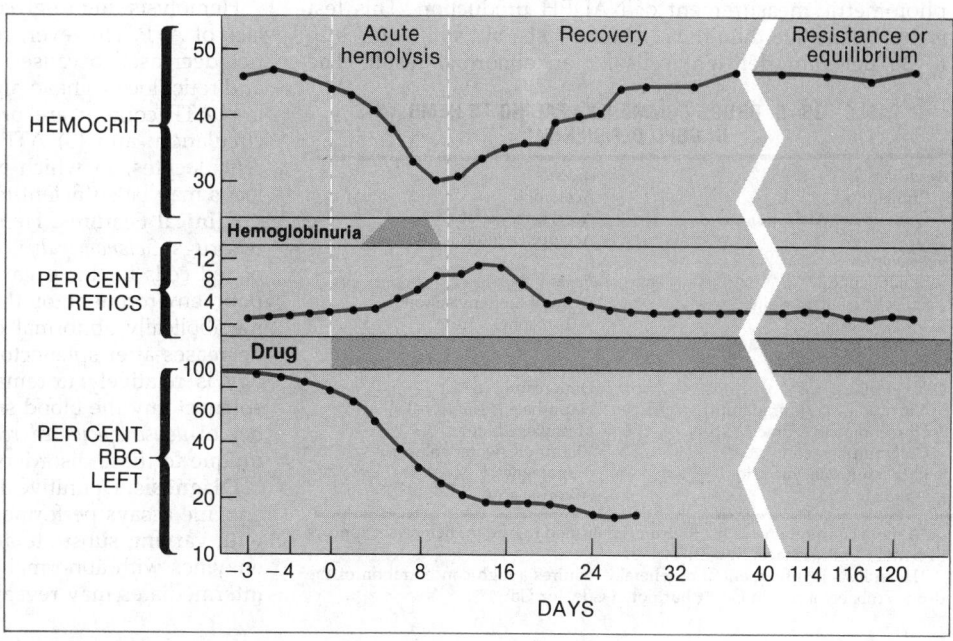

TABLE 138–4. CLINICAL COMPARISON OF THE TWO COMMON FORMS OF G6PD DEFICIENCY

	Gd^{A-}	Gd^{Med}
Frequency	Common in black populations	Common in Mediterranean populations
Chronic hemolysis	None	None
Degree of acute hemolysis	Moderate	Severe
G6PD defect	Old red cells	All red cells
Hemolysis with:		
Drugs	Unusual	Common
Infection	Common	Common
Need for transfusions	Rare	Sometimes

of black males have Gd^B, 20 per cent have Gd^{A+}, and 10 per cent have Gd^{A-}. Black females, however, can be heterozygous for any two of these enzymes. According to the *Lyon hypothesis*, only one X chromosome is active in any somatic cell; thus any given red cell in heterozygous females is either normal or deficient. Mean enzyme activity in females who are heterozygous for G6PD deficiency may be normal, moderately reduced (usual), or grossly deficient, depending on the degree of lyonization. Deficient cells in heterozygous females are just as susceptible to oxidant injury as enzyme-deficient cells in males; however, the overall magnitude of hemolysis is less because of the smaller population of vulnerable cells.

Despite the disadvantages of a gene for G6PD deficiency, it remains common in many geographic areas. Its prevalence has been attributed to a selective advantage it is believed to provide against malaria caused by *Plasmodium falciparum*. This proposal is supported by a large body of data, including epidemiologic studies and observations in heterozygous females demonstrating the resistance of cells containing the abnormal enzyme to malarial infection.

Diagnosis. Several tests for the diagnosis of G6PD deficiency are currently available. Their sensitivity varies and their usefulness is determined by the clinical situation (sex of patient, type of G6PD deficiency, and proximity to the hemolytic episode).

Commonly used screening tests are based on NADPH-mediated dye decolorization or on the reduction of methemoglobin in the presence of methylene blue. These tests are of limited sensitivity, since 30 to 40 per cent of the cells must be abnormal for the deficient state to be detected. This criterion may not be met in patients with Gd^{A-} or Gd^{Canton} after a severe hemolytic episode, since most of their enzyme-deficient, older red cells will have been destroyed.

Definitive assay of the enzyme depends on direct spectrophotometric measurement of NADPH production. This test is more sensitive than the screening tests, but still requires 20 to 30 per cent deficient cells for an abnormal result. The

TABLE 138–5. DRUGS COMMONLY LEADING TO HEMOLYSIS IN G6PD DEFICIENCY*

Antimalarials	*Analgesics*
Primaquine	Acetanilid
Quinacrine (Atabrine)	Acetylsalicylic acid†
	Acetophenetidin (Phenacetin)†
Sulfonamides	
Sulfanilamide	*Sulfones*
Salicylazosulfapyridine (Azulfidine)	Diaminodiphenylsulfone (Dapsone)
Sulfisoxazole (Gantrisin)†	
	Miscellaneous
Other Antibacterials	Dimercaprol (BAL)
Nitrofurantoin (Furadantin)	Naphthalene (moth balls)
Nitrofurazone (Furacin)	Methylene blue†
Chloramphenicol†	Vitamin K (water-soluble
Para-aminosalicylic acid	analogues)†
Nalidixic acid	Ascorbic acid†

*A more comprehensive list of drugs implicated in oxidant hemolysis appears in Beutler E: Pharmacol Rev 21:73, 1969.

†Hemolysis is infrequent and generally requires a high concentration of the drug. Probably a risk in Gd^{Med} but not in Gd^{A-} or Gd^{Canton}.

sensitivity can be enhanced by comparing the level of G6PD to other age-dependent enzymes. With this modification, diagnosis of G6PD deficiency can be made even after a hemolytic episode.

The cyanide-ascorbate test measures the ability of red cells to prevent ascorbate-induced oxidation of hemoglobin. One of the unique aspects of this test is that intact red cells are used instead of hemolysate. Thus each red cell serves as its own cuvette. As a consequence, as few as 10 to 15 per cent of enzyme-deficient cells can be detected. This sensitivity makes the test useful in the diagnosis of G6PD deficiency in female heterozygotes and in males following a hemolytic episode. In addition, this test can detect other abnormalities of the HMP shunt or glutathione metabolism.

Other Defects

Abnormalities of GSH metabolism, the first line of defense against oxidants, can also be associated with hemolysis. Defects in either *glutathione synthetase* or *gamma-glutamylcysteine synthetase*, the two enzymes responsible for the synthesis of GSH, occur in rare patients. Erythrocytes lacking either of these enzymes have very low levels of GSH. Clinically the disorders are similar to G6PD deficiency; they are characterized by mild to moderate hemolytic anemia that is sensitive to drugs. Chronic neurologic disease also occurs in some patients with glutathione synthetase deficiency, but it is not certain that the enzyme disorder and neurologic defect are causally related.

Inherited deficiencies of *GSSG reductase* are thought to exist, but they are rare, and no case of hemolysis due to this disorder has been proved. Many individuals (including all newborn infants) are relatively deficient in *GSH peroxidase*, but they do not have excessive hemolysis. This probably reflects the fact that nonenzymatic reduction of peroxide by GSH occurs at a significant rate.

Defects in Glycolysis

General Features. Abnormalities in nearly every glycolytic enzyme have been described, but pyruvate kinase (PK) deficiency accounts for about 90 per cent of the cases associated with hemolysis.

Almost all of the glycolytic defects are inherited in an autosomal recessive pattern. Hemolysis is observed in homozygotes. Heterozygotes are normal, although their red cells contain less than normal amounts of enzyme. Phosphoglycerate kinase (PGK) deficiency is an exception, since this enzyme is located on the X chromosome.

Hemolysis due to glycolytic defects is thought to be due to lack of ATP. However, red cell ATP concentrations are often not decreased because (1) the mean cell age is very young and reticulocytes have high ATP levels; (2) defective cells with low ATP content are probably removed promptly from the circulation; and (3) ATP may be compartmentalized within reticulocytes, in which case a decline in ATP at one critical locus may be sufficient to cause cell injury.

Clinical Features. Hemolysis is chronic and is not affected by drugs. *Splenomegaly* is usually present because of stagnation of red cells in this organ. The acidic, hypoxic, and nutrient-poor environment of the spleen is an added insult to the metabolically abnormal cells. Thus the hemolytic rate often decreases after splenectomy. In most cases red cell morphology is relatively unremarkable prior to splenectomy. After splenectomy the blood smear typically contains a small number of *dense spiculated red cells*, but this is not invariable or unique to these disorders.

Diagnosis. Definitive diagnosis requires spectrophotometric enzyme assays performed under a variety of conditions (i.e., with varying substrate and cofactor concentrations) to detect enzymes with abnormal kinetics. Measurements of glycolytic intermediates may reveal subtle enzyme abnormalities, since the concentration of an intermediate usually increases proximal to a defect and decreases distal to it.

Pyruvate Kinase (PK) Deficiency

PK catalyzes one of the major reactions responsible for ATP production in glycolysis; it is not surprising, therefore, that deficiency of this enzyme causes hemolytic anemia. Hemolysis can be mild and completely compensated or severe enough to require frequent transfusions. The distal glycolytic block in PK deficiency causes a two- to three-fold increase in red cell 2,3-DPG, which enhances tissue oxygenation and may minimize some of the physiologic consequences of the anemia. In most cases hemolysis improves following splenectomy, although the effect is not as dramatic as in diseases like hereditary spherocytosis. The improvement is related to the fact that PK-deficient reticulocytes depend on mitochondrial oxidative phosphorylation as an ATP source. In vitro incubation of PK-deficient reticulocytes under hypoxic conditions or with inhibitors of oxidative phosphorylation causes ATP levels to fall. The cells subsequently gain Ca^{++}, lose K^+ and water, and become rigid. PK-deficient reticulocytes sequestered in the hypoxic splenic cords presumably undergo similar degeneration. Even when anemia improves following splenectomy, reticulocytes may rise to levels of 50 to 70 per cent. This *paradoxical reticulocytosis* is due to increased reticulocyte survival once the adverse metabolic environment of the spleen is removed.

Defects in Red Cell Nucleotide Metabolism

Deficiency of *pyrimidine-5'-nucleotidase* is the third or fourth most common enzyme deficiency leading to hemolysis. This enzyme degrades pyrimidine nucleotides to cytidine and uridine, which can diffuse out of the cell. Lacking this activity, red cells accumulate partially degraded messenger and ribosomal RNA, and up to 5 per cent of the cells develop *prominent basophilic stippling*. Apparently the basophilic stippling in lead poisoning is produced by a similar mechanism, since pyrimidine-5'-nucleotidase is markedly inhibited by lead. Patients with an inherited (autosomal recessive) deficiency of this enzyme have chronic, moderately severe hemolytic anemia. The mechanism of hemolysis is unknown. Splenomegaly is common, but splenectomy produces little discernible benefit.

Finally, a rare disorder characterized by *overproduction of adenosine deaminase* illustrates the importance of ATP in red cell integrity. In affected patients, excessive deamination of adenosine apparently reduces the amount of this purine sufficiently to impair ATP synthesis. A chronic hemolytic anemia results. The disorder seems to be caused by hyperefficient translation of an adenosine deaminase mRNA that is present in normal amounts and produces a qualitatively normal enzyme. This extraordinary result suggests that a defect will be found in the 5' untranslated region of the mRNA that enhances binding of the message to ribosomes or initiation factors.

Agre P, Asimos A, Casella JF, et al.: Inheritance pattern and clinical response to splenectomy as a reflection of erythrocyte spectrin deficiency in hereditary spherocytosis. N Engl J Med 315:1579, 1986. *By comparing red cell spectrin content with clinical manifestations in 33 HS patients, the authors find that the dominant form of the disease is milder than the nondominant form and that spectrin content correlates closely with spheroidicity, hemolytic rate, and response to splenectomy.*

Becker PS, Lux SE: Hereditary spherocytosis and related disorders. Clin Haematol 14:15, 1985. *Review of the etiology and clinical features of HS.*

Blood cell cytoskeleton: I. Red cell membrane skeleton. Semin Hematol vol 20, no 3, 1983. *Monograph of excellent reviews on normal membrane structure and function and disorders of the membrane skeleton.*

Lux SE: Disorders of the red cell membrane. In Nathan DG, Oski FA (eds.): Hematology of Infancy and Childhood. 3rd ed. Philadelphia, W. B. Saunders Company, 1987. *Comprehensive (1100 references) review of all inherited and many acquired diseases of red cell membranes. Also covers normal membrane structure and function.*

Luzzatto L, Testa U: Human erythrocyte glucose-6-phosphate dehydrogenase: Structure and function in normal and mutant subjects. Curr Topics Hematol 1:1, 1978. *Excellent review of G6PD and G6PD deficiency.*

Palek J: Hereditary elliptocytosis and related disorders. Clin Haematol 14:45, 1985. *A comprehensive review of the etiology and clinical features of HE and HPP.*

Red blood cell membrane. Clin Haematol vol 14, no 1, 1985. *Monograph of excellent reviews covering diseases of the red cell membrane, including HS, HE, permeability defects, PNH, sickle cell anemia, thalassemia, and the red cell storage lesion. Not much information on the normal red cell membrane.*

Schwartz PE, Strioff S, Mucha P, et al.: Postsplenectomy sepsis and mortality in adults. JAMA 248:2279, 1982. *The only good epidemiologic study of postsplenectomy sepsis. Indicates that the risk of serious infection is much lower than previously thought.*

Valentine WN: Hemolytic anemia and inborn errors of metabolism. Blood 54:549, 1979. *Excellent review of the biochemical and clinical abnormalities in the glycolytic enzyme deficiencies.*

139 ACQUIRED HEMOLYTIC DISORDERS

Manuel E. Kaplan

Hemolysis resulting from congenital, intrinsic defects of the red cell has been discussed in Ch. 138. Hemolysis can also result from a variety of acquired abnormalities of the erythrocyte and of the circulatory system in which it functions (see Table 137–1). In these disorders red cells are usually formed normally but are destroyed prematurely as a result of immunologic, physical, or chemical injury. The general manifestations of the acquired hemolytic anemias do not differ from those resulting from inherited intracorpuscular defects.

SEQUESTRATIONAL HEMOLYSIS (HYPERSPLENISM)

By virtue of its unique vascular architecture, the normal spleen carefully sieves circulating red cells (Ch. 164). Arterial blood enters the spleen via arterioles in the white pulp. In the red pulp these arterioles communicate with either endothelial-lined sinuses or with closed, nonendothelialized cords that contain numerous fixed macrophages. To re-enter the venous circulation, red cells in the splenic cords must squeeze through narrow (3µ) fenestrations between epithelial cells that line the splenic sinuses. Poorly deformable red cells are unable to meet this challenge and are destroyed by splenic cord macrophages. The splenic filtration barrier does not significantly jeopardize the survival of normal nonsenescent red cells. However, when the spleen becomes enlarged, it may randomly entrap and destroy normal red cells. This pathologic process is called *hypersplenism*. The differential diagnosis of splenomegaly is discussed in Ch. 164. In patients with hypersplenism the rapidity of hemolysis is poorly correlated with overall spleen size. Indeed, patients with marked splenomegaly may show little or no reduction in red cell survival.

Hypersplenism is best treated by effectively managing the underlying disease process. Splenectomy is rarely indicated; the procedure should be limited to transfusion-dependent patients who are reasonable operative risks and whose condition is refractory to medical therapy. Splenectomized individuals, particularly the young (under age ten), are statistically more likely to develop fulminant bacterial or protozoal infections and are less able to mount an effective primary (IgM) immune response to certain antigens. Consequently the indications for splenectomy and its inherent risks should be carefully weighed before it is recommended.

IMMUNE HEMOLYTIC ANEMIAS

MECHANISMS OF IMMUNE HEMOLYSIS. In patients with immune hemolysis red cell destruction results from the binding of antibodies or complement components or both to the erythrocyte membrane. This may occur as a result of autoimmunization, of alloimmunization, or of exposure to certain drugs.

TYPES OF ANTIBODIES. Antibodies destroy red cells in vivo by mechanisms that are largely determined by their structure, concentration, and immunologic properties (complement fixing activity, the optimal temperature at which they are active) as well as the density and topographic distribution of the membrane antigens with which they combine. IgM red cell antibodies are generally agglutinating, complement fixing, and active at colder temperatures. In contrast, most IgG red cell antibodies are fully active at 37°C, have little or no agglutinating activity, and vary in their ability to fix complement. IgA red cell antibodies usually occur in conjunction with IgG and/or IgM red cell antibodies, have little complement-fixing activity, and destroy red cells poorly.

ROLE OF COMPLEMENT. Most IgM and some IgG red cell antibodies after combining with membrane antigens, activate the classic complement pathway. C1 binds to the Fc region of immunoglobulin heavy chains, develops esterase activity (C1s), and splits C4 into two fragments, C4a and C4b (Ch. 418). Nascent C4b may covalently attach to the red cell membrane and bind C2, which is then cleaved into C2a and C2b by C1s. The C4b, 2a complex acts as the classic pathway C3 convertase, binding and dissociating C3 into C3a and C3b. Nascent C3b may also covalently bind directly to the red cell membrane where it completes assembly of the classic pathway C5 convertase (C4b,2a,3b). After binding to C3b, C5 is cleaved by C2a, thereby activating the terminal "membrane attack complex" (C5-9) of the complement cascade. Insertion of activated terminal complement components into the red cell membrane results in osmotic destabilization of the membrane with egress of hemoglobin from the cell. If complement activation continued unimpeded, life-threatening intravascular hemolysis would invariably ensue. However, the process is restrained by inhibitors and inactivators of complement normally present in the plasma (factor I, factor H, C4-binding protein) and within the red cell membrane itself [CR1 (the receptor for C3b present in plasma immune complexes) and DAF (decay-accelerating factor)]. Red cells bearing covalently bound fragments of activated complement, i.e., C4b, C3b, and C3bi (C3b cleaved by factor I), are removed from the circulation and may be prematurely destroyed, primarily by hepatic macrophages bearing complement receptors (CR1 and CR3). A more detailed description of complement is contained in Ch. 418.

HEMOLYSIS WITHOUT COMPLEMENT ACTIVATION. Red cells sensitized with IgG antibodies that fail to fix complement are sequestered and destroyed primarily within the splenic cords. Here they come into prolonged and intimate contact with macrophages bearing membrane receptors for the Fc component of the IgG molecule. The sensitized cells may be damaged by a cytotoxic process (ADCC), or be totally engulfed, or undergo partial phagocytosis. Partially phagocytized red cells may reseal their membranes and, having lost proportionately more membrane than cytoplasm, assume a microspherocytic configuration. In the cells that survive and re-enter the circulation, their abnormal shape testifies to their previous encounter with splenic macrophages. These spherocytic cells are particularly vulnerable, since their deformability has been impaired and they retain significant membrane antibody.

DETECTION OF ANTIBODIES. The presence of red cell antibodies may be suspected from the appearance of freshly collected venous blood. IgM antibodies induce prompt red cell agglutination at room temperature. IgG antibodies are usually nonagglutinating but may so markedly reduce the negative charge (zeta potential) normally present on red cell surface that the cells are strongly aggregated by fibrinogen and other plasma macromolecules.

The *direct antiglobulin (Coombs') test* is most frequently used to detect immunoproteins present on the red cell membrane. This test measures the ability of a polyspecific antiserum that contains antibodies specific for human immunoglobulins and complement components to agglutinate a washed, dilute suspension of the patient's red cells. More precise identification of the membrane-bound immunoproteins may help to delineate the etiology and pathophysiologic mechanisms underlying a patient's hemolytic disorder. Consequently, when a positive direct antiglobulin test is obtained using a polyspecific reagent, the patient's red cells should be tested with various monospecific antisera that detect individual immunoglobulin classes or complement components. Almost all patients with immune hemolytic disorder exhibit a positive direct antiglobulin reaction. In the small percentage of patients (<5 per cent) in whom this test is negative, more sensitive immunologic techniques may disclose increased concentrations of red cell-associated immunoproteins.

The *indirect antiglobulin test* detects serum antibodies capable of attaching to normal red cells. The serum is first incubated with a panel of serologically defined normal red cells. After the cells are washed, membrane-associated immunoprotein is sought by the antiglobulin reaction. Although in clinical situations the direct and the indirect Coombs' tests are frequently ordered together, only the former provides unequivocal evidence of an immune hemolytic process.

HEMOLYSIS DUE TO ALLOANTIBODIES. Alloantibodies capable of destroying transfused, but not autologous, red cells are products of immunologic responses to (1) bacteria that normally colonize the large intestine (giving rise to so-called natural antibodies that cross-react with allogeneic erythrocyte antigens), (2) transfused, imperfectly matched red cells, or (3) antigens of fetal red cells that entered the maternal circulation during pregnancy or at delivery.

Alloimmune red cell antibodies present in a patient's serum may be detected by agglutination of normal cells or by the indirect antiglobulin reaction. Since these antibodies have specificity for nonself antigens, they are harmless unless the patient is transfused with allogeneic red cells bearing the immunizing antigen. Consequently, it is crucial that these antibodies be detected in patients requiring transfusions and in pregnant women. In the latter, IgG red cell alloantibodies that gain access to the fetal circulation may induce erythroblastosis fetalis.

AUTOIMMUNE HEMOLYTIC ANEMIAS. Autoimmune hemolytic disorders are characterized by antibodies with specificity for autologous red cell antigens. The pathophysiologic mechanisms that result in autoantibody production are not fully understood. B lymphocyte clones capable of producing autoantibodies to red cells probably exist in everyone. They do not normally synthesize detectable quantities of autoantibody because their activities are suppressed by immunoregulatory T lymphocytes. If this suppressor mechanism is deranged, red cell autoantibodies may be produced in quantities sufficient to trigger red cell destruction. Certain diseases—infections, neoplasms, or collagen-vascular disorders—appear to stimulate the development of autoimmune hemolysis. The hemolytic disorders that result are therefore categorized as secondary. In primary or idiopathic autoimmune hemolytic disorders no underlying or predisposing diseases can be detected.

AUTOIMMUNE HEMOLYTIC DISEASE DUE TO IgG WARM-REACTING ANTIBODIES

CLINICAL MANIFESTATIONS. *Disease Associations.* In approximately 40 per cent of patients IgG-mediated autoimmune hemolytic anemia occurs secondary to an underlying disease, usually neoplastic or collagen-vascular in origin. Chronic lymphocytic leukemia and, less frequently, other lymphoproliferative disorders are the most commonly associated malignant disorders. There is a well-documented relationship between ovarian teratoma and warm autoimmune hemolytic anemia. Systemic lupus erythematosus is the most frequently associated collagen-vascular disorder; less common are systemic sclerosis and rheumatoid arthritis. Occasional patients with ulcerative colitis present with warm autoimmune hemolysis.

Symptoms and Signs. Since the rate of red cell destruction, degree of anemia, and presence of underlying disease differ from patient to patient, a highly variable clinical picture can result. If hemolysis occurs suddenly, the patient usually presents with symptoms and signs related to severe anemia, i.e., pallor, fatigue, exertional dyspnea, dizziness, and palpitations. When hemolysis is more gradual, the anemia is usually less severe, and the patient may be relatively asymptomatic. On physical examination mild jaundice and splenomegaly are commonly present.

Laboratory Findings. The degree of anemia is variable, and there are usually normal numbers of white cells and platelets. In occasional patients significant thrombocytopenia, neutropenia, or both occurs in conjunction with immune hemolysis *(Evans' syndrome)*. The mean corpuscular volume (MCV) may be increased, sometimes strikingly so (> 115 fl). When spherocytosis is prominent, the mean corpuscular hemoglobin concentration (MCHC) is usually elevated. The peripheral blood film typically discloses rouleaux formation, significant anisocytosis and poikilocytosis with numerous microspherocytes, and increased numbers of large polychromatophilic reticulocytes. Nucleated red cells may be present, particularly when hemolysis is rapid. The reticulocyte count is almost always elevated. Other typical laboratory findings include hyperbilirubinemia of the unconjugated type, serum haptoglobin that is diminished to absent, normal or slightly elevated plasma hemoglobin levels, and no urine hemosiderin. The direct antiglobulin test discloses only IgG or IgG and complement (C3dg). The indirect antiglobulin test may be positive or negative, a positive result implying that the red cell autoantibody has been produced in excess. Antibody eluted from the patient's red cells may exhibit specificity for well-defined red cell antigens, particularly in the Rh system. More commonly the eluted antibody is found to be a "panagglutinin," reacting with all normal red cells tested.

DIFFERENTIAL DIAGNOSIS. Since underlying diseases are present in almost half the patients with warm autoimmune hemolytic anemia, appropriate diagnostic studies to define them should be undertaken. The possibility of a lymphoproliferative disorder, a collagen-vascular disease, or drug-induced immune hemolysis must be considered. If the hemolytic disorder appears to be acquired but the direct antiglobulin test is negative, a previously undiagnosed congenital hemolytic process, paroxysmal nocturnal hemoglobinuria, and various nonimmunologic causes of hemolysis (hypersplenism, microangiopathy, etc.) must be considered. If there is no evidence for these, the patient may have an immune hemolytic process that can be demonstrated only by immunologic studies more sensitive than the antiglobulin test. Alternatively, this may be inferred from a patient's objective clinical response to an empiric therapeutic trial of steroids.

TREATMENT. If an underlying disease process is identified and treated, marked improvement of the accompanying hemolysis frequently results. Mild hemolysis may require no therapy.

Glucocorticoids. Patients with more rapid hemolysis should be treated with oral steroids equivalent to 1 to 2 mg of prednisone per kilogram per day, in single daily or divided (thrice daily) doses. If the patient is very symptomatic because of severe anemia, initial treatment with intravenous hydrocortisone, 400 to 800 mg per day, may be preferred followed by daily oral prednisone in divided doses. Improvement will usually occur within five to ten days, evidenced by increasing hemoglobin and hematocrit levels and decreasing reticulocytosis. At this time steroid therapy can be given as a single daily dose. Over the succeeding three to four weeks, the daily steroid dosage can usually be tapered, at five- to seven-day intervals, to a daily dose of approximately 20 mg of prednisone. During this time blood counts and reticulocyte counts should be checked periodically. Thereafter, the dose of steroids should be decreased more slowly, every two to three weeks, by 5 mg per day as long as the reticulocyte count does not rise significantly and the hemoglobin level remains stable. In occasional patients it may be possible to discontinue steroids entirely without exacerbating the hemolysis. More commonly, significant hemolysis persists and patients require daily maintenance steroid therapy, 5 to 15 mg of prednisone, or 10 to 30 mg on alternate days, which results in fewer undesirable side effects (Ch. 30).

The mechanism of the corticosteroid effect in warm autoimmune hemolytic disorders is not fully understood. Steroids appear to diminish the number, and possibly the binding strength, of monocyte and macrophage Fc receptors, thereby decreasing the ability of these cells to bind and destroy IgG-sensitized red cells. Prolonged therapy with steroids may suppress antibody synthesis; however, this effect certainly does not explain the prompt, frequently dramatic clinical improvement seen in most patients.

If the response to corticosteroid therapy is unsatisfactory, i.e., if (1) hemolysis and anemia are not significantly improved within two weeks after initiating high-dose steroid therapy or (2) unacceptably large daily doses of steroids (> 15 to 20 mg of prednisone) are required to maintain hematologic improvement, other therapeutic approaches must be considered.

Splenectomy. [51]Cr red cell survival and sequestration studies should be performed, if possible, before splenectomy is undertaken. Typically they will disclose significantly reduced RBC survival (t½ = 5 to 15 days), and the spleen will be the major, if not exclusive, site of red cell destruction. In such a patient splenectomy is advisable and should result in marked hematologic improvement. Occasionally significant hemolysis persists after splenectomy. This usually results from intense red cell sensitization with IgG autoantibody and characteristically responds to small maintenance doses of steroids. If ^{51}Cr sequestration studies reveal the liver to be a major site of red cell destruction, the direct antiglobulin test usually discloses complement (C3dg) as well as IgG. Splenectomy results in less effective control of hemolysis in such patients, favorable responses being achieved in only 30 per cent. Consequently a trial of immunosuppressive therapy may be preferred prior to splenectomy.

Immunosuppressive Drugs. At present either oral azathioprine* (Imuran), 50 to 200 mg per day, or cyclophosphamide* (Cytoxan), 50 to 150 mg per day, is the immunosuppressive agent most frequently employed in patients with warm immune hemolytic anemia. Responses are variable and usually not very dramatic. However, their use in patients whose conditions are refractory to steroids may permit reduction in the excessive steroid dosages required for maintenance.

Transfusion. Before hemolysis is adequately controlled by steroid therapy, severely anemic patients may require red cell transfusions. Transfusion carries an increased risk when the patient has a positive indirect antiglobulin test because donor-patient compatibility cannot be ensured by cross-matching techniques. The serum of such a patient frequently contains a panagglutinating autoantibody reactive with red cells from all prospective donors. More importantly, the serum autoantibody may mask the presence of a red cell alloantibody that may be capable of provoking intravascular hemolysis of transfused red cells. To distinguish these possibilities, patient red cells from which autoantibody has been eluted are used to absorb the autoantibody from the patient's serum. The absorbed serum is then tested for alloantibody activity with potential donor cells. In addition, blood banks usually attempt to identify possible blood group specificity of antibody eluted from a patient's red cells and of the serum antibody. Following these studies, donor red cells "most compatible" with the patient are selected for transfusion. Usually patients with

---

*This use is not listed in the manufacturer's directive.

warm autoimmune hemolysis can be safely transfused when these precautions are taken. Donor cells should be administered slowly, with the patient being closely observed for symptoms and signs suggestive of a possible hemolytic transfusion reaction, the diagnosis and treatment of which are described in Ch. 147.

COURSE AND PROGNOSIS. In patients with secondary autoimmune hemolytic disorders the clinical course and ultimate prognosis are generally determined by the underlying disease process. Autoimmune hemolysis due to warm IgG antibodies is usually well controlled by corticosteroid therapy or splenectomy or both. Uncontrollable hemolysis resulting in death rarely occurs. All evidence of the disease may disappear in some patients. More commonly a positive direct antiglobulin test persists, and the patient experiences recurrent episodes of hemolysis that may require steroid therapy. Splenectomized patients are generally more stable hematologically than are patients managed by medical therapy alone. Major causes of death include thromboembolic complications and sequellae of chronically impaired host defense mechanisms caused by corticosteroids, splenectomy, or immunosuppressive drugs.

AUTOIMMUNE HEMOLYTIC DISEASE DUE TO COLD-REACTING ANTIBODIES

Cold-reacting red cell antibodies combine most avidly with erythrocyte membrane antigens at grossly subphysiologic temperatures (0 to 4° C). They exhibit characteristic "thermal amplitudes," i.e., maximum temperatures beyond which they are unable to combine effectively with their antigens. Pathologically significant cold antibodies produce clinical hemolysis because they retain significant immunologic reactivity at temperatures that are achievable in vivo (30 to 32° C). Thus, if the thermal amplitude of a red cell antibody does not extend to 30° C, the antibody will have no relevance pathophysiologically. IgM cold-reacting antibodies occur most commonly. Because they strongly agglutinate red cells in the cold, they are designated as *cold agglutinins*. Rare IgA cold agglutinins have been described; however, these antibodies do not produce hemolysis in vivo because they lack complement-fixing activity. Cold-reacting IgG red cell autoantibodies are occasionally encountered. They are intensely complement fixing and produce the disease picture of paroxysmal cold hemoglobinuria.

COLD AGGLUTININ DISEASE. *Pathophysiology.* IgM cold agglutinins are normally present in low titer in human serum. They have no known function and may represent byproducts of polyclonal immunologic responses to viruses and other microorganisms. Cold agglutinins in serum are detected and quantified by the cold agglutinin titer, i.e., the maximal serum dilution, at 4° C, that retains red cell agglutinating activity. Normal cold agglutinins are harmless because they are present in low titers (≤ 1:32) and exhibit low thermal amplitudes. Usually, but not always, the higher the patient's cold agglutinin titer, the higher the thermal amplitude of the cold antibody, and the greater the probability that the patient will experience hemolysis.

The synthesis of polyclonal cold agglutinins may increase in response to certain infections, especially mycoplasma, viral (EB, cytomegalovirus), and protozoal (trypanosomiasis, malaria) infections. Titers usually peak within two to three weeks of onset, but rarely do antibody concentrations rise sufficiently to provoke clinically apparent hemolysis.

Cold agglutinin disease occasionally appears in patients with lymphoproliferative disorders, particularly histiocytic lymphoma. Indeed, hemolytic anemia may be the initial manifestation of the lymphoma. In these patients the cold agglutinins are predictably monoclonal, containing either kappa or lambda light chains. Occasionally the antibody may be present in such high concentrations that it is detectable as a spike on serum protein electrophoresis.

TABLE 139–1. RELATIONSHIP BETWEEN COLD AGGLUTININ STRUCTURE AND SPECIFICITY IN VARIOUS DISEASES

Structure	Specificity		
	Anti-I	*Anti-i*	*Anti-PR*
Polyclonal/ oligoclonal (κ + λ)	*Mycoplasma pneumoniae*	Infectious mononucleosis	
Monoclonal κ	Idiopathic cold agglutinin disease	Lymphoma	Idiopathic cold agglutinin disease
λ		Lymphoma	

Idiopathic cold agglutinin disease occurs most frequently in elderly patients in whom, by definition, no underlying infectious or neoplastic process can be identified. The cold agglutinin is almost always monoclonal kappa IgM.

Cold agglutinins react with polysaccharide components of red cell membrane glycolipids and glycoproteins immunochemically related to human ABO blood group antigens. Some of these polysaccharide antigens are better expressed on adult erythrocytes (designated I) and others on fetal red cells (i). Cold agglutinins that react significantly more strongly with adult red cells are said to exhibit anti-I specificity, whereas those that combine better with fetal (cord) erythrocytes show anti-i specificity. I and i are not alleles, and both antigens are usually expressed on adult, as well as on fetal, red cells. However, the red cells of rare, otherwise normal, individuals express only one or the other. Very infrequently patients with cold agglutinin disease have antibodies that exhibit exclusive anti-I or anti-i reactivity. Some cold antibodies that react equally well with adult and cord cells fail to agglutinate red cells pretreated with proteolytic enzymes and are said to show anti-PR specificity. Identification of the major reactivity of a cold agglutinin (anti-I, -i, or -PR) and its clonal diversity may be clinically informative, since cold agglutinins produced in various diseases show different characteristic patterns of reactivity (Table 139–1).

Mechanisms of Hemolysis. High thermal amplitude cold agglutinins bind to red cells in the cooler portions of the circulation and initiate agglutination and complement activation via the classic pathway. Complement-mediated intravascular hemolysis may ensue. However, this occurs minimally, or not at all, in most patients because propagation of the complement cascade is effectively aborted before membrane damage occurs. Activation of the earlier components of the classic pathway (C1, 4, 2, and 3), as previously described, results in the binding of nascent C3b to the red cell membrane (EC3b). EC3b is so rapidly cleaved by the plasma C3 inactivator (factor I) that it is unable to effectively support activation of the membrane attack components of complement (C5–9). Factor I activity is significantly enhanced by cofactors in the plasma (factor H) and in the red cell membrane itself (CRI). EC3b is progressively cleaved into EC3bi and ECdg, which are not able to support further complement activation. Indeed, C3dg appears to inhibit binding of additional cold agglutinin to the red cell membrane. Although significant intravascular hemolysis is prevented, red cells bearing C3b or C3bi are prematurely removed from the circulation and may be prematurely destroyed, primarily by hepatic macrophages.

Clinical Manifestations. In patients with postinfectious cold agglutinin disease, hemolysis is usually self-limited and mild. In contrast, idiopathic and lymphoma-associated cold agglutinin syndromes are accompanied by persistent hemolysis that is usually worse in winter. After exposure to cold, the patient may experience a picture of painful acrocyanosis, similar to Raynaud's phenomenon, induced by intense red cell autoagglutination. Unlike Raynaud's, there is usually no antecedent blanching or reactive hyperemia, and local gangrene does not occur. Severe chilling may accelerate hemolysis to such a degree that hemoglobinuria results.

Diagnosis. On physical examination the patient may be mildly jaundiced. As the patient's blood is drawn, the red cells may clump so rapidly that the blood appears to clot even in the presence of an anticoagulant. Warming of the anticoagulated blood to 37° C rapidly restores its normal appearance. Electronically measured blood counts are frequently inaccurate because of the intense autoagglutination at room temperature. The red count and MCV measurement are particularly affected, leading to distortion of the calculated hematocrit. This situation should be recognized by alert laboratory personnel. Not uncommonly the reticulocyte count is only mildly increased; this suggests suboptimal bone marrow compensation. The cold agglutinin titer is invariably elevated, and the direct antiglobulin test discoses C3dg. Typically, serum haptoglobin levels are decreased, and lactic dehydrogenase (LDH) concentrations increased.

Treatment. When an underlying disease process is identified, it should be treated appropriately. Patients should be told to avoid exposure to the cold and to dress warmly. Treatment with daily chlorambucil,* 2 to 4 mg orally, decreases the hemolysis in some patients with idiopathic cold agglutinin syndrome, probably by reducing the synthesis of cold agglutinin. Glucocorticoids and splenectomy are generally of no benefit. If rapid hemolysis persists despite treatment, it may be advisable for the patient to move to a warmer climate. Although transfusions are not absolutely contraindicated, they should be avoided unless the patient is critically ill, i.e., exhibiting symptoms and signs of vascular decompensation (tachyarrhythmias, angina, congestive failure) or cerebral hypoxia (confusion, visual disturbances, etc.) that respond poorly to bed rest and oxygen therapy. In addition to the transfusion-associated risks previously described in patients with warm autoimmune hemolysis, the following dangers must be considered: (1) Transfused compatible red cells will be hemolyzed as rapidly, or even more rapidly, than the patient's own red cells; the latter, having membrane-associated C3dg, may be more resistant to additional IgM cold agglutinin binding. By increasing the numbers of circulating red cells at risk of complement-mediated destruction, transfusion may exacerbate intravascular hemolysis with hemoglobinemia and hemoglobinuria. This may further jeopardize the patient's renal function and predispose to thromboembolic complications, red cell stroma being thrombogenic. (2) Although theoretically hazardous, the actual danger of transfusing refrigerated donor blood to a patient with cold agglutinin disease has been debated. Some experts strongly advise that a properly functioning, in-line blood warmer be utilized. However, uncontrolled warming of donor erythrocytes may be more hazardous to the patient than the slow administration of refrigerated blood. (3) The usual risks of transfusion therapy (Ch. 147) must be considered. By expanding the patient's blood volume, transfusion may exacerbate congestive heart failure. Transmission of non-A, non-B hepatitis, cytomegalovirus, or HIV infection may occur. When transfusions are administered the patient must be kept warm, a limited volume of red cells (designed to alleviate life-threatening symptoms, not simply to improve the hemoglobin concentration) should be infused slowly, and the patient's response must be monitored carefully.

PAROXYSMAL COLD HEMOGLOBINURIA (DONATH-LANDSTEINER HEMOLYTIC ANEMIA). Paroxysmal cold hemoglobinuria (PCH) is an exceedingly rare autoimmune hemolytic disorder caused by IgG cold-reacting antibodies directed against the ubiquitous P blood group antigen. It was first described in patients with tertiary syphilis who, following exposure to cold, developed paroxysms of chills, fever, headache, and diffuse pain in the abdomen, back, and legs accompanied by hemoglobinuria. PCH now much more commonly occurs as a complication of various viral infections. In this context, hemolysis is rarely paroxysmal, and a history of cold exposure is seldom obtained. Consequently it has been proposed that the syndrome be renamed Donath-Landsteiner hemolytic anemia in honor of the investigators who first described the offending antibody. The diagnosis of PCH (Donath-Landsteiner hemolysis) is made by demonstrating the presence in the patient's serum of a cold hemolysin, an IgG, nonagglutinating antibody, that activates complement so efficiently that intravascular hemolysis results. Normal red cells are mixed with the patient's serum and a source of complement and chilled (0 to 4° C). Thereafter the cell suspension is incubated at 37° C. The appearance of hemolysis is presumptive evidence of the Donath-Landsteiner antibody. The patient's direct Coombs' test is usually weakly positive for IgG and complement. When PCH accompanies a viral infection, hemolysis is usually transient, requiring only supportive therapy and protection of the patient from cold. If hemolysis recurs or becomes chronic, it may respond to treatment with glucocorticoids or to immunosuppressive drugs such as cyclophosphamide.*

IMMUNE HEMOLYSIS DUE TO DRUGS. A number of drugs, or their in vivo metabolic derivatives, may cause immune hemolytic anemia. Three distinct mechanisms have been described:

1. *Drug binding to red cells.* When administered intravenously, certain immunogenic drugs, exemplified by penicillin, bind tightly to erythrocyte membranes. If drug-specific antibodies are produced, they attach to red cells at membrane sites occupied by the drug. In the case of penicillin-induced immune hemolysis, the offending antibody is characteristically IgG and is noncomplement fixing. In vivo, it binds to penicillin-modified red cells and induces their destruction by a mechanism essentially identical to that seen in warm autoimmune hemolytic anemia, i.e., IgG-sensitized red cells are sequestered primarily within the spleen and destroyed by Fc receptor-bearing macrophages. The direct antiglobulin test discloses only IgG. The antipenicillin specificity of the red cell antibody can be demonstrated by indirect antiglobulin testing. IgG eluted from the patient's red cells, as well as antibody that may be present in the patient's serum, fails to combine with normal erythrocytes unless the cells have been pretreated with penicillin. Since hemolysis promptly ceases soon after penicillin is discontinued, corticosteroid therapy is usually unnecessary.

2. *Innocent bystander hemolysis.* Other drugs that induce immune hemolytic anemia in humans (sulfonamides, phenothiazines, quinine, quinidine, etc.) are bound primarily by plasma proteins rather than red cells. Although they are weakly immunogenic, in some patients they stimulate the synthesis of drug-specific, complement-fixing antibodies. As a result, the patient's erythrocytes are bathed in plasma containing drug-antibody immune complexes that activate complement. The nascent C3b generated by these complexes may covalently bind to the red cell membrane. Membrane-bound C3b facilitates activation of the alternative complement pathway by binding factor B, which is then cleaved into Bb by factor D, a proteolytic enzyme normally present in plasma. C3b,Bb complexes represent the alternative pathway C3 convertase, cleaving plasma C3 and thereby generating additional nascent C3b that may covalently bind to the red cell membrane. The C3b,Bb,C3b complexes, acting as the alternative pathway C5 convertase, cleave C5, thereby triggering activation of the terminal (C5-9) membrane attack complex of complement. This process, if unsuccessfully opposed by the complement inactivators and inhibitors previously described, will result in life-threatening intravascular hemolysis. Even if activation of the membrane attack complex is effectively prevented, red cells bearing C4b, C3b, and C3bi are at risk of sequestration and destruction by hepatic macrophages. The direct antiglobulin test reveals only membrane-associated

---

*This use is not listed in the manufacturer's directive.

complement cleavage products, primarily C3dg (the small C3 fragment that remains covalently bound to the red cell membrane after degradation of C3bi by factor I). Efforts to elute immunoprotein from the patient's red cells are usually unsuccessful. The indirect antiglobulin test is characteristically negative; however, if the offending drug, or an appropriate metabolic derivative, is added to normal erythrocytes suspended in the patient's serum with a source of complement, hemolysis may occur, and Coombs' testing of the nonhemolyzed cells may disclose membrane-associated complement fragments. After the drug is discontinued, hemolysis generally subsides promptly, and patients usually require no additional therapy.

3. *Drug-induced autoimmune hemolytic anemia.* A pure IgG direct antiglobulin test appears in approximately 15 per cent of patients undergoing long-term treatment with methyldopa (Aldomet). However, only 10 per cent of these Coombs-positive patients develop clinically apparent hemolysis. Antibodies eluted from the patients' red cells combine readily with normal erythrocytes in the absence of methyldopa, thereby displaying true autoimmune reactivity. Patients treated with levodopa or mefenamic acid (Ponstel), a nonsteroidal anti-inflammatory drug, may develop similar erythrocyte autoantibodies. By unknown mechanisms these agents probably interfere with immunoregulatory processes that suppress the synthesis of red cell autoantibodies. Moreover, it is not clear why hemolysis occurs in only a small percentage of Coombs'-positive methyldopa-treated patients. The mechanism of cell destruction appears identical to that seen in warm autoimmune hemolytic anemia, i.e., splenic sequestration and red cell destruction by Fc receptor-positive macrophages. Hemolysis usually subsides within one to three weeks after methyldopa is discontinued but a positive direct antiglobulin test may persist for many months. Although the hemolysis responds to steroid therapy, it is rarely required. If methyldopa is readministered to a patient who has fully recovered from methyldopa-induced hemolyis, no anamnestic autoimmune response usually occurs. Hemolysis may recur, but only after a prolonged treatment period.

PAROXYSMAL NOCTURNAL HEMOGLOBINURIA

Paroxysmal nocturnal hemoglobinuria (PNH) is an acquired hemolytic disorder resulting from the proliferation of an abnormal clone of stem cells whose progeny are uniquely susceptible to complement-mediated membrane damage. Its etiology is not known. Since patients with PNH are unusually prone to develop aplastic anemia or acute leukemia, it may represent a "preneoplastic" transformation of hematopoietic stem cells. The disease is quite rare; however, it is probably underdiagnosed because its manifestations are frequently protean. It occurs with greatest frequency in early adulthood, but has been described in young children and in the very elderly.

PATHOPHYSIOLOGY. PNH red cells, granulocytes, and platelets are inordinately sensitive to the lytic effects of complement. The patient's peripheral blood frequently contains two or three subpopulations of red cells differing in their sensitivity to complement (I = normally sensitive cells, II = cells of intermediate sensitivity, and III = very sensitive cells). When PNH red cells are exposed to complement activated in vitro by either the classic or the alternative pathway, PNH II and III cells bind much greater quantities of C3b than do normal red cells. The rate of red cell destruction in vivo correlates well with the proportions of circulating red cells that are PNH II and III.

Spontaneous limited in vivo activation of the alternative complement pathway appears to occur normally. This may result in covalent binding of C3b to the red cell membrane. As previously described, membrane-bound C3b exerts posi-

tive feedback on the alternative complement pathway through factors B and D to generate additional nascent C3b available for coupling to the membrane; the assembled C3b,Bb,C3b complexes, representing the alternative pathway C5 convertase, cleave C5, thereby activating the C5-9 membrane attack complex. If unsuccessfully restrained by the complement inactivator/inhibitor substances normally present in plasma and red cell membrane, such complement activation would result in intravascular hemolysis. Normal red cell membranes contain a glycoprotein, designated decay-accelerating factor (DAF), that inhibits assembly of the C3 convertase (C3b,Bb). PNH I and II red cells are deficient in DAF, which may account, in large part, for their marked susceptibility to complement-mediated hemolysis. Similarly, platelets and granulocytes from PNH patients are DAF deficient and also exhibit abnormal sensitivity in vitro to complement activation.

Although the in vivo survival of PNH platelets has been reported to be normal, their enhanced susceptibility to complement activation may underlie the thrombotic diathesis commonly seen in these patients. Functional abnormalities of the PNH granulocyte have also been described.

CLINICAL MANIFESTATIONS. The diagnosis of PNH must be considered in all patients with chronic hemolysis, particularly when associated with hemoglobinuria, pancytopenia, or unusual veno-occlusive events. During episodes of rapid hemolysis, patients commonly experience diffuse abdominal and back pain that has been attributed to ischemia resulting from microcirculatory thrombi. Not infrequently major thromboses occur involving the hepatic, splenic, portal, or cerebral veins. On physical examination pallor and scleral icterus are common. The degree of anemia is highly variable ranging from mild to severe. The reticulocyte count may be inappropriately low, given the severity of the anemia. The MCV may be normal, slightly increased, or diminished, depending upon the degree of reticulocytosis and the presence of accompanying iron deficiency due to prolonged urinary loss. Mild thrombocytopenia and granulocytopenia occur commonly. The peripheral blood smear reveals no autoagglutination, spherocytosis, or red cell fragmentation. The direct antiglobulin test is usually negative. Bone marrow cellularity varies from markedly hypoplastic to profoundly hyperplastic, and iron stores are usually reduced or absent. Erythroid elements predominate, and cell maturation is typically normoblastic.

Because red cell destruction occurs intravascularly, the serum LDH is elevated, serum haptoglobin levels are reduced or absent, and hemosiderinuria is present. Frank hemoglobinuria usually occurs only intermittently and is most apparent after periods of sleep, when the urine is concentrated.

DIAGNOSIS. The diagnosis of PNH requires that the patient's red cells show excessive susceptibility to complement-mediated hemolysis in vitro. This is most frequently demonstrated by mixing the red cells with freshly collected normal human serum that has been mildly acidified (*Ham's test*). Hemolysis, which results from activation of the alternative pathway, is highly specific but unfortunately Ham's test is too insensitive to detect all patients with PNH. The simpler sucrose hemolysis test, which results in complement activation via the classic pathway, is much more sensitive than Ham's test, but is less specific, with positive results occurring in some patients with myeloproliferative disorders. Low levels of neutrophil alkaline phosphatase and red blood cell acetylcholinesterase occur commonly in PNH patients, but are nonspecific. Occasionally these measurements are used to confirm the diagnosis.

Other causes of intravascular hemolysis and hemoglobinuria that should be considered in the differential diagnosis include (1) hemolytic transfusion reactions, (2) paroxysmal cold hemoglobinuria, (3) red cell hemolysins such as those present in snake venoms and *Clostridium welchii* exotoxin,

(4) traumatic intravascular hemolysis as occurs in thrombotic thrombocytopenic purpura or march hemoglobinuria, and (5) G6PD deficiency (Ch. 138).

TREATMENT. Erythropoiesis may be enhanced with folic acid, iron, and androgen therapy. In some patients iron administration may provoke increased hemolysis and hemoglobinuria. This may be prevented by prior transfusion and probably results from the destruction of increased numbers of newly produced, complement-sensitive reticulocytes. Androgen administration may significantly improve the anemia. A six- to eight-week trial of oral fluoxymesterone or oxymesterone (5 to 50 mg per day), or of intramuscular nandralone decanoate (25 to 200 mg once weekly), is usually sufficient to identify androgen-responsive patients.

Steroid therapy (equivalent to 0.25 to 1 mg of prednisone per kilogram per day) significantly slows acute hemolytic episodes in some patients, and prolonged administration of low-dose steroids may reduce ongoing hemolysis. Daily steroids should not be administered except in life-threatening situations because of their unacceptable side effects and the increased danger of overwhelming bacterial or fungal sepsis. Alternate-day prednisone therapy, in dosages ranging from 15 to 40 mg, has been reported to improve more than 50 per cent of patients so treated.

Most patients with PNH eventually require blood transfusions. Initially donor red cells survive normally and suppress the production of the patient's abnormal red cells resulting in marked clinical improvement. Following repetitive transfusions, however, patients are prone to develop hemosiderosis and to produce alloantibodies to red cell, neutrophil, platelet, and even to plasma protein antigens. Once alloimmunization has occurred, further transfusion therapy is difficult, since it may be followed by rapid destruction of recipient (as well as of donor) red cells. Even compatible transfusions may trigger increased hemolysis of patient red cells and hemoglobinuria, probably because the donor packs contain small quantities of activated complement. If evidence of increased hemolysis follows transfusion of packed donor red cells, only washed red cells or frozen and reconstituted red cells should be administered.

PNH patients may require anticoagulation because they are susceptible to major thromboembolic events. Since heparin therapy has been reported to exacerbate hemolysis in some patients, it must be used with caution. Vitamin K antagonists can usually be employed without difficulty, but it is not clear whether continuous prophylactic anticoagulation with Coumadin derivatives is clinically beneficial.

Bone marrow transplantation has successfully eradicated the PNH clone in selected patients.

PROGNOSIS. The course of PNH is exceedingly variable. Most patients survive fewer than ten years from the time of diagnosis. In a small percentage of patients all disease manifestations spontaneously subside, possibly reflecting disappearance of the aberrant clone. More commonly, patients experience waxing and waning hemolysis, which may be exacerbated by immunologic stress such as infection, transfusion, and immunization. Thrombotic events, primarily venous, account for much of the morbidity and mortality. With time, marrow function progressively deteriorates, and a clinical picture more closely resembling aplastic anemia may gradually ensue. In approximately 5 per cent of patients the disease evolves into acute myeloblastic leukemia.

HEMOLYSIS CAUSED BY CHEMICALS

A number of chemicals may directly interact with and injure red cells, resulting in hemolysis. These toxins range in complexity from inorganic cations (arsenic and copper) and simple organic compounds such as chloramine to complex biologic substances produced by microorganisms, plants, and lower animals. Arsenic and copper injure red cells probably by binding to membrane sulfhydryl groups. Copper-induced hemolysis has been observed in hemodialyzed patients, and may be responsible for the transient hemolytic episodes observed in patients with Wilson's disease.

Purification of urban water supplies with alum and chlorine results in the generation of chloramine, a potent oxidant. If chloramine is not efficiently removed from tap water that is used for hemodialysis, it may swiftly induce methemoglobin and Heinz body formation, resulting in rapid hemolysis.

Amphotericin B is a lipophilic fungal product that binds avidly in vitro to red cell membrane lipids. In occasional patients it may provoke hemolysis, presumably by altering red cell membrane stability.

Clostridium welchii, spiders, and snakes produce potent lipolytic toxins capable of damaging red cell membrane integrity, thereby provoking intravascular hemolysis. Marked spherocytosis of circulating red cells is commonly seen. Hemolysis of uncertain etiology may accompany severe infection with other bacteria (*Streptococcus pneumoniae, Escherichia coli, Staphylococcus aureus*). Castor beans and certain species of mushrooms contain hemolysis-inducing toxins.

HEMOLYSIS CAUSED BY METABOLIC ABNORMALITIES

SPUR CELL HEMOLYTIC ANEMIA. Patients with a significant hepatocellular disease are frequently anemic. Blood loss, folate deficiency, alcohol-induced marrow dysfunction, and hypersplenism may contribute to the etiology of the anemia. However, in a small percentage of patients with end-stage cirrhosis, a clinical picture of rapid hemolysis develops with the appearance of numerous acanthocytes (spiculated, occasionally spur-shaped red cells).

Pathophysiology. Red cell membrane cholesterol and phospholipids exist in dynamic equilibrium with plasma lipids. In many patients with severe parenchymal liver disease, abnormal plasma lipoproteins appear to unload cholesterol and phospholipids onto the erythrocyte membrane. As a result the membranes spread and the cells thin out to become target cells. The molar ratio of cholesterol to phospholipids in target cells is normal, and these cells usually survive normally. In patients with spur cell hemolytic anemia, excess cholesterol accumulates in the red cell membrane unaccompanied by parallel increases in phospholipids. This may be caused by an abnormal circulating low-density lipoprotein containing an increased ratio of free cholesterol:phospholipids. Red cell deformability is markedly reduced, and the cells are prematurely destroyed within the congested, hypertrophied spleen.

Clinical Manifestations. Patients with spur cell hemolytic anemia characteristically exhibit marked splenomegaly and signs of advanced cirrhosis including jaundice, ascites, varices, and neurologic manifestations of hepatic encephalopathy. The anemia is usually severe, perhaps in part because of concomitant gastrointestinal blood loss. The peripheral smear contains numerous acanthocytes and polychromatophilic reticulocytes. The direct antiglobulin test is negative. Red cells are sequestered by the spleen and have shortened survival.

Diagnosis. The presence of a significantly elevated reticulocyte count and numerous spur cells on peripheral smear in a patient with end-stage cirrhosis is diagnostic of this syndrome. When normal compatible red cells are incubated with the patient's plasma in vitro, they become acanthocytic.

Prognosis and Treatment. Spur cell hemolytic anemia carries an exceedingly poor prognosis, almost all patients dying within months because of the associated liver disease. The beneficial effects of transfusion are limited since normal cells survive no better than autologous cells in these patients. Splenectomy may slow the rate of hemolysis in selected patients but is exceedingly hazardous because of the severity of the liver disease.

HYPOPHOSPHATEMIA. Hemolysis may occur in patients

with profoundly depressed serum phosphorus levels (< 1 mg per 100 ml) (Ch. 207). Hypophosphatemia of this degree occurs primarily in severely malnourished patients, particularly when they consume excessive quantities of phosphate-binding antacids. Erythrocyte ATP levels fall, the cells become poorly deformable, and hemolysis occurs primarily within the spleen.

HEMOLYSIS CAUSED BY RED CELL PARASITES

MALARIA. *Malarial infections,* particularly with *Plasmodium falciparum,* are probably the most common cause of hemolytic anemia worldwide (Ch. 381). Merozoites parasitize red cells and utilize for their own purposes hemoglobin, enzymes, and substrates, thereby metabolically depriving infected erythrocytes. As a result, the osmotic fragility and cation permeability of parasitized red cells are altered. Infected red cells may display new membrane antigens; this may help to explain the positive direct antiglobulin tests reported in some patients with falciparum malaria. Red cell destruction appears to occur primarily in the spleen and splenomegaly is almost universally present in patients with chronic malarial infection. Rarely, rapid intravascular hemolysis with hemoglobinuria (blackwater fever) occurs soon after antimalarial therapy is initiated. It is not clear whether the infection or the drug plays the more important role in this phenomenon.

BABESIOSIS. *Babesia* are protozoans that parasitize red cells of many animal species (Ch. 389). Several cases of babesia-induced hemolytic anemia have been reported in humans, the disease being particularly fulminant in previously splenectomized individuals. Such patients may present with thrombocytopenia, disseminated intravascular coagulation, and renal insufficiency. Although wood ticks are the usual vector, the disease may be transmitted by transfusion of infected red cells. The disease has been reported most frequently in the northeastern United States (Martha's Vineyard and Nantucket). Intraerythrocytic parasites can usually be seen in Giemsa-stained peripheral blood films.

BARTONELLOSIS. *Bartonella bacilliformis,* a bacterial species endemic to South America, grows on the surface of red cells rather than within them (Ch. 301). The disease is transmitted by the bite of the sand fly. Hemolysis is acute in onset and rapid, the red cells being sequestered by both liver and spleen. The peripheral blood smear typically discloses rod-shaped organisms on the erythrocyte surface and large numbers of normoblasts and reticulocytes. The infection responds well to treatment with penicillin, tetracyclines, streptomycin, or chloramphenicol.

HEMOLYSIS RESULTING FROM TRAUMA TO RED CELLS

When subjected to excessive mechanical stress, circulating red cells may hemolyze. The forces responsible may be generated extracorporeally or intravascularly. For example, fragmentational hemolysis may result from excessive intravascular shear stress originating in critically narrowed heart valves, pathologic shunts (arterial or arteriovenous), cardiac valve prostheses, poorly endothelialized vascular surfaces, or microvascular thrombi. In these situations hemolysis is characteristically accompanied by morphologic evidence of red cell fragmentation. Similarly red cell membranes may be injured by heat with resulting hemolysis. Temperatures higher than 49° C destabilize the normal human red cell membrane. Red cells, when heated in vitro, are observed to undergo membrane budding and fragmentation. Patients who have suffered extensive burns may show evidence of profound red cell membrane damage with prominent spherocytosis on peripheral smear. In some cases hemoglobinemia and hemoglobinuria occur. The major syndromes of traumatic hemolysis will be summarized briefly.

MARCH HEMOGLOBINURIA. As red cells circulate through narrow vessels overlying the bones of the hands and feet, they may be traumatized by repetitive, relatively un-cushioned forces generated by prolonged marching, running, karate blows, and a variety of other activities. Intravascular hemolysis accompanied by hemoglobinemia and hemoglobinuria may result. Interestingly, no red cell morphologic abnormalities are apparent in the peripheral blood film during, or immediately following, the physical activity that precipitated the hemolytic episode.

FRAGMENTATIONAL HEMOLYSIS DUE TO CARDIAC PATHOLOGY OR ABNORMALITIES OF LARGE VESSELS. Cardiac abnormalities involving primarily the left side of the heart, where pressures are high, may predispose to hemolysis. These include aortic stenosis (acquired and congenital), severe aortic regurgitation, and ruptured sinus of Valsalva. Significant red cell fragmentation may also occur as a result of traumatic arteriovenous fistulas, or therapeutic aortofemoral bypass procedures. In patients with these abnormalities hemolysis is usually mild.

More rapid hemolysis occurs, not uncommonly, in patients who have received prosthetic heart valves. Hemolysis is more likely to occur with aortic rather than mitral prostheses, artificial valves rather than those of biologic (porcine) origin, metallic valves rather than Silastic, cloth-covered valves, and with defective or poorly functioning valves that exhibit ball variance or paravalvular leaks.

Clinical Manifestations. Rapid intravascular hemolysis accompanied by hemoglobinemia and hemoglobinuria occurs in occasional patients. More commonly, patients present with increasing anemia, reticulocytosis, and numerous fragmented red cells (schistocytes) on peripheral blood film. Findings typical of significant intravascular hemolysis are usually present, i.e., haptoglobin levels that are low to absent, increased serum LDH concentrations, and hemosiderinuria. Prolonged urinary iron loss may result in iron deficiency. Although the direct Coombs' test is usually negative, a positive result has been found in a few patients with prosthetic heart valves for reasons that are not understood.

Treatment. Patients should be advised to limit their physical activities in an effort to reduce cardiac output and thereby to slow the rate of hemolysis. Oral iron, 300 mg of ferrous sulfate three times a day, should be given to correct iron deficiency, or rarely parenteral iron (iron-dextran) or transfusions may be required. If the rate of hemolysis necessitates recurrent transfusion, it may be preferable to replace the prosthesis.

FRAGMENTATIONAL HEMOLYSIS DUE TO ABNORMALITIES WITHIN THE MICROCIRCULATION (MICROANGIOPATHIC HEMOLYTIC DISORDERS). *Pathophysiology.* Red cells may be fragmented when they are forced to flow through small vessels that have been partially occluded by microthrombi. Excessive shear forces are generated as the cells encounter and become tethered to fibrin strands, which may bisect and fragment the erythrocytes. The microthrombi may be formed as a result of (1) an underlying coagulopathy, i.e., disseminated intravascular coagulation (DIC), (2) injury to the vascular endothelium, or (3) unknown mechanisms. Pathophysiologic processes that trigger DIC commonly induce endothelial injury as well; however, the reverse is frequently not true. Diseases associated with diffuse microvascular pathology may involve none of the characteristic findings of DIC. Consequently, in many patients with microangiopathic hemolytic disorders, the predominant etiologic factor (i.e., coagulation or vascular injury) can be discerned.

DIC results when procoagulant is introduced into the systemic circulation (Ch. 167). Coagulation factors are consumed, thrombus formation occurs, and fibrinolytic mechanisms are secondarily activated. Patients with significant DIC characteristically have thrombocytopenia, abnormally prolonged plasma coagulation studies (prothrombin time, activated partial thromboplastin time) reflecting decreased concentrations of certain clotting factors (particularly V, VIII, and fibrinogen), and increased plasma concentrations of fibrin degradation products, which may prolong the thrombin time. DIC may be triggered by infections, particularly with gram-negative organisms, amniotic fluid embolism, and disseminated neoplasms that synthesize and elaborate potent procoagulants (Trousseau's syndrome). Although patients with severe DIC may be critically ill, hemolysis is usually mild.

Diffuse or localized vascular lesions may induce red cell fragmentation, e.g., cavernous hemangiomas (Kasabach-Merritt syndrome), renal allografts undergoing rejection, malignant hypertension, eclampsia, vasculitic processes (rickettsial infections, periarteritis nodosa, Wegener's granulomatosis), and disseminated neoplasms. The severity of hemolysis ranges from mild to severe. Coagulation abnormalities mimicking those of DIC are usually absent.

Thrombotic thrombocytopenic purpura (TTP) (Ch. 166), the hemolytic uremic syndrome (Ch. 81), and mitomycin C-induced hemolytic uremic syndrome of adult cancer patients are highly fatal disorders of unknown etiology that closely resemble one another clinically. Patients with these disorders develop rapid fragmentational hemolysis, thrombocytopenia, and renal failure. Early there is little or no laboratory evidence of DIC despite the presence of diffuse microvascular thrombi.

Diagnosis. The diagnosis of a microangiopathic hemolytic disorder is based on the demonstration of schistocytes, grossly misshapen, sharply angulated erythrocytes that occasionally appear helmet shaped (Color plate 2J), usually in association with reticulocytosis, serum haptoglobin levels that are diminished to absent, increased serum LDH concentrations, and hemosiderinuria. Hemoglobinemia and hemoglobinuria occur less frequently.

Hemolysis may be accompanied by significant thrombocytopenia, with or without laboratory evidence of DIC (i.e., the prolonged prothrombin, partial thromboplastin, and thrombin times are typically incompletely corrected when an equal volume of normal plasma is mixed with that of the patient). When severe DIC is present, the plasma concentrations of fibrin degradation products are characteristically elevated, and coagulation Factors V, VIII, and I (fibrinogen) are usually decreased.

Treatment. Treatment of the patient with microangiopathic hemolysis must be highly individualized and may be very complex. Efforts should be made to reverse the underlying triggering mechanism (i.e., withdrawal of potentially offending drugs, treatment with antibiotics, etc.) and the patient supported with red cell transfusions, platelet packs, and cryoprecipitate as required. Occasional patients may benefit from anticoagulation with heparin to disrupt the vicious cycle of clotting and fibrinolysis. Vigorous plasma exchange (plasmapheresis combined with infusion of normal plasma) may induce dramatic clinical remissions in TTP. Although antiplatelet drugs and high-dose adrenocorticoid therapy are frequently employed, their efficacy is less certain.

IMMUNE HEMOLYTIC ANEMIA

Nydegger UE, Kazatchkine MD: The role of complement in immune clearance of blood cells. Springer Semin Immunopathol 6:373, 1983. *An interesting and perceptive review of complement activation and complement receptors and their roles in immunologically mediated destruction of peripheral blood cells.*
Petz LD, Branch DR: Drug-induced immune hemolytic anemia. In Chaplin H (ed.): Methods in Hematology. Vol. 18. New York, Churchill Livingstone, Inc., 1985, pp 47–94. *An exhaustive but readily assimilable review of the pathophysiologic mechanisms underlying drug-mediated immune hemolysis and of laboratory techniques useful in the diagnosis of this problem.*
Rosse WF: Autoimmune hemolytic anemia. Hosp Pract 20:105, 1985. *A brief but superb summary of the pathophysiology of autoimmune hemolysis.*
Sokol RJ, Hewitt S: Autoimmune hemolysis: A critical review. CRC Crit Rev Oncol Hematol 4:125, 1985. *A comprehensive and well-integrated review of the pathophysiology, clinical manifestations, and treatment of autoimmune hemolytic disorders.*

PAROXYSMAL NOCTURNAL HEMOGLOBINURIA

Rosse WF: Treatment of paroxysmal nocturnal hemoglobinuria. Blood 60:20, 1982. *A brief review of the treatment of PNH by a physician who has had vast clinical experience with this disease.*
Rosse WF, Parker CJ: Paroxysmal nocturnal haemoglobinuria. Clin Haematol 14:105, 1985. *A probing analysis of the membrane abnormality(ies) in PNH and of the pathophysiologic implications of complement activation on the red cell membrane.*

OTHER

Bowdler AJ: Splenomegaly and hypersplenism. Clin Haematol 12:467, 1983. *A thoughtful, comprehensive review of a topic that has generated controversy for many years.*
Cooper RA: Hemolytic syndromes and red cell membrane abnormalities in liver disease. Semin Hematol 17:103, 1980. *An excellent review of the pathophysiologic mechanisms of red cell membrane changes in liver disease.*

140 HEMOGLOBIN STRUCTURE AND FUNCTION

Alan N. Schechter

The interior of the normal erythrocyte contains a 5 mM solution of hemoglobin, corresponding to about 280 million hemoglobin molecules per cell. Each molecule is a tetramer composed of two pairs of polypeptide chains to which four heme moieties are bound. The ability of the hemoglobin molecule to bind oxygen reversibly allows the erythrocyte to transport oxygen from the lungs to the tissues. The complex structure of the hemoglobin molecule allows it to bind, transport, and release oxygen with extraordinary efficiency. As a result of advances in molecular biology during the last several decades, the relationship between the structure and function of hemoglobin is very well understood. It is now possible to explain the pathophysiology of diseases related to hemoglobin at the molecular, and even atomic, level.

STRUCTURE. The normal hemoglobins of the adult are hemoglobins A (about 97 per cent of the total), A_2 (about 2 per cent), and F (about 1 per cent). The protein, or globin, of each of these is composed of two α polypeptide chains and in addition two β (in hemoglobin A), two δ (in hemoglobin A_2), or two γ (in hemoglobin F) polypeptide chains. An additional α-like globin, the ζ chain, and an additional β-like globin, the ε chain, have been discovered. These chains, with the α and γ chains, form hemoglobins that are detected in the early embryo: hemoglobin Gower 1 ($\zeta_2\epsilon_2$), hemoglobin Portland ($\zeta_2\gamma_2$), and hemoglobin Gower 2 ($\alpha_2\epsilon_2$).

The sequence of appearance, and sometimes disappearance, of the six polypeptide chains known to be synthesized by human beings is illustrated in Figure 140–1. The factors that control the sequential appearance of these polypeptides are poorly understood. The "switching" process from one hemoglobin to another is mainly related to the age of the fetus or infant and has not been clearly shown to be determined by the site of erythropoiesis, humoral factors, or the appearance of different clones of cells.

The chromosomal arrangements of the genes for these six polypeptide chains are shown in Figure 140–2, the α-like genes on chromosome 16 and the β-like genes on chromosome 11. The genes for the α chains appear in two functional copies that code for identical polypeptides. Of the two ζ genes, only the one on the 5' (left) of the gene cluster appears to be functional. Chromosome 11 seems to have but one functional copy of the β, δ, and ε genes but two copies of the γ gene.

The sequence of nucleotides in the regions of DNA corresponding to these genes and in many of the regions separating them has been determined. The nucleotide sequences of the genes that specify amino acids in each of the polypeptides are interrupted by stretches of DNA, or intervening sequences, that do not code for amino acids in the hemoglobin

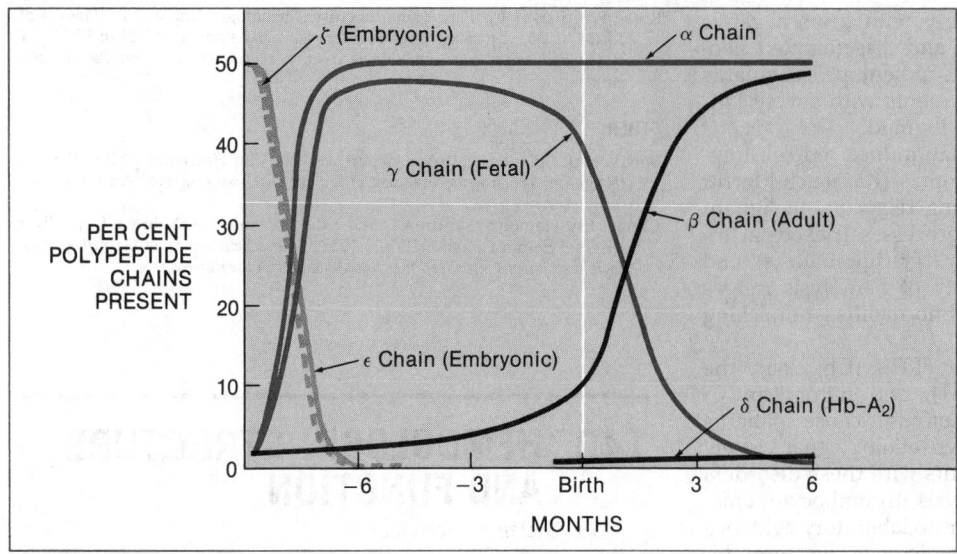

FIGURE 140–1. A diagram of the relative abundance of various human globin chains during development. (From Bunn HF, Forget BG: Hemoglobin: Molecular, Genetic, and Clinical Aspects. Philadelphia, W. B. Saunders Company, 1986.)

molecule (Ch. 141). The elucidation of the anatomy of the human hemoglobin genetic region at this level of detail is providing information about regulatory genetic functions as well as structural genetic elements, as described in Ch. 142.

While globin messenger RNA synthesis reaches a maximum in the early erythroblast series, globin polypeptide synthesis reaches a peak at about the level of the polychromatophilic erythroblast and continues into the reticulocyte stage. There appears to be little enzymatic processing of the globin polypeptides, except for removal of the amino-terminal methionine residue. Each cell contains three or more types of polypeptide chains, and they combine roughly in proportion to their concentrations. As long as synthesis of α (and α-like) chains and β (and β-like) chains is balanced, as it is in the normal person, the hemoglobin in the red cell is formed of two pairs of chains and is largely stable for the lifespan of the erythrocyte. If chain synthesis or degradation is unbalanced as in certain diseases, discussed in Ch. 142, then surplus chains will accumulate. Excess α chains remain monomeric, whereas the excess β chains form tetramers (β_4, hemoglobin H), as do the excess γ chains (γ_4, hemoglobin Barts). All of these surplus chains are unstable compared to normal hemoglobin and precipitate within the erythrocyte, shortening its lifespan and thus causing hemolytic anemias.

The heme prosthetic groups are in four largely hydrophobic pockets, one being formed in each globin polypeptide chain by the amino acid side chains of polypeptide helices on either side of the heme and of other helices at the interior. The iron atoms are at the center of the porphyrin molecules, bound in a square array to the four nitrogen atoms of each pyrrole ring. In addition, the iron is tightly bound to the nitrogen atom of the imidazole side chain of the histidine residue on a nearby helix (the "proximal" histidine). Oxygen or other small molecules such as carbon monoxide bind on the opposite or "distal" side of the heme in a very compact pocket formed by a number of amino acid side chains.

The nonaqueous environment around the iron atom allows it to remain in the ferrous state even in the presence of oxygen molecules, and imparts to the iron-oxygen bond a coordination character that makes its strength intermediate between a noncovalent and a covalent bond. This property is important in allowing the reversibility of oxygen binding. Despite this, some oxidation to the ferric form occurs naturally. A methemoglobin-reduction system exists in the erythrocyte, utilizing reduced nicotinamide adenine dinucleotide and the enzyme methemoglobin reductase, to keep the iron atoms in the ferrous form. This system, and other related enzymatic pathways, will be discussed in more detail in Ch. 146.

FUNCTION. In the range from normal arterial P_{O_2} values (100 mm Hg) to normal tissue P_{O_2} values (thought to be around 40 mm Hg), hemoglobin oxygen saturation decreases from about 100 per cent to about 75 per cent (see Fig. 140–3). Much more oxygen can be released if a further fall in tissue P_{O_2} values occurs. The great physiologic benefit of hemoglobin results from both the sigmoidal shape of the oxygen-binding curve and the fact that the hemoglobin tetramer has relatively

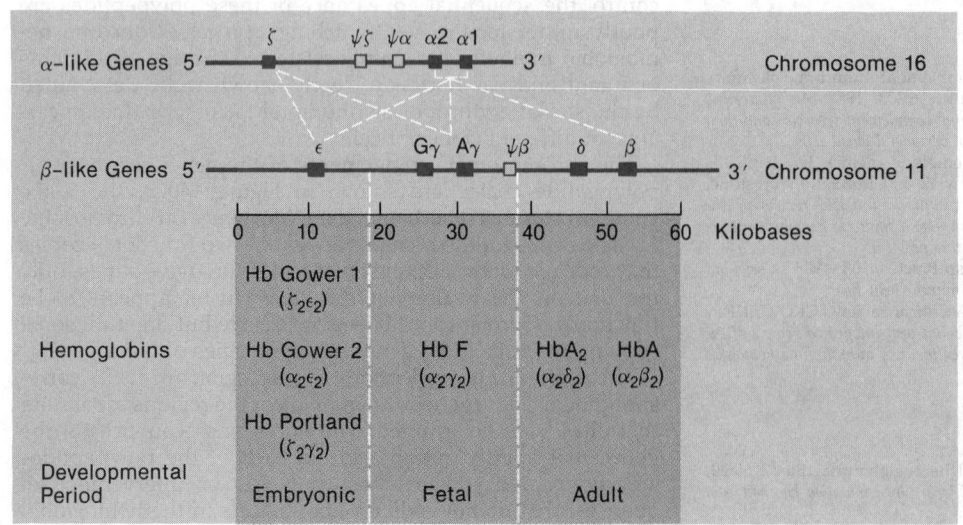

FIGURE 140–2. A diagram of the arrangement of the clusters of human α-like and β-like globin genes on chromosomes 16 and 11 and the embryonic, fetal, and adult hemoglobins that result from the combinations of the various globin chains encoded by these genes. The ψ genes are similar to globin genes but do not code for protein. Distances along the chromosome are expressed in terms of 1000 nucleotide pairs (a kilobase).

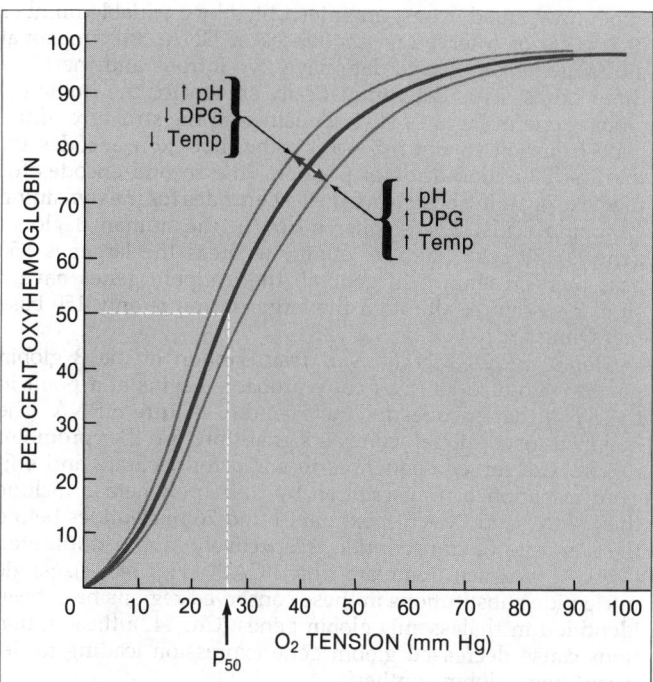

FIGURE 140–3. The oxygen binding curve for human hemoglobin A under physiologic conditions (*dark curve*). The affinity will be shifted by changes in pH, DPG concentration, and temperature as indicated. P_{50} represents the oxygen tension at half saturation. (From Bunn HF, Forget BG: Hemoglobin: Molecular, Genetic, and Clinical Aspects. Philadelphia, W. B. Saunders Co., 1986.)

reduced oxygen affinity (or "shift to the right") as compared to its own subunits or to myoglobin. This allows efficient discharge of oxygen in peripheral tissues.

The normal, relatively low oxygen affinity of hemoglobin is due to the interactions of the subunits with each other and to the binding of protons (the Bohr effect) and the molecule 2,3-diphosphoglyceric acid (DPG) to the hemoglobin tetramer. For reasons that are not completely understood, tetramers of hemoglobin composed of pairs of unlike chains have reduced oxygen affinity as compared to the subunits alone. In the pH region from 7.4 to 7.0, the binding of protons—which increases as pH is lowered—further decreases the oxygen affinity of hemoglobin, i.e., it shifts the oxygen equilibrium curve further to the right (Fig. 140–3). This results in more oxygen being released at a given P_{O_2}, which is very useful since the pH is reduced in the tissues as compared to the capillaries of the lung. Thus the Bohr effect promotes oxygen delivery.

DPG, which is normally roughly equimolar with hemoglobin in the erythrocyte, binds reversibly to the region of the hemoglobin tetramer formed by the amino-terminal ends of each of the β chains. One molecule of DPG binds to each hemoglobin tetramer. The binding affinity of DPG for deoxygenated hemoglobin is much greater than for oxygenated hemoglobin. DPG thus stabilizes the deoxygenated form of hemoglobin, increases its concentration relative to the oxygenated form, and so decreases the overall oxygen affinity, i.e., it causes a shift to the right of the oxygen equilibrium curve (Fig. 140–3). DPG binding to deoxygenated hemoglobin is proportional to its concentration in the erythrocyte, and thus oxygen affinity is inversely related to DPG levels. Variation in intracellular DPG, by mechanisms only poorly understood, appears to be a major physiologic mechanism for adjusting oxygen transport in the human being.

The binding of carbon dioxide to hemoglobin as carbamino complexes also lowers oxygen affinity. This process, however, is a relatively minor one in the red cell, and it is estimated that only 10 per cent of metabolically produced carbon dioxide is transported in this manner.

The sigmoidal nature of the oxygen equilibrium curve itself contributes greatly to the efficiency of hemoglobin by causing a release of much oxygen over a narrow range of tissue P_{O_2} values. (Roughly 250 million molecules of oxygen per red cell are released to the tissues in each cycle.) The shape of the binding curve is due to interactions or cooperativity within and between the dimers of the hemoglobin tetramer. The basis for these interactions at the level of individual atomic groups is still the subject of much debate, but the overall picture seems clear. Deoxygenated hemoglobin exists in a well-defined arrangement of each polypeptide chain with respect to the heme group (tertiary structure) and with respect to each other (quaternary structure), called the T or tense form. Oxygenated hemoglobin has a significantly changed tertiary and quaternary structure, called the R or relaxed form. As oxygenation of each hemoglobin tetramer proceeds, the change in structure occurs in a relatively all-or-none manner, rather than being a gradual structural transition. This property leads to the cooperative or sigmoidal oxygen equilibrium curve.

The trigger for this structural transition is the binding of oxygen to the iron atoms and the resulting changes in the sizes and positions of these iron atoms and the orientations of the heme groups themselves within the polypeptide chains. The most direct result of these changes in the iron atoms and the heme groups is to lead to movements of the proximal histidine residues and the helices to which they are attached. These movements, in turn, cause further changes in the arrangement of the globin polypeptides and interactions among amino acid side chains, within and between subunits. The final result is that the stable quaternary structure of the oxygenated hemoglobin is significantly different from that of the deoxygenated form. The deoxygenated and the oxygenated forms of human hemoglobin have been studied in detail by x-ray crystallography. As described in Ch. 145, this information has been extremely useful in understanding the molecular basis for altered function in certain hemoglobins. In addition, the molecular basis of the polymerization of deoxygenated sickle hemoglobin is explicable with this information, as described in Ch. 143.

Bunn HF, Forget BG: Hemoglobin: Molecular, Genetic, and Clinical Aspects. Philadelphia, W. B. Saunders Company, 1986. *The best single reference to all aspects of the study of hemoglobin.*

Dickerson RE, Geis I: Hemoglobin: Structure, Function, Evolution, and Pathology. Menlo Park, CA, Benjamin/Cummings Publishing Company Inc., 1983. *A sophisticated and magnificently illustrated introduction to hemoglobin structure and function.*

Fermi G, Perutz MF: Haemoglobin and Myoglobin: Atlas of Molecular Structures in Biology. New York, Oxford University Press, 1981, vol 2. *An introduction to information and conclusions from the structure.*

Honig GR, Adams JG: Human Hemoglobin Genetics. New York, Springer-Verlag, 1986. *The first comprehensive treatise on this rapidly moving field of great clinical relevance.*

Perutz MF: Molecular anatomy, physiology and pathology of hemoglobin. *In* Stamatoyannopoulous G, Nienhuis AW, Leder P, et al (eds.): Molecular Basis of Blood Diseases. Philadelphia, W. B. Saunders Company, 1987. *A rigorous but comprehensive analysis of normal and abnormal hemoglobin function in terms of the molecular structure.*

141 HEMOGLOBIN SYNTHESIS

Arthur W. Nienhuis

The red cell is one of the uniquely specialized cells in the body. Lacking a nucleus and therefore devoid of any proliferative potential or even the ability to renew its own protein constituents, the red cell is totally adapted to carrying oxygen and carbon dioxide for its brief lifespan of approximately 120 days. The red cell's unique membrane constituents give it flexibility, allowing passage through even the narrowest capillaries and egress from the red pulp into the sinusoids of the spleen. The oxygen and carbon dioxide transport properties of the red cell depend on its content of hemoglobin. Hemoglobin amounts to more than 95 per cent of the cytoplasmic protein of the red cell; each cell contains 30 pg (approximately 280 million molecules) of this protein. In this chapter we will consider briefly the mechanism of hemoglobin synthesis, beginning with an outline of the flow of genetic information from gene to protein. Also germane are the mechanisms by which red cells come to contain hemoglobin to the virtual exclusion of most other proteins.

FLOW OF INFORMATION FROM GENE TO PROTEIN.

Chromatin Structure. The nuclei of human cells contain chromatin, a complex of histone core particles called nucleosomes around which the DNA double helix is coiled. Nonhistone chromosomal proteins are thought to play a role in establishing higher order structures of chromatin so that the relatively vast amount of DNA may be packed into a cell's small nucleus. Furthermore, nonhistone proteins are thought to include regulatory factors which establish the structure of a restricted number of genes in a specialized cell to allow their exclusive expression. For example, the globin genes in erythroid cells have been shown to be in an active conformation, whereas in brain cells the globin genes are included among those genes whose conformation in chromatin render them inaccessible for transcription. The nature of these regulatory factors and the manner in which they interact with specific genes to promote their expression have only recently become accessible to experimental study.

Gene Structure. The DNA sequences that encode for a specific protein are not co-linear with the messenger RNA (mRNA) for that protein. Rather the coding portions of the gene, now called exons, are interrupted by a variable number of introns or intervening sequences of DNA. All functional globin genes studied to date have two introns and therefore three exons, as is diagrammatically shown for the human β globin gene in Figure 141–1. Considering the structure of the gene from left to right (5' to 3'), the first exon encodes for the first 30 amino acids of β globin, the second encodes for the next 74 amino acids, and the last encodes for the remaining 42 amino acids. The smaller intron in the human β globin gene is 130 base pairs in length, whereas the larger is 850 base pairs in length. In general, the α globin genes have a similar structure, although the larger intron is only 150 base pairs long.

Globin mRNA Metabolism. Transcription of the β globin gene to produce its RNA copy probably begins at a point in the DNA that encodes for the 5' end of mature mRNA. The major transcriptional control signals are in the promoter region. Conserved sequences required for accurate and efficient initiation of transcription by RNA polymerase include the "ATA" and "CAT" boxes at 31 and 76 nucleotides before the start site of transcription, respectively, and a duplicated "CACA" box just upstream from "CAT" (Fig. 141–1). Single nucleotide substitutions in these conserved regions have been identified in thalassemia globin genes (Ch. 142); these mutations cause decreased globin gene expression leading to deficient hemoglobin synthesis.

The entire gene, including its two introns, is copied into a co-linear RNA molecule. Transcription continues beyond those sequences represented in globin mRNA. The nucleotide sequence, "AATAAA," serves as a signal for cleavage of the

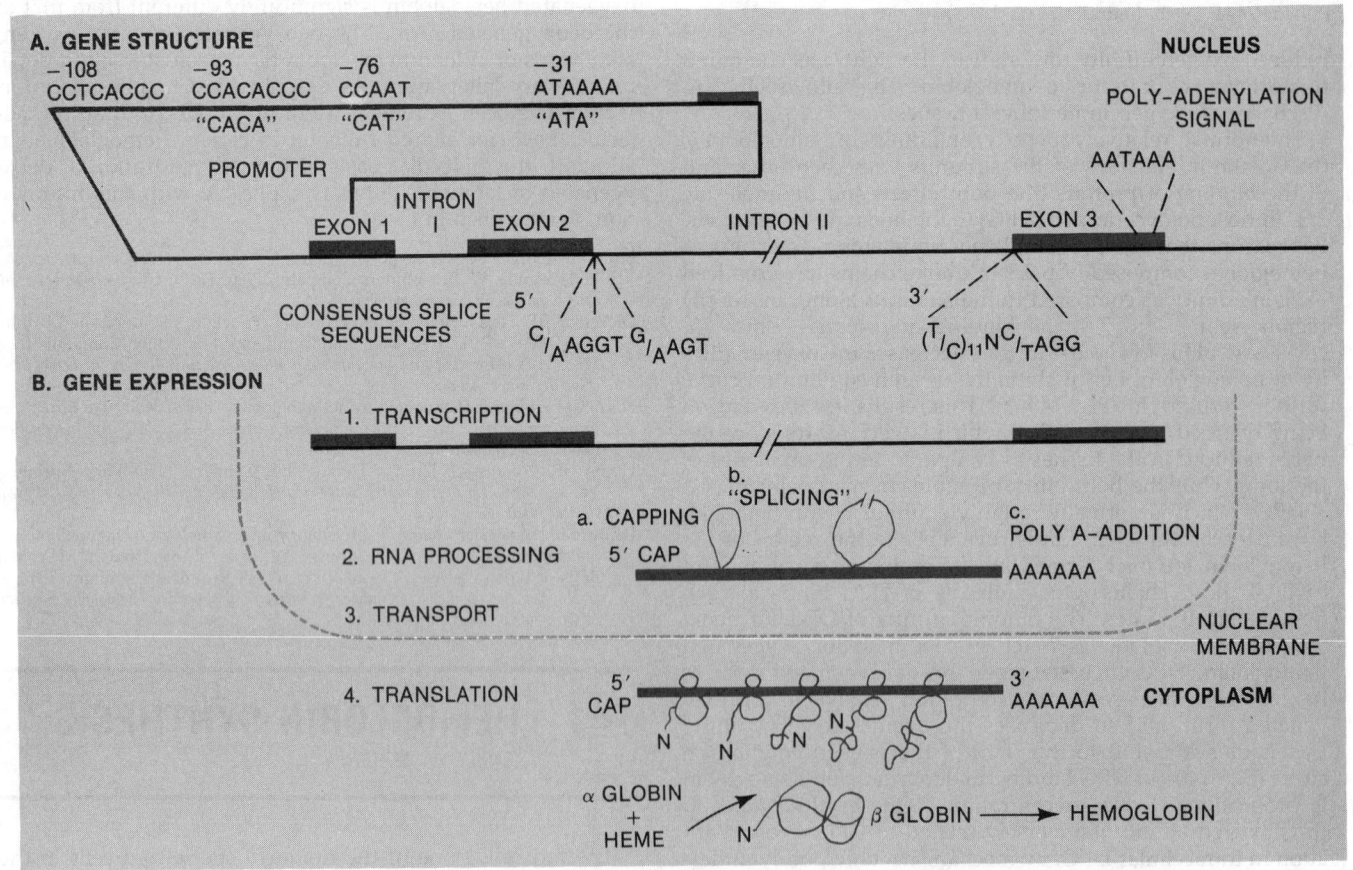

FIGURE 141–1. Structure and expression of the normal human β globin gene. The three exons encode for β globin; these coding sequences are interrupted by two introns or intervening sequences. Certain segments of the promoter region ("boxes") are conserved in many globin genes. The actual sequence of these "boxes" in the β globin gene promoter is shown. The splice sequences shown represent the consensus of those found at many exon-intron boundaries. Those actually found in the β globin gene resemble the consensus sequence but are not identical. C = cytosine, T = thymine, A = adenine, and G = guanine. The processes involved in gene expression include transcription of the gene, processing of the primary RNA transcript, transport of the mRNA from nucleus to cytoplasm, and translation of the mRNA into β globin.

transcription product and addition of a series of adenines to form the poly-A track. The primary transcription product, the β globin mRNA precursor, is a 1600–1700 nucleotide molecule. During transcription, it is also modified at the 5' end by addition of a guanosine diphosphate residue and several methyl groups in a series of reactions referred to as capping (Fig. 141–1).

The DNA sequences found at the exon-intron boundaries, when transcribed into RNA, serve as signals for precise and efficient splicing of the RNA transcript. Comparison of more than 100 exon-intron boundaries has lead to the identification of the consensus splice sequences shown in Figure 141–1. The dinucleotides "GT" and "AG" at the 5' and 3' ends of introns, respectively, are obligatory for functional splicing. The other nucleotides are not invariant and therefore are referred to as *consensus* nucleotides. As discussed in Ch. 142, single nucleotide substitutions in either obligatory or consensus nucleotides at the exon-intron boundaries of thalassemia globin genes cause abnormal RNA splicing, and therefore globin mRNA deficiency. Normally, processing is efficient and rapid; 95 per cent of precursor molecules are thought to become mature mRNA within only a few minutes of their synthesis. Approximately 100 molecules of precursor are present in each erythroblast compared with 20,000 to 50,000 molecules of mRNA.

Globin mRNA Structure. The mature mRNA is 600 to 650 nucleotides in length. Beginning from the cap site, the first 40 to 50 nucleotides represent an untranslated part of the mRNA. The initiation codon (AUG) signals the point at which the beginning of protein synthesis occurs. The next 423 (α) or 438 (β) nucleotides specify the protein sequence of the globin. Next is the terminator or stop codon, UAA in α and β globin mRNA, followed by 80 to 100 nucleotides that make up the 3' untranslated part of the mRNA and then the poly-A track.

The genetic code is the combination of all possible codons that may specify the 20 amino acids that occur in protein. Four nucleotides can be put together in 64 different triplets or codons. The genetic code is degenerate in the sense that all codons are used; each amino acid is specified by more than one codon. Each codon requires a separate transfer RNA (tRNA) to allow it to be translated during protein synthesis.

Protein Synthesis. To translate mRNA into protein, the small and large ribosomal subunits are required along with several protein initiation, elongation, and termination factors and a complement of tRNA molecules. The initiator tRNA carries the amino acid methionine. Protein synthesis begins when this tRNA binds to an initiation factor and then subsequently is bound to the ribosome as specified by its anticodon, TAC, which interacts with the initiator codon. The codon next in line in both human and α and β globin mRNA is GUG, which specifies valine. A tRNA for valine is bound to the ribosome as its anticodon, CAC, recognizes the valine codon in mRNA. A peptide bond is then formed between methionine and valine. The mRNA is then translocated on the ribosome, and the next codon is ready to be read. This series of reactions continues until the terminator codon is encountered, at which point the ribosomal subunits and a completed globin molecule are released from the mRNA by the action of a termination factor. Each mRNA molecule may serve simultaneously as a template for the synthesis of several globin molecules. The protein synthesis mechanism appears to be quite general; no specific factors are required to translate a particular mRNA.

The globins undergo a number of postsynthetic modifications. Removal of the methionine residue, donated by the initiator tRNA, occurs on the polyribosome before synthesis of the globin polypeptide is complete. After assembly into hemoglobin, nonenzymatic glycosylation reactions give rise to a variety of minor electrophoretic variants. The extent of these reactions is proportional to the lifespan of the erythrocyte and to mean blood glucose levels. The major glycosylated form is designated hemoglobin A_{1C}. It has a glucose molecule linked by means of Schiff base to the amino-terminus of the β chain. Since glycosylation varies directly with blood sugar level, measurements of such modified hemoglobins can be used to evaluate control of diabetes mellitus. Perhaps even more important, these modifications of hemoglobin may be the prototype of many other nonenzymatic glycosylation reactions, which could be the pathophysiologic mechanism for damage to various intracellular and extracellular proteins leading to the complications of diabetes mellitus.

IRON ACCUMULATION AND HEMOGLOBIN SYNTHESIS. To obtain the considerable amount of iron required for hemoglobin synthesis, the red cell utilizes membrane receptors specific for the iron transport protein transferrin. The transferrin receptor complex is transiently internalized into the red cell within an endocytic vesicle. The pH within the vesicle is lowered by active ion transport, thereby releasing iron from transferrin. The receptor-apotransferrin complex is then returned to the cell surface, where apotransferrin is released. Synthesis of protoporphyrin is by a series of reactions catalyzed by enzymes found in relatively high concentrations in erythroblasts (see Ch. 203). Excess iron is stored as ferritin and may later become available for heme synthesis or be transferred from erythroid to phagocytic cells in bone marrow.

Nascent or partially completed globin chains may bind heme while still on the polyribosome as soon as that portion of the globin that binds heme is synthesized and folded into an appropriate conformation. The assembly of the individual globins into the hemoglobin tetramer occurs spontaneously by virtue of both their complementary surfaces and their high concentrations within the developing erythroblasts.

Heme has important roles in the process of hemoglobin synthesis in addition to being an essential component of the hemoglobin molecule. Heme deficiency leads to inactivation of a critically required initiation factor, leading to a marked reduction in the rate of protein synthesis. Furthermore, heme may stimulate the synthesis and accumulation of globin mRNA directly and thus may have a regulatory role in modulating globin gene expression.

PRODUCTION OF HEMOGLOBIN DURING ERYTHROBLAST DEVELOPMENT. The erythroblasts in the bone marrow exhibit a series of amplification divisions during which globin mRNA accumulation and hemoglobin synthesis occur (Fig. 141–2). Thus from a very limited number of progenitor stem cells with high proliferative potential are produced a large number of highly specialized but terminally differentiated red cells.

Only 0.1 to 0.5 per cent of the total RNA synthesized in the earliest erythroblasts is globin mRNA, yet the globin mRNA species ultimately represents 95 per cent of the total mRNA present in reticulocytes. This remarkable accumulation of globin mRNA to the exclusion of other mRNA molecules appears to be the result primarily of two factors. First, globin mRNA is remarkably stable during erythroid differentiation. Indeed, there seems to be no degradation of globin mRNA following its synthesis until the reticulocyte stage of maturation. In contrast other mRNA species decay with a half-life of approximately 20 hours and are destabilized to decay even faster toward the end of erythroblast maturation. Also, during the later phases of erythroid maturation, synthesis of other mRNAs declines precipitously, whereas that of globin mRNA appears to continue until just prior to nuclear exclusion. Thus the remarkable stability and the continued synthesis of globin mRNA during all phases of erythroid maturation appear to account for its accumulation to the exclusion of other mRNA species.

MECHANISM OF PRODUCTION OF SPECIFIC HEMOGLOBINS. Fetal red cells contain predominantly Hb F, whereas adult red cells contain Hb A (see Ch. 140). Selective

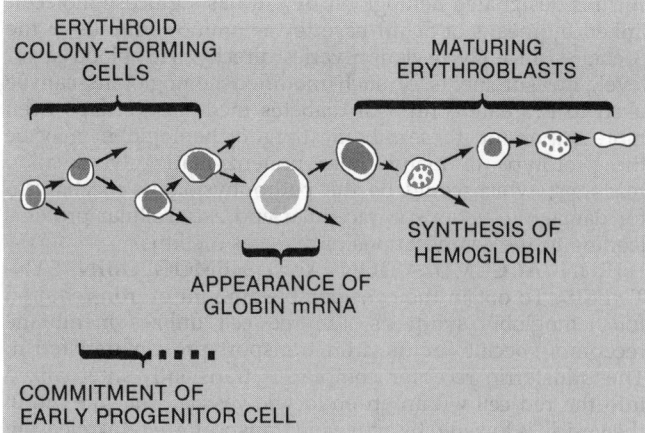

FIGURE 141–2. Regulation of hemoglobin synthesis during erythropoiesis. Two general classes of cells are the precursors of circulating red cells. Erythroblasts at various stages of maturation may be recognized within the bone marrow; these cells and circulating reticulocytes are engaged in hemoglobin synthesis. Erythroid stem cells, the progenitors of erythroblasts, are present within the bone marrow in very small numbers but may be detected by virtue of their ability to form colonies of erythroblasts in semi-solid media in vitro. As discussed in the text, current evidence suggests that commitment to expression of either the γ or β globin genes occurs in erythroid stem cells prior to the initial appearance of globin messenger RNA.

expression of the γ and β genes appears to be modulated at the level of transcription. The precursor to β globin mRNA is present in a lower concentration in fetal erythroblasts than is the precursor to γ mRNA, whereas in adult erythroblasts the β globin mRNA precursor is present in considerably higher concentration than that for γ mRNA. Thus, the pattern of hemoglobin synthesis accurately reflects the relative accumulation of the two mRNA species. Several clues suggest a molecular mechanism(s) that might regulate the transcription of individual globin genes. Nuclease sensitivity studies have shown that the promoter regions of expressed genes are "open" in chromatin, allowing for protein-DNA interactions. The DNA sequences of the promoter region of the individual globin genes are distinctly different, allowing for specific interaction with nonhistone nuclear proteins involved in gene regulation. The frequency of methylation of cytosine residues, a postsynthetic modification of DNA, varies inversely with gene expression and could further alter the interaction of promoter regions with regulatory proteins. Much effort is currently directed at identification of these putative regulatory molecules.

Factors that influence the relative level of expression of individual globin genes appear to be exerted on very primitive erythroid stem cells. Experimental analysis of colonies of erythroblasts formed in vitro indicate that those which develop from the stem cells in fetal liver make Hb F, whereas colonies developing from stem cells in adult bone marrow make predominantly, but not exclusively, Hb A. Thus the primitive stem cells appear to become committed at some very early stage in their differentiation with respect to the pattern of hemoglobin synthesis in their progeny erythroblasts.

Karlsson S, Nienhuis AW: Developmental regulation of human globin genes. Ann Rev Biochem 54:1071, 1985. *A comprehensive review of current knowledge about globin gene structure, expression, and regulation, with particular emphasis on the mechanisms of hemoglobin switching during development.*

Nienhuis A, Wolfe L: The thalassemias: Disorders of hemoglobin synthesis. In Nathan D, Oski F (eds.): Hematology of Infancy and Childhood. 3rd ed. Philadelphia, W. B. Saunders Company (in press). *A detailed account of thalassemic disorders, with a more extensive discussion of gene expression and hemoglobin synthesis than that included here.*

Stamatoyannopoulos G, Papayannopoulou T, Brice M, et al.: Cell biology of hemoglobin switching: I. The switch from fetal to adult hemoglobin formation during ontogeny; Papayannopoulou T, Nakamoto B, Kurachi S,

et al.: Cell biology of hemoglobin switching: II. Studies on the regulation of fetal hemoglobin synthesis in human adults. In Stamatoyannopoulos G, Nienhuis AW (eds.): Hemoglobins in Development and Differentiation. New York, Alan R. Liss, Inc., 1981. *These detailed reviews by major contributors to the problem of hemoglobin switching and erythroid stem cell differentiation should be consulted by those with a serious interest in this topic.*

142 THE THALASSEMIAS
Arthur W. Nienhuis

The thalassemias are hereditary anemias that occur because of mutations that affect the synthesis of hemoglobin. In β thalassemia there is deficient synthesis of β globin, whereas in α thalassemia there is deficient synthesis of α globin. Reduced synthesis of one of the two globin polypeptides leads to deficient hemoglobin accumulation, resulting in hypochromic and microcytic red cells. These red cell abnormalities are the most constant and characteristic features of this group of disorders. Table 142–1 contains a clinical classification of the thalassemias presented in the order in which they will be discussed in this chapter.

The incidence and prevalence of these conditions is highly variable. Most common is thalassemia trait, a mild, clinically insignificant anemia that apparently protects individuals from malaria (see below), and therefore through natural selection it has become extremely common in certain parts of the world. Thalassemia trait generally represents the heterozygous form of either α or β thalassemia. Hence where thalassemia trait is common, homozygous, more severely affected patients will be found frequently. In the United States, the incidence of β thalassemia is highest among ethnic groups originating from the Mediterranean area, parts of Africa, and Asia, whereas the incidence of α thalassemia is highest among those from Asia. Generally the incidence of thalassemia trait in these ethnic groups is 3 to 5 per cent. Approximately 1000 patients with more severe forms of thalassemia are known in the United States.

SEVERE β THALASSEMIA (Cooley's Anemia)

Severe β thalassemia occurs in patients who are homozygous for mutations that lead to a decrease in β globin synthesis. Because both β globin genes are affected, there is marked deficiency in β globin synthesis, but α globin synthesis continues at an approximately normal rate. Accumulation of a large excess of α chains for which there are no β chains with which to combine has several serious deleterious effects. α Globin is highly insoluble and forms large intracellular inclusions. These interfere with the cell cycle in the bone marrow, retard the passage of red cells from the bone marrow, and reduce the survival of red cells in the circulation by virtue of membrane damage and splenic trapping. Marked ineffective erythropoiesis is the hallmark of this disorder because α

TABLE 142–1. CLINICAL CLASSIFICATION OF THE THALASSEMIAS

I. Severe β thalassemia (Cooley's anemia)	Severe anemia, growth retardation, hepatosplenomegaly, bone marrow expansion, and bone deformities
A. Thalassemia major	Transfusion-dependent
B. Thalassemia intermedia	No regular transfusion requirement
II. Thalassemia trait (α or β)	Mild anemia with microcytosis and hypochromia
III. Hb H disease (α-thal)	Moderately severe hemolytic anemia, icterus, and splenomegaly
IV. Hydrops fetalis (α-thal)	Death in utero caused by severe anemia
V. Silent carrier (α or β)	Hematologically normal

inclusions interfere with erythroblast maturation, leading to intramedullary death of many red cell precursors. Severe anemia stimulates erythropoietin production, leading to erythroid stem cell and erythroblast proliferation. The vastly expanded erythroid cell mass results in osteoporosis with a potential for pathologic fractures. Extramedullary hematopoiesis is also often seen, and compression of vital structures, particularly the spinal cord, may occur as a consequence. Because of marrow expansion and bony deformities of the skull and facial bones, patients with severe β thalassemia often have an abnormal appearance with prominent epicanthal folds referred to as a chipmunk facies.

Patients with severe β thalassemia may be divided into two groups on the basis of their requirement for blood transfusion. Those with thalassemia major have an absolute requirement for blood without which severe anemia leads to death in infancy or early childhood. In contrast, patients with thalassemia intermedia are able to maintain their hemoglobin at 6 to 7 grams per deciliter without transfusion. This level is compatible with fairly normal growth and development, and many of these patients survive into adulthood.

Thalassemia Major

CLINICAL FEATURES. At birth patients with thalassemia major are nearly normal hematologically, since γ globin synthesis is normal and Hb F production is therefore adequate. However, as the switch from Hb F to Hb A is completed during the first year of life, the deficiency in β globin production becomes evident. By six to nine months of age, severe anemia reflected by pallor, poor growth, or inadequate food intake leads the anxious parents to bring the infant to the physician, at which time examination reveals the presence of marked hepatosplenomegaly. The hemoglobin may be 3 to 6 grams per deciliter, and the red cells exhibit the characteristic severe microcytosis, hypochromia, and fragmentation (Color plate 2G). Demonstration of thalassemia trait (see below) in both parents is usually sufficient to establish the diagnosis. Study of the infant's blood shows absence of or low Hb A, a large amount of Hb F, and an increase in the amount of Hb A_2 to 4 to 10 per cent of the total (normal <2.5 per cent). Biosynthetic studies, a tool of the research laboratory, may be employed to show the deficiency of β globin production.

CLINICAL COURSE. Prior to the use of regular blood transfusions, these children were grossly deformed because of expansion of the marrow spaces of the skull (see Fig. 130–1). Severe osteoporosis led to pathologic fractures, and anemia caused weakness and inanition. Death by two to three years of age was common. Blood transfusions were initially given infrequently for palliation, but gradually physicians interested in this condition came to recognize that regular transfusion to nearly normal hemoglobin levels could be used to suppress all disease manifestations. Growth and bone development are normal in children who have undergone hypertransfusion, and in fact they are virtually indistinguishable from other children if the hypertransfusion regimen is started at a very early age. If transfusions are given less frequently, the patient may exhibit some stigmata of the untreated disorder—bony deformities, growth retardation, and hepatosplenomegaly.

THE PROBLEM OF IRON OVERLOAD. Because humans have a very limited ability to excrete iron, regular blood transfusions inevitably lead to a vast accumulation. Each unit of packed red cells contains approximately 200 mg of iron, so that by the age of 12 the average thalassemic, having received 125 to 150 units of packed cells, will have accumulated 25 to 30 grams of excess iron. This amount compares to the normal 3 to 4 grams found in adults, 75 per cent of which is present in red cells as hemoglobin. Even in the patient with thalassemia intermedia who has not had transfusions, excess iron absorption leads inevitably to the manifestations of hemochromatosis, although at a later age than in the patient with transfusion-dependent thalassemia. Excess iron deposition occurs in virtually all organs. Most cells have a considerable ability to cope with this extra iron by making ferritin and its partial degradation product hemosiderin. Nonetheless, cell damage occurs by virtue of iron-catalyzed peroxidation of membrane lipids and release of the enzymes from lysosomes rendered labile by their content of hemosiderin granules. Thus tissue hemosiderosis (excess iron) leads ultimately to the clinical condition of secondary hemochromatosis. The liver, endocrine glands, and particularly the heart are the primary target organs (see Ch. 206).

Liver dysfunction is mild in the thalassemic patient with secondary hemochromatosis. Typically the liver is enlarged several centimeters below the right costal margin, and the transaminases are two to four times above the normal limits. Despite a 20- to 30-fold increase in iron concentration over normal, liver biosynthetic function as reflected by the concentration of serum albumin and various clotting factors is preserved. Fibrosis, invariably present on liver biopsy, may progress to frank cirrhosis anatomically, but clinical evidence of cirrhosis is rare.

As noted above, the course of adequately tranfused thalassemic patients is essentially normal until the age of 10 to 12. Then growth failure is a frequent and distressing complication for both the child and parents. The mechanism for this growth failure is not known; growth hormone levels are generally normal, but the serum somatomedin concentration may be low. Failure of growth is accompanied by lack of pubescence. Primary hypogonadism is exceedingly common. The mechanism is usually a failure of the pituitary to produce adequate amounts of FSH and LH. Diabetes mellitus, hypothyroidism, and, rarely, hypoparathyroidism with tetany are additional complications that may occur particularly in patients who are in their late teenage years or early 20's.

Cardiac disease in the patients with severe β thalassemia may take three forms: pericarditis, congestive heart failure, and cardiac arrhythmias. Recurrent attacks of acute pericarditis are manifested by chest pain, often pleuritic and affected by a change of position, accompanied by fever and occasionally a pericardial friction rub. These attacks are usually self-limited, lasting four to seven days. Treatment consists of bed rest, aspirin, and other anti-inflammatory agents such as indomethacin in appropriate doses. Rarely constrictive pericarditis may require a pericardectomy.

Congestive heart failure is to be expected ultimately in patients with secondary hemochromatosis unless death occurs early by virtue of cardiac arrhythmias. Careful echocardiographic studies have suggested that iron deposition begins by the age of five to six years. By ten or twelve years, when the patient has received more than 100 units of blood, left ventricular dysfunction may be demonstrated by radionuclide cineangiography during the physiologic stress of exercise. Clinical congestive heart failure is usually a late complication; most patients die within twelve months of the onset of definite evidence of heart failure. Treatment with digoxin in doses adequate to achieve therapeutic blood levels may be quite helpful. Appropriate use of diuretics and vasodilator therapy may be extremely useful in providing palliation and extending the lifespan of these patients.

Atrial and ventricular ectopy is present in 24-hour electrocardiographic recordings in virtually all patients who have received more than 150 units of packed red cells. High grade ventricular ectopy with couplets, short runs of ventricular tachycardia, and multiple ventricular foci are of ominous prognostic significance. Ectopy may be extremely distressful to the patient, particularly at night when it is often most severe. Tachyrhythmias such as ventricular tachycardia and/or ventricular fibrillation occur despite therapy and are frequent causes of death in patients with severe thalassemia undergoing regular transfusions. The pharmacologic treatment of cardiac arrhythmias is described in Ch. 45.

The prognosis of patients with thalassemia major is determined by the cardiac disease. The average age of death is 17 years, although a few patients may survive to their mid-20's. Because of this grim prognosis, a considerable effort has been focused on attempts to reduce the iron burden in these patients.

THE ROLE OF SPLENECTOMY. Splenic enlargement is frequent and often causes functional hypersplenism as manifested by an increasing transfusion requirement. Careful documentation of the patient's needs will often alert the physician to the development of hypersplenism as the need for blood rises. An average patient on a hypertransfusion regimen designed to maintain the hemoglobin at a level greater than 10 grams per deciliter will require 250 ml of packed cells per kilogram per year. If substantially more blood is required, the spleen should be removed. Leukopenia and thrombocytopenia, if present, are indicators of the presence of hypersplenism and should lead to prompt splenectomy.

The complication of splenectomy in this patient population is a risk of sudden overwhelming sepsis by encapsulated organisms. For this reason delay of splenectomy until after the age of four is highly desirable. Splenectomized patients should receive Pneumovax and may be placed on a regimen of daily penicillin prophylaxis. More important, each patient should be given a small supply of a broad-spectrum antibiotic such as ampicillin to be taken orally in appropriate doses if a high temperature develops and immediate medical attention cannot be obtained.

CHELATION THERAPY. The only drug available for use in removal of iron is deferoxamine (Desferal). This drug has an extremely high affinity for trivalent iron, and despite extensive clinical use it appears to be relatively free of serious toxicity. Its disadvantages are that it must be given parenterally and that it has a very short serum half-life. Thus most drug, given as a single intramuscular injection, is rapidly excreted without binding any iron. To maximize the efficacy of the drug, a technique has been devised to administer it subcutaneously by using a small mechanical infusion pump. A needle is inserted into the subcutaneous tissue of the abdomen, and the drug is infused very slowly over a period of eight to twelve hours. With 1.5 to 2.0 grams of Desferal, two to three times more iron may be removed than by a single daily intramuscular injection. Often daily excretion of 30 to 40 mg of iron may be achieved in older patients and may lead to overall negative iron balance despite continued transfusion therapy, provided that the drug is used at least five times per week. This regimen will retard the rate of iron accumulation in the liver and reduce liver fibrosis.

Clinical evidence indicates that cardiac disease may be delayed. Indeed, reversal of established congestive heart failure with documented left ventricular dysfunction has been observed in patients treated intensively with intravenous deferoxamine. This may be accomplished by placement of a Hickman catheter. Well-motivated patients may be taught to administer the drug daily by the intravenous route in doses of 3 to 4 grams per day given over 18 to 20 hours. Gastrointestinal disturbances and reversible renal dysfunction have been observed. Reduction of dose eliminates these complications. The greatest probability of successfully preventing iron damage is in patients in whom treatment is begun early, preferably by the age of five years. Vitamin C in small doses (150 to 250 mg per day) given orally may increase the amount of iron excretion in response to deferoxamine infusions, although some evidence suggests that this agent may enhance tissue iron toxicity, particularly to the heart, and therefore it should be used with caution in older patients.

Thalassemia Intermedia

Those patients with severe β thalassemia who maintain their hemoglobin levels above 6.0 to 7.0 grams per deciliter have a generally better prognosis. Individual patients with thalassemia intermedia generally have large amounts of Hb F, significant amounts of Hb A_2, and variable amounts of Hb A in their red cells. Iron accumulation may occur because of increased gastrointestinal absorption and ultimately may lead to secondary hemochromatosis with endocrine and cardiac dysfunction, but most patients with thalassemia intermedia survive into adulthood and many have children. Splenectomy may become necessary if evidence of hypersplenism is present. Osteoporosis may be severe, as these patients' erythroid mass is not suppressed. A disabling form of arthritis has been described. Large masses of erythroid tissue in extramedullary sites may cause organ dysfunction. Particularly distressing is spinal cord compression with paraplegia, although usually local radiation will reverse this condition. Any or all of these complications may ultimately lead to the use of a regular transfusion regimen in patients with thalassemia intermedia despite their marginally adequate hemoglobin levels. Such treatment has the added benefit of preventing the disfiguring facial abnormalities.

Genetically this condition is heterogeneous. Often the red cells of both parents exhibit stigmata of thalassemia trait, although frequently one parent may be a silent carrier of the thalassemia gene (see below). In such persons the impairment of β globin synthesis is so mild that the red cells are normal, but when the abnormal β gene is paired with another affected by a more severe β thalassemia mutation, thalassemia intermedia results. Elucidation of any thalassemia mutations at the molecular level has revealed marked quantitative variability ranging from 50 to 100 per cent reduction of β globin mRNA production (see below). Many patients are doubly heterozygous for two different mutations. The clinical heterogeneity of the β thalassemias reflects the many combinations of mutations that may be present in individual patients. Other genetic modifiers of the β thalassemia phenotype include α thalassemia mutations and genetic variants characterized by increased Hb F production. Coinheritance of an α thalassemia gene decreases α globin production leading to partial correction of the highly deleterious imbalance in α and β biosynthesis. Increased γ globin synthesis resulting in increased Hb F production compensates directly for deficient β globin production.

THALASSEMIA TRAIT

CLINICAL CHARACTERISTICS. Common to both α and β thalassemia is a condition referred to as thalassemia minor or trait. This condition generally occurs in individuals who are heterozygous for a mutation affecting α or β globin synthesis (see below). Characteristically the red blood cells are small and contain less hemoglobin than normal; the mean corpuscular volume averages 65 cubic microns (range 56 to 74), whereas the mean corpuscular hemoglobin averages 21 pg (range 20 to 23). Normal values for these parameters are 88 ± 5 and 30 ± 2, respectively. The total red cell count is often increased to 10 to 20 per cent above the normal range, so that anemia, if present, is mild. Rarely the packed cell volume may be as low as 30 per cent; values of 32 to 38 per cent are more typical. Splenomegaly is said to occur but is distinctly unusual, and other causes should be sought if this physical finding is present. No clinical symptoms may be attributed to the presence of thalassemia trait.

DIFFERENTIAL DIAGNOSIS. A characteristic feature of β thalassemia trait is an elevation of the level of Hb A_2. This minor hemoglobin accounts for only 2 or 3 per cent of the total in normal red cells, but in thalassemia trait it may be elevated in the range of 4 to 8 per cent in more than 90 per cent of persons with this condition. Similarly, the level of Hb F is often elevated to 1.5 to 2.5 per cent, although in rare types of thalassemia trait it may be as high as 10 to 15 per cent. In normal red cells, Hb F accounts for less than 1 per cent of the total. The minor hemoglobins, Hb A_2 and Hb F, are either normal or slightly decreased in patients with α thalassemia.

The differential diagnosis of thalassemia trait includes a consideration of iron deficiency. This diagnosis can be excluded only by measurement of the serum iron, total iron binding capacity, and serum ferritin. If these values are normal in patients whose red cells are severely microcytic, but in whom anemia, if present, is mild, the diagnosis of thalassemia trait can be considered established. The distinction between α and β thalassemia depends on the measurement of the minor hemoglobins. If these are normal, the diagnosis of α thalassemia is most likely, although rare subjects with β thalassemia also have normal levels of Hb A_2 and Hb F.

GENE FREQUENCY. Thalassemia trait is thought to protect persons from malaria, particularly during the early years of life when immunity is not yet established and fatal cerebral malaria caused by *Plasmodium falciparum* may occur. This selective advantage accounts for the high frequency of thalassemia genes in regions where malaria has been endemic for the past two millennia. These include the Mediterranean basin particularly, but also large parts of Asia and Africa. The gene frequency may be as high as 20 per cent in certain populations.

HEMOGLOBIN H DISEASE

PATHOPHYSIOLOGY. An anemia of moderate severity characterized by hypochromia, microcytosis, striking red cell fragmentation, and the presence of a fast migrating hemoglobin on electrophoresis occurs in patients who have a moderately severe deficiency in α globin production. The genetics of this condition will be considered later in this chapter. The fast migrating "hemoglobin" has the globin subunit composition β_4. It may account for up to 30 per cent of the total hemoglobin in these patients. Because the β_4 tetramer exhibits no cooperativeness and has an extremely high oxygen affinity, it is functionally useless in oxygen transport. Thus patients with a significant amount of Hb H functionally have a more severe anemia than measurement of the hemoglobin concentration might suggest.

Hb H is an unstable tetramer. Thus as the red cell ages and loses its ability to withstand oxidative stress, Hb H may precipitate, forming inclusions that cause hemolysis. Oxidant drugs such as the sulfonamides may exacerbate hemolysis. Because the β_4 tetramer is soluble during the early phases of the red cell's lifespan, erythropoiesis in the bone marrow is effective and the anemia is generally not as severe as that seen in patients with β thalassemia who have an equivalent impairment in β globin production.

CLINICAL FEATURES. The average patient with Hb H disease maintains gainful employment, marries, and reproduces. Usually the anemia is moderate with a hemoglobin concentration of 7 to 10 grams per deciliter, although occasional patients may have more severe anemia. Moderate splenomegaly is often present. Splenectomy may be considered, but the occurrence of severe postoperative thrombocytosis with a propensity for recurrent pulmonary emboli makes this procedure inadvisable except in patients with unequivocal clinical evidence of hypersplenism as manifested by leukopenia, thrombocytopenia, and a worsening anemia or a transfusion requirement in a previously stable patient. Other therapeutic measures include prescription of folic acid, avoidance of oxidant drugs and iron salts, prompt treatment of infection, and judicious use of transfusions. Acquired Hb H disease has been described as a complication in patients with various forms of myeloproliferative and myelodysplastic disorders. In such patients, treatment and prognosis are related to the primary disorder.

HYDROPS FETALIS

The birth of stillborn infants from parents who both have α thalassemia trait reflects the severest form of α thalassemia.

These infants are grossly edematous or hydropic because of congestive heart failure that occurs as a result of severe anemia. Their failure to produce any α globin results in the production of only Hb Barts (γ_4) and Hb H (β_4) during the later parts of gestation. Both these hemoglobins are nonfunctional in oxygen transport, so that once the embryonic hemoglobins disappear from the circulation early in fetal development, life is no longer possible. A high incidence of toxemia of pregnancy has been noted in mothers of hydropic infants. Prenatal diagnosis of this condition is possible (see below) and should be followed by prompt termination of the pregnancy.

SILENT CARRIER

The silent carrier state was first recognized among the α thalassemia syndromes. One parent of a patient with Hb H disease usually has all the features of α thalassemia trait, whereas the other has normal-appearing red cells with no anemia. Similarly, progeny of persons with Hb H disease fall into two groups: those having α thalassemia trait, and those with apparently normal hemoglobin production. In the silent carrier, the defect in α globin synthesis is so mild that no impairment in hemoglobin synthesis is evident, although when the mutation is paired genetically with a more severe impairment of globin synthesis, e.g., α thalassemia trait, Hb H disease occurs. A similar silent carrier state has also been described among the β thalassemia syndromes. Thalassemia intermedia occurs in those who inherit one thalassemia gene from a silent carrier and a second from a person with thalassemia trait.

THE GENETICS OF THE α THALASSEMIA SYNDROMES

As described in Ch. 140, the α globin genes in humans are duplicated. Thus two genes are found on each chromosome 16, making a total of four in each diploid cell. Four clinical states are seen in α thalassemia: silent carrier, thalassemia trait, Hb H disease, and hydrops fetalis. These conditions occur in persons who have one, two, three, or four α globin genes affected by mutations that reduce α globin synthesis.

The most frequent mutation that leads to α thalassemia is gene deletion. In the silent carrier one of the two genes on one chromosome 16 is missing, whereas the other two genes on the other chromosome 16 are normal. α Thalassemia trait can occur by two mechanisms. Persons who have two chromosomes with only one α gene will exhibit α thalassemia trait. This form is most common in the black population. Hb H disease is distinctly uncommon in this population, since offspring of two persons each of whom is homozygous for the one α gene chromosome can only have α thalassemia trait and not Hb H disease. In the Oriental population, α thalassemia trait occurs most commonly in those who lack both α genes on one chromosome and have the normal two on the other. Mating of such a person with a silent carrier who has one chromosome having only one α gene can lead to children with Hb H disease. Hydrops fetalis occurs among offspring of parents both of whom are heterozygous for chromosomes lacking both normal α globin genes.

In addition to the deletion mutations, many nondeletional types of α thalassemia have been described. Molecular characterization of several has revealed a diversity of defects involving RNA splicing, polyadenylation, mRNA translation, or α globin stability. These mutations are similar to those in β thalassemia globin genes; their effects on RNA metabolism will be discussed in more detail in the next section.

THE MOLECULAR GENETICS OF THALASSEMIA

The β thalassemia mutations may be separated into two classes: β^+ thalassemia, in which there is synthesis of a small amount of normal β globin, and β^0 thalassemia, which in the homozygote is manifested by no β globin production at all.

Similarly, nondeletional types of α thalassemia may abolish (α^0) or decrease (α^+) alpha globin production. Many mutations having specific effects on gene expression have been characterized by molecular cloning, DNA sequencing, and functional characterization. Each of the several steps in RNA metabolism—transcription, processing, transport, and mRNA translation—has been found to be affected by one or more individual mutations. The variable quantitative effect of the individual mutations on globin production has been clarified by these molecular studies.

PROMOTER MUTATIONS. Five globin genes, each of which has a single nucleotide substitution in the promoter region, have been isolated from different individuals with β thalassemia. Three of the mutant genes have substitutions in the "ATA" box (see Fig. 141–1). These mutations reduce promoter function to 20 to 25 per cent of normal, but some β globin mRNA is produced from these genes; hence they cause β^+ thalassemia. The other two promoter mutants characterized to date have substitutions at 86 or 87 nucleotides from the start site for transcription in the first of the conserved "CACA" boxes.

SPLICING MUTATIONS. These are among the most common of mutations that cause thalassemia. Figure 142–1 contains a few illustrative examples classified by the manner in which they affect splicing of the globin mRNA precursor. Mutations that occur within the splice junction sequence decrease or abolish normal splicing at that site and often are accompanied by splicing at other sites that are not normally used. A substitution in the invariant GT, as shown in the example (Fig. 142–1A), abolishes splicing, making this a β^0 gene, whereas substitutions in consensus nucleotides at the splice junction have a quantitative effect on splicing and hence are β^+ mutations.

An interesting class of mutations consists of those that create an alternate site for splicing. These may occur within introns or, as shown in the examples in Figure 142–1B, within coding sequence (exons). These substitutions occur within regions of the precursor RNA molecule that resemble the consensus splice junction sequence (see Fig. 141–1), but lack some critical element necessary for splicing. Nucleotide substitutions that add that element to the potential splice junction sequence lead to its activation, causing abnormal splicing and hence a thalassemic effect. Substitution of A for T in codon 24 of the β globin gene does not alter the amino acid sequence (GGT and GGA both encode for glycine), but creates an alternative splicing site. The other two mutations illustrated in Figure 142–1B (Hb E and Hb Knossos) alter both protein structure and the splicing pattern. Such structural mutants that are also characterized by decreased synthesis are referred to as *thalassemic hemoglobinopathies*.

A class of mutations that has interesting implications for control of splicing is made up of those that create an alternate site and also activate cryptic splice sites remote from the mutation. There is a potential or cryptic splice site in the β globin gene transcript that matches the consensus splice junction sequence nearly perfectly, and yet this site is used rarely if ever during normal splicing. Use of an alternative site, created by a thalassemia mutation, apparently alters the secondary structure of the precursor RNA molecule, leading to splicing at the otherwise cryptic site (Fig. 141–1C).

A POLYADENYLATION MUTATION. The sequence "AATAAA" is one of the signals that leads to cleavage of the globin gene transcript and addition of the poly-A track (see Fig. 142–1). An α thalassemia gene isolated from an individual with Hb H disease has G substituted for A, altering the polyadenylation signal to "AATAGA." Most of the RNA transcript is not processed correctly and is prematurely degraded, although a small amount of normal α globin mRNA is produced by this mutant gene. Thus it is an α^+ thalassemia gene.

MUTATIONS THAT AFFECT mRNA TRANSLATION.

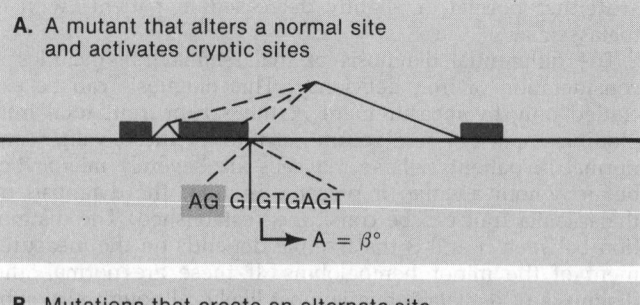

A. A mutant that alters a normal site and activates cryptic sites

AG G GTGAGT

A = β°

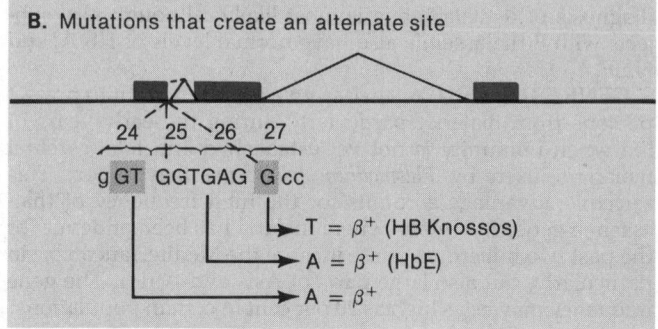

B. Mutations that create an alternate site

24   25   26   27

g GT GGTGAG G cc

T = β^+ (HB Knossos)

A = β^+ (HbE)

A = β^+

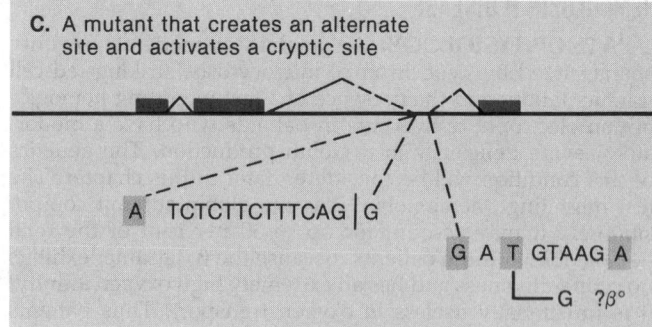

C. A mutant that creates an alternate site and activates a cryptic site

A TCTCTTCTTTCAG G

G A T GTAAG A

G ?β°

FIGURE 142–1. Thalassemia mutations that alter the splicing of the β globin gene transcript. *A*, The nucleotides, guanine (G) and thymine (T), are obligatory for normal splicing. Replacement of the G with adenine (A) abolishes normal splicing and leads to abnormal splicing at otherwise cryptic sites. *B*, Several different mutations at this position in the transcript create an alternate site that leads to abnormal splicing. This segment of the normal transcript includes the obligatory dinucleotide, GT, and matches the consensus sequence in all but the nucleotides in the boxes. Single nucleotide substitutions activate this otherwise inactive site. *C*, A substitution toward the end of intron II creates an alternate splice site. A normally cryptic site further upstream in the intron is also involved in a splicing reaction with exon 2–intron II splice junction, resulting in formation of a processed globin RNA that retains a portion of the sequence transcribed from intron II. Therefore, it cannot be translated into β globin.

Among the more common mutations in thalassemia genes are those that lead to premature termination of mRNA translation. Single nucleotide substitutions or small deletions that alter the mRNA reading frame introduce codons that signal the termination of protein synthesis on the abnormal mRNA. For example, substitution of thymine for cytosine in codon 39 introduces the stop codon UAG at that position. This abnormal β globin mRNA can be read only through codon 38, yielding a small, nonfunctional remnant of β globin. Premature termination mutations cause β^0 (or α^0) thalassemia.

Common mutations that cause α thalassemia are chain termination mutations. As described in Ch. 141, the completed globin molecule is released from the polyribosome when the protein synthetic apparatus encounters the normal terminator codon UAA. A single nucleotide change in this terminator codon will convert it to a codon that is functional for the insertion of any one of several amino acids, depending on the exact nucleotide that is substituted. In this case protein synthesis continues into the part of the mRNA that is usually untranslated, leading to the synthesis of a protein that may be as many as 30 amino acids longer than normal. Such an elongated α globin is found in Hb Constant Spring. This protein accounts for only 1 to 2 per cent of the total α globin in the cells of patients with Hb Constant Spring and their red cells exhibit the stigmata of thalassemia trait.

MUTATIONS THAT AFFECT GLOBIN STABILITY. Certain mutations may alter globin sequence and lead to instability and thus have a thalassemic effect despite a normal rate of synthesis of the mutant globin. Among the more dramatic of this class of mutations is one that leads to substitution of leucine for proline at position 125 of the α globin found in Hb Quong Sze. This mutation was discovered upon sequencing of the abnormal α gene and evidence of α$^{Quong Sze}$ instability was subsequently obtained in vitro. Because of its marked instability, α$^{Quong Sze}$ could not be detected in the red cells of the affected individual. Hb Quong Sze, like Hb E, is another of the thalassemic hemoglobinopathies characterized by both deficient net globin production and a structural abnormality.

DELETION MUTATIONS. Deletions causing α thalassemia have been described earlier. Small deletions that leave one of the two α globin genes intact on a chromosome are classified as α$^+$ mutations, while large deletions that remove both α genes are considered α^0 mutations. In contrast to α thalassemia, in which gene deletion is the most common mutation, gene deletion is rarely the mechanism for β thalassemia. A few patients of Indian ancestry have been found to have a deletion that has removed the 3' half of the β globin gene and a small amount of flanking DNA. A special kind of deletion has resulted in the δβ fusion gene present in a few Italian patients who produce Hb Lepore. An unequal crossover during meiosis has led to the fusion gene that encodes for a globin that has the N-terminal sequence of δ globin and the C-terminal sequence of β globin. This globin is produced in very small amounts; hence this gene leads to thalassemia trait or thalassemia major in heterozygotes or homozygotes, respectively.

Several large deletions that have removed two or more genes from the β cluster have been characterized. The β thalassemia mutations have resulted in loss of the δ and β genes; the $^Aγδβ$ thalassemia deletions include the $^Aγ$ gene in addition. Two interesting forms of γδβ thalassemia have resulted in loss of all but the β gene, and yet this β gene does not function. These observations suggest that the DNA sequences remote from a gene can nonetheless influence its expression. Two deletions have resulted in loss of the entire β-like gene cluster.

MUTATIONS THAT INCREASE Hb F PRODUCTION

About 1 per cent of the hemoglobin in adult blood is Hb F. This fetal hemoglobin is found in 2 to 10 per cent of red cells; these cells—called F cells—contain roughly 4 to 8 pg of Hb F and 24 to 28 pg of adult hemoglobin. As discussed in Chapter 141, these F cells originate during the differentiation of erythroid progenitor cells. F cell number and therefore Hb F levels are genetically determined in man.

Increased Hb F in individuals who are homozygous for β thalassemia mainly reflects amplification of the F cell population. In the bone marrow, those erythroblasts producing small amounts of γ globin have less of an excess in α globin synthesis and therefore are more likely to survive and leave the bone marrow. By this mechanism, the 1 per cent of γ synthesis in the bone marrow cell population may be amplified 10- to 40-fold in the peripheral blood. Of more interest from the aspect of gene control are those mutations that alter Hb F production by genetic mechanisms.

There are two general classes of deletion mutations that increase Hb F production in adults. The δβ thalassemia mutations are characterized by production of 5 to 12 per cent of Hb F in heterozygotes, while *hereditary persistence of fetal hemoglobin* (HPFH) deletion mutations are characterized by production of 25 to 30 per cent. Most of the red cells in

heterozygous individuals with HPFH contain Hb F, whereas heterozygotes with δβ thalassemia mutations have Hb F in only 25 to 30 per cent of their red cells. These mutations have been carefully characterized structurally in an attempt to define the basis at the DNA level for these differing phenotypes. Twenty-eight mutations have been studied, but no common patterns have emerged, with one exception. Deletions that remove the left side of the cluster (ε and γ genes) also inactivate the remaining intact β gene, whereas deletions that remove the right-hand portion of the cluster (δ and β genes) increase expression of the remaining γ globin genes. Removal of sequences within the cluster that normally modulate gene expression or movement of "activating" sequences into the cluster by virtue of deletion are other possible mechanisms that may lead to increased Hb F production as a consequence of these deletions.

Another category of mutations that cause HPFH leave the β-like gene cluster intact and therefore are referred to as *nondeletion mutations*. Nondeletion HPFH mutations are characterized by a heterogeneous distribution of Hb F in red cells (heterocellular) in contrast to the pancellular distribution of Hb F in heterozygotes with the deletion types of HPFH. There may be many different heterocellular HPFH mutations; genetic studies indicate that at least some are not linked to the β-like gene cluster. Five different point mutations within the γ globin gene promoter region have been discovered in individuals with nondeletion HPFH.

PRENATAL DIAGNOSIS

Because of the serious consequences of severe β thalassemia (Cooley's anemia), prenatal diagnosis of this condition with subsequent therapeutic abortion is thought by many to be highly desirable. Two general strategies have made this a feasible undertaking. The first approach is based on the fact that small amounts of β globin synthesis may be detected in the early mid-trimester fetus (see Ch. 140). In fetuses who have inherited two genes for β thalassemia, no β globin or very small amounts are produced at a time when normal fetuses are producing approximately 10 per cent β globin. By using sophisticated obstetric techniques, blood may be obtained from the umbilical vein and used for biosynthetic measurements of the globin synthetic pattern. Absence of or low β globin synthesis occurs in homozygous fetuses, whereas intermediate levels are found in heterozygotes. This strategy has been widely applied in parts of Greece and Italy and has led to a significant reduction in the incidence of the severe form of β thalassemia in certain populations.

A second strategy for prenatal diagnosis relies on the study of DNA prepared from amniotic fluid cells of potentially affected persons. The globin genes in such DNA samples may be characterized by the techniques referred to as restriction endonuclease mapping. The DNA is digested with an enzyme that cuts at a specific nucleotide sequence. Among the million or so fragments generated from human DNA are those few that include the globin genes. The DNA is resolved electrophoretically, transferred to a nitrocellulose paper, and annealed to a radioactive probe specific for globin gene sequences. Depending on the enzyme used, a characteristic set of fragments containing globin gene sequences is generated. In persons who have inherited a mutation reflected by deletion of all or part of a globin gene, a change in a position of a particular fragment will serve to indicate the presence of such a mutation. Many cases of α thalassemia and rare cases of β thalassemia may be diagnosed in this way.

More widely applicable to the prenatal diagnosis of thalassemias are so-called restriction enzyme polymorphisms. A single nucleotide change, in an area within or remote from the globin gene, may result in loss of a restriction endonuclease site and therefore a change in the migration position of a particular fragment containing globin gene sequences. Such a polymorphism, in Hpa I site, was first described by

Kan (1978) in individuals who had inherited the gene for sickle hemoglobin. Other polymorphisms have been discovered and have been found useful for diagnosis of β thalassemia. The unique association or linkage of the Hpa I polymorphism with the β^s gene is unusual; most polymorphisms occur in association with both normal and abnormal β globin genes. Hence a different method of analysis is required rather than simple characterization of a single restriction endonuclease site.

Several restriction endonuclease sites—each of which is polymorphic, either present (+) of absent (−)—may be used to define the haplotype of the β globin gene region on a specific chromosome. Eighty to 90 per cent of the time a single mutation is associated or linked to a single set of restriction endonuclease polymorphisms, a single haplotype. Once the haplotype associated with a particular mutation in an ethnic group is known, haplotype analysis may be used to define the frequency of that mutation in that group. The normal β globin gene is found linked to all haplotypes. Hence, simple haplotype analysis cannot be used for prenatal diagnosis directly. Extensive family studies or study of DNA from an affected or completely normal child is necessary before haplotype analysis can be applied for prenatal diagnosis in that family.

An alternative approach utilizing DNA analysis for prenatal diagnosis is now feasible because several frequent mutations have been defined by DNA sequencing. Synthetic oligonucleotide probes, one specific for the normal gene and one specific for a particular abnormal gene, can be used to discriminate between the normal and abnormal genes in amniotic fluid DNA. This method is simple and direct but requires that several probes be available for each of the mutations that occur frequently in the population for whom prenatal diagnosis is offered. Technical innovations to increase sensitivity and specificity and the ready synthesis of specific probes will undoubtedly make this the method of choice for prenatal diagnosis in the future.

The application of prenatal diagnosis requires appropriate screening and identification of persons at risk. Thalassemia trait can usually readily be identified by virtue of the morphologic changes in the red cells. Confirmation of the diagnosis depends on measurement of hemoglobin A$_2$ and Hb F.

EXPERIMENTAL THERAPY

Knowledge of globin gene structure and regulation has suggested a means to activate the structurally normal but inactive γ globin genes in individuals with severe β thalassemia. Increased γ globin synthesis is desirable because it partially compensates for the deficiency of β globin production and decreases the relative excess of α globin. DNA is modified after synthesis by methylation of cytosine residues. Expressed genes are relatively undermethylated compared to unexpressed DNA sequences. For example, the γ globin genes are undermethylated in fetal erythroid cells, but after the switch to adult hemoglobin synthesis the γ globin genes are fully methylated in adult erythroid cells. 5-Azacytidine* inhibits DNA methylation and has been shown to activate genes in tissue culture cells and in experimental animals. Administration of 5-azacytidine to patients with severe β thalassemia under defined experimental protocols has resulted in increased γ globin synthesis and improvement in red cell production and survival. The effect is transient, lasting only two to three weeks. Reluctance to administer a potentially carcinogenic and toxic drug for longer periods has limited the use of 5-azacytidine to experimental studies of a few severely affected patients. Nonetheless these encouraging results have prompted a search for other effective and less toxic drugs that may make pharmacologic stimulation of the γ globin genes a useful approach for treatment of severe β thalassemia.

*Available from the National Cancer Institute.

Cure of severe β thalassemia can be achieved by bone marrow transplantation from an HLA-identical, unaffected sibling. Several patients have already been cured by this method. This procedure carries a 10 to 40 per cent risk of death or significant graft-versus-host disease (GVHD). Transplantation in infancy, preferably before transfusions are given, increases the probability of successful engraftment and reduces the risk of this disease. However, adequate transfusion therapy and effective chelation may provide 20 or more years of good-quality life for newborns. Thus, the availability of bone marrow transplantation raises a significant ethical dilemma for parents and physicians. In the future, refinements in the treatment of GVHD and transplantation techniques may permit wider application of bone marrow transplantation as treatment for patients with severe β thalassemia.

Insertion of intact globin genes into the bone marrow cells of patients with severe forms of thalassemia has become a feasible research objective. Gene transfer mediated by retroviral vectors is highly efficient and has resulted in the insertion and expression of genes in experimental animals. Many problems remain to be overcome before this strategy becomes clinically feasible, however.

Alter BP: Antenatal diagnosis of thalassemia: A review. Ann NY Acad Sci 445:393, 1985. *A comprehensive description of the methods and results of prenatal diagnosis and its impact on the incidence of severe β thalassemia.*

Ley TJ, Griffith P, Nienhuis AW: Transfusion hemosiderosis and chelation therapy. Clin Haematol 11:437, 1982. *This detailed review describes the pathogenesis of transfusional hemochromatosis and summarizes evidence related to the beneficial effects achieved with chelation therapy.*

Nienhuis AW, Ley TJ, Humphries RK, et al.: Pharmacological manipulation of fetal hemoglobin synthesis in patients with severe beta-thalassemia. Ann NY Acad Sci 445:198, 1985. Ley TJ, Nienhuis AW: Induction of hemoglobin F synthesis in patients with beta thalassemia. Ann Rev Med 36:485, 1985. *Reviews of the results achieved by using drugs in an effort to stimulate fetal hemoglobin synthesis for therapeutic benefit in patients with thalassemia.*

Nienhuis AW, Wolfe L: The thalassemias: Disorders of hemoglobin synthesis. In Nathan DG, Oski F (eds.): Hematology of Infancy and Childhood. Philadelphia, W. B. Saunders Company (in press). *This chapter contains a more detailed exposition of the thalassemia syndromes with a comprehensive account of molecular basis of these disorders and current status of prenatal diagnosis.*

Orkin SH, Kazazian HH Jr, Antonarakis SE, et al.: Linkage of β thalassemia mutations and β globin gene polymorphisms with DNA polymorphisms in human β globin gene cluster. Nature 296:627, 1983. Trisman R, Orkin SH, Maniatis T: Specific transcription and RNA splicing defects in five cloned β thalassemia genes. Nature 302:591, 1983. *These are two classic papers that describe strategies used to identify mutations, to determine their frequencies in populations in which thalassemia genes are common, and to characterize these mutations as to their functional consequences.*

Thomas ED, Sanders JE, Buckner CD, et al.: Marrow transplantation for thalassemia. Ann NY Acad Sci 445:417, 1985. Lucarelli G, Polchi P, Izzi T, et al.: Marrow transplantation for thalassemia after treatment with busulfan and cyclophosphamide. Ann NY Acad Sci 445:428, 1985. *Two papers that represent accounts by leaders in this field of efforts to use bone marrow transplantation to achieve a permanent cure in patients with severe β thalassemia.*

Weatherall DJ, Clegg JB: The Thalassemia Syndromes. 3rd ed. Oxford, Blackwell Scientific Publications, Ltd, 1981. *This superb monograph describes the clinical aspects, genetics, and interactions of the various thalassemia syndromes. It should be consulted by anyone with a serious interest in thalassemia.*

143 SICKLE CELL ANEMIA AND ASSOCIATED HEMOGLOBINOPATHIES

Bernard G. Forget

DEFINITION. The sickle cell syndromes are due to the inheritance of a gene for a structurally abnormal β-globin chain subunit of adult hemoglobin, the β^s-chain of Hb S ($\alpha_2\beta^s_2$). The structural abnormality of the β^s-globin chain consists of a single amino acid substitution or replacement: valine instead of the normal glutamic acid at position number 6 of the β-polypeptide chain. Hb S can be found in the heterozygous state (Hb AS or sickle cell trait), in the homozygous state (Hb SS, sickle cell anemia, or sickle cell disease), in association with other structural hemoglobin variants (i.e., Hb SC and SD disease), in association with β-thalassemia (Hb S/β-thalassemia or sickle/β-thalassemia syndromes), or in association with the thalassemia-like disorder termed hereditary persistence of fetal hemoglobin (Hb SF or Hb S/HPFH). The structural abnormality of Hb C, a nonsickling hemoglobin, also consists of a single amino acid substitution at residue number 6 of the β-globin chain: in the β^C-chain lysine replaces glutamic acid. Clinical syndromes associated with the inheritance of Hb C include Hb SC disease and homozygous Hb C disease.

PREVALENCE AND GENETICS. The sickle cell syndromes are particularly prevalent in black persons of African or Afro-American ancestry. However, the gene is also found at a lower frequency in persons of Mediterranean ancestry (southern Italians, Sicilians, and Greeks), in Saudi Arabia, and in India. The highest gene frequencies occur in equatorial Africa, in the so-called malaria belt. The heterozygous state for Hb S (sickle cell trait) probably confers a biologic advantage against infection with falciparum malaria, and for this reason the gene frequency for Hb S has achieved high levels through natural selection in geographic areas of endemic malaria. In the United States the prevalence of the sickle cell trait in blacks is 8 to 10 per cent and the number of homozygous persons approaches 50,000, or 1 in 400 births. In certain areas of western Africa (Ghana and Nigeria), the prevalence of Hb AS can reach 25 to 30 per cent. The prevalence of Hb AC in black Americans is approximately 3 per cent. Gene-mapping studies, using restriction endonuclease analysis of cellular DNA to identify polymorphisms of nucleotide sequence in the DNA around the β^s globin gene, have disclosed an unexpected heterogeneity of polymorphisms linked to the sickle β-globin genes in different individuals, suggesting multiple independent origins of the sickle gene.

PATHOPHYSIOLOGY. Disease in the sickle syndromes results from aggregation or polymerization of Hb S molecules inside erythrocytes, which causes (1) chronic compensated hemolytic anemia, (2) chronic and progressive tissue and organ damage, and (3) acute painful vaso-occlusive crises. These clinical phenomena are directly related to the physicochemical behavior of the intracellular Hb S molecules and result from alterations of red cell rheology and, possibly, changes in the red cell membrane.

The polymerization process occurs only when the Hb S molecule is in the deoxy conformation (see Ch. 140). When Hb S is in the oxy conformation it has essentially normal physicochemical properties. In the deoxy conformation, Hb S molecules can aggregate with one another into long polymers and are aligned to form a gel of liquid crystals that are also called tactoids. The polymerization process goes through a number of stages, as illustrated diagrammatically in Figure 143–1. In the process of nucleation, Hb S molecules form small aggregates, which then grow by addition of successive Hb S molecules. The larger aggregates then align themselves to form linearly arranged fibers that constitute a paracrystalline gel. These fibers can be detected as helical electron-dense tube-like structures by electron microscopy (Fig. 143–1). The end result of the polymerization process is the transformation of the intracellular contents of the red cell from a fluid liquid to a viscous gel. The amount of Hb S polymer within red cells increases progressively as the percentage of oxygen saturation of the hemoglobin decreases. The viscous polymer decreases the flexibility of the erythrocyte and thus impairs its transit through the microcirculation. When the amount of polymer

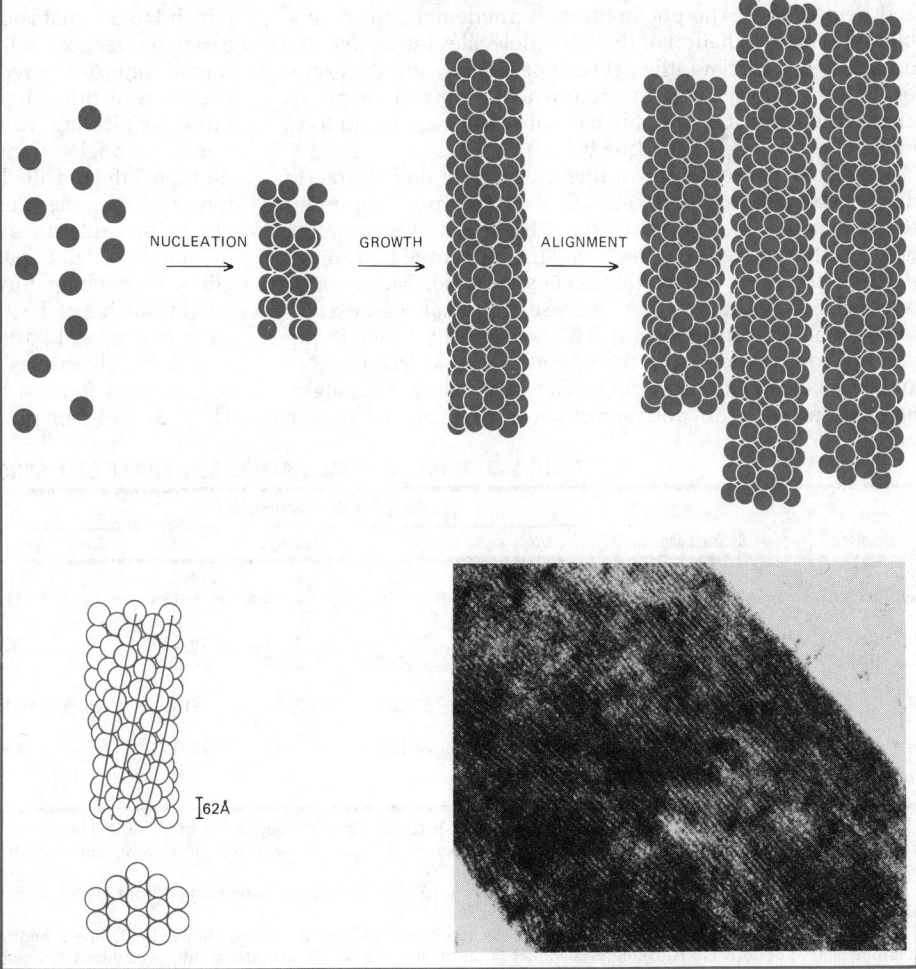

FIGURE 143–1. *Top,* Schematic representation of mechanism of deoxyhemoglobin S polymerization. Each circle represents a deoxyhemoglobin S tetramer: $\alpha_2\beta_2^s$. *Lower left,* Molecular model, based on electron microscopy, of the helical arrangement of deoxyhemoglobin S tetramers in a fiber of polymerized Hb S molecules; side view (above) and cross section or end-on view (below). *Lower right,* Electron micrograph (longitudinal section) of deoxyhemoglobin S gel in a sickled erythrocyte.

NUCLEATION   GROWTH   ALIGNMENT

62A

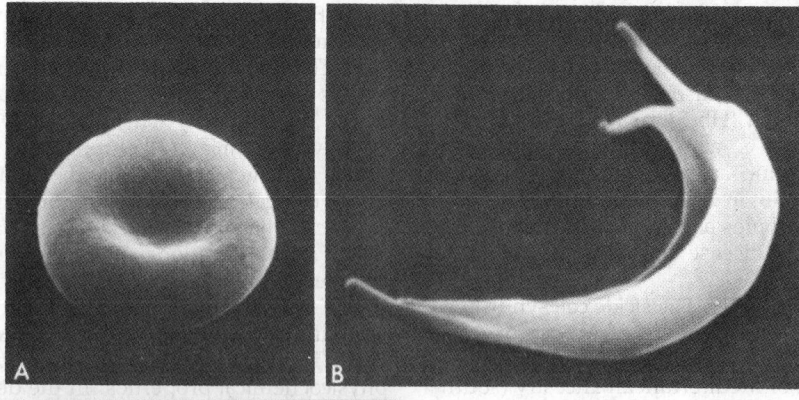

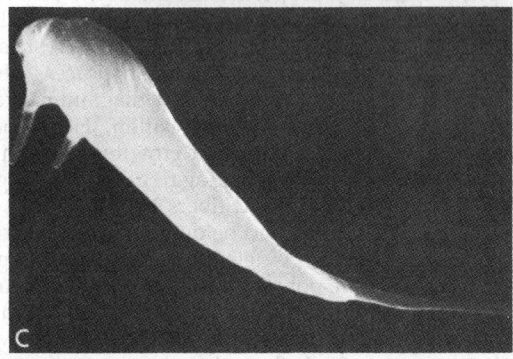

FIGURE 143–2. Scanning electron micrographs of oxygenated (A) and deoxygenated (B and C) SS erythrocytes. (Courtesy of Dr. James White.)

is sufficiently high, the red cells may assume the typical sickle or holly leaf shape associated with sickled erythrocytes (Fig. 143–2). The shape change of the erythrocyte is a passive phenomenon in which the red cell membrane conforms to the shape that is assumed by the intracellular gel of polymerized hemoglobin. The polymerization phenomenon is reversible: With reoxygenation of the Hb S molecules the aggregated molecules disassociate, the gel becomes liquid, and the erythrocyte, if it has sickled, can return to its normal shape, as long as the red cell membrane has not become altered to form an irreversibly sickled cell (see below).

A number of factors can influence the rate and degree of Hb S aggregation in red cells. One of the most important determinants is the concentration of Hb S and of total hemoglobin within the red cell. In general the higher the percentage of Hb S, the more severe the sickle syndrome. Factors such as cellular dehydration that increase the mean corpuscular hemoglobin concentration (MCHC) will greatly facilitate polymerization by increasing the opportunity and frequency of contact between Hb S molecules. The importance of hemoglobin concentration on polymerization is underscored by the

clinical observation that the coinheritance of α-thalassemia together with sickle cell anemia is generally (but not universally) associated with less severe hemolysis. The milder clinical course of Hb S/β-thalassemia is also thought to be due in part to the associated hypochromia. The length of time during which Hb S remains deoxygenated is also very important; Hb S polymerization will be enhanced with any increase in the transit time of the red cell through the microcirculation. The presence of other hemoglobins within the red cell can also influence sickling. In general, at a constant MCHC, any other non-S hemoglobin molecules in the red cell, by a simple dilution effect, will decrease the opportunity of contact between Hb S molecules. In addition, the type of non-S hemoglobin present can differentially affect polymerization: Fetal hemoglobin (Hb F) participates much less readily than normal Hb A in polymer formation, whereas certain mutant hemoglobins such as Hb O Arab and Hb D, although nonpolymerizing per se, will participate in gelation more readily than Hb A. Hb SC disease is associated with a more severe clinical course than is seen in sickle cell trait for two reasons: (1) There is a higher proportion of Hb S in SC than in AS cells

TABLE 143–1. DIFFERENTIAL DIAGNOSIS OF SICKLE CELL SYNDROMES

Genotype	Clinical Condition	Hemoglobin Electrophoresis Findings					Other Associated Findings
		Hb A	Hb S	Hb A$_2$	Hb F	Hb C	
AS	Sickle cell trait	55–60%	40–45%*	2–3%	~1%	—	Asymptomatic; no anemia
SS†	Sickle cell anemia	0	85–95%	2–3%	5–15%	—	Usually clinically severe; Hb F distributed heterogeneously among red blood cells
S/β⁰-thal	Sickle cell/β-thalassemia	0	70–80%	3–5%	10–20%	—	Moderate severity; splenomegaly in over half of the cases; Hb F distributed heterogeneously among red blood cells; hypochromia and microcytosis
S/β⁺-thal	Sickle cell/β-thalassemia	10–20%	60–75%	3–5%	10–20%	—	
SC‡	Hb SC disease	0	45–50%	2–3%	~1%	45–50%	Moderate severity; splenomegaly; many target cells on blood smear
SF (S/HPFH)	Sickle/hereditary persistence of fetal hemoglobin	0	70–80%	1.5–2%	20–30%	—	Uniform distribution of Hb F among all red cells; asymptomatic; no anemia

*Persons with associated α-thalassemia trait have lower levels of Hb S, usually in the range of 26 per cent. The finding of a (nonsickling) hemoglobin with the mobility of Hb S but in much lower amounts (5 to 15 per cent) is suggestive of the Hb Lepore trait (see Ch. 142). Hypochromia and microcytosis are usually associated with these conditions.

†Hb SD disease gives similar electrophoretic findings at pH 8.6, but can be distinguished from Hb SS disease by hemoglobin electrophoresis in citrate agar at pH 6.1.

‡Hb S–O Arab and Hb SE diseases give similar electrophoretic findings at pH 8.6, but can be distinguished from Hb SC disease by hemoglobin electrophoresis in citrate agar at pH 6.1. Hb A$_2$ comigrates with Hb C at pH 8.6 and can be quantitated only by column chromatography.

(Table 143–1); and (2) cells containing Hb C have a higher than normal MCHC, thus facilitating Hb S polymerization. Finally, acidosis can enhance polymerization by decreasing oxygen affinity (see Ch. 140) and thereby increasing the amount of deoxy Hb S in the red cell.

The polymerization phenomenon results in two major red cell disturbances. The first relates to the flow properties of red cells containing substantial amounts of polymerized Hb S. Such cells are much less deformable than normal red cells, and their flow through the microcirculation is greatly retarded. A second major disturbance is damage to the red cell membrane as a result of repeated episodes of aggregation and melting of Hb S polymers. Sickle red cells are "leaky." They tend to lose K^+ and water and eventually become dehydrated, the resulting increase in MCHC probably enhancing further polymerization. The red cell membrane becomes altered in other ways such that it may assume a rigid, abnormal conformation, thus forming an irreversibly sickled cell (or ISC), even when the hemoglobin is not in the aggregated state. As a result of the intracellular polymerization of Hb S, of the increase in MCHC, and of the membrane changes, the red cells become rigid and are sequestered and prematurely destroyed within the reticuloendothelial system. This series of events constitutes the basis for the shortened red cell survival and hemolytic anemia that invariably accompany sickle cell anemia. Occlusion of the microvasculature by viscous erythrocytes leads to ischemia and eventual infarction of the tissue downstream from the obstruction, results in organ damage, and may be the cause of the characteristic painful "crises."

CLINICAL MANIFESTATIONS. *Sickle Cell Trait.* Persons who are heterozygous for Hb S are essentially asymptomatic. They should not have any anemia attributable to the hemoglobinopathy. Any anemia in such persons should be investigated for other secondary causes. Symptoms resulting from vaso-occlusion occur only in extreme circumstances of severe hypoxia such as flying in unpressurized aircraft. However, a universal finding in sickle cell trait is microinfarction of the renal medulla presumably owing to the ambient hyperosmolarity that is thought to lead to dehydration of the red cells, an increased MCHC, and sickling; as a result, in affected persons the urine is unconcentrated and isosthenuria is manifested. Painless hematuria can also occasionally be attributed to microinfarction of the renal medulla, although the other usual causes should be ruled out before painless hematuria in persons with sickle cell trait is attributed to the sickling phenomenon.

Sickle Cell Disease. THE ANEMIA. Patients homozygous for Hb S invariably have a chronic compensated hemolytic anemia of variable severity. In general the hematocrit ranges between 20 and 30 per cent and the hemoglobin between 6.5 and 10 grams per deciliter. The hemolysis is compensated by increased erythropoiesis manifested as an elevated reticulocyte count in the range of 10 to 25 per cent. Mild jaundice and indirect hyperbilirubinemia are also present as a reflection of the hemolysis. The degree of the anemia is usually stable in a given patient, although occasional hypoplastic or aplastic crises can occur owing to suppression of erythropoiesis at the time of infectious episodes and result in a rapid decrease in the reticulocyte count and a precipitous drop in the hemoglobin and hematocrit levels. Infection with a particular parvovirus has been implicated in the pathogenesis of aplastic crises. Another cause of rapid worsening of the anemia is the acute splenic sequestration crisis (a sudden pooling of large volumes of blood in the spleen) that can occur in younger patients with sickle cell anemia before autoinfarction of the spleen or in older patients with Hb SC disease and Hb S/β-thalassemia in whom the spleen is not infarcted and may in fact be enlarged. There is some controversy whether or not a hyperhemolytic state can be associated with sickle cell anemia. From what is known of the basis for the hemolysis in this condition, there is no pathophysiologic mechanism for varia-

ble or accelerated hemolysis resulting from sickling alone. In general, the anemia and hemolysis in sickle cell disease do not increase or worsen during vaso-occlusive painful crises. If hemolysis suddenly worsens, one should look to other secondary causes that may be responsible, such as an associated glucose-6-phosphate dehydrogenase deficiency and exposure to an oxidant stress from drugs or an acute infection. Finally, in patients with marginal nutritional status and increased requirements, such as during pregnancy, folic acid deficiency can develop and aggravate the anemia—the so-called megaloblastic crisis of sickle cell disease.

VASO-OCCLUSIVE CRISES. The major disabilities suffered by patients with sickle cell anemia are related to painful vaso-occlusive crises and to secondary end-organ damage as a direct consequence of the sickling phenomenon and occlusion of the microvasculature of one or another organ, most commonly the bones of the trunk and extremities. The episodes are characterized by sudden onset of excruciating pain in the back, chest, or extremities. There is frequently no identifiable precipitating event, although infections may be associated with the onset of the episode. Other predisposing factors include dehydration, acidosis, or increased hypoxia as during a pulmonary infection. A low grade fever may be associated with the painful attacks, although not necessarily. In general, the onset of fever will occur one or two days after the onset of pain and will parallel the degree of tissue necrosis resulting from the ischemic infarction. The painful attacks last for variable periods, ranging from a few hours to a few days depending on the extent of the vaso-occlusive phenomenon and the rapidity with which treatment is initiated and is successful in reversing the occlusive episode. In general there are no external signs such as heat, swelling, or tenderness of the soft tissues over the affected bones. However, if the bone infarction occurs in proximity to a joint, an effusion can develop. Bone infarction may be difficult to differentiate from osteomyelitis, and definitive diagnosis of the latter must ultimately rely on positive bacterial cultures from aspirated material.

When the vaso-occlusive process occurs in the vasculature (including large vessels) of organs other than bones, the clinical manifestations are primarily related to damage of the affected organ. Common acute vaso-occlusive clinical syndromes include cerebrovascular accidents (i.e., hemiplegia and seizures) caused by involvement of the cerebral vasculature; the acute chest syndrome associated with occlusion of the pulmonary vessels, which can be difficult to differentiate from acute pulmonary infarction caused by emboli or from acute pulmonary infections; hepatic crisis, with marked hyperbilirubinemia and other abnormal liver function tests, which can be difficult to differentiate from acute hepatitis or choledocholithiasis; priapism resulting from vaso-occlusion within the corpus cavernosum; and acute renal papillary infarction with hematuria and/or obstruction of the urinary collecting system.

More chronic complications include refractory skin ulcers of the leg, usually in the vicinity of the medial malleolus, an area that has poor collateral circulation; and variable degrees of renal insufficiency resulting from the combination of repeated infarctions and infectious episodes. All patients manifest the inability to concentrate the urine and have isosthenuria. Microinfarction in the peripheral retina is initially asymptomatic, but may lead to the formation of new blood vessels that are fragile and can hemorrhage, causing retinal detachment and blindness. For this reason periodic eye examinations are important to recognize and treat the early asymptomatic lesion before it progresses to the point of causing visual disturbances. Finally, repeated bone infarcts in the vicinity of joints can lead to secondary degenerative arthritis, and gradual infarction of the head of the femur results in aseptic necrosis of the hip.

OTHER CLINICAL MANIFESTATIONS. Clinical manifestations of

sickle cell anemia not directly related to the sickling phenomenon include increased susceptibility to infections, cholelithiasis, and abnormal growth and development. The increased susceptibility to infections is probably related at least in part to absence of splenic function and in some cases to an abnormality of the properdin opsonization pathway. In early childhood, septicemia and meningitis caused by encapsulated organisms such as *Streptococcus pneumoniae* and *Hemophilus influenzae* are common. In later life common infectious episodes include recurrent pneumonias, urinary tract infections, and osteomyelitis. The predisposition to osteomyelitis is probably related to the repeated bone infarcts that can form a nidus for infection. Although osteomyelitis caused by *Salmonella* occurs almost exclusively in patients with sickle cell anemia or one of the other sickle cell syndromes, *Staphylococcus aureus* is still the most common causative organism of osteomyelitis in these syndromes.

Cholelithiasis is very common, and can be manifested at a young age; it is caused by the chronic hemolysis that results in increased bilirubin production. Episodes of cholecystitis and choledocholithiasis can easily be confused with abdominal and hepatic sickle cell crises. The causes of delayed growth and development are poorly understood. Delayed puberty can result in late closure of the epiphyses and an asthenic habitus.

SICKLE/β-THALASSEMIA AND HB SC DISEASE. The anemia and the hemolysis are less severe in the other sickle syndromes, such as Hb SC disease and sickle/β-thalassemia, in which there is somewhat less propensity for sickling than in homozygous Hb SS disease. The degree of anemia is strongly related to the extent of intracellular Hb S polymerization. In these conditions the anemia frequently ranges between hemoglobin levels of 10 and 12 grams per deciliter, and the reticulocyte counts are usually less than 10 per cent, frequently in the range of 5 per cent.

In general the vaso-occlusive manifestations resulting from sickling are also less frequent and less severe in Hb SC disease and in sickle/β-thalassemia than in sickle cell anemia, although all of the complications previously described for sickle cell anemia can also occur in these conditions. However, in contrast to sickle cell anemia, splenomegaly in adults is usually present in these syndromes, and splenic infarcts and acute splenic sequestration crises can occur. The ocular complications of sickling also tend to occur more frequently in Hb SC disease than in sickle cell anemia and can in fact be the presenting symptoms. There is also increased frequency of aseptic necrosis of the femoral head in Hb SC disease. Sickle/β⁰-thalassemia, in which Hb A is totally absent, is generally more severe than sickle/β⁺-thalassemia and can be as clinically severe as sickle cell anemia.

DIAGNOSIS. The diagnosis of the various sickle syndromes relies on two types of tests: (1) screening tests to detect the presence of Hb S on the basis of its physicochemical properties, and (2) more definitive tests for the precise diagnosis of the particular genetic syndrome involved.

Two types of screening tests for the detection of Hb S are in current use. Both tests simply detect the presence of some Hb S in erythroid cells but do not differentiate sickle cell trait from the other sickle syndromes. The standard "sickle cell preparation" consists of mixing blood with a solution of sodium metabisulfate, which totally deoxygenates the blood and thus induces sickling that can be observed under the microscope. A second screening test is a solubility test which consists of mixing blood with a solution of high ionic strength and observing the mixtures for turbidity; normal hemoglobin will give a clear solution, whereas any Hb S in the solution will precipitate to give a turbid solution through which one cannot see the lines of an indicator card. Both tests, if properly done, are highly specific and accurate. The solubility test has the advantages that a microscope is not needed and that the test solution is relatively stable.

Once Hb S is detected by screening tests, hemoglobin electrophoresis should be carried out for precise diagnosis of the sickle syndrome. Table 143–1 summarizes the results obtained by hemoglobin electrophoresis in the various sickle cell syndromes as well as other associated clinical and laboratory findings that are useful in the differential diagnosis. In general, routine hemoglobin electrophoresis at pH 8.6 will suffice to establish the diagnosis. However, a few exceptions to this rule require additional tests to confirm or establish the suspected diagnosis. Because other hemoglobin variants can have the same electrophoretic mobility as Hb S at pH 8.6, electrophoresis in citrate agar at pH 6.1 should be performed to confirm the diagnosis (see Table 143–1). The distinction between Hb SS disease and Hb S/β⁰-thalassemia can be very difficult to establish, since electrophoretic findings are similar in both cases. The Hb A₂ level should be elevated in Hb S/β-thalassemia, but precise quantitation of Hb A₂ in the presence of Hb S is sometimes unreliable. Findings that should establish the diagnosis of Hb S/β⁰-thalassemia rather than Hb SS disease include (1) the presence of hypochromia and microcytosis indicated by low MCV and MCH; (2) family study showing that one parent or an offspring has β-thalassemia trait rather than sickle cell trait; (3) experimental studies of globin chain synthesis using labeled amino acid precursors (see Ch. 142), demonstrating decreased synthesis of βˢ chains relative to α chains (βˢ/α = 0.5 to 0.6); and (4) gene-mapping studies to distinguish between βᴬ and βˢ globin genes in the patient's DNA (see Fig. 143–3). The rare but interesting syndrome of Hb S/HPFH will also give hemoglobin electrophoretic findings similar to those of Hb SS disease, but with an unusually high level of Hb F in the range of 30 per cent. Such patients, however, are not anemic and should be asymptomatic. The diagnosis can be confirmed by family study showing the absence of sickle cell trait and presence of heterozygosity for HPFH in a parent or offspring. Study of the distribution of Hb F within individual red cells, using the acid elution test of Betke and Kleihauer, will show uniform distribution of Hb F in Hb S/HPFH but heterogeneous distribution of Hb F in Hb SS disease. Inheritance of Hb D (another relatively common β-chain hemoglobinopathy in blacks) along with Hb S can also mimic homozygosity for Hb S, since Hb D comigrates with Hb S on electrophoresis at pH 8.6. Hb SD disease is not as clinically severe as sickle cell disease, and the diagnosis can be established by performing hemoglobin electrophoresis at neutral or acid pH, which separates the two hemoglobins. Similarly, Hb SC disease can be confused with the inheritance of Hb S along with a second hemoglobin variant that has a similar electrophoretic mobility to Hb C at pH 8.6, such as Hb O Arab or Hb E. These syndromes can be distinguished from Hb SC disease by electrophoresis in citrate agar at pH 6 to 7.

The peripheral blood smear in individuals with Hb SS disease shows variable numbers of irreversibly sickled cells (ISC's), usually ranging between 5 and 10 per cent. In general the number of ISC's is relatively stable for a given patient, and there is a rough correlation between the numbers of ISC's and the severity of the hemolytic anemia. There is no correlation between the number of ISC's and the frequency or presence of vaso-occlusive crises. The peripheral blood smear, in addition to ISC's, will usually show variable numbers of target cells and occasional Howell-Jolly bodies owing to absence of spleen function. Other hematologic findings related to functional asplenia include the presence of target cells and somewhat elevated leukocyte counts and platelet counts. Examination of the peripheral blood smear can also be helpful in differential diagnosis of the sickle syndromes. In general, significant numbers of ISC's will be found essentially only in homozygous SS disease and not in the other sickle syndromes. Large numbers of target cells are characteristic of the inheritance of Hb C in either the heterozygous or the homozygous state (Color plate 2I).

TREATMENT. Despite extensive knowledge of the molecular basis and physical chemistry of the polymerization and sickling phenomena, there is still no specific molecular therapy available for the treatment or prevention of sickling. A number of compounds have been tested, and new compounds continue to be sought, that might interfere with sickling in vivo and be useful clinically. Unfortunately no such compound is currently available. Another potential molecular approach to the prevention of sickling would be to reactivate or increase fetal hemoglobin synthesis in the majority of the erythroid cells of affected patients to render them similar to the red cells of patients with Hb S/HPFH, a clinically mild syndrome. Successful enhancement of Hb F levels in patients with sickle cell anemia and homozygous β-thalassemia (see Ch. 142) has been accomplished by the administration of the chemotherapeutic agents 5-azacytidine* and hydroxyurea to a small number of patients. The rationale for 5-azacytidine therapy resided in the findings that the drug causes demethylation of DNA and that active genes are usually hypomethylated, whereas the inactive fetal γ-globin genes of adults are hypermethylated. However, other mechanisms related to cell toxicity, cell selection, and changes in gene expression resulting from disruption of the cell cycle probably also contribute to the increased levels of Hb F following administration of chemotherapeutic agents. These therapies should be considered highly investigational at this time and restricted in their general applicability until the long-term toxicity of these drugs, including carcinogenicity, is established.

The cornerstones of therapy in sickle cell anemia have therefore not changed in recent years and continue to consist of the administration of the following supportive measures: large volumes of intravenous fluids (preferably hypotonic and alkaline); analgesics to control the pain; when indicated, antibiotics to treat any associated bacterial infection; and oxygen to treat hypoxemia. When administering fluids to patients with sickle cell anemia, one should remember that these patients have a fixed renal water loss owing to inability to concentrate urine and that they are frequently dehydrated on presentation because of associated infection and fever. The amounts of intravenous fluids administered should therefore be increased to two to three times what would be considered a normal maintenance volume. Patients with sickle cell disease are frequently hypoxic because of chronic pulmonary disease. Even though they do not appear to be cyanotic, monitoring of arterial P_{O_2} is important, especially if there is an associated chest syndrome, and oxygen should be administered if there is significant hypoxemia. In the absence of arterial hypoxemia, oxygen therapy is probably not beneficial in the treatment of vaso-occlusive crises and may result in suppression of erythropoiesis. The role of alkali is controversial, and certainly if the patient is mildly acidotic, this acidosis should be corrected since it can potentiate the propensity of deoxy Hb S molecules to aggregate.

The role of blood transfusions and partial exchange transfusions is controversial in the treatment of acute vaso-occlusive crises of sickle cell disease. In general there is very little rationale for performing partial exchange transfusions simply for a painful vaso-occlusive crisis in a nonvital organ. Nevertheless such treatment may be occasionally indicated to interrupt an unusually prolonged painful crisis or when a patient is virtually continually disabled by frequent recurrent crises. In cases of life-threatening vaso-occlusive episodes or when there is a threat of severe organ damage as in acute cerebrovascular accidents and priapism, partial exchange transfusions should be promptly carried out because no other effective form of therapy is available. It is also generally agreed that patients who have suffered one cerebrovascular accident are likely to have recurrent life-threatening or debilitating episodes, and a course of long-term maintenance blood transfu-

sions to prevent recurrent sickling is indicated in such cases. Such a program should probably be associated with phlebotomies prior to transfusion and/or the institution of an iron chelation program to prevent or delay the complications of iron overload (see Ch. 142). Use of transfusions during pregnancy is controversial. It is common practice in many centers to give transfusions to pregnant women with sickle cell syndromes during the latter half of pregnancy to prevent fetal wastage and postpartum complications. However, a controlled study has not documented that this practice is clearly beneficial. Finally, it is also general practice for patients with clinically significant sickle cell syndromes to receive a partial exchange transfusion to lower the Hb S value to less than 50 per cent prior to general anesthesia for surgical procedures because of the risk of a fatal or incapacitating sickling episode in the event of an anesthetic accident or transient hypoxia. With the exception of the hypoplastic crises and acute sequestration crises, blood transfusions are not usually required to maintain hemoglobin levels above 6.5 to 7 grams per deciliter, and transfusions are not required on a long-term basis simply to treat the anemia.

Because of the high risk of septicemia and other serious infections caused by *Streptococcus pneumoniae*, young children with sickle cell anemia should receive prophylactic oral penicillin. This approach has been shown to be highly effective in reducing morbidity and mortality in pediatric populations. Pneumococcal vaccines may provide additional protection against such infections.

PROGNOSIS. The prognosis of patients with sickle cell syndromes is variable. A significant number of infants with sickle cell anemia and Hb SC disease may die in the first two to three years because of overwhelming sepsis and/or acute splenic sequestration crises. Cord blood–screening programs and identification of affected individuals with subsequent close medical follow-up, including prophylactic penicillin, should prevent or decrease the incidence of these early fatalities. For the group of patients who survive the early years, improved general medical care has substantially prolonged survival in the last two decades. There are reports of patients surviving to the fifth and sixth decades, although the mean survival is probably to the fourth decade, with death resulting from cardiopulmonary complications and/or renal insufficiency. Other causes of death include sepsis and cerebrovascular accidents. In general, patients with Hb S/β-thalassemia and Hb SC disease have longer survival than patients with sickle cell disease, although there are unexplained cases of relatively mild disease with homozygous inheritance of Hb S.

PREVENTION. Sickle cell disease and other clinically significant sickle syndromes can be prevented in two general ways. First, genetic counseling of identified heterozygotes can alert couples at risk about the possibility of having affected offspring. However, no matter how good the program of genetic counseling and education, it rarely significantly affects the reproductive behavior of identified carriers and generally has little impact on the overall incidence of the disease.

An alternative approach is the availability of prenatal diagnostic services for pregnancies at risk for sickle cell anemia and other sickle hemoglobinopathies. Prenatal diagnosis for sickle cell anemia has gone through many stages in recent years, including fetal blood sampling by fetoscopy for assays of hemoglobin synthesis and analysis by gene-mapping techniques of DNA from amniotic fluid cells, obtained after amniocentesis, for restriction fragment length polymorphisms shown to be linked to the sickle gene by prior study of DNA from family members. A restriction endonuclease enzyme (*Mst* II) can distinguish between a sickle and a nonsickle β-globin gene because the recognition site for this enzyme is specifically abolished by the nucleotide base substitution that is associated with the sickle mutation (Fig. 143–3). Thus the most reliable and acceptable method for prenatal diagnosis of sickle cell anemia is analysis of fetal DNA by the enzyme *Mst*

---

*Investigational agent available from the National Cancer Institute.

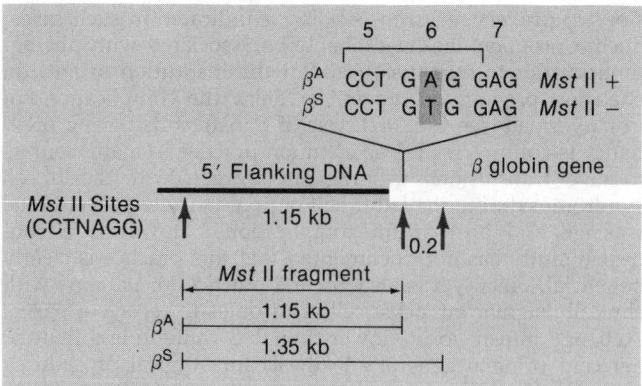

FIGURE 143–3. Direct identification of the sickle cell mutation in cellular DNA by restriction endonuclease digestion using the enzyme *Mst* II. The diagram shows the flanking region and 5′ portion of the beta globin structural gene. Arrows indicate the *Mst* II sites, including the one corresponding to amino acid portions 5, 6, and 7. The 1.15 kilobase (kb) fragment is seen in normal DNA, and the 1.35 kb fragment is seen in sickle DNA.

II. Although amniotic fluid cells obtained after 14 weeks of gestation are currently the source of DNA, it is likely that biopsy of trophoblastic villi in the first trimester will eventually be proved safe and replace amniocentesis.

HOMOZYGOUS Hb C DISEASE. Individuals homozygous for Hb C usually have a mild to moderate hemolytic anemia characterized by splenomegaly and large numbers of target cells on peripheral blood smear. Occasionally intraerythrocytic crystals of Hb C can be visualized in fixed blood smears. The clinical manifestations and general laboratory findngs are those of any mild chronic hemolytic anemia. Diagnosis is established by hemoglobin electrophoresis.

Bunn HF, Forget BG: Sickle cell disease—clinical and epidemiological aspects; and molecular basis of sickle cell disease. In Hemoglobin: Molecular, Genetic and Clinical Aspects. Philadelphia, W. B. Saunders Company, 1986, pp 502–554. Platt O, Nathan DG: Sickle cell disease. In Nathan DG, Oski FA (eds.): Hematology of Infancy and Childhood. 3rd ed. Philadelphia, W. B. Saunders Company, 1987 (in press). *Comprehensive chapters in hematology textbooks covering the pathophysiology as well as the clinical manifestations and therapy of sickle cell disease.*

Dean J, Schechter AN: Sickle–cell anemia: Molecular and cellular bases of therapeutic approaches. N Engl J Med 299:752, 804, 863, 1978. Schechter AN, Noguchi CT, Rodgers GP: Sickle cell disease. In Stamatoyannopoulos G, Nienhuis AW, Leder P, Majerus PW (eds.): Molecular Basis of Blood Diseases. Philadelphia, W. B. Saunders Company, 1987. *Detailed reviews of the physical chemistry and pathophysiology of sickling.*

Fleming AF (ed.): Sickle Cell Disease: A Handbook for the General Clinician. New York, Churchill Livingstone, 1982. Serjeant GR: Sickle Cell Disease. New York, Oxford University Press, 1985. *Comprehensive and detailed clinical descriptions of the manifestations of sickle cell anemia.*

144 UNSTABLE HEMOGLOBINS
Ronald F. Rieder

DEFINITION. The abnormal human hemoglobins manifest their presence by a variety of clinical syndromes of differing severity. One class of mutants, the unstable hemoglobins, is characterized by an increased tendency of the hemoglobin molecule to undergo denaturation. This increased rate of denaturation results in congenital Heinz body hemolytic disease of varying severity.

PATHOGENESIS. The complex three-dimensional arrangement of the four polypeptide subunits of the hemoglobin molecule is maintained primarily by hydrogen bonding and hydrophobic interactions between different amino acids (see Ch. 140). Amino acid substitutions that weaken these forces

holding the molecule together result in decreased thermal stability and an increased tendency for hemoglobin to precipitate, especially when exposed to oxidant compounds. Approximately 100 hemoglobin variants have now been described with such amino acid substitutions. The largest group of unstable hemoglobins consists of those with structural alterations that affect the strength of binding of the heme group to the protein by eliminating a specific heme-globin bond or by altering the configuration of the hydrophobic heme pocket. In some of these hemoglobins the binding of the heme group is so weakened that spontaneous loss of heme groups occurs. Hemoglobin Gun Hill has a deletion of a stretch of five amino acids, including the proximal histidine (β92), which normally forms a covalent bond with the heme iron atom; as a result the β chains of hemoglobin Gun Hill lack heme groups. In other unstable hemoglobins there is interference with the helical structure that provides rigidity to the polypeptide chains. Finally, the structural stability and the physiologic function of hemoglobin depend upon the tetrameric arrangement. In several abnormal hemoglobins an amino acid substitution results in the loss of a hydrogen bond that normally serves to stabilize and reinforce an interchain linkage. In unstable hemoglobin Philly the replacement of tyrosine by phenylalanine results in the loss of a single interchain hydrogen bond, permitting greater ease of separation of the α and β chains and denaturation of the hemoglobin. Hemolysis caused by an unstable hemoglobin is a direct result of the intracellular precipitation of hemoglobin to form multiple insoluble aggregates (Heinz bodies), which attach to the red cell membrane (Fig. 144–1). Clearance from the circulation of erythrocytes containing such inclusion bodies by the reticuloendothelial system or removal of inclusions from the cells by pinching off ("pitting") with reduction in red cell membrane and resultant increased fragility is responsible for decreased red cell life span.

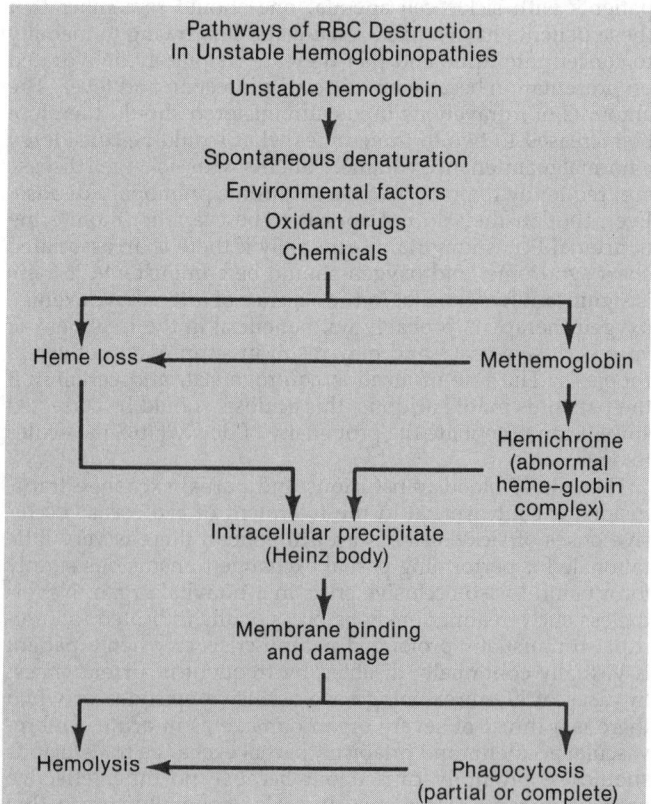

FIGURE 144–1. The presumed mechanisms by which denaturation of hemoglobin leads to erythrocyte destruction are outlined. The rate of travel through the various pathways probably differs for different hemoglobin variants and for a variety of stresses to which the protein is subjected.

CLINICAL MANIFESTATIONS. These disorders are inherited as autosomal dominant traits. Only heterozygotes have been found. The severity of the clinical presentation of patients with unstable hemoglobins is quite varied; some subjects have chronic hemolytic anemia, whereas others with less labile hemoglobins exhibit only mild compensated hemolysis with normal hemoglobin levels. However, exposure of even such mildly affected subjects to a variety of oxidant drugs and chemicals, many of which in large doses can cause methemoglobinemia in normal persons (see Table 146–2), can result in an acute severe hemolysis with the development of pronounced anemia, striking reticulocytosis, and sudden jaundice. Bouts of acute hemolysis may also occur spontaneously during bacterial and viral infections. Some affected subjects exhibit dark urine (pigmenturia) during periods of hemolysis owing to the presence of poorly characterized heme breakdown compounds called dipyrroles.

DIAGNOSIS. Diagnosis of an unstable hemoglobin depends upon the demonstration of a mutant hemoglobin with an increased tendency to precipitate. Intraerythrocytic inclusion bodies (Heinz bodies) can frequently be demonstrated during periods of hemolysis by staining the peripheral blood with a vital dye such as new methylene blue or brilliant cresyl blue. If absent from the circulating red cells, Heinz bodies may appear after incubation of the blood in vitro for two hours at 37° C in the presence of the dye. Instability of the hemoglobin can be demonstrated in hemolysates by formation of a large precipitate with a decrease in the concentration of soluble hemoglobin after heating to 50° C, or to 37° C in the presence of 17 per cent isopropanol. Since similar hemolytic episodes can occur after drug administration in subjects with glucose-6-phosphate dehydrogenase deficiency, this condition should be considered in the differential diagnosis. Hemoglobin electrophoresis may show an abnormal hemoglobin band frequently amounting to less than 25 per cent of the total hemoglobin. Occasionally because of marked preferential destruction of the abnormal molecular species, the unstable hemoglobin may be present in the peripheral blood as only a small percentage of the circulating hemoglobin. Some of the reported unstable hemoglobins are the result of the exchange of one uncharged amino acid for another. Since no alteration in total charge occurs, such mutant hemoglobins may migrate in the same electrophoretic position as hemoglobin A and are therefore difficult to detect by electrophoresis.

TREATMENT. Treatment of subjects with unstable hemoglobins mainly consists of the avoidance of drugs capable of inducing hemolysis (see Table 146–2). Subjects with chronic compensated hemolysis may benefit from prophylactic folic acid administration. Transfusions are required only during periods of profound acute hemolytic anemia. Splenectomy has been helpful when hypersplenism has developed. Special attention should be paid to the possible development of serious hemolytic anemia during episodes of infection.

Bunn HF, Forget BG: Hemoglobin: Molecular, Genetic and Clinical Aspects. Philadelphia, W.B. Saunders Company, 1986. *This authoritative, well-illustrated monograph covers all aspects of human hemoglobins and its disorders. Chapter 13 is devoted to unstable hemoglobin variants.*

Hirano M, Ohba Y, Imai K, et al.: Hb Toyoake: β142(H2O) Ala→Pro. A new unstable hemoglobin with high oxygen affinity. Blood 57:697, 1981. *Chronic hemolytic jaundice, splenomegaly, but no anemia in a subject with an unstable hemoglobin that also has high oxygen affinity.*

Jurićić D, Ruždić I, Beer Z, et al.: Hemoglobin Leiden (β6 or 7 (A3 or A4) Glu→0) in a Yugoslavian woman arisen by a new mutation. Hemoglobin 7:271, 1983. *An example of the way a modern hematology laboratory can investigate a mutant hemoglobin.*

Winslow RM, Anderson WF: The hemoglobinopathies. *In* Stanbury JB, Wyngaarden JB, Fredrickson DS, et al. (eds.): The Metabolic Basis of Inherited Disease. 5th ed. New York, McGraw-Hill Book Company, 1983, pp 1666–1710. *This is a comprehensive treatment of the genetics, structure, function, and clinical properties of the various types of abnormal hemoglobins.*

145 ABNORMAL HEMOGLOBINS WITH ALTERED OXYGEN AFFINITY

Ronald F. Rieder

DEFINITION. The ability of hemoglobin to function as a useful means of transporting oxygen depends upon its becoming fully loaded with oxygen in the lungs and unloading a proportion of this oxygen in the tissues at partial pressures of oxygen that are compatible with cell function and viability. A change in the structure of the hemoglobin molecule can affect this respiratory function. An increase in oxygen affinity can impair the ability of the pigment to donate its oxygen to the cells, whereas a decrease in affinity can prevent it from picking up enough oxygen as it passes through the pulmonary circulation. This affinity for oxygen is frequently expressed as the partial pressure of oxygen at which hemoglobin is half-saturated (P_{50}). Many mutant hemoglobins have some degree of alteration of oxygen-binding properties, but only a few have clinically significant defects. Some of these hemoglobins have increased oxygen affinity (decreased P_{50}), whereas others have a decreased capacity for binding oxygen (increased P_{50}).

PATHOGENESIS. During the process of oxygenation and deoxygenation, hemoglobin undergoes reversible structural changes that involve alterations in the three-dimensional configuration of the individual polypeptide chains, as well as shifts in the way the four chains are arranged in the $\alpha_2\beta_2$ tetramer. When fully deoxygenated, hemoglobin is said to be in the T or tense state and has a relatively low affinity for oxygen. Conversely, when hemoglobin is fully oxygenated, it is in the R or relaxed state and has a high affinity for oxygen. This intramolecular reorganization with its resultant change in oxygen affinity is reflected in the physiologically important sigmoidal shape of the hemoglobin-oxygen dissociation curve (see Ch. 140).

The complex stereochemical changes in molecular structure are accomplished by considerable relative movement of the α and β globin chains along the $\alpha_1\beta_2$ interface and of the C-terminal regions of the β chains. Hydrogen bonds, hydrophobic interactions, and salt bridges between amino acids are broken and new ones are formed during these R-T transitions.

Genetic mutations that affect amino acids situated at the $\alpha_1\beta_2$ interface or that otherwise alter molecular structure to interfere with the R-T equilibrium may affect the respiratory function of hemoglobin. Thus an amino acid substitution that destabilizes the T or low O_2 affinity state would tend to favor the R state and increase the oxygen affinity of a mutant hemoglobin. In abnormal hemoglobin Kempsey, asparagine replaces aspartic acid at position β99. Asparagine, unlike aspartic acid, cannot form the hydrogen bond with tyrosine at α42 that normally stabilizes the deoxyhemoglobin conformation. As a result hemoglobin Kempsey has a high oxygen affinity. In contrast in hemoglobin Kansas, threonine replaces asparagine at position β102. Threonine cannot form the hydrogen bond with aspartic acid at α94 that normally stabilizes the R or high affinity state. Therefore hemoglobin Kansas is shifted toward the T state and has a low oxygen affinity.

2,3-Diphosphoglycerate (2,3-DPG) acts as a physiologic modulator of hemoglobin oxygen affinity and binds to specific amino acid sites on the protein. 2,3-DPG increases the P_{50} (lowers the oxygen affinity), and mutations that inhibit bind-

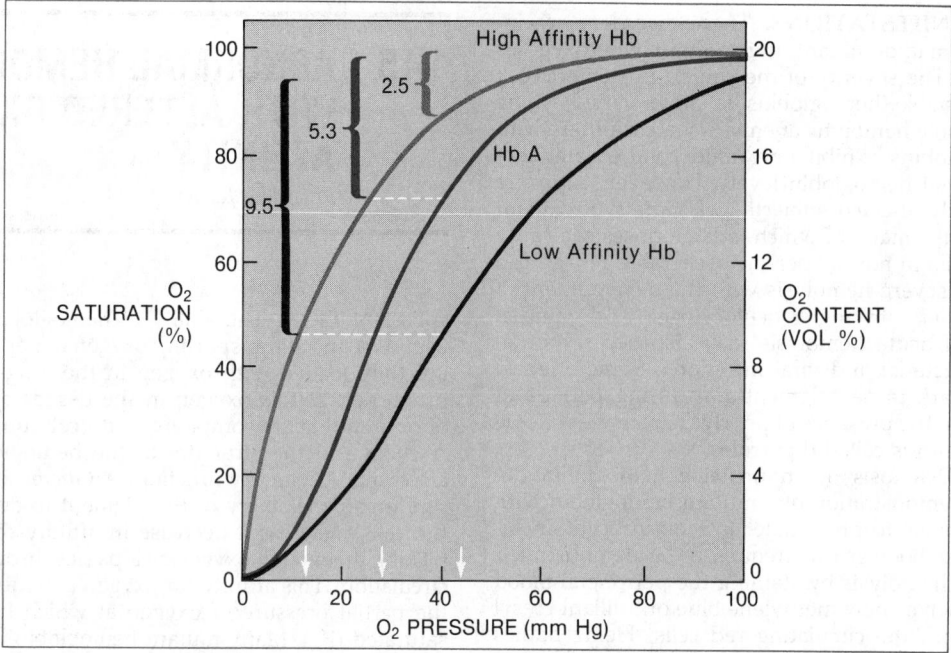

FIGURE 145–1. Hemoglobin-oxygen dissociation curves are illustrated for normal hemoglobin (Hb A) and for model abnormal hemoglobins with high and low oxygen affinities. On the abscissa is indicated the partial pressure of oxygen in millimeters of mercury. On the left ordinate the saturation of hemoglobin with oxygen is indicated as a percentage; on the right ordinate the oxygen content of the hemoglobin is expressed as volumes per cent. The three inverted arrows show the P_{50} for the three hemoglobins (the partial pressure of oxygen at which the hemoglobin is 50 per cent saturated). This value is lowest for the high-affinity hemoglobin. As the partial pressure of oxygen drops from 100 (arterial) to 40 (tissues), hemoglobin desaturates, giving up a portion of its bound oxygen; the numbers on the brackets indicate the amount of oxygen unloaded by the three hemoglobin types expressed in volumes per cent. Note that the high-affinity hemoglobin delivers less than half the oxygen that Hb A gives to the tissues, resulting in tissue anoxia, increased erythropoietin secretion, and erythrocytosis. Conversely, the low-affinity hemoglobin is even more efficient than Hb A in supplying the tissues with oxygen resulting in diminished erythropoietin production and anemia.

ing of this small molecular weight effector result in hemoglobin with increased oxygen affinity.

CLINICAL MANIFESTATIONS. Most of the abnormal hemoglobins with detectable alterations in oxygen-binding characteristics are only minimally affected and of no physiologic significance. However, mutant hemoglobins with greatly increased oxygen affinity tend to unload much less oxygen to the tissues, and this results in relative tissue hypoxia. As a result erythropoietin secretion is increased and erythropoiesis is stimulated with a rise in hematocrit value (Fig. 145–1). Thus subjects with high affinity hemoglobins may have *erythrocytosis.* The disorder is frequently familial and is inherited as an autosomal dominant. No increase in white blood cell or platelet counts occurs. Plasma concentrations of erythropoietin are normal when the subject is polycythemic, but if the hematocrit level is lowered to normal by phlebotomy, an increase in erythropoietin production can be detected.

In subjects with mutant hemoglobins having moderately lowered oxygen affinity, the increased tendency of the hemoglobin to unload oxygen results in enhanced delivery to the tissues. Such persons therefore require less hemoglobin to provide the same volume of oxygen and as a consequence frequently have decreased hematocrit values. In this situation the usually *mild anemia* is not a pathologic condition but is a physiologic response to the increased availability of oxygen at the tissue level.

In some subjects with a hemoglobin with greatly decreased oxygen affinity, *cyanosis* is present owing to the marked inability of the mutant hemoglobin to bind oxygen. Hematocrit values in such cases are normal.

Even in the presence of markedly abnormal hemoglobin function, subjects with hemoglobins with altered oxygen affinity usually are asymptomatic.

DIAGNOSIS. The presence of a hemoglobin with high oxygen affinity should be considered in any patient who has isolated erythrocytosis unaccompanied by increased leukocyte

and platelet proliferation (see Ch. 153). After eliminating causes such as the presence of hypoxemia with secondary erythrocytosis as well as other causes of increased erythropoietin secretion, evidence for an abnormal hemoglobin should be sought. Hemoglobin electrophoresis may reveal an abnormal hemoglobin band, but several of the high affinity hemoglobins have electrophoretic mobilities identical to hemoglobin A. An oxygen-hemoglobin dissociation curve should be determined on whole blood and especially on isolated hemoglobin. The latter can eliminate any contribution of diminished or increased 2,3-DPG levels. By adding back 2,3-DPG to the purified hemoglobin, evidence for diminished 2,3-DPG binding can be detected. A low affinity hemoglobin should be considered in instances of unexplained cyanosis with normal arterial oxygen tension.

TREATMENT. Aside from either erythrocytosis or mild anemia, subjects having these functionally defective hemoglobins are usually asymptomatic and no treatment is indicated. Cyanosis accompanying the rare hemoglobins having very low affinity for oxygen is only a cosmetic problem.

Bunn HF, Forget BG: Hemoglobin: Molecular, Genetic and Clinical Aspects. Philadelphia. W. B. Saunders Company, 1986. *This authoritative, well-illustrated monograph covers all aspects of human hemoglobin and its disorders. Ch. 14 provides an in-depth discussion of hemoglobinopathies with abnormal oxygen binding.*

Charache S, Catalno P, Burns S, et al.: Pregnancy in carriers of high-affinity hemoglobins. Blood 65:713, 1985. *Female carriers of three different high affinity hemoglobins demonstrated no increase in either fetal wastage or intrauterine growth retardation.*

Moo-Penn WF, McPhedran P, Bobrow S, et al.: Hemoglobin Connecticut $\beta 21(B3)(Asp \rightarrow Gly)$: A Hemoglobin variant with low oxygen affinity. Am J Hematol 11:137, 1981. *This hemoglobin with low oxygen affinity was found in three generations of a family and was associated with mild anemia in several individuals.*

Moo-Penn WF, Schneider RG, Shih T-B, et al.: Hemoglobin Ohio $(\beta 142A1a \rightarrow Asp)$: A new abnormal hemoglobin with high oxygen affinity and erythrocytosis. Blood 56:246, 1980. *This high affinity hemoglobin was found in three members of a family, all of whom exhibited erythrocytosis.*

146 METHEMOGLOBINEMIA AND SULFHEMOGLOBINEMIA

Ronald F. Rieder

METHEMOGLOBINEMIA

DEFINITION. The reversible oxygenation and deoxygenation of hemoglobin at physiologic partial pressures of oxygen require that the heme iron of deoxyhemoglobin remain in the ferrous (Fe^{+2}) form. In methemoglobin the iron atom is oxidized to the ferric (Fe^{+3}) form, rendering the molecule incapable of binding oxygen. When hemoglobin is oxygenated during the process of respiration, an electron is partially transferred from the ferrous iron atom to the bound oxygen molecule. Thus in oxyhemoglobin iron possesses some of the characteristics of the ferric (Fe^{+3}) state, whereas the oxygen takes on the characteristics of the superoxide (O_2^-) anion. Under normal circumstances upon deoxygenation of the hemoglobin molecule the electron is returned to the iron atom and the O_2 molecule is released. Interference with the return of the electron to the iron atom results in the formation of methemoglobin. Normally approximately 3 per cent of the hemoglobin is spontaneously oxidized to methemoglobin each day, but the concentration is maintained below 1 per cent by its reconversion to hemoglobin by metabolic processes. A shift in this equilibrium can result in increased amounts of methemoglobin in the peripheral blood and the development of cyanosis. Enzymatic reducing systems in the red cells are responsible for the maintenance of the heme iron of hemoglobin in the ferrous state. An enzyme variously termed NADH-methemoglobin reductase, NADH-dehydrogenase, NADH-diaphorase, or erythrocyte cytochrome b_5 reductase is responsible for over 90 per cent of the hemoglobin reducing capacity of the erythrocyte under physiologic conditions, catalyzing the transfer of an electron from NADH to oxidized cytochrome b_5:

$$NADH + Fe^{+3} - \text{cytochrome } b_5 \xrightarrow{\text{reductase}} NAD^+$$
$$+ Fe^{+2} - \text{cytochrome } b_5$$

Flavine adenine dinucleotide may participate as a prosthetic group on the reductase. Reduced cytochrome b_5 then directly interacts with methemoglobin to result in its reduction to ferrous hemoglobin:

$$Fe^{+2} - \text{cytochrome } b_5 + Fe^{+3} - \text{hemoglobin} \rightarrow$$
$$Fe^{+3} - \text{cytochrome } b_5 + Fe^{+2} - \text{hemoglobin}$$

The reconversion of NAD to NADH depends upon the Embden-Meyerhof glycolytic pathway, primarily at the reaction in which glyceraldehyde-3-phosphate is converted to 1,3-diphosphoglycerate by the enzyme glyceraldehyde phosphate dehydrogenase. An NADPH-dependent methemoglobin reductase is present within the erythrocyte, but normally there is no linked physiologic electron carrier available which is capable of directly donating an electron to reduce methemoglobin. However, when provided with an artificial electron carrier such as methylene blue, this enzyme is of great importance in the therapy of acute toxic methemoglobinemia (see below). Ascorbic acid and reduced glutathione are capable of directly reducing methemoglobin, but these reactions occur quite slowly.

CLASSIFICATION (Table 146–1). Methemoglobinemia may be hereditary or acquired. Hereditary methemoglobinemia may result from an abnormality in the metabolic processes that normally reconvert methemoglobin to hemoglobin (see above) or from an inherited abnormality of the hemoglobin molecule conducive to methemoglobin formation. Acquired

TABLE 146–1. TYPES OF METHEMOGLOBINEMIA

A. Congenital
  1. Defective enzymatic reduction of Fe^{+3}-hemoglobin to Fe^{+2}-hemoglobin
    a. NADH–methemoglobin reductase (cytochrome b_5 reductase) deficiency
    b. Cytochrome b_5 deficiency
  2. Abnormal hemoglobins resistant to enzymatic reduction (M hemoglobins)
B. Acquired
  1. Excessive (toxic) oxidation of Fe^{+2}-hemoglobin
    a. Environmental chemicals
    b. Drugs

methemoglobinemia results from exposure to certain chemical agents that increase the formation of methemoglobin.

Hereditary Methemoglobinemia Caused by Defective Reduction of Methemoglobin

More than 100 subjects with hereditary methemoglobinemia resulting from NADH-methemoglobin reductase deficiency have been described, and several abnormal variant enzymes differing in catalytic activity, structural stability, and electrophoretic mobility are known. The disorder is inherited as an autosomal recessive trait. It occurs with unusually high frequency in Alaskan Eskimos and Indians, Navajo Indians and Puerto Ricans. In certain families with this disorder there has been an associated mental deficiency with neurologic defects. In this form of the disorder the enzyme deficiency is not restricted to the erythrocytes but is widely distributed, including the brain. Patients with methemoglobinemia have persistent slate-gray cyanosis. In contrast to deoxyhemoglobin, which produces cyanosis only when present at levels above 5 grams per deciliter, methemoglobin at a concentration of only 1.5 to 2 grams per deciliter produces significant cyanosis. Homozygotes usually have methemoglobin levels of 15 to 25 per cent, but no deleterious effect is apparent at this concentration. At concentrations of methemoglobin up to 40 per cent, some symptoms of fatigability and malaise have been described. The patients have been characterized as being more blue than sick. No clubbing or cardiopulmonary disease is present, and mild compensatory erythrocytosis has been noted only occasionally. Heterozygotes for the enzyme deficiency have normal concentrations of methemoglobin, but manifest increased susceptibility to the methemoglobin-producing properties of various oxidant drugs and chemicals (Table 146–2). Recently, congenital methemoglobinemia due to deficiency of cytochrome b_5 has been described.

DIAGNOSIS. Persistent cyanosis without hypoxia should suggest the possibility of methemoglobinemia. The peripheral blood is reddish brown and does not become bright red when exposed to oxygen. Methemoglobin has a characteristic absorption peak at 630 nm, which disappears upon addition of cyanide. Several assays are available to quantitate the level of NADH-methemoglobin reductase in erythrocytes, and stain-

TABLE 146–2. DRUGS AND CHEMICALS HAVING TOXIC EFFECT ON HEMOGLOBIN MOLECULE

Agent	Hemoglobin Derivative Observed	
	Methemoglobin	*Sulfhemoglobin*
Acetanilid, phenacetin	+	+
Nitrites (amyl, sodium, potassium, nitroglycerin)	+	+
Trinitrotoluene, nitrobenzene	+	+
Aniline, hydroxylamine, dimethylamine	+	+
Sulfanilamide	+	+
Para-aminosalicylic acid	+	
Dapsone	+	
Primaquine, chloroquine	+	
Prilocaine, benzocaine, lidocaine	+	
Menadione, naphthoquinone	+	
Naphthalene	+	
Resorcinol	+	
Phenylhydrazine	+	+

ing procedures can reveal an abnormal enzyme with altered electrophoretic mobility.

TREATMENT. Treatment of congenital methemoglobinemia caused by reductase deficiency is generally not required, but cosmetic improvement of the cyanosis can be achieved by treatment with methylene blue, 100 to 300 mg per day orally, or ascorbic acid, 500 mg per day orally. Riboflavin, 20 mg per day orally, is also effective. Methylene blue has the disadvantage of producing blue urine. Large doses of ascorbate may lead to oxalate stone production.

Hereditary Methemoglobinemia Due to Abnormal (M) Hemoglobins

Several variant hemoglobins have substitutions in the amino acids that line the heme crevice of the globin chain and contact the porphyrin group or the iron atom. These mutations affect the configuration of the polypeptide chain surrounding the heme group, alter the hydrophobic environment, and often weaken the binding of the porphyrin to the protein. Some of these variant hemoglobins are unstable and lose heme (see Ch. 144), and others are permanently fixed in the methemoglobin state (M hemoglobins). In four of the five described M hemoglobins a histidine is replaced by a tyrosine whose hydroxyl group forms a stable complex with iron in the ferric state. The hemoglobin is thus fixed in the oxidized form. The methemoglobin reductase system of the erythrocyte is ineffective in reducing these abnormal methemoglobins.

CLINICAL MANIFESTATIONS. Subjects inheriting an M hemoglobin are cyanotic but are usually otherwise unaffected by the trait. Mild chronic hemolysis has been observed in association with hemoglobin M Hyde Park, which has a tendency to lose heme and is slightly unstable. The disorder is inherited in a dominant pattern, and families have been reported in which the condition has been noted in several generations.

DIAGNOSIS. The blood has a brown appearance and does not become bright red upon agitation in air. Neither does the addition of cyanide produce the change to the red color that occurs upon such treatment of normal methemoglobin. In subjects with β-chain mutations approximately 50 per cent of the hemoglobin is affected, whereas 20 to 25 per cent of the circulating hemoglobin is methemoglobin in persons with an α Hb M. The presence of an abnormal methemoglobin can be detected by spectrophotometric analysis. The normal absorption peaks of methemoglobin at 630 and 502 nm are shifted to slightly lower wavelengths in the M hemoglobins. In addition, the M hemoglobins have an altered electrophoretic migration; separation from Hb A is most easily demonstrated if first the hemolysate is completely converted to methemoglobin with ferricyanide. No treatment is required for this condition, and methylene blue and ascorbic acid administration are ineffective for significant conversion to reduced hemoglobin.

Acquired or Toxic Methemoglobinemia

A variety of chemical agents and drugs are able to accelerate the oxidation of hemoglobin and produce a significant methemoglobinemia in otherwise normal individuals (Table 146–1). Many of these agents occasionally induce sulfhemoglobinemia and can cause hemolysis in subjects with unstable hemoglobins or glucose-6-phosphate dehydrogenase deficiency. Often these compounds are unable directly to induce the oxidation of hemoglobin in vitro, and thus their toxicity in vivo is probably a result of conversion to intermediate forms that are direct oxidants. Nitrates have been implicated in methemoglobinemia in infants as a result of the use of contaminated well water in the preparation of feeding formulas. They must be converted to nitrite to produce methemoglobinemia. Such conversion may occur as a result of the action of bacteria in the gastrointestinal tract. The ability

of drugs to produce large amounts of methemoglobin depends upon overwhelming the normal pathway in the red cell responsible for maintenance of hemoglobin iron in the ferrous state. In normal subjects large doses of drugs are generally necessary. When the activity of the methemoglobin-reducing system is depressed, susceptibility to these agents is increased. Thus heterozygotes for NADH-methemoglobin reductase variants and newborn infants who normally have low levels of the enzyme until about four months of age are very susceptible to the development of methemoglobinemia. Normal doses of primaquine and dapsone have caused methemoglobinemia in enzyme-deficient adults. Menadione, naphthalene, and aniline dyes used by laundries to mark diapers have been implicated in the induction of methemoglobinemia in very young infants. On the other hand, such agents as prilocaine and sulfanilamide have commonly been reported to cause methemoglobinemia in normal persons.

CLINICAL MANIFESTATIONS. Methemoglobinemia induced by drugs is usually an asymptomatic condition, and any associated ill effects are generally due to other actions of these chemicals. However, severe acute methemoglobinemia with levels of methemoglobin greater than 60 to 70 per cent have been associated with collapse, coma, and death. Affected patients develop severe cyanosis, and upon examination the blood is chocolate brown.

DIAGNOSIS. Diagnosis depends upon demonstration of the presence of methemoglobin (see above) and identification of the causative agent. Erythrocyte reductase levels should be measured to rule out enzyme deficiency.

TREATMENT. With mildly affected patients treatment, aside from discontinuing the offending agent, is not required, and the methemoglobin will be reduced spontaneously to ferrous hemoglobin over a period of two to three days. For severely affected patients therapy with methylene blue is effective. One to 2 mg per kilogram of a 1 per cent solution of methylene blue in saline is administered intravenously over 10 minutes. If there is no adequate response within an hour, a second dose may be administered. This treatment generally results in the prompt conversion of methemoglobin to hemoglobin. Such therapy is not effective in subjects with glucose-6-phosphate dehydrogenase deficiency resulting in inactivity of the hexose monophosphate shunt pathway for the production of NADPH, which is required for the reconversion of oxidized methylene blue to reduced or leuko-methylene blue. Exchange transfusion may be required in severely symptomatic patients. Oral ascorbic acid should not be used in the treatment of acute toxic methemoglobinemia, since its speed of action is slow.

Bunn HF, Forget BG: Hemoglobin: Molecular, Genetic and Clinical Aspects. Philadelphia. W. B. Saunders Company, 1986. *This authoritative, well-illustrated monograph covers all aspects of human hemoglobin and its disorders. Ch. 15 covers the M hemoglobins and Ch. 16 discusses the other forms of methemoglobinemia.*

Jaffé ER: Methaemoglobinemia. Clin Haematol 10:99, 1981. *Review emphasizing enzyme deficiency.*

Mansouri A. Methemoglobinemia. Am J Med Sci 289:200, 1985. *Detailed review covering all forms of methemoglobinemia.*

Schwartz JM, Reiss AL, Jaffe ER: Hereditary methemoglobinemia with deficiency of NADH cytochrome b₅ reductase. In Stanbury JB, Wyngaarden JB, Fredrickson DS, et al. (eds).: The Metabolic Basis of Inherited Disease. 5th ed. New York, McGraw-Hill Book Company, 1983, p 1654. *Authoritative, detailed review of all aspects of the inherited enzyme deficiency.*

SULFHEMOGLOBINEMIA

DEFINITION. Sulfhemoglobin is an incompletely characterized greenish-brown hemoglobin derivative found in the blood of some subjects after exposure to large amounts of various drugs or organic chemicals. The pigment causes cyanosis, makes the blood reddish brown, and has a characteristic optical absorption spectrum with a peak at 620 nm that is not abolished by the addition of cyanide. The precise structure of the abnormal pigment is not known except that a sulfur atom is incorporated into the porphyrin ring.

PATHOGENESIS. Abnormal pigments with similar optical absorption characteristics have been noted in the blood of patients after ingestion of toxic doses of acetanilid, phenacetin, and other drugs, as well as after exposure to large amounts of aromatic amino and nitro compounds. The mechanism for the production of sulfhemoglobin in vivo is not understood. Many of the same compounds that have been noted to cause methemoglobinemia in some patients have been implicated in the appearance of sulfhemoglobin in others (see Table 146–1). Neither the reason for the appearance of one hemoglobin derivative rather than the other nor the relationship in vivo to sulfur is clear. Chronic constipation with the production of excess hydrogen sulfide in the gut has been postulated but never proved to be a contributing factor.

CLINICAL MANIFESTATIONS. Cyanosis is the characteristic feature of subjects with sulfhemoglobinemia. As little as 0.5 gram per deciliter produces a slate-gray discoloration of the skin and mucous membranes. This amount of sulfhemoglobin is much less than the 1.5 and 5 grams per deciliter required for methemoglobin and reduced hemoglobin to cause cyanosis. Patients generally experience no ill effects from the condition, and asymptomatic persons with as much as 10 grams per deciliter have been described.

DIAGNOSIS. Positive identification of sulfhemoglobin as the cause of cyanosis in a patient can be made by observing the characteristic optical absorption spectrum of a hemolysate before and after the addition of a small amount of potassium cyanide. Isoelectric focusing has also been used.

TREATMENT. Treatment consists primarily of identifying the causative agent and eliminating further contact. Reconversion of sulfhemoglobin to hemoglobin is not possible. In symptomatic cases exchange transfusion would be indicated. After cessation of contact with the offending agent, production of sulfhemoglobin ceases, and the compound is eliminated from the blood over a period of weeks during the normal course of erythrocyte aging and clearance from the circulation.

Park CM, Nagel RL: Sulfhemoglobinemia. Clinical and molecular aspects. N Engl J Med 310:1579, 1984. *This is a report of a thoroughly studied case, accompanied by an excellent discussion of diagnosis, chemistry, and pathophysiology.*

147 BLOOD TRANSFUSION

Herbert A. Perkins

A standard unit of blood donated for transfusion consists of 450 ml of blood mixed with 63 ml of a solution that contains citrate to prevent clotting, and glucose, phosphate, and adenine for optimal preservation of red cell viability. Without adenine, storage of red cells is limited to 21 days; with adenine, 35 days is acceptable. Nonviable cells are quickly removed from the circulation of the recipient; the remainder are restored to biochemical normality and live out the rest of their usual life span (up to 120 days).

INDICATIONS FOR BLOOD TRANSFUSION

Blood transfusions have the potential for many harmful side effects. Therefore, blood should never be transfused when the risks to the patient outweigh the expected benefit, or when more specific and safer therapy (e.g., iron, B_{12}) is available. When blood transfusions are indicated, only that fraction of the blood that the patient requires should be administered. Most blood donations are separated into components after collection: red blood cells, platelet concentrates, and/or cryoprecipitates and plasma. The plasma may be subsequently fractionated to provide albumin, gamma globulin, and coagulation factor concentrates.

This discussion will be restricted to the use of red blood cell concentrates and whole blood. The indications for transfusion of platelet concentrates are discussed in Ch. 166, for leukocytes in Ch. 150, and for cryoprecipitates and coagulation factor concentrates in Ch. 167.

The patient who is anemic but has a normal blood volume should receive only red blood cells; therefore whole blood transfusions are rarely justifiable on a medical service. Acute hemorrhage is more common on the surgical services, but even here whole blood is inappropriate in most situations. Patients with acute hemorrhage often have a relatively greater deficit of red cells than of plasma. Transfusing red cells until the blood volume is normalized will result in a higher hematocrit and, in turn, greater oxygen-carrying capacity than would an equal volume of whole blood. Moreover, the usual bleeding patient who loses less than 20 to 25 per cent of the blood volume (1000 to 1500 ml in an adult) can be transfused with red cells supplemented by electrolytes instead of whole blood with no impairment of recovery. It is common practice in many hospitals to provide red cells, not whole blood, for the first three units crossmatched for routine surgery. Whole blood is of greatest value when there has been massive acute blood loss creating need for large-scale red cell and volume replacement.

RED BLOOD CELLS. A variety of red blood cell components can be prepared. These are listed in Table 147–1, together with their usual packed cell volume (PCV) and the proportion of red blood cells (RBC), white blood cells (WBC), and plasma of the original whole blood that remains in the final product.

Red blood cells, often called packed red blood cells, should be the primary component for the treatment of chronic anemia or hemorrhage. This component contains all the red cells of the original unit with enough plasma so that it will flow reasonably rapidly through an intravenous needle.

Red blood cells in additive solution may be stored for 42 days. Preservative solution containing adenine is added after most of the plasma has been removed.

Leukocyte-poor red blood cells are given to patients who have had prior febrile reactions to transfusions caused by recipient alloantibodies reacting with donor leukocytes. Leukocyte-poor red blood cells may be prepared by (1) centrifuging blood with removal of the buffy coat, (2) washing red blood cells with removal of the buffy coat, or (3) transfusing through a special filter red cells that have been refrigerated and then centrifuged to pack the leukocytes into clumps (the spin, cool, filter technique). Removal of 85 to 90 per cent of the donor leukocytes is sufficient to prevent febrile reactions in at least 90 per cent of alloimmunized patients. As much as 20 per cent of red cells may be lost to achieve this level of leukocyte depletion, and the final hematocrit varies with the exact procedure.

Washed red blood cells are rarely indicated. They are required only when a recipient has had prior severe reactions to donor plasma proteins. Although they have often been recommended for patients with paroxysmal nocturnal hemoglobinuria, recent evidence indicates that they are rarely necessary. Washed red blood cells should not be considered to be leukocyte poor unless the washing process was modified to remove the buffy coat.

TABLE 147–1. RED BLOOD CELL COMPONENTS

Component	PCV (%)	RBC (%)	WBC (%)	Plasma (%)
RBC	75	100	100	20
RBC in additive solution	60	100	100	5
Leukocyte-poor RBC				
Centrifuged	95	80	15	5
Washed	75	90	10	0
Spin-cool-filter	75	85	15	20
Washed RBC	75	95	50	0
Frozen RBC	75	90	5	0

Frozen red blood cells are also washed and leukocyte poor by the time they have been readied for transfusion. Red cell loss is inevitable, and the procedures involved are time consuming and expensive. Red blood cells, when prepared with glycerol, can be stored in the frozen state for as long as three years; therefore the most important reason to freeze red cells is for preservation of a type so rare that it would otherwise be unavailable for the patient who must receive it. Frozen red cells are also useful for the patient with antibodies to donor leukocytes so strong that he or she has an uncomfortable febrile reaction to leukocyte-poor red cells.

PROVIDING COMPATIBLE BLOOD FOR TRANSFUSION

BLOOD GROUPS. The external surfaces of all blood cells and plasma proteins contain very large numbers of antigenic determinants whose structures are programmed by genes. Many of these genetic loci have multiple possible alleles, with the result that all blood transfusions expose the recipient to a large number of foreign immunogens. Fortunately, most of these antigenic determinants are poor immunogens or result in antibodies that have no notable clinical effect. In routine transfusions, it is usually sufficient to avoid incompatibility for only three antigens (A, B, and D), all on the red blood cells.

The red blood cell antigenic determinants are divided into blood groups, each blood group consisting of the alleles of a single genetic locus. The most important red blood cell group is the ABO group, with two antigens: A and B. The primary importance of the ABO blood group in transfusion therapy is based on two facts: (1) Anti-A and anti-B are regularly present ("naturally occurring") in the plasma of persons who lack the corresponding antigen on their red cells (Table 147–2), presumably because of previous immunization to crossreacting antigens in bacteria and foods. (2) Anti-A and anti-B are almost always present in high concentration, activate the full complement cascade, and are capable of intravascular destruction of an almost unlimited number of incompatible red blood cells.

The second important red cell blood group is Rh. This is important because one of the antigenic determinants in this group (D) is an unusually potent immunogen, and 15 per cent of Caucasoids lack the D antigen. The term *Rh-positive* indicates the presence of D; *Rh-negative* indicates its absence. There are a large number of additional Rh gene products, but only a few of these commonly stimulate production of alloantibodies: C, E, c, and e. C and c resemble alleles, as do E and e, in that one—but not both—is the product of each normal Rh gene. There is no allele for D, but the symbol "d" is used to indicate its absence.

Altogether, more than 300 different antigenic determinants have been identified on human red blood cells. Some of these have been assigned to blood groups; others have not. In addition to the Rh antigens mentioned, additional important red cell immunogens are found in the Kell, Duffy, and Kidd systems. Antibodies to the Rh, Kell, Duffy, and Kidd antigens are not "naturally occurring" and are found after prior transfusions or pregnancies. Typing donors for these antigens (other than D) is necessary only when the recipient has formed the corresponding antibody. Antibodies to certain other red cell antigens (e.g., M, Lewis, P, I) are relatively common and often naturally occurring, but since these antibodies are generally inactive at body temperature, they are rarely of clinical significance.

COMPATIBILITY TESTING. A hospital transfusion service must type the red blood cells of the patient for A, B, and D and confirm the typing of the donor. Further tests are performed to ensure that the patient has not formed "unexpected" antibodies, i.e., antibodies other than the expected anti-A or B. The search for unexpected antibodies is carried out in two ways: (1) Antibody screening involves testing the serum of the patient with a small number of red cells selected to contain among them all of the antigens which commonly cause trouble. (2) Compatibility testing, or crossmatching, tests the patient's serum with red blood cells from the units intended for transfusion. If unexpected antibodies are detected which appear likely by their specificity and characteristics to impair the survival of transfused red cells containing the corresponding antigen, red cells to be transfused must lack the antigen. In general, a positive crossmatch contraindicates transfusion; exceptions should be approved by someone thoroughly knowledgeable about the possible effects of the antibodies detected.

EMERGENCY TRANSFUSION. Under normal circumstances, transfused red cells are of the same ABO type as those of the recipient; but in urgent situations when ABO-identical red cells are not available, ABO-compatible red cells may be transfused. For example, type O red cells can be given to a recipient of any ABO type, and the type AB recipient can receive red cells of any ABO type. Whole blood should be avoided in these circumstances, since the anti-A and/or anti-B of the donor plasma may destroy recipient red cells.

If Rh negative red cells are not available for an Rh-negative recipient, Rh-positive cells may be transfused in an emergency, but only if the recipient has no anti-D in his or her serum. Special effort should be made to avoid transfusion of Rh-positive cells into Rh-negative recipients who are females and not yet past the childbearing age. The recipient has approximately a 70 per cent chance of being immunized to D, and a subsequent pregnancy with an Rh-positive fetus is very likely to result in severe hemolytic disease of the newborn. If Rh-positive red cells must be transfused into an Rh-negative female of reproductive age, Rh immunoglobulin treatment may prevent immunization.

With sudden massive hemorrhage, it may be necessary to transfuse blood without all of the usual preliminary tests. Type O Rh-negative blood is often reserved for such situations on the grounds that it is likely to be compatible with all recipients. Such blood is in limited supply, however, and it takes only a few minutes to determine the ABO and Rh types of the recipient. Meanwhile, electrolytes or colloid (e.g., albumin) can be used to maintain the patient's circulation. The usual in vitro compatibility tests can be waived if the emergency is sufficiently great, but there must be written documentation of the urgency.

HAZARDS OF BLOOD TRANSFUSIONS

The many potential complications of blood transfusion are listed in Table 147–3.

HEMOLYTIC REACTIONS. Hemolytic reactions correctly attract the most attention, since they can result in serious morbidity or death. Almost all immediate hemolytic transfusion reactions are caused by ABO mismatches, and the cause of the error is almost always clerical. The most common error is incorrect labeling of the patient sample taken for compatibility testing. The patient must be identified without error at the time of sampling, and the correct label must be applied to the crossmatch tube before leaving the patient's side. The other major source of the trouble is transfusion of a unit other than the one intended for that patient. The donor blood label, crossmatch slip, and patient identification must be crosschecked carefully before the transfusion is started.

The most dangerous antibodies are those which activate the complete complement cascade, resulting in intravascular hemolysis. Other antibodies (e.g., Rh, Kell) merely become attached to the red cell, in some instances with subsequent attachment of complement components C3 and C4. The

TABLE 147–2. THE ABO GROUP

Red cell type	O	A	B	AB
Possible genotypes	OO	AA or AO	BB or BO	AB
Antibodies in serum	Anti-A and B	Anti-B	Anti-A	None
Frequency in Caucasoids	45%	40%	10%	5%

TABLE 147–3. HAZARDS OF BLOOD TRANSFUSION

1. Hemolytic reactions
2. Chill-fever reactions
3. Contaminated blood
4. Noncardiac pulmonary edema
5. Post-transfusion thrombocytopenic purpura
6. Transmission of disease
   a. Hepatitis
   b. Malaria
   c. Syphilis
   d. Cytomegalovirus
   e. Acquired immunodeficiency syndrome (AIDS)
7. Allergic reactions
   a. Urticaria
   b. Anaphylaxis
8. Circulatory overload
9. Air embolism
10. Hemosiderosis (see Ch. 142)
11. Massive transfusion problems
12. Graft-versus-host disease

coated red cells may then be destroyed in the reticuloendothelial system by macrophages, which have receptors for the Fc portion of IgG molecules and the C3 and C4.

Intravascular hemolysis (such as that caused by anti-A or anti-B) results in release of free hemoglobin into the plasma, binding of hemoglobin to haptoglobin with subsequent removal of the complex, hemoglobinuria once haptoglobin has been saturated, and later rise of serum bilirubin and possibly methemalbumin. Extravascular hemolysis (typical of Rh antibodies) occurs primarily in the spleen, takes place more slowly, and may be limited by saturation of the reticuloendothelial system. Hyperbilirubinemia is the major laboratory abnormality.

The clinical symptoms associated with hemolytic transfusion reactions are highly variable and range in severity from death to shortened survival of the transfused cells unaccompanied by symptoms. The most frequent complaints are chills, fever, and aching in various parts of the body. Oliguria or anuria caused by acute renal failure may follow these symptoms or in some cases may be the first recognized sign that a hemolytic transfusion reaction has occurred. If the patient is under anesthesia, incompatible red cells may continue to be infused until the magnitude of the intravascular antigen-antibody reaction activates disseminated intravascular coagulation. Under anesthesia, then, generalized bleeding and an unexpected drop in blood pressure may be the first evidence of a hemolytic reaction.

Delayed hemolytic reactions may be recognized when the recipient receives a large volume of red cells containing an antigen to which he was previously immunized. The antibody may have become undetectable by the time of the current crossmatch and too weak to cause a reaction at the time of transfusion. Anamnestic increase in antibody concentration to high levels occurs with obvious effects five to ten days after transfusion. The recipient's hemoglobin falls rapidly, and he or she becomes jaundiced. At this point, the alloantibody is usually easily detectable.

When a hemolytic transfusion reaction is suspected, the transfusion must be stopped and the blood container and attached tubing returned to the laboratory accompanied by a new blood and urine sample from the patient. The laboratory will test for evidence that hemolysis has occurred, recheck the identity of all samples, and retest samples obtained before and after the reaction for evidence of incompatibility. If an antibody is identified, blood lacking the corresponding antigen may then be transfused.

The patient's fluid intake and output must be monitored, and he or she should be well hydrated, avoiding circulatory overload. If oliguria occurs, diuretics may be prescribed. The primary danger comes from rising serum potassium; therefore serial monitoring of electrolytes and electrocardiograms is mandatory. Dangerous levels of potassium may be combated by methods described in Ch. 77. Acute renal failure in these

cases is self-limited, and full recovery can be expected, barring complications, if electrolytes remain under control at all points.

NONHEMOLYTIC FEBRILE TRANSFUSION REACTIONS. Febrile reactions to blood transfusions are far more likely to have been caused by recipient alloantibodies to donor leukocytes than to donor red cells. Alloantibodies to leukocytes develop at some time in at least 20 per cent of women as a result of pregnancy and in 70 to 90 per cent of multitransfused persons. Donor white cells reacting with recipient antibodies will cause a febrile response in proportion to the number of incompatible cells and the rate at which they are transfused.

Mild reactions cause fever alone. If the fever rises rapidly, shaking chills may occur. Severe reactions may be associated with vomiting and collapse. These reactions can be very uncomfortable but are unlikely to cause prolonged morbidity or mortality per se. The febrile response is completed within 12 hours.

If red cell incompatibility has been eliminated as the cause of the reaction, confirmation that white cells were responsible can be obtained by demonstrating antibodies to leukocytes in the serum of the recipient or by showing that the reactions can be prevented by transfusing leukocyte-poor red cells. If leukocyte-poor red cells fail to reduce symptoms adequately, frozen red cells should be tried.

CONTAMINATED BLOOD. Some bacteria are almost inevitably introduced into a small proportion of blood units collected for transfusion, but most fail to multiply at 4°C storage or are killed through the bactericidal effect of blood leukocytes and antibodies. The dangerous organisms are those which grow preferentially at 4°C. These are gram-negative rods which produce endotoxin. If blood heavily contaminated with endotoxin is transfused, shock, generalized bleeding, and death are almost inevitable. Confirmation of the diagnosis is accomplished by a Gram stain of the donor blood.

These contaminated blood reactions are extremely rare, and published reports suggest that many of them could have been prevented by inspection of the blood before transfusion. Contamination of a unit of blood should be suspected if the blood is of abnormal color, if there is evidence of excessive hemolysis, or if clots are readily demonstrable.

NONCARDIAC PULMONARY EDEMA. Rarely blood transfusion has been associated with sudden onset of dyspnea with radiologic evidence of pulmonary opacities. In many of these cases donor antibodies reacting with recipient leukocytes have been detected.

POST-TRANSFUSION THROMBOCYTOPENIC PURPURA. Thrombocytopenic purpura may occur suddenly seven to ten days after transfusion in association with recipient antibodies to donor platelets. In most cases the antibody has been anti-P1^{A1}, and the recipient has been a P1^{A1}-negative female with a history of pregnancies. The patient's own platelets are destroyed by mechanisms that are unclear, and the thrombocytopenia may last for a number of weeks. The most effective treatment has been plasma exchange, presumably through removal of the alloantibody to platelets.

TRANSMISSION OF DISEASE. *Hepatitis* remains the most serious unsolved problem in blood transfusion therapy. It is probable that clinically evident hepatitis follows at least 1 per cent of all transfusions and that ten times as many subclinical cases may occur. Hepatitis B has been greatly reduced by eliminating blood donors who are positive for HBsAg, but it still accounts for at least 10 per cent of post-transfusion cases. Unsuspected hepatitis A is unlikely in a healthy blood donor, because infection with this virus does not result in a chronic carrier state. Non-A non-B hepatitis accounts for almost all of the remaining 90 per cent of cases. Cytomegalovirus explains a minute percentage, and EB virus almost none.

Until the non-A non-B virus(es) is identified and tests to

detect it are available, post-transfusion hepatitis is best prevented by elimination of paid blood donors and other high-risk groups. Elimination of donor units either with anti-HBcAg or an increased level of alanine transferase may reduce the frequency of non-A, non-B post-transfusion hepatitis.

Malaria remains a rare but definite problem despite deferral of blood donors for three years if they have had malaria or have taken prophylaxis. A six-month deferral appears adequate if the donor had exposure to a malaria area but did not take prophylaxis. (Prophylaxis may only prolong the incubation period.)

Syphilis is rarely transmitted at present because of early detection and treatment of infected cases. Regulations still require a serologic test for syphilis on all blood donations, although it serves little purpose and unnecessarily excludes donors with biologic false-positive tests and with previous adequately treated syphilis.

Cytomegalovirus transmission by blood transfusion may have serious consequences in immunosuppressed patients such as premature newborn infants and marrow transplant recipients.

Acquired immunodeficiency syndrome (AIDS) may be transmitted by transfusion of whole blood, red blood cells, platelets, or plasma. The relatively rare occurrence of this complication is overshadowed by the public's concern about the high mortality of this disease. Recipients of clotting factor concentrates were at unusually high risk, but such concentrates are now heat treated to kill the AIDS virus. The risk of AIDS from blood transfusion has been reduced to very low levels by elimination of donors from groups at risk for AIDS and by testing all donations for antibody to the AIDS virus.

ALLERGIC REACTIONS. Urticaria may occur in as many as 3 to 5 per cent of transfusions but is rarely of serious concern and can usually be controlled or prevented by antihistamines. The very rare anaphylactoid reactions are characterized by flushing, tachycardia, wheezing, dyspnea, fall in blood pressure, and unconsciousness. One death has been reported. Most if not all such reactions are caused by recipient antibody to donor IgA globulin. Almost all of the involved recipients have no detectable IgA in their sera and have formed antibodies reacting with all IgA preparations (class specific). Rare persons with normal IgA have produced alloantibodies to an IgA allotype. IgA is absent from the serum of 1 in 900 blood donors; 25 to 50 per cent of these donors have antibodies to IgA. Anaphylactoid reactions are so rare in comparison as to suggest that most of the detected antibodies are not of clinical significance.

Patients with previous anaphylactoid reactions associated with anti-IgA should receive only blood products which lack IgA. Red blood cells can be washed free of plasma proteins. Plasma products should be from donors who lack IgA.

If an anaphylactoid reaction occurs, transfusion should be stopped and intravenous antihistamine given. In most cases, epinephrine and corticosteroids will also be required.

CIRCULATORY OVERLOAD. This is a common side effect of transfusion, especially serious if the patient is in danger of heart failure. The risk is minimized by the use of concentrated components. If the need for red cells is great but the patient is in heart failure, it may be advisable to remove blood from the recipient, discarding the plasma and returning the red cells supplemented with red cells from other donors.

AIR EMBOLISM. This is rarely a problem but if a large amount of air enters the bag as the transfusion set spike is inserted, subsequent external pressure on the bag can embolize air.

MASSIVE TRANSFUSION PROBLEMS. Transfused blood has been altered during collection and storage, and additional problems occur when the volume and rate of blood transfusion introduce abnormalities faster than they can be corrected by the recipient.

Bleeding tendency: Blood stored more than 24 hours is essentially devoid of viable platelets, and dilutional thrombocytopenia becomes possible after transfusion of a volume of blood more than one and a half to two times the blood volume of the recipient. Disseminated intravascular coagulation (DIC) is a frequent complication of conditions requiring massive transfusion. Restoration and maintenance of normal blood volume are essential prerequisites to control of DIC. It will usually be necessary to replace platelets (concentrates), fibrinogen (cryoprecipitates), and possibly other plasma coagulation factors (fresh-frozen plasma).

Citrate intoxication: Although depression of ionized calcium is inevitable when large amounts of citrated blood are rapidly transfused, the recipient has a number of compensating mechanisms. Correction of the hypocalcemia with intermittent intravenous calcium solutions is almost never necessary and may be dangerous.

Hypothermia is a serious risk when large volumes of cold blood are rapidly transfused. Ventricular fibrillation may result. This should be prevented by warming the blood either immediately prior to or during transfusion.

Microaggregates in stored blood can be removed during transfusion using special filters. However, there is no evidence that these filters are required for the usual small volume transfusions, and there is no agreement that microaggregates are harmful during massive transfusion.

Hyperkalemia and *acidosis* are primarily of concern in the transfusion of newborn infants. In fact, the massively transfused adult usually has a low plasma potassium level despite the increased levels of potassium in the plasma of the transfused blood.

GRAFT-VERSUS-HOST DISEASE (GVHD). This is a rare but increasingly recognized complication of blood transfusion. Engraftment of stem cells in the donor blood can result if the immunologic responses of the recipient are sufficiently impaired. Immunocompetent donor lymphoid cells are responsible for GVHD. Recipients with congenital deficiencies of T lymphocytes and those prepared for a marrow transplant are at greatest risk. Others at risk include some patients whose immune apparatus has been suppressed to more than the usual degree by antineoplastic therapy. The risk of engraftment increases with the number of mononuclear cells in the transfused blood component. Granulocyte concentrates appear to carry the highest risk.

The clinical signs of GVHD are nonspecific: dermatitis, gastrointestinal disturbances, and liver dysfunction. The best supportive evidence for GVHD is obtained by demonstrating that the recipient's blood carries genetic markers other than his or her own. HLA typing is most useful for this purpose.

Engraftment can be prevented by irradiating blood prior to transfusion. Doses of 1500 to 5000 rads are used and have no demonstrable effect on red cell viability or on platelet and granulocyte function. Except for patients with severe combined immunodeficiency disease and those prepared for marrow transplantation, the indications for irradiation of blood prior to transfusion are not well established.

SUMMARY. Blood transfusion is a very effective form of therapy but with potential serious side effects. Decisions to transfuse must always consider the risk-benefit ratio. The components prescribed must be appropriate for the indications and selected, when necessary, to avoid repetition of previous transfusion reactions.

The majority of complications of blood transfusion can be avoided by using the patient's own blood whenever possible. Autologous donations may be predeposited prior to elective surgery. Intraoperative salvage of extravasated blood can recover red cells for transfusion.

Mollison PL: Blood Transfusion in Clinical Medicine. 7th ed. Oxford, Blackwell Scientific Publications, 1983. *This is the "bible" of transfusion medicine, emphasizing the laboratory aspects. The answers to most of your questions can be found here; if you need more detailed information, Mollison has probably provided the references.*

Petz LD, Swisher SN: Clinical Practice of Blood Transfusion. New York, Churchill Livingstone, 1981. *This text addresses transfusion problems from the point of view of the clinician, providing not only the necessary background but also addressing specific clinical situations.*

148 FUNCTION OF NEUTROPHILS AND MONONUCLEAR PHAGOCYTES

Bernard M. Babior

Neutrophils and mononuclear phagocytes are essential components of the host defense system. Both are made in the bone marrow, and both accomplish most of their purposes through the act of eating (Gr. *phagein* to eat). Mononuclear phagocytes are versatile cells whose functions include the destruction of invading pathogens, the elimination of debris from the bloodstream and from sites of tissue damage, the remodeling of normal tissues, and the assignment of targets to lymphocytes. Neutrophils, on the other hand, are single-mindedly dedicated to the destruction of invading pathogens.

THE NEUTROPHIL

ORIGIN. Like other cells in the circulation, neutrophils originate from pluripotential stem cells that reside in the bone marrow. Depending on environmental influences, a pluripotential stem cell is capable of giving rise to the committed progenitors of any of the blood cells. Under the influence of a small group of peptides known as *colony-stimulating factors*, this stem cell will proliferate and differentiate to produce a population of neutrophils.

The route from a committed progenitor to a neutrophil involves a series of precursors, some of which can be recognized under the microscope. The earliest identifiable neutrophil precursor is a myeloblast, a relatively large cell with a rim of pale blue cytoplasm surrounding a large nucleus containing dispersed chromatin and multiple nucleoli. As the cell progresses through later stages of differentiation, the chromatin condenses and the nucleoli are lost, while at the same time the cytoplasm acquires its characteristic granules. The various neutrophil precursors are listed in Figure 148–1.

Through the myelocyte stage, neutrophil precursors divide as well as differentiate (Fig. 148–1). These proliferative forms are said to constitute the *mitotic compartment* of the neutrophil precursor pool. Later precursors, which do not divide, constitute the *nonmitotic compartment*. This is also called the *storage compartment*, because cells in this compartment can be released into the bloodstream in response to infections or other stresses. As a rule, the only elements released from the storage compartment are neutrophils and bands. If the stress is sufficiently severe, however, a few metamyelocytes may be liberated as well.

A newly committed stem cell requires approximately eight to ten days to become a mature neutrophil and enter the circulation. In the bloodstream, neutrophils are distributed about evenly between two rapidly exchanging pools: the *circulating pool*, composed of neutrophils suspended freely in the circulating blood, and the *marginated pool*, consisting of cells that have settled onto the endothelium of the capillaries and postcapillary venules. Once having entered the circulation, neutrophils leave for the tissues randomly and rapidly; their half time in the bloodstream is only six hours. In the tissues, however, the cells may sojourn for days.

STRUCTURE. The neutrophil is a terminally differentiated, nondividing cell that is well equipped to perform its function of killing microorganisms. The cell is packed with granules whose contents are used for the destruction and degradation of target microorganisms. The granules are of two types: *azurophil*, which contain proteases and other hydrolytic enzymes, a group of microbicidal peptides known as defensins, and a Cl^--oxidizing enzyme known as myeloperoxidase; and *specific*, which contain among other things a collagenase and an enzyme that releases C5a from the complement component C5. The nucleus is a vestigial structure that can no longer replicate its DNA. The plasma membrane contains an element of the neutrophil's killing apparatus as well as sensors that locate and identify the microorganisms against which the neutrophil acts. The cytoskeleton of the neutrophil is a complex system of tubes and fibers that is responsible for the orderly movement of this highly motile cell.

FUNCTION. Neutrophils undergo radical and abrupt changes in behavior in response to external stimuli. These changes include aggregation, degranulation (i.e., the discharge of granule contents through the plasma membrane), and the initiation of oxidant production. They are provoked by many stimuli, the most important of which are target microorganisms and chemotactic factors at high concentration (see below). These behavioral changes convert the neutrophil from a placid resident of the bloodstream to a powerful weapon. A cell that has undergone these changes is known as an *activated neutrophil*. The destruction of a microorganism by a neutrophil can be divided into three stages: finding the microorganism, ingesting it, and finally killing it and disposing of its remains.

Chemotaxis. The neutrophil finds its target through a chemical sense that enables the cell to detect certain substances known as *chemotactic factors*. These chemotactic factors are continuously released at sites where microorganisms have invaded tissues, diffusing away to set up a concentration gradient. Neutrophils in the circulation are able to sense this gradient and travel toward its source. They begin their journey by marginating on the capillary and postcapillary endothelium. They then migrate outward through the vessel walls, penetrating the subendothelial basement membrane by local digestion, presumably with collagenase. Once outside the

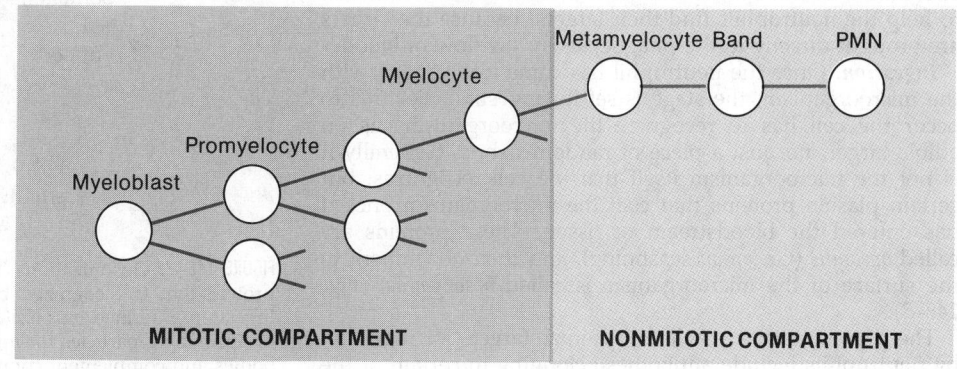

FIGURE 148–1. Neutrophil precursor pool.

Myeloblast

Promyelocyte

Myelocyte

Metamyelocyte   Band   PMN

MITOTIC COMPARTMENT

NONMITOTIC COMPARTMENT

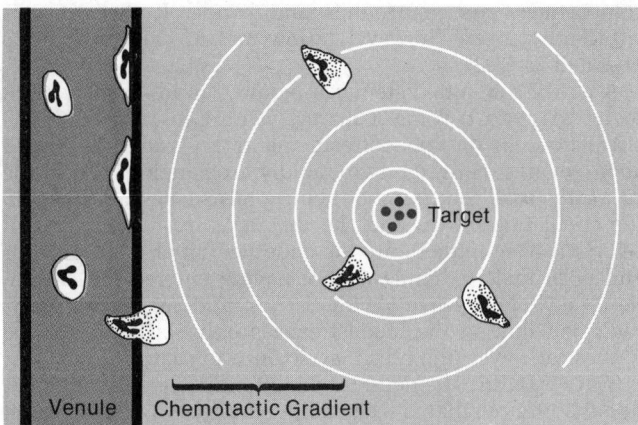

FIGURE 148–2. Chemotaxis. Neutrophils in the venule undergo margination in response to chemotactic factor, then leave the vessel by migrating between the endothelial cells (diapedesis) and travel up the chemotactic gradient toward the target.

capillaries, they continue their directed migration, eventually reaching the site of origin of chemotactic factors—that is, the region of tissue that has been invaded by microorganisms. This process of migrating up a chemical gradient toward the source of the chemical is known as *chemotaxis* (Fig. 148–2).

Neutrophils are able to respond to a very large number of chemotactic factors, but three appear to be of primary importance: (1) *N-formylated oligopeptides*, (2) the complement fragment *C5a*, and (3) a product of arachidonate oxidation known as *leukotriene B_4* (LTB$_4$). These chemotactic factors are produced both by the invading microorganisms (N-formylated oligopeptides and C5a) and by the neutrophils themselves (C5a and LTB$_4$). N-formylated oligopeptides are intermediates in bacterial protein synthesis and are released from bacteria that have been damaged or killed. C5a is produced by the complement system when it interacts with microorganisms and also by activated neutrophils through the release of the C5-splitting enzyme of the specific granules. LTB$_4$ is also produced by activated neutrophils, which manufacture it by liberating and oxidizing arachidonic acid from endogenous phospholipids. The production of C5a and LTB$_4$ by activated neutrophils lends a self-reinforcing character to the process of chemotaxis, since neutrophils that have arrived at a site of inflammation are activated to generate chemotactic factors that attract more neutrophils to the inflamed region.

Bacteria in the circulation are thought to be handled primarily by the mononuclear phagocytes (see below). Neutrophils, however, may play a role in clearing the circulation of microorganisms that enter the bloodstream suddenly and in large numbers. During such episodes of bacteremia, the complement system is activated, releasing C5a into the circulation. Neutrophils react to this pulse of C5a by marginating in the pulmonary capillaries where they may act temporarily (15 to 30 minutes) as a filtration system, removing microorganisms from the blood as they pass through the pulmonary circulation. In this special situation, chemotaxis is not needed to help the neutrophils find their targets, because the targets are brought directly to the phagocytes by the flow of blood.

Ingestion. Once the neutrophil has come into contact with the microorganism, the stage is set for ingestion. For this to occur the cell has to recognize the microorganisms as an edible target, not just a piece of random debris. Generally it is not the microorganism itself that the cell recognizes, but certain plasma proteins that coat the microorganism once it has entered the bloodstream or tissue. These proteins are called *opsonins* (Gr. *opson* seasoning), and their attachment to the surface of the microorganism is called *opsonization* (Fig. 148–3).

The proteins that are able to opsonize targets for ingestion by neutrophils include antibodies belonging to certain of the

IgG subclasses (opsonizing antibodies) and the complement component C3b. Opsonizing antibodies bind to the microbial surface by means of a simple antigen-antibody reaction. C3b binds to the microbial surface by a more complex process that involves the activation of the complement system through either the classic pathway (initiated by the antigen-antibody complex) or the alternative pathway (initiated by certain complex carbohydrates found on microbial surfaces) (see Ch. 418). One of the steps in complement activation by either of these pathways is the cleavage of component C3 into two pieces: C3a, a small fragment that induces capillaries and venules to dilate and become leaky, and C3b, the large opsonizing fragment. Immediately upon release, this opsonizing fragment locks onto the target through a covalent bond. The opsonized target then attaches to the neutrophil surface by means of these opsonins, which are recognized and bound by receptors in the neutrophil membrane: the Fc receptors, which recognize complexes between antigen and opsonizing antibody, and the C3 receptors, which recognize particle-associated C3b.

The attachment of the target to the neutrophil surface is the signal for ingestion (Fig. 148–4). The membrane in the region of the attached particle invaginates into the cell, carrying the particle in with it. When the particle is fully internalized, the invagination closes at its neck to form a vesicle, which detaches from the inner surface of the cell membrane and is released into the cytoplasm of the neutrophil. The end result of the phagocytic event is that a particle initially attached to the surface of the neutrophil is translocated to the cell's interior enclosed in a vesicle lined with what was originally a portion of the neutrophil plasma membrane. This vesicle, known as the *phagocytic vesicle*, is the site of killing of the ingested organism.

Killing. Killing involves two separate actions on the part of the neutrophils: *degranulation* and the *activation of the respiratory burst*. Degranulation refers to a process whereby the granule membrane fuses with another cellular membrane, releasing the granule contents into the compartment on the opposite side of the other membrane (Fig. 148–5). In the case of azurophil granules, degranulation occurs almost exclusively into the phagocytic vesicles, so that the actions of the azurophil granule contents are directed almost entirely against the ingested microorganism. Specific granules degranulate into both the phagocytic vesicles and the external environment, so their contents exert effects exterior to the neutrophils as well as on the ingested microorganisms. Some of the constituents of each of these granules are listed in Table 148–1, together with their actions.

The *respiratory burst* refers to a sequence of metabolic events the purpose of which is the production of potent microbicidal oxidants through the partial reduction of oxygen. The burst

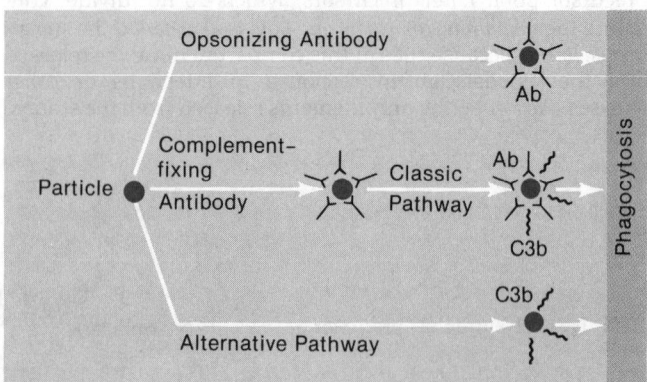

FIGURE 148–3. Opsonization. The coating of a particle by a plasma protein that is recognized by neutrophil receptors as a signal for ingestion is termed *opsonization*. Two classes of proteins are capable of opsonizing particles for ingestion by neutrophils: opsonizing antibodies and complement component C3b.

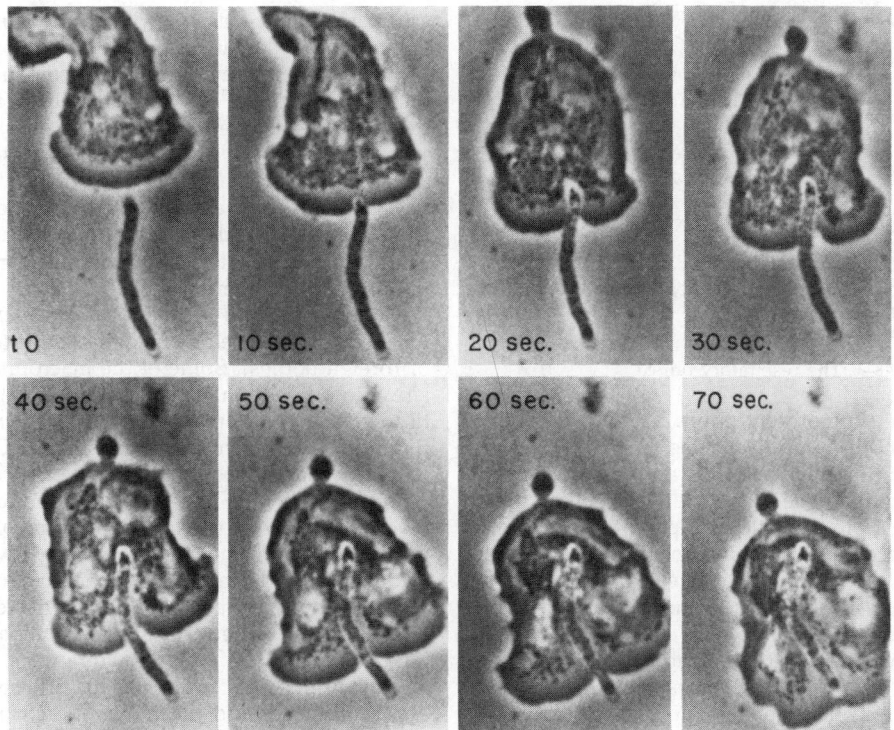

FIGURE 148–4. Ingestion of a target microorganism by a neutrophil. (Reproduced from Hirsch JG: Cinemicrophotographic observations of granule lysis in polymorphonuclear leucocytes during phagocytosis. J Exp Med 116:827, 1962, by copyright permission of the Rockefeller University Press.)

is activated by the same stimuli that provoke degranulation of the specific granules—primarily contact with ingestible particles and exposure to chemotactic factors at high concentrations. These stimuli activate a plasma membrane-bound oxidase dormant in resting cells that catalyzes the one-electron reduction of oxygen to superoxide (O_2^-) at the expense of NADPH (Fig. 148–6). Most of the O_2^- reacts with itself to yield H_2O_2, while at the same time NADPH is regenerated by way of the hexosemonophosphate shunt. These events have nothing to do with respiration as it is usually understood, but they acquired the name *respiratory burst* because of the large increase in neutrophil oxygen uptake that is associated with their onset.

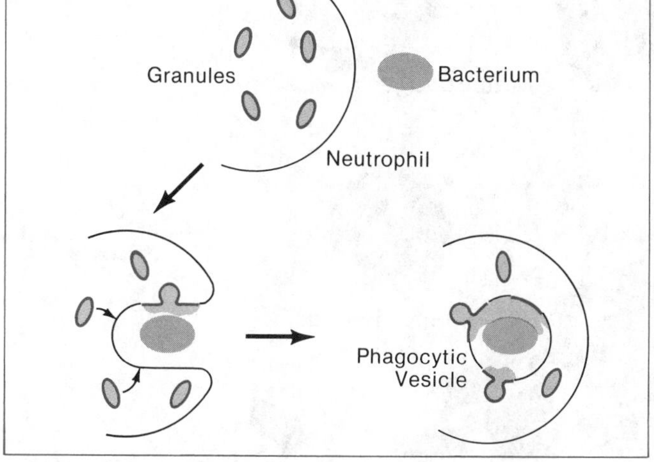

The microbicidal oxidants are derived from the H_2O_2: (1) A portion of the H_2O_2 is used to oxidize Cl^- to the highly microbicidal hypochlorite ion (OCl^-), a reaction catalyzed by myeloperoxidase, an enzyme delivered into the phagocytic vesicle from the azurophil granules. (2) Another portion of the H_2O_2 is converted to the exceedingly reactive hydroxyl radical ($OH\cdot$) in a metal-catalyzed reaction with O_2^-. These and related oxidants attack and kill ingested microorganisms by oxidizing their cellular constituents.

MONONUCLEAR PHAGOCYTES

Mononuclear phagocytes and neutrophils are closely related. Both are descended from the same ancestor, and both share many functions, including the unusual ability to ingest particles as large as half or more their own diameter. There

FIGURE 148–5. Degranulation. Granules migrate toward a phagocytic vesicle, eventually fusing with it. Upon fusion, the contents of the granule are released into the vesicle, while the granule membrane becomes incorporated into the vesicle wall.

TABLE 148–1. CONTENTS OF NEUTROPHIL GRANULES

Component	Function
I. Azurophil granules	
Acid hydrolases (glycosidases, phospholipases, acid proteases)	Degradation of ingested material
Neutral proteases (cathepsin G, elastase)	Destruction of inflamed tissue?
Lysozyme	Digestion of bacterial cell wall
Defensins	Oxygen-independent bacterial killing
Myeloperoxidase	Oxygen-dependent bacterial killing
II. Specific granules	
Lysozyme	Digestion of bacterial cell wall
Cobalamin-binding protein	Binding of bacterial cobalamin analogues
Apolactoferrin	Binding of free iron, control of granulopoiesis
Collagenase	Digestion of connective tissue
C5-splitting enzyme	Release of C5a
III. Indeterminate	
Bactericidal/permeability-increasing protein	Killing of gram-negative bacteria

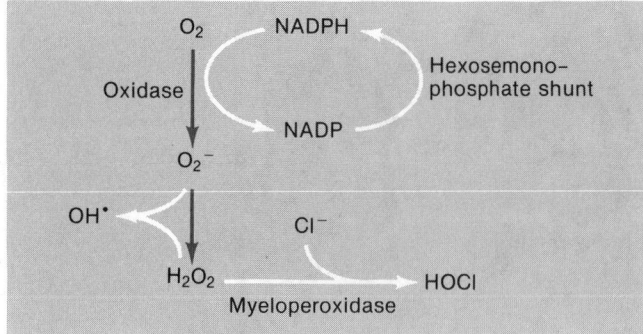

FIGURE 148–6. The respiratory burst.

is, however, only one type of neutrophil, whereas there are many varieties of mononuclear phagocytes.

ORIGIN. All mononuclear phagocytes are derived from a single circulating precursor: the monocyte. This cell and the neutrophil both arise from a single pluripotential stem cell. In the course of differentiation, this stem cell first makes a general commitment to the phagocyte lineage. Later its descendants commit themselves further, some to the neutrophil and others to the monocyte line.

In the monocyte line, the first recognizable precursor is the *monoblast.* In normal marrow, this cell is indistinguishable from a myeloblast; it can be identified, however, in marrow from patients with monocytic leukemia. The next stage is the *promonocyte,* a somewhat larger cell with cytoplasmic granules and an indented nucleus containing finely divided chromatin. Finally, the fully developed *monocyte* appears. It requires about five days to go from a monoblast to a mature circulating monocyte.

STRUCTURE AND FURTHER DIFFERENTIATION. Larger than the neutrophil, and with a large horseshoe-shaped nucleus containing dispersed chromatin, the mature monocyte has cytoplasm that is filled with granules whose contents include hydrolytic enzymes and other proteins necessary for the cell's activities. Unlike the neutrophil, the monocyte seems to have retained a limited capacity to divide and in addition is able to undergo considerable further differentiation.

Monocytes are able to diversify into the many types of cells that constitute the mononuclear phagocyte system. Monocytes circulate in the bloodstream for a time (t½~12 hours)

and then enter the tissue, where they differentiate into mature macrophages that live for weeks to months. The properties of these macrophages are characteristic for the tissues in which they reside. Those in the liver, for example, are the Kupffer cells, spidery phagocytes that bridge the sinusoids separating adjacent plates of hepatocytes (Fig. 148–7A). Those in the lungs are the large ellipsoidal alveolar macrophages (Fig. 148–7B). These and other tissue macrophages are listed in Table 148–2. Little is known about the factors responsible for the various patterns of mononuclear phagocyte differentiation seen in different tissues.

Macrophages are important components of the inflammatory reactions elicited by noxious agents (e.g., microorganisms or foreign bodies). Some of the macrophages that appear at a site of inflammation have been recruited from the surrounding tissues, while others are derived from monocytes that have migrated there from the bloodstream. Once at the inflamed site, the macrophages are exposed to certain stimuli (e.g., *gamma-interferon,* a T lymphocyte product formerly known as macrophage-activating factor, and *lipopolysaccharide,* from the cell walls of gram-negative organisms) which induce them to undergo a sequence of functional and morphologic changes whose purpose appears to be to enable them to deal more effectively with the inciting agent. Initially the cells increase in size, accumulate many new granules, and begin to secrete large quantities of certain specific proteases, including collagenase, elastase, and plasminogen activator, a component of the fibrinolytic system (see Ch. 157). Their capacity for phagocytosis is increased, as is their ability to degrade ingested material. The cells become stickier and more motile and develop the ability to manufacture lethal oxidizing agents. Most important, their microbicidal power is greatly increased, with the result that they become capable of killing pathogens that they were unable to deal with in their former state. Cells that have attained this heightened degree of microbicidal potency are known as *activated macrophages.*

If the inciting agent has not been eliminated within the first few days, the activated phagocytes begin to aggregate into a granuloma. Continued stimulation leads to additional growth of the aggregated cells and further augmentation in secretory capacity; the phagocytes have now turned into epithelioid cells, the characteristic constituents of mature granulomas. Eventually giant cells appear, arising through the fusion of epithelioid cells with each other and with newly arrived macrophages. With the elimination of the inciting agent, the

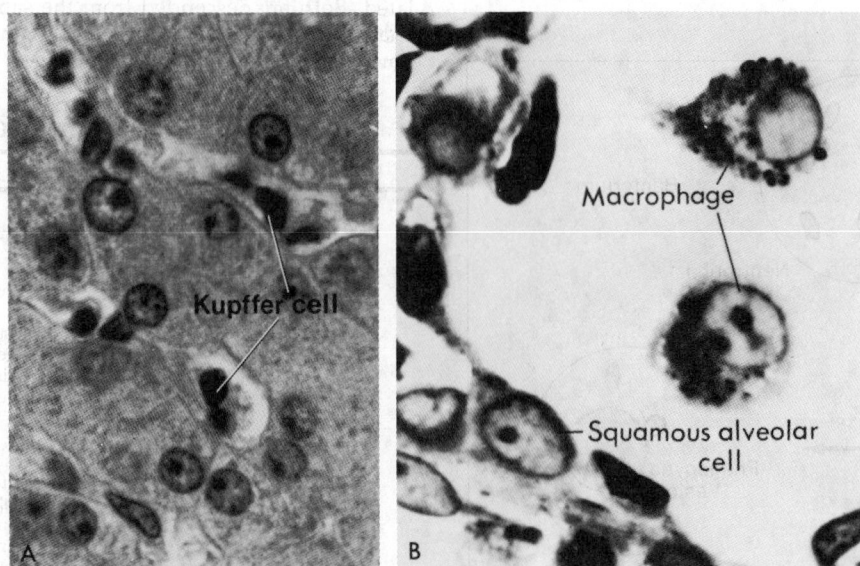

FIGURE 148–7. Some tissue macrophages. *A,* Kupffer cell. (Reprinted with permission from Popper H: Liver Structure and Function. New York, McGraw-Hill Book Company, 1957, p 97.) *B,* Alveolar macrophage. (Reprinted with permission from Sorokin SP: The respiratory system. In Weiss L, Greep RO: Histology. 4th ed. New York, McGraw-Hill Book Company, 1977, p 765.)

TABLE 148–2. TISSUE MACROPHAGES

Fixed
    Kupffer cells
    Microglial cells (central nervous system)
    Macrophages of spleen, lymph nodes, and bone marrow sinusoids
    Mesangial cells (kidney)
    Osteoclasts
Wandering
    Macrophages of serosal cavities (pleural, peritoneal, pericardial)
    Alveolar macrophages

inflammatory process resolves and the macrophages disappear. What becomes of them is not known.

FUNCTIONS. Mononuclear phagocytes carry out three basic functions: secretion, ingestion, and interaction with lymphocytes.

Secretion. Mononuclear phagocytes secrete into the extracellular environment a large number of substances, some protein and others nonprotein in nature (Table 148–3). Lysozyme is secreted by mononuclear phagocytes regardless of their state of activation, whereas proteases active at neutral pH ("neutral proteases") are secreted only by activated cells. Other substances such as O_2^- (superoxide) and leukotrienes are secreted under even more specialized circumstances.

Ingestion. Mononuclear phagocytes received their name from their ability to ingest. These cells use the ability for two separate purposes: to eliminate waste and debris (scavenging) and to kill invading pathogens.

SCAVENGING. Mononuclear phagocytes play a highly important role as general scavengers. They dispose of effete or worn-out cells, remove foreign material from the bloodstream, and clean up debris at sites of infection or tissue damage.

Cell disposal by mononuclear phagocytes is best exemplified by their role in the elimination of outdated red cells. These red cells develop a "senescence antigen" that is recognized by an opsonizing antibody in the circulation. The opsonized cells are then eliminated by splenic macrophages, which internalize and degrade them by a process of phagocytosis, degranulation, and digestion similar to that described for neutrophils. The hemoglobin is converted to bilirubin, iron, and amino acids by lysosomal proteases and other enzymes as described in Ch. 118, while the lipids and complex carbohydrates of the red cell membrane are degraded by lysosomal lipases and glycosidases. Other effete cells are presumably dealt with in a similar manner.

Foreign material is removed from the bloodstream primarily by mononuclear phagocytes in the liver and spleen. In these two organs, the blood is forced to flow through a dense network of mononuclear phagocytes, which ingest foreign matter encountered in the stream. Bacteria and bacterial breakdown products (e.g., lipopolysaccharide) that enter the bloodstream from the large intestine are removed principally by the Kupffer cells of the liver, because these are the first mononuclear phagocytes encountered by the gastrointestinal venous drainage.

Dead cells and tissue fragments are presumably ingested

and degraded at sites of infection or tissue damage by macrophages recruited to the damaged area. Ingestion may be aided by circulating fibronectin, a plasma protein that is able to opsonize denatured collagen for phagocytosis by macrophages. The activated macrophages secrete into the environment neutral proteases that are able to break down damaged connective tissue (collagenase, elastase) and fibrin mesh (plasminogen activator), clearing the way for the reconstruction of the injured tissues.

Mononuclear phagocytes also eliminate from the circulation denatured proteins, protein fragments, and certain native proteins (e.g., activated clotting factors). Some proteins are eliminated through *pinocytosis*, a process in which the material to be eliminated is taken into the cell along with a minuscule quantity of plasma via a tiny invagination of the cell membrane that buds off and enters the cytoplasm as a pinocytotic vesicle. (Mononuclear phagocytes are constantly engaged in pinocytosis; they take in and process several times their own volume of plasma every day.) Other proteins are eliminated by *receptor-mediated endocytosis*, a process similar to pinocytosis except that the ingested protein is bound to a surface receptor before internalization. The lipids of atherosclerotic lesions are derived in part from lipoproteins that had been taken into macrophages by receptor-mediated endocytosis.

KILLING. Like neutrophils, mononuclear phagocytes are able to kill invading microorganisms. Killing by both types of phagocytes involves the same general sequence of events—an initial encounter between the phagocyte and the target microorganism, ingestion, and finally the destruction of the target—but the events differ in detail between the two cell types. Neutrophils, for example, generally find their targets by migrating up a chemotactic gradient, while many mononuclear phagocytes (the fixed tissue varieties such as Kupffer cells and splenic macrophages) have their targets brought to them by the bloodstream. Those mononuclear phagocytes that find their targets by chemotaxis (e.g., monocytes) respond to a wider variety of attractants than neutrophils do. Monocytes, for instance, are attracted by lymphocyte-generated chemotactic factors that have no effect on neutrophils. With respect to ingestion, mononuclear phagocytes can take up particles opsonized by IgE as well as IgG; neutrophils will take up only the latter. Mononuclear phagocytes are also equipped with a mannose receptor that enables them to take up certain bacteria and other particles without the need for opsonization. As to microbial killing, mononuclear phagocytes lose their myeloperoxidase as they develop from monocytes into macrophages, so that oxygen-dependent killing by mature macrophages is accomplished by oxidants that can be generated in the absence of myeloperoxidase (e.g., hydroxyl radical).

Mononuclear phagocytes play a particularly important role in defending against nonviral pathogens that live and grow intracellularly (Table 148–4). For the destruction of these pathogens, macrophage activation is critical. The pathogens are readily killed by activated macrophages, but they are able to infect and multiply within unactivated macrophages, eventually killing them and spreading to infect fresh macrophages. Little is known about how the pathogens evade the microbicidal system of the unactivated macrophages.

TABLE 148–3. SUBSTANCES SECRETED BY MACROPHAGES

Substance	State of Macrophage	Additional Stimulus Needed
Lysozyme	Resident, activated	None
Neutral proteases	Activated	None
Collagenase		
Elastase		
Plasminogen activator		
Interleukin 1	Resident, activated	Lymphokine, endotoxin, others
Superoxide	Activated	Contact with particles or appropriate soluble stimulus
Leukotrienes	Resident, activated	
Complement components		

TABLE 148–4. INTRACELLULAR PATHOGENS AGAINST WHICH MACROPHAGES PLAY A SPECIAL ROLE

Bacteria	*Chlamydia*
Brucella	*Rickettsia*
Listeria	Protozoan parasites
Legionella	*Leishmania*
Salmonella	*Trypanosoma*
Mycobacteria and systemic fungi	*Toxoplasma*
Coccidioides immitis	
Histoplasma capsulatum	
Mycobacterium tuberculosis	
Others	

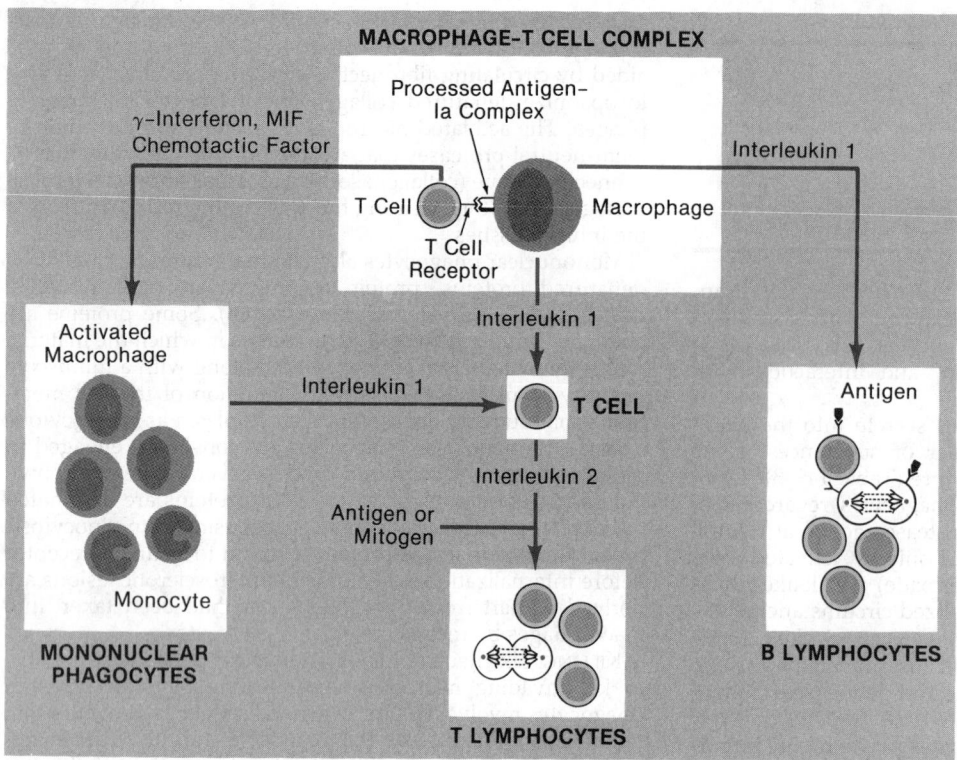

MACROPHAGE-T CELL COMPLEX

FIGURE 148—8. Macrophage-lymphocyte interactions. The macrophage, acting in its capacity as an "accessory cell," presents antigen to a T cell equipped with specific receptors that recognize the Ia-antigen complex on the macrophage surface. The T cell to which the antigen has been presented undergoes activation and begins to secrete lymphokines. These lymphokines include γ-interferon, macrophage-immobilizing factor (MIF), and monocyte chemotactic factor; they cause macrophages to accumulate and undergo activation at the site of the initial macrophage–T cell interaction. Macrophages so activated secrete interleukin 1, a potent mediator capable among other things of inducing the proliferation of both B and T lymphocytes. B cells are directly stimulated by interleukin 1 to proliferate and to differentiate into antibody-secreting plasma cells. T cells, however, proliferate under the influence of a mediator known as interleukin 2 (T cell growth factor), itself a T cell product; interleukin 1 promotes the proliferation of T lymphocytes indirectly by inducing them to secrete interleukin 2.

Mononuclear phagocytes, particularly activated macrophages, are also able to kill malignant cells in vitro. The extent to which they perform this antitumor function in vivo is unknown.

Interactions Between Mononuclear Phagocytes and Lymphocytes. The activation of mononuclear phagocytes by gamma-interferon is one of a series of mutually potentiating interactions between mononuclear phagocytes and lymphocytes that take place at sites of inflammation (Fig. 148–8). Both T cells and B cells participate in these interactions.

The interaction with T lymphocytes begins with a particular type of physical encounter between a T cell and a mononuclear phagocyte. When an antigen-bearing particle is ingested by a mononuclear phagocyte, the antigen is for the most part completely destroyed. A small portion of the antigen, however, is processed to fragments that appear on the surface of the cell in association with the class II histocompatibility antigen known as Ia (the Ia antigen is one of the products of the major histocompatibility complex [see Ch. 417] that controls immune responses to such challenges as foreign proteins, virally infected cells, and tissue allografts). If a T lymphocyte bearing an appropriate receptor should encounter this antigen-primed mononuclear phagocyte, it will recognize the antigen-Ia complex and bind to the phagocyte, and both cells will begin to secrete immunologic mediators. In this interaction, the mononuclear phagocyte is referred to as an *accessory cell* and is said to have "presented" the antigen to the lymphocyte.

The immunologic mediators secreted by the T lymphocytes are called *lymphokines.* They include gamma-interferon, macrophage inhibitory factor, and monocyte chemotactic factor. Their net effect is to cause the accumulation and activation of

mononuclear phagocytes in the region where the initial interaction took place between the antigen-bearing phagocyte and its complementary T lymphocyte. Mediators secreted by mononuclear phagocytes are known as *monokines.* One of these is called *interleukin 1;* among its other effects (for a list, see Table 148–5), it stimulates the proliferation of T lympho-

TABLE 148–5. SOME ACTIONS OF INTERLEUKIN 1

Site of Action	Effect
T lymphocytes	Secretion of interleukin 2 (T cell growth factor)
B lymphocytes	Proliferation, secretion of immunoglobulins
Hepatocytes	Production of acute-phase reactants
Hypothalamus	Fever
Muscle	Catabolism of protein

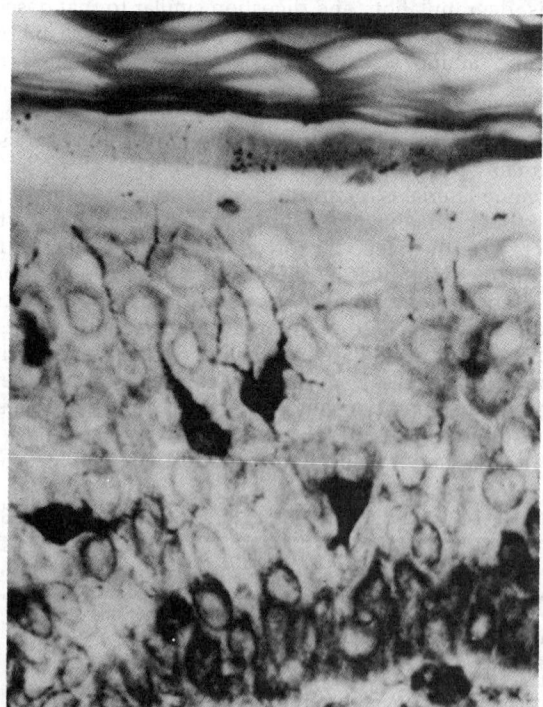

FIGURE 148–9. Langerhans cells in the skin. The darkly stained cells in the acanthocyte layer are the Langerhans cells. Their characteristic branching dendrites are easily seen. (Reproduced with permission from Breathnach AS, Wolff K: Structure and development of the skin. In Fitzgerald TB, Eisen AZ, Wolff K, et al.: Dermatology in General Medicine. 2nd ed. New York, McGraw-Hill Book Company, 1979, p 56.)

cytes indirectly by causing them to secrete *interleukin 2* (also known as T cell growth factor), a substance that promotes their own growth. Another monokine, called *cachectin* or *tumor necrosis factor*, may be responsible for the weight loss seen in patients with chronic wasting illnesses such as tuberculosis and certain forms of cancer.

Macrophages also act upon B lymphocytes. They are not needed for the presentation of antigen to B cells, because B lymphocytes carry surface immunoglobulins that directly recognize the antigens against which the cells are programmed. Rather, the macrophages exert their effects after the antigen-recognition step. They operate through interleukin 1, which they secrete and which causes the antigen-primed B cells to proliferate and differentiate into antibody-secreting plasma cells.

Dendritic Cells. Antigens also appear to be presented by *dendritic cells*. These cells are widely distributed, being found in the follicles of the lymph nodes and spleen, in the thymus, and in the skin, where they are known as *Langerhans' cells* (Fig. 148–9). Like the antigen-presenting class of mononuclear phagocytes, they carry the Ia antigen on their surfaces. They are, however, incapable of phagocytosis. Their role in antigen presentation is not clear, in particular whether they present new antigens or participate only in anamnestic responses and immunologic memory.

Adams DO, Hamilton TA: The cell biology of macrophage activation. Annu Rev Immunol 2:283, 1984. *A complete and clearly written review of this sometimes confusing topic.*

Gallin JI, Fauci AS (eds.): Advances in Host Defense Mechanisms. New York, Raven Press, 1982, vol 1: Phagocytic Cells. *A compilation of authoritative articles on many aspects of phagocyte function. Neutrophils, eosinophils, and mononuclear phagocytes are discussed.*

Ganz T, Selsted ME, Szklarnek D, et al.: Defensins. Natural peptide antibiotics of human neutrophils. J Clin Invest 76:1427, 1985. *The structure and properties of these recently discovered antimicrobial agents.*

Metcalf D: The molecular biology and functions of the granulocyte-macrophage colony-stimulating factors. Blood 67:257, 1986. *An up-to-date survey of this rapidly moving field.*

Steinman RM: Dendritic cells. Transplantation 31:151, 1981. *A short review of dendritic cell structure and function.*

Unanue ER: Cooperation between mononuclear phagocytes and lymphocytes in immunity. N Engl J Med 303:977, 1980. *A concise discussion of the interactions between macrophages and lymphocytes.*

Unanue ER: Antigen presenting function of the macrophage. Annu Rev Immunol 2:395, 1984. *Recent developments in this area, including current views of antigen processing.*

Williams GT, Williams WJ: Granulomatous inflammation: A review. J Clin Pathol 36:723, 1983. *An excellent review of the development and function of granuloma.*

149 DISORDERS OF NEUTROPHIL FUNCTION

Bernard M. Babior

Disorders of neutrophil function are relatively common. For the most part, they are minor manifestations of systemic diseases, rarely diagnosed and of little clinical significance. There are a few disorders, however, in which neutrophil function is defective enough to lead to serious clinical problems. Most of these are inherited disorders in which particular elements of neutrophil function are almost totally deficient.

The principal clinical manifestation of a serious disorder of neutrophil function is the repeated occurrence of major bacterial infections in the affected patient. Such recurrent bacterial infections are most commonly associated with severe neutropenia (<500 neutrophils per cubic millimeter) or an abnormality affecting the immunoglobulins or complement components. In an occasional patient, however, repeated bacterial infections cannot be accounted for by abnormalities in the neutrophil count, the immunoglobulins, or the complement

TABLE 149–1. SCREENING FOR ABNORMALITIES OF NEUTROPHIL FUNCTION

Examination of blood film
Rebuck skin window test
NBT test
Special stains: myeloperoxidase, alkaline phosphatase

system. In such a patient, a qualitative abnormality in neutrophil function is likely to be at the root of the problem.

EVALUATING NEUTROPHIL FUNCTION

A complete evaluation of neutrophil function, including motility, granule content and function, respiratory burst activity, and bacterial killing, requires the services of a specialized laboratory. Screening for functional abnormalities, however, can be carried out relatively simply (Table 149–1). Morphologic abnormalities such as the large malformed granules of Chédiak-Higashi disease can be detected by *examination of a blood film* under the microscope. Chemotaxis and locomotion can be estimated by means of a *Rebuck skin window*, a test in which migration of phagocytes onto a glass coverslip applied to a superficial abrasion is measured over time. The respiratory burst is evaluated by the *NBT test*, in which cells attached to a glass slide are activated in the presence of nitroblue tetrazolium (NBT), a dye that precipitates as a mass of deep blue granules onto any cell that is engaged in the production of O_2^- (superoxide). Neutrophil enzymes can be detected by *special stains for myeloperoxidase and alkaline phosphatase*. One or more of these tests will be abnormal in most symptomatic disorders of neutrophil function.

ACQUIRED DISORDERS

In acquired disorders of neutrophils, functional abnormalities are generally incomplete. Accordingly, signs and symptoms due to neutrophil dysfunction are uncommon in these conditions.

ADHESION (Table 149–2). In the normal course of events, neutrophils undergo frequent alterations in their adhesiveness. These alterations are often expressed as changes in the size of the marginated pool (see Ch. 148). *Corticosteroids* and *epinephrine* reduce neutrophil adhesiveness, releasing the cells from the marginated pool into the circulating pool. Conversely, C5a or agents that cause the release of C5a (e.g., an episode of gram-negative bacteremia) increase neutrophil adhesiveness, causing cells to aggregate into clumps. These tend to be trapped in small vessels, particularly in the lungs.

Besides corticosteroids and epinephrine, certain drugs, notably *aspirin* and *alcohol*, cause decreased adhesiveness of neutrophils. With these agents the decrease in adhesiveness is apparent on testing in vitro, but is not associated with demargination. Evidently neutrophil adhesiveness covers a broader range of functions than merely the ability to attach to an endothelial cell.

In patients undergoing *hemodialysis*, neutrophil counts fall sharply, rising a few minutes later to values that exceed the predialysis counts. Pulmonary symptoms may accompany these changes in neutrophil counts. The fall in the neutrophil count and the accompanying pulmonary symptoms occur because C5a is released when the complement system is

TABLE 149–2. ACQUIRED ALTERATIONS OF NEUTROPHIL ADHESIVENESS

1. Decreased adhesiveness
A. With demargination
Corticosteroids
Epinephrine
B. Without demargination
Aspirin
Alcohol
2. Increased adhesiveness
A. Bacteremia
B. Hemodialysis

**TABLE 149–3. CONDITIONS ASSOCIATED WITH
DEPRESSED NEUTROPHIL CHEMOTAXIS**

Diabetes mellitus	Anergy
Uremia	Hodgkin's disease
Cirrhosis of liver	Leprosy
Severe burns	Sarcoidosis
Bacterial infections	Hypophosphatemia
	Neonates

activated by the passage of blood over the dialysis membrane, causing neutrophils to marginate and be trapped in the lungs. The subsequent neutrophilia reflects the release of cells from the marrow storage pool, possibly another effect of complement activation.

CHEMOTAXIS. Depressed neutrophil chemotaxis is seen in a large number of conditions (Table 149–3). In some of these conditions, chemotactic depression is caused by a circulating inhibitor, while in others the neutrophils themselves are defective. These chemotactic abnormalities contribute in only a minor way to the decreased resistance to bacterial infections characteristic of many of these disorders.

MYELOGENOUS LEUKEMIA AND MYELODYSPLASIA. Variable functional abnormalities are seen in neutrophils from patients with these conditions. Cells in chronic myelogenous leukemia are very sluggish, showing markedly reduced motility and chemotaxis. Granules are often abnormal in number and type (specific granules, for example, may be absent), the respiratory burst is frequently attenuated, and bacterial killing may be depressed. These cells, however, make up in numbers what they lack in function, so infections are unusual in patients with chronic myelogenous leukemia.

In patients with *acute myelogenous leukemia,* neutrophils may arise from residual normal stem cells or by differentiation of the leukemic clone; in the latter case, the neutrophils may show abnormalities similar to those seen in chronic myelogenous leukemia. *Myelodysplasia* is a disease in which hematopoiesis is taken over by a nonmalignant but defective stem cell that gives rise to inadequate numbers of functionally abnormal blood cells. Bilobed nuclei (pseudo Pelger-Huët anomaly) and abnormal granulation are typical of myelodysplastic neutrophils. In both acute myelogenous leukemia and myelodysplasia, bacterial infections are frequent, but their frequency is due more to neutropenia than to functional abnormalities of the phagocytes.

CONGENITAL DISORDERS

CHRONIC GRANULOMATOUS DISEASE. Chronic granulomatous disease (CGD) is the name given to a family of inherited disorders in which phagocytes are unable to express a respiratory burst (Ch. 148). Most cases of the disease are transmitted in an X-linked fashion, but a substantial minority have an autosomal recessive pattern of inheritance. The disorder is caused by a gross impairment in the function of the O_2^--forming NADPH oxidase, whose activity is profoundly reduced in cells from patients with CGD. In some patients the biochemical lesion responsible for the impairment in oxidase activity is in the enzyme itself, while in other patients the lesion affects the system that activates the enzyme. It has not yet been possible to correlate the biochemical lesion with the mode of inheritance of the disorder.

Clinical Picture. The clinical picture of CGD is one of recurrent severe bacterial infections that are slow to heal and difficult to treat. The infections include sinusitis, pneumonia, and abscesses that usually involve the deep subcutaneous tissues, lymph nodes, or liver. Infections generally begin in infancy or early childhood, although the disease is occasionally detected in adolescence or later. In its unmodified form, the course of CGD is characterized by frequent hospitalizations for repeated and protracted infections caused by bacteria that the defective phagocytes are unable to kill (mostly *Staphylococcus aureus* and enterobacteria), with death from infection occurring in the first or second decade. With chronic antibiotic prophylaxis, however, the course of the disease has changed. Hospitalization is much less frequent, and survival seems to be prolonged, but patients develop serious complications due to imperfectly suppressed infections—strictures of the bladder and gastrointestinal tract, for example, and chronic lung disease with fibrosis and bronchiectasis. Death often results from infections by fungi, particularly *Aspergillus.*

Diagnosis. The diagnosis is made by neutrophil function studies. Most of these are normal, but those that measure the respiratory burst are severely deranged: The NBT test is negative (i.e., few if any cells are stained by formazan precipitates) (Fig. 149–1), and O_2^- production and other manifestations of the respiratory burst are greatly reduced or absent. Many microorganisms are handled in a normal fashion by CGD neutrophils (including pneumococci and streptococci, accounting for the rarity of pneumococcal and streptococcal infections in CGD patients), but those, such as *S. aureus,* whose destruction is particularly dependent on oxidant production by phagocytes are poorly killed by these defective cells. In CGD carriers the size of the respiratory burst is decreased by about half, so suspected carriers can often be identified by quantitation of the burst. Female carriers of X-linked CGD are particularly easy to detect. Because these carriers are mosaics, only a fraction of their neutrophils are able to make O_2^-; the NBT test stains only that fraction, leaving the rest of the cells unstained.

A picture similar to CGD has been seen in a few patients with exceptionally severe *glucose-6-phosphate dehydrogenase (G6PD) deficiency.* G6PD is essential for the production of NADPH, the reducing agent used by the O_2^--forming oxidase. In neutrophils that are severely deficient in G6PD, the levels of NADPH may be so low that the O_2^--forming oxidase is starved for substrate, so the cells cannot express an adequate respiratory burst.

Treatment. Management of CGD consists of long-term prophylaxis (trimethoprim-sulfamethoxazole at a trimethoprim dose of 5 to 10 mg per kilogram per day is satisfactory) and vigorous treatment of acute infections with antibiotics in adequate doses, plus surgery if indicated. Leukocyte transfusions may be helpful. Complications should be treated as conservatively as possible, although surgery may be required. Bone marrow transplantation has been performed in a few instances, but with its widely known hazards and the improvement in the outlook of CGD resulting from the use of long-term prophylaxis, marrow transplantation must be regarded as a last resort. Families of CGD patients should be investigated to ascertain the mode of transmission of the disease, and genetic counseling should be offered to them. In pregnant carriers, CGD may be diagnosed prenatally through NBT tests of fetal blood. The recent cloning of the gene responsible for X-linked CGD should soon provide safer methods for the prenatal diagnosis of this condition based on molecular biologic techniques.

CHÉDIAK-HIGASHI DISEASE. Chédiak-Higashi disease is an autosomally inherited defect in the production of lysosomes, the membrane-enclosed granular organelles that are found in almost every type of cell. Normally these organelles are oval bodies of relatively uniform size, but in Chédiak-Higashi disease they are very irregular both in size and shape, ranging from tiny spheres to huge malformed bodies many times larger than normal. The molecular lesion responsible for Chédiak-Higashi disease is unknown, although there is some evidence that the condition may result from an abnormality in microtubule function.

Clinical Picture. The clinical features of Chédiak-Higashi disease result from the malfunction of three types of lysosome-containing cells: the melanocytes, the platelets, and the phagocytes. Melanocyte dysfunction leads to *partial albinism,* a uniform but incomplete loss of pigment from the irises, skin, and hair that can be detected even at birth. The platelet defect

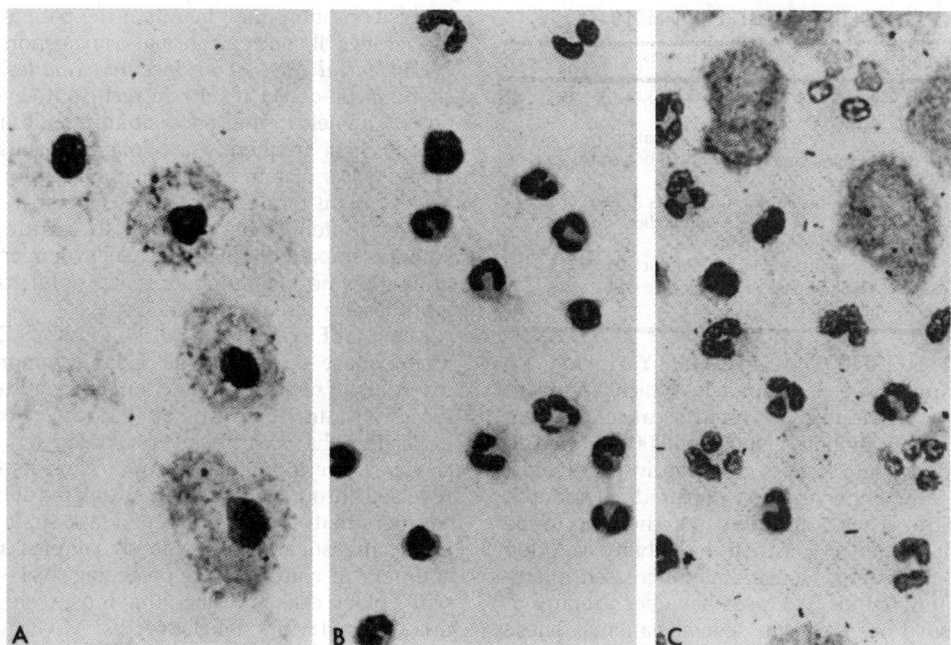

FIGURE 149–1. The NBT test in CGD. Left, normal; center, CGD; right, carrier of X-linked CGD, showing an NBT-positive and an NBT-negative population of neutrophils. (Reprinted with permission from Babior BM, Crawley CA: Chronic granulomatous disease and other disorders of oxidative killing by phagocytes. In Stanbury JB, Wyngaarden JB, Fredrickson DS, et al. [eds.]: The Metabolic Basis of Inherited Disease. 5th ed. New York, McGraw-Hill Book Company, 1983, p 1956.)

causes a mild *bleeding disorder* associated with a prolonged bleeding time. The most serious clinical problems, however, are caused by the abnormalities in the phagocytes. These lead to *marked lowering of resistance to bacterial infections*, so that Chédiak-Higashi patients suffer from frequent deep tissue abscesses as well as recurrent attacks of severe bacterial sinusitis and pneumonia. These infections are difficult to treat and often lead to death in the first or second decade.

Chédiak-Higashi patients who survive into their teens or later are confronted with a further clinical problem, probably the most serious of all. In most of these patients the disease ultimately evolves into a fatal form known as the accelerated phase. This is a peculiar lymphoma-like illness in which the lymph nodes, liver, spleen, and bone marrow become infiltrated with small lymphocytes recently identified as T cells. The lymphocytes look perfectly benign, but they behave in a malignant fashion, causing the infiltrated organs to enlarge and producing through marrow infiltration and splenomegaly a rapid, relentless, and ultimately fatal progression of the mild granulocytopenia seen in the stable phase of the disease. Death from pancytopenia generally occurs within a few months after the onset of the accelerated phase.

In Chédiak-Higashi disease, the white blood cell count is typically low (2000 to 3000 per cubic millimeter), a result of ineffective granulopoiesis (destruction of granulocytes before they leave the marrow). The low white cell count is an important factor in the low resistance to infection that characterizes this condition. Neutrophil chemotaxis and degranulation are depressed, but phagocytosis and the respiratory burst are normal. Bacterial killing is defective, probably because the abnormality in degranulation impedes the delivery of microbicidal substances into the phagocytic vesicles.

Diagnosis. The diagnosis is made by demonstrating under the microscope the presence of giant granules (lysosomes) in neutrophils and eosinophils, a feature that is virtually pathognomonic of Chédiak-Higashi disease (Fig. 149–2) (Color plate 3B). The diagnosis of the accelerated phase depends on finding the characteristic lymphocytic infiltrate in a biopsy of the involved tissue.

Treatment. The management of the early stage of Chédiak-Higashi disease amounts to the management of the infectious

complications. Prophylactic antibiotics (trimethoprim-sulfamethoxazole at the dose given previously) should be used, and infections should be treated vigorously with appropriate antibiotic therapy. Ascorbic acid (20 mg per kilogram per day) has corrected the microbicidal defect in some but not all patients with Chédiak-Higashi disease. Treatment of the accelerated phase is unsatisfactory; splenectomy has been tried, as has chemotherapy with a variety of agents, but neither has proved to be of any benefit. Marrow transplantation has also been used in Chédiak-Higashi disease, though the indications for transplantation (e.g., the question of transplantation in early childhood as opposed to transplantation for the accelerated phase) are not yet clearly established.

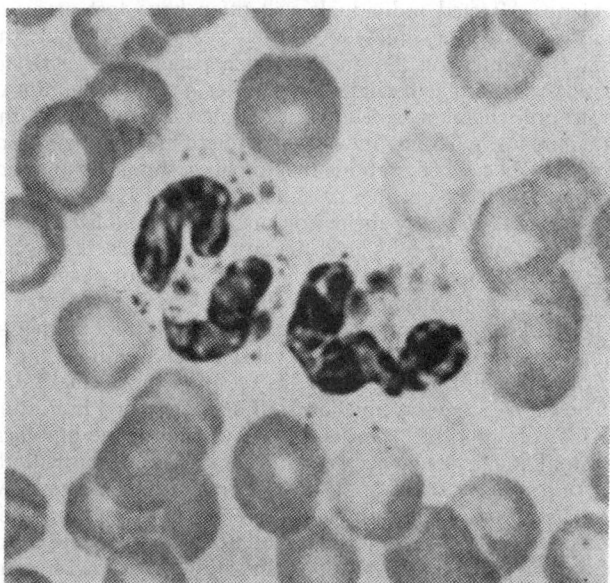

FIGURE 149–2. Neutrophils in Chédiak-Higashi disease, showing the giant granules that are the hallmark of the disease. (Reprinted with permission from Windhorst DB, Zelickson AS, Good RA: Chédiak-Higashi syndrome hereditary gigantism of cytoplasmic organelles. Science 151:81–83, 1966.)

TABLE 149–4. DISORDERS OF NEUTROPHIL MOTILITY

Disorder	Distinguishing Features
Job's syndrome	Cold abscesses, eosinophilia, greatly increased IgE
Juvenile periodontitis	Early severe gingival inflammation, systemic infections only in occasional patients
Leukocyte glycoprotein deficiency	Omphalitis or other infections in newborn, delayed separation of umbilical stump, leukemoid reactions
Congenital absence of specific granules	Abnormal segmentation of nucleus, alkaline phosphatase decreased or absent

DISORDERS OF NEUTROPHIL MOTILITY (Table 149–4). There are a number of conditions in which recurrent abscesses or other bacterial infections occur because of severe impairment in neutrophil mobility. Neutrophils from affected patients migrate poorly onto a glass coverslip in the Rebuck skin window test and show grossly impaired chemotaxis when tested in vitro. These disorders are thought to be inherited, although evidence for their heritability is often weak. For most of them (e.g., congenitally increased microtubule assembly), only one or two cases have been reported. A few, however, have been seen in several patients. These will be discussed here.

Job's Syndrome. This is a condition in which reduced neutrophil motility is associated with bacterial respiratory tract infections and cold staphylococcal abscesses (i.e., abscesses lacking much of the swelling and redness associated with inflammation), eosinophilia, and greatly increased levels of IgE. Patients characteristically have very high blood levels of an antistaphylococcal IgE antibody. Neutrophils from these patients show greatly reduced chemotaxis if assayed immediately after isolation, but chemotaxis returns to normal if the cells are stored for a few hours in the absence of serum prior to assay. This finding suggests that the abnormality lies in the serum, not the cells. The nature of the abnormality is unknown, although a monocyte-derived chemotactic inhibitor has been suggested as the cause of the condition.

Juvenile Periodontitis. In this familial disease neutrophils show a chemotactic defect that is thought to be caused by a serum abnormality. Serious gingival inflammation develops in late childhood or adolescence, similar to but more severe than that seen in normal middle-aged adults with poor dental hygiene. Affected individuals will often have lost many of their teeth by the time they are 30 years old. Among the organisms infecting the gums of such patients is *Capnocytophaga,* an anaerobic bacillus that secretes a potent inhibitor of neutrophil chemotaxis. The antichemotactic agent enters the bloodstream, where in a few patients with juvenile periodontitis it reaches concentrations that impair systemic host defenses and result in repeated bacterial infections. Elimination of the *Capnocytophaga* by means of long-term administration of antibiotics and vigorous local therapy will correct the impairment in host defenses and normalize the patient's resistance against bacterial infections.

Leukocyte Glycoprotein Deficiency. In this inherited disease a chemotactic defect is caused by absence or abnormality of a group of membrane glycoproteins required for normal interaction between neutrophils and surfaces. The first indication of this condition may be delayed separation of the umbilical stump. Patients are subject to recurrent infections, particularly with *Pseudomonas.* The first infection may occur in the newborn as an omphalitis. Infections are generally accompanied by a neutrophilic leukemoid reaction in which the white count may exceed 100,000. The diagnosis can be made with commercially available antibodies (e.g., Mol [Coulter Immunology], OKM1 [Ortho]), which bind to normal but not glycoprotein-deficient white cells. Vigorous and prolonged therapy is necessary for successful treatment of infections in leukocyte glycoprotein deficiency. Prophylactic antibodies are indicated

in this condition; they maintain the patient's health and keep the white cell count at normal or near-normal levels.

Congenital Absence of Specific Granules. In this disorder a chemotactic defect results in recurrent severe bacterial infections. The neutrophils show abnormalities in nuclear segmentation, most frequently a bilobed nucleus (the Pelger-Huët anomaly), and stain poorly or not at all for alkaline phosphatase. Proteins located in the specific granules (e.g., cobalamin-binding protein) are absent from the neutrophils, and bacterial killing is impaired. Under the electron microscope the neutrophils show normal numbers of azurophil granules, but specific granules are rare or absent.

MYELOPEROXIDASE DEFICIENCY. Deficiency of myeloperoxidase (MPO) is the most common of the inherited disorders of neutrophil function. Transmitted as an autosomal recessive trait, it is estimated to affect one person in 500, indicating that nearly one person in ten is a heterozygous carrier. Once thought to be quite rare, its true incidence was revealed through the use of automated white cell differential counters that rely on the peroxidase stain to identify neutrophils. Investigations of blood samples reported by these counters to contain high percentages of "large unidentified white blood cells" revealed that most were from patients with unsuspected MPO deficiency.

Clinically, MPO deficiency is almost completely silent. The only problem that can be attributed to it is an increase in the severity of *Candida* infections seen in a few MPO-deficient patients with coincident diabetes mellitus. The original misconception about the incidence of MPO deficiency can probably be explained by the very low incidence of clinical disease in patients with this condition.

MPO-deficient neutrophils show characteristic functional abnormalities. Chemotaxis, phagocytosis, and degranulation are normal, but the respiratory burst is prolonged because of an increase in the survival of the O_2^--forming oxidase, which is typically destroyed by a myeloperoxidase-dependent process during the course of the respiratory burst. Bacterial killing by MPO-deficient cells is delayed, but eventually reaches completion, indicating that the myeloperoxidase-independent oxidants generated by the deficient cells kill more slowly but just as effectively as the myeloperoxidase-dependent oxidants of normal cells. The completeness of bacterial killing by MPO-deficient cells contrasts with the extensive failure of bacterial killing in CGD, and it explains why bacterial infections are such a serious problem in the latter but not the former condition.

The diagnosis is made from a peroxidase stain of the blood film. The stain normally shows activity in three types of cells: neutrophils, monocytes, and eosinophils. In MPO deficiency the activity is missing from neutrophils and monocytes. Eosinophils, however, stain normally, since their peroxidase is different from the myeloperoxidase found in neutrophils and monocytes and is not affected in myeloperoxidase deficiency. Peroxidase levels can be quantitated spectrophotometrically if desired, but this is usually unnecessary.

No treatment is required for MPO deficiency.

Anderson DC, Schmalstieg FC, Shearer W, et al.: The severe and moderate phenotypes of heritable Mac-1, LFA-1, P150,95 deficiency: Their quantitative definition and relation to leukocyte dysfunction and clinical features. J Infect Dis 152:668, 1985. *A thorough discussion of the clinical and laboratory features of leukocyte glycoprotein deficiency.*

Babior BM, Crowley CA: Chronic granulomatous disease and other disorders of oxidative killing by phagocytes. In Stanbury JB, et al. (eds.): The Metabolic Basis of Inherited Disease. 5th ed. New York, McGraw-Hill Book Company, 1983, pp 1956–1985. *A relatively recent review on disorders of oxygen-dependent killing by neutrophils, including CGD, MPO deficiency, and others.*

Boogaerts MA, Nelissen V, Roelant C, et al.: Blood neutrophil function in primary myelodysplastic syndromes. Br J Haematol 55:217, 1983. *A thorough study of neutrophil dysfunction in myelodysplasia.*

Curnutte JT, Babior BM: Chronic granulomatous disease. Adv Hum Genet 16:229, 1987. *A review of chronic granulomatous disease emphasizing the molecular basis for the disorder. Includes a description of the cloning of the gene for X-linked CGD.*

Donabedian H, Gallin JI: The hyperimmunoglobulin E recurrent infection (Job's) syndrome. A review of the NIH experience and the literature. Medicine 62:195, 1983. *A detailed clinical study of Job's syndrome.*

Gallin JI, Fauci AS (eds.): Advances in Host Defense Mechanisms. New York, Raven Press, 1982, vol 1: Phagocytic Cells. *A multiauthor volume containing several chapters on various abnormalities of neutrophil function.*

Gallin, JI, Wright DG, Malech HL, et al.: Disorders of phagocyte chemotaxis. Ann Intern Med 92:520, 1980. *A brief survey of conditions associated with defective neutrophil chemotaxis and motility.*

Klebanoff SJ, Clark RA: The Neutrophil: Function and Clinical Disorders. Amsterdam, Elsevier/North Holland Biochemical Press, 1978. *This comprehensive treatise includes detailed discussions on many abnormalities of neutrophil function. Separate chapters are devoted to CGD, MPO deficiency, and Chédiak-Higashi disease. Exhaustively referenced.*

Rebuck JW, Crowley JH: A method for studying leukocyte function in vivo. Ann NY Acad Sci 59:759, 1955. *How to perform and interpret the Rebuck skin window test.*

Wolff SM, Dale DC, Clark RA, et al.: The Chédiak-Higashi syndrome: Studies of host defenses. Ann Intern Med 76:293, 1972. *A discussion of Chédiak-Higashi disease emphasizing the abnormalities in neutrophil function seen in this condition.*

150 LEUKOPENIA

Grover C. Bagby, Jr.

The peripheral blood white cell count ranges from 5.0 to 10.0 × 10⁹ per liter in normal individuals. Circulating leukocytes consist of heterogeneous cell types (neutrophils, monocytes, basophils, eosinophils, and lymphocytes), each of which serves a unique purpose and each of which represents a different fractional component of the total peripheral leukocyte population. A rational discussion of leukopenia must therefore focus on specific leukocyte types. Nor can a normal white blood cell count assure that substantial and serious deficiencies of leukocyte components do not exist. Patients may be severely neutropenic or lymphocytopenic despite total white blood counts that fall within the normal range. If there is a reason to order a white blood count, that reason is generally sufficient to justify performance of a differential count as well.

NEUTROPENIA

DEFINITION. Neutropenia exists when the peripheral neutrophil count is less than 2.0 × 10⁹ per liter. Because the normal range in blacks and Yemenite Jews is somewhat lower, neutropenia in these populations is defined as counts less than 1.5 × 10⁹ per liter. The role of the neutrophil in phagocytic defense of the host is generally met if the neutrophil count is above 1.0 × 10⁹ per liter. If the neutrophil count drops below this number, particularly when the count falls below 0.5 × 10⁹ per liter, the incidence of serious, recurrent, and difficult-to-treat infections rises markedly.

ETIOLOGY AND PATHOGENESIS. The multiple causes of neutropenia in pathophysiologic terms are best described in the context of the normal processes of neutrophil production and traffic. Such a description also simplifies the diagnostic and therapeutic approaches to patients with neutropenia. Neutrophils arise from a pool of marrow precursor cells through serial divisions and synchronous maturation steps (Fig. 150–1). The rate of neutrophil production is astonishingly high; more than 10¹¹ cells per day. The bone marrow component of the neutrophil's life consists of a mitotic pool and a storage pool, the latter containing cells that no longer divide. Released after a few days in the bone marrow, neutrophils circulate freely for only a matter of hours before crawling into the extravascular space. For unknown reasons, half of the neutrophils in the peripheral blood are "marginated" along the endothelium and therefore are not measured in the white blood cell count. Accordingly, the true peripheral blood content of neutrophils, consisting of the circulating and the marginated pools, is ordinarily twice that measured by the neutrophil count (Fig. 150–1).

A simple etiologic classification of neutropenia can be derived from the three-compartment model, representing abnormalities in (1) the marrow compartment, (2) the peripheral blood compartment, (3) the extravascular compartment, or (4) combinations of the above (Fig. 150–2).

Abnormalities in the Marrow Compartment. Abnormalities in the marrow account for the majority of neutropenias in clinical practice. Failure of the marrow compartment can occur as a result of direct injury, in which case the marrow usually contains fewer than normal hematopoietic cells, or from maturation defects of hematopoietic cells, principally characterized by normal or increased numbers of morphologically abnormal hematopoietic cells. In either case, neutropenia most frequently occurs along with abnormalities in the number of platelets and red cells. Marrow injury can occur as a consequence of a variety of diseases (Fig. 150–2).

Drug-induced injury is most common (Table 150–1). Antineoplastic and immunosuppressive agents are generally *designed* to inflict injury on a proliferative population of cells; myelo-

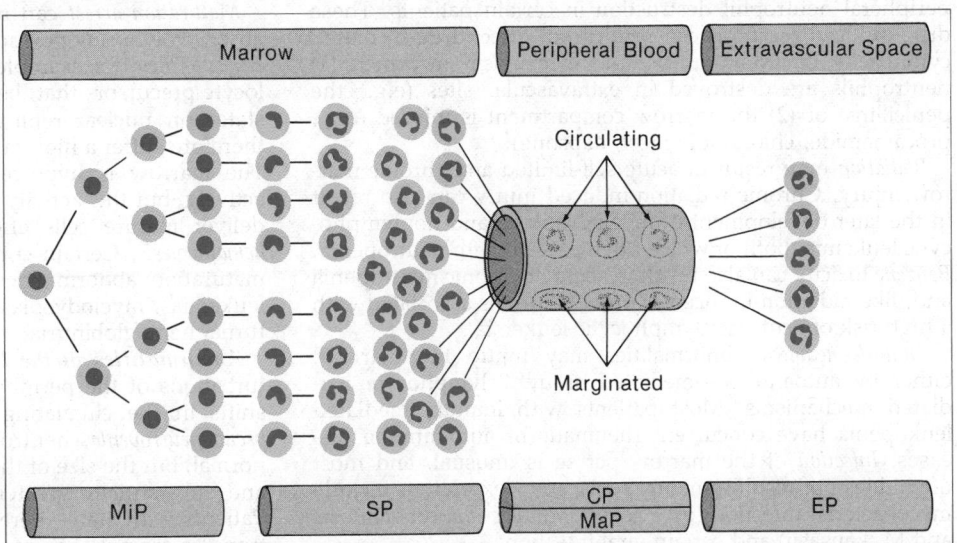

FIGURE 150–1. Production and distribution of neutrophils involves three compartments. Stem cells, committed progenitor cells, and morphologically recognizable precursor cells proliferate and mature (differentiate) under the influence of a variety of humoral regulatory factors, including GM-CSF and G-CSF. These phenomena occur in the "mitotic pool" (MiP). Once the cells reach the intermediate maturation stage known as the metamyelocyte, they stop proliferating but continue differentiating to bands and segmented neutrophils. These cells, although capable of leaving the marrow if needed, generally spend about five days in the marrow, in the "storage pool" (SP). The neutrophils then enter the blood. Half of those cells in the blood circulate and can be measured in a blood sample by counting—the "circulating pool" (CP)—but the other half move about out of the main column of flowing blood, probably in close association with vascular endothelial cells. These latter cells are components of the "marginated pool" (MaP). After their brief sojourn in the peripheral blood, the neutrophils invade the extravascular compartments of most organs, where they are either utilized as defenders or garbage disposal systems or die within one or two days.

Marrow

ABNORMALITIES IN THE BONE MARROW COMPARTMENT

1. Bone Marrow Injury
   A. Drugs
      Cytotoxic and noncytotoxic agents
   B. Radiation
   C. Chemicals
      Benzene, DDT, dinitrophenol, arsenic, bismuth, nitrous oxide
   D. Certain congenital and hereditary neutropenias
   E. Immunologically mediated (largely seen in patients with rheumatic disorders)
      Cytotoxic T cell–mediated (T)
      Antibody–mediated (Ab)
      Mechanisms that require both T and Ab
   F. Infection
      Viral (hepatitis, parvovirus, AIDS)
      Bacterial (*M. tuberculosis, M. kansasii*)
   G. Bone marrow replacement (infiltrative diseases)
      Malignancies (lung, breast, prostate, stomach, lymphomas, and lymphoid leukemias)
      Fibrosis
      Agnogenic myeloid metaplasia
      Long-standing polycythemia vera
      Chronic myelogenous leukemia
      Radiation injury
      Injury from chronic cytotoxic drug therapy
      Acute megakaryocytic leukemia

2. Maturation Defects
   A. Acquired
      Folic acid deficiency
      Vitamin B$_{12}$ deficiency
   B. Neoplastic and other clonal disorders
      Congenital neutropenias
      Acute nonlymphocytic leukemia
      Myelodysplastic syndromes
      Paroxysmal nocturnal hemoglobinuria

Peripheral Blood

ABNORMALITIES IN THE PERIPHERAL BLOOD COMPARTMENT

1. Shift of neutrophils from the circulating to the marginated pool (known as pseudoneutropenia)
   A. Hereditary or constitutional benign pseudoneutropenia
   B. Acquired
      Acute: Severe bacterial infection, frequently associated with endotoxemia
      Chronic: Protein–calorie malnutrition, malaria
2. Intravascular sequestration
   A. In lung (complement–mediated leukoagglutination)
   B. In spleen (hypersplenism)

Extravascular

ABNORMALITIES IN THE EXTRAVASCULAR COMPARTMENT

1. Increased utilization
   A. Severe bacterial, fungal, viral, or rickettsial infection
   B. Anaphylaxis
2. Destruction
   A. Antibody–mediated (rheumatic disorders, drugs)
   B. Hypersplenism

FIGURE 150–2. The causes of neutropenia, arranged according to the compartment in which the abnormality usually resides. The approach to the neutropenic patient should begin by determining which of the three major compartments is likely at fault.

suppressive toxicity is the rule but is generally predictable and dose related. Drugs that are well tolerated in the majority of patients, however, can induce either marrow injury or peripheral neutrophil destruction in certain patients. These drug-induced reactions can result from direct drug-mediated cytotoxicity or from an immune mechanism in which (1) neutrophils are destroyed in extravascular sites (e.g., the penicillins) or (2) the marrow compartment is injured (e.g., procainamide, chloramphenicol, dapsone).

Radiation may result in acute self-limited and chronic marrow injury. Chronic radiation-induced injury can also result in the later development of myelodysplasia and nonlymphocytic leukemia, both of which often present with neutropenia. *Benzene* toxicity can also result in acute or chronic neutropenia and, like radiation-induced marrow failure, is associated with a high risk of acute nonlymphocytic leukemia.

Immune-mediated abnormalities may injure the marrow, either by autoantibody-mediated or by T lymphocyte–mediated mechanisms. Most patients with immune-mediated leukopenia have concurrent rheumatic or autoimmune diseases. *Infection* of the marrow per se is unusual, and most often does not result in neutropenia; some exceptions include mycobacterial infection (especially *Mycobacterium* tuberculosis and M. kansasii) and certain viral infections.

Marrow invasion by abnormal cells can result in neutropenia. Carcinoma of the prostate, breast, stomach, and lung, as well as malignant hematopoietic disorders, can occupy enough of

the medullary space to cause global marrow failure. Similarly, fibroblasts can proliferate in certain disease states to the extent that they dominate the marrow (Fig. 150–2).

Maturation arrest can result in bone marrow failure in the absence of granulopoietic hypocellularity. In *folate* and *vitamin B$_{12}$ deficiency*, for example, the marrow is loaded with granulocyte precursors that, because of the effects of the deficiency states on nuclear replication, fail to mature normally and therefore suffer a high rate of intramedullary death (Ch. 136). The marrow is hypercellular, and hematopoiesis goes on actively, but this activity belies the inability of the marrow to deliver mature cells effectively—hence the term *ineffective hematopoiesis*. Certain congenital neutropenias also represent maturation abnormalities, as do the acute nonlymphocytic leukemias, myelodysplastic syndromes, and paroxysmal nocturnal hemoglobinuria.

Abnormalities in the Peripheral Blood Compartment. Perturbations of the peripheral blood compartment result from shifts in the circulating pool (Figs. 150–1 and 150–2). In *pseudoneutropenia*, neutrophil production and utilization are normal, but the size of the marginated pool is unusually large and substantially greater in size than the circulating pool. Patients with stable hereditary or constitutional pseudoneutropenia are not at increased risk of infection unless a neutrophil function abnormality coexists. Acquired pseudoneutropenia often occurs as an acute or subacute response to systemic infections. It is generally associated with acute

TABLE 150–1. DRUGS THAT CAUSE NEUTROPENIA

Antiarrhythmics
    Procainamide, propranolol, quinidine
Antibiotics
    Chloramphenicol, penicillins, sulfonamides, trimethoprim-sulfa, PAS,
       rifampin vancomycin, isoniazid, nitrofurantoin
Antimalarials
    Dapsone, quinine, pyrimethamine
Anticonvulsants
    Phenytoin, mephenytoin, trimethadione, ethosuximide, carbamazepine
Hypoglycemic Agents
    Tolbutamide, chlorpropamide
Antihistamines
    Cimetidine, brompheniramine, tripelennamine
Antihypertensives
    Methyldopa, captopril
Antiinflammatory Agents
    Aminopyrine, phenylbutazone, gold salts, ibuprofen, indomethacin
Antithyroid Agents
    Propylthiouracil, methimazole, thiouracil
Diuretics
    Acetazolamide, hydrochlorothiazide, chlorthalidone
Phenothiazines
    Chlorpromazine, promazine, prochlorperazine
Immunosuppressive Agents
    Antimetabolites
Cytotoxic Agents
    Alkylating agents, antimetabolites, anthracyclines, vinca alkaloids, *cis*-
      platinum, hydroxyurea, actinomycin D
Other Agents
    Recombinant alpha interferon, allopurinol, ethanol, levamisole, penicillamine

changes in other compartments (Fig. 150–3) and resolves when the infection is appropriately treated or spontaneously abates.

Abnormalities in the Extravascular Compartment. Phagocytes and their precursors respond to infections in a highly coordinated and regulated fashion. The cellular responses are largely controlled by two granulopoietic factors, GM-CSF and G-CSF, and include (1) a rather prompt increase in the rate of production of neutrophils in the mitotic compartment, a response mediated by a complex network of cellular and humoral regulatory interactions, (2) the early release of neutrophils from the marrow storage pool to the peripheral blood pool, (3) an increase in the rate of neutrophil egress from the peripheral blood pool to the invaded tissue or tissues, and (4) increased phagocytic and bactericidal activity of the neutro-

phils. Rarely, increased demand for neutrophils in the extravascular compartment can lead to transient neutropenia, especially in patients with severe infections (Fig. 150–3). In such cases the acute demand for neutrophils completely utilizes the marrow storage pool before it can be restored by increased proliferative activity. The neutrophil count generally rises within a few days. The bone marrow is highly effective in responding to infectious events so that the demand for neutrophils almost never exceeds the capacity of the mitotic pool to supply them. In contrast, neutrophil consumption in patients with autoimmune neutropenia and hypersplenism can outstrip marrow production. Whether this reflects absence in such patients of the complete humoral stimulatory mechanisms that evolve in the infected host, or whether the rate of destruction in these patients actually exceeds the rate of utilization in patients with infections, is not known.

In summary, the causes of neutropenia are heterogeneous and best categorized in pathophysiologic terms (Fig. 150–3).

CLINICAL MANIFESTATIONS. Neutropenia can occur in a wide variety of systemic diseases (Fig. 150–2), the manifestations of which may dominate the clinical picture. Many neutropenic patients remain asymptomatic, most often those whose neutrophil count exceeds 1.0×10^9 per liter or those whose neutropenia is acute and self-limited in duration. When symptoms do occur, they generally result from recurrent, often severe, bacterial infections. This is not surprising in view of the pivotal importance of the neutrophil in the defense of the host against microorganisms (Ch. 148).

This risk of bacterial infection increases significantly as the peripheral neutrophil count falls below 1.0×10^9 per liter but is greatly increased at levels below 0.5×10^9 per liter. The degree to which monocytosis compensates for neutropenia may modify the risk. I have observed a patient with such severe congenital neutropenia that no neutrophil has ever been seen in her blood over a 12-year period. Her leukocyte count is, however, normal because of marked monocytosis; the frequency of infections in this patient has been low.

Lungs, genitourinary system, oropharynx, and skin are the most frequent sites of infection in neutropenic patients. The infecting organisms are the usual pathogens for the given anatomic site. In patients who have recurrent infections and require prolonged and recurrent antibacterial therapy, un-

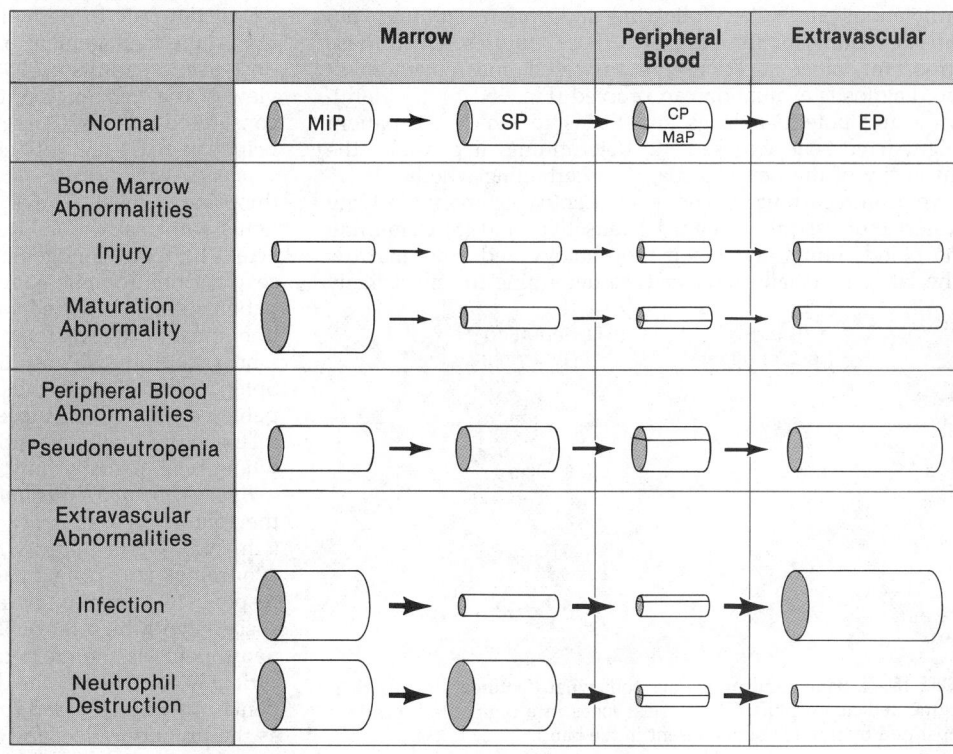

FIGURE 150–3. Pathophysiologic mechanisms of neutropenia. The size of a given compartment is represented by the size of the corresponding cylinder. The number of cells leaving a compartment for the next compartment can vary substantially, but flow between compartments is unidirectional. Notice that, in every case, the circulating neutrophil pool is small, but the size of the other pools is variable. In marrow injury there is a global decline in the size of all pools. A maturation abnormality, however, is characterized by an increase in the number of precursor cells that do not mature. Pseudoneutropenia is characterized by a movement of circulating neutrophils to the marginated pool. In severe infections the acute demand for neutrophils in the infected extravascular site results in a transient loss of storage pool neutrophils before the hypercellular (but as yet immature) mitotic compartments can renew the storage pool. Finally, excessive destruction of neutrophils can result in neutropenia.

usual organisms can colonize and subsequently cause infection. The antibiotic history of patients is important to obtain. *The usual signs and symptoms of infection are often diminished or absent in patients with neutropenia because the cell that mediates much of the inflammatory response to infection is absent.* Thus, neutropenic patients with severe bilateral bacterial pneumonia can present with minimal infiltrates demonstrable by the chest radiograph and nonpurulent sputum; patients with pyelonephritis may not exhibit pyuria; patients with bacterial pharyngitis may not have purulence in the oropharynx; and patients with severe bacterial infection of the skin may present only with erythroderma rather than furunculosis. In the neutropenic patient, infections that in an otherwise normal individual might have been well localized become quickly disseminated. Therefore, not only is the infected neutropenic patient a diagnostic problem, but, in addition, any given infection is more apt to be widespread at the time of diagnosis.

DIAGNOSIS. The diagnostic evaluation of neutropenia is influenced by its severity and the clinical setting in which it occurs. The evaluation in patients with neutrophil counts of less than 0.5 to 1.0×10^9 per liter should obviously proceed briskly. The patient with fever, sepsis, or both, in whom neutropenia is discovered for the first time presents a particularly difficult problem. In such patients it is impossible to determine immediately whether the neutropenia antedated sepsis, a situation with both prognostic and therapeutic implications, or whether the neutropenia is merely a short-lived response to the infection itself (Fig. 150–3). Examination of the peripheral blood smear and differential white blood count can be helpful in such cases. If the blood film has been prepared promptly after obtaining the sample, vacuolization of neutrophil cytoplasm correlates well with the presence of bacterial infection. An increase in the fraction of circulating band forms to levels above 20 per cent suggests that marrow granulopoietic activity is responding appropriately (Fig. 150–4). It is then presumed either that the marrow is recovering from injury or that the neutropenia is derived from a transient shift to the marginated pool or to the extravascular compartment.

The diagnostic evaluation of neutropenia must first address the question of the severity of the disorder and then whether the patient has fever, sepsis, or both. The patient with sepsis and severe neutropenia should be treated promptly with intravenous antibiotics following appropriate cultures, but *without waiting* for the results of those cultures. Once these important initial questions are answered, the remainder of the diagnostic evaluation can proceed (Fig. 150–5): (1) identifying any potential drugs and toxins to which the patient might have been exposed, (2) determining, if possible, the chronicity of the neutropenia, (3) ascertaining whether there have been recurrent infections, (4) identifying any underlying systemic disease that might be causative, and (5) examining the blood counts and blood morphology and bone marrow (the latter is usually indicated) to determine the most likely

pathophysiologic explanation. The latter is important even if a specific, likely causative, underlying disease is promptly identified. Felty's syndrome, for example, is a well-recognized cause of neutropenia, but there are at least two separate pathophysiologic mechanisms in groups of these patients, one mediated by antineutrophil antibodies, the other by T lymphocyte–mediated bone marrow failure. Each mechanism has different therapeutic implications.

One approach to the neutropenic patient is shown in algorithmic form in Figure 150–5. Once the severity of the neutropenia is determined, careful examination of the peripheral blood counts and blood smear is in order. Patients with selective neutropenia are approached differently from those with additional deficiencies of platelets and red cells, although drugs or toxins may be involved in either category. Patients with selective neutropenia but with no drug or toxin exposure, no history of recurrent sepsis, and no underlying chronic inflammatory or autoimmune disease may have stable and benign neutropenia. This category includes some cases of familial and congenital neutropenia and pseudoneutropenia. Any patient with selective neutropenia with a history of sepsis or toxin exposure should have a bone marrow examination to assess (1) the degree of cellularity of each compartment (storage and mitotic pools), (2) the differentiation stages found in each pool, and (3) whether any morphologic abnormality exists in the hematopoietic cells.

In patients with pancytopenia or bicytopenia, bone marrow examination, which must include not only aspiration but biopsy as well, is almost always indicated. The only regular exception to this rule would include patients with unambiguous evidence of vitamin B_{12} or folate deficiency (Ch. 136).

TREATMENT. Rational treatment of the neutropenic patient follows diagnosis and generally involves treatment of the underlying disease or discontinuation of suspected toxins or drugs. The nature of the specific therapy naturally depends on the pathophysiology of the neutropenia in a given patient.

Treatments Specifically Designed to Increase the Neutrophil Count. Trials of the few agents available for the purpose of increasing the neutrophil count must be considered only in patients with severe neutropenia and a history of infections and should be attempted only after the potential risks involved are explained to the patient.

Lithium carbonate, an agent that increases the neutrophil production rate in normal individuals, rarely has been effective in the management of chronic bone marrow failure. The dose used in adults is 300 mg by mouth three times daily. In view of the frequency of toxicity, trials of therapy should be considered only as a last resort. No test to predict individual responsiveness has yet been developed.

Immunosuppressive therapy, including glucocorticoids or azathioprine, almost always elicits a favorable response in patients with marrow failure mediated by cytotoxic T lymphocytes. In vitro clonogenic cultures of bone marrow cells in severely neutropenic patients can aid in the identification of patients apt to respond to such therapy. Some responses to immunosuppressive therapy have also occurred in patients whose neutropenia resulted from antineutrophil antibodies. Splenectomy is rarely helpful in the management of neutropenic patients, even those with Felty's syndrome. It is now reserved for patients with unambiguous hypersplenism in whom bone marrow function is normal.

Bone Marrow Transplantation. In severe aplastic anemia the role of bone marrow transplantation is well established (Ch. 165). Other marrow failure states (e.g., myelodysplastic syndromes and congenital neutropenias) may also prove to respond to transplantation. Allogeneic transplantation is associated with high mortality; its use in patients with **selective** neutropenia is therefore uncertain. Before transplantation is seriously considered, the duration and severity of the neutropenia must be assessed; marrow failure must be established as the primary cause; and immunologically mediated marrow

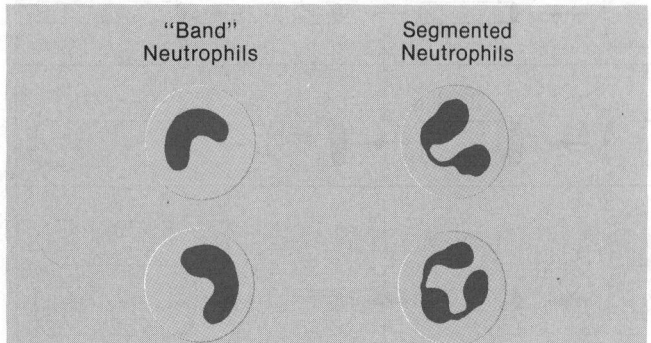

"Band" Neutrophils   Segmented Neutrophils

FIGURE 150—4. Band neutrophils are somewhat "younger" forms than segmented neutrophils. The nuclear lobes in a segmented form are separated by fine filaments absent in the band.

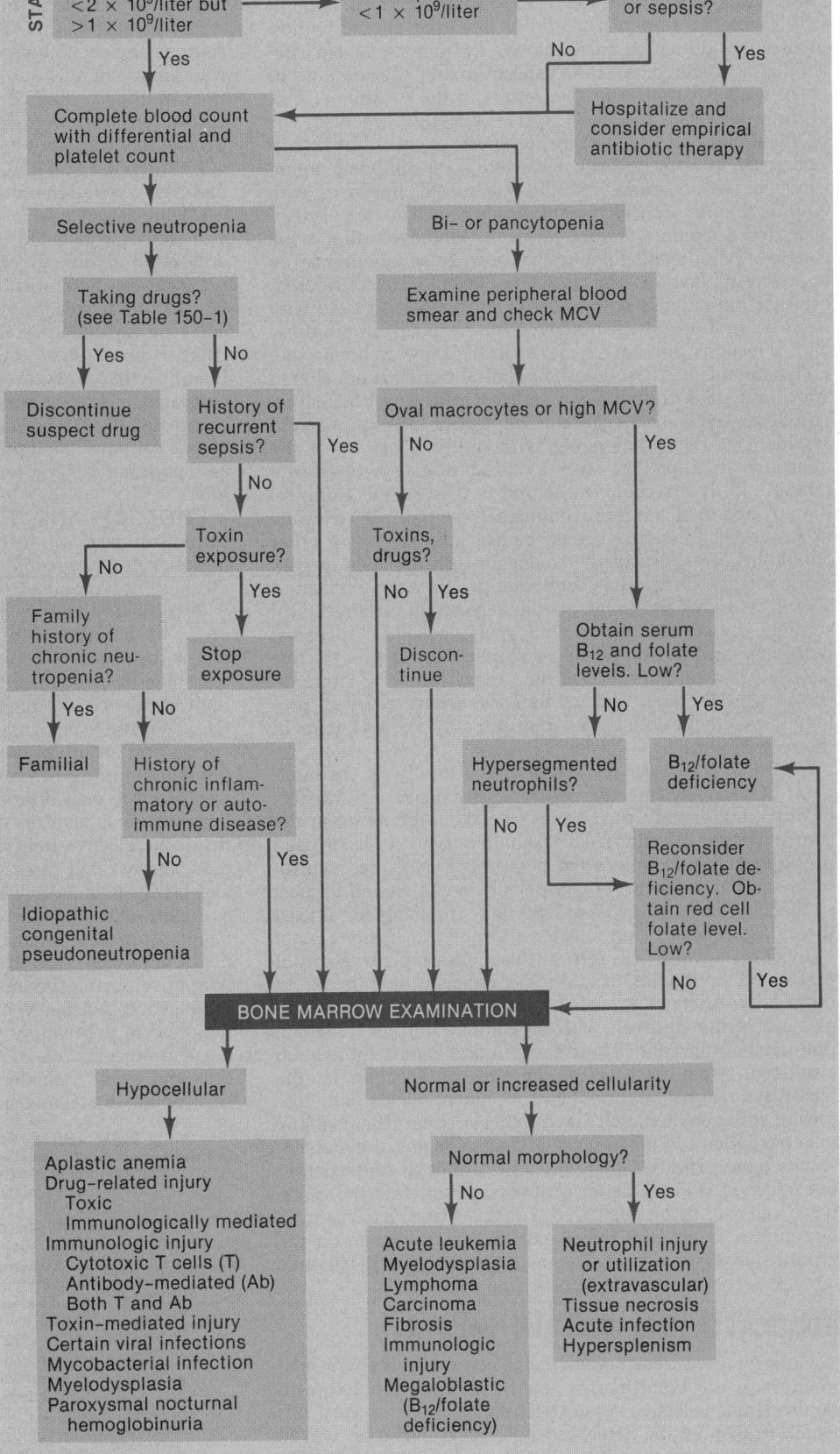

FIGURE 150–5. An algorithm for the evaluation of patients with neutropenia.

failure should be ruled out. If the patient has an identical twin, transplantation might be attempted with fewer constraints, but allogeneic transplantation should always be reserved for individuals with severe and symptomatic neutropenia caused by marrow failure.

Treatment of the Infected Neutropenic Patient. Each patient with neutropenia should understand the function of neutrophils, the consequences of neutrophil deficiency, and the importance of communicating with his or her physician the moment signs and symptoms of infection occur. If a neutropenic patient is afebrile and there is no sepsis, the diagnostic workup should generally take place in the outpatient clinic to avoid unnecessary exposure to nosocomial infections. Patients with severe neutropenia and fever, however, should be hospitalized. Cultures of urine, blood, and other relevant sites should be obtained, but broad-spectrum antibiotics should be given without waiting for the results of these cultures. One of three responses will be seen: (1) A causative organism will be identified, in which case the spectrum of antimicrobial agents can be appropriately narrowed. (2) A candidate organism will not be found, but the patient still improves with empiric therapy. In this type of setting a full course of broad-spectrum antibiotics should be given. Moreover, after a full course of parenteral antibiotics has been given, another seven to fourteen days of oral antibiotics should be considered, especially in patients with invasive infections associated with necrosis, in those whose initial response was slow, or in those with infections that have recurred in the same anatomic site. (3) No organism is found and the clinical picture is not altered after three days of empirical treatment. This unsettling situation occurs with some regularity in practice. The approach to a patient at this point depends on the seriousness of the infection. In a patient with localized disease who is not critically ill, it is sometimes helpful to discontinue empirical therapy and to obtain repeat cultures. If the patient is critically ill, however, antibiotics should be discontinued *only* if other antibiotics are substituted. Among those antibiotics to consider in this situation is amphotericin B. Amphotericin B should be added to the therapeutic regimen in certain clinical settings, i.e., for patients with acute leukemia, diabetes, dysphagia and/or esophagitis, endophthalmitis, or defective cell-mediated immunity (including those receiving immunosuppressive therapy) and for those who have received prolonged treatment with broad-spectrum antibacterial agents in the recent past.

Neutrophil transfusions, when used specifically for the treatment of seriously infected neutropenic patients, are capable of providing enough phagocytes to make a difference in the course of some infections. They should not, however, be used prophylactically in uninfected neutropenic patients. Neutrophils survive briefly in the peripheral circulation and tissues, so that they must be given at least daily, probably for at least three days. The decision to use neutrophil transfusions is not a trivial one. White cells for transfusion are expensive and, if preformed antibodies exist in the recipient, a number of transfusion reactions can occur, including fever, chills, myalgia, and acute dyspnea with or without transient bilateral pulmonary infiltration. These same clinical manifestations can also result from invasion of the sites of infection by the transfused neutrophils and their subsequent release of mediators of inflammation that have hitherto been absent in the infected patient. In the absence of clear-cut signs of hypersensitivity (e.g., urticaria), therefore, one cannot be sure whether the infection is being better controlled or whether the transfused cells are being destroyed. For this reason a decision to discontinue neutrophil transfusions cannot be made on the grounds that such reactions have occurred. Each patient's adverse response must be approached individually.

DEFICIENCIES OF OTHER CIRCULATING PHAGOCYTES

Monocytopenia, eosinopenia, and basophilopenia are seen in most of the bone marrow failure states associated with neutropenia. Selective *monocytopenia,* however, is very unusual. In view of the heterogeneous and critical roles played by the monocyte-macrophage in normal physiology (Ch. 148), complete failure of monocyte production for a period of more than nine to ten months (the estimated lifespan of tissue macrophages) may be incompatible with life.

Eosinopenia and *basophilopenia* are more common than monocytopenia in clinical practice and most often represent redis-

tributional mechanisms resulting from stress, including acute infections, widespread neoplasms, and severe injury (e.g., burns). A variety of humoral factors, including glucocorticoids, prostaglandins, and epinephrine, are released in such settings and are known to induce eosinopenia. In view of the consistency of this stress response, if a patient with sepsis does **not** have eosinopenia, one should consider that adrenal cortical insufficiency or a primary myeloproliferative syndrome may coexist.

LYMPHOCYTOPENIA. The life cycle of the neutrophil involves a well-defined and limited set of compartments and a unidirectional flow of cells from the marrow to the blood and from the blood to the tissues. Lymphocyte production and traffic are difficult to assess: (1) Both T and B lymphocytes replicate in heterogeneous anatomic sites, including the lymph nodes, spleen, tonsils, and bone marrow; (2) lymphocytes are capable of leaving and then later re-entering a given compartment. Given these variables, it is surprising that the lymphocyte counts in the peripheral blood are so tightly regulated; normal counts range from 2 to 4×10^9 per liter. Approximately 20 per cent of these are B lymphocytes, and 70 per cent are T lymphocytes. Lymphocytopenia is defined as a peripheral blood lymphocyte count below 1.5×10^9 per liter.

ETIOLOGY AND PATHOGENESIS. Lymphocytopenia can result from three types of abnormalities: (1) those of lymphocyte production, (2) those of lymphocyte traffic, and (3) those of lymphocyte loss and destruction (Table 150–2).

Reduced Production of Lymphocytes. The most common cause of reduced lymphocyte production in the world is *protein-calorie malnutrition* (Ch. 214). The immunologic paresis resulting from malnutrition contributes substantially to the high incidence of infection in malnourished populations. *Radiation* and *immunosuppressive agents,* including alkylating agents and antithymocyte globulin, can induce lymphocytopenia by injuring the progenitor pool and inhibiting replication of more well differentiated cells. A variety of *congenital lymphocytopenic immune deficiency states* exist, some of which result in selective deficiencies of B lymphocytes, some of T cells, and in other cases, combined deficiencies of both T cells and B cells (Ch. 419). The mechanisms by which production and maturation of B and T lymphocytes are impaired in these patients are heterogeneous; many are ill defined. Immune deficiency states can clearly exist even in the absence of lymphocytopenia, because of abnormal lymphocyte function or selective deficiency of one component of the circulating lymphocyte population. Certain *viruses* are capable of inducing lymphocytopenia; some of these agents infect lymphoid cells and cause their destruction. Such viruses include measles, polio, varicella zoster, and HIV (the acquired immuno-

TABLE 150–2. CAUSES OF LYMPHOCYTOPENIA

Abnormalities of lymphocyte production
  Protein-calorie malnutrition
  Radiation
  Immunosuppressive therapeutic agents
  Congenital immunodeficiency states
    Wiskott-Aldrich syndrome
    Nezelof's syndrome
    Adenosine deaminase deficiency
  Viral infections
  Hodgkin's lymphoma (?)
  Widespread granulomatous infection (mycobacterial, fungal)
Alterations in lymphocyte traffic
  Acute bacterial infection, trauma, stress, glucocorticoids
  Viral infection
  Widespread granulomatous infection
  Hodgkins lymphoma (?)
Lymphocyte destruction or loss
  Viral infection
  Antibody-mediated lymphocyte destruction
  Protein-losing enteropathy
  Chronic right ventricular failure
  Thoracic duct drainage or rupture

deficiency syndrome [AIDS] virus) (Ch. 346). HIV does not frequently cause lymphocytopenia but does infect the helper (T4⁺) subset of T lymphocytes and destroys them, a process that results in a marked decline in the absolute numbers of helper (T4⁺) T cells in the peripheral circulation. Patients with untreated Hodgkin's disease occasionally have lymphocytopenia, especially during the late stages of the disease and with the least favorable histologic subtypes (Ch. 160).

Alterations in Lymphocyte Traffic. Alterations are common and most frequently represent transient responses to a variety of stressful events, including bacterial infections and trauma. These responses are likely mediated by high levels of endogenous glucocorticoids that induce rapid declines in circulating levels of B and T lymphocytes. The lymphocytopenic response to this type of steroid results from a self-limited shift of lymphocytes away from the peripheral blood compartment. Lymphocyte values generally return to normal within 24 to 48 hours. For this reason the transient declines induced by endogenous steroid production are not associated with functional immunologic deficiency. Certain viruses can also bind to lymphocyte populations and cause their departure from the blood compartment into other sites.

More persistent lymphocytopenia has been described in patients with widespread granulomatous disease, a phenomenon that is likely multifactorial, deriving from both inhibition of production and alterations of traffic. Patients with these disorders are often difficult to treat. Establishing a cause-and-effect relationship between the infection and lymphocytopenia is difficult when one considers that the reverse might just as easily be true; consider, for example, the frequency of mycobacterial infection in patients with AIDS.

Increased Destruction of Lymphocytes. Lymphocytopenia can occur as a result of *viral infection*, as outlined above. In some patients lymphocytopenia results from *antilymphocyte antibodies*. As was the case in patients with immunologically mediated neutropenia, the majority of such individuals have underlying autoimmune or rheumatic diseases. Losses of viable lymphocytes can also occur because of *structural defects* in sites of high-density lymphocyte traffic, e.g., via thoracic duct fistulas. In such patients, both T cells and B cells decline in the peripheral blood. Loss of lymphocytes from intestinal lymphatics can occur in protein-losing enteropathies, severe congestive heart failure, or primary diseases of the gut or intestinal lymphatics (Table 150–2).

CLINICAL MANIFESTATIONS AND DIAGNOSIS. There are no specific clinical manifestations of lymphocytopenia per se. The signs and symptoms present in patients with lymphocytopenia are those characteristic of the disease with which the cytopenia is associated. Whether the patient exhibits signs of immunologic deficiency depends on the pathophysiology of the disorder, the duration of the disease, which subsets of lymphocytes are affected most significantly, and the degree to which cellular or humoral immunity is functionally perturbed. Accordingly, unless the clinical setting is clearly one in which transient lymphocytopenia is likely, the approach to diagnosis should involve comprehensive assessment of the integrity of the immune apparatus. Specifically, the subsets of lymphocytes remaining in the circulating blood should be identified and should at least include B cells, helper–inducer T cells, and cytotoxic–suppressor T cells. In addition, quantitative immunoglobulin levels should be measured in the serum, and a series of skin tests performed to detect deficiencies of cell-mediated immunity.

TREATMENT. Because lymphocytopenia ordinarily represents a response to an underlying disease, primary attention must be paid to establishing the nature of that disease and instituting therapy for it. Patients whose lymphocytopenia is accompanied by hypogammaglobulinemia may require immune globulin replacement therapy (Ch. 419). The treatment of severe deficiencies of cell-mediated immunity remains experimental. Responses have been described with transplan-

tation of allogeneic marrow, fetal liver, or thymic epithelial cells.

Abdou NI, Chaiyakiati N, Balentine L, et al.: Suppressor cell mediated neutropenia in Felty's syndrome. J Clin Invest 61:738, 1978. Bagby GC, Gabourel JD: Neutropenia in three patients with rheumatic disorders. Suppression of granulopoiesis by cortisol sensitive thymus dependent lymphocytes. J Clin Invest 64:72, 1979. Bagby GC, Lawrence HJ, Neerhout RC: T - lymphocyte mediated granulopoietic failure: In-vitro identification of prednisone responsive patients. N Engl J Med 309:1073, 1983. *Neutropenic patients with rheumatic and autoimmune diseases had been, until the appearance of these reports, almost as a reflex, classified in pathophysiologic terms as having excessive destruction and/or hypersplenism. The above studies demonstrate that in many patients, immunologically mediated failure of the granulopoietic marrow is the explanation. The third paper documents that among such patients, resolution of neutropenia often occurs upon treatment with immunosuppressive agents.*

Jacob HS, Craddock PR, Hammerschmidt D, et al.: Complement-induced granulocyte aggregation. An unsuspected mechanism of disease. N Engl J Med 302:789, 1980. *This work documents very well the rapidity with which complement-induced aggregation can account not only for neutropenia but for significant respiratory dysfunction as well.*

Lelezari P, Jiang A-F, Yegen L, et al.: Chronic autoimmune neutropenia due to anti-NA2 antibody. N Engl J Med 293:744, 1975. *Despite the difficulties in documenting shortened survival of a cell whose survival is intrinsically short, this paper presents good evidence that chronic neutropenia can be mediated by antibodies directed at antigens expressed by neutrophils.*

Metcalf D.: The molecular biology and functions of the granulocyte macrophage colony-stimulating factors. Blood 67:257, 1986. Donahue RE, Wang EA, Stone DK, et al.: Stimulation of hematopoiesis in primates by continuous infusion of recombinant human GM-CSF. Nature 321:872, 1986. *Since the introduction of the colony-growth assays in 1966, much has been learned about the regulation of phagocyte production by humoral factors. Metcalf's investigative group has shown impressively sustained activity on this subject. This comprehensive and up-to-date paper is one worth reading for a number of reasons, not the least of which is the real possibility that recombinant CSF's will be useful therapeutic agents in certain patients with neutropenia. Indeed, the paper by Donahue et al. documenting the in vivo effects of one of the recombinant factors, GM-CSF, in primates is the first in what will soon be a long list of publications relevant to the therapeutic value of recombinant factors.*

Williams WJ, Beutler E, Erslev AJ, Lichtman MA: Hematology. 3rd ed. New York, McGraw Hill Book Company, 1983. Spivak JL: Fundamentals of Clinical Hematology. 2nd ed. Philadelphia, Harper & Row Publishers, 1984. Wintrobe MM, Lee RE, Boggs DR, et al.: Clinical Hematology. 8th ed. Philadelphia, Lea & Febiger, 1981. *Each of these textbooks of hematology includes a number of chapters on phagocyte and lymphocyte production, traffic, distribution, and function. The reviews of leukopenia are comprehensive, and reference lists are encyclopedic.*

Young GAR, Vincent PC: Drug-induced agranulocytosis. Clin Haematol 9:483, 1980. *This is a concise and comprehensive review of the pathophysiology and clinical features of drug-induced neutropenia.*

151 LEUKOCYTOSIS AND LEUKEMOID REACTIONS

Grover C. Bagby, Jr.

Circulating leukocytes consist of neutrophils, monocytes, eosinophils, basophils, and lymphocytes. Any one or all of these cell types can rise to abnormal levels in peripheral blood in response to various stimuli. Each type of leukocyte is produced in response to specific growth factors. The term *leukocytosis*, an increase in the total leukocyte count to a level above 11.0×10^9 per liter, is less meaningful clinically than are terms that identify the type of leukocyte that is predominantly increased. The terms *neutrophilia* (neutrophilic leukocytosis), *monocytosis, lymphocytosis, eosinophilia,* and *basophilia* suggest specific diagnostic considerations.

Leukocytosis is a common finding in acutely ill patients. When the leukocyte count exceeds 25 to 30×10^9 per liter, it is termed a *leukemoid reaction*. Leukemoid reactions generally reflect the response of healthy bone marrow to signals that evolve in the patient under the influence of trauma, inflammation, and similar stresses. Leukemoid reactions are *not* synonymous with *leukoerythroblastosis*, which indicates the presence of abnormally immature white cells and nucleated red cells in the peripheral blood irrespective of the total

TABLE 151–1. CAUSES OF LEUKOERYTHROBLASTOSIS

Normal Marrow
  Severe acute hemolytic anemia
  Acute infection in hyposplenic patients
Abnormal Marrow
  Multiple fractures
  Marrow infiltration
    Tuberculosis
    Fungal disease
    Fibrosis
    Malignant cells (carcinoma, sarcoma, lymphoma, myeloma,
      acute leukemia)
  Chronic myeloproliferative disorders
    Agnogenic myeloid metaplasia
    Chronic myelogenous leukemia
  Other disorders
    Osteopetrosis
    Gaucher's disease
    Amyloidosis
    Paget's disease of bone
    Severe tissue hypoxia

leukocyte count. Leukoerythroblastosis is less common than leukemoid reactions but often, especially in the adult patient, reflects serious marrow dysfunction (Table 151–1). Consequently the finding of leukoerythroblastosis represents a clear indication to perform bone marrow aspiration and biopsy, unless the clinical setting is acute severe hemolytic anemia, sepsis in a patient with hyposplenism, or massive trauma (with multiple fractures).

NEUTROPHILIA

PATHOPHYSIOLOGY. There are three major anatomic sites of neutrophil traffic: the bone marrow, the peripheral blood, and the extravascular space (Fig. 151–1). Traffic moves unidirectionally from marrow to blood to extravascular space. The number of neutrophils within each site can be independently regulated. The number of neutrophil precursors in the marrow mitotic pool (MiP) is largely influenced by the granulopoietic growth factors: granulocyte-macrophage colony-stimulating factor (GM-CSF), granulocyte colony-stimulating factor (G-CSF), and macrophage colony-stimulating factor (M-CSF, also known as CSF-1). These factors, the products of three separate genes, one on the long arm of chromosome 5, function not only to stimulate the growth and differentiation of granulocyte and/or macrophage progenitor cells but also to assist in activating neutrophils. The marrow storage pool is sufficient to provide the periphery with neutrophils for about five days in the steady state, even if it were unsupported by the MiP. Neutrophils are released from the storage pool into the circulating pool in response to a variety of physiologic stresses, including endogenous glucocorticoids (Fig. 151–1B). Peripheral neutrophils are normally equally divided between the circulating pool and the marginated pool. Neutrophilia can therefore result from a shift of neutrophils from the marginated to the circulating pool—"demargination" (Fig. 151–1C). This response is rapid and can be induced by injections of epinephrine. In patients with acute inflammatory illnesses, both storage pool release and demargination usually occur together (Fig. 151–1D).

A complex regulatory network of mononuclear phagocytes, stromal cells, lymphocytes, and granulocyte progenitors and their progeny responds to acute inflammatory events by augmenting production of the critically important CSF's (Fig. 151–2). The CSF's act on the granulopoietic progenitors to increase mitosis, which expands the storage pool and consequently increases the size of the blood and extravascular pools (Fig. 151–1E). This new state persists until the inflammatory process is resolved.

CAUSES. Neutrophilia (neutrophil counts greater than 7.5 × 10⁹ per liter), a common finding in clinical practice, usually reflects the inflammatory response to acute or subacute illnesses (Fig. 151–2, Table 151–2). Indeed, while the presence of neutrophilia should initiate a search for the cause of this response, it should also be viewed as a sign that the patient is likely responding appropriately to the stimulus.

When neutrophilia occurs in the absence of evidence of acute inflammation or illness, three conditions should be

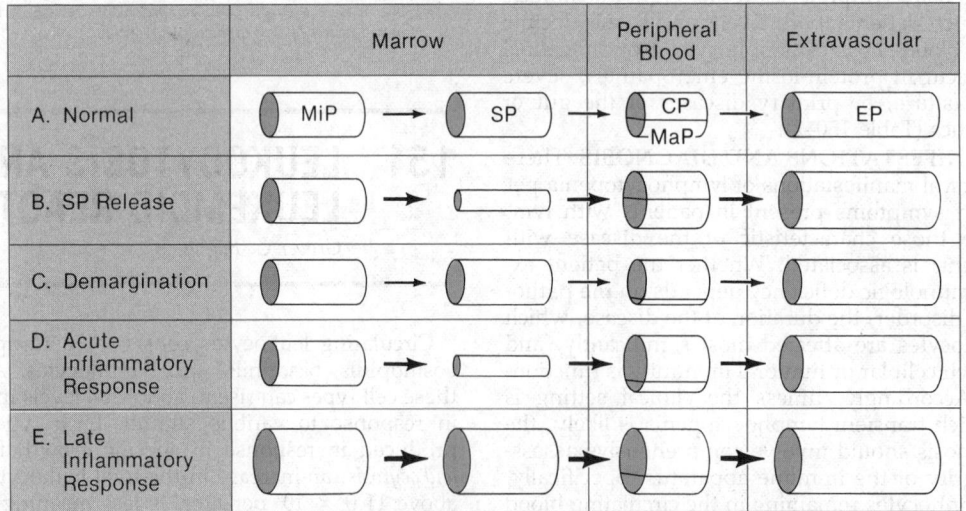

	Marrow		Peripheral Blood	Extravascular
A. Normal	MiP →	SP →	CP / MaP →	EP
B. SP Release				
C. Demargination				
D. Acute Inflammatory Response				
E. Late Inflammatory Response				

FIGURE 151–1. Pathophysiologic mechanisms of neutrophilia. In this figure the size of a given compartment is represented by the size of a given cylinder. The number of cells leaving a compartment for the next compartment is reflected by the size of the arrows between compartments. *A*, MiP = The mitotic pool of granulocyte precursor cells; SP = the granulocyte storage pool; CP = the circulating granulocyte pool; MaP = the marginated pool; EP = the extravascular pool. Notice that, in every case, the circulating neutrophil pool is large, but the size of the other pools is variable. *B*, A variety of stresses on the organism can result, perhaps through the action of glucocorticoid hormones, in the release of storage pool granulocytes. This occurs commonly as an acute response to acute infections. *C*, The circulating granulocyte pool can also increase in size by virtue of a shift of neutrophils from the marginated to the circulating pool. The demargination response can be regularly elicited by the administration of epinephrine and can also result from a variety of stresses, including acute infection. *D*, With most bacterial infections and other inflammatory processes, the acute demand for neutrophils in the infected extravascular sites results in the simultaneous release of storage pool neutrophils and demargination. *E*, Once the hematopoietic growth factor released in response to the inflammatory stimulus (see Fig. 151–2) has induced a few days of proliferation in the mitotic pool, the content of granulocytes in all pools increases and delivery to the tissues becomes maximal.

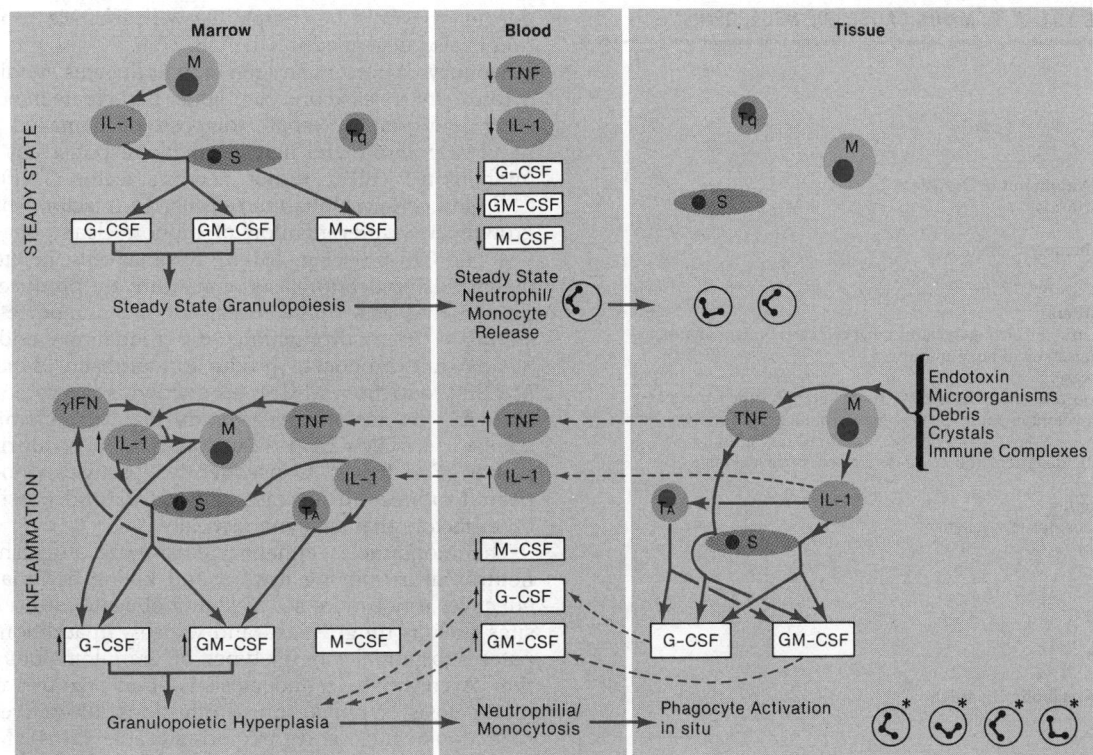

FIGURE 151–2. An intercellular regulatory network controls the production and function of phagocytes in inflammation. The figure represents the likely mechanisms by which neutrophil production and function are enhanced by inflammation. The cells (with nuclei) labeled M, S, and T represent monocytes/macrophages, stromal cells (fibroblasts and endothelial cells), and T lymphocytes, respectively. Tq are quiescent T cells (not activated), and Ta are activated T cells. Two monokines, interleukin-1 (IL-1) and tumor necrosis factor alpha (TNF), are represented by circles labeled IL-1 or TNF. The three lineage-specific granulopoietic growth factors—granulocyte colony stimulating factor (G-CSF), granulocyte/macrophage CSF (GM-CSF), and macrophage CSF (M-CSF)—are represented by rectangles. Relative concentrations of monokines and CSF's are reflected by the size of the circles or rectangles, respectively. In the steady state, stromal cells of the marrow produce all three CSF's. The production of G-CSF and GM-CSF by stromal cells even in the steady state may be under the influence of IL-1 produced by marrow macrophages and monocytes. Blood levels of monokines and growth factors are low. Production of these factors in uninflamed tissues is probably undetectable. In states of inflammation, however, the activation of macrophages by microorganisms, endotoxin, immune complexes, crystals, etc., results in the production of both TNF and IL-1. Both induce the expression of G-CSF and GM-CSF genes by stromal cells and activated T lymphocytes. IL-1 also induces G-CSF expression in macrophages. Production of CSF's in the tissue results in activation of phagocytes in that locale and in increased blood levels of both monokines (the inducers of growth factor expression), and the growth factors themselves. Macrophages, stromal cells and activated T lymphocytes in the marrow also respond to these monokines by producing G- and GM-CSF which stimulate increased growth and differentiation of granulocyte precursors with consequent granulocytic hyperplasia and neutrophilic leukocytosis.

considered: (1) Certain agents such as glucocorticoids, lithium chloride, or epinephrine commonly produce neutrophilia. (2) Malignant tumors may express certain of the CSF genes inappropriately and thereby increase CSF blood levels. When such cancers are effectively treated the neutrophilia resolves. (3) The chronic myeloproliferative disorders—chronic myelogenous leukemia, agnogenic myeloid metaplasia, essential thrombocytosis, and polycythemia rubra vera—may result in substantial neutrophilia. Patients with these diseases can present with few symptoms. When there is an acute inflammatory illness it is most prudent to await its resolution before seeking to rule out one of the myeloproliferative disorders.

DIAGNOSIS. The diagnostic approach to patients with neutrophilia is presented as an algorithm in Figure 151–3. Notice that the diagnostic path leads quickly to the performance of bone marrow aspiration and biopsy for patients with leukoerythroblastosis. In patients without leukoerythroblastosis, neutrophilic leukocytosis generally results from acute toxic, inflammatory, or traumatic stresses, and it is usually best simply to observe the course of neutrophilia to determine its degree of linkage with the underlying disease. If the underlying disease resolves and the neutrophilia does not, other less common explanations must be pursued.

Neutrophil Morphology. Neutrophil morphology can lead to early diagnosis (Fig. 151–3). Toxic granulation of neutrophils, the presence of Döhle bodies, and the presence of vacuoles in the neutrophil cytoplasm suggest that overt or subclinical inflammation, exposure to a toxin, trauma, or neoplasia exists. Because glucocorticoids induce prompt eosinopenia and basophilopenia, these cells are almost universally absent in the blood of the acutely injured or infected patient. Thus their presence should indicate that: (1) the acutely ill patient may have concomitant adrenal cortical insufficiency, (2) the neutrophilia derives from the inappropriate production of GM-CSF (generally by malignant cells), or (3) the neutrophilia is one manifestation of a hematopoietic neoplasm (a chronic myeloproliferative disorder, myelodysplastic syndrome, or certain of the acute nonlymphocytic leukemias).

Leukocyte Alkaline Phosphatase. Leukocyte alkaline phosphatase (LAP) activity is restricted to the neutrophil. Simple histochemical techniques are used to measure LAP levels in neutrophils of the peripheral blood. When neutrophilia represents a reaction to an acute illness, the LAP levels usually increase substantially. In chronic myelogenous leukemia (CML), however, the LAP score is markedly decreased. A

TABLE 151–2. COMMON CAUSES OF NEUTROPHILIA

Infections
Bacteria
Viruses
Fungi
Parasites
Rickettsiae
Rheumatic and Autoimmune Disorders
Rheumatoid arthritis
Vasculitis
Autoimmune hemolytic anemia
Colitis
Gout
Neoplastic Disorders
Pancreatic, gastric, bronchogenic and renal cell carcinoma; melanoma
Any cancer metastatic to bone marrow
Hodgkin's disease
Chronic myeloproliferative disorders (chronic granulocytic leukemia, agnogenic myeloid metaplasia, essential thrombocytosis, polycythemia vera)
Myelodysplastic disorders and acute myelomonocytic leukemia
Chemicals
Mercury poisoning
Venoms (reptiles, insects, jellyfish)
Ethylene glycol
Histamine
Trauma
Thermal injury
Hypothermia
Crush injuries
Electric shock
Endocrine and Metabolic Disorders
Ketoacidosis
Lactic acidosis
Thyrotoxicosis
Hematologic Disorders (non-neoplastic)
Acute hemolytic anemias and transfusion reactions
Postsplenectomy
Recovery from marrow failure
Other Disorders
Tissue necrosis
Pregnancy
Eclampsia
Exfoliative dermatitis
Severe hypoxia
Drugs: Corticosteroids, lithium chloride, and epinephrine

---

low LAP in a patient with neutrophilia should therefore lead to a diagnostic evaluation designed to rule out CML (Table 151–3 and Fig. 151–3).

Differential Diagnosis of Neutrophilic Leukemoid Reactions. Neutrophilic leukemoid reactions generally occur in patients who are obviously systemically ill. When the neutrophil count exceeds 80×10^9 per liter, or when the mildness of the systemic illness seems discordant with the extremely high level of neutrophils in the peripheral blood, the diagnosis most often considered is CML. A number of additional features distinguish leukemoid reactions from CML (Table 151–3). In the past the most definitive test for CML has been a marrow chromosome analysis for the Philadelphia chromosome (see Ch. 155). In the near future even more sensitive tests may be direct DNA analyses to detect structural changes in the bcr (breakpoint cluster region) locus on chromosome 22 or immunoassay for the abnormal c-abl gene product p210 (Table 151–3).

MONOCYTOSIS

Monocytosis is defined as absolute peripheral blood monocyte counts greater than 0.80×10^9 per liter in children and greater than 0.50×10^9 per liter in adults. The monocyte-macrophage is the most evolutionarily conserved blood cell. In fact, its ancestors, found in the circulation or coelomic cavity of marine invertebrates, produce monokines with high degrees of structural and biologic homology to those produced by monocytes of humans. The mononuclear phagocyte plays such an essential role in so many components of biologic life that it seems unlikely that absolute monocyte and macrophage

deficiency would be compatible with life. Macrophage function is also described in Ch. 148.

Monocytes present antigen to lymphocytes, mediate cellular cytotoxicity, release procoagulants, participate in bone remodeling and wound repair, dispose of damaged cells, and regulate immune and hematopoietic responses by producing interleukin-1 (IL-1), tumor necrosis factor (TNF)-alpha, G-CSF, and certain alpha-interferons. Two factors stimulate the growth and differentiation of mononuclear phagocytes: M-CSF and GM-CSF (Fig. 151–3). Stromal cells, including endothelial cells and fibroblasts, constitutively produce M-CSF, a protein that acts only on cells of the monocyte lineage to stimulate their production, differentiation, and survival. Steady-state monocyte production probably depends upon M-CSF production. M-CSF production is not yet known to be inducible by factors released during the inflammatory response, but GM-CSF production is induced during inflammation (Fig. 151–2). Consequently, reactive monocytosis appears to reflect an increase of GM-CSF and possibly also of other factors that act synergistically.

The mononuclear phagocyte is more sluggish than the neutrophil in moving toward and killing bacteria, but is as effective, if not more so, in killing obligate intracellular parasites such as fungi, yeast, and viruses. In addition, it participates substantially in all types of granulomatous inflammation. Accordingly, monocytosis is often seen in patients with tuberculosis, syphilis, fungal infections, ulcerative and granulomatous colitis, and sarcoidosis (Table 151–4). Mild monocytosis is common in patients with Hodgkin's disease and a variety of cancers. High levels of monocytes in the blood are most often seen in patients with myeloid malignant diseases, including acute and chronic myelomonocytic leukemia, acute monocytic leukemia, and chronic myelogenous leukemia of the juvenile type.

EOSINOPHILIA

Eosinophilic leukocytosis (eosinophilia) exists when the esinophil count in the peripheral blood exceeds 0.4×10^9 per

TABLE 151–3. DISTINCTIONS BETWEEN NEUTROPHILIC LEUKEMOID REACTIONS AND CHRONIC MYELOGENOUS LEUKEMIA

Finding/Result	Leukemoid Reaction	CML
Presence of fever or other manifestations of acute or subacute illness	Usual*	Infrequent†
Splenomegaly	Rare	Frequent
Natural course of neutrophilia	Resolution linked temporally with abatement of underlying disease	Progressive slow increase over time
Peripheral blood:		
Basophilia	Rare‡	Common
Leukocyte alkaline phosphatase score	High	Low§
Philadelphia chromosome	Never	Frequent (85%)
Abnormal DNA: Rearrangement of breakpoint cluster region in DNA (chromosome 22)	Absent‖	Frequent (>85%)

*Regular exceptions to this rule are patients with leukemoid reactions associated with certain carcinomas (Table 151–1).

†Patients with CML are not exempt from developing infections. Some patients with infectious processes may be found to have CML. The ideal time to evaluate them diagnostically is after the inflammatory process resolves.

‡Patients with acute allergic reactions and patients with widespread parasitic diseases are frequently exceptions to this rule.

§Leukocyte alkaline phosphatase scores are sometimes normal in CML patients after splenectomy.

‖As described in Ch. 155, the Philadelphia chromosome forms when chromosome 22 breaks in a region called the breakpoint-cluster region (bcr). There are some patients with CML who have no Philadelphia chromosome on karyotypic analysis, yet do have bcr rearrangement on DNA analysis.

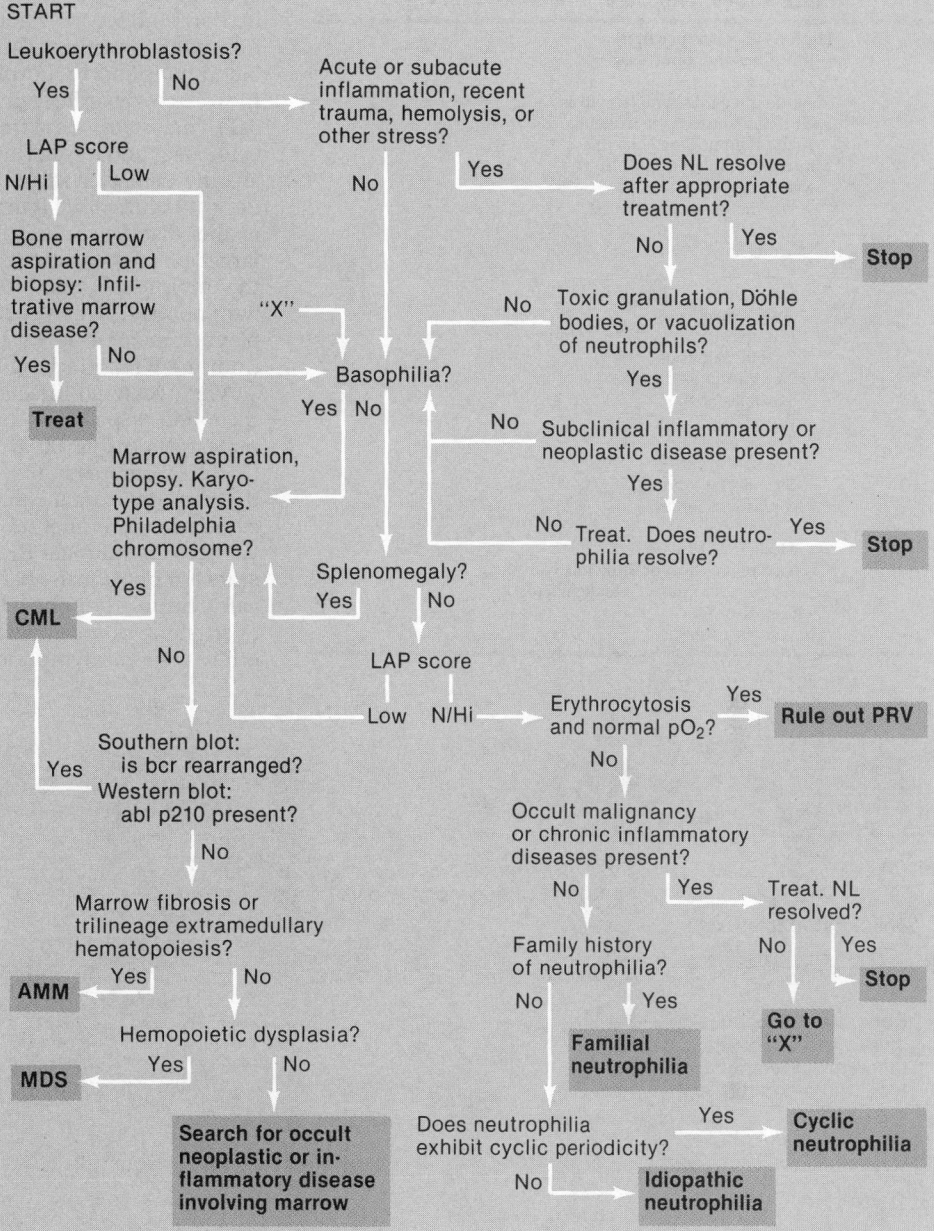

FIGURE 151–3. An algorithm for the evaluation of patients with neutrophilic leukocytosis (NL). LAP = Leukocyte alkaline phosphatase; N/Hi = normal or high; CML = chronic myelogenous leukemia; AMM = agnogenic myeloid metaplasia; PRV = polycythemia vera; MDS = myelodysplastic syndromes; abl p210 = the abnormally large protein that represents the product of the two fused genes, bcr and c-abl. Branch termini are enclosed in boxes.

TABLE 151–4. CAUSES OF MONOCYTOSIS

Infections
  Tuberculosis
  Brucellosis
  Bacterial endocarditis
  Typhoid and paratyphoid fevers
  Listeriosis
  Syphilis
  Fungal infections
  Recovery from acute infections
  Protozoal infections
Neoplastic Disorders
  Hodgkin's disease
  Carcinoma (many)
  Acute and chronic myelomonocytic leukemia, myelodysplastic syndromes, and chronic myelogenous leukemia of the juvenile type
Gastrointestinal Disorders
  Ulcerative colitis
  Granulomatous colitis
  Cirrhosis
Sarcoidosis
Drug Reactions
Recovery from Marrow Suppression
Congenital Neutropenia

liter. Eosinophils are produced by progenitor cells in the marrow under the influence of at least two factors: GM-CSF and another protein that also stimulates the growth and differentiation of B-lymphocytes. Eosinophils function not only as phagocytes, but play an extraordinarily important role in modulating the potentially toxic effects of mast cell degranulation in hypersensitivity reactions.

The eosinophilic syndromes and the causes of eosinophilia are described in Ch. 162.

LYMPHOCYTOSIS

Lymphocytosis is defined as any lymphocyte count in excess of 5.0×10^9 per liter. Atypical lymphocytosis is present when atypical lymphocytes account for more than 20 per cent of the total peripheral blood lymphocyte population (see Ch. 342). The production and traffic of lymphocytes are clearly under tight control. A number of factors induce growth of T lymphocytes (IL-2 and IL-3), natural killer cells (IL-2), and B lymphocytes (IL-2, B cell stimulatory factor [BSF]-1, BSF-2, and B cell growth factor-II).

DIAGNOSIS. Mild to moderate lymphocytosis (lympho-

TABLE 151–5. CAUSES OF LYMPHOCYTOSIS

High (>15 × 10⁹ per liter)
  Infectious mononucleosis
  Pertussis
  Acute infectious lymphocytosis
  Chronic lymphocytic leukemia
  Acute lymphocytic leukemia
Moderate (<15 × 10⁹ per liter)
  Many viral infections
    Infectious mononucleosis
    Measles
    Varicella
    Hepatitis
    Coxsackie
    Adenovirus
    Mumps
    Cytomegalovirus
  Other infectious diseases
    Toxoplasmosis
    Brucellosis
    Tuberculosis
    Typhoid fever
    Syphilis (secondary)
  Neoplastic disorders
    Carcinoma
    Hodgkin's disease
    Acute lymphocytic leukemia (early)
    Chronic lymphocytic leukemia (early)
  Other disorders
    Graves' disease

cyte counts $< 12 \times 10^9$ per liter) is most commonly caused by viral infections, notably infectious mononucleosis and infectious hepatitis. Careful examination of the peripheral blood lymphocyte morphology can help distinguish between these two disorders. In infectious mononucleosis (see Ch. 342), many of the lymphocytes are large, with abundant cytoplasm and a ballerina-skirt-like cytoplasmic border. These are the characteristic "atypical" lymphocytes that exceed 20 per cent of the total lymphocyte population during the course of this disease. Interestingly, while the B lymphocyte is the target of the causative EB virus, the majority of the cells in the peripheral blood of patients with this disease are T lymphocytes. This proliferative response of T cells probably plays a major role in coordinating the process of recovery from the viral infection.

Acute bacterial infections rarely cause lymphocytosis. One exception is pertussis (in children) in which profound lymphocytosis (up to 60×10^9 per liter) is sometimes seen (see Ch. 276). Interestingly, specific soluble factors derived from the causative organism, *Bordetella pertussis*, induce lymphocytosis in experimental animals. In Table 151–5 are listed a variety of additional disorders associated with mild to moderate lymphocytosis. Perhaps with the exception of those with early chronic lymphocytic leukemia, most patients will have overt signs of an underlying illness involving anatomic sites other than the lymphohematopoietic system. This rule also

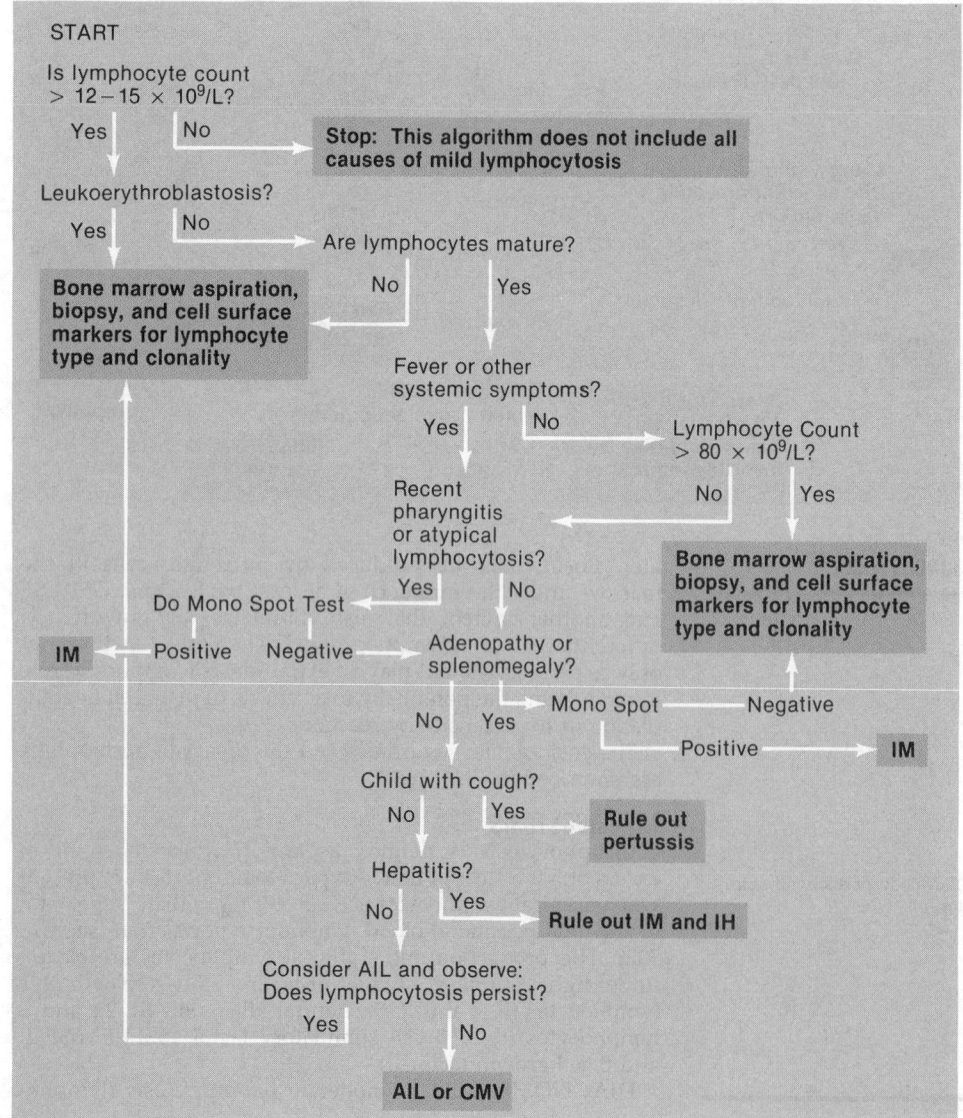

FIGURE 151–4. An algorithm for the evaluation of patients with lymphocytosis in excess of 12×10^9 per liter. IM = Infectious mononucleosis; CMV = cytomegalovirus infection; AIL = acute infectious lymphocytosis; IH = infectious hepatitis. Branch termini are enclosed in boxes.

holds true for patients with substantial lymphocytosis (> 12 to 15 × 10⁹ per liter), the differential diagnosis of which is limited (Table 151–5). The diagnostic approach presented as an algorithm in Figure 151–4 depends simply upon establishing a tissue diagnosis to rule out malignant disease in patients who do not have clear-cut evidence of one of the benign disorders.

An important adjunct to histologic diagnosis is immunophenotypic analysis of the lymphocyte surface. Not only will such studies provide evidence for or against dominance of one lymphocyte type, but they are also capable of determining whether B lymphocytes in the circulation are all members of a single (therefore, likely neoplastic) clone.

Bagby GC, Dinarello CA, Wallace P, et al.: Interleukin 1 stimulates granulocyte macrophage colony-stimulating activity release by vascular endothelial cells. J Clin Invest 78:1316, 1986.

Broudy VC, Kaushansky K, Segal G, et al.: Tumor necrosis factor type alpha stimulates human endothelial cells to produce granulocyte/macrophage colony-stimulating factor. Proc Natl Acad Sci USA, 83:7467, 1986. Zucali J, Dinarello C, Oblon D, et al.: Interleukin 1 stimulates fibroblasts to produce granulocyte-macrophage colony-stimulating activity and prostaglandin E₂. J Clin Invest 77:1857, 1986. *These three papers provide important evidence that the production of granulopoietic factors by stromal cells can be stimulated by the monokines interleukin-1 and tumor necrosis factor-alpha. These in vitro observations provide insight into the importance of mononuclear phagocytes, the producers of monokines, as regulators of phagocyte production and function in inflammatory states. The reader is also referred to Figure 151–2.*

Cory S: Activation of cellular oncogenes in hemopoietic cells by chromosome translocation. Adv Cancer Res 47:189, 1986. *This review reports the pathophysiological significance of bcr gene rearrangement in cells from patients with chronic myelogenous leukemia.*

Donahue RE, Wang EA, Stone DK, et al.: Stimulation of haematopoiesis in primates by continuous infusion of recombinant human GM-CSF. Nature 321:872, 1986.

Fauci AS, Lane HC, Volkman DJ: Activation and regulation of human immune responses: Implications in normal disease states. Ann Intern Med 99:61, 1983. *This is an excellent review of lymphocyte function in health and disease. It covers B cell function and the linkage of T cell function with the function of B cells in a variety of disease states. The references are comprehensive.*

Metcalf D: The molecular biology of the granulocyte-macrophage colony stimulating factors. Blood 67:257, 1986. *This important paper describes the expanding knowledge of the granulocyte-macrophage colony-stimulating factors.*

Williams WJ, Beutler E, Erslev AJ, et al.: Hematology. 3rd ed. New York, McGraw-Hill Book Company, 1983. Wintrobe MM, Lee RE, Boggs DR, et al.: Clinical Hematology. 8th ed. Philadelphia, Lea & Febiger, 1981. *These textbooks of hematology include a number of chapters on phagocyte and lymphocyte production, traffic, distribution, and function. The reviews of neutrophilia, monocytosis, eosinophilia, and lymphocytosis are comprehensive and clinically relevant. Reference lists are encyclopedic and informative.*

152 CLONAL DEVELOPMENT AND STEM CELL ORIGIN OF PROLIFERATIVE DISORDERS

Philip J. Fialkow

Determination of whether a tumor arises from one or many cells can provide important clues about how it develops. For example, a neoplasm resulting from a rare event like mutation in a single somatic cell would by definition have a unicellular (clonal) origin. On the other hand, multicellular origin might be represented by a proliferative process caused by the presence of an abnormal growth factor.

The number of cells from which tumors arise can be conveniently investigated in a person who has at least two genetically distinct types of cells. The normal tissues contain cells of both types, but if the tumor is of clonal origin, it contains only one cell type.

One example of such a model system is the cellular mosaicism present in females heterozygous for the gene on the X chromosome that determines glucose-6-phosphate dehydrogenase (G6PD). In accordance with X chromosome inactivation, only one of the two G6PD genes is active in a given somatic cell. Thus, women who carry a gene for the usual type of G6PD (Gd^B) on one X chromosome and the common variant Gd^A on the other have two cell populations, one producing A type and the other B type G6PD. Since the two enzymes have different electrophoretic mobility, they are easily distinguishable. Cell proliferations with a clonal origin should exhibit only one type of enzyme (A *or* B), whereas those arising from many cells would usually have both A *and* B types. Once it has been determined that a proliferation is clonal, hierarchical relationships of stem cells can be investigated. For example, if both the granulocytes and erythrocytes of a heterozygous female with leukemia have only one and the same G6PD type, it can be inferred that the disease involves a stem cell multipotent for granulocytes and erythrocytes.

MYELOPROLIFERATIVE DISORDERS

Included in this group of diseases are chronic myelogenous leukemia, agnogenic myeloid metaplasia, polycythemia vera, and "essential" thrombocythemia. Although each disorder is characterized by predominance of one cell type (i.e., white cells, red cells, or platelets), there is often evidence of proliferation of other marrow cell types (e.g., in polycythemia vera erythrocytes predominate, but granulocytes and megakaryocytes also often are increased).

CHRONIC MYELOGENOUS LEUKEMIA. This disorder is of particular interest, since about 90 per cent of patients have a very specific and characteristic cytogenetic abnormality, the Philadelphia chromosome rearrangement (Ph) (see Ch. 155). Because Ph is so specific and when present is generally found in over 90 per cent of dividing marrow cells, it is most easily inferred that the disease develops from a single cell containing Ph.

Strong support for the clonal theory of Ph-positive chronic myelogenous leukemia was provided by the finding of only A *or* B G6PD in granulocytes from 32 patients with the disease, whereas both enzyme types were detected in the patients' normal tissues. Conversely, in Gd^B/Gd^A heterozygotes without blood cell abnormalities, with rare exceptions, the granulocytes show both B and A enzymes. The conclusion based on these and other observations that chronic myelogenous leukemia is a clonal disease obviously applies only to the stage at which the disorder is studied. Conceivably, many cells could be affected at an early phase, but when leukemia is clinically evident, only one clone is detected.

Ph has been found in erythroid precursors, suggesting that chronic myelogenous leukemia involves pluripotent stem cells. This postulate has been confirmed with G6PD: The same single-enzyme type found in the leukemic granulocytes was found in erythrocytes, eosinophils, monocytes, platelets, and B lymphocytes. These marker studies in chronic myelogenous leukemia provide definitive evidence for the existence in man of a stem cell pluripotent for lymphoid as well as myeloid cells.

OTHER MYELOPROLIFERATIVE DISORDERS. Although only a few patients have been evaluated with G6PD, the results suggest that the other chronic marrow cell proliferations—agnogenic myeloid metaplasia, polycythemia vera, essential thrombocythemia, and Ph-negative chronic myelogenous leukemia—are also clonal. Furthermore, in each instance, circulating red cells, granulocytes, and platelets displayed only one G6PD type, indicating that pluripotent stem cells were involved.

PATHOGENETIC IMPLICATIONS. The defect in chronic myelogenous leukemia seems to be intrinsic to the leukemic cells. Some workers have proposed that other myeloproliferations such as polycythemia vera or myeloid metaplasia result from proliferation of normal stem cells in response to abnormal stimuli. The G6PD studies suggest that the proliferating hemopoietic cells are very probably clonal and by inference that they are neoplastic in origin. Other points that have emerged from these studies are as follows:

Chromosomal Abnormalities. Specific cytogenetic abnormalities have been described in some patients with polycythemia vera (see Ch. 153). However, in the two studied Gd^B/Gd^A women with this disease, no chromosomal abnormalities were detected, indicating that at least in some patients these aberrations are not a prerequisite for the characteristic clonal proliferation of marrow stem cells. Accordingly, when a chromosomal abnormality occurs, it probably represents emergence of a subclone not required for the initial development of the disease.

G6PD studies of patients with chronic myelogenous leukemia suggest that there are clonally proliferating stem cells that lack Ph. Possibly at least two steps are involved in the pathogenesis of this leukemia—an early event leading to clonal proliferation of hemopoietic stem cells and a later event(s) resulting in the Ph and overt leukemia. The abnormal proliferation of Ph-positive cells is probably related to oncogene expression (see Ch. 169).

Myelofibrosis. Ph has not been detected in most studies of cultured marrow fibroblasts from patients with chronic myelogenous leukemia. It could be argued that the chromosomal abnormality arose in myeloid but not fibroblastic cells after the inception of the disease; however, the finding of normal double-enzyme G6PD types in the cultured fibroblasts indicates that they are not part of the neoplastic process. Similar observations suggest that the myelofibrosis that occurs in polycythemia vera and myeloid metaplasia is secondary. This is especially noteworthy for agnogenic myeloid metaplasia in which myelofibrosis is often the predominant clinical manifestation.

Remission. In clinical remission of chronic myelogenous leukemia or polycythemia vera achieved with conventional therapy, there is persistence of abnormal single-enzyme G6PD types in blood cells, and the percentage of Ph-positive marrow cells generally does not decline. Thus, even though these remissions may be prolonged, they are not accompanied by repopulation of the marrow with normal stem cells.

Residual Normal Stem Cells. In contrast to the results achieved with conventional therapy, about a third of patients with chronic myelogenous leukemia treated with intensive combination chemotherapy have reappearance in their marrows of large populations of Ph-negative cells. Studies of G6PD in one such patient indicated that the Ph-negative cells arose from nonclonal, presumably normal, stem cells. Studies of patients with polycythemia vera also suggest the presence of residual normal stem cells, but with their expression suppressed in vivo.

Summary. The myeloproliferative disorders appear to be clonal proliferations of pluripotent marrow stem cells, i.e., they are neoplasms with varying rates of progression. Myelofibrosis occurs in all of the disorders, but is apparently "reactive" and not part of the abnormal clone. Normal stem cells are present in these patients, and in some cases their expression is suppressed in vivo. Finally, since the clinical manifestations in each disorder are different despite the fact that the diseases all arise in pluripotent stem cells, the clinical variability presumably reflects differences in the responses of cells in the abnormal clones to certain regulatory factors. Determining the nature of these regulatory interactions may permit development of more efficient therapeutic modalities than are currently available.

ACUTE NONLYMPHOCYTIC LEUKEMIA

Many patients with acute nonlymphocytic leukemia have chromosomal abnormalities in marrow cells (see Ch. 156). The data suggest that within a given patient the chromo-

somally abnormal cells are members of a single clone. Findings of single-enzyme G6PD types in 26 heterozygotes with acute nonlymphocytic leukemia indicate that their diseases were clonal.

This leukemia has also been studied with an X chromosome inactivation marker system that has as its basis variations in noncoding intergenic DNA sequences termed restriction fragment length polymorphisms (RFLP's). Studies with RFLP's provide further support for the conclusion that acute nonlymphocytic leukemia develops clonally.

Stem cell relationships have been evaluated with G6PD in 18 patients with this leukemia. The observations in 13 relatively young patients that erythroid cells did not arise from the leukemic clone indicate that the clone did not prevent erythroid differentiation from normal progenitors. Conversely, in five elderly patients the leukemia involved stem cells pluripotent for at least granulocytes, erythrocytes, and platelets. Acute nonlymphocytic leukemia is therefore heterogeneous. In some patients it is expressed in cells with restricted differentiative expression; in others it involves stem cells with multipotent differentiative expression. Perhaps these differences underlie variations in cause and clinical features, including prognosis.

During some clinical remissions of this malignant disease the marrow seems to be repopulated by normal stem cells. For example, normal double-enzyme blood cell G6PD types were observed during remission in nine patients whose leukemia showed restricted differentiative expression. Thus, normal stem cells must have been present, but their proliferation was suppressed during the acute phase of the disease.

Another type of clinical remission, one that was associated with persistence of clonally derived stem cells, was found in two patients whose leukemia involved multipotent stem cells. Evidence that remission granulocytes were clonal was also found in 3 of 13 patients heterozygous for an RFLP.

The demonstration that clonal remissions are not uncommon suggests that this leukemia often has a multistep pathogenesis. Presumably an early event results in clonal proliferation of preleukemic stem cells that can differentiate to normal granulocytes. Overt leukemia evolves after a second step(s) occurs.

LYMPHOPROLIFERATIVE DISORDERS

IMMUNOGLOBULIN MOSAICISM. Immunoglobulin (Ig), as well as G6PD, is a useful marker in lymphoproliferative neoplasms. Since each Ig-synthesizing cell is committed to producing antibody molecules having only one variable region (idiotypic specificity) and only one light chain (κ or λ) and there are thousands of different antibodies, the immune system has extensive cellular mosaicism. The finding that a population of cells synthesizes only one type of Ig suggests that it is clonal. B lymphocytes, the precursors of plasma cells that secrete antibody, synthesize Ig that can be detected in the cytoplasm or on the cell's surface.

CHRONIC LYMPHOCYTIC LEUKEMIA. The proliferating cells in about 95 per cent of patients with this leukemia are B lymphocytes. The supposition that the disease is clonal based on Ig markers has been confirmed with G6PD. The G6PD studies also indicate that chronic lymphocytic leukemia is expressed in progenitors with differentiative expression restricted to the B-lymphocyte pathway and not to myeloid cells or at least to most blood T lymphocytes.

MULTIPLE MYELOMA. With rare exceptions, all the plasma cells in a given myeloma patient secrete Ig with the same light chain and idiotype, indicating clonal development. The total blood lymphocyte count is usually not increased in this disease. However, the fact that the surfaces of many circulating B lymphocytes and the cytoplasm of some pre-B cells have the same Ig molecules as those in the plasma indicates proliferation of a clone of early lymphocytes that ultimately differentiates into Ig-secreting plasma cells. This situation differs from that in chronic lymphocytic leukemia, in which maturation of the clone is restricted, i.e., most such patients do not have high levels of monospecific Ig in their serum.

WALDENSTRÖM'S MACROGLOBULINEMIA. This disease has features in common with chronic lymphocytic leukemia and multiple myeloma (see Ch. 163). As in myeloma, the same monospecific Ig found in the plasma is present on many marrow and circulating lymphocytes. In this sense Waldenström's macroglobulinemia and multiple myeloma might be regarded as forms of chronic lymphocytic leukemia in which the lymphocyte clone continues to mature from the small B cell to the mature plasma cell.

ACUTE LYMPHOCYTIC LEUKEMIA. In those few studied patients whose acute leukemia cells synthesize Ig, the data suggest clonal development. Studies with G6PD in untreated patients with the common form of this leukemia indicate that the disease is clonal and involves progenitors with differentiative expression limited to the lymphoid pathway. Cells in this type of acute lymphocytic leukemia do not have T cell surface markers or Ig synthesis. However, they do have rearranged Ig genes, indicating that they have B cell lineage differentiation potential. In many patients the Ig gene rearrangements are of a single type in all of the blast cells, providing more evidence that the common type of acute lymphocytic leukemia develops clonally. The presence of multiple Ig rearrangements found in some patients with B lymphoid malignant diseases probably results from the origin of the diseases in immature cells that continue to undergo Ig rearrangements as the neoplasms evolve. As differentiation proceeds within this clone, two or more subclones with different Ig gene rearrangements develop.

In 17 patients heterozygous for G6PD tested during remission, there was a return to nonclonal lymphopoiesis, indicating that the marrow was predominantly repopulated by normal cells. However, with a more sensitive Ig gene rearrangement marker technique, residual leukemic cells were found in remission stages of three of seven studied patients. This finding and the fact that the same monomorphic G6PD type found at diagnosis is present in relapse indicates that small numbers of leukemic cells persist during remission.

NON-HODGKIN'S LYMPHOMA. Ig markers in studies of B cell lymphomas indicate clonal development. Burkitt's lymphoma, a disease for which there is much circumstantial evidence of a viral cause, has been evaluated extensively with G6PD and Ig. The results indicate clonal development. Thus, if a virus causes the lymphoma, it either does so by inducing a rare change or constitutes but one of several factors necessary for tumorigenesis.

Burkitt's Tumor Relapses. Although the majority of patients with Burkitt's lymphoma have therapeutically induced clinical remissions, tumors reappear in over half the cases. Clinical and cell marker studies indicate that there are important biologic differences between early and late relapses. Thus, the G6PD and Ig types of early (<5 months) recurrent tumors were the same as those detected in the tumors on initial presentation, indicating re-emergence of the malignant clones. In contrast, the markers in some late (>5 months) Burkitt's tumor relapses were discordant with those originally found, indicating emergence of newly malignant cells or of neoplastic cells present but undetected when the patients were initially studied.

T CELL NEOPLASMS. T lymphocytes have on their surfaces receptors for antibody-bound antigen. In a process analogous to what occurs in B cell differentiation, as T lymphoid cells mature the T cell receptor genes undergo rearrangements. The finding in a neoplasm of such recombinations in the absence of Ig gene rearrangements indicates that the tumor is of T cell origin. The finding of one and the same T cell receptor gene rearrangement in all of the neoplastic cells indicates that the tumor developed clonally. With this system it has been shown, for example, that mycosis fungoides is a clonal neoplasm of T cell origin.

Korsmeyer AJ, Arnold A, Bakhsi A, et al: Immunoglobulin gene rearrangement and cell surface antigen expression in acute lymphocytic leukemias of T cell and B cell precursor origins. J Clin Invest 71:301, 1983.
Raskind WH, Fialkow PJ: The use of cell markers in the study of human hematopoietic neoplasia. In Weinhouse S, Klein G (eds.): Advances in Cancer Research. New York, Academic Press (in press). *A detailed review of studies of blood cell neoplasms with glucose-6-phosphate dehydrogenase, immunoglobulin, and T cell receptor markers; 209 references.*

153 ERYTHROCYTOSIS AND POLYCYTHEMIA

Paul D. Berk

Erythrocytosis, manifested by elevations of the red blood cell count, hematocrit, and hemoglobin concentration, represents a complex problem in differential diagnosis. Accurate diagnosis is crucial to appropriate management, particularly because therapy for certain diagnostic categories would be contraindicated in others.

Early in the evaluation of erythrocytosis it is important to differentiate an increase in the total red cell mass (absolute erythrocytosis) from a decrease in plasma volume (relative erythrocytosis). Patients with absolute erythrocytosis must be further categorized into those in whom excessive production of red cells results from a disorder intrinsic to the erythroid progenitor cells of the bone marrow (primary) or from excessive stimulation of an otherwise normal marrow by substances such as erythropoietin (secondary).

RELATIVE POLYCYTHEMIA

The hemoglobin concentration, hematocrit, and red blood cell count are usually interpreted as indicators of the circulating red blood cell or hemoglobin masses. In fact, these variables are merely measures of the extent to which the red cell mass is diluted in the plasma volume. Both the red cell mass and the plasma volume are regulated by separate and to a considerable extent independent physiologic controls. Hence, a patient with an elevated hemoglobin concentration, hematocrit, or red cell count may have (1) an increase in the red cell mass, i.e., an absolute erythrocytosis; (2) a reduction in the plasma volume; or (3) a combination of a red cell mass at the upper end of the normal range and plasma volume at the lower end of the normal range. These latter two situations have been termed relative or spurious polycythemia, since the elevated hemoglobin concentration, hematocrit, and red cell count do not reflect an absolute increase in the mass of circulating erythrocytes. Strictly speaking, the designation polycythemia should be reserved for conditions involving increased levels of other formed elements (granulocytes, platelets) in addition to erythrocytes; in fact, the term *polycythemia* is also widely applied to disorders characterized solely by abnormalities in erythroid parameters and will therefore be employed in this chapter.

The most frequent cause of relative polycythemia is dehydration. In settings in which dehydration is likely, fluid balance should be corrected before a hematologic evaluation of an elevated hematocrit is done. As an important first step, after dehydration is ruled out, patients with absolute polycythemia can be accurately distinguished from those with relative polycythemia by measurement of both the red cell mass and plasma volume, using ^{51}Cr-labeled erythrocytes and ^{125}I-albumin, respectively. This is especially important because, in the absence of conditions associated with arterial hypoxemia (cyanotic congenital heart disease, chronic pulmonary disease), cases of relative polycythemia are at least as common as cases of absolute polycythemia but need not be subjected to the extensive and expensive investigations that may be required to determine the cause of an absolute increase in the circulating red cell mass.

The normal red cell mass averages 30 ± 3 (SD) ml per kilogram in men and 27 ± 2 ml per kilogram in women. Although some studies indicate that hematocrits as high as 54 per cent in men or 48 per cent in women may be normal, increased red cell masses will be found in a small proportion of individuals of either sex with hematocrits in the upper 40's. As the hematocrit increases into the 50's, the proportion of patients with an increased red cell mass also increases but does not reach 100 per cent until the hematocrit is in excess of 60. Since approximately half of patients with polycythemia vera and other forms of true erythrocytosis and a large majority of those with spurious erythrocytosis present with hematocrits between 50 and 60, the need for direct measurement of the red cell mass to distinguish true polycythemia from spurious erythrocytosis is apparent.

Relative erythrocytosis, also called spurious polycythemia, stress polycythemia, and Gaisböck's syndrome, typically occurs in hypertensive obese middle-aged men, and especially in those who are heavy smokers. The male-female ratio is at least 5:1. Its underlying pathophysiology remains obscure. Both hypertension and its frequent therapy with diuretics may lead to reduction in the plasma volume. Smoking may contribute by two mechanisms. Both nicotine and carboxyhemoglobin, which circulates in smokers because of inhalation of carbon monoxide, may have mild diuretic effects. In addition, the presence of carboxyhemoglobin causes a shift to the left in the oxygen dissociation curve of the remaining hemoglobin, leading to mildly impaired tissue oxygenation. Normal compensatory mechanisms, in turn, lead to a modest increase in the red cell mass that may not always exceed the normal range, particularly when expressed per kilogram of body weight in an obese patient. In some smokers discontinuation of smoking results in cure of the erythrocytosis.

Relative erythrocytosis is not always a benign condition, the incidence of thromboembolic events reaching almost 30 per cent in some series, especially in patients with an absolute reduction in plasma volume. Treatment remains controversial, but maintenance of the hematocrit at no more than 50 per cent by a judicious phlebotomy regimen is often recommended and may be beneficial.

Burge PS, Johnson WS, Prankard TAJ: Morbidity and mortality in pseudo polycythemia. Lancet 1:1266, 1975. *Follow-up study documenting excess morbidity and mortality in patients with relative erythrocytosis.*
Humphrey PRD, Michael J, Pearson TC: Red cell mass, plasma volume and blood volume before and after venesection in relative polycythemia. Br J Haematol 46:435, 1980. *Documents that phlebotomy in relative polycythemia is followed by expansion of the plasma volume, so that hypovolemia does not occur.*
Smith JR, Landaw SA: Smokers' polycythemia. N Engl J Med 293:6, 1978. *A report convincingly linking smoking to polycythemia and suggesting that chain smoking is the link that ties stress to polycythemia.*

ABSOLUTE POLYCYTHEMIA: PATHOPHYSIOLOGY AND CLINICAL EVALUATION

Regulation of the Red Cell Mass

The circulating red cell mass is determined by a balance between the rate at which new erythrocytes are produced and released from the bone marrow and the rate of peripheral red cell destruction. The latter, as measured by studies of the red cell lifespan, is ordinarily fixed, with a normal mean value of about 100 days. While red cell lifespan may be reduced in pathologic states, there are no mechanisms by which it may be increased. Hence, physiologic regulation of the red cell mass occurs entirely by changes in the rate of red cell production.

Alterations in the red cell mass are effected so as to provide for a critical level of tissue oxygenation (Fig. 153–1). The principal sensors of the state of tissue oxygenation in adults are probably located in the kidney, although the existence of extrarenal oxygen sensors has also been proposed. The kidney responds to the perceived adequacy of oxygen delivery by modulating the output of the hormone erythropoietin. The gene for this carbohydrate-rich glycoprotein has been successfully cloned, and its biologic activity has been found to reside in a 166-amino acid polypeptide chain.

The initial commitment of pluripotent bone marrow stem cells to differentiate to the earliest erythroid-committed progenitors, the *erythroid burst-forming units* (BFU$_E$), depends principally on a T cell–derived growth regulator called *burst-promoting activity*. By contrast, erythropoietin, the principal regulator of the subsequent stages of erythropoiesis, appears to stimulate proliferation of the *erythroid colony–forming units* (CFU$_E$), the more differentiated but still morphologically unrecognizable progeny of the BFU$_E$. Since further differentiation of the CFU$_E$ to early, recognizable proerythroblasts is a stochastic process, expansion of the pool of CFU$_E$ results in an increase in the production of recognizable erythroid precursors in the marrow. Erythropoietin also shortens the overall maturation time of developing erythroid precursors and accelerates the release of reticulocytes into the circulation. Hence its net effect is to increase the output of red cells from the marrow and ultimately to expand the circulating red cell mass.

Mechanisms Producing Erythrocytosis

Erythrocytosis or "polycythemia" reflects an increase in marrow red cell production caused by increased proliferation of erythroid progenitors. This proliferation could be either "autonomous" as a result of an intrinsic cellular defect permitting escape from normal regulatory mechanisms or secondary to an external stimulus.

AUTONOMOUS PROLIFERATION. The increased erythroid activity in the primary polycythemias, including polycythemia rubra vera and the more recently described entity of

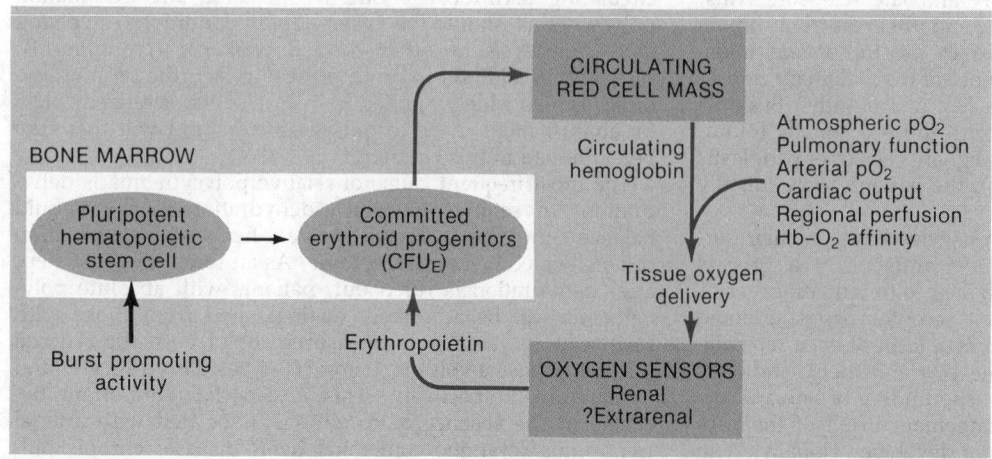

FIGURE 153–1. Relationship between tissue oxygen delivery, erythropoietin output, and the circulating red cell mass.

primary erythrocytosis, is seemingly autonomous in that increased red cell production occurs despite low or undetectable levels of erythropoietin as measured by in vivo bioassay techniques. Moreover, "endogenous colonies" of erythroid progenitors from such patients may be successfully grown in various in vitro tissue culture systems without added erythropoietin, which is otherwise essential for erythroid progenitor growth in vitro. Finally, phlebotomy to low normal or anemic levels produces an increase in erythropoietin production, indicating that the "servomechanism" relating erythropoietin output to tissue oxygen delivery is intact. The apparent erythropoietin independence of erythropoiesis in the primary polycythemias is now recognized to reflect a markedly increased sensitivity of erythroid progenitors to minute amounts of the hormone, rather than total erythropoietin independence.

SECONDARY PROLIFERATION. Alternatively, the proliferation could result from abnormalities in the erythropoietic regulatory mechanism extrinsic to the erythroid progenitors themselves. The increased red cell production in these circumstances is driven by increased levels of erythropoietin or other erythroid stimulatory substances, and erythroid progenitors require exogenous erythropoietin to grow successfully in vitro. These features characterize the various secondary polycythemias.

The secondary polycythemias can be further subdivided into three categories. The *first* is disorders in which the signal resulting in erythrocytosis, most often an increase in erythropoietin production, represents a physiologically appropriate response to poor tissue oxygenation caused by arterial hypoxemia, genetically determined or "acquired" high affinity hemoglobins that release oxygen to tissue inadequately, or reduced tissue perfusion. For these conditions, reduction of the red cell mass by phlebotomy, even to values still substantially greater than normal, may reduce tissue oxygen delivery and result in a further increase in erythropoietin output. The *second* category is disorders characterized by excessive autonomous production of erythropoietic stimulatory substances (erythropoietin, androgens, adrenal corticosteroids). Increased, autonomous erythropoietin production may occur in certain neoplasms, as a result of non-neoplastic lesions in the kidney (hydronephrosis, cysts, tumors, vascular lesions) that produce local ischemia involving the renal oxygen-sensing mechanism, or in certain rare, familial syndromes, without a demonstrable anatomic lesion. For the disorders in this category, erythropoietin production is not influenced by phlebotomy-induced changes in the red cell mass. The *third* category is the entity in which erythropoietin secretion remains under physiologic control in that it responds to phlebotomy, but at a level of production inappropriately high for the level of tissue oxygenation. A classification of the various absolute erythrocytoses, based on underlying mechanisms, is presented in Table 153–1.

Pathophysiology of Absolute Erythrocytosis

Irrespective of underlying etiology, all disorders characterized by an absolute erythrocytosis share certain common clinical manifestations resulting from the expanded blood volume and increased blood viscosity. The increased blood volume leads to generalized vascular expansion and venous engorgement, which are reflected by the characteristic ruddy cyanosis of the skin and mucous membranes. These factors are magnified by the marked decrease in cerebral blood flow that accompanies elevation of the hematocrit and in turn contributes to headaches, tinnitus, a frequently described feeling of fullness in the head and neck, and light-headedness. There appears to be an increase in thrombotic complications, particularly involving the cerebrovascular circulation, in patients with markedly elevated hematocrit and expanded blood volume. Epistaxis and upper gastrointestinal hemorrhage are also more frequent in the hypervolemic patient. The increase in viscosity accompanying hypervolemia and erythrocytosis may result in a decrease in cardiac output, reduction in regional blood flow, and ultimately in an impairment of tissue oxygenation, even in cases in which the underlying initial stimulus was poor oxygen delivery.

In contrast to the consequences of expanded blood volume and blood viscosity, the consequences of bone marrow hyperactivity and of increased red cell destruction are minimal. Because expansion of the red cell mass often occurs very slowly, increases in bone marrow volume, alterations in the myeloid:erythroid ratio, and changes in reticulocyte count or plasma iron turnover may be difficult to appreciate. Similarly, although a doubling of the red cell mass results in a doubling of bilirubin production, this may be insufficient to drive the plasma unconjugated bilirubin concentration outside of its relatively wide normal range.

Clinical Evaluation of the Patient with Erythrocytosis

ROLE OF CONVENTIONAL DIAGNOSTIC METHODS. A systematic approach to the evaluation of the patient with erythrocytosis is illustrated in Figure 153–2. This algorithm ensures the correct classification of patients with relative as opposed to absolute erythrocytosis. In the majority of instances, patients with absolute erythrocytosis can also be appropriately classified as having primary or secondary erythrocytosis, and in the latter case, the specific underlying cause can be identified on the basis of conventional, widely available diagnostic studies. The diagnosis of polycythemia vera is discussed later in this chapter.

SPECIAL STUDIES: ASSAY OF ERYTHROPOIETIN AND ENDOGENOUS COLONY FORMATION. Erythropoietin is most commonly estimated by an in vivo bioassay in polycythemic mice. Injection of patient plasma or urine preparations into such animals stimulates the incorporation of ^{59}Fe into newly produced erythrocytes, to a degree proportional to the erythropoietin content of the injected material. When this assay is applied to urine samples, normal individuals have

TABLE 153–1. CAUSES OF ERYTHROCYTOSIS

I. Relative erythrocytosis (stress, spurious, or pseudopolycythemia; Gaisböck's syndrome)
II. Absolute erythrocytosis
   A. Primary (proliferative bone marrow disorder)
      1. Polycythemia vera
      2. Primary erythrocytosis
   B. Secondary (increased marrow stimulation by erythropoietin, etc.)
      1. Physiologically appropriate increased erythropoietin production
         a. Arterial hypoxemia
           i. High altitude
           ii. Chronic pulmonary disease
           iii. Cardiovascular shunt (right-to-left)
           iv. Massive obesity (pickwickian syndrome)
           v. Postural hypoxemia
         b. Abnormal release of oxygen from hemoglobin
           i. Hereditary high oxygen affinity hemoglobin
           ii. Congenitally decreased red cell 2,3-DPG
           iii. Smoker's polycythemia (carboxyhemoglobinemia)
         c. Interference with tissue oxygen metabolism
           i. Cobalt
      2. Physiologically inappropriate erythropoietin production
         a. Neoplasms
           i. Renal, adrenal, hepatocellular, and ovarian carcinomas
           ii. Cerebellar hemangioblastomas (e.g., von Hippel-Lindau syndrome)
           iii. Adrenal cortical adenoma and/or hyperplasia
           iv. Pheochromocytoma
           v. Large uterine fibroids (rare)
         b. Non-neoplastic renal diseases
           i. Cysts, hydronephrosis
           ii. Bartter's syndrome
           iii. Post-transplantation
         c. Autonomous, fixed increased erythropoietin production without demonstrable anatomic lesion (familial)
        d. Excessive basal erythropoietin output with further augmentation following phlebotomy (familial)
      3. Therapeutic administration or excess production of androgens or certain other corticosteroids

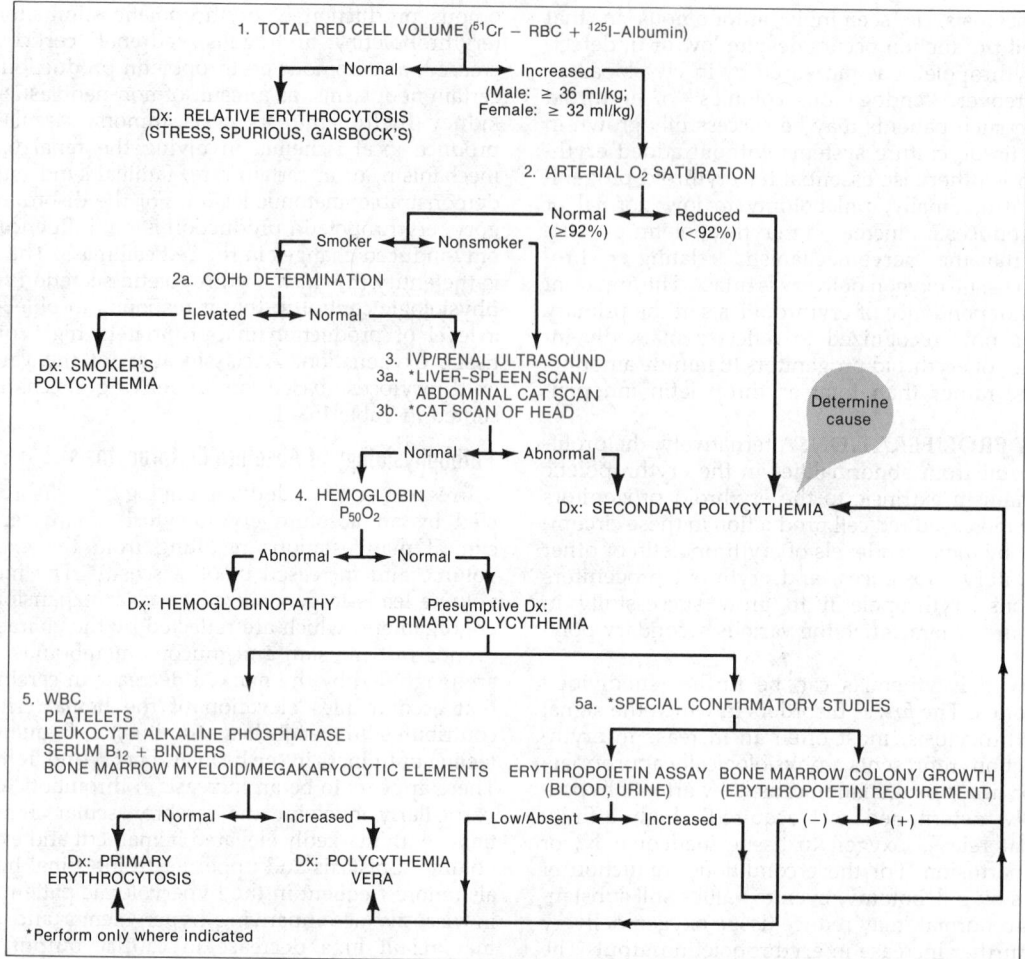

FIGURE 153–2. Algorithm for evaluation of an elevated hematocrit. Laboratory features suggestive of a myeloproliferative disease include elevated platelet and white blood cell counts and increased reticulin and clustered atypical megakaryocytes in a bone marrow biopsy. A careful history (e.g., ? family history of elevated hematocrit, ? heavy smoking) and physical examination (? splenomegaly, evidence of cardiac or pulmonary disease) provide indispensable information.

basal levels of erythropoietin excretion within a well-defined normal range. After phlebotomy urinary erythropoietin excretion increases, and an inverse logarithmic relationship is observed between the hematocrit and the erythropoietin excretion rate. Patients with hypoxic secondary erythrocytosis have variable basal values ranging from normal to increased, but all have increased values following reduction of hematocrit to normal by means of phlebotomy. In contrast, basal urinary erythropoietin excretion is very low in patients with polycythemia vera. Normal human plasma appears to contain 10 to 20 mU of erythropoietin per milliliter. The lower limit of sensitivity of the polycythemic mouse assay is approximately 50 mU per milliliter. Hence, when applied to plasma, this assay cannot distinguish normal subjects from those with polycythemia vera, since both groups fall below this sensitivity limit. The assay can detect the elevated levels seen in some cases of secondary polycythemia. Procedures to concentrate the plasma 40-fold may increase the sensitivity of this technique to approximately 5 mU per milliliter. Using this procedure, patients with polycythemia vera still had undetectable plasma levels of erythropoietin by bioassay, whereas most (but not all) normal subjects had detectable values averaging 7.8 ± 1.1 (SD) mU per milliliter, and the majority of patients with a clinical diagnosis of secondary polycythemia had elevated levels. Unfortunately, the concentration procedure is cumbersome and may introduce artifacts into the in vivo bioassay. Of alternative techniques for measuring erythropoietin, only a hemagglutination inhibition assay is commercially

available, but its reliability has been questioned. Similarly, radioimmunoassay procedures report elevated erythropoietin levels in many cases of secondary polycythemia but equivalent levels in normal subjects and patients with polycythemia vera, possibly reflecting immunoreactive but biologically inert erythropoietin fractions or other materials. Only one experimental assay procedure purports to separate normal serum erythropoietin levels from reduced values in polycythemia vera.

The ability to grow erythroid progenitors from bone marrow or peripheral blood in vitro without added erythropoietin strongly supports the diagnosis of a primary bone marrow disorder of erythroid regulation.

As indicated in the foregoing discussion and in Figure 153–2, when erythropoietin assays and/or studies of in vitro endogenous colony formation are available, they may help to distinguish patients with primary polycythemias from those with secondary polycythemias. In addition, the influence of phlebotomy on erythropoietin output may separate the physiologically appropriate secondary polycythemias from those in which erythropoietin output is autonomous. In the majority of cases, these distinctions can be made on the basis of conventional diagnostic investigations.

Erslev AJ, Caro J: Pure erythrocytosis classified according to erythropoietin titers. Am J Med 76:57, 1984. *Clear demonstration of both the uses and limitations of erythropoietin bioassays in diagnosis of polycythemic states.*
Garcia JF, Ebbe SN, Hollander L, et al.: Radioimmunoassay of erythropoietin: Circulating levels in normal and polycythemic human beings. J Lab Clin

Med 99:624, 1982. *Report on the only erythropoietin radioimmunoassay that distinguishes the reduced values in polycythemia vera from normal levels.*

Golde DW, Hocking WG, Koeffler HP, et al.: Polycythemia: Mechanisms and management. Ann Intern Med 95:71, 1981. *An outstanding review of the pathophysiology, diagnosis, and management of the various polycythemias, with a comprehensive bibliography.*

SECONDARY POLYCYTHEMIAS

In the secondary polycythemias a normal bone marrow is stimulated to produce increased numbers of red blood cells, leading to an increase in the circulating red cell mass, as a result of increased production of erythropoietin or of other erythrostimulatory substances. These disorders all have in common the diverse symptomatic consequences of hypervolemia and increased blood viscosity described earlier. The secondary polycythemias may be classified into those in which the polycythemia is an appropriate physiologic response to inadequate tissue oxygenation and those in which the development of erythrocytosis is inappropriate to the oxygen balance of the patient (Table 153–1).

Physiologically Appropriate Polycythemias

HIGH ALTITUDE. In the presence of normal hemoglobin A and appropriate intraerythrocytic levels of 2,3-diphosphoglyceric acid (DPG), the partial pressure of oxygen in capillaries must be maintained close to 40 mm Hg to ensure adequate off-loading of oxygen to tissues. At sea level, where the atmospheric partial pressure of oxygen is approximately 160 mm Hg, oxygen is readily loaded onto the hemoglobin molecule, and the steep oxygen pressure gradient from the alveoli to the tissue capillaries ensures an adequate driving force for tissue oxygenation. In contrast, at elevated altitudes the atmospheric oxygen tension diminishes, and at approximately 5400 meters, the altitude of the highest permanent human settlement, atmospheric oxygen pressure is only 80 mm Hg, providing a much smaller alveolar–capillary oxygen pressure gradient. To provide adequate tissue oxygenation in the face of this reduced driving force, individuals constantly exposed to high altitude are acclimatized by two principal mechanisms, hyperventilation and the development of erythrocytosis. Hyperventilation causes a reduction in the pulmonary dead space and an increase in the surface area of adequately perfused alveoli. Erythrocytosis increases the oxygen-carrying capacity of circulating blood. Together, these two alterations permit acclimatization to occur without the need for a significant increase in cardiac output. In general, although a shift in the oxygen-hemoglobin dissociation curve to the right would also increase tissue oxygenation at a given capillary oxygen tension, such a change would also impair the on-loading of oxygen in the lungs at high altitudes. The latter appears to take precedence in that direct measurement of oxygen dissociation curves among individuals who live at higher altitudes generally reveals patterns within the normal range.

Approximately 25,000,000 people live at altitudes between 3000 and 5400 meters. The latter, with an atmospheric pressure of approximately one half normal, appears to represent the extreme limit of human long-term physiologic adaptation. Transient adaptation to higher levels is possible, as demonstrated by the successful 1978 scaling of Mount Everest (8848 meters), where atmospheric pressure is approximately one third of normal, without the use of administered oxygen.

Those who dwell for long periods at high altitudes typically develop an increased anteroposterior thoracic diameter, and a ruddy cyanosis secondary to hypervolemia. The increased blood volume is manifested in the engorged capillaries of the conjunctivae, skin, and mucous membranes, and may contribute to all of the classic symptoms of hypervolemia. The hematocrit is elevated, reflecting an increased red cell mass in the presence of a normal plasma volume. White blood cells and platelets are normal, and bone marrow aspirates may appear to be normal or to show modest erythroid hyperplasia.

The acute and chronic effects of living at high altitude are further described in Ch. 537.

CARDIOPULMONARY DISEASE. Arterial hypoxemia, resulting from right-to-left shunts in congenital heart disease (see Ch. 49) or from chronic obstructive pulmonary disease (see Ch. 61), results in expansion of the red cell mass. This may be masked in part in both settings by a concomitant increase in plasma volume.

ALVEOLAR HYPOVENTILATION. Arterial hypoxemia, cyanosis, and secondary erythrocytosis may also result from either centrally mediated or peripheral impairment of alveolar ventilation. One of the settings in which this occurs, Monge's disease (chronic mountain sickness), is described in Ch. 537. Another is the so-called pickwickian syndrome, in which the work load of ventilation in a severely obese individual is aggravated by central hyporesponsiveness to hypoxemia and hypercapnia. In a third group of patients postural hypoxemia occurs during sleep. All of these conditions may be associated with increased erythropoietin production and secondary erythrocytosis.

ABNORMALITIES OF THE OXYGEN-HEMOGLOBIN DISSOCIATION CURVE. Abnormalities in the ability of hemoglobin to release oxygen to tissues, manifested by a shift in the oxyhemoglobin dissociation curve to the left, may occur on either a congenital or an acquired basis. At least 42 such hemoglobins have been described in association with erythrocytosis (Ch. 144). In most an amino acid substitution occurring in the contact area between the α and β chains interferes with the normal conformational changes that facilitate oxygen release from the molecule. The resulting high oxygen affinity hemoglobin results in noncyanotic tissue hypo-oxygenation and ultimately in secondary erythrocytosis. High affinity variants involving both α-chain substitutions (hemoglobin Capetown, hemoglobin Chesapeake) and β-chain substitutions (hemoglobin Ranier, hemoglobin Yakima) have been described. Most of these high affinity mutations are electrophoretically silent because there is no charge difference between the normal and variant hemoglobin. Hence, determination of an oxygen-hemoglobin dissociation curve or determination of the P_{50} is essential in the evaluation of patients suspected of having a high oxygen affinity hemoglobin. This suspicion particularly should be directed toward individuals in whom familial erythrocytosis is observed.

Secondary erythrocytosis may also occur in the presence of certain hereditary methemoglobinemias, disorders in which amino acid substitutions occur in the regions of the heme pockets. Most of these conditions are associated with hemolysis, but, in the few in which the rate of red cell destruction is near normal, compensatory mechanisms may result in a secondary erythrocytosis. Several different congenital disorders involving a decreased ability to synthesize 2,3-DPG have been described. Since reductions in red cell 2,3-DPG content are associated with an increased oxygen affinity for hemoglobin, such patients may behave clinically as if they had a high affinity hemoglobin disorder with resulting secondary erythrocytosis, even though they in fact have hemoglobin A. Finally, prolonged exposure to carbon monoxide, occasionally on an industrial basis but more frequently in chain smokers, results in erythrocytosis because carboxyhemoglobin has the effect of increasing the oxygen affinity of the remaining heme prosthetic groups. The hematocrit is often increased out of proportion to the red cell mass because of secondary effects of carboxyhemoglobin or nicotine or both in reducing the plasma volume.

Physiologically Inappropriate Erythrocytosis

NEOPLASMS AND NON-NEOPLASTIC RENAL DISEASES. Physiologically inappropriate erythrocytosis is seen in a variety of neoplasms, including renal and adrenal carcinoma, cerebellar hemangioblastoma, hepatocellular carcinoma, ovarian carcinoma, pheochromocytoma, and massive uterine fibroids (Ch. 173). The proportion of each of these tumors in which erythrocytosis develops is highly variable. It seems to be particularly high in cases of hepatocellular carcinoma. In most instances, increased erythropoietin production by the tumor is believed to be the underlying mechanism leading to erythrocytosis.

Secondary erythrocytosis also occurs in a variety of nonmalignant disorders of the kidney, including cystic disease and hydronephrosis, and following renal transplantation. Production of increased erythropoietin levels in the presence of renal cystic disease appears likely in view of the frequent documentation of high titers of the hormone in aspirated cyst fluid. Local intrarenal ischemia resulting from various types of renal pathology is believed to mediate an increased erythropoietin output in these disorders. Familial syndromes occur in which autonomous production of increased quantities of erythropoietin has been observed without a demonstrable anatomic lesion. Erythropoietin output in these syndromes does not vary in response to phlebotomy. A single report also describes an inappropriately high level of basal erythropoietin output in an individual in whom phlebotomy resulted in a further increase in hormone production. The nature of the underlying defect in these two syndromes is unclear.

DRUG INDUCED. Testosterone and its various derivatives, and a variety of adrenal corticosteroids, may stimulate red cell production. Testosterone-like compounds are often used therapeutically for this purpose in patients with renal failure who are undergoing dialysis or in patients with aregenerative anemia. In some instances, androgens will also stimulate granulocyte and platelet production. Occasionally, increased levels of steroid hormones, whether administered therapeutically or produced in the course of adrenal disorders, may result in secondary erythrocytosis.

Treatment of the Secondary Polycythemias

Hypervolemia and increased blood viscosity accompany the development of erythrocytosis. Accordingly, when a secondary erythrocytosis is not in response to an appropriate physiologic stimulus, reduction of hematocrit to less than 50 per cent by means of phlebotomy is an appropriate part of the treatment regimen, which should also address itself to the underlying disorder.

The issue is more complex in those secondary erythrocytoses that represent a physiologic response to poor tissue oxygenation. The beneficial effect of expansion of the red cell mass may ultimately be offset by the detrimental effect of increasing blood viscosity on cardiac output, systemic oxygen transport, and local tissue oxygen delivery. In a normovolemic state, oxygen transport is optimal at a hematocrit of 40 to 45 per cent. In the presence of hypervolemia, optimal oxygen delivery may occur at hematocrits close to 60 per cent. However, hematocrits higher than this inevitably impair oxygen delivery. Nevertheless, in a given patient, if an increase in the hematocrit to the region of 60 per cent does not achieve normal tissue oxygenation, a continued increase in erythropoietin output may result in overcompensation. This overcompensation may not only decrease net tissue oxygen delivery but may also impair regional blood flow in a number of organs, particularly within the cerebral circulation. In summary, in the physiologic secondary polycythemias, there is a balance between the beneficial effects of an increasing hematocrit and the negative consequences of an excessive increase in blood viscosity. In general, hematocrits in excess of 60 per cent are detrimental and should be reduced by phlebotomy. In patients with arterial hypoxemia resulting from pulmonary disease or right-to-left cardiac shunts, the optimal level of hemoglobin and hematocrit may be difficult to determine except by trial and error. In some cases, improvement in

cerebral function and decrease in congestive heart failure may follow a reduction in blood volume to hematocrits in the mid 50's or even lower.

Bunn HF, Forget B: Hemoglobin: Molecular, Genetic and Clinical Aspects. Philadelphia, W. B. Saunders Company, 1986, pp 595–622. *This chapter presents an outstanding review of hemoglobin variants with abnormal oxygen binding and their clinical consequences, as well as a comprehensive bibliography.*

Chetty KG, Brown SE, Light RW: Improved exercise tolerance of the polycythemic lung patient following phlebotomy. Am J Med 74:415, 1983. *A detailed clinicophysiologic study documenting that patients with polycythemia due to chronic obstructive pulmonary disease benefit from reduction of hematocrit to the mid 50's by phlebotomy.*

Distelhorst CW, Wagner DS, Goldwasser E, et al.: Autosomal dominant familial erythrocytosis due to autonomous erythropoietin production. Blood 58:1155, 1981. *A well-described family with this rare syndrome. Bibliography includes references to cases with the slightly more common recessive variant.*

Erslev AJ: Blood and mountains. In Wintrobe MM (ed.): Blood, Pure and Eloquent. New York, McGraw-Hill Book Company, 1980, pp 257–280. *A lucid and fascinating review of the evolution of current concepts of human adaptation to the hypoxemia of high altitudes. Excellent bibliography.*

Whitcomb WH, Peschle C, Moore M, et al.: Congenital erythrocytosis: A new form associated with an erythropoietin-dependent mechanism. Br J Haematol 44:17, 1980. *An unusual syndrome characterized by inappropriately high basal erythropoietin output that increased further after phlebotomy.*

POLYCYTHEMIA VERA: A CLONAL STEM CELL DISORDER
Nature of the Defect in Polycythemia Vera

Polycythemia vera is a hematologic malignant disorder characterized by excessive proliferation of erythroid, myeloid, and megakaryocytic elements within the bone marrow, resulting in an increased red blood cell mass and, frequently, elevated peripheral granulocyte and platelet counts. Several lines of evidence, including cytogenetic observations and isoenzyme marker studies in G6PD heterozygotes, indicate that the increased proliferation of all three hematopoietic cell lines can trace its origin to a single abnormal clone, which has presumably developed at the level of the pluripotent stem cell (Ch. 152). B lymphocytes are also derived from the abnormal stem cell clone. Studies of the growth of both erythroid progenitors and granulocyte-macrophage progenitors (CFU-GM) in vitro have demonstrated the presence of residual normal stem cells in the marrow early in the disease, but a steady decline in the proportion of the normal elements as the duration of the illness lengthens.

Thrombotic episodes that are usually attributed to increased blood viscosity and/or thrombocytosis; hemorrhagic episodes associated with thrombopathy and/or the elevated platelet and erythrocyte counts; the development of a "spent" phase characterized by cytopenias, myelofibrosis, and myeloid metaplasia; and the transformation to acute leukemia are among the principal complications of this disorder. Polycythemia vera shares several clinical, pathophysiologic, and histologic features with agnogenic myeloid metaplasia, chronic myelogenous leukemia, and primary (essential) thrombocythemia, which are collectively classified as the myeloproliferative disorders (Ch. 154).

The excessive rate of erythropoiesis in polycythemia vera occurs despite bioassayable erythropoietin levels that are low or absent; endogenous erythroid colonies in this disorder can grow in vitro without added erythropoietin. These observations led to the concept that erythropoiesis in polycythemia vera was "autonomous." The growth of endogenous colonies from patients with polycythemia vera can be markedly reduced or eliminated by adding antierythropoietin antibody to the culture, however, and can be restored by the re-addition of minute quantities of the hormone. This suggests that erythroid progenitors in polycythemia vera, rather than being independent of the hormone, may be uniquely sensitive to trace levels of erythropoietin. In blood and bone marrow of patients with polycythemia vera, increased numbers of pluripotent colony-forming stem cells give rise to mixed colonies of granulocytic, erythroid, macrophage, and megakaryocytic elements (CFU-GEMM). These CFU-GEMM undergo erythroid differentiation without added erythropoietin and, compared to normal CFU-GEMM, exhibit increased megakaryocyte formation. The "endogenous" erythroid differentiation is abolished with antibodies to erythropoietin. Hence, both the increased "erythropoietin-independent" erythropoiesis and increased megakaryopoiesis characteristic of polycythemia vera reflect functional features of an identifiable abnormal pluripotent stem cell population.

The mechanism of malignant transformation in polycythemia vera is unknown. The rare occurrence of documented polycythemia vera in monozygotic twins and the only marginally increased incidence in first-degree relatives of affected patients suggest a minimal genetic role in most cases, and neither toxic chemicals nor exposure to radiation is established as an etiologic factor. Although two documented cases occurred among exposed observers of a 1957 nuclear test explosion, the incidence of polycythemia vera has not been appreciably increased in survivors of the Hiroshima and Nagasaki atomic bomb explosions. The disease is typically one of later life, with the median age at presentation being close to 60 years. Nevertheless, patients in their second through fourth decades are not rare. The disorder is characterized by a slight preponderance in males and a propensity to occur with somewhat increased frequency in patients of Jewish ancestry.

Clinical Manifestations

Multiphasic screening is currently resulting in an increasing percentage of cases being detected prior to the development of symptoms. Alternatively, a routine blood count may demonstrate increased hematocrit and other abnormalities in patients who present with only mild headaches and plethoric facies. Further symptoms as they develop usually will be referable to the combination of hypervolemia and hyperviscosity resulting from the increased red cell mass and blood volume, frequently aggravated by thrombocytosis and platelet dysfunction; to the local consequences of panhyperplasia of the bone marrow; or to the metabolic consequences of increased cell turnover.

SYMPTOMS. Headaches, tinnitus, light-headedness and vertigo, and blurred vision appear to result principally from increased blood viscosity and hypervolemia. Thrombotic complications, which may involve both arterial and venous occlusive events, are usually attributed to a combination of hyperviscosity, thrombocytosis, and platelet dysfunction. An increased incidence of epistaxis, spontaneous bruising, and upper gastrointestinal hemorrhage is also ascribed to the effects of hypervolemia and platelet dysfunction. Peptic ulcer disease seems to occur with increased frequency in patients with polycythemia vera as does pruritus, sometimes aggravated after a hot bath or shower, and occasionally so severe as to be disabling. The increased frequency of both peptic ulcer and pruritus may be related to the increased histamine release caused by excessive turnover of granulocytes and, more specifically, basophils. Approximately one third of patients complain of sweating and weight loss, presumed to be on the basis of a hypermetabolic state. Patients with polycythemia vera often complain of severe pain in their feet, which is characteristically relieved by very low doses of aspirin or nonsteroidal anti-inflammatory agents.

PHYSICAL FINDINGS. In established cases, physical examination typically reveals plethora or dusky cyanosis of the face, hands, feet, and mucous membranes. Engorgement of the conjunctivae and retinal veins is frequently present and, in patients with markedly increased hematocrit, retinal hemorrhages are occasionally seen. Mild hypertension is noted in approximately one third of patients. Ecchymoses are not infrequently observed. The most useful physical finding in terms of differential diagnosis is splenomegaly, which is present in approximately 75 per cent of patients with polycythemia vera and tends to exclude the diagnosis of most of the secondary polycythemias. Procedures such as abdominal computed tomography will demonstrate splenomegaly in a percentage of those patients in whom the spleen is not palpably enlarged. Splenic enlargement appears to reflect principally the development of extramedullary hematopoiesis. Hepatomegaly is present in approximately 40 per cent of patients.

Symptomatic bone pain and tenderness on physical examination, particularly in the ribs and sternum, are occasionally severe and reflect intense panhyperplasia of the bone marrow. In addition to hyperhistaminemia, the cellular proliferation of polycythemia vera results in overproduction of uric acid leading, not infrequently, to either uric acid stone diathesis or overt secondary gout.

Laboratory Data

The characteristic laboratory findings in polycythemia vera reflect the various consequences of increased bone marrow activity.

ERYTHROCYTES. Patients with this disorder typically present with an elevation of the hemoglobin concentration, hematocrit, and red blood cell count. Red blood cell morphology usually reveals hypochromic microcytic cells with a reduced mean corpuscular volume, suggestive of iron deficient erythropoiesis. This suggestion is frequently confirmed by a low serum iron level and absence of bone marrow iron stores. These features may occur prior to the onset of therapeutic phlebotomy and without any history of gastrointestinal blood loss and result from the shift of iron from various body storage pools into the circulating erythron as the red cell mass is expanded. This phenomenon may of course be exaggerated in patients who have gastrointestinal bleeding or in whom therapeutic phlebotomies have been initiated. Of the three conventional parameters reflecting the red cell mass, the red blood count is often most strikingly elevated, and red cell counts of 10×10^6 per microliter may be seen in the newly diagnosed case. In contrast, the hematocrit probably provides the best, although imperfect, simple guide to the size of the circulating red cell mass and to blood viscosity. It is difficult to define the precise upper limit for the normal hematocrit. As noted earlier, increased red cell masses may be found in a small percentage of patients with hematocrits of 48 per cent or above, and an increase in the hematocrit to greater than 60 per cent is required before the hematocrit alone can be taken positively as evidence for an absolute erythrocytosis. The plasma volume in polycythemia vera has variously been reported to be normal, reduced, or increased, and thus has no direct correlation with the red cell mass. The red cell lifespan is normal in the early phases of polycythemia vera, even in the presence of moderate splenomegaly. As the disease evolves, the development of increasingly ineffective erythropoiesis, and a larger element of extramedullary hematopoiesis with hepatomegaly and splenomegaly, results in progressive shortening of the red cell lifespan in some patients. This development is usually associated with the appearance of anisocytosis and poikilocytosis, nucleated red blood cells, and teardrop cells in the peripheral blood. When such studies are available, patients with untreated polycythemia vera will invariably demonstrate very low levels of plasma and urine erythropoietin and the ability to grow endogenous, erythropoietin-independent colonies of erythroid progenitors in vitro from either peripheral blood or bone marrow samples.

LEUKOCYTES. Sixty per cent of patients with polycythemia vera will have an increased granulocyte count in the peripheral blood at the time of diagnosis. Early in the disease, elevations are usually modest and involve the presence of only normal granulocytes and bands. Subsequently, striking elevations in total white count may achieve leukemoid proportions, associated with the appearance of early myeloid forms, particularly myelocytes and metamyelocytes. When the appearance of these cells is accompanied by increasing splenomegaly and the appearance of abnormal erythroid elements in the periphery, a significant element of myeloid metaplasia is likely. The alkaline phosphatase activity of circulating granulocytes is increased in polycythemia vera, in contrast to the reduction observed in chronic granulocytic leukemia. Increased granulocyte turnover is reflected by high serum and urine muramidase (lysozyme) levels, and by an increase in serum B_{12} and unbound B_{12} binding capacity that results from high levels of transcobalamins 1 and 3. The basophil count and, to a lesser extent, the eosinophil count may also be increased in polycythemia vera. Increased excretion of histamine metabolites reflects increased turnover of the former cell line.

PLATELETS. At diagnosis, the platelet count exceeds 500,000 per microliter in approximately half of patients with polycythemia vera, and striking elevations into the millions have been recorded. There is a tendency for the platelet count to increase with time, particularly in patients who are treated principally with phlebotomy. The platelets in polycythemia vera frequently appear morphologically abnormal, with megathrombocytes and megakaryocytic fragments being observed in the peripheral blood smear. An appreciable fraction of patients with polycythemia vera also have abnormalities of conventional studies of platelet function, including aggregation; a prolonged bleeding time may be present. Studies of prostaglandin metabolism also demonstrate decreased lipoxygenase activity and increased thromboxane A_2 production by the platelets of patients with polycythemia vera and other myeloproliferative diseases. However, it has not been possible to correlate either the height of the platelet count or the presence of platelet functional abnormalities with the propensity to thrombosis in these patients. In contrast, there seems to be a crude association between the extent of the elevation of the platelet count and the propensity to hemorrhagic complications.

BONE MARROW. The bone marrow in polycythemia vera is typically hyperplastic and reveals a panmyelosis. Because of the parallel increase in all three cell lines, the myeloid: erythroid ratio may be normal. Megakaryocytes are not merely increased but typically are seen in sheets or clumps, a finding strongly supportive of the diagnosis of a myeloproliferative disease. Bone marrow biopsy as well as aspirate is useful in the assessment of polycythemia vera, both because it gives a better indication of the extent of hypercellularity and because connective tissue staining will illustrate the extent of myelofibrosis. Serum levels of the procollagen III amino terminal peptide, now measurable by commercially available radioimmunoassay, also reflect the extent of myelofibrosis. Cytogenetic studies reveal various abnormalities in as many as 50 per cent of patients with polycythemia vera. Trisomy of chromosomes 8 and 9 or loss of chromosome 7 or its long arm (7q−) is the abnormality most frequently observed in untreated patients; loss of chromosome 5 or of the long arms of chromosome 5 (5q−) or 20 (20q−) has been observed in some patients, especially those treated with myelosuppressives. However, no abnormality is either specific for or diagnostic of polycythemia vera. Interestingly, the presence of cytogenetic abnormalities at the time of diagnosis appears to be of no prognostic significance.

MISCELLANEOUS. Low serum cholesterol concentrations are frequently observed in patients with polycythemia vera; these reflect accelerated catabolism of low density lipoproteins, presumably by the spleen. Hyperuricemia, reflecting a general increase in cell turnover, and an increase in lactic dehydrogenase and the indirect serum bilirubin concentration, reflecting accelerated erythroid turnover, are other commonly found abnormalities.

Diagnosis and Differential Diagnosis

Diagnosis of polycythemia vera is based on the demonstration of an increased red cell mass that is not associated with excessive erythropoietin production, as well as evidence of a concomitant increase in bone marrow production of granulocytes and thrombocytes. Polycythemia vera is one of two disorders characterized by "autonomous" erythropoiesis. It differs from the entity designated *primary erythrocytosis* in its associated increase in granulocyte and megakaryocytic proliferation and the presence of related abnormalities such as elevated levels of leukocyte alkaline phosphatase and serum B_{12}–binding proteins. The abnormalities in primary erythrocytosis are limited to the erythroid series, but within this sphere the low bioassayable erythropoietin levels and the presence of endogenous colonies are similar to those seen in polycythemia vera. Some argue that primary erythrocytosis represents a disorder arising in the committed erythroid stem cell compartment, i.e., at a later stage than the pluripotent stem cell affected in polycythemia vera, but primary erythrocytosis has not yet been demonstrated to be a clonal disorder. Others believe that these patients represent a forme fruste of typical polycythemia vera and that granulocytic or thrombocytic abnormalities will be revealed if patients are observed for sufficient periods.

The diagnosis of a primary bone marrow disorder with autonomous erythropoiesis may be made in accordance with the algorithm illustrated in Figure 153–2 by systematically excluding the various secondary causes of an absolute erythrocytosis. Patients appearing to have increased erythroid proliferation due to a primary bone marrow defect would be classified as having polycythemia vera if they have concomitant granulocytic or platelet abnormalities in the peripheral blood, evidence of a panmyelosis in the bone marrow, or splenomegaly. In the absence of these features, when abnormalities are restricted solely to the erythroid series, the diagnosis of primary erythrocytosis would be made.

The Polycythemia Vera Study Group has developed a set of empiric criteria that permit the diagnosis of polycythemia vera to be established in many patients within one to two office visits (Table 153–2). In patients who meet these criteria, the diagnosis of polycythemia vera is highly likely, the false-positive rate having been found to be less than 0.5 per cent. False-positive results are most likely in patients who are excessive users of both alcohol and tobacco. In this setting, excessive erythroid proliferation associated with carboxyhemoglobinemia and splenomegaly, leukocytosis, and increased leukocyte alkaline phosphatase activity and serum B_{12} associated with alcoholic liver disease may confound the diagnosis. The false-negative rate for the Polycythemia Vera Study Group criteria is unknown. Patients with early disease who do not yet meet these criteria may ultimately prove to have polycythemia vera, or at least a form of primary erythrocytosis, when more extensive evaluation is carried out in accordance with the criteria of Figure 153–2.

TABLE 153–2. PARAMETERS FOR THE DIAGNOSIS OF POLYCYTHEMIA VERA

A1 ↑ Red cell mass
   Male: ≥ 36 ml/kg
   Female: ≥ 32 ml/kg
A2 Normal art. O_2 sat. (≥ 92%)
A3 Splenomegaly
	B1 Thrombocytosis
	   Platelet count > 400,000/μl
	B2 Leukocytosis: > 12,000/μl (no fever
	   or infection)
	B3 ↑ Leuk. alk. p'tase (LAP) (> 100)
	B4 ↑ Serum B_{12} (> 900 pg/ml) or
	   ↑ UB$_{12}$BC (> 2200 pg/ml)*

Dx. acceptable if following combinations are present:
  A1 + A2 + A3
  A1 + A2 + any two from category B
*UB$_{12}$BC = unbound serum B_{12} binding capacity

Course

In the absence of treatment, polycythemia vera is a serious disease in which a high incidence of fatal thrombotic or hemorrhagic complications historically has led to a median survival of 6 to 18 months from diagnosis. Current treatment programs designed to maintain peripheral blood counts and the red cell mass at close to normal levels have achieved median survivals approximating 10 years, during the course of which aspects of the natural history of the disease have become more evident. In many patients, polycythemia vera is a readily managed disorder that remains asymptomatic for long periods. However, inadequate control of the red cell mass predisposes to both thrombotic and hemorrhagic complications, of which cerebrovascular, coronary, and abdominal vascular occlusions involving both arterial (e.g., mesenteric artery) and venous (Budd-Chiari syndrome) thromboses are most frequent. Thrombosis is the major cause of death in polycythemia vera, accounting for approximately one third of all fatalities. Transformation to acute leukemia, the development of other neoplasms, hemorrhage, and myelofibrosis are other major causes of fatality and collectively, along with thrombosis, account for 75 per cent of all deaths. Acute leukemia is clearly a part of the natural history of polycythemia vera, occurring with an incidence of up to 2 to 4 per cent even in patients who have not been exposed either to radiotherapy or to radiomimetic drugs.

Upper gastrointestinal hemorrhage, particularly from bleeding peptic ulcers, occurs with an increased incidence in patients with polycythemia vera. Underlying etiologic factors are believed to be increased acid secretion stimulated by hyperhistaminemia and vascular mucosal ischemia caused by increased blood viscosity and poor regional perfusion.

The complete natural history of polycythemia vera involves the ultimate transition from the proliferative phase, during which therapy is aimed at reducing peripheral blood counts, to a stable phase in which relatively normal blood counts may be maintained without therapy, to the so-called *burned out* or *spent phase*. Transition results predominantly from the gradual development of progressive myelofibrosis and, possibly, from a gradual reduction in the proliferative capacity of the abnormal hematopoietic clone. That myelofibrosis is a complication of polycythemia vera has long been recognized, but the nature of the association has been uncertain. The bulk of current evidence suggests that bone marrow fibroblasts in this setting are not part of the hematopoietic malignant clone. Similar conclusions have been reached in studies of the bone marrow fibroblast following transplantation. Hence, the increasing proliferation of fibroblasts and increased collagen deposition leading to myelofibrosis appear to be reactive phenomena rather than an intrinsic component of the neoplastic process. The clinical features and the management of postpolycythemic myelofibrosis do not differ appreciably from those of idiopathic myelofibrosis with myeloid metaplasia except that the incidence of acute leukemic transformation is markedly increased in the postpolycythemic setting, especially if the myelofibrosis follows treatment with radioactive phosphorus or chlorambucil (see Ch. 154).

Treatment

The initial treatment in any newly diagnosed case of polycythemia vera is phlebotomy. Efforts should be made to reduce the hematocrit to approximately 45 per cent, a level at which the complications of hypervolemia and hyperviscosity will be minimized. In patients with appreciable splenomegaly, the hematocrit no longer reliably reflects the red cell mass, which may continue to be significantly increased despite hematocrits in the upper 40's. The initial phlebotomy regimen may involve removal of 500 ml aliquots of whole blood as often as every two to three days until a normal hematocrit is achieved. Subsequent phlebotomies should be carried out as

frequently as necessary to maintain the hematocrit at or below 45 per cent. As iron deficiency supervenes, red cell production will be retarded such that patients managed by phlebotomy alone may require as few as two or three phlebotomies per year.

Some investigators believe that phlebotomy alone, at rates sufficient to maintain a normal hematocrit and blood viscosity, is adequate to prevent the thrombotic complications of the disease and provides a minimal incidence of leukemic transformation. Others argue that some form of myelosuppression is preferable, in part because this offers an approach to the control of the thrombocytosis that is often a major clinical feature of the illness. Myelosuppression in this disorder has most often been carried out with radioactive phosphorus (^{32}P), with alkylating agents such as chlorambucil or busulfan, and more recently, with the nonalkylating myelosuppressive agent hydroxyurea.

In an ongoing randomized, controlled study in 431 patients, median survivals of 13.9 years with phlebotomy or 11.8 years with radioactive phosphorus therapy were significantly better than those achieved with chlorambucil (8.9 years), although the difference achieved statistical significance only after more than 10 years of treatment. Causes of death varied appreciably as a function of the treatment administered. Patients managed with phlebotomy alone had a significant excess incidence of severe and often fatal thrombotic complications, particularly in the first two to four years of treatment. Thrombotic complications were particularly frequent in more elderly patients (e.g., older than 70 years), in those with a high phlebotomy requirement (more than four to six per year), and in those who had had a prior history of a thrombotic event. Beyond three years the incidence of thrombotic complications became the same in patients treated with phlebotomy alone as in those treated with myelosuppression, suggesting that a subset of patients particularly susceptible to thrombosis had been selected out by this time. By contrast, myelosuppression with either ^{32}P or alkylating agents effectively decreased the risk of thrombotic complications in thrombosis-prone patients early in the disease. However, both chlorambucil and ^{32}P were associated with a statistically significant increased risk of acute leukemia, which became particularly prominent after five to seven years of treatment, and a somewhat later increased incidence of carcinomas of the skin and gastrointestinal tract. Thus, long-term myelosuppression with either of these agents is associated with an increased propensity for malignant transformation of the three rapidly proliferating tissues of the body: bone marrow, skin, and gastrointestinal mucosa. In addition, an increased incidence of intra-abdominal lymphocytic lymphoma has followed long-term treatment of polycythemia vera with chlorambucil.

Radioactive phosphorus, preferably given as an intravenous dose of 3 to 5 mCi, reliably produces a reduction in bone marrow proliferation with few immediate side effects. Chlorambucil or busulfan, administered either continuously or intermittently, also successfully controls peripheral counts in a high proportion of patients. In contrast to ^{32}P, myelosuppression with alkylating agents results in an appreciable incidence of cytopenias, which in the case of busulfan may be prolonged and troublesome. Because of these drug-related cytopenias and the fact that malignant complications occur both earlier and more frequently with chlorambucil than with ^{32}P, long-term treatment of polycythemia vera with alkylating agents can no longer be recommended. Although some argue that complications observed with chlorambucil should not preclude use of other alkylating agents, especially busulfan, there are sufficient anecdotal cases of leukemic transformation with all of the alkylating drugs that the burden of proof must be on those who argue for the safety of any such agent.

Hydroxyurea,* administered at a dose of 0.5 to 1.5 grams

---

*This use is not listed in the manufacturer's directive.

per day, has recently been shown to be an effective nonalkylating chemotherapeutic agent in the management of polycythemia vera. To date, this regimen has not been associated with an increased incidence of malignant transformation. However, the maximal follow-up with this agent, now approximately seven years, is too short for its full mutagenic potential to have been realized.

Since no form of treatment for polycythemia vera is without some risks, the following recommendations would appear to provide the best control of the disease with the fewest treatment-related complications. Because of the increased risk of thrombosis associated with age, patients over 70 are most effectively treated with a combination of ^{32}P and supplemental phlebotomy. Patients below the age of 50, and particularly those in the childbearing years, should be treated with phlebotomy alone whenever possible. Myelosuppression with hydroxyrurea would seem advisable in such younger patients if they are particularly at risk for thrombotic complications because of a high phlebotomy requirement or a history of prior thrombotic events. The role of myelosuppression is most uncertain in the age-group between 50 and 70. In the absence of thrombosis-associated risk factors, it is probably preferable to attempt to manage such patients by phlebotomy alone. If chemotherapy is deemed advisable, hydroxyurea would appear to be the agent of choice. Chlorambucil would now seem to be contraindicated for long-term therapy of polycythemia vera in view of its unacceptably high risk of leukemic and carcinogenic transformation, which may apply as well to other alkylating agents.

Although conclusive data are lacking, many physicians believe that a substantial increase in platelet count (i.e., in excess of 10^6 per microliter) is an indication for myelosuppressive therapy. Excessive splenic enlargement with local symptoms, bone tenderness, intractable pruritus, and poor veins may be other indications for the addition of myelosuppression to the treatment regimen. H_1 (cyproheptadine, 4 mg by mouth three times daily) and H_2 blockers (cimetidine, 300 mg by mouth three times daily), alone or in combination, provide relief from pruritus in some patients.

Attempts to reduce the incidence of thrombotic complications with the prophylactic use of platelet-antiaggregating agents, including aspirin and dipyridamole, have been unsuccessful. Indeed, not only has no significant benefit been achieved in terms of reduction in thrombosis, but these agents have been associated with a statistically significant increase in the incidence of gastrointestinal hemorrhage, particularly with prolonged administration to patients with platelet counts greater than 1 million. Hence, long-term prophylactic use of this group of agents cannot be recommended at this time. Short-term use of platelet-antiaggregating agents may be helpful during transient attacks of digital or cerebral ischemia, but such episodes are an indication for, and often respond to, myelosuppression.

Treatment of the burned-out myelofibrotic stage of polycythemia vera can be extremely difficult but does not differ from that described for idiopathic myelofibrosis. The acute leukemias that develop in polycythemia vera, either spontaneously or following myelosuppressive therapy, may be myeloid, myelomonocytic, lymphoid, or biphenotypic in morphology. In those patients with lymphoid morphology and/or increased levels of terminal deoxyribonucleotidyl transferase (TdT), a trial of vincristine and prednisone is indicated. Nevertheless, response to any form of treatment in these patients is infrequent, and median survival in a relatively recent series of postpolycythemic acute leukemias was approximately 30 days.

Meticulous control of blood volume and viscosity with the use of phlebotomy, supplemented when specifically indicated by judicious use of myelosuppression, can ensure most patients with polycythemia vera a prolonged period of relatively symptom-free survival. Median survival in recent series has exceeded 10 years, and symptom-free survival of 15 to 20 years is no longer uncommon. The longest documented survival following a well-founded diagnosis is 34 years.

Berk PD, Goldberg JD, Donovan PB, et al.: Therapeutic recommendations in polycythemia vera based on Polycythemia Vera Study Group protocols. Semin Hematol 23:132, 1986. *A detailed report on a continuous 19-year randomized control study of a large cohort of patients with polycythemia vera and the therapeutic recommendations derived from it. Part of a useful eight-article symposium on polycythemia vera.*

Caldwell GG, Kelley DB, Heath CW Jr, et al.: Polycythemia vera among participants of a nuclear weapons test. JAMA 252:662, 1984. *A provocative report that illustrates some of the difficulties in conclusively linking relatively uncommon disorders to radiation exposure.*

Conley CL: Polycythemia vera, diagnosis and treatment. Hosp Practice 22:107, 1987. *An excellent overview by a senior hematologist with great experience.*

Ellis JT, Peterson P, Geller SA, et al.: Studies of the bone marrow in polycythemia vera and the evolution of myelofibrosis and second hematologic malignancies. Semin Hematol 23:144, 1986. *An important review of bone marrow findings in polycythemia vera, exploring such issues as the evolution of fibrosis and second malignant disorders.*

Raskind WH, Jacobson R, Murphy S, et al.: Evidence for the involvement of B lymphoid cells in polycythemia vera and essential thrombocythemia. J Clin Invest 75:1388, 1985. *A concise paper illustrating how G6PD–isoenzyme analysis can be used to document that a particular cell line, in this case B lymphocytes, has a clonal origin.*

154 MYELOPROLIFERATIVE DISORDERS

Paul D. Berk

The normal bone marrow contains self-replicating pools of morphologically undifferentiated stem cells, recognizable hematopoietic cells undergoing differentiation and maturation, and connective tissue stromal elements. There is a hierarchy of stem cell populations: (1) a pluripotent stem cell capable under appropriate conditions of producing erythroid, myeloid, megakaryocytic, macrophage, and B lymphocyte progeny; (2) intermediate stem cells capable of producing several but not all of these lineages; and (3) committed, unipotent stem cells giving rise exclusively to erythroid, myeloid, or megakaryocytic offspring. The rate of proliferation, pool size, and rate of transition from less restricted to more restricted potential are carefully regulated so that the bone marrow can respond to the body's need for blood elements in a manner that is both selective in terms of the cell types produced and restricted or self-limited in duration (see Fig. 131–2). Thus in hemolysis, pyogenic infection, and immune platelet destruction, specific needs for increased production of erythrocytes, granulocytes, and platelets, respectively, are met ordinarily by selective erythroid, myeloid, or megakaryocytic hyperplasia of the marrow. Stromal cells such as fibroblasts do not appear to play a significant role in these responses.

In the myeloproliferative disorders, in contrast, each of the three major marrow cell lines proliferates in an unregulated, essentially autonomous and self-perpetuating manner. Four disorders—polycythemia vera, agnogenic myeloid metaplasia, chronic myelogenous leukemia, and essential thrombocythemia—can usefully be classified under this heading. Although the proliferation of one particular cell line may dominate the clinical picture, each of these is a clonal hematopoietic malignant disorder arising at the level of the pluripotent stem cell (Ch. 152). In each disorder erythroid, myeloid, and megakaryocytic elements proliferate excessively, but to varying degrees, in the bone marrow and in sites of extramedullary hematopoiesis (often resulting in splenomegaly). In each disorder there is a variable tendency for reactive proliferation of the otherwise normal bone marrow fibroblast—which is not a part of the malignant clone—with the development of myelofibrosis, and for termination in an acute blastic leukemia. Despite differences in the predominant cell line released into the periphery, bone marrows at the time of presentation show many similarities and may be indistinguishable, with clumps or sheets of abnormal megakaryocytes being common to all. Hyperuricemia secondary to increased cell turnover and abnormal levels of serum B_{12} and its binding proteins and of leukocyte alkaline phosphatase activity are also common to this group. Some investigators include acute leukemias of various types (notably erythroleukemia) and paroxysmal nocturnal hemoglobinuria within the myeloproliferative syndromes; others consider these disorders sufficiently different from the basic four to warrant their exclusion.

The myeloproliferative syndromes have long been considered to exhibit transitions between the various entities. The evolution of polycythemia vera into a disorder characterized by myelofibrosis with myeloid metaplasia is well documented, as is the transition of all entities—albeit with varying frequency—to acute leukemia. Other transitions have been harder to document. Thus, Philadelphia chromosome-positive chronic myelogenous leukemia may present transiently with elevated red cell and platelet counts but does not at this stage represent polycythemia vera. Similarly, a patient with polycythemia vera who has suffered a gastrointestinal hemorrhage may at initial examination have only an elevated platelet count, resembling essential thrombocythemia. Repletion of iron stores with resulting erythrocytosis does not represent a true transition from essential thrombocythemia to polycythemia vera.

Despite the failure to confirm true transitions among several of these disorders, the concept of a myeloproliferative syndrome involving the four basic entities just listed is now firmly supported by their clonal, morphologic, pathophysiologic, and clinical similarities. Various nonspecific cytogenetic abnormalities are also observed in each of these entities. The appearance of the Philadelphia (Ph¹) chromosome, characteristic of chronic myelogenous leukemia, is a late event in the pathogenetic evolution of the disorder and follows the initial development of the malignant clone of pluripotent stem cells.

Adamson JW, Fialkow PJ: The pathogenesis of myeloproliferative syndromes. Br J Haematol 38:299, 1978. *A concise review of cell biologic, cytogenetic, and enzymatic evidence for an analogous clonal origin of the major myeloproliferative disorders.*

Gilbert HS: Myeloproliferative disorders. Clin Geriatr Med 1:773, 1985. *A reassessment of the myeloproliferative disorder concept after 20 years of critical clinical experience.*

MYELOFIBROSIS WITH MYELOID METAPLASIA
Definition and Pathogenesis

Myelofibrosis with myeloid metaplasia is a syndrome in which morphologic evidence of excessive fibroblast proliferation and collagen deposition in the bone marrow is accompanied by myeloid metaplasia of organs such as the liver, spleen, and lymph nodes. These organs, involved normally in fetal but not adult erythropoiesis, become active sites of extramedullary hematopoiesis. Similar clinical syndromes may be seen in three distinct settings. The first of these is progressive hepatosplenomegaly and the evolution of a leukoerythroblastic peripheral blood picture indicative of myeloid metaplasia occurring in the absence of an apparent inciting cause. This disorder, termed *agnogenic myeloid metaplasia*, is a clonal stem cell hemopathy constituting one of the primary myeloproliferative syndromes. Second, a similar picture of myelofibrosis with myeloid metaplasia may evolve in the course of polycythemia vera or chronic granulocytic leukemia, either as a part of the natural history of the illness or as a consequence of the myelosuppressive therapies administered. The third setting is myeloid metaplasia with varying degrees of reactive myelofibrosis that may occur secondary to a wide spectrum of clinical disorders including, among others, severe hemolytic anemia, Hodgkin's disease, various nonhematopoietic neoplasms metastatic to the bone marrow, infections such as tuberculosis, or following bone marrow injury caused by radiation, benzol, fluorine, phosphorus, or strontium.

In myelofibrosis with myeloid metaplasia, the extent of extramedullary hematopoiesis tends to parallel the extent of bone marrow fibrosis. Indeed, it was previously believed that the mesenchymal cells in the liver, spleen, and lymph nodes resumed their embryonic potential for hematopoiesis in an attempt to compensate for myelophthisis. However, in some cases there is a dissociation between the degree of marrow fibrosis and extramedullary hematopoiesis resulting in (1) marrow fibrosis without evidence of significant myeloid metaplasia, or (2) progressive hepatosplenomegaly with a leukoerythroblastic peripheral blood picture in the absence of significant fibrosis. Pluripotent hematopoietic stem cells, presumably of bone marrow origin, are constantly present in the circulation of normal individuals and appear in increased numbers in the peripheral blood of patients with myelofibrosis. It is more likely that these circulating stem cells take up residence in organs such as the liver and spleen to produce extramedullary hematopoiesis than that this represents the reactivation of hematopoietic capabilities in local mesenchymal cells. Except in the secondary setting noted above, the primary pathogenetic event is believed to be a mutation leading to a malignant hematopoietic clone at the level of a pluripotent stem cell. The development of myelofibrosis appears to be a reaction to the presence of this proliferating clone. The release of increased megakaryocyte- and platelet-derived growth factor from the markedly expanded bone marrow megakaryocyte pool of the myeloproliferative syndromes may be in part responsible for the secondary fibroblast proliferation and collagen deposition. Colonization of the liver, spleen, and lymph nodes may, in this setting, represent a form of metastasis of abnormal stem cells to organs that retain an intrinsic potential to support erythropoiesis.

Clinical Features

Myelofibrosis with myeloid metaplasia, whether agnogenic or secondary to another myeloproliferative syndrome, is primarily a disorder of the middle-aged or older adult. At least 60 per cent of cases occur between the ages of 50 and 70, with no predilection for either sex. The onset of symptoms is usually insidious over several years and in most cases disease progression is slow. Most commonly presenting symptoms are referable to anemia with its consequent cardiovascular consequences, or to increased abdominal girth or discomfort resulting from splenic and hepatic enlargement. Bone pain, often migratory, and gouty arthritis occasionally bring the patient to medical attention. Deafness resulting from otosclerosis occurs in a small minority of cases. Increasing numbers of asymptomatic patients are being detected today in the course of routine screening laboratory or physical examinations.

On physical examination, splenomegaly is an almost universal finding. In approximately 85 per cent of cases, the spleen extends 8 cm or more below the left costal margin, and in one third of cases is enlarged more than 16 cm. Occasional patients without palpable splenomegaly will be demonstrated to have splenic enlargement by means of an isotopic or computerized tomographic imaging study. Rarely, significant myelofibrosis with cytopenia occurs, at least initially, without myeloid metaplasia and with no evidence of splenic enlargement. Hepatomegaly occurs in approximately 50 per cent of cases, frequently with mild abnormalities of liver function tests—especially elevation of alkaline phosphatase. Hepatomegaly in the absence of splenomegaly is extremely rare in agnogenic myeloid metaplasia or when the syndrome occurs secondary to another myeloproliferative disease, and points to a diagnosis of secondary myeloid metaplasia. Extramedullary hematopoiesis is frequently demonstrable histologically in lymph nodes, but clinically significant lymph node enlargement occurs in only 10 per cent of cases. Petechiae, caused by both thrombocytopenia and platelet dysfunction, have been reported in up to 25 per cent of patients, and jaundice, edema, and ascites are found in 10 to 20 per cent of cases.

Laboratory Data

At diagnosis, a mild to moderate degree of anemia is typical with the hemoglobin ranging between 9 and 13 grams per 100 ml. Red cells are initially normocytic and normochromic with mild poikilocytosis. Polychromatophilia, a modest reticulocytosis of 2 to 5 per cent, and occasional teardrop erythrocytes are seen (Color plate 3D). The presence of at least a few normoblasts and occasionally even earlier erythroid precursors is extremely common. As the disease progresses and the spleen enlarges, more severe anisocytosis, poikilocytosis, polychromasia, basophilic stippling, and normoblastosis may be sufficiently characteristic to indicate the diagnosis. The white blood cell count is initially normal in about one third of patients, elevated in approximately one half, and low in the remaining 15 per cent. Most typically, the count is in the range of 15,000 to 30,000 per cubic millimeter but counts as high as 70,000 per cubic millimeter are observed. The white count tends to fluctuate with time and often does not show the downward trend observed for the hemoglobin concentration and platelet count. A degree of granulocyte immaturity in the peripheral blood is typical, including the presence of as many as 10 per cent blasts. This does not necessarily suggest the evolution of acute leukemia, particularly when there are proportionate numbers of promyelocytes, myelocytes, and metamyelocytes as well. Basophilia and an acquired Pelger-Hüet anomaly are other typical features of the peripheral blood smear. The leukocyte alkaline phosphatase score is variable but is most often normal or increased. The platelet count initially is most often normal, although reduced or elevated counts are not uncommon. Exceedingly high counts in excess of 10^6 per microliter may cause this condition to be confused with the entity of primary thrombocytosis. Morphologically, megathrombocytes and megakaryocytic fragments are extremely common. Over time, the platelet count gradually tends to decrease, and thrombocytopenia is common late in the disorder. Overall, a peripheral blood smear demonstrating striking teardrop poikilocytosis, leukoerythroblastic nucleated cells, and megathrombocytes and megakaryocytic fragments is highly suggestive of the syndrome of myelofibrosis with myeloid metaplasia. Erythrocyte survival is almost invariably reduced and splenic sequestration often is present. Platelet production is usually increased even in patients with thrombocytopenia, associated with a marked increase in splenic pooling

Normal or slightly elevated serum levels of vitamin B_{12} and B_{12} binding proteins occur both in agnogenic myeloid metaplasia and postpolycythemia myelofibrosis, but the values are not as striking in those seen in chronic granulocytic leukemia. Hyperuricemia, due to increased uric acid production, is common. Miscellaneous laboratory abnormalities include high levels of LDH, modest elevations of serum transaminase and bilirubin levels, increased serum alkaline phosphatase activity caused by both hepatic and bone isoenzyme fractions, and modest increases in muramidase (lysozyme).

Cytogenetic abnormalities occur in up to 50 per cent of patients with agnogenic myeloid metaplasia, with trisomy for a C group chromosome being probably the most common consistent alteration. The Ph^1 chromosome is not present.

Osteosclerosis distributed primarily in the flat bones of the axial skeleton and in the metaphyseal ends of the femur and humerus may be recognized radiographically in up to 70 per cent of patients. Osteosclerosis involving the ear ossicles may result in deafness. The typical radiographic finding is the loss of definition of individual bony trabeculae, leading to a ground glass appearance.

Attempts to aspirate bone marrow almost invariably lead to a dry tap, even when the marrow is very cellular. Accordingly, bone marrow biopsy, either percutaneous or surgical, is usually required for diagnosis. Demonstration of bone marrow fibrosis, often with accompanying osteosclerosis, is the sine qua non. The bone marrow may sometimes be hypercellular, frequently demonstrating a panhyperplasia, in residual focal areas. Even in these areas, in which mature collagen may not be evident, an increase in reticulin fibers can usually be demonstrated by silver impregnation. Extramedullary hematopoiesis is demonstrable in both liver and spleen, but because of the risks involved in percutaneous biopsy of these organs, its diagnosis usually is based on the typical leukoerythroblastic blood picture and occasionally on isotopic erythrokinetic studies. The increase of bone marrow collagen content in myelofibrosis is principally the result of excessive collagen deposition and is reflected in an increase in the serum level of procollagen III amino terminal peptide.

Course of the Disease

The course of both agnogenic and postpolycythemic myelofibrosis is characterized by progressive splenic enlargement and, typically, by slightly less striking enlargement of the liver. The spleen will often fill the entire left side of the abdomen, extending beyond the midline to the right and down into the pelvis. The resulting early satiety, associated with a hypermetabolic state from increased cell turnover, may result in appreciable weight loss. Painful splenic infarcts may also complicate the disease. The marked splenic enlargement and consequent increase in splenic blood flow, coupled with increased resistance to flow within the liver caused by extramedullary hematopoiesis, lead to portal hypertension and its various complications including ascites, edema, and variceal hemorrhage in a small proportion of patients. Hepatic vein thrombosis with Budd-Chiari syndrome is another recognized complication. The progressive splenomegaly is accompanied almost inevitably by progressive anemia and thrombocytopenia, the former occasionally complicated by iron deficiency of blood loss or, less frequently, by folic acid deficiency. Although granulocyte counts are usually better maintained than those of other blood cellular elements, eventually granulocytopenia may develop. In this setting bacterial infections occur with increased frequency and may be a major factor leading to death. The association of myelofibrosis with tuberculosis is well documented, and this infection should be excluded by histologc and bacteriologic examination. When the two disorders coincide it is not clear whether myelofibrosis is always secondary to tuberculous infection of the marrow, or whether, conversely, tuberculosis has supervened in a patient with an underlying clonal hemopathy. Because of the almost inevitable hyperuricemia, attacks of gouty arthritis may develop in untreated patients.

Acute leukemic transformation is an occasional terminal event in agnogenic myeloid metaplasia. About 10 per cent of patients with polycythemia vera will develop a spent phase with advanced myelofibrosis. The likelihood of developing postpolycythemic myelofibrosis does not seem to be influenced by the type of therapy given for the underlying polycythemia, but evolution to the spent phase is a risk factor for subsequent development of acute leukemia. Once myelofibrosis has developed in this setting, the incidence of subsequent leukemic transformation (6 per cent in phlebotomy-treated patients, 45 per cent with chlorambucil, and 25 per cent with ^{32}P) is two and one half to four times greater than in similarly treated polycythemic patients who have not developed myelofibrosis.

Treatment and Prognosis

No agreement has been reached as to the optimal treatment of agnogenic myeloid metaplasia or of postpolycythemic myelofibrosis. There is thus far no effective treatment that inhibits the fibrotic process. Moreover, none of the conventional forms of treatment, including androgen therapy to stimulate erythropoiesis, chemotherapy, or splenectomy, has been shown to prolong life. Because of the relatively indolent progression of the disorder in most patients, a majority of hematologists undertake no specific treatment in the asymptomatic patient except for the administration of allopurinol at doses of 200 to 400 mg per day to avoid the complications of hyperuricemia.

In the presence of symptomatic anemia, androgens may be employed: testosterone enanthate, 200 to 600 mg weekly intramuscularly, or oxymetholone, 50 to 150 mg daily by mouth. Treatment must be continued for at least three months to establish whether a particular preparation is effective, and some hematologists argue that patients who fail to respond to one androgen preparation may ultimately respond to another. Androgens seem most effective in women who have been splenectomized previously or who have never had massive splenomegaly. The doses employed inevitably lead to excessive fluid accumulation and, in female patients, to significant masculinization. The hemolytic anemia almost never responds to corticosteroids; these drugs may, however, increase the risk of infection in granulocytopenic patients. In patients with marked thrombocytosis, busulfan, in an initial dose of 4 mg per day followed by lower doses as the platelet count normalizes, or hydroxyurea, at a dose of 500 to 1500 mg per day, is often effective in obtaining control of the platelet count. Although busulfan is widely used in this setting, its potential mutagenic risks are a cause for concern. These agents may occasionally produce a beneficial reduction in spleen size and/or increase the hemoglobin concentration, but equally frequently will result in suppression of erythropoiesis and thrombopoiesis. Radiation therapy to the spleen has largely been abandoned because the doses required to produce a meaningful reduction in spleen size often cause severe leukopenia and thrombocytopenia.

The role of splenectomy in patients with agnogenic myeloid metaplasia or postpolycythemic myelofibrosis is highly controversial. As a high risk procedure, it should probably be reserved for patients with severe hemolytic anemia, thrombocytopenia sufficient to produce bleeding, portal hypertension, or severe discomfort secondary to pressure symptoms or infarction. Striking thrombocytosis with thrombosis or hemorrhage or both may develop postoperatively and may require aggressive myelosuppression. In some patients splenectomy is followed by progressive enlargement of the liver, with recurrent hemolysis and thrombocytopenia. The diagnosis of acute leukemia is often difficult to make in these patients in whom the percentage of blasts in the peripheral blood may increase slowly and progressively for years.

Survival in agnogenic myeloid metaplasia and in postpolycythemic myelofibrosis is difficult to define with certainty. Several authors suggest that median survival in agnogenic myeloid metaplasia is approximately ten years from the onset of the disease and five years from the time of diagnosis. However, there is considerable heterogeneity, with both shorter and longer survival frequently observed.

Bone marrow transplantation has been attempted both by conventional techniques and after surgical manipulation of bone marrow cavity spaces in attempts to provide an improved microenvironment for the transplanted marrow. Only occasional successes have been reported, and this procedure must be considered highly experimental.

The syndrome of acute myelofibrosis, which is a rapidly progressive and fatal variant, has been shown by various cytologic marker studies to represent a form of acute megakaryocytic leukemia. It is believed that the release of platelet-megakaryocyte–derived growth factor from the malignant megakaryoblasts is responsible for the rapidly progressive marrow fibrosis. Induction chemotherapy may produce temporary hematologic remission, but only partial reversal of marrow fibrosis.

Berk PD, Castro-Malaspina H, Wasserman LR (eds.): Myelofibrosis and the Biology of Connective Tissue. New York, Alan R. Liss, Inc., 1984. *This book contains 29 concise chapters by multiple authors who review the available information about the regulation of fibroblast proliferation, collagen biosynthesis, cell biology of marrow stromal cells, and other aspects of basic biologic science believed to be relevant to the pathogenesis of myelofibrosis.*

Kroopman JE: The pathogenesis of myelofibrosis in myeloproliferative disorders. Ann Intern Med 92:858, 1980. *Excellent brief summary of speculations on the pathogenesis of myelofibrosis.*

Ruiz-Arguelles GJ, Marin-Lopez A, Lobato-Mendizabal E, et al.: Acute megakaryoblastic leukaemia: A prospective study of its identification and treatment. Br J Haematol 62:55, 1986. *An interesting study of diagnostic characterization and response to therapy of acute megakaryoblastic leukemia with myelofibrosis.*

Varki A, Lottenberg R, Griffith R, et al.: The syndrome of idiopathic myelofibrosis. Clinicopathologic review with emphasis on the prognostic variables predicting survival. Medicine 62:53, 1983. *This is a useful review of 88 consecutive patients with bone marrow fibrosis seen at Barnes Hospital. As noted in the title, there is considerable emphasis on prognostic features.*

ESSENTIAL THROMBOCYTHEMIA

Essential thrombocythemia, also known as a hemorrhagic thrombocythemia or essential thrombocytosis, is a primary myeloproliferative disorder in which the predominant laboratory feature is a persistent, striking elevation of the platelet count to values in excess of 1×10^6 per microliter. The disorder shows many features of polycythemia vera including an almost identical distribution of patient ages at the time of diagnosis, similar degrees of leukocytosis, and morphologically similar bone marrow abnormalities. Splenomegaly has been reported to occur in 30 to 75 per cent of cases. The criteria outlined in the following paragraph would restrict the diagnosis to patients who have either normal or reduced hemoglobin concentrations, those with concomitant erythrocytosis being classified as having polycythemia vera.

The Polycythemia Vera Study Group has proposed the following diagnostic criteria for essential thrombocythemia: (1) platelet count persistently greater than 1×10^6 per microliter in the absence of an identifiable cause such as malignant disease, infection, chronic inflammatory disease, or previous splenectomy; (2) normal total red cell volume, the measurement of which may be omitted if the hemoglobin concentration is less than 13 grams per 100 ml; (3) presence of iron in the bone marrow; if iron is absent, failure of the hemoglobin concentration to increase by more than 1 gram per 100 ml after a one-month trial of oral iron therapy; (4) absence of collagen fibrosis in bone marrow biopsy; and (5) absence of the Philadelphia chromosome from unstimulated metaphases obtained from a bone marrow aspirate. Because of both morphologic and clinical similarities, criteria 2 and 3 are necessary to exclude a diagnosis of polycythemia vera, whereas criteria 4 and 5 distinguish the disorder from agnogenic myeloid metaplasia and chronic myelogenous leukemia, respectively.

Clinical Features

The predominant clinical manifestations of essential thrombocythemia result from hemorrhagic and/or thrombotic events. Some patients have easy bruising, epistaxis, unexplained gastrointestinal bleeding, and an excessive tendency to postoperative hemorrhage. Conversely, other patients present evidence for microvascular occlusion in sites such as the extremities, the central nervous system, and the coronary circulation. The commonest manifestation of microvascular occlusion is burning pain in the feet, hands, and digits, which may progress to frank gangrene. Although these symptoms are striking when they occur, large numbers of patients, particularly younger patients, may be asymptomatic for long periods. Hence, the precise incidence of these complications is unknown. Similarly, transition to acute leukemia has been clearly documented, but there is no accurate estimate of its frequency, particularly in patients not previously exposed to mutagenic agents.

Course and Prognosis

The natural history of this disease is poorly appreciated, and most reports in the literature describe very small series of patients with a focus on a particular complication. Descriptions emphasizing hemorrhagic, thrombotic, and embolic episodes and a high fatality rate are directly contradicted by others emphasizing prolonged periods without complications. The largest series suggest a life expectancy perhaps analogous to that of polycythemia vera.

Therapy

Because of uncertainties about its natural history, there is a substantial lack of agreement about appropriate therapy for essential thrombocythemia. Despite strikingly high platelet counts, many hematologists recommend expectant management in asymptomatic patients under the age of 60, while others recommend the use only of platelet-antiaggregating agents (e.g., aspirin 300 mg per day with or without dipyridamole 50 mg three times daily).* However, the experience in polycythemia vera suggests that prolonged administration of platelet-antiaggregating agents may increase the risk of gastrointestinal hemorrhage. Chronic myelosuppression should be attempted in older patients and those who have a history of significant thrombotic episodes. In these cases, prevention of neurologic damage takes precedence over concern about long-term mutagenic effects of myelosuppression. Control of the thrombocytosis can be achieved with melphalan* 6 to 10 mg per day by mouth for one week followed by 4 to 6 mg per day until the platelet count is in the normal range. Subsequent maintenance with 2 to 6 mg per week is continued indefinitely, the appropriate dose depending on the platelet count. Alternatively, hydroxyurea* at an initial dose of 500 to 1500 mg per day, tapered to an individualized maintenance dose as the platelet count falls, or radioactive phosphorus 2.9 mCi per square meter of body surface area intravenously, repeated as necessary at intervals of not less than three months, is highly effective in achieving normalization of the platelet count. Patients presenting with serious thrombotic or hemorrhagic manifestations and uncontrolled thrombocytosis should be treated with platelet-antiaggregating agents, urgent plateletpheresis, and the initiation of a myelosuppressive regimen. Every effort should be made to avoid splenectomy in patients with essential thrombocythemia because of the extreme thrombocytosis and serious complications that often follow this procedure.

---

*This use is not listed in the manufacturer's directive.

Jabaily J, Iland HJ, Laszlo J, et al.: Neurologic manifestations of essential thrombocythemia. Ann Intern Med 99:513, 1983. *A contrary report on the largest series of patients with essential thrombocythemia yet assembled suggesting that approximately two thirds have evidence of at least transient neurologic dysfunction.*

Kessler CM, Klein HG, Havlik RJ: Uncontrolled thrombocytosis in chronic myeloproliferative disorders. Br J Haematol 50:157, 1982. *A retrospective study suggesting that, at least in the younger patient, severe thrombocytosis in myeloproliferative disease may have fewer complications than previously believed.*

Murphy S: Thrombocytosis and thrombocythaemia. Clin Hematol 12:89, 1983. *A detailed review of the pathogenesis, pathophysiology, and management of this puzzling disorder. Excellent bibliography.*

Murphy S, Iland H, Rosenthal D, et al.: Essential thrombocythemia: An interim report from the Polycythemia Vera Study Group. Semin Hematol 23:177, 1986. *A brief but useful update of Murphy's 1983 review.*

155 THE CHRONIC LEUKEMIAS

Bayard Clarkson

CHRONIC MYELOGENOUS LEUKEMIA (Chronic Myeloid Leukemia, Chronic Myelocytic Leukemia, Chronic Granulocytic Leukemia)

DEFINITION. Chronic myelogenous leukemia (CML) is a chronic form of leukemia originating in a primitive myeloid stem cell in which the leukemic cells retain the capacity for differentiation and are able to perform the essential functions of normal hematopoietic cells that they replace in the marrow. The leukemic cells have a pronounced tendency to undergo further malignant transformation with loss of ability to differentiate in later stages of the disease. Although commonly included among other myeloproliferative disorders (see Ch. 154), CML is a distinct entity that is easily recognized because the leukemic cells have a distinctive cytogenetic abnormality, the Philadelphia (Ph¹) chromosome.

ETIOLOGY. The etiology is unknown. The majority of patients with CML have no history of excessive exposure to ionizing radiation or chemical leukemogens, but the incidence increases greatly with exposure to high doses of radiation. This may occur following chronic exposure in radiologists who practice without adequate shielding, in patients who have received radiation treatments for ankylosing spondylitis or other chronic diseases, and in subjects exposed to a single massive dose of radiation as in the atomic bomb explosions in Japan in 1945. After subacute or acute exposure to large radiation doses there is a latent period of several years, after which the incidence of both acute myeloid leukemia and CML increases in an approximately linear relationship to the radiation dose. In the atomic bomb survivors the peak incidence occurred about seven years after the explosion and was about 50 times that of nonexposed subjects. The rate then declined, but still exceeded the national average 15 years later. Radiation hazards are more extensively discussed in Ch. 539.

The contribution of chemicals to the causation of CML is hard to assess. Any chemical capable of causing myelotoxicity or chromosome damage is suspect. However, persons in industrialized societies are exposed to such a wide variety of chemicals with these properties, including solvents, insecticides, hair dyes, and various drugs, that their very prevalence makes it difficult to incriminate specific candidates. Cytotoxic drugs, especially alkylating agents and those used in combination with radiation in the treatment of other neoplastic diseases (such as Hodgkin's disease), are known to increase the incidence of leukemia, usually after a latent period of several years. The most common type of leukemia is one of the variants of acute myeloid leukemia, but CML may also occur rarely. The minimal leukemogenic dose has not been established for any chemical or drug in humans, but it is only prudent to try to minimize unnecessary exposure to any potential leukemogens.

INCIDENCE AND PREVALENCE. The incidence of CML in the United States and most Western countries is about 1.5 per 100,000 population per year and accounts for about 15 per cent of all cases of leukemia. CML is slightly more frequent in men than women, but the course of the disease is the same. The median age is about 45 and the disease is uncommon below the age of 20. In children with CML in whom the Ph[1] chromosome is present, the course of the disease is similar to that of adults. A juvenile form of CML, described in very young children, has a more rapidly progressive course and the leukemic cells lack the (Ph[1]) chromosome.

Although a few instances have been noted of CML occurring in multiple family members, familial occurrence is uncommon, and children born to mothers who have the disease are normal.

PATHOGENESIS AND MECHANISMS. In over 90 per cent of cases the leukemic cells have a unique chromosomal abnormality, the Ph[1] chromosome. The Ph[1] anomaly results from a reciprocal translocation of a portion of the long arm of chromosome 22 to another chromosome, usually the long arm of chromosome 9, although sometimes to another chromosome. Both deletion of the long arm of number 22 and translocation to another chromosome must be demonstrated by appropriate banding studies to confirm Ph[1] positivity.

In Ph[1]-positive CML, the cellular oncogene c-abl, which is normally located on the long arm of chromosome 9 at band q34, is translocated to a small 6 kilobase (kb) region of chromosome 22 designated the breakpoint cluster region or bcr. This translocation results in the transcription of a novel hybrid bcr/c-abl 8.5 kb messenger RNA (mRNA) and its fusion protein product, a 210-kD phosphoprotein (P210). These novel products are larger than the corresponding normal c-abl mRNA (6 and 7 kg) and its protein (145 kD), and the P210 protein has altered tyrosine kinase activity. It is not yet known how these alterations relate to the CML cells' abnormal proliferative behavior. It is strongly suspected, however, that the hybrid bcr/abl gene has a key role in the pathogenesis of the disease because it is such a consistent finding. It is also analogous to a similar fusion protein in mouse cells transformed by the Abelson murine leukemia virus. Some patients present with many clinical features of CML, but do not have the Ph[1] chromosome in their marrow cells. The course of the disease is atypical in these patients, and they generally have a poor response to treatment and shorter survival than Ph[1]-positive patients. It appears that most of them are misdiagnosed as having Ph[1]-negative CML and have other myelodysplastic disorders, most commonly chronic myelomonocytic leukemia (CMMoL).

There is good evidence, based on the occurrence of CML in patients with chromosome mosaicism and in those heterozygous for the enzyme glucose-6-phosphate dehydrogenase, that the leukemic population arises from a single cell because the Ph[1] anomaly has been found to be restricted to just one of their dual cell lines (Ch. 152). The defect is an acquired one, since the Ph[1] marker is not present in nonhematopoietic cells, and monozygous twins of patients with CML do not have the Ph[1] chromosome in their myeloid cells. The presence of the Ph[1] genetic marker in erythrocyte, granulocyte, monocyte, and megakaryocyte precursors indicates that the original transformation occurred in an ancestral cell common to these myeloid cell types, but the exact location of the transforming event within the progenitor cell lineages is still uncertain.

The Ph[1] chromosome is absent in the majority of mature lymphocytes, although in about 20 per cent of patients some of the B cells contain the Ph[1] marker. T lymphocytes are rarely involved, although a few reports indicate some T cell precursors are Ph[1] positive. When one or more of the chronic phase leukemic cells undergo blastic transformation, in about 25 per cent of such cases the blasts have been found to have phenotypic properties associated with lymphocyte precursors, including high levels of terminal deoxynucleotidyl transferase and reactivity with specific antisera prepared against an antigen (cALLA) present on the common type of acute lymphoblastic leukemic cells. Some cases of CML blastic transformation have been reported in which the blasts contain intracellular IgM, a characteristic of pre-B cells. While in most cases of lymphoid blastic transformation detectable cytoplasmic and surface immunoglobulin are lacking, in the majority of cases there is rearrangement of the immunoglobulin heavy chain genes, and in some there is also progression to light chain–gene rearrangements. Since these gene rearrangements are a mandatory early step in B cell development and rarely occur within other human hematopoietic lineages, the findings provide strong evidence that the lymphoid blasts are early B cell precursors.

On the basis of serial hematologic examinations of atomic bomb survivors who developed CML, it has been estimated that about eight years elapse between the original mutational event that results in the first Ph[1]-positive leukemic cell in the marrow and the development of clinical symptoms when the diagnosis is ordinarily made. Since the average survival after diagnosis is three years, the total course of the disease is thus about 11 years. At the time of diagnosis 85 to 100 per cent of the dividing marrow cells contain the Ph[1] marker in the majority of patients. A few patients have lesser degrees of replacement of normal marrow cells by leukemic cells at diagnosis, and in such cases the leukemic and normal populations may coexist in nearly equal balance for a year or more before the leukemic cells eventually replace the normal cells. Cells containing the Ph[1] chromosome have not been found in normal subjects.

Why the leukemic cells have a proliferative advantage is not known. In the chronic stage of the disease the leukemic cells retain the capacity to differentiate almost normally, and the enzymatic and functional defects exhibited by the leukemic cells are not of sufficient severity to prevent them from carrying out their essential functions in supporting life in the absence of normal cells. Many of the defects somehow appear to be related to the increased mass of the leukemic population because such abnormalities as deficient neutrophil alkaline phosphatase, impaired phagocytic capacity of neutrophils, and various platelet and red cell abnormalities return toward normal after the cell density has been reduced by treatment.

There is characteristically a marked shift toward granulocyte differentiation at the expense of erythroid differentiation in untreated CML, but the myeloid-erythroid ratio usually returns toward normal after treatment. In most cases, neutrophilic granulocytes predominate, but eosinophilia and/or basophilia and monocytosis also occur frequently. Increased numbers of megakaryocytes and thrombocytosis frequently accompany the increased granulocyte production, but thrombocytopenia may also be observed. Some degree of anemia is common, and rarely erythrocytosis may occur.

The mass of myeloid tissue is usually greatly increased in CML at the time of diagnosis, sometimes tenfold or more. The leukemic granulocytic precursors in the marrow and spleen divide less rapidly than the corresponding cells in normal marrow, although their rate of proliferation may be nearly normal very early in the disease or after the myeloid mass has been reduced by treatment. In the chronic phase the percentage of myeloblasts is usually not increased compared to that in normal marrow, but their absolute number is greatly increased because of the expanded mass of myeloid tissue in the marrow, spleen, blood, and sometimes other extramedullary sites. There is also a greatly increased incidence of earlier committed granulocyte-monocyte precursors that form colonies and clusters in semisolid culture systems and that show nearly normal in vitro maturation and growth. The primary reason for the expanded myeloid mass is that the leukemic stem cells continue to proliferate after exceeding the cell density limit in the marrow at which normal stem cells arrest cell production. The specific biochemical abnormalities responsible for the failure of the multipotent leukemic stem cells to respond normally to feedback regulation are not yet understood, nor is it known how they may be related to the bcr/abl gene rearrangement.

The leukemic cells in chronic-phase CML have a striking

propensity for further malignant transformation. After a variable duration of the chronic phase, averaging about three years, the disease enters an accelerated or blastic phase. Such malignant progression occurs in about 80 per cent of patients and probably would eventually occur in all of them if they did not die of other complications of the disease or of unrelated causes. The Ph[1] chromosome is preserved, but the transformed cells may acquire additional chromosomal abnormalities such as an additional Ph[1] chromosome, trisomy of chromosome 8 or 17, or trisomy of the long arm of 17. The rapidity with which the transition occurs depends on the degree of further transformation and on the comparative proliferative properties of the chronic and acute phase stem cells. In the accelerated phase the cells retain their capacity for partial differentiation, whereas in the blastic phase they are arrested at the blastic level of differentiation. The direction of differentiation in the accelerated phase is variable as in the chronic phase. Transitional forms may occur among the chronic, accelerated, and blastic phases.

CLINICAL MANIFESTATIONS. Occasionally CML is diagnosed in an asymptomatic patient after incidental detection of splenomegaly or unexplained leukocytosis, basophilia, or thrombocytosis. Common early symptoms are *fatigue* and reduced exercise tolerance resulting from anemia, anorexia, reduction in food capacity, weight loss, and a sense of fullness in the left upper quadrant as a result of progressive splenic enlargement. Headaches, sweating, fever, and bone pain or tenderness may also occur, especially if the leukocyte count is very elevated. *Hemorrhagic manifestations* such as ecchymoses after minor trauma, petechiae, retinal hemorrhages, or hematuria may occur in patients in whom there is severe thrombocytopenia or in those with thrombocytosis with abnormal platelets. *Thrombotic episodes* such as splenic or myocardial infarction and thrombophlebitis are common, and priapism or severe headaches may result from leukostasis in patients with extreme leukocytosis. Acute *gouty arthritis* or *nephrolithiasis* is sometimes associated with elevated uric acid levels. Infections are uncommon in the chronic phase, but occasional patients may have unusual and persistent infections that are difficult to diagnose. Low-grade *fever* in the absence of infection is not unusual in the chronic phase when there is extreme leukocytosis, and the temperature returns to normal when the WBC is lowered by treatment.

PHYSICAL EXAMINATION. The most common finding on physical examination at diagnosis is *splenomegaly*. The spleen may be enormous and fill most of the abdomen, or only minimally enlarged; in less than 10 per cent of cases the spleen is not palpable or enlarged on splenic scan. Slight hepatomegaly is common, but when extreme liver enlargement occurs as a result of leukemic infiltration or there is infiltration of lymph nodes, skin, or other tissues, these are usually indications that the disease will have a rapidly progressive course. Patients who present with the disease already in blastic transformation or in whom this event occurs later in the course of the disease may exhibit any of the clinical findings associated with acute leukemia. Unlike acute leukemia, persistent fever unrelated to infection is common in the blastic phase of CML.

LABORATORY ABNORMALITIES. The most consistent laboratory abnormality at diagnosis is *leukocytosis* (Color plate 3C). The WBC count may range from a minimal elevation to over a million leukocytes per cubic millimeter. The marrow is hypercellular, and differential counts of both marrow and blood show a spectrum of mature and immature granulocytes similar to that found in normal marrow. Increased numbers of eosinophils and/or basophils are often present, and sometimes monocytosis is seen. Increased megakaryocytes are often found in the marrow, and sometimes fragments of megakaryocyte nuclei are present in the blood, especially when the platelet count is very high. The percentage of lymphocytes is reduced in both the marrow and blood in

comparison to normal subjects, but the absolute lymphocyte count is usually normal or increased with normal proportions of B and T cells. The myeloid-erythroid ratio in the marrow is usually greatly elevated. The percentage of blasts in the marrow and blood is usually less than 3 per cent in the chronic phase at diagnosis and less than 1 per cent after the WBC count has been reduced by treatment; a persistent elevation of greater than 10 per cent usually indicates impending transformation. About half of patients present with some degree of *thrombocytosis* at diagnosis; thrombocytopenia is much less frequent. Extreme degrees of thrombocytopenia or thrombocytosis may develop as the disease progresses. In some patients, cyclic fluctuations of the leukocytes and platelets have been observed that are unrelated to treatment.

There may be no anemia at presentation, but variable degrees of *anemia* are common when the WBC count exceeds 50,000 per cubic millimeter. The anemia is normocytic and normochromic, unless complications such as bleeding occur, resulting in iron deficiency. Some patients, especially those with greatly enlarged spleens, have circulating nucleated erythrocyte precursors, but this finding is not usually prominent. There may be shortened red cell survival in patients with severe splenomegaly and/or hepatomegaly, but autoimmune hemolysis is not seen in uncomplicated CML. The reticulocyte count is normal or only slightly increased.

The mature granulocytes in CML usually have markedly diminished neutrophil alkaline phosphatase activity and their content of myeloperoxidase and lactoferrin may also be decreased. Plasma and leukocyte levels of histamine and histamine metabolites are usually elevated. Other common laboratory abnormalities in CML that are associated with the increased rates of cell production and turnover are elevated levels of serum uric acid, lactic dehydrogenase, vitamin B_{12}, the B_{12}-binding protein transcobalamin I, and serum urinary lysozyme. Hyperkalemia resulting from leakage of potassium from leukocytes occurs rarely. Hypercalcemia may also occur, usually in patients with blastic transformation or in those who are entering an accelerated phase and have lytic bone lesions.

Myelofibrosis, demonstrated by special stains of marrow biopsy specimens, may develop in the course of CML. Significant myelofibrosis is more often seen late in the course of disease, but rarely severe acute myelofibrosis is seen prior to treatment in patients with prominent megakaryocytic proliferation. The marrow histiocytes sometimes display prominent phagocytic activity and become engorged with glycolipids, resembling Gaucher cells.

Transition from the chronic phase to the accelerated or blastic phase may occur gradually over a year or longer or abruptly (blast crisis). The disease becomes progressively less responsive to previously effective treatment. Common signs and symptoms heralding such a change are progressive leukocytosis, thrombocytosis, or thrombocytopenia, anemia, increasing and painful splenomegaly, lymphadenopathy, hepatomegaly, or infiltration of other organs, fever, bone pain, development of destructive bone lesions, and thrombotic or bleeding complications. In the accelerated phase, the cells are still completely or partially differentiated, although they usually show increasing morphologic abnormalities. There are no standardized criteria for distinguishing between the accelerated and blastic phases, but most authorities use a persistent elevation of greater than 20 or 30 per cent blasts in the blood and/or marrow or of blasts plus promyelocytes of 30 per cent in blood or 50 per cent in marrow to define the blastic phase. When the spleen is the primary source of the transformed cells, the percentage of blasts in the blood may be higher than in the marrow. The blasts have the morphologic appearance of lymphoblasts in about 25 per cent of cases and contain terminal deoxynucleotidyl transferase, whereas in the remainder they are recognized as primitive myeloid precursors.

DIAGNOSIS. Persistent unexplained leukocytosis with circulating immature granulocytes and an enlarged spleen suggests the diagnosis of CML; some degree of splenomegaly is present at diagnosis in over 90 per cent of patients. A bone marrow aspiration and biopsy should always be done if the diagnosis of CML is suspected. Demonstration of the Ph[1] chromosome in dividing marrow cells provides confirmation of the diagnosis in Ph[1]-positive CML. Occasional patients with complex variant translocations lack a morphologically apparent Ph[1] chromosome, but involvement of chromosomes 9 and 22 can be detected using appropriate molecular techniques.

Leukemoid reactions associated with infections are usually distinguishable in most cases because prominent splenomegaly is absent, neutrophil alkaline phosphatase activity is increased instead of low, and the Ph[1] chromosome is not present (see Ch. 151). Leukemoid or leukoerythroblastic reactions also occur with certain neoplasms, especially when there is involvement of the bone marrow, but sometimes even in the absence of marrow metastases. By appropriate cytochemical tests and analyses of surface antigens it is usually possible to distinguish metastatic tumor cells from immature hematopoietic cells. Leukoerythroblastic reactions may also be associated with hemorrhagic shock or hemolysis or as a rebound phenomenon following cytotoxic or infectious depression of the marrow, but a careful history, appropriate diagnostic tests, and a short period of observation should avoid confusion with CML.

Myelofibrosis, polycythemia vera, and other myeloproliferative variants may present with splenomegaly, leukocytosis, and immature granulocytes in the blood, but the neutrophil alkaline phosphatase activity is usually high in these disorders, and the Ph[1] chromosome is absent. The hematocrit is elevated in polycythemia vera (unless bleeding occurs), whereas it is normal or decreased in CML. Bone marrow biopsy and appropriate stains may reveal some increase in reticulin fibers or fibrosis in CML, but these findings are less prominent than in myelofibrosis. Patients who have the clinical manifestations of CML but without the Ph[1] chromosome may have mixed features of CML and other myeloproliferative disorders. Chronic monocytic or chronic myelomonocytic leukemia (CMMoL) and the chronic form of erythroleukemia are more properly regarded as variants of acute leukemia. Splenomegaly occurs frequently in CMMoL, but the leukocyte count is normal or only moderately elevated, the absolute monocyte count is usually increased, and the serum and urinary lysozyme levels are increased. The Ph[1] chromosome is not present, although other chromosomal abnormalities may occur.

Basophilic leukemia and eosinophilic leukemia may rarely occur as variants of CML or other myeloproliferative diseases and are usually associated with a poor prognosis. Basophilic leukemia should be distinguished from mast cell leukemia, in which urticaria pigmentosa is usually seen concomitantly. Thrombocythemia and megakaryocytic leukemia occur fairly commonly as variants of CML or other myeloproliferative disorders. Infrequently unexplained "essential" thrombocythemia and megakaryocytic hyperplasia are observed as isolated findings without Ph[1]-positive cells in the marrow or other abnormalities of the myeloid elements. Such patients may later develop other manifestations of one of the myeloproliferative diseases.

Chronic neutrophilic leukemia is a rare disease, occurring mostly in older patients, which is characterized by marked splenomegaly, leukocytosis with 90 per cent or more mature neutrophils in the blood, elevated neutrophil alkaline phosphatase, and a chronic course. The absence of immature granulocytes in the blood and of the Ph[1] chromosome in the marrow distinguishes this type of leukemia from CML.

The first clinical manifestations of blastic transformation may occur in extramedullary sites such as the spleen, lymph nodes, meninges, or other tissues, while the marrow and blood are still filled with chronic-phase leukemic cells. If immature granulocytes are the predominant cell type, the extramedullary tumors may have a green hue owing to myeloperoxidase and are sometimes diagnosed as chloromas or granulocytic sarcomas. If the transformed cells resemble lymphoblasts, an erroneous diagnosis of lymphoma is sometimes made. Demonstration of the Ph[1] chromosome in the blasts will lead to the correct diagnosis. Since localized blastic lesions invariably become disseminated, usually within several months, systemic treatment, sometimes in addition to local irradiation, is justified once the diagnosis is made.

The leukemic cells in CML sometimes undergo early blastic transformation without recognition of the chronic phase, and patients may present with what appears to be acute leukemia, either lymphoblastic or one of the myeloid variants. A very large spleen, extreme leukocytosis (>400,000 per cubic millimeter), prominent eosinophilia and/or basophilia, and a normal or elevated platelet count should alert the physician to this possible diagnostic dilemma. However, all of these features may be absent in patients with CML presenting in blastic crisis de novo, and cytogenetic examination of the marrow is necessary to confirm the presence or absence of the Ph[1] chromosome.

All patients with a clinical diagnosis of acute lymphoblastic leukemia (ALL) should have cytogenetic analyses performed prior to treatment because Ph[1]-positive ALL has a worse prognosis than the more common types of ALL. The incidence of Ph[1] + ALL is about 20 per cent and 2 per cent in adults and children, respectively, in patients with a suspected diagnosis of ALL. Ph[1] + ALL has recently been shown to include heterogeneous subtypes: some cases have similar bcr rearrangements as observed in classic CML, whereas in others the leukemic cells express unique abl-derived tyrosine kinases that are distinct from the bcr-abl–derived p210 protein of CML.

TREATMENT. Asymptomatic patients in the chronic phase in whom the WBC count is below 50,000 per cubic millimeter can be observed without treatment until the disease progresses and symptoms develop. When clinical manifestations appear they can usually be controlled with cytotoxic drugs or splenic irradiation, but unlike acute leukemia, true remissions are very rare and the marrow remains largely populated with leukemic cells containing the Ph[1] marker.

Chemotherapy. The most common conventional drug used is *busulfan*, but other alkylating agents such as cyclophosphamide and antimetabolites are also effective. One must be careful to avoid overtreatment of CML, as severe myelosuppression can occur. The usual starting oral dose of busulfan is 4 to 8 mg per day, but doses of 12 to 16 mg or higher may be required initially if the blood leukocyte and/or platelet counts are very high and rapid reduction is necessary. The dose should be reduced as the WBC count falls and the spleen shrinks during the first several weeks, roughly in proportion to halving of the WBC count. For example, if the initial WBC count is 100,000 per cubic millimeter and the initial dose of busulfan is 8 mg per day, when the WBC count reaches 50,000 per cubic millimeter the dose should be lowered to 4 mg per day. The drug should be stopped when the WBC count reaches about 25,000 per cubic millimeter, as it may continue to fall after stopping, and overtreatment can cause prolonged marrow hypoplasia. Other manifestations of chronic busulfan toxicity include sterility, dryness of skin and mucous membrane, hyperpigmentation, and rarely adrenal insufficiency and pulmonary fibrosis. In some patients the WBC count and spleen size may remain nearly normal without further treatment for months after initial control has been achieved, whereas others require continuous treatment. There is considerable variability in responsiveness, and the exact dose must be titrated individually. The dose of busulfan required to maintain control of the chronic phase is usually between 2 mg every other day and 4 mg per day. Some authorities prefer intermittent therapy rather than continuous treatment.

The amount of drug needed for control does not appear to be related to prognosis.

Purine and pyrimidine antagonists and hydroxyurea, a ribonucleotide reductase inhibitor, are also effective in controlling chronic-phase CML. The usual initial oral dose of *hydroxyurea* is between 1 and 3 grams per day, depending on the height of the WBC count and the body surface area. Hydroxyurea should be taken as a single dose at least an hour before eating. After the WBC count and spleen size are reduced to normal, the dose required for maintenance is usually between 0.5 gram every other day and 2.0 grams per day and must be titrated individually. Continuous treatment and close monitoring of the WBC count are necessary with hydroxyurea, as its inhibitory effects on myeloproliferation are much more transient than with busulfan and the WBC count may rise rapidly when it is discontinued. Hydroxyurea is generally well tolerated, but it may cause nausea, vomiting, diarrhea, stomatitis, dermatitis, and megaloblastosis.

Treatment of Acute Leukostatic or Thrombotic Complications. Some patients with CML may present with acute leukostatic or thrombotic complications (e.g., priapism, thrombophlebitis, infarctions of the spleen or other organs, sagittal sinus thrombosis, or other complications affecting the central nervous system), and in such cases it is mandatory to lower the WBC and/or platelet count rapidly with cytotoxic drugs. A continuous intravenous infusion of cytosine arabinoside, 200 mg per square meter of body surface area per 24 hours, or of hydroxyurea, 2 to 3 grams per square meter per day for four or five days, will usually lower the WBC and platelet counts rapidly, relieve the acute symptoms, and prevent additional complications. Leukapheresis and/or plateletpheresis is also effective in rapidly reducing the counts if a continuous flow centrifuge is available. The reduction is usually very transient, however, and chemotherapy should also be begun immediately for sustained control. Thrombocytosis sometimes persists after the WBC has been reduced by chemotherapy, and in such cases melphalan and/or thiotepa may be useful in controlling the platelets.

Tumor Lysis Syndrome. The patient should be well hydrated and allopurinol administered before beginning cytotoxic therapy when rapid cell lysis is anticipated in order to prevent exacerbation of hyperuricemia and development of uric acid nephropathy or acute arthritis. Hyperkalemia, hyperphosphatemia, increase of lactic dehydrogenase, and other biochemical abnormalities may also occur during sudden massive leukemic cell destruction (tumor lysis syndrome), but with adequate hydration to maintain a good urinary output and close monitoring, serious complications resulting from these biochemical alterations can usually be avoided.

Splenic Radiation. Splenic radiation is also effective in reducing the size of the spleen and WBC count. The radiation treatments should be given cautiously in fractionated doses over several weeks because the WBC count may continue to fall after stopping, and, as with busulfan, overtreatment can cause prolonged marrow hypoplasia. The total splenic dose needed for control is usually between 300 and 1200 rads, depending on the size of the spleen and radiation port, but the splenomegaly in some patients may be refractory to even larger doses. Splenectomy performed early in the chronic phase does not significantly affect survival, although in patients who are prone to develop massive splenomegaly it prevents later complications, which become difficult to manage (e.g., hypersplenism, inanition, repeated infarctions).

Aggressive Combination Chemotherapy. Some centers have taken a more aggressive therapeutic approach in chronic-phase CML with the use of combination chemotherapeutic regimens effective in acute myeloid leukemia. Complete remissions with marked reduction or disappearance of Ph[1]-positive leukemic cells in the marrow have been obtained in 20 to 50 per cent of patients, but most of the remissions have been of short duration. Patients having remissions live longer

than nonresponders, but overall survival does not appear to be significantly prolonged by the intensive treatment regimens employed to date.

Interferon Therapy. Both partially purified and recombinant human alfa-interferon have produced hematologic remissions in CML with partial or complete disappearance of Ph[1]-positive metaphases from the marrow, but it is too soon to evaluate the effects of this treatment on survival. Trials of recombinant gamma-interferon have recently been started to determine if this will be equally or more effective, but the eventual role of the interferons and other biologic agents in the treatment of CML is not yet clear.

Marrow Transplantation (see Ch. 165). It has been possible to eradicate the leukemic clone only by administering very high doses of alkylating agents in combination with a supralethal dose of total body irradiation, followed by rescue with transplantation of marrow from a histocompatible donor. More than a dozen patients with CML with identical twins have been so treated, of whom the majority remain free of disease without further treatment with no detectable Ph[1]-positive cells in the marrow for periods of up to ten years. The hazards associated with allogeneic marrow transplantation using histocompatible nonidentical sibling donors are still formidable, especially in older patients, but in the last six years several hundred patients with chronic-phase CML, mostly under the age of 50 years, have received allogeneic transplants at different centers throughout the world. The results are best if performed during the chronic phase, especially within the first year after diagnosis.

The probability of long disease-free survival is 50 to 70 per cent in different series if the transplant is done during the chronic phase; the remaining patients usually die within the first two years of complications related to the procedure, most often of interstitial pneumonia or graft-versus-host disease (GVHD). Depletion of T cells from the donor marrow with lectins or monoclonal antibodies has greatly reduced the incidence of GVHD, but it is not yet clear if overall survival will be improved; in some trials T cell depletion has been associated with an increased incidence of engraftment failure and leukemia relapse. The incidence of leukemic relapse reported so far in different series has varied from 0 to 20 per cent or higher, but because the disease may have a slow evolution, a longer period of observation will be necessary to determine the true incidence. Some patients have evidence of persistent Ph[1]-positive cells in the marrow by karyotype analysis or bcr rearrangement but have not progressed to hematologic relapse.

Treatment of the Accelerated or Blastic Phase. When CML enters an accelerated phase it becomes increasingly refractory to therapy that was previously effective. Increasing doses of busulfan or hydroxyurea are required to control the WBC and spleen size and, in some cases, progressive thrombocytosis. In some cases, severe anemia and/or thrombocytopenia develops, either because of the disease or as a result of drug toxicity.

Therapy of the blastic phase is generally unsatisfactory, and most patients die within a few months after blastic transformation occurs. Hydroxyurea is most commonly used to control myeloid blastic transformation, but multidrug regimens designed for acute nonlymphoblastic leukemia are also used. In the 25 per cent of patients with lymphoblastic transformation, remission can often be achieved with prednisone and vincristine with reversion to the chronic phase, but these are usually of short duration and the average survival in different series was three to eight months. Complete remissions with disappearance of the Ph[1]-positive cells in the marrow have rarely been achieved with intensive combinations of regimens designed for acute lymphoblastic leukemia, but these have all been only temporary and no cures have resulted. The average survival of patients with lymphoblastic transformation who are treated with modern intensive programs designed for ALL

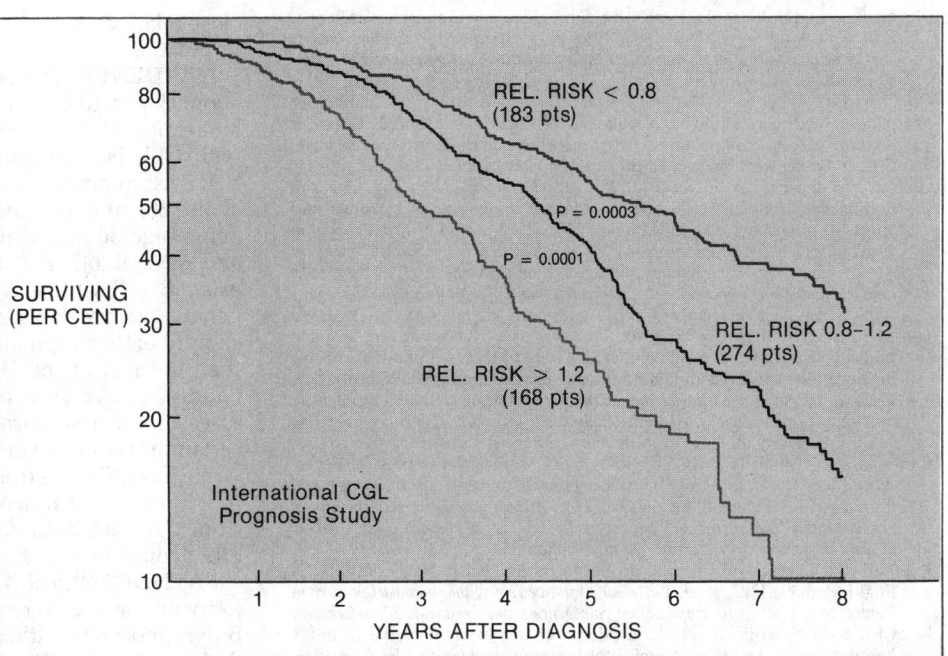

FIGURE 155–1. Actuarial survival of 625 patients with nonblastic Ph¹ chromosome–positive CML, 5 to 45 years old at the time of diagnosis, divided into low-, high-, and intermediate-risk groups, according to a Cox model with five variables, representing sex, spleen size, platelet count, hematocrit, and percentage of circulating blasts. The median survival of the 625 patients was 50.5 months. (From Sokal JE, et al.: Prognostic discrimination among younger patients with chronic granulocytic leukemia: Relevance to bone marrow transplantation. Blood 66:1352–1357, 1985.)

is about a year. The response is not significantly different in patients who initially present in blastic phase (Ph¹ + ALL) compared with those who develop lymphoblastic transformation after a recognized chronic phase. Any of the myriad complications seen in acute leukemia can be encountered during the blastic phase of CML. Meningeal leukemia should be treated with intrathecal methotrexate or arabinosylcytosine and/or cranial irradiation as in acute leukemia.

Since few patients respond satisfactorily to any treatment after myeloid blastic transformation is fully developed, there have been recent attempts to treat such patients aggressively with combination regimens designed for acute myeloid leukemia as soon as early evidence of impending blastic transformation can be detected, such as by appearance of additional chromosomal abnormalities or by a change in the growth pattern of the marrow colony forming cells in vitro. Although this approach may delay overt blastic transformation, it is not clear that survival is significantly affected. The results of aggressive treatment followed by allogeneic marrow transplantation in the accelerated or blastic phases are less favorable than in the chronic phase, with more early deaths due to complications, higher relapse rates, and only 10 to 25 per cent survivors after four years. Intensive treatment of the blastic phase followed by transplantation of stored autologous stem cells obtained from the marrow or blood during the chronic phase has been successful in temporarily restoring the disease to the chronic phase in some patients, but the mortality has been high, and it has not been demonstrated that overall survival is increased. No satisfactory methods have yet been found to selectively purge the marrow ex vivo of Ph¹-positive leukemic progenitors while sparing normal stem cells.

PROGNOSIS. The median survival of patients with Ph¹-positive CML from diagnosis is about three years, with a range of less than a year to over ten years. Although the clinical manifestations of the chronic phase can usually be readily controlled by appropriate treatment and most patients are able to lead normal lives, treatment has not substantially improved survival. Survival after development of an accelerated phase is usually less than a year and after blastic transformation only a few months, although patients with lymphoblastic transformation may live longer with appropriate treatment.

In a multi-institutional study of disease features at diagnosis in more than 800 patients with Ph¹-positive nonblastic CML, the most important characteristics associated with shortened survival were older age, male sex (in patients under 45), large spleen, high platelet count, high percentages of blasts in blood and marrow, high percentages of eosinophils and basophils, presence of nucleated red cells in the blood, a high serum lactic dehydrogenase (LDH) level, and a low hematocrit. Using a Cox model generated with variables representing disease features found on regression analysis to have prognostic significance, the patients could be segregated into three groups with significantly different survival patterns, both for the total population of CML patients studied and for younger patients (aged 5 to 45 years) who might be candidates for bone marrow transplantation. Based on a Cox model using five variables: sex, spleen size, platelet count, hematocrit, and percentage of circulating blasts, the patients could be segregated into a high-risk group who had an actuarial mortality of 30 per cent during the first two years after diagnosis and an annual risk of 30 per cent thereafter, while the most favorable group had a two-year actuarial mortality of 9 per cent, an average annual risk thereafter of 17 per cent, and a median survival of five and one-half years (Fig. 155–1). Additional factors that have been reported to be associated with an unfavorable prognosis in other series are black race, cytogenetic abnormalities in addition to the Ph¹ chromosome, liver enlargement, and myelofibrosis. The predictive models are still undergoing refinement with inclusion of additional features of prognostic values, and they should prove useful in advising patients when to consider alternative forms of treatment, such as bone marrow transplantation.

Ben-Neriah Y, Daley GQ, Mes-Masson A-M, et al.: The chronic myelogenous leukemia-specific P210 protein is the product of the bcr/abl hybrid gene. Science 233:212, 1986. *A report of molecular biology studies demonstrating that the p210 kilodalton phosphoprotein in CML cells is the protein product of the novel 8.5-kilobase bcr/abl fusion transcript.*

Champlin R, Gale RP, Foon KA, et al.: Chronic leukemias: Oncogenes, chromosomes and advances in therapy. Ann Intern Med 104:671, 1986. *An excellent review describing recent developments in understanding the role of oncogenes and chromosomal rearrangements in the chronic leukemias, and including discussion of treatment with biologic agents and bone marrow transplantation.*

Clark SS, McLaughlin J, Crist WM, et al.: Unique forms of the *abl* tyrosine kinase distinguish Ph¹-positive CML from Ph¹-positive ALL. Science 235:85, 1987. *Some Ph¹-positive ALL cells express unique abl-derived tyrosine kinases of 185 to 180 kilodaltons that are distinct from the bcr-abl–derived p210 protein of CML.*

De Klein A, Hagemeijer A, Bartram CR, et al.: *bcr* Rearrangement and translocation of the c-abl oncogene in Philadelphia positive acute lymphoblastic leukemia. Blood 68:1369, 1986. *The pH¹ chromosomes of patients with CML and Ph¹-positive ALL are indistinguishable cytogenetically. However, whereas some of the latter have the same bcr rearrangement as in CML, others do not; Ph¹-positive ALL thus includes several heterogeneous subtypes of leukemia.*

Erikson J, Griffin CA, Ar-Rushdi A, et al.: Heterogeneity of chromosome 22 breakpoint in Philadelphia-positive (Ph+) acute lymphocytic leukemia. Proc Natl Acad Sci USA 83:1807, 1986. *A recent report of molecular biology studies demonstrating heterogeneity in the breakpoints on chromosome 22 in Ph¹-positive ALL.*

Goldman JM, Apperley JF, Jones L, et al.: Bone marrow transplantation for patients with chronic myeloid leukemia. N Engl J Med 314:202, 1986. *The results of allogeneic bone marrow transplantation are described in 52 patients with CML in the chronic phase and 18 patients with more advanced disease.*

Goto T, Nishikori M, Arlin Z, et al.: Growth characteristics of leukemic and normal hematopoietic cells in Ph¹+ chronic myelogenous leukemia and effects of intensive treatment. Blood 59:793, 1982. *Report of a clinical trial in which patients in the chronic phase of CML were treated with a moderately intensive regimen consisting of splenectomy and combination chemotherapy. Although some complete remissions were achieved, these were usually of short duration. The results of other trials of splenectomy and intensive treatment are reviewed.*

Jain K, Arlin Z, Mertelsmann R, et al.: Philadelphia chromosome and terminal transferase positive acute leukemia: Similarity of terminal phase of chronic myelogenous leukemia and de novo acute presentation. J Clin Oncol 1:669, 1983. *A review of the clinical and laboratory features and results of intensive treatment of patients with CML with lymphoblastic transformation either presenting de novo as "Ph¹ + ALL" or as the terminal event after a chronic phase.*

Kantarjian H, Smith TL, McCredie KB, et al.: Chronic myelogenous leukemia: A multivariate analysis of the associations of patient characteristics and therapy with survival. Blood 66:1326, 1985. *An analysis of pretreatment clinical and laboratory features in 303 patients with Ph¹-positive chronic-phase CML to identify the factors of greatest prognostic significance.*

Koeffler HP, Golde DW: Chronic myelogenous leukemia: New concepts. N Engl J Med 304:1201, 1269, 1981. *Authoritative review that summarizes current knowledge of CML, with emphasis on pathogenesis and treatment. 204 references.*

Nitta M, Kato Y, Strife A, et al.: Incidence of involvement of the B and T lymphocytic lineages in chronic myelogenous leukemia. Blood 66:1053, 1985. *Peripheral blood lymphocytes were examined after stimulation in 32 patients with Ph¹-positive CML. Most B cells and T cells were found to be Ph¹-negative in the majority of patients, but about 20 per cent of patients had predominantly Ph¹-positive B cells or a mixture of Ph¹-positive and Ph¹-negative cells that grew as established cell lines after transformation with Epstein-Barr virus.*

Pugh WC, Pearson M, Vardiman JW, et al.: Philadelphia chromosome–negative chronic myelogenous leukemia: A morphological reassessment. Br J Haematol 60:457, 1985. *Twenty-five cases originally classified as Ph¹-negative CML were reexamined, and it was concluded that only one of the 25 was morphologically and clinically indistinguishable from Ph¹-positive CML. The remainder consisted of a heterogeneous group of patients with other myelodysplastic disorders, particularly chronic myelomonocytic leukemia.*

Sokal JE, Baccarani M, Tura S, et al.: Prognostic discrimination among younger patients with chronic granulocytic leukemia: Relevance to bone marrow transplantation. Blood 66:1352, 1985. *A similar regression analysis was conducted in nonblastic CML patients aged 5 to 45 to permit identification of patients at high, intermediate, and low risk for survival. This is the age group usually considered for bone marrow transplantation, and the study may help in deciding when to recommend that the procedure be performed.*

Sokal JE, Cox EB, Baccarani M, et al.: The Italian Cooperative CML Study Group: Prognostic discrimination in "good-risk" chronic granulocytic leukemia. Blood April, 1984. *A multivariate regression analysis of the prognostic significance of disease features at the time of diagnosis in 813 patients with Ph¹ + nonblastic CML collected from six American and European series. With use of the Cox model, four key variables were found that enabled identification of low-, intermediate-, and high-risk groups of patients.*

Talpaz M, Kantarjian HM, McCredie KB, et al.: Hematologic remission and cytogenetic improvement induced by recombinant human interferon alpha in chronic myelogenous leukemia. N Engl J Med 314:1065, 1986. *A preliminary report describing the effects of recombinant human alfa-interferon in 17 patients with Ph¹-positive CML. Fourteen patients responded of whom 13 had a hematologic remission and one a partial remission.*

Thomas ED, Clift RA, Fefer A, et al.: Marrow transplantation for the treatment of chronic myelogenous leukemia. Ann Intern Med 104:155, 1986. *This paper reports the results of the experience of the Seattle group in treating 198 patients with CML using bone marrow transplantation. The probability of long-term survival for allogeneic graft recipients was 49 per cent in the first chronic phase, 58 per cent in the second chronic phase, 15 per cent in the accelerated phase, and 14 per cent in the blastic phase.*

CHRONIC LYMPHOCYTIC LEUKEMIA

DEFINITION. Chronic lymphocytic leukemia (CLL) is a monoclonal neoplasm of slowly proliferating long-lived lymphocytes, usually B lymphocytes, which are immunologically defective.

ETIOLOGY. The etiology is unknown. Unlike the situation in acute and chronic myelogenous leukemia, exposure to ionizing radiation and cytotoxic drugs or chemicals does not result in an increased incidence of CLL. There does appear to be some genetic predisposition, since CLL is the most frequent type of leukemia occurring in multiple family members. There is no clear inheritance pattern, but siblings, especially brothers, appear to have the highest concordance of CLL. Except in rare high-incidence families, the incidence of CLL among close relatives is probably about three times that in the general population.

INCIDENCE. The incidence of CLL in the United States is about 3 per 100,000 population, or about 25 per cent of all leukemias. The incidence in most Western countries is similar, with CLL being slightly more common than CML. CLL is twice as common in males as in females. The mean age is about 60, and the incidence increases with age. It is rare before age 30 and almost never occurs in children. In Japan and several other Asian countries where reliable statistics exist, B cell CLL is very uncommon. This may be due to genetic factors; Japanese living in the United States have a slightly higher incidence than native Japanese, but still lower than the rest of the United States population. On the other hand, T cell variants of CLL and related lymphoproliferative diseases are not uncommon and appear to be endemic in certain areas of Japan. A human T cell leukemia-lymphoma virus (HTLV1) is strongly suspected of having an etiologic role in these T cell neoplasms in Japan, as well as in patients from the Caribbean and less often in the United States and other countries.

PATHOGENESIS AND MECHANISMS. In the great majority of cases, CLL results from a monoclonal proliferation of B lymphocytes, although a slight percentage of cases is derived from T cells. The leukemic B cells have monoclonal surface immunoglobulin (although in lower density than normal B lymphocytes), exhibit Ia-like cell surface antigens, carry receptors for the Fc fragment of IgG (as recognized by the binding of heat-aggregated IgG and several rosetting techniques) and for the C3d and occasionally the C3b complement components, and form spontaneous rosettes with mouse red blood cells. Intracellular crystalline inclusions containing IgM and λ light chains have been observed in the leukemic cells of some patients. A murine monoclonal antibody recognizes a 65,000- to 67,000-dalton antigen (Leu-1) present on B-CLL cells, but not on cells from other types of B cell leukemias or lymphomas. This surface antigen is also expressed by human thymocytes and peripheral T cells, but is absent on normal B cells. Other T cell antigens and the terminal deoxynucleotidyltransferase enzyme are absent on B-CLL cells.

The leukemic lymphocytes in CLL proliferate very slowly, as is also true of normal B lymphocytes and several other low-growth fraction B cell neoplasms such as multiple myeloma and most nodular lymphomas. The great majority of CLL lymphocytes are small cells that are in a quiescent state (G_0). In most cases, only a small fraction of the population consists of intermediate-sized or large lymphocytes, of which some are in various stages of the cell cycle preparing to divide; proliferation may be increased in lymph nodes compared to marrow or blood. Although only a small fraction of the total leukemic population is proliferating at any time, because the leukemic cells have a very long lifespan, they accumulate and continue to recirculate through the body.

The leukemic lymphocytes in CLL appear to be "frozen" in an intermediate stage of the B cell differentiation pathway, but can be induced in vitro with phorbol esters or B cell mitogens to differentiate into more mature B cells, including prolymphocytes, hairy cells, and plasma cells. CLL cells are immunologically defective, and they respond sluggishly to mitogens or immunologic stimuli. CLL cells produce an excess of free light chains, either kappa or lambda, but never both. Only a small percentage of patients secrete sufficient IgM to be detectable as a spike on electrophoresis.

In the early stages of CLL, T lymphocytes are present in the blood in normal or increased absolute numbers, although in reduced proportions. Purified T cells from CLL patients respond normally to mitogens, but form fewer T cell colonies in vitro compared to T cells from normal subjects and are defective in natural killer and antibody-dependent cell-mediated cytotoxicity. Normal T cells can be divided into sub-

TABLE 155–1. RAI'S STAGING SYSTEM FOR CLL*

Stage 0	Absolute lymphocytosis in blood of >15,000 per cubic millimeter
Stage I	Absolute lymphocytosis plus enlarged lymph nodes
Stage II	Absolute lymphocytosis plus enlarged liver and/or spleen (with or without lymph node enlargement)
Stage III†	Absolute lymphocytosis plus anemia (hemoglobin <11 grams per deciliter in males and <10 grams per deciliter in females)
Stage IV†	Absolute lymphocytosis plus thrombocytopenia (platelets <100,000 per cubic millimeter)

*From Rai KR, et al.: Clinical staging of chronic lymphocytic leukemia. Blood 46:219, 1975.

†In stages III and IV, patients may or may not have enlarged lymph nodes, liver, and/or spleen.

populations according to their type of Fc receptor for immunoglobulin: Tμ (IgM), Tα (IgA), and Tγ (IgG), or their reactivities with monoclonal antibodies. In CLL, the proportion of T cells with receptors for IgG (Tγ) is markedly increased, resulting in a decreased T helper cell (Tμ or T4/Leu-3) to T suppressor cell (Tγ or T8/Leu-2) ratio. The decreased T helper function and other immunologic abnormalities that have been described appear to be more pronounced in later stages of CLL.

CLINICAL MANIFESTATIONS. *Staging.* About 25 per cent of patients with CLL are asymptomatic when first seen, and the diagnosis is made following detection of lymphocytosis on an incidental blood count or in the course of investigating the cause of enlarged lymph nodes or splenomegaly. Some cases may have a very benign course, and the patient may remain asymptomatic for many years, whereas in others the disease can progress rapidly. The average survival in CLL is about four to five years. A simple clinical staging system for CLL (see Table 155–1) has proved of prognostic value in several large series. Median survival decreases with advancing stage: stage 0 = 14 (range 12 to 15) years; stage I = 8 (5 to 11) years; stage II = 6 (4 to 9) years; and stages III and IV = 2 (1 to 3½) years. A diagnosis of CLL may be made in some patients with a lesser degree of absolute lymphocytosis than 15,000 per cubic millimeter (i.e., earlier than stage 0) if cell marker studies demonstrate a monoclonal B cell population characteristic of CLL in the blood and marrow. The rate at which the disease progresses from early to late stages is quite variable in individual patients; stage II appears to be especially heterogeneous, and cases tend to diverge into low- or high-risk groups. Other investigators have reported that patients in the intermediate-risk group who had lymphocyte counts over 40,000 per cubic millimeter or diffuse instead of a nodular pattern of marrow involvement had shorter survival. A revised prognostic staging system was proposed by an international workshop on CLL that is based on the number of lymphoid areas involved and the degree of bone marrow failure (Table 155–2). Clinical enlargement of the spleen, of liver, and of lymph nodes in the cervical, axillary, and inguinal regions constitute five separate areas of involvement, each of which is considered one area irrespective of whether the lymphadenopathy is unilateral or bilateral. The advantages of

TABLE 155–2. INTERNATIONAL STAGING SYSTEM FOR CLL*

Clinical Stage†		
A A(0), A(I), or A(II)	No anemia or thrombocytopenia	Less than three areas of lymphoid enlargement
B B(I) or B(II)	No anemia or thrombocytopenia	Three or more involved areas
C C(III) or C(IV)	Anemia and/or thrombocytopenia	Regardless of the number of areas of lymphoid enlargement

*From Binet JL, et al.: A new prognostic classification of chronic lymphocytic leukemia derived from a multivariate survival analysis. Br J Haematol 48:356, 1981.

†It was recommended that the revised classification be integrated with the Rai system by using Roman numerals in parenthesis to represent the latter.

the revised system are that it has fewer stages (which should simplify design and evaluation of comparative therapeutic trials), it recognizes that anemia and thrombocytopenia have a similar prognosis and do not require separate stages, and it recognizes a predominantly splenic form of the disease that may have a relatively favorable prognosis. Survival curves have so far shown distinct differences among the three groups: the median survivals for groups A, B, and C were >10, 7, and 2 years, respectively.

Symptoms. Patients with early-stage disease are often asymptomatic, but increasing symptoms develop with advancing stage and include malaise, easy fatigability, anorexia, weight loss, low-grade fever, and night sweats. Bacterial infections, such as sinusitis, pneumonia, or cutaneous infections, are common and should be treated promptly with appropriate antibiotics. Patients in advanced stages become progressively more immunodeficient, anemic, and neutropenic and are unable to mobilize a normal response to infections. Viral infections such as herpes zoster are also common. Vaccinations for smallpox and other viral illnesses should be avoided because of the danger of generalized vaccinia or other severe reactions. Hyperreactivity to insect bites is common.

Physical Findings. Physical examination in stage 0 CLL (Rai classification) reveals no abnormalities, but in later stages the lymph nodes, spleen, and liver may become progressively enlarged, and there may also be extensive leukemic infiltration of other tissues, including the skin, orbit, conjunctivae, pharynx, lungs, pleura, heart, and gastrointestinal tract. Obstructive jaundice may occur from periportal infiltration or from nodes compressing the bile duct, and venous compression by enlarged nodes may cause edema and/or thrombophlebitis. Pronounced inanition is common late in the disease, and ascites and/or anasarca may develop in association with severe hypoalbuminemia. Leukostasis may cause priapism or infarctions of various organs. Bleeding manifestations such as bruising and epistaxis are common in advanced stages with severe thrombocytopenia. Leukemic involvement of the meninges is rare, but leukoencephalopathy may occur, probably owing to a viral infection.

LABORATORY ABNORMALITIES. The WBC count may range from a slight elevation to over a million per cubic millimeter. The *percentage of lymphocytes is always increased* and may be over 98 per cent (Color plate 3F and G). *Anemia, thrombocytopenia,* and *neutropenia* develop in advanced stages owing to impairment of normal hematopoiesis. The anemia is usually normochromic and normocytic, and the reticulocyte count is normal or reduced. Patients also frequently develop shortened red cell and/or platelet survival resulting from hypersplenism in advanced disease. Autoimmune hemolytic anemia, usually caused by warm reacting IgG antibodies, is common and may be accompanied by reticulocytosis, erythroid hyperplasia in the marrow, a positive direct Coombs antiglobulin test, and hyperbilirubinemia. Autoimmune thrombocytopenia or cold hemagglutinin disease may also occur, and occasionally such autoimmune phenomena may precede other clinical manifestations of CLL or develop shortly after beginning treatment.

Hypogammaglobulinemia is present at diagnosis in about half of patients and eventually develops in almost all of them as the disease advances. Any or all classes of immunoglobulins may be reduced. A small percentage of patients have monoclonal immunoglobulins or light chains demonstrable on electrophoresis or immunoelectrophoresis of the blood or urine. Rarely the abnormal proteins may cause hyperviscosity or cryoprecipitation. Angioneurotic edema may also occur rarely owing to formation of immune complexes.

Unlike CML, until recently no characteristic cytogenetic abnormality was described in CLL, and most studies showed normal karyotypes. Because CLL cells proliferate very slowly, in these earlier studies most of the metaphases analyzed were in normal dividing cells present in the specimen. Using B cell mitogens (e.g., pokeweed mitogen, protein A, or Epstein-Barr virus), chromosome abnormalities have been found in about half of patients with CLL. Trisomy 12 is the most common abnormality, being present in about one third of patients; in advanced disease additional chromosomal abnormalities may develop, probably because of clonal evolution. Abnormalities of chromosome 14 are also common, and several cases of CLL have been reported with translocations between chromosomes 11 and 14 t(11;14) (q13; q32). The heavy-chain immunoglobulin gene is located on chromosome 14, and the oncogenes c-ras-Kirsten and c-ras-Harvey, on chromosomes 11 and 12, respectively, but it is not known how these or other genes might be related to the causation of CLL.

Transformation of CLL cells to a more malignant phenotype is much less common than in CML. The most frequently described transformation is to a large-cell diffuse lymphoma (Richter's syndrome), but other types of transformations may also occur to "prolymphocytoid" leukemia, acute lymphoblastic leukemia (blast crisis), and multiple myeloma. The earlier reports are not informative as to whether the transformed cells arose by malignant evolution of the original CLL clone or were separate neoplasms, but both may occur, with malignant evolution probably being more common.

DIAGNOSIS. The diagnosis of CLL depends on the demonstration of a persistent absolute lymphocytosis in the blood and an increased percentage (usually >50 per cent) of small lymphocytes with round nuclei in the marrow. Pertussis and infectious lymphocytosis and other viral infections can sometimes cause striking lymphocytosis, but these illnesses usually occur in children or young adults, are usually accompanied by fever and other acute symptoms, and are of transient duration. Chronic infections such as tuberculosis may be accompanied by lymphocytosis, but this is usually less prominent than in CLL and appropriate workup should lead to the correct diagnosis. If there is any question about the diagnosis, appropriate cell marker studies should be performed to establish the monoclonality of the lymphocytic population and to distinguish CLL from other lymphoproliferative diseases. A schematic representation of normal B cell differentiation and related B cell neoplasms is shown in Figure 155–2.

If the lymph nodes are involved in CLL, the histologic pattern and immunologic markers characteristic of the cells are identical to those of diffuse well-differentiated lymphocytic lymphoma (DWDL), and these two diagnostic entities appear to be merely different variants of the same type of B cell neoplasia. DWDL may initially be localized in lymph nodes without involvement of the blood or marrow, but in more advanced stages it may be indistinguishable from CLL. Other types of disseminated lymphomas such as diffuse poorly differentiated lymphocytic lymphoma (DPDL), which may involve the blood and marrow, can be distinguished from CLL by differences in morphologic appearance of the tumor cells and appropriate cell marker analysis.

Waldenström's macroglobulinemia may be confused with

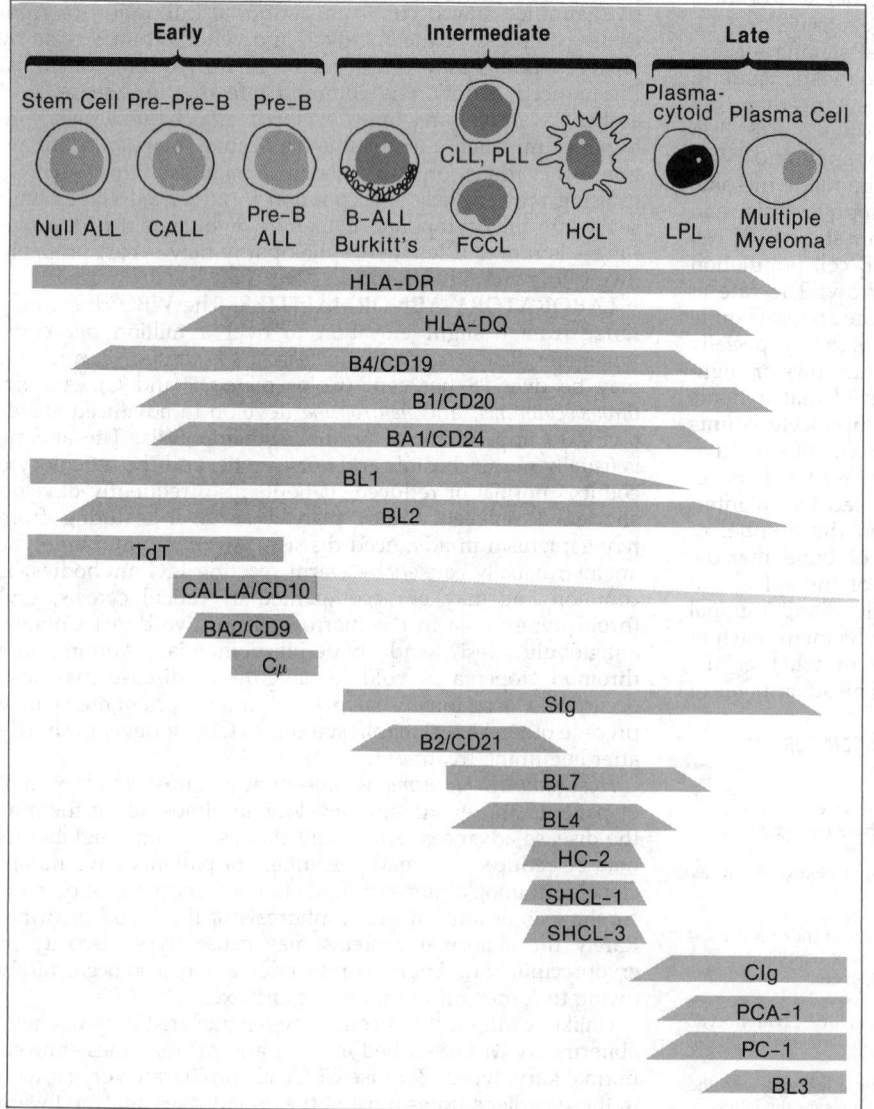

FIGURE 155–2. Schema of B cell differentiation and related B cell lymphoid neoplasms and the ranges of their reactivities with commonly used monoclonal antibodies recognizing B-cell associated antigens. (Prepared by Dr. Benjamin Koziner, Memorial Sloan-Kettering Cancer Center, New York, NY.)

Null ALL = Null acute lymphoblastic leukemia; CALL = common ALL; Pre-B ALL = common ALL with intracytoplasmic immunoglobulin μ heavy chain (Cμ); B-ALL = B cell ALL or Burkitt's lymphoma; CLL = chronic lymphocytic leukemia; PLL = prolymphocytic leukemia; FCCL = follicular center cell lymphoma; HCL = hairy cell leukemia; LPL = lymphoplasmacytoid lymphoma (Waldenström's macroglobulinemia); HLA-DR (Ia) = Dr-related locus of human leukocyte antigens; HLA-DQ = DQ-related locus of human leukocyte antigens; TdT = terminal deoxynucleotidyl transferase; Cμ = intracytoplasmic heavy chain (μ); SIg = surface immunoglobulin; CIg = intracytoplasmic immunoglobulin.

Commonly used monoclonal antibodies recognizing B-cell associated antigens include: anti-B1, B2, B4, CALLA (J-5), PCA-1, and PC-1, available from Coulter Immunology, Hialeah, FL; anti-BA1 and BA2 from Hibertech Inc., San Diego, CA; anti-BL1, BL2, BL3, BL4, and BL7 (Wang CY, et al.: J Immunol 133:684, 1984, and Knowles DM, et al.: Blood 62:191, 1983); anti-HC-2 (Posnett DN, et al.: J Immunol 133:1635, 1984); anti-SHCL-1 (Leu-14) and SHCL-3 (Leu-M5), available from Bectin-Dickinson, Mountain View, CA.

CD refers to antibody/antigen cluster designation defined by the Second International Workshop on Human Leukocyte Differentiation Antigens (Nadler LM: B cell/leukemia panel workshop: Summary and comments. In Reinherz EL, et al. (eds): Leukocyte Typing II. Vol. 2, New York, Springer-Verlag, 1986, p 1).

CLL, but the neoplastic lymphocytes in the former usually have a plasmacytoid appearance, more prominent surface, as well as cytoplasmic immunoglobulin, and they usually do not invade the blood to the same extent as CLL lymphocytes. There is invariably a prominent monoclonal IgM spike in the serum, whereas this is rare in CLL. A few cases may exhibit mixed features of the two entities.

Prolymphocytic leukemia is a rare disease occurring mostly in males in the sixth or seventh decade characterized by prominent splenomegaly, minimal adenopathy, and a poor prognosis. The prolymphocytes differ from CLL lymphocytes in that they are larger and have more cytoplasm, a more prominent nucleolus, and a greater density of surface immunoglobulin, which, again in contrast to CLL cells, exhibits polar migration (capping) after incubation at 37°C.

Hairy cell leukemia is sometimes misdiagnosed as CLL. In the former, the leukocyte count is usually low rather than elevated, and although hairy cells may resemble CLL lymphocytes on Romanowsky-stained smears, close scrutiny will reveal hair-like projections. If there is any doubt, special morphologic and cell marker studies should be performed, as described earlier.

Sézary's syndrome, a cutaneous lymphoma of helper T cell origin closely related to mycosis fungoides, is characterized by a chronic exfoliative erythrodermatitis and circulating atypical lymphocytes with cerebriform nuclei and acid phosphatase activity limited to the cytoplasmic granules instead of the Golgi zone. The prominent skin manifestations and the lesser degree of involvement of the marrow and lymph nodes usually suffice to differentiate Sézary's syndrome from T cell CLL.

Other T cell neoplasms that may be confused with CLL are adult T cell leukemia-lymphoma, T prolymphocytic leukemia, chronic T gamma-lymphoproliferative disease, and T hairy cell leukemia. In contrast to B cell CLL, skin involvement, lytic bone lesions, and hypercalcemia are common in adult T cell leukemia-lymphoma; some patients have been found to be infected with a retrovirus, termed human T cell leukemia-lymphoma virus 1 (HTLV1), which is suspected of causing the disease. The neoplastic cells in T gamma-lymphoproliferative disease are large granular lymphocytes, the WBC count is low with neutropenia, and lymphadenopathy and skin involvement are absent. Appropriate cell marker studies should always be performed to establish the correct diagnosis in CLL and related diseases as it is not always possible to distinguish between the different types on clinical or morphologic grounds.

TREATMENT. Since B cell CLL is a disease mainly affecting older persons, many of whom have a remarkably benign and prolonged course, and since there is no good evidence that early treatment will cure the disease or improve survival, most authorities recommend merely observing asymptomatic patients with early-stage disease until the disease progresses and symptoms develop. Indications for treatment include development of symptomatic or cosmetically disfiguring lymphadenopathy, progressive splenomegaly and/or hepatomegaly, recurrent infections, persistent unexplained fever, weight loss, and development of significant anemia, thrombocytopenia, and/or neutropenia resulting from progressive marrow infiltration, hypersplenism, or autoimmune complications. The rate at which the disease progresses from an early asymptomatic stage to an advanced stage requiring treatment is quite variable, and patients should be observed closely every few months until it can be determined whether their disease is going to remain indolent or become symptomatic. Some patients remain asymptomatic for many years without treatment.

Treatment should be begun when troublesome symptoms develop. *Chlorambucil* (Leukeran) is the most commonly employed drug, but other alkylating agents such as cyclophosphamide are also effective. Because of the slow proliferative rate of the neoplastic cells, antimetabolites are generally less effective, although arabinosyl cytosine has been reported to control the disease in some patients. The usual starting dose of chlorambucil is 6 to 12 mg (0.1 to 0.2 mg per kilogram of body weight) daily for three to six weeks, followed by a maintenance dose of 2 to 6 mg daily, the exact dose depending on the extent of disease, the severity of symptoms, and the patient's weight. The dose should be titrated individually according to the therapeutic response. The drug should be taken at least one hour prior to eating so as not to interfere with its absorption. About 70 per cent of previously untreated patients will show a satisfactory response to chlorambucil with reduction in the WBC count and shrinkage of the enlarged lymph nodes and organomegaly when present. Maintenance treatment is usually continued for six months to a year until a maximal response has been achieved. In some patients the disease may then remain asymptomatic for many months without further treatment, whereas others require continuous treatment for control.

Intermittent administration of chlorambucil has been recommended by some investigators and is probably slightly more effective and convenient than daily therapy. Various dosage schedules have been employed, usually 0.4 to 0.8 mg per kilogram as a single dose every two weeks or 0.4 to 2.0 mg per kilogram once a month. These high intermittent doses sometimes cause gastrointestinal toxicity, which may be partly alleviated by antiemetics. Myelosuppression is the usual dose-limiting toxicity, but immunosuppression, sterility, alveolar dysplasia, pulmonary fibrosis, chromosomal damage, and secondary acute myeloid leukemia may occur following chronic chlorambucil administration.

Corticosteroids are effective in controlling acute symptoms, especially autoimmune complications such as hemolytic anemia or thrombocytopenia. Corticosteroids may also have a pronounced cytolytic effect on the leukemic cells; the WBC count may fall rapidly, or it may rise temporarily concomitantly with regression of the enlarged lymph nodes and spleen. Prednisone is the corticosteroid most commonly prescribed, usually in doses of 10 to 20 mg daily, but larger doses of 50 to 100 mg may be necessary to control hemolytic anemia. Large doses of corticosteroids given over a prolonged period are inadvisable because they may cause severe cushingoid symptoms and increase the risk of infections. Most authorities now recommend that short courses of prednisone in relatively high doses (e.g., 80 mg daily for five days) be given as adjuvant therapy with intermittent chlorambucil, since intermittent steroid therapy produces the desired lymphocytolytic effect and improves the therapeutic response compared to chlorambucil alone while reducing the toxicity associated with continuous steroid administration. Long-term control of autoimmune complications associated with CLL such as hemolytic anemia, thrombocytopenia, or angioneurotic edema is dependent on adequate control of the leukemia. When the leukemic mass has been reduced sufficiently, the autoimmune manifestations usually subside. However, splenectomy is sometimes indicated to control hemolytic anemia, thrombocytopenia, or progressive splenomegaly refractory to drug treatment.

Local radiotherapy is often useful in the treatment of splenomegaly or greatly enlarged lymph nodes resistant to chemotherapy. Whole-body external radiation given cautiously in fractionated doses over several months has been reported to increase the incidence of remissions and prolong survival, and thymic radiation has also been reported to have a good therapeutic effect. However, both thymic and whole-body irradiation have also caused prolonged myelosuppression and fatalities in CLL and must be regarded as experimental forms of treatment that cannot be generally recommended.

Extracorporeal irradiation of the blood has also been shown to be effective in reducing the WBC count and organomegaly, but facilities for this procedure are not available in most centers and leukapheresis is more commonly employed. Leukapheresis is particularly useful in reducing very high lymphocyte counts and organomegaly in advanced disease in the presence of severe thrombocytopenia that limits additional cytotoxic drug therapy. Repeated leukapheresis may reduce the extent of leukemic infiltration of the marrow sufficiently to allow the platelet count to rise and permit resumption of chemotherapy.

In several clinical trials, patients with CLL have been treated more aggressively with various combinations of alkylating agents and other cytotoxic drugs in an attempt to increase the incidence of complete remissions and improve survival. With conventional doses of chlorambucil either alone or with prednisone, complete remissions are rare (0 to 20 per cent in different series), whereas with more intensive treatment higher remission rates have been reported (18 to 45 per cent). The relative effectiveness of the different regimens is difficult to compare, however, because of different patient populations and differing criteria for completeness of remission and durations of observations. Eradication of the leukemic clone has not been possible with any regimen. Patients having remissions live longer than nonresponders, but there is as yet no convincing evidence that overall survival is significantly improved. It is not yet known whether the more intensive regimens will result in a higher incidence of myeloid leukemia or other secondary malignant diseases in CLL.

Hypogammaglobulinemia when present usually persists even after the leukemic mass has been reduced by treatment. Administration of gamma globulin intramuscularly is of little value; clinical trials of various preparations of gamma globulin for intravenous use are currently under way to determine if it is possible to significantly correct the deficiency and reduce the incidence of infections and autoimmune cytopenias. In the rare patient who develops hyperviscosity or circulating autoantibodies, plasmapheresis with replacement by normal plasma is effective in temporarily lowering the abnormal proteins and relieving symptoms. When infections occur, every effort should be made to identify the offending organism and to begin specific antimicrobial treatment promptly.

Various monoclonal antibodies (MoAbs) to the neoplastic cells in B cell or T cell CLL have been investigated to determine their therapeutic efficacy. While some responses have been observed, they have usually been only partial and transient. Additional trials are in progress or planned with new, more specific MoAbs or those coupled with drugs, isotopes, or toxins, cocktails of several MoAbs, and MoAbs in combination with cytotoxic drugs. In contrast to hairy cell leukemia, the clinical trials of alfa-interferon in B cell CLL have shown it to be relatively ineffective, although about half of the patients with cutaneous T cell lymphomas have shown a partial or complete response to this interferon. Investigations of new methods of biologic therapy for CLL are continuing, and it is hoped that these investigations will lead to more selective and effective treatment.

PROGNOSIS. Median survival times of four to five years from diagnosis of CLL have been reported in most series. Since CLL has an extremely variable course, ranging from less than a year to more than 20 years, differences among series are probably due to inclusion of differing proportions of patients with early or advanced disease rather than to differences in treatment. The utility of the proposed clinical staging systems in predicting prognosis was mentioned earlier. There have also been attempts to correlate prognosis with various morphologic, immunologic, or proliferative characteristics of the leukemic cells, but these studies require extension and confirmation before their prognostic value can be accepted. Attempts to eradicate the disease with aggressive treatment have so far been unsuccessful, and there is as yet no convincing evidence that intensive treatment is preferable to more conservative treatment in prolonging overall survival.

Common causes of death in CLL are intercurrent infections,

uncontrollable progressive leukemic infiltration of vital organs, extreme inanition, and bleeding. Since CLL occurs mainly in older persons, some patients also die as a result of unrelated diseases. Patients with CLL have a high incidence of second malignant tumors (3 to 34 per cent in different series), both cutaneous and nondermatologic. Many of the tumors were diagnosed prior to treatment of CLL and cannot be causally related to treatment. The incidence of acute myeloid leukemia is higher than expected in CLL following treatment and is probably related to administration of alkylating agents and/or radiation therapy, as has been reported in Hodgkin's disease and other neoplastic diseases.

Binet JL, Auguier A, Dighiero G: A new prognostic classification of chronic lymphocytic leukemia derived from a multivariate survival analysis. Cancer 48:198, 1981. *A report describing the proposed international prognostic staging system for CLL.*

Byhardt RW, Brace KC, Wiernik PH: The role of splenic irradiation in chronic lymphocytic leukemia. Cancer 35:1621, 1975. *A good review of the indications for splenic irradiation in control of CLL.*

Dillman RO, Shawler DL, Dillman JB, et al.: Therapy of chronic lymphocytic leukemia and cutaneous T-cell lymphoma with T101 monoclonal antibody. J Clin Oncol 8:881, 1984. *Report and brief review of investigational trials of monoclonal antibodies in CLL and cutaneous T cell lymphoma.*

Foon KA, Bottino GC, Abrams PG, et al.: Phase II trial of recombinant leukocyte A interferon in patients with advanced chronic lymphocytic leukemia. Am J Med 78:216, 1985. *Report of a phase II trial of recombinant alfa-interferon in CLL that demonstrated significant dose-dependent toxicity and only a few partial therapeutic responses. It was concluded that alfa-interferon is ineffective, at least in previously treated patients with advanced CLL.*

Foon KA, Todd RF: Immunologic classification of leukemia and lymphoma. Blood 68:1, 1986. *A comprehensive review of advances in the classification of leukemias and lymphomas, using batteries of monoclonal antibodies to define surface antigens, molecular probes to identify immunoglobulin and T cell receptor genes, cytochemical stains, and various other biochemical markers.*

Gale RP, Foon KA: Chronic lymphocytic leukemia. Recent advances in biology and treatment (review). Ann Intern Med 103:101, 1985. *Comprehensive, up-to-date review of developments in investigations of the biology and immunologic defects in CLL and also a good review of the differential diagnosis and conventional and investigational forms of treatment.*

Han T, Ozer H, Sadamore N, et al.: Prognostic importance of cytogenetic abnormalities in patients with chronic lymphocytic leukemia. N Engl J Med 310:288, 1984. *A good review of the cytogenetic abnormalities found in CLL with discussion of their clinical and immunologic significance.*

Juliusson G, Robert H-H, Ost A, et al.: Prognostic information from cytogenetic analysis in chronic B-lymphocytic leukemia and leukemic immunocytoma. Blood 65:134, 1985. *Another review of the cytogenetic abnormalities occurring in CLL with discussion of their prognostic importance.*

HAIRY CELL LEUKEMIA (Leukemic Reticuloendotheliosis)

DEFINITION. Hairy cell leukemia (HCL) is a chronic form of leukemia usually due to clonal proliferation of an unusual type of B lymphocyte. HCL accounts for approximately 2 per cent of all the leukemias. The etiology is unknown.

PATHOGENESIS AND MECHANISMS. Hairy cells are of B cell origin, as they have immunoglobulin gene rearrangements and are capable of monoclonal synthesis of immunoglobulin. Although their level of maturity within the B cell lineage varies, in most patients the neoplastic hairy cells appear to be preplasma cells. A few cases of T cell hairy cell leukemia have been reported.

The hairy cell appears on Wright-Giemsa–stained smears as an intermediate-sized or large lymphocyte (10 to 18 μ in diameter), with fine cytoplasmic projections that give the cell its name. The nucleus may be round, oval, horseshoe shaped, or slightly folded, and it is often eccentrically located. The chromatin can be evenly distributed, moderately coarse, or stippled, and one or more small nucleoli may be present. The cells usually have moderate amounts of pale blue-gray cytoplasm with irregular serrated edges and sometimes pseudopodial extensions (Color plate 3H). The cytoplasmic surface projections are best recognized under the phase-contrast microscope or the scanning electron microscope (Fig. 155–3). The latter reveals a characteristic surface pattern with prominent folds or ruffles that are similar to those present on monocytes but more conspicuous.

Cytochemical reactions are helpful in identifying hairy cells,

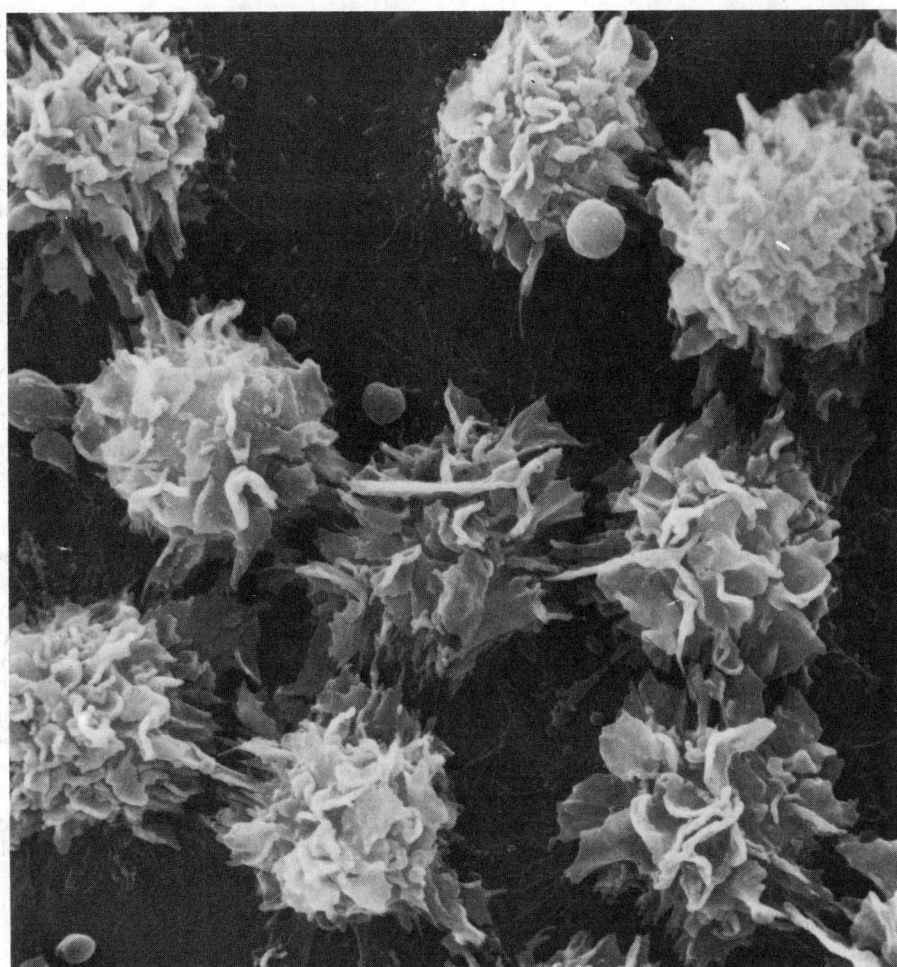

FIGURE 155–3. Hairy cells from the bone marrow as seen in the scanning electron microscope showing characteristic prominent surface ruffles. Magnification × 8750. (Courtesy of Dr. Etienne deHarven and Nina Lampen.)

but show variability in different cases and within the cells of any one population. Hairy cells are almost always positive for *acid phosphatase*, which is commonly, but not invariably, completely or partially resistant to addition of tartaric acid. However, a negative reaction does not exclude the diagnosis of HCL, and a positive reaction is not necessarily diagnostic. Hairy cells in the great majority of patients show varying degrees of positivity for alpha naphthyl acetate or butyrate esterase, and this reaction is usually completely inhibited by sodium fluoride. Cytochemical reactions associated with the granulocytic differentiation pathway (e.g., myeloperoxidase) are invariably negative in hairy cells. Lysozyme activity is absent in hairy cells, which helps to distinguish them from normal or leukemic monocytes.

Surface immunoglobulin (Ig) is present on hairy cells in the great majority of cases. The Ig is usually monoclonal, although in a few cases two different immunoglobulins have been reported. Hairy cells generally lack receptors for the third component of complement (C3), thus providing a helpful diagnostic distinction from monocytes and CLL cells, which carry the C3 receptor. Hairy cells may also frequently exhibit properties characteristic of monocytes (phagocytosis) and T lymphocytes (Tac antigen or interleukin-2 receptor). Several monoclonal antibodies with specificity for hairy cells are now available for confirmation of the diagnosis in difficult cases (see Fig. 155–2).

Hairy cells usually have very low proliferative activity; the percentage of hairy cells in the marrow or blood in DNA synthesis is almost invariably less than 1 per cent. Hairy cells also usually respond poorly in vitro to stimulation with mitogens. Chromosome abnormalities have been difficult to demonstrate because of the low incidence of mitoses, but trisomy of chromosome 12 (similar to CLL) has been reported

in a few cases of HCL, as have abnormalities of the Y chromosome and of chromosomes 3, 6, and especially 14.

CLINICAL MANIFESTATIONS AND DIAGNOSIS. HCL occurs almost exclusively in adults and the median age at diagnosis is about 50 years. Males are affected about four times more frequently than females. Clinical manifestations are usually attributable to hairy cell infiltration of the bone marrow, which can cause suppression of normal hematopoiesis, and of the red pulp of the spleen, which can result in hypersplenism. The onset is usually insidious, and the most common symptoms are weakness caused by *anemia*, development of infections as a result of *neutropenia*, and pain or discomfort in the left hypochondrium owing to *progressive splenic enlargement*.

The liver is enlarged owing to hairy cell infiltration in about 40 per cent of cases, but prominent involvement of the lymph nodes is infrequent. Systemic vasculitis and lytic bone lesions associated with pain and sometimes pathologic fractures may occur. Infiltration of the skin or lungs occurs only rarely, and meningeal involvement is almost never seen.

The majority of patients have *pancytopenia*, but sometimes only one or two of the myeloid cell lines are depressed, most commonly the platelets and neutrophils. Monocytopenia is also frequent and may contribute to the increased susceptibility to infections. In most cases, hairy cells can be identified in smears of the blood or buffy coat, but in some patients they are very rare in the blood. Occasional patients have leukocytosis with numerous circulating hairy cells instead of leukopenia. The bone marrow is always diffusely infiltrated by hairy cells, but it may be difficult to aspirate the marrow in about half of the patients (i.e., "dry tap"). If the diagnosis of HCL is suspected but hairy cells cannot be demonstrated in the blood and bone marrow aspiration is unsuccessful, a marrow biopsy should be performed and imprint preparations made of the freshly obtained biopsy specimen so that the appropriate confirmatory cytologic and cytochemical tests can be done. Reticulin fibers are often increased in the marrow as well as in the spleen, and the marrow may also contain increased numbers of plasma cells. If a splenectomy is performed, experienced pathologists can usually make a definitive diagnosis because involvement of the red pulp by hairy cells and the presence of pseudosinuses are uniquely characteristic of HCL. Sections of liver biopsies show hairy cell infiltration largely confined to the portal areas without destruction of parenchymal hepatic cells. Liver function tests are often normal; the most common abnormality is an elevated serum alkaline phosphatase level that is related to the degree of periportal infiltration.

Other disease entities with which HCL may be confused are CLL, Waldenström's macroglobulinemia, some of the diffuse varieties of non-Hodgkin's lymphomas, histiocytic medullary reticulosis, and monocytic leukemia. The leukocyte count in HCL is usually low instead of elevated as in CLL. The serum immunoglobulins are usually normal or show a polyclonal increase in HCL in contrast to CLL, in which they are often depressed, or to Waldenström's macroglobulinemia, in which there is a monoclonal IgM spike. Histiocytic medullary reticulosis (HMR, malignant histiocytosis, histiocytic leukemia) is a rare, rapidly progressive fatal disease characterized by fever, wasting, jaundice, generalized lymphadenopathy, and hepatosplenomegaly. The involved organs are infiltrated with abnormal histiocytes that commonly show intense erythrophagocytosis, a functional characteristic rarely exhibited by hairy cells. Acute or chronic monocytic leukemia can also be confused with HCL, but the serum or urinary lysozyme levels in HCL are normal or low in contrast to the high levels found in monocytic leukemia.

Although the aforementioned clinical and laboratory features are useful in distinguishing HCL from other disease entities, the essential requirement for the diagnosis is positive identification of the characteristic hairy cells. Their unique features can readily be demonstrated by appropriate morphologic, cytochemical, and immunologic tests, as described under Pathogenesis. Although occasional cells closely resembling or identical to hairy cells have been observed in some varieties of non-Hodgkin's lymphomas, in none of these conditions or in any of the other lymphoproliferative or histiocytic-monocytic neoplasias mentioned earlier is the marrow diffusely infiltrated by characteristic hairy cells.

The diagnosis of HCL is not suspected prior to performing a splenectomy for some ill-defined condition such as "chronic anemia," "primary splenic lymphoma," or "myeloid metaplasia." However, experienced hematopathologists can usually readily diagnose HCL on examination of histologic sections of the spleen and distinguish this entity from lymphomas and other conditions causing splenic enlargement.

PROGNOSIS AND TREATMENT. HCL generally has a chronic course, with a median survival of three to five years and with some patients surviving many years. Rarely the disease is rapidly progressive and may be accompanied by massive infiltration of the skin and multiple internal organs, leading to death within a year. However, early death is most commonly due to infection as a consequence of neutropenia. A large variety of bacteria, fungi, viruses, and mycobacteria have been reported to cause terminal infections.

Patients who are relatively asymptomatic at the time of diagnosis should merely be observed, since the disease may progress very slowly and not require treatment for long periods.

Splenectomy. If there is progressive worsening of the anemia, thrombocytopenia, or neutropenia, splenectomy should be considered, as this has proved to be beneficial in about two thirds of cases and to improve survival in patients who respond favorably. A good response to splenectomy with improvement in one or more of the blood elements is not well correlated with spleen size, but patients with only patchy marrow involvement are more likely to have a favorable response than those whose marrows are densely infiltrated with hairy cells. Improvements in surgical techniques and in prevention of serious infections have greatly reduced the complications of splenectomy in recent years. The majority of patients with HCL will have some hematologic improvement after splenectomy, but the degree and duration of improvement are quite variable. In most cases the improvement will be noted within a few weeks after the operation. About 40 per cent of patients have no response or only a partial response, and in the latter relapse usually occurs within a few months. Forty to 60 per cent of patients in different series have a significant rise in the blood cell counts following splenectomy, with an average duration of response of over a year and with some patients remaining well for several years.

Chemotherapy and Biologic Therapy. Patients in whom the disease progressed after splenectomy heretofore presented a difficult therapeutic problem, but during the last several years two new therapeutic agents, alfa-interferon and pentostatin (2'-deoxycoformycin), have been shown to be highly effective forms of treatment.

In the past, many chemotherapeutic agents have been tried, but most were found to have limited usefulness or even to be deleterious. Glucocorticoids, alkylating agents in low doses, and androgens were employed most frequently. Glucocorticoids sometimes resulted in hematologic improvement and reduction in the size of the spleen, but even in patients who responded, the effect was usually short lived, and glucocorticoids significantly increased the risk of infection, especially fungal infections.

Antimetabolites and other cytotoxic drugs that affect only actively proliferating cells are ineffective and may be harmful in HCL, because the slowly proliferating hairy cells are less sensitive than the residual normal hematopoietic cells to such drugs. Patients with progressive disease who fail to respond to splenectomy or in whom relapse later occurs frequently benefit from treatment with low doses of alkylating agents (e.g., chlorambucil or cyclophosphamide) with a decrease in hairy cell infiltration of the marrow and improvement in the platelet and erythrocyte counts; however, the monocytopenia and granulocytopenia usually persist or may be worsened. Since alkylating agents may cause further myelosuppression, such therapy should be limited to patients whose disease is clearly progressing following splenectomy. Some cases that fail to respond to chlorambucil or that have relapsed show significant hematologic improvement with androgens (e.g., Halotestin* 10 mg three times a day or oxymetholone* 150 mg four times a day), and sometimes the responses are prolonged. However, it is not yet clear what proportion of patients can be expected to have a significant response to androgens, and further trials are indicated. Patients with leukocytosis and large numbers of circulating hairy cells may benefit from intensive leukapheresis, but no significant improvement can be expected in the majority of patients who are leukopenic. A few patients with refractory disease and severe neutropenia and thrombocytopenia secondary to bone marrow replacement by hairy cells have had durable remissions following intensive chemotherapy. However, such aggressive therapy is extremely hazardous and requires intensive supportive treatment, including repeated granulocyte and platelet transfusions during the period of prolonged marrow aplasia; it cannot be recommended except as experimental treatment of patients refractory to conventional treatment in centers specially equipped to provide adequate supportive therapy.

Alfa-interferon is highly effective in the treatment of HCL. The majority of patients show a beneficial response to either

---

*This use is not listed in the manufacturer's directive.

natural or biosynthetic (recombinant) alfa-interferons. The responses are often observed within a month after beginning treatment and may lead to a substantial reduction in hairy cell infiltration of the marrow and normalization of hematopoiesis, including recovery of the monocyte and granulocyte counts, which does not usually occur during treatment with low-dose chlorambucil. Complete remissions with disappearance of all hairy cells from the marrow almost never occur, and there is no evidence that alfa-interferon is curative.

The doses of alfa-interferon have varied in the different clinical trials, but relatively low doses were found to be effective (i.e., 2 million U per square meter of body surface area three times weekly by self-administered subcutaneous injection). Some toxicity was observed in most patients, including fever, fatigue, myalgias, dryness of mucous membranes, myelosuppression, liver function abnormalities, paresthesias, and alopecia, but toxic effects were usually considered acceptable when weighed against the favorable hematologic responses.

Alfa-interferon is already generally considered the treatment of choice in patients with progressive disease after splenectomy, and it is currently being evaluated as first-line treatment, especially in patients whose marrow is densely infiltrated with hairy cells and in whom splectomy is relatively ineffective.

Pentostatin (2'-deoxycoformycin) is also effective in HCL. This drug was originally used clinically in relatively high doses for treatment of T cell neoplasias and various other tumors, but it was largely abandoned because of severe toxicity and the relative lack of antitumor effect. Given in low doses, however, deoxycoformycin is very effective in treating HCL. Some patients have even had complete remission with complete clearing of hairy cells from the marrow. Deoxycoformycin is still considered an investigational agent, and the optimal dosage schedule and response and toxicity patterns are currently being determined in multi-institutional clinical trials.

Bouroncle BA: Leukemic reticuloendotheliosis (hairy cell leukemia). Blood 53:412, 1979. *A review of the manifestations of hairy cell leukemia by the physician who first recognized this disease as a clinical entity.*

Cheson BD, Martin A: Clinical trials in hairy cell leukemia. Ann Intern Med 106:871, 1987. *An excellent review of current therapy for hairy cell leukemia. 71 references.*

Golomb HM: Hairy cell leukemia: Lessons learned in 25 years. J Clin Oncol 1:652, 1983. *Good review of the clinical features, therapeutic options, and biology of HCL with list of pertinent references.*

Jacobs AD, Champlin RE, Golde DW: Recombinant α-2-interferon for hairy cell leukemia. Blood 65:1017, 1985. *The results of a clinical trial of recombinant alfa-interferon are reported that confirm the beneficial therapeutic effects of this agent in HCL as originally reported by Quesada, et al. (see reference below).*

Jansen J, LeBien TW, Kersey JH: The phenotype of the neoplastic cells of hairy cell leukemia studied with monoclonal antibodies. Blood 59:609, 1982. *Eighteen cases of hairy cell leukemia were studied with a battery of polyclonal anti-Ig and monoclonal antibodies. The results support the B cell origin of HCL and suggest that the maturation arrest in HCL is at a more mature stage than in CLL.*

Spiers ASD, Moore D, Cassileth PA, et al.: Remissions in hairy-cell leukemia with pentostatin (2'-deoxycoformycin). N Engl J Med 316:825, 1987.

Westbrook CA, Golde DW: Clinical problems in hairy cell leukemia: Diagnosis and management. Semin Oncol 11 (4 Suppl. 2):514, 1984. *A good general review of the clinical aspects of HCL.*

156 THE ACUTE LEUKEMIAS
Howard J. Weinstein

DEFINITION. The acute leukemias are primary malignant diseases of the blood-forming organs characterized by a predominance of immature myeloid or lymphoid precursors (blasts). The blasts progressively replace normal bone marrow, migrate, and invade other tissues. There is diminished production of normal erythrocytes, granulocytes, and platelets in acute leukemia, and this leads to the most important complications of this disease—anemia, infection, and hemorrhage.

The acute leukemias are classified morphologically by reference to the predominant cell line involved as lymphoblastic (ALL) and myelogenous (AML) forms. If untreated, both forms are universally fatal within a period of months to one year. Therapy has markedly altered prognosis, and many patients with acute leukemia remain free of disease for prolonged periods.

ETIOLOGY. The mechanism of leukemogenesis in humans is unknown, but inciting agents are well established.

Ionizing Radiation. Physicians and scientists exposed to excessive amounts of radiation during the early years of research on medical application of x-rays, patients given low-dose radiation for rheumatoid spondylitis, and persons exposed acutely to radiation during the nuclear attacks on Hiroshima and Nagasaki in 1945 have all been found to have an increased incidence of leukemia. This increase involved chronic myelocytic leukemia (CML), ALL, and AML in survivors of the atomic bombings and has been dose related. The first cases of leukemia were noted two years after irradiation. A peak was reached after five to seven years and diminished to baseline levels by about 1970. Studies of the effects of diagnostic x-ray exposure, including fetal exposure, have not consistently shown an increased incidence of leukemia.

Oncogenic Viruses (see also Ch. 169). Horizontally transmissible RNA viruses (retroviruses) are clearly capable of inducing acute leukemia in mice, domestic cats, cattle, chickens, and gibbon apes. Unequivocal evidence for either an endogenous or a horizontally transmitted human leukemia virus is still lacking. A naturally occurring human type C retrovirus, human T cell leukemia virus (HTLV1), has recently been isolated from malignant lymphocytes of adults with a rare T cell leukemia-lymphoma. HTLV-associated leukemia is prevalent in certain geographic regions such as Southwestern Japan, the Caribbean, and areas of South America. In areas where clustering of adult T cell leukemia-lymphoma occurs, most patients and 10 per cent of healthy individuals have natural antibodies to HTLV, suggesting that HTLV is a common infection. The molecular mechanism of neoplastic transformation of human T cells by HTLV is currently not known.

Genetic and Congenital Factors. The strongest evidence for a genetic predisposition to acute leukemia is the occurrence of this disease in identical twins. If one of a set of identical twins develops leukemia before six years of age, the risk of disease in the other twin is 20 per cent. Leukemia usually develops in a co-twin within months of the first case. Concordant leukemia in monozygotic infant twins may reflect a common prezygotic determinant, shared intrauterine insult, or blood-borne metastases from one twin to the other. For fraternal twins and siblings the risk of developing leukemia is between twofold and fourfold higher than for children in the general population.

Congenital conditions associated with chromosomal instability and a predisposition to acute leukemia include three autosomal recessive disorders: Bloom's syndrome, Fanconi's anemia, and ataxia-telangiectasia. Ataxia-telangiectasia is commonly accompanied by rearrangement of the long arm of chromosome 14 and is one of the inborn immunodeficiency syndromes that predispose to lymphoreticular neoplasms, including acute lymphoblastic leukemia.

Down's syndrome (trisomy 21) is associated with a 10- to 20-fold increased risk of leukemia during the first decade of life. The cell types of leukemia follow the usual distribution, but the age peak is nearly three years earlier than expected. Newborns with Down's syndrome may show a transient proliferation of blast cells (usually myeloblasts) that is often clinically and hematologically indistinguishable from congenital leukemia. In contrast to congenital leukemia, complete permanent recovery occurs within weeks to months without specific antileukemia therapy.

Chemical Agents. Many chemicals have been associated with leukemia. Benzene exposure increases the risk of AML, with bone marrow hypoplasia and/or pancytopenia often preceding the diagnosis of leukemia. Less convincing reports have implicated chloramphenicol and phenylbutazone as leukemogenic agents.

An increased risk for AML and myelodysplastic syndromes has been documented in patients treated with alkylating agents for neoplastic and non-neoplastic diseases. The ten-year cumulative risk ranges from 2 to 10 per cent and has been related to cumulative dose and type of alkylating agent. Many of these secondary leukemias have developed in the absence of radiation or underlying diseases that produce immunologic deficiency.

INCIDENCE. The leukemias account for approximately 3 per cent of all cancer in the United States. The overall frequency of leukemia, as reflected in mortality statistics, increased steadily in developed countries over the first half of the twentieth century and has remained stable during the past three decades. It is believed that this pattern reflected improving ability to diagnose leukemia and increasing accuracy of death records.

The age-adjusted incidence of leukemia is about 8 to 10 per 100,000 persons per year. Acute leukemia accounts for nearly half of all leukemias. The peak incidence of ALL occurs between the ages of two and four years, whereas the incidence of AML progressively increases with advancing age. The ratio of ALL to AML is 4:1 in persons under the age of 15, but this ratio is reversed in adults. Acute leukemia is more common in males than in females and in whites than in blacks.

PATHOPHYSIOLOGY. The molecular basis of leukemic transformation in man is unknown. The fundamental defect in acute leukemia appears to be unregulated proliferation of early precursor cells that have lost their capacity to differentiate in response to normal hormonal signals and cellular interactions. Previously the accumulation of the leukemic cell population was attributed only to rapid and uncontrolled proliferation.

A leukemic transformation may arise at any point during the differentiation of the hematopoietic pluripotential stem cell. Chromosome and glucose-6-phosphate dehydrogenase isozyme studies show that both ALL and AML are of unicellular (clonal) origin (see Ch. 152) and that the cellular level of origin of AML is heterogeneous. In some patients with AML the leukemia is expressed in the erythrocytic and granulocytic pathways, suggesting involvement of the CFU-S (myeloid stem cell). In other patients, the leukemia is expressed in cells restricted to granulocytic and macrophage lineage, suggesting involvement of CFU-GM (committed granulocyte-macrophage progenitor). Acute lymphoblastic leukemia is superimposed on normal hematopoietic cells that are products of normal CFU-S because committed myeloid progenitors in ALL do not contain chromosomal markers that are found in the leukemic lymphoblasts.

In acute leukemia, both normal and malignant cells coexist and compete for ascendancy within the bone marrow. Antileukemic therapy destroys the leukemic clone and allows for return of normal hematopoiesis. This is in contrast to chronic myelogeneous leukemia, in which few normal myeloid stem cells are detectable at any time during the course of the disease.

Certain in vitro investigations and clinical studies provide some evidence that acute leukemia, although clonal, can be influenced by extracellular leukemogenic factors or deficiencies of differentiation factors. Acute leukemia has appeared in the engrafted cells of several leukemic patients who received marrow transplants from histocompatible siblings, for example, suggesting that leukemogenesis may result from unidentified factors that persist in certain susceptible hosts.

CLASSIFICATION. The acute leukemias are extraordinarily heterogeneous, reflecting the complexities of hematopoietic differentiation. The various types of acute leukemia are characterized by multiple methods that include morphology, histochemistry, cell surface and cytoplasmic markers, and cytogenetic and molecular genetic changes.

Morphology and Histochemistry. Blast cells are immature precursors, lacking many of the features for differentiating a lymphoid from a myeloid origin. The capacity to distinguish these blasts is of marked therapeutic and prognostic importance; various cytologic criteria have been established to differentiate between them.

Using the French-American-British (FAB) international morphologic classification, ALL has been divided into subgroups L1 to L3 and AML into subgroups M1 to M7. In L1 the lymphoblasts treated with Wright's stain are small and uniform in size, have smooth, homogeneous nuclear chromatin with indistinct nucleoli, and only a small rim of pale blue staining cytoplasm. L2 blasts are larger and nonuniform in size, have more prominent nucleoli, and a variable amount of cytoplasm. L3 blasts have deeply basophilic, vacuolated cytoplasm and are indistinguishable from Burkitt's lymphoma cells. The majority of L1 and L2 types of lymphoblasts are reactive with periodic acid–Schiff (PAS), and nonreactive with myeloperoxidase. The vacuoles in the L3 blasts are PAS negative, but stain positively for neutral fat (oil red O).

A summary of the AML subtypes and their histochemical reactivity is listed in Table 156–1. Auer rods, which are azurophilic granular cytoplasmic inclusion bodies, are thought to be pathognomonic of AML and are most commonly seen in the M2 and M3 subtypes. Acute leukemias derived from eosinophilic and basophilic precursors, although uncommon, display unique characteristics as well as many features in common with other AML's. Acute megakaryocytic leukemia represents the M7 subtype of AML.

Surface Markers. Four broad subclasses of ALL are defined by leukemic cell surface markers and have prognostic and therapeutic significance. This classification of ALL and the approximate percentage of patients in each subclass is shown in Table 156–2.

The common ALL antigen, or CALLA, is a glycosylated polypeptide that is expressed on the cell surface in approximately 60 and 50 per cent of cases of childhood and adult ALL, respectively. CALLA is also detected in some of the non-Hodgkin's lymphomas, in one third of cases of blast crisis of Ph[1] chromosome–positive CML, on a small percentage of normal bone marrow cells, and on some nonhematopoietic tissues. The early precursor B ALL blasts have undergone immunoglobulin gene rearrangements, indicating a commitment to B cell differentiation.

Patients with T cell ALL have a characteristic clinical presentation—that is, adolescent males with a high white blood cell count and a mediastinal mass. The T lymphoblasts from these patients display markers that characterize their phenotype as early, mid, or late thymocyte.

Blast cells from patients with AML react with many monoclonal antibodies that define antigens at various stages of erythroid, granulocytic, monocytic, and megakaryocytic differentiation. Myeloid leukemic blasts in most instances have Ia antigens, but lack T cell, B cell, and CALLA antigens. A small percentage of cases of ALL and AML express lineage nonspecific markers (e.g., rearranged immunoglobulin genes in a myeloblast) and are referred to as mixed lineage leukemias. It is not clear if these mixed phenotypes represent aberrant differentiation or transformation of an early bipotent stem cell.

Cytoplasmic Markers. At least five cytoplasmic marker enzymes have been used in the classification of acute leukemias: terminal deoxynucleotidyl transferase, hexosaminidase, N-alkaline phosphatase, 5'-nucleotidase, and adenosine deaminase. T lymphoblasts have diminished 5'-nucleotidase and

TABLE 156-1. FAB CLASSIFICATION OF ACUTE MYELOGENOUS LEUKEMIA

FAB Class	Common Name	Morphology	Histochemistry	Unique Clinical or Laboratory Features
M1	Acute myelocytic leukemia without differentiation	Myeloblasts predominate; distinct nucleoli; few granules	MP+	−7/del 7q, +8
M2	Acute myelocytic leukemia with differentiation	Myeloblasts and promyelocytes predominate; further maturation abnormal	MP+	Myeloblastomas, t(8;21)
M3	Acute promyelocytic leukemia	Promyelocytes predominate; hypergranular; may have reniform or bilobed nuclei with small granules	MP+	DIC, t(15;17)
M4	Acute myelomonocytic leukemia	Myelocytic and monocytic maturation evident; peripheral monocytosis	MP+ NSE+	inv 16, +8, eosinophilia, extramedullary leukemia (skin, gums, CNS)
M5	Acute monocytic leukemia	Promonocytes or undifferentiated blasts, cerebriform nuclei, cytoplasmic pseudopods	NSE+	t (——,11), infants, extramedullary leukemia
M6	Erythroleukemia	Bizarre, multinucleated, megaloblastoid erythroblasts predominate; myeloblasts also present	MP+ (myeloblast), PAS+ (erythroblasts)	Complex chromosomal abnormalities
M7	Megakaryocytic leukemia	Pleomorphic, undifferentiated, cytoplasmic blebs	Platelet peroxidase by electron microscopy	Myelofibrosis or increased bone marrow reticulin

FAB = French-American-British classification; MP = myeloperoxidase; NSE = nonspecific esterase; PAS = periodic acid–schiff; t = translocation; S = deletion (loss of entire chromosome or part of the long arm); DIC = disseminated intravascular coagulation; inv = inversion; t (——,11) = translocations with band 11q23 and one of several reciprocating chromosomes (6, 9, 10, 17, 19); t = trisomy.

increased adenosine deaminase activity as useful distinguishing characteristics. For example, deoxycoformycin, an inhibitor of adenosine deaminase, has induced remission in T cell ALL. Terminal deoxynucleotidyl transferase activity provides excellent diagnostic differentiation between ALL and AML, as it is present in 95 per cent of cases of ALL and is mostly absent in AML. It has also correctly defined the lymphoblastic crisis in CML and predicted the efficacy of ALL therapy in its management.

Chromosomal Changes. A detectable nonrandom chromosomal change is usually present in the leukemic cells in over 80 per cent of patients with ALL and AML. A normal karyotype appears with remission, and the original chromosome aberration reappears at the time of relapse. Moreover, specific chromosomal abnormalities correlate with particular FAB subtypes of AML (Table 156–2). Loss of chromosomes 5 or 7 or trisomy 8 has been most consistently observed in patients with myelodysplastic syndromes (preleukemia) or secondary AML (previous history of radiation, cytotoxic drugs, or exposure to strong mutagenic agents).

In ALL the modal chromosome numbers appear to be much higher than in AML. Consistent chromosome translocations have been correlated with various immunophenotypes of ALL (e.g., t(11;14) with T cell, t(8;14) with B cell, and t(1;19) with pre-B cell). An interesting subgroup of patients with ALL include those with a Ph¹ chromosome. It is unclear if Ph¹-positive ALL represents the lymphoblastic crisis of chronic myelogenous leukemia or a different leukemia.

TABLE 156-2. IMMUNOLOGIC CLASSIFICATION OF ACUTE LYMPHOBLASTIC LEUKEMIA

	Early Precursor B	Pre-B	B	T	Unc
Frequency (per cent)	15	60	<5	15	5
Immune phenotype					
Ia	+	+	+	−	−
B4	+	+	+	−	−
CALLA	−	most	rare	rare	−
cIg	−	20–30%	−	−	−
sIg	−	−	+	−	−
Sheep RBC rosettes	−	−	−	most	−
Thymocyte antigens	−	−	−	+	−

Ia = Class II histocompatibility antigen; B4 = early B cell antigen; CALLA = common acute lymphoblastic leukemia antigen; cIg = cytoplasmic immunoglobulin (u heavy chain); sIg = surface immunoglobulin; Sheep RBC rosettes = receptor on T lymphocytes that spontaneously binds sheep erythrocytes; Thymocyte antigens = early to late thymocyte antigens recognized by a series of anti-T monoclonal antibodies; Unc = unclassified.

The mechanism by which cells carrying chromosomal abnormalities gain selective advantage is beginning to be understood. The chromosome position of several cellular oncogenes is now known. The cellular oncogenes are homologous to recognized transforming genes of the acute retroviruses. Little is known about their function in the human genome, but they may be in part responsible for control of cellular proliferation and differentiation. These cellular oncogenes may be perturbed or activated by several mechanisms, including chromosome rearrangement, alteration in gene dosage (gain or loss of a chromosome), or small mutations. Activation or altered expression of cellular oncogenes may turn out to be one of several key steps in neoplastic transformation (see Ch. 169 for a more detailed discussion).

CLINICAL MANIFESTATIONS. The signs and symptoms of acute leukemia relate to decreased numbers of normal hematopoietic cells and invasion of other organs by leukemic cells. Why normal hematopoiesis is suppressed in leukemia is not known. It may result in part from the release of suppressor substances by leukemic blasts.

Anemia. Asthenia, pallor, headache, tinnitus, dyspnea, angina, edema, and congestive heart failure may all indicate anemia. The anemia generally results from decreased erythropoiesis and blood loss. Evidence of specific antibody-mediated hemolysis is uncommon.

Hemorrhage. Hemorrhagic manifestations in newly diagnosed acute leukemia are usually caused by thrombocytopenia. Oozing gums, epistaxis, petechiae, ecchymoses, menorrhagia, melena, and excessive bleeding after tooth extraction are common initial manifestations. Retinal hemorrhages and subarachnoid bleeding are rare. Most thrombocytopenic bleeding occurs when the platelet count is less than 20,000 per microliter.

Intracranial hemorrhages may result from leukostasis, i.e., intravascular clumping of blasts, especially within small vessels of the brain, leading to infarction and hemorrhage. Leukostasis occurs most frequently in acute myelogenous leukemia when the peripheral leukocyte count is in excess of 150,000 per microliter.

In acute promyelocytic leukemia, the abnormal granules in the blast appear to contain tissue thromboplastin activity or fibrinolysins that initiate disseminated intravascular coagulation or fibrinolysis. Massive hemorrhage can occur in this setting (see Ch. 167).

Infection. Most early infections in acute leukemia are presumably bacterial, but specific etiologic agents are often not found. Leukemia may first be recognized by the occurrence of an infection (respiratory, dental, sinus, perirectal abscess, urinary tract, and skin) that never fully clears. These early infections appear to be attributable to granulocytopenia, with the risk of infection being greatest when the absolute granulocyte count is less than 200 cells per microliter. Repeated search for an infectious source of fever is required in all patients, because "leukemic fever" is extremely rare.

Leukemic Infiltration. Although leukemia is primarily a disease of bone marrow and peripheral blood, other tissues may also become infiltrated by the blast cells. The organs most commonly showing initial clinical involvement are the liver, spleen, and superficial lymph nodes. Bone pain is one of the initial symptoms in 25 per cent of patients with acute leukemia, and children with ALL may present with migratory joint pain accompanied by swelling and tenderness that may be confused with juvenile rheumatoid arthritis. These symptoms may be the result of direct leukemic infiltration of the periosteum, periosteal elevation by underlying cortical disease, bone infarction, or expansion of the marrow cavity by leukemic cells.

Central nervous system leukemia (leptomeningeal involvement) is clinically present at the time of diagnosis in about 2 per cent of patients. The most common signs and symptoms include vomiting, headache, papilledema, nuchal rigidity, and cranial nerve palsies. Pleocytosis with the presence of blasts usually makes the diagnosis a simple one, but even with cytocentrifugation techniques, between 5 and 15 per cent of patients with arachnoid infiltration will not have identifiable leukemic cells in the spinal fluid.

Thymic or mediastinal infiltration, most commonly seen in T cell ALL, may cause life-threatening airway or vascular compression. Patients with the monocytic variants of AML frequently have skin and gum infiltration.

Chloromas or myeloblastomas are localized tumors seen in patients with AML that often appear green on the cut surface because of the presence of large amounts of the enzyme myeloperoxidase. These tumors may arise in bones or soft tissues and are frequently seen in the epidural area and around the orbits. Chloromas may appear before the onset of detectable bone marrow disease, or they may herald relapse.

LABORATORY MANIFESTATIONS. Clinical laboratory data often provide a broad spectrum of abnormal findings in the patient with newly diagnosed acute leukemia. Anemia, abnormal white cell and differential blood counts, and thrombocytopenia are common, but as many as 10 per cent of patients may have normal routine blood counts at the time of diagnosis even when the bone marrow is replaced by leukemic cells. Pancytopenia without recognizably abnormal leukocytes is found in a small percentage of patients and has been called aleukemic leukemia.

Blast cells are usually easily detectable in the peripheral blood when the white count exceeds 5000 per microliter (Color plate 3*I* and *J*). The morphology of peripheral blasts may not accurately reflect the status of the bone marrow. For example, normal myeloblasts may be detected in the circulation when lymphoblasts invade the marrow as part of the so-called leukoerythroblastic response to marrow invasion. The definitive diagnosis of leukemia should be made only from a bone marrow aspiration. The marrow specimen is usually hypercellular and contains from 30 to 100 per cent blast cells (Color plate 3*K*). Occasionally bone marrow aspiration results in a "dry tap." This may be attributed to a very packed marrow, reticulum fibrosis, or bone marrow necrosis within the marrow cavity. Marrow needle biopsy will usually produce an adequate specimen. The sample obtained by this technique should be touched to glass slides before it is placed in a fixative, because such touch preparations are very useful in assessing morphology.

Muramidase, or lysozyme, is a hydrolytic enzyme that is present in the primary granules of primitive granulocyte and monocyte precursor cells. Elevated serum and urine levels of this enzyme may be present in AML, with the highest levels in the monocytic and myelomonocytic subtypes. Renal tubular dysfunction and hypokalemia have been reported with increased blood and urine lysozyme. Hyperkalemia, hypocalcemia, and hyperphosphatemia have been associated with hyperleukocytosis and tumor lysis.

DIFFERENTIAL DIAGNOSIS. The diagnosis of acute leukemia is seldom difficult. Infections, neoplasms, and other marrow infiltrations may lead to leukocytosis and to immature cells in the peripheral blood. These leukemoid reactions generally mimic chronic myelogenous leukemia (see Ch. 155). Neutropenia induced by drugs, toxins, or infection may result in bone marrow that is left shifted (filled with myeloblasts and promyelocytes). This normal, early myeloid population can be confused with AML, but it will mature in a few days, thus establishing the diagnosis.

Infectious mononucleosis and other viral illnesses can masquerade as ALL. This differential diagnosis is particularly difficult in the rare patient whose viral illness is complicated by thrombocytopenic purpura or immunohemolytic anemia. Patients with both acute leukemia and aplastic anemia may present with pancytopenia. The bone marrow aspirate in aplastic anemia will be hypocellular, but rarely the two diseases cannot be differentiated initially because a small number of patients with acute leukemia have hypocellular bone marrow.

THERAPY. The possibility of cure for both ALL and AML has become realistic. Complete remission is required to provide a significant prolongation of survival. Such a remission is commonly defined as the reduction of leukemic cells to undetectable levels and the restoration of normal bone marrow function. This includes a return to less than 5 per cent blasts in the bone marrow; normalization of hemoglobin, granulocyte, and platelet counts; resolution of organomegaly; and return of the patient to normal lifestyle.

Initial treatment is directed toward correcting metabolic abnormalities, anemia, and thrombocytopenia and toward controlling infection and preventing hyperuricemia. This may require up to 48 hours, but can usually be achieved in 24 hours. Immediate administration of chemotherapy is necessary to prevent leukostasis in patients with AML and high white cell counts (>200,000 per microliter). Allopurinol is started at diagnosis to decrease the formation of relatively insoluble uric acid from the catabolic products of leukemia cells. Hyperuricemia may occur prior to antileukemic treatment and occasionally may be severe enough to produce impaired renal function before therapy can be started. In this setting, alkalinization and high urine flow should be established before cytotoxic therapy is initiated.

Acute Lymphoblastic Leukemia. Once the patient's condition is stabilized, antileukemic chemotherapy should begin without delay. Therapy is divided into three phases: remission induction, central nervous system prophylaxis, and treatment in remission (maintenance or continuation therapy).

REMISSION INDUCTION. Combinations of two agents have been consistently superior to single agents for inducing complete remission of patients with ALL. The most effective combination has been vincristine and prednisone, which produces complete remission in more than 90 per cent of pediatric patients and 50 per cent of adults with ALL. For patients over 15 years of age, the addition of a third drug (L-asparaginase, doxorubicin, or daunorubicin) increases the remission rate to over 80 per cent. In several studies the remission rates fell to 60 to 70 per cent in patients over 30 years of age.

CENTRAL NERVOUS SYSTEM PROPHYLAXIS. An important advance in the treatment of childhood ALL was CNS prophylaxis. As more children experienced longer bone marrow remission, the CNS became the first site of relapse in over 50 per cent of patients. The risk of relapse in the CNS can be markedly reduced by treatment with irradiation, 2400 rads to the cranial-spinal axis or 2400 rads to the cranium, combined with four doses of methotrexate given intrathecally. Intrathecal methotrexate alone is effective CNS prophylaxis in selected patients with ALL. Treatment of the CNS sanctuary reduces the frequency of subsequent bone marrow relapse and increases the percentage of children whose disease remains in continuous complete remission. CNS prophylaxis is usually administered following completion of the induction regimen and is now routinely used in all childhood and most adult ALL treatment programs. In the adult age group, CNS leukemia is significantly reduced by similar prophylaxis, but this has not resulted in longer bone marrow remission.

Cranial irradiation combined with intrathecal methotrexate is very effective CNS prophylaxis, but carries some risk of CNS damage. For example, irradiation alters vascular permeability to methotrexate, such that subsequent administration of parenteral methotrexate in large doses may result in a demyelinating leukoencephalopathy.

MAINTENANCE OR CONTINUATION THERAPY. After remission induction and CNS prophylaxis, continued therapy is necessary to prevent bone marrow relapse. Standard maintenance regimens have included 6-mercaptopurine, methotrexate, and periodic pulses of the remission-induction drugs. The above type of therapy is of relatively limited value for adults and high-risk children with ALL. Multiple cell cycle–specific and nonspecific agents have been intensively used before maintenance therapy to prevent the emergence of drug-resistant leukemic cells. These newer drug regimens appear to have improved durations of remission for high-risk patients.

How long maintenance therapy should be continued is unclear, in part because of the inability to assess minimal residual disease (less than 10^9 leukemic cells). In the absence of objective evidence, patients are now treated for one and one-half to three years.

RELAPSE. The most common site of relapse is in the bone marrow, with the highest risk during the first two years after diagnosis. CNS relapse has dramatically declined with the routine use of CNS prophylactic therapy; however, the testes are an important extramedullary site of relapse. If testicular relapse occurs during or following cessation of therapy, irradiation in a dose of 2400 rads should be given to both testes. As when CNS relapse occurs, systemic spread must be assumed, and therefore systemic as well as local therapy should be given. The prognosis for males with late testicular relapse appears to be favorable (data apply to children).

Approximately 80 per cent of children and 50 per cent of adults who have relapse will achieve second remissions with the original induction chemotherapy, but these are short lived. A second course of chemotherapy may be curative for a small percentage of patients whose initial remission was greater than two to three years. Bone marrow transplantation, however, is potentially useful therapy for these patients.

BONE MARROW TRANSPLANTATION (see Ch. 165). The initial trials of bone marrow transplantation in ALL involved patients with advanced resistant disease and resulted in long-term survival in 10 per cent. Earlier application of transplantation in patients with ALL has been more successful. Several centers have reported survival of 30 per cent in patients with ALL who underwent transplantation in second or subsequent remission. Marrow transplantation in first remission is now being considered for very high risk patients. Autologous bone marrow transplantation is an interesting approach for patients who lack HLA-identical donors. Bone marrow is obtained in second remission, is treated in vitro by physical, immunologic (e.g., anti-CALLA antibody), or pharmacologic techniques to remove residual leukemia cells, and is cryopreserved. The patient receives supralethal chemoradiotherapy and reinfusion of autologous "treated" bone marrow. The survival rate has been 20 to 30 per cent after autologous transplantation. Recurrent leukemia remains a major problem after allogeneic or autologous transplantation for ALL.

PROGNOSIS. The cure rate for children with ALL now routinely approaches 60 to 70 per cent, but is no more than 30 per cent for adults. In childhood studies, relatively favorable prognostic factors include age of two to ten years, white race, female sex, a white blood count less than 20,000 per microliter, and CALLA positivity. Over 70 per cent of patients in this group remain in continuous complete remission for five or more years after diagnosis. Less favorable prognostic factors include age less than two or greater than ten years, male sex, a mediastinal mass, L3 or Burkitt-type leukemia, Ph^1 chromosome, and an extremely elevated white blood cell count. The presence of T cell disease has a strong correlation with some high-risk clinical features, but is not an independent prognostic variable. The poorer prognosis observed in the older age group may in part be due to a different distribution of biologic subsets of ALL between adults and children.

Acute Myelogenous Leukemia. Progress in the treatment of AML has not equaled that in the management of ALL. More effective antileukemic chemotherapy and more sophisticated supportive care have recently increased the complete remission rate and the duration of remission, however.

REMISSION INDUCTION. Remission induction is now successful in 50 to 85 per cent of patients (adults and children) with AML. The drug dosages necessary to kill myeloblasts come dangerously close to destroying normal marrow cells and cause prolonged bone marrow aplasia until normal hematopoietic progenitors can repopulate the marrow. Therefore, effective remission induction programs are associated with considerable morbidity and mortality. The introduction of cytosine arabinoside (ara-C) and the anthracyclines (daunorubicin and doxorubicin) represented a major advance in the therapy of AML. Remission can be achieved in the majority of patients under 60 years of age with a single course of seven days of cytosine arabinoside and three days of daunorubicin or doxorubicin. In the past, only about one third of patients over age 60 achieved complete remission, but recent results are more encouraging.

CONSOLIDATION AND INTENSIFICATION CHEMOTHERAPY. As in ALL, remission induction therapy reduces but does not eradicate the leukemic clone of cells. Therefore, additional therapy is necessary to achieve prolonged remissions in patients with AML. With most chemotherapy treatment programs, median durations of remission have been 12 to 18 months, but with only 10 to 20 per cent of patients who achieved remission remaining as leukemia-free survivors at five or more years.

In an effort to increase leukemic cell kill during remission, patients have been treated with intensification or consolidation chemotherapy for periods of a few months to one year after induction of remission. This has been based on the steep dose response curve for most chemotherapeutic agents. In some studies, sequential "non-cross-resistant" drug combinations have been administered to circumvent the problem of acquired drug resistance. The chemotherapeutic strategies used have resulted in marked improvements in durations of remission for patients of less than 18 years with AML (life table estimates of 45 per cent leukemia-free survival at five years). For similarly treated adults (18 to 60 years), median durations were longer compared to standard maintenance chemotherapy regimens, but a higher plateau of five-year leukemia-free survival was not achieved. It does not appear that maintenance chemotherapy after consolidation or intensification treatment is of additional therapeutic benefit.

BONE MARROW TRANSPLANTATION (see Ch. 165). Over the past 10 years bone marrow transplantation has become an important therapeutic method in AML. Marrow grafting has been generally limited to persons less than 45 years of age with AML who have HLA-identical donors. Transplantation is ideally performed as soon as the patient enters complete remission. The outcome of bone marrow transplantation for patients with AML with first remission is promising. Leukemia-free survival estimates are as high as 50 to 60 per cent for young patients (<20 years), but decrease in older adults (>35 years). Relapse of leukemia after marrow transplantation has not been a major obstacle to success. Graft-versus-host disease and interstitial pneumonitis account for the major mortality and morbidity in these patients. For children and young adults (<35 years) there is a trend toward improved survival for those receiving a bone marrow transplant compared to chemotherapy in first remission. Bone marrow transplantation is the current treatment of choice for the patient with AML who has had relapse after an initial course of chemotherapy.

CENTRAL NERVOUS SYSTEM LEUKEMIA. CNS relapse is substantially less common (5 to 20 per cent) than in ALL, in part because of earlier death from systemic disease. Patients with myelomonocytic or monocytic leukemia are at increased risk for CNS disease. CNS prophylaxis is not routinely used for adults with AML. It is frequently employed in pediatric patients with AML, but it has not impacted upon overall survival.

PROGNOSIS. The cure rate for children with AML (greater than five years of continuous remission) approaches 30 to 40 per cent, but is no more than 20 per cent for adults. Correlations among age, sex, performance status, morphologic classification, blast cytokinetics, platelet count, splenomegaly, and the response to therapy have been described but are controversial. There is a correlation between the karyotypic abnormality in pretreatment bone marrow samples and response to therapy. Patients with deletions of chromosome 5 or 7 represent a group of patients who are likely to have short survival times.

The terms "myelodysplastic syndromes" or "preleukemia" and "smoldering leukemia" have been applied to a spectrum of abnormalities of bone marrow function characterized by normal to increased marrow cellularity and ineffective hematopoiesis. These patients often have a panmyelopathy, and chromosomal abnormalities are present in up to 75 per cent of cases. Many of these patients will develop AML within 6 to 18 months after diagnosis. The response to chemotherapy is poor, and bone marrow transplantation should be considered for the child or young adult with these diseases.

AML has been reported in patients who received chemotherapy (alkylating agents and nitrosoureas) for neoplastic diseases, including malignant lymphoma, ovarian carcinoma, and gastrointestinal carcinoma. The response of these patients to chemotherapy is also poor, with remission rates of less than 50 per cent in most series.

Immunotherapy. Most studies find immunotherapy to be effective against only relatively small numbers of tumor cells, usually less than 10^5. Because of this limitation the majority of immunotherapy trials have been performed in patients whose disease is in remission. A variety of immunotherapeutic agents have been examined, including BCG, *Corynebacterium parvum*, levamisole, and irradiated allogeneic leukemic blast cells with BCG. In most trials, patients have been randomized to receive chemotherapy alone, immunotherapy alone, or both chemotherapy and immunotherapy. Immunotherapy has almost always failed to increase remission durations in AML and ALL. Recent studies have focused on conjugating monoclonal antibodies to drugs or toxins that can target specific cells, and the use of biologic response modifiers such as the interferons and interleukins.

Supportive Care. Advances in the treatment of acute leukemia, especially AML, have depended on progress in the control of infection and bleeding. Infection is a major complication of induction chemotherapy for AML, with mortality of 20 to 30 per cent. Neutropenia, impaired immunity, central venous catheters, and drug toxicity to nonhematopoietic tissues (gastrointestinal tract) are predisposing factors. Virtually all patients with AML become febrile while receiving induction chemotherapy. Although infection is usually suspected, it is documented in only 50 to 70 per cent of cases. Neverthe-

less, febrile, neutropenic (less than 500 granulocytes per cubic millimeter) patients should receive broad-spectrum antibiotics immediately after appropriate cultures have been obtained. A semisynthetic penicillin and an aminoglycoside are generally included. Enteric gram-negative bacilli colonizing the gastrointestinal tract and gram-positive bacteria (e.g., *Staphylococcus epidermidis*) are responsible for the majority of infections.

Oral nonabsorbable antibiotics, protected environments (laminar airflow), and granulocyte transfusions during induction of remission in patients with AML are not of proven benefit. Oral nonabsorbable antibiotics reduce enteric colonization and have been shown to reduce systemic infection. Several studies indicate a decreased incidence of infections in protected environments, but overall remission rates remain unchanged. Therapeutic granulocyte transfusions in some studies have improved survival in patients with gram-negative bacteremia, but in general they have a limited role because of newer and more potent antibiotics.

In addition to bacteria, a variety of opportunistic organisms invade the immunosuppressed host. Patients receiving "broad-spectrum" antibiotics who remain febrile and granulocytopenic for approximately one week should be carefully observed for fungal infections, and empiric treatment with amphotericin B should be begun. *Pneumocystis carinii* threatens the immunosuppressed host and causes severe interstitial pneumonitis. Infection with this organism can be prevented by prophylactic therapy with trimethoprim-sulfamethoxazole. The severity of chickenpox can be reduced by the prophylactic administration (within 96 hours of exposure) of zoster immune globulin in patients in whom serologic examination indicates lack of varicella-zoster antibody and who are exposed to chickenpox or zoster. Acyclovir is useful for the treatment of varicella-zoster infection.

Platelet transfusions from HLA-mismatched donors are successful in restoring hemostasis in thrombocytopenic patients, but result in alloimmunization in 30 to 50 per cent of patients (see Ch. 166). The alloimmunized patient may be managed by the use of HLA-matched platelets, single-donor platelets obtained by plateletpheresis, or autologous cryopreserved platelets. There is controversy whether platelets should be transfused prophylactically (i.e., when platelet count is less than 20,000 per microliter) or whether they should be used only for active bleeding. The patient's overall clinical status and platelet responsiveness are factors to be taken into consideration in making this decision. The hemorrhagic complications of acute promyelocytic leukemia can be prevented and controlled by administration of heparin.

Transfusion of blood products from normal donors has been associated with graft-versus-host disease in the immunosuppressed and myelosuppressed patient with acute leukemia. Irradiation of blood products at dosages sufficient to destroy T lymphocytes prevents the development of graft-versus-host disease.

Applebaum FR, Dahlberg S, Thomas ED, et al.: Bone marrow transplantation or chemotherapy after remission induction for adults with acute nonlymphoblastic leukemia. Ann Intern Med 101:581, 1984. *One of several studies comparing the outcome of marrow transplantation with that of continued chemotherapy for adults with AML.*

Bennett JM, Catovsky D, Daniel MT, et al.: Proposals for the classification of the acute leukemias. Br J Haematol 33:451, 1976. *Detailed description of the French-American-British (FAB) classification of acute leukemia.*

Casciato DA, Scott JL: Acute leukemia following prolonged cytotoxic agent therapy. Medicine 58:32, 1979. *Includes a complete review of drug-induced leukemia and a complete bibliography.*

Foon KA, Todd RF: Immunologic classification of leukemia and lymphoma. Blood 68:1, 1986. *Detailed review of the cell surface phenotypes in the leukemias and lymphomas.*

Gale RP: Advances in the treatment of acute myelogenous leukemia. N Engl J Med 300:1189, 1979. *Excellent clinical review of current therapies and supportive care for patients with AML. Includes a complete bibliography.*

Gallo RC, Wong-Staal F: Retroviruses as etiologic agents of some animal and human leukemias and lymphomas and as tools for elucidating the molecular mechanism of leukemogenesis. Blood 60:545, 1982. *Review of viral etiology of leukemias including the HTLV retrovirus.*

McCulloch EA: Stem cells in normal and leukemic hemopoiesis. Blood 62:1, 1983. *Good review and bibliography of the nature of differentiation in normal and leukemic process.*

Murphy SB (ed.): Acute Lymphoblastic Leukemia. Semin Oncol 12:79, 1985. *Excellent chapters on the biology and treatment of ALL in both children and adults.*

Prentice HG (ed.): Infections in Haematology. Clin Haematol 13:523, 1984. *Includes chapters on infection prophylaxis and treatment of bacterial, viral, and fungal infections of the immunocompromised host.*

Rowley JD: Biological implications of consistent chromosome rearrangements in leukemia and lymphoma. Cancer Res 44:3159, 1984. *Complete review of consistent chromosomal lesions in the leukemias and oncogene mapping.*

Thomas ED: Bone marrow transplantation in hematologic malignancies. Hosp Pract 22:77, 1987. *Overview of marrow transplantation for acute leukemia.*

157 INTRODUCTION TO NEOPLASMS OF THE IMMUNE SYSTEM

Carol S. Portlock

Neoplasms of the immune system are a heterogeneous group of tumors whose cells of origin may be the lymphocyte, the histiocyte, or other cell components of the immune system. Each neoplasm is thought to be a monoclonal expansion of malignant cells, although this has only been conclusively demonstrated for lymphocytic tumors. Interestingly, these neoplasms often retain many morphologic, functional, and migratory characteristics common to their normal cell counterparts.

With increasing understanding of the normal immune system, it has become possible to classify malignant immune disorders according to their cell of origin. Table 157–1 lists these neoplasms, utilizing current immunologic concepts. Tumors of B lymphocyte lineage are identified by the presence of cell surface immunoglobulin, utilizing fluorescent anti-immunoglobulin antibodies. Each B lymphocytic neoplasm can be immunotyped according to its heavy chain and light chain classes and can be shown to be a monoclonal process. Such immunologic phenotyping may identify distinct groups of patients with different clinical presentations and prognoses. In addition to membrane-bound immunoglobulin, malignant B lymphocytes may have Ia antigen and Fc receptors, as well as receptors for complement.

Tumors of T lymphocyte lineage are identified in vitro by the formation of E rosettes after incubation with sheep erythrocytes. Moreover, monoclonal antibodies that react with normal T cell differentiation antigens can be used to detect distinct malignant T cell subsets. Enzyme determination of

terminal deoxynucleotidyl transferase (TdT) may also identify a T cell lineage, as well as pre-B and lymphoid stem cells.

With utilization of these immunologic techniques, however, some tumors that are of lymphocyte origin morphologically cannot be shown to contain B or T cell surface markers and consequently are termed null cell. Nevertheless, immunoglobulin gene rearrangements may be detected in such null cells, suggesting a pre-B cell origin. Moreover, specific rearrangements of the T cell receptor gene loci identify tumors of T cell origin. Tumors of histiocytic lineage have not yet been identified by monoclonal antibody techniques. These cells lack endogenous immunoglobulin, but may acquire exogenous immunoglobulin on their cell surface. They may be rich in lysozyme or muramidase, and as phagocytic cells, they can be shown to ingest latex particles or sensitized erythrocytes. The cell lineage of the Reed-Sternberg cell in Hodgkin's disease is not known with certainty. It has in vitro characteristics in common with both histiocytes and lymphocytes. It may derive from a dendritic cell or lymphocyte.

In addition to a specific immunologic phenotype, chromosomal abnormalities can be detected in the majority of immune system neoplasms. In many the karyotype appears to be specific (follicular lymphomas, Burkitt's lymphoma, mycosis fungoides). Another marker that appears to be specific is the presence of antibodies to the human retrovirus HTLV-1 (human T cell lymphoma virus) found in patients with mature T cell lymphoma. These and other in vitro methods may provide additional information for defining prognostically important patient subsets.

Each neoplasm of the immune system is a distinct clinicopathologic entity. However, these disorders tend to share some common clinical features. For example, systemic symptoms of fever, night sweats, and weight loss may be present and tend to correlate with advanced stage of disease. The neoplasm usually arises in one or more organs of the hematopoietic system (lymph nodes, spleen, liver, bone marrow) and if untreated or ineffectively treated, it tends to disseminate to all those organs, as well as to other sites. Bone marrow involvement with or without peripheral blood manifestation is common in certain disorders and may be the predominant feature. Meningeal infiltration is often present when aggressive neoplasms involve the bone marrow.

PATHOLOGY AND CLASSIFICATION

Neoplasms of B or T lymphocytic lineage are termed non-Hodgkin's lymphomas. They are a diverse group of diseases with varying clinical presentations, responses to therapy, and prognoses. The Rappaport histopathologic classification of the non-Hodgkin's lymphomas (Table 157–2) has been successfully used in clinical trials and practice. It has permitted the identification of specific clinicopathologic entities and of favorable and unfavorable prognostic groups since 1966. Nevertheless, the Rappaport classification, based exclusively upon morphologic concepts, does not take into account recent information regarding the immune system. For example, the term "histiocytic" lymphoma is generally incorrect because virtually all of the non-Hodgkin's lymphomas are of lymphocytic origin.

Table 157–2 juxtaposes a more recent National Cancer Institute working formulation with the Rappaport classification. Tumor architecture is an important feature in both: Rappaport's "nodular" is replaced by the more immunologically accurate term "follicular." Cell morphology is more descriptive in the working formulation and "histiocytic" is replaced by "large cell." Prognostically favorable and unfavorable groups are termed low, intermediate, and high grade. The low-grade category includes small lymphocytic consistent with chronic lymphocytic leukemia; a miscellaneous category includes mycosis fungoides and true histiocytic lymphoma.

Many non-Hodgkin's lymphomas may exhibit two distinct histologic subtypes. Both the architecture and the cell type

TABLE 157–1. LYMPHOMAS AS NEOPLASMS OF THE IMMUNE SYSTEM

Cell of Origin	Neoplasm
I. B cell	
Medullary B cell	Chronic lymphocytic leukemia, diffuse small lymphocytic lymphoma
Follicular B cell	Follicular lymphomas, diffuse mixed lymphoma, diffuse large cell lymphoma, Burkitt's lymphoma
Immunoblastic B cell	Diffuse immunoblastic lymphoma
II. T cell	
Thymic T cell	Lymphoblastic lymphoma
Mature T cell	Peripheral T cell lymphomas, chronic lymphocytic leukemia (rare), HTLV-I–associated lymphoma, mycosis fungoides, Sézary's syndrome
Immunoblastic T cell	Diffuse immunoblastic lymphoma
III. Histiocytic	
Histiocyte	Malignant histiocytosis, true histiocytic lymphoma (rare)
IV. Unknown	Hodgkin's disease

Modified from Strauchen JA: West J Med 135:276, 1981.

TABLE 157–2. CLASSIFICATION OF THE NON-HODGKIN'S LYMPHOMAS

NCI Working Formulation (1982)	Rappaport Classification (1966)
Low grade	
Small lymphocytic (SLL)	Diffuse lymphocytic, well differentiated (DLWD)
Follicular, small cleaved cell (FSCL)	Nodular lymphocytic, poorly differentiated (NLPD)
Follicular, mixed small cleaved and large cell (FML)	Nodular mixed lymphocytic-histiocytic (NML)
Intermediate grade	
Follicular, large cell (FLCL)	Nodular histiocytic (NHL)
Diffuse, small cleaved cell (DSCL)	Diffuse lymphocytic, poorly differentiated (DLPD)
Diffuse, mixed small cleaved and large cell (DML)	Diffuse mixed lymphocytic-histiocytic (DML)
Diffuse, large cell (cleaved and noncleaved) (DLCL)	Diffuse histiocytic (DHL)
High grade	
Large cell immunoblastic (IBL)	Diffuse histiocytic (DHL)
Lymphoblastic (convoluted and nonconvoluted) (LL)	
Small noncleaved cell (Burkitt and non-Burkitt) (SNCL)	Diffuse undifferentiated (DUL)

may change, usually evolving from a low-grade lymphoma to an intermediate or high-grade lymphoma. Rarely, two histologic subtypes may be present at diagnosis in the same lymph node (composite lymphoma). More often, two histologic subtypes may be seen at diagnosis in two separate biopsy specimens; most frequently, one is seen at diagnosis and a second at relapse or autopsy. It is thought that such "transformation" represents clonal expansion of a more aggressive cell line. Its clinical importance is that both therapy and prognosis may be dramatically altered by its emergence.

DIAGNOSIS AND STAGING

The diagnosis of a neoplasm of the immune system is based upon pathologic classification of biopsy material. This requires adequate tissue (preferably lymph node, so that both architecture and cell type may be assessed), proper handling, and excellent hematopathologic interpretation. Special studies such as imprints, immunotyping, gene rearrangement, karyotyping, TdT determination, and electron microscopy may provide additional information for classification. Since these latter studies require fresh tissue and special handling, it is important that the pathologist be involved *before* biopsy. Likewise, it is important that each case be evaluated jointly by a medical oncologist, radiation therapist, surgeon, and radiologist from the outset.

With the diagnosis established, the extent of disease should be completely defined. Since each neoplasm has distinct clinicopathologic features, the choice of staging studies will be based on that information. All patients should have a complete history, particularly assessing the presence or absence of systemic symptoms, and physical examination. All nodal areas should be examined, including Waldeyer's ring and preauricular, epitrochlear, and popliteal lymph nodes. In addition to liver and spleen, epigastric or other abdominal masses may be found. The lungs, skin, breasts, testicles, and central nervous system should be carefully examined for extranodal involvement. Blood counts and liver and renal function tests are necessary in all patients. In addition to chest radiography, tomography or computed tomography may be indicated in an abnormal chest. Abdominal CT and lymphography are often complementary and not mutually exclusive. Gallium 67 scanning may be useful, but is not a diagnostic method. Liver and spleen scans are of minimal value. Studies of bone or gastrointestinal tract should be performed only when symptoms are present. Bone marrow biopsy is often indicated, particularly if advanced clinical disease is present or the patient has a low-grade lymphoma.

CSF cytology should be determined in all patients with intermediate and high-grade lymphomas who have bone marrow involvement and in all patients with Burkitt's lymphoma, lymphoblastic lymphoma, or malignant histiocytosis.

Several different staging systems are applied to neoplasms of the immune system. Their purpose is to define disease extent, to assist in treatment strategies, to evaluate therapeutic results, and to determine prognosis. In Hodgkin's disease the utility of staging has been elegantly demonstrated, and excellent clinical care demands careful clinical and pathologic staging. Staging laparotomy with splenectomy and biopsy of liver, lymph nodes, and bone marrow was developed for adequate intra-abdominal assessment of Hodgkin's disease. It accurately identifies pathologic stage and its results often dictate treatment strategy. The Ann Arbor staging system for Hodgkin's disease has also been applied to the non-Hodgkin's lymphomas. In this setting it has less value in determining therapy but remains an important prognostic variable. Modified staging systems are used in pediatric lymphomas, chronic lymphocytic leukemia, Burkitt's and lymphoblastic lymphomas, and mycosis fungoides. Since pathologic intra-abdominal assessment is rarely needed to determine treatment in the non-Hodgkin's lymphomas, staging laparotomy is usually unnecessary. Nonetheless, careful clinical staging is imperative in all cases.

DIFFERENTIAL DIAGNOSIS

The differential diagnosis of neoplasms of the immune system is usually that of lymphadenopathy. Reactive processes, infections, other malignant tumors, and collagen-vascular disorders may all cause enlarged lymph nodes or hepatosplenomegaly or both. The location(s) of the lymph nodes, their size, shape, consistency, rapidity of onset, and other characteristics may aid in determining etiology.

Regional lymph node hyperplasia may be seen with acute or chronic infections of the extremities and with vaccinations or insect bites. Diffuse lymphadenopathy may occur following ingestion of phenytoin. Other diffuse reactive processes such as acquired immunodeficiency syndrome, angioimmunoblastic lymphadenopathy, and collagen-vascular disorders may be associated with an increased likelihood of developing lymphoma. Consequently, a single lymph node biopsy may not solve the diagnostic dilemma. That is why pathologic consultation before biopsy is recommended.

Among infectious etiologic factors, viral illnesses predominate and often produce bizarre pathologic material. Infectious mononucleosis may present with features common to Hodgkin's disease. Cytomegalovirus, cat scratch disease, toxoplasmosis, tuberculosis, and syphilis are other considerations. Other malignant neoplasms usually involve lymph nodes by regional spread. For example, cervical lymphadenopathy may be the first symptom of a malignant tumor involving the oropharynx or nasopharynx. Likewise, breast cancer may present with axillary adenopathy and a microscopic primary tumor.

In virtually all instances, the only way to determine conclusively the cause of lymphadenopathy is by pathologic tissue examination. Low cervical and supraclavicular lymph nodes are more likely to yield diagnostic material than axillary and inguinal nodes. When only intrathoracic or abdominal disease is present, bone marrow biopsy may provide diagnostic information and obviate the need for surgery. Fine needle aspiration is of lesser value in neoplasms of the immune system than in solid tumors, because cell morphology and architecture are both important diagnostic parameters.

Berard CW: A multidisciplinary approach to non-Hodgkin's lymphomas. Ann Intern Med 94:218, 1980. *A discussion moderated by Berard of the immunologic concepts pertinent to an understanding of the non-Hodgkin's lymphomas.*

Foon KA, Todd RF III: Immunologic classification of leukemia and lymphoma.

Blood 6:1, 1986. *A comprehensive review of monoclonal antibody and molecular methods of classifying the leukemias and lymphomas.*

Non-Hodgkin's lymphoma pathologic classification project. National Cancer Institute sponsored study of classifications of non-Hodgkin's lymphomas: Summary and description of a working formulation for clinical usage. Cancer 49:2112, 1982. *The working formulation is presented and six pathologic classifications are compared.*

158 THE NON-HODGKIN'S LYMPHOMAS

Carol S. Portlock

The non-Hodgkin's lymphomas are the single largest group of neoplasms of the immune system. Composed of more than ten distinct disease entities, the non-Hodgkin's lymphomas are best understood as a heterogeneous group of malignant diseases whose common link is a characteristic monoclonal expansion of malignant B or T lymphocytes.

EPIDEMIOLOGY

The non-Hodgkin's lymphomas may occur at any age, although they are rarely diagnosed during the first year of life. They occur with increasing frequency throughout adulthood. The incidence is estimated to be approximately 27,000 cases per year in the United States (1986) with males affected more often than females. Moreover, male predominance is most evident among young patients in association with the aggressive histologic subtypes of lymphoblastic and Burkitt's lymphomas.

Geographic clustering is characteristic of some non-Hodgkin's lymphomas: Burkitt's lymphoma in central Africa; adult T cell leukemia/lymphoma in southwestern Japan and the Caribbean; and small intestinal lymphoma with associated immunoglobulin disorders in the Middle East.

Preceding immune dysfunction has been associated with the development of aggressive non-Hodgkin's lymphomas. Congenital immunodeficiency states associated with lymphoma include severe combined immunodeficiency, ataxia-telangiectasia, Wiskott-Aldrich syndrome, X-linked lymphoproliferative syndrome, and common variable immunodeficiency (Ch. 419). Transplant recipients, patients with autoimmune states, and patients with AIDS (acquired immunodeficiency syndrome) also have increased risk of developing lymphoma.

ETIOLOGY AND PATHOGENESIS

The etiology of the non-Hodgkin's lymphomas is unclear. Perhaps the best studied lymphoma is Burkitt's (Ch. 159), with which the Epstein-Barr virus (EBV) has been associated and for which specific chromosomal and oncogene translocations have been implicated in its pathogenesis.

Adult T cell leukemia/lymphoma (ATL), a rare and recently discovered disorder, is associated with a unique human retrovirus, HTLV-I. ATL is endemic in southwestern Japan where 12 to 15 per cent of normal persons have HTLV-I antibodies; it is also found in the Caribbean basin.

The specific chromosomal translocations seen in Burkitt's lymphoma have uniformly involved the *c-myc* oncogene on chromosome 8 and the immunoglobulin heavy- or light-chain genes on chromosomes 14, 2, or 22. Specific chromosomal translocations have also been reported in follicular lymphomas, involving chromosomes 11 and 14 or 18 and 14. The translocation site on chromosome 14 is identical to that in Burkitt's lymphoma, and by analogy, suggests that a transforming gene on chromosome 11 or 18 is activated when brought into proximity with the immunoglobulin heavy-chain

locus. These oncogenes, *bcl-1* (on chromosome 11) and *bcl-2* (on chromosome 18), have been identified and cloned.

In addition to the etiologic considerations of oncogenic viruses and oncogene transformation, other factors that have been associated with an increased incidence of lymphoma include ionizing radiation (whole-body dose greater than 100 rads), hereditary predisposition, and congenital or acquired immunodeficiency.

PATHOLOGY AND CLINICAL FEATURES

Many different pathologic classifications have been proposed for the non-Hodgkin's lymphomas (Ch. 157). Rappaport's classification (Table 157–2) has been the most successfully utilized and applied in clinical trials, while that of Lukes and Collins is more immunologically correct, classifying diseases based on their cell of origin. The National Cancer Institute Working Formulation (1982) is being increasingly accepted, since it is proving both clinically useful and immunologically correct.

Pathologic interpretation of the non-Hodgkin's lymphomas can be supplemented with a variety of complementary studies. Immunophenotyping may identify the cell of origin by demonstrating B cell monoclonal surface immunoglobulin, T cell sheep erythrocyte rosettes (E rosettes), and B or T cell differentiation antigens. Clonality may also be ascertained by detection of the rearrangement of the B cell immunoglobulin genes or of the T cell receptor gene loci. Moreover, the karyotype may reveal a specific chromosomal translocation. The presence of antibody against HTLV-I suggests a T cell lymphoma, whereas HTLV-III antibody suggests an aggressive B cell neoplasm.

Each disease entity of the Working Formulation has a distinct clinical presentation and prognosis, as noted below. The pathologic appearance and some of the clinical characteristics of each category, as outlined in the Working Formulation, are listed in Tables 158-1 and 158-2.

LOW GRADE. The low-grade lymphomas (small lymphocytic [SLL]; follicular, predominantly small cleaved cell [FSCL]; and follicular, mixed, small cleaved and large cell [FML]) have several clinical characteristics in common: (1) Each has a history of waxing and waning or slowly progressive adenopathy. (2) These are rubbery, mobile lymph nodes that are rarely fixed and have no overlying skin infiltration; lymph nodes may be very bulky but are rarely painful. (3) Liver and

TABLE 158–1. PATHOLOGIC CHARACTERISTICS OF THE NON-HODGKIN'S LYMPHOMAS

Subtype	Architectural Pattern	Malignant Lymphocyte Cytology	Immunophenotype/ Immunogenotype
SLL	Diffuse	Small round cells	B cell; rarely T-cell
FSCL	Follicular	Small cleaved cells	B cell
FML	Follicular	Small cleaved cells admixed with large cells, cleaved or noncleaved	B cell
FLCL	Follicular	Large cells cleaved or noncleaved	B cell
DSCL	Diffuse	Small cleaved cells	B cell; occasionally T cell
DML	Diffuse	Admixture of small and large cells cleaved or noncleaved	B cell; T cell
DLCL	Diffuse	Large cells cleaved or noncleaved	B cell; T cell
IBL	Diffuse	Large cells; plasmacytoid, clear, or polymorphic cell variants	B cell; T cell
LBL	Diffuse "starry sky"	Lymphoblasts, convoluted or nonconvoluted nuclei	Thymic T cell
SNCL	Diffuse "starry sky"	Noncleaved cells, round nuclei with prominent nucleoli	B cell

TABLE 158–2. CLINICAL CHARACTERISTICS OF THE NON-HODGKIN'S LYMPHOMAS

Subtype	% of all Lymphomas	Median Age, yr	Sex Ratio M:F	% PS I, II	% PS III, IV	% Bone Marrow Involvement
SLL	3.6	61	1.2:1	11	89	71
FSCL	22.5	54	1.3:1	18	82	51
FML	7.7	56	0.8:1	27	73	30
FLCL	3.8	55	1.8:1	27	73	34
DSCL	6.9	58	2:1	28	72	32
DML	6.7	58	1.1:1	45	55	14
DLCL	19.7	57	1:1	46	54	10
IBL	7.9	51	1.5:1	52	49	12
LBL	4.2	17	1.9:1	27	74	50
SNCL	0.5	30	2.6:1	34	66	14

spleen are frequently involved pathologically and may be enlarged; liver function tests are usually normal, although the alkaline phosphatase may be mildly increased. (4) Bone marrow involvement is common; circulating lymphoma cells may be identified on smear or by cell-sorting techniques. (5) Blood counts are usually normal at diagnosis. Elevation of the white blood cell count with circulating cells, anemia with autoimmune hemolytic anemia, and cytopenias secondary to hypersplenism or bone marrow replacement are uncommon complications. (6) Other extranodal disease sites may include pleura, lung, skin, breast, and gastrointestinal tract. (7) Enlarged lymph nodes may cause lymphedema, ureteral obstruction, or epidural cord compression. (8) Central nervous system (meningeal or parenchymal), renal, or testicular infiltration does not occur.

INTERMEDIATE GRADE AND HIGH GRADE. As a group, the intermediate (follicular, predominantly large cell [FLCL]; diffuse, small cleaved cell [DSCL]; diffuse, mixed small and large cell [DML]; and diffuse, large cell [DLCL]) and high-grade lymphomas (large cell immunoblastic [IBL]; lymphoblastic [LBL]; and small noncleaved cell, including Burkitt's lymphoma and diffuse and undifferentiated lymphoma, non-Burkitt's type [SNCL]) have several general clinical features in common: (1) There is a history of abrupt onset with rapidly enlarging lymph node masses. (2) Lymph nodes may be rubbery and mobile but may also be hard, fixed, and with overlying skin infiltration. Masses may be warm, erythematous, and painful. (3) Bulky lymph node masses (>10 cm) may be present in the mediastinum, retroperitoneum, and/or mesentery. (4) Waldeyer's ring may be involved and is often associated with extranodal disease of the stomach or small bowel or both. (5) Hepatosplenomegaly may be present, and liver function tests may be abnormal. Porta hepatis or even intrahepatic obstructive patterns may be seen. (6) Extranodal involvement is common: stomach, small bowel, lung, skin, bone, and central nervous system (particularly meningeal disease in association with bone marrow involvement). Rarely ovarian, testicular, or renal disease may be present. (7) Bone marrow involvement and circulating cells are less commonly seen at diagnosis than in low-grade lymphomas. A leukemic picture may emerge, however, when progressive disease develops. (8) Lymph node masses may cause lymphedema, ureteral obstruction, vascular obstruction (superior vena cava syndrome, thrombophlebitis), and epidural cord compression.

MISCELLANEOUS. A miscellaneous category of the Working Formulation includes mycosis fungoides—a rare helper T cell lymphoma of the skin; composite lymphoma—multiple histologic subtypes (e.g., FSCL and IBL) occurring simultaneously; and true histiocytic lymphoma.

Since the Formulation's publication in 1982, additional mature T cell lymphomas have been recognized. The peripheral T cell lymphomas are a diverse group of "post-thymic" neoplasms, whose cell of origin is the differentiated T cell. Their morphology includes diffuse small-cell, mixed-cell, large-cell, or immunoblastic lymphoma, as well as subgroups with histologic features of angioimmunoblastic lymphadenopathy, lymphomatoid granulomatosis, Hodgkin's-like disease, or Lennert's lymphoma. Clinical features include a 2:1 male predominance, prominent extranodal disease (particularly lung involvement) in the majority, systemic symptoms, and skin rash. In general, response to treatment and survival appear to parallel their counterparts in the Working Formulation.

HTLV-I associated adult T cell leukemia/lymphoma is characterized by geographic clustering, the presence of antibody to HTLV-I, and a rapidly fatal clinical course. Clinical features include abrupt onset of generalized lymphadenopathy, hepatosplenomegaly, skin infiltration, lytic bone disease, bone marrow involvement with circulating cells, and hypercalcemia. In spite of intensive chemotherapy, median survival is less than one year. Although clinically distinct, this rare T cell lymphoma is not easily distinguishable pathologically from other T cell lymphomas. Diffuse small-cell, mixed-cell, large-cell, and undifferentiated cell types have all been described. Therefore, clinical suspicion and the presence of HTLV-I antibody are necessary to confirm the diagnosis.

DIAGNOSIS AND STAGING

As discussed in Ch. 157, the diagnosis of a non-Hodgkin's lymphoma requires skilled interpretation of adequate tumor tissue, preferably from an involved lymph node, so that tumor architecture as well as cell type may be assessed. B cell and T cell typing studies may complement the pathologic interpretation, but do not supplant it. The clinical history and ancillary studies, e.g., HTLV-I or -III antibody, may also contribute. Once a diagnosis has been established, then it is useful to determine the extent of disease through staging.

The Ann Arbor staging system utilized for Hodgkin's disease (see Ch. 160) is also used in the management of non-Hodgkin's lymphomas. Although of clinical value, this staging system has several shortcomings when applied to non-Hodgkin's lymphomas: Factors such as disease site, disease bulk, and extent of extranodal involvement are not considered. In addition, the presence of systemic symptoms plays a lesser role in influencing treatment planning and prognosis in non-Hodgkin's lymphoma. Nevertheless, thorough pretreatment staging is necessary in all patients.

Noninvasive studies, which should be obtained in all patients, are listed in Table 158–3.

Based on this information, clinical stage of the lymphoma can be determined. Since bone marrow involvement is so common, particularly in low-grade lymphoma, bilateral percutaneous bone marrow biopsies are often the simplest way to establish pathologic stage IV disease.

Pathologic confirmation of other extranodal sites may be appropriate, as when gastroscopic biopsy, pleural cytology, or skin biopsy is obtained. Laparotomy or thoracotomy is indicated only in those patients with no other evident disease or when a gastrointestinal tumor is removed prior to treatment. Staging laparotomy as performed for Hodgkin's disease is rarely if ever indicated.

TABLE 158–3. NONINVASIVE STUDIES IN NON-HODGKIN'S LYMPHOMA

History with assessment of systemic symptoms, predisposing epidemiologic factors
Physical examination
CBC and platelet count; Coombs' test if anemic
Liver and renal function tests
Serum immunoglobulins in low-grade lymphomas
Antibody for HTLV-I or HTLV-III, if indicated
Chest radiograph, PA and lateral
Chest computed tomography, if indicated
Abdominal and pelvic computed tomography
  If unavailable, abdominal ultrasound study
  If normal, lymphography possibly indicated
Bone scan and bone radiographs if clinical involvement suspected
Upper gastrointestinal series, if clinical involvement suspected or if Waldeyer's ring involved
Gallium scan (in SNCL)
CSF cytology (in all patients with intermediate or high-grade lymphomas and known bone marrow disease)

TREATMENT

In defining a treatment approach for the patient with non-Hodgkin's lymphoma, it is necessary to consider such factors as histologic subtype, stage, sites of disease, tumor bulk, thoroughness of initial staging, general medical condition, and age, as well as the goals and effectiveness of therapy. In practical terms the non-Hodgkin's lymphomas can be considered in two broad categories: those diseases that progress slowly and have an indolent natural history (the low-grade lymphomas) and those diseases that present aggressively, progress rapidly, and if unsuccessfully treated are soon fatal (the intermediate and high-grade lymphomas).

LOW-GRADE LYMPHOMAS. As outlined above, low-grade lymphomas infrequently present with truly localized disease (pathologic stage I or II). Only 11 to 27 per cent, depending upon histologic subtype, are therefore eligible for regional treatment with radiation therapy. Although uncommon, this disease presentation appears to be highly favorable, with more than 75 per cent of patients remaining free of disease for ten years or longer after irradiation alone (3500 to 4400 rads to the region).

Many more patients appear to have clinically localized disease after noninvasive staging and bone marrow biopsy, but have not undergone complete laparotomy staging. Under these circumstances, radiation therapy may still accomplish good local control. Many patients, however, will have undetected microscopic disease outside the treatment portal that will slowly progress and lead to disease recurrence several years after initial therapy. Nevertheless, irradiation may still be a reasonable choice, since relapse may occur years later, and salvage treatment at relapse may be effective. Patients eligible for this approach are those with peripheral lymph node presentations (stage I and II) involving cervical, supraclavicular, axillary, or inguinal regions. Abdominal masses usually require whole-abdominal irradiation in which this approach may not be justified. Thoracic presentations are rare.

The majority (74 to 89 per cent) of patients with low-grade lymphomas have advanced stage (III or IV) disease and are therefore ineligible for localized treatment approaches. Optimal management of such patients remains controversial. Complete disappearance of all known tumor (including bone marrow biopsy) may be induced in more than 80 per cent of patients with single or multiagent chemotherapy, with whole-body irradiation, or with combined chemotherapy-irradiation. Unfortunately, remissions are usually limited to two and one half to five years. These seemingly complete responders actually have persistent circulating lymphoma cells in their peripheral blood. The presence of such cells correlates with subsequent relapse.

The most successful current chemotherapy program is C-MOPP (cyclophosphamide, vincristine (Oncovin), procarba-zine, and prednisone). Initially employed in advanced stage FML, ten-year results reveal six of twelve complete responders still in remission. Although a larger prospective study did not confirm the remission durability of C-MOPP in FML, it did show a significant remission advantage in FSCL. Current investigative programs are designed to intensify the chemotherapy-radiation therapy regimens in an attempt to eradicate the malignant clone.

In summary, a standard treatment regimen in advanced low-grade lymphoma has not been established. Daily single-agent cyclophosphamide; daily or pulse chlorambucil; combinations of cyclophosphamide, vincristine, prednisone with or without procarbazine or Adriamycin are reasonable choices depending upon the clinical circumstances. Enrollment in a protocol regimen is encouraged whenever possible, since an optimal treatment regimen has not been identified.

Another management approach in patients with advanced stage low-grade non-Hodgkin's lymphomas is initial treatment deferral with institution of therapy when there is disease progression. This approach is based on the premise that treatment at diagnosis does not appear curative. Many patients have indolent, slowly progressive disease, and treatment deferral does not appear to compromise therapeutic outcome. Approximately one half of all patients may be eligible for observation at diagnosis; the median treatment-free period correlates with histology: more than eight years for SLL, five years for FSCL, and ten months for FML.

Biologic therapies have also been investigated in low-grade lymphomas and appear to have transient efficacy. These include monoclonal antibody therapy directed specifically against the malignant B cell immunoglobulin idiotype, antibody against B cell differentiation antigens, and alpha-interferon.

In up to 50 per cent of patients low-grade lymphomas may change with or without treatment from an indolent to an aggressive form by the eighth year following diagnosis. Most often the transformation presents as rapidly growing disease in one or more sites, while the low-grade component remains stable or progresses slowly. Pathologic study reveals DLCL, IBL, or other aggressive subtypes, and studies of clonality are consistent with the low-grade histology (B cell primarily). Most transformations represent emergence of an aggressive subclone from the original indolent disease, but some cases appear to represent the emergence of a completely new second neoplasm that is a clonally distinct, aggressive lymphoma in the setting of indolent lymphoma.

Histologic transformation is important to recognize, since it has prognostic and therapeutic implications. Median survival is less than one year following its emergence, and intensive treatment programs are necessary to gain disease control. Some patients appear to have the aggressive component eradicated by such measures, often with persistence or later relapse of the indolent histology.

INTERMEDIATE AND HIGH-GRADE LYMPHOMAS. Intensive combination chemotherapy is the mainstay of curative treatment in the aggressive non-Hodgkin's lymphomas. Of the half of all patients who may present with regional disease alone, only that small subset with pathologic stage I presentation may be eligible for radiation therapy alone. This is because the intent and realistic goal of treatment in the aggressive lymphomas is always cure, and relapse must be avoided whenever possible.

The expectation of cure in the vast majority of patients with aggressive lymphomas, regardless of stage, is based upon the following observations in advanced disease: (1) Tumors are rapidly proliferating and initially very sensitive to combination chemotherapy. (2) Survival curves in advanced disease are biphasic, revealing a rapid death rate during the two years (composed of partial and nonresponding patients) and then a plateau of cured cases (composed of complete responders). (3) With intensifying drug regimens the proportion of com-

TABLE 158–4. REPRESENTATIVE DRUG COMBINATIONS FOR INTERMEDIATE AND HIGH-GRADE NON-HODGKIN'S LYMPHOMAS

MACOP-B

Methotrexate	400 mg/m² IV	Weeks 2, 6, 10 with leucovorin
Adriamycin	50 mg/m² IV	Weeks 1, 3, 5, 7, 9, 11
Cyclophosphamide	350 mg/m² IV	Weeks 1, 3, 5, 7, 9, 11
Oncovin	1.4 mg/m² IV	Weeks 2, 4, 6, 8, 10, 12
Prednisone	75 mg PO	Daily, dose tapered over the last 15 days
Bleomycin	10 U/m² IV	Weeks 4, 8, 12
Co-trimoxazole	2 tab PO	Twice daily throughout

ProMACE-MOPP

Prednisone	60 mg/m² PO	Days 1–14
Methotrexate	500 mg/m² IV	Day 15 with leucovorin
Adriamycin	25 mg/m² IV	Days 1 and 8
Cyclophosphamide	650 mg/m² IV	Day 1
Etoposide (VP-16)	120 mg/m² IV	Day 1
Mechlorethamine	6 mg/m² IV	Day 8
Oncovin	1.4 mg/m² IV	Day 8
Procarbazine	100 mg/m² PO	Days 8–14
Prednisone	60 mg/m² PO	Days 8–14

m-BACOD

Methotrexate	200 mg/m² IV	Days 8 and 15 with leucovorin
Bleomycin	4 mg/m² IV	Day 1
Adriamycin	45 mg/m² IV	Day 1
Cyclophosphamide	600 mg/m² IV	Day 1
Oncovin	1 mg/m² IV	Day 1
Dexamethasone	6 mg/m² PO	Days 1–5

CHOP-B

Cyclophosphamide	1 gram/m² IV	Day 1
Hydroxydaunomycin/ Adriamycin	40 mg/m² IV	Day 1
Oncovin	2 mg IV	
Prednisone	100 mg PO	Days 1–5
Bleomycin	15 U IV	Days 1 and 5

plete responders may be increased and, likewise, the proportion cured. (4) Increasing tumor bulk correlates with decreased complete response, the emergence of drug resistance, and poor survival. (5) The highest complete response rates to combination chemotherapy are achieved in patients with regional or disseminated nonbulky disease.

Commonly used agents in combination regimens include: cyclophosphamide, Adriamycin, vincristine, prednisone, methotrexate, bleomycin, etoposide, and cytosine arabinoside. Representative regimens are listed in Table 158–4. Treatment should be initiated promptly after diagnosis and appropriate noninvasive staging; the regimen must be intensive (leading to at least moderate toxicity), administered in high and often escalating doses, on a rigorous schedule; attention must be paid to rapidity of response and any evidence of early drug resistance; and after a defined treatment course, complete restaging is undertaken. Utilizing these guidelines, at least 60 per cent of patients with advanced disease and more than 80 per cent with localized disease will achieve complete response. The majority of complete responses (>70 per cent) are durable, and maintenance chemotherapy is unnecessary.

Intensification of drug treatment has led to further improvement in the results of combination chemotherapy. The MACOP:B drug regimen, for example, delivers high-dose, weekly alternating therapy for 12 weeks followed by no maintenance chemotherapy. Preliminary results reveal 51 of 61 patients (83 per cent) with DLCL achieving complete response and 90 per cent disease free at two years. Another investigative approach has been the use of potentially lethal doses of chemotherapeutic agents with autologous bone marrow rescue in high-risk patients. Preliminary reports suggest that this approach is superior to standard combination chemotherapy.

SPECIAL CONSIDERATIONS. *Histopathologic Subtype.* Lymphoblastic lymphoma and SNCL are often treated with modified intensive drug programs, and all patients require central nervous system prophylaxis.

Mediastinal Disease. Superior vena cava syndrome may be present and is effectively managed with irradiation and/or chemotherapy. Biopsy of undetermined mediastinal masses

must be accomplished with less than 750 to 1000 rads (200 to 250 rad fractions) prophylactic irradiation before biopsy.

Gastrointestinal Disease. Perforation or bleeding or both are frequent complications prior to or following treatment. To avoid this, surgical resection of the involved region is often recommended prior to therapy.

Central Nervous System. All patients with lymphoblastic lymphoma and SNCL, as well as those with other aggressive histologic types and bone marrow involvement, are at risk for meningeal disease. CSF cytology is determined before therapy, and meningeal prophylaxis is given.

Primary brain lymphoma, as often identified in immunodeficient patients, requires high-dose whole-brain irradiation with or without chemotherapy.

Tumor Masses Larger than 10 Cm. Supplementary irradiation is often administered concurrently with or following chemotherapy. Residual fibrosis may occasionally persist after therapy.

Tumor Lysis Syndrome. Rapid tumor shrinkage with excess urate production should be anticipated in all patients and allopurinol administered. With bulky or disseminated tumor or both, rapid cell lysis may lead to hyperkalemia, hypocalcemia, hyperphosphatemia, hyperuricemia, and acute renal failure. Patients with SNCL and lymphoblastic lymphoma are most often affected (see Ch. 159).

PROGNOSIS

The Working Formulation identifies more than ten distinct disease entities and groups them according to prognosis. The survival curves upon which these prognostic groups were initially based are no longer entirely valid because of improved treatment methods. Nevertheless, it is still important to recognize a low-grade category in which the lymphoma progresses slowly and has an indolent natural history, as well as intermediate and high-grade categories in which the disease

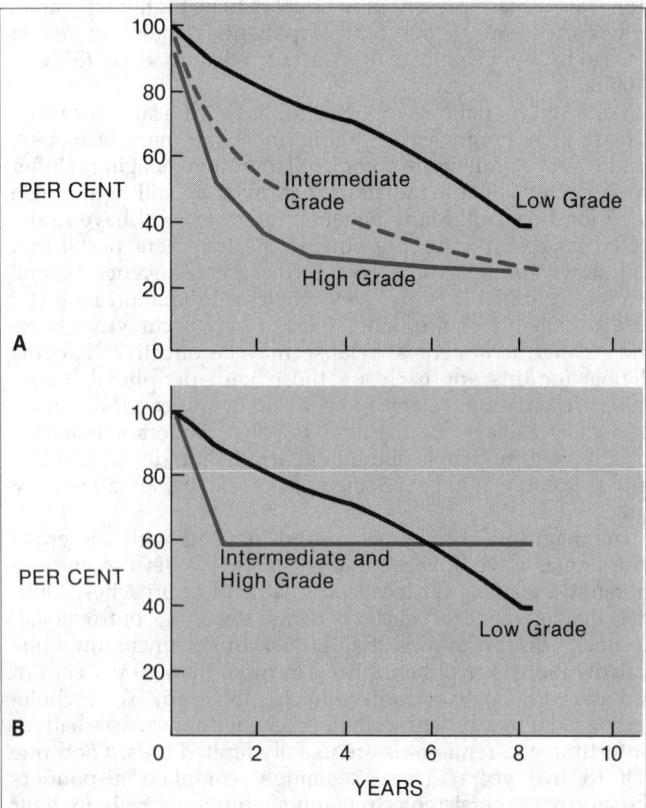

FIGURE 158–1. *A,* Actuarial survival according to histologic grade, based on 1975 data, as reported in the Working Formulation (1982). *B,* Hypothetical actuarial survival according to histologic grade, based on 1985 data (see text).

presents aggressively, progresses rapidly and, if unsuccessfully treated, is soon fatal.

In Figure 158–1A are the overall survival curves of the original Working Formulation (based on 1975 data) according to prognostic category. The median survivals are approximately six and one half years for the low-grade, two and one half years for the intermediate-grade, and one and one half years for the high-grade categories. Figure 158–1B illustrates representative overall survival curves based on 1985 data, according to prognostic category. The median survival in the low-grade category is six and one half years, unchanged from the original Working Formulation; whereas the median survival for the intermediate and high-grade categories has not yet been reached, and at least 60 per cent of all patients remain alive and disease free at five years. Followed to eight years, the curves overlap as patients in the low-grade category succumb to progressive lymphoma, while patients in the intermediate and high-grade categories continue disease free.

This, then, is the prognostic paradox of the non-Hodgkin's lymphomas: Initially favorable and indolent, the low-grade histologic types are, in fact, the unfavorable category with longer observation; and initially unfavorable and aggressive intermediate and high-grade histologic types are, in fact, the favorable categories, since cure may be regularly achieved.

Broder S: T-cell lymphoproliferative syndrome associated with human T-cell leukemia/lymphoma virus. Ann Intern Med 100:543, 1984. *HTLV-I–associated adult T cell leukemia-lymphoma is discussed in detail in this NIH symposium: clinical features, pathology, epidemiology, and molecular biology.*

Klimo P, Connors JM: MACOP-B chemotherapy for the treatment of diffuse large-cell lymphoma. Ann Intern Med 102:596, 1985. *An intensive weekly combination chemotherapy program completed in three months, yielding complete responses in 51 of 61 patients. Relapse-free survival for complete responders was 90 per cent at two years post-therapy.*

Matis LA, Young RC, Longo DL: Nodular lymphomas: Current concepts. CRC Crit Rev Oncol Hematol 5:171, 1986. *A thorough review of low-grade lymphomas: Clinical management, immunobiology, and molecular biology.*

Skarin AT (ed.): Update on treatment for diffuse large-cell lymphoma. In Advances in Cancer Chemotherapy. Park Row Publishers, Inc., 1986. *Proceedings of a symposium updating combination chemotherapy regimens for diffuse large cell lymphoma.*

Sweet DL, Kinzie J, Gaeke ME, et al.: Survival of patients with localized diffuse histiocytic lymphoma. Blood 58:1218, 1981. *Results of radiation therapy alone in pathologic stage I and II patients. At 11 years, disease-free survival was 93 per cent for stages I and IE; 33 per cent for stages II and IIE.*

The Non-Hodgkin's Lymphoma Pathologic Classification Project: National Cancer Institute sponsored study of classifications of non-Hodgkin's lymphomas: Summary and description of a working formulation for clinical usage. Cancer 49:2112, 1982. *The Working Formulation is presented in detail with pathologic and clinical analyses.*

Waldmann TA, Korsmeyer SJ, Bakhshi A, et al.: Molecular genetic analysis of human lymphoid neoplasms: Immunoglobulin genes and the *c-myc* oncogene. Ann Intern Med 102:497, 1985. *Immunoglobulin gene rearrangement is reviewed and its clinical utility assessed; translocations in Burkitt's lymphomas are also discussed.*

Weis JW, Winter MW, Phylikey RL, et al.: Peripheral T-cell lymphomas: Histologic, immunohistologic, and clinical characterization. Mayo Clin Proc 61:411, 1986. *A review of 40 cases of peripheral T-cell lymphomas emphasizing their histologic and clinical diversity as well as the importance of immunophenotyping.*

Ziegler JL, Beckstead JA, Volberding PA, et al.: Non-Hodgkin's lymphoma in 90 homosexual men: Relation to generalized lymphadenopathy and the acquired immunodeficiency syndrome. N Engl J Med 311:565, 1984. *Aggressive histology of non-Hodgkin's lymphomas involving central nervous system, gastrointestinal tract, and other unusual extranodal sites are described in high-risk homosexual males.*

159 BURKITT'S LYMPHOMA

Carol S. Portlock

Burkitt's lymphoma is a rare monoclonal B cell neoplasm of great biologic importance. It was first described in 1958 by Dr. Denis Burkitt, who reported rapidly growing jaw tumors and abdominal masses in Ugandan children. Over the next 25 years, the elucidation of its unique epidemiologic, pathologic, clinical, and laboratory features has pioneered research into the etiology, pathogenesis, and therapy of lymphoma.

EPIDEMIOLOGY

Burkitt's lymphoma is the most common childhood malignant disorder in Uganda. The disease is found along a "lymphoma belt" lying approximately 10 degrees north and 10 degrees south of the African equator. Within the belt there are altitude, temperature, and rainfall restrictions; these climatic conditions are similar to those of Papua, New Guinea, where Burkitt's lymphoma is also commonly identified. Holoendemic or hyperendemic malaria follows the geographic distribution of the lymphoma belt and originally suggested to Burkitt a mosquito-borne vector and/or associated host immune dysfunction.

In addition to its geographic restrictions, endemic Burkitt's lymphoma is associated with time-space clustering. Nonendemic Burkitt's lymphoma, a similar disease occurring rarely and sporadically in other areas of the world (less than one case per million annually in the United States), has also been reported to occur in time-space clusters. Moreover, nonendemic Burkitt's lymphomas may be associated with preceding immune dysfunction (e.g., organ transplantation and acquired immune deficiency syndrome).

ETIOLOGY AND PATHOGENESIS

The Epstein-Barr virus (EBV) is present in almost 90 per cent of African Burkitt's lymphoma but less than half of nonendemic cases. Whether the virus plays an etiologic role or is merely a passenger in Burkitt's lymphoma remains controversial. Typically, primary EBV infection precedes the development of Burkitt's lymphoma by at least seven or more months. Ugandan children with high EBV capsid antigen titers have a 30-fold greater risk of developing Burkitt's lymphoma as compared with controls. Elevated EBV/VCA titers are also associated with a favorable prognosis in both African and nonendemic tumors.

Specific chromosomal translocations have been identified in Burkitt's lymphoma (with or without the concurrent detection of EBV) and involve chromosomes 2, 8, 14, and 22. The most frequent translocation is t(8;14) (q24;q32) and less commonly t(2;8) (p12;q24) and t(8;22) (q24;q11). The immunoglobulin heavy chain maps to chromosome 14, κ light chain to chromosome 2, and λ light chain to 22. In cell culture, there is a direct correlation between the kind of light chain expressed and the type of chromosomal translocation. Moreover, the cellular oncogene *c-myc* maps to chromosome 8 and is involved in each of the three translocations specific to Burkitt's lymphoma. When *c-myc* is translocated to chromosome 14 within the immunoglobulin heavy-chain gene, the break may occur at different nucleotide sequences, e.g., the variable or switch regions, in different Burkitt's cell lines. It is proposed that this transposition of the oncogene to a transcriptionally active site may thus lead to oncogene activation and ultimately, lymphomagenesis. The delineation of the role of *c-myc* and/or other oncogenes in the etiology of Burkitt's lymphoma and the inter-relationship of *c-myc* (if any) with EBV awaits future research.

PATHOLOGY

Burkitt's lymphoma is classified as a high-grade small noncleaved cell malignant lymphoma. It is composed of intermediate-size lymphoid cells containing round nuclei of uniform size and shape, with coarse chromatin and one or more distinct nucleoli. A rim of basophilic cytoplasm is usually present. Large numbers of mitotic figures are invariably seen and a "starry sky" pattern is characteristic. The cells are of monoclonal B cell lineage, expressing IgM of a single light-chain class on their cell surface.

CLINICAL FEATURES

Although similar histologically, African and nonendemic Burkitt's lymphomas are clinically distinct. The African disease affects children aged 2 to 16, average 7 years, with a 2:1 male predominance. Bulky extranodal tumors of the jaw (70 per cent), abdominal viscera (50 per cent), particularly kidneys, ovaries, and retroperitoneum, and meninges (30 per cent) predominate. Nonendemic Burkitt's affects children primarily, average 11 years, but has been documented in adults as old as 70 years. Male predominance is only evident in patients younger than 15 years. Jaw tumors are rare, abdominal disease involves mesenteric lymph nodes rather than viscera, and bone marrow involvement is frequent.

Burkitt's lymphoma has a growth fraction approaching 100 per cent and a tumor doubling time in vivo of less than three days. Patients present with dramatic enlargement of tumors, and these rapidly enlarging masses may obstruct the gastrointestinal tract or ureters or compress nerve roots or spinal cord. Metabolic consequences of rapid tumor growth include excess urate and lactic acid production as well as acute renal failure.

DIAGNOSIS AND STAGING

The diagnosis must be established by biopsy, since the clinical features are not specific. Diseases that may present similarly include other non-Hodgkin's lymphomas, acute myelogenous leukemia with chloromas, plasmacytoma, fibrous dysplasia of bone, disseminated fungal infection, and several pediatric solid tumors (rhabdomyosarcoma, neuroblastoma, retinoblastoma, and Wilms' tumor). In addition to pathologic sections, touch imprints, immunotyping, and tumor karyotype may be of value.

Rigorous staging is of less therapeutic and prognostic importance in Burkitt's lymphoma than in other lymphomas because all patients receive chemotherapy and the rapidity of disease progression demands treatment within 48 hours of presentation. Nevertheless, it is important to document disease extent to evaluate therapeutic efficacy. Studies should include a careful history and physical examination, blood counts, chemistries (including lactate dehydrogenase), chest radiograph, abdominal computed tomography, gallium 67 scan, bone marrow biopsy or aspirate, and CSF cytology.

MANAGEMENT AND PROGNOSIS

The most important prognostic variable in Burkitt's lymphoma is total tumor volume at initiation of chemotherapy. Surgical debulking prior to chemotherapy is clearly of value in those patients with localized disease. On the other hand, radiation therapy does not offer the same benefit. Combination chemotherapy is used in all patients and may be highly effective. High dose cyclophosphamide may be curative as a single agent; however, the complete response rates and remission durability of combination regimens are superior.

Prior to initiation of chemotherapy it is mandatory to carry out anticipatory therapy of uric acid nephropathy and acute tumor-lysis syndrome (rapid rises in serum potassium, phosphate, uric acid, xanthine, and LDH with reciprocal fall in serum calcium).

With current combination chemotherapy programs (which include cyclophosphamide, Adriamycin, vincristine, and methotrexate) virtually all patients achieve complete remission, while approximately half will have relapse. In spite of CNS prophylaxis, meningeal relapse is common. Nevertheless, aggressive second-line approaches, including high dose regimens with bone marrow transplantation, may be curative. Most relapses after discontinuing initial treatment occur during the first three to six months and are unaffected by maintenance therapy. However, in African Burkitt's lymphoma, very late relapses (occurring 12 to 79 months after

discontinuation of treatment) have been reported. Whether some of these relapses represent second neoplasms is not known.

Burkitt DP: The discovery of Burkitt's lymphoma. Cancer 51:1777, 1983. *A personal account.*

Magrath IT, Janus C, Edwards BK, et al.: An effective therapy for both undifferentiated (including Burkitt's) lymphomas and lymphoblastic lymphomas in children and young adults. Blood 63:1102, 1084. *Results of a multiagent intensive drug combination program with intrathecal chemotherapy are described.*

Ziegler JL: Burkitt's lymphoma. N Engl J Med 305:735, 1981. *A complete review of laboratory and clinical data, as well as recommendations for management.*

160 HODGKIN'S DISEASE

John H. Glick

DEFINITION. Hodgkin's disease is a unique malignant disorder, usually arising in lymph nodes, with a characteristic histopathologic appearance. It is defined by the presence of the virtually pathognomonic Reed-Sternberg giant cell in an appropriate cellular background. The disease was first recognized as a distinct clinicopathologic entity in 1832 by Thomas Hodgkin, who described seven patients with a fatal illness involving "hypertrophy of the lymphatic system." Although the etiology is unknown, definitive evidence has emerged that Hodgkin's disease is indeed a malignant neoplasm and not a granulomatous infection or a chronic immunologic disorder. Advances in the pathology, staging, and treatment of Hodgkin's disease during the past two decades have provided a dramatic improvement in the prognosis and potential for cure of all patients with this disease.

ETIOLOGY AND PATHOGENESIS. The cause of Hodgkin's disease is unknown, and the nature of the Reed-Sternberg cell remains an enigma. The Reed-Sternberg giant cell as well as its mononuclear variants is malignant, as established by sustained proliferation in vitro, aneuploidy, and heterotransplantability when inoculated intracerebrally into nude mice. Spleen cells taken from Hodgkin's patients have been grown in tissue culture, with the demonstration of macrophage characteristics, including phagocytic activity and surface receptors for the Fc fragment of immunoglobulins and for the C3b component of complement. Reed-Sternberg cells closely resemble interdigitating reticulum cells found in the interfollicular or T cell region of lymph nodes. Both demonstrate strong expression of human Ia-like antigens, a close physical association with helper/inducer T cells, and a lack of at least two common macrophage antigens. Malignant transformation of the interdigitating reticulum cell to a Reed-Sternberg cell could result in diminished antigen-presenting capacity and could contribute to the known defect in T cell–mediated immunity commonly observed in Hodgkin's disease patients.

The controversy pertaining to the cell of origin is far from resolved. A mouse monoclonal antibody against the Hodgkin cell line L428 has been noted to be specific for both Reed-Sternberg cells and their mononuclear variants, and for a minute and distinct new cell population in normal tonsils and lymph nodes. This observation suggests that a previously unrecognized early myeloid-monocytoid cell may be the progenitor of the Reed-Sternberg cell.

No confirmation of a suggested bacterial, viral, or fungal cause has been obtained. The problem of frequent secondary infections in the immunocompromised patient with advanced Hodgkin's disease continues to thwart investigators searching for an infectious origin. Any theory of the cause of Hodgkin's disease must account for the wide panorama of histopathologic and clinical presentations, the variety of neoplastic giant cells, the signs of an inflammatory reaction and infectious-like symptoms, the characteristic immunologic defects, and the specific epidemiologic patterns.

EPIDEMIOLOGY. Only 7100 new cases of Hodgkin's disease are diagnosed each year in the United States, with approximately 1600 deaths. These patients average 32 years of age and are more commonly male than female. The age-specific distribution curve is an unusual bimodal pattern for both sexes, with the first peak at ages 15 to 35 and the second after age 50. Hodgkin's disease is distributed throughout the world, but the age-specific rates differ markedly in different countries. The developed areas of the United States and Northern Europe have a prominent young adult peak, which is lower in less developed countries and absent in Japan.

There is an inverse risk with family size, with a rate 2.5 times greater among persons without siblings than those with four or more siblings. There is up to a seven-fold increased risk among siblings of young adults with Hodgkin's disease. Increased risk also occurs with early birth order position and improved living conditions. All these factors tend to decrease and delay exposure to infectious agents. It has been suggested that Hodgkin's disease may be an age-dependent host response to a common infection. Population-based studies have failed to document significant "clustering" of cases. No increased risk in medical personnel exposed to large numbers of Hodgkin's patients has been observed. Thus, at the present time, there is no firm evidence for a contagious etiology.

PATHOLOGY. Histologic diagnosis of Hodgkin's disease requires the presence of characteristic Reed-Sternberg giant cells in association with an appropriate stromal background or cellular milieu. The classic Reed-Sternberg cell (Fig. 160–1A) is a large, bilobed cell with prominent eosinophilic nucleoli, perinucleolar clearing, thick nuclear membrane, and relatively abundant cytoplasm. Distinctive multinuclear giant cells in lacunar-like spaces (Fig. 160–1B) are associated with the nodular sclerosis subtype and are considered Reed-Sternberg variants. Mononuclear variants are also found on biopsy but cannot be considered as reliably diagnostic. Although the diagnosis of Hodgkin's disease is rarely made in the absence of Reed-Sternberg cells, the presence of such a cell is not pathognomonic of the disease. Cells indistinguishable from or closely resembling Reed-Sternberg cells may be found in reactive conditions such as infectious mononucleosis in which immunoblasts, or transformed lymphocytes, may mimic Reed-Sternberg cells. The character of the stromal background is as important for the diagnosis of Hodgkin's disease as is the Reed-Sternberg cell. This background consists of a mixed population of cytologically benign cells, including reactive lymphocytes, benign histiocytes, plasma cells, and eosinophils.

Frozen section material should not be used to make a definitive diagnosis when Hodgkin's disease is suspected because of the presence of artifacts. Formalin-fixed tissue is required for careful histologic review. If any uncertainty of diagnosis exists, consultation with an experienced hematopathologist is required. The monoclonal antibody Leu-M1, which reacts with granulocytes, stains Reed-Sternberg cells and their mononuclear variants. This immunodiagnostic marker may be particularly useful in distinguishing Hodgkin's disease from other lymphoproliferative disorders such as peripheral T cell lymphomas. Needle aspiration of lymph nodes for diagnostic purposes is generally not reliable because insufficient tissue is obtained for accurate evaluation.

Hodgkin's disease is subclassified histopathologically into four subtypes according to the Rye classification (Table 160–1). The relative frequency of the four groups is variable in different series, depending on epidemiologic and patient referral factors. The natural history of Hodgkin's disease correlates well with the histopathologic groups. The *lymphocyte predominance type* is the most favorable and is associated with early stage disease in asymptomatic patients with nodal

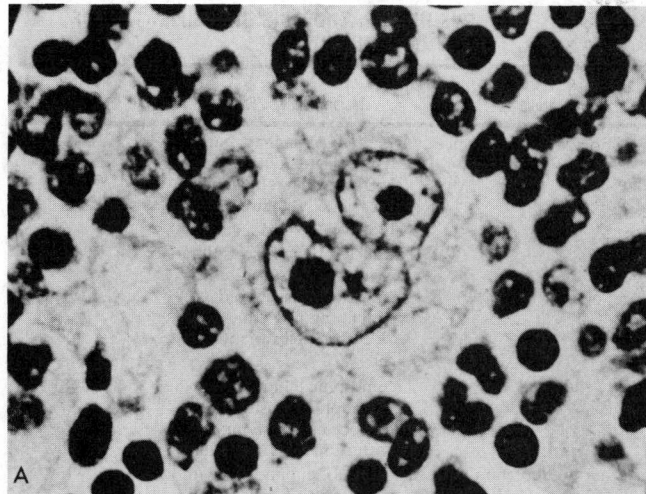

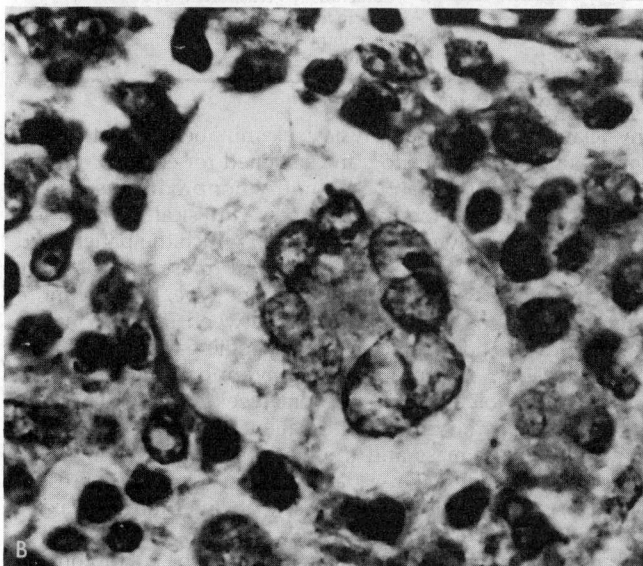

FIGURE 160–1. Pathologic diagnosis. *A,* Diagnostic Reed-Sternberg cell with large inclusion-like nucleoli, high power. *B,* Reed-Sternberg cell variant, lacunar cell type, high power. (Reprinted by permission from Tindle BH: Pathology of Lymphomas. In Bennett JM [ed.]: Lymphomas I. The Hague, Martinus Nijhoff, 1981, p 70.)

presentations. The *nodular sclerosis variety* has a relatively favorable prognosis, usually occurs in young women with multiple node groups, and frequently involves the mediastinum. The *mixed cellularity pattern* tends to occur in middle-aged patients with systemic symptoms and more extensive disease than is first evident on initial presentation. The *lymphocyte depletion subtype* has the least favorable prognosis, as it generally occurs in patients with advanced stage disease, systemic symptoms, and frequently involves the bone marrow. Advances in aggressive therapy, after precise staging, have obscured the prognostic value of histopathologic classification.

CLINICAL MANIFESTATIONS. The initial presentation and subsequent clinical course of patients with Hodgkin's disease can be extremely variable, depending on when in the natural history the patient first seeks medical attention.

Adenopathy. The majority of patients present with a painless and enlarging mass, most commonly in the neck, but occasionally in the axilla or inguinal-femoral region. This lymphadenopathy is usually discovered accidentally by the patient and is often the only manifestation of the disease at the time of diagnosis. Upon examination, this mass is found to be a discrete rubbery usually nontender lymph node or group of surrounding enlarged and matted lymph nodes. Asymptomatic lymphadenopathy also may be noted by the

TABLE 160–1. RYE HISTOPATHOLOGIC CLASSIFICATION OF HODGKIN'S DISEASE*

Subgroup	Major Histologic Features	Relative Frequency
Lymphocyte predominance	Abundant normal-appearing lymphocyte infiltrate with or without benign histiocytes; occasionally nodular; rare Reed-Sternberg (R-S) cells	5–15%
Nodular sclerosis	Nodules of lymphoid infiltrate of varying size, separated by bands of collagen and containing numerous "lacunar" cell variants of R-S cells	40–75%
Mixed cellularity	Pleomorphic infiltrate of eosinophils, plasma cells, histiocytes, and lymphocytes with numerous R-S cells	20–40%
Lymphocyte depletion	Paucity of lymphocytes with numerous R-S cells, often bizarre in appearance; may have diffuse fibrosis or reticulum fibers	5–15%

*Modified from Lukes and Butler.

physician on a routine physical examination. In other instances, a chest roentgenogram, obtained for either a routine purpose or because of a persistent dry nonproductive cough, may demonstrate a mediastinal mass. Physical examination may then disclose lymphadenopathy of which the patient had been unaware. Although these typical presentations may occur at any age with any histopathologic type, they are more common in young patients, usually between 15 and 35 years of age with the nodular sclerosis histologic pattern.

The duration of lymphadenopathy prior to diagnosis is extremely variable. Typically, several weeks to several months elapse between the time of the patient's first observation of an asymptomatic mass and the diagnostic biopsy. However, some patients report that a particular mass has been present for many months to several years, with intermittent waxing and waning in size.

Fever and Systemic Symptoms. Although the asymptomatic presentation is most common, one quarter to one third of patients will present with unexplained and persistent fever and/or night sweats as initial symptoms. Fatigue and weight loss may be associated complaints. Patients with these symptoms tend to be in the older age group, are more often men than women, and are generally discovered to have more widespread disease than the usual patient presenting without symptoms. Although superficial lymphadenopathy is present in most such patients, occasionally palpable lymphadenopathy is absent in the patient past the age of 40 with severe systemic symptoms. These patients present with fever of undetermined origin. Extensive diagnostic efforts may be required to discover the presence of Hodgkin's disease, including lymphangiography, abdominal CT scanning, bone marrow biopsies, or even exploratory laparotomy.

The presence of fever, drenching night sweats requiring the changing of bed clothing, or weight loss exceeding 10 per cent of baseline body weight during the six months preceding diagnosis constitute systemic or B symptoms for staging purposes, and confer an adverse prognosis.

Although fever secondary to Hodgkin's disease is usually low grade, occasional patients have intermittent evening fever lasting several days, alternating with afebrile periods lasting days or weeks. This cyclic fever has been labeled the *Pel-Ebstein type* but is rarely the presenting manifestation of the disease.

Pruritus. Pruritus is another characteristic systemic symptom of Hodgkin's disease. It may be mild and localized, but usually progresses and becomes generalized. Severe pruritus may result in extensive excoriations and inability to sleep. It is rarely relieved by topical medications or antihistamines.

The prognostic significance of pruritus itself is unclear. It rarely occurs in the absence of fever and/or night sweats but is no longer considered as a B symptom because its presence does not correlate with an adverse prognosis. Generalized severe pruritus may occur in patients with non-Hodgkin's lymphomas and in other medical and dermatologic conditions, but its presence should always suggest Hodgkin's disease. Its cause is unknown.

SELECTED CLINICAL PROBLEMS. A wide variety of other symptoms may initially call the attention of patients and their physicians to the disease. These same problems occur more commonly as the course of Hodgkin's disease progresses. In addition, almost all patients receive treatment that profoundly affects the natural history of their illness, resulting in either apparent cure or persistent relapsing Hodgkin's disease, or frequently in complications that become difficult to separate from the manifestations of the disease itself.

Pulmonary involvement occurs in only 10 to 20 per cent of patients at presentation. It appears to arise by spread along lymphatics from ipsilateral hilar lymph nodes. Hodgkin's disease frequently involves the lungs with a patchy pulmonary infiltrate without circumscribed borders. Its appearance is variable, and it must be distinguished from radiation effects, drug reactions, and the wide variety of pulmonary infections that occur in these immunocompromised patients. In a severely ill patient in whom the diagnosis is uncertain, the therapeutic significance of these lesions is so great that bronchoscopy with transbronchial biopsy or diagnostic thoracotomy may be justified. Pleural effusions—transudates, exudates, or chylous—are most frequently caused by central lymphatic and venous obstruction resulting from Hodgkin's disease in the mediastinum or obstruction of the thoracic duct. These effusions are rarely caused by direct pleural involvement, and cytologic examination of the fluid or pleural biopsy infrequently reveals diagnostic Reed-Sternberg cells.

Superior vena caval obstruction or compression of the upper airway by mediastinal Hodgkin's disease may be the initial presentation or a complication in the course of the disease. Myocardial involvement is extremely unusual, but pericardial effusions may occur from direct invasion by adjacent mediastinal Hodgkin's disease. Effusions rarely produce cardiac tamponade, and this complication is more often a consequence of radiation-induced pericarditis.

Spinal cord compression, usually caused by epidural spread of tumor from paravertebral lymph nodes through intervertebral foramina in the thoracic or lumbar regions, may be a devastating acute complication. This syndrome may be seen in patients with an otherwise favorable prognosis, although it usually occurs in patients with progressive tumor in whom primary treatment has failed. Back or neck pain, either directly over the vertebral body or occurring in a radicular pattern, should promptly raise the suspicion of cord compression. Symptoms suggestive of more advanced cord compression include numbness, tingling or weakness of an extremity, motor weakness, and bladder or bowel dysfunction. Prompt diagnostic evaluation, including myelography and/or CT scanning, are mandatory, as is prompt therapeutic intervention with immediate radiotherapy to prevent permanent neurologic damage. Surgical decompression is rarely indicated.

Bone involvement may occur from hematogenous spread in advanced disease or by local nodal spread to adjacent bone. Bone involvement often produces pain but rarely fracture, since the bone lesion is generally osteoblastic or mixed osteoblastic and osteolytic.

Hepatic involvement is present in less than 5 per cent of patients at the time of diagnosis and is generally focal in nature. Liver involvement in Hodgkin's disease is almost always associated with splenic involvement. Massive hepatomegaly or jaundice is rarely seen at the time of initial presentation. However, as the liver becomes progressively involved, diffuse infiltration of the portal spaces may be associated with serious hepatic dysfunction and laboratory features of intrahepatic biliary obstruction. Rarely, enlarged lymph nodes in the porta hepatis may produce extrahepatic biliary obstruction. Direct *renal involvement* is rarely a clinically significant problem, but ureteral obstruction and hydronephrosis, secondary to massive retroperitoneal lymphadenopathy, may be seen in far-advanced disease. The nephrotic syndrome, presenting as lipoid nephrosis, is a rare manifestation of Hodgkin's disease and is occasionally accompanied by evidence of glomerular immune complex deposition.

Infectious complications are common in patients with Hodgkin's disease and may or may not be temporarily related to concurrent treatment. Virtually all patients with uncontrolled Hodgkin's disease who succumb to this disorder will have episodes of serious infections at some point in the course of their disease. Localized or disseminated herpes zoster is the most frequently diagnosed serious viral infection, while cryptococcosis, especially of the lungs and meninges, is the most virulent of the fungal complications. *Pneumocystis carinii* pneumonia causes diffuse pulmonary infiltrates and may appear in patients whose disease is in remission between cycles of chemotherapy, as well as in patients in whom relapse occurs. Toxoplasmosis is being recognized with increasing frequency, while tuberculosis has become distinctly uncommon in this population. Children who have undergone splenectomy are particularly predisposed to overwhelming pneumococcal infections unless prophylactic antibiotics or pneumococcal vaccine is administered.

Immunologic abnormalities are common in patients with Hodgkin's disease even at the time of initial diagnosis and prior to initiation of any treatment. A significantly higher frequency of cutaneous anergy is observed than in a control population. The presence or absence of anergy, however, has been shown to have no influence on the prognosis within a specific stage, given the effectiveness of modern therapy. Thus, there is no role for the routine anergy panel. With refined immunologic techniques, a defect in delayed hypersensitivity and T lymphocyte transformation can be detected even in early stage I disease. These deficits are aggravated by therapy and persist for many years even after successful curative treatment. A serum factor, probably an immune complex, has been identified that interferes with T cell function. This factor can be removed in vitro, can block the usual T cell reactions of normal cells, and is probably different from prostaglandins, which are also increased in the serum of some patients. Therapy for Hodgkin's disease undoubtedly accentuates the T cell abnormality. However, it is still unknown whether the observed immunologic abnormalities contribute to the pathogenesis of the disease or are merely secondary phenomena.

STAGING. The progress achieved in the treatment of Hodgkin's disease has paralleled the improvement in techniques for identifying the extent or stage of disease in the untreated patient. In view of the current choices of therapy, it is essential that all cases of Hodgkin's disease be completely evaluated before therapeutic decisions are made. The primary goals of staging are to assess the extent of disease, facilitate the selection of an appropriate treatment program, provide an accurate determination of prognosis, and establish a baseline for re-evaluation following completion of therapy.

The staging classification in current use is outlined in Table 160–2. Patients are assigned a *clinical stage* (CS) on the basis of their initial biopsy, systemic symptoms, physical examination, laboratory results, and radiologic procedures. However, treatment decisions are generally based on a *pathologic stage* (PS), after the extent of involvement has been documented with appropriate biopsies. The basic staging classification is modified by the adverse prognostic significance of systemic symptoms (B disease) and by the realization that localized contiguous extranodal extension (E disease) gener-

TABLE 160–2. MODIFIED ANN ARBOR STAGING CLASSIFICATION

Stage	
I	Involvement of a single lymph node region (I) or of a single extralymphatic organ or site (I_E)
II	Involvement of two or more lymph node regions on the same side of the diaphragm (II) or localized involvement of an extralymphatic organ or site and of one or more lymph node regions on the same side of the diaphragm (II_E)
III	Involvement of lymph node regions on both sides of the diaphragm (III), which may also be accompanied by involvement of the spleen (III_S) or by localized involvement of an extralymphatic organ or site (III_E) or both (III_{SE})
III_1	Involvement limited to the lymphatic structures in the upper abdomen; that is, spleen, or splenic, celiac, or hepatic portal nodes, or any combination of these
III_2	Involvement of lower abdominal nodes; that is, para-aortic, iliac, inguinal or mesenteric nodes, with or without involvement of the splenic, celiac, or hepatic portal nodes
IV	Diffuse or disseminated involvement of one or more extralymphatic organs or tissues, with or without associated lymph node involvement

E = extralymphatic site; S = splenic involvement.
Note: The presence of fever, night sweats, and/or unexplained loss of 10 per cent or more of body weight in the 6 months preceding diagnosis is denoted by the suffix letter B. The letter A indicates the absence of these symptoms. Each patient is assigned a clinical stage (CS) on the basis of the initial biopsy, physical examination, laboratory and radiologic results, and a pathologic stage (PS) on the basis of subsequent biopsy results, whether normal or abnormal.

ally does not carry the same poor prognosis as hematogenous extranodal involvement (stage IV disease).

Within each stage of Hodgkin's disease there is a spectrum of patients who have a more or less favorable prognosis, depending on the site or sites of disease, size of the tumor masses, and degree of symptoms. The importance of these prognostic factors and substages within the Ann Arbor classification has become increasingly recognized, because treatment methods are now tailored to individual clinical situations. Controversy exists about the prognostic and therapeutic significance of the E lesion, the size of a mediastinal mass, and the substaging of IIIA patients. PS IIIA disease, for example, may be subdivided into a prognostically favorable III_1 group, in which abdominal disease is confined to the upper abdominal nodes and/or the spleen, and a less favorable III_2 group with disease extending to the lower abdomen, including the para-aortic, iliac, or inguinal lymph nodes. A complete knowledge of staging is vital to guide an efficient but thorough diagnostic evaluation. The tests performed as part of a staging evaluation must be individualized rather than obtained automatically.

DIAGNOSTIC EVALUATION. Recommended staging procedures are outlined in Table 160–3. This evaluation should

TABLE 160–3. DIAGNOSTIC EVALUATION

A. Required procedures
  1. Histologic confirmation by biopsy
  2. Detailed history for unexplained fever, weight loss, night sweats, and pruritus
  3. Physical examination to document all areas of lymphadenopathy, including Waldeyer's ring; size of liver and spleen; bony tenderness. Neurologic evaluation
  4. Laboratory studies
    a. CBC and platelet count, ESR
    b. Serum alkaline phosphatase, LDH
    c. Renal function, including uric acid
    d. Liver function
  5. Radiologic studies
    a. Chest roentgenogram
    b. Bipedal lymphangiogram
    c. CT of the chest and whole abdomen including the pelvis
B. Frequently performed procedures under specific clinical conditions
  1. Bone marrow biopsy (needle or open surgical technique)
  2. Bone roentgenography and scanning for areas of bone pain or tenderness
  3. Gallium whole-body scanning
  4. Staging laparotomy and splenectomy, if therapeutic decisions will depend on the identification of subdiaphragmatic disease

commence promptly after the initial biopsy establishes the diagnosis.

History and Physical Examination. A careful history and physical examination are essential to discover characteristic systemic symptoms and to describe all the lymph node areas of the body. Enlarged lymph nodes are not necessarily involved by disease; reactive lymphoid hyperplasia occasionally occurs in some patients with Hodgkin's disease. If confirmation of Hodgkin's disease in suspicious lymph nodes will change the therapeutic approach, then additional biopsies should be obtained. Although Waldeyer's ring involvement is uncommon in Hodgkin's disease, the lymphoid tissues in this region should be evaluated by physical examination. The size of the liver and spleen should be carefully determined, although mild enlargement of either organ may merely be a sign of nonspecific hypertrophy rather than involvement by Hodgkin's disease. A palpable abdominal mass caused by enlarged mesenteric or para-aortic lymph nodes is a rare initial finding. The bones should be examined for areas of tenderness, and a careful baseline neurologic examination performed.

Laboratory Studies. Routine laboratory tests include a complete blood count, erythrocyte sedimentation rate (ESR), urine analysis, renal and liver function tests, and serum alkaline phosphatase. Mild to moderate anemia may be found in patients with widespread disease and is often associated with normal indices, normal or low reticulocyte count, and a negative Coombs' test. Anemia in a patient with Hodgkin's disease is usually caused by the typical chronic anemia of malignancy, and rarely is secondary to hypersplenism, marrow involvement, or a Coombs'-positive hemolytic anemia. A moderate to marked neutrophilic leukocytosis and thrombocytosis are characteristic of active, symptomatic Hodgkin's disease. Occasionally, the granulocytosis may be so marked as to suggest chronic granulocytic leukemia, but more careful evaluation usually demonstrates that this represents a "leukemoid" reaction. Eosinophilia of a mild degree is common. In patients with severe and longstanding pruritus, moderate or marked eosinophilia frequently occurs. Absolute lymphopenia (<1000 per cubic millimeter) may be seen in a small percentage of patients with more advanced disease, and is usually a poor prognostic sign.

The ESR is commonly elevated in patients with active disease, but has limited sensitivity. Other nonspecific laboratory abnormalities include increased levels of serum $alpha_2$-globulin, fibrinogen, haptoglobin, copper, and zinc; depression of serum iron and iron-binding capacity; and increase of leukocyte alkaline phosphatase. An elevated serum alkaline phosphatase level may be a nonspecific finding or secondary to involvement of bone, bone marrow, or liver with Hodgkin's disease. Elevation of the serum uric acid level is rare at the time of initial presentation, except in advanced stages of disease with massive nodal or bone marrow involvement.

Radiologic Studies. Radiologic examinations should include routine chest roentgenograms, which will demonstrate mediastinal involvement in 50 to 60 per cent of patients. In contrast, hilar disease is seen at presentation in less than 20 per cent of cases. In the absence of mediastinal involvement, hilar disease is unusual. Whole lung tomography is of marginal value and has been replaced by computed tomography (CT) of the chest. CT allows better definition of mediastinal, hilar, and paravertebral adenopathy, and pulmonary involvement. CT of the chest is indicated for all patients. Its role is to define more precisely the extent of disease, including possible localized extension into the pulmonary parenchyma, as well as to assist in radiation treatment planning. The presence of a small pleural effusion in the patient with a mediastinal mass does not necessarily indicate malignant involvement of the pleura. Thoracentesis or pleural biopsy is rarely diagnostic of Hodgkin's disease in these situations.

Subdiaphragmatic sites are best evaluated by performing both bipedal lymphangiography and abdominal-pelvic CT. These examinations are complementary, and neither procedure should replace the other. The lymphangiogram is the most reliable means of assessing involvement of retroperitoneal or pelvic lymph nodes, in that abnormalities of intranodal architecture can be demonstrated in up to 25 per cent of cases at presentation (Fig. 160–2). The overall accuracy of this procedure is 80 to 90 per cent. Lymphangiography is also valuable in preparation for exploratory laparotomy, in that it directs the surgeon to potentially abnormal areas for lymph node biopsy. Lymphangiography is also helpful for planning radiotherapy fields, and especially for assessing the degree of response to therapy during serial follow-up evaluation of the involved retroperitoneal lymph nodes.

Abdominal CT can complement lymphangiography by demonstrating lymphadenopathy in the mesentery, porta hepatis, celiac nodes, and para-aortic nodes above the level of those opacified by the lymphangiogram. CT can only assess nodal involvement when there is an increase in lymph node size. In contrast, lymphangiography provides information on abnormal architecture even in unenlarged nodes. Thus, reliance on CT alone may lead to understaging.

Routine bone scans or skeletal x-ray examinations are not indicated in the asymptomatic patient with a normal alkaline phosphatase. However, in those patients with areas of bone pain or tenderness, bone scans complemented by selective x-ray examinations are indicated to detect osseous lesions.

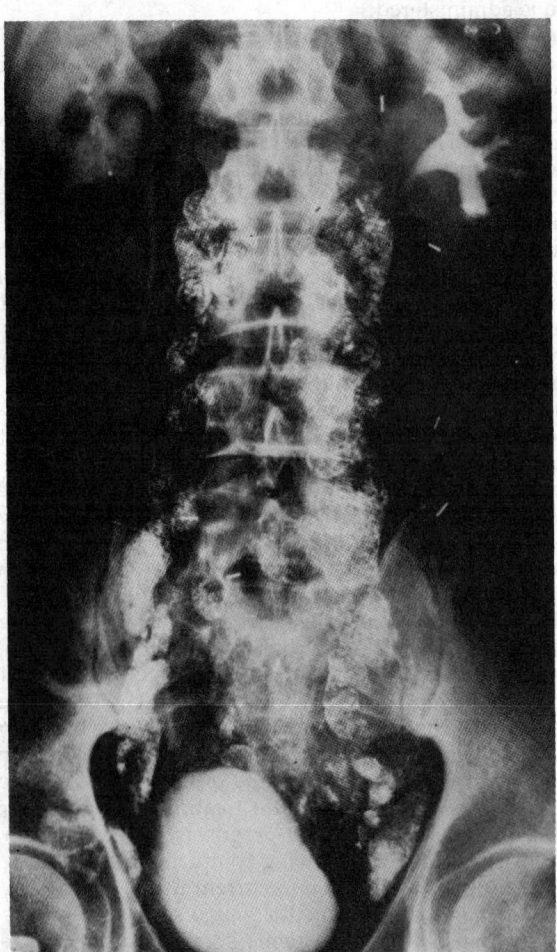

FIGURE 160–2. Abnormal lymphangiogram with enlargement and distortion of the internal architecture in the pelvic, iliac, and paraaortic lymph nodes. Despite the extensive lymphadenopathy, little displacement of the ureters and no obstruction of the upper urinary tracts were seen. (Reprinted by permission from Kaplan HS: Hodgkin's Disease. 2nd ed. Cambridge, Harvard University Press, 1980, p 194.)

Unless the patient has significant hepatomegaly or marked elevations of the liver function tests, liver-spleen scan is not indicated. CT of the liver is more useful in this situation. A single percutaneous needle biopsy of the liver is rarely diagnostic, because of the focal nature of hepatic involvement. Gallium whole-body scans can be helpful in evaluating initial disease as well as potential sites of recurrence, especially in the mediastinum, but cannot be used as evidence of Hodgkin's disease without biopsy confirmation.

Bone Marrow Biopsy. This procedure should be performed in all patients with systemic symptoms or clinical stage III disease or both. It is also useful in patients with significant peripheral blood count abnormalities, increased serum alkaline phosphatase of bony origin, and in those patients with abnormal bone roentgenograms or scans. Hodgkin's disease in the bone marrow is rarely demonstrable by simple marrow aspiration. Involvement is usually focal, often associated with fibrosis, and is diagnosed more readily by either a unilateral or bilateral bone marrow biopsy.

Staging Laparotomy. In the absence of medical contraindications, an exploratory laparotomy with splenectomy is widely employed as part of the routine staging evaluation to identify and confirm the presence of Hodgkin's disease below the diaphragm. The purpose of the laparotomy is diagnostic, the results of which may alter treatment selection significantly. Laparotomy findings that frequently influence both the staging and subsequent treatment include detection of Hodgkin's disease in the spleen, detection of the extent of splenic involvement, and detection of presence of disease in the celiac or retroperitoneal lymph nodes. Secondary benefits from the laparotomy include attempting to preserve ovarian function by means of an oophoropexy when pelvic irradiation is to be utilized in young women, reducing required irradiation fields when the spleen is treated, and improving the peripheral blood counts in the occasional patient with hypersplenism. In one quarter of patients with normal-sized spleens on physical examination, Hodgkin's disease will be found in the spleen removed at surgery. Conversely, approximately 50 per cent of patients with clinical or radiologic enlargement of the spleen do not have histologic involvement. The identification of Hodgkin's disease in the liver is especially difficult. Physical examination, routine liver function tests, and liver scans correlate poorly, if at all, with histologic verification. Liver involvement can be demonstrated at laparotomy on wedge or needle biopsy and is more often found in patients with significant splenomegaly and/or abnormal lymphangiograms.

Staging laparotomy is not a routine diagnostic procedure and should be performed only in those patients in whom the results will potentially modify treatment selection. Discussion of potential treatment options with the radiotherapist or medical oncologist for each stage of Hodgkin's disease should be held prior to the decision to perform a laparotomy. Thus, staging laparotomy with splenectomy is generally recommended for patients with clinical stage I to IIA/B or IIIA disease. Patients with stage IIIB or IV disease are not candidates for laparotomy because combination chemotherapy will be used as their primary method of treatment.

In some cases, staging laparotomy must be deferred or omitted. The patient who presents with massive mediastinal lymphadenopathy should not undergo laparotomy because of the dangers of anesthesia in these patients. In addition, combination chemotherapy is frequently employed in patients with large mediastinal masses, thus eliminating the need for precise staging below the diaphragm.

As a result of staging laparotomy and splenectomy, approximately one third of patients with clinical stages I and II are found to have either subdiaphragmatic lymph node disease or splenic involvement, necessitating extension of the subdiaphragmatic radiation portals. If extensive splenic involvement (> four nodules) is documented, either combination chemotherapy alone or a combined modality program is required. Approximately one quarter of clinical stage IIIA patients (i.e., those with suspicious lymphangiograms or abdominal CT scans) have a negative staging laparotomy that allows their pathologic stage to be downgraded to I or II. Although the results of the laparotomy allow change in the stage in as many as 35 per cent of patients, this change modifies the treatment plan in only approximately 20 per cent, depending on the extent of disease found below the diaphragm. Even in the hands of experienced surgeons, staging laparotomy is associated with a small risk of perioperative morbidity, including infection, fever, and phlebitis, Rare fatalities have been reported. Because of occasional severe bacterial infections occurring after splenectomy, pneumococcal vaccine should be administered preoperatively.

MODE OF SPREAD. Careful mapping of initial sites of involvement of Hodgkin's disease and the use of lymphangiography, staging laparotomy, and splenectomy provide evidence that involvement of various lymph node groups is distinctly nonrandom. Two different theories have been proposed to account for the nonrandom patterns of spread: (1) The *contiguity theory* (Rosenberg and Kaplan) postulates that the disease is unifocal in origin, beginning in an initial focus within the lymphatic system and spreading via lymphatic channels to contiguous lymphatic structures. The contiguity theory has been challenged because of the frequency of cervical, supraclavicular, and retroperitoneal lymph node involvement without intervening mediastinal disease, as well as the common involvement of the spleen, which has no afferent lymphatics. (2) The *susceptibility theory* (Smithers) postulates that the disease is multifocal in origin. The giant cells of Hodgkin's disease are thought to migrate in and out of lymph nodes from the bloodstream but are thought to grow only in preferential sites, presenting an appearance of contiguous spread. Noncontiguous spread is more common in the mixed cellularity and lymphocyte depletion subtypes, when multiple sites are present and when vascular invasion is present. However, the role of vascular invasion in the spread of Hodgkin's disease is not fully understood. Vascular invasion in the spleen may lead to hematogenous dissemination, since the spleen is almost invariably involved when Hodgkin's disease is present in the liver or bone marrow.

TREATMENT. The prognosis for patients with Hodgkin's disease has improved dramatically during the past three decades because of (1) the advances in precise staging and an awareness of the important prognostic factors previously described, (2) the development of supervoltage radiotherapeutic techniques, and (3) the use of effective combination chemotherapy programs.

Radiotherapy. Important factors in determining the success of radiation therapy include the radiation dose per field, the extent of the fields employed, the beam energy, and precision of treatment planning. A tumoricidal dose of 3600 to 4400 rads is required to eradicate the lesions of Hodgkin's disease. Lymphoid regions adjacent to areas of known disease or those that are contiguous via lymphatic channels are usually treated to full dose. Apparently uninvolved areas are treated prophylactically for subclinical disease with dosages of 3600 rads. Large fields, shaped to conform to the patient's anatomy, are designed to treat multiple contiguous lymph node regions. A *mantle* port covers the cervical, supraclavicular, infraclavicular, axillary, mediastinal, and hilar lymph nodes. The *para-aortic* field includes the para-aortic lymph nodes from the level of the diaphragm down to the aortic bifurcation but omits the pelvis and treats the splenic hilar lymph nodes in a patient with a prior splenectomy. An *inverted Y* port includes in one field not only the para-aortic and splenic hilar lymph nodes but also extends into the pelvis to encompass the iliac and inguinal-femoral lymph nodes. The combination of a mantle and a para-aortic field is also referred to as subtotal nodal or extended field irradiation. *Total lymphoid irradiation* implies sequential treatment to both a mantle and an inverted Y field.

The use of sequential large field irradiation minimizes the risk of either overlap or underdosage, which could result in either undue normal tissue toxicity or inadequate therapy. Treatment of these large fields requires supervoltage radiation. This capability is available primarily with contemporary linear accelerators, which have the advantages over cobalt of skin sparing, increased depth dose, and sharp beam edges with reduced lateral scatter. The use of a treatment simulator to plan the radiotherapy fields and proper field verification (portal films) during the treatment process is essential.

Definitive radiation therapy alone is appropriate initial management for the majority of patients with pathologic stage I and II Hodgkin's disease. Mantle and para-aortic radiation is the treatment of choice for stages IA and IIA disease, providing an 85- to 90-per cent chance of cure with irradiation alone. Patients with stage IB and IIB disease are treated with mantle and para-aortic or total lymphoid irradiation and have a 70 to 75 per cent chance of cure with such treatment. Controversy exists about the indications for using both radiotherapy and chemotherapy in stage I or II patients who present with large mediastinal masses, limited contiguous extranodal disease (the E lesion of the Ann Arbor system), or systemic symptoms. In each of these disease settings, the use of radiation alone results in a lower disease-free survival rate than when a combined modality program is employed as the initial treatment, although the use of chemotherapy at relapse may provide an equivalent chance of cure. Patients with III_SA or III_1A Hodgkin's disease and minimal splenic involvement are usually treated with total lymphoid irradiation alone. Controversy exists whether prophylactic hepatic radiation should be delivered to those patients with splenic involvement.

Complications of radiation are related to the technique employed, dosage administered, and irradiated volume. Acute side effects of radiotherapy include transient nausea and vomiting, dysphagia, and marrow suppression. These effects subside shortly after radiation therapy is completed. Late potential side effects of radiation include hypothyroidism, pneumonitis, transient myelitis (generally manifested as electric-like shocks in limbs on neck flexion known as *Lhermitte's sign*), and rarely pericarditis. Persistent myelosuppression is a rare late complication. Radiation-induced decreased bone growth has been noted in children.

Chemotherapy. The major advance in the treatment of stage IIIB and IV Hodgkin's disease was the development of curative combination chemotherapy. The initial studies from the National Cancer Institute demonstrated that a four-drug combination known as MOPP (nitrogen mustard, vincristine, procarbazine, and prednisone) was capable of producing documented complete remissions in 70 to 80 per cent of patients with advanced Hodgkin's disease. At least one half to two thirds of the patients who achieved complete remission with MOPP have not had recurrence after more than 10 to 20 years of observation. Thus, 50 per cent of all patients with stage IIIB and IV who underwent treatment were cured with MOPP chemotherapy alone.

The potential for clinical cure of Hodgkin's disease with chemotherapy exists for all histologic subtypes, stages, and extranodal sites of disease. Patients who have received prior radiotherapy in whom relapse subsequently occurs have an equivalent chance of being cured with "salvage" chemotherapy. Older patients and those with bone marrow involvement, systemic symptoms, bulky disease, and poor performance status have a less favorable long-term response with chemotherapy. The best results have been reported for asymptomatic patients with disease limited to the lymph nodes and/or lung.

It is essential to administer the drugs in the MOPP regimen at full doses and in a timely fashion. Therapy is repeated every four weeks for a minimum of six cycles. An additional two cycles are administered after a complete clinical remission is obtained. At that time, chemotherapy is discontinued only when repeat restaging studies document that a true complete remission has been obtained. The restaging diagnostic evaluation includes repeat radiologic procedures and biopsies as indicated to verify the complete response status. Maintenance chemotherapy beyond the documentation of a restaged complete remission is of no advantage in improving either disease-free or overall survival.

No alternative four- or five-drug combinations have been demonstrated conclusively to be superior to MOPP, considering differences in patient selection, prognostic factors, restaging evaluation, and adequate follow-up. However, comparable results to MOPP have been achieved with a variety of alternative chemotherapy programs that offer significantly less toxicity than MOPP. Combinations that contain cyclophosphamide or chlorambucil instead of nitrogen mustard, vinblastine in place of vincristine, and/or the addition of a nitrosourea appear to be as efficacious as MOPP in producing durable complete responses but have substantially fewer side effects. The BCVPP (BCNU, cyclophosphamide, vinblastine, procarbazine, and prednisone) regimen is one example of an equally effective and less toxic alternative to MOPP.

Patients who have relapsed after definitive irradiation for early stage disease are often salvaged and cured with chemotherapy. Patients who have relapsed after initial chemotherapy have a poorer but not hopeless outlook. Patients who have recurrence after a MOPP-induced complete remission of at least one year may benefit from a second course of the same therapy and achieve a second long-term complete remission, but cure is unlikely. Patients who are definitely MOPP resistant should be treated with chemotherapy regimens that contain different or non-cross-resistant drugs. The ABVD program (Adriamycin, bleomycin, vinblastine, and DTIC) is a widely used second-line regimen that results in complete remission in 30 to 60 per cent of patients. However, the follow-up is still too limited to place confidence in the curative potential of these second-line chemotherapy programs.

The identification of an active non-cross-resistant combination in the patient who has had a relapse led to the investigation of sequential alternating chemotherapy regimens (i.e., MOPP alternating monthly with ABVD or a hybrid of seven drugs MOPP/ABV in one monthly cycle) as primary induction therapy. By exposing tumor cells to more drugs early in the course of disease, drug-resistant clones might be eradicated before growing too large to be cured. The objective is to increase the complete remission rates over that which has been demonstrated with MOPP and, more importantly, to improve relapse-free and overall survival. This approach shows considerable promise, especially for patients with stage IV disease, but longer follow-up will be required before this strategy can be adopted as standard practice for advanced Hodgkin's disease.

The major complication of chemotherapy is bone marrow suppression with increased risk of infection and, rarely, hemorrhage. The peripheral blood counts are monitored carefully during chemotherapy and drug doses are adjusted depending on the degree of myelosuppression. However, drug dose reductions made simply for the purpose of decreasing subjective toxicity are inappropriate because the opportunity for cure is also reduced. Sterility, more commonly seen in males, is a permanent side effect of chemotherapy. Significant nausea and vomiting are seen with the MOPP and ABVD regimens. These drug programs often produce serious psychologic problems that require effective counseling, as well as antiemetic agents. Mild peripheral neuropathy is commonly seen with vincristine, but paresthesias are not an indication to reduce drug dosage. Acute leukemia as a late effect of chemotherapy alone is a recognized but unusual complication.

Combined Modality Therapy. Combinations of irradiation and chemotherapy in the treatment of Hodgkin's disease have been utilized during the past 15 years with the goal of increasing the cure rate. It is logical to assume that combination chemotherapy, effective in curing a significant percentage of patients with advanced disease, should be even more effective for occult disease that might be present after radiation therapy. Patients who have recurrence after receiving MOPP chemotherapy frequently have relapse in sites of major pretreatment involvement, including bulky lymph node areas. An additional rationale for combined modality therapy includes improved management of childhood Hodgkin's disease by reduction of radiation fields that may cause bone growth retardation, decreased requirement for staging laparotomy, and reduced complications from newer radiotherapy techniques involving larger treatment fields.

Adjuvant chemotherapy can substitute effectively for prophylactic irradiation of apparently uninvolved sites, but to date there is no clear justification for the routine use of a combined-modality approach for the overwhelming majority of patients with pathologic stage I or II disease. However, there are certain subsets of patients with early stage Hodgkin's disease for whom combined modality treatment is indicated because of an unacceptably high relapse rate; that is, patients with large mediastinal masses or contiguous extranodal involvement.

The treatment of pathologic stage IIIA Hodgkin's disease remains controversial. Retrospective studies have concentrated on identifying prognostic subgroups in which there is an unacceptably low disease-free survival with radiotherapy alone. At the present time, it would be premature for radiation therapists to abandon total nodal irradiation in III_1A patients in whom the prognosis is favorable and who at laparotomy are found to have minimal involvement of the spleen or upper abdominal nodes. In this subgroup, only those who relapse after primary radiotherapy should receive combination chemotherapy. For patients with clinical stage IIIA/pathologic III_2A disease, and for those with extensive splenic involvement, no one management strategy has been proved superior. Acceptable treatment alternatives for this subgroup include combined modality therapy with total nodal or subtotal nodal radiotherapy plus MOPP, initial chemotherapy followed by irradiation to sites of pretreatment involvement, and chemotherapy alone. Although combination chemotherapy remains the mainstay for stage IIIB disease, both improved disease-free and overall survival may be obtained for these patients in whom initial MOPP chemotherapy followed by or sequenced with total nodal irradiation is utilized.

Significant improvement in survival rates as a result of combined modality programs has not been clearly demonstrated for certain subsets of patients. In part, this is because of the long time (ten or more years) required to establish an overall survival benefit. Combined modality programs generally demonstrate improved disease-free survival, but interpretation of current clinical trials must be tempered by the observation that patients who relapse after radiation alone are frequently salvaged or cured with chemotherapy administered only at the time of relapse. It may be more acceptable to treat patients conservatively at the onset of their disease with one method, reserving the more complicated combined modality programs for those patients with poor prognostic factors and an unacceptably high relapse rate after primary irradiation alone.

The complications and morbidity of combined modality programs are significant. The potential risk of acute complications, including profound and prolonged myelosuppression, sterility of both men and women, and demonstrated risk of second malignant tumors, has modified the enthusiasm for a combined modality approach. The incidence of acute myelomonocytic leukemia is approximately 5 to 7 per cent for patients at risk for seven to ten years following combined modality treatment. Paradoxically, this incidence is greatest in patients over the age of 40 years, the group most likely to have an unfavorable prognosis.

Recommended Therapy. The recommended therapy for a patient with Hodgkin's disease must be individualized. Important management considerations include stage and bulk of disease, age, prior therapy, medical complications, and availability of modern skills in radiotherapy and chemotherapy. The improved results of aggressive therapy after accurate clinical evaluation and pathologic staging are achievable only by experienced teams of physicians working closely together to achieve the excellent cure rates now possible while avoiding the risks of excesses in treatment. The recommended therapeutic approaches for the previously untreated adult patient with various stages of Hodgkin's disease are listed in Table 160–4. Estimated results are expressed as the percentage of patients likely to achieve a disease-free interval of five years. Careful evaluation of their condition and observation of a high proportion of patients, perhaps 90 or 95 per cent, who have survived free from relapse for five years demonstrate that they are cured of their disease.

An early stage patient who has relapsed after radiation therapy alone may be cured with salvage chemotherapy. Thus, freedom from first or even second relapse must be considered in the evaluation of both disease-free and overall survival when the results of current clinical trials are analyzed. With dramatically improved treatment results, the challenge

TABLE 160–4. THE TREATMENT OF HODGKIN'S DISEASE IN ADULTS

Ann Arbor Pathologic Stage	Recommended Therapy	Estimated 5-Year Disease-Free Survival (%)	Investigational Therapy
IA, I_EA, IIA, II_EA*	Mantle and para-aortic radiotherapy	85–90	Limited-field radiotherapy ± combination chemotherapy
IB, I_EB, IIB, II_EB*	Mantle and para-aortic or total lymphoid radiotherapy	70–75	Limited-field or subtotal lymphoid radiotherapy + combination chemotherapy; chemotherapy alone
III_1A, III_SA, III_EA*†	Total lymphoid radiotherapy ± chemotherapy	70–80	Total lymphoid radiotherapy, including hepatic irradiation; combination chemotherapy
III_2A	Combination chemotherapy (i.e., MOPP) ± total lymphoid radiotherapy	65–75	Combination chemotherapy + limited-field radiotherapy to areas of pretreatment involvement
IIIB, III_SB, III_EB	Combination chemotherapy (i.e., MOPP)	60	Combination chemotherapy + either total lymphoid radiotherapy or limited-field radiotherapy to areas of pretreatment involvement
IVA, IVB	Combination chemotherapy (i.e., MOPP)	50	Alternating non-cross-resistant chemotherapy (i.e., MOPP-ABVD); combination chemotherapy followed by limited-field radiotherapy to areas of pretreatment involvement

*Patients with large mediastinal masses (>0.33 of the transverse diameter of the chest) will be controlled by irradiation alone in approximately 40 to 50 per cent of cases and should receive combined modality therapy (chemotherapy and irradiation) as primary management.

†Patients with extensive involvement of the spleen (>4 nodules) will be controlled by irradiation alone in approximately 40 per cent of cases and should receive combined modality therapy (chemotherapy and irradiation), or chemotherapy alone as primary management.

facing physicians and investigators caring for patients with all stages of Hodgkin's disease is to weigh carefully the toxicity-benefit ratio for each new recommended regimen.

PROGNOSIS. Hodgkin's disease is a curable malignant condition. Advances in histopathologic classification, precise diagnostic evaluation, and selection of appropriate aggressive therapy have led to continuous improvement in both disease-free and overall survival. Survival figures and prognostic factors that were acceptable 10 or even 20 years ago are not acceptable today. The five-year survival rate has increased from approximately 25 to 50 per cent 20 years ago to at least 75 per cent today.

The success of modern radiotherapy, chemotherapy, or combined modality programs has obscured the significance of such important prognostic factors as histologic subtype, stage of disease, and the presence of systemic symptoms. In recent years, newer prognostic factors have been identified, including anatomic substage III$_2$A, five or more sites of lymph node involvement, extensive splenic disease, bulky mediastinal lymphadenopathy, and contiguous extranodal extension. Combined modality treatment programs or chemotherapy alone is recommended for patients with these unfavorable prognostic factors. However, any potential disease-free survival advantage seen after combined modality therapy must be balanced by the potential risk of late complications, particularly second malignant conditions, and must be translated into an overall survival benefit before general acceptance.

Table 160–4 presents a reasonable estimate of prognosis, recommended therapy, and current appropriate investigative approaches for the various stages of Hodgkin's disease. These treatment recommendations provide only the broadest of guidelines. Therapy must be individualized, depending on the specific clinical situation and the skill and experience of physicians treating the patient. Any treatment recommendations and estimates of cure must be viewed with the understanding that the management of Hodgkin's disease is dynamic, constantly undergoing change and refinement, and is designed to provide each patient with the best probability of cure and the least possibility of long-term toxicity.

Bakemeier R, Anderson J, Costello N, et al.: BCVPP chemotherapy for advanced Hodgkin's disease: Evidence for greater duration of complete remission, greater survival, and less toxicity than with a MOPP regimen. Ann Intern Med 101:447, 1984. *A large randomized trial that demonstrates that BCVPP is at least as effective as MOPP, but produces significantly less toxicity.*

Bonadonna G, Valagussa P, Santoro A: Alternating non-cross-resistant combination or MOPP in stage IV Hodgkin's disease: A report of 8-year results. Ann Intern Med 104:739, 1986. *An updated report of alternating monthly MOPP-ABVD for stage IV. The patient numbers are small, and the results have not yet been confirmed.*

Canellos G, Come S, Skarin A: Chemotherapy in the treatment of Hodgkin's disease. Semin Hematol 20:1, 1983. *A thorough review of the status of chemotherapy for both early and advanced stages of disease.*

Glick J, Tsiatis A: MOPP/ABVD chemotherapy for advanced Hodgkin's disease. Ann Intern Med 104:876, 1986. *A concise editorial summarizing current results and investigational approaches in advanced Hodgkin's disease. An analysis of the statistical pitfalls of these clinical trials is presented.*

Kaplan H: Hodgkin's disease. 2nd ed. Cambridge, Harvard University Press, 1980. *A detailed, extensively illustrated and referenced volume covering every aspect of the disease as seen by one of the acknowledged experts and pioneers in the field.*

Klimo P, Connors J: MOPP/ABV Hybrid Program: Combination chemotherapy based on early introduction of seven effective drugs for advanced Hodgkin's disease. J Clin Oncol 3:1174, 1985. *A preliminary report of the MOPP/ABV hybrid regimen. Although their results are encouraging, the patient numbers are small and the follow-up too short to allow any conclusions to be drawn as to its superiority over conventionally accepted regimens.*

Leslie N, Mauch P, Hellman S: Stage IA to IIB supra-diaphragmatic Hodgkin's disease. Cancer 55:2072, 1985. *A thoughtful review of the treatment of early stage Hodgkin's disease, emphasizing the experience of the Harvard Joint Center for Radiation Therapy.*

Longo D, Young R, Wesley M, et al.: Twenty years of MOPP therapy for Hodgkin's disease. J Clin Oncol 4:1295, 1986. *A classic and important long-term follow-up report of MOPP-treated patients by the National Cancer Institute group.*

Proceedings of the Symposium on Contemporary Issues in Hodgkin's Disease: Biology, Staging, and Treatment. Cancer Treat Rep 66:601, 1982. *A collection of important papers covering all aspects of Hodgkin's disease. The papers on biology, staging, treatment, and complications are especially worthwhile.*

Rosenberg S, Kaplan H: The evolution and summary results of the Stanford randomized clinical trials of the management of Hodgkin's disease. Int J Radiat Oncol Biol Phys. 11:5, 1985. *An update with long-term follow-up on the important Stanford controlled trials of the use of radiotherapy with or without adjuvant chemotherapy.*

161 LANGERHANS CELL (EOSINOPHILIC) GRANULOMATOSIS

Jerome E. Groopman

The numerous and sometimes confusing classifications of clinical disorders associated with Langerhans cell proliferation reflect our ignorance of both the cause and pathophysiology of many of these diseases. The Langerhans cell belongs to the larger family of cells termed *histiocytes*. Histiocytes are tissue macrophages and include the hepatic Kupffer cell, the alveolar macrophage of the lung, the giant cell of granulomas and the osteoclast in addition to the dermal Langerhans cell. The microglial cell of the brain is probably of macrophage origin as well. All of these tissue macrophages derive from precursor cells that normally reside in bone marrow, mature into circulating blood monocytes, and then egress into tissues and differentiate into a particular type of histiocyte.

A number of benign disorders are associated with proliferation of histiocytes and their fusion into multinucleated giant cells that form granulomas. Langerhans cell (eosinophilic) granulomatosis is an idiopathic benign disease characterized by proliferation and infiltration of tissue by histiocytes and eosinophils. Although this disorder was previously termed eosinophilic granuloma, the proliferating cell that appears primarily responsible for the clinical manifestations of the disorder is the Langerhans cell. The eosinophils may take residence in the lesion because of potent eosinophilic chemotactic factors released secondarily by the histiocytes. Langerhans cell granulomatosis is a distinct disorder unrelated to the eosinophilic syndromes (Ch. 162).

The interaction of "activated macrophages" with surrounding normal tissues may form the pathophysiologic substructure of many of the clinical features of Langerhans cell granulomatosis.

Clinical conditions of unknown cause characterized pathologically by proliferation of tissue macrophages in sheetlike masses with interspersed eosinophils have been difficult to define as specific disease entities. There is great histologic variability within these disorders, and lesions taken from different sites in the same patient may differ pathologically. The clinical course and prognosis do not correlate with histopathologic findings. The concept of Langerhans cell granulomatosis, Hand-Schüller-Christian disease (the classic triad of exophthalmos, diabetes insipidus, and bone destruction) and Letterer-Siwe disease as elements of a continuum termed *histiocytosis X* fails to recognize important differences in clinical course, organ involvement, and therapeutic response. This chapter will discuss unifocal Langerhans cell granulomatosis, multifocal Langerhans cell granulomatosis, and Letterer-Siwe disease. These are the best characterized idiopathic histiocytoses, yet in clinical practice many cases do not readily fit into these categories.

UNIFOCAL LANGERHANS CELL (EOSINOPHILIC) GRANULOMATOSIS

Unifocal Langerhans cell granulomatosis is a benign disorder generally occurring in males during childhood or early adult life. It may occur as late as the sixth or seventh decade of life.

CLINICAL MANIFESTATIONS. The most common presentation of the disorder is a single osteolytic lesion in a long or flat bone, most frequently in the calvarium or femur in children and in a rib in adults. The predilection for skull, femur, rib, pelvis, vertebra, and mandible is not understood. The small bones of the distal extremities are not generally involved. Although the lesions are usually purely lytic, mixed blastic and lytic lesions occur. Pain and swelling over the affected area are common presenting symptoms, although disruption of teeth with mandibular disease, fracture, and otitis media due to mastoid involvement are not infrequent. Many lesions are asymptomatic and diagnosed serendipitously during radiologic evaluation for unrelated problems. Unifocal Langerhans cell granulomatosis of lymph nodes, thymus, or salivary glands is very rare and has the same benign course as that of the more frequent bony lesions. Unifocal Langerhans cell granulomatosis is rarely associated with systemic symptoms and there are no characteristic laboratory findings. Diagnosis is established by biopsy.

DIAGNOSIS. The bone scan is very useful in determining that the lesion is indeed unifocal and in following patients over time for development of new osteolytic lesions. An open biopsy should be performed for diagnosis. Pathologically, an infiltrate with foamy macrophages and admixed eosinophils favors the diagnosis of Langerhans cell granulomatosis. Langerhans' histiocytes contain a cytoplasmic inclusion of unknown composition but with constant thickness and striation termed an X body. They also stain by immunoperoxidase for a cytoplasmic protein termed S-100; detection of S-100 assists the histopathologic diagnosis of Langerhans cell granulomatosis.

TREATMENT. At the time of biopsy, curettage, with or without bone chip packing, should be carried out. This simple surgical approach is almost uniformly successful as definitive therapy for an individual lesion. Lesions in anatomic sites that are difficult to approach surgically, such as weight-bearing bones or cervical vertebrae, are best treated by low-dose (300 to 600 rads fractioned total dose) local supervoltage irradiation. This low-dose radiotherapy generally eradicates the proliferating histiocytes and allows for normal bone repair, while high-dose radiotherapy leads to tissue damage and resultant poor healing. Surgical decompression followed by low-dose irradiation is sometimes indicated for lesions requiring emergency intervention, such as those compressing the spinal cord. Patients should be carefully followed after therapy for the development of new lesions, which generally arise within the first year after diagnosis. Individuals with a lesion in the bones of the head, neck, or pelvis are more likely to have subsequent disease. Bone scans to detect new lesions and plain films to follow the known site of involvement should be obtained every six months for one to two years after therapy. Extraosseous Langerhans cell granulomatosis involving soft tissue is generally successfully managed by complete surgical excision if possible, or by low-dose irradiation.

MULTIFOCAL LANGERHANS CELL (EOSINOPHILIC) GRANULOMATOSIS

CLINICAL MANIFESTATIONS. Similar to the unifocal form, multifocal Langerhans cell granulomatosis generally presents in children, predominantly in males, and often with *bone lesions.* In addition to the calvarium, the sphenoid bone, sella turcica, mandible, and long bones of the upper extremities may be involved. This tropism for the head is unexplained but may indicate local reaction to an inciting agent that enters via the nasopharynx or oropharynx. Complications of this disorder include chronic otitis media caused by destruction of temporal and mastoid bones, proptosis with orbital masses, loose teeth with infiltration of maxilla or mandible, and both anterior and posterior pituitary dysfunction with involvement of the sella turcica. This last complication may occur with focal disease of hypothalamus or pituitary without bone involvement, and growth retardation of the patient may occur. Diabetes insipidus is caused by granulomatous involve-

ment of the hypothalamus or pituitary and may be either transient or permanent. The classic triad of lytic skull lesions, exophthalmos, and diabetes insipidus called *Hand-Schüller-Christian disease* is best viewed as a subset of multifocal Langerhans cell (eosinophilic) granulomatosis. Dermal lesions may appear papulosquamous, seborrheic, eczematous, and rarely xanthomatous. Vulvar lesions with ulceration are not uncommon. Hepatosplenomegaly and lymphadenopathy are unusual in multifocal Langerhans cell granulomatosis.

In *Langerhans cell granulomatosis* the lung is an important extraosseous site of involvement. The disorder mainly affects young adult men and often presents with a chronic cough, pneumothorax, and constitutional symptoms. The chest radiograph usually shows a diffuse micronodular and interstitial infiltrate involving the mid-zones and bases of the lungs with relative sparing of the costophrenic angles. Ultimately a honeycomb appearance may occur; it is caused by coalescence of small parenchymal pulmonary cysts. Fibrosis is a late finding that may lead to chronic cor pulmonale. Pulmonary function tests may show restrictive impairment. Diagnosis is best made by biopsy that shows the mixed histiocytic-eosinophilic infiltrate with a variable degree of fibrosis. Pulmonary Langerhans cell granulomatosis has a highly variable natural history. Spontaneous remissions are not infrequent, but prognosis is poorer at the extremes of age and with involvement of extrapulmonary organs.

DIAGNOSIS. There are no distinctive laboratory abnormalities in multifocal Langerhans cell granulomatosis. The leukocyte count is generally normal and eosinophilia is not present unless it is from another cause. Hypercalcemia generally does not result from bone lesions.

The diagnosis of multifocal Langerhans cell granulomatosis is definitively made by biopsy, usually of a bone lesion. Again, S-100 detected by the immunoperoxidase method may be useful in confirming the diagnosis. The extent of multifocal involvement is established by physical examination, chest radiography, bone scanning, and if indicated, computed tomography of the brain. This last test is useful for hypothalamic or pituitary lesions associated with diabetes insipidus.

TREATMENT. The natural history of multifocal Langerhans cell granulomatosis is relatively favorable when cases best diagnosed as Letterer-Siwe disease (see below) are excluded. Destructive lesions of bone when present early in the clinical course may predict a better outcome. The therapy is guided by the particular organs involved. Diabetes insipidus and growth retardation should be treated by hormonal replacement with vasopressin (Ch. 226) and human growth hormone, respectively. Low-dose irradiation to the suprasellar area may restore endocrine function in certain individuals. The seborrheic dermal eruption is responsive to tar treatments. X-irradiation using doses generally below 600 rads to symptomatic bony lesions is nearly always effective. Surgery may be necessary to relieve spinal cord compression and mastoid problems and to excise skull lesions eroding through skin. Oral granulomatosis can be treated with dexamethasone elixir used as a mouth rinse three times a day. Similarly, topical steroid creams may accelerate the healing of vulvar lesions.

Systemic therapy is indicated when either radiation fails or multiple sites demand treatment. Corticosteroids alone may achieve dramatic results. Prednisone at a single dose of 0.5 to 1.0 mg per kilogram can be used in the acute phase. Alternate day corticosteroid therapy can be initiated after remission is achieved. Use of cytotoxic agents, such as vinblastine or methotrexate, is generally reserved for aggressive and refractory disease.

There is insufficient experience to recommend a single first-line chemotherapeutic regimen. Addition of vinblastine at a dose of 0.1 mg per kilogram intravenously every week for four to eight weeks is generally successful in achieving remission. It is unclear whether maintenance chemotherapy with weekly vinblastine or prednisone is required to sustain remission. Should disease recur within several months after discontinuation of therapy for the acute phase, the patient should be re-treated with the initially successful regimen and receive maintenance therapy. The striking variability in clinical course makes it difficult to generalize with regard to therapeutic guidelines.

LETTERER-SIWE SYNDROME

In 1924 Letterer described a six-month-old child with diffuse purpura, fever, otitis media, lymphadenopathy, and hepatosplenomegaly. Nine years later, Siwe included this case in a series of six similar cases. In all instances, there was diffuse tissue infiltration by histiocytes. The histiocytes of Letterer-Siwe disease have abundant acidophilic cytoplasm and are often vacuolated. There may be prominent hemophagocytosis. Generally there is a relative paucity of eosinophils in the histiocytic infiltrates.

CLINICAL MANIFESTATIONS. Children are usually affected in the first years of life, although an adult form of the syndrome may exist. Liver, spleen, lymph nodes, lung, and bone are the most commonly affected areas. Laboratory evaluation often demonstrates leukocytosis, although pancytopenia caused by hypersplenism or bone marrow infiltration may be seen. The dermal lesion of Letterer-Siwe disease is generally a brown-red, scaly eczematoid or seborrheic eruption, and purpura secondary to thrombocytopenia may be present. Hepatosplenomegaly may occur with or without jaundice or elevated levels of hepatic parenchymal enzymes. There is no familial or hereditary predisposition, and that distinguishes Letterer-Siwe disease from another histiocytic disorder of infants, familial erythrophagocytic lymphohistiocytosis. A clinical pathologic syndrome nearly identical to Letterer-Siwe disease has been described in immunologically compromised children infected with a variety of viruses. In addition, certain cases termed Letterer-Siwe disease may actually be unusual forms of malignant lymphoma.

TREATMENT. The course of Letterer-Siwe disease is commonly fulminant and fatal. Spontaneous remissions are rare. It is important to distinguish Letterer-Siwe disease from disorders of infectious or clearly neoplastic origin before initiating therapy. Systemic symptoms of Letterer-Siwe disease often improve with corticosteroids and focal lesions may be palliated with radiotherapy. Occasionally, clinical remission has been achieved with chemotherapy, particularly vinblastine and prednisone. If this regimen fails, methotrexate and 6-mercaptopurine may be used. Successful allogeneic bone marrow transplantation has been reported in a single case.

Chu T, D'Angio GJ, Favara B, et al.: Histiocytosis syndromes in children. Lancet 1:208, 1987. *This brief article offers an up-to-date classification of this group of disorders "not only as a standard for diagnosis and patient management but also for research and for use in publications on the subject."*

Elema JD, Atmosoerodjo-Briggs JE: Langerhans' cells and macrophages in eosinophilic granuloma: An enzyme-histochemical, enzyme-cytochemical, and ultrastructural study. Cancer 54:2174, 1984. *An excellent description of histopathology of histiocytic disorders with emphasis on diagnostic markers such as the S-100 protein.*

Greenberger JS, Crocker AC, Vawter G, et al.: Results of treatment of 27 patients with systemic histiocytosis (Letterer-Siwe syndrome, Schuller-Christian syndrome and multifocal eosinophilic granuloma). Medicine 60:311, 1981. *A detailed analysis of therapy of histiocytic disorders at a single academic medical center.*

Groopman JE, Golde DW: The histiocytic disorder: A pathophysiologic analysis. Ann Intern Med 94:95, 1981. *Comprehensive review of the histiocytic disorders with emphasis on pathophysiologic mechanisms; extensive bibliography.*

Komp DM: Langerhans cell histiocytosis. N Engl J Med 316:747, 1987. *An informative editorial with an excellent bibliography.*

Risdall RJ, McKenna RW, Nesbit ME, et al.: Virus-associated hemophagocytic syndrome. A benign histiocytic proliferation distinct from malignant histiocytosis. Cancer 44:993, 1979. *Importance of considering infectious causes of clinicopathologic syndromes easily misdiagnosed as histiocytic disorders.*

Sims DG: Histiocytosis X: Follow-up of 43 cases. Arch Dis Child 52:433, 1977. *A large series followed over a long period; illustrates the striking variability in clinical course.*

Zinkham WH: Multifocal eosinophilic granuloma: Natural history, etiology and management. Am J Med 60:457, 1976. *A comprehensive and well-written clinical paper; of great assistance in clinical management.*

162 EOSINOPHILIC SYNDROMES

David A. Bass

Many diseases that cause eosinophilia, such as parasitic infestations, allergies, and drug reactions, are discussed elsewhere in this book. This chapter provides a brief summary of the distinctive qualities of eosinophils and the types of disease that may be associated with eosinophilia in the peripheral blood.

Eosinophils are granulocytic leukocytes and share with neutrophils similar life cycles, morphology, lysosomal enzymes, potent oxidative metabolism, and phagocytic ability. The distinctive qualities of eosinophils become apparent in their responses during specific immunologic and inflammatory processes. Acute inflammation causes stimulation of neutrophil production, inhibition of eosinophil production, and eosinopenia in the peripheral blood. Administration of glucocorticosteroids causes eosinopenia and neutrophilia. Moreover, unlike neutrophils, eosinophils appear closely linked to the immune system. Eosinophil stimulation most commonly follows repeated or prolonged antigenic exposure, especially when the antigens are deposited in tissues and elicit hypersensitivity reactions. Stimulation of eosinophilia in delayed hypersensitivity reactions is T lymphocyte dependent. During immune responses to metazoan parasites, lymphocytes release substances that stimulate eosinopoiesis.

The functions of eosinophils remain a subject of debate. The two currently favored hypotheses appear contrasting, if not contradictory. One hypothesis views the eosinophil as a protective killer cell, similar to the neutrophil, but specifically involved in defense against metazoan parasites. The alternative theory views the eosinophil as an anti-inflammatory modulator of hypersensitivity reactions, serving to constrain the immune response and minimize its unnecessary spread.

Eosinophils may on occasion be harmful rather than beneficial. Prolonged, marked eosinophilia may be associated with Löffler's endomyocardial disease, discussed below. Eosinophils may also contribute to localized tissue damage in specific syndromes. For example, a component of eosinophil granules, the major basic protein, causes cytopathic changes in tracheal epithelium in vitro that are similar to the changes observed in patients with asthma.

EOSINOPHILIC SYNDROMES AFFECTING ORGAN SYSTEMS

HYPEREOSINOPHILIC SYNDROME. This is a myeloproliferative syndrome with persistent, marked eosinophilia (above 1500 per cubic millimeter) and evidence of organ involvement. Eosinophilic infiltrates may cause dysfunction of diverse tissues, including the following: The heart may reveal the changes of Löffler's endomyocardial disease. Most patients have hepatosplenomegaly, although laboratory studies of hepatic functions demonstrate minimal abnormalities, usually limited to a modest elevation of serum alkaline phosphatase. Central nervous system complications may present as diffuse changes (confusion, delusion, psychosis, coma) or localized problems, including peripheral neuropathies or hemiparesis. Gastrointestinal involvement may cause diarrhea, nonspecific abdominal pains, and occasionally malabsorption syndromes. Pulmonary involvement may present as interstitial infiltrates that contain large numbers of eosinophils on biopsy. Pleural effusions may occur. Rashes occur in 25 to 50 per cent of the patients and are usually nonspecific, urticarial, or maculopapular. The presence of angioedema has been suggested to be a favorable indicator of therapeutic responses. Patients often have a mild normochromic normocytic anemia, but severe anemia or thrombocytopenia is rare. Once organ involvement is demonstrated, the prognosis without treatment is poor, with about half dying by nine months.

However, about one third of the patients with this syndrome may respond to corticosteroid therapy; moreover, the majority of the remainder may have a favorable response to hydroxyurea. Death is often due to cardiac involvement with endomyocarditis and congestive failure. Death caused by infections or thrombocytopenia with bleeding is unusual. Rare cases have terminated in a blastic crisis, even following "successful" treatment with hydroxyurea.

EOSINOPHILIC LEUKEMIA. Eosinophilic leukemia is rare. A number of patients have been described with immature eosinophils in the peripheral blood, thrombocytopenia, and severe anemia. In some patients chromosomal aberrations, including the Philadelphia chromosome, have been described.

LÖFFLER'S ENDOMYOCARDIAL DISEASE. This involves a thickening of the endocardium with subendocardial myocardial degeneration and infiltration by eosinophils. Either or both ventricles may be involved; atria are usually minimally affected. It may present as a restrictive cardiomyopathy and/or valvular dysfunction, usually mitral regurgitation, leading to right- or left-sided congestive heart failure. Mural thrombi may further compromise cardiac function or cause embolic events. Over 90 per cent of the patients are males. This disease may be due to the release of some component of eosinophil leukocytes, since it has been observed during diverse illnesses characterized by great and prolonged blood eosinophilia, i.e., an eosinophil count higher than 2000 per cubic millimeter for longer than 12 months, including solid tumors, metazoan parasites, hypersensitivity vasculitis, the hypereosinophilic syndrome, and eosinophilic leukemia.

DISEASES ASSOCIATED WITH EOSINOPHILIA
(Table 162–1)

ALLERGIES AND DRUG REACTIONS. These are discussed in other chapters. Although acute allergic reactions may cause leukemoid eosinophilic responses (eosinophils above 20,000 per cubic millimeter), chronic allergy is rarely associated with eosinophil counts above 2000 per cubic millimeter.

INFECTIONS. Infestations by *invasive metazoan parasites* almost always cause eosinophilia. Noninvasive helminths (e.g., pinworm, whipworm) or encysted parasites (e.g., echinococcus) are less regularly associated with peripheral eosinophilia. Protozoa do not usually cause eosinophilia. Mycobacterial and fungal infections are not usually associated with eosinophilia; however, about 10 per cent of patients with afebrile *tuberculosis* may have a modest increase in blood eosinophils. Acute *coccidioidomycosis* often causes immunologic manifestations, including erythema nodosum, erythema multiforme, urticaria, polyarthritis, and eosinophilia. Acute bacterial and viral infections are usually associated with eosinopenia in the peripheral blood. Exceptions to this rule include the eosinophilias of *chlamydial pneumonia of infancy*, *cat scratch disease*, *infectious lymphocytosis*, and occasional cases of *infectious mononucleosis*. During the convalescent phase of acute infections, occasional patients will develop a transient, usually mild eosinophilia. In scarlet fever, eosinophilia regularly appears coincidentally with the characteristic rash.

SKIN DISEASES. Diverse skin diseases may be associated with eosinophilia. Best documented are the eosinophilias of *atopic dermatitis, eczema, acute urticaria* (but not chronic urticaria or angioneurotic edema), *pemphigus, bullous pemphigoid, herpes gestationis,* and *Wells' syndrome.* Eosinophil counts may be useful in the evaluation of *toxic epidermal necrolysis.* Eosinophil counts are usually elevated when this entity is due to a drug reaction but are usually reduced when staphylococci are the cause.

PULMONARY EOSINOPHILIAS. See Ch. 63.
EOSINOPHILIC GASTROENTERITIS. See Ch. 162.
NEOPLASTIC DISORDERS. A small proportion, about 5

TABLE 162–1. DISORDERS ASSOCIATED WITH EOSINOPHILIA

I. **Allergy**
    A. Allergic rhinitis
    B. Asthma
    C. Atopic dermatitis
    D. Acute urticaria
    E. Drug reactions
II. **Infectious diseases**
    A. Tissue-invasive helminths
       1. Major tropical
          a. Filariasis
          b. Schistosomiasis
       2. North America
          a. Strongyloidiasis
          b. Trichinosis
          c. Toxocariasis
          d. Ascariasis
          e. Occasional in hookworm disease, echinococcosis, cysticercosis
    B. Other infections
       1. Acute coccidioidomycosis
       2. Afebrile tuberculosis
       3. Cat scratch disease
       4. Chlamydial pneumonia of infancy
       5. Convalescent phase of many infections, especially scarlet fever
III. **Other cutaneous diseases**
    A. Bullous pemphigoid
    B. Herpes gestationis
    C. Recurrent granulomatous dermatitis
    D. Scabies
IV. **Other pulmonary diseases**
    A. Transient pulmonary eosinophilic infiltrates (Löffler's syndrome)
    B. Hypersensitivity pneumonitis
    C. Allergic bronchopulmonary aspergillosis
    D. Tropical eosinophilia
    E. Chronic eosinophilic pneumonia
V. **Connective tissue diseases**
    A. Polyarteritis group
       1. Allergic granulomatosis (Churg-Strauss type)
       2. Angiitis with hepatitis B antigenemia
    B. Rheumatoid arthritis (severe)
    C. Eosinophilic fasciitis
    D. Sjögren's syndrome
VI. **Neoplastic and myeloproliferative diseases**
    A. Solid tumors, especially mucin secreting, epithelial cell origin especially when metastatic to serosa or bone
    B. Lymphoid
       1. Lymphomas, especially T cell type and Hodgkin's disease
       2. T cell and acute lymphoblastic leukemias
       3. Occasional with myeloma (heavy chain disease)
    C. Hypereosinophilic syndrome
    D. Other
       1. Histiocytosis with cutaneous involvement
       2. Angiolymphoid hyperplasia (Kimura's disease)
VII. **Immunodeficiency diseases**
    A. Selective IgA deficiency
    B. Swiss-type and sex-linked combined immunodeficiency
    C. Nezelof syndrome
    D. Wiskott-Aldrich syndrome
    E. Hyper-IgE syndrome
    F. Graft versus host reactions
VIII. **Occasional causes of eosinophilia**
    A. Eosinophilic gastroenteritis
    B. Inflammatory bowel disease
    C. Chronic active hepatitis
    D. Long-term dialysis
    E. Acute pancreatitis
    F. Postirradiation
    G. Hypopituitarism
    H. Other localized disorders with occasional blood eosinophilia
       1. Eosinophilic lymphadenitis
       2. Eosinophilic cystitis
       3. Eosinophilic cholecystitis
       4. Eosinophilic meningitis

per cent, of patients with *carcinomas* and *sarcomas* may have eosinophilia. Eosinophilia with solid tumors may be indicative of metastatic dissemination. A mild eosinophilia accompanies *Hodgkin's disease* in roughly one fifth of patients; however, in occasional cases, marked eosinophilia (up to 98 per cent) has occurred. *Immunoblastic lymphadenopathy* is associated with eosinophilia in about one third of cases. Cutaneous involvement with neoplastic disorders, including histiocytic medullary reticulosis, mycosis fungoides, and Sézary's syndrome, may have an associated eosinophilia.

IMMUNE DISEASES. In the absence of pulmonary involvement, polyarteritis is rarely associated with eosinophilia. By contrast, *polyarteritis with pulmonary involvement* (asthma) and the *allergic granulomatosis of Churg and Strauss* are associated with eosinophilia in a great majority of cases. The syndrome of *polyarteritis in association with hepatitis antigenemia* may also be accompanied by eosinophilia. Mild eosinophilia occurs in about 10 per cent of patients with *rheumatoid arthritis* at some time during their disease. Occasional cases, usually those of long standing with nodules and pleuropulmonary involvement, may have marked peripheral blood eosinophilia. The syndrome of *eosinophilic fasciitis* is discussed in Ch. 437. In one large series, about two thirds of patients with *Sjögren's syndrome* had eosinophilia. Mild eosinophilia is often noted in *immune deficiency syndromes*, whether involving the T or B lymphocyte series, and in certain defects of neutrophil production or function. Such patients may respond to pulmonary infection by *Pneumocystis carinii* with marked eosinophilia. The syndrome of *eosinophilic lymphadenitis* is characterized by peripheral blood eosinophilia associated with localized, usually inguinal or axillary, lymphadenopathy. The response appears to follow repeated local exposures to an antigen, such as an insect sting, on a peripheral extremity. Involved lymph nodes may be densely infiltrated with eosinophils.

Many other diseases of presumed immunologic etiology are not associated with eosinophilia; these include systemic lupus erythematosus, systemic sclerosis, glomerulonephritis, acute rheumatic fever, serum sickness, autoimmune hemolytic anemia, thrombocytopenic purpura, Hashimoto's thyroiditis, pernicious anemia, and myasthenia gravis.

RADIATION-RELATED EOSINOPHILIA. About 40 per cent of patients with an intra-abdominal neoplasm exhibit eosinophilia during the first few weeks of radiation therapy. Such patients may also develop proctitis with a marked local infiltration of eosinophils.

INFLAMMATORY BOWEL DISEASE. Local inflammatory lesions of *ulcerative colitis* may be rich in eosinophils, and a slight elevation of blood eosinophils may occur in this disease. Some observers have also reported modest eosinophilia during symptomatic phases of *Crohn's disease*, and this may be a helpful guide in differentiating Crohn's disease from acute appendicitis.

CHRONIC ACTIVE HEPATITIS. About one third of patients with chronic hepatitis have eosinophils in excess of 5 per cent.

DRESSLER'S SYNDROME. Although not mentioned in recent reviews, 20 per cent of the patients in Dressler's original series had eosinophilia.

PANCREATIC DISEASES. A distinctive clinical syndrome associated with acinar cell carcinoma of the pancreas includes polyarthritis, subcutaneous panniculitis, and blood eosinophilia. Similar symptoms and signs may be observed two to six weeks following acute pancreatitis.

DIALYSIS. About one third of patients undergoing long-term hemodialysis develop blood and bone marrow eosinophilia without apparent cause. Similarly, long-term peritoneal dialysis may evoke an eosinophilic peritoneal effusion and occasionally elevated numbers of eosinophils in the blood. This eosinophilic peritonitis may be associated with abdominal pain and fever, and may be mistaken for a bacterial infection unless a differential count of the exudate is obtained.

ADDISON'S DISEASE. Although occasional patients with Addison's disease and eosinophilia have been observed, this is not typical. In one series, the only patients with eosinophilia had hypopituitarism.

Fauci AS, Harley JB, Roberts WC, et al: The idiopathic hypereosinophilic syndrome: Clinical, pathophysiologic, and therapeutic considerations. Ann Intern Med 97:78, 1982. *An excellent up-to-date summary of the eosinophil and hypereosinophilia from the National Institutes of Health.*

Weller PF, Goetzl EJ: Dermatological conditions associated with eosinophilia and eosinophilic diseases. In Kay AB, Goetzl EJ (eds.): Contemporary Issues in Clinical Immunology and Allergy: Immunodermatology. Edinburgh, Churchill Livingstone, 1984. *A general review of the disorders associated with eosinophilia and how they should be approached clinically.*

163 PLASMA CELL DISORDERS
Sydney E. Salmon

GENERAL CONSIDERATIONS

The plasma cell disorders are a group of related neoplastic diseases associated with proliferation of a single clone of immunoglobulin-secreting plasma cells derived from the B cell series of immunocytes. This group of disorders has variously been referred to with a series of synonymous terms: monoclonal gammopathies, plasma cell dyscrasias, gammopathies, immunoglobulinopathies, paraproteinemias, and dysproteinemias.

The plasma cell disorders to be discussed here are monoclonal neoplasms; their secreted immunoglobulin products are electrophoretically and immunologically homogeneous and therefore readily distinguished from the heterogeneous populations of immunoglobulin-antibody molecules secreted by the numerous clones of normal B cells. There are five major classes of immunoglobulins synthesized by B lymphocytes and plasma cells: IgG, IgA, IgM, IgD, and IgE (see Ch. 417). Immunoglobulins are antibody protein molecules that all have a basic monomeric unit structure of two heavy (H) chains and two light (L) chains, which each have "constant" and "variable" regions with respect to amino acid sequence. IgG, IgA, IgD, and IgE are synthesized and secreted as monomers with molecular weights in the range of 150,000 to 190,000; IgM is secreted as a pentameric structure with a molecular weight of 900,000. Class specificity of each immunoglobulin is defined in terms of a series of antigenic determinants on the constant regions of the H chains (γ, α, μ, δ, ϵ). There are also two major types of L chains (κ and λ) defined by antigenic determinants on the constant regions of the L chains. The amino sequence in the variable regions of immunoglobulin molecules corresponds to the zone of the active antigen-combining site of the antibody, whereas the constant regions convey other biologic properties. (Structural and functional properties of immunoglobulins are summarized in Table 417–1 and Figure 417–1).

A homogeneous immunoglobulin, as a sharp peak or "spike" in the beta or gamma globulin zone on electrophoresis, is referred to as an M-component. Electrophoresis and immuno-electrophoresis, respectively, are used to quantitate and qualitatively identify M-components. Definition of an M-component as monoclonal (having a single H chain and a single L chain type) requires immunoelectrophoretic or immunofixation studies or both.

Plasma cells represent the most well-differentiated progeny in the B cell series of immunocytes. They contain substantial quantities of rough-surfaced endoplasmic reticulum that is rich in RNA, and are specialized for production of antibody molecules at a rapid rate. In the normal immune response, individual plasma cells can synthesize and secrete immunoglobulin at rates up to 100,000 molecules per minute. Immunoglobulin secretion rates of neoplastic plasma cells are generally somewhat lower than those for normal plasma cells. Additionally, in neoplastic clones, H and L chain biosynthesis is sometimes "unbalanced" with excessive synthesis of free L chains, which are usually secreted by the cell as L chain dimers of molecular weight 60,000. The relatively low molecular weight of secreted L chains permits them to undergo renal glomerular filtration. While limited amounts of free L chains can be reabsorbed and catabolized by the renal tubule, excessive amounts are excreted in the urine. Monoclonal L chains in the urine in association with B cell neoplasms are referred to as *Bence Jones proteins*, in tribute to the clinical chemist who discovered their differential solubilization on boiling and precipitation on cooling. Electrophoretic and immunologic techniques are now used to assess urinary L chain excretion. The B lymphoid cell precursors of plasma cells have somewhat more limited capability for immunoglobulin synthesis; the immunoglobulin they produce is more frequently displayed on the cell membrane than secreted by the cell. In some instances, individual lymphoid cells may display more than one immunoglobulin on their surfaces (particularly IgD plus IgM). In such instances, both molecules express the identical L chain type and apparent antibody specificity, and the immunoglobulin class expressed is in the course of being "switched" in association with clonal proliferation and differentiation. A number of the B cell neoplasms discussed in this text are manifest as if frozen at various points along this differentiation pathway. Most cases of chronic lymphocytic leukemia, non-Hodgkin's lymphoma, multiple myeloma, macroglobulinemia, and related disorders appear to originate from monoclonal B cell progenitors and are expressed as immunoglobulin-synthesizing neoplasms with either surface membrane or secreted monoclonal immunoglobulin (see Ch. 152). Despite the apparently common origin of these neoplasms, the clinical manifestations, response to treatment, and prognosis of these neoplasms differ substantially. In most instances, the tumor stem cells for one of these neoplasms (those progenitor cells responsible for the metastatic spread and self-renewal of the tumor) give rise to cells that express

the original differentiation state and clinical features of the particular neoplasm (e.g., multiple myeloma). In occasional instances of plasma cell neoplasia (and chronic lymphocytic leukemia and follicular lymphoma) apparent "subcloning" occurs during the patient's clinical course, and the pattern of histology and tumor growth takes on a less differentiated form—e.g., as a poorly differentiated large cell lymphoma. Such transformations are often associated with some change in immunoglobulin synthesis or secretion. Immunologic commonality with the original clone can usually be found, however, by the use of sophisticated techniques. A classification of B cell disorders associated with secretion of an M-component appears in Table 163–1.

Stites DP, Stobo JD, Wells JV: Basic and Clinical Immunology. 6th ed. Los Altos, Lange Medical Publications, 1987. *An excellent and reasonably priced text on immunology for students, house staff, and physicians.*

MULTIPLE MYELOMA

DEFINITION. Multiple myeloma (plasma cell myeloma, myelomatosis) is a disseminated malignant disease in which a clone of transformed plasma cells proliferates in the bone marrow, disrupting its normal functions as well as invading the adjacent bone. The disease is frequently associated with extensive skeletal destruction, hypercalcemia, anemia, impaired renal function, immunodeficiency, and increased susceptibility to infection. Amyloidosis, clotting disorders, and other protein abnormalities are occasional associations. The neoplastic plasma cells usually produce and secrete M-component immunoglobulin, the amount of which in any given case varies proportionally with the total body tumor burden.

ETIOLOGY. The etiology of human myeloma is unknown; however, genetic predisposition, oncogenic viruses, inflammatory stimuli, and chronic antigenic stimulation have all been implicated.

A mouse model of myeloma has provided some basis for the aforementioned hypotheses. Myeloma can be readily induced in the inbred BALB-C strain of mice by intraperitoneal injection of mineral oil. Such mice are known to harbor oncogenic type C RNA viruses. Of interest, BALB-C mice raised in a germ-free environment fail to develop myeloma after oil injection (although other lymphoid neoplasms may arise). This suggests that bacterial antigenic exposure may be required to increase sufficiently the proliferation of populations of immunoglobulin-producing B cells to render them susceptible to myeloma induction. Myeloma appears to be epizootic, having been reported in rats, dogs, cats, horses, and other mammalian species.

INCIDENCE AND PREVALENCE. Multiple myeloma is a disease most frequently observed in the middle-aged and elderly (median age 60), with an incidence that increases with age. Rare cases have been reported in younger persons, including a few teenagers. The annual incidence of myeloma is 3 per 100,000 population (about as common as Hodgkin's disease). It is slightly more common in males than females, and has been reported in all racial groups. Myeloma accounts for about 10 per cent of hematologic malignant tumors and 1 per cent of all forms of cancer.

PATHOPHYSIOLOGY. The symptoms and signs of multiple myeloma and its consequences on the patient are related primarily to (1) the growth kinetics of the neoplastic plasma cells and the total body tumor burden and (2) secreted products of the tumor cells which have physiochemical, immunologic, or humoral effects. The various secreted products can induce a wide variety of clinical syndromes in patients with myeloma.

MYELOMA CELL MASS. Once transformed plasma cells begin to proliferate in a malignant fashion, the clone appears to grow relatively rapidly with a tumor stem cell doubling time of 24 to 48 hours. Although the neoplasm appears to originate from a single transformed cell (10^0 cells) at a single location, progressive myeloma growth is associated with hem-

TABLE 163–1. CLASSIFICATION OF DISORDERS ASSOCIATED WITH MONOCLONAL IMMUNOGLOBULIN (M-COMPONENT SECRETION)

Disorder	M-Component	
1. Plasma cell neoplasms		
A. Multiple myeloma	IgG>IgA>IgD>IgE	
	± free L chain or L chain alone (κ>λ) rarely biclonal or without detectable Ig abnormality	
B. Macroglobulinemia	IgM ± free L chain (κ>λ)	
C. H chain diseases	γ, α, or μ chain or fragment; ?, δ, or ε	
D. Primary amyloidosis	Free L chain (κ>λ) or L chain fragment alone or plus IgG, IgA, IgM, or IgD	
E. Monoclonal gammopathy of unknown significance	IgG, IgM, IgA, or IgD usually without L chain secretion	
2. Other B cell neoplasms	*M-component* (occasionally secreted)	
A. Chronic lymphocytic leukemia	IgM>IgG	
B. B cell non-Hodgkin's lymphomas (any morphologic pattern or lymphoid cell types)		
3. Nonlymphoid neoplasms—Chronic myelogenous leukemia; carcinoma of colon, breast, prostate, or other sites	No consistent patterns	
4. "Autoimmune" or autoreactive disorders	*M-component*	*Antibody activity of M-component*
A. Cold agglutinin disease (some characteristics of Waldenström's macroglobulinemia)	IgMκ most common	Anti-I antigen of RBC membrane
B. Mixed cryoglobulinemia	IgM	Anti-IgG
C. Hypergammaglobulinemia	IgG	Anti-IgG
D. Sjögren's syndrome	IgM	?
5. Miscellaneous inflammatory, storage, or infectious disorders		
Lichen myxedematous	IgGλ	
Gaucher's disease	IgG	
Cirrhosis, sarcoidosis, parasitic diseases, renal acidosis	No consistent pattern	

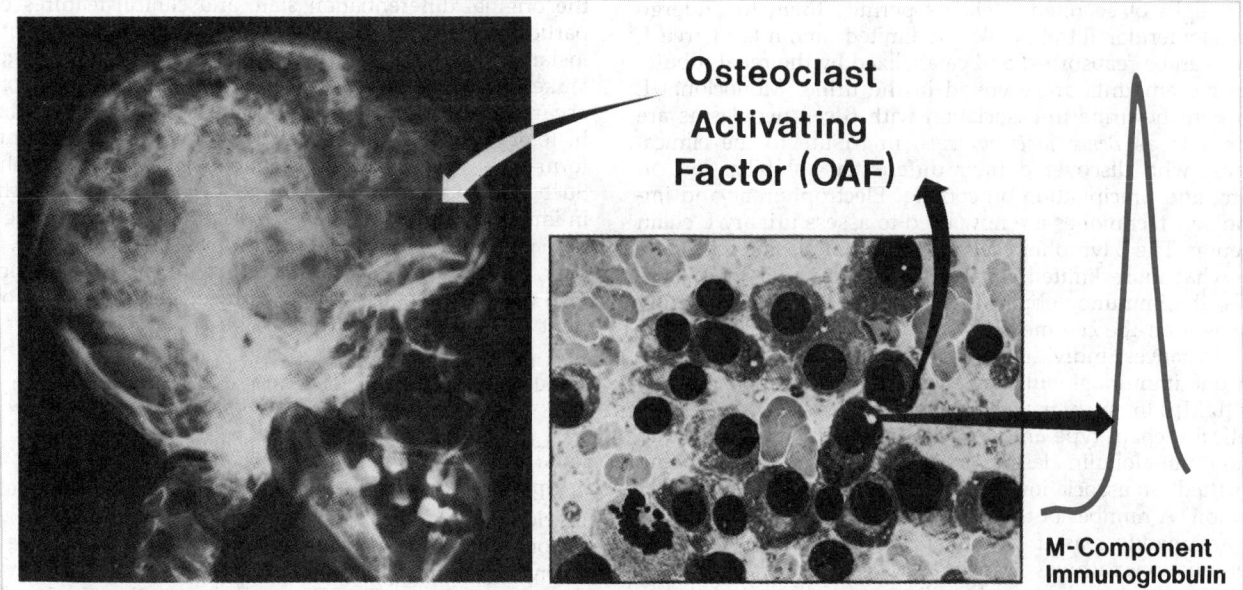

FIGURE 163–1. Clinicopathologic features of multiple myeloma. The type of extensive skeletal destruction ("Swiss cheese"-like lesions) observed in Stage III myeloma patients is represented by the skull at the left of the figure. The patient's bone marrow (center) contains an infiltrate of neoplastic plasma cells which can synthesize and secrete both an osteoclast activating factor (OAF), and a monoclonal immunoglobulin, which appears as a "spike" on protein electrophoresis. Serial measurements of the M-component provide a useful quantitative marker for growth or regression of the neoplasm, as the M-component production rate per myeloma cell remains relatively constant in most cases.

atogenous spread of the neoplastic cells to various skeletal sites, leading to widespread involvement of the bone marrow with nodules or sheets of plasma cells (Fig. 163–1). Marrow involvement leads to development of a normochromic normocytic anemia that is apparent in virtually all patients with myeloma. This appears to be the consequence of tumor-related inhibition of erythropoiesis as well as the disturbance of marrow architecture. A slight shortening of red cell survival, iron deficiency, and blood loss may also contribute to the anemia. High concentrations of a serum M-component may lead to blood sludging and hyperviscosity. Rouleaux formation observed on the peripheral blood smear and an increase in the sedimentation rate are also due to high concentrations of myeloma globulins in the plasma. In addition to monoclonal immunoglobulin, myeloma cells also secrete calcium-mobilizing substances, osteoclast activating factors (OAF's), which stimulate local bone resorption by osteoclasts in the vicinity of foci of myeloma in the bone marrow. Simultaneously, local osteoblastic activity is inhibited. Radiographically, this may result in osteopenia resembling osteoporosis and in discrete osteolytic bone lesions as well as hypercalcemia and hypercalciuria (Fig. 163–2). Several peptides with OAF activity have been isolated. Tumor growth factor alpha (TGF-α) is one of the major growth factors that mobilizes calcium from bone. Secretion of the M-component immunoglobulin appears to occur at a relatively constant rate per myeloma cell in approximately 90 per cent of myeloma patients. Availability of this tumor marker permits quantitation of the total body tumor burden because both the cellular synthetic rate of the M-component and its total body synthetic rate can be determined. "Early myeloma" is associated with a substantial tumor burden $\approx 5 \times 10^{12}$ myeloma cells (about 0.5 kg). As the total body tumor mass reaches the clinical level of detection, its growth rate slows substantially (to a doubling time of two to six months) following a typical gompertzian growth curve (see Ch. 168). Cytokinetically, this slowing of growth is associated with a fall in the fraction of tumor cells traversing the cell cycle, as determined with tritiated thymidine autoradiography. Patients with extensive myeloma who are close to death generally have $>3 \times 10^{12}$ myeloma cells in the body (3.0 kg) as well as extensive lytic bone lesions and fractures and other findings characteristic of myeloma.

M-Components in Myeloma. The monoclonal immunoglobulin types that are secreted as M-component are usually IgG, IgA, or free L chains of Ig. Occasionally, the M-component will be IgD and extremely rarely, IgE. (IgM secretion is characteristically associated with macroglobulinemia.) The frequency of these different immunologic types of plasma cell disorders is roughly proportional to the serum concentration (see Table 417–1) and total body synthetic rate for the various immunoglobulins. When L chains are secreted (as dimers) into the plasma, they are rapidly extracted and metabolized by the kidney and thus are not usually detected on serum electrophoresis. When the renal threshold is exceeded, L chains appear in the urine (Bence Jones proteins). If the patient has renal failure (sometimes induced by L dimers), a serum M-component composed only of L chains may appear. L chains or L chain fragments with high tissue affinity are sometimes deposited as a characteristic infiltrative deposit ("amyloid") in certain tissues (see Immunocytic [Primary] Amyloidosis below).

If an IgG or IgA M-component has a high intrinsic viscosity (related to molecular aggregation or asymmetry) and is present in high concentrations, hyperviscosity and bleeding disorders may develop. These complications are less common in myeloma than in macroglobulinemia. Serum M-components can induce bleeding disorders by complexing or binding immunologically with coagulation factors I, II, V, VII, or VIII. Occasionally, M-components will have narrow thermal amplitude and form cryoglobulins (including mixed cryoglobulin) and lead to Raynaud's phenomenon, impaired circulation, and potential gangrene after cold exposure. Some of these bleeding and circulatory syndromes and other immunologically predicated syndromes (e.g., hemolytic anemia, hyperlipidemia) can now be defined as being due to the M-component's having specific antibody function. These antibodies may have a low binding affinity for a normal antigenic determinant in blood or other tissue, but this may suffice for an interaction in the presence of the large amount of M-component present. Virtually all myeloma immunoglobulins are thought to have some antigen-binding specificity (as the

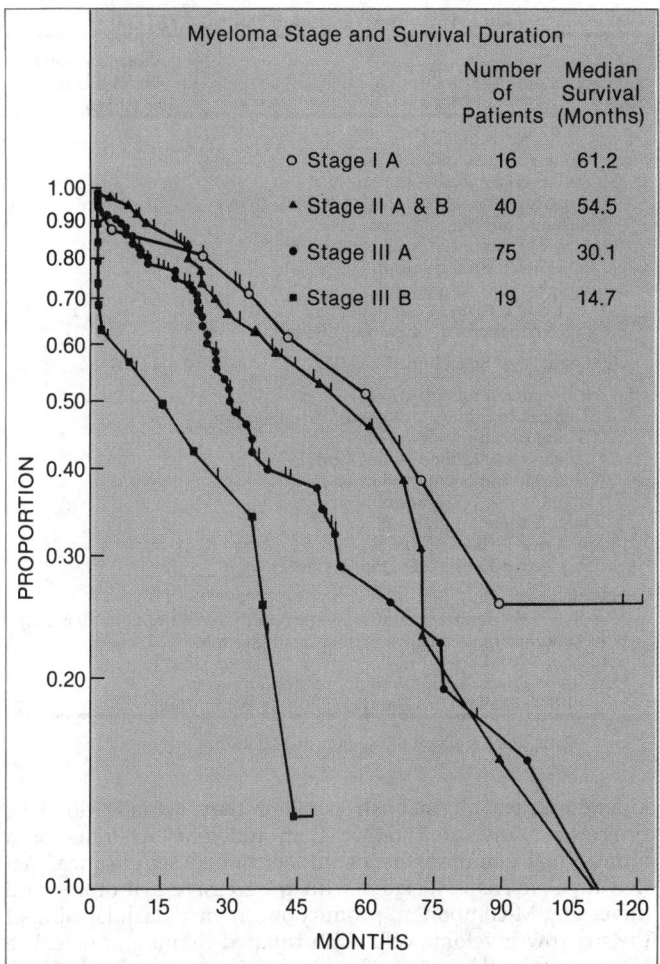

FIGURE 163–2. Life table survival curves for 150 patients with multiple myeloma categorized by stage. (○) Stage IA, (▲) Stages IIA and B, (●) Stage IIIA, and (■) Stage IIIB. Stage IA survival is significantly better than that of Stages IIIA and IIIB. Stages IIA and B are significantly better than Stages IIIA and IIIB. Stages IIIA and IIIB are significantly different from one another. (From Durie BGM, Salmon SE, Moon TE: Blood 55:364, 1980. With permission of the authors and publisher.)

neoplasm arises from a normal committed antibody-producing clone), but in most instances the antibody specificity of any given patient's M-protein remains unknown. Only in the exceptional clinical syndromes (such as those mentioned above) is it likely to be discovered or characterized.

Renal Failure. Renal failure is observed in at least 20 per cent of patients with myeloma and is frequently of mixed pathogenesis. Hypercalcemia leads to calcium nephropathy and is the most common cause of renal failure in myeloma. Second in importance is the presence of heavy Bence Jones proteinuria, which also leads to tubular injury. Additional factors that may also contribute to renal failure in myeloma include hyperuricemia (in association with increased tumor cell DNA turnover), pyelonephritis, and amyloidosis. Functional abnormalities of the kidney in myeloma include acute and chronic renal failure, defects in urine concentration and acidification, and acquired Fanconi syndrome. Histologically the kidneys are usually enlarged; the glomeruli are usually normal. A characteristic "blocked pipe" appearance with eosinophilic casts surrounded by an epithelial syncytium in distal tubules and collecting ducts is the hallmark of "myeloma kidney." This is somewhat more common in patients with lambda L chain excretion.

Immunodeficiency. Patients with myeloma usually have severely depressed serum levels of normal immunoglobulins and a compromised ability to manifest a normal humoral immune response after antigenic stimulation. Consequently,

they are highly susceptible to infection from common encapsulated organisms (e.g., pneumococcus), and pneumonia and other septic episodes are quite common in patients at the time of diagnosis or when the disease has relapsed. A series of mechanisms appears to be responsible for this immunodeficiency syndrome. In the BALB-C mouse model (and presumably in man), myeloma cells secrete an inhibitory substance (not immunoglobulin) that activates macrophage-mediated suppression of proliferation of normal antibody producing B-cell clones. Such macrophage-induced suppression of normal immunoglobulin synthesis has been observed in patients with myeloma. Additionally, in IgG myeloma the secreted IgG M-component accelerates the catabolism of the patient's normal IgG. This is because the IgG fractional catabolic rate increases as the total serum IgG concentration rises, resulting in a shorter half-life for both myeloma and normal IgG. These defects in humoral immunity are often compounded by faulty granulocyte function wherein opsonization and phagocytosis of bacteria may be impaired by the large quantities of M-protein. Finally, the number of available circulating granulocytes may be significantly reduced as a consequence of the disease or myelosuppression secondary to chemotherapy.

CLINICAL MANIFESTATIONS (Table 163–2). Presenting symptoms and signs of myeloma include bone pain (often associated with pathologic fractures of the spine or ribs), weakness resulting from anemia, recurrent infection, hypercalcemia (associated with confusion, polyuria, and constipation), and azotemia, occasionally with paralysis secondary to spinal cord compression or with bleeding disorders. Asymptomatic patients are sometimes identified by the presence of proteinuria in the absence of hypertension, or the presence of increased total serum protein on a multichemistry profile. Not infrequently the presentation is that of back pain, anemia, and a very high sedimentation rate in an older patient. Some patients present with acute renal failure with oliguria, especially following dehydration.

DIAGNOSIS. Patients with one or more of the aforementioned symptoms and signs require laboratory confirmation of the diagnosis of multiple myeloma. Patients may have pallor or focal bone tenderness on examination, but there are no characteristic physical findings. In advanced stages of myeloma, soft tissue plasmacytomas (usually as direct extensions from underlying ribs or other bones) may develop. Lymphadenopathy or splenomegaly is only an occasional finding. The laboratory diagnosis of myeloma includes serum electrophoresis, electrophoresis of a 24-hour urine specimen (with immunologic typing of any serum and/or urine M-components found), and bone marrow aspiration. A complete skeletal x-ray survey should be carried out. Radionuclide bone scans are of little or no value because the suppression of osteoblastic activity associated with myeloma inhibits radionuclide uptake into the lesions. This is also the presumed explanation of the fact that the serum alkaline phosphatase level is usually normal despite severe bony involvement. Typical skeletal x-ray findings appear in Figure 163–1.

TABLE 163–2. CLINICAL MANIFESTATIONS OF MULTIPLE MYELOMA

Bone involvement—osteolysis due to OAF; pain; pathologic fractures; hypercalcemia
Anemia—decreased RBC production plus mild hemolysis
Renal failure—due to calcium nephropathy, L chains, uric acid, amyloid, infection, proteinuria (hypertension is rare), uremia; occasionally acute, oliguric renal failure
Recurrent infections—especially respiratory
Amyloidosis (develops in about 15 per cent)
Plasmacytomas
Rare paraprotein-associated syndromes—hyperviscosity syndrome, cryoglobulinemia, hyperlipoproteinemia
Hemorrhagic diatheses
Very high erythrocyte sedimentation rate and rouleaux formation on blood smear (with serum M-component)

A complete blood count with differential, serum calcium and albumin determinations, one or more tests of renal function, and measurement of serum immunoglobulin and serum beta₂ microglobulin levels are also useful. These tests aid in staging of the disease and distinguishing myeloma from other disorders. Patients suspected of having myeloma on the basis of skeletal and/or bone marrow involvement but lacking a serum M-component generally have L chain myeloma. This is usually identifiable on protein electrophoresis of a 24-hour urine concentrate. Dipsticks for detecting proteinuria are unreliable for detection of urinary L chains, and the heat test for Bence Jones proteins is positive in only about one half of cases of L chain myeloma. Urinary L chains also occur in some patients with primary amyloidosis and about 20 per cent of patients with macroglobulinemia. The rare patients with H chain disease also have urinary or serum M-components on electrophoresis. However, the clinical presentation and immunologic findings are otherwise quite different in those entities.

The definitive diagnosis of multiple myeloma requires the demonstration of plasmacytosis in the marrow (Color plate 3L) or a soft tissue lesion and the presence of significant M-component production plus some evidence of invasiveness. The presence of lytic bone lesions is the best sign of invasiveness. The suppression of normal immunoglobulins, as well as anemia, hypercalcemia, azotemia, bone demineralization, compression fractures, and disease progression, is supportive in making the diagnosis when the major criteria are not all present. Other disorders that must be distinguished from myeloma include monoclonal gammopathy of unknown significance (see under Monoclonal Gammopathies of Undetermined Significance) and metastatic carcinomas. Additionally, indolent myeloma and the occasional case of solitary plasmacytoma (soft tissue) must be distinguished from myeloma because these patients do not require systemic chemotherapy. In patients with myeloma approximately 53 per cent of M-components are IgG, 25 per cent IgA, and 1 per cent IgD. About 20 per cent have apparent pure Bence Jones (L chain) myeloma, with only urinary L chain excretion. Two thirds of patients who have a serum M-component (IgG or IgA) also have concomitant Bence Jones proteinuria. Fewer than 1 per cent of patients have no definable M-component in the serum or urine. Such patients usually have L chain myeloma also, but this is masked by the ability of the kidney to completely catabolize the presented L chains. Immunofluorescent studies of the bone marrow plasma cells with anti-L chain antisera generally identify such patients. One relatively uncommon presentation of myeloma is with plasma cell leukemia. Such patients often have hepatosplenomegaly and occasionally lymphadenopathy as well as an M-component, bone lesions, and a circulating plasma cell count of greater than 2000 per cubic millimeter.

CLINICAL STAGING. As is the case in other neoplasms, quantitative staging information is useful in projecting the prognosis for individual patients and for deciding on the approach and intensity of treatment. A prognostically useful staging system has been developed for myeloma by correlating various pretreatment prognostic factors (hemoglobin, calcium, quantity of M-component secretion, and degree of skeletal involvement on roentgenograms) with the total body tumor cell number as measured immunologically (Table 163–3). Thus, myeloma patients can be categorized as having Stage I (low), II (intermediate), or III (high) disease with respect to tumor burden.

Impairment of renal function has an adverse effect on survival. Cases in which the serum creatinine level is greater than 2.0 mg per deciliter are thus staged with the additional designation B, whereas those with more normal renal function are classed as A. The effect of stage on prognosis is depicted in Figure 163–2. Patients with Stage IA disease sometimes require observation without treatment or, if available, cell

TABLE 163–3. MYELOMA STAGING SYSTEM

Stage	Criteria	Measured Myeloma Cell Mass (Cells × 10^{12} per Square Meter)

I.	*All* of the following:
	1. Hemoglobin value >10 grams/dl
	2. Serum calcium value (≤12 mg/dl)
	3. On x-ray, normal bone structure (scale 0) or solitary bone plasmacytoma only
	4. Low M-component production rates
	  a. IgG value <5 grams/dl
	  b. IgA value <3 grams/dl
	  c. Urine L chain M-component on electrophoresis <4 grams/24 hours
		<0.6 (low)

II.	Fitting neither Stage I nor Stage III	0.6–1.20 (intermediate)

III.	One or more of the following:
	1. Hemoglobin value <8.5 grams/dl
	2. Serum calcium value >12 mg/dl
	3. Advanced lytic bone lesions (scale 3)
	4. High M-component production rates
	  a. IgG value >7 grams/dl
	  b. IgA value >5 grams/dl
	  c. Urine L chain M-component on electrophoresis >12 grams/24 hours
		>1.20 (high)

Subclassification:
A = Relatively normal renal function (serum creatinine value <2.0 mg/dl)
B = Abnormal renal function (serum creatinine value ≥2.0 mg/dl)
Examples:
Stage IA = Low cell mass with normal renal function
Stage IIIB = High cell mass with abnormal renal function

From Durie BGM, Salmon SE: Cancer 36:842, 1975.

kinetic studies to establish whether they actually do have progressive myeloma rather than indolent myeloma or a monoclonal gammopathy of undetermined significance. Active myeloma is associated with progressive symptoms and increasing M-component production. In vitro flash labeling of the marrow myeloma cells with tritiated thymidine reveals a significantly higher proportion of the tumor cells in DNA synthesis in myeloma than in either indolent myeloma or monoclonal gammopathy of unknown significance. Urinary L chain excretion also serves as a signal of an aggressive tumor.

Measurement of serum beta₂-microglobulin can be used as an additional prognostic factor, as its serum concentration appears to reflect myeloma cell burden as well as renal functional impairment. Serum beta₂ microglobulin levels of greater than 6 μg per milliliter are associated with a poor prognosis. However, beta₂-microglobulin does not distinguish between low cell mass myeloma and "monoclonal gammopathies of unknown significance."

TREATMENT AND PROGNOSIS. Some patients with myeloma have relatively indolent disease that, in Stage I cases, is sometimes confused with monoclonal gammopathies of unknown significance. The overwhelming majority of patients have more advanced disease and require active systemic treatment. Two areas of treatment are important: (1) systemic chemotherapy for multiple myeloma, and (2) supportive care for treatment of complications of the disorder (e.g., spinal cord compression, bone pain, hypercalcemia, sepsis, anemia, and renal failure).

Systemic Chemotherapy. Improvements in systemic chemotherapy for multiple myeloma (in the 1960's) resulted in an increased life expectancy for these patients. Prior to this era, the median life expectancy of untreated myeloma patients was less than one year (3.5 to 8.5 months), whereas at present, with optimal chemotherapy, it is about three years on average, and up to five years or more for patients who respond to chemotherapy. Survival is also influenced by the presenting clinical stage and renal function.

Cell cycle nonspecific cytotoxic drugs (alkylating agents, nitrosoureas, and anthracycline antibiotics) have proved to be the most useful agents in the chemotherapy of myeloma. Vinca alkaloids and corticosteroids appear to potentiate the efficacy of the other cytotoxic drugs. Human leukocyte interferons, including the recombinant alfa interferons, are also useful agents in the treatment of myeloma and are currently being evaluated to define their role in combination with other drugs.

Systemic chemotherapy for myeloma traditionally has employed single-agent chemotherapy with an oral alkylating agent plus prednisone. To prevent complications such as hypercalcemia, hyperuricemia, and azotemic patients should be well hydrated before treatment is initiated and ambulated if at all possible. Prevention of treatment-associated hyperuricemia with allopurinol is also of value during the first few months of treatment. (Management of other complications of myeloma is described under Supportive Care.)

The single agents most widely used for the treatment of myeloma are melphalan (Alkeran, L-phenylalanine mustard) and cyclophosphamide (Cytoxan). Either can be given on a chronic low dose daily basis or in intermittent pulsed courses of therapy. Although equivalent therapeutic results appear to be obtained with either of these schedules, the intermittent course necessitates fewer physician visits and may be associated with less late failure of hematopoietic stem cells. For the intermittent pulse schedules, melphalan is generally administered in a total dose of 8 mg per square meter per day orally for four days and repeated every three to four weeks. Alternatively, higher doses may be given with longer intervals between treatments. Cyclophosphamide is given in a dose of 0.8 gram per square meter either intravenously as a single dose or in divided daily oral doses over four days, every three to four weeks. Both of these alkylating agent schedules usually incorporate a course of 60 mg per square meter of prednisone per day for four days. The amounts given of both of the alkylating agents must be monitored closely with regard to the magnitude and duration of toxic side effects, particularly myelosuppression. Oral melphalan seems to vary significantly in bioavailability from patient to patient. In lieu of an assay for its plasma level, it is important to use a sufficient dose to induce some myelosuppression. Both melphalan and cyclophosphamide dosages are generally reduced if the total white blood count at the time of the next treatment is less than 3000 and the granulocyte count less than 2000 or the platelet count less than 100,000. Melphalan, cyclophosphamide, and the nitrosourea carmustine (BCNU) have been combined in various ways, often with the addition of vincristine (Oncovin) and sometimes doxorubicin (Adriamycin). Results with these more intensive regimens, including alternations of a number of active agents, appear better in high tumor burden patients (Stage III) than simple combinations of an alkylating agent and prednisone. Very high intravenous doses of melphalan have been administered to myeloma patients along with aggressive supportive care. While this approach has induced excellent remissions in some patients, it remains quite toxic and experimental. Whether therapy is warranted for Stage I patients remains to be defined, as the treatment often causes toxicity, and therapy can be delayed until clearer evidence of invasiveness is present.

After systemic chemotherapy is initiated, patients with responsive myeloma generally have prompt relief of bone pain and reversal of symptoms and signs of hypercalcemia, anemia, and recurrent infection. Other symptoms frequently improve, and there is often a feeling of general well-being. However, major healing of osteolytic lesions or improvement in the depressed levels of normal immunoglobulins is distinctly uncommon, suggesting some persisting cellular or humoral defect in the recovery from these two myeloma-induced abnormalities. Associated with such symptomatic and general improvement, the quantity of the M-component produced falls progressively as the myeloma cells responsible for its synthesis are killed by the cytotoxic agents. The rate of fall of the serum M-component concentration or of urinary L chain excretion depends both upon the rate of kill of the

myeloma cells and upon the fractional catabolic rate of the immunoglobulin. Inasmuch as L chains have a fractional catabolic rate of about six hours, their excretion can be substantially reduced within three to four days after effective lysis of tumor cells. However, the various serum M-components are metabolized more slowly; reduction in the IgG M-component marker of tumor burden may lag four to six weeks behind symptomatic improvement with chemotherapy. With currently available treatment some 60 to 75 per cent of myeloma patients achieve at least 75 per cent reduction in the total body myeloma cell mass (as calculated from reductions in M-component synthesis). In general, at least this degree of reduction in tumor burden is required to observe significant improvement in survival with chemotherapy. Lesser degrees of tumor regression are observed in the remainder of patients. Although classed as "nonresponders," most achieve some symptomatic benefit. Patients who achieve objective response generally have a persistent and stable low level of monoclonal plasma cells in the bone marrow and M-component secretion despite continued cytotoxic therapy. Cell kinetic studies in remission indicate that the residual tumor cells are hypoproliferative. In some instances, patients can be followed in a remission without continued administration of chemotherapy. However, this is a difficult course to follow in patients who present with Stage III disease or who have Bence Jones myeloma, as these patients tend to relapse quickly (within less than six months) when treatment is discontinued. Most myeloma patients who achieve remission have less than one log of tumor regression (90 per cent) with treatment, and only about 10 per cent of patients have as much as a two log regression (99 per cent). Thus, even in remission, there is a large subclinical residue of tumor cells (greater than 10^{10} tumor cells). Even though many of these cells may not be in the tumor stem cell compartment, there is still a sufficient number of malignant cells present to lead to eventual relapse in virtually all patients with multiple myeloma. Cures will require development of more effective therapy in the future. Patients who present with renal failure and those whose tumor clones produce only L chains (particularly of the λ type) tend to have a poorer response to treatment with more frequent early relapse and shorter survival than those who present with a serum M-component. Outcome in IgG cases also tends to be somewhat better than that in IgA cases. Among Stage III cases, the fraction of the tumor cells in DNA synthesis (growth fraction) also affects prognosis, with the patients with a high growth fraction having relatively brief responses to treatment and short survival. Patients presenting with plasma cell leukemia also have a high growth fraction, poor response to treatment, and short survival.

Patients with tumors exhibiting a high growth fraction tend to respond very quickly to chemotherapy, with a rapid fall in the M-component to remission levels (e.g., within six weeks), but then relapse occurs quickly. More durable responses require three to eight months to achieve. For patients who achieve objective remission, serial monitoring of the quantity of serum and/or urinary M-component on electrophoresis or with nephelometry provides an excellent means for assessing the stability of the remission and for detecting relapse at its earliest stages, often before the patient develops recurrent hypercalcemia or new lytic lesions.

In most patients with myeloma who achieve 75 per cent tumor regression, remission remains for at least three years before relapse occurs, as manifested by a rising M-component or new symptoms. In only occasional Stage III patients is the disease still in remission beyond six years after the diagnosis (Fig. 163–2). Some useful approaches to secondary chemotherapy have been devised that are beneficial to patients in whom relapse results from primary treatment. For example, there is not complete cross-resistance between melphalan and cyclophosphamide, and disease relapsing after treatment with one of these agents will occasionally respond to the other. A more useful approach has been that of the intravenous combination of carmustine (BCNU) and doxorubicin (Adriamycin) with each drug administered at a dosage of 30 mg per square meter every three weeks. Vincristine (Oncovin) and prednisone can be administered along with these drugs in an attempt to potentiate their effect. About one half of patients who initially respond to alkylating agents can achieve second remissions with these agents. Alfa interferons have also been useful for inducing secondary remissions. Second remissions rarely last longer than one year. The terminal phase of myeloma is characterized by symptoms and signs of progressive growth of the drug-resistant tumor (e.g., bone pain, hypercalcemia, fractures, rising M-component, anemia, and renal failure). A late complication of treatment of myeloma (particularly with melphalan) is injury of normal bone marrow stem cells. This injury can result in development of a chronic refractory sideroblastic anemia or acute myelogenous leukemia. It has been projected that well over 5 per cent of myeloma patients may eventually develop leukemia as a result of treatment. However, the risk-benefit ratio for myeloma patients still favors use of systemic chemotherapy. The immediate cause of death is frequently sepsis or renal failure. Recent advances in chemotherapy have resulted in some improvement in the prognosis for patients with myeloma. Better results will require the identification of new drugs with significant antimyeloma activity.

Supportive Care. Patients with newly diagnosed myeloma and those whose disease has relapsed often have problems that require immediate or emergency management that may have to be carried out concomitantly with initiation of chemotherapy.

HYPERCALCEMIA AND OSTEOLYSIS. Hypercalcemia as a metabolic complication of osteolysis is common in myeloma; the serum calcium should be determined initially even in patients lacking the characteristic symptoms of confusion, irritability, and constipation. The effects of hypercalcemia relate to the ionized fraction, which is greater when the serum albumin level is low. When serum calcium is only modestly increased (e.g., 11.5 to 12 mg per deciliter), hydration with several liters of intravenous saline, alone or with furosemide, will often suffice until the effect of systemic chemotherapy can induce a more sustained reduction in the calcium. Ambulation should be encouraged, as it also reduces bone resorption. Oral phosphate solutions (Fleet's phosphosoda enemas) may also prove useful for mild hypercalcemia if renal function is not impaired and the serum phosphate is not increased. Greater degrees of hypercalcemia (serum calcium >12 mg per deciliter) represent a medical emergency because of both cardiac and renal effects, and often require the addition of more aggressive measures, including large doses of corticosteroids. Injections of calcitonin or mithramycin are also indicated if the level of serum calcium is very high (e.g., > 14 mg per deciliter) or if the response to steroids is not rapid. Mithramycin (25 μg per kilogram of body weight) can often normalize the serum calcium in less than 24 hours, but frequently repeated injections are undesirable, as they can induce thrombocytopenia, which may compromise the ability to administer systemic chemotherapy for myeloma. (See Ch. 247 for a further discussion of the treatment of hypercalcemia.)

SPINAL CORD COMPRESSION. Developing neurologic symptoms in the lower extremities plus focal back pain in a patient with myeloma should lead to an emergency evaluation for the possibility of cord compression secondary to an extradural plasmacytoma. Consultations involving neurology, radiation therapy, and neurosurgery should be obtained promptly. If the diagnosis is established with magnetic resonance imaging or myelography before paralysis develops, the chance for recovery of neurologic function with high dose steroids and emergency radiotherapy (with or without laminectomy) is

excellent. Delays in diagnosis or therapy (even 12 hours) can leave the patient with irreversible paraplegia.

BONE PAIN. Bone pain caused by expanding plasmacytomas can usually be managed with analgesics and systemic chemotherapy. In some instances a single bony lesion will be responsible for the patient's pain. Such focal lesions can usually be palliated effectively and quickly with moderate doses of local radiotherapy (2000 to 3000 rads). Radiotherapy generally should be used only if pain is not relieved promptly with chemotherapy, and it should be limited to a relatively small field, as it impairs normal bone marrow function. Long delays in systemic chemotherapy for administration of radiotherapy should be avoided, as new bony lesions often develop during such intervals.

ANEMIA. Transfusion of packed red blood cells is often required in the initial management of Stage III myeloma patients. Occasionally, normal hematopoiesis can be stimulated with androgens. Other hematinics (iron, folic acid, vitamin B_{12}) are not of value. Patients experiencing an objective response to myeloma chemotherapy generally have a rise in hemoglobin of several grams during the first year after initiation of treatment.

INFECTION. Because of the known increased incidence of bacterial infection in myeloma (particularly pneumococcal), various efforts have been made to prevent infection. Immunization with polyvalent pneumococcal vaccine is of limited utility because of the profound defect that myeloma patients have in responding to carbohydrate antigens. Prophylactic administration of large doses of gamma globulin has proved ineffective, in part because of the hypercatabolism of all IgG in patients with IgG myeloma. Prophylactic use of antibiotics (penicillin, ampicillin) is of some benefit in infection-prone patients. If the patient can be depended upon to recognize the earliest signs of infection, prompt treatment at the time of fever or sputum production will usually suffice. When a patient with myeloma has a major septic episode, bactericidal antibiotics must be administered in adequate dosage. Nephrotoxic antibiotics (e.g., aminoglycosides) should be avoided in view of the frequency of overt or subclinical renal impairment in myeloma.

RENAL INSUFFICIENCY. Renal failure is a major cause of death in multiple myeloma. The major causes of renal failure are hypercalcemia and Bence Jones proteinuria. Both are potentially treatable. The patient should be kept well hydrated, and treated promptly for hypercalcemia when it is present. Allopurinol should also be used to prevent hyperuricemia and hyperuricosuria. Intravenous pyelography can precipitate renal failure in myeloma patients (perhaps because of dehydration) and should be approached with caution and with maintenance of hydration. Acute renal failure should be treated aggressively with standard measures, including hemodialysis, with the understanding that it may no longer be required if the injury is not too severe and if a good response is seen to chemotherapy. When the disease is in remission some patients have been supported with long-term hemodialysis. Long-term dialysis is clearly not indicated if the patient fails to achieve clinical remission with systemic chemotherapy.

VARIANT FORMS OF MYELOMA. *Indolent Myeloma.* About 5 per cent of patients under evaluation for multiple myeloma have a more indolent form of the disease with a life expectancy of up to ten years. Such patients are currently difficult to identify prospectively without specialized testing or a period of observation without treatment. Some are asymptomatic patients in whom the diagnosis is made after routine biochemical studies. One or two lytic bony lesions may be present. Most such patients have Stage I myeloma, and significant bone pain, hypercalcemia, azotemia, and Bence Jones proteinuria are absent. The tumor cells in indolent myeloma are hypoproliferative with a tumor cell tritiated thymidine labeling index of less than 0.5 per cent. Patients with indolent myeloma can be followed symptomatically without initiation of systemic chemotherapy. This group is relatively rare, however, and it is probably better to err on the side of treatment if the evidence for indolence is equivocal.

Solitary Myeloma. Occasional patients present with an apparently solitary myeloma. Bilateral core bone marrow biopsies from the iliac spine and a sternal aspirate, as well as electrophoretic studies of the blood and urine, should be performed in all cases thought to involve a solitary lesion. Only about half of patients with solitary myeloma have a demonstrable M-component, and even then a relatively small one. The normal immunoglobulins should also not be depressed in patients with a solitary lesion. Those involving soft tissues (particularly in the head and neck region) have a relatively high probability of being solitary and can often be managed with local surgery and radiation therapy. After effective local treatment of a soft tissue plasmacytoma, myeloma proteins in the blood or urine should disappear promptly. If they do not, occult dissemination can be predicted. In general, patients with a solitary soft tissue plasmacytoma will not require chemotherapy.

In contrast, patients with apparently solitary myeloma of bone generally do have additional occult disease. They also frequently respond unusually well to systemic chemotherapy after the original local lesion is treated with about 4000 rads of radiation. Patients with apparently solitary myeloma of bone can often be followed in unmaintained remission after the initial year of treatment with radiation and chemotherapy.

Barlogie B, Smith L, Alexanian R: Effective treatment of advanced multiple myeloma refractory to alkylating agents. N Engl J Med 310:1353, 1984. *Describes a useful vincristine-doxorubicin-dexamethasone combination treatment of patients with myeloma in relapse.*

Bataille R, Durie BGM, Grenier J: Prognostic factors and staging in multiple myeloma: A reappraisal evaluating new parameters. Blood 64(Suppl 5):152a, 1984. *An assessment of several staging systems for myeloma as well as of serum beta$_2$-microglobulin as a prognostic factor.*

Durie BGM, Dixon DO, Carter S, et al.: Improved survival duration with combination chemotherapy induction for multiple myeloma: A Southwest Oncology Group Study. J Clin Oncol 4:1227, 1986. *Describes an excellent treatment option for remission induction in patients with active myeloma.*

Durie BGM, Salmon SE, Moon TE: Pretreatment tumor mass, cell kinetics and prognosis in multiple myeloma. Blood 55:364, 1980. *A detailed analysis of tumor cell burden, thymidine labeling, response to treatment, and survival in myeloma which identifies kinetically unfavorable patient groups.*

Quesada JR, Alexanian R, Hawkins M, et al.: Treatment of multiple myeloma with recombinant alfa interferon. Blood 67:275, 1986. *A report summarizing the usefulness of interferon in myeloma therapy. Patients receiving this therapy often had improvement in normal immunoglobulin synthesis.*

Salmon SE (ed.): Myeloma and Related Disorders. Clin Haematol Vol 2, 1982. *A review by leading clinical investigators of major clinical and research advances that pertain to multiple myeloma and related entities.*

Salmon SE, Haut A, Bonnet JD, et al.: Alternating combination chemotherapy improves survival in multiple myeloma: A Southwest Oncology Group Study. J Clin Oncol 1:453, 1983. *Evidence supporting the use of aggressive combination chemotherapy for advanced stage myeloma patients.*

MACROGLOBULINEMIA OF WALDENSTRÖM

DEFINITION. Waldenström's macroglobulinemia is characterized by the proliferation and accumulation of malignant cells with lymphoplasmacytic morphology that secrete IgM M-components. Sites of B cell development, including the bone marrow, lymph nodes, and spleen, are usually involved. Major clinical manifestations of the disorder are related to hyperviscosity of the circulating intravascular macroglobulin. The disease has some similarities with myeloma, lymphoma, and chronic lymphocytic leukemia.

ETIOLOGY AND PATHOPHYSIOLOGY. Waldenström's macroglobulinemia is of unknown etiology, but appears to have a slightly increased familial incidence. It has a slight male predominance and increases in incidence with age, usually beginning in the fifth or sixth decade. The neoplasm appears to originate in a plasmacytic lymphocyte in the B cell series, which proliferates in the bone marrow and/or lymph nodes and spleen. Cytogenetic markers are sometimes found but are nonspecific. IgM M-components frequently have phy-

siochemical properties that lead to hyperviscosity, cryoprecipitation, or bleeding phenomena. In contrast to myeloma, osteolysis, renal impairment, and amyloidosis are quite rare in macroglobulinemia.

CLINICAL FEATURES. The clinical onset of macroglobulinemia is often gradual and associated with increasing weakness, fatigue, epistaxis, or other bleeding manifestations. Recurrent infection, visual difficulties, weight loss, or neurologic symptoms are also common. Bone pain is not a symptom of macroglobulinemia, and skeletal x-rays are usually unremarkable. On physical examination, patients often exhibit pallor, lymphadenopathy, and hepatosplenomegaly. Ophthalmoscopic examination usually reveals marked dilatation and vascular segmentation of the retinal veins ("sausage links") secondary to hyperviscosity, and occasional retinal hemorrhages and exudates. About one fourth of macroglobulinemic patients present with neurologic signs secondary to slow blood flow or sludging, including peripheral neuropathy, transient paresis, abnormal reflexes, headache, dizziness, deafness, and/or impaired state of consciousness or coma. Hyperviscosity also leads to bleeding and oozing from mucous membranes. Such symptoms and signs of hyperviscosity are uncommon when the serum viscosity is less than 4 units (normal, 1.4 to 1.8) and increase dramatically in frequency with values above 6 units.

Laboratory findings include a normochromic normocytic anemia, which is partially due to a reduced red cell mass and partially to an expanded plasma volume as a result of hyperviscosity. Rouleaux formation is quite prominent, and the sedimentation rate is increased markedly unless plasma gelation occurs. Plasmacytic lymphocytes are often present on the blood smear and are sometimes present in leukemic proportions. Coombs-positive hemolytic anemia or cold hemagglutinins are occasional findings. (The cold hemagglutinin syndrome is a variant of macroglobulinemia.) An M-component is present on serum electrophoresis in macroglobulinemia and can be shown to be monoclonal IgM with immunoelectrophoresis. Eighty per cent of IgM M-components have κ L chains, and the remaining 20 per cent are λ. Most macroglobulins will precipitate in distilled water (Sia test); however, this test is nonspecific. About 10 per cent of macroglobulins have cryoglobulin properties; some will form gels as the patient's blood is drawn unless a prewarmed syringe is used and subsequent separative procedures are carried out at 37° C. Bence Jones (L chain) proteinuria is also present in 10 per cent of patients with macroglobulinemia. The serum viscosity is usually increased. Normal immunoglobulins (IgG or IgA) are commonly reduced. The bone marrow aspirate usually reveals a substantial infiltrate with plasmacytic lymphocytes and plasma cells.

DIAGNOSIS. The diagnosis of Waldenström's macroglobulinemia requires the presence of typical symptoms and signs, the presence of an IgM M-component of greater than 3 grams per deciliter, and histologic evidence on bone marrow aspirate or biopsy. The differential diagnosis from chronic lymphocytic leukemia, lymphoma, multiple myeloma, and monoclonal gammopathies of undetermined significance depends upon the presence of characteristic immunologic and clinical features. Intermediate forms with characteristics of several of these related B cell disorders occasionally occur. IgM elevations of smaller magnitude are also seen in a variety of infectious and inflammatory disease, including those listed in Table 163–1.

TREATMENT AND PROGNOSIS. Patients with macroglobulinemia who present with a severe hyperviscosity syndrome and marked neurologic findings (e.g., impending coma or paresis) or serious bleeding should be treated by intensive emergency plasmapheresis. This is best accomplished with an intermittent or continuous flow blood cell separator. Red cell transfusion and/or volume replacement is generally required, as 6 to 8 liters of plasma may have to be removed during the first two to four days. Plasmapheresis is quite effective in macroglobulinemia because 90 per cent of the M-component remains in the intravascular compartment as a result of its high molecular weight.

Inasmuch as plasmapheresis removes only a troublesome tumor product and does not alter the underlying tumor, specific therapy requires the suppression of the neoplasm with systemic chemotherapy.

Chlorambucil (Leukeran) is usually administered orally at a dosage of 6 to 8 mg per day, with dosage adjustments made in accord with the WBC and platelet count. Although chlorambucil is well tolerated, the various drug regimens used in the treatment of multiple myeloma are useful in macroglobulinemia and are quite acceptable alternatives. Once patients achieve remission with chemotherapy (at least 80 per cent of cases), intermittent plasmapheresis can usually be discontinued. Systemic treatment is usually continued indefinitely in macroglobulinemia, since treatment, although suppressive, does not eradicate the IgM producing clone. Alfa interferon may be of some use for patients with macroglobulinemia that becomes refractory to alkylating agents.

The median survival in macroglobulinemia is about three years; however, many patients may have an indolent disease and may survive for ten years or more.

MacKenzie MR, Fudenberg HH: Macroglobulinemia: An analysis of 40 patients. Blood 39:874, 1972. *Useful review of clinical and laboratory features of macroglobulinemia of Waldenström.*

Waldenström J: Studies on conditions associated with disturbed gamma globulin formation (gammopathies). Harvey Lect 56:211, 1961. *A lengthy and stimulating discussion of macroglobulinemia and related plasma cell disorders by the clinical investigator who first described macroglobulinemia.*

HEAVY CHAIN DISEASES

The heavy chain diseases are a group of rare lymphoplasmacytic neoplasms associated with secretion of a monoclonal heavy chain or heavy chain fragment by the neoplastic cells. Thus far, H chain diseases related to the three major immunoglobulin classes have been reported (γ, α, μ). The clinical syndromes vary with H chain type but have some similarities with other B cell neoplasms.

GAMMA (γ) CHAIN DISEASE. This syndrome was the first heavy chain disease to be recognized. More than 50 cases have been reported. The symptoms and clinical presentation are similar to those of malignant lymphomas; the patients frequently have recurrent infections, lymphadenopathy, and hepatosplenomegaly. Characteristically, edema of the soft palate and uvula associated with Waldeyer's ring involvement occurs in γ heavy chain diseases. Normochromic normocytic anemia is typical, and many patients are pancytopenic save for an eosinophilia. Several patients have also manifested plasma cell leukemia, but skeletal lesions are uncommon.

Histologic studies of the lymph nodes and bone marrow usually reveal a pleomorphic infiltrate of lymphoplasmacytic and large lymphoid cells and eosinophils, abnormalities reminiscent of Hodgkin's disease.

All patients have free γ heavy chains present in the serum and urine determined by immunologic and electrophoretic techniques. The urinary protein lacks the heat properties of L chains. Immunoelectrophoresis shows the monoclonal peak to have γ chain determinants but to lack κ or λ L chains. Of interest, there is a large deletion (200 amino acids) in the variable region of the γ chain. As in myeloma and macroglobulinemia, normal immunoglobulins are reduced. Although in some patients there has been a rapid downhill course, use of intensive combination chemotherapy (as in diffuse lymphomas) has resulted in long survival in some patients.

ALPHA (α) CHAIN DISEASE. This rare and interesting syndrome has a characteristic genetic and geographic distribution and is about twice as common as γ chain disease. It has been observed predominantly in young Arabs and non-Ashkenazic Jews living in the Middle East ("Mediterranean lymphoma"). However, the disease does occur in patients of

other ethnic backgrounds. Patients usually present with abdominal discomfort and weight loss owing to malabsorption and diarrhea and have extensive mesenteric and small-intestinal lymphatic involvement with lymphoma (see Ch. 104). The lamina propria is extensively infiltrated with neoplastic plasma cells. Cellular morphology is similar to that in γ chain disease; however, marrow involvement is rare. Pulmonary involvement has been observed in two children with α chain disease.

Immunodiagnosis of α chain disease is relatively difficult, as a sharp M-component spike is usually not observed in the serum or urine, and the entity must be thought of in patients with intestinal lymphoma. Alpha chains have a tendency to polymerize and thereby become heterodisperse on electrophoresis, giving the appearance of either a normal serum electrophoresis or diffuse hypergammaglobulinemia. Immunoelectrophoresis, however, demonstrates that only the α chain is present and that L chains are absent. The α chains are monoclonal. Only about half of the patients have free α chain in the urine, presumably because of the tendency for formation of large complexes which do not pass the glomerulus. Although most cases of α chain disease have been fatal, some patients have achieved remissions with chemotherapy. A few patients have achieved remission with antimicrobial therapy, suggesting that an infectious agent may underlie this unusual monoclonal B cell proliferation.

MU (μ) CHAIN DISEASE. Secretion of free μ heavy chains into the plasma is a rare occurrence in chronic lymphocytic leukemia. The seven patients reported have had longstanding disease with retroperitoneal adenopathy and hepatosplenomegaly. Bone marrow aspiration has shown vacuolated lymphoplasmacytic cells. Hypogammaglobulinemia was seen on serum electrophoresis, and immunoelectrophoresis was required to detect the small amount of free μ chains. Most of the patients also had substantial amounts of κ L chain in the urine. The monoclonal lymphoid cells of the neoplasm appear to have a defect in H-L chain assembly, as intracellular L chains are detectable but do not assemble normally into IgM prior to secretion.

Franklin EC: μ-Chain disease. Arch Intern Med 135:71, 1975. *The major clinical features of μ-chain disease are summarized.*

Seligman M: Immunochemical, clinical and pathological features of α chain disease. Arch Intern Med 135:71, 1975. *A clinically relevant immunologic description of α-chain disease.*

IMMUNOCYTIC (PRIMARY) AMYLOIDOSIS
(see also Ch. 210)

DEFINITION. Amyloidosis is not a single disease entity but a term applied to a complex of disorders associated with deposition of insoluble fibrillar proteins in virtually pure form in various tissues of the body. The disease complex was first designated "amyloid" in the 1850's by Virchow, who considered the "waxy, eosinophilic" homogeneous and amorphous tissue deposits to be composed of polysaccharide or starch-like substances. Amyloid stains pink with hematoxylin and eosin and metachromatically with methyl or crystal violet. Congo red stain produces green birefringence under polarized light and is the most specific light microscopic stain for amyloid. Under the electron microscope, amyloid has a characteristic fibrillar B-pleated sheet structure. This structure is not found in normal mammalian tissues.

A complete description of the various forms of amyloidosis is contained in Chapter 210 and a classification based on the chemistry of the amyloid fibrils is presented in Table 210–1. Since immunocytic (primary or AL) amyloidosis may shade into the plasma cell disorders, a further brief summary is given here.

PATHOPHYSIOLOGY (Table 163–4). Amyloid fibrils from primary amyloidosis are homogeneous and homologous to the variable region fragment of either κ or λ L chains (Ig-V_L) and thus have been defined as immunoglobulin amyloid-fibril

TABLE 163–4. CLASSIFICATION OF THE ACQUIRED SYSTEMIC AMYLOIDOSES (β-Fibrilloses)

Classification	Major Protein Component
A. Immunocytic amyloidosis	
1. No evidence of coexisting disease	AL
2. Multiple myeloma	AL
3. Other monoclonal gammopathy	AL
4. Agammaglobulinemia	AL
B. Reactive systemic amyloidosis	AA
1. Acute recurrent and chronic infections	AA
2. Chronic inflammatory conditions (e.g., rheumatoid arthritis)	AA
C. Localized amyloid (involvement of a single organ without generalized involvement)	AL
D. Familial amyloidosis	AA, PA

AL = Amyloid light chain; AA = Amyloid A (protein A); PA = Prealbumin amyloid.

proteins (AL). There is a clear relationship between amyloid-fibril deposits and Bence Jones proteins, which are related to multiple myeloma and related plasma cell disorders. Furthermore, AL appear to be produced in these disorders through a proteolytic mechanism to which only certain free L chains (and not intact Ig components) are susceptible. Such "amyloidogenic" L chains are more frequently of λ than κ L chain type. The characteristic "B-pleated sheet" amyloid fibrils can be produced in vitro by treating certain Bence Jones proteins with proteolytic enzymes. As a result of these studies and the finding of AL type amyloid fibrils in association with virtually all monoclonal gammopathies (including myeloma, macroglobulinemia, H chain diseases, B cell lymphoid neoplasms, and gammopathies of unknown significance) as well as agammaglobulinemia, Glenner proposed that primary amyloidosis be designated *immunocytic amyloid*. This designation clearly has a recognizable relationship to the pathophysiology of amyloid formation in monoclonal B cell disorders.

CLINICAL FEATURES. Patients with immunocytic amyloid present with complaints of weakness, weight loss, ankle swelling, paresthesias, and lightheadedness. Symptoms of multiple myeloma may also be present when the amyloid is associated with that disorder (about 15 per cent of myeloma cases). Major physical findings of immunocytic amyloid include enlargement of the tongue, purpura, hepatomegaly, and occasional splenomegaly. Skin manifestations can include plaques, papules, or nodules. Involvement of periarticular regions can give an appearance similar to that of rheumatoid arthritis. Involvement of the glenohumoral joint leads to a characteristic "shoulder pad sign." Periorbital purpura may appear spontaneously or after straining ("raccoon eyes"). Purpuric bleeding is sometimes associated with an acquired deficiency of factor X. Ankle edema in amyloidosis is often associated with congestive heart failure or the nephrotic syndrome. Heart failure occurs in about 30 per cent of patients, and renal involvement is a leading cause of death. The carpal tunnel syndrome, peripheral neuropathy, and orthostatic hypotension are additional associations with amyloid infiltration.

Laboratory findings include evidence of anemia and/or renal failure in about half of the patients. Ninety per cent have proteinuria. Serum immunoelectrophoresis reveals an M-component in about half of the patients with amyloidosis and in three quarters of those with amyloid associated with myeloma. Addition of urinary immunoelectrophoresis permits detection of an M-component in almost 90 per cent of cases. λ L chain excretion is more common than κ (2 to 1) in amyloidosis. Some increase in marrow plasma cells is common.

Diagnosis of amyloidosis requires tissue biopsy and demonstration of amyloid deposition by the green birefringence of the Congo red stain by polarization microscopy. If easily obtained, the initial biopsy should be of the organ suspected of being infiltrated with amyloid. Alternatively, the first biopsy may be taken from the rectal mucosa, as it is relatively

safe and easy to obtain, and with adequate tissue is positive in more than 75 per cent of cases. Other useful biopsy sites include the gingiva, skin, kidney, and carpal ligament (in patients with the carpal tunnel syndrome). Endomyocardial biopsy via catheter has led to the detection of amyloid in unexplained cases of cardiac failure.

TREATMENT. Because of the relationship of AL amyloid to monoclonal plasma cell proliferation, systemic chemotherapy with alkylating agent-prednisone combinations has been tried with some evidence of improvement or halting in progression of amyloid deposition. Therefore, a trial of therapy similar to that used for myeloma is warranted. Unfortunately, treatment has not yet significantly improved survival. Colchicine has been tried in AL amyloid without proven success. Supportive measures in systemic amyloidosis include management of cardiac and renal failure. Congestive heart failure caused by amyloid does not usually respond to cardiac glycosides, and sudden deaths from arrhythmia have been reported. Diuretics have been useful for relief of edema.

The prognosis in systemic immunocytic amyloidosis is poor. In one review of 236 cases, the average survival was 14.7 months for patients without underlying myeloma (about 50 to 60 per cent of cases) and four months for those with amyloidosis and myeloma (about 20 per cent of cases).

Buxbaum JN, Hurley ME, Chuba J, et al.: Amyloidosis of the AL type: Clinical, morphologic, and biochemical aspects of the response to therapy with alkylating agents and prednisone. Am J Med 67:867, 1979.

Durie BGM, Persky B, Soehnlen BJ, et al.: Amyloid production in human myeloma stem-cell culture, with morphologic evidence of amyloid secretion by associated macrophages. N Engl J Med 307:1689, 1982.

Kyle RA, Greipp PR: Amyloidosis (AL), clinical and laboratory features in 229 cases. Mayo Clin Proc 58:665, 1983. *The best current review of this entity drawing upon the extensive Mayo experience.*

MONOCLONAL GAMMOPATHIES OF UNDETERMINED SIGNIFICANCE

If a patient has an M-component in the serum but lacks other diagnostic findings for myeloma, macroglobulinemia, or one of the other plasma cell neoplasms, the disorder is best classified as monoclonal gammopathy of unknown significance (MGUS). Formerly, the term "benign monoclonal gammopathy" was applied; however, this term is misleading, as some patients in this category do, in fact, develop myeloma or macroglobulinemia after a period of follow-up. Serum M-components without other signs of myeloma or macroglobulinemia occur in about 1 per cent of the population above age 50 and 3 per cent above age 70. Most of these persons never develop signs of a malignant plasma cell disorder. A number of patients have been followed for 15 years or more without developing myeloma.

Patients with monoclonal gammopathy of unknown significance have relatively small M-components present in the serum (usually less than 2 grams per deciliter) and do not excrete urinary L chains (Bence Jones protein). The bone marrow plasma cell percentage is generally less than 5 per cent. Marrow plasma cells from patients with MGUS have an extremely low tritiated thymidine labeling index (less than 0.5 per cent). When anemia, osteolytic lesions, hypercalcemia, Bence Jones proteinuria, or renal failure is present, the patient does not fall in the category of having a monoclonal gammopathy of undetermined significance and should be considered to have a malignant disorder. The levels of nonmonoclonal immunoglobulins are sometimes normal in monoclonal gammopathy of unknown significance, but this does not provide significant differentiation between benign and malignant plasma cell disorders. If there is only a serum M-component and no clear associated disease demonstrable by baseline observations, the patient should be followed without any treatment for the monoclonal gammopathy. In general, the patient should be seen at least every three months during the first year and at intervals of six months thereafter. If the monoclonal protein increases by 50 per cent on repeated serum electrophoresis, then a complete re-evaluation is warranted. In a five-year study of the natural history of 241 cases of monoclonal gammopathy of unknown significance, 57 per cent of patients retained stable protein levels; 9 per cent had a 50 per cent increase in the serum M-component or developed Bence Jones proteinuria; 23 per cent died without five-year serum studies; and 11 per cent developed myeloma, macroglobulinemia, or amyloidosis.

OTHER DISEASES ASSOCIATED WITH MONOCLONAL GAMMOPATHY. Patients with a variety of diseases have a monoclonal gammopathy of unknown significance. Among neoplastic diseases, monoclonal gammopathy has been observed in association with colonic cancer and certain other carcinomas, as well as with several B cell neoplasms (chronic lymphocytic leukemia and various lymphomas). M-components in lymphoid neoplasia may relate to their B cell origin and function. The explanation for an association with nonlymphoid neoplasms remains obscure, and could be coincidental. The incidence of monoclonal gammopathy in this latter group may be no greater than in the general population of that age range.

Among non-neoplastic disorders, a monoclonal gammopathy is regularly associated with the rare skin disorder lichen myxedematosus (papular mucinosis). Patients with this disorder have diffuse progressive deposition of protein in the dermis in association with the presence of a highly cationic IgG M-component, which usually has λ L chains. Monoclonal gammopathies are occasionally associated with other disorders, including Gaucher's disease, hepatitis and other liver diseases, collagen vascular diseases, and myasthenia gravis. Transient monoclonal gammopathies are sometimes observed after bone marrow transplantation, particularly in children with immunodeficiency syndrome.

Kyle RA: Monoclonal gammopathy of undetermined significance. Natural history in 241 cases. Am J Med 64:814, 1978. *An excellent and detailed analysis of the Mayo Clinic experience.*

Miglione PJ, Alexanian R: Monoclonal gammopathy in human neoplasia. Cancer 21:1127, 1968. *These authors analyze the experience at M.D. Anderson Hospital in Houston and suggest that monoclonal gammopathy associated with neoplasms other than myeloma or macroglobulinemia is only coincidental.*

Talerman A, Haije WG: The frequency of M-components in sera of patients with solid malignant neoplasms. Br J Cancer 27:276, 1973.

164 DISEASES OF THE SPLEEN
Douglas V. Faller

PHYSIOLOGY AND FUNCTIONS

The spleen, the largest lymphoid organ in the body, plays a major role in the cellular and humoral immune response to infection and inflammation. In addition, with its unique architecture and network of fixed phagocytic cells, the spleen is the primary filter for circulating senescent cells, antigens, and microorganisms. A spleen of average size (135 grams) receives a blood flow of 300 ml per minute. Splenic vessels from the hilus penetrate into trabeculations formed by invaginations of the splenic capsule (Fig. 164–1). The central arterioles, surrounded by sheaths of lymphoid tissue, have branches (follicular arterioles) that take off at right angles, effectively skimming plasma and circulating antigens from the blood and delivering them directly to the splenic immune system. The terminal arterioles are open ended and dump the remaining concentrated blood cells into the splenic cords. Some cells are shunted rapidly into the venous collection system, but many percolate slowly through the open splenic cords for several minutes before squeezing through 0.5 to 2.5 μm slits between the endothelial cells and the discontinuous

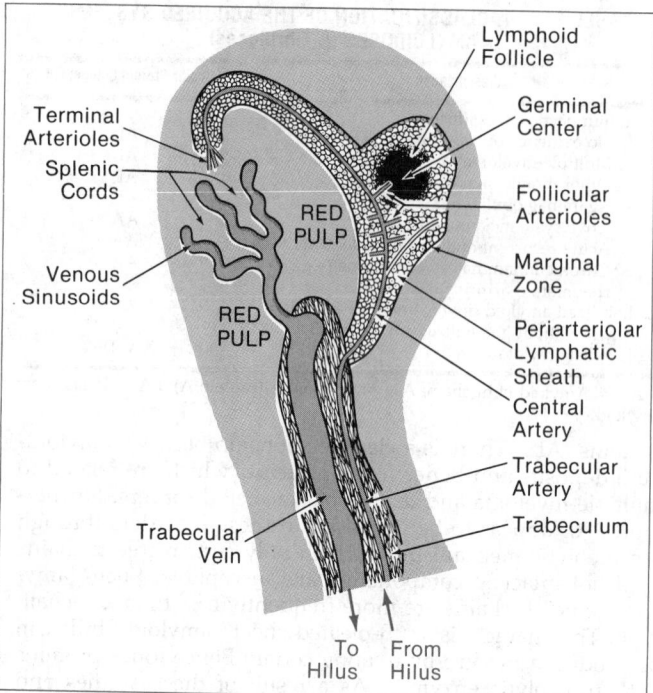

FIGURE 164–1. Diagrammatic representation of the structure of the spleen.

basement membrane of the venous sinusoids and re-entering the splenic venous system. The cut surface of the spleen displays a prominent red pulp, dotted with islands of white pulp, which serve to compartmentalize the filtrative and immunologic functions of the spleen, respectively.

THE WHITE PULP. The white pulp consists of periarteriolar lymphatic sheaths, with a mantle layer of small lymphocytes (predominantly T lymphocytes) surrounding lymphoid germinal centers, which contain B cells and plasmablasts. Blood-borne antigens and pathogens are concentrated and contact immune responder cells in the white pulp. Circulating particulate antigens and opsonized microorganisms are rapidly phagocytized by macrophages in both the white and red pulp and are presented to the lymphocytes surrounding the germinal centers in the white pulp. Reactive plasmablasts secreting IgM appear, and the germinal centers enlarge within 24 hours. Consequently the white pulp component of the spleen hypertrophies in response to infection and antigenic stimulation. The spleen is therefore important in mounting a response to new immune challenges and serves as the major source of IgM production in the body. The marginal zone of the spleen surrounds these periarteriolar lymphatic sheaths of the white pulp with a dense reticulum in which the terminal arterioles end. This marginal zone blends into the red pulp.

THE RED PULP. The splenic cords (of Billroth) make up the red pulp. Erythrocytes slowly traverse these nonendothelialized cords and are subjected to metabolic conditions (including hypoxia, glucose deprivation, and low pH) that stress senescent or even mildly damaged cells. Defective erythrocytes with abnormally stiff cytoplasm (as in the sickle cell hemoglobinopathies), deficient cellular membrane (as in the spherocytic hemolytic diseases), or excessive rigidity of membrane proteins (as in the thalassemia syndromes) are then *culled* from this delayed microcirculation by the avidly phagocytic macrophages, reticular cells, and littoral cells that line the cords. *Pitting* of inclusions from erythrocytes is also performed by these phagocytes as the red cells attempt to squeeze through narrow fenestrations into the venous sinuses. This pitting function removes Howell-Jolly bodies (nuclear remnants), Heinz bodies (denatured hemoglobin), and intraerythrocytic parasites, such as malaria and *Bartonella*. New reticulocytes are *conditioned* in this environment, losing up to 30 per cent of their cell membrane and any remaining mitochondria. Iron from ingested red blood cells is stored by the splenic phagocytes and released to the plasma for *reutilization of iron*. In states of abnormal hemolysis, a buildup of hemosiderin occurs in these cells.

The spleen serves as a *reservoir* for platelets, with up to a third of the total platelet mass being sequestered there at any one time in a freely exchangeable pool. In certain disease states this reservoir function can be exaggerated. Acute entrapment of erythrocytes in the splenomegalic crisis of hemoglobin SC disease or the blackwater fever crisis of falciparum malaria can result in profound shock. Although the spleen is a blood-forming organ until five months of gestation, *hematopoiesis* in the adult spleen occurs only as a result of pathologic, usually neoplastic, conditions. Evidence exists for involvement of the spleen in the *regulation of blood volume* and in the *catabolism of low-density lipoproteins*.

EVALUATION OF THE SPLEEN

The spleen lies against the posterior abdominal wall and the diaphragm. When the spleen enlarges its lower pole moves down, anteriorly and to the right. It is best identified by detection of its movement during respiration. A palpable spleen is nearly always significantly enlarged, except in the very young. Imaging of the spleen and liver can be performed after injection of radiolabeled colloid. To visualize the spleen alone, or to identify accessory spleens, heat- or chemically damaged red blood cells tagged with ^{51}Cr or ^{99m}Tc are used. This test can also be used as an indicator of splenic function.

SPLENOMEGALY

Five general mechanisms may enlarge the spleen: (1) reactive proliferation of lymphoid cells; (2) infiltration by neoplastic cells or lipid-laden macrophages; (3) extramedullary hematopoiesis; (4) proliferation of phagocytic cells; and (5) vascular congestion. Diseases may cause splenomegaly by one or by a combination of these mechanisms (Table 164–1). The causes of massive splenomegaly (greater than 3000 grams) are somewhat more limited (Table 164–2). The myelodysplastic disorders and malignant lymphoid disorders are the most common causes of chronic massive splenomegaly in nontropical countries. Splenomegaly can present as an isolated finding on physical examination, in association with a systemic disorder, or be discovered as a consequence of the secondary hematologic effects of splenic enlargement—the hypersplenism syndrome.

Evaluation of splenomegaly should include examination of the peripheral blood. A spleen scan is recommended to determine the size and shape of the spleen and to look for defects suggestive of tumors, cysts, or nonsplenic masses displacing the spleen. In general, diagnostic tests are not performed on the spleen itself; they are oriented toward the diagnosis of disease states producing splenomegaly. If lymph-

TABLE 164–1. CAUSES OF SPLENOMEGALY

Infection (lymphoid hyperplasia)
  Viral, parasitic, bacterial, fungal
Inflammation (lymphoid hyperplasia)
  Rheumatoid arthritis, sarcoidosis, systemic lupus erythematosus, renal
    dialysis, beryllium
Neoplasms (infiltrative or myeloproliferative)
  Leukemia, lymphoma, polycythemia vera, myeloid metaplasia, cysts,
    metastatic tumors, primary tumors
Hemolytic Disease (phagocytic hyperplasia)
  Spherocytosis, thalassemia major, pyruvate kinase deficiency
Deficiency Diseases
  Iron deficiency, pernicious anemia
Infiltration
  Gaucher's disease, Neimann-Pick disease, amyloidosis, extramedullary
    hematopoiesis
Splenic Vein Hypertension (vascular congestion)
  Cirrhosis, splenic or portal vein thrombosis, hepatic schistosomiasis
Endocrine
  Graves' disease, Hashimoto's thyroiditis
Hemophilia (subsequent to intensive therapy with clotting-factor concentrate)

TABLE 164–2. CAUSES OF MASSIVE SPLENOMEGALY

Acute
  Malaria (falciparum) with splenic sequestration crisis
  Sickle cell anemia with splenic sequestration crisis
Chronic
  Myelodysplastic
    Chronic myelogenous leukemia
    Myeloid metaplasia
    Polycythemia vera (end-stage)
    Primary thrombocythemia
  Neoplastic
    Lymphoma
    Malignant reticuloendotheliosis
    Hodgkins' disease
    Hairy-cell leukemia
  Hematologic
    Thalassemia major
    Sickle cell anemia (rare)
  Inflammatory-infiltrative
    Gaucher's disease
    Sarcoidosis
    Felty's syndrome
  Infectious
    Malaria
    Kala-azar

adenopathy is present, lymph node biopsy may yield a diagnosis. When systemic symptoms accompany splenomegaly but no lymphadenopathy is appreciated, a laparotomy with biopsies of liver, spleen, and lymph nodes is sometimes indicated. Such a study will produce a diagnosis of lymphoma in one third of cases, congestive splenomegaly in one quarter, and an inflammatory state in one fifth.

INFECTION. Systemic infections are the most common causes of moderate and transient splenomegaly. Splenic enlargement is the rule in mononucleosis due to Epstein-Barr virus infection, but is less frequent in the heterophil-negative mononucleosis syndromes associated with cytomegalovirus, adenovirus, or acquired toxoplasmosis. Splenomegaly can be massive, however, in congenital toxoplasmosis or other infectious causes of the TORCH syndrome. A palpable spleen is often detected in the course of viral hepatitis and influenza and less often in association with infectious lymphocytosis, pertussis, and roseola infantum. Bacterial infections causing splenomegaly include secondary syphilis and acute brucellosis. Hematogenous spread of tuberculosis or histoplasmosis can involve the spleen. Splenomegaly is common in tropical populations and is due to malaria, schistosomiasis, leishmaniasis (kala-azar), chronic worm infestation, and other disorders. Rickettsial infection can produce splenic enlargement, a palpable spleen being noted in up to 40 per cent of patients with Rocky Mountain spotted fever. Modest splenomegaly is appreciated in 30 to 80 per cent of patients with the lymphadenopathy accompanying the acquired immunodeficiency disease–related complex (ARC).

INFLAMMATION. Splenomegaly is found in systemic lupus erythematosus (20 per cent), rheumatoid arthritis (5 to 10 per cent), and Behçet's disease and frequently results in production of cytopenias by hypersplenism. Angioimmunoblastic lymphadenopathy, sometimes associated with anticonvulsant administration, is characterized by splenomegaly, autoimmune hemolytic anemia, and dysproteinemia. Regional ileitis is occasionally accompanied by a histiocytic infiltration of the spleen.

NEOPLASMS. The myelodysplastic disorders and leukemias commonly infiltrate the spleen, causing modest to massive enlargement. Splenic involvement is noted in 30 to 40 per cent of adult non-Hodgkin's lymphoma at presentation. Primary malignant tumors of the spleen are rare and include lymphangiosarcomas, hemangiosarcomas, fibrosarcomas, and leiomyosarcomas. They may present with local or systemic problems and are diagnosed by spleen scan and angiography. Metastatic tumor is a rare cause of splenomegaly.

STORAGE DISEASES. Previously undiagnosed Gaucher's disease is a cause of asymptomatic splenomegaly. Niemann-

Pick disease and the sea-blue histiocyte syndrome can also present in this way. Diagnosis can often be made by bone marrow biopsy.

CHRONIC CONGESTIVE SPLENOMEGALY (BANTI'S SYNDROME). This complex is characterized by splenomegaly, pancytopenia as a consequence of hypersplenism, and gastrointestinal bleeding secondary to portal hypertension. The splenic vein hypertension is due to either intrahepatic disease (e.g., cirrhosis or schistosomiasis) or extrahepatic disease (such as portal or splenic vein thrombosis). Splenic vein thrombosis is most commonly caused by compression of the splenic vein by tumor or fibrosis. Pregnancy, trauma, or intravascular coagulation can predispose to portal vein thrombosis. The spleen is markedly enlarged and congested, with distended veins and venous sinuses. Periarteriolar hemorrhage, siderotic nodules, hyperplasia of the red pulp, and progressive fibrosis occur. Symptoms can range from vague gastrointestinal complaints to catastrophic bleeding from esophageal or gastric varices. Hematologic cytopenias may be severe, but are rarely the major medical concern. Etiologic studies of congestive splenomegaly should include evaluation for alcoholism, liver function tests, liver-spleen scan, liver biopsy, and a search for varices. If no liver disease is found, venous obstruction should be considered and splenoportal venography performed. Splenic or hepatic vein thrombosis may be the initial presentation in an occult myeloproliferative disease, particularly polycythemia vera.

HYPERSPLENISM

Hypersplenism is an exaggeration of normal splenic function, with enhanced filtration and phagocytosis of the cellular elements of the blood. The hyperplastic spleen can sequester as much as 90 per cent of the total platelet pool or 45 per cent of the red cell mass. Four criteria support the diagnosis of hypersplenism: (1) cytopenia of one or more hematologic cell lines; (2) compensatory reactive marrow hyperplasia; (3) splenomegaly; (4) correction of abnormalities by splenectomy.

Hypersplenism is frequently secondary to splenic enlargement. Splenomegaly due to infiltrative diseases (lymphoma, chronic leukemia, Gaucher's disease, amyloidosis) is not usually associated with the severe cytopenias of hypersplenism. Enlargement of the spleen due to hypertrophy of the phagocytic elements (inflammatory diseases) or secondary to congestive splenomegaly with slowing of the cellular transit time through the spleen, however, is frequently accompanied by anemia, thrombocytopenia, or granulocytopenia of varying degrees. The erythrostatic environment of hypersplenism is especially threatening to red blood cells with mild intrinsic abnormalities. The patient with well-compensated hereditary spherocytosis or elliptocytosis may experience acute, severe hemolysis from the transient splenic enlargement accompanying mononucleosis. Similarly the anemia of chronic liver disease may worsen as the increasing pressure in the portal system causes stasis and destruction of acanthocytes in the spleen. The harsh metabolic environment of the splenic cords (hypoxia, low glucose levels, and low pH) is exaggerated in the enlarged and congested spleen. In addition, phagocytosis of red cells or platelets stimulates more reactive hyperplasia of splenic histiocytes, begetting more hypersplenism. This is the mechanism underlying *primary hypersplenism*, in which the spleen hypertrophies because of phagocytosis of defective red cells (hereditary spherocytosis), antibody-coated red cells (autoimmune hemolytic anemia), or antibody-coated platelets (autoimmune thrombocytopenia). Hypersplenism can be documented and quantified by demonstrating a decrease in the circulating half-life of labeled erythrocytes along with an increase in the spleen-liver uptake ratio.

INDICATIONS FOR SPLENECTOMY

Splenectomy may be indicated for either of two medical conditions: (1) to stage or control a basic disease process (Hodgkin's disease, hereditary spherocytosis, autoimmune cytopenias) or (2) to alleviate the consequences of hypersplenism secondary to other disease processes. In addition, the spleen may have to be removed because of traumatic or, rarely, spontaneous rupture causing intra-abdominal hemorrhage.

THROMBOCYTOPENIA. *Chronic autoimmune thrombocytopenia* (ITP) refractory to corticosteroid therapy will usually improve (70 to 90 per cent) after splenectomy, with the platelet count becoming normal in 60 per cent. Those who do not respond completely can often be maintained on a lower corticosteroid dose. The thrombocytopenia accompanying *systemic* or *discoid lupus* responds only poorly to splenectomy. *Thrombotic thrombocytopenic purpura* has been treated in the past with splenectomy and steroid therapy, but newer multimodal treatments, including plasmapheresis or plasma exchange, appear more promising (Ch. 166).

HEMOLYTIC ANEMIAS. *Autoimmune hemolytic anemia* caused by warm-reacting antibodies that does not resolve after two months of corticosteroid therapy may be treated by splenectomy. Two thirds of such patients will have complete or partial remission, but the relapse rate is high. Splenectomy is a uniformly effective treatment for the anemia of *hereditary spherocytosis* (Ch. 138). Surgery should be delayed until the age of five years, if possible, to decrease the risk of overwhelming sepsis. Other congenital hemolytic anemias do not respond as consistently to splenectomy, and the decision to remove the spleen should be based on the severity of the anemia and lack of response to alternative treatments.

LEUKEMIAS. Splenectomy is routinely performed for symptomatic cytopenias or splenomegaly in *hairy-cell leukemia* (leukemic reticuloendotheliosis). Improvement occurs in up to 85 per cent of patients, but recurrence of cytopenias is common. Early splenectomy is no longer recommended, and the advent of alpha-interferon therapy for this disease may relegate splenectomy to a secondary role (Ch. 155). In the past, splenectomy was commonly carried out in patients with *chronic myelogenous leukemia* for relief of symptoms or prior to bone marrow transplantation. Any benefit is transient, however; survival is not affected, and the operation in this setting is associated with a high mortality. Splenectomy can provide useful palliation in patients with *chronic lymphocytic leukemia* who have symptomatic splenomegaly or autoimmune hemolytic anemia. Splenectomy improves the hematologic status and the quality of life in cases of severe agnogenic myeloid metaplasia (Ch. 154).

STORAGE DISEASES. Splenectomy can be performed in *Gaucher's disease* when splenomegaly produces mechanical or cytopenic problems. The spleen serves as a storage area for undigested cerebroside, so it is possible that splenectomy might accelerate the disease (Ch. 185).

FELTY'S SYNDROME. Neutropenia of variable degrees and splenomegaly, occasionally accompanied by thrombocytopenia or anemia, occurs in about 1 per cent of patients with rheumatoid arthritis. The spleen appears to be both the source of the antibody coating the neutrophils and the means of their destruction. If the neutropenia is severe enough to cause frequent infections or skin ulcerations, splenectomy is beneficial in 60 to 80 per cent of patients.

THALASSEMIA MAJOR. In the setting of longstanding thalassemia, therapeutic splenectomy is often required. It appears, however, that aggressive transfusion regimens combined with iron chelation therapy may reduce the incidence of severe hypersplenism.

RENAL DIALYSIS HYPERSPLENISM. Up to 10 per cent of uremic patients undergoing long-term dialysis develop signs of hypersplenism. Splenectomy may decrease bleeding tendencies and transfusion requirements in this setting.

ALTERNATIVES TO SPLENECTOMY. Therapy with glucocorticoids inhibits phagocytosis and can provide a useful "chemical splenectomy" in short-term situations. Partial splenectomy is sometimes advocated in children to reduce the risk of postsplenectomy complications. Partial or complete embolization of the spleen using percutaneous catheterization is a relatively safe, effective, and noninvasive approach when surgery is contraindicated. Splenic irradiation (100 to 500 rads) can provide transient therapy for hypersplenism or splenomegaly due to infiltrative diseases.

POSTSPLENECTOMY SYNDROMES AND HYPOSPLENISM

HEMATOLOGIC SEQUELAE. The hyposplenic or post-splenectomy state can often be diagnosed by examination of the peripheral blood smear. In the absence of splenic culling and pitting functions, nucleated red blood cells, Howell-Jolly and Heinz body inclusions, siderocytes, and acanthocytes are found in the circulation. Reticulocytes are no longer conditioned, and their redundant cell membrane produces target cells upon drying and staining.

A transient and modest increase in the leukocyte count occurs after splenectomy and lasts one to two weeks. The bulk of this *leukocytosis* is accounted for by early *neutrophilia*. Later, *lymphocytosis* and *monocytosis* become more prominent.

Splenectomy routinely results in prominent postoperative *thrombocytosis*, often producing platelet counts of 1 million or more per cubic millimeter for weeks to months following surgery. This elevation may persist in 40 per cent of patients. The risk of consequent thromboembolic phenomena is high only after splenectomy in the setting of myeloproliferative disease or paroxysmal nocturnal hemoglobinuria. Attempts should be made to decrease the platelet count with chemotherapy before surgery in such cases. Following surgery, therapy with anticoagulants and antiplatelet agents should be considered, especially if the patient is bedridden.

INFECTION. In the absence of the spleen, or in the setting of functional asplenia, certain inadequacies of immune function can be demonstrated. IgM levels fall, and complement-mediated opsonization is decreased. This is in part due to a fall in the levels of tuftsin and properdin, two opsonic proteins produced by the spleen. The ability to phagocytose circulating antigens is compromised, as is cell-mediated immunity.

The risk of *overwhelming sepsis* following splenectomy or in functional asplenia is especially high in children, being as high as 10 per cent in debilitated infants. The incidence falls in older children (1 per cent) and is rare, but reported, in adults. The etiologic organisms are encapsulated bacteria, predominantly pneumococcus and less commonly meningococcus or *Hemophilus influenzae*. These are poorly opsonized in the body, and the intact spleen, with its slow, tortuous blood flow past avid phagocytes, appears to be the primary site for clearance of these pathogens. All patients with decreased splenic function, whether due to functional hyposplenism or to splenectomy (traumatic or therapeutic) must be warned to take any febrile illness seriously. Prophylaxis with penicillin is recommended for all children with asplenia or splenic hypofunction (e.g., sickle cell anemia). Immunization with polyvalent vaccines to pneumococci, meningococci, and *H. influenzae* is advised for patients over the age of three years. Serologic response to these vaccines is not always normal in hyposplenia or asplenia. The timing of vaccine administration (before or after splenectomy) is not important, but vaccination should precede any chemotherapy, if possible. Serious infections with unusual organisms like *Babesia* or *Bartonella* also occur in asplenic individuals. A concurrent viral infection may predispose hyposplenic patients to fulminant bacteremias.

FUNCTIONAL HYPOSPLENISM. Repeated symptomatic or silent infarction of the spleen in the course of veno-occlusive diseases, like the sickle cell syndromes, results in substantial or total loss of splenic tissue (*autosplenectomy*). The spleen is shrunken and fibrosed. Circulating erythrocytes reflect the loss of the splenic filtration function and are found to contain mitochrondrial remnants and inclusions of nuclear fragments (Howell-Jolly bodies) and denatured hemoglobin (Heinz bodies). Bizarrely shaped red cells, target cells, and large platelets are observed. Hyposplenism can occur even with a large or normal-sized spleen if splenic tissue has been replaced by sarcoid granulomas, amyloid, or multiple myeloma or if splenic phagocytes have been paralyzed by high-dose corticosteroid therapy. Other diseases linked with hyposplenism include ulcerative colitis, celiac disease, dermatitis herpetiformis, systemic lupus erythematosus, primary thrombocythemia, and Graves' disease. Such patients run the same risk of fulminant bacteremia as do those who have had their spleen surgically removed.

CONGENITAL ASPLENIA. This uncommon condition is associated with symmetric development of normally asymmetric organs or pairs of organs. Complex and multiple cardiovascular anomalies are the rule.

OTHER DISEASES OF THE SPLEEN

SPLENIC RUPTURE. Rupture of the capsule may be precipitated by trauma, overly zealous palpation of an enlarged spleen (secondary to mononucleosis, sepsis, or leukemia), or rarely by dissection of a pancreatic pseudocyst into the spleen. The patient presents with left upper-quadrant pain, sometimes radiating to the left scapular region, and abdominal guarding and rigidity and progresses to hypovolemic shock. Usually emergency splenectomy is indicated. In selected cases, nonoperative management or splenorraphy, including wrapping of the ruptured capsule ("hair netting"), is a treatment option to splenectomy.

SPLENIC INFARCTION. Infarction usually occurs in the setting of splenic enlargement secondary to myeloproliferative disease or vascular occlusive phenomena (sickle hemoglobinopathies, including SS, SA, S thal, and SC diseases). These may be silent infarctions or present with severe left upper-quadrant pain.

ARTERIAL ANEURYSMS. These lesions are most common in women beyond middle age. They may be asymptomatic or cause left upper-quadrant pain or vague gastrointestinal complaints. The aneurysm or the spleen is sometimes palpable, and a bruit may be appreciated. Radiologic studies can reveal a calcified aneurysmal wall, and the diagnosis is made by sonography or angiography. Embolization of such aneurysms has been successful in situations in which surgery is contraindicated.

SPLENIC HEMANGIOMATOSIS. Diffuse cavernous hemangiomatosis of the spleen is rare, but the cavernous hemangioma is the most common benign tumor involving the spleen. The patient can present with splenic infarctions, splenomegaly, or thrombocytopenia secondary to platelet destruction within the hemangiomas, or the finding of hemangiomatosis may be incidental. The diagnosis can usually be made by computed tomography or sonography.

SPLENIC CYSTS. Echinococcal infection should be suspected in a patient with an appropriate travel history, single or multiple splenic cysts with calcified walls, and eosinophilia. Serologic studies may be helpful in establishing the diagnosis. True splenic cysts (dermoids and mesenchymal inclusion cysts) are embryonic rests and may be diagnosed by scan and angiography.

SPLENIC ABSCESS. An occult, deep-seated infection, splenic abscess usually follows a bacteremic episode. The source of the septicemia can be infected endocardium; lung (pneumonia, lung abscess, empyema); skin or soft tissue; pelvis (pelvic inflammatory disease or septic abortion); nasopharynx; or ear. Predisposing factors include previous splenic damage by infarction (secondary to sickle cell disease or leukemia), trauma, and infection (malaria, typhoid, amoeba, cysts). Extension of an abscess into the spleen from adjacent perforated abdominal organs (stomach, transverse colon, tail of pancreas) can occur. In most series, streptococci are the most common etiologic agents, followed by staphylococci and, with increasing frequency, by gram-negative organisms (*Salmonella, Enterobacteriaceae, Pseudomonas, Serratia, Bacteroides*) and anaerobes. Presenting symptoms include fever, chills, and left upper-quadrant pain, often accompanied by tenderness, muscle spasm, and subcutaneous edema over the spleen. Infection localized to the upper pole of the spleen can produce pleuritic pain and even left pleural effusion. An abscess in the lower pole may result in signs of peritoneal inflammation. A splenic friction rub may be appreciated. Splenic scan, sonography, and computed tomography aid in the diagnosis. The differential diagnosis must include subphrenic abscess, pulmonary empyema, splenic infarction, perinephric abscess, neoplasms, and pancreatic pseudocyst. A combination of antibiotics and surgical intervention, usually splenectomy, is indicated. Single abscesses respond well, but multiple abscesses, often the result of generalized sepsis in a debilitated or immunocompromised patient, are associated with a high mortality.

Chaikof EL, McCabe CT: Fatal overwhelming postsplenectomy infection. Am J Surg 149:534, 1985. *A review of infection patterns in 776 splenectomized adults and children.*

Chun CH, Raff MJ, Contreras L, et al.: Splenic abscess. Medicine, 59:50, 1980. *Comprehensive review of this often fatal disease, discussing etiology, predisposing factors, diagnosis, and treatment.*

Crosby WH: The spleen. In Wintrobe MM (ed.): Blood, Pure and Eloquent. New York, McGraw-Hill Book Company, 1980, p 96. *Historical review of our understanding of splenic function and hypersplenism.*

Eichner ER: Splenic function: Normal, too much and too little. Am J Med 66:311, 1979. *Useful summary of hypersplenic and hyposplenic states, with recommendations for management.*

Mucha P Jr: Changing attitudes toward the management of blunt splenic trauma in adults. Mayo Clin Proc 61:472, 1986. *Discusses splenic preservation and alternatives to splenectomy.*

165 BONE MARROW TRANSPLANTATION

Rainer Storb

MARROW TRANSPLANT PRINCIPLES. Transplantation of marrow from a donor identical with the recipient at the major histocompatibility complex reduces graft-versus-host disease (GVHD) and improves survival of the recipient. Successful human transplantation using allogeneic, HLA-identical sib donors was carried out first in children with immunodeficiency diseases (reviewed in Ch. 419) and subsequently in patients with severe aplastic anemia and leukemia.

Marrow transplantation differs in several aspects from transplantation of solid organs, in particular kidney (see Ch. 80): (1) the host-versus-graft reaction can generally be abrogated by a single short course of high-dose immunosuppressive therapy given immediately before transplantation; (2) preceding blood transfusions are not beneficial but rather can interfere with subsequent marrow engraftment, particularly in patients with aplastic anemia; (3) donors have mostly been HLA-identical family members; (4) donors do not suffer a permanent organ loss, since the removed marrow is replaced within weeks; and (5) post-grafting immunosuppression of recipients can generally be terminated after 3 to 12 months.

To prepare for marrow transplantation the recipient's immune system must first be destroyed. This is effectively accomplished by use of cyclophosphamide (CY), at 50 mg per kilogram per day for four days, or total body irradiation (TBI), at 800 to 1500 rad midline tissue doses (4 to 25 rad per minute) either alone or combined with CY or other chemotherapeutic agents. This program not only sets the stage for establishment of the allogeneic graft but also serves to kill leukemic cells, if that is the patient's basic disease.

After the conditioning regimen, 2 to 6 × 10⁸ donor marrow cells per kilogram are infused intravenously. Most grafts are initially successful such that within two to four weeks marrow cellularity increases and peripheral blood counts of donor origin rise. Over time, all hematopoietic and immune cells of the recipient are replaced by those from the marrow donor, including plasma cells and tissue macrophages.

COMPLICATIONS. *Graft-versus-host disease* may occur when genetically foreign, immunologically active lymphocytes are transferred into an immunosuppressed recipient incapable of rejecting the lymphocytes. This condition is met within all allogeneic marrow transplant recipients (donors are other than monozygous twins). Donor T lymphocytes present in the marrow inoculum recognize histocompatibility antigens of the host as foreign, become sensitized, proliferate, and attack recipient tissue, thereby producing the clinical syndrome of GVHD. The main targets of GVHD are skin, gastrointestinal tract, and liver. Methotrexate or cyclosporine is given within the first 3 to 12 months after grafting as perhaps the most effective immunosuppressive agent to prevent GVHD. Best results seem to be achieved when both drugs are combined. Once the drugs are discontinued, many patients do well with persisting graft-host tolerance. However, acute GVHD occurs in approximately 35 to 60 per cent of the patients, and as many as 40 per cent of afflicted patients die from associated infections. Xenogeneic antihuman thymocyte globulin (ATG), prednisone, or cyclosporine has been used to treat acute GVHD with some success. Better approaches to prevent or treat acute GVHD are necessary, such as the more imaginative use of known immunosuppressive agents, the use of "germ-free" isolation, or the removal of T cells from the marrow inoculum by antibodies to human T lymphocytes.

Chronic GVHD affects approximately 25 to 45 per cent of patients surviving more than 180 days. It is most frequent in older patients and those who had acute GVHD. It may affect the same organs that are involved in acute GVHD and, additionally, mucous membranes. It resembles collagen vascular diseases and is characterized by severe immune deficiency, impaired granulocyte chemotaxis, and recurrent, sometimes life-threatening bacterial infections. Combination therapy with prednisone and azathioprine, CY, or procarbazine is effective in most patients with chronic GVHD.

Interstitial pneumonias, either of unknown etiology or associated with infectious agents such as cytomegalovirus, are a cause of morbidity and fatality during the first four months after grafting. They are a major problem in patients treated with TBI and then receiving transplants for leukemia and a minor problem in CY-treated patients receiving transplants for aplastic anemia. Probably these infections are the result of deficient immune reactivity of the compromised host (see Ch. 258) although radiation effects may also play a role. Effective methods of accelerating the immune reconstitution and/or the use of antiviral agents or hyperimmune globulin might be of value in obviating the problem of interstitial pneumonia.

CLINICAL RESULTS

SEVERE APLASTIC ANEMIA. Aplastic anemia is most frequently attributable to a stem cell defect (see Ch. 133). In many cases infusion of marrow from a monozygotic twin (syngeneic transplant) has been successful in reconstituting the marrow without immunosuppression of the recipient. Some syngeneic grafts have been successful only after preparation with CY and a second transplant, suggesting that these cases may involve other mechanisms, perhaps of autoimmune etiology, which can be overcome by CY.

Allogeneic marrow transplantation (donors are HLA-identical family members) is often effective therapy for severe aplastic anemia, with significantly better survival.

Marrow graft rejection has been a major problem in aplastic anemia. Two factors have predicted graft rejection: (1) positive in vitro tests of cell-mediated immunity, indicating reaction

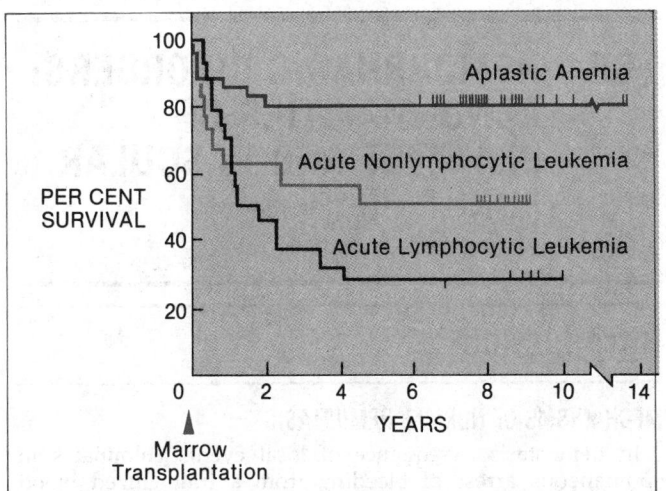

FIGURE 165–1. The survival of 43 untransfused patients with aplastic anemia, 22 patients with acute nonlymphoblastic leukemia having transplants in first remission, and 22 patients with acute lymphoblastic leukemia having transplants in second or subsequent remission after marrow grafts from HLA-identical family members. The surviving patients with leukemia remain in unmaintained remission. Day "0" is the day of marrow transplantation. The tick marks indicate living patients. Survival is as of May 1986.

of recipient lymphocytes against donor cells before transplantation; and (2) a low number of transplanted marrow cells (<3 × 10⁸ per kilogram). Transfusion-induced sensitization is the major cause of graft rejection. In our experience when transplantation is carried out in patients who have not received transfusions before transplantation, graft failure is the exception. Eighty-three per cent of our 43 patients are alive between 4 and 14½ (median 7) years after grafting (Fig. 165–1). We believe that the immunologic mechanisms involved in graft failure are, for the most part, iatrogenic (i.e., induced by previous blood transfusion).

Many programs are being carried out to avoid rejection in multiply transfused patients by using more intensive immunosuppressive conditioning regimens. In all programs CY is used, but other features of the conditioning regimens vary. In Seattle methotrexate and cyclosporine are used after grafting, and viable donor buffy-coat cells are infused together with the marrow inoculum. The donor's peripheral blood is a potential source of additional pluripotent hematopoietic stem cells and/or lymphoid cells capable of overcoming rejection. As a rule, the rejection rates have decreased and survival has increased. Of the last 65 Seattle patients with aplastic anemia who received marrow grafts from HLA-identical siblings following multiple transfusions, 70 per cent are alive after follow-up periods of 4 to 10½ years.

Most of the regimens have associated risks. The addition of buffy-coat cells may lead to an increased risk of chronic GVHD. Radiation regimens carry the potential risk for late malignant disease. Because of these problems and the still existing mortality from rejection, emphasis should be placed on measures to prevent rather than overcome sensitization by blood transfusions. For this the physician should be aware of the possibility of marrow transplantation when aplastic anemia is first diagnosed. If an HLA-identical family member is available, early transplantation before transfusions is the therapy of choice.

LEUKEMIA. Marrow grafting for leukemia presents the same general transplantation problems encountered for aplastic anemia. However, graft rejection is rare. The unique problem is recurrence of leukemia. Formerly marrow transplantation was carried out only after failure of all other therapy when patients were undergoing advanced relapse. Of the first 100 patients with acute leukemia receiving grafts in Seattle after CY and TBI, 12 per cent are alive with the disease in

remission between 11 and 16 years without any maintenance therapy. Approximately 75 per cent of all patients could be expected to have recurrent leukemia unless they died of other causes. Leukemic recurrence usually originated from host-type cells, indicating that it is difficult to kill every leukemic cell once the patient has reached the end-stage of the disease. Current attempts to reduce the rate of leukemic relapse and increase long-term survival in patients with leukemia receiving transplants in the end-stage of their disease involve the use of higher doses of TBI by means of fractionating the radiation and the use of additional chemotherapeutic agents. Perhaps these attempts are doomed to failure since, in an exponential cell kill process, it is difficult to kill the last leukemic cell. Some of the apparent cures may have occurred because of leukemic cell kill by immune mechanisms directed at non-HLA antigens expressed on leukemic cells. This is suggested by the observation of a graft-versus-leukemia effect in man.

It is attractive to carry out marrow transplantation earlier in the course of the disease while the disease is in remission. The advantages of this approach include treatment when the number of leukemic cells in the body is small and before the cells become resistant to therapy, and while the patient is in good clinical condition and therefore better able to tolerate the therapy. Accordingly, we began in 1976 to treat patients with acute nonlymphoblastic leukemia by marrow grafting when the disease was in first or subsequent remission and those with acute lymphoblastic leukemia when it was in second or subsequent remission after conditioning with CY and TBI.

Patients with acute nonlymphoblastic leukemia who received chemotherapy have an approximate median duration of survival of 2 years (see Ch. 156). Only 15 to 20 per cent of patients who received chemotherapy are alive at five years. Of the first 22 patients with *acute nonlymphoblastic leukemia* treated by marrow transplantation during *first remission*, 12 are alive with the disease in unmaintained remission between eight and ten years after transplantation (Fig. 165–1). The survival curve shows a plateau at 55 per cent.

Approximately 50 per cent of patients with acute lymphoblastic leukemia, especially children, can be cured by chemotherapy (see Ch. 156). Once relapse has occurred, another remission can often be induced with chemotherapy, but long-term survival is poor, with very few of the patients alive at two years. Treatment of patients with acute lymphoblastic leukemia during second or subsequent remission by marrow transplantation seems justified in an attempt to change the otherwise grim outlook and perhaps "cure" some of these patients of their disease.

The survival curve of the first 22 patients with *acute lymphoblastic leukemia in second or subsequent remission* receiving marrow grafts in Seattle shows a plateau at 27 per cent 8½ to 10 years after transplantation (Fig. 165–1).

The results of marrow transplantation for the treatment of patients with *chronic granulocytic leukemia* in blast crisis have been similar to those in patients with leukemia in relapse. The projected survival is approximately 15 per cent (Fig. 165–2). The patients' marrows show absence of the Philadelphia chromosome, a unique result.

Transplantation during the *chronic phase of chronic granulocytic leukemia* promises to improve these results. Although follow-up is still short, it appears that long-term disease-free survival will be on the order of 50 per cent (Fig. 165–2).

Marrow transplantation has now also been successfully applied to the treatment of patients with non-Hodgkin's lymphoma, myelofibrosis, multiple myeloma, preleukemia, and hairy cell leukemia.

Common to all results of marrow grafting for leukemia and lymphoma is the problem of recurrence of disease due to host cells that have survived the high-dose chemoradiation therapy. New treatment programs being explored in a number of

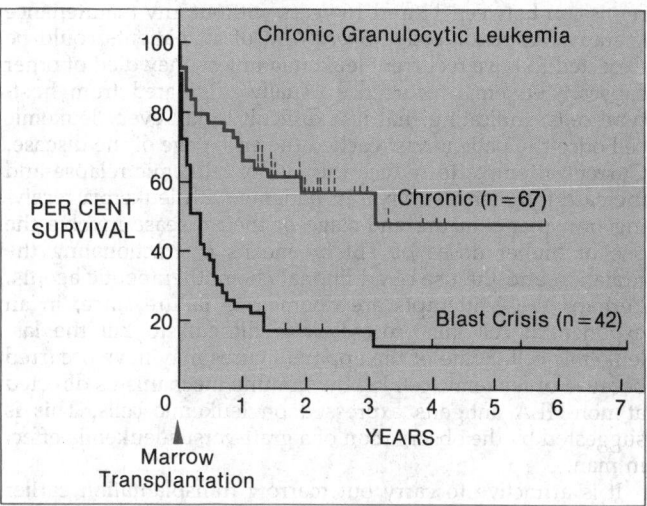

FIGURE 165–2. Survival after marrow grafting in patients with chronic granulocytic leukemia having transplants either in blast crisis or in chronic phase. The tick marks indicate living patients. Survival is as of March 1985.

centers are aimed at more effectively destroying the malignant cells, thereby increasing the success of marrow transplantation.

CONCLUSIONS

Marrow transplantation, once considered a desperate form of therapy in patients with end-stage disease, has now become increasingly successful when used early in the course of aplastic anemia or leukemia. The current success now obliges the physician to identify, soon after diagnosis, those patients who have suitable donors and who may be candidates for transplantation. Marrow grafting has now been extended to the therapy of patients with other hematologic malignant diseases and genetic disorders of hematopoiesis. In the longest survivor with malignant non-Hodgkin's lymphoma, the disease is now in unmaintained remission 16 years after marrow grafting. Cures of congenital Fanconi's anemia, paroxysmal nocturnal hemoglobinuria, thalassemia major, osteopetrosis, and certain genetic storage diseases have been achieved by marrow transplantation.

Many patients do not have HLA-identical sibs, and very few have monozygotic twins. To extend marrow transplantation to a larger number of patients, the use of less well matched family members has been explored with success. Successful human transplants from unrelated donors for the treatment of patients with acute leukemia and aplastic anemia have been carried out.

With the establishment of techniques to "purge" marrow from unwanted malignant cells and to cryopreserve marrow for indefinite periods, in recent years we have seen a renaissance of autologous marrow transplantation for the treatment of malignant diseases. Autologous marrow is attractive, since it avoids the problem of GVHD.

Moller G (ed.): Graft-versus-host reaction. Immunol Rev, Vol 88, 1985. *Reviews by multiple authors of the pathophysiology, immunology, treatment, and prevention of acute and chronic graft-versus-host disease in experimental animals and in man.*

Storb R, Thomas ED: Current state of marrow transplantation. In Silker, R, Gordon AS, Lobue J (eds.): Contemporary Hematology/Oncology, Vol. 3. New York, Plenum Medical, 1984, pp 235–266. *General review with emphasis on GVHD, immunological aspects, opportunistic infections, and recurrence of leukemia.*

Van Bekkum DW, Lowenberg B (eds.): Bone Marrow Transplantation: Biological Mechanisms and Clinical Practice. Vol 3. New York, Marcel Dekker, 1985. *Current state of experimental research and clinical applications in the area of bone marrow grafting. Written by multiple authors.*

Van Rood J, Zwaan F (eds.): Bone Marrow Transplantation. Semin Hematol, Vol 21, 1984. *Multiple-author reviews of marrow transplantation for malignant and nonmalignant hematologic diseases, including late complications and immune reconstitution.*

166 HEMORRHAGIC DISORDERS: ABNORMALITIES OF PLATELET AND VASCULAR FUNCTION

Aaron J. Marcus

Introduction

MECHANISMS OF NORMAL HEMOSTASIS

In hemostasis a sequence of local events culminates in spontaneous arrest of bleeding from a traumatized blood vessel. Three closely linked biologic systems are involved: *blood vessels, platelets,* and *coagulation proteins.* The initial response to interruption of vascular continuity is known as *primary hemostasis* and involves platelets and the vessel surface. Coagulation proteins do not play a role at this juncture. Vascular injury is immediately followed by vessel contraction and platelet adhesion to exposed subendothelial collagen. This adhesive process involves platelet membrane glycoprotein Ib (GPIb) and is mediated by Factor VIII–related von Willebrand factor (Factor VIII: vWF) polymers that adsorb to exposed subendothelial collagen and to platelets. Collagen is an agonist for adherent platelets and induces configurational and biochemical alterations therein. These include (1) secretion of biologically active substances stored in intracellular platelet granules (release reaction); (2) enzymatic liberation of arachidonic acid (by phospholipase[s]) and its oxygenation, mainly to thromboxane A_2 (TXA$_2$) and 12-hydroxyeicosatetraenoic acid (12-HETE); (3) a rearrangement of platelet surface phospholipoprotein, such that it develops procoagulant properties. These include ability to bind and catalyze activation of Factor X and conversion of prothrombin to thrombin. The proteolytic enzyme thrombin is a strong stimulus for further platelet aggregation, TXA$_2$ formation, the release reaction, and further catalysis of fibrin formation.

Platelet secretion can be induced not only by collagen and thrombin, but also by adenosine diphosphate (ADP) and epinephrine. Released platelet products are classified according to their intracellular granule of origin. Thus ADP, serotonin (5-hydroxytryptamine, 5-HT, a powerful vasoconstrictor substance), and calcium originate from dense granules and serve to recruit additional platelets into the hemostatic plug. Alpha-granule components include platelet factor 4 (a heparin-neutralizing protein); beta-thromboglobulin (a platelet-specific protein of unknown function); platelet-derived growth factor (PDGF), which stimulates proliferation of smooth muscle and fibroblasts; Factor VIII: vWF; Factor V; thrombospondin; fibrinogen; albumin; and fibronectin. The threshold for release of alpha-granule components by stimuli is lower than that required for dense body release.

Platelet recruitment, as initiated by released ADP and TXA$_2$, results in further stimulation, aggregation, and augmentation of hemostatic plug formation (Fig. 166–1). In addition, released ADP induces exposure of platelet fibrinogen-binding sites. Exposure of the platelet fibrinogen receptor results from structural transformation of platelet glycoproteins IIb and IIIa during platelet activation. These proteins form a heterodimer complex that expresses fibrinogen receptor activity.

As mentioned, platelet-collagen contact results in liberation of the essential fatty acid, arachidonate, which is oxygenated by two enzymes: a particulate cyclo-oxygenase and a cytoplasmic lipoxygenase. Cyclo-oxygenation of arachidonate (which is inhibited by aspirin acetylation) results in formation of endoperoxides (PGG$_2$ and PGH$_2$), which are transient

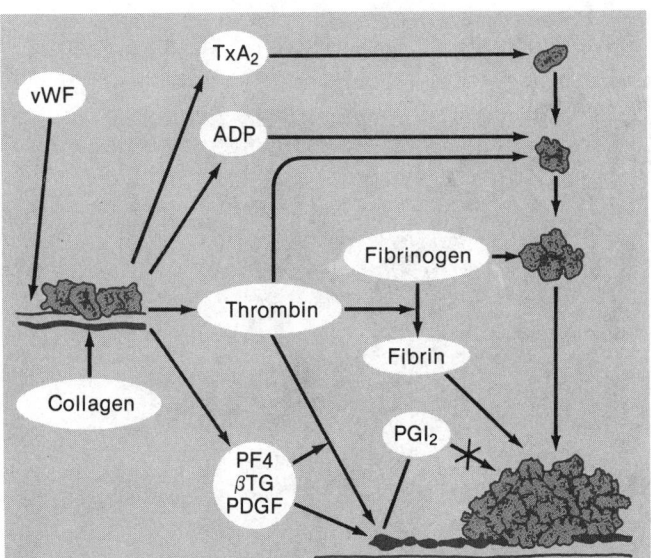

FIGURE 166–1. Reactions of primary (*left*) and secondary (*right*) hemostasis. Following injury of intact vascular endothelium, collagen exposure in the presence of Factor VIII:vWF results in platelet adhesion and activation. These activated platelets release ADP and 5-HT from dense granules and proteins from alpha granules (platelet factor 4, beta-thromboglobulin, and platelet-derived growth factor). Thromboxane is formed from free arachidonic acid and the stimulated platelet phospholipoprotein surface catalyzes activation of Factor X in the formation of thrombin. TxA₂, ADP, and thrombin "synergize" to induce shape change, aggregation, and release in platelets arriving at the injury site. Thrombin formation with consequent conversion of fibrinogen to fibrin comprises secondary hemostasis. Prostacyclin (PGI₂) and other eicosanoids are synthesized by endothelial cells from arachidonate in response to injury, collagen, thrombin, and released platelet endoperoxides. Endothelial cell eicosanoids may regulate the size and extent of platelet deposition in the hemostatic plug (or under pathologic conditions—the thrombus). (Modified from Thompson AR, Harker LA: Manual of Hemostasis and Thrombosis. 3rd ed. Philadelphia, FA Davis Company, 1983.)

intermediates in TXA₂ formation (Fig. 166–2). TXA₂ is rapidly released into the surrounding medium where it induces further platelet aggregation and vasoconstriction. TXA₂ inhibits platelet adenylate cyclase, thereby inducing a fall in cyclic AMP, which in turn increases calcium mobilization. The level of free intracellular calcium is the final determinant of platelet responsiveness. Thrombin and collagen also promote intracellular platelet calcium mobilization independent of, but by comparable mechanisms to, TXA₂. Ionized platelet calcium induces: (1) complex formation with its binding protein, calmodulin, (2) activation of kinases that phosphorylate platelet myosin, (3) activation of phospholipases, and (4) initiation of secretion. In sharp contrast, endothelial cell endoperoxides are converted to prostacyclin (PGI₂) and other eicosanoids. PGI₂ inhibits platelet aggregation and release by increasing platelet cyclic AMP levels, thereby blocking calcium mobilization (Fig. 166–2).

Although primary hemostasis represents a complex sequence of events, its clinical assessment is relatively simple. The bleeding time is a sensitive and reliable index of primary hemostasis. If the bleeding time is prolonged and the platelet count over 100,000 per microliter, primary hemostasis is impaired because of a platelet defect. The qualitative defect can be caused by poor adhesion to the vessel wall or poor platelet cohesion (aggregation). Alternatively, impairment of platelet plug formation as manifested by prolonged bleeding time can be due to thrombocytopenia (platelet count < 100,000 per microliter).

In *secondary hemostasis*, platelets have already aggregated at the site of injury, and the exposed surface membrane phospholipoprotein on activated platelets has catalyzed Factor X

activation and prothrombin conversion to thrombin. Thrombin formation is a critical step that amplifies the reactions of primary hemostasis as well as those leading to fibrin formation and stabilization of the platelet plug (or under pathologic conditions, the thrombus). The actions of thrombin in hemostasis are (1) direct irreversible platelet aggregation with release of ADP, 5-HT, and proteins from alpha-granules; (2) initiation of phospholipase activity culminating in production of TXA₂, thereby indirectly augmenting vasoconstriction, aggregation, and release; (3) conversion of fibrinogen to fibrin strands that consolidate the platelet mass; (4) exposure of platelet receptors for Factor Va to which Factor Xa binds, and enhancement of further thrombin formation; (5) activation of Factor XIII, which catalyzes formation of covalent amide bonds between fibrin polymers, resulting in clot stabilization and completion of the hemostatic process.

Thompson AR, Harker LA: Manual of Hemostasis and Thrombosis. 3rd ed. Philadelphia, F. A. Davis Company, 1983. *This is a compact but very thorough manual that details a pathophysiologic approach to the diagnosis and management of patients with hemostatic and thrombotic disorders. The sequential organization, tables, and figures are presented in a comprehensive manner.*

BLOOD PLATELETS

Platelets are anucleate cytoplasmic fragments derived from marrow megakaryocytes by extension of cytoplasmic processes that undergo attenuation, develop constrictions at their distal ends, and then rupture in the form of free platelets. Production and release of platelets from the marrow may be controlled by two "thrombopoietins"—one regulating the quantity of megakaryocyte-committed stem cells and another modulating megakaryocyte maturation. The presence of large platelets (megathrombocytes) in the circulation may be directly related to the degree of thrombopoietic stimulation. Platelets, which normally circulate for about ten days, are 3.6 ± 0.7 μm in diameter. The normal platelet count is 150,000 to 400,000 per microliter. On a stained blood smear one can visualize about three to ten platelets per oil-immersion field. Approximately 70 per cent of platelets are circulating, and 30 per cent are in the spleen.

Despite its comparatively simple structure the platelet is functionally complex. Stimulated platelets adhere to damaged vessel surfaces (adhesion) as well as to each other (cohesion or aggregation). Stimulation is also a prerequisite for the release reaction and transformation of arachidonic acid to TXA₂, which reinforces hemostatic function. Platelets maintain "vascular integrity" through obscure mechanisms. Rapid onset of thrombocytopenia is often associated with spontaneous hemorrhage into the skin and mucous membranes, whereas in chronic thrombocytopenias there is an ill-defined compensatory mechanism for missing "vascular integrity factor(s)" and hemorrhage is less frequent. Platelets function in the intrinsic coagulation system. The phospholipoprotein surface of stimulated platelets binds and catalyzes interactions between activated coagulation factors culminating in thrombin formation, a property formerly termed platelet factor 3.

Platelets mediate clot retraction, probably via the contractile protein actomyosin. This may play a role in vivo during consolidation of hemostatic plug formation and can be studied in vitro as a well-defined metabolic process.

Platelets, therefore, intrinsically possess multiple mechanisms for responding to and repairing effects of vascular damage. These include a factor(s) for maintaining vascular integrity, the capacity to spontaneously arrest bleeding through plug formation, the ability to catalyze fibrinogen polymerization—thereby stabilizing the plug, and mechanisms for release of growth factors to enhance repair and healing. These processes occur in varying degrees, depending upon strength and concentration of the stimuli. Failure of one mechanism (as in the case of TXA₂ inhibition by aspirin ingestion) results in a minor hemostatic defect, since others such as thrombin responsiveness remain intact. Figure 166–3

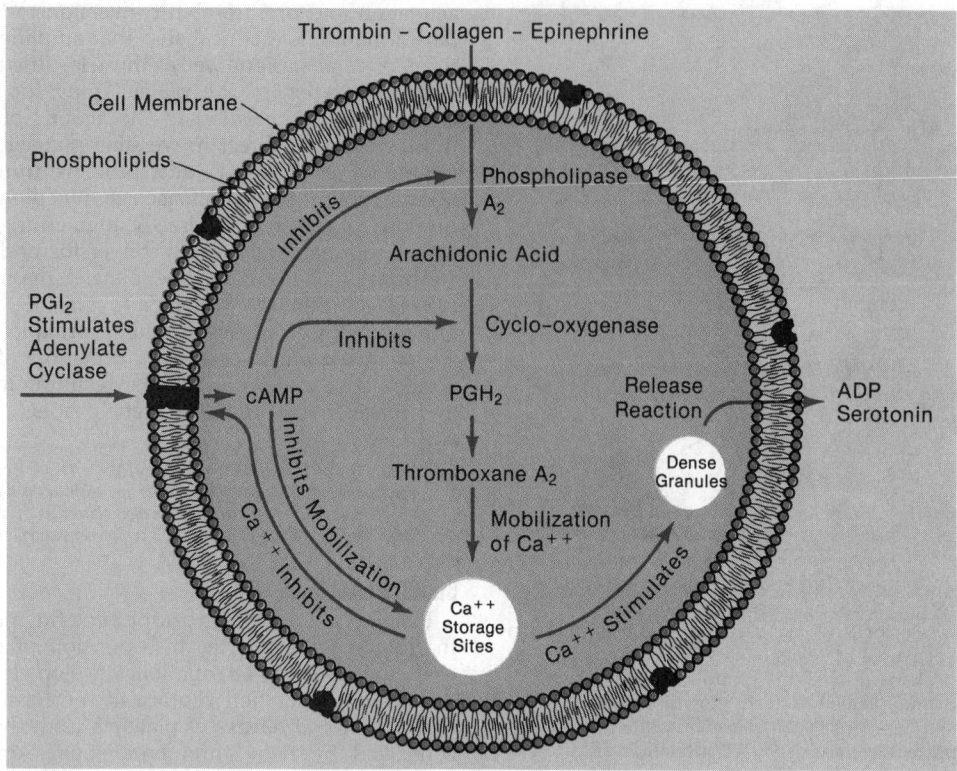

FIGURE 166–2. Diagram of events associated with activation of the platelet arachidonic acid cyclooxygenase pathway. The end product, thromboxane A_2, induces intracellular calcium mobilization and is also released into the microenvironment where it acts as a direct agonist for additional platelet aggregation and vasoconstriction. Mobilized calcium is the major stimulus for initiation of dense granule secretion. ADP and serotonin are among the most important products of the platelet release reaction. The increase in intracellular calcium also inhibits adenylate cyclase, thus lowering cyclic AMP levels, which further promotes aggregation and release. In contrast, PGI_2, the major cyclooxygenase product of endothelial cells, stimulates adenylate cyclase, thus elevating platelet cyclic AMP and blocking calcium mobilization and its consequences. In this manner PGI_2 attenuates platelet responsiveness. Platelets also contain a lipoxygenase pathway of arachidonate metabolism, of which the end product is the chemotactic monohydroxy fatty acid, 12-HETE. In contrast to the cyclooxygenase pathway shown here, the lipoxygenase reactions are not inhibited by aspirin. (From Gorman RR, Marcus AJ: Prostaglandins and cardiovascular disease. Current concepts. A Scope publication. Upjohn Company, 1981.)

depicts platelet ultrastructure with emphasis on functional correlations associated with specific organelles.

Colman RW, Hirsh J, Marder V, et al. (eds.): Hemostasis and Thrombosis: Basic Principles and Clinical Practice. Philadelphia, JB Lippincott Company, 1982. *This book presents the biochemistry and physiology of hemostasis and the pathophysiology of thrombosis in detail. Emphasis is on diagnosis and treatment of hemorrhagic diseases and thrombotic diatheses.*

Marcus AJ: The eicosanoids in biology and medicine. J Lipid Res 25:1511, 1984. *A review and discussion of how eicosanoids and their precursors from multiple cell types exert biologic effects in the microenvironment.*

CLINICAL ASSESSMENT OF PATIENTS WITH POSSIBLE BLEEDING DISORDERS

The physician is required to evaluate the condition of a patient in two clinical settings to determine if a bleeding tendency is present. (1) A screening evaluation is required before the patient undergoes a surgical procedure. (2) The

patient has previously experienced an episode(s) of hemorrhage—either spontaneous or following trauma.

In both instances a meticulous personal and family history, in addition to a physical examination, together with sequentially selected laboratory screening tests, will establish that (1) a hemorrhagic tendency is or is not present; (2) the bleeding diathesis is due to a coagulation abnormality, a vascular defect, or a platelet disorder; (3) the disorder is congenital or acquired (Table 166–1).

MEDICAL, FAMILY, AND DRUG HISTORY. A history of excessive bleeding or bruising occurring spontaneously or following minor trauma is of significance. This is especially true if the bruise is 3 cm or larger. Although such episodes are usually associated with a vascular abnormality, they also occur in coagulation and platelet disorders. The patient should be questioned concerning unusual bleeding following dental extraction or surgery. Characteristically, bleeding in platelet

TABLE 166–1. DIFFERENTIAL CLINICAL DIAGNOSIS OF COAGULATION, PLATELET, AND VASCULAR DISORDERS

	Coagulation Defect	Platelet Disorder	Vascular Abnormality
Family history	Usually positive	Negative	Usually negative
Sex predominance	Males	Frequently females	Mainly females
Nature of symptoms and signs	Visceral, intramuscular and joint hemorrhage; spontaneous and post-mild trauma	Cutaneous, mucous membrane, and CNS hemorrhage; petechiae, purpura, hematuria; hemarthroses rare	Ecchymoses, purpura, frequently spontaneous; melena; no hemarthroses
Time sequence of hemorrhage	Post-traumatic delay followed by persistent oozing	Concomitant with and immediately following trauma; usually of short duration	Post-traumatic or spontaneous localized ecchymoses; generalized bleeding rare
Response to local pressure	Usually ineffective	Usually effective	Effective

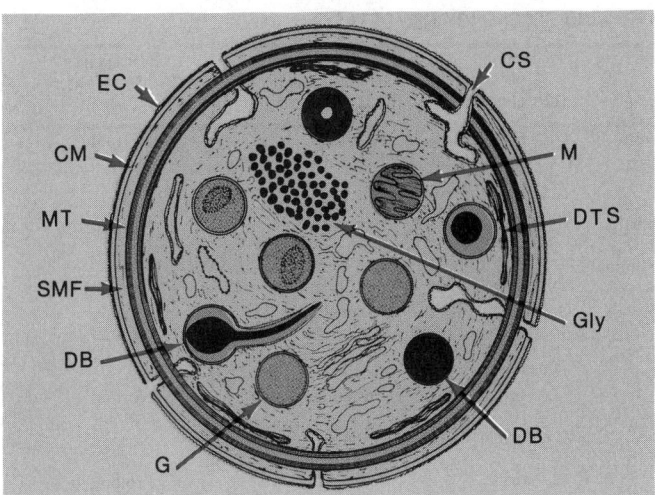

FIGURE 166–3. Diagrammatic representation of platelet ultrastructure. The glycoprotein-rich exterior coat (EC) contains receptors for platelet agonists and inhibitors. Signal transduction also occurs at this site. The cell membrane (CM) consists of the classic lipid bilayer and is rich in arachidonic acid, which is esterified to phospholipid. In activated platelets the CM undergoes a rearrangement to form a catalytic lipoprotein surface for acceleration of coagulation. Concomitantly, membrane calcium release promotes activation of phospholipases for initiation of eicosanoid formation. The submembrane filaments (SMF), now recognized as actin, form parallel structures that induce pseudopod formation upon platelet stimulation. These filaments also line channels of the surface-connected canalicular system (CS). The circumferential microtubule system (MT) constitutes the cytoskeleton, which maintains the disc shape of unstimulated circulating platelets. Platelets also contain mitochondria (M), glycogen (Gly), and dense bodies (DB), which represent sites of storage for ADP, 5-HT, and calcium. Platelet granules (G) are of two types: some are lysosomal, and others contain secretable proteins of the "adhesive" type (fibrinogen, von Willebrand factor, thrombospondin, and fibronectin), as well as PF_4, beta-thromboglobulin, and PDGF. The dense tubular system (DTS) and the surface-connected canalicular system are membrane systems in the platelet, which are counterparts of sarcoplasmic reticulum as defined in other cells. (Courtesy of Dr. James G. White: CRC Critical Reviews in Oncology/Hematology, 4:337, 1986. Copyright CRC Press, Inc., Boca Raton, FL.)

diseases is immediate and transient, and blood loss is minimal to moderate. In coagulation disorders, postoperative or post-traumatic hemorrhage is delayed, prolonged, and moderate to severe. Mucous membrane bleeding such as epistaxis is a common presenting symptom in platelet diseases. Family history is critical, especially in males, since deficiencies of Factors VIII and IX are linked to the X chromosome. Factor VIII deficiency (hemophilia A) accounts for approximately 85 per cent of congenital coagulation disorders. An additional 10 per cent are due to Factor IX deficiency. The other coagulation defects (autosomal recessive) comprise the remaining 5 per cent. In 30 per cent of patients with hemophilia, a family history cannot be elicited.

Acquired abnormalities of platelets, blood vessels, and coagulation factors or a combination of these (including circulating anticoagulants) occur as complications of systemic disorders such as liver disease, malignant disease, systemic lupus erythematosus (SLE), and uremia. A major facet of the history concerns medication. *Aspirin ingestion* during the previous week will interfere with platelet function and will also increase the severity of a hemostatic disorder already present. Drugs known to interfere with platelet function are listed in Table 166–2. Patients taking coumarin anticoagulants or heparin (including those surreptitiously using these drugs) must be identified.

PHYSICAL EXAMINATION. Information from the history is confirmed and extended by physical examination. Presence and distribution of petechiae, purpuric spots, or ecchymoses

should be noted. *Petechiae* are pinpoint lesions resulting from breakage or increased permeability of arterioles, capillaries, or venules. They appear at pressure points and mucosal surfaces. Petechiae are characteristically observed in symptomatic patients with thrombocytopenia. A *purpuric lesion* represents confluent petechiae, also associated with thrombocytopenia. An *ecchymosis* is an extension of the purpuric lesion, indicating that extravasated blood has traversed fascial planes. A *dissecting hematoma* is the most serious form of an ecchymosis. Spontaneous ecchymoses occur in defects in coagulation. *Hemarthroses* or ankylosed joints strongly suggest Factor VIII or Factor IX deficiency. Lesions of Osler-Weber-Rendu disease (hereditary telangiectasia) and spider telangiectasia may resemble petechiae, but blanch on pressure. Cherry hemangioma and angiokeratomas (Fabry's disease) usually do not blanch.

Triplett DA: Hemostasis: A Case Oriented Approach. New York, Igaku-Shoin, 1985. *This text emphasizes prerequisites for diagnosis and care of patients with hemorrhagic or thrombotic disorders. Authentic cases from hospital archives have been utilized for presentation and discussion.*

SEQUENCE OF LABORATORY STUDIES OF HEMOSTATIC FUNCTION

Although a tentative diagnosis of a hemorrhagic diathesis can be made from the history and physical examination, precise characterization requires laboratory studies. Basic screening tests are carried out first. These procedures examine the integrity of platelet, vascular, and coagulation components of hemostasis: (1) microscopic examination of the peripheral blood smear, (2) platelet count, (3) bleeding time, (4) prothrombin time (PT), (5) activated partial thromboplastin time (APTT or PTT), and (6) thrombin time (TT). More sophisticated and expensive assays should not be done unless indicated by abnormal results of screening tests (Table 166–3 and Fig. 166–4).

Platelet numbers and gross morphology can be evaluated from inspection of the peripheral blood smear. In addition, visualization of other formed elements is helpful in patient evaluation. Schistocytes suggest microangiopathic hemolytic anemia as occurs in disseminated intravascular coagulation (DIC). The presence of large platelets indicates increased platelet turnover as seen in immune thrombocytopenia or platelet destruction by artificial cardiac prostheses.

Platelet counts below 100,000 per microliter are the most common cause of serious bleeding. There is an inverse relationship between platelet count and bleeding time. Platelet counts below 50,000 per microliter require phase microscopy for accurate enumeration.

The *bleeding time* is usually determined by a modified Ivy method in which an incision 1 cm long and 1 mm deep is made on the volar surface of the forearm while 40 mm Hg of pressure is maintained on the upper arm with a blood pressure cuff. The bleeding time usually exceeds nine minutes under the following conditions: (1) thrombocytopenia (platelet counts < 100,000 per microliter), (2) qualitative platelet defects, (3) von Willebrand's disease, and (4) vascular defects.

Following aspirin ingestion, the bleeding time may be prolonged from the normal range of two to six minutes to a mean value of nine and one-half minutes. Alcohol and aspirin are synergistic in extending the bleeding time. A prolonged

TABLE 166–2. DRUGS ASSOCIATED WITH ABNORMALITIES IN PLATELET FUNCTION

Aspirin	Low molecular weight dextran
Chlorpromazine	Meclofenamic acid
Clofibrate	Nitrofurantoin
Dipyridamole	Penicillins
Ethanol	Phenylbutazone
Glyceryl guaiacolate (Guaifenesin)	Sulfinpyrazone
Hydroxychloroquine	Tricyclic antidepressants
Indomethacin	*Vinca* alkaloids

TABLE 166–3. SCREENING TESTS FOR PRIMARY AND SECONDARY HEMOSTASIS

Disorder	Platelet Count (~300 × 10³/cu mm)	Bleeding time (<9 minutes)	Clot Retraction	Prothrombin Time (12 seconds)	Activated Partial Thromboplastin Time (33–45 Seconds)	Thrombin Time (3–5 Seconds Above Control)
Thrombocytopenia	Low	Prolonged	Poor to absent	Normal	Normal	Normal
Vascular defects	Normal	Prolonged (tourniquet test positive)	Normal	Normal	Normal	Normal
Qualitative platelet defect	Normal	Prolonged	Normal (poor to absent in thrombasthenia)	Normal	Normal	Normal
Extrinsic coagulation system						
Factor VII deficiency	Normal	Normal	Normal	Prolonged	Normal	Normal
Factor II, V, or X deficiency	Normal	Normal	Normal	Prolonged	Prolonged	Normal
Intrinsic coagulation system						
Factor VIII and IX deficiency	Normal	Normal	Normal	Normal	Prolonged	Normal
von Willebrand's disease	Normal	Prolonged	Normal	Normal	Variable—usually prolonged	Normal
Afibrinogenemia, dysfibrinogenemia	Normal	Variable	Normal	Normal	Normal	Prolonged
DIC, liver failure	Usually low	Variable, often prolonged	Sometimes poor	Prolonged	Prolonged	Prolonged

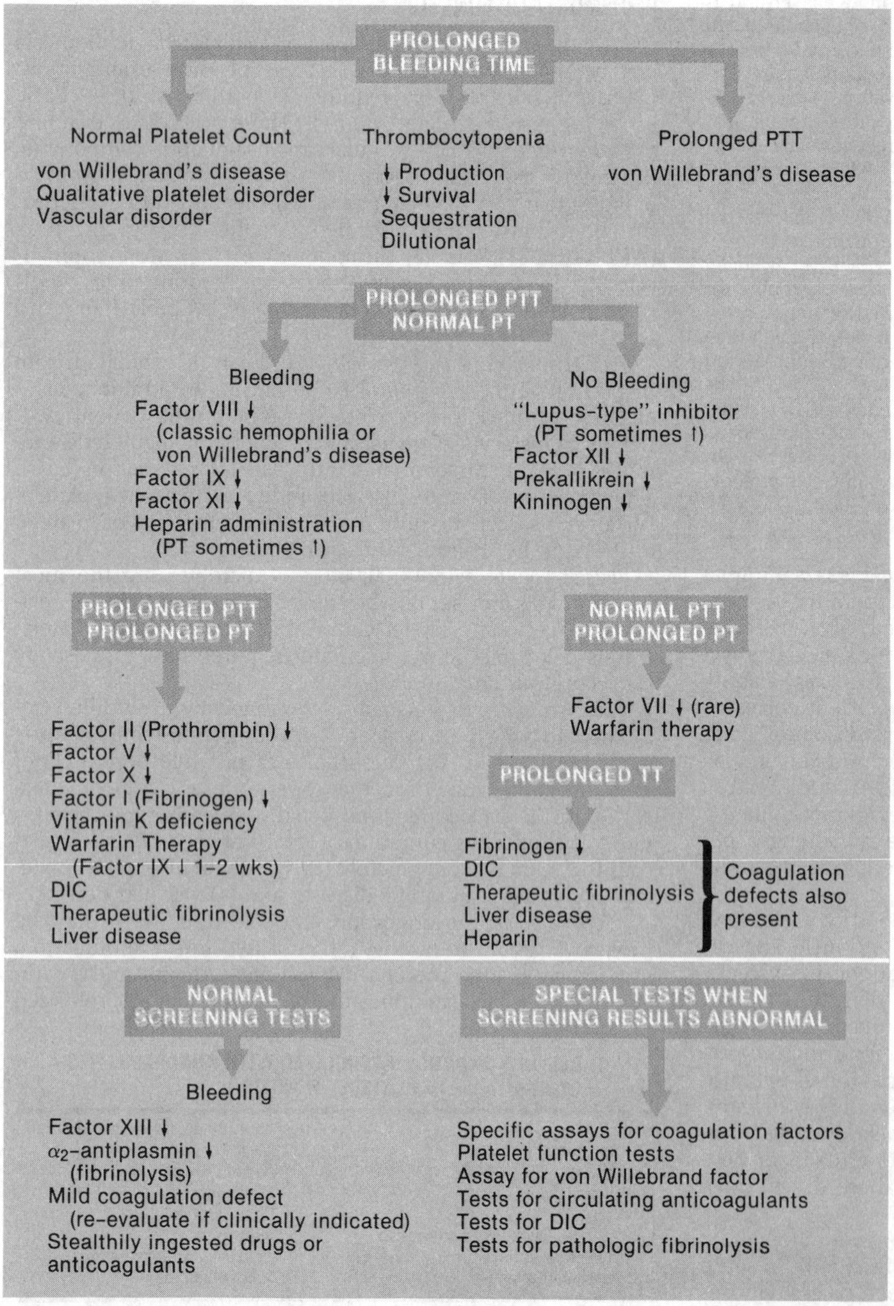

PROLONGED BLEEDING TIME

Normal Platelet Count
von Willebrand's disease
Qualitative platelet disorder
Vascular disorder

Thrombocytopenia
↓ Production
↓ Survival
Sequestration
Dilutional

Prolonged PTT
von Willebrand's disease

PROLONGED PTT NORMAL PT

Bleeding
Factor VIII ↓
(classic hemophilia or von Willebrand's disease)
Factor IX ↓
Factor XI ↓
Heparin administration (PT sometimes ↑)

No Bleeding
"Lupus-type" inhibitor (PT sometimes ↑)
Factor XII ↓
Prekallikrein ↓
Kininogen ↓

PROLONGED PTT PROLONGED PT

Factor II (Prothrombin) ↓
Factor V ↓
Factor X ↓
Factor I (Fibrinogen) ↓
Vitamin K deficiency
Warfarin Therapy
(Factor IX ↓ 1–2 wks)
DIC
Therapeutic fibrinolysis
Liver disease

NORMAL PTT PROLONGED PT

Factor VII ↓ (rare)
Warfarin therapy

PROLONGED TT

Fibrinogen ↓
DIC
Therapeutic fibrinolysis
Liver disease
Heparin
} Coagulation defects also present

NORMAL SCREENING TESTS

Bleeding
Factor XIII ↓
α₂-antiplasmin ↓ (fibrinolysis)
Mild coagulation defect (re-evaluate if clinically indicated)
Stealthily ingested drugs or anticoagulants

SPECIAL TESTS WHEN SCREENING RESULTS ABNORMAL

Specific assays for coagulation factors
Platelet function tests
Assay for von Willebrand factor
Tests for circulating anticoagulants
Tests for DIC
Tests for pathologic fibrinolysis

FIGURE 166–4. Sequential interpretation of screening tests in Table 166–3.

bleeding time in the setting of a normal platelet count defines a vascular abnormality or a qualitative platelet disorder. Approximately 43 per cent of such patients have von Willebrand's disease; 27 per cent will be diagnosed as having vascular purpura (platelets and coagulation normal), 16 per cent have thrombasthenia, 7 per cent have thrombocytopathy with normal-appearing platelets, and 7 per cent have thrombocytopathy with abnormal platelet morphology.

The *prothrombin time* provides an overall assessment of the extrinsic coagulation system. Since factor VII is the first coagulation protein to be depleted by oral anticoagulants, the PT is important for monitoring such patients. In congenital and acquired deficiencies of factors VII, X, V, II, and fibrinogen, the PT will be prolonged.

The *activated partial thromboplastin time* is an excellent screening procedure for the intrinsic coagulation system. The "contact" components of the intrinsic system (Factor XII and cofactors) are activated by particulate ingredients of a reagent such as kaolin or celite. The remaining coagulation proteins are activated by phospholipid in the reagent. If the patient has a normal PT but prolonged PTT, a deficiency of the intrinsic system (Factors XII, XI, VIII, IX, Fletcher factor, and Fitzgerald factor) exists or a circulating anticoagulant is present. Patients with the lupus anticoagulant frequently have a normal PT and prolonged PTT. The PTT is also utilized in monitoring heparin therapy.

The *thrombin time* provides information concerning quantitative and qualitative aspects of plasma fibrinogen and is also influenced by inhibitors. Thus the thrombin time will be prolonged in hypofibrinogenemia, dysfibrinogenemias, during heparin therapy, by the presence of fibrinogen-fibrin split products, and paraproteins. The thrombin time is usually prolonged if the fibrinogen level is below 100 mg per deciliter (Fig. 166–4).

Confirmatory screening tests include procedures for identification of fibrinogen-fibrin degradation products as occur in DIC. When a circulating anticoagulant is suspected on the basis of a prolonged PTT, the patient's plasma is diluted 1:1 with normal pooled plasma. If the PTT is not corrected by this maneuver, a circulating anticoagulant is probably present. Evaluation of clot retraction is simple and inexpensive. If clot retraction is normal, it indicates that platelet numbers, platelet function, the quantity of fibrinogen, and packed cell volume are satisfactory. Clot retraction is defective to absent in thrombasthenia and thrombocytopenia.

An occasional result in routine screening procedures is the combination of normal coagulation tests, normal platelet count and morphology, but a slightly prolonged bleeding time. This mild qualitative platelet defect is most commonly due to ingestion of aspirin or a medication containing aspirin. Another offender is guaifenesin (glyceryl guaiacolate), a component of cough remedies (Table 166–2).

Platelet aggregometry can provide additional information concerning a possible platelet qualitative defect. Aggregation is measured as an increase in light transmission through stirred platelet-rich plasma while a specific agonist is added. Test substances include ADP, collagen, epinephrine, sodium arachidonate, and the agglutinating agent ristocetin. A ristocetin agglutination study for von Willebrand's disease is mandatory if the PTT is prolonged, the bleeding time excessive, and the platelet count normal. In von Willebrand's disease the platelets are unresponsive to ristocetin. In contrast, platelets from patients with thrombasthenia will *agglutinate* upon addition of ristocetin, but will not *aggregate* in the presence of standard stimuli.

Patients with acquired defects in the platelet release reaction (drugs, following cardiopulmonary bypass, uremia) and those with congenital release abnormalities demonstrate a single, reversible wave of platelet aggregation. Platelets from patients who have recently ingested aspirin are unresponsive to arachidonate, and those from patients with myeloproliferative

disorders are unreactive to epinephrine. Correlations between results of in vitro platelet aggregometry may not always be in direct relationship to the hemostatic defect observed clinically. Therefore, aggregometry information should be regarded as largely supportive and correlated with the value obtained for the bleeding time. Further evaluation usually is not required in the patient whose coagulation- and platelet-screening tests are normal. There are instances, however, in which mild clinical and laboratory coagulation or platelet disturbances require further elucidation. This is done by performance of specific assays for coagulation factors or platelet aggregometry or both with an extended group of stimuli at varying concentrations.

Harker LA, Zimmerman TS (eds.): Measurements of Platelet Function. Methods in Hematology Series. Vol. 8. New York, Churchill Livingstone, 1983. *This book is a compilation of recommended methods for evaluating platelet function.*

Sirridge MS, Shannon R: Laboratory Evaluation of Hemostasis and Thrombosis. 3rd ed. Philadelphia, Lea & Febiger, 1983. *This volume covers basic aspects of hemostasis and thrombosis and features detailed descriptions of diagnostic procedures, reagents employed, and interpretations of laboratory tests.*

Quantitative Platelet Disorders

THROMBOCYTOPENIA

Thrombocytopenia is defined as a platelet count below 100,000 per microliter. Except for chronic, longstanding thrombocytopenia, hemorrhage is inversely proportional to the platelet count (especially in disorders of platelet production). Platelet counts in the range of 40,000 to 60,000 per microliter may lead to post-traumatic bleeding, and at 20,000 per microliter, spontaneous hemorrhage can occur. Particularly hazardous are central nervous system and gastrointestinal hemorrhage. Fever, anemia, and chronic inflammation in thrombocytopenic patients render them more susceptible to bleeding and less responsive to platelet transfusions.

There are four basic mechanisms of thrombocytopenia (Table 166–4): (1) decreased or ineffective platelet production, (2) shortened platelet survival time in the circulation due to

TABLE 166–4. CAUSES OF THROMBOCYTOPENIA

I. **Decreased platelet production**
    Reduced megakaryocytes in marrow
        Marrow infiltration—malignant disease, myelofibrosis, chemicals, and drugs
        Marrow hypoplasia—radiation, chemicals, insecticides, drugs, viruses, idiopathic, alcohol
        Congenital—Fanconi's pancytopenia, thrombocytopenia with absence of radius, autosomal recessive thrombocytopenia, cyclic thrombocytopenia, infection (congenital rubella)
    Ineffective thrombocytopoiesis (normal or increased marrow megakaryocytes)
        Hereditary
            Autosomal dominant thrombocytopenia
            May-Hegglin anomaly
            Wiskott-Aldrich syndrome
        Megaloblastic anemias
            Di Guglielmo's syndrome
            Preleukemia
II. **Decreased platelet survival**
    Increased destruction
        Drug-induced thrombocytopenic purpura
        Idiopathic thrombocytopenic purpura
        Post-transfusion purpura
        Isoimmune neonatal purpura
        Secondary immunologic purpura
        HIV infection (AIDS)
    Increased consumption
        Thrombotic thrombocytopenic purpura
        Disseminated intravascular coagulation
        Cavernous hemangioma
        Hemolytic-uremic syndrome
        Acute infections
        Cardiopulmonary bypass
III. **Sequestration (hypersplenism)**
IV. **Dilutional thrombocytopenia**

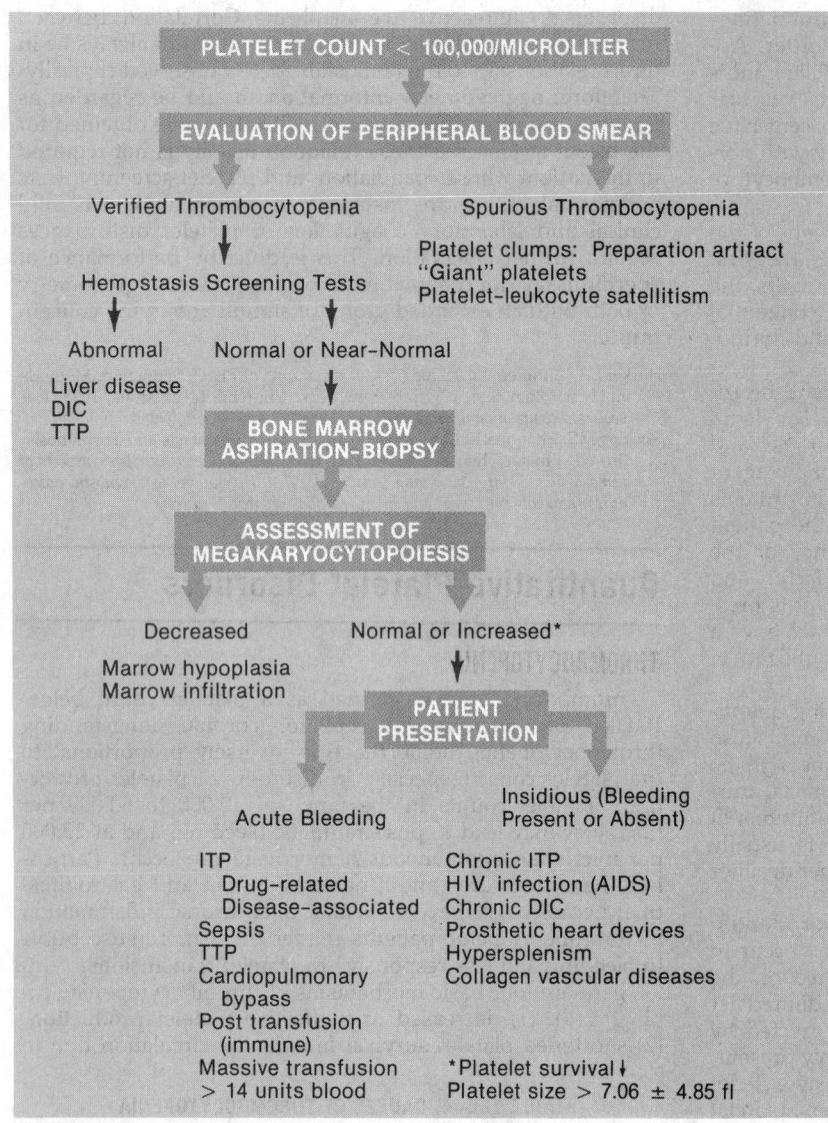

FIGURE 166—5. Evaluation of the thrombocytopenic patient. (Modified from Nathan DG, Oski FA: Hematology of Infancy and Childhood. Philadelphia, WB Saunders Company, 1981.)

increased destruction or consumption or both, (3) splenic sequestration, (4) intravascular dilution of circulating platelets. A diagnostic approach to thrombocytopenic patients is outlined in Figure 166–5.

Decreased Platelet Production

REDUCED MEGAKARYOCYTES. Reduced platelet production by megakaryocytes may result from marrow replacement, chemical injury, or congenital disorders. Compromise of erythroid or myeloid elements may also occur. Since the basic defect is the rate at which platelets enter the circulation, platelet survival is normal or slightly decreased. Mechanical displacement of megakaryocytes in the marrow may be due to metastatic carcinoma, myeloma, leukemias or lymphomas, xanthomatoses, myelofibrosis, and granulomas. Radiation, drugs, or infectious agents may also be responsible for decreased megakaryocytopoiesis. Cancer chemotherapeutic agents predictably induce megakaryocyte damage. Other offending substances include alcohol, anticonvulsants, tranquilizers, thiazides, solvents, and insecticides. Megakaryocytic hypoplasia may occur in congenital diseases such as pancytopenias associated with Fanconi's syndrome—a fatal childhood illness characterized by multiple congenital and skeletal abnormalities. Another autosomal recessive disorder, congenital hypoplastic thrombocytopenia, associated with absent radii (TAR syndrome) is characterized by an early hemorrhagic diathesis. Megakaryocytic hypoplasia also occurs as an autosomal recessive trait in the absence of other somatic abnormalities and as a result of congenital intrauterine rubella infection.

INEFFECTIVE THROMBOCYTOPOIESIS. Ineffective thrombocytopoiesis is characterized by increased marrow megakaryocytes but a decrease in circulating platelets. The defect may involve (1) defective platelet formation, (2) abnormal release of platelets from the marrow, and (3) destruction of platelets in the marrow. An autosomal dominant form of this ineffective thrombocytopoiesis, sometimes in association with increased serum IgA, nephritis, deafness, and "giant" platelets, has been reported. Ineffective platelet production also occurs in the May-Hegglin anomaly (autosomal dominant), the Wiskott-Aldrich syndrome (sex-linked recessive), and DiGuglielmo's disease. Vitamin B_{12} and folate deficiencies are characterized by an increase in megakaryocyte cytoplasmic mass but relatively ineffective platelet production. Thrombocytopenia associated with excessive alcohol ingestion is complex and due to several factors such as megakaryocytic hypoplasia, splenic platelet pooling, shortened platelet survival time, and folate deficiency.

Decreased Platelet Survival Due to Increased Destruction

Drug-Induced Thrombocytopenic Purpura

At least 70 drugs have been implicated in or proven to induce thrombocytopenic purpura (Table 166–5). In these thrombocytopenias, marrow megakaryocytes are increased and platelets are destroyed peripherally. In adults with thrombocytopenic purpura, a drug etiology should be considered

TABLE 166–5. THERAPEUTIC AND CHEMICAL AGENTS THAT MAY PRODUCE THROMBOCYTOPENIC PURPURA

I. Direct marrow suppressants
  Generalized marrow hypoplasia or aplasia
    Antimetabolites
    Antimitotic agents
    Anti-tumor antibiotics
    Benzene and derivatives
    Ionizing radiation
    Nitrogen mustard and congeners
  Occasional association with marrow hypoplasia or aplasia
    Chloramphenicol
    Gold compounds
    Methylphenylethyl hydantoin (Mesantoin), trimethadione (Tridione)
    Phenylbutazone
    Quinacrine
  Selective suppression of megakaryocytes
    Chlorothiazides
    Estrogenic hormones
    Ethanol
    Tolbutamide

II. Production of thrombocytopenia by an immunologic mechanism

Acetazolamide (Diamox)	p-Aminosalicylic acid (PAS)
Carbamazepine	Phenytoin (Dilantin)
Chlorothiazides	Quinidine
Chlorpropamide	Quinine
Desipramine	Rifampin
Digitoxin	Stibophen (Fuadin)
Gold salts	Sulfamethazine
Hydroxychloroquine	Sulfathiazole
Methyldopa	

III. Direct damage to circulating platelets
  Heparin
  Ristocetin

IV. Probable immunologic mechanism; antibodies not always demonstrated

Acetaminophen	Organic hair dyes
Aminopyrine	Nitroglycerin
Aspirin and sodium salicylate	Paramethadione
	Penicillin
Barbiturates	Phenacetin
Bismuth	Phenylbutazone
Carbutamide	Potassium iodide
Cephalothin	Prednisone
Chloroquine	Prochlorperazine
Chlorpheniramine maleate	Promethazine
Chlorpromazine	Propylthiouracil
Codeine	Pyrazinamide
Dextroamphetamine sulfate	Reserpine
Diazoxide	Spironolactone
Digitalis and digoxin	Streptomycin
Disulfiram (Antabuse)	Sulfonamides (sulfadiazine,
Ergot	sulfadimetine, sulfamerazine,
Erythromycin	sulfamethoxazole, sulfisoxazole)
Insecticides	Tetracycline
Iopanoic acid (Telepaque)	Tetraethylammonium (TEA)
Isoniazid	Thiourea
Meperidine	Trimethadione
Meprobamate	Trimethoprim-sulfamethoxazole
Mercurial diuretics	Turpentine

first. This is true even if a medication has been used without previous ill effects.

Typically the patient may become symptomatic with flushing and chills within a few minutes after ingestion of the offending agent. Hemorrhage from the gastrointestinal and urinary tracts may occur 1 to 12 hours later. This is followed or accompanied by petechiae and purpuric lesions in dependent areas, although the palms and soles are usually spared. Hemorrhagic bullae may appear on the oral mucosa, which is pathognomonic of thrombocytopenic purpura. The petechiae are nontender and nonpruritic and do not have an erythematous border—which distinguishes them from allergic skin reactions.

PATHOGENESIS OF DRUG-RELATED THROMBOCYTOPENIAS. A drug rarely induces thrombocytopenia by direct action on circulating platelets. This occurred with the antibiotic ristocetin, which is no longer in clinical use. Many drugs have been suspected, and in some cases they have proven to induce thrombocytopenia by an antibody-mediated immune mechanism.

Heparin, whether administered intravenously or subcuta-

neously, can induce thrombocytopenia with little or no consequences or a thrombocytopenia that is complicated by a thrombotic diathesis. In the mild form, platelet counts are in the range of 100,000 per microliter, and spontaneous bleeding seldom occurs. Patients do not necessarily give a history of receiving heparin in the past. The thrombocytopenic effect may be related to the use of heparin subfractions with a lesser affinity for antithrombin III. This mild syndrome may eventually be eliminated when purified heparin preparations are developed with near-total affinity for antithrombin III. The mild thrombocytopenia occurs within 15 days of heparin administration and is completely reversible upon cessation of heparin therapy. Since the patients are usually asymptomatic, future use of heparin, if required, may be considered. The severe symptomatic heparin-induced thrombocytopenia is slow in onset and increases in severity within a two-week period. The chronology of the event suggests an immune mechanism, and antibodies to the platelet-heparin complex have been identified. The in vivo aggregation of platelets that ensues can result in occlusive vascular lesions in multiple locations. Embolic complications also occur, but hemorrhage is rare. Future therapy with heparin is contraindicated.

Among the most widely studied drug-induced thrombocytopenias is that due to *quinidine*. It serves as a model for chemically related compounds as well as other agents that induce thrombocytopenia.

The immunologic reaction that terminates in platelet destruction occurs in the following manner: (1) The drug (or one of its derivatives or metabolites) acts as a hapten and forms a complex with a plasma protein ("carrier"). (2) The complex formed is antigenic and induces production of high-affinity antibodies. When the drug is reingested the antibody can bind to the drug (hapten) itself. (3) The antigen-antibody complex then adsorbs to platelets via their Fc receptor. (4) Adsorption of the antigen-antibody complex by platelets is nonspecific, i.e., the platelets are "innocent bystanders." (5) Antibody-coated platelets are rapidly and efficiently "recognized" by the reticuloendothelial system and removed from the circulation prematurely, giving rise to thrombocytopenia when bone marrow reserve decompensates.

DIAGNOSIS OF DRUG-INDUCED THROMBOCYTOPENIA. A detailed history concerning drug ingestion or unusual environmental exposure is mandatory. Intake of beverages such as tonic water should also be checked, since it contains quinine, which can induce thrombocytopenia ("cocktail purpura"). If possible, all medications should be withdrawn until a diagnosis has been established. This also serves as a diagnostic test, since the purpura may resolve following removal of an offending drug.

In vitro assays for detection of possible circulating drug-induced antibodies are difficult to perform in most laboratories. No single test (complement fixation, "immunoinjury tests," ^{51}Cr release) will detect all antibodies. Direct binding assays for IgG or complement on the platelet surface are useful but cumbersome and produce variable results. Readministration of the drug, even in smaller doses for confirmation of an etiologic diagnosis, is not recommended. If other hematologic parameters are normal, a bone marrow examination is not necessary. However, if thrombocytopenia persists for more than two weeks after abstinence from the drug, another diagnosis should be considered, and a bone marrow examination is indicated. Exceptions include gold salts and arsenicals, which are excreted slowly.

TREATMENT OF DRUG-INDUCED, ANTIBODY-MEDIATED THROMBOCYTOPENIA. Usually no treatment is necessary, since withdrawal of the offending agent results in recovery. If purpura increases in severity or spontaneous bleeding occurs from mucous membranes, corticosteroid therapy is recommended because it will inhibit phagocytosis of antibody- or complement-coated platelets by macrophages in the spleen. Also, steroids have a beneficial effect on vascular integrity. If the platelet count is below 30,000 per microliter initially, corticosteroids should be administered. Rare instances of life-threatening hemorrhage must be managed with platelet transfusions or, as a last resort, exchange transfusions, on the presumption that the latter would lower plasma concentrations of drug and antibody. Since antibodies in drug-induced thrombocytopenia are specific, alternative pharmacologically equivalent compounds can be substituted. Future use of the offending drug is contraindicated.

King DJ, Kelton JG: Heparin-associated thrombocytopenia. Ann Intern Med 100:535, 1984. *This review discusses the diagnosis and treatment of heparin-induced thrombocytopenia as a laboratory finding in the absence of symptomatology and the syndrome of heparin-associated thrombocytopenia plus arterial thrombosis. The latter can result in stroke, myocardial infarction, and death.*

Idiopathic Thrombocytopenic Purpura

DEFINITION. Idiopathic thrombocytopenic purpura (ITP) refers to thrombocytopenia occurring in the absence of toxic exposure or a disease associated with decreased platelets. In at least 85 per cent of patients with ITP an immunologic mechanism involving IgG-type antibodies can be demonstrated. Since platelet destruction is immune mediated in most cases, the term *autoimmune thrombocytopenic purpura* (ATP) has been suggested. There are two forms of ITP, acute and chronic. Both are characterized by normal or increased marrow megakaryocytes (number and volume), shortened platelet survival, and absence of splenomegaly.

ACUTE ITP. Acute ITP occurs most frequently in childhood (ages two to six) and affects both sexes equally. A history of antecedent upper respiratory viral infection one to three weeks prior to onset can be elicited in 80 per cent of cases. There is a peak seasonal incidence in fall and winter, which may parallel prevalence of viral respiratory infections. Symptomatic patients abruptly develop petechial hemorrhages and purpura. Hemorrhagic bullae in the oral cavity may occur along with epistaxis and gastrointestinal and genitourinary bleeding. Platelet counts of 20,000 per microliter or less are commonly observed. Although the patient is at risk for intracranial hemorrhage, this rarely occurs. If splenomegaly is present it usually reflects the previous viral illness. Peripheral blood smears demonstrate eosinophilia and lymphocytosis. Since 80 per cent of patients recover spontaneously in two weeks to six months, the prognosis of acute ITP in children is excellent. Recurrence after complete recovery is rare, and mortality is less than 1 per cent. In adults, however, spontaneous remission will not occur in 90 per cent of patients with acute ITP.

Therapy is not required unless atraumatic mucous membrane hemorrhage continues and new crops of ecchymoses appear. Some physicians treat all patients with short-term prednisone therapy (1 to 2 mg per kilogram body weight daily) for four weeks when the risk of hemorrhage is maximal. Since spontaneous remission occurs in most children, objective evaluation of corticosteroid therapy is difficult. In rare situations in which life-threatening hemorrhage occurs, platelet transfusions are indicated. Intravenous infusion of high-dose gamma globulin (1.0 to 2.0 grams per kilogram body weight) may induce an increase in platelet counts of patients with ITP. This is due to blockade of Fc receptors on macrophages in the reticuloendothelial system by the immunoglobulin. Thus antibody-coated platelets remain in the circulation. Responses are frequently transient, and a five-day course of treatment costs $6000. However, a single transfusion of gamma globulin (400 mg per kilogram) may be effective in preparation for platelet transfusion or splenectomy in uncontrolled life-threatening acute ITP.

Approximately 10 to 15 per cent of adult patients with acute ITP will not fully recover in six months. If the patient is symptomatic, or if platelet counts are below 100,000 per microliter, treatment with corticosteroids is required. Children who do not respond to a course of prednisone (80 to 100 mg per day) within 6 to 12 months should be considered for

splenectomy. Permanent remission occurs following splenectomy in 85 per cent of patients.

CHRONIC ITP. Chronic ITP in adults can begin insidiously or result from an episode of acute ITP, from which 90 per cent of adults do not undergo spontaneous remission. Although it occurs at any age, chronic ITP is observed most frequently between 20 and 40 years, with women affected more frequently than men (ratio 3:1). In the insidious form there is gradual onset of mucosal petechiae, ecchymoses, epistaxis, and menorrhagia. Cutaneous hemorrhage is more common in distal portions of the extremities. Palpable splenomegaly is not a characteristic of chronic ITP. If present, the diagnosis should be questioned. Platelet counts are in the range of 30,000 to 80,000 per microliter, and bone marrow megakaryocytes are normal or increased in number and volume (Fig. 166–5).

Clinically, chronic ITP undergoes remissions and relapses alternating over long periods. Exacerbations are sometimes cyclic and can be correlated with phenomena such as menstruation. Thus evaluation of treatment is difficult. Although acute ITP in children is not accompanied by immune-type disorders, in adults with chronic ITP periodic evaluation is required for coexistence of diseases such as systemic lupus erythematosus, lymphoproliferative disorders, and autoimmune hemolytic anemia (Evans' syndrome).

THROMBOCYTOPENIA IN THE ACQUIRED IMMUNODEFICIENCY SYNDROME (AIDS). One of the most common hematologic complications of infection with HIV is thrombocytopenia. These patients do not have splenomegaly, and marrow megakaryocytes are normal. The thrombocytopenia is associated with deposition of immune complexes and complement on the platelet surface. This is in contrast to classical ITP (ATP) in which antiplatelet IgG antibody is bound to the platelet surface. Superimposed on this cause of thrombocytopenia, decreased production of platelets may also result from marrow replacement with tumor or infiltration by fungi or mycobacteria (Fig. 166–5).

Thrombocytopenia in patients with AIDS or AIDS-related complex (ARC) may occur early in the course of HIV infections. The use of corticosteroids has resulted in transient improvement in circulating platelet counts, but long-term therapy with steroids in these patients is hazardous. Vincristine or vinblastine has induced temporary improvement, and danazol has been of minimal usefulness. Most patients have been managed conservatively, with splenectomy considered as a last resort. High-dose intravenous gamma globulin has provided benefit over a period of several months.

PATHOGENESIS OF ITP. The pathophysiology and clinical manifestations in 85 to 95 per cent of patients with chronic ITP are due to production of an antiplatelet IgG antibody that binds to platelets and results in premature splenic removal of these platelets. Hepatic removal occurs in highly sensitized patients. Splenic destruction of antibody-damaged platelets occurs because splenic macrophages contain receptors for the Fc portion of the IgG molecule. Platelet-bound IgG has also been identified in patients with malignant tumors, leukemias, thrombotic thrombocytopenic purpura, aplastic anemia, and sepsis. Platelet antigens also fix complement. In ITP, platelets may also contain surface-bound IgM (up to 20 per cent of cases). These platelets are removed by the liver. Hepatic removal of antibody-coated platelets may account for failure of splenectomy to induce complete long-term remissions in about 50 per cent of patients with ITP.

DIAGNOSIS OF CHRONIC ITP. Criteria for diagnosis include (1) evidence of increased platelet destruction as demonstrated by a shortened survival time (in "compensated thrombocytolytic states" the platelet count may be normal or near normal). (2) Increased megakaryocyte size and number in the marrow. (3) Demonstration of antibody bound to platelets by a reliable technique. (4) Other clinical disorders that might meet criteria 1 to 3 should be ruled out. (Drug-induced immunologic thrombocytopenia may be difficult to differentiate from ITP. Platelet counts should return to normal 7 to 14 days following discontinuation of the drug.) (5) Presence of splenomegaly virtually excludes the diagnosis of ITP.

If the patient's platelets *do not contain demonstrable antiplatelet antibody* by available techniques and the other criteria cited above can be met, the term *ITP* should be used (5 to 10 per cent of cases). Patients in whom *platelet antibody can be demonstrated* are classified as *ATP*. Other clinical disorders considered in the differential diagnosis include the thrombocytopenia associated with HIV infection, SLE, lymphomas, and hypersplenism (Fig. 166–5).

TREATMENT. Major therapeutic methods for chronic ITP are: corticosteroids, splenectomy, immunosuppressive agents, and high-dose intravenous gamma globulin. The clinical course of chronic ITP is variable. Spontaneous recovery occurs in less than 10 per cent of cases. Patients whose platelet counts are in the range of 100,000 per microliter and whose hemorrhagic manifestations are minimal may be observed at bimonthly intervals. Maintenance of normal to near-normal hemostasis (occasional cutaneous petechiae or bruising) is more important than the platelet count per se. Hemostasis can be achieved with platelet counts of 40,000 to 60,000 per microliter.

Corticosteroids. If platelet counts remain below 40,000 per microliter and spontaneous bleeding persists, therapy with prednisone is indicated (1 mg per kilogram daily); 70 to 90 per cent of patients respond with an increase in platelets and decrease in hemorrhagic diathesis. The hemorrhagic disorder frequently improves prior to the rise in platelet count. This may be due to a direct effect of corticosteroids on capillaries in improving their physical integrity. Although a clinical response to corticosteroids may occur in 48 hours, beneficial effects become fully evaluable in 1 to 3 weeks. After four to six weeks the corticosteroid dose is gradually tapered and discontinued, especially if no bleeding is present. About 20 per cent of patients have a long-term beneficial response to corticosteroids. If subsequent relapse occurs, readministration of corticosteroids should induce another remission. Over many months only 10 to 15 per cent of patients treated with corticosteroids remain in permanent remission. The subsequent course may become unfortunate, characterized by corticosteroid refractoriness and prohibitive toxicity. The next consideration is splenectomy.

The beneficial effect of corticosteroids in ITP is due to prevention of sequestration of antibody-coated platelets by splenic phagocytic cells. Mononuclear cell phagocytic capacity, chemotaxis, and adherence properties of antibody-coated platelets are all reduced by corticosteroids. Other corticosteroid effects include an increase in platelet production, impairment of immunoglobulin synthesis, and inhibition of antibody-platelet interaction.

Splenectomy. When patients become unresponsive to corticosteroids or require toxic levels to maintain hemostatic balance, splenectomy is indicated. This results in removal of the major site of platelet destruction and a significant source of antiplatelet antibody production. About 70 to 80 per cent of patients improve after splenectomy, and in 60 per cent platelet counts return to normal. In those who respond, there is normalization of platelet survival and decrease in platelet-bound IgG. Interestingly, antiplatelet antibody is still detectable in the plasma and platelets of some patients with ITP in remission. ITP remains in permanent remission in two thirds of splenectomized patients, and in the one third whose platelet counts remain below 100,000 per microliter, bleeding symptoms no longer occur. Over a five-year period, relapse occurs after splenectomy in about 10 to 12 per cent of patients. Many of these patients can be maintained on low-dose prednisone (10 mg or less daily). The presence of an accessory spleen should always be considered in patients who do not

respond completely to splenectomy or in whom relapse occurs soon after a successful splenectomy-induced remission.

Although patients tolerate splenectomy rather well in the setting of severe thrombocytopenia, those with life-threatening bleeding may be prepared for surgery with a single (400 mg per kilogram) intravenous dose of gamma globulin, followed by platelet transfusions preoperatively.

Some observers recommend splenectomy in all patients with ITP of more than 6 months' duration who cannot be maintained therapeutically with 5 to 10 mg prednisone daily. With regard to pneumococcal infection in the postsplenectomy state, prophylactic administration of Pneumovax is recommended 1 to 2 weeks prior to splenectomy in both adults and children.

Management of Patients No Longer Responsive to Corticosteroids and Splenectomy (Refractory ITP). Over a period of years, relapse occurs in the postsplenectomy state in 10 to 12 per cent of patients with chronic ITP. It cannot be managed with corticosteroids, and hemorrhagic manifestations continue to develop. Immunosuppressive drug therapy has been moderately successful in some instances, but the disorder does not lend itself to controlled therapeutic studies. Azathioprine and cyclophosphamide have been useful, and in some cases prolonged remissions have been reported. It may require up to two months to observe a beneficial effect. Vincristine has also been effective, either alone or followed by maintenance therapy with cyclophosphamide. The long-term effects and toxicity of immunosuppressive therapy are not known, so these agents should be used with caution.

High-dose intravenous gamma globulin is an important method for treatment of ITP in children and adults. The induction of temporary reticuloendothelial blockade (Fc receptor) and other, unknown, mechanisms are thought to be responsible for the rise in platelet count. Danazol,* a modified androgen preparation devoid of masculinizing effects, has been used in doses of 200 to 400 mg per day as a substitute for corticosteroids. Partial success in restoration of platelet counts has been reported, as has synergy with corticosteroids.

Platelet transfusions for life-threatening bleeding in ITP were previously ineffective and used only as a last resort. Pretreatment with gamma globulin may facilitate such therapy when required.

In *neonatal ITP*, IgG antibody is passively transferred across the placenta. The disorder can occur whether the mother's disease is in remission or whether she is thrombocytopenic. The infant's platelet count may be normal at birth, but decreases in 12 to 24 hours. Treatment of the mother with prednisone (10 to 20 mg per day) for 10 to 14 days prior to term is recommended, which also permits vaginal delivery.

---

*Four patients receiving danazol therapy for endometriosis developed a reversible ITP-like syndrome. Thus, platelet counts should be closely monitored in patients with ITP receiving danazol therapy (Arrowsmith JB, Dreis M: N Engl J Med 315:585, 1986).

Baumann MA, Menitove JE, Aster RH, et al.: Urgent treatment of idiopathic thrombocytopenic purpura with single-dose gammaglobulin infusion followed by platelet transfusion. Ann Intern Med 104:808, 1986. *Work described here represents an extension of the use of intravenous high-dose gamma globulin for therapy of ITP. Use of a large single dose followed by allogeneic platelet transfusion allows for control of bleeding and preparation for emergency surgery in ITP.*

Harrington WJ: Are platelet-antibody tests worthwhile? N Engl J Med 316:211, 1987. *The author discusses the important role of serologic testing for platelet antibodies in the diagnosis of ITP. Antibody measurements have been less valuable as guides for therapy. Patients with ITP who have normal to increased megakaryocytes in the bone marrow and have not responded to standard conservative therapeutic modalities are candidates for splenectomy.*

Karpatkin S: Autoimmune thrombocytopenic purpura. Semin Hematol 22:260, 1985. *A scholarly monograph that discusses and evaluates all recent clinical and research aspects of autoimmune and idiopathic thrombocytopenia. The concept of "ATP" is developed.*

McMillan R: Chronic idiopathic thrombocytopenic purpura. N Engl J Med 304:1135, 1981. *This review thoroughly encompasses current clinical, laboratory, and therapeutic aspects of ITP.*

Picozzi VJ, Roeske WR, Creger WP: Fate of therapy failures in adult idiopathic thrombocytopenic purpura. Am J Med 69:690, 1980. *An interesting retrospective study in which spontaneous recovery in patients with ITP was surprisingly frequent.*

Post-transfusion Purpura

Post-transfusion purpura is a very rare disorder (approximately 40 cases reported), clinically indistinguishable from fulminant ITP or drug-induced thrombocytopenia. Most cases have occurred in women who had previous pregnancies. The purpuric episode occurs five to eight days following blood transfusion. The patients are thought to have developed an antibody to a genetically determined platelet antigen known as Pl^{A1}, which is present in 98 per cent of the population. It is assumed that the patient became sensitized during pregnancy when fetal platelets (containing Pl^{A1} antigen inherited from the father) became accessible to the maternal circulation. The antigen may then have eluted from the Pl^{A1}-positive fetal platelets and adsorbed to the patient's platelets in a passive manner. Although 1 in 50 recipients is mismatched with respect to the Pl^{A1} antigen, post-transfusion purpura is very rare and production of the antibody is transient. Platelet counts are less than 10,000 per microliter, and thrombocytopenia may persist up to seven weeks. Corticosteroids have been employed for treatment, but frequently the severity of thrombocytopenia and hemorrhagic diathesis has prompted use of exchange transfusions and plasmapheresis. Platelet transfusions are ineffective. Definitive diagnosis is made by detection of the anti-Pl^{A1} antibody by agglutination and complement fixation techniques. Post-transfusion purpura as a syndrome may be heterogeneous and not limited to females or Pl^{A1}-negative individuals.

Isoimmune Neonatal Purpura

If the fetus has inherited a paternal platelet-specific antigen that induces IgG antibody formation by the mother, these antibodies cross the placenta and adsorb to fetal platelets. Frequently the Pl^{A1} system has been implicated (about 50 per cent of cases). Hemorrhage may not be present at birth, but several hours later, petechiae, ecchymoses, and hematomas develop. The most urgent complication is intracranial hemorrhage (mortality 10 to 15 per cent). Therapy has included corticosteroids and, when necessary, platelet transfusions or exchange transfusions. Recovery is usually uneventful, and platelets return to normal within 14 to 21 days. An important differential is that between neonatal ITP and isoimmune neonatal purpura. Thus platelet counts and morphology should be part of prenatal care.

Secondary Autoimmune Thrombocytopenia

Immune-mediated thrombocytopenia, including the presence of platelet-associated IgG (which may not be specific), occurs as a complication of systemic diseases. Most frequent are SLE and lymphoproliferative disorders. About 10 to 15 per cent of patients with SLE develop an ITP-like syndrome in the course of their disease or even have it at initial presentation. The higher incidence of SLE in females and in chronic ITP parallels the increase in frequency of the HLA-DRw2 system in these disorders. Of patients initially presenting with chronic ITP, 25 to 30 per cent may eventually be found to have SLE. Immunologic tests for SLE should be carried out in all new cases of ITP. An ITP-like syndrome may develop in patients with Hodgkin's disease, lymphomas, chronic lymphocytic leukemia, and sarcoidosis. Other reports of this ITP-like illness have appeared in association with thyrotoxicosis, tuberculosis, Hashimoto's thyroiditis, scleroderma, rheumatoid arthritis, and malignancies.

In allergic reactions to insect bites, tetanus toxoid, foods, or vaccines or recovery from viral infections such as rubella or infectious mononucleosis, platelets may be damaged by antigen-antibody complexes and then sequestered in the reticuloendothelial system, rendering the patient thrombocytopenic. In Evans's syndrome, chronic ITP is associated with a Coombs-positive autoimmune hemolytic anemia.

Decreased Platelet Survival Due to Increased Consumption

Thrombotic Thrombocytopenic Purpura (Moschcowitz's Syndrome)

Thrombotic thrombocytopenic purpura (TTP) is a generalized disorder of the microcirculation characterized by thrombocytopenic purpura, microangiopathic hemolytic anemia, transient and fluctuating neurologic signs, renal dysfunction, and a febrile course. More than 400 cases have been reported, of which two thirds have been in women with a mean age of 39. The bleeding is widespread and includes petechiae, ecchymoses, gastrointestinal hemorrhage, retinal bleeding, and hematuria. The neurologic findings are variable and may include an organic mental syndrome, paresis, aphasia, slurred speech, headache, vertigo, and seizures. The renal disease is usually progressive and characterized by hematuria, proteinuria, and an elevated blood urea nitrogen level.

All patients present with thrombocytopenia (platelets less than 50,000 per microliter). The peripheral blood smear demonstrates characteristic abnormalities of microangiopathic hemolytic anemia—fragmented red cells (schistocytes), burr cells, helmet-shaped erythrocytes, and normoblasts. The Coombs test is negative, and there is marked reticulocytosis. In early stages of the disease, laboratory tests do not indicate the presence of disseminated intravascular coagulation (DIC). However, as the illness progresses to hepatic and renal decompensation or onset of sepsis, frank DIC occurs.

The pathologic lesion of TTP is characteristic. Hyaline thrombi occlude arterioles and capillaries of virtually every tissue. Although endothelial cell proliferation may be observed in proximity to the lesions, inflammatory reactions and vasculitis are not observed. The hyaline material is thought to consist of dense platelet aggregates surrounded by thin layers of fibrin.

The etiology of these diffuse occlusive lesions in the microcirculation is unknown. In one third of patients a history of antecedent upper respiratory tract infection can be elicited. TTP has been linked with oral contraceptives, antibiotics, surgery, pregnancy, meningococcal infections, coxsackievirus B, vaccines, and mycoplasmas. An immune mechanism might be involved in the pathogenesis of TTP, since it has been associated with SLE, low levels of serum complement, and identification of complement components in vascular lesions. Successful therapeutic use of plasma, exchange transfusions, and plasmapheresis supports the concept that vascular injury, platelet sequestration, and microvascular thrombosis in TTP could result from deposition of immune complexes in arterioles and capillaries. However, circulating immune complexes in TTP have yet to be identified.

In a typical case the presence of thrombocytopenia, hemolytic anemia, neurologic abnormalities, fever, and renal dysfunction confirm the diagnosis. If the patient is seen late in the course, laboratory tests will indicate DIC. The hemolysis and symptomatology in DIC accompanying other diseases is not as severe, however, as that in TTP. The hemolytic-uremic syndrome (HUS) observed in infants and children may resemble TTP, but neurologic symptoms are rare. TTP involves more organ systems, and HUS is characterized by more serious renal involvement, frequently complicated by severe hypertension. A TTP-like syndrome can occur in patients with malignant disease in association with or following chemotherapy.

Biopsies of marrow, skin, muscle, gingivae, and lymph nodes in TTP have yielded variable results (positive in up to two thirds of cases). Biopsy of petechial sites has been reported to be diagnostic. Hyaline thrombi can be demonstrated in dermal capillaries.

In the past TTP was fatal in 50 to 80 per cent of cases. Therapy has always been difficult to evaluate. It included splenectomy, massive corticosteroids, and inhibitors of platelet function (dipyridamole, aspirin, and dextran)—all with varying degrees of success. Newer therapeutic advances have markedly improved the previously unfavorable prognosis in TTP. Plasma infusions, exchange transfusions, and plasmapheresis have all been utilized with highly encouraging results. Many patients have undergone complete remissions of long duration, and others have been successfully maintained with intermittent plasma infusions. Thus, plasma infusions, plasmapheresis, or both are currently regarded as the treatment of choice. Corticosteroids, aspirin, and dipyridamole may be employed initially, but in the absence of a rapid response, plasma therapy should be initiated. The most adequate trial is 2 to 7 plasma volume exchanges over a two-week interval.

Lian EC-Y, Mui PTK, Siddiqui FA, et al.: Inhibition of platelet-aggregating activity in thrombotic thrombocytopenic purpura plasma by normal adult immunoglobulin G. J Clin Invest 73:548, 1984. *Normal IgG inhibits platelet-aggregating activity present in TTP plasma.*

Marcus AJ: Moschcowitz revisited. N Engl J Med 307:1447, 1982. *Discussion of a new approach to the pathogenesis and treatment of chronic TTP.*

Disseminated Intravascular Coagulation

Disseminated intravascular coagulation (DIC), also known as defibrination syndrome or consumption coagulopathy, represents a complication of medical, surgical, and obstetric situations in which the intrinsic and extrinsic coagulation systems are activated with resulting local and general escape of thrombin into the circulatory system. In DIC fibrinogen is depleted, and platelets are activated and deposited in the microcirculation, leading to thrombocytopenia. The initial thrombotic phase is followed by a hemorrhagic disorder due to depletion of platelet and coagulation factors. Hemorrhage into skin and mucous membranes is followed by bleeding in other tissues and organs. Fibrinolysis ensues, and degradation products formed by the action of plasmin appear as a secondary complication. Thrombocytopenia is usually out of proportion to the coagulation abnormality (platelet counts are well below 100,000 per microliter). The accumulation of fibrinogen-fibrin degradation products due to secondary fibrinolysis further inhibits platelet function. Systemic diseases in which there is tissue damage with release of procoagulant substances and proteases, circulatory stasis, and shock all contribute initiating mechanisms for DIC. The underlying condition should be managed first, and if necessary, plasma, cryoprecipitate, and platelet transfusions are utilized. Heparin should be avoided, except in DIC occurring as a complication of progranulocytic leukemia in which there is intravascular release of tissue factor. Additional features of DIC are discussed in Ch. 167.

Cavernous ("Giant") Hemangioma (Kasabach-Merritt Syndrome)

Approximately 3 per cent of infants with hemangiomas, either subcutaneous or visceral, have thrombocytopenia. Bleeding may occur during the first few days of life or be delayed for several years. The hemangiomas occur subcutaneously or in viscera, but both types of lesions rarely coexist. Although the term *giant* has been used to describe the lesions, size is not correlated with thrombocytopenia. Low platelet counts can be associated with hemangiomas 5 to 6 cm in diameter. Concomitant with development of bleeding complications, the hemangioma may change in size and consistency. Purpura and ecchymoses develop around the lesion per se, followed by DIC. The lesions may regress within five years. Mild thrombocytopenia in the absence of significant bleeding is treated with corticosteroids. Heparin therapy has been used with transient results and is not recommended. Symptomatic patients should be managed with surgical removal of the primary lesion. In vital areas such as the neck and thorax radiotherapy may be required.

Hemolytic-Uremic Syndrome (Gasser's Syndrome)

The hemolytic-uremic syndrome (HUS) occurs mainly in infants and young children and is characterized by a Coombs-negative microangiopathic hemolytic anemia, thrombocytopenia, and acute renal failure. Occasional cases occur in adolescents and young adults. Rarely, HUS complicates immunization procedures or penicillin therapy. A typical episode is preceded by abdominal pain, vomiting, and diarrhea. Anemia, hemorrhage, renal insufficiency, and cardiac decompensation ensue. In contrast to TTP, neurologic signs and symptoms are rare. The thrombocytopenia (85 per cent of cases) is an example of selective platelet consumption without an increase in fibrinogen turnover. Although laboratory features of DIC may be observed early in the course, coagulation factor levels subsequently increase as a "rebound" phenomenon. Thus HUS is not actually an example of DIC.

A syndrome similar to HUS has been reported in women in association with pregnancy, the postpartum period, and ingestion of oral contraceptives. This may be a variant of HUS and is later complicated by nephrosclerosis.

The pathologic lesion of HUS consists of occlusive hyaline deposits closely associated with endothelial cells in the renal microcirculation. Fibrinogen and platelets have also been identified in small blood vessels. HUS may result from an incomplete response to a primary antigenic stimulus with subsequent formation of circulating immune complexes and fibrin deposition in the renal microvasculature.

Therapy in HUS is primarily directed toward management of renal failure with peritoneal dialysis. The combination of packed erythrocyte transfusions, dialysis, and other vigorous supportive measures has reduced the overall mortality from 35 per cent to 5 per cent. Corticosteroids, heparin, fibrinolytic agents, and inhibitors of platelet aggregation have not been consistently beneficial. In analogy with therapy for TTP, plasma infusion, plasmapheresis, and exchange transfusion may be of value.

Kaplan BS, Drummond KN: The hemolytic-uremic syndrome is a syndrome. N Engl J Med 298:964, 1978. *This discussion considers the definition and pathogenesis of the hemolytic-uremic syndrome. The central feature is damage to the vascular endothelium in glomerular capillaries and renal arterioles. Differentiation of this disorder from TTP is discussed.*

Thrombocytopenia in Acute Infections

Bacterial, viral, fungal, rickettsial, and protozoan infections can be associated with thrombocytopenia. In febrile patients with platelet counts below 150,000 per microliter the possibility of gram-negative sepsis or, less commonly, gram-positive sepsis should be evaluated. In some cases platelet production may be suppressed, and in others direct platelet destruction by viruses and bacteria has been demonstrated in vitro. Development of DIC as a complication of infection would further contribute to thrombocytopenia. Toxins produced by microorganisms can bind to platelets and induce aggregation and release. Circulating immune complexes may adsorb to platelets, resulting in their premature removal from the circulation. Only a small percentage of patients with infections develop a hemorrhagic diathesis on the basis of thrombocytopenia. Platelet levels return to normal during recovery.

Thrombocytopenia in Cardiopulmonary Bypass

Thrombocytopenia is one of several hemostatic complications occurring during cardiopulmonary bypass. In some instances it is part of the consumption coagulopathy, but in others it is due to platelet contact with surfaces of oxygenators. This contact may induce platelet activation. Traces of thrombin, which form in the pump or at surgical sites, further stimulate platelets. Currently, platelet transfusions are used to restore hemostasis, but controlled studies to verify their effectiveness have not been carried out. Therapeutic use of platelets may be excessive. Prostacyclin or stable derivatives thereof are currently under study, since they increase platelet cyclic AMP and could block platelet aggregation and release in the extracorporeal circulatory apparatus.

Thrombocytopenia Due to Splenic Sequestration

Splenomegaly accompanying any disease may result in platelet counts of 50,000 to 100,000 per microliter (see Ch. 164). A hemorrhagic diathesis in this setting alone is rare, but trauma or surgery in such patients may be complicated by excessive bleeding. Bone marrow megakaryocytes are normal to increased, and anemia and thrombocytopenia may also occur. In normal subjects 30 per cent of the platelet mass is present in the spleen, but in hypersplenic patients, this may approach 90 per cent. Platelet pooling in the hypersplenic state should be distinguished from actual platelet destruction, as occurs in the immune thrombocytopenias. In chronic ITP the reticuloendothelial system in the spleen prematurely destroys the antibody-coated platelets. In hypersplenism the platelets are essentially normal, but their transit time through the spleen is delayed. This has been verified by studies of platelet survival curves in hypersplenism, in which recovery in the peripheral blood is low but platelet lifespan is normal. The splenic pooling defect does not require therapy unless accompanying anemia mandates splenectomy to decrease transfusion requirements. Splenectomy, if carried out for that reason, will also result in restoration of normal platelet counts. During *hypothermia* there is a reversible thrombocytopenia that is thought to be due to transient sequestration in the spleen and liver.

Thrombocytopenia in the Massively Transfused Patient

In addition to effects of dilution, at least three hemostatic defects occur in patients receiving massive transfusions (10 to 20 units of whole blood or equivalent): (1) thrombocytopenia, (2) platelet dysfunction, and (3) a coagulation defect. If there is concomitant DIC, Factor VIII levels may fall below 25 per cent, necessitating use of cryoprecipitate, which will also provide fibrinogen. Platelet counts fall to 50,000 per microliter, but rarely below this level. Platelet transfusions may be required, but this should be governed by clinical evaluation rather than the platelet count per se. Screening tests for DIC, including thrombin times and measurement of fibrinogen-fibrin degradation products, should be carried out (Table 166–3 and Fig. 166–4). The thrombocytopenia is usually reversible within three to five days.

THROMBOCYTOSIS AND THROMBOCYTHEMIA

Thrombocytosis represents an elevation in platelet count beyond 400,000 per microliter and occurs in three forms: (1) transitory or "physiologic," (2) reactive or "secondary," and (3) autonomous or "primary" (thrombocythemia).

TRANSITORY THROMBOCYTOSIS. This occurs following exercise and physical stress. It may reflect platelet release from the lung, since it occurs in splenectomized individuals. Epinephrine administration produces a 20- to 50- per cent rise in platelet count, which originates from the splenic pool since it does not occur in asplenic persons. Transitory thrombocytosis results from mobilization of preformed platelets rather than from accelerated platelet production, as occurs in the other two forms of thrombocytosis.

SECONDARY OR REACTIVE THROMBOCYTOSIS. This results from accelerated platelet production, via an unknown stimulus. Reactive thrombocytosis occurs in response to hemorrhage, acute and chronic inflammatory disorders, malignant diseases, hemolysis, and the postsplenectomy state. Successful treatment of the underlying disorder reverses the thrombocytosis. It is rarely necessary to employ therapeutic methods to lower platelet counts. Reactive thrombocytosis following splenectomy is observed during the early postoperative period, and platelet levels may reach 1,000,000 per microliter during the ensuing months. Thrombotic or hemorrhagic com-

plications rarely occur, however, and therapy is not required. Reactive thrombocytosis also occurs as a "rebound" phenomenon following a thrombocytopenic state, as in withdrawal of myelosuppressive drugs, recovery from acute alcoholism, and therapy for vitamin B_{12} deficiency. Thrombocytosis also occurs in association with iron deficiency, but may be secondary to blood loss. Iron may in some way regulate thrombocytopoiesis.

PRIMARY THROMBOCYTHEMIA. In primary thrombocythemia increased platelet production is sustained and *independent of normal regulatory processes*. Marrow megakaryocyte mass is markedly increased, and platelet production is correspondingly elevated as much as 15-fold. Platelet counts occur in the range of one to two million per microliter and may be associated with either hemorrhage or thrombosis. The Philadelphia chromosome is absent, and red cell mass is not increased. Importantly, an underlying disorder associated with secondary (reactive) thrombocytosis must be ruled out.

When hemorrhage occurs, it is usually from mucosal surfaces and related to a functional platelet abnormality. Platelets from patients with primary thrombocythemia do not respond normally to epinephrine stimulation in vitro. The thrombotic diathesis could be due to an increased circulating platelet mass per se and excessive TXA_2 production. This is because platelets utilize endoperoxides released from those in proximity for production of additional thromboxane—thereby resulting in enhanced platelet aggregation and vasoconstriction. Along with polycythemia vera, chronic myelogenous leukemia, and agnogenic myeloid metaplasia, primary polycythemia is considered a chronic myeloproliferative disease (see Ch. 154 for a more detailed description of this entity). Primary thrombocythemia also accompanies or evolves into chronic myelogenous leukemia, polycythemia vera, and agnogenic myeloid metaplasia. In common with the latter diseases, primary thrombocythemia is a clonal disorder, originating from a multipotential stem cell. Palpable splenomegaly is present in 80 per cent of cases. Most patients are over 55 years of age, and in this group cardiovascular disease frequently complicates the bleeding or thrombotic diathesis. Splenic infarction and atrophy as a complication of thrombosis occur in 20 per cent of patients. Splenic atrophy is associated with earlier mortality.

In addition to gastrointestinal bleeding, hemorrhage also occurs in skin and mucous membranes. Although episodes of hemorrhage and thrombosis occur in alternating fashion, thromboembolic phenomena, observed in 30 per cent of cases, are the most common cause of death.

Blood smears demonstrate platelet aggregates, giant forms, and fragments of megakaryocytic cytoplasm. Microscopic bone marrow specimens are markedly hypercellular with a background of platelet aggregates. In contrast to polycythemia vera, marrow iron content is normal or increased.

The thrombocytosis gives rise to spurious laboratory values for substances that are normal platelet constituents released into serum upon clotting. Thus there is pseudohyperkalemia and increases in serum acid phosphatase, lactic dehydrogenase, and zinc. These values are normal if the patient's cell-free plasma is retested as a control. Automated laboratory counting devices may estimate large platelets as erythrocytes, rendering the platelet count falsely low. *This emphasizes the importance of monitoring peripheral blood smears.*

The incidence of clinical bleeding or thrombosis does not correlate with laboratory values or in vitro tests of platelet function. However, reducing platelet production (and erythropoiesis, if excessive) is beneficial, especially in symptomatic patients. Some observers believe that patients over 50 years of age with platelet counts greater than 1,000,000 per microliter should be treated with cytoreduction, even if asymptomatic. Alkylating agents are useful for this purpose. These include $^{32}P(2.3$ mCi/m^2), phenylalanine mustard, 1 to 4 mg daily by mouth, or hydroxyurea, 15 to 30 mg per kilogram.

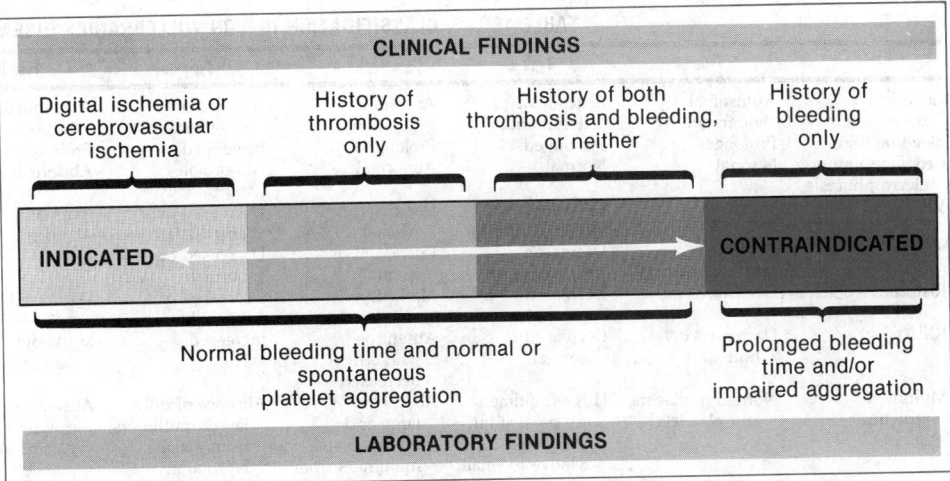

FIGURE 166–6. Correlations between clinical and laboratory results and indications for platelet cyclooxygenase inhibition with aspirin in autonomous thrombocythemia. Inhibition of platelet function may not reduce incidence of thromboembolic complications but may lower the degree of platelet responsiveness. Suggested aspirin dose: 325 mg per day. (Adapted from Schafer AI: Bleeding and thrombosis in the myeloproliferative disorders. Blood 64:1, 1984.)

Re-treatment in 3 to 6 months may be necessary. Platelet counts should be maintained at 600,000 per microliter. In emergency situations involving massive hemorrhage, platelet-pheresis is recommended for an immediate (although transient) therapeutic effect.

About 40 per cent of patients with myeloproliferative disorders have a deficiency in platelet arachidonic acid lipoxygenase. This allows for shunting of free arachidonate through the cyclo-oxygenase pathway and production of excessive TXA_2. Paradoxically, such patients with enhanced TXA_2 production may have a bleeding tendency.

Since the thrombotic diathesis may be a complication of excessive quantities of activated platelets in the circulation, therapy with aspirin (325 mg daily) and dipyridamole* (75 mg three times daily) is recommended as prophylaxis. Since aspirin may also induce bleeding, criteria for its use can be summarized as follows: (1) Aspirin is contraindicated in patients with a previous history of hemorrhage, especially if the bleeding time is prolonged and if in vitro platelet aggregation tests indicate a defect. (2) Patients with no history of previous bleeding who have evidence of thrombosis in the extremities or in the cerebral or myocardial circulation should be treated with aspirin and dipyridamole (in conjunction with cytoreduction). Treatment for patients with a mixed history of bleeding and thrombosis must be individualized. If they have symptoms of thrombosis and the platelet count is between 750,000 and 1,000,000 per microliter, aspirin and dipyridamole are administered with caution, i.e., the patient is observed at monthly intervals and appropriately instructed. These criteria are summarized in Figure 166–6.

Schafer AI: Bleeding and thrombosis in the myeloproliferative disorders. Blood 64:1, 1984. *This review discusses the pathogenesis of autonomous thrombocytosis that occurs in myeloproliferative disorders. Therapeutic efficacy of cytoreduction and inhibition of platelet function are thoughtfully considered.*

---

*This use is not listed in the manufacturer's directive.

Qualitative Platelet Disorders

Patients with a prolonged bleeding time and normal platelet count have a qualitative platelet defect (Fig. 166–4). The abnormality may be intrinsic to the platelet or be due to a deficiency and/or a structural defect of plasma proteins that modulates platelet adhesion to subendothelium or platelet aggregation. One of three aspects of platelet function is abnormal in congenital or acquired qualitative platelet disorders: adhesion, aggregation, or the release reaction.

Coller BS: Disorders of platelets. In Ratnoff OD, Forbes CD (eds.): Disorders of Hemostasis. Orlando, Grune & Stratton, 1984, pp 73–176. *This is an excellent monograph, describing in great detail currently important aspects of platelets in hemostasis, coagulation, and thrombosis. Discussions of each topic, tables, illustrations, and references are excellent.*

BERNARD-SOULIER SYNDROME (Giant Platelet Syndrome)

This very rare congenital bleeding disorder, transmitted as an autosomal recessive trait, is characterized by platelets that vary in size and morphology. Cutaneous, mucous membrane, and visceral hemorrhages occur, and fatalities have been reported. The bleeding time is markedly prolonged because of failure of platelets to adhere to subendothelium. Prothrombin consumption is abnormal, reflecting poor clot-promoting properties of the platelets. This may be due to impaired binding of coagulation proteins to the platelet surface. Platelet aggregation in response to collagen, epinephrine, and ADP is normal, since these are cohesive functions and not related to surface adhesion. There is no agglutination in response to ristocetin, however, because GPIb (missing in the Bernard-Soulier syndrome) is the receptor for von Willebrand factor when platelets are exposed to ristocetin. GPIb-deficient platelets from patients with Bernard-Soulier syndrome cannot bind von Willebrand factor. This is in contrast to patients with von Willebrand's disease in which vWF is deficient or abnormal. In this case ristocetin agglutination is corrected by addition of normal plasma or purified von Willebrand factor, which does bind to their platelets. Platelet transfusions are effective, but may be complicated by development of alloantibodies to GPIb (missing from the patient's platelets), and should be utilized only in urgent clinical situations.

VON WILLEBRAND'S DISEASE (see also Ch. 167)

Von Willebrand factor (vWF) mediates adhesion (via GPIb) between platelets and the vessel wall (Fig. 166–1). vWF is a glycoprotein synthesized in endothelial cells and megakaryocytes and then released into plasma. It circulates as a heterogeneous group of disulfide-linked multimers ranging in molecular weight from 800,000 to 12,000,000 with subunits in the range of 200,000. The pathogenesis of bleeding in von Willebrand's disease (vWD) relates to the absence of platelet adhesion to subendothelium as mediated by vWF. The patient's plasma is also deficient in Factor VIII coagulant activity.

Von Willebrand's disease has been classified into several types and subtypes, all related to defects involving the vWF protein (Table 166–6). *Type IA vWD* (autosomal dominant), the most common form, is associated with a moderate bleeding diathesis. Circulating levels of all vWF multimers are decreased, but their structure is normal. Factor VIII coagulant activity is low, and ristocetin agglutination is absent. *Type IB vWD* is a slight variant of Type IA. All multimers are present, but the large ones are decreased relative to the smaller multimers. *Type IIA vWD* is less common. Multimer assembly from normal subunits is defective, and large and intermediate multimers are missing from plasma and platelets. Congenital inability to assemble intermediate and high-molecular weight multimers is inherited as an autosomal dominant. Ristocetin-induced agglutination activity is markedly decreased, and

TABLE 166–6. CLASSIFICATION OF VON WILLEBRAND'S DISEASE

	Type IA	Type IB	Type IIA	Type IIB	Type IIC	Type IID	Type III
Genetic transmission	Autosomal dominant	Autosomal dominant	Autosomal dominant	Autosomal dominant	Autosomal recessive	Autosomal dominant	Autosomal recessive
Bleeding time	Prolonged	Prolonged	Prolonged	Prolonged	Prolonged	Prolonged	Prolonged
Crossed immuno-electrophoresis	Normal	Normal	Abnormal	Abnormal	Abnormal	Abnormal	Variable (mostly abnormal)
VIIIC	Decreased	Decreased	Decreased or normal	Decreased or normal	Normal	Normal	Markedly decreased
vWF*	Decreased	Decreased	Decreased or normal	Decreased or normal	Normal	Normal	Minute amounts or absent
Ristocetin cofactor	Decreased	Decreased	Markedly decreased	Decreased or normal	Decreased	Decreased	Absent
RIPA†	Decreased or normal	Decreased or normal	Absent or markedly decreased	Increased	Markedly decreased	Decreased	Absent
Multimeric structure	Normal in plasma and platelets	Large multimers are present but are decreased relative to small multimers	Absence of large and intermediate multimers from plasma and platelets	Absence of only larger multimers from plasma. Normal in platelets	Absence of large multimers from plasma and platelets. Triplet structure is aberrant	Absence of large multimers from plasma. Triplet structure is aberrant but different from IIC	Variable

From Ruggeri ZM, Zimmerman TS: Platelets and von Willebrand disease. Semin Hematol 22:203, 1985.
*Measured as antigen by reaction with specific antibodies.
†RIPA = ristocetin-induced platelet aggregation in platelet-rich plasma.

Factor VIII procoagulant activity can be low. In *type IIB vWD* the very largest multimers are absent from plasma, but these multimers have an abnormal affinity for and are present on the patient's platelets and endothelial cells. Platelets that have adsorbed the vWF multimers in type IIB may agglutinate and be cleared from the circulation—thus causing thrombocytopenia. This may also account for the rapid disappearance of large multimers from the plasma and also the prolonged bleeding time. In vitro platelets from patients with type IIB vWD are highly sensitive to ristocetin because of the adsorbed vWF.

Clinically, *type III vWD* patients are the most severely affected. Fortunately this variant is rare, since it represents the homozygotic or double heterozygotic state. Levels of vWF in the circulation, platelets, endothelial cells, and subendothelium are virtually undetectable. Factor VIII:C is also deficient. These patients clinically represent an extreme form of type I vWD.

PSEUDO-VON WILLEBRAND'S DISEASE OR PLATELET-TYPE vWD. Platelets from these patients have an unexplained increased affinity for binding the larger vWF multimers, which are structurally normal. The plasma is almost devoid of large multimers although low molecular weight multimers remain. The bleeding disorder is similar to vWD, but the *abnormality is platelet mediated.* Ristocetin-induced agglutination is enhanced and occurs at low concentrations. Thrombocytopenia and abnormalities of platelet morphology have been reported. In vitro, cryoprecipitate will agglutinate platelets from these patients in the absence of any other agonist, attesting to their sensitivity. This is in contrast to type IIB vWF, in which ristocetin is necessary, albeit at low levels.

Treatment of vWD is directed toward correction of the plasma defect in vWF and Factor VIII, and it differs among the subtypes. For type I vWD the treatment of choice is cryoprecipitate, since this contains high concentrations of vWF, especially the high molecular weight multimers. Fresh or fresh-frozen plasma may be used if cryoprecipitate is not available, and the fluid burden can be tolerated. Cryoprecipitate will shorten the bleeding time to a varying degree for about a 12-hour period. For severe bleeding episodes, as much as 30 to 50 units of cryoprecipitate per kilogram may be required to normalize the Factor VIII level and correct the bleeding time. Epsilon-aminocaproic acid (EACA), which blocks fibrinolysis and stabilizes clot formation, is recommended for prophylactic use prior to dental extraction or minor surgery (50 to 100 mg per kilogram orally or intravenously).

The synthetic analogue of antidiuretic hormone, 1 deamino 8-d-arginine vasopressin (DDAVP), induces a threefold increase in vWF in patients with type I vWD (also Factor VIII). Peak response occurs 30 to 60 minutes after infusion. Prophylactic use of DDAVP and its therapeutic use for mild to moderate bleeding in type I vWD is a major advance, since it can replace therapy with blood components.

Cryoprecipitate should be used for treatment of hemorrhage in type IIA vWD, in which large vWF multimers are absent from plasma and platelets. DDAVP may be tried, since it will increase the low molecular weight vWF components, but it may not improve ristocetin cofactor activity or the bleeding time.

In type IIB vWD, in which there is vWF on the platelets and in endothelial cells, DDAVP infusion may induce release of the abnormal vWF multimers from these tissues with ensuing platelet agglutination in vivo and thrombocytopenia. Thus, DDAVP should not be used in type IIB vWD. For type IIB vWD, cryoprecipitate is recommended. In pseudo-vWD or platelet type vWD there is also platelet-bound normal vWF. In this instance, both DDAVP and cryoprecipitate will elevate plasma levels of large multimers of vWF, but may lead to in vivo agglutination and thrombocytopenia. Thus they should be used with caution. Cryoprecipitate is useful in type III vWD (which clinically resembles severe type I). Use of Factor VIII concentrates is not indicated for treatment of vWD because only low levels of vWF are present and mucosal bleeding is not controlled.

Moroose R, Hoyer LW: Von Willebrand factor and platelet function. Ann Rev Med 37:157, 1986. *This article contains a clear summary of current concepts of vWF-platelet interactions, reviews current research, and presents an update of therapy of von Willebrand's disease.*
Ruggeri ZM, Zimmerman TS: Platelets and von Willebrand disease. Semin Hematol 22:203, 1985. *This review considers recent information on structure-function relationships of von Willebrand factor. Interactions among vWF, platelets, and subendothelium are discussed. Subtypes of vWD are classified in detail.*

THROMBASTHENIA (Glanzmann's Disease)

Thrombasthenia, inherited as an autosomal recessive defect in platelet function, results in a lifelong mild to severe hemorrhagic tendency. Bleeding is of the mucosal type: epistaxis, gastrointestinal hemorrhage, and menorrhagia. Thrombasthenia is characterized by (1) normal platelet count, (2) prolonged bleeding time, (3) clot retraction that is poor or absent, (4) normal agglutination with ristocetin (GPIb, the platelet receptor for vWF is intact), (5) no aggregation in response to ADP, collagen, thrombin, epinephrine, arachidonate, or endoperoxide PGH_2 (although TXA_2 synthesis is normal). In in vitro systems thrombasthenic platelets undergo normal shape change and adhere normally in a single layer to subendothelium. However, "recruitment" of additional platelets to form a normal hemostatic plug is absent. This is in direct contrast to platelets of the Bernard-Soulier syndrome in which there is no adherence to subendothelium because of the absence of GPIb.

PATHOPHYSIOLOGY OF THROMBASTHENIA. Platelet-platelet interactions (cohesion) are grossly defective. The essential modulator of the platelet cohesion reaction is fibrinogen. Whereas unstimulated normal platelets do not bind fibrinogen, platelet activation by agonists such as ADP, thrombin, or epinephrine induces rapid expression of fibrinogen receptors. Platelets in thrombasthenia are incapable of binding fibrinogen, even in the presence of agonists. Solubilized membrane glycoproteins from normal platelets contain approximately 18 per cent of the total protein content as a complex of glycoproteins IIb and IIIa, which forms in the presence of calcium. This complex is diminished to absent in thrombasthenia. The two abnormalities mentioned above, i.e., absence of fibrinogen binding and quantitative deficiency of glycoproteins IIb and IIIa, explain the defect in thrombasthenia. Normally when platelets are stimulated, surface glycoproteins IIb and IIIa change structurally to become the fibrinogen receptor. In thrombasthenia the near-absence of the GPIIb-IIIa complex does not allow for fibrinogen binding. This is presumed to be the cause of the platelet abnormality. In a variant of thrombasthenia the GPIIb-IIIa complex is structurally abnormal so that fibrinogen is not bound. This further verifies the necessity for fibrinogen binding for platelet aggregation. Platelet fibrinogen itself is reduced or absent in thrombasthenia, as are the platelet surface antigens Pl^{A1} and Pl^{A2}.

For treatment of clinically significant hemorrhage, platelet transfusions are indicated. They should be reserved for severe bleeding, however, because of possible development of antibodies to glycoproteins IIb and IIIa. The antibody will interfere with functional integrity of platelets transfused at a later date.

George JN, Nurden AT, Phillips DR: Molecular defects in interactions of platelets with the vessel wall. N Engl J Med 311:1084, 1984. *This Medical Progress article classifies and discusses the pathogenesis and molecular defects of congenital disorders of platelet-vessel wall interactions that result in hemorrhagic disease. Glycoproteins of platelets and plasma are considered in relation to their involvement in primary hemostasis.*

Leung L, Nachman R: Molecular mechanisms of platelet aggregation. Ann Rev Med 37:179, 1986. *A concise analysis of molecular events accompanying platelet stimulation, including assembly of adhesive proteins on the platelet surface.*

ABNORMALITIES OF THE PLATELET RELEASE REACTION

When platelets are stimulated, the initial response results from the direct action of the agonist at its receptor site. The response is recorded in vitro as an initial wave of aggregation. This is normally followed by a "second wave" of aggregation, which is irreversible (in contrast to the first wave). The second wave is fibrinogen dependent, requires release of dense granule constituents such as ADP and 5-HT, and is accompanied by synthesis of TXA_2. Defects in the above processes result in a single reversible wave of aggregation, which is abnormal. Clinically, defects in the release reaction result in a syndrome characterized by mild mucocutaneous, postpartum, and postoperative bleeding and menorrhagia. The bleeding time is slightly prolonged, platelet counts and coagulation profiles are normal. Release reaction disorders can be subdivided as follows: (1) "storage pool" deficiency in which the release defect is due to a paucity of dense granules or alpha-granules within the platelet (a hereditary disorder in which alpha-granules are deficient is known as the gray platelet syndrome); (2) defects due to an abnormality in the release mechanism itself in the setting of a normal granule population

(this is also known as the aspirin-like syndrome); (3) disorders of nucleotide metabolism.

Hereditary deficiency of dense granules, as expected, results in a defect in platelet hemostatic function. This includes the Hermansky-Pudlak syndrome, which is also associated with albinism and the presence of ceroid-like pigment in macrophages. Another example of hereditary dense granule deficiency is the Chédiak-Higashi syndrome (oculocutaneous albinism, infections, and bleeding). In the Wiskott-Aldrich syndrome (thrombocytopenia, infections, and eczema) hemorrhage is disproportionate to the bleeding time. Platelet granule abnormalities have also been reported.

Patients whose platelets appear to have normal dense granule content but deficient release have been classified as having an aspirin-like disorder because of its clinical resemblance to the effects of aspirin ingestion. This disorder must be differentiated from situations in which patients have surreptitiously ingested aspirin or aspirin-containing medications. Reports of cyclo-oxygenase deficiency and TXA_2 insensitivity have appeared, but these are apparently quite rare.

Patients with glycogen storage disease, type I (glucose 6-phosphatase deficiency), can develop a mild hemorrhagic tendency with a long bleeding time. The disorder of nucleotide metabolism resulting from the glucose 6-phosphatase deficiency induces a defect in platelet ADP release, which is more accentuated during periods of hypoglycemia. The syndrome is correctable by intravenous administration of glucose.

In general, patients with abnormalities of the platelet release reaction experience mild to moderate defects in hemostasis. Major surgical procedures and trauma may result in more serious hemorrhage, requiring vigorous therapeutic measures. This emphasizes the importance of preoperative screening as described in Table 166–3 and Figure 166–4. These patients should avoid aspirin or medications containing acetylsalicylic acid, since they will worsen the hemostatic defect.

ACQUIRED DISORDERS OF PLATELET FUNCTION— SYSTEMIC DISEASES

UREMIA. In uremia, patients may develop a hemorrhagic disorder secondary to a defect in platelet function. Abnormalities of adhesion and release as manifested by prolonged bleeding times are observed. Reversal of the clinical and laboratory platelet defects occurs following dialysis. This suggests that platelet dysfunction in uremia is induced by a dialyzable substance(s). Guanidinosuccinic acid, phenols, and urea are compounds implicated in the "uremic platelet defect."

AUTOIMMUNE AND LYMPHOPROLIFERATIVE DISEASES. Acquired von Willebrand's disease has been reported in association with these syndromes. Clinically the bleeding resembles that encountered in mild to moderate vWD. There may be an antibody to the Factor VIII:vWF complex, or the larger vWF multimers may be cleared. Acquired vWD has also been reported in association with SLE, monoclonal gammopathy, hypernephroma, and myeloproliferative disorders.

DYSPROTEINEMIAS. The hemorrhagic diathesis complicating these disorders is multifactorial. The final common denominator is interference with platelet surface-related function. Contributory factors include absorption of paraproteins to platelet and vessel surfaces, plasma hyperviscosity, thrombocytopenia, and coagulation abnormalities. Macroglobulinemia and IgA and IgG myeloma are most frequently associated with these functional disorders. The plasma expander *dextran* can induce defects in platelet function comparable to those seen in the dysproteinemias.

OTHER SYSTEMIC DISEASES. Prolonged bleeding times and platelet functional abnormalities have been reported in many systemic diseases and in association with their treatment. These include acute and chronic leukemias, SLE, pernicious anemia, scurvy, amyloidosis (Factor X deficiency has also been described), homocystinuria, and cirrhosis. Patients with diseases complicated by sepsis and treated with carbenicillin develop a hemostatic defect, as demonstrated by prolonged bleeding time and purpura. The DIC associated with systemic diseases results in platelet dysfunction, which compounds the other coagulation defects. Proteolytic degradation products of fibrinogen-fibrin digestion absorb to platelets and inhibit hemostatic plug formation.

Platelet Transfusions

Platelet transfusions are utilized to control serious hemorrhage in thrombocytopenic patients or in individuals with severe qualitative platelet defects. Major bleeding can be anticipated in patients with platelet counts below 25,000 per microliter; platelet numbers less than 10,000 per microliter are associated with increased morbidity from spontaneous or traumatic bleeding. In the absence of complicating factors such as fever, sepsis, mucosal ulceration, and hypersplenism, patients with megakaryocytic aplasia do not hemorrhage if the platelet count is 5000 per microliter or greater. In the immune thrombocytopenias, platelet counts of 1000 per microliter can be hemostatically sufficient. Patients with thrombocytopenia complicated by platelet dysfunction (neoplasia, drugs, uremia) require platelet counts of 20,000 per microliter or more for prevention of spontaneous hemorrhage. Bleeding time determinations are valuable in the management of individual patients, since it may correlate with the platelet concentration required for adequate hemostasis. As shown in Figures 166–4 and 166–5, coagulation parameters in thrombocytopenic patients are important, since they may contribute to the bleeding diathesis, and obviously coagulation defects do not respond to platelet administration.

If possible, platelets should be transfused approximately 90 minutes following decision and requisition. The usual dose is one unit of platelet concentrate (platelets suspended in 50 ml of plasma) per 10 kilograms of body weight. Clinical and laboratory evaluation is mandatory for judging the effectiveness of a given platelet transfusion and constitutes the major determinant of expected effectiveness of future transfusions. A platelet count should be obtained immediately preceding transfusion and one hour post-transfusion, and a final count should be made approximately 24 hours later. If a concentrate of random donor platelets did not increase the platelet count by 25,000 per microliter, the transfusion was of minimal value, and future transfusions will require quantitatively more platelets or platelets from an HLA-matched donor. After exposure to platelets from approximately 20 separate donors, patients become alloimmunized, and such transfusions are no longer useful therapeutically. This is evidenced by a lack of platelet increment at the one-hour period following transfusion. Thereafter platelets from histocompatible siblings or HLA-matched platelets are required for hemostasis. Thus, platelets are most useful as short-term therapy in hypoproliferative thrombocytopenia and in patients receiving chemotherapy with agents having a temporary marrow-suppressive effect.

Isoimmunization occurs less rapidly in leukemic patients than in patients with aplastic anemia, probably because chemotherapeutic agents are immunosuppressive. Routine use of prophylactic platelet transfusions is controversial, but many oncology centers utilize such treatment in patients whose platelet counts fall below 20,000 per microliter (4- to 6-unit transfusions are recommended).

Although reduction in platelet count and a platelet functional defect associated with cardiopulmonary bypass are documented, the effectiveness of platelet transfusions in this situation is difficult to evaluate. Current consensus is that routine administration of platelets during cardiovascular bypass procedures is probably not indicated.

Possible complications of platelet transfusions should temper decisions to initiate them. Patients receiving platelet concentrates from multiple donors undergo a risk as high as 40 per cent for post-transfusion hepatitis. Evidence of chronic hepatitis will develop in 50 per cent of recipients. Other complications include allergic and febrile reactions, AIDS, malaria, Chagas' disease, several viral infections, and graft-vs.-host (GVH) disease.

When thrombocytopenic bleeding complicates disorders characterized by increased platelet destruction or consumption, platelet transfusions in the past have been rather ineffective, mainly because transfused platelets were rapidly destroyed. High-dose intravenous gamma globulin may improve platelet counts rapidly in disorders such as acute ITP and preoperatively in patients with severe thrombocytopenia requiring splenectomy.

Eisenstaedt R: Blood component therapy in the treatment of platelet disorders. Semin Hematol 23:1, 1986. *This review discusses the therapeutic use of platelet transfusions in quantitative and qualitative platelet diseases. There is also detailed consideration of the ever increasing group of complications associated with platelet administration.*

Vascular Purpuras

As part of the hemostatic response, blood vessels constrict when severed or traumatized. Tests of hemostasis in current use mainly evaluate coagulation mechanisms and platelet function. Aside from the Rumpel-Leede tourniquet test and bleeding time, there are no specific methods to assess a vascular contribution to a hemostatic defect. Thus the diagnosis of vascular purpura is one of exclusion after qualitative and quantitative platelet disorders, coagulation defects, and fibrinolytic disorders have been ruled out. Patients usually present with easy bruisability and spontaneous bleeding from small blood vessels in the form of petechiae, ecchymoses, or both. In addition to a positive Rumpel-Leede vascular fragility test, the bleeding time is prolonged (Tables 166–3 and 166–7 and Figure 166–4).

ALLERGIC PURPURA (HENOCH-SCHÖNLEIN SYNDROME OR "ANAPHYLACTOID PURPURA"). Allergic purpura occurs mainly in children two to seven years of age with male predominance. Onset is sudden with an urticarial lesion, which fades and is replaced by red maculopapular rashes. The latter coalesce to form symmetric ecchymoses, especially over the extensor aspects of the lower extremities and buttocks. Two thirds of children have periarticular joint involvement, characterized by nonmigratory polyarthralgias in the ankles and knees. Abdominal pain with colic, accompanied by melena, occurs as a result of hemorrhage and edema in the small intestine. Occasionally this is complicated by intussusception. Acute glomerulonephritis with hematuria,

TABLE 166–7. VASCULAR PURPURAS

Allergic purpura (Henoch-Schönlein)
Dysproteinemias
   Macroglobulinemia
   Cryoglobulinemia
   Primary hyperglobulinemic (benign) purpura
   Multiple myeloma
   Amyloidosis
Purpura simplex
Drug-induced vascular purpura
Senile purpura
Hereditary disorders of connective tissue
   Ehlers-Danlos syndrome
   Pseudoxanthoma elasticum
   Marfan's syndrome
   Osteogenesis imperfecta
Cushing's syndrome
Scurvy
Autoerythrocyte and DNA sensitivity

proteinuria, and edema can occur during the second or third week. Renal involvement may be accompanied by hypertension with a transient decrease in renal function, which rarely progresses to chronic renal failure (less than 15 per cent). Skin biopsies during the acute episode reveal aseptic vasculitis with perivascular cuffing, fibrinoid necrosis, platelet plugging, and interstitial edema. Substances identified at the site of the inflammatory lesions include IgA, IgM, C3 to C5, and properdin. Similar lesions have been identified in the bowel, and renal biopsies have demonstrated segmental or (rarely) diffuse glomerular proliferation with occlusion of capillaries by fibrinoid material. A possible relationship between Henoch-Schönlein purpura, Buerger's disease, and other forms of IgA nephropathy is discussed in Ch. 81. Although the histopathologic lesions resemble those experimentally induced in immune complex disease, no antigen has been identified in association in Henoch-Schönlein purpura.

Patients with abdominal and joint involvement have been managed with prednisone to reduce the edema and inflammatory response. Corticosteroids, however, have no effect on the renal lesion and do not modify the skin manifestations. The long-term prognosis is good in the absence of chronic renal disease, although a 50 per cent recurrence rate during the initial weeks of recovery has been reported.

PARAPROTEINEMIAS. Vascular-type purpura occurs in paraproteinemias. The hemostatic defect is also attributable to complications of the primary disease such as bone marrow replacement, liver dysfunction, and uremia. Acquired deficiencies of coagulation factors and thrombocytopenia are common. This includes absorption of Factor X to amyloid and coating of the platelet surface and canalicular system with paraprotein. Hyperviscosity and "sludging" of erythrocytes and granulocytes in capillaries, leading to direct endothelial damage inflicted by precipitated paraproteins, also contribute to the vascular purpura.

In *cryoglobulinemia* (and cryofibrinogenemia), exposure of extremities to low temperature can induce purpuric lesions with subsequent ulceration. This is due to cryoglobulin precipitated on the vascular surface, which then interferes with vessel integrity. Complexes among fibrinogen, fibrin, and fibronectin have been identified as cryofibrinogens. These patients fare better in warm climates.

In *macroglobulinemia*, mucosal bleeding is more common than cutaneous hemorrhage. Patients with *primary hyperglobulinemic purpura* develop recurrent episodes of purpura, especially following exertion or physical trauma. The lower extremities are affected more commonly, and the purpuric episodes are preceded by a prodrome of itching and erythema. Progressive pigment deposition with discoloration at the site of the lesion is common. The hyperglobulinemia is monoclonal and of the IgM type. Epistaxis, purpura, and spontaneous bruisability are frequent. *Benign hyperglobulinemic purpura* occurs in systemic diseases such as Sjögren's syndrome, SLE, and rheumatoid arthritis.

In *myeloma*, the most common cause of hemorrhage is thrombocytopenia. Coagulation disorders, a qualitative platelet abnormality, and vascular purpura are also observed (see Ch. 163). Patients with IgA and IgG myeloma are at higher risk for qualitative platelet defects, which are reversible if the immunoglobulin level is reduced following successful therapy. In *amyloidosis* the protein is deposited in skin and subcutaneous tissues. This results in increased vascular fragility, manifested by purpura and subcutaneous hemorrhage (also due to Factor X absorption). Periorbital purpura ("raccoon eyes") is particularly diagnostic in amyloidosis (see Ch. 163).

PURPURA SIMPLEX (SIMPLE BRUISING). The lesions of this disorder are mild, occurring most frequently in women of childbearing age. Hemorrhage is limited to the skin in the form of circumscribed purpura, especially on the lower extremities and trunk. Occurrence during or preceding menstrual periods is frequent. The syndrome, also referred to as devil's pinches, is mainly of cosmetic import and does not require treatment. However, patients should be encouraged to avoid aspirin or aspirin-containing medications.

KAPOSI'S HEMORRHAGIC SARCOMA. Previously observed on the lower extremities of males over 50 years of age, these lesions more recently have been reported in association with immunosuppressive therapy and in patients with HIV infections. The hemorrhagic nodules result from proliferation of vascular elements. Local hemorrhage, followed by hemosiderin deposition, results in the characteristic violaceous or dark brown lesions. In about 10 per cent of cases, lesions are not limited to lower extremities, but appear in the gastrointestinal tract, liver, and lungs.

DRUG-INDUCED VASCULAR PURPURA. Many drugs produce generalized purpura in the absence of thrombocytopenia or a qualitative platelet defect. Examples include iodides, quinine, penicillins, chlorothiazides, sulfa drugs, and coumarin anticoagulants. Upon discontinuance of the offending drug, the purpura subsides. Screening procedures for diagnosis of this entity in contrast to other forms of purpura are outlined in Tables 166-3 and Figure 166-4.

SENILE PURPURA. This disorder should more appropriately be referred to as purpura in the elderly. It results from degeneration and loss of collagen, elastin, and subcutaneous fat in dermal tissues. The purpura most commonly occurs on extensor aspects of the forearms and hands. Anatomic locations that received exposure to actinic radiation are also affected. Lesions consist of red to purple ecchymoses that occur spontaneously. They persist for weeks and may result in residual hemosiderin pigmentation, probably reflecting poor phagocytic function in those anatomic locations. There is no therapy of proven value.

HEREDITARY DISORDERS OF CONNECTIVE TISSUE. Hereditary connective tissue disorders are mesenchymal dysplasias in which connective tissue and perivascular supporting structures of blood vessels are abnormal. This is also manifested by structural defects in larger blood vessels, resulting in increased vascular fragility and abnormal platelet adhesiveness. The hemorrhagic disorder can vary from benign bruisability to serious hemorrhage from viscera or large blood vessels.

CUSHING'S SYNDROME. Vascular purpura on the trunk and extremities occurs as a complication of chronic administration of high-dose corticosteroids or as a feature of Cushing's syndrome (Ch. 230). Bruising occurs spontaneously or following minor trauma. Pathogenesis of the vascular purpura may be related to a catabolic effect of steroids on perivascular supporting tissues. The purpura disappears upon cessation of corticosteroid administration or successful treatment of Cushing's syndrome.

SCURVY. In vitamin C deficiency, collagen synthesis is defective, as is deposition of "intercellular cement" along endothelial linings and perivascular supporting tissues of small vessels. Gingival bleeding and hemorrhage into subcutaneous tissues and muscle occur. Dermal bleeding is conspicuous around hair follicles. Subperiosteal hemorrhage is common in children but rare in adults, who more frequently develop intramuscular hematomas. Other vitamin and nutritional deficiencies usually coexist and complicate the clinical presentation. In adults 1 gram of ascorbic acid daily will terminate the scurvy and its associated hemorrhagic disorder.

AUTOERYTHROCYTE AND DNA SENSITIVITY. Autoerythrocyte sensitivity is characterized by formation of painful ecchymoses on the extremities, preceded by sensations of itching or burning, frequently coincident with emotional stress. The lesions may progressively enlarge and have an erythematous border. Headache, nausea, and vomiting with gastrointestinal, genitourinary, or intracranial bleeding may occur. About 100 patients have been described, of whom 95 per cent are women. Intradermal injection of autologous erythrocytes or erythrocyte stroma results in appearance of similar ecchymoses at the injection site. Thus the purpura may be due to autosensitization to an erythrocyte membrane component. Characteristically there are remissions and exacerbations over long periods.

The syndrome of DNA autosensitivity resembles autoerythrocyte sensitization. The lesions begin as painful nodules on the extremities, which enlarge and become indurated. Ecchymoses occur 24 hours later and may become bullous. Resolution occurs spontaneously. Intradermal injection of the patient's leukocytes or a solution of DNA into the skin will induce an ecchymosis. In some instances chloroquine therapy has been successful.

Ratnoff OD: The psychogenic purpuras: A review of autoerythrocyte sensitization, autosensitization to DNA, "hysterical" and factitial bleeding, and the religious stigmata. Semin Hematol 17:192, 1980. *This is a scholarly summary of the latest information concerning autoerythrocyte sensitization and sensitization to DNA. It also discusses the controversial relationship between emotional stress and the development of a hemorrhagic diathesis.*

Hereditary Hemorrhagic Telangiectasia (Osler-Weber-Rendu Disease)

Hereditary hemorrhagic telangiectasia is a bleeding disorder resulting from a vascular developmental abnormality. It is transmitted as an autosomal dominant trait—thus a family history of bleeding in both sexes is verifiable. The telangiectases result from dilatation and convolution of venules and capillaries in the skin and mucous membranes. Vessel walls are thinned to the level of a single layer of endothelium that has neither anatomic support nor contractile properties. These fragile, angiomatous masses of vascular components bleed spontaneously or following minor trauma. This disease is the most common hereditary vascular disorder associated with a hemorrhagic diathesis. Visible lesions, approximately 3 mm in diameter, occur on nasal mucous membranes, lips, gingiva, buccal mucosa, palate, both sides of the tongue, face, trunk, and palmar and plantar surfaces. The telangiectases are violaceous and flat, blanch on pressure exerted by a glass slide, and are variable in shape from pinpoint to nodular to spider-like. The telangiectases can be seen in children, but their appearance increases with age, peaking between the fourth and fifth decades. This correlates with an increase in the frequency and severity of hemorrhagic episodes. Bleeding is less severe in females. Visceral telangiectases occur in the gastrointestinal, respiratory, and genitourinary tracts.

Mucous membrane bleeding, especially epistaxis, is the most common clinical problem. In any given patient, however, telangiectases in other locations may become the source of chronic, recurrent hemorrhage. Fortunately hemostatic and coagulation values are normal, allowing patients to tolerate surgical procedures when required. Iron deficiency anemia is a common complication.

Vascular malformations in the lung result in pulmonary arteriovenous fistulas in 20 per cent of patients. These malformations, which increase in size and frequency with age, are usually multiple and constitute a source of hemoptysis as well as foci of infection. Shunting of blood through the pulmonary arteriovenous fistulas may induce hypoxemia, digital clubbing, and polycythemia. Recurrent brain abscesses and cerebral embolism have resulted from this pulmonary shunting abnormality. Arteriovenous fistulas also occur in the cerebral, hepatic, and splenic circulation, in addition to hemangiomas in the liver and polycystic kidneys.

The diagnosis is readily made in the setting of repeated episodes of hemorrhage, the presence of multiple telangiectases, and a characteristic family history. The diagnosis may be more difficult when bleeding is mild, telangiectases are absent from the skin or not readily visible, and the family history is unclear. Fiberoptic endoscopy has been helpful in diagnosis. Pulmonary arteriovenous fistulas are demonstrable by pulmonary angiography.

Treatment is mainly supportive and symptomatic. Iron deficiency should be treated by replacement therapy, used parenterally if necessary to maintain the storage pool. The latter is preferable to repeated transfusions. Whenever possible, hemorrhage should be controlled locally. Topical hemostatic agents are useful if the site is accessible. Cautery of bleeding sites not readily accessible is useful mainly as a temporary measure. Estrogens have been utilized to induce squamous metaplasia of the nasal mucosa, but this therapy is controversial. Surgical intervention for uncontrollable bleeding or for removal of arteriovenous fistulas should be considered on an individual basis. Use of oral contraceptives by females is debatable, since it is not known whether the low quantities of estrogen in these agents enhance or reduce the tendency to bleed. Despite the lack of specific therapeutic measures and the potential hazard of spontaneous hemorrhage, the prognosis in hereditary hemorrhagic telangiectasia is relatively good.

167 DISORDERS OF BLOOD COAGULATION
Deane F. Mosher

Normal hemostasis requires interactions among blood vessels, the formed elements of blood, especially platelets and monocytes, and blood coagulation proteins. The general biology of hemostasis and the approach to a patient suspected of having a hemorrhagic diathesis have been discussed in Ch. 166, Hemorrhagic Disorders: Abnormalities of Platelet and Vascular Function. In the present chapter, attention is focused on hemorrhagic and thrombotic disorders that occur as a consequence of abnormalities of blood coagulation proteins.

REVIEW OF BLOOD COAGULATION

Blood coagulation, initiated by substances in injured tissues, is propagated by an interlocking network of enzymic events, the so-called coagulation cascade. These controlled reactions insure that blood coagulation happens quickly and yet remains localized. Blood coagulation results in the formation of a protein scaffolding, the fibrin clot, that controls bleeding and serves as a nidus for subsequent cellular ingrowth and tissue repair. After several days the fibrin clot is lysed and replaced by a more permanent scaffolding of connective tissue matrix molecules. Abnormalities that result in delay of clot formation or in premature lysis of clots are associated with a bleeding tendency. Abnormalities that result in inappropriate activation or localization of blood coagulation are associated with thrombosis.

COAGULATION PROTEINS. Coagulation and fibrinolysis involve many proteins (Table 167–1). This list grows larger as blood coagulation mechanisms are studied in greater depth. Structural and functional similarities allow one to put the proteins into one of several groups. Some are zymogens of serine proteinases and hence members of the serine proteinase family of proteins. Among the serine proteinase family are five proteins (factors II, VII, IX, and X and protein C) that are modified by vitamin K–dependent post-translational carboxylation of glutamic acid residues. A sixth plasma protein, protein S, is also modified by this reaction. The modification allows the six proteins to bind Ca^{++} and phospholipids and thereby participate efficiently in blood coagulation. Factors V and VIII function as helper proteins during blood coagulation

TABLE 167-1. PROTEINS INVOLVED IN BLOOD COAGULATION AND FIBRINOLYSIS

Proteins	Synonym	Size in Kilodaltons*	Plasma Concentrations in mg/dl (μm)*	Kind of Protein	Function†
Fibrinogen	Factor I	340	300(9)	Structural protein, unique	Gels to form clot
Factor II	Prothrombin	72	15(2)	Vit. K–dependent zymogen of serine proteinase	Activates I, V, VIII, XIII, protein C, and platelets
Factor V	Proaccelerin	350	2(0.05)	Ceruloplasmin-like binding protein	Supports X_a activation of II
Factor VII	Stable factor	50	0.1(0.02)	Vit. K–dependent zymogen of serine proteinase	Activates IX and X
Factor VIII	Antihemophilic factor	350	0.1(0.003)	Ceruloplasmin-like binding protein	Supports IX_a activation of X
Factor IX	Christmas factor	57	1(0.2)	Vit. K–dependent zymogen of serine proteinase	Activates X
Factor X	Stuart-Prower factor	59	1(0.2)	Vit. K–dependent zymogen of serine proteinase	Activates II
Factor XI	Plasma thromboplastin antecedent	160	0.5(0.03)	Zymogen of serine proteinase	Activates XII and prekallikrein
Factor XII	Hageman factor	75	2(0.2)	Zymogen of serine proteinase	Activates XI and prekallikrein
Factor XIII	Fibrin-stabilizing factor	320	3(0.08)	Zymogen of transglutaminase	Cross-links fibrin and other proteins
von Willebrand factor	Factor VIII–related antigen	800–20,000	2(0.05)	Structural protein, unique	Binds VIII, mediates platelet adhesion
Prekallikrein	—	88	2(0.3)	Zymogen of serine proteinase	Activates XII and prekallikrein, cleaves HMWK
High molecular weight, kininogen (HMWK)	—	150	2(0.2)	Binding protein, unique	Supports reciprocal activation of XII, XI, and prekallikrein
Fibronectin	—	450	40(1)	Structural protein, unique	Mediates cell adhesion
Major antithrombin	Antithrombin III	60	20(2.5)	Serpin	Inhibits II_a, X_a, and other proteases; cofactor for heparin
Minor antithrombin	Heparin cofactor II	55	5(0.6)	Serpin	Inhibits II_a, cofactor for heparin and dermatan sulfate
Protein C	—	62	0.4(0.06)	Vit. K–dependent zymogen of serine proteinase	Inactivates V and VIII
Protein S	—	69	3(0.4)	Vit. K–dependent binding protein	Cofactor for protein C_a, binds C4b-binding protein
Plasminogen	—	86	10(1.2)	Zymogen of serine proteinase	Lyses fibrin and other proteins
Alpha-2-antiplasmin	—	60	3(0.5)	Serpin	Inhibits plasmin
Prourokinase	—	50	—	Zymogen of serine proteinase	Activates plasminogen
Tissue plasminogen activator	TPA	55	—	Serine proteinase	Activates plasminogen
Plasminogen activator inhibitor I	—	52	—	Serpin	Inactivates TPA
Plasminogen activator inhibitor II	—	55	—	Serpin	Inactivates urokinase

*For comparison, the size of albumin is 68 kilodaltons, and the plasma concentration of albumin is 3500 mg/dl (510 μm).
†For zymogens, the function after activation is given.

and are homologous to one another and to ceruloplasmin, a Cu^{++}-binding plasmin protein. Other proteins are *serine proteinase inhibitors* and hence members of the "serpin" family of proteins. Most of the proteins listed in Table 167–1, including the vitamin K–dependent factors, are synthesized by hepatocytes. A number of the proteins, however, can also be synthesized by other cell types such as megakaryocytes, monocyte-macrophages, and endothelial cells.

GENERAL MECHANISMS. Blood coagulation is activated, propagated, and controlled by mechanisms found in other proteolytic effector systems (e.g., complement). These mechanisms include:

1. Sequential activation by limited proteolytic cleavage
2. Amplification of the response by feedback activation loops
3. Use of binding or helper proteins to bring reactants together
4. Destruction of activated proteins by further proteolytic cleavage
5. Inhibition of activated proteinases by stoichiometric complex formation with specific inhibitor proteins, *i.e.*, the serpins

In addition, there is a mechanism that is so far unique to blood coagulation:

6. Formation of a five-part complex of an activated vitamin K–dependent factor, to-be-activated vitamin K–dependent zymogen, helper protein, Ca^{++}, and phospholipid surface (Fig. 167–1C).

EXTRINSIC AND INTRINSIC PATHWAYS. Blood coagulation can be initiated by exposure of blood to a specific cellular lipoprotein called tissue factor (the "extrinsic system") or by activation of contact factors of plasma (the "intrinsic system"). Both of these initiation pathways lead to a common pathway, which results in the elaboration of thrombin, the master coagulation enzyme. As shown in Figure 167–1A, the concept of the two initiation pathways and the common pathway is useful in understanding two major coagulation tests, the activated partial thromboplastin time (APTT), in which blood plasma is activated by the intrinsic pathway, and the prothrombin time, in which tissue factor is added to plasma so that activation proceeds by the intrinsic pathway. It is unlikely that the two initiation pathways are so clearly delineated in vivo. Activation of factor IX, an intrinsic factor, by factor VII, an extrinsic factor, must be of considerable

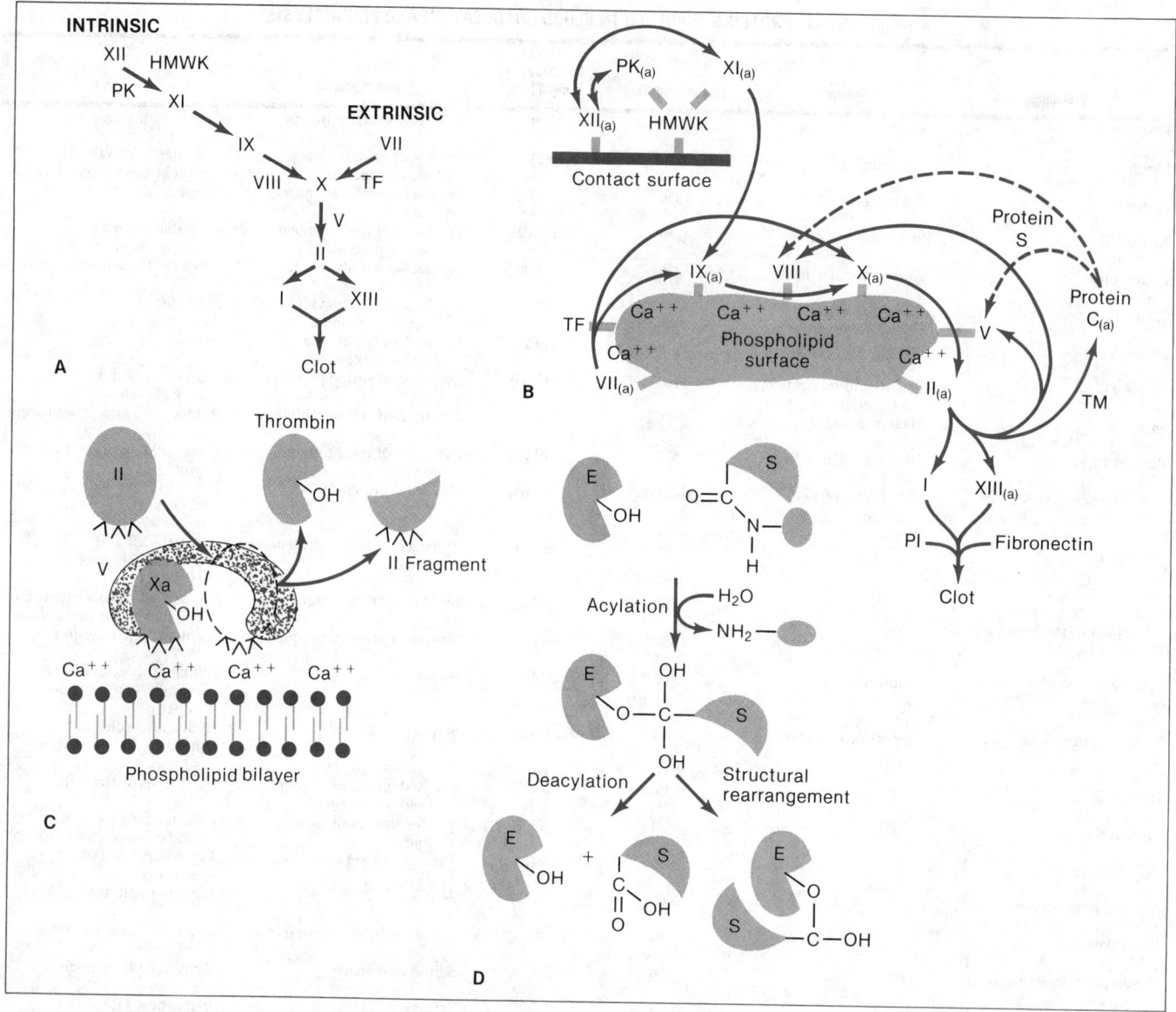

FIGURE 167–1. Diagrams of interactions among coagulation factors. PK = prekallikrein; HMWK = high molecular weight kininogen; TF = tissue factors; PI = alpha-2-antiplasmin; TM = thrombomodulin. *A* (the so-called Y diagram) depicts the intrinsic and extrinsic pathways in their simplest forms. *B* is organized around the contact surface and the phospholipid surface. Solid lines indicate activation. Broken lines indicate inactivation. The stippled patches indicate binding of proteins to surfaces or to one another. The subscript (a) indicates proteins that are zymogens and can be converted to active enzymes. *C* is a close-up of activation of prothrombin (factor II) on a phospholipid surface to which factors X_a and V are also bound. Prothrombin is cleaved, generating thrombin and a large fragment. *D* depicts the reaction of a serine proteinase (E) with a substrate or serpin(s). The proteinase attacks a peptide bond in the substrate or serpin, forming an acylenzyme intermediate. If the attack is on a serpin, it stays bound to the proteinase, and the proteinase is inhibited. With a substrate, the intermediate is deacylated, completing cleavage of the peptide bond and regenerating the proteinase.

importance because deficiencies of factors VII and IX, as well as the factors that follow factor IX in the intrinsic and common pathways, *i.e.*, factors VIII, X, V, II, and I, all are associated with a bleeding tendency. In contrast, deficiency of factor XII, prekallikrein, or high-molecular-weight kininogen does not cause a bleeding problem, and factor XI deficiency is associated with a bleeding tendency in only a minority of cases.

Tissue Factor and the Extrinsic Pathway. Factor VII is unique among coagulation factors because it circulates in an active configuration. To initiate coagulation, however, factor VII requires tissue factor. A major initiating stimulus to coagulation, therefore, is exposure of blood to tissue factor. Tissue factor is present in many types of cells, including fibroblasts, endothelial cells, and monocytes. Normally, tissue factor is cryptic. In response to a variety of stimuli, such as

mechanical disruption in the case of fibroblasts or exposure to lymphokines or monokines in the case of monocytes or endothelial cells, tissue factor becomes expressed on cell surfaces.

In the presence of tissue factor, phospholipid, and Ca^{++}, factor VII can activate factors IX and X (Fig. 167–1*B*). Factor X_a then activates factor II, and factor II_a (thrombin) cleaves fibrinogen to fibrin. The time to clot formation after addition of tissue factor, phospholipid, and Ca^{++} to citrated platelet-poor plasma is called the prothrombin time. When determined with an excess of tissue factor (as is generally done), the prothrombin time measures only factors of the extrinsic and common pathways and does not measure factor IX. When the concentration of tissue factor is low, presumably the more common situation in the body, a considerable portion of the

X-activating capability of factor VII is generated through factor IX, because there is ten times more factor IX than factor VII.

Contact Factors and the Intrinsic System. Activation of contact factors constitutes a second pathway for activating factor X. Negatively charged surfaces, such as sulfatide micelles, glass, kaolin, and celite, bind factor XII and high molecular weight kininogen (HMWK). HMWK, in turn, binds prekallikrein and factor XI. Binding to surfaces initiates a series of reciprocal cleavages of factor XI and prekallikrein by activated factor XII and of factor XII by activated factor XI and kallikrein (Fig. 167-1B). Activated factor XI activates factor IX in a reaction that requires Ca^{++}. Kallikrein also releases bradykinin, a vasoactive and pain-causing octapeptide, from HMWK and low molecular weight kininogen. In the APTT, platelet-poor citrated plasma is allowed to incubate for three to five minutes with kaolin or ellagic acid to optimally activate factor XI. Ca^{++} and phospholipid are then added so that activated factor XI (XI$_a$) can activate factor IX, factor IX$_a$ can activate factor X, and so on.

Amplification of Activation Pathways. Three analogous five-part propagating reactions take place: (1) factor VII activates factor X or IX in the presence of tissue factor, Ca^{++}, and phospholipid; (2) factor IX$_a$ activates factor X in the presence of factor VIII, Ca^{++}, and phospholipid; and (3) factor X$_a$ activates factor II in the presence of factor V, Ca^{++}, and phospholipid. The phospholipid requirement for reaction (1) is satisfied by the surface of the tissue factor–containing cell. For the reactions involving factor VIII or V, the phospholipid requirement is satisfied by platelet phospholipid.

Factor VIII is a trace protein of plasma, and large amounts have become available only recently. The five-part reaction we know most about, therefore, is the one that involves factor V (Fig. 167-1C). Factors X$_a$ and II bind to the phospholipid surface in interactions that require gamma-carboxyl glutamic acid residues; the binding is Ca^{++} dependent. Factor V contains domains for binding factors X$_a$ and II, Ca^{++}, and the phospholipid surface. Stimulated platelets contain discrete binding sites for factor V. The accelerating role of platelets in the X$_a$-V-II reaction is called platelet factor 3 activity. Formation of the five-part complex dramatically increases the rate constant (K$_{cat}$) for activation of factor II by factor X$_a$. In the five-part complex, factor V is most effective after it has been cleaved by factor II$_a$ (thrombin). Thus, thrombin is initially generated at a sluggish rate, but once a small amount of thrombin is generated so that it can cleave factor V to a more active form, subsequent thrombin generation is rapid and efficient, consuming almost all of the factor II in plasma.

LOCALIZATION AND INHIBITION OF BLOOD COAGULATION. Blood coagulation is efficiently activated only on a phospholipid surface (Fig. 167-1), and thus activation is localized to the area of injury. Several mechanisms dampen activation and insure that activated factors do not escape and cause thrombosis at a distant site.

Thrombin acquires altered specificity when complexed to thrombomodulin, a protein on the luminal surface of endothelial cells. Rather than acting upon fibrinogen or factors V and VIII, thrombin cleaves and activates protein C (Fig. 167-1B). Activated protein C, in turn, cleaves thrombin-activated factors V and VIII further so that V and VIII are no longer active. In addition, activated protein C enhances fibrinolysis, probably by neutralizing the major inhibitor of tissue plasminogen activator (see below). Activation of protein C by thrombin-thrombomodulin complex, therefore, is a powerful anticoagulant event, just as the activation of factors V and VIII by thrombin is a powerful procoagulant event. The cleavage of factors V and VIII by activated protein C requires the sixth vitamin K–dependent protein of plasma, protein S. Protein S serves as a cofactor for activated protein C rather than acting as a proteinase.

Two antithrombins in plasma inhibit thrombin and other serine proteinases that are generated during blood coagulation. The antithrombins, members of the serpin family, are substrates for the proteinases. Upon cleavage the antithrombins undergo a structural rearrangement that allows them to form tight one-to-one complexes with the proteinases (Fig. 167-1D). As a result, the proteinases are irreversibly inhibited. The major and minor antithrombins, also called antithrombin III and heparin cofactor II, account for approximately 80 per cent and 20 per cent, respectively, of the inhibitory activity in plasma toward thrombin. The rates at which both antithrombins combine with coagulation proteinases are accelerated manyfold by heparin and by heparan sulfate proteoglycan on the luminal surface of endothelial cells. The acceleration explains the anticoagulant action of heparin. The rate at which the minor antithrombin combines with thrombin is accelerated by dermatan sulfate, a glycosaminoglycan found in the vessel wall.

As described in more detail below, inherited deficiency states of protein C, protein S, the major antithrombin, and the minor antithrombin have all been associated with thrombotic diatheses.

STRUCTURE OF FIBRINOGEN AND FIBRIN. Fibrinogen and fibrin monomer are extended trinodular molecules made up of pairs of three polypeptide chains: alpha, beta, and gamma (Fig. 167-2A). The three chains run through half of the molecule, that is, through half of the central E nodule and the whole of one of the two peripheral D nodules. The chains are thought to adopt a coiled-spring structure between the E and D nodules. This portion of the molecule is particularly susceptible to degradation by the principal fibrinolytic enzyme, plasmin. The nodules resist degradation by plasmin. Thus the products of complete lysis of a clot by plasmin are one E nodule, two D nodules, and small fragments (Fig. 167-2B).

Thrombin cleaves negatively charged small peptides, called fibrinopeptides A and B, from the amino terminals of the alpha and beta chains in the E nodule of fibrinogen. Release of these peptides, which account for less than 3 per cent of the mass of fibrinogen, converts fibrinogen to a clottable derivative called fibrin monomer. At concentrations 1000-fold lower than physiologic, fibrin monomer will assemble to form an infinite branching network of fibrils (Fig. 167-2B). At physiologic fibrin concentrations, this network constitutes a strong gel and immobilizes blood. Fibrinogen is usually completely converted to fibrin during blood coagulation. Thus the concentration of fibrinogen antigen in serum is about 0.02 mg per deciliter, as compared to 200 mg per deciliter in plasma. Fibrinogen, however, forms soluble complexes with fibrin monomer when the concentration of thrombin is low. The soluble complexes can escape from areas of active coagulation and be detected in the circulation.

The fibrin gel is modified by thrombin-activated factor XIII. This enzyme, a transglutaminase, acts upon selected glutaminyl residues in fibrin and other proteins, including fibronectin and alpha-2-antitrypsin, to cause covalent protein-protein cross-linking (Fig. 167-2C). Cross-links are introduced between gamma chains of adjacent D domains, thus ligating the fibrin fibril end to end (Fig. 167-2B). Cross-linking of gamma chains renders the clot insoluble in protein denaturants such as 6 M urea. The alpha chains can ligate side to side among themselves or be cross-linked to fibronectin or alpha-2-antiplasmin. Both the "hardening" of the fibrin clot by cross-linking and the incorporation of other proteins into the clot are probably important. Many cell types have specific receptors for fibronectin that they use to migrate into fibronectin-containing clots. Alpha-2-antiplasmin is a serpin that rapidly forms a one-to-one complex with plasmin. Cross-linked alpha-2-antiplasmin serves to protect the clot from low levels of fibrinolysis. Deficiency of factor XIII or of alpha-2-antiplasmin is associated with a bleeding tendency, and some patients with factor XIII deficiency suffer from poor wound healing.

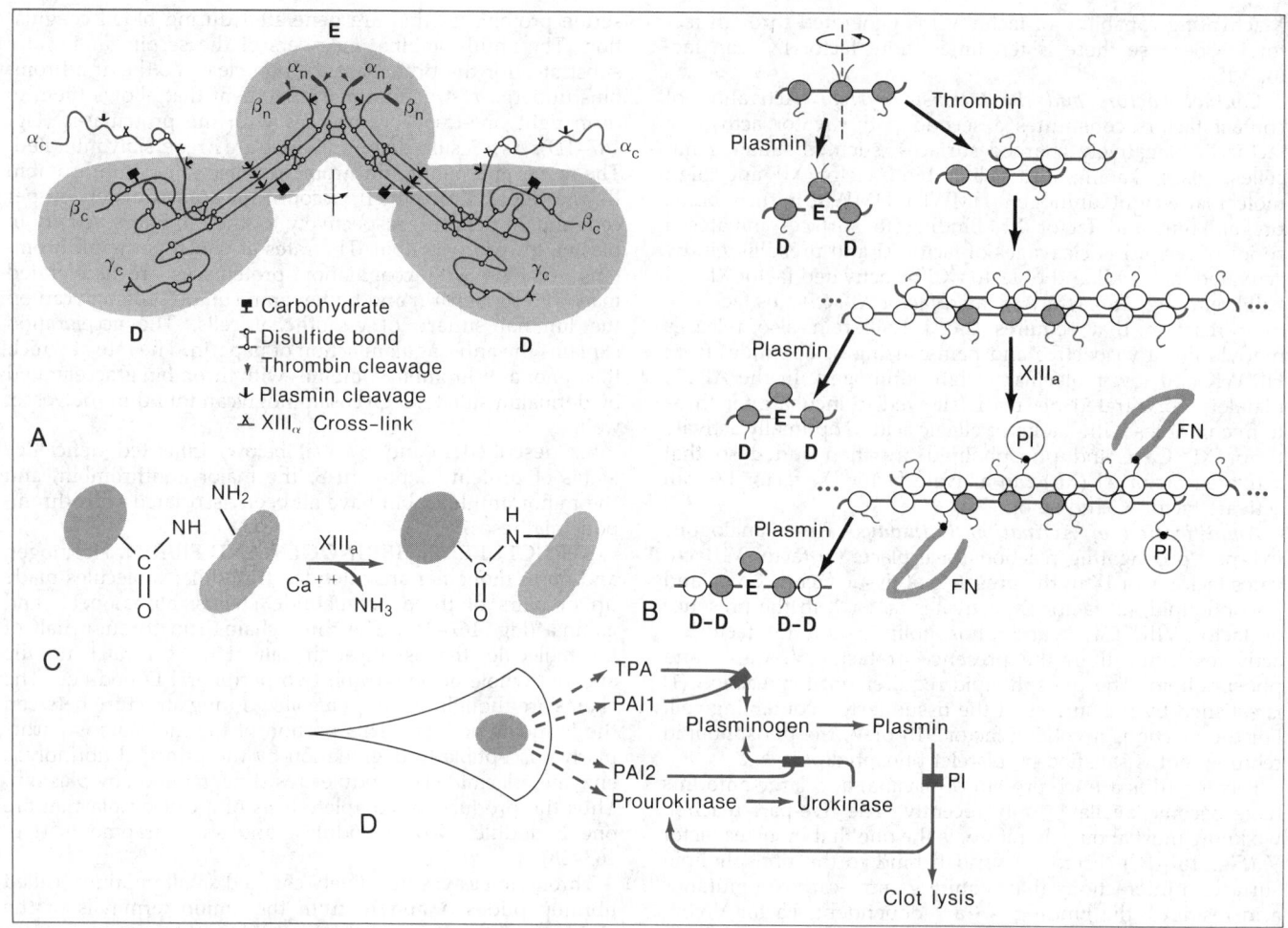

FIGURE 167–2. *A,* Disposition of the six chains of fibrinogen. Fibrinogen is composed of a central E nodule and two peripheral D nodules. One set of three nonidentical chains—alpha, beta, and gamma—runs through half the molecule and is bound to the other set by disulfide linkages in the E domain, where the amino termini of all six chains come together. The strands connecting the peripheral nodules to the central nodule contain all three chains. The carboxyl terminal regions of the three chains constitute the globular D domain. In addition, the extreme carboxyl terminal region of the alpha chain extends out from the D domain. Thrombin releases acidic fibrinopeptides A and B from the E domain to yield fibrin; plasmin cleaves the molecule between E and D. *B,* Activation, assembly, cross-linking, and lysis of fibrinogen and fibrin. Fibrinogen and fibrin are both trinodular proteins. Clotting is initiated by release of the negatively charged fibrinopeptides from the E nodule. Assembly is driven by noncovalent E nodule–D nodule interaction. End-to-end covalent cross-linking occurs between gamma chains. Alpha-2-antiplasmin (PI) and fibronectin (FN) cross-link to the extended carboxyl terminal portion of the alpha chain. Plasmin cleaves this portion of the alpha chain and separates the D and E nodules. *C* diagrams the cross-linking reaction catalyzed by factor XIII. *D* depicts the activation of plasminogen by its physiologic activators, urokinase and tissue plasminogen activator (TPA), and the control of the activation by plasminogen activator inhibitors (PAI1 and PAI2). These four molecules are secreted by cells. Plasmin is inhibited by alpha-2-antiplasmin (PI).

FIBRINOLYSIS. Cleavage of plasminogen to the active proteinase plasmin is carried out by two plasminogen activators: tissue plasminogen activator (TPA) and urokinase (Fig. 167–2D). TPA is secreted as an active serine proteinase, whereas urokinase can be activated from a somewhat active precursor, prourokinase. Among the activators of prourokinase is plasmin. TPA, plasminogen, and plasmin all bind to fibrin, and it is in a fibrin clot that TPA can activate plasminogen to plasmin most efficiently. Prourokinase does not bind to fibrin. However, small amounts of plasmin already bound to fibrin can activate prourokinase to urokinase, which then can activate more plasminogen to plasmin.

Localization of fibrinolysis to the fibrin clot is further insured by an efficient array of inhibitors. Cells secrete specific inhibitors of TPA and urokinase, presumably to regulate fibrinolysis in their local environment. Indeed, tightly controlled secretion of activator and inhibitor may allow a cell to localize plasminogen activation to volumes that are only nanometers across. Anti-TPA is present in the circulation in

low concentrations. Also in the circulation is alpha-2-antiplasmin, which inhibits plasmin extremely rapidly and efficiently.

Plasmin degrades a variety of proteins in addition to fibrin, especially connective tissue proteins, and undoubtedly has other physiologic functions besides lysis of fibrin clots. For instance, ovarian follicular cells secrete plasminogen activator in response to hormonal stimulation just prior to ovulation and thereby initiate degradation of the follicular wall.

Epsilon-aminocaproic acid (EACA) and its cyclic analogue, tranexamic acid, bind to a single site on plasminogen and plasmin and inhibit binding of these molecules to fibrin. As a result, the molecules are good inhibitors of plasminogen activation.

Streptokinase, a bacterial protein, forms a complex with plasminogen and causes a conformational change that opens up the active site of plasminogen. The streptokinase-plasminogen complex can degrade fibrin and activate free plasminogen to plasmin. The complex is not inhibited by alpha-2-antiplasmin.

Colman RW, Hirsh J, Marder VJ, Salzman EW (eds.): Hemostasis and Thrombosis: Basic Principles and Clinical Practice. 2nd ed. Philadelphia, J. B. Lippincott Company, 1987. *Extensive information about the structure and function of blood coagulation proteins with earnest attempts to relate biochemical facts to clinical problems.*

APPROACH TO PATIENTS WITH COAGULATION DISORDERS

HISTORY AND PHYSICAL EXAMINATION. There are three components to effective hemostasis: the blood vessel, platelets, and the network of soluble factors. Abnormal bleeding occurs with much greater frequency when two of the three components are compromised as, for example, in a hemophilic patient who suffers trauma or takes aspirin, or in a patient with peptic ulcer and thrombocytopenia. Disorders of platelets or blood vessels often cause mucosal or superficial bleeding; deficiency of a coagulation factor results in a tendency to form soft tissue hematomas or to suffer from repeated hemarthroses. Thrombosis tends to occur when there is inflammation, abnormalities of the luminal surface of a large blood vessel, or stasis.

A personal history, family history, and physical examination are important parts of the evaluation of a possible coagulation problem. In taking a history, it is not enough simply to ask: "Do you or your close relatives bleed or clot abnormally?" One must also determine how the hemostatic system has been stressed: "Have you had any operations or tooth extractions? If so, did you bleed abnormally or require blood transfusions afterward? Are your menstrual periods heavy? Do you bruise easily? Do you take iron tablets? Have you ever had a limb immobilized?" And so on. A formal family tree indicating how many family members are at risk and which ones have symptoms or laboratory evidence of a coagulation disorder should be constructed.

LABORATORY SCREENING TESTS. When a bleeding disorder is suspected a group of reproducible and fairly inexpensive laboratory tests should detect most clinically significant abnormalities of platelets, blood vessels, and the coagulation factor network:

1. A complete blood count and examination of the blood smear screen for abnormalities in bone marrow function or platelet number and morphologic changes in red cells caused by intravascular thrombosis or microangiopathy.

2. A quantitative platelet count provides more definitive information about platelet number.

3. A template bleeding time screens for abnormalities of blood vessels and platelets.

4. The prothrombin time and APTT screen for abnormalities of the extrinsic and intrinsic coagulation pathways, respectively. Both tests are sensitive to abnormalities of the common pathway. The prothrombin time or APTT should be abnormally long if a single factor is below 20 to 40 per cent of its normal plasma concentration.

5. The solubility of the fibrin clot in concentrated (6 M) urea will detect clinically significant deficiency of factor XIII. In the absence of factor XIII the clot will not be covalently cross-linked and therefore will be soluble.

Evaluation of a Prolonged Prothrombin Time or APTT. The first step is to perform mixing experiments of normal plasma and the abnormal plasma to decide whether the abnormal plasma is deficient in a coagulation factor or contains an inhibitor of coagulation. If the screening test of the mixture is normal, it is likely that the abnormal plasma is deficient in one or more factors, and specific factor assays can be done to identify the deficiency. If the screening test of the mixture is abnormal, it is likely that the abnormal plasma contains an inhibitor. Inhibitors may be of the so-called lupus type and directed against the phospholipid used in the assays or more rarely may be directed against a single coagulation factor. Lupus-type inhibitors rarely cause clinical bleeding. Indeed, as described below, some patients with lupus-type inhibitors suffer from repeated episodes of venous and arterial throm-

bosis. Inhibitors directed against single factors, especially VIII and IX, may cause serious bleeding.

SPECIFIC TESTS OF INDIVIDUAL PROTEINS. A plasma protein can be measured as the protein per se, usually with an immunoassay, or for protein activity. Plasma contains many different proteins, some of which will influence the activity of the coagulation factor of interest and others of which may influence the end point of the assay. Activity assays for coagulation proteins are therefore less straightforward than many laboratory measurements. In general, there are two approaches for such activity assays: use of factor-deficient plasmas and use of chromogenic substrates.

Use of Factor-Deficient Plasmas. Normal and patient's plasma are compared for their ability to correct the prothrombin time or APTT of plasma from an individual severely deficient in the factor of interest. Thus factor VIII can be measured, using plasma from an individual with severe classic hemophilia. If the patient has a factor VIII deficiency, the patient's plasma should correct the APTT of the hemophilic patient's plasma less well than does normal plasma. By convention, the normal plasma is said to have 100 per cent or 1 unit per milliliter of activity. If a 1/10 dilution of the patient's plasma has the correcting power of a 1/100 dilution of normal plasma, the patient will be said to have a factor VIII activity of 10 per cent or 0.1 unit per milliliter. Such an assay should be accurate to within 10 to 20 per cent of the reported value.

Use of Chromogenic Substrates. A chromogenic substrate is a small peptide that is cleaved rapidly and relatively specifically by an activated proteinase to yield a colored product. The rate of cleavage can be measured with high precision in a spectrophotometer, using dilute solutions of plasma. As an example, plasminogen can be assayed by addition of streptokinase to diluted plasma and quantification of cleavage of a chromogenic substrate by streptokinase-plasminogen complexes. Alternatively, antiplasmin can be assayed by addition of plasmin to diluted plasma and quantification of the loss of the ability of plasmin to cleave the same substrate due to formation of plasmin-inhibitor complexes. Such assays should be accurate to within 3 to 5 per cent of the reported value, but may be subject to artifact. For instance, a patient with a recent streptococcal infection could have artifactually low apparent plasminogen activity due to neutralizing antibodies to streptokinase.

Indications for Specific Tests. When there is a suspicious bleeding history but normal screening tests, several specific assays should be considered. Mild factor VIII or IX deficiency (10 to 40 per cent of normal) is clinically significant, but may result in a screening APTT that is at the upper limits of normal but still within the normal range. Deficiency of plasma alpha-2-antiplasmin can be diagnosed only with a specific assay.

Evaluation of a possible thrombotic diathesis, at present, can be done only with specific assays for proteins C and S, the two antithrombins, plasminogen, and perhaps other components of the fibrinolytic system.

Diagnosis of a 50 Per Cent Deficiency State. Laboratory studies of family members are often crucial to the evaluation, especially when the diagnosis centers around a heterozygous (50 per cent of normal) deficiency. The normal level (i.e., the value in 99 per cent of normal individuals) of a coagulation factor is typically 70 to 140 per cent; the level of the factor in individuals with heterozygous deficiency is typically 35 to 70 per cent; and the assay for the factor is accurate to within only 5 to 10 per cent of the reported value. The problem of distinguishing the 50 per cent deficiency state from normal is therefore a formidable one. If the apparent deficiency is found in other family members at risk, one can be much more confident that a true deficiency state exists. For example, a random woman with a 50 per cent factor VIII level is probably not a carrier of classic hemophilia. If the sister of a hemophilic patient has a 50 per cent factor VIII level, however, the sister has a 95 per cent chance of being a carrier. Heterozygous deficiency states associated with thrombosis (i.e., deficiency of the major antithrombin, the minor antithrombin, protein C, or protein S) present a similar problem. The most important facet of the care of a patient with heterozygote deficiency is appropriate counseling. Therefore a physician should not be reluctant to arrange extensive family studies. To give an example, it would be much more efficient (and cost-effective) to identify a patient with antithrombin deficiency as part of a family study and counsel that patient that he or she is at risk for thrombosis after surgery than to screen all patients prior to surgery with a specific assay for antithrombin. In the future it is likely that informative protein or restriction fragment length polymorphisms will be identified that will allow most deficiency states to be traced in families with more than 99 per cent confidence.

Suchman AL, Griner PF: Diagnostic uses of the activated partial thromboplastin time and prothrombin time. Ann Intern Med 104:810, 1986. *Critical evaluation of when these tests should be ordered and how the tests should be interpreted.*

INHERITED DISORDERS OF BLOOD COAGULATION
General Comments

The plasma protein coagulation factors that are named with Roman numerals, with the exception of factor XII, were identified as a consequence of patients presenting with bleeding disorders, eventually recognized as unique and familial. Bleeding may be due to a structural defect in a coagulation factor or to a lack of its synthesis. In the former situation there will be immunologically cross-reacting material (CRM) present in the patient's plasma, and the patient is said to be CRM +. In the latter situation the patient is said to be CRM −. Genetic material for most of the coagulation factors has been cloned, and considerable information about the exact genetic defects that underlie inherited bleeding disorders is being generated. It is likely that a number of different genetic defects will be demonstrated for each coagulation factor, in analogy to the many defects in the β globin gene in patients with hemoglobinopathy or thalassemia. In other words, Murphy's law of genetic disease—"Whatever can go wrong with a gene will go wrong"—will be proven again and again. Future studies of genetic defects of coagulation proteins will undoubtedly give important new insights into the functions of these proteins, will allow deficient patients to be separated into subgroups in ways that are clinically relevant, and, as described above, will allow more definitive diagnosis of heterozygous deficiency states.

GENETICS. Deficiencies of factors VIII and IX are inherited as X-linked traits with bleeding occurring in the male hemizygotes. Von Willebrand disease is usually an autosomal dominant disorder, although rare patients have severe autosomal recessive disease. Deficiencies of all of the other coagulation factors are transmitted as autosomal recessive traits, with clinically significant bleeding usually manifested only in patients with homozygous deficiency. Heterozygous carriers may have reduced plasma levels of a coagulation factor activity, but the deficiency seldom affects hemostasis. In the case of protein deficiencies associated with familial tendency to thrombosis, however, heterozygotes with 50 per cent of the normal level of the protein are at risk. Inherited deficiencies may be combined. Most frequently cited are patients with combined factor V and factor VIII deficiencies that appear to be familial. The reason for the association is not known, although it is intriguing that factors V and VIII are homologous to one another and perform analogous functions (Fig. 167–1). Combined deficiencies in the functions of factors II, VII, IX, and X have been observed in patients with congenitally defective vitamin K–dependent gamma-carboxylation.

TREATMENT STRATEGIES. The most obvious treatment is replacement of the missing factor. Concentrates of factors VIII and IX are readily available at a cost of 12 to 20 cents per unit. Because of its large size, factor VIII distributes mainly in the blood plasma. There is approximately 40 ml of plasma per kilogram of body weight. Thus it would take 1400 units of factor VIII (at a cost of $168 to $280) to raise the plasma factor VIII level of a 70-kg patient with severe classic hemophilia from less than 1 per cent (<0.01 unit per milliliter) to 50 per cent (0.5 unit per milliliter) as calculated by the following formula:

$$0.5 \text{ unit/ml} \times 40 \text{ ml/kg} \times 70 \text{ kg} = 1400 \text{ units}$$

Because of its smaller size, factor IX distributes in a volume 1½-fold to 2-fold greater than the plasma volume. Thus, proportionately more factor IX than factor VIII must be infused to achieve a similar response in a patient with hemophilia B. Because of its longer half-life in the body, however, factor IX needs to be given less often than factor VIII to maintain a therapeutic level.

The above calculation points out one of the drawbacks of replacement therapy: cost. A shortage of concentrates is a potential problem, but at present there is enough source plasma to supply the needs of hemophilic patients. The most important, indeed overriding, problem with purified factor concentrates is with contaminating viruses. Each batch of concentrate is made from thousands of units of plasma, some of which come from commercial plasmapheresis centers. There is a high likelihood that recipients will be infected with hepatitis B, non-A, non-B hepatitis, and/or human immunodeficiency virus (HIV). This likelihood can be minimized by use of source plasma that does not contain antibodies to the viruses and has a normal level of transaminase. The infectivity of concentrates can be further decreased and perhaps eliminated by subjecting the concentrates to treatment (e.g., heating or extraction with an organic solvent) that will inactivate the viruses but preserve the activity of the factor of interest. It will be some time before efficacies of the attenuation processes are completely known or before products made by recombinant DNA techniques are available. In the meantime the clinician and patient must weigh the convenience and effectiveness of potentially infective factor concentrates against treatments that are more cumbersome but minimize exposure to multiple donors (e.g., use of cryoprecipitate rather than factor VIII concentrate) or do not require exposure to blood products at all (e.g., use of desmopressin to transiently raise the level of factor VIII and EACA to minimize mucosal bleeding).

When elective procedures are contemplated that require prophylactic therapy to raise factor levels, it is wise to test the proposed therapy prior to the procedure to be sure that target levels can be achieved.

HEMOPHILIA A (FACTOR VIII DEFICIENCY)

Hemophilia A, the most frequently encountered serious inherited disorder of blood coagulation, occurs in 1 of 10,000 males. Some patients lack plasma factor VIII, whereas others have a nonfunctional factor VIII molecule present in normal concentrations. The majority of hemophilic patients give a positive family history with an X-linked inheritance pattern. In the remainder the mutation of the factor VIII gene may be new. A hemophilic patient's daughters will all be carriers, but all his sons will be normal. A carrier woman has a 50 per cent chance of producing a hemophilic male or a female carrier. Because of random inactivation (lyonization) of the X chromosome, the carrier is a genetic mosaic with two populations of cells containing either a normal X chromosome or an abnormal X chromosome (bearing the hemophilic gene). Therefore, a carrier should have about 50 per cent of the normal level of factor VIII activity. The range of factor VIII levels in carriers is broad, probably because inactivation of one of the X chromosomes is often disproportionate. If extreme lyonization occurs so that the preponderance of cells in the carrier female contains the X chromosome with the hemophilic gene and the factor VIII level is less than 40 per cent of normal, the woman may have clinical features of mild hemophilia.

CLINICAL MANIFESTATIONS. In general, the degree of factor VIII deficiency correlates with the frequency of clinically significant bleeding. Furthermore, the degree of deficiency and bleeding severity tend to be similar in affected members of a given family. Hemophilia, therefore, is often classified as severe (<1 per cent normal activity), moderate (1 to 5 per cent normal activity), or mild (5 to 25 per cent normal activity). Bleeding from the umbilical cord is rare at birth, presumably because the extrinsic limb of the coagulation system functions normally in the presence of high concentrations of tissue factor.

Hematomas and Internal Hemorrhage. Depending on the severity of the deficiency, soft tissue hematomas may develop in early infancy. More difficulties begin when the child becomes physically active, and these continue throughout life. Hematomas often occur in muscles and soft tissues. Considerable blood loss can occur into thigh muscles or the retroperitoneum; extent of blood loss in these areas may be difficult to discern clinically and is frequently underestimated. The bleeding of hemophilia can involve virtually any anatomic area and give rise to secondary symptoms and signs caused by compression. If bleeding occurs in the pharynx or neck, airway obstruction can result. Severe bleeding may occur from peptic ulcerations. Partial intestinal obstruction may result from hemorrhage into the bowel wall. Mesenteric bleeding can lead to the development of bowel ischemia and necrosis. Hematuria can be painless or may present as ureteral colic due to formation of clots that obstruct the ureter. Subdural hematomas and other central nervous system hemorrhages are uncommon, but represent a major cause of death and disability. Many bleeding episodes appear to develop spontaneously without a history of trauma or other provoking causes. Such spontaneous bleeding may occur during periods of stress, as before school examinations or following family dissension. When bleeding follows trauma, it may be delayed, since the primary hemostasis furnished by vessels and platelets is intact (see Ch. 166).

Hemarthroses. Bleeding occurs in joints, usually in the elbows, knees, and ankles and less often in the wrist and hand. In about half of hemophilic patients, repeated hemarthroses result in eventual deformity and crippling. These patients have factor VIII activity levels well below 5 per cent of normal and usually less than 1 per cent of normal. The patient experiences considerable pain with bleeding into joints due to distension of the joint capsule. Movement is severely limited, causing disuse atrophy of the muscles about the joint. Pressure erodes the ends of long bones, causing periosteal pain, eventual necrosis, and pseudocyst formation. Hemarthrosis causes proliferation of the synovium. Thus a vicious cycle is set in play in which a joint, once weakened, may experience hemorrhage again and again in a seemingly spontaneous manner.

Bleeding after Surgery. Major or minor surgery, including dental extractions, can result in marked blood loss in a hemophilic patient and therefore must be carried out in conjunction with factor VIII replacement therapy to assure adequate hemostasis. Even those patients with mild hemophilia, factor VIII levels of 5 to 25 per cent of normal, may develop clinically significant bleeding with surgery or trauma and require replacement therapy.

DIAGNOSIS. A history of joint and soft tissue bleeding, a family history compatible with X-linked inheritance, and the presence of arthropathy on physical examination would all point to the diagnosis of sex-linked hemophilia. Factor VIII deficiency is most likely, although IX deficiency (hemophilia B) must also be considered. Laboratory screening tests should show a normal prothrombin time and prolonged APTT. The abnormal APTT should be corrected by all deficient plasmas

except those from individuals with known factor VIII deficiency. In particular, the abnormal APTT should be corrected by plasma from a patient with factor IX deficiency. If plasmas from patients with known deficiencies are not available, correction can be attempted with normal plasma absorbed with barium salts (which will remove factor IX but not factor VIII) and serum (which contains factor IX but not active factor VIII). Absorbed plasma, but not serum, will correct the abnormal APTT of a patient with factor VIII deficiency. As described above, a quantitative assay for factor VIII can be done by testing the ability of dilutions of the patient's plasma to correct the defect in factor VIII–deficient plasma.

Von Willebrand factor (see below) stabilizes factor VIII in the circulation; severe deficiency of von Willebrand factor is therefore accompanied by severe deficiency of factor VIII, and hemophilia A can be confused with von Willebrand disease. Unlike hemophilia, however, von Willebrand disease is inherited as an autosomal dominant trait and may present with a history of vascular type bleeding. Upon screening, the bleeding time should be grossly prolonged in von Willebrand disease, whereas the bleeding time is usually at the upper limit of normal or only slightly prolonged in hemophilia. Further investigation should demonstrate deficiency or abnormality of von Willebrand factor and defective platelet aggregation mediated by the antibiotic ristocetin in von Willebrand disease but not in hemophilia. If the diagnosis remains in doubt, it may be helpful to perform laboratory tests on family members to determine the inheritance pattern of the deficiency.

TREATMENT. The patient and family must learn about the nature of hemophilia, the anticipated severity of the patient's disease, the recognition and management of various types of bleeding episodes, the difference the disorder may make in the patient's future life style, and the genetics of its transmission.

General Considerations. A major goal of patient, family, and physician is to have the patient lead as normal a life as possible. This will entail some restrictions of activities as a child and limitations on career choices. The physician, guided by the medical history, the degree of physical impairment, the severity of bleeding in affected family members, and the plasma level of factor VIII, should advise the patient to participate in activities commensurate with the severity of his disease. A hemophilic child should be reared in a protective environment until he understands the consequences of hemophilia and can take responsibility for his actions. The physician should be alert for denial mechanisms sometimes constructed by patient and parents about the disease. For example, the patient may develop a willingness and receive unconscious encouragement from the parents to participate in dangerous activities or to forgo needed treatments. With maturity, the patient usually accepts the constraints imposed by his disease. He should be encouraged to develop his education and interests as fully as possible and counseled to adopt a career that does not expose him to undue hazards, is compatible with his physical capabilities, and allows him access to adequate health insurance coverage.

To be free to develop as normal a life as possible, the patient must participate in a major way in his medical care. This has led to the widespread adoption of home care programs in which the patient treats himself at home with the backup of a primary physician, a nurse coordinator, and a multidisciplinary team of a hematologist, orthopedic surgeon, dentist, social worker, financial counselor, and so on. It is reasonable to expect a responsible patient in a home care program to work or go to school full time, to require a minimum of emergency room visits, and to be hospitalized only for major trauma, medical illness, or elective surgery. The major cost of such a program is replacement therapy: A 70-kg patient who has severe hemophilia and needs to give himself an infusion every other week would consume approximately $6000 (25 × $250) in blood products per year. Home care programs, however, are cost effective because bleeding episodes are treated when first symptomatic and do not proceed to the point at which hospitalization is required for aggressive replacement therapy and pain management. About 50 per cent of patients with hemophilia A have enough problems to make home care worthwhile.

Patients receiving long-term replacement therapy need regular evaluation at 6- to 12-month intervals. The clinic visit should include a physical examination with special attention paid to joints, an inhibitor screen, a chemistry panel with special attention paid to liver function, and tests for antibodies to hepatitis viruses and HIV.

Factor VIII Preparations. Bleeding episodes are managed primarily by administration of factor VIII, either in the form of cryoprecipitate or as a commercially prepared lyophilized concentrate. The use of cryoprecipitate or factor VIII concentrate avoids the complication of volume overload that would occur with the large amount of plasma that would be necessary to attain acceptable levels of factor VIII activity.

Blood banks prepare cryoprecipitate by freezing individual bags of fresh normal plasma, each containing approximately 200 units of factor VIII activity in 200 ml of plasma, at $-90°C$ and then thawing at 4°C. Approximately 50 per cent of the factor VIII contained in the plasma remains as a precipitate, which is separated from the bulk of the plasma and stored frozen in individual bags containing approximately 100 units of factor VIII activity in 20 to 40 ml of residual plasma. When needed, the appropriate number of bags is thawed at 37°C, and the contents are pooled and administered intravenously to the patient.

Lyophilized factor VIII concentrate has been taken through several purification steps and is available in vials containing different amounts of factor VIII activity (exact amounts stated on the labels). The concentrates are readily soluble upon addition of diluent and thus can be prepared and administered intravenously within 30 minutes.

The major advantage of cryoprecipitate, especially for the patient who needs only occasional infusions of factor VIII, is that it exposes the recipient to fewer donors and thus minimizes the chance of blood-transmitted viral infection. Indeed, individuals have been supported from infancy to young adulthood with cryoprecipitate prepared from plasma donated sequentially by the same donor. The major disadvantages of cryoprecipitate are the inconvenience of thawing and pooling bags prior to administration and the need for the bags to stay frozen at $-20°C$ until the time of administration in a home freezer that does not have a frost-free cycle and preferably has a device that graphs temperature over time.

The major advantages of lyophilized concentrates are stability on storage and convenience of administration. Another major advantage of concentrates in the future will be the knowledge that the concentrates have been processed to totally inactivate HIV and possibly also hepatitis B and the agent(s) of non-A, non-B hepatitis.

Patients should be vaccinated against hepatitis B at the time of diagnosis and will be prime candidates for vaccines that may be developed in the future for non-A, non-B hepatitis viruses and HIV.

Replacement Therapy. Intensity of replacement therapy depends on the estimated plasma level of factor VIII required to halt the bleeding and the disappearance rate of the infused factor VIII. Very early hemarthrosis can be managed with a single infusion to attain a peak factor VIII level of 25 to 50 per cent of normal. For more extensive hemorrhage, factor VIII infusions are usually continued for two days after cessation of symptoms or signs of bleeding. Early hemarthrosis or hematuria can be managed by maintenance of the plasma factor VIII level at 25 to 50 per cent of normal for two to three days. Muscle hematomas require a longer period of sustained factor VIII levels, in the range of 40 to 60 per cent of normal

for four to six days. Major trauma or surgery requires that the factor VIII level be maintained at more than 70 per cent of normal until hemostasis is achieved and then in the range of 25 to 50 per cent of normal for 10 to 14 days. Plasma factor VIII can be measured after administration of the calculated dose to document that the desired peak level has been achieved and prior to subsequent scheduled doses to determine whether desired levels have been sustained. If a low factor VIII level persists despite replacement therapy, it may be that simply not enough factor VIII is being given, that the factor VIII concentrates contain less than their stated activity, or that the patient has developed an inhibitor that neutralizes infused factor VIII.

The amount of concentrate needed to achieve and maintain a desired level of factor VIII activity can be estimated by knowing (1) that the patient's plasma volume is about 40 ml per kilogram of body weight, (2) the amount of factor VIII activity in the average bag of cryoprecipitate (usually about 100 units) or in available vials of lyophilized concentrate factor VIII activity, and (3) that factor VIII has a half-life of about 10 to 12 hours in the circulation. Therefore replacement therapy is ordinarily given three times a day when tight control of the level is needed and twice a day when deeper troughs in the level can be tolerated.

Treatment of Hemarthroses. In addition to replacement therapy, joint bleeding is initially managed by immobilization of the affected limb and application of ice packs to diminish swelling and discomfort of the joint. Because of the risk of introducing infection or of causing additional bleeding, hemarthroses should not be aspirated unless such acute pain and tension are present that pressure necrosis is a major possibility. Aspiration should be performed only after administration of replacement factor VIII. Splinting or using elastic bandages over a hemarthrosis may make the patient more comfortable and insure that a position of joint function is maintained during the acute stage. When pain and swelling have subsided, the patient should begin rehabilitation to regain motion and strength in conjunction with prophylactic replacement therapy. Patients with joint disease may benefit from periodic assessment by an orthopedic surgeon. In properly selected patients, synovectomy and artificial joint replacement have been very successful in improving the usefulness of severe chronic joint deformity.

Dental Care. The patient should be instructed about the importance of dental hygiene and should have frequent dental examinations. Bleeding in deep tissues of the oropharynx can be life threatening. Therefore, a local anesthetic should be administered by needle puncture only after prophylactic administration of factor VIII concentrate. Extraction also requires prior administration of factor VIII concentrate. For patients with mild or moderate hemophilia, it is likely that adequate levels of factor VIII can be achieved with use of desmopressin, as described below for patients with von Willebrand disease. Administration of EACA by mouth, also described below, is useful in prevention of rebleeding after tooth extraction.

Use of Analgesics. Bleeding can cause extraordinary pain, especially in joints. Injudicious use of narcotics can lead to addiction in hemophilic patients. Aspirin must be avoided by the hemophilic because it decreases platelet aggregation and accentuates bleeding. Acetaminophen and codeine are recommended as the first choices of analgesics. In selected cases, ibuprofen can be given for chronic joint pain. The likelihood that ibuprofen will cause increased bleeding can be assessed by a template bleeding time after the patient has received the drug for several days. If the bleeding time is prolonged compared to the bleeding time before therapy, the drug should be discontinued.

Factor VIII Inhibitors. The possibility that the patient has acquired neutralizing antibodies to factor VIII (factor VIII inhibitor) should be of constant concern. An inhibitor may initially appear at almost any time in the life of a hemophilic patient and need not be associated with any obvious change in the clinical severity of the disorder. Patients with inhibitors present special problems. Much depends on the titer of the inhibitor, which is commonly expressed in Bethesda units: 1 Bethesda unit, by definition, inhibits 1 unit of factor VIII, i.e., the factor VIII in 1 ml of normal plasma. If one calculates the amount of factor VIII required to neutralize the inhibitor and achieve a 50 per cent normal level of circulating factor VIII in a patient who weighs 70 kg and has a plasma volume of 2,800 ml and an inhibitor titer of 10 Bethesda units per milliliter, the amount (and cost) is immense:

2800 ml × 10.5 units/ml = 29,400 units (cost = $3528 to $5880)

Several strategies are available, all expensive and none totally adequate. Because some inhibitors take up to several hours to complex with and inhibit factor VIII, it may be possible to maintain factor VIII levels at a therapeutic level by constant infusion. If the inhibitor is of modest titer (1 to 10 Bethesda units per milliliter), it may be possible to remove enough inhibitor by plasmapheresis to make therapy feasible with lower amounts of factor VIII. A patient receiving factor VIII concentrate may have an anamestic immune response with an increase in the titer and avidity of his inhibitor. Therefore, everything possible should be done to achieve permanent hemostasis in the four- to six-day "golden period" during which replacement therapy is possible. Patients with high titers of rapidly acting inhibitor can be given activated factor IX concentrate that also contains activated factor X and therefore "bypasses" factor VIII in the coagulation cascade. Such a concentrate, unfortunately, is expensive and has considerable thrombogenic potential.

AIDS. Regardless of whether they have antibodies to HIV, patients who have used significant quantities of blood products must take proper precautions to protect their close contacts and loved ones. They can be assured that the virus is not transmitted by casual household contact. They must be taught safe disposal procedures for needles and other injection paraphernalia. It should be strongly recommended that condoms be used during all sexual intercourse. This raises an irreconcilable conflict for couples considering pregnancy. There is a high likelihood of transmission of HIV to the newborn of a virus-positive mother. Thus, wives of men with hemophilia who are considering pregnancy should receive specific education and counseling and be tested for antibodies to HIV before pregnancy occurs.

PROGNOSIS. Factor VIII concentrate is a two-edged sword. The major long-term complications of moderate and severe hemophilia are (1) progressive joint deformity and crippling, (2) development of inhibitors to factor VIII activity, (3) hepatitis and cirrhosis, and (4) acquired immune deficiency syndrome.

Despite the availability of replacement therapy, many hemophiliacs, for a variety of reasons, are treated inadequately or haphazardly and become severely crippled and, ultimately, chronic invalids. The last three of the four complications listed above are seen more often in patients who receive frequent replacement therapy. Up to 15 per cent of hemophilic patients develop inhibitory antibodies to factor VIII activity, usually in childhood. The tendency to develop antibodies may be genetic. If so, the accumulating information about lesions in hemophilic factor VIII genes should lead to knowledge that will allow identification of patients at high risk for development of inhibitors. Most patients who have received factor VIII concentrate in the past have been exposed to hepatitis viruses and HIV. The risks of chronic hepatitis and AIDS in exposed individuals are both probably greater than 10 per cent. On the whole, the availability of concentrates has been beneficial and has improved the prognosis of all forms of hemophilia A—mild, moderate, and severe. With the elimination of viruses in concentrates and a better understanding

of inhibitor formation, it is reasonable to hope that future cohorts of hemophiliacs will enjoy the benefits of replacement therapy without the complications. Patients who have been treated in the past, however, are at risk for these complications, especially AIDS, and thus their prognosis is guarded.

CARRIER DETECTION. Women who have relatives with hemophilia frequently seek help to determine whether they may pass the disorder to their children. Daughters of men with the disorder, mothers of more than one hemophilic son, and mothers who have a hemophilic son and another hemophilic male relative in their pedigree are obligate carriers of the hemophilic gene. Only about 15 per cent of the instances of hemophilia arise because of spontaneous mutation. Determination of factor VIII procoagulant activity is of limited usefulness in the identification of carrier women, because low-normal levels overlap with factor VIII levels found in obligate heterozygotes. A major reason for scatter in factor VIII levels is scatter in the levels of von Willebrand factor, which functions as a carrier protein for factor VIII. Therefore the overlap between normal persons and obligate carriers is decreased considerably if the factor VIII level is corrected for the level of immunoreactive von Willebrand factor (sometimes called factor VIII–related antigen). When the ratios of these two proteins are analyzed by logarithmic discriminant analysis, greater than 95 per cent of carriers can be identified. Such an analysis is best done by a laboratory that is highly experienced with the assays and has proven the validity of the analysis in an adequate number of obligate carriers.

Several restriction fragment length polymorphisms close to the gene for factor VIII have been shown to be useful in tracing hemophilia A in families. In families in which the polymorphisms segregate with hemophilia, the polymorphisms can identify carriers with greater than 99 per cent confidence. The polymorphisms also can be used to diagnose hemophilia in fetuses in the first trimester, whereas assays of factor VIII per se can only be done in the second trimester when the fetal circulation is accessible for blood sampling by fetoscopy.

Graham JB, Green PP, McGraw RA, et al.: Application of molecular genetics in prenatal diagnosis and carrier detection in the hemophilias: Some limitations. Blood 66:759, 1985. *Summarizes the initial cloning literature on factor VIII and the potential application to patients.*

Levine PH: The clinical manifestations and therapy of hemophilias A and B. In Colman RW, Hirsh J, Marder VJ, et al. (eds.): Hemostasis and Thrombosis: Basic Principles and Clinical Practice. 2nd ed. Philadelphia, J. B. Lippincott Company, 1987, pp 97–111.

VON WILLEBRAND DISEASE

This disorder, named for the Finnish physician who described it in 1926, is due to a deficiency or abnormality of a plasma protein, von Willebrand factor, that is required for the stabilization of factor VIII in the circulation and for the normal adherence of platelets to sites of vascular injury. The gene for von Willebrand factor is on chromosome 12. The hallmarks of von Willebrand disease historically have been a low factor VIII level, a long bleeding time, and autosomal inheritance. The last two characteristics distinguish von Willebrand disease from hemophilia A. With extensive characterization of von Willebrand factor over the last decade has come a broadening of the definition of von Willebrand disease so that the name now encompasses a heterogeneous group of defects of von Willebrand factor.

FUNCTION OF VON WILLEBRAND FACTOR. Factor VIII and von Willebrand factor circulate in normal plasma as a complex. Endothelial cells and megakaryocytes-platelets synthesize, store, and secrete von Willebrand factor. Secretion increases when endothelial cells are stimulated or injured. Therefore the concentration of plasma von Willebrand factor is labile and can be increased by stimuli as innocuous as a vigorous Valsalva maneuver, and it is common to find levels of von Willebrand factor elevated twofold to tenfold in ill patients. Von Willebrand factor exists as a series of multimers ranging in size from 850,000 to 12,000,000 daltons. The largest multimers, which have a half-life in the circulation of only several hours, are most active in mediation of platelet adhesion. Both large and small multimers complex with factor VIII. Von Willebrand factor can interact with platelets in two different ways. It binds to platelet glycoprotein Ib in a reaction that is greatly enhanced by ristocetin (an antibiotic that cannot be used because it causes thrombocytopenia). It also binds to platelet glycoprotein IIb-IIIa complex, but only when platelets are activated. Von Willebrand factor binds to collagen and other components of the vessel wall and thus mediates attachment and spreading of platelets to the subendothelium of damaged vessels. The role of von Willebrand factor in platelet adhesion is especially important when blood passes through the blood vessel at high shear rate and the red blood cell count is normal or increased.

PATHOGENESIS OF VON WILLEBRAND DISEASE. In classic (type I) von Willebrand disease, patients have prolonged bleeding time, abnormal platelet aggregation in response to ristocetin, and parallel decreases in plasma factor VIII activity, immunoreactive von Willebrand factor, and ristocetin cofactor activity. Patients with severe, usually homozygous, disease can have less than 1 per cent of normal von Willebrand factor in plasma and platelets and no detectable von Willebrand antigen in endothelial cells. Their factor VIII levels may be less than 5 per cent of normal. Intravenous infusion of small amounts of normal plasma, hemophilic plasma, or normal serum into patients with severe von Willebrand disease results in a prolonged increase in factor VIII that is out of proportion to the factor VIII content of the transfused plasma or serum. This probably results from stabilization of the patients' endogenously produced factor VIII by infused von Willebrand factor.

A number of qualitative abnormalities of von Willebrand factor result in variant diseases called type IIA, type IIB, and so on. In type IIA disease the large and intermediate-sized multimers are not present in plasma or platelets. Von Willebrand factor function (e.g., ristocetin cofactor activity) is decreased more than von Willebrand factor antigen. These patients have abnormal platelet adhesion and long bleeding times, but normal factor VIII activity. Abnormal multimer patterns can be ascertained by probing separated plasma proteins with antibodies to von Willebrand factors after agarose gel electrophoresis. Subtypes IIC, IID, etc., of von Willebrand disease have been identified, based on additional subtle abnormalities in the electrophoretic pattern of the multimers. In type IIB disease the largest multimers are missing from plasma but not from platelets, and the abnormal von Willebrand factor causes platelet aggregation at lower than usual ristocetin concentration. It is thought that the largest multimers are missing from plasma because the multimers bind spontaneously to platelets. In principle, such a spontaneous interaction could be due to defects in the patient's von Willebrand factor or in the patient's platelets ("platelet von Willebrand disease"), and indeed patients have been identified in whom the defect is in the platelets.

CLINICAL MANIFESTATIONS. Von Willebrand disease has a broad spectrum of clinical and laboratory features. It can range from a severe hemorrhagic disorder, in which the level of factor VIII is low enough and the bleeding problems severe enough that the disease must be differentiated from classic hemophilia, to an asymptomatic condition that is a laboratory curiosity. The severity of symptoms due to von Willebrand disease can vary considerably even among afflicted family members, probably because there are a number of factors that control the synthesis and secretion of von Willebrand factor.

Patients with severe disease usually have inherited it from both parents, as either a true homozygous or as a double heterozygous disease. The principal bleeding problems are of the superficial type. Epistaxis is a frequent complaint, especially early in life, as is easy bruising. Hematuria and gastrointestinal bleeding occur less frequently, and hemarthroses are quite rare. Without adequate replacement therapy, postoperative bleeding is a major hazard. In patients with heterozygous type I or II disease, the hemorrhagic tendency usually becomes evident or troublesome only with trauma, surgery, or dental extractions. Women with the disorder commonly experience excessive menses and postpartum bleeding. In all forms of the disease, the frequency and severity of bleeding tend to lessen with age.

DIAGNOSIS. The classic findings in type I von Willebrand disease are prolonged bleeding time and a low level of factor VIII. Confirmatory testing should reveal a low level of immunoreactive von Willebrand factor and absence or diminished platelet aggregation when ristocetin is added to the patient's platelet-rich plasma. The analysis using ristocetin can be made more sensitive and quantitative by testing the ability of dilutions of the patient's plasma to support agglutination of washed platelets; this is often called the ristocetin cofactor titer. Patients with severe type I disease lack von Willebrand factor antigen when endothelial cells of skin biopsies are stained by immunofluorescence or platelets are lysed and subjected to immunoassay.

Electrophoretic analysis of the site distribution of von Willebrand factor multimers should be done in patients who are suspected of having type II von Willebrand disease on the basis of bleeding problems, prolonged bleeding time, and abnormal ristocetin-induced platelet aggregation but normal or only slightly decreased levels of von Willebrand factor and factor VIII. In type IIA disease the larger multimers are missing in both plasma and platelets. In type IIB disease (hypersensitivity to ristocetin) the larger multimers are missing in plasma but not in platelets.

It may be very difficult to know for sure whether someone with mild decreases in von Willebrand factor and factor VIII, say to 50 per cent of normal, has von Willebrand disease. A number of factors influence the plasma concentration of von Willebrand factor. For instance, people with type O blood have lower levels than people with types A and B. As another example, hypothyroidism causes the level of von Willebrand factor to fall. As mentioned above, endothelial cells can be stimulated to release von Willebrand factor. Thus, one must worry about both overdiagnosis and underdiagnosis. Serial studies of the same patient and studies of other family members can be helpful. Because symptoms in such patients are mild and tend to decrease with age, however, it may suffice to be honest with such patients about the ambiguities of the laboratory tests and counsel them to alert their physician about the possibility of von Willebrand disease in the event of trauma or major surgery.

TREATMENT. Indications for therapy in von Willebrand disease include surgery, severe epistaxis, severe menorrhagia, and recurrent gastrointestinal bleeding.

Replacement Therapy. Cryoprecipitate is equally rich in factor VIII and von Willebrand factor and therefore will correct both the deficiency of factor VIII and the long bleeding time of type I von Willebrand disease. Factor VIII concentrates are poor in von Willebrand factor and will not correct the bleeding time defect. Hence, replacement therapy in von Willebrand disease should be with cryoprecipitate rather than factor VIII concentrate. Because the largest multimers of von Willebrand factor are cleared rapidly after infusion, the bleeding time is usually corrected only transiently. The smaller multimers allow the patient's own factor VIII to circulate, and the factor VIII level may remain elevated for considerably longer than would be predicted, based on the amount of infused factor VIII. In the case of ongoing hemorrhage or major surgery, cryoprecipitate should be given, using the guidelines described above for factor VIII replacement in hemophilia A. The infusion should be given immediately prior to maneuvers designed to achieve hemostasis. This will insure that the bleeding time as well as the factor VIII level is maximally corrected. It is not practical to give cryoprecipitate often enough to keep the bleeding time continuously corrected or to quantify the correction with serial bleeding times. Therefore, once hemostasis is achieved, therapy should be directed toward keeping the level of factor VIII in the appropriate therapeutic ranges as described above for hemophilia A. This probably will require less cryoprecipitate than if one were treating a hemophiliac.

Desmopressin. There are difficulties in obtaining an effective virus-free purified concentrate of von Willebrand factor. The largest multimers are hard to purify, and the potential market is small enough that there is no economic incentive to develop such a product by recombinant DNA techniques. Therefore, considerable attention has been devoted to the therapeutic potential of desmopressin (1-desamino-8-D arginine vasopressin, DDAVP), especially in patients with mild von Willebrand disease. Desmopressin causes release of von Willebrand factor and plasminogen activator from endothelial cells. EACA suppresses baseline and desmopressin-stimulated fibrinolysis and may be useful as an adjunctive therapy. Desmopressin, 0.3 μg per kilogram of body weight in 50 ml of saline, is given over 15 minutes. In type I disease, severalfold increases of both factor VIII and von Willebrand protein occur 15 to 30 minutes after infusion, with a concomitant decrease in the bleeding time. The effect may last for several hours. The magnitude and duration of the response vary among individual patients, especially among those with type IIA disease. Desmopressin is contraindicated in type IIB disease because appearance of the large multimers in the circulation can cause thrombocytopenia.

To learn if the treatment is feasible in a given patient, one should quantify the response to a test dose of desmopressin at the time of diagnosis or five to seven days prior to a planned procedure. For oral surgical procedures, EACA is given orally in a dosage of 75 mg per kilogram every six hours for seven to ten days beginning the evening before the procedure. It is controversial whether an antifibrinolytic agent should be given with major surgery.

Menstruation and Pregnancy. Excessive menstrual blood loss can be managed with hormonal suppression. Levels of factor VIII, von Willebrand factor, and ristocetin cofactor activity may become normal during pregnancy. Therefore, these tests, along with determination of the bleeding time, should be repeated during the third trimester to plan for replacement therapy during delivery. Cryoprecipitate should be given if the factor VIII level remains low. If the factor VIII level is greater than 50 per cent, but the bleeding time remains long, cryoprecipitate should be on call, because postpartum blood loss is frequently severe enough to require replacement infusion.

Complications of Therapy. Chronic arthropathy is less common in von Willebrand disease than in hemophilia A. The complications of replacement therapy for severe von Willebrand disease are the same as those described above for hemophilia A. Rarely, antibodies that inhibit the activity of von Willebrand protein develop. Patients receiving blood products should be vaccinated against hepatitis B and monitored for the acquisition of hepatitis viruses and HIV.

Moroose R, Hoyer LW: Von Willebrand factor and platelet function. Ann Rev Med 37:157, 1986. *Review of recent advances in knowledge of von Willebrand factor.*

Richardson DW, Robinson AG: Desmopressin. Ann Intern Med 103:228, 1985. *Review of the effectiveness of this drug in a variety of situations, including mild hemophilia, von Willebrand disease, liver disease, and uremia.*

HEMOPHILIA B (FACTOR IX DEFICIENCY)

Factor IX deficiency is inherited as an X-linked disorder that presents with the historical and clinical features of classic hemophilia (hemophilia A). The deficiency is most often quantitative, but can be due to qualitative defects of factor IX structure. The severity of bleeding is usually similar in members of a single family. In general, for a given degree of deficiency, factor IX–deficient patients have fewer symptoms than do patients with factor VIII deficiency, e.g., patients with severe (<1 per cent of normal) factor IX deficiency have the symptoms of patients with mild (1 to 5 per cent of normal) factor VIII deficiency. Nevertheless, factor IX deficiency causes serious bleeding problems. Patients with factor IX deficiency can be more cavalier about their disease than can patients with factor VIII deficiency, and therefore they are not as quick to seek medical attention when they need it—sometimes to their detriment.

CLINICAL MANIFESTATIONS. Many patients with low levels of factor IX are asymptomatic until the hemostatic system is stressed by surgery or trauma. Patients with the most severe disease may develop muscle hematomas, gastrointestinal hemorrhage, and bleeding into large joints with progression to crippling joint deformities.

DIAGNOSIS. This disorder is suspected with the finding of a normal prothrombin time and prolonged APTT that can be corrected by normal serum but not by barium sulfate–adsorbed plasma. The inability of the patient's plasma to correct the prolonged APTT of plasma from a patient with known factor IX deficiency establishes the diagnosis.

TREATMENT. The care and long-term goals of therapy for the patient with factor IX deficiency are similar to those described above for the patient with hemophilia A. Most patients will need less care than if they had hemophilia A, but they require the same intensity of education and counseling.

Replacement Therapy. Fresh frozen plasma is used to treat mild to moderate bleeding, especially in those patients who have hemorrhagic episodes infrequently. Ordinarily, transfusion of 500 ml of plasma twice daily is sufficient to maintain a level of factor IX activity 10 to 12 per cent above baseline. EACA can be used as an adjunct to transfusions of plasma in patients with mucosal bleeding or dental work.

Patients with moderate to severe hemorrhage, such as large hemarthroses or muscle hematomas, and patients being prepared for surgery can be treated with commercially prepared factor IX concentrate, aiming for levels that are approximately two-thirds as high as those described above for factor VIII replacement therapy. Because the volume of distribution and the half-life of factor IX are both greater than for factor VIII, a greater loading dose of factor IX must be given than for factor VIII, but subsequent doses can be given less frequently. The length of therapy is dependent on the severity of the hemorrhage and the patient's response. Therapy is generally continued for two days after bleeding and related symptoms have subsided.

Complications of Therapy. Presently available factor IX concentrates are a mixture of all of the vitamin K–dependent factors—factors II, VII, IX, and X and proteins C and S—and are heat treated. Factor IX stands up to heat treatment better than factor VIII, and therefore the concentrates are heated more vigorously and should be freer of infectious HIV than are factor VIII concentrates. However, the concentrates are not free of infectious hepatitis viruses. Patients therefore should be immunized against hepatitis B.

Factor IX concentrates contain trace amounts of activated vitamin K–dependent factors and therefore are thrombogenic and carry a risk for thromboembolism, especially when used in high dosage in patients who have liver disease or are immobilized after surgery. EACA greatly enhances the risk of thromboembolism and should never be used as an adjunct to factor IX concentrates. Indeed, some advocate that low-dosage heparin (5000 units every 12 hours) and plasma (as a source of antithrombins) be given to surgical patients receiving factor IX concentrate. Because of these potential complications, it is advisable to reserve the use of factor IX concentrates for patients who have acquired antibody to hepatitis B surface antigen as a result of prior exposure or immunization and for whom the benefits of treatment outweigh the risks of thromboembolism. In a situation in which levels greater than 10 to 15 per cent above baseline are desired but use of factor IX concentrate is contraindicated, plasmapheresis can be used to prevent volume overload.

Antibody inhibitors to factor IX occur in 5 to 10 per cent of treated patients.

CARRIER DETECTION. The normal range for factor IX is narrower than the normal range for factor VIII, and therefore carrier testing based on coagulation assays is better for hemophilia B than for hemophilia A. Nevertheless, laboratory definition of the carrier state is still an exercise in probabilities and is best done with genetic markers. The factor IX gene is more polymorphic than the factor VIII gene, and it seems likely that informative genetic markers will be found in most families. However, it is worthwhile doing factor IX activity assays in known and potential carriers, because women who are carriers may have factor IX levels that are sufficiently low to cause mild bleeding, especially after trauma or surgery.

Thompson AR: Structure, function, and molecular defects of factor IX. Blood 67:565, 1986. *Comprehensive summary of information about factor IX and hemophilia B.*

DEFICIENCIES OF CONTACT FACTORS

Deficiencies of factor XII, prekallikrein, or high molecular weight kininogen are clinically benign, and deficiency of factor XI may sometimes be benign. Patients with these abnormalities, however, have APTT's that are as prolonged as are those of patients with factor VIII or IX deficiency. Therefore it is important to establish the correct diagnosis and to counsel the patient that he or she has a laboratory abnormality that carries no risk for bleeding.

Deficiency of Factor XII, Prekallikrein, or High Molecular Weight Kininogen

These autosomal recessive disorders are almost always asymptomatic and are usually identified as a result of delayed coagulation times in routine laboratory assays. The deficiencies should be suspected when the APTT is prolonged in a patient who does not have a history of any bleeding tendency. The APTT of a mixture of patient's plasma and normal plasma should be normal, i.e., with no inhibitor demonstrable. The plasma concentrations of factors VIII and IX should be normal. The coagulation defect can be identified by the inability of the patient's plasma to correct the APTT of plasma from a patient known to have a deficiency of factor XII, prekallikrein, or high molecular weight kininogen.

Deficiency of Factor XI

Factor XI deficiency is fairly common among Ashkenazi Jews, and the prevalence of homozygous factor XI deficiency in cities with a sizable Jewish population is comparable to the prevalence of hemophilia A. The defect is usually asymptomatic, but it does occasionally cause spontaneous bleeding. Major bleeding into muscles or joints is rare. The inheritance pattern is autosomal recessive so that the deficiency is found with equal frequency in men and women. The APTT is prolonged. The prothrombin time and bleeding time are normal. Normal serum or barium sulfate–adsorbed plasma will both correct the APTT. Specific assays for factors VIII and IX are normal. The diagnosis is established by demonstrating that the patient's plasma does not correct the APTT of plasma known to be deficient in factor XI.

Clinically significant bleeding usually occurs in association with trauma, surgery, or dental extractions. Fresh frozen plasma, 10 to 20 ml per kilogram, should be given as treatment of bleeding or as prophylaxis for surgery. One infusion should suffice, because factor XI has a half-life of about 72 hours.

Silverberg M, Kaplan AP, Colman RW: Contact activation and its abnormalities. In Colman RW, Hirsh J, Marder VJ, et al. (eds.): Hemostasis and Thrombosis: Basic Principles and Clinical Practice. 2nd ed. Philadelphia, J. B. Lippincott Company, 1987, pp 18–38. *Well-referenced description of the biochemistry of factor XI and the deficiency state.*

DEFICIENCIES OF THE EXTRINSIC AND COMMON PATHWAYS

Deficiencies of factors VII, X, V, and II are all associated with clinically significant bleeding. The hemorrhagic diathesis is not as predictable or severe as in hemophilia A, but replacement therapy probably will be required at some point in a patient's lifetime, especially to control bleeding from mucous membranes, after dental extractions, or during menses.

Deficiency of Factor VII

This is a rare autosomal recessive defect, having been reported in fewer than 100 patients. Both qualitative and quantitative abnormalities of factor VII occur, and patients can be either mixed heterozygotes or true homozygotes.

CLINICAL MANIFESTATIONS. Patients have a history of bleeding, usually beginning in infancy or early childhood. Bleeding, however, is frequently mild, even in patients with severe deficiency. Heterozygous relatives have no bleeding tendency. Mucous membrane bleeding, epistaxis, intramuscular hemorrhage, hemarthroses, and menorrhagia are the most common problems; gastrointestinal bleeding is less common, hematuria occurs only occasionally, and central nervous system bleeding is rare. Bleeding after dental extractions is predictable, and such extractions should be done with prophylactic replacement therapy. Clinical manifestations of bleeding can vary from mild to severe in the same patient. In fact, patients with impressive bleeding histories have undergone major surgery without accompanying hemorrhage. This phenomenon is unexplained and not consistent with the central role assigned to factor VII in the physiologic initiation of blood coagulation. Also incongruent are observations of thromboembolism in factor VII–deficient patients.

DIAGNOSIS. A diagnosis of factor VII deficiency should be considered if the prothrombin time is prolonged whereas the APTT is normal. The coagulation time of the patient's plasma in response to Russell's viper venom, which directly activates factor X, is normal. The diagnosis is established by the inability to correct the patient's prothrombin time with plasma from a person known to have factor VII deficiency.

TREATMENT. Bleeding is treated with plasma, not necessarily fresh frozen because factor VII is very stable. The half-life of factor VII is two to six hours, and therefore frequent treatment is needed during a bleeding episode. Levels of 15 to 20 per cent of normal can be obtained with a loading dose of plasma of 10 to 20 ml per kilogram followed by 3 to 6 ml per kilogram every 12 hours and should suffice to stop bleeding or as prophylaxis for surgery. Commercially available factor IX concentrates, which contain factors VII, IX, X, and II, can be used if it is essential to avoid any possibility of intravascular volume overload; such concentrates carry the risk of thromboembolism and hepatitis. Menorrhagia may require treatment with oral contraceptive agents.

Deficiency of Factor X

This is also a rare autosomal recessive disorder secondary to absence of or reduced synthesis of a normal molecule and/or production of a normal amount of antigen that has little or no function. Clinical symptoms include epistaxis, occasional mucous membrane, joint, and muscle hemorrhages, and gastrointestinal bleeding. Women may have severe, life-threatening menses and postpartum hemorrhage. The diagnosis is suspected when both the prothrombin time and APTT are prolonged. The abnormal tests correct with normal serum, but not with barium sulfate–adsorbed plasma.

The clotting time of plasma in response to Russell's viper venom is usually prolonged, although an abnormal factor X has been described that is activated normally by Russell's viper venom but not by the intrinsic or extrinsic systems of blood coagulation. The diagnosis is established by demonstration that the abnormal plasma does not correct plasma known to be specifically deficient in factor X. Bleeding episodes are treated with plasma as described above for factor VII deficiency; plasma needs to be given less often because the plasma half-life of factor X is 24 to 48 hours.

Deficiency of Factor II (Prothrombin)

Like deficiency of factors VII and X, factor II deficiency (hypoprothrombinemia) is a rare recessive disorder due to decreased synthesis of factor II and/or synthesis of a dysfunctional molecule. Bleeding ranges from mild to severe and generally occurs only if the factor II activity level is less than 20 per cent of normal. Symptoms include umbilical bleeding at birth, epistaxis, menorrhagia, postpartum hemorrhage, and bleeding after trauma or minor surgical procedures. The diagnosis is suspected if the prothrombin time and APTT are prolonged and the thrombin time is normal. Neither serum nor barium sulfate–adsorbed plasma will correct the abnormalities. A specific assay can be done based on the relative ability of the unknown to correct the prothrombin time of known factor II–deficient plasma. Alternatively, a test can be done in which clotting of plasma is initiated with Taipan venom, a specific activator of factor II. Bleeding is treated with infusions of fresh frozen plasma as described above for factor VII deficiency. Infusions are necessary only every two days, since the half-life of factor II is about 72 hours.

Global Deficiency of Vitamin K–Dependent Factors

Several patients have been described who presented as infants with bleeding, grossly prolonged prothrombin time and APTT, and low levels (<5 per cent of normal) of factors II, VII, IX, and X even though there was no evidence of liver disease, malabsorption, or ingestion of coumarin drugs. The levels of the vitamin K–dependent factors increased to 30 to 40 per cent of normal when the patients were given pharmacologic doses (10 mg per day) of vitamin K, and the patients did well with minimal symptoms. This syndrome is probably due to some abnormality of vitamin K metabolism, such as an abnormality of vitamin K epoxide reductase.

Deficiency of Factor V

This disorder usually is inherited as an autosomal recessive trait, although families in which there is dominant transmission have been identified. Most patients lack factor V antigen.

CLINICAL MANIFESTATIONS. As with deficiencies of the other common pathway components, severity of bleeding symptoms is variable, and hemorrhage most often involves the mucous membranes of the nose and oral cavity. Hemarthroses are unusual. Menorrhagia may be so severe as to be life threatening. Some women with factor V deficiency, however, have normal menses or only mild menorrhagia. Obstetric deliveries may occur with little or no bleeding, but postpartum hemorrhage is frequent and requires replacement therapy.

DIAGNOSIS. Both the APTT and prothrombin time are prolonged. The prothrombin time can be corrected by barium sulfate–adsorbed fresh plasma, but not by serum. Definitive diagnosis is established if the patient's plasma does not correct the deficiency of a patient known to lack factor V activity. For unknown reasons, the bleeding time is prolonged in about one third of factor V–deficient patients.

THERAPY. Factor V is an extremely labile protein. Treatment, therefore, should be with plasma that is either fresh or was frozen while fresh and has not been stored for more than several months. The therapeutic goal should be a factor V

activity level greater than 25 per cent of normal. Because factor V is larger than the vitamin K–dependent factors, it should be possible to achieve such a level with the doses of plasma described above for factor VII deficiency. The plasma half-life of factor V activity is 12 to 36 hours. Cryoprecipitate and factor VIII concentrate are not enriched in factor V. Surgery should be done under the "cover" of prophylactic replacement therapy.

Platelets contain 10 to 20 per cent of the factor V in blood, and therefore platelet concentrates are a good source of factor V. Several patients have responded well to platelet transfusion after developing neutralizing antibodies to factor V.

Combined Deficiencies of Factors V and VIII

A number of patients have mild deficiencies of both factors V and VIII inherited as an autosomal recessive trait. The basis of the syndrome is unknown, but it probably is related to some post-translational modification of the two homologous proteins which is necessary for their function. Therapy should be directed toward replacement of both proteins.

Roberts HR, Foster PA: Inherited disorders of prothrombin conversion. In Colman RW, Hirsh J, Marder VJ, et al. (eds.): Hemostasis and Thrombosis: Basic Principles and Clinical Practice. 2nd ed. Philadelphia, J. B. Lippincott Company, 1987, pp 162–181. *Thoroughly referenced, and an excellent source of more detailed information about the diagnosis and management of patients with rare but clinically important factor deficiencies.*

ABNORMALITIES IN CONVERSION OF FIBRINOGEN TO FIBRIN

Disorders of Fibrinogen

These fall into two categories: absence (afibrinogenemia) or a low content (hypofibrinogenemia) of plasma fibrinogen and abnormally functioning plasma fibrinogen (dysfibrinogenemia). Afibrinogenemia and hypofibrinogenemia are autosomally recessive traits. Dysfibrinogenemia can be autosomally dominant or recessive.

AFIBRINOGENEMIA. In patients with absence of or low content of fibrinogen, the bleeding tendency may be noted at birth as continued oozing from the umbilical stump. The intensity and frequency of bleeding after trauma or surgery vary from mild to severe. Death from intracranial hemorrhage may occur in infancy or early childhood. It is not understood why some patients have a minimal bleeding tendency whereas others are very symptomatic. All assays that require formation of fibrin as an endpoint are abnormal. Plasma fibrinogen cannot be detected by immunologic or chemical (salting out) methods. The bleeding time may be markedly prolonged. Bleeding episodes should be treated with cryoprecipitate, which contains eightfold to tenfold more fibrinogen than does an equivalent amount of plasma. Plasma fibrinogen concentrations greater than 100 mg per deciliter are generally adequate and can be achieved by administration of one bag of cryoprecipitate for each 10 kg of body weight.

DYSFIBRINOGENEMIA. Dysfibrinogenemias are usually named after the cities in which they were discovered. The clinical features are very variable. Most individuals are asymptomatic. Some have mild to moderate bleeding tendencies, usually manifest only after surgery or trauma. Wound dehiscence is a problem in some. Some have a tendency for thrombosis. The abnormal proteins have a fascinating array of defects. For instance, several of the abnormal fibrinogens are poor substrates for thrombin, so that the fibrinopeptides are released slowly. Other abnormal fibrinogens, once converted to fibrin monomer by thrombin, display impaired aggregation into a fibrin gel. The diagnosis of these disorders should be suspected when delayed or poorly formed fibrin endpoints are observed in the prothrombin time, APTT, and thrombin time assays. The fibrinogen level, measured immunologically or chemically, is normal to low-normal. The majority of patients do not require treatment. In instances of bleeding or before surgical procedures on a patient known to have a propensity to bleed, replacement therapy in the form of cryoprecipitate should be given to attain a functioning plasma fibrinogen level of 100 to 150 mg per deciliter. Because the half-life of fibrinogen is four days, such infusions need to be given only once every several days. There are no absolute guidelines for how long therapy must be continued, but infusions of cryoprecipitate should be administered for two days after bleeding stops.

Deficiency of Factor XIII

Bleeding symptoms in factor XIII deficiency occur in individuals with less than 1 to 2 per cent of normal plasma factor XIII activity. The symptomatic deficiency state is an autosomal recessive trait. The bleeding diathesis is commonly apparent at birth as umbilical stump hemorrhage and continues throughout life. Wounds ooze slowly for days and heal poorly with scar formation. Intracranial hemorrhage after inapparent or only minor trauma is common. Males tend to be sterile, and women with the disorder have a high incidence of fetal loss unless they receive replacement therapy during pregnancy. Thrombin formation or conversion of fibrinogen to fibrin is not impaired. Consequently the prothrombin and APTT are normal. Platelet function tests are also normal. The laboratory diagnosis consists of demonstrating that a fibrin clot, made by recalcification of the patient's plasma, dissolves overnight at room temperature in 5 M urea or 1 per cent monochloroacetic acid. Fibrin clots formed in the presence of greater than 1 to 2 per cent of the normal concentration of factor XIII remain intact indefinitely in these solvents.

Treatment consists of giving fresh frozen plasma. Correction of the plasma concentration of factor XIII to 5 to 10 per cent of normal will provide normal hemostasis. The half-life of factor XIII is approximately 12 days, and thus prophylactic replacement therapy is feasible. Because central nervous system hemorrhage is a major risk, factor XIII–deficient patients are commonly given 5 to 10 ml per kilogram of fresh frozen plasma every three weeks. Extra plasma should be given in preparation for surgery or other head trauma. Development of inhibitory antibody to factor XIII as a consequence of transfusion therapy is apparently rare.

Deficiency of Alpha-2-Antiplasmin

Congenital homozygous deficiency of alpha-2-antiplasmin is associated with a severe, hemophilia-like, bleeding tendency. Heterozygous family members with plasma concentrations of the inhibitor 50 per cent of normal have a mild bleeding tendency characterized by postoperative bleeding, excessive bleeding after tooth extraction, and easy bruising after trauma. Levels of alpha-2-antiplasmin can be quantified with an activity assay. Patients with severe homozygous deficiency have fewer bleeding episodes when they receive long-term treatment with tranexamic acid. Heterozygotes would probably also benefit from treatment with tranexamic acid or EACA when symptomatic or when their antiplasmin level is depleted by stresses such as major surgery.

Gralnick HR: Congenital disorders of fibrinogen. In Williams WJ, Beutler E, Ersley AJ, et al. (eds.): Hematology. New York, McGraw-Hill Book Company, 1983, pp 1399–1410. *Detailed information about inherited fibrinogen abnormalities.*

Kitchens CS, Newcomb TF: Factor XIII. Medicine 58:413, 1979. *A comprehensive review.*

Kluft C, Vellenga E, Brommer JP, et al.: A familial hemorrhagic diathesis in a Dutch family: An inherited deficiency of alpha-2-antiplasmin. Blood 59:1169, 1982. *Description of a fairly large kindred.*

INHERITED TENDENCIES TOWARD THROMBOSIS

There has been considerable progress in the biochemical definition of hypercoagulability. Quantitative or functional deficiencies of four plasma proteins—protein C, protein S, the major antithrombin, and the minor antithrombin—have been reported to be associated with a tendency toward throm-

bosis in affected families. Abnormalities of homocysteine metabolism have been shown to be associated with arterial thrombosis (Ch. 194). As more is learned about fibrinolysis, it is likely that genetic abnormalities of plasminogen, plasminogen activators, and plasminogen activator inhibitors will be identified that are associated with a thrombotic diathesis.

APPROACH TO THE PATIENT WITH A SUSPECTED THROMBOTIC TENDENCY. Patients with the recently described deficiency syndromes are fairly rare. It is therefore difficult to make firm guidelines about when or how to search for deficiency states and how to treat or counsel affected individuals. In general, it is worthwhile to evaluate the status of patients with family histories of thrombosis, young (<40 years old) patients, and patients with rare types of thrombosis (e.g., dural sinus or mesenteric vein thrombosis). Patients should be questioned and their status evaluated to ascertain whether they or family members have or have had conditions that would put them at risk for thrombosis (obesity, prolonged immobilization, injury to or abnormalities of vessels) or causes for secondary hypercoagulability (myeloproliferative syndrome, paroxysmal nocturnal hemoglobinuria, malignant disease, lupus anticoagulant). It has been estimated that of patients with "unexpected thrombosis," 1 to 2 per cent will have deficiency of the major antithrombin, 5 per cent will have deficiency of protein C, and 5 per cent will have deficiency of protein S. In my practice the laboratory evaluation in individuals with a possible thrombotic diathesis includes activity assays of total antithrombin and plasminogen (readily available) and immunoassays of proteins C and S (available in coagulation reference laboratories). Plasma is also frozen at −70°C with the anticipation that new tests may become available in the future. For especially suspicious cases, plasma can be sent to reference or research laboratories for functional assays of proteins C and S and immunoassay and functional assay of the minor antithrombin. Patients with premature peripheral or cerebral occlusive arterial disease should be screened for excessive homocysteine accumulation after a standardized methionine-loading test.

The number of assays that could be done on a patient with a probable thrombotic diathesis is seemingly endless. Consider just the example of protein C. If protein C antigen is normal, protein C function could be impaired. Functional activities of protein C that could be impaired include: ability to generate an active site; ability to become activated by thrombin-thrombomodulin complex; ability once activated to cleave its physiologic substrates, factors V and VIII; ability to interact with protein S; and so on. In the future it is likely that screening assays will be developed to evaluate the protein C–protein S system, the antithrombins, and the fibrinolytic system. These screening assays, unfortunately, are unlikely to be as simple, inexpensive, and comprehensive as are the screening assays that we have for the coagulation cascade. And until the assays are developed, we must make do with the present laboratory tests, which, although not totally satisfactory, are extremely useful in selected situations.

Deficiency of Protein C

Two syndromes of hereditary protein C deficiency have been described: (1) heterozygous deficiency in which half-normal concentrations of protein C are associated with an increased risk of venous thromboembolism and (2) homozygous deficiency in which total lack (<1 per cent of normal) of protein C is associated with neonatal purpura fulminans (ischemic necrosis of skin and digits) and massive venous thrombosis. Not all individuals with heterozygous deficiency have thrombosis. In families in which there is thrombosis, some family members with 50 per cent levels are asymptomatic, i.e., the phenotype displays autosomal dominance with incomplete penetrance. In several large kindreds ascertained because of infants with homozygous deficiency, none of more than 30 individuals with heterozygous deficiency had a history of venous thrombosis, i.e., in some families heterozygous deficiency apparently does not increase the risk for thrombosis. It is likely, however, that homozygous deficiency is invariably associated with problems. Indeed, the syndrome of coumarin-induced skin necrosis recapitulates the syndrome of homozygous deficiency. Upon initiation of warfarin therapy, the plasma concentration of protein C, which has a half-life of six hours, falls more quickly than the concentrations of factors II, IX, and X, thus causing a hypercoagulable state.

The diagnosis of protein C deficiency is usually based on decreased amounts of antigen in plasma. For patients receiving long-term therapy with warfarin, other vitamin K–dependent proteins, e.g., factors X and II, are also measured with an immunoassay to correct for the 35 to 50 per cent drop in the level of circulating vitamin K–dependent proteins due to undercarboxylation. As discussed above, the antigenic measurements will not detect individuals with dysfunctional protein C.

Because not everyone with heterozygous protein C deficiency has thrombosis, long-term anticoagulation should be reserved for individuals who have had a thrombotic episode unless the family history is so striking that the physicians and affected members agree that prophylactic treatment is warranted. Asymptomatic family members should be counseled that they are at greater risk for thrombosis and advised about the dangers of prolonged immobilization of limbs, obesity, and smoking. When warfarin therapy is started in a patient with heterozygous deficiency, the anticoagulant effect should be achieved at a leisurely pace by daily administration of the predicted maintenance dose rather than by administration of a loading dose of drug. It is preferable to begin warfarin therapy while the patient is being treated with heparin. However, one should be aware that heparin induces thrombocytopenia and thrombosis in some patients, especially those who have received heparin for more than ten days.

Infants with homozygous protein C deficiency respond acutely to administration of plasma or factor IX concentrate, which is rich in protein C. Oral anticoagulants can be used to decrease the frequency of thrombotic events.

Deficiency of Protein S

In a number of families, decreased levels of plasma protein S antigen or activity are associated with venous thrombosis. Correlation between antigen and activity is poor, probably because a fraction of protein S in plasma is complexed with C4b-binding protein, and only the protein S that is free has anticoagulant activity. The tendency toward thrombosis is inherited as an autosomal dominant trait with incomplete penetrance. Affected individuals tend to have levels of protein S that are 50 per cent of normal, i.e., they are heterozygous for the deficiency. The incidence of symptomatic heterozygous protein S deficiency is probably the same as the incidence of symptomatic protein C deficiency. Pending further information about this recently described syndrome, it seems reasonable to approach and treat heterozygous protein S deficiency using the guidelines described above for heterozygous protein C deficiency.

Deficiency of the Major Antithrombin (Antithrombin III)

The average concentration of the major antithrombin in deficient patients is approximately 50 per cent of normal. The most frequent manifestation of thromboembolism is lower extremity thrombophlebitis, often bilateral and recurrent and often with pulmonary embolism. Patients may develop venous insufficiency and chronic leg ulcers. Upper extremity thrombophlebitis and mesenteric vein thrombosis are less common. Rare patients may develop retinal or cerebral vein thrombosis, thrombosis of the renal vein or inferior vena cava, Budd-Chiari syndrome, priapism, or widespread clotting and defibrination syndrome. The cumulative incidences of throm-

boembolism are estimated to be 15 per cent by age 19, 50 per cent by age 29, and 85 per cent in individuals over 40 years. Complete, i.e., homozygous, lack of the major antithrombin has not been described. Patients homozygous for a dysfunctional antithrombin, however, have been reported.

Antithrombin deficiency can be ascertained by an activity assay in which diluted plasma and heparin are mixed with a known concentration of thrombin, and the amount of uninhibited thrombin is quantified with a chromogenic substrate. Ongoing thrombosis and heparin therapy both lower the concentration of plasma antithrombin. Therefore the diagnosis of antithrombin deficiency is best made after the patient has recovered from a thrombotic event.

A patient with acute thrombosis should be treated with heparin. Because of depletion of the major antithrombin, the level of antithrombin may become so low that the patient is resistant to heparin. In this case, a source of antithrombin should be infused, in the form of either fresh frozen plasma or, if available, antithrombin concentrate. The half-life of antithrombin is 16 to 24 hours. Administration of warfarin should be started promptly, and the patient probably should receive warfarin indefinitely.

Prophylactic use of anticoagulants should be considered in view of the spontaneous and unpredictable occurrence of thromboembolism with the potential for a fatal outcome. At the very least, affected individuals should be counseled about the risks of the disorder. Pregnancies should be managed in high-risk clinics prepared to cope with the difficult questions of how, when, or whether anticoagulants should be administered during the pregnancy.

Deficiency of the Minor Antithrombin (Heparin Cofactor II)

Two families have been reported in which half-normal plasma concentrations of the minor antithrombin were associated with venous and arterial thrombosis. The number of family members studied was not large enough to prove formally that the deficiency state segregates with the thrombotic deficiency, but the reports certainly are suggestive. If the association is confirmed in larger kindreds, low concentrations of minor antithrombin in a patient who has had a thrombotic event would be an indication for long-term warfarin therapy.

Boers GHJ, Smals AGH, Trijbels FJM, et al.: Heterozygosity for homocystinuria in premature peripheral and cerebral occlusive arterial disease. N Engl J Med 313:709, 1985. Mudd SH: Vascular disease and homocysteine metabolism. N Engl J Med 313:751, 1985. *Descriptions and discussions of homocystinuria as a cause of premature arterial disease.*

Clouse LH, Comp PC: The regulation of hemostasis: The protein C system. N Engl J Med 314:1298, 1986. *Summary of the biochemical and clinical evidence for the importance of proteins C and S, especially protein C, in prevention of thrombosis.*

Cosgriff TM, Bishop DT, Hershgold EJ, et al.: Familial antithrombin III deficiency: Its natural history, genetics, diagnosis and treatment. Medicine 62:209, 1983. *Comprehensive review of deficiency of the major antithrombin.*

Kamiya T, Sugihara T, Ogata K, et al.: Inherited deficiency of protein S in a Japanese family with recurrent venous thrombosis: A study of three generations. Blood 67:406, 1986. Comp PC, Doray D, Patton D, et al.: An abnormal plasma distribution of protein S occurs in functional protein S deficiency. Blood 67:504, 1986. *Studies of two large kindreds that point out some of the clinical and laboratory features of protein S deficiency.*

Rodgers GM, Shuman MA: Congenital thrombotic disorders. Am J Hematol 21:419, 1986. *Particularly good for its summary of the literature concerning the fibrinolytic system.*

Schafer AI: The hypercoagulable states. Ann Intern Med 102:814, 1985. *Balanced and well-referenced overview of primary and secondary causes of thrombosis.*

Tran TH, Marbet GA, Duckert F: Association of hereditary heparin co-factor II deficiency with thrombosis. Lancet 2:413, 1986. Sie P, Dupouy D, Pichon J, et al.: Constitutional heparin co-factor II deficiency associated with thrombosis. Lance 2:414, 1986. *Initial reports that deficiency of the minor antithrombin in plasma may predispose individuals to thrombosis. Representative of the tenuous but provocative arguments found in papers describing new deficiency syndromes associated with thrombosis.*

ACQUIRED DISORDERS OF BLOOD COAGULATION

GENERAL COMMENTS. In a number of clinical situations, the APTT and/or prothrombin time are prolonged because of acquired deficiencies: vitamin K deficiency secondary to malabsorption or dietary deficiency, severe liver disease, use of coumarin anticoagulants to lower the activity of vitamin K–dependent factors, and consumption coagulopathy associated with severe illness. Rarer causes of acquired deficiencies include selective urinary loss of a coagulation factor in nephrotic syndrome, selective adsorption of a coagulation factor, especially factor X, to amyloid, and selective depletion of a clotting factor due to development of a non-neutralizing antibody to the factor.

Vitamin K Deficiency

METABOLISM AND FUNCTION OF VITAMIN K. Vitamin K is required for the post-translational gamma-carboxylation of specific glutamyl residues in factors VII, IX, X, and II and of proteins C and S and certain other proteins, e.g., osteocalcin, which constitutes 1 per cent of the protein in bone. In vitamin K–deficient states, levels of the vitamin K–dependent plasma proteins are near normal; however, the functions of these proteins in reactions and assays (e.g., the prothrombin time) that require a phospholipid surface are severely impaired. As vitamin K deficiency develops, the activities of factor VII and protein C decrease rapidly, followed by diminished activities of factors IX, X, and II.

There are limited body stores of vitamin K. A normal diet containing green leafy vegetables provides 300 to 500 μg of vitamin K, more than enough to meet the adult daily requirement of 1 μg per kilogram of body weight. In addition, vitamin K synthesized by normal gastrointestinal bacterial flora contributes to the daily requirement. Vitamin K is a fat-soluble vitamin, and solubilization of fat must occur before vitamin K can be absorbed (Ch. 104). Hence, vitamin K deficiency may occur in bile salt–deficient states, in all malabsorptive disorders, or with an inadequate dietary intake combined with gastrointestinal sterilization by orally administered antibiotics. Vitamin K occurs naturally in two forms, vitamin K_1 (phylloquinone) and vitamin K_2 (menaquinones), both of which require lipid for absorption. A synthetic water-soluble form, vitamin K_3 (menadione), is commercially available. Despite its ready absorption from intestine, menadione must be converted to vitamin K_2 by the liver and therefore is not as rapidly effective as vitamin K_1 in promoting the gamma-carboxylation reaction.

VITAMIN K DEFICIENCY OF THE NEWBORN. At birth, vitamin K levels are low, and production of vitamin K by intestinal bacteria is insufficient to meet an infant's requirements for production of normally functioning coagulation factors. The vitamin K–deficient state lasts for three to five days and may be the reason Israelites did not circumcise their babies until the eighth day (Leviticus 12:3). Cow's milk contains some vitamin K, but human milk contains essentially none (1 to 2 μg per liter). Unless vitamin K is given, the physiologic state of neonatal hypoprothrombinemia can lead to hemorrhagic disease of the newborn in the following high-risk groups: premature infants; breast-fed infants; infants of mothers who are receiving vitamin K antagonists, especially hydantoin anticonvulsants; and infants with malabsorption. If the prothrombin time is prolonged to greater than twice normal, it is common to encounter bleeding from the umbilicus, ecchymoses and hematomas, hematuria, and, most importantly, intracranial hemorrhage. Prophylactic intramuscular administration of a 1-mg dose of vitamin K_1 at delivery virtually eliminates the risk of subsequent hemorrhage. Excessive administration (5 mg or more) of vitamin K_3 may cause hemolytic anemia and kernicterus in the newborn and should be avoided.

MALABSORPTION SYNDROMES. Malabsorptive states (Ch. 104) with impaired absorption of fat, such as adult celiac disease, regional enteritis, use of cholestyramine or neomycin, or deficient intraluminal bile salts (obstruction of biliary ducts, cholestatic liver disease), are often associated with vitamin K deficiency. Similarly, various chronic diarrheas can cause vitamin K deficiency, presumably because of decreased transit time and relative malabsorption of fats. The hallmark of vitamin K deficiency is prolonged prothrombin time. If the prothrombin time is longer than twice normal, the patient likely will have ecchymoses, gingival bleeding, hematomas, hematuria, and/or melena. Daily oral administration of vitamin K_1 in supraphysiologic doses (2 to 10 mg) prevents the deficiency and should be routine in patients with malabsorption of fat. The bleeding tendency, once developed, is easily corrected by giving 10 to 25 mg of vitamin K_1 intramuscularly. In cases in which the bleeding diathesis is so severe that intramuscular injections are contraindicated, 20 to 40 mg of vitamin K_1 may be infused intravenously. It should be infused slowly at a rate of 1 mg per minute because the vehicle in which the vitamin is dissolved can cause an adverse reaction. If this does not correct the prothrombin time, it is unlikely that additional vitamin K will have any effect.

DEBILITATED PATIENTS WHO MAY BE RECEIVING ANTIBIOTICS. Patients who are without oral intake for more than several days and receiving antibiotics should be given parenteral vitamin K_1 at a dosage of 150 μg per day because they are likely to become vitamin K deficient. Patients with uremia or malignant disease are at special risk and may become vitamin K deficient on the basis of poor oral intake alone.

Some third-generation cephalosporins have a hypothrombinemic effect that is greater than would be expected from elimination of bowel flora. It has been suggested that the N-methylthiotetrazole side chain shared by cefamandole, moxalactam, and cefoperazone is cleaved from the antibiotic and interferes with the action of vitamin K, especially in patients who are borderline deficient in vitamin K.

COUMARIN ANTICOAGULANTS. Warfarin and other coumarin anticoagulants competitively inhibit the effects of vitamin K in the post-translational gamma-carboxylation of vitamin K–dependent plasma proteins. Upon initiation of therapy, the activities of the proteins with the most rapid half-lives will be lost first. Thus the activities of the vitamin K–dependent proteins become depressed in the following order: factor VII and protein C, factor IX, factor X, and factor II. Coumarin anticoagulants are administered for a long time for the prevention of recurrent thromboembolism in patients who have experienced deep vein thrombosis and pulmonary embolism or myocardial infarction. Patients should be reliable, able to be supervised, and without known potential sources of hemorrhage in the central nervous, gastrointestinal, or genitourinary systems. The art of administration of warfarin involves balancing drug intake against vitamin K intake so as to prolong the prothrombin time about one and one-half times as compared to a normal control, e.g., 17 to 19 seconds as compared to a control of 12 seconds. Ratios below this value are less effective in preventing thrombosis, whereas values twice normal or greater carry a high risk for hemorrhage. An adult receiving a normal diet will usually need 5 to 10 mg of warfarin per day to achieve the desired ratio. After initiation of therapy, it will take three to four days before the chosen dose of warfarin will cause its maximal effect on the prothrombin time. The dose can then be altered to maintain the prothrombin time in the therapeutic range.

Once the prothrombin time is stabilized, it needs to be checked only every three to four weeks if the patient is on a stable diet and in usual health. The therapeutic dose of warfarin may change dramatically if the diet is changed or if changes are made in the intake of one of the many drugs that enhance or depress the effect of warfarin (Table 167–2). Patients should wear a bracelet or neck tag stating that they are receiving an oral anticoagulant. They should not take aspirin in any of its forms.

It is not uncommon for patients to experience slight gingival bleeding, purpura with minimal trauma, or trace hematuria

TABLE 167–2. DRUGS AND CONDITIONS THAT INFLUENCE RESPONSE TO WARFARIN

Increased Resistance to Warfarin

Hereditary warfarin resistance	Increased warfarin metabolism
Increase in vitamin K	Barbiturates
Reduced drug absorption	Primidone
Malabsorption syndrome	Carbamazepine
Liquid paraffin laxatives	Ethchlorvynol (Placidyl)
Cholestyramine resin	Glutethimide (Doriden)
Magnesium trisilicate	Meprobamate
	Griseofulvin
	Rifampin
	Nafcillin

Increased Sensitivity to Warfarin

Vitamin K deficiency	Synergism with warfarin
Malabsorption syndrome	Vitamin E
Wide-spectrum antibiotics	Anabolic steroids
Liquid paraffin	Danazol
Clofibrate	Blocking of warfarin metabolism
Displacement of albumin binding	Phenytoin sodium (Dilantin)
Phenylbutazone	Chloramphenicol
Aspirin	Clofibrate
Indomethacin	Tricyclic antidepressants
Sulindac	Erythromycin
Mefenamic acid	Cimetidine
Tolmetin	Sulfamethoxazole-trimethoprim
Ibuprofen	Sulfinpyrazone
Naproxen	Unknown mechanism
Fenoprofen	Quinine
Phenytoin sodium (Dilantin)	Quinidine
Oral hypoglycemic agents	Phenothiazine
Nalidixic acid	Disulfiram (Antabuse)
Estrogen	Sulfisoxazole
Miconazole	Amiodarone

From Peterson CE, Kwaan HC: Current concepts of warfarin therapy. Arch Intern Med 146:581, 1986.

while receiving anticoagulants in the therapeutic range. These symptoms become more marked when there is overanticoagulation, and the patient is at risk for severe gastrointestinal or genitourinary hemorrhage, bleeding or hematoma formation after trauma, and intracranial bleeding. If the prothrombin time is prolonged and increased bleeding is not a clinical problem, warfarin, which has a half-life of 35 hours, can be omitted until the desired prothrombin time is obtained. When overanticoagulation results in clinically significant bleeding, the physician can give fresh frozen plasma, 10 to 20 ml per kilogram, as a source of normal vitamin K–dependent proteins, and/or give vitamin K, depending on the immediacy of the problem and whether continuation of warfarin is necessary. The effect of plasma on the prothrombin time is immediate but temporary. The use of factor IX concentrates to treat warfarin overdose should be avoided because of occasional thrombotic complications and the risk of hepatitis. Oral or intramuscular vitamin K_1, 5 to 25 mg, should correct the prothrombin time within 8 to 24 hours. Slow intravenous infusion of vitamin K, 20 to 40 mg, should correct the prothrombin time in four to six hours. Administration of more than 5 mg of vitamin K will make the patient warfarin resistant and necessitate a round of re-anticoagulation. Therefore the best strategy for the patient who needs continued anticoagulation is to give plasma and small doses (1 to 2 mg) of vitamin K while closely monitoring the prothrombin time and clinical state.

Patients occasionally present with bleeding complications after ingestion of a coumarin compound, either surreptitiously or as a suicide attempt. Patients who take coumarins surreptitiously are usually depressed and receive gain from medical attention. They often belong to a health profession. The coumarin compounds in rat poisons are much more powerful than warfarin and can cause extreme resistance to vitamin K for weeks and even months.

Coumarin anticoagulants should not be given from the 6th to the 12th week of gestation because of the high likelihood that characteristic facial and skeletal malformations, the so-called coumarin embryopathy, will be induced. Use of cou-marin drugs in the second and third trimesters is associated with an increased incidence of CNS malformations presumed to be due to sporadic intracranial hemorrhages. If anticoagulation is needed during pregnancy, one approach is to switch to subcutaneous heparin between the 6th and 12th week and after the 38th week.

Barza M, Furie B, Brown AE, et al.: Defects in vitamin K–dependent carboxylation associated with moxalactam treatment. J Infect Dis 153:1166, 1986. *Interim summary of the moxalactam story.*

Hull R, Hirsh J, Ray R, et al.: Different intensities of oral anticoagulant therapy in the treatment of proximal-vein thrombosis. N Engl J Med 307:1676, 1982. *Good data in support of less intensive therapy.*

Iturbe-Alessio I, Fonseca MdC, Mutchinik O, et al.: Risks of anticoagulant therapy in pregnant women with artificial heart valves. N Engl J Med 315:1390, 1986. *One group's approach to a difficult subject.*

Lipton RA, Klass EM: Human ingestion of a "superwarfarin" rodenticide resulting in a prolonged anticoagulant effect. JAMA 252:3004, 1984. Jones EC, Growe GH, Naiman SC: Prolonged anticoagulation in rat poisoning. JAMA 252:3005, 1984. *Illustrative case reports.*

O'Reilly RA: Vitamin K antagonists. In Colman RW, Hirsh J, Marder VJ, et al. (eds.): Hemostasis and Thrombosis: Basic Principles and Clinical Practice. 2nd ed. Philadelphia, J. B. Lippincott Company, 1987, pp. 1367–1372.

Peterson CE, Kwaan HC: Current concepts of warfarin therapy. Arch Intern Med 146:581, 1986. *A concise review.*

Suttie JW: Vitamin K–dependent carboxylase. Ann Rev Biochem 54:459, 1985. *Update on the biochemistry of vitamin K action and the opposing effect of the coumarin anticoagulants.*

Liver Disease

The liver is the major site of synthesis of fibrinogen, plasminogen, the vitamin K–dependent proteins, the antithrombins, and many other plasma proteins. The mechanisms by which steady state concentrations of these proteins in plasma are regulated are obscure. As part of the "acute phase reaction" in response to interleukin-1 and tumor necrosis factor, the synthesis of many plasma proteins, especially fibrinogen, increases at the expense of albumin synthesis. The normal liver seems to have a considerable reserve for production of fibrinogen but to be working at near maximal capacity in the synthesis of vitamin K–dependent proteins.

Patients with liver disease occasionally develop petechiae, ecchymoses, prolonged bleeding from venipunctures, and/or gastrointestinal hemorrhage. Clinically significant bleeding may occur with biopsies and surgery. The causes of these problems are diverse.

In patients with alcoholic liver disease, bleeding can be secondary to dietary *vitamin K deficiency* and will respond promptly to oral vitamin K. With more advanced disease, patients may become vitamin K deficient on the basis of fat malabsorption as well as poor nutrition, and parenteral vitamin K must be given. The synthesis of vitamin K–dependent factors becomes impaired as hepatocytes are lost, rendering the patient resistant to parenteral vitamin K. A poor prognosis is associated with a prolonged prothrombin time (greater than 1½ times normal) that does not become corrected after intravenous vitamin K. If the patient no longer responds to parenteral vitamin K, abnormal bleeding or correction of the prothrombin time prior to invasive procedures will require transfusions of fresh frozen plasma. In fulminant hepatocellular disease, *hypofibrinogenemia* can be profound enough to be considered the cause of bleeding; in such cases, both fresh frozen plasma and cryoprecipitate should be given.

Acquired dysfibrinogenemia, manifested by abnormal fibrin polymerization, has been observed in a number of patients having hepatic diseases such as alcoholic cirrhosis, postnecrotic cirrhosis of unknown cause, drug-induced hepatic failure, and hepatoma. The fibrinogen in these patients has about twice the normal content of sialic acid, indicating an overall increase in the amount of attached carbohydrate. The clotting of these fibrinogens by thrombin is delayed in proportion to the increase of sialic acid. If the liver disease improves, the defect may disappear.

Patients with liver disease commonly have *increased fibrinolysis*, because of an inability to maintain normal levels of alpha-2-antiplasmin and/or decreased hepatic clearance of plasminogen activators. Enhanced fibrinolysis, however, is rarely the primary cause of bleeding. Occasionally, chronic, smoldering *disseminated intravascular coagulation* may develop, in which case the platelet count is decreased and levels of several coagulation factors fall because of consumption. These patients do not require therapy unless they exhibit clinically significant bleeding, in which case the approach should be the same as for patients with other causes of diffuse intravascular coagulation (see below). Patients in whom LeVeen peritoneovenous shunts have been placed and women with acute fatty liver of pregnancy and marked deficiency of the major antithrombin (<25 per cent of normal) are at particular risk to develop disseminated intravascular coagulation.

Efforts should be made to normalize the prothrombin time, fibrinogen concentration, and platelet count in patients with liver disease prior to surgery, biopsy, or other invasive procedures. Factor IX concentrates are not recommended for prophylaxis in patients in whom the prothrombin time will not correct with parenteral vitamin K because such patients are likely to be deficient in plasma antithrombin, to have decreased hepatic clearance of activated clotting factors, and therefore to be at risk for thromboembolism. Platelet concentrates should be given if the platelet count is less than 75,000 per microliter. If hypersplenism is the cause of thrombocytopenia, however, it may be difficult to achieve a satisfactory platelet count.

Blanchard RA, Furie BC, Jorgensen W, et al.: Acquired vitamin K–dependent carboxylation deficiency in liver disease. N Engl J Med 305:242, 1981. *Interesting clinical study of circulating levels of normal and abnormal factor II.*
Liebman HA, McGehee WG, Patch MJ, et al.: Severe depression of antithrombin III associated with disseminated intravascular coagulation in women with fatty liver of pregnancy. Ann Intern Med 98:330, 1983. *Presents argument that acquired deficiency of the major antithrombin can cause widespread thrombosis.*
Joisr JH: Hemostatic abnormalities in liver disease. In Colman RW, Hirsh J, Marder VJ, et al. (eds.): Hemostasis and Thrombosis: Basic Principles and Clinical Practice. 2nd ed. Philadelphia, J. B. Lippincott Company, 1987, pp 861–872. *Review with good references.*

Renal Disease

Patients with uremia occasionally develop purpura, mucous membrane bleeding, gastrointestinal hemorrhage, and prolonged bleeding from venous and arterial needle puncture sites. Such patients usually have a prolonged bleeding time. The pathogenesis of the bleeding tendency is complex. The platelet count may be low. More importantly, platelet function is abnormal because of accumulation of a dialyzable substance in the circulation (Ch. 166). Anemia contributes to platelet dysfunction in vivo, because the stirring action of red cells causes a large increase in the diffusivity of platelets and allows platelets to be transported efficiently to areas where the vessel wall is injured. Daily infusion of cryoprecipitate has been useful in correcting the bleeding tendency in uremia. Although uncertain, the correction may be related to the high molecular weight von Willebrand factor multimers contained in cryoprecipitate. Desmopressin, which is effective in raising the plasma level of von Willebrand factor in patients with von Willebrand disease (see above), temporarily corrects the bleeding time in patients with uremia. Daily intravenous administration of conjugated estrogens may also correct the bleeding time over a period of days. Thus a number of therapeutic maneuvers can be tried in a symptomatic uremic patient: dialysis to restore platelet function; transfusion to normalize red cell and platelet number; and administration of cryoprecipitate, desmopressin, or conjugated estrogen.

Coagulation factors, especially vitamin K–dependent factors and factor V, tend to be at low concentration in chronic renal disease, although not to levels that should cause bleeding. Some of these deficiencies probably result from hepatic insufficiency or from vitamin K deficiency secondary to oral antibiotic therapy, malabsorption caused by uremic enteritis, and diminished dietary intake. Very low plasma factor IX levels

(10 per cent of normal) have been observed in patients with severe nephrotic syndrome and preferential loss of factor IX into the urine. Subclinical disseminated intravascular coagulation occasionally occurs in patients with chronic renal disease, as evidenced by elevated amounts of fibrin degradation products in serum and urine. It has been suggested that loss of the major antithrombin in nephrotic syndrome may cause renal vein thrombosis. There are no clear guidelines as to when and how to treat such deficiencies. If the prothrombin time is long or the factor IX level is low in a patient who is bleeding, fresh frozen plasma is the replacement product of choice, although it may be difficult to give enough to someone who cannot compensate for the large volume.

di Minno G, Martinez J, McKean, M-L, et al.: Platelet dysfunction in uremia: Multifaceted defect partially corrected by dialysis. Am J Med 79:552, 1985. Castillo R, Lozano T, Escolar G, et al.: Defective platelet adhesion on vessel subendothelium in uremic patients. Blood 68:337, 1986. *Two studies of platelet function in uremic patients.*
Janson PA, Jubelirer SJ, Weinstein MJ, et al.: Treatment of the bleeding tendency in uremia with cryoprecipitate. N Engl J Med 303:1318, 1980. Mannucci PM, Remuzzi G, Pusineri F, et al.: Deamino-8-D-arginine vasopressin shortens the bleeding time in uremia. N Engl J Med 308:8, 1983. Livio M, Mannucci PM, Vigano G, et al.: Conjugated estrogens for the management of bleeding associated with renal failure. N Engl J Med 315:731, 1985. *Contain results of three different but possibly related approaches to improvement of the bleeding time in uremic patients. The mechanisms of the favorable clinical effects are enigmas.*
Livio M, Gotti E, Marchesi D, et al.: Uraemic bleeding: Role of anaemia and beneficial effect of red cell transfusions. Lancet 2:1013, 1982. *Evidence that patients with higher hematocrits have more normal bleeding times.*

Sporadic Acquired Factor Deficiency

A number of patients with amyloidosis have factor X deficiency because of its removal from the circulation through binding of zymogen factor X to the amyloid deposits. Patients present with mild to severe bleeding just as do individuals with the inherited form of factor X deficiency. Replacement therapy can be given with plasma or factor concentrates. However, the in vivo half-life of factor X is shortened.

Occasionally a patient is seen with isolated factor deficiency but no evidence of a neutralizing antibody, e.g., when the patient's plasma is mixed 1:1 with normal plasma, the factor level in the mixture is 50 per cent. Such a patient with factor II deficiency was recently studied in depth and shown to have a non-neutralizing antibody to factor II. Administration of corticosteroids was associated with a rise in factor II activity and cessation of bleeding, but circulating factor II was bound to antibody. These observations suggested that non-neutralizing antibodies to factor II cause plasma factor II deficiency because of rapid clearance of the antigen-antibody complexes, which is slowed by corticosteroids. Demonstration of non-neutralizing antibodies requires special techniques and takes some time. Therefore, in a patient who is bleeding seriously, one may need to begin administration of corticosteroids, possibly supplemented with fresh frozen plasma, before the diagnosis is established.

Bajaj SP, Rapaport SI, Barclay S, et al.: Acquired hypoprothrombinemia due to nonneutralizing antibodies to prothrombin: Mechanism and management. Blood 65:1538, 1985. *Although this paper describes only one patient, it illustrates what may be a fairly common happening.*
Greipp PR, Kyle RA, Bowie EJ: Factor X deficiency in amyloidosis: A critical review. Am J Hematol 11:443, 1981. *Well-documented description of the cause of this deficiency.*

Syndromes of Disseminated Intravascular Coagulation (DIC)

GENERAL COMMENTS. In the following discussion, DIC is divided into four clinical syndromes: (1) *compensated DIC,* which may be associated with thrombosis but does not result in bleeding; (2) *defibrination syndrome,* in which the mechanisms that localize blood coagulation are overwhelmed by release of tissue factor, leading to massive utilization and depletion of fibrinogen, other clotting factors, and platelets and resultant thrombosis and/or bleeding; (3) *primary fibrin-*

olysis, in which the mechanisms that localize fibrinolysis are overwhelmed by release of plasminogen activators, leading to bleeding; and (4) *microangiopathic thrombocytopenia*, in which platelet microthrombi are widespread, leading to depletion of platelets, ischemic necrosis of tissues, and microangiopathic changes in red cells. The causes of DIC syndromes are many, and there is considerable overlap among syndromes. Patients with DIC often have multiple medical problems, including bone marrow failure, liver failure, renal failure, vitamin K deficiency, and the like, which may complicate the clinical and laboratory analysis in a given patient. Much of the controversy that surrounds DIC undoubtedly stems from attempts to lump diverse conditions and patients together. Despite its oversimplicity, the following scheme is useful because the treatments of the four paradigm syndromes are quite different. For many of the diseases associated with DIC, specific descriptions of the DIC and recommendations for treatment can be found under individual diseases elsewhere in this textbook.

COMPENSATED DIC. Patients with serious underlying diseases (trauma, infection, malignant tumor, etc.) usually have increased production and consumption of platelets, fibrinogen, and other coagulation proteins. Patients with traumatized or inflamed tissues manifest an "acute phase reaction" mediated by interleukin-1 and tumor necrosis factor in which hepatic plasma protein synthesis is altered. A number of plasma alpha-1, alpha-2, and beta globulins, including alpha-2-antiplasmin and fibrinogen, increase in concentration, whereas other plasma proteins, including transferrin and albumin, decrease in concentration. In areas of trauma or inflammation, there is ongoing coagulation and fibrinolysis. Under such conditions, unclottable fibrin degradation products can be detected by immunoassay in serum. However, the prothrombin time is normal, the platelet count is normal or only minimally decreased, and plasma fibrinogen concentration is elevated. There is speculation that low-grade DIC is associated with microemboli and microthrombi that contribute to the organ failure commonly found in patients with severe illnesses. At this point, however, the only indication to use heparin or other anticoagulants in such patients is as prophylaxis or treatment of thrombosis in large vessels. An outstanding example of the need for anticoagulation is in the Trousseau syndrome of "migratory" venous thrombosis in patients with malignant disease (Ch. 171). Warfarin therapy is often ineffective in such patients, and they must instead be started on a long-term regimen of heparin therapy.

DEFIBRINATION SYNDROME. The prototype of defibrination syndrome is the rapid onset of generalized bleeding that occurs when tissue factor is released into the circulation after massive brain trauma or during amniotic fluid embolization. Laboratory tests in such patients demonstrate gross depletion of platelets and fibrinogen, increase in fibrin degradation products, prolongation of prothrombin time, and variable decreases in factors V and VIII, factor II and the other vitamin K–dependent factors, the antithrombins, and plasminogen. Defibrination syndrome occurs most frequently with shock, sepsis, cancer, burns, and obstetric complications. Patients with sepsis, especially due to meningococcus, may develop purpura fulminans or the Waterhouse-Friderichsen syndrome (hemorrhagic necrosis of vital organs, including the adrenals). The patient's hemostatic system must be supported while the patient is resuscitated and the underlying cause is treated. Thus the patient should receive platelet concentrates, cryoprecipitate as a source of fibrinogen, and fresh frozen plasma as a source of other plasma proteins, especially the antithrombins. An appropriate mix is 10 bags of cryoprecipitate for every 2 to 3 units of plasma. One's goals should be a platelet count of more than 50,000 per microliter, a fibrinogen concentration greater than 100 mg per deciliter, a prothrombin time that is within 2 to 3 seconds of normal, and a concentration of antithrombins that is greater than 40

per cent of normal. The role of heparin is controversial. It is my view that, unless the patient improves quickly or active bleeding cannot be controlled, heparin should be infused in low dosages (10 to 15 units per kilogram per hour after a loading dose of 30 to 40 units per kilogram) with the goal of dampening further defibrination as the patient's clotting components are replenished with cryoprecipitate and plasma. If the patient has overt thrombosis, the dose of heparin can be increased. The low dose of heparin should not cause lengthening of the prothrombin time or APTT or exacerbate the bleeding diathesis. Patients who are severely ill and have defibrination syndrome are at high risk of becoming vitamin K deficient and therefore should receive parenteral vitamin K.

PRIMARY FIBRINOLYSIS. Primary fibrinolysis, in its pure form, is rare and results from massive release of plasminogen activator. Conditions associated with DIC that cause "primarily" fibrinolysis, if not primary fibrinolysis, include carcinoma of the prostate, acute promyelocytic leukemia, hemangiomas, and sustained release of plasminogen activator by endothelial cells due to injection of venoms. A critical point is reached when enough plasmin is activated to deplete the circulation of alpha-2-antiplasmin. This allows plasmin to work unopposed on a variety of substrates in blood. Fibrinogen is lysed to fibrinogen degradation products. Because of the lack of fibrinogen and the inhibitory effect of degradation products on fibrin polymerization, the prothrombin time is prolonged. The platelet count, however, is appropriate for the state of the bone marrow, and antithrombin levels are normal. Ecchymoses, mucosal bleeding, and bleeding from needle puncture sites can be extensive. It is usually possible to give enough cryoprecipitate to keep plasma fibrinogen at a concentration greater than 100 mg per deciliter. There is, however, no concentrated source of alpha-2-antiplasmin. EACA, 1 gram per hour in an adult, may be effective in minimization of bleeding, and in my view it should be given a therapeutic trial in a symptomatic patient if the activity of alpha-2-antiplasmin in plasma is less than 35 to 40 per cent of normal. If there is a worry about induction of thrombosis with EACA, heparin in a low dose can be infused simultaneously as described above.

THERAPEUTIC FIBRINOLYSIS (THROMBOLYSIS). Intravenous administration of streptokinase, urokinase, or tissue plasminogen activator is accepted useful therapy for deep vein thrombosis, pulmonary embolism, acute myocardial infarction, and peripheral arterial thromboembolism. These agents re-establish patency of vessels more quickly than does heparin. The dosage and method of administration of the agents are specific for the different conditions, and in some instances the agent is administered by selective catheterization of the involved vessel.

In the case of streptokinase or urokinase administered systemically, therapeutic effectiveness requires that systemic fibrinolysis be achieved, i.e., that the patients develop iatrogenic primary fibrinolysis. Prolongation of the thrombin time to twice normal is often taken as evidence that the desired effect has been achieved. Such patients also have decreased plasma fibrinogen, plasminogen, and alpha-2-antiplasmin. In the case of streptokinase administered locally or TPA administered systemically or locally, thrombi can be lysed with variable and sometimes minimal evidence of systemic fibrinolysis.

If the level of plasminogen falls to zero, the patient will be relatively resistant to further infusion of fibrinolytic agents. At that point, or at the end of the planned infusion, there is hypercoagulability, and anticoagulation with heparin should be carried out.

The main complication of fibrinolytic therapy is hemorrhage, usually in the form of continuous, slow oozing at sites of invasive procedures. If a pressure dressing does not control this bleeding, administration of the agent can be discontinued with the anticipation that fibrinolytic activity will subside within a few hours. Fresh frozen plasma can be given if the bleeding is severe.

MICROANGIOPATHIC THROMBOCYTOPENIA. The hallmarks of microangiopathic thrombocytopenia are a low platelet count and fragmented red cells on blood smear. Although the serum may contain fibrin degradation products, the prothrombin time is generally not elevated, and the fibrinogen concentration is normal or increased. Microangiopathic thrombocytopenia can be seen in patients with sepsis, malignant disease, immune complex disease, vasculitis, malignant hypertension, eclampsia, vascular malformations, and intravascular aspergillosis. The prototype conditions, however, are hemolytic uremic syndrome (HUS) and thrombotic thrombocytopenic purpura (TTP) (Ch. 81). HUS involves mainly the vessels of the kidney, usually occurs in children, and usually is self-limited. TTP involves many organs, including the brain, usually occurs in adults, and usually causes death unless aggressively treated. Acute neurologic symptoms are the most striking feature of full-blown TTP. The pathogenesis of HUS and TTP is obscure. It has been suggested that patients lack prostacyclin; have von Willebrand factor multimers that are extra large and cause spontaneous platelet aggregation; have autoantibodies that damage endothelial cells; or have a circulating substance, possibly of microbial origin, that causes spontaneous platelet aggregation and that is neutralized by immunoglobulin present in normal plasma. There are intriguing instances in which HUS or TTP occurs in small clusters, is recurrent, or is familial. Whatever the cause(s), both HUS and TTP respond in the majority of cases to infusion of fresh frozen plasma. In some cases the requirement for plasma is so great that plasma exchange is necessary. In other cases, occasional infusion of 1 to 2 units of plasma will suffice. If extensive plasmapheresis fails, therapeutic options include use of drugs that inhibit platelet aggregation, splenectomy, and use of vincristine.

SNAKE BITES. Venoms from various snakes, especially the vipers and rattlesnakes, contain proteins that can, depending on the species, clot fibrinogen, activate factor II, factor X, protein C, or platelets; or cause release of plasminogen activator from endothelial cells. Fortunately the clinical problems associated with DIC's from venoms are not as striking as the laboratory abnormalities displayed by the victims. Treatment in most instances can be conservative: administration of antivenoms, transfusion of platelets and/or plasma, and general supportive therapy. In some instances, hypofibrinogenemia and thrombocytopenia persist for weeks.

Aster RH: Plasma therapy for thrombotic thrombocytopenic purpura: Sometimes it works, but why? N Engl J Med 312:985, 1985. *Interim analysis of a perplexing question.*

Marder VJ, Martin SE, Frances CW, Colman RW: Consumptive thrombohemorrhagic disorders. In Colman RW, Hirsh J, Marder VJ, et al. (eds.): Hemostasis and Thrombosis: Basic Principles and Clinical Practice. 2nd Ed. Philadelphia, J. B. Lippincott Company, 1987, pp 975–1015. *Richly referenced, well-organized discussion of DIC in its many guises.*

Schwartz BS, Williams EC, Conlan MG, et al.: Use of epsilon aminocaproic acid (EACA) in treatment of patients with acute promyelocytic leukemia and acquired alpha-2-antiplasmin deficiency. Ann Intern Med 105:873, 1986. *Emphasizes the importance of plasma alpha-2-antiplasmin concentration in the evaluation of fibrinolytic states.*

Verstraete M, Collen D: Thrombolytic therapy in the eighties. Blood 67:1529, 1986. *A review of a rapidly evolving field.*

ANTICOAGULANTS

GENERAL COMMENTS. An anticoagulant is any substance that, when added to blood, decreases the ability of the blood to clot. By this definition the coumarin antagonists of vitamin K are not anticoagulants, because their effect is to interfere with the hepatic synthesis of normal clotting factors. The four general categories of anticoagulation important to human clinical disease are (1) heparin and heparin-like substances, (2) factor VIII inhibitors, (3) anticoagulants associated with lupus erythematosus (so-called lupus anticoagulant), and (4) miscellaneous rare inhibitors of other clotting factors.

Heparin

Heparin is used commonly for its anticoagulant properties in the prevention of and therapy for thromboembolism and to keep blood fluid during extracorporeal circulation. By definition, 1 unit of heparin will render 1 ml of sheep blood incoagulable. The therapeutic concentration in a human (i.e., a patient with an APTT 1½ times longer than normal) is 0.1 to 0.3 units per milliliter.

Bleeding is the most common complication of heparin therapy. This can be minimized by (1) administration of the drug by continuous infusion rather than in boluses; (2) quantification of the anticoagulant effect at regular intervals by whole blood clotting times or APTT; (3) selection of patients who do not have an occult bleeding site or underlying bleeding diathesis; and (4) prohibition of aspirin and intramuscular injections. Despite this, purpura, ecchymoses, hematomas, gastrointestinal hemorrhage, hematuria, retroperitoneal bleeding, or bleeding at sites of invasive procedures may occur. Heparin is cleared from the circulation within two to four hours. Therefore if bleeding is minimal and can be controlled by local measures, discontinuation of heparin may be all that is necessary. If bleeding is severe, the effects of heparin can be counteracted by giving 1 mg of protamine sulfate for each 100 units of heparin estimated to be in the patient's circulation.

After seven to ten days of heparin therapy, thrombocytopenia sometimes occurs, subsiding when heparin is discontinued. Mild thrombocytopenia is likely due to a direct effect of heparin on platelets. In some patients the thrombocytopenia can be severe and associated with venous and/or arterial thrombosis and DIC. In these patients the thrombocytopenia is probably immunologically mediated. It is important to be alert for such a patient, because one's tendency is to treat the thrombosis by increasing the dose of heparin, only to make the situation worse. Heparin therefore should be discontinued if the platelet count drops precipitously. Low-molecular-weight heparin holds the promise of providing anticoagulant activity without undesirable reactions with platelets and may be a therapeutic option in the future for patients with heparin-induced thrombocytopenia. For the present, however, the best defense is prophylactic, i.e., to initiate warfarin therapy early so that a stable anticoagulant effect is achieved during the first week of heparin therapy.

Several patients with neoplastic plasma cell disorders have had clinical bleeding due to a circulating heparin-like proteoglycan that required the major antithrombin for its function and could be neutralized by protamine sulfate.

Turpie AGG, Levine MN, Hirsh J, et al.: A randomized controlled trial of a low-molecular-weight heparin (enoxaparin) to prevent deep-vein thrombosis in patients undergoing elective hip surgery. N Engl J Med 315:925, 1986. Salzman EW: Low-molecular-weight heparin: Is small beautiful? N Engl J Med 315:957, 1986. *Good update and review of trends in heparin therapy.*

Factor VIII Inhibitors

An endogenously produced anticoagulant, usually referred to as a circulating anticoagulant or a circulating inhibitor, is an antibody that interacts with a clotting factor in a manner that neutralizes the functional activity of the factor. Production of such an antibody is pathologic and often results in hemorrhage. Factor VIII inhibitors are commonly observed in hemophilia A (factor VIII deficiency), but are rare in nonhemophilic patients. Conditions in which sporadic factor VIII inhibitors occur include the postpartum state, diseases of immunologic dysfunction, and old age. The sporadic inhibitors induce a hemophilia-like state, i.e., a significant bleeding diathesis, but are unlike the inhibitors of hemophilic patients in several ways. They tend to be of low titer (<1 to 20 Bethesda units) and to bind factor VIII weakly. Titers often drop when patients are treated with cytoxan, 1 gram intravenously, and prednisone, 80 mg per day to be tapered once an effect is seen. Such a therapeutic response is rare in patients with hemophilia and an inhibitor. Acute bleeding episodes can be managed with variable success by continuous infusion of factor VIII concentrate or cryoprecipitate.

When a factor VIII inhibitor is present, the prothrombin time is normal but the APTT is prolonged. If the patient's plasma is incubated for several hours with an equal quantity of normal plasma, the APTT of the mixture should be prolonged. The factor VIII level in the patient's plasma and in the mixture of patient's plasma and normal plasma should be low no matter what dilutions are tested, whereas the factor IX level should be normal. These characteristics distinguish factor VIII inhibitors from the antiphospholipid inhibitors associated with lupus erythematosus (lupus-type inhibitors). A lupus-type inhibitor may cause prolongation of the prothrombin time, especially when the test is done with diluted thromboplastin; does not require an incubation period to express inhibitory activity in mixtures of patient's and normal plasma; and may interfere with the assays for both factors VIII and IX when the patient's plasma is tested at a 1:10 dilution but not when the patient's plasma is tested at a 1:200 or 1:500 dilution. The implications of having a factor VIII inhibitor versus a lupus-type inhibitor are very different, and the physician and laboratory must be sure that the correct diagnosis is made, even though there is no single test with which to make the distinction.

Herbst KD, Rapaport SI, Kenoyer DG, et al.: Syndrome of an acquired inhibitor of factor VIII responsive to cyclophosphamide and prednisone. Ann Intern Med 95:575, 1981. *Good description of six nonhemophilic patients with inhibitors.*

Lupus-Type Inhibitors

Patients with systemic lupus erythematosus sometimes develop a circulating anticoagulant unrelated to the severity or duration of disease. A similar inhibitor sometimes occurs in patients who do not have lupus. Patients who have the lupus-type inhibitor also may have anticardiolipin antibodies and thrombocytopenia. Only rarely is the inhibitor associated with clinically significant bleeding. When patients with the inhibitor do bleed, it is due to thrombocytopenia, platelet dysfunction, and/or acquired factor II deficiency. Instead, patients with the lupus-type inhibitor are at increased risk of having recurrent thromboembolic events. Thrombosis can involve both veins and arteries. There is probably accelerated atherosclerosis. Women with the inhibitor have a greatly increased incidence of spontaneous abortion. Some patients have neurologic abnormalities that may be due to cerebral thrombosis or myelitis or both. In short, the problems associated with a lupus-like inhibitor can be devastating.

Inhibition of clotting tests is thought to be a consequence of binding of the inhibitor to the acidic phospholipids used in the prothrombin time and APTT. The prolongations of both assays can be very impressive. Presumably, platelet membranes, rather than phospholipid micelles, provide the surface for activation of factors X and II, thus accounting for the fact that clinically significant bleeding does not occur. The pathogenesis of the thrombotic diathesis associated with lupus-type inhibitors is unknown. A reasonable hypothesis is that the lupus-type inhibitor and the anticardiolipin are members of a cross-reacting family of antiphospholipid antibodies, and within the family are antibodies that react in a noxious fashion with endothelial cells, e.g., to block prostacyclin production or to inhibit the cofactor activity of thrombomodulin in the protein C–protein S pathway.

Without knowledge of the pathogenesis of the thromboembolism there is no rational approach to treatment. Anticoagulants should be given, but may not be effective. It also is reasonable to try immunosuppressive therapy or plasmapheresis. Administration of corticosteroids and low-dose aspirin during pregnancy had favorable laboratory and clinical effects in a group of women with the inhibitor and impressive histories of spontaneous abortion.

Branch DW, Scott JR, Kochenour NK, et al.: Obstetric complications associated with the lupus anticoagulant. N Engl J Med 313:1322, 1985. Feinstein DI: Lupus anticoagulant, thrombosis, and fetal loss. N Engl J Med 313:1348, 1985. *Article and accompanying editorial that illustrate well the dilemmas of lupus-type inhibitors.*

Miscellaneous Inhibitors of Clotting Factors

Approximately 5 per cent of patients with factor IX deficiency (hemophilia B) develop inhibitors to factor IX after repeated transfusion. Inhibitors to factor V have been reported in about eight patients, only one of these being a factor V–deficient patient. Acquired inhibitors to von Willebrand factor activity have developed in a very few patients. An IgG inhibitor was found in a factor XIII–deficient patient following transfusion. A few patients receiving isoniazid have developed an inhibitor directed toward the fibrin cross-linking sites; this results in defective fibrin polymerization.

Myeloma or macroglobulinemia may give rise to defective fibrin polymerization as a result of interference by high concentrations of gamma globulin. If overt bleeding occurs, plasmapheresis may restore adequate hemostasis by reducing serum protein concentration.

A very interesting inborn error of alpha-1-antiproteinase (alpha-1-antitrypsin) has been reported in which the mutant serpin is a rapid, specific inhibitor of thrombin, thus causing a severe hemorrhagic diathesis.

168 INTRODUCTION

John Laszlo

HISTORICAL BACKGROUND AND DEFINITIONS

Cancer is an English term derived from the Greek word for crab, *Karkinos*, which was believed to be first used by Hippocrates, who attributed this affliction to an excess of black bile. Cancer was known in antiquity, being described in the early writings of Greeks and Romans. Tumors in Egyptian mummies dating back 5000 years represent the first known human malignant growths, although there is pathologic evidence of bone tumors occurring in dinosaurs and other prehistoric animals.

Peyton Rous, a Nobel laureate for his pioneering work on viral causes of animal tumors, wrote: "Tumors destroy man in an unique and appalling way, as flesh of his own flesh, which had somehow been rendered proliferative, rampant, predatory and ungovernable."

Cancer is a prevalent group of diseases, with more than 900,000 new cases diagnosed annually in the United States and more than 600,000 deaths. Trends in the cancer death rates for males and females are shown in Figures 168–1 and 168–2. More than five million Americans have survived cancer; in more than three million of these the diagnosis was established five or more years ago.

Any definition of cancer must consider (1) the property of an uncontrollable growth of cells originating from normal tissues and (2) the property of killing the host by means of local extension or distant spread (metastasis). Cancer has been defined in terms of an autonomous growth that is unresponsive to normal regulatory factors; in terms of the irreversibility with which cancer cells progressively lose the differentiated characteristics and functions of the normal tissue of origin; on the basis of morphologic or cytogenetic features; and on the basis of reversion to growth and antigenic properties characteristic of fetal cells. All of these qualities are typical of most cancer cells, but they are not universally characteristic. The exceptions make any single definition suspect. Some endocrine-related tumors, for example, not only closely resemble the morphologic features of the tissue of origin but also mimic its functions. They may even be at least partially responsive to hormonal control.

Certain animal and human tumors are capable of differentiation and even spontaneous remission. The embryonal cell carcinoma, for example, may begin with a single type of undifferentiated cell and give rise to highly differentiated teratoid tumors containing tissues such as cartilage and hair. Human leukemic cells can be stimulated to undergo terminal differentiation in vitro, and there is the potential to accomplish this by pharmacologic means in patients. Even the property of rapid growth is not characteristic of most tumors, nor does it distinguish a tumor from rapidly growing fetal tissues or certain normal adult tissues such as bone marrow cells or

gastrointestinal epithelium. For example, chronic lymphocytic leukemia results from the accumulation of a slowly proliferating clone of small (B) lymphocytes that are identifiable because they share characteristic enzymatic and cell membrane properties. Etiology is not useful as a means of separating cancers from normal tissues, since the etiology is usually unknown. Indeed, different causes of a single type of malignant tumor may give rise to varying behavior. For example, acute myelogenous leukemia arising de novo differs in its behavior from a morphologically similar leukemia caused by exposure to ionizing radiation.

Shimkin MB: Contrary to Nature. Washington, D.C., US Department of Health, Education and Welfare, 1977. *An outstanding and eminently readable work on the development of knowledge about cancer from earliest records to modern times. This well-illustrated book traces the impact of the scientists and institutions that have contributed to cancer research throughout the world.*

ETIOLOGY

Many chemicals (benzpyrene, aflatoxin, arsenicals, asbestos), viruses, and physical agents (ionizing radiation, ultraviolet light) can serve as carcinogenic stimuli capable of inducing malignant transformation in animals or humans (Ch. 170). Some cancers are iatrogenic in origin, as in patients who develop acute leukemia or other cancers years after being cured of systemic cancer by the use of cytotoxic chemotherapeutic drugs, or in patients who receive prolonged immunosuppressive therapy as part of their renal transplantation program.

Substances that are not themselves carcinogens may serve as co-carcinogens in that they promote tumor formation when given in conjunction with or following exposure to specific carcinogens. The major public health hazard relating to cancer in the United States is from the use of *tobacco products. The incidence, time to occurrence, and site of cancer depends upon the frequency and mode of use (smoking, chewing), as well as on exposure to potentiating factors such as alcohol or asbestos.* About one third of cancers in the United States and Europe are related to the use of tobacco products. Additionally, *host susceptibility* is a critical determinant in the carcinogenic process, for a known carcinogen may cause cancer, premalignant changes, or no detectable effect in a given person. This is partly explained by genetic (or acquired) differences in the metabolism of a precursor to the proximate carcinogen and by differences in hormonal milieu and immunologic resistance.

In addition to the use of tobacco, other aspects of lifestyle appear to be important contributors to human carcinogenesis. A high intake of dietary fat increases susceptibility of numerous forms of cancer. Low fiber and low calcium intake appear to increase the risk for colon cancer. High alcohol intake increases oral cancer. All of these are common in most industrialized nations of the Western world. Sexual lifestyle also can be etiologic, as with the high incidence of cervical cancer among women who have many sexual partners (presumably due to papilloma virus) and the high incidence of Kaposi's sarcoma among male homosexuals with AIDS.

Fundamental mechanisms that govern the etiology of human cancer, a subject devoid of new ideas for many years, have recently become enormously exciting as new information

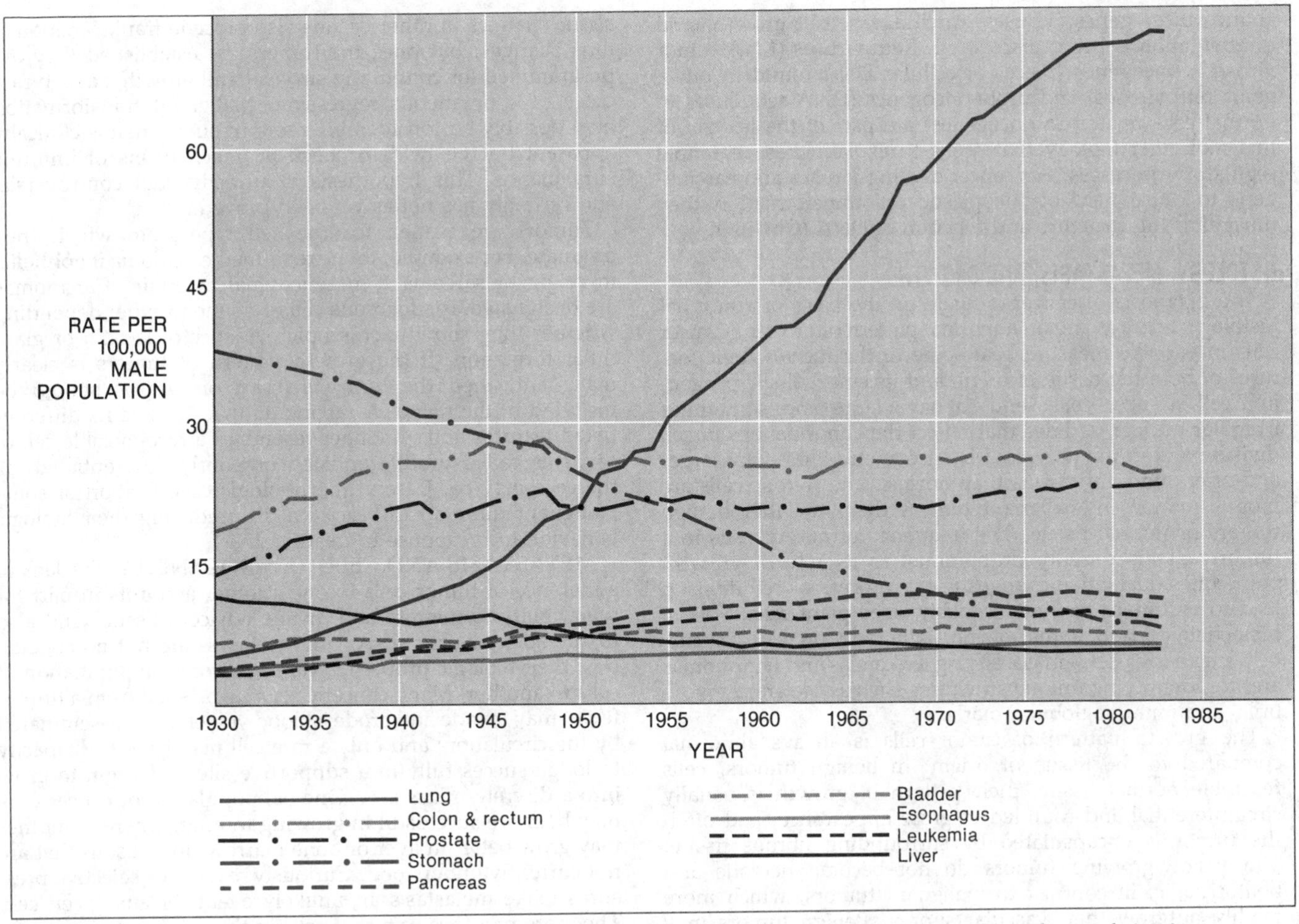

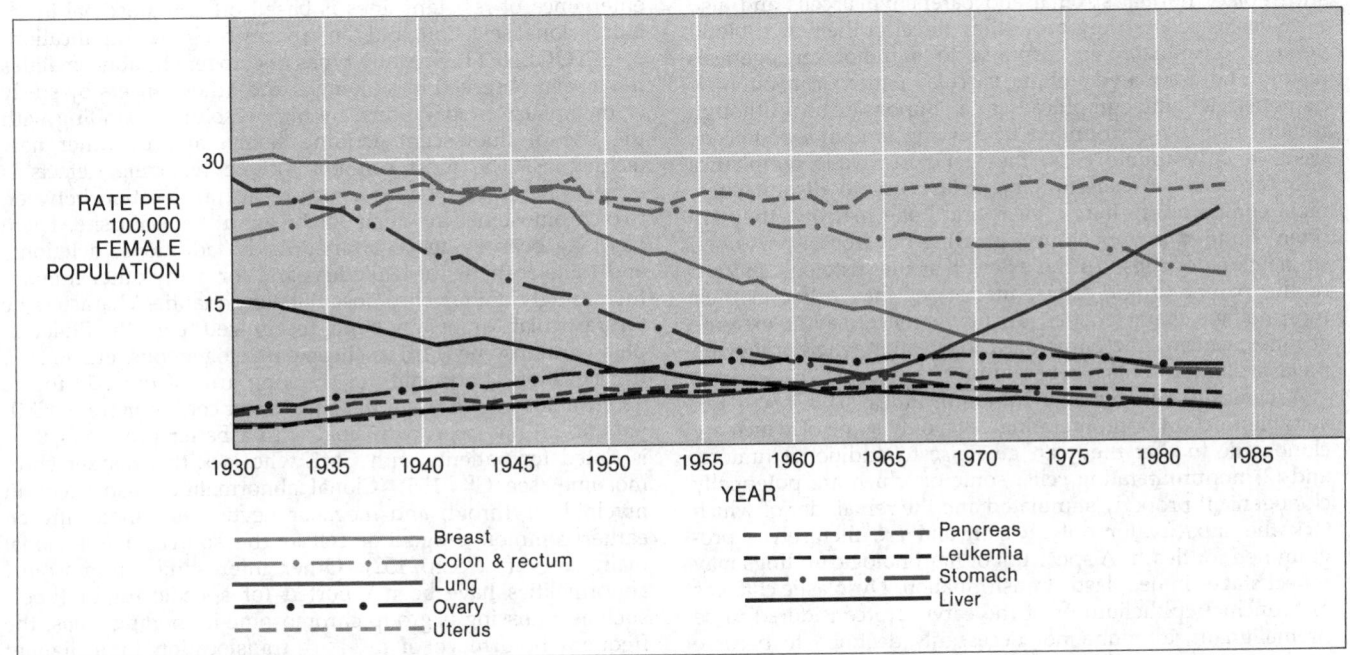

FIGURE 168–1. Male cancer death rates by site in the United States, 1930 to 1983. The rate for the male population is standardized for age on the 1970 United States population. Sources for statistics are the National Vital Statistics Division and Bureau of the Census, United States. (Courtesy of the Epidemiology and Statistics Department, American Cancer Society.)

FIGURE 168–2. Female cancer death rates by site in the United States, 1930 to 1983. The rate for the female population is standardized for age on the 1970 United States population. Sources for statistics are the National Vital Statistics Division and Bureau of the Census, United States. (Courtesy of the Epidemiology and Statistics Department, American Cancer Society.)

about cancer genes, viruses, carcinogens, cell growth, and differentiation is being discovered. Retroviruses (RNA tumor viruses), oncogenes (pieces of cellular DNA found in oncogenic retroviruses) and proto-oncogenes (DNA sequences in normal cells related to oncogenes) are part of the lexicon of this molecular biology that seeks to explain these essential regulatory processes. For cancer-causing viruses and carcinogens to cause heritable neoplastic cell transformation they must alter the structure and function of DNA (Ch. 169).

HISTOLOGY, METASTASIS, AND GROWTH

The diagnosis of cancer is made on the basis of abnormal histologic features and an abnormal pattern of growth. Cancer cells in variable measure bear some of the morphologic features of both the tissue of origin and its embryologic progenitor cell. Cancer cells tend to have large and sometimes irregular nuclear outlines that reflect the abnormalities in cell division and in the polyploid DNA content. Nuclei are larger and often more numerous than normal, and mitotic cells are more common in malignant tumors than in either benign tumors or normal tissue. The frequency of mitotic cells in a tumor mass is roughly proportional to its rate of growth. Sometimes qualitative changes in the process of cell division lead to multinucleated and variably sized giant cells. Special histochemical and immunologic stains and procedures may be particularly useful in classifying leukemias and lymphomas and for identifying unique structures such as melanin, myofibrils, and immunoglobulin markers.

The growth pattern of tumor cells is always abnormal compared to the tissue of origin. In benign tumors, cells resemble normal tissue; their pattern of growth is usually circumferential and rounded in gross appearance, and often the tumor is encapsulated by surrounding fibrous tissue. These slow-growing tumors do not become necrotic and hemorrhagic, in contrast to malignant tumors, which more readily outgrow their vascular supply. Benign tumors may show a spectrum of variation from normal, and on occasion the distinction between a benign and a malignant lesion on the basis of histology alone may be subtle. Malignant tumors are more deviant in their cellular and organizational characteristics, and the cells adhere less to one another. Aided by the elaboration of proteases, they thus tend to spread locally and replace normal stromal and parenchymal cells and also to metastasize. As they grow they develop their own blood vessels, presumably in response to a tumor angiogenesis factor. The associated unique vascular pattern can often be demonstrated angiographically as a "tumor blush." Although tumors may be surrounded by varying amounts of fibrous tissue and lymphoid cells, they tend to invade lymphatics and capillaries. When tumors metastasize to distant sites, most commonly to lungs, liver, and bone marrow, they are often rounded in appearance, growing out from a presumed single clone of cells. To the extent that the histologic pattern of the parent tumor varies, metastases may differ in their morphologic characteristics. This divergence may be extreme at times, causing the pathologist to question whether a given metastasis represents a separate primary tumor.

A clinically recognizable tumor includes (1) a small but variable fraction of proliferating cells, only some of which are clonogenic in that they can give rise to additional tumors, and (2) nonproliferating cells, some of which are potentially clonogenic if properly stimulated and the remainder of which lack the capacity for cell division and are themselves programmed for death. A spectrum of morphologic findings may reflect stages in neoplastic transformation. Dysplastic changes of bronchial epithelium or of the cervix are considered to be premalignant, although not necessarily destined to become cancerous, particularly if the inciting stimulus is removed. As cells become more anaplastic in appearance, they may begin to show microscopic invasion, progressing from carcinoma in situ to microscopic invasion to overt invasive disease. *Dys-*

plastic changes in other organs also precede frank carcinomatous changes, but once the tumors are established they are programmed for continuing survival and growth, save in rare cases of spontaneous regression. Malignant transformation may possibly be considerably more frequent than is clinically apparent but be held in check by mechanisms of immune surveillance. This hypothesis is attractive but controversial and certainly has not as yet been proved.

Tumors are named for the cell type from which they originate. For example, they are termed carcinoma if epithelial in origin or sarcoma if mesenchymal in origin. Carcinomas are designated as squamous cell or adeno in type, depending whether they show microscopic evidence of keratin or glandular formation. If the growth pattern of tumors is clearly malignant, then the term *carcinoma* or *sarcoma* should be included in the name. A carcinoma that has lost its differentiated features and no longer resembles a recognizable cell of origin is called undifferentiated or poorly differentiated, as the case may be. Careful morphologic classification of some malignant tumors can be critical in predicting their biologic behavior and response to treatment.

METASTASIS AND CELL HETEROGENEITY. The lack of adherence of tumor cells to one another accounts in part for their ability to migrate and invade adjacent tissues and also to spread to distant sites. Tumor masses are not homogeneous; their biologic properties vary from one subpopulation of cells to another. Many cancer cells may be shed from a tumor; fewer may invade and erode a blood vessel to be disseminated by the circulation; and only a rare cell may have the capacity to lodge successfully in a supportive site and begin to grow into a discrete metastasis. One subpopulation of cancer cells may be more successful in growing in lung, whereas another may grow better in liver or bone marrow, for reasons that are not currently understood. Curiously, extensive selective pressures make metastasis an unlikely event for any given cell. The mere presence of tumor cells in the venous drainage of a tumor specimen does not necessarily presage the development of a metastasis. Metastases, like the primary tumor, may cause pressure symptoms or replace normal tissues to damage the host further. The phenotypic heterogeneity of tumors may explain the emergence of resistant lines following chemotherapy, radiation therapy, or hormonal therapy. The emergence of resistant lines is based on chromosomal instability, clonal selection, and the capacity for gene amplification.

CYTOGENETICS. Many types of cytogenetic abnormalities have been observed in leukemias and other cancers by study of metaphase preparations, by high resolution banding with the use of fluorescent acridine stains, and by other new techniques. The most common of the recurring defects is either a band deletion or a reciprocal translocation between two chromosomes in which one breaks at a specific site. There has long been evidence of aneuploidy, additions, deletions, and translocations for leukemias and for many other tumors. Increasingly unique chromosomal abnormalities characteristic for particular tumors are being recognized, e.g., the Philadelphia chromosome (Ph[1]) in chronic myelogenous leukemia, a translocation abnormality of the long arm of the G22 to the C9 chromosome. Present in some 85 per cent or more of CML patients, it has been correlated with a better prognosis than is noted for patients with CML who lack this marker chromosome (see Ch. 155). Clonal abnormalities also occur in myeloid, erythroid, and megakaryocytic cells, indicating an earlier common progenitor cell as the source of this clonal malignancy (see Ch. 152). Other interesting chromosomal abnormalities have been reported for specific tumor types, such as a missing G group chromosome in meningiomas, the frequent occurrence of a 14 q+ translocation in malignant lymphomas, and the aneuploid cytogenetic characteristics of adult leukemia. A series of chromosomal abnormalities are found in Burkitt's lymphoma, Wilms' tumor, neuroblastoma, and small cell lung cancer.

Pierce GB, Fennell RH: Pathogenesis of cancer: In Holland JF, Frei E III (eds.): Cancer Medicine. Philadelphia, Lea & Febiger, 1982, p 149. *A lively discussion of the properties of cancer cells and how they relate in histology and growth to the normal cells of origin. Subsequent chapters on tumor invasion, metastases, cell kinetics, and cytogenetics also give details to supplement this introductory chapter.*

Yunis JJ: The chromosomal basis of human neoplasia. Science 221:227, 1983. *Summarizes evidence obtained by newer techniques that chromosomal abnormalities exist in most malignant neoplasms. It integrates the emerging oncogene story with findings of consistent morphologic evidence of chromosomal deletion, translocation, and so on.*

GROWTH KINETICS. Oncologists endeavor to quantify the growth rate of tumors as objectively as possible, using such parameters as the growth fraction of tumors, the duration of the cell cycle, the number of cells in the resting (G_0) phase, and the rate of cell death and removal (Fig. 168–3). The kinetics of tumor growth are crucial in determining prognosis and are also factors in determining response to chemotherapy. "Doubling time" tends to be characteristic of particular tumors. *A tumor that has reached the size of clinical detectability (ca. 1 cm) has already undergone approximately 30 doublings to reach 10^9 cells. Only 10 further doubling cycles are required to produce a tumor burden of approximately 1 kg, which is usually lethal.*

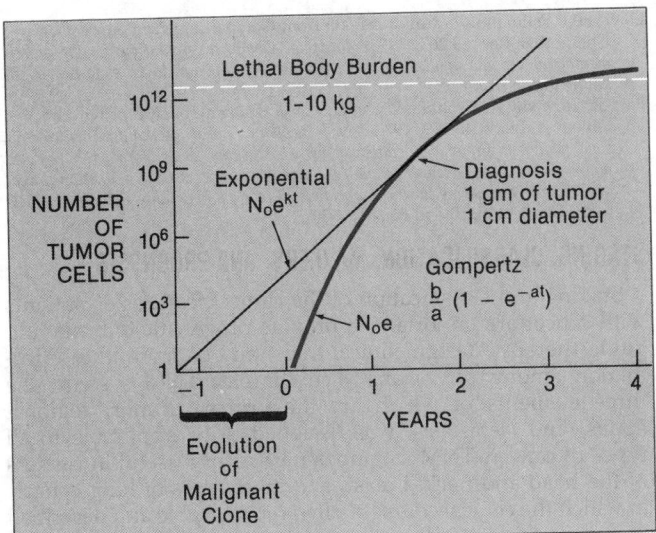

FIGURE 168–4. A schematic log-linear plot to describe models of exponential and gompertzian growth curves. Over any short span of observation it is not possible to distinguish between the two, but conclusions drawn about the latent period, prognosis, and susceptibility to treatment may be quite different between the two models. (Courtesy of Dr. Edwin Cox.)

The simple exponential growth curve is a useful first approximation to the growth of tumors (Fig. 168–4). Deviation of the growth rate from a simple exponential expression has important implications for early diagnosis and for explaining difficulties in curing bulky tumors. As most tumors grow, the generation time of dividing cells remains fairly constant, but an ever increasing percentage of daughter cells enters a nonproliferating state, G_0, from which they may (potentially) be recruited back into cell cycle if the tumor cell population is reduced (Fig. 168–3). In many instances, less than 10 per cent of the cells constituting the tumor mass are actively proliferating by the time the tumor is detected; thus the remaining 90 per cent of cells are not susceptible to most antimetabolites because they are not engaged in DNA synthesis. The progressive movement of cells into G_0 and the increasing relative death rate of cells as the tumor grows larger combine to produce a slowing of the relative growth rate, reflected in a deviation of the growth curve away from a simple exponential function.

Tumor growth curves are often better described by the Gompertz equation, which has also been found useful to describe biologic growth, such as the growth of the human fetus, of individual organs, and of transplantable tumors. Tumors described by the Gompertz curve appear to be growing exponentially over any short span of observation, up to three or four doublings. Observation over a longer time span reveals the gradual slowing of relative growth rate (Fig. 168–4), to an eventual plateau level at which the rate of new cell production just equals the rate of cell loss. Fitting an exponential curve to tumors that show a Gompertz growth characteristic is somewhat misleading in that it underestimates the underlying growth rate, overestimates the latent cell line, and predicts more rapid progression and death than are observed.

A number of concepts for cancer treatment based on this kinetic model have been suggested (see Ch. 176). One of these is surgical "debulking" of tumors to reduce them to a small size at which their growth rate increases and the cells are more susceptible to chemotherapy as a function of increased cell division. The availability of more potent and potentially curative chemotherapy programs has given this added importance. A second and related notion is that of deriving comparable equations for expressing cell killing by drugs, in order to predict how many courses of treatment would be required to achieve a total cell kill.

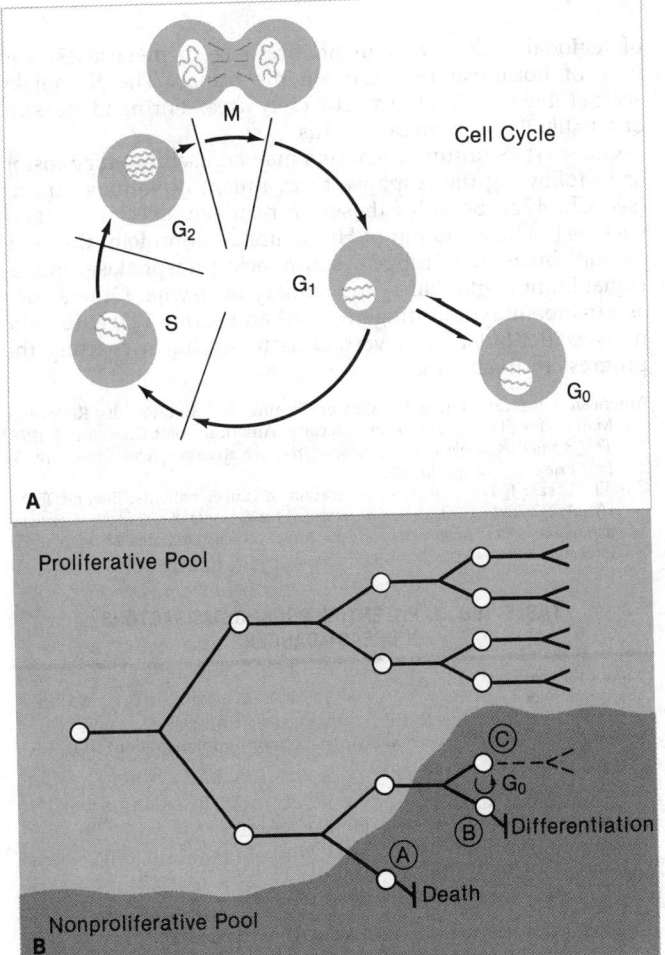

FIGURE 168–3. *A,* A diagrammatic representation of the events during the cell cycle. M is the period of mitosis—approximately one hour from prophase to cell division. G_1 reflects normal cell metabolism prior to DNA synthesis and usually constitutes more than half of the total cell generation time. Cells not actively undergoing replication are described as being G_0; here they may remain indefinitely or be recruited back into the cycle. The DNA synthetic (S) phase is generally 6 to 24 hours. *B,* A schematic representation of tumor growth. As the cell population expands, a progressively higher percentage of cells leave the proliferative pool by death (A), by differentiation (B), or by entering resting phase G_0 (C) from which they may be recruited back into the proliferative pool if the population site is reduced.

Lloyd HH: Estimation of tumor cell kill from Gompertz growth curves. Cancer Chemother Rep 59:267, 1975. *Illustrates Gompertz growth curves for experimental tumors and applies theories on tumor growth rates to estimate tumor cell killing due to treatment.*

Rai KR, Sawitsky A, Cronkite DP, et al.: Clinical staging of chronic lymphocytic leukemia. Blood 46:219, 1975. *Tumor burden and prognosis can be predicted for some malignant growths by statistical analysis of simple descriptors. More complex and sophisticated systems for multiple myeloma have also been developed that depend upon estimating the mass of malignant cells by its immunoglobulin products (e.g., Durie et al.: Blood 55:364, 1980).*

STAGING, CLASSIFICATION, MARKERS, AND PROGNOSIS

Staging and classification of the clinical features of patients with cancer are important to provide prognostic information, guide therapy, design clinical trials, and communicate information among physicians. The complex TNM system, the three elements of which are the primary *tumor*, regional *nodes*, and *metastasis*, was designed to be applicable to all types of cancer. TNM staging is particularly useful in cancers of the head and neck, breast, and most types of lung cancer, in which the clinical course is often reproducible and described by progression of disease as a local growth, followed by increasing regional node involvement, and finally by distant metastasis (Table 168–1). By contrast, it is less useful for tumors such as small cell lung cancer, which tend to metastasize early. The size of the primary tumor ranges up to 2 cm for T_1 lesions, 2 to 4 cm for T_2, and larger than 4 cm for T_3 (these criteria vary slightly for some other tumors). Progressive involvement of regional nodes is clinically assessed from the nondemonstrable N_0 to the large and fixed nodes of an N_3 lesion. Metastases are either clinically unsuspected, M_0, or are present beyond the cervical lymph nodes, M_1, in the case of head and neck cancer. Related staging systems based on anatomic extent of disease are also useful for tumors such as cervical cancer and Hodgkin's disease. Indeed, the combined contribution of careful morphologic classification, clinical staging, and substaging together with systematic treatment is best demonstrated in Hodgkin's disease, in which these concerted studies have raised the overall curability from 10 per cent to over 80 per cent during the past 25 years.

The use of the TNM system by practicing physicians is still the exception rather than the rule. In addition to anatomic extent of disease, other determinants affect prognosis, response to treatment, and quality of life (Table 168–2). Table 168–3 relates the general factors listed in Table 168–2 to specific prognostic factors in breast cancer, and is designed to include almost all factors potentially relevant to outcome. Not all of these are equally important, or even comparable for different tumors. In breast cancer the most commonly used information includes the characteristics of the local lesion (size, location, fixation, skin or nipple involvement), extent

TABLE 168–1. THE TNM SYSTEM

Primary Tumor (T)	
T_0	No evidence of primary tumor
T_{1b}	Carcinoma in situ
T_1, T_2, T_3, T_4	Progressive increase in tumor size and involvement, e.g., for breast cancer, 0–2 cm, 2–5, >5, any size plus skin or chest wall
Regional Lymph Nodes (N)	
N_0	Regional nodes not demonstrable
N_{1a}, N_{1b}	Homolateral regional nodes (breast): metastases not suspected (a), suspected (b)
N_2, N_3	Homolateral regional nodes: fixed axillary (N_2), homolateral supraclavicular (N_3), or edema of arm; metastases suspected
N_x	Regional lymph nodes cannot be assessed clinically
Distant metastasis (M)	
M_0	No known distant metastasis
M_1	Distant metastasis present
Specific site _____	

The Manual for Staging of Cancer may be obtained free of charge from the American Joint Committee, 55 East Erie Street, Chicago, Ill. 60611.

TABLE 168–2. POSSIBLE DETERMINANTS OF RESPONSE TO TREATMENT AND LENGTH AND QUALITY OF SURVIVAL

I. Biologic characteristics of tumor
  a. Growth fraction
  b. Generation time
  c. Rate of spontaneous cell loss
  d. Degree of differentiation, cell-cell interaction
  e. Propensity to metastasis
II. Host resistance
  a. Status of immune competency
  b. Nutrition
  c. Co-morbid medical conditions
III. Host-tumor interaction
  a. Microenvironment, invasiveness
  b. Location of tumor
    (1) Interference with function of vital organs
    (2) Extirpation without harm to vital functions
  c. Systemic effects of tumor, paraneoplastic syndromes
  d. Occurrence of metastasis (regional node involvement)
  e. Site of metastasis, multiple versus single
  f. Endocrine and other metabolic modulation of tumor growth
IV. Effect of treatment on the tumor versus effect on host
  a. Completeness of extirpation of primary tumor
  b. Timing of primary extirpation with respect to occurrence of metastasis
  c. Dose-response relationship to tumor cell killing
  d. Toxicity, therapeutic ratio
  e. Reinforcement of normal host defense mechanisms (immunostimulation, fibrosis in irradiated area)

of regional node involvement, presence of metastases, and type of hormonal receptors on the tumor. The Karnofsky scale (Table 168–4) is the most widely used shorthand measure of a patient's performance status.

Other types of tumor markers may be useful in diagnosing or in following the response to treatment of various cancers (see Ch. 172). Some of these are relatively specific markers such as the beta subunit of HCG, alpha-fetoprotein, thyrocalcitonin, breast cyst antigen, serum acid phosphatase, monoclonal immunoglobulins, and urinary lysozyme. Others such as carcinoembryonic antigen (CEA) and serum LDH are quite nonspecific, but may nevertheless be useful in charting the progress of treatment.

American Joint Committee for Cancer Staging and End-Results Reporting: Manual for Staging of Cancer. Chicago, American Joint Committee, 1978. *This manual is available free of charge from the American Joint Committee, 55 East Erie St., Chicago, Ill. 60611*

Cox EB, Laszlo J, Freiman A: Classification of cancer patients: Beyond TNM. JAMA 242:2691, 1979. *A critical review of the elements of classification systems, with a discussion of how computers can help to expand clinicians' ability to assess individual patients.*

TABLE 168–3. POTENTIAL PROGNOSTIC FACTORS IN BREAST CANCER*

Primary disease
  Epidemiology
    Familial occurrence (I, II, III)
    Endocrine milieu (menstrual history, hormone administration) (IIIf)
  Primary lesion
    Size (IVb)
    Location (IIIb, IIId, IVa)
    Histologic type and grade (Ia, Id, IIIa)
    Ulceration, invasion, fixation (IIIa, IIIb)
    Kinetic analysis, thymidine labeling (Ia, Ib, Ic)
    Pathology description of surgical specimen (IVa)
  Extraprimary
    Involvement of regional lymph nodes (Ie, IIId, IIIe, IVb)
    Metastatic involvement—history and physical examination, screening and selected special studies (Ie, IIId, IIIe, IVb)
Recurrent disease
  Time to first recurrence (Ia, Ib, Ic, IIIf, IVa)
  Site(s) of metastasis (Ie, IIIa, IIIb, IIIf)
  Hormone receptors and hormonal responsiveness (IIIf, IVd)
  Doubling time, kinetic studies (Ia, Ib, Ic)
  Response to chemotherapy (IVc, IVd)
  Response to radiation therapy (IVc, IVd, IVe)
  Serum calcium (IIIc)
General
  Skin testing, immunoglobulin levels, macrophage chemotaxis (IIa)
  General medical history and physical (IIb, IIc)

*Numerals refer to Table 168–2.

TABLE 168–4. "PERFORMANCE STATUS" (KARNOFSKY SCALE)

Criteria of Performance Status (PS)

Able to carry on normal activity; no special care is needed	100	Normal; no complaints; no evidence of disease
	90	Able to carry on normal activity; minor signs or symptoms of disease
	80	Normal activity with effort; some signs or symptoms of disease
Unable to work; able to live at home and care for most personal needs; a varying amount of assistance is needed	70	Cares for self; unable to carry on normal activity or to do active work
	60	Requires occasional assistance but is able to care for most needs
	50	Requires considerable assistance and frequent medical care
Unable to care for self; requires equivalent of institutional or hospital care; disease may be progressing rapidly	40	Disabled; requires special care and assistance
	30	Severely disabled; hospitalization is indicated although death not imminent
	20	Very sick; hospitalization necessary; active supportive treatment is necessary
	10	Moribund, fatal processes progressing rapidly
	0	Dead

DIAGNOSIS OF CANCER AND ITS COMPLICATIONS

GENERAL EVALUATION. The diagnosis of cancer can be simple or it can tax all of the skills of clinical investigation, depending on the site and extent of the disease The challenge is to detect cancer as early as possible, when it is most likely to be curable. In large cancer centers one third of new patients are found to have in situ or localized cancer, one quarter to have regional disease, and one third to have distant disease. The rest of the cancers are unknown or unstaged. Early detection of localized, malignant disease is aided by an awareness of risk factors in the family history, personal habits (tobacco, alcohol, sun exposure) and occupational exposure (e.g., asbestos, chromium, plastic factory). It also requires attention to subtle and nonspecific symptoms of fatigue, weakness, weight loss, depression, headache, pain, changes in bowel habits, persistent cough or hoarseness, and other clues from the history. The frequency with which the diagnosis of cancer results from attention to such nonspecific manifestations is obviously much less than if the patient presents with physical evidence such as masses in the skin or abdomen, enlargement of nodes or organs, evidence of lymphatic or venous obstruction, or pleural or ascitic effusions.

The physician should carefully examine the nose, oral cavity, pelvis, and rectum for masses or ulcerated lesions as part of any complete evaluation, and these should not be "deferred." More subtle clues may be seen in the skin with petechiae, with hyperpigmentation of skin folds (acanthosis nigricans), rarely with herpes zoster that can antedate the finding of certain cancers such as lymphoproliferative cancers, or with peculiar types of neuromyopathies (see Ch. 174 and 175). Leads from laboratory testing may be found in unexplained anemia, thrombocytopenia, hypercalcemia, or elevation of serum LDH and alkaline phosphatase, or by specific search for tumor markers.

INITIAL DIAGNOSIS. There are two major categories of diagnostic problems: obtaining the original diagnosis, and correctly identifying the many types of complications or intercurrent illnesses which may arise during the course of the disease. The former is usually the simpler of the two, requiring a tissue diagnosis, for example, in a patient who has a signal lesion in the lung, an enlarging lymph node, or a skin lesion. Intra-abdominal disease is more difficult to find—for example, in the patient with anorexia and extensive weight loss who has a pancreatic neoplasm. Fortunately, advances in imaging techniques (ultrasound, CT scanning,

liver and spleen scanning) frequently help to demonstrate pancreatic tumor tissue when it exists (see Ch. 109). Radionuclide bone scanning is a powerful tool for detecting metastases that are not yet visible on standard bone radiographs, although bone scans may also be abnormal owing to arthritis or previous trauma. *Indirect diagnostic techniques are not a substitute for a histologic or cytologic diagnosis of cancer.* Occasionally it may not be possible to obtain tissue for histologic diagnosis, e.g., when there is a deep-seated brain tumor.

Physicians often face the diagnostic dilemma posed by the discovery of a metastatic lesion when the primary site of tumor is unknown. For example, a mass on the arm is excised and found to be an adenocarcinoma, but radiographic studies of lung, bowel, and kidneys are normal. The most common sources of such lesions are tumors of the lung and pancreas. Even so, the majority of primary sites are never found. It is of dubious value to perform blind and invasive diagnostic procedures in the absence of some directive clues. One constructive action that can be taken is to consider the possibility of extragonadal germ cell tumors in patients under 50 years of age. The finding of mediastinal, retroperitoneal, or lymph node involvement and high HCG or alpha-beta protein levels may be indicative of germ cell tumors. These may respond dramatically to cisplatin-based chemotherapy programs.

DETECTION AND SCREENING. How can the presence of cancer be detected at a curable stage in asymptomatic people? It is not sufficient to make an earlier diagnosis unless that knowledge prolongs life. Detailed discussion of the cost-benefit factors of various screening techniques is beyond the scope of this chapter. It is almost impossible to prove that a detection test decreases mortality. Simple and inexpensive measures such as self-examination of the breasts or testes, routine cervical cytology, and examination of stools for occult blood seem more likely to be of value, particularly in high risk groups, than frequent chest x-ray examinations, routine proctoscopy, and widespread mammography. The latter procedures are better advised for specific high-risk groups, but even some of these points are highly debatable. For example, mammography is the most effective means of detecting small (<0.5 cm) cancers, and the cost of this procedure is falling, which improves the risk-benefit ratio. The routine use of mammography leads to additional biopsies, however, which are costly, and usually the results show the lesion is benign. This creates a dilemma of some magnitude, as does screening stool specimens for occult blood. (The American Cancer Society is a good source of guidelines for various screening procedures.)

Diagnostic approaches taken for the *symptomatic patient* are relatively direct compared to the question of cost-effectiveness of mass screening, which is more difficult and controversial. How much testing is advisable for a concerned asymptomatic patient who can afford noninvasive procedures even if they have a lower yield than would seem appropriate for mass screening? There are no good sources or valid generalizations about this subject, and the answer will depend on the information and attitude of the doctor and relationship with the patient. It comes down to the doctor recommending what would be optimal and the patient selecting on the basis of all information.

DIAGNOSTIC PROBLEMS DURING CONTINUING CARE OF THE PATIENT WITH CANCER. The physician who undertakes the continuing care of a patient with cancer must be vigilant in promptly identifying complications arising from the progression of tumor, and in detecting curable intercurrent illness which may be mistaken for manifestations of cancer itself. The patient with a known tumor who develops anorexia, weight loss, and jaundice may have cholecystitis and biliary obstruction, rather than metastatic cancer, and may die from that disorder unless the correct diagnosis is established. Furthermore, some potentially treatable conditions are actually caused by the cancer therapy—as in postoperative adhesions or radiation-induced strictures leading to bowel obstruction, or chemotherapy-induced immunosuppression leading to an opportunistic fungal infection. Certain drugs may even produce complications that simulate paraneoplastic syndromes, such as inappropriate secretion of ADH, neuromyopathy, or cerebellar degeneration. Although errors in diagnosis of intercurrent medical and surgical illness sometimes seem almost inevitable, the best way to minimize these problems is to *assume that each new condition is due to a nonmalignant process, until it is proven otherwise.*

Eddy DM: Finding cancer in asymptomatic people. Cancer 51:2440, 1983. *The author reviews the degrees of evidence that early detection tests are effective in reducing mortality, with emphasis on the two areas (breast, lung) in which randomized controlled studies exist.*

Greco FA, Vaughn WK, Hainsworth JD: Advanced poorly differentiated carcinoma of unknown primary site: Recognition of a treatable syndrome. Arch Intern Med 104:547, 1986. *A positive approach to treatment of patients who have cancer of unknown origin.*

PRINCIPLES OF MANAGEMENT OF THE PATIENT WITH CANCER

APPROACHES TO TREATMENTS. A therapeutic strategy should be clearly defined for each patient with cancer, once the diagnosis has been firmly established, staging of the tumor has been carried out, and careful assessment has been made of the patient's overall physical, physiologic, and social situation. Such a strategy is often best devised by a multidisciplinary team, including medical, surgical, and radiation oncologists who will weigh the possibilities of cure or significant palliation, consider the various treatment options and their expected untoward effects, and then embark on a therapeutic trial. Fortunately the therapeutic horizons are constantly changing. For example, patients with disseminated testicular cancer, acute lymphocytic leukemia, Ewing's sarcoma, Wilms' tumor, ovarian carcinoma, Hodgkin's disease, and histiocytic lymphoma now have an excellent chance for a cure, whereas this would have been impossible even in the recent past. Since the outcome for an individual patient cannot be precisely predicted, the initial treatment plan must often be updated on the basis of changing circumstances or after restaging procedures, in order to provide the broadest chance of response to therapy. Obviously surgery or localized radiation therapy with the aim of cure is a desirable option if the clinical circumstances are appropriate. Surgery is used as the sole initial treatment for over 50 per cent of patients with *all* types of localized cancer, the remainder being treated either with radiation alone or in various combinations with or without chemotherapy. Local or regional recurrences may still permit localized radiotherapy with the intent of cure, but systemic disease requires chemotherapy if all tumor cells are to be reached. The difficulty of attempting to predict tumor response to chemotherapy may one day be overcome through in vitro sensitivity tests, but for the present the selection process depends upon prior reports of clinical trials for particular types of cancer.

Forty to fifty per cent of all patients with cancer are potentially curable at the time of diagnosis. It is more important to understand the principles underlying the various types of treatment, the order in which they are used, and how aggressively they are to be applied than to remember their dosage schedules. The risk of serious side effects may be much more acceptable to a patient who stands a good chance for a cure than to one who does not. A limited trial of therapy in patients who have tumors that are unlikely to respond is usually warranted, with a careful look for changes in tumor size or tumor markers. At least such an approach gives patients an opportunity for palliation, without committing them to many months of ineffective treatment. These judgmental decisions must bridge the gap between careful assessment of the individual patient and knowledge concerning current therapeutic methods. After careful explanation by the physician of all options, it is the competent patient who must make the ultimate decisions about treatment. Therefore, it is essential to develop a meaningful therapeutic alliance in dealing with such choices.

SUPPORTIVE CARE. In its broadest sense, "supportive care" refers to all types of medical care required to provide for the needs of the patient with cancer. Certain specific supportive care programs for patients receiving aggressive chemotherapy for leukemia and other conditions have led to gratifying improvements in cure rates by anticipating and/or counteracting potentially fatal complications such as *infection and bleeding.* Early detection and vigorous treatment with newer antibiotics can be lifesaving for infected patients during periods of severe granulocytopenia. It has become unusual to see a fatal infection during the first few such episodes in the treatment of cancer. Similarly, platelet transfusions can minimize the risk of hemorrhage during periods of profound thrombocytopenia. These two advances, together with aggressive systemic and intrathecal chemotherapy, are responsible for the 50 per cent cure rate that can now be achieved in childhood leukemia, for example.

Severe *nausea and vomiting* induced by combination chemotherapy may be major, even limiting, factors in patient compliance because of the serious deterioration in the quality of life induced by these potent drugs. The woman receiving adjuvant chemotherapy for breast cancer or the man being treated for testicular cancer may endure a year of these exhausting side effects unless an effective antiemetic program is administered. Many patients fail to respond to conventional antiemetics, such as large doses of phenothiazines, but may respond very well to high dose metoclopramide and steroids, haloperidol, delta-9-tetrahydrocannabinol (THC) and other antiemetics. The effectiveness of antiemetic drugs varies, depending on the type of chemotherapy, with high dose cisplatinum therapy being the most potent and difficult emetic stimulus to control. Anxiety is a very important part of the whole symptom complex. It frequently leads to anticipatory nausea and vomiting. The anxiety portion can be alleviated by benzodiazepines such as lorazepam.

General supportive care also involves meeting nutritional, rehabilitative, psychosocial, and analgesic requirements (see below). Anorexia and weight loss are almost invariably associated with advanced cancer; occasionally profound *cachexia* may occur in a patient with only a small and apparently localized lesion such as lung cancer. There are several potential explanations for the varying *nutritional problems*—anatomic causes such as abdominal pressure or head and neck surgery, liver disease, paraneoplastic syndromes, effects of chemotherapy, depression, or the release of peptides such as cachectin. In the individual patient it is often difficult to sort out the factors that contribute to anorexia and hypercatabolism, and frequently they occur together. Regardless of etiology it is important to reverse this catabolic trend, since malnourished patients tolerate the usual courses of chemotherapy or radiation therapy very poorly and may die prematurely of complications related to treatment toxicity. Thus, in the case of a patient with recurrent cancer of the head and neck, improvement in nutrition is often a necessary prerequisite to the use of chemotherapeutic drugs. Increasingly, oncologists are using parenteral or tube feedings prior to major cancer surgery, radiation therapy, or chemotherapy. The dietitian familiar with the practical problems faced by these patients is an essential member of the team working with the patient and family.

Hyperuricemia and *hyperuricosuria* have the potential of producing acute urate nephropathy in patients in whom tumors are rapidly destroyed by chemotherapy. This complication can be effectively prevented by the use of allopurinol to block urate synthesis and by vigorous hydration prior to and during administration of cytotoxic therapy for lymphocytic leukemia or lymphoma, for example.

Every physician caring for patients with cancer must appreciate the cumulative debilitating effects of bed rest, continuous intravenous infusions, weight loss, and cytotoxic chemotherapy. Losses of muscle mass and bone structure are predictable in patients with advanced cancer, and they predispose to further immobility, hypercalcemia, and fractures. A simple and useful exercise program developed by Rosenbaum and associates can be done at home or in the hospital. The program also contributes to a feeling of well-being and preservation of body image.

The *psychosocial problems* that may be encountered by patients with cancer are profound and varied. Many of these are not unique to cancer and occur in age-matched patients with other types of chronic illness and shortened life expectancy. Shock, bereavement, anger, denial, withdrawal, and depression are common responses of people faced with such overwhelming problems. Disfigurement, feelings of shame and disgrace, loss of sexual activity, and job discrimination are problems that are more prevalent in patients with cancer than in those with many other illnesses. *The attitude of the physician and staff* is of key importance in helping the patient make the best possible adjustment, given all of the premorbid factors and limitations imposed by the illness. The physician who (verbally or nonverbally) conveys the impression that "There is nothing further that I can do" is sentencing his patient to untold misery or forcing him into the waiting arms of enthusiastic cancer quacks. All patients need help. Most patients respond positively to it, and they appreciate a gently supportive role that stresses honesty, trust, and a willingness simply to be available to help both patient and family with their fears and needs.

The *care of the patient who is dying of cancer* is the most sensitive issue for both patient and family. This is also commonly the period in which patients feel abandoned by physicians who themselves are frustrated by their inability to cure or cause remission of the illness and by the tragic human circumstances that often accompany such illnesses. Indeed, these take their toll on doctors and nurses as well as on relatives and friends, and busy cancer clinics recognize the need for support groups for their staff. (Indeed, unless there is an active self-renewing effort, oncology workers are subject to "burnout," an insidious syndrome difficult to recognize.) The physician must always prepare a reassuring setting so that when specific therapy is no longer warranted, patient comfort will be attended to in a considerate and thoughtful manner. In the final weeks of the illness, family members may require even more attention than the patient, and the team of doctor, nurse, social worker, and chaplain should provide the necessary support for all concerned including staff.

Patients fear *pain* perhaps more than any other aspect of cancer, and there are many misconceptions about this subject by the public. Yet adequate techniques are available to control pain in most patients, if these are used in a timely and appropriate fashion. Here again a carefully obtained history is an important initial step in diagnosis, for a patient with pain may have anything from cord compression or bone metastasis to a benign condition such as arthritis. The complaint of pain may even reflect the fear of abandonment. Relatively simple radiotherapy or neurosurgical procedures employed sufficiently early for localized pain and the *liberal use of narcotics for severe generalized pain* are usually successful in alleviating cancer-related pain. One need not be concerned with potential narcotic addiction in dying patients. Patients themselves are often reluctant to take adequate doses of analgesics and should be encouraged to take them with sufficient frequency to alleviate pain *before* it becomes very severe.

Depending on the wishes of the family, it is often preferable to provide for the care of the dying patient in his or her own home. This can be done with a home care program supple-

mented by visiting nurses and volunteers. *Hospice programs* are rapidly developing in the United States, and these can provide the supportive ingredients for both the patient and family that others cannot supply. The patient is often much more comfortable in familiar surroundings and near to loved ones. Family and friends usually respond willingly to their duties when properly directed. Finally, the savings in costly hospitalizations can conserve already depleted financial resources. Indeed, careful curbing of unnecessary costly tests and interventions can make an enormous financial difference over the course of the illness.

DeVita VT, Hellman S, Rosenberg SA (eds.): The Principles and Practice of Oncology. Philadelphia, J. B. Lippincott Company, 1985. *A major text of oncology that is particularly useful for looking up specific tumors and treatment.*

Holland JF, Frei E III (eds.): Cancer Medicine. Philadelphia, Lea & Febiger, 1982. *Excellent textbook with resource materials for all levels of study. It is an oncology textbook with general articles on diagnostic procedures and principles of treatment, as well as hard-to-find highly technical and basic articles related to various aspects of cancer research.*

Laszlo J: Antiemetics and Cancer Chemotherapy. Baltimore, Williams & Wilkins Company, 1983. *The first detailed study of the neurophysiology, fluid balance, drug therapies, and behavioral therapy of the nausea and vomiting produced by chemotherapeutic drugs.*

Laszlo J: Physician's Guide to Cancer Care Complications: Prevention and Management. New York, Marcel Dekker, 1986. *Careful review of the complications of surgery, radiation therapy, and chemotherapy from experts who have special interests in minimizing predictable problems in management of patients with cancer.*

Rosenbaum EH, Rosenbaum IR: A Comprehensive Guide for Cancer Patients and Their Families. Palo Alto, CA, Bull Publishing Co., 1980. *A sensitive and practical manual describing the attitudes, stresses, and losses of the patient who has cancer, and a helpful guide to rehabilitative services, nutrition, and bed care management. Encompasses the range of personal support services to patients in a book that is suitable for the entire health team.*

169 ONCOGENES
J. Michael Bishop

CANCER AS A GENETIC DISEASE

Astute observers have long nurtured the thought that cancer might be at its heart a genetic disease. The thought was at first vague and arose from seemingly disparate discoveries that included the existence of heritable diatheses to cancer, the presence of abnormal chromosomes in cancer cells, and the likelihood that many carcinogens act by inducing mutations in cellular DNA. Medical geneticists and epidemiologists first conceived the possibility of "cancer genes," prompted by occasional examples of human tumors whose occurrence seemed dictated by recessive or dominant inherited traits. Now the long-imagined cancer genes have been brought to view, unearthed by two experimental strategies: the use of viruses that cause tumors in animals and the search for tumorigenic genes in the DNA of cancer cells. From these studies we have learned that the human genome contains a set of genes (more than 20 loci but perhaps less than 100) that may lie at the heart of every cancer. These genes are called *proto-oncogenes* (to designate them as precursors to oncogenic determinants) or *cellular oncogenes* (to designate them as potentially oncogenic determinants that are part of the genetic dowry of all normal cells), and their value to cancer research is beyond measure. They are our present best hope of achieving an understanding of the molecular mechanisms by which cancer arises, a keyboard on which many different carcinogens may play, the possible components of a final common pathway to neoplastic growth.

FIRST DESCRIPTIONS: VIRAL ONCOGENES

Documentation that specific genes can elicit cancerous growth emerged first from the study of viruses that cause tumors in animals. By the use of formal genetic analyses, and

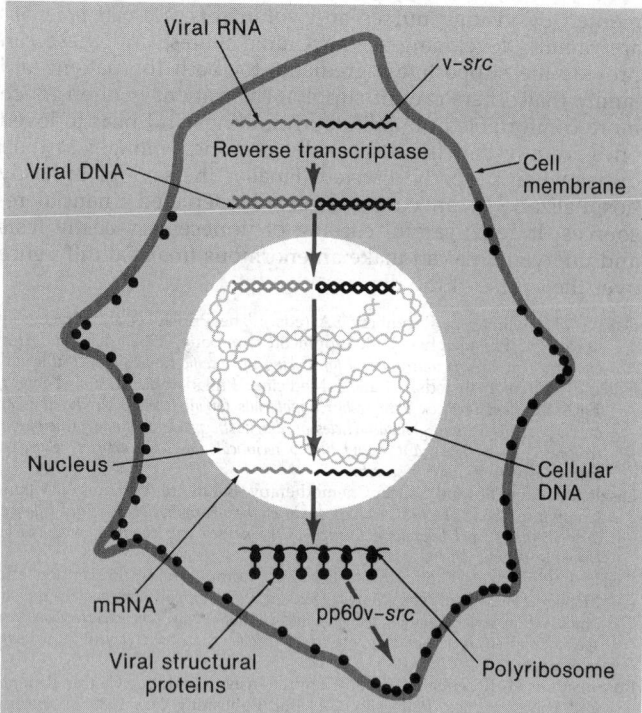

FIGURE 169–1. The molecular life cycle of retroviruses leads to insertion of viral genes into the chromosome of the host cell and the subsequent production of viral proteins that can transform the cell to neoplastic growth. In the example illustrated, the protein encoded by the *src* oncogene of the Rous sarcoma virus attaches to the inner surface of the plasma membrane and catalyzes phosphorylation of tyrosine residues in cellular proteins. (Modified from Bishop JM: Oncogenes and proto-oncogenes. Hosp Pract 18:68, 1983, with permission from HP Publishing Co., Inc.)

later of recombinant DNA, investigators were able to show that the tumorigenicity of many viruses can be attributed to domains within the genomes of the viruses. In time, these domains became known as oncogenes because they are oncogenic and are coincident with active viral genes that encode proteins produced in infected cells.

The most decisive paradigm for the genetic origins of cancer emerged from the study of retroviruses, whose genes are carried in RNA but are copied into DNA by reverse transcriptase early in viral replication. The life cycle of retroviruses provides a microcosm of carcinogenesis (Fig. 169–1). The viral DNA produced by reverse transcriptase is inserted (or "inte-

grated") into the chromosomal DNA of the host cell. Thereafter, the cell uses its own machinery to express the integrated viral genes. These events hold two possibilities for carcinogenesis. First, the integration of viral DNA is potentially mutagenic: It can damage vital cellular genes, and it can influence their expression by bringing them under the sway of powerful viral signals. Virologists call this *insertional mutagenesis*; it may indeed be tumorigenic (see below), and the cellular genes perverted by viral DNA are candidate "proto-oncogenes." Second, some (but not all) retroviruses carry oncogenes whose expression is sufficient to give rise to cancerous growth. The oncogenes of retroviruses make no apparent contribution to viral replication; therefore, their presence in viral genomes posed a puzzle. The puzzle was solved with the discovery that retroviral oncogenes are not viral genes at all, but wayward copies of cellular genes acquired during the course of viral replication by a process known formally as transduction, and carried as mere passengers in the viral genome. It is likely that transduction by retroviruses is a rare accident of nature, without design for the virus, and attributable to details of the curious means by which retroviruses replicate. There is no reason to believe that the transduction is limited to genes with tumorigenic potential. However, transduction by retroviruses is of profound consequence because it has brought to view cellular genes whose activities may be central to all forms of carcinogenesis. Many decades might have been necessary to find these genes in the morass of the mammalian genome; instead, the genes were manifested in viruses, excerpted, and made available for close scrutiny.

THE PATHOGENIC MECHANISMS OF RETROVIRAL ONCOGENES

The study of viral oncogenes began with the hope that the mechanisms by which these genes act might help to reveal the inner workings of the cancer cell, to elucidate the biochemical abnormalities that prompt cancerous growth. This is now a burgeoning prospect because the number of retroviral oncogenes has grown to at least 20, each inducing specific forms of malignancy, each encoding a protein whose action apparently causes harm (Table 169–1). The first hint of how informative these genes might be came with the discovery that several retroviral oncogenes encode protein kinases, located on the plasma membrane of the cell and possessing a previously unencountered substrate specificity for tyrosine. It would be difficult to envision a better explanation for neoplastic transformation: By phosphorylating numerous cellular proteins, a single enzyme could rapidly change myriad aspects of cellular structure and function. If the phosphorylated

TABLE 169–1. THE PROTEINS ENCODED BY RETROVIRAL ONCOGENES

Oncogenes	Tumorigenicity	Biochemical Properties	Subcellular Location	Cellular Homologue
abl	Lymphoma	Protein kinase	Plasma membrane	
erb-A*	?	?	?	
erb-B	Erythroleukemia	Glycosylated	Intracellular and plasma membranes	Receptor for EGF
ets*	?	?	?	
fgr	Sarcoma	Protein kinase	Plasma membrane	
fms	Sarcoma	Glycosylated	Plasma membrane	Receptor for CSF-I
fos	Osteosarcoma	?	Nucleus	
fps/fes†	Sarcoma	Protein kinase	Plasma membrane	
kit	Sarcoma	Protein kinase	Plasma membrane	
mos	Sarcoma	?	Cytoplasm	
myb	Myelomonocytic leukemia	?	Nucleus	
myc	Carcinomas, leukemia and sarcoma	Binds to DNA	Nucleus	
raf/mht/mil†	Sarcoma	Glycosylated	Membranes	
ras	Sarcoma and erythroleukemia	Binds and hydrolyzes GTP	Plasma membrane	G/N regulatory proteins
rel	Lymphoma	?	?	
ros	Sarcoma	Protein kinase	Plasma membrane	Subunit 2 of PDGF
sis	Sarcoma	Growth factor	Cytoplasmic	
ski	Sarcoma	?	Nucleus	
src	Sarcoma	Protein kinase	Plasma membrane	
yes	Sarcoma	Protein kinase	Plasma membrane	

*The exact contribution of *erb-A* and *ets* to tumorigenesis by the viruses in which they occur is not yet apparent.
†Multiple names denote genes isolated from different species but later proved to be homologous.

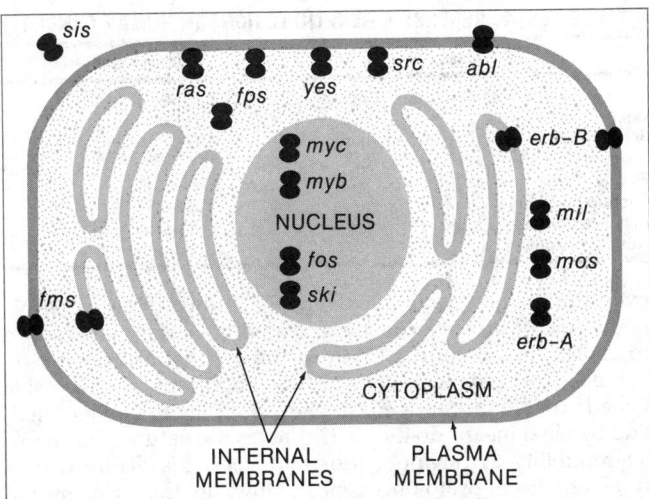

FIGURE 169–2. The products of oncogenes assume diverse locations within the cell, where they perform functions involved in the regulation of cellular growth and differentiation. (Modified with permission from Hunter T: The proteins of oncogenes. Sci Am 251:78, 1984.)

proteins can be found (only a few have been, to date), a door will be opened to the secrets of neoplastic growth.

Protein phosphorylation is not the only means by which retroviral oncogenes may act (Table 169–1). As more and more of the proteins encoded by oncogenes came into view, a provocative diversity emerged: Some of the proteins are protein kinases, others are not (one is a component of the growth factor normally released by platelets); some attack in the nucleus of the cell, some in the cytoplasm, some at the plasma membrane (Fig. 169–2); and there is little correlation between what we now know of how oncogenes function and the character of their tumorigenicities. What does this diversity signify? The growth of cells is regulated by an interdigitating network that spans from the surface of the plasma membrane to the depths of the nucleus. If that network were to be touched at any point by an adverse influence and tilted out of balance, cancerous growth might ensue. Perhaps the diverse means by which different oncogenes act may mirror various components of the regulatory network, revealing how the network performs its task. By studying oncogenes, we are likely to be learning of both cancerous and normal growth at one and the same time. It is an old adage of medical science that study of the abnormal can reveal the normal.

PROTO-ONCOGENES AND ONCOGENES

The cellular genes whose transduction engenders retroviral oncogenes provided the first glimpse and the first definition of proto-oncogenes. By all available criteria, these are cellular genes, not viral genes in disguise. They can be found in every member of every vertebrate species examined, probably in all metazoan organisms. Evolutionary conservation of this magnitude signifies that the proto-oncogenes serve essential functions for the species in which they are harbored. Proto-oncogenes are expressed in normal cells and tissues, and their expression can vary from one tissue to another, from one embryologic lineage to another, from one time in embryogenesis to another. It is widely assumed that, in their normal guise, proto-oncogenes help to control the growth and development of cells and organisms. This assumption has been strengthened by the discovery that several of the proto-oncogenes encode proteins known to participate in the regulation of cellular proliferation, including platelet-derived growth factor (PDGF) and the receptors for epidermal growth factor (EGF) and colony-stimulating factor I (CSF-I) (Table 169–1).

Why are the transduced forms of proto-oncogenes tumorigenic? What converts a proto-oncogene, a compliant member of the cellular citizenry, to an oncogene—an unruly and

potentially lethal enemy? The possible answers to these questions have taken two general forms: Transduction may have unleashed the genes from their usual controls and outlandish or inappropriate expression of otherwise normal genes might be the fatal flaw; alternatively, mutation during or after transduction could change the structure of the genes and the proteins they encode, giving rise to abnormal function. For the moment, it appears that either explanation may on occasion apply. There is no question but that transduction by retroviruses mandates relatively vigorous gene expression. Comparisons of retroviral oncogenes to their cellular progenitors have revealed a variety of structural changes sufficient to evoke anomalous function. These issues are not arcane: they prefigure the debate over whether, and if so how, proto-oncogenes might be the intrinsic "cancer genes" of human cells.

PROTO-ONCOGENES AS CANCER GENES

Do proto-oncogenes participate in many or all forms of tumorigenesis? Are they a common keyboard for all the players in carcinogenesis? Since these questions were first raised, the pertinent evidence has grown from a thin thread to a rich and provocative fabric of experimental observation.

1. Direct manipulation of proto-oncogenes isolated by molecular cloning has revealed that some (but not all) of these ostensibly normal genes can elicit neoplastic growth if they are first attached to viral signals that command vigorous gene expression and then inserted into cells in culture.

2. There is evidence that retroviruses without oncogenes of their own initiate tumorigenesis by the mutation of proto-oncogenes. The mutations may be of two sorts: those that enhance expression of a gene and those that change the structure of the protein(s) encoded by a gene.

3. Some human tumors (the exact number is not yet clear) display karyotypic evidence of gene amplification (double-minute chromosomes and homogeneously staining regions in marker chromosomes) and contain one or another proto-oncogene whose number has been multiplied as much as 200-fold over normal. As a consequence of amplification, the proto-oncogene is expressed in inordinately large amounts. Amplification of proto-oncogenes has been found in two patterns: as sporadic and occasional features of diverse tumors and as a common feature of particular tumors. The latter pattern gives promise of being clinically useful. For example, amplification of a proto-oncogene known as N-*myc* is a frequent feature of human neuroblastomas and appears to connote an ominous prognosis that will justify attempts at new therapeutic regimens.

4. At least several of the chromosomal translocations that typify a substantial variety of human tumors move a proto-oncogene from one chromosome to another. As a consequence, expression of the proto-oncogene may be altered, or the gene may sustain mutations within the domain that encodes a protein. Present examples include Burkitt's lymphoma (translocation of the proto-oncogene c-*myc*) and chronic myelogenous leukemia (translocation of c-*abl*), in which the Philadelphia chromosome (Ph[1]) raised the possibility many years ago that consistent forms of chromosomal damage might figure in tumorigenesis.

BIOLOGICALLY ACTIVE ONCOGENES IN THE DNA OF HUMAN TUMORS

The frequency with which proto-oncogenes first identified through the use of retroviruses have been implicated in the genesis of human tumors is not easy to dismiss as coincidence. The incriminating evidence remained entirely circumstantial, however, until a direct assault revealed biologically active oncogenes in human tumors. Application of DNA from a variety of human tumors to cells in culture can elicit neoplastic growth, as if the DNA contained oncogenes of the sort once found only in viruses. Approximately 20 per cent of all human tumors demonstrate activity of this type, no matter what their histopathology. The responsible genes have now been identified for a substantial variety of tumors. With remarkable frequency, they have proved to be one or another member of a family of proto-oncogenes known as *ras* genes and already familiar to us from the study of retroviruses. But other genes have been found as well—some that were known to us before from the study of retroviruses, others that are entirely new to us. Many of the oncogenes appear to be active because they have suffered mutations that change single amino acids in the protein products of the genes.

ONCOGENES AND THE MULTIPLE STEPS IN CARCINOGENESIS

The attribution of tumorigenesis to oncogenes seemed at first glance simplistic, since the genesis of tumors has long been described as a protracted and complex sequence of events. However, the identification of oncogenes and the proto-oncogenes from which they are derived has given us a tool with which to recognize several separate steps in tumorigenesis. In at least some human and animal tumors, it is possible to point to at least two coexistent genetic lesions afflicting proto-oncogenes in various ways. For example, two oncogenes have been incriminated in the genesis of Burkitt's lymphoma: a proto-oncogene that has been relocated and possibly activated by chromosomal translocation, and another gene whose action transforms rodent cells in culture, perhaps because a mutation has altered the protein encoded by the gene.

The manner in which such pairings might exemplify distinct steps in carcinogenesis has been demonstrated by experiment. Two oncogenes can be combined to elicit a tumorigenic phenotype in cultures of embryonic rodent cells that could not be rendered tumorigenic by either of the oncogenes alone. Medical geneticists have in the past suggested that at least some tumors may owe their origins to no more than two genetic lesions. These suggestions now appear more credible than ever before.

RECESSIVE GENETIC DAMAGE IN TUMORS

The oncogenes considered so far are thought to be genetically dominant: Their abnormalities have an impact even when a normal allele of the same gene is also present in the cell. But at least some human tumors (and perhaps all) also bear lesions that are recessive, that make their presence known only when no normal counterpart is present. By inference from karyotypes and by the use of restriction endonucleases, substantial evidence has been obtained for the presence of recessive mutations in a variety of tumors. The examples of retinoblastoma and Wilms' tumor are presently the most celebrated, but other (and more common) examples are now emerging as well (Table 169–2). In each instance, the faulty chromosome—and sometimes the responsible region of that chromosome—is known. But no particular gene has yet been incriminated, nor do we know how recessive mutations might interact with dominant oncogenes.

Recessive mutations explain hereditary diatheses to several forms of neoplasm (again, retinoblastoma and Wilms' tumor are the seminal examples). By contrast, there is as yet no evidence to implicate any of the dominant oncogenes in the inheritance of cancer.

THE FUTURE

By one means or another, at least 11 proto-oncogenes have been implicated in different types of tumorigenesis. In some instances, expression of the gene is enhanced; in other instances, the structure of the protein encoded by the gene has been changed. In a few instances, both of these events may have occurred. These are remarkable conclusions, reached within a decade of the discovery of proto-oncogenes. How-

TABLE 169–2. RECESSIVE GENETIC LESIONS IN HUMAN CANCER

Tumor	Chromosomal Locus
Retinoblastoma (and secondary tumors)	13(q14)
Wilms' tumor	11(p13)
Beckwith-Wiedemann syndrome (embryonal tumors)	11p
Bladder carcinoma	11p
Carcinoma of lung	3(p14–23)
Renal carcinoma (hereditary)	t3;8(p12;q24) or t3;11(p;p)
Neuroblastoma	1(p32-pter)

ever, the unknown still outweighs the known. How extensive is the role of proto-oncogenes in tumorigenesis? How are we to explain the majority of human tumors that as yet offer no evidence of genetic lesions? How important are recessive genetic traits in tumorigenesis, how are they to be identified, and by what means do they act? What is the nature of heritable susceptibility to carcinogenesis and does this diathesis ever originate from proto-oncogenes? How do the proteins encoded by oncogenes conduct their nefarious business? After all, will we be able to parlay the growing information about oncogenes into devices for the prevention, diagnosis, and treatment of human cancer? It is too early to foretell how quickly the answers to these questions may come, but there now seems little reason to doubt that we have laid hold of cancer with a grip that should eventually extract the deadly secrets of the disease.

Bishop JM: The molecular biology of RNA tumor viruses: A physician's guide. N Engl J Med 303:675, 1980.
Bishop JM: Oncogenes. Sci Am 246(3):80, 1982.
Bishop JM: Cellular oncogenes and retroviruses. Ann Rev Biochem 52:301, 1983.
Bishop JM: Oncogenes and proto-oncogenes. Hosp Pract 18:67, 1983.
Bishop JM: Trends in oncogenes. Trends Genet 1:245, 1985.
Hunter T: The proteins of oncogenes. Sci Am 251(2):70, 1984.
Varmus HE: The molecular genetics of cellular oncogenes. Ann Rev Genet 18:553, 1984.
Weinberg RA: A molecular basis of cancer. Sci Am 249(5):126, 1983.
Weinberg RA: The action of oncogenes in the cytoplasm and nucleus. Science 230:770, 1985.
All of these references offer general reviews of this rapidly expanding area of medical research.

170 EPIDEMIOLOGY OF CANCER

Joseph F. Fraumeni, Jr.

Epidemiology has contributed substantially to knowledge about the origins of human cancer, and provides the foundation for measures designed to prevent cancer. The approach dates from the eighteenth century, when the occupational physician Bernardino Ramazzini reported that nuns were at high risk of breast cancer, and the surgeon Percivall Pott observed that chimney sweeps exposed to soot were prone to scrotal cancer. The initial leads to epidemiologic investigation have often come from astute clinicians who noted an excessive number of patients with the same tumor and traced the "cluster" to a particular cultural, occupational, or iatrogenic exposure. Major insights into cancer etiology are provided also by experimental approaches to detect carcinogens in laboratory animals or mutagens in short-term test assays, and to clarify basic mechanisms of carcinogenesis. In recent years the pace of epidemiologic and experimental research in cancer etiology has accelerated, including efforts to identify environmental factors, which are generally held responsible for a large proportion of cancers in the general population.

PATTERNS OF CANCER OCCURRENCE

Cancer is second only to heart disease as a cause of death in the United States, and accounts for 22 per cent of all deaths.

It is estimated that in 1986 about 930,000 Americans developed cancer, excluding in situ carcinomas and nonmelanoma skin cancer, and that about 472,000 died from the disease. The most common cancers occur in the lung in males, the breast in females, and the colon and rectum in each sex.

It has been widely claimed that 80 to 90 per cent of all cancer is related to environmental influences, particularly those related to life style practices. These estimates are derived from the substantial international variation in cancer incidence, in which rates for the lowest-risk countries are subtracted from the rates prevailing in the United States. The resulting difference is attributed to environmental causes, and the lowest risk is assumed to represent the baseline level for tumors that develop "spontaneously" and cannot be prevented. Around the world the reported age-adjusted incidence rates for total cancer vary by a factor of about three, whereas the rates for certain anatomic sites, particularly the esophagus and liver, vary by more than 100-fold. Even the risks for the more common tumors in Western countries differ by factors of about 8 to 40. Although some of this variation may have a genetic basis, evidence supporting a major role for environmental factors can be found in the experience of migrant populations, such as the Japanese who moved to Hawaii and California. Generally, as migrant groups adopt customs of the new land, their risk of various cancers shifts away from the rate prevailing in the country of origin to approximate that of the host country. The change in incidence for some cancers, notably cancer of the colon, is often evident within two to three decades of migration, whereas the change for other cancers, notably cancer of the breast, requires more than one generation. Although variations within countries are not as great as those seen internationally, the mapping of cancer death rates in the United States at the county level has revealed geographic clustering that provides leads to the investigation of environmental exposures.

Variations in cancer incidence and mortality over time may also reflect environmental factors, although some fluctuations can be explained by changing medical practices and reporting procedures. Most dramatic has been the increase in lung cancer rates in the United States and other countries; in the 1950's cigarette smoking was determined to be responsible. Upward trends have been noted also for thyroid cancer resulting from x-ray therapy to the head and neck during childhood, malignant melanoma from changing clothing styles and recreational exposures to sunlight, and endometrial cancer from the use of menopausal estrogens. The increases in prostatic cancer and multiple myeloma, however, are at least partly due to improvements in diagnostic measures. In the black population of the United States, sharp increases over time have been reported for cancers of the lung, esophagus, prostate, and pancreas and multiple myeloma, and these tumors are now more common in blacks than whites. Several cancers have shown little change, while a few have displayed downward trends, including cancers of the stomach, cervix, and liver.

THE CAUSES OF CANCER

Although much remains to be learned about the factors responsible for variations of cancer in the general population, several environmental exposures have been identified as causes of cancer (Table 170–1). The evidence is based primarily on case-control studies (comparing the past experience of persons with and without a particular cancer) or cohort studies (following-up individuals whose experiences and characteristics are already defined). There is a growing recognition, however, that most cancers result from the combined effects of multiple exposures and susceptibility states. This is consistent with multistage models in which different risk factors accelerate the transition rates at various stages of carcinogenesis. Some affect early stages as initiators, others act at late stages as promoters, and still others influence both early and late stages.

TABLE 170–1. ENVIRONMENTAL CAUSES OF HUMAN CANCER

Agent	Type of Exposure	Site of Cancer
Alcoholic beverages	Drinking	Mouth, pharynx, esophagus, larynx, liver
Alkylating agents (melphalan, cyclophosphamide, chlorambucil, semustine)	Medication	Leukemia
Androgen-anabolic steroids	Medication	Liver
Aromatic amines (benzidine, 2-naphthylamine, 4-aminobiphenyl)	Manufacture of chemicals	Bladder
Arsenic (inorganic)	Mining and smelting of certain ores, pesticide manufacturing and application, medication and contaminated drinking water	Lung, skin, liver (angiosarcoma)
Asbestos	Manufacturing and application	Lung, pleura, peritoneum, gastrointestinal tract
Benzene	Leather, petroleum, and other industries	Leukemia
Bis(chloromethyl)ether	Manufacture of ion exchange resins	Lung
Chlornaphazine	Medication	Bladder
Chromium compounds	Manufacturing	Lung
Estrogens	Medication	
Synthetic (DES)		Vagina, cervix (adenocarcinoma)
Conjugated (Premarin)		Endometrium
Steroid contraceptives		Liver (benign)
Immunosuppressants (azathioprine, cyclosporin)	Medication	Lymphoma (histiocytic), skin (squamous carcinoma), soft tissue sarcoma
Ionizing radiation	Atomic blasts, medical use, radium dial painting, uranium and metal mining	Nearly all sites
Isopropyl alcohol production	Manufacturing by strong acid process	Nasal sinuses
Mustard gas	Manufacturing in wartime	Lung, larynx, nasal sinuses
Nickel dust	Refining	Lung, nasal sinuses
Phenacetin-containing analgesics	Medication	Renal pelvis
Polycyclic hydrocarbons	Coal carbonization products and some mineral oils	Lung, skin (squamous carcinoma)
Tobacco chews and powder	Snuff dipping and chewing of tobacco, betel, lime	Mouth
Tobacco smoke	Smoking, especially cigarettes	Lung, larynx, mouth, pharynx, esophagus, bladder, pancreas, kidney
Ultraviolet radiation	Sunlight	Skin, including melanoma
Vinyl chloride	Manufacture of polyvinyl chloride	Liver (angiosarcoma)
Wood dusts	Furniture manufacturing	Nasal sinuses

late stages. It is generally thought that cumulative environmental exposures, long latency periods, and multistage processes account for the increasing risk of most cancers with advancing age.

TOBACCO. The principal carcinogenic hazard in western countries is tobacco smoking, which produces cancers of the lung, larynx, mouth, pharynx, esophagus, bladder, pancreas, kidney, and possibly cervix. It is estimated that smoking, especially cigarettes, contributes to about 30 per cent of all cancer in men and women combined. The greatest impact is on lung cancer, with the risk for male smokers of two or more packs per day being about 20 times that of nonsmokers. However, the rates for lung cancer are now rising more sharply in women than in men, reflecting the growing popularity of cigarettes among women in the past 20 to 30 years. Smokers of filter-tipped cigarettes with reduced tar and nicotine have a lower risk of lung cancer than do smokers of nonfilter cigarettes, but still a much higher risk than do nonsmokers. Smokeless tobacco products are also of concern, since oral cancer has been linked with snuff dipping, a common practice in rural southern areas of the United States. In parts of Asia, oral cancer is very common in people exposed to various tobacco chews, which are often mixed with betel, lime, and other agents that may enhance the risks.

ALCOHOL. Consumption of alcoholic beverages has been shown to multiply the effects of tobacco smoking on cancers of the mouth, pharynx, esophagus, and larynx. Heavy drinking also increases the risk of liver cancer, particularly among cirrhotic patients. Ethanol is not carcinogenic in laboratory animals, so the mechanism by which alcohol promotes carcinogenesis is not clear. Under suspicion are nutritional deficiencies associated with heavy drinking, the effects of congeners or contaminants (e.g., nitrosamines, hydrocarbons) in alcoholic beverages, and the capacity of alcohol to solubilize carcinogens or enhance their penetration into tissue.

SOLAR RADIATION. The dominant risk factor for non-melanoma skin cancer (squamous and basal cell carcinomas) and for malignant melanoma is ultraviolet (UV) radiation from the sun. The evidence is based on the tendency for skin cancers to arise on sun-exposed surfaces, the high rates among outdoor workers, the inverse correlation between skin cancer incidence and distance from the equator, the predisposition of light-skinned and especially fair-complexioned populations who sunburn easily, the resistance of dark-skinned populations with protective melanin pigment, the exceptional risks of skin cancer among persons with genetic diseases exacerbated by sunlight (e.g., xeroderma pigmentosum, albinism), and the capacity of UV radiation in repeated doses to induce skin cancer in experimental animals.

IONIZING RADIATION. Although ionizing radiation probably accounts for less than 3 per cent of all cancer, it appears that virtually no site of the body is spared from its carcinogenic effects. It is difficult to measure directly the effects of low doses of sparsely ionizing radiation, such as x- or gamma rays, but extrapolations are possible by studying populations who have been exposed to high and moderate doses for medical, occupational, or military reasons. In general, the breast, thyroid, and bone marrow are the most radiosensitive organs. Radiogenic leukemia shows a wave-like pattern with the excess risks starting about two to four years after exposure, peaking at six to eight years, and declining to normal within 25 years. In contrast, radiogenic carcinomas have a minimal latent period of five to ten years and a temporal distribution that resembles the natural incidence curve, suggesting that age-dependent factors influence tumor expression. Surveys of medically irradiated populations have revealed an excess risk of leukemia and other cancers among patients treated for ankylosing spondylitis, benign gynecologic diseases, and various neoplasms; breast cancer among women treated for postpartum mastitis or who received fluoroscopies to monitor pneumothorax treatment of tuberculosis; thyroid cancer among children treated for thymus enlargement, benign head and neck disease, or tinea capitis; leukemia and other childhood cancers following prenatal x-ray exposure; and various cancers following use of radioactive compounds (osteosarcoma with radium-224, leukemia with phosphorus-32, and leukemia and liver angiosarcoma with Thorotrast).

OCCUPATIONAL HAZARDS. Occupational exposures are usually reported to account for less than 5 per cent of all cancer in men, but the percentage is higher for certain tumors, such as the bladder. Most occupational carcinogens have been first detected through clinical and epidemiologic observations with subsequent confirmation by laboratory studies. However, inorganic arsenic has not been shown to be carcinogenic in laboratory animals. In the case of mustard gas and vinyl chloride, the risks were detected in humans after the substances had been shown to induce tumors in laboratory animals, although little attention was given to the experimental studies when first reported. The effects of some agents, particularly asbestos and radon, are greatly potentiated by cigarette smoking, so that programs to reduce either the workplace exposure or smoking would significantly lower but not eliminate the occupational risk. A number of manufacturing industries (e.g., furniture, leather, rubber) are associated with cancer risk, although the specific carcinogens have not been identified. Industrial hazards and their detection have important implications beyond the work force, since most agents are not confined to the plant but ultimately become part of the general environment to which large segments of the population may be inadvertently exposed.

ENVIRONMENTAL POLLUTION. Pollutants in the urban air have long been suspected in the etiology of lung cancer, with fossil fuel combustion products, especially polycyclic hydrocarbons, being of special concern. In several studies the rates for lung cancer have shown correlations with measurement of benzo(a)pyrene in the ambient air, yet the available evidence suggests that the urban excess of lung cancer is mainly due to cigarette smoking and partly to occupational exposures. In the large-scale survey of the American Cancer Society, age- and smoking-standardized rates for lung cancer were computed among men not occupationally exposed to dust, fumes, or vapors. No major differences in mortality were seen between urban and rural areas, or between cities characterized by indices of pollution. Another approach has been to extrapolate from studies of workers heavily exposed to hydrocarbons, with the results suggesting only small effects from urban air pollutants. In some studies the effects of smoking a particular amount were greater in urban than rural areas, suggesting that tobacco smoke may interact with carcinogens in the ambient atmosphere.

Asbestos bodies and calcified pleural plaques have been reported in large segments of the urban population, but the carcinogenic effects following nonoccupational exposures are uncertain. It is clear, however, that mesotheliomas may result from neighborhood exposures to asbestos industries and from household contact with asbestos dust, particularly through laundering of work clothing. Another hazard may result from airborne levels of arsenic, since high mortality from lung cancer has been reported among male and female residents in communities with arsenic-emitting smelters.

Recent interest has centered on contaminants in drinking water, since several halogenated organic compounds produced during chlorination are carcinogenic and mutagenic in laboratory tests. Levels of these compounds in drinking water have shown correlations with the rates for cancers of the bladder, colon, and rectum in the same area.

MEDICATIONS. Several carcinogens have been detected by studies of patients exposed to medicinal agents. Some drugs have been withdrawn from clinical practice, while others are retained since risk-benefit considerations may warrant their use in certain conditions. A major discovery in this area was that synthetic estrogens given during pregnancy produce adenocarcinomas of the vagina and cervix several years later in daughters exposed in utero. This was the first demonstration of transplacental carcinogenesis in humans. Endometrial cancer was then firmly linked to the use of conjugated estrogens for menopausal symptoms, and further studies suggested that the occurrence of breast cancer might also be excessive in long-term users. Oral contraceptives have been related to benign liver tumors, to endometrial cancer among users of the sequential type of contraceptives, and possibly to cervical cancer and to breast cancer among some high-risk women (e.g., with benign breast disease). A reduced risk of endometrial and ovarian cancers has been reported with the use of combined oral contraceptives.

An excess risk of acute nonlymphocytic leukemia, and perhaps other cancers, has been seen among patients receiving certain alkylating agents. These risks may be acceptable when treating conditions with a poor prognosis such as metastatic cancer, but for conditions with a favorable long-term prognosis the benefits of treatments should be carefully weighed against the risks. These drugs may exert their action in part by breaking chromosomes, since other leukemogens (radiation, benzene) have a similar effect.

Immunosuppressive agents have been assessed primarily by studies of renal transplant recipients, most of whom have had azathioprine and corticosteroids. The risk of histiocytic lymphoma is very high, and first appears within months of transplantation. This explosive onset has suggested that a latent oncogenic virus may be activated by immunologic mechanisms. For all other cancers combined, the excess risk is about two-fold and first becomes evident about two years after transplantation. It has not affected all forms of cancer, as might be predicted by the hypothesis of "immunologic surveillance," but increased risks have been noted for cancers of the liver, biliary system, and bladder, and for soft-tissue sarcomas, adenocarcinoma of the lung, squamous carcinoma of the skin, and malignant melanoma. Recently, other groups of patients receiving immunosuppressants have shown an excess of lymphomas, squamous carcinoma of the skin, and soft-tissue sarcomas, but at lower rates than those seen in transplant patients. It is noteworthy that the predominance of lymphomas with drug-induced immunosuppression is seen also among patients with primary immunodeficiency syndromes.

INFECTIOUS AGENTS (see also Ch. 169). Evidence is increasing that both DNA and RNA viruses are causally related to certain forms of human cancer. The epidemiologic patterns of cervical cancer have long suggested venereal transmission of an infectious agent, with human papillomaviruses and herpes simplex virus type 2 being chief suspects. The Epstein-Barr virus (EBV) is linked to nasopharyngeal cancer and Burkitt's lymphoma, particularly in areas of the world where these tumors are highly prevalent. Hepatitis B infection is related to hepatocellular carcinoma, especially in endemic regions of Africa and Asia. Outbreaks of adult T cell leukemia in certain areas, especially in Japan and the Caribbean, have been linked to infection with the human T-lymphotropic virus type I (HTLV-I). Another human retrovirus (HTLV-III), also known as lymphadenopathy-associated virus (LAV) or human immunodeficiency virus (HIV), has been shown to cause the acquired immunodeficiency syndrome (AIDS). Recognized in epidemic form since 1981, AIDS affects mainly homosexual men, hemophiliacs, and intravenous drug abusers and is often accompanied by Kaposi's sarcoma and non-Hodgkin's lymphoma (Ch. 158).

If viruses are oncogenic in humans, it seems likely that predisposing factors are operating. Thus, EBV may interact with certain histocompatibility antigens to produce the high rate of nasopharyngeal cancer in Chinese populations, with persistent malarial infections to induce African Burkitt's lymphoma, or with a genetic immunodeficiency trait to cause family clusters of lymphoma. Hepatitis B infection may combine with dietary aflatoxin to produce liver cancer in endemic regions. In animal models the production of immunodeficiency enhances viral carcinogenesis, so that the narrow range of tumors complicating immunodeficiency states of humans suggests that viruses play only a limited role in human cancer.

Parasitic infections affect the risk of cancer in certain areas of the world. In Africa and Papua New Guinea, the geographic patterns of malaria and Burkitt's lymphoma are closely correlated; in the Middle East and North Africa schistosomiasis produces squamous carcinoma of the bladder; and in Asia infestation with liver flukes (clonorchiasis and opisthorchiasis) predisposes to cholangiocarcinoma.

NUTRITION. International correlations and migrant studies have suggested that certain features of the affluent Western diet contribute to a sizable proportion of all cancers. Various nutritional hypotheses are under study, although the mechanisms appear complex and difficult to unravel. For example, high dietary fat may affect the risk of colonic cancer by increasing the concentration of bile acids in the bowel, which are then metabolized by bacterial flora into carcinogens or co-carcinogens, and it may promote the development of breast cancer by increasing estrogen production and prolactin release. Dietary fat and caloric excess may also contribute to endometrial cancer and the associated manifestations of obesity, diabetes, and hypertension.

It appears also that a low intake of certain food classes may predispose to cancer. In several studies, the risk of colonic cancer has been inversely related to the consumption of fiber, which may protect against intestinal carcinogens or precursors by dilutional or other effects. Micronutrients and trace metals may also have a protective influence, since cancers of the lung and other sites have been associated with a low intake of vitamin A, beta-carotene, and selenium. The risk of stomach cancer has been related to a deficiency of fruits and vegetables containing vitamin C, which may act by inhibiting the formation of carcinogenic nitrosamines in the stomach. In a study of colonic cancer, patients ingested smaller than usual amounts of cruciferous vegetables (e.g., broccoli, cabbage, Brussels sprouts, cauliflower), containing indole compounds, which can inhibit carcinogenesis in laboratory animals. In esophageal cancer, the high rate among black males has been attributed to heavy alcohol consumption and generalized poor nutrition.

A variety of other dietary factors, including additives and contaminants, have fallen under suspicion. The consumption of aflatoxin, a carcinogenic metabolite of the fungus *Aspergillus flavus*, correlates closely with the distribution of liver cancer

TABLE 170–2. HEREDITARY NEOPLASMS

	Inheritance*	Features
Retinoblastoma	AD	Susceptibility to second primary tumors, including osteosarcoma of leg and radiogenic sarcoma of orbit; chromosome deletion (13q14) in some cases
Nevoid basal cell carcinoma syndrome	AD	Basal cell cancers of skin increased by UV and ionizing radiation; medulloblastoma, ovarian fibromas, and developmental defects in some cases
Multiple endocrine neoplasia I (Wermer's syndrome)	AD	Adenomas of anterior pituitary, parathyroid, pancreatic islet cells, thyroid, and adrenal cortex; carcinoid tumors of intestine and bronchus in some cases
Multiple endocrine neoplasia II (Sipple's syndrome)	AD	Pheochromocytoma and medullary thyroid carcinoma; parathyroid tumors and neurofibromas in some cases
Chemodectomas	AD	Paragangliomas from chemoreceptor system
Polyposis coli	AD	Multiple adenomatous polyps and adenocarcinomas of large bowel; some families feature osteomas, fibromas, lipomas, and epidermal cysts (Gardner's syndrome)
Tylosis with esophageal carcinoma	AD	Squamous cell carcinoma of esophagus with keratoses of palms and soles
Dysplastic nevus syndrome	AD	Hereditary melanomas derived from nevi, especially after sun exposure

*AD = autosomal dominant.

TABLE 170–3. HEREDITARY PRENEOPLASTIC SYNDROMES

	Inheritance*	Neoplasms
Phacomatoses		
Neurofibromatosis	AD	Sarcomatous change in 10% of cases; gliomas of brain and optic nerve, acoustic neuromas, meningiomas, and acute leukemia
Tuberous sclerosis	AD	Hamartomatous growths in several organs; brain tumors, chiefly giant-cell astrocytoma, in 1–3% of patients
von Hippel-Lindau syndrome	AD	Angiomatosis of retina and cerebellum; renal adenocarcinoma, pheochromocytoma, and ependymoma in some cases
Multiple exostoses (diaphyseal aclasis)	AD	Chondrosarcoma in 5–11% of patients
Peutz-Jeghers syndrome	AD	Rare malignant change in hamartomatous polyps of gastrointestinal tract; ovarian neoplasms in 5% of female patients
Cowden's multiple hamartoma syndrome	AD	Oral papillomas, cystic mastopathy and breast cancer, thyroid and colonic neoplasms
Genodermatoses		
Xeroderma pigmentosum	AR	Various skin cancers in all patients exposed to sunlight; defective cellular repair of DNA damage induced by UV light
Albinism	AR	Skin cancers, chiefly squamous, in sun-exposed areas
Epidermodysplasia verruciformis	AR	Skin cancers, chiefly squamous, in multiple warts induced by papillomavirus
Polydysplastic epidermolysis bullosa	AR	Skin cancers, chiefly squamous, in scars
Dyskeratosis congenita	AR	Squamous carcinomas of skin and mucous membranes; features of Fanconi's anemia in several cases
Werner's syndrome (adult progeria)	AR	Soft tissue sarcoma, other tumors
Chromosome instability		
Bloom's syndrome	AR	Acute leukemia, lymphoma, other cancers
Fanconi's anemia	AR	Acute myelomonocytic leukemia and squamous carcinoma of mucous membranes; hepatoma reported after androgen-anabolic steroids
Immune deficiency		
Ataxia telangiectasia	AR	Lymphoma, lymphocytic leukemia, stomach cancer, other tumors; chromosome fragility and ineffective DNA repair reported; heterozygous carriers prone to leukemia, lymphoma, and carcinomas of biliary tract, stomach and ovary
Common variable immunodeficiency	?AR	Lymphoma, stomach cancer
Wiskott-Aldrich syndrome	XR	Lymphoma, acute leukemia
X-linked (Bruton's) agammaglobulinemia	XR	Lymphoma, acute leukemia
X-linked lymphoproliferative syndrome	XR	Abnormal response to infection by Epstein-Barr virus, resulting in severe infectious mononucleosis, immunoblastic sarcoma, B cell lymphoma, or plasmacytoma

*AD = autosomal dominant; AR = autosomal recessive; XR = X-linked recessive.

in Africa. Coffee intake has been associated with bladder and pancreatic cancers in some studies, but causal relationships have not been established. The artificial sweeteners saccharin and cyclamate are weak bladder carcinogens or co-carcinogens in laboratory animals, but a recent large-scale study of bladder cancer indicated that the risk in humans is very small if present at all. Cooking practices may generate hydrocarbons or other carcinogens at high temperatures, although no epidemiologic observations are available.

GENETIC SUSCEPTIBILITY. Compared to environmental factors in cancer, genetic determinants are less conspicuous and more difficult to identify by clinical and epidemiologic means. Although racial and ethnic differentials for most cancers appear largely modulated by environmental influences, genetic factors may contribute to some high rates (e.g., nasopharyngeal cancer among Chinese and gallbladder cancer among American Indians and certain Hispanic groups) and some low rates (e.g., testicular cancer and Ewing's sarcoma among blacks in Africa and the United States). Genetic susceptibility is most evident for skin cancer, since ethnic variations correspond to the degree of protective skin pigmentation.

Although only a small percentage of cancer is inherited in a mendelian fashion, over 200 single-gene disorders have been linked to neoplasia. Table 170–2 lists some cancers that occur as an inherited trait (hereditary neoplasms), and Table 170–3 presents those arising as a complication of inherited precursor lesions (preneoplastic states). In some syndromes environmental factors contribute to the development of cancer. Neoplasms of a hereditary nature tend to occur earlier in life than do nonfamilial occurrences of the same tumor, and usually arise from multiple foci within the affected organ.

In contrast to the hereditary syndromes, the common human cancers show small familial risks, on the order of two- to three-fold. However, the familial risks for breast and colonic cancers are as high as 20- to 30-fold among subgroups of patients with early onset and bilateral or multifocal origin. Familial susceptibility also appears to enhance the effects of environmental exposures, such as smoking in lung cancer, and sunlight exposure in melanomas derived from dysplastic nevi. In some families there are remarkable aggregations of cancer consistent with an autosomal dominant mode of inheritance. These "cancer families" may display either a single type of cancer or a constellation of multiple cancers, especially adenocarcinomas of the colon and endometrium, or the breast and ovary. Other families are prone to diverse cell types of childhood and adult cancers, particularly soft-tissue and bone sarcomas, breast carcinoma, brain tumors, adrenocortical neoplasms, and leukemia. The delineation of genetic and familial syndromes is helpful in applying laboratory probes to clarify the heritable component and basic mechanisms of carcinogenesis, and in targeting screening and prevention programs designed to protect high risk individuals.

Chaganti RSK, German JL (eds.): Genetics in Clinical Oncology. New York, Oxford University Press, 1985. *A concise guide to the heritable aspects of cancer and the application of cancer genetics to clinical medicine.*

Doll R, Peto R: The causes of cancer: Quantitative estimates of avoidable risks of cancer in the United States today. J Natl Cancer Inst 66:1191, 1981. *A critical review of carcinogenic hazards with emphasis on quantitative risk assessment and the preventable nature of most forms of cancer.*

Schottenfeld D, Fraumeni JF Jr (eds.): Cancer Epidemiology and Prevention. Philadelphia, W. B. Saunders Company, 1982. *A detailed survey of cancer epidemiology, with 70 chapters covering virtually all aspects of the field. The contribution of epidemiology to the development and evaluation of preventive measures is emphasized.*

Vessey MP, Gray M (eds.): Cancer Risks and Prevention. New York, Oxford University Press, 1985. *A review of cancer risk factors and the methods used to apply this information to cancer prevention.*

171 PARANEOPLASTIC SYNDROMES

Paul A. Bunn, Jr.

The paraneoplastic syndromes are a heterogenous group of signs and symptoms indirectly caused by cancers at a distance from the primary tumor or its metastases. These "remote" or "biologic" effects of malignancy are not a direct effect of the primary or metastatic cancer. Distinguishing between the tumor and the paraneoplastic syndrome is the most important step in the differential diagnosis. The majority of paraneoplastic syndromes are caused by proteins secreted by these tumors. In some instances (e. g., endocrine paraneoplastic syndromes), the proteins (hormones) are well characterized, and the pathophysiology is well understood. These paraneoplastic syndromes invariably improve with effective antineoplastic therapy. In addition, drugs that interfere with the hormone action may be useful in severe cases or when the tumor fails to respond to therapy. In other instances the etiology of the syndrome is not clear, and the syndrome may not improve even with effective antitumor therapy. This is often true of the neurologic syndromes, perhaps because the nervous system cannot regenerate and damage is often permanent. Some of these syndromes may be caused by an immunologic reaction to tumor antigens that are shared with normal cells.

Recognizable paraneoplastic syndromes, other than wasting of the host or tumor cachexia, occur in a minority of cancer patients. They may be extremely important, however, in the early detection of the original cancer or may be the first sign of recurrence. They may also simulate metastatic disease and thus prevent patients from receiving curative therapy. Conversely, signs and symptoms of metastatic disease may be falsely ascribed to a paraneoplastic syndrome and thus lead to the withholding of appropriate therapy. Paraneoplastic syndromes may be disabling but treatable with proper recognition. Thus, establishing a diagnosis is extremely important. True paraneoplastic syndromes must be distinguished from those caused by the primary tumor or its metastases, infections, toxicities of therapy, vascular abnormalities, obstruction caused by a tumor or its products, and fluid and electrolyte abnormalities. It is also important to understand which paraneoplastic syndromes respond to primary antitumor therapy. Alternative forms of therapy aimed at symptomatic control should be considered in those syndromes in which response to primary antitumor therapy is unlikely.

WASTING OF THE HOST. Wasting of the host, sometimes called tumor cachexia or the cachexia of malignant disease, is the most common of the paraneoplastic syndromes. The catabolic phase that usually accompanies malignant disease may be out of keeping with the size of the tumor and may be complex in its pathogenesis—decreased caloric intake (there is often a perverted sense of taste and smell with aversion to specific foods), malabsorption, loss of protein (e.g., hemorrhage or effusions), fever, and possibly a change in metabolic pathways. For example, increased anaerobic glycolysis with enhanced gluconeogenesis from amino acids and partial insulin resistance have been described. Possibly factors capable of distorting metabolism are secreted by the tumor, for example, cachectin, a macrophage-derived factor that is capable of inhibiting the activity of certain lipogenic enzymes. Certainly the caloric expenditure tends to remain high, and the basal metabolic rate is increased, despite the reduced intake of calories, suggesting a deranged metabolism.

Treatment of the underlying tumor is the major approach to therapy. Replacement alimentation is reserved for patients undergoing surgical treatment or for patients with severe nutritional deficiency but for whom there is hope for significant remission or cure.

ENDOCRINE PARANEOPLASTIC SYNDROMES. The original description of a paraneoplastic syndrome was that of ectopic Cushing's syndrome, as reported by Brown in 1928. The endocrine neoplastic syndromes are listed in Table 173–1 and are described in detail in Ch. 173, to which the reader is referred.

NEUROLOGIC PARANEOPLASTIC SYNDROMES (Table 174–1). Neurologic signs and symptoms appear frequently in cancer patients and are most often directly related to metastases, fluid and electrolyte abnormalities, vascular abnormalities, infections, or toxicity of therapy. True paraneoplastic syndromes are generally diagnosed by exclusion of these other conditions (Ch. 174). Subacute cerebellar degeneration, subacute motor neuropathy, sensory neuropathy, Eaton-Lambert syndrome, and dermatomyositis in older males are so strongly associated with cancer that their presence should lead to a search for a primary tumor when none is evident.

HEMATOLOGIC PARANEOPLASTIC SYNDROMES. Cancers may indirectly affect any of the hematopoietic cell lines, producing increases or decreases in either individual cell lineages or multiple lineages. Increased cell numbers are generally produced when the tumor secretes a stimulatory hormone/growth factor.

Erythrocytosis most often results from erythropoietin production by renal or liver tumors. In a large review, paraneoplastic erythrocytosis when found was most often associated with hypernephromas (35 per cent), benign renal abnormalities (14 per cent), hepatomas (19 per cent), cerebellar hemangioblastomas (15 per cent), uterine tumors (7 per cent), adrenal tumors and pheochromocytomas (3 per cent), and miscellaneous tumors (3 per cent). In rare cases, induction of local kidney or systemic hypoxia by tumors may also result in erythrocytosis.

Leukemoid reactions, granulocytosis, eosinophilia, and/or basophilia are most often produced when the tumor secretes a colony-stimulating factor (CSF) and thus are corrected by effective treatment of the primary tumor. Granulocytosis is most often associated with lung, gastric, pancreatic, and brain cancers; melanomas; and Hodgkin's and non-Hodgkin's lymphomas. Eosinophilia is most often associated with lymphomas, especially Hodgkin's disease, and gastrointestinal carci-

TABLE 171–1. PARANEOPLASTIC SYNDROMES

1. Wasting of the host—"tumor cachexia"
2. Endocrine/hormone—see Table 173–1
3. Neuromyopathies—see Table 174–1
4. Hematologic
    Erythrocytosis, granulocytosis, thrombocytosis
    Anemia (chronic disease, pure red cell aplasia, hypersplenic, autoimmune hemolytic anemia, microangiopathic hemolytic anemia)
    Granulocytopenia, thrombocytopenia
5. Thromboembolic
    Venous thrombosis (Trousseau's syndrome)
    Disseminated intravascular coagulation
    Nonbacterial thrombotic endocarditis (murantic endocarditis)
6. Renal
    Secondary to hormonal or metabolic effects
    Glomerulopathies—including the nephrotic syndrome
    Miscellaneous—myeloma kidney, amyloidosis, uric acid nephropathy, etc.
7. Dermatologic—see Table 175–4
8. Gastrointestinal
    Anorexia, nausea, vomiting
    Protein-losing enteropathy
    Malignant hepatopathy
9. Miscellaneous
    Lactic acidosis
    Clubbing/hypertrophic pulmonary osteoarthropathy
    Hyperlipidemia
    Hypertension—hypotension
    Hyperamylasemia
    Amyloidosis
    Arthritis

nomas. These syndromes must be differentiated from chronic myelogenous leukemia and other causes of leukemoid reactions such as infection, inflammatory diseases, metabolic diseases, and certain drugs (Ch. 151).

Anemia is frequently associated with malignant disease, and granulocytopenia and thrombocytopenia may also be paraneoplastic in nature. *Autoimmune hemolytic anemia* is most often associated with B cell lymphoproliferative neoplasms and less often with ovarian and lung cancers (Ch. 139). Successful treatment of the primary tumor often leads to improvement; corticosteroids are usually unsuccessful. *Pure red cell aplasia* is found in association with thymomas (50 per cent) and a variety of other cancers.

Microangiopathic hemolytic anemia, a rare cause of anemia in patients with cancer, is diagnosed by the presence of severe hemolytic anemia with fragmented erythrocytes seen in the blood smear and a negative Coombs test. Most often this syndrome is associated with mucin-producing adenocarcinomas, especially those from the stomach (55 per cent), breast (13 per cent), lung (7 per cent), and unknown primary site (10 per cent). It is often abrupt in onset and associated with thrombocytopenia and disseminated intravascular coagulation.

Granulocytopenia is usually the result of chemotherapy, radiation therapy, severe infection, or marrow involvement, but has been reported rarely in association with thymoma. A syndrome resembling *idiopathic thrombocytopenic purpura (ITP)* may occur in association with lymphomas (especially chronic lymphocytic leukemia, Hodgkin's disease, and immunoblastic lymphadenopathy) and less frequently with other malignant disorders.

THROMBOEMBOLIC PARANEOPLASTIC SYNDROMES. A *hypercoagulable* state is frequent in cancer patients and may manifest as: (1) *migratory thrombophlebitis* (Trousseau's syndrome); (2) subacute or overt *disseminated intravascular coagulation* (DIC); and (3) *nonbacterial thrombotic endocarditis* (NBTE, murantic endocarditis); or (4) a combination of these three.

Thrombophlebitis occurs in as many as 1 to 11 per cent of cancer patients and is most often associated with mucin-producing adenocarcinomas of the gastrointestinal tract. It may also be seen with lung, breast, ovarian, and prostate cancers. The treatment of migratory thrombophlebitis is difficult; acute episodes require heparin. Long-term therapy with warfarin is generally unsuccessful, but long-term administration of subcutaneous heparin has had some limited success.

DIC may present as an acute hemorrhagic diathesis or be discovered incidentally as chronic laboratory abnormalities. Coagulation abnormalities by laboratory test may be seen in as many as 90 per cent of patients with cancer, but most of these never develop overt bleeding episodes. Acute episodes are most frequently associated with acute promyelocytic leukemia (APL) and adenocarcinomas (especially prostatic). Identification and treatment of all precipitating factors are the keystones to the management of DIC. This includes therapy for the primary tumor as well as for infection, acidosis, and other factors. Heparin is often used prophylactically in APL although this is not mandatory if all coagulation parameters are normal and are monitored closely. For overt DIC, heparin appears to be superior to warfarin; spontaneous remission of DIC may occur in adenocarcinomas without any therapy.

NBTE is characterized by sterile verrucous lesions on the left-sided heart valves; these thrombi may embolize to the brain and other vital organs. These occur most often with mucin-producing adenocarcinomas. Therapy is directed to the primary tumor. The therapeutic role of heparin and warfarin is uncertain.

RENAL PARANEOPLASTIC SYNDROMES. Most renal abnormalities that occur in patients with cancer are due to metatases, obstruction, electrolyte and fluid imbalances, toxicity of therapy, or infection. The most common renal paraneoplastic syndrome, other than those linked to hormones

(e.g., SIADH), is the nephrotic syndrome. In one report 10 per cent of patients with nephrotic syndrome had underlying malignant disease, with Hodgkin's disease being the most frequently associated disorder. Most of these patients have lipoid nephrosis (minimal change glomerulopathy). In contrast, patients with non-Hodgkin's lymphomas often have immunoglobulin deposits suggesting an immune complex etiology. In both instances the nephrotic syndrome resolves if there is a response to antitumor therapy. Patients with carcinomas most often have membranous glomerulonephritis with subepithelial electron-dense deposits. Other renal abnormalities associated with cancer include (1) the host of abnormalities associated with multiple myeloma and amyloidosis (Ch. 163); (2) the potassium wasting and hypokalemia syndrome caused by lysozyme secreted by patients with acute myelogenous leukemia (M4 or M5); (3) the syndrome of intrarenal obstruction preceded by mucoprotein secreted by patients with pancreatic carcinoma; and (4) the syndrome of nephrogenic diabetes insipidus found in some patients with leiomyosarcoma.

DERMATOLOGIC PARANEOPLASTIC SYNDROMES. This group of syndromes is summarized in Ch. 175. The strongest dermatologic associations with malignant disease are with acanthosis nigricans, erythema gyratum repens, tylosis, dermatomyositis in older males, flushing in the carcinoid syndrome and with the hereditary syndromes (Gardner's syndrome, Peutz-Jegher's syndrome, etc).

GASTROINTESTINAL PARANEOPLASTIC SYNDROMES. *Protein-losing enteropathy* may be produced by inflammation and ulceration of the mucosa, obstruction of intestinal lymphatics (lymphomas), congestive heart failure (carcinoid, pericardial constriction), and by undefined mechanisms. While hypoalbuminemia is common in cancer patients, true protein-losing enteropathy is rare.

Malignant *hepatopathy* (Stauffer's syndrome) is characterized by biochemical abnormalities (increased alkaline phosphatase, hypercholesterolemia, prolonged prothrombin time) and hepatosplenomegaly in association with hypernephroma or malignant schwannoma without liver metastases. These abnormalities improve following resection of the primary tumor.

MISCELLANEOUS PARANEOPLASTIC SYNDROMES. *Fever* is a common finding in cancer patients and is often idiopathic. This is most common in lymphomas (where it is associated with a poor prognosis), hypernephromas, osteogenic sarcomas, and myxomas, although it may be found with other tumors. It almost always disappears with successful antitumor therapy. *Lactic acidosis* may be associated with acute leukemias and lymphomas and responds to successful antitumor therapy. *Hyperlipidemias* have been reported in association with multiple myeloma, hepatoma, and colon cancer.

Hypokalemia and hypertension with tumor production of renin have been reported with lung cancer, hypernephroma, and Wilms' tumor. *Hypotension* has been reported in association with a prostaglandin A–secreting hypernephroma and with intrathoracic tumors secondary to abnormal baroreceptor responses. *Hyperamylasemia* may be caused by lung cancers, especially adenocarcinomas, and is generally not associated with symptoms.

Hypertrophic pulmonary osteoarthropathy is characterized by clubbing, periostitis of the long bones, and occasionally polyarthritis. Involved bones include the distal ends of the tibia, fibula, humerus, radius, or ulna. It is associated most frequently with lung cancer (except small-cell), mesothelioma (especially the benign form), and other cancers when they metastasize to the lungs or mediastinum. The abnormalities improve with successful treatment of the primary tumor. The etiology is unknown.

Amyloidosis occurs in association with multiple myeloma, lymphoma, or carcinomas (especially hypernephroma) in about 15 per cent of cases. The amyloidogenic protein is monoclonal light-chain (AL) in the case of B cell tumors; other proteins (AA) are associated with other tumors (Ch. 210). Amyloidosis causes signs and symptoms by deposition in nerves, heart, kidney, and joints. Prognosis is poor, and there is no specific therapy. *Polyarthritis* has been reported in association with breast and other cancers. *Polymyalgia rheumatica* may precede development of several forms of cancer, and *systemic lupus erythematosus* (SLE) is associated with lymphomas, leukemias, thymomas, and testicular, lung, and ovarian cancers. Remission of SLE may occur with successful antitumor therapy.

Antman KH, Skarin AT, Mayer RJ, et al.: Microangiopathic hemolytic anemia and cancer: A review. Medicine 58:377, 1979. *Reviews the clinical manifestations and etiology of this syndrome.*

Barnes BE: Dermatomyositis and malignancy. A review of the literature. Ann Intern Med 84:68, 1976. *This review evaluates the association of dermatomyositis and malignant disease and shows the strong association in older males.*

Bunn PA Jr, Minna JD: Paraneoplastic syndromes. In DeVita VT, Hellman S, Rosenberg SA (eds.): The Principles and Practice of Oncology. Philadelphia, JB Lippincott Company, 1985, pp 1797–1842. *This chapter is an extensive review of all types of paraneoplastic syndromes with a complete bibliography*

Crowthers D, Bateman CJT: Hematologic aspects of systemic disease—malignant disease. Clin Hematol 1:447, 1972. *This review discusses the various hematologic paraneoplastic syndromes in more detail.*

Markham M: Response of paraneoplastic syndromes to antineoplastic therapy. West J Med 144:5, 1986. *A thorough review of the paraneoplastic syndromes that improve or disappear in response to effective antitumor therapy*

McKinney TD (ed.): Renal Complications of Neoplasia. New York, Praeger, 1986. *A thorough review of all of the renal paraneoplastic syndromes.*

Rickles FR, Edwards RL: Activation of blood coagulation in cancer: Trousseau's syndrome revisited. Blood 63:14, 1983. *Reviews the possible causes of the hypercoaguable state in cancer.*

Sack GH, Levin J, Bell WR: Trousseau's syndrome and other manifestations of chronic disseminated coagulopathy in patients with neoplasms. Medicine 56:1, 1977. *A thorough review of the various manifestations of the hypercoagulable state associated with cancer.*

Torti FM, Dieckmann B, Beutler B, et al.: A macrophage factor inhibits adipocyte gene expression: An in vitro model of cachexia. Science 229:867, 1985. Theologides A: Anorexins, asthenins, and cachectins in cancer. Am J Med 81:696, 1986. *These two articles suggest that "cachectin"–"tumor necrosis factor" and/or other monokines may play a role in the cachexia of malignant disease.*

172 TUMOR MARKERS

Paul A. Bunn, Jr.

In malignant disease there is aberrant expression of a number of genes. Many of the products of these genes, including hormones, enzymes, immunoglobulins, and a variety of other proteins, may be secreted by the tumor cell. If there is sufficient secretion (dependent on the tumor burden and the secretory capacity of each cell) without rapid metabolic degradation, the secreted protein may be detectable in the serum. These proteins or biomarkers are potentially useful for (1) screening populations, (2) early detection of patients with suspected disease, (3) assessing tumor burden and prognosis, (4) assessing response to therapy, and (5) evaluating early recurrence. Currently available radioimmunoassays can often detect minute amounts (nanograms) of the marker substance. All of the marker proteins, however, are products of normal cells and may be present in small amounts in normal serum. Furthermore, the levels of some marker proteins may also increase with inflammation. Thus the specificity of each marker must be well defined. Very few tumor markers are sufficiently sensitive and specific to be useful for each of these above purposes. The most established tumor markers include the beta subunit of human chorionic gonadotropin (beta-HCG), alpha fetoprotein (AFP), idiotypic immunoglobulins, and carcinoembryonic antigen (CEA). A list of currently used markers is shown in Table 172–1.

HORMONES. Human chorionic gonadotropin *HCG* is a two-chain (alpha and beta subunits) glycoprotein hormone secreted by the trophoblastic epithelium of the placenta. The beta subunit is normally present in maternal serum during pregnancy, but its presence in males and nonpregnant females is indicative of cancer. Measurement of HCG has been used

TABLE 172–1. TUMOR CELL MARKERS

Marker	Tumor Types
Hormones	
Beta subunit of chorionic gonadotropin	Testicular cancers, choriocarcinoma, hydatidiform mole
AVP, ACTH	Small-cell lung; APUD tumors
Calcitonin	Medullary thyroid carcinoma, small-cell lung and APUD tumors
Gastrin-releasing peptide (bombesin)	Small-cell lung cancer
Placental lactogen	Trophoblastic tumors, various carcinomas
Oncofetal Proteins	
Alpha-fetoprotein	Hepatoma, testicular cancers
Carcinoembryonic antigen (CEA)	Gastrointestinal tract, breast, lung, ovarian cancers
Enzymes	
L-dopa decarboxylase	Small-cell lung cancer
Creatine phosphokinase (BB)	Prostate cancer, small-cell lung cancer
Neuron-specific enolase	Prostate cancer, small-cell lung cancer, others
Acid phosphatase (prostate specific)	Prostate cancer
Placental alkaline phosphatase	Uterus, ovary, breast, lung cancers
Lysozyme	Acute nonlymphatic leukemia (myelomonocytic and monocytic types)
Serum galactosyltransferase	Gastrointestinal carcinoma, breast and prostate cancers
Lactic dehydrogenase (LDH)	Lymphomas, Ewing's sarcoma, various carcinomas
Secreted Tumor Antigens	
CA 125	Ovarian cancer, other epithelial cancers
CA 19-9	Various carcinomas
Other glycosphingolipids	Various carcinomas
β_2 microglobulin	Multiple myeloma
Miscellaneous	
Vitamin B_{12}–binding proteins	Acute or chronic myelogenous leukemia, myeloproliferative disease
Immunoglobin	B cell lymphoproliferative diseases
Polyamines	Various carcinomas
Chromogranin A	Small-cell lung cancer
Proton NMR spectroscopy	All malignant tumors

for the diagnosis and management of trophoblastic tumors (choriocarcinoma, hydatidiform mole), and certain germ cell tumors of the testes. Its level has prognostic importance. The rate of decline may be used to assess the effectiveness of therapy, and its reappearance is direct evidence of tumor recurrence. Extragonadal germ cell tumors often secrete beta-HCG and it can be used to help confirm the origin of undifferentiated mediastinal or retroperitoneal tumors. Beta-HCG may also be secreted by adenocarcinomas of the ovary, pancreas, stomach, and lung and by hepatomas.

A variety of other hormones may be useful tumor markers. Human placental lactogen is secreted by the majority of trophoblastic tumors and a minority of lung cancers, hepatomas, endocrine tumors, leukemias, and lymphomas.

Polypeptide hormones such as adrenocorticotropic hormone (*ACTH*) and arginine vasopressin (*AVP*) may be useful markers when produced by small-cell lung cancer or other tumors with properties of amine precursor uptake and decarboxylation (APUD tumors). Similarly, *calcitonin* is used to predict medullary carcinoma of the thyroid in families or it can be used as a marker in APUD tumors that secrete it. *Gastrin-releasing peptide* (bombesin-like protein) is produced by the majority of small-cell lung cancers. It is not an ideal tumor marker, however, because it is rapidly degraded in plasma. Elevated levels in the cerebrospinal fluid (CSF) may be useful for predicting leptomeningeal metastases.

ONCOFETAL PROTEINS. *Alpha-fetoprotein* (AFP) is normally secreted in large amounts during the twelfth through fifteenth weeks of gestation and then declines to low levels (<40 ng per milliliter) by the age of one year. Elevated levels occur in the majority (75 per cent) of patients with embryonal and teratocarcinomas of the testes and ovary, as well as in those with extragonadal germ cell tumors. Like beta-HCG, the level has prognostic implications; the rate of decline predicts the effectiveness of therapy, and a rising titer is direct evidence of tumor progression. Elevated AFP levels are present in 70 to 95 per cent of hepatomas. The incidence is highest in areas where hepatoma is endemic. AFP is increased in a minority of patients with cancers of the pancreas, stomach, colon, and lung. Since AFP is produced by normal cells, there are instances of "false positives." AFP may be produced by benign liver tumors, by cirrhotic livers, or during hepatitis, although these entities usually produce levels less than 500 ng per milliliter. AFP may be increased in patients with ataxia-telangiectasia.

Carcinoembryonic antigen (CEA) is normally secreted during the second to sixth months of gestation. In nonsmoking adults, serum levels are less than 2.5 ng per milliliter, whereas smokers have normal levels up to 5 ng per milliliter. Serum levels of CEA may increase in a variety of inflammatory conditions (e.g., cirrhosis, pancreatitis, inflammatory bowel disease, and rectal polyps) as well as in a variety of human cancers.

Elevated levels of CEA are reported in patients with colon cancer (60 to 90 per cent), pancreatic cancer (80 per cent), gastric cancer (60 per cent), lung cancer (75 per cent), breast cancer (50 per cent), and many other malignant tumors in lower frequency. The frequency with which the level of CEA is elevated and the level attained are dependent on the extent of disease, the degree of differentiation (well-differentiated tumors produce more), and the presence of liver metastases. Because of the high false positive rate in inflammatory diseases, the principal use of CEA is in monitoring response to therapy and disease progression, especially for carcinoma of the colon (Ch. 107). Elevated levels should return to normal following complete resection of the primary tumor. A persistent elevation or an increasing concentration is highly suggestive of residual or recurrent tumor. Surgical reexploration in the face of increasing CEA without clinical evidence of disease may lead to discovery of surgically resectable recurrences. These patients may then have a long disease-free survival.

Radiolabeled antibodies to CEA and AFP are being evaluated for their ability to detect metastatic disease and for therapy. Preliminary studies show sensitivities in the range of 60 to 80 per cent.

ENZYMES. A variety of enzymes are also useful tumor markers in some settings. The key APUD enzyme, L-dopa decarboxylase, is often increased in patients with small-cell lung cancer and other APUD tumors. The serum level of the BB isoenzyme of creatine phosphokinase is elevated in the majority of patients with small-cell lung cancer or cancer of the prostate. Serum levels of neuron-specific enolase are often elevated in patients with these same tumors.

Prostatic epithelium also produces a specific *acid phosphatase* (*prostatic acid phosphatase*) whose serum level is elevated in about one third of patients with occult prostatic cancer and in 75 per cent of patients with more advanced prostatic cancers. *Placental alkaline phosphatase* is secreted by a minority of cancers of the female reproductive organs and breast and lung cancers. *Lysozyme*, a monocyte-derived enzyme, is frequently increased in patients with acute monocytic and myelomonocytic leukemia. An isoenzyme of *serum galactosyltransferase* is present in the serum of patients with gastrointestinal carcinomas (75 per cent), and breast cancer (78 per cent), as well as in a minority of patients with prostatic cancer and lymphoproliferative cancers. Serum lactic dehydrogenase (LDH) levels are elevated in a variety of malignant diseases, including lymphomas (especially Burkitt's), Ewing's sarcomas, and a variety of carcinomas. The extent of elevation may provide prognostic information as well as a useful measure of antitumor response.

SECRETED TUMOR ANTIGENS. The development of monoclonal antibody technology has led to recognition of many new glycoprotein and glycolipid antigens on tumor cells that may be secreted into the plasma. The antigen recognized by the monoclonal antibody *CA 125* is a useful marker for the majority of patients with ovarian cancer. *CA 19-9* recognizes an antigen secreted by many epithelial carcinomas, including colon cancer, but this marker is probably less useful than CEA. Many epithelial carcinomas, especially adenocarcinomas, secrete glycosphingolipids such as Lewis blood group antigens and human milk fat globule antigens. The value of these markers remains to be established. β_2 microglobulin, an HLA class I antigen, is present on the cell surface of most nucleated cells. It is secreted into the plasma in excess amounts in patients with multiple myeloma, where its level has prognostic value and may be useful in assessing response to therapy.

MISCELLANEOUS. *Vitamin B_{12}*–binding proteins are frequently increased in myeloproliferative disorders and occasionally in acute or chronic myelogenous leukemias. The idiotypic *immunoglobulins* produced by B cell lymphoproliferative malignant disorders are excellent tumor markers and may be used to assess tumor burden as well as to follow response to therapy. More than 99 per cent of patients with multiple myelomas and Waldenstrom's macroglobulinemia secrete a heavy chain or a light chain (Ch. 163). Occasionally these tumors secrete globulins of more than one idiotype. Monoclonal antibodies to the idiotypic immunoglobulin are being evaluated as therapeutic agents. *Polyamines* are generally secreted in direct relation to the rate of proliferation. In many malignant diseases their quantitation has proven to be useful for prognosis and in assessing response. They are not sufficiently sensitive or specific for widespread use. *Chromogranin A* is a 68,000-dalton protein found in the neurosecretory granules of normal and malignant APUD cells. Serum measurement by radioimmunoassay may be a useful marker of small-cell lung cancer disease activity. *Water-suppressed proton nuclear magnetic resonance spectrum* of plasma is dominated by the resonances of plasma lipoprotein lipids. This spectrum narrows in patients with all types of cancer evaluated and is thus a potentially valuable approach to the early detection of cancer and the monitoring of therapy.

Aroney RS, Dermody WC, Aldernderfer P, et al.: Multiple sequential biomarkers in monitoring patients with carcinoma of the lung. Cancer Treat Rep 68:859, 1984. *Reviews the variety of proteins secreted by small-cell lung cancers that can be used as tumor markers.*

Fossel ET, Carr JM, McDonagh J: Detection of malignant tumors. Water suppressed proton nuclear magnetic resonance spectroscopy of plasma. N Engl J Med 315:1369, 1986. *This stimulating novel technique was valuable in the early diagnosis and follow-up of a variety of malignant tumors.*

Hakomori S: Glycosphingolipids. Sci Am 254(5):44, 1986. *This article reviews the various glycosphingolipid antigens present on cancer cells.*

Novis BH, Gluck E, Thomas P, et al.: Serial levels of CA 19-9 and CEA in colonic cancer. J Clin Oncol 4:987, 1986. *An article comparing the utility of these markers.*

Rosen SW, Weintraub BD, Vaitukaitus JL, et al.: Placental proteins and their subunits as tumor markers. Ann Intern Med 82:71, 1975. *A review of the value of placental proteins as tumor markers.*

Sobol RE, O'Connor DT, Addison J, et al.: Elevated serum chromogranin A concentrations in small cell lung cancer. Ann Intern Med 105:698, 1986. *This article is an example of one of several markers of neuroendocrine cells that are useful in following the course of small-cell lung cancer patients.*

Wanebo HJ, Rao B, Pinsky CM, et al.: Preoperative carcinoembryonic antigen level as a prognostic indicator in colorectal cancer. N Engl J Med 299:448, 1978. *This article shows the value of oncofetal markers as prognostic indicators.*

173 ENDOCRINE MANIFESTATIONS OF TUMORS: "ECTOPIC" HORMONE PRODUCTION

William D. Odell

Cancers often produce symptoms by means of the elaboration of humoral or hormonal substances in addition to those symptoms produced directly by tumor mass or invasion.

Although several chemical classes of hormones exist, these cancer humoral or hormonal substances are usually protein or peptide in nature. These protein substances are so ubiquitously distributed in noncancerous tissues that it is difficult to determine whether they are ectopic or eutopic. Furthermore, all cancers appear to be associated with production of such proteins, usually in markedly increased amounts over normal tissues. These proteins are usually biologically inactive or weakly bioactive and produce no recognizable clinical symptoms. When biologically active substances are produced, clinical symptoms result. A very large number of proteins are produced by cancers; those that are hormones or hormone precursors are listed in Table 173–1. Steroids or thyronines seem not to be secreted as part of ectopic endocrine syndromes, although rarely a cancer may convert a bioinactive steroid such as dehydroepiandrosterone to a bioactive one. As discussed under hypercalcemia, some malignant tumors may convert 25-hydroxyvitamin D to 1,25-dihydroxyvitamin D.

ECTOPIC ACTH PRODUCTION. The association of Cushing's syndrome with carcinoma is the most common ectopic endocrine syndrome. Fifty per cent of reported patients have carcinoma of the lung (predominantly oat cell or small round cell), 10 per cent have carcinoma of the thymus, 10 per cent have carcinoma of the pancreas (including carcinoids and islet cell tumors), 5 per cent have medullary carcinoma of the thyroid (which also produces calcitonin), and 5 per cent have neoplasms derived from the neural crest (pheochromocytoma, neuroblastoma, paraganglioma, and ganglioma). Considered conversely, about 3 per cent of patients with oat cell carcinoma of the lung have clinical or laboratory evidence of Cushing's syndrome—often extremely subtly manifested. Although other carcinomas are associated with Cushing's syndrome less frequently, numerous isolated case reports suggest that any carcinoma may show this association.

Immunoactive ACTH can be detected universally in extracts prepared from carcinomas of the lung, colon, stomach, pancreas, or esophagus. In fact, a large glycoprotein containing immunoactivities of both ACTH and beta-melanocyte-stimulating hormone may be extracted from all normal nonendocrine tissues. This material, present in small quantities in normal tissues, is present in large quantities in extracts of carcinomas, regardless of histologic type. It has no biologic activity in sensitive dispersed adrenal cell assays in vitro, but is converted to a 4500 MW bioactive ACTH by exposure to trypsin. Presumably this material in both normal tissue extracts and carcinomas is *proopiomelanocortin* (POMC). An identical material is detectable in the blood of 70 per cent of patients with carcinoma of the lung, regardless of histologic type, using immunoassays. However, only some carcinomas enzymatically convert this biologically inactive POMC to biologically active ACTH. This conversion process is preferentially associated with the histologic types of neoplasms previously listed as being associated with clinical Cushing's syndrome.

POMC, in addition to the ACTH sequence, also contains the sequence of the endorphins, lipotropin, and beta-melanocyte-stimulating hormone. Previous reports of MSH and lipotropin production by cancers are best explained by detection of circulating POMC per se or its cleavage products, lipotropin and/or MSH.

The symptoms produced by the ectopic production of *bioactive* ACTH are varied, ranging from none—simply the laboratory data of increased cortisol—to full features of Cushing's syndrome. Often they are subtle, consisting only of mild weakness or the laboratory finding of hypokalemia without physical abnormalities. Hypokalemia is uncommon in Cushing's disease of pituitary origin. The classic Cushing's syndrome is not commonly associated with cancer, for such physical changes usually require from months to years to be produced and often the neoplasm is present but a short while.

TABLE 173–1. HORMONES REPORTED TO BE SECRETED BY CANCERS

Proopiomelanocortin	Calcitonin
ACTH	Growth hormone
Chorionic gonadotropin	Prolactin
Alpha peptide chain	Gastrin
Beta peptide chain	Secretin
Vasopressin	Glucagon
Somatomedins	Corticotropin releasing hormone
Hypoglycemia-producing factor	Growth hormone releasing hormone
Growth factors	Gastrin-releasing peptide
Osteoclast-activating factor	Somatostatin
1,25-Dihydroxyvitamin D	Chorionic somatotropin
Parathormone-like-factors	Neurophysins
Erythropoietin	Eosinophilopoietin
Hypophosphatemia-producing factor	

The occurrence of psychosis, weakness, hypokalemia, or an abnormal glucose tolerance curve in a patient with known cancer suggest ectopic bioactive ACTH production. Plasma ACTH concentrations are often extremely high, unlike those in Cushing's disease, which are usually "normal" but in association with an elevated cortisol concentration. In addition, suppression with high doses of oral dexamethasone (8 mg per day) usually does not occur in ectopic ACTH syndrome, but does occur in Cushing's disease (of pituitary origin). Adrenal carcinomas or adenomas producing excess cortisol are associated with undetectable or very low levels of plasma ACTH in conjunction with elevated plasma cortisols (see Ch. 230).

Approximately 50 to 60 per cent of patients with bronchial adenoma and ectopic Cushing's syndrome show cortisol or ACTH suppression with administration of large doses of dexamethasone. The most likely explanation is that these neoplasms produce corticotropin-releasing hormone (CRH) (a 41-amino acid peptide normally produced by the hypothalamus to control pituitary ACTH secretion). The tumor CRH stimulates secretion of ACTH by the normal pituitary. In such patients dexamethasone inhibits CRH action directly at the pituitary gland. Although this hypothesis is untested with respect to bronchial adenoma–ACTH syndrome, the production of CRH-like material by tumors has been described.

Treatment of Cushing's syndrome caused by cancer depends upon resection of the tumor or effective chemotherapy. If this is not possible, treatment with drugs that interfere with adrenal steroid synthesis prevents the continued ACTH production from stimulating excess adrenal secretion of cortisol—e.g., metyrapone, aminoglutethimide, or ketoconazole.

In summary, POMC is probably produced in small quantities by all normal nonendocrine tissues. It may be an autocrine or paracrine substance. Cancers produce increased quantities of POMC that can often be detected by immunoassay in increased quantities in the blood of patients with cancer. Selected carcinomas, related to histologic type, metabolize POMC to biologically active ACTH and occasionally MSH or lipotropin, producing the so-called ectopic ACTH-MSH syndrome. These and similar data concerning chorionic gonadotropin (CG) have led to the belief that ectopic humoral syndromes are not ectopic. Why some cancers metabolize POMC and most do not remains an important unanswered question.

HYPERCALCEMIA AND CANCER. Hypercalcemia is a common finding in patients with cancer. In a large series of patients with bronchogenic carcinoma, 12.5 per cent were hypercalcemic. The frequency of hypercalcemia varied with histologic type: 23 per cent with epidermoid carcinoma, 12.5 per cent with anaplastic carcinoma, and 2.5 per cent with adenocarcinoma. When carcinoma-associated hypercalcemia occurs, the tumors most frequently found are carcinoma of the lung (approximately 35 per cent), carcinoma of the kidney (24 per cent), and carcinoma of the ovary (8 per cent). However, any carcinoma may produce hypercalcemia. The cause of hypercalcemia in the majority of patients remains controversial. Multiple substances appear to be involved. Most of these factors appear to stimulate osteoclast activity with resultant increased bone resorption. This increased resorption is not associated with increased bone formation. Such "uncoupling" of resorption and formation is characteristic of cancer hypercalcemia.

The mechanisms of hypercalcemic caused by solid tumors are different from those caused by malignant hematologic disease. The malignant hematologic diseases appear to produce one or more factors that act locally (paracrine effects) to stimulate bone resorption. In contrast, solid tumors causing hypercalcemia act by producing factors that circulate as a hormone and stimulate osteoclastic activity. In addition, the hypercalcemia caused by both solid tumors and hematologic malignant disease is commonly associated with decreased renal clearance of calcium.

Hematologic Malignant Disease and Hypercalcemia. Most patients with multiple myeloma have extensive bone destruction, and 20 to 40 per cent develop hypercalcemia. This hypercalcemia is produced by increased osteoclast activity caused by locally acting factors produced by the myeloma cells. These factors probably include (1) osteoclast-activating factor (OAF), a bone-resorbing protein produced by activated normal lymphocytes; (2) lymphotoxin (produced by lymphocytes); and (3) tumor necrosis factor, also called cachectin (produced by monocytes). All of these proteins stimulate bone resorption in vitro. Decreased renal excretion of calcium is also important in the development of hypercalcemia in these patients.

Many patients with adult T cell lymphoma develop hypercalcemia. Most of the hypercalcemic patients have lymphoma caused by a type C retrovirus, HTLV-I. These cells produce several factors that increase osteoclast activity, including OAF, colony-stimulating factors, and gamma interferon. These tumor cells also produce lymphokines, and thus additional possibilities include lymphotoxin and/or tumor necrosis factor. In addition, these tumor cells hydroxylate 25-hydroxyvitamin D to 1,25-dihydroxyvitamin D, which may also contribute to hypercalcemia by increasing bone resorption in patients with HTLV-I lymphoma.

Solid Tumors and Hypercalcemia. Solid tumors produce a humoral substance or substances that stimulate osteoclast activity. This syndrome of solid-tumor hypercalcemia is usually associated with increased renal cyclic AMP production, inhibition of renal tubule phosphate reabsorption, and increased renal calcium reabsorption, all consistent with the effects of parathormone (PTH). There is no renal bicarbonate wasting, however, as is observed in primary hyperparathyroidism.

Contrary to previous concepts, the hypercalcemia is not due to the ectopic production of PTH: (1) With current assays, PTH is either suppressed or undetectable in this syndrome. (2) PTH messenger RNA is not detectable in such tumors. (3) Anti-PTH antibodies do not inhibit the biologic action of the hypercalcemic factor(s) in in vitro assays of tumor and blood extracts of patients with solid tumors and hypercalcemia. This PTH-like factor does bind to PTH receptors in in vitro cell systems, and its binding is abolished by specific PTH antagonists acting at the receptor level. Purification and characterization of this PTH-like factor are being actively pursued.

Several other proteins that stimulate osteoclastic activity in in vitro assays are also produced: transforming growth factor alpha (TGF-alpha), platelet derived growth factor (PDGF), transforming growth factor beta (TGF-beta). The *sis* oncogene codes for a peptide with homology to PDGF. In vitro PDGF enhances the osteoclast-stimulating potency of TGF-beta and -alpha.

Prostaglandins. Several reports describe hypercalcemia produced by carcinomas that were associated with increased prostaglandin excretion or production. In a few patients, treatment with indomethacin returned elevated serum calcium levels to normal. However, as large numbers of patients were studied, no investigators have reported success with routine use of indomethacin as treatment for hypercalcemia caused by cancer. Production of prostaglandins by cancer with release systemically is probably not a common cause of hypercalcemia in patients.

Concurrent Primary Hyperparathyroidism. Hyperparathyroidism per se is a common disorder and has repeatedly been described in patients with known cancers. The presence of hyperparathyroidism in a patient with cancer may be suggested by a high plasma PTH level (which is very rare in cancer), using amino terminal PTH immunoassays.

Summary. Hypercalcemia is a common abnormality produced by cancer. Since hypercalcemia may itself produce considerable morbidity or even death, recognition and prompt treatment are essential, and the diagnosis should be considered in any patient with cancer who develops polyuria, constipation, lethargy, or personality change. Patients with known carcinomas may be eucalcemic when active and ambulatory, but may rapidly develop dangerous hypercalcemia when immobilized. The nonspecific treatment of severe hypercalcemia is described in Ch. 247. It generally depends on infusions of saline, diuresis with furosemide, and ambulation. If this does not suffice, treatment with mithramycin, which inhibits bone resorption, may be necessary as an emergency procedure. The administration of calcitonin and glucocorticoids has been used for short-term treatment. Diphosphonate or phosphate, given orally, has been used for long-term treatment. Obviously therapy directed toward the tumor itself should be concomitantly employed, but this is much more slowly effective, if at all.

HYPOPHOSPHATEMIA. A rare syndrome of profound hypophosphatemia, with normal serum calcium, in association with an unusual variety of neoplasms, has been described in perhaps 20 patients. The neoplasms producing this syndrome include pleomorphic sarcomas, hemangiomas, giant cell tumors of bone, or benign osteoblastomas. This syndrome may be more common than previously recognized, being sometimes erroneously reported as adult-onset vitamin D–resistant rickets. Recently, patients with prostatic carcinoma were reported to have hypophosphatemia. The syndrome is associated with dramatic phosphaturia, normal or undetectable plasma PTH, normal serum calcium, and, often, severe muscle spasms. There is severe osteomalacia with bone pain and fractures that occur with minimal trauma. In some (perhaps all) patients, the profound phosphaturia is also associated with aminoaciduria and glucosuria. Blood concentrations of 25-hydroxyvitamin D are normal; 1,25-dihydroxyvitamin D concentrations are low. The serum phosphorus returns to normal following resection of the tumor or following treatment with 1,25-dihydroxyvitamin D. These tumors apparently elaborate a material that inhibits 1-hydroxylation of vitamin D by the kidney.

CHORIONIC GONADOTROPIN. A substance similar but probably not identical to normal chorionic gonadotropin (CG) is elaborated by all normal human tissues and is extractable from all carcinomas. In about 5 to 15 per cent of patients with carcinomas of all kinds, this gonadotropin is detectable in blood. The difference between CG secreted by the trophoblast and that contained in normal tissues lies in the carbohydrate composition. Carbohydrate constitutes about a third of the molecular weight of trophoblast CG. Normal tissue CG contains little or no carbohydrate. The degradation rate or metabolic clearance rate of CG from plasma is inversely related to its carbohydrate content. Thus, presumably, carbohydrate-free CG has extremely little biologic activity in vivo and is cleared from plasma with a half-life of minutes. Carbohydrate-rich CG is cleared slowly with a half-life of hours. All carcinomas also secrete CG. However, those associated with detectable blood concentrations also glycosylate this material, increasing biologic activity and slowing metabolic clearance sufficiently to reach detectable blood concentrations. Approximately 10 per cent of patients with a wide variety of carcinomas have elevated blood CG (e.g., carcinoma of the lung, stomach, pancreas, colon). Men with such tumors often have mild gynecomastia. A rare syndrome produced by CG is precocious puberty in boys with hepatoblastoma.

HYPOGLYCEMIA AND CANCER. Tumor-associated hypoglycemia occurs most frequently with neoplasms that can be loosely termed mesotheliomas. They include more specifically fibrosarcomas, neurofibromas, neurofibrosarcomas, spindle cell carcinomas, rhabdomyosarcomas, and leiomyosarcomas. Such tumors are usually large when hypoglycemia is noted, ranging in size from 800 to 10,000 grams, and are found mainly in the abdomen. They may also develop within the thorax. In the remaining one third, the most frequent tumors are hepatic carcinomas (21 per cent), adrenal cortical carcinomas (6 per cent) and a variety of anaplastic adenocarcinomas, pseudomyxomas, and cholangiomas. Studies utilizing both tumor extracts and blood samples can be summarized as follows: (1) A hypoglycemic factor that mimics insulin activity by in vitro bioassay is often demonstrable; (2) insulin itself is usually not demonstrable by insulin radioimmunoassay; and (3) a substance is often detectable in increased concentrations as measured by radioreceptor assays that quantify somatomedins and so-called nonsuppressible insulin-like activity or insulin-like growth factors (IGF-I and IGF-II). Thus, hypoglycemia associated with cancer may be caused by one or more of the somatomedins, a family of protein substances normally elaborated by the liver that differ structurally from insulin but that have many of its biologic properties. Current assay systems indicate that such substances are increased in blood and tumor extracts from some (perhaps 50 per cent), but not all, of the patients with this syndrome.

GROWTH HORMONE AND GROWTH HORMONE RELEASING HORMONE. Acromegaly associated with bronchial carcinoid or pancreatic islet cell tumor occurs in a small number of patients. In at least five of these patients, growth hormone (GH) secretion was restored to normal or the clinical signs of acromegaly subsided after the extrapituitary tumor was removed without any therapy being directed toward the pituitary gland. Extracts from such an adenoma were found to contain a potent substance capable of releasing GH from dispersed pituitary cells in culture. This GH releasing hormone (GHRH) has been shown to be probably identical to that produced by the hypothalamus normally to control secretion of GH. Elaboration of GHRH by a peripheral tumor may therefore have the potential of leading to a pituitary tumor. The presence of an extrapituitary tumor should be excluded in any patient with acromegaly.

In addition to elaboration of GHRH, tumors could elaborate GH per se. High concentrations of GH have been found in extracts of ovarian carcinomas in patients without acromegaly.

CALCITONIN. Calcitonin is normally secreted by the parafollicular cells of the thyroid gland and serves as an excellent hormonal marker of tumors developing from these cells—medullary carcinomas (Ch. 248). Calcitonin is also secreted ectopically by a variety of carcinomas, but since this hormone has little or no biologic effect in normal adults, no symptoms are produced. Elevated plasma concentrations of calcitonin have been described in patients with carcinomas of the lung (regardless of histologic type), colon, breast, and pancreas. Direct synthesis of calcitonin by the tumor or an arteriovenous gradient of the hormone across a tumor has not been reported.

VASOPRESSIN. Schwartz and Bartter first described the syndrome of cancer associated with hyponatremia, hypervolemia, renal sodium loss, and inappropriately high urine osmolality to which their name is sometimes attached (see Ch. 77). The associated symptoms are those of decrease in mental acuity, confusion, or even seizures. This syndrome has been attributed to secretion of arginine vasopressin (AVP)

by the tumor; vasopressin has been demonstrated by bioassay and radioimmunoassay in extracts of such neoplasms, and synthesis of AVP (incorporation of tritiated amino acids) by extracts of lung cancer has been found in vitro. Ectopic production of vasopressin is very common in patients with carcinoma of the lung (found in 42 per cent in one series). Excess vasopressin produces no symptoms unless the patient continues to drink "excess" water. In normal persons thirst is suppressed by a fall in plasma osmolality. Possibly the smaller percentage of patients with excess vasopressin who develop symptoms of water intoxication and hyponatremia have both a sustained hypersecretion of vasopressin and a defect in thirst control. The treatment of the syndrome of inappropriate secretion of antidiuretic hormone, sometimes called SIADH, is considered in Ch. 77.

A single larger precursor molecule contains the amino acid sequence of both neurophysin II and arginine vasopressin (see Ch. 227). Normally enzymatic cleavage releases neurophysin II and vasopressin on a mole-for-mole basis. Elevation of plasma neurophysin has been found in approximately 40 per cent of unselected patients with lung carcinoma, a value similar to that found for vasopressin.

ERYTHROPOIETIN. This glycoprotein hormone is normally secreted by the kidney and stimulates differentiation of early red cell stages, resulting in increased red cell production (see Ch. 153). A variety of benign and malignant conditions involving the kidney are associated with erythrocytosis. About two thirds of patients with erythropoietin-induced erythrocytosis have hypernephroma, renal cysts, or hydronephrosis. These are not examples of ectopic hormonal syndromes, but represent retained properties of a neoplasm derived from the tissue normally producing the hormone. About one third of patients have neoplasms derived from tissues not known to produce erythropoietin normally. These include hemangioblastomas (21 per cent), uterine fibromas (6 per cent), adrenal cortical neoplasms (3 per cent), ovarian neoplasms (3 per cent), hepatomas (3 per cent), and pheochromocytomas (1 per cent). The biochemical characteristics of the tumor-produced erythropoietin are indistinguishable from erythropoietin produced by the normal kidney.

EOSINOPHILOPOIETIN. Eosinophilia occurs in an occasional patient with malignant disease. Eosinophilia, irrespective of cause, is in turn often associated with endocardial fibrosis, mural thrombus development, and embolic phenomena. An undifferentiated lung carcinoma that produced this syndrome was found to contain large amounts of an eosinophilopoietin-like material, measured by an in vitro eosinophil colony growth assay. In proximity to fibrotic cardiac endothelium were masses of aggregated eosinophils. These eosinophils were shown to generate large amounts of toxic oxygen species, demonstrated to be toxic to cultured endothelial cells in vitro.

SUMMARY. A large variety of protein hormones or protein hormone-like materials are produced by cancers. Most are biologically inert or weakly bioactive. Similar or identical substances are often produced by most or all normal tissues (e.g., POMC, CG) or by a selected group of normal tissues (e.g., erythropoietin, IGF-I and II). Selected carcinomas, correlated with histologic type, metabolize some of these substances into bioactive forms, producing humoral syndromes. It may presently be hypothesized that ectopic hormone production is not ectopic. Detection and quantification of the biologically inactive or weakly bioactive proteins have been useful in early tumor diagnosis and in following response to therapy.

GENERAL REFERENCES

Frohman LA: Ectopic hormone production. Am J Med 70:995, 1981. *An editorial overview of current concepts concerning production of hormones by tumors. There is a short but useful list of references.*

Mundy GR: Ectopic hormonal syndromes in neoplastic diseases. Hosp Prac 22:113, 1987. *A recent useful review.*

Odell WD: Humoral manifestations of cancer. *In* Williams RH (ed.): Textbook of Endocrinology, 7th ed. Philadelphia, W.B. Saunders Company, 1984, Chapter 31. *A more detailed review of humoral syndromes produced by cancer.*

PROOPIOMELANOCORTIN, LIPOTROPIN, MSH

Saito E, Iwasa S, Odell WD: Widespread presence of large molecular weight adrenocorticotropin-like substances in normal rat extrapituitary tissues. Endocrinology 113:1010, 1983. *This paper shows for the first time that proopiomelanocortin is extractable from all normal nonendocrine tissues.*

HYPERCALCEMIA

Bender RA, Hansen H: Hypercalcemia in bronchogenic carcinoma. A prospective study of 200 patients. Ann Intern Med 80:205, 1974. *An analysis of the frequency of hypercalcemia in patients with various histologic types of lung cancer.*
Breslau NA, McGuire JL, Zerwekh JE, et al.: Hypercalcemia associated with increased serum calcitriol levels in three patients with lymphoma. Ann Intern Med 100:1, 1984. *Evidence for another interesting mechanism for tumor-associated hypercalcemia—that of production of the most active form of vitamin D.*
Goltzman D, Stewart AF, Broadus AE: Malignancy-associated hypercalcemia: Evaluation with a cytochemical bioassay for parathyroid hormone. J Clin Endocrinol Metab 53:899, 1981.
Merendino JJ Jr, Insogna KL, Milstone LM, et al.: A parathyroid hormone-like protein from cultured human keratinocytes. Science 231:388, 1986.
Mundy GR: Pathogenesis of hypercalcemia of malignancy. Clin Endocrinol 23:705, 1985. *This is an outstanding review of hypercalcemia caused by cancer.*
Simpson EL, Mundy GR, D'Souza SM, et al: Absence of parathyroid hormone messenger RNA in nonparathyroid tumors associated with hypercalcemia. N Engl J Med 309:325, 1983.

HYPOPHOSPHATEMIA

Weidner N, Cruz DS: Phosphaturic mesenchymal tumors: A polymorphous group causing osteomalacia or rickets. Cancer 59:1442, 1987. *This is an excellent review of this intriguing topic of the production of reversible metabolic bone disease by tumors.*

CHORIONIC GONADOTROPIN

Yoshimoto Y, Wolfsen AR, Odell WD: Glycosylation, a variable in the production of hCG by cancers. Am J Med 67:414, 1979. *This study demonstrates that hCG-like material is present in extracts of all carcinomas and of all normal human tissues. The hCG in most carcinomas and in all normal tissues except the placenta is very low in or free of carbohydrate. The hCG extracted from placenta or present in cancers or blood of patients with cancer associated with detectable hCG is carbohydrate rich.*

HYPOGLYCEMIA

Gordon P, Hendricks CM, Kahn CR, et al.: Hypoglycemia associated with non-islet-cell tumor and insulin-like growth factors. N Engl J Med 305:1452, 1981.

GROWTH HORMONE AND GROWTH HORMONE RELEASING HORMONE (GHRH)

Frohman LA, Szabo M, Berelowitz M, et al.: Partial purification and characterization of a peptide with growth hormone-releasing activity from extrapituitary tumors in patients with acromegaly. J Clin Invest 65:43, 1980. *This manuscript is a good source of reference for this syndrome. In addition, this offers the first chemical characterization of GHRH extracted from extrapituitary tumors causing pituitary tumors and acromegaly.*

CALCITONIN

Schwartz KE, Wolfsen AR, Forster B, et al.: Calcitonin in the nonthyroidal cancer. J Clin Endocrinol Metab 49:438, 1979. *This report offers a good review of earlier publications and itself indicates the frequency of elevated blood calcitonin in patients with a wide variety of carcinomas. Fluctuations in calcitonin in parallel with removal and relapse of the tumor are shown.*

VASOPRESSIN

Robertson GL, Berl T.: Water metabolism. In Brenner BM, Rector FC Jr (eds.): The Kidney, 3rd ed. W.B. Saunders Co., Philadelphia, 1986, pp. 385–432. *This is an excellent and up-to-date review of the SIADH in the context of a more general discussion of the control of water metabolism.*

EOSINOPHILOPOIETIN

Slungaard A, Ascensao J, Zanjani E, et al.: Pulmonary carcinoma with eosinophilia: Demonstration of a tumor-derived eosinophilopoietic factor. N Engl J Med 309:778, 1983.

174 NONMETASTATIC EFFECTS OF CANCER ON THE NERVOUS SYSTEM

Jerome B. Posner

When patients with systemic cancer develop nervous system dysfunction, metastasis is usually the cause. However, cancer exerts deleterious effects on the nervous system by mechanisms other than metastases. Recognition of these nonmetastatic neurologic complications can prevent inappropriate and perhaps harmful therapy directed at a nonexistent metastasis. Since at times the nervous system symptoms precede the discovery of the cancer, they can also lead the physician to the diagnosis of an otherwise occult neoplasm.

An almost bewildering variety of neurologic disorders have been ascribed to effects of systemic cancer (Table 174–1). Most patients with nervous system dysfunction not caused by metastases are eventually found to be suffering from infection, vascular or metabolic disorders, or from unwanted side effects of chemotherapy. This chapter discusses two other types of nervous system damage related to cancer not described elsewhere in this book: "remote effects" or paraneoplastic syndromes (Table 174–2), and radiation injury.

REMOTE EFFECTS

Remote effects of cancer on the nervous system, paraneoplastic syndromes, are terms that refer to nervous system dysfunction of unknown cause occurring almost exclusively or at higher frequency in patients with cancer. These syndromes are not common. In a series of 1465 patients with cancer, about 7 per cent were found to have unexplained neurologic dysfunction, usually weakness and wasting of proximal muscles associated with absence of or diminished deep tendon reflexes. The more classic paraneoplastic syndromes, cerebellar degeneration and myelopathy, occurred three times each; there was no instance of sensory neuronopathy. Therefore, excluding patients with mild peripheral neuropathy or myopathy possibly associated with cachexia, remote effects probably occur in less than 1 per cent of unselected patients with cancer. Lung cancer, particularly small cell cancer, accounts for more than 50 per cent of cases; the incidence is greatest among patients with ovarian and small cell lung cancer. Because of its rarity, the diagnosis of remote effects should never be

TABLE 174–1. NONMETASTATIC EFFECTS OF CANCER ON THE NERVOUS SYSTEM

Remote Effects or Paraneoplastic Syndromes (see Table 174–2)
Side Effects of Therapy
  Chemotherapy
  Radiation therapy (see Table 174–3)
Metabolic and Nutritional Abnormalities
  Destruction of vital organs (e.g., liver)
  Elaboration of hormonal substances by tumor
  Competition between tumor and brain for essential substrates (e.g., glucose)
  Malnutrition
Infections (usually associated with lymphomas)
  Parasites (e.g., toxoplasmosis)
  Fungi (e.g., cryptococcosis, aspergillosis, mucormycosis)
  Bacteria (e.g., *Listeria monocytogenes* infection)
  Viruses (e.g., herpes zoster)
Vascular Disease
  Intracranial hemorrhage
  Cerebral infarction

TABLE 174–2. REMOTE EFFECTS OF CANCER ON THE NERVOUS SYSTEM (PARANEOPLASTIC SYNDROMES)

Brain and Cranial Nerves
Subacute cerebellar degeneration
Opsoclonus-myoclonus
Limbic encephalitis
Brain stem encephalitis
Optic neuritis
Retinal degeneration
Spinal Cord
Necrotizing myelopathy
Subacute motor neuronopathy
Motor neuron disease
Myelitis
Dorsal Root Ganglia
Subacute sensory neuronopathy
Peripheral Nerve
Subacute or chronic sensorimotor peripheral
neuropathy
Acute polyradiculoneuropathy (Guillain-Barré
syndrome)
Remitting and relapsing peripheral
neuropathy
Mononeuropathies
Mononeuritis multiplex
Brachial neuritis
Autonomic neuropathy
Peripheral neuropathy associated with
paraproteinemia
Neuromuscular Junction and Muscle
Lambert-Eaton myasthenic syndrome
Myasthenia gravis
Dermatomyositis, polymyositis
Acute necrotizing myopathy
Carcinoid myopathies
Myotonia
Cachectic myopathy
"Neuromyopathy"

accepted until a thorough evaluation has excluded metastatic or other nonmetastatic causes of neurologic dysfunction. In particular, infiltration of nerve roots by tumor in the leptomeninges may mimic paraneoplastic peripheral neuropathy.

The etiology of remote effects is unknown. Hypotheses have included opportunistic viral infections, competition between tumor and nervous system for essential metabolites, and secretion by tumor of a neurotoxin. The hypothesis for which there is most evidence is that remote effects are autoimmune responses. The evidence includes the demonstration of autoantibodies reactive with specific neurons in the serum of patients with paraneoplastic cerebellar degeneration (see below), subacute sensory neuronopathy (see below), and some other paraneoplastic disorders. Plasma and IgG from patients suffering from Lambert-Eaton myasthenic syndrome (see below) passively transfer that neuromuscular defect to experimental animals. It seems likely that remote effects of cancer are a heterogeneous group of disorders in which different pathogenetic mechanisms play a role. Furthermore, although the disorders described in this chapter are separated by their clinical signs into anatomic categories, more than one clinical syndrome may be present in a given patient. This is particularly true of the dementias, which are often lumped together with brain stem, cerebellar, and spinal cord lesions as carcinomatous encephalomyelitis, and also of myopathy and peripheral neuropathy associated with cancer, often called carcinomatous neuromyopathy.

Brain and Cranial Nerves

CEREBRUM. Cerebral remote effects are usually characterized by dementia with or without other neurologic findings. Dementia usually begins insidiously and progresses. Loss of recent memory and affective alterations, either anxiety or depression, characterize the disorder. Seizures are prominent in some patients, and others have a fluctuating confusional state. When other abnormal neurologic signs are present, they usually point to brain stem, cerebellar, or peripheral nerve involvement. The electroencephalogram is diffusely slow, and the cerebrospinal fluid sometimes contains 10 to 40 lymphocytes per cubic milliliter and a slight elevation of the protein concentration.

Pathologically, there are two main groups. In some patients, no significant pathologic changes are found in the cerebrum despite unequivocal clinical dementia. Other patients demonstrate widespread cerebral neuronal loss and perivascular collections of lymphocytes, particularly in the medial temporal lobes (limbic encephalitis) or the thalamus. The differential diagnosis includes brain or leptomeningeal metastases, fungal or parasitic infections (including multifocal leukoencephalopathy), and metabolic encephalopathy. Focal cerebral signs other than dementia, CT and MRI (Ch. 456), and cerebrospinal fluid studies support the diagnosis of infection or metastatic disease. Metabolic encephalopathy can usually be diagnosed by appropriate laboratory tests, as indicated in Ch. 457. Progressive dementia in middle age accompanied by cerebellar, brain stem, or peripheral nerve dysfunction but no other focal cerebral signs suggests dementia as a remote effect of cancer. There is no specific treatment for these dementias, but they may improve with successful therapy of the cancer.

BULBAR ENCEPHALITIS. Brain stem dysfunction associated with dementia, which develops insidiously or subacutely and is progressive, may be a remote effect of the cancer. The brain stem signs include vertigo, nystagmus, dysphagia, ophthalmoplegia, and at times ataxia and extensor plantar reflexes. The pathologic changes, predominantly in the lower pons and medulla, are those of neuronal loss and perivascular lymphocytic cuffing. The lymphocytic infiltration is responsible for the term *encephalitis*. The cause is unknown, and there is no effective treatment.

CEREBELLUM. Paraneoplastic cerebellar degeneration is clinically sufficiently characteristic to suggest cancer even when neurologic symptoms predate diagnosis of the tumor. Symptoms usually evolve over weeks, with bilateral and symmetric cerebellar dysfunction, the patient being equally ataxic in arms and legs. Severe dysarthria is usually present, and vertigo and diplopia are common, but nystagmus may be absent. Many patients have neurologic signs pointing to disease outside the cerebellum: extensor plantar responses are common; tendon reflexes may be either diminished or exaggerated; and dementia occurs in about half. The cerebrospinal fluid is usually normal, but there may be as many as 40 lymphocytes per cubic milliliter and an elevated protein content. The disease, which may be associated with any cancer, precedes the discovery of the neoplasm by periods of from weeks to three years in more than half the patients. Cerebellar atrophy may be seen on a CT scan, particularly if done late in the course of the illness. Characteristic pathologic changes consist of diffuse or patchy loss of Purkinje cells in all areas of the cerebellum. There may be lymphocytic cuffs around blood vessels, particularly in the deep nuclei. This illness can be distinguished from cerebellar metastases by the symmetry of its signs and the absence of increased intracranial pressure, and from alcoholic-nutritional cerebellar degeneration because dysarthia and ataxia in the upper extremities are prominent in the carcinomatous cerebellar degenerations, and are usually mild or absent in the alcoholic variety. The hereditary cerebellar degenerations rarely run so rapid a course. At times the disorder stabilizes or improves with successful treatment of the tumor. Autoantibodies that react to cytoplasm of Purkinje cells have been identified in the serum of women with paraneoplastic cerebellar degeneration and breast or ovarian cancer. The antigen identified by the antibody has been identified in the tumor of at least one patient suffering cerebellar degeneration. The role of the autoantibody in the pathogenesis of the disease is not established.

Another, less common, cerebellar syndrome is that of opsoclonus (spontaneous, conjugate, chaotic eye movements most severe when voluntary eye movements are attempted). Opsoclonus is frequently associated with cerebellar ataxia and myoclonus of the trunk and extremities. It is most common in children as a remote effect of neuroblastoma. In children, the neurologic symptoms may respond to adrenocorticosteroids or to treatment of the tumor.

Spinal Cord

Two rare but distinct myelopathies complicate cancer: The first, *subacute motor neuronopathy*, affects anterior horn cells, usually in patients with Hodgkin's disease or other lymphomas. The course is subacute, with progressive painless asymmetric lower motor neuron weakness of legs and arms. Some patients complain of sensory symptoms, but sensory loss is mild or absent despite profound weakness. The major pathologic finding is neuronal degeneration of anterior horn cells. Sometimes there is inflammation in the anterior horns and demyelination in the white matter of the spinal cord. The clinical course is different from most remote effects in that many patients improve spontaneously, independent of the course of the underlying lymphoma. The etiology is unknown, but a similar disorder in mice harboring lymphomas appears to be caused by a virus. Rarely, gray matter myelopathies with clinical courses resembling syringomyelia or autonomic insufficiency (q.v.) complicate systemic cancer.

The second complicating condition is *subacute necrotic destruction of the spinal cord*, a myelopathy in which both gray and white matter are affected equally. Clinically, there is rapidly ascending sensory and motor loss, usually to midthoracic levels, the patient becoming paraplegic and incontinent within hours or days. The neurologic symptoms often precede the discovery of the neoplasm, and the illness is clinically and pathologically indistinguishable from idiopathic subacute necrotic myelopathy. Since epidural spinal cord compression from metastatic tumor or arteriovenous spinal cord anomalies may present similar clinical signs, a myelogram is essential. In addition to the two aforementioned entities, many patients with paraneoplastic cerebellar degeneration develop extensor plantar responses, mild sensory changes, and reflex asymmetries and weakness associated with degenerations of long tracts and anterior horn cells of the spinal cord. However, spinal cord symptoms do not predominate in these patients. Amyotrophic lateral sclerosis has been reported as a remote effect of cancer, but it is doubtful that it occurs in patients with cancer more often than in the general population.

Peripheral Nerves and Dorsal Root Ganglia

Four clinical peripheral nerve disorders occur in association with cancer. Characteristic of carcinoma is a *subacute sensory neuronopathy* marked by loss of sensation with relative preservation of motor power. The illness sometimes precedes the appearance of the carcinoma and progresses over a few months, leaving the patient with moderate or severe disability. The cerebrospinal fluid protein is usually elevated. Pathologically, there is destruction of posterior root ganglia with perivascular lymphocytic cuffing and wallerian degeneration of sensory nerves. Many of the patients have inflammatory and degenerative changes in brain and spinal cord as well. The disorder is usually associated with small cell carcinoma, and in some such patients serum autoantibodies reacting against the nuclei of neurons but not other cells have been identified. The antibody is specific for the disorder, but its role in pathogenesis is not known. There is no treatment.

More common than sensory neuropathy is a *distal sensorimotor polyneuropathy* characterized by motor weakness, sensory loss, and absence of distal reflexes in the extremities. The illness is pathologically characterized by either segmental demyelination or wallerian degeneration (or both) of sensory and motor peripheral nerves. Pathologically and clinically, the sensorimotor neuropathy is indistinguishable from polyneuropathies not associated with cancer. Indeed, some have suggested that the late or terminal polyneuropathy may be due to nutritional deprivation associated with cancer. Its etiology, however, is not clear, and it does not respond to treatment with vitamins and other nutritional supplements.

A *polyneuritis* clinically and pathologically indistinguishable from acute postinfectious polyneuropathy (Guillain-Barré syndrome) also complicates cancer, particularly Hodgkin's disease, with impaired immunity. A few patients with *neuropathy limited to the autonomic nervous system* have been reported.

Neuromuscular Junction and Muscles

NEUROMUSCULAR JUNCTION. *Myasthenia gravis* is associated with thymomas, but usually not other systemic tumors. The Lambert-Eaton myasthenic syndrome is characterized by weakness and fatigability of proximal muscles, particularly of the pelvic girdle and thighs. The cranial nerves and respiratory muscles are usually spared. Patients often complain of dryness of the mouth, impotence, pain in the thighs, and peripheral paresthesias. On examination there is weakness of the proximal muscles, but strength increases over several seconds of a sustained contraction. The deep tendon reflexes are diminished or absent. The diagnosis is made by electromyographic studies in which repeated nerve stimulations at rates above ten per second cause a progressive *increase* in the size of the muscle action potential (the opposite of myasthenia gravis). About two thirds of patients with this syndrome either have or will develop cancer, usually small cell carcinoma of the lung. The neuromuscular defect in this illness is believed to be deficient release of acetylcholine. Similar findings have been produced in experimental animals by injection of either serum IgG or extract of tumor in patients with the disorder, suggesting an autoimmune etiology. Plasmapheresis and immune-suppressant drugs may relieve symptoms. The illness responds poorly to anticholinesterase drugs, but does respond to guanidine hydrochloride given in doses of 15 to 40 mg* per kilogram per day.

MUSCLE. Typical *dermatomyositis* or *polymyositis* may occur as a remote effect of cancer (Ch. 443). Fewer than 10 per cent of patients with this disorder have cancer, but the figure is higher in older patients. The clinical picture of polymyositis associated with cancer (i.e., subacute development of weakness, particularly involving proximal muscles and sometimes bulbar muscles) is indistinguishable from that of dermatomyositis or polymyositis not associated with cancer. Pathologically, there may be two groups: one with the typical inflammatory lesions of polymyositis and one with little inflammation but severe muscle necrosis. The latter group may suffer an explosive clinical course. The patients respond somewhat less well to corticosteroid therapy than do those with dermatomyositis unaccompanied by cancer, although substantial improvement with steroid treatment does occur in some.

Muscle Weakness. Some patients with cancer complain of *weakness* and *fatigability* that seem worse than can be accounted for by their cancer alone. Cachexia and weight loss alone do not usually cause measurable muscle weakness. The weakness is usually proximal and produces particular difficulty climbing stairs or getting out of low chairs. Ankle reflexes may be diminished or absent. Further neurologic evaluation does not yield findings diagnostic of one of the remote effects of cancer described above. Brain and his colleagues have labeled this entity a neuromyopathy because its exact anatomic locus is unclear, but others have suggested that it is a nonspecific accompaniment of cachexia and systemic illness. Specific (type II) muscle fiber atrophy develops early in patients with systemic cancer. The cause and treatment of the weakness are unknown.

Anderson NE, Cunningham JM, Posner JB: Autoimmune pathogenesis of paraneoplastic neurological syndromes. CRC Crit Rev Clin Neurobiol. (in

---

*May exceed manufacturer's recommended maximum dosage.

press) *A comprehensive review of paraneoplastic syndromes, with emphasis on the evidence for autoimmune pathogenesis.*

Henson RA, Urich H: Cancer and the Nervous System. Oxford, Blackwell Scientific Publications, Ltd., 1982. *Comprehensive descriptions of all of the paraneoplastic disorders affecting the nervous system.*

NERVOUS SYSTEM INJURY FROM THERAPEUTIC RADIATION

Adverse effects of ionizing radiation on the nervous system (Table 174–3) are related to the total dose of radiation, the size of each fraction, the total duration over which the dose is received, and the volume of nervous system tissue irradiated. Other factors, such as underlying nervous system disease (e.g., brain tumor, cerebral edema), previous surgery, concomitant use of chemotherapeutic agents, and individual susceptibility make it impossible to define precisely a safe dose of radiation therapy for a given individual. However, guidelines allow the radiation therapist to calculate generally safe nervous system doses. Adverse effects may involve any portion of the central or peripheral nervous system and may occur acutely or be delayed weeks to years following irradiation.

CLINICAL MANIFESTATIONS. *Acute encephalopathy* may follow large radiation doses to the brains of patients with increased intracranial pressure, particularly in the absence of corticosteroid prophylaxis. Immediately following treatment, susceptible patients develop headache, nausea and vomiting, somnolence, fever, and occasionally worsening of neurologic signs, rarely culminating in cerebral herniation and death. Acute encephalopathy usually follows the first radiation fraction and becomes progressively less severe with each ensuing fraction. This disorder is believed to result from increased intracranial pressure and/or brain edema from radiation-induced alteration of the blood-brain barrier. It responds to corticosteroids. Acute worsening of neurologic symptoms does not occur after spinal cord irradiation.

Early delayed reactions appear 6 to 16 weeks after therapy and persist for days to weeks. A transient, diffuse encephalopathy commonly follows prophylactic irradiation of the brain for leukemia in children and for small cell lung cancer in adults. The disorder is characterized by somnolence, often associated with headache, nausea, vomiting, and sometimes fever. The electroencephalogram may be slow, but there are no focal signs. Whole-brain irradiation for brain tumor sometimes causes lethargy and worsening of focal neurologic signs, simulating progression of the brain tumor. CT may also indicate worsening. Both disorders usually respond to steroids, but if untreated will resolve spontaneously. A brain stem disorder characterized by diplopia, ataxia, dysarthria and dysphagia, and associated with foci of demyelination resembling acute multiple sclerosis, rarely follows irradiation to the brain stem. *Early delayed myelopathy* follows radiation therapy to the neck or upper thorax and is characterized by Lhermitte's sign (an electric shock–like sensation radiating into various parts of the body when the neck is flexed). The symptoms resolve spontaneously. Early delayed radiation syndromes are believed to result from demyelination, possibly due to radiation-induced damage to oligodendroglia.

Late delayed radiation injury appears after months to years and may affect any part of the nervous system. In the brain, there are two clinical syndromes. The first follows whole-brain irradiation either prophylactically or in some patients with primary and metastatic brain tumors. The disorder is characterized by dementia without focal signs. There is cerebral atrophy on CT scan, pathologic changes are nonspecific, and there is no treatment. The second disorder affects patients who receive either focal brain irradiation during therapy of extracranial neoplasms or whole-brain irradiation for intracranial neoplasms. Neurologic signs suggest a mass and include headache, focal or generalized seizures, and hemiparesis. Brain CT scans reveal a hypodense mass, sometimes with contrast enhancement. Neuropathologic features include coagulative necrosis of white matter, telangiectasia, fibrinoid necrosis and thrombus formation, and glial proliferation and bizarre multinucleated astrocytes. The clinical and CT findings cannot be distinguished from brain tumor, and the diagnosis can be made only by biopsy. Corticosteroids sometimes ameliorate symptoms. The treatment, if the disorder is focal, is surgical removal. *Late delayed myelopathy* is characterized by progressive paralysis, sensory changes, and sometimes pain. A Brown-Sequard syndrome (weakness and loss of proprioception in the extremities of one side with loss of pain and temperature sensation on the other) is often present at onset. Patients occasionally respond transiently to steroids, and the disorder may stop progressing, but generally patients become paraplegic or quadriplegic. Pathologic changes include necrosis of the spinal cord. *Late delayed neuropathy* may affect any cranial or peripheral nerve. Common disorders are blindness from optic neuropathy and paralysis of an upper extremity from brachial plexopathy after therapy for lung or breast cancer. The pathogenesis is probably fibrosis and ischemia of the plexus. There is no treatment.

Radiation-induced tumors, including meningiomas, sarcomas, or, less commonly, gliomas, may appear years to decades after cranial irradiation and may follow even low doses. Malignant or atypical nerve sheath tumors may follow irradiation of the brachial, cervical, and lumbar plexuses. The central nervous system may also be damaged when radiation alters extraneural structures. Radiation therapy accelerates *atherosclerosis*, and cerebral infarction associated with carotid artery occlusion in the neck may occur many years after neck irradiation. *Endocrine* (pituitary, thyroid, parathyroid) dysfunction from radiation may be associated with neurologic signs. Hypothyroidism often presents as a neurologic disorder, and hyperthyroidism or hyperparathyroidism from radiation may also cause an encephalopathy.

Gilbert HA, Kagan AR (eds.): Radiation Damage to the Nervous System. A Delayed Therapeutic Hazard. New York, Raven Press, 1980. *A comprehensive description of all of the nervous system side effects of therapeutic irradiation.*

TABLE 174–3. RADIATION INJURY TO THE NERVOUS SYSTEM

Time After RT	Organ Affected	Clinical Findings
Primary injury		
Immediate (min to hrs)	Brain	Acute encephalopathy
Early delayed (6–16 wks)	Brain	Somnolence, focal signs
	Spinal cord	Lhermitte's sign
Late delayed (mos to yrs)	Brain	Dementia, focal signs
	Spinal cord	Transverse myelopathy
	Peripheral nerves	Paralysis, sensory loss
Secondary injury (years)	Several	Brain, cranial and/or peripheral nerve sheath tumors
	Arteries (atherosclerosis)	Cerebral infarction
	Endocrine organs	Metabolic encephalopathy

175 CUTANEOUS MANIFESTATIONS OF INTERNAL MALIGNANCY

Frank Parker

Cutaneous changes associated with internal malignant disease are diverse. Some skin alterations are clear indicators of underlying malignant disease. Others, less specific, arise in either the presence or absence of malignancy, but occur with sufficient frequency to arouse suspicion and the need to search for underlying carcinoma or lymphoma. These various skin findings may precede any signs associated with the internal malignant disease; they are therefore of crucial importance in early identification and cure of internal neoplasms.

Skin manifestations of internal malignant disease can be classified into two major groups: (1) those in which malignant cells can be found in the skin on biopsy (specific skin lesions) and (2) those in which malignant cells cannot be identified on a skin biopsy (nonspecific skin lesions). The specific lesions are diagnostic of the internal malignant disease, while the nonspecific skin alterations may or may not be associated with an internal neoplasm. Some of the nonspecific skin changes are clear indicators of underlying tumor; others merely arouse concern.

SPECIFIC SKIN LESIONS ASSOCIATED WITH INTERNAL MALIGNANT DISEASE

Carcinomas, leukemia, lymphoma, plasma cell dyscrasias, and sarcomas can all affect the skin specifically in clinically identifiable patterns. A biopsy of a suspicious skin lesion is helpful because the tissue of origin (primary underlying neoplasm) can often be identified.

Skin Metastases (Table 175–1 and Color plate 6A)

Metastases to the skin are comparatively rare (approximately 1 to 5 per cent of internal malignancies), but when present are readily diagnosed by biopsy. Cutaneous metastases usually appear as flesh-colored to red-purple or brownish solitary papules or nodules, stony-hard to the touch, and often innocent in appearance. There is no relationship between site of origin and size, color, and consistency of the metastatic deposit. Lung cancer in men and breast cancer in women most commonly involve the skin; other sources include malignant tumors of the gastrointestinal tract, kidney, ovary, uterus, and urinary bladder and oral cavity carcinomas.

Clinical patterns of metastatic spread to skin depend on several factors such as the organ of origin and whether tumor is disseminated by lymphatics or blood. In general, those neoplasms that spread via lymphatics, such as breast and oral cavity carcinoma, localize in the skin late in the clinical course. Tumors that often embolize through venous channels, such as those arising in the lung, kidney, and ovary, can appear early in the skin and thus may be the first indication of the internal malignant disease.

Certain areas of the skin are predisposed to metastases, localizing near the site of the primary cancer (Table 175–1). Thus, abdominal wall metastases, especially around the um-

bilicus (Sister Mary Joseph's nodules), arise from neoplasms of the stomach, kidney, and ovary. The lower abdominal wall and external genitalia metastases arise from cancers of the genitourinary systems; face and neck skin metastases, from carcinomas of the oropharynx; and the scalp is a favorite site for metastases from breast, lung, and the genitourinary system.

Some patterns of metastatic disease are characteristic. For example, metastases to the scalp simulate wens or turban (pilar) tumors that may ulcerate. More distinctive is "alopecia neoplastica"—that is, areas of scarring alopecia in the scalp with induration and atrophy that simulate alopecia areata. Metastases from the breast and, less commonly, from the stomach, prostate, lung, uterus, and pancreas can produce dramatic changes in the chest wall: carcinoma en cuirasse. This scirrhous form of cutaneous metastatic spread produces extensive fibrosis of the dermis as a result of lymphatic involvement and obstruction by the cancer cells so that large areas of the chest are girdled by a thick, rigid encasement to which pink to flesh-colored papules and nodules evolve to form morphea-like plaques. The distinctive skin lesion of inflammatory carcinoma, or "carcinoma erysipeloides," is usually caused by breast cancer (less frequently by malignant tumors of the uterus, lung, and gastrointestinal tract) and simulates cellulitis over the ipsilateral chest wall anteriorly. Renal cell carcinoma and medullary and anaplastic forms of thyroid cancer, which are highly vascularized tumors, may simulate hemangiomatous nodules that pulsate on palpation when deposited in the skin. *Inflammatory oncotaxis* is a term describing the attraction of cancer cells to an area of tissue trauma resulting presumably because trauma (surgery and radiation) causes inflammation and capillary disruption, thus predisposing cancer cells to settle in these areas. For example, cutaneous metastases from colon, kidney, and cervix have been known to localize in abdominal wall surgical incisions.

Prognosis among patients with cutaneous metastases is poor, as they imply metastases elsewhere internally. If a cutaneous metastatic lesion is discovered years after the primary cancer is diagnosed, a second internal cancer should be ruled out, since only 10 per cent of internal cancers (mostly breast carcinoma) spread to the skin after five years' time. Clearly any skin nodule or papule of obscure origin and uncertain diagnosis should undergo biopsy, especially if there are reasons to suspect malignancy.

Lymphomas

Specific cutaneous involvement (neoplastic cellular proliferation in the skin) is seen less frequently in the lymphoma-leukemia group of neoplasms when compared with carcinomas. Rather, cutaneous manifestations are more often nonspecific (i.e., pruritus, petechiae, purpura, infections) in patients with leukemias and lymphomas, occurring in 25 to 40 per cent of such patients (see below, Nonspecific Skin Lesions Associated with Internal Malignant Disease). The specific skin lesions that are seen are similar in patients with lymphoma and leukemia, regardless of the various types of these neoplasms. Thus, skin lesions in all forms of lymphomas and leukemias appear as red, blue, and violaceous asymptomatic macules, nodules, and plaques that may ulcerate. Particularly suggestive are thickened, beefy-red arcuate lesions as well as poikilodermatous plaques (hyperpigmentation and hypopigmentation with telangiectasis throughout the thickened patches).

Cutaneous T Cell Lymphomas (Table 175–2)

These lymphomas are lymphoproliferative disorders of helper T lymphocytes with an affinity for skin (epidermotropism) in which atypical lymphocytes accumulate in clusters in the epidermis to form so-called Pautrier's abscesses. They represent at least three types of lymphoma: mycosis fungoides, Sézary syndrome, and adult T cell lymphoma, each

TABLE 175–1. INTERNAL MALIGNANCIES METASTATIC TO SKIN CLINICAL FEATURES AND AREAS OF DISTRIBUTION

Primary Internal Malignancy	Cutaneous Clinical Features	Areas of Distribution
Breast	Papules, nodules—rock hard En cuirasse—scirrhous form Erysipelatoides—cellulitis form Alopecia neoplastica	Chest wall Trunk Scalp
Lung	Papules, nodules Scirrhous—morpheic form Erysipeloides—cellulitis form Alopecia neoplastica	Chest wall Scalp Face
Kidney	Angiomatous, pulsatile nodules Scirrhous—en cuirasse form Alopecia neoplastica	Abdominal wall, trunk Scalp Face External genitalia
Stomach, bowel, pancreas	Nodules Scirrhous—en cuirasse form Cellulitis—erysipelatoides	Anterior abdomen Periumbilical
Ovary, uterus	Nodules Cellulitis form—erysipelatoides	Umbilicus, abdomen
Oral cavity	Nodules	Face and neck
Thyroid	Pulsatile angiomatous nodules	Anywhere

TABLE 175–2. CUTANEOUS T CELL LYMPHOMAS

Lymphoma	Skin Lesions	Other Features
Mycosis fungoides	Erythematous patches, plaques, tumors, erythroderma	Late involvement of lymph nodes, internal organs
Sézary syndrome	Erythroderma with ectropion and leonine facies; often spares body folds	Sézary cells in blood with high WBC, hepatosplenomegaly, lymphadenopathy
Adult T cell lymphoma	Erythroderma, papules, nodules	HTLV 1 virus antibodies, hepatosplenomegaly, osteolytic bone lesions, hypercalcemia
T immunoblastic lymphoma	Plaques, tumors	Arise from pre-existing mycosis fungoides or Sézary syndrome
Chronic lymphoblastic leukemia, T cell type	Erythroderma, plaques, nodules	Prolonged course
T lymphoblastic lymphoma	Tumors of skin	Rapidly fatal with bone marrow and mediastinal involvement

of which presents with variable clinical characteristics and biologic behavior.

Mycosis fungoides (Color plate 6*B*) usually follows a prolonged course, beginning with nonspecific skin lesions (socalled premycotic stage) that, after a variable number of years, evolve into histologically specific skin lesions (cutaneous patches, plaques—the mycotic stage) and then into ulcerative nodules and tumors (tumor stage).

Extracutaneous disseminated disease involves first lymph nodes and then, in advanced stages, liver and spleen and other internal organs. Less commonly the disease may begin with cutaneous nodules and tumors without evolving from patches and plaques. Several types of clinical lesions (patches, plaques, and tumors) may coexist in any one patient. The premycotic stage (biopsy of lesions is nonspecific) can persist from a few months to more than 40 years, the morphology of the skin lesions resembling a number of banal dermatoses: psoriasis or eczema or poikilodermatous telangiectatic, stippled pigmented patches. In the plaque stage the premycotic lesions become infiltrated, although indurated, red-purple plaques also arise from previously uninvolved skin. The lesions usually are oval to round, but they may also be arciform or annular or assume a horseshoe shape, or the entire integument may be infiltrated, producing a thickened, red hide (erythroderma). In the final stage, tumors develop from pre-existing plaques, erythroderma, or previously uninvolved skin. Tumors may be a few centimeters to 10 cm in size and often ulcerate. It is difficult to diagnose mycosis fungoides in the premycotic stage; it requires multiple skin biopsies over extended periods.

The *Sézary syndrome* (Color plate 6*C*), the leukemic variant of mycosis fungoides, consists of generalized exfoliative dermatitis with edema, redness, and thickening of the skin associated with ectropion, leonine facies, keratoderma of the palms and soles, hepatosplenomegaly, and lymphadenopathy associated with large numbers of atypical T lymphocytes in the circulation. The latter, so-called Sézary cells, represent T cells with highly convoluted nuclei identical to the cells infiltrating the skin in mycosis fungoides. The immediate source of the circulating Sézary cells appears to be the skin, as the bone marrow is rarely involved. In many patients mycosis fungoides pursues a chronic course, and the patients die of unrelated causes; some experience rapid progression to cutaneous tumors and ulcerative lesions and disseminated disease (visceral involvement is frequently diffuse and resembles leukemic infiltrates). Sézary syndrome has a particularly poor prognosis. Staphylococcal or *Pseudomonas* septicemia is the most common terminal event, accounting for half of the deaths.

Adult T cell lymphoma, which is associated with a retrovirus, human T cell lymphoma virus (HTLV), occurs mainly in blacks in the United States. Cutaneous findings are prominent in 70 per cent of patients and may be the presenting feature. Flesh-colored papules, nodules, and tumors as well as generalized erythroderma may be present. The papules are diffusely disseminated over the trunk and coalesce to form plaques. Patients also display peripheral and mediastinal lymphadenopathy, and hepatosplenomegaly is found in half of the patients. A unique feature of this lymphoma is trabecular and bone marrow involvement with multiple "punched-out" osteolytic lesions in the axial skeleton and long bones associated with extreme hypercalcemia.

Several other forms of T cell lymphomas occur with skin involvement and are outlined in Table 175–2.

Non-Hodgkin's Lymphomas and Cutaneous B Cell Lymphomas (see Ch. 158)

Red, blue, or violaceous skin lesions occur in all forms of non-Hodgkin's lymphoma. They appear as papules, nodules, and plaques with occasional large, ulcerated tumors that evolve in the skin after lymph node involvement. Skin involvement can be seen as the initial presentation, or it may occur late in the course of the disease. It appears to have no impact on prognosis.

Hodgkin's Disease (see Ch. 160)

The skin is not commonly involved in a specific way, but when it is, the erythematous papules, nodules, and plaques that often ulcerate are indistinguishable from the skin lesions found in non-Hodgkin's lymphoma. The site of predilection is the thoracic wall, spread being via retrograde lymphatic drainage pathways from massively enlarged axillary and cervical lymph nodes. Specific cutaneous involvement is seen in those patients with extensive and highly aggressive Hodgkin's disease.

Leukemias

Leukemia cutis usually develops months after the diagnosis of leukemia (55 per cent of patients) or at the time of diagnosis (38 per cent), but it can occasionally precede systemic disease and be the first sign of the underlying condition. Red to violaceous papules, nodules, and thickened plaques are the usual forms that leukemic infiltrates take, but rarely is erythroderma found. When chronic myelogenous leukemia (CML) enters the blast phase, greenish tumors may develop in the skin, forming chloromas or granulocytic sarcomas (see Ch. 155). Skin lesions in acute leukemias and chronic lymphocytic leukemia (CLL) are found on the face and extremities, while those associated with CML are more commonly seen on the trunk. In monocytic leukemia, widespread leukemia skin infiltrates occur, and oral mucosal involvement (gingival hyperplasia) is commonplace. In general, the histology of leukemic cells in skin for various forms of leukemia mimics that seen in the blood and bone marrow, but it is difficult to diagnose the type of leukemia from skin biopsies.

Plasma Cell Dyscrasias

Specific skin manifestations of multiple myeloma, extramedullary plasmacytoma, and Waldenström's macroglobulinemia consist of lymphoplasmacytoid cell infiltrates or deposition of monoclonal paraprotein immunoglobulins (see Ch. 163). Bluish-red and flesh colored nonulcerated nodules and plaques on the trunk are observed in 4 per cent of patients with multiple myeloma, representing in most instances extensions from underlying medullary plasma cell proliferation.

Cutaneous Histiocytic Malignant Tumors

Malignant tumors of histiocytes may be solitary or present as disseminated disease. *Malignant histiocytosis* (histiocytic medullary reticulosis), a systemic, progressive proliferation of atypical histiocytes, produces wasting, fever, lymphadenopathy, hepatosplenomegaly, pancytopenia, and skin lesions. Children and adults are affected, and skin lesions are an integral part of the disease, especially in children (up to 90 per cent have cutaneous changes). The reddish-purple papulonodular and ulcerative plaques occur over the trunk and face early in the clinical course. Malignant histiocytosis is fatal in adults, but is somewhat less aggressive in children.

Angioblastic Lymphadenopathy

Immunologically mediated, this often fatal disorder is characterized by proliferation of plasmacytoid immunoblasts and plasma cells. Fever, malaise, weight loss, hepatosplenomegaly, and generalized lymphadenopathy are accompanied in 40 per cent of cases by generalized, maculopapular, purpuric, and, at times, exfoliative erythroderma. Biopsy findings of involved lymph nodes are diagnostic (proliferation of plasma cells, arborizing vessels, and deposition of amorphous material), while skin biopsy reveals a lymphohistiocytic vasculitis composed of plasma and immunoblast-like cells.

Neuroblastoma

Neuroblastoma, a poorly differentiated tumor derived from primordial neural crest cells, arises within the sympathetic ganglion (cervical, thoracic, and pelvic tumors) and adrenal glands of children. It frequently metastasizes to bone, lymph nodes, liver, and skin. Bluish nodules appear over a wide area (causing these children to be called blueberry-muffin children). A helpful clinical sign occurs after rubbing these lesions: They blanch with a halo of surrounding erythema, probably related to the release of catechols contained in the cells of the tumors. Even though patients with neuroblastoma are not hypertensive, 85 per cent have increased urinary catecholamine metabolites.

Kaposi's Sarcoma (Color Plate 6D–F)

Kaposi's sarcoma, a multifocal, vascular malignant tumor, can occur in four major clinical settings: African Kaposi's, classic Kaposi's in elderly Jewish or Mediterranean males, Kaposi's secondary to immunodeficiency conditions, and Kaposi's sarcoma occurring as a complication of acquired immunodeficiency syndrome (AIDS). In each instance the skin lesions are identical histologically and clinically; they present as purplish-brown macules, plaques, papules or nodules. The distribution and course of these sarcomatous lesions, however, vary according to the clinical setting (Table 175–3). Thus, classic Kaposi's sarcoma occurs in elderly males of

Mediterranean background as purplish macules that may progress to infiltrative plaques and nodules on the distal extremities, following an indolent course. The Kaposi's sarcoma occurring in young homosexuals and others with AIDS is characterized by widely distributed, red-brown macules, papules, nodules over the upper body and progresses in a fulminant course. The Kaposi's lesions in AIDS often follows skin cleavage lines and frequently involve the oropharyngeal mucosa, appearing as purple hemorrhagic plaques. The importance of the immune status in the evolution of Kaposi's sarcoma is dramatically illustrated in renal transplant patients who are immunosuppressed. Kaposi's sarcoma develops after 9 to 16 months following transplantation and initiation of immunosuppressive drugs. Rapidly progressive, widespread, red to purple papules ensue, but they may regress when immunosuppressive therapy is withdrawn.

NONSPECIFIC SKIN LESIONS ASSOCIATED WITH INTERNAL MALIGNANT DISEASE (Table 175–4)

Malignant cells cannot be identified in the skin in a wide variety of cutaneous manifestations of internal malignant disease. The pathogenesis of these disparate skin reactions is obscure. Often the only evidence that malignancy and cutaneous changes are related is the observation that following removal of the tumor or treatment of the neoplasm the skin change subsides or disappears and may subsequently exacerbate if the neoplasm recurs. Skin manifestations may coincide with, antedate, or follow the clinical diagnosis of internal malignant disease.

Although nonspecific manifestations are often highly suggestive of underlying malignant disease, they are more frequently seen with other nonmalignant conditions. When these skin changes are observed, therefore, an internal neoplasm is only one of several possibilities in the differential diagnosis.

Nonspecific skin manifestations can be considered under two major headings: (1) skin changes common to many skin diseases, including internal malignancy and (2) syndromes and entities commonly associated with internal neoplasia.

Skin Changes Common to Many Skin Conditions, Including Internal Malignancy

Pruritus, unassociated with detectable abnormalities of the skin except for secondary lesions such as excoriations or prurigo-like papules, may be an important manifestation of various internal malignant diseases, including Hodgkin's disease, lymphocytic leukemia, carcinoid, polycythemia vera (in

TABLE 175–3. KAPOSI'S SARCOMA: COMPARISON OF VARIOUS FORMS

	Classic Form	African Form	Immunologic Deficiency State	AIDS Associated
Age	40–70 years	Middle age	Any age	20–50 years
Sex	M:F, 10–15:1	—	M or F	Mostly males
Social characteristics	Mediterranean or Jewish ancestry	Blacks in equatorial Africa	Patients taking immunosuppressive drugs—renal transplant, etc.	Homosexuals, drug addicts, hemophiliacs
Occurrence	0.2% cancers in USA	10% of all malignant tumors in Africa	400% greater incidence than population at large	Increasing; 35% of AIDS patients
Clinical appearance of skin lesion	Multiple purple-brown macules, papules, plaques, nodules	Nodules, exophytic lesions, infiltrative, burrowing plaques	Papules, nodules	Multiple purple-brown macules, papules, nodules; follow cleavage lines of skin
Cutaneous location	Lower legs most often, occasionally arms	Extremities	Trunk, neck—widespread lesions	Widespread—upper body, face, neck
Mucosal involvement	Rare	Rare	—	Common
Node and systemic involvement	Rare—occasionally nodes, GI tract, liver in 10% of patients	Uncommon	—	Frequent; 75% with visceral involvement; 5% visceral lesions only
Course and prognosis	Indolent course, 15% mortality within 10 years	Indolent course	Good; may regress if immunosuppressive drugs can be stopped	Fulminant condition, poor prognosis
Response to therapy	Excellent	—	Good	Poor

TABLE 175–4. NONSPECIFIC SKIN LESIONS ASSOCIATED WITH INTERNAL MALIGNANCIES

I. Skin lesions common to many skin conditions, including internal malignancy
II. Syndromes and entities commonly associated with internal malignancy
  A. Nongenetic syndromes
    1. High incidence of association with internal malignancy
      Paget's disease
      Stewart-Treves syndrome
      Acanthosis nigricans
      Dermatomyositis
      Leser-Trélat syndrome
      Glucagonoma syndrome
      Bazex syndrome
      Pulmonary osteoarthropathy
      Carcinoid syndrome
    2. Low incidence of association with malignancy
      Sweet's syndrome
      Amyloid
      Urticaria pigmentosa and mastocytosis syndrome
      Bowen's disease
  B. Genetic syndromes
    1. High incidence of association with malignancy
      Torre's syndrome
      Gardner's syndrome
      Cowden's syndrome
      Multiple endocrine neoplasia III
      Ataxia-telangiectasia
    2. Low incidence of association with malignancy
      Neurofibroma
      Peutz-Jeghers
      Basal cell carcinoma nevus syndrome
      Bloom's syndrome

which pruritus often occurs after exposure to heat), and, less commonly, carcinoma. The itching may be mild or severe, localized or generalized, intermittent or constant. In Hodgkin's disease, itching is usually continuous and may be localized to the feet and lower part of the body, only later to become generalized. Up to 30 per cent of patients with Hodgkin's disease may itch. Pruritus of leukemia has a greater tendency to be generalized and may evolve into generalized erythroderma. Carcinomas of the gastrointestinal tract, lung, ovary, and prostate may also be associated with itching, which may precede recognition of these cancers by a year. Although dry skin (xerosis) is the most common cause of pruritus, other systemic causes of this bothersome symptom should be sought in addition to malignant disease, including drug reactions, cholestatic liver disease, uremia, diabetes, and thyroid disease.

Erythroderma, or exfoliative dermatitis, is a cutaneous reaction pattern with various causes. In 10 per cent of patients, total-body cutaneous redness, edema, scaling, and lichenification are associated with malignancy. In clinical practice the usual cause of exfoliative dermatitis is either a drug reaction or a generalized exacerbation of a pre-existing dermatosis such as atopic dermatitis, psoriasis, or contact dermatitis. When it is due to malignant disease, erythroderma is most pathognomonic of Hodgkin's disease, less frequently seen in lymphocytic leukemia, or rarely associated with underlying carcinoma. Erythroderma may be the first sign of Hodgkin's disease or leukemia. Skin biopsies do not reveal lymphomatous or leukemic infiltrates, although the patients clinically look similar to those with Sézary's syndrome (in which skin biopsies display diagnostic Sézary cells).

Figurate erythemas are red, gyrate, serpiginous, and annular bands that take on a pattern reminiscent of a wood grain and have been given descriptive names such as erythema gyratum repens and erythema annular centrifugum. These lesions are occasionally associated with neoplasia, especially breast and lung cancer.

Urticaria-like lesions, flesh-colored to red pruritic papules, nodules, and plaques, at times accompany leukemia, so-called leukemids. They may precede the development of leukemia by many months, and biopsy of the lesions does not show malignant cells. Treatment and control of leukemia often result in clearing.

Acquired hypertrichosis lanuginosa (malignant down), the sudden onset of excessive growth of fine, long, unpigmented fetal hair (lanugo) over the face, trunk, and limbs, has been associated with breast, uterine, pancreatic, pulmonary, and gastrointestinal carcinomas as well as lymphomas.

Herpes zoster is increased in incidence in patients with Hodgkin's disease and chronic lymphocytic leukemia as well as with a variety of neoplasms that are being managed with chemotherapy. This is evidence of the important role that impaired cellular immunity plays in activating viral replication. The painful, unilateral, grouped, clear, and often hemorrhagic umbilicated vesicles in a dermatomal distribution are readily recognized (see Ch. 343).

A number of miscellaneous dermatoses have occasionally been associated with internal malignant disease, but it is not entirely clear whether these associations are real or fortuitous. Table 175–5 lists some of these.

Syndromes and Entities Associated with Internal Neoplasia

A number of unique cutaneous syndromes, both genetic and nongenetic, are associated with internal neoplasms with sufficient frequency to alert the clinician to look for these potentially curable neoplasms early in their evolution. In some instances there is a high incidence of associated neoplasms, while in others this association is less clear.

Nongenetic Syndromes and Entities Associated with Internal Malignant Disease

HIGH INCIDENCE OF CUTANEOUS LESIONS ASSOCIATED WITH MALIGNANCY. *Paget's disease* of the breast is invariably found with an underlying intraductal mammary carcinoma. Erythematous scaling or weeping, sharply marginated patches on the nipple and areola of one breast should alert the clinician to examine the breast carefully. A breast mass may not be palpable or may not be definitely found with mammography, but in virtually every case an underlying carcinoma is present. Paget's disease can also occur in the anogenital region (extramammary Paget's disease). In this disorder, eczematous, pruritic, crusted, lichenified, well-demarcated patches may involve the lower abdominal wall, inguinal regions, genitalia, or perianal area. In up to 50 per cent of such patients, an underlying carcinoma of the rectum, prostate, urethra, other parts of the genitourinary tract, or apocrine gland is found. Biopsies taken from mammary and extramammary Paget's disease show the same diagnostic features, namely, large, round cells with clear cytoplasm in the epidermis (Paget's cells).

Stewart-Treves syndrome is the occasional occurrence of lymphoangiosarcoma as a complication of chronic lymphedema of the arm after radical mastectomy for carcinoma of the breast. Angiomatous, livid, or dusky red blebs and nodules exuding fluid may evolve from 2 to 20 years following mastectomy and the onset of the lymphedema. Angiosarcoma has also developed in congenital lymphedema as well as in lymphedema of the legs following surgery for cervical cancer.

TABLE 175–5. DERMATOSES ASSOCIATED WITH INTERNAL MALIGNANT DISEASE

Dermatosis	Associated Cancer
Bullous lesions: pemphigoid, pemphigus, dermatitis herpetiformis	Rectal, breast, larynx, lymphoma
Tylosis: palmar hyperkeratosis	Esophagus
Acquired ichthyosis	GI leiomyosarcoma, lymphoma, multiple myeloma, lung, breast
Palmar fasciitis and polyarthritis: palmar fascial thickening with erythema, swelling of palms and dorsum of hands	Ovary

Acanthosis nigricans (Color plate 6G) presents as soft, velvety, verrucous, brown hyperpigmentation of the body folds, especially those of the neck, axillae, and groin. When it occurs in patients over the age of 40 years, it is often a sign of an underlying malignant tumor, usually adenocarcinoma (most often stomach, gastrointestinal tract, and uterus; less commonly, ovary, prostate, breast, and lung) and rarely lymphoma. Acanthosis nigricans involving the tongue and oral mucosa is highly suggestive of underlying malignancy. Acanthosis nigricans may appear before the malignant neoplasm 20 per cent of the time. Regression of the skin sign following therapy for the tumor and reappearance with reactivation of the tumor have been observed, suggesting that the underlying tumor secretes an as yet unidentified substance that is responsible for the verrucoid skin lesions. Acanthosis nigricans is more commonly found in individuals under 40 years of age, and then it is not usually associated with malignancy but rather with obesity or a variety of endocrinopathies (Cushing's disease, acromegaly, polycystic ovaries, hypothyroidism and hyperthyroidism, insulin-resistant diabetes). It also occurs on a familial basis. Special concern must be given to nonobese adults who have recently developed the verrucous areas in body folds. In 80 to 90 per cent of all instances the cancer arises in the stomach.

Dermatomyositis (Color plate 6H) developing in individuals over 40 years of age also calls for a careful search for underlying carcinoma (see Ch. 443). Although there is disagreement whether the incidence of internal malignant disease is increased in dermatomyositis, numerous cases have been reported with this association. Not uncommonly the dermatomyositis resolves upon removal of the carcinoma, but the syndrome recurs if the tumor reappears. In some instances the dermatomyositis precedes the cancer by several years. The search for neoplasm should be continued, therefore, even if the initial evaluation fails to find it, especially with (1) failure of the dermatomyositis to respond to conventional therapy (i.e., after systemic steroids), (2) a history of previous malignant disease, or (3) presence of atypical symptoms of the dermatomyositis. Malignant tumors of the breast and lung are those most commonly associated with dermatomyositis. Dermatomyositis is recognized by proximal muscle pain and weakness and a characteristic dermatitis that includes heliotrope rash (edematous, dusky, violaceous discoloration of the eyelids) along with a brilliant violaceous, erythematous telangiectatic scaling rash over the cheeks, forehead, V of the neck, elbows, and knees. Gottron's papules, slightly elevated red to violaceous papules or small plaques over the knuckles, are also an important finding in dermatomyositis.

The *Leser-Trélet sign*, the sudden appearance and growth of multiple seborrheic keratoses, occurs with underlying cancer in the elderly. This sign has been the subject of controversy, since seborrheic keratoses of the same histologic type are common in the elderly. Nevertheless, several case reports have described new and enlarging keratoses in association with cancer of the lung, adenocarcinoma of the bowel, mycosis fungoides, and Sézary's syndrome and, in some of these patients, the keratoses regressed when the malignant tumor was treated.

Necrolytic migratory erythema, associated with alpha-cell tumors of the pancreas and elevated glucagon levels, evolves as gradually enlarging erythematous patches with central, superficial blister formation progressing to central crusting and healing. Annular and figurate lesions result, with exudative, erosive, and crusting areas most pronounced in the perineum, groin, and perioral areas. Painful glossitis may be another prominent sign of the glucagonoma syndrome. The skin rash and stomatitis often resolve within a week after the tumor is removed. The pathogenesis of the skin and mucous membrane lesions is unclear. The glucagonoma syndrome is discussed more completely in Ch. 233. Similar skin lesions may be seen in association with severe zinc deficiency.

Bazex syndrome, or acrokeratosis paraneoplastica, is a unique cutaneous marker of carcinomas of the upper respiratory tract, especially seen with squamous cell carcinomas of the oral, pharyngeal, laryngeal, esophageal, and bronchial areas, primarily in males. When the tumor is asymptomatic, red to violaceous, scaling, psoriasis-like patches are found confined to the bridge of the nose, the fingers, toes, and margins of the ear helices. The nail folds are often red, scaling, and tender with grooving of the nails and onycholysis. Later the eruption on the acral areas becomes more extensive, spreading from the fingers to the palms and soles, which, in turn, become red and scaling and form a honeycomb-like thickening. The fingers and toes become violaceous and bulbous, and the rash evolves on the nose. In the last stage, if the tumor has not been treated and has progressed, new scaling lesions resembling psoriasis spread over the face, trunk, knees, arms, and scalp. Nail dystrophy (ridged, brittle, crumbling nails) is extensive.

Clubbing of the fingers is a well-known manifestation of bronchogenic carcinoma, mesothelioma, metastatic carcinoma to the thorax (from the colon, larynx, breast, or ovary) and occasionally Hodgkin's disease. *Hypertrophic pulmonary osteoarthropathy* is the term used when clubbing is accompanied by subperiosteal new bone formation along the shafts of the long bones of the extremities and digits. Joints of the ankle, knees, wrists, and hand may be painful and swollen. In some patients cutaneous thickening of the forearms and legs produces cylindric enlargement of the limbs, and the facial features become coarse with deep facial furrows simulating acromegaly. At times, deep confluent skin wrinkles evolve over the forehead and scalp, a condition termed *pachydermoperiostosis* when the skin changes accompany acromegaloid features.

Carcinoid, malignant tumor of the chromaffin cells of the gastrointestinal tract and, less frequently, the bronchus, may be associated with intermittent scarlet to violet red flushing of the head, neck, and upper part of the trunk. Eventually the erythema becomes permanent, and telangiectasis and tortuous veins evolve in the flushed areas. This syndrome and its cutaneous manifestations are described more fully in Ch. 243.

LOW INCIDENCE OF CUTANEOUS LESIONS ASSOCIATED WITH MALIGNANCY. *Amyloid deposits* in the skin may occur without obvious cause (cutaneous amyloidosis), as part of an inherited syndrome or secondary to plasma cell dyscrasias—either primary systemic amyloidosis or multiple myeloma. In the case of plasma cell dyscrasias, shiny, translucent, waxy, firm purpuric papules and plaques occur on the mucocutaneous junctions of the eyes, nose, and mouth along with macroglossia. Occasionally, infiltrated papules are not apparent, and only purpuric lesions evolve around the eyes ("raccoon eyes").

Urticaria pigmentosa consists of skin lesions that appear as numerous red-brown macules and papules on the trunk and extremities. Light stroking of the skin lesions causes urtication with edema and a red flare due to the release of histamine from the mast cells infiltrating the skin (Darier's sign). These skin lesions are sometimes associated with systemic mastocytosis (see Ch. 427) or, more rarely, with mast cell leukemia or myeloproliferative disorders (myelofibrosis, myeloid metaplasia, polycythemia, and granulocytic leukemia) with extensive infiltration of mature mast cells in the marrow and mast cells or basophils in the peripheral blood.

Bowen's disease of the skin consists of multiple superficial squamous cell cancers occurring in non–sun-exposed areas of the body, particularly in individuals with a history of long-term ingestion or exposure to arsenicals (drinking of well water, exposure to insecticides or industrial arsenicals). Bowen's skin lesions appear as discrete, red, scaling, flat to slightly raised patches that mimic eczematous or psoriatic patches. These skin lesions should be removed to prevent progression to invasive squamous cell carcinoma. The relationship of these lesions to internal malignancy is controversial, but a careful search for cancers of the larynx, lung, esophagus, liver, and bladder is warranted.

Sweet's syndrome (acute febrile neutrophilic dermatosis) is associated rarely with underlying chronic myelogenous leukemia. Red, tender, infiltrated plaques and annular lesions are distributed asymmetrically on the face, neck, and upper arms. The skin lesions consist of massive polymorphonuclear infiltration of the dermis, of unknown cause. Patients with Sweet's syndrome also suffer from fever, malaise, peripheral leukocytosis, arthralgias and arthritis, and conjunctivitis and episcleritis. Peripheral leukocyte counts generally range from 15,000 to 20,000 with 80 to 90 per cent mature polymorphonuclear leukocytes. Careful evaluation of the peripheral cells and occasionally of the bone marrow is indicated because of the possibility of coincident myelogenous leukemia.

Genetic Syndromes Associated with Internal Malignant Disease

HIGH INCIDENCE OF ASSOCIATION WITH INTERNAL MALIGNANCY. *Gardner's syndrome* consists of multiple epidermoid and sebaceous cysts of the face and scalp, fibrous tissue tumors of the skin (desmoid tumors, fibromas and fibrosarcomas), osteomas of the membranous bones of the face and head, and polyps of the colon and rectum (Ch. 107). No patients with this syndrome live beyond the seventh decade without developing adenocarcinoma of the bowel.

Cowden's disease, a condition in which there are numerous hamartomas of the skin, mucous membranes, and internal organs, is associated with malignant neoplasms of the breast and thyroid in a high percentage of patients. The hamartomas present on the skin as keratotic, warty papules and nodules on the central area of the face and on the hands and arms. Papular, cobblestone lesions may appear on the gingiva, palate, tongue, and larynx.

Torre's syndrome, another autosomal dominant condition, consists of multiple sebaceous gland tumors, sebaceous adenomas, sebaceous hyperplasia, and basal cell cancers with sebaceous differentiation. It is associated with cancers of the colon, duodenum, ampulla of Vater, uterus, and genitourinary tract. The skin tumors in this condition are yellowish or red papules and nodules.

Multiple endocrine neoplasia type III (see Ch. 241). Medullary carcinoma of the thyroid and pheochromocytoma are found in association with a marfanoid habitus and multiple whitish to pink papular mucosal neuromas studding the lips, tip of the tongue, and, less often, the buccal mucosa, gingivae, palate, and pharynx. Neuromas also develop on the conjunctivae and corneas, and thickened corneal nerves may be found with slit lamp examination.

Ataxia-telangiectasia, an autosomal recessive disorder associated with lymphomas, is recognized by telangiectasias over the ears, eyelids, nose, butterfly area of the face, and conjunctivae in association with progressive cerebellar ataxia, profound immunologic deficiency, and sinopulmonary infections (see Ch. 419). Hodgkin's disease, non-Hodgkin's lymphoma, or leukemia develops in 10 per cent of patients, with other malignant neoplasms such as ovarian dysgerminomas, gliomas, cerebellar medulloblastomas, and gastric adenocarcinomas occurring less frequently. Persons with *Wiskott-Aldrich syndrome* also display a propensity to malignant lymphomas (79 per cent) or leukemias (13 per cent) by the age of ten years, probably related to widespread immunologic abnormalities of both the humoral and cell-mediated systems found in this condition. The skin changes are similar to atopic dermatitis (and are associated with petechiae due to thrombocytopenia).

LOW INCIDENCE OF ASSOCIATION WITH INTERNAL MALIGNANCY. Some dominant inherited conditions are associated with internal malignancy, but the relationship is not frequently found. Thus, patients with *neurofibromatosis* have café au lait spots, axillary freckles, and multiple neurofibromas. They are prone to develop pheochromocytomas (10 per cent of patients by the age of 60 years), acoustic neuromas, and neurofibrosarcomas.

Patients with the *Peutz-Jeghers syndrome* have numerous brown-black macules on the lips, perioral regions, hands, and feet in association with hamartomatous polyps of the small bowel, stomach and, less commonly, colon (see Ch. 107). Malignancy occasionally develops in the polyps. *Nevoid basal cell carcinoma syndrome* is occasionally associated with the development of medulloblastoma or fibrosarcoma of the jaw.

Bloom's syndrome (telangiectatic redness of the skin in photoexposed areas and stunted growth) and the *Chédiak-Higashi syndrome* (light coloration of skin and hair) are autosomal recessive conditions associated with a propensity to develop leukemias and lymphomas.

Braverman IM: Skin Signs of Systemic Disease. Philadelphia, W. B. Saunders Company, 1981. *This classic book, on all skin signs associated with systemic disease, has many useful pictures of the cutaneous lesions related to internal malignant disease.*

Callen JP: Cutaneous Aspects of Internal Disease. Chicago, Year Book Medical Publishers, 1981. *This book, written by a number of authoritative authors, reviews in detail the varied manifestations of cutaneous signs of internal malignancy. Part 3 is especially useful in covering the hematologic and oncologic cutaneous signs of systemic lymphomas and carcinomas.*

Thiers BH, Maize C (eds.): Symposium on Cutaneous T Cell Lymphoma and Related Disorders. Dermatol Clin Vol. 3, No. 4, 1985. *A series of articles relating to the basic scientific and clinical features of cutaneous lymphomas by a number of authorities in the field.*

176 PRINCIPLES OF CANCER THERAPY

Bruce A. Chabner

During the past two decades, fundamental changes have taken place in the treatment of cancer. Once an undertaking with limited expectations, the treatment of cancer is now increasingly effective because of the development of new drugs and more effective radiotherapy and surgery. Many advanced malignant diseases affecting younger age groups, such as the lymphomas, choriocarcinoma, testicular cancer, and childhood leukemia, can often be cured by drug therapy with or without irradiation. The solid neoplasms of later life, particularly adenocarcinomas originating in the gastrointestinal tract and lung, remain a formidable therapeutic challenge in which the potent toxicities and risks of aggressive therapy must be carefully weighed against the limited benefits likely to result. Here the major hope is for the cure of patients at initial presentation through aggressive use of all methods of treatment, including drugs. This chapter will consider the basic biologic and pharmacologic principles that govern the selection of a therapeutic plan for cancer patients. The treatment of specific tumors will be discussed elsewhere.

The objectives of cancer treatment are not the same for all patients and all diseases. They are conditioned by an appreciation of the potential for cure or palliation and an assessment of the patient's tolerance to the side effects of possible treatments. For potentially curable patients, it is imperative that an optimal regimen be selected and pursued without compromise or dosage reduction. On the other hand, curative regimens may not be appropriate for some patients. For example, although curative chemotherapy exists for the majority of patients with diffuse histiocytic lymphoma, not all patients with this diagnosis are appropriate candidates for intensive therapy. Older patients, for example, may have serious medical problems, such as cardiac or pulmonary disease, that preclude aggressive treatment. In such cases, the physician must weigh the chances of successful treatment against the probability of life-threatening side effects and must discuss these conditions frankly with the patient and family. At times, less intensive treatment or only supportive care with pain control and psychologic support may be the wisest therapeutic choice.

Palliation of symptoms and attention to the details of good medical care are often neglected in patients who have reached an incurable phase of their illness. Detection and treatment of complications such as intestinal obstruction, brain metastases, and hypercalcemia, although not affecting the ultimate outcome of disease, may allow the patient extended periods of functional and pain-free life. Thus, it is vital for the physician to listen to the patient's complaints, to conduct periodic physical examinations, and to maintain a concerned and supportive relationship, despite knowledge of the likely eventual outcome.

DETERMINANTS OF TREATMENT PLAN

The primary determinants in the choice of treatment are (1) the histologic diagnosis of the malignant tumor, (2) the stage or extent of disease (including specific sites of organ involvement), and (3) an assessment of the biologic features or specific growth characteristics of the individual tumor.

DIAGNOSIS AND CLASSIFICATION. Accurate pathologic diagnosis and classification of a tumor are obviously crucial. Correct subtyping of tumors is important for many tumors, such as the lymphomas, carcinoma of the lung, and ovarian carcinoma. These general categories encompass disease types with variant patterns of clinical progression and response to treatment. *Histologic grading* is also required for an accurate prognosis and as a guide to therapy in some tumors. Biochemical characterization may be required to identify tumors, e.g., mediastinal malignant teratomas that contain marker proteins (beta-subunits of human chorionic gonadotropin or alpha-fetoprotein); these features assist in distinguishing these from other undifferentiated carcinomas. Similarly, histiocytic lymphoma may be difficult to distinguish from an unusual primary occurrence of acute myeloid leukemia arising in lymph node or bone or from undifferentiated carcinomas unless appropriate touch preparations, histochemical stains, and patterns of reactivity with monoclonal antibodies are examined. The subclassification of lymphoid leukemias, such as B and T cell chronic lymphocytic leukemia (CLL) and childhood acute lymphocytic leukemia, may require the use of cell-surface immunologic typing, in addition to the usual histologic evaluation. The prognosis and treatment of each of these disorders are distinct and different. Genetic techniques, such as chromosomal or oncogene analysis, may be required to distinguish neuroblastoma from neuroepithelioma (Table 176–1). *The internist must always consider the possibility of an alternative, treatable diagnosis, and must seek expert pathologic clarification before committing the patient to a plan of treatment.*

STAGING. In general, knowledge of the extent of a malignant disease (*staging*) is essential to plan effective treatment. In selected cases, staging procedures may pose inappropriate risks to the patient and should never take precedence over necessary therapeutic intervention. For patients with life-threatening local complications of disease, such as upper airway obstruction, superior vena cava obstruction, or biliary obstruction, definitive staging should be delayed to administer surgical or local radiation therapy or chemotherapy.

Staging strategies are based on a knowledge of the natural history of disease, specifically its likely patterns of dissemination to regional and distant sites. In development of a staging plan, the morbidity of a given procedure must be balanced against its probable yield of positive information (the risk-benefit ratio). The procedure should be performed only if the results obtained would affect the treatment decision. For example, a procedure such as lymphangiography, which has low morbidity in the absence of compromised pulmonary function, has great usefulness in lymphomas because of its high yield of positive results and the major impact of these results on treatment choice. In contrast, the staging laparotomy frequently employed to define intra-abdominal disease in Hodgkin's disease has only limited utility in non-

Hodgkin's lymphomas. The latter diseases are usually disseminated at presentation and in advanced stages are not appropriately treated for cure with local therapeutic measures such as radiation therapy. For patients with solid tumors of epithelial origin (carcinomas), an orderly progression of disease occurs, first with involvement of local lymph nodes, and then dissemination to distant sites such as lung, bone, and liver. In such patients, the initial diagnostic workup usually includes bone and liver scans and chest x-ray; if these sites are free of tumor, a definitive surgical procedure is undertaken, with removal of the primary mass and adjacent lymph nodes. In general, the physician should resist the temptation to order batteries of duplicative tests, such as CT and ultrasound evaluations, or tests that have low yield in the absence of localizing symptoms, such as bone scans in asymptomatic patients with clinically localized breast cancer.

BIOLOGIC CHARACTERISTICS OF THE TUMOR. In planning a treatment program, the physician must also take into account the biologic characteristics of the tumor, and in particular its growth rate. Aggressive treatment is likely to be least beneficial and effective in tumors that contain a small fraction of actively dividing cells. Thus, certain patients with chronic lymphocytic leukemia may give a clinical history indicating extremely indolent clinical behavior of the tumor over a period of several years. These patients are unlikely to be cured by aggressive treatment, and many can be safely observed without treatment. In contrast, other patients with the same diagnosis but with the prolymphocytic leukemia variant may have a more aggressive clinical course indicating a need for early aggressive combination chemotherapy. In summary, although the clinical impression of tumor growth rate is not frequently used as a determinant of a therapeutic choice, it may be an important criterion in determining when to begin chemotherapy in patients with chronic lymphocytic leukemia, multiple myeloma, and other "indolent" types of malignant disease.

The foregoing information concerning pathology, stage, and clinical progression must then be synthesized to yield a clear understanding of the clinical circumstances at the time of making a decision about treatment. At this point, certain questions must be faced: (1) Is cure possible and, if so, by what therapies? What are the possible short-term and long-term side effects of the various alternative therapies? (2) If cure is impossible, is significant prolongation of survival possible and, if so, at what cost to the patient's sense of well-being and his or her ability to derive satisfaction from daily life? (3) Is palliation of symptoms a more reasonable objective than undertaking life-threatening treatment? In no other specialty of medicine is the treatment decision more influenced by the personal philosophies of physician and patient and

TABLE 176–1. ANALYSIS OF ONCOGENE EXPRESSION, KARYOTYPE, AND NEURAL ENZYMES ALLOWING SUBCLASSIFICATION OF HISTOLOGICALLY INDISTINGUISHABLE FORMS OF PERIPHERAL NERVOUS SYSTEM TUMORS*

Genetic Alterations	Neuroblastoma	Peripheral Neuroepithelioma
Cytogenetic		
Double-minute chromosomes or homogeneously staining regions	+	−
Reciprocal translocation involving chromosomes 11 and 22	−	+
Molecular Genetic		
Amplified N-*myc* oncogene	+	−
High-level N-*myc* expression (RNA)	+	−
Neurotransmitter-associated Enzymes		
Dopamine hydroxylase ⎫ Tyrosine hydroxylase ⎬	+	−
Choline acetyltransferase ⎭	−	+

*Peripheral neuroepithelioma is highly responsive to combined-method therapy, whereas neuroblastoma is more refractory to treatment. (See Israel MA: The evolution of clinical molecular genetics. Am J Pediatr Hematol/Oncol 8:163, 1986.)

TABLE 176–2. COMBINED-METHOD THERAPY OF PRIMARY BREAST CANCER

Aim	Therapeutic Procedure	Rationale
Control of primary tumor	1. Local excision	Removal of bulk tumor and preservation of breast
	2. High-dose local irradiation	Sterilization of residual microscopic tumor implants of radiosensitive tumor
Prevention of distant recurrence	Adjuvant chemotherapy with 5-fluorouracil, cyclophosphamide, methotrexate	Treatment for occult metastases in patients with positive lymph nodes

their assessment of potential risks and benefits. Increasingly, conclusions from prospective clinical trials are providing a rational basis for making these decisions. While there is no single simple answer for all patients with the same diagnosis, no patient should be discouraged from aggressive therapy if there exists a reasonable chance for cure.

MANAGEMENT OF LOCAL-REGIONAL DISEASE

CANCER SURGERY. Prior to the advent of radiotherapy in the 1920's and chemotherapy in the 1950's, cancer treatment was the exclusive province of the surgeon. Cancer surgery for localized tumors is based on the principle of first establishing a diagnosis, secondly determining the extent of local disease, and thirdly establishing tumor-free surgical margins whenever possible. Current treatment often calls for integration of surgery with radiotherapy or chemotherapy to preserve bodily function and to prevent distant metastases. As examples, limited, limb-sparing surgery with high-dose irradiation may be used for soft tissue sarcomas of the extremities (Table 176–2) and surgical biopsy followed by local irradiation for primary breast cancer less than 5 cm diameter (see Ch. 240). The medical oncologist and radiotherapist should participate in treatment planning before definitive surgical procedures are undertaken.

Surgical resection of regional lymph nodes is performed for both diagnostic and, less frequently, therapeutic reasons. In some instances—e.g., testicular carcinoma with occult retroperitoneal lymph node metastases and in carcinomas of the head and neck—radical lymphadenectomy may be curative. In most other carcinomas (breast carcinoma, malignant melanoma, and colon carcinoma), lymph node dissection provides important staging information, but, if lymph nodes are positive, the operation is usually not curative because of the strong association between nodal metastases and later relapse in distant sites. This prognostic information is of particular benefit for diseases in which effective adjuvant therapy is available. In breast cancer, gastric carcinoma, and rectal carcinoma, lymph node dissection has become a staging, rather than a purely therapeutic, procedure. Its findings are critical in making the decision whether to use adjuvant chemotherapy.

While the role of surgery for treatment of local and regional disease has been modified to accommodate multimethod strategies, its employment in patients with disseminated disease has expanded. Early and aggressive resection of pulmonary metastases in patients with osteogenic sarcoma or soft tissue sarcoma has led to improved survival rates and occasional cures. Surgical resection of solitary intracranial metastases is clearly indicated for patients with breast cancer or malignant melanoma if this lesion is the sole site of metastatic disease. Reduction of tumor bulk by surgery, while not curative in its own right, may increase recruitment of previously dormant cells into active DNA synthesis and thereby render the residual tumor more susceptible to chemotherapy or radiotherapy.

In summary, the specific indications for surgery vary with clinical diagnosis and circumstances and need not be restricted to primary curative treatment of nonmetastatic disease.

RADIATION THERAPY. As an alternative to surgery, radiation therapy possesses significant advantages for locoregional treatment of malignant disease, because it produces less acute morbidity and loss of function of the affected body part. Radiotherapy exerts its biologic effect through the formation of ion pairs or reactive oxygen metabolites such as superoxide, H_2O_2, or hydroxyl radicals. These products cause breaks in DNA, which, if not repaired, may lead to cell death. Mutagenesis and carcinogenesis, resulting from sublethal effects of radiation on DNA, are other recognized late effects of radiation therapy. Radiation therapy may be delivered in the form of electromagnetic waves, such as x-rays or gamma rays, or as particle streams, such as heavy ions, protons, neutrons, pi mesons, or electrons. The characteristics of these forms of radiation have important implications for their clinical use. Electron-beam irradiation deposits its energy at the skin. Low energy x-rays, or *kilovoltage* x-rays, yield their energy readily as they pass through tissue, and consequently cause considerable damage to skin and normal tissues overlying deep-seated tumors. Higher energy x-rays, generated by linear accelerators, and gamma radiation generated by a ^{60}Co-machine, cause less skin damage, a significant advantage in the treatment of visceral tumors such as gastrointestinal carcinomas, brain tumors, or carcinoma of the lung. Charged particle beams, particularly protons, heavy ions, and pi mesons, have the further advantage of depositing their energy in a sharply focused peak below the skin surface (Fig. 176–1).

The biologic effects of conventional x-ray therapy in both the kilovoltage and megavoltage energy range are greatly enhanced by the presence of oxygen. Hypoxic cells, as found in the poorly vascularized centers of large tumors, are relatively insensitive to x-rays. In contrast, high-energy particle beams, such as neutrons, heavy ions, and protons, are less dependent on oxygen in their cytotoxic action. Thus, with respect to biologic action and dose-distribution characteristics,

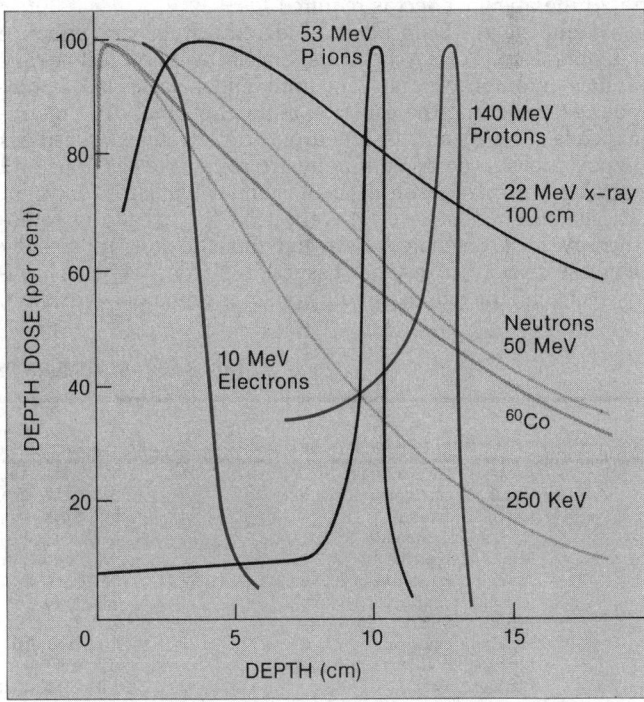

FIGURE 176–1. Penetration of various types of x-rays. Percentage of radiation dose absorbed at indicated depth below skin surface. MeV = Million electron volts; KeV = thousand electron volts. (From Becker FF [ed.]: Cancer, A Comprehensive Treatise. Vol VI. New York, Plenum Press, 1977.)

TABLE 176–3. NORMAL TISSUE TOLERANCE TO RADIOTHERAPY

Tissue	Toxic Effect	Dose Limit (Rads)*
Bone marrow	Aplasia	250
Liver	Hepatitis	2500
Intestine	Ulceration, perforation, fibrosis	4500
Brain	Infarction, necrosis	5000
Spinal cord	Infarction, necrosis	4500
Heart	Pericarditis	4500
Lung	Pneumonitis, fibrosis	1500
Kidney	Nephrosclerosis	2000
Skin	Sclerosis, dermatitis	5500

*Radiation delivered in 200-rad fractions, to whole organ, five days per week, will produce a 5 per cent incidence of toxicity.

TABLE 176–4. TUMORS CURABLE WITH CHEMOTHERAPY

	Agent(s)	Long-Term Disease-Free Survival (%)
Curable with Single-Agent Chemotherapy		
Choriocarcinoma (low-risk patients)	MTX	90
Burkitt's lymphoma (Stage I)	Alk	90
Curable with Combination Chemotherapy		
Acute lymphocytic leukemia	Vin, Pred, Anth, MTX, 6-MP	60
Hodgkin's disease (stages III and IV)	Alk, Vin, Pro, Pred	60
Diffuse histiocytic lymphoma (stage II–IV)	Alk, Vin, Pro, Pred, MTX, Anth	70
Nodular mixed lymphoma (stage II–IV)	Alk, Vin, Pro, Pred	75
Testicular carcinoma (stage II–III)	Vel, Plat, Bl, VP-16	70–90
Childhood sarcomas (with radiation and surgery)	Act-D, Alk, Vin	70–90
Childhood lymphomas	Alk, Vin, Pred, Anth	75

Act-D = actinomycin D; Alk = alkylating agent; Anth = anthracycline; Bl = bleomycin; 6-MP = 6-mercaptopurine; MTX = methotrexate; Plat = cis-platinum; Pred = prednisone; Pro = procarbazine; Vel = vinblastine (Velban); Vin = vincristine.

particle therapy has significant theoretic advantages for treating large, poorly vascularized visceral tumors.

Radiotherapy is typically administered in fractionated doses of 150 to 250 rads per day, four or five days per week, for four to seven weeks. Fractionation produces an improved therapeutic index as compared with single large doses, possibly because of the greater capacity of normal cells to repair radiation-induced damage as compared to tumors. For single doses of radiation, a shoulder is observed in the curve that relates dose to cell kill. The width of this shoulder is believed to reflect the ability of the cell to repair DNA breaks. In general, normal cells have a broader radiation dose-response shoulder and therefore tolerate individual doses of radiation with less damage than do malignant cells. Fractionation of doses has the further advantage of allowing time for death of tumor cells in the interval between fractions; the reduction in tumor size is associated with improved oxygenation of formerly hypoxic tumor cells, rendering them more sensitive to subsequent radiation. The choice of fraction size and total dose is determined by the relative radiosensitivity of the tumor and the tolerance of normal tissue in the irradiated field (Table 176–3). Less sensitive tumors, such as malignant melanoma or sarcomas, are usually treated with larger individual fractions. Fraction size may be increased if a more rapid therapeutic effect is required.

Attempts have been made to identify drugs that enhance radiation effect (radiosensitizers) or selectively protect normal tissues (radioprotectors). The nitroimidazole class of compounds, including the common antitrichomonal drug metronidazole (Flagyl) and less neurotoxic derivatives, sensitizes hypoxic cells in tissue culture by accepting free electrons and forming toxic free-radicals in a manner similar to oxygen. These compounds have little effect on the toxicity of radiotherapy for oxygenated cells and thus do not appreciably increase toxicity to normal tissues. A second class of radiosensitizers, the halopyrimidines such as bromodeoxyuridine,

is incorporated into DNA, which sensitizes the nucleic acid to strand breakage by irradiation. Clinical trials of such compounds have not been completed at this writing. An alternative approach is the use of protective compounds such as sulfhydryl compounds that interact with and detoxify the free-radicals produced by irradiation. These compounds would have to be selectively taken up by normal tissues to create a therapeutic advantage. Their use is still experimental.

Nonpharmacologic measures may also enhance radiation effects; these measures include hyperbaric oxygenation, which decreases the proportion of anoxic, and thus radioresistant, cells, and hyperthermia, which enhances toxicity to both normal and malignant cells. Neither of these ancillary measures has received thorough clinical trial.

THE MANAGEMENT OF METASTATIC CANCER. Approximately 40 per cent of patients with cancer are cured by local or regional forms of treatment. For the remainder, systemic therapy is used at some time during their illness, and in selected diseases and selected clinical situations this therapy may be curative (Table 176–4). In other diseases (Table 176–5), drug therapy produces partial or complete regression in the majority of patients, and treatment is associated with prolongation of survival for some patients. However, few of these patients are cured by chemotherapy, and relapse eventually leads to death. It has been estimated that approximately 40,000 cancer patients each year are cured by chemotherapy, either by treatment of clinically apparent metastatic disease

TABLE 176–5. TUMORS RESPONSIVE TO CHEMOTHERAPY

	Agents*	Partial or Complete Response (%)	Long-Term Disease-Free Survival (%)
Breast carcinoma (Stage III–IV)	MTX, FU, Alk, Anth	75	rare
Small cell carcinoma of the lung	Alk, MTX, Pro, Anth, VP-16	90	10
Gastric carcinoma	FU, Anth, Mit	50	rare
Ovarian carcinoma	MTX, FU, Alk, Plat, Hex	75	10–20
Multiple myeloma	Alk, Pred, Vin, Anth	75	rare
Acute nonlymphocytic leukemia	Ara-C, Anth, Alk	75	20
Chronic lymphocytic leukemia	Alk, Pred	75	rare
Prostate cancer	H T	75	rare
Head and neck cancer	Bl, MTX, Plat	75	rare
Mycosis fungoides	Alk, MTX	75	rare
Bladder cancer	Alk, MTX, Plat, Vel	60	rare

*Combination therapy yields responses in majority of patients, but less than 25% have long-term disease-free survival. Median survival of treated patients is prolonged.

Act-D = actinomycin D; Alk = alkylating agents; Anth = anthracycline (Adriamycin or daunomycin); Ara-C = cytosine arabinoside; Bl = bleomycin; FU = 5-fluorouracil; Hex = hexamethylmelamine (investigational drug available from National Cancer Institute); H T = hormonal therapy; Mit = mitomycin C; MTX = methotrexate; Plat = cis-platinum; Pred = prednisone; Pro = procarbazine; Vel = vinblastine (Velban); Vin = vincristine.

or by adjuvant chemotherapy. The therapeutic index, or margin of safety between therapeutic and toxic drug doses, is extremely narrow for many of the effective compounds; thus, small changes in pharmacokinetics or increased patient sensitivity to drug action may lead to unacceptable toxicity. In this setting, the clinician requires as much information as possible concerning the determinants of tumor cell kill, prediction of antitumor effects, pharmacokinetics, and drug interactions to maximize the effectiveness of therapy and to avoid needless toxicity.

The Kinetic Basis of Drug Therapy

FRACTIONAL KILL HYPOTHESIS. The kinetics, or growth cycle, of mammalian cells have been summarized in Ch. 168. In treating experimental tumors, a constant fraction of the total cell population is killed by a given dose of drug. Since each treatment cycle kills a specific fraction of the remaining cells, the results of treatment are a direct function of the dose of drug administered and the frequency with which treatment is repeated. However, because tumors in humans are large and are composed of heterogeneous cell populations, the "fractional kill" hypothesis does not apply as well in this situation. Treatment will eliminate sensitive cells, leaving behind the more drug-resistant population. In addition to the problem of drug resistance, most human neoplasms contain a large fraction of slowly dividing or nondividing cells (termed G_0 cells) (Fig. 176–2). Since many antineoplastic agents are most effective against rapidly dividing cells, the initial kinetic stage is unfavorable for drug treatment. However, if the number of tumor cells can be reduced by surgical treatment or radiotherapy, the remaining cells are recruited into active proliferation and become increasingly susceptible to therapy with drugs. Through this mechanism, an initially slowly responding tumor may actually become more responsive to therapy as its size is reduced by treatment.

HETEROGENEITY OF HUMAN TUMORS. The fractional kill hypothesis assumes that tumors are composed of a uniformly sensitive population of cells. Most human tumors do evolve from a single clone of malignant cells, as judged by the presence of unique chromosomal markers or by G6PD typing (see Ch. 152). However, as tumors grow, significant mutation takes place, and advanced tumors are composed of multiple cell types that differ in their biochemical and morphologic characteristics and, most importantly, in their sensitivity to treatment. Drug-resistant cells are believed to arise from a parent-sensitive population by random mutation. The probability that a drug-resistant cell exists in a tumor is a function of the mutation rate for the drug-resistance gene and the absolute number of tumor cells. Thus, the chances for cure are greatest when the tumor population is smallest and least likely to contain treatment-resistant mutants. Also, com-

bination therapies employing drugs with differing mechanisms of action are more likely to eradicate a tumor population than single-agent treatment, since a given cell is less likely to be simultaneously resistant to more than one agent.

PREDICTION OF DRUG RESPONSE. The selection of drugs for treating individual patients is primarily based on past experience in treating patients with the same histologic diagnosis and the same stage of disease. It would be highly desirable to be able to predict the sensitivity of individual tumors to treatment, and thus avoid needless toxicity of ineffective agents. The most successful laboratory aid for predicting response is the measurement of hormone receptors as a guide for hormonal therapy of breast cancer. This topic will be considered in detail later in this chapter. Biochemical tests based on the mechanism of drug action or mechanisms of drug resistance are able to predict response in animal tumors, but have not been used extensively in clinical trials. A notable exception is the treatment of acute myeloblastic leukemia with cytosine arabinoside. The duration of complete remission in this disease may be predicted prior to treatment by the ability of leukemic cells to activate this drug and retain its triphosphate form. Attempts to develop drug sensitivity testing based on in vitro cultures of primary human tumors have met with mixed success; in general, these assay systems are too unreliable and too labor-intensive to be useful for routine clinical use.

PHARMACOKINETIC DETERMINANTS OF RESPONSE

The outcome of cancer chemotherapy depends in large part on the inherent sensitivity of the tumor under treatment to the agents being used. However, pharmacokinetic factors such as drug absorption, metabolism, and elimination also influence response and are extremely variable from one patient to the next. The oral route of drug administration is sparingly used in cancer chemotherapy. Up to tenfold variability in the bioavailability of orally administered 6-mercaptopurine, methotrexate, hexamethylmelamine,* 5-fluorouracil, and melphalan has been reported.

Most agents are given intravenously to assure adequate drug entry into the bloodstream. A few agents can be administered by other routes. Cytosine arabinoside, an antileukemic drug, may be given subcutaneously, a route that produces slow absorption and more prolonged drug concentrations in plasma than observed by the intravenous route. Methotrexate or cytosine arabinoside may be administered into the lumbar space for treatment of meningeal leukemia, lymphoma, or carcinoma, although neurotoxic side effects (coma, seizures, meningeal irritation) are observed with methotrexate, particularly at doses above 12 mg.

Several drugs have been administered by the intraperitoneal route, including methotrexate, 5-fluorouracil, and *cis*-platinum, for treatment of malignant disease confined to the peritoneal surfaces, such as ovarian cancer. The advantage of this route is that drug, instilled in a volume of 2 liters of dialysate, exits slowly from the peritoneal space, producing a marked concentration gradient of 100- to 1000-fold between the peritoneal fluid and plasma. Metabolism of drug in the liver as it exits from the peritoneum through the portal circulation further reduces drug concentrations reaching the systemic circulation. This type of therapy has produced documented remissions in ovarian cancer resistant to conventional regimens, but it is complex to administer, does not effectively treat disease outside the peritoneum, and thus has uncertain value in the general management of this disease.

For metastatic tumor confined to the liver, as often occurs in patients with previously resected colon cancer, hepatic arterial perfusion with 5-fluorouracil or 5-fluorodeoxyuridine appears to produce a higher response rate than intravenous therapy with the same agents; continuous infusions of two

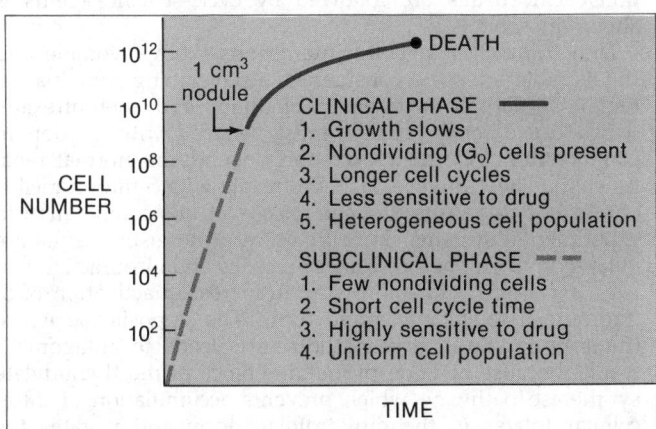

FIGURE 176–2. Kinetic phases of tumor growth.

---

*Investigational drug available from National Cancer Institute.

TABLE 176–6. DOSE ADJUSTMENTS FOR ALTERED RENAL OR HEPATIC FUNCTION

Condition	Agent	Dose Adjustment*
Altered renal function	Methotrexate *cis*-Platinum VP-16 Hydroxyurea Bleomycin	Decrease dose in proportion to decrease in creatinine clearance
Altered hepatic function	Adriamycin Vincristine Velban Vindesine	Decrease dose by 50% in patients with serum bilirubin >3.0 mg/dl

*Guidelines are approximations. Doses should be further adjusted on the basis of toxicity resulting from the initial dose.

weeks' duration, or longer, are well tolerated, since the drugs are degraded in their flow through the liver before they can enter the systemic circulation. Disadvantages of this therapy are local catheter complications, the need for a constant infusion device, and the failure to treat disease outside the liver. Biliary sclerosis is a known complication. Intra-arterial perfusion of extremity sarcomas and melanomas has been performed in experimental studies but has uncertain efficacy.

Elimination rates for commonly used drugs vary considerably and are not always predictable on the basis of renal or hepatic function. Alterations in drug dosage are necessary for patients with compromised ability to excrete or metabolize specific drugs (Table 176–6). For agents not listed in the table, reductions in drug dosage should not be made unless mandated by leukopenia, thrombocytopenia, serious infection, or other life-threatening complications, as dose reduction can only compromise the chances for response.

Drug-level monitoring has not been used as a standard guide to dose adjustment, except for the monitoring of high-dose methotrexate therapy (see below). The high reactivity, complex metabolism, and low plasma concentrations of anticancer drugs in general have made such monitoring difficult for other agents, except in investigative settings.

ASSESSMENT OF RESPONSE

An objective assessment of the response of a tumor to treatment is of central importance. Too often subjective impressions of improvement based on a patient's sense of well-being or performance status are not borne out by objective criteria. The standard criterion for partial response is a 50 per cent or greater reduction in the sum of the product of perpendicular diameters of all lesions measurable by physical examination or by radiologic techniques. A complete response denotes complete disappearance of disease, and in most diseases *should be documented by pathologic restaging if possible.* Pathologic restaging requires rebiopsy of previously involved organ sites. For tumors that secrete quantifiable marker proteins, such as gestational choriocarcinoma or germ cell tumors of the testis, a fall of these markers to normal levels and a persistence at this level for two to three months is necessary for a judgment of complete remission. Even in the presence of normal markers, persistent abnormalities on chest film or computed scanning may still require biopsy. For example, in patients with testicular carcinoma who present with intra-abdominal tumor, the induction of remission must be verified by repeat biopsy of retroperitoneal lymph nodes, even if radiographs and markers are negative. Partial responses rarely lead to significantly improved survival.

STRATEGIES OF CLINICAL CHEMOTHERAPY

COMBINATION CHEMOTHERAPY. *Background.* The first effective drugs for treating cancer were introduced in the mid and late 1940's, but initial therapeutic results were disappointing. Although impressive regressions of acute lymphocytic leukemia and adult lymphomas were obtained with nitrogen mustard, antifolates, corticosteroids, and the vinca

alkaloids, responses were only partial in degree and of short duration. Attempts at retreatment usually met with a diminished response or frank resistance to further therapy. Increased doses could not be given because of prohibitive bone marrow toxicity or neurotoxicity, and few patients derived lasting benefit. The single exception was the cure of choriocarcinoma by methotrexate. The introduction of combination chemotherapy for acute lymphocytic leukemia of childhood in the early 1960's marked a turning point in the effective treatment of neoplastic disease. Such combinations of chemotherapeutic agents are now the standard for the treatment of most advanced cancers.

Rationale. The principal rationale for combination chemotherapy derives from an appreciation of the reasons for failure of single-agent treatment: (1) De novo resistance to any given single agent is frequent, even in the most responsive tumors. (2) Initially responsive tumors rapidly acquire resistance after drug exposure. Drugs either induce resistance or select resistant mutants from an initially heterogeneous tumor cell population. However, since the various anticancer drugs have diverse mechanisms of action, cells resistant to one agent might still be sensitive to the several other drugs in the regimen. If drugs have different, nonoverlapping toxicities, each can be used in full dosage in a combination regimen. For example, drugs such as vincristine, prednisone, bleomycin, and hexamethylmelamine, which lack bone marrow toxicity, are particularly valuable for combination with myelosuppressive agents. On the basis of these principles, curative combinations have been devised for acute lymphocytic leukemia (vincristine-prednisone ± Adriamycin and L-asparaginase), Hodgkin's disease (nitrogen *m*ustard-vincristine [Oncovin]-*p*rednisone-*p*rocarbazine; called MOPP), histiocytic lymphoma (C-MOPP), and testicular carcinoma (bleomycin-vinblastine-*cis*-platinum). The cure of advanced malignancy, when possible, is primarily achieved with combination regimens (Table 176–5).

Scheduling. The scheduling of drugs in combinations was initially based on convenience and empirical experience. Intermittent cycles of therapy allow for periods of recovery of host bone marrow and immune function. More recent combinations have incorporated nonmyelosuppressive agents in the "off period" between doses of myelotoxic drugs. High-dose methotrexate with leucovorin rescue has proved to be particularly useful in this capacity in the off period because of its minimal effect on white blood cell and platelet counts. Logic dictates the initial use of drugs that kill in all phases of the tumor cell growth cycle, such as the alkylating agents or nitrosoureas (if active against the disease in question), to reduce tumor bulk and thereby recruit slowly dividing cells into active DNA synthesis, then to be followed by cell cycle–dependent agents (such as methotrexate or the fluoropyrimidines) that kill preferentially in the DNA synthetic phase. An example of such a regimen in which the cycle-nonspecific drugs are followed by cycle-specific agents is shown in Table 176–7.

Drug Interactions. Drug interactions, both favorable and unfavorable, must be considered in developing combination regimens. Drugs such as *cis*-platinum and methotrexate, which cause renal toxicity, must be used with caution in combination since their excretion depends on normal renal function. The sequence of methotrexate with 5-fluorouracil is critical in determining the cytotoxicity of this combination in experimental systems. In cell culture, synergistic results are obtained when methotrexate precedes 5-fluorouracil by at least one hour, probably owing to increased activation of 5-fluorouracil to its nucleotide form. The opposite sequence (fluoropyrimidine, then methotrexate) leads to antagonistic results because of fluoropyrimidine block of the thymidylate synthetase pathway, which prevents accumulation of intracellular folates in the dihydrofolate form and negates the effect of inhibition of dihydrofolate reductase by methotrexate

TABLE 176–7. STRATEGIES FOR COMBINATION CHEMOTHERAPY: USE OF NON–CROSS-RESISTANT DRUGS IN SEQUENCE IN MACOP-B REGIMEN

	Week											
	1	2	3	4	5	6	7	8	9	10	11	12
Doxorubicin 50 mg/m²	x		x		x		x		x		x	
Cyclophosphamide 350 mg/m²	x		x		x		x		x		x	
Methotrexate 400 mg/m²		x				x				x		
Vincristine 1.4 mg/m²		x		x		x		x		x		x
Bleomycin 10 U/m²				x				x				x
Prednisone 75 mg daily												→
Leucovorin, 15 mg every 6 hr for 6 doses, beginning 24 hr after methotrexate												

Adapted from Ann Intern Med 102:596, 1985.

Notable features:

1. Early use of all six agents discourages outgrowth of resistant tumor cells.
2. Therapy begun with drugs that are not cell cycle–specific, followed by cycle-specific agents in week 2.
3. Nonmyelosuppressive drugs in weeks 2, 4, 6, 8, 10, and 12 allow recovery from drugs in odd-numbered cycles.

(Fig. 176–3). Similarly, L-asparaginase prior to methotrexate aborts the toxic effect of the antifolate, and is therefore avoided in clinical scheduling. *cis*-Platinum, a drug that covalently binds to DNA, markedly enhances the toxicity of antimetabolites, such as 5-fluorouracil and cytosine arabinoside. Methotrexate and 6-mercaptopurine are highly synergistic; methotrexate blocks de novo purine biosynthesis, thus augmenting the uptake and utilization of preformed purines such as 6-mercaptopurine.

Adjustments Within Combinations. All drug combination regimens require dose adjustment scales to allow increases or decreases of dose according to toxicity. It becomes difficult to determine which of the several agents is responsible if overlapping toxicity patterns are present. In this setting, arbitrary scales of dose adjustment according to bone marrow toxicity or other readily identifiable and quantifiable toxicity are usually provided with protocols.

New Strategies. In the first combination chemotherapy trials, such as MOPP chemotherapy of Hodgkin's disease, the overall strategy was to deliver intensive therapy over a finite time period and then to restage the condition to rule out the presence of occult residual disease. Treatment was discontinued in those patients having complete remission. The duration of unmaintained complete remission then served as an index of the completeness of response. In an effort to improve the long-term disease-free survival rate associated with cyclic chemotherapy, this basic strategy has been modified in the following ways:

1. Alternative combinations to the primary regimen have been identified by trials in patients resistant to the primary treatment. An example is the ABVD regimen for Hodgkin's disease, which incorporates four agents (Adriamycin, bleomycin, vinblastine, and DTIC) that are non–cross-resistant with the MOPP drugs. The second regimen can then be used in alternating cycles of treatment with the primary combination, or one set of drugs can be used on day 1 and a second set on day 8 of a 28-day cycle. The day 1–day 8 alternation has the better chance of discouraging the development of drug-resistant cells (see Table 176–7).

2. An alternative is to use non–cross-resistant agents for maintenance therapy, after induction of complete remission with the standard combinations, as is standard practice in childhood leukemia.

COMBINED RADIATION AND CHEMOTHERAPY. Chemotherapy can often be usefully combined with other forms of treatment, such as irradiation or surgery. As an example, surgical resection of residual testicular carcinoma following chemotherapy leads to cure of a fraction of patients who would otherwise be only partial responders. There is evidence that the combination of irradiation and chemotherapy may improve the complete response rate and survival in children with Wilms' tumor and embryonal rhabdomyosarcoma.

Unfortunately, chemotherapy and radiotherapy have synergistic actions on *both* normal and malignant tissue, and this may lead to problems in their integrated use. The normal tissue of greatest concern is the bone marrow. Radiation given to the pelvic or midline abdominal areas produces a decline in blood counts and a decrease in bone marrow reserve. Appropriate shielding of the pelvic structures and the use of megavoltage radiation with limited scatter can preserve a significant portion of this marrow-bearing tissue. The sequence of administration may be of crucial importance. For example, chemotherapy followed by total nodal irradiation is less well tolerated because of severe myelosuppression in the radiation phase of treatment. One must anticipate cumulative effects of both chemotherapy and irradiation on bone marrow reserve.

High-dose chemotherapy (usually cyclophosphamide) and total-body irradiation have been used to eradicate residual acute myelocytic leukemia in children and young adults. These patients are rescued from lethal toxicity by allogeneic bone marrow transplantation (see Ch. 165). Similar therapy for solid tumors, using BCNU, alkylating agents, or combinations of drugs with autologous bone marrow reconstitution, has been successful in selected cases of lymphoma, but remains experimental because of its extreme toxicity to bone marrow, liver, and lung, and the high rate of tumor recurrence.

Other examples of interactions between chemotherapeutic agents and irradiation are as follows: (1) Adriamycin and concurrent mediastinal irradiation enhance toxicity for the heart, esophagus, and lung. (2) Bleomycin enhances x-ray damage to pulmonary tissue. (3) Methotrexate may produce recall reactions in previously irradiated skin. (4) Prednisone suppresses the immediate reaction to pulmonary irradiation, but withdrawal of steroids may be associated with a serious flare in radiation-induced pneumonitis. Reduction of radiation dose or an alteration in drug dose or schedule may be necessary to avoid untoward effects.

The *carcinogenicity* of both radiotherapy and chemotherapy is another negative consideration in their combined use. Agents listed in Table 176–8 are strongly suspected of being carcinogenic, based on (1) association with a high incidence of second malignant tumors in humans, (2) proven carcinogenicity in animals, or (3) strongly positive mutagenicity in bacterial assays. Irradiation is also strongly mutagenic and carcinogenic. The combination of alkylating agents and procarbazine with irradiation has led to an estimated 5 per cent incidence of second malignant disease (most frequently acute myelocytic leukemia) in patients with Hodgkin's disease. The carcinogenic potential of specific regimens is difficult to quantitate because of the brief survival of many patients undergoing such treatment and uncertainty as to the number of patients at risk in retrospective studies. Nonetheless, there is sufficient evidence of irradiation-drug synergy to warrant caution in accepting combinations of irradiation and carcinogenic drugs, particularly for patients who have an excellent chance of cure or long-term survival by single-method treatment.

Both irradiation and chemotherapy are capable of producing *infertility*. Cyclophosphamide, chlorambucil, busulfan, mel-

**TABLE 176–8. CARCINOGENICITY
OF ANTINEOPLASTIC AGENTS**

	Second Tumors in Humans	Carcinogen in Animals	Mutagen*
High risk			
Cyclophosphamide	+	+	+
Melphalan	+	+	+
Chlorambucil	+	+	NR
Procarbazine	+	+	–
Methyl CCNU	+	+	NR
6-Mercaptopurine	+	+	+
Adriamycin	NR	+	+
Low risk			
Methotrexate	–	–	–
Cytosine arabinoside	–	–	–
5-Fluorouracil	–	NR	–
Risk unknown			
Bleomycin	NR	–	–
Cis-platinum	NR	NR	+
Actinomycin D	NR	–	+
Vincristine	NR	–	–
Vinblastine	NR	+	–

*Mutagen in Ames assay using *Salmonella typhimurium* testor strain and rat liver microsomes.
NR = not reported.

phalan, and procarbazine, as well as combination regimens, cause infertility in both males and females, often with permanent sterility in males and in women over 40 years. Adriamycin, *cis*-platinum, the vinca alkaloids, the antimetabolites, and the nitrosoureas have not been carefully studied in this respect. In men, the development of azoospermia is usually but not always irreversible.

ADJUVANT THERAPY. Adjuvant therapy is treatment given after surgical resection of a primary tumor in an effort to prevent recurrence at distant sites. The need for adjuvant therapy arises from two sources: (1) the high recurrence rate of certain tumors following surgery for apparently localized disease (e.g., breast cancer, soft tissue sarcoma, osteogenic sarcoma, Dukes' B and C colon and rectal cancer, and various solid neoplasms of childhood), and (2) the failure of chemotherapy or combined-method treatment to cure patients after recurrence of disease. Tumors are generally most susceptible to chemotherapy at their earliest stages of growth. This increased sensitivity of small tumors is based on a higher growth fraction, a shorter cell cycle time, and a decreased probability of there being drug-resistant cells in the population; these factors allow for a greater fractional cell kill for a given drug dose. As a tumor enlarges, its growth fraction decreases, the cell cycle time lengthens, and the probability of drug-resistant mutations arising increases. In addition, patients are able to accept chemotherapy best when they are not debilitated by metastatic disease.

There are disadvantages of adjuvant therapy related to both short-term and long-term risks. An unidentifiable fraction of patients receiving adjuvant treatment will have been cured by the primary surgical procedure and therefore will be experiencing needless risks and toxicity. In considering adjuvant therapy, late complications such as carcinogenicity (Table 176–8) and sterility assume greater importance. Nonetheless, intensive treatment in the adjuvant setting offers a higher probability of cure than treatment at later stages of disease.

ANTINEOPLASTIC DRUGS

The effective and safe use of cancer chemotherapeutic agents requires a fundamental understanding of their action, interactions, pharmacokinetics, and toxicity in man. Primary reviews of antineoplastic drugs should be consulted for more detailed information.

ANTIMETABOLITES. *Antifolates.* Antimetabolites act as fraudulent substrates for vital biochemical reactions. Most of the effective antimetabolites used in cancer treatment inhibit the synthesis of DNA or its precursors. The first antimetabolite to be used clinically was aminopterin. It has since been replaced by another folate analogue, *methotrexate*, which has more predictable clinical toxicity and at least equal clinical activity. Tetrahydrofolates, among other functions, provide one-carbon groups used in the synthesis of the purine nucleotides and thymidylate, which are precursors of DNA (Fig. 176–3). In the synthesis of thymidylate, N^{5-10} methylenetetrahydrofolate donates its one-carbon methylene group and at the same time is oxidized to dihydrofolate, an inactive form of folic acid. Methotrexate and its polyglutamate metabolites inhibit dihydrofolate reductase (DHFR) (Fig. 176–3), the enzyme responsible for reducing inactive dihydrofolate back to the active tetrahydrofolate form. The block in DHFR depletes folate cofactor pools, leads to a buildup of toxic dihydrofolate, and shuts down the synthesis of purine nucleotides and thymidylate. The polyglutamate forms of methotrexate, particularly those with three or four additional glutamates, are preferentially retained within tumor cells and are potent inhibitors of a number of folate-dependent enzymes in addition to dihydrofolate reductase.

The biochemical effects of methotrexate can be reversed by administration of the reduced folate leucovorin. This leucovorin "rescue" prevents methotrexate toxicity to bone marrow and gastrointestinal epithelium if administered in sufficient doses within 36 hours after infusions of high doses of methotrexate. Methotrexate infusion of 6 to 36 hours in duration, and in total doses of 1500 mg per square meter* or greater, can be given safely if followed by leucovorin rescue. The dose of leucovorin required (usually 15 to 50 mg per square meter every 6 hours for 48 hours) depends on the methotrexate

*Exceeds manufacturer's recommended maximum dose.

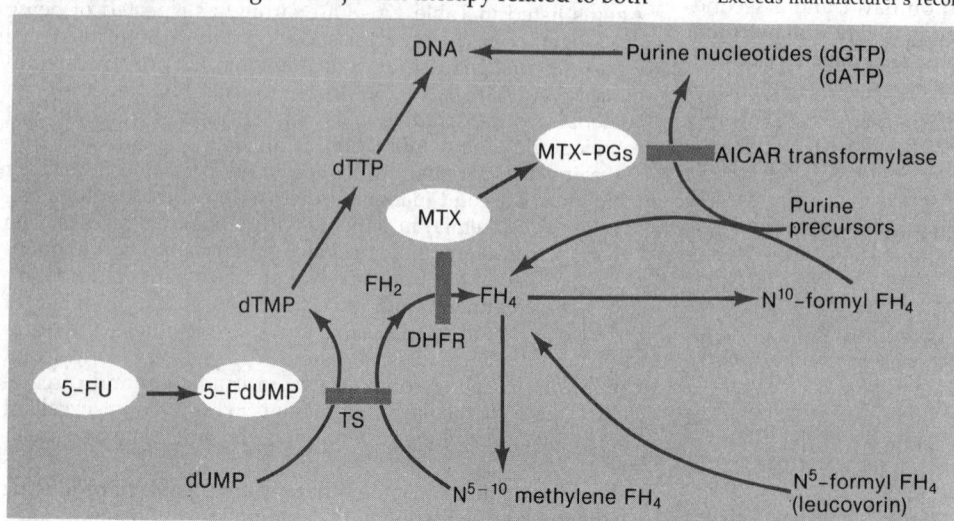

FIGURE 176–3. Sites of action of methotrexate (MTX) and 5-fluorodeoxyuridylate (5-FdUMP). DHFR = Dihydrofolate reductase; TS = thymidylate synthase; AICAR transformylase = aminoimidazolecarboxamide ribonucleotide transformylase; FH₂ = dihydrofolic acid; FH₄ = tetrahydrofolic acid. Note that MTX-PG's (MTX polyglutamates) directly inhibit AICAR transformylase and TS (not shown), in addition to inhibition of DHFR.

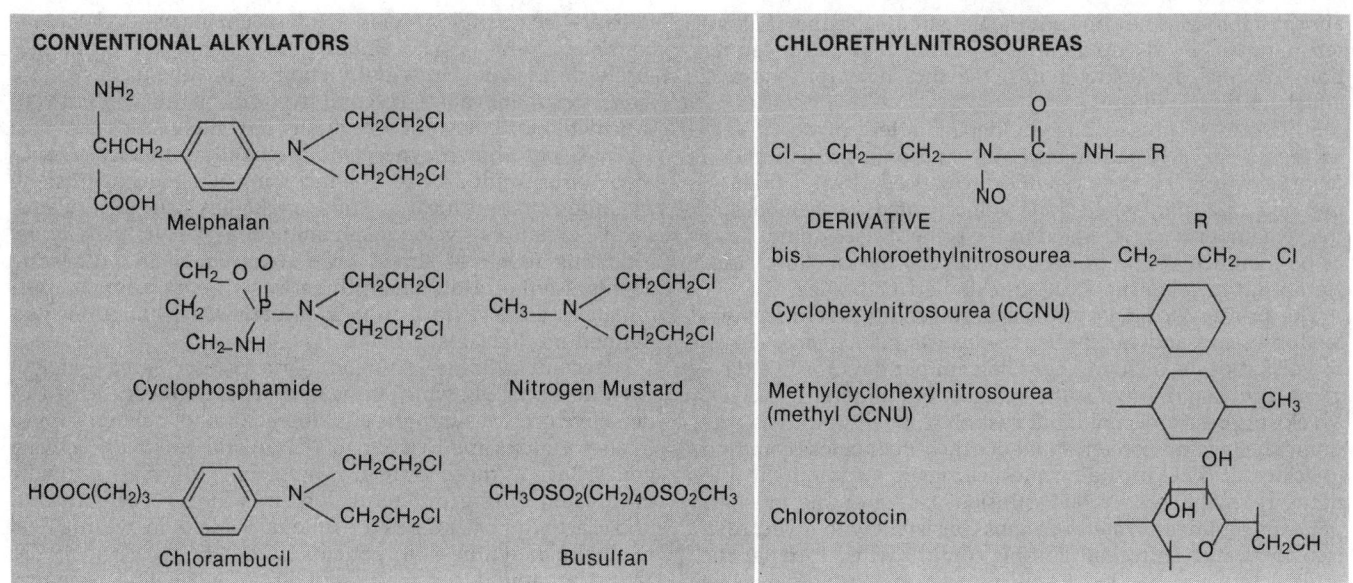

FIGURE 176–4. Chemical structure of clinically useful alkylating agents and the related class of nitrosourea compounds.

concentration at the time of rescue and may have to be increased in patients with inadequate renal function and delayed drug elimination.

Tumor cells acquire resistance to antifolates by several different biochemical mechanisms: (1) deletion of a high-affinity, carrier-mediated transport system for reduced folates, shared by methotrexate; (2) an increase in the concentration of DHFR; (3) an altered reductase that fails to bind methotrexate; and (4) decreased thymidylate synthesis activity. An increase in enzyme concentration owing to amplification of the reductase gene is readily induced by exposure of cells to gradually increasing drug concentration in tissue culture and has been documented to occur in the clinical setting. In attempts to overcome resistance, high doses of methotrexate (1500 mg per square meter* or greater) are given in 6- to 36-hour infusions, followed by repeat doses of the rescue agent leucovorin. This therapy is designed to provide sufficiently high drug concentrations to penetrate the cell membrane by passive diffusion and to saturate increased concentrations of enzyme. Methotrexate may be administered intravenously in doses ranging from 25 to 7500 mg per square meter.* Its primary plasma half-life is approximately two to three hours with excretion largely by the kidney (90 per cent). In patients with abnormal renal function or in those receiving doses above 1000 mg per square meter, monitoring of drug concentration in plasma is recommended to avoid serious toxicity. Methotrexate concentrations in plasma can be measured accurately with a competitive binding assay or radioimmunoassay and are useful for detecting patients at high risk of toxicity, who should then receive leucovorin rescue doses.

Methotrexate distributes slowly into "third spaces" such as ascites, pleural effusions, or cerebrospinal fluid. In patients with effusions or ascites the slow reentry of drug into the systemic circulation has been associated with a prolonged terminal half-life and unexpected toxicity. Systemic methotrexate enters spinal fluid poorly with concentrations only 3 per cent of those simultaneously in plasma. Only with high-dose methotrexate therapy are cytotoxic concentrations achieved in the spinal fluid. Alternatively, methotrexate may be injected directly into the lumbar intrathecal space or directly into the ventricle through an indwelling reservoir.

Acute methotrexate toxicity results from its effects on rapidly proliferating tissues (bone marrow and intestinal and oral epithelium). Drug concentrations of 1×10^{-8} M or greater in plasma produce myelosuppression and mucositis, which peak

5 to 14 days following a bolus dose or short-term infusion, with rapid recovery. More prolonged toxicity may be observed in patients who fail to eliminate the drug normally. High-dose therapy with methotrexate may lead to acute renal injury, believed to result from intrarenal precipitation of methotrexate or methotrexate-derived material. This can be prevented by vigorous pretreatment hydration, urine alkalinization (pH≥7), and, in patients with underlying renal disease, dose reduction proportional to the decrease in renal function. Renal toxicity and delayed drug excretion are aggravated by concomitant use of nonsteroidal anti-inflammatory drugs. Both acute and chronic hepatotoxicity may be caused by methotrexate with acute increase of serum levels of hepatic enzymes and, in patients receiving long-term oral treatment, hepatic fibrosis and cirrhosis. An acute pneumonitis, possibly of hypersensitivity origin, and rare episodes of anaphylaxis have been described.

Various manifestations of neurotoxicity are observed in up to 30 per cent of patients receiving intrathecal methotrexate, including motor dysfunction, cranial nerve palsies, coma, or seizures. Symptoms are accompanied by increased spinal fluid pressure and protein concentration and a reactive pleocytosis. Continued methotrexate treatment in this setting may be fatal.

Fluoropyrimidines. 5-Fluorouracil (5-FU), an analogue of thymine, inhibits thymidylate synthesis (Fig. 176–4). 5-FU has activity against many solid tumors, including breast, colon, head and neck, and ovarian carcinoma, and is now commonly used in combination therapy. Two biochemical actions may account for its cytotoxicity. 5-FU is converted to its corresponding ribose-triphosphate (5-FUTP) which, in turn, is incorporated in RNA and inhibits RNA processing and function. A second metabolite, 5-FdUMP, binds tightly to thymidylate synthase and inhibits the eventual formation of dTTP, one of the four necessary precursors of DNA. Resistance to 5-FU develops through deletion of one of the several key enzymes required for its activation (uridine kinase, nucleoside phosphorylase, and orotic acid phosphoribosyl transferase) or through amplification of thymidylate synthetase.

5-FU is usually given intravenously or intra-arterially because of erratic oral absorption and rapid first-pass metabolism in the liver. It may be given with leucovorin to enhance its binding to thymidylate synthase. Leucovorin increases 5-FU gastrointestinal toxicity and may enhance its therapeutic activity in breast and colon cancer. After intravenous administration of 10 to 15 mg per kilogram, peak plasma concentrations reach 0.1 to 1 mM, but rapid metabolism to dihydrofluorouracil in the liver and other tissues leads to an

*Exceeds manufacturer's recommended maximum dose.

abrupt fall in plasma concentrations with a half-time of about ten minutes. By six hours after injection, plasma concentrations of 5-FU are below 1 μM, the threshold for cytotoxic effects in tissue culture.

5-FU can be infused into the hepatic artery or portal vein for treatment of hepatic metastases, and only small amounts of drug will reach the systemic circulation. Greater than 80 per cent of administered 5-FU is inactivated by metabolism, the remainder being excreted in the urine. Doses do not have to be modified in the presence of hepatic dysfunction, since significant metabolism occurs in extrahepatic tissues.

The primary toxicities of *bolus* intravenous 5-FU are myelosuppression and mucositis. *Continuous intravenous infusion* of 5-FU at doses of 30 mg per kilogram per day* for five days gives equivalent therapeutic results, but different toxicity. Myelosuppression is mild, but gastrointestinal symptoms predominate (again, stomatitis and diarrhea). Other less common toxicities of 5-FU include acute neurologic symptoms in patients receiving intracarotid infusions, a syndrome of chest pain and serum enzyme elevations consistent with myocardial ischemia, and acute and chronic conjunctivitis. Intrahepatic arterial infusion has led to biliary sclerosis and progressive jaundice.

Cytosine Arabinoside. Cytosine arabinoside (ara-C, cytarabine) is an analogue of deoxycytidine, differing only in the substitution of the sugar arabinose for deoxyribose. Ara-C readily penetrates cells by a carrier-mediated process and then is converted to its active form, ara-CTP. Ara-C is incorporated into DNA and causes premature termination of the growing strand of newly synthesized DNA. Two inactivating enzymes, cytidine deaminase and dCMP deaminase (which degrade ara-C and ara-CMP, respectively), are present in high concentration in some tumors and are thought to exert an important negative influence on drug action. Ara-C kills cells selectively during the S phase of the cell cycle and has little activity against slowly growing solid tumors.

Resistance to ara-C is not well understood, but may relate to (1) deletion of deoxycytidine kinase, a necessary enzyme for activation, (2) an increased intracellular pool of dCTP (the nucleotide that competes with ara-CTP), (3) increased cytidine deaminase, or (4) a deficiency of the membrane transport process. In patients with leukemia, clinical response to ara-C may be predicted by the ability of leukemic cells to form and to retain ara-CTP after exposure to ara-C in vitro.

Ara-C is administered intravenously and is distributed rapidly into total body water, including cerebrospinal fluid. Owing to rapid inactivation (half-time of seven to twenty minutes) and its S-phase specificity, ara-C is given by continuous infusion in dosages of 100 mg per square meter per day or in a bolus of 50 to 100 mg every eight to twelve hours, for five to ten days. More than 70 per cent of administered ara-C is excreted in the urine as its inactive metabolite ara-U, which is formed in liver, plasma, granulocytes, and other sites. Alternatively, ara-C has been given in very high doses (up to 3 grams per square meter*) every 12 hours for six days, a regimen that appears to improve the response rate in refractory types of acute myelocytic leukemia. Alternatively in patients with preleukemic syndromes or in elderly patients, ara-C has been administered in low doses of 10 to 20 mg per square meter per day subcutaneously. Responses in preleukemic patients have been ascribed to an induction of tumor differentiation by low levels of ara-C.

Ara-C may also be administered intrathecally for treatment of meningeal leukemia or carcinomatosis. Because spinal fluid contains little cytidine deaminase, intrathecal doses of 50 mg per square meter yield high peak levels (1 mM), which decline with a half-time of two hours.

The primary side effects of ara-C are myelosuppression and gastrointestinal epithelial injury (nausea, vomiting, diarrhea).

Patients frequently develop mild serum enzyme elevations consistent with hepatocellular damage, but these changes rarely necessitate a discontinuation of treatment. High-dose ara-C treatment causes cerebral dysfunction, ataxia, and conjunctivitis, toxicities not seen with conventional doses.

Ara-C has shown synergistic biochemical interaction with many other antitumor agents, including alkylating agents, *cis*-platinum, thiopurines, uridine analogues, and antifolates. Ara-C enhances cyclophosphamide and BCNU activity by inhibiting repair of strand breaks caused by the alkylating agents. Methotrexate given three to six hours prior to ara-C enhances ara-CTP formation in experimental tumors by undefined mechanisms.

A second cytidine analogue, *5-azacytidine (5-azaC)*, is activated to 5-azaCTP, which is incorporated into RNA and causes defective protein synthesis and degradation of polyribosomes. It also inhibits methylation of DNA and thus can activate genes, such as those for fetal hemoglobin, which are normally inactivated during differentiation. In addition to its antileukemic activity, 5-azaC has the unique action of increasing fetal hemoglobin synthesis in patients with beta-thalassemia (Ch. 142). The rapid decomposition of 5-azaC in alkaline or neutral solution necessitates either fresh mixing prior to administration or formulation at a slightly acid pH in Ringer's lactate (pH 6.2). The drug undergoes rapid removal from the plasma, either through metabolism or chemical decomposition. Less than 2 per cent of an administered dose remains in plasma as parent compound 30 minutes after administration. The primary toxicities of 5-azaC are myelosuppression and severe and prolonged nausea and vomiting. The latter symptoms are lessened by a prolonged or continuous infusion, with no apparent change in its therapeutic efficacy.

Purine Analogues. 6-Mercaptopurine (6-MP) and 6-thioguanine (6-TG) have the single substitution of a thiol group in place of the 6-hydroxyl group found in the basic purine nucleus. Both require activation to the nucleotide level by hypoxanthine-guanine phosphoribosyltransferase (HGPRT'ase) to inhibit de novo purine biosynthesis and block the conversion of the purine precursor inosinic acid to adenylic acid or to guanylic acid. The triphosphate nucleotides of 6-TG and 6-MP are incorporated into DNA and produce delayed toxicity after several cell divisions. Biochemical resistance to these agents in human leukemic cells is commonly associated with increased concentrations of a degrading enzyme, a membrane-bound alkaline phosphatase, or decreased concentrations of the activating enzyme HGPRT'ase. 6-MP is not reliably absorbed orally; 6-TG is erratically absorbed, and is thus administered by intravenous infusion. 6-MP is rapidly eliminated (plasma half-time 20 to 45 minutes) by oxidation to 6-thiouric acid catalyzed by xanthine oxidase. This reaction is inhibited by allopurinol; thus the dose of orally administered 6-MP must be reduced 75 per cent in the presence of the xanthine oxidase inhibitor. 6-TG is degraded by desulfuration and by oxidation with a plasma half-time of 80 to 90 minutes. No reduction in 6-TG dosage is required for patients who are also receiving allopurinol. Both agents are well tolerated in doses of approximately 100 mg per square meter for at least five days. 6-MP is used at reduced doses for maintenance of remission.

The primary toxicity of both thiopurines is myelosuppression and epithelial injury. Myelosuppression is maximal within seven days of drug administration, and recovery occurs in one to two weeks. Both drugs produce reversible hepatotoxicity with enzyme and bilirubin increases in a pattern suggesting cholestatic jaundice. Mucositis, esophagitis, and gastrointestinal complaints are usually mild.

The 6-thiopurines and the related compound azathioprine, which is metabolized to 6-mercaptopurine by the liver, are potent suppressors of cell-mediated immunity and thus find numerous applications for treating autoimmune diseases and preventing transplant rejection. Immunosuppression with

---

*Exceeds manufacturer's recommended maximum dose.

these agents can be achieved at doses that produce little decrease in the white blood cell count. Long-term immunosuppressive therapy with azathioprine, prednisone, and other immunosuppressive agents in renal transplantation is associated with an increased risk of squamous carcinomas of skin and histiocytic lymphoma and predisposes patients to bacterial and opportunistic infections.

An unusual purine analogue, deoxycoformycin, has the ability to induce remissions in hairy cell leukemia (see Ch. 155) and chronic lymphocytic leukemia. When used in low dosages of 4 mg per square meter every two weeks, this drug effectively blocks adenosine deaminase activity leading to dATP accumulation and cell death. In high-dose regimens, it causes somewhat unpredictable, but occasionally severe, neurotoxicity or renal failure.

ALKYLATING AGENTS. Alkylating agents kill tumor cells and normal dividing tissues by forming covalent bonds with nucleic acids. The alkyl groups attach to DNA, interfere with its integrity, and thereby produce significant cytotoxic, mutagenic, and carcinogenic effects.

Alkylating agents spontaneously form positively charged carbonium ions in aqueous solution. In the case of chloroethyl derivatives, the alkylating intermediate is $R-CH_2CH_2^+$, which attacks nucleophilic (electron-rich) sites on nucleic acids, proteins, sulfhydryls (glutathione), and amino acids. It is likely that the primary cytotoxic and mutagenic effects of alkylating agents result from binding to guanine (which accounts for about 90 per cent of alkylated sites), adenine, and cytosine. Based alkylation leads to misreading of the DNA code, but also single-strand breakage. Cross-linkage of DNA occurs when bifunctional alkylating agents are employed. These agents, such as nitrogen mustard, possess two chloroethyl groups, each capable of forming a reactive carbonium ion. The formation of cross-links correlates closely with the lethality of alkylating agents and nitrosourea derivatives in cell culture. Alkylating agents such as nitrogen mustard and cyclophosphamide kill cells in all phases of the cell cycle, but have quantitatively greater activity against rapidly dividing cells.

Alkylating agents share a common mechanism of action, but they differ in their pharmacokinetic features, lipid solubility, chemical reactivity, metabolism, and membrane transport properties (Table 176–9). Tumors may therefore differ in their response or resistance to agents in this class. For example, nitrosoureas and *cis*-platinum may be effective against tumors resistant to cyclophosphamide. The structures of commonly used alkylating agents are shown in Figure 176–4.

Nitrogen mustard (mechlorethamine), the first alkylating agent to receive clinical trial, is used primarily for treatment of malignant lymphomas and as a topical solution for treatment of mycosis fungoides. Nitrogen mustard enters cells through an active transport mechanism shared with the physiologic amine choline. Resistance is believed to result from enhanced repair of DNA alkylation or inactivation by cellular thiols. The primary clinical toxicities of nitrogen mustard consist of myelosuppression and gastrointestinal symptoms (nausea and vomiting). Minor cholinergic side effects occur

at high doses and include lacrimation, diarrhea, and diaphoresis. The high chemical reactivity of this compound causes severe local tissue injury when infiltrated into the skin. It is used to ablate the pleural space in patients with chronic pleural effusion (0.2 to 0.4 mg per kilogram into the pleural space after draining the effusion).

Cyclophosphamide (Cytoxan) has largely replaced nitrogen mustard in clinical use. The drug requires hepatic activation in a multistep process to yield the active compound, phosphoramide mustard, and a side product, acrolein. Acrolein may be responsible for the common side effect of hemorrhagic cystitis, a complication that can be reduced by orally administered thiols. Cyclophosphamide is well absorbed orally, but is usually given by intravenous infusion. It produces only mild thrombocytopenia in comparison with leukopenia. Nausea, vomiting, and alopecia are common side effects. Attempts to prevent cystitis by vigorous hydration of patients carry the risk of inducing symptomatic hyponatremia, since in high-dose infusion regimens (doses of 50 mg per kilogram) cyclophosphamide causes inappropriate water retention owing to direct effects on the renal tubule. Hyponatremia, seizures, and death have occurred as a consequence of water retention. Other toxicities associated with cyclophosphamide treatment include suppression of humoral and delayed immunity, acute myocardial necrosis (after high-dose administration associated with bone marrow transplantation), and, after prolonged courses of treatment, acute myeloblastic leukemia and pulmonary fibrosis.

Melphalan (L-phenylalanine mustard, Alkeran) has activity similar to that of cyclophosphamide (lymphomas, breast and ovarian cancer, multiple myeloma) but does not cause hemorrhagic cystitis. The drug has variable bioavailability by the oral route; thus, the average dose of 0.1 to 0.2 mg per kilogram must be adjusted according to bone marrow tolerance. Melphalan enters cells by active transport, utilizing amino acid transport systems. After intravenous administration, the parent compound disappears from plasma with a half-life of approximately two hours. Less than 15 per cent of the drug is excreted in the urine intact.

Chlorambucil (Leukeran), a close structural congener of melphalan, is also stable in aqueous solution and is given orally. Thus, it is a convenient alkylating agent for treating chronic lymphocytic leukemia, nodular lymphomas, or multiple myeloma, which require long-term management. It has suppressive effects on both granulocytes and platelets, but few other side effects. Like cyclophosphamide and melphalan, chlorambucil therapy has been linked to late occurrences of acute myeloblastic leukemia.

Busulfan (Myleran) consists of two labile methane-sulfonate groups attached at opposite ends of a four-carbon alkyl chain. This compound is sufficiently stable for oral administration, but it rapidly forms carbonium ions leading to alkylation of DNA. It is primarily used for the treatment of chronic granulocytic leukemia, in which its myelosuppressive action provides effective, long-term regulation of the white blood cell count. Myelosuppression is not quickly reversible and may be permanent if excessive doses are used. In addition to myelosuppression, busulfan causes diffuse pulmonary fibrosis and an addisonian-like state characterized by cutaneous hyperpigmentation and weakness, but without abnormal adrenal function.

The *chloroethylnitrosoureas* form a structurally distinct group of alkylating agents. These highly lipid-soluble, chemically reactive compounds have clinical activity against the lymphomas, malignant melanoma, brain neoplasms, and gastrointestinal carcinomas. A new glycosylated nitrosourea, chlorozotocin,* has a similar spectrum of activity but less bone marrow toxicity. Chemical decomposition of these agents yields a reactive chloroethyl carbonium ion ($ClCH_2CH_2^+$) that alkylates DNA. Decomposition of nitrosoureas also yields isocyanates

TABLE 176–9. ALKYLATING AGENTS

Agent	Route (IV/PO)	Schedule	Dose (mg/m²)	Plasma t½ (hr)
Cyclophosphamide	IV	q.d. × 5	400	6–12
	PO	q.d.	50–100	
Chlorambucil	PO	q.d.	1–2	1.5
Melphalan	IV	q.d. × 5	4	1.8
	IV	q. 4 w.	8	
	PO	q.d. × 5	8	
Nitrosoureas				
BCNU	IV	q. 6 w.	150–225	RCD
CCNU	PO	q. 6 w.	100–150	RCD
Methyl CCNU	PO	q. 6 w.	150–200	RCD

RCD = rapid chemical degradation.

*Investigational drug.

of differing reactivity that may attack NH_2 groups in a carbamylation reaction and are believed to inhibit DNA repair and to alter maturation of RNA. Because of the extreme clinical reactivity of these compounds in aqueous solution, intact parent compounds (BCNU, CCNU, or methylCCNU) have not been detected in plasma, and little is known about their disposition in man. The high lipid solubility of the nitrosoureas may account for their activity against intracranial tumors, in which the chloroethyl portion of CCNU reaches concentrations 30 per cent of those found simultaneously in plasma. The primary toxicity of the nitrosoureas is delayed and cumulative myelosuppression. Nadir leukopenia and thrombocytopenia occur six to eight weeks after dosage. These compounds are strongly carcinogenic in animal test systems, and methylCCNU has been associated with acute myeloblastic leukemia in humans. Pulmonary fibrosis and renal failure are observed in patients after prolonged courses of treatment (greater than 1500 mg per square meter of BCNU or its congeners). High doses of BCNU (above 500 mg per square meter*) have been used to eradicate tumors such as malignant melanoma or lymphoma, followed by autologous bone marrow transplantation, and are associated with severe, and at times fatal, hepatic and pulmonary toxicity.

CIS-PLATINUM. *Cis* (II) platinum diamminedichloride (cis-DDP), the only heavy metal compound used as a cancer chemotherapeutic agent, has a unique mechanism of action and spectrum of biologic effects. It possesses important therapeutic activity against testicular tumors, ovarian carcinoma, bladder cancer, and head and neck cancer. The cis-dichloro structure has cytotoxic activity by virtue of its ability to form covalent bonds and cross-links with DNA. The chloride ions of the coordinate complex are readily displaced by water, generating two positively charged sites. This activated complex then interacts with a nucleophilic site on DNA, RNA, or protein to form covalent cross-links in a manner similar to alkylating reactions. The formation of cross-links continues for hours after drug exposure, and is opposed by repair processes that excise and rebuild damaged segments of DNA. It is likely that the ability to repair DNA is an important determinant of sensitivity to this drug. *cis*-Platinum causes profound cumulative nephrotoxicity due to the reactivity of the parent compound excreted in glomerular filtrate. This toxicity can be prevented by maintaining a high urine flow and a high chloride concentration in urine.

Cis-platinum is usually administered after a four- to six-hour period of hydration and diuresis with 1 liter of a sodium chloride solution. The intravenous dose administered is 40 to 75 mg per square meter and varies according to frequency of administration and individual patient tolerance. An alternative schedule is 20 mg per square meter per day for five days, a regimen that causes less nephrotoxicity and nausea. The renal toxicity of high doses of *cis*-platinum (up to 120 mg per square meter) can be prevented by chloride diuresis with 250 ml of hypertonic saline, given over a one-hour period. The clearance of total platinum from plasma proceeds rapidly during the first few hours after injection (half-time 20 to 60 minutes), but slowly thereafter, owing to covalent binding of drug to serum proteins. The drug bound to protein is inactive. Between 20 and 75 per cent of administered drug is excreted in the urine in the 24 hours after administration. The remainder is probably bound to tissues or plasma protein. *Cis*-platinum penetrates poorly into the central nervous system, the plasma-cerebrospinal fluid ratio being 21:1 or greater. There is considerable interest in the use of *cis*-platinum by intraperitoneal instillation, 90 mg per square meter in 2 liters of dialysate, for treatment of ovarian cancer.

Cis-platinum causes nephrotoxicity in 30 per cent of patients treated with 50 to 75 mg per square meter per course unless preventive pretreatment hydration is undertaken. The primary pathologic findings are coagulative necrosis of the distal

tubular epithelium and collecting ducts. In patients with platinum nephrotoxicity, changes in tubular function include magnesium wasting and the excretion of high molecular weight proteins. Hypomagnesemia, a common finding in patients treated with *cis*-platinum, is usually asymptomatic but may lead to tetany. Nausea and vomiting are distressing symptoms in patients taking *cis*-platinum and are poorly relieved by standard antiemetics. These symptoms may be lessened by giving smaller doses once daily for five days. *Cis*-platinum causes only moderate myelosuppression. Leukopenia, thrombocytopenia, and anemia may develop in patients after extended treatment or during high-dose therapy. Other toxicities include a distal, sensory neuropathy after prolonged treatment; hypersensitivity reactions such as urticaria, wheezing, and hypotension (which can be prevented in some patients by pretreatment with antihistamines and corticosteroids); and a progressive loss of high frequency hearing, particularly in older patients.

Analogues of *cis*-platinum, such as CBDCA [carboplatin], appear to cause less nephrotoxicity and ototoxicity and are undergoing clinical evaluation at this time. CBDCA causes greater myelosuppression than *cis*-platinum, perhaps because higher doses are tolerated without renal toxicity.

ANTITUMOR ANTIBIOTICS. *Bleomycin.* Bleomycin, a mixture of antibiotic peptides, is widely used for treating lymphomas, testicular cancer, and head and neck cancer. Bleomycin produces single- and double-strand breaks in DNA through a complex sequence of reactions, beginning with its binding to DNA. Ferrous ion (Fe^{2+}), which is intimately bound to bleomycin, then undergoes spontaneous oxidation to the Fe^{3+} state, liberating an electron that is accepted by oxygen to form reactive oxygen species such as the superoxide or hydroxyl radicals, which in turn attack the deoxyribose backbone of DNA, releasing free bases and leading to strand breaks.

Bleomycin kills cells preferentially during the premitotic, or G_2, phase or in the mitotic phase of the cell cycle. The possibility of increasing cell kill by exposing cells during the G_2 phase or mitosis has led to continuous infusion of bleomycin. The determinants of bleomycin sensitivity are poorly understood. There is indirect evidence that the same processes required to repair radiation damage to DNA also repair bleomycin-induced lesions.

Bleomycin is administered by subcutaneous, intramuscular, or intravenous injection with no obvious difference in clinical response rates. Following an intravenous bolus injection of 15 units per square meter, bleomycin has a biphasic plasma disappearance with half-times of 24 minutes and two to four hours. The drug is primarily excreted unchanged in the urine. Bleomycin pharmacokinetics are therefore markedly altered in patients with abnormal renal function. A half-time of 21 hours has been reported in a patient with a creatinine clearance of 11 ml per minute; a decreased dosage of bleomycin (25 to 50 per cent of normal) is indicated for patients with compromised renal function.

Bleomycin has myelosuppressive toxicity only at high doses (above 25 units per square meter*) or in patients with hypoplastic bone marrow. The most important toxicity of bleomycin is progressive interstitial pulmonary fibrosis, manifested first by cough, dyspnea, and bibasilar pulmonary infiltrates on a chest radiograph. The diffusion capacity of the lung progressively decreases with increased total doses of the drug. The decline becomes more rapid above doses of 250 units, and the incidence of significant pulmonary toxicity is 10 per cent at total doses above 450 units. Toxicity is more likely to occur in patients over 70 years of age, in patients with underlying lung disease, in patients receiving high concentrations of oxygen during anesthesia subsequent to bleomycin therapy, and in those previously treated with pulmonary irradiation. Anti-inflammatory agents such as corticosteroids have not been proved to prevent or effectively treat this

*This exceeds the manufacturer's recommended dosage.

*This exceeds the manufacturer's recommended dosage.

fibrosis. The clinical symptoms and x-ray findings of bleomycin pulmonary toxicity are difficult to distinguish from other pulmonary syndromes observed in cancer patients, such as progressive tumor, infectious processes such as *Pneumocystis carinii* or cytomegalovirus, or radiation pneumonitis. Open lung biopsy, often required to rule out these other processes, reveals an acute inflammatory infiltrate, interstitial and intraalveolar edema, pulmonary hyaline membrane formation, and interstitial fibrosis.

Bleomycin also causes cutaneous toxicity with erythema, induration, thickening, and eventual peeling of skin over the fingers, palms, and extremity joints. Many patients develop hyperpigmentation of skin creases and a general skin darkening. Raynaud's phenomenon has also been reported during bleomycin therapy. Other less frequent toxicities include acute hypertension (at doses greater than 25 units per day), hyperbilirubinemia, fever, and hypersensitivity reactions with urticaria and bronchospasm.

Anthracyclines. Daunomycin and doxorubicin (Adriamycin) belong to the anthracycline class of antibiotics produced by *Streptomyces* species. Anthracyclines have a wide spectrum of clinical activity, including breast cancer, leukemia, and sarcomas. Anthracyclines have many biologic and biochemical effects, including (1) chelation of divalent cations, especially Fe^{2+}, with production of oxygen radicals and superoxide, (2) cyclic oxidation-reduction of the quinone-hydroquinone functional group; and (3) intercalation between strands of the DNA double helix. Intercalation results in inhibition of DNA, RNA, and ultimately protein synthesis. The generation of free radicals of either the drug itself or oxygen is responsible for cytotoxicity.

The anthracyclines induce single-stranded DNA breaks. These breaks are believed to result either from drug-induced cleavage mediated by the enzyme topoisomerase II or from free radicals initiated by reduction of the anthracyclines. Tocopherol (vitamin E), a known free-radical scavenger, lessens oxygen radical generation by doxorubicin in vitro and in animals lessens the cardiac toxicity of Adriamycin without diminishing its antitumor activity. The reason for the particular susceptibility of the heart to doxorubicin action is not clear, but may be due to the lack of free-radical detoxifying enzymes, particularly glutathione peroxidase in that organ.

Assay methods for the anthracyclines have been developed but are not routinely available. The pharmacokinetics of the parent drug include half-lives of 11 minutes, 3 hours, and 25 to 28 hours. The liver is the main site of metabolism of both doxorubicin and daunorubicin. As a result, drug dosages are often modified in the face of abnormal liver function, but precise guidelines based on pharmacokinetics are not available.

Myelosuppression and mucositis are the dose-limiting acute toxicities of the anthracyclines. Alopecia is also common. Extravasation of these agents leads to severe local reaction, beginning as erythema and pain that progress over weeks to deep ulcerative lesions requiring surgical debridement and grafting.

Cardiac damage is the most serious toxicity caused by these agents. In rare instances, an acute syndrome develops hours to days after a dose of doxorubicin or daunorubicin and consists of arrhythmias or pump failure, but clinically significant acute effects are unusual (supraventricular arrhythmias, heart block, and ventricular tachycardia). A more serious toxicity is cumulative, dose-dependent cardiomyopathy, which leads to congestive heart failure in 1 to 10 per cent of the patients who receive more than 550 mg per square meter of doxorubicin or daunomycin. A progressive decrease in cardiac contractility is observed with increasing total dose and is associated with progressive pathologic changes on endocardial biopsy. Congestive heart failure may not appear until up to nine months after cessation of anthracycline therapy. There are no proven methods for preventing acute or chronic

anthracycline-induced cardiac damage. Various doxorubicin analogues, many of which have less cardiac toxicity than the parent compound in animals, are undergoing evaluation in humans. The most promising appear to be 4¹-epidoxorubicin and mitoxantrone, the latter a related anthracenedione. Both of these agents have activity in lymphomas and breast cancer.

Mitomycin. Mitomycin C is an antibiotic with clinical activity in gastrointestinal tumors, breast cancer, and ovarian cancer. Its mechanism of action is unclear, but may be the result of free radical generation or alkylation. Only when metabolically activated does the drug alkylate DNA, producing intrastrand and interstrand cross-links, inhibition of DNA synthesis, and cell death.

There is little information on the pharmacokinetics and disposition of this agent. Bolus intravenous doses of 22.5 to 45 mg per square meter* produce peak plasma levels of 0.4 µg per milliliter. Metabolic activation occurs in many tissues and may account for its rapid clearance from the plasma. The liver does not play a necessary role in metabolic activation, and dose modification is not indicated in the presence of liver disease.

The major dose-limiting toxicity of mitomycin C is myelosuppression, which is delayed in onset and cumulative with successive cycles of therapy. Leukocyte and platelet counts usually reach a nadir four to six weeks after treatment. Doses often require modification by the third course of treatment. This drug has been implicated in unusual instances of interstitial pneumonitis, nephrotoxicity, and a syndrome characterized by intravascular hemolysis and renal failure (the hemolytic-uremic syndrome). Mitomycin C may accelerate the development of anthracycline-induced cardiomyopathy.

Actinomycin D. Actinomycin D has activity in the treatment of Wilms' tumor, Ewing's sarcoma, embryonal rhabdomyosarcoma, and gestational choriocarcinoma. This antibiotic intercalates with DNA by virtue of a specific interaction between its cyclic polypeptide chains and deoxyguanosine, causing inhibition of DNA-directed RNA synthesis. Actinomycin D also causes single-stranded DNA breaks.

Actinomycin D is primarily excreted unchanged in bile and urine. Clearance of the drug from plasma is rapid initially, but a slow phase (half-time of 36 hours) of drug disappearance predominates, corresponding to slow release of drug from tissues. Human pharmacologic data are inadequate to allow rational dose modification in the face of liver or renal failure. The dose-limiting toxicity of this agent is myelosuppression, but gastrointestinal side effects are also prominent, and include abdominal pain, cramps, diarrhea, and mucositis. Actinomycin D also enhances x-irradiation toxicity to skin, the gastrointestinal tract, and other sites. A cutaneous recall reaction may occur in patients treated with actinomycin D several months after x-irradiation.

PLANT PRODUCTS. The Vinca alkaloids vincristine and vinblastine, derived from the ornamental shrub *Vinca rosea* (periwinkle), and the epipodophyllotoxins VM-26† and VP-16, derived by modification of a product of the mandrake plant, are among the few plant products with clinically useful cytotoxic activity. Resistance to these agents, as well as to the anthracyclines and actinomycin D, may develop through amplification of a drug-binding glycoprotein, the P-170 glycoprotein, a change that confers multidrug resistance to natural product agents of diverse structure. This pattern of multidrug resistance is believed to result from increased efflux of the anticancer drugs from the tumor cell.

Vinca Alkaloids. The vinca alkaloids bind to tubulin, an intracellular protein that polymerizes to form the microtubular apparatus. Microtubules are components of the mitotic spindle, but also play an important role in maintaining cell

---

*This exceeds the manufacturer's recommended dosage.
†Investigational drug that has been recommended for approval by FDA Oncologic Drug Advisory Committee.

structure and in providing channels for movement of cellular secretions and neurotransmitters. The vinca alkaloids inhibit the assembly of microtubules and cause dissolution of the mitotic spindle. Vincristine and vinblastine are given intravenously in dosages of 1.0 to 1.4 mg per square meter and 2 to 4 mg per square meter, respectively, at weekly intervals. Only minute concentrations of these alkaloids (less than 0.01 μM) are required to kill sensitive cells. Both alkaloids undergo hepatic metabolism and biliary excretion. Very little parent drug is excreted in the urine. A 50 per cent reduction in dose of either vinca alkaloid is recommended for patients with hepatic dysfunction and a serum bilirubin above 3 mg per deciliter; no dose adjustment is necessary for patients with altered renal function.

Total doses of vincristine greater than 2 mg often cause a progressive neurotoxicity, particularly in older patients and in those receiving weekly treatment. Patients experience a decrease in deep tendon reflexes, paresthesias of the fingers and lower extremities, and, at more advanced stages, cranial nerve palsies, and profound weakness of the dorsiflexors of the foot and extensors of the wrist. The sensory changes may improve with discontinuation of vincristine, but motor deficits usually show little improvement. Vincristine causes little myelosuppression. The platelet count may actually rise during treatment as a result of endoreduplication of megakaryocytes. In contrast, vinblastine is highly toxic to bone marrow, producing leukopenia and thrombocytopenia. Mucositis is also a frequent side effect, but neurotoxicity is rare. Vindesine,* another vinca alkaloid, causes both myelosuppression and moderately severe neurotoxicity. Vincristine promotes release of antidiuretic hormone and may rarely cause symptomatic dilutional hyponatremia. This syndrome is easily treated by fluid restriction.

Podophyllotoxins. Two glycosidic derivatives of podophyllotoxin, VP-16 and VM-26, have important clinical activity in the treatment of lymphomas, small-cell carcinoma of the lung, leukemia, and testicular cancer. They promote DNA strand breaks mediated by the enzyme topoisomerase II. VP-16 and VM-26 have no effect on microtubular assembly and arrest cells in G_2 rather than in mitosis. VP-16 and VM-26 are given intravenously. VP-16 has a shorter terminal half-life, less metabolic alteration, and greater renal excretion (30 per cent unchanged in urine) than VM-26. VP-16 dosage should be reduced by at least 50 per cent in patients with serum creatinine of 2 mg per deciliter or higher. Both drugs penetrate poorly into the cerebrospinal fluid despite their high lipid solubility. The primary route of elimination for VM-26 is metabolic.

Typical well-tolerated intravenous dosages of VP-16 are 45 mg per square meter per day for seven days, 86 mg per square meter per day twice weekly, and 290 mg per square meter once weekly. VM-26 is usually given in weekly dosages of 67 mg per square meter. The dose-limiting toxicity for both drugs is leukopenia. Nausea, vomiting, and neurotoxicity (paresthesias or tendon reflex depression) occasionally occur in patients receiving these drugs.

OTHER AGENTS. *Hexamethylmelamine.* Hexamethylmelamine (HMM) exhibits significant activity against ovarian cancer, breast cancer, the lymphomas, and small-cell carcinoma of the lung. The methylamines can be converted by enzymatic hydroxylation to methylol ($R-CH_2OH$) analogues, which are cytotoxic in tissue culture and may be the active alkylating form of the drug. Because of its limited aqueous solubility, HMM can be given only by the oral route. Usual dosages of 4 to 12 mg per kilogram per day are given for courses of 14 to 21 days. However, the bioavailability of HMM by this route is highly variable. The parent compound has a half-time of 4.7 to 10.2 hours in plasma. HMM produces nausea and vomiting as its dose-limiting toxicity. HMM also produces neurotoxic symptoms, such as mood alterations, hallucinations, and peripheral neuropathy. These effects gradually increase in severity during a protracted course of treatment and disappear upon drug withdrawal.

Dacarbazine (DTIC). DTIC, an imidazole-4-carboxamide derivative, was first synthesized as an inhibitor of purine biosynthesis but, in fact, functions as an alkylating agent. It is active against Hodgkin's disease, malignant melanoma, and soft tissue sarcomas. The metabolic activation of this agent by hepatic microsomes leads to production of an active methyl cation (CH_3^+), which binds to nucleic acid bases. This alkylation is believed to be responsible for the cytotoxic action of DTIC. Schedules of intravenous administration vary from 150 to 300 mg per square meter per day for five to ten days, depending on prior treatment history, concurrent therapy, and patient tolerance. There is no accurate information on its pharmacokinetics or metabolism in man. Severe nausea and vomiting occur during the first days of treatment but may be lessened by reducing the initial dose and gradually increasing the dose during the course of treatment. Mild myelosuppression may occur two to three weeks following treatment. Other toxicities include a flu-like syndrome and a possible enhancement of doxorubicin cardiac toxicity.

Procarbazine. Procarbazine has become an important agent in the treatment of Hodgkin's disease, brain tumors, and lung cancer. It undergoes metabolic activation, yielding a methyldiazonium ion ($^+CH_2-N=NH$), which becomes bound to nucleic acids, phospholipids, and protein. The pharmacokinetics of procarbazine in humans have been incompletely characterized. The parent drug disappears from plasma with a rapid half-time of seven minutes following intravenous administration. Procarbazine is usually administered orally in daily doses of 100 mg per square meter per day for 10 to 14 days.

Procarbazine may produce a number of adverse reactions. It causes moderate nausea and decreased appetite, mild to moderate leukopenia and thrombocytopenia, and, less frequently, neurotoxicity (paresthesias of the extremities, drowsiness, or depression). The mental status changes may be related to inhibition of monoamine oxidase; therefore, patients taking procarbazine should avoid foods containing tyramine, such as wine, bananas, yogurt, and ripe cheese, since these may provoke a hypertensive crisis. Other monoamine oxidase inhibitors should not be used with this drug. Procarbazine has an Antabuse-like action, which may lead to sweating, flushing, and headache upon ingestion of alcohol. It also causes hypersensitivity reactions, most prominently a maculopapular rash or pulmonary infiltrates. In addition to its cytotoxic action, procarbazine is a potent immunosuppressant, teratogen, and carcinogen. The compound is highly mutagenic in bacterial assays and produces both carcinomas and acute myelocytic leukemia in rodents and monkeys. An increased incidence of second tumors, most prominently acute leukemia, has been observed in patients receiving MOPP combination chemotherapy with irradiation for Hodgkin's disease, and procarbazine is suspected of being the responsible carcinogen in this combination. Thus, its use for non-neoplastic diseases should be carefully weighed with these late toxicities in mind.

L-*Asparaginase.* L-Asparagine is a nonessential amino acid synthesized by transfer of an amine group to L-aspartic acid. The synthetic reaction is catalyzed by the enzyme L-asparagine synthetase, which is found in many tissues but is lacking in certain human malignant diseases, particularly lymphoid tumors. In tumor cells lacking L-asparagine synthetase, the amino acid can be obtained only from the plasma pool of amino acids. The enzyme L-asparaginase, obtained from *Escherichia coli* or *Erwina carotovora*, degrades asparagine and has potent activity against childhood acute lymphocytic leukemia.

---

*Investigational drug that has been recommended for approval by FDA Oncologic Drug Advisory Committee.

Resistance to L-asparaginase arises through an increase in L-asparagine synthetase activity in tumor cells. Preparations of L-asparaginase from different bacterial strains have slightly different properties and are not cross-reactive in immunologically sensitized patients. Thus, preparations from *Erwinia* may be used in patients who are hypersensitive to the *E. coli* L-asparaginase. Most L-asparaginase preparations contain L-glutaminase activity, which is 3 to 5 per cent of the L-asparaginase activity. The usual doses are 6000 IU per square meter every other day for three to four weeks, or 1000 to 2000 IU per square meter daily for ten to twenty days.

The half-life of L-asparaginase in plasma is 14 to 22 hours, but there is considerable variation among different preparations. Plasma clearance is greatly accelerated in hypersensitive patients, and enzyme activity may disappear from plasma within four hours. The enzyme distributes primarily within the intravascular space. However, the cerebrospinal fluid concentration of asparagine falls rapidly, and an antileukemic effect is exerted in this sanctuary. The primary toxicities of L-asparaginase are related to immunologic sensitization or result from decreased protein synthesis. Positive skin tests to L-asparaginase are rarely observed in untreated persons, but anaphylaxis may occur with the first dose of drug. Allergic reactions, such as urticaria, laryngeal edema, bronchospasm, or hypotension, occur following multiple courses of the enzyme. Passive hemagglutinating antibodies are observed in patients who subsequently develop anaphylaxis, and complement-fixing antibodies are found in serum after an anaphylactic episode. Toxic effects resulting from inhibition of protein synthesis include hypoalbuminemia and decreased serum fibrinogen, prothrombin, antithrombin III, and other clotting factors, leading to either hemorrhagic or thrombotic episodes; decreased serum insulin with hyperglycemia; decreased serum lipoproteins; and, in 25 per cent of patients, cerebral dysfunction with confusion, stupor, or frank coma. Other toxicities not explained by inhibition of protein synthesis include acute pancreatitis and abnormal liver function tests (increased serum bilirubin, SGOT, and alkaline phosphatase). Approximately 65 per cent of patients receiving L-asparaginase experience nausea, vomiting, and chills as an immediate reaction, but these side effects are controlled by antiemetics, antihistamines, or corticosteroids. L-Asparaginase has no known toxicity to gastrointestinal mucosa or bone marrow and thus is easily used in combination chemotherapy. The only well-established drug interactions are its ability to terminate methotrexate action and its enhancement of ara-C cytotoxicity. Large doses of the antifolate are well tolerated if followed at 24 hours by L-asparaginase rescue because the duration of effective exposure of the bone marrow and gastrointestinal mucosa to methotrexate is limited. The combination of methotrexate and L-asparaginase may have value in the treatment of acute lymphocytic leukemia.

HORMONAL THERAPY

Steroid hormones, like the polypeptide hormones, initiate their action at the cellular level by their binding to discrete receptors. These receptors are present in tumors derived from steroid-responsive normal tissues, such as endometrium, prostate, or breast, and can be assayed in tumor homogenates by competitive binding methods. The correlations between estrogen steroid receptor content and clinical response is strong. For example, the response rate to hormonal manipulation in estrogen receptor–positive (ER⁺) patients with breast cancer is approximately 65 per cent, whereas it is less than 10 per cent in ER⁻ patients. Thus ER⁻ patients can safely be excluded from consideration for endocrine therapy on the basis of the assay. At least three factors must be kept in mind in assessing the value of the steroid receptor assay: (1) The laboratory performing the test should conform in its methods to nationally established standards. (2) Repeat evaluation of receptor status should be undertaken with each change in therapy, if possible, since receptor status may evolve with time and with intervening treatment. For example, changes from ER⁺ to ER⁻ status clearly occur in approximately 20 per cent of patients having sequential analyses of metastatic breast cancer. (3) Multiple sites should be evaluated if accessible, since biopsy results will differ in receptor content in 10 to 20 per cent of patients with metastatic breast cancer.

The general mechanism of action of steroid hormones is described in Ch. 221. In brief, this action is initiated by binding of the hormone to cytoplasmic receptor, followed by transformation of the steroid-receptor complex to an "active" form, translocation of the receptor-steroid complex to the nucleus, and binding of the complex to an acceptor site on chromatin. Nuclear binding then affects the transcription of messenger RNA coding for specific protein, such as growth-promoting or growth-inhibiting factors, leading ultimately to cell death. In experimental systems, many possible mechanisms of steroid resistance, in addition to absence of the receptor protein, have been identified involving defects in receptor binding, complex transformation and translocation, and nuclear binding. Steroid antagonists, such as the anti-estrogen tamoxifen, bind to receptor and undergo translocation but fail to initiate the transcriptional changes produced by the native steroids or elicit growth-inhibiting proteins. A list of commonly used steroid hormones and antagonists, as well as their major pharmacologic properties, is provided in Table 176–10.

Surgical or radiotherapeutic ablation of an endocrine gland presents an alternative to hormonal therapy in some cases, but has the obvious disadvantage of the ablative procedures itself, and produces in some cases undesirable hormonal deficiencies. For example, adrenalectomy for metastatic breast cancer leads to glucocorticoid and mineralocorticoid deficiency which necessitates replacement therapy. Ablative procedures currently represent first-line therapy only in prostatic cancer, male breast cancer, and premenopausal female breast cancer. As an alternative to adrenalectomy, the production of estrogenic steroids by the adrenal may be inhibited by aminoglutethimide, plus a glucocorticoid (added to suppress pituitary ACTH production).

Analogues of luteinizing hormone releasing hormone (LHRH) are capable of inducing a fall in plasma testosterone levels to castration values. These analogues are effective in producing remission in patients with prostatic cancer, and are an effective alternator to orchiectomy or estrogens.

BIOLOGIC THERAPIES

Surgery, irradiation, and cytotoxic chemotherapy are the principal methods of cancer treatment, but they have the inherent disadvantage of damaging normal tissues. As the result of advances in understanding cancer biology and immunologic defenses against cancer, attention has turned to biologic substances that modify or augment the host response. These biologic response modifiers (BRMs) offer the promise of greater specificity and fewer side effects and are depicted in Figure 176–5.

The basis for immunologic approaches to cancer treatment arises from the knowledge that both cellular and humoral defenses exist against cancer. The cellular defenses include at least three classes of naturally occurring cytotoxic lymphocytes (natural killer cells, lymphokine-activated killer [LAK] cells, and natural cytotoxic cells) that are capable of recognizing and killing tumor cells. These cells can be stimulated to proliferate, and their antitumor activity can be enhanced by administration of biologic substances such as the interferons and interleukins. In addition, humoral substances secreted by

TABLE 176–10. HORMONES AND HORMONE ANTAGONISTS IN CANCER TREATMENT

Agent	Route	Dose and Schedule	Acute Toxicity	Late Complications	Uses
Estrogen					
Diethylstilbestrol	PO	5 mg t.i.d. (breast) 1–3 mg q.d. (prostate)	Nausea, vomiting, sodium and fluid retention, uterine bleeding, hypercalcemia (in patients with bone metastases)	Feminization, risk of death from cardiovascular disease	Prostate cancer, postmenopausal breast cancer
Estrogen antagonist					
Tamoxifen	PO	10 mg b.i.d.	Hypercalcemia, nausea, thrombocytopenia (transient), mild estrogenic action, hot flashes	Retinal degeneration, cataracts in high doses (above 40 mg/day)	Breast cancer
Progestins					
Hydroxypro-gesterone	IM	1 gram b.i.w.	Fluid retention, hypercalcemia, cholestatic jaundice		Breast, endometrial, renal cancer
6-Methyl hydroxy-progesterone	IM PO	200–600 mg b.i.w. 100–200 mg q.d.			
Megestrolacetate	PO	160 mg q.d.			
Androgens					
Fluoxymesterone	PO	10–20 mg q.d.	Cholestatic jaundice (fluoxymesterone), virilization, fluid retention, ureteral obstruction (males), hypercalcemia (in patients with bone metastases)	Hepatic adenomas, hepatoma	Breast carcinoma in ER+ patients who have prior response to estrogen or anti-estrogen therapy
Glucocorticoids					
Prednisone	PO	40 mg/m² q.d.	Fluid retention, hyperglycemia, euphoric state, hypokalemia	Osteoporosis, immunosuppression, cushingoid habitus, gastrointestinal ulcers, hypertension, suppression of pituitary-adrenal axis	Lymphomas, leukemia, multiple myeloma, breast cancer
Hydrocortisone hemisuccinate	IV	200 mg/m² q.d.			
Dexamethasone	PO	2–10 mg/m² q.d. in divided doses		Same as above	Cerebral edema

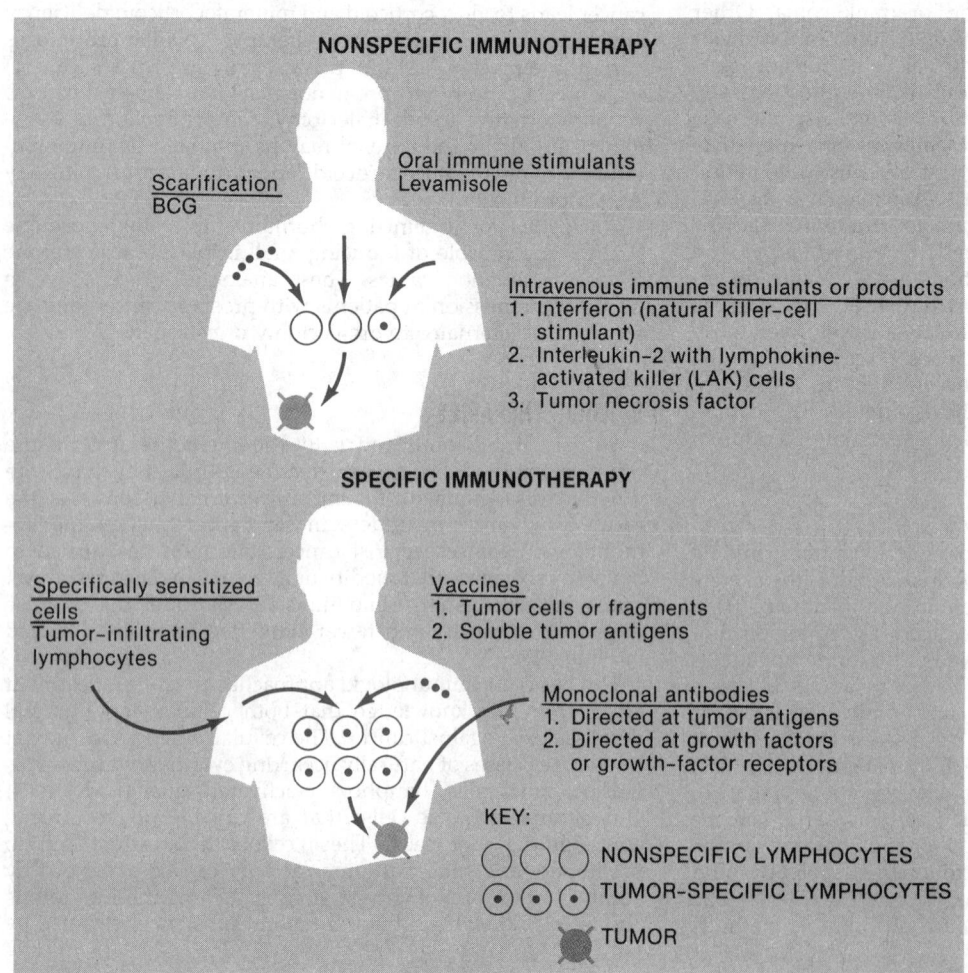

FIGURE 176–5. Concepts of tumor immunotherapy. Nonspecific therapies cause proliferation of a broad range of immune cells, some of which have inherent antitumor activity, such as natural killer cells or LAK cells. Specific immunotherapies employ products that have specificity for a particular tumor based on the tumor's surface antigens or based on its growth factor requirements. These antigens, or growth-factor requirements, may be shared by normal cells derived from the same tissue.

TABLE 176–11. PROMISING BIOLOGIC APPROACHES FOR CANCER THERAPY

Target	Role in Cancer Progression	Therapeutic Concept
Epidermal growth factor (EGF)	Stimulates cancer cell proliferation of epithelial–derived cancers	Employ monoclonal antibody to EGF receptor
Bombesin	Stimulates proliferation of small-cell carcinoma of the lung	Employ monoclonal antibody to bombesin
Laminin	Basement membrane protein to which cancer cells attach during invasion and metastasis	Prevent attachment with administration of soluble laminin fragments
Interleukin-2 (IL-2)	Stimulates proliferation of neoplastic T cells	Employ monoclonal antibody to IL-2 receptor

lymphocytes, such as the interferons and tumor necrosis factor, have direct antitumor activity. The most successful use of biologic substances has been in the treatment of hairy cell leukemia, chronic granulocytic leukemia, and non-Hodgkin's lymphoma with alfa-interferon. An early trial of LAK-cell therapy—using cells taken from the host, expanded in vitro in the presence of IL-2, and reinfused in the presence of IL-2—has produced responses in patients with renal carcinoma, malignant melanoma, and colon cancer, but this treatment is compromised by significant host toxicity related to IL-2, including marked fluid retention.

An alternative approach is to develop antibodies that recognize antigens specific for a malignant tissue, such as the anti–B-cell antibodies used to clear bone marrow cells of B cell lymphomas in bone marrow autotransplantation. While tumor-specific antigens have been identified in experimental neoplasms, such antigens have been difficult to isolate in human tumors. However, in at least one setting, a tumor-specific antigen has been used as the target for monoclonal antibody therapy in man; the idiotypic immunoglobulin found on the surface of lymphoma cells has been used as the antigen to elicit antibody specific for that tumor. While patients with lymphoma have shown consistent tumor regression with such therapy, preparation of such anti-idiotypic antibody is arduous, and most responses have been only temporary. Radiolabeled monoclonal antibodies have proven capable of localizing to tumor deposits, but in early clinical trials these antibodies have little cytotoxic effect. Attempts to arm anti-

bodies with alpha- or beta-particle emitters, or with toxins such as the ricin-A chain, are in progress.

Other, less-well-understood immunotherapies have been tested, including tumor vaccines, nonspecific immunostimulants such as BCG (bacillus Calmette-Guerin), and macrophage stimulators such as muramyl dipeptide. None has an established place in cancer therapy, with perhaps the exception of intravesicular instillation of BCG in patients with bladder carcinoma is situ.

Biologic properties of tumor, including dependence on specific factors for growth and metastasis, are also being examined as targets for biologic therapies; promising ideas are listed in Table 176–11.

CONCLUSIONS

In perhaps no other specialty of internal medicine is the physician faced with more crucial choices and a smaller margin for error than in the treatment of a patient with cancer. Because of the potency of the drugs used and the fact that vital-organ function may be compromised by the malignant process, the physician must take into account physiologic and pharmacologic factors in choosing regimens, doses, and duration of therapy. In addition, the physician must never lose sight of the reality that poorly conceived or inadequately administered treatment carries with it the certainty of a fatal outcome.

Chabner BA: The Pharmacologic Basis of Cancer Treatment. Philadelphia, W. B. Saunders Company, 1982. *A text covering both the clinical and experimental pharmacology of anticancer drugs, with particular emphasis on clinical pharmacokinetics, cell kinetics, and drug interactions.*

De Vita VT Jr, Hellman S, Rosenberg SA: Cancer: Principles and Practice of Oncology. 2nd ed. Philadelphia, J. B. Lippincott Company, 1986. *A detailed consideration of three treatment methods of cancer: surgery, irradiation, and chemotherapy.*

Goldie JH, Goldman AJ: A mathematic model for relating the drug sensitivity of tumors to their spontaneous mutation rate. Cancer Treat Rep 63:1727, 1979. *The most useful and illuminating analysis of the relationship of spontaneous mutation rate to drug resistance.*

Pinedo HM, Chabner BA: Cancer Chemotherapy. Amsterdam, Elsevier-North Holland, 1986. *A yearly update of drug research and clinical chemotherapy, with detailed and critical evaluation of important new papers.*

Rosenberg SA, Lotze MT, Muul LM, et al.: Observations on the systemic administration of autologous lymphokine—activated killer cells and recombinant interleukin-2 to patients with metastatic cancer. N Engl J Med 313:1485, 1985. *A landmark study describing the response of patients with various solid tumors to LAK cells with a recombinant growth factor, interleukin-2. This is the first positive trial of an anticancer therapy based on cell-mediated immunity.*

Tannock I: A presentation of classical cell kinetics and its application to cancer chemotherapy: A critical review. Cancer Treat Rep 62:1117, 1978. *A lucid discussion of the basic principles of cellular kinetics and their application, or lack thereof, in the design of current clinical chemotherapy regimens.*

PART XIV

METABOLIC DISEASES

177 INTRODUCTION
James B. Wyngaarden

The term *metabolism* encompasses the numerous chemical transformations that occur within living organisms. These are often divided into two large categories. Those reactions or processes that are synthetic, and in general result in a larger molecule than any of the reactants, are called *anabolic*. Such reactions are usually energy requiring. Those reactions that are degradative and involve the breakdown of large molecules into smaller products are termed *catabolic*. Such processes are essentially energy yielding. The term *intermediary metabolism* refers to all changes that take place between the moment of entry of a nutrient into the organism and the discharge of all of the chemical products into the environment. It is customary to consider separately the intermediary metabolism of carbohydrates, lipids, and proteins, although no sharp lines can be drawn among these three areas of knowledge. The term *basal metabolism* refers to energy requirements for maintenance and conduct of cellular and tissue processes under conditions in which the effects of muscular activity and the work of digestion and metabolism of foodstuffs are minimal.

Part XIV of this textbook is concerned with Metabolic Diseases. A disorder is classified as a metabolic disease when the fundamental pathogenetic mechanism involves a chemical transformation or process. Many diseases of metabolism involve specific enzyme or other protein abnormalities. When these can be attributed to an underlying genetic abnormality, they are termed *inborn errors of metabolism* (see Ch. 34). Disorders associated with specific enzyme defects have been described for more than 100 individual enzymes. Most of these are described somewhere in this textbook, but not all have been collected into Part XIV. For example, hemolytic anemias attributable to specific enzyme defects are included with the other hemolytic anemias in Part XII, Hematologic Diseases, and adrenal hyperplasia attributable to specific enzyme defects is discussed in Part XVI, Endocrine and Reproductive Diseases. The disorders included in this Part are chiefly those whose manifestations are multisystemic or in which the biochemical and genetic factors dominate the description.

PATHOGENESIS OF HEREDITARY METABOLIC DISEASES. The etiology of an inborn error of metabolism is a mutant gene. The alteration in DNA structure produces a disturbance in protein structure and function, which in turn affects cell and organ function. Hereditary metabolic diseases can be considered in terms of these three sequential levels.

Altered DNA Structure. The nature of mutations can be deduced from changes in amino acid sequences in the mutant proteins and the genetic codes (see Ch. 33). This approach has been applied most extensively in studies of variant hemoglobins and glucose-6-phosphate dehydrogenases. DNA restriction enzyme analyses and DNA sequencing techniques now permit direct analysis of alterations in DNA structure. By these methods, point mutations, deletions, and insertions are now readily identified, and hybrid proteins or prematurely terminated or aberrantly extended proteins or totally deleted proteins explained in terms of genetic mechanisms. Restriction endonucleases identify variations in gene structure as fragment-length polymorphisms. The latter approach has provided first clues to the genetic abnormality in Huntington's disease and cystic fibrosis. With the availability of DNA cloning techniques it is now possible to study directly the altered DNA sequence in many human mutations, even those that involve genes that code for quantitatively minor proteins such as enzymes. These techniques also disclose mutations in noncoding regions of DNA that affect rate of synthesis, processing, or stability of specific messenger RNAs.

Altered Protein Function. Abnormalities in the synthesis or structure of a specific enzyme protein result in absence of or reduced or (occasionally) enhanced rates of a specific enzyme-catalyzed reaction. In most genetic enzyme deficiency states, a reduced but detectable level of enzymatic activity can be measured by sensitive assays. The residual enzyme activity can frequently be attributed to a catalytically abnormal enzyme, which may exhibit decreased affinity for substrates, cofactors, or inhibitors. In the most extensively studied series of enzyme defects, those involving glucose-6-phosphate dehydrogenase, most of the enzyme deficiencies reflect unstable enzymes whose activities decay as the erythrocyte ages. This is a common mechanism of enzyme deficiency in the anucleated red blood cell, but has not been demonstrated to be an important cause of enzyme deficiency in disorders that affect primarily nucleated cells. The most interesting example of mutations leading to increased enzyme activities involves phosphoribosylpyrophosphate synthetase. Different mutations in an X-linked structural gene lead to four discrete subtypes exhibiting (1) reduced sensitivity to nucleotide regulators, (2) increased affinity for substrate, (3) increased specific activity per enzyme molecule, or (4) a combination of (1) and (3). Relatively few lesions, other than hemoglobinopathies, have been attributed to mutations in genes coding for nonenzymic proteins. One example is the ZZ variant of alpha$_1$-antitrypsin deficiency, in which an altered protein is not susceptible to normal post-translational processing (glycosylation), with the result that the defective glycoprotein cannot be secreted by the liver. In some nonenzymic proteins, a structural abnormality leads to aggregation (e.g., sickle cell hemoglobin). In others, the mutation affects the affinity of a receptor for a specific ligand (e.g., the low-density lipoprotein [LDL] receptor in familial hypercholesterolemia and the cytoplasmic androgen receptor in complete testicular feminization).

Disrupted Cell and Organ Function. Most genetic diseases first come to clinical attention because of disturbances at the level of cell and organ function. Several types of derangements occur:

1. Altered flux through metabolic pathways. This is the most frequent basis of recognition of an inborn error of metabolism. The product may be missing (albinism), or a

precursor may accumulate (mucopolysaccharidoses) or be shunted into a toxic metabolite (phenylketonuria).

2. Disordered feedback regulation of synthetic pathways. Decreased synthesis of a regulatory end-product may result in faulty control of an early step of the pathway with excessive production of intermediates. The classic example is acute intermittent porphyria, in which a deficiency of uroporphyrinogen synthetase leads to diminished production of heme, a normal feedback inhibitor of porphyrin synthesis. Decreased production of heme leads to overactivity of δ-aminolevulinic acid synthetase, overproduction of nonheme porphyrins, and acute intermittent porphyria.

3. Disordered membrane function. This is the basis for a large group of genetic diseases in which there is impairment of a specific function of a plasma membrane protein. In one type, transmembrane transport of specific small molecules is defective, apparently because a membrane carrier protein is nonfunctional. The affected substrates can be amino acids (cystinuria), carbohydrates (renal glycosuria), or ions (renal tubular acidosis). In another type, receptor-mediated endocytosis of a macromolecule is defective. In familial hypercholesterolemia a mutation in the gene that codes for a receptor results in defective uptake and degradation of LDL by body cells, resulting in accumulation of LDL and its cholesterol in plasma and arterial walls. Still another type involves a defect in a plasma membrane protein whose action is required for hormone action. In pseudohypoparathyroidism, the guanosine triphosphate (GTP)–sensitive N protein is defective, and parathyroid hormone cannot stimulate adenylate cyclase in the target cell. The latter two types of defects are inherited as dominant traits, in contrast to those that involve transmembrane transport of small molecules which behave as recessive traits.

4. Disordered intracellular compartmentation. A few examples of primary genetic defects in cell compartmentation are known. The ZZ variant of alpha₁-antitrypsin deficiency, discussed above, is one. Another is I-cell disease, in which there is a deficiency of a processing enzyme that is normally responsible for the occurrence of mannose-6-phosphate residues in lysosomal enzymes. In the absence of mannose-6-phosphate residues, enzymes do not bind to a specific receptor that directs them to the lysosome, and these enzymes pass through the cell into the plasma like a secretory protein. An additional example is a rare form of familial hypercholesterolemia in which there is an abnormal cell surface receptor that can bind LDL but cannot transport it into the cell.

5. Distorted cell or tissue architecture. The distorted shapes of erythrocytes in sickle cell diseases and in hereditary spherocytosis are examples of this type. Another example is illustrated by the immotile cilia syndrome (Kartagener's syndrome), in which a structural protein of cilia, dynein, is defective. In consequence the "dynein arms" that cross-link microtubules are missing, they cannot slide properly, and cilia cannot undulate. Still another type is exemplified by Type VI Ehlers-Danlos syndrome, in which collagen is deficient in hydroxylysine and does not cross-link normally.

ACQUIRED METABOLIC DISEASES. There are many examples of metabolic diseases that are acquired rather than hereditary. Gout exists in primary and secondary varieties. The secondary types occur because of excessive nucleic acid turnover in myeloproliferative diseases or chronic hemolytic anemias, or because of impaired renal excretion of uric acid resulting from drug effects upon the kidney or acquired renal disease. Certain varieties of porphyria can be attributed to acquired intoxications. Hyperlipoproteinurias are common accompaniments of other diseases: hypothyroidism, the nephrotic syndrome, acute and chronic alcoholism, biliary obstruction. In many conditions there is a prominent interaction between hereditary and environmental factors: obesity and diabetes mellitus, ingestion of phenylalanine-containing proteins in phenylketonuria, ingestion of milk in galactosemia. Without the environmental stress these conditions would remain silent.

Some of the diseases of metabolism are very common, such as diabetes, with a prevalence in the United States of about 2.5 per cent, and the hyperlipidemias. Others are quite rare, and a few are perhaps more properly regarded as biochemical anomalies rather than diseases—pentosuria, for example. The study of rare metabolic disorders has provided a better understanding of normal metabolic processes, and in some instances has allowed early recognition of a disorder whose manifestations are preventable simply by adjustment of diet (galactosemia, phenylketonuria). The identification of specific enzyme defects has led to attempts at replacement therapy with inklings of success following enzyme infusion (Gaucher's disease, Fabry's disease) or organ transplantation (bone marrow in immunologic deficiency states; kidney in cystinosis, Fabry's disease, Gaucher's disease).

Bondy PK, Rosenberg LE (eds.): Metabolic Control and Disease. 8th ed. Philadelphia, W. B. Saunders Company, 1980. *An excellent general text.*
Stanbury JB, Wyngaarden JB, Fredrickson DC, et al. (eds.): The Metabolic Basis of Inherited Disease. 5th ed. New York, McGraw-Hill Book Company, 1983. *An authoritative text that presents detailed discussions of various hereditary diseases of metabolism by recognized experts on each topic.*

Disorders of Carbohydrate Metabolism

178 GALACTOSEMIA
Stanton Segal

The galactosemias are toxicity syndromes exhibited by patients with an inherited inability to metabolize the sugar, galactose, which is a constituent of the disaccharide lactose found in milk and milk products. There are three disorders, each of which results from a deficiency of one of the enzymes that catalyze the normal conversion of galactose to glucose: galactokinase, galactose-1-phosphate uridyltransferase, and uridine diphosphate-4-epimerase. A defect in galactokinase is manifested primarily by cataract formation early in life. Uridyltransferase deficiency, which is the most prevalent and commonly referred to as classic galactosemia, results in a syndrome of nutritional failure, liver disease, abnormal renal tubule function, cataracts, mental retardation, and ovarian abnormalities in affected females. A deficiency of epimerase activity clinically resembles transferase deficiency, but may exist in a more benign form when the enzyme defect is limited to red blood cells. For all three disorders, the elevations of the level of galactose and its metabolites in blood, urine, and tissues can be corrected and the clinical manifestations alleviated by omission of dietary galactose.

ETIOLOGY. Galactokinase, galactose-1-phosphate uridyltransferase, and uridine diphosphate-4-epimerase deficiencies are all autosomal recessive genetic disorders. The individual human genes have been located on chromosomes 17, 9, and 1 respectively. The tissues of obligate heterozygotes contain about 50 per cent of the normal enzyme activity, while homozygotes exhibit absence of or very little activity. Immunoelectrophoretic analysis has shown that patients with transferase deficiency produce a protein similar to the normal, but with severely reduced enzyme activity or reduced stability, suggesting single amino acid substitution defects in the majority rather than deletion mutations.

PREVALENCE. Uridyltransferase deficiency has a prevalence of 1 per 40,000 births and a carrier rate of about 1 per cent in the U.S. population. A gene known as the Duarte variant is allelic to the normal transferase and codes for a protein that is electrophoretically different and enzymatically less active. The gene frequency of the Duarte variant is about 0.05 per cent, and homozyotes for the Duarte variant have about 50 per cent of normal transferase activity in their red blood cells. With widespread neonatal screening a number of babies have been detected with low red cell transferase activity who are compound heterozygotes with one gene for defective transferase and another for the Duarte variant. Such infants have only 10 to 25 per cent of red cell enzyme activity, but rarely have impaired galatose utilization that requires treatment.

Galactokinase deficiency is quite rare, having a prevalence of one in 500,000 to one in one million births. Epimerase deficiency is also rare. The benign type has mainly been described in Swiss and Japanese populations, while only a few cases of symptomatic epimerase deficiency have been detected.

PATHOGENESIS. Galactose is converted to glucose by a unique series of three enzyme reactions. The first enzyme in the pathway, galactokinase, causes galactose to react with ATP to form galactose-1-phosphate:

$$\text{Galactose} + \text{ATP} \rightarrow \text{Galactose-1-P}$$

Next, galactose-1-P reacts with UDP-glucose to form UDP-galactose in a reaction catalyzed by uridyltransferase:

$$\text{Galactose-1-P} + \text{UDP-glucose} \rightleftharpoons \text{Glucose-1-P} + \text{UDP-galactose}$$

The third enzyme, epimerase, performs the spatial change of the hydroxyl group about the fourth carbon to convert galactose to glucose:

$$\text{UDP-galactose} \rightleftharpoons \text{UDP-glucose}$$

In the presence of pyrophosphate, UDP-glucose pyrophosphorylase cleaves UDP-glucose to glucose-1-phosphate, which is converted to glucose-6-phosphate by phosphoglucomutase and then enters various other pathways of glucose metabolism. Normally this pathway functions efficiently. Galactose rapidly disappears from blood after intravenous infusion, even faster than a comparable amount of glucose. In normal individuals liver extraction of galactose results in a rise in the level of blood glucose.

In each of the three forms of galactosemia, diminished enzyme activity produces an accumulation of the substrates proximal to the metabolic block: galactose in galactokinase deficiency, galactose and galactose-1-phosphate in transferase deficiency, and galactose, galactose-1-phosphate plus UDP-galactose in epimerase deficiency. When galactose is increased, alternative pathways form large amounts of otherwise trace metabolites. In one reaction galactose is reduced to form the sugar alcohol, galactitol, while in another galactose is oxidized to galactonic acid. These metabolites accumulate in tissues and are excreted in considerable amounts in the urine.

Identification of accumulated metabolites and the elucidation of alternative pathways have provided insights into the relationship of biochemical toxicity and clinical manifestations of the disorders. In galactokinase deficiency, in which galactose and metabolites of alternative pathways are increased,

the principal clinical finding is cataracts, without multiple organ involvement. These findings implicate galactose-1-phosphate as causing the severe multisystem disease of transferase deficiency and systemic epimerase deficiency. Cataract formation appears to be due to the formation of galactitol by lens aldose reductase. Galactitol, which cannot be further metabolized, accumulates in the lens and produces osmotic changes with imbibition of fluid, lens swelling, and protein precipitation. The exact biochemical alterations in target organs affected by transferase deficiency have not been defined. There are no structural alterations of the brain associated with mental retardation in cases of transferase deficiency, but liver dysfunction is accompanied by altered architecture of liver characterized by pseudoacinar formation of hepatic cells. The ovaries of females afflicted with hypogonadism may be small, fibrotic, or streaked.

The fact that galactose-1-phosphate can be increased in red cells of transferase-deficient patients and that mental retardation and ovarian abnormalities can occur in patients with no exposure to galactose has fostered the concept that there is continuous self-intoxication in this disorder. This could occur as a result of the formation of UDP-galactose from UDP-glucose via epimerase activity and subsequent pyrophosphorolysis of UDP-galactose to liberate galactose-1-phosphate. The pyrophosphorylase plays a dual role in the process, since it is also responsible for the formation of UDP-glucose from uridine triphosphate and glucose-1-phosphate.

CLINICAL MANIFESTATIONS. Cataracts are the principal finding in patients with galactokinase deficiency, who otherwise are healthy. The cataracts are usually discovered in infants and children examined for other medical reasons. Pseudotumor cerebri has been described in some galactokinase-deficient patients as well as those with transferase deficiency. Cataracts have been observed in some heterozygous carriers, and patients under 40 years with cataracts frequently have lower than normal red cell galactokinase levels.

Uridyltransferase deficiency usually manifests itself shortly after birth or within the first few weeks of life with growth failure, vomiting, diarrhea, hepatomegaly, ascites, jaundice, hemolytic anemia, hypoglycemia, proteinuria, and a renal Fanconi syndrome. Cataracts may not be easily observed with an ophthalmoscope in young infants, but are found on slit lamp examination. Infants with this disease may die in the first few days of life from overwhelming *Escherichia coli* sepsis before other manifestations are evident. Without elimination of galactose from the diet, severely affected infants will die of inanition and liver failure. Occasionally, because of vomiting, the infant's formula will be changed to one that is galactose free, with subsequent cessation of the toxicity syndrome. Later in childhood these patients have severe mental retardation and cataracts after milk is reintroduced into the diet. Mental retardation is frequent if therapy is not initiated within the first two to three months of life. Postpubertal females have a high incidence of hypergonadotropic hypogonadism expressed as either primary or secondary amenorrhea, but the testes of male patients are normal. There is no correlation of the clinical course with ovarian function, but the frequency of hypogonadism appears to be higher where diet therapy was delayed.

Black patients with transferase deficiency may have a milder toxicity syndrome and in some cases have no symptoms. This has been called the Negro variant. Such patients have been found to metabolize some galactose because of the presence of 10 per cent of normal transferase activity in liver and intestinal mucosa. A toxicity syndrome resembling transferase deficiency occurs in cases of systemic epimerase deficiency.

DIAGNOSIS. Galactokinase deficiency should be suspected in any infant or child with cataracts and the diagnosis confirmed by assay of red blood cell or cultured fibroblast galactokinase. A presumptive diagnosis is possible by detection of reducing sugar in urine that is glucose oxidase negative (galactose) or by chromatographic analysis for galactitol in the urine. These urinary findings also obtain in transferase deficiency, whose definitive diagnosis require the assay of red cell transferase activity. Since severely affected babies may be given blood transfusions before a diagnosis of galactosemia is considered, red cell transferase assay should be delayed until transfused blood has been replaced by the infant's own cells. However, assay of transferase in parents' red cells and the findings of 50 per cent of normal activity in both may be helpful in making a presumptive diagnosis in such infants or in those who may have died before specimens for assay were obtained.

In the differential diagnosis, hereditary fructose intolerance with hepatomegaly, liver dysfunction, hypoglycemia, renal Fanconi syndrome, and nonglucose reducing substance in the urine should be considered. Lactosuria, a common finding in a variety of gastrointestinal disorders, also causes a positive test result for reducing substance. However, many laboratories use glucose oxidase-based tests for blood and urinary sugar determination, and in such instances, galactosemia and galactosuria would go undetected. The greatest confusion in differential diagnosis is the distinction between transferase deficiency and primary liver disease. Because the liver is the major organ metabolizing galactose, any disruption of hepatocellular function may result in galactosemia and galactosuria. Red cell transferase assay should be employed to make the distinction. Patients with clinical findings resembling classic transferase deficiency galactosemia who have normal red cell transferase activity should also be tested for red cell epimerase activity.

Besides the quantitative assay of red cell transferase, the performance of starch gel electrophoresis or isoelectric focusing to determine isoenzyme banding may be useful in distinguishing the carrier for classic galactosemia, the homozygous Duarte variant whose red cell enzyme activity is comparable to carriers for the classic disease, and mixed Duarte–classic galactosemia carriers who have 10 to 25 per cent of normal activity, as well as the Rennes and Chicago variants of transferase deficiency. In addition to these variants with diminished red cell activity and electrophoretic abnormalities, there are other variant forms. The Indiana variant has typical symptoms of transferase deficiency galactosemia and unstable red cell activity, while clinical disease in the Munich variant is caused by abnormal inhibition of transferase by glucose-1-phosphate, the product of the reaction.

Many cases are presently diagnosed as a result of neonatal screening. More than one half of the states in the United States and several foreign countries test all newborns by analysis of heel-stick-blood spots on filter paper. All of the procedures used will detect transferase deficiency. Some will also detect galactokinase or epimerase deficiency. All positive test results require confirmation by quantitative assay of the individual enzymes. Such screening has resulted in delineation of the benign form of epimerase deficiency in which galactose-1-phosphate appears to accumulate only in red blood cells. Subsequent studies have indicated the epimerase in such cases is unstable because of increased requirement for cofactor NAD, which can be supplied by other cells but not red blood cells.

TREATMENT. The institution of a galactose-free diet is the cornerstone of treatment. With galactose elimination, early cataracts may regress. Liver dysfunction and renal tubule abnormalities disappear, and growth and development are normal. Besides the banning of milk and all milk products, care should be taken to eliminate foods in which milk is used in cooking and baking or lactose has been added. There is no indication that the ability to metabolize galactose increases with age, so that dietary restrictions should not be relaxed in older children.

PROGNOSIS. Untreated patients with transferase deficiency may not survive. Those who do will be severely retarded mentally. The best prognosis for normal mentation occurs in those treated at birth or shortly thereafter. Those treated after three months of age have a poorer outcome. Despite excellent treatment from birth, patients with a normal IQ may not do well in school and may have diminished attention span and visual-perceptual difficulties. A significant number may have abnormal EEG patterns. The possibility exists that continuous self-intoxication with endogenous galactose-1-phosphate formation underlies the less than perfect mental outcome and ovarian atrophy in transferase deficiency, even with excellent dietary treatment.

PREVENTION. The best outcome results from the earliest dietary treatment. Heterozygote mothers of known galactosemic patients should receive a galactose-free diet to prevent any intrauterine exposure of a fetus who may be affected. Prenatal diagnosis can be performed by enzyme assay of cultured amniotic cells.

Fishler, Koch R, Donnell GN, et al.: Developmental aspects of galactosemia from infancy to childhood. Clin Pediatr 19:38, 1980. *Data describing outcome of dietary treatment of uridyltransferase-deficient patients in relation to age of diagnosis reveals normal IQ but abnormal visual-perceptual status and EEG in patients well treated before three months of age.*

Kaufman FR, Kogut MD, Donnell GN, et al.: Hypergonadotropic hypogonadism in female patients with galactosemia. N Engl J Med 304:944, 1981. *Describes amenorrhea and ovarian abnormalities in patients with uridyltransferase deficiency.*

Levy HL, Hammersen G: Newborn screening for galactosemia and other galactose metabolic defects. J Pediatr 92:871, 1978. *Details of methods and results of worldwide screening of about six million infants.*

Segal S: Disorders of galactose metabolism. In Stanbury JB, Wyngaarden JB, Fredrickson DS, et al. (eds.): The Metabolic Basis of Inherited Disease. 5th ed. New York, McGraw-Hill Book Company, 1983, pp. 167–192. *A comprehensive treatise of the enzymology and metabolism of galactose, the biochemical basis of galactose toxicity, and the clinical aspects of inherited disorders.*

179 THE GLYCOGEN STORAGE DISEASES

R. Rodney Howell

Glycogen is the principal storage form of carbohydrate in man and is found in varying concentrations in virtually all cells. Glycogen is composed exclusively of glucose molecules, and differs from starch in having a highly branched structure that greatly enhances its solubility.

In the glycogen storage diseases the tissue concentration of glycogen is most commonly elevated, but in certain of these disorders the significant abnormality is in the structure of glycogen. Although liver glycogen content reflects to some extent the nutritional status of the subject, excessive alimentation does not lead to abnormal accumulation of hepatic glycogen in the normal subject in the absence of corticosteroid treatment.

The glycogen storage diseases are of historic importance in that the first direct demonstration of a liver enzyme deficiency in man was made in glycogen storage disease by the Coris over 35 years ago.

As new specific enzyme defects were recognized, the Coris began a numbering system for the glycogen storage diseases that has been in wide use. However, we will not refer to the numbering system here; its use is to be discouraged, because the numbers beyond VI vary considerably from author to author and the existence of some of the conditions defined by recent numbers is in doubt.

Although most of the glycogen storage diseases produce fairly widespread accumulation of glycogen, in large part the diseases present clinically as either hepatic or muscular forms.

THE HEPATIC FORMS OF GLYCOGEN STORAGE DISEASE. Hepatorenal glycogen storage disease (von Gierke's disease) is the prototype of the hepatic forms of glycogen storage disease. Glucose-6-phosphatase deficiency is the basic defect. Children with this disorder have proportionately short stature with a very prominent abdomen and massive enlargement of the liver. The hepatic enlargement is due to both glycogen and lipid accumulation. Although the kidneys are enlarged because of the deposition of glycogen, this cannot be appreciated clinically except by radiographic examination. The eyes reveal multiple bilateral, symmetric, yellowish, discrete, paramacular lesions, which are specific for this form of glycogen storage disease. Xanthomas are common over the extensor surfaces of the arms and legs; bleeding may present major clinical problems.

Prominent hypoglycemia on fasting and a reduced rise in blood sugar after subcutaneous injection of epinephrine or glucagon are typical. The response to glucagon and epinephrine is rarely "flat," because the degradation of branch points of glycogen leads to glucose release even in the absence of glucose-6-phosphatase. Dramatic increases of blood lactate, pyruvate, triglycerides, cholesterol, and uric acid are usual.

After puberty the hyperuricemia with complicating clinical gouty arthritis (see Ch. 195) and the occurrence of multiple benign hepatic adenomas (and very rarely hepatic carcinoma) become the main clinical problems. Death from renal disease, possibly related to uric acid, has occurred in several adult patients.

The precise diagnosis must be routinely established by a liver biopsy and the demonstration of deficient activity of the enzyme glucose-6-phosphatase. Patients are recognized in whom no glucose-6-phosphatase activity is demonstrated on a fresh biopsy sample, but completely normal activity is demonstrated on the frozen sample. This condition represents a defect in glucose-6-phosphate translocase, a specific protein that shuttles glucose-6-phosphate across the membrane.

Other prominent forms of hepatic glycogen storage disease appear clinically similar to glucose-6-phosphatase deficiency glycogen storage disease except that they are milder. In the deficiency of the debrancher enzyme there is excessive accumulation of glycogen of abnormal structure. The stored glycogen has short outer branches. These patients generally have much milder hypoglycemia and much milder growth retardation and do not present with hyperuricemia or the severe lipid problems that are seen in glucose-6-phosphatase deficiency glycogen storage disease. Hepatic adenomas are not known to occur.

The typical patient with debrancher deficiency glycogen storage disease tends to achieve more normal height, and following puberty the liver will frequently appear normal in size. Because of the generalized nature of the enzyme defect in these patients (including liver as well as muscle), some of these patients have had significant myopathy in adulthood related to storage of abnormally structured glycogen. Muscle weakness and wasting can be the predominant findings in the older patient. The diagnosis is usually established by assaying liver, muscle, white cells, or red cells for the specific debranching enzyme. Direct liver assay is often required.

A genetic deficiency of the branching enzyme presents as liver failure in early infancy. These children display the usual hallmarks of liver failure (jaundice, ascites), usually by age two years. Muscle weakness can be prominent. A deficiency of the branching enzyme can be demonstrated in leukocytes and in fibroblasts as well as in liver tissue. The glycogen content of the liver is usually within or below normal range, but the structure demonstrates very long outer branches secondary to deficiency of the branching enzyme.

A group of patients has been recognized with very mild clinical symptoms of hypoglycemia and growth retardation but with substantial hepatomegaly. Some lack clinical symptoms. On biochemical examination they have a significant increase of normally structured liver glycogen and a deficiency of the enzyme phosphorylase. The deficiency in all instances has been partial (perhaps total deficiency would be lethal). The outlook in phosphorylase-deficient patients is good, and ordinarily no specific treatment is required.

Further study of patients with defects in the phosphorylase system has demonstrated a substantial number of males who are genetically deficient in the enzyme phosphorylase b kinase. This glycogen storage disease is different from all others (which are inherited as autosomal recessive traits), in that phosphorylase b kinase activity is inherited in an X-linked recessive manner. Females who carry this gene (heterozygotes) may have modest hepatomegaly, whereas affected males (hemizygotes) have substantial hepatomegaly without the other major symptoms of hypoglycemia or hyperlipidemia. Their response to epinephrine and glucagon is variable, but they routinely have significant plasma elevations of liver enzymes such as SGOT and SGPT. Leukocyte phosphorylase b kinase assays can usually establish the diagnosis.

Treatment of the Hepatic Forms of Glycogen Storage Disease. A variety of hormonal treatments, such as thyroxine and glucagon administration, have been ineffective in the hepatic forms of glycogen storage disease. Some patients have benefited from portacaval shunting, most specifically in restoration of growth. Because of substantial morbidity this treatment is no longer recommended.

At present, the most appropriate treatment for the symptomatic forms of hepatic glycogen storage disease is nasogastric infusion of a high carbohydrate diet. Continuous nasogastric feeding overnight with either carbohydrate alone or carbohydrate plus protein is of great benefit not only in restoring growth toward normal but also, importantly, in restoring the lipid and carbohydrate abnormalities toward normal. Oral cornstarch during the day is helpful. These treatments, currently in wide use, are safe and their clearest benefit is on growth.

The adult patient with hyperuricemia and gout is effectively treated with allopurinol and is usually not responsive to uricosuric drugs. Liver transplantation has been performed in patients with glucose-6-phosphatase, debrancher, and brancher enzyme deficiency. This treatment is likely to be of increasing importance in seriously affected persons.

THE MUSCULAR FORMS OF GLYCOGEN STORAGE DISEASE. The most dramatic of the muscular forms of the glycogen storage diseases is generalized glycogen storage disease (Pompe's disease). There is prominent deposition of glycogen in all muscular tissues and a genetic deficiency of the lysosomal enzyme alpha-1,4-glucosidase.

This condition was originally described in infants, with the typical child dying of cardiorespiratory disease in the first two years of life. In recent years, additional patients with muscular glycogen storage disease, secondary to deficiency of alpha-1, 4-glucosidase, have presented with muscular weakness in late childhood or in adulthood. Patients presenting as young adults have commonly been diagnosed as having muscular dystrophy. Respiratory failure has been the presenting symptom in certain adults. Cardiac involvement has been either minimal or absent in the older patients.

The diagnosis of this form of glycogen storage disease depends on a muscle biopsy that demonstrates an increased concentration of glycogen, which on electron microscopy is seen within the lysosome. Alpha-1,4-glucosidase deficiency is transmitted in an autosomal recessive manner. Specific enzyme analyses of leukocytes may demonstrate an absence of an acid alpha-1,4-glucosidase, but such studies are not always reliable. The presence in white cells of a neutral maltase that has considerable activity in the range of pH 4 can lead to relatively normal white cell activities for alpha-1,4-glucosidase, although the acid maltase characteristic of the lysosome is deficient. There is a consistent deficiency of alpha-1,4-glucosidase activity in cultured skin fibroblasts. Patients with myopathy appearing in late adulthood must be considered as potential candidates for alpha-1,4 glucosedase deficiency glycogen storage disease, as well as for debrancher deficiency glycogen storage disease, as mentioned above.

Muscle phosphorylase deficiency or McArdle's disease is perhaps the rarest of the glycogen storage diseases. Patients with this disorder are probably under-recognized, for their symptoms appear functional. Patients are usually asymptomatic until adolescence or early adulthood when they develop painful muscle cramps after exercise. If exercise is continued, myoglobinuria and renal failure may ensue.

These patients demonstrate absence of the increase in venous lactate that follows anaerobic exercise. The condition should be suspected in healthy, well-developed adults with painful muscle cramps after exercise who demonstrate no increase in lactate after exercise. A specific diagnosis is made on muscle biopsy, which demonstrates an increased concentration of structurally normal glycogen and a deficiency of phosphorylase activity. This condition is inherited as an autosomal recessive trait.

Patients with a genetic deficiency of muscle phosphofructokinase activity appear clinically identical to patients with an absence of muscle phosphorylase activity. The diagnosis is established in a similar fashion; they have painful muscle cramps after exercise, demonstrate no increase in venous lactate after anaerobic exercise, and show increased concentration of glycogen in the muscle, but absence of muscle phosphofructokinase activity.

Isolated patients have been reported in whom activities of phosphohexoisomerase, phosphoglucomutase, or cyclic 3',5'-AMP-dependent kinase have been deficient, but these conditions need further clarification. Reported deficiencies of UDPGlc-glycogen transferase activity probably represent defects in gluconeogenesis; the low enzyme activity is likely a reflection of the well-known instability of the enzyme when tissue glycogen content is low.

Treatment of the Muscular Glycogen Storage Diseases. Patients with deficiencies of phosphofructokinase or of phosphorylase in muscle can be benefited by avoiding strenuous exercise. There is some suggestion that isoproterenol (which increases blood flow to the muscle) may be helpful by making more glucose available for direct utilization by muscle.

At present there is no specific treatment for Pompe's disease (alpha-1,4-glucosidase deficiency glycogen storage disease). A strain of cattle in Australia affected with a condition identical to Pompe's disease in man is proving valuable as an experimental model. Bone marrow transplants have been tried; they are not likely to be effective in man.

PRENATAL DIAGNOSIS OF THE GLYCOGEN STORAGE DISEASES. Glucose-6-phosphatase deficiency glycogen storage disease cannot be diagnosed by amniocentesis because the enzyme deficient in this condition (glucose-6-phosphatase) is not present in normal cultured human fibroblasts. New techniques of molecular genetics (e.g., restriction mapping) should permit prenatal diagnosis in the near future. However, the enzyme alpha-1,4-glucosidase is active in normal cultured skin fibroblasts, and Pompe's disease can be reliably diagnosed in utero. Debrancher deficiency glycogen storage disease is difficult to establish in utero. Although the debranching enzyme is present in normal fibroblasts, widespread tissue variability of the inherited deficiency makes the prenatal diagnosis of this disorder difficult. Brancher deficiency glycogen storage disease can be diagnosed in utero.

Phosphorylase b kinase deficiency can be diagnosed in cultured human fibroblasts. The mildness of this condition, however, makes prenatal diagnosis inappropriate.

Beratis NG, LaBadie GU, Hirschhorn K: Genetic heterogeneity in acid alpha-glucosidase deficiency. Am J Hum Genet 35:21, 1983. *Study examines differences at the molecular level among the several clinical forms of acid alpha-glucosidase deficiency.*

Chen YT, Cornblath M, Sidbury JB: Cornstarch therapy in Type I glycogen storage disease. N Engl J Med 310:171, 1984. *The usefulness of oral cornstarch to maintain blood sugar concentrations is demonstrated.*

Folk CC, Greene HL: Dietary management of Type I glycogen storage disease. J Am Diet Assoc 84:293, 1984. *A detailed approach to the nutritional treatment of the hepatic glycogen storage diseases.*

Howell RR, Williams JC: The glycogen storage diseases. In Stanbury JB, Wyngaarden JB, Fredrickson DS, Goldstein JL, Brown MS et al. (eds.): The Metabolic Basis of Inherited Disease. 5th ed. New York, McGraw-Hill Book Company, 1983. *This is a thorough coverage of the clinical and biochemical aspects of the glycogen storage diseases. This article is extensively referenced.*

Narisawa K, Otomo H, Igarashi Y, et al.: Glycogen storage disease type Ib: Microsomal glucose-6-phosphatase system in two patients with different clinical findings. Pediatr Res 17:545, 1983. *This article summarizes current information about the microsomal glucose-6-phosphatase system and the glucose-6-phosphate translocase.*

Starzl TE, Iwatsuki S, Shaw BW Jr, et al.: Analysis of liver transplantation. Hepatology 4:47S, 1984. *A review of liver transplantation in genetic as well as other diseases.*

180 PENTOSURIA
(Essential Pentosuria)
R. Rodney Howell

Pentosuria is an innocuous, rather common heritable abnormality of carbohydrate metabolism that occurs almost exclusively in Jews and Lebanese. It is transmitted in an autosomal recessive fashion with an estimated prevalence of 1:2000 to 1:5000 in these populations. Affected persons excrete between 1 and 4 grams of the pentose L-xylulose in the urine daily. Loading of the glucuronic acid cycle by the oral administration of glucuronolactone will cause an increase in urinary L-xylulose excretion in the homozygote and a lesser response in the heterozygote. Red blood cells of normal persons contain two L-xylulose reductases: a major and a minor isozyme. The residual enzyme activity in red cells of pentosuric persons and the normal minor isozyme have similar Michaelis constants for L-xylulose and xylitol and also possess other similar biochemical properties. Homozygosity for the pentosuria allele results in absence of the major isozyme and in a residual isozyme that is identical to the minor isozyme of normal persons. The presence in the urine of L-xylulose, a reducing sugar, has in the past led to false diagnoses of diabetes. The sugar can easily be distinguished from others by paper or thin-layer chromatography. Glucose oxidase, which is the reagent in the commonly used dipstick type of urine test, does not react with this sugar, whereas reducing agents will.

Hiatt HH: Pentosuria. In Stanbury JB, Wyngaarden JB, Fredrickson DS (eds.): The Metabolic Basis of Inherited Disease. 4th ed. New York, McGraw-Hill Book Company, 1978, p 110. *This is a detailed review of the history and biochemistry of essential pentosuria.*

Lane AB: On the nature of L-xylulose reductase deficiency in essential pentosuria. Biochem Genet 23:61, 1985. *This reference summarizes our current understanding of the L-xylulose reductases and their deficiency in pentosuria.*

181 ESSENTIAL FRUCTOSURIA AND HEREDITARY FRUCTOSE INTOLERANCE
R. Rodney Howell

ESSENTIAL FRUCTOSURIA (FRUCTOSURIA). Fructosuria is a rare asymptomatic condition caused by a deficiency of the enzyme fructokinase. It is inherited in an autosomal recessive manner and has a recognized prevalence of 1:130,000. Fructokinase activity is normally present only in liver, kidney, and intestinal mucosa and catalyzes the first reaction in the major pathway of fructose utilization in man.

The diagnosis of fructosuria is established indirectly by a fructose loading test. Following such a load, an excessive rise in fructose concentration in the blood and the chromatographic identification of significant amounts of fructose in the urine are diagnostic. In normal persons after fructose loading the blood fructose concentration will peak at one hour and does not exceed 25 mg per deciliter, with no significant concentration of fructose in the urine. Hepatic fructokinase activity is undetectable in tissue from patients with essential fructosuria. Fructose is a reducing sugar and reacts with Clinitest tablets and other reducing agents, so confusion with diabetes must be avoided. Since fructose does not react with glucose oxidase in the urine dipstick utilized in most clinical laboratories, the confusion of this benign condition with diabetes is less of a problem now than in the past.

HEREDITARY FRUCTOSE INTOLERANCE. Hereditary fructose intolerance is a potentially life-threatening disorder and can be suspected from a detailed nutritional history. This condition is due to a structural mutation of the liver enzyme fructose-1-phosphate aldolase (aldolase B) and is transmitted in an autosomal recessive fashion. In humans there are three types of aldolases (A, B, and C) that are tetrameric molecules that may form hybrids. They differ in their tissue distribution and in their activity ratios toward their two substrates fructose-1,6-diphosphate (FDP) and fructose-1-phosphate (F1P). Aldolase B is characterized by an activity ratio of 1 and is present in large amounts in liver, renal cortex, and small intestine. Tissue from patients with hereditary fructose intolerance exhibits profound deficiency of activity against fructose-1-phosphate and modest reduction in activity against fructose-1,6-diphosphate.

Symptoms are present only after the ingestion of fructose. Immediately after fructose ingestion there is a brisk reduction in blood glucose and serum phosphorus concentrations and a marked increase in serum uric acid concentration. There is a striking deterioration of renal tubular function as manifested by the inability to acidify the urine, bicarbonaturia, aminoaciduria, and phosphaturia in the presence of a falling serum phosphorus concentration. Hypokalemia may occur. The infant who continues to ingest fructose will exhibit vomiting, failure to thrive, hypotonia, jaundice, hepatosplenomegaly, ascites, bleeding disorders, abnormal liver function test results, hypoglycemia, acidosis, proteinuria, and fructosuria. The differential diagnosis includes galactosemia and tyrosinemia, and diagnosis can be difficult.

The acidosis is due primarily to excess lactic acid and to a lesser extent to proximal renal tubular dysfunction. The fructosemia and fructosuria are secondary to the inhibition of fructokinase by its accumulated reaction product fructose-1-phosphate. The hypoglycemia following ingestion of fructose results from a defect in the phosphorolysis of glycogen to glucose-1-phosphate.

Liver biopsies show early stages of cirrhosis. The brain may show diminished neurons. In spite of the recurrent hypoglycemia in infancy, affected adults have normal intelligence.

The dose-dependent reduction of ATP and the accumulation of fructose-1-phosphate within the renal cortex have been thought to explain the Fanconi-like syndrome observed in these patients. The reduction of phosphate is, however, of greatest importance. The hyperuricemia results from the increased conversion of adenine nucleotides to urate induced by fructose and from decreased renal clearance of urate in the presence of elevated blood lactate concentrations.

In patients with hereditary fructose intolerance, clinically important chronic fructose intoxication can occur after infancy without causing symptoms of acute fructose intoxication. This is expressed as isolated, reversible retardation of somatic growth. Older affected children and adults are protected by the development of an aversion to sweets and a self-imposed fructose-free diet.

If the diagnosis of hereditary fructose intolerance is suspected the immediate elimination of fructose from the diet is recommended. The diagnosis is established by the intravenous fructose tolerance test after several weeks of fructose withdrawal; should the diagnosis still be uncertain, liver biopsy is advised for assay of aldolase and reference enzymes and for histologic study.

The treatment is the exclusion of fructose from the diet. With a fructose-free diet the patient's outlook is favorable.

Cox TM, O'Donnell MW, Camilleri M: Allelic heterogeneity in adult hereditary fructose intolerance. Detection of structural mutations in the aldolase B molecule. Mol Biol Med 1:393, 1983. *Molecular studies in aldolase B in hereditary fructose intolerance; structural defects are shown.*

Gregori C, Besmond C, Odievre M, et al.: DNA analysis in patients with hereditary fructose intolerance. Ann Hum Genet 48:291, 1984. *Molecular genetic studies in 11 patients with hereditary fructose intolerance; major deletion of the gene was not observed.*

Gitzelmann R, Steinmann B, van den Berghe G: Essential fructosuria, hereditary fructose intolerance, and fructose-1,6-diphosphate deficiency. In Stanbury JB, Wyngaarden JB, Fredrickson DS, et al. (eds.): The Metabolic Basis of Inherited Disease. 5th ed. New York, McGraw-Hill Book Company, 1983. *This review covers in detail the clinical and biochemical aspects of hereditary fructose intolerance and essential fructosuria.*

Mock DM, Perman JA, Thaler M, et al.: Chronic fructose intoxication after infancy in children with hereditary fructose intolerance. A cause of growth retardation. N Engl J Med 309:764, 1983. *Reviews and focuses on growth retardation as a feature of chronic, rather than acute, fructose intoxication.*

Morris, RC, McInnes RR, Epstein CJ, et al.: Genetic and metabolic injury of the kidney. In Brenner BM, Rector FC (eds.): The Kidney. Philadelphia, W. B. Saunders Company, 1976, pp 1214–1218. *This chapter details the mechanism of renal injury in hereditary fructose intolerance.*

Steinmann B, Gitzelmann, R: The diagnosis of hereditary fructose intolerance. Helv Paediatr Acta 36:297, 1981. *Excellent review of diagnostic tests for hereditary fructose intolerance.*

182 PRIMARY HYPEROXALURIA
Lloyd H. Smith, Jr.

Primary hyperoxaluria is a general term for two rare genetic disorders of glyoxylate metabolism productive of excessive synthesis and urinary excretion of oxalic acid. Both disorders are transmitted as autosomal recessive traits. The diseases are characterized by the onset in childhood of recurrent calcium oxalate nephrolithiasis or nephrocalcinosis, or both, usually leading to early death secondary to renal failure. In addition to the usual clinical features of uremia, severe peripheral vascular insufficiency may complicate the course of the disease. At postmortem examination calcium oxalate may be found widely deposited in extrarenal sites, a condition known as *oxalosis*. More rarely, milder forms of the disease may be found in adults. Although oxalate is an important constituent in approximately two thirds of all kidney stones, most adult patients with calcium oxalate nephrolithiasis excrete normal amounts of urinary oxalate (Ch. 90).

Primary hyperoxaluria Type I (glycolic aciduria) represents a genetic defect in the activity of peroxisomal alanine: glyoxylate aminotransferase. The resulting accumulation of glyoxylate leads to its excessive oxidation to oxalate and its reduction to glycolate, both of which are excreted in increased amounts in the urine (more than 60 mg per 1.73 square meters per 24 hours each). In *primary hyperoxaluria Type II* (L-glyceric aciduria) there is a defect in the enzyme D-glyceric dehydrogenase. Hydroxypyruvate accumulates and is reduced by lactic dehydrogenase (LDH) to L-glyceric acid, a compound that is undetectable in normal urine. The reduction of hydroxypyruvate to L-glycerate is probably coupled to the oxidation of glyoxylate to oxalate, both catalyzed by LDH. Each disease can be diagnosed by the characteristic pattern of metabolites in urine: Type I, oxalate and glycolate; Type II, oxalate and L-glycerate. Pyridoxine deficiency in laboratory animals and man also leads to hyperoxaluria and even oxalosis with a urinary pattern similar to that of the genetic disease Type I. With the onset of renal failure the clearance of oxalate is reduced (its clearance is normally about 1.2 times that of creatinine) so that its urinary excretion may return to normal. The diagnosis may then be difficult to establish because of the unreliability of currently available methods for measuring serum oxalate.

No specific methods of treatment are now available. Efforts are directed toward reducing the amount of oxalate excreted and increasing its solubility. Large amounts of pyridoxine (200 to 400 mg per 24 hours) may decrease oxalate excretion in the Type I disease. More physiologic doses of pyridoxine (2 to 10 mg) may be effective in some patients. Dilute urine should be maintained by forcing fluids, and a phosphate or magnesium oxide supplement may offer partial protection against stone formation. Renal homotransplantation has been disappointing because of rapid deposition of calcium oxalate in the transplanted kidney, but there have been some reports of success. Long-term dialysis and pyridoxine are therefore indicated when renal failure is severe. Nitroglycerin has been reported to be effective in treatment of the peripheral vascular insufficiency associated with oxalosis. A search for an inhibitor of oxalate synthesis is highly indicated.

Increased urinary excretion of oxalate and stone diathesis (in the absence of glycolic aciduria or L-glyceric aciduria) occur in many patients who have small bowel disease and malabsorption. Normally oxalate and fatty acids of the small intestine compete for available calcium ion, and calcium oxalate is poorly absorbed. This important form of acquired hyperoxaluria results from excessive absorption of dietary oxalate in the presence of significant steatorrhea. It can be controlled by a low oxalate diet.

Danpure CJ, Jennings PR, Watts RWE: Enzymological diagnosis of primary hyperoxaluria type I by measurement of hepatic alanine: Glyoxylate aminotransferase activity. Lancet 1:289, 1987. *In contrast to the previous suggestion of a carboligase defect, this new study seems to establish this disorder as a specific transaminase defect. This is more consistent with the therapeutic response to pyridoxine.*

Earnest DL: Enteric hyperoxaluria. Adv Intern Med 24:407, 1979. *An excellent general review of the clinical features, pathogenesis, and treatment of the most frequent cause of hyperoxaluria, that associated with its excessive absorption from dietary sources.*

Yendt ER, Cohanim M: Response to a physiological dose of pyridoxine in Type I primary hyperoxaluria. N Engl J Med 312:953, 1985. *This article describes varying degrees of sensitivity in the reduction in oxalate excretion during pyridoxine therapy and raises the intriguing possibility that in some patients the diagnosis may be obscured by small amounts of the vitamin.*

Disorders of Lipoprotein Metabolism

183 THE HYPERLIPOPROTEINEMIAS

John D. Brunzell

Disorders of lipoprotein metabolism are related to abnormalities in the synthesis and degradation of plasma lipoproteins. These abnormalities may result from primary inborn errors of metabolism or may be secondary to a variety of other disease states. Hyperlipidemia, the elevation of plasma cholesterol and/or triglyceride concentrations, is the hallmark of the lipoprotein disorders. Clinical delineation of these disorders is important because of the association of some with premature coronary artery disease and others with recurrent pancreatitis.

The classification of disorders of lipoprotein metabolism was first based on the varieties of xanthomas that occur and the appearance of plasma turbidity due to the accumulation of large, light-scattering lipoprotein particles in plasma. With the discovery of relatively discrete lipoprotein species, classification of these disorders was based on separation of lipoproteins by ultracentrifugation or by electrophoresis. Understanding of lipoprotein physiology has allowed classification of lipoprotein disorders according to pathophysiologic defects, with specific discrete apoprotein, enzyme, or receptor abnormalities identified in some disorders.

PHYSIOLOGY OF LIPOPROTEIN TRANSPORT
Structure and Function of Lipoproteins

The structure of the lipoprotein macromolecule is well suited for the solubilization of lipids in plasma. The nonpolar lipids—cholesteryl ester and triglyceride—are present in the lipoprotein core surrounded by a monolayer composed of specific proteins and the polar lipids, unesterified cholesterol and phospholipid. This monolayer allows the lipoprotein to remain miscible in plasma.

The lipoproteins function as an efficient vehicle for site-to-site transport of triglyceride and cholesterol of both exogenous and endogenous origin. Although caloric need is fairly constant throughout the day, food is ingested only periodically. The excess calories that enter the circulation with each meal are transported mainly as triglyceride to be stored in adipose tissue for future utilization between meals as free fatty acids. Ingested and synthesized cholesterol also needs to be transported to extrahepatic tissues to serve as a source of membrane cholesterol and as substrate for steroid hormone synthesis. The transport of triglyceride and cholesterol is accomplished by a spectrum of lipoproteins that have been classified by arbitrary operational boundaries according to either their density by ultracentrifugation or mobility by electrophoresis (Fig. 183–1). Fortunately the lipoproteins, as separated by ultracentrifugation or electrophoresis, are so similar that the synonyms based on each of these methods of separation are essentially interchangeable.

The triglyceride-rich lipoproteins can enter the plasma as chylomicrons derived from dietary fat adsorbed from the gut or endogenously as triglyceride-rich very low density lipoprotein (VLDL) synthesized from glucose or circulating free fatty acids in the liver. After removal of some of their triglycerides and surface components, the remaining lipoprotein remnant of the chylomicron is taken up by the liver and degraded. The remnant of endogenous triglyceride-rich lipoprotein probably also requires the liver for further processing. In contrast to the chylomicron, however, only some components of VLDL are removed, resulting in formation of the low-density cholesterol-rich lipoprotein.

This is likely to be an oversimplification, as there is a continuous spectrum of particles, and lipoproteins enter and exit at many sites along this spectrum of varying lipoprotein sizes. High-density lipoproteins interact with this system for transport of triglyceride and cholesteryl ester, as will be noted later.

Both the physiology and the pathophysiology of lipoproteins can be evaluated by examining the sites of lipoprotein production and the multiple steps in lipoprotein catabolism. Most pathophysiologic abnormalities leading to hyperlipi-

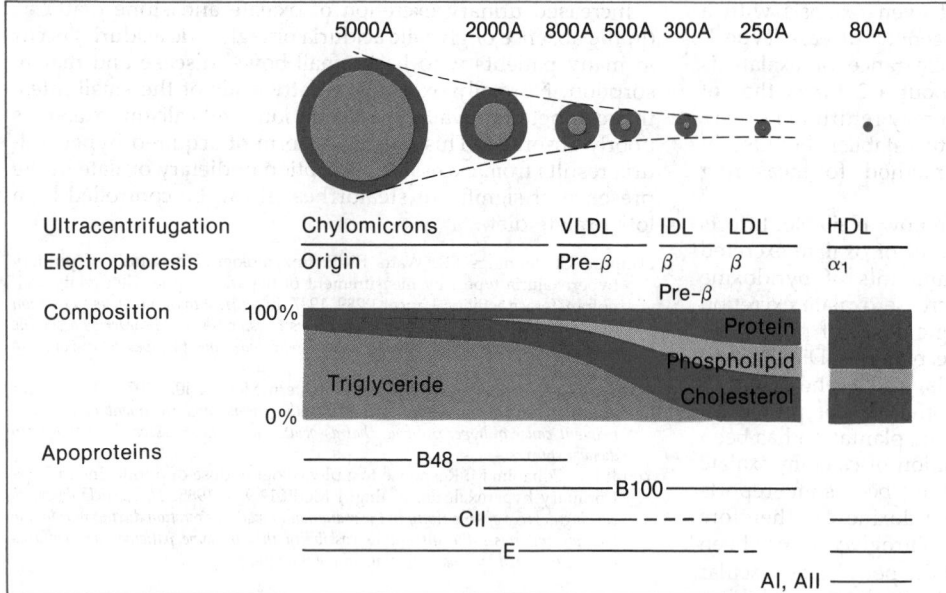

FIGURE 183–1. Classification of plasma lipoproteins by physical and chemical properties. (Modified from Bierman EL: Current Concepts: Hyperlipoproteinemia. The Upjohn Company, 1984.)

demic states can be understood by examining four sites of regulation of plasma lipoprotein transport: (1) triglyceride-rich lipoprotein input, (2) lipoprotein lipase–mediated triglyceride catabolism, (3) remnant catabolism, and (4) cholesterol-rich lipoprotein catabolism (Fig. 183–2).

Production of Triglyceride-Rich Lipoproteins

After hydrolysis of dietary triglycerides in the small intestine, the resulting fatty acids and monoglycerides are taken up by the absorptive cells of the small intestine and incorporated into large triglyceride-rich lipoproteins with a specific

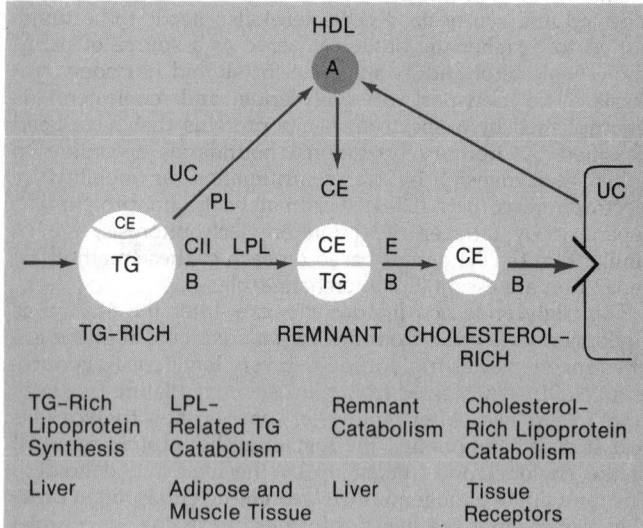

FIGURE 183–2. The triglyceride-rich lipoprotein (VLDL) is synthesized in the liver and contains apo-B, which remains with the particle through its subsequent catabolism. The triglyceride-rich lipoprotein core contains triglyceride (TG) and cholesteryl ester (CE) and surface unesterified cholesterol (UC) and phospholipid (PL). Upon entering plasma, acquired apo CII activates lipoprotein lipase (LPL) to catabolize TG core. The resulting remnant acquires apo-E, which interacts with hepatic receptors to catabolize remnant to cholesterol-rich low density lipoprotein (LDL). The LDL binds to high-affinity receptor, with subsequent intracellular degradation of the lipoprotein. High density lipoproteins with apoproteins AI and AII (A) acquire surface components of lipoproteins and plasma membranes of cells and form cholesteryl esters. These cholesteryl esters exchange with other lipoproteins or are delivered directly to the liver and may be the primary source of biliary cholesterol and bile acids.

form of apoprotein B (apo B-48), phospholipid, and a small amount of cholesterol. These chylomicrons are secreted from the absorptive cells into the lymphatics and subsequently enter the plasma via the thoracic duct. Chylomicron secretion and transport represent a system of high-capacity energy transport, allowing calories ingested at one time, over and above immediate needs, to be transferred to sites of storage for use between meals. The chylomicron remnant taken up and degraded by the liver suppresses synthesis of components of endogenous triglyceride-rich lipoproteins.

Input into plasma of triglyceride-rich lipoproteins also occurs from endogenous sources. During meals, plasma free fatty acids enter the liver, where they may be esterified with glycerol to form triglyceride. Between meals, free fatty acids are mobilized from adipose tissue triglyceride stores. These serve as a potential source for hepatic triglyceride synthesis. Lipogenesis, synthesis of fatty acids de novo from carbohydrate, also occurs in the liver. Fatty acids in the cytosol of the hepatocyte can either enter mitochondria, where oxidation occurs, or can remain in the cytosol, where they are esterified to form triglyceride. These processes appear to be regulated by changes in insulin and glucagon levels that occur with feeding: glucagon enhances and insulin prevents mitochondrial fatty acid uptake by regulating long-chain acyl carnitine transferase. Insulin also induces lipogenic enzymes in the hepatocytes that regulate the synthesis of fatty acids.

Triglyceride synthesized in the liver, together with cholesteryl ester, is combined with the lipoprotein monolayer composed of phospholipid, unesterified cholesterol, and apoprotein B, and secreted into the hepatic venous outflow as triglyceride-rich VLDL. Hepatic apoprotein B (apo B-100) in VLDL has a larger molecular weight than intestinal apoprotein B (apo B-48) found in chylomicrons.

In normal individuals, the majority of triglyceride input into the plasma is of dietary origin. While the average American diet contains about 100 grams of triglyceride per day, less than 30 grams of triglyceride are secreted endogenously.

Lipoprotein Lipase-Mediated Triglyceride Catabolism

The triglyceride that enters the plasma in chylomicrons and endogenously synthesized triglyceride-rich lipoproteins is transported to adipose tissue for storage or to muscle for utilization. The enzyme in adipose tissue and muscle that catalyzes this triglyceride uptake is lipoprotein lipase. In adipose tissue the enzyme is synthesized in the fat cell, and following secretion and transport to the capillary endothelial cell, hydrolyzes the triglyceride in these lipoproteins at the endothelial surface. At least two of the three fatty acids potentially releasable from triglyceride hydrolysis are then transported to the fat cell where they are re-esterified with glycerol and stored as intracellular adipocyte triglyceride. The vast majority of the triglyceride in the adipocyte enters by this mechanism; little lipogenesis de novo from glucose occurs in adipose tissue in humans. The functional activity of lipoprotein lipase in adipose tissue is increased during and after meals. In humans, most of this increase in function is due to the increase in triglyceride-rich lipoproteins that serve as enzyme substrate. Although insulin is required to maintain lipoprotein lipase levels in adipose tissue, little change in enzyme levels occurs with normal meals. Between meals, calories stored as triglyceride are released from the adipocyte as free fatty acids. This hydrolysis of intracellular adipocyte triglyceride is mediated by "hormone-sensitive" lipase of the fat cells. Between meals, when insulin levels are low and glucagon is increasing, hormone-sensitive lipase activity increases, and free fatty acids are released to be used for energy utilization by most tissues of the body.

The interaction of lipoprotein lipase with triglyceride in triglyceride-rich lipoproteins requires a cofactor, apoprotein CII. When secreted from the absorptive cell of the gut and from the liver, chylomicrons and VLDL do not contain this activator. Shortly after entering plasma these lipoproteins pick up apoprotein CII from a reservoir in circulating high-density lipoprotein (HDL). Thus the triglyceride-rich lipoproteins contain both substrate and activator for their hydrolysis by lipoprotein lipase. Following hydrolysis of the triglyceride in these lipoproteins, the apoprotein CII is released and again picked up by HDL. Thus, HDL appears to serve as a shuttle for apoprotein CII (as well as other lipoprotein components) (see below). Other apoproteins (CI and CIII) are transferred bidirectionally between triglyceride-rich lipoproteins and HDL and may play a role in lipoprotein lipase triglyceride hydrolysis, as well as other lipoprotein interactions.

Remnant Lipoprotein Catabolism

Following hydrolysis of the triglyceride in triglyceride-rich lipoproteins and the simultaneous removal of surface components, "remnant" lipoproteins are formed from chylomicrons and endogenous triglyceride-rich lipoproteins. The intermediate-density lipoprotein fraction isolated by ultracentrifugation consists largely of remnant particles of VLDL. Those remnants formed from chylomicrons and large endogenous VLDL often distribute, however, in the density range

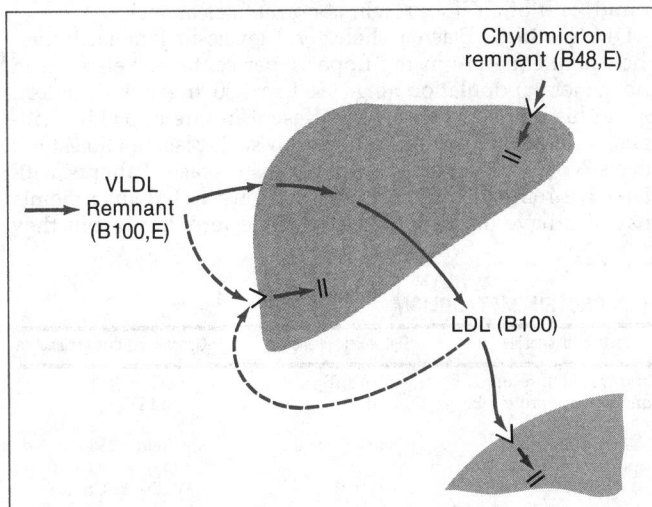

FIGURE 183–3. The liver is involved in the conversion of VLDL remnants containing apo B-100 and apo E to LDL, which are terminally catabolized via the LDL receptor in peripheral or hepatic tissue. The chylomicron remnant containing apo B-48 and apo E is processed completely in the liver via the apo E or chylomicron receptor.

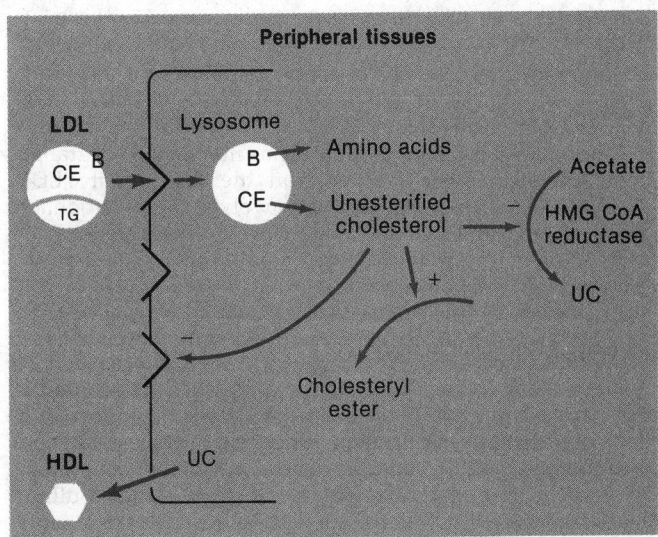

FIGURE 183–4. LDL containing apo B are removed from plasma by a high-affinity receptor and are processed in the lysosome. The resulting unesterified cholesterol regulates the cellular homeostatic mechanisms.

of small VLDL. Thus, remnants and endogenously synthesized triglyceride-rich lipoproteins cannot be separated completely by ultracentrifugation. Once formed, the remnant has a short half-life in plasma and appears to be taken up by the liver (Fig. 183–3). The endogenous triglyceride-rich lipoprotein remnant is further processed into the cholesterol-rich low-density lipoprotein (LDL). During this catabolic process, further triglyceride and cholesterol as well as some surface proteins are removed. The remnant lipoprotein contains apoprotein B, and several forms of apoprotein C and apoprotein E. The apoprotein E that accumulates as the remnant lipoproteins are formed appears to be important for hepatic uptake of those remnants. There is a complex interaction of hepatic receptors specific for apoprotein E and other receptors that bind both apoprotein B and apoprotein E, with the apoproteins in the remnant lipoproteins regulating their hepatic uptake. By the time the cholesterol-rich LDL has been formed, apoprotein B is the only apoprotein of the triglyceride-rich lipoproteins remaining.

Cholesterol-Rich Low-Density Lipoprotein Catabolism

As the cholesterol-rich LDL normally arises from the remnant lipoprotein of VLDL, it contains the same amount of apoprotein B per lipoprotein particle as endogenous triglyceride-rich VLDL, while other apoproteins have been almost entirely removed, together with much of the phospholipid and some cholesterol. The cholesterol-rich lipoprotein can be removed from plasma by extrahepatic tissues where it functions as the chief source of cholesterol for membrane synthesis or steroid hormone synthesis by these tissues. Alternatively the lipoprotein may be taken up by the liver and degraded if not utilized peripherally. Apoprotein B in the cholesterol-rich lipoprotein appears to be recognized by a specific, high-affinity binding site in tissues (Fig. 183–4). Once bound, the lipoprotein is internalized by the cell in an endocytotic vesicle that fuses with a primary or pre-existing secondary lysosome. The protein moiety is degraded and the cholesteryl ester hydrolyzed to unesterified cholesterol by a lysosomal acid cholesteryl ester hydrolase. Hydrolysis of the triglyceride and phospholipid may also occur in the lysosome. The cell is able to regulate its own cholesterol content through a feedback control system in which intracellular free cholesterol suppresses endogenous cholesterol production by inhibiting the rate-limiting enzyme in cholesterol synthesis (HMG-CoA reductase). Furthermore, accumulation of intracellular free cholesterol limits the further uptake of cholesterol-rich lipoproteins by inhibiting synthesis of the lipoprotein receptor itself and stimulates its own re-esterification to cholesteryl ester by activating an acyl CoA:cholesterol transferase in the cytosol. Cholesterol content in the cell is regulated by a receptor-mediated system involving HDL as a vehicle for cholesterol.

Apoprotein B containing lipoproteins may also be degraded by a scavenger system other than the high-affinity LDL receptor. This scavenger pathway involves the macrophage system and assumes greater importance in lipoprotein catabolism when defects in the LDL receptor or other abnormalities in lipoprotein catabolism exist.

Lipoprotein Surface Catabolism

Newly synthesized lipoproteins with their hydrophobic triglyceride and cholesteryl ester core are surrounded by a monolayer composed of protein, unesterified cholesterol, and phospholipid. As the core is removed and the lipoprotein decreases in size, several mechanisms process the resulting "excess" surface. The catabolism of these surface components involves HDL and the enzyme lecithin-cholesterol-acyl-transferase (LCAT). HDL synthesized by the liver and the intestine, is composed of phospholipid and two major structural apoproteins, apoprotein AI and apoprotein AII. This HDL serves as an acceptor for the phospholipid (mainly lecithin) and unesterified cholesterol from the triglyceride-rich lipoprotein surface. LCAT associated with HDL then removes a fatty acid from lecithin and transfers it to cholesterol, producing cholesteryl ester and lysolecithin. The cholesteryl ester is transferred from HDL to the liver directly or after transfer to other lipoproteins via lipid transfer protein, making the HDL apoproteins available to shuttle more lipoprotein surface components. HDL, LCAT, and transfer proteins may also play a role in the regulation of intracellular cholesterol content by enhancing the efflux of free cholesterol from extrahepatic tissues. Thus, HDL may play a role in the transport of cholesterol from cells to liver where it is ultimately excreted. In addition, HDL serves as the shuttle for apoprotein CII and apoprotein E to and from triglyceride-rich lipoproteins as part of their catabolism.

Cholesterol Excretion

Cholesterol and phospholipids are excreted as such in the bile, or after conversion of cholesterol into bile acid. A large proportion of the secreted bile acids is reabsorbed in the enterohepatic circulation and recycled. However, a net loss of bile acid, cholesterol, and phospholipid in the stool occurs by this pathway.

The definitive source of the cholesterol for output in the bile and for bile acid formation has not been determined. Cholesterol excreted into the bile may be synthesized directly in the liver. Alternatively, cholesterol may be secreted from the liver and gut in triglyceride-rich lipoproteins and may be esterified by the LCAT-HDL system, and may reenter the liver directly with HDL or via remnant lipoproteins.

INBORN ERRORS OF LIPOPROTEIN METABOLISM

The primary, or inborn, errors of lipoprotein metabolism leading to hyperlipidemia generally can be grouped into disorders associated with overproduction of triglyceride-rich lipoproteins or disorders due to defects in one of three catabolic steps in lipoprotein degradation (see Fig. 183–2). Much more is known about defects in lipoprotein catabolism than about defects leading to lipoprotein overproduction (Table 183–1).

Defective Low-Density Lipoprotein Catabolism: Familial Hypercholesterolemia

DEFINITION. Familial hypercholesterolemia is an autosomal dominant trait with defective receptors for plasma LDL. An increase in LDL cholesterol is associated with characteristic xanthomas in the Achilles tendons, the patellar tendons, the extensor tendons of the hands, and with early coronary artery disease.

ETIOLOGY AND PATHOGENESIS. This disorder in LDL catabolism is caused by one of several alleles producing an abnormal LDL receptor. One of these alleles is associated with absence of LDL receptor synthesis and the others with the production of receptors of abnormal composition. These nonfunctional receptors are associated with decreased LDL catabolism and, in the heterozygote, with an approximate twofold increase in LDL levels. In the very rare homozygote, no receptor degradation occurs, and LDL is removed by a lower-affinity "scavenger" pathway with a sixfold or greater increase of cholesterol-rich lipoproteins in plasma.

CLINICAL MANIFESTATIONS. This disorder often manifests as coronary artery disease in a young male, who then is noted to have elevated cholesterol levels. The mean age of the first myocardial infarction in males with familial hypercholesterolemia who develop atherosclerosis is about 41 years. Affected women without additional risk factors often go through life without clinical manifestations of atherosclerosis. Low HDL cholesterol levels and cigarette smoking have marked effects on accelerating coronary artery disease and may be the major determinants of clinical disease in females. Peripheral vascular disease and cerebrovascular disease do not seem to be increased as much as coronary artery disease in this disorder. Lipid deposits in tendons are pathognomonic for this disorder. These xanthomas, usually bilateral, may be nodular irregularities in the Achilles tendons or extensor tendons of the hands, but can extend to diffuse, generalized thickening. Corneal arcus and xanthalasma may occur but are found with other lipoprotein abnormalities as well.

DIAGNOSIS. Plasma cholesterol levels in familial hypercholesterolemia are in the upper 1 per cent of levels seen in the general population (e.g., 300 to 500 mg per deciliter). Since this disease seems to be present in one in 500 individuals, at least one person in five with such plasma cholesterol levels would be expected to have this disease. Patients with defective remnant removal and those with chylomicronemia may also have markedly elevated cholesterol levels, but they

TABLE 183–1. INBORN ERRORS OF LIPOPROTEIN METABOLISM

Name	Prevalence	Physiologic Abnormality	Protein Abnormality	Lipoprotein Phenotype	Lipoproteins that Accumulate
Familial hypercholesterolemia	1/500	↓ LDL catabolism	Abnormal LDL receptor	IIA (IIB)	LDL ± VLDL
Familial dysbetalipoproteinemia	1/10,000	↓ Remnant catabolism	Abnormal apoprotein E	III	β VLDL
Lipoprotein lipase or Apo CII deficiency	Very Rare	↓ TG catabolism	Absence of LPL or apoprotein CII	I (V)	Chylo ± VLDL
Familial hypertriglyceridemia	? 1/200	↑ VLDL-TG and bile acid synthesis	?	IV (V)	VLDL ± Chylo
Familial combined hyperlipidemia	? 1/100	↑ Apoprotein B synthesis	? Apoprotein B	IIA, IIB, IV	LDL and/or VLDL

Phenotypes based on World Health Organization recommendations.
Chylo = chylomicron.

can be distinguished by the degree of coincident hypertriglyceridemia. Hypothyroidism and the nephrotic syndrome are also associated with elevated cholesterol levels. The increase in LDL in familial hypercholesterolemia uniquely is persistent, is almost always present in a parent, and is detectable at birth. The coexistence of tendon xanthomas and hypercholesterolemia is diagnostic of this disorder. Unilateral Achilles tendon thickening may be the result of injury.

TREATMENT. Discontinuation of smoking should be the first consideration for those who smoke. A low saturated fat, low cholesterol diet should be initiated in all affected individuals with this disorder, even though only a 5 to 15 per cent reduction in LDL levels occurs. Normalization of LDL levels occurs with the combination of a bile acid-binding resin (15 to 30 grams per day in divided doses with meals) and very high dose nicotinic acid with meals and at bedtime (2 to 7.5 grams per day). Compliance with each drug regimen has been poor. Fat-soluble vitamins should be given at bedtime, since the resins (colestipol or cholestyramine) prevent their absorption. Some recommend therapy with nicotinic acid and resins for all affected individuals. More conservatively, treatment can be restricted to postadolescent males and women with additional risk factors for coronary artery disease. Drugs that suppress hepatic HMG-CoA reductase and hepatic cholesterol synthesis may be available soon and should simplify the treatment of this disorder.

Remnant Removal Disease: Dysbetalipoproteinemia

DEFINITION. This disorder is due to the interaction between (1) an autosomal recessive defect in apoprotein E with abnormal remnant catabolism and (2) independent overproduction of triglyceride-rich lipoproteins. This results in the accumulation of postlipoprotein lipase remnants from both chylomicrons and endogenously synthesized VLDL that cause xanthomas and coronary artery and peripheral vascular disease.

ETIOLOGY AND PATHOGENESIS. About 1 per cent of individuals have two genes leading to an abnormal apoprotein E. Multiple alleles exist for apoprotein E; those producing amino acid substitutions in a critical region of the apoprotein have abnormal apoprotein E binding to hepatic membranes. Affected individuals either have two identical abnormal genes or are compound heterozygotes with two different abnormal genes. Most of these individuals do not have hyperlipidemia but rather have low plasma cholesterol and LDL levels, presumably because of defective conversion of VLDL remnants to LDL. VLDL remnants that are cholesteryl ester enriched are present, but plasma triglyceride levels are usually normal. About one in 100 individuals with this abnormal apoprotein E has hyperlipidemia with remnant removal disease. These individuals appear to have an independent abnormality leading to hypertriglyceridemia in addition to the defect in apoprotein E, and accumulate significant levels of chylomicron and VLDL remnants. Much rarer forms of remnant removal disease are caused by total absence of apoprotein E or an absence of postheparin plasma hepatic triglyceride lipase.

CLINICAL MANIFESTATIONS. This disorder may present initially as premature clinical atherosclerosis or as planar or tuberous xanthomas, or it may be detected as hyperlipidemia on routine laboratory screen. This disorder is usually not manifested as an abnormality in triglyceride or cholesterol levels in men until the third or fourth decade or in women until after menopause. The coexistent apoprotein E abnormality can be detected at birth. The onset of the xanthomas also is late. Planar xanthomas of the palmar crease and tuberous or tuberoeruptive xanthomas are highly suggestive of this disorder, although both can occur in severe, chronic obstructive liver disease with residual hepatocellular function. Atherosclerosis often is first noted in men around age 50 years. Peripheral vascular disease often predominates, but coronary artery disease is increased as well. In females, development of peripheral vascular and coronary artery disease after menopause is rapid as compared with nonaffected females. The presence of estrogen in the premenopausal state seems to minimize the defect in remnant catabolism.

DIAGNOSIS. The presence of palmar or tuberous xanthomas in the absence of liver disease is diagnostic. Plasma cholesterol and triglyceride are increased to similar levels. A method for separation of VLDL from the remainder of the more dense lipoproteins is necessary to demonstrate that these VLDL are cholesteryl ester enriched and have beta mobility on electrophoresis ("beta VLDL") rather than the typical pre-beta mobility of VLDL. An abnormal apoprotein E can usually be demonstrated by isoelectric focusing. The concentration of LDL is typically low, and HDL is often normal or slightly depressed. Hypothyroidism can aggravate this disorder or rarely can lead to remnant accumulation by itself.

TREATMENT. In obese individuals with this disorder, weight loss should be considered in lowering triglyceride and cholesterol levels. In postmenopausal females, low-dose ethinyl estradiol seems to normalize the defect in remnant removal and to correct the hypercholesterolemia. Clofibrate (1 gram twice a day) or gemfibrozil (0.6 gram twice a day) also is effective in decreasing lipid levels. Alternatively, high-dose nicotinic acid is considered by some investigators as the drug of choice for treatment of this disorder. There is evidence that the form of atherosclerosis occurring with this disorder may be partially reversible with treatment.

Defective Lipoprotein Lipase–Related Triglyceride Catabolism

DEFINITION. Familial lipoprotein lipase (LPL) deficiency is a rare autosomal recessive trait characterized by complete absence of active enzyme protein in all tissues leading to massive hypertriglyceridemia from birth and recurrent episodes of pancreatitis. Similar syndromes also are caused by inborn defects in other aspects of the LPL system.

ETIOLOGY AND PATHOGENESIS. Hydrolysis of triglyceride from chylomicrons and endogenous VLDL in vivo requires both lipoprotein lipase and its activator apo CII. A defect of either of these proteins is associated with severely decreased triglyceride removal and massive hypertriglyceridemia. In infants and young children the triglyceride accumulates primarily as chylomicron triglyceride of dietary origin. As the patient gets older, a defect in VLDL triglyceride removal becomes more apparent as well. Both LPL and apoprotein CII deficiency are autosomal recessive disorders; often consanguinity can be documented. Individuals also exist who have LPL activity missing from only selected tissues or have a familial inhibitor of LPL activity. These latter groups usually have less severe hypertriglyceridemia and become symptomatic later in life than in the classic form of LPL deficiency.

CLINICAL MANIFESTATIONS. Infants with LPL deficiency rapidly manifest intolerance to fatty foods. As these children grow, they learn to avoid certain high fat foods such as whole milk. Abdominal pain, often with pancreatitis, occurs in association with the high levels of chylomicron triglyceride. Eruptive xanthomas occur on extensor surfaces, notably the elbows, knees, and the buttocks, and are pathognomonic for chronic chylomicronemia. Hepatomegaly and occasionally splenomegaly occur because of the accumulation of lipid-laden foam cells. The hepatosplenomegaly rapidly diminishes on a fat-free diet, which clears the chylomicronemia. Eruptive xanthomas also disappear with time after lowering of chylomicron levels. Other signs and symptoms seen with chronic chylomicronemia may also occur (see below).

DIAGNOSIS. A young child with abdominal pain and milky, lactescent plasma should be studied for a genetic abnormality in LPL. Other causes of chylomicronemia before adulthood relate to the occurrence of a common form of hypertriglyceridemia with diabetes or glucocorticoid therapy. Absent or diminished activity of lipoprotein lipase can be demonstrated in adipose tissue or muscle tissue, or in plasma after intravenous heparin. Apoprotein CII deficiency can be detected by radioimmunoassay or by gel electrophoresis of the protein components of lipoproteins.

TREATMENT. In all the inborn errors of the LPL-related triglyceride removal system associated with chylomicronemia, a decrease in total dietary fat is absolutely indicated. A total of polyunsaturated and saturated fat as low as 10 to 20 per cent of calories is often required. Medium-chain triglycerides can be used to prepare some foods, since their fatty acids leave the gut unesterified via the portal vein rather than via the thoracic duct as chylomicron triglyceride. The goal is to decrease the amount of dietary fat to a level low enough to eliminate the occurrence of abdominal pain. These individuals can also be sensitive to agents that raise endogenous VLDL levels, such as alcohol or glucocorticoids, and to the effects of pregnancy.

Other Genetic Disorders with Mild to Moderate Hypertriglyceridemia

A number of less well characterized disorders associated with persistent or intermittent elevated VLDL levels exist. Some may be associated with increased hepatic secretion of VLDL, others with defective VLDL catabolism. It has been useful to classify those conditions into several relatively homogenous groups on the basis of the existence of large, well-characterized families for each.

FAMILIAL HYPERTRIGLYCERIDEMIA. This apparently autosomal dominant trait may be quite common. Individuals with familial hypertriglyceridemia appear to have a defect leading to enhanced hepatic triglyceride synthesis with subsequent secretion of triglyceride-enriched, large VLDL. These individuals may also have increased cholesterol and cholic acid synthesis. LPL-related triglyceride removal and remnant lipoprotein catabolism appear to be normal. LDL levels are normal, while HDL is triglyceride-enriched with depletion of HDL cholesterol.

Most individuals with this disorder do not have an increased predisposition for coronary artery disease, remain asymptomatic, and are detected by routine lipid screen. Occasionally with the onset of another disorder associated with elevated triglyceride levels, they will develop the chylomicronemia syndrome (see below). These individuals develop no characteristic xanthomas. There is no increase in obesity in this disorder, and no increase in the frequency of diabetes.

Individuals with this disorder have persistent hypertriglyceridemia once they become adults. Below the age of 20, the abnormality is not manifest. Some of the increase in VLDL may persist after weight loss. Increased levels of LDL do not occur. One parent is characteristically affected, as are half of the siblings. These individuals appear to be quite sensitive to other factors that cause only mild hypertriglyceridemia in normal adults: obesity and alcohol, and estrogen, diuretic, beta-adrenergic blocker, and glucocorticoid therapy.

Treatment with clofibrate or gemfibrozil usually leads to significant decreases in VLDL levels. In families without evidence of increased atherosclerosis, no known benefit accrues from this therapy, and it should be discouraged. Drugs causing elevation of triglyceride levels should be avoided because they may precipitate massive chylomicronemia and pancreatitis.

FAMILIAL COMBINED HYPERLIPIDEMIA. This disorder was first suggested in 1973 to be very common in those with premature coronary heart disease, to be inherited as an autosomal dominant trait, and to be characterized by different "combinations" of hyperlipidemia: elevated cholesterol level alone, elevated triglyceride level alone, or elevations in levels of both lipids (familial multiple lipoprotein-type hyperlipidemia). It now appears that this disorder is better characterized as one with elevated plasma apoprotein B levels with variable lipid phenotype even in the same individual at different times, in contrast with familial hypercholesterolemia. The increase in apoprotein B, whether in VLDL or in LDL, appears to be caused by increased hepatic synthesis of the apoprotein. These individuals also have abnormalities in HDL with a mild decrease in HDL cholesterol and apoprotein AI.

Males with this disorder have premature coronary artery disease with mean age of infarct at about 40 years. Smoking has a marked effect on the prevalence of clinical heart disease. Individuals with this disorder are slightly more obese and may have more systemic hypertension. They have no characteristic xanthomas, but occasionally have nonspecific xanthalasma.

OTHER FORMS OF HYPERTRIGLYCERIDEMIA. Individuals with chylomicronemia and triglyceride levels between 1000 and 2000 mg per deciliter are said to aggregate in families. In addition, there are individuals with primary hypertriglyceridemia noted to have a defect in VLDL removal not characterized by one of the above defects in the lipoprotein lipase system.

APPROACH TO THE PATIENT WITH MILD TO MODERATE HYPERTRIGLYCERIDEMIA. The major concern for the individual with hypertriglyceridemia relates to a possible increase in risk for atherosclerosis. When an individual is identified with elevated plasma triglyceride levels, acquired forms of hyperlipidemia should be identified and treated, and the primary forms of hypertriglyceridemia associated with defective remnant catabolism or LPL deficiency should be ruled out.

Elevations in plasma triglyceride levels often serve as a marker for associated abnormalities potentially related to atherosclerosis. A strong family history of early coronary artery disease in the father or mother's male relatives helps to identify such a hypertriglyceridemic individual at risk for early atherosclerosis.

The hypertriglyceridemic individuals who intermittently develop hypercholesterolemia caused by increased LDL levels as well as those who have elevated LDL apoprotein B levels with normal LDL cholesterol also seem to be ones with increased risk for atherosclerosis.

The level of HDL cholesterol is often low in the presence of hypertriglyceridemia. This can occur with familial LPL deficiency and with familial hypertriglyceridemia and does not seem to be associated with the increase in coronary risk seen with a low HDL cholesterol level in the absence of hypertriglyceridemia. However, a decrease in the level of the major apoprotein of HDL, apoprotein AI, seems to be a good predictor of risk, even in the presence of hypertriglyceridemia.

The aforementioned abnormalities characteristic of the hypertriglyceridemic subject at risk for atherosclerosis are similar to those in familial combined hyperlipidemia, which may account for a significant portion of this group.

While weight loss and clofibrate (or gemfibrozil) therapy lower VLDL levels, those at risk for early coronary disease may respond with an increase in LDL levels. Preferred therapy for the hypertriglyceridemic individual at risk, in particular the one with familial combined hyperlipidemia, may be like that used to treat elevated LDL levels in familial hypercholesterolemia: combined bile acid resin and high-dose nicotinic acid therapy, in addition to a diet low in saturated fat and cholesterol. Because of the uncertainty of the significance of elevated triglyceride levels and the unknown risks of lifelong drug therapy, many authorities have recommended diet therapy alone for hypertriglyceridemia.

TABLE 183–2. ACQUIRED DISORDERS OF LIPOPROTEIN METABOLISM

A. Hypertriglyceridemia
  1. Mild to moderate hypertriglyceridemia
    a. Diabetes mellitus*
    b. Uremia and/or dialysis*
  2. Minimal hypertriglyceridemia alone
    a. Obesity
    b. Estrogen*
    c. Alcohol*
    d. Beta-adrenergic blocking agents*
  3. Rare forms of moderate to marked hypertriglyceridemia
    a. Systemic lupus erythematosus
    b. Dysgammaglobulinemias
    c. Glycogenosis type I
    d. Lipodystrophy
B. Combined hyperlipidemia
  1. Hypothyroidism*
  2. Nephrotic syndrome
  3. Glucocorticoid excess*
  4. Diuretics*
C. Hypercholesterolemia
  1. Acute intermittent porphyria
  2. Anorexia nervosa

*Can be associated with chylomicronemia syndrome when it occurs with the familial forms of hypertriglyceridemia.

ACQUIRED DISORDERS OF LIPOPROTEIN METABOLISM

Some disease states are associated with mild to moderate hyperlipidemia in the absence of primary forms of hyperlipidemia, while others seem to have a significant effect only in the presence of a familial form of hyperlipidemia. In general, these can be divided into conditions associated with increased levels of triglyceride-rich lipoproteins and those associated with multiple lipoprotein-type expression (acquired combined hyperlipidemia) (Table 183–2).

Hypertriglyceridemia

DIABETES MELLITUS. Persons with untreated insulin-dependent diabetes and untreated symptomatic non-insulin-dependent diabetes have low adipose tissue or muscle lipoprotein lipase activity with a mild to moderate increase in triglyceride levels and decreased HDL cholesterol levels. With insulin resistance and milder degrees of insulin deficiency, hypertriglyceridemia is caused by excess free fatty acids mobilized from adipose tissue that are re-esterified in the liver and secreted as endogenous VLDL. Treatment with insulin or oral sulfonylurea agents will correct the abnormality in LPL over a period of weeks. In the treated diabetic, variability in free fatty acid mobilization and hepatic triglyceride synthesis, related to the degree of diabetic control, accounts for most of the variation in triglyceride levels.

CHRONIC UREMIA AND DIALYSIS. Many individuals with chronic uremia have elevated VLDL levels with hypertriglyceridemia and low HDL cholesterol levels. This persists after initiation of maintenance hemodialysis or peritoneal dialysis. These lipoprotein abnormalities appear to be related to defects in LPL-mediated triglyceride removal and, with smoking and hypertension, account for the marked atherosclerosis in the dialysis population.

OTHER. Obesity, estrogen use, and alcohol are associated with minimal to mild increases in triglyceride levels, usually not to levels considered abnormal, which appear to be caused by modest increases in hepatic VLDL secretion. Diuretic agents and beta-adrenergic blocking agents are also associated with small increases in triglyceride levels. The diuretics often raise LDL levels, while the beta-blocking agents decrease HDL.

Moderate to marked hypertriglyceridemia occurs extremely rarely in systemic lupus erythematosus or dysgammaglobulinemia caused by an immunoglobulin lipoprotein interaction. Moderate hypertriglyceridemia can also occur in rare disorders such as glycogenosis (type I), lipodystrophy, and carnitinepalmitoyl transferase deficiency.

Combined Hyperlipidemia

HYPOTHYROIDISM. Thyroid hormone appears to be necessary for proper functioning of most steps in lipoprotein metabolism. Thyroxine is necessary for maintenance of the LDL receptor; in hypothyroidism LDL levels are elevated because of defective catabolism. Remnant removal is impaired, resulting in the accumulation of chylomicron with VLDL remnants, and finally the LPL level is low, resulting in hypertriglyceridemia. Thyroxin replacement corrects all of these defects.

NEPHROTIC SYNDROME. With urinary loss of albumin and the development of hypoalbuminemia, increases in levels of VLDL or LDL or both occur. These lipoprotein abnormalities are associated with increased hepatic lipid synthesis and defective catabolism of triglyceride-rich lipoproteins. The latter defect may be related to the loss in the urine of cofactors required for LPL function.

GLUCOCORTICOID EXCESS. Excess glucocorticoid levels caused by Cushing's syndrome or exogenous steroid therapy are associated with elevated VLDL and/or LDL levels. The best studied situation is in the glucocorticoid-treated renal transplant subject, who in the absence of uremia or proteinuria has combined hyperlipidemia.

Hypercholesterolemia

Elevated LDL levels may occur in occasional individuals in response to high saturated fat and cholesterol feeding. Much of the hypercholesterolemia in the population has remained unexplained and has been termed multifactorial, suggesting that it is due to interaction of multiple genes (polygenic) with the environment. Elevated LDL levels occur in acute intermittent porphyria and have been reported with hepatomas and in anorexia nervosa.

CHYLOMICRONEMIA SYNDROME

DEFINITION. Marked chylomicronemia with plasma triglyceride levels in excess of 2000 mg per deciliter is associated with a constellation of signs and symptoms called the chylomicronemia syndrome.

ETIOLOGY AND PATHOGENESIS. This syndrome can occur because of one of several inborn errors in the lipoprotein lipase system for plasma triglyceride removal as noted earlier. Much more commonly, the marked hypertriglyceridemia occurs as a result of the interaction of two common forms of hypertriglyceridemia, usually one genetic and one acquired. Untreated symptomatic diabetes mellitus in the presence of familial hypertriglyceridemia, familial combined hyperlipidemia, or, less commonly, remnant removal disease is a frequent cause of chylomicronemia. Commonly used drugs that interact with these inborn errors are the estrogens, diuretics, beta-adrenergic blocking agents, alcohol, and glucocorticoids. The effects of these drugs are often markedly exaggerated in patients with pre-existing hyperlipidemia. Hypothyroidism and uremia may also occasionally contribute.

CLINICAL MANIFESTATIONS. For unexplained reasons, some individuals are asymptomatic with plasma triglyceride levels as high as 29,000 mg per deciliter. More commonly, abdominal pain and/or pancreatitis or even chest pain is present. Impairment of recent memory can often be detected and the patient may complain of paresthesias of the extremities, similar to the carpal tunnel syndrome. Lipemia retinalis can often be observed, hepatomegaly is common, splenomegaly can occur, and eruptive xanthomas are evidence of chronic chylomicronemia. All of these symptoms and signs clear when triglyceride levels are decreased below 1000 or 2000 mg per deciliter. Marked hypertriglyceridemia may cause insulin resistance and impair control of diabetes. Also, many routine laboratory tests are invalid in the presence of milky plasma. Simple removal of chylomicrons from plasma by short-term ultracentrifugation helps to avoid this problem.

DIAGNOSIS. It is very simple to make a presumptive diagnosis of chylomicronemia syndrome by visual examination of the patient's plasma. Milky plasma always indicates the presence of chylomicrons, as does a plasma triglyceride level above 1000 mg per deciliter. In the presence of symptoms and signs of the chylomicron syndrome, a definitive diagnosis is made if these clear when the triglyceride level is lowered.

TREATMENT. With pancreatitis, the discontinuation of oral intake will rapidly decrease triglyceride levels. With refeeding, fat must be avoided initially and replaced slowly. Often, mild to moderate abdominal pain can be treated by lowering dietary fat content and avoiding alcohol. The mainstay of treatment is to identify the causes of the elevation in triglyceride levels. A genetic form of hypertriglyceridemia is invariably present and may need to be treated with clofibrate, gemfibrozil, or nicotinic acid. The last drug is difficult to use in diabetic patients because it impairs insulin sensitivity. The acquired disease or agent contributing to the hypertriglyceridemia should be treated or removed. Slowly, the patient can be refed while the plasma is watched for turbidity and the patient's symptoms and signs are observed. With appropriate therapy, the chylomicronemia syndrome should rarely recur.

HYPERLIPIDEMIA AND ATHEROSCLEROTIC VASCULAR DISEASE

Although the etiology of atherosclerosis is multifactorial, the development of premature coronary artery disease and peripheral vascular disease is strongly dependent on abnormalities in plasma lipoprotein metabolism. Thus, coronary artery disease in men under the age of 50 years and in women of any age is more likely to occur in the presence of one of the inborn errors or acquired forms of hyperlipidemia. Independently, HDL may protect against atherosclerosis. Differences in HDL cholesterol levels between men and women may explain a large part of the sex difference in development of atherosclerosis.

Familial hypercholesterolemia unequivocally is associated with premature coronary artery disease and aggravated by cigarette smoking and low HDL cholesterol levels. Remnant removal disease is also associated with peripheral vascular disease and coronary artery disease. Familial hypertriglyceridemia may impose some increased risk for atherosclerosis in a few families, but atherosclerosis is generally not increased in this form in hypertriglyceridemia. The increased atherosclerosis seen in diabetics and in patients undergoing long-term hemodialysis may also be related in part to abnormalities in lipoprotein metabolism. One must be concerned that the lipoprotein changes seen with diuretic and beta-adrenergic blocking therapy for elevated blood pressure may contribute to coronary artery disease.

Nonetheless, all of these factors still account for only a minor part of premature atherosclerosis. Mildly elevated levels of LDL, apoprotein B, or triglyceride and low levels of HDL cholesterol and apoprotein AI have been suggested to be present in the majority of patients with premature coronary artery disease. The frequency of familial combined hyperlipidemia in this undefined heterogeneous group of individuals has yet to be determined.

The goal of therapy aimed at correcting hyperlipidemia is to prevent the progression of atherosclerosis. Direct evidence now suggests this may be possible in some individuals with specific lipoprotein abnormalities. Young individuals at risk can be identified as those with a family history of premature coronary artery disease or known acquired causes of hyperlipidemia (Table 183–2). After consideration of the acquired causes of hyperlipidemia, individuals with plasma cholesterol levels in the upper 25th percentile of the normal distribution should be treated with a low-saturated fat, low-cholesterol diet. Young and middle-aged men whose LDL cholesterol remains in the upper fifth to tenth percentile should be

considered for therapy with a bile acid–binding resin, high-dose nicotinic acid, or neomycin. Combinations of a resin with nicotinic acid or with a fibric acid derivative (clofibrate or gemfibrozil) may be of further benefit. The use of the fibric acid drugs alone does not seem warranted because of the tendency for LDL to increase in those with hyperlipidemia who are at risk for premature coronary disease.

RARE DISORDERS OF LIPOPROTEIN METABOLISM

Several rare inherited disorders of lipoprotein metabolism are of considerable theoretical importance because they assist in understanding normal lipoprotein physiology. Each of these disorders is an autosomal recessive trait.

Abetalipoproteinemia presents in early childhood and is associated with absence of apoprotein B–containing lipoproteins due to defective synthesis. Intestinal fat malabsorption, ataxia, neuropathy, retinitis pigmentosa, and acanthocytosis result. *Tangier disease* presents in childhood with absence of HDL and extremely low levels of apoproteins AI and AII. Cholesteryl esters deposit in tonsils and other lymphoid tissues and corneal opacities develop. *Lecithin-cholesterol acyltransferase deficiency* presents in the young adult as hemolytic anemia and renal failure. Although the free cholesterol level in plasma is variable, the cholesteryl ester level is very low. Other even rarer disorders are described in recent reviews.

Disorders of lipoprotein and lipid metabolism. In Stanbury JB, Wyngaarden JB, Fredrickson DS, et al. (eds.): The Metabolic Basis of Inherited Disease. 5th ed. New York, McGraw-Hill Book Company, 1983, pp 589–747. *Seven extensive reviews in great detail about the inborn errors leading to abnormalities in plasma lipoproteins.*
Havel RJ: Symposium on lipid disorders. Med Clin North Am 66:317, 1982. *Contains 12 review articles by experts in the field concerning basic biochemistry and physiology of lipoproteins, pathophysiology of specific diseases, and therapy of these disorders.*
Journal of Lipid Research 25:1425–1634, 1984. *Series of articles ranging from basic biochemistry of lipids to clinical lipoprotein disorders.*

184 FABRY'S DISEASE (Glycosphingolipidosis)

James B. Wyngaarden

DEFINITION. Fabry's disease is an inborn error of glycosphingolipid metabolism characterized by telangiectatic skin lesions, hypohidrosis, corneal opacities, acral pain and paresthesias, intermittent fevers, renal failure, and cardiovascular, gastrointestinal, and central nervous system disturbances.

PREVALENCE. The disease has an estimated prevalence of 1:40,000 births.

ETIOLOGY AND PATHOGENESIS. Fabry's disease is an X-linked condition, fully manifest in the hemizygous male. Heterozygous females may exhibit the disease in an attenuated form, and usually show corneal clouding; occasionally a female may have most of the features of the full syndrome, including renal failure.

The biochemical defect is a deficiency of the lysosomal enzyme, alpha-galactosidase-A. The enzymatic defect leads to a progressive deposition of neutral glycosphingolipids with terminal alpha-galactosyl moieties in most visceral tissues and fluids of the body. The most prominent of these is a trihexosylceramide called globotriaosylceramide, a degradation product of a constituent of membrane called globoside. The majority of anatomic and physiologic abnormalities observed in Fabry's disease can be related to the cumulative deposition of glycosphingolipid, particularly in the lysosomes of the cardiovascular-renal system.

PATHOLOGY. Morphologically, Fabry's disease is characterized by widespread tissue deposits of a crystalline glyco-sphingolipid that shows birefringence under polarized light. The glycosphingolipid is deposited in all areas of the body, predominantly in the lysosomes of endothelial, perithelial, and smooth muscle cells of blood vessels. Lipid deposits are also prominent in epithelial cells of the cornea, in glomeruli and tubules of the kidney, in muscle fibers of the heart, and in ganglion cells of the dorsal roots and autonomic nervous system. The skin lesions are telangiectases or small superficial angiomas. Capillaries, venules, and arterioles show pathologic lipid storage, and there is marked dilatation of the capillaries of the dermal papillae just below the epidermis. The larger lesions are usually located in the upper dermis, where they may produce elevation, flattening, or hypertrophy of the epithelium, with keratosis; hence the term *angiokeratoma.* On electron microscopy lipid inclusions show a concentrically arranged lamellar structure with alternating light- and dark-staining bands. Peripheral nerves show densely stained inclusions in the cytoplasm of perineurial fibroblasts and the endothelial cells of the endoneurial blood vessels. There is loss of unmyelinated neurons but not of myelinated neurons. Some neurons contain ceramide trihexoside.

CLINICAL MANIFESTATIONS. *Telangiectases* may occur in childhood and lead to early diagnosis. They increase in size and number with age, and range from barely visible to several millimeters in diameter. The lesions are punctate, dark red to blue-black, and flat or slightly raised. They do not blanch with pressure, and the larger ones may show slight hyperkeratosis. The lesions tend to occur in the "bathing trunk area," but may occur anywhere, including the oral mucosa. The hips, thighs, buttocks, umbilicus, lower abdomen, scrotum, and glans penis are common sites, and there is a tendency toward bilateral symmetry. In some patients skin lesions are absent and lesions are entirely visceral. Sweating is often decreased, and hair may be sparse; shaving may be required only infrequently. Ocular lesions may be present in all elements of the eye. The most prominent are in the cornea, conjunctiva, and retina. Corneal opacities, observed by slit lamp examination, are present in most heterozygotes. The conjunctival and retinal vessels may show mild to marked tortuosity, with aneurysmal dilatations of thin-walled venules, as well as angulation and segmental, sausage-like dilatation of veins.

Pain is the most debilitating symptom. Fabry's crises, lasting from minutes to several days, consist of agonizing, burning pain in palms, soles, and proximal extremities, associated with fever. The pain may become more severe with age, or may disappear. Attacks of abdominal or flank pain may simulate appendicitis or renal colic. In addition, there may be chronic troublesome paresthesias of hands and feet.

With increasing age progressive infiltration of the cardio-vascular-renal system with glycosphingolipid gives rise to anginal chest pain, myocardial infarction, cardiomegaly, or congestive heart failure. Involvement of renal parenchymal vessels leads to hypertension. During childhood and adolescence protein, red cells, casts, and desquamated kidney and urinary tract cells appear in the urine. Azotemia is common in the second to fourth decade. Birefringent lipid globules with characteristic Maltese crosses within and without cells can be observed in the urine sediment by polarized light microscopy. Other features may include chronic bronchitis and dyspnea, lymphedema of the legs without hypoprotein-emia, episodic diarrhea, osteoporosis, retarded growth, and delayed puberty. The mean age at death is 41 years, but survival may extend into the sixties.

DIAGNOSIS AND DIFFERENTIAL DIAGNOSIS. The diagnosis in hemizygous males is most readily made from the history of painful paresthesias and episodic crises with fever, and the observation of characteristic skin lesions, corneal opacities, and conjunctival lesions. The disorder is often misdiagnosed as rheumatic fever, erythromelalgia, or neu-rosis. The skin lesions must be differentiated from the benign angiokeratomas of the scrotum of older men (Fordyce's disease) or from angiokeratoma circumscripta. Angiokeratomas identical to those of Fabry's disease have been reported in fucosidosis and sialidosis. The diagnosis is confirmed biochemically by demonstration of markedly alpha-galactosidase-A activity in plasma or serum, leukocytes, tears, biopsied tissue, or cultured skin fibroblasts. Increased levels of globo-triaosylceramide are found in urinary sediment, plasma, or cultured fibroblasts.

Suspect heterozygotes may show corneal opacities, isolated skin lesions, and lipid-laden cells in skin or other tissues or in urinary sediment. Intermediate activities of alpha-galacto-sidase-A can usually be demonstrated.

Prenatal diagnosis of Fabry's disease may be made by amniocentesis at approximately 14 weeks of gestation and demonstration of deficient alpha-galactosidase-A activity and XY karyotype in cultured amniotic cells, and accumulated trihexosylceramide in amniotic acid.

TREATMENT. Pain may be relieved with phenytoin or carbamazepine in some patients. Maintenance administration of phenytoin, carbamazepine, or both, or corticosteroid therapy has also provided symptomatic relief. Renal insufficiency is treated with long-term hemodialysis or renal transplantation. In some recipients biochemical and clinical regression, with relief of pain, has followed placement of renal allografts. Alpha-galactosidase-A purified from human placenta has been administered to several hemizygotes. The enzyme was rapidly cleared from plasma and taken up by liver. There was a reduction in level of circulating trihexosylceramide. Current research centers on target delivery of enzyme and methods of protecting it from rapid inactivation.

Case Records of the Massachusetts General Hospital: Case 2–1984 (Fabry's Disease). N Engl J Med 310:106, 1984. *Excellent presentation of nervous system involvement in Fabry's disease.*
Desnick RJ, Klionsky B, Sweeley CC: Fabry's disease (α-galactosidase A deficiency). In Stanbury JB, Wyngaarden JB, Fredrickson DS, et al. (eds.): The Metabolic Basis of Inherited Disease. 5th ed. New York, McGraw-Hill Book Company, 1983. *A definitive chapter describing clinical, pathologic, and biochemical manifestations of Fabry's disease; 400 references.*
Goldman ME, Cantor R, Schwartz MF, et al.: Echocardiographic abnormalities and disease severity in Fabry's disease. J Am Coll Cardiol 7:1157, 1986. *Echocardiographic evidence of Fabry's disease appears to correlate with age-related severity of disease.*

185 GAUCHER'S DISEASE

Edwin H. Kolodny

DEFINITION. This relatively common familial disorder results from progressive accumulation of glucocerebroside within phagocytic cells of the monocyte-macrophage system involving principally the liver, spleen, bone marrow, and lymph nodes. Three genetically distinct clinical types have been differentiated: type 1, a chronic non-neuronopathic or "adult" form that may appear at any age and is associated with hypersplenism and bone lesions; type 2, an acute neuronopathic or "infantile" form that presents in infancy with multiple brain stem signs; and type 3, a "juvenile" subacute neuronopathic form that presents in childhood and causes seizures and mental deterioration. The activity of glucocere-brosidase is deficient in all three types, but each is due to a different mutation.

PATHOLOGIC PHYSIOLOGY AND PATHOGENESIS. Glucocerebroside contains equimolar amounts of spingosine, fatty acid, and glucose. Considerable quantities of this compound are generated daily by the turnover of senescent red and white blood cells. In the central nervous system, glucocerebroside is produced in the course of ganglioside metabolism. A deacylated derivative, glucosylsphingosine, also accumulates in Gaucher's disease. This highly cytotoxic compound is probably responsible for the nerve cell destruction that occurs in the neuropathic forms of the disease. Both of these glycolipids are degraded by acidic glucosylceramide-β-D-glucosidase (glucocerebrosidase; E.C. 3.5.1.2.1), a lysosomal enzyme with multiple molecular forms. Its catalytic efficiency is increased by a low molecular weight, heat-stable protein that combines with the enzyme-lipid complex. The gene for glucocerebrosidase has been mapped to the q21 region of chromosome 1, and its cloned cDNA has been used as a molecular probe to identify the catalytic site of the enzyme and variations in restriction pattern of genomic DNA from Gaucher patients.

A distinctive morphologic feature is the *Gaucher cell*, a large round or polyhedral phagocyte, 20 to 100 μ in diameter, containing one or more small eccentrically placed nuclei and a pale, striated cytoplasm resembling wrinkled tissue paper or crumpled silk (Fig. 185–1A). Under the electron microscope, this fibrillary network consists of numerous dilated saclike structures resembling lysosomes containing tubules; these are similar to the twisted bilayers characteristic of glucocerebroside deposits. The reaction of the Gaucher cell cytoplasm with the periodic acid–Schiff stain is strongly positive. Stains for iron and acid phosphatase are also positive, but the reaction with lipid stains is weak. The bone marrow of patients with chronic myelogenous leukemia often contains cells with a similar appearance; the deposits in these "pseudo-Gaucher" cells are linear rather than twisted.

Glucosylceramide is increased two- to three-fold in plasma and more than 200-fold in the spleen and liver. Gaucher cells are present in virtually all organs surrounding small blood vessels and as sheets infiltrating their parenchyma. The spleen

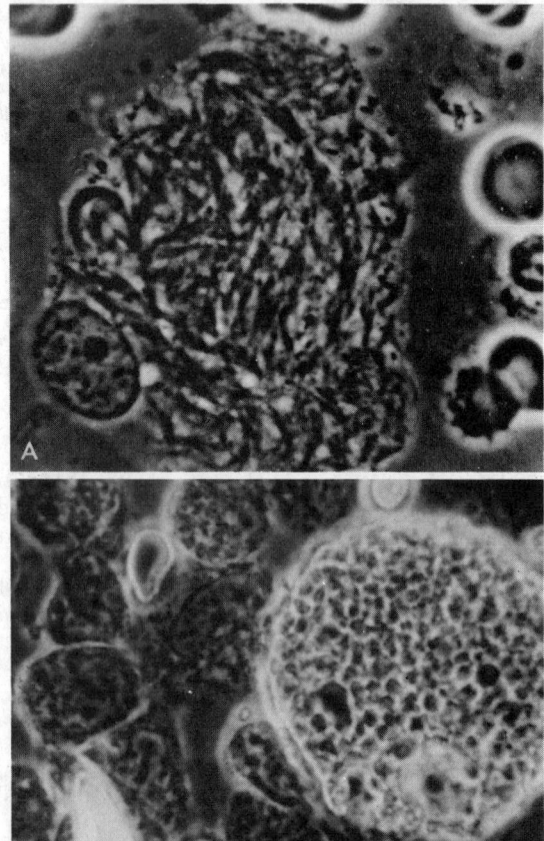

FIGURE 185–1. Appearance of the typical Gaucher cell (*A*) and a foam cell seen in Niemann-Pick disease (*B*). Both are viewed under phase microscopy in unstained smears of aspirated bone marrow. Magnification can be estimated from adjacent red cells.

may become massively enlarged and develop multiple infarcts and fibrosis. The red pulp of the spleen appears white because of lipid infiltration by Gaucher cells; foci of extramedullary hematopoiesis can occur. In most patients the liver is also enlarged, the Kupffer cells of their sinusoids transformed into Gaucher cells. Fibrosis is present, but there is no proliferation of the bile ducts and liver failure is rare. Excretion of glucosylceramide into the bile probably prevents more massive accumulation within the liver. In some cases, portal hypertension develops.

Gaucher cells may completely fill the medullary cavity of bone, cause thinning of the cortex, loss of its normal trabeculation, patchy myelosclerosis, bone infarcts, and osteonecrosis. The metaphyseal plate in the long bones is especially prone to damage. An *Erlenmeyer flask deformity* of the distal femur is an early radiographic sign of bone involvement. With progression of the disease, spontaneous fractures and painful lytic lesions are found. Diffuse pulmonary infiltration can occur with direct involvement of the alveoli, pleura, and interstitium resulting in dyspnea and cor pulmonale. Renal involvement with severe proteinuric nephropathy and glomerulonephritis occurs in a few cases.

Central nervous system pathology has been found in all three types. Perivascular collections of Gaucher cells, nerve cell loss, neuronophagia, and infiltration of microglia are the principal changes observed. The most affected area in type 2 are the deeper layers of the frontal cortex and the nuclei of the basal ganglia, midbrain, and brain stem. The high concentrations of glucosylsphingosine, a cytotoxic compound, present in the brain, liver, and spleen of type 2 patients probably contribute to the necrosis that occurs in these tissues.

The activity of tartrate-resistant acid phosphatase and angiotensin converting enzyme and concentrations of several serum proteins, including the immunoglobulins, are increased, especially in type 1 patients. The increased acid phosphatase is the type 5 isozyme and therefore of osteoclastic origin and indicative of bone involvement. Some older patients develop a monoclonal gammopathy with multiple myeloma. Leukemias and other forms of malignant neoplasms are also more frequent in elderly patients with type 1 disease.

CLINICAL MANIFESTATIONS. *Chronic Non-neuropathic Type.* This disease is transmitted as an autosomal recessive trait and affects both sexes equally. It has been observed in whites, blacks, and Asians, but more than one half of cases are found in Ashkenazic Jews. Since one in 20 of this population is a carrier, it is not unusual for the disease to appear in two successive generations of the same family. Clinical symptoms in this so-called adult form may appear at any age, from the first year of life to the ninth decade. One third of all cases are diagnosed in the first decade. The majority of these children are not of Jewish ancestry. They develop massive enlargement of the spleen and evidence a delay in somatic growth that may severely hamper their intellectual and social development. The condition in another 25 per cent of patients is not diagnosed until after age 30. These patients have a much more benign course. Only rarely do these individuals have serious hematologic or osseous complications.

The most common presenting symptom is excessive fatigue associated with a hypochromic anemia and splenomegaly. Frequently there is a long history of bleeding tendency such as repeated epistaxis and ecchymoses, but this rarely attracts medical attention unless it is associated with a major hemorrhage such as splenic rupture, bleeding from esophageal varices, subdural hematoma, or hemopericardium. The first indication in some patients may be the appearance of bone or joint pain or a pathologic fracture. Lytic lesions develop in the shafts of the long bones, vertebrae, ribs, and pelvis. This produces osteosclerosis and, in the most virulent cases, osteonecrosis and eventually collapse of bone. In the acute crises affecting bone or joints there is severe incapacitating pain, erythema, swelling, tenderness, and occasionally joint effusion. While only 20 per cent of all type 1 patients have significant clinical involvement of bone, more than one half have radiologic evidence of the Erlenmeyer flask deformity with tapering of the midshaft of the femur and failure of normal trabeculation causing a widening of the distal end.

The clinical course is variable. In response to an acute infection, the size of the spleen may increase dramatically and then regress, but slowly progressive splenomegaly is the usual pattern. Anemia, thrombocytopenia, and leukemia are frequent but rarely cause significant morbidity. Bleeding may occur if the platelet count falls below 50,000 to 70,000 per cubic millimeter; however, the count usually rises again spontaneously within a few weeks. Hepatomegaly with a firm liver edge is common, and in a few severe cases liver failure and portal hypertension occur.

Acute Neuronopathic Type. This form of the disease is much rarer than the adult type 1 variety. It is observed in infants of different ethnic groups and does not show any predilection for Jews. The disease usually presents a few months after birth with retroflexion of the head, strabismus, increasing muscular hypertoncity, and marked increase in the size of the liver and spleen. In some cases, developmental milestones are normal until the second or third year. The major central nervous system signs reflect brain stem and and cranial nerve involvement. There are extreme arching of the neck, retraction of the lips, trismus, laryngeal spasm with a chronic cough and stridor, and spastic rigidity of the extremities. Seizures and psychomotor retardation also occur. Death results from respiratory infection within a few months to two years after signs appear.

Juvenile Type. This includes a heterogeneous group of patients with signs of the chronic adult type combined with progressive neurologic disease that begins in childhood or adolescence. A subtype of this disease that occurs in Swedish youngsters is referred to as the Norrbottnian variant. Their growth is retarded, and there are hypersplenism and skeletal changes of the type that occurs in the chronic non-neuropathic form. In addition, they develop oculomotor apraxia, convergent squint, seizures, and a delay in motor development. In splenectomized patients, white retinal infiltrates may appear, the infiltration of glucosylceramide into the central nervous system is accelerated, and the pace of mental deterioration is faster than in nonsplenectomized patients. In other patients with the juvenile type, the principal manifestations are medication-resistant myoclonic seizures and slow intellectual decline.

DIAGNOSIS. Gaucher's disease should be suspected in any patient with unexplained splenomegaly and a bleeding tendency, bone or joint pains, or pathologic fractures. A radioisotope scan of the liver and spleen will reveal the extent of the hepatosplenomegaly and the presence of infarcts. Radionuclide scintigraphy or magnetic resonance imaging is useful for locating lytic changes in bone. The bone marrow may demonstrate Gaucher cells. The diagnosis is established by assaying the activity of glucosylceramide-β-D-glucosidase in leukocytes or cultured fibroblasts. The artificial fluorogenic substrate, 4-methylumbelliferyl-β-glucoside, is commonly employed as a substitute for the natural lipid substrate. The degree of enzyme deficiency is similar in all three clinical subtypes of Gaucher's disease. Within the same family, expression of the disease may vary considerably so that enzyme assays should be done on all close relatives of the patient, whether or not they are symptomatic. Heterozygotes have approximately one half the normal enzyme activity; however, with current methods the range of values overlaps with the normal range. Therefore, carrier detection cannot be done with 100 per cent certainty. Prenatal diagnosis is possible using cultured amniotic cells.

TREATMENT AND PROGNOSIS. Iron therapy may partially correct the anemia, but the persistent use of iron in the presence of adequate iron stores increases the risk of hemo-chromatosis. Splenectomy is performed for severe and persistent thrombocytopenia or when mechanical factors cause massive swelling, abdominal pain, or gastrointestinal dysfunction. Correction of the thrombocytopenia occurs immediately after the operation with a less dramatic improvement noted in the anemia. In children, the growth curve usually improves. However, splenectomy may hasten the pace of lipid deposition into the liver and bones, and osteolytic lesions may appear within a few months after the operation. Therefore, the surgeon may elect to leave in place any accessory spleen tissue that is present or to perform a partial splenectomy. Acute lesions in bone and joints are initially treated with immobilization and the prevention of weight bearing. However, as soon as possible a graduated program of exercises is introduced to maintain joint mobility and prevent further loss of bone. Fractures of the head and neck of the femur are usually treated by prosthetic hip replacement. Enzyme replacement therapy and bone marrow transplantation have been tried in a few patients without long-term benefit. The prognosis in children with the early onset form of the type 1 disease is poor because of the severe lung, liver, and bone involvement in these cases. In milder cases of later onset, longevity is normal. Children with the infantile neuronopathic form do not survive beyond age two to three years, whereas those with the juvenile subacute neuronopathic variant may live into their third decade.

Brady RO, Barranger JA: Glucosylceramide lipidosis: Gaucher's disease. In Stanbury JB, Wyngaarden JB, Fredrickson DS, et al. (eds.): The Metabolic Basis of Inherited Disease. 5th ed. New York, McGraw-Hill Book Company, 1983. *A review of the clinical and metabolic abnormalities in Gaucher's disease.*

Desnick RJ, Gatt S, Grabowski GA (eds.): Gaucher Disease: A Century of Delineation and Research. New York, Alan R. Liss, 1982. *A complete review of all aspects of Gaucher's disease based on reports presented at the First International Symposium on Gaucher Disease held in July, 1981.*

Ginns EI, Choudary V, Tsuji S, et al.: Gene mapping and leader polypeptide sequence of human glucocerebrosidase: Implications for Gaucher disease. Proc Natl Acad Sci USA 82:7101, 1985. *This report describes the mapping of the structural gene for glucocerebrosidase to chromosome 1 band q21 using radiolabeled human glucocerebrosidase cDNA. For other reports describing the cDNA see Proc Natl Acad Sci USA 82:5442 and 7289, 1985, and J Biol Chem 261:50, 1986.*

Rosenthal DI, Scott JA, Barranger J, et al.: Evaluation of Gaucher disease using magnetic resonance imaging. J Bone Joint Surg 68:802, 1986. *The sensitivity of MRI in detecting bone lesions is documented in this study of 24 patients.*

Rubin M, Yampolski I, Lambrozo R, et al.: Partial splenectomy in Gaucher's disease. J Pediatr Surg 21:125, 1986. *A review of the surgical outcome in 11 children with type 1 Gaucher's disease.*

Stowers DW, Teitelbaum SL, Kahn AJ, et al.: Skeletal complications of Gaucher disease. Medicine 64:310, 1985. *Description of bone findings in 327 patients with Gaucher's disease.*

186 NIEMANN-PICK DISEASE

Edwin H. Kolodny

DEFINITION. The eponym Neimannn-Pick disease originally referred to the classic infantile form of lipid storage disease described more than a half century ago. The lysosomal enzyme sphingomyelinase is absent in this disease; this causes widespread deposition of sphingomyelin, a ceramide phospholipid. Foam cells proliferate within the liver, spleen, and bone marrow, and there is nerve cell loss within the central nervous system. This acute neuronopathic form was subsequently designated as type A to distinguish it from other variants of sphingomyelin lipidosis which have since been described. These variants are distinguished by their age of onset, degree of central nervous system involvement, and sphingomyelinase activity (Table 186–1).

PATHOLOGY. *Foam Cell.* The cytoplasm of this large histiocyte contains numerous uniform-sized lipid-staining droplets that create a fine reticulated web resembling a hon-

TABLE 186–1. THE SPHINGOMYELIN LIPIDOSES

Type	Descriptive Name	Racial and/or Geographic Predilection	Affects Brain	Deficiency
A	Acute neuronopathic	Ashkenazic Jewish	Yes	Sphingomyelinase
B	Chronic non-neuronopathic	No	No	Sphingomyelinase
C	Subacute neuronopathic or juvenile dystonic lipidosis	No	Yes	Cholesterol esterification
D	Nova Scotian	Yarmouth County, Nova Scotia	Yes	Unknown
E	Adult non-neuronopathic	No	No	Unknown

eycomb or mulberry (see Fig. 185–1*B*). Under the electron microscope these cytosomes consist of both concentrically laminated membranous arrays and dense homogeneous bodies. Foam cells are present in the tissues of the reticuloendothelial system.

Sphingomyelin. The ceramide and phosphorylcholine portions of this lipid are linked by a phosphodiester bond that under normal circumstances is cleaved by sphingomyelinase. Sphingomyelin is increased 15- to 45-fold in the liver and spleen of patients with type A Niemann-Pick disease, and about half as much in type B patients. The organs of type C patients exhibit a three- to six-fold increase in sphingomyelin, but it is not the major accumulating lipid in this variant. Sphingomyelin storage occurs in the brain of type A but not type B patients. Patients with every variety of Niemann-Pick disease also accumulate bis (monoacylglycero) phosphate, unesterified cholesterol, glucosylceramide, and other neutral glycolipids.

Sphingomyelinase. Patients with type A and type B Niemann-Pick disease are totally deficient in sphingomyelinase, the acid hydrolase that removes the phosphorylcholine moiety from sphingomyelin. The absence of this phosphodiesterase probaby explains the simultaneous increase of bis (monoacylglycero) phospate. In type C patients, sphingomyelinase may be normal or partially deficient, but the principal finding is a defect in esterification of nonlipoprotein cholesterol. A low molecular weight protein, SAP-2, stimulates spingomyelinase by binding to the enzyme. The gene for this activator has been mapped to chromosome 10, but no cases of SAP-2 deficiency associated with Niemann-Pick disease have been reported.

CLINICAL MANIFESTATIONS. *Type A.* Hepatosplenomegaly, diffuse pulmonary infiltration, and developmental delay are noticeable as early as one to two months of age. Weight gain is poor partly because of vomiting associated with feedings. Lymphadenopathy, opisthotonic posturing, and seizures develop. Eye signs include periorbital puffiness, clouding of the corneas, yellowish discoloration of the lens, and cherry-red maculae. The skin becomes brownish-yellow, and xanthomas may appear. The affected child becomes emaciated with very thin extremities, a protuberant abdomen, and ascites. Developmental milestones normal for a one-year-old are never attained, and after the child lingers in a vegetative state for many months, death occurs, usually before the fourth year. Postmortem studies reveal a large yellow liver and atrophic brain with widespread nerve cell loss and gliosis. The cytoplasm of remaining neurons and of the glial cells is ballooned with lipid inclusions. A high percentage of patients with this rare autosomal recessive disorder are of Ashkenazic Jewish ancestry.

Type B. Severe early involvement of the lungs, liver, and spleen also characterizes type B Niemann-Pick disease, but mental development in this variant is normal. The chest radiograph reveals nodular densities throughout the lung fields and thickening of the interlobar fissures. Signs of hypersplenism such as mild anemia, leukopenia, and thrombocytopenia with easy bruising often occur. A few patients have been described with a brownish-red spot in the macula, and sea-blue histiocytes are sometimes found in the bone marrow. These cells contain ceroid that confers on them a bluish cast when stained with Giemsa. Normal longevity is

possible but may be limited by chronic pulmonary insufficiency and the mechanical effects of the enlarged spleen and liver on other abdominal organs.

Type C. This diagnosis has been applied to a heterogeneous group of patients with a variable age of onset. In some cases, jaundice is present during the first three months, but this subsides despite the progression of the disease. A liver biopsy in these instances may show chronic hepatitis with giant cells. One group of type C patients, between one and one-half and three years of age, exhibits slowing of speech and motor development and then develops blindness and spasticity. The condition of these children deteriorates rapidly over a two-year period and they die at age five to six years. Other type C patients may not develop overt neurologic symptoms until after age five years. These consist of a decline in intellect, progressive impairment of vertical gaze, dysarthria, dysphagia, incoordination, seizures, and involuntary movements. A few have also developed cataplexy. These patients usually survive into adult life.

Type D. This designation is used for cases similar to type C occurring in descendents of an Acadian couple born in Yarmouth, Nova Scotia, in the 1600's. No sphingomyelinase deficiency has been reported in these cases.

DIAGNOSIS. Niemann-Pick disease should be suspected whenever foam cells are present in the bone marrow of a patient with hepatosplenomegaly. The infant of Ashkenazic Jewish heritage who develops slowly would suggest the type A variant. Early jaundice and a subsequent period of normal development might stimulate a work-up for type C Neimann-Pick disease. The foam cell, a lipid-laden histiocyte, should not be confused with the Gaucher cell, which also contains lipid, but of a different morphologic appearance. Foam cells also occur in hypertriglyceridemia and certain other lysosomal storage diseases such as fucosidosis, mannosidosis, GM₁ gangliosidosis, Sandhoff's disease, Wolman's disease, and I-cell disease. In long-standing cases of type B disease, sea-blue histiocytes containing a ceroid-like material are also observed in the bone marrow. The definitive diagnosis of Niemann-Pick disease types A and B is based upon the assay of sphingomyelinase activity. Homogenates of cultured skin fibroblasts or leukocytes from these patients, when incubated with sphingomyelin labeled with ^{14}C in the choline portion of the molecule, have less than 5 per cent of control activity. Intermediate values are obtained for type A and type B heterozygotes. Type C homozygotes may exhibit a partial deficiency, but type C heterozygotes cannot be determined enzymatically. The defect in cholesterol esterification present in type C patients can be demonstrated in fibroblast culture by incubating the cells with LDL protein and ^3H-labeled oleate and then analyzing their content of unesterified and esterified cholesterol. Prenatal diagnosis of type A and type B Niemann-Pick disease is accomplished by determining the enzyme activity of cultured amniotic fluid cells.

TREATMENT. There is no specific treatment available for any of the sphingomyelin storage diseases. In type B patients splenectomy may be done to relieve mechanical pressure within the abdomen or to correct a thrombocytopenia with hemorrhagic diathesis. Neither replacement with exogenous enzyme nor organ transplants have been successful, but it is possible that bone marrow transplantation will in the future prove beneficial to patients without central nervous system involvement. Animal models of Niemann-Pick disease are available for laboratory trials of potential new therapies.

Besley GTN, Moss SE: Studies on sphingomyelinase and β-glucosidase activities in Niemann-Pick disease variants. Phosphodiesterase activities measured with natural and artificial substrates. Biochim Biophys Acta 752:54, 1983. *Sphingomyelinase activity in cultured skin fibroblasts and liver is characterized and the deficiency in types A, B, and C Neimann-Pick disease described.*

Brady RO: Sphingomyelin lipidosis: Neimann-Pick disease. In Stanbury JB, Wyngaarden JB, Fredrickson DS, et al. (eds.): The Metabolic Basis of Inherited Disease. 5th ed. New York, McGraw-Hill Book Company, 1983. *A comprehensive review of the different clinical forms of sphingomyelin lipidoses.*

Details of their pathology, metabolic disturbance, and enzymatic aspects are provided, as well as a complete bibliography.

Breen L, Morris HH, Alperin JB, et al.: Juvenile Niemann-Pick disease with vertical supranuclear ophthalmoplegia. Arch Neurol 38:388, 1981. *A comprehensive review of the clinical features in the later-onset form of type C. References to the sea-blue histiocyte syndrome are included.*

Pentchev PG, Comly ME, Kruth HS, et al.: A defect in cholesterol esterification in certain patients designated as Niemann-Pick disease type C. Proc Natl Acad Sci USA 82:8247, 1985. *Description of the enzyme defect in type C Niemann-Pick disease.*

Winsor EJ, Welch JP: Genetic and demographic aspects of Nova Scotia Niemann-Pick disease. Am J Hum Genet 30:530,1978. *A useful source of references to type D Niemann-Pick disease.*

Inborn Errors of Amino Acid Metabolism

187 HYPERAMINOACIDURIA (With a Classification of the Inborn and Developmental Errors of Amino Acid Metabolism)

Charles R. Scriver

Study of the inborn errors of amino acid metabolism has improved our knowledge of metabolism, and in several instances has improved diagnosis and treatment of specific diseases. The inborn errors of renal transport are important "probes" of the mechanisms dedicated to amino acid reabsorption. They identify either the carriers or the metabolic processes that are coupled to the transcellular flux that achieves net reabsorption.

A certain amount of L-aminoaciduria, representing less than 2 to 3 per cent of the total urinary nitrogen, is a normal phenomenon. A small fraction, usually less than 5 per cent, of the filtered load of the amino acids in plasma is not reabsorbed completely by the proximal portion of the renal tubule and is excreted in the urine. In the healthy person, the efficiency of renal tubular transport of the individual amino acids is related to their chemical and steric structure, the amount in the glomerular filtrate, and the sex, age, and physiologic state of the subject.

Abnormal aminoaciduria will result when there is an ac-

quired or hereditary disturbance of cellular metabolism or transport of amino acids. The known hyperaminoacidurias (see Table 187–1, which also includes several inborn errors of amino acid metabolism not necessarily associated with hyperaminoaciduria per se, but identified by organic acid and fatty acid derivatives) can be classified according to four basic mechanisms (Fig. 187–1):

1. *Saturation:* Amino acid is at elevated concentration and approaches or exceeds the capacity of the system to reabsorb it ("overflow" aminoaciduria).

2. *Competition:* One amino acid at elevated concentration competes with others sharing access to a transport system ("combined" aminoaciduria).

3. *Modification of reactive site(s):* Amino acid(s) is (are) not transported efficiently because access to the system is impaired ("renal" aminoaciduria).

4. *Inhibition of substrate transfer:* Energy-dependent processes coupled to the carrier and transfer of substrates across membranes are impaired ("renal" aminoaciduria).

The individual mechanisms required for transport of each amino acid can be grouped into at least five major gene-controlled and non-overlapping systems, each having a preference for a particular group of amino acids normally found in plasma and revealed by a mendelian phenotype (see Table 187–1, Group III). Another series of carriers appears able to recognize individual free amino acids, with perhaps one site for each of the protein amino acids. (Yet another series permits transepithelial absorption of oligopeptides, with hydrolysis following uptake of the peptides.)

Text continued on page 1155

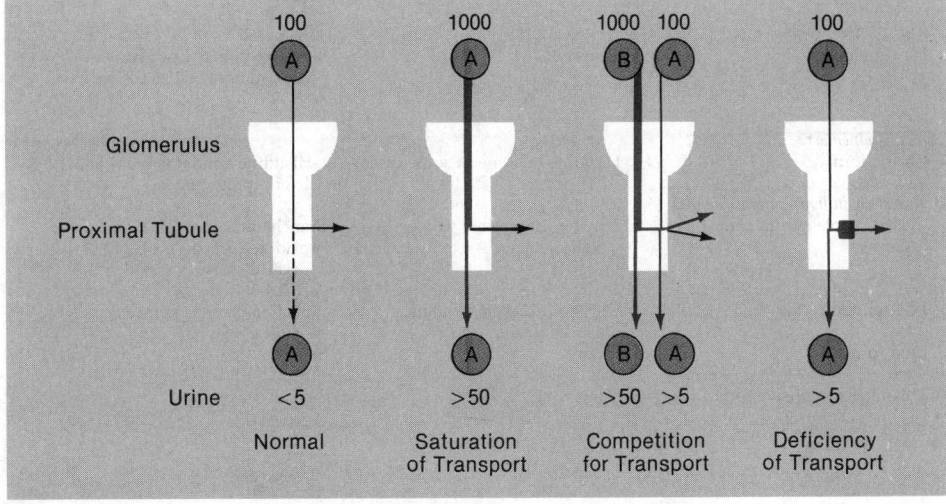

FIGURE 187–1. Mechanisms of hyperaminoaciduria. *Panel 1:* Normal reabsorption reclaims > 95 per cent of filtered amino acid molecules. Hyperaminoaciduria can occur if (*Panel 2*) filtered load increases (10× increase shown) and transport mechanism is saturated, or (*Panel 3*) amino acid in excess competes with another on a shared carrier, or (*Panel 4*) carrier is modified (mutant) or coupling of energy to carrier is impaired.

TABLE 187–1. HEREDITARY AND ACQUIRED AMINOACIDOPATHIES

The aminoacidurias presented in this table are divided into acquired and inherited types. Disturbances related to perinatal adaptive phenomena of multifactorial origin are included. The classification recognizes physiologic factors affecting amino acid distribution between plasma and urine, and whether the disorder primarily affects catabolism or membrane transport of the amino acid(s).

Thus the disorders are grouped according to mechanism and preferred fluid for detection. The data refer to those conditions associated with perturbation of the normal content of ninhydrin-reactive metabolites in plasma or urine; some exceptions have been made to include ninhydrin-negative metabolites.

GROUP IA

The primary defect is in catabolism. There is a low renal clearance of amino acid but a hyperaminoaciduria by saturation of transepithelial transport. Detection in the plasma is preferable unless otherwise indicated, but the use of urine for screening (or diagnosis) is not precluded; assignment to this group implies primarily that diagnosis (or screening) of the condition is feasible by virtue of significant metabolite accumulation in blood (or plasma).

Amino Acid Affected:
↓ = decreased; ↑ = increased. Source of enzyme number is *Enzyme Commission*. IP = apparent inheritance pattern; AR = autosomal recessive; AD = autosomal dominant; (AR) = probably autosomal recessive; XL = X-linked. *Remarks*: CNS = central nervous system; CoA = coenzyme A; CSF = cerebrospinal fluid.

Condition or Disease	Amino Acid Affected	Enzyme Affected (Synonym) In Group A	IP	Remarks
		*Common Perinatal (Adaptive) Traits**		
Neonatal hyperphenylalaninemia	Phenylalanine	Phenylalanine 4-monooxygenase (phenylalanine-hydroxylating system) [1.14.16.1]	—	Benign; may respond to folic acid; often occurs with tyrosinemia
Neonatal tyrosinemia	Tyrosine	4-Hydroxyphenylpyruvate dioxygenase (*p*-hydroxyphenyl pyruvic acid hydroxylase) [1.13.11.27]	—	Benign; responds to ascorbic acid and reduced protein intake
Hypermethioninemia	Methionine	? Methionine adenosyltransferase (ATP:L-methionine S-adenosyltransferase) [2.5.1.6]	—	Benign; usually found with high protein intake
Hyperhistidinemia	Histidine	? L-Histidine ammonia-lyase [4.3.1.3]	—	Benign; related to high protein intake
		Inherited Traits		
Hyperphenylalaninemia				
Classic phenylketonuria	Phenylalanine	Phenylalanine 4-monooxygenase (L-phenylalanine, tetrahydropteridine:oxygen oxidoreductase [4-hydroxylating]) [1.14.16.1]	AR	Plasma phenylalanine > 16 mg/100 ml; causes mental retardation; when untreated, L-phenylalanine tolerance in diet is 250–500 mg/day
Atypical phenylketonuria	Phenylalanine	Same	(AR)	Plasma phenylalanine > 16 mg/100 ml; similar to entry above, but dietary tolerance for L-phenylalanine is > 500 mg/day
Transient phenylketonuria	Phenylalanine	Same	(AR)	Plasma phenylalanine > 16 mg/100 ml; change in status to that of next entry or normal, several months or years after birth
Benign hyperphenylalaninemia	Phenylalanine	Same	AR	Plasma phenylalanine < 16 mg/100 ml on normal diet; benign trait
Dihydropteridine reductase deficiency	Phenylalanine	Dihydropteridine reductase [1.6.99.7]	AR	Deficient tetrahydrobiopterin cofactor also impairs biosynthesis of L-DOPA and 5-HT in CNS; low phenylalanine diet does not correct this
Biopterin synthesis defect	Phenylalanine	Various enzymes in synthesis pathway	AR	See preceding entry
Hypertyrosinemias				
Tyrosinosis (Medes)	Tyrosine	? Tyrosine aminotransferase (L-tyrosine:α-ketoglutarate aminotransferase) [2.6.1.5]	(AR)	One case known; myasthenia gravis probably incidental finding
Hypertyrosinemia I	Tyrosine (and methionine in acute stage)	Fumarylacetoacetate hydrolase [3.7.1.2]	AR	Hepatic cirrhosis and renal tubular failure; usually fatal in absence of tyrosine restriction
Hypertyrosinemia II	Tyrosine	Soluble (cytosol) tyrosine aminotransferase [2.6.1.5]	AR	Associated with developmental retardation; Richner-Hanhart syndrome in some patients
Hawkinsinuria	Tyrosine	4-Hydroxyphenyl pyruvate dioxygenase [1.13.11.27]	AD	Disease signs are variable and include failure to thrive; reflect formation of epoxides and adducts of glutathione
Hyperhistidnemia†				
Classic form	Histidine (alanine in some cases)	L-Histidine ammonia-lyase [4.3.1.3]; liver, epidermis	AR	Harmless condition in majority
Branched-chain hyperaminoacidemia‡				
Classic maple syrup urine disease	Leucine, isoleucine, valine, alloisoleucine	Branched-chain α-ketoacid lipoate oxidoreductase (probably decarboxylase component) [1.2.4.3(4)]	AR	Postnatal collapse; mental retardation in survivors; diet therapy can be effective
Intermittent form	Leucine, isoleucine, valine, alloisoleucine	Branched-chain α-ketoacid oxidase(s)§ [1.2.4.3(4)]	(AR)	Intermittent symptoms; development may be otherwise normal
Mild form	Same	Same	(AR)	Unremittent; milder than classic form
Thiamine-responsive form	Same	Same	(AR)	Mild form; responsive to thiamine (vitamin B₁)

TABLE 187–1. HEREDITARY AND ACQUIRED AMINO ACIDOPATHIES *Continued*

Condition or Disease	Amino Acid Affected	Enzyme Affected (Synonym) In Group A	IP	Remarks
		Inherited Traits (Continued)		
Multiple dehydrogenase form	Same (plus pyruvate and α-ketoglutarate)	Dihydrolipoamide dehydrogenase [1.8.1.4]	(AR)	Congenital lactic acidosis plus branched-chain amino-keto acid disorder
Hypervalinemia	Valine	Branched-chain amino-acid aminotransferase (valine aminotransferase) [2.6.1.66]	AR	Retarded development and vomiting; responds to diet
Type I hyperlysinemia	Lysine	Deficient "aminoadipic semialdehyde synthase" (bifunctional enzyme with lysine-ketoglutarate reductase [1.5.1.8] + saccharopine reductase [1.5.1.9] activities)	AR	Associated with mental retardation, hypotonia
Type 2 hyperlysinemia	Lysine, methionine and homocyst(e)ine	Only saccharopine reductase activity of bifunctional enzyme is deficient	AR	Same as above
Homocyst(e)inuria (methylene THF reductase deficiency)	Methionine (low) and homocyst(e)ine (high)	5,10-Methylenetetrahydrofolate reductase [1.7.99.5]	AR	Defective remethylation of homocysteine to methionine; neurologic and behavioral symptoms associated
Homocyst(e)inuria (with methylmalonic aciduria)	Homocyst(e)ine (high), methionine (low); plus methylmalonate	a. Defective cobalamin coenzyme biosynthesis b. Defective cobalamin transport (lysosomal)	AR (AR)	Defective remethylation of homocysteine and methylmalonyl-CoA mutase (MMA mutase) activity; severe neurologic signs and acidosis after birth
Cystathioninuria†	Cystathionine	Cystathionine γ-lyase [4.4.1.1]	AR	Probably benign trait; vitamin B_6 corrects biochemical trait in most patients
Hyperglycinemias Ketotic form	Glycine and other glucogenic amino acids	Propionyl-CoA carboxylase (ATP-hydrolyzing) propanoyl-CoA:carbon-dioxide ligase [ADP-forming]) [6.4.1.3]	AR	Ketosis, neutropenia, mental retardation; often fatal; detectable in skin fibroblasts
Ibid.	Ibid.	Methylmalonyl-CoA mutase [5.4.99.2]	AR	Symptoms are those of methylmalonic aciduria with acidosis (some mutase-affected patients are responsive to vitamin B_{12})
Ibid.	Ibid.	Acetyl-CoA acyltransferase (β-ketothiolase) [2.3.1.16] deficiency¶	AR	Signs are those of α-methyl-β-hydroxybutyric aciduria (with or without tiglic aciduria) and acidosis
Nonketotic form	Glycine	Glycine cleavage reaction (CO_2, NH_3, and hydroxymethyltetrahydrofolate formed) [1.4.4.2, 2.1.2.10]	AR	Severe CNS depression soon after birth; high CSF:plasma glycine ratio; benzoate decreases plasma glycine; no effect on CNS prognosis; strychnine improves seizures
Sarcosinemia†	Sarcosine	Sarcosine oxidase (sarcosine:oxygen oxidoreductase [demethylating]) [1.5.3.1]	AR	Benign trait (probably)
"Sarcosinemia" (glutaric aciduria, type II)	Sarcosine (glutaric acid and multiple fatty acids)	? Electron transfer flavoprotein (affecting multiple aryl-CoA dehydrogenases) [1.3.99.2-3]	AR	Postnatal lethargy, vomiting, coma, and acidosis; odor; multiple abnormalities of fatty acid oxidation
Hyperprolinemias Type I	Proline	L-Proline dehydrogenase (oxidase) [1.5.99.8]	AR	Benign trait
Type II	Proline	1-Pyrroline dehydrogenase (Δ¹-pyrroline-5-carboxylate:NAD⁺ oxidoreductase) [1.5.1.12]	AR	Benign trait; Δ¹-pyrroline-5-carboxylate and 3-hydroxy-1-pyrroline-5-carboxylate excreted in urine
Hyperhydroxyprolinemia	Hydroxyproline	4-Hydroxy-L-proline dehydrogenase (oxidase) [1.1.1.104]	AR	Benign trait
Hyperlysinemias, Hypertryptophanemias, and Related Diseases Type I	Lysine (and glutamine)	Saccharopine dehydrogenase (NADP⁺, lysine-forming) [1.5.1.8]	AR	Associated with mental retardation and hypotonia
Saccharopinuria†	Lysine, saccharopine, citruline	? Saccharopine dehydrogenase (NADP⁺, L-glutamate-forming) (saccharopine dehydrogenase) [1.5.1.10]	AR	Associated with mental retardation
Pipecolic acidemia†	Pipecolic acid	L-Pipecolate dehydrogenase (pipecolate oxidase) [1.5.99.3]	AR	Hepatomegaly and mental retardation (peroxisomal dis.)
α-Aminoadipic aciduria	α-Aminoadipic acid	? Mitochondrial α-aminoadipate amino transferase [2.6.1.39]	(AR)	Variable clinical features
α-Ketoadipic aciduria	α-Aminoadipic and α-ketoadipic acids	? α-Ketoadipic decarboxylase	(AR)	Mental retardation
Glutaric aciduria type I	Glutaric acid	? Glutaryl-CoA dehydrogenase [1.3.99.7]	(AR)	Mental retardation
Glutaric aciduria type II (multiple acyl-CoA dehydrogenase deficiency)	Glutaric acid, complex organic aciduria, sarcosine	Electron transport flavoprotein [1.3.99.2-3]	AR	Severe form, neonatal metabolic disease; adult form, recurrent hypoglycemia
Hydroxylysinemia	Free hydroxylysine	? Hydroxylysine kinase [2.7.1.81]	(AR)	Mental retardation
Tryptophanemia	Tryptophan (with indoleketonuria)	? Formamidase [3.5.1.9]	(AR)	Variable, probably benign

Table continues on following page. See page 1154 for footnotes.

TABLE 187–1. HEREDITARY AND ACQUIRED AMINOACIDOPATHIES *Continued*

Condition or Disease	Amino Acid Affected	Enzyme Affected (Synonym) In Group A	IP	Remarks
Inherited Traits (Continued)				
Hyperammonemias				
Carbamyl phosphate synthetase (CPS) deficiency	Glycine, glutamine	Carbamate kinase (ATP:carbamate phosphotransferase) [2.7.2.2]	AR	Group of diseases with ammonia intoxication, protein intolerance, hepatomegaly, vomiting, etc.; argininosuccinic aciduria also has trichorrhexis nodosa
Ornithine transcarbamylase (OTC) deficiency	Glutamine	Ornithine carbamoyltransferase (carbamoylphosphate:L-ornithine carbamoyltransferase [2.1.3.3]	XL	Same as above
Citrullinemia	Citrulline	Argininosuccinate synthetase (L-citrulline:L-aspartate ligase [AMP-forming]) [6.3.4.5]	AR	Same as above
Argininosuccinicaciduria†	Argininosuccinic acid	Argininosuccinate lyase (L-argininosuccinate arginine-lyase) [4.3.2.1]	AR	Same as above
Hyperargininemia	Arginine	Arginase (L-arginine amidinohydrolase) [3.5.3.1]	AR	Deterioration of CNS function and IQ in childhood; hyperammonemia (inconstant) aggravated by protein
Hyperornithinemia	Ornithine	Unknown (mitochondrial ornithine transport system?)	AR	Associated with hyperammonemia and homocitrullinemia (HHH syndrome)
Hyperornithinemia (without hyperammonemia)	Ornithine	L-Ornithine; 2-oxoacid aminotransferase [2.6.1.13]	AR	Associated with gyrate atrophy of choroid and retina but no hyperammonemia
Hyperalaninemia	Alanine	Pyruvate dehydrogenase (lipoate) (pyruvate dehydrogenase) [1.2.4.1] deficiency, pyruvate carboxylase [6.4.1.1] deficiency, and other defects	AR	Lactic acidosis, intermittent ataxia, mental retardation
			AR	Intermittent lactic acidosis, intermittent hypoglycemia
Aspartylglucosaminuria	Glycoasparagines	Aspartylglucosylaminase (2-acetamido-1[β¹-L-aspartamido]-1,2-dideoxyglucose amidohydrolase) [3.5.1.26]	AR	Lysosomal disease; mental retardation
Glutathionemia†	Glutathione or related peptides	γ-Glutamyltransferase (γ-glutamyltranspeptidase) [2.3.2.2]	AR	Mental retardation associated with finding
Hyperthreoninemia	Threonine	Unknown	(AR)	Seizures
Other Conditions Which May Affect Amino Acids in Plasma				
Protein-calorie malnutrition	Tryptophan/leucine/isoleucine/ valine ↓; tyrosine/glycine/proline ↑	—	—	Severity of change related to severity of malnutrition
Prolonged fasting	Alanine ↓; threonine, glycine ↑	—	—	Early fasting does not show same pattern
Obesity	Leucine/isoleucine/valine/ phenylalanine/tyrosine ↑; glycine ↓	—	—	Reflects insulin insensitivity
Hepatitis	Methionine/tyrosine ↑	—	—	Reflects severity of liver disease

*These conditions have been detected by screening methods applied in the newborn period of life. They should not be misdiagnosed as permanent disorders of amino acid metabolism also identifiable by screening.

†Urine screening is as efficient as, or even more reliable than, blood screening in these conditions.

‡A number of disorders of branched-chain amino acid catabolism cause accumulation of substances that are ninhydrin negative. These compounds can usually be detected by gas-liquid chromatographic methods (see Goodman SI: Am J Hum Genet 32:781, 1980).

§Partial activity; more than 2 per cent of normal.

¶Hyperglycemia observed only in some patients with this enzyme deficiency.

GROUP IB

The primary defect is in catabolism. There is a high renal clearance of amino acid and a hyperaminoaciduria by saturation of transepithelial transport. Detection in the urine is preferable.

Source of enzyme number is *Enzyme Commission*. IP = apparent inheritance pattern; AR = autosomal recessive; (AR) = probably autosomal recessive; AD = autosomal dominant.

Condition or Disease	Substance Affected (Synonym)	Enzyme Affected (Synonym) [Enzyme Commission No.]	IP	Remarks
Hypophosphatasia	Phosphoethanolamine	? Deficiency of ethanolaminephosphate phospho-lyase (O-phosphorylethanolamine phospho-lyase) [4.2.99.7]	AR	"Rickets" unresponsive to vitamin D; craniosynostosis; hypercalcemia
Pseudohypophosphatasia	Phosphoethanolamine	? Same as above; activity present but altered	(AR)	Same as above
β-Aminoisobutyric-aciduria	β-Aminoisobutyric acid	?	AD/AR	Benign polymorphic trait

TABLE 187–1. HEREDITARY AND ACQUIRED AMINOACIDOPATHIES *Continued*

Condition or Disease	Substance Affected (Synonym)	Enzyme Affected (Synonym) *In Group A*	IP	Remarks
4-Hydroxybutyric aciduria (γ-amino butyrate pathway)	γ-OH butyrate	Succinic semialdehyde dehydrogenase [1.2.1.24]	AR	Mental retardation, hypotonia. Detectable by GC/MS analysis of urine, plasma, CSF
Hyper-β-alaninemia	β-Alanine	? β-Alanine-pyruvate aminotransferase (β-alanine transaminase) [2.6.1.18]		Seizures; somnolence; mental retardation
Carnosinemia	Carnosine	Aminoacyl-histidine dipeptidase (carnosinase) [3.4.13.3]	AR	Seizure and mental retardation; or benign possibly
Pyroglutamic aciduria*	L-Pyroglutamic acid (5-oxo-L-proline; pyrrolidone-2-carboxylic acid)	Glutathione synthetase [6.3.2.3]	AR	L-Pyroglutamic acid (5-oxo-L-proline) results from overproduction via modified γ-glutamyl cycle

*Urine screening is as efficient as, or even more reliable than, blood screening in these conditions

GROUP II

There is a primary defect in catabolism and a secondary defect in transport. Hyperaminoaciduria is of combined origin—saturation and competition. Detection is possible in both plasma and urine.

Disease	Amino Acids Affected in Plasma	Amino Acids Present in Urine	Remarks
Hyperprolinemia, types I and II	Proline	Proline, + hydroxyproline and glycine	See entries in Group IA; competition occurs on iminoglycine transport system (see Group III)
Hyper-β-alaninemia	β-Alanine	β-Alanine, + β-aminoisobutyric acid and taurine	See Hyper-β-alaninemia in Group IB; competition occurs on β-amino transport system
Hyperlysinemia	Lysine	Lysine, + ornithine and arginine	See entries in Group IA; competition occurs on "dibasic" transport system (see Group III)
Hyperargininemia	Arginine	Ornithine and lysine, and sometimes generalized hyperaminoaciduria	See entry Hyperargininemia in Group IA; competition occurs on "dibasic" transport system (see Group III); pathogenesis of generalized aminoaciduria unknown

GROUP III

The primary defect is in the renal membrane transport site. There is a high renal clearance of amino acid, and detection is possible only in the urine. *Activity Affected:* Presumed gene product activity affected by mutant gene. IP = apparent inheritance pattern; AD = autosomal dominant; (AD) = proba-

bly autosomal dominant; AR = autosomal recessive; (AR) = probably autosomal recessive; XL = X-linked. *Remarks:* PTH = parathyroid hormone.

Trait	Substance Affected	Activity Affected	Other Tissues Affected	IP	Remarks
Common Perinatal (Adaptive) Trait					
Neonatal iminoglycinuria	Proline, hydroxyproline, glycine	Specific proline and specific glycine transport (probably)	—	—	Benign adaptive trait; prolinuria subsides at ~ 100 days, glycinuria at ~ 200 days after full-term birth
Neonatal cystine-lysinuria	Cystine and dibasic amino acids (lysine, ornithine, and arginine)	Specific dibasic transport system	—	—	Transient; evident in newborn period in some but not all infants
Inherited Hyperaminoacidurias					
Selective					
Hyperdibasic aminoaciduria type 2 (Lysinuric-protein intolerance)	Lysine, ornithine, arginine ("dibasic" group)	Shared "dibasic" amino acid transport system in basolateral membrane	Intestine (basolateral membrane, efflux defect). Fibroblasts (plasma membrane; efflux defect on γ⁺ system)	AR	Associated with protein intolerance, failure to thrive, hyperammonemia basolateral membrane defect; silent carrier
Hyperdibasic aminoaciduria type I	Lysine, ornithine, arginine	Shared "dibasic" amino acid transport system (brush-border membrane)	Intestine	AR/AD	Associated with mental retardation in one reported patient; carriers have hyper dibasic aminoaciduria
Isolated hyperlysinuria	Lysine	Lysine-specific system (brush border)	Intestine	AR	One proband reported
Classic cystinuria	Lysine, ornithine, arginine, and cystine	Shared membrane system in brush-border membrane	Intestine	AR	"Negative" reabsorption of affected amino acid can occur; three alleles (? same locus), each causing different phenotypes: in type I carrier (vs. types II and III) no excess of amino acids in urine ("silent"); in type III patient, intestinal transport intact (or partial defect)
Hypercystinuria	Cyst(e)ine	Specific system for cyst(e)ine	?	(AR)	One pedigree only
Iminoglycinuria	Proline; hydroxyproline; glycine	Shared system for imino acids, glycine (and sarcosine)	Intestine	AR	Four alleles (? same locus); I and II are silent carriers; III and IV are hyperglycinuric carriers; I associated with intestinal defect; IV with K_m mutant

Table continues on following page. See page 1154 for footnotes.

TABLE 187–1. HEREDITARY AND ACQUIRED AMINOACIDOPATHIES *Continued*

Trait	Substance Affected	Activity Affected	Other Tissues Affected	IP	Remarks
Inherited Hyperaminoacidurias (Continued)					
Hartnup disorder	Neutral amino acids (excluding imino acids, glycine, cyst(e)ine and β-amino acids	Shared system for large neutral amino acid group (luminal membrane)	Intestine	AR	Three alleles (? same locus); I, intestine affected; II, intestine normal; III, kidney normal; carrier "silent" in all
Hyperhistidinuria	Histidine		Intestine	AR	Associated with mental retardation in siblings
Hyperdicarboxylic aminoaciduria (glutamate-aspartate transport defect)	Glutamic acid, aspartic acid	Shared dicarboxylic acid transport system (brush-border membrane)	Intestine ±	AR	Benign
Idiopathic (primary genetic) Fanconi syndrome	Generalized effect on all solutes and water	? Coupling of energy; ? tight junction integrity	Secondary to renal phenotype	AR (and AD)	Adult onset and infantile-childhood forms are differentiated; basic defect unknown; probably several alleles
Secondary genetic forms of Fanconi syndrome					
Cystinosis; type I, type II	Same as above (secondary response)	Cystine storage (lysosomal defect), with secondary damage to tubule and glomerulus (later)	Secondary to renal phenotype	AR*	Several alleles; infantile (type I) and adolescent (type II) forms have differing rates for onset of nephropathy; "adult" form (type III) has no nephropathy
Hereditary fructose intolerance	Same as above, + fructose	Fructose-1-phosphate aldolase (fructose bisphosphate aldolase) (with secondary effects on cellular ATP)	Secondary to renal phenotype (hepatic cirrhosis)	AR	Nephropathy dependent on intact PTH-cAMP axis in kidney; responds to fructose withdrawal
Galactosemia	Same as above, + galactose	Galactose-1-phosphate uridylytransferase (with secondary effects on cellular ATP)	Secondary to renal phenotype (cataracts, CNS effects)	AR	Fanconi's syndrome responds to galactose withdrawal; "Galactosemia" due to galactokinase deficiency does *not* have Fanconi's syndrome
Hereditary tyrosinemia	Same as above, + tyrosine metabolites	Unknown (with secondary effects on cellular ATP)	Secondary to renal phenotype (hepatic cirrhosis)	AR	Fanconi's syndrome responds to tyrosine restriction
Wilson's disease	Same as above, with proximal and distal renal tubular acidosis	Unknown (? secondary effects on cytochrome oxidase system)	Hepatolenticular degeneration	AR	Fanconi's syndrome responds to depletion of copper storage
Lowe's oculocerebrorenal syndrome	Generalized dysfunction with defective urinary NH₃ production	Unknown	An oculocerebro-intestinal-renal syndrome (? involving tissues with high γ-glutamyl cycle activity)	XL†	Basic defect still unknown: treatment for tubular reclamation defects does not improve mental retardation or the cataracts and hydrophthalmia
Vitamin D dependency (pseudodeficiency rickets)	Generalized defect (secondary response)	Type I: 25-Hydroxyvitamin D-1-α-hydroxylase Type II: Defective binding of hormone	Deficiency of synthesis or binding affects intestinal absorption of calcium and initiates PTH response	AR	Nephropathy dependent on PTH excess and hypocalcemia (phenocopy occurs in vitamin D deficiency)
Miscellaneous					
Glycoglycinuria	Glucose and glycine	Unknown (the two solutes do *not* share a common carrier)	—	(AD)	Asymptomatic; normal-Tm (type B) glucosuria; possibility that there is a heterozygous manifestation of a Fanconi-like tubulopathy merits consideration
Luder-Sheldon syndrome	Generalized amino acids, glucose, and phosphate	Unknown	—	AD	Symptoms of Fanconi's syndrome have occurred in probands
Rowley-Rosenberg syndrome	Generalized aminoaciduria	Unknown	—	(AR)	Associated components of syndrome; growth retardation, muscular hypoplasia, pulmonary involvement, and right ventricular hypertrophy

*For each type
†Recessive.

Benson PF, Fensom AH: Genetic Biochemical Disorders. Oxford Monographs on the Medical Genetics No. 12. Oxford, Oxford University Press, 1985. *A "handbook," leaner than* The Metabolic Basis of Inherited Disease *(the standard "encyclopedia"), that covers, in short essays, nearly all entries in Table 187–1.*

Scriver CR, and Tenenhouse HS: Mendelian phenotypes as "probes" of renal transport systems for amino acids and phosphate. Handbook of Physiology (Renal Section, 1987). *A review of the amino acid transport systems (in kidney and other tissues) delineated by mutations in man and of their relative importance in metabolic homeostasis.*

Wellner D, Meister A: A survey of inborn errors of amino acid metabolism and transport in man. Annu Rev Biochem 50:911, 1981. *A crisp review of events in a field that now moves more slowly than it once did.*

The *group-specific sites* are classified into the β-amino system and the α-amino systems. Within the following list, the representative inborn error of amino acid metabolism that reveals the system is also indicated.

1. *The β-amino system*: β-alanine, β-aminoisobutyric acid, and taurine (viz., hyper-β-alaninemia)
2. *The α-amino systems*:
   a. "Dibasic" systems
      i. System I: lysine, arginine, ornithine, and cystine in brush border membrane (viz., cystinuria)
      ii. System II: lysine, arginine, ornithine in basal-lateral membrane (viz., lysinuric-protein intolerance)
   b. "Acidic" system: aspartic, glutamic (viz., dicarboxylic aminoaciduria)
   c. "Neutral" systems
      i. System I: proline, hydroxyproline, and glycine (viz., hyperprolinemia and renal iminoglycinuria)
      ii. System II: the remaining neutral α-amino acids (viz., Hartnup disorder)

It is usually possible to classify the aminoaciduria and its pathogenesis by analyzing the amino acid content of plasma and urine collected conjointly (see Table 187–1 and Fig. 187–1). Elution chromatography and gas chromatography–mass spectrometry will reveal the details of hyperaminoaciduria and any related organic aciduria. The recognition of a specific disorder of amino acid metabolism may provide an opportunity for treatment and, by genetic counseling, could prevent disease in relatives.

Rosenberg LE, Scriver CR: Disorders of amino acid metabolism In Bondy PK, Rosenberg LE (eds.): Metabolic Control and Disease. Philadelphia, W. B. Saunders Company, 1980, pp 583–776.

Scriver CR, Rosenberg LE: Amino Acid Metabolism and Its Disorders. Philadelphia, W. B. Saunders Company, 1973.

Wellner D, Meister A: A survey of inborn errors of amino acid metabolism and transport in man. Annu Rev Biochem 50:911. 1981

188 THE HYPERPHENYLALANINEMIAS
Lloyd H. Smith, Jr.

Phenylalanine is an essential amino acid. In its main metabolic pathway phenylalanine is irreversibly hydroxylated in the 4 position of its phenyl ring to form tyrosine, a reaction catalyzed by phenylalanine hydroxylase (Fig. 188–1). In addition to its role in protein synthesis, tyrosine is necessary as a precursor of the biogenic amines dopamine and norepinephrine in the central nervous system, of thyroxine and triiodothyronine in the thyroid gland, and of melanin in melanocytes. The hydroxylation of phenylalanine to form tyrosine is a complex reaction that requires the apoenzyme phenylalanine hydroxylase, oxygen, and a specific cofactor, tetrahydrobiopterin, as an electron donor. In the process of the reaction tetrahydrobiopterin is oxidized to dihydroquinone and must be regenerated by dihydropteridine reductase (and NADH) before it is again functional in phenylalanine metabolism (Fig. 188–1). In this system there are several sites for possible metabolic errors, and in fact a number of disorders have been described characterized by hyperphenylalaninemia (greater than 1.2 mg per deciliter of plasma). When phenylalanine accumulates there is increased shunting into its minor metabolites: phenylpyruvate, phenyllactate, phenylacetate, and phenylacetylglutamine.

CLASSIC PHENYLKETONURIA

Phenylketonuria was one of the first metabolic abnormalities to be established as a cause of mental deficiency, being discovered in 1934 by Følling with the use of the ferric chloride test (for phenylpyruvate). Phenylketonuria is an autosomal recessive disorder, which in the homozygote results in a severe deficiency of phenylalanine hydroxylase activity secondary to an abnormality of the apoenzyme. Heterozygotes have partial activity, which is sufficient to maintain normal plasma levels of phenylalanine in most circumstances. Phenylketonuria occurs with a prevalence of approximately 1 in each 10,000 to 12,000 births in whites and Orientals with a carrier rate of 2 per 100, but it occurs much less frequently in blacks.

CLINICAL MANIFESTATIONS. Patients with phenylketonuria are usually normal at birth. If the disease is unrecognized and untreated, however, the infant during the first year of life gradually develops mental retardation, delayed psychomotor maturation, tremors, seizures, eczema, a tendency to hypopigmentation, and hyperactivity. Impairment of mental function is usually severe, with I.Q. scores less than 50, and this taken with the other neurologic problems leads to the need for the majority of untreated patients to be institutionalized. There may be a "mousy odor" to the patient, and especially to the urine, which has been attributed to phenylacetic acid. Early diagnosis and treatment of phenylketonuria, within the first month of life, will prevent the development of these clinical complications.

PATHOGENESIS. The marked reduction in phenylalanine hydroxylase activity in classic phenylketonuria results in hyperphenylalaninemia with concentrations usually exceeding 16 mg per deciliter of plasma (approximately 1 mM). In addition, the shunting of phenylalanine into its transamination pathway leads to the excessive production and urinary excretion of phenylpyruvate and the other metabolites listed earlier. The mechanism of the neurologic deficit in phenylketonuria has not been established, but it is clearly related to the accumulation of phenylalanine (or its metabolites) rather than to a deficiency of tyrosine or its metabolites, since control of the hyperphenylalaninemia by diet prevents complications. Phenylalanine may inhibit the transport and therefore the availability of other amino acids to the brain during a critical time in its growth and maturation. Phenylalanine has been shown to be a competitive inhibitor of tyrosinase in the pathway of melanin synthesis, which is the probable explanation for the pigment dilution seen in untreated patients. In phenylketonuria tyrosine becomes an essential amino acid, but this requirement for tyrosine is usually adequately met from dietary sources.

DIAGNOSIS. The diagnosis of phenylketonuria is now usually made by screening techniques during the neonatal period. These techniques depend upon the demonstration of hyperphenylalaninemia rather than urinary phenylketonuria, since the transaminase necessary for the formation of phenylpyruvate may not be fully active in the neonatal period. The most widely used test is the Guthrie bacterial inhibition assay, which can detect excess levels of phenylalanine from a single drop of capillary blood collected from a heel prick onto a special type of filter paper. An abnormal result must be followed up with more specific determinations of plasma phenylalanine, which is usually found to be more than 16 mg per deciliter when there is normal protein ingestion after the first few days of life. The differentiation of phenylketonuria from the other forms of the hyperphenylalaninemias depends upon the level of amino acid measured, whether it is sustained with time, and the biochemical and clinical response to dietary therapy. The recent cloning of the human phenylalanine hydroxylase gene now allows for the prenatal detection of about 87 per cent of either the carrier state or the homozygous disease in white families based on locus–specific DNA polymorphisms. The involved gene is on chromosome 12.

TREATMENT. In the absence of any method to replace the missing phenylalanine hydroxylase apoenzyme, treatment is dependent upon dietary restriction of phenylalanine. By the

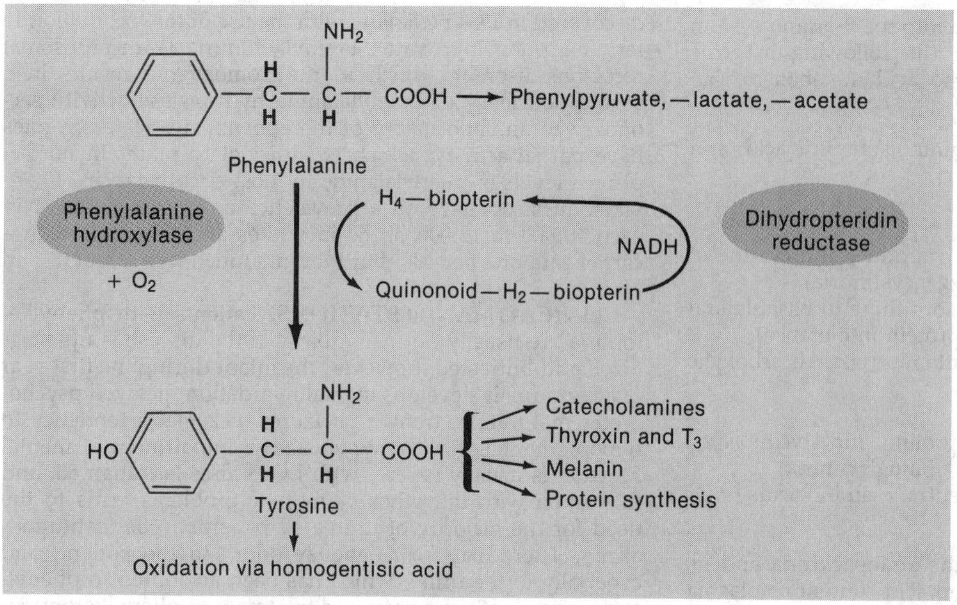

FIGURE 188–1. Pathways of phenylalanine and tyrosine metabolism.

use of special semisynthetic diets, such as Lofenalac or PKUaid in the United States, it is possible to reduce phenylalanine intake to 250 to 500 mg per day while maintaining good nutrition for all other dietary requirements. Phenylalanine ingestion is monitored to maintain its plasma level in the range of 3 to 12 mg per deciliter. This regimen has been found to be highly successful in preventing the clinical manifestations of the disease. Scrupulous adherence to such a dietary regimen is of particular importance during the early months of life. In the absence of clearly established guidelines, it is probably wise to continue dietary therapy at least through the first decade and perhaps indefinitely. It is particularly important that a woman with phenylketonuria maintain careful dietary control of her plasma levels of phenylalanine during pregnancy in order that the developing central nervous system of the fetus may not be damaged during intrauterine life.

HYPERPHENYLALANINEMIC VARIANTS

A number of variants from classic phenylketonuria may also be associated with increased concentrations of plasma phenylalanine in newborns. This is not surprising in view of the usual heterogeneity of genetic disorders and also the number of factors in the complex reaction catalyzed by phenylalanine hydroxylase (Fig. 188–1). It is important to distinguish these variants from classic phenylketonuria because they may have different prognoses and require different treatment programs. The benign disorders must also be carefully distinguished from "malignant hyperphenylalaninemia," as noted below.

TRANSIENT PHENYLKETONURIA. A number of patients exhibit the chemical findings of phenylketonuria at birth but have disappearance of these abnormalities over the following few weeks. It has been assumed that this syndrome represents a maturational delay in the development of some component of the phenylalanine hydroxylase system, although this has not been established. Dietary control of hyperphenylalaninemia is indicated during the initial phases of this syndrome (when it may not be distinguishable from classic phenylketonuria), but can later be discontinued.

PERSISTENT HYPERPHENYLALANINEMIA. Some patients exhibit milder forms of phenylketonuria and probably represent variants with higher residual activities of phenylalanine hydroxylase. Even in the absence of dietary control, their plasma levels of phenylalanine may be in the range of 4 to 16 mg per deciliter, levels not ordinarily associated with mental deficiency. Many of these patients do not require

therapy and would never have come to attention were it not for mass screening programs for newborns. This is a heterogeneous group of patients with varying degrees of impairment in the metabolism of phenylalanine.

MALIGNANT HYPERPHENYLALANINEMIA. A small number of patients in whom phenylketonuria is diagnosed by the criteria just outlined fail to respond clinically to dietary restriction of phenylalanine. The hyperphenylalaninemia responds to diet as anticipated, but despite this chemical response they develop progressive neurologic deficits and seizures and usually die in the first few years of life. These patients, who represent between 1 and 3 per cent of all infants with a positive Guthrie test, are missing dihydropteridine reductase, necessary for the regeneration of the tetrahydrobiopterin cofactor of phenylalanine hydroxylase (Fig. 188–1). Activity of dihydropteridine reductase can be assayed in skin fibroblasts and in peripheral blood cells (lymphocytes, granulocytes, and platelets). More rarely they may retain the reductase but exhibit a block in the biosynthesis of the cofactor. Although the adverse effects of the resulting defect in phenylalanine metabolism can be largely circumvented by diet, tetrahydrobiopterin is also a cofactor for at least two other hydroxylations important in the production of neurotransmitters in the central nervous system: the hydroxylation of tryptophan to 5-hydroxytryptophan and of tyrosine to L-dopa. It is assumed that these deficits, or deficits of other reactions not yet demonstrated that require the cofactor, explain the progressive neurologic abnormalities. A rapid test for malignant hyperphenylalaninemia is available in that a single oral dose of tetrahydrobiopterin* (2 mg per kilogram) will reduce the plasma phenylalanine to normal in six hours in these patients. Classic phenylketonuria, as expected, shows no response. Treatment of these patients is being attempted with 5-hydroxytryptophan and L-dopa as well as with a low phenylalanine diet. These patients can be treated with tetrahydrobiopterin and neurotransmitters without dietary restriction of phenylalanine. Tetrahydrobiopterin is not transported in significant amounts into the brain, so treatment with it alone does not suffice as replacement in malignant hyperphenylalaninemia.

*Investigational drug.

Daiger SP, Lidsky AS, Chakroborty R, et al.: Polymorphic DNA haplotypes at the phenylalanine hydroxylase locus in prenatal diagnosis of phenylketonuria. Lancet 1:229, 1986. *Description of the current status of using restriction fragment length polymorphisms for this purpose, with accuracy of diagnosis of approximately 87 per cent for siblings at risk.*

Danks DM, Schlesinger P, Firgaira F, et al.: Malignant hyperphenylalaninemia—clinical features, biochemical findings and experience with administration of biopterins. Pediatr Res 13:1150, 1979. *This report presents four patients with this most recently described variant of hyperphenylalaninemia and summarizes current clinical and biochemical knowledge concerning the effects of biopterin deficiency.*

Kaufman S, Woo S, Scriver CR: Disorders of phenylalanine metabolism. In Scriver CR, Beaudet A, Sly W, et al. (eds.): The Metabolic Basis of Inherited Disease. 6th ed. New York, McGraw-Hill Book Company, 1988, in press. *Although the emphasis in this review is on the pathogenesis of the various forms of the hyperphenylalaninemias, there is a reasonable clinical description and an extensive and useful bibliography.*

Ledley FD, Levy HL, Woo SL: Molecular analysis of the inheritance of phenylketonuria and mild hyperphenylalaninemia in families with both disorders. N Engl J Med 314:1276, 1986. *Demonstration of multiple and distinct mutations in the phenylalanemia hydroxylase gene.*

189 ALCAPTONURIA

James B. Wyngaarden

DEFINITION. Alcaptonuria is a rare hereditary disease in which homogentisic acid oxidase activity is missing. Homogentisic acid produced during the metabolism of phenylalanine and tyrosine accumulates and is excreted in the urine. It causes pigmentation of cartilage and other connective tissue (ochronosis) and in later years a degenerative arthritis of the spine and the larger peripheral joints. The disease has historic significance, for it was chiefly on the basis of study of families with alcaptonuria that Sir Archibald Garrod developed the concept of inborn errors of metabolism. The disease is inherited as an autosomal recessive trait. No method of detection of heterozygotes has been found.

INCIDENCE AND PREVALENCE. At least 600 cases have been reported, including one in an Egyptian mummy 3500 years old. A prevalence of three to five per million individuals was found in Northern Ireland.

PATHOGENESIS. The activity of homogentisic acid oxidase in the normal adult human liver is sufficient to metabolize over 1600 grams of homogentisic acid per day. Normally, no homogentisic acid can be detected in plasma or urine. In alcaptonuric individuals there is no detectable activity of this enzyme in liver or kidney tissue. Plasma levels of homogentisic acid rise to about 3 mg per deciliter, and the urinary excretion ranges from 4 to 8 grams per day. Mammalian tissue contains an enzyme called homogentisic acid polyphenoloxidase that catalyzes the oxidation of homogentisic acid to an ochronotic pigment, but pigment can also be produced nonenzymatically in the presence of oxygen and alkali, as for example in urine. The homogentisic acid polymer has a high affinity for cartilage and connective tissue macromolecules. The stained tissue is fragile and eventually may break down, leading to degenerative intervertebral disc or joint disease. Homogentisic acid may also have a direct effect upon collagen synthesis through inhibition of lysyl hydroxylase.

PATHOLOGY. In an adult alcaptonuric patient cartilage in many areas, particularly the costal, laryngeal, and tracheal cartilage, is densely pigmented, sometimes being coal-black in appearance. Pigmentation is also present throughout the body in fibrous tissue, fibrocartilage, tendons, and ligaments. To a lesser degree it is also found in the endocardium, in the intima of larger vessels, in various organs such as kidney and lung, and in the epidermis.

CLINICAL MANIFESTATIONS. Homogentisic acid is present in urine from birth, but urine is colorless when passed. Before the days of disposable diapers the diagnosis was sometimes made when diapers turned brown in alkaline soaps. Pigment may appear in perspiration and stain clothing in the axillary and genital regions. Generally, the earliest change that can be detected externally is a slight pigmentation of the sclerae or the ears, beginning at 20 or 30 years of age.

The cartilage of the ears may be slate blue or gray and feel irregular and thickened. Sometimes dusky discolorations of underlying tendons can be seen through the skin over the hands. In many patients, however, pigment is scarcely evident. The arthritis usually presents with limitation of motion of the hips, knee joints, or shoulders. There may be periods of acute inflammation, and later there is usually rather marked limitation of motion and ankylosis in the lumbosacral region. The arthritic complications are often severe and painful and may lead to extensive crippling. In addition, alcaptonuric patients appear to have a high incidence of cardiovascular disease, including generalized arteriosclerosis and chronic mitral and aortic valvulitis, with calcification of valves and annulus. At least one degenerated pigmented aortic valve has been replaced with a prosthesis. Myocardial infarction is a common cause of death. Other reported complications include ruptured intervertebral discs, prostatitis, and renal stones.

X-RAY CHANGES. These may be almost pathognomonic of alcaptonuria. The vertebral bodies of the lumbar spine show degeneration of the intervertebral discs with narrowing of the space and dense calcification of remaining disc material. There is variable fusion of vertebral bodies, but little osteophyte formation and minimal calcification of intervertebral ligaments. The degenerative changes of ochronotic arthritis are most severe in the hip, shoulder, and knee, and there may be calcific deposits in the tendons. The sacroiliac joints and smaller joints of the extremities usually show little or no abnormality. Ear cartilage may be calcified.

DIAGNOSIS AND DIFFERENTIAL DIAGNOSIS. The diagnosis is suggested by the history of pigmentary changes of urine, the presence of non-glucose reducing substance, the pigmentation of sclerae or cartilage, the arthritic episodes, and especially the typical x-ray changes of the lumbar spine. Specific identification of homogentisic acid in urine can be accomplished by chromatographic or enzymatic assays.

The ochronotic changes of skin and cartilage may be confused with pigmentary changes resulting from prolonged use of Atabrine, or use of carbolic acid dressings for chronic cutaneous ulcers. The arthritis must be differentiated chiefly from rheumatoid arthritis, osteoarthritis, and gout.

TREATMENT. There is no effective treatment. Dietary restriction of phenylalanine and tyrosine of the degree necessary to reduce homogentisic aciduria is impractical and potentially deleterious. Large amounts of ascorbic acid have been given in an effort to reduce pigment formation. Ascorbic acid protects lysyl hydroxylase from inhibition by homogentisic acid in vitro. It does not alter the metabolic defect.

Justesen P, Anderson PE Jr: Radiologic manifestations in alcaptonuria. Skeletal Radiol 11:204, 1984. *Characteristic radiologic findings are demonstrated.*

La Du BN: Alcaptonuria. In Stanbury JB, Wyngaarden JB, Fredrickson DS (eds.): The Metabolic Basis of Inherited Disease. 4th ed. New York, McGraw-Hill Book Company, 1978, p 268. *A detailed discussion of the history, clinical features, and biochemical derangements of alcaptonuria and ochronosis.*

190 HISTIDINEMIA

Lloyd H. Smith, Jr.

Histidinemia is a rare genetic disorder, probably transmitted as an autosomal recessive trait, in which the activity of histidase is markedly diminished. As a result there is a block in the conversion of histidine to urocanic acid. Histidine accumulates in the blood and is transaminated in increased amounts to imidazolepyruvic acid. In a screening program of urine specimens from newborns in Massachusetts, a prevalence of 1 in 14,190 was found for histidinemia. The diagnosis is established by demonstrating fasting hyperhistidinemia (four to ten times increased over the normal of approximately

1 mg per deciliter), histidinuria, and urinary imidazolepyruvic acid (which will give a positive ferric chloride test or Phenistix test for phenylketonuria). The enzyme defect can be demonstrated in biopsy specimens from skin and liver. In several patients low levels of platelet serotonin have been noted. In the past, varying degrees of mental retardation and of speech defects have been attributed to this genetic disorder. More recent evidence suggests that these represented the bias of ascertainment and that histidinemia has no demonstrated biologic disadvantage.

191 THE HYPERPROLINEMIAS AND HYDROXYPROLINEMIA
Lloyd H. Smith, Jr.

The imino acids proline and hydroxyproline are nonessential; proline is readily synthesized in the body from glutamate and ornithine and hydroxyproline from proline. The synthesis of hydroxyproline occurs uniquely in peptide linkage largely as a constituent of collagen. Three rare genetic disorders of the degradative pathways of the acids have been described.

HYPERPROLINEMIAS. Two distinct disorders of proline metabolism, both transmitted as autosomal recessive traits, are associated with hyperprolinemia. In Type I hyperprolinemia there is a block in the metabolism of proline to Δ'-pyrroline-5-carboxylate because of decreased activity of the enzyme proline oxidase. In Type II hyperprolinemia there is a block at the second step in the degradative pathway, the conversion of Δ'-pyrroline-5-carboxylate to L-glutamate, because of decreased activity of Δ'-pyrroline-5-carboxylate dehydrogenase. In both disorders the accumulation of proline in the blood leads to prolinuria and, through competition for a common renal tubular transport mechanism, to hydroxyprolinuria and glycinuria as well. In the Type II disorder there is also excessive urinary Δ'-pyrroline-5-carboxylate. The disorders can be diagnosed by finding the characteristic changes of hyperprolinemia and iminoaciduria as noted above. Although various forms of renal disease have been described with the Type I disorder and neurologic abnormalities and seizures in some patients with either Type I or Type II hyperprolinemia, these may represent the bias of ascertainment. Since no clinical entity has been clearly established, there is no indicated therapy for either form of hyperprolinemia.

HYDROXYPROLINEMIA. An increased plasma level of free hydroxyproline associated with hydroxyprolinuria has been described in members of several families, but this disorder has not resulted in prolinuria or glycinuria. The disorder is assumed to be an autosomal recessive trait in which the homozygote has deficient activity of hydroxyproline oxidase. There is no associated abnormality of collagen metabolism, and the urinary excretion of peptide-bound hydroxyproline is normal. As in the case of the hyperprolinemias, no clinical entity has been demonstrated and no treatment is indicated.

192 DISEASES OF THE UREA CYCLE
Lloyd H. Smith, Jr.

Humans are ureotelic; they are dependent upon the synthesis of urea for nitrogen excretion. The only source of net urea formation is through the urea cycle (Fig. 192–1), which consists of five enzymes necessary for the sequential synthesis of carbamyl phosphate, citrulline, argininosuccinate, arginine, and urea. When the function of this pathway is impaired, ammonia tends to accumulate. The associated clinical abnormalities show certain common features such as mental retardation and severe neurologic dysfunction. Genetic diseases associated with blocks at each of these five steps have been discovered and will be described briefly below. In addition, one patient has been described with deficiency of N-acetylglutamate synthetase, which catalyzes the formation of acetylglutamate, which is required for the activation of carbamyl phosphate synthetase in step 1, as shown in Figure 192–1.

CARBAMYL PHOSPHATE SYNTHETASE (CPS) DEFICIENCY. Carbamyl phosphate (CAP) channeled for urea synthesis, in contrast to pyrimidine-channeled CAP, is synthesized in mitochondria from ammonia, bicarbonate, and ATP in a reaction catalyzed by CPS in the presence of N-acetylglutamate as an enzyme activator. Approximately 19 patients with deficiency of CPS have been discovered, usually presenting with hyperammonemia, protein intolerance, and neurologic symptoms during the neonatal period. The diagnosis is established by measuring carbamyl phosphate synthetase in a liver biopsy or in peripheral leukocytes. There are no characteristic changes in amino acids in blood or urine.

ORNITHINE CARBAMYL TRANSFERASE (OCT) DEFICIENCY. OCT catalyzes the mitochondrial carbamylation of ornithine by CAP to form citrulline. Approximately 40 to 50 patients have been described with hyperammonemia and neurologic abnormalities secondary to deficient activity of OCT. The disorder seems to be transmitted as a sex-linked dominant trait with hemizygous males rarely surviving the neonatal period; females manifest varying degrees of protein intolerance. As in the case of CPS deficiency, there are no detectable abnormalities of amino acid metabolism. Mitochondrial CAP accumulates, however, and spills over into the cytosol to drive pyrimidine synthesis (Fig. 192–1). This results in orotic aciduria as a constant finding. The enzyme defect can be shown in biopsy specimens from liver or intestinal mucosa or in leukocytes. Prenatal diagnosis of the disease is now possible using a gene-specific probe.

ARGININOSUCCINATE (ASA) SYNTHETASE DEFICIENCY (CITRULLINEMIA). Citrulline synthesized in mitochondria normally diffuses into the cytosol, where it is condensed with L-aspartic acid in the presence of ATP to form argininosuccinic acid. This reaction is catalyzed by ASA synthetase. Approximately 20 patients who have been documented as having neonatal citrullinemia have exhibited marked heterogeneity in the severity of their clinical and

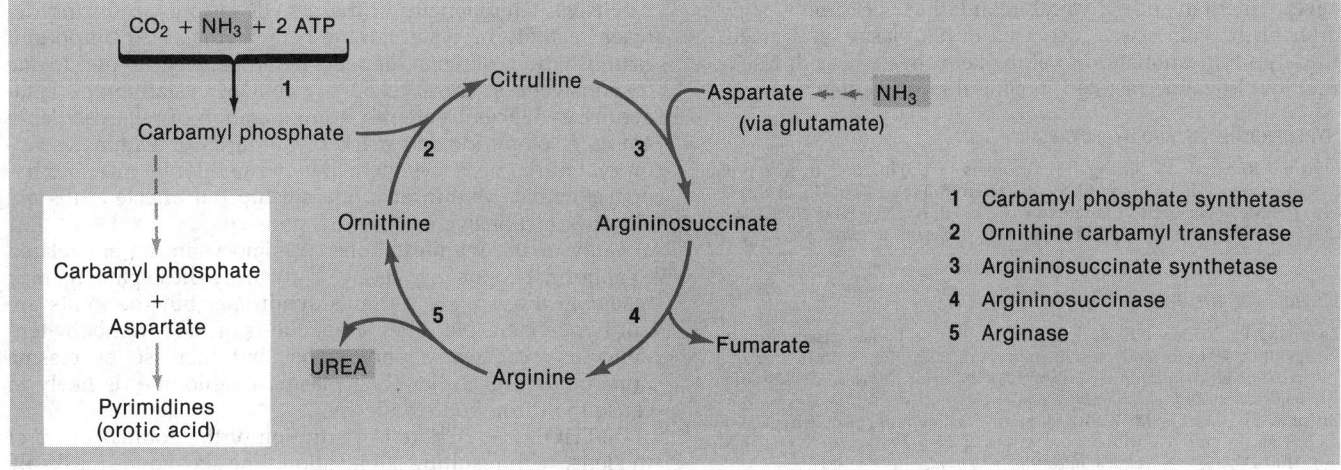

FIGURE 192–1. The urea cycle.

chemical manifestations. The associated hyperammonemia is in general less severe than in deficiency of CPS or OCT, but does occur after protein ingestion. Citrulline is increased in blood and urine, and secondary orotic aciduria has been noted, presumably reflecting excess CAP. Patients with a late onset form of presentation have been described, especially from Japan.

ARGININOSUCCINASE (ASase) DEFICIENCY (ARGININOSUCCINIC ACIDURIA). Cytosolic argininosuccinic acid undergoes reversible cleavage to arginine and fumarate catalyzed by ASase. Approximately 60 patients have been described with argininosuccinic aciduria. Clinical findings, which vary widely in severity, have included mental retardation, seizures, ataxia, hepatomegaly and hepatic fibrosis, and friable hair (trichorrhexis nodosa). In addition to large amounts of ASA in blood, urine, and cerebrospinal fluid (readily demonstrable by chromatography), patients with ASase deficiency may have citrullinemia.

ARGINASE DEFICIENCY (HYPERARGININEMIA). Arginine is hydrolyzed to urea and ornithine, catalyzed by arginase, in the last step of the urea cycle. Only 13 patients have been described with deficiency of arginase, which has been associated with mental retardation and spasticity. Arginine is increased in blood and urine and may occasionally cause secondary cystinuria owing to competitive inhibition of the renal tubular transport of dibasic amino acids. Hyperammonemia may be found after protein ingestion. The absence of arginase can be conveniently demonstrated in circulating erythrocytes.

193 BRANCHED-CHAIN AMINOACIDURIA

Lloyd H. Smith, Jr.

Leucine, isoleucine, and valine are essential, so-called branched-chain amino acids, which have certain structural resemblances and share some common metabolic pathways. Three rare genetic disorders in the degradative pathways of the branched-chain amino acids will be described briefly.

MAPLE SYRUP URINE DISEASE. This disorder, also called *branched-chain ketonuria*, derives its name from the characteristic odor of the urine of affected infants. The disease is transmitted as a rare (1 in 120,000 to 290,000 births) autosomal recessive trait in which the affected homozygote exhibits deficient activity in the complex oxidative decarbox-

ylation pathway of the keto acids of leucine, isoleucine, and valine. As a consequence these three amino acids and their corresponding keto acids accumulate in excess in blood and urine and presumably throughout the body. A few patients have a variant disorder that responds to treatment with large amounts of thiamine (20 times the normal daily requirement). These patients have a dehydrogenase enzyme with a decreased affinity for alpha-ketoisovalerate and thiamine pyrophosphate. The pathogenesis of the deleterious effects in maple syrup urine disease has not been firmly established and may be complex, but probably relates mostly to the accumulation of leucine.

Severe hypotonia, lethargy, feeding difficulties, and hypoglycemia develop in the first week in an infant who seemed normal at birth. Convulsions and decorticate rigidity may develop, and most patients die, often of intercurrent infection, within the first year of life (often within the first few weeks). The diagnosis can usually be suspected from the characteristic odor of the urine and is confirmed by the abnormal pattern of amino acids and keto acids in blood and urine. The enzyme defect is demonstrable in leukocytes and fibroblasts. Treatment—by careful dietary control of leucine, isoleucine, and valine—is simple in theory but difficult in practice because of the necessity to balance three individual essential amino acids that are not easily analyzed. In those few cases in which rigid dietary control with careful monitoring of plasma levels has been instituted early, the results have been gratifying. A few patients have been described with milder variants of maple syrup urine disease. Thiamine therapy should be tried, as noted.

ISOVALERIC ACIDEMIA. This rare genetic disorder in the degradative pathway of leucine is due to a block in the conversion of isovaleric acid to beta-methylcrotonic acid, which is catalyzed by isovaleryl-CoA dehydrogenase. Isovaleric acid accumulates in blood and urine and gives rise to an odor that has been described as like sweaty feet. The pathogenesis of the associated clinical features has not been established. Symptoms, which usually begin in the first week of life, consist of attacks of vomiting, acidosis, tremors, lethargy, or even coma. Leukopenia, anemia, and thrombocytopenia have been observed during acute attacks. Patients who survive have generally exhibited mental retardation. As in the case of maple syrup urine disease, which it may clinically resemble, isovaleric acidemia may be suspected from the associated odor. The diagnosis is established by the demonstration of excess isovaleric acid in the serum by gas-liquid chromatography or of isovalerylglycine in the urine. Treatment is by strict control of dietary leucine.

HYPERVALINEMIA. This disorder has been described only in one Japanese infant who exhibited vomiting and severe mental and physical retardation, beginning shortly after birth. Valine was increased in his plasma and failed to undergo transamination to alpha-ketoisovaleric acid. Use of a diet low in valine resulted in clinical improvement.

HYPERPROLINEMIA AND HYDROXYPROLINEMIA

Scriver CR, Smith RJ, Phang JM: Disorders of proline and hydroxyproline metabolism. In Stanbury JB, Wyngaarden JB, Fredrickson DS, et al. (eds.): The Metabolic Basis of Inherited Disease. 5th ed. New York, McGraw-Hill Book Company, 1983, p 360. *An extensive analysis of the chemical derangements in these rare disorders.*

DISEASES OF THE UREA CYCLE

Beaudet AL, O'Brien WE, Bock H-GO, et al.: The human argininosuccinate synthetase locus and citrullinemia. Adv Hum Genet 15:161, 1986. *An excellent general review of this rare disorder, with particular emphasis on the molecular analysis of the defective gene.*
Brusilow SW, Danney M, Waber LJ, et al.: Treatment of episodic hyperammonemia in children with inborn errors of urea synthesis. N Engl J Med 310:1630, 1984. *A review of interesting new therapeutic approaches.*
Brusilow SW, Horwich AL: Disorders of the urea cycle. In Scriver CR, Beaudet A, Sly W, et al. (eds.): The Metabolic Basis of Inherited Disease. 6th ed. New York, McGraw-Hill Book Company, 1988, in press. *A large number of disorders are associated with derangements in urea synthesis. This chapter gives a lucid summary of the biochemistry of urea synthesis and the pathogenesis of the various disorders associated with that pathway. As always in* The Metabolic Basis of Inherited Disease, *there is a large and useful bibliography.*
Rowe PC, Newman SL, Brusilow SW: Natural history of symptomatic partial ornithine transcarbamylase deficiency. N Engl J Med 314:541, 1986. *Studies of the disease in a series of symptomatic female heterozygotes with a description of clinical manifestations, therapy, and outcome.*

BRANCHED-CHAIN AMINOACIDURIA

Danner DJ, Armstrong N, Heffelfinger SC, et al.: Absence of branched-chain acyl-transferase as a cause of maple syrup urine disease. J Clin Invest 75:858, 1985. *The demonstration of a specific enzyme defect in the 4-enzyme complex that normally decarboxylates these keto acids.*
Elsas LJ: Disorders of branched chain amino acid metabolism. In Scriver CR, Beaudet A, Sly W, et al. (eds.): The Metabolic Basis of Inherited Disease. 6th ed. New York, McGraw-Hill Book Company, 1988, in press. *This is the most sophisticated general presentation of the pathogenesis of this group of disorders. Although the emphasis is on the biochemical basis, there is a useful clinical discussion and an extensive bibliography.*

194 HOMOCYSTINURIA

S. Harvey Mudd

DEFINITION. The term *homocystinuria* designates a biochemical abnormality, not a disease entity. Several known genetic disorders lead to homocystinuria. Most common is cystathionine beta-synthase deficiency. In this condition ectopia lentis, mental retardation, bony abnormalities, osteoporosis, and thromboembolic phenomena are frequent.

PREVALENCE. More than 600 adequately documented cases of cystathionine beta-synthase deficiency have been reported. Screening of newborn infants indicates a *minimal* prevalence of 1 in 200,000 worldwide.

ETIOLOGY AND PATHOGENESIS. Cystathionine beta-synthase deficiency is inherited as an autosomal recessive trait. Deficient activity of this enzyme has been demonstrated in liver extracts, in brain, and in cultured skin fibroblasts and lymphocytes. The enzyme deficiency results in failure of homocysteine to react with serine to form cystathionine on the pathway to cysteine. Homocystine is the disulfide oxidation product formed from two molecules of homocysteine. Normally homocystine is not detected in human plasma by methods of the usual sensitivity. In cystathionine beta-synthase-deficient patients fasting plasma concentrations up to 0.2 μmol per milliliter of homocystine have been reported. The urine may contain up to 1 mmol of homocystine per day. Plasma methionine levels are also raised, and plasma cystine is low. Detailed studies, chiefly of cultured fibroblasts, suggest

extensive heterogeneity in the genetic lesions producing deficient activity of cystathionine beta-synthase. An important manifestation of such genetic heterogeneity is pyridoxine responsiveness. In 40 to 50 per cent of cystathionine beta-synthase–deficient patients, administration of relatively large amounts of pyridoxine markedly reduces or eliminates homocystinuria, homocystinemia, hypermethioninemia, and hypocystinemia. Within any one sibship, all affected sibs are either B_6 responsive or B_6 nonresponsive.

Many of the manifestations of homocystinuria are related to abnormal connective tissue. Outwardly these patients may resemble those with Marfan's syndrome, but the joints are not hyperextensible. The pathogenesis of the thrombotic tendency is not clearly understood, but increase of plasma homocyst(e)ine, rather than plasma methionine, is likely to cause the thrombotic tendency.

PATHOLOGY. There is disruption of the zonular fibers of the lens, with resulting subluxation. The skeleton is markedly osteoporotic, and the vertebrae show rarefaction with biconcave compression. Thrombi and emboli have been reported in almost every artery or vein. These result in brain infarcts, coronary occlusion, and myocardial infarction, pulmonary infarcts, renal infarcts, and thrombophlebitis with pulmonary emboli.

CLINICAL MANIFESTATIONS. Among individuals with cystathionine beta-synthase deficiency there is marked variation with regard to the major clinical features of this condition, their time of onset, and severity. Clinical manifestations tend to be less prevalent, slower in onset, or less marked among B_6-responsive patients than among nonresponsive ones. A survey of 629 patients showed that mental capabilities ranged from severely retarded to IQ's as high as 130. Median IQ for B_6-responsive patients was 78; for B_6-nonresponsive patients, 56. Mental retardation, when present, most commonly becomes manifest during the first few years of life.

The incidence of dislocated optic lenses increases with age. By the age of 10 years, 55 per cent of B_6-responsive patients have dislocated lenses; 82 per cent of B_6-nonresponsive patients. Acute glaucoma and reduced visual acuity may result.

Thromboembolism is the life-threatening complication of cystathionine beta-synthase deficiency. By age 15, chances of having had a clinically detected thromboembolic event are 12 per cent among B_6-responders and 27 per cent among B_6-nonresponders. Large and small arteries and veins may be affected. Major cerebral vascular thrombosis may occur. Venous thrombosis with pulmonary emboli is common. By age 30 years, 4 per cent of B_6-responsive patients had died and 23 per cent of B_6-nonresponsive patients.

The spine is the most common site of osteoporosis, followed by the long bones. By age 15, chances of having radiologically detected spinal osteoporosis are 36 per cent among B_6-responders and 65 per cent among B_6-nonresponders. Scoliosis occurs in many individuals, although kyphosis is infrequent. Vertebral collapse and pathologic fractures of long bones may occur. The long bones are generally thin and excessively lengthened. Pectus carinatum or excavatum is common.

DIAGNOSIS AND DIFFERENTIAL DIAGNOSIS. The diagnosis is suggested by ectopia lentis and thromboembolic phenomena, together with other aforementioned features. The urinary cyanide-nitroprusside reaction is positive. Other disulfidurias, for example, cystinuria, also produce a positive cyanide-nitroprusside reaction, so homocystinemia and homocystinuria distinguish cystathionine beta-synthase deficiency from alternative forms of disulfiduria. Cystathionine beta-synthase deficiency is confirmed by demonstration of markedly reduced enzyme activity with cultured skin fibroblasts or phytohemagglutinin-stimulated lymphocytes or in a liver biopsy specimen.

Heterozygotes may be identified by assay of cystathionine beta-synthase activity in liver biopsy tissue. Cystathionine beta-synthase activities in cultured fibroblasts or phytohemagglutinin-stimulated lymphocytes from most heterozygotes are below the control range, but there is some overlap. For unequivocal identification such studies are best accompanied by methionine loading tests. In some young adults premature peripheral or cerebral occlusive arterial disease may be due to heterozygosity for cystathionine beta-synthase deficiency.

Rarer forms of homocystinuria are caused by decreased 5-methyltetrahydrofolate-dependent homocysteine methylation, owing either to decreased 5,10-methylenetetrahydrofolate reductase activity or to a variety of lesions that interfere with the ability to produce methylcobalamin. In all of these, plasma methionine levels are low. The condition is first noted in childhood. Homocystinuria also occurs following 6-azauridine triacetate administration.

TREATMENT. Management is directed toward the biochemical abnormality with the aim of preventing or ameliorating clinical manifestations, and toward the clinical treatment of complications.

Newborns known to have the abnormality have almost always been treated with a low-methionine diet (usually accompanied by cystine supplementation). Such therapy prevents mental retardation and may decrease the rate of lens dislocations and reduce the incidence of seizures. It is too early to assess the effects on thromboembolic events, osteoporosis, or mortality. When the condition is diagnosed at later ages in B_6-responsive patients, pyridoxine treatment (doses up to 500 to 1000 mg per day) accompanied by folate repletion has been shown to produce a statistically significant reduction in the rate of initial thromboembolic events. When diagnosis is made at later ages in B_6-nonresponsive patients, strict methionine limitation, if accepted and carefully adhered to, may be beneficial in preventing thromboembolic events. Re-

cently, in early studies of such patients, betaine, which lowers homocysteine by accelerating its methylation, has appeared useful. Antithrombotic therapy with aspirin and dipyridamole has also been advocated.

Boers GHJ, Fowler B,. Smals AGH, et al.: Improved identification of heterozygotes for homocystinuria due to cystathionine synthase deficiency by the combination of methionine loading and enzyme determination in cultured fibroblasts. Hum Genet 69:164, 1985. *When liver tissue is not available.*

Boers GHJ, Smals AGH, Trijbels FJM, et al.: Heterozygosity for homocystinuria in premature peripheral and cerebral occlusive arterial disease. N Engl J Med 313:709, 1985. *A possible cause of early, otherwise unexplained, thromboembolic events.*

Carson NAJ: Homocystinuria: Clinical and biochemical heterogeneity. In Cockburn F, Gitzelmann R (eds.): Inborn Errors of Metabolism in Humans. Lancaster, Eng., MTP Press, 1982. *Successful treatment of late-diagnosed B_6-nonresponsive patients by methionine restriction.*

Mitchell GA, Watkins D, Melancon SB, et al.: Clinical heterogeneity in cobalamin C variant of combined homocystinuria and methylmalonic aciduria. J Pediatr 108:410, 1986. *Contains a useful brief summary of other causes of homocystinuria.*

Mudd SH, Skovby F, Levy HL, et al.: The natural history of homocystinuria due to cystathionine-β-synthase deficiency. Am J Hum Genet 37:1, 1985. *An international questionnaire study covering 629 patients. The natural history of the untreated disease is defined for the major clinical manifestations and the effects of therapies evaluated statistically.*

Mudd SH, Levy HL: Disorders of transsulfuration. In Stanbury JB, Wyngaarden JB, Fredrickson DS, et al. (eds.): The Metabolic Basis of Inherited Disease. 5th ed. New York, McGraw-Hill Book Company, 1983. *A detailed review of the clinical features of 350 confirmed cases of cystathionine β-synthase deficiency, with a discussion of metabolic factors in homocystinuria.*

Wilcken DEL, Wilcken B, Dudman NPB, et al.: Homocystinuria—the effects of betaine in the treatment of patients not responsive to pyridoxine. N Engl J Med 309:448, 1983. *Eleven patients responded with a substantial decrease in plasma homocysteine levels and an increase in total cysteine levels. In six there was prompt clinical improvement, such as darkening of new hair and improvement in behavior.*

Disorders of Purine and Pyrimidine Metabolism

195 GOUT
James B. Wyngaarden

Gout is a term representing a heterogeneous group of genetic and acquired diseases manifested by *hyperuricemia* and a characteristic *acute inflammatory arthritis* induced by *crystals* of monosodium urate monohydrate. Some patients develop aggregated deposits of these crystals (*tophi*) in and around the joints of the extremities that can lead to severe crippling. Many patients develop a *chronic interstitial nephropathy*. In addition, uric acid *urolithiasis* is common in gout.

Some patients develop all of the features of the disease described above, but these manifestations can occur in different combinations. However, essential hyperuricemia alone, even when complicated by uric acid lithiasis, should not be called gout; gout signifies inflammatory arthritis or tophaceous disease.

A classification emphasizing the heterogeneity of gout is presented in Table 195–1.

PREVALENCE AND INCIDENCE. The prevalence of gout varies from about 0.13 to 0.37 per cent in Europe and the United States to 10 per cent in adult male Maori of New Zealand. Exceptionally high prevalences are also found in Filipinos (in the United States, but not in the Philippines) and in the natives of the Mariana Islands. During World Wars I and II acute gouty arthritis was uncommon in Europe. When

dietary protein again became plentiful, its frequency returned to prewar levels. Although formerly rare in Japan, gout has now become common in parallel with the increase in protein consumption in that country.

Primary gout is chiefly a disease of adult men; only about 5 per cent of cases are found in women, largely in the postmenopausal group. The frequency of gout is increased in patients taking diuretics, especially of the thiazide group; in certain nephropathies; and in polycythemia vera, myeloid metaplasia, or chronic hemolysis. Gout in all of its forms makes up about 5 per cent of arthritis cases.

GENETICS OF GOUT. A family history of clinical gout is generally found in 6 to 18 per cent of patients in the United States and Denmark. Figures of 40 to 80 per cent have been reported from England, and also from the United States following tenacious family studies. About 25 per cent of first-degree relatives of gouty subjects are hyperuricemic, and about 20 per cent of these have symptomatic gout. Familial hyperuricemia is polygenic and multifactorial. Hyperuricemia is correlated with maleness, surface area, obesity, ponderal index, protein intake, social status, and educational level. Thus many variables affect the phenotypic expression of hyperuricemia. In primary gout associated with hypoxanthine-guanine phosphoribosyltransferase (HGPRT) deficiency and phosphoribosylpyrophosphate (PP-ribose-P) synthetase variants, the genetic transmissions are X linked. Glycogen storage disease type I, which is associated with a specific form of secondary gout, is an autosomal recessive trait.

PATHOGENESIS AND PATHOLOGY. The hallmark of gout is hyperuricemia. The risk of gout increases with the

TABLE 195–1. CLASSIFICATION OF HYPERURICEMIA AND GOUT

Type	Disturbance in Uric Acid Metabolism	Inheritance
Primary		
I. Idiopathic (>99% of primary gout)		
A. Normal urinary excretion (80–90% of primary gout)	Decreased renal clearance ± overproduction	Polygenic
B. Increased urinary excretion (10–20% of primary gout)	Overproduction ± decreased renal clearance	Polygenic
II. Associated with specific enzyme or metabolic defects (<1% of primary gout)		
A. Increased activity of PP-ribose-P synthetase	Overproduction; increased synthesis of PP-ribose-P	X-linked
B. "Partial" deficiency of hypoxanthine-guanine phosphoribosyltransferase	Overproduction; increased PP-ribose-P concentration	X-linked
Secondary		
I. Associated with increased purine biosynthesis de novo		
A. "Complete" deficiency of hypoxanthine-guanine phosphoribosyltransferase	Overproduction; Lesch-Nyhan syndrome	X-linked
B. Glucose-6-phosphatase deficiency	Overproduction and decreased renal clearance; glycogen storage disease, type I (von Gierke)	Autosomal recessive
II. Associated with increased nucleic acid turnover	Overproduction, e.g., chronic hemolysis; polycythemia; myeloid metaplasia	—
III. Associated with decreased renal clearance of uric acid	Reduced renal functional mass; inhibition of secretion and/or enhanced reabsorption by drugs, toxins, or endogenous metabolic products	—

TABLE 195–3. SOLUBILITY OF URATE ION AS A FUNCTION OF TEMPERATURE IN THE PRESENCE OF 140 mM Na$^+$*

Temperature (° C)	Maximal Equilibrium Concentration of Urate in the Presence of 140 mM Na$^+$ (mg/dl)
37	6.8
35	6.0
30	4.5
25	3.3
20	2.5
15	1.8
10	1.2

*From Loeb: Arthritis Rheum 15:189, 1972.

is toxic; all of the features of gout derive from responses to the urate crystal.

The solubility of urate in body fluids is strongly influenced by pH and temperature (Table 195–3). At pH 7.4 and 37°C, the solubility of urate in fluid having the sodium composition of plasma is 6.4 to 6.8 mg per deciliter. An additional 0.4 mg per deciliter is protein bound, chiefly to an alpha$_1$-alpha$_2$-globulin. Thus 7.0 mg per deciliter is about the solubility limit of urate in plasma at normal central body temperature. But solubility is considerably less at the temperature of peripheral joints, which may be 32°C in the knee, and 29°C in the ankle (Hollander, 1949). Concentrations of plasma urate above 7 mg per deciliter at 37°C define hyperuricemia in a physicochemical sense. Urate forms stable supersaturated solutions, but such solutions are poised for crystal formation when perturbed.

Mechanisms of Hyperuricemia. The concentration of urate in plasma is determined by the balance between absorption and production of purines on the one hand and destruction and excretion on the other. Exogenous purines contribute substantially to body uric acid stores. Purine restriction leads to a reduction of serum urate of 0.6 to 1.8 mg per deciliter in normal subjects. Similar regimens have little effect on hyperuricemia of gouty subjects who greatly overproduce purines, but exhibit comparable effects in patients with reduced renal urate clearance. Abnormalities of purine absorption have not been implicated as a cause of hyperuricemia.

Human beings lack uricase; therefore uric acid is the end-product of purine metabolism. In normal subjects approximately one third of the uric acid disposed of each day is degraded by bacteria in the gut, and two thirds is excreted unchanged by the kidney. Decreased uricolysis has been excluded as a mechanism for hyperuricemia. In fact, with high urate concentrations in body fluids, enteric uricolysis is enhanced; with the onset of renal insufficiency, intestinal uricolysis assumes increased importance and in extreme instances may account for 80 per cent of daily urate disposition. By contrast, both increased purine biosynthesis and decreased renal excretion of uric acid play important roles in the pathogenesis of primary hyperuricemia.

Random urine samples in normal men commonly contain 500 to 1000 mg per 24 hours. On a purine-restricted diet these values average 418 ± 70 mg per 24 hours. Gouty subjects show slightly higher average values, 497 mg per 24 hours, but the overlap with the normal range is extensive. From 10 to 20 per cent of gouty subjects show basal values above the upper limits of normal. Because of the insensitivity of urinary urate measurements in the assessment of purine production, isotopic tracer studies have been employed for this purpose. With labeled uric acid the miscible pool of uric acid in normal man averages 1200 mg, and the daily rate of production averages 750 mg. From one half to three fourths of the pool turns over each day. The difference between the rate of production and the rate of excretion of urate ranges from 100 to 365 mg per day and represents the amount of intestinal uricolysis.

A second method of study involves measurement of incorporation of an isotopically labeled purine precursor, usually glycine, into urinary uric acid. The incorporation can be

degree of hyperuricemia and also with age (Table 195–2). Virtually all patients with gout have serum urate values above 7.0 mg per deciliter. An occasional patient will have a lower value at the time of attack, perhaps attributable to the urate diuresis that sometimes accompanies the inflammatory response. Repeat analyses will almost always show hyperuricemia during quiescent periods.

In normal prepubertal children, serum urate values average 3.6 mg per deciliter in both sexes. At puberty these levels increase, and thereafter mean values are 5.1 mg per deciliter in males and 4.1 mg per deciliter in females. After the menopause, mean values in females increase to approximate levels in males. In the United States the central 95 per cent segment of the distributions encompasses values of 2.2 to 7.5 mg per deciliter in adult males and 2.1 to 6.6 mg per deciliter in adult premenopausal females. Definitions of hyperuricemia based on distributions of serum urate are useful for epidemiologic studies. But statistical expressions are not adequate definitions of the pathophysiologic significance of hyperuricemia, for it is the *solubility* of urate in plasma and body fluids that is important. There is no evidence that urate in solution

TABLE 195–2. PREVALENCE OF GOUTY ARTHRITIS IN MEN IN RELATION TO SERUM URATE CONCENTRATION AND AGE

Serum Urate Level (mg/dl)	Mean Age 49 Years* (%)	Mean Age 58 Years† (%)
6.0–6.9	2	2
7.0–7.9	4	17
8.0–8.9	11	25
9.0–9.9	30	90
10 +	48	90

*Zalokar et al.: Chron Dis 25:305, 1972.
†Hall et al.: Am J Med 42:27, 1967.

corrected for extrarenal disposal to give total incorporation values. By use of these methods, evidence of some degree of excessive production of uric acid has been obtained in about two thirds of gouty patients studied. The most extreme values are found in subjects with HGPRT deficiency or PP-ribose-P synthetase variants, but these represent fewer than 1 per cent of gouty subjects. Many patients whose 24-hour urinary uric acid values fall within the normal range show modest increases in the rate of turnover of an enlarged uric acid pool and/or overincorporation of glycine into urate. Studies of the intramolecular distribution of ^{15}N in uric acid following administration of ^{15}N-glycine show excessive labeling of position 9, which is derived from the amide-N of glutamine and from ammonia. Thus many more gouty subjects show evidence for mild overproduction of purine than would have been deduced from urinary uric acid measurements alone.

The first unique reaction of purine biosynthesis and the site of metabolic regulation by purine ribonucleotide inhibitors is that which synthesizes phosphoribosylamine, catalyzed by amidophosphoribosyltransferase:

$$\text{Glutamine} + \text{PP-ribose-P} + H_2O \xrightarrow{Mg^{2+}}$$
$$\text{phosphoribosylamine} + \text{glutamic acid} + PP_i$$

There are several possible mechanisms for loss of regulation at this site and acceleration of purine biosynthesis. These include (1) excessive concentrations of the substrates PP-ribose-P, glutamine, or both; (2) a structural alteration or increased amount of the enzyme, rendering it more active or less sensitive to inhibition by purine ribonucleotides; or (3) a reduced concentration of one of the regulatory nucleotides (AMP or GMP) which exert cooperative allosteric inhibition of enzyme activity. Intracellular levels of PP-ribose-P are strikingly raised in HGPRT deficiency and also in PP-ribose-P synthetase overactivity. The increased concentration of PP-ribose-P drives purine biosynthesis both by furnishing more of the rate-limiting substrate and by allosteric activation of amidophosphoribosyltransferase. PP-ribose-P turnover is accelerated in gouty patients in whom uric acid is overproduced. However, erythrocyte PP-ribose-P levels are normal in gouty patients without specific enzyme defects. Plasma glutamate values are slightly raised in gouty subjects, both in the fasting state and after oral glutamate loads, but plasma glutamine levels are normal. Although reduced activities of glutaminase and of glutamic dehydrogenase have been postulated in gout, no direct evidence for such enzyme deficiencies exists. Any process that results in accelerated breakdown of intracellular adenyl nucleotides may lead to hyperuricemia by prompt degradation of daughter purine compounds to uric acid and to secondary acceleration of purine synthesis de novo through release of inhibition of amidophosphoribosyltransferase. This biphasic mechanism has been implicated in glycogen storage disease type I following fructose infusion, following alcohol ingestion, and in a gouty patient with a variant AMP deaminase that showed reduced sensitivity to GTP, its normal regulator. The last example has been proposed as a possible general mechanism in idiopathic gout. There are no examples of gout attributable to intrinsic alterations of the amidophosphoribosyltransferase itself.

In the normal turnover of nucleic acids and nucleotides some are degraded to free purine bases, chiefly hypoxanthine and guanine. Nucleotides synthesized de novo in excess of nucleotide and nucleic acid requirements are promptly degraded to hypoxanthine. Guanine is deaminated to xanthine by guanase. Hypoxanthine and xanthine are oxidized to uric acid by xanthine oxidase (Fig. 195–1). Hepatic xanthine oxidase activity is increased in gouty overproducers, but this appears to be an induced rather than a primary change. Nevertheless this is an additional factor contributing to accelerated uric acid synthesis in these patients.

In a substantial fraction of gouty subjects the immediate

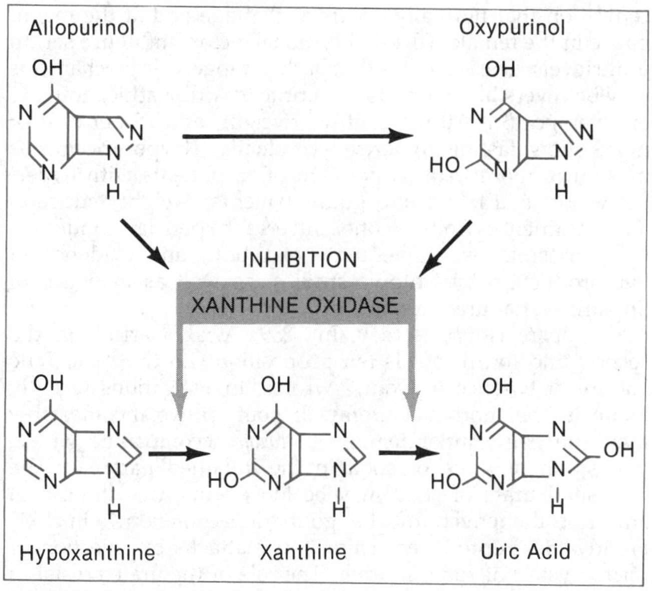

FIGURE 195–1. Pathway of uric acid synthesis catalyzed by xanthine oxidase and the site of action of allopurinol.

pathogenetic mechanism of hyperuricemia appears to be a decreased renal tubular clearance of urate. Renal excretion of urate is a complex function of glomerular filtration, tubular reabsorption, and tubular secretion. Filtration of plasma urate is assumed to be complete, on the basis of micropuncture studies in animals and ultrafiltration studies of human plasma in vitro. Less than 5 per cent of plasma urate is protein bound in man under physiologic conditions at 37°C. Filtered urate appears to be almost completely reabsorbed in the proximal tubule (presecretory reabsorption). Some of the secreted urate is also reabsorbed in the distal portion of the proximal tubule and to a lesser extent in the ascending portion of the loop of Henle and in the collecting ducts (postsecretory reabsorption). The urate that is excreted is thought to arise almost entirely by tubular secretion. These conclusions rest on clearance studies with and without inhibitors of reabsorption, such as probenecid, or of secretion, such as pyrazinamide, which have major limitations.

Studies in gouty patients have been interpreted as indicating reduced secretion of urate per nephron, but enhanced postsecretory reabsorption would also explain the data. The difference in renal tubular handling of urate in gout is small, and conclusions rest upon statistical analysis of clearance data on groups of patients. On this basis the renal contribution to hyperuricemia is most marked in patients with normal 24-hour excretion values of urate, normal turnover values of the uric acid pool, and normal values of glycine incorporation into uric acid. But reduced renal urate clearances per nephron are not restricted to this group. With the exception of patients with HGPRT deficiency or PP-ribose-P synthetase variants, overproducer gouty subjects as a group also show reduced renal urate clearance (Simkin). Thus, although some investigators have separated the large group of patients with an undefined biochemical lesion, idiopathic gout, into two discrete subgroups termed metabolic (overproducer) and renal gout, the evidence does not support such a categoric distinction, inasmuch as many subjects show both defects. Since chronic excessive alcohol consumption is common in gouty subjects and causes excessive turnover of adenine nucleotides and increased urate production and excretion, it is possible that some of the metabolic contributions to hyperuricemia in idiopathic gout are alcohol related.

The complexity of the pathogenesis of hyperuricemia is illustrated by two additional observations. The first is that asymptomatic hyperuricemia begins at puberty in the male as an exaggeration of the modest increase in serum urate concentration that normally occurs at that age and at the menopause in the female. Clearly hormonal factors influence serum urate levels. The second is that both pathogenetic mechanisms may be reversible. Subjects with primary (idiopathic) gout are on average 15 to 30 per cent overweight, and 75 per cent or more show fasting hypertriglyceridemia. (Hyperuricemia is present in more than 80 per cent of all patients with hypertriglyceridemia.) In some gouty patients, weight reduction and abstinence from alcohol reverse hypertriglyceridemia, hyperuricemia, excessive urate excretion, and evidence of overproduction by isotopic studies, as well as evidence of impaired renal urate clearance.

The Acute Gouty Attack. In 1859, A. B. Garrod, in the second and fourth of his ten propositions on the "The True Nature of Essence of Gout," wrote: "Investigations recently made in the morbid anatomy of gout, prove incontestably that true gouty inflammation is *always* accompanied with a deposition of urate of soda in the inflamed part. . . . The deposited urate of soda may be looked upon as the cause, and not the effect, of the gouty inflammation." In 1899 Freudweiler reproduced acute gouty attacks by injection of microcrystals of sodium urate. The role of the urate crystal in acute gout was rediscovered in 1961 by McCarty and Hollander. In laboratory animals experimental gouty arthritis requires the presence of leukocytes. However, synovitis can also be produced experimentally by other crystals of similar size and shape, and occurs in pseudogout caused by calcium pyrophosphate dihydrate crystals.

Although a number of cellular mechanisms are activated by the urate crystal, the exact sequence by which inflammation is initiated is uncertain. Hagemen factor, kallikrein, kinin-like peptides, and the complement system all participate in the response, but each has also been excluded as an obligatory factor in the inflammatory reaction. Urate crystals are leukotactic. Leukocytes and synovial lining cells ingest the urate crystals. Within minutes leukocytes release leukotriene B_4 (LTB_4) and a glycoprotein chemotactic factor (mw = 11,500). Production of these chemoattractants is blocked by colchicine. The acute inflammatory response to injected urate crystals is also blocked by prior treatment with colchicine, but the inflammatory response to purified crystal-induced chemotactic factor is not. Thus this factor and LTB_4 may be important mediators of the inflammatory reaction in gout. Monocytes are also stimulated by urate crystals in vitro, with release of interleukin-1. IL-1 may also contribute to initiation and amplification of gouty inflammation.

Crystal-cell interactions may be modulated by proteins adherent to the crystals. Crystals from patients with acute gout have surface coats of IgG, and to a lesser extent of IgM, IgA, C_3, and fibrinogen, but not of albumin. In studies in vitro, IgG coating enhances neutrophil responsiveness to urate crystals, whereas certain other proteins inhibit. Such modulating factors may account for the variable inflammatory responses to urate crystals in gouty subjects.

Phagocytosis of the crystal leads to rapid destruction of the phagolysosome membrane with release of hydrolytic enzymes into the cell. This results in cell necrosis and release of the crystal and lysosomal and cytoplasmic enzymes into the surrounding tissue. In a simulated system (liposomes) phospholipid membranes are susceptible to urate-induced lysis if they contain cholesterol or testosterone and refractory if they contain beta-estradiol. These observations suggest obvious interpretations, based upon the relative preference of gout for men and postmenopausal women.

The events leading to the putative burst of microcrystals of urate that initiates the acute attack are largely speculative. Three major theories have been advanced. The first postulates that trauma may result in shedding of crystals from preexisting cartilaginous tophi into the synovial fluid. The second emphasizes the ability of organized proteoglycans of cartilage to absorb (solubilize) urate. Disruption and increased turnover

of proteoglycans are postulated to occur following trauma, with release of additional urate into the already supersaturated synovial fluid, and resulting crystallization. The third postulates a joint effusion with trauma, followed by a more rapid rate of reabsorption of water than of solute, resulting in further supersaturation of synovial fluid with urate, and precipitation of crystals. The first metatarsophalangeal joint is exposed to the greatest pressure per unit area of any joint in the body during walking, and it and other lower extremity joints, which are the joints predominantly involved in gout, are especially susceptible to trauma. In addition, the low temperature of peripheral leg joints will favor crystallization of urate from supersaturated synovial fluid. Thus each of these theories, which are not mutually exclusive, has merit.

Tophi. The pathognomonic lesion of gout is the *tophus*, a deposit of fine acicular crystals of monosodium urate monohydrate, surrounded by a mononuclear reaction and a foreign body granuloma of epithelial and giant cells, some of which may be multinucleate. Urate crystals are water soluble, but when tissues are treated with nonaqueous fixatives (e.g., absolute alcohol) the crystals are preserved and are brilliantly anisotropic and negatively birefringent in compensated polarized light. Tophi are commonly found in articular and other cartilage, synovia, tendon sheaths and other periarticular structures, epiphyseal bone, the subcutaneous layers of the skin, and the interstitial areas of the kidney. The articular cartilages are the most common and at times the exclusive sites of urate deposition. The deposits, although superficial, are actually embedded in the intercellular matrix. In the joint, cartilaginous degeneration, synovial proliferation and pannus, destruction of subchondral bone, proliferation of marginal bone, and sometimes fibrous or bony ankylosis develop. The punched-out lesions of bone commonly seen on roentgenograms represent marrow tophus deposits, which may communicate with the urate crust on the articular surface through defects in the cartilage. In vertebral bodies, urate deposits involve the marrow spaces adjacent to the intervertebral discs, as well as the discs themselves.

All of these sites of urate deposition are rich in proteoglycans, and the postulated role of these substances in attracting and solubilizing urate when organized, and of releasing urate during metabolic turnover, cited above, may serve to explain both localization and occurrence of tophi. Curiously, the process in the tissues evokes only a minimal inflammatory response in comparison with the violence of the acute gouty attack brought about by crystals within the synovial space. Urate crystals stimulate mesenchymal cells of joints to produce collagenase and prostaglandin E_2, both of which may play roles in articular destruction.

The Gouty Kidney. The only distinctive histologic feature of the gouty kidney is the presence of sodium urate crystals in the medulla or pyramids and surrounding round cell and giant cell reaction. These are found in a high percentage of gouty patients at autopsy and are associated with acute and chronic interstitial inflammatory changes, fibrosis, tubular atrophy, glomerular sclerosis, and arteriolar nephrosclerosis. The earliest change in the kidney is an interstitial reaction, maximal near the loops of Henle, associated with tubular damage. In kidneys without tophi the interstitial reaction tends to spare the medulla and juxtamedullary cortex. Although renal disease is common in gout, it is generally mild and only slowly progressive. The origin of the interstitial nephropathy is not known. It is not even certain that in the absence of crystalline deposits it is related to hyperuricemia. Other possibilities include nephrosclerosis, uric acid stone disease, urinary infection, aging, and lead poisoning. Crystalline deposits may occur within the distal tubules and collecting ducts and are probably composed of uric acid and related to the intratubular concentration of uric acid and the acid pH of the urine; they lead to dilatation and atrophy of the more proximal tubules. Deposits within the interstitium are composed of sodium urate and are believed to be related to the elevated urate concentration of plasma and interstitial fluid.

Uric Acid Urolithiasis. The overall incidence of renal stones in gout is about 20 per cent, about 200-fold higher than in the general population. In 84 per cent of gouty subjects, the stones are pure uric acid (not sodium urate); in 4 per cent, uric acid and calcium oxalate; and in 12 per cent, calcium oxalate or phosphate alone. The incidence of stones rises with the degree of hyperuricemia and approximates 50 per cent at serum urate values above 12 mg per deciliter. Marked hyperuricemia probably influences stone formation primarily by increasing uric acid *excretion*. The incidence of stones rises above 20 per cent in gouty subjects when the uric acid excretion exceeds 700 mg per 24 hours, and reaches 50 per cent at values above 1100 mg per 24 hours. Patients with increased uric aciduria also have an increased incidence of calcium oxalate stones. Urate (not uric acid) can participate in "heterogeneous nucleation" with calcium oxalate.

Other factors in the pathogenesis of uric acid stones include the *concentration of uric acid in urine,* the *acidity* of urine, and possibly the availability of stone *matrix* and the level of *solubilizing substances* in the urine. The solubility of urate decreases with fall of pH because of the shift to free uric acid. The pKa of uric acid is 5.75. In plasma at pH 7.4 more than 99 per cent is present in ionized form (urate), whereas in urine at pH 5.0 about 85 per cent is un-ionized (uric acid). At this pH only 15 mg of uric acid per deciliter of urine are soluble at 37°C, so supersaturation is required to excrete an average uric acid load in a normal urine volume. The solubility increases more than 10-fold at pH 7.0 and more than 100-fold at pH 8.0 over pH 5.0.

Both gouty and nongouty uric acid stone formers exhibit unusually low urinary pH values when fasting and throughout the day. The persistently acid urine has been attributed to subnormal ammonium production with a compensatory increase in titratable acidity. There is debate whether these data reflect occult or measurable renal damage (e.g., interstitial nephropathy), aging, or an intrinsic renal defect. Regardless of the explanation, the tendency toward persistently acid urine favors uric acid stone formation.

CLINICAL MANIFESTATIONS. The clinical manifestations of gout are conveniently described in four categories: acute gouty arthritis, tophaceous gout, gouty nephropathy, and uric acid urolithiasis.

Clinical gout is extraordinarily rare before puberty, when males at risk for primary idiopathic gout first develop hyperuricemia. Exceptions occur in the juvenile gout of the Lesch-Nyhan syndrome or glycogen storage disease type I, in which marked hyperuricemia is present from infancy. Only about 20 per cent of hyperuricemic subjects ever develop acute gout, although this figure rises as the degree of hyperuricemia increases (Table 195–2). The peak age of onset of gout is about 45 years in men. Thus the usual gouty male is exposed to 30 years of hyperuricemia before an attack occurs. In women gout usually occurs some years after the menopause, when serum urate values rise to hyperuricemic levels in those genetically at risk for gout.

Acute Gouty Arthritis. When acute gouty arthritis develops, it often appears as a fulminating arthritic attack of incapacitating severity. Acute gout is predominantly a disease of the lower extremity. Seventy-five to 90 per cent of initial attacks are monoarticular, and at least half of first attacks involve the metatarsophalangeal joint of the great toe (podagra). Next in order of frequency as sites of initial involvement are the instep, ankle, heel, knee, wrist, finger, and elbow. Later attacks are more often polyarticular and may include the shoulder or hip, or rarely such joints as the sacroiliac, sternoclavicular, mandibular, or even the spine. The more distal the site of involvement, the more typical are the attacks.

Some patients report short trivial episodes of "ankle sprains" or sore heels or twinges of pain in the great toe prior to the first attack, sometimes going back over several years. More often the first attack occurs with explosive suddenness during apparent excellent health, often at night. Within minutes to hours the affected joint becomes hot, dusky red, and exquisitely painful. Lymphangitis may be evident. Systemic signs of inflammation may include fever, leukocytosis, and elevation of the erythrocyte sedimentation rate. The inflammatory reaction may suggest a cellulitis or septic joint, and on occasion a joint is erroneously incised by an unwary physician.

Acute gouty arthritis often follows a precipitating event, such as trauma, surgery, alcohol or dietary overindulgence, starvation, or infection. Attacks may follow a long walk, golf, or hunting trip (e.g., "pheasant hunter's toe"). Postoperative gout usually occurs on the third to the fifth day and has been attributed to the subsidence of the adrenal alarm by analogy with the recrudescence of acute gout that may follow cessation of steroid therapy. Alcohol intoxication and starvation increase serum urate levels by inhibition of renal excretion by the accompanying lactic acidosis and ketosis, respectively. Regular ingestion of alcohol also increases urate production by stimulating purine nucleotide catabolism. Thus the legendary association of gout with imbibition has now acquired a sound metabolic explanation. Experimentally, urate crystals coated with endotoxins are particularly inflammatory; a subthreshold dose of injected uncoated crystals becomes violently inflammatory when endotoxin is given intravenously. Perhaps these observations bear upon the role of infection in precipitating attacks. It is postulated that uricosuric agents and allopurinol may induce acute attacks by lowering synovial fluid urate and favoring shedding of synovial crystals during dissolution.

The course of an untreated attack is highly variable. Initial attacks are usually self-limited. Mild attacks may subside in several hours or a few days. Severe attacks may last many days to several weeks. As the attack subsides, the inflamed skin may desquamate. Once the attack has broken, recovery is generally rapid and complete. The patient then re-enters an asymptomatic phase, often termed *intercritical* gout in recognition of the tendency of acute attacks to recur. The subsequent course of gout is difficult to predict. Some patients never have a second attack. Others never fully recover from the first episode and suffer a series of exacerbations leading directly to chronic gouty arthritis. More commonly a pattern of recurrences develops. In an extensive series, 62 per cent of patients had recurrences within the first year, 16 per cent in one to two years, 11 per cent in two to five years, and 4 per cent in five to ten years; 7 per cent had no recurrence during prolonged follow-up. In the untreated patient the frequency of attacks often increases, and they may become more severe, last longer, and eventually resolve less completely. The patient may reach a state in which he or she is rarely free of gouty inflammation, and in which residual swelling, stiffness, and joint pain give permanent disability not responsive to measures usually effective in acute attacks.

Tophaceous Gout. Before effective control of hyperuricemia became possible, more than one half of gouty patients developed visible tophi. The incidence now ranges from 13 to 25 per cent. In noncompliant patients it still exceeds 50 per cent. Development of tophi is correlated with the degree of hyperuricemia, severity of renal involvement, and duration of disease. The time from initial attack to visible tophaceous involvement ranged from 3 to 42 years in one large series, with an average of 11.6 years. In 0.5 per cent of patients, tophi are present at the time of the initial attack; virtually all such patients have gout secondary to a myeloproliferative disease.

Chronic gouty arthritis is a consequence of the progressive inability to dispose of urate as rapidly as it is produced. Crystalline deposits of urate appear in and around joints.

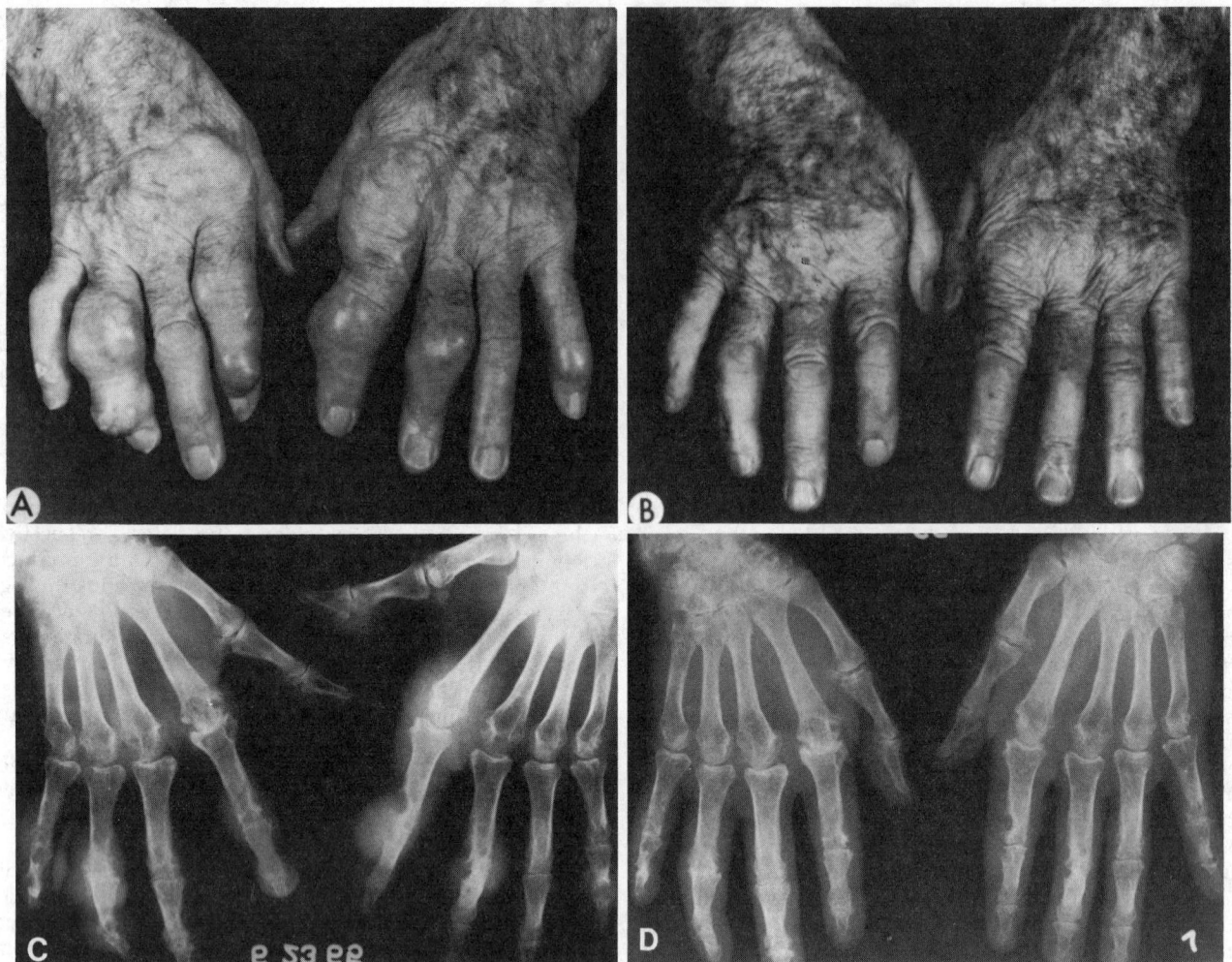

FIGURE 195–2. Chronic gouty arthritis (*A*) with tophaceous destruction of bone and joints (*C*), and improvement after three years of treatment with allopurinol, prophylactic colchicine, and a moderately low purine diet (*B* and *D*). (Courtesy of R. Wayne Rundles, Duke University Medical Center.)

Destruction of tissue is particularly evident in cartilage and bone, leading to radiolucent "punched-out" lesions, and to cortical erosions with characteristic "overhanging margins" (Fig. 195–2). A frequent site of tophaceous deposits is the external ear, especially in the helix and antihelix. Subcutaneous deposits, especially of fingertips, palms, and soles, may be visible as yellowish-white infiltrates. Tophaceous deposits may produce irregular asymmetric tumescences over joints. The classic gout shoe has a window cut to accommodate a tender prominent joint, usually the first metatarsophalangeal. At later stages, fusiform or nodular enlargements of Achilles tendons, or saccular distensions of olecranon bursae, are common and characteristic.

The process of tophaceous deposition advances insidiously, and although the tophi themselves are relatively painless, often progressive stiffness and persistent aching limit the use of affected joints. Eventually extensive destruction of joints and large subcutaneous tophi may lead to grotesque deformities and progressive crippling (Fig. 195–2). The tense, shiny, thin skin overlying the tophus may ulcerate and extrude white chalky or pasty material composed of myriads of fine, needle-like crystals. The olecranon bursa may be massively distended with "urate milk." Rarely tophi may involve the tongue, epiglottis, vocal cords, arytenoid cartilage, corpus cavernosum and prepuce of the penis, aorta, aortic or mitral valves, and cardiac conducting system, causing rhythm disturbances. They do not involve the liver, spleen, lungs, or central nervous system.

As chronic gouty changes and renal disease advance, acute attacks occur less frequently and are milder. No joint is exempt from chronic gouty involvement, although those of the lower extremity and hand are most commonly involved. The hip and spinal joints are rarely affected by tophaceous changes in the absence of extensive disease elsewhere. Radiographic changes of the sacroiliac joint and aseptic necrosis of the hip are sometimes attributable to gout.

Gouty Nephropathy. Renal disease is common in gout. One third of patients show isosthenuria and moderate proteinuria. The glomerular filtration rate is well preserved in many gouty subjects, but in others it gradually falls. Decline in renal function appears to be correlated with aging, renal vascular disease and hypertension, renal calculi, pyelonephritis, or independently occurring nephropathy, including that of lead poisoning. Only occasionally is it ascribable to gout alone. Hyperuricemia alone had no deleterious effect upon renal function during follow-up studies of gouty subjects ranging up to 12 years (Berger and Yu). Renal dysfunction does not shorten life expectancy in the average gouty subject, even though uremia is the eventual cause of death in 17 to 25 per cent of subjects. The majority of gouty patients die of cardiac or cerebral vascular disease (60 per cent) or malignant disease, which occur in about the same incidence and at about the same time of life as in nongouty American males.

Hypertension is present in one third to one half of patients and may be severe (diastolic pressure >130 mm Hg) in 10 per cent. Arterial and arteriolar nephrosclerosis are frequently prominent post mortem. There are no characteristic clinical or laboratory features to distinguish gouty kidney from other causes of chronic renal failure, except for the association of gout with the former. Renal failure from gouty nephropathy in the absence of gouty arthritis, tophi, or stones is extraordinarily rare; indeed, the entity is open to question.

Gouty nephropathy, sometimes referred to as *urate nephropathy* to emphasize the identity of the interstitial crystals, must be distinguished from *uric acid nephropathy*, an entirely different entity leading to acute renal failure from tubular obstruction by uric acid crystals.

Urolithiasis. The incidence of urolithiasis in gout is correlated with both the degree of hyperuricemia and the magnitude of the 24-hour uric acid excretion. Above serum levels of 12 to 13 mg per deciliter or excretion values of 1100 mg per 24 hours, the incidence is 50 per cent. Many of these subjects will have secondary gout, with a myeloproliferative disease such as polycythemia vera or myeloid metaplasia. The incidence of stones in such patients is 35 to 40 per cent. Of gouty subjects who pass stones, about one third have their first episode of urolithiasis before the onset of gouty arthritis, sometimes more than a decade earlier. Pure uric acid stones are radiolucent and are demonstrable in the body only by use of contrast media. Renal stones are reduced in frequency in gouty patients given allopurinol.

GOUT ASSOCIATED WITH SPECIFIC ENZYME DEFECTS. Gout occurring on the basis of specific enzyme defects has special clinical features. These forms of gout are rare, accounting for fewer than 1 per cent of cases.

Glycogen Storage Disease Type I (see Ch. 179). Over 50 cases of von Gierke's glycogen storage disease (glucose-6-phosphatase deficiency) and gout have been recorded. Gout does not complicate other forms of glycogen storage disease. Affected subjects may develop gouty arthritis by the end of the first decade of life. Chronic tophaceous gout and gouty nephropathy may account for a major portion of morbidity when these patients become adults. The sexes are involved equally. Avoidance of nocturnal hypoglycemia by a diet high in starch or by continuous intragastric feeding may markedly reduce or even correct hyperuricemia and ameliorate gout. The hyperuricemia also responds to allopurinol, less well to uricosuric agents because of renal disease.

Hypoxanthine-Guanine Phosphoribosyltransferase Deficiency. Deficiency of HGPRT gives rise to two different X-linked syndromes. A complete deficiency is associated with the Lesch-Nyhan syndrome (see Ch. 196). There is extreme exaggeration of uric acid production, and the greatly increased excretion leads to crystalluria, renal stones with ureteral colic, and sometimes uric acid nephropathy. Death from renal failure usually occurs by age ten; if allopurinol therapy is begun early, the patients may live into their 20's. A few of the more than 100 reported patients, all males, have had typical attacks of gouty arthritis.

An incomplete deficiency of HGPRT is associated with renal stones and recurrent acute gouty arthritis. Erythrocytes show from 0.2 to 50 per cent of normal HGPRT activity; the disorder is heterogeneous. Fifteen per cent of patients show minimal to moderate neurologic dysfunction resembling spinocerebellar ataxis or cerebral palsy. A few have survived neonatal episodes of uric acid nephropathy. Gout usually begins in the second or third decades; tophi develop early. Three quarters of patients have renal stones, half of these before age ten. These subjects have more marked hyperuricemia (usually >10 mg per deciliter) and uricaciduria (usually >1 gram per 24 hours) than most gouty subjects. Fewer than 100 cases—again, all males—have been described. HGPRT normally catalyzes a reaction between hypoxanthine or guanine and PP-ribose-P in reconstituting ribonucleotides, often called a "salvage" reaction. In HGPRT deficiency intracellular PP-ribose-P levels are raised and drive the first reaction of purine biosynthesis to excess. The female heterozygous carriers of complete HGPRT deficiency are not hyperuricemic, and their erythrocytes show normal HGPRT assay values. Carriers of the partial defect may be hyperuricemic and may show intermediate levels of HGPRT activity. Presumably, only cells possessing at least minimal HGPRT activity survive lyonization. Heterozygotes for the partial defect may develop uric acid stones or typical gout, which may occur before the menopause. Partial HGPRT deficiency should be considered in all females with gout or uric acid stones who exhibit raised urinary uric acid excretion values.

Phosphoribosylpyrophosphate Synthetase Variants. These patients resemble those with partial HGPRT deficiency in showing marked hyperuricemia and uricaciduria, and in developing uric acid stones or gout, and sometimes uric acid nephropathy, at an early age. They do not have neurologic abnormalities. Purine overproduction is prodigious. The enzyme abnormalities, of which there are four different types leading to increased activity, result in increased intracellular concentrations of PP-ribose-P and excessive purine biosynthesis. This, too, is an X-linked disorder, and all gouty patients are males. Fewer than 20 families have been identified with this disorder.

SECONDARY GOUT. Any acquired hyperuricemic state may be complicated by secondary gout. This disorder occurs in 5 to 10 per cent of patients with polycythemia vera or myeloid metaplasia, occasionally in secondary polycythemia complicating congenital heart disease or chronic pulmonary disease, in chronic myelogenous leukemia, in multiple myeloma, or in chronic hemolytic anemias. In such instances the mean age of onset is later (59 years), women are more commonly involved (16 per cent), and both serum and urinary uric acid values tend to be higher than in idiopathic primary gout. Acute gouty arthritis may occasionally antedate evidence of the myeloproliferative disorder by many months, or even by several years. A syndrome of coexisting sarcoidosis, psoriasis, and gout has been described but may represent fortuitous concurrence of common diseases.

In all the instances mentioned above, hyperuricemia appears to result from an increase in turnover of nucleic acid. Hyperuricemia may also result from reduced renal excretion of urate, either because of drug effects or because of parenchymal disease.

Hyperuricemia frequently follows the use of potent diuretic agents. Mean increases in serum urate concentrations are less than 2 mg per deciliter, but some subjects exhibit rises of 4 to 5 mg per deciliter. The hyperuricemic effect of diuretic agents results from salt and water loss, volume contraction, and avid solute reabsorption (including urate) in the proximal tubule. Typical gouty attacks may occur in patients receiving such drugs as hydrochlorothiazide, ethacrynic acid, or furosemide. In the 14-year study of the adult population of Framingham, Massachusetts, one half of the new cases of gout occurred in subjects taking potent diuretics. Three to five per cent of patients with gout have diabetes, but this incidence is not far from that of diabetes in the population of equivalent age. In markedly obese patients, total caloric restriction may result in extreme hyperuricemia, which is correlated with serum levels of beta-hydroxybutyric acid and may be associated with severe attacks of acute gouty arthritis, especially of knees and ankles.

Chronic renal disease is a frequent cause of hyperuricemia, but only about 1 patient per 1000 develops gout. Uremia appears to interfere in some way with the inflammatory response to urate crystals. Gout continues to be found in patients who survive lead exposure early in life and go on to develop slowly progressive lead nephropathy. In addition, saturnine gout is particularly prevalent in the southeastern United States, where it is attributed to the chronic ingestion of moonshine whiskey of high lead content with resulting renal tubular damage. Lead nephropathy and polycystic renal disease predispose to gout more often than do other forms of chronic renal disease.

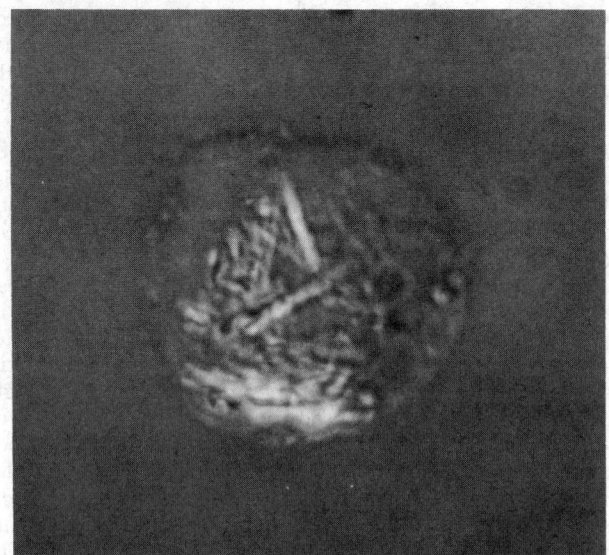

FIGURE 195–3. Sodium urate monohydrate crystals phagocytized by leukocyte in synovial fluid from acute gouty arthritis, examined by polarized light. (Courtesy of Edward W. Holmes, Duke University Medical Center.)

DIAGNOSIS. The diagnosis of acute gouty arthritis is not difficult when there is an explosive onset of a typical inflammatory attack of characteristic severity in a peripheral joint, especially of the lower extremity. The diagnosis is established by the demonstration of typical negatively birefringent needle-shaped crystals of sodium urate in the leukocytes of synovial fluid (Fig. 195–3). With proper technique, including the use of a polarizing microscope, intraleukocytic sodium urate crystals are found in over 95 per cent of aspirates from joints in acute gout. The leukocyte count may range from 1000 to more than 50,000, depending on the acuteness of the inflammation. A Gram stain should always be obtained to evaluate infection, which may coexist. In the rare event of failure to find crystals on the first attempt, a second aspirate obtained some hours later is usually positive. Urate crystals must be distinguished from calcium pyrophosphate dihydrate crystals of pseudogout. The latter are weakly positively birefringent under polarized light and usually more rectangular than urate crystals. Every patient suspected of having gout should have the diagnosis confirmed by crystal demonstration. It is not necessary to repeat the procedure in later attacks, unless they are atypical and other diagnoses (trauma, infection) are also under consideration. A rapid response of pain and inflammation to the administration of colchicine is so characteristic as also to be of diagnostic value. Responses of rheumatoid arthritis and sarcoid arthritis to colchicine are not so dramatic or complete as those in gout. The finding of hyperuricemia is anticipated and helpful, but since hyperuricemia is common (13 per cent of hospitalized male patients), it may coexist with other acute arthropathies. The presence of tophi or of typical roentgenographic findings of punched-out, destructive bony lesions will help establish the diagnosis of chronic tophaceous gout, but does not prove that the current event is acute gout. Only the demonstration of a large proportion of intraleukocytic crystals of sodium urate in the synovial fluid of the involved joint will do that. In 70 per cent of patients with crystal-proven gout, extracellular urate crystals are demonstrable in asymptomatic first metatarsophalangeal joints. Such crystals are rare (5 per cent) in hyperuricemic subjects who have never had clinical gout.

Each gouty patient should also have a determination of the 24-hour urinary excretion of uric acid. The sample should be collected after three days of moderate purine restriction, during an intercritical period. Values of greater than 600 mg per 1.72 square meters per day under these conditions prob-

ably indicate overproduction, and those of over 800 mg per day warrant additional studies for a specific subtype of primary gout, such as HGPRT deficiency of PP-ribose-P synthetase overactivity, or of secondary gout, such as a myeloproliferative disorder. Elevated urinary uric acid values also signify that the patient is at higher risk for renal stone and represent an indication for allopurinol rather than uricosuric drug therapy for gout.

Chronic gouty arthritis may be diagnosed by the presence of urate deposits in or near the affected joints or bursae or of soft-tissue deposits in the helix of the ear, the fingertips, the Achilles tendon, or other locations. The diagnosis may be confirmed by removal of the chalky contents of a tophus, by microscopic identification of sodium urate crystals by optical means, by chemical identification by the murexide test, or, preferably, by ultraviolet spectrophotometry and degradation by uricase.

DIFFERENTIAL DIAGNOSIS. Acute gout must be differentiated from acute rheumatic fever, rheumatoid arthritis, traumatic arthritis, osteoarthritis, pyogenic arthritis, sarcoid arthritis, cellulitis, bursitis, tendinitis, and thrombophlebitis. Podagra, the most common initial presentation of gout, can be mimicked by trauma, degenerative arthritis, acute sarcoidosis, psoriatic arthritis, pseudogout, palindromic rheumatism, Reiter's syndrome, or infection. Acute monoarticular arthritis of the great toe in the immediate postoperative period following parathyroidectomy can be caused by hydroxyapatite crystals. These various forms of "pseudopodagra" may be suggested by a negative examination of synovial fluid for urate crystals. Pseudogout (see Ch. 444), which is manifested by acute attacks of arthritis of knees and other joints, is usually accompanied by calcification of joint cartilage; the synovial fluid contains nonurate crystals of calcium pyrophosphate. However, gout and pseudogout may coexist, and both types of crystals will then be found in synovial fluid leukocytes.

Chronic gouty arthritis must chiefly be differentiated from rheumatoid arthritis, osteoarthritis, traumatic arthritis, and residua of pyogenic arthritis. The history of onset, progression, response to colchicine, and demonstration of hyperuricemia, asymmetric tumescences, typical roentgenographic changes, and tophi or crystals of urate in synovial fluid and leukocytes should establish the diagnosis.

TREATMENT. The therapeutic aims in gout are (1) to terminate the acute gouty attack as promptly and gently as possible, (2) to prevent recurrences of acute gouty arthritis, (3) to prevent or reverse complications of the disease resulting from deposition of sodium urate in joints and kidneys, and (4) to prevent formation of uric acid kidney stones. The therapeutic program differs according to the stage of the disease and the complications present. In the majority of patients it is possible to abort or prevent acute attacks, to control hyperuricemia, and to prevent chronic gouty arthritis, nephropathy, and stones.

Acute Attack. The affected joint should be placed at rest, and an anti-inflammatory agent administered promptly. Three types of agents are available: colchicine, nonsteroidal anti-inflammatory agents, and glucocorticoids (or ACTH). *Colchicine* is the only agent of specific diagnostic value in acute gout. It should be given as soon as the diagnosis is suspected. The initial dose of 0.6 to 1.2 mg of colchicine is followed by 0.6 mg every hour for eight hours and then every two hours until pain is relieved or until nausea, vomiting, cramping, or diarrhea develops. Maximum tolerated doses range from 4 to 8 mg. In many patients dramatic relief of pain and onset of gastrointestinal side effects occur simultaneously. The diarrhea may be treated with paregoric, 4 ml, or Kaopectate, 30 ml, after each loose stool. Colchicine should be discontinued until gastrointestinal symptoms subside. Since the effective dose of colchicine varies, each patient should learn his or her own tolerance dose and stop just short of this in treatment of subsequent attacks. If started promptly, colchicine affords relief over 90 per cent of the time; if treatment is delayed beyond 12 hours, only 75 per cent of patients will respond within 24 to 48 hours. Since colchicine is concentrated within cells and turns over with a half-life of about 30 hours, repeated courses of colchicine carry a higher risk of toxicity; treatment failures should be treated with a nonsteroidal anti-inflammatory drug (NSAID).

Colchicine may also be given intravenously (subcutaneous infiltration may result in tissue necrosis). The usual initial dose is 1 to 2 mg in 20 ml saline solution given slowly, and if a single dose is not effective, the injection may be repeated once in four to five hours (maximum intravenous dose, 3 to 5 mg). Gastrointestinal symptoms are uncommon with intravenous administration, although occasionally nausea will occur.

Dose-related toxic responses to colchicine include alopecia (reversible), bone marrow suppression (leukopenia, thrombocytopenia, anemia), and hepatocellular damage. The drug should not be used in patients with advanced hepatic or renal disease.

NSAID's are equally effective in acute gout, and are usually preferred over colchicine because they are so much milder for the patient. Indomethacin has been most widely used. It is given orally in initial doses of 50 mg three or four times a day. When pain is relieved, doses are tapered over another 48 to 72 hours. Larger doses may cause severe headache, gastric distress, or a transient depersonalization reaction in some patients, but these side effects have been noted only rarely in gouty patients receiving short courses of the drug. *Phenylbutazone* and *oxyphenbutazone* (Tandearil) are also effective in acute gouty arthritis and may be preferred when the gouty attack has proceeded for some time or when the attack does not abate completely with colchicine or indomethacin. The initial dose is 400 mg orally, followed by 100 mg every four to eight hours for two to three days. Bone marrow suppression may rarely occur, even after a short course of either drug. Other NSAID's, such as *naproxen* and *ibuprofen*, can also be used, especially in patients with a history of peptic ulcer. With all NSAID's, renal function should be monitored, especially in hypertensive patients.

If full doses of colchicine or NSAID's are contraindicated (e.g., in postoperative gout) or ineffective, *ACTH* may be employed by intravenous drip (40 units per day) or as intramuscular gel (40 to 80 units per day), or systemic glucocorticoids may be given for two to three days, rarely longer, following which the doses are reduced in stepwise fashion and discontinued. Unfortunately, rebound attacks of gout are rather common after such therapy. *Triamcinolone hexacetonide* in a dose of 5 to 20 mg injected intra-articularly into the involved joint is useful in treating acute gout limited to a single joint or bursa, particularly in patients in whom the standard drugs cannot be used, and relief from pain is usually prompt and complete within 24 to 36 hours. Steroid hormones are not recommended for parenteral use in acute gout, as the effects are inconsistent and rebound attacks frequent.

Uricosuric agents and allopurinol are of no value in treatment of the acute attack.

Interval Phase. The patient with gout should avoid high purine foods so as to lessen the burden of uric acid excretion. A severe limitation of purine-containing foods is rarely indicated, unless renal function is poor. Gradual weight reduction is indicated if the patient is overweight, and may of itself reduce hyperuricemia and the tendency to develop attacks of gout. Sudden weight reduction may precipitate gouty attacks and should be avoided. In general, diets of moderate protein content, somewhat low in fat, are preferred. Hypertension should be treated vigorously, even if antihypertensive agents worsen hyperuricemia; the result can be countered with appropriate antihyperuricemic drug therapy.

A high fluid intake is advisable to maintain a urinary output of 2000 ml per day. Uric acid excretion is thus promoted, and the dangers of crystal formation in the kidney or ureter are reduced. Beer, ale, and wine should be avoided, as they may precipitate attacks. Distilled alcoholic beverages in moderation generally have little influence on the gouty process. Illicit liquor (moonshine) should be prohibited. Excessive alcohol use in any form should be avoided, as it enhances purine production and also leads to hypertriglyceridemia.

Patients who recognize prodromal symptoms may abort acute attacks by prompt institution of colchicine, phenylbutazone, or indomethacin therapy; they frequently require only a few tablets to achieve success. The daily ingestion of 0.6 to 1.8 mg of colchicine is generally effective in reducing the number of acute gouty attacks in patients who are subject to frequent episodes. Toxicity is rare, but may include alopecia, bone marrow suppression, and hepatocellular damage. Maintenance colchicine therapy is particularly important during the first months or year after institution of uricosuric drugs or of allopurinol. Daily ingestion of indomethacin, 25 or 50 mg has also been employed for this purpose and appears to be effective. The risks of renal and gastrointestinal toxicity make use of indomethacin undesirable as a prophylactic agent or as therapy for chronic gouty arthritis.

Chronic Gouty Arthritis. Use of a drug to lower the serum level of uric acid to 6 mg per 100 ml or less is indicated in all gouty patients with visible tophi, with roentgenographic evidence of urate deposits, or with a history of two or more major attacks of acute gouty arthritis. Allopurinol is the drug of choice unless the patient is already well managed with a uricosuric agent. With either type of agent the number of acute gouty attacks may be increased during the first few months unless maintenance colchicine therapy is given, whereas after 12 to 18 months the number may be decidedly reduced.

Allopurinol controls serum urate levels by inhibiting xanthine oxidase and thereby regulating production of uric acid (Fig. 195–1). Allopurinol is converted to oxipurinol in the body, and the latter compound has a longer biologic half-life (28 hours), ultimately being largely excreted in the urine. Inhibition of conversion of hypoxanthine and xanthine to uric acid permits these precursors to be excreted instead. In gouty subjects other than those with HGPRT deficiency, the increment in hypoxanthine plus xanthine excretion is only about two thirds of the decrement in uric acid excretion, presumably because of enhanced feed-back inhibition of purine synthesis de novo by nucleotides reconstituted from hypoxanthine. The induced xanthinuria has not resulted in xanthine stone formation in the usual gouty subjects, but has done so in a rare patient with HGPRT deficiency and in patients being treated with antineoplastic agents. Use of allopurinol results in reduction of levels of uric acid in serum *and in urine*. The drug is effective even in the presence of renal failure, when uricosuric agents generally are not. Its action is not blocked by salicylates. The usual dose is 300 mg, given orally once a day. In the presence of moderate nitrogen retention the dose of allopurinol should be reduced by one half or more (see Ch. 24), as the biologic half-life of the active metabolite, oxipurinol, is prolonged. Allopurinol is usually well tolerated, but may cause gastric irritation, diarrhea, or skin rash or induce an attack of gout. Toxic hepatitis, epidermal necrolysis, and vasculitis may occasionally be severe, even fatal. Toxic effects are more frequent and more severe in the presence of renal failure. Intramuscular crystals of xanthine and oxipurinol have been described in patients receiving allopurinol, but their significance in terms of toxicity is not clear. Uricosuric agents may be used concurrently with allopurinol to hasten mobilization of urate deposits, but combined therapy may require larger doses of allopurinol because uricosuric drugs also enhance the excretion of oxipurinol. Since allopurinol decreases uric acid excretion, it is also very useful in controlling uric acid stone formation, especially in patients who are overproducers of uric acid. If the serum urate values can be controlled at levels below saturation of urate in body fluids, extensive resolution of soft tissue tophi and modest reduction in size of bony erosions may be achieved, together with some recalcification of bony lesions (Fig. 195–2). Joint mobility and comfort may be greatly improved.

Uricosuric drugs block tubular reabsorption of filtered urate. Those of use in gout are probenecid and sulfinpyrazone. These agents begin to lose effectiveness when the creatinine clearance falls below 80 ml per minute and are completely ineffective when the clearance falls below 30 ml per minute. *Probenecid* is given in doses of 0.5 gram to 3 grams daily in two or three evenly spaced doses (average dose, 1 to 1.5 grams). This drug may produce gastrointestinal upsets, headaches, or skin rash. *Sulfinpyrazone* may be given in doses of 100 to 600 mg daily in three or four divided doses (average dose, 300 mg). This drug is related to phenylbutazone and may cause untoward reactions, but is generally somewhat better tolerated than probenecid. *Salicylates* block the uricosuric action of both probenecid and sulfinpyrazone and must not be used concurrently. Salicylates are uricosuric when given in high doses (4 to 6 grams daily), but few patients can tolerate these quantities.

With all uricosuric agents the doses should be low initially, to avoid sudden excretion of large quantities of urate, and increased at weekly intervals to maintenance levels. Fluids should be forced to prevent formation of concentrated urine, especially during the late hours of the night. During the first days or weeks of therapy the urine should be kept at pH 6 or above, by administration of sodium bicarbonate or sodium citrate–citric acid (Shohl's solution); this may be difficult to achieve, as acid urine tends to be produced in gouty patients. In patients in whom urate is being mobilized, and especially those in whom uric acid gravel is formed, alkalinization during the night, when fluid intake is reduced, is important. A single 250-mg tablet of acetazolamide (Diamox) taken at bedtime will serve to keep the urine alkaline and dilute throughout the night.

In selected patients surgical removal of large extra-articular urate deposits, such as those in olecranon bursae, may be advisable. Occasionally amputation of irreparably damaged digits, especially those containing draining sinuses, is indicated. Physical therapy and appropriate self-help devices are valuable in patients who are partially disabled.

Asymptomatic Hyperuricemia. Asymptomatic hyperuricemia is frequent in family members of patients with gout and in the general population. It usually requires no therapy, as only about one fifth of patients will ever develop articular attacks, and adequate therapy can be instituted when these supervene. Exceptions may exist in patients with markedly elevated serum levels of uric acid, especially if urinary urate excretion is low and there is a family history of tophaceous disease. In such circumstances the asymptomatic subject should be treated with allopurinol before articular or renal complications develop. It is essential that the physician maintain frequent close observation of the patient.

Berger, L. Yu T-F: Renal function in gout: IV. An analysis of 524 gouty subjects including long-term follow-up studies. Am J Med 59:605, 1975. *An important study showing that deterioration of renal function in gout is largely associated with aging, renal vascular disease, hypertension, renal calculi with pyelonephritis, or independently occurring nephropathy. Hyperuricemia alone had no deleterious effect on renal function over periods up to 12 years.*

Cherian PV, Schumacher HR Jr: Immunochemical and ultrastructural characterization of serum proteins associated with monosodium urate crystals (MSU) in synovial fluid cells from patients with gout. Ultrastruct Pathol 10:209, 1986. *Various proteins associated with intracellular urate crystals, IgG > IgM or IgA > C3 or fibrinogen, may influence the inflammatory properties of those crystals.*

Reibman J, Haines KA, Rich AM, et al.: Colchicine inhibits ionophore-induced formation of leukotriene B₄ by human neutrophils: The role of microtubules. J Immunol 136:1027, 1986. *The mechanisms of colchicine action in inhibiting production of leukotriene B₄ by neutrophils appears to depend upon its effect upon the number and integrity of the microtubules.*

Simkin PS: Uric acid excretion in patients with gout. Arthritis Rheum 22:98, 1979. *An analysis of six published studies relating the rate of urate excretion to*

plasma urate levels in normal and gouty subjects. The kidneys of the average gouty person lag significantly behind the normal in their response to any concentration of plasma urate. The kidneys of overproducers (38 of 73 gouty subjects) were no less handicapped than those of other gouty subjects.

Spillberg I, Mandell B, Mehta J, et al.: Mechanism of action of colchicine in acute urate crystal-induced arthritis. J Clin Invest 64:775, 1979. *Phagocytosis of urate crystals by neutrophils induces the synthesis and release of a glycoprotein that is chemotactic both in vitro and in vivo. Colchicine decreases production and release of this factor. Colchicine abrogates the acute arthritis produced by urate crystals in rabbits, but has no effect upon the arthritis induced by injection of purified cell-derived chemotactic factor.*

Wyngaarden JB, Kelley WN: Gout. In Stanbury JB, Wyngaarden JB, Fredrickson DS, et al. (eds): The Metabolic Basis of Inherited Disease. 5th ed. New York, McGraw-Hill Book Company, 1983. *A detailed account of purine metabolism and the pathogenesis of primary gout.*

Wyngaarden JB, Kelley WN: Gout and Hyperuricemia. New York, Grune & Stratton, 1976. *Everything you have always wanted to know about gout but never dared to ask, condensed into 500 pages.*

---

196 OTHER DISORDERS OF PURINE METABOLISM

Edward W. Holmes

XANTHINURIA

Classic xanthinuria, which is inherited as an autosomal recessive trait, is the consequence of an isolated deficiency of xanthine oxidase. As a result of this enzyme deficiency, uric acid is replaced by xanthine and hypoxanthine as the end products of purine metabolism. Serum urate concentrations in these patients range from 0 to 1.4 mg per deciliter and urinary uric acid excretion ranges from 0 to 8 mg per day; serum oxypurine (xanthine plus hypoxanthine) concentrations and urine oxypurine excretion are increased in this disorder.

More than 50 patients with classic xanthinuria have been described, and the prevalence of this disorder is estimated to be approximately 1 in 45,000. Over 50 per cent of individuals with classic xanthinuria are asymptomatic, the diagnosis being suspected by the incidental finding of a very low serum urate concentration during evaluation of presumably unrelated medical problems. The diagnosis is virtually established by the demonstration of low serum and urinary uric acid levels in association with increased urinary oxypurine excretion, and it is confirmed by assaying liver or intestinal mucosa for xanthine oxidase activity. One third of patients develop radiolucent renal calculi composed of xanthine. Four adult patients have had myopathic symptoms characterized by muscle cramps following exercise, and crystalline deposits of xanthine and hypoxanthine have been found in skeletal muscle. Recurrent polyarthritis has been described in three patients, and it has been suggested but not established that this symptom may represent crystal-induced synovitis.

A new subtype of xanthinuria has been described in which the deficiency of xanthine oxidase is associated with a deficiency of sulfite oxidase. Both of these enzymes require a molybdenum cofactor for catalytic activity, and absence of this cofactor has been demonstrated in the liver of a patient with this combined enzyme defect. Five patients have been reported with an inherited deficiency of these two enzymes, and all five presented in the first weeks of life with a severe neurologic disorder characteristic of isolated sulfite oxidase deficiency. Symptoms include feeding difficulties from birth, tonic-clonic seizures, nystagmus, enophthalmus, ocular lens dislocation, and Brushfield spots. As in isolated sulfite oxidase deficiency, urinary excretion of sulfate is low while that of sulfite, thiosulfate, S-sulfocysteine, and taurine is increased. Characteristic biochemical findings of xanthinuria are also present.

An acquired phenocopy of the combined defect has been

described in a 20-year-old male with short-bowel syndrome maintained for 18 months with total parenteral nutrition. In addition to hypouricemia and hypouricaciduria, urinary excretion of sulfite and thiosulfate was increased while excretion of sulfate was decreased. Following infusion of commercially available amino acid solutions the patient experienced headaches, night blindness, irritability, lethargy, and then coma.

The prognosis in classic xanthinuria is excellent, as shown by the high percentage of patients who are asymptomatic. Therapy for xanthine calculi includes high fluid intake, and on occasion allopurinol has been used in patients with residual xanthine oxidase activity to increase the excretion of hypoxanthine relative to xanthine, the former being more soluble than the latter. In patients with the inherited form of combined xanthine oxidase and sulfite oxidase deficiency, the neurologic symptoms have been refractory to therapy with a number of agents, including oral ammonium molybdate. With the acquired form of this combined disorder, treatment with ammonium molybdate reversed the biochemical abnormalities and the neurologic symptoms were markedly ameliorated.

Holmes EW, Wyngaarden JB: Hereditary xanthinuria. In Stanbury JB, Wyngaarden JB, Fredrickson DS, et al.: (eds.): The Metabolic Basis of Inherited Disease. 5th ed. New York, McGraw-Hill Book Company, 1983, pp 1192–1201. *A thorough coverage of the clinical and biochemical abnormalities found in classic xanthinuria, as well as the inherited and acquired forms of the combined deficiency of xanthine oxidase and sulfite oxidase.*
Wadman SK, Duran M, Beemer FA, et al.: Absence of hepatic molybdenum cofactor: An inborn error of metabolism leading to a combined deficiency of sulfite oxidase and xanthine dehydrogenase. J Inherited Metab Dis 6:78, 1983. *Metabolic and clinical observations on five patients with this disorder.*

THE LESCH-NYHAN SYNDROME AND PARTIAL DEFICIENCY OF HYPOXANTHINE-GUANINE PHOSPHORIBOSYLTRANSFERASE

The Lesch-Nyhan syndrome, caused by a virtually complete deficiency of hypoxanthine-guanine phosphoribosyltransferase (HGPRT) activity, is manifested clinically by hyperuricemia, excessive production of uric acid, and neurologic features including self-mutilation, choreoathetosis, spasticity, and mental retardation. Partial deficiency of HGPRT activity is associated with uric acid overproduction, severe gout, and occasionally neurologic abnormalities, but self-mutilation is absent. The Lesch-Nyhan syndrome occurs in about one in 100,000 births, and partial deficiency of HGPRT is noted in less than 1 per cent of the gouty population.

ETIOLOGY AND PATHOGENESIS. Studies have demonstrated a single but different amino acid substitution in 16 mutant forms of HGPRT documenting marked genetic heterogeneity in this disorder. Failure to reutilize hypoxanthine in the salvage pathway as a result of HGPRT deficiency leads to increased oxidation of this purine base to uric acid. An increase in the intracellular concentration of phosphoribosylpyrophosphate, which also results from reduction in hypoxanthine reutilization, leads to an increase in the rate of purine biosynthesis de novo. The combined effect of these abnormalities is increased uric acid production resulting in hyperuricaciduria, which predisposes to uric acid crystal and stone formation, and hyperuricemia, which leads to gouty arthritis and tophaceous deposits. The biochemical basis for the unusual and devastating neurologic abnormalities seen in the Lesch-Nyhan syndrome is not clearly understood, but abnormalities in dopamine neuron function have been described. Position emission tomography has demonstrated a selective decrease in glucose utilization in the caudate.

CLINICAL MANIFESTATIONS. The gene for HGPRT is located on the X chromosome, and consequently the deficiency of HGPRT activity is fully expressed only in affected males. Females heterozygous for HGPRT deficiency may have subtle abnormalities in purine metabolism, but they are generally asymptomatic.

Infants with the Lesch-Nyhan syndrome are normal at birth,

and the earliest consistent abnormality is a delay in motor development noted at three to four months of age. Between eight and twelve months extrapyramidal signs develop leading to choreoathetosis, and at about one year of age signs of pyramidal tract involvement, such as hyper-reflexia, clonus, and scissoring of the legs, appear. Compulsive self-destructive behavior appears any time between early childhood and adolescence. This is the most distinctive neurologic feature of the syndrome, and is manifested by biting of the fingers, lips, and buccal mucosa. Repeated attempts at self-injury, such as placing extremities in dangerous areas and self-inflicted head trauma, are also common. Sensation is intact in these children. Mental retardation is noted in most cases, but it is unclear whether the enzyme deficiency per se causes this or whether it is the result of poor performance on formal testing in children with dysarthria and choreoathetosis. Growth retardation is also a prominent feature of the syndrome. Uric acid crystalluria may be noted as orange crystals on the diaper during the first weeks of life and in untreated patients progresses to uric acid nephrolithiasis, obstructive uropathy, and azotemia. Hyperuricemia is usually present and may attain levels of 18 mg per deciliter, but the serum urate concentration may be normal, especially before puberty. Gout is unusual in the Lesch-Nyhan syndrome before 12 to 15 years of age. Death usually occurs in the second or third decade from infection or renal failure.

Patients with partial deficiency of HGPRT develop uric acid crystalluria and renal calculi in childhood, and gouty arthritis often occurs before 20 years of age. Neurologic manifestations, including mental retardation, mild spastic quadriplegia, dysarthria, cerebellar ataxia, and seizures, are noted in 20 per cent of patients with partial HGPRT deficiency, but self-mutilation does not develop. Patients with partial HGPRT deficiency may seek medical attention with the only symptom being the passage of a renal calculus or an attack of gouty arthritis. Life expectancy is normal in these patients.

DIAGNOSIS. Self-destructive behavior is the most distinguishing clinical feature of the Lesch-Nyhan syndrome; whereas retarded children with other disorders will bite their fingers, mutilation to the point of tissue destruction is rare in any disorder other than the Lesch-Nyhan syndrome. Severe self-biting in other neurologic disorders is usually associated with a loss of pain sensation. As pointed out, hyperuricemia is usually present, but this is not an invariable finding. The diagnosis is established by demonstrating a virtual absence of HGPRT activity in readily accessible tissues such as erythrocytes. Analyses of erythrocyte lysates are not useful in identifying heterozygous female carriers, but this can be accomplished with cell culture of skin fibroblasts or through analysis of hair follicles.

Partial deficiency of HGPRT should be suspected in male patients with the onset of gouty arthritis before 20 years of age and in young males with uric acid crystalluria or uric acid nephrolithiasis. Uric acid overexcretion is found invariably in patients with normal renal function, and the diagnosis is confirmed by enzyme assay. Patients with partial HGPRT activity will have erythrocyte lysate values that are usually in the range of 0.1 to 5 per cent of control values, rarely up 30 to 50 per cent of control values, while Lesch-Nyhan patients will have values less than 0.01 per cent of control values.

TREATMENT. Uric acid stone formation, tophi, and gouty arthritis can be controlled in both the Lesch-Nyhan syndrome and partial deficiency of HGPRT with drugs that inhibit xanthine oxidase activity. However, a few patients have developed xanthine stones with this therapy. No drugs have been found that correct the neurologic deficits, but supportive measures such as restraints that reduce the tendency to self-mutilation are well accepted by the patient. Drugs such as diazepam help control the movement disorder. Given the devastating neurologic complications of the Lesch-Nyhan syndrome, therapeutic abortion has been used as a preventive measure following heterozygote identification and intrauterine diagnosis.

Edwards NL, Recker D, Fox IH: Overproduction of uric acid in hypoxanthine-guanine phosphoribosyltransferase deficiency. J Clin Invest 63:922, 1979. *A careful analysis of the basis for uric acid overproduction in patients with HGPRT deficiency.*

Kelley WN, Wyngaarden JB: Clinical syndromes associated with hypoxanthine-guanine phosphoribosyltransferase deficiency. In Stanbury JB, Wyngaarden JB, Fredrickson DS, et al. (eds.): The Metabolic Basis of Inherited Disease. 5th ed. New York, McGraw-Hill Book Company, 1983, pp 1115–1143. *A detailed description of the clinical and biochemical consequences of HGPRT deficiency.*

Wilson JM, Stout JT, Palella TD, et al.: A molecular survey of hypoxanthine-guanine phosphoribosyltransferase deficiency in man. J Clin Invest 77:188, 1986. *A description of specific mutations at the molecular level in patients with HGPRT deficiency.*

2,8-DIHYDROXYADENINE RENAL STONES

Deficiency of adenine phosphoribosyltransferase, an enzyme in the salvage pathway of purine nucleotide synthesis, leads to the accumulation and increased urinary excretion of 2,8-dihydroxyadenine, the product of adenine oxidation by xanthine oxidase. Because of the insolubility of this purine, patients with this autosomal recessive disorder are predisposed to development of renal calculi composed of 2,8-dihydroxyadenine. Six individuals homozygous for this enzyme deficiency have presented with acute renal failure, and three of these patients suffered permanent renal damage. Renal colic may occur within the first months of life, as late as 40 years of age, or individuals with this disorder may be asymptomatic. 2,8-Dihydroxyadenine stones are usually radiolucent. The diagnosis is confirmed by analysis of the stone with ultraviolet, infrared, or mass spectrometry or x-ray crystallography, or by demonstrating the absence of adenine phosphoribosyltransferase activity in erythrocyte lysates. Except for the excessive excretion of adenine and its metabolites with the consequent development of renal calculi, no other biochemical or clinical abnormalities have been reported in individuals homozygous for this enzyme deficiency.

The prevalence of the homozygous state is not documented, but it is calculated to occur once in 35,000 to 250,000 births, since the prevalence of heterozygosity for adenine phosphoribosyltransferase deficiency varies from 0.4 to 1.0 per 100. Individuals heterozygous for the enzyme deficiency have no recognized clinical abnormalities.

Prognosis depends on renal function at the time of diagnosis. Therapy with dietary purine restriction, high fluid intake, and allopurinol—to prevent oxidation of adenine to 2,8-dihydroxyadenine—is effective in reducing stone formation and preserving renal function.

Simmonds A, Van Acker KL: Adenine phosphoribosyltransferase deficiency. In Stanbury JB, Wyngaarden JB, Fredrickson DS, et al. (eds.): The Metabolic Basis of Inherited Disease. 5th ed. New York, McGraw-Hill Book Company, 1983. *A detailed review of all known cases of complete APRT deficiency and discussion of the metabolic defect.*

Van Acker KJ, Simmonds A, Potter C, et al.: Complete deficiency of adenine phosphoribosyltransferase. Report of a family. N Engl J Med 297:127, 1977. *Adenine, 8-hydroxyadenine and 2,8-dihydroxyadenine amounted to 25 per cent of urinary purines in two homozygous male children, one of whom had "pure uric acid stones" later correctly identified as 2,8-dihydroxyadenine.*

MYOPATHY ASSOCIATED WITH MYOADENYLATE DEAMINASE DEFICIENCY

Deficiency of myoadenylate deaminase has been noted in approximately 2 per cent of muscle biopsies submitted for routine investigation in some centers. This isozyme of adenosine monophosphate (AMP) deaminase is found only in skeletal muscle, and this is the only organ affected by this enzyme deficiency. In approximately half of the cases that have been carefully studied, AMP deaminase deficiency is not associated with other neuromuscular pathology, and in these individuals the enzyme deficiency is marked (<1 per cent of normal). In cases in which the residual enzyme activity

is higher (1 to 10 per cent of normal) the patients have a broad spectrum of neuromuscular diseases. Three quarters of patients with primary myoadenylate deaminase deficiency report exercise-related symptoms of easy fatigability, cramps, and myalgias, usually beginning in childhood or young adulthood. Weakness without exercise is noted in less than one third of patients. Hypotonia has been described in two patients. Reduced AMP deaminase activity has occasionally been reported in patients with other neuromuscular disorders, but no definite association of this enzyme deficiency has been established with any symptom complex other than easy fatigability, cramps, and myalgias. Since a few individuals with myoadenylate deaminase deficiency have been reported to be asymptomatic, factors in addition to AMP deaminase deficiency may contribute to the exercise-related manifestations described above.

Serum creatine kinase activity is mildly and variably increased in about one half of patients with this disorder, and routine laboratory studies including electromyography and histochemistry of muscle are not diagnostic. In the patient with exercise-related symptoms the specific diagnosis of myoadenylate deaminase deficiency is suggested by the finding of reduced NH_3 production in a forearm ischemic exercise test. NH_3 is a product of AMP deamination, a normal consequence of ATP catabolism in skeletal muscle. However, not all patients with reduced NH_3 production following ischemic forearm exercise will have myoadenylate deaminase deficiency, and the diagnosis needs to be confirmed by direct assay of AMP deaminase activity in skeletal muscle.

AMP deaminase is one of the components of the purine nucleotide cycle, a series of reactions that is potentially important in energy production and utilization in skeletal muscle. Deficiency of myoadenylate deaminase activity may impair energy generation through diminished production of citric acid cycle intermediates, and it may adversely affect energy utilization through a reduction in the rate of adenosine triphosphate (ATP) hydrolysis by myofibrillar ATPase.

Prognosis in myoadenylate deaminase deficiency is generally good. Present experience suggests the symptoms are slowly progressive, and the disorder leads to mild disability in most cases, although there have been exceptions to these generalizations. No effective therapy is available at this time.

Fishbein WN: Myoadenylate deaminase deficiency: Inherited and acquired forms. Biochem Med 33:158, 1985. *Review of biochemical data supporting primary and secondary forms of AMP deaminase deficiency.*

Sabina RL, Swain JL, Olanow CW, et al.: Myoadenylate deaminase deficiency: Functional and metabolic abnormalities associated with disruption of the purine nucleotide cycle. J Clin Invest 73:720, 1984.

Swain JL, Sabina RL, Holmes EW: Myoadenylate Deaminase Deficiency. In Stanbury JB, Wyngaarden JK, Fredrickson DS, et al. (eds.): The Metabolic Basis of Inherited Disease. 5th ed. New York, McGraw-Hill Book Company, 1983, pp 1184–1191. *Discussion of the clinical and biochemical findings in 26 patients with myoadenylate deaminase deficiency, as well as a review of the role of the purine nucleotide cycle in skeletal muscle function.*

IMMUNE DYSFUNCTION ASSOCIATED WITH PURINE ENZYME DEFICIENCIES

Adenosine deaminase deficiency is an uncommon disorder, approximately 100 to 150 families having been identified, that leads to a clinical syndrome of severe combined immunodeficiency, i.e., a defect in both T cell and B cell function. About one fifth of patients with severe combined immunodeficiency, in which the disorder is inherited as an autosomal recessive condition, or more rarely as an X-linked recessive disorder, will have this enzyme deficiency. Approximately 85 per cent of patients with adenosine deaminase deficiency come to medical attention at one to two months of age with recurrent infections of the skin and the gastrointestinal and respiratory systems. Both ordinary and opportunistic pathogens are encountered, and candidiasis is almost invariably present. Diarrhea is common, as well as delayed physical growth and development. Physical findings are for the most part unremarkable except for the absence of lymph nodes and pharyngeal lymphoid tissue. A rachitic rosary, or prominence of the costochondral junctions, has been noted in some patients. Laboratory tests show absence of a thymic shadow, lymphopenia, negative skin test results for delayed hypersensitivity, attenuated lymphocyte responses to lectins and antigens in vitro, and hypogammaglobulinemia. The diagnosis is established by documenting adenosine deaminase deficiency in erythrocyte lysates or other cell extracts. Approximately 15 per cent of individuals with this disorder have a milder disease with later age of onset and relative sparing of humoral immunity. In the severe form of this disorder, if untreated, overwhelming infection and sepsis lead to death before two years of age.

Current mechanisms favored to explain the immune defects observed in adenosine deaminase deficiency are deoxy-ATP accumulation leading to inhibition of ribonucleotide reductase with resultant decrease in DNA replication, and S-adenosylhomocysteine accumulation leading to inhibition of transmethylation reactions. Either or both of these proposed mechanisms could reduce lymphocyte proliferation and function.

Treatment of adenosine deaminase deficiency by bone marrow transplantation has resulted in virtually complete immune reconstitution in some patients, and at present this is the preferred therapy if compatible donors are available. Enzyme replacement with repeated transfusions of irradiated red blood cells (to prevent graft-versus-host disease) has improved immune function in some patients.

Purine nucleoside phosphorylase deficiency is less common than adenosine deaminase deficiency, approximately 15 to 20 patients having been recognized with this disorder. Purine nucleoside phosphorylase deficiency is also inherited as an autosomal recessive disorder, but it leads to a defect in cell-mediated immunity with little if any abnormality in humoral immunity. In patients with this disorder diagnosis has been made as early as four months and as late as nine years of age, with infections involving skin, lung, middle ear, mastoids, and urinary tract. Infections with nonbacterial agents have been most common, reflecting the primary defect in cellular immunity. Laboratory tests show lymphopenia, diminished number of circulating T cells, reduced lymphocyte response to antigens, and negative skin test results for delayed hypersensitivity. Immunoglobulin levels are normal, but several patients have exhibited signs of immunoregulatory abnormalities as shown by autoimmune hemolytic anemia, antinuclear antibodies, and rheumatoid factor. In addition, patients with purine nucleoside phosphorylase deficiency have hypouricemia, a finding of no clinical consequence in itself, but one that suggests the diagnosis of this enzyme deficiency in a child with recurrent infections.

Confirmation of the diagnosis is obtained by assay of erythrocyte lysate or other cell extracts for purine nucleoside phosphorylase activity. It has been proposed that accumulation of deoxyguanosine triphosphate in T lymphocytes with resultant inhibition of ribonucleotide reductase and DNA replication is responsible for the immune defect in this disorder. Prognosis in purine nucleoside phosphorylase deficiency is generally better than that for adenosine deaminase deficiency, but therapy with bone marrow transplantation and erythrocyte transfusion has been less successful.

Adenosine deaminase in disorders of purine metabolism and in immune deficiency. Ann NY Acad Sci vol. 451, 1985. *A collection of papers dealing with clinical, metabolic, and immunologic aspects of adenosine deaminase deficiency.*

Giblett ER: Adenosine deaminase and purine nucleoside phosphorylase deficiency: How they were discovered and what they may mean. In Elliot K, Whelan J (eds.): Enzyme Defects and Immune Dysfunction. Ciba Found Symp 68:3, 1979. *An interesting story about scientific serendipity and discovery of a new group of clinical disorders.*

Kredich N, Hershfield MS: Immunodeficiency diseases caused by adenosine deaminase deficiency and purine nucleoside phosphorylase deficiency. In Stanbury JB, Wyngaarden JB, Fredrickson DS, et al. (eds.): The Metabolic Basis of Inherited Disease. 5th ed. New York, McGraw-Hill Book Company, 1983, p 1157. *An authoritative review of the clinical, laboratory, and biochemical abnormalities in these disorders. This chapter also includes a detailed discussion of purine nucleoside metabolism in normal and pathological situations.*

197 DISORDERS OF PYRIMIDINE METABOLISM

Lloyd H. Smith, Jr.

Pyrimidine nucleotides share equally with purine nucleotides the chemical chore of transmitting genetic information for reproduction or for phenotypic expression within the cell. They also function in the intermediary metabolism of lipids and carbohydrates. Only a few disorders of pyrimidine metabolism have been recognized.

Hereditary orotic aciduria is a rare genetic disorder of pyrimidine metabolism characterized by megaloblastic anemia resistant to the usual hematinic agents, leukopenia, failure of normal growth and development, and the continued excessive urinary excretion of orotic acid. Patients also have impaired cellular immunity with intact humoral immunity. Orotic acid is highly insoluble and often forms a heavy sediment of urinary crystals that may on occasion result in ureteral or urethral obstruction. The disorder, which is transmitted as an autosomal recessive trait, is usually characterized by reduced activities of two consecutive enzymes in pyrimidine biosynthesis, orotate phosphoribosyltransferase (OPRT) and orotidine 5'-phosphate decarboxylase (ODC). Both enzymatic activities may reside in a single multifunctional protein for which the gene is located on the long arm of chromosome 3. A single patient has been described with isolated deficiency of ODC. There is a prompt and sustained hematologic and general clinical response to oral uridine (2 to 4 grams per day), which must be continued indefinitely as replacement therapy. The disease has attracted special attention because it represents a block in the de novo pathway of pyrimidine synthesis, is an example of a double enzyme defect, and produces a requirement for replacement of a normal metabolic intermediate, uridine.

Orotic aciduria, without the characteristic hematologic abnormalities, also occurs in *ornithine transcarbamylase deficiency.* It is presumed that this results from the overflow of carbamyl phosphate from urea synthesis (partially blocked in this disease) to pyrimidine synthesis. Orotic aciduria has also been found in purine nucleoside phosphorylase deficiency and in PP-ribose-P synthetase deficiency (see Ch. 419).

Excessive urinary excretion of orotic acid and orotidine occurs during treatment with *allopurinol* or *6-azauridine.** Metabolic products of both compounds inhibit orotidine 5'-decarboxylase activity.

Beta-aminoisobutyric aciduria is a benign hereditary disorder of thymine catabolism that occurs in 5 to 10 per cent of Caucasians and in a much higher percentage of Asians. The defect presumably lies in the transamination of beta-aminoisobutyric acid to methylmalonic acid semialdehyde. The aminoaciduria that results, representing the only known disorder of pyrimidine catabolism, has no known biologic disadvantage.

Pyrimidine 5'-nucleotidase deficiency is a rare form of hereditary hemolytic anemia, transmitted as an autosomal recessive trait. The erythrocytes exhibit prominent basophilic stippling owing to aggregates of undegraded ribosomes and on analysis contain very high concentrations of cytidine and uridine nucleotides. The mechanism by which the nucleotidase deficiency leads to hemolysis is unclear. Lead inhibits pyrimidine 5'-nucleotidase activity and leads to a similar anemia with basophilic stippling, possibly through this mechanism.

Becoft DMO, Suttle DP, Webster DR: Orotic aciduria. In Scriver CR, Beaudet A, Sly W, et al. (eds.): The Metabolic Basis of Inherited Disease. 6th ed. New York, McGraw-Hill Book Company, 1988, in press. *This is the most*

*Investigational drug.

complete description of normal pyrimidine metabolism in man and the derangements that occur in hereditary orotic aciduria.

Girot R, Hamet M, Perignon J-L, et al.: Cellular immune deficiency in two siblings with hereditary orotic aciduria. N Engl J Med 308:700, 1983. *Two children with orotic aciduria exhibited impaired cellular immunity but normal humoral immunity, analogous to that seen with purine nucleoside phosphorylase deficiency.*

Smith LH Jr: Purine and pyrimidine metabolism in man. In Smith LH Jr, Thier SO (eds.): Pathophysiology: The Biological Principles of Disease. 2nd ed.

International Textbook of Medicine, Vol 1. Philadelphia, W. B. Saunders Company, 1985. *This chapter in the companion textbook of pathophysiology gives a classification and general survey of the currently recognized diseases involving the synthesis or degradation of pyrimidines.*

Valentine WN, Fink K, Paglia DE, et al.: Hereditary hemolytic anemia with human erythrocyte pyrimidine 5'-nucleotidase deficiency. J Clin Invest 54:866, 1974. *This is the original and still the best description of the altered pyrimidine metabolism leading to hemolytic anemia in this rare but interesting genetic disease.*

Inherited Disorders of Connective Tissue

198 THE MUCOPOLYSACCHARIDOSES
William S. Sly

The mucopolysaccharidoses are a group of lysosomal storage diseases, each of which is produced by an inherited deficiency of an enzyme involved in degradation of acid mucopolysaccharides (now called glycosaminoglycans and abbreviated GAG's). They are clinically progressive and have many common features that result from accumulation of partially degraded GAG's in various tissues. They produce disability primarily from storage-related abnormalities of the connective tissue, the heart, the bony skeleton, and the central nervous system.

Delineation of this group of diseases on the basis of clinical features, radiologic findings, and biochemistry of the urinary GAG's led to the famous classification of McKusick into MPS I to VI in 1966. Over the next six years, an exciting series of investigations from the laboratories of Neufeld and co-workers led to the discoveries that fibroblasts from patients with these disorders show storage abnormalities in culture, that fibroblasts from genetically different patients could "cross-correct" each other in culture, and that this "cross-correction" was due to secretion and recapture of lysosomal enzymes by the complementing fibroblast cell lines, each of which could secrete the enzyme the other was missing and take up the "corrective factor" for which it was deficient. These complementation studies served for nearly a decade as means for clinical diagnosis, for segregation of the disease into complementation groups (e.g., segregation of Hurler's and Scheie's syndromes into one complementation group, and separation of Sanfilippo's syndrome into several complementing groups), and also guided the purification of the corrective factors, each of which was eventually identified as a specific GAG degradative enzyme. Although still useful in certain situations, the complementation assays have largely been replaced by direct assays for the enzymes listed in Table 198–1 as deficient for each of the disorders.

ETIOLOGY OF GLYCOSAMINOGLYCAN STORAGE. The GAG's are long linear polysaccharide molecules composed of repeating dimers, each of which contains a hexuronic acid (or galactose in the case of keratan sulfate) and an amino sugar. They are usually found in covalent linkage to a core protein on which they are synthesized and from which they branch like bristles from a brush. The individual GAG's differ from each other in the hexuronic acid-amino sugar combinations in the repeating dimers, in the linkages between these components, in the linkages between repeating dimers, and in the degree to which individual sugar components are N-acetylated or sulfated. The major GAG's and their respective repeating dimers are chondroitin sulfate (glucuronic acid β1-3 N-acetylgalactosamine-4/6-sulfate); dermatan sulfate (iduronic acid α1-3 N-acetylgalactosamine-4-sulfate); heparan sulfate, which has both glucuronic acid and iduronic acid linked β1-4 and α1-3, respectively, to either N-acetylglucosamine or glucosamine N-sulfate; and keratan sulfate (galactose β1-4 N-acetylglucosamine-6-sulfate). The large proteoglycan molecules made up of protein cores and their GAG branches are secreted by cells and make up a significant fraction of the extracellular matrix of connective tissue. Their turnover depends on their subsequent internalization by endocytosis, their delivery to lysosomes, and their digestion by lysosomal enzymes. Lysosomal proteases digest the core protein, endoglycosidases reduce the size of the GAG's to oligosaccharides of varying length, and many exoglycosidases act sequentially to degrade the GAG's to their monosaccharide components. Each lysosomal enzyme is specific for a specific linkage. An inherited deficiency for any enzyme involved will disrupt the sequential degradative process and lead to accumulation in lysosomes of partially degraded GAG. The accumulation is progressive and eventually disrupts cellular architecture and disturbs cell function. The tissues and organs most affected and the severity depend on the degree of enzyme deficiency, i.e., whether partial or complete. Severity also depends on which enzyme is missing, since individual GAG's vary in their tissue distribution and their rate of turnover.

The enzyme deficiencies, the major storage products, and the clinical features for the mucopolysaccharidoses are summarized in Table 198–1. There is marked genetic heterogeneity within this group of disorders, with many different clinical phenotypes resulting from the different enzyme deficiencies (see MPS I–VII, Table 198–1). It is now clear also that quite different phenotypes can result from the same enzyme deficiency, depending on whether it is partial or complete (see MPS I-H, MPS I-S, and MPS I-H/S in Table 198–1).

GENETICS OF THE MUCOPOLYSACCHARIDOSES. Except for Hunter's syndrome (MPS II), in which the missing enzyme is specified by a gene on the X chromosome and the inheritance is X linked, all of the mucopolysaccharidoses result from deficiencies of enzymes specified by autosomal genes. Thus the inheritance pattern is autosomal recessive. In most cases, affected offspring can be shown to be the products of heterozygous carrier parents, both of whom have about half normal levels of the enzyme for which the affected patient is deficient. Even though the enzymes can now be measured for most of these disorders, the disorders are too rare to make screening for carriers practical. However, carrier status can be determined by enzyme assays in high-risk individuals, and prenatal diagnosis for most of these disorders is available to high-risk mothers, such as mothers of an affected offspring, who face a 25 per cent chance of another affected offspring in a subsequent pregnancy.

CLINICAL AND PATHOLOGIC CONSEQUENCES OF GLYCOSAMINOGLYCAN STORAGE. Connective tissue storage produces connective tissue laxity in most of these disorders, manifest by inguinal and umbilical hernias. Connective tissue thickening also occurs, owing in part to GAG storage and in part to excessive collagen deposition. This combination leads to coarse facial features, peripheral nerve entrapments, thickened meninges that may lead to cord compression and hydrocephalus, and thickened joint capsules. Connective tissue deposition in valve leaflets, the endocardium, and the myocardium produces symptomatic heart disease, a common cause of death in these patients to which coronary vascular insufficiency also contributes. Most of these disorders produce short stature, partly because of impaired long bone growth and partly because of vertebral abnormalities. These and many other changes in the bony skeleton are collectively referred to as *dysostosis multiplex*. Central nervous system storage may produce progressive mental retardation, especially in disorders involving impaired degradation of heparan sulfate (MPS I, II, and III). Corneal clouding and visual handicap result from storage of the partially degraded GAG's in the corneal stroma, especially in disorders involving impaired degradation of dermatan sulfate and keratan sulfate (MPS I, IV, and VI). Hepatomegaly is common and may be massive, but rarely is important clinically. Excessive urinary excretion of incompletely degraded GAG's (mucopolysacchariduria) is a constant finding of considerable diagnostic significance (Table 198–1) but has little pathologic significance.

HURLER'S SYNDROME (MPS I-H). *Pathology.* The basic defect is a deficiency of alpha-L-iduronidase, an enzyme that participates in degradation of dermatan sulfate and heparan sulfate. Accumulation of membrane-bound storage material in parenchymal and mesenchymal cells is the chief pathologic finding. It affects every organ. Vacuolated cells distended with storage material distort normal cell and tissue architecture. In most cells this storage material is granular and composed of GAG's. In neurons, lipids are also present, presumably because stored GAG's inhibit sphingolipid degradation.

Clinical Features. Although patients are thought to be normal until six months of age, they develop persistent nasal discharge, noisy breathing, frequent upper respiratory infections, stiff joints, a thoracolumbar gibbus, and some degree of chest deformity in the last half of the first year of life. Over the second year, the classic syndrome develops with large head, coarse features, corneal clouding, hypertelorism, prominent eyebrows, thick lips, and broad flat nose with depressed nasal bridge. The hands are short and stubby, and joint limitation produces a clawhand deformity. Abdominal protuberance results from hepatosplenomegaly and lax abdominal musculature, often with inguinal and umbilical hernias. Dwarfism is obvious by the end of the second year, by which time cardiac murmurs are present.

Developmental delay is obvious before 18 months of age, and mental retardation progresses slowly. Limitation of joint movement leads to contractures of the hands, the elbows, and the knees. Death usually occurs by the age of 10 from pneumonia or heart failure, after about five years of steady regression and nearly total loss of acquired skills. Hearing loss is usually moderate to severe, and coronary insufficiency and peripheral vascular insufficiency are important late findings.

Radiologic abnormalities of dysostosis multiplex are striking. The skull is large and scaphocephalic, and the calvarium is thickened. The sinuses are poorly developed. The sella is enlarged anteriorly and referred to as J shaped. The ribs are oar shaped, being narrow posteriorly and greatly expanded anteriorly. The medial third of the clavicle is thickened. The vertebrae are initially rounded and appear ovoid. One or two lower thoracic and upper lumbar vertebrae are often hypoplastic and wedge shaped, producing the gibbus deformity. The pelvis shows flared iliac wings, a small body of the ilium,

and shallow oblique acetabula. The hips show coxa valga deformities. The metatarsals and phalanges are short and wide; the proximal ends of the metacarpals taper sharply, a classic finding called proximal pointing. The long tubular bones have expanded diaphyses. There is loss of normal angulation of the humerus at the shoulder. The radiologic changes are progressive, but the changes vary considerably from patient to patient at a given age. The lower extremities are generally more mildly affected than the upper extremities, except for the hips, which often show changes resembling aseptic necrosis of the femoral heads that correlate with severe hip disability clinically.

Diagnosis. The diagnosis can be suspected on clinical and radiologic grounds, supported by demonstration of mucopolysacchariduria (DS>HS), and established definitively by demonstration of the enzyme deficiency, using the commercially available phenyl-L-iduronide substrate. Enzyme activity can be measured in extracts of leukocytes or cultured fibroblasts.

Treatment. Only supportive and symptomatic treatment can be offered to patients, as no effective treatment for the storage abnormality is available.

SCHEIE'S SYNDROME (MPS I-S). This rare disorder is also due to a deficiency of alpha-L-iduronidase and is characterized by severe corneal clouding, deformity of the hands, and aortic valve disease. Symptoms appear between the ages of 5 and 15. The height is normal, as is the intelligence. The striking joint stiffness of the hands is similar to that seen in Hurler's syndrome but is complicated by the carpal tunnel syndrome with median nerve entrapment. Aortic stenosis, regurgitation, or both are present but are usually not symptomatic in early life. Life expectancy may be nearly normal. Diagnosis depends on the same criteria as for Hurler's syndrome. Corneal transplant and aortic valve replacement are reasonable, since intelligence is normal.

THE HURLER-SCHEIE COMPOUND (MPS I-H/S). Some patients with a phenotype that is intermediate between that of Hurler's and Scheie's syndromes are thought to represent compound heterozygotes, having inherited one Hurler and one Scheie gene from each parent.

HUNTER'S SYNDROME (MPS II). Hunter's syndrome is distinguished from Hurler's syndrome by three features: (1) slower progression with longer survival, (2) lack of corneal clouding, and (3) X-linked rather than autosomal recessive inheritance. A severe and a mild form exist. The severe form has most of the features of Hurler's syndrome, but they are slightly milder except for hearing impairment, which is more severe. The patients usually die by age 15. A much milder form has been reported with near-normal intelligence and near-normal survival. Diagnosis is made on the basis of the clinical findings, radiologic evidence of dysostosis multiplex, increased urinary GAG's, and demonstration of sulfoiduronate sulfatase deficiency on serum or on extracts of leukocytes or cultured fibroblasts. Carrier detection is still imperfect, but prenatal diagnostic tests are reliable.

SANFILIPPO'S SYNDROME (MPS III). This syndrome can be produced by a deficiency of at least four different enzymes, all of which participate in degradation of heparan sulfate (Table 198–1). Early development is normal but slows or halts between the ages of two and six years, after which mental deterioration is often rapid. Gait becomes unsteady, muscles atrophy, and the patient becomes bedridden. Death usually occurs by puberty. The head is large, the hair coarse, and hirsutism common. Visceromegaly is mild to absent. Cardiac involvement is rare. Height may be normal through the first decade and then falls behind. Skeletal findings of dysostosis multiplex are mild and include thickened calvarium, ovoid vertebral bodies, mild dysplasia of the pelvis, and mild rib changes. The clinical diagnosis may be suspected from the severe mental retardation, which appears disproportionate with relatively mild somatic and radiologic abnor-

TABLE 198–1. THE MUCOPOLYSACCHARIDOSES (MPS STORAGE DISEASES I TO VII)

Abbreviation	Eponym	Enzyme Deficiency	Major Storage Product	Urinary GAG's	Clinical Features
MPS I-H	Hurler's	α-L-Iduronidase	DS + HS	↑ 5–25X DS > HS	Onset 6–12 months, coarse features, rhinorrhea, grunting respiration, corneal clouding, cardiac disease, visceromegaly, dwarfism, dysostosis multiplex, progressive mental retardation after the first year; death by 5–10 years
MPS I-S (formerly MPS V)	Scheie's	α-L-Iduronidase	DS + HS	↑ 5–25X DS > HS	Onset 5–15 years, corneal clouding, stiff joints, clawhand, genu valgum, dysostosis multiplex, aortic valve disease; however, normal height, normal intelligence, and long survival (difficult to distinguish clinically from mild MPS VI)
MPS I-H/S	Hurler-Scheie	α-L-Iduronidase	DS + HS	↑ 5–25X DS > HS	Onset 2–4 years, all findings of MPS-H but milder, slower progression, and survival into 20's
MPS II, severe	Hunter's severe form	L-Sulfoiduronate sulfatase	HS + DS	↑ 5–25X DS = HS	Onset 2–4 years, clear corneas, deafness, all other features of MPS I-H, but milder; mental retardation progresses to profound state; death by 10–15 years
MPS II, mild	Hunter's mild form	L-Sulfoiduronate sulfatase	HS + DS	↑ 5–25X DS = HS	Onset in first decade, short stature, clear corneas, joint stiffness, dysostosis multiplex, visceromegaly, cardiac disease, nerve entrapments, near-normal intelligence; survival to 30's–60's, depending on heart involvement
MPS III-A	Sanfilippo's, type A	Heparan sulfate sulfamidase	HS	↑ 5–20X 85% HS	Onset 2–6 years, large head, normal height; Hurler-like features, dysostosis multiplex, hepatomegaly are all mild; mental retardation is rapidly progressive and severe; death at end of puberty
MPS III-B	Sanfilippo's, type B	N-acetyl-α-D-glucosaminidase	HS	↑ 5–20X 85% HS	Clinically indistinguishable from MPS III, type A
MPS III-C	Sanfilippo's, type C	Acetyl CoA: α-glucosamide N-acetyltransferase	HS	↑ 5–20X 85% HS	Clinically indistinguishable from MPS III, type A
MPS III-D	Sanfilippo's, type D	N-acetyl-α-D-glucosamine-6-sulfatase	HS	↑ 5–20X 85% HS	Clinically indistinguishable from MPS III, type A
MPS IV-A	Morquio's, classic form	N-acetylgalactosamine-6-sulfatase (gal-6-sulfatase)	KS + Ch 6-S	↑ 3–5X KS + Ch-S	Characteristic facies, short-trunk dwarfism, deformed thorax, corneal clouding, hearing deficit, aortic valve disease, unstable neck, spinal cord transection; intelligence is normal; death usually in 20's from cardiorespiratory problems
MPS IV-B	Morquio-like syndrome	β-Galactosidase deficiency	KS + Ch 4-S	↑ 2–5X KS = Ch-S	Short stature, corneal clouding, mild dysostosis multiplex, prominence of lower face, pectus carinatum, hip deformity, normal intelligence
MPS VI	Maroteaux-Lamy, severe	N-acetylgalactosamine-4-sulfatase (arylsulfatase B)	DS + ?Ch 4-S	↑ 4–20X 70–90% DS	Onset age 2–4 years, growth failure from age 4 slowly progressive, joint stiffness, corneal clouding, aortic valve disease, and severe hip deformity; dysostosis multiplex, striking white cell inclusions; intelligence normal; death in 20's
	Maroteaux-Lamy, mild	N-acetylgalactosamine-4-sulfatase (arylsulfatase B)	DS + ?Ch 4-S	↑ 4–20X 70–90% DS	Onset 5–7 years, short stature, severe osseous changes, especially in the hips; nerve entrapment, corneal clouding, aortic valve disease; normal intelligence, long survival; difficult to distinguish from MPS I-S
MPS VII	Sly	β-Glucuronidase	HS, DS, Ch-S	↑ 6–8X HS, DS Ch 4/6-S	Onset 1–2 years, mild to moderate Hurler-like features, dysostosis multiplex, pectus carinatum, visceromegaly, cardiac murmurs, short stature, moderate mental retardation; slowly progressive after infancy; striking granulocyte inclusions; milder forms exist, as does a more severe form with neonatal ascites and death within two years.

DS = dermatan sulfate; HS = heparan sulfate; Ch-S = chondroitin sulfate; KS = keratan sulfate.

malities, supported by the presence of heparan sulfaturia, and established definitively by demonstration of the specific enzyme deficiency.

MORQUIO'S SYNDROME, CLASSIC FORM (MPS IV-A). The predominant clinical features relate to skeletal abnormalities and to symptoms of spinal cord compression resulting from instability of the neck. Intelligence is normal. By the age of two years, pigeon chest deformity, genu valgum, and gait disturbance appear. Knees and wrists enlarge. The neck appears short, and the head seems to sit on the deformed thorax. Universal platyspondylisis, evident on x-ray examination, kyphoscoliosis, and contractures at the knees and hips all contribute to dwarfism. The face is unusual because of mid-face hypoplasia, depressed nasal bridge, flared nares, and prominence of the lower third of the face on side view. The teeth are wide spaced and the dental enamel thin. Corneal clouding is mild but slowly progressive. Long survival is rare, with death between the ages of 20 and 40 from cardiopulmonary complications. The cardiac disease is valvular (aortic regurgitation). The respiratory problems arise from thoracic deformities and from neurotrophic myelopathy caused by atlantoaxial subluxation. Diagnosis depends on the clinical and radiologic features, which are characteristic; the finding of keratan sulfaturia (which may disappear in adolescence); and the deficiency for N-acetylgalactosamine-6-sulfatase,

which is active on both GalNAc 6-S in chondroitin sulfate and Gal 6-S in keratan sulfate. The enzymatic assay is available in only a few laboratories. Treatment is symptomatic. Posterior cervical fusion should be done early in the disease to prevent spinal cord damage. Correction of the genu valgum requires a single operation at about six years.

THE MORQUIO-LIKE SYNDROME WITH BETA-GA-LACTOSIDASE DEFICIENCY (MPS IV-B). Short stature, mild pectus carinatum, corneal clouding, odontoid hypoplasia with cervical instability, mild dysostosis multiplex, moderate lumbar kyphosis, and mild genu valgum are all features that are found in this Morquio-like disease resulting from beta-galactosidase deficiency. Absent are hearing deficit, dental abnormalities, cardiac murmurs, hepatomegaly, and joint laxity. Keratan sulfaturia is present. The diagnosis is based on normal N-acetylgalactosamine-6-sulfatase levels and reduced beta-galactosidase levels. Presumably this disorder reflects a mutation that impairs the activity of the enzyme on galactose linkages in keratan sulfate but spares its activity on GM_1 ganglioside. Thus the findings of chondrodystrophy predominate, and the neurologic manifestations of GM_1 gangliosidosis are absent.

THE MAROTEAUX-LAMY SYNDROME, SEVERE AND MILD TYPES (MPS VI). Maroteaux and colleagues recognized a new form of mucopolysaccharidosis in 1963 that resembled Hurler's syndrome but differed in that intelligence of the dwarfed, deformed patients was spared; the urinary GAG was almost exclusively dermatan sulfate; and the leukocytes exhibited striking metachromatic inclusions. Affected patients often die in their 20's with cardiac failure. Many suffer cervical cord compression and hydrocephalus resulting from thickened meninges. Since specific enzymatic assays have become available both for arylsulfatase B, missing in MPS VI, and alpha-L-iduronidase, missing in MPS I, it has become clear that many patients with milder forms of MPS VI exist who might previously have been thought to have Scheie's syndrome. No specific treatment is available for the storage abnormality. However, shunting for hydrocephalus, spinal fusion for atlantoaxial subluxation, corneal transplants for visual handicap, and cardiac valve and hip replacement are all reasonable when required, because intelligence is preserved and patients with milder forms of the abnormality have the potential for long survival.

BETA-GLUCURONIDASE DEFICIENCY MUCOPOLY-SACCHARIDOSIS (MPS VII). Most patients present by age three with a Hurler-like illness manifest by frequent upper respiratory infections, chest deformities, cardiac murmurs, hepatosplenomegaly, hernias, dysostosis multiplex, and mild to moderate mental retardation. Many develop corneal clouding. About 20 patients, showing a wide range of clinical severity, have been recognized. Most of the patients have shown slow progression in clinical abnormalities after the age of six. The natural history beyond the teens is yet to be determined. Urinary GAG's have been increased, and heparan sulfate, dermatan sulfate, and chondroitin sulfate have all been reported to be increased in urine. Striking inclusions in leukocytes are typical, as in MPS VI. The diagnosis depends on the demonstration of the enzyme deficiency. Carrier detection and prenatal diagnosis are available.

OTHER DISORDERS RELATED TO THE MUCOPOLY-SACCHARIDOSES. Mucolipidosis II (also called I-cell disease) and mucolipidosis III (also called pseudo-Hurler polydystrophy) are severe and milder forms, respectively, of a Hurler-like disease with many features in common with the mucopolysaccharidoses. However, these patients do not have mucopolysacchariduria.

These disorders result, not from a deficiency for a single lysosomal enzyme like the mucopolysaccharidoses, but from a defect in the processing N-acetylglucosaminyl phosphotransferase that normally targets acid hydrolases to lysosomes. Failure to add the phosphomannosyl-recognition marker that normally directs their segregation into lysosomes allows acid hydrolases to be secreted instead. As a consequence, there is an intracellular deficiency of most of the enzymes involved in the degradation of GAG's (and an extracellular excess), which is part of a general pattern of deficiency involving nearly all lysosomal enzymes. The absence of mucopolysacchariduria, and the 10- to 50-fold elevations of levels of acid hydrolases in serum, distinguish these two disorders from the single-enzyme deficiency mucopolysaccharidoses.

Another group of disorders, not classified with the mucopolysaccharidoses, may produce a Hurler-like picture, including mental retardation, visceromegaly, and dysostosis multiplex. These disorders result from single-enzyme deficiencies for enzymes involved in the catabolism of the oligosaccharide components of glycoproteins. Included are mannosidosis, fucosidosis, and the more recently delineated group of sialidoses (one of which has been described under the name mucolipidosis I). The sialidoses result from a deficiency of oligosaccharide N-acetylneuraminidase. The primary storage products in these disorders are oligosaccharides derived from glycoproteins. However, there is some storage of keratan sulfate as well. It appears that these enzymes are required for degradation of some oligosaccharide side chains on keratan sulfate. Impaired degradation of keratan sulfate may explain

the dysostosis multiplex that mimics the skeletal findings of the mucopolysaccharidoses in these disorders.

Kelly TE: The mucopolysaccharidoses and mucolipidoses. Clin Orthop 114:116, 1976. *A nice summary of clinically relevant information.*

McKusick VA, Neufeld EF, Kelly TE: The mucopolysaccharide storage diseases. In Stanbury JB, Wyngaarden JB, Fredrickson DS, et al. (eds.): The Metabolic Basis of Inherited Disease. 5th ed. New York, McGraw-Hill Book Company, 1983. *A comprehensive chapter with good historical perspective.*

Neufeld EF, Muenzer J: The mucopolysaccharide storage diseases. In Scriver CR, Beaudet AL, Sly WS, et al. (eds.): The Metabolic Basis of Inherited Disease. 6th ed. New York, McGraw-Hill Book Company, 1988. *A current, comprehensive treatment of biochemical and genetic information.*

---

199 THE MARFAN SYNDROME

Peter H. Byers

DEFINITION. The Marfan syndrome is a dominantly inherited connective tissue disorder characterized by musculoskeletal abnormalities (arachnodactyly, tall stature, scoliosis, pectus deformities, and ligamentous laxity), cardiovascular abnormalities (mitral valve prolapse and regurgitation, aortic valve insufficiency, and aortic dilatation, aneurysm, and dissection), lens dislocation, and myopia.

ETIOLOGY AND PATHOGENESIS. For most patients the molecular defect is not known. However, increased production of hyaluronic acid by cultured fibroblasts, the synthesis of an α2(I) chain of type I collagen that contains a small insertion, and alterations in the cross-linking of collagen and elastin in the aorta have each been identified in at least one patient.

PREVALENCE. The Marfan syndrome affects about 1 in 15,000 individuals without racial or ethnic predilection.

PATHOLOGY. The mitral and aortic valves are characterized by "myxomatous degeneration" or the appearance of large pools of nonfibrous material that separates the normal cells of the valves. The valves may be thickened. In the absence of dissection there is accumulation of metachromatic material in the aortic media and disruption of the normal elastic laminae. Aortic dissection characteristically begins in the ascending aorta and may proceed in both directions. Death frequently results from cardiac tamponade due to hemopericardium, coronary occlusion, occlusion of the arteries to the brain, internal hemorrhage, or loss of perfusion of multiple abdominal organs.

CLINICAL MANIFESTIONS. The Marfan syndrome is highly variable in its clinical manifestations, and affected members within the same family may differ in the degree to which they express the mutation; the differences between families may be explained, in part, by different mutations in connective tissue genes. The diagnosis can be made occasionally in newborns because of lens dislocation, mitral valve prolapse, scoliosis, and tall stature with arachnodactyly. More commonly, affected infants may be tall, but cardiac findings are minimal. Many have mild to moderate scoliosis with pectus deformities (excavatum or carinatum); progression of scoliosis or pectus deformities may be rapid during the adolescent growth spurt. About half the patients with the Marfan syndrome have ocular lens dislocation, usually in a superior and nasal direction and generally nonprogressive. Cataract formation and glaucoma are occasional complications of ectopia lentis. Mitral prolapse is seen in virtually all patients with the Marfan syndrome and in some progresses to symptomatic mitral regurgitation; associated rhythm disturbances may be symptomatic.

The major life-threatening complication of the Marfan syndrome is aortic dissection and rupture, and most deaths result from cardiovascular disease. The risk of dissection is well correlated with aortic diameter. In some children aortic root diameters, measured by echocardiography, are greater than normal but, more commonly, aortic diameters do not exceed the normal range (20 to 37 mm) until adulthood and usually enlarge gradually, although the rate may vary. Aortic dissection in the Marfan syndrome is occasionally asymptomatic, but usually there is prolonged, severe substernal chest pain of a tearing or searing quality, often with radiation into the neck, back, and arms. It is often accompanied by diaphoresis, hypotension, and shock. Blood pressure in the two arms may differ. Rarely, pregnancy may be complicated by dissection, even in the presence of a normal aortic diameter.

DIFFERENTIAL DIAGNOSIS. The Marfan syndrome is one of several disorders in which the characteristic habitus is seen. *Contractural arachnodactyly* is a dominantly inherited disorder characterized by arachnodactyly, joint contracture rather than joint laxity, small cup-shaped ears, pectus deformity, mild scoliosis, and mitral valve prolapse, but lens dislocation is absent, and aortic dilatation is not a complication. *Homocystinuria* (see Ch. 194) is characterized by autosomal recessive inheritance, tight joints, peripheral vascular disease, thrombosis of arterial vessels, and, often, mild mental retardation. The diagnosis is confirmed by detection of excessive homocystine in the urine. In the *nonasthenic form* of the Marfan syndrome, body habitus is normal, but lens dislocation and mitral prolapse are common, and death from aortic aneurysm and dissection often establishes the diagnosis. Aortic dissection generally occurs in the fifth to seventh decades; the disorder is inherited in an autosomal dominant fashion. The *mitral valve prolapse syndrome* is commonly mistaken for the Marfan syndrome because of the presence of mitral valve prolapse, tall stature, and some of the mild skeletal features of the Marfan syndrome. The disorder is inherited in an autosomal dominant fashion; the absence of lens dislocation and progressive aortic root dilatation distinguish it from the Marfan syndrome. Patients with the *Stickler syndrome* may have a marfanoid habitus, degenerative arthritis of multiple joints, cleft palate, and, generally, vitreal degeneration. The *marfanoid habitus* may be seen in some patients with sickle cell disease, the Klinefelter syndrome (the 47 XXY karyotype, see Ch. 36), and multiple endocrine adenomatosis type IIB (see Ch. 241).

TREATMENT. Treatment of the Marfan syndrome has several objectives: control of excessive height, prevention of glaucoma, regulation of blood pressure, and prevention of aortic dissection. Excessive height may be controlled by administration of testosterone (to boys) and estrogens (to girls) prior to puberty to hasten epiphyseal closure. Routine ophthalmologic examination is important to assure that dislocation of the lens into the anterior chamber does not occur and to treat any retinal detachment (the consequence of the high myopia that accompanies the syndrome). Rarely the lenses must be removed because of recurrent anterior chamber displacement or because the lens edge is in the center of the visual field and adequate correction cannot be achieved. Blood pressure should always be maintained in the normal range because hypertension is known to increase the risk of dissection, even in normal persons. There is some indication that treatment with agents that decrease cardiac contractility (beta-adrenergic blockers, for example) may delay the rate of aortic progression, but this is an area of controversy, and appropriate controlled studies have not yet been published; nonetheless, in some centers such treatment is routine.

Recently, the advances in surgical technique have made replacement of diseased portions of the aorta a routine treatment that appears to provide increased life expectancy. Replacement should be considered when aortic root diameter reaches approximately 55 mm and prior to decompensation of the left ventricle as a result of aortic valve insufficiency. A composite graft that includes an aortic valve is now used. In some patients, mitral valve function is compromised and the valve requires replacement. Techniques for replacement of large portions of the aorta have also helped to prolong survival.

PROGNOSIS. The prognosis in the Marfan syndrome depends largely on the vascular complications. In one major study the mean age of death for all affected individuals was in the early 40's, and virtually all died of the cardiovascular complications. The judicious use of surgical replacement of the ascending aorta and, if needed, of additional parts of the aorta appears to prolong survival. If the controlled studies of treatment with beta-adrenergic blockage demonstrate effectiveness, then another treatment of the cardiovascular complications will be available.

Patients with the Marfan syndrome should be observed yearly by an internist, a family physician, or a geneticist. Echocardiography should be performed yearly to follow aortic root diameter and the magnitude of mitral regurgitation and aortic insufficiency. Patients should see an ophthalmologist regularly and should consult with a cardiac surgeon as the aortic root diameter passes 50 to 55 mm.

Pregnancy usually is completed without complication, but women in whom the aortic diameter is greater than 40 mm (above the upper limits of normal) may be at greater risk for complications. All pregnancies should be followed in a high-risk center.

Prenatal diagnosis, the only form of prevention, is not currently available. Genetic counseling is important for all members of the proband's family to identify those who are affected.

Gott VL, Pyeritz RE, Magovern GJ Jr, et al.: Surgical treatment of aneurysms of the ascending aorta in the Marfan syndrome: Results of composite-graft repair in 50 patients. N Engl J Med 314:1070, 1986. *A review of the surgical approach to the patient with the Marfan syndrome; outcome, complications, criteria for selection, and longevity.*

Maumenee IH: The eye in the Marfan syndrome. Trans Am Ophthalmol Soc 79:684, 1981. *The most comprehensive review of the eye findings in the Marfan syndrome and their differential diagnosis.*

McKusick VA: Heritable Disorders of Connective Tissue. 4th ed. St. Louis, CV Mosby Company, 1972, pp 61–200. *Still the most comprehensive description of patients with the Marfan syndrome. Many case histories, easy and interesting to read; anecdotal.*

Pyeritz RE, McKusick VA: The Marfan syndrome: Diagnosis and management. N Engl J Med 300:772, 1979. *A more formal statistical compilation of the frequency of physical findings and complications in patients with the Marfan syndrome. Recommendations for management and follow-up.*

200 EHLERS-DANLOS SYNDROME

Peter H. Byers

DEFINITION. Ehlers-Danlos syndrome (EDS) is a group of more than ten inherited connective tissue disorders characterized by abnormalities of the skin, ligaments, and internal organs. The clinical manifestations include skin fragility, abnormal scar formation, excessive bruising, joint laxity, and, in one variety, rupture of viscera and arteries (Table 200–1).

ETIOLOGY. EDS results from mutations in the synthesis and processing of types I and III collagens, the major proteins of skin, ligaments, tendons, blood vessels, and viscera. The molecular bases of EDS types I, II, III, V, and VIII are not known. The known defects include mutations affecting the structure, synthesis, processing, or stability of type III collagen (EDS type IV); deficient hydroxylation of lysyl residues in type I and type III collagen (EDS type VI); defective conversion of type I procollagen to collagen (EDS type VII); defective collagen cross-linking and abnormal cellular utilization of copper (EDS type IX); and a functional defect in fibronectin (EDS type X).

PREVALENCE. The aggregate frequency of EDS is about one in 5000 births. EDS type III, benign familial hypermobility,

TABLE 200–1. CLINICAL FEATURES, MODE OF INHERITANCE, AND BIOCHEMICAL DISORDERS OF THE EHLERS-DANLOS SYNDROME

Type	Clinical Features	Inheritance	Biochemical Disorders
I. Gravis	Soft, velvety, hyperextensible skin; easy bruising; "cigarette-paper" scars; hypermobile joints; varicose veins; prematurity	AD	Not known
II. Mitis	Similar to type I, but less severe	AD	Not known
III. Familial hypermobility	Soft skin, no scarring, marked large and small joint hypermobility	AD	Not known
IV. Arterial	Thin, translucent skin with visible veins; marked bruising; skin and joints have normal extensibility; arterial, bowel and uterine rupture	AD (AR)	Abnormal type III collagen synthesis, secretion or structure
V. X linked	Similar to type II	XLR	Not known
VI. Ocular	Soft, velvety, hyperextensible skin; hypermobile joints, scoliosis; ocular fragility and keratoconus	AR	Lysyl hydroxylase deficiency
VII. Arthrochalasis multiplex congenita	Congenital hip dislocation, joint hypermobility; soft skin with normal scarring	AD	Abnormal structure of the aminoterminal cleavage site in pro $\alpha 1(I)$ and pro $\alpha 2(I)$
VIII. Periodontal	Generalized periodontitis; skin similar to type II	AD	Not known
IX. Cutis laxa, bladder diverticula	Soft, extensible, lax skin; bladder diverticula and rupture; short arms, limited pronation and supination; broad clavicles; occipital horns	XLR	Abnormal copper utilization with defect in lysyl oxidase
X. Fibronectin defect	Similar to type II	AR	Defect in fibronectin

accounts for most patients identified as having EDS; some forms are uncommon (EDS types IV, VI, VII, and VIII); others have been found in only a few families (EDS types IX and X). There is no racial or ethnic predisposition for any of the common types of EDS.

PATHOLOGY AND PATHOGENESIS. Dermal collagen fibrils in patients with EDS types I, II, and III are larger than normal and irregular in outline when viewed by electron microscopy. In EDS type IV, skin is thin and collagen fibril diameter is frequently smaller than normal. Arterial wall thickness is usually less than normal, and tensile strength is diminished. Fibroblastic cells in dermis frequently have marked dilatation of the rough endoplasmic reticulum as a result of defective secretion of type III procollagen. Death results from arterial rupture (with the presenting signs depending on the site of rupture), bowel rupture with sepsis, and rupture of the gravid uterus during late gestation or delivery. In EDS type VI the ultrastructural abnormalities of collagen fibrils are similar to those seen in EDS types I, II, and III. There are no specific pathologic features of the other types of EDS.

CLINICAL MANIFESTATIONS. The clinical manifestations of each type of EDS are different (Table 200–1); it is important to identify patients with EDS type IV because of the grave consequences of the disease and to identify those with EDS types VI, V, and IX because of the risk of recurrence in their families.

EDS types I and II are characterized by marked joint laxity, soft, velvety, and hyperextensible skin, easy bruising, and "cigarette-paper" scars in areas of trauma. They differ in severity. Prematurity is common in EDS type I but rare in EDS type II. The major complications of both are the recurrent joint dislocations, skin fragility, and a high frequency of early-onset osteoarthritis. Many of the manifestations are more severe in childhood and decrease following puberty. At present the diagnosis depends on recognition of the appropriate clinical findings; electron microscopic studies of dermis may be confirmatory but are not specific. Patients with EDS type III are commonly seen by rheumatologists because of the joint discomfort and early onset degenerative joint disease.

EDS type IV, the most severe form, usually results from heterozygous (dominant) mutations in the genes of type III collagen; autosomal recessive inheritance has been described but is rare. The diagnosis is confirmed by finding decreased amounts of type III collagen in skin or by identifying a defect in the structure, synthesis, or secretion of type III procollagen by cultured dermal fibroblasts. In the newborn period some infants already have bruising, but most affected infants are difficult to identify. By adolescence the veins are readily visible on the trunk and extremities, and bruising is common. Vascular or bowel rupture is rare during childhood. Arterial fragility may manifest as sudden death, stroke, shock from retroperitoneal or intra-abdominal bleeding, or compartmental

syndromes, depending on the site of vessel rupture. Prompt surgical intervention may be lifesaving, although tissue friability may make repairs difficult. Pregnancy may be complicated by arterial or uterine rupture, either of which is often fatal. Recurrent abdominal pain may result from repeated mural hemorrhage in the small intestine. Survival beyond the fifth decade is rare.

EDS type VI is an autosomal recessive disorder characterized by a marfanoid habitus, skin and joint findings similar to those in EDS type II, ocular fragility, and scoliosis. The diagnosis is made by finding decreased amounts of hydroxylysine in skin and confirmed by low levels of lysyl hydroxylase measured in cultured dermal fibroblasts. Late complications may include vascular rupture, and blindness from retinal detachment or globe rupture.

The initial presentation of EDS type VII is often in the newborn period, the patient having bilateral hip dislocation and marked joint laxity. The hips are often difficult to stabilize, and recurrent dislocation may continue at the hips and other joints. When suspected clinically the diagnosis can be confirmed in some patients by identifying intermediates in the conversion of type I procollagen to collagen in skin and confirming the defect in cultured dermal fibroblasts.

EDS type VIII is characterized by the combination of non-inflammatory gingival loss (often leading to loss of teeth) and the cutaneous and joint signs of the EDS type II phenotype.

EDS type IX is noted in childhood with skin hyperextensibility and laxity, drooping facies, and minor skeletal anomalies. Evidence of bladder dysfunction may be present by the age of six years, and diverticula of the bladder and hydronephrosis may be apparent by that age. Mild chronic diarrhea, orthostatic hypotension, short upper arms with limited pronation and supination, and the growth of occipital inferior horns become apparent during adolescence. Intelligence is usually in the normal range; inheritance is X-linked recessive. The diagnosis is made by the low serum copper and ceruloplasmin levels and confirmed by low lysyl oxidase levels in cultured dermal fibroblasts. Maintenance of normal urinary drainage is important to prevent renal failure, and continuing bladder drainage may be essential to prevent rupture. There is some variation in severity among families.

DIFFERENTIAL DIAGNOSIS. The differential diagnosis is generally limited to the varieties of EDS, although some patients with the Marfan syndrome have marked joint laxity and others with forms of osteogenesis imperfecta have joint laxity and easy bruising. Patients with EDS type IV and EDS types I and II are often investigated for a bleeding diathesis before the correct diagnosis is made. Because of joint instability and laxity many patients with EDS types I, II, III, VI, and VII are investigated for developmental delay before it is recognized that they have a form of EDS.

TREATMENT. The gaping skin wounds that occur in some forms of EDS should be approximated carefully, and the removable sutures should be left in place for twice the usual time. Recurrent dislocations can often be repaired surgically although further recurrence is more common than in unaffected individuals. Arterial rupture in patients with EDS type IV needs to be treated surgically unless bleeding is controlled by compartmental limitation (e.g., some retroperitoneal bleeding). The repair of affected arteries is often difficult because of extreme friability. If colon rupture recurs, the colon should be excised to prevent further episodes. Rupture of the small bowel is very rare. Some patients with EDS type VI respond to ascorbic acid (1 to 4 grams per day) with some symptomatic improvement and increased excretion of hydroxylysine in the urine. There is no metabolic treatment for other forms of EDS, and management is largely symptomatic.

PROGNOSIS. The prognosis in EDS depends on the specific type with which the patient is affected. Life expectancy is considerably shortened in EDS type IV because of organ and vessel rupture and may be decreased in EDS type VI; in all others, life expectancy is normal. With the exception of EDS type VI, no specific therapy is available that affects the natural history of the condition.

Prevention by prenatal diagnosis is feasible for some types of EDS. Heterozygosity for the EDS type VI mutation has been recognized by examination of amniotic fluid cells in a family at risk for recurrence. The structural mutations in EDS type VII and in EDS type IV should be recognizable by studies of collagens synthesized by chorionic villus cells in culture, but this approach has not yet been used. Analysis of copper uptake and distribution by amniotic fluid cells should facilitate prenatal diagnosis of EDS type IX. All families should have genetic counseling once a proband is identified.

Byers PH, Holbrook KA: Molecular basis of clinical heterogenity in the Ehlers-Danlos syndrome. Ann NY Acad Sci 460:298, 1985. *The most comprehensive and up-to-date review of the molecular lesions in EDS.*

Hollister DW, Byers PH, Holbrook KA: Genetic disorders of collagen metabolism. Adv Hum Gene 12:1, 1982. *Detailed biochemical and clinical description of the different forms of EDS.*

McKusick VA: Heritable Disorders of Connective Tissue. 4th ed. St Louis, C. V. Mosby Company, 1972, pp 292–371. *Although the classification is not up to date, the richness of clinical detail is unsurpassed. A delight to read because of the many case histories and the personal touch.*

201 OSTEOGENESIS IMPERFECTA

David W. Rowe

Osteogenesis imperfecta is a heritable disorder of connective tissue that results primarily in fragile bones that break with minimal trauma. The disease may be limited to a few fractures in childhood, cause 50 to 100 fractures by adulthood with severe long-bone deformity, or cause death in the newborn. The prevalence is 5 per 100,000 live births, and there is no known racial or ethnic predilection. Interest in this disease is increasing as advances in molecular biology are applied to defining the underlying abnormalities within the type I collagen genes. There is also the hope that understanding the mutations of mild osteogenesis imperfecta will give insight into certain forms of osteoporosis that have a familial or genetic component.

PATHOGENESIS. The tissues that are abnormal in osteogenesis imperfecta are composed primarily of type I collagen. This collagen type is a triple helical molecule formed by two genetically distinct but related polypeptide chains in a ratio of two alpha-1 (I) and one alpha-2 (I) chains. The mildest form of osteogenesis imperfecta (type I—see below) appears to result from underproduction of type I collagen owing to reduced accumulation of alpha-1 (I) collagen mRNA within

the cytoplasm. In the more severe forms of osteogenesis imperfecta (types II, III, and IV), there are mutations within the helical regions of either the alpha-1 (I) or the alpha-2 (I) chain. These changes result from either a partial gene deletion or a nucleotide point mutation that alters an amino acid essential for the helical conformation of the alpha chains. Molecules containing a mutant alpha chain do not form normal triple helical molecules. A molecule containing a mutant chain can interfere with the interactions of adjacent molecules, thus weakening the entire structure. The severity of the clinical defect is probably related to the qualitative nature of the mutation and the extent to which the abnormal chains accumulate within specific tissues (Table 201–1).

TYPES AND CLINICAL MANIFESTATIONS. The terms *osteogenesis imperfecta tarda* or *congenita* have been replaced by a classification scheme based on relatively distinct syndromes that reflect *fundamentally different defects in type I collagen* biosynthesis. Osteogenesis imperfecta type I is the mildest form and is associated with nondeforming fractures during childhood which cease after puberty. Fractures can reappear with trauma and in postmenopausal women. In most cases a dominant family history can be elicited having the associated features of blue sclerae, joint laxity, and thin skin, findings that are less obvious in older affected individuals. More variable are hearing abnormalities, short stature, and dentinogenesis imperfecta. Sporadic cases occur and presumably reflect a new mutation. By contrast, the most severe form of osteogenesis imperfecta (type II) results in infants that do not survive the newborn period. Their bones have a crumpled appearance on roentgenography and are so weak that dismemberment may occur. The disorder is usually acquired as a sporadic new mutation, although cases have been observed that suggest a recessive mode of inheritance. In osteogenesis imperfecta type III, there are severe deformities of long bones, marked short stature, and moderate joint laxity. Gray sclerae, impaired hearing, and dentinogenesis imperfecta are frequently present. Fractures and deformity are usually present at birth such that ambulation is never possible. Severe scoliosis can progress to cause respiratory failure. The inheritance is recessive. Osteogenesis imperfecta type IV is less severe, but usually results in moderate long-bone deformity. Ambulation is possible but may require external bracing or internal fixation of the long bones. Blue sclerae, lax joints, and hearing impairment are less common, while dentinogenesis imperfecta is more frequently found. Both dominant and recessive modes of inheritance occur. This is the most heterogeneous group and any individual case may have features of either type I or type III.

DIAGNOSIS. The diagnosis of each form of osteogenesis imperfecta is based on the history, physical examination, family pedigree, and x-ray features. The bone biopsy is not usually of diagnostic aid. Only the milder forms of this disease should pose a diagnostic problem with other disorders that cause minimal bone deformity or fractures. The bowing and fractures associated with osteomalacia or rickets are differentiated by roentgenography and the biochemical measures of calcium, phosphorus, PTH, and vitamin D. Juvenile, disuse,

TABLE 201–1. CLINICAL CLASSIFICATION OF OSTEOGENESIS IMPERFECTA

Type	Description	Inheritance	Suspected Mutation
I	Mild, nondeforming	AD	Deficient amounts of alpha-1 (I) mRNA
II	Lethal	NM, AR	Mutation within helical domain of alpha-1 (I)
III	Severe long-bone deformity and scoliosis	NM, AR	Poorly defined
IV	Mild with long-bone deformity	AD	Mutation within helical domain of alpha-2 (I)

AD = autosomal dominant; AR = autosomal recessive; NM = new mutation.

and steroid-induced osteoporosis can be distinguished by history. Other rare diagnoses to be considered are infantile cortical hyperostosis (Caffey's disease) and hypophosphatasia. Studies of collagen synthesis and collagen mRNA in cultured fibroblasts plus analysis of restriction fragment length polymorphisms for the type I collagen genes are beginning to provide the means for a specific diagnosis for the various forms of the disease. However, most of these methods remain experimental, and one must rely primarily on ultrasonography for intrauterine diagnosis of the severe forms (type II and type III) of the disease.

TREATMENT. The use of supplemental calcium, vitamin D, fluoride, anabolic steroids, calcitonin, and pyrophosphate has not been shown to provide a satisfactory response. Since many of these drugs were used in heterogeneous groups of patients with osteogenesis imperfecta, there may be subgroups of patients who could benefit from certain medical regimens. At present, therapy is primarily orthopedic with external bracing, and surgical straightening with intramedullary splinting (rodding) of the long-bone deformities. Use of lightweight plastic bracing will assume a greater role in promoting ambulation. However, attempts to halt the progression of scoliosis in osteogenesis imperfecta have not been successful. In all forms of osteogenesis imperfecta maintenance of good muscle tone and range of motion is crucial for the optimal use of the extremities. Creative use of physical therapy, especially in the form of swimming, may be the most useful preventive measure in this disorder.

Akeson WH, Bornstein P, Glimcher MJ: Symposium on Heritable Disorders of Connective Tissue. St. Louis, C. V. Mosby Company, 1982. *See Chapters 20–23 for a general review of clinical, morphologic, and biochemical aspects of osteogenesis imperfecta.*

Albright JA, Millar EA: Osteogenesis imperfecta. Clin Orthop 159:2, 1981. *A collection of numerous articles on the pathology and treatment of this disease.*

Byers PH, Bonadio JF: The molecular basis of clinical heterogeneity in osteogenesis imperfecta: Mutations in type I collagen genes have different effects on collagen processing. In Lloyd JK, Scriver CR (eds.): Genetic and Metabolic Disease in Pediatrics. London, Butterworths International Medical Reviews, 1985. *Most current and best-written review of the molecular basis of osteogenesis imperfecta.*

Smith R, Francis MJO, Houghton GP: The Brittle Bone Syndrome. London, Butterworth Co., 1982. *A comprehensive review by one group of investigators having a large experience with osteogenesis imperfecta. Chapter 7 has a good differential diagnosis.*

202 PSEUDOXANTHOMA ELASTICUM

Jouni Uitto

Pseudoxanthoma elasticum (PXE) (synonyms: Grönblad-Strandberg syndrome, systemic elastorrhexis) is a generalized progressive connective tissue disorder primarily affecting the elastic fibers. Clinically, PXE manifests as characteristic cutaneous lesions, ocular changes, and widespread vascular abnormalities. The relative severity of these changes results in a variety of clinical pictures. The onset of the disease may be in early childhood, and in most cases the cutaneous changes are evident before the age of 30 years. The exact incidence of PXE is not known, although estimates are about 1 in 160,000 persons. The male-female ratio is probably 1:1.

CLINICAL MANIFESTATIONS. *Skin.* The primary cutaneous lesions are relatively small (1 to 3 mm) yellowish papules that give the affected area a pebbly, "plucked chicken skin" appearance. The primary lesions tend to coalesce into larger plaques, and the skin of the involved areas becomes thickened and leathery (Fig. 202–1). Gradually, the affected skin becomes redundant, lax, and inelastic. The predilection sites are the face, neck, axillary folds, lower abdomen, and

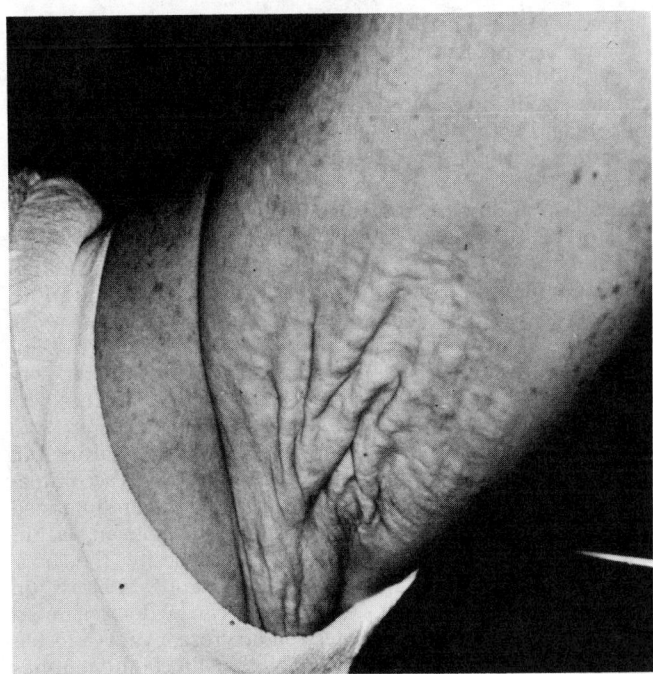

FIGURE 202–1. Typical cutaneous manifestations of pseudoxanthoma elasticum. The lesion demonstrates redundant and inelastic skin in the axillary fold.

thighs. The nasolabial folds and chin creases may be strikingly accentuated. Yellowish lesions similar to those noted on the skin can also be seen on the mucous membranes.

Eye. The ocular changes are characterized by angioid streaks, i.e., grayish or brownish-red, poorly defined streaks radiating across the fundus of the eye. Their development usually starts later than that of the cutaneous lesions, often during the third or fourth decade. The ocular changes are commonly bilateral and include hemorrhages and exudates in Bruch's membrane, an elastin-rich structure located between the retina and the choroid. The degenerative changes of the eye frequently lead to impaired vision, and complete blindness, although rare, is one of the major complications of PXE. Angioid streaks may be present without noticeable cutaneous changes, but other accompanying observations, such as vascular changes, may lead to correct diagnosis of PXE. Angioid streaks can also be associated with other diseases—for example, Paget's disease of bone, sickle cell anemia, tumoral calcinosis, lead poisoning, and idiopathic thrombocytopenia.

Vascular Manifestations. The early manifestations of arterial involvement include hypertension, weak peripheral pulses, and, occasionally, intermittent claudication. The most devastating complications develop as a result of coronary occlusion or cerebral hemorrhage; the most frequent complication is recurrent bleeding from the gastrointestinal tract. A common site of the gastrointestinal bleeding is the gastric mucosa, where the elastic fibers of the arteries are particularly affected. Bleeding from the urinary tract can also occur.

INHERITANCE. Most cases of PXE are inherited as an autosomal recessive disease. However, autosomal dominant inheritance has been documented in a few families. The classification proposed by Pope divides the dominantly inherited form of PXE into two categories. The type I dominant form is characterized by classic cutaneous changes associated with severe vascular complications. The type II dominant form, which is more frequent than type I, is characterized by focal cutaneous involvement associated with hyperextensible skin, blue sclerae, high arched palate, and loose-jointedness. The type I recessively inherited form is the classic, most frequently encountered type of pseudoxanthoma elasticum, characterized by typical cutaneous, vascular, and ocular manifestations. The type II recessively inherited disease, characterized by generalized cutaneous involvement and by the absence of vascular and ocular manifestations, is very rare.

In addition to the inherited forms, several cases with cutaneous findings consistent with PXE but without family history and without vascular or ocular involvement have been reported. In some of these cases, the development of skin lesions is related to external trauma, such as exposure to Norwegian saltpeter. Patients with an unusual perforating variant of cutaneous PXE have been described. In these patients the lesions are confined to the abdomen, most often in a periumbilical distribution. Periumbilical perforating PXE appears to be a distinct acquired form of the disease.

PATHOLOGY. Histopathologic examination of the involved skin demonstrates an accumulation of structures in the middle or lower dermis that stain positively with stains specific for elastic fibers, e.g., Verhoeff stain. In contrast to the elastic fibers in normal skin, the elastic material in PXE appears irregularly clumped and fragmented. The accumulation of elastic fibers has also been quantitated by computerized morphometric analyses and by assay of desmosine, an elastin-specific cross-link compound. Characteristically the fragmented elastic fibers contain calcium that appears bluish on routine hematoxylin-eosin stain and that can be demonstrated by calcium-specific stains. Electron microscopy of affected skin demonstrates that the amorphous elastin component has been replaced by bundles of granular material with staining properties different from normal elastin. Also, foci containing

calcium hydroxyapatite crystals can be detected in the elastic fibers. These morphologic findings thus provide evidence for derangement in the organization of the elastic structures in PXE. Biochemical proof of the exact molecular defect in the structure or metabolism of elastin is, however, lacking, and it is unclear whether the calcification of elastic fibers is a primary or secondary event.

THERAPY. No specific treatment is available, and the primary prevention entails genetic counseling. Although treatment with vitamin E, vitamin C, or a low calcium diet has been advocated in isolated case reports, no clinical proof of their efficacy is available in the form of controlled clinical trials. In selected cases, plastic surgery may be helpful in improving the cosmetic appearance of the skin.

Neldner KH, Martinez-Hernandez A: Localized acquired cutaneous pseudoxanthoma elasticum. J Am Acad Dermatol 1:523, 1979. *Clinical description of a distinct acquired form of pseudoxanthoma elasticum.*

Pope FM: Two types of autosomal recessive pseudoxanthoma elasticum. Arch Dermatol 110:219, 1974. *A clinical study establishing the genetic heterogeneity of this condition.*

Rosenbloom J: Elastin: Relation of protein and gene structure to disease. Lab Invest 51:605, 1984. *A comprehensive review on elastin structure and metabolism.*

Uitto J: Elastic fibers in cutaneous diseases. Curr Concepts Skin Dis 6:19, 1985. *A review of the molecular defects of elastin in heritable connective tissue diseases, including pseudoxanthoma elasticum.*

Uitto J, Paul JL, Brockley K, et al.: Elastic fibers in human skin: Quantitation of elastic fibers by computerized digital image analyses and determination of elastin by a radioimmunoassay of desmosine. Lab Invest 49:499, 1983. *Demonstration of increased elastin concentrations in the lesional skin in pseudoxanthoma elasticum.*

Disorders of Porphyrins or Metals

203 PORPHYRIA

D. Montgomery Bissell

Porphyrias are characterized clinically by neurologic and/or cutaneous manifestations and chemically by overproduction of porphyrins or the porphyrin precursors, delta-aminolevulinic acid (ALA) and porphobilinogen (PBG). The most important members of this group of diseases are hereditary, but acquired porphyria occurs also; in all instances, porphyria must be distinguished from simple porphyrinuria, which accompanies a variety of common conditions and is without clinical significance.

BIOSYNTHESIS OF HEME. Heme is a metalloporphyrin, a member of a group that includes chlorophyll and vitamin B_{12}. These have been termed the molecules of life, in view of their importance to aerobic metabolism. Heme is formed from succinyl CoA and glycine in a series of enzyme-catalyzed steps (Fig. 203–1). The initial enzyme of the pathway, ALA synthetase, is rate-determining for the overall synthesis. Its activity is regulated in a "feedback" manner, so that it responds rapidly to the changing needs of the tissue for heme. When a relative deficiency of heme occurs—from increased heme-protein formation or impaired heme synthesis or both—ALA synthetase is stimulated, and the flow of heme precursors into the pathway increases. With formation of the initial porphyrin-like intermediate uroporphyrinogen, a branch point occurs involving different porphyrin isomers. While there are four possible isomers of uroporphyrinogen, only I and III occur in nature, isomer III being the physiologic intermediate. The isomer I pathway is abortive, proceeding only as far as coproporphyrin I, and normally is inconsequential. Metabolism of uroporphyrinogen III involves modifications of porphyrin side chains that render the molecule

progressively more lipophilic and redirect its excretion from the body. Whereas the water-soluble ALA, PBG, and uroporphyrin are excreted entirely or very largely in urine, coproporphyrin is excreted in both urine and feces and protoporphyrin solely in feces. The porphyrinogens constitute the true intermediates of heme synthesis. The porphyrins—with the exception of protoporphyrin—are side products of the pathway that are irreversibly oxidized and must be excreted. Although loss of heme precursors from the pathway occurs and is measurable in urine or stool, it normally represents less than 1 per cent of heme synthesis. Increased excretion of these compounds implies an underlying disturbance of heme formation, either hereditary or acquired.

TISSUE SITES OF PORPHYRIN PRODUCTION. Heme serves as the prosthetic group for mitochondrial cytochromes as well as for other heme proteins and therefore is required by all cells in the body; presumably each tissue provides its own heme by endogenous synthesis. This requirement, however, varies widely among individual tissues, reflecting large differences in the concentration and turnover of specific heme proteins. Relatively high rates of heme synthesis are characteristic of both bone marrow and liver. In bone marrow, heme synthesis is devoted very largely to formation of hemoglobin; in liver, heme is required for several relatively short-lived heme proteins, in particular a group of microsomal cytochromes known as P-450. In rat liver, turnover of these cytochromes appears to account for 60 to 70 per cent of heme utilization. Synthesis of hepatic cytochrome P-450 is inducible by numerous drugs and possibly also by endogenous lipophilic substances, and administration of an inducing drug results in stimulation of ALA synthetase and a consequent increase in the rate of heme formation. In extrahepatic tissues (including bone marrow), the regulatory role of ALA synthetase remains poorly defined, and inducing effects of administered drugs have not been documented.

CLASSIFICATION, GENETICS, AND PREVALENCE. In the hereditary porphyrias, the specific genetic defect presum-

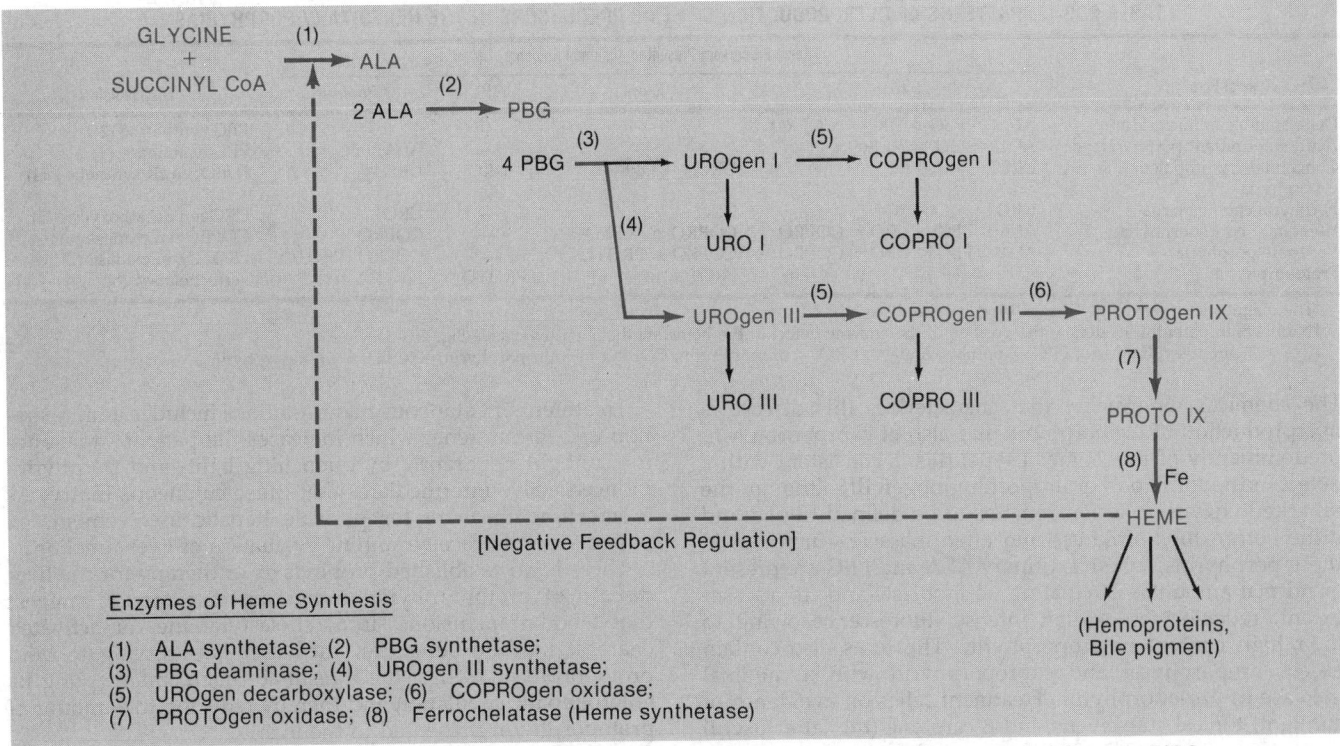

FIGURE 203–1. Pathway of heme biosynthesis (ALA = δ-aminolevulinic acid; PBG = porphobilinogen; URO = uroporphyrin; COPRO = coproporphyrin; PROTO = protoporphyrin).

ably is present in all cells of the body. However, for reasons as yet unclear, abnormal porphyrinogenesis is confined largely to either bone marrow or liver, with the possible exception of protoporphyria, which may involve both tissues. Accordingly, the classification presented in Table 203–1 separates the porphyrias into erythropoietic and hepatic types. Other tissues may be affected by the porphyria-producing lesion, but their contribution to total body production of heme precursors is small. Congenital erythropoietic porphyria and delta-aminolevulinic aciduria are rare autosomal recessive diseases; the other hereditary porphyrias are dominant disorders, and the sexes are equally affected. Although their distribution appears to be worldwide, accurate prevalence figures are not available because many carriers in the general population are asymptomatic. Clinically manifest hepatic porphyria appears to be much more common in whites than in blacks or Asians; whether this reflects differences in carrier rates or only variable clinical expression of the defect among these populations is unknown.

BIOCHEMICAL CHARACTERIZATION. While the porphyrias as a group represent disturbances of heme synthesis, they may be differentiated on the basis of the specific enzymatic defect in each type and the unique pattern of excretion of heme precursors (ALA, PBG, or porphyrins) associated with each defect (Table 203–2). This pattern is determined with quantitative tests; qualitative tests such as the Watson-Schwartz test for PBG are best reserved for urgent circumstances or when quantitative determinations are unavailable. With examination of the entire array of heme precursors in

TABLE 203–1. CLASSIFICATION OF THE PORPHYRIAS

Erythropoietic
   Congenital erythropoietic porphyria (Günther's disease)
   Protoporphyria (erythropoietic or erythrohepatic protoporphyria)
Hepatic
   Acute intermittent porphyria (pyrroloporphyria)
   Hereditary coproporphyria
   Variegate porphyria (South African porphyria)
   Delta-aminolevulinic aciduria
   Porphyria cutanea tarda (symptomatic porphyria)
   Toxic porphyria

urine and feces, true porphyrias are readily differentiated from asymptomatic porphyrinuria, which may accompany acute liver disease, various tumors (hepatoma, Hodgkin's disease), and neurologic diseases. Porphyrinuria in these instances generally involves an isolated increase in urine coproporphyrin, with or without a modest increase in uroporphyrin. In lead poisoning, urine exhibits a significant increase in ALA with a lesser increase in coproporphyrin; PBG and fecal porphyrins are normal. None of these patterns resembles those associated with porphyria (Table 203–2).

Overproduction, with excess excretion, of ALA and PBG or porphyrins is associated with specific clinical manifestations. Increased circulating ALA and PBG are linked to a variety of neurologic problems that may include psychosis, seizures, and paresis. A neuropathic effect of ALA or PBG has been postulated. By contrast, overproduction of porphyrins is associated predominantly with cutaneous photosensitivity; no effect on neurologic function has been observed. The dermatologic effects of porphyrins are proportional to their approximate concentration in subcutaneous tissues and depend on excitation of porphyrins by visible light (peak effective wavelength, ca. 400 nm).

CONGENITAL ERYTHROPOIETIC PORPHYRIA

Fewer than 100 patients with this condition have been described. Pink urine and cutaneous photosensitivity are the principal manifestations and, classically, are present from early childhood. While the diagnosis usually is made at this time, a first presentation has been described also in adults, whose clinical state resembled that of relatively severe porphyria cutanea tarda (see below). Acute attacks of abdominal pain with neurologic manifestations do not occur. Cutaneous lesions consist of bullae, vesicles, and shallow ulcers on light-exposed skin. Repeated injuries are accompanied by hypertrichosis, and, in patients surviving beyond childhood, may cause disfiguring scars with loss of portions of the nose, ears, eyelids, and digits. Erythrodontia, reflecting accumulation of porphyrins in teeth and bones, and splenomegaly also have been present in a high proportion of cases, associated with a compensated hemolytic anemia, which may be intermittent.

TABLE 203–2. PATTERNS OF OVERPRODUCTION OF HEME PRECURSORS IN THE HEREDITARY PORPHYRIAS

Type of Porphyria	Heme Precursors Present in Abnormal Amounts				Enzyme Defect
	Urine	Feces	RBC	Plasma	
Delta-aminolevulinic aciduria	ALA* > PBG > URO < COPRO	—		—	PBG synthetase (2)†
Acute intermittent porphyria	ALA < **PBG** > > URO	—		ALA, PBG	PBG deaminase (3)
Congenital erythropoietic porphyria	URO > > COPRO	URO > COPRO	**URO**	URO	?UROgen III synthetase (4)
Porphyria cutanea tarda	**URO** > > COPRO	URO	—	URO	UROgen decarboxylase (5)
Hereditary coproporphyria	ALA < PBG < URO < COPRO	**COPRO** > > PROTO	—	COPRO	COPROgen oxidase (6)
Variegate porphyria	ALA < PBG < URO < COPRO	COPRO < **PROTO**	—	COPRO, PROTO	PROTOgen oxidase (7)
Protoporphyria	—	PROTO	**PROTO**	PROTO	Ferrochelatase (8)

*The diagnostic abnormality for each type is in boldface type.
†Numbers in parentheses denote the position of the enzyme defect in the heme synthetic pathway (see Fig. 203–1).
ALA = δ-aminolevulinic acid; PBG = porphobilinogen; URO = uroporphyrin; COPRO = coproporphyrin; PROTO = protoporphyrin.

The chemical abnormality that characterizes this disease is overproduction of uroporphyrin and also of coproporphyrin, predominantly of the isomer I type; this is consistent with a defect in the formation of uroporphyrinogen III, although the inherited enzymatic lesion remains to be defined. Blood and urine both exhibit striking—and often massive—increases in these porphyrins, whereas urinary ALA and PBG are present in normal amounts. Circulating normoblasts and, to a lesser extent, reticulocytes, exhibit intense fluorescence owing to their high content of uroporphyrin. The feces also contain excess uroporphyrin and coproporphyrin with a minimal increase in protoporphyrin. Treatment relies on avoidance of sunlight; topical sunscreens and β-carotene (the latter useful in protoporphyria) are of no proven value. In patients with hemolysis, splenectomy may lead to prolongation of red cell lifespan and diminished porphyrin excretion.

PROTOPORPHYRIA

A relatively common condition, in most patients this is manifest solely as cutaneous photosensitivity. Within minutes of exposure, sunlight causes a burning, stinging sensation or pruritus of unprotected skin, followed by erythema and/or edema (solar urticaria). Attacks subside over a period of hours, often without sequelae; in some patients, repeated episodes lead to thickening of the skin (solar eczema). The cutaneous manifestations associated with other types of porphyria (bulla formation, mechanical fragility, or hypertrichosis) are absent in protoporphyria. The disease is characterized chemically by excess protoporphyrin IX in erythrocytes, plasma, and feces. Excretion of ALA, PBG, and uroporphyrin is normal, whereas fecal coproporphyrin may be moderately increased. Diffusion of protoporphyrin from red cells to plasma and cutaneous tissues appears to be responsible for the observed photosensitivity and distinguishes protoporphyria from other, acquired conditions with elevation of the level of red cell porphyrin. In iron deficiency, lead intoxication, and certain refractory chronic anemias, excess protoporphyrin is present in erythrocytes but is bound within the cell; plasma protoporphyrin levels invariably are normal, and cutaneous symptoms are absent.

The hereditary defect is a partial deficiency of ferrochelatase, which is the final enzyme of the heme synthetic pathway, catalyzing the conversion of protoporphyrin to heme. In some patients, the excess protoporphyrin appears to be derived entirely from the bone marrow, whereas in others the liver has been implicated as well. The clinically latent carrier state is frequent. About 10 per cent of patients form protoporphyrin-containing gallstones, and subclinical liver disease also appears to be relatively common, presumably because of deposition of protoporphyrin in the liver. In rare instances, the presenting manifestation is cholestasis, with inflammation, fibrosis, and crystalline protoporphyrin inclusions in bile canaliculi and liver cells. Progression to portal hypertension and death may be rapid. Fatal hepatic involvement has been associated with markedly elevated plasma protoporphyrin concentrations (>1000 μg per deciliter).

Treatment of cutaneous manifestations includes administration of beta-carotene, which increases the patient's tolerance for sunlight apparently by quenching light- and porphyrin-induced active intermediates that cause cutaneous injury. As a screening measure for possible hepatic involvement, all patients should receive routine evaluation of liver function.

There is no established prophylaxis or therapy for the liver disease of protoporphyria. Individual case reports suggest that blood transfusions, iron, cholestyramine, or activated charcoal may be beneficial, the latter two serving to bind protoporphyrin within the intestinal lumen, interrupting its enterohepatic circulation and thereby reducing the amount of protoporphyrin presented to the liver.

HEPATIC PORPHYRIA WITH NEUROLOGIC MANIFESTATIONS

DEFINITIONS. *Acute Intermittent Porphyria.* This disease is caused by a hereditary partial deficiency of PBG deaminase and is characterized by excretion of excess ALA and PBG in urine. Acute neurologic attacks occur; cutaneous symptoms are not a feature of this type of porphyria.

Hereditary Coproporphyria. A partial deficiency of coproporphyrinogen oxidase is present, leading to excretion of excess ALA, PBG, uroporphyrin, and coproporphyrin in urine and excess coproporphyrin in feces. In addition to acute neurologic attacks, approximately 30 per cent of patients experience cutaneous manifestations consistent with overproduction of porphyrins.

Variegate Porphyria. This type results from a partial deficiency of protoporphyrinogen oxidase and is characterized by excess excretion of the entire series of heme precursors; excretion of protoporphyrin in feces is characteristically high. Erythrocyte porphyrin levels are normal. Cutaneous photosensitivity or unusual fragility of sun-exposed skin is present in a majority of affected individuals and may be a chronic manifestation; the lesions are similar to those present in porphyria cutanea tarda (see below). However, as in the two preceding types, the occurrence of acute neurologic attacks is the most important clinical feature.

Delta-aminolevulinic Aciduria. There is profound deficiency of PBG synthetase in this condition, associated with excess ALA in the urine. Coproporphyrin also is increased, for reasons as yet unclear. The urinary findings are similar to those in persons with heavy metal intoxication, which must be excluded. The clinical presentation is identical to that of acute intermittent porphyria, except that symptoms occur only in homozygotes.

PATHOGENESIS. The individual genetic defect in each type appears to limit the flow of heme precursors and to be responsible for potential or actual heme deficiency in the liver. Circumstances that increase the demand for heme synthesis—the classic example being induction of cytochrome P-450 by barbiturates—cause the deficiency to be expressed, leading to derepression of ALA synthetase, overproduction of heme precursors preceding the genetic defect, and clinical symptoms. In addition to drugs, changes in endogenous factors have also been implicated in precipitating acute attacks. Involvement of steroid hormones is suggested by the fact that symptoms are rare prior to puberty, and disease is expressed clinically in women more often than in men. Estrogens (including oral contraceptives) are among the drugs that precipitate attacks, and cyclic premenstrual exacerbations occur in some women, resolving with onset of menstruation. The effect of pregnancy on disease activity is unpredictable. Infection or fasting (deliberate or as a result of concurrent illness) also predisposes carriers to acute attacks.

CLINICAL PRESENTATION. Acute neurologic attacks are common to all of the porphyrias cited above, and their identical presentations and management justify treating these types as a group. An acute attack consists of abdominal, back, or extremity pain, initially subacute but increasingly intense over a period of 24 to 48 hours until it may suggest acute cholecystitis, appendicitis, or other surgical diagnosis. Anorexia, nausea, and vomiting are frequent. Constipation typically is longstanding and worsens at the onset of an attack. In evaluating pain, the examiner may be impressed that the severity of the symptoms is out of proportion to the abdominal findings; rebound tenderness is seldom present. Tachycardia is a frequent finding and a useful parameter of disease activity. Fever is unusual and suggests a concurrent infectious process. X-ray examination of the abdomen may show dilated loops of small bowel consistent with paralytic ileus. In general, the abdominal manifestations are believed to represent a neurogenic motility disturbance of the bowel. They often occur in association with frank neurologic dysfunction: Generalized seizures or mental abnormalities that range from confusion to psychosis may be presenting features of an acute attack. With prolonged attacks, motor and sensory deficits appear and may progress to quadriplegia, respiratory paralysis, and death. The neuropathic changes are variable; patchy demyelination of peripheral nerves and focal degeneration of the autonomic nervous system have been described. Routine laboratory tests generally are unremarkable. Anemia is not a feature of the hepatic porphyrias, and blood loss does not precipitate acute attacks. Liver function test results similarly are normal, apart from slight increase of serum transaminase activity. Hyponatremia occurs in a minority of patients but occasionally is striking; it may reflect inappropriate secretion of antidiuretic hormone, complicated in some instances by aggressive intravenous fluid therapy with glucose and water.

Apart from acute episodes, in which the diagnosis is obvious, carriers of these genetic defects may complain of mood swings and bodily pains, which fail to suggest a specific diagnosis and may be without associated physical findings. The porphyric nature of such symptoms often is difficult to resolve. Although excretion of heme precursors is uniformly increased in acute attacks, it varies widely among asymptomatic carriers and thus does not provide a secure basis for differentiating porphyric from nonspecific manifestations. Treatment is empiric, with due regard for those drugs that may induce acute attacks (see below). There is no evidence that dietary manipulations (e.g., excess carbohydrate) are useful.

DIAGNOSIS. Urinary PBG is increased in these porphyrias during acute attacks (except in delta-aminolevulinic aciduria) and remains increased while symptoms persist. This may be documented by rapid qualitative methods (Watson-Schwartz or Hoesch tests) in which PBG reacts with Ehrlich's reagent (dimethylaminobenzaldehyde in HCl) to form a red complex that is not extractable with *n*-butanol. Positive test results should be confirmed by quantification of urinary PBG by ion-exchange column chromatography. With quantification of urinary and fecal porphyrins, the specific type of porphyria usually can be established. Uroporphyrin often is reported as increased in acute intermittent porphyria, despite the fact that its formation theoretically is compromised by the genetic defect of this type. This apparently reflects nonenzymatic conversion of PBG to a dark uroporphyrin-like compound

(porphobilin), which may occur in the urinary bladder. The conversion is accelerated by exposure of urine to light, accounting for the visible darkening of voided urine from patients with acute intermittent porphyria. A "urine porphyrin screen" does not measure PBG and therefore could be misleading in the investigation of patients with acute abdominal pain.

In the absence of clinical symptoms, increase of urinary PBG is inconstant. In 20 to 30 per cent of asymptomatic carriers of acute intermittent porphyria, PBG in urine is within the normal range. In these cases, assay of erythrocyte PBG deaminase may be used to identify carriers. This activity is significantly reduced in affected persons and is abnormal regardless of the age or clinical state of the person. Many asymptomatic carriers with hereditary coproporphyria or variegate porphyria excrete PBG in normal amounts. Identification of carriers requires measurement of fecal coproporphyrin in the case of hereditary coproporphyria and fecal protoporphyrin for variegate porphyria. While the inherited defects in these types of porphyria are known, the enzymes are intramitochondrial; therefore, their assay requires nucleated cells (leukocytes or cultured skin fibroblasts) and at present is a research procedure.

MANAGEMENT. Emphasis is on the prevention of acute neurologic attacks. In families with a known case of porphyria, identification of carriers is mandatory, using the appropriate screening procedure for the type of porphyria involved (see above). Carriers should be instructed as to the hazards of fasting and of taking drugs that may precipitate acute attacks (Table 203–3). Carriers of hereditary coproporphyria or variegate porphyria who experience cutaneous manifestations in the absence of a porphyrogenic drug should minimize their exposure to sunlight and wear protective clothing.

The management of neurologic exacerbations includes immediate withdrawal of possible offending drugs, administration of carbohydrate, correction of electrolyte abnormalities, and general supportive care. Carbohydrate is given to reverse the fasting state, usually as intravenous dextrose because of nausea or vomiting, and in amounts approaching 400 grams per day. To avoid administration of a water load, hypertonic solutions may be infused by a central line. Seizures, when present, generally occur early in the course of an attack and respond to parenteral diazepam. For analgesia, chlorpromazine may be used, although the specificity of its action is uncertain; excessive sedation is a troublesome side effect. In many patients, meperidine will be required despite the danger of addiction. Propranolol counters the tachycardia of acute attacks; it should be introduced at very low doses (e.g., 10 mg twice daily).

If acute manifestations fail to respond to these measures within 48 hours, treatment with hematin (hydroxyheme) is

TABLE 203–3. HAZARDOUS AND SAFE DRUGS IN PORPHYRIA WITH NEUROLOGIC MANIFESTATIONS

May Precipitate Acute Attacks	Believed to Be Safe
Apronalid	Aspirin
Barbiturates	Bromides
Chlordiazepoxide	Chlorpromazine
Chloroquine	Corticosteroids
Chlorpropamide	Diazepam
Dichloralphenazone	Dicumarol
Ergot preparations	Digoxin
Estrogens	Diphenhydramine
Ethanol	Ether
Glutethimide	Guanethidine
Griseofulvin	Meperidine
Hydantoins	Morphine
Imipramine	Neostigmine
Meprobamate	Nitrous oxide
Methsuximide	Penicillins
Methyldopa	Propranolol
Methyprylon	Tetracyclines
Novonal	
Sulfonamides	

indicated with the rationale that it compensates for the genetic impairment of endogenous heme synthesis. The solution consists of pyrogen-free hemin (ferriprotoporphyrin IX chloride) dissolved in aqueous sodium carbonate (10 grams per liter), adjusted to pH 8.0 with HCl and sterilized by membrane filtration. It is infused slowly (over 10 to 15 minutes) into the largest available vein. A dose of 2 mg per kilogram body weight at 24-hour intervals usually is effective, as shown by a decline in urinary PBG to less than 10 per cent of the pretreatment level. If the response to this regimen is unsatisfactory, the frequency of the dose may be doubled. However, the total administered hematin should not exceed 6 mg per kilogram body weight per day. Subjective improvement parallels the chemical response and is evident 72 to 96 hours after the initial hematin infusion. Improvement in neurologic deficits depends on the underlying pathologic condition. Hematin may arrest a progressive neuropathy, but has no effect on established lesions involving demyelination. With cessation of hematin treatment, a rise in urinary PBG may occur, although the patient's condition usually remains stable (Fig. 203–2).

Hematin is available commercially as a powder (Panhematin), which is reconstituted for use with sterile water. The prepared solution is unstable and should be infused promptly. It may be stored at 4°C for up to 12 hours, but then should be discarded. Side effects of hematin administration include chemical phlebitis at the site of infusion (4 per cent of cases) and reduced clotting activity. Abnormal coagulation tests and reduced platelets have been observed in several patients receiving hematin. These effects are dose related and may be due to decay product(s) of dissolved hematin rather than to hematin itself. They are minimized by the use of freshly prepared material. When present, they are maximal 10 minutes after injection of hematin, diminished at 5 hours, and undetectable at 48 hours. Clinically significant bleeding has not occurred except in patients also receiving another anticoagulant. The findings suggest that hematin should not be used in patients with impaired coagulation or in those undergoing surgical procedures. At doses substantially in excess of the recommended maximum, hematin has caused renal toxicity, which was reversible. Similar problems have not been observed with the usual doses, despite the fact that

patients with acute hepatic porphyria may exhibit reduced renal function.

For women with regular and disabling premenstrual porphyric symptoms, prophylactic hematin (administered one or two days prior to the expected onset of symptoms) and ovulatory suppression with oral contraceptives have been tried. From the limited experience to date, neither therapy can be considered established. Ovulatory suppression by means of peptide analogues of luteinizing hormone releasing hormone (LH-RH) is logical, because such analogues lack the porphyria-inducing properties of contraceptive steroids, and this approach is being evaluated at the present time.

PROGNOSIS. The vast majority of carriers remain asymptomatic, provided that they avoid drugs associated with exacerbations, and their longevity appears to be unaffected. Acute neurologic attacks formerly carried a substantial mortality. However, as a result of hematin therapy and modern intensive care for complications such as respiratory failure, the outlook for these patients is much improved. Neurologic deficits may require months or years to resolve, but complete recovery is observed in many instances. Although mental abnormalities occur in acute attacks, these are neither persistent nor progressive.

PORPHYRIA CUTANEA TARDA

This relatively common condition is characterized by mechanical fragility and blistering of light-exposed skin. Acute neurologic attacks do not occur. The onset of manifestations is insidious, patients often failing to associate cutaneous lesions with sun exposure. Seemingly trivial trauma to the dorsa of the hands, arms, face, or feet leads to vesicles that rupture to an open sore, eventually healing with scar formation. Sclerodermoid changes and hypertrichosis may occur. A history of ethanol abuse and/or chronic liver disease can be obtained from a majority of patients with this type of porphyria. The pathologic changes seen in liver biopsies are nonspecific and do not correlate with the severity of the porphyria. In a few patients, hepatomas containing a high concentration of porphyrin have been diagnosed and presumably were the cause of cutaneous manifestations. Almost all liver biopsy specimens exhibit an increase in stainable iron, and freshly obtained tissue is fluorescent under ultraviolet light because of its high content of uroporphyrin. Associations of this disease with systemic lupus erythematosus, diabetes mellitus, and hemochromatosis (heterozygous state) have been reported.

Urine from patients is red-orange or brown. Its uroporphyrin content (predominantly isomer I) is strikingly elevated; cutaneous manifestations are associated with levels greater than 800 μg per 24 hours (normal, <50 μg per 24 hours). Urinary coproporphyrin excretion is moderately increased, whereas fecal coproporphyrin and protoporphyrin are normal. This pattern clearly distinguishes patients with porphyria cutanea tarda from those with variegate porphyria and cutaneous manifestations (Table 203–2).

The *pathogenesis* of porphyria cutanea tarda is incompletely understood. The pattern of porphyrin excretion, with predominance of isomer I compounds, suggests a partial defect at the level of uroporphyrinogen III synthetase; on the other hand, excretion of uroporphyrin is greater than that of coproporphyrin, consistent with deficient activity of uroporphyrinogen decarboxylase. A partial deficiency of the latter activity appears to be present in the liver of all patients with porphyria cutanea tarda. Whether or not this represents a hereditary abnormality in all cases is controversial at present. In some patients the defect is expressed not only in liver but also in erythrocytes; first-degree relatives of these patients also exhibit the defect in a pattern consistent with autosomal dominant inheritance. On the other hand, in some patients the defect is detectable solely in liver tissue. The erythrocyte

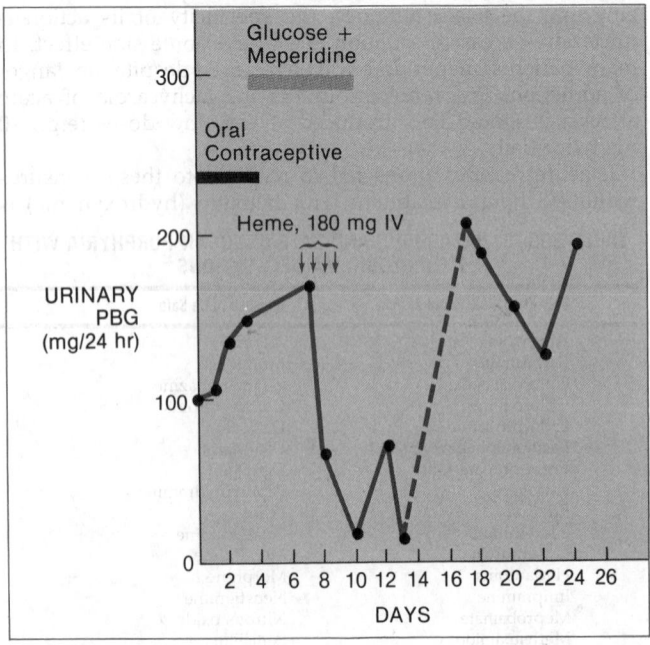

FIGURE 203–2. Acute intermittent porphyria in a patient taking oral contraceptive medication: response of urinary PBG (porphobilinogen) to administered heme (hematin). Normal PBG less than 2 mg per 24 hours.

enzyme of the patient and family members is normal. The latter has been termed *sporadic* porphyria cutanea tarda. The available data are insufficient for determining whether this is an acquired disease or a hereditary variant of porphyria cutanea tarda. Because of the regular association of porphyria cutanea tarda with hepatic siderosis and moderately increased transferrin saturation (averaging 60 per cent), testing for the hemochromatosis gene has been carried out (see Ch. 206). Heterozygosity for hemochromatosis (by HLA testing) appears to occur frequently in persons with clinically evident porphyria cutanea tarda and may be required for its expression. Regardless of the genetic component, it is clear that environmental or purely acquired factors play a central role in the pathogenesis of symptoms. Dietary iron, ethanol ingestion, and certain drugs (notably, estrogens) all may provoke increased porphyrin production, apparently acting in concert with the underlying genetic defect to compromise heme synthesis at the level of uroporphyrinogen III formation. The cutaneous manifestations of porphyria cutanea tarda have been observed in a few patients with renal failure receiving hemodialysis, and increase of plasma uroporphyrin has been noted; the pathogenesis is obscure.

Management involves attention to possible aggravating factors: administered iron, estrogen, ethanol, or occupational exposure to noxious chemicals should be eliminated, and this alone may lead to a reduction in porphyrin excretion and remission of cutaneous manifestations. However, phlebotomy, to remove iron from the liver and accelerate resolution of the disease, usually is indicated. With monitoring of the patient's hemoglobin level, 500 to 1000 ml of blood may be removed once or twice monthly, until urine porphyrin levels begin to decline. The time-course of the response varies widely among patients, averaging six months. For patients with disabling cutaneous disease and unable to tolerate phlebotomy, chloroquine* at low doses may be introduced. However, this carries a definite risk of a hepatotoxic reaction, and close monitoring of liver function is required. Plasmapheresis also may be useful for directly reducing the concentration of circulating uroporphyrin. Topical sunscreens and beta-carotene offer little or no protection against light-induced damage in this disease. When pathogenic environmental factors have been eliminated, a clinical response is observed in virtually all patients treated with serial phlebotomies and usually is long lasting.

TOXIC PORPHYRIA

Cutaneous porphyria on a large scale occurred in Turkey in 1959, when several thousand persons consumed grain that had been treated with a fungicide (hexachlorobenzene). Other cases have resulted from accidental or industrial exposure to hepatotoxins, epidemiologic considerations indicating that the disease is acquired rather than hereditary. The clinical manifestations and laboratory abnormalities are indistinguishable from those of porphyria cutanea tarda.

Anderson KE, Spitz IM, Sassa S, et al.: Prevention of cyclical attacks of acute intermittent porphyria with a long-acting agonist of luteinizing hormone-releasing hormone. N Engl J Med 311:643, 1984. *Premenstrual porphyric attacks and a possible new treatment for them.*

Bissell DM: Haem metabolism and the porphyrias. In Wright R, Millward-Sadler GH, Alberti KGMM, Karran S (eds.): Liver and Biliary Disease. 2nd ed. London, Balliere, Tindall & Cox, 1985, pp 387–413. *The hepatic porphyrias, with emphasis on the clinical aspects.*

Goetsch CA, Bissell DM: Instability of hematin used in the treatment of acute hepatic porphyria. N Engl J Med 315: 235, 1986. *A discussion of hematin therapy, with evidence that some treatment failures and side effects of hematin result from the use of decayed material.*

Kappas A, Sassa S, Anderson KE: The porphyrias. In Stanbury JB, Wyngaarden JB, Fredrickson DS, et al. (eds.): The Metabolic Basis of Inherited Disease. 5th ed. New York, McGraw-Hill Book Company, 1983, pp 1301–1384. *A detailed review of genetic and biochemical aspects of the porphyrias.*

Kushner JP, Edwards CQ, Dadone MM, et al.: Heterozygosity for HLA-linked hemochromatosis as a likely cause of the hepatic siderosis associated with sporadic porphyria tarda. Gastroenterology 88:1232, 1985. *A discussion of familial and sporadic porphyria cutanea tarda and of the possible involvement of the hemochromatosis gene in the expression of this porphyria.*

Ridley A: The neuropathy of acute intermittent porphyria. Q J Med 38:307, 1969. *Neurologic manifestations in 25 patients.*

204 ACATALASIA

James B. Wyngaarden

DEFINITION AND SYNONYMS. Acatalasia is a rare inherited deficiency of catalase in erythrocytes (acatalasemia) and other tissues. In some subjects acatalasia is associated with severe gangrenous lesions of the oral cavity and destruction of alveolar bone (Takahara's disease).

EPIDEMIOLOGY. Acatalasia was discovered in Japan in 1946. Takahara's disease occurs chiefly among Japanese and Koreans but has also occurred in Peru. Asymptomatic acatalasemia has been reported from Japan, Korea, Switzerland, Israel, Mexico, and Peru, and hypocatalasemia from several additional countries, including the United States.

ETIOLOGY AND PATHOGENESIS. Acatalasia is inherited as an autosomal recessive condition and is often associated with consanguinity. In Japan the estimated frequencies of homozygotes and heterozygotes are 4×10^{-6} and 1.7×10^{-3}, respectively. The distribution of blood catalase values among homozygous affected, heterozygous, and normal subjects is triphasic, without overlap. Residual catalase activity among Japanese with acatalasia is very low; the enzyme is electrophoretically normal, of normal stability, and low specific activity. Among Swiss homozygotes, residual catalase activity is higher, and the enzyme is electrophoretically abnormal and heat labile. Swiss heterozygotes have normal blood catalase levels.

Takahara's disease results from oral sepsis with hydrogen peroxide–producing bacteria and appears to be restricted to subjects with very low catalase activities. Acatalasemic Japanese with Takahara's disease have 0.23 per cent of normal catalase activity; those without have 0.57 per cent. Homozygotes from Switzerland, Israel, and Mexico have higher values and are clinically normal. Homozygotes have been classified into five subtypes by Aebi and Wyss, on the basis of genetic and clinical heterogeneity.

CLINICAL MANIFESTATIONS. About one half of acatalasemic subjects remain asymptomatic throughout life. Takahara's disease usually begins before age ten, sometimes during infancy. Over 50 cases have been reported. Mild disease consists of ulcers in the dental alveoli or in tonsillar crypts. In moderate disease (the most common) there is alveolar gangrene, recession of alveolar bone, and loss of teeth. In severe cases there is widespread destruction with gangrene of the maxilla and soft tissue, similar to noma. After healing, extensive scarring may limit opening of the mouth. Gangrenous lesions of the oral cavity are rare after puberty.

DIAGNOSIS. The disease should be suspected in any child with shaggy discolored ulcers of dental alveoli or gangrenous lesions of the mouth. A presumptive diagnostic test is easily performed as follows: When hydrogen peroxide is added to acatalasemic blood, it turns brown-black because of formation of methemoglobin, whereas normal blood bubbles vigorously and remains pink. Asymptomatic acatalasemic and hypocatalasemic subjects have been diagnosed in family studies or in population surveys by quantitative assays of blood catalase activity.

TREATMENT. Curettage and excision of granulating tissue, drainage, irrigation of septic areas, extraction of teeth, and antibiotic therapy have been employed. Reconstructive

---

*This use is not listed in the manufacturer's directive.

surgery and bone grafts have been required. Direct application of crystalline catalase suspensions and transfusions of normal catalase-rich whole blood have been suggested. Once healing has taken place the disease does not recur.

Aebi HE, Wyss SR: Acatalasemia. In Stanbury JB, Wyngaarden JB, Fredrickson DS, et al. (eds.): The Metabolic Basis of Inherited Disease. 5th ed. New York, McGraw-Hill Book Company, 1983. *An authoritative review of genetic, metabolic, and clinical features of acatalasia.*

Matsunaga T, Segar R, Höger P, et al.: Congenital acatalasemia: A study of neutrophil functions after provocation with hydrogen peroxide. Pediatr Res 19:1187, 1985. *Chemotaxis of neutrophils is depressed by H_2O_2 in vitro. This mechanism may contribute to the formation of mucosal ulcers in acatalasia.*

205 WILSON'S DISEASE

Andrew Deiss

DEFINITION. Wilson's disease (hepatolenticular degeneration) is a hereditary disorder characterized by the accumulation of copper in the body, especially in the liver, brain, kidneys, and corneas. The excess copper leads to tissue injury and ultimately, if effective treatment is not instituted, to death.

ETIOLOGY AND PREVALENCE. Wilson's disease is inherited as an autosomal recessive trait. The gene responsible for the disturbance in copper metabolism is closely linked to the locus for esterase D on the long arm of chromosome 13. The prevalence of the disease is approximately 30 per million.

PATHOGENESIS. Normally, loss of copper from the body occurs primarily through the bile. Much of biliary copper is secreted in a poorly absorbable form and thus is lost in the feces. Copper balance is normally maintained by this mechanism. In Wilson's disease biliary excretion of copper is impaired, and as a consequence total body copper is progressively increased. The specific nature of the metabolic abnormality that causes this defect is not known.

Positive copper balance begins in infancy in Wilson's disease and continues thereafter unless appropriate therapy is given. However, the distribution of copper changes as the disease progresses. Liver copper is actually greater in presymptomatic homozygotes than in symptomatic ones. Thus not only does net deposition of liver copper cease, but a portion of previously deposited copper is lost from the liver and deposited elsewhere. This copper redistribution probably takes place when liver injury occurs. If this injury occurs abruptly in many hepatocytes, liver disease may be clinically manifested and a large amount of copper may be released over a short period, creating the potential for acute erythrocyte injury and hemolytic anemia as well. However, if hepatocyte injury is more gradual, acute liver disease will not occur, and the patient will remain asymptomatic as the important site of copper deposition shifts to the brain. With the latter course, most patients will present at a later time with neurologic or psychiatric symptoms, usually with clinically inapparent cirrhosis.

The serum concentration of the copper-containing protein ceruloplasmin is low in 95 per cent of patients with Wilson's disease. The mechanism for the hypoceruloplasminemia is not known, but it is not believed to play a pathogenetic role in the disease.

PATHOLOGY. The diagnosis cannot be made on the basis of histologic sections of the liver. Fatty change and glycogen-filled nuclei are present early, followed later by piecemeal necrosis, lymphocytic infiltration, erosion of limiting plates, parenchymal collapse, and fibrosis. Ultimately these abnormalities evolve into postnecrotic cirrhosis. Stains for copper are unreliable, being negative most frequently during the early stages of the disease when diagnostic help is most needed.

In the brain abnormal astrocytes and neuronal necrosis are widely distributed, and there is atrophy or cavitation of the basal ganglia and occasionally the cerebral cortex.

CLINICAL MANIFESTATIONS. Wilson's disease is a disorder of young persons. Although the disease may occur at any time from the age of five years into the sixth decade, two thirds of patients seek medical attention between the ages of eight and twenty. The physician should suspect the disorder in children under the age of 15 years with signs of progressive hepatic dysfunction or in young people over that age with characteristic neurologic abnormalities.

The hepatic symptoms are quite diverse. Commonly a brief illness characterized by malaise, anorexia, jaundice, and increased aminotransferases is mistaken for viral hepatitis. Similar episodes may recur at intervals of months or years, or a latent period may occur during which the patient is asymptomatic until neurologic symptoms begin. If clinically overt hepatocyte injury persists over a longer period, a syndrome resembling chronic active hepatitis results. Occasionally liver injury occurs precipitously; without rapid institution of appropriate treatment, death is likely in these patients and the need for prompt diagnosis is urgent. More commonly, however, hepatocyte injury is gradual and is not accompanied by symptoms of liver disease; nevertheless cirrhosis develops ultimately in all patients. This liver injury may not be recognized until neurologic disease is evaluated.

Episodes of hemolytic anemia occur when massive release of copper from the liver takes place. Thus hemolysis is usually accompanied by overt liver disease; it occurs regularly in patients with fulminant hepatic failure. Hemolysis usually lasts only a short period and disappears spontaneously.

The neurologic signs at onset may take a variety of forms. Patients may start with a slightly dystonic facies in which the upper lip is drawn tightly over the teeth. Shortly afterwards they develop awkward, dystonic postures in the upper extremities and often an unsteady gait. Once recognized by prior experience, these particular neurologic manifestations are seldom mistaken. In other patients, tremor may be the initial sign, often a characteristic "wing-beating" rhythmic oscillating tremor of the upper extremities that in severe cases gradually extends to the trunk. Frequently loss of coordination of fine movements, such as those required for handwriting, is the earliest neurologic sign. As the disease progresses, patients may develop combinations of these abnormalities. Dysarthria, rigidity, drooling, and titubation are late features. Seizures are infrequent and sensory abnormalities absent. The Kayser-Fleischer (K-F) ring, described below, is definitively diagnostic in the neurologic variety and nearly so in the hepatic form of the disease.

Psychological symptoms of Wilson's disease are prominent and consist of early development of intellectual deterioration, personality changes, and unstable behavior. Children begin to fail at school, and young adults may show difficulty in performing jobs once considered routine. Schizophreniform symptoms and other forms of bizarre behavior may appear, but the mental status examination always shows signs of organic dementia. Effective removal of excess copper often improves but usually fails to eliminate these symptoms completely.

Kayser-Fleischer rings are golden brown or greenish rings or arcs in Descemet's membrane at the limbus of the cornea. They are composed of copper-containing granules and develop primarily after redistribution of liver copper. They may be visible with the unaided eye, but slit-lamp examination should always be obtained. K-F rings are present in all or nearly all patients in the neurologic or psychiatric stage of the disease, but are not present in about one third of those with hepatic symptoms.

Rare symptoms ascribable to Wilson's disease include cholelithiasis, sunflower cataracts, arthropathy, renal calculi, and the Fanconi syndrome.

DIAGNOSIS. The classic diagnostic features of K-F rings, low serum ceruloplasmin concentration (<20 mg per deciliter) and increased amounts of liver and urine copper (>250 μg per gram of dry weight and >100 μg per 24 hours, respectively) are present in nearly all patients with fully evolved neurologic Wilson's disease, but only in about two thirds of those presenting with liver disease. In these patients, K-F rings often have not yet formed, and the serum ceruloplasmin concentration may be difficult to interpret. Even in Wilson's disease, serum ceruloplasmin increases during inflammation, estrogen administration, and pregnancy and may decrease during liver failure. Measurement of the copper content of the liver should resolve the problem. Hepatic copper is often greater than normal (50 μg per gram of dry weight) in a variety of chronic liver diseases, but it seldom reaches the concentration seen in most patients with Wilson's disease (>250 μg per gram of dry weight). In a patient with a disease clinically suggestive of Wilson's disease, hepatic copper of this magnitude is essentially diagnostic. All measurements of copper metabolism should be entrusted only to laboratories experienced with their determination, and the normal values of that laboratory should be used.

In primary biliary cirrhosis and chronic cholestasis, diseases with acquired abnormalities of copper excretion, liver copper may be greatly increased and K-F rings occur rarely. The age, symptoms, and laboratory abnormalities of patients with these diseases help distinguish them from Wilson's disease.

Early during the hemolytic anemia the urinary copper excretion is very great. The Coombs test result is negative. When hemolysis and acute liver disease occur concurrently in a young person, Wilson's disease is the most probable cause.

Examination of all siblings of patients with Wilson's disease is mandatory to identify presymptomatic homozygotes. K-F rings will be absent. Serum ceruloplasmin concentration is reduced in 95 per cent of homozygotes and 10 per cent of heterozygotes. If it is low, liver copper content should be measured. Hepatic copper is slightly increased in most heterozygotes. If the copper is greater than 250 μg per gram of dry weight, Wilson's disease is present, and it should be treated as in symptomatic patients. Heterozygotes never become symptomatic and should not be treated. Some homozygotes will be missed by this evaluation, so continued follow-up is necessary.

TREATMENT. Without effective lifetime therapy, Wilson's disease is inevitably fatal. If treatment is begun early enough, symptomatic recovery usually is complete, and a life of normal length and quality can be expected. If treatment is begun too late, death may not be prevented, or recovery will be only partial.

Effective therapy depends upon establishing negative copper balance, thereby preventing deposition of more copper and mobilizing for excretion excess copper already deposited. The copper chelating agent, D-penicillamine, should be given to all patients initially. The usual dose is 1 to 1.5 grams per day, given in divided doses before meals and at bedtime. Response typically is quite slow, occurring over months, but it may occur more rapidly. A year or more is often required to obtain maximum improvement. About 10 per cent of patients experience a worsening of their neurologic symptoms during the first month or two of treatment, and this phenomenon should not suggest that the diagnosis is in error. Compliance and the effectiveness of therapy must be monitored at one- to two-month intervals with measurements of urine copper, serum ceruloplasmin, and serum non-ceruloplasmin copper (total serum copper minus ceruloplasmin copper). Non-ceruloplasmin copper should decrease early and ceruloplasmin more gradually if treatment is adequate. Urine

copper will increase at once to 1 to 5 mg per 24 hours during the first few months, then gradually decrease as the excess of copper decreases.

Toxic effects are frequent. Rash, fever, adenopathy, neutropenia, or thrombocytopenia often occurs during the first two weeks of treatment. In such circumstances, penicillamine should be discontinued; when the symptoms have cleared, prednisone should be begun at a dose of 40 mg per day and penicillamine resumed at 250 mg per day and gradually increased to full dose over a period of a few weeks. The steroids can then be tapered and stopped. Side effects that occur later after initiation of penicillamine administration include proteinuria, nephrotic syndrome, systemic lupus erythematosus, Goodpasture's syndrome, and a variety of chronic skin diseases. These side effects can often be reversed by temporarily stopping penicillamine and resuming it after the symptoms have abated, sometimes with the addition of steroids. Suspension of treatment should never be permitted for more than a few months.

If penicillamine toxicity is intolerable, trientine (250 mg four times a day) is an effective alternative. Zinc acetate also produces a negative copper balance with tolerable side effects, but there is little experience with its use.

Some patients, especially those with fulminant hepatic failure, are so severely ill that the benefits of medical treatment cannot occur rapidly enough to prevent death. In these patients, liver transplantation, if successful, is curative.

Cartwright GE: Diagnosis of treatable Wilson's disease. N Engl J Med 298:1347, 1978. *An excellent description of the protean and often confusing clinical presentations of Wilson's disease and a few illustrations of what happens when the diagnosis is missed.*

Deiss A, Lynch RE, Lee GR, Cartwright GE: Long-term therapy of Wilson's disease. Ann Intern Med 75:57, 1971. *The natural history of Wilson's disease is related to the evolving pattern of copper deposition.*

Scheinlieb IH, Sternlieb I: Wilson's Disease. Philadelphia, W. B. Saunders Company, 1984. *The authoritative monograph based on the authors' vast experience with all aspects of Wilson's disease.*

Sternlieb I, Scheinberg IH: Prevention of Wilson's disease in asymptomatic patients. N Engl J Med 278:352, 1968. *An important report defining the criteria for identifying homozygotes and heterozygotes in families of patients with Wilson's disease.*

206 HEMOCHROMATOSIS (Iron Storage Disease)

Arno G. Motulsky

DEFINITION. The most common generalized iron storage disease in the United States and in persons of European origin is a genetic disorder known as primary or idiopathic hemochromatosis that is linked to the HLA locus. Massive iron deposits in parenchymal cells may develop after years of increased iron absorption, and functional organ impairment of the liver, heart, and other organs ensues. Secondary hemochromatosis with parenchymal cell involvement also occurs in a variety of anemias associated with both ineffective erythropoiesis and increased iron absorption—most commonly in homozygous beta-thalassemia. Blood transfusions contribute further to the pathologic iron overload. In these patients, clinical signs and symptoms of excessive iron storage develop in adolescence or even earlier.

Hemochromatosis affecting parenchymal tissues needs to be differentiated from iron loading of macrophages of the reticuloendothelial system that is relatively benign. If severe and generalized, the latter condition is known as hemosiderosis and typically occurs after multiple blood transfusions in patients with aplastic anemia in whom iron absorption is not increased. Iron overload of parenchymal liver cells is rarely observed under such conditions and occurs only with massive iron deposits after considerable time has elapsed to permit redistribution of iron.

ETIOLOGY, GENETICS, AND PATHOGENESIS. "Idiopathic" hemochromatosis is caused by an autosomal recessive gene that causes increased iron absorption in the gut. The nature of the metabolic abnormality remains unknown but may relate to failure of iron storage in gastrointestinal and reticuloendothelial cells. Thus, instead of being stored normally in such cells, iron enters the bloodstream to be deposited in parenchymal cells of the liver and other organs. Clinical signs and symptoms will develop after many years of excessive iron absorption when total body iron stores have reached levels of 15 to 40 grams as compared with normal iron stores of 0.2 to 2.0 grams.

The gene for hemochromatosis is located on the short arm of chromosome 6 and is linked to the HLA locus. The hemochromatosis gene is physically close to the HLA-A allele of the HLA complex. About 70 per cent of hemochromatosis patients carry the HLA-A$_3$ allele as compared to 25 to 30 per cent of the general population.

Recombination between the hemochromatosis gene and the HLA-A allele is very rare. Since these genes are separate, hemochromatosis is not likely to be a direct effect of HLA-A gene action. An increased frequency of HLA B$_7$ and HLA B$_{14}$ is also observed and is caused by "hitchhiking" of each of these determinants on the chromosome carrying the hemochromatosis gene (linkage disequilibrium). The development of clinical hemochromatosis in the vast majority of cases requires the "double dose" of the mutant gene, and affected patients are homozygotes. Among sibships that include at least one affected homozygote with hemochromatosis, additional homozygotes as well as heterozygote carriers can often be defined by HLA testing using the principles of genetic linkage. Thus, the HLA status of the affected patient who has inherited a hemochromatosis gene from each parent is determined (Fig. 206–1). Sibs with both HLA haplotypes identical to that of the affected patient will carry the linked hemochromatosis allele on the maternal as well as the paternal chromosome 6. Such persons are homozygous, are at high risk to develop iron overload, or may already be affected. Sibs who share only one HLA haplotype are heterozygotes, and sibs who share none are normal, not having inherited any hemochromatosis gene. No test to detect heterozygotes in the general population exists. Detection of homozygotes in the population at large must utilize measures of iron status (transferrin saturation, serum ferritin) and nonspecific indices of liver damage (e.g., transaminase). HLA testing is not useful for detection in the population.

Homozygotes for hemochromatosis absorb increased iron. The actual amount of stored iron at a given time depends upon additional factors such as age, sex, iron content of food, caloric intake, degree of alcohol ingestion, and unknown factors. Not enough iron to produce clinical findings will have been absorbed in younger persons. Males generally eat larger quantities of food than females and therefore absorb more iron. Most importantly, females lose iron periodically during menstruation and occasionally during pregnancy. Therefore, while the prevalence of homozygotes for the hemochromatosis gene is identical in both sexes, *clinically* apparent hemochromatosis occurs about ten times more frequently in males. Excessive alcohol intake further contributes to liver damage, and many patients with the clinical disease give a history of excessive alcohol intake. Alcohol may stimulate iron absorption, and certain alcoholic beverages such as red wines contain increased amounts of iron. Ingestion of iron-containing medications—particularly over prolonged periods—would cause additional iron absorption.

Excessive iron in various parenchymal organs, particularly the liver and the heart, is required before clinical manifestations develop. There is a fairly good correlation between the quantity of iron stored and the development of clinical signs

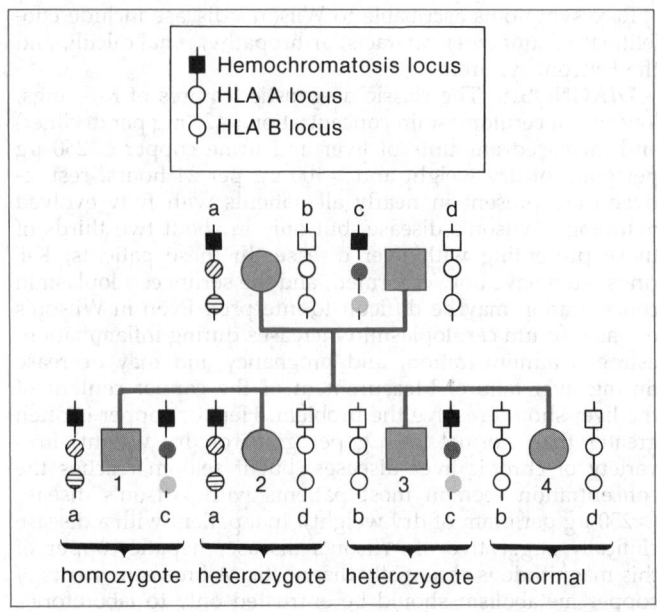

FIGURE 206–1. Hypothetical distribution of iron-loading alleles, each designated by an HLA haplotype, among family members of a patient (1) with fully developed idiopathic hemochromatosis. The "topographic" relationships between the gene (■) and the HLA loci (○) are diagrammatic approximations. The mother of the patient has two number 6 chromosomes, designated a and b, of which chromosome a carries the mutant allele of the hemochromatosis locus. In the father the mutant allele occurs on the sixth chromosome that is designated c. The patient inherited both mutant genes and is a homozygote. (From Bothwell TH, Charlton RW, Motulsky AG: Idiopathic hemochromatosis. In Stanbury JB, Wyngaarden JB, Fredrickson DS, Goldstein JL, Brown MS [eds.]: The Metabolic Basis of Inherited Disease. 5th ed. New York, McGraw-Hill Book Company, 1983.)

and symptoms. Heterozygotes for the hemochromatosis gene may absorb somewhat increased amounts of iron, and minor abnormalities of iron loading have sometimes been detected. Test results of iron status in heterozygotes are closer to those found in normals than to those in homozygotes for hemochromatosis; clinical manifestations rarely if ever occur. It is conceivable that heterozygotes are at higher risk to develop iron overload under conditions at which normal persons would not be affected. However, iron overload in alcoholic liver disease appears not to be associated with the heterozygote state for hemochromatosis. Not all homozygotes develop clinical disease. The fraction of those who do so depends upon the various circumstances affecting iron balance already discussed. It is clear that full-blown clinical findings are the "tip of the iceberg" and that many homozygotes may have no symptoms or exhibit only mild clinical findings that are not recognized as being related to the underlying iron storage disease.

PATHOLOGY. Although iron in reticuloendothelial cells is relatively harmless, parenchymal cell deposits are noxious to tissues. Iron in hemochromatosis is stored mostly in parenchymal cells as insoluble granular gold-brown aggregates known as *hemosiderin*. Normally, most iron is stored as ferritin, but with increasing iron overload the proportion of hemosiderin increases. With advancing hemosiderosis, fibrosis increases, and cirrhosis is frequent in fully developed cases. In such patients wide fibrotic bands characteristically separate liver lobules to cause monolobular cirrhosis.

Skin pigmentation is caused by melanin in the deeper epidermis while the slate-gray appearance in some cases is caused by hemosiderin. Pancreatic iron deposits are more marked in exocrine than in endocrine cells, and fibrosis is the rule. Iron pigment may be deposited in myocardial fibers. Synovial linings as well as various endocrine glands, including thyroid, parathyroid, and anterior pituitary, may be heavily infiltrated with hemosiderin. Testicular atrophy without hemosiderin deposits is frequent. These descriptions refer to fully developed cases. Early cases exhibit significantly fewer pathologic findings.

PREVALENCE. Studies in Utah, Brittany (France), and Sweden suggest homozygote frequencies varying between 1/200 and 1/600. This implies a high frequency of the heterozygote state for the disease, ranging from 8 to 13 per cent. Such frequencies make hemochromatosis one of the most common genetic diseases. Since only a certain portion of homozygotes will develop typical clinical findings, the frequency of the clinical disease will be lower and was estimated to be roughly 1/5000 in the Pacific Northwest of the United States and 1/500 and 1/1000 in autopsy series in Scotland and Southern Sweden, respectively. More prevalence studies are required.

CLINICAL MANIFESTATIONS IN THE FULL-BLOWN DISEASE. Because of the long time required to produce organ damage, the onset of clinical disease is usually, but not always, delayed to the age of 40 to 60. Males are more frequently and earlier affected than menstruating females. The most important clinical signs and symptoms in the fully developed disease include hepatomegaly, skin pigmentation, weakness and lethargy, chronic abdominal pain, diabetes, arthralgia, loss of libido, and impotence. However, more and more patients are being discovered in the early stages of the disease with few or no clinical findings.

The *skin pigmentation* causes browning of the skin that is most pronounced in exposed areas and scars. With increasing hemosiderin deposits, the skin takes on a slate-gray appearance.

Hepatomegaly is the most common physical finding and may occur without symptoms and with normal liver function test results. Portal hypertension and esophageal varices are seen less frequently than in Laennec's cirrhosis. Episodes of hepatic failure are rare, but may be precipitated by blood loss or surgical procedures. *Splenomegaly* occurs. Chronic aching *abdominal pain* is common once cirrhosis has developed and may be the presenting symptom. Carcinoma of the liver is a relatively frequent late complication. Unfortunately, *once cirrhosis has developed, the risk of a malignant hepatoma appears undiminished by iron removal and emphasizes the importance of early case detection and initiation of iron-removing therapy* (see below). Dysrhythmia and refractory cardiac failure may occur and may present clinically as *congestive cardiomyopathy*.

Insulin-dependent diabetes is often seen. A family history of diabetes unrelated to iron storage is more common among patients with hemochromatosis than among controls, suggesting expression of a genetic predisposition to diabetes in persons with liver and pancreatic injury. *Arthralgia* and *arthropathy* different from rheumatoid arthritis and osteoarthritis are common. The second and third metacarpophalangeal joints are usually first involved. Knees, hips, shoulders, and lower back may be affected and acute synovitis with pseudogout of the knees has been observed. Roentgenograms show chondrocalcinosis with small cysts characteristically affecting the second or third metacarpophalangeal joints. Osteoporosis is sometimes observed. *Loss of libido* and sexual impotence with testicular atrophy are common. Scanty body hair may be present long before significant hepatic impairment. Clinically manifest *hypogonadism* is usually of hypogonadotrophic origin. Marked lethargy, increased sleep requirements, and inability to think clearly are frequent complaints.

DIAGNOSIS. The clinical diagnosis of hemochromatosis requires a high index of suspicion and needs to be sought more frequently. Many patients are being detected fortuitously after discovery of abnormally saturated transferrin levels during general workups. Iron overload should be carefully considered among patients (particularly males) who present with any one or a combination of the following: hepatomegaly, weakness and lethargy, abnormal skin pig-

mentation, atypical arthritis, diabetes, impotence, unexplained chronic abdominal pain, or idiopathic cardiomyopathy. Excessive alcohol intake increases the diagnostic probability. A careful history of such illness among sibs should be obtained, and diagnostic suspicions should be particularly high when the family history is positive for the various clinical findings that might suggest this disease.

The diagnosis requires laboratory testing of iron status. The most practical screening test is the determination of serum iron and of transferrin saturation. Serum iron is characteristically elevated in patients with hemochromatosis, and there is increased iron saturation of transferrin, ranging between 60 and 100 per cent (normal, less than 50 per cent). However, abnormally high transferrin saturation can occur as a result of sample contamination, physiologic plasma iron fluctuation, iron therapy, liver disease, and red cell disorders. An abnormal value for transferrin saturation is seen early in the course of the disease and does not reflect the extent of iron storage. In contrast, a valuable noninvasive test to assess iron stores is the measurement of serum ferritin, which correlates reasonably well with the extent of iron storage in the absence of excessive alcohol consumption, inflammation, rheumatoid arthritis, neoplasia, and liver disease such as that induced by drugs or viral hepatitis. Without such complications, a level above 300 μg per liter in males and above 200 μg per liter in females indicates increased iron stores and requires further investigation. Patients with fully developed hemochromatosis have ferritin levels ranging between 700 and several thousand micrograms per liter. However, rare families with significant iron overload and normal ferritin values have been described. Various imaging techniques such as hepatic computerized tomography and nuclear magnetic resonance may become useful for the assessment of hepatic iron stores.

Because of problems with specificity and sensitivity with all laboratory and imaging tests, the definitive test for hemochromatosis is a *liver biopsy*. Parenchymal hemosiderin deposits can be demonstrated histochemically, and the actual concentration of iron should be estimated biochemically. The extent of liver damage and cirrhosis can be determined by histologic examination.

DIFFERENTIAL DIAGNOSIS. The most common differential diagnostic problem is raised by alcoholic liver disease not associated with HLA-linked hemochromatosis. Many such patients have an increased amount of stainable liver iron but no increased iron stores (usually less than 3 grams). Unlike genetic hemochromatosis, the iron in this disease is mostly located in reticuloendothelial cells. Liver function abnormalities are more severe than in hemochromatosis. Appropriate tests (including serum ferritin, liver biopsy, and even a trial of phlebotomies) can establish whether there is increased generalized iron storage. HLA testing and studies of iron status in family members may be helpful, since familial aggregation is not seen in patients with alcoholic liver disease. Iron overload due to chronic anemias (see below) such as beta-thalassemia major rarely raises diagnostic problems, although occasional patients with thalassemia intermedia or sideroblastic anemia with only slightly depressed hematocrit may give diagnostic difficulties.

FAMILY DETECTION FOR PREVENTION. Early treatment can remove increased iron stores that ultimately cause disease. Most importantly, treatment before the onset of cirrhosis most likely prevents the high frequency of hepatoma observed in hemochromatosis. All efforts should therefore be made to detect the disease as early as possible. Since the disease is an autosomal recessive trait, there is a 25 per cent chance that sibs of a patient will be similarly affected. Ideally all family members require a single determination of their HLA status to ascertain which sibs share all HLA determinants with the index case and therefore are homozygotes for the disease. Functional testing includes transferrin saturation, and serum ferritin. If full identity in HLA status and the characteristic iron metabolism abnormalities are found, a liver biopsy should be performed to assess the extent of iron storage. With iron overload, phlebotomies to remove iron should be initiated. Sib testing should be initiated at about puberty for males and after the age of 20 years for females. HLA-identical male sibs found to have a normal iron load should be restudied every two to three years, females somewhat less frequently. Frequent blood donations (three times a year) will prevent potentially toxic iron accumulation and are recommended for HLA-identical sibs. Parents and children of affected patients are obligate heterozygote carriers. Since the gene frequency of hemochromatosis appears to be high, matings of homozygotes with heterozygote carriers are not uncommon, and one half of the offspring of such couples will be homozygotes (pseudodominant vertical transmission). Thus, a parent or a child of a patient with hemochromatosis may also be a homozygote. Family detection therefore should include the entire family.

Occasionally, differentiation of heterozygotes from affected homozygotes may be difficult by serum ferritin and transferrin testing alone. HLA status may aid in such cases, since heterozygotes usually share only one half their HLA haplotypes with their homozygote sibs. Treatment to remove iron is rarely if ever required in heterozygotes.

TREATMENT. Excess iron can usually be removed by periodic venesections. The removal of one unit (approximately 500 ml) of blood depletes the body of 200 to 250 mg of iron. Weekly venesections are required for about two to three years to return iron stores to normal levels in patients with the full-blown disease and for lesser periods for those with early disease. Even though there is no scientific or medical contraindication to using blood from hemochromatic patients for blood transfusions, many blood banks do not use such blood.

Treatment should be monitored by frequent hematocrit determinations and plasma iron and ferritin levels six to ten times per year (Fig. 206–2). After an initial fall, hematocrit levels stabilize at approximately 90 per cent of pretreatment levels. Indicators of iron status do not change until significant depletion of iron stores has occurred. After iron stores have been normalized as shown by ferritin and transferrin levels,

venesections are required at two- to three-month intervals to prevent reaccumulation of iron. An iron-free diet is not necessary at any time during treatment. Treatment of hepatic, cardiac, endocrinologic, and metabolic complications is along conventional lines. Many manifestations of hemochromatosis *except* arthropathy, portal hypertension, and cirrhosis and hepatoma are dramatically improved by phlebotomy therapy.

PROGNOSIS. The five-year survival rate after diagnosis in untreated patients with the fully developed disease is 18 per cent and the ten-year survival rate 6 per cent. The principal cause of death in such patients relates to liver complications: hepatic failure and portal hypertension (30 per cent) and malignant hepatoma (30 per cent). An additional one third of patients die of cardiac failure.

Recently 163 treated patients whose disease was diagnosed between 1959 and 1983 were studied in West Germany. There were 53 deaths. Kaplan-Meier plots indicated cumulative survival of 92 per cent at 5 years, 76 per cent at 10 years, 59 per cent at 15 years, and 49 per cent at 20 years. Life expectancy was reduced significantly further in patients who had cirrhosis, diabetes, or required more than 18 months of venesection for iron depletion. Death was due to cirrhosis in 25 per cent and to hepatoma in 25 per cent. By contrast, in *treated patients without cirrhosis survival expectation was identical to that of the unaffected control population.* It is noteworthy that hepatoma has never been reported in any series among individuals with hemochromatosis who had not developed cirrhosis.

SECONDARY HEMOCHROMATOSIS. Classic hemochromatosis with iron deposits in parenchymal cells of the liver and other organs is observed in several anemias associated with erythroid marrow hyperplasia and ineffective erythropoiesis. Beta-thalassemia major and beta-thalassemia–hemoglobin E disease are the most common anemias of this type. Severe iron loading already occurs before transfusion therapy. Repeated blood transfusions produce further iron overload. In contrast to the HLA-linked hemochromatosis, iron overload in beta-thalassemia major occurs more rapidly and causes clinical symptoms early in life. Hepatic fibrosis is already common in children as is retarded growth and delayed puberty. Cardiac death usually occurs in adolescence or early adulthood unless iron removal is carried out.

Phlebotomies cannot be done since these patients are severely anemic. Chelation therapy with desferrioxamine together with frequent transfusions has improved the prognosis markedly. Death due to complications of iron storage can be prevented if iron removal can be initiated before clinical signs and symptoms of iron overload appear.

Patients with hypoplastic anemias do not absorb increased amounts of iron, but often require blood transfusions over prolonged periods. The transfused iron is largely stored in macrophages. No clinical signs or symptoms occur with storage of iron in macrophages. Redistribution to parenchymal cells with development of hepatic cirrhosis and/or other typical organ involvement occurs rarely.

Bothwell TH, Charlton RW, Motulsky AG: Idiopathic hemochromatosis. In Stanbury JB, Wyngaarden JB, Fredrickson DS, et al. (eds): The Metabolic Basis of Inherited Disease. 5th ed. New York, McGraw-Hill Book Company, 1983, pp 1269–1298. *A full discussion of all aspects of iron metabolism and genetics in HLA-linked and secondary hemochromatosis.*

Edwards CQ, Dadone MM, Skolnick MH, et al.: Hereditary haemochromatosis. Clin Haematol 11:411, 1982. *A comprehensive review of the disease based on the extensive Utah experience.*

Fairbanks VF, Baldus WP: Hemochromatosis: The neglected diagnosis. Mayo Clin Proc 61:296, 1986. *A succinct summary of this underdiagnosed disease and practical advice regarding laboratory tests.*

Halliday JW, Powell LW: Iron overload. Semin Hematol 19:42, 1982. *A balanced discussion of all aspects of idiopathic and secondary hemochromatosis.*

Milder MS, Cook JD, Stray S, et al.: Idiopathic hemochromatosis, an interim report. Medicine 59:34, 1980. *Clinical features and treatment of idiopathic hemochromatosis based on 34 cases.*

Niederau C, Fischer R, Sonnenberg A, et al.: Survival and causes of death in cirrhotic and in noncirrhotic patients with primary hemochromatosis. N Engl J Med 313:1256, 1985. *A detailed account of the natural history of treated hemochromatosis in 163 patients with 53 deaths.*

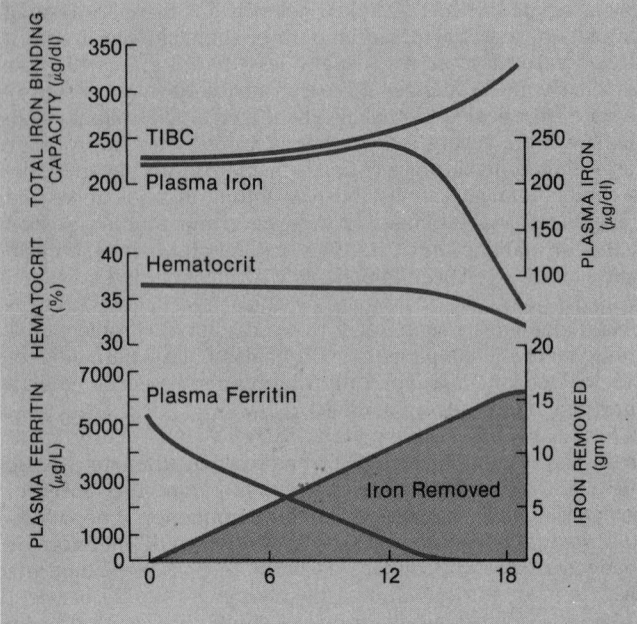

FIGURE 206–2. Serial changes in the hematocrit, plasma iron concentration, total iron-binding capacity, and plasma ferritin concentration in a subject with idiopathic hemochromatosis on repeated venesection therapy. (From Bothwell TH, Charlton RW, Cook JD, Finch CA: Idiopathic haemochromatosis. In Iron Metabolism in Man. Oxford, Blackwell Scientific Publications, 1979.)

Simon M, Bourel M, Genetet B, et al.: Idiopathic hemochromatosis. Demonstration of recessive transmission and early detection by family HLA typing. N Engl J Med 297:1017, 1977. *Data to support HLA linkage and review of the inheritance of hemochromatosis with practical recommendations.*

Valberg LS, Ghent CN: Diagnosis and management of hereditary hemochromatosis. Annu Rev Med 36:27, 1985. *A useful review of the current status of diagnosis and management.*

207 PHOSPHORUS DEFICIENCY AND HYPOPHOSPHATEMIA

Lloyd H. Smith, Jr.

Phosphorus is necessary for the structural and functional integrity of all living things. In hydroxyapatite it is a key constituent of bone; as a part of phospholipids (lecithin, sphingomyelin) it is necessary for the structure of all cell membranes, both external and internal (endoplasmic reticulum, lysosomes, nuclear membranes). It furnishes the backbone of nucleic acids, captures and stores metabolic energy (~P), serves as a second messenger in endocrinology (cAMP, cGMP), regulates the release of O_2 by hemoglobin (2,3-diphosphoglycerate), and buffers urine. Even this partial list indicates that a severe deficiency of phosphorus would lead to widespread and serious consequences.

In an adult of average size there are approximately 700 to 800 grams (25 moles) of phosphorus, of which 80 to 85 per cent is in the skeleton and 10 per cent in muscle. Phosphate is the major anion of intracellular fluid (about 100 mM), where it is found mostly as phosphoproteins, phospholipids, or phosphosugars rather than as free orthophosphate. In extracellular fluid the normal concentration of phosphorus in adults is 2.7 to 4.5 mg per deciliter (0.9 to 1.5 mM), of which most is free; perhaps 10 per cent is protein bound. Serum phosphorus is normally higher in children (4.0 to 7.0 mg per deciliter). (It is conventional to express serum phosphate as the amount of elemental P, since pH influences the relative amounts of $H_2PO_4^-$ and HPO_4^- present.) The average American diet contains about 1000 mg P, most of which is absorbed by active transport, increased by 1,25-dihydroxycholecalciferol. Approximately 90 per cent of that absorbed from the diet is excreted in the urine by a process involving filtration and partial renal tubular reabsorption. The tubular reabsorption of phosphate is diminished by parathyroid hormone (PTH), acting with cAMP as a second messenger. Through vitamin D, PTH, calcitonin, and the mineralization of osteoid, phosphate metabolism is closely linked with that of calcium. These interrelationships are discussed more completely in Ch. 244.

Hyperphosphatemia that is sustained occurs almost exclusively in three clinical conditions: (1) renal insufficiency (see Ch. 78), (2) hypoparathyroidism (including various types of pseudohypoparathyroidism) (see Ch. 247), and (3) acromegaly or gigantism (see Ch. 226). When severe, hyperphosphatemia may contribute to the acidosis of uremia, further reduce the extracellular fluid concentration of ionized calcium, or lead to metastatic calcification in extraosseous sites. Transient hyperphosphatemia may occur with acute tissue destruction, such as the tumor lysis syndrome or rhabdomyolysis.

CAUSES OF HYPOPHOSPHATEMIA. Hypophosphatemia (serum P <2.7 mg per deciliter) may be associated with a normal total body phosphate (representing a transient intracellular shift) or with phosphate deficiency. The two most common causes of transient hypophosphatemia are (1) ingestion of carbohydrates, which deplete phosphate in extracellular fluid in the process of their intracellular transport and metabolism, and (2) acute respiratory alkalosis, which leads to an intracellular shift of phosphate through mechanisms not fully explained.

TABLE 207–1. CAUSES OF HYPOPHOSPHATEMIA*

I. Moderate hypophosphatemia (P 1.0 to 2.5 mg per deciliter)
Hyperparathyroidism
Osteomalacia (usually with hyperparathyroidism), malabsorption, deficiency of vitamin D, familial hypophosphatemic rickets, vitamin D dependent rickets, oncogenic rickets
Carbohydrate administration or ingestion or enhanced metabolism—glucose, fructose, glycerol, lactate, insulin administration
Hypomagnesemia
ECF volume expansion
Acute alkalosis—bicarbonate infusion or moderate hyperventilation
Hemodialysis

II. Severe hypophosphatemia (P less than 1.0 mg per deciliter)
Chronic alcoholism and alcoholic withdrawal
Diabetic ketoacidosis, recovery phase
Enteric phosphate binding—excessive use of agents binding phosphate in the gut
Hyperalimentation
Nutritional recovery syndrome
Uptake by rapidly proliferating malignant tumors (rare)

*Modified from Knochel JP: Hypophosphatemia. West J Med 134:15, 1981.

It is convenient to summarize the causes of hypophosphatemia as those that usually result in only moderate reductions in serum P (1.0 to 2.5 mg per deciliter) and those that may result in severe hypophosphatemia (P <1.0 mg per deciliter) (Table 207–1). The latter may also be associated with lesser degrees of phosphate depletion as well.

Moderate hypophosphatemia may occur transiently during carbohydrate metabolism or alkalosis, as noted above, in the absence of phosphate depletion. Increased PTH, associated with either primary or secondary hyperparathyroidism, reduces the renal tubular reabsorption of phosphate and leads to renal phosphate wasting. In familial hypophosphatemic rickets there may be a primary defect in the renal tubular reabsorption of phosphate. The association of hypophosphatemia with hyperparathyroidism and the various types of osteomalacia or rickets is discussed more fully in Ch. 246 and 247. Hypomagnesemia and extracellular fluid volume expansion may result in reduced renal tubular reabsorption of phosphate and mild hypophosphatemia. Hemodialysis with equilibration against a dialysate deficient in phosphate may lead to overshoot hypophosphatemia. There are no well-defined acute metabolic consequences of moderate hypophosphatemia. Prolonged hypophosphatemia in this range may result in the defective mineralization of bone characteristic of osteomalacia or rickets.

Severe hypophosphatemia may cause serious metabolic consequences as described below. The most frequent cause of severe hypophosphatemia in clinical practice is *alcoholism*, especially during the withdrawal phase. The causes of phosphate depletion in alcoholics are complex and may include (1) poor dietary intake, (2) vomiting, (3) diarrhea, (4) the use of antacids which bind phosphate and reduce its absorption, (5) a possible phosphaturic effect of ethanol itself, (6) magnesium deficiency with phosphaturia, and (7) calcium deficiency with secondary hyperparathyroidism. The serum P level may be further reduced by the hyperventilation characteristic of alcohol withdrawal and by the therapeutic infusion of glucose. Patients with *uncontrolled diabetes mellitus* often become phosphate depleted through catabolism of intracellular organic phosphates and phosphaturia secondary to osmotic diuresis. Initial serum P levels are often normal or even high during diabetic ketoacidosis, but rapidly fall to hypophosphatemic levels during the first six to twelve hours of treatment with volume expansion, glucose, and insulin. Hyperventilation with *marked respiratory alkalosis* can cause profound hypophosphatemia within minutes; metabolic alkalosis of the same degree causes only moderate hypophosphatemia. Excessive ingestion of *phosphate binding antacids*, such as aluminum hydroxide, may inhibit phosphate absorption from the intestine sufficiently to cause chronic depletion, especially when combined with reduced dietary ingestion of phosphate. Excessive utilization of phosphate during tissue repletion may

TABLE 207–2. CONSEQUENCES OF SEVERE HYPOPHOSPHATEMIA

Acute—"metabolic"
Hematologic
    Red cell dysfunction and hemolysis
    Leukocyte dysfunction
    Platelet dysfunction
Muscle
    Weakness
    Rhabdomyolysis
    Myocardial dysfunction
Central nervous system dysfunction
Peripheral neuropathy
Hepatic dysfunction

Chronic—"structural"
Osteomalacia or rickets

occasionally result in severe hypophosphatemia during *hyperalimentation* (without adequate supplementary P) and during the *nutritional recovery syndrome* of refeeding patients with protein-calorie malnutrition or starvation. Whatever its cause, severe hypophosphatemia requires early attention because of its potential consequences.

CONSEQUENCES OF SEVERE HYPOPHOSPHATEMIA

(Table 207–2). The long-term consequences of severe hypophosphatemia are largely structural, those of metabolic bone disease (see Ch. 246). The short-term consequences may be considered to be metabolic, although the distinction is an arbitrary one.

Red cell dysfunction in severe hypophosphatemia may result from two biochemical abnormalities, depletion of intracellular 2,3-diphosphoglycerate (2,3-DPG) and of ATP. Phosphate is a cofactor for glyceraldehyde-3-phosphate dehydrogenase, an enzyme in the pathway of the synthesis of 2,3-DPG. When intracellular erythrocytic phosphate decreases, a block in the glycolytic pathway results with accumulation of triose phosphates and depletion of 2,3-DPG. This molecule normally exercises a unique allosteric effect on the dissociation curve of oxyhemoglobin, shifting it "to the right" and thereby enhancing the tissue availability of oxygen (see Ch. 140). Reduction of erythrocytic 2,3-DPG, conversely, impairs effective oxygen delivery to the periphery. The same block in the glycolytic pathway reduces ATP synthesis. The degradation of AMP to inosine 5′-phosphate (IMP) by AMP deaminase is enhanced when the restraining influence of phosphate is reduced, further depleting the intracellular concentration of adenine nucleotides. As a result the concentration of erythrocytic ATP tends to fall in parallel with the reduction of serum phosphorus. At a critical level of ATP (usually with serum P <0.5 mg per deciliter), the energy metabolism of the erythrocyte may become inadequate to maintain the integrity of its membrane and *hemolysis* may occur.

Leukocyte dysfunction has been demonstrated during phosphate depletion in experimental animals, characterized by impaired chemotaxis, phagocytosis, and bactericidal function. These defects presumably result from inadequate ATP for normal cellular functions, possibly including the synthesis of phospholipids in membranes. Similarly *platelet dysfunction* occurs in experimental phosphate depletion, but no hemorrhagic diathesis has been attributed to phosphate deficiency in man.

Many patients with severe hypophosphatemia complain of *weakness*. This is often nonspecific and difficult to delineate from that caused by the associated disorder, but improved diaphragmatic contractility has been noted following the treatment of hypophosphatemia in patients with respiratory failure. *Rhabdomyolysis* is an occasional complication of severe

hypophosphatemia, perhaps being somewhat analogous to hemolytic anemia in its pathogenesis, i.e., related to deficiency of ATP. The severity of rhabdomyolysis varies from that manifested solely by an elevated serum level of "muscle enzymes" (aldolase and creatine phosphokinase) to a full-fledged syndrome of muscle weakness, pain, tenderness, and stiffness associated with myoglobinuria. Interestingly, the release of phosphate from the necrosis of muscle may suffice to return the serum P level to normal. A few patients with severe phosphate depletion have exhibited congestive cardiomyopathy, which has seemed to respond to phosphate repletion. These clinical observations are strengthened by the demonstration of decreased myocardial contractility during experimental phosphate depletion in dogs.

Severe hypophosphatemia may result in *central nervous system dysfunction* with a constellation of symptoms and signs designated as metabolic brain disease or metabolic encephalopathy (see Ch. 457). These abnormalities may vary from irritability, weakness, and paresthesias to obtundation, seizures, and coma. It is presumed that this CNS dysfunction results from deranged energy metabolism of the brain secondary to ATP depletion. Observations have suggested that hepatic function is further impaired in alcoholics with severe hypophosphatemia, with early improvement during replacement therapy, but a clinical entity of *hypophosphatemic hepatic dysfunction* has not yet been well established.

TREATMENT OF HYPOPHOSPHATEMIA. The treatment of hypophosphatemia depends upon its cause, its acuteness, and its severity. Hypophosphatemia caused by acute respiratory alkalosis or the infusion of carbohydrates does not require replacement therapy. Chronic hypophosphatemia associated with aluminum hydroxide therapy, for example, may require reduction of the antacid and an oral source of supplemental phosphate such as milk (1 gram of P or 30 to 35 mmol per quart) or a balanced solution of phosphate salts (sodium or potassium salts as in Fleet enema solution or Neutra-Phos). It is rare that hypophosphatemia is so acute and severe as to require parenteral replacement therapy. When such treatment is undertaken it is well to remember that (1) it is unusual for hypophosphatemia to cause metabolic disturbances at concentrations greater than 1.0 mg per deciliter, so full parenteral replacement is neither necessary nor desirable; and (2) if hyperphosphatemia results, there is a danger of producing a decrease in ionized calcium (with tetany or convulsions) and/or metastatic calcification of soft tissues. It is usually safe and sufficient to administer intravenously 1 mmol of phosphate per kilogram of body weight evenly over a 24-hour period in the treatment of acute, severe hypophosphatemia associated with phosphate depletion. Since potassium depletion is so frequently associated with phosphate depletion both in alcoholics and in patients with diabetic ketoacidosis, it may be useful as a guideline to give half of parenterally administered potassium as its phosphate salt. Obviously parenteral phosphate should not be given in the face of hyperphosphatemia.

Agus ZS: Oncogenic hypophosphatemic osteomalacia. Kidney Int 24:113, 1983. *A description of the interesting syndrome of tumor-associated renal phosphate wasting.*

Janson D, Birnbaum G, Baker FJ: Hypophosphatemia. Ann Emerg Med 12:107, 1983. Knochel JP: Hypophosphatemia. West J Med 134:15, 1981. Yu GC, Lee DBN: Clinical disorders of phosphorus metabolism. West J Med (in press). *These three articles give excellent general reviews of the clinical and pathophysiologic aspects of phosphate deficiency syndromes in man and related disorders produced in experimental animals. They have useful bibliographies that allow the reader to pursue in depth the available information about each specific syndrome described above.*

Knochel JP: The clinical status of hypophosphatemia. N Engl J Med 313:447, 1985. *This useful editorial emphasizes the adverse effect of phosphate depletion on muscle function.*

208 DISORDERS OF MAGNESIUM METABOLISM

Lloyd H. Smith, Jr.

Magnesium is the fourth most common cation in the human body (after sodium, potassium, and calcium) and the cation in second highest concentration intracellularly. The average adult body contains about 25 grams (1000 mmol) of magnesium, of which 50 to 60 per cent is in bone. The normal serum magnesium concentration is 1.6 to 2.1 mEq per liter, approximately one fourth to one third being protein bound. The average American diet contains approximately 500 mg (20 mmol) of magnesium, much of this in chlorophyll. It has been estimated that about 0.15 mmol (3.5 to 4.5 mg) of dietary magnesium per kilogram per day is necessary to maintain a positive balance in adults. More is required in children. Magnesium is actively absorbed in the small intestine by a process that is enhanced by 1,25-dihydroxycholecalciferol, resulting in a net absorption of about 30 to 40 per cent of that ingested. This net absorption is balanced at equilibrium by renal excretion, which reflects filtration of the 65 to 75 per cent not protein bound followed by net renal tubular reabsorption of approximately 95 per cent. The kidney can control the excretion of magnesium over a wide range—from more than 250 mmol to less than 1 mmol per day. The factors that control the renal tubular reabsorption of magnesium are not completely understood, but include sodium excretion, calcium excretion, parathyroid hormone, and extracellular fluid volume. Excretion is also increased by ethanol and by many diuretic agents.

Magnesium has a structural role in bone crystal. It also serves as an activator of a large number of specific enzymes. Of particular importance it is a cofactor in all transphosphorylation reactions involving ATP, so that it is intimately involved in energy metabolism and the synthesis of macromolecules, for example. Perhaps even more basic in biology is its obligate role in the function of chlorophyll. By and large it has not been possible to correlate the signs or symptoms of magnesium deficiency or excess with any one of its specific biochemical functions.

HYPERMAGNESEMIA. Because of the ability of the normal kidney to excrete a magnesium load, significant hypermagnesemia is rarely seen in clinical practice. In the past magnesium ion was occasionally infused as a hypotensive agent in the treatment of acute hypertension with the secondary production of symptomatic hypermagnesemia. In patients with renal insufficiency the excessive use of magnesium, as in magnesium-containing antacids, may cause hypermagnesemia. The manifestations of hypermagnesemia are largely in the central nervous system and the cardiovascular system. Ionized magnesium is a sedative that depresses the function of the central nervous system and exerts a curare-like effect on the neuromuscular junction at high concentrations (>10 mEq per liter). The cardiovascular effects of hypermagnesemia are those of peripheral vasodilatation resulting in hypotension, generalized depression of the cardiac conduction system, bradyrhythmias, and asystole with cardiac arrest in diastole. The cardiac effects of Mg^{++} are usually manifested at serum concentration greater than 10 mEq per liter with asystole at levels greater than 25 mEq per liter, but a few patients have exhibited exceptional sensitivity with cardiotoxicity at levels of 4.5 to 5.5 mEq per liter. Factors that augment the cardiotoxicity of Mg^{++} include hypocalcemia, hyperkalemia, acidosis, digitalis therapy, and renal insufficiency (beyond its effect on the serum Mg^{++} level). Treatment of hypermagnesemia is usually limited to discontinuing its exogenous source.

In severe hypermagnesemia, intravenous treatment with calcium may temporarily reverse many of the toxic effects because of the pharmacologic antagonism of ionized calcium and magnesium in the central nervous system.

HYPOMAGNESEMIA. Hypomagnesemia is a much more frequent metabolic derangement than hypermagnesemia, and usually occurs as one component of a complex deficiency state, affecting many minerals, vitamins, and nutrients.

Causes of Hypomagnesemia. Magnesium deficiency and hypomagnesemia result from decreased absorption or from increased excretion (Table 208–1). Very rarely it may result from "loss" into bone during excessive osteogenesis, the "hungry bone syndrome," during the repair of osteitis fibrosa generalisata following the removal of a parathyroid tumor (see Ch. 247). Serum levels may also fall, as do those of calcium, during acute pancreatitis. In general, decreased absorption of magnesium occurs in the same circumstances as does decreased calcium absorption, especially caused by dietary deficiency and malabsorption syndromes of whatever origin. Decreased absorption in uremia may result from deficiency of 1,25-dihydroxycholecalciferol. A few infants have been described with convulsions associated with hypocalcemia and hypomagnesemia in the absence of renal magnesium wasting. They have responded to continued high ingestion of magnesium, but not of calcium, and are thought to have a selective defect in gut absorption of magnesium. It is not clear whether ethanol diminishes magnesium absorption directly or only through diminished ingestion or vitamin D deficiency.

Increased loss of magnesium can occur from excessive vomiting, from diarrhea, or via the kidney. Rarely patients may exhibit what appears to be an inherited renal tubular defect in magnesium reabsorption. These patients have tended to have potassium wasting as well and to present with hypokalemia, hypomagnesemia, and hypocalcemia (secondary to hypomagnesemia). In general, magnesium clearance tends to parallel that of sodium and calcium and may be increased by diuretics (osmotic, thiazides, ethacrynic acid, furosemide), by ionized calcium, and possibly by ethanol. Renal magnesium wasting also occurs as a result of the renal tubular effect of certain drugs, especially aminoglycosides, amphotericin B, and cisplatin. The magnesium wasting of uncontrolled diabetes mellitus probably results from tissue catabolism and osmotic diuresis. Lactation hypomagnesemia is well described in cattle and has been documented in one woman whose serum Mg^{++} fell to 0.4 mEq per liter.

Consequences of Hypomagnesemia. Hypomagnesemia rarely occurs as a single deficiency so that it is not always possible to distinguish its signs and symptoms from those of associated deficiency states. Selective magnesium deficiency has been produced experimentally in man, however, and it is based on these observations, together with clinical correlations in patients, that the spectrum of manifestations listed in Table

TABLE 208–1. CAUSES OF HYPOMAGNESEMIA (SEEN MOST FREQUENTLY CLINICALLY IN ALCOHOLISM AND MALABSORPTION)

I. **Decreased absorption from dietary sources**
   Diet poor in magnesium
   Parenteral feeding without magnesium
   Ethanol effect on absorption
   Malabsorption syndromes
   Uremia
   Selective intestinal defect for magnesium absorption (rare)
II. **Increased loss of magnesium from the body**
   Gastrointestinal tract—diarrhea, fistulas, suction
   Kidney
     Primary renal tubular defects
     Secondary—diuretics, Ca^{++}, ethanol, expansion of ECF, diabetes mellitus, treatment with gentamicin, cisplatin, or amphotericin B
   Breast—lactation hypomagnesemia (mostly in cattle, rarely in humans)
III. **Internal redistribution**
   Acute pancreatitis
   Increased loss into bone ("hungry bone syndrome")

TABLE 208–2. CONSEQUENCES OF MAGNESIUM DEFICIENCY

Neuromuscular
Lethargy, weakness, fatigue, decreased mentation, paresthesias
Neuromuscular irritability, in part due to associated hypocalcemia
Hyaline and vacuolar degeneration of myofibers with segmental necrosis
Gastrointestinal
Anorexia, nausea, vomiting
Paralytic ileus
Cardiovascular
Increased sensitivity to digitalis glycosides
Cardiac arrhythmias
Metabolic
Hypocalcemia—probably due to the combined result of decreased PTH secretion and decreased end-organ responsiveness to PTH
Hypokalemia—tendency toward renal potassium wasting

208–2 has been described. Patients with magnesium deficiency are lethargic, weak, and irritable with decreased attention span. They may have tetany with positive Chvostek and Trousseau signs because of associated hypocalcemia (see below). In experimental magnesium deficiency, muscles are weak and may show hyaline and vacuolar degeneration of myofibers, sometimes followed by leukocytic infiltration, segmental necrosis, and early calcification. Patients with hypomagnesemia are generally anorectic and may have nausea, vomiting, and poor intestinal mobility. Hypomagnesemia may occur in congestive heart failure because of anorexia, malabsorption, and the excessive use of diuretic agents. Magnesium deficiency increases the sensitivity of the heart to digitalis glycosides so that digitalis toxicity occurs at a lower serum level and also tends to persist longer. Hypomagnesemia has also been associated with cardiac arrhythmias independent of digoxin–ventricular premature beats, ventricular tachycardia, and ventricular fibrillation. This association is often difficult to establish because other abnormalities generally coexist, especially hypokalemia.

Magnesium metabolism has a number of interesting interrelationships with that of calcium: (1) both are absorbed by the gut through mechanisms enhanced by vitamin D; (2) excess magnesium may inhibit calcium absorption, but not vice versa; (3) calcium and magnesium may compete for renal tubular reabsorption; (4) calcium and magnesium are physiologic antagonists in the central nervous system; and (5) magnesium is necessary for the normal secretion of parathyroid hormone (PTH) in response to hypocalcemia and also for the activity of PTH as a hormone at the site of its target organs. *Hypocalcemia* is one of the most consistent and important findings in magnesium deficiency with hypomagnesemia. Hypocalcemia responds promptly to magnesium replacement and is accompanied by a rise in plasma PTH. A burst of PTH secretion occurs within minutes after the infusion of magnesium intravenously into patients with combined hypocalcemia

and hypomagnesemia. Many of these patients show evidence of resistance to exogenous PTH as well. Hypomagnesemia therefore results in a complex combination of hypoparathyroidism and acquired pseudohypoparathyroidism. This entity should be suspected especially in alcoholics or patients with malabsorption who present with hypocalcemia. *Hypokalemia* is frequently found with hypomagnesemia. Although some of the conditions that cause magnesium depletion also produce potassium depletion, there is evidence that magnesium deficiency itself enhances renal excretion of potassium. This associated hypokalemia is usually resistant to potassium replacement unless magnesium is replaced first.

Treatment of Hypomagnesemia. The treatment of hypomagnesemia is rarely an acute emergency. When rapid replacement therapy is judged to be vital (convulsions, tachyrhythmias), 2 grams of $MgSO_4$ (16.3 mEq) can be given intravenously over several minutes. This can be followed by a constant intravenous infusion of approximately 1 mEq of magnesium per kilogram per 24 hours, which usually suffices for initial replacement therapy. Ampules often contain 1 gram of $MgSO_4 \cdot 7H_2O$ which is 8.1 mEq Mg, so that initial replacement therapy usually requires 8 to 10 grams of $MgSO_4$ given either intravenously as above or intramuscularly as 2 grams every four hours for five doses. After the first day approximately 0.5 mEq of Mg per kilogram per 24 hours should be given intravenously or intramuscularly for two to five days, based on the return of the serum magnesium level to normal. Parenteral replacement therapy is often preferable to oral therapy because of the tendency of magnesium salts to cause diarrhea. When renal function is impaired, the aforementioned schedules for magnesium replacement must be followed with extra caution and with careful monitoring of serum levels. When there is chronic loss of magnesium (renal wasting, for example), oral therapy is preferred and can be carried out with various preparations as tolerated without diarrhea—magnesium hydroxide tablets, magnesium acetate solution, or liquid milk of magnesia.

Berkelhammer C, Bear RA: A clinical approach to common electrolyte problems. 4. Hypomagnesemia. Can Med Assoc J 132:360, 1985. *This succinct review is a very useful starting point from which to read more extensively about magnesium metabolism in man.*
Cronin RE, Knochel JP: Magnesium deficiency. Adv Intern Med 28:509, 1983. *An excellent general review of magnesium metabolism and the pathophysiology of magnesium deficiency (102 references).*
Dirko JH: The kidney and magnesium regulation. Kidney Int 23:771, 1983. *A succinct review of the role of the kidney in magnesium metabolism and of the causes of hypomagnesemia (36 references).*
Levine BS, Coburn JW: Magnesium, the mimac/antagonist of calcium. N Engl J Med 310:1253, 1984. *An editorial about the complex interactions of these important cations.*
Whang R: Magnesium deficiency: Pathogenesis, prevalence, and clinical implications. Am J Med 82(Suppl. 3A):24, 1987. *A succinct general review with a useful up-to-date list of 43 references.*

Other Hereditary Disorders

209 FAMILIAL MEDITERRANEAN FEVER
Daniel G. Wright

DEFINITION. Familial Mediterranean Fever (FMF) is an inherited, recurrent inflammatory disease of unknown cause. The disease is characterized by acute self-limited attacks of fever and peritonitis, sometimes accompanied by pleuritis, arthritis, and erythematous skin lesions. Among affected individuals in the Middle East and Europe, FMF is frequently

complicated by amyloidosis and progressive renal failure. FMF has been given a number of other names: familial paroxysmal polyserositis, benign paroxysmal peritonitis, periodic peritonitis, and periodic disease. The first of these is descriptively accurate and an appropriate alternative name for the disease; the other terms, however, are misleading and should not be used. FMF is not a benign condition, given the potentially lethal complication of amyloidosis. Moreover, attacks of acute serositis in FMF affect sites other than the peritoneum, and they recur at irregular, unpredictable intervals that do not reflect true periodicity.

INCIDENCE, PREVALENCE, AND GENETICS. Although FMF has been recognized in many parts of the world, it is largely restricted to ethnic groups originating in the eastern

Mediterranean area. It is an uncommon disease, even in Israel where the largest number of cases are seen. Half the reported cases of FMF are in patients of Sephardic Jewish ancestry; approximately 20 per cent of patients are Armenian, and another 20 per cent are of Turkish or Arabic descent. Most of the remaining patients are of Italian, Greek, or Ashkenazic Jewish ancestry. However, the disease has also been recognized rarely in individuals with Anglo-Saxon or northern European origins. The disease is familial, and in well-studied, affected kindreds it appears to be inherited as an autosomal recessive trait. Nonetheless, nearly 50 per cent of patients do not give a positive family history for the disease. Among reported cases males predominate by a ratio of 3:2.

ETIOLOGY. Many pathogenetic explanations have been proposed for the acute inflammatory episodes of FMF. However, the etiology of this disease remains unknown. Extensive studies have failed to establish an infectious or allergic basis for the disease, and there is no good evidence to support suggestions that FMF represents a hormonal or psychosomatic disturbance. Recently, it has been suggested that FMF might be caused by a genetically determined defect in the normal regulation of acute inflammatory responses. Abnormalities of suppressor T lymphocytes, altered metabolism of lipoxygenase products of arachidonic acid, and absence of a normal inhibitor of the complement-derived anaphylatoxin C5a have been described in FMF. However, the etiologic significance (if any) of these observations remains to be clarified and confirmed.

PATHOLOGY. Pathologic findings in FMF are those of nonspecific, acute inflammation. Neutrophilic infiltration predominates in exudates recovered from peritoneal, pleural, or joint spaces at the time of acute attacks. Serosal thickening and secondary adhesions may occur, which in the abdomen can lead to mechanical bowel obstruction. Amyloidosis is the most serious histopathologic finding in FMF. In affected individuals, amyloid is deposited in the intima and media of arterioles and in the subendothelium of venules in all major organs. There is also parenchymal deposition of amyloid, particularly in the renal glomeruli, adrenals, spleen, and alveolar septa of the lung, while the liver and heart are characteristically spared.

CLINICAL MANIFESTATIONS. In most patients the signs and symptoms of FMF begin during the first two decades of life, usually between the ages of 5 and 15 years. Rarely, however, onset of the disease may occur in infancy or as late as the fifth or sixth decade. There is considerable variability in the duration and frequency of attacks even in the same patient. Acute attacks typically last for 24 to 48 hours and recur once or twice a month. However, attacks may recur as frequently as several times a week or as infrequently as once a year, and symptoms may persist for as long as a week during individual episodes. Some patients experience spontaneous remission that persists for years, followed by recurrence of frequent attacks. Pregnancy is often associated with remission of attacks, which then resume postpartum. Some patients relate the occurrence of attacks to cold weather and find that they experience attacks more frequently during winter than during summer. Recurrent attacks may also become less severe and/or less frequent as patients age or as they develop amyloidosis. Between attacks, patients typically feel entirely well.

Temperatures as high as 39° to 40°C occur with almost all attacks. Fevers may occur without concomitant evidence of serositis, but this is unusual. The rise in temperature is sometimes preceded by chills and typically peaks by 12 to 24 hours; diaphoresis frequently accompanies defervescence.

More than 95 per cent of patients experience abdominal pain and signs of peritonitis during acute attacks. Pain often begins in one quadrant and then becomes diffuse, sometimes with distension, rigidity, rebound tenderness, and ileus with nausea and vomiting. Pain may radiate to the back or to the shoulders, and upright abdominal roentgenograms may show small air-fluid levels and edema of the bowel. Although these signs and symptoms are self-limited, they can be indistinguishable from those of an acute abdominal emergency, and patients may undergo one or more exploratory laparotomies before the true nature of their disease is recognized. Potential uncertainties about the clinical management of acute abdominal episodes have led to the recommendation that elective appendectomy be carried out during a symptom-free period so that acute appendicitis will not confuse patients' subsequent care.

Pleuritic pain occurs during acute attacks in 75 per cent of patients. Symptoms of pleuritis may sometimes precede abdominal pain, and a few patients experience pleuritic attacks without abdominal symptoms. Chest pain is usually one sided and may be associated with diminished breath sounds, a friction rub, and transient pleural effusion.

Nonspecific, mild arthralgia is a common feature of febrile attacks, and acute, monoarticular or oligoarticular arthritis may occur. Although arthritis is unusual among patients in the United States, it is a frequently observed manifestation of FMF among Israeli patients. Arthritis usually affects large joints, the knee in particular, and effusions are common. While arthritic episodes are typically short lived, joint symptoms may also be protracted and follow a course that is distinct from the acute abdominal and/or pleuritic attacks. Roentgenographic findings are nonspecific.

As many as a third of patients experience transient, erysipelas-like skin lesions that appear typically on the lower leg, ankle, or dorsum of the foot. These lesions are well-circumscribed, painful, erythematous areas of swelling, 5 to 20 cm in diameter, that subside spontaneously within 24 to 48 hours.

Self-limited pericarditis, conjunctivitis, aseptic meningitis, and other forms of serositis have been reported as manifestations of this disease, but are very unusual. Migraine-like headaches and emotional lability have also been observed during acute attacks, but it is unclear whether there are primary or secondary manifestations.

The most serious complication of FMF is amyloidosis. The natural history of amyloidosis in this disease is one of relentless progression to renal failure and death, which may occur in adolescence or even earlier. While a high proportion of Turkish and Israeli patients develop amyloidosis, this complication has been very unusual among patients in the United States and in several well-studied Armenian kindreds. The genetic and/or environmental factors that explain these differences in the incidence of amyloidosis remain unclear. In Israel, 90 per cent of patients who develop amyloidosis (particularly common in Sephardic Jews) do so after first experiencing typical attacks of FMF (phenotype I); however, amyloidosis may also occur in asymptomatic siblings of FMF patients, or it may precede the onset of typical FMF attacks (phenotype II).

Laboratory findings in FMF are nonspecific. During acute attacks there is prominent leukocytosis (up to 30,000 per cu mm), and the erythrocyte sedimentation rate and acute phase reactants are increased. These values return to normal between attacks. With amyloidosis, laboratory abnormalities reflect the associated nephrotic syndrome and renal failure.

DIAGNOSIS. The diagnosis of FMF is based primarily upon clinical presentation and history, for there is as yet no clearly proven laboratory measurement or test that is specific for this disease. In individuals of appropriate ethnic background with typical recurrent, self-limited attacks, diagnosis should not be difficult; in such individuals, delay in recognizing the disease is usually because the diagnosis is not considered. Nonetheless, when a patient is first seen or when attacks are infrequent, a variety of other acute febrile conditions must be considered and excluded by appropriate diagnostic studies and follow-up, in particular appendicitis, pancreatitis, cholecystitis, and intestinal obstruction. Familial hyperlipidemia and porphyrias associated with abdominal symptoms must also be considered.

The diagnosis is usually most elusive when patients have a limited or atypical symptom complex. Isolated pleural attacks may closely mimic acute infections or pulmonary emboli. Arthritis, when it is a prominent manifestation, can at first be clinically indistinguishable from various infectious and noninfectious arthritides, and skin lesions on the lower legs may resemble cellulitis or superficial thrombophlebitis. Rare patients have febrile episodes without serositis, and these may require orderly evaluation to determine their origin. Recently it has been reported that infusion of metaraminol diluted in normal saline provokes acute signs and symptoms of FMF with a high degree of specificity for the disease. However, the appropriate role of such a test in establishing the diagnosis remains unclear. At present this procedure, which carries intrinsic risks from catecholamine effects and salt load, should be considered experimental and not for use in general practice.

Once FMF is diagnosed, a degree of diagnostic vigilance must be maintained, for patients are not immune to the more common acute illnesses that FMF mimics. Of note, these patients appear to be particularly prone to develop gallbladder disease.

TREATMENT. Colchicine treatment is effective in FMF. Several controlled clinical trials, together with extensive, uncontrolled clinical experience since the mid 1970's, have shown that prophylactic colchicine,* 0.6 mg orally two to three times a day, prevents or substantially reduces the acute attacks of FMF in 75 to 90 per cent of patients. Treatment failures are often associated with noncompliance and/or intolerance to the drug.

Some patients can abort attacks with intermittent courses of colchicine, beginning at the onset of attacks (0.6 mg orally every hour for 4 hours, then every 2 hours for 4 hours, then every 12 hours for 2 days). In general, patients who benefit from intermittent colchicine therapy are those who experience a recognizable, albeit vague, prodrome before developing fever and clear-cut acute symptoms. Colchicine does not alter fully developed attacks. Patients who experience gastrointestinal intolerance to colchicine may benefit from reduced doses. Although definite chronic complications from colchicine have not become apparent with its long-term use in FMF, it is still recommended that a trial of intermittent colchicine therapy be attempted, particularly in young patients, before long-term colchicine prophylaxis is used. Azoospermia and chromosomal nondisjunctions have been associated with use of this drug. This recommendation does not apply to individuals from ethnic groups and in geographic regions associated with a high risk of amyloidosis, for it is now evident that long-term colchicine therapy not only prevents the development of amyloidosis but may also arrest its progression in FMF.

Symptomatic and supportive treatment is indicated for patients who do not respond to colchicine. However, every effort should be made to avoid the use of narcotics. In the United States, addiction to narcotics has been the major long-term complication among FMF patients.

PROGNOSIS. The prognosis for normal longevity for patients in the United States with FMF is excellent, and since the recognition of colchicine's efficacy in this disease, most patients can be maintained almost entirely symptom-free. Except in very rare cases, this disease does not affect the physical growth and development of children. Long-term colchicine therapy has also clearly improved the prognosis of patients in the Middle East who are prone to develop amyloidosis, even those whose symptomatic attacks continue. However, among patients who are unable to tolerate colchicine or in whom amyloidosis has led to nephrotic syndrome or uremia, the likelihood of eventual death from renal failure remains great.

Sohar F, Gafni J, Pras M, et al.: Familial Mediterranean fever. A survey of 470 cases and review of the literature. Am J Med 43:227, 1967.

Schwabe AD, Peters RS: Familial Mediterranean fever in Armenians. Analysis of 100 cases. Medicine 53:453, 1974.

Meyerhoff J: Familial Mediterranean fever: Report of a large family, review of the literature, and discussion of the frequency of amyloidosis. Medicine 59:66, 1980. *These three articles provide extensive reviews of the clinical and pathologic manifestations of FMF. The last two discuss differences in the incidence of amyloidosis.*

Dinarello CA, Wolff SM, Goldfinger SE, et al.: Colchicine therapy for familial Mediterranean fever. A double-blind trial. N Engl J Med 291:934, 1974. *One of several controlled trials that clearly established the efficacy of prophylactic colchicine therapy in preventing FMF attacks.*

Wright DG, Wolff SM, Fauci AS, et al.: Efficacy of intermittent colchicine therapy in familial Mediterranean fever. Ann Intern Med 86:162, 1977. *A double-blind study that shows that intermittent courses of colchicine can successfully abort attacks in some patients with FMF.*

Zemer D, Pras M, Sohar E, et al.: Colchicine in the prevention and treatment of the amyloidosis of familial Mediterranean fever. N Engl J Med 314:1001, 1986. *A retrospective review of 1070 patients that provides convincing evidence that long-term colchicine therapy arrests the development of amyloidosis.*

210 THE AMYLOID DISEASES

Joel N. Buxbaum

DEFINITION. The amyloid diseases comprise a group of conditions of diverse causes characterized by the accumulation of ultrastructurally fibrillar material in various tissues such that vital organ function is compromised. The associated disease states may be inflammatory, hereditary, or neoplastic, and the deposition can be local or systemic. The clinical outcome may be benign or as malignant as the most aggressive of neoplasms. In many senses, amyloid deposition is a symptom of an underlying disorder, much as anemia is a symptom of a variety of pathologic states. The symptoms of the amyloidoses depend upon the amount and localization of deposition of amyloid.

In tissue sections with conventional staining techniques, all amyloid appears homogeneous and eosinophilic. All types bind Congo red and under polarized light emit an apple-green fluorescence when stained with this dye. Viewed with the electron microscope, all amyloid contains two discrete structures, a major fibrillar component with a characteristic periodicity and a minor rodlike component that, viewed on end, has the appearance of pentamer with a hollow core (the P-component). The P-component appears to be physically and chemically identical in all amyloids and normally circulates as a soluble serum protein. Its role in the process of tissue infiltration has not been established.

The deposited fibril, regardless of its chemical nature, when isolated and analyzed has the x-ray diffraction pattern characteristic of a beta-pleated sheet. It is insoluble at physiologic salt concentrations, but can be released from tissue deposits by extraction with distilled water. The latter observation, made in the early 1970's, allowed the chemical analysis of fibrils obtained from many preparations of amyloid from tissues of individuals with different diseases. These studies have, in turn, permitted a more precise, chemically based, classification of the various amyloid syndromes (Table 210–1).

The ability to analyze the deposited proteins has also allowed the identification of circulating precursors of the insoluble fibrils and given general insight into processes that may be common to all types of amyloid deposition. It appears that all amyloid fibrils have a soluble precursor. In those individuals with pathologic deposition, either the amount of precursor is increased or the precursor is processed in such a way as to render it insoluble under physiologic conditions. It is not clear when or how processing takes place vis-à-vis

---

*This use of colchicine is not listed in the manufacturer's directive.

TABLE 210–1. CHEMICAL CLASSIFICATION OF THE AMYLOIDOSES

Clinical Syndrome	Fibril Precursor	Fibril	Common	Chemical
Primary or Myeloma, with Amyloid	Ig L chain	L chain or fragment	AL	Aλ (1-n) or Aκ (1-n)
Secondary*	SAA	AA	AA	$AA_{prototype}$ $AA_{(trp) var}$
Hemodialysis-Associated	β2m	β2m monomer or dimer	β2m	$A_{β2m}$
Senile				
Cardiac	TBPA or TT	TBPA or TT	AS_{cl}	A_{TBPA} (var) or A_{TT} (var)
Brain (Alzheimer's)	Unknown	β-protein	$AS_{β}$	$A_{β-protein}$
Pancreas	? Proin	? Proin	AS_{P}	—
Familial				
Neuropathic	TBPA (TT)	TBPA (TT)	AF†	A_{TBPA} (var)
Cardiomyopathic	TBPA (TT)	TBPA (TT)	AF_{Da}	A_{TBPA} (var)
Nephropathic	SAA	AA	AF†	AA
Vascular HCHWA (Iceland)	Cystatin‡ (gamma-trace)	Cystatin	AF_{HCHWA}	Cystatin (var)
Localized				
Endocrine			AE	
Medullary carcinoma, thyroid	(?) Procal	(?) Procal	AE_{t}	A_{procal}
Islet cell tumor	(?) Proins	(?) Proins	AE_{P}	A_{proins}
Skin	?	?	AD	?
Papular	?	?	AD_{P}	?
Macular	?	?	AD_{m}	?
Nodular	?	?	AD_{n}	?

*Inflammation associated.

†Familial amyloids have been designated by the geographic locale in which they have been found. The fibrils are identified by the notation AF with the country of origin indicated by a subscript, e.g., AF_P for the Portuguese.

‡Cystatin is a lysosomal proteinase inhibitor formerly known as gamma-trace.

β2m = beta-2-microglobulin; AF = amyloid fibril; Procal = procalcitonin; Proins = proinsulin; SAA = serum AA; TBPA = thyroxine-binding prealbumin; TT = transthyretin.

deposition. In some instances, it appears that structurally normal proteins, e.g., some intact Ig light chains, may be amyloidogenic even without extensive processing, and it is excessive production that leads to tissue deposition. In other conditions, synthesis of normal amounts of a structurally aberrant molecule leads to deposition with or without cleavage. It is also not certain what controls the site and rate of deposition. While some molecules undergo the entire process of synthesis, processing, and deposition in a confined locale, other equally amyloidogenic substances are deposited far from the site of synthesis.

Over the years, numerous attempts have been made to classify the amyloidoses. Histologic distribution, specific organ involvement, and the presence or absence of other overt disease have served as distinguishing parameters. Each of these classifications had some merit, but none of them was without overlap or inconsistencies. The currently utilized chemically based scheme is the result of the analysis of the structure of proteins making up the deposited fibrils (Table 210–1). What has become obvious is that the same protein may constitute the fibril in diseases of apparently different causes.

PATHOGENESIS. *AA Amyloidosis.* AA amyloid is most frequently found when deposition takes place in the course of chronic inflammatory disease. In the past, chronic infectious processes, such as tuberculosis and osteomyelitis, were the usual precipitating diseases. In recent years, the most commonly associated conditions have been the chronic noninfectious inflammatory diseases. Rheumatoid arthritis has a reported prevalence of up to 20 per cent in autopsy series with somewhat lower prevalence clinically (5 to 7 per cent). The prevalence in juvenile rheumatoid disease varies considerably in different countries (e.g., 0.14 per cent in the United States to 10 per cent in Poland). Other inflammatory joint diseases including the seronegative spondyloarthropathies, gout, and psoriasis as well as inflammatory bowel disease, even without arthritis, have been associated with amyloid deposition. Also at high risk for the development of AA disease are those individuals who inject foreign substances intracutaneously or subcutaneously. The chronic or recurrent skin inflammation found in these patients seems to be particularly effective in the induction of amyloidosis.

Renal deposition of the AA protein has been the ultimately fatal event in the course of some groups of patients with

familial Mediterranean fever (FMF) (Ch. 209). In the past, approximately 90 per cent of North African patients with this disease succumbed to renal failure by the age of 40.

AA deposition is also seen with a variety of nonlymphoid tumors and some nonimmunoglobulin producing lymphomas. Renal and gastric carcinomas and Hodgkin's disease have been the tumors most frequently associated with AA amyloid.

Kidneys, liver, and spleen are the most important sites of AA deposition. The renal disease is characterized initially by proteinuria of the glomerular type. Early in the disease, the kidneys may be enlarged but with time they shrink and the ultimate course is one of progressive renal failure. A variety of tubular disorders have also been described, including renal tubular acidosis, because of impaired bicarbonate reabsorption, nephrogenic diabetes insipidus, glycosuria, and hyperkalemia caused by decreased potassium exchange. The liver disease is relatively nonspecific, usually resulting in only moderate hepatomegaly and liver function test abnormalities.

In the past, when chronic infections were the most frequent stimuli to amyloid deposition, a small number of cases were reported in which eradication of the infection resulted in arrest of progression or actual regression of the amyloidosis as documented by biopsy. In general, even without treatment the course of AA disease is more chronic than that of AL amyloid.

The deposited AA protein appears to be a discrete proteolytic product of the serum AA protein (SAA) that has a monomer molecular weight of 12,500, but circulates as a molecule of 220,000 to 235,000 molecular weight complexed to high-density lipoprotein. It has also been found complexed to albumin. It behaves as an acute phase protein, rising rapidly in the course of inflammation (infectious or noninfectious) and peaking and falling to normal levels with resolution of the inflammation. SAA levels are generally higher in the elderly, and high levels have also been noted in patients with myeloma. Its synthesis is stimulated by the monokine interleukin 1. It appears that the predisposition to develop AA deposition resides in the production of an amyloidogenic isotypical form of SAA, the inability to degrade SAA completely, or both occurring in the same individual.

AL Amyloidosis. AL (or light chain-related) deposition is the most common form of amyloidosis seen in current clinical practice. The proportion of the total number of cases that represents multiple myeloma or primary amyloid is difficult to judge, since marrow plasmacytosis may be significant in both and the diagnostic distinctions between the primary disease and myeloma blurred (Ch. 163). Functionally, both diseases are malignant. In the case of myeloma, the outcome is related primarily to the proliferative capacity of the neoplastic clone. When AL deposition is present, it contributes to the poor prognosis. In primary amyloid disease the growth of a dominant plasma cell clone appears to be limited, but the amyloidogenicity of its homogeneous product results in the ultimately fatal compromise of organ function, most commonly renal or cardiac.

AL deposition is more likely to occur in tongue, heart, lymph nodes, spleen, carpal ligaments, joints, peripheral nerves, and skin than in the AA type. Hence, cardiac failure, arrhythmias, carpal tunnel syndrome, peripheral neuropathy, and ecchymoses are more frequent in AL disease. A deficiency of clotting factor X has been reported with an attendant bleeding diathesis. There is evidence to suggest that some AL proteins may have affinity for the clotting factor with resultant lowering of the plasma levels. Removal of an amyloid-laden spleen has reversed the deficiency in some patients. Blood vessels tend to be fragile in AL patients, since the amyloid is deposited in vessel walls. When vessel walls become rigid, not only are they sensitive to trauma but they do not respond well in the reflex-mediated changes in body position. When this occurs, orthostatic hypotension may become a major clinical problem. Coronary artery amyloid deposition can result in clinical angina pectoris or myocardial infarction.

A large number of studies have now documented that the deposited fibrillar protein is related to the excess monoclonal light chain produced by the expanded plasma cell clone and found in the patient's serum, urine, or both. The actual tissue protein may represent the whole light chain or a fragment thereof, usually containing at least the variable region. Amino acid sequence analyses of tissue AL protein and the isolated light chain obtained from the same patient have demonstrated chemical identity.

Despite several detailed analyses, it is still not clear what makes a given light chain amyloidogenic. Of light chain types associated with either primary amyloid or myeloma-associated amyloid, it appears that lambda chains are more frequent than kappa, and that the $V\lambda_{VI}$ light chain subgroup is overly represented. It has been suggested that tissue affinity could be charge related or that the interaction between light chain and tissues could represent an autoantibody antigen interaction. Neither of these hypotheses has conclusive experimental support. Further, it has not been established whether amyloidogenesis involves only the processing of intact light chains to fragments or if some of the molecules are synthetic fragments that are predisposed to deposition. It is possible that both phenomena occur.

Most AL patients, even those with primary amyloid, have a detectable M-component, usually free light chains of a single class, found in the serum or urine. However, 5 to 15 per cent have not had such proteins detectable. Analyses of a small number of these patients indicate that in tissue culture their bone marrow cells synthesize an excess of free monoclonal light chains. Because of their low concentration in the serum and their presumed high affinity for tissues they cannot be detected by conventional immunochemical techniques. In no instance yet reported has an immunoglobulin heavy chain been found to make up the fibril isolated from human amyloid tissue.

Recently a number of patients have been reported in whom organ compromise has taken place because of infiltration with monoclonal light chains without discrete fibril formation. Some of these patients have had clinical multiple myeloma; others have not. It is likely that this condition is analogous to AL amyloid, but that the deposited proteins do not have the intrinsic properties necessary to form beta-pleated sheets of sufficient size and stability to make fibrils. While these proteins have been identified in tissue deposits by immunofluorescence, chemical studies of the circulating and tissue forms have not yet been carried out; therefore, formal proof of their identity is lacking.

Senile Amyloidosis. The term *senile amyloid* has been used to describe Congo red–binding material found at autopsy in the tissues of elderly individuals. The material is most commonly found in the heart but has also been noted in the pancreas and brain. It is likely that it represents a variety of tissue-specific proteins.

The cerebral plaques identified in Alzheimer's disease are congophilic. It is not yet clear whether these are primary or secondary in the pathogenesis of the condition. Nonetheless, material isolated from the plaques and from amyloid-containing cerebral vessels of these patients, using techniques that allowed the characterization of other amyloids, has been found to consist of a polypeptide containing 28 amino acids that has no homology to any other sequenced protein. The material does not share antigenic determinants with the paired helical filaments that are also characteristic of Alzheimer's disease; hence the role of the sequenced "beta-protein" in the pathogenesis of the diseases is presently uncertain.

Amyloid material has also been noted in the brain lesions of Jakob-Creutzfeldt patients (Ch. 488.2) and animals suffering from scrapie. Immunohistochemical and nucleotide sequence analyses have indicated that the Alzheimer and Jakob-Creutzfeldt proteins are separate entities.

While many individuals in their eighth and ninth decades have scattered atrial deposits, clinically significant cardiac disease, characterized by either congestive heart failure or arrhythmia, appears to occur rarely. Once it does, the prognosis is poor. The presence of a chronic inflammatory disease (e.g., rheumatoid arthritis) or multiple myeloma does not increase the incidence of senile cardiac amyloid (SCA) deposition; this suggests an independent pathogenesis for all three diseases.

Recent studies have indicated that the fibril of SCA isolated from ventricular myocardium has an amino acid sequence homologous with serum thyroxine-binding prealbumin (transthyretin). Since prealbumin is not known to be synthesized by myocardial cells, SCA suggests that the precursor is produced at a remote site and localizes in its target organ by some unknown mechanism. Clinical studies have suggested that pulmonary involvement may also be associated with cardiac deposition, implying that deposition of the SCA protein may be more systemic than previously appreciated.

AL, AA, and SCA make up the bulk of the amyloid diseases encountered in clinical practice; however, there are additional, less common forms, the analysis of which has yielded insight into the genesis of these deposits. Localized forms have been noted in medullary carcinoma of the thyroid, in which the fibrillar protein is related to procalcitonin, and in insulinomas, in which the material appears to be antigenically related to insulin.

Congo red–binding structures are also seen in the pancreas of elderly patients with type II diabetes mellitus. Immunochemical analysis suggests that these may also be related to insulin.

Hemodialysis-Associated Amyloidosis. During the last decade a syndrome has been recognized in patients who have been maintained with long-term hemodialysis. It is characterized by carpal tunnel syndrome, i.e., compression of the median nerve by a thickened carpal ligament, and arthropathy, frequently severe enough to require joint replacement. Examination of the surgically removed ligaments and synovial and rectal biopsies from affected individuals have revealed amyloid. Chemical analysis of the fibrils shows that they consist of monomers and dimers of beta-2–microglobulin, the light chain of cell surface major histocompatibility antigens A, B, and C.

TABLE 210–2. FAMILIAL AMYLOID SYNDROMES*

Syndrome	Onset	Clinical	Fibril
Neuropathic			
Portuguese-Japanese (I)†	20–40	Lower limbs, autonomic	TPBA‡; Val 30→Met
Swiss-Indiana (II)	>40	Upper extremities, vitreous opacities	TBPA; Ile 84→Ser
Swedish	30–50	Upper and lower extremities, pupillary abnormalities, renal disease, autonomic and CNS dysfunction	TBPA; Val 30→Met
Iowa (III)	20–40	Upper and lower extremities, pupillary abnormalities, renal disease	Not known
Israel	20's	Upper and lower extremities, autonomic dysfunction, vitreous opacities	TBPA; Phe 33→Ile (?) Thr 49→Gly
Finland	40's	Facial, renal disease, lattice corneal dystrophy	Not known
Appalachian	40–60	Peripheral neuropathy, autonomic, cardiac	TBPA; Thr 60→Ala
Non-neuropathic			
Familial Mediterranean fever	10–30	Inflammatory serositis, nephropathy	AA
Derbyshire	10–30	Deafness, urticaria, fever, renal disease	Not known
Polish	40–60	Splenomegaly, hypertension, renal disease	Not known
Irish-American	40–60	Lung, renal	Not known
Iceland	20–40	Cerebral hemorrhage	Cystatin (var)
Denmark	30–70	Cardiac failure	TBPA (var)

*All appear to be autosomal dominants except for FMF, which is autosomal recessive.
†Roman numerals represent old clinical classification that applied when these were all called familial amyloidotic polyneuropathy.
‡Thyroxine-binding prealbumin or transthyretin (see Table 210–1).

Familial Amyloidosis. A series of genetically transmitted amyloid deposition diseases with characteristic clinical syndromes has been described; they are summarized in Table 210–2. The majority are primarily neuropathic with autosomal dominant inheritance. Other hereditary forms of primary nephropathic, cardiopathic, or cutaneous nature have also been described. The best studied of the renal forms, Familial Mediterranean Fever, is discussed in Ch. 209.

CLINICAL MANIFESTATIONS. Regardless of the type of protein, the clinical manifestations of amyloid deposition in a given organ are similar. The renal disease is primarily manifested by proteinuria, reflecting the glomerular localization of the deposition. Renal tubular defects have also been reported. Azotemia and renal failure usually occur late. The latter may be associated with vascular involvement. There is a 5 to 15 per cent incidence of renal vein thrombosis, particularly in patients with AA disease and the nephrotic syndrome. Amyloid renal disease may be associated with hypertension. The kidneys may be small, normal sized, or enlarged. Contraction of the kidneys usually occurs late in the disease.

The most characteristic cardiac presentation is that of a restrictive cardiomyopathy with congestive heart failure. Supraventricular arrhythmias are common, as are varying degrees of A-V block. Echocardiographic studies usually show a thickened ventricular wall without a dilated ventricle and may reveal a characteristic sparkling of the myocardial echoes. Patients with myocardial amyloidosis tend to be sensitive to digitalis glycosides, and these drugs are generally not used. Pulmonary involvement tends to mirror cardiac involvement both in frequency and extent, but rarely it becomes a dominant clinical syndrome with impairment of both the mechanics of respiration and gas exchange. Localized upper and lower airway amyloid infiltration can present major mechanical problems requiring surgical intervention.

Gastrointestinal involvement is most frequently manifested by bleeding, although diarrhea and malabsorption due to either submucosal infiltration or autonomic neuropathy have been reported.

DIAGNOSIS. The diagnosis of amyloidosis is made by the demonstration of the characteristic tissue deposits. Over the years the choice of appropriate tissue for biopsy has become wider. In patients in whom the diagnosis is suspected on clinical grounds, recent data suggested that subcutaneous fat aspiration will yield Congo red-positive material in 90 to 95 per cent of cases of AL disease and two thirds of cases of AA deposition. Rectal biopsy in similar patients yields positive

results in 75 to 85 per cent, if adequate mucosal and submucosal tissue is obtained. Gingival tissue will be positive in approximately one half of cases. Bone marrow biopsies have been positive in 40 to 50 per cent of patients with AL disease. These sites can be sampled with little chance of serious complications.

When there is evidence of involvement of a particular organ, diagnostic yields improve considerably. Operative specimens from carpal tunnel releases performed on patients with AL or hereditary neuropathic disease may show 95 per cent positivity. Renal biopsies in individuals with proteinuria have been reported to be positive in more than 90 per cent of patients. Liver biopsies also have a high yield; however, as with closed renal biopsies, significant, even fatal, bleeding has occurred. Hence these procedures are performed only after evaluation of bleeding tendencies and clotting factors. Liver biopsy is generally not carried out if a coagulopathy is present

In recent years it has become possible to distinguish the chemical types of amyloid in biopsy material. In the past a diagnosis of the AL type of disease could be inferred by the presence in the serum and urine of monoclonal Igs or light chains. With the use of potassium permanganate to bleach Congo red staining it is now possible to distinguish AA from AL in about two thirds of cases, AA staining being permanganate sensitive and the AL type resistant. More recently, antisera to the different light chain classes, AA proteins, beta-2-microglobulin, and prealbumin have been utilized either in the immunofluorescent or immunoperoxidase staining of biopsy samples. Since each of the deposited proteins arises from a different precursor, presumably in response to a different stimulus, it is reasonable to assume that these distinctions will eventually have therapeutic implications.

TREATMENT AND PROGNOSIS. AL deposition associated with multiple myeloma has been treated in the course of treating the neoplastic process. While 50 to 60 per cent of patients with myeloma will respond to treatment with alkylating agents and prednisone with extension of survival, the disease has not yet been cured nor has the amyloid deposition been reversed.

A number of patients with AL disease but without overt myeloma have been reported to show prolonged survival after therapy with myeloma-like protocols. However, these are anecdotal results at best and a single attempt at a randomized trial of alkylating agent therapy did not provide convincing evidence of prolonged survival. Nonetheless, it appears that some patients may respond to these regimens. There have also been occasional reports of improvement in AL disease during administration of the organic solvent dimethyl sulfoxide,* usually with concurrent alkylating agent therapy.

The most successful therapy of amyloid has been the prophylactic use of colchicine* in patients with North African Familial Mediterranean Fever (see Ch. 209). As a result of this experience and the observation that colchicine will also prevent experimental casein-induced murine AA deposition, several groups have instituted large-scale trials of colchicine in both AA and AL disease. Apart from the experience with Familial Mediterranean Fever, to date no regimen has been uniformly successful in the treatment of any form of amyloid deposition once it has become established.

Browning MJ, Banks RA, Tribe CR, et al.: Ten years' experience of an amyloid clinic. Q J Med 54:213, 1985. *The experience of a large British referral clinic, worth comparing with the Mayo experience in the last two references below.*

Glenner GG: The β-fibrilloses. N Engl J Med 302:1283; 1333, 1980. *A comprehensive review of the amyloidogenic proteins and the pathology of the disease in the context of newer information concerning the chemical structure of the fibrils.*

Glenner G, Osserman EF, Benditt EP, et al. (eds.): Amyloidosis. New York, Plenum Press, 1986. *The proceedings of the Fourth International Symposium, summarizing current work and thinking of most of the workers in the field, with the first formal interchange between individuals working primarily in Alzheimer's disease and those whose main interests lie in amyloid per se.*

Husby G, Sletten K: Chemical and clinical classification of amyloidosis 1985. Scand J Immunol 23:253, 1986. *An integrated review of the pathogenesis and molecular biology of the amyloidoses.*

Kyle RA: Amyloidosis: Review of 236 cases. Medicine 54:271, 1975. *The Mayo Clinic experience from 1960 to 1972 is described retrospectively. This is a very good review of the clinical features of the major syndromes seen in a large referred population.*

Kyle RA, Greipp PR: Amyloidosis (AL), clinical and laboratory features in 229 cases. Mayo Clin Proc 58:665, 1983. *This more recent reference extends the Mayo Clinic experience with an excellent description of the relevant features of this type of amyloidosis (117 references).*

*This use is not listed in the manufacturer's directive.

211 HEREDITARY SYNDROMES INVOLVING MULTIPLE ORGAN SYSTEMS

Arno G. Motulsky

The emergence of clinical genetics as a specialty has led to the definition of a large number of previously undifferentiated birth defects and syndromes. In some of these diseases the origin is monogenic, and multiple organ involvement is caused by the action of the mutant gene in various tissues. In other cases, a detectable chromosomal error or a known teratogen (such as Dilantin) causes multiorgan birth defects. Most frequently, neither a specific genetic nor environmental cause can be identified. Clinical genetics has grown rapidly, and most physicians are unable to keep abreast of the many newly described syndromes. While most of these conditions become manifest in infancy or childhood, adolescent and adult patients with such conditions often initially come to internists and primary care physicians, who should be aware of the various diagnostic, genetic, and management problems. A vague diagnosis of "multiple birth defects" or "genetic syndrome" usually is not sufficient. Appropriate genetic counseling ideally must be based on a definite diagnosis, optimal care often requires knowledge of the specific diagnosis and natural history of a given syndrome. The reader is referred to various textbooks and compendia for orientation and diagnostic approaches. Because of phenotypic variability in most syndromes, diagnosis may be difficult and new syndromes continue to be described. In this chapter a few selected syndromes are discussed briefly.

Cohen MM Jr: The Child with Multiple Birth Defects. New York, Random Press, 1982. *An excellent analytical introduction of approaches to syndromes and multiple birth defects.*

de Grouchy J, Turlean J: Clinical Atlas of Human Chromosomes. 2nd ed. New York, John Wiley & Sons, 1984. *A good general reference volume for standard syndromes associated with cytogenetic abnormalities.*

Emery AEH, Rimoin DL: Principles and Practice of Medical Genetics. 2 vol. New York, Churchill Livingstone, 1983. *The standard reference text in clinical genetics with full descriptions of disease entities and their genetics.*

Gorlin RJ, Pindborg JJ, Cohen MM Jr (eds.): Syndromes of the Head and Neck. 2nd ed. New York, McGraw-Hill Book Company, 1976. *Helpful for reference and differential diagnosis.*

McKusick V: Mendelian Inheritance in Man. 7th ed. Baltimore, Johns Hopkins University Press, 1986. *Standard reference book listing definite and possible monogenic disease, traits, and syndromes with short descriptions and literature citations.*

Schinzel A: Catalogue of Unbalanced Chromosome Aberrations in Man. New York, W. de Gruyter, 1984. *The definitive detailed reference for unbalanced chromosomal aberrations.*

Smith D: Recognizable Patterns of Human Malformation. 3rd ed. Philadelphia, W. B. Saunders Company, 1982. *The "bible" for description of malformation syndromes. Many photographs and short accounts of many different types of defects. Practically useful.*

WERNER'S SYNDROME

Werner's syndrome is a rare disorder with some clinical features that resemble early aging. Onset of clinical findings is usually in the second or third decade. Affected patients are short because of absence of the adolescent growth spurt and have slender limbs. There is premature graying and then loss of hair. Atrophy and hyperkeratosis of the skin with ulcerations around the feet are often seen. A characteristic squeaky voice and atrophy of muscle, fat, and bone of the extremities are the rule. Soft tissue calcifications usually develop. Atherosclerosis is premature with coronary heart disease and medial calcification of peripheral vessels. Juvenile cataracts and osteoporosis are typical. Hypogonadism occurs in both sexes, and mild diabetes is common. Malignant tumors occur in about 10 per cent of cases, with an unusually high occurrence of meningiomas and sarcomas. Mean age of death is in the early 40's. The phenotype of Werner's syndrome has been considered as a "caricature" of senescence rather than as a model of the normal aging process. The condition is inherited as an autosomal recessive trait. Altered glycosaminoglycan turnover in various tissues with increased excretion of hyaluronic acid in the urine has been frequently noted and suggests a fundamental abnormality affecting connective tissue. However, hyaluronic aciduria is not specific for Werner's syndrome. Fibroblasts from skin biopsies of patients with Werner's syndrome are difficult to culture. They grow more slowly, assume a senescent morphology more rapidly, and demonstrate a markedly reduced lifespan in vitro. DNA repair is normal. Karyotype preparations show a normal number of chromosomes, but variable stable chromosomal rearrangements such as translocations involving several chromosomes (variegated translocation mosaicism) are seen in over 90 per cent of cells (fibroblasts or lymphocytes). Werner's syndrome therefore can be classified among the group of chromosomal instability syndromes. No single enzymatic defect has been discovered yet to explain the multiple clinical, biochemical, and cytogenetic manifestations. Werner's syndrome is sometimes termed adult progeria, but it is entirely unrelated to the pediatric syndrome of progeria (Hutchinson-Gilford), in which death occurs in early adolescence from cardiac or cerebrovascular disease.

Epstein CJ, Martin GM, Schultz AL, et al.: The Werner's syndrome. Medicine 45:177, 1966. *A detailed summary of clinical and laboratory characteristics of 125 cases of Werner's syndrome.*

Salk W: Werner's syndrome. A review of recent research with an analysis of connective tissue metabolism, growth control of cultured cells, and chromosomal aberrations. Hum Genet 62:1, 1982. *A review of the current status of Werner's disease.*

SYNDROMES ASSOCIATED WITH HYPOGONADISM AND VARIOUS CONGENITAL ANOMALIES

LAURENCE-MOON-BARDET-BIEDL SYNDROME AND RELATED DISORDERS. The Laurence-Moon-Bardet-Biedl syndrome clinically exhibits the pentad of retinal dystrophy (usually pigmentary retinopathy), truncal obesity, mild to severe mental retardation, polydactyly, and hypogonadism. When not all of the five cardinal findings are seen, the diagnosis may be difficult. Electroretinography is useful for early diagnosis of the retinal dystrophy. Loss of central vision is gradual, and total blindness usually occurs after the age of 30 years. Although primary and secondary hypogonadism have been reported, hypogonadism is less frequently found in females. Interstitial nephritis may lead to renal failure.

Some investigators (the "splitters") distinguish between the Bardet-Biedl and the Laurence-Moon syndrome by the presence of spastic paraplegia and the absence of polydactyly and obesity in the latter condition. However, others (the "lumpers") believe that these distinctions relate to variable expression of a single disorder.

Alstrom's syndrome appears distinct and is also associated with retinal dystrophy and obesity. Affected patients are usually blind in early childhood and develop moderately severe deafness before age 10. Diabetes mellitus and slowly progressive chronic nephropathy in young adults are seen. Mental retardation and digital anomalies are not encountered.

Carpenter's syndrome (acrocephalopolysyndactyly) is a syndrome characterized by acrocephaly, syndactyly, and a characteristic facial appearance associated with polydactyly of the feet, obesity, mental retardation, and hypogonadism. The various characteristic skeletal findings should cause few diagnostic difficulties.

All these conditions (the syndromes of Laurence-Moon-Bardet-Biedl, Alstrom, Carpenter) are inherited as autosomal recessive traits.

PRADER-WILLI SYNDROME. In this not uncommon condition, infants are born with severe hypotonia and feeding difficulties; boys exhibit a small penis and cryptorchidism, and hypoplastic labia are seen in girls. Thin, turned-down upper lips and almond-shaped and up-slanting palpebral fissures are often seen. Skin and hair color tends to be fair. The feeding difficulties of infancy give way to compulsive hyperphagia with development of severe central obesity in later childhood. The limbs are relatively thin, and the hands and feet are characteristically small (acromicria). Young adults may present with pickwickian syndrome manifesting as cardiopulmonary compromise and somnolence. Severe obesity is the major cause of morbidity and mortality in this disorder. Affected patients are short, and there is hypogonadotrophic hypogonadism with sterility. Scoliosis and strabismus are common. Mild to severe mental retardation with behavioral and personality problems are the rule. Mild diabetes mellitus is often seen. Retinal abnormalities and polydactyly do not

occur. In many cases a chromosome abnormality affecting band q11-12 of the long arm of chromosome 15 has been detected by high-resolution methods. The defect usually is a small deletion in the paternal chromosome 15, but more complex rearrangements affecting the relevant chromosomal segment have also been seen. Although the syndrome usually occurs as a sporadic event, rare familial cases have been reported. Parental chromosomes are usually normal. It is likely that an as yet undetectable chromosomal defect exists in those cases in which no visible chromosomal abnormality has been found. The relationship of the unique and specific chromosomal deletion to the pathogenesis of the syndrome remains unknown.

NOONAN'S PHENOTYPE. This phenotype is often diagnosed, but its boundaries are not sharply defined because of marked clinical variability. Its frequency has been estimated as 1 in 1000 to 1 in 2500. There are no chromosomal abnormalities, in contrast to the Turner syndrome (XO) that it somewhat resembles ("male" Turner syndrome). However, females can be affected as well. Previously suspected etiologic heterogeneity is contested by recent studies that suggest marked changes in the Noonan phenotype with age. Affected adolescents and adults are often but not always short and have a triangular micrognathic facial appearance with frequent hypertelorism, occasional ptosis, and posteriorly angulated low-set ears with a thick helix. A short webbed neck is common. The simultaneous presence of superior pectus carinatum and inferior pectus excavatum is helpful diagnostically. Pulmonary valve stenosis is seen frequently and can be accompanied by other types of congenital heart defects. Mild mental retardation is occasionally found. Lymphatic dysplasia causing lymphedema occurs sometimes.

Autosomal dominant inheritance can be frequently documented, but many cases are sporadic and presumably caused by new mutations. Careful examination of first-degree relatives often shows minor signs of the condition.

Allanson JE, Hall JG, Hughes HE, et al.: Noonan syndrome: The changing phenotype. Am J Med Genet 21:507, 1985. *Describes changes in Noonan phenotype from infancy to adulthood.*

Bray GA, Dahms WT, Swerdloff RS, et al.: The Prader-Willi syndrome. A study of 40 patients and a review of the literature. Medicine 62:59, 1983. *A comprehensive review of the syndrome.*

Cassidy SB: Prader-Willi syndrome. Curr Probl Pediatr 44:1, 1984. *An extensive review of the clinical, cytogenetic, behavioral, and management aspects, with many references.*

Goldstein J, Fialkow PJ: The Alstrom syndrome. Medicine 52:53, 1973. *Classic summary of the clinical, genetic, and pathophysiologic aspects of the syndrome.*

Klein D, Amman F: The syndrome of Laurence-Moon-Bardet-Biedl and allied disorders. J Neurol Sci 9:470, 1969. *Clinical description and differential diagnosis.*

Ledbetter DH, Mascarello JT, Riccardi VM, et al.: Chromosome 15 abnormalities and the Prader-Willi syndrome: A follow-up report of 40 cases. Am J Hum Genet 34:278, 1982. *Current status of the chromosomal defect affecting chromosome 15 q11-12.*

Mendez HMM, Opitz JM: Noonan syndrome: A review. Am J Med Genet 21:493, 1985. *Recent review of various manifestations with many references.*

PART XV
NUTRITIONAL DISEASES

212 NUTRIENT REQUIREMENTS

Robert M. Russell

Recommended Dietary Allowances

Recommended Dietary Allowances (RDA's) have been established for most essential nutrients by the Food and Nutrition Board of the National Academy of Sciences. A nutrient is defined as essential if its absence from the diet results in a deficiency disease. For some nutrients, essentiality is uncertain. The United States RDA's are but one set of many recommendations put out by various countries and organizations (e.g., World Health Organization, Food and Agriculture Organization). In the United States the RDA's are used as a standard upon which several food assistance programs are based. For example, the school lunch program must meet 33 per cent of the RDA's for 12-year-old children in its meal planning. It is necessary in meeting such standards, however, that planners choose foods that will be eaten and enjoyed. The RDA's (Table 212–1) do not represent nutrient requirements for individuals; they are designed as guidelines for the daily intake of nutrients sufficient to ensure that almost all members of the population are not at risk of developing nutrient deficits. Thus, the RDA's exceed the nutrient requirements for most healthy individuals. Recommendations for energy intakes are an exception in that they represent averages ± 1 SD for particular age and sex groups. There have been efforts to link the RDA values for specific nutrients to the prevention of certain chronic diseases, such as cancer. At the present time, knowledge of such linkages is rudimentary.

RDA's have been determined by balance studies, measurement of the amount of a nutrient needed to result in tissue saturation, examination of the food supplies of healthy populations, examination of minimal nutrient intakes required to prevent or correct either a naturally occurring deficit or an experimentally produced deficit, epidemiologic observations, and animal studies. Precise RDA's have not been established for some nutrients (e.g., vitamin K, selenium, etc.) because of limited experimental data. However, ranges of safe intakes of these nutrients have been determined by the National Academy of Sciences and are provided in Table 212–2. Continued consumption of trace minerals above the upper limit of the recommended ranges can lead to toxic effects, as in the case with most individual nutrients.

The RDA's should be met by a variety of foods for two major reasons. First, certain dietary components (e.g., carotene, fiber, and possibly others as yet undefined) that are not considered "required" may nevertheless have a beneficial effect on body functioning. For example, if an individual is limited to a diet containing only preformed vitamin A, he or she could be deprived of the alleged beneficial effects of carotene (a vitamin A precursor). Second, a monotonous diet over a prolonged period may not supply a beneficial ratio of individual nutrients (e.g., a diet of very high carbohydrate content may increase the body's need for thiamine). Although other nutrient interactions have been defined (vitamin B_{12} is necessary for the demethylation of 5-methyl tetrahydrofolate; zinc is needed for the oxidation of retinol to photochemically active retinaldehyde), many such interactions are not fully known at present.

Body growth, body size, pregnancy, and lactation alter the RDA's. Pregnancy increases nutrient needs for the expansion of blood volume and for the growth and development of the fetus, placenta, uterus, and breasts. Similarly, lactation increases nutrient needs in proportion to the quantity of milk produced. Pregnancy and lactation RDA adjustments are provided in Table 212–1. Other factors that result in an alteration of dietary needs include environmental temperature, fever, menstruation (an increased requirement for iron), disease, and medication. Disease and/or drugs may change nutrient requirements by altering nutrient absorption or bioavailability, storage capacity, or excretion or by changing a nutrient's metabolism. For example, kidney disease may result in a decreased ability to change 25-hydroxyvitamin D to its active 1, 25-dihydroxylated form (Ch. 245); drugs that stimulate microsomal cytochrome P450–mediated enzyme activities (e.g., alcohol) cause an increased hepatic metabolism of vitamin A. The physician should remember that the RDA's were not designed for sick or traumatized patients or for individuals with metabolic disorders such as hyperthyroidism. Despite all of these caveats, the RDA's do serve as useful guidelines for the practitioner to judge the adequacy of an individual's diet. Table 212–3 provides a guide to the possible effects of medication on nutrient requirements and the mechanisms by which these interactions occur.

Nutrient requirements and dietary recommendations for adults are defined in broad age classes in Table 212–1, namely 19 to 22 years, 23 to 50 years, and 51 years and older (76 years and older for energy). In the absence of adequate information, the present recommendations for the elderly are the same as for the young adult population with few exceptions. Calcium may be needed in greater amounts in postmenopausal women in order to achieve positive calcium balance. Moreover, aging is characterized by body composition changes, resulting in less metabolically active tissue or lean body mass. Old people eat fewer calories than young people, and accompanying this diminished calorie intake is a concomitant reduction in intake of almost all other nutrients. For nutrients whose requirements are fixed (rather than relative to calories), such across-the-board reductions may result in intakes that are insufficient to meet metabolic demands; for example, the amount of dietary protein needed for nitrogen equilibrium is not reduced with age. Age-related changes affect the absorption, metabolism, and excretion of many nutrients, so that age-specific standards for the elderly are needed. In addition, chronic disability, illness, and the increased use of medications in the elderly introduce other variables. Suffice it to say that the elderly person's diet should be of high quality in terms of nutrient density (i.e., quantity of nutrients/calorie).

TABLE 212–1. FOOD AND NUTRITION BOARD, NATIONAL ACADEMY OF SCIENCES—NATIONAL RESEARCH COUNCIL RECOMMENDED DAILY DIETARY ALLOWANCES,* Revised 1980

Designed for the maintenance of good nutrition of practically all healthy people in the U.S.A.

	Age (years)	Weight (kg)	Weight (lb)	Height (cm)	Height (in)	Protein (g)	Fat-Soluble Vitamins — Vitamin A (µg RE)†	Vitamin D (µg)‡	Vitamin E (mg α-TE)§	Water-Soluble Vitamins — Vitamin C (mg)	Thiamine (mg)	Riboflavin (mg)	Niacin (mg NE)¶	Vitamin B_6 (mg)	Folacin** (µg)	Vitamin B_{12} (µg)	Minerals — Calcium (mg)	Phosphorus (mg)	Magnesium (mg)	Iron (mg)	Zinc (mg)	Iodine (µg)
Infants	0.0–0.5	6	13	60	24	kg × 2.2	420	10	3	35	0.3	0.4	6	0.3	30	0.5††	360	240	50	10	3	40
	0.5–1.0	9	20	71	28	kg × 2.0	400	10	4	35	0.5	0.6	8	0.6	45	1.5	540	360	70	15	5	50
Children	1–3	13	29	90	35	23	400	10	5	45	0.7	0.8	9	0.9	100	2.0	800	800	150	15	10	70
	4–6	20	44	112	44	30	500	10	6	45	0.9	1.0	11	1.3	200	2.5	800	800	200	10	10	90
	7–10	28	62	132	52	34	700	10	7	45	1.2	1.4	16	1.6	300	3.0	800	800	250	10	10	120
Males	11–14	45	99	157	62	45	1000	10	8	50	1.4	1.6	18	1.8	400	3.0	1200	1200	350	18	15	150
	15–18	66	145	176	69	56	1000	10	10	60	1.4	1.7	18	2.0	400	3.0	1200	1200	400	18	15	150
	19–22	70	154	177	70	56	1000	7.5	10	60	1.5	1.7	19	2.2	400	3.0	800	800	350	10	15	150
	23–50	70	154	178	70	56	1000	5	10	60	1.4	1.6	18	2.2	400	3.0	800	800	350	10	15	150
	51+	70	154	178	70	56	1000	5	10	60	1.2	1.4	16	2.2	400	3.0	800	800	350	10	15	150
Females	11–14	46	101	157	62	46	800	10	8	50	1.1	1.3	15	1.8	400	3.0	1200	1200	300	18	15	150
	15–18	55	120	163	64	46	800	10	8	60	1.1	1.3	14	2.0	400	3.0	1200	1200	300	18	15	150
	19–22	55	120	163	64	44	800	7.5	8	60	1.1	1.3	14	2.0	400	3.0	800	800	300	18	15	150
	23–50	55	120	163	64	44	800	5	8	60	1.0	1.2	13	2.0	400	3.0	800	800	300	18	15	150
	51+	55	120	163	64	44	800	5	8	60	1.0	1.2	13	2.0	400	3.0	800	800	300	10	15	150
Pregnancy						+30	+200	+5	+2	+20	+0.4	+0.3	+2	+0.6	+400	+1.0	+400	+400	+150	‡‡	+5	+25
Lactation						+20	+400	+5	+3	+40	+0.5	+0.5	+5	+0.5	+100	+1.0	+400	+400	+150	‡‡	+10	+50

*The allowances are intended to provide for individual variations among most normal persons as they live in the United States under usual environmental stresses. Diets should be based on a variety of common foods in order to provide other nutrients for which human requirements have been less well defined.

†Retinol equivalents. 1 retinol equivalent = 1 µg retinol or 6 µg β-carotene.

‡As cholecalciferol. 10 µg cholecalciferol = 400 IU of vitamin D.

§α-tocopherol equivalents. 1 mg d-α-tocopherol = 1 α-TE.

¶1 NE (niacin equivalent) is equal to 1 mg of niacin or 60 mg of dietary tryptophan.

**The folacin allowances refer to dietary sources as determined by *Lactobacillus casei* assay after treatment with enzymes (conjugases) to make polyglutamyl forms of the vitamin available to the test organism.

††The recommended dietary allowance for vitamin B_{12} in infants is based on average concentration of the vitamin in human milk. The allowances after weaning are based on energy intake (as recommended by the American Academy of Pediatrics) and consideration of other factors, such as intestinal absorption.

‡‡The increased requirement during pregnancy cannot be met by the iron content of habitual American diets nor by the existing iron stores of many women; therefore the use of 30 to 60 mg of supplemental iron is recommended. Iron needs during lactation are not substantially different from those of nonpregnant women, but continued supplementation of the mother for two to three months after parturition is advisable in order to replenish stores depleted by pregnancy.

TABLE 212–2. ESTIMATED SAFE AND ADEQUATE DAILY DIETARY INTAKES OF SELECTED VITAMINS AND MINERALS*

| | Age (years) | Vitamins | | | Trace Elements† | | | | | | Electrolytes | | |
		Vitamin K (μg)	Biotin (μg)	Panthothenic Acid (mg)	Copper (mg)	Manganese (mg)	Fluoride (mg)	Chromium (mg)	Selenium (mg)	Molybdenum (mg)	Sodium (mg)	Potassium (mg)	Chloride (mg)
Infants	0–0.5	12	35	2	0.5–0.7	0.5–0.7	0.1–0.5	0.01–0.04	0.01–0.04	0.03–0.06	115–350	350–925	275–700
	0.5–1	10–20	50	3	0.7–1.0	0.7–1.0	0.2–1.0	0.02–0.06	0.02–0.06	0.04–0.08	250–750	425–1275	400–1200
Children	1–3	15–30	65	3	1.0–1.5	1.0–1.5	0.5–1.5	0.02–0.08	0.02–0.08	0.05–0.1	325–975	550–1650	500–1500
and	4–6	20–40	85	3–4	1.5–2.0	1.5–2.0	1.0–2.5	0.03–0.12	0.03–0.12	0.06–0.15	450–1350	775–2325	700–2100
Adolescents	7–10	30–60	120	4–5	2.0–2.5	2.0–3.0	1.5–2.5	0.05–0.2	0.05–0.2	0.10–0.3	600–1800	1000–3000	925–2775
	11+	50–100	100–200	4–7	2.0–3.0	2.5–5.0	1.5–2.5	0.05–0.2	0.05–0.2	0.15–0.5	900–2700	1525–4575	1400–4200
Adults	—	70–140	100–200	4–7	2.0–3.0	2.5–5.0	1.5–4.0	0.05–0.2	0.05–0.2	0.15–0.5	1100–3300	1875–5625	1700–5100

*Because there is less information on which to base allowances, these figures are not given in the main table of RDA and are provided here in the form of ranges of recommended intakes.

†Since the toxic levels for many trace elements may be only several times usual intakes, the upper levels for the trace elements given in this table should not be habitually exceeded.

From National Research Council: Recommended Dietary Allowances. 9th ed. Washington DC, National Academy of Sciences, 1980.

Since parenteral administration of some nutrients bypasses any problems due to limited absorption, nutrient requirements are generally less when delivered by the parenteral route than by the enteral route. However, the underlying cause (e.g., disease, catabolism) that necessitates parenteral delivery in a patient often dictates overall higher nutrient requirements (see Ch. 220).

WATER

Owing to a high ratio of surface area to volume, infants are more prone to dehydration than adults. The average adult needs a minimum of 700 to 1000 ml of water per day in order to survive, but 2000 ml per day (1 ml per Kcal intake) provides a safe and adequate basal maintenance amount. Approximately 100 ml per day of water is lost in feces, 500 to 1000 ml in evaporation and exhalation (insensible loss), and the remainder in urine. Diets providing a high renal solute load (e.g., diets high in protein, sodium, potassium, chloride) will result in higher urinary water losses. In a sick patient additional water must be supplied if body temperature is elevated (each 1° C elevation over normal results in an additional obligatory water loss of 200 ml per day), if diarrhea is present, or if polyuria is present (e.g., from uncontrolled diabetes mellitus or kidney disease). In such cases, measured losses may be added to the maintenance requirements. Elevated environmental temperature and exercise will increase insensible losses (for each 2°C rise in temperature above 32°C, 500 ml of extra water should be provided). Acute alterations in water balance can be estimated by rapid changes in body weight.

ENERGY

Energy needs vary with body size, growth phase, age, sex, and activity. Factors that increase energy requirements are cold exposure, pregnancy, lactation, infection, fever, hyperthyroidism, and trauma. Recommended energy allowances

for all ages are presented in Table 212–4. In pregnancy, energy allowances should be increased 150 Kcal per day for the first trimester and 300 Kcal per day for the remainder of pregnancy. Lactation increases energy requirements by 500 Kcal per day. The energy allowances for children are based on median heights of American children at different ages. The allowances for young adults are based on so-called desirable weights of American men and women engaged in moderate work (e.g., walking, shopping, playing golf, etc.). In addition to the age groups 19 to 22 and 23 to 50 years energy recommendations for older people are divided into 51 to 75 and 75+ years. The aging process normally results in a progressive decrease in energy needs, primarily as a result of a decrease in energy expenditure.

Protein and carbohydrate supply approximately 4 Kcal per gram, alcohol 7 Kcal per gram, and fat 9 Kcal per gram. Basal energy expenditure (BEE) is the amount of oxygen consumed under resting, fasting conditions extrapolated to 24 hours. A simple rule of thumb to estimate BEE is 25 Kcal per kilogram body weight. However, this formula is not useful in overweight people. Since adipose tissue is relatively inert from a metabolic point of view, the relationship between BEE and body weight becomes nonlinear in overweightness. A more accurate estimate of BEE for healthy individuals is the Harris Benedict equation:

Men: BEE = 66 + (13.7 weight in kg)
          + (5 × height in cm) − 6.8 (age in years)

Women: BEE = 655 + (9.6 × weight in kg)
            + (1.7 × height in cm) − 4.7 (age in years)

Depending on factors such as activity level, illness, etc., energy needs may be increased many times over the basal level. Ingestion and metabolism of food increase the caloric requirement by about 7 per cent of the BEE, provided that a mixed diet is being consumed. Activity increases energy

TABLE 212–3. EXAMPLES OF DRUG-NUTRIENT INTERACTIONS

Drug	Increased Requirement	Potential Mechanism	Deficiency Symptoms
Antacids (aluminum and magnesium hydroxides)	Phosphate	Formation of insoluble salts	Malaise, paresthesias, anorexia
Anticonvulsants (phenobarbital, phenytoin)	Vitamin D	Induction of hepatic microsomal enzymes resulting in inactive vitamin D metabolites	Rickets, osteomalacia
Oral contraceptives (norethindrone/mestranol)	Folic acid	Inhibition of polyglutamic folate absorption	Megaloblastic anemia
Antituberculous drugs (isoniazid, cycloserine)	Vitamin B_6	Excretion of pyridoxal hydrazone complex	Peripheral neuropathy
Anticoagulants (coumarin, warfarin)	Vitamin K	Inhibition of vitamin K recycling	Hypoprothombinemia
Diuretics (benzothiadiazides)	Potassium	Enhancement of renal excretion	Hypokalemia

TABLE 212–4. MEAN HEIGHTS AND WEIGHTS AND RECOMMENDED ENERGY INTAKE*

Category	Age (years)	Weight (kg)	Weight (lb)	Height (cm)	Height (in)	Energy Needs (Kcal)
Infants	0.0–0.5	6	13	60	24	kg × 115
	0.5–1.0	9	20	71	28	kg × 105
Children	1–3	13	29	90	35	1300 ± 400
	4–6	20	44	112	44	1700 ± 400
	7–10	28	62	132	52	2400 ± 400
Males	11–14	45	99	157	62	2700 ± 400
	15–18	66	145	176	69	2800 ± 400
	19–22	70	154	177	70	2900 ± 400
	23–50	70	154	178	70	2700 ± 400
	51–75	70	154	178	70	2400 ± 400
	76+	70	154	178	70	2050 ± 400
Females	11–14	46	101	157	62	2200 ± 400
	15–18	55	120	163	64	2100 ± 400
	19–22	55	120	163	64	2100 ± 400
	23–50	55	120	163	64	2000 ± 400
	51–75	55	120	163	64	1800 ± 400
	76+	55	120	163	64	1600 ± 400
Pregnancy						+300
Lactation						+500

*Adapted from National Research Council: Recommended Dietary Allowances. 9th ed. Washington DC, National Academy of Sciences, 1980.

requirements over a wide range (1.1 to 10.3 Kcal per kilogram per hour) depending on the intensity and type of work being done. The number of daily calories that should be provided in addition to the BEE are 400 to 800 Kcal for sedentary activity, 800 to 1200 Kcal for light activity (e.g., sewing, desk work), and 1200 to 1800 Kcal for moderate work (e.g., walking). The number of kilocalories to be added for heavy work (e.g., running, swimming) ranges from 1800 to 4500 Kcal per day. Although fasting and malnutrition reduce energy expenditure, the stress of illness increases caloric requirements. For each 1°C of fever, a 13 per cent increase in calories is required. In catabolic patients, 50 to 100 per cent of the BEE may be necessary to prevent further tissue breakdown.

PROTEIN

A constant supply of protein (i.e., amino acids) is needed to maintain body function and structure. On a protein-free diet, the average net loss of body protein by males is about 0.34 gram per kilogram of body weight. However, when allowance is made for incomplete utilization of dietary protein and for variability in needs, the allowance recommended for adults rises to 0.8 gram of protein per kilogram. Protein needs are dependent, in part, on energy intake. Increased energy intake results in protein conservation and decreased energy intake results in the diversion of protein to meet energy needs. Pregnancy and lactation increase the body's protein requirement.

There is a continuum of food protein quality depending on the digestibility of the protein and its amino acid composition. Nine essential amino acids must be provided in the diet, since the human body lacks the ability to synthesize them. These amino acids are lysine, leucine, isoleucine, valine, methionine, phenylalanine, tryptophan, threonine, and possibly histidine, especially for infants.

High-quality proteins have a high degree of bioavailability (i.e., they are easily digested and absorbed) and have a high biologic value (a measure of the efficiency of utilization of absorbed protein, which in turn is dependent on adequate amounts and proportions of essential amino acids). The highest quality proteins are found in eggs and milk. Seeds and nuts, rice, corn, and grain proteins are of lesser quality. It is recommended that 10 to 15 per cent of caloric intake be derived from protein. Amino acids supplied in excess of the body's requirement are not stored but are degraded to metabolic products (urea, uric acid), and the carbon skeleton is converted to carbohydrate and fat or oxidized for energy. It is important that a mixed diet be consumed so that adequate amounts of each essential amino acid are received. Some amino acids are complementary; for example, tyrosine may in part meet the body's requirement for phenylalanine, and cystine may in part meet the body's requirement for methionine. The ability of the body to utilize protein is impaired if one essential amino acid is missing, underscoring the need for mixed sources of dietary proteins.

In parenterally fed patients, zero nitrogen balance may be achieved with as little as 0.5 gram per kilogram per day of mixed amino acids (including all essential amino acids). However, patients with abnormal losses or increased demands (burns, trauma, wound repair) may require 1.2 to 1.6 grams per kilogram of amino acids per day.

In the clinical setting, the state of nitrogen balance can be crudely estimated by measuring the 24-hour urinary urea nitrogen excretion:

$$\text{Nitrogen balance} = \frac{\text{protein intake}}{6.25} - (\text{urinary urea nitrogen} + 4)$$

CARBOHYDRATE

Protein and fat alone can provide all the energy needs of the body; there is no fixed requirement for carbohydrate in the diet. However, carbohydrates help to make the diet palatable and comprise the main energy source for most people in the world. Carbohydrate supplies 65 per cent of the world's food energy (50 per cent in developed countries, 75 per cent in developing countries), and of this 10 to 50 per cent is from simple sugars. Further, a diet low in carbohydrate would be likely to result in ketosis. Carbohydrate may be divided into available (i.e., digestible and utilizable as sugars) and unavailable (i.e., dietary fiber). The primary sources of both available and unavailable carbohydrates are of vegetable origin. Dietary fiber reaches the large intestine intact but then may undergo fermentation by bacteria, with the subsequent absorption of breakdown products and some "rescue" of calories. Dietary fiber is made up of crude fiber (cellulose, lignin), mucilages, pectins, hemicellulose, and water-soluble gums. Each type of fiber has different characteristics with regard to water holding, cation exchange, and adsorptive properties (e.g., for bile acids and drugs). For example, mucilages have a high capacity for water holding, and pectins avidly adsorb bile acids. Increases in stool weight and faster intestinal transit result from increases in dietary fiber. Primarily because of epidemiologic disease patterns (e.g., for colon cancer and diverticulitis), an increase of dietary fiber has been suggested. At least 20 to 25 grams of dietary fiber per day are needed for a therapeutic effect in the irritable bowel syndrome. Gums and pectins have been shown to have a beneficial effect on diabetes by delaying the absorption of glucose. As with most dietary components, too much fiber may be harmful: large amounts of dietary fiber may contribute to trace metal deficiency in certain parts of the world by adsorbing divalent cations (e.g., zinc) and making them unavailable for gastrointestinal absorption.

FAT

Fat, a concentrated source of calories, serves as a carrier for fat-soluble vitamins. All body cells with the exception of the central nervous system and erythrocytes can directly utilize fatty acids as a source of energy. Polyunsaturated essential fatty acids (linoleic, linolenic) and their derivatives serve as precursors for eicosanoids, which include the leukotrienes, prostaglandins, and thromboxanes. They are also needed for membrane structure and integrity. Polyunsaturated fatty acids have been shown to promote carcinogenesis in experimental animals, however, and may reduce circulating HDL cholesterol and promote gallstone formation. Thus, an upper limit of 10 per cent of calories taken in as polyunsaturated fats is advised. Monounsaturated fatty acids appear to be preferable (but neutral) to saturated fatty acids for optimizing plasma lipoproteins. There is recent interest in the role of N-3 polyunsaturated fatty acids, derived from linolenic acid or from fish oils, in the prevention of ischemic heart disease. Eskimos with a high consumption of N-3 polyunsaturated fatty acids and a low consumption of N-6 (e.g., linoleic) polyunsaturated fatty acids are relatively free from cardiovascular disease. More investigation is needed on the interaction between N-6 and N-3 fatty acids in human tissue before sound dietary recommendations can be made. Linoleic acid is a prominent component of dietary fats, but deficiency has been recognized only among patients on prolonged parenteral feedings containing no fat. Two per cent of calories in the form of linoleic acid and 0.5 per cent as linolenic acid are recommended for the average daily diet.

VITAMINS AND MINERALS

Requirements for vitamins and minerals are discussed in Ch. 217 and 218.

NUTRITIONAL RECOMMENDATIONS

See Ch. 13 concerning the judicious diet.

The United States dietary goals, prepared and published in 1977, attempt to outline a prudent diet for the relatively affluent United States public in order to avoid diseases and disabilities that appear to have a relation to diet. Other sets of similar recommendations have been proposed by organizations such as the American Heart Association and the National Cancer Institute. These goals recommend a reduction in the percentage of calories ingested as fat by the United States public from 42 per cent to 30 per cent (<10 per cent saturated, 20 per cent mono- and polyunsaturated). At least 12 per cent of total calories should be ingested as protein. It further recommends that total calories ingested as carbohydrate be increased from 40 per cent to 58 per cent, with an increase in complex carbohydrates (e.g., starches, fiber) and naturally occurring sugars from 28 per cent to 48 per cent. Refined and processed sugar ingestion should be decreased to 10 per cent of the total caloric intake. With a view toward reducing coronary artery disease, the American Heart Association recommends, in addition, a restriction of dietary cholesterol to 300 mg per day and of sodium to 3 grams per day. As more knowledge becomes available, these guidelines may be altered in the future.

Energy and Protein Requirements, Report of a Joint FAO/WHO/UNU Expert Consultation. Geneva, WHO, 1985.

Goodhart RS, Shils ME (ed.): Modern Nutrition in Health and Disease. Philadelphia, Lea and Febiger, 1980.

National Research Council: Recommended Dietary Allowances. 9th ed. Washington DC, National Academy of Sciences, 1980.

Present Knowledge in Nutrition. 5th ed. Washington, DC, The Nutrition Foundation, Inc., 1984.

Roe DA: Drug Induced Nutritional Deficiencies. Westport, AVI Publishing Company, Inc., 1976.

Select Committee on Nutrition and Human Studies, United States Senate: Dietary Goals for the United States. US Government Printing Office, 1977.

All of the above are general references that give a broad overview of human nutrition and of recommended dietary allowances. As such they provide excellent background information as well as references concerning more specific topics.

213 NUTRITIONAL ASSESSMENT
Robert M. Russell

The recognition and treatment of malnutrition that accompanies illness plays an important role in optimizing patient care. New modes of delivering nutrients to sick patients by both the parenteral and enteral routes may result in improvements in morbidity and mortality and shorten the length of hospitalization for both medical and surgical patients.

Methods of nutritional assessment that have been used for some time to judge the severity of malnutrition among populations in lesser developed countries (e.g., anthropometric measures) are now being applied to hospitalized patients in North America and Western Europe. An unexpectedly high prevalence (up to 40 per cent) of protein energy malnutrition has been identified among Western patients. Some of the reasons for the lack of recognition of malnutrition in hospitalized patients include preoccupation with the treatment of the disease process, neglect of the overall nutritional status of the patient (e.g., failure to obtain regular weights or to observe a patient's dietary intake), lack of sensitivity of casual observation in the recognition of protein energy malnutrition, absence of a single indicator for diagnosis of malnutrition, and latent onset of clinical signs of malnutrition and relative lack of specificity of these signs. A single nutrient deficiency rarely occurs in a patient; rather, a complex and confusing array of deficiencies is most often present.

The diagnosis of malnutrition should be made on the basis of dietary information, anthropometric and laboratory measurements, and clinical examination. By using all of this information, a more accurate diagnosis of the malnourished can be achieved, and an effective plan of treatment can be instituted.

DIET

It is not expected that the physician will interpret dietary records of a patient in detail. However, a physician should be able to perform a dietary evaluation by assessing the intakes of major food groups (dairy, meat-poultry-fish, fruits-vegetables, grains) and the quality of selection within these groups. A mixed diet is a desirable goal, when advising patients on healthful diets. Moreover, the clinician should be aware of the key questions to ask patients, which provide clues about whether or not the patient's dietary intake requires adjustment (Table 213–1). A detailed medical and social history can alert the physician to an existing dietary problem or the likelihood of a dietary problem occurring in the future. For example, poverty, physical or mental disability, complaints of dysphagia, anorexia, nausea, abdominal pain while eating, ill-fitting dentures, and alcoholism may all be factors that prevent adequate dietary intake. Increased nutritional requirements can result from diarrhea, fever, open wounds or burns, malabsorption, diabetes, and hyperthyroidism. The physician should be able to counsel patients regarding general dietary guidelines and recognize cases for referral to a dietitian for more detailed counseling.

TABLE 213–1. KEY QUESTIONS TO ASK AS PART OF THE NUTRITIONAL ASSESSMENT OF THE ADULT

1. Is there recent weight gain or weight loss? How much?
2. Are there alterations in appetite, sense of smell, or taste?
3. Are there problems with chewing or swallowing? Does the patient have poor dentition or poorly fitting dentures?
4. Are there symptoms of gastrointestinal disorders: diarrhea, constipation, nausea, vomiting, early satiety?
5. Does the patient live alone? If not, who prepares meals? Does he/she know how to cook?
6. What type of cooking facilities and refrigeration are in the patient's home?
7. Does the patient purchase a variety of food? If not, is it due to financial difficulties?
8. How many meals are eaten per day? How many snacks? Are one or more meals eaten outside of the home? If so, where?
9. Is the patient physically or mentally handicapped? Does this prevent the individual from shopping, cooking, or feeding herself or himself?
10. Does the patient take any dietary supplements (e.g., vitamins)?
11. How much alcohol does the patient consume?
12. Does the patient use prescription or nonprescription drugs?
13. Are there any religious or ethnic beliefs or food intolerances that prevent adequate food intake?
14. Does the patient follow a dietary restriction? Is it prescribed or self-imposed?
15. Is the patient depressed?

The elderly are a group with an increased risk of malnutrition. The reasons for this include poverty, the inability to move around easily, the cumulative effects of chronic disease necessitating multiple medications, social isolation, and the lack of knowledge for adequate preparation of meals (particularly among elderly men). Problems often arise when interviewing the elderly person for dietary habits (e.g., by 24-hour dietary recall, food frequency questionnaires) if the individual is senile or has impaired short-term memory. Even a three- to seven-day dietary record, wherein the patient records everything eaten during that period, has proven difficult for the elderly patient to keep. A family member may therefore be of great assistance when obtaining dietary information. Finally, appropriate standards for judging the elderly person's diet are not currently available. The Recommended Dietary Allowances (see Table 212–1) were developed as population standards (not individual requirements) and are set to meet the needs of most healthy individuals. The standards for adults are based only on young adults. As a result, they may not be appropriate for meeting the needs of the elderly patient who has an array of chronic diseases or aging disorders, or both.

ANTHROPOMETRIC MEASUREMENTS

Sophisticated and specialized methods to assess body composition are available, e.g., underwater weighing for body density, CT scanning, neutron activation analysis, and K^{40} counting. However, none of these methods is available for widespread clinical use. Anthropometric reference values derived from measurements on normal populations provide inexpensive, quick, and convenient estimates of a patient's nutritional status in terms of protein and fat reserves. The most useful anthropometric measures include height, weight, triceps skinfold (actually fatfold) thickness, and midarm area. Accurate measurements require only three simple pieces of equipment: a beam or lever balance scale with a vertical measuring rod and a headpiece, a constant tension skinfold caliper, and a flexible measuring tape, preferably with an insertion.

WEIGHT FOR HEIGHT. Single reference weights for each inch of height have been derived from United States life insurance actuarial data on longevity and have been termed "ideal" or "optimal" by some investigators. However, these single weights should not be interpreted as "ideal," since they represent the midpoint of an acceptable range for a person of medium frame and were derived from the mortality experience of only those men and women between the ages of 20 to 59 years who could afford life insurance. These weights are neither age- nor race-specific and do not represent all cultural groups. Further, these reference weights cannot be applied to patients with peripheral edema or ascites. Despite the recognized flaws in using such single reference weights as standards, clinicians have found the 1983 Metropolitan Life Insurance Reference Weights for Height useful for judging a patient's nutritional status reflecting caloric sufficiency. These reference weights (corrected to the nude state) are provided in Table 213–2 and may be used for judging underweightness or overweightness for the population age group 20 to 55. For people over the age of 55 it is recommended to use age-specific weight-for-height median values (medium frame size) derived from the combined data sets of the Health and Nutrition Examination Surveys of 1971 to 1974 and 1976 to 1980 (Table 213–3). Body mass index (weight ÷ height squared) is another means of assessing relative body weight which has the advantage of minimizing height as a factor in estimating overweightness and underweightness. Body mass index thus partially compensates for the shrinkage in height which takes place during the adult life span (Ch. 216). In children, weight and height are often used as separate measures to indicate malnutrition and are expressed as per-centiles of a cross-section of American children. Weight and height tables for children can be found in most pediatric textbooks.

The amount of weight lost and the rate at which it was lost by a patient are also important for judging an individual's nutritional status. A weight loss of 1 kg represents approximately a 7000 calorie deficit. A history of unintentional weight loss of 10 per cent or greater (6 per cent in an overweight patient) over a six-month period can be indicative of malnutrition.

TRICEPS SKINFOLD THICKNESS. This measurement provides an estimate of the body's fat reserves. The measurement should be taken at a marked point on the right arm, halfway between the acromial process of the scapula and the olecranon process of the elbow. The patient's arm should be relaxed when the fatfold is grasped posteriorly between the thumb and forefinger of the examiner. The fold should be raised, allowing underlying muscle to fall back to the bone, and the calipers applied. The measurement is useless if arm edema or paralysis is present. Age- and sex-specific standards for triceps skinfold (TSF) thickness for all ages through 75

TABLE 213–2. REFERENCE WEIGHT/HEIGHT FIGURES DERIVED FROM ACTUARIAL (MORTALITY EXPERIENCE) DATA OF THE 1979 BUILD AND BLOOD PRESSURE STUDY FOR USE IN AGES 20 TO 55*

| Height | | Weight | | | |
| | | Male | | Female | |
in	cm	lb	kg	lb	kg
58	147.3	—	—	114	51.7
59	149.9	—	—	116.5	52.8
60	152.4	—	—	119	53.9
61	154.9	—	—	122	55.3
62	157.5	133	60.3	125	56.7
63	160.0	135	61.2	128	58.0
64	162.6	137.5	62.4	131	59.4
65	165.1	140	63.5	134	60.8
66	167.6	143	64.9	137	62.1
67	170.2	146	66.2	140	63.5
68	172.7	149	67.6	143	64.9
69	175.3	152	68.9	146	66.2
70	177.8	155	70.3	149	67.6
71	180.3	158.5	71.9	152	69.0
72	182.9	162	73.9	—	—
73	185.4	166	75.3	—	—
74	188.0	169.5	76.9	—	—
75	190.5	174	78.9	—	—

*Weights represent the midpoint of the middle frame for each height. These values correct the 1983 Metropolitan Tables to nude weights and heights.

TABLE 213–3. AVERAGE WEIGHT FOR HEIGHT FOR AGE 55 to 74 FROM COMBINED HANES I AND II DATA SETS

| Height | | Weight | | | |
| | | Male | | Female | |
in	cm	lb	kg	lb	kg
58	147	—	—	125.4	57
59	150	—	—	136.4	62
60	152	—	—	143.0	65
61	155	—	—	140.8	64
62	157	149.6	68	140.8	64
63	160	154.0	70	143.0	65
64	163	156.2	71	145.2	66
65	165	158.4	72	147.4	67
66	168	162.8	74	145.2	66
67	170	171.6	78	158.4	72
68	173	171.6	78	154.0	70
69	175	169.4	77	158.4	72
70	178	176.0	80	160.6	73
71	180	184.8	84	—	—
72	183	178.2	81	—	—
73	185	193.6	88	—	—
74	188	209.0	95	—	—

Adapted from Frisancho AB: Am J Clin Nutr 40:808, 1984.

TABLE 213–4. SUGGESTED CRITERIA TO JUDGE MALNUTRITION AND OBESITY IN THE UNITED STATES POPULATION

Weight/Height	Standard Male/Female	At Risk for Malnutrition (% of standard)	At Risk for Obesity (% of standard)
Age 20–55	Table 213–2	<80	>130
Age >55	Table 213–3	<80	>120
Triceps skinfold			
Age 25–54	12/23	<50	>170
Age 55–75	12/25	<50	>150
Mid-arm muscle area (cm²)			
Age 25–54	55/31	<70	NA
Age 55–75	52/35	<65	NA

The percentage below and above the given standards for assessing malnutrition and obesity correspond to less than the 15th percentile and greater than the 85th percentile, respectively, on the combined data sets of HANES I and II normative values.

years are summarized in Table 213–4. A wide range on either side of the standard is considered an acceptable TSF measure, since large variances are found for fatfold thicknesses in the normal population. A patient whose TSF thickness is less than 50 per cent of the HANES standard is considered to have depleted body fat stores, whereas the patient whose TSF thickness is more than 150 to 170 per cent of standard is considered obese.

MIDARM MUSCLE AREA. This derived value is used to estimate lean body or skeletal muscle mass. To calculate this value, the midarm circumference must first be measured at the same site as the triceps fatfold with the patient's right arm in a relaxed posture. The formula to calculate bone-free, upper-arm midarm muscle area is:

$$\frac{[\text{midarm circumference (cm)} - (0.314 \times \text{TSF mm})]^2}{4\pi} \begin{array}{l} - 10 \text{ (males)} \\ - 6.5 \text{ (females)} \end{array}$$

Median values are summarized in Table 213–4. Thirty to thirty-five per cent below this standard (depending upon age) is indicative of a depletion of lean body mass. Neither TSF nor midarm muscle area standards have been derived for the very elderly (i.e., older than 75 years). A summary of criteria to judge malnutrition and obesity by anthropometric measurements is presented in Table 213–4.

CLINICAL ASSESSMENT

By noting certain physical changes in the patient (e.g., temporal muscle wasting, hair depigmentation, edema, etc.), the clinician may have the clinical impression of protein calorie malnutrition, which objective anthropometric and laboratory measurements can confirm. However, early clinical symptoms and signs of malnutrition are rather vague and often include weakness, lethargy, irritability, and lightheadedness. Many of the symptoms and signs are nonspecific for a single nutrient deficit and may be caused by insufficiency of one of several nutrients. For example, flaking dermatitis may accompany deficiencies of protein, riboflavin, or linoleic acid. On the other hand, when certain clinical signs appear, the nutrient deficit may be very severe (e.g., scleromalacia, a leading and rapidly progressive cause of blindness due to vitamin A deficiency). Table 213–5 contains a listing of clinical presentations and the associated nutrient deficits that may cause them.

Functional and end organ testing has been advocated for diagnosis of specific nutrient deficits (e.g., dark adaptation for vitamin A, taste and smell for zinc, bone density for vitamin D, and so on). However, functional tests are not available to assess the status of most nutrients, and, as with clinical signs, the functional tests are often nonspecific. For example, impairment of dark adaptation may be caused by zinc deficiency as well as vitamin A deficiency. Taste and smell may be affected by age, smoking, and drugs as well as by zinc nutriture. Bone density is diminished in both osteoporosis and osteomalacia due to vitamin D deficiency.

TABLE 213–5. CLINICAL SIGNS AND SYMPTOMS OF NUTRITIONAL INADEQUACY IN ADULT PATIENTS

	Clinical Sign or Symptom	Nutrient
General	Wasted, skinny	Calorie
	Loss of appetite	Protein-energy
Skin	Psoriasiform rash, eczematous scaling	Zinc
	Pallor	Folate, iron, vitamin B$_{12}$, copper
	Follicular hyperkeratosis	Vitamin A
	Perifollicular petechiae	Vitamin C
	Flaking dermatitis	Protein-energy, niacin, riboflavin, zinc
	Bruising	Vitamin C, vitamin K
	Pigmentation changes	Niacin, protein-energy
	Scrotal dermatosis	Riboflavin
	Thickening and dryness of skin	Linoleic acid
Head	Temporal muscle wasting	Protein-energy
Hair	Sparse and thin, dyspigmentation	Protein
	Easy to pull out	
Eyes	History of night blindness (also impaired visual recovery after glare)	Vitamin A, zinc
	Photophobia, blurring, conjunctival inflammation	Riboflavin, vitamin A
	Corneal vascularization	Riboflavin
	Xerosis, Bitot spots, keratomalacia	Vitamin A
Mouth	Glossitis	Riboflavin, niacin, folic acid, vitamin B$_{12}$, pyridoxine
	Bleeding gums	Vitamin C, riboflavin
	Cheilosis	Riboflavin
	Angular stomatitis	Riboflavin, iron
	Hypogeusia	Zinc
	Tongue fissuring	Niacin
	Tongue atrophy	Riboflavin, niacin, iron
	Scarlet and raw tongue	Niacin
	Nasolabial seborrhea	Pyridoxine
Neck	Goiter	Iodine
	Parotid enlargement	Protein
Thorax	Thoracic rosary	Vitamin D
Abdomen	Diarrhea	Niacin, folate, vitamin B$_{12}$
	Distention	Protein-energy
	Hepatomegaly	Protein-energy
Extremities	Edema	Protein, thiamin
	Softening of bone	Vitamin D, calcium, phosphorus
	Bone tenderness	Vitamin D
	Bone ache, joint pain	Vitamin C
	Muscle wasting and weakness	Protein, calorie, vitamin D, selenium, sodium chloride
	Muscle tenderness, muscle pain	Thiamin
	Hyporeflexia	Thiamin
	Ataxia	Vitamin B$_{12}$
Nails	Spooning	Iron
	Transverse lines	Protein
Neurologic	Tetany	Calcium, magnesium
	Paresthesias	Thiamin, vitamin B$_{12}$
	Loss of reflexes, wrist drop, foot drop	Thiamin
	Loss of vibratory and position sense	Vitamin B$_{12}$
	Dementia, disorientation	Niacin
Blood	Anemia	Vitamin E, B$_{12}$, folate, iron, pyridoxine
	Hemolysis	Phosphorus

As with dietary assessment, the elderly present a particular problem when evaluated for the presence or absence of clinical signs or symptoms of malnutrition. Some of the changes associated with malnutrition may also be a function of normal aging (e.g., hypogeusia, dry skin, sparse hair, atrophy of the tongue, bleeding gums from ill-fitting dentures). Nevertheless, as with younger patients, clinical signs should be assessed for possible nutritional implications.

LABORATORY ASSESSMENT

Laboratory measurements are another tool that can aid the physician in making a diagnosis of malnutrition, although, once again, certain laboratory abnormalities that could reflect malnutrition can also have a non-nutritional cause (e.g., calcium, albumin, hematocrit, etc.). Modern analytical instruments (e.g., high-performance liquid chromatography), techniques (e.g., radio or enzyme immunoassays), and computerization have greatly increased the capability of nutritional biochemical testing. Currently available biochemical tests for assessing nutritional status include the direct measurement of a nutrient or nutrient metabolite in blood, other body fluid (e.g., urine, saliva), or tissues (e.g., white blood cells, hair, liver) and the measurement of a biochemical function that is nutrient specific. For example, laboratory tests for pyridoxine status may include the direct measurement of pyridoxal 5'-phosphate in plasma or the enzymatic activity of erythrocyte transaminase, for which pyridoxal 5'-phosphate is a cofactor. The latter test involves the calculation of an activity coefficient whereby red blood cell transaminase activity is determined before and after the addition of pyridoxal 5'-phosphate. An activity coefficient of greater than 1 is indicative of pyridoxine deficiency.

The establishment of normal nutrient values in body fluids or tissues for each sex varies from laboratory to laboratory, and the normal range usually represents a mean ± 2 SD of a normal population. Optimally, a low biochemical nutrient value in body fluids or tissue should be coupled with a specific functional abnormality before making the diagnosis of a nutrient deficiency. However, in practice this is rarely done. One guide for interpretation of laboratory values that reflects the status of various nutrients in the blood or serum of adults is presented in Table 213–6. For some nutrients (e.g., vitamin A) children have a different normal range than adults. The reader is referred to a pediatric or nutrition text for detailed information on age-specific normal values. Normal biochemical ranges have not been established for the very old (i.e., over 75 years). The physician must rely upon values derived from younger populations to judge the nutritional biochemical parameters for this group.

Many nutrient biochemical diagnostic tests are not readily available in a hospital clinical chemistry laboratory. Nevertheless, there are several laboratory tests that are routinely performed (e.g., hemoglobin level, serum protein level) that may aid the physician in assessing the nutritional status of his or her patients. In the absence of liver disease, a low serum albumin may be used as an indicator of protein nutriture. In sick patients who are obese, silent kwashiorkor (protein malnutrition) may develop, as reflected by low serum protein values, although the patient may continue to look overnourished and anthropometric measures may be normal or exceed the normal range. Other proteins that are synthesized in the liver and that have a more rapid turnover than albumin (e.g., transferrin, transthyretin) may also be used to diagnose protein malnutrition at an earlier stage, provided that the patient does not have liver damage. The transferrin in serum, if not directly measured, may be estimated from the total iron binding capacity (TIBC) according to the formula: $(0.8 \times TIBC) - 43$. Protein values that are more than 20 per cent below the lower limit of the normal range are generally regarded as severely substandard. It has been suggested that elderly people have a somewhat lower normal serum albumin value and that age-specific standards for serum protein values are needed.

Muscle protein can be estimated from urinary creatinine excretion; this complements the anthropometric indicator MAMA. The amount of creatinine appearing in the urine over 24 hours is proportional to muscle mass. A crude standard for creatinine excretion can be derived by multiplying an individual's reference weight-for-height by 23 or 18 (for males and females, respectively). Twenty per cent below these derived values may represent muscle protein depletion. However, several factors are known to affect creatinine excretion (e.g., kidney disease, diet, fever, strenuous exercise, menstrual cycle), and the interpretation, therefore, must be carried out cautiously.

In protein-energy malnutrition, the number of circulating lymphocytes diminishes, and the patient demonstrates impaired delayed hypersensitivity to common skin antigens (e.g., mumps, *Candida*, tuberculin). Thus, these tests also may be used in assessing the patient's nutritional status, although anergy may result from many non-nutritional factors as well (e.g., disease, drugs). A lymphocyte count of fewer than 1200 per cubic millimeter is regarded as severely substandard. The effect of advanced age on these parameters is uncertain.

The value of nutritional assessment parameters in predicting patient outcome is unproven. A prognostic nutritional index has been derived from various nutritional assessment indices (e.g., albumin, transferrin, triceps skinfold, delayed hypersensitivity) and applied to surgical patients to predict postoperative complications and mortality. In one study a higher prognostic nutritional index score correlated with greater postoperative problems, but further evaluation is necessary. Moreover, it is not known if this index has any value in predicting outcomes in medical patients.

TABLE 213–6. GUIDE FOR INTERPRETATION OF SERUM AND/OR BLOOD INDICES FOR SELECTED NUTRIENTS

Nutrient	Normal*	Deficient	Marginal
Albumin	3.5–5.5 grams/dl	2.8–3.2	3.2–3.5
Transferrin	200–400 mg/dl	< 200	
Transthyretin	10–40 mg/dl	< 10	
Ferritin	12–300 ng/ml	< 12	
Retinol	30–90 µg/dl	< 15	15–30
Carotene	40–240 µg/dl	< 40	
Vitamin E	0.5–1.8 mg/dl	< 0.5	0.5–0.7
Vitamin D (25-OH-D₃)	15–40 ng/ml		
Thiamin (erythrocyte)	0.9–1.25†	> 1.25	1.25–1.20
Riboflavin	0.9–1.39†	> 1.40	1.30–1.40
Pyridoxine	0.9–2.2†	> 2.2	
Niacin (urine 2-pyridone/N'-methyl nicotinamide—metabolite ratio)	1.0–4.0	< 1.0	
Serum folate	6–20 ng/ml	≤ 3.0	3–6
Red cell folate	150–450 ng/ml	< 150	
Vitamin B₁₂	> 200 pg/ml	< 150	150–200
Vitamin C	0.3–2.0 mg/dl	< 0.2	0.2–0.3
Calcium	8.5–10.5 mg/dl	< 8.5	
Phosphorus	2.5–4.5 mg/dl	< 2.5	
Iron	50–170 µg/dl		
Zinc	70–130 µg/dl	≤ 65	65–70
Copper	70–160 µg/dl	< 70	
Magnesium	1.4–2.5 mg/dl	≤ 1.4	

*These normal values will vary with the method used and in different laboratories.

†An enzymatic assay. Values represent an activity coefficient.

Frisancho AR: New norms of upper limb fat and muscle areas for assessment of nutritional status. Am J Clin Nutr 34:2540, 1981. *This article presents American standards for anthropometric measures for ages 1 to 75 years, derived from the HANES survey of 1971–1974.*

Frisancho AR: New standards of weight and body composition by frame size and height for assessment of nutritional status of adults and the elderly. Am J Clin Nutr 40:808, 1984. *This article presents American standards for weight and height from ages 1 to 75, derived from the combined data sets of HANES I (1971–1974) and II (1976–1980).*

214 PROTEIN-CALORIE UNDERNUTRITION

Robert B. Baron

Protein-calorie undernutrition occurs when inadequate protein and/or calories are ingested to meet an individual's nutritional requirements. For many parts of the developing world, protein-calorie undernutrition is the most important nutritional problem and one of the most significant health problems. Protein-calorie undernutrition is usually described as two distinct syndromes: (1) *Kwashiorkor* is the clinical syndrome that develops when protein intake is deficient despite adequate or nearly adequate energy intakes. (2) *Marasmus* is the clinical syndrome that results from inadequate intake of both protein and calories.

In industrialized nations, these distinct syndromes are rarely observed, yet protein-calorie undernutrition is quite common. Not a syndrome confined to postweaning children or victims of famine, protein-calorie undernutrition is most commonly a consequence of severe illness. Extreme poverty can also lead to undernutrition in industrialized societies, particularly among the elderly, young children, pregnant women, the homeless, substance abusers, and patients with chronic psychiatric illnesses.

In North America and Europe 28 to 80 per cent of hospitalized medical and surgical patients have been reported to have protein-calorie undernutrition. These studies probably used overly sensitive diagnostic criteria; the true prevalence in those populations is probably closer to 20 per cent. This chapter will emphasize the forms of protein-calorie undernutrition most commonly seen in industrialized nations.

Pathogenesis

In industrialized nations, protein-calorie undernutrition is caused by decreased intake of calories and protein, increased nutrient losses, or increased nutrient requirements (Table 214–1). It can develop slowly owing to chronic illness or chronic semistarvation or quite rapidly owing to acute illness.

In uncomplicated starvation and semistarvation, metabolism adapts to reduce the breakdown of lean body mass. Fat and fat-derived fuels gradually replace glucose as the major energy sources in order to preserve body protein. During the initial phase of a complete fast, glucose requirements for the brain, bone marrow, renal medulla, and peripheral nerves are provided by glycogen. Glycogen stores, however, last for only 12 to 24 hours. As glucose levels decline slightly, insulin levels also decline and glucagon levels increase. Amino acids, particularly alanine, are released by muscle. Hepatic gluco-

TABLE 214–1. CAUSES OF PROTEIN-CALORIE MALNUTRITION IN HOSPITALIZED PATIENTS

Decreased Oral Intake

Anorexia	Poverty
Nausea	Old age
Dysphagia	Social isolation
Pain	Substance abuse
Gastrointestinal obstruction	Depression
Poor dentition	

Increased Nutrient Losses

Malabsorption	Nephrosis
Diarrhea	Fistula drainage
Bleeding	Protein-losing enteropathy
Glycosuria	

Increased Nutrient Requirements

Fever	Trauma
Infection	Burns
Neoplasms	Medications
Surgery	

neogenesis from amino acids provides glucose for the central nervous system and other glycolytic tissues. The changes in insulin and glucagon also favor lipolysis. Mobilized fatty acids provide the fuel for the remaining tissues. By the second week of a complete fast, fatty acids are less completely oxidized and more of them form ketone bodies. Ketones become the primary energy source for the brain and reduce the need for glucose. The muscles catabolize less protein, release less alanine, thus conserving their protein content.

Adaptation also decreases the body's total energy requirement, by as much as 40 per cent in severe chronic undernutrition. Absolute requirements decrease as body weight diminishes owing to a decrease in body mass. More importantly, however, energy requirements also decrease per unit of body mass. Both ingested food and circulating endogenous substrates, are utilized more efficiently. More endogenous amino acids, for example, are utilized for protein synthesis than for oxidation. In addition, virtually all of the body's biochemical and physiologic processes are curtailed. Quantitatively, the most important of these processes is the sodium-potassium ATPase system. This pump is thought to account for approximately one third of the basal energy requirement, so that a change in its activity can have a major impact on total energy requirements. Less energy is also expended for protein turnover, temperature regulation, the inflammatory response, and the function of most body organs during chronic undernutrition.

During a severe acute illness, the body is unable to adapt in this manner, and undernutrition can develop quite rapidly. In this instance, circulating levels of catecholamines, glucocorticoids, and glucagon are elevated. While necessary to optimize the body's response to injury, these hormones stimulate release of amino acids and stimulate gluconeogenesis. In this manner the body's protein mass can be rapidly depleted. Similarly, energy requirements are typically increased and changes in body weight and body composition can occur quite rapidly.

Physiologic Consequences of Malnutrition

Virtually every organ and organ system of the body can undergo marked morphologic and functional changes during protein-calorie undernutrition.

The most obvious manifestation in chronic undernutrition is loss of body weight. Most patients can tolerate a loss of 5 to 10 per cent of body weight without significant consequences, but losses greater than 40 per cent below ideal weight are almost always fatal. Both adipose tissue and the lean body mass are depleted, but losses of adipose tissue are greater. Extracellular water remains nearly constant, resulting in its relative increase. In severe undernutrition, the body's organs also decrease in size. In experimental animals, for example, a seven-day fast results in a 40 per cent decrease in liver mass, 28 per cent decrease in the gastrointestinal tract, 20 per cent decrease in the kidneys, and 17 per cent decrease in cardiac mass. Changes in organ function parallel these changes in organ size.

BODY WEIGHT. During acute malnutrition caused by severe acute illness, changes in body weight and adipose stores may be less marked despite severe changes in organ morphology and function. Many patients may actually gain weight owing to retention of sodium and therefore of body water, despite the development of severe undernutrition. In this setting, cardiac mass is decreased but cardiac index and contractility may increase owing to a relative hyperdynamic state.

HEART. In the "Minnesota experiment," in which 32 male volunteers were semistarved for six months, a 24 per cent decrease in body weight was associated with an 18 per cent decrease in cardiac stroke volume and a 38 per cent decrease in cardiac index. Studies of starved dogs have demonstrated similar findings, as well as decreases in left ventricular contractility and compliance, decreased myocardial glycogen, myofibrillar atrophy, and interstitial edema.

LUNG. The lung parenchyma is minimally affected during malnutrition, but marked changes in pulmonary function can occur as a result of the loss of mass and strength of the muscles of respiration. In the "Minnesota experiment," vital capacity, tidal volume, and minute volume were decreased by 8 per cent, 19 per cent, and 30 per cent, respectively, after 24 weeks of semistarvation. The ventilatory response to hypoxia is also decreased during semistarvation. After 10 days of semistarvation, normal volunteers showed a 42 per cent decrease in the hypoxic ventilatory response.

GASTROINTESTINAL TRACT. During severe malnutrition, gastric motility is slowed and gastric acid secretion is decreased. The most significant effects of undernutrition on the luminal gastrointestinal tract are seen in the small intestine. Total small bowel mass is decreased, primarily owing to mucosal atrophy and loss of villi. Lymphocytic infiltration of surface epithelial cells can occur, and epithelial cell renewal is decreased. Both disaccharidase enzyme activity and the rate of absorption of amino acids are decreased. Although pancreatic endocrine activity is spared, exocrine insufficiency can also be seen in severe undernutrition.

LIVER. In typical protein-calorie undernutrition, liver mass decreases but the liver histology remains normal. Fat, protein, and glycogen are depleted, but the number of hepatocytes is preserved. In contrast, patients with kwashiorkor have enlarged livers with fatty infiltration and excess glycogen. In both instances, serum levels of albumin and other serum transport proteins are commonly decreased owing to diminished hepatic synthesis.

KIDNEY. Renal mass is also decreased during undernutrition, but renal histology remains normal. Renal function is well preserved except for an impaired concentrating ability due to a lowering of the medullary osmotic gradient.

ENDOCRINE. The endocrine response to undernutrition is complex and greatly affected by concurrent illnesses. In uncomplicated protein-calorie undernutrition, hypothalamic-pituitary function is also altered. Growth hormone levels are most often increased, although somatomedins may be low. Serum thyroxine is typically at the lower limits of normal or slightly decreased. Peripheral conversion of thyroxine (T_4) to triiodothyronine (T_3) is commonly decreased, favoring the conversion to reverse triiodothyronine (Ch. 229). Serum TSH and the TSH response to TRH, however, are unaltered. Gonadal hormones are also affected. In men, testosterone levels are decreased and LH and FSH levels are appropriately increased. In women, however, gonadotropin release is depressed despite low levels of circulating estrogens.

IMMUNE SYSTEM AND DEFENSE AGAINST INFECTIONS. The effects of severe malnutrition on the immune system are among its most important consequences. Virtually all components of the immune system are adversely affected in rough proportion to the degree of nutritional impairment. Peripheral blood lymphocyte counts are commonly decreased, with values often less than 1200 per cubic millimeter. Both the percentage of T cells and T cell function are depressed. Skin tests for delayed hypersensitivity reactions are often nonreactive, and lymphocyte response to phytohemagglutinin and poke weed mitogens is decreased. Atrophy of the thymus gland occurs in malnourished children.

Humoral immunity is also affected, but in a more variable fashion. Specific antibody responses are depressed in some instances and preserved in others. For example, antibody production following administration of poliovirus, tetanus, diphtheria, measles, and pneumococcal polysaccharide antigens is normal, whereas impaired responses have been observed after the administration of yellow fever and influenza A vaccines. In some instances, the affinities and binding capacity of antibodies are reduced.

Slight neutropenia may occur during uncomplicated protein-calorie undernutrition, but leukocytosis results in the usual fashion during concurrent bacterial infections. Neutrophils are normal morphologically, but some measures of neutrophil function, including chemotaxis and bacterial killing, are abnormal. Phagocytosis is usually normal.

Levels of individual complement components, other than C4, and total serum hemolytic complement activity are commonly decreased. Other nonspecific host defense mechanisms, including interferon production, opsonization, and plasma lysozyme production, may also be adversely affected by protein-calorie undernutrition. Acute phase reactants such as C-reactive proteins, alpha$_2$-macroglobulin, alpha$_1$-antitrypsin, and haptoglobin tend to be elevated. Changes in the body's anatomic barriers to infection, including atrophy of the skin and gastrointestinal mucosa, may contribute to an increased risk of infection.

It is not possible to define the exact mechanisms of enhanced susceptibility to infections observed with protein-calorie undernutrition. Each of these abnormalities of the immune response probably contributes in part. Micronutrient deficiencies may occur concurrently with protein-calorie undernutrition and can also cause significant abnormalities in the immune response. Zinc deficiency, for example, can lead to abnormalities in cellular immunity, whereas iron deficiency can result in impaired bacterial killing by phagocytes.

WOUND HEALING. Almost all aspects of wound healing are adversely affected in patients with severe protein-calorie undernutrition. Neovascularization, fibroblast proliferation, collagen synthesis, and wound remodeling are delayed. Local factors, such as edema associated with hypoalbuminemia and micronutrient deficiencies, may contribute to poor wound healing in undernourished patients. In mild protein-calorie undernutrition, however, wound healing is relatively well-preserved despite negative nitrogen balance. Even during complete starvation, endogenous substrates can be effectively utilized for collagen synthesis during the early phases of wound healing.

Clinical Manifestations

The clinical manifestations of protein-calorie undernutrition are complex, changing markedly with the severity of the nutritional deficiency and the relationship between energy and protein intake. In addition, the clinical manifestations can be greatly affected by the patient's age, other concurrent nutrient deficiencies, and the presence of other associated illnesses.

In cases of severe protein undernutrition, particularly in children in the developing world, the clinical manifestations of protein-calorie undernutrition may follow the classic patterns of kwashiorkor and marasmus. Intermediate syndromes of protein-calorie undernutrition are much more common, however, and mild and moderate cases predominate, particularly in industrialized nations.

KWASHIORKOR. The child with severe kwashiorkor commonly has a decreased blood pressure, bradycardia, and hypothermia. Body weight is usually low but may be normal owing to edema and anasarca. The child is usually apathetic, lethargic, and anorectic, with decreased spontaneous movement of the extremities. The cry may be weak and present only if the child is disturbed. The skin demonstrates a "flaky paint" dermatitis with dry, hyperpigmented, hyperkeratotic lesions over the face, extremities, and perineum. The lesions may be excoriated and secondarily infected. The hair is typically sparse, dry, and brittle and may be reddish or yellowish. The abdomen is distended owing to hepatomegaly and ascites. The extremities are commonly wasted and edematous. Clinical signs of concurrent micronutrient deficiency may also be present (Ch. 218).

The serum albumin is typically less than 2.8 grams per deciliter and the lymphocyte count less than 1200 cells per cubic millimeter. A mild anemia is common; it is usually normochromic and normocytic unless other deficiencies are also present. The serum transferrin is usually decreased but may be normal or slightly elevated if iron deficiency is also present. Other serum transport proteins, including ceruloplasmin, retinol-binding protein, and hormone-binding proteins, are decreased. Immunoglobulins are typically normal, or elevated if infections are present. Serum glucose and lipids are decreased. Serum levels of liver enzymes are most often normal and may be low. Blood urea nitrogen and urinary urea nitrogen are low. Electrolyte disorders are common, particularly hypokalemia, hypomagnesemia, and hypophosphatemia. The serum calcium is usually low owing to hypoalbuminemia but with normal levels of ionized calcium. A hyperchloremic metabolic acidosis is also frequently present.

MARASMUS. Patients with marasmus have less characteristic manifestations. Although the pulse, blood pressure, and body temperature may be low, patients tend to be less apathetic and lethargic and to have a good appetite. Growth is retarded and the weight is low. There is obvious muscle wasting and loss of body fat and the patient looks emaciated, but there is no edema. The skin is dry and loose with decreased turgor. The dermatitis of kwashiorkor is usually absent. The hair is thin, dry, and dull. The abdomen is thin without signs of hepatomegaly or edema. Typically, there are fewer laboratory abnormalities than in patients with kwashiorkor. Serum albumin and other transport proteins are often normal. A mild anemia is common. Any of the other laboratory abnormalities of kwashiorkor may be present but are usually absent.

INTERMEDIATE FORM OF PROTEIN-CALORIE UNDERNUTRITION. Patients with protein-calorie undernutrition in industrialized nations typically have an intermediate form that is more similar to marasmus than to kwashiorkor. The clinical picture tends to be dominated by the associated illness that has caused the undernutrition. Nevertheless, any of the clinical features of kwashiorkor and marasmus may be present and should suggest the diagnosis of secondary protein-calorie undernutrition. In mild cases, growth retardation in children and weight loss in adults may be the only manifestation.

Diagnosis

The absence of distinct clinical manifestations can make the diagnosis of protein-calorie undernutrition quite difficult. A high index of suspicion based on the patient's risk factors for undernutrition and the overall clinical setting and close observation of the patient over time are often necessary.

BODY WEIGHT. The most sensitive diagnostic measure is a documented history of weight loss. Weight loss should be quantified as a per cent of body weight lost. Weight loss can also be reported as a per cent of ideal body weight, but this may obscure significant weight loss in previously obese patients. Significant changes in weight, however, may also be obscured by changes in total body water in edema-forming conditions. Some patients, particularly those with a severe acute illness such as sepsis, burns, or multiple trauma, can develop severe protein depletion rapidly without significant weight loss. Unfortunately, no standard amount of weight loss occurring over an established period of time clearly indicates clinically significant undernutrition. Nevertheless, most authors consider a 10 per cent loss of body weight occurring during the present illness to be clinically significant.

LABORATORY TESTS. Each of the clinical abnormalities seen in patients with severe protein-calorie undernutrition can be used as a diagnostic test to detect undernutrition. Most commonly used for this purpose are the serum albumin, other serum transport proteins, anergy to skin test antigens, total lymphocyte count, blood urea nitrogen, urinary excretion of creatinine, and anthropomorphic measures of body composition such as skinfold thickness and mid-arm muscle circumference. Each of these tests when abnormal, like a history of weight loss, has been shown to predict poor clinical outcomes in patients in a wide variety of clinical settings. Combining these tests into indices further improves their predictive accuracy. Unfortunately, it remains unclear whether the poor outcomes predicted by excessive weight loss or by abnormalities in these tests reflect the consequences of undernutrition or the severity of the underlying illness.

CLINICAL ASSESSMENT. A thorough, nutritionally focused history and physical examination predict outcomes as well as any of the above tests and indices. The initial assessment is often equivocal; that is, the presence of clinically significant undernutrition is uncertain. In such cases, serial evaluations of the clinical examination, body weight, and laboratory parameters and close observation of the patient's nutrient intake as a function of their estimated requirements is necessary to make the diagnosis of protein-calorie undernutrition.

Treatment

The goals of treatment of protein-calorie undernutrition are to provide adequate energy, protein, and micronutrients to restore body composition to normal and to treat the underlying process that caused the deficiency to develop.

STRATEGY. Treatment should proceed in two stages. In severe undernutrition, the first priority should be correction of fluid and electrolyte abnormalities and treatment of acute medical problems, most commonly infections. Although any combination of electrolyte and acid-base abnormalities can occur, most common are hypokalemia, hypocalcemia, hypophosphatemia, hypomagnesemia, and a hyperchloremic metabolic acidosis.

In the second phase one must provide adequate nutritional substrate to begin repletion. Nutrients should be provided quite slowly to prevent complications of overfeeding. In most adult patients no more than 0.8 gram of protein per kilogram and 30 Kcal per kilogram of actual body weight should be provided. As the patient becomes stabilized, protein and energy intake can be increased to 35 to 40 Kcal per kilogram and 1.0 to 1.5 grams of protein per kilogram per day. Adequate micronutrients must also be simultaneously provided. Patients with severe, life-threatening undernutrition should be fed even more cautiously.

ROUTE OF THERAPY. Nutrients can be provided either enterally or parenterally. Patients whose gastrointestinal tract is functioning and who can protect their airway should be fed enterally, either by mouth, feeding tube, or tube enterostomy (Ch. 219). Patients with contraindications to enteral feeding can be given required nutrients parenterally via either peripheral or central veins (Ch. 220). An algorithm for selecting the most appropriate method of nutritional support is shown in Figure 214–1.

COMPLICATIONS OF THERAPY. Particular care must be taken to avoid complications of refeeding. Many deaths attributable to protein-calorie undernutrition occur not during starvation but during repletion.

Electrolyte abnormalities, for example, are common during refeeding. The provision of energy and protein to a severely undernourished patient may convert a catabolic state to an anabolic one. As new tissues are synthesized and old tissues replenished, potassium and other electrolytes are transported intracellularly and may precipitate an acute drop in serum levels and result in life-threatening cardiac arrhythmias.

Congestive heart failure and pulmonary edema can be precipitated by refeeding. As noted above, undernutrition is associated with decreased cardiac mass, decreased cardiac index and stroke volume, a slowing of the metabolic rate, and hypovolemia. The acute provision of carbohydrate, fluid, and sodium may correct the metabolic and volume abnormalities more rapidly than the depressed myocardium can handle and

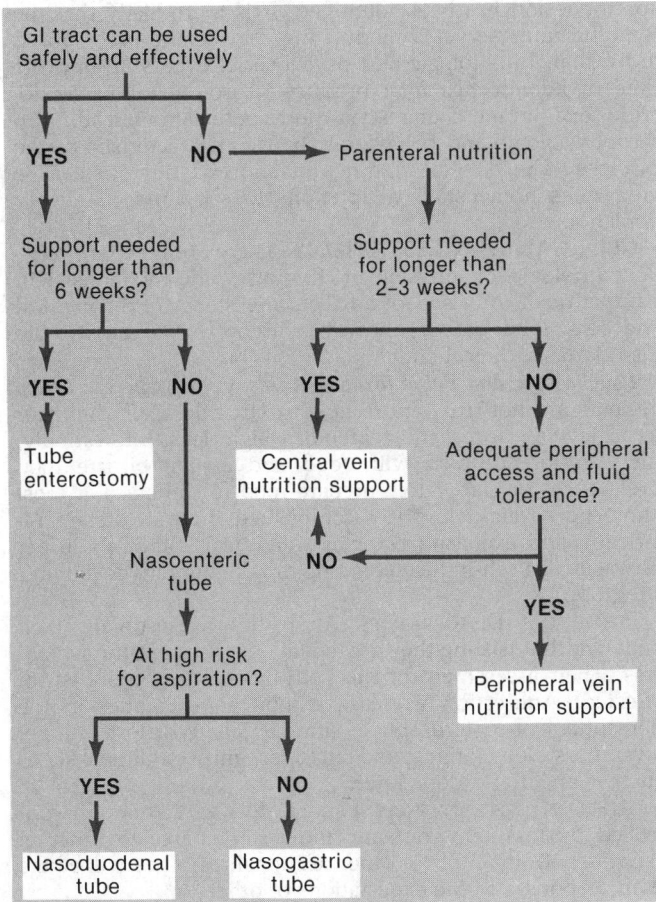

FIGURE 214–1. Decision tree concerning method of nutritional support.

result in fluid overload. Should this complication occur, standard measures for the treatment of congestive heart failure should be used together with a slowing of the rate of nutritional repletion.

Benign refeeding edema must be differentiated from refeeding congestive heart failure. Many severely undernourished patients develop edema in dependent areas during refeeding without an associated increase in left ventricular filling pressures. The cause of refeeding edema is unclear. Changes in renal sodium retention, in part due to increased serum insulin, and poor venous tone have both been implicated. Treatment should include reassurance, elevation of dependent areas, and modest sodium restriction. Diuretics are rarely effective and may result in intravascular volume depletion.

Diarrhea may result from enteral refeeding. Severely undernourished patients have atrophy of the gastric mucosa, decreased disaccharidase activity, and a mild deficiency of the exocrine pancreas. The provision of intraluminal nutrients can thus result in malabsorption and diarrhea. Gradual refeeding and restriction of lactose and lipid during the early refeeding phase will decrease the risk of diarrhea.

REHABILITATION. Treatment of patients with protein-calorie undernutrition requires more than the provision of nutrients. Physical therapy and other measures to improve the patient's functional status are effective adjuncts to nutritional treatment. Physical therapy may result in greater repletion of muscle mass and smaller adipose tissue stores than nutritional repletion without muscle contraction.

The most important non-nutritional factor in the treatment of these patients is the resolution of the disease or social process that caused the undernutrition. In most instances, if the underlying process cannot be effectively treated, little benefit is derived from treating the patient's nutritional deficiencies. In particular, patients with terminal illnesses who become progressively malnourished as they near death will obtain little benefit from aggressive nutritional treatment. In these instances, nutritional therapy can be withheld using the same criteria as for other life-sustaining treatments.

Prevention

In industrialized societies protein-calorie undernutrition is best prevented by the early identification of high-risk patients during admission to the hospital. Each patient admitted to the hospital should be screened for predisposing risk factors for protein-calorie undernutrition (Table 214–1). Those patients at risk should receive more formal assessment of their nutritional status. Patients identified early in the course of their illness, while undernutrition is still mild, can often be treated with less invasive forms of nutritional support, preventing both the consequences of undernutrition and the complications of nutritional support. Patients who require prolonged hospitalization, including those in chronic care facilities, should be regularly re-evaluated for the development of new risk factors for protein-calorie undernutrition.

The prevention of protein-calorie undernutrition in the developing world is much more complex and difficult. Poverty and underdevelopment, not overpopulation or world food shortages, are the primary causes of undernutrition in the developing world. Although the direct transfer of food during periods of famine can be lifesaving, the development of agricultural techniques, food distribution systems, and other public health improvements is more important for the long-term prevention of undernutrition.

The identification and early treatment of individual cases of protein-calorie undernutrition among children of the developing world are also of great importance. Programs that monitor growth and development, that provide nutritional information and supplements to pregnant and lactating women, infants, and children, and that provide family planning and prenatal care are also important measures. Of particular importance is the abolition of programs that distribute infant formulas and discourage traditional breast feeding practices.

Baron RB: Malnutrition in hospitalized patients: Diagnosis and treatment. West J Med 144:63, 1986. *Brief review of current controversies in the diagnosis and treatment of malnutrition in hospitalized patients.*

Golden MNH, Jackson AA: Chronic severe undernutrition. In Nutrition Reviews: Present Knowledge in Nutrition. Washington, DC, The Nutrition Foundation, 1984. *Review of severe undernutrition in children in the developing world.*

Siberman H, Eisenberg D: Parenteral and Enteral Nutrition for the Hospitalized Patient. E. Norwalk, CT, Appleton-Century-Crofts, 1982. *Excellent brief textbook on theoretical and practical aspects of nutrition support.*

Viteri FE, Torun B: Protein-calorie malnutrition. In Goodhart RS, Shils ME (eds.): Modern Nutrition in Health and Disease. 6th ed. Philadelphia, Lea & Febiger, 1980. *Balanced review of the classic syndromes of protein-calorie undernutrition.*

215 THE EATING DISORDERS

Douglas A. Drossman

The eating disorders—anorexia nervosa, bulimia, and rumination—attract much public attention and scientific inquiry. Diagnosis and treatment require an understanding that these disorders result from a combination of biologic, psychologic, and social influences.

ANOREXIA NERVOSA

DEFINITION. Anorexia nervosa is a chronic disorder characterized behaviorally by self-induced weight loss, psychologically by body-image and other perceptual disturbances, and biologically by physiologic alterations (e.g., amenorrhea) that result from nutritional depletion.

HISTORICAL NOTE. The disorder was first reported 300 years ago by Morton in describing an 18-year-old patient as a "skeleton only clad with skin" with "total suppression of her monthly courses." In 1874, Gull first used the term *anorexia nervosa* in reporting a "nervous, morbid disease" associated with loss of appetite and severe wasting. It is now recognized that these patients are not truly anorectic; they are *preoccupied* with food and struggle against hunger to achieve the desired goal of thinness.

EPIDEMIOLOGY. Anorexia nervosa afflicts predominantly young, affluent white females (95 per cent). The incidence may be increasing. In one community study the number of new cases per year over a 10-year period rose from 0.55 per 100,000 to 3.26 per 100,000. The disorder is associated with higher social class, occurring in up to 1 in 250 adolescent students in private school and with a prevalence of 1 per cent.

ETIOLOGY AND PATHOGENESIS. *Sociocultural Factors.* The cultural ideal for women's bodies has shifted in the last century from that of plumpness (formerly representing wealth, abundance, maternalism, and fertility) to a slimmer female image (representing independence, assertiveness, and success). Thinner women predominate on prime-time television and among beauty pageant contestants and high-fashion models. Social pressures from peers, particularly during adolescence, seem to influence young women and girls to engage in anorectic behaviors. These factors are probably not sufficient for the disorder to develop but may create the proper environment for its expression in the predisposed individual.

Psychologic Factors. It is believed that anorectics have an incompletely developed personal identity and struggle to maintain a sense of control over their environment. Psychiatric interviews suggest that the patient develops within a family that values outward appearance, proper behavior, and achievement more than self-actualization. In response to parental expectations, the pre-anorectic child learns to be hard working, eager to please, and attentive to family needs. In turn, the parents support and indulge in the behaviors of their model child ("best little girl in the world"). Therefore, these actions are mutually reinforced, leading to interdependence among the family members (enmeshment). However, the high standards within the family are rarely achieved by the child, who obsessively struggles for parental approval.

It follows that "negative" childhood behaviors (e.g., assertiveness, rebellion) are not permitted. These behaviors are believed necessary for the development of individual identity. As a result, the pre-anorectic child comes to rely on externally imposed ideal values to maintain self-esteem, but at the expense of self-actualization and a sense of autonomy.

It is not surprising that a distressing period for the pre-anorectic child occurs during or soon after puberty, when physical, social, and psychologic events (menarche, growth spurt, school, and adolescent peer pressure) encourage separation from the family and individuation. Over 80 per cent of anorectic patients develop the disorder within seven years of menarche. The compounded life events at this time are experienced with feelings of helplessness and ineffectiveness. The decision to diet, while not fully understood, may be a desperate attempt for control of one's body, at least, in a distressing new environment.

Biologic Factors. There is an increased risk of anorexia nervosa among siblings (6 per cent), with a four to five-fold difference in concordance rates for monozygotic twins, suggesting a predisposing role for genetic factors. Also, there are more perinatal complications reported among anorexia nervosa patients. The higher birth weight and the increased prevalence of obesity preceding the onset of illness suggest that premorbid obesity is an influencing factor. Abnormalities in satiety, temperature regulation, and endocrine function suggest that a hypothalamic abnormality exists, although no specific lesion has been identified. It is more likely that the hypothalamus serves a modulating role. In the predisposed individual, the biologic and psychosocial events around the time of adolescence may produce neurotransmitter, endocrine, or immune changes via the hypothalamus, leading to the physiologic and behavioral changes characteristic of the disorder. The biologic findings of anorexia nervosa can be viewed as homeostatic adaptations to self-imposed energy depletion.

CLINICAL MANIFESTATIONS. There are no characteristic pathologic or physiologic findings, and no consistent psychiatric diagnosis is found. The consistency of the medical and behavioral features, however, argues for classifying the disorder as a clinical entity.

Psychologic and Behavioral Features. PURSUIT OF THINNESS. Patients are not truly anorectic, but struggle against hunger to achieve an unrealistic degree of weight loss. Interestingly, they are preoccupied with food and exhibit bizarre food preferences or elaborately prepare food for others. For most anorectics, weight loss is accomplished through dietary restriction and exercise (restrictor subgroup), although 20 per cent will also self-induce vomiting or take purgatives (bulimic subgroup).

PERCEPTUAL DISTURBANCES. Anorectics overestimate their body width, insisting they are too fat despite profound weight loss. Their assessment of the body habitus of others is not affected. Anorectics may also exhibit abnormalities in the perception of enteroceptive stimuli. They distort hunger awareness, deny fatigue, and fail to recognize emotional states such as anger and depression.

SENSE OF INEFFECTIVENESS. Patients feel as if they are controlled by their environment and seem unable to function separately from family or other relationships. They will gauge their responses to the expectations of others.

COGNITIVE DEFICITS. Patients may exhibit deficits in conceptual thought and abstract reasoning. They may be unable to view situations in anything but extremes, and they interpret events in a rigid and highly personalized form.

Medical Features. Most of the physical, metabolic, and endocrine abnormalities of anorexia nervosa are also seen in starvation secondary to other conditions. The severity of the findings correlate with the nutritional state.

PHYSICAL SIGNS. Patients will have severe loss of subcutaneous fat and exhibit bony prominences. Core temperature, blood pressure, and pulse are decreased. Examination of the skin may reveal acrocyanosis, downy hair (lanugo), and a yellow discoloration (hypercarotenemia). Elevated serum carotene and vitamin A levels are due either to an excess intake of dietary carotenoids or to an acquired defect in the utilization or metabolism of these compounds. Secondary sexual features will be absent in the patient who develops anorexia nervosa before puberty.

ENDOCRINE ABNORMALITIES. *Gonadal.* The endocrine hallmark is gonadal dysfunction, and for women this presents as amenorrhea. Male anorectics lose libido and are infertile. Patients have decreased follicle-stimulating (FSH) and luteinizing hormone (LH) and do not exhibit secretory bursts of LH throughout the day in response to endogenous luteinizing hormone-releasing factor (LHRF), indicating an abnormality in hypothalamic regulation. This "immature" secretory pattern, characteristic of prepubertal girls, may result from the loss of a critical amount of body fat content or from the psychophysiologic effects of stress in the absence of significant weight loss. Normal menses usually recur with weight gain, when body fat content reaches 22 per cent.

Thyroid. Patients may exhibit clinical features suggestive of hypothyroidism, such as decreased vital signs, dry skin, constipation, cold intolerance, and a delayed ankle jerk, although lethargy is not usually observed. T_3 levels tend to be low, with a corresponding increase in reverse T_3, the relatively inactive isomer of T_3 (Ch. 229). Under the stress of malnutrition, the liver preferentially deiodinates T_4 to rT_3. The clinical findings of mild hypothyroidism may arise from a decreased availability of the more active T_3 isomer, which preferentially binds to the thyroid receptor. However, free thyroxine, total T_4 levels, and the TSH response to TRH are normal. Clinically significant hypothyroidism does not occur, and treatment with exogenous thyroid is not indicated.

Adrenal. Anorectic patients usually have normal or slightly elevated plasma cortisol levels with decreased urinary excretion of 17-hydroxycorticosteroids. This is due to a decrease in the metabolic clearance of cortisol from plasma with an increase in cortisol-binding capacity. The 24-hour cortisol production rate and basal ACTH secretion are normal. The response to ACTH stimulation may be increased, and the response to metyrapone stimulation is normal. Decreased libido and delayed virilization in males may be due to a shift of androgen metabolism from the 5 α-reductase enzyme system (yielding testosterone and its congeners) to the 5 β-reductase system, producing the weaker androgen etiocholanolone (Ch. 235).

Growth Hormone. Human growth hormone (hGH) levels are normal or slightly elevated. Concurrently there is a decrease in somatomedin levels. This growth-promoting peptide is produced by the liver and other tissues under the influence of hGH. Somatomedin mediates the anabolic effects of hGH but not its lipolytic effects. Thus, anorectic patients and other malnourished individuals maintain their adipose tissue breakdown (increased hGH) without growth effects.

CARDIOVASCULAR ABNORMALITIES. Patients exhibit depressed cardiovascular function with a decreased cardiac O_2 consumption, left ventricular wall thickness, cardiac chamber size, and blood pressure. These are adaptive responses to malnutrition and decreased catecholamine levels. Electrocardiographic changes include bradycardia, decreased QRS amplitude, prolonged QT interval, nonspecific ST segment changes, and U waves. Patients may also develop arrhythmias (tachycardia, sinus arrest, and ectopic atrial, junctional, or ventricular rhythms) due either to the primary disorder or to metabolic disturbances secondary to purgation. Sudden death has been reported among severely emaciated patients.

HEMATOLOGIC FINDINGS. Leukopenia and decreased white cell function, anemia, thrombocytopenia, and hypocomplementemia may occur. Anorectic patients do not seem to have a greater susceptibility to infection, however.

GASTROINTESTINAL FINDINGS. Constipation, delayed gastric emptying, pancreatic fibrosis, and jejunal dilatation may occur. Malabsorptive diarrhea and acute gastric dilatation may develop with rapid refeeding.

DIAGNOSIS. It is difficult to know when the diagnosis should be made, since social and cultural factors promote and maintain anorectic behaviors. Five per cent of college women without weight loss display attitudes and behaviors consistent with the diagnosis. Within some population groups (e.g., high-fashion models, ballerinas) low body weight is *de rigeur* and the associated anorectic behaviors are accepted. The diagnosis of anorexia nervosa should be considered when the person voluntarily restricts food intake in the face of hunger to achieve an unrealistic degree of weight loss and becomes psychosocially dysfunctional. The diagnosis is confirmed by identifying the described behavioral features and by excluding any treatable medical disorders.

The use of clinical criteria such as those proposed by the American Psychiatric Association (Table 215–1) is recommended. The differential diagnosis in this young population will include primary endocrine disorders (panhypopituitarism, Addison's disease, hyperthyroidism, diabetes mellitus), gastrointestinal disease (Crohn's disease, celiac sprue), chronic infection (tuberculosis), neoplastic disorders (lymphoma), and, rarely, CNS disorders (hypothalamic tumor, vascular malformation).

TABLE 215–1. DIAGNOSTIC CRITERIA FOR ANOREXIA NERVOSA*

Intense fear of becoming obese, which does not diminish as weight loss progresses.
Disturbance of body image, e.g., claiming to "feel fat" even when emaciated.
Weight loss of at least 25 per cent of original body weight or, if under 18 years of age, weight loss from original body weight plus projected weight gain expected from growth charts may be combined to make the 25 per cent.
Refusal to maintain body weight over a minimal normal weight for age and height.
No known physical illness that would account for the weight loss.

*Used by permission from the American Psychiatric Association Diagnostic and Statistical Manual of Mental Disorders. 3rd ed. Washington, D.C., copyright APA, 1980.

All patients should receive a nutritional assessment to determine the severity of the malnutrition and to establish a baseline for follow-up. Height and weight are usually sufficient. Patients with marked weight loss should have other nutritional measures obtained (serum transferrin, albumin, measurement of triceps skin fold thickness, skin test reactivity to *Candida* antigen) in order to gauge the approach to nutritional treatment.

TREATMENT. There are two goals in the treatment of patients with anorexia nervosa: nutritional restitution with alleviation of medical complications, and modification of the psychologic and environmental factors that promote anorectic behavior. No single treatment is superior, and a multidisciplinary approach involving medical, psychiatric/psychologic, and nutritional (dietitians, pharmacists) personnel is needed.

General Medical Care. The medical physician performs the initial clinical assessment, is responsible for the medical and nutritional care of the patient, and provides psychologic support. The general approach should include (1) fostering a sense of autonomy in the patient by encouraging her to take personal responsibility in the treatment plan, (2) remaining objective, consistent, and honest in order to maintain the patient's trust, (3) involving the family as part of the treatment program, (4) serving as liaison and patient advocate with the various consultants and counselors.

Nutritional Care. All anorectic patients will require some dietary management, although nutritional supplementation is not needed unless the patient is at risk of medical complications. With mild degrees of weight loss (e.g., weight 80 per cent of ideal or better), nutritional and psychologic counseling is sufficient. The physician's role includes personal support, education about adolescent body development and its relationship to diet, and scheduling of periodic visits to observe for clinical deterioration. With moderate malnutrition (weight 65 to 80 per cent of ideal) nutritional supplements may be necessary, but hospitalization usually is not required. Oral replacement with a palatable, nutritionally complete formulation (e.g., Ensure Plus) may help, with the goal being intake of 250 to 500 calories above daily energy requirement. In some cases metoclopramide or bethanechol may be used to improve gastric emptying and the patient's tolerance of larger meals. With severe malnutrition (weight less than 65 per cent of ideal) hospitalization is usually required. Oral replacement may be attempted, but if the patient is unable or unwilling to comply, tube feeding into the duodenum may be necessary. The patient can receive 400 to 600 calories above daily caloric need, with the goal being no more than 1 to 2 kg weight gain per week.

If the patient is severely malnourished and tolerates a feeding tube poorly or refuses to eat, parenteral nutrition may be considered. The peripheral venous route is preferred, since central hyperalimentation is more expensive and is associated with a greater frequency of complications. If a central venous route is chosen, it should be supervised by an experienced hyperalimentation team. Caloric delivery should begin with one half of the daily requirement, progressing to full requirement by day three or four. Electrolytes, serum chemistries, and hepatic and renal function must be monitored.

The goal of enteral or parenteral supplementation is to *slowly* get the patient to a body weight out of the range of medical risk. Rapid refeeding produces excess water stores and edema, secondary metabolic disturbances, and possibly cardiac failure. Continued nutritional intervention beyond achieving a "dry weight" of 80 per cent of ideal is not recommended. These procedures are psychologically invasive and minimize the patient's involvement in treatment, thereby increasing anxiety and resistance. Furthermore, supplements interfere with appetite and with attempts to re-establish normal eating patterns.

Pharmacotherapy. No pharmacologic agent is of proven value. Chlorpromazine, amitriptyline, lithium carbonate, and cyproheptadine have been reported effective in small, short-term inpatient treatment trials. Their use should be ancillary to the long-term nutritional and behavioral approaches.

Psychotherapy. Psychotherapy is used to help the patient modify the aberrant eating behavior and to improve psychosocial function. Behavior modification is an effective means of achieving short-term weight gain. Family therapy offers the best potential for long-term benefit, since treatment is directed toward modifying the family interactions that maintain the anorectic behavior. Insight therapy may occasionally help the motivated patient.

PROGNOSIS. The short-term prognosis is generally favorable; over 75 per cent of patients will attain a body weight above 75 per cent of ideal. Menses will resume in at least half; however, less than one third of patients will resume normal eating patterns. The long-term prognosis is variable, and relapses requiring hospitalization occur in about half of the patients. The mortality rate among hospitalized patients averages 6 per cent, with the main causes of death being inanition and severe electrolyte disturbances; suicide occurs in 1 per cent. A poorer prognosis is associated with a late age of onset, self-induced vomiting or laxative abuse, long duration of illness, male sex, and the presence of associated psychiatric disturbance. It appears that anorexia nervosa is a lifelong behavioral disorder with periodic exacerbations requiring medical, psychologic, and nutritional intervention.

BULIMIA

DEFINITION. Bulimia, derived from the Greek meaning "ox-eating," is a behavioral disorder characterized by episodes of overeating (binging), usually followed by acts to "undo" the threatened weight gain with self-induced vomiting, cathartic or diuretic abuse (purging), fasting, or excessive physical activity. Bulimia nervosa is sometimes used to distinguish the behavior of patients who binge and purge from that of other bulimics who binge but do not purge. Compared to anorectics, bulimics have normal body weight and tend to have less distortion of body image. Bulimics are more aware that their behavior, although secretive, is aberrant, and they may therefore be more accepting of treatment.

EPIDEMIOLOGY. Although bulimia was only first reported as a diagnostic entity in 1979, its prevalence is very high and it has probably existed a long time. Binge eating, at least once, occurs in half of the population, and weekly binge eating is reported by up to 15 per cent. Self-induced vomiting or laxative/diuretic abuse associated with binge eating occurs in up to 20 per cent of college students, and 4 per cent report this type of behavior at least weekly. Bulimia is almost exclusively diagnosed in young (< 30 years) women (> 95 per cent). Most bulimics carry on their activity secretly; less than one third have discussed their behavior with their physician, and in one survey only 2.5 per cent were under medical care.

ETIOLOGY AND PATHOGENESIS. Patients commonly report obesity during childhood or adolescence, and the onset of bulimia is associated with a conscious decision to diet. At some point the patients lose control of their compulsion to eat large amounts of "forbidden foods" and will binge. Self-induced vomiting is discovered as a convenient method of reestablishing weight control. Thus, a binge-purge cycle becomes established.

As with anorexia nervosa, societal influences seem to play a prominent role in the desire to be thin. Also, there are historical and social precedents for self-induced vomiting. The ancient Romans ate lavishly and then induced vomiting at feasts. Socialites who must attend many dinner parties will sometimes induce vomiting. Bulimics report coming from families that emphasize hearty eating and where food is used to celebrate happy times and to console during sad times. For these patients eating takes on greater meaning than simply to achieve nutritional benefit, and this may help to explain the emotional and behavioral investment present in food and eating.

CLINICAL MANIFESTATIONS. *Psychologic and Behavioral Features.* The characteristic behavioral feature is the binge-purge cycle: an eating compulsion with a failure to achieve or to respond to normal satiety. These episodes occur secretly and are often associated with feelings of frustration, loneliness, or the sight of tempting foods. Binges are usually planned, and the preparation is associated with anxiety and excitement. During the binge, high-calorie "junk" foods are pleasurably consumed. The binge is usually terminated when feelings of guilt or physical discomfort such as nausea, abdominal pain, or headache occurs. At this point the patient will self-induce vomiting and/or take cathartics or laxatives. Bulimics generally look healthy, and their behaviors are unnoticed by friends and family. They are more outgoing than their anorectic counterparts. Some patients may exhibit impulsive or antisocial behaviors such as drug abuse, kleptomania, and sexual promiscuity. The patient who seeks help does so because of feelings of guilt, anxiety, or depression, or she is no longer able to continue the habit and still function in daily activities.

Medical Features. The medical findings of bulimia are consequences of the vomiting and laxative abuse. The physical examination may reveal parotid or salivary gland swelling due to vomiting, bruising of the knuckles from their rubbing against the upper incisors during the induction of vomiting, pharyngitis and dental erosions from reflux of gastric acid, or conjunctival hemorrhages from retching.

Frequent vomiting may also be complicated by esophagitis, Mallory-Weiss tears, or aspiration pneumonitis. Hypokalemic hypochloremic metabolic alkalosis due to loss of H^+, Cl^-, and K^+ is the most common metabolic complication, and this may lead to cardiac arrhythmias or renal injury. Secondary metabolic disturbances may produce weakness, tetany, and seizures. Emetics such as ipecac may produce cardiac conduction defects and arrhythmias. Stimulant laxatives can produce a "cathartic colon' with degeneration of Auerbach's plexus.

The majority of patients are clinically depressed by the time of clinical presentation, and 5 per cent have attempted suicide. It is believed that bulimia may be a manifestation of an underlying depressive disorder, since a large proportion of patients have first-degree relatives with major affective disorders.

DIAGNOSIS. The diagnosis of bulimia is based on recognition of the binge eating pattern and the exclusion of other medical diseases that might explain the behavior. The differential diagnosis, which is limited in this young population group, would include schizophrenia, use of oral contraceptives, seizures, and rare neurologic disorders (Klüver-Bucy syndrome, Kleine-Levin syndrome).

TREATMENT. The goal of treatment is to help the patient overcome the urge to overeat. Bulimic patients recognize their behaviors as maladaptive. Compared to anorectics, they are more aware of associated psychologic difficulties and are more willing to work with physicians and counselors in a treatment plan.

The current psychotherapeutic technique is cognitive-behavioral treatment in which the patient identifies the abnormal behaviors and then uses behavioral techniques to extinguish them, thereby accomplishing greater self-control. The treatment is safe and probably effective.

Antidepressants have been reported to be successful in decreasing the binge activity and in increasing the patient's sense of well-being.

RUMINATION SYNDROME

Rumination syndrome, or merycism, is an eating disorder in which the person repetitively regurgitates small amounts of food from the stomach, rechews the food, and then reswallows it. The disorder has been recognized as a medical curiosity for over 300 years, and ruminators have been known for their tendencies to offer public performances.

Infants frequently ruminate, and the disorder is described among institutionalized adults and children with emotional and intellectual deficits. No characteristic psychologic profile or psychiatric diagnosis has been reported. There may be two subpopulations with the disorder, those in whom the behavior develops in childhood as a learned maladaptive habit worsening at times of stress, and those in whom rumination is associated with bulimia. A familial association is reported, although the role for genetic factors in the pathogenesis is not established.

The prevalence of rumination in adults is unknown, since generally physicians are unfamiliar with the clinical features. Patients who seek treatment report symptoms of weight loss, regurgitation, or vomiting and may express concern about there being an underlying medical disorder. Parents may bring the adolescent child to the doctor because of halitosis or dental problems.

Rumination in humans is not the same physiologic event as in ruminant animals, since reverse peristalsis does not occur. Radiographic and manometric studies indicate that an episode is initiated by a belch or swallow, at which time the lower esophageal sphincter pressure is lowered, creating a common channel between the stomach and esophagus. At the same time diaphragmatic and rectus muscle contractions raise the intra-abdominal pressure, thereby leading to regurgitation. When the upper esophageal sphincter is relaxed, food is ejected into the mouth, where it is expectorated or reswallowed.

The diagnosis depends on identifying the characteristic clinical features in the absence of other organic or psychiatric disease. Medical conditions such as esophageal stricture, reflux esophagitis, intestinal obstruction, or esophageal motor disorders (achalasia, diffuse esophageal spasm) should be excluded by radiography, video-fluoroscopy, and manometry. Since the disorder appears to be a learned maladaptive habit, behavioral modification and biofeedback techniques are recommended as approaches to treatment. However, cure may be difficult because the act is pleasurable and patients may not be motivated to change.

Balaa MA, Drossman DA: Anorexia nervosa and bulimia: The eating disorders. DM 31:1, 1985. *This monograph comprehensively reviews the epidemiology, pathophysiology, medical and psychosocial characteristics, diagnosis, and treatment of the two major eating disorders.*

Diagnostic and Statistical Manual of Mental Disorders. 3rd ed. Washington, DC, American Psychiatric Association, 1980. *This manual provides the standards of nomenclature and diagnostic criteria for anorexia nervosa and bulimia.*

Harris R. T.: Bulimarexia and related serious eating disorders with medical complications. Ann Intern Med 99:800, 1983. *Provides a good review of the medical complications in bulimia.*

Hsu LKG: The treatment of anorexia nervosa. Am J Psychiatry 143:573, 1986. *A review of treatment, including discussion of the approach to the patient, pharmacotherapy, psychotherapy, and behavior modification.*

Mitchell JE, Seim HC, Colon E, et al.: Medical complications and medical management of bulimia. Ann Intern Med 107:71, 1987. *This is an excellent general review documented with 86 useful references concerning this common disorder.*

Levine DF, Wingate DL, Pfeffer JM, et al.: Habitual rumination: A benign disorder. Br Med J 287:255, 1983. *Presents some of the clinical features of nine patients with rumination syndrome.*

216 OBESITY

F. Xavier Pi-Sunyer

Obesity is a frustrating problem for the patient and the physician alike. Its underlying cause is rarely clear, and its treatment is fraught with difficulty and failure. Management of obesity therefore requires much understanding and persistence.

About 34 million adult Americans (26 per cent of those aged 20 to 75 years) are overweight, 12.4 million severely so. The per cent of adult women who are overweight (27.1 per cent) is somewhat greater than that of men (24.2 per cent).

DEFINITION

Visual inspection of a patient can give a subjective but fairly accurate estimate of the degree of obesity. More objective measures are height-weight tables, weight-related indices, and other anthropometric measurements.

The three most commonly used indices are (1) tables of average weights by height and age; (2) tables of desirable weights for height associated with lowest mortalities in insured populations; and (3) indices derived from height and weight, of which the body mass index is the most useful.

TABLES OF AVERAGE WEIGHTS. National Health and Nutrition Examination Surveys (NHANES) are periodically conducted on a representative United States population and then compiled in percentile tables as weights for height for sex. These cross-sectional data can be used for defining obesity, with a commonly made arbitrary decision that above the 85th percentile is "overweight." This comparison to a reference population makes no statement as to health risk involved at any weight level. The biggest problem is that of finding an appropriate reference population, particularly for minorities.

IDEAL WEIGHT TABLES. The Metropolitan Life Insurance Company Tables of Heights and Weights indicates the weight at which longevity is greatest, based on those insured. The 1983 tables were derived from the pooled data of 25 insurance companies in the United States and Canada, including about 4.2 million policies issued between 1950 and 1971. People with major diseases were screened out. The tables show weights based on lowest mortality for men and women at ages 25 to 59 by height and body frame.

The Metropolitan tables have been criticized as being inaccurate because (1) insured subjects do not represent a random sample of the population; (2) insured subjects are screened for illness and so are healthier than average; (3) no actual body frame measurements were taken when data were gathered so that the division into three frame categories (small, medium, and large) was a post hoc manipulation of the data; (4) about 20 per cent of the subjects used in the tables reported their heights and weights but were not actually measured (the bias being that women tend to under-report their weight and men to over-report their height; (5) the tables do not distinguish between obesity and overweight.

BODY MASS INDEX (BMI). In an effort to clear the

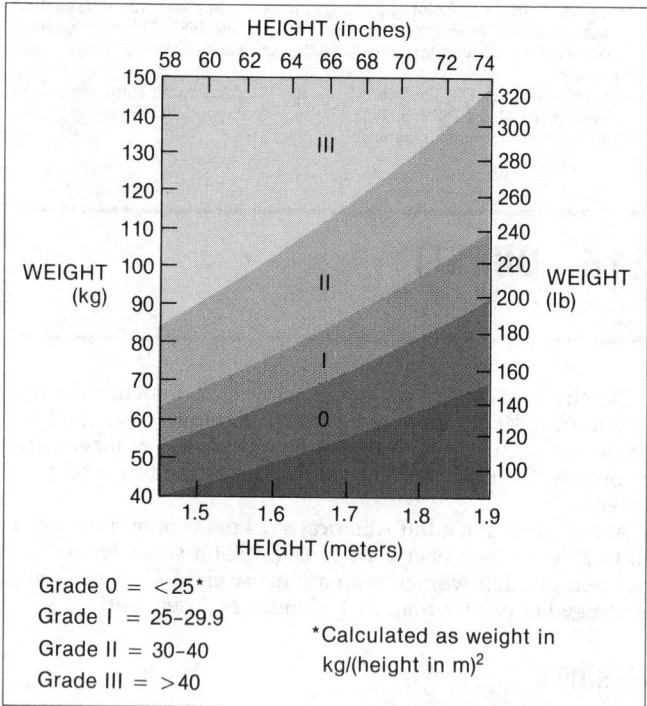

Grade 0 = <25*
Grade I = 25–29.9
Grade II = 30–40
Grade III = >40

*Calculated as weight in
kg/(height in m)²

FIGURE 216–1. Grades of obesity as defined by body mass index. (Reproduced with permission from Garrow JS: Treat Obesity Seriously. Edinburgh, Churchill Livingstone, 1981, p 3.)

confusion about how to classify overweight, the BMI has been computed:

$$BMI = kg/(ht \ in \ M)^2$$
$$or \ BMI = lb/(ht \ in \ inches)^2 \times 703.1$$

This simple measurement correlates quite highly with other estimates of fatness, although some very muscular individuals

may be classified as obese when they are not. It is also a somewhat more accurate index of fatness for males than for females.

The mean BMI (weighted for the height distribution of the United States population) taken from the mid-point of the medium frame of the 1983 Metropolitan tables is 22.4 kg/M² for men and 22.5 kg/M² for women. Patients can be divided for degree of obesity as shown in Figure 216–1. Patients can also be defined in relative weight units (RW), using the BMI of 22.4 for men and 22.5 for women as a RW of 1.00.

Aging is a fattening process, so that a young and old person of comparable body weight are not comparably obese (Fig. 216–2). This has led to controversy concerning whether it is the total weight of an individual that should stay constant from 25 years to 70 years or the fat-free mass, that is, the working cellular mass of the body plus the skeleton. The average weight data from the United States population show a gradually increasing weight with age, more pronounced and sustained for women than for men (Fig. 216–3).

Whereas many studies suggest that an increase from one's weight at 25 years old may increase mortality, a number have suggested that for the lowest mortality, the pattern of body weight should be leanness in the twenties followed by a very moderate weight gain as one gets older. The minimal mortality points in relation to BMI for each age-sex grouping have been calculated. The regression lines, computed separately for men and women, are presented in Figure 216–4. Clearly, age strongly affects the BMI associated with the lowest mortality in this study. Also, the regression lines for men and women are nearly the same. The "best" BMI gradually increases with age in both sexes, with no consistent difference between men and women. As a result, a single set of weight goal tables (Table 216–1) can be constructed as applicable for both men and women. The goals, which are somewhat more liberal for certain age groups than are the Metropolitan tables, are given by decade of age, with generally higher allowable weights as persons get older. Until the issue is further clarified, these goals seem to be reasonable for a physician to utilize in counseling patients in preventive medicine. Two caveats must be added. First, these tables have been derived from and are applicable primarily to white men and women. Second, the tables have been derived from populations without risk fac-

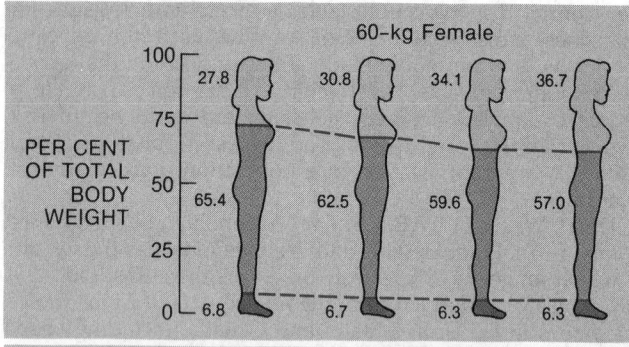

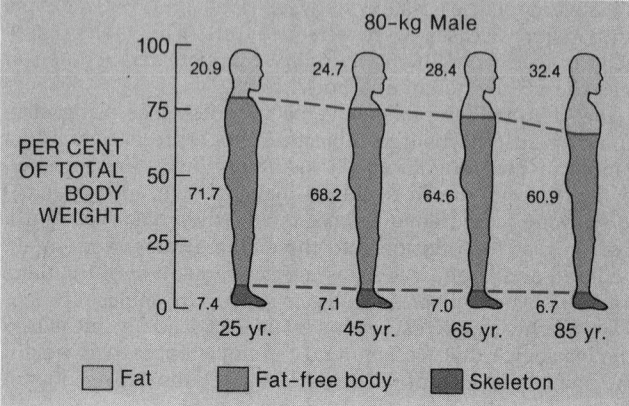

FIGURE 216–2. Body composition change with aging. (Adapted from Moore FD, Olesen KH, McMurrey JE, et al.: The Body Cell Mass and Its Supporting Environment. Philadelphia, W. B. Saunders Company, 1963.)

TABLE 216–1. AGE-SPECIFIC WEIGHT-FOR-HEIGHT TABLES*
(GERONTOLOGY RESEARCH CENTER)

Height	Weight Range for Men and Women by Age (Years)†				
	25	35	45	55	65
ft–in	←		lb		→
4–10	84–111	92–119	99–127	107–135	115–142
4–11	87–115	95–123	103–131	111–139	119–147
5–0	90–119	98–127	106–135	114–143	123–152
5–1	93–123	101–131	110–140	118–148	127–157
5–2	96–127	105–136	113–144	122–153	131–163
5–3	99–131	108–140	117–149	126–158	135–168
5–4	102–135	112–145	121–154	130–163	140–173
5–5	106–140	115–149	125–159	134–168	144–179
5–6	109–144	119–154	129–164	138–174	148–184
5–7	112–148	122–159	133–169	143–179	153–190
5–8	116–153	126–163	137–174	147–184	158–196
5–9	119–157	130–168	141–179	151–190	162–201
5–10	122–162	134–173	145–184	156–195	167–207
5–11	126–167	137–178	149–190	160–201	172–213
6–0	129–171	141–183	153–195	165–207	177–219
6–1	133–176	145–188	157–200	169–213	182–225
6–2	137–181	149–194	162–206	174–219	187–232
6–3	141–186	153–199	166–212	179–225	192–238
6–4	144–191	157–205	171–218	184–231	197–244

*Values in this table are for height without shoes and weight without clothes. To convert inches to centimeters, multiply by 2.54; to convert pounds to kilograms, multiply by 0.455.

†Data from Andres R: Gerontology Research Center, National Institute of Aging, Baltimore, MD.

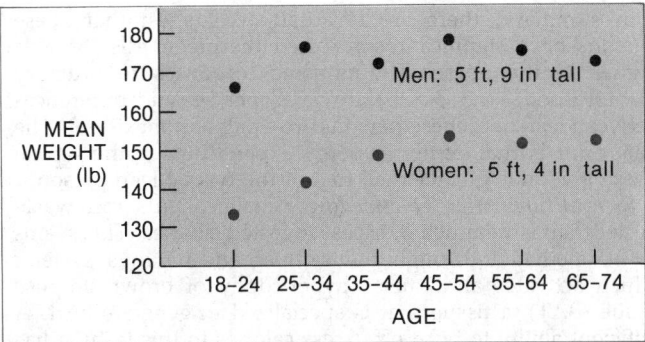

FIGURE 216–3. Weight change with aging for men and women. (Adapted from National Center for Health Statistics: Weight by height and age for adults 18–74 years, United States, 1971–1974. DHEW Publication No. [PHS] 79-1656, Series 11, No. 208, 1979.)

tors. Patients with significant risk factors such as coronary artery disease, hypertension, and diabetes mellitus are better counseled on stricter tables, such as the Metropolitan Life ones.

OTHER METHODS. Over half of the fat in the body is deposited under the skin. Its thickness can be measured at various sites using standard skin calipers. It is not difficult to become adept in the use of the calipers, and a running record of a patient's estimated body fat can be easily kept. The most useful and accurate tables are based on the measurement of four skinfold thicknesses—biceps, triceps, subscapular, and suprailiac. For such tables, see the British Journal of Nutrition 2:77, 1974.

Other methods of defining obesity are more difficult and expensive and therefore are used mostly for research purposes: (1) Total body water can be measured by dilution with tritiated or deuterated water. Water is then assumed to be a fixed proportion of fat-free mass (FFM = water mass/0.73), and FFM is subtracted from total body weight to obtain total body fat. (2) Body density can be measured by underwater

weighing (with accurate correction for lung and abdominal air) and the amount of fat-free mass and body fat can be calculated. (3) The amount of body potassium can be estimated by measuring the amount of its naturally radioactive isotope ^{40}K in a whole body counter. From this figure the lean body mass can be calculated as LBM = total K^+ (mmol)/68.1. Total body fat can be calculated as total weight minus LBM.

ETIOLOGY

Very little is known about the etiology of obesity. There are probably many different causes, and some may even co-exist in one individual. Obviously excess lipid deposition occurs because energy intake exceeds energy expenditure. An obese individual may have increased intake, decreased expenditure, or both.

FAMILIAL OBESITY. Obesity tends to run in families. The children of fat parents tend to be fatter. Whether this is environmental or genetic is unclear, and the likelihood is that both play a significant part. Recent twin and adoption studies indicate that human fatness is under strong genetic control. From 64 to 88 per cent of the variance in skinfold thickness, body mass index, and relative weight has been attributed to genetic factors. Environment is also clearly important, although the environmental impact in children seems to recede as they become adults.

A number of rare genetic diseases are associated with obesity, but through unknown mechanisms: the Prader-Willi syndrome, the Laurence-Moon-Biedl syndrome, the Alstrom syndrome, the Cohen syndrome, the Carpenter syndrome, and Blount's disease. The reader is referred to textbooks on genetic disorders for further descriptions of these entities.

ENERGY INTAKE. Hyperphagia is the striking cause of obesity in a number of animal models (both genetic and brain-lesioned). The cause of human obesity is usually much less straightforward, however. Obesity has been regarded as an eating disorder for centuries, but the presumed eating abnormality has been difficult to document. Measuring food intake in a free-living environment is subject to large errors. It is also difficult to agree on what constitutes abnormal intake, since the range of caloric intake varies greatly even in lean individuals. Most studies have suggested that obese persons do overeat (at least in their weight-gaining phases). There are numerous examples of individuals who categorically deny overeating but who lose weight when brought into a metabolic ward and placed on a calculated weight-maintaining diet for their height and age.

Possibly obese persons are unduly attracted by the hedonic aspects of food, or they have impaired feedback signals registering satiety, or they have insensitive central reception centers for the feedback signals. It has also been suggested that feeding behavior is learned and that satiety is a conditioned response. Maladaptive conditioning is said to occur in obese persons. None of these theories has been scientifically validated.

ENERGY EXPENDITURE. *Basal Metabolic Expenditure.* Obese individuals may gain weight because they are "thrifty"; i.e., less ingested nutrient is spent as heat and thus more is available for storage. This argument has been put forward by those who contend that obese individuals do not eat more than lean ones and may actually eat less. Impaired thermogenesis seems to exist in certain animal models of obesity, but it has been more difficult to document in humans.

Thermogenesis can be defined as *intrinsic*, that is, the basal metabolic rate (BMR), or as *extrinsic*, that occurring in response to specific stimuli, such as changes in the ambient temperature, the acute ingestion of food, chronic overfeeding, muscular work, certain hormones, or a combination of these factors. All of these are possible loci of impaired thermogenesis and therefore of obesity.

BMR is the energy expended in the postabsorptive state to drive basic life-supporting processes under thermoneutral

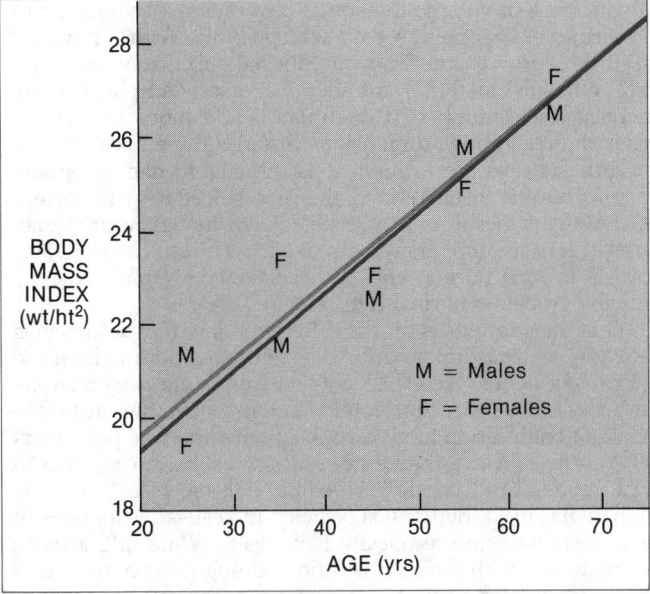

FIGURE 216–4. The effect of age on the body mass index (BMI) associated with lowest mortality. Minimal mortality points were computed for each age-sex group. The regression lines were computed separately for men (dark red line) and for women (light red line). Note that there is a strong effect of age on the BMI associated with lowest mortality and that the regression lines for men and women are nearly identical. (From The Build Study, 1979. Adapted by Andres R: In Andres R, Bierman EL, Hazzard WR (eds.): Principles of Geriatric Medicine. New York, Mc Graw-Hill Book Company, 1985.)

conditions. BMR, expressed as total amount of energy spent per unit time, is higher in obese persons than in lean ones. BMR can be well correlated with total weight but can be better correlated with LBM. This explains why men have higher BMR's than women and why BMR's decrease with age. The LBM contributes three to five times more per kilogram to the BMR than does fat.

Obese individuals have a higher LBM that those who are lean, since they require an extra amount of sustaining cell mass to maintain the extra fat. When BMR is expressed per unit of body weight, obese persons often have values below those who are lean. This is because per unit of weight they have a relatively lower amount of metabolizing cell mass and a larger amount of stored fat, which is relatively inert in energy utilization. In terms of basal or resting energetics, therefore, the obese do not have impaired BMR's and are not more "efficient" than lean persons.

The BMR varies as much as 25 to 30 per cent from individual to individual, even when they are matched for age, sex, and surface area. If a difference in metabolic rate between individuals can be as high as one third, it is clear that at a given caloric intake one individual may gain weight and another may lose it. Energy balance depends on matching intake to expenditure. It is not surprising that different individuals will maintain weight on widely differing caloric intakes.

Expenditure in Activity. The obese expend more energy during physical activity, since an obese person is moving a greater load through space, whether walking, running, or climbing stairs. This is true even when body weight is supported, as in cycle ergometer exercise, probably because of the higher cost of moving the larger leg mass. Thus, more kilowatts of energy are expended. Increases in energy expenditure relative to increases in work are similar in obese and lean individuals, however. That is, if lean and obese individuals are given the same amount of work to do, once the constant amount of extra energy related to the extra cost of moving the extra weight is accounted for, they will expend an equivalent amount of energy.

Studies of obese persons, however, show most of them to be less active, both in engaging in physical activities and in moving about once engaged. The amount of energy expended over 24 hours in physical activity is very variable, however, and it is difficult to generalize.

Expenditure After Food. Food is an important thermogenic stimulant, since it generates heat as it is metabolized. Because of this, a fed person has a higher metabolic rate than a fasting one. This elevation of postcibal metabolic rate above basal has been called the thermic effect of food (TEF). With a mixed diet, about 10 per cent of the metabolizable energy ingested is lost as heat.

Obese persons may have TEF responses equivalent to lean persons, or they may have a somewhat depressed response. The impaired response appears to be related to insulin resistance. Obese persons with insulin resistance have a slower glucose disposal. The impaired utilization of glucose by the cells of the body slows down heat production. Thus, glucose loads in an insulin-resistant obese person can generate lesser amounts of heat per calorie ingested. This impaired thermogenic effect can be normalized by giving insulin, so that an equivalent thermic response to that of insulin-sensitive persons occurs. Thus, it seems likely that a thermogenic defect relating to carbohydrate disposal is found in obese patients who are insulin resistant and not found in those who are equivalently obese but insulin sensitive. Despite this, the evidence for an overall diminished thermic effect of food in obese as compared to lean individuals is meager. Also, even insulin-resistant obese persons with a decreased TEF have an overall energy expenditure greater than do lean persons for the three- to four-hour period after the meal, since the slight decrease in TEF is less than the inherent elevation in their BMR.

In summary, there are few data to suggest that obese persons have significantly impaired thermogenesis. BMR is higher in the obese. Thermogenic responses to ordinary stimuli (food, stress, cold) are small per se, and differences between lean and obese persons are small to nonexistent. The net result is that 24-hour energy expenditure in the typical obese person is greater than that of the typical lean person.

Expenditure After Overfeeding. Small rodents can waste rather than store much of excess ingested calories. This seems to be mediated through the sympathetic nervous system, which activates and causes hypertrophy of brown adipose tissue (BAT), a tissue that is specialized to generate heat. A deficient ability to burn off excess calories in this fashion has been documented in a number of genetically obese rodents. There is little evidence that humans have an adequate amount of brown fat to mount a similar excess of heat production, however.

In studies in lean humans, significant overfeeding (of the order of 2000 extra calories per day) for a sufficient length of time (about 10 days or more) may lead to energy wastage. In the few studies of overfeeding done in obese volunteers, no evidence of similar energy wastage has been found, but very few long-term studies are available.

The number of calories required to maintain a previously lean individual at an overweight level is much higher than that required to maintain an already obese individual at the same overweight level. While the reason for this is unclear, it does suggest an increased "efficiency" of at least some obese subjects.

Do obese people lack a protective mechanism, i.e., heat dissipation, that lean people possess if they overeat? There is not much convincing experimental evidence to date, although it is a tempting hypothesis that needs to be further investigated.

PATHOPHYSIOLOGY

FAT CELLS. Fat cells (adipocytes) form a reservoir of energy that expands or contracts according to the energy balance of the organism. Fat cells develop from precursor preadipocytes to accommodate excess nutrient calories. Adipocytes gradually increase in volume to about 1 μg of mass, at which point no further enlargement seems to be possible. With continuing positive energy balance, new adipocytes form from precursor cells and the total cell number increases. Adipocytes can increase their number in an unlimited fashion, so that fat mass can reach huge dimensions through hyperplasia.

Once fat cells are formed, it is difficult to dedifferentiate them. This has been termed the "ratchet effect," because a ratchet turns in only one direction. Even though weight may be lost, fat cell numbers remain fixed. As a result, fat cell size reverts toward normal and with sustained weight loss may actually go below normal (Fig. 216–5).

What the stimulus is for the differentiation of preadipocytes into adipocytes is unknown. Adipose tissue lipoprotein lipase (LPL) may be involved. LPL acts on circulating chylomicrons and very low density lipoprotein (VLDL), activating the breakdown of triglyceride to glycerophosphate and free fatty acids (FFA). The FFA can then enter adipocytes, be re-esterified to triglycerides, and be stored. Adipose tissue LPL activity is high in obesity. Whether it is primary and causative for obesity or is secondary to the obesity is unclear. While LPL activity seems to rise with weight loss and is thought to be important in the accelerated weight regain of many patients, it seems to drop after the maintenance of weight loss for a time, suggesting that its elevation in the obese patient may be secondary rather than primary.

REGIONAL DISTRIBUTION OF ADIPOSE TISSUE. Fat mass is distributed differently in men and women. The android, or male, pattern is characterized by fat distributed predominantly in the upper body above the waist, whereas the gynecoid, or female, pattern shows fat predominantly in

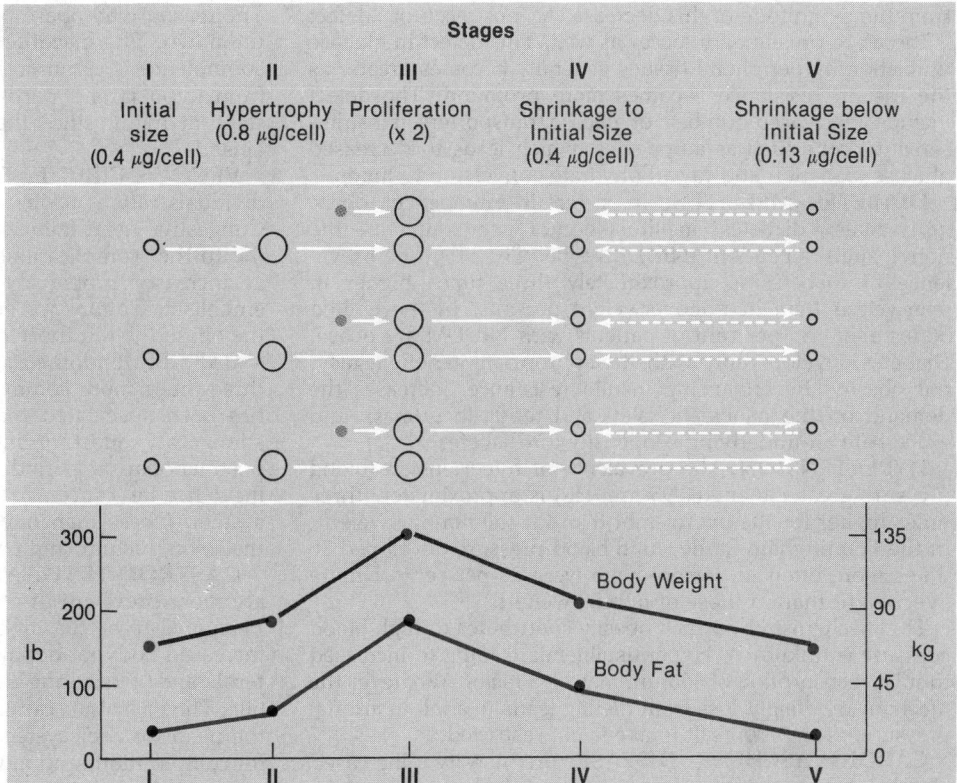

Stages

I	II	III	IV	V
Initial size (0.4 µg/cell)	Hypertrophy (0.8 µg/cell)	Proliferation (x 2)	Shrinkage to Initial Size (0.4 µg/cell)	Shrinkage below Initial Size (0.13 µg/cell)

FIGURE 216—5. Fat cell hypertrophy, proliferation, and shrinkage to and below initial size. (Adapted from Van Itallie TB: The enduring storage capacity of fat. In Stunkard AJ, Stellar E (eds.): Eating and Its Disorders. New York, Raven Press, 1984.)

the lower body, that is, lower abdomen, buttocks, hips, and thighs. Upper body fat has a significantly worse prognosis for morbidity and mortality than does lower body fat. The regional distribution can be measured in a variety of ways. The easiest, most common, and very useful way is by measuring body circumference at the hips and at the waist and calculating a waist: hip ratio. Normally, the ratio is 0.7 to 0.8.

Fat cells from the upper body seem to be functionally different from fat cells in the lower body. They are more sensitive to catecholamines and insulin. It is likely that the greater lipolytic and lipogenic potential of the upper body cells is related to an underlying difference in sex-hormone response of the two tissues. Thus, testosterone and estrogen influences may be important and may act differently on upper and lower body fat cells.

Abdominal or android fatness carries a greater risk for hypertension, cardiovascular disease, hyperinsulinemia, and diabetes mellitus. Since more men than women have the android distribution, they are more at risk for these conditions. Also, women who deposit their excess fat in a more android manner have a greater risk than women whose fat distribution is more gynecoid. Upper body fat deposition tends to occur primarily by hypertrophy of the existing cells, whereas lower body fat deposition is by differentiation of new fat cells, i.e., hyperplasia. Reducing a normal number of enlarged fat cells to normal size is easier than reducing large numbers of the cells in the lower body hyperplastic depot to normal or below normal sized cells. This may explain the weight loss difficulties of many women with lower body obesity.

SET POINT. The concept of a "set point" of body weight suggests that each person has a control system that "sets" how much weight, or alternatively how much fat, he or she should have. How the control system is regulated, that is, where the feedback signals from "weight" or "fat" originate and how they might be transmitted (humoral, neural, both?) to the hypothalamic feeding and satiety areas are totally unknown.

This set-point theory suggests that people are at a given weight because they are "set" there. That is, one's set point is the weight one normally maintains. Although this is circular thinking, set-point theory has been used to suggest that weight loss programs are misguided and that the effort to lose weight is inevitably fraught with failure because set point will bring individuals up to their pre-weightloss weight.

Animals with ventromedial hypothalamus (VMH) lesions seem to "set" themselves at a higher prevailing weight, from which they then once more regulate their weight normally. That is, once they have attained their plateau higher weights, they gain more weight if overfed but return to normal weight if they are allowed to eat ad lib; if they are food-deprived, they lose weight and when fed ad lib return to their plateau weight. In a similar manner, animals with lesions in the lateral hypothalamus are hypophagic and lose weight to a new lower weight "set point," which they then return back to from either overweight if they have been overfed or underweight if they have been further underfed. Genetically obese animals, such as the Zucker rat, also seem to defend elevated weights.

If and how these models relate to human obesity is unclear. The set point theory has been used to suggest that exercise and some drugs lower set point and most palatable foods raise it. Once these statements have been made, however, no closer understanding of the regulation of body weight and of food intake has been attained. Certainly, if there is a "set point," it is a very movable one that seems to change easily under the influence of a number of environmental conditions.

CLINICAL MANIFESTATIONS

INSULIN RESISTANCE. Obesity induces an insulin-resistant state in man, one that is associated with both basal and stimulated hyperinsulinemia. This is a change in insulin release rather than in the threshold to glucose stimulation. The enlarged fat cell is less sensitive to the antipolytic and lipogenic actions of insulin. While a decreased number of insulin receptors contributes to the insulin resistance, the resistance is generally much greater than would be predicted from the magnitude of this decrease. A "postreceptor" defect is therefore presumed to occur as well. This defect in glucose utilization by peripheral tissues generally becomes greater as the insulin resistance becomes more profound. The defect includes decreased numbers of glucose transporters in insulin-sensitive cells such as adipocytes, which leads to decreased glucose oxidation and to carbohydrate conversion to lipids.

DIABETES MELLITUS. In a certain number of obese individuals, diabetes mellitus occurs, generally as the non–insulin-dependent (NIDDM) type (Ch. 231). The prevalence of diabetes is approximately three times higher in overweight than in nonoverweight persons. In the United States about 85 per cent of patients with NIDDM are obese. Diabetes develops only with the appropriate genetic legacy, but obesity, by enhancing insulin resistance, increases the demand on the pancreatic islets and tends to unmask and exacerbate an underlying propensity for diabetes.

HYPERTENSION. The prevalence of hypertension (blood pressure greater than 160/95 mm Hg) is approximately three times higher for the overweight than for the nonoverweight. In the Framingham Study, high blood pressure developed 10 times more often in persons who were 20 per cent or more overweight than in those of normal weight.

The mechanism by which obesity contributes to high blood pressure is unknown. Hyperinsulinemia leading to increased tubular reabsorption of sodium may be a factor. Whatever the mechanism, weight loss from dieting leads to a fall in arterial pressure, even when salt intake is not restricted.

CARDIOVASCULAR DISEASE. In obesity, increased blood volume, stroke volume, left ventricular end-diastolic volume, and filling pressure result in a high cardiac output. This can lead to predominantly left ventricular hypertrophy and dilatation. Hypertension will also contribute to left ventricular hypertrophy. Thus, obese hypertensive patients are at greater risk for congestive heart failure.

BLOOD LIPIDS. The correlation between hypercholesterolemia and obesity has been only marginally significant (Ch. 183). Hypertriglyceridemia is more prevalent in obese persons, possibly because the insulin resistance and hyperinsulinemia of obesity lead to increased hepatic production of triglycerides. This hypertriglyceridemia generally improves with weight loss, but if a true genetic lipoprotein disorder coexists, more intensive therapy specific for the lipoprotein abnormality may be required.

RESPIRATORY PROBLEMS. Severe obesity can lead to chronic hypoxia with cyanosis and hypercapnia. Associated with this are an increased demand for ventilation, an increased breathing workload, respiratory muscle inefficiency, and decreased functional reserve capacity and expiratory reserve volume. Peripheral lung units can close, resulting in a ventilation-perfusion mismatch.

The end-stage associated with severe obesity is the Pickwickian syndrome, in which the hypoventilation is so marked that the hypoxia leads to long periods of somnolence. In these patients, pulmonary hypertension occurs and cardiac failure may supervene.

SLEEP APNEA. Sleep apnea is very common in severely obese patients (Ch. 72). The relationship between obesity and sleep apnea is unclear, since the most morbidly obese individuals are not necessarily the most severely affected. Apnea can be obstructive or central, and both are more prevalent in obese persons. In obese persons the upper airways may be obstructed by the large local accumulation of fat tissue, often in combination with micrognathia and enlarged tonsils and adenoids. The obstruction leads to hypoventilation and hypoxia, which somehow trigger apneic episodes that then make the hypoxia and hypercapnia worse. These patients benefit from weight loss and sometimes from surgical removal of some of the obstructive tissues. Central apnea is characterized by a cessation of ventilatory drive from brain centers, so that diaphragmatic excursions stop for periods of 10 to 30 seconds.

The reason why obese persons are prone to this condition is unknown. Pharmacotherapy is sometimes helpful. Daytime somnolence is common in obese patients with apnea, partly from hypoxia and partly from the continual disturbance of sleep at night, since they tend to awake after each apneic episode.

VENOUS CIRCULATORY DISEASE. Severely obese individuals often have varicose veins and venous stasis. Congestive heart failure may add to dependent edema, with the further complications of trophic changes of the skin and an increased propensity for thrombophlebitis and thromboembolism. Pulmonary embolism is much more common in the obese than in those of normal weight (Ch. 67).

CANCER. Endometrial cancer and breast cancer are two to three times more common in obese than in lean women. It has been speculated that this increased risk is due to the stimulatory effect of increased levels of estrogens in the postmenopausal period. Obese women also have a higher incidence of cancer of the gallbladder and of the biliary system. Obese men have a higher mortality from cancer of the colon, rectum, and prostate for reasons that are unknown.

GASTROINTESTINAL DISEASE. Cholesterol gallstones are more prevalent in obesity. The pathogenetic sequence is presumed to be that of greater cholesterol production in the increased body fat depots, greater biliary excretion of cholesterol, and a resulting supersaturation of the cholesterol in bile. The gallstones can lead to cholecystitis (see Ch. 130) and the need for cholecystectomy. The obese carry a greater risk for complications and mortality from such abdominal surgery.

Many obese patients have fatty livers with modest abnormalities of liver function tests, but hepatic diseases in general are not more common in obese than in lean persons.

ARTHRITIS. As the severity of obesity increases, joint symptoms related to osteoarthritis become common. Excess stress is particularly placed on joints of the lower extremities and the lower back.

There is a strong correlation between body weight and serum uric acid level. Urate clearance is decreased and urate production increased. Since hypertension and diabetes mellitus also are correlated with elevated uric acid levels, the relationship between hyperuricemia and obesity is multifactorial.

SKIN. Skin problems are common in obesity, particularly intertrigo in redundant folds of skin. Fungal and yeast infections of skin are common. Acanthosis nigricans occurs in a minority of morbidly obese patients.

PSYCHOLOGIC MANIFESTATIONS

The psychologic toll of severe obesity is large. Poor self-image and impaired social relationships are common. Obese individuals are often discriminated against in educational and professional settings, engendering anxiety, anger, and self-doubt. There is no evidence, however, of any particular neurotic or psychotic character in obese individuals. The depression and anxiety seem to be situational rather than endogenous and often improve if the obesity can be ameliorated.

MORTALITY

Obesity is associated with increased mortality. The effect of obesity on cardiovascular mortality has generally not been found to be an independent variable, but rather occurs through linkage with other risk factors such as hypertension, diabetes, and hyperlipidemia. In the Framingham Study, for every 10 per cent rise in relative weight, systolic blood pressure rose 6.5 mm Hg, plasma cholesterol 12 mg per deciliter, and fasting blood glucose 2 mg per deciliter. The causes of increased mortality for those 20 per cent or more overweight include coronary heart disease, cerebral "hemorrhage" (stroke), diabetes, digestive diseases, and cancer (Table 216–2).

TABLE 216–2. PATTERN OF EXCESS MORTALITY VARIATION WITH EXCESS WEIGHT (MEN AGES 15–34 YRS AT ENTRY)

Weight Relative to Average Weight (per cent)	Mortality Ratio
105–115	110
115–125	127
125–135	134
135–145	141
145–155	211
155–165	227

Adapted from 1979 Build Study.

OBESITY AND THE ENDOCRINE SYSTEM

Although it has been tempting to describe obesity as an "endocrine" disease, less than 1 per cent of obese patients have any significant endocrine dysfunction. Hypothalamic, pituitary, thyroid, adrenal, ovarian, and possibly pancreatic endocrine syndromes have been related to obesity.

HYPOTHALAMIC DISEASE. In this type of obesity, the appetite centers or tracts located in the hypothalamus are affected. Bilateral damage in the ventromedial hypothalamus produces obesity in the rat; conversely, bilateral damage in the extreme lateral portion of the hypothalamus causes aphagia. Rather than a single balance of a "feeding center" and a "satiety center," however, it is now clear that diffuse excitatory and inhibitory neuronal systems controlling feeding course through the limbic system and the whole brain. Following trauma, inflammation, or a tumor in the hypothalamus, a few patients develop hyperphagic obesity, most of them after surgery for tumors in the hypothalamic area. Craniopharyngioma has been most commonly associated with rapidly progressive obesity. The diagnosis is usually based on history and physical findings, which may or may not include focal neurologic defects, depending on the nature and extent of the injury.

PITUITARY AND ADRENAL DYSFUNCTION. Cushing's disease is the most common form of pituitary dysfunction leading to obesity (Ch. 230). ACTH is excessively produced either by a pituitary tumor or by hyperactive pituitary cells, which leads to excess production of cortisol by the adrenal cortex. Cushing's syndrome can also have a variety of other causes, including exogenous glucocorticoids, primary disorders of the adrenal, and paraneoplastic syndromes of excess ACTH production. The hypercortisolism causes adipocytes located primarily at the center of the body to proliferate and fill, while those at the extremities do so much less. With this central obesity comes hypertension and diabetes.

THYROID DISEASE. Obesity is often ascribed to "hypometabolism" caused by underactivity of the thyroid gland, but this is in fact seldom true. Severe hypothyroidism can lead to increased fat, but most of the excess weight is actually edema, which is lost with the institution of thyroid hormone replacement.

POLYCYSTIC OVARIAN SYNDROME (Ch. 237). Mild hirsutism, irregular menses or amenorrhea, and obesity have been linked in the "polycystic ovarian syndrome." In this syndrome the ovaries have atretic follicles, the patient is anovulatory, and menstrual disturbance (long-term amenorrhea to oligomenorrhea) is the rule. The ovaries overproduce androgens, some of which are converted to estrogens peripherally, primarily in adipose tissue. Hirsutism is common, but virilization is not. The relation of obesity to the polycystic ovarian syndrome is not clear, but the two conditions often coexist.

ENDOCRINE CONSEQUENCES OF OBESITY. One of the pathophysiologic consequences of obesity may be certain endocrine abnormalities. The sex-hormone abnormalities associated with obesity are different in males and females. Severely obese men have mild hypogonadotropic hypogonadism, with less than two thirds the normal mean plasma levels of total testosterone, free testosterone, and follicle-stimulating hormone. Gonadotropic hormones are suppressed by elevated plasma estrogens derived from increased aromatization of adrenal precursors in the excessive body fat. Obesity seems to be associated with increased metabolic clearance rates of testosterone, caused partly by decreased sex hormone–binding globulin (SHBG). Spermatogenesis, libido, and potency, however, are normal.

Estrogens are not elevated in obese premenopausal women, probably because the amount of estrone conversion by the adipose tissue is small in comparison with regular ovarian estradiol production. Estrogens are elevated, however, in postmenopausal obese women, most likely owing to increased peripheral conversion of the prehormone androstenedione to estrone.

In obesity, insulin resistance develops and hyperinsulinemia results. Whether impaired glucose tolerance or frank diabetes ensues depends on the degree of insulin resistance and the underlying genetic make-up of the individual. Triiodothyronine (T_3) may be elevated to high normal in conditions of high caloric intake with adequate carbohydrate, while thyroxine levels and TSH levels are normal. Slightly low blood cortisol levels may be present in obesity, probably because of enhanced turnover rates of cortisol. The circadian rhythm of cortisol secretion is usually normal in obesity. Urinary free cortisol levels are normal if related to the lean body mass or urinary creatinine. Also, these obese patients usually suppress normally with dexamethasone (Ch. 230).

Pseudotumor cerebri (benign intracranial hypertension) (Ch. 495) occurs most commonly in young women who are frequently obese. No intracranial pathology has been found, although headache and blurred vision occur. Why obesity is common in so many of these patients is unclear. It is possible that altered function of the ventromedial or paraventricular region of the brain occurs owing to the increased intracranial pressure.

Hypothalamic control of prolactin and growth hormone is often defective in obesity, with poor response to insulin hypoglycemia. These abnormalities generally revert to normal with significant weight loss, but not always. Whether these pituitary abnormalities reflect altered hypothalamic control due to obesity or abet the obesity in some way is unclear.

TREATMENT

Obesity is very difficult to treat, because the primary emphasis must be on active patient self-control rather than on passive drug therapy. The responsibility of the physician is to be as supportive and helpful as possible. The three approaches to weight control are diet, exercise, and drugs.

DIET. A truly motivated individual will generally stay on a diet for a long time, initially for weight loss and then for weight maintenance. Crash diets for a few days or weeks generally accomplish little of permanent value. Because of the long-term requirement for a diet, it must be tailored to a person's tastes and habits.

The diet must be nutritionally adequate. It is not possible to calculate a diet under 1100 calories that contains adequate amounts of vitamins and minerals. If the diet is lower in calories than this, vitamin and mineral supplements are necessary. The goal of weight loss is loss of as much fat as possible while losing as little lean body mass as possible. A mixed, balanced diet is a sensible approach to long-term weight reduction. A diet of at least 0.8 to 1.2 grams of protein per kilogram of desirable body weight will minimize nitrogen losses. The protein should be of high quality, so that essential amino acids can be utilized to maintain lean body mass.

It is a common strategy in many popular weight-reduction programs to use very unbalanced diets that focus on particular food groups at the expense of others. The high-fat–low-carbohydrate diets are ketogenic, whereas the low-fat–high-carbohydrate diets are much less so. These diets have in common a marked imbalance of macronutrients, with a concomitant imbalance of micronutrients. They cannot be recommended. If such diets are used, careful calculations for nutritional adequacy must be made, and appropriate supplements must be taken daily by the patient. These supplements require a number of tablets and capsules each day, so that compliance becomes a greater problem that must be strictly monitored.

VERY LOW CALORIE DIETS. Very low calorie diets (VLCD) severely limit daily intake to 300 to 700 calories. Some diets are strictly limited to protein and have been called protein-supplemented modified fasts (PSMF). Others allow both protein and carbohydrate. The concept of protein-supplemented fasting arose because this regimen improves nitrogen balance over fasting programs. There is little evidence, however, that at equicaloric levels protein alone is better than protein with carbohydrate. The extra weight lost early in the diet when protein alone is given is that of water. With this water diuresis there is electrolyte loss as well. The calories can be given either in liquid formula form or as natural foods. High-quality protein must be given, as a number of deaths from intractable cardiac arrhythmias have occurred in association with poor-quality protein intake on these VLCD. It is also imperative that adequate supplements of vitamins and minerals be taken. Although these very severe diets have been given for extensive periods of time, it is dangerous to allow them for longer than 16 weeks. These diets, especially those relying on liquid formulas, have been popular because of their relative ease and because, since they are so hypocaloric, the weight loss is more rapid.

Side effects of these severe diets include orthostatic hypotension (secondary to both sodium loss and impaired norepinephrine secretion), fatigue, cold intolerance, dry skin, hair loss, and menstrual irregularities. Rarely, cholecystitis and pancreatitis occur. Unfortunately, most individuals rapidly regain weight after being on these crash programs, perhaps in large measure because the very low caloric content and the liquid form of the diet do not educate the patient to make the adjustments in lifestyle and eating behavior necessary to maintain the weight loss.

BEHAVIOR MODIFICATION. Psychoanalysis and psychotherapy have not been very helpful in weight control. An extended change in eating behavior requires a great change in life style, however, so behavior modification programs have proliferated. Behavior therapy is a fundamental departure from the traditional "dietary" training of the past, in which a list of foods, the allowable quantities, and specific menus were supplied. In behavior modification the patient is first made aware of what and how much he or she eats as a background for changing that behavior. Many persons eat quite unconsciously, with little thought of how much they eat and with little or no knowledge of its caloric content. Initially, in the education process, careful food intake diaries are kept. Patients record not only what was eaten, but where, with whom, how, their feelings, and their degree of hunger. These diaries are analyzed, and nutrient densities of foods are discussed. New modes of eating are suggested, including not eating between meals, eating always at table, eating only three times per day, watching the portions of food eaten, not doing other activities while eating, and eating slowly with concentration. Behavior modification also strives at stimulus control and environmental management. The aim is to break learned associations between environmental cues and food intake. Particular situations that trigger eating are avoided or controlled. Behavior modification therapy is usually done in groups, with continued dialogue between the trained group leader (psychologist, nutritionist, physician), the other group members, and the patient.

EXERCISE. Obesity is a consequence of greater energy intake than energy expenditure. To lose weight, the imbalance must be tipped the other way, with expenditure becoming greater than intake. This is done not only by hypocaloric

TABLE 216–3. APPROXIMATE ENERGY EXPENDITURE IN SELECTED ACTIVITIES FOR PEOPLE OF DIFFERENT WEIGHTS (CALORIES PER 30 MINUTES)*

Activity	Weight (pounds)					
	110	130	150	170	190	210
Aerobic dancing						
"walking pace"	99	114	132	150	168	186
"jogging pace"	159	186	213	243	270	300
"running pace"	204	240	276	315	351	387
Basketball	207	243	282	318	357	396
Canoeing—leisure	66	78	90	102	114	126
Canoeing—racing	156	183	210	237	267	294
Carpentry	78	93	105	120	135	147
Cycling—5.5 mph	96	114	132	147	165	183
Cycling—9.4 mph	150	177	204	231	258	285
Dancing—ballroom	78	90	105	117	132	144
Dancing—disco	156	183	210	237	267	294
Gardening	150	177	204	231	258	285
Golf	129	150	174	195	219	243
Judo	294	345	399	450	504	558
Lying or sitting down	33	39	45	51	57	63
Mopping floor	96	105	120	138	153	171
Running						
11.5 minutes per mile	204	240	276	315	351	387
9 minutes per mile	291	342	393	447	498	552
7 minutes per mile	366	417	468	522	573	624
5.5 minutes per mile	435	513	591	669	747	828
Skiing, cross-country	216	252	291	330	369	408
Standing quietly	39	45	51	57	66	72
Swimming						
backstroke	255	300	345	390	435	486
crawl	192	228	261	297	330	366
Table tennis	102	120	138	156	174	195
Tennis	165	192	222	252	282	312
Walking						
3 mph	102	114	126	138	153	165
4 mph	120	141	162	186	207	228

*Adapted from Gutin B: The High Energy Factor. New York, Random House, 1983.

dieting, but also by increasing activity. Obese persons tend to be inactive; it is therefore important to increase caloric utilization. The patient should be taught the approximate number of calories being expended over basal level in individual activities. Most patients are surprised at how much exercise it takes to expend just a few calories (Table 216–3).

Moderate exercise only transiently increases the metabolic rate. The calories expended are the calories of work done. In the obese, moderate exercise does not actually lower food intake, but they do not seem to increase intake to keep pace with the extra expenditure, as do lean persons. This is helpful in inducing weight loss.

DRUG THERAPY. The only place for drugs in weight control is as short-term adjunctive therapy to that of diet and exercise. Over the long term the use of drugs has been disappointing, owing to the development of tolerance or of adverse side effects. In general, drugs affect appetite modestly, and tolerance often develops, requiring an increase in dosage. The anorectic drugs act centrally through brain catecholamine, dopaminergic, or serotoninergic pathways. For example, amphetamine and its derivatives seem to produce anorexia through stimulating the central hypothalamic neurochemical pathways in which norepinephrine and/or dopamine is the principal neurotransmitter.

Amphetamine not only decreases appetite; it also elevates mood and increases arousal, probably mediated through making norepinephrine and dopamine more abundant at synapses. In contrast, fenfluramine is thought to increase brain serotonin. Mazindol probably works through a dopaminergic mechanism. It therefore appears that increasing the activity of norepinephrine, dopamine, and/or serotonin at certain central nervous system sites can lead to anorexia and weight loss.

All of the drugs mentioned have a greater effect on appetite control than do placebos. Problems arise, however, from abuse potential and side effects. Amphetamine has clearly addictive properties. Amphetamine and phenmetrazine have disturbing side effects, such as sleep disturbances, agitation, and psychosis. Irritability and insomnia have been reported with diethylpropion, mazindol, and phentermine. Fenfluramine often causes depression, sedation, and diarrhea. Contraindications include severe hypertension, coronary artery disease, glaucoma, and history of drug abuse.

These drugs are generally prescribed for short periods of time, in an effort to help patients over difficult weight "plateaus" or crisis periods. Some experts, however, suggest that certain of the drugs lower "set point" of weight and should be given chronically. This is not, however, generally accepted practice.

GOALS. Very often the patient, and sometimes the physician, has unrealistic goals of what can be accomplished. One pound of fat is equivalent to 4000 calories. With a deficit of 400 calories per day, losing one pound takes 10 days. The more accurate the knowledge of daily energy expenditure and energy intake is, the closer a physician can predict the rate of weight loss. This may prevent unrealistic goals and disappointment by both patient and therapist.

SURGERY. Certain patients have severe obesity (greater than 100 per cent of desirable weight), have tried weight control programs without success, and often have complications like sleep apnea, heart failure, phlebitis, and arthritis. Their life expectancy is much lower than normal. These patients may be candidates for surgery for obesity, since nonoperative management rarely leads to permanent weight reduction.

Surgery for obesity should be considered experimental, as there is no one accepted procedure and all carry significant risks and complications. Short bowel procedures (jejunoileal bypass) generally leave about 50 cm of small bowel between the ligament of Treitz and the ileocecal valve, with the bypassed portion of bowel draining directly into the ileal remnant (end-to-end or end-to-side) or into the colon. Jejunoileal bypass generally produces weight loss but is fraught with complications, including diarrhea, electrolyte losses, vitamin deficiencies, hepatic toxicity, calcium oxalate kidney stones, intestinal pseudo-obstruction, and polyarthritis. As a result, it has largely been abandoned.

Because of the severe side effects of intestinal surgery, gastric surgical procedures have become popular. In these operations, no part of the stomach is resected, so that the operation is theoretically reversible. A small fundic pouch or reservoir is created so that the individual will be severely limited in the amount of food that he or she can eat. The pouch is generally created by stapling across the stomach, leaving a reservoir of about 50 ml. The distal stoma created for the pouch has variably been designed to empty into the rest of the stomach or into a loop of jejunum, with the rest of the stomach and duodenum becoming a blind loop. Alternatively, in vertical banded gastroplasty, as opposed to horizontal banding, only a small tubular reservoir remains for food entering from the esophagus. Side effects include gastric distress and vomiting. If vomiting is severe enough, electrolyte disturbances can occur. Also, some patients do not lose much weight, because many eat "around" the small reservoir with frequent servings of liquid or semisolid foods. A mean weight loss of two thirds of excess weight has been reported, but failure is not uncommon. Dilatation of the gastric pouch, stomal dilation, stomal obstruction, and staple line dehiscence can occur as complications.

Surgery is still unsatisfactory and experimental, but it may be advisable in some cases. Because life-long follow-up and vitamin and mineral supplementation are necessary, a responsible and cooperative patient and an interested surgeon are a requisite duo.

WEIGHT REGAIN

The most difficult problem in the treatment of obesity is the maintenance of a reduced body weight. The ability to maintain weight loss may depend on the severity of obesity and the amount of hypercellularity of the adipocytes in a given individual.

A person who is modestly overweight with enlarged adipocytes but little proliferation of extra adipocytes can more easily maintain weight loss. The adipocyte hyperplasia of greater obesity is likely to create a much greater problem in maintenance of weight loss. The degree of filling of adipocytes is very likely a regulated factor in energy balance. Obese persons with adipocyte hyperplasia begin to decrease the mass of each adipocyte as they lose weight. If the adipocyte mass drops below a normal lower level of about 0.5 μg per cell, individuals seem to have greater difficulty in maintaining weight reduction. Adipocyte mass seems to be a regulated factor with a feedback effect on energy intake, so that the reduced obese seem to experience strong food intake cues that they have trouble resisting.

Lipogenic enzyme activities increase when a hypocaloric diet is liberalized as a patient goes from a weight-loss to a weight-maintenance period. This is consequent to an increase in caloric intake rather than being primarily caused by the reduction in weight. It is not clear whether an increased food efficiency is present, but reduced obese individuals have been reported to require about 25 per cent fewer calories per square meter of surface area to maintain their body weight than do either normal persons or obese individuals who have not dieted and lost weight. Thus, reduced obese persons have energy requirements typical of a semifasted state despite their taking sufficient calories to maintain weight at a level that is still above normal.

PREVENTION

The propensity toward obesity is partially inherited, but a large component is also environmental. Obesity leads to an increased morbidity and mortality from a number of diseases, especially for those who are under 45 years old. Being overweight in early adult life is more dangerous than it is at older ages.

It is incumbent on physicians to make their patients aware of these risks and try to keep patients at a body mass index of grade 0 to grade 1 (see Fig. 216–1). This is particularly true for those patients who already have, or have a family history of, the diseases that are precipitated and abetted by obesity.

Hubert HB, Feinleib M, McNamara PM, et al.: Obesity as an independent risk factor for cardiovascular disease: A 26-year follow-up of participants in the Framingham Heart Study. Circulation 67:968, 1983. *A re-examination of the relationship of the degree of obesity and the incidence of cardiovascular disease over 26 years in more than 5200 men and women indicates that obesity is a significant independent predictor, particularly among women.*

Kissebah AH, Vydelingum N, Murray R, et al.: Relation of body fat distribution to metabolic complications of obesity. J Clin Endocrinol Metab 54:254, 1982. *A study in women of the sites of fat predominance as an important prognostic marker for glucose intolerance, hyperinsulinemia, and hypertriglyceridemia.*

Krotkiewski M, Bjorntorp P, Sjostrom L, et al.: Impact of obesity on metabolism in men and women. Importance of regional adipose tissue distribution. J Clin Invest 72:1150, 1983. *A study of the regional differences between the sexes with regard to adipose tissue distribution and of the differential risk of upper and lower body obesity as it relates to lipid and carbohydrate metabolism.*

Lew EA, Garfinkel L: Variations in mortality by weight among 750,000 men and women. J Chron Dis 32:563, 1979. *A description of the mortality experience of men and women in a long-term prospective study by the American Cancer Society, documenting that individuals 30 to 40 per cent heavier than average had a mortality rate 50 per cent higher than those of average weight. Mortality comparisons as a function of weight for all common diseases are included.*

National Institutes of Health Consensus Development Panel on the Health Implications of Obesity: Health implications of obesity. Ann Intern Med 103:147, 1985. *A statement on the risks of obesity.*

Olefsky JM: Insulin resistance and insulin action. An in vitro and in vivo perspective. Diabetes 30:148, 1981. *A discussion of the pathophysiology of insulin resistance with an emphasis on obesity.*

Ravussin E, Bogardus C, Schwartz RS, et al.: Thermic effect of infused glucose and insulin in man. Decreased response with increased insulin resistance in obesity and non–insulin dependent diabetes mellitus. J Clin Invest 72:893, 1983. *An investigation and discussion of the impaired thermogenic effect on glucose in patients with abnormal glucose tolerance and its improvement with adequate insulinization.*

Segal KR, Pi-Sunyer FX: Exercise, resting metabolic rate, and thermogenesis.

Diabetes/Metab Rev 2:19, 1986. *A review of the differences in thermogenic response to food and to exercise in lean and obese persons.*

Sims EA: Mechanisms of hypertension in the overweight. Hypertension 4:43, 1982. *A review of the pathophysiology of hypertension in the obese.*

Sims EAH, Danforth E: Expenditure and storage of energy in man. J Clin Invest 79:1019, 1987. An excellent, up-to-date review of energy balance in man with a useful bibliography of 71 references.

Stunkard AJ, Sorensen TIA, Harris C, et al.: An adoption study of human obesity. N Engl J Med 314:193, 1986. *A study of the contributions of genetic factors and the family environment to human fatness, concluding that genetic influences have an important role in determining human fatness in adults.*

Van Itallie TB, Yang MU: Diet and weight loss. N Engl J Med 297:1158, 1977. *A review and a careful metabolic study of the effects of macronutrient composition of low-calorie reducing diets on body composition.*

Wadden TA, Stunkard AJ, Brownell KD: Very low calorie diets: Their efficacy, safety, and future. Ann Intern Med 99:675, 1983. *A comprehensive review of very low calorie diets for weight loss.*

217 DISORDERS OF VITAMIN METABOLISM: DEFICIENCIES, METABOLIC ABNORMALITIES, AND EXCESSES

Richard S. Rivlin

In approaching disorders of vitamin metabolism, several considerations should be kept in mind about the properties of vitamins, their roles in biochemistry, and the shifting nature of their deficiencies that have evolved over a period of years. In general most vitamins must be acquired from dietary sources because they cannot be synthesized in the body. There are several exceptions to this rule in that certain vitamins can be synthesized in the body but in very small amounts. An example is niacin, which is formed in vivo from an essential amino acid, tryptophan. A tryptophan-poor diet cannot provide sufficient precursor to meet the metabolic needs for niacin, and niacin would have to be obtained from dietary sources in order to avoid deficiency. Other examples of vitamins synthesized by the body, or more correctly by the intestinal microflora, are vitamin K and biotin. Deficiency of these vitamins may result from long-term antibiotic therapy, which eliminates the bacterial sources. Under normal circumstances, however, endogenous supplies are not sufficient, and some must be obtained from food sources. Vitamin D can be synthesized in the skin in considerable amounts after exposure to light (Ch. 245).

The group of B vitamins functions as essential coenzymes required in intermediary metabolism. The dietary form of the vitamin is first converted into its active derivatives before it can serve as a coenzyme. Examples include dietary thiamin and its coenzyme derivative thiamin pyrophosphate, pyridoxine and pyridoxal phosphate, and riboflavin and flavin adenine dinucleotide. Vitamin deficiencies may arise not only because of dietary deficiencies but also because conversion of the dietary form of the vitamin to its coenzyme derivatives is diminished by drugs, diseases, or other factors. Vitamin deficiencies may also be caused by abnormalities of intestinal absorption, plasma transport, tissue storage, binding to proteins, or excretion. Assuring adequate vitamin status involves *exogenous* factors, such as dietary adequacy and food processing, preparation, and storage, as well as *endogenous* factors, that is, those that control vitamin utilization by the body.

Overt vitamin deficiencies caused by diet are seldom isolated. Although generations of students are familiar with scurvy caused by vitamin C deficiency and pellagra resulting from niacin deficiency, in common clinical practice in the United States these classic syndromes are encountered only rarely. Rather, the typical picture one encounters in hospitalized patients with protein-calorie malnutrition is that of mul-

tiple deficiencies, because a diet poor in one vitamin is usually poor in several others. Furthermore, one vitamin is often required for the metabolism of another. An example is riboflavin, which is involved in the metabolism of folic acid, pyridoxine, vitamin K, and niacin.

The clinical development of vitamin deficiencies is generally gradual; the physical examination is usually not useful in detecting deficiencies of specific vitamins early in their course. For example, by the time that perifollicular hemorrhages characteristic of scurvy have developed, vitamin C deficiency is already far advanced. Even the abnormalities detected by physical examination late in the course of the deficiency state are often not pathognomonic. Cheilosis and glossitis, typically attributed to deficiency of riboflavin, can be observed with deficiencies of a number of other B vitamins. Finding an abnormality of this kind on physical examination helps to establish the diagnosis of malnutrition but does not identify a specific nutrient as missing from the diet.

Increasing attention is now being paid to drugs and alcohol as significant causes of specific vitamin deficiencies. Drug-induced vitamin deficiencies often are poorly recognized and become evident most frequently in chronically ill long-term drug users on a marginally adequate diet. The elderly are particularly vulnerable to the deleterious effects of ethanol. This commonly used and abused substance is now established as the major cause of deficiencies of folate and thiamin among individuals 65 years of age and older, and this is probably true in younger age groups as well.

The rate at which vitamin stores are depleted following restriction of dietary intake varies widely among vitamins. The body stores of some vitamins, such as B_{12}, may not be depleted for years, whereas folic acid, thiamin, and niacin may be depleted within weeks or months. In general, the body's capacity for storage of water-soluble vitamins is limited, and when the storage capacity is exceeded, the excess is usually excreted rapidly; their tissue concentrations often cannot be increased even by massive doses given parenterally. By contrast, body stores of fat-soluble vitamins may become very great, and toxicity often develops with prolonged administration of doses greatly exceeding the recommended dietary allowances (RDA).

At present, many individuals are consuming vitamins in doses far in excess of the RDA. More than one third of individuals 65 years of age and older in the United States are estimated to be taking some kind of nutritional supplement. The supplements used are often poorly selected. Supplement use is greater among females than males, whites than blacks, and well educated than poorly educated; vitamin C is the most commonly consumed supplement. Toxicity frequently develops with prolonged use of megadoses of vitamins A and D. Individuals vary considerably in the rate at which they develop toxicity with prolonged use of megadoses of vitamins. Certain conditions predispose to early symptomatology. For example, individuals with a gouty diathesis may be at increased risk for renal toxicity caused by megadoses of vitamin C, and the onset of acute liver disease may precipitate vitamin A toxicity in a previously stable patient who has taken megadoses of this vitamin. Vitamins may play specific roles in prevention of disease. Examples include vitamin A and beta carotene in possible prevention of certain malignancies and B vitamins and C in the prevention of neural tube defects when consumed during pregnancy.

Under certain circumstances vitamins may be used appropriately as drugs. For example, ascorbic acid is widely employed to acidify the urine in cases of refractory urinary tract infections. Certain derivatives of vitamin A, in particular the 13-cis isomer of retinoic acid, have potent antikeratinizing effects that have been applied to the treatment of cystic acne. Nicotinic acid is utilized in the management of severe hyperlipoproteinemia. Certain pyridoxine dependency syndromes require pharmacologic doses of vitamin B_6. In these and other vitamin-responsive inborn errors of metabolism, therapy must be specific and targeted. Thus, the therapeutic applications of vitamins extend far beyond their roles in correcting dietary deficiency.

Elsas LJ, McCormick DB: Genetic defects in vitamin utilization. Part 1: General aspects and fat-soluble vitamins. Vitam Horm 43:103, 1986.

Rhoads GG, Mills JL: Can vitamin supplements prevent neural tube defects? Current evidence and ongoing investigations. Clin Obstet Gynecol 29:569, 1986.

Suter PM, Russell RM: Vitamin requirements of the elderly. Am J Clin Nutr 45:501, 1987. *Review of special needs of older persons.*

VITAMIN B₁ (THIAMIN)

Structure and Biochemical Function

The thiamin molecule is shown in Figure 217–1. The principal biochemical role of thiamin is that of precursor of thiamin pyrophosphate, a coenzyme required for oxidative decarboxylation of α-ketoacids to aldehydes. These reactions are widely distributed and are an important source of energy generation. In addition, thiamin pyrophosphate serves as the coenzyme for transketolase, which catalyzes the conversions of the two 5-carbon sugars, xylulose-5-PO_4, and ribose-5-PO_4, to the 7-carbon sugar, sedoheptulose-7-PO_4, and the 3-carbon sugar glyceraldehyde-3-PO_4. This reaction is used as a functional index of thiamin nutritional status, as discussed later in this chapter.

In addition to serving as coenzyme, thiamin may have a role in the neurophysiology of facilitating conduction in peripheral nerves. The initiation of nerve impulses is associated with hydrolysis of thiamin pyrophosphate or thiamin triphosphate or both.

Normal Physiology

Dietary thiamin is absorbed from the intestinal tract both by passive diffusion (high concentrations) and by active transport (low concentrations). The absorptive process is associated with phosphorylation of the thiamin molecule within the mucosal cell. In folate deficiency the absorption of thiamin is diminished. About 30 per cent of thiamin is bound to serum proteins normally. Muscle serves as the major storage organ for thiamin; most of the body stores are in the form of thiamin pyrophosphate, with lesser amounts stored as thiamin triphosphate, thiamin monophosphate, and thiamin itself. The degradation and excretion pathways of thiamin are not known with certainty, and more than 25 metabolites of the vitamin have been recovered from urine.

Requirements and Dietary Sources

The RDA for thiamin in adult males is 1.2 to 1.5 mg per day and in adult women, 1.0 to 1.1 mg per day, depending upon age, with a 50 per cent increase during pregnancy and lactation. The allowance is generally related to caloric intake as 0.5 mg per 1000 Kcal, although it is recommended that thiamin intake not go below 1.0 mg per day even with a caloric intake reduced below 2000 Kcal. The best dietary sources of thiamin are beef, pork, whole grains, enriched cereal grains, peas, beans, and nuts. Thiamin is rapidly destroyed at alkaline pH and is also heat-sensitive when not under strongly acid conditions. Some food items, particularly raw fish and seafood, are believed to contain thiaminases, which destroy the dietary supply of thiamin. A number of antithiamin factors have been identified from both plant and animal sources.

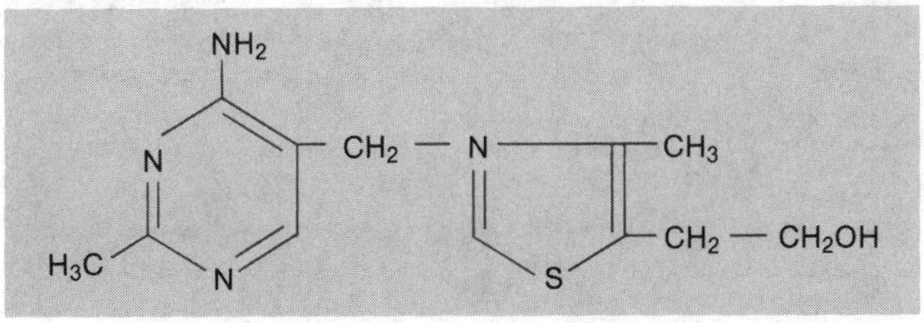

Deficiency

PATHOGENESIS. In addition to being caused by a poor diet, thiamin deficiency in the United States most commonly occurs as a result of *alcoholism*. Thiamin absorption is exquisitely sensitive to ingested ethanol, which significantly interferes with thiamin absorption even in healthy individuals. Repeated drinking throughout the day prevents most of the dietary thiamin from being absorbed, particularly in alcoholics, in whom some degree of malabsorption is quite common. Approximately 25 per cent of alcoholics admitted to general hospitals in the United States have evidence of thiamin deficiency by either clinical or biochemical criteria. Alcoholism is clearly the most important cause of thiamin deficiency in older age groups and probably in younger age groups as well. There is some evidence that alcohol also adversely affects the intermediary metabolism of thiamin, and chronic liver disease secondary to alcoholism may diminish the conversion of thiamin to thiamin pyrophosphate. Refeeding an alcoholic patient without thiamin may precipitate thiamin deficiency.

It is likely that other factors, such as heavy coffee consumption, possibly may diminish the intestinal absorption of thiamin. Thiamin deficiency is also observed with diabetes, cancer, other chronic illnesses, and with long-term parenteral nutrition or use of intravenous fluids not containing thiamin.

CLINICAL FEATURES. Early thiamin deficiency is characterized by anorexia, irritability, and weight loss. Later, individuals experience weakness, peripheral neuropathy, headache, and tachycardia. Advanced thiamin deficiency presents with involvement of two major organ systems predominantly: the cardiovascular system (the syndrome known as "wet beriberi," i.e., beriberi heart disease) and the nervous system, both central and peripheral (known as "dry beriberi").

The following criteria are generally accepted for the diagnosis of beriberi heart disease: absence of other known etiologic factors, history of at least three months of documented dietary thiamin deficiency, associated peripheral neuritis, enlarged heart with normal sinus rhythm (usually tachycardia), peripheral edema, nonspecific ST- and T-wave changes, and rapid therapeutic response to thiamin administration. Beriberi heart disease is well recognized as a cause of high output failure, which is a consequence of the profound peripheral vasodilatation. Resting tachycardia, weakness, and weight loss often resemble the clinical features of apathetic hyperthyroidism, with which it is frequently confused.

The central nervous system manifestations of thiamin deficiency consist primarily of the Wernicke-Korsakoff syndrome (Ch. 467). The Wernicke's component is an acute disorder consisting of variable degrees of vomiting, horizontal nystagmus, ophthalmoplegia caused by weakness of the rectus muscles, fever, ataxic gait, and progressive mental impairment. Patients have died when the disease has been unrecognized and allowed to progress. The Korsakoff syndrome typically has loss of memory and confabulation as prominent features.

The peripheral nervous system abnormalities of thiamin deficiency typically consist of a symmetric lesion that involves motor, sensory, and reflex responses. The legs are usually involved earlier and more completely than the arms. Pain and paresthesias may be particularly disabling to afflicted patients. An abnormal transketolase with high Km for thiamin pyrophosphate has been described, which may predispose certain alcohol abusers to severe thiamin deficiency diseases.

DIAGNOSIS. Thiamin status can be evaluated using bioassays, microbiologic techniques, chemical analyses, and functional enzyme assays. The most sensitive method for analyzing thiamin in small quantities in body fluids, tissues, and

FIGURE 217–1. Structural formula of thiamin.

foods is high-performance liquid chromatography (HPLC). In actual practice, the two most widely used assays are urinary thiamin excretion and the transketolase activity coefficient. Urinary thiamin can be determined accurately, but the results may be misleading if there has been recent thiamin intake in a previously deficient patient or if the patient has recently taken diuretics, which promote thiamin excretion. The results obtained under those circumstances would not yield the expected low value. Transketolase, as noted previously, requires thiamin pyrophosphate as its coenzyme. In vitamin deficiency, the erythrocyte apoenzyme is not fully saturated with its cofactor, and addition of the cofactor in vitro to an erythrocyte hemolysate results in an increase in measured enzyme activity. The degree of increase in the activity coefficient (i.e., enzyme activity after incubation with the coenzyme in vitro compared to that before incubation in vitro, expressed as a per cent) is an indication of the degree of unsaturation of the apoenzyme with thiamin pyrophosphate. The degree of unsaturation, in turn, is indicative of the magnitude of depletion of body stores of thiamin. An activity coefficient of 15 to 20 per cent or greater is generally regarded as reflecting significant thiamin deficiency. If these assays are unavailable, a therapeutic trial of thiamin, which provides rapid improvement (in 12 hours or less) in cardiovascular function and in ophthalmoplegia, may be regarded as supportive evidence for the diagnosis of thiamin deficiency. Cardiac output may diminish and vascular resistance increase within 30 minutes of intravenous administration of a single 100-mg dose of thiamin given to a patient with beriberi.

TREATMENT. If thiamin deficiency is suspected, rapid treatment with large doses of the vitamin is essential. Generally, 50 to 100 mg are administered intramuscularly or intravenously every day for the first few days, after which lower doses in the range of 5 to 10 mg may be given orally. Other therapeutic applications for which pharmacologic doses of thiamin are required include several rare inborn errors of metabolism: thiamin-responsive megaloblastic anemia, thiamin-responsive lactic acidosis, and thiamin-responsive branched-chain ketoaciduria (maple syrup urine disease), as well as subacute necrotizing encephalomyelopathy (Leigh's syndrome), a condition in which thiamin triphosphate is deficient in the brain.

Toxicity

Thiamin can be given safely by mouth in very large amounts without fear of toxicity, although the intestinal absorptive capacity is limited. When given by the intravenous route, large doses of thiamin on very rare occasions have been associated with poorly understood reactions resembling anaphylactic shock. Fortunately, these reactions occur so rarely that intravenous therapy with thiamin should not be withheld from a seriously ill thiamin-deficient patient.

Breen KJ, Buttigier R, Iossifidis S, et al.: Jejunal uptake of thiamin hydrochloride in man: Influence of alcoholism and alcohol. Am J Clin Nutr 42:121, 1985. *Study of how alcohol causes thiamin deficiency.*

Iber FL, Blass JP, Brin M, et al.: Thiamin in the elderly—Relation to alcoholism and to neurological degenerative disease. Am J Clin Nutr 36:1067(Suppl), 1982. *Discussion of effects of alcohol and drugs upon thiamin bioavailability.*

Mukherjee AB, Svoronos S, Ghazanfari A, et al.: Transketolase abnormality in cultured fibroblasts from familial chronic alcoholic men and their male offspring. J Clin Invest 79:1039, 1987. *Description of an inborn error of transketolase predisposing to thiamin deficiency.*

Neal RA, Sauberlich HE: Thiamin. In Goodhart RS, Shills ME (eds.): Modern Nutrition in Health and Disease. 6th ed. Philadelphia, Lea & Febiger, 1980, pp 191–197. *Discussion of structure, function, requirements, and toxicity of thiamin.*

VITAMIN B₂ (RIBOFLAVIN)
Structure and Biochemical Functions

Riboflavin (Fig. 217–2) must be converted to its coenzyme derivatives, flavin mononucleotide (FMN) and flavin adenine dinucleotide (FAD), in order to be metabolically active. These coenzymes are formed sequentially from dietary riboflavin after reacting with ATP and function as cofactors for a wide variety of enzymes in intermediary metabolism, particularly those involving oxidation-reduction reactions. FAD-dependent enzymes include α-glycerophosphate dehydrogenase, xanthine oxidase, and NADPH-cytochrome c reductase. A small fraction of tissue flavin is found in covalent linkage with protein and includes the enzymes monoamine oxidase (MAO), succinic dehydrogenase, and sarcosine dehydrogenase.

Normal Physiology

Riboflavin and FMN are absorbed from the upper gastrointestinal tract by a specific and saturable transport process. FAD, the predominant form in foods such as meat, must first

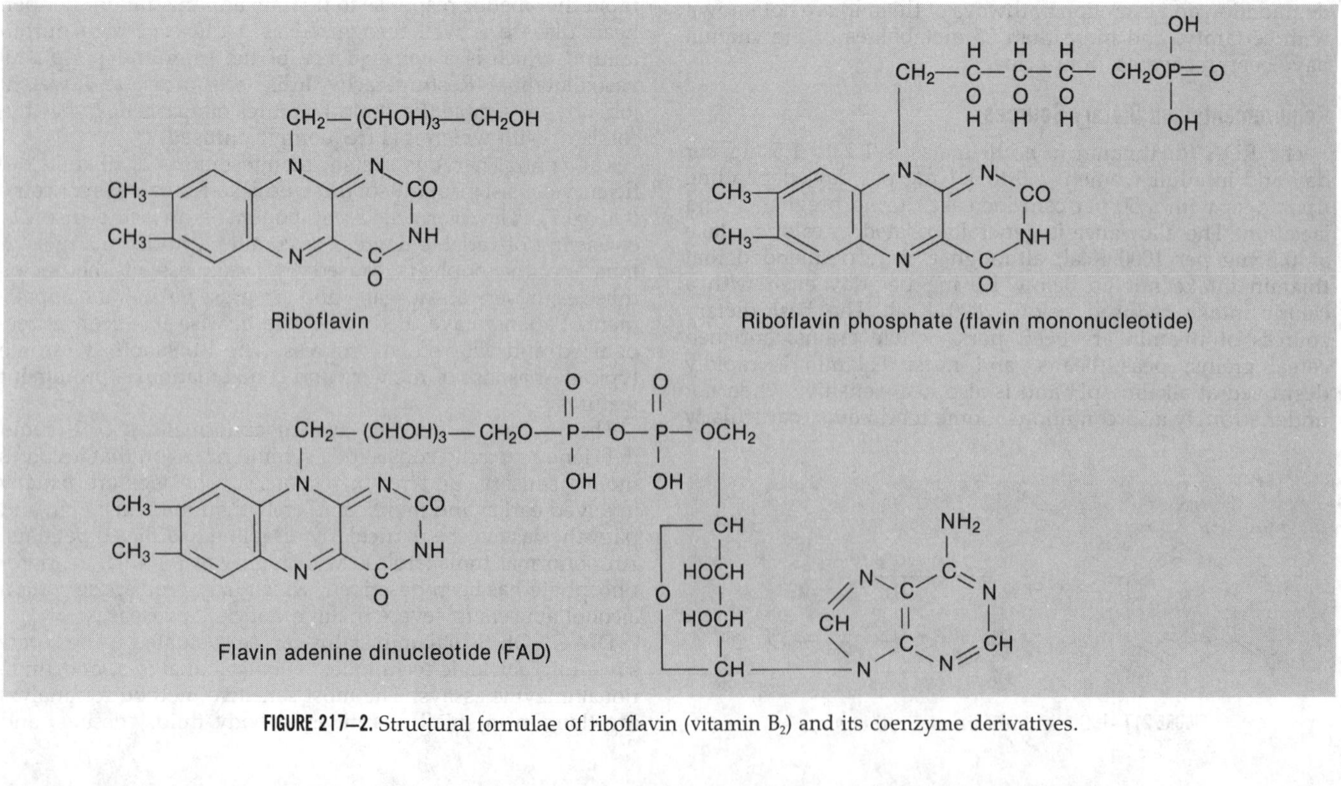

FIGURE 217–2. Structural formulae of riboflavin (vitamin B₂) and its coenzyme derivatives.

be degraded to riboflavin and FMN prior to being absorbed. Covalently bound flavins are largely unavailable as nutritional sources of riboflavin. A number of metals and drugs form complexes or chelates with dietary riboflavin and may influence the bioavailability of this vitamin. Such agents include copper, zinc, iron, saccharin, tryptophan, and ascorbic acid. After absorption, riboflavin is bound to several serum proteins, particularly to IgA and IgG. The amount of riboflavin bound to serum proteins varies widely in normal individuals. The renal tubule transports riboflavin in both directions, and in urine the predominant form detected is riboflavin rather than the coenzyme derivatives. Additional metabolites of riboflavin in human urine include 7α- and 8α-hydroxyriboflavin.

Thyroid and adrenal hormones regulate the conversion of riboflavin to FMN, FAD, and covalently bound flavins. Analogues of riboflavin interfere with certain actions of aldosterone and may possibly have potential as antihypertensive agents.

Requirements and Dietary Sources

The RDA for riboflavin in adult males is 1.4 to 1.7 mg per day and in adult females, 1.2 to 1.3 mg per day, depending upon age. Allowances are increased during pregnancy and lactation and probably should be increased with heavy exercise. When riboflavin is consumed in amounts greater than the RDA, increased urinary excretion occurs promptly. In the United States, milk and milk products supply close to half the daily intake of riboflavin, with meat, fish, poultry, eggs, and legumes providing another 30 per cent; the remainder comes largely from fruits, vegetables, and grain products. In developing countries, the principal sources are cereals, roots, and tubers. Riboflavin is light-, acid-, and alkali-sensitive and rapidly loses biologic activity when exposed to sunlight or when treated with sodium bicarbonate, a common but unfortunate practice used to retain the color of green vegetables.

Deficiency

PATHOGENESIS. Riboflavin deficiency arises not only because of an inadequate diet, but also when hormones, drugs, or diseases impair the absorption, utilization, metabolic transformations, binding, or excretion of this vitamin. In experimental animals, the psychotropic drugs chlorpromazine, imipramine, and amitriptyline and the antitumor agent Adriamycin, all diminish the conversion of riboflavin to its active coenzyme derivatives, FMN and FAD. Chlorpromazine treatment greatly accelerates the development of riboflavin deficiency. The underlying mechanism of this effect appears to be inhibition of flavokinase, the enzyme that converts riboflavin to FMN, the first of two steps in the biosynthesis of FAD. Phototherapy of newborn infants with hyperbilirubinemia may lead to some decomposition of riboflavin because of its light sensitivity. Ethanol may diminish both the intestinal absorption of riboflavin and its bioavailability from food sources. Deficiency of riboflavin likely results also after severe trauma, burns, surgery, chronic debilitating diseases, and severe and prolonged diarrhea. Increased riboflavin excretion may occur under conditions of negative nitrogen balance, including diabetes after withdrawal of insulin. Hypothyroidism impairs riboflavin metabolism.

Riboflavin deficiency has particularly important effects upon fat metabolism and alters the plasma and tissue concentrations of phospholipids. The rate of biosynthesis of renal prostaglandins, PGE_2 and $PGF_{2\alpha}$ is increased in riboflavin deficiency.

CLINICAL FEATURES. Early symptoms of riboflavin deficiency include soreness of the mouth, burning and itching of the eyes, and personality deterioration. Advanced riboflavin deficiency produces a constellation of findings that include cheilosis, angular stomatitis, seborrheic dermatitis, glossitis, corneal vascularization, reticulocytopenia and anemia, and retarded intellectual development (see Color plate

8A). Cheilosis and angular stomatitis, once thought to be specific for riboflavin deficiency, are now known to occur frequently in other nutritional deficiencies. The clinical picture of riboflavin deficiency isolated from other deficiencies is rarely observed. Riboflavin deficiency is a major cause of congenital malformations in experimental animals, but it is unclear at present whether malformations result from human maternal riboflavin deficiency. The rate of metabolism of a number of drugs is altered in riboflavin deficiency, at least in part because the microsomal hydroxylase system requires flavin coenzymes. There is evidence that riboflavin deficiency provides protection against infection with *Plasmodium* in both animals and humans.

DIAGNOSIS. In riboflavin deficiency, there is a reduction in urinary excretion of riboflavin as well as a reduction in the concentrations of various flavins in plasma and in erythrocytes. A functional test of riboflavin status is the activity coefficient of erythrocyte glutathione reductase, an FAD-requiring enzyme. When FAD is added in vitro to an erythrocyte hemolysate, the increase in activity produced is much greater in erythrocytes from riboflavin-deficient than from riboflavin-replete individuals. As with transketolase and thiamin pyrophosphate (referred to above), this assay reflects the lesser degree of saturation of the apoenzyme with its cofactor in deficient compared with normal individuals. Results are expressed as the activity coefficient, i.e., the ratio of enzyme activity after incubation with FAD in vitro to that before incubation. Activity coefficients greater than 1.2 to 1.3 are generally considered to be indicative of a riboflavin-deficient state.

TREATMENT. Riboflavin deficiency can be treated satisfactorily with food sources high in riboflavin, such as milk, liver, meat, eggs, and certain vegetables, or with the vitamin itself. Deficient patients treated with 10 to 15 mg per day of riboflavin undergo healing of skin lesions within days to weeks of initiation of therapy. The intravenous administration of riboflavin, which may be needed in debilitated patients or in those with serious disorders of the gastrointestinal tract, is greatly restricted by its limited solubility in aqueous solution.

Riboflavin in large doses has been utilized to treat several rare inborn errors of metabolism, including congenital methemoglobinemia, pyruvate kinase deficiency, glutaryl-CoA dehydrogenase deficiency, and defects of β-oxidation. In some instances both clinical improvement and correction of the biochemical lesions have occurred.

Toxicity

Riboflavin, FMN, and FAD are completely free of any known toxicity.

Dutta P, Pinto, J, Rivlin R: Antimalarial effects of riboflavin deficiency. Lancet 2:1040, 1985. *New hypothesis that agents interfering with riboflavin metabolism have antimalarial effects.*

Massey V, Williams CH (eds.): Flavins and Flavoproteins. Seventh International Symposium. North Holland, NY, Elsevier, 1983, 890 pp. *Volume covering the latest conference proceedings of subjects related to biochemistry, chemistry, and medical aspects of riboflavin and its coenzyme derivatives.*

Pinto JT, Huang YP, Rivlin RS: Mechanisms underlying the differential effects of ethanol upon the bioavailability of riboflavin and flavin adenine dinucleotide. J Clin Invest 79:1343, 1987. *New study showing how alcohol causes riboflavin deficiency.*

Rivlin RS: Riboflavin. In Olson RE (ed.): Present Knowledge in Nutrition. 5th ed. Washington DC, The Nutrition Foundation, 1984, pp 285–302. *Discussion of the physiology, sources, functions, and metabolic roles of riboflavin.*

NIACIN

Structure and Biochemical Function

The term niacin is used here to refer to two compounds, nicotinic acid and nicotinamide, and other biologically active pyridine derivatives, as shown in Figure 217–3. The term niacin is sometimes restricted to nicotinic acid only. Niacin is a precursor of two coenzymes, nicotinamide adenine dinucleotide (NAD) and nicotinamide adenine dinucleotide phos-

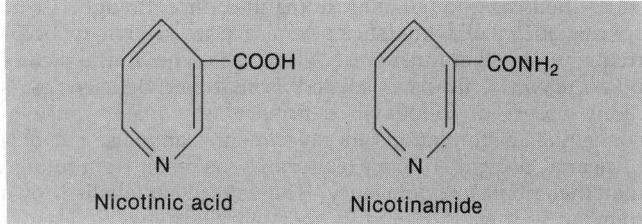

FIGURE 217–3. Structural formulae of nicotinic acid and nicotinamide.

phate (NADP), which function in a wide number of oxidation and reduction reactions. NAD and NADP are involved in glycolysis, pyruvate metabolism, pentose biosynthesis, and lipid, amino acid, protein, and purine metabolism. These coenzymes also have other functions, some of which are discussed in the following paragraphs. Niacin is stable both to light and to heat.

Normal Physiology

Niacin given by itself appears to be nearly completely absorbed by diffusion from the stomach and small intestine in amounts as high as 3 grams. When present in a bound form in certain foods such as corn, however, niacin has only limited bioavailability. A portion of dietary niacin occurs in a bound form (as niacinogen) in cereal grains but remains biologically available. Normally, approximately 1.5 per cent of dietary tryptophan is converted to niacin. The efficiency of this conversion is regulated by a number of hormonal and nutritional factors and is greater under conditions of niacin deficiency. Vitamin B_6 is required for this conversion. Niacin is present in all cells, and only small amounts can be stored in the body. Both nicotinic acid and nicotinamide, as well as certain of their metabolites, particularly N-methylnicotinamide and 2-pyridone, are excreted in urine.

Requirements and Dietary Sources

The RDA for niacin in adult males is 16 to 19 mg and in adult females, 13 to 14 mg, depending upon age, with an additional 2 mg recommended for pregnancy and 5 mg for lactation. The allowance is expressed in terms of niacin equivalents, because approximately 60 mg of dietary tryptophan are needed to form 1 mg of niacin. Proteins of animal origin such as meat, milk, and eggs have a relatively high tryptophan content and therefore are good sources of endogenously generated niacin. Vegetable proteins also supply tryptophan, but the concentration is lower than in animal proteins. Diets dependent heavily upon corn are a particular problem because not only is the tryptophan content low but also the availability of niacin is poor. Niacin from wheat sources also has limited bioavailability. Pyridoxine deficiency increases the dietary requirement for niacin, because it is required for the biosynthesis of niacin from tryptophan.

Deficiency

PATHOGENESIS. Niacin deficiency may develop because of a number of factors. First, dietary deficiency develops when corn is the major staple of the diet. Pellagra caused by consumption of corn was once very common in parts of the United States but fortunately has largely disappeared at the present time. Secondly, niacin deficiency may arise as a result of alcoholism, a condition in which diet is often poor and erratic. It is likely that in prolonged alcoholism, particularly in the presence of other nutrient deficiencies, the absorption and metabolism of niacin may be impaired. In addition, certain drugs interfere with niacin metabolism to a clinically significant degree, the best known of which is isonicotinic acid hydrazine (INH). The neurologic symptoms occurring with INH treatment can be ameliorated by administration of pyridoxine. Certain anticancer drugs, particularly 6-mercap-

topurine, may produce niacin deficiency. In the rare inborn error of Hartnup's disease, pellagra may develop because of a defect in the intestinal and renal tubular transport of tryptophan and of several other amino acids (Ch. 84). Malnourished patients with the malignant carcinoid syndrome have been known rarely to exhibit manifestations of pellagra because of diversion of dietary tryptophan to serotonin (Ch. 243). Under certain conditions, excess leucine in the diet produces a deficiency by inhibiting the conversion of tryptophan to niacin.

CLINICAL FEATURES. In the early stages of niacin deficiency, clinical findings may be vague and nondiagnostic. Patients often complain of decreased appetite, loss of weight, abdominal aching and discomfort, weakness, irritability, inability to concentrate, and other nonspecific indications of illness. As the deficiency progresses, there may be epithelial changes that include glossitis, stomatitis, soreness and pain in the mouth (particularly the tongue), and eventually development of the characteristic skin lesions. These lesions, when well established, are dark, scaling, and cracking and occur prominently over the areas of skin that are exposed to sunlight, frequently leaving a sharp line of demarcation at the unexposed skin surfaces, although these may be affected also. The lesion may resemble a necklace and is described as Casal's necklace (see Color plate 8B and C).

In addition to the dermatitis, patients with the advanced form of niacin deficiency, that is, pellagra, have diarrhea and dementia. The diarrhea is often severe and intractable and may have a component of malabsorption that appears to be related to villous atrophy. The latter likely results from the long period of minimal food intake. Neuropsychiatric manifestations are mild at first but in advanced cases may progress to confusion, disorientation, seizures, hallucinations, and frank psychosis. Death may result in very advanced cases, usually preceded by major confusional states. Pellagra is popularly known for the four D's: dermatitis, diarrhea, dementia, and death.

Niacin deficiency secondary to drugs is generally mild and often unrecognized by clinicians. The consequences of drug-induced deficiencies of niacin and of other vitamins are much greater in the presence of a marginal or frankly deficient diet.

DIAGNOSIS. The diagnosis of advanced deficiency can often be made on clinical grounds alone if the patient exhibits the classic findings. Such patients are very unusual, however. In the early stages of the illness or in the absence of all the classic features, diagnosis may be difficult and is often missed without a high index of suspicion. Blood concentrations of NAD and NADP are reduced but may not be indicative of niacin deficiency, because reduced levels also occur in other severe, constitutional illnesses that are unrelated to niacin status. Attention has therefore turned to assay of urinary metabolites of niacin as indices of niacin nutriture. The most widely used is N-methylnicotinamide. Low urinary levels are interpreted as indicative of niacin deficiency. The excretion of another metabolite, 2-pyridone, is less widely used and requires a cumbersome assay. Some investigators have considered the ratio of these two metabolites in urine to be the most accurate index of niacin nutriture. Urinary metabolites can now be measured accurately by high performance liquid chromatography (HPLC).

TREATMENT. The treatment of advanced pellagra has been accomplished satisfactorily by administering large oral doses (approximately 50 to 150 mg) of niacin as nicotinamide (the form present in most commercial vitamin formulations). The exact dose given is somewhat empirical. The therapeutic response is often dramatic, and patients may show marked improvement within several days after the start of therapy. Maintenance levels are then given together with dietary repletion. Nicotinamide is usually well tolerated.

Other therapeutic applications of niacin include its use as nicotinic acid in the control of elevated serum cholesterol and triglyceride levels in daily doses of 3 grams or more (Ch. 183). Nicotinic acid may be useful in treating patients of types II, IV, and V hyperlipoproteinemia. The mechanism of the therapeutic effect on lipid metabolism is not known, and this property is not shared by nicotinamide. With nicotinic acid treatment, HDL levels rise because of a slight decrease in synthetic rate with a large decrease in degradative rate. Because of the toxicity of nicotinic acid at high doses, treatment with this agent is generally reserved for patients with severe lipid abnormalities.

Doses in the range of those used to treat pellagra are also needed to treat niacin deficiency in Hartnup's disease and in the carcinoid syndrome. Massive doses of niacin have not proven useful in the treatment of schizophrenia and other psychiatric disorders, despite the claims of food faddists and so-called "orthomolecular" therapists.

Toxicity

At the doses of nicotinamide used to treat niacin deficiency (described previously) there is little if any toxicity. When nicotinic acid in doses of 3 grams or more is used in the treatment of a lipid disorder, the most common side effect observed is flushing of the face due to vascular dilatation. Other common side effects of nicotinic acid may include dryness, itching and increased pigmentation of the skin, and abdominal pain. Rarely, hepatotoxicity, hyperuricemia, and worsening of peptic ulcer and glucose tolerance have been observed. The abnormalities in liver function may be severe, but both biochemical and histologic findings regress with discontinuation of nicotinic acid.

Henderson LaVM: Niacin. In Darby WJ, Broquist HP, Olson RE (eds.): Annual Review of Nutrition. Vol. 3. Palo Alto, Annual Reviews Inc, 1983, pp 289–307. *This review covers transport, metabolism, and physiologic and pharmacologic effects of niacin.*
Moran JR, Greene HL: The B vitamins and vitamin C in human nutrition. II. "Conditional" B vitamins and vitamin C. Am J Dis Child 133:308, 1979. *Discussion of physiology, metabolic disorders, and toxicity of niacin.*
Narasinga Rao BS, Gopalan C: Niacin. In Olson RE (ed.): Present Knowledge in Nutrition. 5th ed. Washington DC, The Nutrition Foundation, 1984, pp 318–331. *Review stressing metabolism, function, pathogenesis of deficiency, and therapeutic uses of niacin.*

VITAMIN B₆ (PYRIDOXINE)
Structure and Biochemical Function

The term vitamin B_6, or pyridoxine, is used to refer to three closely interrelated compounds, pyridoxine, pyridoxamine, and pyridoxal, together with their phosphate derivatives. Of all these compounds, pyridoxal-5-phosphate (Fig. 217–4) is the most important, because it constitutes the major coenzyme involved in the intermediary metabolism of amino acids, including aminotransferases, decarboxylases, racemases, and synthetases. Pyridoxal phosphate is also involved in biosynthesis of heme and sphingosine. In certain circumstances, pyridoxamine phosphate can also fulfill a coenzyme function. Pyridoxine is the major dietary source found in plants, whereas pyridoxal and pyridoxamine constitute the major forms in foods from animal sources. Pyridoxine is stable in

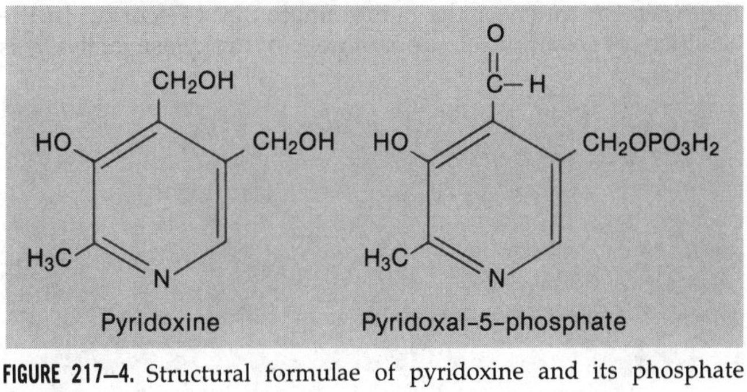

FIGURE 217–4. Structural formulae of pyridoxine and its phosphate derivative.

acid solutions in the absence of light but is highly light-sensitive in acid or neutral solutions. Pyridoxal and pyridoxamine are destroyed at high temperatures, particularly by autoclaving.

Normal Physiology

Dietary pyridoxine and related compounds are absorbed from the upper gastrointestinal tract, probably by simple diffusion. The vitamin is widely distributed in the body; muscle constitutes an important storage organ, in which it is bound to phosphorylase a, thus serving to stabilize the enzyme molecule. The various forms of pyridoxine are readily interconverted to one another by the liver. Only very small amounts of dietary pyridoxine are converted to pyridoxal phosphate. In urine, pyridoxine, pyridoxal, and pyridoxamine can all be detected but at low concentrations; the major metabolite of pyridoxine, 4-pyridoxic acid, is found in urine in high concentrations, particularly in alcoholic patients.

Thyroid hormones reduce the concentrations of vitamin B_6 in various tissues, and increased sensitivity to insulin is demonstrable during B_6 deficiency.

Requirements and Dietary Sources

The RDA for vitamin B_6 is 2.2 mg per day for adult males and 2.0 mg per day for adult females, regardless of age, with a 0.5 to 0.6 mg per day increase during pregnancy and lactation. The requirement for vitamin B_6 is greater with a higher protein intake.

Vitamin B_6 is widely distributed in the food supply and can be derived from both plants and animals. Sources of vitamin B_6 are similar to those of other B vitamins and include liver, meat, wheat, nuts, beans and other vegetables, fruits, and cereals. Considerable losses occur during prolonged cooking, particularly pressure cooking. The bioavailability of vitamin B_6 from dietary sources varies widely depending upon storage, processing, and composition of food.

Deficiency

PATHOGENESIS. Dietary deficiency of pyridoxine may occur occasionally despite its widespread sources in the food supply. Deficiency of pyridoxine is recognized increasingly as a consequence of prolonged therapy with certain medications. Foremost among these drugs is isoniazid, which complexes with pyridoxal phosphate to a clinically significant degree. Individuals with the genetic trait of inactivating isoniazid at a slow rate are particularly susceptible to B_6 deficiency from this drug. Isoniazid induces peripheral neuritis and diarrhea in adult patients; in children it produces anemia and seizures that can be prevented by coincident administration of pyridoxine. Cycloserine, another drug widely used for tuberculosis, is also a vitamin B_6 antagonist. With the widespread use of penicillamine for the treatment of rheumatoid arthritis, its B_6-antagonistic properties are of increasing clinical importance. Pyridoxine deficiency occurs frequently in alcoholism in association with deficiencies of other vitamins, particularly folic acid. The increased urinary excretion of certain tryptophan metabolites, particularly xanthurenic acid, in women treated with oral contraceptives has been interpreted as indicating vitamin B_6 deficiency because B_6 is needed for conversion of tryptophan to niacin. L-dopa, used for Parkinson's disease, may also cause B_6 deficiency over a prolonged period of time.

CLINICAL FEATURES. Deficiency of vitamin B_6 is not thought to produce a characteristic syndrome. As with deficiencies of other B vitamins, dermatitis, glossitis, cheilosis, and stomatitis may be manifestations of pyridoxine deficiency. Markedly deficient patients may have irritability, weakness, depression, dizziness, peripheral neuropathy, and seizures. As noted previously, deficiency in infants and children is typically characterized by diarrhea, anemia, and seizures. The rapidity with which drug-induced deficiency of B_6 occurs depends upon the adequacy of the patient's diet as well as the dosage and duration of drug therapy. Chronic vitamin B_6 deficiency also leads to secondary hyperoxaluria, increasing the risk of kidney stone formation (Ch. 90).

In addition to the deficiency syndromes of vitamin B_6 caused by diet or drugs or both, there is a group of disorders in which the affected patients do not display manifestations of deficiency, yet require pharmacologic doses of this vitamin for adequate treatment. These disorders are known as dependency syndromes and include such diverse entities as pyridoxine-dependent convulsions, pyridoxine-responsive anemia, homocystinuria caused by cystathionine synthetase deficiency, cystathioninuria, xanthurenic aciduria, and some cases of primary hyperoxaluria.

Of these, pyridoxine-responsive anemia requires special mention because it is often confused with iron-deficient anemia; both disorders are characterized by hypochromic, microcytic red cells. In the pyridoxine-responsive anemia, however, serum iron is elevated with an increase in saturation of transferrin and an increase in iron absorption from the intestinal tract. There is evidence of iron overload, with hemosiderin deposits in bone marrow, liver, and other organs. Many patients have hepatosplenomegaly, and a hemolytic component may contribute to the anemia. It is important to differentiate this syndrome from iron-deficient anemia, because in the former inadvertent administration of iron worsens pyridoxine-responsive anemia. The blood count rises satisfactorily in response to pharmacologic doses of vitamin B_6. In patients with cystathionine synthetase deficiency, the greatly elevated serum concentrations of homocysteine and methionine can be normalized with doses of pyridoxine of several hundred milligrams per day.

DIAGNOSIS. The diagnosis of pyridoxine deficiency can be made by direct assay of vitamin B_6 in blood (normal levels generally are greater than 50 ng per milliliter) or by determining the urinary excretion of the main metabolite of pyridoxine, 4-pyridoxic acid. The excretion of less than 1.0 mg per day of this compound is generally considered suggestive of deficiency. Less frequently, the excretion of pyridoxine in urine is also determined. Functional enzyme assays, similar to those in use for diagnosing thiamin and riboflavin deficiencies, have also been developed for vitamin B_6 using aspartate aminotransferase or alanine aminotransferase in erythrocyte hemolysates. Enzyme activity is determined with and without the addition of pyridoxal phosphate in vitro. When activity coefficients (as defined previously) are greater than 1.5 for aspartate aminotransferase and 1.2 for alanine aminotransferase, they are considered to be indicative of pyridoxine deficiency. These procedures have generally supplanted the tryptophan load test, in which the increased excretion of xanthurenic acid is taken as an index of B_6 nutriture. Probably the most widely accepted index of vitamin B_6 nutriture at present is the direct measurement of pyridoxal phosphate concentrations in blood.

TREATMENT. Dietary deficiency of pyridoxine can be treated satisfactorily with oral doses in the general range of 2 to 10 mg per day; doses of 10 to 20 mg per day may be needed in pregnancy. Pyridoxine deficiency occurring in association with specific drugs that inhibit pyridoxine metabolism, such as isoniazid, cycloserine, and penicillamine, requires higher doses, perhaps up to 100 mg per day, to ameliorate peripheral neuropathy. Rather than administer B_6 when symptoms develop, it is much more effective to prevent these side effects by administering vitamin B_6 when therapy with a B_6-antagonizing drug is initiated and particularly when a prolonged course of treatment is anticipated. Since iatrogenic vitamin B_6 deficiency is entirely preventable, B_6 is now routinely prescribed for patients receiving INH. Treatment with high doses of vitamin B_6 is contraindicated in patients receiving L-dopa, however, as it may interfere with the efficacy of the drug.

Treatment of a pyridoxine-dependency syndrome requires much higher doses of B_6, and amounts in the range of 300 to 500 mg per day generally have been prescribed. The possible effectiveness of pyridoxine in the management of the carpal-tunnel syndrome and premenstrual tension is controversial. In some women on contraceptive steroids, vitamin B_6 has appeared to benefit depression. Pyridoxine is regarded as ineffective in treating schizophrenia, autism, and childhood hyperactivity, as well as peripheral neuropathies in which there is no known B_6 deficiency, such as in diabetes.

Toxicity

A sensory neuropathy has been described in a small number of patients receiving 2 grams or more of pyridoxine per day, and some subjects have had symptoms on only 500 mg per day. This potentially important finding requires confirmation and extension. At the present time, there are probably no indications for treatment of any disorder, even a pyridoxine-dependency syndrome, with doses of this magnitude. Thus, pyridoxine appears to be safe when prescribed in the appropriate milligram amounts needed to correct deficiency and to treat dependency states.

Henderson LM: Vitamin B_6. In Olson RE (ed.): Present Knowledge in Nutrition. 5th ed. Washington DC, The Nutrition Foundation, 1984, pp 303–317. *Review of B_6 stressing absorption, transport, and human requirements.*
Reynolds RD, Leklem JE: Vitamin B_6: Its Role in Health and Disease. New York, Alan R. Liss, 1986, 526 pp. *Volume covering the proceedings of a conference on this vitamin in nutrition and metabolism.*
Schaumburg H, Kaplan J, Winderbank A, et al.: Sensory neuropathy from pyridoxine abuse. A new megavitamin syndomre. N Engl J Med 309:445, 1983. *New description of B_6 toxicity.*
Sturman JA, Rivlin RS: Pathogenesis of brain dysfunction in deficiency of thiamine, riboflavin, pantothenic acid, or vitamin B_6. In Gaull GE (ed.): Biology of Brain Dysfunction. Vol. 3. New York, Plenum Press, 1975, pp 425–475. *Discussion of the pyridoxine-dependent syndromes.*

VITAMIN B_{12} (COBALAMIN)

The structure, function, pathophysiology, and therapeutic use of vitamin B_{12} are discussed in Ch. 136 in association with the megaloblastic anemias.

VITAMIN C (ASCORBIC ACID)
Structure and Biochemical Function

Ascorbic acid resembles glucose in having several polyhydroxyl groups adjacent to one another (Fig. 217–5). Ascorbic acid can be oxidized to dehydro-L-ascorbic acid, which is also biologically active, and can be generated from the latter by reacting with reduced glutathione.

Ascorbic acid participates in oxidation-reduction reactions and in hydrogen ion transfer. This vitamin is a powerful reducing agent or anti-oxidant, particularly in lipid and vitamin metabolism, and is especially important in preventing oxidation of tetrahydrofolate. In addition, ascorbic acid enhances the intestinal absorption of nonheme iron. This vitamin is required in collagen metabolism, specifically for the synthesis of chondroitin sulfate and of hydroxyproline from proline. Defects in collagen biosynthesis are believed to be the basis for much of the symptomatology of scurvy. In the absence of vitamin C, dopamine-β-hydroxylase activity is

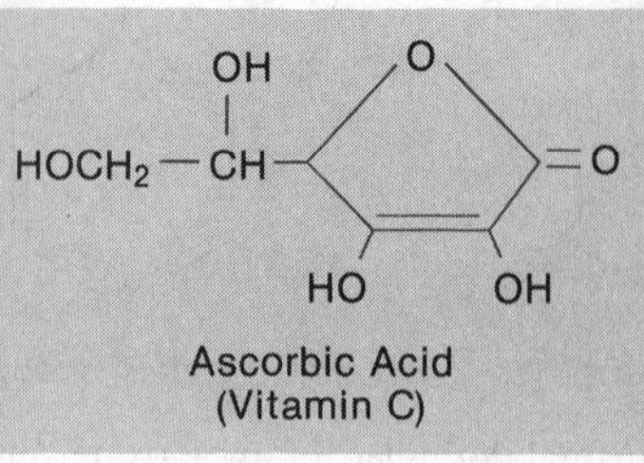

FIGURE 217–5. Structural formula of ascorbic acid.

reduced, impairing the biosynthesis of neurotransmitters. Ascorbic acid is also involved in carnitine biosynthesis, tyrosine metabolism, wound healing, and immune function and is a component of drug-metabolizing enzyme systems.

Prolonged storage or excessive cooking diminishes the biologic activity of ascorbic acid. This highly water-soluble vitamin is also destroyed by oxidation, particularly by exposure to air in the presence of copper ion and an alkaline medium.

Normal Physiology

Ascorbic acid is absorbed by a limited-capacity mechanism in the distal small intestine. As dietary intake of ascorbic acid increases, a progressively smaller proportion is absorbed, that is, about 95 per cent at 100 mg, 75 per cent at 1 gram, but only 20 per cent at 5 grams. Within the usual range of dietary ascorbic acid intake of 10 to 130 mg per day, the plasma level is proportional to the amount ingested. Ingestion of massive amounts of ascorbic acid has only a very small effect upon elevating plasma levels of this vitamin. As the dietary intake increases further, however, the low renal threshold for excretion assures that excess plasma levels of ascorbic acid are promptly excreted. Another mechanism protecting against excessive accumulation of ascorbic acid is the microsomal enzyme NADPH monodehydro-ascorbate transhydrogenase, which is induced by its substrate, ascorbic acid; in response to a large dietary load of ascorbic acid, degradative capacity is rapidly and substantially increased.

The body pool of ascorbic acid in adult males consuming about 80 mg per day is estimated to be approximately 1500 mg, and the rate of catabolism is about 3 per cent of the pool size per day. Increasing the dietary intake of ascorbic acid to more than 80 mg per day seems not to increase significantly the saturation of tissues with this vitamin. Similar to most B vitamins, the storage capacity for vitamin C is limited. Urinary excretion is in the form of ascorbic acid and dehydro-L-ascorbic acid, as well as several metabolites, including a sulfated derivative, ascorbate-2-sulfate, and oxalic acid.

Requirements and Dietary Sources

The RDA for ascorbic acid is 60 mg per day for all healthy adult males and females regardless of age. This allowance is generally regarded as quite generous inasmuch as 10 mg per day prevents scurvy. As noted, amounts greatly in excess of the RDA do not increase tissue stores significantly. The dietary allowance is increased by 20 mg per day during pregnancy and 40 mg per day during lactation. Human milk contains 30 to 55 mg per liter. It is especially important to maintain an adequate intake of ascorbic acid during lactation, because the vitamin concentration in milk is closely dependent upon dietary intake.

Serum ascorbic acid levels are lowered in smokers, possibly as a result of accelerated metabolism or diminished intake, and in users of oral contraceptive drugs, but the implications of these findings are unclear. The decreases are quantitatively small and can be corrected with a modest increase in consumption of ascorbic acid from dietary sources (about 40 mg for smokers). Patients who are exposed to cold or heat stress or who are febrile, undergoing surgery, or subjected to trauma have increased requirements for vitamin C. Patients receiving parenteral nutrition have higher requirements because of urinary losses.

The best dietary sources of ascorbic acid appear to be citrus fruits and green vegetables, especially broccoli, green peppers, tomatoes, cabbage, oranges, grapefruits, and lemons. Care must be taken during food preparation in order to avoid losses of the vitamin. Much smaller amounts are contained in milk, meats, and cereals. As noted above, ascorbic acid is heat-sensitive and is destroyed by alkali. Some decreased vitamin content is also observed with prolonged storage.

Deficiency

PATHOGENESIS. Urban poor, particularly the elderly, are at increased risk for dietary deficiency of ascorbic acid, in large measure because economic deprivation prevents them from obtaining the richest sources, namely citrus fruits, leafy vegetables, and tomatoes.

An increasingly important cause of ascorbic acid deficiency is food faddism and bizarre nutritional practices. The strict macrobiotic diet may lead to scurvy, particularly with pressure cooking of food items that have little ascorbic acid to begin with. Elderly individuals following a "tea and toast" diet are vulnerable to a number of deficiencies, particularly of ascorbic acid, as these sources are grossly inadequate. Children develop scurvy when fed unsupplemented cow's milk for the first year of life. Vitamin C deficiency progressing to scurvy is common in chronic alcoholics, probably because the diet is notably deficient in vitamin C–containing food items. Vitamin C deficiency, however, is not generally as prevalent as deficiencies of B vitamins in chronic alcoholism.

CLINICAL FEATURES. In the early stages of deficiency, symptoms and signs may be fairly nonspecific and include general malaise, lethargy, and weakness. As the disease progresses, probably one to three months after onset, patients may complain of dyspnea and pain in bones and joints, due predominantly to hemorrhages below the periosteum. Perifollicular hemorrhages, particularly about hair follicles, are indicative of advanced deficiency. Petechiae often are prominent and may appear over the arms after application of a sphygmomanometer. This finding is known as the Rumpel-Leed test. With progressive vitamin C depletion, there are ecchymoses and purpura initially at areas of trauma, irritation, or pressure. Joints, muscles, and subcutaneous tissues may become sites of hemorrhage. Swollen, bleeding gums are characteristic manifestations of advanced deficiency. Pallor and anemia may be the result of prolonged bleeding or associated folic acid deficiency, with which scurvy commonly occurs. In children, disturbances of growth occur, and teeth, bones, blood vessels, and other collagen-rich structures develop abnormally. Preformed teeth may become loose and fall out because of alveolar bone resorption.

Wounds heal poorly, and previously healed wounds may open up again. In very advanced deficiency, edema, oliguria, and neuropathy are prominent. Should intracerebral bleeding occur, serious neurologic sequelae and even death may result.

DIAGNOSIS. The diagnosis of advanced scurvy is often made on clinical grounds alone because the skin changes may be quite characteristic. Capillary fragility is commonly abnormal. X-rays are used in demonstrating subperiosteal elevation, disturbances of calcification of the cartilage matrix, fractures and dislocations, ground glass appearance of the cortex, alveolar bone resorption, and other findings.

Plasma ascorbic acid levels are greatly reduced in scurvy, usually to 0.1 mg per deciliter or lower. Some depression of plasma ascorbic acid levels occurs, however, in a variety of other conditions, including cigarette smoking, tuberculosis, rheumatic fever, many chronic disorders, and in some women using oral contraceptive drugs. These conditions must be considered when a low ascorbic acid level is detected.

The assay of ascorbic acid in serum or plasma can be accomplished with titrimetric, spectrophotometric, or fluorometric methods. Some laboratories prefer to make the diagnosis of scurvy by assay of platelet ascorbic acid.

TREATMENT. As little as 10 mg per day of ascorbic acid can completely prevent the clinical manifestations of scurvy. Even far-advanced cases of scurvy respond rapidly to ascorbic acid in the range of 100 to 200 mg per day. Marked improvement is to be expected within several days. Patients should also be instructed in the importance of a proper diet to prevent further recurrences.

Patients with rare inborn errors of metabolism, including tyrosinemia, osteogenesis imperfecta, and Chédiak-Higashi syndrome, have had some apparent benefit from the use of ascorbic acid in the range of 50 to 200 mg per day. Certain forms of the Ehlers-Danlos syndrome are the only disorders in which pharmacologic doses (4 grams) have been reported to be effective.

Special mention must be made of two conditions in which the use of megadoses of ascorbic acid has attracted wide attention: the common cold and advanced cancer. Many studies have been performed on the possible benefits of 2 grams and higher per day of ascorbic acid on the prevention of colds and on the alleviation of symptoms once they develop. On balance, the predominance of evidence favors the view that while some individuals may receive slight benefit in terms of symptoms, probably as a result of a mild antihistamine action of ascorbic acid, no consistent, reproducible improvement occurs in the frequency, duration, or severity of illness in the great majority of cases.

Vitamin C at a dose level of approximately 0.5 to 3 grams per day has been used to acidify the urine in cases of refractory urinary tract infections. Ascorbic acid is only a weak acidifying agent, and its efficacy under these circumstances is difficult to evaluate.

Ascorbic acid in amounts ordinarily contained in food may be useful in facilitating the intestinal absorption of nonheme iron. To be effective, the ascorbic acid and the iron sources must be consumed together. As little as 100 ml of orange juice, which contains 40 to 50 mg of ascorbic acid, has been reported to increase the absorption of nonheme iron more than three-fold.

With respect to advanced cancer, there is some theoretical basis for the view that maintenance of immune function may depend upon the adequacy of vitamin C nutriture, as may wound healing, collagen formation, and cytotoxicity of a number of chemotherapeutic drugs. Nevertheless, treatment of colon cancer patients with megadoses of vitamin C after chemotherapy and radiation has been ineffective when evaluated in an objective manner. The use of vitamin C under no circumstances should replace established methods of treating cancer with chemotherapy, surgery, or radiation.

A potentially useful application of ascorbic acid lies in its ability to inhibit the conversion of nitrites and secondary amines to the carcinogenic nitrosoamines in vitro, and, under certain circumstances, in vivo. Whether ascorbic acid can achieve this effect in vivo under ordinary circumstances of food consumption is important to determine. It is of interest that foods high in vitamin C are associated with reduced risk of gastric and esophageal cancer.

Toxicity

At the dose range of approximately 1 gram per day and higher there is potential for toxicity. There is great variability among individuals in regard to susceptibility to the side effects of megadoses of ascorbic acid and the doses necessary to cause toxicity. In the intestinal tract, large doses (2 grams and higher) of ascorbic acid may produce pain, discomfort, and an osmotic diarrhea. Doses of ascorbic acid above 1 gram give a false-negative guaiac test for blood, thereby obscuring recognition of occult bleeding. Urine tests for glucose also may be misleading when very large doses of ascorbic acid are ingested, producing a false-negative glucose oxidase reaction (Tes-Tape) and false-positive copper-reduction reaction (Clinitest), and making urine strips more difficult to read. At daily doses of 3 grams and higher, automated measurements of alanine aminotransferase, lactate dehydrogenase, and uric acid may be affected.

As oxalate is a degradative product of ascorbic acid, large amounts of this vitamin will be expected to increase renal excretion of oxalate, posing the potential risk of oxalate stones in susceptible individuals. The increase in oxalate excretion is small in magnitude, however, and in most cases still falls within the normal range. There is recent evidence that patients with recurrent formation of kidney stones exhibit increased production and urinary excretion of oxalate following a 2-gram load of ascorbic acid. Uricosuria and uric acid stones are also believed to occur with increased frequency. Nevertheless, the frequency of kidney stone formation in users of megadose ascorbic acid is not known at present.

There is a likelihood of exacerbating systemic acidosis in those disorders with failure of urinary acidification, such as chronic renal disease and renal tubular acidosis. Certain patients with diminished glucose-6-phosphate dehydrogenase activity may be at increased risk for hemolytic episodes with megadose ascorbic acid therapy. Scurvy has been reported in several infants of mothers who consumed large amounts of ascorbic acid during pregnancy, presumably as a result of a dependency state developing in the infant. Therefore, it is probably not advisable to treat pregnant women with large doses of vitamin C. There is some concern that ascorbic acid, which increases intestinal absorption of iron, may also increase absorption of heavy metals such as lead and mercury and accelerate the development of toxicity from these metals.

Burns, JJ, Rivers JM, Machlin LJ (eds.): Vitamin C. New York, New York Academy of Sciences, in press. *Proceedings of a recent symposium on advances in vitamin C metabolism.*

Levine M: New concepts in the biology and biochemistry of ascorbic acid. N Engl J Med 314:892, 1986. *Important update of biochemistry, physiology, and nutrition applications of vitamin C.*

Sauberlich HE: Ascorbic acid. In Olson RE (ed.): Present Knowledge in Nutrition. 5th ed. Washington DC, The Nutrition Foundation, 1984, pp 260–272. *Comprehensive discussion of ascorbic acid in nutrition and medicine.*

Wooliscroft JO: Megavitamins: Fact and fancy. DM 29(5):1, 1983. *Discussion of the hazards of misuse of large doses of vitamin C and other vitamins.*

VITAMIN A
Structure and Biochemical Function

Vitamin A refers to retinol, although the term is often used loosely to indicate all related compounds (Fig. 217–6). The term retinoids has been used to designate all the natural and synthetic isomers and derivatives of vitamin A. Retinol is oxidized to vitamin A aldehyde (retinal), which is critical to

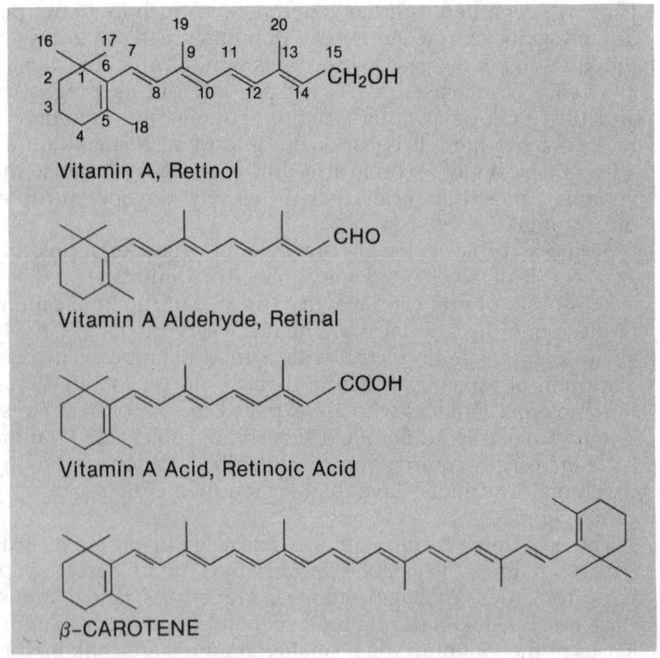

FIGURE 217–6. Structural formulae of retinol, retinal, retinoic acid, and β-carotene.

vision. Retinoic acid (vitamin A acid) is the major oxidative metabolite of retinol. Retinoic acid can fulfill the growth-promoting and epithelium-differentiating roles of retinol but cannot fully maintain its function in reproduction, nor can retinoic acid fulfill the functions of retinal in vision. Carotenoids are larger precursor molecules that undergo cleavage to yield retinal. The most important of the more than 30 carotenoids with pro-vitamin A activity is β-carotene (Fig. 217–6).

Of the various metabolic roles of vitamin A, the best understood is the visual process. Retinal is the prosthetic group of all the visual pigments that capture light. The human retina contains four kinds of visual pigments: rhodopsin in rods and three iodopsins in cones. In the dark-adapted retina, rhodopsin is activated by photons of light. This event initiates the visual cycle, during which retinal changes its conformation from a cis to a trans isomer, and other conformational changes occur in the protein. During dark adaptation, these processes are reversed and rhodopsin is regenerated. In view of the absolute requirement for retinal, it is not surprising that loss of highly sensitive night vision is an early symptom of vitamin A deficiency. Vitamin A probably serves additional roles in the normal functioning of the retina.

The mechanism of action of vitamin A in growth and differentiation is not known. One hypothesis is that vitamin A is similar to steroid hormones in influencing events in the genome following attachment to specific cellular binding proteins. An alternative hypothesis is that vitamin A participates in the synthesis of glycoproteins, which in turn mediate metabolic events. The striking effects of vitamin A upon differentiation, particularly of epithelial tissues, underlie the current concept that this vitamin and its derivatives may possibly have a role in the prevention of certain cancers, particularly of epithelial origin.

Retinol is fat soluble, sensitive to acid and heat, and is rapidly oxidized upon exposure to light and oxygen. Beta-carotene is relatively less heat-sensitive than retinol.

Normal Physiology

Foods containing retinol or carotenoids are digested by gastric pepsin and intestinal enzymes, and then both forms are absorbed by the intestinal mucosa. About 80 to 90 per cent of dietary vitamin A is absorbed. The rate of absorption of dietary β-carotene is much slower, and only 40 to 60 per cent is absorbed. Within the intestinal mucosa, β-carotene is cleaved to two molecules of retinal, which are then reduced to retinol. The retinol generated from β-carotene, as well as that absorbed directly, is esterified with palmitic acid. The retinyl esters formed are incorporated into chylomicra and transported via lymph to the general circulation, where the triglycerides in the chylomicra are degraded by lipoprotein lipase. The smaller chylomicra remnants remaining are then cleared by the liver, the major storage organ for vitamin A, which contains approximately 90 per cent of the total body reserves. Retinyl esters, mostly in the form of retinyl palmitate, are stored in the liver as a complex; hydrolysis of the retinyl esters in the liver generates retinol, which binds to a specific apo-retinol binding protein (RBP). The holo-RBP is secreted into the plasma, where it forms a 1:1 molar complex with prealbumin, a tetrameric serum protein that also binds thyroxine and triiodothyronine. In recognition of both roles, this protein is now called transthyretin.

Cell surfaces recognize the RBP-retinol complex rather than retinol, and once inside the cell, all trans-retinol binds to a specific protein, cellular retinol binding protein (CRBP). CRBP may deliver retinol to intranuclear binding sites that mediate genomic expression and/or transport retinol across cellular membranes. CRBP concentrations are increased in certain animal and human tumors. A cellular retinoic acid binding protein (CRABP) has also been detected in a number of

neonatal tissues and epithelial tumors that are sensitive to retinoic acid therapeutically.

In vitamin A deficiency, total plasma RBP levels fall to about half their normal levels and consist primarily of apo-RBP. At the same time, the liver concentration of apo-RBP is greatly increased. With vitamin A repletion, the liver apo-RBP becomes saturated, and levels of holo-RBP begin to rise in blood.

The degradative metabolism of retinol and its derivatives proceeds by a series of chain-shortening steps to yield a group of compounds of little if any intrinsic biologic activity. These compounds can be detected in urine but have not been generally utilized diagnostically to characterize vitamin A nutriture.

Requirements and Dietary Sources

The RDA for vitamin A is currently 1000 μg of retinol equivalents (RE) for adult males and 800 μg for adult females. One RE is defined as 1 μg retinol or 6 μg β-carotene. The allowances are calculated in this fashion because the overall utilization of β-carotene is only about one sixth that of retinol, as a result of the relative inefficiency with which β-carotene is absorbed and converted to vitamin A.

Vitamin A allowances were formerly expressed in terms of international units (IU), and this nomenclature still appears on most commercial vitamin bottles. One retinol equivalent is equal to 3.33 IU retinol and 10 IU β-carotene. The RDA for vitamin A expressed in terms of IU is 5000 for adult males and 4000 for adult females. These figures are based upon the estimate that the U.S. diet contains approximately equal amounts of β-carotene (2500 IU = 250 RE, for males) and retinol (2500 IU = 750 RE, for males).

Beta-carotene is derived predominantly from plant sources, including vegetables such as carrots and sweet potatoes, leafy green vegetables, and some fruits. Palm oil is a particularly rich source of carotenes. Preformed vitamin A is derived almost exclusively from animal sources. Liver obviously is the richest source, followed by kidney, milk and milk products, and eggs. Fish liver oils have unusually high concentrations of vitamin A.

Deficiency

PATHOGENESIS. Vitamin A deficiency is a very common problem world wide, particularly in developing countries, as a consequence of famine or shortages of vitamin A–rich foods. The ocular manifestations of vitamin A deficiency are such a serious problem that they now constitute the leading cause of blindness in young children throughout the world. In such situations, a diet high in rice, wheat, maize, and tubers contains little if any β-carotene. Breast and cow's milk do not provide enough vitamin A to meet the needs of the growing child.

In the United States, vitamin A deficiency is encountered among the urban poor, the elderly, alcoholics, patients with malabsorption, and those individuals on a marginal diet. Individuals chronically using laxatives, particularly mineral oil, and certain other drugs may be vulnerable to vitamin A deficiency. In alcoholism, vitamin A deficiency may develop for several reasons. Zinc deficiency, which frequently occurs in alcoholism, impairs the release of holo-RBP from liver and probably interferes with the conversion of retinol to retinal needed in vision. Thus, alcoholism-associated zinc deficiency may intensify night blindness and other sequelae of dietary vitamin A deficiency. Also, in alcoholism it has been suggested that the degradative enzyme, alcohol dehydrogenase, which converts retinol to retinal in the retina, may be so saturated with ethanol that retinal production is sharply diminished. Furthermore, as malabsorption develops in chronic alcoholism, dietary carotenes and vitamin A may be lost in increasing amounts in the stool.

Vitamin A deficiency may occur after long-term use of mineral oil because this fat-soluble vitamin is dissolved in the oil. Other laxatives may result in vitamin A deficiency because of rapid intestinal transit and diminished intestinal absorption. Vitamin A deficiency may result also after prolonged use of drugs, such as cholestyramine, colestipol, neomycin, and colchicine.

CLINICAL FEATURES. Night blindness, as noted previously, may be an early manifestation of vitamin A deficiency. It has been suggested that the frequent episodes of falling and of traffic accidents involving chronic alcoholics at night may be due to some degree to underlying night blindness. In addition, dryness or xerosis of the conjunctivae and later of the cornea may develop, leading to softening and perforation of the cornea and development of Bitot's spots (small, white patches) on the sclerae (see Color plate 8D and E). Because of the role of vitamin A in maintaining differentiated epithelium, deficiency leads to abnormal development of epithelial tissue and keratinization, particularly in the eye, lung, sweat glands, and gastrointestinal tract. Loss of taste may also occur.

It has been suggested that decreased intake of β-carotene or vitamin A–rich foods or both may be associated with an increased prevalence of epithelial cancers, particularly lung cancers, among smokers. In some studies, intake of β-carotene but not vitamin A has had a strong negative correlation with cancer risk. Also, vitamin A–deficient animals have an increased risk of chemical carcinogenesis; administration of retinoids can prevent chemically induced cancers in animals.

DIAGNOSIS. The demonstration of abnormal dark adaptation is important evidence for the diagnosis of vitamin A deficiency. Techniques are being developed that can be carried out under field conditions without expensive equipment. Retinol can be detected directly in serum by immunoassay. Normal levels are in the approximate range of 30 to 65 μg per deciliter. Serum levels may be increased by hypothyroidism, nephrotic syndrome, oral contraceptives, and other disorders of lipid metabolism. By the time serum levels of retinol begin to decrease in dietary deficiency, liver reserves are already seriously depleted.

TREATMENT. The extensive eye problems of vitamin A deficiency encountered in developing countries are best approached through a systematic plan of prevention. Such programs are increasing in scope and magnitude. Injections of vitamin A in large doses (50,000 to 100,000 IU), every four to six months, are highly effective and are tolerated remarkably well. In children from population groups that have a high prevalence of vitamin A deficiency, capsules containing 200,000 IU given every six months markedly reduced mortality, particularly from infectious diseases. In the United States, when dietary deficiency is advanced, it should be treated with doses similar to these but for several days only, and then maintenance doses should be administered. Water-soluble forms of vitamin A should provide great assistance in patient management.

Derivatives of vitamin A (referred to as retinoids), particularly 13-cis-retinoic acid (isotretinoin), have been used to treat cystic acne with considerable success. Investigations are continuing in other dermatologic disorders, including psoriasis, actinic keratosis, leukoplakia, and pityriasis rosea. The mechanism of action of this derivative may lie in inhibition of keratinization, suppression of sebaceous gland secretion, or possibly a direct anti-inflammatory effect.

The use of β-carotene or retinoids or both, especially the less toxic forms, for the possible prevention of epithelial cancers is under intense study. Smokers should be expected to benefit particularly by increasing their intake of vitamin A and/or carotenoids, but no amounts of these agents are large enough to protect completely against the harmful effects of smoking. Consumption of foods rich in carotenes and vitamin A is not a substitute for failure to stop smoking. The exact doses necessary to achieve preventive effects are not known,

and it is possible that major benefits can be obtained simply by increasing the intake of foods rich in carotenoids or vitamin A without additional supplementation.

Toxicity

The carotenoids are generally without toxicity. Consumption of β-carotene in large amounts from foods, for example, carrots, may stain the skin a curious yellow-orange color, but this phenomenon is believed to be entirely benign. The sclerae remain white in carotenemia; thus the condition can easily be differentiated from jaundice.

Vitamin A (retinol), on the other hand, is quite toxic when taken continuously in large amounts, particularly at the level of 50,000 IU and higher, for periods of three months or more. The skin may become dry, pruritic, coarse, and scaly with fissures; hair loss may occur. Both vitamin A excess and deficiency have adverse effects upon the skin. Sore mouth, anorexia, and vomiting may ensue. The most serious side effects of vitamin A overdosage pertain to the central nervous system: patients may develop severe headaches, drowsiness, irritability, failure to concentrate, increased intracranial pressure, and papilledema. The liver may enlarge, rarely progressing to fibrosis and cirrhosis. Generalized lymph node enlargement may become evident. There may be painful hyperostoses, and there are preliminary indications that long-term use of vitamin A in large amounts possibly may accelerate the bone loss of aging. Hypercalcemia may occur after large doses. Congenital malformations have occurred in the infants of several women consuming 50,000 IU per day during pregnancy.

In cases of vitamin A toxicity, serum vitamin A levels are increased, particularly in the form of retinyl esters. In an asymptomatic patient receiving megadoses of vitamin A, the onset of liver disease such as hepatitis may precipitate overt clinical toxicity, presumably by releasing stored retinol into the general circulation. With discontinuation of megadoses of vitamin A, the symptoms will gradually recede.

The development of synthetic retinoids with lower toxicities and greater uptake in target organs is expected to facilitate the application of these agents in the possible chemoprevention of cancer.

Goodman DS: Vitamin A and retinoids in health and disease. N Engl J Med 310:1023, 1984. *This comprehensive review highlights advances relating vitamin A and retinoids to clinical medicine and public health, particularly ophthalmology, nutrition, dermatology, and cancer.*

Menkes MS, Comstock GW, Vuilleumier JP, et al.: Serum beta-carotene, vitamins A and E, selenium, and the risk of lung cancer. N Engl J Med 315:1250, 1986. *Study relating risk of lung cancer with serum levels of vitamins.*

Olson JA: Vitamin A. In Olson RE (ed): Present Knowledge in Nutrition. 5th ed. Washington DC, The Nutrition Foundation, 1984, pp 176–191. *Review of physiology, binding proteins, metabolism, and function of vitamin A.*

Ong DE, Chytil F: Vitamin A and cancer. Vitam Horm 40:105, 1983. *Review of underlying basis for use of vitamin A and derivatives (retinoids) in chemoprevention of cancer.*

Sporn MB, Roberts AB: The role of retinoids in differentiation and carcinogenesis. Cancer Res 43:3134, 1983. *Discussion of the recent application of vitamin A and its related compounds to the chemoprevention of certain forms of cancer.*

VITAMIN D

Vitamin D is discussed in Chapter 245 in association with calcium metabolism and metabolic bone diseases.

VITAMIN E

Structure and Biochemical Function

Vitamin E activity is derived from a series of dietary tocopherols and tocotrienols, the most potent of which is d-α-tocopherol (Fig. 217–7). At least eight compounds with vitamin E activity have been isolated from plants. The most widely accepted function of this vitamin is as an antioxidant, protecting polyunsaturated fatty acids in membranes and other cellular structures from attack by free radicals. Vitamin E deficiency in animals increases the likelihood of membrane and cellular damage from ozone, nitrogen dioxide, and hy-

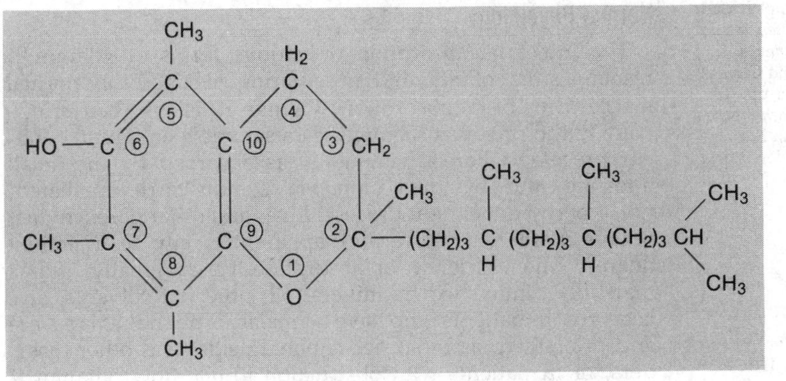

FIGURE 217–7. Structural formula of D-alpha tocopherol (vitamin E).

perbaric oxygen. Dietary selenium is a precursor of selenide, a cofactor for glutathione peroxidase, which also provides important protection against lipid peroxidation in vivo, working in conjunction with vitamin E and other enzymes, including superoxide dismutase and catalase. Dietary selenium under certain circumstances may spare the requirement for vitamin E.

Normal Physiology

Intestinal absorption of tocopherols requires normal mechanisms of digestion and absorption of fat, particularly bile acids. Tocopherols are transported to the general circulation in chylomicra. Levels of tocopherols in blood correlate with those of lipoproteins to which they are bound both normally and in various disease states. In contrast to vitamin A, there does not appear to be a specific carrier protein in blood for vitamin E, nor a specific organ in which it is stored. Some vitamin E is also transported in erythrocytes. The most important storage sites of the vitamin are fat, liver, and muscle. Vitamin E undergoes little metabolic transformation after absorption. The major excretory route is through the feces. Since dietary deficiency occurs only under very unusual circumstances, cases of vitamin E deficiency have usually been identified with prolonged and severe fat malabsorption. Vitamin E deficiency has also been detected in patients receiving parenteral nutrition.

Requirements and Dietary Sources

The dietary allowance for vitamin E is expressed in terms of mg α-tocopherol equivalents (α-TE) and is 10 mg per day (15 IU) for adult males and 8 mg per day (12 IU) for adult females, with increases of 2 mg per day for pregnancy and 3 mg per day for lactation. The increased requirement for vitamin E with diets high in polyunsaturated fatty acids is thought not to be clinically relevant, since the items highest in vitamin E content—soybean, corn, cottonseed, wheat germ, and safflower oils and their derivatives—are also high in polyunsaturated fatty acids. As a group, the tocopherols and tocotrienols are widely distributed in the food supply. The natural tocopherols are relatively unstable and lose significant activity during storage and cooking.

Deficiency

PATHOGENESIS. Clinical deficiency of vitamin E is generally encountered in the setting of severe malabsorption. The most serious deficiency is associated with a genetic disorder, abetalipoproteinemia, in which there is failure both of intestinal absorption and of serum transport. Vitamin E deficiency occurs in children with biliary atresia, cystic fibrosis, and chronic cholestasis, as well as in adults who survive these diseases or who have celiac disease, Crohn's disease, or other serious forms of malabsorption (Ch. 104).

CLINICAL FEATURES. Deficiency of vitamin E has generally not been recognized as a clearly definable syndrome.

The red cell half-life may be shortened, although anemia is uncommon in the absence of other precipitating causes. Most importantly, clinical and neuropathologic evidence of posterior column and spinocerebellar tract abnormalities have been described, with areflexia, ophthalmoplegia, and disturbances of gait, proprioception, and vibration. In premature infants, vitamin E deficiency is associated with hemolytic anemia, thrombocytosis, edema, intraventricular hemorrhage, and increasing risk of retrolental fibroplasia and bronchopulmonary dysplasia, both of which are related to oxygen toxicity.

DIAGNOSIS. Diagnosis of vitamin E deficiency is usually made by measurement of plasma E levels; normal levels are generally 0.50 to 0.70 mg per deciliter and higher. In several of the hemolytic anemias, such as sickle cell anemia and G-6-PD deficiency, serum vitamin E levels tend to be low. Serum vitamin E levels correlate with those of serum cholesterol and β-lipoprotein and are elevated in diabetes and other lipid disorders. The serum vitamin E concentration should be viewed in relation to serum lipid levels when vitamin E nutritional status is being evaluated.

TREATMENT. The therapeutic role of vitamin E remains controversial at the present time. Although vitamin E has been advocated by food faddists as an "anti-aging" vitamin, there is no evidence that it prolongs life in man. This vitamin has been claimed to enhance sexual performance, an attribute that also has not been substantiated. Some patients with intermittent claudication appear to have improved after therapy with vitamin E. Hemolytic anemia in the premature newborn is generally benefited by vitamin E therapy, and the severity but not the incidence of retrolental fibroplasia may be reduced. Administration of vitamin E has reduced the incidence of intraventricular hemorrhage in premature infants. Large doses of vitamin E have diminished the neurologic complications in abetalipoproteinemia and cholestatic liver disease.

There are a number of other effects of vitamin E demonstrable in vitro in experimental animals and in some instances in man, but their clinical relevance remains unresolved. These effects include reducing platelet aggregation, inhibiting conversion of nitrites to nitrosoamines, inhibiting prostaglandin synthesis, improving erythrocyte formation, and protecting against environmental toxicants and pollutants.

Toxicity

Vitamin E is far less toxic than the other fat-soluble vitamins, and a daily intake in the range of 200 to 800 mg per day (20 to 80 times the RDA) is generally considered safe. Nausea, flatulence, and diarrhea have been reported at doses in excess of 1000 mg. In animals the intestinal absorption of vitamin A and K is reduced at high doses, which possibly may be clinically significant in patients on marginal diets. Vitamin E appears to increase the vitamin K requirement, and megadoses of vitamin E administered together with the anticoagulant drug warfarin may result in overt bleeding.

Bieri JG, Corash L, Hubbard VS: Medical uses of vitamin E. N Engl J Med 308:1063, 1983. *This article reviews the rationale for treatment with vitamin E in various clinical disorders, limitations of treatment, and toxicities encountered.*

Lubin B, Machlin LJ (eds.): Vitamin E: Biochemical, Hematological and Clinical Aspects. New York, New York Academy of Sciences, 1982, 506 pp. *This volume covers the proceedings of a conference dealing with cellular biochemistry, relation to human diseases, deficiencies, and therapeutic doses of vitamin E.*

Machlin LJ: Vitamin E. In Machlin LJ (ed.): Handbook of Vitamins. New York, Marcel Dekker, 1984, pp 99–145. *Up-to-date review of physiology and medical uses of vitamin E.*

VITAMIN K

Structure and Biochemical Functions

Vitamin K occurs naturally in two forms, differing from one another only in their side chains. Vitamin K_1 (now called phylloquinone) is made by plant sources; vitamin K_2 (menaquinone) is synthesized by normal intestinal flora. It is also contained in some animal tissues. Vitamin K_3 (menadione) is an artificial provitamin that can be converted to menaquinone (K_2) by the liver (Fig. 217–8).

The mechanism of action of vitamin K consists of a post-translational γ-carboxylation of glutamic acid moieties in inactive precursor proteins, which confers calcium-binding properties to the proteins. The most widely known of these proteins are involved in blood coagulation. Four clotting factors are dependent upon vitamin K for this important action: prothrombin (Factor II), proconvertin (Factor VII), Christmas factor (Factor IX), and Stuart-Prower factor (Factor X). Lack of vitamin K may result in death from uncontrolled hemorrhage.

The anticoagulant drugs warfarin and dicoumarol inhibit the vitamin K–dependent γ-carboxylation by interfering with activation of vitamin K to its metabolically active hydroquinone form. As a result of this inhibition, the activation of the four clotting factors is greatly reduced.

Proteins that are involved in the mineralization of bone (osteocalcin) and possibly also in calcium resorption from the renal tubule also require vitamin K for their synthesis. Other vitamin K–dependent proteins have been identified (protein C, protein S). The vitamin K antagonists, warfarin and dicoumarol, cause a marked decrease in formation of osteocalcin, presumably by interfering with γ-carboxylation.

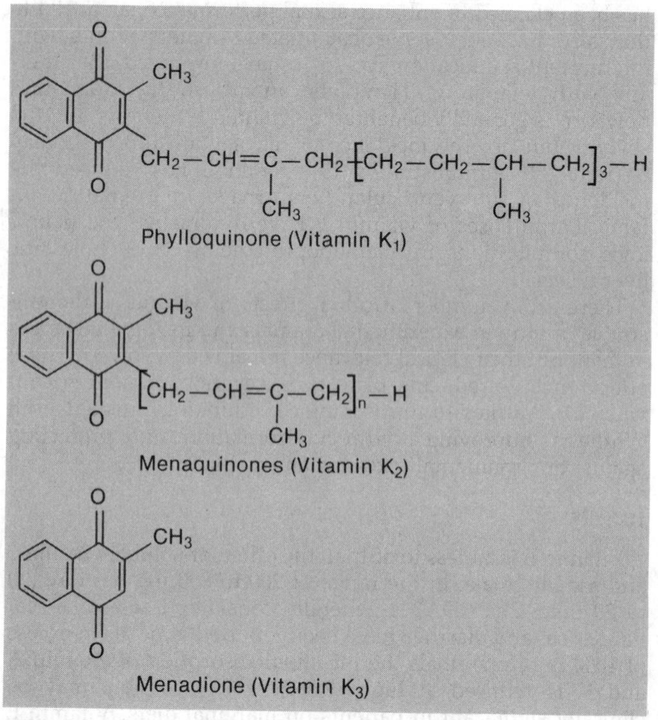

FIGURE 217–8. Structural formulae of vitamin K_1, vitamin K_2, and vitamin K_3.

Normal Physiology

The intestinal absorption of various forms of vitamin K resembles that of vitamin E in requiring bile and other normal mechanisms of fat absorption. Vitamin K_1 is absorbed principally in the proximal segment via a saturable energy-dependent process, whereas vitamin K_2 is absorbed by the small intestine and by the colon via a non–carrier-mediated, non–energy-dependent process. Liver and other parenchymal organs store vitamin K, but apparently only to a limited degree. The efficiency of absorption varies greatly and is markedly diminished by mineral oil, other fat solvents, and laxatives. In patients who have fat malabsorption that is severe and prolonged, as in sprue, regional ileitis, and other disorders, or in patients with obstruction to bile flow, vitamin K deficiency commonly develops. Deficiency also may occur after prolonged antibiotic therapy, destroying the intestinal synthesis of vitamin K.

After absorption, vitamin K is transported via the lymphatic system in association with chylomicrons. The main excretory products of vitamin K in urine are derivatives that have undergone chain shortening and oxidation.

Requirements and Dietary Sources

The best sources of vitamin K are green, leafy vegetables, particularly turnip greens, broccoli, brussels sprouts, spinach, and lettuce. There are moderate amounts in liver, bacon, cheese, butter, coffee, and green tea. No single recommended dietary allowance is made for vitamin K because of the important and variable contribution made by intestinal bacteria. It is recommended only that normal adults consume 70 to 140 μg per day. Dietary deficiency based upon consuming less than this amount is uncommon at the present time in the United States, because the usual diet contains ample amounts of vitamin K.

Deficiency

PATHOGENESIS. Vitamin K deficiency occurs frequently in newborn infants for several reasons. First, fetal stores tend to be low because very little of this vitamin is transported across the placenta. In addition, the fetal gut is sterile, and therefore the newborn lacks the supply of vitamin K that can be provided by normal intestinal flora. As the intestinal tract becomes colonized postnatally, the synthesis of vitamin K becomes appreciable. Deficiency generally does not develop unless there is an abnormality of intestinal function or antibiotic therapy, as noted above.

CLINICAL FEATURES. Vitamin K deficiency may be manifested clinically as increased tendency to hemorrhage. Such bleeding episodes may be particularly severe in newborn infants.

DIAGNOSIS. The only practical and reliable method for diagnosis of vitamin K deficiency is by direct assay of one or more of the four vitamin K–dependent clotting factors.

TREATMENT. Vitamin K deficiency responds rapidly to the administration of vitamin K, provided that liver function is normal. A number of preparations of vitamin K are available, some of which are water soluble, for example, menadiol sodium diphosphate. These forms are more toxic than the lipid-soluble phylloquinone form. In patients with advanced liver disease, the serum prothrombin is decreased and responds poorly if at all to administration of vitamin K. Patients with low serum prothrombin caused by vitamin K deficiency can be distinguished from those with low prothrombin caused by liver disease because in vitamin K deficiency the prothrombin precursor in blood is not γ-carboxylated; usually γ-carboxylated prothrombin is found in patients with liver disease.

Toxicity

Consumption of large quantities of foods rich in vitamin K is not believed to produce clinical toxicity. Certain water-soluble derivatives administered parenterally have caused hemolytic anemia and jaundice.

Olson RE: Vitamin K. In Goodhart RS, Shils ME (eds.): Modern Nutrition in Health and Disease. 6th ed. Philadelphia, Lea & Febiger, 1980, pp 170–180. *Thorough discussion of nutritional aspects of vitamin K, with emphasis upon biochemical mechanisms.*

Suttie JW: Current concepts of the mechanism of action of vitamin K and its antagonists. In Lindenbaum J (ed.): Nutrition in Hematology. Contemporary Issues in Clinical Nutrition. Vol. 5. New York, Churchill Livingstone, 1983, pp 245–270. *Discussion of the basic biochemistry of vitamin K and its relation to clotting factors.*

Suttie JW: Vitamin K Metabolism and Vitamin K–Dependent Proteins. Baltimore, University Park Press, 1980, 592 pp. *Comprehensive volume dealing with biochemical, nutritional, and functional aspects of vitamin K.*

218 DISTURBANCES OF TRACE MINERAL METABOLISM

Clifford Tasman-Jones

The bulk of living matter is formed by eleven elements, all of which are from the lowest part of the periodic table (H, C, N, O, Na, Mg, P, S, Cl, K, and Ca). In addition to these, there are essential minerals that are present in trace amounts. These latter include F, Si, V, Cr, Mn, Fe, Co, Ni, Cu, Zn, Se, Mo, Sn, and I.

While deficiencies of trace minerals and vitamins are uncommon in humans eating a normal diet, there is a likelihood of trace mineral deficiencies developing with the use of enteral and parenteral feeding. Deficiencies developing during parenteral nutrition have focused attention on trace mineral function in human metabolism.

Trace minerals essential for life act as essential cofactors of enzymes and as organizers of the molecular structures of the cell (e.g., mitochondria) and its cellular membrane. There is an optimal tissue concentration for trace minerals; excess can be toxic and insufficiency leads to metabolic failure.

Trace mineral bioavailability is affected by the physiologic status of the person (intrinsic factors), as well as by dietary availability (extrinsic factors). Absorbed through the intestine, trace minerals in the plasma are bound either to a specific protein or to albumin for transportation. The excretory path varies, but most are excreted into the gastrointestinal tract, many by way of bile; some are excreted in the urine and some by the sweat glands. Not all trace minerals have been shown to be clinically important. Some, such as iron and iodine, are so important in specific disorders that they are covered separately in this volume.

METABOLISM. Although zinc represents only 0.003 per cent (1.4 to 2.3 grams) of the human body, it is an intrinsic part of at least 110 metalloenzymes and other cellular components and is essential for the synthesis of protein, DNA, and RNA.

Zinc is absorbed from the small intestine, although the exact mechanism for this remains uncertain. A low-molecular-weight zinc-binding ligand, possibly secreted from the pancreas, is a postulated mechanism for absorption.

The highest concentrations of zinc are in the prostate, the skin and its appendages, the brain, choroid, liver, pancreas, bone, and blood. In blood approximately 80 per cent of zinc is in erythrocytes, 16 per cent in plasma, 3 per cent in leukocytes, and the remaining 1 per cent in platelets. Plasma zinc is normally 12 to 20 μmol per liter. Zinc is excreted mainly in the feces, but small amounts (between 4.0 and 12.0 μmol per 24 hours) are secreted in the urine.

DEFICIENCY SYNDROMES. In man zinc deficiency has been described in a chronic form and in an acute form. In Iran and Egypt hypogonadal dwarfism in males is associated with zinc deficiency and a deficiency of dietary protein. Additionally, these children usually eat clay, which may bind zinc, making it unavailable for absorption.

Acrodermatitis enterohepatica, a rare autosomal recessive inherited disorder of zinc metabolism, represents a chronic form of pure zinc deficiency. This entity is characterized by diarrhea; an unpleasant skin rash of the extremities, face, and perineum; alopecia; mental irritability; muscle wasting; and depression. Although the nature of the disease remains in doubt, it may be caused by an absence of the ligand essential for zinc absorption. This ligand is present in human milk but not in cow's milk.

Acute zinc deficiency has been described in patients receiving parenteral nutrition. This syndrome is characterized by diarrhea; disturbance of the central nervous system with mental irritability and depression; skin lesions of the face, perineum, limbs, and skin folds; alopecia; loss of taste; and defects in the immunologic mechanisms. Treatment with zinc supplementation, usually in the form of zinc sulfate, results in a dramatic response.

Zinc deficiency may occur in inflammatory bowel disease, malabsorption, cirrhosis, and high alcohol intake, probably because of an increased excretion of zinc in the urine. In Crohn's disease, when there is severe catabolism, zincuria may be severe, depleting body stores that are needed during anabolism. Although the alcoholic has increased zinc loss, there appears to be increased absorption to compensate.

In sickle cell anemia, delayed puberty, decreased hair, poor growth, and roughened skin are related to zinc deficiency.

Zinc taken in excess may cause gastrointestinal upset with nausea and vomiting.

COPPER

METABOLISM. An average healthy adult has 12.6 to 18 mmol of body copper. Copper is absorbed from the stomach and proximal duodenum by complexing with amino acids. In the presence of excess intraluminal micronutrients such as zinc or calcium, copper absorption may be reduced. Absorbed copper is bound to albumin, and after circulating through the liver, it is complexed to ceruloplasmin for distribution to body tissues. The plasma concentration of copper is 13 to 22 μmol per liter, 90 per cent of which is bound to ceruloplasmin. Plasma copper may not adequately reflect copper stores but rather reflect plasma ceruloplasmin concentrations.

The best known function of copper is its effect on erythropoiesis. It is essential for hemoglobin formation. Many copper enzymes are known. Copper is necessary for collagen formation, the functioning of the central nervous system, and skin pigmentation.

Usually copper is excreted in the bile as a metallocomplex. There is an additional copper loss in the urine (0.16 to 0.95 μmol per day) and saliva (0.006 to 0.008 μmol per day).

The highest concentrations of copper occur in the liver, brain, heart, spleen, kidneys, and blood. The mean daily requirement of copper is estimated to be between 5 and 15 μmol when given intravenously and between 30 and 40 μmol when given orally.

DEFICIENCY SYNDROMES. Hypocupremia occurs in a number of inherited disorders such as Wilson's disease (a disease of copper excess), Menkes' kinky hair syndrome (a syndrome of neurologic disorder with hypocupremia), and familial hypoceruloplasminemia. It may also be found with decreased copper intake, as in parenteral nutrition, or with the poor absorption or increased loss associated with protein-losing enteropathy, the nephrotic syndrome, cystic fibrosis, and other malabsorptive diseases such as celiac disease and sprue.

Menkes' kinky hair disease is a rare X-linked genetic disorder in which there is defective connective tissue formation, gross mental retardation, imperfect keratinization of the skin, and depigmentation of the hair. Serum copper and ceruloplasmin levels are very low and return to normal with parenteral but not when oral copper is given. This therapy has no demonstrated benefit in the disease, however.

Chronic copper deficiency causes anemia, usually of a microcytic type, but sometimes is associated with megaloblastic changes in the marrow, leukopenia, and neutropenia.

EXCESS. Hypercupremia occurs in response to inflammation and has been described in rheumatoid arthritis. The rise in copper is most probably caused by the rise in ceruloplasmin—an acute-phase reactant protein. Copper in excess may produce nausea, vomiting, myalgia, and hemolysis. *Wilson's disease*, the most important human disorder of excess copper, is described in detail in Ch. 205.

MANGANESE

METABOLISM. Manganese, a trace element essential for life, is present in an amount of approximately 12 to 20 mg in the average adult. Maximally absorbed in the duodenum by an unknown transport mechanism, magnesium is bound to transmanganin, a specific beta$_1$-globulin transport protein. Manganese is concentrated in tissues rich in mitochondria and is widely distributed in the body with maximal concentrations in the brain, kidneys, pancreas, bone, and liver. The blood and serum levels vary widely. Manganese is principally excreted in bile.

Manganese is an activator of many enzymes, but only one manganese metalloenzyme is known—pyruvate carboxylase. Manganese appears to be intimately involved in the synthesis of DNA, RNA, and protein.

DEFICIENCY. The syndrome associated with deficiency of manganese includes the following features: impaired growth, skeletal abnormalities, abnormal reproductive function, ataxia, convulsions, and anomalies of fat metabolism. In the best described patient with manganese deficiency there were weight loss, a transient dermatitis, nausea and vomiting with changes in the color and growth of hair, and hypocholesterolemia.

EXCESS. Manganese poisoning, which usually occurs after industrial exposure, induces a syndrome that closely resembles Parkinson's disease.

CHROMIUM

METABOLISM. Chromium is an essential micronutrient required for the maintenance of normal blood glucose levels. The recommended daily intake is 50 to 200 µg, and the normal serum level is 0.5 to 9.0 µg per liter. Chromium is present in yeast, meat, and grain. Chromium complexes with nicotinamide to form the glucose tolerance factor. This factor acts as a facilitator for insulin to react at receptor sites on insulin-sensitive tissues.

DEFICIENCY. Chromium deficiency is characterized by impaired glucose tolerance, encephalopathy, and neuropathy. Because of impaired insulin activity, patients may develop hyperglycemia with hyperosmolar nonketotic coma. Chromium deficiency may give a confusional state similar to hepatic encephalopathy with ataxia and peripheral neuropathy. A suggested association between chromium deficiency and coronary artery disease awaits confirmation.

EXCESS. If too much chromium is given, symptoms of nausea, vomiting, gastrointestinal ulceration, liver damage, kidney damage, and central nervous system abnormalities with convulsions may occur.

SELENIUM

METABOLISM. Selenocysteine in the enzyme glutathionine peroxidase is important in protecting lipids of cell membranes, proteins, and nucleic acids against oxidant damage.

In the United States, the blood level of selenium is 1.90 to 3.17 µmol per liter. A low blood selenium concentration reflecting a low soil content has been noted in Finland, China, New Zealand, Sweden, and Denmark.

The daily requirement for selenium is estimated to be 0.73 µmol for women and 1.02 µmol for men. It is probably dependent on the supply of other trace minerals, including zinc, copper, magnesium, and iron and also the supply of other antioxidant substances, such as vitamin E and vitamin C. In the United States the intake is 0.76 to 2.79 µmol per day.

DEFICIENCY. *Keshan disease* is a syndrome of endemic cardiomyopathy in the People's Republic of China that is alleviated by giving oral sodium selenite. In the areas of China where Keshan disease is prevalent the dietary intake is estimated at less than 0.38 µmol. A New Zealand woman receiving intravenous feeding developed muscle pains and tenderness and a very low blood selenium level. The symptoms were alleviated by giving selomethionine. In Finland a reduced serum selenium concentration has been shown to correlate with cardiovascular death and acute coronary heart disease. In a prospective study the selenium level in the serum of those patients who subsequently developed malignant disease was found to be significantly lower than that of controls.

EXCESS. Excess selenium is a cell toxin and, as such, selenium should be given with considerable care. Selinosis occurs with daily intake in excess of 6.35 µmol.

MAGNESIUM

METABOLISM. Magnesium is of great physiologic importance. It is second only to potassium as the most abundant intracellular cation. The amount of magnesium in the human body is about 1000 mmol, of which about 60 per cent is in bone, 20 per cent in muscle, and only 1 per cent is extracellular.

The recommended intake, about 15 mmol, comes from green vegetables, meat, and fish. Normally 35 to 40 per cent of dietary magnesium is absorbed, mostly in the middle and lower small bowel.

Magnesium is an essential part of some 300 different enzymes and is necessary for cell membrane permeability; neuromuscular excitability; protein, nucleic acid, and fat synthesis; muscle contraction; and so on. While there is no laboratory test that unequivocally reveals magnesium deficiency, the serum magnesium level is not without value. Normal values for serum magnesium are 0.8 to 1.0 mmol per liter. Magnesium deficiency is often present without low serum magnesium levels. Analysis of urinary magnesium may be of some value; it is usually 3 to 5 mmol per day.

Mild hypomagnesemia is not uncommon, and its clinical importance is often missed. The disorder should be thought of when hypokalemia and/or hypocalcemia is present.

Disorders of magnesium metabolism are described in detail in Ch. 208.

VANADIUM

Analysis of vanadium is difficult. The total body vanadium is about 100 µg. Blood levels are very low, 0.005 to 8.4 µmol per liter.

Vanadium depresses plasma cholesterol levels, Na$^+$/K$^+$ ATPase, myosin, Ca^{++} ATPase, adenylate kinase, and phosphofructokinase, and it stimulates adenyl cyclase. Vanadium deficiency has been postulated to play a role in nutritional edema, and vanadium excess has been postulated to be a factor in manic-depressive illness. Neither of these suggestions has been confirmed.

COBALT

Cobalt in human metabolism is related to vitamin B_{12}, a topic that is covered in Ch. 136 in the discussion of pernicious anemia.

NICKEL

Nickel is present in the serum in three forms: a nickel-histamine complex, nickel bound to albumin, and nickel bound to alpha$_2$-macroglobulin. With short-term nickel administration the highest concentrations occur in the kidneys and urine; with long-term administration nickel accumulates in the lungs. Nickel workers have increased risk of cancers of nose, lung, and possibly kidney.

SILICON

Silicon is found in high concentrations in tendons, aorta, and eye tissues. It is necessary for mammalian bone growth and calcification. In experimental animals, silicon appears to inhibit atheroma development. Chronic inhalation of silicon as silica (SiO_2) produces lung disease, as described in Ch. 536.

Brenton DP, Gordon TE: Fluid and electrolyte disorders. Magnesium. Br J Hosp Med 32:60, 1984. *A practical review of magnesium and its deficiency syndrome.*

Cousins RJ: Absorption, transport and hepatic metabolism of copper and zinc: Special reference to metallothionein and ceruloplasmin. Physiol Rev 65:238, 1985. *A comprehensive review of copper and zinc metabolism, with particular reference to the key role of the liver.*

Fitzgerald FT, Tierney LM: Trace metals in human disease. Adv Intern Med 30:337, 1984. *An overall introduction to trace metals in human disease.*

Nève J, Vertongen F, Molle L: Selenium deficiency. Clin Endocrinol Metab 14:629, 1985. *A useful review emphasizing the current knowledge and areas of poor understanding.*

O'Dell BL: Bioavailability of trace elements. Nutr Rev 42:301, 1984. *A useful review of problems of determining and understanding trace mineral availability.*

Prasad AS: Clinical manifestations of zinc deficiency. Am Rev Nutr 5:341, 1985. *A full review of the etiological and clinical features of zinc deficiency.*

Wallach S: Clinical and biochemical aspects of chromium deficiency. J Am Coll Nutr 4:107, 1985. *A comprehensive readable review of chromium metabolism indicating its importance in clinical medicine.*

Williams DG: Copper deficiency in humans. Semin Hematol 20:118, 1983. *Major features of normal copper metabolism and copper deficiency are summarized in a very readable form.*

219 PRINCIPLES OF NUTRITIONAL SUPPORT: ENTERAL NUTRITIONAL THERAPY

David H. Alpers

Enteral nutrition therapy implies modification of the usual diet and is used for two major general indications. The first is supplementation of protein and calories in a wide variety of situations with the intention of providing part or all of the daily requirements. This use is not disease-specific. The second and more traditional indication involves the use of diets for specific diseases or pathophysiologic situations. The diets used involve restricting a particular element of the diet (e.g., fat, lactose), adding a nutrient that may be required in larger amounts than are available from a well-balanced diet (e.g., calcium, potassium), or altering the consistency of the diet (e.g., high-fiber, full-liquid). These two major indications will be discussed in this chapter. Also included is a discussion about formulating a plan for calorie and protein supplementation, which will place this and the following chapter on parenteral nutrition in proper perspective.

PROTEIN AND CALORIE SUPPLEMENTATION

Initial Decisions: Completeness of Nutrient Provision and Route of Administration

The range of methods for providing protein and calorie supplements has expanded greatly beyond table foods in recent years, and likewise the range of available products for this use is very great. For many patients all that may be needed is a careful history of dietary intake, estimation of protein and caloric requirements, and adjustment of the diet to provide the needed nutrients. Whether table foods or commercial supplements are used, there are two major considerations for the physician to provide the most appropriate therapy for each patient: (1) Is the supplement intended as a partial fulfillment of daily needs (incomplete provision) or a total replacement of calories and protein (complete provision)? (2) Are the nutrients to be delivered by the enteral or the parenteral route? Table 219–1 summarizes these major choices. Forced enteral feeding refers to the delivery of nutrients to the small intestine via a small (7 to 8 French) polyurethane or silicone catheter placed through the nose or percutaneously via the endoscope (percutaneous endoscopic gastrostomy) or by a surgical procedure. Parenteral supplementation by peripheral or central vein will be discussed in Ch. 220. The options listed in Table 219–1 are not mutually exclusive. For example, sometimes forced enteral feeding can be used together with peripheral vein feeding; nutritionally complete commercial supplements can be used orally in some patients to supply total macronutrient requirements; central vein feeding can be supplemented by oral intake.

Formulating a Protein-Calorie Support Plan

Figure 219–1 illustrates a flow diagram used for selecting patients in negative protein and calorie balance for intensive nutritional support. The correct choice for nutritional support (enteral vs. parenteral, oral vs. forced enteral) depends largely upon the four key questions outlined in the figure. The physician should estimate protein and caloric requirements for the individual patient. Methods for making these estimates are available in a number of handbooks. While the estimates are fairly crude, they are clinically useful, since they provide some quantitative guidelines for deciding the magnitude of supplementation needed. The most commonly used formulas for determining basal requirement are those of Harris and Benedict:

$$BMR_{women} = 655 + (9.6 \times W) + (1.8 \times H) - (4.7 \times A)$$
$$BMR_{men} = 66 + (13.7 \times W) + (5 \times H) - (6.8 \times A)$$

where W is ideal weight in kg; H is height in cm; A is age in years. For ambulatory patients the basal requirements can be estimated at two thirds of their total caloric need. Most ill

TABLE 219–1. STRATEGY FOR CALORIE AND PROTEIN SUPPLEMENTATION

Route of Delivery	Incomplete Provision	Complete Provision
Enteral	Oral supplementation Table foods, e.g., milk, peanut butter, egg Commercial supplements Individual macronutrients (e.g., protein, fat, carbohydrate) Nutritionally complete supplement	Forced enteral feeding Nutritionally complete commercial diets Blenderized formulas
Parenteral	Peripheral (e.g., 3 per cent amino acids, 5 to 10 per cent dextrose, 10 per cent lipid emulsion)	Central (e.g., 4.25 per cent amino acid, 25 per cent dextrose, vitamins, minerals, fatty acids)

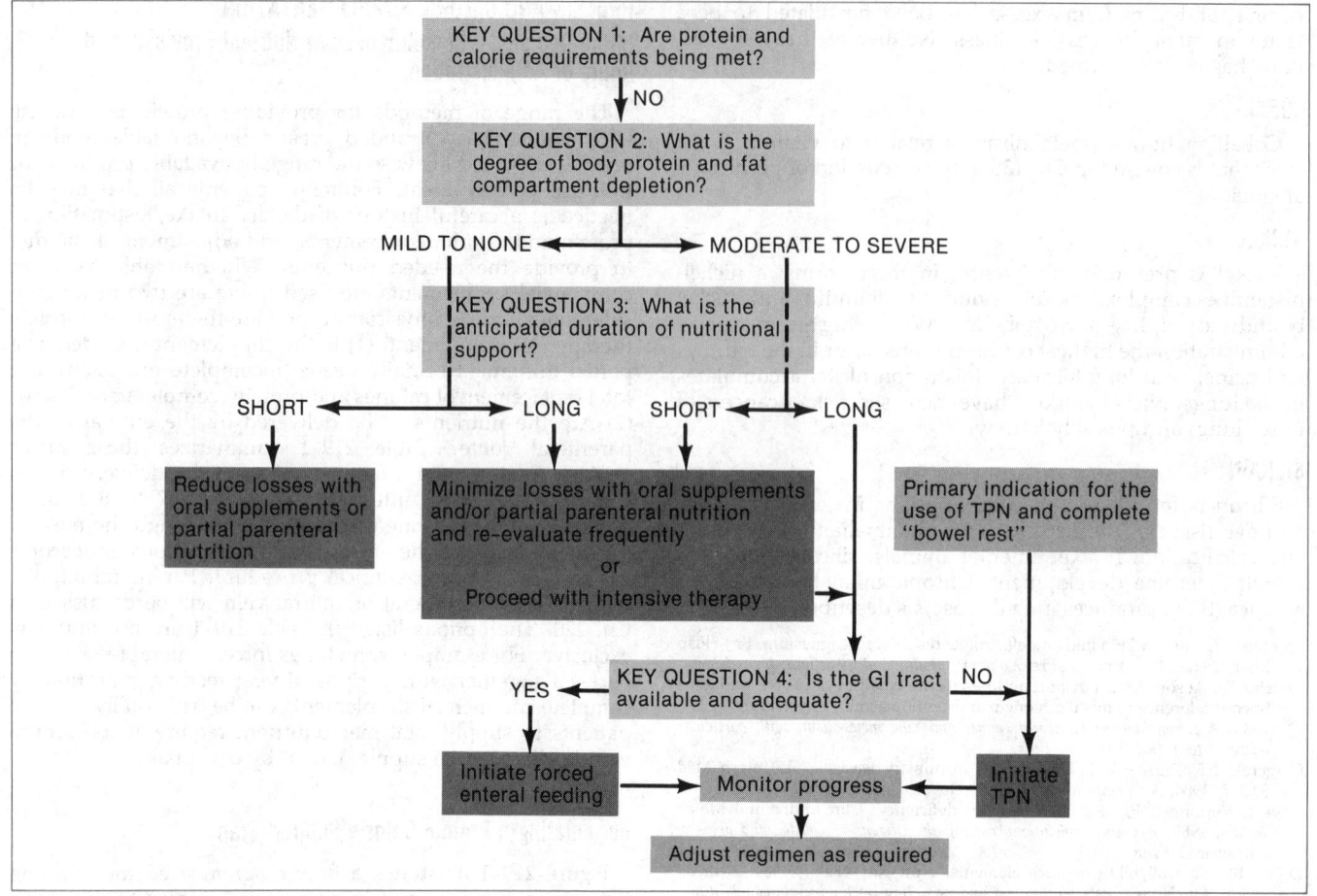

FIGURE 219–1. Flow diagram useful for selecting patients in negative protein and calorie balance for intensive nutritional support. TPN = total parenteral nutrition; GI = gastrointestinal.

hospitalized patients will not require calories in excess of their estimated basal requirement, based on their usual weight. Hospitalized patients receiving protein of high biologic value (egg, milk, meat) need only 0.5 gram per kilogram body weight per day for mild illness. For ambulatory patients this figure becomes 0.8 gram per kilogram per day to allow for the protein content of a mixed animal and vegetable diet. For severely ill patients the requirement rarely exceeds 1 gram per kilogram per day. Larger amounts of protein cannot be assimilated by sick patients, largely because of the high caloric requirement needed to fix the protein in the body. In general, calorie and protein requirements for ill or hospitalized patients have been overestimated in the past.

If the diet is meeting requirements (question 1), no further therapy is needed. If the diet is inadequate, an assessment of the patient's present nutritional status is then obtained. Caloric reserves are monitored most easily by body weight and protein reserves by serum albumin levels. Other available methods are discussed in Ch. 213. If the degree of depletion (question 2) as assessed by body weight is mild (about 5 per cent decreased) and the gastrointestinal tract is intact, oral supplements may be used. If the degree of depletion is moderate (5 to 10 per cent decreased) to severe (over 10 per cent decreased) and the anticipated duration of support is long (question 3), intensive therapy may be needed. As is apparent in the algorithm in Figure 219–1, the definition of *long* is crucial for decision making. If the patient can be expected to lose up to 10 per cent of body weight during the illness, the needed duration of treatment is considered to be long. Alternatively, an arbitrary number of days with inadequate intake can be considered "long": seven to ten days for normally nourished patients, three to five days for poorly nourished patients. Whether forced enteral feeding or total

parenteral nutrition (TPN) via a central vein is chosen depends on the availability or adequacy of the gastrointestinal tract (question 4). The gastrointestinal tract is usually evaluated by history (the presence or absence of diarrhea or malabsorption), physical examination (normal motility or ileus), and barium radiographs. Some patients are selected for TPN because of the need for complete bowel rest. Data to support the use of this therapy have been obtained in Crohn's disease, ulcerative colitis, the postoperative adaptive period of the short-bowel syndrome, and severe pancreatitis (see Ch. 200). Some patients with these disorders can be treated with forced enteral feeding. Often, however, bowel rest will control symptoms more rapidly. Other considerations (social, economic) may play a role in the final choice of therapy for a given patient. The patient may be unwilling to maintain a nasal feeding tube, or hospitalization may not be possible because of cost restrictions. Finally, an occasional patient may need to be fed via gastrostomy or jejunostomy.

The percutaneous gastrostomy has allowed relatively simple establishment of this feeding route and has expanded the indications for gastrostomy. Gastrostomy feeding is now used when the anticipated time for enteral supplementation is long, and the patient cannot swallow. The tube is placed endoscopically if the esophagus is patent (e.g., stroke) or surgically if it is not. A more detailed discussion of the indications for TPN can be found in the following chapter (Ch. 220).

The following categories of patients are commonly considered for enteral nutrition therapy: (1) chronically ill patients with anorexia, (2) patients with chronic inflammatory illnesses who have increased requirements but a usual caloric intake for their size, (3) poor or marginally nourished patients preparing for tests or intestinal surgery, and (4) patients with specific dietary needs that benefit from the special characteristics of some commercial supplements (e.g., low-residue, lactose-free). Forced enteral feeding typically is used for those patients who have moderate to severe anorexia, those who cannot maintain a calorie and protein intake commensurate with their needs (e.g., burn patients), or those whose illnesses prevent them from satisfactory oral feeding (e.g., patients with neck fractures or swallowing disorders).

Delivery of Enteral Supplements

Table Foods

If requirements are not great and appetite is good, table foods can be recommended as protein and calorie supplements. Each ounce of meat, fish, poultry, or cheese contains about 7 grams of protein, an egg 6 to 7 grams, and one cup of milk 8 grams. One half cup of dried beans, peas, or nuts contains 5 grams or more of protein, but these sources contain protein of a lower biologic value (sustains growth less well) and are not usually recommended for "catch up" therapy. Milk products are very useful, provided that lactose intolerance is not a problem. Meat and fish are helpful if fat is well tolerated. Otherwise, poultry without skin or tuna canned in water should be selected. Peanut butter contains 8 grams of fat and 4.2 grams of protein per tablespoon and is a good source of concentrated calories and protein. Table foods remain an excellent choice for oral supplementation, since they are tasty, esthetically and socially appealing, reasonable in cost, easily obtained, and available in a wide variety of choices. They should not be supplemented by commercial supplements unless the supplements exhibit specific properties that make them preferable.

Commercial Supplements

Commercial supplements, like table foods, display a diversity of characteristics that help the physician determine the choice for each patient. They are available as sources of single macronutrients (protein, carbohydrate, or lipid) or as nutritionally complete supplements, containing all necessary macronutrients and micronutrients. These products are of high caloric density and precisely defined nutrient composition but have the disadvantages of limited esthetic and taste appeal, taste fatigue with constant use, frequent occurrence of diarrhea, and higher cost than table foods. The nutritionally incomplete supplements can be used when the deficiency is specific (protein or calorie) or the deficiency is anticipated only for a short time, as in preparation for surgery. Protein is not wisely provided without another source of calories, since about 25 to 40 Kcal of nonprotein are needed per gram of protein to maintain positive nitrogen balance. Otherwise, a portion of the amino acids in the protein is converted to carbohydrate to provide the energy needed for assimilation.

The nutritionally complete supplements are largely distinguished by four major characteristics: (1) the presence or absence of lactose, (2) the use of intact protein or hydrolyzed protein (or amino acids), (3) the presence of small or large amounts of fat as caloric sources, and (4) isotonic or hypertonic osmolality. Supplements that are isotonic or nearly so contain less available carbohydrate and more lipid, which is osmotically less active. This characteristic is of greatest importance when forced enteral feeding is used, but any of the hypertonic solutions may be diluted or infused at a slower rate. The other three characteristics are more important for patients with abnormal intestinal absorption. Hydrolyzed protein may be useful for patients with pancreatic insufficiency, lactose-free supplements for patients with lactose intolerance, and low-fat supplements for those with limited intestinal fat absorption. The nutritionally complete supplements just described are designed to be the sole source of daily nutrients and thus contain all needed micronutrients in adequate quantities, if deficiencies are not present and if requirements are usual. Nonprescription milk-based products also provide good sources of protein and calories in a wide variety of flavors. If the patient is lactose tolerant, they may be used very successfully.

COMPLICATIONS OF ENTERAL FEEDING USING COMMERCIAL SUPPLEMENTS. The use of enteral feeding with highly concentrated supplements can be limited by side effects. The most common is diarrhea, which can be due to intolerance to one of the macronutrients (fat, lactose) or intolerance to the osmotic load. Altering the rate of delivery or the concentration of the supplement is often helpful. Complications of forced enteral feeding alone include esophagitis and tracheobronchial aspiration. Volume or sodium overload can occur, especially in the edema-prone patient.

THERAPEUTIC DIETS FOR SPECIFIC DISORDERS OR PATHOPHYSIOLOGIC STATES

The diets most commonly used to control systems are those that restrict one or another element in the diet. Diets restricted for each of the major macronutrients (fat, carbohydrate, and protein) have their individual uses (Table 219–2). As expected, these diets are helpful in altering pathophysiologic states and are not specific for any disease. Any condition causing steatorrhea can be improved symptomatically by limiting fat intake. Care must be taken with any restrictive diet to supplement any nutrients that have been secondarily limited. Thus, a fat-restricted diet must be made isocaloric by increasing carbohydrate intake. For this diet to be successful the patient must not have any generalized carbohydrate intolerance. Similarly, the low-lactose or low-available-carbohydrate diet is low in calcium. Most restrictive diets do not eliminate the nutrient whose content is altered. A low-lactose diet is much easier to achieve than a truly lactose-free one and is usually sufficient to relieve symptoms. Control of symptoms is the usual goal of dietary management, and restriction of the appropriate nutrient to the point at which symptoms are altered is an acceptable goal. Thus, a low-protein diet for hepatic encephalopathy should still deliver the estimated daily protein allowance (0.5 to 0.8 gram per kilogram of body weight) to avoid protein deficiency. This concept is especially important in the management of chronic renal failure, a situation in which the protein requirement may be actually increased. When the glomerular filtration rate (GFR) falls below 25 ml per minute, the protein allowance should be not more than 1.3 grams per kilogram per day (referring to ideal body weight) and falls to 0.6 gram per kilogram per day for a GFR of 4 to 10 ml per minute. Over 50 per cent of the protein intake should be of high biologic value (with high essential amino acid content). Requirements actually increase with dialysis because of the loss of amino acids in the dialysate. The allowance rises with hemodialysis to 1 gram per kilogram per day, and to 1.2 to 1.5 grams per kilogram per day with chronic peritoneal dialysis.

TABLE 219–2. THERAPEUTIC DIETS CHARACTERIZED BY RESTRICTION OF DIETARY COMPONENTS

Diet	Typical Indication
Low fat (60–75 grams/day)	Steatorrhea, mild
Low fat (40–60 grams/day)	Steatorrhea, severe
Low oxalate	Enteric hyperoxaluria
Low lactose	Lactose intolerance
Low available carbohydrate	Reactive hypoglycemia
Gluten free	Celiac sprue (see Ch. 104)
Low fiber	Acute diarrhea, bowel preparation
Low protein	Hepatic encephalopathy (see Ch. 128)
	Chronic renal failure (see Ch. 79)
Elimination	Food allergies
Controlled carbohydrate	Diabetes mellitus (see Ch. 231)
Calorie restricted	Obesity
Low sodium	Edematous states
Low fat, cholesterol, or carbohydrate according to type	Hyperlipidemia (see Ch. 183)
Low copper	Wilson's disease
Low phosphate	Chronic renal failure (see Ch. 79)

Some of the diets used for therapy actually control or modify the content of macronutrients rather than restrict them. The diet for diabetes mellitus is a good example of this principle (see Ch. 231). Successful management of the obese diabetic combines a weight reduction diet with regulation of the carbohydrate content. The prudent diet recommended by the American Diabetes Association still contains 40 to 50 per cent of calories as carbohydrates, but there is much less simple sugar (requiring no pancreatic digestion) and more starch than in normal diets. There is also less cholesterol and saturated fats to reduce blood lipids. These latest recommendations contain relaxed restrictions on carbohydrate intake. High-starch diets are well tolerated by diabetics as long as total caloric intake is controlled. Many patients require diets that may utilize elements from diets designed specifically for weight reduction, diabetes mellitus, hyperlipidemias, and chronic renal failure.

Diets That Supplement Dietary Components

Although less commonly required, diets that add a component to the normal diet are often employed (Table 219–3). A high fiber intake has not been clearly shown to have a beneficial effect on the symptoms of the irritable bowel syndrome and on the recurrence of attacks of acute diverticulitis, although supplementation with fiber is now commonly used for these disorders. The reasons for the uncertainty are that (1) these disorders are identified mostly by clinical criteria, (2) the irritable bowel syndrome is probably a heterogeneous group of motility disorders, (3) the definition of fiber and estimation of its intake are imperfectly developed, and (4) many types of fiber supplements are used, containing different components of dietary fiber. There are limited data on the food content of the major components of dietary fiber, i.e., cellulose, hemicelluloses, pectin, mucilage and gums, and lignins. Thus, it is not always clear when an individual patient is ingesting a low-fiber diet. Most often fiber is supplemented by ingestion of commercial preparations containing psyllium seed or by the use of bran. Psyllium is rich in hemicelluloses, while bran contains more cellulose. Present practice recommends the addition of 6 to 10 grams of fiber per day (2 teaspoons of psyllium seed or three quarters cup of bran) for the irritable bowel syndrome (characterized by alternating diarrhea and constipation) and for recurrent diverticulitis. Benefits of high fiber intake (type and amount variable) have been reported for diabetes mellitus, maintenance of lower calorie intake, and lowering of serum cholesterol. At present the data do not clearly support a required role for a fiber-supplemented diet in any of these disorders.

A diet low in fiber (Table 219–2) is useful in acute diarrheal illness and as a preparation for barium enema, colonoscopy, and intestinal surgery. The diet is then additionally modified in the form of a clear liquid diet for further reduction in ileal residue.

The best treatment for postmenopausal osteoporosis is still debatable, but it is generally agreed that increased calcium intake is an important component of the treatment plan (Ch. 249). Milk products serve this role best, as they provide protein as well as calcium. In the patient who is lactose-

TABLE 219–3. THERAPEUTIC DIETS CHARACTERIZED BY SUPPLEMENTATION OF DIETARY COMPONENTS

Diet	Typical Indication
High fiber	Irritable bowel, prevention of recurrent diverticulitis
High calcium (milk products, CaCO₃, or combination)	Postmenopausal osteoporosis
High protein (high biologic value)	Chronic hemodialysis or peritoneal dialysis
High protein	Malabsorption
Supplemental potassium	Diuretic use
High calorie	Weight loss due to illness

TABLE 219–4. SODIUM AND POTASSIUM CONTENT OF COMMON FOODS

Food	Portion	Sodium Content (mg)	Potassium Content (mg)
Milk	cup	120	350
Meat, fish, poultry	ounce	25	100–180
Most fruits and their juices	cup	4–10	300–490
Most vegetables	½ cup	5–9	300–500

intolerant or who does not like milk, calcium carbonate (40 per cent calcium by weight) may be used. In some patients a more water-soluble form of organic calcium (e.g., glubionate or gluconate) should be used, since the carbonate salt is not always well absorbed.

When diuretics and low-sodium diets are used, potassium is frequently replaced as an inorganic salt, but dietary supplementation can often be used and would be more palatable. For instance, the salt substitutes often used with low-sodium diets contain about 12 mEq of potassium per gram, and potassium is present in fairly high concentration in most fruits and vegetables and their juices (Table 219–4). Eight ounces of frozen orange or tomato juice contains 12 mEq potassium and one medium orange or banana 6 to 8 mEq. Milk is also a good source of potassium, but because of its high sodium content would be an inappropriate supplement for a patient taking diuretics. Only a minority of patients taking diuretics daily will develop hypokalemia. Therefore, for most patients, advice on dietary potassium supplements will be more than sufficient.

Protein supplements are needed for conditions characterized by excessive protein loss, such as protein-losing enteropathy, dialysis, and burns. These supplements can be supplied as table food or as commercial supplements. For each 10 grams of protein added, another 250 Kcal from nonprotein sources must also be ingested to ensure that the amino acids will be converted into body protein.

Diets That Alter the Consistency of Food

One of the most common dietary manipulations used in hospitalized patients is the *liquid diet*. The clear liquid diet provides the daily requirement for water and requires minimal digestion and intestinal motility, but it does not provide adequate amounts of protein or calories. It is also a low-fiber diet. If the patient who requires such a diet is already protein and calorie malnourished, the diet needs to be supplemented with carbohydrate, protein, or both. Even so, it is difficult to provide much more than 1000 Kcal per day. For long-term use the full liquid diet is more often prescribed. If table foods from all food groups are used or the diet is enriched with commercial supplements, the diet can be nutritionally complete. Care should be given to determining the actual food ingested, however, since a full liquid diet is often used for a patient who has some difficulty in swallowing table food. Thus the ingested food may not equal what is ordered. This precaution of course should be exercised when any diet is used for therapy, but it is particularly important when impairment of food ingestion or anorexia is the reason for the prescribed diet.

The *bland diet* is often combined with a mechanical soft diet for the treatment of peptic ulcer disease. Despite this widespread use, there are no data that clearly support the value of such a diet for any clinical condition, and present practice does not favor its use (see Ch. 100). Restriction of seasonings makes the food less palatable and discourages the successful use of whichever diet is being presented.

Alpers DH, Clouse RE, Stenson WF: Manual of Nutritional Therapeutics. 2nd ed. Boston, Little, Brown and Company (in press). *A detailed practical account of the use of diets and enteral therapy. Includes nutritional characteristics of most commercial supplements and diets.*

American Dietetic Association: Handbook of Clinical Dietetics. New Haven, Yale University Press, 1982. *A comprehensive and carefully outlined source for obtaining the details of most diets.*

Avioli LV: Calcium and osteoporosis. Ann Rev Nutr 4:471, 1984. *A well-reasoned review of the available information on the value of calcium supplementation in elderly women.*

Garrow JS: Treat Obesity Seriously. London, Churchill Livingstone, 1981. *A sensible and multifaceted approach to the therapy of obesity, especially for use of diet.*

Grundy SM: Recommendation for the treatment of hyperlipidemia in adults: A joint statement of the Nutrition Committee and the Council on Arteriosclerosis of the American Heart Association. Arteriosclerosis 4:445A, 1984. *The most definitive statement available on altered fat diets for atherosclerosis.*

Kabadi UM: Nutritional therapy in diabetics. Postgrad Med 79:145, 1986. *A balanced review of carbohydrate restriction.*

Paige DM (ed.): Lactose Digestion. Baltimore, Johns Hopkins University Press, 1981. *A symposium covering all aspects of lactose intolerance.*

Trowell H, Burkitt D, Heaton K (eds.): Dietary Fiber Depleted Foods and Disease. London, Academic Press, 1985. *Summarizes the evidence for the role of fiber in human disease.*

220 PARENTERAL NUTRITION
Ray E. Clouse

Parenteral nutrition includes delivery of micronutrients and macronutrients. Those nutrients that can rapidly become depleted in disease, such as water and major minerals, are administered routinely by vein to the hospitalized patient. The technical feasibility of providing nutrients that become depleted more slowly, such as amino acids and essential fatty acids, has resulted in the ability to deliver total parenteral nutrition support in the hospital and at home. Parenteral delivery of protein and calories can serve to partially meet, to totally meet, or to exceed the daily nutritional requirements. Thus, parenteral nutrition can be utilized in much the same way as enteral supplements or forced enteral feeding when an appropriate nutritional support plan is designed (see Ch. 219). The technique of delivery, morbidity (physical and psychological), and cost of such methods are more important considerations in the choice of parenteral or enteral nutrition routes than are differences in basic concepts of energy or specific nutrient requirements.

PARENTERAL ENERGY AND PROTEIN DELIVERY

Protein and calorie requirements are closely linked. Positive nitrogen balance, reflecting net positive endogenous protein synthesis, is most successfully accomplished if positive energy balance has been achieved. If parenteral nonprotein calories are provided for the average hospitalized patient in a ratio of calories to amino acid nitrogen (in grams) of greater than or equal to 150:1, delivered amino acids are likely to be utilized for protein synthesis. The ratio decreases in more intense catabolic states (e.g., major burns) and increases in less stressed situations.

ENERGY (CALORIE) SOURCES. Both carbohydrate and lipid are used as parenteral calorie sources (Table 220–1). The monohydrate form of dextrose used in most commercial intravenous solutions provides 3.4 kcal per gram, in contrast to 4 kcal per gram for the carbohydrate alone. Dextrose can be used as the sole nonprotein calorie source. Approximately 50 per cent of patients will require insulin supplementation in the parenteral infusion if dextrose is used to meet all daily calorie requirements. Lipid emulsions contain a source of calories in the form of emulsified droplets of soybean or safflower oil, which provide 9 kcal per gram, supplemented slightly by the caloric contribution of the emulsifiers (Table 220–1). Lipid emulsions may be used to supply the essential fatty acid linoleic acid as well as up to 70 per cent of the daily caloric requirement. A contraindication to the use of the emulsions is pre-existing hyperlipidemia. Complications related to the lipids are uncommon, but may limit their use (see below).

The preferred parenteral energy source or combination of sources is controversial. Positive energy balance as well as positive nitrogen balance can be achieved if dextrose is used alone to provide daily calories, as long as adequate amino acids are also supplied. However, lipid emulsions reduce the likelihood of hyperglycemia, the volume of fluid needed, and the metabolic response to the infusion. The lower respiratory quotient for lipids (0.7) compared with carbohydrates (1.0) indicates reduced carbon dioxide production from fat metabolism for isocaloric infusion of these energy sources. Thus, lipids have theoretic (and practical) advantages in patients with respiratory compromise. Lipid emulsions are somewhat more expensive than dextrose and usually necessitate additional intravenous equipment. The use of a combination of lipid and dextrose with other nutrients in a single infusion bag has eliminated some of the cumbersome equipment required for lipid infusion, but not all patients are in stable enough condition to make this technique practical. Lipid emulsions are utilized for their essential fatty acid content at least several times per week; thus many institutions currently use lipids daily as a component of their energy provision.

PROTEIN DELIVERY. Protein requirements are met in parenteral nutrition by infusion of amino acids. Amino acid profiles in standard commercial products are based largely on normal plasma amino acid concentrations, with modifications observed to stimulate anabolism. The amino acid content (in grams) is roughly comparable to the dietary protein in the RDA, except for differences due to absorption efficiency and slight differences related to dissimilarities of amino acid profiles in average dietary proteins and in the solutions.

Amino acid ratios in specialized commercial products have been modified for specific disease conditions. Solutions with increased branched-chain amino acids (isoleucine, leucine, valine) and decreased aromatic amino acids (phenylalanine, tyrosine, tryptophan) are promoted for use in liver failure. Such solutions will often improve encephalopathy due to portal-systemic shunts, but have not consistently been shown to have a favorable impact on survival from liver disease. Essential amino acids are reduced in concentration in the plasma of patients with renal failure. Specialized formulas with an increased proportion of essential amino acids are available. Blood urea nitrogen will be reduced and positive nitrogen balance attained when dietary protein contains a larger percentage of essential amino acids. Infusion of essential amino acids will retard accumulation of urea nitrogen. However, at least in acute renal failure, both essential and nonessential amino acids are necessary for sustained anabolism. Clinical success in protein delivery in the management of many patients with renal failure is similar with standard and specialized amino acid formulas as long as a protein restriction is maintained (generally not less than 0.5 gram per kilogram per day) and positive energy balance is established.

PRACTICAL APPLICATIONS. A combination of dextrose, amino acids, and water provides the base solution to which vitamins and minerals can be added. Parenteral nutrition solutions that provide all energy and protein requirements usually have to be administered through the central vein, since they are so hyperosmotic. For example, a formulation

TABLE 220–1. PROTEIN AND CALORIE SOURCES UTILIZED IN PARENTERAL NUTRITION

Macronutrient Category		Parenteral Form of Macronutrient	Nonprotein Caloric Value
Protein		Crystalline amino acids	
Calories	Carbohydrate	Dextrose monohydrate	3.4 Kcal/g
	Fat	Lipid emulsion	10% emulsion—1.1 Kcal/ml
			20% emulsion—2.0 Kcal/ml

made from 500 ml of 50 per cent dextrose (2500 mOsm per liter) and 500 ml of 8.5 per cent amino acids (850 mOsm per liter) would provide 850 kcal (from nonprotein sources) and 42.5 grams of amino acids with a resultant osmolarity of 1675 mOsm per liter. Vitamin and mineral additives will further raise the final osmolarity. Lipid emulsions are run in parallel with the base solution. Macronutrient delivery can be shortened for patients in stable condition to a 10- to 12-hour period, e.g., at night. Both methods of calorie and protein delivery are effective in achieving positive energy and nitrogen balance. Gradual conversion over two to three days is required from a 24-hour schedule to the cyclic schedule. Once conversion is effected, the base solution (and lipid emulsion, if used as a daily energy source) is discontinued each morning by reducing the rate in two or three 30-minute steps. The rate is similarly increased at the reinitiation of infusion in the evening. These precautions are effective in preventing hypoglycemia and hyperglycemia for most patients. Patients on cyclic regimens are then free from infusion in the daytime.

Macronutrients may also be provided through peripheral veins. Lesser concentrations of dextrose and amino acids are required to keep the final osmolarity less than 600 to 800 mOsm per liter and thereby reduce the likelihood of thrombophlebitis. Continuous coadministration of isotonic lipid emulsion will reduce the osmolarity yet allow for the total energy and protein requirement to be infused. For this reason, lipid emulsions are regularly used as daily energy sources in peripheral vein parenteral nutrition. Parenteral prescriptions that provide less calories than the daily energy requirement can serve as supplements to an inadequate enteral regimen or can be used alone to reduce negative nitrogen balance. Even with excessive amino acid infusion (greater than 2 grams per kilogram per day), however, sustained positive nitrogen balance will not be accomplished without adequate energy supply. Thus this parenteral nutrition practice is not a substitute for more intensive support, if nutritional restoration is the goal.

TOTAL PARENTERAL NUTRITION

Besides amino acids and calorie sources, all other recognized nutrients can be provided by a parenteral route. Total parenteral nutrition (TPN) is required for short or long periods by patients with either temporarily or permanently unusable or inadequate small intestines. TPN can be administered through catheters in central or peripheral veins; in most instances, the central venous route is utilized. Detailed techniques of TPN are beyond the scope of this textbook and are described in many monographs and handbooks. The most successful TPN programs involve the direction of a knowledgeable physician and the cooperation of informed and interested colleagues in the pharmacy, nursing, and dietetics departments.

INDICATIONS. A small number of patients require lifelong TPN because of extensive resection (e.g., from mesenteric vascular accidents, Crohn's disease, trauma) or advanced small-bowel disease (e.g., scleroderma, radiation enteritis). The majority of patients with short-bowel syndrome from resection, however, can eventually be managed with oral feeding after an initial adaptation period. TPN is indicated as a temporary nutritional therapy mainly for two patient groups: (1) those selected for intensive nutritional support in whom the intestinal tract is not usable for forced enteral feeding (see Ch. 219) and (2) those in whom a nothing-by-mouth regimen ("bowel rest") would be beneficial to a primary gastrointestinal disease. The majority of patients placed on a TPN regimen are those with the first indication. Figure 219–1 gives a flow diagram incorporating the various questions used in deciding which patients are indeed candidates for intensive nutritional support. In general, this group has moderate to severe protein-compartment depletion at the initial evaluation

and is expected to suffer significant additional losses with the current illness.

Gastrointestinal Diseases. In the nothing-by-mouth regimen TPN is used for both *parenteral nutrition* and *bowel rest* in an attempt to assist in disease regression. Prior to the availability of TPN, regression had been observed in some patients who were not allowed to eat or who minimized input for brief periods, especially those with Crohn's disease, ulcerative colitis, enterocutaneous fistulas, and pancreatitis (Table 220–2). With TPN, regression of disease is variable, but is most frequent in patients with uncomplicated Crohn's disease of the small bowel who have failed usual regimens (Table 220–2). In a prospective randomized trial, patients with acute ulcerative colitis who were managed with TPN and bowel rest in addition to usual medical measures did no better than those given oral feedings and standard intravenous fluids as the nutritional adjuvants, as judged by the number requiring colectomy in each group. However, nutritional benefits that are gained by the severely malnourished patient or nutritional deterioration that is prevented by initiating TPN in the healthier patient preoperatively will not be reflected in a small number of patients if colectomy is the only endpoint. TPN allows total bowel rest to be carried on for longer periods without the fear of nutritional deterioration, possibly improving the chances that bowel rest will be successful in aiding disease regression. An adequate TPN plan will also uniformly replenish the malnourished patient in the process; any additional beneficial effects of nutritional repletion on the primary disease are difficult to assess.

TPN with or without bowel rest is also often indicated in gastrointestinal disorders that have severe symptoms, especially if the patient would also be selected for intensive nutritional support. Such conditions include severe diarrhea, intractable vomiting, and small-intestinal disorders that interfere significantly with enteral feeding (e.g., radiation enteritis, obstruction from inflammatory adhesions, following small-bowel resection).

Other Diseases. When TPN is utilized in management of patients with disease not involving the gastrointestinal tract, bowel rest is not enforced. Use of TPN with modified amino acid formulas in patients with hepatic and renal disease has been mentioned. Despite intuitive impressions that TPN should reduce mortality and could improve organ function in these disorders, results from clinical studies have not been conclusive. In patients with cancer, nutritional status can be maintained or improved with an adequate TPN program, but

TABLE 220–2. SUMMARY OF THE EFFECTS OF TOTAL PARENTERAL NUTRITION (TPN) WITH BOWEL REST IN VARIOUS DISEASES

Disease	Nutritional Maintenance or Repletion Achieved	Short-Term (In-Hospital) Disease Regression	Long-Term Disease Regression
Ulcerative colitis*	Majority	30–50%	20–30%
Crohn's disease*	Yes	60–80%	50–60%
Subgroup with fistulas†	Yes	30–40%	10–30%
Subgroup with colitis†	Yes	60%	NA‡
Enterocutaneous fistulas (not Crohn's disease)	Yes	30–70% closure§	NA
Severe pancreatitis	Yes¶	NA	NA

*Many patients in reported series are treated with corticosteroids as well as TPN and bowel rest.

†Small patient series; subgroups not always designated.

‡Adequate data not available.

§Many patients eventually managed with surgical therapy; wide range of reported success rates.

¶Parenteral nutrition is successful and does not contribute to morbidity of pancreatitis despite theoretical concern regarding pancreatic stimulatory effects.

this has not proved to be of overall benefit in enhancing tumor responsiveness to antineoplastic agents. The best candidates for intensive nutritional support are those who have tumors potentially responsive to anticancer therapy, but who could not receive optimal management because of the combined detrimental effects of the planned therapy and malnutrition. Patients undergoing allogeneic bone marrow transplantation for leukemia often typify this situation. Some patients can be managed with forced enteral nutrition rather than TPN. Patients who are severely catabolic or who will likely need major surgery may also be candidates for intensive nutritional support. Such candidates would be selected by following the algorithm outlined in Ch. 219.

Home TPN. Home administration should be considered for patients with irreversible gastrointestinal disease or for patients whose conditions are relatively stable and who need TPN for a month or more. The cyclic method of macronutrient delivery and long central catheters burrowed through a subcutaneous tunnel on the anterior chest are employed. Approximately one third of patients requiring home TPN have malignant disease or intestinal complications related to therapy for malignant disease (resection or radiation). One third have inflammatory bowel disease, and the remainder have a variety of intestinal disorders, including severe gastrointestinal motility disturbances (such as scleroderma bowel) and short-bowel syndrome following trauma or ischemic insult.

NUTRIENTS PROVIDED DURING TPN (Table 220–3). Protein requirements (as described in Ch. 212) are met with crystalline amino acids in commercially available solutions. Nonprotein calories are provided by concentrated dextrose and by lipid emulsions. Two liters of a base solution composed of equal amounts of 8.5 per cent amino acids and 50 per cent dextrose in conjunction with 500 ml of a 10-per cent lipid emulsion is a feasible daily protein-calorie prescription. This would provide approximately 80 grams of protein as amino acids, 1680 carbohydrate calories, and 550 fat calories. The resultant nonprotein calorie-nitrogen ratio is 170:1, with 25 per cent of the daily calories provided by fat. An alternate regimen would provide all the nonprotein calories as dextrose. The daily protein and calorie prescription should be tailored to a patient's requirements or exceed them by 20 to 40 grams of protein and 500 to 1000 kcal, if restoration of depleted compartments is a goal. Water requirement varies, depending on the capability of the patient to excrete an osmotic load, 30 ml per kilogram (or approximately 1 ml per kilocalorie delivered) being typical. Increased water delivery is necessary for fever (360 ml per day per degree centigrade elevation) and anabolism (300 to 400 ml per day).

Major mineral requirements vary considerably from patient to patient and during any one patient's course of TPN. In particular, potassium requirements may be initially large because of extracellular to intracellular fluxes with glucose (and possibly insulin) infusion and because of reversal of the catabolic state. The ranges of major mineral requirements listed in Table 220–3 are typical for the average adult patient, but careful monitoring of serum levels is always necessary to determine the correct provision, especially in the first few weeks of TPN.

Deficiencies of trace minerals are rarely observed in patients receiving oral feedings because these nutrients are widely distributed among foods and the requirements are low. Deficiencies of zinc, chromium, copper, and selenium may occur during long courses of TPN, however. Such deficiencies are now prevented by supplementing TPN fluid with trace minerals from the outset. Zinc, copper, chromium, and manganese are commonly provided; selenium and iodine (and occasionally molybdenum) are usually given only to patients receiving very long courses of TPN, as during home TPN. Manganese and molybdenum deficiencies have not yet been reported in TPN patients. See Ch. 218 for further discussion of the trace minerals.

TABLE 220–3. TYPICAL DAILY NUTRIENT PROVISIONS DURING TOTAL PARENTERAL NUTRITION (TPN) FOR STABLE ADULT PATIENTS WITHOUT CARDIAC, HEPATIC, OR RENAL FAILURE

Calories	Dextrose	60–80% of requirement (see Ch. 212)
	Lipid emulsion*	20–40% of requirement
Protein	Crystalline amino acids	100% of requirement (see Ch. 212)
Minerals	Sodium	90–120 mEq
	Potassium	90–150 mEq
	Chloride	90–150 mEq
	Calcium	12–16 mEq
	Phosphorus	20–40 mmol
	Magnesium	12–16 mEq
	Iron†	
	Zinc‡	2–8 mg
	Copper	1–1.6 mg
	Chromium	10–16 μg
	Manganese	0.4–0.8 mg
	Selenium§	120 μg
	Iodine§	50–80 μg
	Molybdenum§	20 μg
Vitamins¶	A	3300 IU
	D	200 IU
	E	10 IU
	B_1 (thiamin)	3.0 mg
	B_2 (riboflavin)	3.6 mg
	B_3 (pantothenic acid)	15.0 mg
	B_5 (niacin)	40.0 mg
	B_6 (pyridoxine)	4.0 mg
	B_7 (biotin)	60.0 μg
	B_9 (folic acid)	400.0 μg
	B_{12} (cobalamin)**	5.0 μg
	C (ascorbic acid)	100.0 mg††
	K	5 mg/wk‡‡
Essential Fatty Acid§§	Linoleic acid	4% of total calories

*See text for a discussion of the use of lipid emulsion as a daily calorie source. May be co-administered with the base solution.

†The daily requirement (not taking phlebotomy losses into consideration) is about 1.5 mg and can be met by giving 1 ml (50 mg Fe) of iron-dextran solution intramuscularly per month. Replacement is usually dictated by indices of iron stores.

‡Requirements are increased if intestinal fluid losses are great (see Ch. 218).

§Additive usually reserved for patients on long courses of TPN.

¶Based on guidelines from the American Medical Association/Nutrition Advisory Group, 1975. These guidelines do not take into account increased requirements during metabolic stress.

**May be given by monthly intramuscular injection.

††Daily provision often increased to 500 mg or more during periods of catabolic stress.

‡‡Not provided by multivitamin preparation; given by separate injection.

§§Provided by lipid emulsions on a biweekly or triweekly basis. Linolenic acid is also present in some emulsions and may be required during long-term TPN (see text).

Recommendations for vitamin supplementation are given in Table 220–3; few detrimental effects have appeared when these guidelines have been followed. More commonly, vitamin deficiency results from the inadvertent omission of folate or cobalamin, which may not be included in the multivitamin preparation used, or from omission of vitamin K, which is not included in any parenteral multivitamin formulation. Less vitamin D than the recommendation is necessary for patients undergoing long-term therapy.

Linoleic, linolenic, and arachidonic acids cannot be synthesized by humans. However, essential fatty acid (EFA) deficiency can usually be prevented by supplying adequate quantities of linoleic acid alone. EFA deficiency is rarely observed as an isolated deficiency except during TPN. A large amount (8 to 10 per cent) of the fat in adipose tissue contains the EFA's. However, the high insulin levels observed during TPN with concentrated dextrose are believed to impair access to this store through inhibition of lipolysis. Manifestations of EFA deficiency include dry, cracked skin, coarsening of the hair, hair loss, and impaired wound healing. It is estimated that 4 to 5 per cent of the daily energy requirement should be provided by linoleic acid to prevent deficiency, and lipid emulsions (500 ml of 10 per cent emulsion triweekly) will satisfy this requirement. A report of linolenic acid deficiency in a child receiving a lipid emulsion low in this fatty acid during long-term TPN suggests that linoleic acid alone may not always be adequate to prevent EFA deficiency in humans. Use of a lipid emulsion with both linoleic and linolenic acid is currrently recommended to avoid EFA deficiency during long courses of TPN.

COMPLICATIONS OF PARENTERAL NUTRITION

Both administration-related and metabolic complications may occur with parenteral nutrition (Table 220–4). *Thrombophlebitis* from hyperosmolar solutions is the most frequent complication when a peripheral vein is used. Several complications will be detected by a chest radiograph (in expiration if pneumothorax is suspected) after central-vein catheter insertion, a practice that should always be followed. Some degree of clinically inapparent catheter-related thrombosis may occur in as many as 50 per cent of patients. At present, only symptomatic patients (certainly less than 5 per cent of those with subclavian vein catheters) are observed and treated for noninfected thrombosis along the catheter path.

Catheter-related sepsis should also occur in no more than 5 per cent of patients treated with TPN of varying course length in a typical hospital-based program if maximal efforts are being made to prevent infection. Contamination from the catheter hub is often responsible for catheter-related infection. Culturing of material from removed catheter tips will indicate if the source of fever was actually an infected catheter.

Metabolic complications include the appearance of nutritional deficiencies resulting from inadequately prescribed TPN. Figure 220–1 shows the relative time to appearance of deficiencies under these circumstances. Each deficiency, of course, will become more quickly apparent if body stores of that nutrient were originally depleted. Deficiencies are rare if nutrients are attentively prescribed.

Hyperglycemia is common in patients given concentrated dextrose by central vein. Regular insulin added to the base solution should be used to keep serum glucose below 200 mg per deciliter. *Hypoglycemia* is not likely to occur if (1) exogenous insulin is added to the base solution rather than given subcutaneously, (2) the base solution is not interrupted ab-

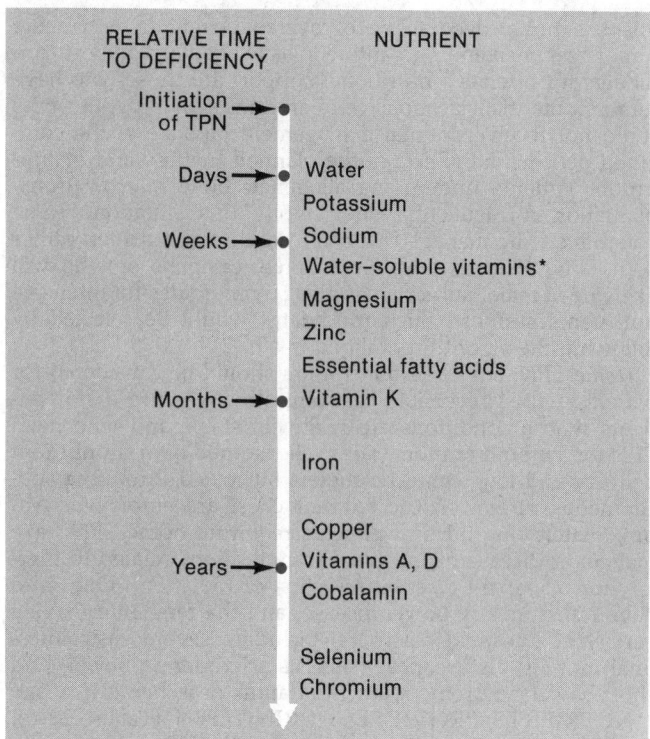

FIGURE 220–1. Relative time to the development of nutrient deficiencies during inadequately supplemented total parenteral nutrition (TPN). The time is proportional to body stores and inversely related to the fractional catabolic rate of the nutrient in an individual patient. Thus, the relative times given are only estimates. (*Excluding cobalamin.)

ruptly, and (3) parenteral nutrition is terminated slowly over 24 hours or more with a stepwise reduction in the rate of glucose delivery. Incorrect provisions of major minerals can also be detected by regular laboratory monitoring, especially during the first two weeks of parenteral nutrition therapy.

Hepatic dysfunction not infrequently occurs. Increases in serum levels of liver enzyme are frequently noted following initiation of TPN. Transaminase increases usually do not persist. Delayed or persistent increases (> 20 days) may indicate toxic hepatitis related to the amino acid infusion, or more likely, a process not related to parenteral nutrition. Elevations of alkaline phosphatase values (up to two times normal) are noted in half of patients receiving TPN for more than 20 days. In some patients this represents fat accumulation from excessive carbohydrate feeding. Painful hepatomegaly may occur in these circumstances; fatty liver may be detected by computed tomography. Prevention or correction of increases of liver enzymes has been observed in some patients treated with metronidazole. Reduction in overgrowth of intestinal organisms and their toxic by-products in the portal stream has been speculated as the mechanism of this effect.

Periarticular, long-bone, and back pain, a syndrome that usually appears months into a course of TPN, is of unclear cause, but is likely related to altered vitamin D metabolism. Other factors contributing to bone disease include hypercalciuria observed during the TPN infusion (probably related to glucose loading and/or increased organic sulfate burden) and possibly improper trace mineral administration. Patients respond to discontinuation of TPN and removal of vitamin D from the TPN fluid.

Early or immediate *reactions to lipid emulsions* (dyspnea, cyanosis, cutaneous allergic phenomena, nausea, headache, back pain, autonomic discharge) occur with an incidence of less than 1 per cent. Hyperlipidemia resulting from the infusion should clear within four hours after the infusion. Poor lipid clearance is common with renal or hepatic failure. Delayed adverse reactions include hepatomegaly, jaundice,

TABLE 220–4. COMPLICATIONS OF PARENTERAL NUTRITION

Administration-Related Complications
More frequent
  Thrombophlebitis (peripheral vein)
  Infection
  Inappropriate tip placement
  Pneumothorax
  Central vein thrombosis
Rare
  Hemothorax
  Air embolus
  Arterial laceration
  Brachial plexus injury
  Central venous catheter fragmentation and embolization

Metabolic Complications
More frequent
  Hyperglycemia and hyperosmolarity
  Hypoglycemia
  Electrolyte disturbances
  BUN elevation
  Liver dysfunction
  Fatty liver
  Hypercapnia
  Cholelithiasis (long-term treatment)
  Hyperlipidemia from lipid emulsion
Rare
  Vitamin and trace mineral deficiency (Fig. 220–1)
  Essential fatty acid deficiency
  Metabolic bone disease
  Other adverse reaction to lipid emulsion
  Hyperammonemia

splenomegaly, thrombocytopenia, and leukopenia. Alterations in pulmonary function studies may occur in patients receiving lipid emulsions. A reduction in pulmonary diffusing capacity may be the most significant change, a change that has been seriously detrimental to premature infants with hyaline membrane disease, but less clinically significant to adults with respiratory disease.

As many as one third of patients treated with TPN for a period of two years have detectable *gallstones*. The prevalence is even higher (50 per cent) in the subset with ileal disease (Crohn's disease or prior resection or both). Gallbladder stasis and an increase in bile saturation with fasting are possible explanations for these higher than expected prevalences. Other metabolic complications resulting from alteration of normal physiology are likely to be recognized as more patients with potentially catastrophic small-bowel resections or disease are maintained with long courses of TPN at home.

Alpers DH, Clouse RE, Stenson WF: Manual of Nutritional Therapeutics. 2nd ed. Boston, Little, Brown and Company (in press). *This manual outlines parenteral nutrient requirements and describes techniques of parenteral nutrition in a chapter devoted to the subject. It is also a reference source for nutrient composition of proprietary products.*

A.S.P.E.N. Board of Directors: Guidelines for use of local parenteral nutrition in the hospitalized adult patient. J Parent Enteral Nutr 10:441, 1986. *A more comprehensive list of current recommendations for the use of parenteral nutrition in various disease settings.*

Bengoa JM, Rosenberg IH: Parenteral nutritional therapy in gastrointestinal disease. Adv Intern Med 28:363, 1983. *Provides a critical review and summary of the use of these techniques in patients with inflammatory bowel disease and other gastrointestinal disorders.*

Brennan MF: Total parenteral nutrition in the cancer patient. N Engl J Med 305:375, 1981. *The many studies examining various effects of parenteral nutrition on cancer management are reviewed. The author summarizes reasonable expectations of the use of this form of nutritional support in cancer patients. Correspondence regarding this review should also be read (N Engl J Med 305:1589, 1981).*

Grant JP: Handbook of Total Parenteral Nutrition. Philadelphia, W. B. Saunders Company, 1980. *A well-referenced monograph with a detailed review, particularly of uses and complications, of parenteral nutrition.*

Kaminski MV Jr (ed.): Hyperalimentation: A Guide for Clinicians. New York, Marcel Dekker, 1985. *Contributions from many experts in the field of parenteral nutrition make this book a comprehensive reference. The chapters on principles of parenteral nutrition in various diseases are useful.*

PART XVI
ENDOCRINE AND REPRODUCTIVE DISEASES

221 PRINCIPLES OF ENDOCRINOLOGY

John D. Baxter

Multicellular organisms must communicate among their cells to maintain homeostasis, to carry out normal growth and development, and to allow for effective adaptations to stress. The endocrine system and the nervous system, both separately and through their interactions, have evolved to meet that need.

The term *endocrine* refers to the process of secretion of biologically active substances in the body; by contrast, the term *exocrine* refers to external secretion, as into the gastrointestinal tract. The endocrine glands, usually of mesodermal or entodermal origin, release hormones into the systemic circulation for more universal distribution, whereas the nervous system, of ectodermal origin, in general informs by the local release of neurotransmitters in the immediate vicinity of the target cell. However, hormones also may have more restricted pathways of effective distribution; this occurs, for instance, in the portal systems of the abdomen and of the hypothalamic-hypophyseal region. Finally, both hormones and neurotransmitters can act on the same cells that release them (autocrine communication) or can migrate to nearby target cells through the interstitial fluid without entering the circulation (paracrine communication).

In the nervous system there is physical continuity with complex arcades of integration; the endocrine system is multifocal in form and function. Strictly speaking, it is not one "system" but a series of systems for intercellular chemical communication. There can be integration among glands in the flow of information, as illustrated by the sequential responses that follow the release of corticotropin releasing factor (CRF) by the hypothalamus. CRF triggers corticotropin (ACTH) release from the adenohypophysis (anterior pituitary gland), which stimulates cortisol release from the adrenal cortex to effect physiologic responses in numerous target tissues. Other endocrine glands are more freestanding. The parathyroid glands and their hormone, parathyroid hormone (PTH), function in a closed circuit to maintain extracellular calcium homeostasis independent of the nervous system, and have no known direct interactions with the pituitary gland, although they are indirectly linked to the endocrine systems of calcitonin and of vitamin D and its products.

In spite of these distinctions, the endocrine and nervous systems overlap in their functions and are closely interrelated. Thus the ectodermal posterior pituitary gland (neurohypophysis) and adrenal medulla are arguably parts of the nervous system, although they release vasopressin and epinephrine, respectively, for systemic distribution. Nervous impulses can trigger hormone release and vice versa. The same chemicals (e.g., dopamine, norepinephrine) can serve as both hormones and neurotransmitters. Further, neurotransmitters and hormones also share common mechanisms in eliciting their actions.

Neuroendocrinology has emerged as a discipline that focuses on the interrelationships between the nervous and endocrine systems. The central role of the hypothalamus as a neuroendocrine organ has long been known, as summarized in Ch. 225. Several of its secretory products that trigger the release of hormones (e.g., ACTH, gonadotropins) from the anterior pituitary gland have been characterized and synthesized for clinical use. The peptides with opiate activity found in both the pituitary and central nervous system are discussed in Ch. 222. Even hormones previously thought to be strictly gastrointestinal (gastrin, cholecystokinin) are now known to be abundant in the central nervous system. Thus the two major systems for communications are interrelated directly and in more subtle ways. Perhaps it is more appropriate to think instead of a single neuroendocrine integrating system with subspecialization of delivery systems into neurons, gland cells, and various mixed forms in between.

A *hormone* therefore is a substance that is released in one tissue and travels through the circulation (usually) to the target tissue, where it elicits a particular response. There are interesting variations in this simple schema. The potential autocrine and paracrine functions of hormones are mentioned above. Estradiol, for instance, can affect ovarian granulosa cells. In addition, a precursor to a hormone may be released with the final effector molecule being formed in the circulation, the target tissue, or even another organ. Renin substrate (angiotensinogen) is synthesized in the liver as a prohormone to be subsequently converted in the plasma to the effector substance angiotensin II by two successive modifications catalyzed by renin (from the kidney) and angiotensin-converting enzyme (from the lung and other tissues), respectively. Testosterone is converted to dihydrotestosterone, which is responsible for many androgenic actions, by 5α-reductase in the target tissue. The endogenous biosynthesis of the most active form of vitamin D_3, 1,25-dihydroxycholecalciferol, requires steps that are sequentially carried out in the skin, liver, and kidney.

The *target cell* for hormone action must possess special mechanisms for recognizing and responding to these particular chemical signals, accepting those that are appropriate and rejecting those that are inappropriate from among the jumble of substances to which it is exposed. This specificity of recognition exists in the three-dimensional structure of unique macromolecules termed *receptors* that bind the hormone selectively and with high affinity. The target cell must also contain mechanisms to couple the hormone-receptor interaction with the subsequent steps in the cellular response to the information received.

Receptors are also useful for classifying hormone action. For example, cortisol, the major glucocorticoid in man, elicits glucocorticoid actions such as on gluconeogenesis and inflammatory reactions by binding to glucocorticoid receptors. Cortisol can also bind to mineralocorticoid receptors and promote sodium retention and potassium loss. However, aldosterone is the major mineralocorticoid in man and also binds to mineralocorticoid receptors. Thus, when cortisol or aldosterone binds to mineralocorticoid receptors the steroid acts as a mineralocorticoid. Similarly, catecholamines can bind to alpha$_1$, alpha$_2$, beta$_1$, and beta$_2$ receptors and elicit their respective adrenergic actions; this use of receptors to classify hormone action avoids problems encountered when a given hormone can bind to more than one type of receptor and when several different hormones bind to the same receptor.

What then are the limits of endocrinology? They are not always easy to define. The brain (endorphins, gastrin, releasing factors), liver (renin substrate, 25-hydroxycholecalciferol), heart (atrial natriuretic factor), and kidney (erythropoietin, renin, and 1,25-dihydroxycholecalciferol) are endocrine glands. Nevertheless the definitions become arbitrary and conventional. The prostaglandins are important intercellular regulators with receptors on the cell surface. Although they are not often considered to be hormones in the strict sense, their function is autocrine and/or paracrine. They are discussed together with other arachidonate metabolites in Ch. 223. By convention the major islet cell hormones have been translocated into "metabolism," and the extensive gastrointestinal hormone system has been woven into gastroenterology. Various polypeptide growth factors (nerve, epidermal, platelet derived) for specific target tissues have been identified, but are not yet generally sanctified as hormones. Further, whereas oncology is not generally considered a discipline of endocrinology, certain products of cancer genes are similar to growth factors, growth factor receptors, or steroid or thyroid hormone receptors. The thymus has emerged more into immunology than endocrinology, but thymosin might properly be considered a hormone, and, more remotely, the various lymphokines are recognized as chemical messengers as well. Since *hormone* derives from a Greek verb meaning "to set in motion" or "to spur on," what better candidate can there be than a chemotactic factor?

A communication system must be coupled for both emission (signal) and reception that lead to an appropriate response. Classic endocrinology has been signal oriented. Attention has been devoted mostly to the release and transport of hormones and the arcades of control that govern those phenomena. This has been enormously productive in the study of normal physiology and of the pathophysiology, diagnosis, and treatment of human endocrine diseases. It seemed at one time that endocrinology, almost by definition quantifiable by measurements of hormone levels in the circulation, could be reduced to a Mendeleev-type periodic table of syndromes representing all possible combinations of "too much" or "too little" of the known hormones. As such it might be considered largely a laboratory endeavor. More recently, attention has been increasingly shifted to the reception-response domain of the discipline. Pseudohypoparathyroidism was recognized as a syndrome of resistance to hormone action as early as 1942 by Fuller Albright and his colleagues. Many examples of such resistance, both genetic and acquired, are now known that involve not only rare but also common conditions. Situations also occur when increased sensitivity to hormones contributes to the pathophysiology of disease. These will be described below and in specific detail in other chapters of Part XVI. The structures of hormone receptors and how they are linked to cellular responses are now becoming understood. The mechanisms that have been detected and the experimental approaches merge into cellular and molecular biology without sharp distinction. Endocrinology *within the cell* increasingly is being pursued through receptor and postreceptor mechanisms to the point of response generation. Perhaps Albright with his whimsy would have called this endoendocrinology.

HORMONE SYNTHESIS AND RELEASE

Over 50 different hormones are produced by the body. As usually defined, these are represented by several types of molecules: (1) amino acid analogues and derivatives (thyroid hormones, catecholamines), (2) polypeptides, and (3) lipids (steroids and arachidonic acid metabolites). The arachidonic acid system (prostaglandins, prostacyclins, thromboxanes, and hydroxy fatty acids) will not be discussed here, but is presented in Ch. 223. Endocrine glands synthesize and to some extent store their hormones for subsequent release into the circulation. This function is similar whether it is found in an anatomically separate gland (pituitary, thyroid, adrenal, parathyroids) or in specialized cells or cell clusters within other host tissues (islets of Langerhans, testis, ovary, small intestine, kidney). In some cases the endocrine function has not been found to be isolated to cells specialized for that function—e.g., the production of somatomedins or renin substrate by liver or of erythropoietin or 1,25-dihydroxycholecalciferol by the kidney.

AMINO ACID ANALOGUES AND DERIVATIVES. Tyrosine is the unique amino acid precursor of these hormones. In the thyroid gland, tyrosine moieties within the large protein thyroglobulin are iodinated to form monoiodotyrosine (MIT) and diiodotyrosine (DIT) while still in peptide linkage. These iodotyrosines undergo oxidative condensation, which couples the respective phenolic groups through ether linkage to form the iodinated thyronines, thyroxine (T$_4$), and triiodothyronine (T$_3$). The thyroglobulin of colloid is then taken up by the cuboidal cells of the thyroid follicle in which the actions of proteases and peptidases release T$_3$ and T$_4$ to be delivered into the circulation. The major secretory product, T$_4$, serves largely as a prohormone, since it is then further converted to the more active T$_3$ in the peripheral tissues by the removal of an outer ring iodine. These steps are detailed in Ch. 229 (see Fig. 229–1).

Catecholamines and dopamine, in contrast, are synthesized from free tyrosine in a series of reactions that enzymatically hydroxylate and decarboxylate the parent molecule. These reactions are summarized in Ch. 242.

POLYPEPTIDE HORMONES. The polypeptide hormones are synthesized by the steps outlined in Figure 221–1. The polypeptide gene contains sequences whose transcripts code for the hormones; these are flanked by DNA sequences important for directing the initiation and termination of transcription and in many cases the level of expression of the gene. Between the flanking sequences are "exon" sequences in the DNA whose transcripts contain the RNA sequences that are contained in the mature mRNA product of the gene. The exon sequences are usually interrupted in one or more places in the gene by intervening sequences termed introns. When the gene is transcribed, a large precursor messenger RNA (pre-mRNA) is made. This is then processed by the removal of the sequences transcribed from the introns, and splicing together of the exon sequences in the RNA and the cleavage of sequences from the end of the transcript with polyadenylation of the terminus to form the mature mRNA that is transported to the cytoplasm. The polypeptide hormones, like other secreted proteins, are synthesized in a larger precursor form termed a prehormone as the direct product translated from the mRNA. In addition to the amino acids of the hormone (or "prohormone" [see below]), the prehormone contains a "signal peptide" sequence at the amino terminus that is important for transfer of the protein

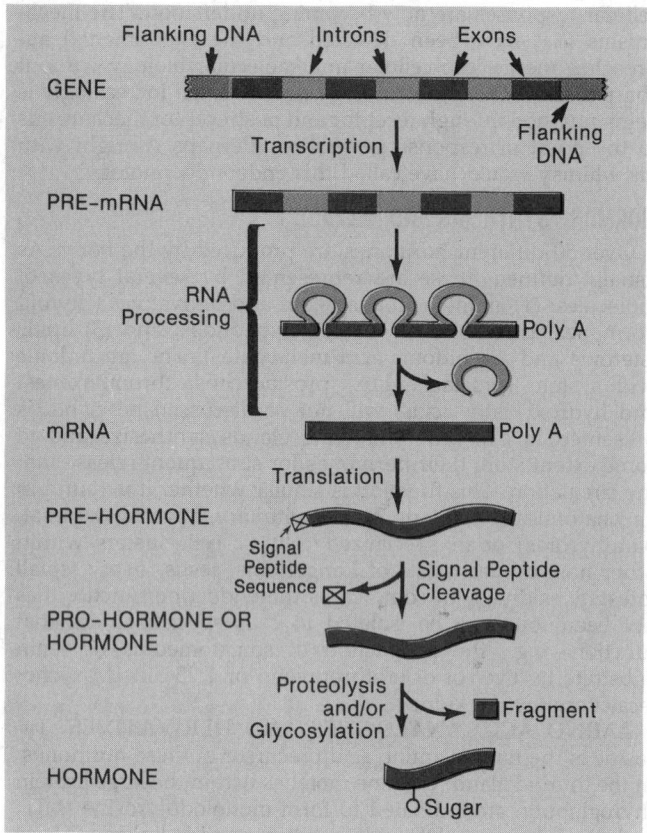

FIGURE 221-1. Steps in polypeptide hormone biosynthesis.

from the surface of the endoplasmic reticulum in the cytoplasm, where it is synthesized, into the endoplasmic reticulum. The signal peptide sequence is responsible for binding of the polyribosome complexes, containing mRNA, ribosomes, and nascent protein chains being synthesized, to the rough endoplasmic reticulum. The signal peptide sequence is subsequently removed by proteolysis, leaving either the hormone (e.g., growth hormone, prolactin) or a prohormone (e.g., proinsulin, proparathyroid hormone, proopiomelanocortin, procalcitonin). Further proteolysis of the prohormone in the endoplasmic reticulum or the secretory vesicles derived from it occurs to yield the hormone itself. Insulin is formed, for example, by the excision of a C peptide that connects the A and B chains in the nascent molecule. In the mature molecule, the latter chains are linked through disulfide bonds. ACTH is cleaved from the center of a much larger protein (proopiomelanocortin) that contains several other hormones, including β-endorphin and α- and β-melanocyte-stimulating hormone. Some hormones are further modified by glycosylation prior to their release; these include thyroid-stimulating hormone (TSH), luteinizing hormone (LH), chorionic gonadotropin (hCG), and follicle-stimulating hormone (FSH). These hormones consist of two subunits, each encoded by a separate gene. The subunits bind together following their synthesis.

Variations in this scheme can sometimes result in different hormones arising from the same gene. For instance, growth hormone pre-mRNA is processed in two ways that differ in the size of one of the intervening sequences that is removed. These differences result in two growth hormone mRNAs and consequent protein forms that differ somewhat in their biologic activities. The pre-mRNA that yields mRNA coding for preprocalcitonin is alternatively processed primarily in the brain to yield an mRNA that codes for a different peptide. At the post-translational level, proopiomelanocortin can be processed to yield in some cases predominantly ACTH and β-lipotropin (β-LPH) and in other cases predominantly corticotropin-like intermediate lobe peptide (CLIP) and β-endorphin.

The hormones within the cisternae of the endoplasmic reticulum are transported to the Golgi complex. This occurs either by direct transfer through the cisternae, which are in continuity with the membrane channels of the Golgi complex, or by the formation of vesicles (transition elements). Secretory vesicles (and/or secretory granules) with more condensed protein contents are formed in the Golgi complex. The hormones are then released into the extracellular fluid by exocytosis, which involves a fusion of the membrane of the granules with the plasma membrane.

STEROIDAL HORMONES. The steroid hormones are derived from cholesterol, and 7-dehydrocholesterol is the precursor to vitamin D. In a series of modification reactions, the side chain of cholesterol is cleaved to yield the 21-carbon steroid pregnenolone. The functioning steroidal hormones are then derived through a series of specific hydroxylations and other modification reactions. For example, there is placement of a 4-5 double bond in the A ring with progesterone, testosterone, cortisol, and aldosterone and aromatization of the A ring in the case of estrogens. Most of these reactions take place in the specific endocrine gland, although in some cases final modifications occur in the target tissue (testosterone→dihydrotestosterone) or in other peripheral tissues (testosterone in the female; estradiol in the male). As an example, the biosynthetic pathway for cortisol is shown in Ch. 230. Specificity in the production of steroidal hormones depends upon the presence of the appropriate enzymes. Through this mechanism almost all of the aldosterone is produced in the adrenal glomerulosa, most cortisol in the adrenal fasciculata-reticularis, and most estradiol in women in the ovary.

HORMONE STORAGE AND RELEASE. Endocrine cells store hormones to a varied extent. For example, the steroid hormones, although predominantly hydrophobic in nature, still are polar enough not to accumulate in large supply in lipid stores. By contrast, vitamin D and its metabolites accumulate in appreciable quantities in lipid stores. With many of the polypeptide hormones, the glands can store substantial quantities of the hormones. For example, a five-day supply of insulin can be stored in the pancreatic islets. Although the thyroid gland does not store thyroxine per se in appreciable quantities, the gland can have about a two-week supply of this hormone stored as precursors in thyroglobulin. Also, nerve endings usually contain several days' supply of norepinephrine.

The stimuli to hormone production can trigger both the release of stored hormone and the synthesis of new hormone. The various mechanisms for hormone release have received relatively little attention in comparison with the extensive studies on hormone synthesis (with which it is closely linked). Some of the polypeptide hormones (insulin, glucagon, growth hormone) are released by active exocytosis of granules in which they are stored in response to regulatory stimuli. The cells that release these hormones are said to contain a regulated secretory pathway. By contrast, proteins in other tissues (liver) are released shortly following their synthesis; this release is mostly insensitive to regulatory stimuli (constitutive secretory pathway). Thyroid hormones are released by proteolysis of thyroglobulin derived from follicular stores by pinocytosis. Steroidal hormones seem only to diffuse down concentration gradients.

The pattern of release of hormones shows marked variations. The release of some hormones (ACTH, cortisol) is predominantly pulsatile in nature. The mechanisms by which this occurs are not clear; nor is it established whether these irregular bursts of secretion reflect predominantly changes in synthesis promoting release or in secretion alone. It is especially important to be aware of such episodic changes in evaluating the significance of random blood samples assayed for hormones released in this way. By contrast, the release of other hormones (PTH, prolactin) is more steady. Some hormones (e.g., insulin) display both pulsatile and steady release characteristics. Finally, a few hormones also have an overall pattern of release that is circadian (e.g., ACTH and cortisol).

REGULATION OF HORMONE PRODUCTION (Fig. 221–2)

For the endocrine system to serve effectively its function of communicating information among cells, it must have mechanisms for regulating the release of hormones. These include not only mechanisms that affect basal and circadian release of hormones but also those that allow hormone levels to increase or decrease in response to physiologic or pathologic stimuli. The system also makes use of mechanisms that monitor whether the hormonal signal has been appropriate to attain its goals of maintenance of homeostasis, stimulation of growth and development, and response to stress.

For the most part, three types of influences govern hormone release: (1) There can be spontaneous release of hormone from the gland at a relatively constant rate (e.g., thyroxine) or in a circadian rhythm (e.g., cortisol). These patterns may be due to intrinsic activity of the gland, or to extrinsic factors that affect hormone release. (2) Hormone release can be affected by a variety of physiologic or pathologic influences that act through the same mechanisms that affect the basal release or through separate pathways. (3) "Sensor" mechanisms monitor the appropriateness of the hormonal levels or responses and provide further regulation. Three major modulators of hormone release that can act at any of the levels discussed above are other hormones, the central nervous system, and the physiologic responses produced.

HORMONES THAT STIMULATE THE RELEASE OF OTHER HORMONES. The primary function of several hormones is to stimulate or inhibit the release of other hormones. This is the case with the "tropic" hormones of the anterior pituitary gland (ACTH, TSH, LH) and the hypothalamic releasing factors (CRF, thyrotropin releasing hormone [TRH], gonadotropin releasing hormone [GnRH]). Some of these factors are essential for the release of the respective hormones under their control. For instance, with TSH or ACTH deficiency, thyroxine and cortisol production, respectively, drop to negligible levels and there is atrophy of the corresponding glands. By contrast, with chronic excess of these hormones

there can be hyperplasia and hypertrophy of the target gland that, in addition, increases its capacity to produce hormones. Other factors are inhibitory of hormone release; their disappearance leads to increased production of hormone by the gland. Lesions of the pituitary stalk can block the inhibitory influence of dopamine on the prolactin-producing cells of the anterior pituitary gland, resulting in an increase in the secretion of this hormone. The production of tropic hormones is usually modulated by the hormones whose production they stimulate; thus these hormones themselves measure the appropriateness of the response to the tropic hormone. For instance, feedback inhibition of ACTH release occurs in response to cortisol, inhibition of TSH release occurs in response to thyroxine, and inhibition of LH release occurs in response to testosterone. Conversely, during the menstrual cycle, the rising concentration of estradiol triggers the surge of LH and FSH release prior to ovulation (see Ch. 237). The feedback influences can be exerted either directly at the level of the pituitary or more indirectly at the level of the hypothalamus to block production of the releasing factor that stimulates the pituitary gland. Most commonly the stimulatory influences as well as the feedback-inhibitory effects occur rapidly, within minutes to hours, although the tropic and certain other effects require a longer time. These simple servomechanisms, which are essentially chemostats, maintain the level of the free—i.e., the active—hormone at a "normal" level. These mechanisms alone would not allow for alterations in hormone secretion according to changing need, since they do not measure the ultimate physiologic response. For example, they would not call forth the increased secretion of ACTH to elevate plasma cortisol during stress. Nevertheless, much of endocrinology depends upon an understanding of these relationships. The interpretation of the plasma level of a tropic hormone or its linked target organ hormone can be made logically only in the context of these relationships, as described below.

INFLUENCES OF PHYSIOLOGIC RESPONSES OR EXTRACELLULAR SUBSTANCES. Hormones whose production is controlled by the physiologic responses that they regulate are predominantly those that maintain homeostatic control over key substances in extracellular fluids. For example, increases in plasma glucose levels increase insulin and depress glucagon release. Increases in Ca^{++} decrease PTH release, increase calcitonin release, and decrease 1,25-hydroxycholecalciferol production. Increases in extracellular Na^+ and decreases in plasma K^+ decrease aldosterone release, and an increase in the plasma osmolality increases vasopressin antidiuretic hormone (ADH) release. Changes in the effector substances in the converse direction have the corresponding opposite effect on hormone secretion. In each case the effect of the change in the hormone concentration is to "correct" the changes in the extracellular substance toward "normal." These mechanisms most often operate rapidly (minutes to hours), and they provide an exquisitely sensitive system for the maintenance of homeostasis. The regulation by the effector substance can occur directly on the hormone-producing cell, as with the effect of glucose on insulin or glucagon release or of K^+ on aldosterone release, or it can occur indirectly. As an example of the latter, an increase in plasma sodium (probably through its associated Cl^-) depresses the release of renin by the kidney. The decreased renin level results in less angiotensin production, which in turn results in lower aldosterone production.

CENTRAL NERVOUS SYSTEM. The central nervous system (CNS) participates in the regulation of hormone release in several ways. It not only directs spontaneous patterns of hormone secretion, but also mediates stress-stimulated secretion and other responses that interrupt the spontaneous (basal) rhythms. These influences occur through effects on the hypothalamus with consequent changes in the delivery of releasing factors to the pituitary, and they also occur through influences on the sympathetic nervous system. The

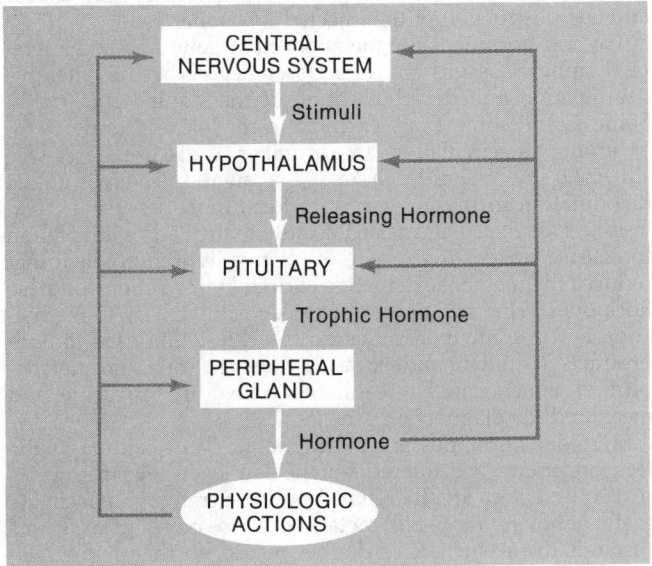

FIGURE 221–2. Organization of a set of endocrine glands, with interrelated regulatory elements. Shown is the flow of information from the central nervous system through the hypothalamus to the pituitary and then to the peripheral glands. Also indicated is that either the hormone product of the peripheral gland or the physiologic actions induced by the hormone can feedback-inhibit the stimuli to hormone release at any of several loci. As a rule, all of the potential regulatory influences do not operate with respect to a given set of glands, nor do all of the components shown operate for all endocrine glands.

influences of the CNS on the hypothalamus govern the circadian release of CRF that stimulates ACTH release, the surges in growth hormone during REM sleep, events surrounding the onset of puberty, the release of prolactin during suckling, and the release of growth hormone and ACTH with "stress." Little is known about how the spontaneous patterns are determined, although in some cases they may be due to the influences of extrinsic factors on the CNS. The circadian rhythm of ACTH release in rodents appears to be "set" predominantly by the feeding cycle. Events influenced by the CNS through the sympathetic nervous system include the release of insulin by the pancreas, of renin by the kidney, and of epinephrine by the adrenal medulla. These can be considered as part of "fight or flight" responses. Thus the CNS is able to determine the needs of the organism for normal physiology and development, to sense when there is a need for intervention for specific purposes, and to dictate the appropriate response.

There are many aspects of the regulation of hormone synthesis and release that remain poorly understood in terms of both the mechanisms involved and why certain stimuli are effective. For instance, the release of growth hormone is influenced by the level of blood sugar or certain amino acids, but these may not be the most important physiologic determinants for its secretion. What are the function and the control of prolactin secretion in the male?

HORMONE TRANSPORT

The polypeptide hormones circulate largely as free entities. By contrast, the steroid and thyroid hormones circulate largely bound by plasma proteins. For most of these (aldosterone is an exception), specific plasma proteins bind the hormones with high affinity such that only a small amount of the hormone (<1 to 10 per cent) is free. Thyroxine-binding globulin (TBG), thyroid hormone–binding prealbumin (TBPA), and corticosteroid-binding globulin (CBG) are examples of such specific proteins. The hormones rapidly equilibrate with their protein carriers and also rapidly dissociate from them when the free hormone concentration is lowered. The function of these proteins is unknown. They do not appear to have an obligatory role in hormone action, and genetic disorders in which the binding proteins are markedly reduced or increased are not associated with abnormal endocrine function. They do not appear to be required to "transport" the hormones, which are soluble enough at concentrations at which they are active. The plasma proteins serve to some extent as a reservoir that "buffers" the plasma against rapid fluctuations in hormone release and also tend to decrease the clearance of the circulating hormones, making them less accessible to degradative enzymes and to loss through glomerular filtration. CBG-like proteins also exist within some cell types; in the kidney, these may serve to sequester cortisol and prevent it from occupying mineralocorticoid receptors that mostly bind aldosterone. In addition to the association with high-affinity plasma-binding proteins, hormones also bind with lower affinity to other proteins, particularly to albumin.

Free hormone rather than the plasma-bound hormone appears to be responsible for eliciting hormone action. Furthermore, the physiologic regulatory mechanisms that are sensitive to the concentration of hormones in plasma respond to the free rather than to the total hormone concentration.

The concentrations of the plasma binders of hormones vary both on a genetic basis and as the result of the effects of certain drugs or other factors. For instance, estrogens increase CBG and TBG. In contrast, the synthesis of these binding proteins tends to be diminished by androgens and in patients with severe liver disease, and they may be lost in the urine in the nephrotic syndrome. As noted, there are rare persons who have a genetic deficiency of a specific binding protein.

It is particularly important to be aware of plasma binding in the clinical evaluation of endocrine excess and deficiency states. Since the free hormone is biologically active and is maintained by homeostatic mechanisms, this fraction rather than the total hormone concentration reflects the state of endocrine function. Plasma assays of free hormone concentrations have been developed but are not commonly available; instead, the total plasma hormone concentration is usually measured. The total plasma concentration of a hormone will be elevated or depressed in parallel with any change in the level of its binding protein, even though the free hormone concentration will usually be maintained normal by homeostatic control mechanisms. Conversely, a patient with low binding protein levels could have a high free hormone level and endocrine hyperfunction in the face of a low total hormone concentration, and a patient with a high binding protein level could have an elevated total but a low free hormone concentration and therefore endocrine hypofunction. The evaluation of thyroid function, for example, relies heavily on assessing both the total hormone levels and the plasma hormone–binding capacity (Ch. 229).

METABOLISM OF HORMONES

For the endocrine system to be able to adapt to physiologic needs, there must be a turnover of the circulating hormones. This requires mechanisms for removal of active hormones, which may be very rapid (a few minutes for most protein hormones) or comparatively prolonged (over a week for thyroxine). As might be expected, the rapidity of removal tends to parallel the rapidity with which the specific endocrine gland is called upon to adapt its secretion to various stimuli.

The polypeptide hormones are broken down to their component amino acids in the plasma and by tissue proteases and peptidases. To some extent this occurs intracellularly after the hormone is taken up (internalized). Inactive fragments of polypeptide hormones may circulate (e.g., fragments of PTH) and thereby constitute a problem in radioimmunoassay procedures (see Ch. 247). At present, there are no known endocrine syndromes caused by abnormalities in the metabolism of polypeptide hormones, although sometimes insulin resistance in diabetes can be due to excessive subcutaneous destruction of the injected hormone.

Thyroid hormones are metabolized largely by deiodination in peripheral tissues and to a lesser degree by the oxidative deamination and decarboxylation of the alanine side chain. Some T_4 and some T_3 are excreted in the bile and undergo an enterohepatic circulation. In a number of disease states (see Ch. 229) the metabolism of T_4 is altered to favor initial deiodination in the inner ring to form more reverse T_3, and less T_3 is formed. This may contribute to the body's adaptation to disease by creating a state of relative hypothyroidism that reduces the metabolic demands elicited by the actions of these hormones. The metabolism of catecholamines, by O-methylation and oxidative deamination (see Ch. 242), leads to endproducts (vanillylmandelic acid, metanephrine, normetanephrine) which can be readily identified in the urine and measured for diagnostic purposes.

Steroidal hormones are hydrophobic. Thus, although the free hormones are filtered by the kidney, they are mostly reabsorbed and are therefore poorly excreted. To facilitate their removal, they are metabolized to more polar forms through the reduction of double bonds, further hydroxylations, and conjugation with glucuronide or sulfate prior to excretion into the urine and to a lesser extent into the gut. As an example, the metabolic pathway for inactivation of cortisol is described in Ch. 230. An important step in this pathway, the reduction of ring A by specific hepatic enzymes, may be impaired in severe liver disease such that the half-life of cortisol and of estradiol, for instance, is significantly prolonged. Whereas plasma cortisol is maintained at a normal level, in this case by appropriate reduction in its rate of secretion by the adrenal cortex, the abnormality results in elevated estradiol levels. The obverse obtains in thyrotoxicosis: Cortisol is more rapidly metabolized; however, the plasma cortisol level is maintained normal by enhanced secretion. Sometimes drugs can increase the rate of steroid metabolism although homeostatic mechanisms ordinarily normalize the hormone concentration by compensatory changes in output. Such variations can be important when hormones are used in therapy either for replacement of an endocrine deficiency or for treating nonendocrine diseases with pharmacologic doses.

MECHANISMS OF HORMONE ACTION

The action of a hormone is initiated by its binding to a specific receptor protein. The polypeptide and catecholamine hormones bind to receptors that are located on the cell surface; the steroid and thyroid hormones bind to receptors within the cell. The polypeptide or catecholamine hormone-receptor interaction usually triggers changes in the production and levels of intracellular mediators, which in turn are responsible for eliciting the hormone effect. The steroid and thyroid hormone-receptor interactions stimulate or inhibit the transcription of particular genes with consequent changes in the levels of their mRNA products. The altered levels of proteins translated from these mRNAs then mediate the hormonal effect. There are exceptions to these generalities. Certain actions of thyroid and steroid hormones may not be mediated through nuclear events, for example. Furthermore, the possibility that polypeptide hormones act by binding to receptors inside the cell is a subject of active inquiry.

HORMONE RECEPTORS. Receptor proteins bind hormones specifically and with high affinity; this binding then triggers subsequent reactions that result in the hormone response. The binding is noncovalent in nature, is driven predominantly by hydrophobic interactions, and is facilitated by electrostatic and other ionic interactions between the hormone and the receptor. Since the hormone-receptor interaction is reversible, the laws of mass action may be applied to its study. The initial binding reaction usually conforms to the relationship:

$$\text{Hormone (H) + receptor (R)} \rightleftharpoons \text{[HR] complex}$$

Thus, the equilibrium dissociation constant (K_d), which is the reciprocal of the equilibrium association constant (K_a), conforms to:

$$K_d = \frac{[H][R]}{[HR]} = \frac{[H][R_{TOTAL} - HR]}{HR}.$$

Rearrangement of this and substituting bound (B) for HR, free (F) for H, and R_T for R_{TOTAL} yields the Scatchard equation:

$$\frac{B}{F} = \left(-\frac{1}{K_d}\right)B + \frac{R_T}{K_d}.$$

This is the equation of a straight line of which the slope is $-1/K_d$ and the intercept of the abscissa equals R_T. Thus, in a plot of B/F as a function of B, the finding of a straight line indicates that the reaction is bimolecular, and the slope and intercept of that line indicate, respectively, the affinity (K_d) and the total concentration of binding sites.

For most hormone-receptor interactions a straight line is obtained. There are exceptions, however, and these generally indicate either the presence of several independent classes of sites or of negative cooperativity. For example, with insulin and aldosterone binding, concave Scatchard plots can be generated. With insulin (especially at temperatures below

physiologic), there is negative cooperativity whereby binding of the first molecule of insulin lowers the affinity of other unoccupied receptor units for binding subsequent molecules. By contrast, aldosterone binds to two molecular species, exhibiting a higher affinity binding to "mineralocorticoid" receptors that mediate sodium-retaining actions and lower affinity binding to "glucocorticoid" receptors that mediate glucocorticoid actions.

The structure of the binding site on the receptor is such that it exhibits a high specificity for binding the major hormones that act through it. For example, glucagon receptors have a high affinity for glucagon but not for insulin, and vice versa. However, there are several circumstances in which different hormones have overlapping associations. This is illustrated by the weak binding of aldosterone to glucocorticoid receptors; this is probably of little consequence physiologically, since the concentration of aldosterone relative to its affinity for these receptors is too low to result in appreciable occupancy. Conversely, as mentioned earlier, cortisol can bind significantly to mineralocorticoid receptors that are the primary mediators of aldosterone action. Even though cortisol has only 1 to 2 per cent of the affinity of aldosterone for these receptors, it circulates at concentrations much higher than aldosterone, and consequently cortisol does play some role as a salt-retaining hormone. As another example, epinephrine as a catecholamine binds to and acts through both alpha- and beta-adrenergic receptors.

In most, if not all, cases the hormone-receptor interaction results in conformational changes in the receptor that lead to the cascade of events in the hormone response. These properties of receptors distinguish them from other hormone-binding proteins such as those present in plasma. However, in some cases the function of cell surface receptors is not to initiate hormone action at the cell surface, but to facilitate the uptake and internalization of the macromolecules that bind to them. The low-density lipoprotein (LDL) receptor that internalizes LDL particles (Ch. 183) is an example of this class of receptor, sometimes referred to as a class II receptor to distinguish it from the traditional class I receptors.

The primary structures of the receptors for thyroid hormone and for several of the steroid hormones have been elucidated. These receptors, each products of a single gene, are comprised of single polypeptide chains ranging from 456-777 amino acids. Each chain consists of an amino terminal domain of unknown function, a central DNA-binding domain, and a carboxy terminal hormone–binding domain. The receptors have divergent structures in their amino terminal domains, marked homology in their DNA-binding domains (45 to 90 per cent), and modest (20 to 55 per cent) homology in their carboxy terminal domains. The DNA-binding and carboxy terminal domains also have homology to the avian erythroblastosis virus oncogene, erb-A. These similarities imply that the viral oncogene and steroid and thyroid hormone receptor genes are part of a family of genes that are evolutionarily related.

The steroid hormone receptor gene sequences have been transferred into cells with low endogenous receptor levels and have been shown to function in these cells in that their products both bind the hormone and confer hormone responsiveness to the recipient cells. Experiments of this nature comprise formal proof that the proteins in question are receptors. When the amino acids of the carboxy terminal domain are deleted, hormone-binding activity is lost in certain cases, but the resulting protein with its DNA-binding domain activates hormone responses in a hormone-independent manner. This suggests that ordinarily the carboxy terminal steroid–binding domain represses the activity of the DNA-binding domain and that steroid binding promotes a conformational change in the receptor that inhibits the suppression of the DNA-binding domain by the steroid-binding domain. Mutations of the DNA-binding domain can abolish receptor activity. The function of the amino terminal domain is not clear. Whereas it has been deleted without abolishing receptor function, in other cases mutations in this domain result in decreased receptor function.

The primary structures of several of the polypeptide hormone receptors have also been elucidated. The epidermal growth factor (EGF) receptor, a single-chain glycoprotein, contains (1) an amino terminal EGF-binding domain exposed to the outside surface of the cell, (2) a transmembrane domain that spans the cell membrane, and (3) a domain on the internal surface of the cell membrane that contains both a tyrosine kinase function that is activated by hormone binding and sites for autophosphorylation by the tyrosine kinase activity. The insulin receptor is derived from a single glycosylated precursor that yields alpha and beta subunits. The receptor contains two alpha subunits and two beta subunits that are joined by disulfide bonds to form the cross-linked heterodimer (alpha-beta)$_2$ of molecular weight 350,000 to 400,000. The receptor has a symmetric immunoglobulin-like structure and probably binds more than one molecule of the hormone. Insulin binds predominantly to the alpha subunits that are on the outside surface of the cell. The beta subunits may participate in binding and span the cell membrane; these subunits contain hormone-activated tyrosine kinase domains located in the cytoplasmic portion.

HORMONE AGONISTS AND ANTAGONISTS. A hormone agonist is capable of eliciting the actions of the hormone; a hormone antagonist can directly block agonist actions. Antagonists bind to receptors, but they do not (in contrast to agonists) trigger the subsequent steps in the hormonal response. If present in sufficient concentrations, antagonists occupy hormone binding sites on the receptors and thereby block the binding and actions of agonists. Some compounds are partial agonists in that they bind to receptors and elicit a response that is less than that of a full agonist. If present in sufficient concentration, the partial agonist can block the binding and actions of an agonist, but in this case it serves as a "partial antagonist," since its partial agonist response will be observed. Hormone antagonists (e.g., the antimineralocorticoid spironolactone and the beta-adrenergic blocker propranolol) can have important clinical uses.

POLYPEPTIDE AND CATECHOLAMINE HORMONES. The binding sites for receptors that mediate polypeptide and catecholamine hormone action are exposed to the outside surface of the cell. Binding of the hormone by the receptor alters the conformation of the receptor in a manner such that intracellular mediators are affected; these in turn are responsible for eliciting the hormonal responses. These mediators include cyclic AMP that activates serine and threonine kinases, other kinases, phospholipids and their metabolic products, and calcium ion. Examples of hormones that appear to act through particular mechanisms are shown in Table 221–1. In numerous instances hormones utilize more than one mechanism, and, as described below, these effector systems have extensive interrelations. Knowledge in this area is evolving rapidly, and the list in Table 221–1 will probably be modified.

In many cases, occupancy of only a small proportion of the receptors for polypeptide and catecholamine hormones results in a full hormonal response. In these cases, "spare receptors" are said to be present. This situation arises because the limiting factor in determining the magnitude of the hormonal response resides in some step distal to the initial hormone-receptor interaction. The spare receptors are hardly spare, however, as they are functional and allow for a greater receptor occupancy (and, as a consequence, a greater hormonal response) at lower concentrations of the hormone. This derives from the fact that the quantity of hormone-receptor complexes is proportional not only to the hormone but also to the receptor concentration.

Cyclic AMP (cAMP) and Kinase Activation. cAMP is the intracellular mediator for the actions of many hormones.

TABLE 221–1. MEDIATORS OF POLYPEPTIDE AND CATECHOLAMINE HORMONE ACTIONS

Elevate cAMP	Stimulate Phospholipid Turnover and/or Synthesis
ACTH	
β-adrenergic agonists	ACTH
Calcitonin	Angiotensin II
HCG	α-adrenergic agents
CRF	HCG
Dopamine D$_1$	EGF
FSH	GnRH
GRF	LH
Glucagon	Muscarinic agents
LH	PTH
PTH	TRH
Prostaglandin E$_1$	TSH
Serotonin 5-HT$_1$	Vasopressin
TSH	
Vasopressin V$_2$	**Increase Intracellular Ca^{++}**
	ACTH
Lower cAMP	α-Adrenergic agents
	Angiotensin II
Acetylcholine	HCG
Adenosine A$_1$	EGF
α$_2$-adrenergic agents	GnRH
Angiotensin II	LH
Insulin	TSH
Muscarinic agents	Vasopressin
Opiates	
Oxytocin	**Increase cGMP**
Somatostatin	
	ANF
Stimulate Tyrosine Kinase	**Sodium Channel Activation**
EGF	Nicotinic acetylcholine
Insulin	
Platelet-derived growth factor	**Chloride Channel Activation**
Insulin-like growth factor 1	
	GABA
	Glycine

ACTH = corticotropin; ANF = atrial natriuretic factor; HCG = chorionic gonadotropin; CRF = corticotropin releasing factor; EGF = epidermal growth factor; FSH = follicle-stimulating hormone; GABA = gamma aminobutyric acid; GRF = growth hormone releasing factor; GnRH = gonadotropin releasing hormone; LH = luteinizing hormone; PTH = parathyroid hormone; TRH = thyrotropin releasing hormone; and TSH = thyroid-stimulating hormone. The classification in this table is meant to reflect current thinking rather than established fact.

These increase or decrease cAMP levels by affecting the production or, rarely, the degradation of the nucleotide. cAMP is formed from ATP by adenylate cyclase (Fig. 221–3).

At least three components are necessary for the activation or inactivation of adenylate cyclase (Fig. 221–3): the hormone receptor, a guanine nucleotide–binding regulatory protein, and a catalytic unit of the cyclase enzyme itself. There are two regulatory proteins (N$_s$ and N$_i$, or G$_s$ and G$_i$) that are actually heterotrimers. One N$_s$ or G$_s$ stimulates and the other N$_i$ or G$_i$ inhibits the activity of the enzyme in response to the hormone-receptor complex (Fig. 221–3). For activation of the cyclase the hormone binds to the membrane receptor, and the resulting receptor-hormone complex associates with N protein. This stimulates the alpha subunit of the N protein to bind GTP and the dissociation of the alpha subunit-GTP complex from the beta-gamma subunit complex. The alpha subunit-GTP complex then associates with and activates the catalytic moiety of adenylate cyclase to convert ATP to cAMP. A GTPase activity of the alpha subunit then converts GTP to GDP. This and perhaps reassociation of the alpha subunit with the beta-gamma subunit results in a loss of activity of the regulatory protein, which terminates the activation. In addition, GTP can act to reduce receptor affinity for the hormone, thereby terminating the response by promoting hormone dissociation. Analogous steps occur when hormones inhibit adenylate cyclase; in these cases the hormone-receptor complex binds to the inhibitory protein trimer leading to steps that in turn inhibit the activity of the cyclase.

cAMP is formed inside the cell and acts intracellularly. Some cAMP may leak into the extracellular fluid, but there is no evidence that it has any extracellular function. This extracellular cAMP can occasionally be of diagnostic usefulness;

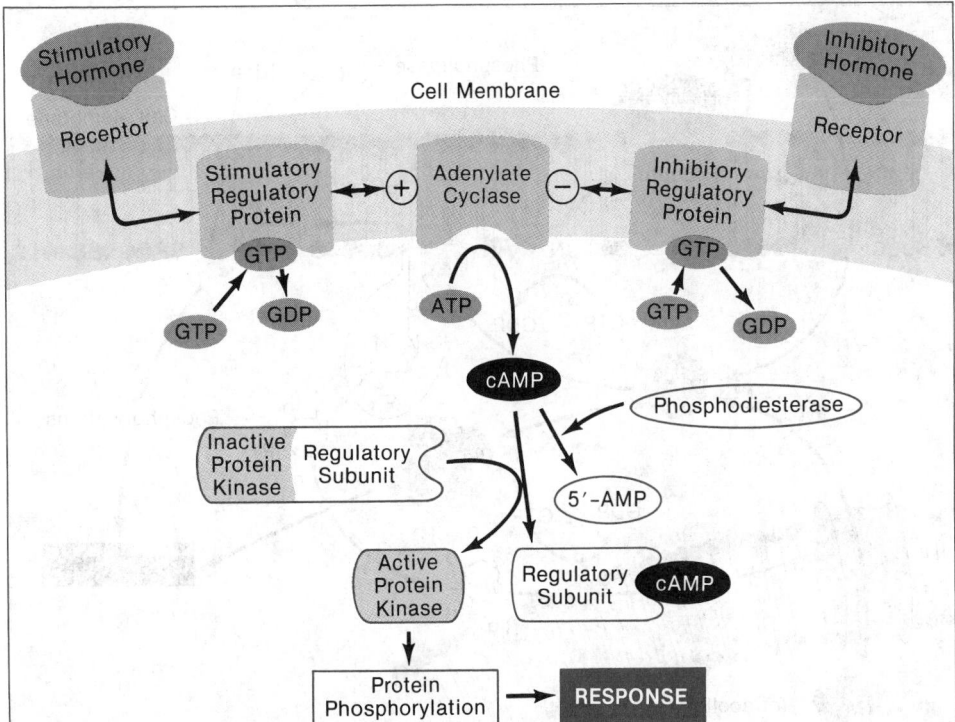

FIGURE 221–3. Steps in the hormonal activation or inactivation of adenylate cyclase and in the actions of cAMP. In several cases the proteins indicated have several subunits (see text).

urinary cAMP measurements can provide an index of the actions of PTH on the kidney (see Ch. 247).

Most if not all of the actions of intracellular cAMP are mediated through its activation of intracellular protein kinases (Fig. 221–3). There are two major forms of these cAMP-activated protein kinases (only a small subset of the total cellular kinases) that exist in an inactive basal state with two regulatory subunits associated with two catalytic subunits. cAMP binds to and promotes dissociation of the regulatory subunits from the catalytic subunits, thereby activating them to stimulate the phosphorylation of specific serine and, to a lesser extent, threonine residues on proteins. Some of these phosphorylations alter the conformation and thus the enzymatic activities of proteins that in turn affect metabolic events in the cell.

cAMP is degraded by phosphodiesterases (Fig. 221–3). Since the concentration of intracellular cAMP represents a balance between its synthesis and degradation, regulation could occur at either step. Although it appears that regulation of cAMP synthesis is the predominant mechanism, there are circumstances in which phosphodiesterase is regulated; for example, insulin in some cases can increase phosphodiesterase activity. Certain pharmacologic agents, such as the methylxanthines (caffeine, theophylline), can inhibit phosphodiesterase (although they may also have other actions) and thereby elevate cAMP levels.

Calcium as a Second Messenger. Ionized calcium also plays a role in mediating the actions of many hormones. The hormone-receptor interaction affects the intracellular calcium concentration either by promoting its uptake through the cell membrane or by stimulating its release from intracellular organelles (e.g., mitochondria or sarcoplasmic reticulum) into the cytoplasm (Fig. 221–4). In the case of cell membrane–stimulated uptake, the hormone-receptor complex may directly, or indirectly, open calcium channels, permitting the influx of ionized calcium into the cell from the extracellular space. A major stimulant for increasing the cytoplasmic calcium ion concentration from extracellular or intracellular sources appears to be inositol-1,4,5-triphosphate, generated from hormone-receptor complex activation of phospholipase C, as discussed in the following section.

The actions of calcium ion as a hormonal second messenger are often mediated through its interactions with an intracel-

lular calcium receptor termed calmodulin (Fig. 221–4). When calmodulin binds calcium, the protein changes to a configuration in which it activates a number of enzymes, including Ca^{++}- Mg^{++}-dependent ATPase, adenylate cyclase, cAMP phosphodiesterase, and several protein kinases such as glycogen phosphorylase kinase and myosin light-chain kinase.

One of the best-studied actions of Ca^{++} is the activation of glycogen phosphorylase kinase that activates glycogen phosphorylase that catalyzes the breakdown of glycogen to glucose-1-phosphate. Catecholamines bind to alpha-adrenergic receptors in cell membranes of hepatocytes and thereby stimulate an increase in intracellular Ca^{++}. In this case, calmodulin is an integral part of the glycogen phosphorylase kinase enzyme complex, binds calcium, and is induced to activate the enzyme.

Several other Ca^{++}-binding proteins also participate in metabolic control. For example, troponin C, a calcium-binding protein, facilitates the interactions between actin and myosin in muscular contraction. Protein kinase C is a serine and threonine kinase whose functions are being elucidated, but include roles in platelet activation and inhibitory actions on certain peptide hormone receptors. This enzyme is activated by diacylglycerol (DAG) produced from inositol phospholipids (discussed below) in response to hormonal and other stimuli. DAG increases markedly the affinity of protein kinase C for calcium ion and activates the enzyme. In this case, unlike that with proteins such as calmodulin and troponin C, the activation can occur in the absence of changes in cytosolic calcium ion concentration. In addition, many receptors activate both protein kinase C through DAG and increase cytosolic calcium ion, and there are synergisms between the actions of the kinase and those due to the increased calcium ion.

There are common interrelationships between the actions of calcium ion and cAMP. These are typically of two general types. In monodirectional systems the control is in one direction (off versus on), and the two types of second messengers give the same response, with one messenger commonly augmenting the response of the other messenger and vice versa. In these systems the same hormone may increase the levels of both messengers. The tissues controlled by the pituitary tropic hormones illustrate this type of control. In bidirectional systems cAMP and calcium ion act antagonisti-

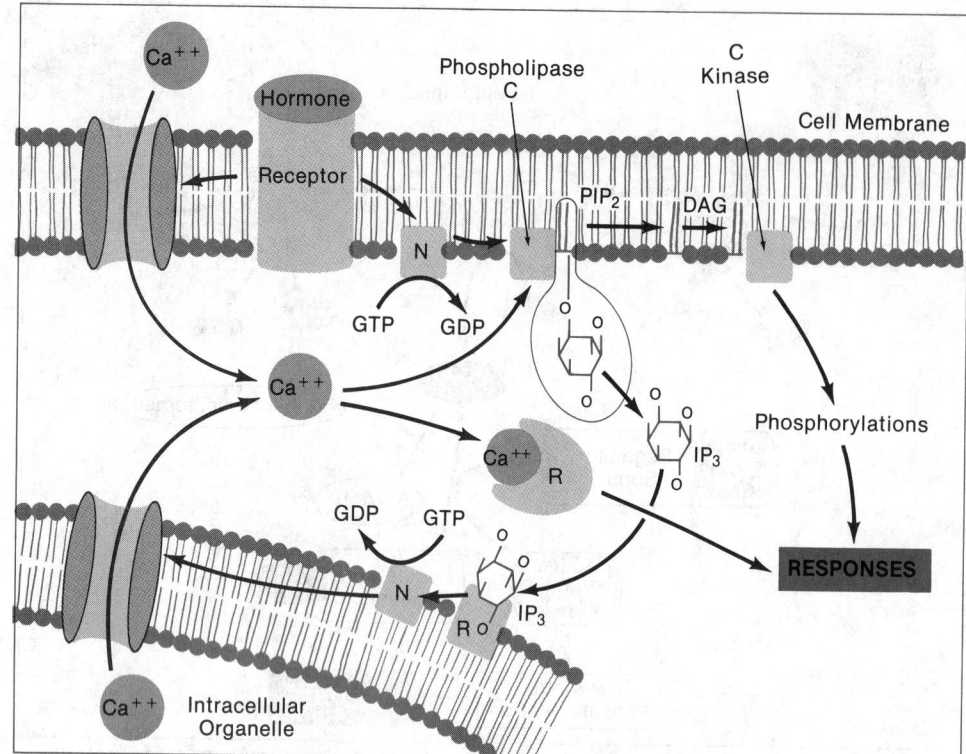

FIGURE 221–4. Actions of hormones on PIP$_2$, breakdown to IP$_3$ plus DAG with consequent activation of C kinase by DAG and elevation of cytosolic Ca^{++} by IP$_3$. Hormone-receptor actions on Ca^{++} influx can occur by IP$_3$-independent mechanisms. Receptors for IP$_3$ occur as shown in intracellular organelles and also (not shown) on the plasma membrane. Abbreviations are cited in the text.

cally and are controlled by separate stimuli. In smooth muscle, for example, acetylcholine increases cytosolic calcium ion concentrations, leading to contraction, whereas catecholamines increase cAMP levels, leading to decreased calcium ion levels and relaxation.

Phospholipids. Membrane phospholipids and their metabolic products participate in hormone action in at least three ways: (1) as a source of arachidonic acid precursors for synthesis of prostaglandins and related compounds that secondarily have target-tissue effects; (2) by stimulating increased turnover of inositol phospholipids and formation of polyphosphoinositides and their products that influence target-cell metabolism; and (3) by increasing phospholipid methylation with formation of phosphatidylcholine and consequent changes in receptor properties within the plasma membrane.

STIMULATION OF PRODUCTION OF ARACHIDONIC ACID AND OTHER PRECURSORS OF PROSTAGLANDINS AND RELATED COMPOUNDS. Arachidonic acid, a precursor to the eicosanoids (prostaglandins, prostacyclins, thromboxanes, and hydroxy fatty acids), is released from phospholipids by phospholipase A$_2$. Several hormones (ACTH, hypothalamic releasing factors) activate such membrane-associated phospholipases that catalyze arachidonic acid release, leading to an increase in eicosanoid synthesis. These compounds can then elicit other actions on target cell metabolism to form important links between hormone action and eicosanoid action (see Ch. 223). The mechanisms by which phospholipase A$_2$ is activated are not clear, although they may be indirect. The activation in many cases is Ca^{++} dependent, and it may be the result of hormone-induced changes in intracellular Ca^{++}. Other sites in the pathway of phospholipid metabolism may also be activated. In ovarian granulosa cells, for example, prostaglandin production is increased by LH, not by increasing arachidonic acid formation but by increasing prostaglandin synthetase activity.

STIMULATION OF PHOSPHOINOSITIDE TURNOVER (Fig. 221–4). Phosphoinositides make up a minor proportion of the membrane phospholipids. The breakdown and resynthesis and/or the synthesis of these phospholipids is enhanced by a number of hormones (Table 221–1). Phosphatidylinositol is converted to phosphatidylinositol 4-phosphate that is converted to phosphatidylinositol 4,5-bisphosphate (PIP$_2$). The latter is con-

verted into DAG plus inositol 1,4,5-triphosphate (IP$_3$) by phospholipase C (Fig. 221–4). The activation of this enzyme is characteristic of the actions of hormones such as vasopressin and angiotensin II that increase the intracellular calcium ion concentration. The hormone-receptor activation of phospholipase C is mediated by a guanyl nucleotide–binding protein that acts analogously to but apparently differs from those involved in regulating adenylate cyclase. The activation by the resulting DAG kinase of protein C and the actions of this kinase are described in the preceding section. The tumor-promoting phorbol esters such as tetradecanoylphorbol acetate (TPA) can also activate protein kinase C, an effect that may contribute to their tumor-promoting activities. DAG can also be converted to phosphatidic acid that has been proposed to have calcium ionophore activity. As stated above, IP$_3$ increases intracellular Ca^{++} by stimulating its release from intracellular organelles and its influx from extracellular fluid (Fig. 221–4). These actions of IP$_3$ are believed to be mediated through its binding to microsomal and membrane receptors that are coupled to calcium channels through an as yet uncharacterized guanyl nucleotide–binding regulatory protein.

STIMULATION OF PHOSPHOLIPID METHYLATION. Several hormones such as beta-adrenergic agonists can stimulate phospholipid methylation. This may influence membrane proteins and exert actions such as enhancing receptor coupling to postreceptor events and activating certain enzymes.

Activation of Tyrosine Kinase. The binding of several classes of hormones (Table 221–1) to their receptors results in activation of tyrosine kinase activity of the receptor. This results in phosphorylation of tyrosine moieties on the receptors and other cellular proteins. These phosphorylations may mediate subsequent events in the actions of these hormones, although in most cases it is not known what the specific sequelae of the phosphorylations are or whether these reflect the major action of the hormone. The products of certain oncogenes also have similar tyrosine kinase activity, providing another example of similar actions of growth factors and oncogene products.

Activation of Guanylate Cyclase. In one case, a hormone has been shown to activate guanylate cyclase with consequent cGMP production and activation of a cGMP-dependent serine

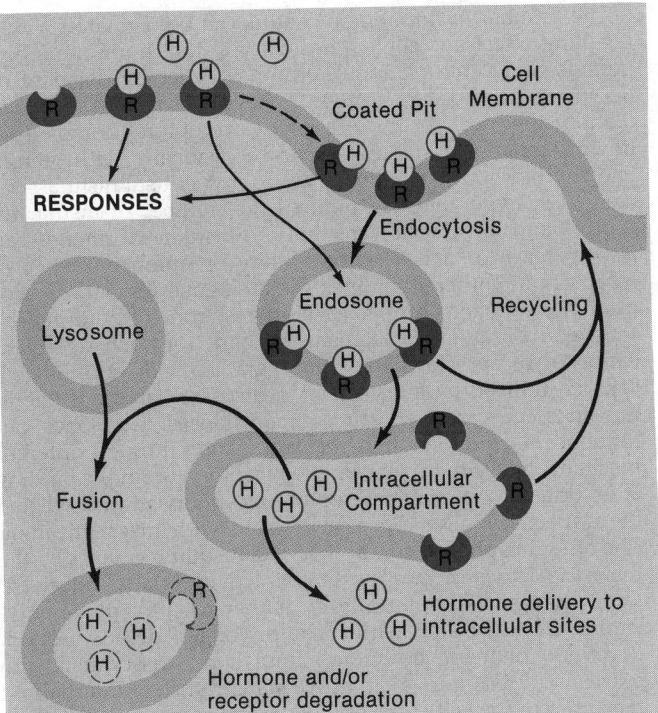

FIGURE 221–5. Internalization of hormone-receptor complexes and intracellular trafficking and metabolism of hormones and receptors. H = Hormone; R = receptor.

and threonine kinase. For example, such an activation may mediate the vasorelaxant actions of atrial natriuretic factor (ANF).

Other Possible "Second Messengers." A number of other factors are currently under consideration as possible second messengers for hormones. These include other ions (K^+, Cl^-), certain other enzymes that may modify protein structure by other phosphorylations, acetylation, or methylation, for example, and peptide mediators, as for instance with insulin or prolactin action.

INTERNALIZATION OF SURFACE RECEPTORS FOR HORMONES. Cell surface receptors and their complexes are internalized by invagination of the cell membrane into vesicles, particularly at specialized regions of the cell membrane termed coated pits (Fig. 221–5). At these distinctive regions the protein clathryn accumulates on the inside portion of the membrane. Endocytotic vesicles from coated pits undergo conversion into vacuoles called endosomes or receptosomes in which the hormone-receptor complexes can then have a variety of fates. The endosome appears to have specialized functions such as a proton pump that can decrease the intraendosomal pH. This promotes in some cases the dissociation of the hormone from the receptor. The endosome can be returned to the cell membrane or can fuse with and/or differentiate into other cellular compartments such as the Golgi apparatus where the hormones and receptors can be separated. Membranes of these compartments can then pinch off and either be returned to the membrane to deliver the receptors and sometimes the hormone-receptor complex back to the cell surface or can be fused with the lysosome wherein the hormone or the receptor or both can be degraded.

The quantitative aspects of these pathways vary considerably with different hormones. For instance, most of the internalized insulin is degraded, whereas some of the receptors are returned to the membrane. With EGF, most of the receptors and hormone are degraded. This provides one of the mechanisms whereby hormones can down-regulate the levels of their receptors. With iron bound to transferrin, the metal is released inside the cell, and both transferrin and its receptor are returned to the membrane. With the LDL receptor, cholesterol bound to lipoprotein is released inside the cell where its metabolic products feedback-inhibit cholesterol biosynthesis.

STEROID HORMONES. Steroid hormones penetrate cells readily (Fig. 221–6). The existence of transport systems has not been excluded, but if they exist, they do not appear appreciably to affect the accessibility of the hormone to the soluble intracellular receptors. In some cases (estrogens), the hormone-free receptors appear to be concentrated in the nucleus, whereas in other cases (glucocorticoids) at least some of the free receptors may be in the cytoplasm. Binding of the active steroid induces conformational changes in these receptors, termed activation or transformation, that may stimulate their binding to the DNA of the nuclear chromatin. This presumably occurs by the release of inhibitory actions of the carboxy terminal domain on the DNA-binding domain as described above. This DNA binding then influences the rates of transcription of specific genes, with consequent changes in the mRNA's encoded by them. Changes in the levels of the translation products of these mRNA's then mediate the response to the steroid hormone. For instance, glucocorticoids increase the synthesis of certain hepatic enzymes involved in gluconeogenesis and decrease the synthesis of proopiomelanocortin. Mineralocorticoids induce proteins that facilitate Na^+ reabsorption in the cortical collecting tubules of the kidney.

Steroid hormone-responsive genes contain specific DNA sequences on which receptor-steroid complexes act. These regulatory sequences, termed glucocorticoid regulatory elements or GRE's, in the case of glucocorticoid control sequences, act as receptor-responsive "enhancer" sequences. Thus, they are distinct from the promoter sequences where DNA transcription is initiated by RNA polymerase, but they modulate (usually positively) the activity of the promoter.

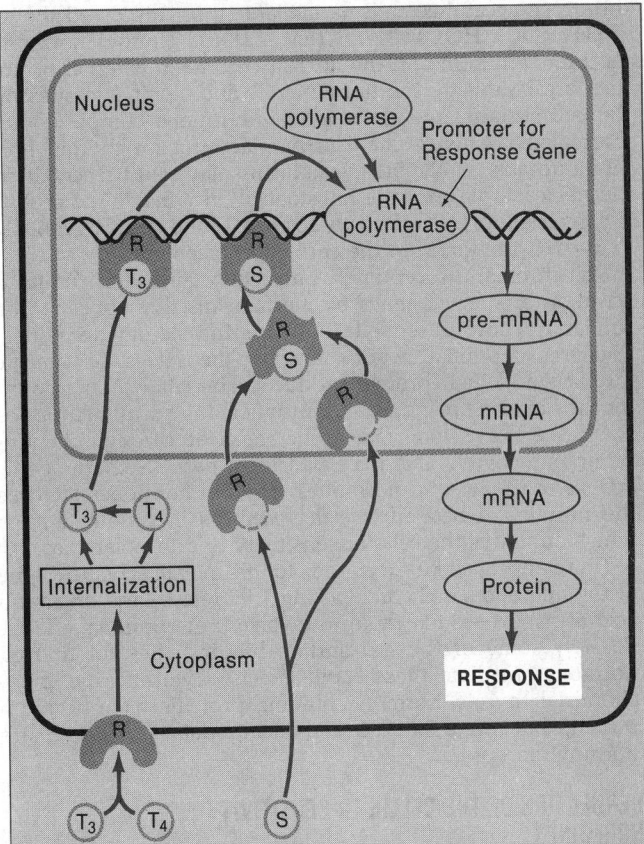

FIGURE 221–6. Steps in steroid and thyroid hormone action. S = Steroid; T_3 = triiodothyronine; T_4 = thyroxine; R = receptor. The arrow between the steroid-receptor complex and the RNA polymerase indicates that the complex increases RNA polymerase activity.

They can be located either fairly close to or at least up to several hundred nucleotides away from the promoter (Fig. 221–6). The regulatory sequences bind the receptor-steroid complexes (alone or in conjunction with other factors) with a much higher affinity than does random DNA. This DNA binding then results in an influence on the rate of initiation of transcription at the promoter of the steroid-responsive gene. The mechanisms by which the stimulation occurs are not known, but may involve a receptor-induced perturbation of chromatin structure that increases RNA polymerase accessibility to the promoter.

In some cases, steroid hormones can regulate mRNA levels through influences on mRNA stability. The mechanisms by which this occurs are not understood, but the steroids could, through transcriptional mechanisms, regulate other proteins that secondarily have effects on mRNA stability.

There is usually a close correlation between steroid binding by the receptor and the relative magnitude of the hormone response. This implies that the receptor rather than other elements of the response is limiting in determining the magnitude of the response.

Responses to steroid hormones are ordinarily observed several hours after administration of the hormone. This latent period represents the time required for the steroid-induced mRNA's and proteins to accumulate. Similarly, following removal of the steroid, the effect may last for a considerable time (hours to days). Again, this prolonged effect probably reflects the time required for degradation of the induced mRNA's and proteins. There are exceptions to these general mechanisms, but they are probably rare. Glucocorticoids inhibit ACTH release within a very few minutes, too rapidly for the effect to be due to an influence of the hormones on the transcription of DNA and its ultimate phenotypic expression. Even in this system, however, the hormone elicits other slower actions on ACTH mRNA that probably are mediated through nuclear mechanisms similar to those discussed above.

THYROID HORMONES (Fig. 221–6). Thyroid hormone receptors are found on the nuclear chromatin whether or not they are bound by the hormone. T_4 and T_3 bind to sites on the cell surface, and these protein-hormone complexes are internalized. This mechanism may account for thyroid hormone uptake. Transport mechanisms may also participate in the nuclear uptake of the hormones. Once inside the cell, T_4 is converted to T_3. This newly formed T_3 and the exogenously derived T_3 then bind to the chromatin receptors.

The chromatin receptor–T_3 interaction stimulates the transcription of specific genes by mechanisms that appear to be similar to those described above for the steroid hormones. The transcriptional actions change the levels of specific mRNA's and their protein products. The latter then account for the hormone response. For instance, the hormones induce Na^+/K^+ ATPase that may generate heat through its ion-pumping activity. This may explain in part the thermogenic actions of the thyroid hormones. Thyroid hormones increase the number of beta-adrenergic receptors in certain tissues, which enhances the cellular sensitivity to catecholamines.

There appear to be exceptions to this overall scheme. Some of the influences of T_3 on blocking TSH release and on amino acid transport are too rapid to involve transcriptional effects. Possibly some of the cell surface–binding sites for thyroid hormones mediate these rapid effects. Cytosolic and mitochondrial thyroid hormone–binding proteins have been reported, but there are no convincing data that these are hormone receptors.

REGULATION OF THE CELLULAR SENSITIVITY TO HORMONES

The sensitivity of target cells to hormones can show striking variations. These can occur in disease states (discussed later) or as normal physiologic or developmental events.

The number of hormone receptors can be regulated with a resulting effect on cellular sensitivity to that hormone. Polypeptide and catecholamine hormones generally decrease or down-regulate (desensitization, tachyphylaxis, negative regulation) the levels of their respective receptors (homologous down-regulation) and this occurs occasionally with steroid and thyroid hormones. For instance, hyperinsulinism associated with hyperglycemia reduces the number of insulin receptors and lowers the sensitivity to insulin. Hormones can also increase or decrease the affinity or number of sites of receptors for other hormones (heterologous regulation). For example, estrogens can increase progesterone receptor levels.

Several different mechanisms account for such desensitization of receptor activity. The degradation of hormone receptors induced by internalization discussed above is operative in some cases. In other circumstances, hormones can influence receptor synthesis or degradation through different mechanisms. With catecholamine receptors, hormone binding is associated with rapid receptor phosphorylation mediated by a specific kinase that is correlated with desensitization. The autophosphorylation of EGF and insulin receptors by the hormone-activated tyrosine kinase activity is also correlated with decreased receptor affinity. Other receptor phosphorylations are associated with more prolonged desensitization. Recovery following hormone stimulation is associated with recycling of receptors to an active state, return of internalized receptors to the cell surface, and/or new receptor synthesis.

Both homologous and heterologous regulation of the cellular sensitivity to hormones also occurs extensively owing to modulation of postreceptor mechanisms. Both synergisms and antagonisms also exist in postreceptor regulation of hormone responsiveness among different classes of hormones. As examples, glucocorticoids are required for certain actions of the catecholamines and vice versa; glucagon, glucocorticoid hormones, and growth hormone have actions that lead to decreased sensitivity to insulin; insulin-induced insulin resistance is due in part to postreceptor mechanisms.

ACTIONS OF HORMONES: INTEGRATED RESPONSES

The endocrine system controls metabolic events in individual tissues and coordinates effects that occur simultaneously or sequentially in many tissues. The actions of hormones are diverse, affecting every tissue in some way, but with substantial selectivity in terms of the particular functions that are affected. Some tissues respond to only a few hormones, whereas others respond to many. The actions of some hormones are predominantly directed at one or a few tissues (e.g., aldosterone), whereas other hormones (cortisol, epinephrine) affect many tissues, commonly in a highly coordinated manner. Whereas the stimuli to hormone release sometimes affect only one hormone, in other cases they affect many hormones whose actions can also be highly coordinated with both complementary and counterbalancing effects. Some examples of the actions of hormones have been provided previously in this chapter, with emphasis on tropic hormones and the regulation of responsiveness to hormones. Although any attempt to list the actions of hormones represents an oversimplification, some of the more prominent types of influences deserve emphasis.

Hormones exert major control of intermediary metabolism. Many of the responses are due to integrated influences on several tissues and can involve several different hormones. The actions on carbohydrate metabolism are illustrative. In liver, glucagon and epinephrine promote glycogen breakdown and inhibit glycogen synthesis. These hormones and cortisol stimulate glucose production by enhancing gluconeogenesis. In fat cells, epinephrine, cortisol, and growth hormone stimulate lipolysis, providing free fatty acids (an alternative to glucose as an energy source) and glycerol, which may be converted to glucose. Epinephrine and cortisol inhibit glucose uptake by fat cells, and epinephrine stimulates glycogenolysis in muscle. Cortisol inhibits glucose uptake in lymphoid and fibroblastic tissues, and inhibits protein synthesis and stimulates protein breakdown in several tissues. The amino acids released increase the substrate available for gluconeogenesis. All of these responses tend to elevate the blood sugar and can make glucose available, for instance during fasting. By contrast, insulin lowers the blood sugar by stimulating glycogen synthesis, lipogenesis, and protein synthesis, and by inhibiting lipolysis. Thus, through its ability to recruit several different hormones and to affect multiple tissues in an integrated way, the endocrine system can be highly effective in the maintenance of homeostasis. Such an integrated system may reduce dependency on only one hormone or tissue, a feature that can facilitate compensation in disease states.

Many hormones affect growth. Prominent among these is growth hormone, which stimulates the production of yet other growth factors termed somatomedins. EGF, fibroblast growth factor, multiplication-stimulating activity (MSA), nonsuppressible insulin-like activity (NSILA), sex steroids, thyroid hormones, erythropoietin, and the tropic hormones that affect endocrine glands are also growth factors. Although in some cases the physiologic roles of these hormones are understood, in other circumstances considerable additional clarification is needed.

Hormones affect water and mineral metabolism. Thus, aldosterone regulates sodium, potassium, and hydrogen ions; vasopressin regulates water; PTH, vitamin D, and calcitonin affect calcium and phosphate ions; and prolactin affects milk production.

Hormones affect the cardiovascular and respiratory systems. The catecholamines have numerous effects. Glucocorticoids can promote bronchodilation in asthma and can increase the blood pressure. Angiotensin II and vasopressin cause vasoconstriction. Bradykinin produces vasodilation. Atrial natriuretic factor has a constellation of actions that produce vasodilation and natriuresis. Some hormonal actions on the cardiovascular system are indirect. For instance, sodium retention induced by an excess of aldosterone can cause hypertension.

Hormones are important in development and differentiation. Deficiency of thyroid hormone in childhood results in the serious and irreversible intellectual impairment of cretinism. Abnormalities in sexual maturation result from deficient androgenic effects during development. In fact, most classes of hormones have some developmental actions.

Hormones are crucial for controlling reproductive functions. These include the gonadotropins of pituitary (FSH, LH) or placental (HCG) origin, prolactin, hypothalamic releasing substances, and the sex steroids.

Hormones vary considerably in the rapidity with which they act. Some hormones act quickly and are more important in the minute-to-minute control of metabolism. Epinephrine, glucagon, and other "surface-active" hormones are representative of this type of hormone. Other classes of hormones regulate more long-term responses and thus tend to provide more long-term types of adaptations. Steroid and thyroid hormones generally fall into this latter category. These patterns are not surprising, based on the molecular mechanisms of action of these hormones (activation of enzymes by surface-active hormones and induction of macromolecular synthesis by steroid and thyroid hormones). Exceptions to these generalities occur.

DISORDERS OF THE ENDOCRINE SYSTEM (Fig. 221–7)

Endocrinology has traditionally been signal oriented, concerning itself largely with whether hormones are secreted appropriately or inappropriately (in excess or deficit). Indeed, most recognizable disorders of the endocrine system are due to an excess or a deficiency of particular hormones, whether caused by abnormalities of endocrine glands, ectopic produc-

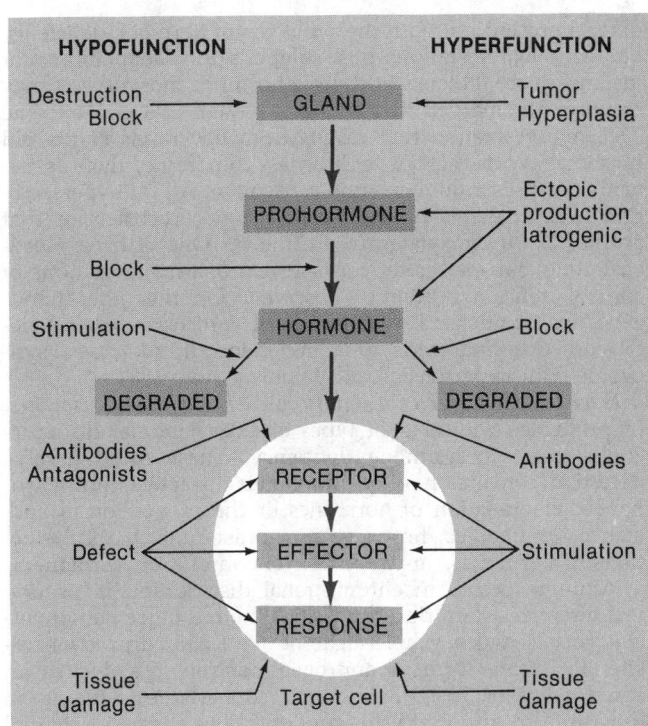

FIGURE 221–7. Causes of hypofunction or hyperfunction of the endocrine system.

tion of hormones, abnormal conversion of prehormones to their active forms, or iatrogenic factors. Endocrine abnormalities can also be due to changes in the responsiveness (either enhanced or diminished) of target tissues to hormones. These disorders can occur by a variety of mechanisms.

HORMONE DEFICIENCY SYNDROMES. *Hypofunction of Endocrine Glands.* Endocrine glands may be injured or destroyed by neoplasia, infections, hemorrhage, autoimmune disorders, and other causes. The destruction can be acute, but commonly it is chronic with normal basal hormone production until late in the disease. The gland is usually compromised in its reserve capacity before the basal level of secretion falls and cannot respond normally in circumstances in which an increase in hormone production is needed. Such partial defects may therefore not be detected by measurement of basal hormone levels, but require other testing of the reserve function of the gland. Since many manifestations of endocrine disease require weeks or even months to develop, there can be considerable differences in the clinical presentation, depending on the rapidity of glandular destruction. In acute endocrine deficiency, chronic manifestations of the disease may not be present.

As would be expected, a deficiency of a hormone that controls the synthesis and release of another hormone may result in a syndrome which simulates a primary deficiency of that target organ. Thus, hypothalamic lesions resulting in impaired secretion of releasing hormones can be manifested by pituitary dysfunction, and the latter can result in abnormalities in the function of its various target organs (gonads, thyroid, adrenal).

Genetic defects can cause endocrine hypofunction, usually because of abnormalities in hormone synthesis, but rarely because of the production of an abnormal hormone (as documented for insulin in a rare form of diabetes melitus). These genetic defects in hormone synthesis can be partial or complete. For example, a rare form of growth hormone deficiency is due to deletion of the growth hormone gene. A partial defect may be somewhat analogous to incomplete destruction of the gland—i.e., basal hormone production may be normal, but reserve may be inadequate. In fact, sometimes genetic defects present not with the problems of hormone deficiency but with manifestations of a compensatory adaptation. For instance, partial blocks in thyroid hormone biosynthesis may result in an enlarged thyroid gland (goiter) that is due to the TSH hypersecretion that results from low levels of thyroid hormone. With the 17α-hydroxylase syndrome, there is defective cortisol production and consequent ACTH hypersecretion with excessive production of adrenocorticosteroids that are not 17α-hydroxylated (see Ch. 230). One of these (corticosterone) substitutes for cortisol such that manifestations of cortisol deficiency are not observed. On the other hand, excessive compensatory synthesis of corticosterone and deoxycorticosterone leads to a mineralocorticoid excess syndrome with hypertension and hypokalemia.

Hormone Deficiency Secondary to Extraglandular Disorders. In principle, a number of types of extraglandular disorders could result in hormone deficiency. These could involve defective conversion of prohormones to active forms, enhanced degradation of hormones or the production of substances (antibodies, hormone antagonists) that block the actions of hormones. Impaired conversion of a prohormone to a hormone occurs in chronic renal disease and in pseudo vitamin D–resistant rickets in which there is defective conversion of 25-hydroxycholecalciferol to 1,25-hydroxycholecalciferol. A rare form of androgen deficiency is due to an abnormality of 5α-reductase that converts testosterone to dihydrotestosterone. In this condition, there is only a partial loss of androgenic effects since testosterone itself is weakly active in some target tissues. Rare forms of diabetes mellitus result from antibodies to the insulin receptor that block insulin action. Antibodies to insulin develop during insulin therapy and can affect its availability. Although there are no syndromes known to be due to enhanced hormone degradation, this can vary, as discussed earlier, and can affect the response to exogenously administered hormones (e.g., phenytoin and thyroid hormone increase the metabolism of certain glucocorticoids). Also, such influences can unmask or aggravate a partial hormonal deficiency; for example, the development of thyrotoxicosis can unmask latent Addison's disease.

Hyporesponsiveness to Hormones. Hormone levels may be normal or even elevated in the presence of manifestations of endocrine deficiency. The conditions can be due to some of the problems listed above (e.g., antibodies to the insulin receptor and decreased conversion of testosterone to dihydrotestosterone). They can also be due to a decreased capability of the endocrine target gland to respond to the hormone. Such disorders can be acquired or genetic, and they can be due to abnormalities at any step in the cascade of the hormone response from the receptor to the effect generated.

Several syndromes are due to receptor abnormalities. The most commonly recognized abnormality of this type occurs in type II diabetes mellitus. In this case, chronic hyperinsulinemia induced by increased food intake induces insulin resistance by down-regulating the concentration of insulin receptors and by postreceptor influences. Recognition of this problem also affects the therapy, since treatment is directed not only at correcting the hyperglycemia with insulin or other drugs but also at decreasing insulin need and levels by dietary maneuvers. This form of diabetes also exhibits the abnormality by which the pancreatic islets do not release insulin normally in response to glucose. In the testicular feminization syndrome there is unresponsiveness to androgens. As a consequence, a female phenotype occurs in a person with a male genotype. Most persons with this X-linked disorder have a defect in the androgen receptor.

At least one disorder is due to an abnormality in the coupling of hormone-receptor complexes to effector mechanisms. In pseudohypoparathyroidism there are symptoms and chemical derangements of hypoparathyroidism associated with elevated PTH levels and insensitivity to this hormone (see Ch. 247). In some such patients this insensitivity is due to decreased levels of the guanyl nucleotide–binding regulatory protein that couples the PTH-receptor complex to adenylate cyclase.

Overall damage to the hormone target tissue can result in insensitivity to hormones. For instance, renal disease can lead to insensitivity to vasopressin, and liver disease can lead to insensitivity to glucagon.

There are several forms of target organ insensitivity in which the molecular mechanisms have not been elucidated. One form of dwarfism (Laron) is due to impaired ability of growth hormone to generate somatomedin production. Vasopressin-resistant diabetes insipidus is not associated with frank renal disease.

Abnormal Production or Administration of Antagonists. Rarely, endogenously produced or exogenously administered substances can produce a hormone-deficient state. Antibodies to the insulin receptor can produce insulin resistance with functional insulinopenia. Cimetidine given for peptic ulcer disease can act as an androgen antagonist and produce an androgen-deficient state.

HORMONE EXCESS SYNDROMES. Hormone excess syndromes can result from hyperfunctioning endocrine glands, "ectopic" hormone production by tumors, less commonly from influences on target tissues that enhance hormone sensitivity, autoimmune disease in which antibodies cause hypersecretion of hormones or act as hormone agonists, defects in hormone biosynthesis in which precursor hormones produced in excess have deleterious consequences, and iatrogenic or therapeutic administration of hormones or substances that act like hormones.

Hyperfunction of Endocrine Glands. The most common cause of hormone excess syndromes is hyperfunction of endocrine glands secondary to tumors of the glands or to hyperplasia of several causes. Hyperfunctioning tumors of endocrine glands are usually well-differentiated adenomas (although carcinomas also occur) so that the prognosis is usually favorable with an early diagnosis. In addition to the manifestations of hormone excess, local extension of the tumor can produce symptoms. For instance, pituitary tumors can destroy the normal gland or extend into the suprasellar region to cause headaches or visual impairment.

Hyperplasia is a cause of hyperfunction of several of the endocrine glands (thyroid, adrenals, parathyroids). The most common form of thyroid hyperplasia appears to be due to an immunologic abnormality in which antibodies stimulate the gland in a manner similar to TSH. Hyperplasia of the zonae fasciculata and reticularis of the adrenal with consequent cortisol hypersecretion is usually due to ACTH hypersecretion by a pituitary tumor or an ectopic hormone-secreting tumor. The etiology in other cases of endocrine gland hyperplasia is less clear, as with hyperplasia of the adrenal zona glomerulosa with excessive aldosterone production, or of chief cell hyperplasia of parathyroid glands with PTH hypersecretion.

Ectopic Hormone Production by Tumors (see Ch. 173). Sometimes hormones are produced in excess by cells of endocrine or nonendocrine origin that are not normally the primary source of the hormone. In most cases, hormones produced ectopically by tumors are those that arise from a single gene (e.g., ACTH, growth hormone, prolactin, PTH, calcitonin, gastrin, erythropoietin), or two genes (hCG). This may be due to the fact that for other hormones (e.g., steroids, thyroid hormones, catecholamines) a large number of genes not ordinarily expressed by the tumor but whose products participate in hormone biosynthesis would need to be activated to produce the hormone. Although a large number of different types of tumors can produce hormones, specific cell types are more commonly associated with certain tumors (see Ch. 173). For instance, certain cells of entodermal origin, termed *a*mine *p*recursor *u*ptake and *d*ecarboxylation (APUD) cells, are more commonly associated with ectopic hormone production. These cells are found in oat cell carcinoma of the lung, carcinoid tumors, thymomas, and others. Although a number of molecular mechanisms are now understood that could explain how genes that are ordinarily not expressed are activated in tumors, those actually causing ectopic hormone production are not understood.

Iatrogenic Causes. When hormones are used to treat non-endocrine diseases, when hormone replacement therapy is excessive, and sometimes when patients self-administer hormones (or their analogues), iatrogenic endocrine disease may occur. Patients will sometimes take excessive doses of glucocorticoids or thyroxine because these hormones produce a feeling of well-being. Rarely, administration of nonhormonal substances can cause hormone-like effects. Licorice ingestion can produce a syndrome mimicking primary aldosteronism, for example.

Tissue Hypersensitivity. Endocrine excess syndromes caused by hypersensitivity of target tissues are uncommon. Thyroid hormones increase the catecholamine receptors in certain tissues and thereby lead to excessive beta-adrenergic stimulation. In this case the hyperresponsiveness is actually part of the syndrome of hyperthyroidism. Many of the manifestations of primary aldosteronism are simulated in a rare syndrome with low plasma renin and aldosterone levels in which the kidney responds as if it is excessively stimulated by aldosterone. Finally, disease of the target tissue itself can render it excessively sensitive to a hormone. For instance, cardiac arrhythmias, such as atrial fibrillation in thyrotoxicosis, probably occur most frequently in an already damaged heart.

A lingering question is whether subtle abnormalities in the sensitivity to hormones contribute to the pathogenesis of disease more than is generally perceived. With more refined methods for measuring alterations in sensitivity to hormones, it may be possible to detect more subtle abnormalities. For instance, are some forms of essential hypertension due to increased sensitivity to pressor substances or decreased sensitivity to vasodilator substances? Are some forms of osteoporosis due to abnormalities in sensitivity to estrogens or to calcium-regulating hormones? Why do glucocorticoids increase the intraocular pressure (and even precipitate glaucoma) in some persons but not in others?

Autoimmune Disease. Autoimmune disease can result in the production of antibodies that act as hormones. The most frequent situation in which this occurs is Graves' disease, discussed in Ch. 229. Rarely, antibodies to the insulin receptor have insulin-like actions.

Hormone Biosynthetic Defects. Certain adrenal steroid biosynthetic defects (for example, the 21α- and 11β-hydroxylase syndromes) result in overproduction of hormones proximal to the block; these syndromes are discussed in Ch. 230.

Secondary Causes of Hormone Hypersecretion. Hypersecretion of hormones may be due to excessive physiologic stimulation of glands that are basically normal. The secondary hyperaldosteronism of hepatic disease and ascites, congestive heart failure, the nephrotic syndrome, and other conditions is illustrative. The excess aldosterone can aggravate the tendency to edema in these conditions. Secondary hyperparathyroidism occurs in azotemia (see Ch. 249).

MULTIPLE ENDOCRINE SYNDROMES (see also Ch. 241). Simultaneous involvement of more than one endocrine gland can result in syndromes of hyperfunction or hypofunction. The most common syndrome of multiple endocrine deficiencies, sometimes termed Schmidt's syndrome, can involve the pancreatic islets, thyroid, adrenals, parathyroid glands, and gonads. The disease appears to be caused by immunologic destruction of the glands. This may result from common antigenic determinants in the affected glands, caused possibly by a common development origin of the glands.

At least three syndromes of multiple endocrine hyperfunction result from hyperplasia, adenomas, or carcinomas of endocrine tissues, termed multiple endocrine neoplasia

(MEN) types 1, 2, and 3. Type 1 is associated with hyperfunction of the parathyroids, pancreatic islets, pituitary, adrenal cortex, and thyroid. In some cases more than one hormone may be produced by the tumor; islet cell tumors can produce insulin, glucagon, gastrin, vasoactive intestinal peptide (VIP), prostaglandins, ACTH, PTH, ADH, somatostatin, and serotonin. MEN type 2 is associated with pheochromocytoma (sometimes bilateral and extra-adrenal), medullary carcinoma of the thyroid, and parathyroid hyperplasia. MEN type 3 is associated with medullary thyroid carcinoma, pheochromocytoma, and other features such as neuromas. These syndromes are often familial with a dominant transmission, but the basic pathogenesis is unknown.

ABNORMALITIES OF ENDOCRINE GLANDS NOT ASSOCIATED WITH HORMONAL IMBALANCE. Tumors, nodules, cysts, infiltrative diseases, and other abnormalities may involve endocrine glands without impairing their secretory functions significantly. For instance, nodules of the thyroid gland are common but usually nonfunctioning. The major problem is that malignancy may develop in them. Sometimes particular processes have a propensity for affecting an endocrine tissue. This is the case with tuberculosis and the adrenals.

CLINICAL ASSESSMENT OF ENDOCRINE STATUS

The assessment of the endocrine status of a patient relies on findings from the history and physical examination and on laboratory testing. The latter can involve measurements of levels of hormones or their metabolites in plasma or urine either in the basal state or in response to provocative testing. Laboratory tests may also be used to measure abnormalities that result from derangements in hormonal secretion and to evaluate the patient's sensitivity to hormones.

HISTORY AND PHYSICAL EXAMINATION. Many syndromes of hormonal excess or deficiency display manifestations that are readily apparent at the time of the initial presentation, e.g., severe thyrotoxicosis or Cushing's syndrome. In other instances, the clinical presentation can be more subtle and the physician must rely on laboratory testing to establish a diagnosis. This is especially true in the early stages of most endocrine problems, in elderly persons (e.g., with thyrotoxicosis or myxedema), or when the disease presents acutely and has not been present long enough for chronic manifestations to develop. Since it is beneficial to treat these diseases early, it is important for the physician to consider endocrine diseases in patients without full-blown manifestations, despite the fact that in the early stages of many of these disorders (e.g., adrenal insufficiency, hypothyroidism, Cushing's syndrome, hyperparathyroidism) the presenting symptoms and signs are sufficiently vague to suggest more common problems. Thus, endocrine diseases should be considered in the differential diagnosis of many common problems, such as weakness, tiredness, vague gastrointestinal discomfort, hypertension, or weight loss or gain. Once the diagnosis is considered, it is usually relatively easy to establish whether or not the disorder is present. Since endocrine diseases can be caused by primary processes external to the endocrine systems, the physician should consider these in taking the history and performing the physical examination. Sometimes, the primary process (e.g., carcinoma of the lung producing ACTH, tuberculosis causing adrenal insufficiency) will dominate the clinical presentation such that hormonal abnormalities are more difficult to detect clinically.

LABORATORY TESTING. *Hormone Levels.* Over the past few decades, assays have been developed to measure the levels of most of the hormones in body fluids. These vary in the ease with which they can be performed and their overall reliability; some assays are generally available, whereas others are performed only in certain research institutions.

RADIOIMMUNOASSAY. The advent of radioimmunoassay, first developed for measuring plasma insulin levels, was a major breakthrough in endocrinology. Antibodies that are relatively specific for certain chemical groups or conformations on the hormone can be developed for the polypeptide hormones and also for the smaller ligands such as thyroid and steroid hormones. The success of the assay depends on the specificity of the antibody as well as its affinity for binding the hormone.

In the radioimmunoassay, the plasma or urine sample or an extract of it is incubated with the antibody to the hormone along with a tracer of radiolabeled hormone. Then the antibody-tracer complexes are quantified in a variety of ways. For instance, charcoal can be used to adsorb the hormone that is not bound by the antibody, and the remaining radiolabeled hormone–antibody complexes can then be assessed. The extent to which the hormones in the sample block the binding of the radiolabeled hormone by the antibody is then related to a standard curve prepared from reactions in which known quantities of the hormone are present to yield the concentration of the hormone in the sample.

In most cases, radioimmunoassay yields extremely accurate information. However, there are problems that the physician should consider in interpreting the results. The antibody may cross-react with related hormones or with precursors or metabolites of the hormone. If these compounds are present in sufficient concentration, they can give spuriously high values. For instance, some antibodies are specific for the carboxy terminal portion of PTH. This part of the molecule is present in certain circulating fragments of PTH that are biologically inactive. This is especially true in chronic renal disease, in which PTH levels by radioimmunoassay are extremely high. This problem can be obviated by the use of antibodies that are specific for other parts of the PTH molecule (see Ch. 247).

More recently there has been increasing usage of nonradiologic means for immunoassay. For example, with the enzyme-linked immunoabsorbent assay (ELISA), hormone-antibody complexes are measured by binding them to anti-antibody antibodies to which enzymes are linked. In this case the enzyme activity bound to the complexes provides an estimate of their concentration.

COMPETITIVE PROTEIN-BINDING AND RADIORECEPTOR ASSAYS. These assays depend on the availability of a protein that binds the hormone with high affinity and specificity. The protein can be the normal receptor for the hormone, or it can be another protein, usually a plasma hormone–binding protein (e.g., CBG, TBG, sex hormone–binding globulin [SHBG]). The assay is performed in a manner analogous to that of the radioimmunoassay.

These assays provide an indication of summed products of the affinities times the concentrations of all compounds in the sample that bind to the protein. Typically, however, only one hormone accounts for most or all of the activity that is present. Radioreceptor assays are not widely used currently, in part because it is difficult to work with receptor preparations. By contrast, several competitive protein-binding assays have come into general use. Noteworthy are the CBG-isotope and TBG assays for cortisol and thyroxine, respectively, that depend on the fact that the major chemical species in plasma that binds to CBG is cortisol and to TBG is thyroxine.

CHEMICAL ASSAYS. Many hormones can be assayed by chemical means. For example, the fluorimetric assay for cortisol depends on the fluorescence of steroids with Δ^4-3-ketone, 20-ketone, and 11β- and 21-hydroxyl groups. However, these techniques have mostly been supplanted by the other methods described.

HIGH-PERFORMANCE LIQUID CHROMATOGRAPHY (HPLC). The development of more sophisticated HPLC techniques has increased their capability for routine measurements. Although these methods are not commonly used for hormone measurements, they will probably be used increasingly for the measurement of smaller molecules such as steroids, catecholamines, and small peptides.

LEVELS OF FREE HORMONE. Free hormone, rather than that which is protein bound, is usually the best index of its effective concentration in plasma. The problems with assessment of total hormone concentrations due to potential variations in the concentrations of plasma steroid and thyroid hormone–binding proteins have been emphasized earlier in this chapter.

Levels of free hormone can be assessed in several ways: (1) The free hormone can be physically separated from that which is plasma bound and measured directly, although these methods have not yet come into general use. (2) The plasma concentration of the binding protein can be measured directly. Again this approach has not been applied widely. (3) The saturation of the binding protein can be assessed. When plasma levels of binding proteins are high, the protein will be undersaturated and less of the total hormone is free, whereas the converse occurs when plasma levels are low. This approach is now used in the case of TBG. Thus, the T_3 uptake assay measures the capacity in plasma for T_3 binding, which mostly reflects the extent of saturation of TBG. Combined knowledge of the total T_4 levels with the extent of saturation of TBG provides a reasonable estimate of the plasma free T_4 concentration (see Ch. 229). (4) An index of the free hormone concentration can sometimes be obtained by measuring its urinary excretion (or that of one of its metabolites). For instance, a small fraction (less than 1 per cent) of the secreted cortisol is excreted unchanged into the urine. A measurement of the 24-hour urine free cortisol usually provides a reasonable estimate of the integrated levels of free plasma hormone. In essence this method uses the glomerular basement membrane to separate hormone that is bound from that which is free.

SECRETION AND PRODUCTION RATES. Hormone production can be assessed by more complicated assays that involve either the injection of radioactive tracers or a combined assessment of plasma levels and hormone excretion. These techniques can circumvent many of the problems in interpretation associated with sole measurements of plasma or urinary hormones. Unfortunately, these procedures are cumbersome and not generally available.

SELECTIVE SAMPLING. Sometimes more accurate indications of a hormone-excess state and the site of hormone hypersecretion can be obtained by assaying the venous effluent from a given gland or organ. For example, in renovascular hypertension, peripheral renin levels may be normal, but sampling from a catheter inserted into the renal veins may reveal renin hypersecretion from one side and hyposecretion from the other side. Pituitary venous effluent sampling from the petrosal sinuses can be useful to determine whether ACTH hypersecretion results from a pituitary adenoma or from ectopic sites.

CLINICAL INTERPRETATION. With marked hormone excess or deficiency states, plasma or urinary hormone measurements commonly provide a clear indication of the abnormality. Nevertheless, it is important to be aware of the limitations of such tests. Hormone levels increase and decrease owing to physiologic stimuli, the presence of which must be considered when evaluating the significance of a hormone determination. For instance, plasma insulin levels should be evaluated in relation to the plasma glucose concentration, and PTH levels should be considered in relation to the serum calcium levels. Basal hormone secretion may not reflect the functional capacity of the gland, as considered in more detail under Dynamic Testing, below. Hormone levels should be evaluated in relation to target cell sensitivity. For example, in maturity-onset diabetes of the obese, plasma insulin levels are often elevated, but may still be inappropriately low in view of the associated insulin resistance. Since the release of many hormones is not constant, random readings can be particularly misleading. Cortisol, for example, is released episodically. In Cushing's syndrome the number of these releases is increased. Although this commonly results in an elevation of the plasma cortisol throughout the day, the morning plasma levels of this steroid may be normal. Since cortisol production integrated over a 24-hour period is increased in Cushing's syndrome, the 24-hour urine free cortisol will provide a more accurate index of whether there is cortisol hypersecretion.

Although urinary measurements can sometimes be more useful than plasma assays for obtaining an integrated assessment of the production of certain hormones (especially steroids), they cannot be used in this way for other hormones (e.g., thyroid hormones) whose metabolites are not predominantly secreted into the urine. Further, urinary metabolites of steroids can sometimes be derived from several sources (e.g., 17-ketosteroids from the adrenal and gonads), and hormone excretion can be influenced by changes in renal function. There are also circumstances in which the quantities of metabolites (e.g., of aldosterone) can be primarily affected by factors that do not affect the production or plasma levels of the hormone.

Sometimes the significance of hormone levels can be evaluated only by the simultaneous measurement of more than one hormone. For instance, with progressive damage to the thyroid gland and impaired release of thyroid hormones, secretion of TSH increases in a compensatory fashion such that normal plasma levels of the thyroid hormones may be maintained. By simultaneously measuring thyroid hormone levels and TSH, an indication of the compensatory response can be obtained. Such a simultaneous assessment of linked hormones can also provide an indication of the site of a primary defect. Plasma estrogens are low in ovarian failure. If ovarian failure is due to disease of the ovary, plasma gonadotropins will be increased. If ovarian failure is secondary to pituitary or hypothalamic disease, plasma gonadotropin levels will be decreased.

Dynamic Testing. Provocative testing assesses the ability of a gland to respond to stimuli as an index of its reserve capacity. This is especially useful when plasma or urinary hormone measurements are borderline. It can also yield information about the site of the endocrine defect. In some cases, a hormone is given that stimulates the release of another hormone(s). For example, the administration of GnRH stimulates LH and FSH release, and TRH stimulates TSH and prolactin release. In other cases hormone production is blocked to interrupt normal feedback inhibition. Metyrapone blocks cortisol production by inhibiting 11β-hydroxylation, thereby stimulating ACTH release. The elevated ACTH levels increase the release of adrenal steroids proximal to the block (e.g., 11-deoxycortisol). A normal increase in 11-deoxycortisol signifies not only a normal adrenal but also a normal hypothalamic-pituitary axis. Sometimes a physiologic stimulus to hormone release is given. Insulin-induced hypoglycemia is used to assess the ability of cells that produce ACTH and growth hormone to respond. With endocrine hyperfunction, provocative tests can assess the extent to which the normal physiologic mechanisms that control hormone release are suppressed or the degree of autonomy of the hormone-producing tumor or hyperplastic gland. In primary aldosteronism resulting from an aldosterone-producing adenoma, the plasma renin levels that are suppressed by excessive sodium retention will not rise with acute postural, salt restriction, or diuretic stimuli. In Cushing's syndrome resulting from ectopic secretion of ACTH by a tumor, the glucocorticoid dexamethasone will not ordinarily suppress the elevated ACTH levels.

Tests That Provide Indirect Information. Useful information can frequently be obtained from laboratory tests that provide an index of the actions of the hormones (or a lack of them) or else an indication of the primary process causing the endocrine disease. Thus, it is helpful to follow the blood sugar levels in diabetes, the serum calcium levels in hyperparathyroidism, and the serum potassium levels in primary aldosteronism. Such tests often provide indices of the severity of the condition even more important than the hormone level.

In conditions in which immunologic processes are important, assessment of antibody levels can be particularly helpful. Other tests provide information that is more of a corroborative nature, but which nonetheless can be useful. For instance, the serum sodium is almost always greater than 139 mEq per liter in patients with an aldosterone-producing adenoma; the plasma cholesterol tends to be high in hypothyroidism and low in hyperthyroidism; the serum potassium tends to be high in Addison's disease; the alkaline phosphatase tends to be elevated in osteomalacia; and the serum phosphorus levels tend to be elevated in acromegaly.

Evaluation of the Sensitivity of Target Cells to Hormones. Suspicion of hyposensitivity to a hormone is raised when manifestations of deficiency of the hormone occur in the presence of elevated hormone levels. In type II diabetes mellitus there is hyperglycemia with hyperinsulinism; in pseudohypoparathyroidism, hypocalcemia and symptoms resulting from this with elevated PTH levels; and in pseudo-hermaphroditism caused by the testicular feminization syndrome, decreased androgenicity with elevated plasma testosterone levels. The existence of hyposensitivity can be confirmed by administering the hormone in question and determining the presence or extent of response, although commonly it is not necessary to do this. In some cases, such as with insulin or androgen resistance, it is possible to obtain further confirmation of the hyposensitivity state by isolating cells from the patient and measuring receptors or responses, although these techniques are not generally available. Conversely, hypersensitivity to hormones is characterized by low hormone levels relative to the response. In low-renin "essential" hypertension the adrenal glomerulosa is excessively sensitive to angiotensin II. This is reflected by normal to elevated plasma aldosterone levels in the presence of low angiotensin II levels. This sensitivity can be documented by measuring the plasma aldosterone levels following an infusion of angiotensin.

TREATMENT OF ENDOCRINE DISEASES

For endocrine deficiency syndromes, hormones are generally administered to replace the deficiency. In general the hormone that is deficient is replaced. In some cases this is not possible or expedient, and other hormones are given that help compensate for the defect. For instance, vitamin D is given instead of PTH to treat hypoparathyroidism since it can increase the extracellular Ca^{++}. In cases in which hormone resistance is present, steps are taken when possible to alleviate this, as through diet restriction in diabetes.

In hormone-excess syndromes, a variety of approaches is used. Hyperfunctioning tumors are removed when possible, and sometimes hyperplastic glands are removed. In other cases drugs are given to block hormone production (propylthiouracil in thyrotoxicosis and bromocriptine for prolactin-producing adenomas). Antagonists such as spironolactone in primary aldosteronism due to hyperplasia can sometimes be useful.

For both excess and deficiency syndromes adjunctive therapy is frequently important. Thus multiple measures are used to treat the complications to diabetes mellitus, and patients with Addison's disease are cautioned to avoid stress.

SUMMARY

Endocrinology is increasingly an open-ended discipline for the study of molecule-mediated communication and response. New systems are still being elaborated (opioids, prostaglandins, leukotrienes, vitamin D, cell growth factors); older systems are increasingly being defined in molecular terms. In addition, the clinical abnormalities that occur are being understood and the means to evaluate them are being refined to allow more rational, accurate, and beneficial approaches to diagnosis and treatment. This introductory chapter has presented a general overview of this discipline as a background for the following chapters, which will be devoted to its specific components and the disorders that occur in human endocrine diseases.

Alberts B, Bray D, Lewis J, et al.: Molecular Biology of the Cell. New York, Garland Publishing, Inc., 1983. *Reviews in detail advances in cell and molecular biology, including information on gene structure and function, protein synthesis, internalization, and hormone action.*

Cohen P: The role of protein phosphorylation in neural and hormonal control of cellular activity. Nature 296:613, 1982. *An overview of the role of phosphorylation in hormone action.*

Felig P, Baxter JD, Broadus AE, et al. (eds.): Endocrinology and Metabolism. 2nd ed. New York, McGraw-Hill Book Company, 1987. *Provides an extensive analysis of the topics included in this chapter. The chapters by Gertz and Baxter on gene expression and recombinant DNA; by Gill on biosynthesis, secretion, and metabolism of hormones; by Viatukaitis on hormone assay; and by Catt on hormone action provide much detailed information.*

Ganong WF: The brain as an endocrine organ. Acta Physiol Lat Am 32:31, 1982. *Provides an excellent discussion of neuroendocrine relationships.*

Green S, Chambon P: A superfamily of potentially oncogenic hormone receptors. Nature 324:615, 1986. *A brief review of studies of the genes and actions of steroid and thyroid hormone receptors.*

Greenspan FS, Forsham PH (eds.): Basic and Clinical Endocrinology. 2nd ed. Los Altos, Lange Medical Publications, 1986. *An excellent general reference on endocrinology and metabolism.*

Gustafson J-Å, Carlstedt-Duke J, Poellinger L, et al.: Biochemistry, molecular biology and physiology of the glucocorticoid receptor. Endocr Rev 8:185, 1987. *A comprehensive review of glucocorticoid hormone action with reference to other classes of steroid hormones.*

Hopkins CR: The importance of the endosome in intracellular traffic. Nature 304:684, 1983. *A concise update of the events in hormone and receptor internalization, recycling, and degradation.*

Wilson JD: Disorders of androgen action. Clin Res 35:1, 1987. *A discussion of the problems of hyposensitivity to androgens as illustrative of the general problem of hormone resistance.*

Wilson JD, Foster DW (eds.): Williams' Textbook of Endocrinology. 7th ed. Philadelphia, W. B. Saunders Company, 1985. *An excellent general reference on endocrinology and metabolism.*

222 THE ENDORPHIN FAMILY OF OPIOID PEPTIDES: BIOCHEMISTRY, ANATOMY, AND PHYSIOLOGY*

Stanley J. Watson

Many structures throughout the central and peripheral nervous systems contain cells that secrete peptides. Major among these is a family of endogenous neuropeptides capable of mimicking many actions of opiate alkaloids, such as morphine. These peptides have a common pentapeptide sequence at their amino terminus [Tyr-Gly-Gly-Phe-Met (or-Leu)], which is important for their opiate activity. All such *endogenous opioid peptides* carry the generic name of endorphins (*endogenous morphines*). There are actually three main families of endorphins, each with its own separate protein precursor, mRNA, and gene (Fig. 222–1). (1) *Pro-Opio-Melano-Cortin* (or POMC), (2) *Pro-Enkephalin*, and (3) *Pro-Dynorphin/Neo-Endorphin*. POMC produces one opiate peptide, beta-endorphin, and several nonopioid products, e.g., ACTH and alpha-, beta-, and gamma-melanocyte-stimulating hormones (MSH). In contrast, pro-enkephalin has seven repeated opioid sequences, and pro-dynorphin has three.

The discovery of three families of endorphins with their many active peptides grew out of a rich set of pharmacologic tools and behavioral paradigms. Briefly, the structural pharmacology of the opiate alkaloids allowed the description of active and inactive stereoisomers of both opiate agonists and antagonists. The introduction of radiolabeled versions of the

active alkaloids made it possible, in the early 1970's, to describe the existence of opiate receptors in brain. A search for their natural ligands followed, and more than 20 active peptide fragments were extracted and sequenced during the next decade. The first active peptides were the methionine- and leucine-enkephalin pentapeptides (derived from pro-enkephalin); they were very soon followed by alpha-, beta-, and gamma-endorphin (derived from POMC). A few years later the dynorphin family of peptides was discovered. The use of molecular genetics allowed the description of mRNA and gene structures for all three peptide families. Such structural information radically improved our knowledge of the sequences of the endorphins within their precursors and provided better understanding of their relationships with their nonopiate fragments. The availability of peptide and precursor sequences then allowed the production of antibodies and nucleic acid probes for studying the anatomy, peptide biochemistry, nucleic acid biochemistry, receptors, and physiology of all three endorphin families.

Anatomic studies have provided a clearer view of the complexity of these peptide-secreting cells and their related fiber projections. Figure 222–2 shows a diagram of each of the endorphin systems in rat brain (human brain is very similar in pattern). It is clear that these systems are widespread, with several cell groups and complex projections throughout the neuraxis. All three endorphin systems commonly innervate some of the same areas, as well as project to unique areas. No single pattern emerges from this rich anatomy; rather, one is impressed with the involvement of endorphins in many major systems (e.g., motor, endocrine, limbic, autonomic).

As the structure of the endorphin peptides and precursors became clear, major questions arose concerning the biosynthetic processing of the peptides in different neural and endocrine tissue. The most obvious example of tissue-specific processing of the endorphins is found with POMC in the pituitary of the rat. In the anterior lobe the corticotrophs produce, among other things, the full ACTH molecule (1–39). In contrast, in the intermediate lobe (found in most species, but in humans present only in pregnant women and fetuses) that same molecule is further processed to make alpha-melanocyte-stimulating hormone [or N acetyl ACTH 1–13 amide and ACTH (18–39)]. Similar tissue-specific processing patterns are found for other POMC peptides, such as beta-endorphin as well as for pro-dynorphin– and pro-enkephalin–produced peptides. For example, pro-enkephalin in adrenal is cleaved into larger fragments, whereas in brain it is actively processed to much smaller peptides.

From these findings, several principles are beginning to emerge about the processing of neuropeptides. A given precursor can give rise to one set of products in one tissue and a different set of products in another tissue. General processing differences are due to the cleavage site chosen, indicated by the presence of a dibasic peptide bond (see above about alpha-MSH versus ACTH). A second type of processing variant involves post-translational processing in which other chemical moieties are added to a given site in a peptide sequence. Amidation, acetylation, sulfation, and phosphorylation have all been described for the endorphin peptides. Both types of processing choices can alter the nature and potency of these molecules. For example, the addition of an acetyl group to the amino terminal tyrosine of beta-endorphin decreases its opiate activity by more than 1000-fold. Thus, two of the largest problems in peptidergic systems, especially in brain, are in understanding the precursor-processing pathways and the final structure of the peptides produced by each precursor, in a tissue of interest. Figure 222–1 provides a simplified version of this information for each precursor.

Given what we have just described (post-translational processing and tissue-specific processing) it is clear that these peptidergic cells have a range of control over the materials

---

*I want to express my appreciation for the important contributions of Dr. Huda Akil in the preparation of this chapter.

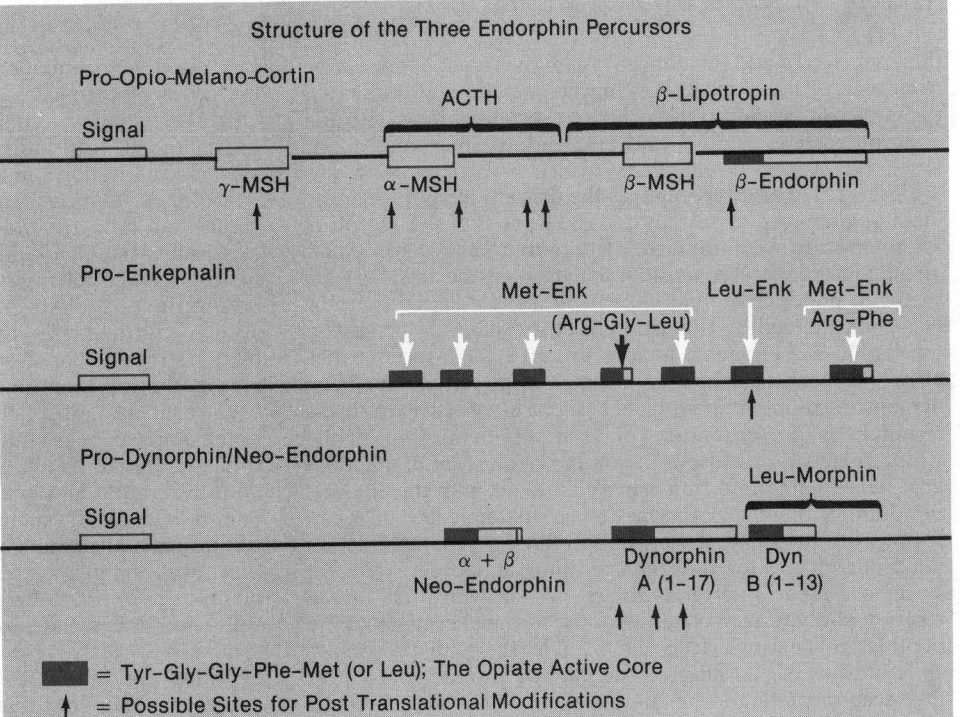

FIGURE 222–1. Simplified schematic of the precursors for all three endorphin families. Note the many peptides produced from each precursor, their similar size, and in the case of pro-enkephalin and pro-dynorphin, the multiple copies of opioid peptides produced by each.

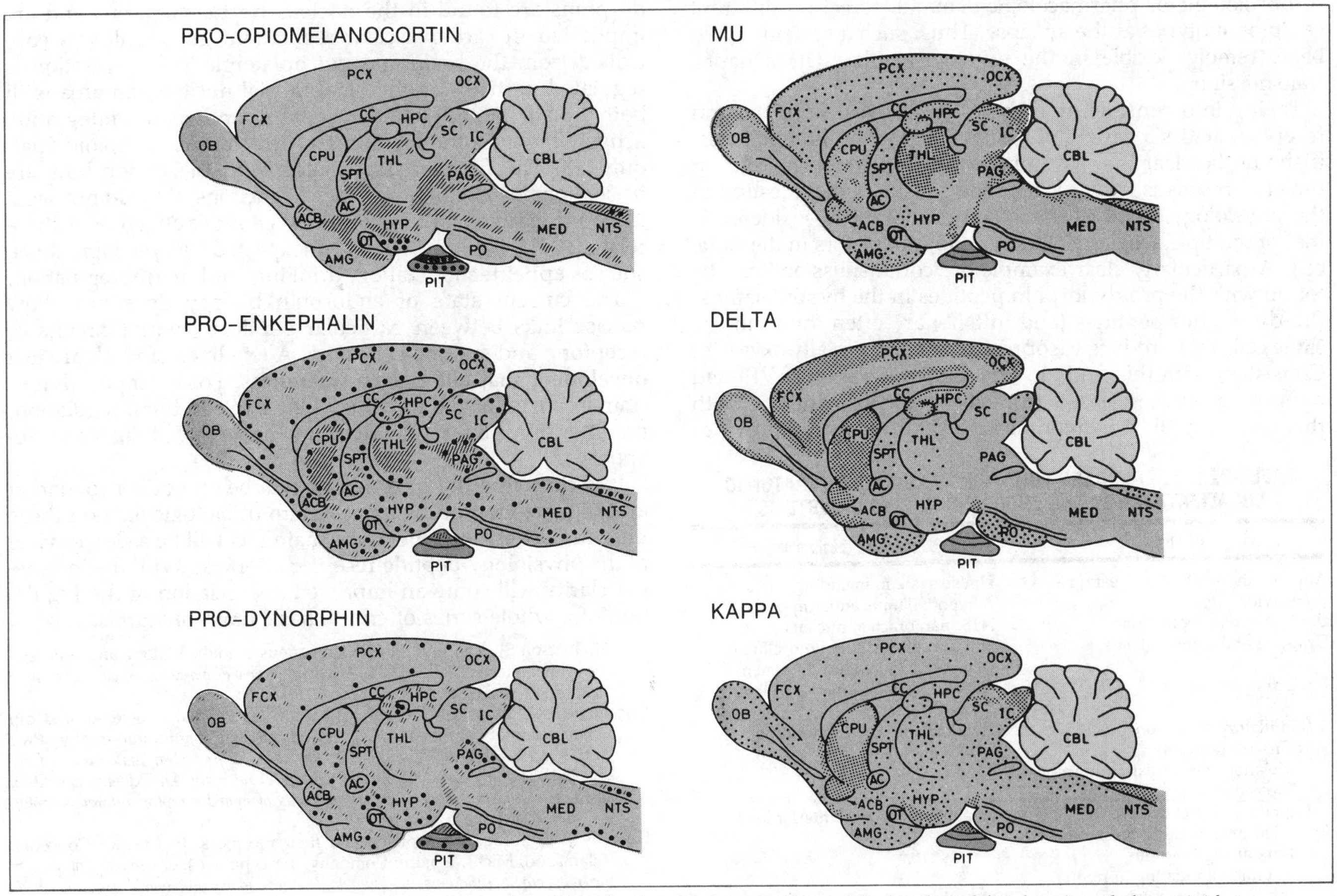

Structure of the Three Endorphin Percursors

Pro-Opio-Melano-Cortin

Signal

γ-MSH α-MSH β-MSH β-Endorphin

ACTH β-Lipotropin

Pro-Enkephalin

Signal

Met-Enk Leu-Enk Met-Enk Arg-Phe
(Arg-Gly-Leu)

Pro-Dynorphin/Neo-Endorphin

Signal

Leu-Morphin

α + β Neo-Endorphin Dynorphin A (1–17) Dyn B (1–13)

▬ = Tyr-Gly-Gly-Phe-Met (or Leu); The Opiate Active Core

↑ = Possible Sites for Post Translational Modifications

PRO-OPIOMELANOCORTIN

MU

PRO-ENKEPHALIN

DELTA

PRO-DYNORPHIN

KAPPA

FIGURE 222–2. Schematic representations of the distribution of the opioid peptide families (*left column*) and the opioid receptor subtypes (*right column*) in the rat brain and pituitary. All three opioid families are differentially distributed with POMC cell bodies (*large closed circles*) being localized in the hypothalamus and NTS and sending fibers (represented by hatch marks) to numerous limbic and brain stem nuclei. Pro-enkephalin and Pro-dynorphin cell bodies are more widely distributed and can be seen in numerous nuclear groups and in cortex. The opioid receptor subtypes are also differentially localized one from the other (*right column*) and can be seen in the vicinity of the opioid peptides. Note the fairly complicated possible relationship that may exist between the opioid peptides and receptors. For instance, within the NTS, all three opioid peptides and receptors can be observed. AC = Anterior commissure; ACB = nucleus accumbens; AMG = amygdala; CBL = cerebellum; CC = corpus callosum; CPU = caudate-putamen; FCX = frontal cortex; HPC = hippocampus; HYP = hypothalamus; IC = inferior colliculus; MED = medulla; NTS = nucleus tractus solitarius; OB = olfactory bulb; OCX = occipital cortex; OT = optic tract; PAG = periaqueductal gray; PCX = parietal cortex; PIT = pituitary; PO = pons; SC = superior colliculus; SPT = septum; THL = thalamus.

they secrete. To add further complexity, several peptides arise from each of the three endorphin precursors, and nonopioid peptides can be co-produced and co-secreted along with the endorphins (e.g., ACTH and beta-endorphin from anterior lobe).

Figure 222–2 also schematizes the distributions of the three main opiate receptor subclasses. The three types of receptors are referred to with the Greek letters mu, kappa, and delta. The mu receptor is very sensitive to morphine; the delta receptor seems to prefer enkephalin-like peptides; the kappa receptor was characterized by the action of ethyl ketocyclazocine and dynorphin-like peptides. In addition, an epsilon receptor has been suggested for beta-endorphin, although it has been demonstrated only in peripheral tissue. The selectivity of these receptors is not absolute. For example, dynorphin, while kappa preferring, is also a potent mu agonist, and enkephalins, while delta preferring, can also interact with the mu site. In addition, there is not a one-to-one anatomic link between kappa receptors and dynorphin-producing cells and fibers; nor is there one for the delta receptor and pro-enkephalin systems. Rather, one tends to see two or even three opiate receptor subtypes associated with the terminal systems of the peptidergic neurons. It is conceivable that the processing choices of a cell, by altering the peptide products, can alter the receptor preference of the materials secreted. In effect, it is possible that the cell modulates its products as a function of physiologic or pharmacologic demand, to act on different receptor subtypes at the synapse. Thus, such a system would be extremely flexible in the way it modulates its synaptic transmission.

Taking into consideration the multiplicity of peptides and receptors across a variety of tissues, each with different roles, it should be clear that assuming a single physiologic role for the endorphins is naive. When one considers the question of the physiology, another factor that needs to be considered is that of multiple active transmitters and modulators in the same cell. A particularly clear example of "cotransmission" can be found with the pro-dynorphin peptides in the hypothalamus. Pro-dynorphin peptides (and mRNA) are often found in the same cells that produce vasopressin and occasionally oxytocin. Consistent with this finding, arginine vasopressin (AVP) and dynorphin are coreleased from the posterior pituitary with the same stimuli. It is hypothesized that dynorphin provides local feedback inhibition on further AVP secretion. Other examples of cotransmission among the endorphins include enkephalin and catecholamines in the adrenal medulla, enkephalin and catecholamines in the sympathetic nervous system, and dynorphin and LH/FSH in the anterior pituitary.

Table 222–1 summarizes the main physiologic observations associated with the endorphins. The endorphins have been classically associated with modulation of stress and pain. The neuronal and endocrine systems involved in these responses are, in the case of stress, the hypothalamic-pituitary-adrenal system and the limbic system. In fact, each major component of the stress-response system contains endorphins. For example, the hippocampus, a main site of corticosteroid feedback, contains enkephalin and dynorphin neurons; the hypothalamus contains all three opioid families; the anterior pituitary contains POMC; and the adrenal medulla produces both dynorphin and enkephalin. A similar pattern is seen in pain-modulatory systems in the spinal cord, periaqueductal central gray, thalamus, and the limbic system. It seems clear that stress and pain responses are, in several ways, dependent on endorphin physiology.

If one studies the physiology of the endorphins, as presented in Table 222–1, a few patterns become clear: (1) These peptides are implicated in a wide variety of physiologic events. (2) Many of these events correlate fairly well with the anatomy of the opioid peptides. For example, all three endorphins are found in the nucleus tractus solitarius and are implicated in cardiovascular regulation; gut motility is controlled from the brain and gut opiatergic loci; respiration is regulated partially by the parabrachial nucleus, an area with both opiate peptides and receptors; and motor integration actively involves the nigrostriatal system, rich in opioid anatomy. (3) The functions associated with the endorphins are basic, homeostatic, limbic, "core" functions; they do not seem to be primarily cognitive, but may be more affective or drive related. (4) There are a few "unexpected" physiologic links, such as appetite modulation, drinking, and thermoregulation.

The current state of endorphin biology does not allow precise links between particular peptides, neural circuits or receptors, and specific behaviors. A few lines of work are just developing that allow such inferences. For example, dynorphin in posterior pituitary may play a role in thirst regulation, or anterior pituitary POMC may be involved in stress responses.

It is clear that the next decade will be one of consolidation and organization of the great wealth of biologic data on these important systems. One of the main foci will be a clearer view of the physiology-peptide-receptor interface. With the increasing clarity will come an improved appreciation of the regulation of a whole series of critical basic brain functions.

TABLE 222–1. PROPOSED FUNCTIONS AND KNOWN ANATOMIC LOCALIZATIONS OF THE ENDOGENOUS OPIOID SYSTEMS

Function	Anatomic Localization
Appetite modulation and eating behavior	Limbic system, including hypothalamus and amygdala
Cardiovascular regulation	NTS, parabrachial nucleus
Drinking and water balance	Subfornical organ, magnocellular hypothalamic-pituitary system
Endocrine responses	Hypothalamic-pituitary-peripheral axis
Stimulatory effects on Growth hormone Melanocyte-stimulating hormone Prolactin	Hypothalamus and anterior lobe
Inhibitory effects on Follicle-stimulating hormone Luteinizing hormone Thyroid-stimulating hormone	Hypothalamus and anterior lobe
Inhibition of release of vasopressin and oxytocin	Hypothalamus and posterior lobe
Gastrointestinal motility	NTS, area postrema, and GI nervous plexi
Pain inhibition	Thalamus, periaqueductal gray, substantia gelatinosa, NTS, spinal cord
Respiration	Parabrachial nucleus, NTS
Response to stress	Hypothalamic-pituitary-adrenal axis
Sensory-motor integration	Nigrostriatal system, globus pallidus, inferior and superior colliculi
Thermoregulation	Hypothalamus

NTS = Nucleus tractus solitarius.

Akil H, Watson SJ, Young E, et al: Endogenous opioids: Biology and function. Ann Rev Neurosci 7:223, 1984. *A general review of many issues associated with the biology of the endorphins.*

Goodman RR, Snyder SH, Kuhar MJ, et al: Differentiation of delta and mu opiate receptor localizations by light microscopic autoradiography. Proc Natl Acad Sci USA 77:6239, 1980. *Provides the first clear dissociation of the distributions of mu and delta opioid receptors in rat brain. Dr. Kuhar's laboratory has been a leader in developing the methods of opioid receptor autoradiography, and this paper is a good example of their work.*

Holaday JW: Endogenous opioids and their receptors. In Current Concepts. Kalamazoo, Mich., Upjohn Company, 1984, pp 4–64. *A summary of some of the physiologic functions attributable to the endogenous opioid systems. It is particularly recommended for the novice who wishes to have a general summary of opioid systems and their possible function.*

Loh YP, Brownstein MJ, Gainer H: Proteolysis in neuropeptide processing and other neural functions. Ann Rev Neurosci 7:189, 1984. *A thorough overview of the issue of processing in neuropeptide precursors.*

Martin WR: Pharmacology of opioids. Pharmacol Rev 32:283, 1984. *An authoritative and comprehensive review of opiate pharmacology. The author presents an in-depth analysis of how different classes of opiates may influence analgesia, respiration, cardiovascular function, pupil dilation, temperature, EEG, and dependence.*

Millan MJ, Herz A: The endocrinology of the opioids. Int Rev Neurobiol 26:1, 1985. *A comprehensive review of the role of the opioid peptides and receptors in neuroendocrine responses. The authors have worked many years in this area and provide a thoughtful review of this field.*

223 PROSTAGLANDINS AND RELATED COMPOUNDS

Garret A. FitzGerald

Arachidonic acid, a natural constituent of the phospholipid component of cell membranes, is released in response to specific stimuli, as well as to nonspecific chemical and physical perturbations of membranes. Subsequent oxygenation by either the cyclooxygenase or lipoxygenase enzymes gives rise to biologically active compounds. A third pathway of metabolism via cytochrome P450 has recently been identified (Fig. 223–1). The capacity to release arachidonic acid is common to all cells, but the predominant enzymatic products that are formed are highly cell specific. Because they are derived from a polyunsaturated eicosanoic (C_{20}) fatty acid, these compounds—thromboxane A_2, the prostaglandins (PG's), epoxygenases, leukotrienes, and lipoxins—are collectively known as eicosanoids. Because of their diverse biologic properties and rapid metabolism to inactive products, the eicosanoids have been implicated as local mediators in a range of physiologic processes and in diverse human diseases, including bronchial asthma, inflammation, and unstable coronary disease.

THE CYCLOOXYGENASE PATHWAY (Fig. 223–2)

The biotransformation of arachidonic acid into thromboxane (Tx)A_2, prostacyclin (PGI$_2$), PGE$_2$, PGF$_{2\alpha}$, and PGD$_2$ is catalyzed by a common enzyme, the fatty acid cyclooxygenase. The product of the cyclooxygenase reaction is an unstable endoperoxide, PGG. A second oxygen molecule is then introduced at C_{15}, resulting in the 15-hydroperoxy endoperoxide PGH, and liberating a free radical. The cyclooxygenase and peroxidase activities reside in a single membrane-associated protein. PGH is then metabolized by cell-specific enzymes to form either the "classic" prostaglandins of the D, E, and F series, PGI$_2$, or TxA$_2$. Arachidonic acid contains four double bonds ($\Delta^{5, 8, 11, 14}$). It is apparent from the sequence of biosynthesis (Fig. 223–2) that two double bonds remain in its (bisenoic) cyclooxygenase products. This is denoted by the *subscript 2*, as in TxA$_2$ and PGE$_2$. Analogous metabolism of other fatty acid substrates gives rise to monoenoic or trienoic prostaglandins and thromboxanes (Fig. 223–3). For example, metabolites of eicosatrienoic acid ($C_{20:3}$ n-6) contain only one (Δ^{13}) double bond. Eicosapentaenoic acid (EPA) ($C_{20:5}$ n-3), which is prevalent in certain fish and aquatic mammals, is transformed by cyclooxygenase to metabolites with three ($\Delta^{5, 13, 17}$) double bonds such as PGI$_3$ and TxA$_3$. Structurally, prostaglandins of the D, E, and F series possess a cyclopentane ring and differ only in their substituent groups. Treatment of E prostaglandins with sodium borohydride reduces the C_9 ketone groups to give two C_{10} hydroxyl isomers, the alpha-isomer of which is identical with PGF. Thus, the F series prostaglandins are referred to as PGF$_{1\alpha}$, PGF$_{2\alpha}$, and PGF$_{3\alpha}$. In man, many of the metabolites formed from PGD$_2$ contain an F ring, and one of these, $9_\alpha, 11_\beta$-PGF, contracts bronchial and vascular smooth muscle and inhibits platelet aggregation.

THROMBOXANE A$_2$. TxA$_2$, the predominant cyclooxygenase product formed by platelets, stimulates aggregation of these cells and constricts vascular and bronchial smooth muscle. These biologic properties are shared by the PG endoperoxides. TxA$_2$ and the PG endoperoxides seem to produce their effects via shared receptors. TxA$_2$ is very evanescent at physiologic pH; its half-life has been estimated at 30 seconds.

In addition to initiating aggregation of platelets, TxA$_2$ that is generated by platelets aggregated in response to epinephrine, adenosine diphosphate (ADP), and platelet-activating factor (PAF) is responsible for a "secondary wave" of aggregation. Aspirin inhibits platelet aggregation by preventing the formation of TxA$_2$, although the capacity of platelets to form TxA$_2$ must be inhibited by greater than 95 per cent for even modest inhibition of platelet function.

PROSTACYCLIN. Prostacyclin (PGI$_2$) is the predominant cyclooxygenase product of arachidonic acid formed by vascular endothelium and also by subendothelium. PGI$_2$ both inhibits the aggregation of platelets by all recognized agonists and disaggregates previously aggregated platelets. PGI$_2$ also inhibits the adherence of platelets and neutrophils to foreign surfaces and damaged endothelium. These receptor-mediated events are transduced via an increase in intraplatelet cyclic AMP. Two other important properties of prostacyclin are the dilation of both bronchial and vascular smooth muscle and the modulation of cholesterol efflux from arterial walls. Nanomolar quantities of PGI$_2$ stimulate the activity of both the lysosomal and cytoplasmic cholesterol ester hydrolases when added experimentally to vascular smooth muscle cells, but have no effect on the microsomal acyl-CoA cholesterol acyl transferase (ACAT), which re-esterifies free cholesterol.

PGI$_2$, like TxA$_2$, is evanescent at physiologic pH (half-life of 3 minutes). Although prostacyclin differs from other prostaglandins in undergoing minimal metabolism during transit through the lung, circulating concentrations are rarely, if ever, sufficient to mediate a systemic response. Many factors associated with thrombogenesis, such as trauma, thrombin, ADP, PAF, and platelet-derived growth factor, stimulate PGI$_2$ formation by endothelial cells in vitro. This would suggest that local formation might serve both to limit the deposition of platelets and leukocytes following vascular injury and to prevent their further recruitment. PGI$_2$ generation might also antagonize the attendant vascular spasm induced by platelet-derived vasoconstrictor compounds, such as TxA$_2$. Consistent with such a local homeostatic role, PGI$_2$ biosynthesis is increased in several human diseases in which evidence of platelet activation is present. These include severe peripheral arterial disease and unstable coronary disease.

PROSTAGLANDIN D$_2$. Prostaglandin D$_2$, the principal cyclooxygenase product of the mast cell, is released, together with histamine and other mediators, by IgE-dependent and other stimuli. Infusion of PGD$_2$ in humans results in nasal stuffiness, systemic hypotension, and flushing. These symptoms are characteristic of the syndrome of systemic mastocytosis in which there is diffuse mast cell infiltration of tissues (Ch. 427). A minority of patients with this disorder exhibit a rise in blood pressure rather than hypotension in association with flushing. One possible explanation for this observation is preferential conversion of PGD$_2$ to its $9_\alpha, 11_\beta$-PGF metabolite, which contracts vascular smooth muscle in vitro. The role of PGD$_2$ in the normal immunologic response is unclear. PGD$_2$ is increased in bronchoalveolar lavage fluid following antigen challenge in atopic individuals, suggesting that it may contribute to the bronchomotor response in allergic asthma. PGD$_2$

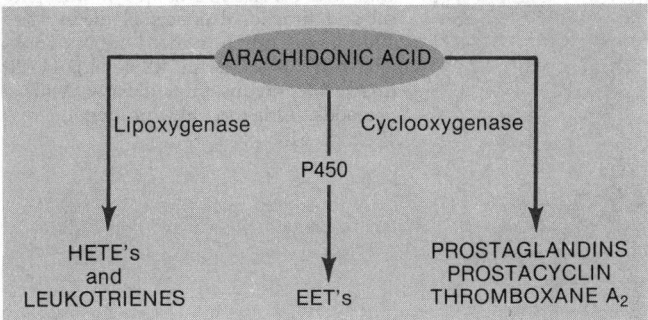

FIGURE 223–1. Major pathways of metabolism of arachidonic acid.

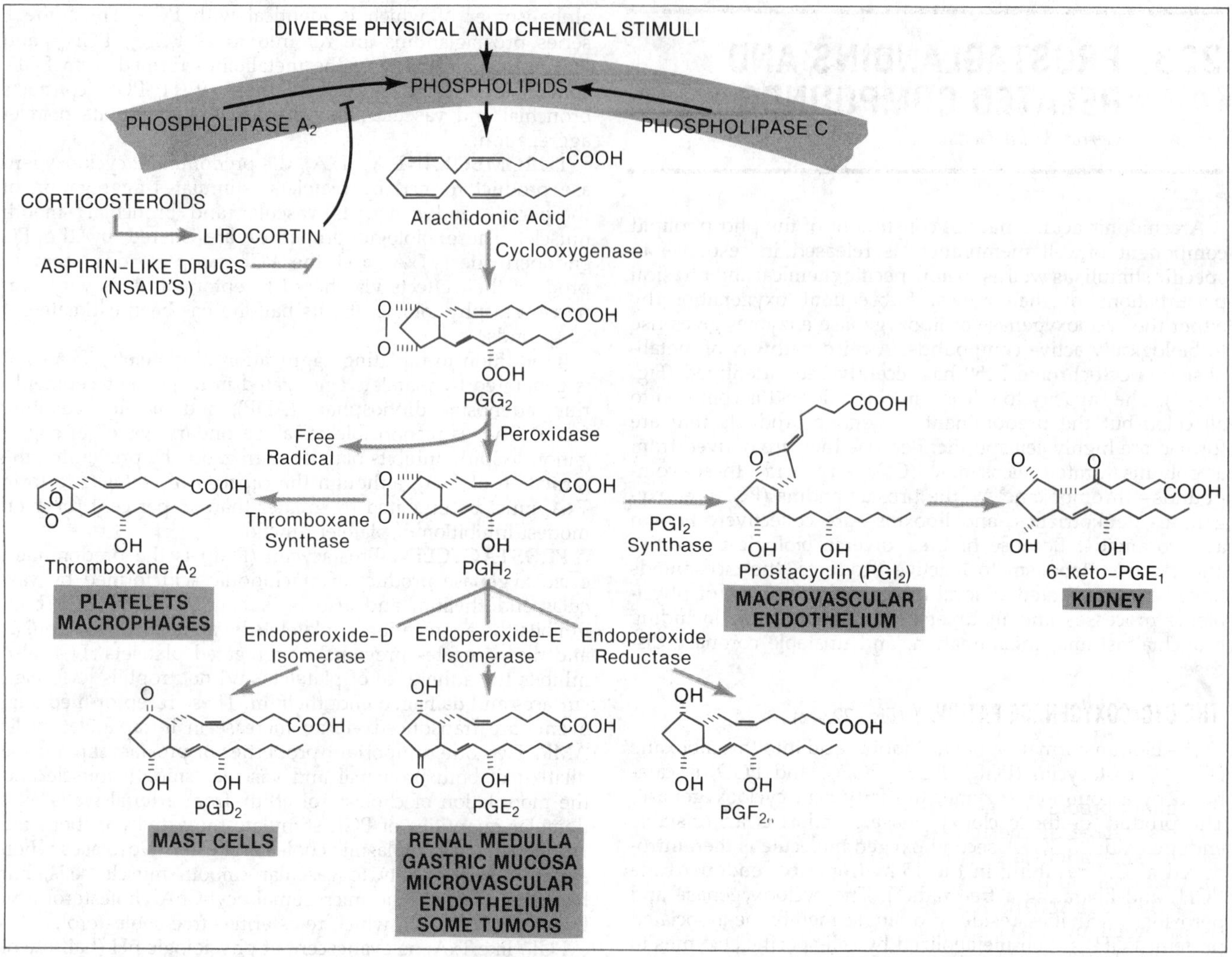

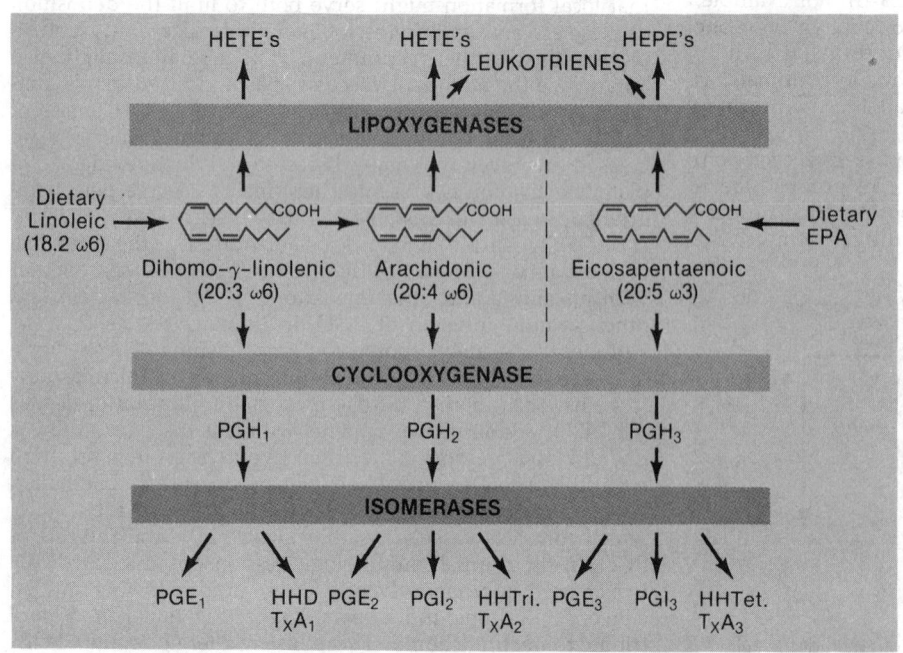

FIGURE 223–2. Metabolism of arachidonic acid by fatty acid cyclooxygenase. The major tissues of origin of the eicosanoids are shown.

FIGURE 223–3. Analogous formation of mono-, bis-, and trienoic prostaglandins. (Reproduced with permission from Fitz-Gerald GA, Price P, Knapp HR: Biochemical and functional effects of dietary substrate modification in man. In Simopoulos AP, Kifer RR, Martin RE (eds.): Health Effects of Polyunsaturated Fatty Acids in Seafoods. Orlando, FL, Academic Press, 1986, pp 61–80.)

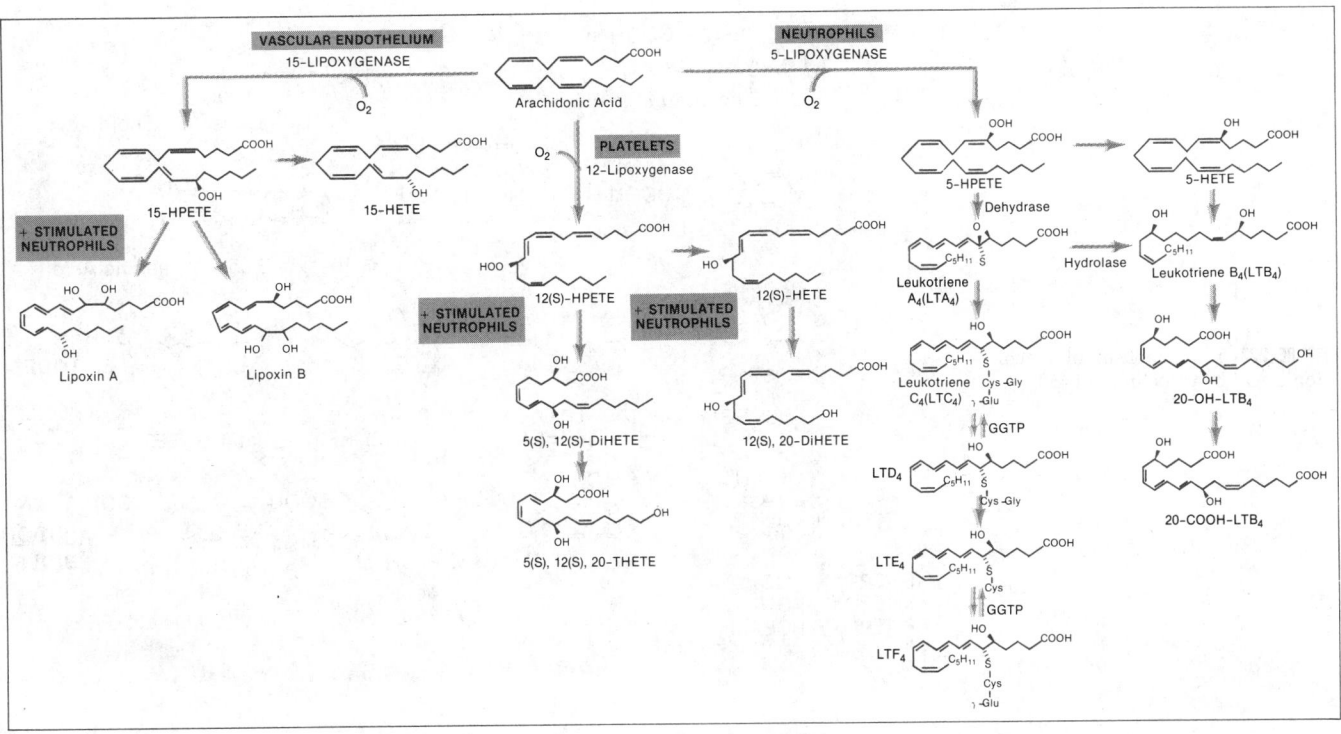

FIGURE 223–4. Metabolism of arachidonic acid by lipoxygenase enzymes.

is a minor product of the platelet cyclooxygenase. Both PGD$_2$ and its 9$_\alpha$,11$_\beta$-PGF metabolite inhibit platelet aggregation by stimulating adenylate cyclase, thereby increasing intraplatelet cyclic AMP.

PROSTAGLANDIN E$_2$. The formation of PGE$_2$ from PGH$_2$ is catalyzed by a PGE$_2$ isomerase that is present in renal medulla, gastric mucosa, and platelets. PGE$_2$ rather than PGI$_2$ may be the predominant prostaglandin formed by microvascular endothelium. In the kidney PGE$_2$ can act both as a vasodilator and as an inhibitor of tubular sodium absorption. PGE$_2$ is the predominant cyclooxygenase product of arachidonic acid formed in gastric mucosa. It participates in the regulation of gastric blood flow and limits the effects of diverse physical and chemical insults to the gastric mucosa. This "cytoprotective" property is shared by PGI$_2$, but the mechanism by which this protection occurs is unknown. Other biologic properties of PGE$_2$ include relaxation of bronchial smooth muscle, contraction of uterine smooth muscle (19-hydroxylated E prostaglandins are the major arachidonic acid products in human semen), inhibition of platelet aggregation (albeit considerably less potently than PGI$_2$), and modulation of lymphocyte function. PGE$_2$ also modulates neurotransmission via presynaptic receptors on adrenergic neurons in vitro.

In a minority of patients with solid tumors, PGE$_2$ production by the tumor causes hypercalcemia via stimulation of osteoclast activity. In such cases, suppression of PGE$_2$ biosynthesis will lower the level of serum calcium. However, when metastases to bone occur, local mechanisms for hypercalcemia supervene. High concentrations of PGE$_2$ are found in the joint fluid of patients with rheumatoid arthritis. The role of PGE$_2$ in this setting is unknown although the clinical response to cyclooxygenase inhibitors suggests that eicosanoids are of relevance to the local inflammatory process.

PROSTAGLANDIN F$_{2\alpha}$. PGF$_{2\alpha}$, formed from PGH$_2$ by the action of an endoperoxidase reductase, contracts bronchial and uterine smooth muscle and is a vasoconstrictor in some uterine beds. Neither a unique site of its formation nor a clearly defined pathophysiologic role for PGF$_{2\alpha}$ has been identified.

THE LIPOXYGENASE PATHWAY (Fig. 223–4)

Arachidonic acid is also widely subject to lipoxygenation reactions (Fig. 223–4). In neutrophils, insertion of an oxygen molecule adjacent to one of the double bonds yields the hydroperoxy derivative, 5-hydroperoxyeicosatetraenoic acid (5-HPETE). This can undergo further metabolism to either a 5-hydroxyeicosatetraenoic acid (5-HETE) or by dehydration to an unstable 5,6-epoxide intermediate, leukotriene (LT)A$_4$. This compound can be hydrolyzed to 5,12-dihydroxyeicosatetraenoic acids, of which one is LTB$_4$. The *subscript 4* refers to the number of double bonds. Thus, analogous to the nomenclature for cyclooxygenase products, substitution of eicosapentaenoic acid for arachidonic acid as a substrate would result in formation of LTB$_5$. The site of the initial lipoxygenation reaction tends to vary with cell type. Thus 12-HETE is predominantly formed in platelets, 5-HETE by polymorphonuclear leukocytes, and 5-HETE, 11-HETE, and 15-HETE by endothelial cells in culture.

LTA$_4$ also is conjugated enzymatically with glutathione to yield LTC$_4$. This compound is metabolized to LTD$_4$ and LTE$_4$ by successive elimination of a gamma glutamyl residue and glycine. The cysteinyl-containing leukotrienes are powerful bronchoconstrictors and vasoconstrictors. In addition they have been shown to be identical with "slow-reacting substance of anaphylaxis"—a product first identified following immunologic challenge or addition of cobra venom to guinea pig ileum. These compounds also dilate microvessels, increase vascular permeability, and stimulate mucus secretion. LTC$_4$ causes pulmonary bronchoconstriction, an effect that is partially blocked by cyclooxygenase inhibitors. This implies that LTC$_4$ may mediate this effect via the release of a bronchoconstrictor prostaglandin, such as thromboxane A$_2$. LTC$_4$ may cooperate with luteinizing hormone-releasing hormone (LHRH) in the control of LH release by cells of the anterior pituitary, judged by in vitro studies.

LTB$_4$ stimulates adhesion, migration, aggregation, enzyme release, and generation of superoxide by polymorphonuclear leukocytes. These biologic properties strongly suggest a role

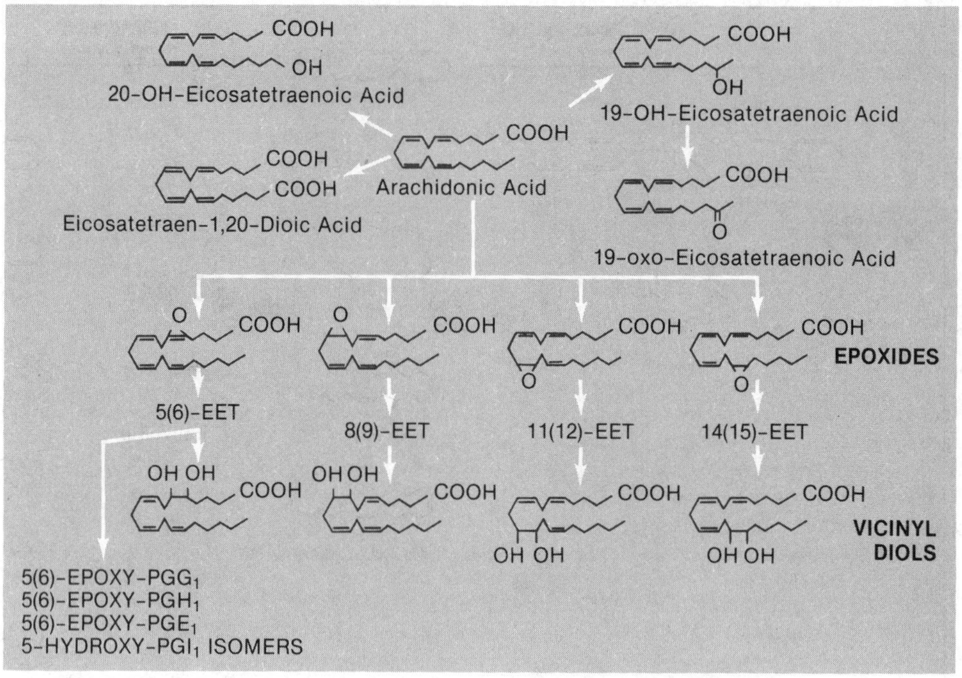

FIGURE 223–5. Metabolism of arachidonic acid by cytochrome P450.

for lipoxygenase products in both inflammation and antigen-evoked bronchoconstriction, although this remains to be definitively established in man. Di-HETE's can be formed via transcellular metabolism, at least in vitro. Examples include 12,20-di-HETE formed by a mixed suspension of platelets and polymorphonuclear leukocytes. Leukocytes can utilize erythrocyte LTA_4 to generate LTB_4, and endothelial cells can utilize platelet-derived PGH_2 to generate PGI_2, as shown in in vitro studies.

Stimulated human leukocytes can convert 15-HPETE to products termed lipoxins (LX) containing a characteristic tetraenoic structure (Fig. 223–4). The two major products identified are LXA and LXB. LXA is a potent stimulus to superoxide generation by neutrophils and contracts pulmonary tissue. Both LXA and LXB inhibit natural killer cell cytotoxicity in vitro, by a mechanism distinct from that of PGE_2, which decreases the binding between target and effector cells.

THE EPOXYGENASE PATHWAY (Fig. 223–5)

In addition to metabolism by cyclooxygenase and lipoxygenase enzymes, arachidonic acid is subject to omega and omega-1 oxidation by cytochrome P450 enzymes in microsomal preparations. This results in the formation of 19-OH and 19-oxo-eicosatetraenoic acid (by omega-1-oxidation) and 20-OH-eicosatetraenoic and eicosatetraene-1,20-dioic acids (by omega oxidation). In addition a series of epoxides 14(15)-epoxy-, 11(12)-epoxy-, 8(9)-epoxy-, and 5(6)-epoxy-eicosatrienoic acids (EET's) can be formed by this enzyme from arachidonic acid. These compounds can then be further transformed to vicinyl-diols by epoxide hydrolases. One such compound 11,12-dihydroxyeicosatrienoic acid inhibits the Na^+K^+-ATPase enzyme in vascular smooth muscle. It has been reported that 5(6)-EET inhibits sodium absorption and potassium secretion by the rabbit cortical collecting duct, and synthetic 5(6)-EET stimulates the release of LH and somatostatin by pituitary cells in culture. Interestingly, 8,9-EET and 14,15-EET stereospecifically inhibit human platelet cyclooxygenase. By contrast, all EET's studied inhibit platelet aggregation in vitro by a nonspecific mechanism independent of an effect on thromboxane formation. Finally, 5(6)-EET is metabolized to epoxides of PGG_1, PGH_1, and PGE_1 and to the 5S, 6S, and 5R, 6R isomers of 5-hydroxy-PGI_1. It remains to

be determined whether these compounds are formed in humans and, if so, whether they are of physiologic or pathologic importance in vivo.

PHARMACOLOGIC AND DIETARY REGULATION OF BIOSYNTHESIS

None of the oxygenated products of arachidonic acid is stored in significant quantities for subsequent release by cells. Release is equivalent to biosynthesis. Arachidonate release may occur by several mechanisms. Phosphatidylinositol (PI) may be hydrolyzed by a PI-specific phospholipase C (PLC), yielding diacylglycerol (DAG) and inositol phosphate. DAG is then further hydrolyzed, yielding free arachidonic acid and other fatty acids. Alternatively, phosphatidylcholine (PC) may be hydrolyzed by phospholipase $A_2(PLA_2)$, yielding arachidonic acid from the sn-2 position. Phospholipase A_2 may also liberate arachidonic acid from phosphatidylethanolamine.

CORTICOSTEROIDS. Corticosteroids appear to modify the production of prostaglandins, TxA_2, and leukotrienes by the induction of a phospholipase-inhibitory protein, variously named lipocortin, macrocortin, lipomodulin, and renomodulin (Fig. 223–2). It is hypothesized that initially steroids bind to specific cell surface receptors and that the complex is then transferred to the nucleus where steroids regulate the expression of genes and, subsequently, the synthesis of a PLA_2-inhibitory protein. The lipocortin family is now known to be derived from a monomeric 40 kD protein that contains two disulfide bridges, a glycosylation site, and two potential phosphorylation sites. Phosphorylation of this protein by protein kinases results in its activation as an inhibitor. Interestingly, there is a striking sequence homology between this protein and the 40 kD protein that is phosphorylated following the binding of epidermal growth factor to its receptor. Prevention of protein synthesis blocks the inhibitory effect of steroids on the release of radiolabeled arachidonate by neutrophils with the chemoattractant peptide f-Met-Leu-Phe. A cDNA has been isolated and cloned that encodes for a 40 kD protein that inhibits arachidonic acid release from prelabeled cells. At present there is little evidence that corticosteroid administration depresses formation of oxygenated metabolites of arachidonic acid in vivo or by cellular systems ex vivo in humans. However, the dependence of lipocortin induction on the presence of steroid receptors would imply that not all cells would be targets for this aspect of steroid activation. Further studies will be necessary to elucidate the contribution of this mechanism to the therapeutic efficacy of corticosteroids in man.

CYCLOOXYGENASE INHIBITORS. Nonsteroidal antiinflammatory drugs (NSAID's) prevent the formation of prostaglandins by inhibiting the enzyme cyclooxygenase. This group of drugs includes aspirin, salicylate, indomethacin, ibuprofen, piroxicam, fenoprofen, paracetamol, phenylbutazone, oxyphenbutazone, tolmetin, sulfinpyrazone, and sulindac. Paracetamol (acetaminophen) is a considerably less potent inhibitor than the other compounds, except perhaps in the brain. Aspirin is also unlike the other compounds in that it acetylates the active site of the cyclooxygenase and inhibits it irreversibly. This accounts for the unique effects of aspirin on the platelet. While other cells have the capacity for de novo protein synthesis, the anucleate platelet does not; thus inhibition of TxA_2 formation by aspirin persists for the lifetime of the platelet. By contrast, the effects of aspirin on eicosanoid formation by other cells (e.g., prostacyclin biosynthesis by vascular endothelium) may not be so prolonged. The irreversible actions of aspirin on platelet cyclooxygenase also account for the cumulative inhibition of platelet TxA_2 formation by the repeated administration of low dosages of aspirin (20 to 40 mg per day: A regular aspirin capsule contains 325 mg). This results in partial inhibition of platelet cyclooxygenase after single-dose administration. Even though low doses of aspirin tend to depress PGI_2 formation, its effect is more pronounced in platelet TxA_2 biosynthesis during long-term dosing. This relative "biochemical selectivity" for TXA_2 may result from partial recovery of PGI_2 formation, differential sensitivity of the platelet and vascular enzymes to aspirin inhibition, or pharmacokinetic properties of the drug. Aspirin is subject to extensive first-pass metabolism by the liver, and its deacylated product, salicylic acid, is a weak inhibitor of platelet cyclooxygenase. Lower doses of aspirin may approach the threshold for complete hepatic extraction. This would still permit cumulative inhibition of platelet cyclooxygenase in the presystemic circulation while protecting the cyclooxygenase in the systemic vasculature from aspirin exposure.

Tissue-selective inhibition of cyclooxygenase may also be possible with sulindac and sulfinpyrazone. These compounds are pro-drugs that are converted by the intestinal flora to their sulfide derivatives, which are potent cyclooxygenase inhibitors. Renal tissue possesses the capacity to retroconvert these sulfides to their inactive sulfones, and evidence suggests that renal prostaglandin synthesis may be spared by doses of these drugs that completely inhibit TXA_2 formation by platelets.

THROMBOXANE SYNTHASE INHIBITORS AND RECEPTOR ANTAGONISTS. Many imidazole and pyridine analogues selectively inhibit thromboxane synthase. These compounds depress TxA_2 formation without coincidental inhibition of PGI_2 synthesis, as seen with NSAID's. Indeed, following Tx synthase inhibition, accumulated platelet PGH_2 can be utilized by vascular PGI_2 synthase. Tx synthase inhibitors have been shown to increase the biosynthesis of platelet-inhibitory, vasodilator prostaglandins such as PGI_2 and PGE_2 at the platelet-vascular interface in man. Although limited clinical trials have failed to demonstrate benefit from these compounds, this may reflect incomplete suppression of TxA_2 biosynthesis throughout the dosing interval with these reversible inhibitors and/or substitution for the action of TxA_2 by accumulated PGH_2. In this regard, antagonists of the shared TxA_2-PGH_2 receptor are currrently under study in man. Synergy of these compounds with Tx synthase inhibitors has been demonstrated in animal models of thrombosis.

DIETARY SUBSTRATE MODIFICATION. Mortality from coronary heart disease seems to be lower in populations that consume large quantities of n-3 fatty acids, such as EPA, from aquatic mammals or fish. One hypothesis has been that a shift toward the formation of TxA_3 (which is biologically

inactive) and PGI_3 (which is a platelet-inhibitory, vasodilator compound like PGI_2) may favorably influence platelet-vessel wall interactions (Fig. 223–3). Although fish oil supplementation of the Western diet has only modest effects on platelet function, it has caused apparent regression of atherosclerosis in several animal models. The biologic properties of many icosanoids suggest their relevance to the evolving atherosclerotic lesion. It is possible that the altered biologic activity of their trienoic analogues, together with other properties of marine oils, such as their ability to influence plasma lipids and cell membrane fluidity, may facilitate plaque regression. Similarly, it has been hypothesized that marine oils might modulate inflammatory or immune diseases by altering the profile of lipoxygenase product formation.

LIPOXYGENASE INHIBITORS AND ANTAGONISTS. Specific inhibitors of the 5-lipoxygenase pathway have yet to be studied extensively in humans. In addition, while initial experiments have been performed with sulfidopeptide leukotriene antagonists, the available compounds possess additional pharmacologic properties, such as phosphodiesterase inhibition. No pharmacologic inhibitors of epoxygenase product formation are currently available for use in humans. The availability of such pharmacologic probes will facilitate the elucidation of the functional role of lipoxygenase and epoxygenase products of arachidonic acid in human disease.

FUNCTIONS OF ARACHIDONIC ACID METABOLITES IN VIVO

The evidence implicating arachidonate metabolites in mechanisms of some human diseases include measurements of their biosynthesis and the effects of drugs that prevent their formation or antagonize their actions. Because of the evanescence of the primary compounds, estimates of in vivo synthesis have largely been based upon measurement of long-lived, but biologically inactive, metabolites. The capacity of tissues to generate arachidonic acid metabolites greatly exceeds the actual production rates in vivo. Thus, artifacts related to sample collection—for example, platelet activation ex vivo during blood sampling or catheter-induced vascular trauma—can seriously confound attempts to measure these compounds in the bloodstream. For this reason, measurement of metabolite excretion in urine has been favored as a noninvasive, albeit indirect, approach.

THE CARDIOVASCULAR SYSTEM. TxA_2 is one of many platelet agonists generated in vivo. While aspirin inhibits Tx-dependent aggregation, other agonists, such as thrombin and high doses of collagen, can induce aggregation in vitro despite the presence of aspirin. In view of these properties it is perhaps surprising that aspirin has been shown to influence outcome in a variety of clinical trials in cardiovascular disease, presumably because of its effects on TxA_2 formation.

Aspirin has been shown to reduce significantly the incidence of stroke in patients suffering transient ischemic attacks, the incidence of thrombotic occlusion following coronary artery bypass graft implantation, and the incidence of myocardial infarction and death in patients with unstable coronary disease. Pooled analysis of clinical trials designed to study the effects of aspirin in the secondary prevention of myocardial infarction suggests that the risk of a second infarct is reduced by about 20 per cent in aspirin-treated patients. However, aspirin significantly influenced a predetermined endpoint (nonfatal myocardial infarction and death) within only one of the seven clinical trials designed to address this question. The more clearcut results in unstable angina may reflect the earlier initiation of aspirin therapy and the more prominent role of thrombosis in determining outcome in these patients. Angioscopic and angiographic evidence of thrombosis is present in unstable angina, and phasic increases of TxA_2 formation coincide with episodes of cardiac ischemia. By contrast, the alteration in TxA_2 formation after myocardial infarction is transient, and there is no evidence for platelet activation in patients with chronic stable angina. Thus, after myocardial infarction, patients represent a more "dilute" population potentially susceptible to benefit from antiplatelet therapy. Although aspirin has been used in combination with dipyridamole in many of these studies, there is little evidence that this drug contributes to the antithrombotic efficacy of aspirin in humans.

The lowest dose of aspirin shown to be effective as an antithrombotic agent in a large-scale clinical trial has been 324 mg in unstable angina. Because of cumulative inhibition of platelet cyclooxygenase it is likely that long-term administration of lower doses would inhibit TxA_2 formation to a comparable degree. Indeed, such regimens may eventually be shown to be preferable, because of reduction of dose-related side effects and preservation of the capacity to augment PGI_2 biosynthesis.

The use of PGI_2 itself as a platelet inhibitory drug has been restricted by the need to administer it as an infusion and the steep dose-response relationship. Doses that inhibit platelet function are close to those that cause side effects such as gastric cramping and hypotension. Nonetheless, its potential efficacy as a platelet inhibitor is illustrated by its marked effects on platelet adhesion and aggregation in extracorporeal circuits such as pump oxygenators and hemodialysis units, a setting in which aspirin is markedly less effective. Infusion of PGE_1, a synthetic PGE_2 analogue, which is an inhibitor of platelet function, may reduce the incidence of reocclusion following coronary angioplasty. Potential refinements of this approach will include the development of stable, orally administered PGI_2 analogues, the development of PGI_2 receptor agonists, and the use of long-lived Tx synthase inhibitors in combination with receptor antagonists to counteract the effects of accumulated PGH_2.

THE RESPIRATORY SYSTEM. While many of the oxygenated metabolites of arachidonic acid have biologic actions on respiratory tissue, their contribution to the asthmatic response to inhaled antigens in humans is currently unknown. A minority of asthmatics, perhaps 10 per cent, exhibit bronchoconstrictive hypersensitivity reactions to aspirin. This appears to reflect a role for prostaglandins, TxA_2, or leukotrienes, as these attacks are provoked by a range of structurally distinct inhibitors of cyclooxygenase but rarely by salicylate, which resembles aspirin but is a weak inhibitor of that enzyme. No evidence presently supports an allergic basis for this condition. Drug-induced reactions in such patients may be quite severe and often feature profuse rhinorrhea and flushing, in addition to bronchospasm. Whether such attacks are mediated by differential inhibition of bronchoconstrictor versus bronchodilator prostaglandins, by a shunting of the arachidonate substrate toward lipoxygenation and the formation of bronchoconstrictor leukotrienes, or by reduced formation of a prostaglandin that normally inhibits release of other mediators of bronchoconstriction is unknown.

Aspirin may also trigger a hypersensitivity response in which alterations in blood pressure, flushing, tachycardia, and diarrhea predominate over bronchospasm. Some of these patients have systemic mastocytosis.

THE GASTROINTESTINAL SYSTEM. Both PGI_2 and PGE_2 are cytoprotective of gastric mucosa in vitro and are thought to contribute to the regulation of mucosal blood flow. The dose-related gastrointestinal side effects of NSAID's are thought to reflect increased susceptibility to local injury (e.g., H^+ back diffusion) due to inhibition of these prostaglandins. Oral dimethyl PGE analogues have been used in the treatment of peptic ulcers. The watery diarrhea associated with multiple endocrine neoplasia often responds to treatment with prostaglandin inhibitors. Excessive formation of LTB_4 has been demonstrated in colonic mucosa and rectal dialysates obtained from patients with inflammatory bowel disease. Whether this mediator contributes to symptomatology is unknown.

RENIN RELEASE AND RENAL FUNCTION. While sympathoadrenal activity is the principal regulator of renin re-

lease, it appears to be via a cyclooxygenase metabolite of arachidonic acid. PGI_2 is the most potent of the prostaglandins as a renin secretagogue. 6-Keto-PGE_1, a putative metabolite of PGI_2, shares this biologic property. Inhibition of cyclooxygenase by NSAID's has implications for the diagnostic application of renin measurements. The associated reduction in aldosterone production may be deleterious for patients with hyperkalemia.

Metabolites of arachidonic acid contribute little to the regulation of renal blood flow under physiologic circumstances. Under conditions of increased vasoconstrictor tone, however, preservation of renal blood flow becomes increasingly dependent upon the generation of vasodilator prostaglandins. This is particularly so in patients with chronic glomerulonephritis, Bartter's syndrome, the nephropathy of systemic lupus erythematosus, congestive heart failure, or combined hepatic and renal dysfunction. It has been proposed that the decline in renal function in such patients following administration of NSAID's is less likely to occur with sulindac as a result of retroconversion of the sulfide to the sulfone.

The kidney possesses the capacity to generate TxA_2, in addition to vasodilator prostaglandins. Renal biosynthesis of TxA_2 is increased in some patients with severe nephropathy in association with systemic lupus erythematosus, and infusion of a PGH_2-TxA_2 receptor antagonist improves indices of renal function in such patients. Increased TxA_2 biosynthesis by the kidney has been demonstrated in animal models in response to ureteric obstruction, renal vein thrombosis, development of hypertension following partial renal ablation and coincident with the development of cyclosporine-induced nephrotoxicity. Increased Tx formation during renal allograft rejection has been reported in humans; however, it is unknown whether this is an epiphenomenon or of primary importance in the rejection process.

In addition to its potential significance as a vasodilator, PGE_2 is the major product formed from arachidonic acid in the renal medulla, where it appears to inhibit sodium reabsorption in the distal tubule. The consequent sodium retention caused by administration of a cyclooxygenase inhibitor persists only for a day or two, after which sodium balance is reversed despite continued treatment. Prostaglandins may also influence free water clearance. Indomethacin will diminish the excessive water elimination in nephrogenic and lithium-induced diabetes insipidus.

THE REPRODUCTIVE SYSTEM. Both PGE_2 and $PGF_{2\alpha}$ are potent stimulants of myometrial contraction. Both they and their methylated analogue have been utilized as abortifacients and in the induction of labor, usually as an adjunct to low amniotomy. Cyclooxygenase inhibitors are currently being evaluated in the treatment of premature labor. A potential hazard of this approach has been premature closure of the ductus arteriosus. Indeed, closure of a persistent ductus arteriosus can be achieved with indomethacin in the neonatal period. This implies that a cyclooxygenase metabolite contributes to ductal patency. Infusion of PGE_1 has been used to maintain an open ductus in infants with pulmonary atresia until corrective surgery is performed.

Biosynthesis of the prostaglandins increases during pregnancy, particularly during labor. In the case of PGI_2, biosynthesis is increased markedly from as early as the first trimester. Interestingly, this increment is less pronounced in patients with pregnancy-induced hypertension (PIH). Indeed, diminished PGI_2 biosynthesis is apparent prior to the rise in blood pressure. Studies of TxA_2 biosynthesis indicate that platelet activation is present in normal pregnancy and may be enhanced in the presence of PIH. Administration of aspirin to patients at risk may both reduce the incidence of PIH and limit its fetal sequelae.

FEVER AND INFLAMMATION. Cyclooxygenase inhibitors share antipyretic, analgesic, and anti-inflammatory actions. Paracetamol differs from the other compounds in being an efficient antipyretic despite weak anti-inflammatory properties in the periphery. The prostaglandins that mediate fever are unknown. Vasodilator prostaglandins seem to act in concert with other mediators to augment the inflammatory response. Among these may be the leukotrienes, which enhance capillary permeability and function as chemoattractants and leukocyte activators. These properties suggest that combined cyclooxygenase inhibitors may be more effective anti-inflammatory agents than aspirin-like drugs. Clearly, inhibition of products from both pathways may account for the anti-inflammatory action of corticosteroids, although this remains to be definitively established.

FitzGerald GA, Pedersen AK, Patrono C: Analysis of prostacyclin and thromboxane A₂ in cardiovascular disease. Circulation 67:1174, 1983. *A review of the various approaches to estimating the biosynthesis of metabolites of arachidonic acid in man.*

Lewis RA, Austen KF: The biologically active leukotrienes: Biosynthesis, metabolism, receptors, functions and pharmacology. J Clin Invest 73:889, 1984. *A review that concentrates on the pharmacology of these compounds.*

Needleman P, Turk J, Jakshik BA, et al.: Arachidonic acid metabolism. Ann Rev Biochem 55:69, 1986. *A comprehensive review with emphasis on the epoxygenases.*

Prostaglandins, thromboxane A₂ and the leukotrienes. Br Med Bull 39(3):1, 1983. *This issue provides a comprehensive overview of the biologic actions of these compounds.*

Reilly IAG, FitzGerald GA: Aspirin in cardiovascular disease. Drugs (in press). *A review of the pharmacology of aspirin and the clinical trials that underlie its use in cardiovascular disease.*

Samuelsson B: Leukotrienes: Mediators of immediate hypersensitivity and inflammation. Science 220:568, 1983. *A review that concentrates on the biosynthesis and metabolism of these compounds and their role in inflammation.*

Schlondorff D: Renal prostaglandin synthesis: Sites of production and specific actions of prostaglandins. Am J Med 81(2B):1, 1986. *A review of eicosanoid formation within the kidney.*

Serhan CN, Hamberg M, Samuelsson B: Lipoxins: A novel series of biologically active compounds. In Bailey JM (ed.): Prostaglandins, Leukotrienes and Lipoxins. New York, Plenum Press, 1985, pp 3–16. *An account of the discovery of these compounds.*

Vane JR: The road to prostacyclin. Adv Prostaglandin Thromboxane Leukotriene Res 15:11, 1985. *An account of the discovery and pharmacology of this prostaglandin.*

224 NATRIURETIC FACTORS

Philip Needleman

Two intrinsic natriuretic substances capable of modifying sodium homeostasis have been described. The cardiac (atrial) derived peptide has been isolated, the structure elucidated, and the peptide synthesized. The availability of appropriate molecular probes, antisera, and chemically synthesized material has permitted a rapid analysis of the biosynthesis, storage, release, response, and potential for therapeutics. Much of this chapter will focus on the properties of the atrial peptides.

A second natriuretic (ouabain-like) factor has not yet had its structure elucidated. As a result, the physiology, pathophysiology, and potential for pharmacologic manipulation of this hormonal factor are still unclear. The evidence in support of the existence and the actions of the endogenous ouabain-like factor remains circumstantial and at the level of biologic activities of extracts of biologic fluids and tissues.

NATRIURETIC HORMONE. Expansion of the extracellular fluid volume leads to (1) enhanced urinary sodium excretion, which is independent of changes in glomerular filtration rate, aldosterone, or vasopressin, and (2) the appearance of a factor that increases sodium excretion when extracted from urine or plasma and then injected into assay animals. It is therefore referred to as "natriuretic hormone." It was initially noted that cross-circulation of blood from a volume-expanded donor animal causes recipient natriuresis, and that extracts of urine or plasma from volume-expanded subjects produces a natriuresis in assay rats. The natriuretic hormone(s) is believed to act as a ouabain-like inhibitor of Na-K-ATPase (the enzymatic expression of the Na-K pump), which in the kidney results in natriuresis and increases vascular resistance. Inhibition of vascular smooth muscle Na-K-ATPase increases intracellular sodium, which is believed to result in elevated intracellular calcium by reversal of a membrane Na-Ca exchange mechanism. Such ionic events would be expected to enhance the sensitivity to such intrinsic vasoconstrictors as norepinephrine, angiotensin, and vasopressin.

An endogenous Na-K-ATPase inhibitor has been hypothesized to contribute to the pathogenesis of hypertension; its presence has been demonstrated in some patients with essential hypertension. One theory suggests that suppressed sodium excretion in essential hypertensives causes an elevation in circulating ouabain-like factor which increases peripheral resistance. An alternate theory suggests that the natriuretic hormone inhibits neural Na-K-ATPase, which suppresses the ouabain-sensitive catecholamine reuptake system, thereby enhancing vascular smooth muscle tone by exaggerating regional adrenergic transmitter levels.

Plasma or urine extracts from volume-expanded dogs, patients with chronic renal failure, pregnant women, patients on a high-salt diet, and hypertensive patients and animals have been demonstrated (a) to inhibit sodium transport in frog skin, toad urinary bladder, and rabbit renal collecting tubule segments (suggesting inhibition of distal sodium transport) and in red and white blood cells; (b) to displace labelled ouabain from its receptor sites; (c) to cross-react with antidigoxin antibodies; and (d) to stimulate glucose-6-phosphate dehydrogenase activity in intact cells. The source of the material is unclear, but the hypothalamus, possibly localized or influenced by the anteroventral third ventricle (AV3V) area, has been implicated. The chemical nature of the material is unresolved. Some believe the factor to be a low molecular substance, but there is no agreement as to whether it is a lipid, a peptide, or some other chemical entity. It is important at this point to determine the similarity of material derived from such sources as brain, plasma, urine, and amniotic fluid, since different assays and reagents are being employed in the analyses. A comparison of various materials in the same assays and based on careful, complete concentration dependency curves, duration, and reversibility would allow establishment of the parallelism and relative quantities of the natriuretic hormone. Such studies would resolve whether a single or multiple factors exist.

At this point it is not possible to determine the interrelationship between the atrial peptides (described below) and the "natriuretic hormone." Clearly, the substances are quite different. The atrial peptides do not inhibit Na-K-ATPase, compete in [³H]-ouabain radioreceptor assays, or cross-react with digoxin antisera. The natriuretic hormone constricts blood vessels, whereas the atrial peptides are vasorelaxants. The two factors may be released into the circulation by similar stimuli, and one system may modulate the other.

ATRIOPEPTIN: A CARDIAC-DERIVED NATRIURETIC HORMONE

OVERVIEW. The discovery of this cardiac hormone had its origin in a number of earlier physiologic, clinical, and morphologic observations. Stimulation of the atria by distention causes diuresis, bradycardia, hypotension, and decreased vascular resistance. Increased plasma volume has been proposed to stimulate the atria to release a substance into the circulation that stimulates target organs to reduce the plasma volume.

Recently, a peptide hormone has been characterized which we termed atriopeptin based on its origin and its multiple effects distinct from causing natriuresis. It is intimately involved in the regulation of renal and cardiovascular homeostasis. Granules present in atrial (but not in ventricular) cardiocytes alter their density with dietary changes in sodium

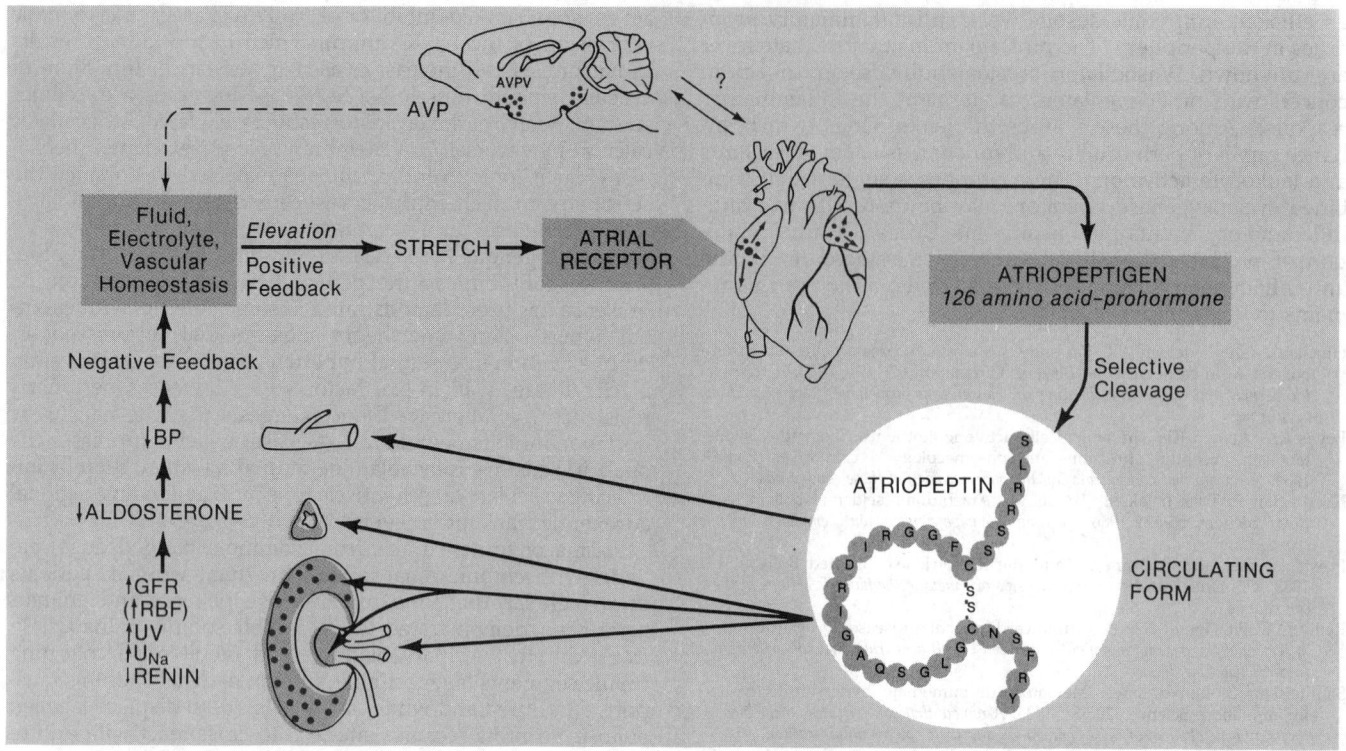

FIGURE 224–1. Schematic diagram of the atriopeptin hormonal system. The 126 amino acid–prohormone, atriopeptigen, is stored in granules in perinuclear atrial cardiocytes. Elevated vascular volume results in the release of atriopeptin, which acts on the kidney (glomeruli and papilla) to increase the glomerular filtration rate (GFR), renal blood flow (RBF), urine volume (UV), and sodium excretion (U_{Na}) and to decrease plasma renin activity. Natriuresis and diuresis are also facilitated by the suppression of aldosterone and the release of arginine vasopressin (AVP). Diminution of vascular volume provides a negative feedback that suppresses circulating levels of atriopeptin. (From Needleman P, Greenwald JE: Atriopeptin: A cardiac hormone intimately involved in fluid, electrolyte, and blood-pressure homeostasis. N Engl J Med 314:828, 1986, with permission.)

and water, suggesting that the atria may be involved in the physiology of electrolyte and fluid balance. Extracts from rat atria produce a profound natriuresis and diuresis in recipient rats and relax isolated strips of blood vessel. Purification of atrial extracts has identified a number of small peptides (21 amino acids and longer) that have natriuretic, diuretic, and vasodilator activities. The various peptides, which arise from a single 126-residue prohormone, all contain the same core sequence of 17 amino acids within a cystine disulfide bridge (Fig. 224–1), but the lengths of their N-termini differ. A carboxy-terminal, phe-arg on the atrial peptide, appears to be essential for full biologic activity as a natriuretic-diuretic, spasmolytic agent.

Figure 224–1 schematically shows how atriopeptin links the heart, kidneys, adrenals, blood vessels, and brain in a hormonal system involved in volume and pressure homeostasis. The human atrial gene codes for a preprohormone with 152 amino acids. Loss of a hydrophobic leader sequence generates the 126-amino acid prohormone, the storage form of the atrial peptide in granules of the atrial myocytes. Release of peptides with natriuretic-diuretic and vasodilator properties from isolated perfused hearts can be demonstrated by bioassay and radioimmunoassay. Increases in the plasma level of atriopeptin in experimental animals can be elicited by atrial stretch caused by volume expansion, vasoconstrictor agents that elevate atrial pressure, immersion in water, atrial tachycardia, and high-salt diets. Although the peptide is stored as the high molecular weight prohormone, the primary form in the plasma is the low molecular weight carboxy-terminal fragment atriopeptin-28. Thus, a very selective enzymatic cleavage of the prohormone occurs during the release process.

Once in the circulation, the peptide exerts a number of effects (which often are associated with increased cellular

levels of cyclic guanosine monophosphate) through specific receptors, to produce a multiplicity of actions involved in renal and cardiovascular functions. The combined effects that alter salt and water metabolism arise from direct renal effects: pronounced natriuresis and diuresis, inhibition of aldosterone secretion by the cells in the adrenal zona glomerulosa, suppression of vasopressin release, and inhibition of the angiotensin-induced drinking response.

Atriopeptin affects blood pressure by suppressing elevated plasma levels of renin and relaxing blood vessels directly, thereby reducing vascular resistance. Atriopeptin is somewhat selective as a renal vasodilator; it decreases renal resistance at doses that do not influence coronary, iliac, or mesentery blood flow. Atrial peptides dilate vessels, especially when vascular tone is elevated.

Atriopeptin-immunoreactive neurons have been observed in brains from rats, especially in the hypothalamus in the anteroventral periventricular nucleus (AV3V), adjacent to the anterior tip of the third ventricle. This hypothalamic region of the brain has extensive connections with structures that are important in cardiovascular regulatory functions. Animals with lesions that include the anteroventral periventricular nucleus show profound alterations in the regulation of fluid balance, and neither renal hypertension nor salt-induced hypertension develops. Thus, atriopeptin may serve as both a central neuromodulator and a peripheral hormone in the regulation of cardiovascular and renal function.

A CARDIAC ENDOCRINE SYSTEM. Proof that atrial peptides function as an endocrine system that regulates fluid and electrolyte homeostasis requires demonstration and validation of the release of atriopeptin from the heart into the circulation. Atriopeptin immunoreactivity has been detected in rat plasma. Rats on a high-salt diet have plasma atriopeptin immunoreactivity that is twice that of control rats, a finding consistent with the hypothesis that an increase in vascular volume stimulates an increase in the release of atriopeptin from the heart. Such an increase is needed to meet the greater fluid challenge. In addition, the changes in right atrial pressure that are produced by volume expansion have been found to cause increases in atriopeptin immunoreactivity in the plasma. Right atrial appendectomy markedly attenuates the natriuresis and diuresis produced by acute volume expansion without altering the renal response to exogenous atriopeptin or furosemide. Pharmacologic doses of vasopressin can produce a profound and sustained release of atriopeptin immunoreactivity into the circulation of anesthetized rats. We have also observed a direct correlation between increased right atrial pressure and increased plasma atriopeptin levels in anesthetized rats immersed to their heads in water. When plasma from vasopressin-stimulated rats was purified by high-performance liquid chromatography, two distinct peaks (in a ratio of 10:1) were resolved, and these peaks migrated with the standards of atriopeptin-28 and atriopeptin-24, respectively. The presence of these structures was confirmed by demonstrating their biologic activity as vasorelaxants on pre-contracted rabbit aorta strips and by gas-phase sequence analysis. The direct demonstration of the peptide in the circulation supports the proposal that atriopeptin is a hormonal participant in the regulation of fluid and electrolyte balance.

EFFECTS ON RENAL FUNCTION. Infusion of AP into experimental animals produces a dramatic increase in salt and water excretion. The renal mechanisms whereby AP induces natriuresis and diuresis are unclear. High-affinity receptor sites for AP are present on the glomeruli and in the papilla. Such novel and unique sites of action might indicate that AP could act when conventional diuretics, which act through tubular sites, are ineffective. Glomerular filtration rate and filtration fraction are elevated during peptide infusion. These effects diminish abruptly when the peptide infusion is terminated. Micropuncture studies suggest that the increase in filtration caused by AP results from a rise in glomerular capillary hydraulic pressure, which appears to arise from afferent arteriolar vasodilation and efferent arteriolar vasoconstriction. However, the threefold increase in sodium delivery to the last accessible portion of the distal tubule cannot account for the 10- to 50-fold increase in urinary solute excretion produced by the peptide. Thus, the AP-induced salt and water loss would not appear to be entirely due to increased glomerular ultrafiltration. Transport of sodium and chloride by isolated renal epithelial cells or in discrete perfused rabbit nephron segments was unaffected by AP. A clue to the possible mchanism is the finding that AP infusion produced a urinary sodium concentration that exceeds plasma levels. A likely source for the high urinary sodium concentration is the hypernatriuretic renal papillary interstitium. Specific AP receptors have been localized on medullary collecting duct cells, and AP has been found to increase cyclic GMP and to inhibit Na$^+$ entry-dependent oxygen consumption.

HUMAN PHYSIOLOGY AND PATHOPHYSIOLOGY. In normal volunteers, the basal plasma levels of atriopeptin range from 10 to 70 pg per milliliter. Posturally induced elevations in venous return and right atrial pressure increase plasma levels of atriopeptin. Normal subjects undergoing a three-hour head-out water immersion exhibited a prompt and marked increase in plasma AP and a concurrent marked diuresis and suppressed plasma renin and aldosterone. Certain pathophysiologic states induced by specific organ dysfunction cause a central hypervolemia and an increase in atriopeptin levels. In children with volume overload secondary to end-stage renal disease, predialysis plasma levels of atriopeptin were double the postdialysis levels, whereas normovolemic children with end-stage renal disease did not have significantly elevated levels of the peptide. Similarly, plasma atriopeptin was elevated in adults with chronic renal failure

but not in patients with cirrhosis of the liver with or without ascites. Plasma atriopeptin levels were also increased in patients with congestive heart failure in direct correlation with cardiac filling pressure; furthermore, plasma AP levels fell toward normal with successful diuretic therapy. The paradox of high circulating plasma AP and fluid retention in congestive failure may suggest a renal insensitivity, perhaps due to down-regulation of AP receptors. Atrial arrhythmias produce elevations in right atrial pressure, and they are frequently associated with polyuria. Patients with either paroxysmal atrial tachycardia or atrial tachycardia produced by atrial pacing were found to have increased levels of plasma atriopeptin. The atriopeptin levels decreased significantly when the tachycardia was terminated.

In early clinical studies, intravenous infusion of atriopeptin in normal subjects has been shown to markedly increase urinary volume and the excretion of sodium, chloride, calcium, magnesium, and phosphate but not potassium. Glomerular filtration rate increases only transiently, but the filtration fraction rises markedly. Atriopeptin-induced natriuresis would be expected to spare potassium excretion because it inhibits aldosterone synthesis. Intravenous administration of human atriopeptin to normal or hypertensive persons causes a moderate but transient and dose-dependent decrease in arterial blood pressure with an increased heart rate and a transient increase in skin blood flow.

THERAPEUTIC POTENTIAL. Atriopeptin may have a unique role as a therapeutic agent, especially in critical care situations in patients who are undergoing parenteral therapy.

With its glomerular action, the peptide may be useful in maintaining diuresis in cases in which conventional diuretics lose effectiveness, such as in patients with ischemic renal injury. A major problem in aggressively treating severe volume overload with conventional methods is the marked urinary potassium loss. Parenteral administration of atriopeptin can produce an impressive loss of sodium and water without inducing a significant kaliuresis.

A potent natriuretic and diuretic agent that is a somewhat selective renal vasodilator would have therapeutic potential in pathophysiologic states involving fluid and electrolyte imbalances. Some obvious clinical targets for atriopeptin therapy might include acute or chronic renal failure. Parenteral administration of a peptide would be practical in such critical care situations. Furthermore, endogenous AP appears to be directly involved in the adaptive increase in sodium excretion in chronic renal failure. A possible use of atriopeptin is illustrated by experiments in rats with a surgical model of chronic renal failure (i.e., a five-sixths nephrectomy and salt water ingestion). Infusion of very low concentrations of atriopeptin into these severely azotemic rats markedly increased urine volume and sodium excretion (there was a 12-fold increase in the fractional excretion of sodium) and lowered mean arterial blood pressure at doses that produced little response in control rats. Even though the rats with a reduced renal mass had an elevated single-nephron glomerular filtration rate, the atriopeptin infusion produced a further increase in their total glomerular filtration rate. The exaggerated sensitivity in the salt-loaded uremic rats may reflect the additive response of the elevated endogenous peptide levels and the infused exogenous AP. If comparable results can be achieved in patients, atriopeptin might provide a useful approach to the treatment of volume overload and salt retention in those with chronic renal failure. The discovery and characterization of atriopeptin provides a unique opportunity for the development of new pharmacologic agents for the therapeutic manipulation of circulatory, volume, and electrolyte homeostasis.

Ballerman BJ, Brenner BM: Role of atrial peptides in body fluid homeostasis. Circ Res 58:619, 1986. *Comprehensive review of the renal properties of atriopeptin.*
Buckalew VM Jr, Gruber KA: Natriuretic hormone. Ann Rev Physiol 46:343, 1984. *Comprehensive review of the ouabain-like factor.*

Cole BR, Kuhnline MA, Needleman P: Atriopeptin III: A potent natriuretic, diuretic and hypotensive agent in rats with chronic renal failure. J Clin Invest 76:2413, 1985. *Animals in chronic renal failure are exquisitely sensitive to the effects of atriopeptin.*

de Bold AJ, Borenstein HB, Vereso AT, et al.: A rapid and potent natriuretic response to intravenous injection of atrial myocardial extract in rats. Life Sci 28:89, 1981. *This seminal paper first demonstrated that crude atrial extracts contained a potent natriuretic-diuretic substance.*

DeWardener HE, Clarkson EM: Concept of natriuretic hormone. Physiol Rev 65:658, 1985. *Comprehensive review of the ouabain-like factor.*

Needleman P, Adams SP, Cole BR, et al.: Atriopeptins as cardiac hormones. Hypertension 7:469, 1985. *Review of the discovery and characterization of atriopeptin.*

Needleman P, Greenwald JE: Atriopeptin: A cardiac hormone intimately involved in fluid, electrolyte, and blood pressure homeostasis. N Engl J Med 314:828, 1986. *Review of the biochemistry, pharmacology, and therapeutics of atriopeptin.*

Smith S, Anderson S, Ballerman BJ, et al.: Role of atrial natriuretic peptide in the adaptation of sodium excretion with reduced renal mass. J Clin Invest 77:1395, 1986. *Exhibits the effectiveness of atriopeptin in rats with chronic renal failure.*

225 NEUROENDOCRINE REGULATION AND ITS DISORDERS

Lawrence A. Frohman

NEUROENDOCRINE REGULATION

The central nervous system exerts profound regulatory control over hormonal secretion and metabolic processes. The integration of this control is focused in the region of the ventral hypothalamus and consists of three major systems:

1. A classic neuronal pathway traveling through the base of the brain, through the autonomic nervous system pathways of the spinal cord, and terminating in the liver, gastrointestinal tract, pancreas, adrenal medullae, and adipose tissue. The pathway, which consists of bidirectional fibers, is involved in neurometabolic regulation, and its greatest effects are on blood glucose and fatty acid regulation and on metabolic homeostasis, i.e., appetite control (satiety), temperature control (thermoregulation), and body fat stores (nutrient regulation).

2. A neurosecretory pathway from the anterior hypothalamus that traverses the floor of the ventral hypothalamus and pituitary stalk and terminates in specialized neuronal elements called pituicytes, located in the posterior pituitary. The system is involved in osmoregulation, through the production of vasopressin, and in parturition and nursing, through the secretion of oxytocin. A detailed discussion of this system is provided in Ch. 227.

3. A neuroendocrine system involving clusters of peptide- and monoamine-secreting cells in the anterior and mid-portion of the ventral hypothalamus whose products are transported along nerve fibers to terminals in the outer layer of the median eminence, from where they are released into the capillary vessels of the hypothalamic-hypophyseal portal system and transported to the pituitary to regulate the secretion of the hormones of the anterior pituitary.

Neuroendocrine Anatomy

The *neurometabolic function* of the hypothalamus can be divided into those components associated with the sympathetic or the parasympathetic branches of the autonomic nervous system. Medial sympathetic and lateral parasympathetic zones of the hypothalamus have been defined, but the cellular elements (neuronal perikarya) involved in a particular function cannot be precisely localized to one specific nuclear region. Neurons involved in the inhibitory control of food

intake (satiety) are located more medially, and those responsible for appetite stimulation are located more laterally. This distinction probably explains why destructive lesions of the hypothalamus, which frequently occur in the midline, are more likely to result in obesity than in starvation. A second reason is that fibers from the hypothalamic controlling centers cross the midline, and thus bilateral hypothalamic destruction is necessary for interruption of normal regulatory control.

Neurons of the *neurohypophyseal system* represent a more anatomically distinct entity with cell bodies located in the paraventricular and supraoptic hypothalamic nuclei. Within these areas there are also neurons producing a variety of other neuropeptides. The posterior pituitary hormones, oxytocin and vasopressin, are synthesized in the cell bodies as part of a precursor molecule, which also contains specific carrier proteins (neurophysins), and transported along axonal fibers through the ventral hypothalamus and pituitary stalk, during which time the hormones are cleaved from the precursor. In the pituicytes of the posterior pituitary they are packaged into storage granules to be released in response to stimulation (e.g., osmotic, barometric) of receptors on the cell bodies in the hypothalamus. The posterior pituitary is therefore functionally an integral part of the brain.

The cell bodies of the neuroendocrine system are diffusely distributed throughout the mediobasal hypothalamus in an area known as the hypophysiotropic region. Although the releasing hormone–secreting neurons receive input from other brain regions in response to changes in the external environment, they continue to function even in the absence of extrahypothalamic input, indicating that their most important homeostatic stimuli are blood borne. Cells secreting thyrotropin releasing hormone (TRH) and somatotropin release inhibiting factor (SRIF) that regulate pituitary function are located in the anterior hypothalamus, while those secreting growth hormone releasing hormone (GRH) are concentrated in the region of the arcuate and ventromedial nuclei. Cells secreting gonadotropin releasing hormone (GnRH) are more widely distributed, with cell bodies in both the anterior hypothalamus and the arcuate nuclei. Cell bodies of corticotropin releasing factor (CRF) neurons terminating in the median eminence are located predominantly in the paraventricular nucleus. A prolactin inhibiting factor (PIF) exhibits a distribution identical to that of GnRH.

The releasing and inhibiting hormones are stored in nerve terminals in the median eminence where their concentrations are 10 to 100 times as great as elsewhere in the hypothalamus. Since the portal blood flow to the pituitary is not compartmentalized, i.e., various cells types in the pituitary are distributed throughout the gland, releasing and inhibiting factors secreted into the portal system have access to all cell types of the anterior pituitary. Specificity of action is achieved not by anatomic segregation but by the presence of specific receptors on individual pituitary cell types.

The cells of both the neuroendocrine and neurohypophyseal systems have been called transducer cells, containing both neuronal and endocrine characteristics. They respond to classic neurotransmitter-mediated signals, yet they respond by releasing peptide hormones into a regional or systemic circulation.

PORTAL VASCULAR SYSTEM. The vascular supply of the anterior pituitary is unique in that there are no direct connections with the arterial system. All of the arterial blood flows through the hypothalamic arteries and forms a capillary plexus within the outer layer of the median eminence in juxtaposition to nerve terminals of the hypophysiotropic neurons. In contrast to most other brain regions, the blood-brain barrier in the area of the median eminence is incomplete, permitting protein and peptide hormones as well as other charged particles access to the intercapillary spaces and the nerve terminals contained therein. These terminals (and/or their perikarya) respond to changes in concentrations of

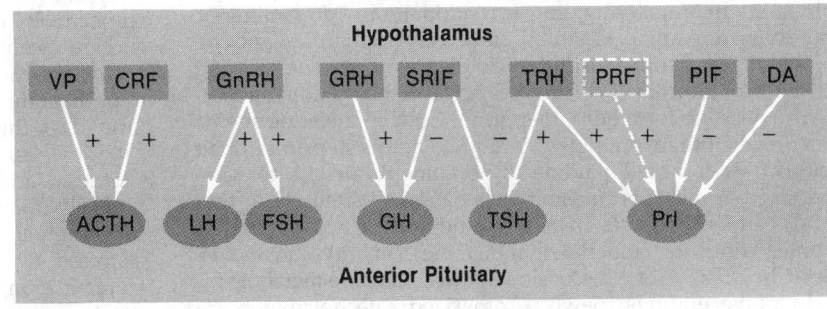

FIGURE 225–1. Interrelationships between hypothalamic and pituitary hormones. Solid lines denote hormones, the structures of which have been determined. Interrupted line indicates factors, the identity of which is still unknown.

circulating hormones and metabolic signals as well as to classic neuronal stimuli by secreting releasing and inhibiting factors into the portal system.

The portal capillaries coalesce into a series of veins that descend through the pituitary stalk and form a second capillary plexus that bathes the cells of the anterior pituitary. Venous drainage from the anterior pituitary passes through the posterior pituitary and from there into systemic veins.

Releasing and Inhibiting Hormones

The hypothalamic hormones that control the secretion of anterior pituitary hormones and their effects on pituitary hormone secretion are shown in Figure 225–1. Several different patterns of control exist: (1) a single hypothalamic hormone stimulating release of a single pituitary hormone (CRF: ACTH), (2) a single hypothalamic hormone stimulating release of several pituitary hormones (GnRH: luteinizing hormone [LH] and follicle-stimulating hormone [FSH], TRH: thyroid-stimulating hormone [TSH] and prolactin), and (3) several hypothalamic hormones affecting a single pituitary hormone (GRH and SRIF: growth hormone [GH]).

With one exception, the predominant influence of the hypothalamic hormones of the pituitary is stimulatory. Interference with the integrity of the hypothalamic-pituitary connection results in decreased secretion of pituitary hormones. The exception is prolactin, the secretion of which is increased when hypothalamic influence is removed.

All of the recognized hypothalamic hormones whose structures have been determined are, again with one exception, peptides with sequence length ranging from 3 to 44 amino acids. As the complexity of the structures increases, both multiple forms of the peptide (see section on somatostatin and GRH) and marked species variation in sequence occur. Whereas the structures of TRH, GnRH, and SRIF are identical in all mammalian species studied to date, and for TRH in amphibia as well, those of GRH and CRF exhibit marked species specificity. The structure of human CRF is identical to that of rat CRF. The existence of a separate PRF is still controversial, though a candidate for this title is vasoactive intestinal polypeptide (VIP). The one nonpeptide hypophysiotrophic hormone is dopamine. In addition to its major role as a neurotransmitter, dopamine is the most important physiologic inhibitor of prolactin. A 56-amino acid prolactin-inhibiting peptide has been identified as a carboxy-terminal extension on the GnRH precursor. The physiologic role of this GnRH-associated peptide (GAP) awaits further study.

ROLE OF BIOGENIC AMINES AND NEUROPEPTIDES IN THE REGULATION OF HYPOTHALAMIC HORMONE SECRETION. The major neurotransmitter systems utilized for intercellular communication within the central nervous system consist of monoamines and peptides. Neurotransmitters can influence the hypothalamic hormone–secreting neurons at several sites (Fig. 225–2). These include axodendritic connections (site 1) and axoaxonic connections involving presynaptic receptors on the hormone-containing nerve terminals (site 3). Multiple neurotransmitters may also participate in the

regulation of hormone secretion through intermediary neurons (site 2), and neurotransmitters may be released directly into the portal system to modify the effect of hypothalamic hormones on the pituitary (site 4). Major advances in the understanding of hypothalamic-pituitary function have occurred as a consequence of the availability of neuropharmacologic compounds that selectively alter neurotransmitter function.

Catecholamines (Dopamine, Norepinephrine, Epinephrine). The common precursor for the catecholamines is tyrosine, which is actively transported from the blood into catecholaminergic neurons in the CNS. Tyrosine is converted to dihydroxyphenylalanine (L-dopa) by tyrosine hydroxylase, which, because of its low concentration, represents the rate-limiting step in catecholamine biosynthesis. It is therefore the enzyme most susceptible to pharmacologic blockage by tyrosine analogues such as alpha-methylparatyrosine. L-dopa is rapidly decarboxylated by aromatic L-amino acid decarboxylase to dopamine (5-hydroxytryptamine). This enzyme can be inhibited by L-dopa analogues such as alpha-methyldopa and

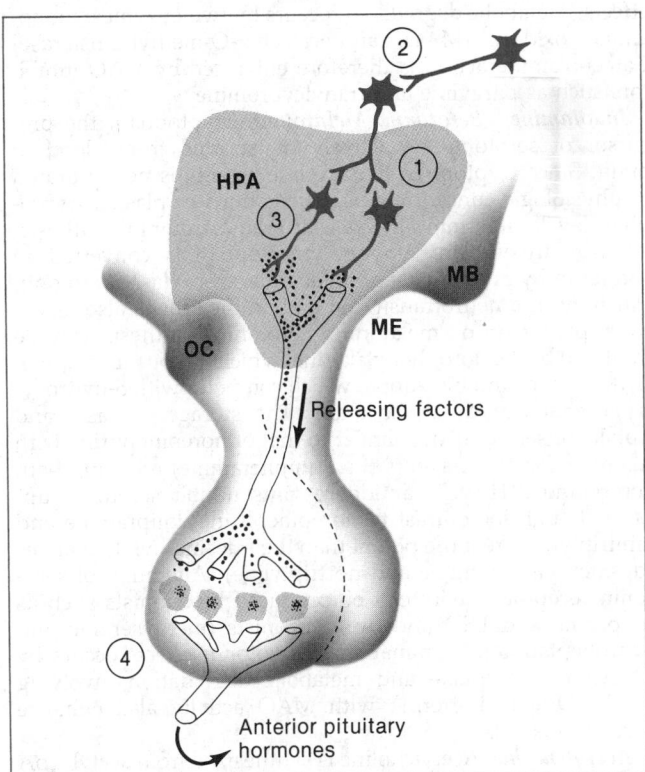

FIGURE 225–2. Sites of potential neurotransmitter effects on hypothalamic releasing and inhibiting hormone secretion and function. HPA = Hypophysiotropic area; OC = optic chiasm; ME = median eminence; MB = mamillary body. Refer to text for description of effects at each site. (Reprinted with permission from Frohman LA: Clinical neuropharmacology of hypothalamic releasing factors. N Engl J Med 286:1391, 1972.)

alpha-methyldopahydrazine (carbidopa). In dopaminergic neurons, dopamine is stored in secretory granules and released as a neurotransmitter, while in noradrenergic and adrenergic neurons it is further hydroxylated by dopamine β-hydroxylase to form norepinephrine. Copper-chelating agents such as disulfiram are potent inhibitors of this step and impair the conversion of dopamine to norepinephrine. In noradrenergic neurons, this transmitter is packaged similarly to that of dopamine, whereas in selective neurons it is converted to epinephrine by phenylethanolamine-N-methyltransferase. See Ch. 242 also for a discussion of catecholamine metabolism.

In nerve endings, newly synthesized catecholamines are stored in secretory granules that protect them from enzymatic degradation. There are at least two distinct pools of neurotransmitters that are differentially susceptible to releasing stimuli. A long-lasting depletion of catecholamines can be produced by reserpine, which causes a slow but constant release of the monoamines and inhibits reuptake. Catecholamine release occurs in response to nerve stimulation by fusion of the secretion vesicle membrane with the cell membrane and extrusion of the amine directly into the intercellular space. Once released, catecholamines bind to postsynaptic receptors that appear to be similar in the hypophysiotropic neurons to those demonstrated in other neural sites. In addition, they bind to presynaptic receptors on the nerve terminals to effect a feedback regulation. Alterations in presynaptic and postsynaptic receptor activity are accomplished by the use of receptor agonists and antagonists. The specificity of most of the available agents, however, is not absolute. Catecholamine action terminates primarily by reuptake of the neurotransmitter into the presynaptic neuron, but also by removal into the circulation and metabolic degradation. Drugs such as cocaine, tricyclic antidepressants, or nomifensine inhibit reuptake, resulting in enhancement of catecholamine effects. Metabolic degradation occurs by two enzymes: monoamine oxidase (MAO) and catechol-O-methyltransferase. Catecholamine action is therefore enhanced by MAO inhibitors such as pargyline and tranylcypromine.

Indolamines (Serotonin, Melatonin). Tryptophan, the precursor of serotonin, is actively transported from blood to brain. Since tryptophan hydroxylase activity is not saturated at physiologic concentrations, fluctuations in plasma tryptophan levels determine the rate of brain serotonin synthesis. After hydroxylation, 5-hydroxytryptophan is converted to serotonin by aromatic L-amino acid decarboxylase. Serotonin functions as a neurotransmitter and, in the pineal, also serves as a precursor of melatonin. Serotonin synthesis can be inhibited by p-chlorophenylalanine, which inhibits tryptophan hydroxylase, and by L-dopa, which competes with 5-hydroxytryptophan for decarboxylation. The storage, release, and uptake of serotonin are similar to that of norepinephrine with many of the same agents (i.e., amphetamine) releasing both compounds. Tricyclic antidepressants inhibit serotonin uptake, though in contrast to norepinephrine, imipramine and amitriptyline are more potent than their desmethyl derivatives (desmethylimipramine and nortriptyline). Alteration of serotonin receptor activity can be produced by agonists such as quipazine and LSD and by antagonists (methysergide and cyproheptadine). Termination of serotonin effects occurs by presynaptic reuptake and metabolic degradation involving MAO. Drugs interfering with MAO activity also enhance serotonin effects.

Acetylcholine. Acetylcholine is synthesized from acetyl-CoA and choline. The source of choline is probably phosphatidylcholine which, after crossing the blood-brain barrier, is partially degraded to choline. Choline is then converted to acetylcholine by choline acetyltransferase. There are two types of acetylcholine receptors, muscarinic and nicotinic, which have different anatomic distribution and physiologic function. Arecoline and atropine, a muscarinic agonist and antagonist,

respectively, cross the blood-brain barrier and modify acetylcholine receptor activity.

Gamma-Aminobutyric Acid (GABA). In the mammalian hypothalamus GABA is an inhibitory neurotransmitter. It is formed by the decarboxylation of L-glutamate and is metabolized by transamination. Numerous agents inhibit GABA synthesis and degradation, but none is specific or useful clinically in altering neuroendocrine function.

Histamine. Histamine is synthesized within the CNS from histidine by a specific decarboxylase and the nonspecific aromatic L-amino acid decarboxylase. Alteration of histamine effects is brought about primarily by histamine receptor antagonists. There are two classes of histamine receptors: H_1 and H_2. Drugs such as diphenhydramine and cyproheptadine inhibit H_1 receptors, while cimetidine and ranitidine inhibit H_2 receptors.

Neuropeptides. A large number of neuropeptides have been identified in the hypothalamus, and their role in the regulation of neuroendocrine function is, at present, only incompletely understood. A list of neuropeptides with potential effects on releasing and inhibiting hormones is provided in Table 225-1. Many of these peptides are widely distributed in extrahypothalamic CNS and function as neurotransmitters or neuromodulators in other pathways. Of particular significance is a group of peptides common to both the CNS and the gastrointestinal tract. Although the function of these peptides within the CNS remains to be determined, they may have a role in the number of integrative systems relating to homeostatic mechanisms. Their presence throughout evolution and as far back as unicellular organisms underscores their essential role in intercellular communication. With the exception of analogues of enkephalin capable of crossing the blood-brain barrier and of TRH, neuroendocrine effects of peptides other than hypophysiotropic hormones have not been documented in man. Limited information is available concerning biosynthesis, storage, secretion, and local metabolism of hypothalamic neuropeptides. Peptidases capable of degrading neuropeptides have been demonstrated, though their specificity and physiologic importance are not yet known.

MECHANISM OF ACTION OF HYPOTHALAMIC HORMONES. Hypophysiotropic hormones affect pituitary hormone secretion by several mechanisms. Specific, high-affinity receptors are present on the anterior pituitary target cells, and evidence now points to the participation of several intracellular mediator or second messenger systems, including adenylate cyclase–cyclic AMP, calcium-calmodulin, and phosphatidylinositol-protein kinase C. In addition, releasing hormones stimulate RNA and protein synthesis, and excessive stimulation can lead to cellular hyperplasia and even tumor formation.

The mechanism of action of the inhibitory hormones somatostatin and dopamine is less well understood. Somatostatin inhibits adenylate cyclase formation and enhances phosphodiesterase activity, both of which actions would impair cyclic AMP–mediated hormone release. Somatostatin also inhibits transmembrane Ca^{++} transport and may have other

TABLE 225–1. NEUROPEPTIDES WITH POTENTIAL EFFECTS ON HYPOTHALAMIC RELEASING HORMONES

Somatostatin	Pancreatic polypeptide
Thyrotropin releasing hormone	Methionine/leucine-enkephalin
Vasoactive intestinal polypeptide	Dynorphin
Cholecystokinin	Beta-endorphin
Gastrin	Alpha-melanocyte–stimulating
Substance P	hormone
Neurotensin	Neuropeptide PYY
Bombesin/gastrin releasing peptide	Neuropeptide PHI/PHM
Secretin	Calcitonin
Motilin	Angiotensin
Insulin	Bradykinin
Glucagon	Galanin

effects on exocytosis. The inhibitory effects of dopamine appear to be independent of cyclic AMP levels, and, like somatostatin, occur at a late stage in the secretory process.

The effects of all the hypophysiotropic hormones studied to date are modified by target gland hormones, i.e., thyroxine, cortisol, estrogens, androgens, inhibin, and insulin-like growth factors. The hormones act primarily by altering the number of receptors on pituitary cells for releasing or inhibiting hormones, but also exhibit effects at postreceptor sites.

Regulation of Hypophysiotropic and Pituitary Hormone Secretion

The control of hypophysiotropic hormone secretion is best appreciated when considered in conjunction with that of the five major pituitary hormone systems they regulate: ACTH, LH and FSH, TSH, GH, and prolactin. Each consists of feedback (closed loop) systems involving primarily blood-borne signals on which are superimposed other signals mostly originating within the CNS (open loop), mediated by neurotransmitters, and representing environment (temperature, light-dark), stress (pain, fear, psychic) and intrinsic rhythmicity (ranging from ultradian or short-term to diurnal, monthly, and seasonal). Thus, both internal and external environmental factors are important determinants of the activity of these systems. A summary of neurotransmitter effects on pituitary hormone secretion is provided in Table 225–2.

HYPOTHALAMIC-PITUITARY-ADRENOCORTICAL AXIS. Nearly all of the monoamine neurotransmitters affect CRF release. Acetylcholine stimulates CRF release predominantly through nicotinic receptors and appears to be the primary neurotransmitter mediating stress-induced CRF release. Serotonin also stimulates CRF release, but the effect is likely mediated through a cholinergic interneuron, since it can be blocked by atropine. Norepinephrine inhibits the cholinergic effects on CRF release through an alpha-adrenergic receptor, and GABA exerts a similar effect. Melatonin inhibits CRF release and may be responsible for the circadian pattern of CRF release that is entrained to the light-dark cycle. Enkephalins exert inhibitory effects on the pituitary-adrenal axis. This effect is believed to occur within the hypothalamus at the level of CRF release, though an additional action on the pituitary has not been excluded.

CRF stimulates ACTH release, which in turn stimulates the secretion of glucocorticoids and mineralocorticoids from the adrenal cortex. Glucocorticoids inhibit ACTH secretion by a concentration-dependent rapid feedback (minutes) and a concentration-independent delayed feedback (hours). The rapid feedback occurs primarily at the pituitary by inhibiting the response to CRF but also by inhibiting CRF release. The delayed feedback also occurs at both pituitary and hypothalamic levels and appears to reflect inhibitory effects on CRF and ACTH synthesis. In addition, ACTH exerts a "short-loop feedback" on CRF release.

Plasma ACTH secretion exhibits a diurnal pattern, with lowest levels occurring between 6 and 11 P.M. followed by a rise in the early morning, peaking between 6 and 8 A.M. The pattern appears independent of sleep stage. Superimposed on this regulatory system are the stimulatory effects of stress, including severe trauma, pyrogens, hypoglycemia, and anxiety. Considerable interaction exists between the feedback influence of circulating corticosteroids and neurotransmitters. Phenytoin administration, for example, decreases CNS sensitivity to steroid feedback, thereby diminishing the ACTH response to metyrapone (which reduces circulating glucocorticoid levels) but also enhances pulsatile ACTH secretion while not affecting the ACTH response to stress and vasopressin. Vasopressin, once believed to be CRF, stimulates ACTH release directly as well as through a CNS-mediated mechanism and potentiates the effects of CRF. A role for endogenous vasopressin and possibly other peptides as additional CRF's is suggested by the fact that only 80 per cent of the ACTH response to stress is mediated by CRF.

HYPOTHALAMIC-PITUITARY-GONADAL AXIS. The major neurotransmitter effects on GnRH identified to date involve dopamine and serotonin. Dopamine stimulates the release of GnRH, though it is not clear whether this involves the tonic or cyclic release of GnRH. Serotonin exerts an inhibitory effect on both cyclic and tonic GnRH secretion. Norepinephrine may also stimulate GnRH release.

The regulation of the hypothalamic-pituitary-gonadal axis is complex, varying with age and sex. LH and FSH are present in circulation from birth, and through the early stages of puberty FSH levels gradually increase to a greater degree than do LH levels. During this period, FSH responses to GnRH are greater than LH responses, a pattern opposite to that seen after puberty, and the hypothalamus is exceedingly sensitive to the suppressive effects of gonadal steroids. In the later prepubertal period (seven to nine years) sleep-related pulsatile LH secretion begins, and synchronization occurs between LH and FSH pulses, particularly in girls. These pulses stimulate the secretion of testosterone in boys and estradiol in girls that initiates the clinical characteristics of puberty. At the same time, evidence for lessening sensitivity of hypothalamic GnRH secretion in response to steroid feedback can be demonstrated. In women, development of positive feedback on LH and FSH by gonadal steroids permits the cyclic preovulatory gonadotropin surge resulting in the establishment of cyclic ovulation by the mid teens. In adult males the LH secretory pattern is characterized by eight to ten pulses occurring randomly through the day, and the teenage relationship to the sleep-wake pattern disappears. Similar pulsatile secretion of LH and FSH occurs in mature women, the frequency and magnitude of the pulses varying with the phase of the menstrual cycle. When ovarian follicles disappear at menopause, secretion of the major ovarian hormones decreases, and the loss of negative feedback of these hormones enhances secretion of FSH and, to a lesser extent, LH. A similar increase in LH and FSH is observed in men in the seventh and eighth decades in response to decreasing testicular function.

In men, surgical stress results in a transitory rise in the level of LH followed by a prolonged fall, accompanied by a fall in testosterone levels. No changes have been observed in

TABLE 225–2. EFFECTS OF AMINERGIC AND PEPTIDERGIC NEUROTRANSMITTERS ON ANTERIOR PITUITARY HORMONE SECRETION

	Norepinephrine	Dopamine	Serotonin	Acetylcholine	Histamine	GABA	Other
ACTH	α ↑	–	↑	↑	–	–	Enkephalins ↓
LH and FSH	(↑)	↓	–	–	–	–	Neurotensin ↓
TSH	↑	↓	↑	↑	–	(↑)	Neurotensin ↓
GH	α ↑ β ↓	↑	↑	–	–	–	Substance P ↓ Enkephalins ↓ Neurotensin ↓
Prolactin	–	↓	↑	–	↑	↑	Neurotensin ↓ Enkephalins ↑ VIP ↑

NOTE: ↑ = stimulates; ↓ = inhibits; – = no effect or insufficient data; ( ) = conflicting data exist. All effects reflect CNS rather than pituitary sites of action (with the exception of dopamine). The data are derived (whenever possible) from studies in humans.

women, although hypothalamic anovulation is frequently seen during periods of stress. Pheromones or other environmental factors have been implicated as the cause for the synchronization of menstrual cycles seen in women living in close association.

Steroid hormones regulate LH and FSH secretion by two major mechanisms. Gonadal steroids regulate tonic secretion by a negative feedback mechanism. Testosterone appears to be more potent than estrogen in this negative feedback effect, while progesterone has an intermediate effect. Inhibin, a peptide produced by germinal epithelium, has a selective action in inhibiting FSH release, possibly by impairing the effects of GnRH. Cyclic release of LH and FSH is stimulated by a positive feedback effect of ovarian steroids during the final phases of follicular growth prior to ovulation. The preovulatory surge of LH is preceded by an increase in circulating estrogen levels in the presence of low or decreasing progesterone levels. The positive effects occur at both the hypothalamic and pituitary levels, though the latter appear to be more important. GnRH is released in a tonic pulsatile manner by the hypothalamus approximately every 90 minutes, and this pattern of secretion is critical for its effects on the pituitary. In an individual deficient in GnRH secretion, pulsatile administration of GnRH allows restoration of normal cyclic ovulation. In contrast, constant infusion of GnRH leads to down-regulation of pituitary GnRH receptors and a loss of gonadotropin secretion. This phenomenon has resulted in major advances in therapy aimed at enhancing or preventing fertility. In contrast to its stimulatory effects on GnRH release, dopamine inhibits tonic LH secretion. The physiologic significance of this observation is unclear, since inhibitory effects on the midcycle LH surge can also be blocked by dopamine receptor blockers.

HYPOTHALAMIC-PITUITARY-THYROID AXIS. TSH secretion by the pituitary is regulated by TRH and somatostatin. For a discussion of the control of somatostatin secretion, the reader is referred to the section on the regulation of GH secretion. TRH secretion is stimulated by norepinephrine and dopamine and is inhibited by serotonin. TRH stimulates TSH secretion, which in turn enhances the release of thyroxine and triiodothyronine by the thyroid. The feedback effects of these hormones, primarily triiodothyronine, occur principally in the pituitary where they inhibit the TSH response to TRH. A reduction in circulating thyroid hormone levels leads to a prompt rise in TSH levels. TRH is not required for this acute response, though it is necessary for the full expression of TSH hypersecretion over a long time. In addition, TRH is required for maintaining basal TSH secretion. In contrast to its effects on the pituitary, triiodothyronine exerts a stimulatory effect on TRH secretion from the hypothalamus.

Acute changes in environmental conditions requiring increased metabolic activity, such as cold exposure, lead to a TRH-mediated increase in TSH secretion. This effect is readily demonstrable in infants but not in adults, in whom other mechanisms of thermogenesis (mediated by the autonomic nervous system and resulting in shivering and free fatty acid mobilization) are more important. Agents inhibiting adrenergic neurotransmission block the TSH response to cold.

Dopaminergic agents exert an inhibitory effect on TSH release by the pituitary that is most pronounced in patients with elevated TSH levels but also seen in normal individuals. A role of endogenous dopamine in suppressing TSH secretion has also been demonstrated.

Somatostatin inhibition of TSH secretion exerts a relatively minor physiologic role under normal circumstances, but increases in hypothalamic somatostatin release as a result of elevated GH levels can suppress TSH secretion to subnormal levels. Somatostatin, however, is a less potent inhibitor of TSH than of GH.

HYPOTHALAMIC-PITUITARY-SOMATOTROPH AXIS. GH secretion is regulated by releasing and inhibiting hormones: GRH and SRIF (somatostatin). GH secretion is characterized by a diurnal pattern with stable basal levels, superimposed on which are occasional surges of GH related to an inherent neural rhythmicity, the greatest of which occurs about one hour after the onset of sleep and is associated with sleep stages 3 and 4. With age, GH secretion changes dramatically, both qualitatively and quantitatively. Extremely high levels seen in the first few days of life decrease by two weeks of age. During the pubertal period levels indistinguishable from those of adults are seen, though the GH surges occur more frequently. By the fifth and sixth decades, GH surges, both during the day and in association with sleep, are diminished. Similarly, responses to GH releasing stimuli decrease with age. Neurotransmitter regulation of GH secretion has been extensively defined. Dopamine, norepinephrine (through the alpha receptor), epinephrine, serotonin, GABA, and acetylcholine have all been shown to stimulate GH secretion. Melatonin has both stimulatory and inhibitory effects, TRH and neurotensin exhibit inhibitory effects, and endorphins-enkephalins have stimulatory effects, all mediated within the CNS. The mechanism by which these neurotransmitters affect the secretion of GRH and SRIF is not completely understood, though several neurotransmitters and/or agonists have been reported to directly stimulate GRH or SRIF release.

GH secretion is profoundly affected by nutrients. Elevations of amino acid levels, decreases in free fatty acids, and hypoglycemia all stimulate GH secretion, while hyperglycemia inhibits GH release. GH secretion is increased by exercise, anxiety, and emotional or physical stress. Many hormones affect GH responsiveness. Estrogen administration increases GH responsiveness, while excesses of corticosteroid and thyroid hormone decrease responsivity. GH secretion is also decreased in states of thyroid hormone deficiency. In pubertal and prepubertal males, androgen administration also enhances GH responses. GH secretion is sexually dimorphic: Women have higher basal levels and smaller pulses than do men. These differences may, in part, contribute to sex-related differences in growth patterns.

In addition to these "open-loop" stimuli, a closed-loop feedback system also exists. GH stimulates the production of somatomedin C (insulin-like growth factor [IGF-I]) by numerous tissues, and both GH and IGF-I exhibit feedback effects. IGF-I stimulates the release of somatostatin and also inhibits basal and GRH-stimulated GH release by the pituitary. GH itself stimulates SRIF secretion at concentrations that are achieved during secretory pulses. The effects of GH and IGF-I on GRH secretion remain to be clarified.

HYPOTHALAMIC-LACTOTROPH-BREAST AXIS. Prolactin secretion is predominantly controlled by inhibitory CNS influences, with dopamine being the major prolactin inhibiting factor. Two peptides, TRH and vasoactive intestinal polypeptide (VIP), appear to have physiologic prolactin releasing factor (PRF) activity, though their relative importance is not yet clear. Neurotransmitter influences on prolactin secretion are extensive. Serotonin stimulates prolactin release by effects on PRF. Melatonin and histamine have stimulatory effects within the CNS as do opioid peptides and GABA. The effect of the latter two agents appears due to their inhibitory effects on the tuberoinfundibular dopaminergic system.

Prolactin secretion is increased by tactile stimulation of the breast via receptors in the nipple and areola that reach the spinal cord by the intercostal nerves. During pregnancy, prolactin levels increase as a result of estrogen stimulation. Following parturition, the rapid decline in estrogen and progesterone levels allows the unopposed action of prolactin to stimulate lactation from the estrogen-primed breast. The suckling stimulation of prolactin secretion is in part controlled by VIP. Prolactin levels return to normal after several months even during continual lactation. Prolactin is a stress-responsive hormone, and increased secretion is observed after surgical stress, exercise, and insulin hypoglycemia. Prolactin secretion is increased in states of thyroid hormone deficiency and decreased in the presence of thyroid hormone excess.

Frohman LA, Krieger DT: Neuroendocrine physiology and disease. In Felig P, Baxter JD, Broadus AE, et al. (eds.): Endocrinology and Metabolism. 2nd ed. New York, McGraw-Hill Book Company, 1987, pp 185–247. *A systematic in-depth presentation of the anatomy and physiology of human neuroendocrinology, along with the clinical manifestations, diagnosis, and therapy of anatomic and functional disorders. Designed for the medical student, clinical trainee, and practicing physician.*

Krieger DT, Brownstein M, Martin JB (eds.): Brain Peptides. Vol 2. New York, John Wiley & Sons, 1987. *A comprehensive collection of monographs on the role of brain peptides as transmitters, hypophysiotropic hormones, and messengers throughout the nervous system. This is a definitive reference volume. Of interest to the medical student, neurobiologist, and clinical trainee.*

Morley JE, Levine AS, Gosnell BA, et al.: Control of food intake. In Muller EE, MacLeod RM, Frohman LA (eds.): Neuroendocrine Perspectives. Vol. 4. Amsterdam, Elsevier, 1985, pp 145–190. *An integrative approach to the regulation of feeding behavior with emphasis on neuropeptides, biogenic amines, and hormones. Principles of basic physiology are applied to clinical disorders of food intake.*

Nikolics K, Mason AJ, Szonyi E, et al.: A prolactin-inhibiting factor within the precursor for human gonadotropin-releasing hormone. Nature 316:511, 1985. *A classic paper describing the use of molecular biologic techniques to identify, synthesize, and characterize a new hypothalamic hypophysiotropic hormone. While there is still some uncertainty concerning the physiologic importance of this peptide, it is of major scientific interest.*

Voles T, Robertson GL: Clinical effects of altered vasopressin secretion. In Muller EE, MacLeod RM, Frohman LA (eds.): Neuroendocrine Perspectives. Vol 4. Amsterdam, Elsevier, 1985, pp 1–42. *A clearly written review of the neuroendocrine regulation of salt and water metabolism with emphasis on disorders of vasopressin secretion in humans.*

DISEASES OF THE CENTRAL NERVOUS SYSTEM WITH ALTERED NEUROENDOCRINE AND NEUROMETABOLIC FUNCTION

The frequent association of altered hormone secretion with disorders of the CNS has been recognized for many decades. The hypothalamus was the initial focus of attention because of its crucial role in neuroendocrine regulation. Diseases localized to extrahypothalamic brain regions as well as non-localized CNS disorders can also produce disturbances in neuroendocrine function. The clinical and laboratory manifestations of these disorders are frequently indistinguishable from those of hypothalamic origin, since their mediation is usually via the hypothalamus. Similarly the distinction between hypothalamic and pituitary causes of certain pituitary hormone secretory disorders may be difficult for other reasons.

Because of the reticular organization of the anatomic structure of the hypothalamus, only certain functions can be localized to a precise site. In addition, neurons within a specific hypothalamic locus may be involved in several separate regulatory functions. Consequently the extent of endocrine or metabolic disturbance is more dependent on the location than the size of the hypothalamic lesion. Furthermore, slowly growing lesions tend to be silent until they have reached considerable size, whereas rapidly enlarging lesions, depending on location, can cause dramatic clinical and laboratory manifestations even when quite small.

Acute hypothalamic damage is associated with impairment of consciousness, sustained hyperthermia, and severe disturbances of cardiovascular, gastrointestinal, or respiratory function. In contrast, persistent disease in the hypothalamus results in alterations in cognition and complex homeostatic functions. Although disorders of neuroendocrine regulation can be produced by acute lesions destroying the median eminence or the pituitary stalk, they generally tend to be seen with chronic disorders and often result in inability of the endocrine system to adapt to environmental changes rather than in alteration of basal hormone secretion. Because hypothalamic neuronal projections, in contrast to those involving sensory and motor function, are generally not lateralized, unilateral damage seldom results in significant or prolonged symptoms. Thus disturbances of hypothalamic function are most commonly seen with infiltrative or inflammatory diseases that affect the region diffusely, with tumors of the midline that expand bilaterally, or with disorders affecting the median eminence, the final common effector pathway to the pituitary.

Etiology of Hypothalamic Disease

Anatomically defined disorders of the hypothalamus vary in frequency with age groups and are summarized in Table 225–3. In addition, disturbances of neuroendocrine or neurometabolic function are frequently unassociated with anatomic evidence of hypothalamic disease. Many have been attributed to disorders of neurochemical function, though it is currently not known whether they represent defects in receptor binding, postreceptor mechanisms, biosynthetic defects, or other disorders.

TUMORS. Hypothalamic tumors are frequently located in the region of the third ventricle. Those tumors located in the inferior portion of the third ventricle or the anterior mediobasal hypothalamus commonly produce disturbances in neuroendocrine and neurometabolic regulation. The most frequent hypothalamic tumors are craniopharyngiomas (see next section) and their variants (ependymomas and epidermoid cysts), followed by astrocytomas and dysgerminomas. Two other tumor types, hypothalamic pinealomas and hamartomas, will be considered separately because of their association

TABLE 225–3. ETIOLOGY OF HYPOTHALAMIC DISEASE

Neonates
Intraventricular hemorrhage
Meningitis: bacterial
Tumors: glioma, hemangioma
Trauma
Hydrocephalus, hydranencephaly, kernicterus

1 Month–2 Years
Tumors: glioma, especially optic glioma, histiocytosis X, hemangiomas
Hydrocephalus, meningitis
"Familial" disorders: Laurence-Moon, Bardet-Biedl, Prader-Labhart-Willi

2–10 Years
Tumors: craniopharyngioma, glioma, dysgerminoma, hamartoma, histiocytosis X, leukemia, ganglioneuroma, ependymoma, medulloblastoma
Meningitis: bacterial, tuberculous
Encephalitis: viral and demyelinating, various viral encephalitides and exanthematous demyelinating encephalitides, disseminated encephalomyelitis
"Familial" disorders: diabetes insipidus, etc.
Damage from nasopharyngeal radiation therapy

10–25 Years
Tumors: craniopharyngioma, pituitary tumors, glioma, hamartoma, dysgerminoma, histiocytosis X, leukemia, dermoid, lipoma, neuroblastoma
Trauma
Subarachnoid hemorrhage, vascular aneurysm, arteriovenous malformation
Inflammatory diseases: meningitis, encephalitis, sarcoidosis, tuberculosis
Associated with midline brain defects: agenesis of corpus callosum
Chronic hydrocephalus or increased intracranial pressure

25–50 Years
Nutritional: Wernicke's disease
Tumors: glioma, lymphoma, meningioma, craniopharyngioma, pituitary tumors, angioma, plasmacytoma, colloid cysts, ependymoma, sarcoma, histiocytosis X
Inflammatory: sarcoidosis, tuberculosis, viral encephalitis
Subarachnoid hemorrhage, vascular aneurysms, arteriovenous malformation
Damage from pituitary radiation therapy

50 Years and Older
Nutritional: Wernicke's disease
Tumors: sarcoma, glioblastoma, lymphoma, meningioma, colloid cysts, ependymoma, pituitary tumors
Vascular: infarct, subarachnoid hemorrhage, pituitary apoplexy
Infectious: encephalitis, sarcoidosis, meningitis

Adapted from Plum F, Van Uitert R: Non-endocrine diseases of the hypothalamus. In Reichlin S, Baldessarini RJ, Martin JB (eds.): The Hypothalamus. New York, Raven Press, 1978, p 415.

with specific neuroendocrine disorders. Since they are frequently of developmental origin, the majority of hypothalamic tumors occur in patients under 25 years of age. Endocrine disturbances generally result from destruction of those neuronal elements required for normal pituitary function. The most frequently occurring manifestations are diabetes insipidus, hypogonadism, and growth retardation. Disturbances in thyroid and adrenal function are less common. The diagnosis of a hypothalamic tumor is made by standard neuroradiologic and neuro-ophthalmologic procedures, computed tomography, magnetic resonance imaging, and visual field measurement. The combination of an atypical visual field defect (i.e., loss of inferior visual fields), normal sellar anatomy, and intact responses to releasing hormones in a patient with hypopituitarism points to primary hypothalamic disease. The surgical treatment of hypothalamic tumors generally precludes complete removal without destruction of normal tissue critical for maintaining homeostasis. Many of these tumors, because of their developmental origin, tend to be slow growing and may even undergo spontaneous growth arrest or regression. Cystic tumors can be aspirated or marsupialized into the cerebroventricular system. Radiotherapy is also effective in many of these tumors. The loss of endocrine function is, however, rarely reversible, and replacement hormone therapy is required.

Hamartomas. One type of hypothalamic tumor, the hamartoma, has been associated with increased, rather than decreased, hypothalamic function. Hamartomas consist of masses of redundant, partially disoriented glial and neuronal cells or an abnormally lodged collection of normal nerve tissue. Hamartomas associated with precocious puberty consist of encapsulated nodules in the posterior hypothalamus containing membrane-bound secretion granules similar to those in hypothalamic neurosecretory cells. Vessels in the hamartoma have fenestrations characteristic of those in the median eminence, suggesting a secretory process similar to that in the median eminence. These vessels are presumed to connect to the pituitary portal system. The secretion granules contain GnRH, which is found in high concentrations in CSF from patients with this disorder. Hamartomatous cells are believed to secrete GnRH in a pulsatile manner, but are not under normal prepubertal inhibitory influences. The resultant hormonal effects produce pubertal changes that in girls lead to menarche and cyclic ovulatory menses as early as the second year of life.

Hamartomas are present in one third of all children with this form of precocious puberty. Specific therapy aimed at the hamartoma appears unnecessary, since its course is benign with no other neuroendocrine disturbances and no loss of nonendocrine hypothalamic structure or function. Therapy of the precocious puberty, however, is of greatest importance both for psychologic reasons and for prevention of premature epiphyseal fusion and stunted growth. This disorder has in the past been treated with long-acting progesterone or a mild androgen to suppress the gonadotropin responses to GnRH, but with less than full effectiveness in retarding the accelerated rate of bone growth. Optimal therapy is currently achieved with the use of a GnRH agonist to down-regulate pituitary GnRH receptors, resulting in diminished gonadotropin secretion and suppression of bone growth.

Hypothalamic hamartomas have also been associated with acromegaly and GH-secreting pituitary tumors. They have been shown to contain GRH, which is secreted into the portal system, resulting in GH hypersecretion and somatotroph tumor formation.

Gangliocytomas. A closely related tumor, the gangliocytoma, consists of randomly oriented large ganglion cells similar to those in the hypothalamic magnocellular (large cell) nuclei. Intrapituitary gangliocytomas are also seen in association with acromegaly and GH-secreting tumors of the pituitary and contain GRH. In contrast to hypothalamic hamarto-

mas, the axons of the intrapituitary tumors directly contact the somatotropic cells. A CRF-containing pituitary gangliocytoma has also been described in association with ACTH hypersecretion and Cushing's disease.

Pineal Tumors. Pineal tumors constitute less than 1 per cent of all intracranial neoplasms and consist of three separate tumor types: pinealomas (pineal parenchymal tumor [20 per cent]), glial tumors (25 per cent), and germinomas (also called ectopic pinealomas or teratomas [55 per cent]). The neuroendocrine effects (precocious puberty) of the first two types are most likely a consequence of destruction of the normal pineal by tumor, leading to loss of pineal secretory products (possibly melatonin, arginine vasotocin, or another factor) that normally inhibit the initiation of sexual maturation. Only a small percentage of pineal tumors cause sexual precocity and usually not until they extend beyond the pineal region. Some pineal tumors are associated with delayed puberty, which may be mediated by production of an antigonadotropic factor. Precocious puberty associated with germinomas, which are similar both histologically and functionally to ovarian and testicular germ cell tumors, is caused by the production of chorionic gonadotropin. Levels as high as those seen during the first month of pregnancy are often present. Many of the "ectopic" pinealomas occur in the midline of the ventral hypothalamus and result in loss of other endocrine functions. Surgical treatment of pinealomas is generally unsatisfactory though the tumors consisting of germinal elements are exquisitely radiosensitive. Many tumors, however, contain nongerminal elements (teratomas) that are relatively radioresistant. See also Ch. 228.

INFILTRATIVE AND INFLAMMATORY DISEASES. *Histiocytosis X* (see also Ch. 161). This granulomatous disease of the histiocytic type, with eosinophilic elements, involves the ventromedial hypothalamus and is associated with diabetes insipidus, anterior hypopituitarism due to destruction of releasing hormone–secreting neurons, or both. The three clinical subgroups of the disease are Hand-Schüller-Christian disease, the most common type, characterized by polyuria, exophthalmos, and skull defects; Letterer-Siwe disease, a more rapidly progressive form; and eosinophilic granuloma, in which similar pathologic findings are present in isolated bones. The disease may begin with diabetes insipidus, which is present in nearly 50 per cent of patients with Hand-Schüller-Christian disease. Less commonly, growth failure, hypogonadism, and panhypopituitarism are seen. The diagnosis is established by bone or intracranial biopsy. The CNS forms of the disease may respond to high-dose glucocorticoid therapy or chemotherapy, but the impairment in neuroendocrine function appears irreversible.

Sarcoidosis (see Ch. 69). Involvement of the CNS by sarcoidosis is uncommon. When it is present, however, the hypothalamus and pituitary are frequently involved with infiltrating granulomatous nodules. Patients may develop diabetes insipidus, galactorrhea due to hyperprolactinemia, partial or total anterior pituitary insufficiency, and neurometabolic and neurovegetative symptoms such as somnolence or hyperphagia. In general, the usual treatment with glucocorticoids does not improve the endocrine dysfunction.

TRAUMA. Basal skull fractures are frequently accompanied by shearing of the pituitary stalk, leading to panhypopituitarism and diabetes insipidus. In patients who become comatose following skull fractures, impairment in the pituitary-thyroid and pituitary-gonadal axes has been reported in the absence of stalk damage. Gonadal and thyroid hormones generally return to normal upon recovery.

RADIATION-INDUCED HYPOTHALAMIC DYSFUNCTION. Radiation therapy for intracranial neoplasms, including pituitary tumors, and for nasopharyngeal and maxillary sinus carcinomas frequently leads to hypopituitarism. The interval between therapy and appearance of hormone deficiencies ranges from one to ten years or possibly longer.

Children appear more susceptible than adults, and the critical dose is believed to be about 4000 rads. In children, growth failure associated with reduced GH secretion, hypogonadotropic hypogonadism, and hypothyroidism is seen. The site of the defect appears to be variable, with some patients exhibiting hypothalamic and others pituitary damage. In some, but not all, patients, pituitary hormone responses to the injection of hypothalamic releasing hormones may distinguish the anatomic site of the defect.

FUNCTIONAL DISEASES OF THE CENTRAL NERVOUS SYSTEM WITH NEUROENDOCRINE DISTURBANCES

Disturbances in neuroendocrine function manifested by both decreased and increased pituitary hormone secretion can occur in the absence of structurally detectable disease in the pituitary or CNS. With the aid of releasing hormones to test specifically the pituitary component and other stimuli to test the hypothalamic-pituitary unit, some degree of discrimination can be made as to the source of the disordered hormone secretion. The following are recognized functional disturbances that have been attributed to hypothalamic (or possibly other CNS) disease. The specific biochemical defect responsible remains to be determined.

HYPOTHALAMIC HYPOGONADISM. This disorder is defined as an impairment in pituitary-gonadal function caused by deficient or disordered secretion of GnRH. The manifestations vary according to the age at presentation (see also Ch. 235 and 237).

Prepubertal. The presence of hypothalamic hypogonadism prior to puberty results in failure of normal sexual maturation. Other pituitary hormone deficiencies, also attributed to hypothalamic dysfunction, may coexist. A major subgroup of this disorder, most frequently seen in boys, includes anosmia or hyposmia (*Kallmann's syndrome* or olfactory-genital dysplasia). This syndrome may be associated with other neurologic defects such as color blindness and nerve deafness. The disorder is frequently familial, though sporadic cases have also been reported. Midline developmental defects occasionally occur, and hypoplasia in the region of the anterior commissure, olfactory bulb, and hypothalamus has been found. In some patients there is an additional defect characterized by decreased testicular response to LH. The gonadotropin responses to a single injection of GnRH are markedly impaired or absent, indicating a lack of prior GnRH function. Repeated administration of GnRH, given to prime the gonadotrophs, eventually produces a normal or supranormal gonadotropin response and serves to differentiate this disorder from that of primary gonadotroph failure. Standard therapy consists of the use of gonadal steroids for the development and maintenance of secondary sexual characteristics and gonadotropins for promoting fertility. GnRH itself can produce both effects if administered by an intermittent infusion pump to simulate endogenous gonadotropin secretion.

Postpubertal. Postpubertal hypothalamic hypogonadism affects primarily women. It is manifested clinically by secondary amenorrhea or oligomenorrhea and occasionally by infertility associated with anovulatory cycles. The terms *functional* or *psychogenic amenorrhea* and *infertility* have also been used for this disorder. Patients may exhibit normal basal levels of gonadotropins and estradiol, resulting in maintenance of secondary sexual characteristics, although pulsatile secretion of LH, seen in normal women, is absent, and the cyclic ovulatory surge of gonadotropins does not occur. The gonadotropin responses to a single injection of GnRH reveal enhancement of the FSH rather than the LH response. These women respond normally to clomiphene, an estrogen receptor antagonist, suggesting the defect is related to a functional derangement in the positive estrogen feedback mechanism. The disorder is usually self-limited.

Hyperprolactinemia exerts an inhibitory effect on the positive feedback effect of estradiol on GnRH secretion that has been attributed to enhanced tuberoinfundibular dopamine secretion. The negative estrogen feedback mechanism appears intact, since elevated FSH and LH levels are maintained in postmenopausal women with hyperprolactinemia. In men, hyperprolactinemia produces hypogonadism, manifested most frequently by diminished libido and potency.

In severe cases, basal estradiol levels and serum gonadotropin responses to GnRH are reduced, implying a defect in tonic as well as cyclic GnRH secretion. Similar physiologic disturbances are seen in some patients with hyperprolactinemia irrespective of cause. Marked increases and decreases in body weight are often accompanied by amenorrhea, as occurs in professional ballet dancers and female athletes; anorexia nervosa (see details later in this section); and severe obesity. Evidence for decreased GnRH secretion has also been found in male athletes.

Treatment of this disorder depends on the extent of hypogonadism and the patient's desire for fertility. Restoration of ovulatory menses may be accomplished by cycles of clomiphene administration, cyclic estrogen-progestin (oral contraceptive) therapy, gonadotropin administration, or GnRH infusions, depending on the desired goal. In hypoestrogenemic women, decreased vaginal secretions, leading to dyspareunia and decreased libido, and the long-term consequences of osteopenia and metabolic bone disease warrant replacement therapy. In men, testosterone replacement therapy is indicated if endogenous hormone levels are subnormal.

Polycystic Ovary Syndrome (see also Ch. 237). The polycystic ovary (Stein-Leventhal) syndrome is characterized by amenorrhea, obesity, hirsutism, and consistently elevated LH levels. It is occasionally associated with a history of childhood CNS injury or "encephalitis." The altered hormonal secretory pattern of polycystic ovaries appears to be secondary to the increased LH secretion. This syndrome is occasionally seen in patients with hyperprolactinemia, but the causal relationship remains to be established.

HYPOTHALAMIC HYPOTHYROIDISM. This is an uncommon disorder manifested by hypothyroidism, a low or normal plasma TSH level, and an exaggerated and delayed response of TSH to TRH. In patients with this disorder, peak TSH responses occur at 90 to 120 minutes, in contrast to the 15- to 30-minute peak response time seen in normal subjects. Children of one subgroup have shown elevated basal TSH levels with decreased biologic activity, but in most subjects basal levels are normal. Hypothalamic hypothyroidism can occur as an isolated defect or, more commonly, is seen in association with deficiencies of gonadotropin, GH, or ACTH secretion. Treatment of this disorder is with thyroxine.

HYPOTHALAMIC-ADRENAL DYSFUNCTION. Decreased ACTH secretion on the basis of hypothalamic or other CNS disorders is relatively rare. It is seen most commonly in association with other pituitary hormone deficiencies during childhood and, by inference, has been attributed to a CNS cause. Disturbances of ACTH diurnal rhythm and suppressibility of ACTH are common in patients with a variety of intracranial diseases and reflect disturbances in neuroendocrine control mechanisms. They do not have major clinical significance, but subtle effects on behavior cannot be excluded. In particular, patients with affective disorders (unipolar depression) or experiencing bereavement exhibit a lack of normal glucocorticoid suppressibility similar to that seen in Cushing's disease.

IDIOPATHIC HYPERPROLACTINEMIA. Idiopathic hyperprolactinemia (IH) is a disorder in which prolactin levels are elevated in the absence of demonstrable pituitary or CNS disease and of any other recognized cause of increased prolactin secretion (see Ch. 239). The clinical manifestations of IH consist of galactorrhea and amenorrhea. In some patients, oligomenorrhea is present, and in a few, sporadic ovulation persists. Prolactin levels are elevated, but rarely exceed 150 ng per milliliter. The disease is confined to women of childbearing age. The diagnosis remains inferential and based on exclusion of a pituitary microadenoma.

Many patients in whom IH was previously diagnosed have subsequently been found by computed tomography to harbor microadenomas. Extensive testing using neuropharmacologic probes has failed to distinguish patients with IH from those with microadenomas, suggesting that the same pathophysiologic mechanism underlies both disorders. IH has been attributed to a CNS neurotransmitter defect related to dopamine metabolism, based on the observations that drugs impairing dopaminergic neurotransmission (i.e., neuroleptic dopamine receptor antagonists) increase prolactin secretion. The major action of these drugs in elevating prolactin levels, however, appears to be at the pituitary rather than within the CNS. IH is a benign condition, since less than 5 per cent of patients observed over a period of years will subsequently show evidence of a pituitary tumor.

Therapy depends on the level of symptoms and the degree of inconvenience they produce. Bromocriptine (2.5 mg two or three times a day) is a dopamine receptor agonist that suppresses prolactin levels, eliminates galactorrhea, and restores cyclic menses and fertility. Nearly 80 per cent of patients will experience menses within two months of initiating therapy, and 65 per cent will become fertile. The effect of the drug is of short duration, however, and hyperprolactinemia recurs following its discontinuation. In some patients, hyperprolactinemia may remit spontaneously or following a pregnancy subsequent to bromocriptine administration. There is no evidence that long-term bromocriptine therapy per se restores prolactin secretory dynamics to normal. Even in the absence of a desire for fertility, the increased risk of osteopenia in hyperprolactinemic, hypoestrogenemic women provides the rationale for therapy.

HYPOTHALAMIC DISORDERS OF GROWTH HORMONE SECRETION. *Idiopathic Growth Hormone Deficiency.* Idiopathic GH deficiency (IGHD) occurs as either an isolated hormone deficiency or in association with other anterior pituitary hormone deficiencies and as both a familial and sporadic disorder. It is a disease of childhood, the diagnosis frequently being made because of impaired linear growth when the child is between two and three years of age. Impairment in GH secretion may be complete, with basal levels barely detectable, or partial, with subnormal responses to stimuli. The absence of radiologic abnormalities of the pituitary and the frequent coexistence of TRH- and GnRH-responsive deficiencies of TSH and gonadotropins suggest the defect is located in the hypothalamus. Limited histologic studies of the pituitary or hypothalamus are available because of the generally benign nature of the disease. It is assumed to be due to a deficiency of GRH secretion, most likely on the basis of a neurotransmitter or biosynthetic abnormality, rather than to a structural defect in the hypothalamus. Approximately 75 per cent of patients with IGHD exhibit an intact GH response to GRH, indicating that the disorder has a heterogeneous etiology. Several other subgroups of GH deficiency are now also recognized, including one in which partial deletion of the GH gene results in complete absence of the hormone and another in which there is spontaneous recovery of GH secretion. Therapy of IGHD should be initiated as soon as the diagnosis is established and consists of administration of biosynthetic human GH. Preliminary results using GRH as therapy indicate that this releasing hormone may effectively substitute for GH in at least half of the patients with IGHD. Hypothyroidism, if present, must also be treated. If gonadotropin deficiency is present, therapy with gonadal steroids is postponed as long as possible to avoid accelerating bone growth and producing epiphyseal closure before acceptable linear bone growth is achieved by GH.

Psychosocial Dwarfism. A pattern indistinguishable from IGHD is seen occasionally in children reared in environments with deficient maternal care and affection. Children with this disorder, also termed the emotional deprivation syndrome, exhibit impaired GH responses to stimuli when studied. Within a short time in an improved environment, however, GH secretion returns to normal, and linear growth is restored. It is presumed that the impaired GH secretion is secondary to a behaviorly associated alteration in neurotransmitter metabolism impairing normal GRH-SRIF interrelationships.

Cerebral Gigantism. This childhood disease is characterized by rapid growth, accelerated bone age, and mental retardation. Ventricular enlargement is present, although no focal CNS lesions have been detected. GH secretion has been normal in the few patients described with this disorder. A variant of the syndrome is associated with lipodystrophy, hyperpigmentation, hypertrichosis, hepatosplenomegaly, increased adrenal steroid production, and hyperlipemia.

CENTRAL NERVOUS SYSTEM DISORDERS OF WATER REGULATION. Organic lesions of the CNS and drug therapy can lead to "cerebral hyponatremia" or "cerebral hypernatremia," which are entities distinct from diabetes insipidus (see Ch. 227, Posterior Pituitary).

Hyponatremia. The syndrome of inappropriate secretion of antidiuretic hormone (ADH) results from the autonomous secretion of vasopressin, resulting in hyponatremia, renal sodium loss, and inability to excrete dilute urine in the presence of normal renal, pituitary, adrenal, and thyroid function; resistance to correction by hypertonic saline; and reversibility following restriction of water (see Ch. 77). The increased renal sodium excretion occurs secondary to expanded extracellular volume. When measured, plasma vasopressin levels have been increased.

This syndrome has been reported in patients with carcinoma metastatic to the brain, primary brain tumors, cerebral infarction, basal skull fracture, subarachnoid hemorrhage, meningoencephalitis, and acute intermittent porphyria, but it may also occur in the absence of any underlying structural disease. Certain hypoglycemic and antineoplastic drugs can produce the same syndrome. The former, including chlorpropamide and tolbutamide, augment ADH action on the renal tubule and also stimulate ADH release. Vincristine and cyclophosphamide have direct neurotoxic effects on neurohypophyseal tissue. Other agents such as carbamazepine (Tegretol), amitriptyline (Elavil), thioridazine (Mellaril), and clofibrate (Atromid-S) also produce the syndrome, presumably by affecting endogenous vasopressin release.

Hypernatremia. Patients with intracranial lesions with or without disturbances of consciousness may exhibit hypernatremia in the presence of normal renal function, adequate fluid intake, absence of thirst, and failure of forced fluid intake to correct the hyperosmolality. This syndrome has been attributed to impaired regulation of thirst as well as vasopressin secretion, and has been described in association with histiocytosis, craniopharyngioma, optic nerve glioma, pineal tumor, encephalitis, and ruptured intracranial aneurysm. The treatment of this disorder, above and beyond that of the specific causative lesion, is similar to that for diabetes insipidus.

DISORDERS OF NEUROMETABOLIC REGULATION. *Acute Disorders.* Acute disturbances of metabolic regulation occur most commonly in states of stress that activate the sympathetic nervous system. Thus, patients with hyperthermia, trauma, sepsis, and burns, and undergoing general anesthesia, may exhibit hyperglycemia and hyperglucagonemia along with impaired insulin secretion. In most instances these changes represent merely an extension of normal physiologic processes, do not result in significant clinical problems, and resolve spontaneously when the stress disappears. However, when stress is prolonged, as in severe burns, the responses can produce a severe catabolic state that can be life threatening.

Stress diabetes, seen frequently in the same clinical disorders, may have several causes. Some patients may manifest true diabetes mellitus for the first time under circumstances in which there is enhanced secretion of cortisol, glucagon, catecholamines, and GH, but in other patients the marked hyperglycemia may be unrelated to true diabetes. A syndrome indistinguishable from nonketotic hyperglycemia with or without coma is associated with severe head injury, cerebral thrombosis, encephalitis, and heat stroke. The severity of the hyperglycemia and its duration predict the probability of survival following head injury. Treatment consists of hydration and small doses of insulin. Beta-adrenergic blockade has been used in some patients, but should not be considered standard therapy.

Hypoglycemia is seen only rarely with hypothalamic disease. It has been reported in association with subdural hemorrhage.

Chronic Disorders. Destruction of the ventromedial hypothalamus leads to a syndrome of obesity, while damage to the ventrolateral hypothalamus results in anorexia and inanition. Because bilateral destruction is necessary, inanition is infrequently observed, since the concomitant loss of other important homeostatic mechanisms is usually incompatible with prolonged survival. An anatomically identifiable hypothalamic lesion is present in only a small percentage of patients with extensive obesity or inanition. However, the remarkable similarity of clinical and biochemical features in patients with and without definable lesions suggests that many "functional" disorders of caloric homeostasis ("essential" obesity and anorexia nervosa) are caused by biochemical disturbances in hypothalamic function that are presently undefined.

HYPOTHALAMIC OBESITY. Ventromedial hypothalamic destruction resulting from encephalitis, infiltrative diseases (leukemia or histiocytosis X), trauma, vascular accidents, and tumors has been associated with obesity. Oxygen consumption, insulin secretion, body composition, and adipose metabolism are similar in patients with hypothalamic obesity and in those with essential obesity. Adipose tissue mass increases primarily as the result of hypertrophy rather than hyperplasia. Marked insulin resistance is present, and diabetes may develop in some patients. GH secretion is impaired, and hypogonadism is common.

A number of familial disorders (Laurence-Moon, Bardet-Biedl, Alstrom-Hallgren, Prader-Willi) are associated with extreme obesity and evidence of other hypothalamic disturbances, including hypogonadism, temperature intolerance, and loss of diurnal rhythms; and of extrahypothalamic disturbances, such as deafness, pigmentary retinopathy, hypotonia, and mental retardation.

Therapy of hypothalamic obesity is not very successful. Once true destruction has occurred, the functional alterations are almost always irreversible. In children with hypothalamic leukemic infiltrates, successful chemotherapy can lead to cessation of hyperphagia and reduction of weight to normal. In general, therapeutic measures are aimed at treatment of the morbidly obese patient.

ANOREXIA NERVOSA. This disorder has been recognized for more than 300 years, is seen almost exclusively in young women, and consists of weight loss, amenorrhea, and behavioral disturbances. See Ch. 215 for a detailed description.

Almost every neuroendocrine system is affected by the disorder. Gonadotropin secretion "regresses" to a prepubertal stage characterized by absence of pulsatile secretion of LH and altered FSH-LH responses to GnRH. GH levels are normal or, at times, elevated, particularly in the presence of severe malnutrition, in which a paradoxic response to glucose may be observed. TSH responses to TRH are reduced, but thyroid function tends to be normal. Plasma cortisol levels are elevated, but diurnal variation is generally preserved. Patients tend to be poikilothermic, exhibiting difficulty in maintaining body temperature in response to changes in the environment. Impaired vasopressin secretion can be demonstrated, but is rarely of clinical importance.

Most of the endocrine metabolic disturbances can be attributed to the severe malnutrition, and successful therapy resulting in weight gain is usually accompanied by restoration of normal neuroendocrine responses. One exception is gonadotropin secretion, which frequently remains abnormal and results in persistence of amenorrhea in up to one third of patients. Another appears to be osmoregulation, which remains discoordinated, with vasopressin being secreted for prolonged periods.

Prognosis for the reversal of cachexia and weight loss is reasonably good. Mortality is currently less than 5 per cent, and the majority of patients return to within 10 per cent of original body weight. Only 40 per cent of patients maintain their weight over a long term; the remainder exhibit moderate to severe weight loss with time.

CENTRAL NERVOUS SYSTEM BEHAVIORAL DISORDERS AFFECTING NEUROENDOCRINE FUNCTION. Disturbances of endocrine function have been observed in patients with a variety of psychiatric illnesses. The association is presumably through disordered neurotransmitter metabolism, although it is still unclear whether the same defect underlies both the behavioral and neuroendocrine dysfunction or whether altered behavior itself secondarily affects neuroendocrine function.

Of all the conditions studied, depressive affective behavior and the manic-depressive state have been most clearly shown to exhibit endocrine changes. Cortisol secretion in depressed patients is enhanced, and they are relatively resistant to dexamethasone suppression. This abnormality reverts to normal with successful treatment. In manic-depressive patients, cortisol secretion tends to be decreased during manic states and elevated during depressive periods.

Brown GM, Koslow SH, Reichlin S (eds.): Neuroendocrinology and Psychiatric Disorder. New York, Raven Press, 1984. *Neuroendocrine disturbances have been detected in many types of behavioral disorders. This excellent book reviews the new insights gained from the large-scale effort to link specific neuroendocrine response alterations with specific psychiatric diagnoses.*

Gold PW, Kaye W, Robertson GL, et al.: Abnormalities in plasma and cerebrospinal fluid arginine vasopressin in patients with anorexia nervosa. N Engl J Med 38:1117, 1983. *A careful investigation of the disturbances in water regulation in patients with anorexia nervosa. Insight is provided into some of the previously recognized features of a mild diabetes insipidus-like state.*

Gold PW, Loriaux DL, Roy A, et al.: Responses to corticotropin-releasing hormone in the hypercortisolism of depression and Cushing's disease. N Engl J Med 314:1329, 1986. Gold PW, Gwirtsman H, Avgerinos PC, et al.: Abnormal hypothalamic-pituitary-adrenal function in anorexia nervosa. N Engl J Med 314:1335, 1986. *The authors have used the CRF stimulation test to uncover specific abnormalities of the hypothalamic-pituitary-adrenal axis in patients with two different psychiatric disorders. The extrapolation of their findings to a generalized disorder of extrahypothalamic CRF is still controversial but, nevertheless, an intriguing possibility.*

Hoffman AR, Crowley WF Jr: Induction of puberty in men by long-term pulsatile administration of low-dose gonadotropin-releasing hormone. N Engl J Med 307:1237, 1982. *Description of the use of pulsatile administration of GnRH to stimulate gonadotropin secretion in subjects with hypogonadotropic hypogonadism. A classic example of the transfer of information from animal physiologic studies to treat human disease.*

Jeffcoate WJ, Laurance BM, Edwards CRW, et al.: Endocrine function in the Prader-Willi syndrome. Clin Endocrinol 12:81, 1980. *A human model of hypothalamic obesity with careful neuroendocrine studies that provide an important characterization of the disorder.*

Lieblich JM, Rogol AD, White BJ, et al.: Syndrome of anosmia with hypogonadism (Kallmann's syndrome). Clinical and laboratory studies in 23 cases. Am J Med 73:506, 1982. *An excellent clinical study of Kallmann's syndrome with detailed endocrine studies very lucidly presented.*

Pescovitz OH, Cutler GB Jr, Loriaux DL: Precocious puberty. In Muller EE, MacLeod RM, Frohman LA (eds.): Neuroendocrine Perspectives. Vol 4. Amsterdam, Elsevier, 1985, pp 73–94. *This is an excellent review of a disorder caused in most patients by premature activation of the neuroendocrine portion of the reproductive system. The use of a GnRH agonist arrests the process by decreasing gonadotropin secretion as a consequence of down-regulation of pituitary GnRH receptors, which forms the basis for therapy of a number of other disorders of reproductive physiology.*

226 THE ANTERIOR PITUITARY
Lawrence A. Frohman

ANATOMY

The pituitary is located in a saddle-shaped cavity, the *sella turcica*, which is an integral portion of the sphenoid bone. Its anterior boundary is the midline *tuberculum sellae* and the anterior clinoid processes that project posteriorly from the sphenoid wings. The posterior limit is the *dorsum sellae*, which projects laterally to form the posterior clinoid processes. The lateral boundaries of the sella are nonosseous and consist of the medial wall of the cavernous sinus, in which is contained the internal carotid artery. The *diaphragma sellae*, a thickened reflection of the *dura mater*, forms the roof of the sella and is attached to the clinoid processes. Only the external layer of the dura extends into the sella as a periosteal lining, and thus the pituitary is normally extradural and not in direct communication with cerebrospinal fluid. The pituitary stalk and its blood vessels pass through a foramen in this membrane that may be incomplete or fenestrated.

The shape of the sella varies from ovoid to spheroid, resulting in considerable variation in normal pituitary dimensions. The average dimensions of the pituitary are 10 mm (anterior-posterior) by 13 mm (transverse) by 6 mm (height). Pituitary weight varies from 0.5 to 0.7 gram, being slightly greater in women. The anterior lobe constitutes about 75 per cent of the total pituitary weight and during pregnancy can increase up to twofold in size.

The arterial blood supply of the pituitary originates from the internal carotid artery via branches from the circle of Willis and hypophyseal arteries. Whereas the posterior lobe is supplied directly by the inferior hypophyseal artery, the blood supply of the anterior lobe is derived entirely from the portal vascular system (see Ch. 225). Venous drainage from the anterior lobe enters the posterior pituitary capillary bed and then the cavernous sinus. The nerve supply of the anterior pituitary consists almost exclusively of postganglionic sympathetic fibers that accompany and terminate on arteriolar vessels. The importance of these fibers in regulating pituitary blood flow is unknown. There are also nerve fibers connecting the posterior and anterior lobes, and their function is also unknown.

EMBRYOLOGY

The glandular portion of the pituitary (*adenohypophysis*) is derived from Rathke's pouch, an ectodermal evagination of the oropharynx that fuses with an outpouching of the region of the third ventricle in the developing embryo. This portion of the diencephalon eventually differentiates into the *neurohypophysis*, or posterior lobe. That portion of Rathke's pouch not in contact with the diencephalon differentiates to form the *pars anterior*, or anterior lobe. Two lateral outgrowths from the anterior lobes fuse in the midline and extend forward along the hypophyseal stalk to form the *pars tuberalis*, which in humans is limited to a small group of cells along the anterior region of the stalk. The portion of Rathke's pouch contiguous with the neurohypophysis develops less extensively and forms the *pars intermedia*, or intermediate lobe. This structure is not well defined in humans and tends to become intermingled with the anterior lobe. This combined structure has been called the *pars distalis*.

Cells of the pars anterior differentiate into cells that secrete growth hormone (GH), prolactin, corticotropin (ACTH), thyroid-stimulating hormone (TSH), luteinizing hormone (LH), and follicle-stimulating hormone (FSH). Cells of the pars intermedia secrete ACTH, lipotropin, and endorphins. Pituitary tumors developing in various regions of the pars distalis tend to reflect the predominant cell types in each region.

The lumen of Rathke's pouch is obliterated during development, although remnants may persist at the boundary of the neurohypophysis as either a cleft or small colloid-filled cysts. The connection with the oropharynx disappears early in development, because of growth of the sphenoid bone, although a few cells in the lower portion of the pouch may persist along the tract, occasionally within the sphenoid bone, and are known as the pharyngeal pituitary. These cells contain secretory granules for GH and prolactin, can be a source of "ectopic" pituitary tumor development, and conceivably could exhibit significant endocrine function subsequent to destruction or removal of the pars distalis.

Pituitary hormones are detected immunochemically as early as the seventh week, and some CNS control of anterior pituitary hormone secretion occurs early in gestation. In contrast, true functional maturation, including aspects of feedback regulation, do not develop until well into postnatal life.

CELL TYPES

The anterior pituitary contains many cell types, the predominant function of which is the synthesis, storage, and release of a specific hormone(s). Immunohistochemical stains have permitted distinction of specific hormone-containing granules, leading to identification of individual cell types.

SOMATOTROPHS. Originally identified as acidophilic cells, these cells secrete GH. Tumors of the cell type lead to acromegaly. The cells are located predominantly in the lateral portions of the anterior lobe.

LACTOTROPHS. Lactotrophs are also acidophilic and secrete prolactin. They tend to be located more peripherally than somatotrophs, and their secretion granules are smaller. During pregnancy and fetal life, lactotrophs are increased in number, reflecting the effects of increased estrogen levels. Virtually all of the increase in pituitary size during pregnancy can be accounted for by lactotroph proliferation. Both lactotrophs and somatotrophs appear to be derived from a common stem cell, tumors of which may secrete both GH and prolactin.

THYROTROPHS. The basophilic staining cells that secrete TSH occur most frequently at the anterior edge of the pituitary near the midline, although they are also present in deeper portions of the gland. Their secretory granules are smaller than GH and prolactin granules and exhibit considerable heterogeneity. Under normal conditions, thyrotrophs constitute only about 6 per cent of anterior lobe cells. In primary hypothyroidism they undergo marked hypertrophy and exhibit changes indicative of increased secretory activity.

GONADOTROPHS. These cells are located deep in the lateral portion of the gland in association with lactotrophs and secrete both LH and FSH. Although constituting only 3 to 4 per cent of anterior pituitary cells normally, they increase in number following castration and decrease during pregnancy as a result of placental gonadotropin production.

CORTICOTROPHS. Cells of this type, which can exhibit chromophobic or basophilic characteristics, are found in two separate locations. One group of cells resides most commonly in the medial mucoid region of the anterior lobe. A second group migrates during development to the junctional region of the anterior and posterior lobes and also to the pars tuberalis. Anterior lobe corticotrophs exhibit sparse granulation, whereas those in the pars tuberalis–posterior lobe region contain large and electron-dense granules. The same precursor molecule is present in both cell types, although processing enzyme activity varies, resulting in different ratios of hormones derived from the precursor (ACTH, melanocyte-stimulating hormone [MSH], lipotropins, and endorphins) in the two different regions. Increases in glucocorticoid levels produce degranulation and microtubular hyalinization of corticotrophs (Crooke's changes). Anterior lobe corticotrophs increase in number with glucocorticoid deficiency, while those in the intermediate-posterior lobe region decrease, suggesting that only the former are physiologically important ACTH-secreting cells.

OTHER CELL TYPES. As many as 15 to 20 per cent of anterior pituitary cells cannot be stained by antibodies to any of the recognized anterior pituitary hormones. Some of these may represent resting degranulated cells or undifferentiated primitive secretory cells. However, some may be responsible for the secretion of other as yet uncharacterized pituitary hormones such as tissue-specific growth factors. In addition, a few cells are stellate, with cellular processes extending into the perivascular spaces in a manner suggestive of primitive follicle formation. These cells generally do not contain secretory granules, and their function is unknown.

ANTERIOR PITUITARY HORMONES

The anterior pituitary secretes six well-recognized hormones for which specific and sensitive radioimmunoassays are available. They can be divided into three general categories: corticotropin and related peptides, glycoprotein hormones, and somatomammotropin hormones. The chemical characteristics of these hormones are given in Table 226–1.

CORTICOTROPIN-RELATED PEPTIDES. ACTH and its related family of peptides are synthesized as a single precursor molecule, pro-opiomelanocortin, with a molecular weight of approximately 29,000. Following glycosylation, the molecule is differentially cleaved into an NH_2-terminal fragment, the biologic activity of which remains uncertain; a midportion, which contains ACTH; and a COOH-terminal portion, beta-lipotropin (LPH). Subsequent processing, which varies in the different groups of corticotrophs and also in the brain, may also cleave ACTH into alpha-MSH and corticotropin-like intermediate lobe peptide. Beta-LPH is also differentially processed further to beta-endorphin and other endorphin-related peptides (see Ch. 225). Although the structures of beta-MSH and met-enkephalin are contained within the beta-LPH sequence, the former is not synthesized in postnatal human pituitaries, and the biosynthesis of the latter occurs through a separate precursor.

ACTH. The primary effects of ACTH are stimulation of secretion of glucocorticoid, mineralocorticoid, and androgenic steroids by the adrenal cortex. ACTH binds to specific receptors on adrenocortical cell membranes and stimulates steroidogenesis by enhancing cholesterol conversion to pregnenolone. ACTH also stimulates adrenal protein synthesis, leading to cellular growth and hyperplasia.

Extra-adrenal effects of ACTH include stimulation of lipolysis in adipose tissue, insulin-releasing effects on the pancreatic B cell, stimulation of GH secretion, enhancement of glucose and amino acid transport into muscles, and prolongation of cortisol half-life in plasma. Except in patients with ACTH-secreting tumors, it is unlikely that plasma ACTH levels sufficient to produce these effects are ever achieved. Although ACTH has less potent pigmenting effects than alpha-MSH or beta-MSH, it has long been considered the major pigmenting hormone in man. Recent studies, however, have indicated control of pigmentation to be a complex process, and the importance of ACTH has come under question.

ACTH is the most difficult of the pituitary hormones to measure, and plasma levels exhibit the greatest variability, in part because of its episodic secretion. Plasma ACTH levels in normal adults range from undetectable to 80 pg per milliliter (the lower limit of detection in most assays is approximately 10 pg per milliliter). In addition to its episodic secretion, a diurnal rhythm can be detected with lowest levels in the evening and peak levels in the early morning. Changes in plasma ACTH levels can be shown to precede those of plasma cortisol with a short lag period. With stress, plasma ACTH levels can reach several hundred picograms per milliliter. In patients with ectopic ACTH production, immunoreactive ACTH levels may be exceedingly high and consist in part of larger molecular sized forms ("big" ACTH) believed to represent partially processed but biologically inactive precursor molecules. ACTH is rapidly eliminated from plasma; its half-life is 3 to 9 minutes, leading to an estimated secretion rate of 25 μg per day, which represents approximately 5 per cent of pituitary hormone content.

Beta-LPH, Endorphins, and Related Peptides. Beta-LPH and beta-endorphin are secreted in an equimolar ratio to ACTH in response to all types of stimulation. The presence of both molecules in the same precursor as ACTH, with enzymatic cleavage immediately prior to or concomitant with the secretory process, provides an explanation for this observation. The plasma levels of beta-LPH and beta-endorphin, however, do not necessarily parallel those of ACTH because of slower metabolic clearance rates. Beta-LPH is cleared primarily by the kidneys, and its levels rise disproportionately to those of ACTH in renal failure. Since ACTH secretion is normal in this disorder, beta-LPH must exert relatively little feedback effect on its own secretion or that of ACTH. Beta-LPH and beta-

TABLE 226–1. ANTERIOR PITUITARY HORMONES IN HUMANS

Class	Members	Molecular Weight	Amino Acids	Carbohydrate	Other Features
Corticotropin-lipotropin	ACTH	4,500	39		All members of class derived from a single precursor
	α-MSH	1,800	13		N-terminal 13 amino acids of ACTH. In humans, found only in fetal life and in tumors
	β-Lipotropin	11,200	91		
	β-Endorphin	4,000	31		C-terminal (amino acids 61–91) portion of β-LPH
Glycoprotein	LH	29,000	α subunit: 89 β subunit: 115	1% sialic acid	All have two subunits, with the α subunit being identical or nearly identical and the β subunit conferring biologic specificity
	FSH	29,000	α subunit: 89 β subunit: 115	5% sialic acid	
	TSH	29,000	α subunit: 89 β subunit: 112	1% sialic acid	
	Chorionic gonadotropin*	46,000	α subunit: 92 β subunit: 139	12% sialic acid	
Somatomammotropin	Growth hormone	21,800	191		All single-chain proteins with two or three disulfide bridges
	Prolactin	22,500	198	†	
	Placental lactogen*	21,800	191		

Adapted from Frohman LA: Diseases of the anterior pituitary. In Felig P, Baxter JD, Broadus AE, Frohman LA (eds.): Endocrinology and Metabolism. 2nd ed. New York, McGraw-Hill Book Company, 1987.
*Of placental origin and included for comparison purposes.
†Carbohydrate-containing forms of prolactin have recently been identified.

endorphin have not been shown to have any effects peripherally at the levels normally seen in plasma.

GLYCOPROTEIN HORMONES. The pituitary glycoprotein hormones consist of an alpha and beta subunit, each containing a peptide core with branched carbohydrate side chains that are required for biologic activity and for stability in plasma. The alpha subunits of the glycoprotein hormones are identical, whereas the beta subunits vary, thereby providing the biologic specificity of each hormone. There is considerable homology between beta subunits of the different hormones as well as cross-species homology of both alpha and beta subunits, which explains why bovine or ovine glycoprotein hormones are active in humans. The isolated subunits have no intrinsic biologic activity. Evidence of hormone heterogeneity, related to the degree of glycosylation, has been detected and may explain the reported variations in glycoprotein bioactivity at different times in the menstrual cycle. The individual subunits are synthesized separately, and the rate-limiting step in glycoprotein hormone secretion is controlled by beta subunit production. Elevations in plasma alpha subunit levels can be seen after both TRH and GnRH stimulation and occasionally in pituitary tumors.

TSH. TSH effects on the thyroid cells are largely analogous to those of ACTH on the adrenal cortex. High-affinity receptors are present on cell membranes, and TSH binding leads to activation of adenylate cyclase, enhanced iodine transport and binding to protein, increased thyroglobulin and thyroid hormone synthesis, and increased thyroglobulin proteolysis with release of thyroid hormones. RNA and protein synthesis are also stimulated, leading to an increase in thyroid size and vascularity.

TSH is measured by a specific assay utilizing an antibody directed to antigenic determinants on the beta subunit that exhibit little or no cross-reactivity with other glycoprotein hormones. Normal levels of plasma TSH are generally reported as under 6 μU per milliliter, with most assays being unable to detect levels less than 1 μU per milliliter. Some of the more recently developed assays appear to have greater sensitivity and specificity, resulting in an upper limit of 3 μU per milliliter and the ability to discriminate normal from low levels. In primary hypothyroidism, TSH levels may increase to greater than 100 μU per milliliter. A few patients have been described with hypothyroidism and slightly elevated TSH levels in whom administration of thyrotropin releasing hormone (TRH) results in an exaggerated TSH increase and a concomitant increase in thyroxine. Evidence for a biologically less potent TSH has been found in such individuals. TSH is cleared from circulation with a half-life of 75 to 80 minutes, and the secretion rate of the hormone is 100 to 200 mU per day. In hypothyroidism, secretion rates may be increased 10 to 15 times that in normals.

LH and FSH. Gonadal function is regulated by two pituitary hormones: (1) FSH, which stimulates ovarian follicular growth, testicular growth, and spermatogenesis, and (2) LH, which promotes ovulation and follicular luteinization, stimulates testicular interstitial cell function, and enhances production of steroids in both ovary and testis. In the ovary, FSH promotes growth and maturation of the primordial follicle cell, and LH stimulates progesterone production by the corpus luteum by enhancing the conversion of cholesterol to pregnenolone. In the testis, FSH acts on the Sertoli cell, where, in conjunction with testosterone, the production of an androgen-binding protein is stimulated. The target cell of LH is the Leydig cell, leading to enhanced testosterone production. The androgen binding protein serves to transport testosterone in high concentrations into tubular cells to stimulate spermatogenesis. (See also discussion in Ch. 235.)

The gonadotropin assays exhibit a slight degree of cross-reactivity between the hormone and its subunits, though this is not a practical problem. Of importance, however, is the cross-reactivity due to the great similarity between LH and chorionic gonadotropin. Most LH assays do not discriminate between the two hormones.

Plasma levels of FSH and LH in women vary with the menstrual cycle. FSH levels rise slightly and then decline progressively during the early follicular phase of the cycle, during which time LH levels are generally stable or rise slightly. An abrupt rise in LH at midcycle, initiated by increasing estrogen secretion by the developing follicle and accompanied by an FSH rise, triggers ovulation. Both hormone levels decline during the luteal phase. Levels of FSH and LH in males are similar to those in females during the follicular phase. FSH and LH levels increase in response to age-related decreases in gonadal function in both sexes. In women this occurs at menopause, and in men a gradual increase is seen during the sixth to eighth decades. The half-life of LH in circulation is approximately 30 minutes, whereas that of FSH is twice as long, the difference being attributed to the varying sialic acid content of the hormones.

SOMATOMAMMOTROPIC HORMONES. This hormonal class consists of GH, prolactin, and a structurally similar placental hormone, chorionic somatomammotropin, or placental lactogen. Extensive interspecies homology exists for both GH and prolactin, suggesting relatively limited changes in gene duplication during evolution. Despite the similarity, subprimate growth hormones are biologically inactive in humans. GH and placental lactogen exhibit 83 per cent homology, in contrast to only 16 per cent homology between GH and prolactin. Despite these differences, each hormone has both intrinsic lactogenic and growth-promoting activity. Large-molecular-weight–sized hormones ("big" GH and prolactin) have been identified in both pituitary and plasma. The big hormones appear to be dimers connected by interchain disulfide linkages. They are secreted by the pituitary, bind to the hormone target cell receptors, and exhibit reduced biologic activity as compared to the monomer. There are four or five additional GH variants, including proteolytically modified forms, electrophoretic variants, and a smaller molecule ("20K variant") lacking amino acids 32 to 46, which is encoded by a separate mRNA species derived from the authentic GH gene and formed by differential splicing of pre-mRNA to mRNA. This variant, while representing 10 per cent of pituitary GH, constitutes less than 5 per cent of secreted GH, and levels in circulation do not change in response to GH secretagogues. It appears to have the same biologic effects as 22K GH, with the possible exception of reduced diabetogenic activity.

Growth Hormone. GH exhibits an important role in production of linear growth and regulation of metabolic processes. GH administration to GH-deficient patients results in positive nitrogen balance, decreased urea production, decreased body fat stores, and enhanced carbohydrate utilization. Biphasic effects on circulating glucose, amino acid, and free fatty acid levels occur in response to GH with an initial decrease and subsequent return to normal or an increase. The acute effects of GH in isolated tissues resemble those of insulin and include increased amino acid uptake and incorporation into protein, stimulation of new RNA synthesis, and enhanced glucose utilization. GH also antagonizes the lipolytic effect of catecholamines in adipose tissue. These acute effects disappear within three to four hours, by which time a series of delayed effects appears. These include enhanced triglyceride lipolysis, increased sensitivity to catecholamine-mediated lipolysis, and inhibition of glucose uptake and utilization secondary to impaired pyruvate decarboxylation. These effects form the basis of the diabetogenic action of the hormone. GH also exhibits multiphasic effects on insulin secretion. There is an acute direct stimulatory effect on the beta cell, a subsequent inhibitory effect, and a late and persistent stimulation of insulin release that occurs secondary to the impairment of carbohydrate utilization. The last effect has the greatest pathophysiologic significance in the development of diabetes secondary to GH hypersecretion.

Many GH effects cannot be produced by acute exposure of tissues to the hormone and are mediated by a group of GH-dependent growth factors that are synthesized in numerous tissues. GH binds to specific cell-membrane receptors to stimulate their production. The most important of these factors is somatomedin C or insulin-like growth factor I (IGF-I), a peptide of about 7500 daltons that has many similarities to insulin, including structural resemblance to proinsulin and binding to insulin receptors. Somatomedin C receptors are present in many tissues, including cartilage, where sulfate incorporation into proteoglycan and amino acid uptake incorporation are stimulated. The importance of IGF-I in the growth-promoting effects of GH is illustrated by the Laron dwarf in whom impairment of GH stimulation of IGF-I production results in severe growth retardation. Although the question whether IGF-I is synthesized in the same cell in which it acts (autocrine) or in neighboring cells (paracrine) is unsettled, it is now widely regarded as a GH second messenger rather than as a true hormone. Thus, while circulating IGF-I levels are a measure of GH secretion, they most likely reflect local IGF-I production rather than serving as a source for tissue uptake. It is currently believed that cell differentiation and growth require both GH and IGF-I, with GH serving to commit a precursor cell to a specific pathway of differentiation and IGF-I enhancing growth and replication. Other growth factors, such as IGF-II platelet-derived growth factor and epidermal growth factor, do not appear to be GH dependent. GH also stimulates cardiac and renal hypertrophy and production of specific hormones such as renin and aldosterone and conversion of thyroxine to triiodothyronine.

Immunoreactive measurements of GH are considered valid indicators of GH bioactivity. Mean GH levels during adolescence and adult life are generally less than 3 ng per milliliter, although the spontaneous secretory pulses of GH can produce elevations as great as 30 to 50 ng per milliliter in young adult subjects. Levels in women during the childbearing age are generally greater than in men, particularly in response to exercise or other stimuli. GH is cleared from plasma primarily by the liver and to a lesser extent by the kidney. The half-time of GH disappearance from circulation is 20 minutes, and the overall secretion in normal adults ranges from 300 to 500 µg per square meter per day.

Prolactin. The major effect of prolactin is to stimulate the synthesis of milk constituents, including lactalbumin, casein, lipids, and carbohydrates (see Ch. 239). Prolactin receptors are present on alveolar surfaces of mammary cells and, in addition, have been identified in liver and kidney. Prolactin is not required for normal breast development in humans, and pathologic elevations of the hormone are not generally associated with an increase in breast size. During pregnancy, prolactin, in conjunction with estrogen, progesterone, and placental lactogen, results in further breast development and milk formation. Following parturition, the abrupt decrease in estrogen and progesterone derived from the placenta permits initiation of lactation. This effect underlies the use of estrogens to inhibit lactation in the postpartum period and explains the frequent development of galactorrhea in hyperprolactinemic women after discontinuance of oral contraceptives. Continued prolactin secretion is required to maintain lactation once it is initiated, and the return of prolactin to normal levels in the postpartum period is delayed in women who nurse for prolonged periods. The actual milk let-down reflex is mediated by the release of oxytocin in the posterior pituitary rather than by prolactin. Oxytocin stimulates contraction of myoepithelial cells surrounding the terminal acinar lobules that expel their milk into the lobular ducts. Although prolactin has numerous effects on behavior and on fluid and electrolyte metabolism in lower species, no such effects have been convincingly demonstrated in humans.

Normal prolactin levels do not exceed 15 ng per milliliter in men or 20 ng per milliliter in women. There are no significant changes during the menstrual cycle, but levels decrease at menopause. During pregnancy, prolactin levels rise continuously from early gestation to values of 150 to 200 ng per milliliter at term. Prolactin is cleared from circulation with a half-time of approximately 50 minutes. The liver and, to a lesser extent, the kidney are the major sites of prolactin removal.

TESTS OF ANTERIOR PITUITARY HORMONE FUNCTION

ACTH. Since ACTH levels in normal subjects may be undetectable at times, random measurements of the hormone are of limited value. In a patient with signs and symptoms of adrenocortical insufficiency and low plasma cortisol levels, a low or even normal ACTH level is suggestive of hypothalamic-pituitary disease. The most useful test for evaluating ACTH function is that of insulin hypoglycemia. A dose of insulin calculated to decrease the fasting blood glucose to 40 mg per deciliter is administered, and plasma cortisol levels are measured over a two-hour period. A rise greater than 10 µg per deciliter or a peak level greater than 20 µg per deciliter is indicative of a normal hypothalamic-pituitary-adrenal axis. The standard dose of insulin is 0.1 U per kilogram (intravenously), although the dose should be decreased by 50 per cent when the diagnosis of hypopituitarism is strongly suspected and increased by 50 per cent in patients with anticipated insulin resistance (i.e., obesity). No treatment is necessary for mild symptoms of hypoglycemia (catecholamine-mediated phenomena), but symptoms of central glucopenia (impaired mentation or altered states of consciousness) require immediate therapy. This test must not be performed in patients with suspected primary adrenal insufficiency.

Corticotropin releasing factor (CRF) is currently being evaluated as a diagnostic agent for assessing ACTH function and, when available for general use, is expected to provide a valuable adjunct. A normal response to CRF and an impaired response to insulin hypoglycemia, for example, would suggest hypothalamic rather than pituitary disease. Impairment of normal cortisol feedback using metyrapone, an 11β-hydroxylase inhibitor, at a dose of 750 mg orally every four hours for six doses, with measurement of plasma 11-desoxycortisol or urinary 17-hydroxycorticoids, is an alternative way to test the entire hypothalamic-pituitary-adrenal axis. This test is less useful than insulin hypoglycemia in predicting normal responsiveness of the axis to stress.

The best test of suspected excessive ACTH and cortisol secretion is by dexamethasone suppression. The rapid dexamethasone suppression test involves administration of 1 mg dexamethasone orally at 11 P.M. and measurement of plasma cortisol at 8 o'clock the following morning. A level of less than 5 µg per deciliter indicates normal suppressibility. In patients in whom normal suppression is not demonstrated, a standard low-dose dexamethasone suppression test (0.5 mg orally every six hours for 48 hours) is performed. Plasma cortisol will be suppressed to less than 5 µg per deciliter, and urinary free cortisol levels will be suppressed to less than 20 µg per 24 hours in normal subjects but not in patients with pituitary ACTH hypersecretion or primary adrenocortical hypersecretion. In patients in whom suppression fails, a high-dose dexamethasone suppression test (2 mg orally every six hours for 48 hours) is then used to distinguish between pituitary and adrenal causes.

TSH. Impairment of TSH secretion should be suspected in patients with hypothyroidism in whom plasma TSH levels are not elevated. Differentiation of pituitary from hypothalamic causes of TSH deficiency can usually, but not always, be accomplished by administering TRH, 500 µg (intravenously), and measuring plasma TSH levels. In normal persons, plasma TSH increases to at least 8 µU per milliliter after TRH administration, and peak levels usually occur at 15 to 30 minutes. In patients with hypothalamic hypothyroidism, the response may be exaggerated and is frequently prolonged, with peak values occurring at 90 to 180 minutes. Since thyroxine impairs the TSH response to TRH, it is not possible to assess TSH function in patients receiving thyroid hormone replacement therapy until at least a month after discontinuation of medication.

LH AND FSH. LH and FSH deficiency should be suspected in patients with clinical evidence of hypogonadism and subnormal testosterone or estradiol levels in whom gonadotropin levels are not elevated. An increase of at least three- to fivefold in LH is seen in normal subjects. A single injection, however, may not distinguish between hypothalamic and hypopituitary causes, since impaired responses may be seen in both disorders and only after repeated injections does a response occur in patients with hypothalamic hypogonadism. Clomiphene, an estrogen antagonist, will stimulate gonadotropin levels in some patients with hypothalamic hypogonadism.

GROWTH HORMONE. The most frequently employed stimulus for GH secretion is insulin hypoglycemia. The details of testing and the cautions required are as described under ACTH testing. Peak growth hormone levels usually occur at 60 or 90 minutes, and a peak level of 9 ng per milliliter or greater is required for a normal response. Up to 30 per cent of normal subjects may not respond to insulin hypoglycemia. L-arginine (0.5 gram per kilogram intravenously during a 30-minute period), L-dopa (0.5 gram orally), and clonidine (25 μg orally) are other effective stimuli used to test GH secretory reserve. The responses are comparable in magnitude to those after insulin. Although other stimuli have been used (glucagon plus propranolol, endotoxin, vasopressin, ACTH), none has any advantage over those described. Although still investigational, GRH appears to be useful in distinguishing between hypothalamic and pituitary causes for GH deficiency in some patients. Lack of an adequate GH response, however, may also be due to excessive somatostatin secretion.

Suppressibility of GH secretion in patients with elevated GH levels is evaluated with a standard glucose tolerance test. A decrease in GH levels to less than 2 ng per milliliter is seen in normal subjects. TRH is also used in distinguishing between types of suspected GH hypersecretion. TRH has no effect on GH levels in normal subjects, whereas in 80 to 90 per cent of patients with acromegaly a rapid increase in GH levels occurs.

PROLACTIN. Impaired prolactin secretion is rarely a clinical problem. Prolactin deficiency should be suspected in patients with levels of less than 2 ng per milliliter, and the diagnosis is confirmed by the absence of a response to TRH. Elevated prolactin levels in nearly all patients, with the exception of occasional patients with prolactin-secreting tumors and patients with chronic renal failure, can be suppressed by dopamine infusions, L-dopa, or other dopaminergic agents. These tests have limited usefulness in determining the cause of hyperprolactinemia and are generally not used.

Chrousos GP, Schuermeyer TH, Doppman J, et al.: Clinical applications of corticotropin-releasing factor. Ann Intern Med 102:344, 1985. *An excellent clinical discussion of the role of CRF in diagnosis of pituitary-adrenal disease.*

Ezrin C, Horvath E, Kovacs K: Anatomy and cytology of the normal and abnormal pituitary gland. In DeGroot LJ, Cahill GF Jr, Martini L, et al. (eds.): Endocrinology. Vol 1. New York, Grune & Stratton, 1979, pp 103–121. *A well-organized and referenced presentation of pituitary structure with emphasis on the changes in human disease.*

Frohman LA: Diseases of the anterior pituitary. In Felig P, Baxter JD, Broadus E, et al. (eds.): Endocrinology and Metabolism. 2nd ed. New York, McGraw-Hill Book Company, 1987, pp 247–338. *A detailed systematic description of the chemistry, physiology, and pathophysiology of the pituitary. Of particular use to the clinical trainee and practicing physician.*

Frohman LA, Jansson J-O: Growth hormone-releasing hormone. Endocr Rev 7:223, 1986. *A review of basic and clinical aspects of GRH, its use as a diagnostic and therapeutic agent, and disorders of GRH secretion.*

Jaffe RB, Monroe SE: Hormone interaction and regulation during the menstrual cycle. In Ganong WF, Martini L (eds.): Frontiers in Neuroendocrinology. Vol 6. New York, Raven Press, 1980, pp 219–248. *A comprehensive review of hormonal interactions responsible for the cyclical reproductive cycle in women. Provides a firm basis with which to understand pathophysiologic conditions.*

Kolesnick RN, Gershengorn MG: Thyrotropin-releasing hormone and the pituitary. New insights into the mechanism of stimulated secretion and clinical usage. Am J Med 79:719, 1985. *An excellent, readable review of basic and clinical aspects of TRH effects on the pituitary.*

Peters JR, Foord SM, Dieguez C, et al.: TSH neuroregulation and alterations in disease states. Clin Endocrinol Metab 12:669, 1983. *A comprehensive review of the regulation of TSH secretion stressing the interaction of neurotransmitters, TRH, and thyroid hormones.*

Raiti S, Tolman RA (eds.): Human Growth Hormone. New York, Plenum Medical, 1986, pp 1–662. *A review of basic and clinical aspects of growth hormone with emphasis on regulation of secretion and mechanism of action.*

Sheldon W Jr, DeBold CR, Evans WS, et al.: Rapid sequential intravenous administration of four hypothalamic releasing hormones as a combined anterior pituitary function test in normal subjects. J Clin Endocrinol Metab 60:623, 1985. *Description of a rapid, simple, and safe method of testing pituitary hormone secretory reserve.*

HYPOPITUITARISM

DISEASE STATES ASSOCIATED WITH HYPOPITUITARISM (Table 226–2). The subject's age, rapidity of onset of the disorder, and the extent of impaired hormone secretion as well as the specific pathologic process all influence the clinical manifestations. When acute and complete, the disease can be life threatening, but in a mild form it can remain undetected for many years. Hypopituitarism can occur as a result of a *primary* disorder due to absence or destruction of anterior pituitary cells or *secondary* to CNS disease. In the latter, pituitary hormone deficiency occurs because of a lack of appropriate releasing hormones.

The classic example of *primary hypopituitarism* is ischemic postpartum pituitary necrosis, first associated with the clinical features of hypopituitarism by Simmonds and characterized by Sheehan. The mechanism of acute ischemic necrosis is believed to relate to vasospasm of hypophyseal vessels, possibly influenced by estrogen-induced sensitivity to the vasoconstrictive stimulus of hypoxia. This disorder occurs most

TABLE 226–2. ETIOLOGY OF HYPOPITUITARISM

A. Primary
    Pituitary tumors
        Primary intrasellar (chromophobe adenoma, craniopharyngioma)
        Parasellar (meningioma, optic nerve glioma)
    Ischemic necrosis of the pituitary
        Postpartum (Sheehan's syndrome)
        Diabetes mellitus
        Other systemic diseases (temporal arteritis, sickle-cell disease and trait, arteriosclerosis, eclampsia)
    Aneurysm of intracranial internal carotid artery
    Pituitary apoplexy (almost always related to a primary pituitary tumor)
    Cavernous sinus thrombosis
    Infectious disease (tuberculosis, syphilis, malaria, meningitis, fungal disease)
    Infiltrative disease (hemochromatosis)
    Immunologic (granulomatous or lymphocytic hypophysitis)
    Iatrogenic
        Irradiation to nasopharynx
        Irradiation to sella
        Surgical destruction
    Primary empty sella syndrome
    Metabolic disorders (chronic renal failure)
    Idiopathic (frequently monohormonal and occasionally familial)

B. Secondary
    Destruction of pituitary stalk
        Trauma
        Compression by tumor or aneurysm
        Iatrogenic (surgical)
    Hypothalamic or other central nervous system disease
        Inflammatory (sarcoidosis)
        Infiltrative (lipid storage diseases)
        Trauma
        Toxic (vincristine)
        Hormone induced (glucocorticoids, gonadal steroids)
        Tumors (primary, metastatic, lymphomas, leukemia)
        Idiopathic (frequently congenital or familial, often restricted to one or two hormones, and may be reversible)
        Nutritional (starvation, obesity)
        Anorexia nervosa
        Psychosocial dwarfism

Adapted from Frohman LA: Diseases of the anterior pituitary. In Felig P, Baxter JD, Broadus AE, Frohman LA (eds.): Endocrinology and Metabolism. 2nd ed. New York, McGraw-Hill Book Company, 1987.

frequently in the immediate postpartum period and is associated with severe hemorrhage and hypotension. Some degree of hypopituitarism occurs in up to one third of women experiencing severe hemorrhage during delivery. The disorder is recognized by absence of lactation in the postpartum period and failure of normal cyclic menstruation to resume. Because of the slowly progressive nature of this disease the presence of postpartum lactation does not preclude development of the disorder at a later time. Since complete hypopituitarism requires at least 90 per cent destruction of the pituitary, the diagnosis may never be made in many patients with pituitary necrosis and minimal evidence of hypopituitarism. The disease is currently much less common than previously, because of the marked improvement in obstetric care during the past half century. Ischemic pituitary necrosis can be seen with other disorders, though much less commonly.

The most common cause of hypopituitarism is a pituitary tumor (discussed in the following section). Other parasellar mass lesions, including CNS tumors and internal carotid aneurysms, can also invade the sella and destroy the pituitary. Intrapituitary hemorrhage (*pituitary apoplexy*) associated with pituitary tumors may produce varying degrees of hypopituitarism. If bleeding occurs gradually, the pituitary is compressed and symptoms of hypopituitarism predominate. If the hemorrhage is sudden, presenting symptoms include headache, visual field defects or blindness, ophthalmoplegia, and subarachnoid irritation. Furthermore, a pre-existing pituitary tumor may suddenly expand. Immediate glucocorticoid therapy is essential in such patients. Most will recover without the need for surgical intervention, but it may be necessary in some to restore visual function.

Radiation therapy for treatment of malignant tumors of the head and neck frequently causes primary or secondary hypopituitarism. Growth disturbances are the most common manifestations in children, whereas hypogonadism is more common in adults. Hypopituitarism may occur within 6 to 12 months after a dose of 3000 rads or greater, and children appear to be more susceptible than adults. The disorder may not appear until several years following irradiation. Lymphocytic hypopituitarism, a recently recognized disorder, tends to occur in the postpartum period and may present as an expanding pituitary mass lesion associated with hypopituitarism (and occasionally hyperprolactinemia). Destruction of pituitary tissue with lymphocyte infiltration has been found histologically, but the cause is unknown. Hypopituitarism may occur without detectable underlying disease and may be limited to one or two hormones rather than involving all of them. There are reports of both autosomal and X-linked recessive varieties of the disease. Partial hypopituitarism also occurs in patients with chronic renal failure and is reversible after renal transplantation.

Secondary hypopituitarism can be caused by diverse CNS disorders, all of which disrupt the delivery of releasing factors to the pituitary. The distinction between CNS and pituitary causes can frequently, but not always, be made on the basis of responses to the hypothalamic releasing hormones. Diseases of the pituitary stalk are most frequently due to trauma. Basilar skull fractures often shear the stalk, rupturing both neural and vascular connections. Parasellar tumors and aneurysms can compress the stalk sufficiently to impair blood flow to portal vessels. Disorders of the CNS, primarily the hypothalamus, that impair releasing hormone secretion are described in Ch. 225.

CLINICAL FEATURES. In the most dramatic form of hypopituitarism, panhypopituitarism occurring after surgical hypophysectomy, severe pituitary apoplexy, or withdrawal of hormone therapy, clinical features are noted within a few hours (diabetes insipidus) to a few days (adrenal insufficiency). In partial hypopituitarism the signs and symptoms develop slowly and may be vague and nonspecific. The clinical features are best considered in terms of the deficiencies of individual pituitary hormones.

Hormone-specific Features. ACTH. Manifestations of ACTH deficiency are similar to those of adrenocortical deficiency. Weakness, postural hypotension, malaise, dehydration, and cold intolerance are common, though a true addisonian crisis is infrequent because some aldosterone secretion is maintained through the renin-angiotensin mechanism, which is independent of ACTH. Nausea, vomiting, and severe hypothermia can occur, and hypoglycemia associated with prolonged fasting or alcohol ingestion may be seen as a result of impaired gluconeogenesis. In contrast to Addison's disease, in which hyperpigmentation occurs, patients with ACTH deficiency frequently exhibit depigmentation and decreased tanning after exposure to sunlight. If ACTH secretion is only partially impaired, symptoms may be experienced only during periods of stress. Adrenal androgen deficiency occurs and contributes to decreased libido and to loss of axillary and pubic hair in women. In men the deficiency is of little consequence if testicular function is preserved.

TSH. The features of primary and secondary TSH deficiency are quite similar with the exception of severity. Patients experience cold intolerance, dry skin, pallor, mental slowing, bradycardia, hoarseness, and constipation. True myxedema and hypercholesterolemia are seen only infrequently. Menstrual flow may be increased or more likely decreased because of associated gonadotropin deficiency. During childhood, TSH deficiency results in growth retardation that is unresponsive to GH treatment.

LH AND FSH. In women, gonadotropin deficiency results in amenorrhea and signs of estrogen deficiency, including breast atrophy, skin dryness, decreased vaginal secretions, and, occasionally, decreased libido. In males, the testes decrease in size and become softened. Decreased androgen production results in a loss of libido and potency, decreased rate of growth of secondary sexual hair, and reduced muscular strength. If the deficiency occurs prior to puberty there is total or partial impairment of secondary sexual development. If GH secretion is unaltered, failure of sex steroid–induced epiphyseal closure of the long bones produces excessive growth of limbs, leading to a eunuchoid appearance.

GROWTH HORMONE. GH deficiency in the adult is unassociated with clinically recognized symptoms. Carbohydrate tolerance is impaired in GH-deficient subjects, but this disorder is distinct from diabetes mellitus and is not associated with microangiopathy. In children, GH deficiency results in growth retardation. Fasting hypoglycemia is often seen, particularly when ACTH deficiency is also present.

PROLACTIN. Prolactin deficiency results only in the absence of postpartum lactation.

VASOPRESSIN. Deficiency of vasopressin results in diabetes insipidus, described in detail in Ch. 227. The impairment of water reabsorption by the kidneys results in polyuria and polydipsia, and, if fluid intake is not maintained, severe dehydration. Extreme thirst may be present that is preferentially relieved by ice water. Polyuria may not be present when ACTH deficiency coexists because of the requirement of cortisol for free water excretion. The appearance of polyuria during ACTH or glucocorticoid administration is highly suggestive of a combined vasopressin and ACTH deficiency.

OXYTOCIN. Oxytocin deficiency is unassociated with any clinically apparent disease in humans. In particular, in women with panhypopituitarism who become pregnant, initiation of labor is normal, as is parturition.

General Clinical Features. The skin of hypopituitary patients often exhibits decreased turgor and a waxy character. Perioral and periorbital wrinkling is common, giving the appearance of premature aging. Nutrition, in general, is quite well preserved. Moderate anemia commonly occurs; it is usually normochromic and normocytic, but it may be hypochromic or macrocytic and is attributed to a combination of thyroid, testosterone, and erythropoietin deficiencies. Mental slowing and apathy are quite common, as are other psychiatric symptoms, including delusions and occasionally paranoid psychosis. Carbohydrate metabolism is generally intact in nondiabetics, but in insulin-requiring diabetics, hypopituitarism necessitates reduction of insulin dosage, frequently to less than half of the original level; there is also an increased tendency for hypoglycemic reactions. These changes may persist even with full glucocorticoid replacement therapy.

The sequence of pituitary hormone loss varies among patients with hypopotuitarism. In general, deficiencies of GH and gonadotropins are the earliest to occur and thus the most frequently observed. ACTH and TSH deficiencies are less common and are seen at a later stage in the natural history of the disease. The pattern, however, is not predictable in individual patients, thus precluding the usefulness of evaluating pituitary function by measurement of only one or two hormones.

DIFFERENTIAL DIAGNOSIS. The major categories of diseases with which hypopituitarism can be confused include (1) disorders of multiple target glands or of the CNS and (2) diseases that share the generalized features of hypopituitarism that are unassociated with endocrine dysfunction.

While measurement of pituitary hormones is indispensable in the differential diagnosis, certain clinical features have discriminatory value. Primary adrenal insufficiency is associated with hyperkalemia, hyperpigmentation, and salt craving, all of which are absent in hypopituitarism. Some patients with primary gonadal failure exhibit a discrepancy between the loss of gonadal steroid production and the loss of spermatogenesis or ovulation. Both components of gonadal function are diminished to the same extent in hypopituitarism. Primary ovarian failure often results in characteristic symptoms (hot flashes) that are usually not seen when ovarian failure is secondary to gonadotropin deficiency.

Patients with chronic malnutrition or liver disease exhibit weakness, lethargy, cold intolerance, and decreased libido, frequently raising the possibility of hypopituitarism. The presence of cachexia is important in suggesting a nonpituitary disease. Although anorexia nervosa may often be confused with hypopituitarism, the severe weight loss, psychiatric symptoms, and preservation of axillary and pubic hair are all useful discriminating factors (see Ch. 215).

DIAGNOSIS. The diagnosis of hypopituitarism should be carefully and appropriately established since therapeutic decisions imply lifelong hormonal replacement therapy. In addition, studies directed at determining the etiology of the hypopituitarism (neuroanatomic studies) are an integral part of the workup and are discussed in the section on pituitary tumors.

Functional studies of each of the anterior pituitary hormones have been described in the previous section, where the specific testing details are provided. Certain general concepts used in testing are described here.

In evaluation of ACTH secretion, it is important to consider the practical implications. Testing is performed to identify patients with suspected partial adrenal insufficiency in whom an inadequate response to stress may occur. The best stimulus for this purpose is insulin hypoglycemia, in which the response to cortisol correlates well with that to surgical stress. The same test can also be used to evaluate GH responsiveness. Insulin hypoglycemia can be dangerous and should not be used in patients with primary adrenal insufficiency. Recent administration of glucocorticoid therapy can complicate the workup of a patient with suspected hypopituitarism. The suppressive effects of glucocorticoids on the hypothalamic pituitary-adrenal axis can result in a subnormal response or absence of response to any of the stimuli used. Glucocorticoids should be discontinued for at least one month, if possible, prior to definitive testing.

A similar problem occurs in evaluating TSH function in patients who have been receiving long-term thyroid hormone therapy, which can impair the TSH response to TRH for at least one month.

In patients with gonadotropin deficiency, distinguishing between hypothalamic and pituitary causes is often difficult. A single GnRH challenge is frequently of little help in making this distinction and is useful primarily when neuroanatomic evidence of pituitary disease is present and the status of the gonodotrophs is being questioned.

Documentation of GH deficiency is important primarily in children of short stature when therapy with exogenous GH is being considered. The high frequency (> 75 per cent) of GH responses to GRH in children with no anatomic evidence of hypothalamic-pituitary disease argues for a hypothalamic etiology in most GH-deficient children. Decisions concerning GH therapy require careful assessment because of the effort and expense involved. Failure of response to at least two stimuli, usually insulin hypoglycemia and arginine, is generally required before institution of GH therapy. In addition, hypothyroidism, if present, must be corrected prior to GH testing. In adults, GH deficiency serves as a marker for acquired hypopituitarism, particularly for pituitary tumors. In children and adults with obesity, GH responses to all stimuli tested are impaired, even in the presence of seemingly normal growth.

THERAPY. Hormonal replacement therapy must be determined individually and treatment goals specifically defined. The therapeutic use of pituitary hormones is restricted to GH for correcting growth retardation and gonadotropins for inducing fertility. GnRH may be used for introduction of puberty and treatment of infertility and GRH can be substituted for GH when the cause of hormone deficiency is hypothalamic rather than pituitary. For the most part, target organ hormones are used because of their cost advantage, ease of administration, and prolonged action.

ACTH. ACTH deficiency is treated with glucocorticoids. Cortisone (25 mg orally), hydrocortisone (20 mg orally), or prednisone (5 mg orally) given as a divided dose provides adequate therapy for most patients under normal conditions. Supplemental mineralocorticoid therapy is unnecessary because of the partial preservation of aldosterone secretion. The use of predisone is preferred because of its reduced cost. Occasional patients may require full glucocorticoid replacement therapy (a dose 50 per cent greater that those listed), but in most patients this dose is excessive. The clinical assessment of the adequacy of therapy relates to the patient's sense of well-being and the absence of excessive weight gain. During stress, the dose should be increased two- to threefold and then gradually tapered. If oral medication cannot be retained, injectable steroids (hydrocortisone hemisuccinate [Solu-Cortef] for initial emergency use, 100 mg intramuscularly or intravenously), or cortisone acetate for long-term use (50 to 100 mg intramuscularly every 12 hours) is indicated. Treatment of the acutely ill hypopituitary patient requires the same dosage of hydrocortisone (100 to 300 mg per day) as used in primary adrenal insufficiency. Preoperatively, patients should receive hydrocortisone hemisuccinate 50 mg intramuscularly every 6 hours beginning the night prior to surgery and continuing through the immediate postoperative period, followed by gradual tapering to maintenance dosage. Treatment of patients with partial ACTH deficiency without symptoms in the nonstressed state is more controversial. With adequate education, many patients will not need maintenance replacement therapy except in times of stress. Such patients in particular should wear appropriate medical identification bracelets.

TSH. TSH deficiency is treated with L-thyroxine 0.15 mg per day, though a lower dose may suffice in occasional patients. Clinical assessment of the patient and serum thyroxine levels during initiation of therapy are used to establish the appropriate dose. Adrenal insufficiency must be corrected prior to instituting thyroid hormone replacement therapy, and patients with partial adrenal insufficiency may require glucocorticoid replacement only after thyroid hormone replacement is started. In the presence of severe or longstanding hypothyroidism a small dose of thyroxine (0.05 mg per day) should be used initially and increased slowly to a maintenance dose. The use of triiodothyronine, particularly as long-term therapy, is not recommended, because its shorter biologic half-life results in more rapid appearance of thyroid deficiency in the event therapy is omitted.

LH and FSH. Treatment of gonadotropin deficiency requires consideration of both gonadal steroid replacement and treatment of infertility. The subjects are considered in greater detail in Ch. 235 and 237.

WOMEN. Estrogen replacement therapy is indicated in premenopausal women to maintain secondary sex characteristics and to prevent osteoporosis and possibly coronary artery disease. This can be accomplished with ethinyl estradiol 5 to 20 μg per day or conjugated estrogens (Premarin) 0.6 to 1.25 mg per day. The lowest possible dose that produces the desired clinical effects should be used. To induce cyclic bleeding, estrogen should be given for 25 days each month, accompanied on the last five days by a progestinic agent such as medroxyprogesterone 5 to 10 mg per day. Alternatively, an oral contraceptive preparation containing no more than the equivalent of 25 μg estradiol per day can be used. The advantage of replacement therapy after the menopause is still controversial, and the potential risks and benefits should be discussed with the patient to help make an appropriate decision. Estrogen therapy usually corrects the dyspareunia attributable to local estrogen deficiency in women with hypopituitarism, but decreased libido due to the absence of adrenal androgens often persists. This can be corrected by injection of a small dose of long-acting androgen such as testosterone enanthate 50 mg every one to two months or by oral administration of fluoxymesterone 5 to 10 mg once or twice weekly.

Restoration of fertility is possible in a large percentage of women with clomiphene or GnRH therapy (the latter given in a pulsatile manner by an intermittent subcutaneous infusion pump) if the cause of the disorder is hypothalamic or with combined FSH-LH preparations if pituitary disease is present. An FSH-rich preparation from postmenopausal urine is used to initiate follicular growth and maturation; it is monitored by measurement of plasma estradiol levels. Human chorionic gonadotropin is then injected to induce ovulation. This therapy is expensive, entails the risk of superovulation and multiple pregnancy, and should be undertaken only under the direction of an experienced physician.

MEN. Testosterone replacement therapy in adult males is accomplished by intramuscular injection of a long-acting testosterone preparation (testosterone enanthate or cypionate, 200 mg every three to four weeks). The endpoints are restoration of full androgenization, including beard growth, improvement in muscular strength, libido and potency. Androgen therapy should be withheld as long as possible in the adolescent with growth retardation to avoid premature epiphyseal closure, which limits the potential for future linear growth. Testosterone therapy may be required for many months before full restoration of libido and performance. If gonadotropin deficiency has developed before puberty, full androgenization may never occur. In patients with longstanding hypogonadism, psychosocial behavioral changes affecting the patient's entire lifestyle may be disrupted by initiation of testosterone therapy, leading to major adjustment problems with both sexual and nonsexual relationships.

Infertility in men with hypopituitarism can be corrected with a combination of FSH and human chorionic gonadotropin (HCG), though therapy is required for several months, and the success rate is less than 50 per cent. In the future,

GnRH, given intermittently as in women, may serve as an alternate method of therapy in individuals with hypothalamic hypogonadism.

Growth Hormone. GH therapy is indicated for the correction of impaired linear growth, and its use is thus confined almost exclusively to childhood and adolescent years. Early establishment of the diagnosis is critical, since the probability of successful long-term therapy is inversely related to the extent of growth retardation. Treatment requires the use of human GH, which was traditionally extracted and purified from human pituitaries obtained at autopsy. Recognition of the association of pituitary GH therapy with Creutzfeldt-Jakob disease led to an abrupt discontinuation in the use of this form of GH in 1985 and substitution of GH produced by recombinant DNA technology, which has comparable biopotency. GH is administered intramuscularly or subcutaneously at a dose of 0.1 mg per kilogram three times weekly; its use is continued until the final height is achieved, coincident with long-bone epiphyseal closure. A goal of 5 feet 4 inches is generally pursued but not always achieved. Careful attention must be given to concomitant hormone deficiencies, particularly thyroid. Glucocorticoids should be used sparingly because of their interference with growth-promoting effects of GH. Some physicians have proposed that small doses of oral androgens be used simultaneously to increase growth velocity, though this has not gained widespread acceptance. Estrogens are to be avoided because of their greater effect on epiphyseal closure. Gonadal steroid therapy is usually initiated during the years of puberty to avoid psychosocial problems. However, if significant catch-up growth is required, its use should be delayed. GH therapy increases height age more rapidly than bone age, may initially be associated with a decrease in body fat, and also corrects the fasting hypoglycemia of GH-deficient children. GRH, or one of its analogues, may be useful in treatment of at least 50 per cent of children with isolated GH deficiency and in the future may be administered by noninjectable routes.

Asa SL, Bilbao JM, Kovacs K, et al.: Lymphocytic hypophysitis of pregnancy resulting in hypopituitarism: A distinct clinicopathologic entity. Ann Intern Med 95:166, 1981. Baskin DS, Townsend JJ, Wilson CB: Lymphocytic adenohypophysitis of pregnancy simulating a pituitary adenoma: A distinct pathological entity. Report of two cases. J Neurosurg 56:148, 1982. *Two reports of a pregnancy-related syndrome diagnosed by histologic examination of pituitary tissue. Clinical differentiation from pituitary tumors is difficult, and the pathogenesis is unclear.*

Gharib H, Frey HM, Laws ER Jr, et al.: Coexistent primary empty sella syndrome and hyperprolactinemia. Report of 11 cases. Arch Intern Med 143:1383, 1983. *The empty sella syndrome is being recognized with greater frequency, and coexisting hyperprolactinemia does not necessarily imply the presence of a pituitary microadenoma.*

Hintz RL, Rosenfeld RG: Clinical uses of synthetic growth hormone. Hosp Prac 18:115, 1983. *A clinically oriented presentation of the use of human growth hormone produced by recombinant DNA technology.*

Hurley DM, Brian R, Outch K, et al.: Induction of ovulation and fertility in amenorrheic women by pulsatile low-dose gonadotropin-releasing hormone. N Engl J Med 310:1069, 1984. *The use of intermittent GnRH injections as a practical and effective technique for treatment of infertility.*

Phillips JA, Parks JS, Hjelle BL, et al.: Genetic analysis of familial isolated growth hormone deficiency type I. J Clin Invest 70:489, 1982. *Analysis of nuclear DNA from patients with familial isolated GH deficiency has suggested the presence of genetic mutations. Similar studies can be expected in the future that may explain the pathogenesis of many isolated hormonal deficiencies.*

Sheehan HL, Summers VK: The syndrome of hypopituitarism. Q J Med 42:319, 1949. *The classic monograph describing the clinical-pathologic correlations of hypopituitarism. Its lucid and detailed presentation make it worthwhile reading even after nearly four decades.*

Stackpoole PW, Interlandi JW, Nicholson WE, et al.: Isolated ACTH deficiency: A heterologous disorder. Critical review and report of four new cases. Medicine 61:13, 1982. *The pathogenesis of this disorder is heterologous despite similar clinical manifestations. Detailed endocrine testing is required to differentiate the various causes.*

PITUITARY TUMORS

Classification. Pituitary tumors are subdivided by their histologic characteristics and also by their functional activity. Specific considerations of hormone-secreting pituitary tumors will be found in the next section. The two major histologic types of primary pituitary tumors are the adenoma and the craniopharyngioma. In addition, parasellar tumors such as optic nerve glioma, meningioma, sphenoid wing sarcoma, as well as metastatic tumors, can also be present within the sella turcica.

Pituitary Adenomas. This cell type constitutes greater than 90 per cent of all pituitary tumors. The classic subdivision into chromophobic and chromophilic tumors has given way to more specific identification on the basis of immunohisto-chemical stains for individual hormones. Using these techniques, only 10 to 20 per cent of pituitary adenomas appear to be nonfunctioning. Pituitary tumors account for 6 to 18 per cent of all brain tumors, and small adenomas, many of which are functioning, have been detected in up to 30 per cent of unselected autopsy series. The growth pattern of pituitary adenomas appears unrelated to hormone secretion. Rapidly enlarging tumors are generally recognized because of their mass effects, whereas slowly growing tumors tend to allow for greater expression of the hormone hypersecretory effects. The peak incidence of nonfunctioning pituitary adenomas is between 40 and 50 years, and the frequency is uninfluenced by sex. Some "nonfunctioning" tumors may actually produce portions of hormones (e.g., the glycoprotein alpha subunit common to TSH, LH, and FSH) or may synthesize but be incapable of releasing the hormone. Although pituitary adenomas are almost always histologically benign, they may exhibit aggressive growth behavior with invasion of surrounding structures, making their surgical removal impossible. Adenomas are generally solid with a well-defined capsule, although they may on occasion be cystic and hemorrhagic. Calcification, if present, results from organization of a previous hemorrhage.

Craniopharyngiomas. These tumors are of congenital origin, may be partly or entirely cystic, and are always benign. The cyst fluid may be cholesterol rich. Calcification, generally concentric, is present in 50 per cent. The tumors grow at variable rates and may remain dormant for many years. Although half of the tumors are seen during childhood, they may appear at any time during life. The site of origin of most tumors is in the midline at the upper portion of the pituitary stalk, and approximately 15 per cent involve the upper portion of the anterior lobe and are therefore intrasellar. Variations of craniopharyngiomas include ependymomas and epidermoid cysts.

CLINICAL FEATURES. The manifestations of pituitary tumors are neuroanatomic, endocrinologic, and radiologic. Presenting symptoms of piuitary tumors have changed in frequency over the years with refinements in diagnostic procedures. Whereas in nearly 90 per cent of cases diagnosed 30 years ago patients exhibited visual disturbances, only 25 per cent do so at present. In contrast, the most common presentation today relates to impaired gonadal function, frequently associated with prolactin-secreting pituitary tumors. A small percentage of patients (less than 5 per cent) are discovered accidentally on review of head-imaging procedures obtained for other purposes.

Neuroanatomic manifestations occur secondary to tumor growth causing pressure on the overlying dura and the diaphragma sellae. This results in headaches that are variable in nature, imprecisely located, generally of dull quality, unassociated with nausea or visual symptoms, unrelated to position, and inconsistently relieved by analgesics. Disappearance of headache is frequently a sign of rupture of the dura. With continued expansion the tumor exerts pressure on the optic chiasm, leading to the classic findings of bitemporal hemianopsia. At earlier stages the field defects may be asymmetric and involve only the superior temporal fields. Eventually, blindness and optic atrophy will occur. Anterior growth of the tumor may cause symptoms limited only to one eye. Papilledema occurs in one fourth of craniopharyn-

giomas but rarely in pituitary adenomas. Further growth results in hypothalamic compression leading to temperature instability, hyperphagia, altered sleep patterns, and emotional disturbances. Pressure on the third ventricle results in internal hydrocephalus. Rarely, temporal or frontal lobe compression may cause behavioral changes and seizures, and midbrain compression may produce long-tract signs. Lateral extension is more common and leads to compression of the third, fourth, and sixth cranial nerves in the cavernous sinus, resulting in ophthalmoplegia and diplopia. Expansion inferiorly into the sphenoid sinus may result in cerebrospinal fluid rhinorrhea. Hemorrhage into the tumor, *pituitary apoplexy*, may result in rapid expansion of the tumor and lead to the sudden appearance of headache of varying intensity that subsides after a few days. If the tumor is intrasellar, hypopituitarism often results; if extrasellar, there may be rapid deterioration of vision. "Spontaneous" cures of hormone-secreting pituitary tumors may also occur as the result of hemorrhagic tumor necrosis.

Neuroradiologic presentations consist of a deformed or enlarged sella seen on standard skull roentgenography or a mass lesion seen on computed tomography (CT) or magnetic resonance imaging (MRI) performed for unrelated reasons.

Endocrine symptoms include diminished function secondary to destruction of normal pituitary tissue by tumor or interference with portal blood supply and hyperfunction due to tumor or hyperplasia. The two may be combined. In addition, diminished function may occur secondary to the effects of hormone hypersecretion (i.e., hypogonadism secondary to hyperprolactinemia). The frequency of presentation and the manifestations have been described in the previous section.

DIAGNOSTIC PROCEDURES. Diagnosis of a pituitary tumor necessitates differentiation from other parasellar disorders, determination of the tumor size and extent of sellar and extrasellar destruction, and assessment of the extent of hormone deficiencies. Endocrine evaluation should be performed prior to definitive therapy, if possible, since the extent of hypopituitarism may influence the type and extent of therapy. When this is not possible, because of rapidly deteriorating vision or progressive neurologic symptoms, the patient must be considered to have panhypopituitarism and immediate treatment with glucocorticoids must be initiated.

Neuroradiologic procedures have improved remarkably during the past decade, and until very recently the definitive study has been CT, performed with intravenous contrast media, using a fourth-generation scanner (Fig. 226–1). The best views are obtained using coronal sections. This technique permits evaluation of the contents of the sella as well as the

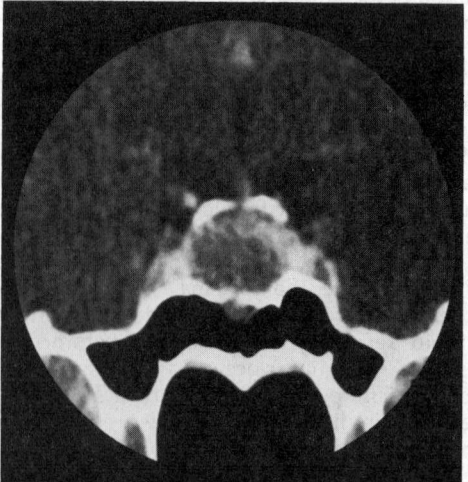

FIGURE 226–1. Computerized axial tomographic (CT) scan of pituitary (coronal view) demonstrating a pituitary tumor with suprasellar extension and erosion of the sellar floor with inferior extension of the tumor into the sphenoid sinus.

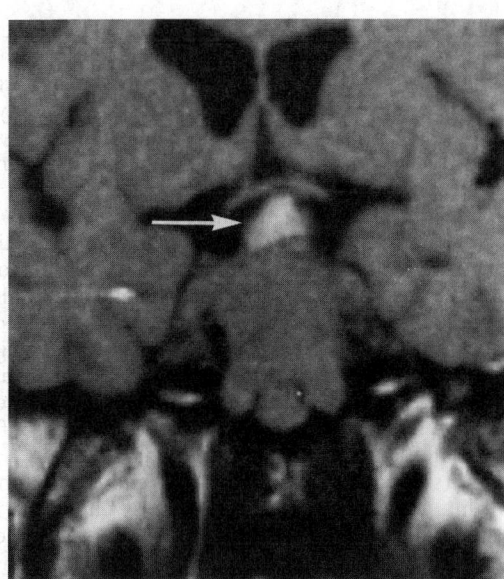

FIGURE 226–2. Magnetic resonance image (MRI) of a pituitary adenoma (coronal view). The large tumor mass extends inferiorly and superiorly. The intense (white) signal (*arrow*) in the dorsal portion of the tumor represents recent hemorrhage. The superiorly displaced optic chiasm is seen just above the tumor.

surrounding bony structures. CT can also indicate the degree of extension of pituitary tumors in all directions and has precluded the need for invasive procedures such as pneumoencephalography. Digital vascular imaging is also useful as an adjunct in determining the position of the carotid arteries in relation to the tumor prior to surgical intervention and has almost entirely replaced carotid angiography. The use of MRI has resulted in pituitary imaging quality that is comparable to that of CT, except perhaps in microadenomas. The advantage of MRI relates to the absence of radiation exposure as well as improved anatomic definition (Fig. 226–2).

The most important neuro-ophthalmologic study is evaluation of visual fields. Test objects of varying sizes and colors can provide an excellent assessment of both central and peripheral fields. The technique is reproducible and sensitive and useful in observing patients for serial changes. Bitemporal field defects are, however, not specific for pituitary tumors; they may occur with parasellar tumors, vascular abnormalities, arachnoiditis, or rarely with chiasmal prolapse into the sella associated with the empty sella syndrome. Atypical field defects may also occur, even those suggesting superior rather than inferior pressure. Another useful test is the visual evoked response (VER), which measures the pattern and latency of the response from the occipital cortex produced by photic stimulation. Chiasmal pressure produces a delayed or reduced response in the crossed pathways as compared with uncrossed pathways and may provide evidence of abnormalities before they are evident on visual field examination.

DIFFERENTIAL DIAGNOSIS. Disorders that must be differentiated from pituitary tumors include the empty sella syndrome, parasellar diseases, and pituitary enlargement associated with other endocrine disorders.

The *empty sella* is partly or nearly completely filled with CSF and results from extension of the subarachnoid space into the intrasellar region. The pituitary gland is flattened along the posterior portion of the floor and the dorsum. Primary empty sella syndrome is unassociated with prior surgical or irradiation therapy and has been found in up to one quarter of autopsy series, usually unassociated with endocrine disease. The etiology is unknown, but the syndrome has been postulated to be due to incomplete formation of the diaphragma sella, permitting CSF pressure to be transmitted to the sella and gradually leading to herniation of the arachnoid and remodeling of the sella. Nearly all patients are asymptomatic,

though some may have nonspecific headaches. The syndrome is seen commonly in obese women and in association with systemic hypertension, benign intracranial hypertension (pseudotumor cerebri), and CSF rhinorrhea. The sella is usually symmetrically enlarged or ballooned and may be deformed. Endocrine function is generally normal, though diminished TSH and gonadotropin secretion, hyperprolactinemia, and rarely panhypopituitarism or diabetes insipidus may be present. The diagnosis is established by CT or MRI. The empty sella may coexist with a pituitary tumor, which is usually hyperfunctional. The secondary empty sella syndrome is seen in patients following pituitary surgery or irradiation.

The signs and symptoms of parasellar disorders may mimic those of pituitary tumors. Parasellar disorders include inflammatory and granulomatous diseases (sarcoidosis, eosinophilic granuloma), degenerative disorders (aneurysms), and neoplasms (meningiomas, hamartomas, metastatic tumors). Suprasellar tumors usually present with the neurologic manifestations of increased intracranial pressure, hypothalamic symptoms, and internal hydrocephalus. Endocrine manifestations tend to follow rather than precede neurologic symptoms. CT and MRI are extremely valuable in differentiating these disorders from primary pituitary tumors.

Longstanding primary hypothyroidism or hypogonadism can result in sellar enlargement, increased TSH or gonadotropin secretion, hyperplasia of tropic hormone–producing cells, and in some patients, hormone-secreting tumors. Institution of appropriate replacement hormone therapy can reverse the hypersecretory and hyperplastic changes.

THERAPY. Treatment of nonfunctioning pituitary tumors is required to prevent or limit the loss of pituitary function and the consequences of extrasellar extension. The two therapeutic methods are surgery and radiation therapy.

Pituitary surgery is the conventional therapy for pituitary tumors. The transsphenoidal approach is currently used for all tumors except those with extensive suprasellar extension, particularly when separated from the intrasellar portion by a narrow neck. Tumors encircling optic nerves or encasing cerebral vessels can be removed only by a transfrontal approach. Currently the operative mortality is less than 1 per cent. The transsphenoidal approach includes the use of modern fluoroscopic aids and microsurgical techniques. It provides better visualization of the sellar contents and has been instrumental in permitting selective adenomectomy to be performed. If preoperative evaluation reveals preservation of anterior pituitary function, a more conservative approach is indicated to preserve remaining pituitary hormone secretion. A small rim of adenohypophyseal tissue is often sufficient to maintain adequate pituitary function. Glucocorticoid coverage is essential for the perioperative period even for patients with intact pituitary-adrenal function and is accomplished with parenteral administration of hydrocortisone, 50 mg intramuscularly every six hours. Postoperatively the patient must be carefully observed for the development of diabetes insipidus, particularly since an obtunded patient may not perceive thirst. Transient polyuria and increased plasma osmolality commonly occur in the immediate postoperative period as a result of mild trauma to the pituitary stalk. Persistence of these findings beyond the first 48 hours usually indicates significant destruction of the stalk or posterior pituitary and permanent impairment of function. However, fluctuations in posterior pituitary function may occur for a period of several weeks, and recovery has been observed as late as many months postoperatively. Initially the patient should be treated with aqueous vasopressin (5 U subcutaneously) or desmopressin (DDAVP) (1 or 2 μg subcutaneously) rather than with a long-acting preparation so the natural history of the process can be observed.

Radiation therapy can be used as an alternative to surgical excision of the pituitary tumor or as adjunct therapy. Although less popular as primary therapy, because of its delayed effects, radiation therapy using conventional high-energy sources (supravoltage) or heavy-particle (proton beam) sources is an effective method of treatment. Radiation therapy is to be avoided in patients with significant suprasellar extension or in the presence of marked visual field defects.

The recurrence rate of pituitary tumors following surgical treatment alone ranges from 25 to nearly 100 per cent in different series. Since postoperative radiographic and endocrine studies indicate that intraoperative assessment of the extent of pituitary tumor removal is often inaccurate, postoperative irradiation is indicated in all patients with nonfunctioning pituitary adenomas unless specifically contraindicated. The dose currently employed is 4500 to 5000 rads, which can be given with minimal side effects. Some late loss of pituitary function occurs in 15 to 25 per cent of patients.

Baskin DS, Wilson CB: Surgical management of craniopharyngiomas. J Neurosurg 65:22, 1986. *Presentation, manifestations, and therapy of this relatively uncommon tumor are succinctly described and discussed.*

Burrow GN, Wortzman G, Rewcastle NB, et al.: Microadenomas of pituitary and abnormal sellar tomograms in unselected autopsy series. N Engl J Med 304:156, 1981. *Clinically unrecognized microadenomas were found in one third of an autopsy series. Many were hormone containing but without manifestations of hypersecretion.*

Cardoso ER, Peterson EW: Pituitary apoplexy: A review. Neurosurgry 14:363, 1984. *A thorough discussion of the varied manner in which this disorder presents and a rationale for management.*

Cook DM: Pituitary tumors: Diagnosis and therapy. CA 33:215, 1983. *An excellent, well-referenced review of the recent literature that compares therapeutic effectiveness of methods as reported by others. Very readable.*

Crane TB, Yee RD, Hepler RS, et al.: Clinical manifestations and radiologic findings in craniopharyngiomas in adults. Am J Ophthalmol 94:220, 1982. *A comprehensive review of the clinical features in 51 patients emphasizing the predominance of visual findings.*

Daniels DL, Williams AL, Thornton RS, et al.: Differential diagnosis of intrasellar tumors by computed tomography. Radiology 141:697, 1981. Chambers EF, Turski PA, LaMasters D, et al.: Regions of low density in the contrast enhanced pituitary gland: Normal and pathologic processes. Radiology 144:109, 1982. *The use of CT in diagnosis of pituitary tumors is now well established. Subtleties in interpretation of the results, however, must be carefully assessed.*

Kaufman B: Magnetic resonance imaging of the pituitary gland. Radiol Clin N Am 22:795, 1984. Glaser B, Scheinfeld M, Benmair J, et al.: Magnetic resonance imaging of the pituitary gland. Clin Radiol 37:9, 1986. *Descriptions of the most current techniques of imaging the pituitary gland.*

Max MB, Deck MD, Rottenberg DA: Pituitary metastasis: Incidence in cancer patients and clinical differentiation from pituitary adenoma. Neurology 31:998, 1981. *A careful analysis of both autopsy and clinical series in which differentiation was facilitated by the clinical rather than the radiologic characteristics.*

Valenta LJ, Sostrin RD, Eisenberg H, et al.: Diagnosis of pituitary tumors by hormone assays and computerized tomography. Am J Med 72:861, 1982. *Analysis of 170 patients with endocrine abnormalities by dynamic testing and CT examination demonstrating the value of each in the diagnosis or exclusion of tumors.*

PITUITARY HYPERFUNCTION: HORMONE-SECRETING PITUITARY TUMORS

Except in the case of certain hormone-secreting tumors, pituitary hormone hypersecretion generally involves overproduction of only a single hormone. Physiologically, hormone overproduction occurs in response to altered feedback signals (i.e., hyperprolactinemia due to increased estrogen secretion in pregnancy; ACTH, TSH, and gonadotropin hypersecretion in response to diminished target organ feedback in primary hypofunction of the adrenal, thyroid, and gonads; and GH hypersecretion associated with chronic and severe caloric malnutrition). Whereas these changes begin as functional alterations, prolonged stimulation can result in hyperplastic as well as hypersecretory changes. Pathologic hyperfunction occurs in association with pituitary hyperplasia or tumor unrelated to regulatory feedback mechanisms. These disorders involve, almost exclusively, somatotrophic, lactotrophic, and corticotrophic cells.

Growth Hormone–Secreting Tumors: Acromegaly

GH hypersecretion is most commonly associated with a pituitary somatotroph tumor or rarely somatotroph hyperplasia. These tumors previously were considered eosinophilic

(due to GH storage granules) or chromophobic (when little hormone was stored). Tumors with abundant hormone storage tend to be better differentiated and more slowly growing, resulting in more pronounced clinical features of GH hypersecretion whereas the less differentiated non-hormone–storing tumors tend to grow more rapidly, leading to more pronounced effects of an expanding tumor mass.

CLINICAL FEATURES. The clinical manifestations of GH hypersecretion depend on the age at which the disorder begins. During childhood and prior to epiphyseal fusion, GH hypersecretion produces proportional skeletal growth leading to gigantism. Hypogonadism is frequently present, leading to delayed epiphyseal closure and thus a more prolonged growth period. The tallest reported patient with gigantism reached a height of nearly 9 feet. It is more common for patients to exhibit features of both gigantism and acromegaly, reflecting persistence of GH hypersecretion into adult life.

Signs and symptoms of GH hypersecretion beginning during adult life develop slowly. Soft tissue swelling and hypertrophy involving the extremities and face are the earliest findings (Fig. 226–3). These changes are usually best documented by comparing photographs taken over a one- to two-decade span. Spadelike changes develop in the fingers, and increased soft tissue volume necessitates ring enlargement and increases in glove and shoe sizes. The skin becomes thickened and leathery, and skin folds increase in prominence. A generalized increase in hair growth and pigmentation often occurs. Fibroma molluscum (pedunculated epithelial tags) and acanthosis nigricans are common. The skin becomes oily, and sebaceous cyst formation is common. Increased sweating occurs in most patients and is a sensitive biologic indicator of disease activity.

Bony changes occur more slowly and include cortical thickening, tufting of terminal phalanges, and osteophyte proliferation. Degenerated articular cartilages and ligamentous hypertrophy produce a hypertrophic arthropathy that eventually leads to deforming and crippling arthritis. Prognathism results

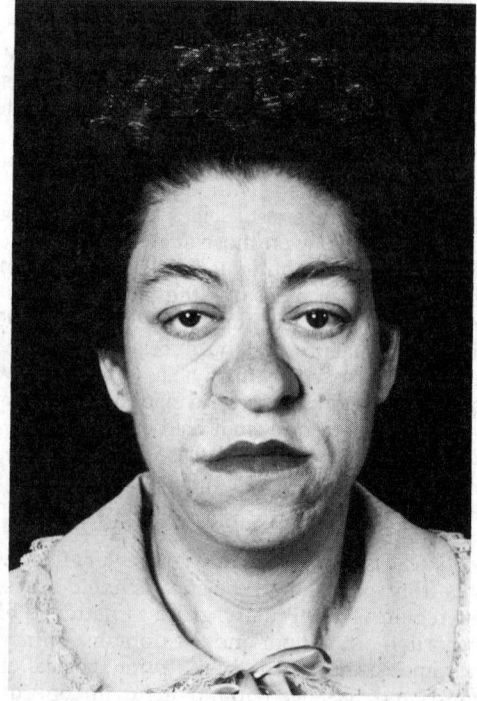

FIGURE 226–3. Clinical features of a 43-year-old patient with acromegaly of 15 years' duration. Coarsened features result from soft tissue overgrowth about the eyes, nose, and mouth. Lacrimal overgrowth, thickening of skin folds, and fibroma molluscum are also present. (Reprinted with permission from Frohman LA: In Felig P, Baxter JD, Broadus AE, Frohman LA (eds.): Endocrinology and Metabolism. 2nd ed. New York, McGraw-Hill Book Company, 1987, p 302.)

from mandibular enlargement and causes a significant over-bite of the lower incisors and increased spacing of the teeth. Bony overgrowth of the frontal, malar, and nasal bones occurs; increase in size of the paranasal sinuses together with vocal cord hypertrophy leads to deepening of the voice. Eustachian tube mucosal hypertrophy often produces obstruction and serous otitis media.

Peripheral neuropathy commonly occurs because of nerve entrapment by surrounding tissue overgrowth, most commonly affecting the median nerve and producing the carpal tunnel syndrome. Axonal demyelinization of peripheral nerves associated with perineurial and subepineurial proliferation results in palpable nerve fibers. Paresthesias, sensory losses, and proximal muscle weakness occur frequently.

Prolonged hypersecretion leads to generalized visceromegaly involving salivary glands, liver, spleen, and kidneys. Salivary gland enlargement is detectable clinically whereas that of the other organs is not, and significant hepatosplenomegaly usually implies the presence of a coexisting disease. Both secretory and reabsorptive functions of the kidney are increased in acromegaly.

Thyroid enlargement with nodule formation is common, but true hyperfunction is infrequent. Parathyroid hyperplasia and adenoma are frequently associated, explaining the hypercalciuria and nephrolithiasis often observed. Mild elevations of prolactin levels occur in one third of patients, resulting in galactorrhea, amenorrhea, and decreased libido.

The effects of GH on the cardiovascular system are controversial. Hypertension is common but generally mild and responsive to drug therapy. Cardiomegaly is routinely found, but there is no characteristic form of acromegalic heart disease. Cardiac failure, when it occurs, appears related to hypertension and not to the effects of GH hypersecretion. Yet the incidence of cardiovascular disease is increased in acromegalics, as is mortality. Weight gain is uncommon, but carbohydrate intolerance and diabetes are seen in 25 per cent of acromegalics, primarily in those with a family history of diabetes. Insulin resistance is common and the development of ketosis is occasionally noted. Diabetic microangiopathy, however is extremely uncommon, even in longstanding disease.

LABORATORY STUDIES. The diagnosis of acromegaly is established by the finding of elevated plasma GH levels that do not respond normally to physiologic suppression and stimulation; in adults, a GH value greater than 2 ng per milliliter in males or 5 ng per milliliter in females after oral glucose administration is confirmatory. Randomly obtained samples with markedly elevated levels are also diagnostic. However, in normal children and young adults, GH levels as high as 50 ng per milliliter are sporadically exhibited, thereby necessitating dynamic studies of GH secretion in many patients. TRH stimulates GH secretion in 70 to 80 per cent of acromegalics but not in normal subjects, and this procedure is useful in following up the patient after therapy as well. GH secretion in acromegalics differs in other ways from that in normal persons, including absence of a sleep-associated increase in GH and a tendency for wide spontaneous fluctuations in GH levels, indicating intermittent secretory activity. Plasma GH levels increase after GRH in most acromegalics, but the test is not of diagnostic help.

Plasma IGF-I (somatomedin C) levels are also increased in acromegaly and provide good correlation with the clinical manifestations of GH hypersecretion. Determination of IGF-I levels for assessing disease activity after therapy is useful, particularly when GH levels are borderline.

DIFFERENTIAL DIAGNOSIS. The clinical features of acromegaly are not confused with other diseases. The question commonly raised is whether features suggestive of the disease are associated with active disease, inactive disease, or no disease. Dynamic studies of GH secretion are required to differentiate these possibilities. Gigantism during childhood

occasionally occurs in the absence of GH hypersecretion (cerebral gigantism) through a yet to be determined mechanism. GH levels are elevated in patients with renal failure, cirrhosis, protein calorie malnutrition, and anorexia nervosa and in the Laron dwarf (growth retardation caused by a defect in IGF-I production associated with diminished GH binding to plasma membranes), but in these conditions the clinical features of acromegaly are absent.

PATHOGENESIS. Acromegaly can occur as a primary disorder due to neoplastic transformation of somatotrophs within the pituitary or, rarely, as secondary to excessive somatotroph stimulation by an ectopic GRH-secreting tumor or to an ectopic GH-secreting tumor. Selective removal of the GH-secreting adenoma is followed in most patients not only by restoration of normal GH values but by normal responses to dynamic testing. In some patients, however, GH-secreting pituitary tumors have been associated with carcinoid tumors of the bronchus and foregut, pancreatic islet tumors, and small-cell carcinoma of the lung. Removal of the extrapituitary tumor has resulted in a return of GH levels to normal and regression of the pituitary tumor. GRH has been isolated from several of these tumors, and its sequence was first determined from a pancreatic islet tumor rather than from the hypothalamus. Pituitary histology in patients with secondary acromegaly ranges from local or generalized somatotroph hyperplasia to actual tumor formation. In addition, neuronal tumors present in the hypothalamus (hamartomas) or in the pituitary, contiguous with the somatotroph adenoma (gangliocytoma or choristoma), may also be the source of GRH production in a few patients with acromegaly. Since excessive stimulation by GRH is capable of inducing adenomas as well as hyperplasia, it is possible that some patients now considered to have primary pituitary disease actually have a hypothalamic disorder characterized by excessive GRH production from nontumorous tissue.

Comparison of the limited numbers of reported patients with secondary acromegaly does not provide any evidence of differences in either clinical manifestations or responses to dynamic studies of GH secretion, with the possible exception of decreased frequency of GH responses to GRH. In patients with ectopic GRH production, immunoreactive plasma GRH levels are readily detectable, in contrast to patients presumed to have primary pituitary disease in whom levels are near or beneath the limits of detectability.

THERAPY. Therapy for patients with acromegaly involves three potential methods: surgery, irradiation, and medical (pharmacologic). Considerations of the space-occupying mass and of hypopituitarism are similar to those described for nonfunctioning pituitary tumors. Prior to initiation of therapy to the pituitary itself, consideration should be given to the possibility of an extrapituitary tumor, removal of which may reverse the GH hypersecretion.

Surgical treatment of GH-secreting pituitary tumors is currently the treatment of choice. Transsphenoidal or, if necessary, transfrontal adenomectomy is indicated once the presence of the disease has been established, even though the radiologic findings are minimal. The results in published series vary, some reports indicating up to 90 per cent cure rates with small tumors. The success in returning GH levels to normal is inversely related to the size of the tumor; less favorable results occur with tumors greater than 2 cm in diameter or plasma GH levels greater than 100 ng per milliliter. The clinical features of GH, however, are frequently improved dramatically even without complete restoration of GH values to normal. In patients whose GH levels return to the normal range, tumor recurrence is infrequent (approximately 5 per cent), but with incomplete removal the recurrence rate is greater than 50 per cent if no further therapy is administered.

Radiation therapy, using methods similar to those for nonfunctioning tumors, is effective as a primary means of treatment of acromegaly. The reduction in GH hypersecretion is, however, slow, and return to normal levels may require five or even ten years, although 70 to 80 per cent of patients will exhibit normal GH levels after two years. Postoperative irradiation is indicated when GH levels remain elevated and, used in conjunction with surgery, offers the best prognosis.

Pharmacologic therapy in acromegaly is of limited value. Bromocriptine, a dopamine receptor agonist, is effective in lowering GH levels to normal in only 25 per cent and in decreasing tumor size in only 5 per cent of patients. Dosages of up to 60 mg per day may be required, and side effects are frequent. A somatostatin analogue, SMS 201-995, is effective in reducing GH levels to normal in more than half of acromegalics and tumor size slightly in some patients. The drug must be injected three or four times daily and at the present time is still investigational. Both drugs are effective only during continued administration and should be considered only as adjunct therapy or in patients who are not surgical candidates.

Arosio M, Giovanelli MA, Riva E, et al.: Clinical uses of pre- and postsurgical evaluation of abnormal GH responses in acromegaly. J Neurosurg 59:402, 1983. *Responses to dynamic testing of GH secretion indicate that persistence of abnormal responses postoperatively even when the basal GH levels are within the normal range should be considered evidence of residual neoplastic tissue. The studies may help distinguish between reactivation of disease and true recurrence.*

Baskin DS, Boggan JE, Wilson CB: Transsphenoidal microsurgical removal of growth hormone-secreting pituitary adenomas. A review of 137 cases. J Neurosurg 56:634, 1982. *The largest published series of GH-secreting tumors to date indicating that the greatest success occurs in patients with tumors confined to the sella and with GH levels less than 40 ng per milliliter.*

Dons RF, Rieth KG, Gorden P, et al.: Size and erosive features of the sella turcica in acromegaly as predictors of therapeutic response to supervoltage irradiation. Am J Med 74:69, 1983. *Size and basal GH levels tended to parallel one another and formed a rough predictor of the response to therapy. In all patients the decrease in GH levels occurred in proportion to the initial value.*

Frohman LA, Thominet JL, Szabo M: Ectopic growth hormone releasing factor syndromes. In Raiti S, Tolman R (eds.): Human Growth Hormone. New York, Plenum Publishing, 1986, p 347. *Acromegaly secondary to ectopic GRH secretion is described, with particular attention to differential diagnosis.*

Lamberts SWJ, Uitterlinden P, Verschoor L, et al.: Long-term treatment of acromegaly with the somatostatin analogue SMS 201–995. N Engl J Med 313:1576, 1985. *The use of a long-acting analogue of somatostatin in acromegaly offers the potential of medical suppression of growth hormone hypersecretion.*

Melmed S, Braunstein GD, Chang RJ, et al.: Pituitary tumors secreting growth hormone and prolactin. Ann Intern Med 105:238, 1986. *A well-balanced review of the current literature on hormonally active pituitary tumors.*

Prolactin-Secreting Tumors: Amenorrhea-Galactorrhea Syndrome

Hyperprolactinemia is the most common form of pituitary hyperfunction. It is present in as many as 25 per cent of infertile women. The incidence in men is much lower. In patients with pituitary tumors the incidence of elevated prolactin levels ranges from 60 to 80 per cent and is greater than that of any other pituitary hormone. The distinction between patients with *idiopathic hyperprolactinemia* and those with *prolactin-secreting tumors* is currently made on the basis of CT or MRI examination of the pituitary. Thus, changes in the relative frequency of the two diseases reflect primarily recent improvements in radiologic technology.

CLINICAL FEATURES. In women, hyperprolactinemia causes galactorrhea, oligomenorrhea or amenorrhea, and infertility (see Ch. 239 for a discussion of galactorrhea). Galactorrhea requires near-normal levels of ovarian steroids and is therefore not seen in all patients. It frequently occurs in association with oral contraceptive use, usually following their discontinuation. The reported incidence of galactorrhea in patients with prolactin-secreting tumors varies from 50 to 90 per cent. Oligomenorrhea or amenorrhea occurs in a similar percentage of patients and in nearly all with radiographic evidence of a pituitary tumor. The development of amenorrhea and the development of galactorrhea are not necessarily related to one another and are of no diagnostic importance. The cause of amenorrhea is related to effects of altered CNS neurotransmitters, principally dopamine, as a result of hy-

perprolactinemia, which interferes with a normal positive feedback effect of estradiol on GnRH secretion and with the self-priming effect of GnRH. The effects of anovulation include hypoestrogenemia, which results in decreased vaginal secretion, and dyspareunia, which may be responsible for diminished libido. Mild hirsutism may also occur in association with increased dehydroepiandrosterone sulfate production by the adrenals. Longstanding hyperprolactinemia has, in some women, been associated with decreased bone density, only part of which may be attributed to the hypoestrogenemia.

In men, hyperprolactinemia results in impotence and diminished libido. A defect in endogenous GnRH secretion is present, along with diminished testosterone secretion. The decreased libido is, however, not explained entirely on this basis, since it often persists despite testosterone replacement therapy. In some men oligospermia is also present.

LABORATORY STUDIES. Plasma prolactin levels in patients with prolactin-secreting tumors vary from slightly above normal (15 to 20 ng per milliliter) to values greater than 10,000 ng per milliliter. Levels less than 200 ng per milliliter are of little use in distinguishing between the various causes of the disorder, whereas levels greater than 200 ng per milliliter are invariably associated with prolactin-secreting tumors. Since prolactin is a stress-responsive hormone and levels fluctuate in normal subjects, repeated sampling in patients with moderate degrees of hyperprolactinemia is essential.

A large number of dynamic studies of prolactin secretion reveal differences between normal persons and pathologic hyperprolactinemics, but none is reliable in distinguishing between idiopathic hyperprolactinemia and prolactin-secreting tumors. Prolactin responses to submaximally suppressive infusions of dopamine are impaired in such patients, as compared to those with known extrapituitary disorders using hyperprolactinemia, though the latter can usually be distinguished on clinical grounds. Patients with prolactin-secreting tumors and idiopathic hyperprolactinemia have impaired responses to dopamine receptor–blocking agents, to stimulation with TRH, and to a combination of L-dopa plus the dopa decarboxylase inhibitor, carbidopa.

In some patients with pituitary tumors and mild hyperprolactinemia (i.e., less than 100 ng per milliliter) the tumor does not secrete prolactin, but rather appears to interrupt hypothalamic-pituitary portal blood flow, resulting in increased prolactin secretion by normal lactotrophs.

DIFFERENTIAL DIAGNOSIS. Consideration should be given to an extrapituitary cause for hyperprolactinemia in all patients, since subtle changes on CT studies may not always indicate the presence of a pituitary tumor. This is particularly true in patients with prolactin levels less than 200 ng per milliliter. The differential diagnosis of hyperprolactinemia is given in Table 226–3. If none of the disorders listed is present and there is no history of drug ingestion, the patient with a normal radiographic examination is considered to have idiopathic hyperprolactinemia.

The many similarities between patients with idiopathic hyperprolactinemia and those with small prolactin-secreting pituitary tumors (microadenomas) have led to the belief that these entities represent different stages of the same disorder. Follow-up evaluation of idiopathic hyperprolactinemia suggests that only a small percentage of cases (under 5 per cent) progress to demonstrable pituitary tumor formation and that among cases of microadenoma the vast majority remain stable for years with respect to both prolactin levels and tumor size.

Some patients with galactorrhea have normal or borderline elevation of prolactin levels, normal dynamic studies of prolactin secretion and ovulatory menses, and normal fertility. These patients represent the most common type of nonpuerperal galactorrhea, termed *normoprolactinemic galactorrhea*, which is attributed to enhanced sensitivity of the breast to prolactin. It can be seen as persistence of postpartum galactorrhea or following discontinuation of oral contraceptives.

TABLE 226–3. DIFFERENTIAL DIAGNOSIS OF NONPHYSIOLOGIC HYPERPROLACTINEMIA

A. Pharmacologic Agents
　Monoamine synthesis inhibitors (alpha-methyldopa)
　Monoamine depletors (reserpine)
　Dopamine receptor antagonists (phenothiazines, butyrophenones, thioxanthines)
　Estrogens (oral contraceptives)
　Narcotics (morphine, heroin)

B. Central Nervous System Disorders
　Inflammatory/infiltrative (sarcoidosis, histiocytosis)
　Traumatic (stalk section)
　Neoplastic (hypothalamic or parasellar tumors)

C. Pituitary Disorders
　Prolactin-secreting tumors
　　Macroadenomas
　　Microadenomas
　Empty sella syndrome

D. Idiopathic Hyperprolactinemia

E. Other
　Hypothyroidism
　Renal failure
　Cirrhosis
　Granulomatous or lymphocytic hypophysitis
　Chest wall/breast disease or surgery
　Thoracic spinal lesions

PATHOGENESIS. As with GH-secreting tumors, a controversy currently exists whether prolactin-secreting tumors represent a primary pituitary disease or are secondary to altered hypothalamic influence. Prolactin-secreting tumors also occur in association with other tumors, in particular pancreatic islet tumors and parathyroid tumors/hyperplasia as part of the multiple endocrine neoplasia syndrome type I (Ch. 233).

A hypothalamic etiology is supported by a large number of pharmacologic studies suggesting impaired CNS dopaminergic tone. However, evidence for prolactin resistance to dopamine has also been demonstrated, though this appears to be unrelated to altered dopamine receptors. Careful studies appear to have excluded a pathogenic role of oral contraceptives. However, the possibility of a role for a yet unidentified prolactin-releasing factor still exists.

THERAPY. The treatment of prolactin-secreting tumors has undergone considerable change in the past decade. Although surgery has been the therapy of choice in the past, many prolactinomas can now be treated as effectively by medical (pharmacologic) means. Prolactinomas should be divided into three subgroups when therapy is considered:

1. *Macroadenomas with only slightly elevated prolactin levels* (i.e., <100 to 150 ng per milliliter). This tumor is composed primarily of nonprolactin–secreting cells and should be managed similarly to the nonfunctioning tumor, i.e., surgical removal of tumor mass with preservation of pituitary function.

2. *Microadenomas.* Primary surgical therapy of microadenomas has resulted in up to 90 per cent "cure" rates as judged by restoration of cyclic menses and fertility. However, growth of microadenomas is infrequently observed (5 to 10 per cent become macroadenomas), and this, plus their presence in one third of unselected autopsies, raises the question whether their removal is indeed necessary in all patients. Furthermore, long-term follow-up of presumably cured patients indicates recurrence of hyperprolactinemia in at least 25 per cent. The most frequent reason for treatment of microadenomas is infertility. The most rapid and effective means of reducing prolactin levels to normal in such patients is by use of the dopamine agonist bromocriptine, which suppresses prolactin secretion in all forms of hyperprolactinemia by an action directly on the lactotroph. Prolactin levels are decreased by more than 90 per cent, and galactorrhea is improved or eliminated in most patients, even if prolactin levels remain slightly elevated. Similarly, cyclic menses and fertility may return without complete normalization of prolactin levels. The dosage required for most patients is 2.5 to 7.5 mg per day in divided doses. Some patients may require up to 15 mg per day. Side effects consist primarily of nausea and vomiting due to stimulation of the emesis center, occasionally of hypotension due to a CNS-mediated mechanism, and of mood changes. The side effects may be minimized by initiating therapy with a small dose and gradually increasing it, though 5 to 10 per cent of patients are unable to tolerate the drug. The incidence of congenital abnormalities in infants of women who have conceived while taking bromocriptine is not increased, and even when given throughout pregnancy the drug appears to be safe. It is, in fact, the recommended therapy for women who develop signs and symptoms of a prolactin-secreting tumor during pregnancy. Even when fertility is not of concern, reduction of prolactin levels is warranted in an attempt to correct osteopenia and prevent subsequent symptomatic osteoporosis. The same rationale is used for treating idiopathic hyperprolactinemia.

3. *Macroadenomas with markedly elevated prolactin levels.* This tumor is composed almost exclusively of lactotrophs. In addition to the above considerations, the size of this tumor can be markedly decreased by bromocriptine, most dramatically when the tumor is very large. In about two thirds of patients, bromocriptine will reduce tumor size by 50 to 75 per cent. The effects are usually quite rapid, occurring within days, but in some patients, tumor shrinkage may require several months. The reduction in size continues for as long as therapy is continued, even up to 10 years. Discontinuation of the drug after one year or less of therapy is often associated with rapid regrowth of the tumor, and symptoms may recur within days. However, after several years, drug dosage can be markedly reduced and in occasional patients, discontinued without evidence of tumor regrowth. This drug is useful in reducing the size of very large tumors prior to surgery, in postoperative treatment of patients in whom partial tumor removal was accomplished, and in patients who are not candidates for surgery.

Bromocriptine is also effective in males with prolactinomas. Restoration of serum testosterone levels and of libido and potency follows institution of therapy and normalization of prolactin levels.

Glickman SP, Rosenfield RL, Bergenstal RM, et al.: Multiple androgenic abnormalities including free testosterone, in hyperprolactinemic women. J Clin Endocrinol Metab 55:251, 1982. *Adrenal androgens are increased in women with hyperprolactinemia, and an increase in free testosterone is also present, related to decreased testosterone-binding globulin. These alterations explain the increased androgenization seen in some hyperprolactinemic patients.*

Klibanski A, Greenspan SL: Increase in bone mass after treatment of hyperprolactinemic amenorrhea. N Engl J Med 315:542, 1986. *The first demonstration that suppression of hyperprolactinemia can lead to correction of decreased bone mass, which has been known to occur with this disease.*

Liuzzi A, Dallabonzana D, Oppizzi G, et al.: Low doses of dopamine agonists in the long-term treatment of macroprolactinomas. N Engl J Med 313:656, 1985. *Long-term therapy with dopamine agonists is a practical and effective alternative to surgery in the treatment of prolactinomas.*

Molitch ME: Pregnancy and the hyperprolactinemic woman. N Engl J Med 312:1364, 1985. *A review of the risk of pregnancy in women with macroadenomas, microadenomas, and with no evidence of a pituitary tumor.*

Molitch ME, Elton RL, Blackwell RE, et al.: Bromocriptine as primary therapy for prolactin-secreting macroadenomas: Results of a prospective multicenter study. J Clin Endocrinol Metab 60:698, 1985. *A carefully planned prospective study showing the effectiveness of bromocriptine in decreasing tumor size in patients with prolactinomas.*

Randall RV, Laws ER Jr, Abboud CE, et al.: Transsphenoidal microsurgical treatment of prolactin producing adenomas. Results in 100 patients. Mayo Clin Proc 58:108, 1983. Wilson CB, Dempsey LC: Transsphenoidal microsurgical removal of 250 pituitary adenomas. J Neurosurg 48:13, 1978. *Two large series of patients with prolactinomas treated surgically show similar results in that the cure rate is highest in microadenomas and considerably lower in large tumors and in patients with prolactin levels above 200 ng per milliliter.*

Schlechte JA, Sherman BM, Chapler FK, et al.: Long term follow-up of women with surgically treated prolactin-secreting pituitary tumors. J Clin Endocrinol Metab 62:1296, 1986. *Recurrence of hyperprolactinemia after transsphenoidal adenomectomy occurs commonly and forms the basis for attempting other treatment methods.*

Spark, RF, Wills C, O'Reilly G, et al.: Hyperprolactinaemia in males with and without pituitary macroadenomas. Lancet 2:129, 1982. *The major clinical manifestation of hyperprolactinemia in males is impotence. Bromocriptine is effective in restoring normal testosterone levels and potency in most subjects with or without tumors.*

von Werder K, Eversmann T, Rjosk H-K, et al.: Treatment of hyperprolactinemia. In Ganong WF, Martini L (eds.): Frontiers in Neuroendocrinology. Vol 7. New York, Raven Press, 1982, pp 123–160. March CM, Kletzky OA, Davajan V, et al.: Longitudinal evaluation of patients with untreated prolactin-secreting pituitary adenomas. Am J Obstet Gynecol 139:835, 1981. *These two studies report on the natural history of idiopathic hyperprolactinemia and microadenomas, followed without specific treatment. They indicate that in the vast majority (> 90 per cent) size and prolactin levels remain relatively stationary for many years, concluding that immediate surgical intervention is not required in many patients.*

ACTH-Secreting Tumors: Cushing's Disease

Basophilic adenomas of the pituitary associated with bilateral adrenocortical hyperplasia and the features of hypercortisolism constitute a disorder first described by Cushing. The tumors, which tend to be located in the midline or near the anterior-posterior pituitary junction, are usually benign, but in contrast to other pituitary tumors, often exhibit more aggressive growth behavior, may have true malignant potential, and on rare occasions metastasize within and without the CNS. Corticotroph tumors may first become clinically apparent following bilateral adrenalectomy in patients with Cushing's disease (Nelson's syndrome). Corticotroph tumors may also be chromophobic and are found in 5 to 7 per cent of pituitaries at autopsy in patients without evidence of ACTH hypersecretion during life. Defects in the hormone secretory process may be responsible for these nonfunctioning tumors.

CLINICAL FEATURES. The clinical features of corticotroph tumors consist of those related to hypercortisolism and those caused by hypersecretion of ACTH and related peptides. The signs and symptoms of hypercortisolism are indistinguishable from those associated with adrenocortical adenomas or exogenous hormone administration and include centripetal obesity, hypertension, diabetes, amenorrhea, hirsutism, acne, osteoporosis and compression fractures, muscle atrophy, violaceous striae, capillary fragility, impaired wound healing, decreased resistance to infection, and behavioral changes. These are discussed in greater detail in Ch. 230. Increased secretion of ACTH and beta-LPH produces pigmentation similar to that seen in Addison's disease. In addition to generalized pigmentation, the pressure points (knuckles, elbows, knees, belt or brassiere strap regions), areolae, genitalia, mucous membranes, and recently healed scars are particularly affected. Because ACTH production is only partially autonomous in this disease, hyperpigmentation is mild or moderate in the early stages, but may be more pronounced after adrenalectomy or in very large tumors.

LABORATORY STUDIES. Randomly obtained plasma cortisol levels are elevated in only about half of the patients with Cushing's disease. The 24-hour urinary free cortisol is the most reliable measurement for distinguishing patients with increased adrenocortical function. Normal values are less than 100 µg per 24 hours. Of the dynamic tests, dexamethasone suppressibility is the most reliable and widely used. In normal subjects, low-dosage dexamethasone (0.5 mg every six hours for two days) decreases urinary free cortisol to less than 20 µg per 24 hours and plasma cortisol to less than 5 µg per deciliter. Patients with corticotroph tumors exhibit impaired suppression with the low dosage but at least 50 per cent suppression with the high dosage (2.0 mg every six hours for two days). In some patients, however, larger doses may be required to demonstrate suppression. Dexamethasone does not suppress cortisol secretion fully at any dose in patients with adrenal adenomas or ectopic ACTH secretion. These conditions can be distinguished by measurement of plasma ACTH levels, which are absent in the former and exceedingly high in the latter. Patients with Cushing's disease exhibit ACTH hyperresponsiveness to CRF; those with adrenal adenomas or ectopic ACTH production do not exhibit a response. High-quality CT of the pituitary will demonstrate the presence of a tumor in only 60 per cent of patients with Cushing's disease.

DIFFERENTIAL DIAGNOSIS. ACTH-secreting tumors are responsible for approximately 80 per cent of cases of endogenous hypercortisolemia. Adrenal tumors are present in about 15 per cent, and the remainder are caused by ectopic ACTH-secreting or, rarely, by CRF-secreting tumors. The differential diagnosis of these disorders is discussed in greater detail in Ch. 230. Ectopic ACTH production can occur in a variety of tumors, most commonly small-cell lung carcinomas, carcinoids, and pancreatic islet tumors (see Ch. 173). The disease can mimic that of corticotroph tumors, though in patients with malignant diseases, weight gain is often absent and severe hypokalemia is a prominent feature. Some of these tumors have been shown to secrete CRF alone or in combination with ACTH, explaining the occasional similarity in responses to dynamic hormone testing to those in patients with corticotroph tumors. Ectopic ACTH secretion should be suspected when the clinical and biochemical features of hypercortisolism occur on a periodic or intermittent basis.

Mild elevations of plasma cortisol, loss of diurnal variation, and absence of dexamethasone suppressibility are seen in patients under stress, during periods of bereavement, and in patients with depressive illness. Biochemically it is frequently impossible to distinguish these patients from those with ACTH-secreting tumors, though the clinical features of hypercortisolism are generally absent.

PATHOGENESIS. Arguments have been made for both a hypothalamic and a pituitary cause of ACTH-secreting tumors. Hypothalamic tumors have been identified in association with Cushing's disease, suggesting tumorous overproduction of CRF. Patients with ACTH-secreting tumors generally respond to CRF, as does tumor tissue tested in vitro. Basophilic hyperplasia, rather than tumor, is occasionally found in patients with Cushing's disease. In addition, cyproheptadine, a serotonin-receptor blocker, suppresses ACTH secretion in some patients with the disorder, providing strong support for a primary CNS role. The major argument for a primary pituitary disorder is based on the successful treatment by transsphenoidal adenomectomy, which includes reestablishment not only of normal quantitative cortisol secretion but of diurnal periodicity and glucocorticoid suppressibility. It is possible that two subgroups of the disease exist that are not readily distinguishable by clinical or laboratory methods currently available. Several lines of evidence suggest the presence of two subgroups, including the ultradian pattern of ACTH and cortisol secretion and the biochemical responses of the tumor in vivo and in vitro. Both groups, however, have a common characteristic: diminished sensitivity to feedback inhibition by cortisol.

THERAPY. Definitive treatment of ACTH-secreting pituitary tumors is indicated as soon as the diagnosis has been established. Once ectopic ACTH or CRF production has been excluded, surgical removal of the pituitary ACTH-secreting tumor is indicated. Tumors may be extremely small and difficult to identify. If the tumor cannot be located or if the patient remains hypercortisolemic following surgery, anterior hypophysectomy or bilateral total adrenalectomy is necessary, the decision being influenced by the patient's age, desire for subsequent pregnancy, and overall general health. Following pituitary adenomectomy, adrenocortical hypofunction requiring glucocorticoid replacement therapy may persist for as long as two years. A success rate of up to 85 per cent has been reported in patients with small ACTH-secreting tumors, although in those with large tumors this figure is reduced to about 30 per cent.

Radiation is also effective as primary therapy in ACTH-secreting tumors. Cure rates have been reported of 80 per cent in children and 60 per cent in adults with either conventional radiotherapy or proton beam therapy. Some long-term loss of other pituitary function has been noted after radiotherapy.

Pharmacologic therapy of Cushing's disease is directed at suppression of cortisol biosynthesis by the adrenals, using aminoglutethimide, metyrapone, or mitotane (o,p'-DDD) or ketoconazole; at neurotransmitter metabolism within the CNS; or at the pituitary directly. Detailed discussion of drugs acting on the adrenal is provided in Ch. 230. They have been used, together with radiotherapy, as an alternative to surgical treatment in selected patients. The serotonin-receptor blocker cyproheptadine and the GABA agonist sodium valproate have been successful in a small number of patients with Cushing's disease in restoring both ACTH and cortisol secretion to normal. Responses have also been seen in patients with Nelson's disease. A few patients will also exhibit decreases in ACTH secretion during bromocriptine therapy. There is no evidence for regression of tumor size by these agents to date.

Carey RM, Varma SK, Drake CR, et al.: Ectopic secretion of corticotropin-releasing factor as a cause of Cushing's syndrome. N Engl J Med 311:13, 1984. *Although uncommon, ectopic secretion of hypothalamic hormones must be considered when dealing with pituitary hormone hypersecretory states.*

Cauter EV, Refetoff S: Evidence for two subtypes of Cushing's disease based on the analysis of episodic cortisol secretion. N Engl J Med 312:1343, 1985. *One of a number of approaches attempting to separate patients with Cushing's disease into different subgroups.*

Chrousos GP, Schulte HM, Oldfield EH, et al.: The corticotropin-releasing factor stimulation test. N Engl J Med 310:622, 1984. *Patients with Cushing's disease respond to CRF while those with ectopic ACTH secretion do not. Thus the test is quite useful in the differential diagnosis.*

Dornhorst A, Jenkins JS, Lamberts SW, et al.: The evaluation of sodium valproate in the treatment of Nelson's syndrome. J Clin Endocrinol Metab 56:985, 1983. *This GABA agonist reduced ACTH levels, produced clinical improvement, and in one patient decreased pituitary tumor size. The site of action is believed to be the hypothalamus, where it increases GABA activity, thereby inhibiting CRF release.*

Findling JW, Aron DC, Tyrrell JB, et al.: Selective venous sampling for ACTH in Cushing's syndrome: Differentiation between Cushing's disease and the ectopic ACTH syndrome. Ann Intern Med 94:647, 1981. *The selective sampling procedure used was capable of identifying the source of elevated ACTH levels when other procedures failed to differentiate between pituitary and extrapituitary sources.*

Fitzgerald PA, Aron DC, Findling JW, et al.: Cushing's disease: Transient secondary adrenal insufficiency after selective removal of pituitary microadenomas: Evidence for a pituitary origin. J Clin Endocrinol Metab 54:413, 1982. *Temporary adrenal insufficiency is observed after successful removal of an ACTH-secreting tumor, providing evidence for suppression of residual pituitary corticotrophs.*

Krieger DT: Physiopathology of Cushing's disease. Endocr Rev 4:22, 1983. *A detailed review presenting the arguments pro and con for both pituitary and CNS causes of Cushing's disease. Evidence for multiple causes is supported by the author's arguments.*

Lamberts SW, de Lange SA, Stefanko SZ: Adrenocorticotropin-secreting pituitary adenomas originate from the anterior or the intermediate lobe in Cushing's disease: Differences in the regulation of hormone secretion. J Clin Endocrinol Metab 54:286, 1982. *ACTH-secreting tumors can be subdivided into two subgroups with different sites of origin, responses to dynamic testing, and probabilities of surgical cure.*

Sonino N, Boscaro M, Merola G, et al.: Prolonged treatment of Cushing's disease by ketoconazole. J Clin Endocrinol Metab 61:718, 1985. *A new approach to the treatment of Cushing's disease by inhibiting enzymes involved in adrenal steroidogenesis.*

Other Hormone-Secreting Tumors

TSH and gonadotropin secretion by pituitary tumors is extremely rare. TSH-secreting tumors are detected during the workup of hyperthyroid patients with elevated rather than suppressed TSH levels. The clinical manifestations consist of hyperthyroidism and a pituitary tumor mass. Occasionally mixed pituitary cell types are present with coexisting GH or prolactin hypersecretion. TSH secretion is not completely autonomous, since suppression of thyroxine production by methimazole frequently results in an increase of TSH secretion. Treatment must be directed to removal of the tumor mass, though medical therapy to suppress the elevated thyroxine levels is required preoperatively.

FSH and FSH/LH-secreting pituitary tumors are very rare and often associated with longstanding hypogonadism. Occasionally tumors otherwise considered to be nonfunctioning may produce the isolated glycoprotein alpha subunit that is devoid of any clinical manifestations and serves primarily as a tumor marker.

Beckers A, Stevenaert A, Mashiter K, et al.: Follicle-stimulating hormone-secreting pituitary adenomas. J Clin Endocrinol Metab 61:525, 1985. Vance ML, Ridgway EC, Thorner MO: Follicle-stimulating hormone and alpha-subunit-secreting pituitary tumor treated with bromocriptine. J Clin Endocrinol Metab 61:580, 1985. *There is now convincing evidence for production of FSH by pituitary tumors, and preliminary evidence suggests that bromocriptine may be effective in therapy.*

Klibanski A, Ridgway EC, Zervas NT: Pure alpha subunit-secreting pituitary tumors. J Neurosurg 59:585, 1983. *Six patients with otherwise "nonfunctioning" pituitary tumors are described with elevated glycoprotein alpha subunit levels that can be used as a marker for monitoring the effects of therapy. No clinical manifestations of the secretory product have yet been recognized.*

Smallridge RC, Smith CE: Hyperthyroidism due to thyrotropin-secreting pituitary tumors. Diagnostic and therapeutic considerations. Arch Intern Med 143:503, 1983. *In a review of 33 reported cases the authors describe the characteristic laboratory findings and provide recommendations for therapy.*

227 THE POSTERIOR PITUITARY

Thomas E. Andreoli

ANTIDIURETIC HORMONE

The neurohypophysis of humans elaborates two hormones: *arginine vasopressin* (AVP), which exhibits vasopressor and antidiuretic activity, and *oxytocin*, which is galactobolic and uterotonic. Both hormones are octapeptides of approximately 1100 daltons, with a 20-member ring structure created by disulfide bonds. The antidiuretic and vasopressor activities of AVP are each approximately 100 times as great as those of oxytocin, a difference that is related to the different tertiary conformations of the two peptides.

The posterior pituitary gland contains terminal axons whose cell bodies lie in hypothalamic cell clusters known as the *supraoptic* and *paraventricular nuclei*. Synthesis of posterior pituitary hormones occurs in these hypothalamic nuclei rather than in the posterior pituitary gland: (1) AVP can be demonstrated immunochemically in cells of both the supraoptic and the paraventricular nuclei; and (2) neurosecretory granules accumulate only on the hypothalamic side of a sectioned hypophyseal stalk.

The cardinal steps in the biosynthesis of antidiuretic hormone (ADH) are illustrated in Figure 227–1. Neurohypophyseal hormones, including vasopressin, are synthesized as prohormones in conjunction with specific carrier proteins called neurophysins. Vasopressin, specifically, is synthesized as a prohormone in conjunction with neurophysin II, and the complex is sometimes termed the van Dyke protein. It is then transported to the posterior pituitary gland in discrete neurosecretory granules by axonal streaming within the cytoplasm of pituicytes. In the posterior pituitary gland, these granules rest in terminal projections of axonal plasma membranes, juxtaposed to systemic circulation capillaries. Other pituicyte nerve fibers terminate in the median eminence and along the third ventricle, thus allowing access of vasopressin to cerebrospinal fluid.

There are two pools of AVP-containing neurosecretory granules in pituicytes: one adjacent to the cell membrane and therefore available for immediate release, and a second storage pool removed from immediate contact with the plasma membrane. Release of hormone occurs by an exocytotic process involving fusion of neurosecretory granules with pituicyte plasma membranes. In other words, AVP release is quantal. A stimulus to the hypothalamic pituicyte cell body is transmitted to the site of granule storage, where it causes cell membrane depolarization, an associated increase in calcium permeability, and rapid calcium entry into the pituicytes. This

Form	Molecular Weight	Synthetic Step
Preprohormone ↓	≃21,000	Protein synthesis; magnocellular neuron ribosomes
Prohormone ↓	≃23,000	Glycosylation and membrane packaging; magnocellular neuron; Golgi apparatus
Neurosecretory Granule (NSG) ↓	$(23,000)_n$	Transport down supraopticohyophyseal tract as osmotically inactive granules
Neurophysin + Hormone	≃10,000 ≃1,100	Storage in posterior pituitary; cleavage within NSG

FIGURE 227–1. Flow diagram for the pathway of posterior pituitary hormone biosynthesis. (From Hebert SC, Culpepper RM, Andreoli TE: The posterior pituitary and water metabolism. In Foster DW, Wilson JD (eds.): Textbook of Endocrinology. 7th ed. Philadelphia, W. B. Saunders Company, 1985, pp 614–652.)

influx of calcium activates the exocytosis of AVP-containing neurosecretory granules.

RELEVANT PHYSIOLOGY. Detailed accounts of the renal and pituitary processes resulting in the formation of dilute or concentrated urine are presented in Ch. 75 and 77. ADH exerts major physiologic effects on discrete regions of the nephron and also affects vascular smooth muscle tone. In all epithelia that respond to ADH, the hormone binds to specific receptors on the basolateral plasma membrane of the cell and, in so doing, activates the enzyme adenylate cyclase. Adenylate cyclase increases the production of 3',5'-cyclic adenosine monophosphate (cAMP) from its substrate adenosine triphosphate (ATP). Cyclic AMP then acts as a second messenger to activate a cell-specific protein kinase, which induces the final cellular response to the hormone (see Ch. 221). ADH-stimulated adenylate cyclase is present in the collecting duct and in the medullary, but not cortical, thick ascending limb of Henle (mTALH) of mammalian kidneys.

The *cardinal* physiologic effect of ADH is to promote the formation of hypertonic urine. The formation of hypertonic urine depends particularly on two sets of events operating in parallel within the renal medulla. First, in the thick ascending limb of Henle, approximately 15 to 20 per cent of the filtered load of sodium chloride is absorbed. Since the mTALH is water impermeable, this process contributes simultaneously to the maintenance of a hypertonic medullary interstitium and to the formation of dilute urine. Under normal circumstances, the osmolality of the renal medullary interstitium rises from isotonic, at the corticomedullary junction, to very hypertonic, approximately 1200 mosm per kilogram of H_2O, at the papillary tip. Since the enrichment of medullary interstitial osmolality and dilution of tubular fluid both depend on sodium chloride absorption by the water-impermeable mTALH, the latter region of the nephron is commonly termed the medullary diluting segment. Approximately 10 per cent of fluid filtered at the glomerulus, or about 18 liters daily, reaches the early distal tubule with an osmolality of approximately 50 mosm per kilogram of H_2O.

When ADH is absent, the water permeability of collecting ducts is at a minimum. Thus there is reduced osmotic equilibration of fluid passing through collecting ducts with the medullary interstitium, and most of the fluid escapes unchanged as hypotonic urine. Since only 10 per cent of filtered water normally reaches the collecting duct system, the maximal degree of polyuria in a patient with complete pituitary diabetes insipidus (or complete nephrogenic diabetes insipidus) is therefore approximately 18 liters daily. During normal antidiuresis, ADH, by way of cAMP, increases the water permeability of luminal (urinary) cell membranes of cortical and outer medullary collecting ducts. Thus in the presence of ADH, there is osmotic equilibration of hypotonic luminal fluid

in collecting ducts with the hypertonic medullary interstitium and, consequently, water absorption, a reduction in urine volume, concentration of urine, and conservation of body water.

The ADH-dependent increase in the water permeability of collecting ducts is due to a hormone-dependent increase in the number of water-specific channels available for water transport through luminal membranes. These channels are rather narrow, approximately 2 Å in radius, and therefore exclude urea and NaCl. As a consequence, the luminal fluid concentrations of these two solutes increase when water is abstracted from cortical and outer medullary collecting ducts during antidiuresis. In turn, the increase in luminal urea concentration creates a favorable gradient for passive urea diffusion out of inner medullary (papillary) collecting ducts into the interstitium, thereby maintaining interstitial hypertonicity. ADH also causes a slight increase in papillary duct urea permeability, thus favoring passive movement of urea down its concentration gradient for recirculation through the medullary interstitium.

A *second ADH-mediated* event in the antidiuretic response is to increase the rate of NaCl transport in medullary, but not cortical, mTALH. This process involves a furosemide-sensitive electroneutral cotransport of $Na^+:K^+:2Cl^-$ from luminal fluid into cells; virtually all of the potassium entering cells through this process is recycled back into luminal fluid via potassium-specific channels in luminal membranes. Consequently, ADH increases urinary concentrating power in two ways: by enhancing the water permeability of collecting ducts and by increasing the net rate of salt absorption by the mTALH, thus enriching medullary interstitial osmolality.

This latter effect of ADH on medullary diluting segments is opposed by at least three other factors. (1) As interstitial NaCl concentrations increase, the backleak of NaCl into the tubular lumen of the mTALH also increases and thereby tends to reduce net NaCl absorption by the mTALH. (2) Increases in interstitial osmolality down-regulate the ADH stimulation of NaCl cotransport. (3) Prostaglandins of the E series, which are produced in the renal medullary interstitium in response to increasing interstitial osmolality, inhibit competitively the ADH-mediated increases in the rate of intracellular cAMP formation.

These three processes have a negative feedback on ADH enhancement of active NaCl absorption in the mTALH, so that the diluting power of the mTALH remains constant during either antidiuresis or water diuresis.

Finally, prostaglandins of the E series also antagonize the ADH-dependent enhancement of collecting-duct water permeability. This effect may be produced either by prostaglandins synthesized endogenously by collecting-duct cells or by prostaglandins synthesized within the medullary interstitium. Thus prostaglandins blunt urinary concentrating power by offsetting ADH effects in at least two loci, the mTALH and the collecting duct.

At levels of hormone that exceed those necessary for antidiuresis, ADH also has pressor activity (this was the first known effect of posterior pituitary extract and provided the basis for the name vasopressin) that is the result of a direct constricting effect on vascular smooth muscle. At all but high pharmacologic doses, this pressor effect is easily overcome by compensatory vasodilatory reflexes, so that hypertension is not routinely seen during AVP replacement therapy. Lesser doses may, however, cause significant vasoconstriction of coronary arteries. Another effect of vasopressin, seen at levels that supersede those necessary for antidiuresis, is stimulation of intestinal motility. Finally, AVP released into the CSF and thalamic centers may play a role in such diverse processes as memory and regulation of corticotropin release.

OSMOTIC REGULATION OF ADH RELEASE. Verney's elegant studies demonstrated a strong antidiuretic response to perfusion of carotid vessels with hypertonic solutions of various solutes, including sodium salts and glucose; hypertonic urea solutions elicited no such response. Therefore he concluded that specific cells that acted as osmoreceptors were present within the distribution of the carotid circulation and that the plasma membranes of these cells were impermeable to sodium salts and glucose, but permeable to urea. In the presence of extracellular hyperosmolality induced by impermeable species, these osmosensing cells reached osmotic equilibrium by losing water to the hypertonic plasma. In other words, Verney deduced that osmoreceptor shrinkage, produced by raising plasma osmolality with solutes restricted to the extracellular compartment, was the stimulus for ADH release.

When the anterior wall of the third ventricle is exposed to hypertonic saline, neurons in both the anterior hypothalamus and the preoptic area have increased rates of depolarization. Concomitantly, about half of the pituicytes in hypothalamic nuclei show a characteristic depolarization pattern, and plasma antidiuretic activity increases. Therefore it is probable that the neurons in the anterior hypothalamus and preoptic areas, which depolarize in response to hypertonic saline, represent Verney's osmoreceptors.

In normal man, plasma AVP levels are undetectable below a plasma osmolality of 280 mosm per kilogram of H_2O. Since the usual plasma osmolality in man is approximately 287 mosm per kilogram of H_2O, secretion of AVP is tonic; the average circulating hormone levels are between 2.0 and 2.5 pg per milliliter. Vasopressin levels increase in a linear fashion with increasing plasma osmolality, such that a rise in plasma osmolality of only 1 per cent (2.9 mosm per kilogram of H_2O) evokes a 1 pg per milliliter rise in AVP. Parallel examinations of plasma AVP and urine osmolality indicate that each unit increase in AVP allows an increase of 250 mosm per kilogram of H_2O in urinary concentration. Since the maximal concentrating ability of the human kidney is approximately 1200 mosm per kilogram of H_2O, maximal water conservation is therefore achieved at a plasma AVP level of 5.0 pg per milliliter.

Combining these relations yields a measure of the efficiency of the water homeostatic mechanism: for each 1 mosm per kilogram of H_2O change in plasma osmolality there is a change in urinary concentration of 95 mosm per kilogram of H_2O, which represents a gain of almost 100-fold. The ingestion of water sufficient to decrease plasma osmolality by only 1 mosm per kilogram of H_2O will reduce urinary concentration by 95 mosm per kilogram of H_2O, thus allowing the water to be excreted and osmotic balance to be restored. The opposite effect, water loss, results in stimulation of ADH release, increase in urinary concentration, and conservation of body water by the same magnification phenomenon.

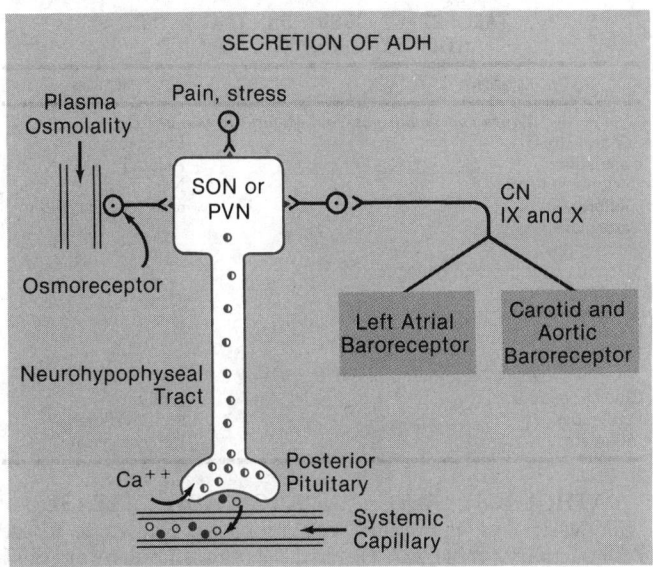

FIGURE 227–2. Secretory stimuli for calcium-dependent ADH release: van Dyke protein (◑), vasopressin (●), neurophysin II (○). SON = supraoptic neuron, PVN = paraventricular neuron.

NONOSMOTIC REGULATION OF ADH RELEASE. Isotonic or hypotonic volume depletion results in an antidiuretic state. Evidence now exists for stretch receptors, or baroreceptors, that sense changes in vascular wall tension in both the venous (low pressure) and arterial (high pressure) circulations. Immersion and negative pressure breathing, i.e., maneuvers that augment intrathoracic blood volume, as well as balloon distension of the left atrium, all produce water diuresis that can be overcome by administering ADH. Conversely, positive pressure breathing and upright posture, which reduce intrathoracic blood volume, or left atrial collapse, produce antidiuresis. These observations indicate that the left atrium and the pulmonary vasculature are the major loci for low pressure baroreceptors that modulate ADH release.

Hypotension, or selective clamping of major systemic arterial vessels, also produces profound antidiuresis. These data indicate the presence of a baroreceptor system in the arterial circulation, localized to the carotid bifurcations and aortic arch, that also modulates ADH release. This type of nonosmotic ADH release is modulated by stimulatory or inhibitory signals arriving from the baroreceptors via parasympathetic pathways in the vagus and glossopharyngeal nerves. The low pressure baroreceptors are more sensitive regulators of ADH release than those in high pressure regions of the circulation. These relations are summarized in Figure 227–2.

Circulating levels of ADH rise with vascular volume depletion. However, volume-mediated, nonosmotic ADH release has a "threshold" requiring more than 7 per cent blood volume depletion, with greater degrees of blood volume contraction eliciting exponential rises in circulating ADH levels. Thus nonosmotic ADH release differs strikingly from osmotically mediated ADH release, which occurs with only a 1 to 2 per cent increase in plasma osmolality and rises linearly with further increases in plasma osmolality. With less than a 7 per cent decrease in blood volume, ADH release is governed wholly by plasma osmolality. At greater reductions in blood volume, ADH release is increasingly dominated by nonosmotic, volume-dependent stimuli. This observation explains the finding of progressive fluid dilution in patients with hypovolemia or states of decreased cardiac output.

Input from higher cortical functions also appears to influence ADH release. Pain, emotion, stress, and some psychotic states are associated with ADH stimulation or inhibition. Most common is the transient antidiuresis that occurs postoperatively.

TABLE 227–1. CONDITIONS THAT ALTER ANTIDIURETIC HORMONE ACTIVITY

Enhance	Suppress
Drugs and Conditions That Modify Release of ADH	
Surgical stress	Phenytoin
Vincristine	Alcohol
Cyclophosphamide	Narcotic antagonists
Clofibrate	α-Adrenergic agents
Carbamazepine	
Barbiturates	
Morphine and narcotic analogues	
Nicotine	
β-Adrenergic agents	
Hypoxia	
Hypercapnia	
Drugs That Modify the ADH Effect on Collecting Ducts	
Chlorpropamide	Lithium
Biguanides	Methoxyflurane
Indomethacin	Demeclocycline

PATHOLOGIC ALTERATION OF ADH RELEASE. A wide variety of agents and conditions are known to affect ADH activity (Table 227–1). Nicotine, as a stimulant of ADH release, and acute alcohol ingestion, as an inhibitor of ADH release, have figured prominently in devising means to assess neurohypophyseal integrity. Stimulatory drugs such as clofibrate and chlorpropamide have been utilized to treat states of partial ADH insufficiency. Other drugs, such as lithium and demeclocycline are prominent for their effect on the renal collecting duct, making it unresponsive to ADH, and thereby producing nephrogenic diabetes insipidus.

The syndrome of inappropriate antidiuretic hormone secretion (SIADH) is characterized by persistent hyponatremia, an inappropriately elevated urine osmolality, and no discernible stimulus for ADH release. A common cause for this condition is neoplastic, most notably oat cell carcinoma of lung; SIADH is due to ectopic production of ADH by the tumor, with persistent release of hormone independent of regulatory influences. Inflammatory disorders of the lung, such as pneumonia or cavitary tuberculosis, provide other sites for ectopic ADH production. The syndrome also occurs in patients with head trauma or with other diseases of the central nervous system and often terminates with recovery of neurologic function. The SIADH syndrome is discussed in detail in Ch. 77.

THIRST REGULATION. Body water content is governed not only by ADH modulation of renal water excretion but also by regulation of water intake through thirst. Both systems operate in parallel under the influence of osmotic and volume mediators. Thirst also requires an intact cerebral cortex, which transforms the urge to drink into appropriate behavior to secure water.

Hyperosmolality, and presumably shrinkage of thirst receptors, is the primary stimulus for thirst, and requires only a 2 per cent rise in plasma osmolality. The thirst "threshold" in conscious humans is about 294 mosm per kilogram, the same osmolality at which maximal urinary concentration under ADH is achieved. Hypovolemia also stimulates thirst via an angiotensin II-mediated mechanism. Indeed, hyperreninemic states such as malignant hypertension are often accompanied by pathologic thirst. Phenothiazines enhance thirst and contribute to the hyponatremia seen in some patients treated with these drugs for affective disorders. Finally, prostaglandin E also stimulates thirst. The polydipsia that accompanies hypokalemia probably depends on increased production of prostaglandin E.

WATER REPLETION REACTION. The details of the water repletion reaction are presented in Figure 6 of Ch. 76. The positive limb of the water repletion reaction has two cardinal features—redundancy and variable gain. Thus two sets of stimuli—osmotic and nonosmotic—stimulate both thirst and antidiuresis. The osmotic stimuli represent, especially for antidiuresis, the system that is activated by 2 per cent changes

in effective plasma osmolality, and has a linear gain. In contrast, nonosmotic stimuli enhance thirst and antidiuresis only in response to rather large (that is, more than 7 per cent) reductions in effective circulatory volume. Moreover, particularly with respect to antidiuresis, greater degrees of volume contraction provide exponential rather than linear increases in concentrating power.

Atrial natriuretic peptide, or atriopeptin, may have a central role in the negative feedback limb of the water repletion reaction. The factors responsible for the biosynthesis and release of atriopeptin are described in detail in Ch. 224. Stated briefly, atriopeptin is released from atrial granules in response to increases in effective circulating volume. Moreover, immunoreactive atriopeptin is produced in the anterolateral periventricular areas of the hypothalamus. In the present context, two actions of either circulating or centrally released atriopeptin have particular relevance: blunting of ADH release in response to osmotic or nonosmotic stimuli and suppression of angiotensin-mediated thirst. These effects suggest a central role for atriopeptin in negative feedback regulation of the water repletion reaction.

Hebert SC, Culpepper RM, Andreoli TE: The posterior pituitary and water metabolism. In Foster DW, Wilson JD: Textbook of Endocrinology. 7th ed. Philadelphia, WB Saunders Company, 1985, pp 614–652. *A complete analysis of the physiology of the water repletion reaction.*

Needleman P, Greenwald JE: Atriopeptin: A cardiac hormone intimately involved in fluid, electrolyte, and blood-pressure homeostasis. N Engl J Med 314:828, 1986. *A review of the role of atriopeptin in the physiology and pathophysiology of volume and electrolyte homeostasis.*

Verney EB: The antidiuretic hormone and the factors which dsetermine its release. Proc R Soc Lond (Biol) 135:25, 1947. *A classic treatise describing a series of elegant studies which led to the notion of a central nervous system osmoreceptor for ADH secretion.*

DIABETES INSIPIDUS
Pituitary Diabetes Insipidus

DEFINITION. Pituitary diabetes insipidus is a polyuric syndrome that results from a lack of sufficient ADH to effect appropriate concentration of the urine or water conservation. The disease is identified by the persistence of an inappropriately dilute urine in the presence of strong osmotic or nonosmotic stimuli to ADH secretion, and in the absence of renal concentrating defects, and a rise in urine osmolality upon the administration of vasopressin. Pituitary diabetes insipidus may result either from destruction of the centers of ADH synthesis or from failure of the mechanisms effecting ADH release.

ETIOLOGY. Trauma to the neurohypophysis, either accidental or as a result of hypophysectomy, is the major identifiable cause of diabetes insipidus. A second major cause for pituitary diabetes insipidus is an intracranial tumor, which may be primary, as in craniopharyngioma, or metastatic, among which breast carcinoma is the most likely cause. Less frequent causes of pituitary diabetes insipidus are granulomatous lesions of the central nervous system, including tuberculosis and sarcoidosis, the histiocytoses, encephalomeningitis, or vascular lesions. There is a rare familial form of pituitary diabetes insipidus which affects either sex, occurs at any age, and is associated with extensive gliosis of neurohypophyseal nuclei. Finally, 30 to 40 per cent of all patients with pituitary diabetes insipidus have no identifiable cause for the disorder.

PATHOGENESIS. Pituitary diabetes insipidus depends on one of two different pathogenic mechanisms. Most commonly the disorder occurs when there is atrophy or destruction of the hypothalamic centers responsible for hormone production. Neither removal of the posterior pituitary gland alone nor low section of the neurohypophyseal tract with preservation of hypothalamic nuclei is sufficient to produce a permanent polyuric state. Rather, direct trauma to the pituitary gland or low section of the neurohypophyseal tract results in transient diabetes insipidus; for example, the polyuric state following low stalk section lasts for only one to two weeks postsurgery. Since the anterior and posterior lobes of the pituitary gland have totally separate blood supplies, infarction of the anterior pituitary gland does not disrupt posterior pituitary function.

A second group of cases has been identified, often classed under the heading essential hypernatremia, in which osmotic stimuli fail to elicit ADH release, while nonosmotic stimuli result in antidiuresis. Although euvolemic, these patients are polyuric and excrete hypotonic urine, and water deprivation alone fails to elicit an antidiuretic response. However, when volume contraction occurs in these patients, significant antidiuresis ensues. Thus, in this disorder there is selective failure of osmoreceptors to stimulate ADH release. The intact response of ADH release to nonosmotic stimulation verifies the integrity of the hypothalamic centers that produce ADH.

Nephrogenic Diabetes Insipidus

DEFINITION. The term *nephrogenic diabetes insipidus* should be applied to disorders in which renal tubular unresponsiveness to ADH, without disturbances either in solute delivery to the loop of Henle or in countercurrent multiplication or exchange processes, is responsible for polyuria and hyposthenuria. Thus nephrogenic diabetes insipidus may be due to inability of ADH to raise cellular cAMP concentrations, to inability of cAMP to increase the water permeability of luminal membranes of collecting ducts, or to a combination of these two disorders.

FAMILIAL NEPHROGENIC DIABETES INSIPIDUS. This familial disorder occurs primarily in males and exhibits a hereditary pattern of X-linked transmission with variable penetrance in females. In normal individuals or patients with pituitary diabetes insipidus, exogenous ADH can increase the rate of urinary cAMP excretion. In some patients with familial nephrogenic diabetes insipidus, comparable doses of ADH do not increase rates of urinary cAMP excretion. However, in two groups of children with nephrogenic diabetes insipidus, both basal and ADH-stimulated rates of urinary cAMP excretion exceeded those of normal children. These disparate results led to the postulate that familial nephrogenic diabetes insipidus is a heterogeneous disorder produced by either a defect in hormone receptor adenylate cyclase stimulation or a defect beyond the generation of cAMP. In patients with familial nephrogenic diabetes insipidus, however, plasma cortisol concentrations can rise in response to ADH, a finding interpreted to indicate that vasopressin stimulation of extrarenal, i.e., pituitary, cAMP formation is intact in the disease.

ACQUIRED NEPHROGENIC DIABETES INSIPIDUS. Vasopressin-resistant hyposthenuria associated with otherwise normal or nearly normal renal function may occur as a complication of drug therapy or in association with systemic diseases. This acquired nephrogenic diabetes insipidus is to be distinguished from the rare familial disorder described earlier.

Vasopressin-unresponsive hyposthenuria occurs in patients receiving demeclocycline; both the concentrating defect and vasopressin-unresponsiveness are reversible and disappear shortly after discontinuance of antibiotic therapy. The glomerular filtration rate in these patients is generally normal, as is the ability for maximal urinary dilution (positive free water formation), indicating that solute abstraction from the loop of Henle is probably unimpaired.

In human renal medulla, demeclocycline noncompetitively inhibits basal adenylate cyclase activity, ADH-stimulated adenylate cyclase activity, and cAMP-dependent protein kinase activity. Thus demeclocycline-induced nephrogenic diabetes insipidus may be due in part to inhibition of cAMP accumulation in collecting duct cells.

Nephrogenic diabetes insipidus may also be produced by volatile fluorocarbon anesthetics. Methoxyflurane anesthesia is complicated by a full spectrum of renal injury, ranging from vasopressin-resistant polyuria and hyposthenuria to acute tubular necrosis. Both fluoride and oxalic acid, which are

metabolic products of methoxyflurane, contribute to the nephrotoxicity of the anesthetic. However, the polyuric state is related to the markedly increased serum concentration and urinary excretion of inorganic fluoride. Sodium fluoride causes vasopressin-resistant polyuria in dogs, and in rats inorganic fluoride seems to reduce collecting duct water permeability without affecting salt transport in the ascending limb.

Serum lithium concentrations of 0.5 to 1.5 mEq per liter, which are generally regarded as being in the therapeutic range for affective disorders, produce vasopressin-resistant diabetes insipidus. Nephrogenic diabetes insipidus has been observed in 12 to 30 per cent of patients receiving lithium therapy; the defect is usually reversible, and urinary concentrating ability returns toward normal when lithium is discontinued. Finally nephrogenic diabetes insipidus characterized by persistent, vasopressin-resistant hyposthenuria and polyuria occurs rarely in certain systemic diseases, including most notably sarcoidosis and Sjögren's syndrome.

ACQUIRED POLYURIC STATES. Other disorders may present with polyuria and relative vasopressin resistance, although not necessarily with profound hyposthenuria. Rather, these polyuric disturbances are generally characterized by inability to concentrate urine maximally in response to vasopressin, either stimulated endogenously or administered exogenously; random urine samples are ordinarily not profoundly hypotonic but are usually only slightly hypotonic or modestly hypertonic.

In general, such polyuric disorders occur most commonly in association with hypokalemic nephropathy (Ch. 77) or hypercalcemic nephropathy (Ch. 247), or as a consequence of diseases that disrupt medullary architecture and consequently impair the generation and maintenance of a hypertonic medullary interstitium. The latter disorders include those diseases that affect particularly the renal interstitium, such as sickle cell disease, pyelonephritis, analgesic nephropathy, and multiple myeloma. These diseases are considered in Ch. 82.

Finally, states characterized by osmotic, or solute, diuresis, for example, in diabetic ketoacidosis and hyperglycemic nonketotic states, may result in polyuria with isotonic urine formation and unresponsiveness to vasopressin. In these disorders, the fraction of isotonic glomerular filtrate delivered to the loop of Henle is greatly increased because of failure to absorb solute, for example, glucose, in the proximal nephron. Thus the amount of solute and water reaching the loop of Henle becomes large with regard to the diluting or concentrating ability of the loop of Henle and collecting ducts, respectively, and vasopressin-resistant polyuria and isosthenuria ensue. Consequently the polyuric state in osmotic diuresis differs from that in nephrogenic diabetes insipidus in two respects; urinary solute excretion is dramatically increased in osmotic diuresis but not in nephrogenic diabetes insipidus; and the urine osmolality is nearly isotonic in solute diuresis but rather hypotonic in nephrogenic diabetes insipidus.

Pituitary or Nephrogenic Diabetes Insipidus

CLINICAL MANIFESTATIONS. The foremost clinical feature of either pituitary or nephrogenic diabetes insipidus is *polyuria*, with urine volumes ranging from 3 to 15 liters per day. Along with polyuria there is near-continuous thirst, often with a preference for ice cold water. The disease is almost always accompanied by *nocturia*, in contrast to persons with primary polydipsia (compulsive water drinking), in whom nocturia is usually absent. The onset of polyuria in pituitary diabetes insipidus is most often abrupt, with peak urine flow reached in one or two days. Therefore, polyuria developing over weeks or months suggests a disease other than pituitary diabetes insipidus. The polyuria of familial nephrogenic diabetes insipidus is present from birth.

The polyuria in complete diabetes insipidus, either pituitary or nephrogenic, has an upper limit of approximately 18 liters daily, or about 10 per cent of filtered water, since 90 per cent of the glomerular filtrate is normally absorbed by the nephron prior to reaching the collecting system. In partial pituitary diabetes insipidus, the daily urine volume may be considerably smaller. In contrast, persons afflicted with compulsive water drinking, often referred to as primary or psychogenic polydipsia, not infrequently ingest more than 20 liters of fluid daily. Therefore, the daily urine volume in these patients may also exceed 20 liters.

Modest degrees of volume depletion may curtail polyuria, even in complete diabetes insipidus, for two reasons. First, volume contraction will increase the fraction of glomerular filtrate absorbed by the proximal nephron, so that a smaller volume of hypotonic fluid reaches the collecting duct system. Second, even in the absence of ADH, or when collecting ducts are unresponsive to ADH, collecting ducts have a slight permeability to water; consequently, a small fraction of the water reaching the collecting duct system can be absorbed even without ADH. Since the volume of glomerular filtrate reaching the collecting duct system is reduced during volume contraction, the further absorption of relatively small volumes of water by collecting ducts during the volume-contracted state can result in dramatic reductions in polyuria.

Aside from the discomfort and inconvenience of polyuria and polydipsia, patients with pituitary or nephrogenic diabetes insipidus suffer no ill effects unless they are *deprived of access to water*. When this happens, *circulatory collapse* or *hypertonic encephalopathy* may occur. Because of the high rates of urine flow in some patients with diabetes insipidus, these complications may develop in a period of hours. For example, a patient with pituitary diabetes insipidus might excrete 5 per cent of his glomerular filtrate daily, or about 9 liters of urine. In a 70-kg man having 42 kg of body water, this loss, if not continually replenished, would result in a 20 per cent reduction in body water in only 24 hours.

Hypertonic Encephalopathy. Acute increases in intracellular fluid osmolality to levels exceeding 350 mosm per kilogram of H_2O produced by solutes such as NaCl or glucose (in diabetes), which cross cell membranes poorly, result in central nervous system dysfunction ranging from lethargy to frank coma. Since comparable elevations of plasma osmolality produced by urea, which permeates cell membranes freely, do not produce the disorder, it is evident that hyperosmolality per se is not the basis for the disturbance. Rather, acute hypertonic encephalopathy occurs because cell membranes, being freely permeable to water, are in virtually constant osmotic equilibrium with extracellular fluid. When hypernatremia develops acutely, cellular water loss produces brain shrinkage, and the increase in brain solute content is accounted for entirely by a rise in intracellular Na^+, K^+, and Cl^- concentrations.

In children who develop acute hypernatremia and attain a serum sodium concentration above 160 mEq per liter in 24 hours, the mortality exceeds 40 per cent; about two thirds of the survivors have permanent neurologic sequelae. At autopsy, cerebral vessels are markedly congested and engorged, hemorrhages are evident both in subcortical brain parenchyma and subarachnoid spaces, and venous thrombosis occurs.

When hypernatremia develops gradually, the incidence of hypertonic encephalopathy is greatly reduced, both in man and in experimental animals. This occurs because brain cells adapt to gradually developing hypernatremia by accumulating solutes intracellularly. The sum of brain Na^+, K^+, and Cl^- accounts for approximately 75 per cent of intracellular solutes; the remaining solutes, as yet unidentified, are commonly referred to as idiogenic osmoles. Thus in chronic hypernatremia, the accumulation of idiogenic osmoles in the brain minimizes the extent of water loss and consequently brain shrinkage. This in turn reduces the frequency with which encephalopathy develops.

Posthypophysectomy Course. The acute diabetes insipidus following hypophysectomy has a characteristic triphasic response. For a few hours to days following the insult, there exists a polyuric, hyposthenuric phase which depends on inhibition of ADH release. Next, there follows a period with reduced urine volume and a rise in urine osmolality. During this phase, there is persistent release of ADH from atrophying neurons, an inability to excrete a water load, and the risk of progressive hypotonicity with continued parenteral administration of large volumes of hypotonic fluids. The final phase, if the diabetes insipidus becomes permanent, is marked by recurrence of polyuria and hyposthenuria.

LABORATORY MANIFESTATIONS. Persistent hyposthenuria, with urine specific gravity of 1.005 or less and urine osmolality less than 200 mosm per kilogram of H_2O, is the hallmark of the diabetes insipidus syndromes. In euvolemic patients, the glomerular filtration rate (GFR) is normal. Since patients with diabetes insipidus ingest water in response to plasma hypertonicity, random plasma osmolality determinations in these patients will be, on the average, above the usual norm of 287 mosm per kilogram of H_2O. The serum sodium concentrations are also elevated and account quantitatively for the increases in plasma osmolality. In contrast, persons with primary polydipsia have a primary aberration of the thirst mechanism and ingest water independent of physiologic stimuli. These patients often have mild dilutional hyponatremia.

In patients whose diabetes insipidus, either pituitary or nephrogenic in origin, begins in childhood, considerable dilation of the urinary bladder, ureters, and renal pelvis may occur. This dilation has led to a reduction in GFR in some patients.

DIAGNOSIS. Based on the underlying pathophysiology, the polyuric syndromes may be grouped into the following general categories: (1) pituitary diabetes insipidus, in which there is absence or diminished production and secretion of ADH; (2) solute diuresis, in which excessively high rates of solute delivery to the loop of Henle overwhelm quantitatively the ability of distal nephron segments to dissociate solute and water absorption; (3) nephrogenic diabetes insipidus, either familial or acquired, in which collecting duct cells are partially or completely unresponsive to ADH; (4) renal concentrating disorders, in which there is impaired generation of a hypertonic medullary interstitium by renal countercurrent multiplication and exchange processes; and (5) primary polydipsia, in which the ingestion of unusually large volumes of water results in polyuria, the appropriate physiologic response.

Disorders such as diabetes mellitus, which produces solute diuresis, are characterized by isotonic urine and by glycosuria. The history and laboratory data are adequate to identify disorders such as sickle cell disease or interstitial nephritis, both of which impair the ability to generate a hypertonic medullary interstitium. Routine laboratory screening readily identifies the presence of hypercalcemia or hypokalemia. Finally, congenital nephrogenic diabetes insipidus is identified by a history of having been present since birth, generally in males, and by *persistent* unresponsiveness to exogenous ADH. Acquired nephrogenic diabetes insipidus is recognized by ADH unresponsiveness combined with a history of exposure to agents, such as lithium, demeclocycline, or methoxyflurane anesthesia, which antagonize the action of ADH on collecting ducts.

The more difficult diagnostic problem is the differentiation of patients with partial or complete deficiency of ADH from those with primary polydipsia. Certain factors may point toward the most likely diagnosis. For example, a 24-hour urine volume greater than 18 liters, a random plasma osmolality determination below 285 mosm per kilogram of H_2O, and a history of episodic polyuria all suggest compulsive water drinking as the underlying disorder. A history of head trauma or neoplasm, a history of sudden onset of unrelenting polyuria, and a random plasma osmolality determination greater than 290 mosm per kilogram of H₂O all suggest pituitary diabetes insipidus.

The basis of all tests for pituitary diabetes insipidus rests on the ability of the kidney to excrete hypertonic urine after an osmotic stimulus. The simplest maneuver is to produce hypertonicity of body fluids by water deprivation. The absolute level of urine concentration achieved with water deprivation is nondiagnostic, since maximal concentrating ability depends on the degree of medullary hypertonicity as well as the presence of adequate amounts of ADH. For example, the maximal urine osmolality produced by water deprivation in a group of randomly selected hospitalized patients was found to be 764 mosm per kilogram of H₂O as compared with 1067 mosm per kilogram of H₂O in healthy volunteers. Presumably the lower value for maximal urine concentrating ability in hospitalized patients reflects a reduction in medullary interstitial hypertonicity with respect to that present in normal volunteers.

Even in patients with a reduced medullary interstitial tonicity, the maximal urine osmolality achieved with water deprivation depends on maximal degrees of endogenous ADH release in response to dehydration. Therefore, in those with intact mechanisms for ADH production and release, the administration of exogenous ADH will not produce an increase in the maximal urine osmolality achieved via water deprivation. This rationale forms the framework for a test scheme, illustrated in Figure 227–3, for distinguishing complete or partial pituitary diabetes insipidus from other polyuric syndromes.

In patients with mild polyuria, water deprivation may begin the night preceding the test; patients with severe polyuria should have water restricted during the day, to allow for close observation. The test begins with paired measurements of urine and plasma osmolality. All water intake is then withheld and hourly measurements of urine osmolality and body weight are made. When two sequential urine osmolalities vary by less than 30 mosm per kilogram of H₂O, or when 3 to 5 per cent body weight is lost, 5 units of aqueous vasopressin is injected subcutaneously. A final urine osmolality is measured 60 minutes later.

The time required to achieve a maximal urine concentration varies from 4 to 18 hours. In normal persons, water deprivation results in urine osmolality two to four times greater than that of plasma. More important, the subsequent administration of exogenous ADH results in a less than 5 per cent further increase in urine osmolality. In patients with primary polydipsia, who have reduced medullary interstitial tonicity as a result of prolonged water diuresis, the urine may con-

centrate only slightly after water deprivation. However, they too will have stimulated endogenous ADH release maximally and will exhibit a less than 5 per cent rise in urine osmolality with supplemental ADH.

In patients with complete pituitary diabetes insipidus urine osmolality will not rise above that of plasma in response to water deprivation, but will show a greater than 50 per cent increase in response to injection of ADH. In patients with partial pituitary diabetes insipidus the urine may concentrate to some degree in response to water deprivation, but urine osmolality will also increase by at least 10 per cent after ADH injection. An interesting observation is that patients with partial pituitary diabetes insipidus often show a peak urine osmolality that decreases with further water restriction. This suggests a limited reserve of neurohypophyseal hormone that is depleted after an initial secretory burst. Finally, in patients with nephrogenic diabetes insipidus deprived of water, the urine osmolality fails to rise above that of plasma even when they are given exogenous ADH. When a diagnosis of pituitary diabetes insipidus is made, a careful evaluation for neoplasm involving the hypothalamus or neurohypophyseal tract is mandatory.

Levels of circulating vasopressin measured by radioimmunoassay have heretofore been available only for research purposes. A commercial assay is now marketed for clinical use, but its utility is, as of now, undefined. Hypertonic saline infusions have also been utilized to test for release of ADH. This procedure is hazardous in patients with limited cardiac reserve, in whom volume expansion may precipitate cardiac decompensation. Moreover, the results of the test are uninterpretable if the patient develops salt diuresis, thus fixing urine osmolality near isotonicity.

Nicotine, a nonosmotic stimulus to ADH secretion, has been used to elicit antidiuresis in those patients who have "essential hypernatremia," i.e., ADH release in response to volume contraction but not to hypertonicity. A better diagnostic approach in these patients is to assess the antidiuretic response to mild volume contraction.

TREATMENT. Patients with diabetes insipidus, either pituitary or nephrogenic, may require emergency treatment of hypertonic encephalopathy or maintenance therapy for polyuria.

Hypertonic Encephalopathy. The goal in treating this medical emergency is to replenish body water, thereby restoring osmotic balance and replenishing cell volume, at a rate that avoids significant complications. Since the brain adjusts to hypertonicity, at least in part, by increasing intracellular osmolar content via accumulation of "idiogenic osmoles," rapid repletion of body water with extracellular fluid dilution

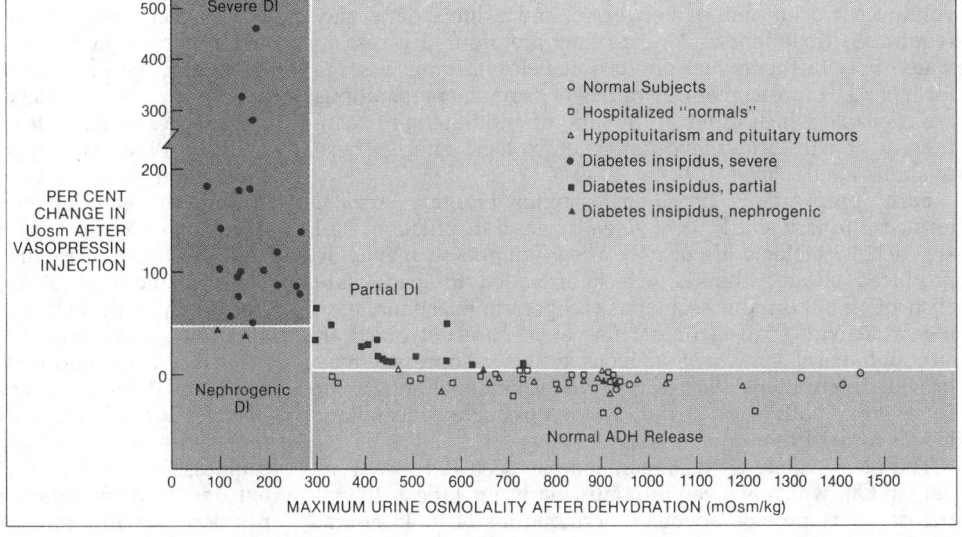

FIGURE 227–3. Maximal urine osmolality after dehydration versus the percentage change in urine osmolality induced by subsequent vasopressin injection. DI = diabetes insipidus; ADH = antidiuretic hormone. (From Miller M, et al.: Ann Intern Med 73:721, 1970. Reprinted with permission of the publisher.)

TABLE 227–2. COMPARISON OF NEUROHYPOPHYSEAL HORMONES AND SYNTHETIC ANALOGUES

Preparation	Activity					Duration of Activity	Route of Administration
	Antidiuretic	*:*	*Vasopressor*	*:*	*Oxytocic*		
8-Arginine vasopressin							
Pitressin, aqueous	100	:	100	:	5	2–6 hours	Intravenous
Pitressin tannate in oil						24–48 hours	Intramuscular
8-Lysine vasopressin							
Lypressin	60	:	70	:	1	2–6 hours	Nasal insufflation
1-Deamino, 8-D-arginine vasopressin							
(dDAVP), desmopressin	290	:	0.14			6–20 hours	Nasal insufflation
Oxytocin	1	:	1	:	100		

will cause translocation of water into cells to achieve osmotic equilibrium. The result of this water movement is cell swelling and cerebral edema. Seizures occur in up to 40 per cent of patients treated for severe hypernatremia by rapid infusions of hypotonic solutions. If water repletion is undertaken at a slower rate, brain cells lose the accumulated intracellular solutes and osmotic equilibration can occur without cell swelling. Consequently, a good rule of thumb is to administer fluids at a rate which reduces the serum sodium concentration to normal over a 36- to 48-hour period, or to reduce the serum sodium concentration by about 1 mEq per liter every two hours.

The choice of fluid to be administered in the diabetes insipidus syndromes depends in large part on three factors: the extent to which circulatory collapse may be present; the rate at which hypernatremia has developed; and the magnitude of hypernatremia. Hypotonic NaCl solutions are best used as initial therapy in patients with modest volume contraction and only modest elevations of serum sodium concentrations, that is, less than 160 mEq per liter. However, in more advanced cases of hypernatremia, particularly if the hypernatremia has developed gradually, that is, over a period greater than 24 hours, and is accompanied by signs of circulatory collapse, more prudent initial therapy is to administer normal saline solutions. The reasons for this choice are twofold: in advanced hypernatremia, a normal saline solution is dilute relative to the patient's body fluid osmolality and thus will dilute the latter while minimizing the risk of iatrogenic cerebral swelling; at the same time, the normal saline solution provides an effective means of volume expansion. Finally, 5 per cent glucose solutions may be used to replenish body water in acute hypernatremia without significant circulatory collapse. However, the glucose infusion rate must be less than the rate of glucose metabolism to avoid glycosuria. Otherwise, the resulting osmotic diuresis will thwart attempts to replenish body free water. The treatment of drug-induced nephrogenic diabetes insipidus consists of removal of the offending agent.

Polyuria. Patients with partial hormonal deficiency and volumes of urine output between 2 and 6 liters daily may require no treatment as long as they are assured access to water. Specific therapy for pituitary diabetes insipidus is some form of ADH replacement. A variety of hormone preparations are available which differ in the ratio of antidiuretic to vasopressor activity and the duration of biologic effect. These relations are depicted in Table 227–2.

Early preparations of dried posterior pituitary extract, termed pituitary snuff, were given by nasal insufflation, had an effective biologic life of only a few hours, and inevitably produced chronic rhinitis, which often led to inadequate absorption of hormone. Aqueous vasopressin injections, having an activity span of only a few hours, are not practical, although nasal sprays of aqueous lysine vasopressin may provide intermittent relief of polyuria. Rhinitis, although not so severe as with dried extract, is also a frequent concomitant to this form of therapy.

The most widely used preparation has been Pitressin Tannate in Oil, which is given intramuscularly, As little as 0.5 ml per day may provide adequate hormone for 24 to 48 hours.

Great care must be exercised in preparing the injection by careful warming and mixing of the ampule so as to suspend the pellet of hormone in the oil. Failure to do so may result in injection of the oil vehicle alone and apparent "vasopressin resistance." Pain at injection sites and sterile abscesses are frequent complaints with this preparation. Persistent abdominal pain from the effect of ADH on intestinal motility is a not uncommon problem.

A synthetic analogue of vasopressin, dDAVP (1-deamino,8-D-arginine vasopressin), provides antidiuretic activity for 8 to 20 hours with negligible pressor effect, can be taken as a nasal spray, and is the current drug of choice. The drug is best started at night to find the lowest dose that will prevent nocturia. This dose, usually 5 to 10 μg, can be given twice daily or doubled as a single morning dose. A nasal catheter is provided, which is measured for convenient dosing in the 5 to 24 μg range. Headache may be a troublesome side effect with large doses but usually disappears with a reduction of dosage.

For patients having some residual ADH production, the oral hypoglycemic agent chlorpropamide may provide adequate amelioration of symptoms. This drug stimulates ADH secretion and augments the activity of residual ADH on the collecting duct. Doses of 250 to 500 mg daily are sufficient to reduce polyuria in most patients with partial pituitary diabetes insipidus, but the side effect of hypoglycemia limits the drug's usefulness.

Thiazide diuretics may reduce the volume of urine in patients with all forms of diabetes insipidus, that is, either pituitary or nephrogenic, by causing a state of mild salt depletion. This results in a secondary increase in isotonic proximal tubular fluid absorption and a decrease in the volume of fluid delivered to the collecting duct. The effect is produced by 50 to 100 mg of hydrochlorothiazide daily, is sustained even in the absence of diuretics by salt restriction, and can be abolished by salt loading even with continued diuretic administration.

Vasopressin infusions have also been used to treat bleeding esophageal varices by reducing splanchnic blood flow. Desmopressin, a synthetic analogue of arginine vasopressin, stimulates the production of clotting factor VIII. These other actions are discussed elsewhere in this textbook.

Nephrogenic Diabetes Insipidus. The therapeutic considerations outlined above, particularly with respect to the treatment of hypertonic encephalopathy and to the value of a chronic mild salt-depleted state in minimizing polyuria, apply equally well to the care of patients with pituitary or nephrogenic diabetes insipidus. In patients with nephrogenic diabetes insipidus acquired as a consequence of drug therapy (for example, lithium or demeclocycline), the offending agent should be discontinued.

Finally, it is important to stress the need to minimize the extent of polyuria in children with congenital nephrogenic diabetes insipidus, since there is a close correlation between repeated bouts of dehydration during childhood and mental dullness in adulthood. Alternatively, in patients in whom episodes of dehydration have been minimal, both mental and physical growth retardation can be avoided.

Barlow ED, DeWardener HE: Compulsive water drinking. Q J Med 28:235, 1959. *A thorough examination of the clinical course and pathophysiology of urinary concentration in a group of patients with primary polydipsia.*

Baylis PH, Gill GV: The investigation of polyuria. Clin Endocrinol Metab 13:295, 1984. *A brief discussion of the approach to the diagnosis and treatment of the polyuric states.*

DeRubertis FR, Michelis MF, Beck N, et al.: "Essential" hypernatremia due to ineffective osmotic and intact volume regulation of vasopressin secretion. J Clin Invest 50:97, 1971. *A description of patients having intact neurohypophyseal function but lacking normal regulation of ADH because of a specific defect in osmoregulation.*

Hebert SC, Culpepper RM, Andreoli TE: The posterior pituitary and water metabolism. In Foster DW, Wilson JD (eds.): Textbook of Endocrinology. 7th ed. Philadelphia, W.B. Saunders Company, 1985, pp 614–652. *A full review of the polyuric syndromes, their differential diagnosis and treatment; extensively referenced.*

Miller M, Dalakos T, Moses AM, et al.: Recognition of partial defects in antidiuretic hormone secretion. Ann Intern Med 72:721, 1970. *A concise guide to testing procedures for states of ADH insufficiency and a rational scheme for interpreting the test results.*

Robertson GL: Thirst and vasopressin function in normal and disordered states of water balance. J Lab Clin Med 101:351, 1983. *A detailed account of the physiology and pathophysiology of ADH secretion and thirst in normal patients and those with polyuric disorders.*

Schrier RW (ed.): Vasopressin. New York, Raven Press, 1985. *A comprehensive multiauthored text covering many aspects of vasopressin chemistry, cellular actions, neural control, and pathophysiology.*

THE SYNDROME OF INAPPROPRIATE ADH PRODUCTION (SIADH)

For convenience SIADH has been discussed in Ch. 77 as a major disorder producing hyponatremia.

OXYTOCIN

Oxytocin is produced in the same hypothalamic nuclei and by the same synthetic mechanism as vasopressin. AVP and oxytocin are produced in both the paraventricular and the supraoptic nuclei of the hypothalamus. However, a given neuron in these nuclei produces only one hormone. Neurophysin I is the specific carrier protein synthesized with oxytocin and has been used as a marker for oxytocin release.

PHYSIOLOGY. The primary stimuli for oxytocin secretion are nipple stimulation (suckling) and deformation of the reproductive tract (especially the vagina) in females and muscular contraction of the reproductive organs in the male. The neural arcs serving these stimuli are not well defined, but some evidence suggests that the final synaptic transmitter is dopamine. Estrogens appear to influence secretion directly, based on observations of increased neurophysin I in blood during estrogen peaks of the menstrual cycle, or permissively, based on findings of a graded response to vaginal distension over the period of a menstrual cycle and an enhanced response with exogenous estradiol. Progesterones inhibit response to mechanical stimuli. Hypertonicity of body fluids also appears to cause oxytocin secretion. For example, in congenitally vasopressin-deficient Brattleboro rats, hypertonicity causes degranulation of the neurohypophysis, indicating sustained secretion of oxytocin, a relatively weak antidiuretic principle.

BIOLOGIC ACTIVITY. In females, oxytocin initiates its primary effect by binding to specific myometrial receptors, the affinity of which increases strikingly in the presence of estrogen. Exogenously administered oxytocin elicits contractions of the fundus indistinguishable from those of labor. However, the initiation of labor is apparently oxytocin independent, with increasing secretions seen only with dilation of the birth canal. Oxytocin may play a key role in final expulsion of the fetus and placenta. The total absence of oxytocin does not prevent parturition, although prolonged labor is seen in such women. The cellular events leading to uterine contraction are unknown, but parallel an oxytocin-induced increase in ion permeability with depolarization of the myometrial cell membrane.

The mild-ejection reflex is also mediated via oxytocin.

Contraction of mammary myoepithelium is stimulated, leading to a rise in intramammary pressure and expulsion of milk from alveolar channels to large sinuses, where it is accessible to the suckling infant. A true galactogenic effect of oxytocin leading to increased milk production has not been convincingly demonstrated. Absence of oxytocin abolishes the milk-ejection reflex.

In the male, oxytocin increases ejection of sperm into the semen in response to stimulation of the reproductive organs. Oxytocin retains some antidiuretic activity, about 1 per cent that of AVP, but exerts no significant antidiuretic effect at physiologic levels of secretion. Vascular smooth muscle is relaxed by oxytocin, causing a decrease in blood pressure, cutaneous flushing, and increased limb blood flow. Reflex tachycardia and sympathetic responses quickly restore hemodynamics to normal except when such reflexes are rendered inactive as in deep anesthesia.

THERAPEUTIC USE. The primary use of oxytocin (Pitocin) is to induce or to improve the quality of labor. The uterus is relatively resistant to oxytocin in early pregnancy, but infusions given with hypertonic saline injections may speed abortions of later pregnancy.

With long-term infusion of oxytocin, patients may experience sufficient antidiuretic effects to be at risk of water intoxication. Antidiuresis may be detected at oxytocin infusion rates of 15 mU per minute, and maximal urinary concentration is usually attained at rates of 45 mU per minute. Infusions for delivery and control of postpartum uterine hemorrhage may reach 20 to 40 mU per minute, and infusions for therapeutic abortions range from 20 to 100 mU per minute.

Roberts JS: Oxytocin, Vol I. Montreal, Eden Press, 1977. *This review covers the extensive work in oxytocin physiology and chemistry; very readable and fully referenced.*

228 THE PINEAL
Seymour Reichlin

The pineal gland was discovered more than 20 centuries ago, and its function has long been a matter of scientific and philosophic speculation. Arising embryologically from ependyma lining the roof of the third ventricle, the pineal consists of parenchymal cells supported by a meshwork of neuroglia.

In the adult, the gland weighs between 100 and 180 mg and is a cone-shaped organ lying in the groove formed by the superior colliculus. Although connected to the epithalamus by a peduncle, the pineal does not receive a direct nerve supply from this source. Rather, it is innervated by postganglionic nerve fibers that arise in the cervical sympathetic ganglia and travel along the great vein of Galen (the blood vessel into which pineal secretions drain). The sympathetic inflow to the pineal is in turn regulated by impulses arising in the suprachiasmatic nuclei, paired structures lying just above the optic chiasm (Fig. 228–1). This nucleus is innervated by a direct nerve pathway from the retina termed the retinohypothalamic tract. Changes in external lighting influence pineal activity (and other endocrine functions) via this pathway even when pathways mediating conscious light perception have been severed. The suprachiasmatic nucleus is also believed to serve as an internal "clock" (or biologic oscillator), regulating a number of endogenous endocrine rhythms. Circadian changes can occur even in the absence of external sensory cues, including light changes, thus indicating that there is a mechanism for determining intrinsic rhythms. The rhythm of the endogenous oscillator can be modified by external signals such as normal light-dark cycles.

SECRETIONS OF THE PINEAL. Many different neurotransmitter substances, including norepinephrine, serotonin,

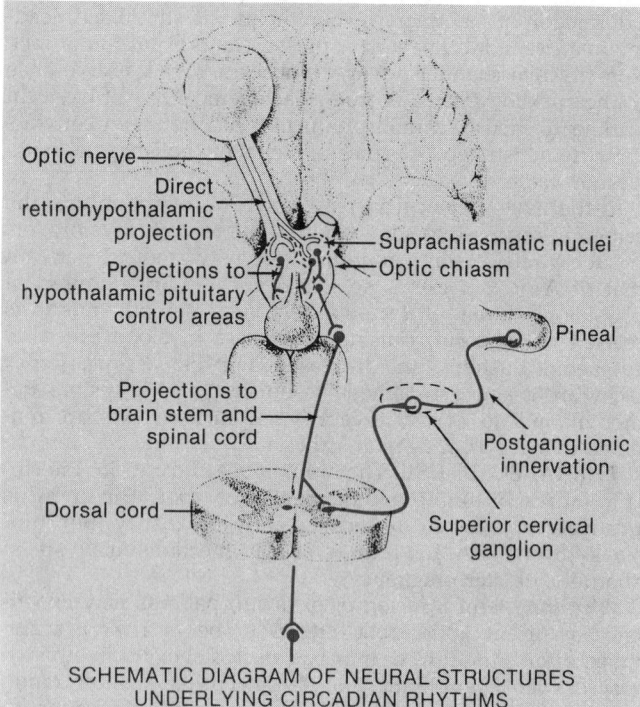

Optic nerve
Direct retinohypothalamic projection
Projections to hypothalamic pituitary control areas
Suprachiasmatic nuclei
Optic chiasm
Pineal
Projections to brain stem and spinal cord
Postganglionic innervation
Dorsal cord
Superior cervical ganglion

SCHEMATIC DIAGRAM OF NEURAL STRUCTURES UNDERLYING CIRCADIAN RHYTHMS

FIGURE 228–1. Control system for pineal regulation. Light impinging upon the retina is transduced into neural signals that reach the brain, giving both visual and nonvisual responses. This diagram outlines the nonvisual component. Those involved in endocrine regulation are mainly conducted by the direct retinohypothalamic projection to the suprachiasmatic nuclei (located in the hypothalamus). From the suprachiasmatic nuclei, nerve pathways project to the hypophysiotropic control areas of the hypothalamus and also to the spinal cord, where they influence the primary neurons of the sympathetic nerve outflow tract that terminate in the superior cervical ganglia. From the superior cervical ganglia, postganglionic sympathetic nerves (noradrenergic in function), accompanying the venous drainage of the pineal gland, enter the gland to innervate the pineal parenchymal cells. Suprachiasmatic nuclei are responsible for endogenous rhythms as well as those influenced by external lighting (see text). (Redrawn from Moore RY: In Yen SSC, Jaffe RB (eds.): Reproductive Endocrinology: Physiology, Pathophysiology and Clinical Management. Philadelphia, W. B. Saunders Company, 1978, pp 3–33.)

histamine, melatonin, dopamine, octopamine, and gamma-aminobutyric acid (GABA), and the peptides somatostatin and TRH are contained in the pineal. Of these biologically active substances, only melatonin appears to be the principal secretion. It is present in blood, cerebrospinal fluid, and urine of many species of animals, including humans. Hormone levels at night are higher than day values. Light to dark is a potent stimulus to melatonin release. Melatonin is believed to exert suppressive effects on a number of endocrine functions in experimental animals, the most important of which is on the release of gonadotropic hormones. Important effects of melatonin injection in humans are the production of sleepiness and changes in the electroencephalogram, mainly an increase of alpha waves.

Melatonin is formed by a series of enzymatic steps from tryptophan in which one of the intermediates is serotonin. Enzymatic activity of the pineal gland and its secretory function are regulated by noradrenergic nerve endings on pinealocytes. Beta-catecholamine receptors activate adenyl cyclase with the formation of cyclic AMP through the classic second-messenger mechanism. The activated ATP-protein kinase is believed to promote the formation of the melatonin-synthesizing enzymes. Norepinephrine also stimulates pineal uptake of the precursor tryptophan.

ABNORMALITIES OF THE PINEAL: CALCIFICATION. The pineal gland has no known function in man, but becomes of clinical significance because of the occurrence of calcification and of tumor formation. Calcific nodules form in a matrix of ground substance secreted by pinealocytes. This process begins in early childhood and becomes increasingly evident by roentgenography, beginning in the second decade of life. Calcification has no known effect on pineal function.

DISEASES OF THE PINEAL. Diseases of the pineal are rare. A few cases of hypoplasia and aplasia have been reported, and these have been associated in a relatively high proportion with genital precocity. Less than 1 per cent of intracranial neoplasms are tumors of the pineal gland, and they are seen almost exclusively in young males. The term *pinealoma* refers to a tumor of the pineal parenchymal cell, called pinealoblastoma or pinealocytoma according to its degree of differentiation. In one series of pineal tumor cases, only 9 of 53 fitted this category, and there were 13 glial tumors, including astrocytomas and glioblastomas. The most common tumor (approximately 50 per cent) is best termed germinoma and is really not a tumor of pineal parenchymal cells. Rather these tumors are believed to be due to embryologic rests of germ cells. Identical tumors are found in the testis and anterior mediastinum. Approximately 10 per cent of intracranial germinomas metastasize to the spinal cord. Germinomas arising in the pineal gland may infiltrate the third ventricle and the floor of the hypothalamus, producing a characteristic triad: diabetes insipidus, hypogonadism, and optic atrophy. An identical clinical presentation can be due to germinomas arising from midline tissues at the base of the brain. Teratomas may also arise in the pineal region and rarely give rise to choriocarcinomas. Several cases of precocious puberty have been reported to be caused by gonadotropin-secreting choriocarcinomas of the pineal, an abnormality associated with detectable human chorionic gonadotropin (HCG) in the spinal fluid and blood.

Pineal tumors also cause sexual precocity by hypothalamic damage that destroys structures normally inhibitory to the development of puberty. Precocious puberty caused by pinealomas occurs almost exclusively in males. The most important local manifestations of pineal neoplasms are due to pressure on the quadrigeminal plate of the midbrain. An enlarging mass in the pineal region compresses the aqueduct of Sylvius and distorts the structure, giving rise to headache, vomiting, papilledema, and disturbed consciousness. Pressure on the superior colliculi causes paralysis of conjugate upward gaze (Parinaud's syndrome). The characteristic wide-based gait may be due to pressure on the cerebellum or brain stem.

DIAGNOSIS OF TUMORS OF THE FLOOR OF THE THIRD VENTRICLE. Pinealoma and other tumors of the floor of the third ventricle are relatively safe to approach surgically for biopsy, which is generally recommended unless a tissue diagnosis of choriocarcinoma can be inferred by demonstrating elevated blood or cerebrospinal fluid levels of HCG and/or alpha-fetoprotein. If one or both of these tumor markers are positive, it is not necessary to obtain a surgical biopsy, and one can proceed directly to treatment by local irradiation.

If a diagnosis of parasellar pinealoma cannot be made by tumor markers, it should be approached as any other parasellar lesion in which a tissue specimen is essential for proper management.

TREATMENT OF TUMORS OF THE PINEAL REGION. The management of tumors of the pineal region is somewhat complex because the surgical approach to the pineal gland is difficult. Prior to the introduction of microsurgery under dissecting microscopic control, it also carried a high risk. Surgical biopsy is indicated because of the wide variety of lesions encountered in this region, because some can be completely removed surgically and because some are radioresistant. If the patient presents with internal hydrocephalus, a shunt procedure may be a necessary first step, but it should be recalled that tumor implants may be carried into the spinal cord by such shunts.

Radiotherapy has achieved 5-year survival rates of 60 to 88 per cent among a group of patients with heterogeneous pineal tumors. Local recurrence rates have been reduced even further by increasing radiation dosage to 5500 rads. A good initial radiation response may not be indicative of curability.

Surgical treatment of pineal tumors was, for many years, associated with extremely high mortality, but with the introduction of microsurgery, operative mortality has fallen dramatically. For example, in one series of 128 cases subjected to direct surgical approach there were only two operative deaths. These rare tumors are best treated surgically in a center with much experience in this approach.

Chemotherapy should be considered in cases that fail to respond to radiotherapy or that relapse after an initial good response. The extensive and favorable experience for therapy of testicular choriocarcinoma has led to similar approaches in treatment of central germ-cell tumors.

Ahmed SR, Shalet SM, Price DA, et al.: Human chorionic gonadotropin secreting pineal germinoma and precocious puberty. Arch Dis Child 58:743, 1983. *Case report and literature review of endocrine-secreting pineal tumors.*

Ehrenkranz JR, Tamarkin L, Comite F, et al.: Daily rhythms of plasma melatonin in normal and precocious puberty. J Clin Endocrinol Metab 55:307, 1982. *Study of pineal in determining onset of puberty in the human.*

Ehrlich SS, Apuzzo MLJ: The pineal gland: Anatomy, physiology, and clinical significance. J Neurosurg 63:321, 1985. *Comprehensive review of the pineal in man.*

Jennings MT, Gelman R, Hochberg F: Intracranial germ-cell tumors: Natural history and pathogenesis. J Neurosurg 63:155, 1985. *Comprehensive review of germ cell tumors, including pineal teratoma.*

Lieberman HR, Waldhauser F, Garfield G, et al.: Effects of melatonin on human mood and performance. Brain Res 323:201, 1984. *Detailed study of melatonin effects on psychological function.*

Reichlin S: Neuroendocrinology. In Williams R (ed.): Textbook of Endocrinology. 7th ed. Philadelphia, W. B. Saunders Company, 1985, pp 535–539, 541–544. *Review of pineal function and anatomy. Detailed account of clinical aspects, including diagnosis and management. Designed for medical students and fellows.*

Schmidek HH, Waters A: Pineal masses: Clinical features and management. In Wilkins RH (ed.): Neurosurgery, 1985. Review of Surgical Management. New York, McGraw-Hill Book Company, 1984, Vol I, pp 688–694. *The definitive monograph for the clinician responsible for the care of the patient with a pinealoma.*

229 THE THYROID

P. Reed Larsen

The thyroid gland secretes thyroxine, 3,5,3′,5′-tetraiodothyronine (abbreviated T_4) and small amounts of 3,5,3′-triiodothyronine (abbreviated T_3). The principal role of these substances is to regulate tissue metabolism. In infants, adequate supplies of thyroid hormone are necessary for the development of the normal central nervous system in the first one to two years of life. The absence of thyroid hormone during this period results in irreversible mental retardation, a syndrome known as *cretinism*. The hormone is also required for normal growth and bone maturation in children. Despite these important functions, the body can withstand marked reductions in thyroid hormone for long periods, although at the cost of abnormal function of many organ systems.

EMBRYOLOGY AND ANATOMY

The thyroid develops from a combination of pharyngeal midline and bilateral primitive tissues from the fourth branchial pouch. These primitive thyroid cells migrate from the pharyngeal floor, leaving behind a residual thyroglossal duct that normally becomes obliterated. The major portion of the thyroid cell mass is derived from the median mid-pharyngeal tissue. The lateral thyroid anlagen migrate medially to fuse with median-derived thyroid tissue, but primarily contribute the *parafollicular* or *C-cells*. The C cells secrete calcitonin, not thyroid hormone, and do not play a role in thyroid physiology (see Ch. 248). The evolution of thyroid function occurs over the first 10 to 12 weeks of fetal life, with definite appearance of T_4 in the gland by 10 to 11 weeks. The placenta is impermeable to T_3 and T_4; the fetus depends on its own thyroid for its supply of these hormones. The adult size (15 to 20 grams) of the thyroid is reached at about age 15. The thyroid gland has the configuration of a butterfly, with the two lobes measuring about 5×2 cm. The lobes are composed of spherical structures called *follicles*, consisting of *colloid* surrounded by a single layer of epithelial cells enclosed by a basement membrane. Colloid consists predominantly of the protein *thyroglobulin*, which is the storage form of T_4 and T_3.

THYROID PHYSIOLOGY

The structures of the thyroid hormones and their precursors, monoiodotyrosine and diiodotyrosine (MIT and DIT), are shown in Figure 229–1. Iodine accounts for 65 per cent of the weight of T_4. Since this is a relatively scarce element in the earth's crust, the thyroid cell has mechanisms to concentrate and conserve iodine.

IODINE METABOLISM. The daily intake of iodine in man varies markedly in different areas of the world. It ranges from extremely low levels (20 μg or less per day) to as high as 600 or 700 μg per day in certain areas of the United States. The optimal iodine intake for adults is thought to be 150 to 300 μg per day. Levels appreciably below this lead to the condition known as *endemic goiter*, which is discussed later in this chapter. The high level of iodine intake in the United States is, in part, due to iodination of salt. Iodine in all forms is reduced to iodide (I^-) in the gastrointestinal tract and absorbed within 30 minutes of ingestion. I^- leaves the blood via two mechanisms. It is concentrated by the thyroid or excreted in the urine. There is a wide variation in the fraction of I^- concentrated by the thyroid per 24 hours, depending on iodine uptake. In the United States, iodine uptake by the thyroid varies from about 5 to 30 per cent.

INTRATHYROIDAL IODIDE METABOLISM. In Figure 229–2 are shown the steps involved in the synthesis of the thyroid hormones. Because the concentrations of I^- in the plasma are so low, the thyroid cell concentrates I^-, the cell-plasma ratio being about 20 to 40:1. The trapped I^- is rapidly oxidized and incorporated into protein. As a consequence, there is little I^- per se in the thyroid gland. The process of I^- oxidation and its incorporation into tyrosine is known as *organification*. The substrate for iodine is the 660,000 molecular weight glycoprotein thyroglobulin. Only about 25 per cent of the tyrosine residues of this specialized protein are available for iodination. Both MIT and DIT are formed. In a typical molecule of fully iodinated human thyroglobulin, there are approximately 6 to 7 residues of MIT, 4 to 5 DIT, 3 to 4 of T_4 and 0.2 to 0.3 of T_3. The T_4 and T_3 arise from the coupling of either 2 DIT residues or 1 MIT and 1 DIT residue, a reaction that requires thyroid peroxidase. This process is known as *coupling*. Both organification and coupling are inhibited by *thiourea compounds*, which are used in the treatment of patients with hyperthyroidism (see below). The thyroglobulin is iodinated at the apical border of the cell and is then exocytosed into the colloid. Under normal circumstances, T_4 and T_3 secretion occurs from this pool. The thyroid secretory process starts with phagocytosis of thyroglobulin by the apical cell membrane, leading to the formation of a *colloid droplet*. This is combined with a lysosome, and as the colloid droplet traverses the thyroid cell, proteolysis occurs with eventual release of T_4 and T_3 at the basal cell border. Deiodination of T_4 to T_3 also occurs during this process, resulting in a ratio of

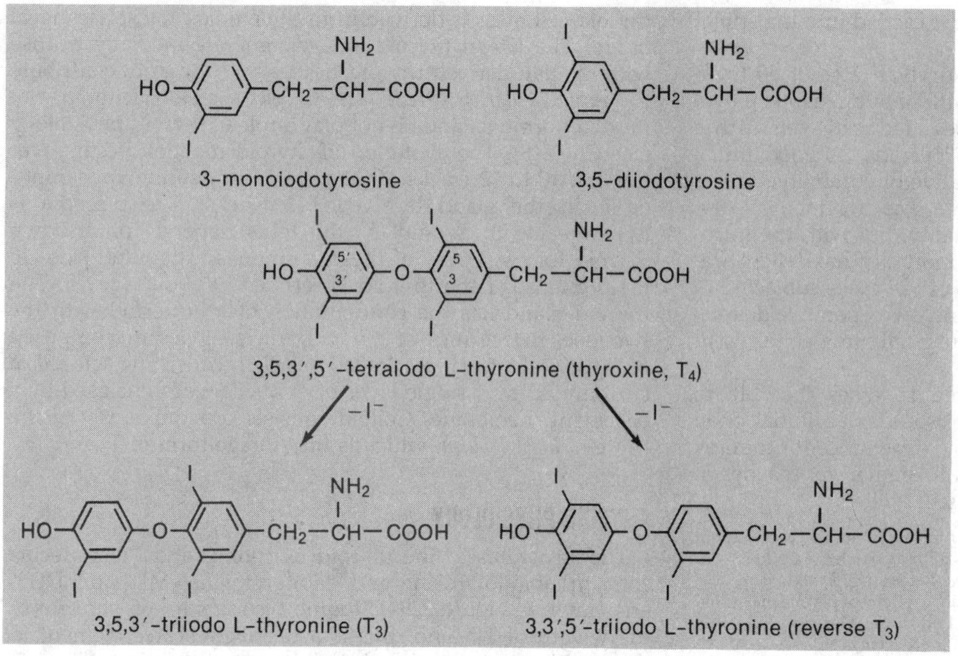

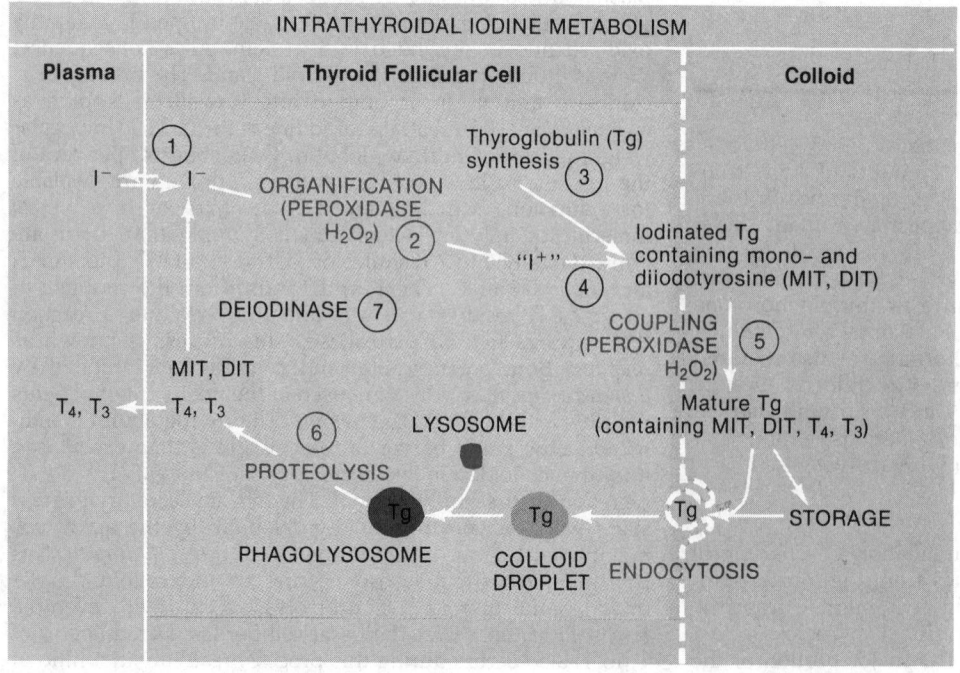

FIGURE 229–1. Structure of the thyroid hormones and their precursors.

T_4 to T_3 in thyroid secretion that is somewhat less than the 15:1 value found in the thyroglobulin itself. To conserve iodine for reuse in the thyroid cell, a *deiodinase* is present that removes the iodine from MIT and DIT, allowing it to recycle.

CIRCULATING T_4 AND T_3. Thyroid hormones in plasma exist in two forms, free and protein bound. Although only about 0.02 per cent of total plasma T_4 and 0.3 per cent of plasma T_3 are free, it is the free hormone concentration that is maintained constant by the feedback regulatory system and that appears to parallel the rate of cellular uptake of these hormones. It is, therefore, the free hormone concentration that determines the thyroid status irrespective of the total plasma concentration. In the euthyroid person the total hormone is determined by the quantity and affinity of certain thyroid hormone-binding proteins, which are *thyroxine-binding globulin* (TBG), transthyretin (formerly termed thyroxine-binding prealbumin), and albumin. TBG is by far the most important of these, transporting about 75 per cent of serum T_4 and T_3. It is a glycoprotein, with a molecular weight of 55,000,

which is synthesized in the liver. TBG has a high affinity for both T_4 and T_3, although the affinity for T_4 is about 10- to 15-fold higher than that for T_3. There is normally sufficient TBG in serum to bind approximately 20 μg of T_4 per deciliter at a molar ratio of 1:1. The serum TBG concentrations change under many circumstances, which are listed in Table 229–1. It is important to recognize these conditions, since the resultant changes in total T_4 and T_3 may duplicate abnormalities that are found in patients with thyroid dysfunction. For example, during pregnancy, serum total T_4 and T_3 are increased but serum free T_4 and T_3 concentrations remain constant. The relationships are described in the following equation:

$$[TH] \text{ is proportional to } \frac{[TH\text{—}TBG]}{[TBG]}$$

where TH = free T_4 or T_3, [TH—TBG] = TBG-bound T_4 or T_3, and TBG = unoccupied TBG. When [TBG] increases, the

FIGURE 229–2. Principal steps in the synthesis and secretion of thyroid hormones. MIT = Monoiodotyrosine; DIT = diiodotyrosine. The steps denoted by the numbers are those in which defects have been identified in patients with inherited abnormalities in thyroid hormone biosynthesis (see Sporadic and Endemic Goiter, below).

TABLE 229–1. CIRCUMSTANCES ASSOCIATED WITH CHANGES IN THE CIRCULATING CONCENTRATION OF THYROXINE-BINDING GLOBULIN (TBG)

Increased TBG
1. Pregnancy
2. Treatment with supraphysiologic amounts of estrogens, including oral contraceptives
3. In some patients with cirrhosis or acute hepatitis
4. As a congenital abnormality
5. In acute intermittent porphyria
6. After administration of heroin, methadone
7. After administration of clofibrate

Decreased TBG
1. Protein malnutrition, hepatic failure, chronic illness
2. Nephrotic syndrome
3. After administration of L-asparaginase
4. As a congenital abnormality (usually X-linked)
5. During treatment with androgenic steroids or pharmacologic doses of glucocorticoids.

TABLE 229–3. DRUGS THAT CAN INFLUENCE THYROID FUNCTION OR ALTER TEST RESULTS

Type of Effect	Common Examples
Suppress TSH secretion	Dopamine, L-dopa, glucocorticoid excess
Inhibit thyroid hormone synthesis or release	Iodide, lithium carbonate, phenylbutazone, sulfonylureas
Decrease hormone-protein binding	Salicylates, phenytoin, fenclofenac, furosemide
Inhibit T_4 to T_3 conversion	
Type I 5'-deiodinase	Propylthiouracil, not methimazole (Tapazole)
	Propranolol (not other beta-adrenergic antagonists)
	Glucocorticoid excess
Types I and II 5'-deiodinase	Amiodarone (Cordarone), Iopanoic acid (Telepaque), ipodipic acid (Oragrafin)

bound hormone also increases until a new steady state is achieved at which [TH] is again normal. This occurs through both decreased metabolism and increased secretion of T_4 and T_3. To interpret a total serum T_4 or T_3 measurement accurately it is necessary to know the fraction of the hormone that is free; alternatively the free hormone can be measured directly or estimated (see Direct Tests of Thyroid Function later in this chapter). Certain compounds compete with T_4 and T_3 for binding to TBG. Two such drugs are salicylates and phenytoin. About a 20 to 30 per cent reduction in serum T_4 and T_3 is observed when 300 mg of phenytoin or salicylates in excess of 2.4 grams per day are given.

KINETICS OF T_4 AND T_3. Deiodination of the iodothyronines is the most significant metabolic transformation of the thyroid hormones. In the case of T_4, deiodination of the distal ring, occurring predominantly in liver and kidney, gives rise to T_3, which has approximately three to four times the metabolic potency of the parent hormone (Fig. 229–1). About 30 to 40 per cent of the 80 μg of T_4 produced per day is metabolized via this pathway (Table 229–2), giving rise to about 80 per cent of the T_3 produced daily. Loss of an iodine in the proximal ring of T_4 leads to formation of *reverse T_3* (3,3',5'-triiodothyronine), a compound that appears to have no metabolic effect. About 40 per cent of T_4 is metabolized via this pathway, the remainder being excreted via the biliary tract into the feces following conjugation with glucuronide. T_3 and reverse T_3 are, in turn, deiodinated in both proximal and distal rings, giving rise to the predicted monoiodothyronines and diiodothyronines, none of which has physiologic effects. T_4 to T_3 conversion and reverse T_3 deiodination appear to be catalyzed by the same enzyme. If this reaction is inhibited, as it is under diverse circumstances, a reduction in serum T_3 and an increase in the serum reverse T_3 concentrations occur.

The differences between T_3 and T_4 in terms of distribution volume, the intracellular fraction, and half-life can be attributed principally to the differences in the affinities of these two hormones for the plasma-binding proteins (Table 229–2).

TABLE 229–2. COMPARISON OF T_3 AND T_4 IN HUMANS

	T_3	T_4
Serum concentration		
Total (μg/dl)	0.14	8
Free (ng/dl)	0.4	1.6
Fraction of total serum hormone that is in the free form (%)	0.3	0.02
Distribution volume (liters)	35	10
Fraction intracellular (%)	64	10–20
Half-life (days)	1	7
Production rate (μg/day)	33	80
Fraction directly from thyroid (%)	20	100
Relative metabolic potency	1	0.3

The higher intracellular T_3 content explains in part its higher potency relative to T_4. Given the 3 to 4:1 ratio of metabolic potency of T_3 and T_4 and the fact that approximately one third of T_4 is converted to T_3, it appears that T_4 has little intrinsic metabolic activity in man.

REGULATION OF T_4 TO T_3 CONVERSION. Two classes of enzymes convert T_4 to T_3 (iodothyronine 5'-deiodinases). One of these (type I), most active in liver and kidney, provides the bulk of the T_3 to the plasma pool. A second enzyme (type II), present in the central nervous system, pituitary, brown adipose tissue (BAT), and placenta, selectively provides T_3 to the cells of these tissues. For example, about 80 per cent of intracellular T_3 in cerebral cortex and 50 to 60 per cent of T_3 in the anterior pituitary or BAT is provided by the type II deiodinase. The type I enzyme is readily inhibited by propylthiouracil (PTU) and decreases with hypothyroidism, whereas the type II enzyme is resistant to PTU-inhibition, and its activity increases when T_4 is reduced. In BAT the deiodinase activity is also stimulated by the sympathetic nervous system. Type I activity is reduced during fasting, severe illness, in patients with significant hepatic disease, and in the human fetus. One or both deiodinases may be inhibited by various drugs (Table 229–3). Inhibition of type I activity is the likely cause of the reduction in serum T_3 and the rise in serum reverse T_3 in sick patients. The latter occurs because 5'-deiodination by the type I enzyme is a rate-limiting step in reverse T_3 degradation. The increase in type II activity during hypothyroxinemia acts as a homeostatic mechanism to maintain normal intracellular T_3 concentrations when T_4 production is reduced. The capacity for PTU and glucocorticoid to inhibit type I activity is important in short-term treatment of severe hyperthyroidism.

MECHANISM OF ACTION OF THYROID HORMONE. Thyroid hormone regulation of protein synthesis is thought to occur through effects on transcription, messenger RNA stabilization, or both. A DNA- and T_3-binding nucleoprotein, the putative T_3 receptor, has about tenfold higher affinity for T_3 than for T_4, explaining in part why T_3 is the active hormone. Effects of thyroid hormone in many tissues can be related to the degree of saturation of these receptors by T_3. Other direct effects of thyroid hormone at the cell membrane or mitochondria may also occur. The regulation of the type II deiodinase by T_4 does not require protein synthesis, but the mechanism for this action is not understood. The human thyroid hormone nuclear receptor has recently been identified as the gene product of the c-erb-A oncogene.

REGULATION OF THYROID FUNCTION. The feedback loop for regulation of thyroid function is presented in Figure 229–3. *Thyrotropin-releasing hormone* (TRH) is secreted by hypothalamic cells and stimulates synthesis and release of thyrotropin (TSH, thyroid-stimulating hormone). This hormone in turn stimulates all of the steps involved in thyroid hormone synthesis and release through activation of adenylate cyclase.

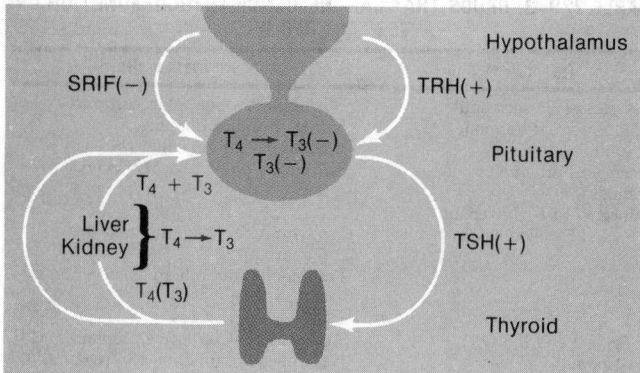

FIGURE 229–3. Current concepts of hypothalamic-pituitary-thyroid inter-relationships.

T_4 and smaller amounts of T_3 are released from the gland with monodeiodination of T_4 to T_3 in liver and kidney. Both serum T_3 and T_4 (via its intrapituitary conversion to T_3) suppress the synthesis and release of TSH competing with TRH to complete the feedback loop. *Somatostatin* (SRIF) and possibly other substances such as neuropeptides and dopamine also inhibit TSH release (see Ch. 225). T_3 may also have a direct effect on TRH synthesis and/or release.

DeGroot LJ, Larsen PR, Refetoff S, et al.: The Thyroid and Its Diseases. 5th ed. New York, John Wiley & Sons, 1984. *A basic text.*

Ingbar SH, Braverman LE: In Werner's The Thyroid. 5th ed. Philadelphia, J. B. Lippincott Company, 1986. *A basic text.*

Kaplan MM, Larsen PR (eds.): Symposium on thyroid disease. Med Clin North Am 69:847, 1985. *This issue contains chapters directed at the most important clinical aspects of thyroid disease authored by experts in their respective fields.*

Larsen PR: Feedback regulation of thyrotropin secretion by hormones. N Engl J Med 306:23, 1982. *A detailed, but clinically oriented, discussion of the feedback regulation of TSH secretion by thyroid hormones.*

Larsen PR, Silva JE, Kaplan MM: Relationships between circulating and intracellular thyroid hormones: Physiological and clinical implications. Endocr Rev 2:87, 1981. *A review of the physiologic significance of intracellular T_4 to T_3 conversion and nuclear binding in various tissues.*

TESTING FOR SUSPECTED THYROID DYSFUNCTION

The thyroid gland is unique among the endocrine organs in that symptoms may arise from two general types of problems. Hyperfunction of the thyroid (*hyperthyroidism* or *thyrotoxicosis*) or decreased secretion of thyroid hormone (*hypothyroidism* or *myxedema*) may cause the patient to seek medical help. Alternatively, physical enlargement of the thyroid (*goiter*) may cause respiratory embarrassment or dysphagia or, more commonly, cosmetic abnormalities. Goiter may exist in the absence of any functional abnormality. Although the most severe forms are dramatic and unmistakable, milder degrees of thyroid dysfunction lead to many symptoms that are nonspecific, requiring biochemical tests for diagnostic confirmation.

PHYSICAL EXAMINATION OF THE THYROID

The high incidence of thyroid disease, particularly in the female (5 to 10 per cent), makes a careful examination of the thyroid gland an important part of the general physical examination. Thyroid enlargement may be the first clue to thyroid functional abnormalities in a patient with otherwise nonspecific symptoms. A cup of water is a necessity, and the patient should first be asked to swallow with the neck moderately extended while the anterior area of the neck is inspected. Significant thyroid enlargement and thyroid nodules can often be discerned by this maneuver. The position of the trachea should then be determined, followed by palpation of the thyroid. The isthmus of the thyroid is first identified and is usually found just inferior to the cricoid cartilage. The left and right thumbs are then employed in turn to palpate the left and right lobe of the gland as the patient swallows. The normal thyroid gland is palpable in a large proportion of

younger persons, although in the elderly patient it is not surprising to find the cricoid cartilage at or below the sternal notch. The pyramidal lobe, a small cylinder of tissue extending vertically from the isthmus to the thyroid cartilage to the left or right of the midline, can often be palpated as well.

DIRECT TESTS OF THYROID FUNCTION

MEASUREMENT OF TOTAL SERUM THYROID HORMONE CONCENTRATIONS. Serum T_4 and T_3 are both readily quantitated by specific radioimmunoassays that require 200 μl or less of serum. Typical normal ranges for the total T_4 and T_3 concentrations are presented in Table 229–4, as well as the values in patients with alterations in TBG and in those with thyroid dysfunction.

SERUM FREE T_4 AND T_3 AND THE FREE T_4 INDEX. Since the concentration of free, rather than total, thyroid hormones parallels the thyroid status, the ideal thyroid function test would be the direct determination of free thyroid hormones. The absolute serum free T_4 and T_3 can be measured either by immunoassay of a dialysate of human serum or by estimating the dialyzable (free) fraction of T_3 and T_4, multiplying this by the total hormone concentration (Table 229–2). In patients who have abnormal total T_4 and T_3 concentrations caused by changes in serum TBG concentration but who are euthyroid, the free hormone concentrations are normal. Unfortunately, such determinations are time consuming.

An indirect estimate of the free fraction of T_4 and T_3 can be obtained by estimating the thyroid hormone-binding ratio (THBR). These tests, formerly termed T_3 or T_4 uptake tests, are performed by analyzing the distribution of tagged T_3 or T_4 in a sample of dilute serum. A common method has been to add charcoal or resin to this sample and quantitate the fraction of the tagged iodothyronine bound to this matrix. The result should be expressed as the ratio of matrix-bound counts to serum protein–bound counts, with a typical normal range of 33 to 50 per cent. To improve reproducibility, this result should be normalized to that obtained in samples of normal sera assayed simultaneously, such that the normal range is 0.85 to 1.15. The ratio of tracer thyroid hormone bound to the inert matrix to that bound to serum protein is directly proportional to the free fraction of thyroid hormone. While the relative distribution of T_3 on the serum binding-proteins is slightly different from that of T_4 (T_3 is only weakly bound to transthyretin), its distribution is sufficiently similar so that in many laboratories it is used instead of T_4. The similarity between the free fraction of thyroid hormones and the THBR can be formalized by calculating the free T_4 (or T_3) index. This is the product of a normalized THBR value and the total serum T_4 or T_3 concentration. The normal range for these indices in units is approximately the same as the total thyroid hormone concentrations. In my laboratory, the normal free T_4 index is 4.7 to 10.5. The free T_4 index is an excellent approximation of the free T_4.

An alternative estimate of the free T_4 may be obtained by using one of several commercial kits. While there are some technical advantages to these tests, they do not measure the free T_4 directly, but provide only an estimate of its concentra-

TABLE 229–4. SERUM THYROID HORMONE CONCENTRATIONS IN NORMAL PERSONS AND PATIENTS WITH THYROID DISEASE

	Serum T_4 (μg/dl)		Serum T_3 (ng/dl)	
	Mean	*Range*	*Mean*	*Range*
Euthyroid				
Normal TBG	8	5–11	140	80–220
Increased TBG	12	8–20	190	120–320
Reduced TBG	2	<1–5	60	20–100
Infants				
Cord serum	11	8–15	48	20–80
Age six weeks	10	7–14	163	120–220
Hyperthyroidism	21	8–35	480	200–1600
Hypothyroidism	2	<1–5	50	<20–150

tion, as does the free T_4 index. One notable clinical situation in which both methods often provide falsely high estimates of the free T_4 is in patients with congenital T_4 binding.

In patients with this syndrome a portion of the serum albumin binds T_4, but not T_3, with abnormally high affinity. The total T_4 value is elevated, but the free fraction of T_4 by dialysis is reduced; therefore the free T_4 concentration is normal. Since T_3 does not bind to the abnormal albumin with increased avidity, estimation of THBR employing T_3 is normal, and therefore a free T_4 index calculated using this value is elevated. Other artifacts in the analogue method kits result in the same falsely high estimate of free T_4. The use of T_4 in estimation of THBR would solve the problem in this syndrome and in other situations such as severe illness in which the changes in the binding of T_3 and T_4 are not identical. The terms T_3 *uptake* and T_3 *resin* are sometimes confused with the direct immunoassay of serum T_3 concentrations, and these terms should be discarded in favor of the THBR.

COMPARISON OF THE UTILITY OF T_4 AND T_3 DETERMINATIONS. The free T_4 index is the best screening test for thyroid dysfunction. It is superior to the free T_3 index by virtue of the fact that the principal thyroid secretory product is T_4. About 80 per cent of circulating T_3 derives from T_4 to T_3 conversion. Therefore, in patients who are sick or who have received any of the drugs listed in Table 229–3, which inhibit T_4 to T_3 conversion, the serum T_3 will invariably be reduced relative to the serum T_4, but this does not imply thyroid disease. In hypothyroidism, serum T_3 may be normal despite significant impairment of thyroid function. On the other hand, in hyperthyroidism there is a small fraction of patients in whom serum T_4 is not elevated but the concentration of serum T_3 is. This condition is called T_3 *thyrotoxicosis* (see below).

SERUM REVERSE T_3 AND OTHER IODOTHYRONINES. The normal concentration of reverse T_3 is 15 to 30 ng per deciliter. It derives exclusively from peripheral metabolism of T_4, and its concentration in the blood reflects a combination of that process and the rate of its degradation. Its measurement is not generally useful clinically, although it is an excellent barometer of the rate of T_4 to T_3 conversion. Immunoassays have been developed for both monoiodinated and diiodinated thyronines, but these measurements do not have clinical applicability.

SERUM THYROID HORMONE-BINDING PROTEIN CONCENTRATIONS. The normal concentration of circulating TBG and transthyretin can be measured by immunoassay or by determination of the binding capacity. The normal concentration of TBG is 1.5 mg per deciliter. This quantity of protein will bind approximately 20 μg of T_4 (1 mole T_4 per 1 mole TBG). The binding capacity of transthyretin is approximately 250 μg T_4 per deciliter. These measurements are rarely necessary for clinical purposes.

RADIOACTIVE IODINE UPTAKE (RAI UPTAKE). The normal 24-hour thyroidal uptake of radioiodine ranges from 5 to 30 per cent. All the radioiodine in the thyroid at this time is in the organified form. Because of the broad normal range for this test, it is not a reliable method for determining thyroid status. Its major diagnostic use is in separating patients who have hyperthyroidism caused by subacute thyroiditis in whom the uptake is reduced or absent from those with Graves' disease (see next section). It is contraindicated in pregnancy.

TESTS OF THYROID REGULATION

SERUM THYROTROPIN. The normal range for serum TSH is 0.5 to 5.0 μU per milliliter. In patients with thyroid hypofunction, TSH increases, and when thyroid function is autonomous, TSH is reduced, as expected from the normal feedback relationships (Fig. 229–3). Newer TSH assays can discriminate between normal TSH concentrations and those that are reduced. Previously it was necessary to employ the TRH infusion test to make this differentiation. With this immunometric assay (TSH-IMA), so called because a combination of monoclonal antibodies is usually employed, serum TSH values less than 0.1 μU per milliliter usually correlate well with absence of a TSH increase in response to TRH (see below). The TSH-IMA should prove to be useful in monitoring the status of hypothyroid patients receiving replacement therapy and those patients in whom TSH suppression is desired, such as those with thyroid carcinoma or TSH-dependent nodular goiter. It may also be used as a screening test in patients suspected of thyroid disease as an alternative to the free T_4 index (Fig. 229–4). Virtually all patients with clinical symptoms attributable to primary hypothyroidism will have serum TSH concentrations greater than 20 μU per milliliter, and many subjects with minimal symptoms or goiter alone will have results between 10 and 20 μU per milliliter. An elevation of the serum TSH concentration almost always indicates that thyroid function is impaired. It is also the critical test for separating patients with primary thyroid disease from those with hypothyroidism resulting from hypothalamic or pituitary dysfunction.

THYROTROPIN RELEASING HORMONE INFUSION TEST. TRH can be infused intravenously and TSH measured in serum to determine whether TSH is present in the pituitary. Pituitary TSH is reduced in patients with hyperthyroidism and in those with autonomous thyroid hormone production and often in patients with hypothalamic pituitary disease. This test may soon be superseded by the TSH-IMA described above. Typical normal and pathologic responses are shown in Figure 229–5. In practice, a basal serum sample is obtained, followed by intravenous infusion of 400 μg of TRH over one minute. A second serum sample is obtained 30 minutes after the infusion, and both are assayed for TSH. In normal persons the minimal TSH increment is 2 μU per milliliter except in males over the age of 40, in the seriously ill, or in patients with depression or exogenous or endogenous glucocorticoid excess in whom the normal response can be lower. The response is amplified (30-minute value greater than 25 μU

FIGURE 229–4. Proposed schema for evaluation of patients based on the TSH-IMA. The TSH-IMA is capable of differentiating the lower limit of normal from the TSH concentration in the sera of patients with autonomous thyroid hyperfunction as well as quantifying elevated levels. The current experience suggests that this approach would not be useful in patients with nonthyroidal illness in whom TSH may be suppressed by factors other than thyroid hyperfunction.

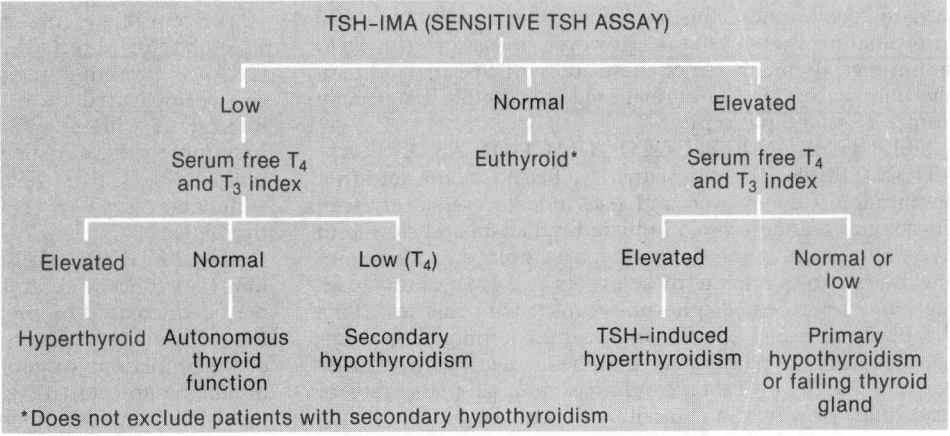

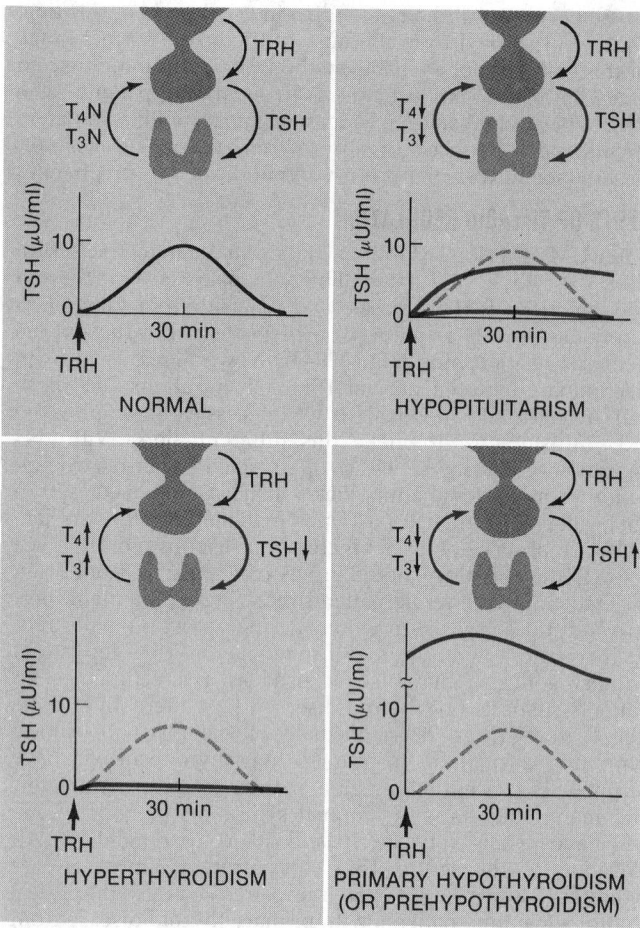

FIGURE 229–5. Typical responses to the infusion of TRH in patients with hyperthyroidism and primary and secondary hypothyroidism. In patients with hypopituitarism or hypothalamic disease virtually any TRH response pattern can be seen. The most pertinent diagnostic information is that serum TSH is not increased in a patient with a reduced serum free T_4 index.

per milliliter) in patients with primary hypothyroidism. A significant increment in TSH eliminates the diagnosis of hyperthyroidism except in the extremely rare patient with the TSH-induced form of this disease.

T_3 **SUPPRESSION TEST.** This test is used to determine what fraction of thyroid function can be accounted for by endogenous TSH (which is suppressible) and what fraction is autonomous. It has been largely replaced by the TRH test or TSH-IMA, and at present its utility is quite limited.

METABOLIC INDICES OF THYROID STATUS

BASAL METABOLIC RATE (BMR). Since thyroid hormone is an important factor in the regulation of the rate of oxygen consumption, this test should theoretically be useful in evaluating thyroid status. However, it has given way to serum measurements, since these are more specific and usually more accurate. The normal range for the BMR is usually from -15 to $+5$ per cent.

DEEP TENDON REFLEX CONTRACTION AND RELAXATION TIMES. Thyroid status is reflected in the rate (not amplitude) of contraction and relaxation of skeletal muscle. These rates are more rapid in hyperthyroidism and slowed in hypothyroidism. Some clinicians have employed a kinemometer tracing to quantitate these events and have observed as high as 70 per cent diagnostic accuracy with this test. Like the BMR, it is less specific than serum hormone measurements, since hypothermia, peripheral neuropathy, gross edema, and many other conditions may slow the rate of relaxation. However, a clinically apparent delay in the relax-

ation phase of the deep tendon reflexes is almost invariably present in patients with significant hypothyroidism, although the more rapid relaxation in hyperthyroidism is difficult to appreciate visually.

ANATOMIC EVALUATION OF THE THYROID GLAND

THE THYROID SCAN. The capacity of the thyroid gland to trap ions such as I^- or molecules with a similar charge and configuration has provided a useful method for correlating structure and function. Of the iodine isotopes either ^{123}I or ^{131}I can be used. ^{123}I, although more expensive, is to be preferred for scanning, particularly in younger persons, since the radiation dose to the thyroid is 7.5 mrads per microcurie administered, as opposed to 800 mrads per microcurie for ^{131}I. Another isotope that gives a low radiation dose is $^{99m}TcO_4^-$ (pertechnetate), which is trapped, but not organified, by the thyroid. For this reason, a scan is obtained 30 minutes after intravenous injection of this isotope. The thyroid scan is usually used to determine the functional state of a palpable thyroid nodule (see later in chapter) or in evaluating masses in the neck or upper part of the chest to see if thyroid tissue is present.

THYROID ULTRASOUND. Whether a given thyroid mass is solid or cystic can be determined by ultrasonography. Ultrasound is now sufficiently sensitive to allow identification of 1- to 3-mm nodules that are too small to be palpated. Such nodules are present in as many as 40 per cent of the population and have unknown clinical significance. Ultrasound may serve as a useful objective method for following the response of a thyroid nodule to TSH suppressive therapy.

NEEDLE BIOPSY OR ASPIRATION. Either a fine (21 to 26 gauge) or cutting needle (Vim-Silverman) can be used to obtain a sample of thyroid cells for histologic examination. These techniques have received increased attention in recent years as a method for evaluation of thyroid nodules. Accurate interpretation of a fine-needle aspirate requires an experienced cytologist.

OTHER TESTS SPECIFICALLY RELATED TO THYROID FUNCTION OR DISEASE

ANTITHYROID ANTIBODIES. In autoimmune thyroid disease (Hashimoto's thyroiditis or Graves' disease), antibodies that bind to various antigens of thyroid tissue are present in the serum. The most important of these is the *thyroid microsomal antibody (TMAb)*. Thyroid peroxidase may be the principal antigen in thyroid microsomes. TMAb is found in approximately 95 per cent of patients with Hashimoto's thyroiditis and in only about 10 per cent of adults with no apparent thyroid disease. The test is generally performed by a tanned red cell hemagglutination technique, and the results are reported as the highest titer causing agglutination. Titers in excess of 1:100 are significant. About 55 per cent of patients with Graves' disease also have circulating TMAb's. *Thyroglobulin antibodies* (TgAb's) are also present in the serum of about 60 per cent of patients with Hashimoto's disease.

Antibodies directed against the thyroid TSH receptor (TRAb's), present in the sera of patients with Graves' disease, can be measured by many techniques that quantitate their interaction with the TSH receptor on thyroid cells. These immunoglobulins are usually stimulatory at the receptor level, but may block TSH-TSH receptor interaction without causing stimulation (see Graves' Disease and Other Causes of Hyperthyroidism).

SERUM THYROGLOBULIN. The normal serum thyroglobulin (Tg) concentration is 2 to 20 ng per milliliter. Serum Tg may be increased in any patient with an enlarged thyroid or following acute trauma to the thyroid, whether a consequence of inflammation, surgery, or radiation. Thyroglobulin determinations are most useful in the follow-up of patients with metastatic thyroid carcinoma following thyroidectomy. An increase in serum Tg indicates the presence of tumor tissue, although a normal value does not eliminate this possibility. Serum thyroglobulin concentrations are generally reduced in patients who have *thyrotoxicosis factitia,* and this measurement may be useful in separating this group of patients from those with hyperthyroidism due to thyroid inflammation.

THE EFFECTS OF NONTHYROIDAL ILLNESS AND COMMON DRUGS ON THYROID FUNCTION TESTS

ILLNESS. Patients with nonthyroidal illnesses can have abnormalities in serum T_4 and T_3 concentrations that may suggest underlying thyroid dysfunction. All such patients will have impaired T_4 to T_3 conversion and, accordingly, have low serum T_3 and raised serum reverse-T_3 concentrations. Most will also have slight reduction in total serum T_4 concentrations. A portion of this decrease is a result of a reduced serum TBG, especially if severe liver disease or proteinuria is present. However, about 10 per cent of patients with typical medical illnesses will have a subnormal serum T_4. This may be due to the release of a substance that inhibits the binding of T_4 to TBG. The fraction of T_4 free, as measured by equilibrium dialysis, is usually increased in such patients. Thus, the free T_4 is normal, indicating that hypothyroidism is not present. Occasionally a patient may have severe illness and an elevated level of serum T_4. Such patients should be suspected of having underlying autonomous thyroid function and often must be treated for hyperthyroidism. This phenomenon may also occur in patients with *acute psychiatric illness* and *hyperemesis gravidarum.* Strategies for dealing with these potentially confusing situations are presented later in the chapter.

DRUGS. Many therapeutic agents interfere (or appear to interfere) with thyroid function. The most commonly used and troublesome agents are listed in Table 229–3. Dopamine or pharmacologic administration of glucocorticoids can transiently suppress TSH concentrations and may contribute to the reduced serum T_4 often seen in the seriously ill patient. Lithium carbonate may cause goiter or hypothyroidism, especially in individuals with mild underlying Hashimoto's thyroiditis. Phenylbutazone and sulfonylurea drugs inhibit normal thyroid gland function if given in sufficient dosage. In addition to the agents listed in Table 229–1, salicylates (>2 grams/day), phenytoin, fenclofenac, and furosemide all inhibit thyroid hormone–protein binding. Because these agents are weak binding inhibitors, they do not usually cause an abnormality in the THBR, and therefore the free T_4 index is mildly reduced. Agents that inhibit the type I 5'-deiodinase generally cause a reduction in serum T_3. If this is severe and prolonged enough, a compensatory increase in TSH secretion occurs, and the serum T_4 concentration rises. In patients receiving more than 200 mg propranolol, mild elevations in the serum free T_4 index are not uncommon.

Amiodarone has complex effects on thyroid function. Since this drug is about 30 per cent iodine by weight, it may produce all of the effects of iodide, that is, either hypothyroidism or hyperthyroidism. Even after discontinuation of this agent, tissue stores of iodine are significantly increased for six to nine months. In addition, amiodarone seems to inhibit both pathways for T_4 to T_3 conversion and causes compensatory hyperthyroxinemia. There is some question whether it might also be a peripheral antagonist of thyroid hormone action, a further stimulus to a compensatory increase in TSH secretion. Iopanoic acid and ipodate, radiographic agents used for visualization of the gallbladder, are also effective inhibitors of T_4 to T_3 conversion. Their effect is transient and disappears within three to four weeks. All agents that inhibit peripheral T_4 to T_3 conversion will raise the ratio of serum T_4 to T_3. In a patient receiving these agents, a TSH-IMA assay or a TRH test may be required to determine if hyperthyroidism is present.

Chopra IJ, Hershman JM, Pardridge WM, et al.: Thyroid function in nonthyroidal illnesses. Ann Intern Med 98:946, 1983. *A review of many of the effects of systemic illness on thyroid function.*

Docter R, Bos G, Krenning EP, et al.: Inherited thyroxine excess: A serum abnormality due to an increased affinity for modified albumin. Clin Endocrinol 15:363, 1981. *An explanation of the thyroid hormone-binding abnormalities in families with congenital T₄-binding albumin elevation.*

Kaplan MM: Clinical and laboratory assessment of thyroid abnormalities. Med Clin North Am 69:863, 1985. *A detailed examination of the clinical application of thyroid function tests and a review of the effects of drugs that can influence these.*

Spencer CA, Lai-Rosenfeld AO, Guttler RB, et al.: Thyrotropin secretion in thyrotoxic and thyroxine-treated patients: Assessment by a sensitive immunoenzymometric assay. J Clin Endocrinol Metab 63:349, 1986. *The performance of a TSH-IMA in monitoring patients undergoing thyroid hormone replacement or with thyrotoxicosis.*

Wiersinga WM, Endert E, Trip MD, et al.: Immunoradiometric assay of thyrotropin in plasma: Its value in predicting response to thyroliberin stimulation and assessing thyroid function in amiodarone-treated patients. Clin Chem 32:433, 1986. *An example of the utility of the TSH-IMA in that most challenging diagnostic situation, the patient with amiodarone-induced thyroid dysfunction.*

GRAVES' DISEASE AND OTHER CAUSES OF HYPERTHYROIDISM

DEFINITION. The clinical syndrome of hyperthyroidism is one of the most dramatic in clinical medicine. The major symptoms associated with this syndrome are predominantly a reflection of the hypermetabolism resulting from excessive quantities of circulating thyroid hormone. The many disorders that can be associated with this syndrome are listed in Table 229–5 in their approximate order of frequency. Graves' disease accounts for more than 85 per cent of such patients. Toxic nodular goiters, both multinodular (*Plummer's disease*) and uninodular, and subacute thyroiditis account for the bulk of the remainder.

Graves' Disease

In 1835, Robert Graves described a clinical syndrome including hypermetabolism, diffuse enlargement of the thyroid gland, and *exophthalmos* (forward displacement of the eyes). In continental Europe, the same condition is known as Basedow's disease after von Basedow's description in 1840. In addition to thyroid involvement and ophthalmopathy, patients may have a dermatologic condition, *pretibial myxedema.* As Graves' disease is presently defined, patients may have only one of these three major clinical manifestations, and the only common denominator is likely to be the presence of TSH receptor antibodies in the serum. *Jodbasedow's* disease refers to hyperthyroidism (Basedow's disease) in iodine-deficient patients after iodine (jod) replacement.

ETIOLOGY AND PATHOGENESIS. The precise etiology of Graves' disease is still not known, but it seems likely that it is an autoimmune disorder. Hyperthyroidism is its principal manifestation, yet TSH is suppressed and no intrinsic regulatory abnormalities in the thyroid have been identified. Thus the thyroid stimulation seems likely to be a consequence of a circulating, non-TSH, thyroid stimulator. This "stimulator" is now thought to be a gamma globulin or a family of gamma globulins.

TABLE 229–5. DISEASES OR CLINICAL SYNDROMES ASSOCIATED WITH THYROTOXICOSIS

Graves' disease
Toxic multinodular goiter
Toxic adenoma
Iodide-induced hyperthyroidism
Subacute thyroiditis
Factitious (exogenous) thyrotoxicosis
Neonatal thyrotoxicosis (mother with Graves' disease)
TSH-secreting pituitary tumor
Nontumorigenic pituitary-induced hyperthyroidism
Choriocarcinoma (uterine or testicular origin) or hydatidiform mole
Struma ovarii
Hyperfunctioning thyroid carcinoma (usually metastatic)

It is postulated, with increasing evidence, that in Graves' disease, for reasons as yet unclear, B lymphocytes secrete antibodies directed against the TSH receptor. These antibodies, termed TRAb, are generally polyclonal and may be stimulatory or inhibitory at the receptor, depending on the nature of their interaction with the receptor site. The reason for the appearance of TRAb and their perpetuation in Graves' disease has not been elucidated. Assays for the presence of TRAb depend either on the capacity of the serum to activate adenylate cyclase in thyroid cell membranes or thyroid cell lines or to compete with labeled TSH for binding to the TSH receptor on thyroid cells or on guinea pig adipocyte membranes. TRAb are found in 85 to 90 per cent of patients with clinical evidence of Graves' disease.

The etiology of Graves' ophthalmopathy is not known. Patients with exophthalmos and particularly those with dermopathy almost invariably have high titers of circulating TRAb, suggesting that these two clinical manifestations represent the most severe form of this disease. Antibodies to soluble human eye muscle antigens were found in 17 of 23 patients with Graves' ophthalmopathy, but not in Graves' patients without this manifestation and rarely in those with Hashimoto's thyroiditis. This suggests a similar autoimmune etiology for ophthalmopathy and for hyperthyroidism. It has also been proposed that Tg–anti-Tg circulating immune complexes may bind to eye muscles and play a pathogenic role. Further studies will be required to resolve this question.

Emotional Factors in the Etiology of Hyperthyroidism. The emotional lability of the patient with hyperthyroidism has led many clinicians to question the role of psychologic trauma in the pathogenesis of this disease. Numerous anecdotes have been cited to suggest that emotional trauma may somehow trigger the onset of overt hyperthyroidism. If this is so, it would still appear to require participation of the immune system, since circulating TRAb are such a constant feature of the clinical picture. In my mind, it seems more likely that an episode of physical or emotional trauma brings the patient to medical attention, at which time pre-existing hyperthyroidism is recognized.

INCIDENCE. Graves' disease is common, affecting as many as 1.9 per cent of the female population and about a tenth that number of males, according to a population survey in northern England. It reaches its peak incidence in the third and fourth decades. The reason for the female predominance in this as in all thyroid diseases is not known. There is a strong familial component to Graves' disease with a family history of autoimmune thyroid disease (Graves' disease, Hashimoto's thyroiditis, or "goiter") in a significant fraction of patients. The importance of genetic inheritance in the predisposition to this syndrome has been confirmed by finding a higher relative risk of this condition in patients with the histocompatibility antigens HLA-B8 (Caucasians), HLA-B35 (Japanese), and HLA-Bw46 (Chinese).

PATHOLOGY. The thyroid of the patient with Graves' disease is diffusely enlarged and hypercellular. In patients undergoing thyroidectomy without prior treatment with antithyroid drugs or iodine, a diffusely hyperplastic epithelium is noted with little or no colloid present and often with lymphocytic infiltration, varying from minimal to extensive. In some specimens it is impossible to distinguish the microscopic picture from Hashimoto's thyroiditis (a condition sometimes called hashitoxicosis). If the patient receives iodide preoperatively, the gland contains large amounts of colloid, cells are of normal height, and the vascularity is markedly reduced. Other tissues show no specific changes except in severely hyperthyroid patients. In those situations there may be edema and focal necrosis in the liver with cellular infiltration.

In hyperthyroid patients with mild eye manifestations of Graves' disease such as lid retraction and stare, no significant orbital pathology is found, and these changes probably are due to the hyperthyroidism per se. In more severe cases, edema of the extraocular muscles occurs in association with infiltration with lymphocytes, plasma cells, and neutrophils. In addition, hydrophilic mucopolysaccharide collects in the orbital tissues. The conjunctivae may show perivascular lymphocytic infiltration and edema (*chemosis*). The end stage of these processes is fibrosis, which most often involves the inferior eye muscles, causing restriction of upward globe movement.

CLINICAL PICTURE. The common clinical symptoms of thyrotoxicosis are listed in Table 229–6. These occur in any patient with excessive thyroid hormone secretion whether due to Graves' disease or some other cause. They are a consequence of the stimulatory effect of thyroid hormone on the metabolic rate and on many other tissues, especially the heart and central nervous system. The typical patient with Graves' disease is in her mid-20's with symptoms that can often be dated to six to twelve months previously. The patient is nervous, anxious, and fidgeting, and speaks rapidly. She will complain of her agitated fatigue, palpitations, and, in warmer climates, heat intolerance. There may be weight loss despite increased appetite, or the patient may merely report success in her efforts at weight control. An increased frequency of bowel movements and, rarely, diarrhea, may be noted. Emotional lability is often apparent during the interview, and a history of deteriorating domestic or occupational relationships may be obtained. A history of neck swelling (often not noted first by the patient) may be present. Amenorrhea or oligomenorrhea is not uncommon. Rarer manifestations of hyperthyroidism include pruritus and urticaria. About 5 per cent of males may experience gynecomastia, and even less commonly *hypokalemic periodic paralysis* may occur. For unknown reasons, this condition is much more common in males of Oriental extraction.

Apathetic or Masked Hyperthyroidism. The symptoms given in Table 229–6 are those generally found in the younger patient. The clinician should be aware that in some patients, particularly the elderly, the clinical symptoms and signs of hypermetabolism may not be so dramatic. Rather than appearing agitated, the elderly patient with hyperthyroidism may be depressed. Weight loss and symptoms of congestive heart failure can be the predominant manifestations of the hypermetabolic syndrome. Often this is complicated by atrial fibrillation or other supraventricular tachyarrhythmia, leading to suspicion that the heart, rather than the thyroid, is the source of the problem. Because of the subtlety of this clinical form of hyperthyroidism it is recommended that any patient with the recent onset of atrial fibrillation have tests of thyroid function. In this way a reversible cause of congestive heart failure and/or recurrent arrhythmias may be recognized and appropriate treatment instituted.

Graves' Ophthalmopathy. Eye symptoms are present in more than 50 per cent of patients with Graves' disease but, except for modest lid lag and stare, are rare in patients with other causes of hyperthyroidism. This is a useful point in establishing the diagnosis. Common complaints are protruding eyes, easy tearing, especially on exposure to wind or cold, photophobia, a gritty foreign body sensation in the eyes, and,

TABLE 229–6. COMMON SYMPTOMS AND SIGNS OF HYPERTHYROIDISM (THYROTOXICOSIS)

Symptoms	Signs
Nervousness and/or tremor	Tachycardia or atrial fibrillation
Weight loss (usually with increased appetite)	Widened pulse pressure with increased systolic and decreased diastolic pressures
Palpitations	
Heat intolerance and excessive perspiration	Hyperdynamic precordium and accentuated S1
Emotional lability	Warm, smooth skin
Muscle weakness	Tremor
Hyperdefecation	Proximal muscle weakness
	Thyroid enlargement or abnormality

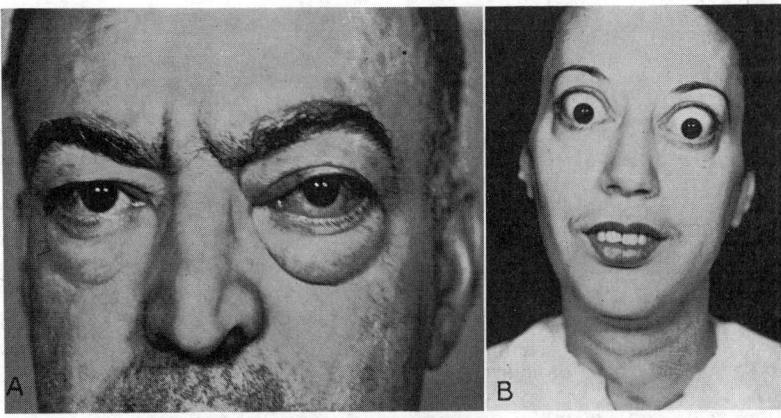

FIGURE 229–6. Two patients showing the typical ophthalmopathy characteristic of Graves' disease. Patient A demonstrates marked periorbital swelling, exophthalmos, chemosis, and conjunctival injection. The proptosis, limitation of extraocular movements, and other manifestations of ophthalmopathy are much more severe in Patient A than in Patient B. Patient B has marked widening of the palpebral fissures owing to lid retraction and also has significant proptosis. Patient A is euthyroid; Patient B is mildly hyperthyroid. (From Williams RH (ed.): Textbook of Endocrinology. 6th ed. Philadelphia, W. B. Saunders Company, 1981, p 189.)

less commonly, diplopia. (Fig. 229–6). The patient with significant *proptosis* (exophthalmos) may complain of irritation, particularly on arising, since the eyelids do not completely cover the sclera when the patient is sleeping *(lagophthalmos).* Rarely, severe chemosis, inflammation, and periorbital edema occur (malignant exophthalmos). Eye complaints are usually bilateral, but may be unilateral, and Graves' disease is one of the most common causes of unilateral exophthalmos.

Pretibial Myxedema. In a few patients with Graves' disease (1 to 2 per cent) a brawny, nonpitting swelling of the pretibial area, ankles, and/or feet is present. This can appear in plaques. It has an orange-skin appearance and is usually not tender. This dermopathy, found exclusively in Graves' disease, is termed *pretibial myxedema.* The name derives from the histologic similarity of the mucopolysaccharide infiltration of the subcutaneous tissues to that found in advanced hypothyroidism (myxedema).

Euthyroid Graves' Disease. In a small fraction of patients with Graves' disease, eye manifestations (unilateral or bilateral) with or without pretibial myxedema appear, but hyperthyroidism is not present. This can arise because of destruction of the thyroid as a result of coexistent Hashimoto's disease, or hyperthyroidism may be delayed in its appearance for months or years after the first eye symptoms. In many such patients, appropriate testing will often reveal subtle evidence of thyroid dysfunction.

PHYSICAL SIGNS. In younger patients, tachycardia is almost universal. The systolic blood pressure is elevated primarily because of the increased inotropic effect of thyroid hormone on the heart. The diastolic pressure is reduced owing to a decrease in peripheral vascular resistance associated with increased skin capillary blood flow. Body temperature is usually normal. The skin is smooth, warm, and moist, and the patient may radiate heat. A fine tremor of the outstretched hands and occasionally *onycholysis* of the fourth and fifth fingers or clubbing *(thyroid acropachy)* are observed. The thyroid is almost always diffusely enlarged from 1.5 to 5 to 6 times normal. One third of elderly patients will not have a detectable goiter. The gland may be soft or firm, depending on the degree of hyperthyroidism and the level of iodine intake. Auscultation of the neck may reveal a multitude of sounds. In the younger patient a *venous hum* may be heard over the external jugular vein, particularly with the patient in the sitting position. Third or fourth heart sounds are heard easily in the neck, and a carotid bruit is not uncommon. In addition, a bruit over the thyroid gland is present in some patients, a manifestation of the high blood flow to this organ. A diffuse lymphadenopathy may be present in hyperthyroidism, and splenomegaly is found in 10 per cent of patients. The liver is not enlarged except in elderly patients with congestive failure. The neurologic examination shows tremor and proximal muscle weakness. Eye signs include lid lag, a failure of the upper lid to cover the upper margin of the iris as the globe traverses from upward to downward gaze, a

widened palpebral fissure so that the sclera is visible above and/or below the iris, conjunctival injection and chemosis, periorbital swelling, and proptosis. The last-named finding is determined by measuring the distance from the lateral portion of the bony orbit to the cornea, using the *exophthalmometer*. In the white population this distance is 17 mm or less, with an upper limit of normal of 20 mm (22 mm for the black population). The difference between the two eye measurements should not be more than 3 mm. In addition to these moderate abnormalities, there may be impairment of globe movement. The most common restriction is in upward and/or outward gaze. This is due not to weakness of the superior eye muscles but to swelling and fibrosis of the inferior rectus and inferior oblique muscles beneath the globe. In addition, abduction and convergence may also be affected. Eye signs may be absent or mild, are usually bilateral when present, but may be asymmetric.

Laboratory Diagnosis of Hyperthyroidism

The various steps to be followed in establishing the laboratory diagnosis of hyperthyroidism are outlined in Figure 229–7. The initial screening test is to determine the free T_4 index. In virtually all patients an elevation in the free T_4 index is present. In the hospitalized patient the diagnosis may be somewhat more complicated if the patient is severely ill or has received any of the agents listed in Table 229–3, which cause inhibition of T_4 to T_3 conversion. In these patients an impairment of T_4 clearance or inhibition of T_4 to T_3 conversion may lead to an elevation in the serum free T_4 index without hyperthyroidism. Other causes of an elevated free T_4 index not necessarily indicating hyperthyroidism are *congenital elevation of T_4-binding albumin* (see Direct Tests of Thyroid Function), hyperemesis gravidarium, and acute psychosis. In the last two conditions the increase in the free T_4 index is usually transient. An alternate approach is to use the strategy depicted in Figure 229–4. Except in seriously ill patients this approach should be equally effective.

In such patients and in patients in whom the clinical suspicion of hyperthyroidism is present but the free T_4 index is normal or equivocal, serum T_3 determination is required. The ratio of T_3 to T_4 is increased in the thyroid gland in patients with Graves' disease. As a consequence, the T_3 production rate and the fraction of T_3 coming directly from the thyroid are increased. Thus the serum T_3 is elevated to a greater extent than is the serum T_4 (see Table 229–4). Patients in whom serum T_3 is elevated but the serum free T_4 index is not have T_3 *thyrotoxicosis*, which occurs in 3 to 5 per cent of patients in the United States but is more common in areas where dietary iodine is lower. The diagnosis of hyperthyroidism cannot be eliminated until the free T_3 index (as well as the free T_4 index) has been found to be normal. Even in hyperthyroidism, a substantial fraction of T_3 derives from peripheral T_4 to T_3 conversion. Impairment of this process from any cause (illness or drugs) can lead to a reduction in

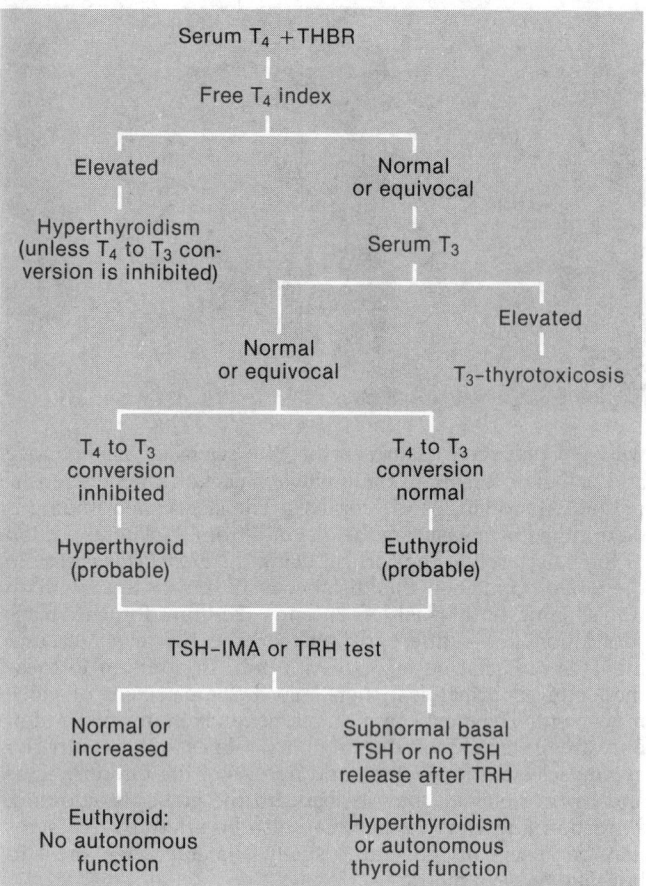

FIGURE 229–7. Laboratory diagnosis of hyperthyroidism. THBR refers to the thyroid hormone binding ratio (formerly termed T_3 or T_4 uptake). TSH-IMA refers to the serum TSH measured by an immunometric assay that can discriminate between normal and suppressed as well as elevated TSH concentrations.

serum T_3. However, in hyperthyroidism, even with severe illness, the serum T_3 is rarely depressed to less than 100 ng per deciliter.

In equivocal situations a TSH-IMA or a TRH infusion test will be helpful. A normal TSH-IMA or a normal increase in TSH after TRH administration eliminates all forms of hyperthyroidism except the extremely rare case with increased TSH secretion (Fig. 229–4). Since patients with fixed or autonomous, but not supranormal, thyroid hormone production will also have reduced serum TSH, an abnormal test does not indicate the presence of hypermetabolism and the need for treatment.

In patients with a classic history and laboratory abnormalities, an RAI uptake and thyroid scan are not necessary to establish the diagnosis. However, if the hyperthyroidism is of brief (less than three months') duration, if the thyroid is not enlarged or palpable, or if it is tender, subacute thyroiditis must be considered, and an uptake and scan should be performed after pregnancy has been excluded. These tests are also required when nodular goiter or factitious thyrotoxicosis is suspected (Table 229–5).

Unilateral Ophthalmopathy. Since Graves' ophthalmopathy may be unilateral and not associated with frank hyperthyroidism, local pathology such as orbital tumor, pseudotumor of the orbit, cavernous sinus–carotid aneurysm, and sphenoid ridge meningioma must be considered. In addition to the free T_4 index, serum T_3, and TRH test, such patients require orbital x-ray examinations, ultrasound examination, and computed tomography. In almost all patients with Graves' ophthalmopathy, bilateral involvement of the extraocular muscles will be found even though clinically the process appears unilateral.

Positive serum tests for TRAb or TMAb will provide further support for this diagnosis.

OTHER CHEMICAL ABNORMALITIES ASSOCIATED WITH HYPERTHYROIDISM. In 5 to 20 per cent of patients with hyperthyroidism any of the following may be found: modest hypercalcemia, increased alkaline phosphatase (bone or hepatic isozyme), increased direct bilirubin, and a mild anemia of "chronic disease." Modest neutropenia may occur (1000 to 2000 per cubic millimeter).

Differential Diagnosis of Hyperthyroidism

Few clinical syndromes mimic hyperthyroidism. Pheochromocytoma and neurocirculatory asthenia may cause some clinical confusion, but appropriate laboratory testing will eliminate these from consideration. Differentiation of patients with Graves' disease from those with other forms of hyperthyroidism is rarely difficult based solely on the history and physical examination (Table 229–5). The use of the RAI uptake and scan to identify patients with subacute thyroiditis or nodular disease has been discussed. Iodine-induced hyperthyroidism is due to either multinodular goiter or Graves' disease (jodbasedow). Factitious thyrotoxicosis, the ingestion of excess thyroid hormone, should be considered particularly in paramedical personnel in whom symptoms and laboratory manifestations are associated with a nonpalpable thyroid gland. TSH-induced hyperthyroidism is often diagnosed retrospectively after treatment has begun. It is so rare that it is not cost-effective to screen all hyperthyroid patients for this disease. Chorionic gonadotropin-induced hyperthyroidism is confirmed by the elevation in serum HCG in association with molar pregnancy or choriocarcinoma.

Treatment

TREATMENT OF HYPERTHYROIDISM OF GRAVES' DISEASE. The treatment of patients with Graves' disease must be considered in the context of its natural history. In 10 to 50 per cent of patients, depending on the series, thyroid function returns to normal (remission) in association with (but probably not because of) drug treatment directed at the thyroid, not at the apparent primary defect in the immune system. If the patient destined for remission could be identified, a rational treatment approach for this disease could be developed. At present this is not possible, although a reduction in circulating TRAb titers generally accompanies remission, and it may be possible to employ such assays in the future to guide therapy. Early studies suggested that if patients were given antithyroid drugs for 12 to 18 months, approximately 50 per cent would remain euthyroid after discontinuation of the drugs. More recently that fraction may have decreased to 10 to 20 per cent. The reason for the apparent change in the natural history of hyperthyroidism in the United States is not clear. One possible explanation is the recent increase in iodine intake. Since antithyroid drugs markedly deplete thyroidal iodine, the capacity to re-establish excessive secretion of thyroid hormone could be influenced by the iodine supply. In patients with Graves' disease who undergo a remission, hypothyroidism may occur some 20 to 30 years later. This is presumably autoimmune in origin, further emphasizing the similarities between Graves' disease and Hashimoto's thyroiditis. Lastly, in patients whose condition is in remission, relapse may occur months to years later.

As the underlying cause for Graves' disease is not known, no specific therapy for this condition is available. There are two phases of the treatment of the hyperthyroidism of Graves' disease. The first is acute therapy with the goal of re-establishing euthyroidism. The second phase is definitive therapy, the induction of a permanent alteration in thyroid function.

Short-term Treatment of Hyperthyroidism. ANTITHYROID DRUGS. In a typical patient with hyperthyroidism caused by

Graves' disease, the first step in management is to suppress the elevated thyroid hormone secretion rate. The drugs of choice for this purpose are derivatives of thiourea. In the United States, propylthiouracil (PTU) and methimazole (Tapazole) are used. Both inhibit the organification of iodine by the thyroid gland as their major mechanism of action. Neither drug affects I^- trapping, nor does either inhibit the release of preformed thyroid hormone. PTU, but not methimazole, is an inhibitor of T_4 to T_3 conversion, giving it a modest therapeutic advantage over the latter agent. This drug has special importance in the short-term treatment of hyperthyroidism. Carbimazole, rapidly converted to methimazole in the body, is used in Europe and is equal in potency to methimazole.

PTU and methimazole are rapidly absorbed and are probably concentrated by the hyperactive thyroid. Although the plasma half-life is relatively short, suggesting the need for frequent dosage, in practice it is often possible to maintain satisfactory suppression of thyroid hormone synthesis by administration of these drugs twice or even only once per day. Methimazole is approximately 15 times as potent as PTU. Initial treatment consists of 300 to 450 mg of PTU per day (or the equivalent of methimazole) divided into three doses. Rarely as much as 1600 mg per day of PTU is required, but problems with compliance are common at such dosages. Since there is a five- to ten-day half-time for the disappearance of the metabolic effects induced by excess thyroid hormone, it is not unusual for the serum level of T_4 to fall before the patient begins to obtain relief from the symptoms of hyperthyroidism. It is my practice to see the patient three to four weeks after the initial visit, obtaining a free T_4 index and serum T_3 at that point to ascertain the progress of therapy. If clinical improvement has not occurred, the serum T_4 has not decreased, and compliance has been maintained, the dose of antithyroid drug should be increased. After the first months of treatment, the dose of antithyroid drug can be reduced to a level of 100 to 300 mg per day of PTU, and the patient seen at two- to three-month intervals. In patients to be treated for six to eighteen months, therapy can be monitored by both clinical and laboratory parameters. The serum T_3–T_4 ratio will be increased because of intrathyroidal iodine deficiency and the increased thyroidal T_3–T_4 ratio in Graves' disease. Therefore both serum T_3 and the free T_4 index should be monitored. Serum TSH may increase if the serum T_4 falls below normal even if serum T_3 is normal. This is undesirable, since it can lead to further thyroid enlargement and possibly an exacerbation of eye symptoms.

Thiourea derivatives have several side effects. A maculopapular rash occurs in 2 to 8 per cent of patients, but does not usually require discontinuation of the drug. Both agents can rarely cause hepatocellular damage, and PTU can cause vasculitis. The most serious side effect of both agents is agranulocytosis. This occurs in 2 to 5 of 1000 patients and can be fatal if not recognized. Since this reaction may be abrupt in onset and is so rare, it is not, in the opinion of many experts, necessary to monitor the white blood count at frequent intervals. Instead, a baseline WBC and differential are obtained, and the patient is cautioned on each visit about the symptoms and significance of agranulocytosis. The patient is instructed to report immediately if infection occurs and to stop the medication. The WBC and differential are repeated and the drug discontinued permanently if indicated. The reaction may appear at any time during therapy and does not appear to be dose related (except at extremely high doses). It is seen most commonly in the first few months of therapy. If such a reaction occurs, the drug should be withdrawn and appropriate supportive care provided. Recovery occurs in almost all patients, and an alternative treatment method should then be used. Special precautions about the use of antithyroid drugs in pregnancy are discussed below. Iodide (saturated solution of potassium iodide, 1 gram KI per milliliter) 3 drops twice a day or Lugol's solution (125 mg I^- per

milliliter) 10 drops three times a day is the most effective antithyroid drug for short-term use, since it inhibits both thyroid hormone release and thyroid hormone synthesis (through the Wolff-Chaikoff effect). Iodide alone can be given to patients with allergies to thiourea drugs to suppress thyroid function for periods of 10 to 28 days. Since the initially depressed hormone release will increase gradually during treatment, iodide administration should not be prolonged beyond two to three weeks. Iodide is often used to decrease the vascularity of the thyroid gland in the preparation of patients who are to have surgery. Since it will interfere with the subsequent administration of ^{131}I, it should not be used in the weeks prior to this treatment.

The benefits of bed rest, adequate diet, and the extrication of the patient from the usual occupational or domestic pressures cannot be overemphasized. Remarkable clinical improvement is often noted within one to two days simply as a result of hospitalization. The short-term treatment of severe hyperthyroidism is discussed below under Thyroid Storm.

BETA-ADRENERGIC BLOCKING AGENTS AND OTHER DRUGS. The similarity of the symptoms of hyperthyroidism to those of catecholamine excess is striking. The molecular basis for this similarity is not clearly established. Although animal studies have shown thyroid hormone-induced increases in beta-adrenergic receptors in cardiac tissue, the receptor number is normal in lymphocytes from patients with thyrotoxicosis. Plasma catecholamine concentrations are normal in hyperthyroidism. Nevertheless, blockade of beta-adrenergic receptors by propranolol or other beta-receptor antagonists may result in symptomatic improvement prior to a decrease in serum thyroid hormones. A dose of 20 to 40 mg of propranolol every four to six hours may be used, but patients with congestive heart failure or bronchial asthma should not receive this therapy. In most patients with mild to moderate hyperthyroidism this adjunctive therapy is not necessary and may complicate the therapeutic regimen. In patients with more profound tachycardia or with thyroid storm (see below), it may have an important beneficial effect. Propranolol, although decreasing pulse rate and cardiac output in patients with hyperthyroidism, does not alter the elevated basal metabolic rate. Therefore the tissues continue to consume oxygen at a high rate in the presence of a decrease in cardiac output.

Lithium inhibits release of preformed thyroid hormone from the thyroid gland, probably by inhibiting hydrolysis of thyroglobulin, and may also inhibit peripheral T_4 degradation. In patients with allergies to thiourea drugs and iodide, lithium carbonate 0.9 to 1.5 grams per day (serum lithium concentrations of 0.5 to 1.0 mEq per liter) may be of value in the treatment of acute hyperthyroidism. Serum lithium levels must be closely monitored, as some of the toxic effects of lithium are similar to those of thyrotoxicosis.

Iopanoic acid (Telepaque) and ipodate (Oragrafin) contain iodide and also are potent inhibitors of type I and type II 5'-deiodinase activities. These agents would therefore appear to be ideal for short-term treatment of hyperthyroidism. However, both remain in the body for long periods, which may prohibit subsequent ^{131}I therapy. They can be used in emergency situations, especially if surgery is contemplated as definitive therapy, and might also be as effective as PTU for blocking T_4 to T_3 conversion, such as might be required in the rare patient with severe exogenous thyrotoxicosis.

The Second Phase of Hyperthyroidism Treatment. If the symptoms of hyperthyroidism are not severe or after short-term treatment of symptoms with thiourea drugs, a decision must be made as to long-term therapy. There are three choices: further antithyroid drugs with hopes of a spontaneous remission, surgery, or radioiodine. None of these is ideal, and the choice for each patient must be made individually.

LONG-TERM ANTITHYROID DRUG THERAPY. If long-term antithyroid drug therapy is undertaken in anticipation of a remission, it should be continued for six to eighteen months. If the quantities of drug required to maintain euthyroidism remain relatively large (e.g., 200 mg of PTU or greater) and serum T_3 and T_4 rise when the dosage is reduced, then a remission has not occurred. If the thyroid becomes smaller and the required amount of antithyroid drug lower, then a remission is probable. Some authorities recommend a TSH assay at this juncture, but I prefer to determine serum T_3 and T_4, to discontinue the treatment, and to repeat these tests in four weeks. The serum T_3 is especially important, since it may become elevated prior to the T_4 when a relapse occurs. If thyroid hormones remain normal, the patient should be seen at bimonthly intervals for one year, at which time the visits can be reduced in frequency.

SURGERY. Surgical removal of a portion of the thyroid gland to regulate hyperthyroidism is a time-honored and effective treatment in the hands of expert surgeons. Hyperthyroidism rarely recurs, although roughly 50 to 60 per cent of patients will eventually become hypothyroid. In most patients, hyperthyroidism is controlled by antithyroid drugs for one to two months prior to surgery. About seven to ten days before surgery, saturated solution of potassium iodide or Lugol's solution should be given to reduce the vascularity of the thyroid (see above).

Alternatively, propranolol alone may be used to prepare the patient, or it may be combined with I⁻. One to two weeks of pretreatment with 40 mg of propranolol every six hours has been given. This approach should not be employed for patients who can undertake standard preoperative therapy with thiourea drugs. Aside from hypothyroidism, other potential complications of surgery include neck hemorrhage, recurrent laryngeal nerve damage, and hypoparathyroidism. In highly experienced clinics, such complications are quite rare (<1 per cent).

RADIOIODINE. Treatment of hyperthyroidism with ¹³¹I has been used since the late 1940's. The principal complication of this treatment is hypothyroidism, which occurs in about 10 per cent of patients in the first year and increases about 5 per cent per year thereafter over 20 years. Depending on the dose given, about 20 per cent of patients require a second treatment. No increased risk of thyroid carcinoma or leukemia occurs after such treatment. For many years, there was a reluctance to employ ¹³¹I in the treatment of women in the childbearing age group, but the ovarian dose from a typical 10 mCi treatment is approximately 2 to 4 rads, which is in the same range as that from hysterosalpingography or a barium enema. Although any unnecessary radiation is to be avoided, the calculated increase in the gamete mutation rate from exposure in this range is only a small fraction of the spontaneous mutation rate. Thus ¹³¹I therapy does not appear to offer a significant risk of fetal malformation, although it is recommended that pregnancy not be undertaken for six months after this therapy to avoid transient radiation-induced changes in the gametes.

I will generally pretreat patients who are to have ¹³¹I therapy with thiourea derivatives to provide symptomatic relief and avoid the remote chance of an exacerbation of hyperthyroidism from radiation thyroiditis. These are discontinued four days prior to determining the 24-hour ¹³¹I uptake. My practice is to administer orally an amount of ¹³¹I which when multiplied by the RAI uptake will result in thyroidal accumulation of 5 mCi ¹³¹I. This will result in an average dose of 80 to 90 μCi per gram or 6000 to 7000 rads, which is associated with resolution of hyperthyroidism in about 80 per cent of patients within six months. Therapy with thiourea drugs may be restarted after one week, although it is not usually required. Patients are seen monthly thereafter with appropriate diagnostic and therapeutic measures to maintain the euthyroid state. At least six months is allowed to elapse before considering a second treatment. Since radioiodine crosses the pla-

centa and would be concentrated by the thyroid of the fetus at 12 weeks and older, it is imperative that possibility of pregnancy be eliminated before radioiodine is administered.

The therapist administering radioiodine is committed to the planning of adequate follow-up. This consists of thoroughly informing the patient about the risks of delayed hypothyroidism (occurring in 80 to 100 per cent), providing written documentation of the treatment and its complications, and maintaining proper communication with referring physicians as to the need for indefinite follow-up. Patients are alerted to the symptoms of hypothyroidism and instructed that after the acute phase of treatment they should be seen at least every four to six months for appropriate thyroid function testing until hypothyroidism appears and treatment is initiated.

Choice of Therapy. None of the three long-term therapies for hyperthyroidism is ideal. Some thyroidologists will not use radioiodine in patients under the age of 35 or 40 because of the fear of long-term complications, whereas others employ radioiodine routinely in the treatment of hyperthyroidism in children. On balance, from the point of view of lack of immediate complications and effectiveness, radioiodine treatment is the most effective approach currently available. My approach is to inform the patient of all treatment options and to recommend antithyroid drugs only to patients who have goiters less than three times normal or in patients who are hesitant regarding radioiodine therapy. In women in whom pregnancy is planned, a requirement for high doses of antithyroid drugs indicates the need for definitive treatment prior to undertaking pregnancy. Surgery is recommended only for patients with extreme thyroid enlargement or those who have coexisting nonfunctioning thyroid nodules. The physician advising patients regarding this decision must consider not only these theoretical arguments and the patient's preferences but also the availability of an experienced surgeon.

Graves' Disease and Pregnancy. The peak incidence of Graves' disease occurs in women during the reproductive period. Therefore, it is not uncommon to find hyperthyroidism in a pregnant patient or for pregnancy to occur during therapy with antithyroid drugs. There is a tendency for Graves' disease to exacerbate during the first trimester of pregnancy and to ameliorate during the third trimester. One to two months after delivery, an exacerbation is not uncommon. Since PTU and methimazole cross the placenta, whereas thyroid hormones do not, minimal quantities of these agents must be used during pregnancy. PTU crosses the placenta less well than does methimazole. While pregnant patients tolerate moderate degrees of hyperthyroidism quite well, uncontrolled thyrotoxicosis is associated with an increased risk of spontaneous abortion and may be associated with thyroid storm at the time of delivery.

With these facts in mind, pregnant patients with hyperthyroidism should be seen at monthly intervals, with careful clinical examination supplemented by measurements of serum T_3, T_4, and THBR. It should be recalled that the normal range for both serum T_4 and T_3 is higher during pregnancy (see Table 229–4). PTU should be given at the lowest dosage that maintains the patient at an acceptable euthyroid state. I do not employ supplemental thyroid hormones in the treatment of the pregnant hyperthyroid patient, as has been recommended by some. An attempt to reduce the antithyroid drug dose should be made as the third trimester approaches. If the patient's hyperthyroid symptoms cannot be controlled on less than 300 mg of PTU per day, then subtotal thyroidectomy should be considered during the second trimester. Iodides can be given for seven to ten days in preparation for surgery but should not be given over a long period during pregnancy, since the fetus may develop hypothyroidism because of transplacental iodide transfer and the Wolff-Chaikoff effect.

The newborn infant of the mother with Graves' disease

should be examined carefully for either hypothyroidism as a consequence of excessive antithyroid drug or hyperthyroidism resulting from transplacental passage of TRAb. In either situation goiter may be present, which may lead to respiratory embarrassment. Even the most meticulously managed patients will often have infants with modest reductions in serum T_4 that quickly normalize in the first week of life. Neonatal hyperthyroidism is transient, but occasionally must be treated with antithyroid drugs and digitalis for tachycardia.

The quantities of PTU in the milk of mothers receiving 200 to 300 mg PTU per day are not great enough to cause impairment of an infant's thyroid function. It seems likely that nursing mothers could take PTU at low doses, though the infant could still be at risk for nonthyroidal complications of this drug. Methimazole (and presumably carbimazole) is present in milk in significant amounts and should not be given to nursing mothers.

Thyroid Storm. Some patients with hyperthyroidism develop severe manifestations that are exaggerations of many of the symptoms listed in Table 229–6. Often these occur because of superimposed stress or infection. The patient may be febrile, have abdominal pain, and become delirious, obtunded, or psychotic. This condition, called *thyroid storm,* has a mortality of 20 to 40 per cent. Such patients should be hospitalized and treated with a protocol such as is outlined in Table 229–7. I^- is the most effective agent for inhibiting release of preformed thyroid hormone. If it is felt that the patient has a so-called surgical abdomen, intravenous propranolol may be used intraoperatively to control tachycardia, assuming that there are no contraindications. The line between severe hyperthyroidism and thyroid storm is nebulous. In patients with severe symptoms but without fever, I^- should be added to PTU therapy to achieve a more rapid decrease in thyroid hormones. The I^- can be discontinued after one week.

Treatment of Ophthalmopathy. In most patients with ophthalmopathy no specific therapy is needed. Return of the hyperthyroid state to euthyroidism will often result in amelioration of many of the minor symptoms, including stare and

TABLE 229–7. MANAGEMENT OF PATIENTS WITH THYROID STORM

Diagnostic
1. Serum T_3 and T_4 concentrations, THBR
2. Appropriate evaluation for underlying precipitating causes such as infection, acute surgical abdomen, central nervous system lesions, or psychologic trauma
3. Baseline WBC and differential, electrolytes, Ca, P
4. Plasma cortisol

Therapeutic
1. Intravenous fluids—dextrose with or without electrolytes as indicated, multivitamins
2. Propylthiouracil, 400 mg every six hours (by nasogastric tube, if necessary), to inhibit thyroid hormone synthesis and block T_4 to T_3 conversion
3. Sodium iodide, 250 mg every six hours (orally or intravenously)
4. Hydrocortisone, 50 to 100 mg every six hours intravenously
5. External cooling and acetaminophen (300 to 600 mg) every four to six hours for severe hyperpyrexia (do not use salicylates, which increase free thyroid hormones and oxygen consumption)
6. Propranolol—in patients without asthma, chronic bronchitis, or non-arrhythmia-related, congestive heart failure, 10–40 mg may be given every four to six hours orally; a slow intravenous infusion of 1 mg per minute for two to ten minutes with careful monitoring of blood pressure and ECG may be used if oral therapy is not feasible; propranolol may precipitate pulmonary edema in a few patients with hyperthyroidism; reserpine or guanethidine would not appear to have any advantages over propranolol in this situation
7. Oxygen may be helpful
8. Digitalis glycosides should be employed for therapy of congestive failure and for blockade of a rapid ventricular response to an atrial tachyrhythmia
9. Appropriate treatment of precipitating event if any

lid lag. It is important to avoid hypothyroidism, as anecdotal data suggest that this may be associated with an exacerbation of eye symptoms. The patient may note periorbital edema, especially on arising in the morning. An extra pillow or elevation of the head of the bed will relieve this. Alternatively, a diuretic can be administered at bedtime. In patients with more severe symptoms, artificial tears (1 per cent methylcellulose) are prescribed.

A small fraction of patients with Graves' disease will have more severe problems than can be relieved by these minor therapeutic measures. In patients with severe proptosis, desiccation of the sclera or even cornea may occur at night because of lagophthalmos. Taping the lids closed at night may alleviate this symptom, although lateral tarsorrhaphy is a more permanent solution. Diplopia may be treated by prisms or, if permanent, by muscle repositioning or relief of fibrous adhesions. This procedure should not be performed until the eye disease has stabilized, often a matter of two to three years. In the patient with severe inflammation and chemosis (*malignant exophthalmos*), prednisone is required. Although 15 to 20 mg per day may be sufficient, in many patients as much as 100 mg per day is necessary with the attendant complications of treatment. Such patients should have frequent measurements of visual acuity and visual fields. Deterioration of either test is an emergency requiring steroid treatment and ophthalmologic consultation. An alternative treatment is orbital irradiation, 2000 rads being given to the retro-orbital region to suppress local lymphocytic infiltration. This is usually used in conjunction with glucocorticoid administration. In the case of optic compression or persistent corneal ulceration, surgical decompression may be required. Fortunately, in most patients the severity of the eye manifestations will abate after 12 to 18 months, although in many the proptosis will never revert to normal.

Pretibial Myxedema. The lesions of pretibial myxedema are not generally incapacitating but may be cosmetically disfiguring. They may be treated with topical application of glucocorticoids, with enhancement of absorption by occlusive dressings if necessary.

PROGNOSIS. In most patients, Graves' disease is a benign disorder in which the physician can play an important role in providing considerable relief to the patient. Because of the complications of treatment and the possibility of hypothyroidism even in patients with a spontaneous remission, patients with Graves' disease require lifelong observation.

TREATMENT OF OTHER CAUSES OF HYPERTHYROIDISM. The short-term treatment of hyperthyroidism associated with toxic multinodular goiter or toxic adenoma does not differ from that of patients with Graves' disease. These entities are discussed in detail later in the chapter. The hyperthyroidism associated with subacute thyroiditis (particularly the lymphocytic variety) is discussed in the section Thyroiditis.

TSH-secreting pituitary tumor must be treated by surgery or x-ray. Patients with this condition are identified and separated from the group with nontumorigenic TSH-induced hyperthyroidism by finding elevation of the value of the serum alpha-TSH subunit as well as elevation of TSH. Nontumorigenic hypersecretion of TSH is thought to be due to a reduction in feedback sensitivity to T_3 and T_4 at the pituitary level. Such patients are treated with antithyroid drugs. In patients with choriocarcinoma or hydatidiform mole, removal of the tumor will relieve these symptoms. Extremely rare is the ovarian teratoma containing thyroid tissue, *struma ovarii.* This should be treated surgically. In general, thyroid carcinoma does not function well enough to lead to hyperthyroidism. Hyperthyroidism can occur if extensive metastases are present that retain a significant degree of function, as may be seen occasionally in follicular carcinoma. This condition is readily diagnosed and is treated with ^{131}I.

Borst GC, Eil C, Burman KD: Euthyroid hyperthyroxinemia. Ann Intern Med 98:366–378, 1983. *The differential diagnosis in individuals with an elevated serum T₄.*

Burrow GN: The management of thyrotoxicosis in pregnancy. N Engl J Med 313:562, 1985. *A review of factors to be considered when managing the pregnant patient with active Graves' disease.*

Davis PJ, Davis FB: Hyperthyroidism in patients over the age of 60 years. Medicine 53:161, 1974. *An excellent summary of the clinical syndrome of hyperthyroidism in the elderly patient.*

Henneman G, Krenning EP, Sankaranarayanan K: Place of radioactive iodine in treatment of thyrotoxicosis. Lancet 1:1369, 1986. *The author makes a persuasive argument for the use of radioiodine as the first-line treatment for patients with Graves' disease. A brief but thorough review of the pros and cons of this approach to therapy.*

Morley JE, Jacobson RJ, Melamed J, et al.: Choriocarcinoma as a cause of thyrotoxicosis. Am J Med 60:1036, 1976. *Three typical cases of this syndrome are presented with complete thyroid evaluation.*

Silva JE: Effects of iodine and iodine containing compounds on thyroid function. Med Clin North Am 69:881, 1985. *The author reviews all aspects of iodine excess and deficiency. The discussion of iodide-induced hyperthyroidism is particularly relevant for this section.*

Wall JR, Kuroki T: Immunologic factors in thyroid disease. Med Clin North Am 69:913, 1985. *A discussion of the immunopathology in patients with Graves' disease and Hashimoto's thyroiditis.*

Weintraub BD, Gershengorn MC, Kourides IA, et al.: Inappropriate secretion of thyroid-stimulating hormone. Ann Intern Med 95:339, 1981. *A review of the pathophysiology, diagnosis and treatment of TSH-induced hyperthyroidism.*

HYPOTHYROIDISM AND MYXEDEMA

DEFINITION. *Hypothyroidism* is the clinical syndrome that results from a deficiency of thyroid hormone. In severe hypothyroidism a hydrophilic mucopolysaccharide substance accumulates in subcutaneous tissues, causing a nonpitting edema referred to as *myxedema*. Some authorities use the terms *hypothyroidism* and *myxedema* interchangeably, whereas others reserve the latter term for the severe form of this syndrome.

ETIOLOGY. A list of causes to be considered in patients with hypothyroidism is given in Table 229–8. *Primary hypothyroidism*, that caused by thyroid gland malfunction, accounts for over 95 per cent of such cases, of which Hashimoto's thyroiditis, idiopathic myxedema (probably a variant of Hashimoto's thyroiditis), and thyroid destruction resulting from ¹³¹I therapy or surgery for hyperthyroidism account for the

TABLE 229–8. CAUSES OF HYPOTHYROIDISM

I. **Primary hypothyroidism**
  A. Acquired
    1. Destructive lesions
      a. Hashimoto's thyroiditis
      b. Idiopathic myxedema (probably the end-stage of Hashimoto's thyroiditis)
      c. ¹³¹I therapy for hyperthyroidism
      d. Subtotal thyroidectomy, especially for Graves' disease
      e. Therapeutic external x-ray treatment to the neck for other diseases
      f. After subacute thyroiditis (may be transient)
      g. Cystinosis
    2. Impaired function of a normal or near-normal gland
      a. Endemic goiter—iodine deficiency or naturally occurring goitrogens
      b. Iodine excess (>6 mg per day) in patients with underlying thyroid disease
      c. Drug-induced: lithium carbonate, para-aminosalicylic acid, thiourea drugs, sulfonamides, phenylbutazone, and others
  B. Congenital
    1. Defects in enzymes required for thyroid hormone synthesis (congenital goiter)
    2. Thyroid agenesis
    3. Thyroid dysgenesis or ectopy
    4. Maternal iodide or antithyroid drugs
II. **Secondary hypothyroidism**
  A. Hypothalamic dysfunction
    1. Neoplasms
    2. Eosinophilic granuloma
    3. Therapeutic irradiation
  B. Pituitary dysfunction
    1. Neoplasms
    2. Pituitary surgery or irradiation
    3. Idiopathic hypopituitarism
    4. Sheehan's syndrome (postpartum pituitary necrosis)
    5. Dopamine infusion and/or severe illness(?)
III. **Tissue resistance to thyroid hormone**

greatest proportion. Hashimoto's and subacute thyroiditis are discussed in the next section. Hypothyroidism after therapeutic irradiation to the thyroid area for lymphoma or Hodgkin's disease is found in 10 to 30 per cent of these patients, usually within one to two years of treatment.

Hypothyroidism can also occur with normal or near-normal thyroid tissue when there is a superimposed stress on thyroid hormone synthesis. Hypothyroidism may be caused either by severe iodine deficiency (<25 μg iodine per day) or by naturally occurring goitrogens such as have been found in Colombia or are generated by eating the cassava plant in Africa (see Sporadic Goiter and Endemic Goiter). In patients with Graves' disease, especially after RAI treatment, or in those with mild Hashimoto's thyroiditis, iodine excess may cause hypothyroidism through the Wolff-Chaikoff effect (I⁻-induced inhibition of organification). These glands are unable to reduce I⁻ uptake in the presence of an elevated plasma I⁻ as normally occurs. The drugs listed in Table 229–8 inhibit organification of thyroidal I⁻. In most cases the hypothyroidism associated with these drugs is mild.

Screening of newborns for hypothyroidism is now widely practiced, and the incidence of this condition is about 1 in 4000 births. About 65 per cent of infants with congenital hypothyroidism in North America have thyroid agenesis or hypoplasia, 25 per cent have ectopic thyroid glands, and about 10 per cent have defects in one of the steps required for thyroid hormone synthesis (see Sporadic Goiter and Endemic Goiter).

Secondary hypothyroidism occurs as a result of hypothalamic or pituitary dysfunction. Dopamine infusion and/or severe illness may suppress TSH release sufficiently to cause a modest, transient hypothyroidism. A rare cause of hypothyroidism is tissue resistance to thyroid hormones, which may be due to an abnormality in the nuclear receptor for these hormones.

INCIDENCE. Hypothyroidism is common in adults. In one epidemiologic survey, 1.4 per cent of adult females and about 0.1 per cent of adult males were affected. Autoimmune destruction of the thyroid gland is the most common cause of thyroid gland failure in adults. This generally affects women over the age of 40, but can occur at any age. Hypothyroidism is also a common congenital disease, occurring in about 1 of 4000 neonates in North America and Western Europe and more frequently in areas of iodine deficiency.

PATHOLOGY. The pathology of the thyroid gland in hypothyroidism depends on the etiology of the syndrome. In "idiopathic myxedema," the thyroid tissue is generally replaced by fat with few intact follicles and lymphocytic infiltration (see also Thyroiditis). When the thyroid cells remain partly functional, the elevated serum TSH leads to hyperplasia and hypertrophy. In secondary hypothyroidism, the number of follicular cells is low and considerable colloid is present. The gland is small in contrast to the goiter found when thyroid cell dysfunction is present and TSH secretion is increased.

The nonthyroidal pathology of the hypothyroid state is the same regardless of its etiology. The longer the duration and the more severe the deficiency, the greater are the changes. The accumulation of mucopolysaccharide in connective tissues has already been mentioned. This material may also appear in muscle. Effusions, which often have a high protein content, occur in various serous cavities.

CLINICAL MANIFESTATIONS. The common clinical manifestations of this syndrome in the adult are summarized in Table 229–9. These symptoms and signs can be attributed to either deceleration of cellular metabolic processes or the accumulation of the hygroscopic mucopolysaccharide in the vocal cords or oropharynx, as well as the more obvious changes in the subcutaneous tissues. The symptoms are nonspecific, particularly in the early phases, and may either pass unnoticed by the patient or be attributed to advancing

TABLE 229–9. COMMON SYMPTOMS OF HYPOTHYROIDISM

Weakness, fatigue, lethargy
Dry, coarse skin
Swelling of the hands, face, and extremities
Cold intolerance, decreased sweating
Coarsening or huskiness of the voice
Modest weight gain (~10 lbs) with anorexia
Decreased memory, hearing impairment
Arthralgia, paresthesias
Constipation
Muscle cramps

age. Characteristically, the patient becomes aware of their multiplicity and severity only after thyroid hormone replacement leads to a return of normal function. This is particularly true of younger patients. In the elderly, hearing impairment, somnolence, and decreased memory and ability to calculate may occur. These may lead to an apparent psychologic withdrawal and paranoia at times requiring hospitalization. The term *myxedema madness* has been used to describe this syndrome, which can be mistaken for cerebrovascular insufficiency or senile dementia. Alternatively, the patient may confabulate or respond with humorous non sequiturs to draw the interviewer's attention from his or her limited recall of recent events. This behavior has been termed *myxedema wit*. A variety of menstrual disorders may be present, although menorrhagia is said to be the most common pattern. Pregnancy may occur in patients with hypothyroidism, and the increased hormone requirements of that condition may cause a previously borderline functioning thyroid to decompensate. Despite the developmental abnormalities associated with congenital hypothyroidism, the symptoms of hypothyroidism in infants are few. Severe thyroid hormone deficiency is associated with growth retardation in the older infant and child. In the adolescent, thyroid enlargement, *adolescent goiter*, may be the only manifestation and is usually seen in the pubertal female. In some patients in whom the hypothyroidism is of rapid onset, cramps in large muscle groups may be a prominent symptom. Such symptoms usually occur after a rapid change from a hyperthyroid to a hypothyroid state, such as after surgery for Graves' disease, a second RAI treatment for hyperthyroidism, or even vigorous antithyroid drug therapy.

Many of the common signs of hypothyroidism are the opposite of those seen in the hyperthyroid patient. Bradycardia is common and is sometimes associated with hypothermia. Systolic pressure is generally reduced and diastolic pressure increased, the latter resulting from increased peripheral vascular resistance. Myxedema is manifested by a puffy, nonpitting swelling of the subcutaneous tissue, which may particularly collect in the periorbital area. Body and scalp hair are reduced; the skin may be coarse, the texture of sandpaper, and is usually cool and sallow. The yellow complexion is due to the accumulation of carotene in the serum in patients with significant hypothyroidism. The thyroid may be enlarged, of normal size, or not palpable, depending on the cause. The heart sounds are distant, and the heart shadow is often enlarged. The latter can be a manifestation of pericardial effusion, which is common but rarely leads to tamponade. In addition to the cortical dysfunction previously mentioned, cerebellar ataxia may be present. Other neurologic signs, including delayed relaxation of the deep tendon reflexes, peripheral neuropathy, and carpal tunnel syndrome, can completely resolve with treatment.

Certain physiologic abnormalities are characteristic of hypothyroidism. Cardiac output is reduced, although not out of proportion to the decrease in O_2 consumption. Glomerular filtration is also subnormal, leading to an impairment of the capacity to excrete free water. In addition inappropriate ADH secretion may lead to hyponatremia. Gastrointestinal motility is reduced, and occasionally the patient may develop an apparent obstruction, *myxedema megacolon*. There are important abnormalities in the respiratory center. The sensitivity to both hypercarbia and hypoxia is reduced, and such patients may readily develop CO_2 narcosis or cardiac arrhythmias associated with hypoxia. This is one of the chief causes of death in the severe form of myxedema, *myxedema coma*. Pituitary function is impaired in severe hypothyroidism even of the primary variety. Hypoglycemic stress does not elicit normal growth hormone or cortisol responses in such patients, so that testing pituitary function must be delayed until the hypothyroid state has been corrected. Serum prolactin is increased in moderate to severe primary hypothyroidism, and this may lead to galactorrhea in a small percentage of patients.

LABORATORY DIAGNOSIS. The diagnosis of hypothyroidism can be easily confirmed by using the scheme outlined in Figures 229–4 and 229–8. When the diagnosis is not made, it is usually because the nonspecificity of signs and symptoms does not immediately suggest this cause. This disease is one of the "great imitators," and a high index of suspicion should be maintained, as the condition is so readily diagnosed and treated. In all patients with hypothyroidism, the free T_4 index will be reduced. Serum T_3 concentrations are often in the normal range in hypothyroid patients, and this test is not useful in the diagnosis of this condition. It is unlikely that significant symptoms will be present in patients with an equivocal reduction in this hormone. Once a reduced free T_4 index has been found, it is imperative to determine whether the cause of the disease is primary, i.e., owing to thyroid disease, or secondary, involving the hypothalamic-pituitary axis. An increase in serum TSH establishes the diagnosis of primary hypothyroidism. If the serum TSH concentration is normal or borderline, then the diagnosis of pituitary or hypothalamic hypothyroidism is made, and further steps are taken to evaluate the possibility of a deficiency of other pituitary hormones. It is extremely important that this be done prior to the onset of therapy, since thyroid replacement will exacerbate mild ACTH insufficiency associated with hypothalamic or pituitary disease. *If unrecognized, such patients may have an Addisonian crisis provoked by thyroid hormone replacement.* There are two circumstances in which primary hypothyroidism is not associated with TSH elevation. This may be the case when hypothyroidism follows shortly after a period of hyperthyroidism, since the latter causes suppression of pituitary TSH synthesis lasting four to five weeks. Dopamine infusion may also cause suppression of an elevated TSH concentration into the normal range.

In the patient whose symptoms are nonspecific or borderline and in whom an equivocally reduced free T_4 index is obtained, the serum TSH may be significantly elevated. Elevated serum TSH is the most sensitive index of impairment of thyroid gland function. Whether or not such patients are actually metabolically hypothyroid cannot be determined by using present tests. This condition has been called *subclinical hypothyroidism*.

There are a few clinical situations in which the free T_4 index is reduced but serum TSH is not elevated in the absence of hypothalamic or pituitary disease. This may occur in severely ill patients without thyroid disease, but who presumably have transient hypothalamic-pituitary hypothyroidism. In such patients, a serum cortisol determination is indicated to eliminate the possibility of ACTH deficiency. If clinically indicated, therapy can then be initiated with both thyroxine and glucocorticoid. Patients receiving 2 to 3 grams per day of salicylate or 300 mg per day of phenytoin may have a reduction in the free T_4 index without hypothyroidism (see Table 229–3), and also patients ingesting replacement quantities (25 µg or more) of triiodothyronine (Cytomel) will have reduced serum T_4 due to suppression of TSH, even if the thyroid gland is normal. A 24-hour RAI uptake test may not separate hypothyroidism from the euthyroid state and is not useful in diagnosis.

Other Biochemical Abnormalities and Associated Diseases in Patients with Hypothyroidism. Serum cholesterol and triglycerides, creatine phosphokinase (MM isozyme), aldo-

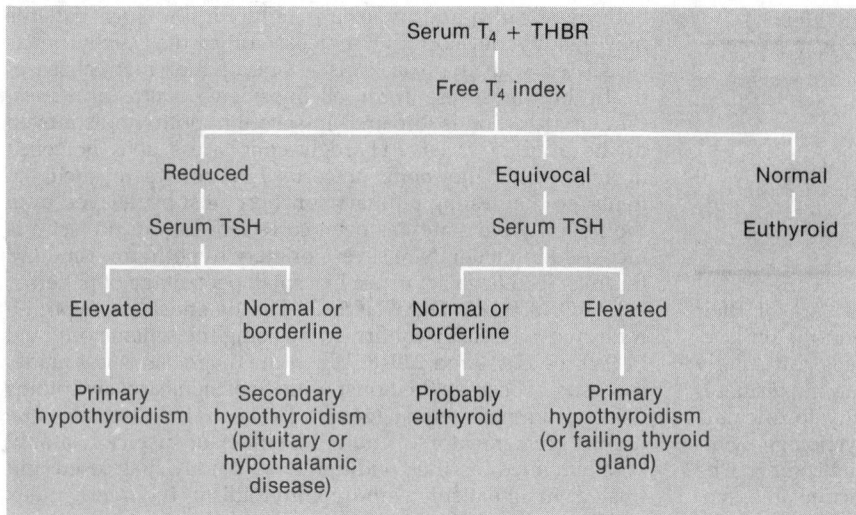

FIGURE 229—8. Laboratory diagnosis of hypothyroidism. THBR refers to the thyroid hormone binding ratio (formerly termed T_3 or T_4 uptake).

lase, lactic dehydrogenase, and SGOT may all be elevated in the patient with moderate to severe hypothyroidism. Hyponatremia with or without the inappropriate ADH syndrome is seen. There is often a modest anemia of chronic disease that may be macrocytic. Serum vitamin B_{12} should be measured in these patients because of the 3 to 6 per cent coexistence of pernicious anemia with Hashimoto's thyroiditis. Other conditions found with increased frequency in patients with autoimmune thyroid disease include idiopathic adrenocortical deficiency, diabetes mellitus, hypoparathyroidism, myasthenia gravis, vitiligo (Ch. 241), and mitral valve prolapse.

DIFFERENTIAL DIAGNOSIS. There are few conditions that can masquerade as hypothyroidism in its classic form. However, patients with nephrotic syndrome or hypoalbuminemia and associated peripheral edema may be suspected of this diagnosis. Although the serum T_4 in these conditions is reduced because of hypoproteinemia, the THBR is generally quite elevated with a consequent normal free T_4 index. Patients with chronic renal disease may have symptoms entirely similar to those of hypothyroidism (including hypothermia), and laboratory tests are required to evaluate the possible coexistence of these two diseases. In patients with spontaneous primary hypothyroidism, the tests for autoantibodies to either thyroglobulin or microsomal components of the thyroid cell are generally positive. This is true even if the typical thyroid enlargement of Hashimoto's thyroiditis is not present. The other causes of hypothyroidism have already been discussed (Table 229–8), and reversible causes should be eliminated.

THERAPY. Hypothyroidism is a readily treatable disease. The preparations available for thyroid replacement are listed in Table 229–10. Levothyroxine is most frequently used as replacement therapy, since it provides stable and easily measureable serum concentrations for use in monitoring therapy and allows physiological regulation of extrathyroidal T_3 production. Ideally, both serum T_3 and T_4 concentrations should be normalized for satisfactory replacement. Since in the euthyroid individual, 20 per cent of T_3 is derived directly from the thyroid gland (Table 229–2), one would predict that normalization of serum T_3 in hypothyroid individuals would be associated with a serum free T_4 index that is about 60 per

cent above the euthyroid value. Because intrapituitary T_3 is derived independently from both serum T_4 *and* serum T_3, this could well result in a subnormal TSH-IMA. At present the data are too incomplete to allow an informed decision whether serum T_3 or serum TSH concentrations should be normalized, assuming that both goals could not be achieved simultaneously. It is recognized that excessive thyroid hormone replacement may be deleterious to cardiac function and to bone mineralization. At present, I use a combination of clinical evaluation and the TSH-IMA test as the guidelines for adequate replacement, although serum T_3 is measured periodically. The dose of levothyroxine required to achieve symptomatic and biochemical replacement in most patients is about 1.8 μg T_4 per kilogram (about 0.8 μg T_4 per pound). This is a significantly lower requirement than previously used because of improvements in tablet formulation. In most female patients a dose of 100 μg is quite adequate. The difference between this amount and the T_4 production rate of 1.1 μg per kilogram per day is due to the incomplete absorption of orally administered levothyroxine. In patients who become hypothyroid after ^{131}I treatment for Graves' disease, the requirement may be lower because of residual, nonsuppressible T_4 or T_3 secretion.

In patients who are in good health otherwise or whose hypothyroidism is very modest, therapy can be initiated with half-replacement doses immediately on establishment of the diagnosis. This can be increased to full replacement after one month. In patients with more severe hypothyroidism, elderly patients, or those with a history of cardiovascular disease, I prefer to begin therapy with smaller amounts (25 μg of thyroxine per day) and to increase these by 25-μg increments at four-week intervals (with due attention to symptoms) until a replacement dose is achieved. In patients with primary hypothyroidism there may rarely be associated primary autoimmune hypoadrenalism *(Schmidt's syndrome)*. Such patients will require adequate replacement of glucocorticoid prior to institution of thyroid hormone replacement. A similar procedure must be employed in patients in whom hypothalamic-pituitary disease is a cause of hypothyroidism.

Long-term monitoring of thyroid hormone replacement should include annual measurements of the serum free T_4

TABLE 229–10. HORMONE CONTENT OF THYROID REPLACEMENT PREPARATIONS
(AMOUNTS APPROXIMATELY EQUIVALENT TO 1 GRAIN (65 mg) DESICCATED THYROID)

| | Levothyroxine | Liotrix | | Desiccated Thyroid (1-Grain Tablets) | | Levotriiodothyronine |
		Euthroid-1	Thyrolar-1	Armour	Proloid	
T_4 (μg)	100	60	50	63	55	0
T_3 (μg)	0	15	12.5	12	16	25

index, TSH, and serum T_3. The replacement dose of T_4 may be 20 to 40 per cent lower in elderly patients.

Special Problems in Hypothyroid Patients. The patient who presents simultaneously with angina and hypothyroidism poses a serious therapeutic problem. In some patients with coronary artery disease, reintroduction of thyroid hormones results in increased myocardial oxygen demands without an adequate increase in myocardial blood flow. A trial of propranolol with small increments of thyroxine may reduce myocardial oxygen consumption without decreasing the pulse rate to unacceptably low levels. If an exacerbation of angina occurs during thyroxine therapy, T_4 to T_3 conversion may be acutely reduced in peripheral tissues with propylthiouracil (see Graves' Disease and Other Causes of Hyperthyroidism). In patients with localized coronary artery disease in whom bypass graft surgery is indicated, the frequent adverse effects of thyroxine replacement have raised the possibility that surgery should be performed prior to thyroid hormone replacement. The overall morbidity may be lower in patients operated on in the hypothyroid state than in patients in whom replacement is attempted prior to surgery.

While theoretical considerations suggest that hypothyroidism would impair the physiologic response to surgical stress, patients with mild to moderate hypothyroidism do not appear to have more perioperative complications with major surgery than do euthyroid patients, at least as assessed in retrospective studies. While elective surgery should not be performed in the untreated hypothyroid patient, a moderate degree of hypothyroidism does not preclude carefully managed emergency procedures.

Patients with subclinical hypothyroidism (low-normal free T_4 index and TSH >10 μU per milliliter) may benefit from therapy even though their symptoms are not obvious. This biochemical pattern together with a small goiter and positive antithyroid microsomal antibodies indicates the presence of Hashimoto's thyroiditis (see below), and it is my practice to treat such patients to prevent further thyroid enlargement.

Treatment of Myxedema Coma. In severe myxedema the patient may lapse into coma. This serious complication (mortality, 20 to 50 per cent) occurs most commonly in patients with severe hypothyroidism who are subjected to an additional physiologic stress. This may occur spontaneously, following cold exposure, or during infection, but in all too many instances it is iatrogenic. The administration of sedatives to hypothyroid patients may precipitate coma, as drugs are not metabolized as rapidly in these patients. The reduced sensitivity of the respiratory center to changes in blood gases may lead to inappropriately small ventilatory responses. In other situations, surgery may be performed in a patient who is not recognized to be severely hypothyroid, and postoperative opiates or sedatives lead to clinical deterioration. In Table 229–11 are shown the important steps in management of patients with myxedema coma. In these emergent situations

TABLE 229–11. MANAGEMENT OF PATIENTS WITH MYXEDEMA COMA

Diagnostic
1. Serum T_4, T_3 uptake, THBR
2. CBC, glucose, electrolytes, blood gases, BUN, creatinine, CPK
3. Plasma cortisol before and 30 and 60 minutes after Cortrosyn, 0.25 mg, intravenous bolus
4. Careful evaluation for concomitant disease; continuous ECG and temperature monitoring

Therapeutic
1. Levothyroxine, 2 μg per kilogram intravenously over five to ten minutes initially, and 100 μg intravenously every 24 hours thereafter
2. Cover to conserve body heat; do not rewarm externally
3. Tracheal intubation and mechanical ventilation as required
4. Intravenous fluids as determined by initial blood glucose and electrolytes and by the state of hydration; watch for water retention
5. Hydrocortisone, 100 mg by intravenous bolus, then 25 mg every six hours as a continuous intravenous drip
6. Vigorous treatment of associated and precipitating conditions such as infection

it is important to institute treatment immediately. If the serum free T_4 index is reduced, treatment is begun even if the cause of the hypothyroidism (primary versus secondary) has not been identified. Accordingly, testing for adrenal function is carried out immediately, followed by institution of glucocorticoid replacement. Because of the irregularities of either intramuscular or gastrointestinal absorption in hypothyroidism, medications should be given intravenously. Glucocorticoid replacement should not be given in pharmacologic quantities, since this will impair T_4 to T_3 conversion.

PROGNOSIS. The prognosis of hypothyroidism is excellent, provided that thyroid hormone replacement is maintained at an appropriate level.

Withdrawal of Thyroid Hormone After Prolonged Replacement. The question sometimes arises whether thyroid hormone therapy is indicated in a patient already receiving it. If, based on the history, the physician is skeptical of the need for replacement, such a patient is instructed to discontinue the medication completely and return for serum free T_4 index and TSH determinations in three weeks. The patient is advised that there may be mild manifestations of low thyroid function and to notify the physician sooner if these become severe. Three weeks after cessation of treatment, a patient with normal thyroid function will have a low normal serum free T_4 index, but the serum TSH will not be elevated. If this correlates with the clinical symptomatology, the patient is instructed to return after a further three-week interval for repeat testing. The results after six weeks can be used as a reliable index of the underlying thyroid functional capacity. If the free T_4 index and TSH are normal at that time, one can exclude the diagnosis of significant hypothyroidism.

Gow SM, Caldwell G, Toft AD, et al.: Relationship between pituitary and other target organ responsiveness in hypothyroid patients receiving thyroxine replacement. J Clin Endocrinol Metab 64:364, 1987. *A correlation of serum TSH-IMA and thyroid hormones with various other markers of thyroid status in hypothyroid patients receiving levothyroxine.*

Hennessey JV, Evaul JE, Tseng Y-C, et al.: L-Thyroxine dosage: A reevaluation of therapy with contemporary preparations. Ann Intern Med 105:11, 1986. *Evidence supporting lowered dose requirements when using the reformulated levothyroxine preparation, Synthroid.*

Rees-Jones RW, Rolla AR, Larsen PR: Hormonal content of thyroid replacement preparations. JAMA 243:459, 1980. *Analyses of desiccated thyroid tablets show that some generic preparations have reduced quantities of T_4 and T_3 relative to those contained in brand-name products.*

Refetoff S: Syndromes of thyroid hormone resistance. Am J Physiol 243 (Endocrinol Metab 6:88, 1982. *A review of the various ways in which thyroid hormone resistance may present and of the pathophysiology of these disorders.*

Weinberg AD, Brennan MD, Gorman CA, et al.: Outcome of anesthesia and surgery in hypothyroid patients. Arch Intern Med 143:893, 1983. *Results of this experience at the Mayo Clinic suggest that patients with mild to moderate primary hypothyroidism withstand nonelective general surgery as well as do euthyroid patients.*

THYROIDITIS

Thyroiditis is classified into three types: acute, subacute, and chronic. Despite the common factor of inflammation in all of these entities, there are marked differences in their clinical presentations and etiology.

Acute Thyroiditis

Acute thyroiditis results from a bacterial infection of the thyroid gland with typical symptoms of such involvement, including a fever, local tenderness, and swelling. This condition is quite rare. The infection may involve the whole gland or only a portion of it. Laboratory studies generally show normal thyroid function, but there is an elevated leukocyte count with a polymorphonuclear predominance. The thyroid scan may show an area of decreased uptake corresponding to the involved portion, but the 24-hour RAI uptake is usually normal. Treatment of this condition requires proper identification of the causative agent and appropriate antimicrobial drugs. This may require a needle aspiration. If localized abscess formation occurs, the abscess should be drained. The process usually responds rapidly to these measures.

Subacute (Nonsuppurative) Thyroiditis

This condition is also referred to as *giant cell thyroiditis*, *granulomatous thyroiditis*, or *de Quervain's thyroiditis*. In the classic form of this disease the patient presents with an exquisitely tender thyroid, which is pathologically characterized by follicular cell destruction and by a lymphocytic and polymorphonuclear leukocyte infiltration, together with multinucleate giant cells. In recent years, a different type of subacute thyroiditis has appeared, which is often painless and associated with hyperthyroidism. It shares some pathologic features with Hashimoto's thyroiditis (see below). This condition, which will be denoted *subacute lymphocytic thyroiditis*, is discussed separately below because of its unique features. The disease described by de Quervain will be referred to as *subacute granulomatous thyroiditis*.

INCIDENCE. The incidence of subacute granulomatous thyroiditis is not known, but it is not rare. It is most common in the third to fifth decades, and females are affected about three to four times more commonly than males. It occurs with increased frequency in HLA-B35–positive individuals.

ETIOLOGY. The granulomatous form of subacute thyroiditis often follows a viral infection by several weeks. At the time of the acute illness, elevated titers of antibody to influenza virus, coxsackievirus, or adenovirus can be found. Over the next few months these fall in many patients, suggesting that an acute infection has recently occurred. In only two cases has a virus been cultured from thyroid tissue, which in both cases was mumps. Some authorities interpret the thyroiditis as being a consequence of a process set in motion by the viral illness but not representing a direct infection of the gland. The precise etiology is unknown.

PATHOLOGY. The classic pathologic picture includes the cellular infiltrate described above, along with severe destruction of the normal follicular architecture. Fibrosis appears in the latter phases. Despite the extensive destruction, complete restoration of the normal thyroid structure generally occurs.

CLINICAL MANIFESTATIONS. Subacute granulomatous thyroiditis is characterized by an often exquisitely painful two- to three-fold enlargement of the thyroid gland together with systemic symptoms, including fever, chills, and malaise. Patients often complain of neck or ear pain or dysphagia and may have had evaluation for pharyngeal infection. Symptoms of hyperthyroidism may also be present. The patient may report a prior viral illness. If symptoms of hyperthyroidism are present, they are generally of very short duration (less than two months) and are due to the release of thyroid hormones resulting from thyroid destruction. Physical examination may show fever, tachycardia, and exquisite tenderness of the slightly enlarged thyroid gland. This generally involves the whole gland but may be asymmetric.

DIAGNOSIS. The leukocyte count is mildly elevated, but there is characteristically a marked elevation of the erythrocyte sedimentation rate (ESR). This has been one of the hallmarks of this disease. The free T_4 index may be normal or increased. As would be expected from the pathology, the RAI uptake is low and the thyroid is poorly visualized on scan. The RAI uptake is the principal test for separating patients with this disease from those with hyperthyroidism resulting from Graves' disease. There may be an asymmetric involvement of the thyroid with decreased function in that area. Antimicrosomal and antithyroglobulin antibodies are absent or low in titer, although the serum thyroglobulin may be increased, reflecting the destructive process.

TREATMENT. Since this is a self-limited disease, treatment is symptomatic. Mild analgesics such as aspirin (2 to 4 grams per day) should be given for neck discomfort. In a significant fraction of patients, this will not be sufficient, and prednisone, 20 to 40 mg per day, is required. The immediate relief associated with this therapy is almost diagnostic. The glucocorticoid should be continued for two to three weeks and then tapered over the next three weeks. There may be an exacerbation of the original symptoms during discontinuation of glucocorticoid requiring reinstitution of this therapy. Eventually this will not occur. The hyperthyroidism is usually mild but may require propranolol. Antithyroid drugs are of no use, as the serum T_4 and T_3 will decrease when the glandular supply is exhausted.

There may be transient hypothyroidism following subacute granulomatous thyroiditis, and this may be severe enough to require treatment in some patients. Therefore it is important for these patients to be followed closely during the recovery period to ascertain whether or not this complication has occurred. Replacement thyroxine can be discontinued after three to six months with appropriate biochemical monitoring to establish that thyroid function has returned to normal. In 5 to 10 per cent of patients, permanent hypothyroidism supervenes. Occasionally a patient will be seen initially in the hypothyroid phase of this illness. An elevation in serum TSH and low thyroid hormones in the absence of antimicrosomal or antithyroglobulin antibodies should alert the physician to this possibility.

Subacute Lymphocytic Thyroiditis

This disease has been referred to by a variety of descriptive terms, including *painless thyroiditis, lymphocytic thyroiditis, lymphocytic thyroiditis with spontaneously resolving hyperthyroidism, hyperthyroiditis,* and *atypical subacute thyroiditis*. This confused nomenclature reflects the principal clinical and pathologic features of the disease: hyperthyroidism that is self-limited and lymphocytic infiltration of the thyroid.

ETIOLOGY. The etiology of the disease is unknown. There is little suggestion of a prior viral illness in these patients. The pathologic features are much closer to those of Hashimoto's disease than to those of granulomatous thyroiditis, suggesting an autoimmune etiology.

INCIDENCE. The precise incidence is not known, but one suspects that it has been increasing over the last five to ten years. This condition may account for 5 to 20 per cent of patients with hyperthyroidism. About two thirds of reported cases are in women, with patients ranging from 13 to over 80 years of age.

PATHOLOGY. Lymphocytic infiltration is the common feature in all specimens studied. Destruction of follicular architecture and fibrosis similar to that of subacute granulomatous thyroiditis is seen, but foreign body giant cells are rare. Germinal centers characteristic of Hashimoto's disease are rarely seen.

CLINICAL MANIFESTATIONS. The principal symptoms of this form of subacute thyroiditis are those of hyperthyroidism, as described in the section Graves' Disease and Other Causes of Hyperthyroidism. Nonthyroidal stigmata of Graves' disease, exophthalmos and pretibial myxedema, are not present, although a stare and widened palpebral fissure may occur as a consequence of the hyperthyroidism per se. The duration of the hyperthyroid phase is short (usually less than three months), and it is generally modest in severity. Physical signs include those typical of hyperthyroidism and a normal or slightly enlarged thyroid gland which is not tender. The gland may be firm.

The natural history of thyroid function in a patient who had a typical episode of this disease is presented in Figure 229–9. The acute phase of hyperthyroidism resolved rapidly and spontaneously and was followed by a period of transient hypothyroidism requiring treatment. This was discontinued after three months, and after an initial period of thyroidal resistance to TSH, normal function returned. A phase of significant hypothyroidism such as this follows the hyperthyroidism in about one third of patients. For obscure reasons, this form of thyroiditis occurs with increased frequency in the first few months post partum.

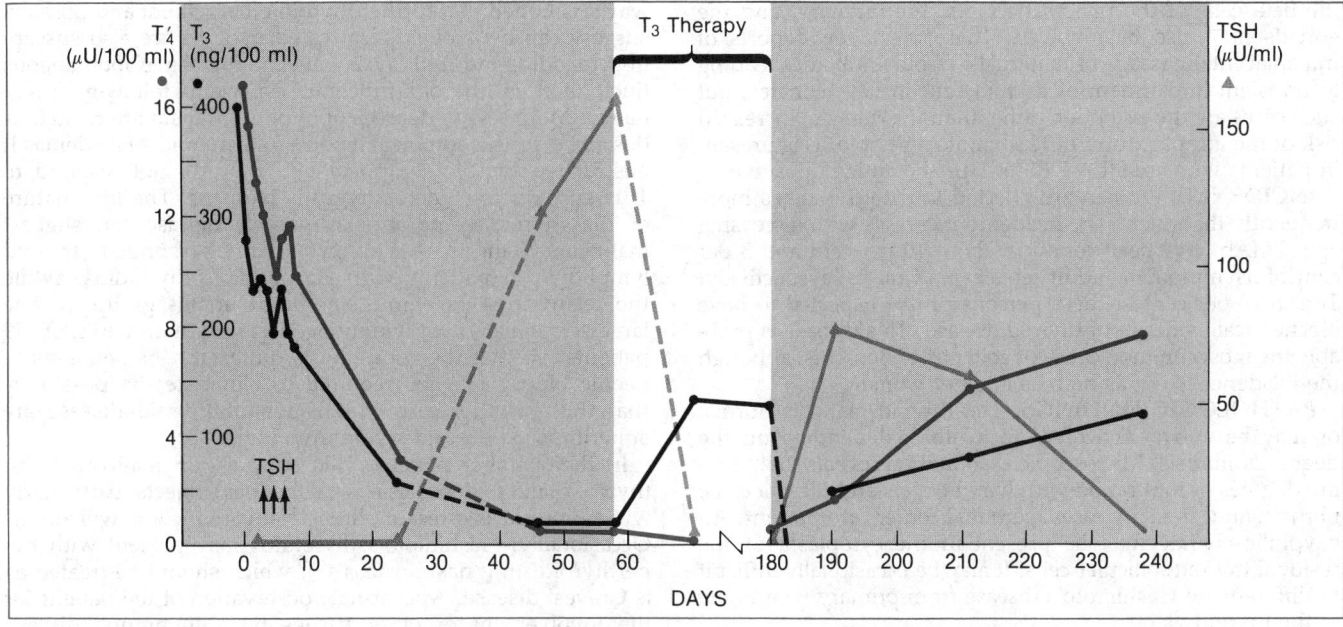

FIGURE 229–9. Changes in serum T$_3$, T$_4$, and TSH in a patient with subacute lymphocytic thyroiditis. The rapid decrease in serum T$_3$ and T$_4$ in the first five days is due to exhaustion of thyroidal stores as a consequence of the destructive process. Transient T$_3$ replacement was employed because of prolonged hypothyroidism. Normal thyroid function had returned by eight months after the initial episode. (From Larsen PR: Metabolism 23:467, 1974.)

LABORATORY DIAGNOSIS. Serum T$_4$ and T$_3$ concentrations are generally elevated, the leukocyte count normal, and the ESR normal or only slightly elevated (<50 mm at 1 hour, Westergren). This is in marked contrast to the results in the granulomatous form of the disease. The 24-hour RAI uptake is reduced and will not increase even after TSH injection. Serum thyroglobulin is increased in the acute phase of the disease, and the titers of TMAb and TgAb may be low or elevated, depending on the clinical pattern. In postpartum thyroiditis, these antibody titers are elevated, and the condition appears to be associated with underlying Hashimoto's thyroiditis. In such patients, repeated episodes of hyperthyroidism followed by transient hypothyroidism should be anticipated with each pregnancy.

This disease must be separated from other causes of hyperthyroidism, notably Graves' disease. The best test for this is the 24-hour RAI uptake. A low uptake may occasionally also be observed in a patient with Graves' disease who has received excess iodide. This may be obvious from the history or can be eliminated by measuring the urinary iodide, which must be considerably elevated (>2 mg per 24 hours) to suppress the uptake in hyperthyroidism associated with thyroid hyperfunction. A needle biopsy will also be diagnostic. To distinguish this condition from factitious hyperthyroidism, 10 units of bovine TSH can be injected, followed in one day by a 24-hour RAI uptake. No change in the uptake is found in patients with subacute lymphocytic thyroiditis.

TREATMENT. As with subacute granulomatous thyroiditis, treatment is symptomatic. Beta-adrenergic blockade may be required for the hyperthyroid phase, but propylthiouracil is of no value except to inhibit T$_4$ to T$_3$ conversion. Glucocorticoid is not required since there is no tenderness, but more rapid resolution of the hyperthyroidism has been reported in patients given a four-week course of prednisone starting at 40 mg per day. A hypothyroid phase should be treated for three to six months, followed by withdrawal of the therapy.

PROGNOSIS. The hyperthyroid phase usually remits within a few months, and the entire history of this disease lasts less than a year. However, the potential for subsequent hypothyroidism indicates the need for annual examination of thyroid function in these patients.

CHRONIC THYROIDITIS

There are two types of chronic thyroiditis: Hashimoto's and Riedel's thyroiditis (*Riedel's struma*).

Hashimoto's Thyroiditis

This is an apparently autoimmune disease of the thyroid gland. It appears to be closely related to Graves' disease. Synonyms for this condition are *chronic lymphocytic thyroiditis* and *lymphadenoid goiter*.

ETIOLOGY. The sera of patients with this condition contain antibodies to one or more thyroid antigens, including thyroid peroxidase (antithyroid microsomal antibodies), thyroglobulin, or a colloid antigen that can be separated from thyroglobulin. At present it is not certain whether these antibodies are the cause or the result of this disease. The pathologic features of the condition can be reproduced in laboratory animals by immunization with thyroid tissue. However, the experimental disease is not sustained once immunizations have been discontinued, nor can the injury be induced by serum from immunized animals. Since the disease can be transferred by sensitized lymphocytes, it has been proposed that the destruction is produced by cell-mediated processes. On exposure to thyroid tissue antigens in vitro, lymphocytes of patients with Hashimoto's thyroiditis (and Graves' disease) will produce substances causing inhibition of leukocyte migration. This response is not found in patients with other forms of thyroid disease or by exposure to extracts of other tissues. Similar observations have been made in patients with idiopathic myxedema, suggesting that the atrophic thyroid found in this condition is affected by a similar process. Other evidence supporting the autoimmune hypothesis is the increased prevalence of many of the so-called autoimmune diseases in patients with Hashimoto's thyroiditis. These include Sjögren's syndrome, lupus erythematosus, idiopathic thrombocytopenic purpura, and pernicious anemia. As many as 6 per cent of patients with Hashimoto's disease have been reported to have pernicious anemia. Although rare, involvement of endocrine glands by this immunopathologic process may occur. Idiopathic Addison's disease and Hashimoto's disease may appear in the same patients. This combination is called Schmidt's syndrome (see Ch. 241). The parathyroids, the beta cells of the pancreatic islets, the pituitary, and the gonads may also be involved. There are a few reports of transplacental passage of maternal thyroid antibodies leading to transient impairment of thyroid function in neonates, but such cases are the exception rather than the rule. An increased risk of the atrophic form of Hashimoto's thyroiditis is present in patients who are HLA-DR3 or HLA-B8 antigen positive.

INCIDENCE. Women are affected four to five times more frequently than men. The incidence increases with increasing age. TMAb have been found in about 10 per cent and 3 per cent of asymptomatic adult females and males, respectively. Ten to 20 per cent of these persons can be expected to have biochemical evidence of thyroid disease. This disease is probably the most common cause of goiter in adolescents, although the incidence is not as high as in older women.

PATHOLOGIC FINDINGS. The thyroid gland is normal or may be enlarged twofold to fivefold, depending on the degree of fibrosis. Microscopic examination reveals that varying degrees of infiltration with lymphocytes and plasma cells, fibrosis, and, in many cases, germinal centers are present. An oxyphilic change may be present in the cytoplasm of the residual thyroid follicular cells. It may be occasionally difficult to differentiate Hashimoto's disease from primary lymphoma of the thyroid gland.

CLINICAL MANIFESTATIONS. Two clinical forms of thyroid involvement are described. In the so-called atrophic form the gland is normal or reduced in size, and hypothyroidism is the prominent symptom (Table 229–9). This may well be the same syndrome as idiopathic myxedema. In other patients, variable degrees of thyroid enlargement and hypothyroidism occur, but goiter is the most common chief complaint. The gland is generally symmetrically enlarged, and often the pyramidal lobe is quite prominent, suggesting generalized hypertrophy. The thyroid is firm and may feel lobular or diffusely enlarged. Occasionally Hashimoto's disease presents as a single nodule in the thyroid gland, which represents the residual functioning thyroid tissue in a gland the remainder of which has been destroyed by this disease. The patient may have a family history of Graves' or Hashimoto's disease, pernicious anemia, or other autoimmune phenomena. As mentioned in the discussion of *lymphocytic thyroiditis,* as many as 5 to 10 per cent of women may have postpartum episodes of transient hyperthyroidism followed by transient hypothyroidism associated with elevated TMAb.

LABORATORY DIAGNOSIS. The serum free T$_4$ index is reduced and serum TSH increased in many patients with this syndrome. Approximately 95 per cent of patients have positive TMAb tests, and about 50 to 60 per cent have positive TgAb. The PBI may be normal or elevated even in the presence of a reduced free T$_4$ index as a result of the presence of iodoproteins circulating in the blood. The RAI uptake may be reduced, normal, or even increased, depending on the residual thyroid cell function and the serum TSH. The thyroid scan generally reveals a heterogeneous uptake of the isotope. Occasionally a single island of functioning tissue remains. This can be differentiated from a functioning adenoma of the thyroid only by appropriate tests of thyroid function. If the diagnosis remains in doubt, a needle biopsy can be performed, which will reveal the characteristic changes of lymphocytic infiltration in the majority of cases.

TREATMENT. In the early phases of Hashimoto's thyroiditis, goiter may be present and the serum TSH mildly increased, but the free T$_4$ index is in the lower normal range. Nevertheless, the presence of an elevated serum TSH suggests substantial decompensation of the thyroid, since in the presence of normally responsive thyroid tissue such TSH levels are quite stimulatory. Accordingly, even though the patient may have few symptoms of hypothyroidism, it is my practice to initiate treatment in the patient with thyroid enlargement once a secure serologic diagnosis has been established. In this

way it is hoped that further thyroid enlargement and possibly surgery can be avoided. Untreated patients are also susceptible to iodide-induced myxedema and may have spontaneous fluctuation in thyroid function, especially following pregnancy. More severe degrees of hypothyroidism are treated as described in the section, Hypothyroidism and Myxedema. If obstructive symptoms appear and they do not respond to TSH suppression, then surgery is required. The firm nature of the thyroid gland in Hashimoto's disease can suggest malignancy, and there is an increased risk of primary thyroid lymphoma in patients with Hashimoto's thyroiditis. While the relative risk is highly significant in this group, in one large series malignant lymphoma occurred in only four of 829 patients, so that the condition is quite rare. Nonetheless, a needle biopsy may be required to eliminate the possibility that this or other forms of malignant thyroid disease are superimposed on underlying thyroiditis.

In the younger patient, TSH suppression may cause the thyroid gland to decrease in size. In older subjects, particularly when fibrosis is present, little if any reduction will occur. Occasionally, Hashimoto's thyroiditis may present with hyperthyroidism ("hashitoxicosis"), which should be treated as is Graves' disease. Appropriate observation of the patient for the involvement of other tissues by autoimmune disease should be carried out as indicated.

PROGNOSIS. The prognosis of this condition is excellent as long as thyroid hormone therapy is provided when indicated. In patients with serologic evidence of Hashimoto's thyroiditis but normal thyroid function, an annual evaluation for hypothyroidism is indicated.

Riedel's Thyroiditis

This is a rare disorder of unknown cause in which a sclerosing fibrous infiltration of the thyroid gland occurs, causing the gland to become extremely firm. As the disease progresses, local muscles in the neck and the trachea are infiltrated and hypothyroidism appears. This condition may be difficult to differentiate from carcinoma of the thyroid. It is clinically associated with both retroperitoneal fibrosis and sclerosing cholangitis. Obstruction of the trachea may occur as the fibrosis proceeds, and a surgical approach is the only satisfactory method of treatment to relieve tracheal obstruction. Glucocorticoid therapy can be beneficial to some patients.

Amino N, Mori H, Iwatani Y, et al.: High prevalence of transient post-partum thyrotoxicosis and hypothyroidism. N Engl J Med 306:14, 849, 1982. *A prospective survey showing a 5.5 per cent incidence of transient thyrotoxicosis or hypothyroidism post partum.*

Holm L-E, Blomgren H, Lowhagen T: Cancer risks in patients with chronic lymphocytic thyroiditis. N Engl J Med 312:601, 1985. *An extensive epidemiologic study showing that while the relative risk of lymphoma is increased in individuals with chronic lymphocytic thyroiditis, the incidence of this complication is extremely low.*

Nikolai TF, Brosseau J, Kettrick MA, et al.: Lymphocytic thyroiditis with spontaneously resolving hyperthyroidism (silent thyroiditis). Arch Intern Med 140:478, 1980. *Clinical and laboratory results in 62 episodes of subacute lymphocytic thyroiditis, which these authors estimate is the cause of hyperthyroidism in 10 to 20 per cent of their patients.*

Tunbridge WMG, Evered DC, Hall R, et al.: The spectrum of thyroid disease in a community: The Whickham survey. Clin Endocrinol 7:481, 1977. *The epidemiology of thyroid disease in an English community; this study provides a firm basis for estimates of the prevalence of Hashimoto's and Graves' disease as well as nodular goiter.*

BENIGN AND MALIGNANT TUMORS OF THE THYROID: THE SOLITARY THYROID NODULE

In this section are discussed those benign and malignant tumors that usually present as a solitary thyroid nodule. Multinodular goiter is discussed in the next section, Sporadic and Endemic Goiter. Virtually all tumors of the thyroid arise from glandular cells and are therefore adenomas or carcinomas. A scheme for evaluation of the patient with a solitary thyroid nodule is presented at the end of this chapter.

ETIOLOGY. The fundamental cause of thyroid tumors is unknown. However, two factors, exposure to ionizing radiation and the presence of TSH, have been found to be important for inducing thyroid tumors in animals. Similar data are available with respect to radiation exposure in humans, which is responsible for an increased incidence of both benign and malignant thyroid neoplasms. A significant proportion of patients presenting with thyroid carcinoma have a history of radiation delivered to the upper thorax 10 to 15 years earlier for treatment of "status thymolymphaticus," enlarged tonsils and adenoids, acne, eustachian tube dysfunction, facial hemangiomas, pertussis, and tinea capitis. In patients who receive at least 300 to 400 rads of thyroidal irradiation at less than five years of age, the incidence of thyroid carcinoma is approximately 6 per cent 10 to 20 years later. Benign thyroid tumors are about three to four times as prevalent in the same patients. For doses of external thyroid irradiation in this range, the expected incidence of carcinoma is three cases per rad per year per 1 million persons exposed. TSH stimulation per se does not appear to cause thyroid carcinoma, as this disease is not increased in areas of iodine deficiency; however, it plays a permissive role.

There are two types of familial thyroid carcinoma. The first is medullary carcinoma occurring in families with the syndrome of multiple endocrine neoplasia Type II (pheochromocytoma, parathyroid hyperplasia) or Type III (pheochromocytoma, mucosal neuroma) (Ch. 241). Papillary or follicular carcinoma may occur as part of the familial multiple hamartoma syndrome (Cowden's disease).

INCIDENCE AND PREVALENCE. Solitary palpable thyroid nodules are common. The estimated incidence is about 1 to 3 per cent of the adult population, with a 2 to 1 preponderance of females. There is some difficulty in obtaining precise figures in this area, since a significant number of nodules that seem to be solitary by palpation are found to be dominant nodules in multinodular goiters at surgery or autopsy. This estimate represents a relatively small fraction of the true prevalence of thyroid nodules, which is about 40 to 50 per cent as revealed by autopsy studies or high-resolution ultrasonography. Such nodules are rarely true neoplasms. The estimated incidence of thyroid nodules is 0.1 per cent per year, but since many nodules are found at autopsy that were not suspected clinically the true incidence may be higher. The incidence of thyroid carcinoma is estimated to be 36 new cases per year per 1 million persons. These two estimates would suggest that about 3 or 4 per cent of patients who develop solitary thyroid nodules have thyroid carcinoma. Many surgical series report thyroid carcinoma in 10 to 30 per cent of resected solitary nodules, which indicates that the screening procedures employed to identify high-risk patients are effective. Various autopsy series have reported an incidence of thyroid carcinoma ranging from 0.1 to 6 per cent. The higher figures are from studies in which an extremely careful search was made for microscopic carcinomas, virtually all being less than 5 mm in diameter. The clinical significance of such lesions is negligible, and this "background" of asymptomatic microscopic lesions should be kept in mind when evaluating this literature.

Benign Neoplasms

PATHOLOGY. The *follicular adenoma* is by far the most common benign thyroid tumor. It varies from microscopic to 8 to 10 cm in size and is composed of a normal-appearing thyroid epithelium arranged in a follicular structure. An intact capsule surrounds these tumors, and there is often evidence of compression of surrounding normal thyroid tissue. The follicles may range from extremely small with little colloid (*fetal adenoma* or *microfollicular adenoma*) to large distended

structures (*macrofollicular adenoma*). The *embryonal* adenoma is an even more primitive-appearing structure possessing very little colloid. On occasion, the tumors may be composed of oxyphils (*oxyphil adenoma* or *Hürthle cell adenoma*). None of these differences in microscopic picture appear to bear on the functional characteristics of these nodules, nor do such nodules appear to become malignant. The hypercellular adenomas may be extremely difficult to differentiate from follicular carcinomas, especially when only a needle biopsy sample is available. Follicular adenomas have specific receptors for TSH, and these cells respond to TSH normally. However, many of these tumors do not possess the capacity for concentrating iodide or other similar substances. Since such nodules do not concentrate isotopes, they are referred to as *nonfunctioning* or *cold*.

CLINICAL MANIFESTATIONS. Thyroid adenomas fall into two categories: those that produce significant quantities of thyroid hormones, and those that do not. The latter are the more common (90 to 95 per cent). Patients with these tumors present with an asymptomatic mass in the neck. The patient may be discovered to have this tumor on routine physical examination and often is completely unaware of its existence. The tumor usually becomes palpable by the time it reaches 1 cm in diameter, but it may reach 5 to 10 cm without being noticed by the patient. Thyroid function studies in patients with nonfunctioning follicular adenomas are normal, and the thyroid scan will generally reveal an area of decreased or absent uptake of $^{123}I^-$ or $^{99m}TcO_4^-$ (a "cold" nodule). The precise diagnosis can be made only by obtaining a tissue specimen by aspiration biopsy, cutting needle biopsy (Vim-Silverman needle or its equivalent), or excision of the nodule. As these nodules may outgrow their blood supply, cystic degeneration may occur. Ultrasonography of such a lesion will reveal a cystic cavity within the nodule.

Functioning follicular adenomas may present with or without symptoms of hyperthyroidism, largely depending on their size. Lesions over 3 cm in diameter tend to cause thyrotoxicity and constitute about 50 per cent of these adenomas in patients 60 years and older. T_3 thyrotoxicosis was found in 46 per cent of such patients in one large series. More commonly the patient is asymptomatic, and a thyroid scan shows that the only area concentrating radioactivity is the nodule itself. Such patients generally have normal or high-normal serum thyroid hormone levels, the serum TSH-IMA is subnormal, and TRH infusion will not cause TSH release. Such nodules are functioning autonomously at a rate sufficient to suppress TSH synthesis in the pituitary (hence the lack of function in the remainder of the thyroid) but not at a sufficiently high level as to cause metabolic hyperthyroidism. Functional lesions that have suppressed TSH synthesis but not caused hyperthyroidism are denoted *warm* nodules, whereas those associated with hyperthyroidism are called *hot* nodules. Assessment of the thyroid functional state is necessary for proper evaluation of these lesions, since the thyroid scan is identical. This is especially important, since Hashimoto's disease may present as a solitary focus of functioning thyroid tissue, as may congenital absence of one lobe of the thyroid. The presence of potentially functioning thyroid tissue can be demonstrated by injection of 10 units of bovine TSH, followed in 24 hours by a thyroid scan. Unlike multinodular goiters, follicular adenomas of the thyroid rarely grow large enough to cause significant physical encroachment on the trachea or esophagus.

TREATMENT. The finding of an autonomously functioning nodule virtually eliminates the diagnosis of thyroid carcinoma. Treatment at that point depends on the thyroid status. If the patient is euthyroid (a warm thyroid nodule), nothing more than an annual follow-up with appropriate thyroid function tests (including a serum T_3) is necessary. In the hyperthyroid patient, surgery or ^{131}I is available for definitive treatment, although antithyroid drugs may be necessary to control symptomatic hyperthyroidism prior to definitive therapy. The choice of treatment depends on the age of the patient and the size of the nodule. In patients under the age of 20, surgical resection should be performed, as the radiation delivered to extranodular tissue after radioiodine therapy may reach a level that is considered carcinogenic. In older patients with cosmetically disfiguring lesions or those that are compressing vital structures in the neck, surgery is also preferred. For the rest, ^{131}I is indicated. I attempt to deliver 10 mCi of ^{131}I into the nodule. Following either surgery or radioactive iodine treatment, a period of four to six weeks is required for re-establishment of pituitary TSH secretion, following which function of the previously suppressed normal thyroid tissue should occur. The patient may need to receive thyroxine supplementation during this interim period, but may not require indefinite replacement. The approach to the *nonfunctioning thyroid nodule* is described below under Clinical Manifestations and Diagnosis of Thyroid Carcinoma—The Solitary Nodule.

Malignant Thyroid Tumors

Four types of malignancy are found in the thyroid gland. *Papillary carcinoma* comprises the largest fraction, about two thirds of all cases of thyroid malignancy. *Follicular carcinoma* accounts for another 20 per cent, including the *Hürthle cell* variant with *medullary*, and *poorly differentiated* carcinomas about 5 per cent each. Another 5 per cent is accounted for by *non-Hodgkin's lymphoma* which has become more common in recent years. Medullary carcinoma is a tumor of calcitonin producing C cells and has no relationship to the thyroid follicular epithelium.

PATHOLOGY AND NATURAL HISTORY. *Papillary carcinoma* is the most benign and the most common form of thyroid carcinoma. It is two to three times more common in women than in men and occurs with equal frequency in the third to seventh decades. Since the less well differentiated forms of carcinoma increase with age, papillary carcinoma is the most common malignant thyroid tumor in younger patients. The size of these tumors varies from microscopic to several centimeters in diameter. Of the clinically apparent variety, the *occult* tumors (defined as those less than 1.5 cm in diameter) are differentiated from the *intrathyroidal* tumors, which are larger but do not extend through the thyroid surface. The tumor is classified as *extrathyroidal* if it extends through the thyroid capsule and involves surrounding tissues. Microscopically, papillary carcinoma consists of well-differentiated thyroid epithelium covering papillary fibrovascular stalks. The nuclei are frequently clear, as opposed to the denser appearance of normal nuclei. A virtually pathognomonic feature in about 40 per cent of papillary thyroid carcinomas is the so-called *psammoma body*. These calcific globules are 5 to 100 microns in diameter and are often present in the tips of the papillary projections. Their etiology is unknown, but their presence in the thyroid tumor raises the high likelihood of its carcinomatous nature. Cervical lymphatic involvement even with occult thyroid tumors is common, occurring in as many as 50 per cent. Blood-borne metastases are uncommon. The presence or absence of lymph node metastases does not seem to alter the prognosis. In a large series studied at the Mayo Clinic, the 20-year survival of patients with occult or intrathyroid papillary carcinoma was not significantly different from that of a control group. However, the 20-year survival for patients with extrathyroidal carcinoma was about 40 per cent, and this dropped to 20 per cent over the next ten years. Many thyroid cancers have areas of follicular as well as papillary structure, and blood-borne metastases may occur that have a follicular pattern even though the primary tumor is papillary. Thus, many predominantly papillary tumors have follicular elements, but the biologic behavior of these lesions seems to be a function of the predominant microscopic appearance.

Follicular carcinomas also are more common in women than in men, but tend to increase in incidence with increasing age. The tumors vary from well-differentiated, virtually normal-appearing thyroid tissue to nearly solid sheets of follicular epithelium with little evidence of follicle formation. The former are differentiated from follicular adenomas only by demonstration of capsular and vascular invasion. Such a diagnosis generally cannot be made without the entire nodule for examination, and even at frozen section the carcinomatous nature of the lesion may not be recognized. Cyst formation may occur as it does in benign follicular tumors, and calcification may occur centrally. Follicular carcinomas tend to metastasize via blood vessel invasion and not, in general, via lymphatics. Metastases may not be evident at the time of initial evaluation, but may appear years later despite apparent complete excision of the tumor. It is not unusual for the follicular carcinoma to concentrate radioiodine, although it does so considerably less well than does normal thyroid tissue. Thus, it is only in the absence of normal thyroid tissue and in the presence of increased TSH that this potential is appreciated. However, it is useful in treatment in some of these tumors (see below). Patients who have had removal of well-encapsulated, noninvasive follicular carcinomas appear to have a normal lifespan. On the other hand, patients with tumors that show extensive local involvement and angioinvasion at the time of initial surgery have an approximately 30 per cent ten-year survival, which is decreased to less than 20 per cent at 20 years.

The most aggressive form of thyroid epithelial carcinoma, anaplastic or undifferentiated, may appear in *giant* or *spindle cell* forms. The small-cell variety of this lesion has proven to be a lymphoma in most cases. Undifferentiated thyroid carcinoma is the most highly malignant tumor of the thyroid gland. It is found almost exclusively in patients over the age of 60. The average prognosis from diagnosis to death in the giant cell tumors is less than six months, whereas patients with small-cell carcinoma may have five-year survival of 20 to 25 per cent. Both tend to extend locally and often cause tracheal obstruction. Distant metastases may occur with either type.

Medullary carcinoma of the thyroid is a malignant tumor of the C cell and produces thyrocalcitonin. Its occurrence in association with multiple endocrine neoplasia syndromes has been mentioned. It may also occur spontaneously. These tumors are characterized by sheets of tumor cells separated by a hyaline-amyloid-containing stroma. The amyloid is formed by the tumor cells and deposited in the stroma. The tumors may also produce ACTH, prostaglandin, or carcinoembryonic antigen. In familial syndromes, the penetrance of this tumor is complete, so that screening of family members is indicated by use of calcium and/or pentagastrin infusions to stimulate calcitonin release from pathologic cells (see Ch. 248).

Lymphoma is usually the nodular histiocytic form and generally arises in a gland affected by Hashimoto's thyroiditis. It should be considered diagnostically in patients with Hashimoto's disease who present with a rapidly enlarging mass in the thyroid gland, and a core or aspiration biopsy should be performed with appropriate cytochemical stains. Depending on the clinical stage, these lesions may respond quite well to radiotherapy, with or without chemotherapy. Complete cure by surgical resection of small lesions has also been reported.

CLINICAL MANIFESTATIONS AND DIAGNOSIS OF THYROID CARCINOMA—THE SOLITARY NODULE. The approach to the patient with a solitary thyroid nodule is a matter of considerable disagreement among clinicians. For some, thyroid carcinoma is sufficiently serious to require a surgical approach to all potentially carcinomatous lesions; others feel that considerable selection should be used prior to surgery. The benign nature of the common forms of thyroid carcinoma and the relatively large number of benign nodules make a conservative approach rational. There are several clinical characteristics that dictate an open surgical approach to a nonfunctioning thyroid nodule. This includes a history of prior irradiation. Nodules in such patients carry a 20 to 25 per cent risk of carcinoma. A history of rapid growth, evidence of recurrent nerve paresis, obvious involvement of lymph nodes, or fixation of the nodule to surrounding tissues should also lead to serious consideration of immediate surgery. Statistically, the risk of a solitary cold nodule being malignant is higher in a male than in a female, since benign disease of the thyroid is much more common in females. Thyroid nodules in children are more likely to be carcinoma than those in adults.

In the absence of specific signs pointing to a diagnosis of thyroid carcinoma, there are two avenues of approach (Fig. 229–10A and 10B). If there is no obvious thyroid dysfunction (either hyperthyroidism or hypothyroidism) and an experienced cytopathologist is available, a needle aspiration can be performed (Fig. 229–10A). If the lesion is a simple cyst this will be curative; otherwise the cytologic report guides therapy. If carcinoma is found, surgical exploration is indicated. If a cellular follicular aspirate is obtained that is consistent with a

benign or a malignant lesion, a ^{123}I (or ^{131}I) scan is performed. If the lesion is hypofunctional, surgical exploration is advised. If it is warm or hot, management is as discussed earlier under autonomous nodules. If the cytologic report indicates that the lesion is benign, thyroxine is given to suppress TSH, and this is monitored by TSH-IMA measurement. The need for surgery is then determined by the natural history of the individual case. Aspiration biopsy cytology yields false-positive results very rarely, and false-negative results, that is, a benign diagnosis in a patient with a malignant lesion, should occur in only 2 to 3 per cent of patients. This figure, however, may be higher during the early experience with this technique in a given center. A number of patients are referred for surgery because of a cytologic picture that is suspicious but not clearly diagnostic. Nonetheless, in most clinics, aspiration cytology has reduced the apparent need for surgical exploration by 50 to 60 per cent. In other words, approximately 40 per cent of patients with solitary nodules will require surgical exploration because of frankly or suspiciously malignant lesions.

If a trained cytopathologist is not available, then thyroid scanning is performed followed by ultrasonography if the nodule is not hyperfunctioning (Fig. 229–10B). Rarely a malignant nodule will be warm by ^{99m}TcO$_4^-$ but cold by iodide scan. This should be suspected and tested for when warm lesions do not suppress function in the remainder of the gland. Ultrasonography of hypofunctioning nodules is performed. A cystic lesion can be treated by aspiration and the procedure repeated twice more if the fluid reaccumulates before surgery is indicated. In the nonfunctioning solid nodule, needle aspiration cytology, cutting needle biopsy, or surgical exploration is advised. I recommend surgical excision for patients under 20, for all males, and for those high-risk patients with familial carcinoma and radiation exposure. The availability of experienced thyroid surgeons plays an important role in this approach, since serious morbidity attends inadvertent resection of the parathyroid glands or recurrent laryngeal nerve paresis. In older women and men in whom other illnesses make surgery less desirable, a diagnosis may be obtained by needle biopsy or aspiration cytology.

Alternatively, thyroxine may be given to suppress TSH. Most nodules will not change in size, and therapy is individualized, whereas patients with nodules that increase during TSH suppression are referred for surgery, and those patients with nodules that decrease in size are followed with continued suppression. None of these responses clearly differentiates a benign from a malignant lesion.

At the time of initial surgery a frozen section should be obtained from all solitary thyroid nodules and an attempt made to provide definitive treatment. A reasonable approach to intrathyroidal papillary carcinoma is to perform a lobectomy with isthmectomy and explore for and remove any involved lymph nodes. An examination of the other lobe should be made for tumor, but, except in the irradiated patient, bilateral lobectomy is not required. With extrathyroidal extension of papillary carcinoma and bilateral lymph node metastases, a total thyroidectomy is performed with great care to preserve the recurrent laryngeal nerves and parathyroid glands. A follicular carcinoma is approached as are the papillary lesions, except that the presence of distant lymph node metastases or extensive capsular and vascular invasion in the initial frozen section should lead to consideration of bilateral thyroidectomy. This is done to remove residual normal tissue to facilitate radioiodine therapy (see below). Radical neck dissection does not offer any advantage over the less-mutilating procedures described above. Medullary carcinoma of the sporadic variety may be treated as papillary carcinoma, but the familial form requires bilateral lobectomy. It is, of course, important to determine that pheochromocytoma and hyperparathyroidism are not present before undertaking surgery. Anaplastic carcinoma is rarely restricted enough to lend itself

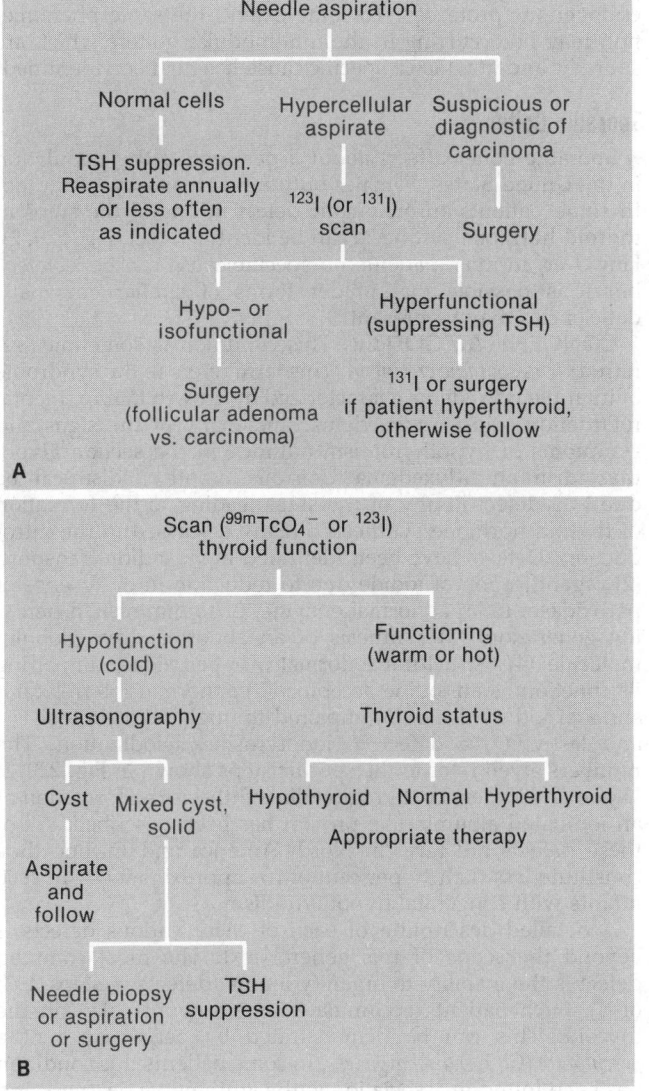

FIGURE 229–10. *A* shows a schema for the diagnostic evaluation of patient with a solitary thyroid nodule based on aspiration biopsy cytology. *B* presents an alternative solution to the same problem starting with a thyroid scintiscan.

to surgical therapy, except for palliation to prevent tracheal compression. Lymphoma should be treated by radiotherapy and chemotherapy in consultation with a hematologist.

RADIATION THERAPY. I⁻ may be concentrated to a sufficient degree to be useful by as many as 50 to 60 per cent of well-differentiated thyroid tumors. This can be demonstrated only after the establishment of hypothyroidism with an increase in serum TSH. In general, prophylactic therapy with radioiodine in patients with papillary carcinoma does not appear to be beneficial, although metastases may respond to this method. In follicular carcinoma with evidence of vascular invasion or in patients with follicular metastases, particularly to the lungs, significant amelioration of symptoms and dramatic changes in the x-ray picture may be associated with this therapy. It does not appear to be as useful for patients with bone metastases. To be weighed against these beneficial effects is the increased incidence of leukemia in patients treated with large doses of ¹³¹I (300 mCi and more).

The usual approach to evaluation of the feasibility of this therapeutic method is to remove residual functioning thyroid tissue surgically or by ¹³¹I administration. After this, the patient is switched to triiodothyronine (50 μg per day) for a period of approximately three weeks, following which administration of the hormone is discontinued. Within two to three weeks, most patients will show the maximal uptake in metastatic tissue. At that time, a tracer dose of ¹³¹I should be given with appropriate dosimetry of the tumor mass, bone marrow, and lungs. Following this, the maximal tolerable ¹³¹I dose should be given and the patient started on TSH-suppressive therapy with thyroxine one day later. Local recurrences of papillary carcinoma can often be treated surgically by removal of involved lymph nodes. In such patients this is preferable to ¹³¹I, which should be reserved for a nonresectable lesion.

Despite the poor function of thyroid tumors in terms of radioiodine trapping, carcinomatous thyroid cells have TSH receptors and respond to TSH in vitro. Accordingly, efforts should be made to suppress TSH below normal, as monitored by TSH-IMA or by demonstrating that TRH does not increase TSH into the measurable range of a conventional assay. In patients who have had total thyroidectomy and radioiodine ablation, serum thyroglobulin concentrations should be monitored, since normal or increased levels of this protein will then indicate the presence of residual thyroid tumor.

Kaplan MM, Garnick MB, Gelber R, et al.: Risk factors for thyroid abnormalities after neck irradiation for childhood cancer. Am J Med 74:272–280, 1983. *This study shows that both benign and malignant thyroid nodules, as well as hypothyroidism, may appear 5 to 35 years after therapeutic irradiation to the neck.*

McConahey WM, Hay ID, Woolner LB, et al.: Papillary thyroid cancer treated at the Mayo Clinic 1946 through 1970: Initial manifestations, pathologic findings, therapy, and outcome. Mayo Clin Proc 61:978, 1986. *An update of a large retrospective evaluation of the results of various treatment modalities in patients with well-differentiated thyroid carcinoma.*

Miller JM: Evaluation of thyroid nodules: Accent on needle biopsy. Med Clin North Am 69:1063, 1985. *A discussion of the extensive experience of a clinical group active in the care of patients with nodular thyroid disease.*

Schneider AB, Recant W, Pinsky SM, et al.: Radiation-induced thyroid carcinoma: Clinical course and results of therapy in 296 patients. Ann Intern Med 105:405, 1986. *Follow-up study of several hundred patients with radiation-induced thyroid carcinoma that examines risk factors and provides guidelines for appropriate treatment of these individuals.*

SPORADIC AND ENDEMIC GOITER

DEFINITION. *Sporadic goiter* refers to thyroid enlargement, which is found in a relatively small fraction of a given population. The cause for the thyroid enlargement may be different from patient to patient. The term *endemic goiter* refers to a condition seen in a much larger fraction of the population, which is presumably a consequence of one or several environmental influences, most commonly iodine deficiency. Although the causes of sporadic and endemic goiter are, by definition, different, the pathophysiology and pathology underlying these conditions are probably quite similar, and they will therefore be grouped together.

ETIOLOGY. The common factor that is thought to lead to thyroid enlargement is *hypersecretion of TSH*. TSH increases in response to decreased production of thyroid hormones, especially T_4, as a consequence of an intrinsic abnormality in the process of thyroid hormone synthesis in the case of sporadic goiter, or the lack of adequate quantities of iodine in the diet or the presence of a goitrogen in the environment in endemic goiter. TSH increases as T_4 falls. As a consequence of the increased TSH secretion, iodine turnover by the thyroid is accelerated, the T_3 to T_4 ratio in thyroid secretion is increased, and serum T_3 may remain entirely normal. Such patients appear to be clinically euthyroid at the expense of an elevated serum TSH concentration and an enlarged thyroid gland.

PATHOLOGY. In the early phases, the thyroid gland may be diffusely enlarged with cellular hyperplasia as a result of TSH stimulation. Later, large follicles form with low epithelium. As the process continues, there is further stimulation of some thyroidal areas and atrophy of others with concomitant fibrosis. These multiple nodules have markedly varying activity. The accumulation of thyroglobulin, particularly in the iodine-deficient patients, may occur because poorly iodinated thyroglobulin is relatively resistant to digestion by endogenous proteases. To some extent, the same phenomenon may be occurring in the multinodular goiters which are sporadic and in which a specific cause has not been identified.

Sporadic Goiter

Sporadic goiter affects about 5 per cent of the population in the United States. Females outnumber males by a 3:1 ratio. In some patients an enzymatic defect in one of the steps in thyroid hormone synthesis can be identified (see Fig. 229–2). However, in most patients no specific cause can be isolated, but it is possible that milder forms of similar enzymatic deficiencies may be present.

CONGENITAL GOITER. This condition is sometimes referred to as *sporadic cretinism*. This term refers to the syndrome of infantile myxedema characterized by growth failure, mental retardation, diffuse myxedema, and many of the signs and symptoms of hypothyroidism outlined in the section Hypothyroidism and Myxedema. Goitrous hypothyroidism can be due to a defect in any of the steps leading to the formation of thyroid hormone synthesis already discussed in the introduction. Defects have been identified in (1) iodide transport; (2) organification of iodide due to reduction in or absence of peroxidase, to an abnormal enzyme, or to diminished peroxide generation; (3) synthesis of an abnormal thyroglobulin molecule; (4) a structural abnormality in peroxidase, impairing its function as an iodine acceptor; (5) abnormal interrelationships of iodotyrosine; (6) impaired thyroglobulin proteolysis; and lastly, (7) a defect in iodotyrosine deiodination. The numbers given refer to the specific steps shown in Fig. 229–2. In some disorders of thyroglobulin synthesis the formation of an iodinated albumin-like protein has been described. All of these defects are rare. In North America and Europe they constitute less than 10 per cent of the approximately 1 in 4000 infants with congenital hypothyroidism.

A detailed description of each of these various defects is beyond the scope of this general text. The most common defect is the inability to organify iodine (defects in steps 2, 3, or 4). Such patients accumulate large amounts of I⁻ in the thyroid. This can be demonstrated by performance of a *perchlorate (ClO_4^-) discharge test*. In some patients this condition has been found in association with eighth nerve deafness and has the eponym *Pendred's syndrome*.

Regardless of the specific defect, these patients present with goiter and hypothyroidism, the serum T_4 index is reduced, and serum TSH is elevated. Further evaluation for the type of biochemical defect requires careful laboratory investigation. The treatment of such patients is with exogenous thyroid hormone. Thyroxine treatment will cause regression of the enlarged thyroid, and mental retardation may be ameliorated or prevented if treatment is started before three months of age. Genetic counseling is desirable so that these patients will be aware of the risk of hypothyroidism in subsequent offspring.

MULTINODULAR GOITER IN THE ADULT. The hypothesis that adults with multinodular goiter have mild defects in thyroid hormone synthesis similar to the more complete forms found in infants remains to be proved. If this is the case, then the goiter could be explained by modest increases in TSH, which is secreted by the pituitary in response to the reduced serum T_4. A significant physiologic increase in TSH may be as little as 2 to 3 μU per milliliter, often below the sensitivity of the TSH immunoassay which is clinically available. The compensatory increase in the size of the thyroid gland under these circumstances results in adequate rates of thyroid hormone formation, so that the vast majority of patients with this abnormality are euthyroid.

CLINICAL MANIFESTATIONS. Patients with multinodular goiter may come to the physician because of respiratory obstruction or dysphagia. More often the patient is asymptomatic and the enlarged multinodular thyroid is discovered on a routine physical examination. Such patients should be questioned carefully for symptoms of respiratory obstruction. The goiter often extends retrosternally; this may be demonstrated by having the patient extend the arms directly over the head. If a significant substernal goiter is present, jugular venous distention and suffusion of the face occurs (*Pemberton's sign*). Aside from physical obstruction, the most significant clinical aspect of the multinodular goiter is the tendency for hyperthyroidism to develop late in life (*Plummer's disease*). It is postulated that after decades of stimulation by TSH one or more of the nodular hyperplastic areas become autonomous. Since this condition generally appears in the elderly patient, the resulting hyperthyroidism may be of the apathetic variety (see the section Graves' Disease and Other Causes of Hyperthyroidism). In one series, administration of 50 to 100 mg of KI per day to eight patients with multinodular goiter resulted in hyperthyroidism in four patients, which required definitive treatment. The etiology of this form of iodide-induced thyrotoxicosis (probably not jodbasedow) is not clear, but caution is needed before the administration of iodide or iodine-containing drugs, such as amiodarone, to patients with multinodular goiter.

LABORATORY DIAGNOSIS. The physician must investigate both the anatomic and the functional nature of the thyroid pathology. Anatomic information is gained by chest or esophageal radiography, from a scintiscan, and when indicated by computed tomography of the neck and upper thorax. ^{131}I is recommended for thyroid scanning of these patients since the γ rays emitted by $^{99m}TcO_4^-$ and $^{123}I^-$ may not be strong enough to penetrate the sternum. The scintiscan image shows patchy focal uptake of radioactivity in an enlarged thyroid gland. The significance of the nonfunctioning areas in such scintiscans is discussed below. Measurements of serum free T_4 index, T_3, TSH, and TMAb and TgAb should be obtained, especially since Hashimoto's thyroiditis may present as a multinodular goiter. A TSH-IMA assay or a TRH test is indicated if Plummer's disease is suspected.

TREATMENT. The proper treatment depends on the clinical manifestations in the individual patient. Hyperthyroidism associated with multinodular goiter is best treated with radioactive iodine. However, because of the heterogeneity of the tissue uptake of radioiodine, a larger dose of radioiodine will be necessary (180 μCi per gram) or 10 mCi in a typical gland. The not uncommon coexistence of cardiac or pulmonary disease in this age group, together with the large size of the thyroid gland and the possibility of radiation thyroiditis, has

led me to pretreat most elderly hyperthyroid patients with antithyroid drugs prior to radiotherapy. The antithyroid drugs are discontinued approximately four to five days prior to treatment. If a high plasma I^- (low RAI uptake) does not permit the use of radioiodine, then surgical treatment must be undertaken after appropriate preparation with antithyroid drugs.

Hypothyroid patients require treatment with thyroxine as described in the section Hypothyroidism and Myxedema. Young euthyroid patients with diffuse thyroid enlargement may be started on thyroxine replacement therapy to suppress TSH, particularly if this is slightly elevated. One may block further thyroid enlargement by this treatment as well as cause regression of goiter in some. In patients over the age of 40, it is unlikely that significant amelioration in physical symptoms will occur with TSH suppression, but this hormone may be administered on a trial basis. Great care must be exercised, particularly in the elderly, since one or more of the hyperplastic thyroid nodules may be functioning autonomously. In all patients with multinodular goiter it is suggested that a TSH-IMA assay or TRH test be performed prior to initiation of therapy with thyroid hormone to avoid iatrogenic hyperthyroidism. In such circumstances, well-meaning attempts to suppress TSH can cause iatrogenic hyperthyroidism. If physical symptoms of obstruction are present or there is evidence of recurrent laryngeal nerve dysfunction, surgical treatment is generally in order.

The Multinodular Goiter and Thyroid Carcinoma. Nodular disease of the thyroid is common and thyroid carcinoma is relatively rare. Poorly functioning areas may be present in the thyroid scintiscans of multinodular goiters, but this is not an indication for surgery for malignant disease. As heterogeneity of function is the rule, other criteria must be employed for recognition of malignancy in the multinodular goiter. Factors that raise this possibility include previous exposure to therapeutic thyroidal irradiation in childhood, a family history of thyroid carcinoma or enlargement of cervical lymph nodes, recurrent laryngeal nerve palsy, or the continuing enlargement of a single "cold" nodule in an otherwise stable gland. In situations in which doubt exists, needle biopsy may provide the requisite microscopic diagnosis to reassure the patient and the physician that conservative therapy is the appropriate course of action.

PROGNOSIS. Patients with euthyroid multinodular goiter should have thyroid function and physical findings evaluated at annual intervals. Most do not require surgery.

Endemic Goiter

Iodine deficiency is the most common cause of thyroid disease in the world population, although iodination of salt has eliminated this problem in North America. Areas in which iodine intake remains low include mountainous regions such as the Andes and Himalayas. In addition, there are areas of endemic goiter in central Africa, New Guinea, and Indonesia. Iodine prophylaxis, either in foodstuffs or in the form of iodized oil injection, has been successful in many of these countries, but iodine deficiency remains a considerable public health problem. In a few geographic locations, ingestion of a goitrogen has been implicated in the high incidence of goiter. Examples include a thiocyanate derivative from the cassava, which is eaten in large quantities in central Africa, and a goitrogenic hydrocarbon found in the water supply in parts of Colombia and in Chile.

CLINICAL MANIFESTATIONS IN ADULTS. The minimal quantity of iodine required for normal thyroid function is approximately 100 μg per day. As the level of iodine in the diet decreases below this level, there is a progressive fall in serum T_4 and a progressive rise in serum TSH. Serum T_3 concentrations remain normal or slightly elevated, a persistently elevated TSH being required for this compensation. Serum TSH concentrations may exceed 100 μU per milliliter.

In the presence of lifelong stimulation of this degree, enormous hypertrophy and hyperplasia of the thyroid gland can occur. Such glands may weigh 1 to 5 kg, producing considerable physical impairment.

EFFECTS OF IODINE DEFICIENCY IN INFANTS. In areas of endemic goiter, cretinism is not uncommon. Despite the capacity of the placenta to transport I⁻, in areas where iodine intake is severely reduced (25 μg per day or less) the 24-hour maternal RAI uptake is virtually 100 per cent. Infants in these areas may be born with congenital hypothyroidism as a consequence of iodine deficiency.

In areas such as the Andes or New Guinea where iodine intake may be less than 20 μg per day, a different form of *endemic cretinism* may be seen. As opposed to dwarfism and mental retardation, some children in these areas have spastic diplegia, squint, and deafness. The etiology of this syndrome is still not clarified. It may be a manifestation of the effect of iodine deficiency per se on the embryologic development of the central nervous system. Fetal or maternal hypothyroidism as a consequence of severe iodine deficiency may also contribute to this problem.

TREATMENT. The treatment of iodine deficiency is to supply this element either as a food additive or by direct injections of iodinated oil. This has often been difficult because of the inaccessibility and restricted governmental resources of those countries in which iodine deficiency is a problem. The *jodbasedow phenomenon* (iodine-induced hyperthyroidism) will occur in some patients receiving iodine supplementation. These presumably are patients with underlying Graves' (Basedow's) disease who are given adequate supplies of the substrate for thyroid hormone synthesis.

Lever EG, Medeiros-Neto GA, DeGroot LJ: Inherited disorders of thyroid metabolism. Endocr Rev 4:213, 1983. *A comprehensive review of this topic.*

Stanbury JB, Dumont JE: Familial goiter and related disorders. *In* Stanbury JB, Wyngaarden JB, Fredrickson DS, et al. (eds.): The Metabolic Basis of Inherited Disease. 5th ed. New York, McGraw-Hill Book Company, 1983, pp. 231–269. *A thorough review of the literature in this area with 327 references. The emphasis is on the emzymology of pathogenesis.*

Stanbury JB, Hetzel BS (eds.): Endemic Goiter and Endemic Cretinism. New York, John Wiley & Sons, 1980. *A detailed discussion of this worldwide problem by many authorities.*

Thilly CH, Delange F, Lagasse R, et al.: Fetal hypothyroidism and maternal thyroid status in severe endemic goiter. J Clin Endocrinol Metab 47:354, 1978. *The effects of iodine deficiency on mother and newborn are described, comparing treated and untreated patients.*

Wolff J: Congenital goiter with defective iodide transport. Endocr Rev 4:240, 1983. *The clinical, pathophysiological, and biochemical findings in patients with this form of sporadic goiter.*

230 DISORDERS OF THE ADRENAL CORTEX

J. Blake Tyrrell and John D. Baxter

230.1 Structure and Development of the Adrenal Cortex

John D. Baxter

The major function of the adrenal cortex is to produce glucocorticoid and mineralocorticoid hormones, of which cortisol and aldosterone, respectively, are the most important in humans. The glucocorticoids, named for their carbohydrate-regulating properties, are essential for survival, at least in times of stress, and regulate intermediary metabolism, hemodynamic functions, and developmental processes. The mineralocorticoids regulate sodium, potassium, and hydrogen ion balance and secondarily affect the blood pressure. Either an excess or deficiency of these steroids can have deleterious effects. Glucocorticoid excess and deficiency are termed Cushing's syndrome and Addison's disease, respectively. Aldosterone excess and deficiency are referred to as aldosteronism and hypoaldosteronism, respectively. Whereas diseases of the adrenal cortex are relatively uncommon, their clinical stigmata are part of the differential diagnosis of common problems. In addition, iatrogenic glucocorticoid excess is a common clinical problem due to the widespread usage of glucocorticoids in therapy. Secondary hyperaldosteronism is also a common problem requiring antimineralocorticoid therapy.

The human adrenal cortex produces at least 50 other steroids. This gland is a major source of androgenic steroids in the female (see Ch. 237), but is a trivial source of these steroids in the male compared to the testes (see Ch. 235). The adrenal produces only minute quantities of estrogens and progestins. Some adrenal steroids ordinarily produced in physiologically insignificant quantities can result in clinical abnormalities when they are produced in excess in certain pathologic states.

STRUCTURE. There are two adrenal glands, located extraperitoneally at the upper poles of each kidney lateral to the eleventh thoracic to first lumbar vertebrae. The right gland tends to be higher and more lateral than the left. The average gland weighs 4 grams and is 2 to 3 cm wide and 4 to 6 cm long. A series of small arteries arising from the abdominal aorta, renal and phrenic arteries, and occasionally from ovarian or spermatic arteries, feed the gland. Because of this, arterial infarction is unusual. The venous drainage of the gland on the left is ordinarily into the renal vein and on the right into the inferior vena cava. The gland is innervated by autonomic fibers.

The adrenal cortex comprises about 90 per cent of the gland and surrounds the centrally located medulla that produces catecholamines. The cortex has three zones. The ill-defined zona glomerulosa, about 15 per cent of the cortex, is present under the capsule and contains foci of cells, with a small cytoplasmic volume and lipid content, that produce aldosterone. The remainder of the cortex, the zonae reticularis and fasciculata, can be considered as a single unit involved predominantly in cortisol and androgen production. Cells of the zona fasciculata, about 75 per cent of the cortex, appear vacuolated or clear on stained sections because of their high cholesterol content. The cells of the inner zona reticularis are more compact with less lipid.

The morphology of the gland is influenced by ACTH, angiotensin II, and potassium. Elevations of ACTH levels increase adrenal blood flow within minutes and adrenal weight within hours; the clear fasciculata cells lose their lipid, attain the compact morphology and ultrastructural features of reticularis cells, and produce cortisol. With prolonged stimulation there is hyperplasia and hypertrophy that can double the adrenal weight. Similar increases in angiotensin II and potassium result in hypertrophy and hyperplasia of the glomerulosa cells and increased aldosterone production. Deficiency of angiotensin II leads to atrophy of the zona glomerulosa, and deficiency of ACTH to atrophy of the zonae fasciculata-reticularis; this is reversible upon restimulation. Occasionally, accessory adrenal glands may be present in a variety of locations in the abdomen or pelvis and can assume significant function in states of ACTH excess.

DEVELOPMENT. The adrenal cortex is derived from mesenchymal tissue. Cortical cells emerge to form a primitive fetal cortex around the sixth week of development. This then evolves into a fetal zone that is involved predominantly in the synthesis of androgen and estrogen precursors, and a definitive zone destined to become the adult gland. The fetal zone constitutes the major bulk of the adrenal cortex at birth; it begins to recede by the last intrauterine month and disappears around the end of the first year. The permanent cortex is formed from cells of the outer portion of the fetal gland and is not developed completely until around 3 years of age.

230.2 Synthesis, Circulation, and Metabolism of Adrenal Steroids

John D. Baxter

SYNTHESIS

The structures and steps in biosynthesis of a number of steroid hormones are shown in Figure 230–1. The letter designation for the carbon rings and the number designation of the carbon atoms are shown for pregnenolone, a key biosynthetic intermediate. α- and β- are used to designate the positions of the side groups above (β) or below (α) the plane of the molecule. The various steroids differ in (1) the saturation of the A ring (Δ indicates a double bond); (2) hydroxyl and ketone groups at positions 3, 11, 17, and 21; (3) the presence of a 3-carbon side chain at position 17; and (4) an aldehyde group at position 18. Since the chemical nomenclature is cumbersome, trivial names for the steroids are used most frequently.

All steroids are derived from cholesterol that is obtained mostly by receptor-mediated internalization of plasma low-density lipoproteins and to a lesser extent from synthesis by the gland. This uptake mechanism is increased when the adrenal is stimulated.

Subsequent steps occur in the mitochondrion or endoplasmic reticulum. The first step is the conversion of cholesterol to pregnenolone. This step is rate limiting and is regulated by the major factors (ACTH, angiotensin II, and potassium) that stimulate steroid biosynthesis. This conversion involves several steps, catalyzed by the enzyme 20,22-desmolase (cholesterol side chain cleavage enzyme). Pregnenolone is then modified either (1) by converting its 5,6 to a 4,5 double bond with the use of 3β-hydroxysteroid dehydrogenase and Δ^5-oxysteroid isomerase, resulting in progesterone; or (2) by addition of a 17α-hydroxyl group with the use of 17α-hydroxylase, resulting in 17α-hydroxypregnenolone. The former pathway occurs in the glomerulosa, which lacks 17α-hydroxylase activity; although controversial, the latter pathway probably predominates in the fasciculata-reticularis, with subsequent conversion of 17α-hydroxypregnenolone to 17α-hydroxyprogesterone.

CORTISOL. Cortisol is synthesized by two successive hydroxylations of 17α-hydroxyprogesterone. The first is at the 21 position, catalyzed by 21-hydroxylase and results in 11-deoxycortisol (also called compound S). The second, at the 11 position of 11-deoxycortisol, is catalyzed by 11β-hydroxylase and yields cortisol (also called hydrocortisone or compound F). These hydroxylations also require a flavoprotein dehydrogenase and a cytochrome P450.

ALDOSTERONE. Aldosterone is produced by 21-hydroxylation of progesterone to form deoxycorticosterone (DOC); 11β-hydroxylation of DOC to form corticosterone; 18-hydroxylation of the latter to form 18-hydroxycorticosterone; and oxidation of the 18 CH$_2$OH group to an aldehyde to form aldosterone with the use of 18-hydroxycorticosteroid hydroxylase. This step is unique to the glomerulosa, explaining why aldosterone is not made by the zonae fasciculata and reticularis.

ANDROGENS. The adrenal androgens have 19 carbon atoms (C-19 steroids) and serve as precursors for more potent androgens produced in peripheral tissues. These are dehydroepiandrosterone (DHEA) and its sulfate (DHEA-S), androstenedione and testosterone. DHEA is derived from 17α-hydroxypregnenolone by removal of its C-17 side chain, that leaves a keto group, with the use of C-17,20-lyase, and 17β-hydroxysteroid dehydrogenase. The sulfation of DHEA at the

TABLE 230–1. SECRETION RATES AND PLASMA CONCENTRATIONS OF ADRENAL STEROIDS*

Steroid	24-hr Secretion (mg)	Mean Plasma Concentration (ng/ml)
Aldosterone	0.15	0.16
Androstenedione	2.4	1.5
Corticosterone	2.5	3
Cortisol	16	100
11-Deoxycorticosterone (DOC)	0.6	0.16
11-Deoxycortisol	0.4	1.7
DHEA	0.7(F), 3.0(M)	5.4
DHEA-S	7	1200
Progesterone	nil	0.2(M,F), 12(F)†
17α-Hydroxyprogesterone	nil	0.2(M), 0.6(F),2.0(F)†
Testosterone	0.2	5.6(M), 0.5(F)

Modified from Baxter JD, Tyrrell JB: The adrenal cortex. In Felig P, Baxter JD, Broadus AH, et al. (eds.): Endocrinology and Metabolism. 2nd ed. New York, McGraw-Hill Book Company, 1987, p 521, where references to primary source material can be found.

*Mean values are reported for adults. Individual female (F) and male (M) values are reported only when these differ by more than twofold.

†Refers to the luteal phase of the menstrual cycle.

3 position to DHEA-S is catalyzed by a sulfokinase. Androstenedione can be derived from either 17α-hydroxyprogesterone or DHEA, as illustrated. The adrenal synthesizes minute quantities of the C-18 steroids estradiol and estrone as outlined in Figure 230–1. However, DHEA and DHEA-S synthesized by the fetal adrenal account for substantial amounts of maternal production of estriol, estradiol, estrone, testosterone, and androstenedione.

PRODUCTION RATES. The production rates and the blood levels under basal conditions of the major adrenal steroids are shown in Table 230–1. More cortisol is produced than any other steroid; much less aldosterone is produced. The production of DHEA plus DHEA-S is nearly as high as cortisol; although the plasma levels of DHEA are only a fraction of those of cortisol, plasma levels of DHEA-S are severalfold higher than those of cortisol because of the slow metabolism of DHEA-S. Corticosterone has substantial glucocorticoid activity, but is produced at much lower levels than cortisol. Similarly, DOC has substantial mineralocorticoid activity, and more DOC than aldosterone is produced, but free levels of this steroid in plasma are much lower than those of aldosterone even though total levels are similar. The adrenal production of progesterone and 17α-hydroxyprogesterone is minimal. The production of testosterone is at levels similar to those of aldosterone.

INHIBITORS. Several compounds can inhibit adrenal steroid biosynthesis at various steps in the biosynthetic pathway. They can be useful for diagnosis and therapy of adrenal disorders (discussed below). Of these, metyrapone (SU-4885), aminoglutethimide, and mitotane (o,p'-DDD) have been used most commonly. Metyrapone predominantly inhibits 11β-hydroxylation and to a lesser extent 21-hydroxylation. Aminoglutethimide blocks the early steps in conversion of cholesterol to pregnenolone (cholesterol to 20α-hydroxycholesterol). Mitotane blocks adrenal mitochondrial functioning and results in generalized inhibition of steroid biosynthesis and adrenal atrophy. Spironolactone can block aldosterone biosynthesis by inhibiting the 11β- and 18-hydroxylation steps; these actions may add to the antimineralocorticoid actions of this compound.

PLASMA BINDING OF ADRENAL STEROIDS

GLUCOCORTICOIDS. Approximately 90 to 93 per cent of the circulating cortisol is bound by plasma proteins. About 80 per cent of this binding is due to specific and high-affinity association of cortisol with corticosteroid-binding globulin (CBG, also termed transcortin). A lesser quantity is bound by albumin, and a negligible amount by other plasma proteins.

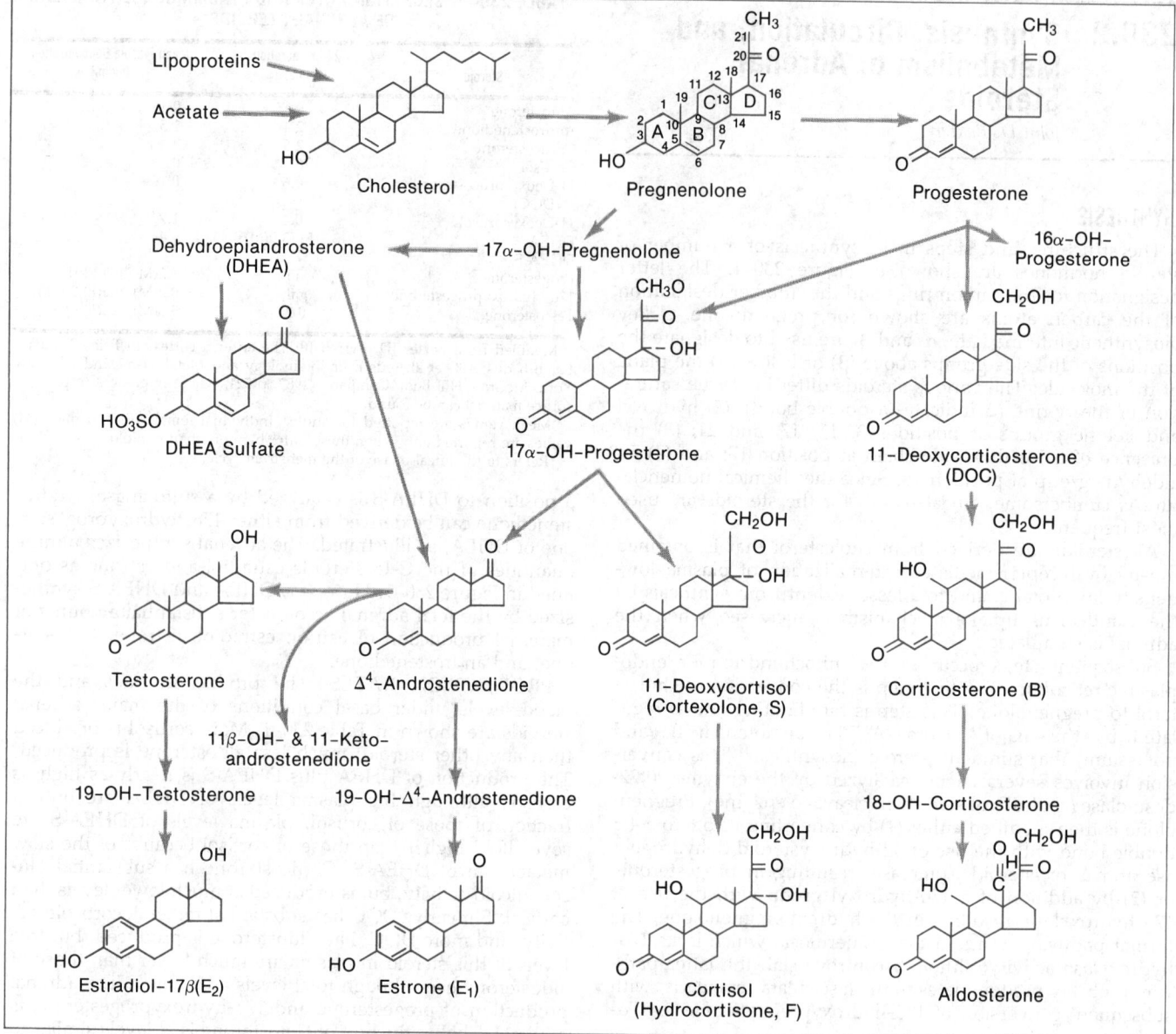

FIGURE 230–1. Steps in adrenal steroid biosynthesis. The numbers for the carbon atoms and the letters designating the rings of the steroid molecule are shown for pregnenolone. Arrows indicate the conversion pathways; the use of two arrows between intermediates indicates that more than one step is involved in the interconversion. (Adapted from Baxter JD, Tyrrell JB: In Felig P, Baxter JD, Broadus AE, et al. (eds.): Endocrinology and Metabolism. 2nd ed. New York, McGraw-Hill Book Company, 1987, p 516.)

CBG is synthesized in the liver, and at its usual concentrations in plasma has a capacity for binding cortisol of around 25 μg per deciliter; thus, when cortisol levels begin to exceed this saturation capacity, the proportion of free cortisol is increased. Although several other steroids (e.g., corticosterone, progesterone) can bind to CBG, under most circumstances such occupancy is minimal.

CBG concentrations in plasma vary on a genetic basis and are also regulated by hormones and other factors. CBG levels are increased in pregnancy (by almost twofold during the third trimester), in hyperthyroidism, in diabetes, and by estrogens and oral contraceptives. Such effects can be maximal in three to five days and reversed by two to three weeks after cessation of the stimulus. CBG levels can be low congenitally and in liver disease (decreased protein production), multiple myeloma, obesity, hypothyroidism, and the nephrotic syndrome (through urinary loss).

The physiologic role of the plasma steroid-binding proteins has not been determined. Although these have been called transport proteins, there is no obligatory need for this as cortisol is soluble at concentrations spanning its physiologic effectiveness. Similarly there appears to be no obligatory role for CBG in glucocorticoid hormone action. For instance, tissue culture cells respond to cortisol in the absence of detectable CBG. Further, the free rather than the plasma-bound steroid is physiologically active, and physiologic stimuli that regulate cortisol levels respond to the free rather than the total steroid concentration. Thus, when the CBG levels are primarily elevated or depressed, there are elevations or depressions, respectively, of the total cortisol in plasma, but the free cortisol concentration remains the same. This point is critical for evaluation of states of glucocorticoid excess or deficiency.

That CBG may have some importance is suggested by its ubiquity in mammals, even though plasma levels vary enormously, and by the fact that congenital absence of CBG in humans has never been found. CBG or CBG-like proteins are located intracellularly, and in the kidney they may sequester and therefore prevent cortisol from occupying the mineralocorticoid receptors. This would preserve the latter for occupancy by aldosterone as the major salt-regulating hormone.

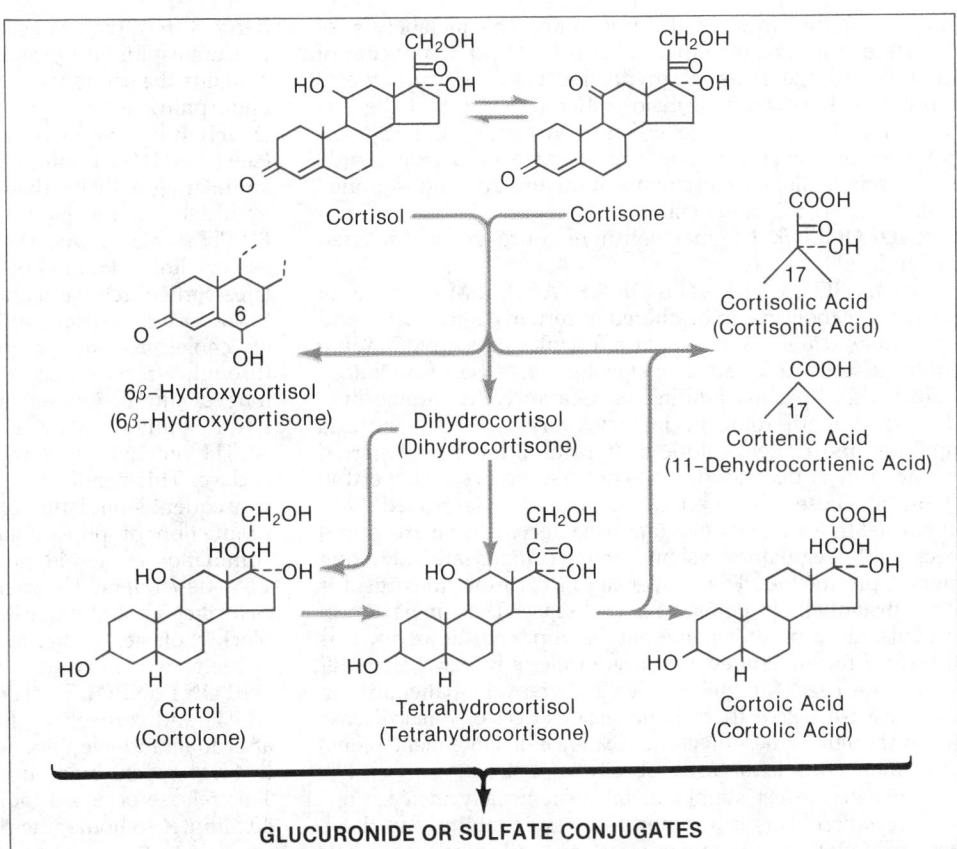

FIGURE 230-2. Metabolism of cortisol. See text. The interconversion of cortisol to cortisone is shown. The other steroid metabolites can be derivatives of either cortisol or cortisone. Structures shown and names are for the cortisol derivatives. The names of the cortisone derivatives are shown in parentheses. In some cases, only part of the steroid molecule is shown; in these cases numbers refer to the steroid carbons for orientation. For tetrahydrocortisol, tetrahydrocortisone, and their derivatives, the 3-hydroxyl and 5-hydrogen are shown in the α and β configurations, respectively, but both α and β orientations occur at both positions. For a more extensive discussion and references, see Baxter JD, Tyrrell JB: In Felig P, Baxter JD, Broadus AE, et al. (eds.): Endocrinology and Metabolism. 2nd ed. New York, McGraw-Hill Book Company, 1987, p 544.

By contrast, these intracellular proteins are not present in high concentrations in certain regions of the brain where these mineralocorticoid receptors are probably largely occupied by cortisol. Furthermore, the protein binding of steroids in the blood may buffer rapid changes in plasma free cortisol levels that would otherwise occur as a result of episodic release of cortisol from the adrenal gland.

MINERALOCORTICOIDS. Under physiologic conditions, about 60 per cent of the total plasma aldosterone is protein bound, largely to albumin. The binding is weaker than that of cortisol with CBG, and the free plasma aldosterone seems to be physiologically active.

DOC has potent mineralocorticoid activity, and its plasma levels are similar to those of aldosterone. However, DOC is not normally a physiologically important mineralocorticoid since over 95 per cent of it is bound to plasma proteins and thus its free levels are much lower than those of aldosterone.

METABOLISM OF ADRENAL STEROIDS

The hydrophobic steroids, although filtered by the renal glomerulus and excreted into the urine, are mostly reabsorbed. For example, only about 1 per cent of the cortisol produced daily is excreted unchanged in the urine. Nevertheless, the kidneys account for over 90 per cent of the excretion of metabolized steroids (DOC and corticosterone are exceptions); the remainder is lost in the gut. To render them capable of renal elimination, the steroids are inactivated and made more water soluble through enzymatic modifications. These involve hydroxylation of the keto groups, reduction of the double bond in the A ring, and conjugation at the 3 or 21 position with glucuronide or sulfate. These conversions occur mostly in liver, although during pregnancy the placenta assumes metabolic importance. The conversions alter the steroids so that the renal clearance of a major cortisol metabolite, tetrahydrocortisone glucuronide, is around 70 per cent that of the creatinine clearance. More than 50 metabolites of cortisol and aldosterone have been detected in humans. The pathways shown in Figure 230-2 appear generally to be dominant.

GLUCOCORTICOIDS. Cortisol is cleared from the plasma with a half-life of 80 to 120 minutes. About 70 per cent of infused cortisol, and presumably of that secreted, will be eliminated within 24 hours. The 11β-hydroxyl group of cortisol can be oxidized to the ketone, forming cortisone. The reaction is reversible. These two steroids have similar subsequent metabolic fates, and roughly equivalent quantities of metabolites of these steroids are produced. Quantitatively the most important subsequent modification involves reduction of the 3-keto moiety to form dihydrocortisol and dihydrocortisone, followed by a reduction of the 4,5 double bond to form tetrahydrocortisol and tetrahydrocortisone. When the 3-hydroxyl group is formed, over 95 per cent of the products are conjugated at this position to form the glucuronide and to a lesser extent the sulfate derivatives. Conjugates of these two steroids make up around 30 per cent of the urinary cortisol metabolites. The second major site for modification involves the reduction of the 20-ketone to a hydroxyl, with subsequent reduction of the A ring, resulting in cortol (11-OH) or cortolone (11-keto). These account for approximately 25 per cent of the cortisol metabolites. Alternatively, there can be conversion of the 21-hydroxyl to a COOH; cortoic (11-hydroxyl) or cortolonic (11-keto) acid results when the A ring is reduced and the C-20-hydroxyl is formed, and they account for about 10 per cent of the cortisol metabolites. Other minor pathways involve the C-17 modifications discussed above without A-ring reduction, removal of the C-17 side chain with formation of 17-keto or 17-COOH moieties, formation of the C-21 COOH (without C-20-keto) and 6β-hydroxylation. The latter modifications constitute a major pathway in infants in whom the esterification mechanism has not been developed and for the synthetic glucocorticoids used in therapy.

MINERALOCORTICOIDS. Aldosterone is cleared with a half-life of around 15 minutes. Its conversion to metabolites is so effective that very little aldosterone survives passage through the liver. Less than 0.5 per cent of the aldosterone appears in the urine in the free state. The metabolism of aldosterone is similar to that of cortisol. About 35 per cent of the steroid appears as tetrahydroaldosterone glucuronide (3 position). However, two major differences are that there is much less 11β-hydroxy to 11-keto conversion, and 15 to 20 per cent of the aldosterone appears as a C-18 glucuronide that is acid labile; measurements of the urinary "aldosterone" usually reflect this metabolite.

ANDROGENS. The metabolism of androgens is discussed in Ch. 235.

VARIATIONS IN RATES OF METABOLISM. The rate of steroid metabolism can be altered in certain clinical states and by various drugs. Agents that affect plasma steroid-binding proteins secondarily affect metabolism because of inhibitory influences of plasma binding on clearance. In chronic liver disease, hypothyroidism, infancy, very old age, anorexia nervosa, and protein calorie malnutrition, the rate of steroid metabolism is decreased. The converse occurs in hyperthyroidism. These states are in general not associated with abnormal free steroid levels (anorexia nervosa is an exception) because the regulatory systems tend to compensate by altering steroid production. The conversion of cortisone to cortisol is not substantially impaired in liver disease. The conversion of prednisone to prednisolone may be impaired, however. It is therefore recommended that prednisolone rather than prednisone be used for glucocorticoid therapy in patients with liver disease. Also, there is no major effect of renal disease (even though it does affect the clearance of some metabolites) or of most chronic diseases, obesity, and stress.

Drugs that affect steroid metabolism usually increase 6β-hydroxylation. This is a minor pathway in adults, and these drugs do not have a major effect on endogenous cortisol. They have a greater effect on the clearance of synthetic glucocorticoids such as dexamethasone and prednisone, and this is therefore an important consideration with steroid therapy or with the use of glucocorticoids to assess the hypothalamic-pituitary-adrenal axis. These drugs include mitotane, phenytoin, rifampicin, aminoglutethimide, and barbiturates.

230.3 Regulation of Adrenal Steroid Production

John D. Baxter

Adrenal cortisol and androgen production is regulated by the hypothalamic-pituitary-adrenal axis, whereas aldosterone production is regulated predominantly by the renin-angiotensin system and by potassium (Fig. 230–3). These systems allow for basal and circadian steroid production, regulation of plasma steroid levels in normal circumstances, and increased or decreased steroid production in response to a number of specific stimuli.

REGULATION OF GLUCOCORTICOID PRODUCTION

The hypothalamus, pituitary, and adrenal comprise a neuroendocrine axis concerned with regulation of cortisol production (see Ch. 225). Corticotropin releasing factor (CRF) and arginine vasopressin (AVP) are elaborated by the hypothalamus, travel through its portal system to the anterior pituitary where they stimulate the release of corticotropin (ACTH), which in turn increases adrenal cortisol production.

Three major types of mechanisms are involved in regulating cortisol release: (1) circadian rhythms of secretion are established by the brain, (2) a number of types of excitatory factors can increase cortisol production, and (3) production of CRF and ACTH are regulated negatively by glucocorticoids.

ACTH AND RELATED PEPTIDES. ACTH circulates free in the plasma with a half-life of around 10 minutes. It is derived from the proteolysis of proopiomelanocortin, a larger precursor pituitary protein of about 290 amino acids that also contains the sequences of several other proteins, including β-endorphin, α-, β-, and γ-melanocyte-stimulating hormones (MSH), β-lipotropin (β-LPH), and an amino-terminal fragment (see Ch. 221). Although MSH itself has the greatest pigment-stimulating activity, this activity in humans is due predominantly to MSH sequences contained within ACTH (α-MSH), β-LPH (β-MSH), and the amino-terminal fragment (γ-MSH), as very little MSH is present in the circulation. ACTH stimulates cortisol release within two to three minutes. This is due to increased cortisol synthesis primarily through stimulation of cholesterol to pregnenolone conversion, rather than through effects on secretion of stored hormone. More prolonged stimulation results in increased protein, RNA, and DNA synthesis with both hypertrophy and hyperplasia. ACTH binds to surface receptors and activates adenylate cyclase. This results in increased cyclic AMP generation with consequent stimulation of protein phosphorylation and of the production of phospholipids that may be involved in the stimulation of steroidogenesis. The actions of ACTH are also Ca^{++} dependent. These effects increase cholesterol side chain cleavage, cholesterol esterase and lipoprotein uptake, and block cholesterol ester synthesis with a resulting stimulation of the conversion of cholesterol to pregnenolone.

SPONTANEOUS RHYTHMS. The circadian rhythm of ACTH and cortisol results in decreasing release through the afternoon and evening. Secretion begins to increase around 3 to 4 A.M., peaks by around 8 A.M., and then begins to decline. This release occurs in pulses with intervals between them of 40 minutes to hours; the changes in overall cortisol production are due to the number of pulses that occur. These result in cortisol levels that vary enormously within minutes; thus, single plasma cortisol determinations may not give an adequate integrated assessment of overall cortisol production.

The spontaneous rhythm of cortisol secretion can be interrupted acutely by a variety of psychologic and physical factors. These can vary from seemingly mild stresses such as the confrontation for venipuncture to more severe ones such as the preparation for cardiac surgery or severe anxiety. However, there are major individual variations. Major trauma or surgery, severe illness, hypoglycemia, fever, burns, and intensive exercise are illustrative of physical stresses that increase cortisol production by up to sixfold. Minor illnesses such as upper respiratory infections or minor surgery have minimal or no influence. Variations in cortisol levels can be blunted by chronic diseases such as congestive heart failure with hepatic congestion due to delayed cortisol clearance and with central nervous system disease and pituitary tumors even when they do not affect basal ACTH release. In depression there is a circadian rhythm, but there can be increased cortisol secretion and impaired suppression by glucocorticoids. Serotonin antagonists such as cyproheptadine inhibit both spontaneous and stimulated changes in ACTH release.

FEEDBACK INHIBITION OF ACTH RELEASE. Glucocorticoids feedback-inhibit the release of both CRF and ACTH (see Ch. 221). ACTH levels are increased up to 10-fold to 20-fold in primary adrenal insufficiency. Conversely, endogenous levels and stress-induced increases of cortisol and ACTH are depressed with exogenous glucocorticoid administration. The feedback inhibition in response to glucocorticoids occurs within a few minutes, is progressive with continual exposure in a dose- and time-dependent fashion, affects both basal and stress-stimulated release, and is reversible. Although there are considerable individual variations, administration of a large dose of glucocorticoids for a few days does not, in general, result in suppression of pituitary function for more than a few hours; more prolonged exposure is accompanied by substantial suppression. Thus after several years of glucocorticoid therapy and then withdrawal of steroid administration, a year may be required for the hypothalamic-pituitary-

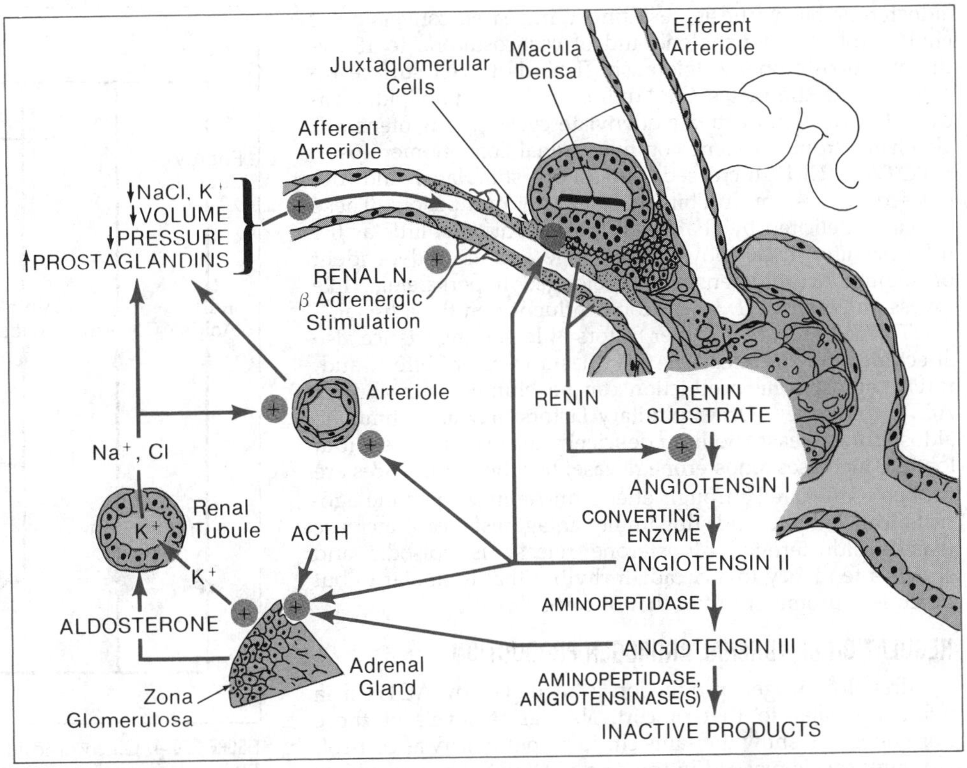

FIGURE 230–3. Renin-angiotensin system. The plus and minus signs indicate stimulation and inhibition, respectively. (Reprinted from Baxter JD, Perloff D, Hsueh W, et al.: In Felig P, Baxter JD, Broadus AE, et al. (eds.): Endocrinology and Metabolism. 2nd ed. New York, McGraw-Hill Book Company, 1987, p 701.)

adrenal axis to return to normal functioning. Although significant suppression occurs at both the hypothalamic and pituitary levels, the quantitative contribution of each of them has not been clarified.

REGULATION OF MINERALOCORTICOID PRODUCTION

Aldosterone production is controlled predominantly by the renin-angiotensin system and potassium, although other factors such as sodium, ACTH, dopamine, and serotonin also affect aldosterone secretion (Fig. 230–3). The renin-angiotensin system is important for adaptive blood pressure changes and is involved in the pathogenesis of some forms of hypertension.

RENIN. Renin, a glycoprotein of 274 amino acids, is produced in the juxtaglomerular cells of the afferent renal arteriole as a precursor protein (prorenin) that is cleaved to yield active renin. These cells release renin into the circulation where it has a half-life of around 15 minutes. Although prorenin is also made in other tissues, the biologic role for this is uncertain, and extrarenal prorenin does not contribute to the plasma renin. The release of renin is stimulated by lowering the blood pressure, assumption of the erect posture, salt depletion, β-adrenergic or central nervous system stimulation, and certain prostaglandins. It is inhibited by increases in blood pressure (except with malignant hypertension), salt loading, angiotensin II, vasopressin, potassium, calcium, β-adrenergic antagonists, α-methyldopa, clonidine, and inhibitors of prostaglandin synthesis such as indomethacin.

Three types of influences mediate changes in renin release: (1) Changes in renal tubular sodium chloride concentration are detected by the macula densa, a specialized segment of the distal tubule that makes contact with the juxtaglomerular cells of the afferent arteriole just before it enters the glomerulus. This information is transmitted to the juxtaglomerular cells so that factors that reduce volume or lower the plasma sodium and chloride levels (e.g., dehydration, fluid or blood loss) increase renin release. (2) Renal baroreceptors stimulate renin release in response to decreases in renal perfusion pressure as with fluid loss or decreases in blood pressure. These receptors can function independently of innervation and salt delivery and respond more to changes in pressure

than to the absolute pressure. (3) Renal sympathetic nerves that terminate in the juxtaglomerular cells and smooth muscle cells of the renal afferent arterioles secrete norepinephrine, which in turn stimulates renin release through β-adrenergic receptors. Blockage of this mechanism by agents such as propranolol probably explains how they decrease renin release. However, catecholamines can have other indirect effects on renin release through influences on renal blood flow and glomerular filtration.

Renin acts in the plasma and cleaves renin substrate (angiotensinogen) to yield the decapeptide angiotensin I. Angiotensinogen contains over 400 amino acids, is secreted by the liver, and its level can be increased by estrogens and glucocorticoids. Angiotensin I is not known to have physiologically important actions; instead it serves as a substrate for production of angiotensin II. Normally the production of angiotensin I is rate limiting for angiotensin II generation.

CONVERTING ENZYME. The conversion of angiotensin I to the octapeptide angiotensin II is catalyzed by converting enzyme that is present in a number of tissues and in high concentrations in the lung. In certain pulmonary diseases there can be decreases or increases in the plasma levels of the enzyme, although these changes do not appear to have a physiologically important effect on angiotensin II generation. Converting enzyme also catalyzes other reactions; important among these is the inactivation of bradykinin. Inhibitors of converting enzyme, captopril and enalapril, have come into widespread usage in the treatment of hypertension and heart failure.

ANGIOTENSIN II. Angiotensin II is a potent vasoconstrictor with direct effects on arterioles. It inhibits directly the release of renin by the juxtaglomerular cells. Finally it is a potent stimulator of aldosterone release. The hormone also has other complex effects on the kidney that affect salt balance, possibly through influences on kallikreins and prostaglandins. Plasma concentrations of angiotensin II can vary up to 25-fold; the hormone has a half-life of only one to two minutes. There are several breakdown products of angiotensin II. One of these, angiotensin III, a polypeptide of seven amino acids, has angiotensin II activity, but its biologic importance is probably less than that of angiotensin II.

Angiotensin II stimulates both early and late steps in

aldosterone biosynthesis, resulting in increased conversion of cholesterol to pregnenolene and of corticosterone to 18-hydroxycorticosterone. Angiotensin II binds to cell surface receptors and stimulates Ca++ influx and phospholipid turnover, but does not activate adenylate cyclase. Angiotensin II also has a tropic influence on the adrenal zona glomerulosa.

POTASSIUM. Increased potassium stimulates and decreased potassium inhibits aldosterone production. These effects are elicited by changes in potassium of as little as 0.1 mEq per liter in the physiologic range and are independent of sodium or angiotensin II. Prolonged hyperkalemia, like excess angiotensin II, has a tropic influence on the adrenal.

OTHER FACTORS. Other factors of lesser importance also affect aldosterone release. ACTH has a transient effect, and, rarely, aldosterone production can be blunted with chronic ACTH deficiency. Other pituitary factors may also stimulate aldosterone release. Sodium deficiency decreases and sodium loading increases aldosterone release, but these influences are probably mediated through effects on renin. Dopamine agonists can inhibit and dopamine antagonists can increase plasma aldosterone. Aldosterone release is episodic and shows a tendency to a circadian rhythm that is similar to but much less prominent than that of cortisol.

REGULATION OF ADRENAL ANDROGEN PRODUCTION

Adrenal androgen production is regulated by ACTH in a manner similar to that of cortisol. Plasma levels of these hormones also show the same circadian periodicity as cortisol, although this is masked in the case of DHEA-S because of its prolonged plasma half-life. Adrenal androgen release is also altered during prepuberty (adrenarche) by poorly understood mechanisms. Further, it should be remembered that androgens released by the testes and ovaries contribute to plasma androgen levels.

230.4 Actions of Adrenal Steroids

John D. Baxter

GLUCOCORTICOIDS

Glucocorticoids have diverse actions that affect most mammalian tissues and are also essential for survival, at least in times of stress.

INTERMEDIARY METABOLISM. Glucocorticoids have multiple influences on glucose metabolism with diverse secondary effects (Fig. 230–4). In most tissues these steroids inhibit glucose uptake. Liver, heart, brain, and erythrocytes are exceptions. In many of these tissues the steroids also block protein and nucleic acid synthesis and stimulate turnover of these macromolecules. In adipose tissue the steroids inhibit lipolysis and block lipogenesis. In liver the steroids stimulate glycogen deposition, gluconeogenesis, the ability of other hormones to stimulate gluconeogenesis, and lipoprotein synthesis. Gluconeogenesis is further facilitated because of increased availability of glycerol and amino acid substrate due to the effects in peripheral tissues. The steroids also tend to stimulate the appetite, and in adrenal insufficiency there is anorexia. Finally, glucocorticoids tend to blunt the actions of insulin and decrease the affinity for insulin binding to its receptors.

The net effect of these influences is a glucocorticoid-induced tendency to hyperglycemia, ketosis, and hyperlipidemia. However, in normal subjects the elevated levels of glucose increase insulin release that in turn blunts the effects of the steroid. However, in diabetes or latent diabetes, significant hyperglycemia and insulin resistance can ensue. Lipogenesis induced by secondary increases in plasma insulin levels along with the increased food intake due to appetite stimulation

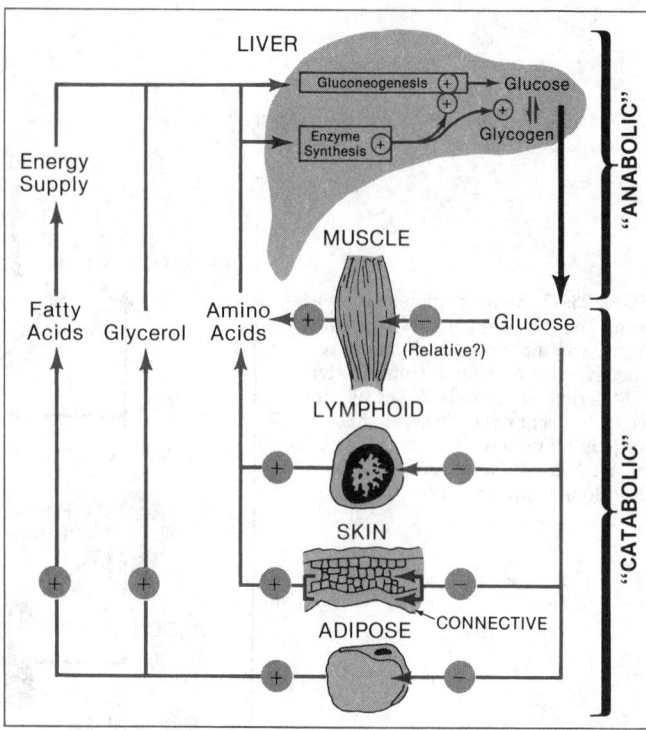

FIGURE 230–4. Glucocorticoid influences on intermediary metabolism. Plus and minus signs refer to stimulation and inhibition, respectively. (Modified from Baxter JD, Forsham PH: Tissue effects of glucocorticoids. Am J Med 53:579, 1972.)

may explain the truncal and sometimes generalized obesity seen in Cushing's syndrome. Conversely, in adrenal insufficiency there is a tendency to hypoglycemia; usually this is not marked in the adult, but it can be significant if there is concomitant fasting. Many of the actions of glucocorticoids on intermediary metabolism can be perceived as a protection against fasting; there is peripheral catabolism with sparing of essential tissues (heart, brain, blood cells) to make available substrate for maintenance of the blood sugar levels.

These actions of glucocorticoids on intermediary metabolism also explain many other effects of glucocorticoid excess. Thus inhibition of metabolic functions in peripheral tissues may explain glucocorticoid-induced myopathy, inhibition of immunologic and inflammatory responses, poor wound healing, thinning of the skin, striae, and osteoporosis.

INFLAMMATORY AND IMMUNOLOGIC RESPONSES. In excess, glucocorticoids suppress inflammatory and immunologic responses, but it is not clear whether they normally modulate immunologic systems. In excess, glucocorticoids inhibit antigen processing; T cell function; synthesis of cellular mediators of the inflammatory response such as interleukins, plasminogen activator, lymphokines, other active peptides, and prostaglandins and other eicosanoids; cellular migration and action at sites of inflammation; and inflammatory reactions themselves. In general they do not affect most antibody responses, although there are a few exceptions. Some populations of lymphocytes are killed by glucocorticoids; this explains the efficacy of these steroids in treating certain leukemias such as acute lymphoblastic leukemia of childhood. The steroids also affect mononuclear cell trafficking and tend to decrease blood monocyte, lymphocyte, and eosinophil levels and increase polymorphonuclear leukocytes; there are reciprocal changes during adrenal insufficiency. Interestingly, glucocorticoids do not produce any permanent impairment of the immunologic system.

OTHER ACTIONS. Glucocorticoids can also elevate the circulating levels of erythrocytes and platelets, and decreases in these elements are seen with adrenal insufficiency.

Glucocorticoids affect the cardiovascular system. There is a tendency to hypertension and increased atherosclerosis in Cushing's syndrome and to hypotension and decreased cardiac output in Addison's disease. Some of these effects can be due to mineralocorticoid actions of glucocorticoids (discussed below), but there are separate glucocorticoid actions on the heart, the production of vasoactive substances, elements of the renin-angiotensin system, ion balance, and the glomerular filtration rate.

Glucocorticoids have complex actions on calcium metabolism. Hypercalcemia can occur in Addison's disease. Hypocalcemia does not result from glucocorticoid excess (probably because of compensatory changes in parathyroid hormone), but these steroids can be used to ameliorate certain types of hypercalcemia. They affect the cellular distribution of calcium, and also block calcium uptake by the intestine and certain bone cell functions. The steroids decrease renal calcium and phosphate reabsorption, and hypercalciuria and an increased incidence of renal stones occur in Cushing's syndrome. These actions result in negative calcium balance and osteopenia in glucocorticoid excess states.

Glucocorticoids penetrate the blood-brain barrier and have complex actions on the brain. These include a number of effects on brain enzymes and on the permeability of the blood-brain barrier. Changes in mood and occasionally psychosis are observed in both glucocorticoid excess and deficiency states. However, with glucocorticoid therapy, euphoria is common. Addisonian subjects commonly have increased sensitivity to a variety of sensory stimuli such as smell or taste. The mechanisms of these influences are poorly understood. Glucocorticoids increase the intraocular pressure, probably by blocking fluid uptake by the trabecular meshwork. Glucocorticoid therapy can precipitate glaucoma in susceptible individuals and can enhance cataract formation.

In the gastrointestinal tract glucocorticoids inhibit DNA synthesis and tend to enhance stimuli to gastric acid secretion. They probably also enhance the tendency to form duodenal ulcers and, in high doses, the tendency to develop gastritis.

In excess, glucocorticoids inhibit linear growth, as a result of their inhibitory influences on a number of tissues. However, glucocorticoid action is required for a number of developmental processes. One particularly important process is the synthesis of surfactant in the lung. Lack of glucocorticoid induction of this factor in premature birth contributes to the respiratory distress syndrome of the newborn.

Complex interrelationships exist between glucocorticoids and other hormones. Glucocorticoids inhibit vasopressin release; conversely, ACTH deficiency can lead to hyponatremia with water intoxication. Glucocorticoids secondarily increase insulin and parathyroid hormone (PTH) levels, and in some cases blunt the production of growth hormone, prolactin, insulin, glucagon, thyroid-stimulating hormone (TSH), and testosterone. Multiple synergisms and antagonisms between glucocorticoids and other hormones also exist at the cellular level. For example, they are synergistic with epinephrine and glucagon in stimulating hepatic gluconeogenesis. These effects are sometimes termed permissive glucocorticoid actions.

STRESS. Why glucocorticoids are essential for survival in times of stress is poorly understood. Two factors are probably operative. First, stress increases the production of a number of biologically active substances such as catecholamines, prostaglandins and other arachidonic acid metabolites, proteases, and kinins. Glucocorticoids, by contrast, tend to blunt the production and actions of these substances, which, if left unchecked during stress, would lead to shock and vascular decompensation. Second, the stimulation of cardiovascular functions by glucocorticoids may be critical in times of stress when other compensatory systems may be less effective.

MOLECULAR MECHANISMS OF ACTION. Glucocorticoids penetrate cells and bind to intracellular receptors; the resulting hormone-receptor complexes then bind to specific sites on the DNA where they enhance the ability of RNA polymerase to stimulate transcription of glucocorticoid-responsive genes (see Ch. 221). The protein products of the resulting mRNA's then mediate the glucocorticoid responses. In some circumstances the steroids probably block transcription by similar mechanisms. Also, some glucocorticoid effects occur by mechanisms that do not involve stimulation of transcription.

MINERALOCORTICOIDS

Mineralocorticoid hormones act on kidney, gut, salivary glands, and sweat glands to affect the balance of electrolytes. Direct actions on other tissues including brain, mammary gland, placenta, and pituitary have been reported, but with less complete evidence. Thus the spectrum of mineralocorticoid action is more restricted than that of glucocorticoid action.

In the kidney, the most important target organ, mineralocorticoids promote the reabsorption of sodium ion and secretion of potassium ion in the cortical collecting tubules, and possibly in the connecting segment of the nephron, and stimulate the secretion of hydrogen ion in the medullary collecting tubules. Thus, with mineralocorticoid excess, there is sodium retention, hypokalemia, and alkalosis. In primary mineralocorticoid excess, hypertension develops with time. With mineralocorticoid deficiency there is sodium ion loss and a tendency to hyperkalemia and acidosis. The overall effects of mineralocorticoids on both sodium and potassium ions also depend on the level of salt intake. Increased sodium intake results in more tubular sodium for reabsorption; this enhances potassium secretion. Conversely, sodium restriction diminishes aldosterone-induced kaliuresis. In most circumstances with persistent mineralocorticoid excess, the sodium retention that occurs reaches a limit such that the body "escapes" from further sodium retention. This is due to secondary increases in the secretion of other factors or hormones such as atrial natriuretic factor (ANF) and changes in renal hemodynamics with compensating influences of sodium excretion. Exceptions are the secondary hyperaldosteronism of heart failure and of cirrhosis with ascites in which sodium retention is progressive. As noted, hyperkalemia directly stimulates aldosterone secretion, which in turn enhances renal potassium excretion. This servomechanism forms an important component of the body's defense against hyperkalemia.

Mineralocorticoid actions are probably mediated through molecular mechanisms similar to those described above for cortisol and in Ch. 221. The mineralocorticoid receptors bind aldosterone and DOC with high affinity; they also bind cortisol with 1 to 2 per cent of the affinity for aldosterone. Since plasma free cortisol concentrations are around 100-fold higher than those of aldosterone, there is probably some occupancy of mineralocorticoid receptors by cortisol, although they may be blunted by other cellular proteins that sequester cortisol. The synthetic steroid 9α-fluorocortisol binds tightly to mineralocorticoid receptors and is used for mineralocorticoid replacement therapy, since it is more stable than aldosterone after oral administration. Mineralocorticoid antagonists such as spironolactone bind to these receptors and block aldosterone action.

Aldosterone stimulates the synthesis of several renal proteins that result in increases in (1) sodium permeability in the apical membrane exposed to the tubular lumen; (2) various mitochondrial enzymes that increase cellular ATP and thereby enhance the actions of the Na^+-K^+ ATPase; (3) the Na^+-K^+ ATPase; and (4) probably other as yet unidentified factors of the basolateral membrane. These combined actions result in Na^+ reabsorption. Potassium ion secretion increases secondarily to the Na^+-K^+ exchange because of the pumping action of the Na^+-K^+ ATPase; however, other mechanisms must also operate since there can be independent actions of aldosterone on Na^+ and K^+.

Aldosterone-stimulated renal tubular transport of hydrogen ion, about which little is known, can probably occur independently of the effects on Na⁺ and K⁺. However, potassium ion deficiency decreases Na⁺-K⁺ exchange, which in turn increases the Na⁺-H⁺ exchange and hydrogen ion excretion. As in the case of potassium, hydrogen ion loss can be blunted with sodium restriction. The mineralocorticoid-induced alkalosis is also promoted by hydrogen ion movement into cells in exchange for losses in potassium.

The major known extrarenal targets for aldosterone are the sweat and salivary glands, ileum, and colon where the steroid promotes potassium loss and sodium retention. These actions are ordinarily minor in terms of overall salt balance.

230.5 Laboratory Evaluation of Adrenocortical Function

J. Blake Tyrrell

The function of the adrenal cortex is best assessed by plasma steroid assays. Certain urinary assays remain useful, however, despite the disadvantage of 24-hour collections. Assays for plasma levels of tropic hormones, e.g., ACTH, and related peptides, renin and angiotensin, can also be useful. The following considerations must be remembered when using these assays. (1) Current assays for plasma steroids measure total hormone concentration, not bioactive free hormone. (2) Plasma levels of cortisol and ACTH vary greatly because of episodic secretion and many other factors (see below); thus single determinations should not in general be relied upon for a definitive diagnosis. (3) In assessing adrenal function, stimulation and suppression testing provide the most definitive information.

GLUCOCORTICOID FUNCTION

ACTH AND RELATED PEPTIDES. Immunoassays for ACTH are extremely useful but are technically difficult. ACTH is unstable in plasma and adheres to glass; specimens should be collected in anticoagulated plastic or silicon-coated tubes on ice, centrifuged in the cold without delay, and frozen until assayed. The normal range of plasma ACTH in the morning (8 to 9 A.M.) is 20 to 100 pg per milliliter in most assays. Values at other times of the day are lower, and consideration of this episodic secretion is important in interpretation.

Plasma ACTH levels are primarily used to differentiate pituitary, adrenal, and other causes of adrenal dysfunction. Thus, in patients with cortisol deficiency elevated ACTH levels (generally greater than 250 pg per milliliter) confirm the diagnosis of primary adrenal insufficiency (Addison's disease). Conversely, with secondary adrenal insufficiency due to hypothalamic or pituitary disease, or steroid therapy, ACTH levels will be low normal or subnormal (<50 pg per milliliter). In states of cortisol excess (Cushing's syndrome), a suppressed or undetectable ACTH level (<20 pg per milliliter) is diagnostic of an adrenal tumor hypersecreting cortisol or of exogenous glucocorticoid administration. With ACTH-producing pituitary tumors (Cushing's disease), plasma ACTH levels are normal to modestly elevated (40 to 200 pg per milliliter), whereas in the ectopic ACTH syndrome they are usually elevated markedly (100 to >1000 pg per milliliter). ACTH levels in the two latter conditions may overlap, but very high (>300 pg per milliliter) values point to an ectopic tumor. Plasma ACTH levels are also elevated in congenital adrenal hyperplasia proportional to the extent of cortisol deficiency, and are markedly elevated in pituitary tumors that arise following bilateral adrenalectomy (Nelson's syndrome).

Immunoassays for other peptides derived from proopiomelanocortin are also available. The antisera usually measure both β-LPH and β-endorphin. Reported normal morning values of immunoreactive β-LPH/β-endorphin are 20 to 200 pg per milliliter. Levels of these peptides vary similarly to those of ACTH, but because of its longer plasma half-life, β-LPH levels show less episodic variability than ACTH, and β-LPH is considerably more stable than ACTH in plasma.

PLASMA CORTISOL AND RELATED STEROIDS. Plasma cortisol is most frequently measured by radioimmunoassay; current antisera show little cross-reactivity with other natural or synthetic steroids. Competitive protein binding and high-performance liquid chromatography assays are also in use. Normal values of plasma cortisol vary with the circadian rhythm of ACTH. Mean levels at 8 A.M. are 10 to 12 μg per deciliter with a range of 3 to 20 μg per deciliter. Values at 4 to 6 P.M. are approximately 50 per cent of the morning levels, although there is great variability. Values obtained between 10 P.M. and 2 A.M. are less than 3 μg per deciliter and may be unmeasurable. Episodic variability and the numerous conditions increasing cortisol secretion or CBG concentrations (Table 230–2) limit the utility of single cortisol determinations.

Measurement of plasma 11-deoxycortisol (compound S) is used in metyrapone testing of pituitary-adrenal reserve (see below).

URINARY CORTICOSTEROIDS. Measurements of urinary steroids have been traditionally used to evaluate adrenal function and provide an integrated assessment of steroid production and excretion. With the exception of urinary free cortisol, these methods are less advantageous and have been largely supplanted by measurements of plasma cortisol or ACTH levels.

Urine free cortisol, although less than 1 per cent of total adrenal cortisol secretion, is a useful measurement in the diagnosis of hypercortisolism. The urine is extracted and the steroid is then measured by radioimmunoassay or competitive protein binding. Normal values range from 20 to 100 μg per 24 hours. Elevated levels are almost always present in Cushing's syndrome but not in simple obesity; this ability to separate these conditions is a major advantage. Urinary cortisol excretion is increased by any condition that increases adrenal cortisol secretion (Table 230–2) and is decreased in renal failure.

Urinary 17-hydroxycorticosteroids (17-OHCS) and 17-ketogenic steroids (17-KGS) measure steroid metabolites, predominantly those of cortisol and 11-deoxycortisol. These methods are currently not recommended in most situations, since the levels are altered in many disease states and the assays are subject to interference by commonly used drugs and medications.

SUPPRESSION TESTS. Suppression tests evaluate the ability of dexamethasone, a potent synthetic glucocorticoid not measured in current cortisol assays, to inhibit ACTH and cortisol secretion. In Cushing's syndrome glucocorticoids do not normally inhibit ACTH release, and this abnormality is diagnostic. There are two types of dexamethasone suppression tests: (1) Low-dose tests are used to document the presence of Cushing's syndrome. (2) High-dose tests are used to distinguish the various causes of Cushing's syndrome. The techniques for performing these tests and the expected responses are summarized in Table 230–3.

TABLE 230–2. CONDITIONS CAUSING ELEVATED CORTISOL LEVELS

Increased CBG	Increased Secretion
Estrogen therapy	Spontaneous Cushing's syndrome
Pregnancy	Exercise
Hyperthyroidism	Physical stress
Diabetes mellitus	Anxiety
Hematologic disorders	Depression
Congenital	Starvation
	Anorexia nervosa
	Alcoholism
	Chronic renal failure

TABLE 230–3. DEXAMETHASONE SUPPRESSION TESTS

Low-Dose Tests

Overnight test
Dexamethasone 1 mg p.o. at 11 P.M.; plasma cortisol at 8 to 9 A.M.
Normal response—plasma cortisol <5 μg/dl

Two-day test
Dexamethasone 0.5 mg p.o. q6h for 8 doses; plasma cortisol 1 hr after last dose and 24-hr urine free cortisol and/or 17-OHCS during second day of dexamethasone

Normal response—plasma cortisol <5 μg/dl; urine free cortisol <25 μg/24 hr; urine 17-OHCS <4 mg/24 hr or <1 mg/gram urine creatinine

High-Dose Tests

Overnight test
Dexamethasone 8 mg p.o. at 11 P.M.; plasma cortisol before and at 8 to 9 A.M. after dexamethasone

Response—Cushing's disease; suppression of cortisol to <50% of baseline; ectopic ACTH/adrenal tumors: no cortisol suppression

Two-day test
Dexamethasone 2.0 mg p.o. q6h for 8 doses; plasma cortisol before dexamethasone and 1 hr after last dose; 24-hr urine free cortisol and/or 17-OHCS before dexamethasone and during second day
Response—Cushing's disease; suppression of plasma or urine steroids to <50% of baseline; ectopic ACTH/adrenal tumors: no steroid suppression

Low-Dose Dexamethasone Tests. The overnight 1 mg dexamethasone suppression test is an excellent screening procedure for Cushing's syndrome. The test can be used on an ambulatory basis, and in this setting abnormal responses occur in about 95 per cent of patients with Cushing's syndrome. False positive responses occur in 25 per cent of hospitalized and chronically ill patients, in 15 per cent of obese patients, and in a number of other conditions, including acute illness, anxiety, depression, alcoholism, anorexia nervosa, estrogen therapy, and uremia. Drugs that accelerate dexamethasone metabolism, especially phenytoin and phenobarbital, also cause false positive results. The two-day low-dose test provides the same information as the 1 mg overnight test, but is more time consuming.

High-Dose Dexamethasone Tests. Glucocorticoids in pharmacologic doses suppress ACTH and cortisol secretion in most patients with ACTH-producing pituitary tumors, but not in patients with adrenal and ectopic tumors. Two tests are available (Table 230–3). The overnight high-dose test is simpler and more accurate than the two-day high-dose test. Approximately 90 per cent of patients with pituitary ACTH-producing tumors have suppression of cortisol levels to less than 50 per cent of baseline levels, whereas about 95 per cent of those with adrenal tumors or the ectopic ACTH syndrome do not achieve this degree of suppression. The two-day high-dose test is more time consuming and less reliable in that 15 to 30 per cent of patients with Cushing's disease fail to achieve greater than 50 per cent suppression of urine 17-OHCS, urine free cortisol, or plasma cortisol.

STIMULATION TESTS. These procedures assess the reserve capacity of the hypothalamic-pituitary-adrenal axis and its ability to respond appropriately to stressful situations. These tests act at different sites of the axis and thus can be used to assess its different functions.

CRF Testing. Corticotropin releasing factor (CRF) testing may have future utility in the diagnosis of adrenal insufficiency and Cushing's syndrome. CRF is generally administered intravenously in a dose of 1 μg per kilogram of body weight. ACTH and cortisol secretion peak at 30 to 60 minutes and may be sustained for several hours. Flushing and occasionally hypotension have been observed, and thus the test should be performed with the patient supine. Subnormal ACTH and cortisol responses occur in secondary adrenocorticoid insufficiency due either to hypothalamic-pituitary dis-

orders or to glucocorticoid therapy, and a subnormal cortisol response with high ACTH levels occurs in primary adrenocortical insufficiency. Most but not all patients with pituitary ACTH-producing tumors have abnormally increased ACTH and cortisol responses, whereas there is no response in patients with cortisol-producing adrenal tumors and in most patients with ectopic ACTH-producing tumors.

ACTH Testing. The administration of ACTH, which allows direct assessment of adrenal glucocorticoid reserve, is useful in the diagnosis of both primary and secondary adrenal insufficiency. The rapid ACTH stimulation test is performed with synthetic human α1–24 ACTH (Cortrosyn), which has full biologic potency and a lesser incidence of allergic reactions than previously used ACTH preparations. The test is performed by administering 250 μg of Cortrosyn intravenously or intramuscularly; plasma cortisol levels are obtained prior to and at 30 or 60 minutes after ACTH administration. Normally the peak plasma cortisol level is greater than 15 to 20 μg per deciliter, depending on the laboratory, and will increase by at least 5 μg per deciliter. Subnormal responses to ACTH stimulation establish the diagnosis of adrenal insufficiency. A normal response excludes primary adrenal failure and complete secondary insufficiency, but it does not exclude partial secondary adrenal insufficiency. A normal response to ACTH in the latter case occurs when there is sufficient basal ACTH secretion to prevent adrenal atrophy but not enough pituitary reserve to respond to stress. When this infrequent situation is suspected, the issue can be resolved with the use of metyrapone or insulin hypoglycemia testing.

The rapid ACTH stimulation test gives no information regarding the cause of adrenal dysfunction. This distinction can be made by measuring either the basal plasma ACTH level, which is elevated in primary adrenal insufficiency and is low in secondary adrenal insufficiency, or the aldosterone response to ACTH stimulation (normally an increment in the plasma aldosterone of at least 4 ng per deciliter above baseline). The latter test is based on the fact that the zona glomerulosa responds acutely to ACTH and that this response is preserved in secondary adrenal insufficiency, but is deficient in the primary form in which the entire adrenal cortex is destroyed.

Metyrapone Testing. Metyrapone inhibits the synthesis of cortisol predominantly by blocking 11β-hydroxylation. As a result, ACTH secretion increases and drives the production of steroids proximal to the site of the block. Thus, measurement of plasma 11-deoxycortisol following metyrapone administration can be used to assess the functional reserve of both the adrenal and pituitary. The test is mostly used when secondary adrenal insufficiency is suspected in the setting of a normal ACTH stimulation test. The overnight test is most commonly used because of its rapidity and simplicity; because of the short duration of inhibition of cortisol synthesis there is little risk of precipitating acute adrenal insufficiency. Metyrapone is given at midnight with food, and plasma for 11-deoxycortisol and cortisol determinations is obtained at 8 A.M. The dose of metyrapone* is 2 grams for patients less than 70 kg; 2.5 grams for those 70 to 90 kg; and 3 grams for patients weighing more than 90 kg. A plasma cortisol value less than 10 μg per deciliter indicates adequate 11β-hydroxylase inhibition, and in normal persons plasma 11-deoxycortisol increases to greater than 7 μg per deciliter. A normal response to metyrapone indicates adequate function of both the pituitary and adrenals. A subnormal response establishes the diagnosis of adrenal insufficiency and correlates well with deficient responses to stress and hypoglycemia. The test per se does not differentiate primary and secondary causes. However, in the presence of a normal response to the rapid ACTH stimulation test a subnormal response to metyrapone indicates secondary adrenal insufficiency.

---

*This dose is not listed in the manufacturer's directive.

Insulin Hypoglycemia Testing (see Ch. 232). Hypoglycemia elicits a stress response that stimulates ACTH secretion and, as a consequence, cortisol release. A normal cortisol response to hypoglycemia indicates a normal hypothalamic-pituitary-adrenal axis and rules out adrenal insufficiency or decreased pituitary ACTH reserve. This test is most often utilized in the evaluation of suspected hypothalamic or pituitary disorders, since growth hormone reserve can be assessed simultaneously with that of ACTH.

MINERALOCORTICOID FUNCTION

PLASMA RENIN. Assessment of plasma renin is essential in the diagnosis of states of excess and deficient mineralocorticoid secretion; it is also helpful in the evaluation of other types of hypertension (see Ch. 47). Currently used assays do not measure the plasma renin concentration directly, but instead measure the plasma renin activity (PRA) by quantifying the amount of angiotensin I (AI) generated over time in the patient's plasma. The normal values of PRA depend on the salt intake and postural status. In subjects with moderate salt intake (around 110 mEq Na+ per day) and in the supine and standing positions, for one hour, the plasma renin activity ranges, respectively, from 1 to 3 and 3 to 6 ng of AI generated per milliliter per hour. In individuals in whom salt has been restricted (20 mEq Na+ per day) for four days and who have been in the upright posture for two hours the values range from 5 to 10 ng AI per milliliter per hour. In clinical practice, diuretic therapy is the most commonly observed factor that increases the PRA. In patients with primary hyperaldosteronism the PRA is characteristically suppressed. With aldosterone-producing adenomas, the PRA is unresponsive or only weakly responsive to provocative stimuli, whereas in those with primary aldosteronism with bilateral hyperplasia, the PRA, although suppressed, does respond to such stimuli.

In patients with borderline low PRA in whom primary aldosterone excess is suspected, stimulation tests with measurement of PRA may be necessary. Patients can be subjected to salt restriction (10 to 20 mEq of sodium per day for five days), or given 40 to 60 mg of furosemide intravenously, or 50 mg of captopril, orally; blood samples are then taken after one to four hours in the upright posture. If the plasma renin does not increase under these conditions primary aldosteronism is probable. Caution should be exercised in performing these tests, since severe and life-threatening volume depletion or hypokalemia could ensue; these risks must be weighed before the test is performed.

ALDOSTERONE AND 18-HYDROXYCORTICOSTERONE MEASUREMENTS. These measurements are utilized in the diagnosis of primary aldosteronism and in the differentiation of its subtypes of adenoma and hyperplasia. Plasma measurements ordinarily involve extraction and chromatography of the steroid followed by radioimmunoassay. The urine measurements ordinarily quantify by radioimmunoassay the 18-glucuronide metabolite of aldosterone (about 15 per cent of the total aldosterone production). Less commonly, urinary tetrahydroaldosterone is measured.

Measurements should be made after adequate sodium repletion (a sodium intake of at least 120 mEq per 24 hours for four days) and withdrawal of diuretics for at least two to three weeks, and in the case of plasma measurements after at least six hours of recumbency. Normal values for aldosterone excretion are 4 to 17 μg per 24 hours; elevated values are typically seen with both adrenal adenoma and hyperplasia causing primary aldosteronism. Basal plasma values in the supine patient are usually 4 to 12 ng per deciliter. Plasma aldosterone levels are almost always elevated above 20 ng per deciliter in patients with an aldosterone-producing adenoma. By contrast, with primary aldosteronism due to bilateral adrenal hyperplasia, plasma aldosterone levels are usually less than 20 ng per deciliter and are commonly in the normal

range. Plasma and urinary aldosterone values must be interpreted with caution in the presence of hypokalemia that results in decreased aldosterone production; normal aldosterone levels may be found in patients with primary aldosteronism and hypokalemia.

Plasma 18-hydroxycorticosterone (18-OHB) measurements (normal range 10 to 30 ng per deciliter) are also especially useful in the differential diagnosis of primary aldosteronism. When sampled at 8 A.M. after overnight recumbency and during a high-salt diet as described above, plasma 18-OHB levels almost always exceed 100 ng per deciliter in patients with an aldosterone-producing adenoma. Levels are less than this with primary aldosteronism due to bilateral hyperplasia.

The use of both aldosterone and 18-OHB measurements has greatly simplified the diagnosis and differential diagnosis of primary aldosteronism. However, in circumstances in which plasma renin values are suppressed and aldosterone values are normal or borderline, suppression tests can be performed. These include (1) high-sodium diet (300 mEq per day for five days), (2) fludrocortisone acetate (9α-fluorocortisol) 0.3 mg per day for three days, or (3) 2 liters of saline intravenously over 4 hours. These maneuvers reduce plasma aldosterone levels to less than 5 ng per deciliter in normal subjects, but the levels ordinarily exceed 10 ng per deciliter in patients with primary aldosteronism.

Two additional methods for differentiating primary aldosteronism due to an adenoma from that due to hyperplasia take advantage of the fact that plasma aldosterone and 18-OHB levels in hyperplasia, but not adenoma, are under control of the renin-angiotensin system. The first involves postural studies. The plasma aldosterone is initially measured in the supine position at 8 A.M. after four days of a sodium intake of at least 120 mEq per 24 hours and then subsequently after two to four hours in the upright posture. In patients with an adenoma there is generally either no increase or an actual decrease in plasma aldosterone in the upright position, whereas with hyperplasia, there is almost always an increase in plasma aldosterone concentrations after two to four hours in the upright position. The second test involves a saline infusion. Patients receiving 120 mEq of sodium per day receive an intravenous infusion of 1250 ml of isotonic saline between 8 A.M. and 10 A.M. after overnight recumbency. The ratio of 18-OHB to cortisol is measured in plasma samples taken before and immediately after the infusion. This ratio increases in patients with an aldosterone-producing adenoma, but decreases in patients with hyperplasia.

ADRENAL ANDROGENS

Plasma levels of the predominant adrenal androgens, DHEA, DHEA-S, and androstenedione, can be measured. These assays plus that of testosterone are most frequently used for the evaluation of hirsutism. Stimulation and suppression tests have not been as useful as in other pituitary and adrenal disorders. Plasma free testosterone measurements usually provide a better index of total androgenicity than total levels of the hormone, since androgen excess decreases sex hormone–binding globulin and can result in a normal total level in the presence of an elevated free testosterone concentration. Measurement of androstanediol and its glucuronide, metabolic products of dihydrotestosterone, provides an index of peripheral androgen production and may provide the best index of androgen excess.

Urinary 17-ketosteroids are measured to assess adrenal androgen production and reflect metabolites of DHEA and DHEA-S. However, this test has limited utility, since the more potent androgens such as testosterone and dihydrotestosterone contribute less than 1 per cent of the total urinary 17-ketosteroids. Furthermore, 17-ketosteroids are increased in obesity without androgen excess, and there is interference by multiple drugs and medications.

230.6 Adrenocortical Hypofunction

John D. Baxter

Adrenal insufficiency is defined by deficient production of glucocorticoids or mineralocorticoids or both. Primary adrenocortical insufficiency (Addison's disease) is due to destruction of the adrenal cortex, whereas in secondary adrenocortical insufficiency impaired cortisol production is due to deficient ACTH production. Hyporeninemia causes selective aldosterone deficiency. Selective adrenal defects due to congenital enzyme deficiencies also occur (see Ch. 234).

PRIMARY ADRENOCORTICAL INSUFFICIENCY

ETIOLOGY. Primary adrenocortical insufficiency has multiple causes. In the United States over 80 per cent of the cases are due to autoimmune destruction of the adrenal. Tuberculosis is the second most frequent cause and remains a common cause of the disease in underdeveloped countries. Other rare causes include hemorrhage due to sepsis, anticoagulation, coagulopathies, trauma, surgery, and pregnancy; bilateral infarction, e.g., due to thrombosis or arteritis; fungal infection; invasive disorders such as lymphoma, metastatic tumors, amyloidosis, sarcoidosis, and hemochromatosis; surgery; cytotoxic agents such as mitotane; and congenital hypoplasia and hyporesponsiveness to ACTH. Primary adrenocortical insufficiency due to any cause is a rare disease with an estimated incidence in Western countries of around 50 per million population.

The idiopathic autoimmune form of adrenal insufficiency is two- to three-fold more common in females and is usually diagnosed in the third to fifth decades of life. Early in the disease there is lymphocytic infiltration of the gland, and there is a high association (40 to 53 per cent of patients) with disorders of other endocrine glands or with pernicious anemia or vitiligo. Antibodies to the gland are commonly present, and there is evidence for abnormal cell-mediated immunity.

The association of Addison's disease with the other disorders has been referred to as *Schmidt's syndrome*, autoimmune endocrine failure, and the polyglandular failure syndrome (Ch. 241). Approximate associations are ovarian failure, 25 per cent of female patients (testicular failure in males is unusual); hyperthyroidism, 7 per cent (mostly female); hypothyroidism or Hashimoto's thyroiditis with goiter, 9 per cent; subclinical thyroiditis, up to 80 per cent; diabetes mellitus (type I), 12 per cent; vitiligo, 9 per cent, presumably due to immunologic destruction of melanocytes; hypoparathyroidism, 6 per cent; and, pernicious anemia, 4 per cent. The development of autoimmune adrenocortical insufficiency shows some hereditary predisposition, and an autosomal recessive pattern of inheritance has been suggested. About 40 per cent of patients have first- or second-degree relatives with one of the associated disorders. Further, there is an increased incidence of histocompatibility antigen (HLA) types B8, Dw3 and of the haplotype HLA-A1,B8.

CLINICAL MANIFESTATIONS. The development of clinical manifestations of adrenocortical insufficiency requires loss of more than 90 per cent of the adrenal cortices. The rate of destruction varies, depending on the cause, but with the idiopathic variety this usually requires several months. With gradual destruction, increases in ACTH secondary to the lower cortisol levels tends to stimulate the gland maximally. Thus in the period prior to complete destruction there may be normal plasma cortisol levels but absence of responsiveness to stress. In about 25 per cent of patients symptoms first appear in a crisis or impending crisis. However, in the majority of cases destruction becomes more complete, and the patient experiences symptoms that lead to medical evaluation before a crisis occurs. The destruction of the gland

results in loss of both glucocorticoid and mineralocorticoid functions and secondary increases in ACTH and in renin.

The clinical presentation depends on the rate and degree of adrenal destruction, the presence of stressful influences, and the pathology of associated or causative conditions. For these reasons it is convenient to discuss separately the chronic and acute presentations.

Chronic primary adrenocortical insufficiency develops gradually over months to years. The major clinical features (Table 230–4) are generalized weakness and fatigue, weight loss, anorexia, hyperpigmentation, hypotension, gastrointestinal upset (including vague discomfort, nausea, vomiting, and less commonly diarrhea), salt craving, and postural dizziness. Weight loss is due both to dehydration secondary to salt loss, and to anorexia. The blood glucose concentration is ordinarily in the low-normal range, although hypoglycemia can occur with fasting, vomiting, or illness and in children. Female patients can also have amenorrhea and loss of axillary hair, the latter due to decrease of adrenal androgens. Although dehydration can be significant, this is typically compensated for by increased salt intake. Hyponatremia is present in most patients, although it may be masked somewhat if there is dehydration. Mild hyperkalemia is also usually present; the presence of severe hyperkalemia should suggest concomitant renal or other disease. A normocytic, normochromic anemia is common, but can also be masked by dehydration and hemoconcentration. There tends to be neutropenia, lymphocytosis, and eosinophilia. Dehydration when present leads to increases in blood urea nitrogen and creatinine, and there may be mild acidosis. The heart tends to be small and vertical on radiographic examination; the abdominal radiograph is usually normal, but can show adrenal calcification in about 50 per cent of those cases due to tuberculosis. Calcification of the ear lobes sometimes occurs in longstanding cases.

Hyperpigmentation, an important diagnostic feature, may precede other manifestations. It is generalized, but is accentuated in sun-exposed areas, pressure points such as the elbows, knees, knuckles, and toes, and on palmar creases, nail beds, buccal mucosa, tongue, nipples, areolae, and perivaginal or perianal mucosa, and in recent surgical scars. In blacks, pigmentation of the tongue is of diagnostic helpfulness. Hyperpigmentation is commonly misinterpreted as an excessive sun tan and the "healthy" appearance of the patient may lead to a dismissal of other symptoms.

Acute adrenocortical insufficiency is seen most commonly in a patient with either undiagnosed or diagnosed adrenocortical insufficiency who is exposed to one of the stresses discussed earlier and who therefore has an increased requirement for glucocorticoids. It can also be seen with acute adrenal destruction secondary to hemorrhage, most commonly associated with septicemia or anticoagulant therapy (adrenal apoplexy). In these cases, anorexia is often profound with nausea and vomiting that exaggerates volume depletion and dehydration. Abdominal pain is frequent and may mimic a surgical condition of the abdomen; however, these symptoms are usually vague. The blood pressure falls, and hypovolemic shock

TABLE 230–4. CLINICAL FEATURES OF CHRONIC PRIMARY ADRENOCORTICAL INSUFFICIENCY

Feature	%	Feature	%
Weakness and fatigue	100	Hypotension	88
Weight loss	100	Gastrointestinal symptoms	56
Anorexia	100	Salt craving	19
Hyperpigmentation	92	Postural symptoms	12

Modified from Nerup J: Acta Endocrinol 76:127, 1974 and Thorn GW: The Diagnosis and Treatment of Adrenal Insufficiency. Springfield, IL, Charles C Thomas, 1951, and reprinted in Baxter JD, Tyrrell JB: The adrenal cortex. In Felig P, Baxter JD, Broadus AH, et al. (eds.): Endocrinology and Metabolism. 2nd ed. New York, McGraw-Hill Book Company, 1987, p 587.

develops that is incompletely responsive to fluid replacement. Fever is common and may or may not be due to the precipitating event. Hyperpigmentation will be present or absent, depending on the duration of the disease; when present it is an important diagnostic sign. The presence of hyperkalemia, lymphocytosis, and eosinophilia should also suggest the diagnosis. Severe hypoglycemia is uncommon and is more likely to occur in children or in adults with secondary adrenal insufficiency (see below). The diagnosis of acute adrenocortical insufficiency should be considered in any patient with unexplained shock, and the consideration of this should not be diverted by the presence of an accompanying disorder such as infection or diabetic ketoacidosis.

SECONDARY ANDRENOCORTICAL INSUFFICIENCY. Secondary adrenocortical insufficiency results from inadequate ACTH production. The causes are discussed in Ch. 226. Pituitary and hypothalamic tumors are the most common spontaneous cause. In these cases there is progressive loss of ACTH such that cortisol production and responses to stress are decreased, but mineralocorticoid production is usually normal. Chronic suppression of ACTH production with exogenous glucocorticoids followed by their withdrawal also causes the syndrome and is by far the most frequent cause.

The development of clinical manifestations is usually gradual, but like primary adrenocortical insufficiency can be acute. The presenting features are similar to those of primary adrenocortical insufficiency with four exceptions: (1) Since hypersecretion of ACTH and related peptides is absent, there is no hyperpigmentation; in fact, patients with hypopituitarism commonly exhibit pallor of the skin. (2) The electrolyte abnormalities of hyponatremia, hyperkalemia, and mild acidosis are absent because of preservation of aldosterone secretion. Hyponatremia, if present, is due to decreased glomerular filtration rate, hypothyroidism, or increased vasopressin release. (3) Other features of hypopituitarism (see Ch. 226) may be present. (4) Hypoglycemia are more common because of the combined ACTH and growth hormone deficiency.

DIAGNOSIS. The clinical suspicion of Addison's disease should be confirmed by laboratory testing. However, in seriously ill patients, in whom the diagnosis is suspected, therapy should not be delayed by prolonged diagnostic measures; if means for a rapid diagnosis are unavailable, therapy should be initiated and diagnostic testing performed at a later date. Although an elevated plasma cortisol level (e.g., greater than 25 μg per deciliter) makes the diagnosis unlikely, normal random cortisol levels can be present with impaired adrenal responsiveness to stress. Thus the adrenal reserve should be tested.

Figure 230–5 shows a diagnostic strategy. If adrenocortical insufficiency is suspected, the rapid ACTH stimulation test should be performed. This test requires only 30 minutes and can be done even in most acute situations. A normal response excludes the diagnosis of primary adrenocortical insufficiency; an abnormal response establishes the presence of adrenocortical insufficiency. Rare patients with secondary adrenocortical insufficiency will respond normally. The basal plasma ACTH level, determined prior to ACTH administration, is measured to distinguish between primary and secondary adrenocortical insufficiency. In primary adrenocortical insufficiency, the levels exceed 250 pg per milliliter and usually are greater than 400 pg per milliliter. By contrast, plasma ACTH levels in secondary adrenocortical insufficiency are inappropriately low, ranging from 0 to 50 pg per milliliter. The plasma aldosterone response to ACTH can also be used to differentiate primary from secondary adrenocortical insufficiency, but there is less extensive experience with this procedure.

Further diagnostic procedures are needed only in exceptional cases, for example, in suspected secondary adrenocortical insufficiency with a normal response to ACTH or in cases in which plasma ACTH measurements are unavailable. In these cases the metyrapone or insulin hypoglycemia tests can be helpful. The latter test is usually performed in suspected

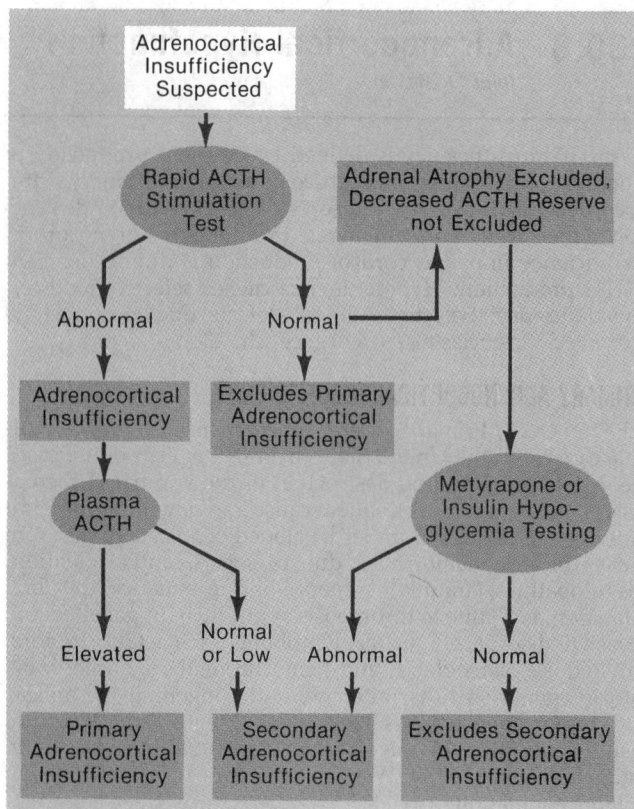

FIGURE 230–5. Evaluation of suspected primary or secondary adrenocortical insufficiency. Boxes enclose clinical decisions and ovals enclose diagnostic tests. (Reprinted from Baxter JD, Tyrrell JB: The adrenal cortex. In Felig P, Baxter JD, Broadus AE, et al. (eds.): Endocrinology and Metabolism. 2nd ed. New York, McGraw-Hill Book Company, 1987, p 593.)

hypopituitarism, since simultaneous assessment of both growth hormone and ACTH can be carried out (see Ch. 226). The metyrapone test is performed in patients in whom hypoglycemia is contraindicated or in those who have had prior glucocorticoid therapy, since it provides essentially the same information and is of less potential risk to the patient. An abnormal response to metyrapone or insulin hypoglycemia establishes the diagnosis of secondary adrenocortical insufficiency when the primary form has been excluded by the ACTH stimulation test. The presence of low-normal or low ACTH levels further confirms this diagnosis.

In spontaneous adrenocortical insufficiency of any type, the clinical evaluation should include an assessment of associated disorders or precipitating factors. In primary adrenocortical insufficiency the laboratory evaluation should include blood glucose and serum calcium and phosphorus; thyroid function tests, including TSH and thyroid antibody determinations; and testing for tuberculosis. If there is oligomenorrhea or amenorrhea, FSH and LH levels should be determined. First- and second-degree relatives should be screened for endocrine deficiency syndromes because of the increased risk in these individuals. In secondary adrenocortical insufficiency, patients should be examined for other pituitary dysfunction, pituitary or hypothalamic tumors, and prior glucocorticoid therapy (see Ch. 226). In acute adrenocortical insufficiency, the precipitating cause should be determined, since this is often infectious.

TREATMENT. *Acute Adrenocortical Insufficiency.* In an acute crisis, therapy should be instituted as soon as the diagnosis is suspected (Table 230–5). A soluble glucocorticoid, such as cortisol hemisuccinate or phosphate, should be given intravenously. Volume depletion, electrolyte abnormalities, and hypoglycemia should be corrected and general supportive measures instituted. Precipitating factors should be assessed

TABLE 230–5. THERAPY OF ADRENAL INSUFFICIENCY

Acute Crisis

1. Cortisol (hydrocortisone) 100 mg IV, every 6 hr for 24 hr. If stable, reduce to 50 mg every 6 hr and then taper to oral maintenance in 4 to 5 days. Maintain or increase dose to 200 to 400 mg per 24 hr if complications persist or occur.
2. Correct volume depletion, dehydration, hypotension, and hypoglycemia with intravenous saline and glucose.
3. Correct precipitating factors, especially infection.

Maintenance

1. Cortisol 15 to 20 mg p.o. q A.M.; 5 to 10 mg at 4 to 6 P.M.
2. 9α-Fluorocortisol 0.05 to 0.1 mg q A.M. (primary).
3. Follow weight, blood pressure, and electrolytes.
4. Educate patient to increase cortisol dosage during stress.

Modified from Tables 12–17 and 12–18 in Baxter JD, Tyrrell JB: The adrenal cortex. In Felig P, Baxter JD, Broadus AH, et al. (eds.): Endocrinology and Metabolism. 2nd ed. New York, McGraw-Hill Book Company, 1987.

and corrected. If recovery is satisfactory, the glucocorticoid dose can then be reduced on the second day and then tapered to oral maintenance doses by the fourth to fifth days. Mineralocorticoid replacement is unnecessary when high doses of cortisol are given, but should be given when the cortisol dose has been tapered to near-maintenance levels.

Chronic Adrenocortical Insufficiency. The treatment of the primary form of this condition requires both glucocorticoid and mineralocorticoid replacement, whereas the secondary form usually requires only glucocorticoid replacement (Table 230–5). Patients must be made aware that a lifetime of replacement is necessary and of the need to increase glucocorticoid replacement in times of stress. Each patient should carry an identification bracelet or card. Cortisol at levels similar to physiologic production is given in a way that approximates the circadian rhythm. Thus, for ordinary maintenance, 15 to 20 mg of cortisol are given in the early morning and 5 to 10 mg in the late afternoon. An equivalent amount of prednisolone or prednisone (about 5 mg per day) or cortisone acetate (37.5 mg per day) is also acceptable; however, the potency of dexamethasone has probably been underestimated, and this steroid is not recommended. For mineralocorticoid replacement, 9α-fluorocortisol (fludrocortisone) 0.05 to 0.1 mg orally per day is recommended. Follow-up is mainly by clinical assessment of a feeling of well-being, examination of signs of glucocorticoid or mineralocorticoid excess or deficiency, and measurements of serum electrolytes. Measurements of plasma cortisol, ACTH, and renin are usually not helpful. The doses may need to be adjusted somewhat. Many of the subjective complaints of Addison's disease can be reversed within a few days; a somewhat longer time is required before strength returns to normal and hyperpigmentation subsides.

In times of stress, it is sometimes difficult to predict the need for increased glucocorticoid administration. It is best to err on the side of overreplacement rather than underreplacement. For minor illnesses such as significant upper respiratory infections, the cortisol dose should be doubled or tripled and then tapered as soon as possible. It is not usually necessary to change the 9α-fluorocortisol dose. Patients with vomiting and substantial diarrhea should seek medical attention and

TABLE 230–6. STEROID COVERAGE FOR SURGERY

1. Correct electrolytes, blood pressure, and hydration if necessary.
2. Hydrocortisone phosphate or hemisuccinate, 100 mg IM, on call to operating room.
3. Hydrocortisone phosphate or hemisuccinate, 50 mg IM or IV, in recovery room and every 6 hr for the first 24 hr.
4. If progress is satisfactory, reduce dosage to 25 mg every 6 hr for 24 hr; then taper to maintenance dosage over 3 to 5 days. Resume previous 9α-fluorocortisol dose when patient is taking oral medications.
5. Maintain or increase cortisol dosage to 200 to 400 mg per 24 hr if fever, hypotension, or other complications occur.

Modified from Baxter JD, Tyrrell JB: The adrenal cortex. In Felig P, Baxter JD, Broadus AH, et al. (eds.): Endocrinology and Metabolism. 2nd ed. New York, McGraw-Hill Book Company, 1987, p 596.

receive parenteral cortisol. Patients who may not have early access to medical attention should keep injectable cortisol available and be instructed in its use.

In the event of major trauma, treatment should be similar to that for adrenal crisis discussed above. In the case of elective major surgery the protocol described in Table 230–6 had been shown to be effective.

PROGNOSIS. Survival of patients in whom adrenocortical insufficiency is adequately diagnosed and treated now approximates that of the normal population. This is in sharp contrast to the period before steroids were available or when only mineralocorticoid replacement was available, at which time the survival rate was usually two years or less.

HYPOALDOSTERONISM

PATHOGENESIS. Hypoaldosteronism can occur in association with hypocortisolism or as an isolated defect. The major cause of isolated hypoaldosteronism is defective renal renin secretion (hyporeninemic hypoaldosteronism) (see Ch. 77). Other rarer causes include isolated adrenal biosynthetic defects (18-hydroxylase syndrome) and focal destruction of the adrenal glomerulosa (hyperreninemic hypoaldosteronism), transient deficiency following removal of an aldosterone-producing tumor, unresponsiveness to aldosterone (pseudohypoaldosteronism) with normal or increased aldosterone production, marked potassium depletion, and heparin administration.

HYPORENINEMIC HYPOALDOSTERONISM. This is seen generally in older patients with renal disease due to a variety of causes such as diabetes mellitus, interstitial nephritis, or multiple myeloma. It has also been observed following removal of an aldosterone-producing tumor or rarely without any apparent cause in association with hypertension. The hyporeninemia leads to decreased aldosterone production and impaired ability of the zona glomerulosa to respond to stimuli. However, the gland usually retains some capacity to secrete aldosterone through stimulation by potassium. Hypoaldosteronism results secondarily in hyperkalemia, which is disproportionate to the extent of renal disease. Chronic renal disease per se ordinarily does not lead to hyperkalemia unless the glomerular filtration rate is severely impaired (e.g., less than 15 ml per minute). In fact, hyporeninemic hypoaldosteronism is probably a common cause of hyperkalemia in patients with renal disease and creatinine clearance rates greater than 15 ml per minute. Although these patients can develop hyponatremia, in adults this is less common, probably because of the fact that the primary disease tends to favor sodium retention. These patients also tend to develop a metabolic acidosis due to the lack of H^+-secreting actions of aldosterone; this can be accentuated by a decreased glomerular filtration rate. This form of acidosis has been classified as type IV renal tubular acidosis (see Ch. 84).

TREATMENT. The treatment of hypoaldosteronism involves therapy for the primary condition plus mineralocorticoid replacement as described above for primary adrenocortical insufficiency. However, in some patients with hypertension, treatment with 9α-fluorocortisol is not indicated and diuretics are used instead. Conversely, some patients require higher doses of mineralocorticoids, probably because the renal disease renders them more refractory to the steroid.

230.7 Cushing's Syndrome

J. Blake Tyrrell

Cushing's syndrome is the result of chronic glucocorticoid excess. It occurs most commonly in patients receiving supraphysiologic doses of glucocorticoids. Spontaneously occurring Cushing's syndrome, a rare disorder, occurs as a result of either primary tumors of the adrenal gland that hypersecrete cortisol or from excess ACTH secretion that may be of pituitary or nonpituitary (ectopic ACTH syndrome) sources.

Cushing's disease (spontaneous hypercortisolism due to excessive pituitary ACTH secretion) accounts for two thirds of reported cases. This disorder is most common in women 20 to 40 years old, with a female-male ratio of 8:1.

Secretion of ACTH from ectopic tumors accounts for about 15 per cent of cases of Cushing's syndrome. The true incidence of this disorder is probably higher, since many patients lack the typical clinical features of cortisol excess because of the dominance of the manifestations of cancer and the rapidity of progression. Because of the current predominance of oat cell carcinoma of the lung in males, the ectopic ACTH syndrome has a female-male ratio of 1:3 and an age of onset most frequently between 40 and 60 years.

Primary adrenal tumors secreting cortisol cause approximately 15 per cent of cases of Cushing's syndrome. In adults there is an equal frequency of adenoma and carcinoma. In childhood prior to the age of ten years, adrenal carcinoma is the most frequent cause of Cushing's syndrome. Both adenomas and carcinomas secreting cortisol are more prevalent in women than in men. The average age at diagnosis is approximately 40 years, and 70 per cent of cases occur in adults.

PATHOLOGY. Pituitary adenomas (see Ch. 226) are present in over 90 per cent of patients with Cushing's disease. These tumors are usually small; 50 per cent are 5 mm or less in diameter. They are typically basophilic and unencapsulated and contain ACTH, β-LPH, and β-endorphin. The patients with Cushing's disease who do not have pituitary adenomas have (1) diffuse hyperplasia; (2) hyperplasia with multiple nests of adenomatous cells; (3) an adenoma or adenomatous hyperplasia of the intermediate lobe of the pituitary; or (4) no obvious pituitary disorder.

Adrenocortical hyperplasia in Cushing's disease results in modest increases in combined adrenal weight due to hyperplasia of the zonae reticularis and fasciculata. In the ectopic ACTH syndrome, adrenal enlargement and hyperplasia of the zona reticularis are usually more marked with a concomitant reduction in the number of zona fasciculata cells. Bilateral nodular hyperplasia occurs in approximately 20 per cent of cases of ACTH excess and in some cases may be due to more prolonged stimulation of the adrenal cortex by ACTH. In this case, in addition to diffuse hyperplasia of the zonae reticularis and fasciculata, there are multiple nodules that vary from microscopic to several centimeters in diameter and that contain clear cells similar to those of the zona fasciculata.

Cortisol-secreting adenomas are usually encapsulated, range from 2 to 6 cm in diameter, typically secrete cortisol alone, and are usually composed of zona fasciculata-like cells. Adrenal carcinomas that secrete cortisol are usually large at the time of diagnosis, may be palpable as abdominal masses, and usually secrete a number of steroids. Histologically these tumors may appear benign or exhibit considerable pleomorphism, and the histologic appearance does not predict benign or malignant behavior. Therefore the diagnosis of adrenal carcinoma is dependent on the demonstration of either local tumor invasiveness or metastatic spread. Extension of these tumors occurs locally, and common sites of metastases are the liver and lung.

ETIOLOGY AND PATHOGENESIS. The etiology of Cushing's disease is unknown. It is possible that primary pituitary tumors arise spontaneously. In cases in which diffuse or adenomatous hyperplasia is present, excessive secretion of CRF or some other factor may stimulate the pituitary. Rarely CRF-producing tumors have been reported. The ectopic ACTH syndrome occurs in a relatively small number of tumor types. Oat cell carcinoma of the lung accounts for approximately 50 per cent of cases. The greatly increased production of cortisol and 11-deoxycorticosterone stimulated by very high ACTH levels commonly results in manifestations of both mineralocorticoid and glucocorticoid excess.

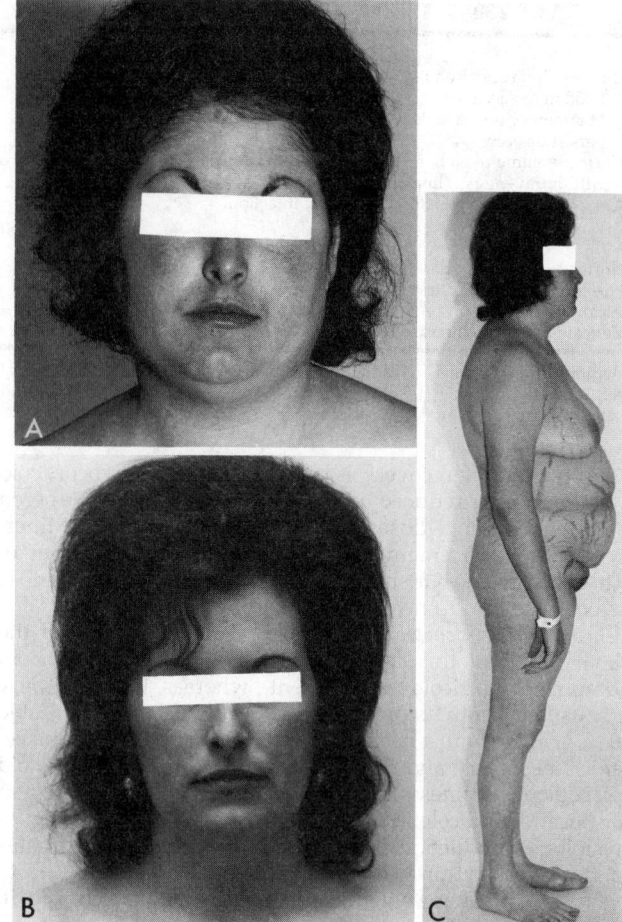

FIGURE 230–6. The appearance of a patient with Cushing's syndrome (A) before and (B) one year after removal of an adrenal adenoma. (C) Profile, before treatment.

Other ACTH-secreting tumors include thymomas, islet cell tumors of the pancreas, carcinoid tumors, medullary carcinomas of the thyroid, and pheochromocytomas. Many other tumors may secrete ACTH, but this occurs very rarely.

Cortisol-producing adrenal tumors arise spontaneously and are not under normal control by the hypothalamic-pituitary axis; their secretion of cortisol and the other steroids is autonomous, episodic, and random.

CLINICAL FEATURES. The classic features, most typically seen in Cushing's disease (Fig. 230–6, Table 230–7) usually

TABLE 230–7. INCIDENCE OF CLINICAL FEATURES OF CUSHING'S SYNDROME

Feature	%
Obesity	94
Facial plethora	84
Hirsutism	82
Menstrual disorders	76
Hypertension	72
Muscular weakness	58
Back pain	58
Striae	52
Acne	40
Psychologic symptoms	40
Bruising	36
Congestive heart failure	22
Edema	18
Renal calculi	16
Headache	14
Polyuria/polydipsia	10
Hyperpigmentation	6

Modified from Plotz CM, et al.: Am J Med 13:597, 1952, and Ross EJ, et al: Q J Med 35:149, 1966, and reprinted from Baxter JD, Tyrrell JB: The adrenal cortex. In Felig P, Baxter JD, Broadus AE, et al. (eds.): Endocrinology and Metabolism. 2nd ed. New York, McGraw-Hill Book Company, 1987, p 606.

develop insidiously over several years. The most common manifestation is central obesity with rounding of the face and fat accumulation around the trunk, supraclavicular areas, and dorsocervical spine. Serial photographs are helpful in recognizing these gradual changes. Classically this pattern of obesity spares the extremities; however, generalized obesity including the extremities occurs in about 50 per cent of patients. Atrophy of the skin and underlying connective tissue is frequent. This leads to facial plethora, easy bruisability, and red to purple depressed striae. The last occur most commonly over the lower abdomen, but can also be more generalized on the trunk and upper legs. Patients also have poor healing of minor or major injuries and abrasions and an increased incidence of superficial fungal infections. Hirsutism is present in approximately 80 per cent of female patients as a result of excessive adrenal androgen secretion. Hypertension is present in the majority of patients; it is rarely accompanied by hypokalemia in Cushing's disease, although this is common in the ectopic ACTH syndrome or adrenal carcinoma. Hypertension contributes greatly to the mortality of untreated Cushing's syndrome.

Additional common manifestations include hypogonadism in both male and female patients, psychologic disturbances (usually depression), which occur in the majority, and proximal muscle weakness. Osteopenia is present in virtually all patients and may progress to frank osteoporosis (see Ch. 250). Back pain is common, and compression fractures of the spine occur in approximately 20 per cent. Renal stones, secondary to hypercalciuria, and thirst and polyuria, which may be due to hyperglycemia, can also occur. Routine laboratory abnormalities include high normal or modestly elevated values for the hematocrit, slightly elevated white cell counts, and a depressed percentage of lymphocytes and eosinophils. Electrolyte abnormalities occur only rarely in Cushing's disease, and the presence of hypokalemia should suggest the ectopic ACTH syndrome or adrenal carcinoma.

DIAGNOSIS. A suggested plan for the evaluation of suspected Cushing's syndrome is shown in Figure 230–7. If the syndrome is suspected the 24-hour urine free cortisol should be measured and the overnight 1 mg dexamethasone suppression test performed.

If results of both of these tests are normal, the diagnosis of Cushing's syndrome is excluded, with two exceptions: (1) Rare patients whose disease activity is episodic can have normal tests during periods of inactivity. In these cases, repeated evaluation during periods of disease activity will establish the diagnosis. (2) Rare patients with Cushing's disease have delayed clearance of dexamethasone, and therefore have normal responses to low-dose dexamethasone. However, these patients have elevated urine free cortisol levels.

If the 24-hour urine free cortisol level is elevated and the 1 mg overnight dexamethasone suppression test is abnormal, then spontaneous Cushing's syndrome is present provided that several abnormalities that lead to false positive responses can be excluded. Results of the dexamethasone suppression test can be abnormal in obesity, estrogen therapy, drug therapy that increases dexamethasone metabolism (listed in Ch. 30), and chronic renal failure, although the 24-hour urine free cortisol is almost always in the normal range. In the case of obesity or estrogen therapy, the two-day low-dose dexamethasone test should be performed; the results are almost always normal in the absence of Cushing's syndrome. Response to both the 24-hour urine free cortisol and the 1 mg dexamethasone suppression tests can be abnormal in alcoholism, acute and chronic illness, depression and other states of substantial emotional stress, and anorexia nervosa. In these cases, in the absence of spontaneous Cushing's syndrome the abnormalities will subside following cessation of the condition.

ETIOLOGIC DIAGNOSIS. Once the diagnosis of Cushing's syndrome has been established, it is essential to deter-

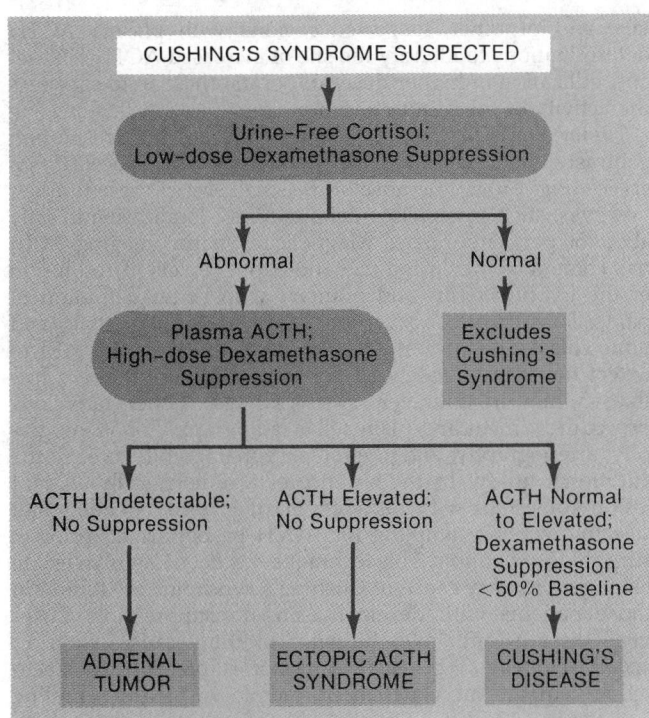

FIGURE 230–7. Evaluation of Cushing's syndrome. Boxes enclose clinical decisions and ovals enclose diagnostic tests. See the text for details and the potential for false-positive and false-negative results. (Reprinted from Baxter JD, Tyrrell JB: The adrenal cortex. In Felig P, Baxter JD, Broadus AE, et al. (eds.): Endocrinology and Metabolism. 2nd ed. New York, McGraw-Hill Book Company, 1987, p 609.)

mine its specific cause. The two most useful procedures are (1) the measurement of basal plasma ACTH levels and (2) the high-dose dexamethasone suppression test. In Cushing's disease, ACTH levels are normal to modestly elevated (50 to 200 pg per milliliter), and in 90 per cent of these patients, plasma or urinary steroid levels are suppressed to less than 50 per cent of baseline values in response to the high-dose dexamethasone test. In the ectopic ACTH syndrome, plasma ACTH values are often markedly elevated and are more than 200 pg per milliliter in two thirds of patients. In about 95 per cent of these patients, hypothalamic-pituitary control of ACTH and cortisol secretion is absent, and there is no response to high-dose dexamethasone suppression. Exceptions occur mostly in patients with relatively benign carcinoid tumors or thymomas in whom ACTH levels may be only modestly elevated and in whom the high dose of dexamethasone may suppress ACTH release. With glucocorticoid-secreting adrenal tumors, plasma ACTH levels are suppressed to either low normal or undetectable levels, and dexamethasone suppression testing produces no reduction in cortisol levels.

Two major problems are encountered in determining the cause: (1) In approximately 10 per cent of patients with Cushing's disease the cortisol levels are not suppressed adequately in response to dexamethasone, and (2) approximately 5 per cent of patients with ectopic tumors have suppression in response to high-dose dexamethasone and thus may appear to have Cushing's disease. No advantage of CRF testing over current procedures has been demonstrated. In some cases, lack of suppression with pituitary adenomas occurs with larger tumors that are apparent when computed tomographic (CT) scanning is performed. Also, this problem is more frequent when there is nodular adrenal hyperplasia. With these cases it is necessary to use additional procedures to establish the diagnosis. These include the use of head and body CT to search for an ectopic tumor, selective venous sampling of the petrosal sinuses that drain the anterior pituitary and of other suspected regions with plasma ACTH determinations to identify the site of increased ACTH release, and utilization of higher doses of dexamethasone to suppress the activity of the pituitary tumor.

Tumor Localization. In Cushing's disease high-resolution contrast-enhanced CT of the pituitary is the procedure of choice (Fig. 230–8). Because of the small size of these tumors, however, such scans allow definite tumor localization in only about 50 per cent of cases. Magnetic resonance imaging (MRI) has come into increasing use and allows excellent resolution of the hypothalamus and pituitary with better definition of parasellar structures (cavernous sinuses, pituitary stalk, and optic chiasm) than does CT. However, the ability of MRI to detect the approximately 50 per cent of tumors that are less than 5 mm in diameter is still limited. Other radiologic procedures, including plain sellar radiographs, polytomography, arteriography, and pneumoencephalography, are of little additional utility. In the absence of a radiologically evident lesion consistent with an adenoma it is recommended that selective venous sampling for ACTH be performed prior to surgical intervention. This technique has been useful in establishing a pituitary cause of Cushing's syndrome, including in those patients with dexamethasone-nonsuppressible Cushing's disease, and in excluding a pituitary cause when an occult ectopic ACTH-secreting tumor is present. The technique requires an experienced radiologist, since sampling from the inferior petrosal sinuses is required to assess pituitary ACTH secretion adequately. A gradient of 2:1 of central to peripheral ACTH levels establishes the presence of Cushing's disease.

CT and ultrasonography of the adrenal (Fig. 230–9) should be used in patients with suspected adrenal tumors or in whom the cause is in doubt. Adrenal tumors are usually larger than 2 cm in diameter when diagnosed and thus are readily visible with those procedures. Adrenal scanning should also be performed when ACTH levels or dexamethasone studies are inconclusive. In this case they will help differentiate hyperplasia from primary adrenal tumors and may help to establish the diagnosis of nodular adrenal hyperplasia.

TREATMENT. Pituitary microsurgery with a transsphenoidal approach is the current method of choice for the initial therapy of Cushing's disease. It is critical that it be performed by a surgeon with substantial experience with the technique as it is not a common procedure. Under ideal circumstances, pituitary tumors can be located at surgery in 90 per cent of patients, and successful responses to surgery occur in approximately 80 per cent of all the patients, including those with larger tumors. Surgical mortality is rare, and significant complications occur in less than 2 per cent of patients. Heavy-particle irradiation is also effective therapy for Cushing's disease, with long-term correction of cortisol hypersecretion occurring in approximately 80 per cent of patients. Unfortunately this therapy is currently available in only one center in the United States. Conventional radiotherapy is successful in only 15 to 25 per cent of adults and should not be used as initial therapy because it precludes any further radiation therapy. In contrast, an 80 per cent response rate to conventional radiation has been reported for Cushing's disease in childhood; the reason for this discrepancy is unclear. Bilateral adrenalectomy, previously an accepted initial therapy for Cushing's disease, should be limited to patients in whom other therapies are unsuccessful. In the past, this procedure was accompanied by a high degree of surgical morbidity and mortality and the subsequent development of Nelson's syndrome (discussed below). Reserpine, bromocriptine, cyproheptadine, and valproate sodium have been used to suppress ACTH and treat Cushing's syndrome, but only a minority of patients respond. In general their use is recommended for adjunctive therapy in patients who have had unsuccessful responses to other therapy.

Drugs that inhibit adrenal cortisol secretion can also be used as adjunctive therapy or in patients in whom more definitive treatments have been unsuccessful. Most com-

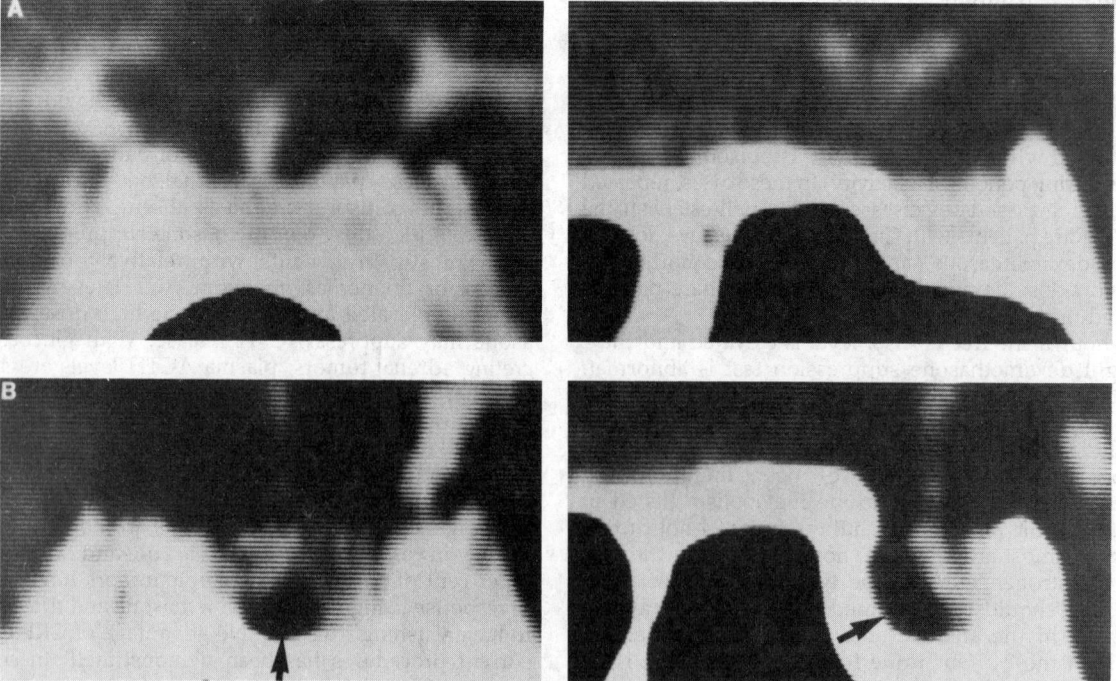

FIGURE 230–8. CT scans of normal and abnormal pituitary glands. The sections shown are computer re-formations derived from 1.5-mm axial sections through the sella turcica. Coronal re-formations are shown on the left and sagittal ones on the right. *A,* Normal pituitary gland. The upper border is flat; the pituitary stalk (seen on the coronal section) is midline; and the gland is relatively homogeneous in density. The lateral margins of the sella turcica (see coronal section) are formed by the contrast-enhancing cavernous sinuses. *B,* In a patient with Cushing's disease, a 3- to 4-mm pituitary adenoma is visualized as a low-density lesion in the anterior inferior portion of the anterior lobe (*arrows*). (Reprinted from Findling JW, Tyrrell JB: In Greenspan FS, Forsham PH (eds.): Basic and Clinical Endocrinology. 2nd ed. Los Altos, Lange Medical Publications, 1986, p 65.)

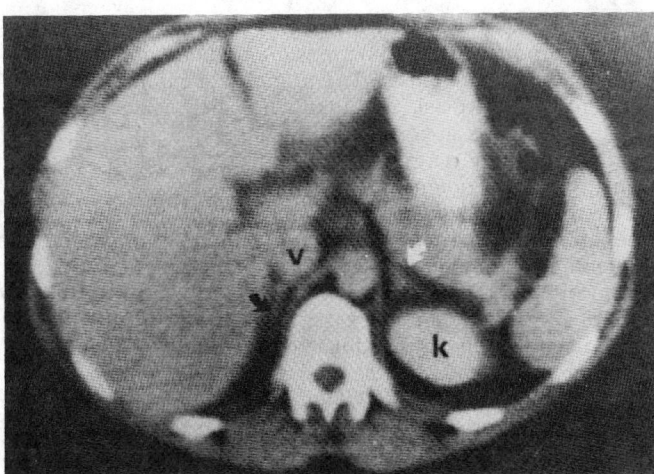

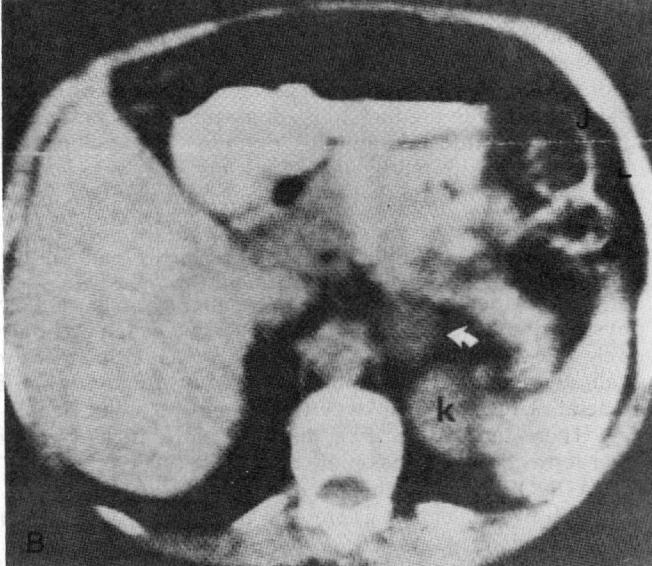

FIGURE 230–9. CT scans in Cushing's syndrome. *A*, Patient with ACTH-dependent Cushing's syndrome. The adrenal glands are not detectably abnormal by this procedure. The curvilinear right adrenal (*black arrow*) is shown posterior to the inferior vena cava (v) between the right lobe of the liver and the right crus of the diaphragm. The left adrenal (*white arrow*) has an inverted Y appearance anteromedial to the left kidney (k). *B*, A 3-cm left adrenal adenoma (*white arrow*) anteromedial to the left kidney (k). (From Korobkin M, White EA, Kressel HY, et al.: Computed tomographs in the diagnosis of adrenal disease. Am J Roentgenol 132:231, 1979.)

monly, metyrapone* (ordinarily 2 grams per day) and aminoglutethimide (1 gram per day) are given simultaneously in four divided doses. These drugs are expensive, have frequent side effects (predominantly gastrointestinal) and result in secondary increases in ACTH levels that sometimes are sufficient to overcome the enzyme inhibition. They are not usually used for long-term therapy of Cushing's disease. Ketoconazol* in doses of 800 to 1000 mg per day inhibits cortisol secretion in Cushing's syndrome; however, current experience is limited. Alternatively, mitotane, 3 to 6 grams per day in divided doses, can be used if tolerated. Although remission rates with the drug in Cushing's disease are approximately 80 per cent, relapse usually occurs following discontinuation of therapy. In addition, the response to mitotane is slow, requiring weeks to months to control cortisol excess, and side effects that include nausea, vomiting, diarrhea, somnolence, and skin rash occur in the majority of patients. Since the use of these drugs may produce hypoadrenalism, careful monitoring of steroid levels and glucocorticoid replacement may be required.

---

*This use is not listed in the manufacturer's directive.

In the ectopic ACTH syndrome the tumor hypersecreting ACTH should be removed. This may be possible in the minority of patients with the more benign tumors such as thymoma, bronchial carcinoid, or pheochromocytoma. Unfortunately in the majority of patients the tumors are malignant and metastasize prior to the diagnosis of cortisol excess. In such patients, drug therapy as discussed above is used to control cortisol excess. Metyrapone and aminoglutethimide are preferred to mitotane because of their more rapid onset of action. Also hypokalemia should be corrected as required, and spironolactone therapy may be useful in blocking the mineralocorticoid effects of cortisol and 11-deoxycorticosterone. Bilateral adrenalectomy might be considered in a rare patient in whom drug therapy is inadequate and the cortisol excess rather than the tumor is life threatening.

The treatment of adrenal tumors is primarily surgical. Patients with unilateral adrenal adenoma should undergo resection of the affected adrenal. Although surgical cure of adrenocortical carcinoma is unusual, surgical removal of the primary tumor is indicated to reduce cortisol secretion even when metastases are present. Mitotane 6 to 12 grams per day in divided doses, if tolerated, is recommended for patients with residual or nonresectable carcinoma, and approximately 75 per cent of patients achieve reduced steroid secretion. Only about one third of patients undergo reduction in tumor bulk, however, and it is not clear whether the drug prolongs survival. Metyrapone and aminoglutethimide can be used in patients who do not respond to or tolerate mitotane. The prognosis is poor with adrenal carcinoma; most patients survive less than five years following the onset of symptoms.

The normal hypothalamic-pituitary-adrenal axis is suppressed in Cushing's syndrome of all causes, and months to sometimes two years are required for it to recover following removal of an adrenal, pituitary, or ectopic tumor. Thus, following the resection of a cortisol or ACTH-producing tumor, glucocorticoid replacement therapy, as described above for secondary adrenocortical insufficiency, is required until normal pituitary and adrenal function recovers.

NELSON'S SYNDROME. Defined as the clinical progression of an ACTH-secreting pituitary adenoma following bilateral adrenalectomy for Cushing's disease, this syndrome appears to occur in at least one third of such patients. Fortunately the incidence of this disorder has dropped dramatically because of the decreased use of bilateral adrenalectomy for treatment of Cushing's disease.

The syndrome probably results when cortisol feedback inhibition is removed by bilateral adrenalectomy, thus allowing progression of the adenoma. Nelson's syndrome is characterized by increasing hyperpigmentation, usually within one to two years following adrenalectomy. In addition, these patients frequently exhibit local manifestations, including hypopituitarism, visual loss, headache, cavernous sinus invasion with extraocular muscle palsies, and rarely malignant changes with metastatic spread. Plasma ACTH levels are dramatically elevated and usually range from 1000 to 10,000 pg per milliliter. The majority of these tumors are greater than 1 cm in diameter and are readily localized by CT or MRI of the sella turcica.

The treatment of Nelson's syndrome is considerably less successful than that of Cushing's disease because of the large size and aggressive nature of these tumors. Although pituitary microsurgery is the preferred initial therapy, complete tumor resection is usually not possible. Heavy-particle irradiation may be utilized either as primary therapy or after surgery in patients with intrasellar tumors; however, in those with extrasellar extension, conventional postoperative radiation therapy should be undertaken. Although pharmacologic inhibition of ACTH secretion has been attempted with cyproheptadine, bromocriptine, and valproic acid, it appears that only a minority of patients respond. Nevertheless, trials of these medications are indicated if surgical treatment and radiotherapy are unsuccessful.

230.8 Mineralocorticoid Excess States

John D. Baxter

PRIMARY ALDOSTERONISM

Increased and inappropriate production of aldosterone from the adrenal is known as primary aldosteronism and leads to sodium retention with hypertension, suppression of plasma renin, and hypokalemia and its manifestations. It is due mainly to an adrenocortical adenoma, bilateral adrenocortical hyperplasia, or rarely to an adrenal carcinoma. The disease occurs in all age groups, with a peak incidence during the third and fourth decades. About 70 per cent of the adenomas occur in women. Although primary aldosteronism almost always results in hypertension (normotensive primary hyperaldosteronism is extremely rare), the syndrome is present in less than 2 per cent of patients with hypertension. Nevertheless, this largely reversible form of hypertension should be considered in all hypertensive patients.

ALDOSTERONE-PRODUCING ADENOMAS. With an aldosterone-producing adenoma (Conn's syndrome), aldosterone excess leads to sodium retention and to potassium and hydrogen loss. Other steroids that are normally synthesized in the zona glomerulosa (i.e., deoxycorticosterone, corticosterone, and 18-hydroxycorticosterone) are also produced in excess, although they are probably not important in the overall pathophysiology. Sodium retention expands the extracellular fluid volume, increases total body sodium content, elevates the serum sodium concentration and ultimately results in an increased intracellular sodium content that increases vascular reactivity. With time, the sodium retention leads to hypertension. It has been proposed that aldosterone may have other hypertensive actions as well. The hypokalemia results in muscular weakness, a tendency to cardiac irritability and arrhythmia, carbohydrate intolerance, resistance to vasopressin (nephrogenic diabetes insipidus), and abnormalities in baroreceptor function. The last results in a more volume-dependent hypertension. The expansion of the extracellular fluid and plasma volume is registered by the stretch receptors at the juxtaglomerular apparatus and by sodium chloride flux at the macula densa with suppression of renin release, low plasma renin levels, and unresponsiveness of renin release to provocative stimuli. Thus, increased aldosterone production with a suppressed renin system defines the disorder.

The sustained hypertension leads to compensatory effects that act to decrease the plasma volume, which can be normal or increased. However, an increased sodium and extracellular fluid volume persists, and the hypertension continues to be aldosterone dependent. The hypertension can also lead to many of the complications of hypertension such as renal damage, stroke, and myocardial infarction.

BILATERAL ADRENAL HYPERPLASIA. Bilateral adrenal hyperplasia can be diffuse or nodular, and selectively involves the glomerulosa cells. It accounts for perhaps 20 per cent of the patients in whom primary aldosteronism is diagnosed; however, its precise incidence is not known, since there is a gradient between what is termed low-renin essential hypertension without frank aldosterone excess and this syndrome. Adrenal hyperplasia does not appear to precede development of an adenoma.

The pathophysiology of hyperplasia shows several differences from that of adenoma: (1) Although the plasma renin is suppressed, it does respond to postural and other stimuli. (2) The adrenal is hypersensitive to angiotensin II, exhibiting a marked increase in aldosterone production rather than insensitivity. (3) The aldosterone hypersecretion is less than with the adenoma, a feature that is useful in the differential diagnosis. By contrast the blood pressure in the two groups tends to be similar. (4) The hypertension in most patients does not respond to adrenalectomy, implying that common factors produce both hypertension and enhanced adrenal sensitivity to angiotensin II. The mechanisms for the development of hyperplasia are unknown. There is active inquiry whether there is abnormal production (or loss) of factor(s), perhaps of pituitary origin, that enhance adrenal and vascular sensitivity to angiotensin II.

There are also subgroups of hyperplasia. In a few patients the hypertension does respond to adrenalectomy. In rare patients the hypertension and aldosterone excess respond to glucocorticoid therapy. In some patients the suppression tests described earlier can decrease aldosterone levels. In rare patients with unilateral nodular hyperplasia, the dynamics of aldosterone release can resemble more those of adenoma.

CLINICAL PRESENTATION. Patients present with elevated blood pressure detected on routine screening or, less commonly, because of hypokalemia. The blood pressure elevations range from mild to severe, with mean presenting pressures in the range of 200 mm Hg systolic and 120 mm Hg diastolic. Malignant hypertension is rare. A history of hypertension in pregnancy is common with female patients who develop the disorder. When present, symptoms of hypokalemia include tiredness, loss of stamina, weakness, nocturia, and lassitude. Symptoms of more severe depletion include alkalosis; rarely tetany with a positive Trousseau or Chvostek sign; increased thirst and polyuria with low urine specific gravity and unresponsiveness to vasopressin; paresthesias; cardiac arrhythmias such as ventricular tachycardia; and postural hypotension with dizziness. Headache is a frequent incidental complaint. There are no characteristic physical findings. In spite of fluid overload, edema is only rarely present. The heart is usually only mildly enlarged, if at all, and electrocardiographic changes are usually those of moderate left ventricular hypertrophy and potassium depletion. There tend to be fewer funduscopic changes than in other forms of hypertension of comparable severity.

DIAGNOSIS. The hallmarks of the disorder are hypertension with hypokalemia, suppression of the renin-angiotensin system, and increased aldosterone production. The serum sodium is rarely less than 139 mEq per liter in the absence of diuretic therapy. A suggested evaluation plan is shown in Figure 230–10. The initial step is to determine whether hypokalemia is present, since this is the primary clue to mineralocorticoid excess. All patients with hypertension should be screened, especially those with spontaneous hypokalemia, after diuretics have been withheld for at least three weeks.

The evaluation of hypokalemia requires control of the sodium balance, since sodium depletion from decreased intake or diuretics can decrease urinary potassium excretion and thus mask hypokalemia. Random serum potassium levels may be normal in up to 20 per cent of patients with primary aldosteronism, but salt loading will unmask hypokalemia in virtually all patients with adenoma and in most patients with hyperplasia. In the latter group the serum potassium levels will almost always be below 4 mEq per liter. If according to the dietary history the patient's usual sodium intake is 120 mEq or greater per 24 hours, measurement of normal potassium levels on three occasions obviates the need for further evaluation. If dietary intake is inadequate or unclear, the patient is instructed to consume a normal diet supplemented with 1 gram of NaCl with each meal for four days, and the serum potassium is then measured.

If the plasma potassium value is low, other causes of hypokalemia should be ruled out: diuretic therapy, gastrointestinal loss due to vomiting or diarrhea, other mineralocorticoid excess syndromes (discussed below), starvation, insulin and glucose therapy, metabolic acidosis, renal disease, and renovascular and accelerated hypertension.

Random unstimulated plasma renin activity (PRA) or plasma renin concentration (PRC) should be determined as the next step in diagnosis. In primary aldosteronism this will

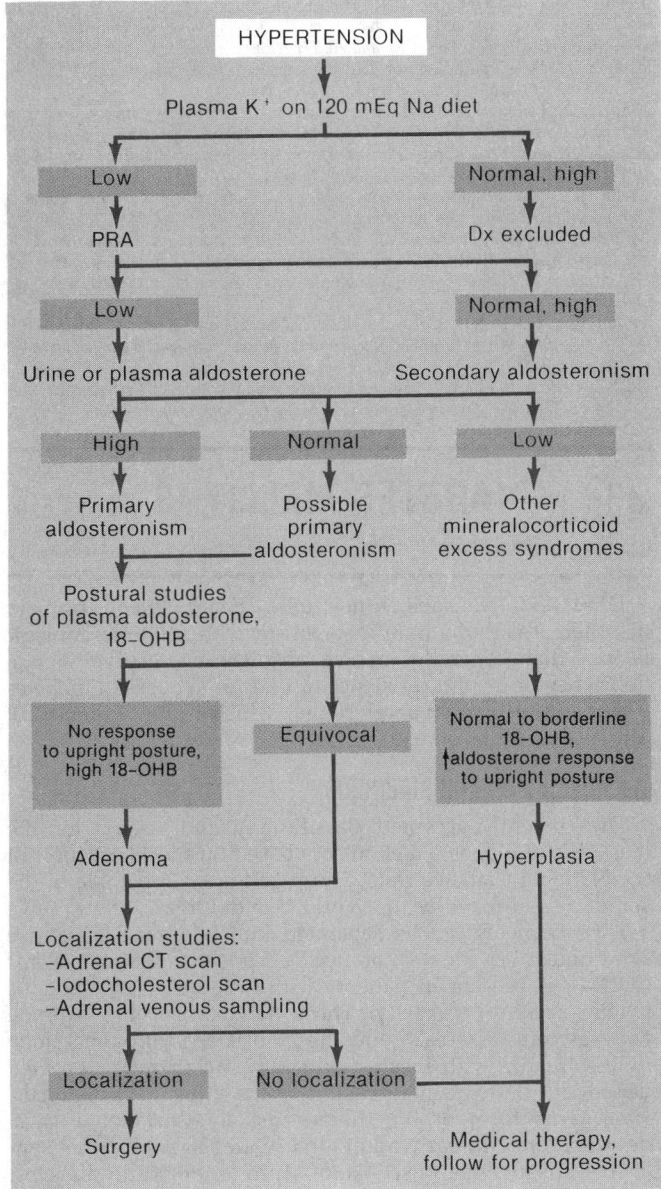

FIGURE 230–10. Flow diagram for diagnosis of primary aldosteronism and differentiation of adrenal adenoma from hyperplasia. (Adapted from Baxter JD, Perloff D, Hsueh W, et al.: In Felig P, Baxter JD, Broadus AE, et al. (eds.): Endocrinology and Metabolism. 2nd ed. New York, McGraw-Hill Book Company, 1987, p 756.

be suppressed even after short-term diuretic therapy, salt restriction, assumption of erect posture, or exercise, although other causes of low renin must be excluded. If PRA is normal or high, primary aldosteronism is unlikely.

If the plasma renin value is low or marginally low, 24-hour urinary aldosterone and plasma aldosterone levels should be measured. It is critical to monitor the salt intake and posture, as discussed earlier, because patients with essential hypertension and a low-salt intake have increased aldosterone levels. As discussed in the Laboratory Evaluation section, the urinary aldosterone is increased to over 17 µg per 24 hours in most cases of primary aldosteronism. With an adenoma the overnight recumbent plasma aldosterone levels almost always exceed 20 ng per deciliter. In hyperplasia the plasma aldosterone levels are ordinarily less than 20 ng per deciliter and frequently are in the normal range. Hypokalemia decreases aldosterone secretion; therefore with hypokalemia and suppressed PRA, aldosterone levels in the normal range are inappropriately high and thus abnormal.

In the presence of marginally suppressed PRC and mild

elevation of plasma or urinary aldosterone, one of the stimulation tests (discussed earlier) may be necessary to diagnose primary aldosteronism. Marginal cases are usually due to primary aldosteronism with hyperplasia, in which case antimineralocorticoid therapy is indicated. In many patients such therapy can be initiated and the patient re-evaluated at a later time.

If the diagnosis of primary aldosteronism is made, it is important to distinguish between adenoma and hyperplasia. As discussed above and in the Laboratory Evaluation section, the levels of plasma aldosterone provide an initial indication, but 18-OHB measurements provide an even better discrimination and should be performed. An 18-OHB level of over 100 ng per milliliter indicates adenoma; below this value it indicates hyperplasia. In situations in which these tests do not give a clear answer, the postural studies or the saline infusion tests will usually be helpful in reaching a decision.

Once an adenoma is suspected, CT scanning of the adrenals should be performed. In most cases this will permit localization of the tumor. In the less than 20 per cent of patients in whom an adenoma is not found, usually those with tumors less than 1.4 cm in diameter, selective venous sampling with measurements of aldosterone-cortisol ratios is usually helpful, can determine whether adenoma or hyperplasia is present, and can lateralize an adenoma. In addition, an iodocholesterol scanning technique can localize an adenoma accurately and detect the presence of hyperplasia in cases in which the diagnosis remains uncertain. For this technique dexamethasone is given to suppress adrenal fasciculata and reticularis function, and Lugol's solution is given to suppress thyroid uptake of radiolabeled iodide prior to the infusion of ^{131}I-6β-10-iodomethyl-19-nor-cholesterol. Adrenal uptake of radioactivity is then assessed by scanning.

TREATMENT. Unilateral adrenalectomy is indicated for aldosterone-producing adenomas. Prior to surgery the blood pressure and serum potassium should be normalized by treatment with the mineralocorticoid antagonist spironolactone (200 to 400 mg per day) or the potassium-sparing diuretic amiloride (20 to 40 mg per day). These dosages of spironolactone can be reduced to around 100 to 150 mg per day once normalization of blood pressure and hypokalemia has occurred. Medical therapy can be continued in the rare patient in whom surgery is contraindicated. This form of treatment also tends to reactivate the suppressed renin-angiotensin system so that the incidence of postoperative hypoaldosteronism is reduced. Also the response of the blood pressure to this therapy provides an excellent indication of the anticipated response to surgery.

Following surgery the blood pressure returns to normal in around 50 per cent of patients with reduction of hypertension in another 25 per cent. However, hypertension, but not hyperaldosteronism, returns in about 40 per cent by ten years postoperatively.

Most patients with bilateral hyperplasia will not respond to surgery; therefore medical therapy is recommended. These patients should be given spironolactone or amiloride in doses described above; this will correct the hypokalemia, but will not correct the hypertension in most cases. Additional antihypertensive medications are usually necessary. There is also a rare subgroup of patients with hyperplasia whose hyperaldosteronism is responsive to glucocorticoids; treatment of these patients with a glucocorticoid in normal replacement amounts or slightly above such amounts is recommended. Whether all patients with hyperplasia should be screened for this responsiveness is controversial.

OTHER FORMS OF HYPERTENSION ASSOCIATED WITH MINERALOCORTICOID EXCESS

There are several other mineralocorticoid-excess conditions. DOC excess can occur in the 11β- and 17α-hydroxylase syndromes (see Ch. 234), in patients with Cushing's syndrome, especially with ectopic ACTH-producing carcinoma and with adrenal adenomas and carcinoma. In these cases the PRC is suppressed as it is in primary aldosteronism; however, plasma aldosterone levels are usually suppressed as well. Rarely mineralocorticoid-excess hypertension results from excessive ingestion of licorice, carbenoxolone (for ulcer treatment), 9α-fluorocortisol for postural hypotension, or mineralocorticoid-containing nasal sprays. It can be present in rare cases of relative generalized insensitivity to glucocorticoids when elevated cortisol levels have mineralocorticoid actions. There are some rare syndromes in which there are hypertension, hypokalemia, and suppressed PRC with no detectable elevations of known mineralocorticoids (e.g., Liddle's syndrome; see Ch. 84). Some of these syndromes could represent primary hypersensitivity to mineralocorticoids. In all of these conditions there are hypertension, hypokalemia, and suppression of PRC without an associated increase of aldosterone.

SECONDARY HYPERALDOSTERONISM

Secondary hyperaldosteronism results from stimulation of the adrenal glomerulosa by extra-adrenal factors, usually the renin-angiotensin system. It can be physiologic or contribute to the pathology of disease states. A physiologic increase occurs during excessive potassium intake as part of the body's defense against hyperkalemia. Secondary hyperaldosteronism can occur during the luteal phase of the menstrual cycle and occasionally during oral contraceptive use. Aldosterone secretion increases progressively during normal pregnancy; levels reach ten times those of nonpregnant women by the third trimester. This is presumably due to an increase in renin and angiotensin, possibly due to a decrease in blood pressure. Interestingly, renin levels are more elevated during the first trimester, whereas plasma aldosterone levels are highest during the third trimester. This may be due to a progressive increase in sensitivity of the adrenal glomerulosa to angiotensin II. Aldosterone secretion increases when there is excessive sodium loss and when there is dietary restriction of sodium. Aldosterone increases in some patients with congestive heart failure and with significant hypoalbuminemia. In heart failure the aldosterone levels result from counterbalancing influences of decreased renal perfusion secondary to reduced cardiac output that increases renin and aldosterone release, and of sodium retention that suppresses renin and aldosterone levels. Renin and aldosterone levels are commonly elevated in cirrhosis when ascites is present; this is accentuated by decreased clearance of aldosterone. The increased aldosterone further promotes sodium retention and potassium loss. Elevated aldosterone levels are found in Bartter's syndrome (see Ch. 84). Finally, secondary hyperaldosteronism and hypertension can occur with renal artery stenosis, unilateral renal ischemia, accelerated hypertension, and renin-secreting tumors.

Aron DC, Tyrrell JB, Fitzgerald PA, et al.: Cushing's syndrome: Problems in diagnosis. Medicine 60:25, 1981. *An analysis of the problems and approaches when results do not conform to the usual norms.*

Baxter JD, Tyrrell JB: The adrenal cortex. In Felig P, Baxter JD, Broadus AE, et al. (eds.): Endocrinology and Metabolism. 2nd ed. New York, McGraw-Hill Book Company, 1987, pp 511–650. *An extensive review of the physiology and pathology of the adrenal cortex.*

Baxter JD, Perloff D, Hsueh W, et al.: The endocrinology of hypertension. In Felig P, Baxter JD, Broadus AE, et al. (eds.): Endocrinology and Metabolism. 2nd ed. New York, McGraw-Hill Book Company, 1987, pp 693–788. *An analysis of the pathophysiology and approaches to diagnosis and treatment of not only primary aldosteronism but also of other types of endocrine hypertension.*

Chrousos GP, Schuermeyer TH, Doppman J, et al.: Clinical applications of corticotropin-releasing factor. Ann Intern Med 102:344, 1985. *A review of the diagnostic utility of CRF.*

Crapo L: Cushing's syndrome: A review of diagnostic tests. Metabolism 28:955, 1979. *A detailed evaluation of the many diagnostic approaches to Cushing's syndrome. Required reading for a background in this area.*

Hall PF: Tropic stimulation of steroidogenesis: In search of the elusive trigger. Recent Prog Horm Res 41:1, 1985. *A review of the mechanisms regulating steroid biosynthesis.*

Keeton TK, Campbell WB: The pharmacologic alteration of renin release. Pharmacol Rev 31:81, 1980. *An overview of renin release with emphasis on pharmacological factors that alter it.*

Keller-Wood ME, Dallman M: Corticosteroid inhibition of ACTH secretion. Endocr Rev 5:1, 1984. *A review of the kinetics and mechanisms whereby glucocorticoids block both CRF and ACTH release.*

Krieger DT: Physiopathology of Cushing's disease. Endocr Rev 4:22, 1983. *This analysis of Cushing's disease emphasizes its possible causes.*

Marver D, Kokko JP: Renal target sites and the mechanism of action of aldosterone. Min Elect Metab 9:1, 1983. *A review of the actions of aldosterone.*

May RE, Carey RM: Rapid adrenocorticotrophic test in practice. Am J Med 79:679, 1985. *An assessment of the usefulness of this test.*

Melby JC: Primary aldosteronism. Kidney Int 26:769, 1984. *An overview of mineralocorticoid-excess syndromes.*

Munck A, Guyre P, Holbrook NJ: Physiological functions of glucocorticoids in stress and their relation to pharmacological actions. Endocr Rev 5:25, 1984. *A new proposal that explains how glucocorticoids are useful in the body's response to stress.*

Parker LN, Odell WD: Control of adrenal androgen secretion. Endocr Rev 1:392, 1980. *An excellent examination of the factors that regulate adrenal androgen production.*

Re NJ: Cellular biology of the renin-angiotensin systems. Arch Intern Med 144:2037, 1984. *An excellent overview of the renin-angiotensin system.*

231 DIABETES MELLITUS

Jerrold M. Olefsky

DEFINITION. Diabetes mellitus is a heterogeneous primary disorder of carbohydrate metabolism with multiple etiologic factors that generally involve absolute or relative insulin deficiency or insulin resistance or both. All causes of diabetes ultimately lead to hyperglycemia, which is the hallmark of this disease syndrome.

CLASSIFICATION AND DIAGNOSIS

The currently accepted classification and criteria for the diagnosis of diabetes mellitus are based on the 1979 report of the National Diabetes Data Group and are comparable to the standards set forth by the World Health Organization (Table 231–1). Diabetes can be separated into two general disease syndromes: (1) *Type 1*, or *insulin-dependent diabetes mellitus* (IDDM), is present in patients with little or no endogenous insulin secretory capacity. These patients develop extreme hyperglycemia, ketosis, and the associated symptomatology unless treated with insulin, and they are therefore entirely dependent on exogenous insulin therapy for immediate survival. This form of the disease usually, but not always, develops prior to early adulthood. Older terms for this syndrome are juvenile onset, ketosis prone, or brittle diabetes. (2) *Type II*, or *non–insulin-dependent diabetes mellitus* (NIDDM), occurs in patients who retain significant endogenous insulin secretory capacity. Although treatment with insulin may be necessary for control of hyperglycemia, these patients do not develop ketosis in the absence of insulin therapy and are not dependent on exogenous insulin for immediate survival. Previous terms for this form of the disease are maturity or adult onset, nonketotic, and stable diabetes. The diagnosis of diabetes in patients with the insulin-dependent form of the disease is usually unequivocal, and the distinction between

TABLE 231–1. CLASSIFICATION OF DIABETES

1. Insulin-dependent, or type I diabetes (IDDM). Formerly called juvenile-onset or ketosis-prone diabetes.
2. Non–insulin-dependent, or type II diabetes (NIDDM). Formerly called adult-onset, maturity-onset, or nonketotic diabetes.
   A. Obese (~80%)
   B. Nonobese (~20%)
3. Secondary diabetes
   A. Pancreatic disease (e.g., pancreatectomy, pancreatic insufficiency, hemochromatosis)
   B. Hormonal (excess counterinsulin hormones, e.g., Cushing's syndrome, acromegaly, pheochromocytoma)
   C. Drug-induced (e.g., thiazide diuretics, steroids, phenytoin)
   D. Associated with specific genetic syndromes (e.g., lipodystrophy, myotonic dystrophy, ataxia-telangiectasia)
4. Impaired glucose tolerance (IGT). Formerly called chemical, latent, borderline, or subclinical diabetes.
5. Gestational diabetes: glucose intolerance with onset during pregnancy.

type I and type II diabetes can usually be made on clinical grounds. However, there are occasional patients with minimal, but clearly detectable, endogenous insulin secretion in whom the disease is difficult to categorize initially. Usually these are lean adult, sometimes elderly, patients who at the time of initial diagnosis retain sufficient insulin secretory function so that the disease meets the classification of type II diabetes; with time, insulin secretion diminishes to the point that the disease merges into the category of type I diabetes.

The diagnosis of NIDDM is based on a distinction between normal and abnormal levels of glycemia and therefore is less precise. Prior to the report of the National Diabetes Data Group, oral glucose tolerance tests were commonly used to establish this diagnosis. This approach is fraught with difficulties because oral glucose tolerance is affected by numerous other variables that can cause mild abnormalities of glucose metabolism independent of diabetes. Concomitant illness, stress, physical inactivity, hypocaloric or low carbohydrate intake, various drugs, and aging are among those factors that can adversely influence glucose tolerance. Therefore, when employed, glucose tolerance testing must be rigorously controlled by administering a standard oral glucose load (75 grams), insuring an appropriate antecedent diet (eucaloric with at least 200 grams carbohydrate per day), adequate physical activity, and the absence of drugs affecting carbohydrate metabolism. Even with these precautions, only a minority (15 to 25 per cent) of individuals who have normal fasting plasma glucose levels with abnormal glucose tolerance tests go on to develop overt diabetes. In recognition of the above facts, the National Diabetes Data Group recommended relatively stringent criteria for establishing the diagnosis of NIDDM: (1) fasting venous plasma glucose concentration greater than 140 mg per deciliter on at least two separate occasions, or (2) in the absence of fasting hyperglycemia, a diagnosis of NIDDM can be made following ingestion of the standard 75-gram oral glucose tolerance test if the two-hour venous plasma glucose and one other sample (the 30-, 60-, or 90-minute sample) exceed 200 mg per deciliter.

Impaired glucose tolerance exists if the fasting plasma glucose level is less than 140 mg per deciliter and if the 30-, 60-, or 90-minute plasma glucose concentration exceeds 200 mg per deciliter along with a two-hour plasma glucose level between 140 and 200 mg per deciliter. Microvascular complications of diabetes rarely occur in individuals with impaired glucose tolerance, and the great majority of these cases do not deteriorate to overt diabetes in long-term follow up. Most instances of impaired glucose tolerance, therefore, are probably unrelated to the disease syndrome of NIDDM. Almost all patients who meet the criteria for NIDDM during oral glucose tolerance testing show fasting hyperglycemia (greater than 140 mg per deciliter) when evaluations are repeated. Furthermore, in those few patients who meet the criteria for NIDDM in the absence of fasting hyperglycemia, many do not develop fasting hyperglycemia during prolonged follow-up, and clinical symptoms of diabetes are unusual. Thus the clinical significance of impaired glucose tolerance is unclear. As previously mentioned, only a minority (2 to 35 per cent, depending on the population examined) of these patients go on to develop overt NIDDM when followed for up to 20 years. In evaluating the meaning of impaired glucose tolerance, the real challenge is to develop markers to detect which patients with impaired glucose tolerance have a benign nonprogressive abnormality of glucose intolerance and which have a prediabetic state. Patients with impaired glucose tolerance who secrete low amounts of insulin, compared to normal individuals, have a much higher risk of developing overt diabetes (perhaps up to 40 per cent), whereas those who secrete high amounts of insulin seldom (about 5 per cent) progress to frank diabetes. In view of the above, it would seem that glucose tolerance testing is unnecessary for patient management in the absence of clinical signs and symptoms of diabetes, although this is still a highly useful procedure for epidemiologic or research purposes. An exception to this would be in a pregnant subject suspected of having gestational diabetes, since criteria for this diagnosis are less stringent and vigorous management of minimal degrees of hyperglycemia are deemed important.

Serum and plasma glucose concentrations are identical and run 10 to 15 per cent higher than whole blood determinations (the latter are infrequently performed nowadays). The glucose concentration in capillary blood is essentially identical to that in venous blood during the fasting state, but under postprandial conditions, tissues readily take up glucose and capillary blood glucose concentrations can be 10 to 30 mg per deciliter greater than concomitant venous blood glucose levels.

There is an age-related decline in glucose tolerance that has been extensively studied. Insulin secretion is not decreased in aging, whereas insulin resistance is a common finding in aged populations. This insulin resistance is due to a postreceptor defect in insulin action. Age-related variables such as inadequate diet, increasing adiposity with decreased lean body mass, and physical inactivity can contribute to this insulin-resistant state, but the aging process itself also plays a significant role. The glucose intolerance of aging tends to be mild and is most easily detected following an oral glucose challenge. When mild abnormalities of oral glucose tolerance tests were used to diagnose diabetes, age-adjusted criteria for these tests had to be employed. However, with the current more stringent criteria noted above, this problem is largely obviated, since the glucose intolerance of aging does not cause significant fasting hyperglycemia (more than 140 mg per deciliter) and only rarely would cause glucose intolerance severe enough to meet the new criteria in the absence of fasting hyperglycemia.

EPIDEMIOLOGY AND CLINICAL PRESENTATION

The prevalence of diabetes has been difficult to quantitate accurately because the criteria for the diagnosis of NIDDM have varied from survey to survey over the years; the less stringent the criteria the greater the prevalence and vice versa. It is hoped that the widely accepted, uniform, WHO and National Diabetes Data Group standards will successfully address this problem. Furthermore, the prevalence of diabetes differs widely among different populations, depending on ethnic group constituents, age, economic conditions, and probably other environmental factors. For example, the prevalence of diabetes is extremely high among Pima Indians (about 35 per cent) and certain Micronesian cultures (about 35 per cent). Indians, particularly after emigrating from their country, have a higher rate of diabetes than other ethnic groups. Thus, Indians living in South Africa, Trinidad, Singapore, Malaysia, and Fiji exhibit a higher prevalence of diabetes than the local population and than those living on the Indian subcontinent. A low prevalence of diabetes has been noted in Eskimos, Athabascan Indians (Alaska), and Chinese (although prevalence increases in Chinese populations living in Western countries). The proportion of IDDM to NIDDM also differs widely among different populations; IDDM is extremely rare in Pima Indians, Micronesians, and Eskimos, but is more common in Caucasian populations. *Overall, in the United States the prevalence of diabetes is probably between 2 and 4 per cent, with IDDM comprising 7 to 10 per cent of all cases.* The prevalence of IDDM (0.2 to 0.3 per cent) is probably more accurate than the estimates for NIDDM, because of the relative ease of ascertainment and the fact that many patients with NIDDM are asymptomatic and the disease is undiagnosed.

A few facts concerning the prevalence of major diabetes-related complications serve to underscore the enormous impact of this disease. Approximately 25 per cent of all new cases of end-stage renal failure occur in patients with diabetes. About 20,000 amputations (primarily of toes, feet, and legs) are carried out in patients with diabetes, representing approximately half of the nontraumatic amputations performed in the United States. Furthermore, diabetes is the leading cause of new cases of blindness, with approximately 5000 new cases occurring each year.

INSULIN-DEPENDENT DIABETES MELLITUS (IDDM, TYPE I). These patients have little or no endogenous insulin and usually present with relatively abrupt clinical symptoms of *polyuria, polydipsia,* and *polyphagia. Weight loss,* fatigue, and infection can often accompany the initial presentation. Because of the extreme hypoinsulinemia and hyperglucagonemia, these patients readily develop *ketosis,* and the initial onset of this disease may be clinically evident as full-blown ketoacidosis. At the time of the first clinical presentation, symptoms can usually be traced back for several days to a few weeks; however, in most cases beta cell destruction began months and often years prior to the onset of clinical symptoms. In some cases, detection of this preclinical state may be possible by assessing the presence of circulating antibodies to islet cells or insulin. Unfortunately, proven methods to delay or prevent the full-blown disease are not available. The peak age of onset of IDDM is 11 to 13 years, coinciding with early adolescence and puberty. A secondary peak is noted at age 6 to 8 years, and by the third decade of life the incidence falls to a steady, but still substantial level. It is unusual for IDDM to begin past age 40. Once IDDM is diagnosed, insulin therapy is required to achieve initial metabolic control. In many patients a "honeymoon" period follows initial treatment in which the disease remits and little or no insulin is required. This remission is due to a partial return of endogenous insulin secretion, which may last for several weeks or months and occasionally 1 to 2 years; ultimately, however, the disease recurs, and insulin therapy is required permanently.

NON–INSULIN-DEPENDENT DIABETES MELLITUS (NIDDM, TYPE II). Patients with NIDDM typically present with polyuria and polydipsia of several weeks' to months' duration. Polyphagia can occur but is less common, whereas weight loss, weakness, and fatigue are frequent. Dizziness, headaches, and blurry vision are common accompanying complaints. In many patients no symptoms are apparent and the disease is diagnosed by routine blood or urine testing. In others, diabetes is advanced, and the presenting complaints are related to neuropathic, retinopathic, or vascular complications. NIDDM patients are usually but not always older than 40 at presentation and 70 to 90 per cent are overweight. Endogenous insulin secretion is relatively preserved and may even be excessive; thus, ketosis is rare, explaining why NIDDM is categorized as nonketotic or ketosis resistant.

SECONDARY DIABETIC STATES. In addition to the major categories of diabetes (IDDM and NIDDM), a large number of secondary forms of diabetes have been described. Secondary diabetes exists when some other readily identifiable primary disease entity or pathophysiologic state causes or is strongly associated with the diabetic state (Table 231–1). In general, these cases are unusual and comprise only a small proportion of the total cases of diabetes. Any disease process that limits insulin secretion or impairs insulin action can cause secondary diabetes, and numerous syndromes exist. Disorders that lead to pancreatic destruction such as chronic pancreatitis, cystic fibrosis, or hemochromatosis can reduce insulin secretion enough to cause diabetes. Conditions in which excess amounts of counterinsulin hormones are secreted, such as Cushing's disease, acromegaly, pheochromocytoma, and glucagonoma, can also produce diabetes. A number of drugs such as thiazide diuretics, glucocorticoids, and adrenergic agents can lead to, or at least exacerbate, diabetes. Many unusual genetic diseases are associated with a higher than normal incidence of diabetes through unknown mechanisms; these include muscular dystrophy, myotonic dystrophy, Friedreich's ataxia, Turner's syndrome, and others.

Finally, several rare syndromes have been identified, the biochemical mechanisms of which are well described and which primarily involve abnormalities of insulin-glucose physiology. Certain patients with extreme insulin resistance, acanthosis nigricans, and diabetes have been identified with circulating anti-insulin receptor antibodies. These antibodies are part of a more generalized autoimmune process, since proteinuria, leukopenia, and antinuclear and anti-DNA antibodies also exist. Other patients with the triad of acanthosis nigricans, insulin resistance, and diabetes do not have anti-receptor antibodies, but instead have a profound decrease in cellular insulin receptors. Typically these are young females with hirsutism and polycystic ovaries. In one such patient, several family members were also found to have decreased insulin receptors and insulin resistance, suggesting that this disorder is due to a genetically mediated decrease in insulin receptors. Patients have been reported in whom abnormal insulin products are synthesized and secreted and the specific molecular lesions identified. Familial hyperproinsulinemia involves a defect in the proinsulin molecule that prevents normal cleavage of proinsulin to insulin in the pancreatic B cell. This leads to the secretion of large amounts of proinsulin (which is biologically less active than insulin) instead of insulin. This disorder can lead to impaired glucose tolerance, but has not yet been associated with overt fasting hyperglycemia. Rarely patients carry mutations in the insulin structural gene itself that lead to the secretion of insulin species with single amino acid substitutions resulting in markedly reduced biologic activity. These patients have a clinical picture of typical NIDDM. These mutant insulins are immunologically reactive and are secreted in large quantities in response to the hyperglycemic state. The clinical hallmark of this condition is the presence of hyperglycemia and marked hyperinsulinemia in a patient with normal sensitivity to exogenous insulin.

GENETICS

Diabetes has long been termed a geneticist's nightmare. The disease clearly aggregates in families and has a strong familial component. However, the precise genetic contribution to diabetes has been difficult to ascertain for at least four reasons: (1) no specific genetic marker has been identified. Glucose tolerance is the currently used method of diagnosis, but because of differences in the way tests are performed and the criteria used, it is difficult to compare one study to another; (2) There is a great deal of etiologic heterogeneity between IDDM and NIDDM and within these categories. This indicates genetic heterogeneity even though the phenotype (hyperglycemia) is comparable. It is also possible that, depending on environmental factors, there can be variable phenotypic expression of a common genotype; (3) It is likely that a "diabetogenic gene" interacts with external factors as well as with other genetic components, making the specific genetic influences underlying the final phenotypic expression of the diabetes hard to detect; (4) Actual transmission rates of diabetes from generation to generation are low.

Genetic factors are clearly important in the etiology of diabetes. This is demonstrated by classic twin studies. When twins below the age of 40 years are studied, if one twin has diabetes (mostly IDDM based on age) then the other twin develops diabetes only 50 per cent of the time. If the two pairs are concordant, the second twin usually develops diabetes within a couple of years of the first. For a purely genetic disease, concordance should be 100 per cent. This suggests that while genetic factors are important in IDDM, they are only predisposing and must interact with environmental influences if diabetes is to develop. This does not exclude the possibility that in some patients IDDM occurs entirely because of genetic or environmental factors. In twins over 40 years the concordance rate for diabetes (almost all NIDDM based on age) approaches 100 per cent. This suggests that genetic factors are more important in this form of diabetes and may be causal or closely associated with causal mechanisms.

Despite the contribution of genetic factors, direct transmission of diabetes from parent to offspring is surprisingly low. If one parent has IDDM the risk to the offspring of developing IDDM is on the order of 2 to 5 per cent. If one child has IDDM the average risk for another sibling is 5 to 10 per cent. However, the risk is much greater if the second sibling is HLA (human leukocyte antigen)-identical to the first, intermediate if HLA-haploidentical, and very low if HLA-nonidentical. The type of diabetes tends to run true in families, and the incidence of NIDDM in the offspring of an IDDM parent is probably not greater than normal. If one parent has NIDDM the risk is 10 to 15 per cent for offspring developing the disease. When both parents have NIDDM, the transmission risk increases, but adequate data are not available to quantitate the increase in risk. If one sibling has NIDDM, the risk for another sibling is 10 to 15 per cent. These low rates of transmission make it difficult to trace models of inheritance in family studies, but the facts are clinically important in counseling and reassuring diabetic patients who wish to have children.

Strong associations have been identified between IDDM and specific HLA's coded by the major histocompatibility complex region located on the short arm of the sixth chromosome (see Ch. 425). Four loci, designated A, B, C, and D, are now recognized in this region. Loci A, B, and C are defined serologically while the D locus is detected by the mixed lymphocyte (MLC) reaction. A DR locus can also be identified and typed using a serologic test. Although not proven, antigens at the D locus detected by MLC may be identical to the antigens at the DR locus identified serologically. At each of these loci numerous alleles (genes) exist, some of which confer increased risk for the development of IDDM. These high risk alleles include: HLA-DR3, HLA-Dw3, HLA-DR4, HLA-Dw4, HLA-B8, and HLA-B15 (the small w means that the antigen identified at the D locus by MLC has been provisionally accepted by the International Histocompatibility Workshop; the w is deleted when identification is considered definite). The HLA-A, B, and C antigens are present on virtually all nucleated cell types, whereas the HLA-D or DR antigens or both show tissue restriction and are predominantly expressed on B lymphocytes and macrophages. It is possible that D/DR antigens are also expressed on islet cells, but this is unproven at the current time.

An HLA haplotype refers to a particular set of alleles at the four closely linked HLA loci A, B, C, and D, on one of the sixth chromosomes (each person inherits two haplotypes, one from each parent). In this system, some of the alleles are in linkage disequilibrium. This means that certain HLA antigens encoded by alleles at the different HLA loci occur together more frequently within the same haplotype than would be predicted by random statistical chance, taking gene (allele) frequency into account. The antigens encoded by the HLA alleles associated with higher risk for IDDM do not directly cause or predispose to the disease. Rather, these alleles are felt to be in linkage disequilibrium with genes in the HLA region (possibly certain immune response genes) that are directly related to the etiology of IDDM. In other words, through linkage disequilibrium one "looks" at the "diabetogenic gene" via the more easily measured HLA antigens.

Current evidence indicates that the D locus is more important than the B locus because it is more closely linked to the etiologically important genes. In this event, the predictive value of the HLA-B antigen is through its linkage disequilibrium to the D locus. The relative risk for IDDM conferred by HLA-B8 or HLA-B15 is two to four times normal and is four to ten times normal for DR3/Dw3 or DR4/Dw4. Interestingly, homozygosity at any of these alleles (i.e., DR3/DR3) does not lead to greater risk than when the allele occurs on only one haplotype. However, if both sixth chromosomes bear two different diabetes-associated alleles at a particular locus (i.e., DR3/DR4) the increase in risk is more than additive.

It should be kept in mind that the diabetes-associated HLA antigens are quite frequent in the nondiabetic population (although, clearly less frequent than in IDDM). For example, 30 to 35 per cent of normal persons are positive for DR3 or DR4. Thus, far more people who are positive for these antigens are normal than have IDDM (e.g., if the average risk for IDDM in a population is 0.2 per cent, and if a particular HLA haplotype confers a ten-fold increase in risk, then the risk would still be only 2 per cent for those with this haplotype). This is an important point to realize in thinking about HLA typing for screening or predictive value in a practical or clinical sense.

Despite all this information, the model of inheritance for IDDM is obscure, although it is clearly not autosomal dominant. The low penetrance of the diabetes-associated genes combined with the relative degrees of HLA associations suggests that the genetic predisposition must interact with specific environmental factors for IDDM to occur. Additionally, the disease could be multigenic, with at least two genes necessary (allelic or nonallelic) for IDDM to develop. With this model environmental factors would still be necessary.

In NIDDM no HLA associations have been identified, demonstrating the differences in etiology between the two major forms of diabetes. Although the location of the genetic component for NIDDM is not known, possible changes have been noted on the eleventh chromosome, which contains the insulin gene. A 1.5 to 3.4 kilobase insertion of extra DNA, about 500 base pairs upstream from the 5' flanking end of the insulin gene, has been described by some workers as a polymorphism more frequent in patients with NIDDM compared to normal persons or patients with IDDM. The association is slight and the meaning currently uncertain. If this insertion (or some other polymorphism) proves to be an accurate marker for NIDDM, however, this will be of great value in predicting subjects at risk and in tracing inheritance patterns. Furthermore, if this insertion influences gene regulation, it might have causal significance in terms of insulin biosynthesis. However, since NIDDM patients usually have adequate amounts of insulin within B cells, it is not readily apparent how this potential gene abnormality could influence functional dynamics of insulin secretion.

PATHOGENESIS

Before discussion of the pathogenetic aspects of diabetes it is important to review briefly some of the essential features of insulin and glucose physiology. Insulin is produced in the pancreatic B cell as the primary biosynthetic product preproinsulin containing 109 amino acid residues (MW ~ 11,500). This peptide is rapidly converted to proinsulin (86 amino acid residues, MW ~ 9000) by cleavage of the amino terminal 23 amino acid "pre" sequence. Within the B cell secretory granules, proinsulin is converted by proteolytic cleavage to insulin (51 amino acids, MW ~ 6000) and C peptide (31 amino acids, MW ~ 3000). Thus, the final B cell secretory product is 95 per cent insulin and C peptide in equimolar amounts and 5 per cent unconverted proinsulin. In familial hyperproinsulinemia, mutations in the proinsulin sequence prevent proteolytic conversion within the secretory granule, leading to release of large amounts of proinsulin having only 7 to 10 per cent of insulin's biologic activity. The regulation of insulin release is extremely complex, being influenced by glucose, amino acids, gut insulinogenic hormones, glucagon, neural influences, and other factors. However, glucose is the most important stimulus for insulin secretion.

After a brief circulating time (t½ 4 to 8 minutes) insulin interacts with target tissues to exert its biologic effects. At the target cell, insulin action is initiated by binding of the hormone to specific cell surface insulin receptors. In an important advance, the complete amino acid structure of the insulin receptor has now been elucidated. Following formation of the insulin receptor complex one or more signals are propagated (second messengers) that interact with a variety of cellular effector systems such as enzymes and glucose transport proteins to produce insulin's ultimate biologic effects. Insulin exerts its major effects on carbohydrate homeostasis by stimulating peripheral glucose disposal and inhibiting hepatic glucose production. A variety of abnormalities in insulin biosynthesis, secretion, and action can lead to diabetes.

A number of other hormones affect carbohydrate homeostasis termed anti-insulin or counterregulatory hormones (glucagon, growth hormone, cortisol, and catecholamines). Among these, glucagon is probably most important in terms of the pathophysiology of diabetes. Glucagon is 29 amino acids (MW ~ 3000) in length and is synthesized in the pancreatic alpha cells as proglucagon (MW ~ 9000 to 11,000). Its release is stimulated by hypoglycemia, amino acids, neural influences, and stress. Its major effect on glucose metabolism is exerted at the liver where it binds to surface receptors, stimulates cyclic AMP generation, and promotes glycogenolysis, gluconeogenesis, and ketogenesis. Its lipolytic effects are minimal in man, and glucagon has little if any effect on peripheral glucose uptake. Thus, glucagon affects glucose metabolism by influencing hepatic glucose production, and glucagon levels are absolutely or relatively increased in both IDDM and NIDDM.

NIDDM. Abnormalities of insulin and, to a lesser extent, glucagon secretion and action are central to the pathogenesis of NIDDM. Syndromes involving abnormalities of insulin biosynthesis have already been discussed. These include familial hyperproinsulinemia and mutations in the structural gene for insulin leading to secretion of a biologically defective insulin molecule. These rare syndromes lead to mild degrees of glucose intolerance or a clinical picture indistinguishable from NIDDM. Beyond these unusual syndromes, however, insulin biosynthesis is qualitatively normal in NIDDM.

Secretion of insulin is not normal in NIDDM. In some patients with impaired glucose tolerance, substantially reduced amounts of insulin are secreted in response to a glucose load. These subjects are not insulin resistant and the defect in insulin secretion appears adequately to account for their abnormal glucose metabolism. These patients have a relatively high propensity to develop overt NIDDM (up to 50 per cent) and should be followed for progression. Other patients with impaired glucose tolerance secrete normal or increased amounts of insulin, although in some cases the dynamics of secretion may be altered with a delay in release of insulin following a glucose stimulus. These patients are insulin resistant primarily because of decreased insulin receptors. This is true in both the obese and nonobese categories of this classification. In relatively few (about 5 per cent) of the hyperinsulinemic insulin-resistant patients with impaired glucose tolerance is there progression to fasting hyperglycemia.

The great majority of patients with NIDDM are both insulin deficient and insulin resistant. The decrease in insulin action exists whether they are obese or nonobese (although approximately 80 per cent are obese). Patients with NIDDM may have normal or elevated fasting insulin levels, but they almost always secrete decreased amounts of insulin following oral glucose or meals. Other functional abnormalities that have been identified include a marked decrease in early release of insulin (first phase) after intravenous administration of glucose, and much greater blunting of the insulin response to glucose compared to other insulin stimuli (amino acids, sulfonylureas, glucagon, or B agonists). These latter findings have given rise to the idea that B cell dysfunction in NIDDM may be characterized by a defect in glucose recognition by islet cells.

In addition to these abnormalities of insulin secretion, patients with NIDDM are also insulin resistant. Insulin action is a complex sequence of events beginning with binding to surface receptors; insulin resistance can be due to any abnormality at any step along the insulin action pathway. For convenience, the cellular causes of insulin resistance can be broadly divided into binding and postbinding defects (Fig. 231–1). A binding defect involves a decrease in insulin binding due to a decrease in either receptor number or affinity or to both. A postbinding defect refers to any biologically significant abnormality in the activity of effector proteins (such as insulin-sensitive enzymes or transport proteins) or an impairment in

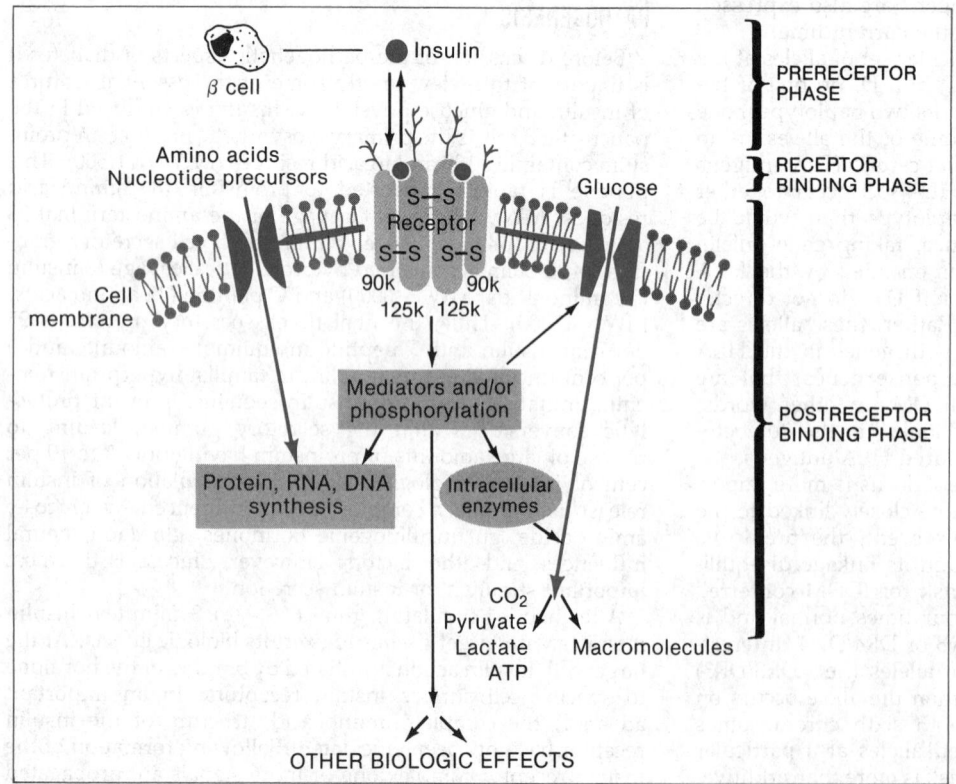

FIGURE 231–1. Model of insulin action and categories of insulin resistance. Abnormalities can occur at the prereceptor phase, involving biosynthesis and secretion of abnormal beta cell products; at the receptor binding phase, involving decreased insulin binding to receptors due to decreased receptor number or affinity; or at the postreceptor binding phase, involving any defect in the insulin action cascade distal to the initial binding event.

the coupling or transducing mechanisms between insulin receptor complexes and effector units. In subjects with impaired glucose tolerance who are insulin resistant, binding defects exist (decreased receptor number), but postbinding function is normal. In NIDDM, insulin resistance exists in the great majority of patients. Although a receptor defect (decreased number) is present in most insulin-resistant NIDDM patients, this does not appear to be the major abnormality. Postbinding defects also exist, and these appear to play the predominant role in causing the insulin-resistant state. As far as glucose homeostasis is concerned, at least one type of postbinding defect has been biochemically defined in NIDDM; that is, these patients exhibit a decrease in the intrinsic activity of the glucose transport effector system.

Insulin deficiency and insulin resistance both contribute to the hyperglycemia of NIDDM. In addition, another abnormality also contributes to the hyperglycemia. Hepatic glucose production rates are increased in NIDDM, and the magnitude of this increase is proportional to the level of fasting hyperglycemia. This hepatic abnormality is, at least partially, due to resistance to insulin's normal restraining effect on liver glucose production. Additionally, glucagon levels are often elevated, either absolutely or relatively, in NIDDM, and it is possible that excess glucagon stimulation also contributes to the increase in glucose production.

Thus, insulin deficiency, insulin resistance, and accelerated hepatic glucose production all exist in NIDDM, and all contribute to the hyperglycemia (Fig. 231–2). It is tempting to suggest a unifying pathogenetic hypothesis in which one metabolic lesion is primary and the others secondary. Unfortunately it is not possible to choose any particular sequence at this time. All three abnormalities can be generated in animal models by inducing hyperglycemia and hypoinsulinemia, and all three are at least partially reversible with weight loss, oral sulfonylureas, or insulin therapy.

IDDM. A strong genetic component is involved in the etiology of IDDM, but extragenetic factors must also contribute, at least in most patients. Several lines of evidence suggest a role for *viruses* in IDDM: (1) Autopsies of IDDM patients dying within a few months of the disease's onset have revealed an "insulitis" consisting of round cell infiltration of islet tissue. (2) A modest seasonal variation to the incidence of IDDM has been noted in some studies. (3) A clinical history of preceding viral-type illness, particularly Coxsackie B and mumps, is often reported at the onset of IDDM. (4) Increased viral titers, including coxsackievirus B4, have been reported in IDDM patients at or near the time of the disease's onset. (5) Certain diabetogenic viruses (encephalomyocarditis M,

coxsackievirus B, and rheovirus) can cause diabetes when inoculated into rodents. Further, the susceptibility of different rodent strains to develop viral-induced diabetes appears to be under genetic control. (6) Diabetogenic viruses can also directly infect B cells in culture, causing cell lysis and death. (7) Finally, direct support for virus-induced diabetes has been obtained in humans. Coxsackievirus B4 was isolated from the pancreas of a boy with new-onset IDDM who died of severe ketoacidosis closely following a flulike illness associated with rising serum titers of neutralizing antibody to the virus. The viral isolate was inoculated into experimental animals, producing diabetes, and viral antigens could be demonstrated in the B cells from the infected animals.

Autoimmunity may also play a role in the etiology of IDDM. Circulating antibodies to thyroid, gastric mucosa, and the adrenal are far more common in patients with IDDM than in normal persons. More importantly, up to 90 per cent of patients with new-onset IDDM have demonstrable titers of plasma islet cell antibodies. These antibodies are heterogeneous, some binding to cytoplasmic antigens common to all islet cells and others directed against the B cell surface. The latter lyse B cells in culture in the presence of complement, consistent with a pathophysiologic role in vivo. These islet cell antibodies are also observed in BB rats, an animal model that spontaneously develops an IDDM-like syndrome. In humans, titers of islet cell antibodies fall after the onset of clinical disease; by five years only 20 per cent of patients have demonstrable titers, and by 10 to 20 years the prevalence falls to 5 to 10 per cent. Patients who continue to demonstrate antibodies after several years may be examples of heterogeneity within IDDM. In these patients IDDM may represent a primary autoimmune disease, since they are largely female, show a great prevalence of other organ-specific antibodies, and have a strong family history of autoimmune disease. Patients with onset of IDDM at an older age tend to fall in this group. Genetically, they may also be different, since they have a greater prevalence of HLA-B8 and DR3. In cases of IDDM in which islet cell antibodies are cleared within one year of the disease's onset, patients are more often male, do not typically show signs of other autoimmune phenomena, experience onset of disease at a younger age, and have a higher association with HLA-B15 and HLA-DR4. Circulating antibodies may not be the only component of the immune response associated with IDDM; a cell-mediated immune response may also be involved. Increased K cells (killer lymphocytes) have been reported in IDDM along with alterations in T lymphocyte subpopulations. Both antibody-induced and cell-mediated immune phenomena may be involved in the pathogenesis of IDDM.

Strong arguments can be made for the role of genetic susceptibility, viruses, and altered immunity in the etiology of IDDM (Fig. 231–3). However, the contribution of these factors and the sequential relationship among them cannot be stated at this time. Clearly, immune responses could provide the causal link between the HLA associations and clinical IDDM, since the HLA alleles are thought to be associated through linkage disequilibrium to immune response genes. One way to integrate these factors would be to postulate that susceptibility to IDDM is inherited through genes closely associated with the HLA loci. Given this proper genetic background, environmental agents such as certain viruses exhibiting B cell tropism and possibly chemical agents can injure and in some cases destroy B cells. Following B cell injury, an immune response (possibly antibody and cell mediated) directed against B cells occurs owing to release of B cell antigens into the circulation, alteration of B cell antigens, cross-reactivity with viral antigens, or primary modulation of the immune response. In any event, the immune response would then exacerbate or complete the initial viral or chemical B cell injury. Of course this is only one of several sequences that can be proposed. IDDM is probably heterogeneous, and

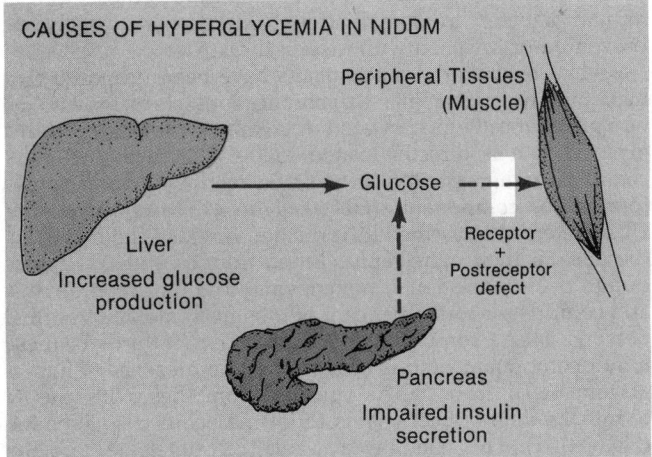

FIGURE 231–2. Summary of the metabolic abnormalities in NIDDM which contribute to the hyperglycemia. Increased hepatic glucose production, impaired insulin secretion, and insulin resistance due to receptor and postreceptor defects all combine to generate the hyperglycemic state.

In the figure: CAUSES OF HYPERGLYCEMIA IN NIDDM — Peripheral Tissues (Muscle), Glucose, Receptor + Postreceptor defect, Liver, Increased glucose production, Pancreas, Impaired insulin secretion

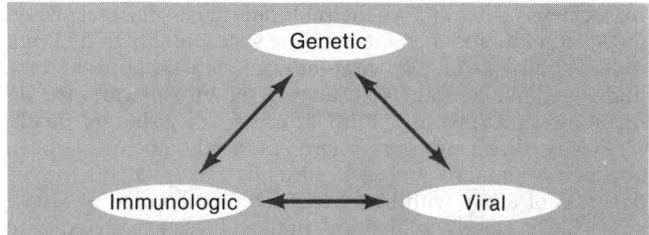

FIGURE 231–3. An interplay of genetic, immunologic, and viral etiologies contributes to the pathogenesis of NIDDM. The importance of each factor probably differs in subpopulations of IDDM, demonstrating the heterogeneity of this disease.

no single sequence of pathogenetic events will necessarily explain all cases. For example, IDDM patients who are HLA-B8/DR3 display other organ-specific autoantibodies and probably have a primary autoimmune disease and do not need an environmental factor to develop the disease. Based on the intertwining of genetic, viral, and immune influences, it also follows that B cell destruction in IDDM does not usually occur acutely. It is likely that this process is gradual over months to years, even though the clinical onset of metabolic decompensation is usually abrupt when destruction of B cell mass reaches a critical point or an intercurrent illness occurs. Indeed, the presence of circulating islet cell antibodies has been detected several years prior to the clinical onset of IDDM in a number of patients. This raises the possibility of intervention therapies (immune or other) following the onset of B cell injury but prior to clinical manifestations of IDDM, since by the time IDDM appears B cell destruction may be too far advanced for effective therapy. Such an approach would require a method to detect preclinical IDDM.

C peptide is secreted in equimolar amounts compared to insulin. Since C peptide has a much longer half-life than insulin, it provides an excellent measure of insulin secretory capacity, especially in those patients with circulating anti-insulin antibodies that interfere with usual insulin radioimmunoassays. In patients with type I diabetes who have been treated with insulin for longer than five years, C peptide levels are usually undetectable. However, C peptide may be measured in many of these patients during the first years of their disease. This suggests that the loss of beta cell secretion in IDDM is not abrupt, but continues for several years after the diabetes becomes clinically apparent. For the most part, ease of diabetic management and stability of metabolic control in IDDM are correlated with the degree of the residual insulin

TABLE 231–2. SOME FEATURES DISTINGUISHING INSULIN-DEPENDENT FROM NON–INSULIN-DEPENDENT DIABETES

	IDDM	NIDDM
Synonym	Type I	Type II
Age of onset	Usually <30	Usually >40
Ketosis	Common	Rare
Body weight	Nonobese	Obese (80%)
Prevalence	0.2%–0.3%	2%–4%
Genetics		
HLA association	Yes	No
Monozygotic twin studies	40%–50% concordance rate	Concordance rate near 100%
Circulating islet cell antibodies	Yes	No
Associated with other autoimmune phenomena	Occasional	No
Treatment with insulin	Always necessary	Usually not required
Complications	Frequent	Frequent
Insulin secretion	Severe deficiency	Variable: moderate deficiency to hyperinsulinemia
Insulin resistance	Occasional: with poor control or excessive insulin antibodies	Usual: due to receptor and postreceptor defects

secretion. Those patients with the highest levels of circulating C peptide are easier to treat, and in those with undetectable levels the disease is more unstable. Some of the major clinical and pathophysiologic distinctions between IDDM and NIDDM are listed in Table 231–2.

TREATMENT

In this section, details concerning the various methods of diabetic management will be discussed. However, since the severity and clinical picture of diabetes are quite variable, therapeutic methods are also varied. In particular, major differences exist in the approach to NIDDM versus IDDM, and whenever possible therapeutic distinctions for these two forms of diabetes will be made.

RELATIONSHIP BETWEEN HYPERGLYCEMIA AND COMPLICATIONS. It is important to start with more general principles and to identify overall therapeutic goals. A consideration of therapeutic goals involves one of the most important questions in the field, that is, what is the relationship between hyperglycemia and the development of diabetic complications? Simply put, are complications due to hyperglycemia or are they due to genetic or other factors independent of hyperglycemia? This is the central clinical question in diabetes concerning which a voluminous literature exists.

Hyperglycemia is the most obvious metabolic abnormality in diabetes. It is therefore reasonable to suspect that elevated glucose levels play a role in diabetic complications. Consistent with this is a large body of retrospective evidence showing that better control is usually associated with fewer complications. Unfortunately, in the absence of randomized, prospective studies in which significant differences in glycemic control are achieved between matched experimental and control groups over an extended period, current clinical studies can provide only nonconclusive evidence. Classic diabetic complications can occur in secondary diabetes (in which genetic aspects of diabetes are presumably missing) and in normal kidneys following transplantation into diabetic patients. Furthermore, in twin studies the degree of retinopathy is comparable in twins concordant for IDDM, whereas in discordant pairs the nondiabetic twin does not have retinopathy. Certain abnormalities seen in diabetes, such as retinal capillary leakage (as demonstrated by fluorescein angiography), slowed motor nerve conductive velocity, and microalbuminuria, can be reversed by intensive insulin therapy, but the relationship between these physiologic abnormalities and clinically significant complications has not been demonstrated. In animal experiments a number of studies have shown good correlation between the level of hyperglycemia and microvascular complications similar (but perhaps not identical) to those seen in human diabetes. In animals, these complications can also be prevented or reversed with insulin therapy.

Several biochemical mechanisms have been proposed that may link hyperglycemia to complications. Proteins can be nonenzymatically glycosylated in vivo, and the degree of this glycosylation is directly related to the degree of hyperglycemia. Chromatography of red blood cell hemolysates shows four minor components (HbA_{1a1}, HbA_{1a2}, HbA_{1b1}, HbA_{1c}) of HbA, referred to as the HbA_1 fraction or "fast" hemoglobins (because of their more rapid elution from columns). HbA_1 is due to post-translational, nonenzymatic modification of HbA and comprises about 6 per cent of total hemoglobin in normal persons. HbA_{1c} comprises approximately two thirds of these minor components and is increased in the presence of hyperglycemia. To form HBA_{1c}, glucose combines with the N terminal valine of beta chains to form a Schiff base aldimine (Fig. 231–4). This compound is relatively unstable, and the reaction is readily reversible. The aldimine undergoes an Amadori rearrangement to form the more stable ketoamine. HbA can also be glycosylated through the same chemical reaction at the N terminus of the alpha chain and epsilon amino groups of lysines. HbA_{1c} can be measured by various

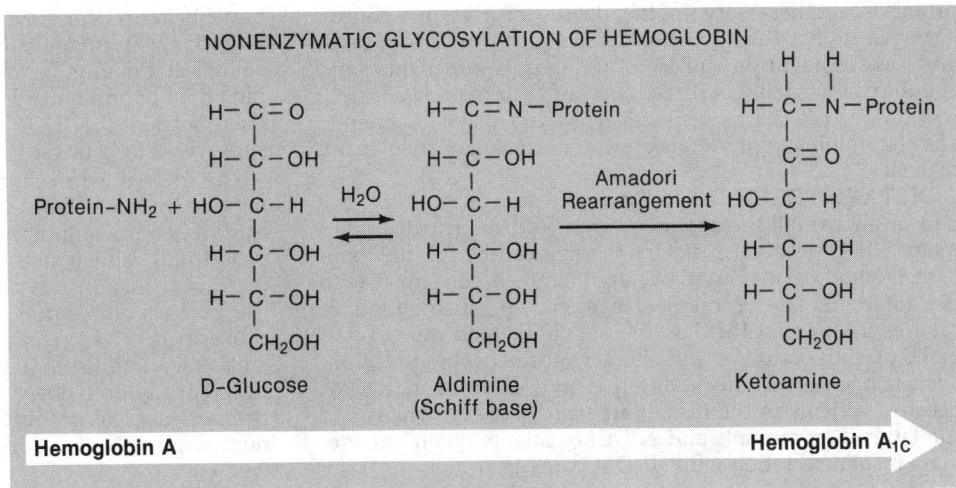

FIGURE 231–4. Chemical reactions underlying the nonenzymatic glycosylation of hemoglobin A to hemoglobin A_{1C}

chromatographic techniques, and total glycosylated hemoglobin can be measured chemically. Glycosylation occurs continuously within the red cell and is a direct reflection of the average glucose concentration in which the cell is exposed throughout its 120-day lifespan. Measurement of glycosylated hemoglobin content therefore provides a useful means to assess the chronic degree of hyperglycemia that existed in a given patient over the preceding several weeks and is not affected by acute changes in plasma glucose level. Additionally, the nonspecific and nonenzymatic nature of hemoglobin glycosylation raises the possibility that glycosylation of other body proteins can occur, leading to structural or functional changes that may be related to chronic diabetic complications. Increased amounts of glycosylated low-density lipoprotein (LDL) molecules, for example, circulate in hyperglycemic diabetic patients and do not bind normally to LDL receptors. Since abnormal glycosylation may affect all tissues, this mechanism could be related to a variety of diabetic complications.

Additional biochemical lesions related to hyperglycemia have been proposed for nervous tissue. *Sorbitol* is a polyhydroxyl alcohol (polyol) produced from glucose by aldose reductase in nerve tissue; once formed, sorbitol can be converted to fructose (Fig. 231–5). It is theorized that this polyol pathway is particularly active in diabetes because of the hyperglycemia. This could lead to increased intracellular osmolarity (due to accumulation of sorbitol and fructose) with water influx, swelling of Schwann cells, anoxia, and demyelination. Consistent with this, an increase in sorbitol content has been found in nerve tissue of diabetic rats, and it is reversible with insulin therapy. However, Schwann cell swelling and increased water content have not yet been demonstrated, and further testing of the polyol pathway hypothesis is necessary. Another hyperglycemia-related metabolic lesion in nervous tissue has been proposed involving *myoinositol*. Concentrations of this compound are decreased in peripheral nerves of diabetic rats, and this is associated with a decrease in nerve conduction velocity. These abnormalities can be prevented by insulin or oral myoinositol supplements. It is possible that uptake of myoinositol by nerves is inhibited by hyperglycemia, leading to depletion and pathologic sequelae. A link may exist between polyol and myoinositol metabolism in that increased activity of the polyol pathway contributes to the reduction in nerve myoinositol content.

The above discussion cites clinical and biochemical evidence supporting the relationship between hyperglycemia and complications. On the other hand, there is evidence against this relationship. For example, patients have been reported with diabetic complications at the time of onset of IDDM, when hyperglycemia should not have preexisted for a significant time. Additionally, some patients with very poor glycemic control never develop complications. Perhaps, independent of IDDM, patients have differing genetic susceptibilities to complications related to hyperglycemia. Ultimately, however, the main argument against the relationship is simply that it has not been proven with certainty by well-controlled, prospective studies in humans. An NIH-sponsored multicenter study called the Diabetes Control and Complications Trial (DCCT) is now under way to answer this important question.

Taking all factors into account, it seems reasonable to conclude that although a definitive relationship between hyperglycemia and complications has been neither established nor disproved at present, the bulk of evidence weighs in favor of such a relationship. With this in mind it seems prudent to establish as a therapeutic goal the maintenance of plasma glucose levels as close to normal as possible in diabetic patients. The major complication of aggressive antidiabetic therapy is hypoglycemia, which, if severe enough, can unequivocally produce immediate and irreversible CNS damage. Therefore, diabetic management should be pushed until glucose levels are normal or near normal, unless recurrent, overt episodes of hypoglycemia develop. If this occurs, then com-

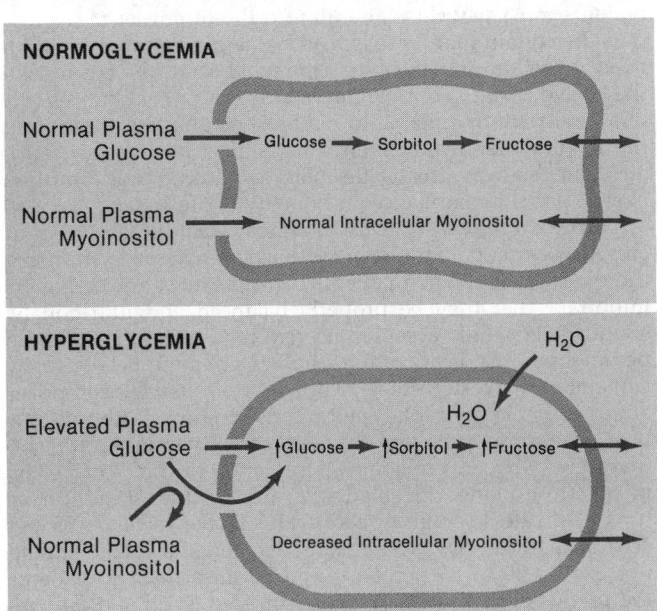

FIGURE 231–5. Metabolic theories for the pathogenesis of diabetic neuropathy secondary to hyperglycemia. This demonstrates the suggested effects of hyperglycemia to increase intracellular sorbitol and fructose concentrations, leading to an osmotic increase in intracellular water content. In addition, it has been suggested that hyperglycemia depletes intracellular myoinositol content by competitively inhibiting the uptake of myoinositol from the extracellular space.

promises are necessary in the degree of glycemic control achieved. Other therapeutic goals include (1) normal growth and development in children, (2) normal pregnancy and childbirth in females, (3) reduction of diabetes-related atherosclerosis risk factors, especially in adult diabetic patients, and (4) minimal interference with normal life style in all diabetics.

DIETARY TREATMENT. Dietary treatment is an integral part of the overall therapeutic plan in all diabetic patients. In many NIDDM patients dietary therapy can be the predominant method of treatment. Dietary therapy is concerned with the total number of calories ingested, the distribution of calories throughout the day, the individual food sources that make up these calories, and maintenance of proper nutrition. Dietary therapy is much different in NIDDM and IDDM, because patients in the former are usually obese, whereas in the latter they are not, and NIDDM patients retain endogenous insulin secretion while IDDM patients do not.

Total Caloric Intake. Since most NIDDM patients are overweight, caloric restriction is advisable and can be of great benefit. The essential tenet of weight reduction is straightforward: if caloric expenditure exceeds intake, weight will be lost. There are many ways to calculate daily caloric expenditure, but on the average this amounts to 30 to 35 kcal per kilogram in normal humans; 25 kcal per kilogram is attributed to the basal metabolic rate and the rest to physical activity. Daily caloric requirements are about 30 kcal per kilogram in sedentary individuals and approximately 35 kcal per kilogram in moderately active subjects. For those who engage in brisk physical exertion for prolonged intervals throughout the day caloric expenditure can exceed 35 kcal per kilogram. Another factor affecting caloric requirements (at least on a per kilogram basis) is the degree of adiposity. Adipose tissue is predominantly storage triglyceride, which is relatively inert metabolically with a decreased caloric need per unit weight. Thus the greater the degree of adiposity, the lower an individual's caloric requirement per kilogram. In very obese, sedentary individuals, daily caloric requirements can be as low as 25 kcal per kilogram of body weight.

A number of approaches to weight reduction exist that vary in the degree of caloric restriction and rate of weight loss, dietary constituents, as well as behavioral and psychological support measures. These include nutritionally sound and modestly restricted diets that achieve slow gradual weight loss over several months, nutritionally balanced and very low calorie diets for rapid weight loss, and behavior modification, pharmacologic aids, and even surgical procedures (i.e., gastric plication) in the morbidly obese patient in whom medical therapy fails. These approaches are discussed in detail in Ch. 216.

For all these methods, inducing the initial period of weight loss is not the major problem in weight reduction, but, rather, the major problem is weight regain or recidivism. Motivated patients can usually successfully lose weight over the initial dietary period, but it is the unusual patient who successfully keeps the pounds off. The major challenge in weight reduction therapy is to develop a proper supportive environment and patient motivation to maintain weight loss after it has been achieved. In the NIDDM patient, significant caloric restriction is usually successful in lowering plasma glucose levels even before significant weight loss is achieved. Depending on the degree of obesity that was present initially and the amount of weight loss, continued beneficial effects on glycemic control can be maintained after the goal weight is achieved and a eucaloric diet is initiated. In general, the more recent the onset of NIDDM, the more responsive the patient will be to the beneficial effects of weight reduction. In patients with pronounced fasting hyperglycemia, very low calorie diets (300 to 600 kcal per day) are often useful in achieving rapid glycemic control as well as an initial rapid rate of weight loss (which can often be of important psychological and motiva-

tional benefit). Very low calorie diets usually consist of liquid formula meals and should not be utilized unless they contain adequate amounts (a minimum 30 to 40 grams per day) of high quality protein and are supplemented with vitamins and micronutrients. NIDDM patients on such diets should be supervised by a physician.

The mechanisms whereby weight reduction improves hyperglycemia in NIDDM are not completely clear. Weight loss leads to a reduction in the accelerated rates of hepatic glucose production, ameliorates the degree of insulin resistance by increasing insulin receptors and reducing the magnitude of the postreceptor defect in insulin action, and possibly improves beta cell secretion. However, the precise cellular mechanisms leading to these effects are not known. Patients with IDDM are seldom obese, and an important nutritional goal is maintenance of adequate nutrition, particularly to assure normal growth and development in children and pregnant women.

Distribution of Calories. In addition to total caloric consumption, attention should also be paid to the distribution of calories throughout the day in any dietary prescription. Two principles should be kept in mind: (1) calories should be spread as evenly as possible throughout the major daily meals to avoid a large concentration of calories at any one meal and not to overwhelm the diabetic patient's impaired capacity to metabolize food; and (2) in those patients receiving exogenous insulin, caloric intake should be temporally adjusted to coincide with the time course of action of the administered insulin. The latter point highlights a major difference in dietary consideration between patients with IDDM and NIDDM. In NIDDM, endogenous insulin secretion is still present and the beta cell can respond at the appropriate times (albeit to a limited degree) to food ingestion, regardless of when it occurs throughout the day. This is even true, although to a lesser extent, in NIDDM subjects who are treated with insulin. Thus, in these patients it is sufficient to balance calories throughout the day, but the patient has a good deal of leeway to determine the timing of specific meals as long as calories are ingested at times of peak exogenous insulin action. For practical purposes, the only insulin present in patients with IDDM is that which is administered exogenously. Therefore, patients must pay close attention to the timing of meals and must be certain that there is reasonable concordance between meal ingestion and the time course of action of the insulin they have taken. To a certain extent the patient can elect a temporal pattern suitable to his lifestyle and preference and the insulin therapy regimen can then be tailored appropriately. In this way greater flexibility is allowed that improves overall patient compliance and quality of life.

Nutrient Content of Diet. A great deal of attention is currently being paid to the individual components comprising the diabetic diet. When patients consume eucaloric diets, it is important that they be properly balanced and nutritionally sound. A generally accepted protein requirement is 0.8 gram per kilogram per day for adults, but larger amounts are usually consumed in Western diets. Thus, protein usually comprises about 15 per cent of total caloric consumption. With this as a base, the proportions of fat and carbohydrate (CHO) are inversely related. Previous attempts to restrict total CHO intake are no longer deemed advisable, and most authorities now advocate liberalization of CHO intake to 50 to 55 per cent of total calories. This means that total fat intake should not exceed 30 to 35 per cent, and because diabetic patients are predisposed to macrovascular disease, saturated fat (primarily animal fat) intake should be reduced so that the polyunsaturated-saturated fat ratio is equivalent to 1:0. Ideally, cholesterol intake should not exceed 450 mg per day. The makeup of the CHO portion of the diet also requires attention. In the past it was felt that diabetics should rigorously avoid sucrose because it is rapidly absorbed and raises the blood glucose level inordinately. While this may be true when sucrose is consumed as the sole nutritive component, as in soft drinks or certain candies, it is less of a problem when modest amounts of sucrose are eaten in a mixed meal setting. Because of this, up to 5 per cent of total CHO can be consumed as added sucrose, as long as it is taken in the context of a mixed meal and spaced out through the day. This allows the diabetic a wider variety of food choices, making the diet more palatable; a side benefit of this approach is that it improves patient adherence to the dietary prescription and to the other elements of the overall therapeutic plan. The remainder of the CHO should consist predominantly of starches. All complex CHO cannot be lumped together as a single food group because the glycemic response to different starches differs widely, being lowest for lentils and pasta and highest for wheat and potatoes. More work needs to be done to determine the glycemic potency of a large number of foods, singly and together, in diabetic patients before the precise composition of the CHO in the diet can be recommended with certainty. At this stage it is advisable for the diabetic to consume 50 to 55 per cent of calories as CHO with a modest restriction in sucrose intake and emphasis on ingestion of those complex CHOs with low glycemic potency.

Fructose is a nutritive sweetener that may also have a place in the diabetic diet. This simple CHO is somewhat sweeter than sucrose and has similar properties when prepared in foods. Thus, fructose can be substituted for sucrose in most foods with little change in taste or texture. The advantage is that fructose is absorbed from the gastrointestinal tract more slowly than sucrose and is predominantly taken up and metabolized by the liver through non-insulin–dependent mechanisms. Within the liver, fructose is phosphorylated and eventually converted to glycogen or triglyceride through the triose phosphate intermediates. Thus, little fructose escapes hepatic uptake to enter peripheral circulation, and only a small amount of fructose is converted to glucose for release from the liver. Ingestion of fructose leads to a minimal postprandial rise in plasma glucose or insulin levels in normal persons and in diabetics when taken alone or as part of a mixed meal. For these reasons, fructose offers some advantage in the diabetic diet, and amounts up to 75 grams per day can be safely consumed. The major exception occurs in patients with severely uncontrolled NIDDM or in poorly insulinized IDDM patients. In these conditions glycogen production is inhibited and fructose enters the gluconeogenic pathway and is ultimately released as glucose, causing hyperglycemia.

Dietary fiber can also influence CHO absorption. Glycemic excursions are reduced and insulin secretion diminished when normal persons and subjects with NIDDM consume fiber-enriched diets. This effect is mediated through delayed gastric emptying and overall slowing of the rate of CHO digestion and absorption. Since large amounts of fiber (10 to 15 grams per meal) are needed to observe these effects, major changes in dietary patterns would be necessary to achieve beneficial results. Nevertheless, when fiber is consumed as natural foods, there do not seem to be any untoward effects of increased fiber ingestion, and some studies indicate that increased fiber intake can lower serum triglyceride levels. The only potential caveat to this statement involves growing children and pregnant women, since subtle undesirable changes in micronutrient absorption due to high fiber ingestion have not been ruled out.

A minority of diabetic patients adhere to the recommended dietary regimens. To a large extent this is due to inadequate understanding on the part of the patient as well as the physician regarding dietary goals and methods. An additional factor is that dietary therapy must be individualized, taking into account each patient's life style, economic status, food preferences, and social needs. This can be a time-consuming process, and few physicians have the time or training to participate with patients in this type of detailed dietary management. For this reason it is critical to incorporate a dietitian or nutritionist trained in the principles of dietary therapy of diabetes as part of the health care team. One cannot simply give pamphlets, instructional aids, and meal plans and expect even motivated patients to adhere to the necessary regimens. Detailed instruction by a nutrition counselor is necessary to tailor the diet to each patient's special needs. Dietary therapy is a means of long-term treatment, and therefore the longer view is important. Occasional deviations from recommended meal plans for special occasions are acceptable, providing the patient has a clear understanding of how this should be managed. Often this allows for better patient compliance with the overall diet plan. Periodic meetings with a nutrition counselor are necessary to implement and maintain individualized dietary regimens.

ORAL HYPOGLYCEMIC AGENTS. Oral hypoglycemic agents are often therapeutically effective in NIDDM patients. In patients who do not respond satisfactorily to diet and do not have severe hyperglycemia (i.e., plasma glucose levels consistently greater than 250 mg per deciliter), oral agents are an appropriate therapeutic choice. In patients with severe hyperglycemia, insulin therapy is preferable, at least initially, to gain more rapid control of clinical symptoms and to prevent hyperosmolarity. While sulfonylureas are effective in patients with NIDDM, they are ineffective in IDDM. Some have suggested that combinations of oral agents with insulin can reduce insulin requirements of IDDM; however, this has not been proven, and would be of minor clinical importance anyway.

The mechanism of action of sulfonylureas is complex. In the short term, they augment B cell insulin secretion. However, after several months of therapy, insulin levels return to pretreatment values while glucose levels remain improved. These findings led to the demonstration that sulfonylureas exert extrapancreatic effects on glucose metabolism: (1) They reduce the accelerated rates of hepatic glucose production in NIDDM; (2) they partially reverse the postbinding defect in insulin action; and (3) they increase the number of cellular insulin receptors. These all represent significant components of the insulin resistance of NIDDM, so sulfonylureas can improve glycemia by improving insulin's effectiveness at target cells. The relative importance of each of these actions in ameliorating hyperglycemia is unclear, but it is likely that the pancreatic and extrapancreatic effects of these agents combine to produce the hypoglycemic action of these drugs.

There are several different kinds of sulfonylureas, differing primarily in potency, pharmacokinetics, and modes of metabolism as outlined in Table 231–3. *Tolbutamide* is metabolized to inert products by the liver and has a relatively short half-life, necessitating administration two to three times a day. Although it is the least potent of the available sulfonylureas on a weight basis, it has not been clearly demonstrated that any sulfonylurea produces greater hypoglycemic potency at maximal doses in diabetic patients. Therefore, for practical purposes, the differences in relative potency of the different drugs simply mean that more or less of a given agent should be used. *Tolazamide* and especially *acetohexamide* are metabolized by the liver to biologically active products that are then excreted by the kidneys. These drugs have intermediate half-lives and are usually given twice (but sometimes once) a day. *Chlorpropamide* also undergoes considerable hepatic degradation into less active metabolites excreted in the urine. This compound can cause significant water retention and hyponatremia by potentiating ADH action on the kidney. Chlorpropamide has the longest circulating half-life and duration of action (about 60 hours) and is given only once a day. Hypoglycemia is the major complication of sulfonylureas, and this can be particularly severe with chlorpropamide because of its long duration of action. Elderly NIDDM subjects are more susceptible to hypoglycemia, especially those prone to skip meals. The route of metabolism of the different compounds may influence the choice of agent. One should be

TABLE 231–3. CHARACTERISTICS OF SULFONYLUREAS

Generic Name	Brand Name	Dosage Range (mg)	Duration of Action (hr)	Comments
Tolbutamide	Orinase	500–3000	6–12	Metabolized by liver to inert products, given 2–3 ×/day
Chlorpropamide	Diabinase	100–500	60	Metabolized by liver (~70%) to less active metabolite, and excreted intact (~30%) by kidneys; can potentiate ADH action, given 1×/day
Acetohexamide	Dymelor	250–1500	12–24	Metabolized by liver to active metabolite, given 1–2×/day
Tolazamide	Tolinase	100–1000	10–18	Metabolized by liver to active product, given 1–2×/day
Glyburide	Micronase	2.5–30	10–30	Metabolized by liver to inert products, given 1×/day
Glipizide	Glucotrol	5–40	18–30	Metabolized by liver to inert products, given 1×/day

cautious about the use of chlorpropamide, acetohexamide, and, to a lesser extent, tolazamide in patients with compromised renal function because of the route of excretion. Second-generation sulfonylureas, such as *glibenclamide* and glipizide were released for use in the United States in 1984 and are rapidly finding increased use in practice. These agents are metabolized by the liver and have relatively long duration of action and can be given once a day. It is claimed, but not rigorously demonstrated, that the second-generation sulfonylureas are more effective than the first-generation drugs.

The other major category of oral hypoglycemic agents consists of the biguanides, such as *phenformin*. The exact mechanism of action of these drugs is not clear, although they may interfere with hepatic gluconeogenesis. However, these drugs were strongly implicated in the development of lactic acidosis and have been prohibited from clinical use in the United States by the Food and Drug Administration.

In NIDDM, the usual practice is to begin with a low dose of a given sulfonylurea, advancing the dose until the therapeutic response is satisfactory or a maximal dose is reached. Occasionally patients who do not respond to one drug can be switched to another with beneficial effect. Most patients who do not achieve a therapeutic response with a given sulfonylurea will not respond satisfactorily by switching to another. Enough patients do respond to this approach, however, so that it is an appropriate tactic before it is concluded that oral hypoglycemic drugs are not effective in a specific patient. Certain drug interactions occur with sulfonylureas, that is, phenylbutazone and anticoagulants compete for hepatic removal mechanisms with sulfonylureas. A disulfiram (Antabuse)-like reaction can occasionally occur following alcohol consumption by patients taking sulfonylureas. This is most frequently reported with chlorpropamide and has not yet been noted with the second-generation agents. Potential interactions of this sort should always be kept in mind in the appropriate clinical context.

Approximately 10 to 20 per cent of NIDDM patients do not respond to oral agents, and treatment is termed primary failure. Secondary failure occurs when a patient responds initially to an oral agent, but then ceases to respond in the next year or two. This occurs in 5 to 20 per cent of patients, but these proportions obviously depend on the particular NIDDM population studied. For example, patients with new-onset diabetes respond better than those with longstanding disease. In some cases, secondary failure is due to dietary noncompliance in a patient who previously successfully adhered to a dietary regimen. However, this is often not the case, and the mechanisms of secondary failure in many patients with NIDDM remain unknown.

Debate exists as to which patients with NIDDM are appropriate candidates for oral sulfonylurea therapy. In view of the evidence implicating hyperglycemia with diabetic complications, the therapeutic goal with oral agents should be the maintenance of glucose levels as near to normal as possible. In patients with mild to moderate fasting hyperglycemia (140 to 230 mg per deciliter), dietary therapy should be tried first;

if the above therapeutic goals are not achieved with this approach, then a sulfonylurea can be added. The problem arises in patients with more severe fasting hyperglycemia (more than 230 mg per deciliter) who have pronounced clinical symptoms despite dietary treatment. In these patients, some would advise an initial period of sulfonylurea therapy, and if satisfactory control is not achieved, then insulin treatment should be substituted. Others would suggest an initial period of insulin therapy following which the patient is switched to sulfonylureas: if satisfactory control is achieved, the drug is continued. Alternatively, insulin can be used indefinitely in these patients. Clearly this is a gray area, and the particular approach should be individualized to each patient, taking into account the total clinical context of the patient's disease, acceptance of the various therapeutic methods, level of diabetes education, and motivation. In a patient in whom severe fasting hyperglycemia is maintained, with marked clinical symptoms and incipient hyperosmolarity, oral agents are probably not appropriate, at least initially. In these patients insulin therapy should be the primary mode of treatment and can be continued indefinitely, or a therapeutic trial of sulfonylureas can be substituted once the hyperglycemia has been brought under control by the initial period of insulin treatment. In general, response to sulfonylurea therapy is best if the onset of diabetes is recent and the patient is over 40 years of age and not thin.

INSULIN TREATMENT. Insulin is the primary mode of therapy in all patients with IDDM and in many with NIDDM (see above). The goals of therapy include: (1) normal growth and development in children, (2) normal pregnancy, delivery, and conceptus in women, (3) minimal interference with psychosocial adjustment, (4) acceptable glycemic control, with minimal hypoglycemia, and (5) prevention of complications. Little disagreement exists concerning goals 1 to 3; however, different views exist of how best to achieve goals 4 and 5. There are many different methods of insulin therapy, and the method chosen is highly dependent on one's views of goals 4 and 5. If a physician holds closely to the important relationship between control and complications, then "acceptable control" will be much more rigorously defined and a method of insulin treatment that is designed to produce the desired response will be chosen. On the other hand, those who question the link between hyperglycemia and complications are advocates of looser control and will utilize a less intensive method of insulin delivery. In general, it is quite easy to eliminate overt symptoms of hyperglycemia with any method of insulin therapy, but it is extremely difficult, and probably impossible, to achieve euglycemia on a 24-hour basis. How close one comes to this ideal depends on the method of insulin delivery chosen, which in turn depends on one's philosophy of diabetic management.

Insulin Preparations. To begin a discussion of the methods of insulin treatment, let us first consider the many different kinds of insulin available. Commercial insulin comes in concentrations of 100 units per milliliter (U-100) and 500 units per milliliter (U-500). The various insulin preparations differ in their time course of action (rapid, intermediate, and long acting), degree of purity, and source (beef, pork, beef-pork, or human synthetic insulin); these properties are outlined in Table 231–4. By adjustment of pH during preparation, the size of the zinc-insulin crystal can be modified; the larger the crystals, the slower the release after subcutaneous injection, and this accounts for the differences in time of action between semilente (rapid-acting) and ultralente (long-acting) insulin. Lente (intermediate-acting) insulin is simply a 30:70 mixture of semilente and ultralente, respectively. The other method to delay the onset of action of injected insulin is to mix it with a protein (protamine) and adjust the pH. This results in NPH (intermediate-acting) and PZI (long-acting) preparations. It should be cautioned that the values for peak onset and duration of action listed in Table 231–4 are simply estimates. There is a great deal of variability in these values from patient to patient as a result of circulating anti-insulin antibodies that alter the pharmacokinetics of insulin, variation in subcutaneous absorption, individual responses, and other factors. Additionally, absorption of insulin may be quite variable within a single patient from day to day, since absorption of subcutaneous insulin is markedly increased by vigorous exercise of the injected extremity, or by heating or massage of the injection site. Differences in purity also exist. Conventional insulin preparations contain less than 10,000 parts per million (ppm) of impurities; improved single peak insulin, less than 50 ppm; and "purified" insulin, 1 to 10 ppm. The impurities mentioned are predominantly proinsulin, with smaller amounts of insulin dimers, proinsulin-like products, glucagon, pancreatic polypeptide, somatostatin, and vasoactive polypeptide. For practical purposes, commercially available insulin preparations are labeled as purified (1 to 10 ppm); if they are not specifically labeled, they contain 20 to 50 ppm. The older less pure forms are no longer widely distributed. Essentially all preparations can be obtained as purified pork, beef, or beef-pork mixtures. Finally, highly purified human insulin is now available as a product of recombinant DNA biosynthesis or chemical conversion of pork to human insulin.

Methods of Treatment. The insulin regimen can be more or less intensive, depending on the number of injections per day, types of insulin used, and frequency and method of assessing control. Many NIDDM patients, and occasional IDDM patients, can achieve excellent glycemic control with a single daily (morning) injection of an intermediate-acting insulin. Because of postbreakfast hyperglycemia, it is often necessary to mix a short-acting preparation with this single dose. In most patients who realize excellent control with this regimen, endogenous insulin secretion is retained. A somewhat more intensive method to regulate glycemia involves a split-dosage regimen. This includes morning (before breakfast) and evening (before dinner) injection of mixtures of intermediate- and rapid-acting insulin. About two thirds of the total daily dose is usually given in the morning and about one third in the evening; the proportion of intermediate- to rapid-acting insulin at each injection is usually two thirds to one third. In patients receiving single-dose therapy who require more than 50 to 60 units per day a split-dose regimen should usually be tried. In a 70-kg man, normal 24-hour

insulin output has been estimated at 25 units per day. Therefore, in normal-sized diabetic subjects starting insulin therapy, it is reasonable to begin with a total daily dose of about 20 units per day with upward adjustments every several days based on the level of blood glucose. In mildly obese IDDM patients, starting doses can be 5 to 10 units per day higher. Because of insulin resistance, obese NIDDM patients requiring insulin will often need 60 to 90 units per day. With the availability of highly purified insulins (both human and animal) that are less antigenic, it is probably advisable to start all new patients with one of these insulin preparations. With the above methods of insulin delivery, assessment of glycemic control can be carried out in several ways. Measurements of urinary glucose and ketones can be obtained before breakfast and once or twice throughout the day. Patients should be instructed to void 30 minutes before obtaining urine for glucose determination (double voiding), particularly for the morning sample, so that the urinary glucose is more representative of the corresponding blood glucose. Regardless of how carefully urinary glucose is determined, it provides only a rough approximation of blood glucose levels. Factors such as renal threshold, renal blood flow, and urine volume greatly affect the meaning of urine glucose measurements (i.e., a 4+ reaction in a concentrated urine sample is of little significance compared to a 4+ reaction in a dilute sample). For these reasons, urinary glucose is a poor way to monitor diabetic control and if at all possible should not be relied upon as the sole guide on which to base the insulin regimen. Twenty-four hour urinary glucose excretion can be periodically assessed to provide a better estimate of daylong control (less than 5 grams per day is excellent control), or glycosylated hemoglobin can be measured to assess the overall state of glycemic control during the preceding few weeks. The best current method to assess glycemic control is home-, or self-, monitoring of glucose (see below). This requires the patient to assess his own blood glucose level daily and to make appropriate adjustments in insulin dosage. This approach places a large part of the management responsibility in the hands of the patient and emphasizes the need for a continuous outpatient education program.

When patients with new-onset IDDM are started on insulin therapy, after an initial period of stabilization, insulin requirements frequently decrease dramatically over the ensuing few weeks. This is the so-called honeymoon phenomenon, and it is sometimes possible to maintain near-normal levels of glycemia without administering any insulin. This honeymoon phase may last for a few weeks and sometimes as long as one to two years. It is invariably followed by worsening of metabolic control with permanent recrudescence of the insulin-dependent state. Some experts have recommended that during this honeymoon period insulin administration should never be completely stopped, even if dosages have to be reduced to homeopathic levels. The reason for this is the fear that if there is a prolonged period in which insulin is not administered, once insulin therapy is reinstituted an anamnestic response with rising titers of anti-insulin antibodies might occur. However, with use of the highly purified insulin preparations now available, or with biosynthetic human insulin, this may be less of a problem.

If more intensive insulin management is required to achieve closer to normal glycemic control, then multiple daily injections of insulin or continuous subcutaneous insulin infusion (CSII) are used. At the current time these approaches are generally limited to patients with IDDM. However, if ideal control of glycemia is the therapeutic goal, there is no reason these methods could not be used in patients with NIDDM whose disease cannot be satisfactorily controlled by other means. Multiple injections involve administration of regular insulin before each meal, with the dose adjusted to the anticipated meal size. This is usually combined with either a long-acting or an intermediate-acting preparation in the evening.

TABLE 231–4. PROPERTIES OF VARIOUS INSULIN PREPARATIONS

Class	Type	Peak Effect (hr)	Duration of Action (hr)
Rapid	Regular crystalline insulin (CZI)	2–4	6–8
	Semilente	2–6	10–12
Intermediate	Neutral protamine (NPH)	6–12	18–24
	Lente	6–12	18–24
Long Acting	Protamine zinc (PZI)	14–24	36
	Ultralente	18–24	36

The most intensive method of insulin delivery is CSII. This consists of constant insulin delivery into a subcutaneous site in the abdominal wall via an open loop delivery device consisting of a small insulin pump that must be worn by the patient essentially 24 hours a day. The key to this method of therapy is the constant delivery of basal insulin. The basal insulin infusion is supplemented by a preprandial bolus of insulin given 15 minutes prior to meal ingestion. This gives the patient a fair degree of flexibility in the timing and content of meals, since the preprandial bolus is given at the patient's discretion in an amount picked to match meal size. In general, the basal insulin infusion accounts for about 50 per cent of the total daily insulin dose and usually averages 0.5 to 1 unit per hour. Typically, preprandial boluses are 5 to 10 units, depending on meal size, time of day, and proximity to time of exercise. To be successful, intensive insulin therapy regimens must be combined with home- (or self-) glucose monitoring. This requires the patient to obtain capillary blood by finger prick for glucose measurement, using a reflectance meter. There are numerous devices and algorithms for constant insulin delivery and various approaches to the frequency and method of self-glucose measurements. A detailed discussion of these issues is beyond the scope of this chapter. With properly motivated and educated patients and physicians, excellent control can be achieved in nearly all subjects. Patients generally accept this mode of therapy quite well and report an increased feeling of well-being. However, CSII should not be used indiscriminantly, since pump dysfunction does occur, and hypoglycemia is a real problem, especially nocturnally. Additionally, a great deal is asked of patients when they participate in these programs in terms of dedication, education, and changes in life style.

Many other insulin treatment schedules have been proposed, all of which represent variations on the above common themes. Some of these are listed in Table 231–5. No single method is inherently superior to any other, and it is probably best for a physician to become accustomed to one or two methods and use them more or less exclusively so that he will be familiar with problems associated with insulin therapy and its individualization. All of these approaches are meant as guidelines rather than rigid algorithms.

Regardless of the insulin regimen employed, an established daily dose in a given patient must not be considered to be fixed. Even long-established insulin dosages may need to be increased because of changes in growth status, subtle intercurrent illness or stress, or development of anti-insulin antibodies. Dosages may need to be decreased because of consistent increases in physical activity, dietary changes, or changes in concomitant drug therapy (e.g., stopping steroids). Additionally, absorption may vary from one anatomic site to another, and the rate of absorption of insulin can be augmented by exercise involving a particular injection site. This simply means that the physician and the patient must constantly review the treatment program and be prepared to make changes when indicated.

Complications of Insulin Therapy. The most significant complication of insulin treatment is *hypoglycemia*. This is because even the best mode of insulin delivery is still an imperfect method to mimic the homeostatic mechanisms in normal subjects. Normal persons respond to food ingestion, exercise, and stress in such a way as to keep the blood glucose level within narrowly defined limits. One can hope to approach this, but not match it, with the methods used for delivery of exogenous insulin. For example, when normal individuals exercise, peripheral glucose uptake increases, and this is matched by a corresponding increase in hepatic glucose production. A decrease in insulin secretion allows the increase in hepatic glucose production to occur. Obviously this degree of fine tuning is difficult to achieve with exogenous insulin administration. Consequently hypoglycemia is a common complication of insulin therapy as the result of overzealous insulin administration or inappropriate timing. Most often this occurs in a situation in which tight control is attempted. Occasional mild episodes of hypoglycemia are probably acceptable if they appear in a patient in whom excellent control is generally achieved and who is fully aware of their occurrence and of methods to abort them. However, frequent and severe hypoglycemic reactions are unacceptable. These are serious and occasionally can be fatal. Furthermore, the long-term effects on the central nervous system of frequent hypoglycemic episodes have not been determined. If satisfactory control cannot be achieved without recurrence of such reactions, then compromises in the overall therapeutic plan must be made. It would seem imprudent to expose patients to known complications of hypoglycemia in the hope that superior control will prevent chronic diabetic complications in the future. Some IDDM patients are particularly susceptible to hypoglycemia, seemingly because of impaired secretion of counter-regulatory hormones, particularly glucagon.

An interesting aspect of hypoglycemic episodes is the so-called *Somogyi phenomenon*. This involves rebound hyperglycemia due to excessive secretion of counter-regulatory hormones following a previous episode of hypoglycemia. The classic situation involves nocturnal hypoglycemia followed by marked hyperglycemia prior to breakfast. This can induce a self-defeating cycle in which the insulin dose is progressively raised in response to the fasting hyperglycemia when a reduction in insulin dose, to prevent the nocturnal hypoglycemia, would be more appropriate.

A minority of patients beginning insulin therapy experience a variety of local allergic reactions at the injection site. Manifestations include local itching, erythematous, indurated lesions, and occasional small, discrete subcutaneous nodules. These local reactions are usually self-limited and eventually disappear with continued insulin treatment. Antihistamines may be used for symptomatic relief if necessary. The frequency of these problems has decreased significantly with the use of the newer more highly purified insulins. Rare patients may develop systemic reactions, including generalized urticaria and even anaphylactic reactions. This usually occurs when insulin therapy has been stopped for a time and then reinstituted. If these symptoms cannot be controlled by antihistamines, and if insulin treatment is mandatory for the patient's well-being, then formal desensitization regimens are necessary. Other local reactions at the injection site include lipoatrophy and hypertrophy. Lipoatrophy at the injection

---

TABLE 231–5. DIFFERENT INSULIN REGIMENS

Split dose intermediate (NPH or lente) + regular insulin
A.M. dose:	⅔ TDD
	~70% intermediate
	~30% regular
P.M. dose:	⅓ TDD
	50%–70% intermediate
	30%–50% regular

Intermediate + preprandial regular insulin
Breakfast:	Regular, 25%–40% TDD
Lunch:	Regular, 25%–30% TDD
Dinner:	Regular, 25%–30% TDD
Night:	NPH or lente, 15%–25% TDD

Ultralente + preprandial regular insulin
Breakfast:	Regular, 15%–25% TDD
Lunch:	Regular, 15%–25% TDD
Dinner:	Regular, 15%–25% TDD
	Ultralente, 40%–60% TDD

Triple A.M. mixture: regular, lente + ultralente insulin

Double A.M. mixture: regular + NPH (or lente) insulin

TDD = total daily dose

site is a benign condition usually due to impurities in the insulin preparation. It can usually be corrected by changing to a highly purified pork insulin and injecting this into the lipoatrophic areas, which then fill in with subcutaneous fat in a normal fashion. Most likely the new highly purified human insulin preparations will also be suitable for this purpose. Insulin hypertrophy is attributed to the local lipogenic effects of the injected insulin. In advanced cases the underlying tissue can be fibrous and less vascular, making the overlying skin anesthetic. This explains why many patients prefer these areas as sites of injection. This problem can usually be corrected by carefully rotating injection sites.

FUTURE MODES OF THERAPY

Even with the most meticulous mode of insulin therapy in the most motivated patients, euglycemic control is difficult to achieve for prolonged periods. Thus the search for better, more effective, and, in some cases, curative forms of therapy continues. Transplantation of the pancreas or islet cells continues to receive extensive study. Numerous logistic, immunologic, and technical problems need to be overcome before such therapies become available for routine clinical purposes, but there are signs that some positive results might be seen in the next several years. This is the one mode of therapy that might actually be considered curative.

Efforts continue to be expended in developing newer and better external or implantable insulin-delivery devices. Unquestionably the mechanical and engineering aspects of insulin-delivery devices will continue to improve dramatically over the next several years, and pumps that are smaller, safer, and more flexible will be produced. It also seems likely that reliable implantable devices are in the offing. However, unless such devices can be used to administer insulin via the portal route, the advantage of implantable pumps appears to be mostly esthetic. An additional hope for internal devices is that a closed-loop system can be designed. This would require development of a reliable, fail-safe glucose sensor integrated into the appropriate algorithms for insulin delivery. If such artificial pancreases become readily available, they would obviously have wide applicability. Finally, since hyperglucagonemia has been implicated in the pathogenesis of the hyperglycemia in diabetes, agents that specifically suppress glucagon secretion have been sought. Attempts to develop a glucagon-specific somatostatin derivative continue; such a compound might be a useful adjunctive therapy in the management of diabetes.

ACUTE COMPLICATIONS

The acute metabolic complications of diabetes are diabetic ketoacidosis, hyperosmolar nonketotic coma, lactic acidosis, and hypoglycemia.

Diabetic Ketoacidosis (DKA)

DKA is due to insulin deficiency. Before consideration of the pathogenesis of the metabolic derangement, it is important to review the normal physiologic effects of insulin on carbohydrate, protein, and fat metabolism, since DKA simply represents a reversal of these normal insulin-stimulated processes.

PHYSIOLOGY OF FED AND FASTED STATE. When food is ingested, insulin functions as the major anabolic hormone facilitating the disposition of carbohydrate, protein, and fat and their synthesis into macromolecules for storage (Fig. 231–6A). Glucose is absorbed into the portal vein, and approximately 60 per cent of the ingested glucose-derived carbons end up in liver glycogen in the postprandial period. A significant portion of this is probably not a result of direct hepatic glucose uptake, but is due to peripheral metabolism of glucose to three-carbon fragments (lactate, pyruvate) that are then recycled to the liver where they enter the gluconeo-

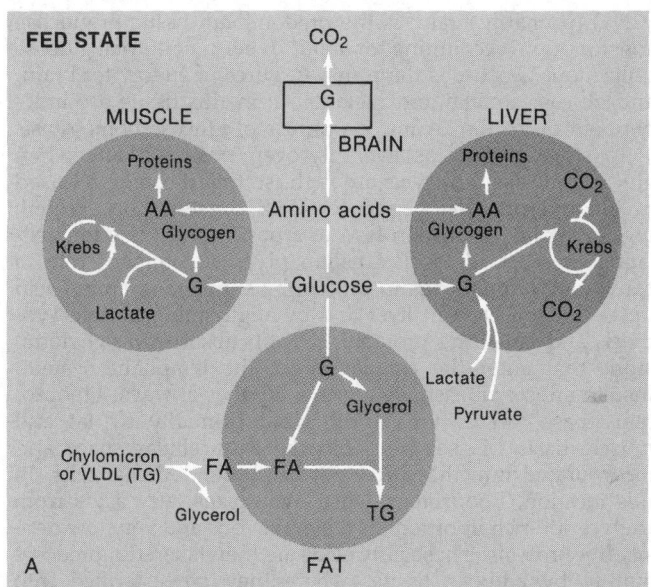

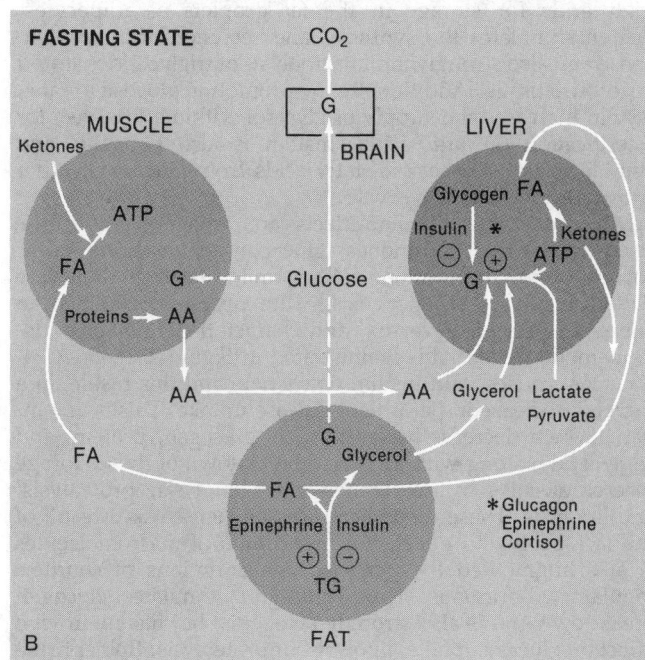

FIGURE 231–6. *A,* Fuel homeostasis during the immediate postprandial fed state. The key features of this diagram are the storage of glucose, amino acids, and fatty acids as the macromolecules glycogen, protein, and triglyceride in tissue depots; each of these processes is facilitated by the anabolic effects of insulin. *B,* Reversal of the anabolic effects of insulin during the insulinopenic fasting state. The major purpose of these homeostatic responses is to maintain a supply of glucose for obligate glucose uptake by the CNS while other tissues cease their consumption of glucose in favor of fatty acids from adipose tissue depots.

genic pathway and are synthesized into glycogen. Glycogen then serves as the storage form of carbohydrate for later release. When glucose is metabolized via the glycolytic (anaerobic) pathway, 2 moles of ATP are generated per mole of glucose. Aerobic, or oxidative, metabolism (Krebs' cycle) is far more efficient as an energy-producing process and generates 12 moles of ATP per mole of glucose. Insulin exerts multiple anabolic effects on this process. It stimulates glucose uptake and glycogen synthesis by muscle and inhibits glycogenolysis. In liver, insulin does not directly stimulate glucose uptake, but it does actively promote glycogenesis and inhibit glycogenolysis. Although most of the ingested glucose, or glucose-derived carbon, ends up in the liver in the postprandial period, over a 24-hour day the central nervous system

(CNS) (primarily brain) is the predominant tissue of glucose consumption, accounting for about 70 per cent of total glucose utilization. Glucose is the primary source of energy for brain, and glucose uptake and metabolism in this tissue are independent of insulin. A major purpose of glucose homeostasis is to store glucose as liver glycogen postprandially when glucose and insulin levels are high, so that it can be released in the interprandial period for CNS consumption. Protein digestion and absorption lead to a postprandial rise in circulating amino acid levels. Insulin plays a dominant role in converting amino acids to protein by stimulating amino acid uptake in muscle and liver and by augmenting protein synthesis and inhibiting proteolysis. Fat is absorbed as chylomicrons that enter the circulation via the lymphatic system. Insulin affects fat assimilation in a number of ways. Lipoprotein lipase, an enzyme synthesized primarily by fat and muscle tissue, is secreted into the extracellular space and incorporated into the surface of nearby endothelial cells. In this location, lipoprotein lipase hydrolyzes fatty acids from triglyceride-rich lipoproteins (chylomicrons and very low density lipoproteins). These fatty acids are then taken up, predominantly by adipose tissue, where they are esterified into triglyceride for storage in the fat droplets of adipocytes. Insulin stimulates the synthesis and secretion of lipoprotein lipase and also strongly inhibits lipolysis of triglycerides stored in adipose tissue. Additionally, by promoting glucose uptake, insulin increases the supply of glycerol within adipocytes for esterification of fatty acids. Insulin is also lipogenic and stimulates the synthesis of fatty acids from glucose or other substrates that form pyruvate.

Many of these insulin effects are antagonized by the counter-regulatory hormones, glucagon, epinephrine, cortisol, and growth hormone. When mild (fasting) or severe (DKA) insulin deficiency exists, the processes outlined in Figure 231–6A are reversed, and characteristic metabolic derangements occur. This is illustrated in Figure 231–6B. A 24-hour fast causes mild insulin deficiency, and this results in a marked decrease in peripheral glucose uptake. This is accompanied by a decrease in synthesis of glycogen, protein, and triglyceride, along with increased breakdown of these storage macromolecules by accelerated glycogenolysis, proteolysis, and lipolysis. These catabolic processes increase as a result of the lack of insulin effect, but breakdown of macromolecules is also augmented by increased concentrations of counter-regulatory hormones. Thus, glucagon stimulates glycogen breakdown and is also strongly ketogenic, but has no in vivo effect on glucose uptake, lipolysis, or proteolysis. Epinephrine promotes glycogenolysis and lipolysis and also inhibits peripheral glucose uptake. Cortisol probably has effects that are additive or possibly synergistic with the other counter-regulatory hormones and may independently stimulate proteolysis. Growth hormone probably plays a minor role in these events mediated through inhibition of glucose uptake. Taken together fasting-induced insulin deficiency plus increased counter-regulatory hormones lead to a marked decrease in glucose metabolism by insulin-sensitive tissues, "sparing" glucose for the obligate CNS utilization. The source of glucose in this setting is the liver. For the initial 12 to 24 hours, hepatic glucose production is largely due to breakdown of stored glycogen. After this time, hepatic glycogen stores are depleted and hepatic glucose output is sustained by gluconeogenesis. Hepatic gluconeogenesis is supported by the increased supply of gluconeogenic substrates flowing from the periphery, that is, muscle proteolysis, leading to an increased supply of gluconeogenic amino acids (mainly alanine) and increased lipolysis resulting in enhanced glycerol release from adipose tissue. Some lactate and pyruvate are supplied from anaerobic metabolism of glucose in peripheral tissues (Cori cycle). Thus the liver is the central clearing house in this process by converting the breakdown products of stored fat and protein to supply glucose for the CNS in a

setting (fasting) in which exogenous glucose is unavailable. In this situation the predominant energy source for non-CNS tissues is circulating free fatty acids (FFA) derived from breakdown of adipose tissue triglyceride (the CNS cannot utilize FFA as a metabolic fuel). FFA also supply the liver with the energy necessary to drive gluconeogenesis. Ketone bodies are produced in the liver from fatty acid oxidation under conditions of insulin deficiency and glucagon excess. In fasting this serves an important homeostatic purpose, since ketone bodies can be utilized by the CNS and muscle for energy, markedly reducing the need for protein breakdown to supply gluconeogenic precursors for liver glucose production. Ketone bodies provide a mechanism to convert adipose tissue energy stores into a substrate that can be metabolized in the CNS; this spares critical body proteins, allowing humans to survive relatively long-term fasts.

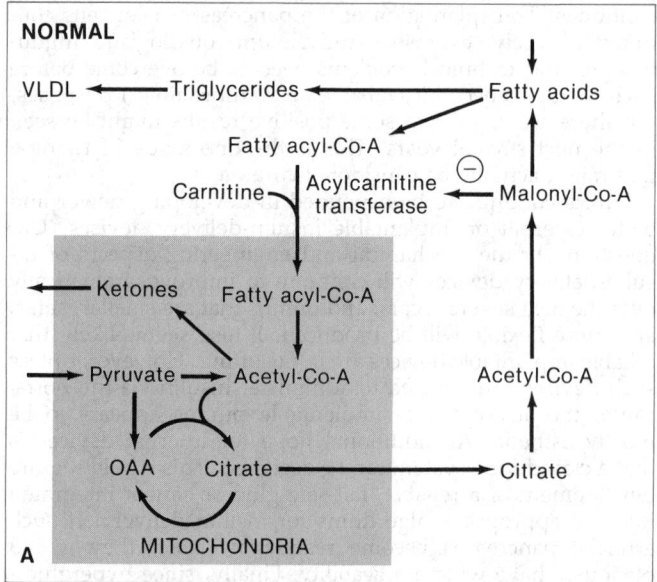

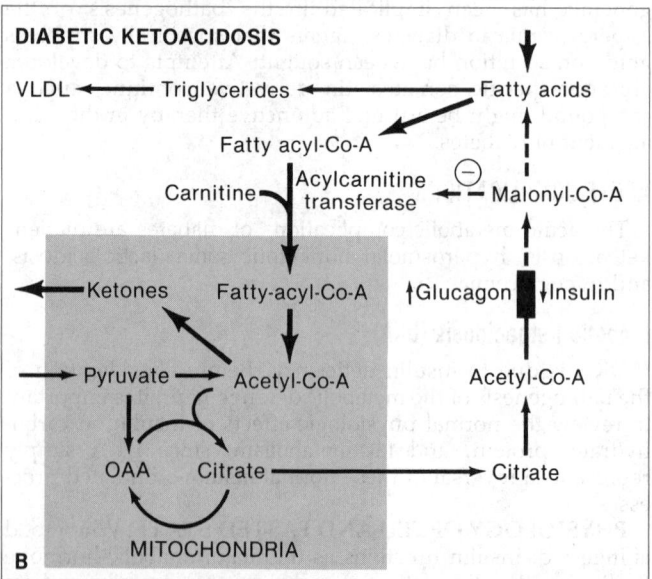

FIGURE 231–7. Hepatic fatty acid and ketoacid metabolism in the normal state (upper panel) and insulinopenic diabetic ketoacidotic state (lower panel). Malonyl-Co-A is a key regulatory intermediate in this scheme, competitively inhibiting the ability of acyl carnitine transferase to translocate fatty acyl-Co-A molecules from the cytosol to the intramitochondrial space in the normal state. In diabetic ketoacidosis, glucagon excess and insulin deficiency inhibit the generation of malonyl-Co-A, releasing the inhibition of acyl carnitine transferase. See text for further details.

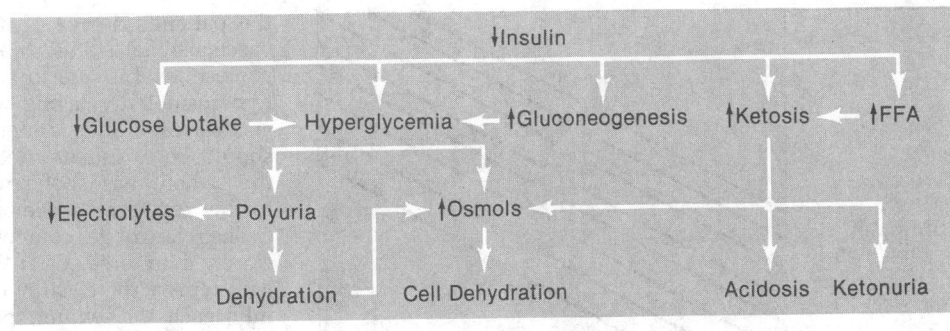

FIGURE 231–8. Pathophysiology of diabetic ketoacidosis. Severe insulin deficiency leads to hyperglycemia and ketonemia, and from this all of the other pathophysiologic sequelae result.

PATHOPHYSIOLOGY OF DKA. In DKA, all of these homeostatic processes are out of control, leading to pronounced hyperglycemia and ketonemia. The hyperglycemia is due to a combination of increased hepatic glucose production and decreased peripheral glucose uptake. The biochemical mechanisms underlying the hyperketonemia are somewhat more complex, as seen in Figure 231–7. Ketone bodies are produced in hepatocyte mitochondria by beta oxidation of fatty acids, and glucagon is the primary hormone responsible for inducing the hepatic ketogenic state. It does this by lowering malonyl coenzyme A levels, the first committed substrate in fatty acid synthesis, which leads to a marked increase in the activity of carnitine acyl transferase I. This enzyme translocates fatty acids from the cytosol to the intramitochondrial space, where they are converted to ketones. Hepatic carnitine levels are also increased, which further drives this transfer step by mass action. The key regulatory point in understanding ketogenesis is that in the fed state, entry of fatty acids into the mitochondria is low, limiting fatty acid oxidation and ketogenesis in favor of fatty acid and triglyceride synthesis; thus the liver is rate limiting in ketone body formation. When the level of insulin is low and glucagon high (as in starvation or DKA), fatty acids freely enter mitochondria to be converted to ketones, and therefore the supply of fatty acids to the liver is rate limiting for ketogenesis. Fatty acids are freely permeable across the hepatocyte plasma membrane, and thus the plasma concentration of FFA drives ketogenesis. In starvation, fatty acid levels are only moderately increased, leading to enhanced, but controlled, ketogenesis; in DKA, FFA levels are much higher, leading to uncontrolled ketogenesis. Another factor enhancing ketonemia in DKA is related to ketone body utilization. Insulin normally stimulates ketoacid uptake by peripheral tissues, and this is inhibited in DKA; additionally, very high levels of ketones may saturate the uptake mechanisms, further limiting utilization.

All of the pathophysiologic sequelae of DKA follow from hyperglycemia and hyperketonemia (Fig. 231–8). Thus, acidosis and ketonuria are directly due to the buildup of the ketoacids beta-hydroxybutyrate and acetoacetate. The hyperglycemia and hyperketonemia produce an osmotic diuresis that causes intravascular volume depletion and dehydration and urinary electrolyte loss. The hyperosmolarity further exaggerates intracellular dehydration.

CLINICAL PICTURE. Diabetic ketoacidosis can be a life-threatening situation, and the clinical presentation is often dramatic. An antecedent history of polyuria and polydipsia for one to several days is typical, and nausea, vomiting, and anorexia are frequent accompanying symptoms. Occasionally, abdominal pain is a predominant feature, sometimes mimicking an acute abdominal condition. Often this is due to gastric stasis and distension. In the obtunded patient with gastric distension, nasogastric suction should be considered to avoid vomiting with aspiration. Physical findings include tachypnea, dehydration, and disorientation, or even coma. If systemic acidosis is severe, Kussmaul respirations are present. Precipitating causes of DKA include failure of the patient to take insulin, infection, intercurrent illness, trauma, or emo-

tional stress. When a known diabetic presents with signs and symptoms of DKA, the diagnosis is usually straightforward. However, DKA can also be the initial presenting episode of diabetes. DKA is a disease of IDDM, only rarely occurring in NIDDM, and only when precipitating causes are extreme.

Although the diagnosis of DKA can be strongly suspected on a clinical basis, confirmation is based on laboratory analyses. The diagnosis is made by demonstrating hyperglycemia and hyperketonemia in the presence of acidosis. However, the severity of these abnormalities can vary over a wide range. Occasionally the presenting episode may be severe ketonemia and acidosis and only mild hyperglycemia (200 to 400 mg per deciliter). Other patients may have severe hyperglycemia and only mild ketonemia and acidosis. Occasionally, alcoholic patients have ketonemia and hyperglycemia, and this condition, termed alcoholic ketoacidosis, must be differentiated from DKA (see next section). Direct quantitative measurements of acetoacetate and beta-hydroxybutyrate are not usually readily available, and most physicians rely on reagent strips (Ketostix) or tablets (Acetest) for measurements. With this method, a nitroprusside reaction is the indicator; nitroprusside reacts mainly with acetoacetate, to a lesser extent with acetone, and not at all with beta-hydroxybutyrate. Since beta-hydroxybutyrate levels are much higher than acetoacetate levels in DKA, this method can sometimes be confusing. For example, when concomitant lactic acidosis exists, acetoacetate production may be inhibited in the presence of very high levels of beta-hydroxybutyrate. In this setting the nitroprusside reaction may not be strongly positive. During the course of insulin therapy for DKA, beta-hydroxybutyrate levels may fall out of proportion to acetoacetate levels, giving the impression that therapy is less effective than it actually is. Serum sodium levels are usually mildly decreased. This is due to the hyperglycemia- and hyperketonemia-induced hyperosmolarity, which attracts extracellular water from the intracellular space, leading to dilution of serum sodium. It should be kept in mind that the osmolar contribution of the hyperketonemia can often approach the contribution of the hyperglycemia. Serum bicarbonate levels are depressed, and the magnitude of decrease is in proportion to the degree of acidosis. BUN levels are usually modestly elevated as a result of dehydration and a component of prerenal azotemia. Serum potassium levels can be high, low, or normal, depending on the degree of dehydration and acidosis. In all cases, severe total body and intracellular potassium depletion exists. Because of cellular buffering mechanisms, which exchange intracellular potassium for extracellular hydrogen ion, extracellular potassium levels are often maintained in acidotic states. Nevertheless, greater than 95 per cent of total body potassium is intracellular, so in the presence of acidosis, extracellular potassium levels do not reflect total body potassium stores unless the potassium concentration is plotted on a nomogram related to serum pH (Fig. 231–9).

TREATMENT OF DKA. The treatment of DKA should be started as soon as it is diagnosed. The goals of therapy are to increase the rate of glucose utilization by insulin-dependent tissues, to reverse ketonemia and acidosis, and to correct the depletion of water and electrolytes. To accomplish this, treat-

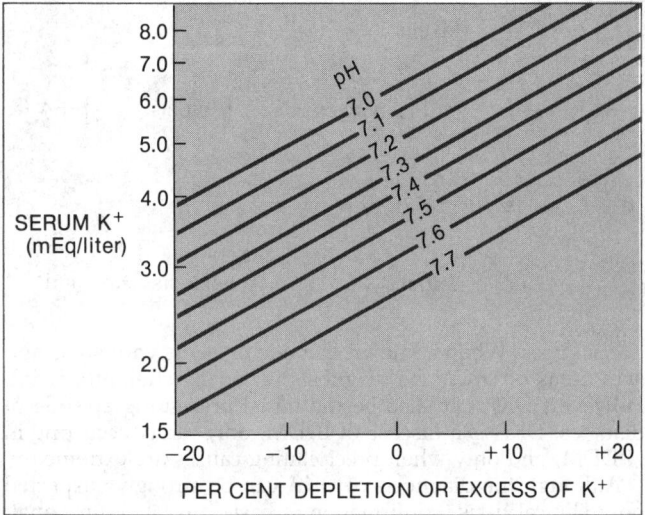

FIGURE 231–9. Nomogram depicting the relationship between total body potassium depletion, serum potassium, and serum pH. Per cent potassium depletion or excess is calculated by drawing a horizontal line from the ordinate intercept of the serum potassium concentration to the intersection of the diagonal line corresponding to the coexisting serum pH. From this intersection a vertical line is dropped to the abscissa and per cent potassium depletion or excess is read from the abscissal intercept. For example, at a serum potassium concentration of 4.0, at a concomitant serum pH of 7.2, an approximate 10 per cent depletion of total body potassium stores exists.

ment can be divided into four general areas: (1) insulin administration, (2) replacement of fluid and electrolytes, (3) treatment of any precipitating problems, and (4) avoidance of complications.

A variety of *insulin* regimens are possible, ranging from constant intravenous infusion to intermittent administration of intravenous, subcutaneous, or intramuscular boluses. The aim of all forms of insulin administration is to achieve a rapid and maximal insulin effect. In vivo insulin action is near maximal at an insulin concentration of about 200 μU per milliliter, and achieving higher levels has little further benefit. Since insulin is rapidly cleared from the circulation ($t\frac{1}{2}$ = 7 minutes), boluses must be given frequently (every 30 to 60 minutes) to maintain maximally effective insulin levels. With constant intravenous administration, serum insulin levels are maintained at a steady state throughout the infusion. In normal subjects, an infusion rate of 10 units per hour will result in an insulin level of approximately 200 μU per milliliter by 30 minutes, and if this mode of treatment is chosen a priming dose (10 to 20 units) should be given initially. Advocates of constant intravenous infusion maintain that the rate of metabolic improvement is smoother and more predictable and hypoglycemia is less common. Additionally, problems of variable or inadequate absorption from subcutaneous or intramuscular sites are avoided. One difficulty with this method occurs in the occasional patient with severe insulin resistance due to sepsis or high titers of insulin antibodies. If clear-cut metabolic improvement is not seen within the first few hours of constant insulin infusion, a bolus of insulin (20 to 30 units) should be given and the rate of insulin infusion increased.

Fluid replacement should also be started immediately. Patients with DKA are dehydrated and hypovolemic and usually have fluid deficits of 5 to 8 liters or more. Thus, rapid expansion of intravascular volume is essential, and this is achieved by an initial infusion of 1 to 2 liters of normal saline, or equivalent, over the first one to two hours. Of course, caution should be used in those patients with underlying cardiovascular or oliguric renal disease. Following initial rapid fluid administration, the rate of replacement can be slowed to restore estimated losses by 16 to 24 hours, depending on

the patient's degree of dehydration and underlying cardiovascular-renal status. Much of the initial decline in plasma glucose level is due to volume expansion with reduction of hyperosmolarity, along with increased glomerular filtration and corresponding urinary glucose loss. In general, the aim should be to initiate metabolic correction rapidly, but once the patient has shown clear-cut substantial improvement, further replacement therapy can proceed more cautiously.

The electrolyte content of administered fluids must be closely monitored. Over the entire course of therapy the goal is to replace the electrolyte deficit, which averages 200 to 400 mEq each for sodium, potassium, and phosphate. Patients are usually ingesting some form of calories by 16 to 24 hours, and this provides the most physiologic replacement method. Potassium replacement requires the most attention. Regardless of the initial serum potassium level, total body reserves are depleted and serum levels will fall dramatically as acidosis and hyperglycemia are corrected. As glucose is taken up by cells under the influence of insulin, potassium is also transported intracellularly, and as acidosis is reversed the cellular buffering process exchanging intracellular potassium for extracellular hydrogen ion diminishes. To prevent hypokalemia, potassium should be included in the intravenous fluids once it is established that renal perfusion and urine flow are adequate following initial intravascular fluid expansion. To accomplish this, 40 mEq of potassium can be added to each liter of intravenous fluids as the phosphate salt. Phosphate depletion is also uniform in DKA, and some replacement is advisable, particularly if serum phosphate levels are low. This can be accomplished by administering 10 to 20 mmol per hour and can be accomplished along with potassium replacement by giving potassium phosphate. Since excessive phosphate repletion can cause hypocalcemia, ongoing phosphate administration should be guided by the serum phosphorus and calcium levels. Bicarbonate replacement should be initiated in patients with severe acidosis (pH < 7.0). This can be administered at the rate of 44 mEq per liter with appropriate monitoring of pH until it rises above 7.0. Three to four ampules of bicarbonate (44 mEq per ampule) will usually suffice to achieve this goal. Excessive bicarbonate replacement is contraindicated since this will exacerbate the tendency toward hypokalemia and may also result in rebound CNS acidosis. The latter occurs because carbon dioxide is more rapidly diffusible across the blood-brain barrier than is bicarbonate ion, causing CNS pH to fall at a time when peripheral pH is rising. This can lead to stupor and worsening of CNS status at a time when metabolic improvement is occurring.

Therapy should be monitored by frequent assessment of clinical status and laboratory measurements of urine and serum glucose and ketone levels. A fall in plasma glucose level is the earliest sign of effective therapy, and therefore plasma glucose should be frequently monitored. Once plasma glucose levels fall to approximately 250 mg per deciliter, 5 per cent glucose should be added to the intravenous fluids. Occasionally children or adolescents with DKA exhibit marked mental deterioration, including development of coma 4 to 6 hours after therapy has begun. Usually this is associated with a marked fall in hyperglycemia and serum osmolality, and cerebral edema has been noted in a few autopsy cases. Overall this is probably a rare complication of therapy. Because of the importance of plasma glucose monitoring in assessing the effectiveness of therapy, administration of glucose has no place in the initial stages of DKA treatment.

While insulin and fluid and electrolyte replacement therapy are being administered, a concomitant search for underlying precipitating factors should be undertaken. Leukocytosis often accompanies uncomplicated DKA and so should be viewed appropriately when one is searching for underlying infection. Hypothermia can be associated with DKA, and therefore fever should be a strong impetus to screen rigorously for a site of infection.

The major complications of DKA are mostly the result of treatment and include *hypokalemia, late hypoglycemia, rebound CNS acidosis,* and *CNS deterioration* (possibly due to cerebral edema). However, with proper attention to therapeutic details the former two can always be avoided, and the latter are fortunately rare. Recurrence of DKA can occur in the hospital if the vigorous phase of therapy is relaxed too soon. Maintenance of a flow chart with all therapies and laboratory tests recorded is an important means of coordination so that unexpected results do not go undetected and inappropriate therapies are not given.

Alcoholic Ketoacidosis

Alcoholic ketoacidosis can sometimes present a problem in the differential diagnosis of DKA when the patient is not a known diabetic or when a diabetic patient ingests large amounts of alcohol. This syndrome is characterized by hyperketonemia, acidosis, and dehydration. Serum glucose levels can be normal or sometimes elevated to the lower range of values seen in DKA. In the latter case a diagnostic problem can occur. The clinical picture of alcoholic ketoacidosis occurs in alcoholics following a recent, and sometimes prolonged alcoholic debauch; abstinence during the immediately preceding 12 to 24 hours is a common finding. The patient is usually anorexic, sometimes with nausea and vomiting, and some degree of starvation over the preceding one to three days is always present. The starvation, perhaps accompanied by stress-related hyperglucagonemia, creates a ketogenic state in the liver. This is accompanied by elevated FFA levels similar to those seen in starvation, which are perhaps augmented by adrenergic activation related to alcohol withdrawal, creating the metabolic environment for ketoacidosis. It is unusual for these patients to have hyperglycemia, but it can occur. When it does, the pathogenesis is unclear. In some patients, abnormalities of glucose tolerance exist after therapy, and thus the hyperglycemia may be stress related in previously glucose-intolerant patients. Alternatively, adrenergic mechanisms related to alcohol withdrawal could suppress residual endogenous insulin secretion, facilitating mild hyperglycemia. Regardless of the underlying mechanisms, the metabolic abnormalities are rapidly reversed by intravenous administration of fluids and glucose. Only occasionally is insulin needed in the early stages of treatment.

Nonketotic Hyperosmolar Syndrome

The term *nonketotic hyperosmolar coma* has frequently been applied to this syndrome, but by no means do all patients display coma or even mental obtundity. Rather, this syndrome comprises a spectrum ranging from mild degrees of hyperosmolarity with minimal CNS symptoms to severe hyperosmolarity with minimal CNS symptoms to severe hyperosmolarity with accompanying coma. The biochemical hallmarks are extreme hyperglycemia (mean 1000 mg per deciliter, range 600 to 2400 mg per deciliter) in the absence of overt ketoacidosis. Dehydration, hypovolemia, and disorientation are accompanying features. This syndrome usually develops over a much longer interval than DKA, with symptoms of polyuria antedating clinical presentation by several days and sometimes weeks. This syndrome usually occurs in elderly patients with NIDDM (often not previously diagnosed) who for some reason are unable to keep up with the osmotic diuresis by adequate water ingestion and this results in severe dehydration. The severe hyperglycemia is at least partly caused by decreased renal glucose excretion due either to intrinsic underlying renal disease or to decreased glomerular filtration and prerenal azotemia secondary to the marked hypovolemia and dehydration. Frequently this condition is associated with steroid, diuretic, or phenytoin therapy as a precipitating cause. Other precipitating factors include infections, cerebrovascular events, or therapeutic maneuvers such as hypertonic peritoneal dialysis or parenteral nutrition.

Serum sodium and potassium levels are usually normal while serum bicarbonate levels are often somewhat depressed. This is usually not associated with significant ketonemia and probably reflects an underlying component of lactic acidosis due to hypovolemia. The BUN is uniformly elevated because of hypovolemia and prerenal azotemia. In these cases, though, acidosis is mild, and serum osmolality can be approximated by the formula:

$$\text{serum osmolality (mOsm per liter)} = 2 \times [\text{Na}^+ + \text{K}^+ \text{ (mEq/L)}] + \frac{\text{plasma glucose (mg/dl)}}{18} + \frac{\text{BUN (mg/dl)}}{2.8}$$

Since urea is freely diffusible across cell membranes it does not alter the effective serum osmolality, which is the clinically important factor to consider in this hyperosmolar condition. Most experts do not consider BUN levels in this calculation and prefer to estimate effective serum osmolarity as:

$$\text{Osm}_E = 2 \times [\text{Na}^+ + \text{K}^+ \text{ (mEq/L)}] + \frac{\text{plasma glucose (mg/dl)}}{18}$$

Values above 300 mOsm per liter are abnormal and above 320 mOsm per liter are indicative of clinically significant hyperosmolarity.

The reason ketosis is not a feature of this condition has not been satisfactorily explained. FFA levels are not as high in this syndrome as they are in DKA, and most investigators attribute the relatively lower FFA levels and decreased rates of ketogenesis to higher residual insulin levels in patients with the hyperosmolar syndrome. This answer is not entirely satisfactory, however, since measured peripheral insulin levels overlap with those reported in DKA. On the other hand, peripheral insulin levels do not always reflect portal insulin concentrations, and significant differences in portal insulin levels may exist in DKA versus hyperosmolar syndrome, with the higher levels in hyperosmolar syndrome restraining hepatic ketogenesis.

In some series, the mortality has ranged up to 50 per cent. However, the relatively high mortality reflects selection criteria since mortality tends to be higher with greater severity of the hyperosmolality. The first priority of treatment should be intravascular volume expansion to restore circulatory integrity. This is accomplished by infusion of 1 to 2 liters of normal saline, or equivalent, over one to two hours, provided absolute cardiovascular contraindications do not exist. Even normal saline is hypotonic relative to serum in these patients, and therefore this therapy will initiate the correction of the hyperosmolality. As in DKA, insulin can be administered by constant intravenous infusions or bolus therapy. Since absorption of insulin administered subcutaneously or intramuscularly is variable because of dehydration and hypovolemia, and since late hypoglycemia is a more common complication of the hyperosmolar syndrome, constant intravenous administration of insulin can be very effective in this condition, leading to a predictable and fairly constant, smooth decline in plasma glucose levels. Once plasma glucose begins to decrease, and provided acceptable volume expansion and urine flow have been established, potassium phosphate salts should be added to the intravenous fluids. Subsequent to the initial volume expansion, intravenous fluids can consist of 0.5 normal saline with added potassium phosphate. Once plasma glucose levels decline to approximately 250 mg per deciliter, 5 per cent glucose should be added to the intravenous fluids. The above comments are meant more as guidelines than hard and fast rules, since, as in DKA, therapy must be individualized as far as replacement of fluids and electrolytes is concerned. This is best done by maintaining an organized flow chart with frequent measurements of plasma glucose, electrolytes, blood pressure, and urine volume. Despite even the best therapy, morbidity and mortality are high in this condition. Thrombosis and embolic events as well as infections, particularly pneumonia with accompanying adult respiratory distress syndrome, contribute significantly to adverse outcomes. In summary, rigorous but carefully monitored hydration and reestablishment of circulatory integrity are critical for successful therapy. These goals should be pursued while hyperosmolarity is corrected by administration of relatively hypotonic fluids with adequate free water along with insulin to reduce the hyperglycemia. Concomitantly a careful workup should be instituted to uncover precipitating factors with appropriate therapy when necessary.

CHRONIC OR LATE COMPLICATIONS OF DIABETES

Retinopathy (Color plate 1)

Eye disease is common in diabetes, and permanent loss of vision is one of the most striking and feared complications. Approximately 25 per cent of all newly reported cases of blindness are attributed to diabetes. When diabetics of all ages and types are considered together, the incidence of blindness from diabetic retinopathy is 0.2 per cent per year in all diabetics and 0.6 per cent per year in diabetics with retinopathy. This is 11 and 29 times greater, respectively, than the incidence of blindness from all other causes combined in the general population.

The major form of diabetic eye disease is diabetic retinopathy. Two general categories exist: nonproliferative or background retinopathy and proliferative retinopathy. Nonproliferative retinopathy can include venous abnormalities, microaneurysms, retinal hemorrhages, retinal edema, and exudates. This may progress to proliferative retinopathy, characterized by neovascularization, glial proliferation, and vitreoretinal traction. In general, diabetic retinopathy is progressive and tends to worsen with the duration of disease. However, most diabetics do not develop proliferative retinopathy. The incidence of this complication is substantially lower in NIDDM then in IDDM, even when corrected for duration of disease. However, since there are many more patients with NIDDM than IDDM, the absolute numbers of NIDDM and IDDM patients with proliferative retinopathy are roughly comparable.

NONPROLIFERATIVE RETINOPATHY. Probably the earliest retinal change is increased capillary permeability seen on fluorescein angiography. This abnormality can be readily reversed by effective glycemic control, but the relationship of this form of capillary permeability to retinopathy is unknown. Nonperfusion of retinal capillaries occurs early in diabetic retinopathy (so-called capillary dropout), and this leads to areas of retinal ischemia and infarction. Microaneurysms are small (15 to 50 μm diameter) excrescences along capillaries and are particularly prominent along the edges of areas of capillary nonperfusion. Fusiform aneurysms, or general dilatation of capillary loops, can also occur. Retinal veins are often tortuous and dilated; dilatation can be segmental, giving rise to a beaded or "sausage string"appearance. Exudates can be of two types: (1) Hard, *waxy exudates* are white to yellowish, shiny, with defined borders but without surrounding pigmentation. These exudates are due to lipid- and protein-containing fluid that has leaked from surrounding capillaries. (2) *Cotton-wool, or soft, exudates* are really areas of nonperfusion representing retinal microinfarcts and are often surrounded by microaneurysms. Clinically, an increase in cotton-wool areas indicates progressive capillary dropout and is a poor prognostic sign. Subretinal hemorrhages tend to be small and dot shaped and may resorb within a few weeks. Larger, flame-shaped hemorrhages occur in the superficial retinal layers and resorb more slowly. Preretinal hemorrhages are more serious and can impair vision if they are large or if they impinge on the macula. Following resorption, scarring and vitreous retraction or retinal detachment can occur. Edema of the retina is due to abnormal capillary permeability and ischemia. When persistent macular edema exists, vision is seriously impaired, and usual forms of therapy (photocoagu-

lation) may not be effective. The primary pathogenetic events underlying these changes of nonproliferative background retinopathy are unclear, but loss of supporting capillary pericytes, endothelial proliferation, and hyperviscosity with red cell aggregation, together or alone, have all been proposed.

PROLIFERATIVE RETINOPATHY. The hallmark of proliferative retinopathy is new vessel formation or neovascularization. These capillary fronds or loops can grow on the surface of the retina or extend into the vitreous. Often this is accompanied by proliferation of glial elements in the region of the optic disc or along the new vessel arcades. Traction between the vitreous and the neovascular and glial elements can ultimately develop, leading to retinal detachment or large-scale hemorrhage into the vitreous. These events will lead to serious loss of vision or blindness. It has been suggested that the stimulus for neovascularization is retinal ischemia with local release of growth-promoting factors.

Photocoagulation is the therapy of choice for proliferative diabetic retinopathy. With this therapy, a light beam is focused on the retina to produce a burn or coagulum in a precisely defined area. By this means, one can selectively destroy microaneurysms, leaky vessels, neovascular elements, and areas of microinfarction or edema. Destruction of vessels prone to hemorrhage or causing traction directly prevents further deterioration. Destroying areas of retina that are poorly perfused and hypoxic may curtail the ischemic stimulus for neovascularization, preventing further proliferative changes. Regardless of the mechanism, the cooperative trial of the Diabetic Retinopathy Study Research Group clearly showed that photocoagulation decreases the incidence of retinal detachment, hemorrhage, and loss of vision. Thus, photocoagulation involves selective treatment of new vessels as well as panretinal treatment to destroy 20 to 30 per cent of the remaining retinal tissue. Photocoagulation therapy may also be useful for proliferative retinopathy as indicated by results from the Early Diabetic Retinopathy Treatment Study. All patients with significant diabetic retinopathy should be followed by an ophthalmologist and photocoagulation considered when new vessel formation or preretinal hemorrhage occurs. Photocoagulation early in the course of diabetic retinopathy can also be advisable. In the past, hypophysectomy was used as treatment for proliferative retinopathy. However, the therapeutic responses to this maneuver are quite variable, and significant complications exist. With the advent of photocoagulation, use of hypophysectomy has been largely abandoned. In patients with severe vitreal involvement, total vitrectomy may offer some possibility of improvement and preservation of vision.

Other Complications of Diabetes Affecting Vision

In addition to retinopathy, the eyes are affected in other ways by diabetes mellitus. Diabetics may experience temporary blurring of vision and *changes in refraction,* most likely due to osmotic changes in lens shape as a result of fluctuations in hyperglycemia. These changes can be disconcerting, but patients should be advised not to seek new refractions until a stable period of metabolic control is produced. It may take six to eight weeks before the hyperglycemia-induced changes in visual acuity subside. *Glaucoma* is also more frequent in diabetics. Rubeosis iridis is due to capillary neovascularization of the iris, which can produce closed-angle glaucoma. Usually occurring when diabetic retinopathy is advanced, this form of glaucoma is generally refractory to treatment. Open-angle glaucoma is also more frequent in diabetics, and this may relate to fibrosis or scarring of the canals of Schlemm, which drain the anterior chamber. Although *cataracts* are common in diabetes, it has not been rigorously demonstrated that the incidence of cataracts is increased in this condition. For the most part, cataracts in diabetics are indistinguishable from senile cataracts in nondiabetic patients, and the indications for surgery are the same as in nondiabetics. It is possible that the presence of diabetes accelerates the development of senile cataracts so that they occur at an earlier age than in nondiabetics. It has been postulated that hyperglycemia leads to increased sorbitol production in the lens, resulting in osmotic changes that accelerate cataract formation. While evidence in favor of this theory exists, it still remains to be proved. Opacities in the lens termed snowflake cataracts are occasionally noted in young patients whose diabetes is in poor control. This form of cataract is more specific for diabetes but can occur in other conditions and, unlike the senile cataract, can regress when glycemic control is achieved.

Nephropathy

Kidney disease is common in diabetes (see also Ch. 85 for an extensive discussion of the kidney in diabetes), and renal failure is one of the major causes of death.

PATHOLOGY. The dominant form of diabetic nephropathy is microvascular disease affecting the renal glomerulus. A number of distinct morphologic and functional abnormalities characterize diabetic glomerulopathy. Early in diabetes the kidney increases in size, and the associated glomerular hypertrophy leads to an increased glomerular filtration rate with hyperfiltration and microalbuminuria in up to 50 per cent of patients with new-onset IDDM. The hyperfiltration and increased kidney size revert to normal following effective insulin therapy and are unassociated with other glomerular lesions. Later in the disease, diffuse thickening of the glomerular basement membrane is noted along with increased mesangial volume. Patients with substantial histologic changes can exhibit normal renal function; however, impaired renal function probably does not occur in the absence of morphologic changes. Later in the disease, when decreased renal function is evident, the mesangium further expands and occupies a greater proportion of the glomerular volume while the thickness of the glomerular basement membrane is not necessarily increased. Glomerular occlusion accompanies this picture. Often characteristic nodular hyaline-like deposits, termed nodular glomerulocapillary sclerosis or Kimmelstiel-Wilson lesions, are evident in the center of peripheral glomerular capillary lobules.

CLINICAL AND FUNCTIONAL ASPECTS. The manifestations of diabetic nephropathy are quite heterogeneous. Asymptomatic, mild proteinuria can remain constant for many years. In other patients proteinuria may increase and be followed by progressive reduction in glomerular filtration and renal function. Persistent proteinuria (3 to 5 grams per day or greater) is a poor prognostic sign, usually heralding renal failure within five years. However, exceptions exist. The proteinuria may progress to include all of the classic features of the nephrotic syndrome. Once azotemia develops, progression to renal failure and uremia is inevitable within a few months to two to three years.

The diagnosis of diabetic nephropathy is usually made on clinical grounds, and renal biopsy is rarely indicated. Invasive diagnostic procedures should be aimed at detection of reversible features such as infection or obstruction. Contrast studies should not be conducted without clear indications, since rapid deterioration of renal function with acute renal failure sometimes follows intravenous pyelography or angiography in azotemic diabetic patients. When the study is performed, patients should be well hydrated before testing.

If renal failure develops in a diabetic, dialysis or transplantation must be considered. As recently as 10 to 15 years ago, uremic diabetics were thought to be extremely poor risks for dialysis with very low survival rates and high rates of complications, particularly infections and deterioration of vision. However, in recent years, results have been much better with a first-year survival of over 80 per cent and three-year survival of over 60 per cent. Additionally, far fewer cases of progressive visual impairment and blindness occur. Thus, in the absence of other negative factors, the presence of diabetes should not be considered a contraindication to dialysis, and decisions to initiate this form of therapy should generally proceed as in nondiabetic uremic patients. Chronic ambulatory peritoneal dialysis (CAPD) has been tried in some patients, but overall experience is still limited. Indications for CAPD vary widely among treatment centers, as does enthusiasm for this mode of therapy. Recent experience with renal transplantation has also been encouraging. Regardless of donor source (cadaver or related donor), survival rates after renal transplantation in diabetics approach those in nondiabetics. Interestingly, diabetic-type glomerular changes have been noted in biopsy specimens from the transplanted kidney in many of these patients.

Neuropathy (See Also Ch. 507)

Diabetic neuropathy is perhaps the most common disabling chronic complication of diabetes. Although death seldom results from neuropathic changes alone, a great deal of morbidity and reduced quality of life can be attributed to diabetic neuropathy. The incidence and severity of neuropathy generally progress with duration of diabetes, and severe neuropathy can often exist in the absence of other chronic diabetic complications. A number of different classification schemes have been proposed, but none is entirely satisfactory, primarily because the causes of diabetic neuropathy are not known, and therefore classification must be descriptive in nature rather than based on pathogenetic mechanisms. Table 231-6 provides a simplified method of classification that may prove useful. Polyneuropathy is a diffuse symmetric disorder of peripheral nerve function. Asymmetric neuropathy implies a cluster of signs and symptoms that can be anatomically related to dysfunction of a single nerve trunk (mononeuropathy) or to more than one nerve trunk (mononeuropathy multiplex) either simultaneously or successively. It has been proposed that the symmetric or diffuse neuropathies are due to "metabolic" abnormalities of the neurons or the Schwann cells, whereas the asymmetric or focal neuropathies are due to vascular occlusion and ischemia. Diabetic neuropathy is very common in both IDDM and NIDDM, and mild to severe disease can exist in up to 50 per cent of patients. The incidence of symmetric neuropathy is comparable in IDDM and NIDDM when corrected for duration of disease, but focal neuropathies are more common in older NIDDM patients, suggesting a vascular contribution to the etiology.

NEUROPATHIC LESIONS AND THE DIABETIC FOOT. Loss of sensation can lead to the development of a Charcot joint as a result of repeated undetected trauma. More commonly, neuropathic ulcers develop, particularly on the plantar aspect of the foot. This can be due to weakness of the intrinsic muscles of the foot secondary to neuropathy, leading to abnormal pressure distribution. Weight bearing is then accentuated on the metatarsal heads, causing degeneration of the underlying fat pads and eventually leading to the typical open, draining neuropathic ulcer. Ulcers can also result from penetrating wounds caused by stepping on tacks or other sharp objects the patient does not feel. The best therapy is preventive. All diabetics should be trained to examine their feet daily for callous formation, blisters, or trauma. Shoes should be properly fitted; orthotic or other devices to aid in proper weight distribution are sometimes helpful. Patients should be advised never to walk barefoot. In all cases the feet should be kept clean and dry, and professional trimming of

TABLE 231-6. CLASSIFICATION OF DIABETIC NEUROPATHY

1. Symmetric distal polyneuropathy
2. Asymmetric neuropathy
    A. Cranial mononeuropathy and mononeuropathy multiplex
    B. Peripheral mononeuropathy and mononeuropathy multiplex
    C. Neuromuscular syndromes
3. Autonomic neuropathy

toenails and callosities is often advisable. Neuropathic foot ulcers can lead to gangrene and the requirement for amputation. Meticulous foot care substantially decreases the incidence of these ulcers and is a major form of preventive therapy that all diabetics should receive. Once open ulcers develop, healing can still occur if peripheral circulation is adequate. A high index of suspicion should be maintained for underlying osteomyelitis. Treatment is supportive with bed rest, elevation of the foot, warm (but not hot) foot soaks, debridement, and in some cases antibiotics. Protective plaster casts are sometimes advised. If these therapies fail and gangrene develops, amputation is the only recourse.

SYMMETRIC DISTAL POLYNEUROPATHY. This form of diabetic neuropathy can be divided into two types: (1) relatively asymptomatic and (2) painful. The first form is diffuse, distal, usually in the lower extremities with a stocking type of distribution. It is characterized by numbness, tingling, or pins-and-needles sensation, often worse at night. Although the course may wax and wane, it is generally progressive and irreversible. Symptoms of the painful form can range from burning or dull aching sensations to cramping or excruciating, lancinating pain. The pain is often worse at night and partially relieved by movement. Hyperesthesia can be so marked that even light touch is so painful that the patient cannot tolerate bed covers. Physical examination is similar in both types and is often rather unremarkable. The single most common finding is absence of deep tendon reflexes in the lower extremities (i.e., loss of knee and ankle jerks).

ASYMMETRIC NEUROPATHY. Diabetic mononeuropathies of the cranial nerves usually involve the third, sixth, or fourth cranial nerve in order of frequency. This gives rise to extraocular muscle paralysis with diplopia. The most common syndrome is isolated third nerve palsy accompanied in 80 per cent of cases by sparing of the pupillary reflex. Mononeuropathies of peripheral nerves most frequently occur at sites of external pressure or entrapment (i.e., carpal tunnel). Manifestations include footdrop, wristdrop, or other symptoms related to the particular nerve involved.

Another diabetic neuropathic syndrome involves *radiculopathy.* This syndrome is characterized by dysesthesias and painful hyperesthesia localized to the anatomic distribution of one or more spinal nerves. Symptoms can resemble herpes zoster, although skin lesions are seldom noted.

Diabetic neuropathic cachexia is a syndrome of elderly male diabetics characterized by marked weight loss, painful peripheral polyneuropathy, and depression. The weight loss is so marked that patients appear cachectic, leading to a diagnosis of suspected underlying malignant disease. Other complications of diabetes are typically absent, and patients spontaneously recover in about one year.

For a thorough discussion of diabetic symmetric distal polyneuropathy, asymmetric neuropathy, and autonomic neuropathy see Ch. 507.

Cardiovascular Disease

Cardiovascular disease is the major cause of death in diabetic patients and is far more prevalent than in the nondiabetic population because of accelerated atherogenesis. Not only is cardiovascular disease more frequent, but onset is at an earlier age, and manifestations are more severe. The etiology of the accelerated atherosclerosis in diabetes is incompletely understood, but the causes are probably multifactorial. Most forms of hyperlipoproteinemia are more common in diabetic subjects, and high-density lipoprotein levels tend to be decreased in patients with uncontrolled diabetes. Furthermore, in patients with chronic hyperglycemia, circulating lipoproteins become glycosylated, adversely altering their turnover and sites of tissue deposition. This phenomenon might contribute to the increased risk of atherosclerosis in the absence of grossly elevated circulating lipid levels. Abnormalities of endothelial cell function have also been proposed that would enhance the susceptibility of arterial walls to injury. Increased platelet aggregation and hyperviscosity have also been proposed. Medical management of these risk factors is similar to that in nondiabetic subjects. Thus, specific diet and drug therapy for the various hyperlipoproteinemias should be used when indicated (Ch. 183). On occasion, lipid-lowering drugs such as nicotinic acid may accentuate glucose intolerance. Because of the high risk for atherogenesis, diabetics should be strongly encouraged to abstain from cigarette smoking. Arterial hypertension is a frequent concomitant of diabetes and should be treated promptly. Interestingly, epidemiologic studies have suggested that the existence of hypertension causes little in the way of additive risk for atherosclerosis in diabetics. The diabetic has a substantially greater risk for the development of all forms of cardiovascular disease even when hypertension and hyperlipoproteinemia are taken into account.

The pattern of coronary artery disease (CAD) has been reported to be different in diabetics and nondiabetics, exhibiting in diabetics a greater tendency toward diffuse distal lesions in addition to the usual proximal lesions. However, systematic studies have not uniformly confirmed this notion, suggesting that if this is a feature of CAD in diabetes, then only a minority of patients show diffuse distal occlusive disease. This is important, since one would expect coronary artery bypass surgery to be less successful in patients with distal disease and poor runoff. Overall the indications for myocardial revascularization are probably no different in diabetics and nondiabetics, although a greater incidence of postoperative complications is seen in diabetics. The presence of diabetes substantially eliminates the sex differences in CAD, since the incidence of CAD is roughly comparable in premenopausal diabetic women and age-matched diabetic men. Complications of myocardial infarction are more frequent in diabetics, and postinfarction survival is less. Although angina pectoris is common in diabetic patients, atypical anginal syndromes are seen more frequently than in nondiabetics. Various atypical pain patterns have been described. Painless myocardial infarction has been described in diabetes, probably due to disturbance of afferent nerve fibers. The diagnosis should be suspected in diabetic patients with the sudden onset of left ventricular failure. A syndrome of diabetic cardiomyopathy has been described and is characterized by congestive heart failure in the absence of proximal CAD. It is thought that this syndrome is due to small-vessel occlusive disease. Whether a distinct cardiomyopathy exists in diabetes in the absence of any CAD is still being debated.

Peripheral vascular disease is far more frequent in the diabetic than in the nondiabetic population, and this is particularly so for distal vascular insufficiency of the lower limbs. When combined with the neuropathic complications of diabetes, this unfortunately presents an ideal setting for the development of ischemia and gangrene, necessitating amputation. Because of the marked distal small-vessel disease, vascular bypass surgery is often satisfactory. Most forms of cerebrovascular disease and stroke are also seen more frequently in diabetes.

Dermatologic Lesions

Dermatologic abnormalities are common in diabetes. For example, these patients are more prone to various skin infections such as carbuncles and furuncles. These can often be extensive and difficult to treat. Vaginal candidiasis is frequent in hyperglycemic glycosuric women. Antifungal agents are effective in treating this disorder, but recurrences are common until glycosuria is effectively controlled. Necrobiosis lipoidica diabeticorum consists of round or oval, sharply defined, plaque-like lesions on the anterior surface of the lower legs. The borders of these lesions are frequently elevated, and the center may be depressed. The centers tend to be yellowish, while the borders are hyperpigmented. Although this lesion is uncommon in diabetics, when it does occur, the plaques can ulcerate upon minimal trauma. Diabetic dermopathy (shin spots) is the most frequent dermatologic lesion seen in diabetic patients, occurring in 60 per cent of males and 30 per cent of females. These lesions are common over the tibial area, but also can be observed on forearms and thighs. They begin as small reddish papules that gradually heal, leaving thin hyperpigmented atrophic areas behind. Typical xanthomatoses can occur secondary to hyperlipoproteinemia. In insulin-dependent diabetic subjects, tight waxy skin over the dorsum of the hands in conjunction with joint contractions has been observed. This may be an important clinical observation, since these patients appear to have accelerated development of other microangiopathic complications.

CONCLUSIONS

Diabetes mellitus is a chronic disease and therefore the approach to the patient and methods of management must encompass a long-term view. Patients with diabetes will be interacting with health care providers for the remainder of their lives. The patient must become well educated concerning the disease and eventually learn to individualize all the various components of therapy to his or her own personal circumstances. Ultimately many of the day-to-day therapy and management decisions rest in the hands of the patient. Since much of the treatment of diabetes involves intensive self-care, in a very real sense the patient may be his or her own most important physician. This requires education, motivation, and psychological adjustment.

Brand PW: The diabetic foot. In Ellenberg M, Rifkin H (eds.): Diabetes Mellitus. Theory and Practice. 3rd ed. New Hyde Park, NY, Medical Examination Publishing Co., 1983, pp 829–849. *An in-depth review of the clinical manifestations and management of diabetic foot problems.*

Bunn HF: Evaluation of glycosylated hemoglobin in diabetic patients. Diabetes 30:613, 1981. *A review of the biochemistry, clinical significance, and use of glycosylated hemoglobin in diabetes.*

Cudworth AG, Wolf E: The genetic susceptibility to type I (insulin-dependent) diabetes mellitus. Clin Endocrinol Metab 11:389, 1982. *A discussion of the HLA associations in type I diabetes mellitus.*

Early Treatment Diabetic Retinopathy Study Research Group: Photocoagulation for diabetic macular edema. Arch Ophthalmol 103:1796, 1985. *A report of the multicenter study designed to determine at what point photocoagulation is appropriate therapy for diabetic retinopathy.*

Feig PU, McCurdy DK: The hypertonic state. N Engl J Med 297:1444, 1977. *A discussion of the pathophysiology and clinical treatment of the hyperosmolar syndrome.*

Feingold KR: Hypoglycemia: A pitfall of insulin therapy. West J Med 139:688, 1983. *An excellent clinical discussion of this important complication of the therapy of diabetes, with 56 references.*

Foster DW, McGarry JD: The metabolic derangements and treatment of diabetic ketoacidosis. N Engl J Med 309:159, 1983. *A thorough and current review of the pathogenesis and treatment of this disorder.*

Geffner ME, Lippe BM: The role of immunotherapy in Type I diabetes mellitus. West J Med 146:337, 1987. *A recent review covering the pros and cons of the various forms of immunotherapy which have been used or considered for the early treatment of IDDM.*

Given BD, Mako ME, Tager H, et al.: Circulating insulin with reduced biological activity in a patient with diabetes. N Engl J Med 302:129, 1980. *The first description of a patient producing a biologically defective insulin molecule.*

Goetz FC: Recent progress in the management of end-stage diabetic nephropathy. Clin Endocrinol Metab 11:579, 1982. *A good discussion of the relative success rates of dialysis and transplantation in end-stage diabetic neuropathy.*

Greene DA, Lattimer S, Ulbrecht J, Carroll P: Glucose-induced alterations in nerve metabolism: Current perspective on the pathogenesis of diabetic neuropathy and future directions for research and therapy. Diabetes Care 9:290, 1985. *A comprehensive review article discussing current concepts about the pathogenesis of diabetic neuropathy with a view toward therapy.*

Grogen CH, Lernmark A: Islet cell antibodies in diabetes. Clin Endocrinol Metab 11:409, 1982. *A literature review of islet cell antibodies in diabetes mellitus.*

Kroc Collaborative Study Group: Blood glucose control and the evolution of diabetic retinopathy and albuminuria. N Engl J Med 311:365, 1984. *A report of a well-designed multicenter clinical trial to examine the effect of intensive diabetic control on diabetic complications.*

Lernmark A, Baekkeskov S: Islet cell antibodies—Theoretical and practical implications. Diabetologia 21:431, 1981. *A discussion of the potential role of autoantibodies directed against beta cells in the pathogenesis of diabetes.*

L'Esperance FA Jr, James SA Jr: The eye and diabetes mellitus. In Ellenberg M, Rifkin H (eds.): Diabetes Mellitus. Theory and Practice. 3rd ed. New Hyde Park, NY, Medical Examination Publishing Co., 1983, pp 727–757. *A general review of the ocular complications of diabetes mellitus with particular emphasis on retinopathy.*

McGarry JD, Foster DW: Regulation of hepatic fatty acid oxidation and ketone body production. Ann Rev Biochem 49:395, 1980. *Detailed review of the intermediary metabolism of ketogenesis and the pathogenesis of diabetic ketoacidosis.*

National Diabetes Data Group: Classification and diagnosis of diabetes mellitus and other categories of glucose intolerance. Diabetes 63:843, 1977. *A description of the unified classification system and methods and criteria for diagnosis of diabetes mellitus.*

Olefsky JM, Kolterman OG: Mechanisms of insulin resistance in obesity and noninsulin dependent (type II) diabetes. Am J Med 70:151, 1981. *A review of the pathogenesis and contribution of insulin resistance in NIDDM.*

Peacock I, Tattersall R: Methods of self monitoring of diabetic control. Clin Endocrinol Metab 11:485, 1982. *A review of the rationale and technique of self-monitoring of glucose in diabetes mellitus.*

Rotter JI, Rimoin DL: The genetics of diabetes. Hosp Pract 22:79, 1987. *A useful general discussion of the genetics of the various types of diabetes mellitus, with a tabular summary of a large number of genetic syndromes associated with it.*

Rotter JI, Anderson CE, Rimoin DL: Genetics of diabetes mellitus. In Ellenberg M, Rifkin H (eds.): Diabetes Mellitus. Theory and Practice. 3rd ed. New Hyde Park, NY, Medical Examination Publishing Co., 1983, pp 481–503. *A review of the inheritance patterns and the genetic contributions to the etiology of type I and type II diabetes mellitus.*

Schade DS, Santiago JV, Skyler JS, et al.: Intensive insulin therapy. Princeton, Excerpta Medica, 1983. *A recent monograph outlining the physiologic principles and methods of administering intensive therapy by multiple injections as well as CSII.*

Skyler JS: Complications of diabetes mellitus: Relationship to metabolic dysfunction. Diabetes Care 2:499, 1979. *A discussion of the value of glycemic control in the late complications of diabetes mellitus.*

Unger RH, Orci L: Glucagon and the A cell. Physiology and pathophysiology. N Engl J Med 304:1518, 1575, 1981. *A review of the physiology of glucagon secretion and action as well as its role in the pathophysiology of diabetes.*

Yoon J-W, Austin M, Onodera T, et al.: Virus-induced diabetes mellitus. N Engl J Med 300:1173, 1979. *A report of a well-documented case of viral-induced diabetes.*

Zata R, Brenner BM: Pathogenesis of diabetic microangiopathy. Am J Med 80:443, 1986. *A discussion of the role of hemodynamic abnormalities in the pathogenesis of diabetic microangiopathy.*

---

232 HYPOGLYCEMIC DISORDERS

F. John Service

Hypoglycemia is a pathophysiologic state and not a disease. Just as pain, fever, or vomiting requires identification of the underlying condition, hypoglycemia warrants diagnosis of the primary disorder causing the low plasma glucose level.

Hypoglycemia can be defined as a glucose concentration below the lower limit of normal. Since hypoglycemic disorders are clinical syndromes almost invariably associated with symptoms from the low concentration of glucose, hypoglycemia is usually considered to be a glucose concentration in the range below the level at which symptoms could be expected to occur.

PHYSIOLOGY

The plasma glucose concentration is maintained within narrow bounds, in spite of intermittent food ingestion and periods of fasting, as the net balance between the rates of glucose production and utilization. Following food ingestion the increase in plasma glucose, in concert with an incretion effect from enteric factors, results in an increase in plasma insulin, which accelerates glucose utilization and suppresses hepatic glucose production. As the plasma glucose concentration falls postprandially, plasma insulin decreases, which restores glucose utilization and production to the preprandial rates. There is then a transition from a state of glucose storage to one of carefully husbanded glucose production at rates designed to satisfy the obligatory needs of the body. In the postabsorptive period four to six hours after food ingestion, plasma glucose concentrations are generally 80 to 90 mg per deciliter with rates of glucose production and utilization of approximately 2 mg per kg^{-1} per min^{-1}. About half of the glucose produced is metabolized by the central nervous system.

GLYCOGENOLYSIS. In the postabsorptive period glucose production is primarily from hepatic glycogenolysis (70 to 80 per cent), with a small contribution from gluconeogenesis (20 to 25 per cent). Hepatic glycogen stores become exhausted after 24 to 36 hours of fasting. Glycogenolysis is stimulated by epinephrine and glucagon and inhibited by insulin. Several enzymes are involved in the cleavage of glucose moieties from glycogen and the final appearance of free glucose in the circulation. Abnormalities of these enzymes may result in hypoglycemia. For example, deficient activity of glucose-6-phosphatase (von Gierke's disease) may cause severe hypoglycemia, whereas deficient activities of glycogen phosphorylase and debrancher enzyme cause milder degrees of hypoglycemia (see Ch. 179). Deficiency of glycogen synthetase results in severe hypoglycemia in newborns.

GLUCONEOGENESIS. The generation of new glucose from non-carbohydrate substrates is termed gluconeogenesis. Defects in this process result in hypoglycemia after prolonged fasting when glycogen stores have been depleted. Lactate and pyruvate, glycerol, and amino acids account for approximately 58 per cent, 13 per cent, and 29 per cent respectively of the glucose produced via gluconeogenesis. Defects in gluconeogenesis may arise from (1) diminished substrate availability, e.g., ketotic hypoglycemia in children; (2) altered redox state, which inhibits several important gluconeogenic enzymes, e.g., alcohol hypoglycemia; and (3) inhibition of fatty acid oxidation, which diminishes the energy source for gluconeogenesis, e.g., poisoning from the unripe akee fruit.

Alanine and glutamine are the most important amino acids that act as glucose precursors. The carbon source of alanine is muscle-derived pyruvate, and the nitrogen source for the transamination of pyruvate to alanine is thought to be branched-chain amino acids. Impaired metabolism of leucine, a branched-chain amino acid, observed in maple syrup urine disease (see Ch. 193), is associated with reduced alanine production and sometimes with hypoglycemia. After three days of fasting, glucose production is primarily derived from hepatic gluconeogenesis; after prolonged fasting, renal gluconeogenesis may account for approximately 50 per cent of glucose production.

HORMONAL CONTROL OF GLUCOSE HOMEOSTASIS. The effects of insulin, glucagon, catecholamines, cortisol, and growth hormone on glucose homeostasis and recovery from hypoglycemia are shown in Table 232–1. Insulin is the primary hypoglycemic hormone; the others act by a variety of mechanisms to elevate glucose concentrations. Although plasma glucagon, catecholamines, cortisol, and growth hormone increase in response to insulin-induced hypoglycemia, glucagon makes the major contribution to the quick recovery from hypoglycemia. Catecholamines can result in a modest elevation of glucose concentration in the presence of glucagon deficiency or severe hypoglycemia.

TABLE 232–1. HORMONAL CONTROL OF GLUCOSE HOMEOSTASIS

Hormone	Hepatic Glucose Production	Extrahepatic Glucose Utilization	Basal Glucose Production	Relative Importance to Recovery from Insulin-Induced Hypoglycemia
Insulin	↓	↑	↓	
Glucagon	↑	–	↑	+ + +
Catecholamines*	↑	↓	–	+
Cortisol	↑	↓	↑	–
Growth hormone†	↑	↓	–	–

NOTE: ↑ = increase; ↓ = decrease; – = no effect.
*Epinephrine is approximately ten times more potent than norepinephrine. Its action is primarily through a beta-adrenergic mechanism. In the presence of glucagon deficiency, catecholamines make a modest contribution to the recovery from hypoglycemia.
†Has an acute and transient hypoglycemic effect.

CLINICAL EVALUATION

Defects of many of the mechanisms that maintain plasma glucose in the normal range are associated with readily recognizable clinical syndromes. In some instances the symptoms and signs of the primary disorder predominate over those of hypoglycemia, or at least point to the existence of the primary disorder causing hypoglycemia. In some patients with multisystem disease, poor nutrition, or multiple drug use, the bases for hypoglycemia may be uncertain and the patient too ill to undergo extensive evaluation. Common causes of hypoglycemia are listed in Table 232–2.

In the majority of patients with symptoms of hypoglycemia who appear healthy, screening laboratory tests should include plasma glucose, serum insulin, calcium, phosphorus, uric acid, lipids, creatinine, liver function, insulin antibodies, and plasma and urine corticosteroids. Documentation of drug-induced hypoglycemia may be difficult. A detailed history must be obtained, and every medication used by the patient, including nonprescription drugs, must be examined.

When a patient is observed with symptoms of hypoglycemia, 10 to 20 ml of blood in addition to that for glucose determination should be withdrawn. The specific analyses can be determined by the clues generated from the history and physical examination. Such an opportunity may provide sufficient data to establish the cause of the hypoglycemic disorder or narrow the diagnostic possibilities. Glucose should be administered following blood withdrawal to any patient suspected of being hypoglycemic. Prompt treatment will shorten the duration of hypoglycemia, and if the patient is not hypoglycemic, no harm will have been done.

In patients with asymptomatic hypoglycemia one must be alert to artifactual hypoglycemia. Whole-blood glucose values may be spuriously low in polycythemia vera because of the unequal distribution of glucose between erythrocyte and plasma or because of excessive glycolysis by erythrocytes, or both, and in leukemia because of excessive glycolysis by leukocytes. Prompt measurement of glucose in plasma in these conditions should provide accurate results.

An uncommon and challenging problem is the low plasma glucose concentration in an asymptomatic patient in whom laboratory error and spurious result have been ruled out. Such patients may have adapted to longstanding hypoglycemia or have mild symptoms that have been completely unrecognized.

A flow diagram of a clinical approach to the evaluation of a suspected hypoglycemic disorder is presented in Figure 232–1. Note that the evaluation is directed to patients who appear healthy. For those who do not appear healthy the results of the history and physical examination will determine the direction of the investigation.

Hypoglycemic disorders cause a constellation of symptoms that usually recur as discrete episodes at irregular intervals. A useful but not infallible historical aid is the timing of symptoms in relation to food intake: Those occurring within five hours of food intake are the *food-stimulated hypoglycemias* and those occurring beyond five hours of food intake are the *food-deprived hypoglycemias*.

Considerable effort should be expended to obtain from the patient and family members a detailed description of symptoms, careful attention being paid to their occurrence in relation to food intake. The food-stimulated hypoglycemias usually cause symptoms of catecholamine release—sweating, shakiness, anxiety, palpitations, and weakness—and rarely

TABLE 232–2. COMMON CAUSES OF HYPOGLYCEMIA

Medications	Non-islet cell tumors
Ethanol	Multifactorial in sick patient
Factitial	Islet dysplasia of infancy
Insulinoma	Ketotic hypoglycemia

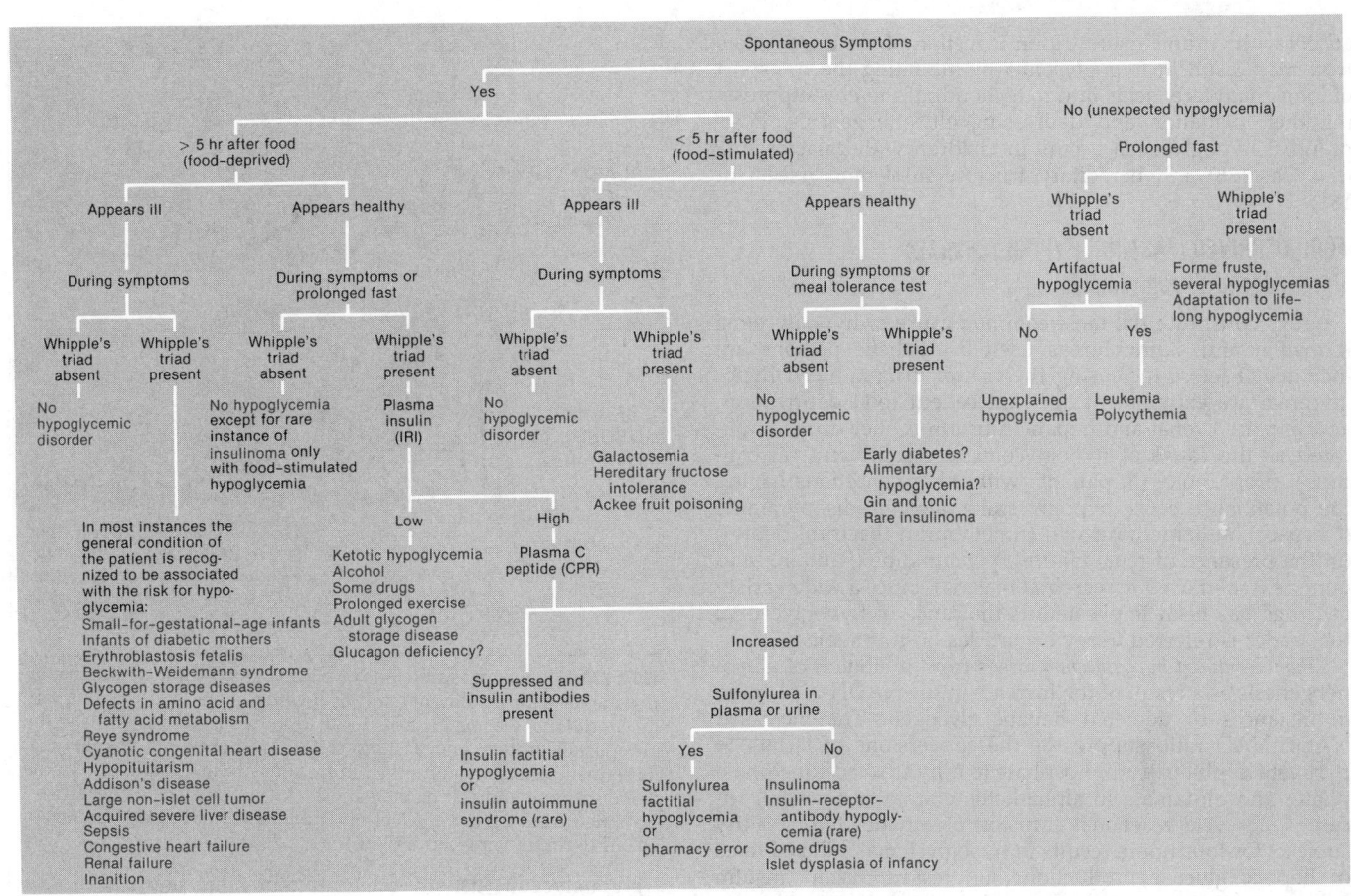

FIGURE 232–1. Evaluation of hypoglycemic disorders.

those of impairment of central nervous system function. The food-deprived hypoglycemias, on the other hand, usually result in impairment of central nervous system function—reduced intellectual capacity, confusion, irritability, abnormal behavior, convulsions, and coma. Sometimes there is complicating hypothermia. Often the symptoms of catecholamine release that precede the central nervous system symptoms go unrecognized. Symptoms of hypoglycemia usually occur at plasma glucose concentrations of about 45 mg per deciliter or less (whole-blood glucose, 40 mg per deciliter or less). Although some studies suggest that a rapid fall in glucose concentration results in symptoms even when plasma glucose does not decrease below 45 mg per deciliter, the weight of evidence does not support this relationship. The symptoms of hypoglycemia are nonspecific. For this reason it is necessary to demonstrate a low plasma glucose value concomitant with symptoms and subsequent relief of symptoms by correction of the hypoglycemia, i.e., *Whipple's triad.* This triad should be demonstrated before hypoglycemia can be considered to be the basis for a patient's symptoms. Although food, especially free carbohydrate, will relieve symptoms regardless of the cause of the hypoglycemia, persons without a hypoglycemic disorder may feel better after eating. It is therefore imperative to confirm that symptoms are due to hypoglycemia.

FOOD-STIMULATED (POSTPRANDIAL) HYPOGLYCEMIAS

Subsequent to the conceptualization of hyperinsulinism as a disease, after insulin became available for the treatment of diabetes, many patients with postprandial symptoms were found to have concomitant blood sugar concentrations within or even above the normal range. For such cases the term *functional hypoglycemia* was coined. Eventually reliance on a subnormal glucose concentration at the time of spontaneous symptoms came to be replaced by the oral glucose tolerance test. Reproduction of those symptoms experienced during ordinary daily activities and documentation of a plasma glucose nadir less than or equal to 50 mg per deciliter (or its equivalent) during the oral glucose tolerance test have been considered confirmation of the presence of a food-stimulated hypoglycemic disorder. Use of the oral glucose tolerance test is fraught with risk of misdiagnosis, since (1) in at least 10 per cent of healthy persons the plasma glucose nadir is less than 50 mg per deciliter; (2) there is no correlation between the nadir of plasma glucose concentration and the occurrence of symptoms of hypoglycemia in patients with symptoms suggestive of food-stimulated hypoglycemia; (3) the results of oral glucose tolerance tests are variable upon repeated testing; (4) subjects with symptoms during an oral glucose tolerance test may have similar symptoms during a placebo oral glucose tolerance test; and (5) glycemia less than 50 mg per deciliter after ingestion of glucose cannot usually be reproduced after a mixed meal despite the presence of symptoms following both. Measurement of plasma cortisol responses, calculation of rates of glucose descent, and hypoglycemic indices have not improved the accuracy of the oral glucose tolerance test.

Unfortunately, reliance on the oral glucose tolerance test for the diagnosis of food-stimulated hypoglycemia has led to extensive literature not on disorders of hypoglycemia but on the oral glucose tolerance test. Although there undoubtedly are patients with true postprandial hypoglycemia, most persons with symptoms following meals have been shown to have psychoneurosis. Low-carbohydrate–high-protein diets, sulfonylureas, biguanides, or anticholinergic agents have not been proven to be effective treatment.

Hypoglycemia following the ingestion of substances that are toxic to susceptible persons may be considered in the category of postprandial hypoglycemias. The ingestion of large amounts (equivalent to three highballs) of ethanol and carbohydrate (gin and tonic) may cause hypoglycemia within three to four hours in some healthy persons. In children or adults with chronic malnutrition ingestion of the unripe akee fruit may result in hypoglycemia by inhibiting the transport of long-chain fatty acids into mitochondria, thereby suppressing their oxidation and depressing gluconeogenesis. Postprandial hypoglycemia occurs in children with galactosemia (see Ch. 178) and hereditary fructose intolerance (see Ch. 181).

FOOD-DEPRIVED (FASTING) HYPOGLYCEMIAS
Drug-Induced Hypoglycemias

Drugs constitute the most common cause of hypoglycemia if insulin and sulfonylureas used by diabetic persons are included. Factors increasing the risk of drug-induced hypoglycemia are extremes of age, antecedent food deprivation, and impaired renal and hepatic function. Other drugs implicated as the cause of hypoglycemia are salicylates (in children), propranolol (in patients with other conditions having the potential to cause hypoglycemia), alcohol, disopyramide (Norpace), sulfamethoxazole, trimethoprim (Bactrim, Septra) (in the presence of renal failure), pentamidine (Pentam), and quinine (when used for cerebral malaria). Since a wide variety of drugs has been implicated as the cause of hypoglycemia, the reader is referred to review articles on this subject.

Ethanol-induced hypoglycemia arises from inhibition of gluconeogenesis as a result of the increase in the NADH-NAD ratio in instances of depleted hepatic glycogen. The increased NADH-NAD ratio suppresses the conversions of lactate to pyruvate, alpha-glycerophosphate to dihydroxyacetone phosphate, and glutamate to alpha-ketoglutarate and several tricarboxylic cycle reactions. Infusion of ethanol into healthy subjects for four hours results in hypoglycemia; reduced rates of hepatic glucose production; suppressed plasma insulin concentrations; increased plasma lactate, beta-hydroxybutyrate, glycerol, and free fatty acid concentrations; and increased lactate-pyruvate and beta-hydroxybutyrate–acetoacetate ratios. Hypoglycemia usually develops within 6 to 36 hours of the ingestion of even moderate amounts of alcohol by persons chronically malnourished or by healthy persons who have missed one or two meals. Children are especially susceptible to alcohol-induced hypoglycemia. Blood alcohol levels may not be elevated when the patient is hypoglycemic.

Insulinoma

Approximately 60 per cent of patients with insulinoma are women. Insulinomas are uncommon in persons less than 20 years of age and rare in those less than 5 years of age. The median age at diagnosis is about 50 years, except in patients with multiple endocrine neoplasia (MEN) syndrome, in which it is in the mid 20's. Ten per cent of patients with insulinoma are older than 70 years of age.

Of patients with insulinoma 80 per cent have single benign tumors, 11 per cent have multiple benign tumors, 6 per cent have single malignant tumors, and the remainder have multiple malignant tumors or islet hyperplasia. Ten per cent of insulinoma patients have MEN syndrome type 1 (Ch. 241), and 80 per cent of these patients with multiple insulinomas have MEN syndrome.

Some insulinomas secrete other hormones in addition to insulin: gastrin, 5-hydroxyindoles, ACTH, glucagon, and somatostatin. In rare instances, insulinomas have occurred in non–insulin-dependent diabetic persons, but have never been documented in an insulin-dependent patient.

CLINICAL PICTURE. Symptoms may be present for many years prior to the diagnosis. In one series 85 per cent of patients had various combinations of diplopia, blurred vision, sweating, palpitations, or weakness; 80 per cent had confusion or abnormal behavior; 53 per cent had unconsciousness or amnesia; and 12 per cent had grand mal seizures. Twenty per cent of cases may be misdiagnosed, the belief being that the patient has a neurologic or psychiatric disorder.

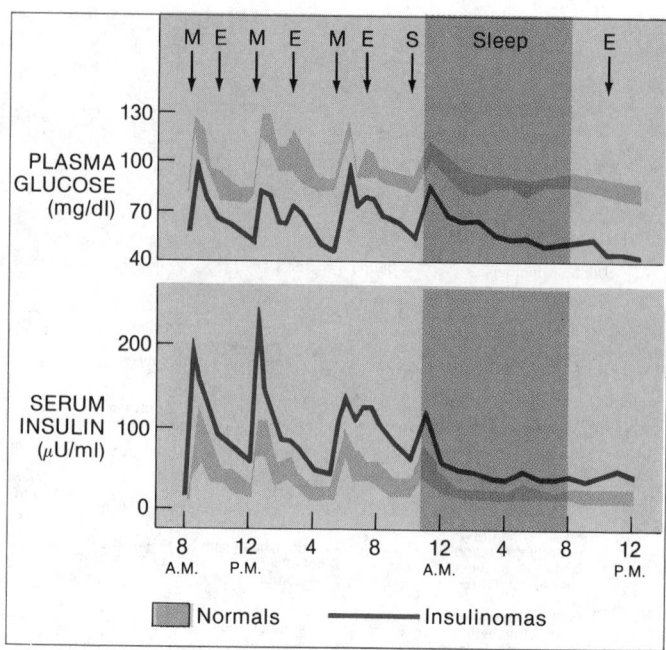

FIGURE 232–2. Serial measurements of plasma glucose and serum insulin in patients with insulinoma and in healthy subjects under ordinary life conditions. Plasma glucose declined to hypoglycemic levels in the late postabsorptive and fasting states in those with insulinoma. Hyperinsulinemia was observed in response to meals and also in the postabsorptive and fasting states. (M = Meal; S = snack; E = exercise.) (Modified from Service FJ, Nelson RL: Insulinoma. Comp Ther 6:70, 1980. Reprinted with permission.)

Hypoglycemia usually occurs five or more hours after any meal (Fig. 232–2). In rare instances, symptoms may occur solely in the postprandial period (two to four hours after eating) and never during fasting. Symptoms may be aggravated by exercise, alcohol use, a high-protein–low-carbohydrate diet, treatment with sulfonylureas, and fasts. Less than 20 per cent of patients with insulinoma gain weight.

DIAGNOSIS. The diagnosis of insulinoma is based on the demonstration of Whipple's triad and hyperinsulinemia or an inappropriately normal insulin level for a low glucose value. Insulin antibodies are usually undetectable, but may be present in low titers in some patients. Useful diagnostic tests are daily fasting plasma glucose and insulin determinations and the intravenous tolbutamide test and C-peptide suppression test. These tests should be performed only in persons for whom the fasting plasma glucose is known to exceed 50 mg per deciliter on the day of the test and who have not been food deprived for several days preceding the test.

Prolonged Supervised Fasting. This is a highly reliable test for the diagnosis of insulinoma. During the fast the patient should be active during the day. Noncaloric beverages can be consumed. The frequency of blood sampling should be guided by the patient's history of tolerance to food withdrawal and be increased as the plasma glucose approaches the hypoglycemic range. Whenever blood is withdrawn for glucose determinations, a sample should also be drawn for determination of serum insulin and, if factitial hypoglycemia is suspected, of C peptide and sulfonylurea. The patient's intellectual status should be checked regularly by simple mathematic tasks such as serial sevens. During prolonged fasting healthy women experience lower plasma glucose concentrations than do healthy men: Values as low as 42 mg per deciliter in men and 34 mg per deciliter in women may be unaccompanied by symptoms. Therefore it is essential to continue the fast to the point at which symptoms develop, or to 72 hours. Serum insulin concentrations may be in the "normal" range in about 50 per cent of determinations when the plasma glucose is in the hypoglycemic range (Fig. 232–3); 10 per cent of patients with insulinoma may have all insulin

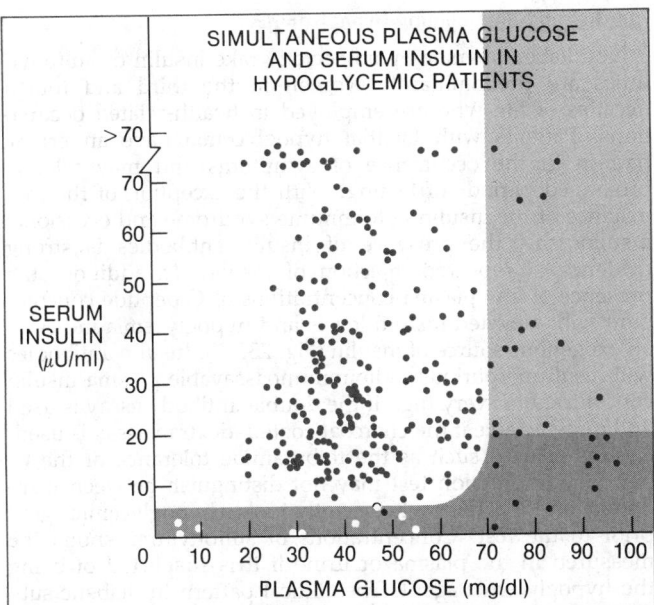

FIGURE 232–3. Simultaneously measured serum insulin and plasma glucose in 72 patients with insulinomas (red circles) and six patients with non–insulin-mediated hypoglycemia (white circles). Ten per cent of patients with insulinoma for whom multiple simultaneous insulin and glucose determinations were made had insulin values in the normal range (0 to 20 µU/ml) during concomitant hypoglycemia. Serum insulin concentrations greater than 6 µU/ml during hypoglycemia are diagnostic of insulin-mediated hypoglycemia. (Modified from Service FJ (ed.): Hypoglycemic Disorders: Pathogenesis, Diagnosis, and Treatment. Boston, GK Hall, 1982. Reprinted with permission.)

values in this normal range during hypoglycemia; however, this normal serum insulin concentration is probably excessive if it is above 6 µU per milliliter and certainly excessive if it is above 10 µU per milliliter during hypoglycemia. Various glucose-insulin ratios provide less diagnostic accuracy.

In a large series, Whipple's triad was demonstrated within 12 hours of the last meal in 29 per cent of patients, within 24 hours in 71 per cent, within 36 hours in 79 per cent, within 48 hours in 92 per cent, within 60 hours in 97 per cent, and within 72 hours in 98 per cent. In rare instances, patients with insulinoma may not develop hypoglycemia during prolonged fasting of even up to 96 hours. At the time of hypoglycemic symptoms, plasma glucose concentrations were less than or equal to 46 mg per deciliter in 100 per cent of patients, 39 mg per deciliter in 75 per cent, 35 mg per deciliter in 50 per cent, and 28 mg per deciliter in 25 per cent.

Tolbutamide Test and C-Peptide Suppression Test. Diagnostic criteria for the tolbutamide test and for the C-peptide suppression test are illustrated in Figures 232–4 and 232–5, respectively. Diagnostic criteria will reflect local laboratory procedures and so should be generated at each institution. If the plasma glucose responses to intravenous tolbutamide are normal, the insulin values give little additional information.

Miscellaneous Tests. The intravenous glucagon test, which is considered to be positive if the peak insulin response exceeds 130 µU per milliliter, has a diagnostic accuracy of 50 to 80 per cent. The utility of other tests such as glycosylated hemoglobin, human pancreatic polypeptide, and infusions of alcohol, calcium, epinephrine and propranolol, diazoxide, and somatostatin-tolbutamide in the diagnosis of insulinoma is unproven or inadequate. Human chorionic gonadotropin or one of its subunits may be a marker for functioning malignant insulinomas. Eighty per cent of patients with insulinoma may have elevated proinsulin concentrations (>20 per cent of total immunoreactive insulin).

LOCALIZATION. Only after the diagnosis of insulinoma has been confirmed biochemically should a localization procedure be done. Pancreatic angiography has been reported to have a high rate of success if stereoscopy, magnification, and subtraction are used. Insulinomas appear as homogeneous, intensely vascular, sharply circumscribed masses within the substance of the pancreas.

Computed tomography has had limited success in localization. Real-time high-resolution ultrasonography done both preoperatively and especially intraoperatively is currently demonstrating a high degree of accuracy (Fig. 232–6). The indications for and value of selective venous sampling for insulin determinations done either by the percutaneous transhepatic route or directly at the time of surgery remain undetermined. Failure to localize an insulinoma by any of these techniques should not deter pancreatic exploration in a patient for whom the diagnosis has been firmly established. Surgeons experienced in insulinoma surgery are highly successful in finding the tumor even when it has not been localized preoperatively.

TREATMENT. Surgical removal is the preferred form of treatment for insulinoma. In a large series, 54 per cent of subjects underwent successful enucleation of the tumor; 38 per cent, partial pancreatectomy; and the remainder, a variety of other procedures. In the series, 84 per cent were cured, 7 per cent had diabetes, and the remainder required medical treatment to control persistent hypoglycemia from malignant insulinoma, islet hyperplasia, or a tumor missed during surgery. There was no operative mortality, and the postoperative complication rate was 10 per cent.

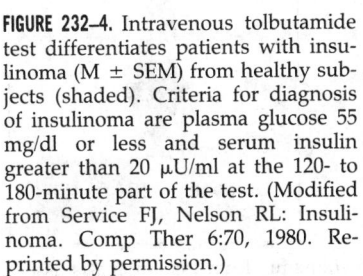

FIGURE 232–4. Intravenous tolbutamide test differentiates patients with insulinoma (M ± SEM) from healthy subjects (shaded). Criteria for diagnosis of insulinoma are plasma glucose 55 mg/dl or less and serum insulin greater than 20 µU/ml at the 120- to 180-minute part of the test. (Modified from Service FJ, Nelson RL: Insulinoma. Comp Ther 6:70, 1980. Reprinted by permission.)

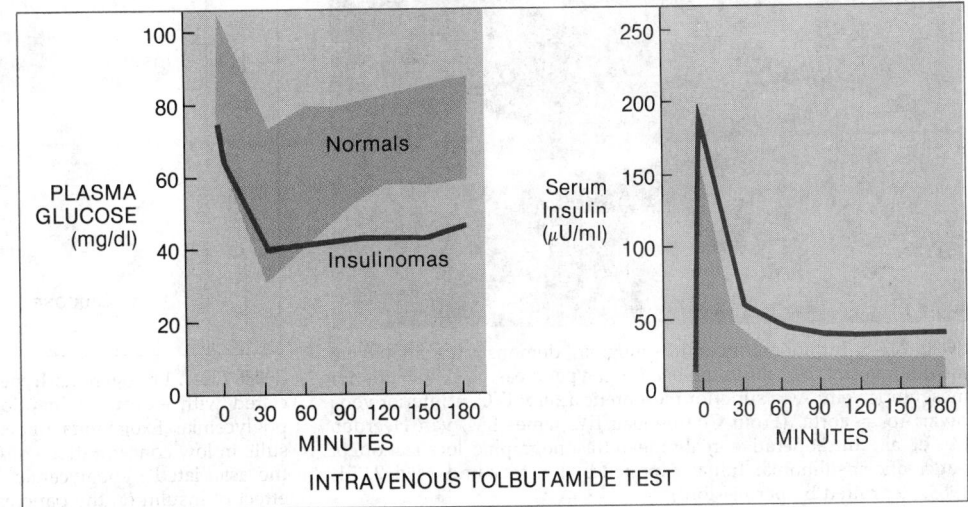

INTRAVENOUS TOLBUTAMIDE TEST

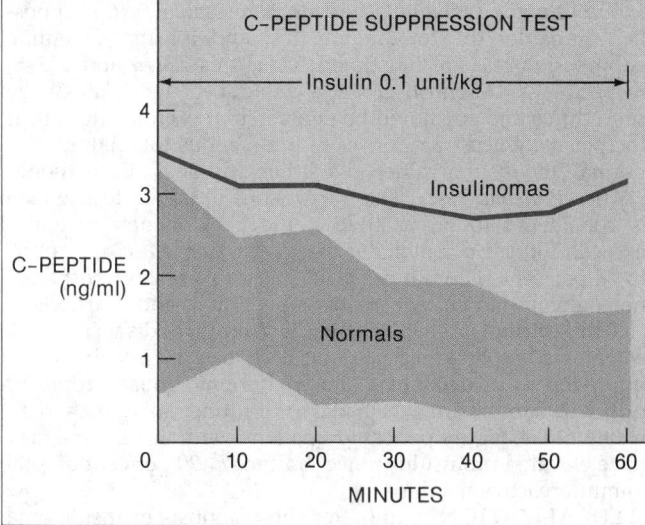

FIGURE 232–5. In response to insulin-induced hypoglycemia, insulinomas fail to suppress C-peptide normally. (Modified from Service FJ, Nelson RL: Insulinoma. Comp Ther 6:70, 1980. Reprinted with permission.)

Intraoperative glucose monitoring should not be relied upon for surgical management, since there is a high (23 per cent) incidence of failure of plasma glucose to increase after successful insulinoma removal.

The median diameter of benign tumors is 1.5 cm. Malignant tumors are usually large. Tumors are evenly distributed throughout the pancreas whether benign or malignant, single or multiple. Ectopically located insulinoma and islet hyperplasia are very rare. There is no correlation between the severity of symptoms and size of the insulinoma.

Treatment of persistent hypoglycemia in a patient with malignant insulinoma, in a patient in whom insulinoma cannot be found at pancreatic exploration, or in one who refuses surgery is best accomplished with diazoxide, which inhibits insulin release, although phenytoin, propranolol, somatostatin, and verapamil have been used successfully in some cases. Malignant insulinoma metastasizes primarily to local structures such as regional lymph nodes and liver; distant metastases are uncommon. The chemotherapeutic regimen of choice consists of streptozotocin and 5-fluorouracil. Survival exceeds that in adenocarcinoma of the pancreas.

Factitial and Autoimmune Hypoglycemia

Nondiabetic persons who secretly take insulin or sulfonylureas are predominantly women in the third and fourth decades of life who are employed in health-related occupations. Patients with factitial hypoglycemia have an erratic pattern in the occurrence of symptoms and may tolerate prolonged periods of fasting. With the exception of the rare instance of the insulin autoimmune syndrome and occasional insulinomas, the presence of insulin antibodies is strong evidence of repeated injection of insulin. In addition, the presence of low plasma concentrations of C peptide concomitant with elevated insulin levels and hypoglycemia indicates an exogenous source of insulin (Fig. 232–7). Insulin antibodies will result in spurious radioimmunoassayable plasma insulin concentrations: very high if the double-antibody assay is used and undetectable if the charcoal-coated–dextran assay is used. Results of tests such as the tolbutamide tolerance or the C-peptide suppression test may not distinguish between insulinoma and a patient who secretly took a hypoglycemic agent prior to the test. Concentrations of sulfonylurea should be measured in the plasma or urine if it is suspected of being the hypoglycemic agent. The clinical pattern in diabetic subjects consists of increased frequency of hypoglycemia during treatment and persistence of hypoglycemic episodes after complete cessation of use of the agent. The presence of insulin antibodies is of no help in the diagnosis in the insulin-treated patient. An inverse relation between C-peptide and insulin levels during hypoglycemia is diagnostic of surreptitious insulin administration. Insulin has been used for suicide, homicide, and child abuse. Errors in filling prescriptions by substitution of a sulfonylurea for the intended medication have led to hypoglycemia.

In rare instances, patients who apparently have never had an insulin injection but have insulin antibodies may have hypoglycemia. These patients may range in age from a few days to elderly. Hypoglycemia may be severe, occur during fasting or postprandially, and is often self-limited. Too few cases have been adequately described to ascertain whether free insulin concentrations are abnormal during episodes of hypoglycemia; free C-peptide concentrations appear to be appropriately suppressed. Discrimination between autoimmune and factitial hypoglycemia rests on demonstrating differences in the characteristics of the insulin antibodies and the absence of bovine and porcine proinsulin and C-peptide specific antibodies. Neither the biochemical characteristics of this syndrome nor the mechanism of the hypoglycemia has been fully elucidated. Hypoglycemia has been observed in a

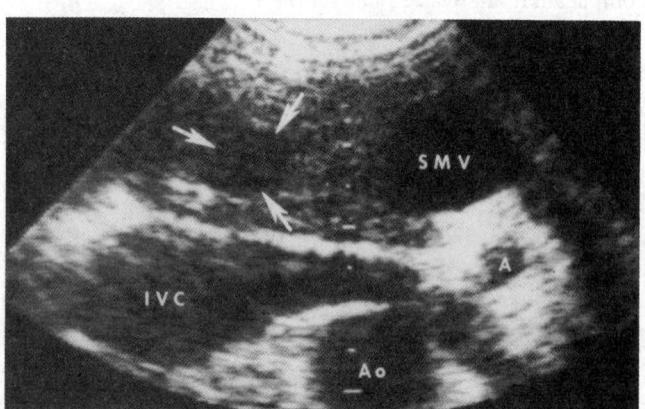

FIGURE 232–6. Intraoperative ultrasonogram demonstrates an 0.8-cm insulinoma (*arrows*) within the head of the pancreas. SMV = Superior mesenteric vein; A = superior mesenteric artery; IVC = inferior vena cava; Ao = aorta. (From Charboneau JW, James EM, van Heerden JA, et al.: Intraoperative real-time ultrasonographic localization of pancreatic insulinoma: Initial experience. J Ultrasound Med 2:251, 1983. Reprinted by permission.)

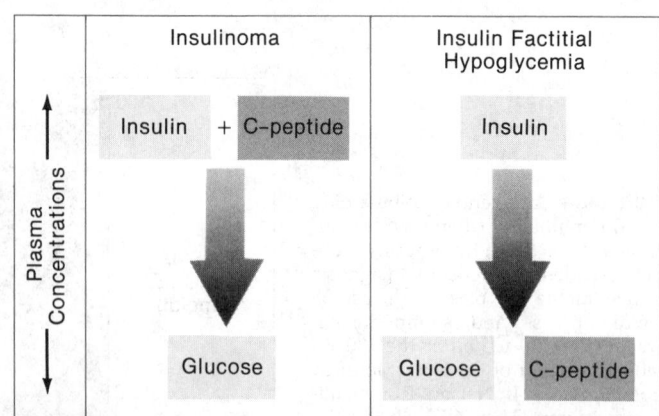

FIGURE 232–7. Endogenous hyperinsulinemia from insulinoma is associated with elevated C-peptide concentrations with concurrent hypoglycemia. Exogenous hyperinsulinemia from injected insulin results in low concentrations of C-peptide both because of the effect of the associated hypoglycemic and because of the direct suppressive effect of insulin on the pancreatic beta cell.

few persons with insulin receptor antibodies that presumably act like insulin agonists. Most of the reported patients had pre-existing insulin-resistant diabetes and evidence for autoimmune disease prior to the development of hypoglycemia. This syndrome may respond to glucocorticoid therapy but not to immunosuppressive agents or plasmapheresis.

Non—Beta-Cell Tumor Hypoglycemia

A wide variety of tumors of mesenchymal or epithelial origin and some malignant hematologic diseases have been associated with hypoglycemia.

Mesenchymal tumors account for 45 to 64 per cent of the reported cases. Approximately one third of the tumors are located in the chest and two thirds are in the abdomen, usually in the retroperitoneum. They usually are large and therefore readily detectable. Hepatomas account for 22 per cent of cases.

No single pathogenetic mechanism satisfactorily explains all cases of tumor-related hypoglycemia. In some, more than one mechanism may be involved. Metastatic destruction of the adrenals or pituitary and extensive metastatic involvement of the liver can impair glucoregulatory mechanisms. Some tumors evince a high rate of glucose utilization. In others, substances such as tryptophan metabolites may impair gluconeogenesis. The conflicting data regarding the presence or absence of elevated concentrations of insulin-like growth factors in the serum of these patients may be due to methodologic differences in measuring the substances. Total or partial surgical removal of the tumor usually results in amelioration of the hypoglycemia.

Hypoglycemia in Hepatic, Renal, and Endocrine Disorders

Symptomatic hypoglycemia is uncommon in liver disease because glucose homeostasis can be maintained with as little as 20 per cent of healthy parenchymal cells, but biochemical hypoglycemia has been reported in a wide variety of acquired hepatic diseases. The hypoglycemias of congestive heart failure, sepsis, and Reye's syndrome are considered to be due to hepatic mechanisms.

Hypoglycemia is uncommon in adrenocortical insufficiency. Hypoglycemia in hypopituitarism is common in children under six years of age, but less so beyond that age. Asymptomatic hypoglycemia has been observed in isolated growth hormone deficiency after prolonged fasting. Spontaneous hypoglycemia has been reported to be a frequent finding in isolated ACTH deficiency. Adults surgically deprived of epinephrine are not subject to hypoglycemia.

Hypoglycemia in nondiabetic persons with renal failure may be due to inadequate gluconeogenic substrate availability. Glucagon deficiency is a theoretical mechanism for hypoglycemia, but the existence of this disorder has not been confirmed.

Froesch ER, Zopf J, Widmer U: Hypoglycemia associated with non-islet cell tumor and insulin-like growth factors (letter). Gorden P, Kahn CR, Roth J, et al.: (response to letter). N Engl J Med 306:1178, 1982. *The letter and response describe the controversy regarding the concentrations of insulin-like growth factors in non-beta cell tumor hypoglycemia.*

Hogan MJ, Service FJ, Sharbrough F, et al.: Oral glucose tolerance test compared with a mixed meal in the diagnosis of reactive hypoglycemia. A caveat on stimulation. Mayo Clin Proc 58:491, 1983. *The authors demonstrate the inadequacy of the oral glucose tolerance test for the diagnosis of postprandial symptoms. Patients considered to have food-stimulated hypoglycemia after oral glucose tolerance testing had no hypoglycemia after a mixed meal despite the presence of postprandial symptoms. In addition, EEG monitoring during postprandial symptoms showed no changes.*

Le-Ran A, Anderson RW: The diagnosis of postprandial hypoglycemia. Diabetes 30:996, 1981. *The authors report the results of oral glucose tolerance testing in a large group of healthy persons, in 10 per cent of whom the glucose nadir was ≤47 mg per deciliter. In addition, the nonspecificity of the post-oral glucose symptoms is underscored by the observation of symptoms following administration of a placebo.*

Marks V: Hypoglycemia. Oxford, Blackwell Scientific Publications, 1981. *This is an authoritative reference work on hypoglycemic disorders.*

Scarlett JA, Mako RE, Rubenstein AH, et al.: Factitious hypoglycemia. Diagnosis and measurement of serum C-peptide immunoreactivity and insulin-binding antibodies. N Engl J Med 297:1029, 1977. *Seven cases of surreptitious injection of insulin are described. The authors emphasize the importance of the triad of low plasma glucose and high plasma insulin levels and suppression of plasma C peptide for diagnosis of this condition. In addition, there is a useful discussion of characteristics of antibodies to insulin, proinsulin, and C peptide of human, porcine, and bovine origin for the distinction between factitial and autoimmune hypoglycemia.*

Seltzer HS: Severe drug-induced hypoglycemia: A review. Comp Ther 5:21, 1979. *This review is an excellent reference source regarding the drugs implicated and the conditions conducive to drug-induced hypoglycemia.*

Service FJ: Hypoglycemic Disorders: Pathogenesis, Diagnosis, and Treatment. Boston, G. K. Hall, 1983. *This book is recommended for those desiring more detailed description of hypoglycemic disorders. For those interested in hypoglycemias in the pediatric age range the chapter, Hypoglycemia in Infants and Children, by Drs. Tsalikian and Haymond, is an excellent reference source.*

Taylor SI, Greenberger G, Marcus-Samuels B, et al.: Hypoglycemia associated with antibodies to the insulin receptor. N Engl J Med 307:1422, 1982. *The authors report a nondiabetic patient with fasting hypoglycemia ascribed to the action of autoantibodies to the insulin receptor. Although the few other patients with this syndrome had a history of prior diabetes, evidence for coexistent autoimmune disease is a clue to the presence of antireceptor antibodies.*

233 PANCREATIC ISLET CELL TUMORS

Carl Grunfeld

THE ISLETS OF LANGERHANS

Dispersed throughout the exocrine pancreas are nests of endocrine cells, the islets of Langerhans. The islet itself is a miniature organ with a distinctive organization of individualized cells, each of which produces a single hormone (Fig. 233–1). Insulin-containing B cells form the core of the islet

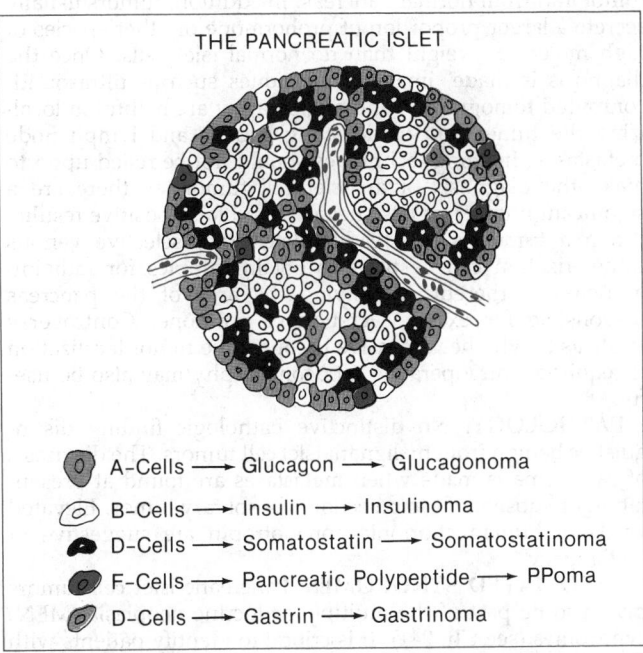

FIGURE 233–1. Morphology of the islets of Langerhans. This schematic representation of a typical islet demonstrates the distinctive distribution of hormone-secreting cells within the islet. Insulin-containing B cells, forming the core of the islet, are surrounded by glucagon-containing A cells. D cells are interspersed. In the posterior portion of the head of the pancreas, the proportion of cells containing pancreatic polypeptide is increased and the number of glucagon-secreting cells is strikingly decreased. (Modified from Unger RH, Orci L: Glucagon and the A cell: Physiology and pathophysiology. N Engl J Med 304:1518, 1981. Reprinted with permission.)

and make up 60 per cent of the endocrine pancreas. They are surrounded by a rim of A cells that secrete glucagon or F cells containing pancreatic polypeptide. D cells containing somatostatin or gastrin are primarily found between the A and B cells. The location and function of cells containing other hormones, such as vasoactive intestinal polypeptide, have not yet been precisely defined.

Cells of the islets may become hyperplastic in response to prolonged stimulation of hormone secretion. Thus, A cells containing glucagon are often increased in diabetes mellitus. B cells increase after prolonged excessive caloric ingestion or in the presence of insulin resistance.

ISLET CELL TUMORS

Tumors can arise from any of the hormone-producing cells of the islets of Langerhans. Patients with islet cell tumors may seek help either because of distinct syndromes due to the hypersecretion of hormones by the tumors or because of mass effects of local or metastatic tumor spread. Nearly all benign islet cell tumors and more than 80 per cent of carcinomas secrete clinically significant amounts of hormone. Some tumors have been shown to produce multiple hormones. Clinical presentation usually reflects the dominance of one hormone.

The tumor is named after the hormone responsible for the syndrome or, in asymptomatic patients, the hormone found in highest concentration in the circulation or in the tumor. For example, a tumor producing insulin is known as an insulinoma, and one producing glucagon is a glucagonoma. The tumors also retain the morphologic characteristics of the cell of origin.

DIAGNOSIS. Diagnosis of islet cell tumors is usually made by detecting elevated basal or fasting levels of the suspected hormone in the presence of the characteristic syndrome. Provocative tests have also been developed that use pharmacologic agents to discriminate between secretion from a tumor and from normal pancreas. In addition, tumors usually secrete a larger proportion of prohormone or other species of high molecular weight than do normal islet cells. Once the diagnosis is made, imaging techniques such as ultrasound, computed tomography, and angiography are helpful in localizing the tumor and in detecting hepatic and lymph node metastases. Imaging techniques should not be relied upon to make the diagnosis of an islet cell tumor, as there are a significant number of false negative and false positive results. When a tumor is not readily detectable, selective venous catheterization can be used to obtain samples for radioimmunoassay, thereby identifying the area of the pancreas responsible for excess secretion of hormone. Controversy exists as to whether extensive preoperative tumor localization is required. Intraoperative ultrasonography may also be useful.

PATHOLOGY. No distinctive pathologic finding distinguishes benign from malignant islet cell tumors. The diagnosis of carcinoma is made when metastases are found at presentation or subsequent to resection of a solitary tumor. Elevated levels of human chorionic gonadotropin are suggestive of malignancy.

ASSOCIATED SYNDROMES. Pancreatic islet cell tumors may also be part of the multiple endocrine neoplasia (MEN) syndromes (see Ch. 241). It is critical to identify patients with these syndromes as they may have multiple islet cell tumors. Identification of the tumor or area of the pancreas responsible for excess secretion is essential to allow limited pancreatic resection. Unfortunately in patients with an MEN syndrome, tumors may recur, necessitating total pancreatectomy. The presence of hypercalcemia in patients with islet cell tumors is suggestive of the MEN 1 syndrome, as 85 per cent of patients with MEN type 1 have hyperparathyroidism at some time.

THERAPY. The primary therapy of solitary islet cell tumors is surgical resection. When a patient has islet cell carcinoma

with metastasis, therapy is directed toward ameliorating the symptoms of the presenting syndrome and may include pharmacologic inhibitors of hormone secretion and action, chemotherapeutic agents, radiotherapy, or surgical debulking. The specific agents are discussed under each tumor.

Similar syndromes resulting from hypersecretion of pancreatic hormones occasionally occur secondary to diffuse hyperplasia of islet cells. The treatment of hyperplastic syndromes is partial or near-total pancreatectomy.

The characteristic syndromes associated with islet cell tumors are outlined in Table 233–1.

Insulinoma

The most common islet cell tumor is the insulinoma, which may produce life-threatening hypoglycemia. Insulinoma is reviewed in Ch. 232.

Gastrinoma

The second most common islet cell tumor is the gastrinoma associated with Zollinger-Ellison syndrome, producing recurrent peptic ulcers due to hypersecretion of gastric acid. This syndrome is discussed in Ch. 100.6.

VIPoma or the Diarrheogenic Syndrome

CLINICAL PRESENTATION. VIP (vasoactive intestinal polypeptide)-oma or the diarrheogenic syndrome, associated with islet cell tumors, severe watery diarrhea, and hypokalemia, is also called pancreatic cholera, Verner-Morrison syndrome, WDHA (watery diarrhea, hypokalemia, achlorhydria) syndrome, or WDHH (water diarrhea, hypokalemia, hypochlorhydria) syndrome. Patients have profound but intermittent secretory diarrhea, with peak diarrhea output exceeding 3 liters per day in 80 per cent. A more general discussion of secretory diarrhea is contained in Ch. 103. Unlike the diarrheal discharge of long-term laxative abuse, in this diarrhea the discharge is rich in electrolytes; fecal potassium loss can reach 300 mEq per day. Serum potassium is usually less than 3 mEq per liter and is accompanied by acidosis due to severe losses of bicarbonate.

The severe hypokalemia may lead to profound weakness, to flaccid paralysis, and to renal failure due to hypokalemic nephropathy. More than half of the patients have frank diabetes or glucose intolerance, which is probably secondary to hypokalemia, a known inhibitor of insulin secretion (see Ch. 77 for a discussion of hypokalemia). Hypercalcemia is found in half of the patients during attacks and is not usually indicative of hyperparathyroidism (and the MEN 1 syndrome), as parathyroid hormone levels are suppressed and the hypercalcemia remits with resection of the primary islet cell tumor. Despite hypercalcemia, tetany due to hypomagnesemia has been described. Dilation of the gallbladder or small intestine may be seen during radiographic examination, and flushing of the skin has been reported.

DIFFERENTIAL DIAGNOSIS. Secretory diarrhea may result from three other endocrine tumors: gastrinoma, carcinoid, and somatostatinoma. However, peak volume of diarrhea rarely exceeds 3 liters per day in these syndromes. Further, the diarrhea in Zollinger-Ellison syndrome is caused by hypersecretion of gastric acid and can be reversed by gastric suction or with cimetidine. The diarrheogenic syndrome is almost always accompanied by achlorhydria or hypochlorhydria; decreased gastric acid secretion persists when the diarrhea is in remission and the serum potassium is normal.

PATHOLOGY. Eighty per cent of the patients with the diarrheogenic syndrome are found to have islet cell tumors. Nearly half are malignant. When the diarrhea is constant, the probability of malignancy is increased. Patients without islet cell tumors often have diffuse islet cell hyperplasia. The diarrheogenic syndrome has also been reported with bronchial tumor, pheochromocytoma, and ganglioneuroblastoma.

TABLE 233–1. SYNDROMES ASSOCIATED WITH ISLET CELL TUMORS

Tumor	Major Findings	Minor Findings	Other Hormones in Tumor or Plasma	Per Cent Malignancy	Hyperplasia	MEN Syndrome
Insulinoma	Adrenergic: palpitations, tremor, hunger, sweating Neuroglycopenic: confusion, seizures, transient focal deficit, coma	Ischemic cardiovascular disease, permanent neurologic deficits	Gastrin, glucagon, pancreatic polypeptide, somatostatin, GRF*	10	Occasional	10%
Gastrinoma	Peptic ulcers, enhanced acid secretion	Diarrhea, malabsorption, weight loss, dumping	ACTH, insulin, glucagon, VIP, 5-HIAA, MSH, somatostatin, calcitonin, pancreatic polypeptide	40–60	10%	25%
VIPoma	Watery diarrhea, hypokalemia, hypochlorhydria	Hypercalcemia, hyperglycemia, weakness, hypomagnesemia	PHM, pancreatic polypeptide, prostaglandins (?), GRF	40	20%	Rare
Glucagonoma	Rash, diabetes, weight loss, anemia	Diarrhea, abdominal pain, thromboembolic disease	Pancreatic polypeptide, VIP, 5-HIAA, gastrin, insulin	60	Occasional	Occasional
Somatostatinoma	Diabetes, cholelithiasis, steatorrhea, malabsorption, weight loss	Indigestion, abdominal pain, anemia, diarrhea, ductal obstruction, hypoglycemia	ACTH, gastrin, calcitonin, PGE$_2$, glucagon, GRF, pancreatic polypeptide, VIP, 5-HIAA, substance P	66	None reported	One case (MEN 3)
PPoma	None	Watery diarrhea, hypokalemia, achlorhydria; abdominal pain, weight loss	Glucagon, insulin, SRIF, VIP	40	Occasional	25%

*GRF = growth hormone releasing factor.

The diarrhea probably results from excess secretion of VIP. Infusion of VIP into laboratory animals and humans results in secretory diarrhea, hypokalemia, inhibition of gastric acid secretion, and hypercalcemia. Increased plasma VIP levels have been found in patients in whom islet cell tumor, islet cell hyperplasia, bronchogenic carcinoma, ganglioneuroblastoma, or pheochromocytoma was found to be the cause of the syndrome. VIP is difficult to detect in the circulation of normal humans; therefore the absence of VIP does not rule out the diagnosis. VIPomas also synthesize and secrete peptide histidine methionine (PHM), a peptide produced by the same mRNA as VIP that also enhances intestinal fluid secretion. Islet cell tumors producing only pancreatic polypeptide (another presumed hormone of unknown normal function) or prostaglandin E$_2$ have also been reported to be associated with this syndrome.

THERAPY. Treatment of the diarrheogenic syndrome is primarily by surgery. Because of the profound systemic effects of this tumor, resection is considered even in the presence of metastases. When no tumor is found, subtotal pancreatectomy is usually attempted. If hyperplasia is then identified on histopathologic examination and symptoms persist, total pancreatectomy should be considered. The tumors may be transiently responsive to steroids, indomethacin, somatostatin, metoclopramide, lithium carbonate, or trifluoperazine, which may be useful in preparing patients for surgery or as a palliative for metastatic disease. Radiotherapy, streptozotocin and alfa-interferon have been reported to reduce the size of metastases and volume of diarrhea.

Glucagonoma

CLINICAL PRESENTATION. The glucagonoma syndrome is characterized by a waxing and waning skin rash (necrolytic migratory erythema), diabetes, hypoaminoacidemia, weight loss, and anemia. The classic cutaneous lesion begins as an erythematous base, becomes indurated, and develops superficial central blistering. The blisters then erode and crust over. Healing may be accompanied by hyperpigmentation. This process takes 7 to 14 days with lesions developing in one area while others are resolving. The rash is most prominent on the perineum, along intertriginous folds, and around the mouth and nose. Liquefaction necrosis of the granular cell layer and subcorneal blistering may be seen on biopsy. Glossitis, stomatitis, and cheilitis are common. Onycholysis and brittle nails may be present.

Although cutaneous lesions were the hallmark of the first reported cases, the rash is actually present in only two thirds of patients with glucagonoma. The remaining patients usually present because of widespread metastatic disease. Rarely, patients are found during the evaluation of diabetes mellitus or the MEN 1 syndrome.

Frank diabetes occurs in 60 per cent of patients with glucagonoma, and an additional 30 per cent have glucose intolerance. Even in patients with severe hyperglycemia, diabetic ketoacidosis is rarely observed in the glucagonoma syndrome, despite the known ability of glucagon to stimulate hepatic ketogenesis. It is thought that the presence of normal or elevated levels of insulin suppresses lipolysis, limiting the free fatty acid substrates for hepatic ketone production.

Weight loss and anemia are found at the time of diagnosis in half of the patients with glucagonoma. Gastrointestinal symptoms include diarrhea, abdominal pain, and nausea and vomiting. Thromboembolic disease has also been described.

Glucagonoma is infrequently found in the MEN 1 syndrome. However, rare MEN 1 kindreds have been reported in which some members have glucagonoma and others have hyperglucagonemia without clinically detectable tumors. In addition, a familial glucagonoma syndrome has been reported in the absence of other endocrine tumors.

DIAGNOSIS. The diagnosis of glucagonoma is made by detecting elevated levels of glucagon and excluding other conditions associated with hyperglucagonemia, including diabetic ketoacidosis and hyperosmolar syndromes, chronic renal failure, cardiovascular collapse, and cirrhosis of the liver. Normal circulating levels of glucagon are 50 to 150 pg per milliliter. Most patients with glucagonoma have levels in excess of 500 pg per milliliter (occasionally as high as 10,000 pg per milliliter), while glucagon levels in the previously mentioned syndromes average 200 to 500 pg per milliliter.

Once the diagnosis of glucagonoma is confirmed, computed tomography or angiography may be helpful in localizing the tumor and detecting the presence of metastases. At the time of presentation 60 per cent of glucagonomas have metastasized, most commonly to the liver and local lymph nodes.

THERAPY. Surgery is the treatment of choice for glucagonoma confined to the pancreas. Surgery may also be indicated with metastatic disease, as debulking of the tumor mass may ameliorate the glucagonoma syndrome. Streptozotocin, with or without 5-fluorouracil and dacarbazine (DTIC), may induce significant remission. Somatostatin and its long-acting analogues consistently decrease glucagon secretion from glucagonomas and improve the rash. Phenoxybenzamine may also inhibit glucagon secretion from tumors.

The skin rash resolves within a few days of successful

surgery and may improve during tumor remission induced by chemotherapy. The immediate cause of the cutaneous lesions is thought to be hypoaminoacidemia, found in 90 per cent of patients with glucagonoma, secondary to enhanced hepatic catabolism of amino acids. An impressive improvement of the rash may occur with hyperalimentation of amino acids, suggesting that amino acid deficiency rather than hyperglucagonemia per se may be the basis of the skin lesion.

Somatostatinoma

CLINICAL PRESENTATION. Somatostatinomas are not common; most are found incidentally during laparotomy or during the workup of obstructive jaundice or abdominal pain with identification made retrospectively on the basis of elevated concentrations of somatostatin in the tumor or in the patient's plasma. The tumors contain granules characteristic of D cells. The primary tumor is located in the duodenum or jejunum in 40 per cent of cases.

A syndrome associated with hypersomatostatinemia has been proposed that includes diabetes mellitus, cholelithiasis, steatorrhea with malabsorption, dyspepsia, and significant weight loss. Patients may also have hypochlorhydria, watery diarrhea, anemia, and flushing. The diabetes is usually mild.

The pathophysiology of the syndrome is consistent with the known effects of somatostatin. Infusion of somatostatin in humans inhibits the release of multiple hormones, including insulin, glucagon, secretin, gastrin, and motilin. Hyperglycemia results from suppression of insulin secretion, but ketosis is infrequent, presumably because of the concomitant inhibition of glucagon secretion. Suppression of secretin, motilin, and gastrin, which decreases hydrochloric acid secretion, gastric emptying, and duodenal motility, may cause indigestion and abdominal pain. Inhibition of gallbladder contraction is thought to predispose to cholelithiasis. Malabsorption is produced by inhibition of pancreatic exocrine function.

It is difficult to make the prospective diagnosis of somatostatinoma, as all of these symptoms are nonspecific and are found more commonly in other disorders. The incidence of cholelithiasis is increased in patients with diabetes. Malabsorption may occur in diabetics with chronic pancreatitis. This diagnostic difficulty is further compounded, as most patients with documented somatostatinoma have none of the components of the proposed syndrome. Three patients had severe hypoglycemia and were suspected of having insulinomas. Their tumors also contained insulin, and it was proposed that secretion of small amounts of insulin from the tumors with concomitant suppression of compensatory release of glucagon from the normal pancreas resulted in hypoglycemia.

Somatostatinomas may secrete additional hormones that modify the clinical syndrome. Striking elevations of serum calcitonin can cause watery diarrhea due to the effects of calcitonin on water and electrolyte transport in the gut. Somatostatinomas can produce ACTH, causing Cushing's syndrome, or prostaglandin E_2, causing flushing. A patient with Zollinger-Ellison syndrome was found to have an endocrine tumor of the gut secreting both gastrin and somatostatin. Hyperplasia of cells containing pancreatic polypeptide (resulting in excess secretion of this hormone) has been reported in the presence of somatostatinoma.

DIAGNOSIS. The diagnosis of somatostatinoma is made by detecting elevated basal or stimulated levels of circulating somatostatin. Tolbutamide or calcium-pentagastrin infusion results in marked elevation of somatostatin in patients with somatostatinoma and normal basal somatostatin levels but not in controls.

THERAPY. Two thirds of patients with somatostatinoma have metastases at presentation; this may reflect the difficulty in the clinical diagnosis of this syndrome. Surgical resection should be performed if possible. Streptozotocin therapy reduces tumor size and plasma somatostatin levels.

Other Hormones Produced by Islet Cell Tumors

PANCREATIC POLYPEPTIDE. Many endocrine tumors of the pancreas and gut produce pancreatic polypeptide (PP) as a secondary hormone, allowing it to serve as a marker for islet cell tumors. Increasing numbers of islet cell tumors that produce PP as their major hormone are being identified; these may account for a substantial percentage of the tumors previously identified as "nonfunctional." The role of PP in normal islet physiology is not apparent, and no clinical syndrome has been definitively associated with PPomas. A few cases of islet cell tumors associated with watery diarrhea, hypokalemia, and achlorhydria have been accompanied by elevated serum levels of PP with normal VIP levels.

ACTH. Pancreatic islet cell tumors producing ACTH account for nearly 10 per cent of cases of Cushing's syndrome due to ectopic ACTH production. Such tumors are usually found to secrete multiple hormones, including insulin, gastrin, serotonin, or somatostatin. However, it is more common to find Cushing's *disease* due to a pituitary adenoma associated with other islet cell tumors in patients with MEN type 1.

GROWTH HORMONE RELEASING FACTOR. Acromegaly has been reported in patients with islet cell tumors secreting growth hormone releasing factor. Although these patients often have hyperplasia of the growth hormone-secreting cells of the pituitary, it is very difficult to distinguish them from patients with classic acromegaly due to a pituitary adenoma (see Ch. 226). In either case the sella may be normal or enlarged, and growth hormone levels may show paradoxic responses to provocative testing.

Bloom SR, Polak JM: Glucagonoma syndrome. Am J Med 82(5B):25, 1987. *A comprehensive and useful general review, with 44 references.*

Berelowitz M: Somatostatin-producing tumors. Adv Exp Med Biol 188:475, 1985. *Only 6 of 21 patients with pancreatic somatostatinoma and none of 13 patients with a small-intestine primary tumor showed clinical symptoms of the proposed somatostatinoma syndrome.*

Krejs GJ: VIPoma syndrome. Am J Med 82(5B):37, 1987. *An excellent general review of this interesting entity, with 120 references. A good place to start.*

Moossa AR: Tumors of the Pancreas. Baltimore, Williams & Wilkins, 1980. *Includes detailed chapters on the pathology, pathophysiology, radiology, and surgical treatment of islet cell tumors.*

234 DISORDERS OF SEXUAL DIFFERENTIATION
Julianne Imperato-McGinley

NORMAL SEXUAL DIFFERENTIATION

The fetus is bipotential for sexual differentiation. The bipotentiality includes the gonad, the internal sex structures, and the external genitalia.

Development of the Bipotential Gonad

In fetuses of both sexes an undifferentiated gonad develops during the fifth week of fetal life. A thickened area of coelomic or germinal epithelium appears on the medial aspect of the mesonephros, and proliferation of germinal epithelium cells and underlying mesenchyme produces a prominence on the medial side of the mesonephros designated the gonadal ridge. Following this, cords of cells known as primary sex cords proliferate from the epithelium into the mesenchyme. The gonad at this stage consists primarily of mesodermal cells of coelomic epithelial origin. The primordial germ cells are visible

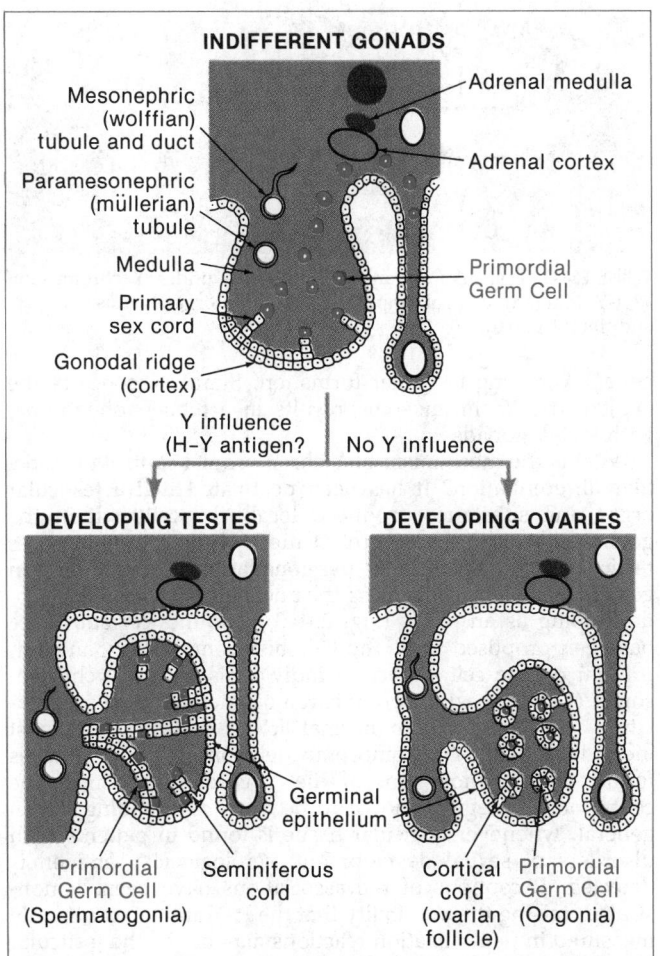

FIGURE 234–1. Development of the bipotential gonad from coelomic epithelium (primary sex cords) underlying mesenchymal tissue and primordial germ cells and its differentiation to either a testis or an ovary.

early in the third week among the endodermal cells of the wall of the yolk sac near the origin of the allantois. During folding of the embryo, the primordial germ cells migrate by a combination of ameboid movement and passive transfer along the dorsal mesentery to the gonadal ridges. During migration the germ cells multiply by mitosis. By the fifth week of fetal life they begin to migrate into the underlying mesenchyme, and by the end of the sixth week the undifferentiated or bipotential gonad is formed (Fig. 234–1). The primordial germ cells develop into spermatogonia in the male and ova in the female, the sex cords become either seminiferous tubules or primary ovarian follicles, and the mesenchymal cells form either the Leydig cells or the theca and stromal cells in the female.

Gonadal Differentiation—Development of the Testes and Ovaries

Testicular or seminiferous cords evolve from primary sex cords of the indifferent gonad at approximately the seventh week of gestation (Fig. 234–1). The Sertoli cells differentiate within each cord, enlarge, aggregate, and engulf the germ cells. The distal ends of the seminiferous cords then interconnect to form a network of solid cords, the rete testes, which is in direct contact with the wolffian (mesonephric) ducts. By the sixth month the ends of the rete testes develop a lumen continuous with the mesonephric tubules, which later develop into the ductuli efferentia. The fetal Leydig cells are apparent by 8 weeks of fetal life, and at 3 months of gestation they completely fill the interstitial spaces.

Ovarian differentiation from the indifferent gonad begins at approximately 50 days of gestation (Fig. 234–1). The primary sex cords form irregular groups of cells called medullary cords containing primitive granulosa cells that engulf primordial oogonia. The oogonia are in the prophase of meiosis at day 50 to 55. The leptotene stage begins at day 60, the pachytene stage at approximately day 80, and by day 90 the oogonia enter the diplotene stage. As the oogonia differentiate the primitive granulosa cells organize around them and form a single layer constituting the primordial follicle. Primary follicles are formed when the primordial follicle containing oocytes of the diplotene stage becomes separated by connective tissue. At 18 to 20 weeks of gestation, there are approximately 7 million oogonia and oocytes, whereas at birth the number decreases to approximately 2 million.

Phenotypic Differentiation

Ductal Development

Every fetus has both *wolffian (mesonephric) ducts*, which develop into epididymis, vas deferens, and seminal vesicles in

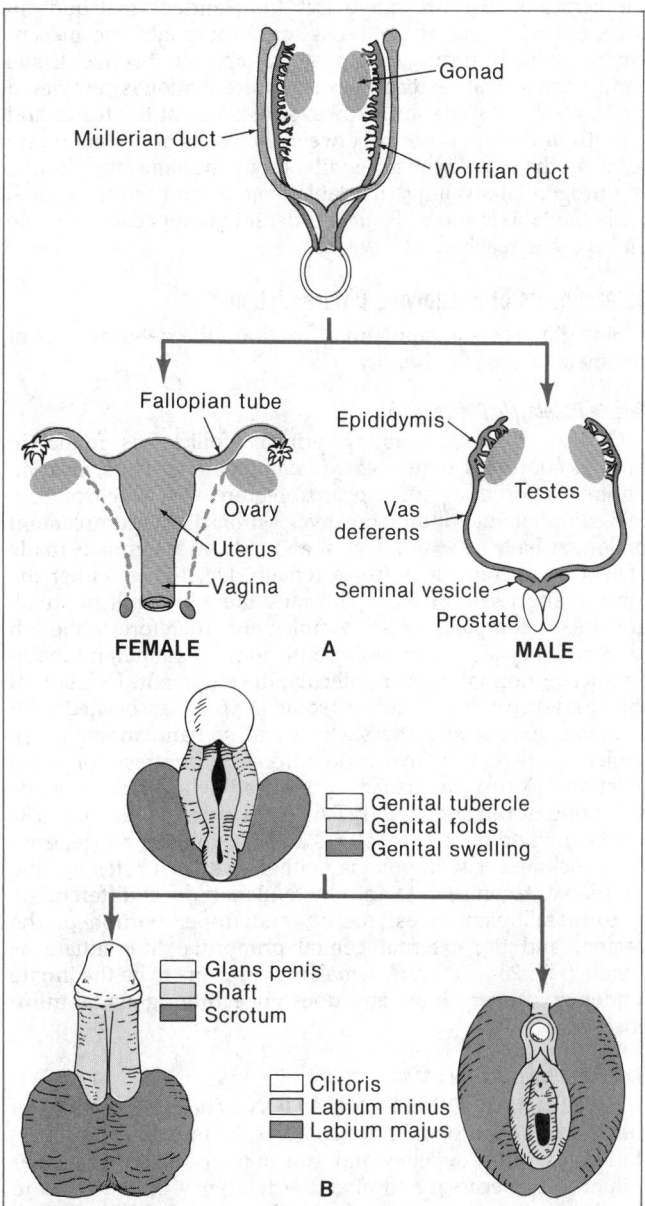

FIGURE 234–2. Summary of male and female sexual differentiation. *A*, Internal sexual differentiation from wolffian and müllerian ducts. *B*, Development of male and female external genitalia from common primordia.

the male, and *müllerian (paramesonephric) ducts,* which develop into fallopian tubes, uterus, and upper third of the vagina in the female (Fig. 234–2). The wolffian ducts appear at 25 to 30 days of gestation, and the müllerian ducts at 44 to 48 days. In the male the initial event is regression of the müllerian ducts, completed at about 7½ weeks of gestation, followed by stabilization and differentiation of the mesonephric wolffian ducts to form the epididymis, vas deferens, seminal vesicles, and ejaculatory ducts. In the female the wolffian ducts regress at approximately 10½ weeks, and the müllerian ducts differentiate to form the fallopian tubes, uterus, and upper portion of the vagina.

Development of the External Genitalia

The external genitalia of both sexes (like the gonad) develop from common primordia, the urogenital tubercle, urogenital folds, and urogenital swellings (Fig. 234–2). In the male, external genital masculinization begins shortly after wolffian ductal differentiation. The urogenital tubercle elongates to become the glans penis, the urogenital folds fuse and become the shaft of the penis, and the urogenital swellings become the scrotum. The prostate arises from endodermal buds in the urethral lining at 10 weeks and grows into the mesenchyme, which forms the muscular and connective tissue components. Male external sexual differentiation is completed by 14 weeks of gestation. However, descent of the testes and growth of the penis occur between 20 weeks of gestation and term. In the female the urogenital tubule becomes the clitoris, the urogenital swellings the labia majora, and the urogenital folds the labia minora. Female differentiation occurs after the embryo has reached 10½ weeks.

Determinants of Phenotypic Differentiation

Since the fetus is bipotential, what are the determinants of the male or female phenotype?

Female Phenotypic Differentiation

Ovarian tissue containing primary follicles is found in human abortuses with a 45 XO complement. Thus, ovarian differentiation does not appear to require a 46 XX chromosomal complement. Adults, however, with a 45 XO complement no longer have ovarian follicles, and only streak gonads made of whorls of connective tissue remain. Deletion of either the long or short arm of the X chromosome will result in streak gonads. A complete 46 XX complement, therefore, although not necessary for ovarian differentiation, is essential for maintenance of normal ovarian follicular development. Deletion of the short arm of the X chromosome (XXp-) is associated with streaked gonads and the skeletal and somatic anomalies of subjects with 45 XO Turner's syndrome. In contrast, long arm deletions (XXq-) are usually associated with streak gonads and none of the stigmata of Turner's syndrome. See Ch. 237 for a complete discussion of XO and XX gonadal dysgenesis.

In the absence of gonads, either ovaries or testes, the wolffian anlagen regress and the müllerian ducts differentiate to form fallopian tubes, uterus, and upper portion of the vagina, and the external genital primordia differentiate as female (Fig. 234–2). Thus, femaleness appears to be the innate tendency of every fetus and does not require gonadal influence.

Male Phenotypic Differentiation

TESTICULAR DIFFERENTIATION. The development of the male phenotype is more complex; to initiate the process the testes must develop and function normally. Testicular influence is necessary to alter the tendency of the fetus to develop as female. In man, normal testicular differentiation is controlled by the Y chromosome. Analysis of Y chromosome structural abnormalities in man suggests that the short arm (Yp) of the chromosome near the centromere carries the

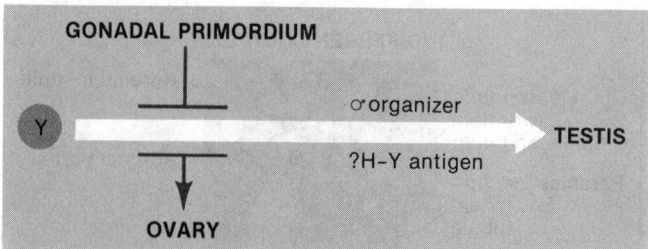

FIGURE 234–3. Testicular organizing substance under Y chromosome (?H-Y antigen) control imposing testicular organogenesis on the indifferent gonad.

gene(s) directing testicular formation. Simple absence of the (Yp) of the Y chromosome results in a female phenotype, with streak gonads.

What is the mechanism of Y chromosomal control of testicular differentiation? It has been postulated that a testicular organizing substance produced locally by cells within the gonad and under the control of the Y chromosome imposes testicular organogenesis on the gonadal primordium early in gestation, thereby preventing the undifferentiated gonad from developing as an ovary (Fig. 234–3). The inducer substance has been proposed to be the H-Y histocompatibility antigen, present on the cell surface of individuals with a Y chromosome: (1) Males with two Y chromosomes have more circulating H-Y antigen than normal 46 XY males. (2) In most individuals with Y chromosome deletions the H-Y gene is found on the short arm of the Y chromosome near the centromere, a region known to be testis determining. (3) In general, whenever testicular tissue is found in patients with disorders of sexual development, serologic H-Y antigen is detected. Exceptions of the associations have been demonstrated, raising the possibility that the H-Y antigen commonly measured in neutralization reactions may not be the testicular organizing factor, but may be located in proximity to the testicular organizing factor. In certain mice that develop a male phenotype and testes, H-Y antigen is absent.

DIFFERENTIATION OF MALE GENITAL STRUCTURES. Two secretions from the developing fetal testes are essential for male phenotypic differentiation, testosterone and müllerian inhibiting factor. Responsiveness to both hormones is present only during the critical period of male sexual differentiation, from the eighth to the fourteenth weeks of gestation. In the male fetus at eight weeks of gestational age the histologic appearance of differentiated Leydig cells and the onset of testosterone formation are temporally related and appear to be under the stimulation of placental chorionic gonadotropin. The initiation of testicular testosterone formation from the Leydig cells coincides with wolffian differentiation and differentiation of the male external genitalia. However, for differentiation of the external genitalia, testosterone acts as a prohormone and is converted to 5α-dihydrotestosterone by the microsomal enzyme, steroid Δ⁴ 5α-reductase.

Thus, testosterone and its metabolite dihydrotestosterone are essential for sexual differentiation in the male fetus, with selective roles for each hormone during embryogenesis. Testosterone acting locally mediates differentiation of the wolffian ductal system to the vas deferens, epididymis, and seminal vesicles, while the local conversion of testosterone to dihydrotestosterone mediates development of male external genitalia and prostate (Fig. 234–4). Male pseudohermaphrodites with 5α-reductase deficiency and decreased dihydrotestosterone production (see Male Pseudohermaphroditism) have defined the necessity for dihydrotestosterone in the formation of male external genitalia and prostate and have delineated specific actions for the two androgens in utero.

Both testosterone and dihydrotestosterone bind to the same high-affinity androgen receptor protein within the cells of androgen-dependent target areas. Testosterone enters the

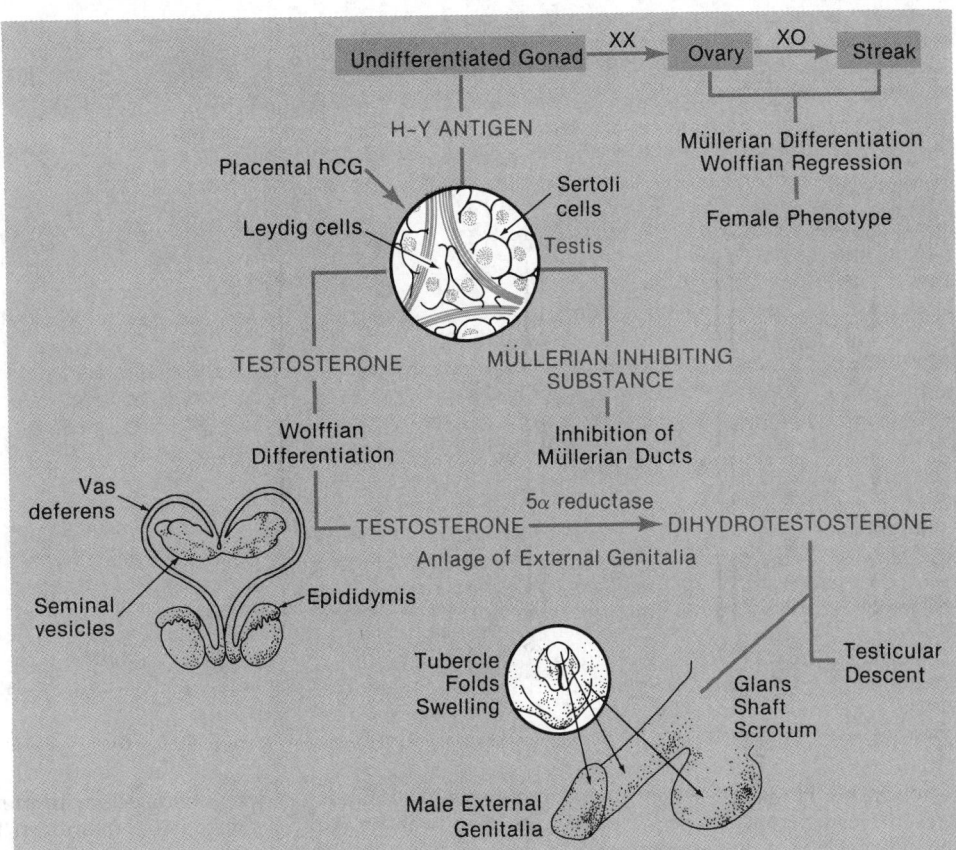

FIGURE 234–4. Schematic representation of the factors involved in male and female sexual differentiation.

target cell by a process of passive diffusion and either binds to a cytoplasmic receptor or is converted to dihydrotestosterone, which binds to the receptor. This androgen receptor complex then binds to acceptor sites in nuclear chromatin and ultimately initiates transcription of messenger ribonucleic acid (mRNA), resulting in the complex metabolic processes of androgen action (Ch. 221).

The inhibition of the müllerian anlage is not under androgen control; müllerian inhibiting factor, a high-molecular-weight glycoprotein, is a product of the Sertoli cells of the seminiferous tubules. Its secretion begins shortly after the initiation of seminiferous tubular differentiation and continues through the perinatal period.

In summary, normal male phenotypic development requires that the testes differentiate and function normally, so that at a critically sensitive period in utero (8 to 14 weeks) müllerian inhibiting factor, secreted by the Sertoli cells, and testosterone, secreted by the Leydig cells, are produced in sufficient amounts. Müllerian inhibiting factor, acting locally, suppresses the müllerian anlage, and testosterone, also acting locally, causes differentiation of the wolffian anlage to epididymis, vas deferens, and seminal vesicles. Testosterone circulates and is converted by the enzyme 5α-reductase to dihydrotestosterone in the cells of the urogenital tubercle, urogenital sinus, and urogenital folds, resulting in differentiation of the male external genitalia (Fig. 234–4). Depending upon specific target tissue, either testosterone or dihydrotestosterone complexes with the cytoplasmic receptor, and this receptor-hormone complex is transferred to the nucleus to initiate androgen action.

Genetic Control of Male Sexual Differentiation

The multifactorial process of male sexual differentiation is under complex genetic control. Testicular differentiation requires the presence of gene(s) normally found on the Y chromosome. The enzymes involved in testosterone biosyn-

thesis, as well as the enzyme 5α-reductase converting testosterone to dihydrotestosterone, are known to be regulated by genes located on the autosomes. Genes located on the X chromosome control the cytoplasmic receptor at the androgen-dependent target areas. Inherited forms of müllerian inhibiting factor deficiency are transmitted as a recessive trait, either autosomal or X linked. Thus, normal male phenotypic development is regulated by multiple genes located on the autosomes as well as on both X and Y chromosomes.

Byskov AG: Differentiation of mammalian embryonic gonad. Physiol Rev 66:71, 1986. *All aspects of gonadal differentiation are covered, from formation of the gonadal primordium to theories of gonadal differentiation. Excellent bibliography.*

ABNORMALITIES OF SEXUAL DIFFERENTIATION
Male Pseudohermaphroditism

The known etiologic factors in male pseudohermaphroditism or incomplete masculinization can be divided into three basic categories: (1) disorders of testicular differentiation and development; (2) disorders of testicular function; and (3) disorders of function at the androgen-dependent target areas. Table 234–1 lists the specific clinical entities within each category.

Disorders of Testicular Differentiation and Development

XY GONADAL DYSGENESIS. *Clinical Presentation.* Subjects with pure gonadal dysgenesis have a 46 XY chromosomal complement, but are phenotypic females with primary amenorrhea, tall stature, eunuchoidal proportions, and scant axillary and pubic hair. The uterus and fallopian tubes are present, and streak gonads are found. In the incomplete forms of this condition, variable amounts of functional testicular tissue are found, and consequently at birth the subjects frequently have clitoromegaly, ambiguous genitalia, or, rarely, a penile urethra. Virilization at puberty is also variable. In pure gonadal dysgenesis, postpubertal gonadotropins are increased and in the castrate range with female levels of

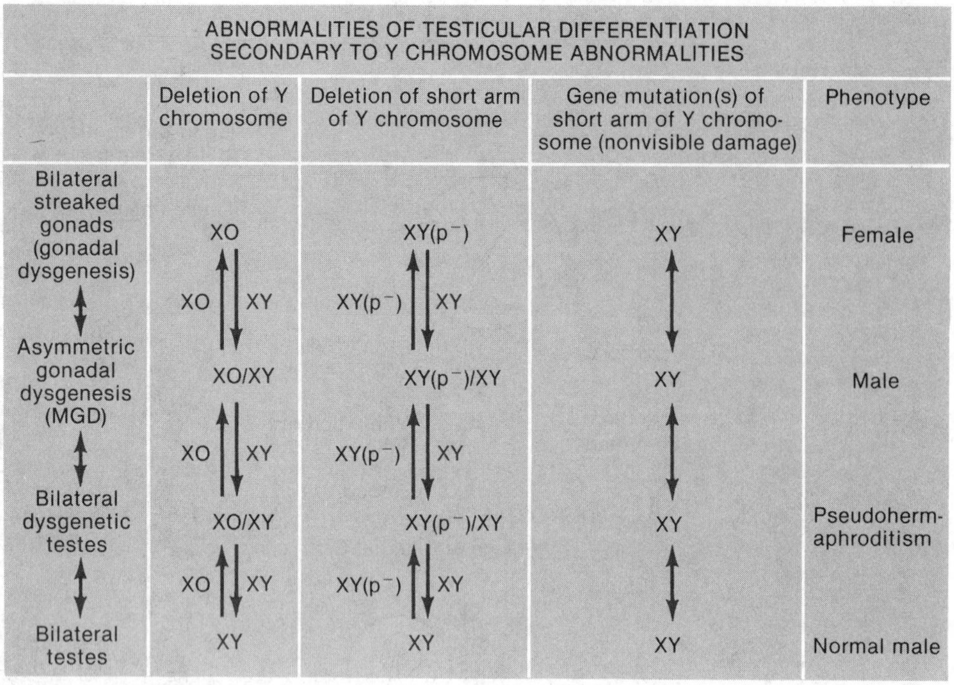

ABNORMALITIES OF TESTICULAR DIFFERENTIATION
SECONDARY TO Y CHROMOSOME ABNORMALITIES

	Deletion of Y chromosome	Deletion of short arm of Y chromosome	Gene mutation(s) of short arm of Y chromosome (nonvisible damage)	Phenotype
Bilateral streaked gonads (gonadal dysgenesis)	XO	XY(p⁻)	XY	Female
Asymmetric gonadal dysgenesis (MGD)	XO ↑↓ XY XO/XY	XY(p⁻) ↑↓ XY XY(p⁻)/XY	XY	Male
Bilateral dysgenetic testes	XO ↑↓ XY XO/XY	XY(p⁻) ↑↓ XY XY(p⁻)/XY	XY	Pseudoherm-aphroditism
Bilateral testes	XO ↑↓ XY XY	XY(p⁻) ↑↓ XY XY	XY	Normal male

FIGURE 234–5. The abnormalities of testicular differentiation may be thought of as a spectrum of disorders that can be produced by more than one genotype.

testosterone. However, when functioning testicular tissue is present, testosterone can be increased from slightly above the female level to a low-normal male level. Additionally, if müllerian inhibiting factor is produced there may be partial or complete absence of müllerian structures (Fig. 234–5).

Pathophysiology. In pure gonadal dysgenesis the testes do not differentiate at all, and in the absence of a functional testis phenotypic development is female, with wolffian duct regression and müllerian differentiation. In the incomplete forms there is variable testicular development with varying degrees of fetal masculinization. The etiology of this condition is unknown, but it could be due to a number of theoretical causes involving testicular organizing substance. There could be a lack of or decreased secretion of testicular organizing substance, abnormalities in its structure, or lack or decrease in its gonadal specific receptor. Interestingly, serologic anal-

TABLE 234–1. CLASSIFICATION OF THE CAUSES OF MALE PSEUDOHERMAPHRODITISM

I. Disorders of testicular differentiation and development
  A. Testicular dysgenesis, affecting both Leydig cell and seminiferous tubule development
    1. Y chromosomal abnormalities
    2. XY gonadal dysgenesis
    3. XO/XY gonadal dysgenesis
    4. Testicular regression syndrome
  B. Leydig cell agenesis or dysgenesis—selective absence or decrease in Leydig cell differentiation and function—seminiferous tubule embryogenesis occurring normally
    1. Abnormality of the HCG-LH receptor: absence of precursor Leydig cell

II. Disorders of testicular function
  A. Abnormalities of müllerian inhibiting factor synthesis or action—persistent müllerian duct syndrome
  B. Enzyme deficiencies affecting testosterone biosynthesis
    1. Cholesterol 20,22-desmolase
    2. 17α-Hydroxylase
    3. 17,20-Desmolase
    4. 3β-Hydroxysteroid dehydrogenase:Δ$^{5-4}$ isomerase
    5. 17β-Hydroxysteroid dehydrogenase

III. Disorders of function at the androgen-dependent target areas
  A. Disorders of androgen action (complete and partial androgen insensitivity)
    1. Cytosol androgen-receptor binding abnormalities
    2. Post cytosol androgen-receptor binding abnormalities
  B. Disorders of testosterone metabolism
    1. 5α-Reductase deficiency

yses of subjects with pure gonadal dysgenesis have revealed a negative H-Y antigen titer in some subjects, while others have a positive titer. Future studies using Y-specific DNA probes should yield some interesting findings in subjects with this condition.

Approximately 13 familial cases of pure gonadal dysgenesis have been described, and inheritance appears to be either X-linked recessive or autosomal dominant-sex limited. Within families there may be variable expressivity of the gene defect, with some sibs having the pure form and a female phenotype and others with ambiguous genitalia.

Management and Therapy. The streak gonads should be removed since approximately 20 to 30 per cent of subjects will develop gonadoblastomas or dysgerminomas within the streak gonads. Dysgerminomas may be malignant, and approximately 5 to 8 per cent of gonadoblastomas also contain malignant elements. In pure gonadal dysgenesis, infants are invariably reared as female and come to the attention of the physician at puberty because of lack of secondary sexual development. Estrogen and progesterone replacement therapy should be instituted after prophylactic removal of the streak gonads. In complete forms, the child should be reared in the sex that will be more functional, and appropriate surgical correction of the genitalia carried out. Intra-abdominal testicular tissue should always be removed because of the increased risk of malignancy.

MIXED GONADAL DYSGENESIS. *Clinical Presentation.* Classically, subjects with mixed gonadal dysgenesis have a streak gonad on one side and a testis on the contralateral side. Most demonstrate XO/XY mosaicism on chromosomal analysis. The phenotypic spectrum ranges from phenotypic females, with or without the clinical characteristics of Turner's syndrome, to subjects with ambiguous genitalia, to normal phenotypic males. The genitalia are sufficiently ambiguous in most affected subjects that approximately two thirds are raised as girls, with the stigmata of Turner's syndrome occurring in one third. Affected subjects have a uterus, and most have bilateral fallopian tubes. The vas deferens, if present, is on the side of the testis, and frequently a fallopian tube also exists adjacent to the vas deferens. Virilization generally occurs at puberty. The testes appear histologically normal before puberty. However, after puberty the seminiferous tubules demonstrate thickened walls and contain few if any germ cells. Consequently, affected subjects are infertile. If pubertal gynecomastia occurs, a gonadal tumor should be suspected.

Pathogenesis. XO/XY mosaicism in subjects with this condition can be best explained as resulting from mitotic nondisjunction or anaphase lag, resulting in loss of the Y chromosome. Perhaps the lack of testicular differentiation of the streak gonad is related to the preponderance of the XO cell line in that gonad. Despite good Leydig cell function with virilization at puberty, the testis must have been functionally dysgenetic (between the eighth and fourteenth weeks of gestation—the critically responsive period), as evidenced by absence of or incomplete virilization of the external genitalia. Theoretically a delay in testicular differentiation and function in utero could result in delayed secretion of testosterone and müllerian inhibiting factor, completely or partially missing the critically responsive period and resulting in the presence of female or ambiguous genitalia and müllerian structures.

There are subjects with an XO/XY chromosomal complement and bilaterally streaked gonads as well as XO/XY subjects with bilateral testes. Thus the classic clinical syndrome of mixed gonadal dysgenesis may be one clinical entity in a spectrum ranging from streaked gonads and a female phenotype to varied abnormalities of testicular development (symmetric or asymmetric) and genital ambiguity, possibly depending upon the preponderance of a particular cell line, either XO or XY, within the gonad at the time of differentiation (Fig. 234–5).

Management and Therapy. Because of the increased incidence of tumor formation, an intra-abdominal testis that cannot be brought into the scrotum should be removed as well as the streak gonad. If the subject is being raised as male, a scrotal testis should be preserved. In instances in which the testes cannot be brought to the scrotum and must be removed, or the external genitalia are severely ambiguous, or both conditions exist, the sex of rearing should be female and appropriate genital surgery performed.

XY AGONADISM, TESTICULAR REGRESSION, OR VANISHING TESTES SYNDROME. *Clinical Presentation.* Typically these subjects are 46 XY phenotypic females presenting with a total absence of gonads and no müllerian or wolffian internal structures. The lack of müllerian structures, together with a total lack of gonadal remnants, separates this entity from pure XY gonadal dysgenesis. The condition appears to be secondary to regression of the differentiating testis before the onset of androgen secretion, resulting in lack of wolffian differentiation, but after the onset of secretion of müllerian inhibiting factor, resulting in inhibition of female internal structures. There is, however, a phenotypic spectrum of agonadal subjects perhaps related to testicular regression occurring at various times, during or after the critical period of male sexual differentiation. Affected subjects can therefore vary widely in phenotypes: from those with total absence of internal sex structures and female external genitalia, to subjects with ambiguous genitalia, to normal males with absence of testes but a microphallus.

Pathophysiology. The etiology of the testicular regression is unknown. These subjects are unequivocally 46 XY, and chromosomal abnormalities have never been demonstrated. Familial cases of agonadism in XY subjects occur, however, suggesting that in some cases it may be an inherited condition. Variable phenotypic expression in agonadal siblings from the same kindred also occurs, suggesting that this condition is a clinical spectrum due to the time of regression of the embryonic testes.

LEYDIG CELL AGENESIS OR DYSGENESIS, GONADOTROPIN UNRESPONSIVENESS. *Clinical Characteristics.* Adult subjects with Leydig cell agenesis or dysgenesis have either normal female external genitalia or slight posterior fusion of the labia majora and have been raised as females.

Two prepubertal cases have been described, one with totally female genitalia and the other with a bifid scrotum, a clitoral-like phallus, and a urogenital sinus. An epididymis and vas deferens are present in all affected subjects, indicating that little testosterone is needed at a critical period to initiate wolffian differentiation. No müllerian structures are found, confirming the fact that müllerian inhibiting factor is not secreted by the Leydig cells, but is secreted by the Sertoli cells of the seminiferous tubules. In the adults, normal appearing Sertoli cells with few spermatogonia and few or no Leydig cells are present in the testis.

Pathophysiology. In adult cases, plasma androgen levels are in the female range and do not significantly change with administration of human chorionic gonadotropin (HCG). Luteinizing hormone (LH) levels are significantly elevated, while follicle-stimulating hormone (FSH) levels are in the normal range. In the children, there is no demonstrable plasma androgen response to administration of HCG.

Theoretically the absence or decrease in Leydig cells can result from (1) an absence of or decrease in precursor cells destined to become functioning Leydig cells under HCG-LH stimulation or (2) a decrease in the HCG-LH receptor or receptor response of the precursor Leydig cells. It can also be theorized that the HCG-LH receptor mediates Leydig cell differentiation, and without these receptors, precursor Leydig cells are not formed. A complete phenotypic spectrum of subjects with this disorder can be anticipated, dependent upon the severity of the developmental defect.

Management and Therapy. Those subjects in whom the diagnosis is made in infancy or early childhood should be raised in the sex in which they will be more apt to function normally. In most instances this would be as female because of the severe genital ambiguity. Thus the testes should be removed and corrective genital surgery performed.

Those subjects in whom the diagnosis is made in adulthood who were raised as females and have a female gender identity should have the testes removed, and female sex hormone therapy should be instituted to induce and maintain breast development.

Disorders of Testicular Function

In disorders of testicular function, the testes have differentiated normally, but there is an abnormality in the secretion of either müllerian inhibiting factor or testosterone.

MÜLLERIAN INHIBITING FACTOR DEFICIENCY. *Clinical Presentation.* Males with this condition have a uterus and bilateral fallopian tubes. They have bilateral testes with normal male differentiation of wolffian structures and external genitalia and undergo normal male puberty. This entity most frequently occurs as unilateral cryptorchidism with a contralateral inguinal hernia containing müllerian structures, "uteri inguinale," and a testis. The incidence of testicular tumors is approximately 13 per cent, a figure similar to that found in cryptorchidism. The presence of the inguinal hernia most often brings affected males to a physician's attention. Although fertility has been described, azoospermia is frequently noted. More than 70 cases of this entity have been reported, including at least eight families with two affected sibs. The majority of pedigree studies suggest an X-linked or autosomal recessive inheritance. In one family study, however, inheritance was compatible with X-linked or autosomal dominant inheritance. In approximately 5 per cent of affected patients, either seminomas or other germ cell tumors occur.

Pathogenesis. This entity could be due to a number of abnormalities affecting the synthesis, structure, timing of secretion, or action of müllerian inhibiting factor. Documentation of the actual biochemical abnormality will have to await characterization of the factor or its receptor. The ultimate effect is lack of suppression of the müllerian anlage resulting in the presence of a uterus. Androgen secretion is adequate during the critical period of sexual differentiation, with normal sexual differentiation of the wolffian ducts and external genitalia.

Management and Therapy. In affected males the müllerian structures should be surgically removed if they are in the inguinal canal. Since malignant change in müllerian structures have never been reported, surgical removal is not necessary if they are located in the abdomen. The cryptorchid testes should be brought into the scrotal sac as early as possible and the patient examined frequently for the development of testicular tumors.

Imperato-McGinley J: Sexual differentiation—Normal and abnormal. Curr Top Exp Endocrinol 5:231, 1983. *Of particular interest in this review is the section on male pseudohermaphroditism, including an extensive bibliography for each clinical entity described.*

DEFICIENCIES OF TESTOSTERONE BIOSYNTHESIS.

Clinical Features. Five enzymatic reactions convert cholesterol to testosterone; deficiencies of all have been described. These enzyme deficiencies constitute the nonvirilizing forms of the adrenogenital syndrome. The five enzymatic steps include (1) cholesterol 20,22-desmolase, (2) 3β-hydroxysteroid dehydrogenase:Δ^{5-4} isomerase, (3) 17α-hydroxylase, (4) 17,20-desmolase, and (5) 17β-hydroxysteroid dehydrogenase (Fig. 233–6). A deficiency of the enzymes cholesterol 20,22-desmolase and 3β-hydroxysteroid dehydrogenase:Δ^{5-4} isomerase also impairs production of aldosterone and cortisol. 17α-Hydroxylase deficiency impairs cortisol production, while 17,20-desmolase and 17β-hydroxysteroid dehydrogenase deficiencies affect only androgen biosynthesis. Since androgens are the precursors of estrogens, it follows that estrogen production is also low in all of the enzyme deficiencies except 17β-hydroxysteroid dehydrogenase (Table 234–2). These disorders appear to be inherited as autosomal recessive traits. Genotypic females are phenotypically normal at birth, with the exception of females with 3β-hydroxysteroid dehydrogenase deficiency, who may be mildly virilized.

The testes differentiate normally, and normal amounts of müllerian inhibiting factor are secreted, so that no müllerian structures are present. However, the impaired secretion of testosterone by Leydig cells at the critical period of sexual differentiation in utero (8 to 14 weeks of gestation) causes ambiguity of the external genitalia. Wolffian differentiation is usually normal. In general, the severity of the enzyme defect is reflected in the degree of external genital ambiguity at birth and the amount of virilization at puberty. Each specific enzyme deficiency, however, may show considerable variation in clinical presentation, and affected males with the same enzyme deficiency may present with totally female external genitalia or as males with mild hypospadias and cryptorchidism.

The possible causes for the abnormalities of enzymatic function include mutant genes at structural loci coding for the amino acid sequences of the enzymes changing the enzyme structure and altering its catalytic efficiency, or mutations at sites other than the structural loci. These mutations can be classified as *regulatory*, altering the rate of synthesis or degradation of the enzyme; *architectural*, affecting incorporation of enzyme molecules into active sites in the cell; or *temporal*, affecting the development of the tissue or the time of activation of regulatory systems.

Congenital Lipoid Adrenal Hyperplasia (Cholesterol 20,22-Desmolase Deficiency). In 1957, a genetic male from a consanguineous marriage was described with wolffian differentiation but with female external genitalia. The infant died in adrenal crisis at six days of age, and at autopsy the adrenals showed enormous accumulation of lipids in the cortical cells. Consequently the disorder was labeled congenital lipoid adrenal hyperplasia. Subsequent autopsy reports of other affected genotypic male infants have confirmed that the large, yellowish adrenals contain cells with foamy, spongy cytoplasm and stain positively for lipids.

The affected genotypic males have abdominal or inguinal testes with wolffian differentiation. There are no müllerian structures. The external genitalia are either female or severely ambiguous. As would be expected, genotypic female infants have normal female internal and external accessory sex organs.

Approximately 20 cases have been described with equal numbers of both sexes affected. Most of the affected have died in adrenal crisis in infancy, because of severe deficiencies of glucocorticoid and mineralocorticoid production.

PATHOGENESIS. A deficiency in the conversion of cholesterol to pregnenolone results in decreased glucocorticoid, mineralocorticoid, and sex steroid production (Fig. 234–6). All plasma steroid values are low to unmeasurable, and little or no urinary 17-ketosteroids, 17-hydroxysteroids, or aldosterone is found (Table 234–2). In the conversion of cholesterol to pregnenolone, at least three enzymes are involved: 20α-hydroxylase, 22α-hydroxylase, and 20,22-desmolase. These reactions are mitochondrial mixed-function oxidase reactions.

In a study of adrenal tissue from a child who died with this condition, a deficiency of the enzyme 20α-hydroxylase was suggested as the cause. In another study of adrenal tissue from an affected infant, partial deficiency of cytochrome P-450, with decreased cholesterol 20,22-desmolase activity, was demonstrated. Thus there may be genetic heterogeneity in the expression of this disorder.

MANAGEMENT AND THERAPY. In the newborn, signs of adrenal insufficiency with hyperkalemia and hyponatremia occur within the first two weeks, and this condition must be distinguished from 3β-hydroxysteroid dehydrogenase deficiency or congenital adrenal hypoplasia. In a phenotypic female infant, or an infant with ambiguous genitalia and

TABLE 234–2. XY MALE PSEUDOHERMAPHRODITISM WITH AN ENZYMATIC DEFECT IN TESTOSTERONE BIOSYNTHESIS

Enzyme Deficiency	External Genitalia		Secretion			Puberty	Comments
	Female or Urogenital Sinus	Ambiguous	Cortisol	Aldosterone	Androgens		
Cholesterol 20,22-desmolase	++++	+	↓	↓	↓	↓	
3β-Hydroxysteroid dehydrogenase:Δ^{5-4} isomerase	+	++++	− ↓	− ↓	↑ DHEA ↑ 17OH preg	Gynecomastia despite low estrogens	Intact peripheral 3βHSD with conversion of Δ^5 to Δ^4 steroids
17α-Hydroxylase	++++	++	− ↓	B ↑ DOC ↑	↓	Gynecomastia despite low estrogens	Hypertension due to ↑ DOC with ↓ renin and aldosterone
17,20-Desmolase	++++	+	−	−	↓		
17β-Hydroxysteroid dehydrogenase	++++	++	−	−	↓ T ↑ Δ^4	Gynecomastia due to increased estrogen and decreased T	Peripheral conversion of androstenedione to E$_1$

↑ elevated; ↓ decreased; − normal; + relative frequency of occurrence; B = corticosterone; DOC = desoxycorticosterone; DHEA = dehydroepiandrosterone; 17OH Preg = 17α-hydroxypregnenolone; T = testosterone; Δ^4 = androstenedione; 3βHSD = 3β-hydroxysteroid dehydrogenase; E$_1$ = estrone.

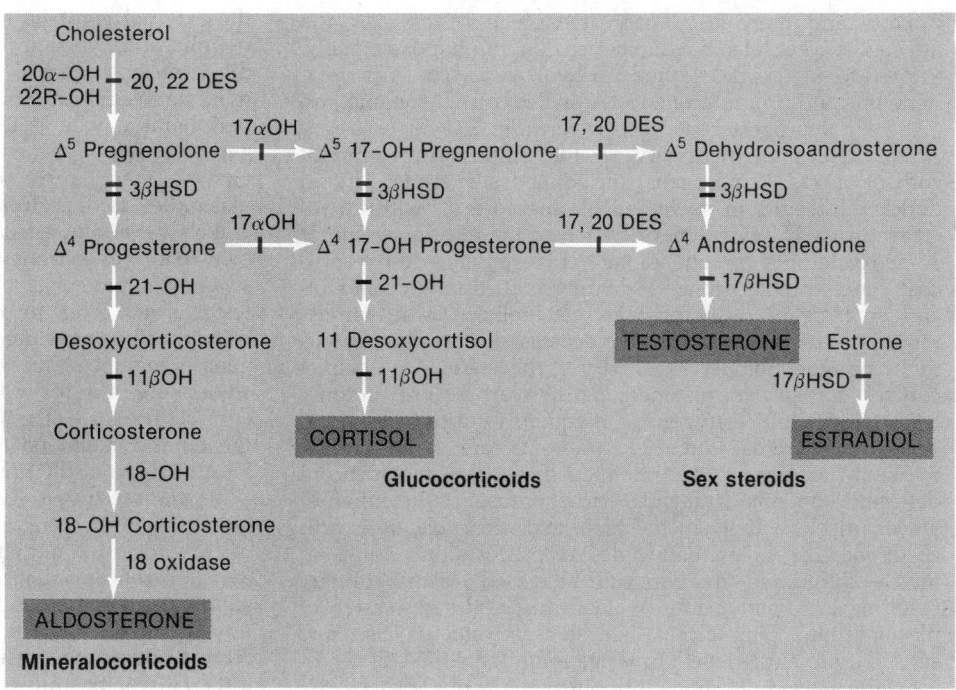

FIGURE 234–6. Congenital adrenal hyperplasia. *Left,* Enzyme deficiencies resulting in male pseudohermaphroditism. Cholesterol 20,22-desmolase, 17α-hydroxylase, 3β-hydroxysteroid dehydrogenase:Δ⁵⁻⁴ isomerase, 17,20-desmolase, 17β-hydroxysteroid dehydrogenase. *Center and right,* Enzyme deficiencies resulting in female pseudohermaphroditism. 21-Hydroxylase, 11β-hydroxylase, 3β-hydroxysteroid dehydrogenase:Δ⁵⁻⁴ isomerase. (DES = desmolase; OH = hydroxylase; HSD = hydroxysteroid dehydrogenase.)

adrenal insufficiency, demonstration of a 46 XY karyotype or demonstration of enlarged adrenals by a radiographic technique will help distinguish this condition from congenital adrenal hypoplasia. The finding of low urinary 17-ketosteroid and low plasma dehydroepiandrosterone levels will distinguish it from 3β-hydroxysteroid dehydrogenase deficiency. Once the diagnosis is established, glucocorticoid and mineralocorticoid therapy should be immediately instituted and is essential for survival. In genotypic males, sex hormone therapy should be instituted at puberty in accordance with the sex of rearing. In most instances, because of the severity of the genital defect, the sex of rearing would be female. Genotypic females will also require appropriate female sex hormone therapy at puberty.

3β-Hydroxysteroid Dehydrogenase:Δ⁵⁻⁴ Isomerase Deficiency. CLINICAL PRESENTATION. In 1961 the first three cases of 3β-hydroxysteroid dehydrogenase:Δ⁵⁻⁴ isomerase deficiency were described in both males and females. Affected 46 XY subjects had genital ambiguity, although mild to moderate hypospadias is more common than severe perineoscrotal hypospadias. Internal male sexual differentiation is normal, with wolffian differentiation and müllerian ductal inhibition. Curiously, genetic males who reach puberty develop gynecomastia, the etiology of which is not known. At birth affected females have normal or slightly virilized external genitalia, with clitoral hypertrophy and slight labial fusion.

Severely affected children have adrenal insufficiency and die in infancy as a result of salt-losing crisis if not adequately treated. In the milder cases sufficient cortisol and aldosterone are synthesized, and consequently adrenal insufficiency is not present in infancy.

PATHOGENESIS. In the adrenal the enzyme deficiency ultimately results in decreased cortisol production, which causes increased ACTH secretion and consequent increased production of Δ⁵,3β-hydroxysteroids (Fig. 234–6). Plasma levels of pregnenolone, 17α-hydroxypregnenolone, and dehydroepiandrosterone and their sulfate conjugates are usually increased, with decreased levels of aldosterone and cortisol. The slight virilization of the external genitalia in the female is most probably due to the mild androgenic effect of the excess plasma dehydroepiandrosterone or its subsequent peripheral conversion to Δ⁵-androstenediol and other androgens (Table 234–3). Surprisingly, plasma Δ⁴ steroids, i.e., progesterone, 17α-hydroxyprogesterone, androstenedione, and occasionally

testosterone, may be normal or even increased. These findings have been interpreted as reflecting intact hepatic and peripheral 3β-hydroxysteroid dehydrogenase:Δ⁵⁻⁴ isomerase enzyme activity. Also in some affected subjects, the gonadal defect is not as severe as the adrenal defect. Thus the same enzyme may be under different genetic control in different areas, or there may be different isoenzymes within the adrenal, gonad, and liver.

MANAGEMENT AND THERAPY. In infancy the diagnosis is suggested in a 46 XY male with ambiguous genitalia and adrenal insufficiency. In distinction to an infant with cholesterol 20,22-desmolase deficiency, urinary 17-ketosteroid values are normal to high with increased plasma dehydroepiandrosterone. Treatment involves mineralocorticoid and glucocorticoid replacement therapy, as in cholesterol 20,22-desmolase deficiency. If needed, sex steroid therapy should be instituted at puberty to induce sexual development in accordance with the sex of rearing.

17α-Hydroxylase Deficiency. CLINICAL PRESENTATION. The first case of 17α-hydroxylase deficiency was in a 35-year-old genetic and phenotypic female with a lack of secondary sexual development, hypertension, and hypokalemic alkalosis. Since then, many cases have been reported in both genetic males and females. In 46 XY subjects the defect of the external genitalia is usually severe, resulting in completely female external genitalia at birth. Müllerian structures are absent, and wolffian structures are either developed or hypoplastic. Often gynecomastia develops at puberty with little or no virilization. Thus, males with this enzyme deficiency can have the same phenotype in adulthood as subjects with the complete androgen insensitivity syndrome. In 46 XX females with this condition secondary sexual development is absent at

TABLE 234–3. CLASSIFICATION OF CAUSES OF FEMALE PSEUDOHERMAPHRODITISM

I. Androgenic influences
  A. Fetal
    1. Congenital adrenogenital syndrome:
      a. 21-Hydroxylase deficiency;
      b. 11β-Hydroxylase deficiency;
      c. 3β-Hydroxysteroid dehydrogenase:Δ⁵⁻⁴ isomerase deficiency
  B. Maternal
    1. Excess maternal androgen production
    2. Maternal ingestion of virilizing substances
II. Idiopathic

puberty and there is primary amenorrhea. Classically the affected subjects also have hypertension and hypokalemia.

PATHOGENESIS. The enzyme 17α-hydroxylase converts pregnenolone and progesterone to 17α-hydroxypregnenolone and 17α-hydroxyprogesterone, respectively (Fig. 234–6). These enzymatic steps are necessary for the ultimate formation of cortisol and C19 androgens, including testosterone. Thus a deficiency results in decreased plasma cortisol, with an increase in ACTH and hypersecretion of the plasma precursor 17-deoxysteroids (pregnenolone, progesterone, desoxycorticosterone, corticosterone, 18-hydroxycorticosterone) and increased excretion of their urinary metabolites. Those steroids requiring 17α-hydroxylation are decreased, i.e., plasma 17α-hydroxypregnenolone, 17α-hydroxyprogesterone, 11-deoxycortisol, cortisol, androstenedione, dehydroepiandrosterone, testosterone, and estrogen. Consequently, urinary levels of 17-hydroxysteroids and 17-ketosteroids are low. Despite markedly impaired cortisol production, signs of glucocorticoid deficiency do not generally occur, because of the inherent glucocorticoid activity in the high levels of circulating corticosterone. Excess circulating desoxycorticosterone results in increased sodium retention with increased plasma volume, resulting in hypertension, hypokalemia, and suppression of plasma renin. The plasma aldosterone value is also low secondary to a low level of plasma renin (Table 234–2).

In affected adults, gonadotropin values are elevated, sex steroid levels are low, and in the male there is little or no testicular 17α-hydroxyprogesterone and testosterone response to HCG administration. Consanguinity has been documented in some cases, as has an occurrence of the disorder in siblings of both the same and opposite sex, supporting an autosomal recessive mode of inheritance.

MANAGEMENT AND THERAPY. Hypertension associated with hypokalemic alkalosis in an XY individual with female external genitalia or ambiguous genitalia should suggest the diagnosis. It should also be suspected in any XX female with the same symptom complex who has primary amenorrhea and lack of secondary sexual development. Glucocorticoid replacement therapy is administered to reverse the metabolic abnormality and lower the blood pressure. Appropriate sex steroid therapy concordant with the sex of rearing should be administered at puberty.

17β-Hydroxysteroid Dehydrogenase Deficiency. CLINICAL PRESENTATION. This condition, described only in 46 XY males, is characterized by either female external genitalia or mild ambiguity of the genitalia. With few exceptions, those affected have been raised as girls. In subjects with totally female appearing external genitalia at birth, the abnormality is not noted until puberty, when virilization frequently occurs with clitoral enlargement. At puberty there are two distinct clinical presentations. Some subjects develop gynecomastia in addition to virilization, while others undergo strong virilization with a male pattern of body hair, deep voice, android build, and no gynecomastia. All subjects raised as females throughout childhood who were castrated prior to or during their teenage years have maintained a female gender identity.

PATHOGENESIS. 17β-Hydroxysteroid dehydrogenase catalyzes the conversion of androstenedione to testosterone, the final step in the synthesis of testosterone (Fig. 234–6), and the oxidation-reduction of estrone and estradiol, dehydroepiandrosterone, and Δ5-androstenediol. In affected 46 XY subjects, the enzyme deficiency results in increased circulating plasma levels of androstenedione, while plasma levels of testosterone are low to low normal (Table 234–2). Plasma luteinizing hormone is increased, while plasma follicle-stimulating hormone is normal to increased. Approximately 90 per cent of circulating testosterone arises from the extragonadal conversion of androstenedione. Thus in the adult the defect appears to affect the testes while peripheral enzyme activity appears to be intact. However, for masculinization of

the external genitalia to be minimal or absent in the fetus, peripheral conversion of androstenedione to testosterone and dihydrotestosterone in the anlage of the external genitalia must be insignificant or absent during early gestation. Thus, peripheral as well as testicular 17β-hydroxysteroid dehydrogenase activity appears deficient in utero, whereas peripheral enzyme activity appears to be intact in the adult. The elevated plasma levels of androstenedione result in increased peripheral conversion to estrone (Table 234–2). In some subjects the conversion of estrone to estradiol also appears to be as severely impaired as the conversion of androstenedione to testosterone, while in others it is impaired to a lesser degree or not at all, suggesting that the 17β-hydroxysteroid dehydrogenase enzyme(s) converting estrone to estradiol and androstenedione to testosterone may be under different regulatory control. The lower the plasma testosterone-estradiol ratio, the greater the likelihood of gynecomastia developing in an affected subject at the time of puberty.

MANAGEMENT AND THERAPY. 46 XY affected subjects with female external genitalia should be raised as females and castration carried out either before or during early puberty to avoid significant virilization. Female sex hormone therapy should be instituted at puberty. In those subjects with ambiguous genitalia that can be surgically corrected, a male sex of rearing should be considered. If the diagnosis is made peripubertally or postpubertally, careful psychosexual evaluation should be performed to determine the gender identity before any therapy is instituted. If a gender change from female to male has occurred with puberty, corrective male genital surgery is needed.

17,20-Desmolase Deficiency. CLINICAL PRESENTATION. In 1972 a child with male ambiguous genitalia was described with a defect postulated to be secondary to 17,20-desmolase deficiency. A male pseudohermaphroditic cousin and maternal 46 XY "aunt" were included in the report. Since then nine cases of the enzyme deficiency in 46 XY males have been reported, all phenotypic females or subjects with severely ambiguous genitalia. More recently the first case of a genetic female with primary amenorrhea and lack of secondary sexual development has been reported.

PATHOGENESIS. Partial or complete lack of the enzyme 17,20-desmolase in the adrenal and gonads results in decreased cleavage of the two-carbon side chain from either 17α-hydroxyprogesterone or 17α-hydroxypregnenolone with a resultant decrease in androstenedione and dehydroepiandrosterone production, respectively (Fig. 234–6). This step is essential for the ultimate formation of testosterone and estrogens.

It is not known why the basal plasma levels of progesterone, pregnenolone, 17α-hydroxyprogesterone, and 17α-hydroxypregnenolone are elevated, particularly in prepubertal subjects with this enzyme deficiency. Since the enzyme 17,20-desmolase is not involved in cortisol biosynthesis, ACTH levels should be normal with subsequent normal amounts of the C21 precursor steroids mentioned above (Fig. 234–6).

MANAGEMENT AND THERAPY. In genotypic males the sex of rearing will depend upon the degree of ambiguity of the external genitalia. In the more severe cases, patients should be raised as females, with castration carried out in early childhood. Sex hormone therapy at puberty will invariably be necessary. In genotypic females, estrogen and progesterone supplementation will invariably be needed at the time of puberty.

White PC, New MI, Dupont B: Congenital adrenal hyperplasia. N Engl J Med 316:1519, 1580, 1987. *An all-encompassing review of the biochemical aspects of nonvirilizing and virilizing forms of congenital adrenal hyperplasia. A gem.*
Peterson RE, Imperato-McGinley J: Male pseudohermaphroditism due to inherited deficiencies of testosterone biosynthesis. In Serio M, Motta M, Zanisi M, et al. (eds.): Sexual Differentiation: Basic and Clinical Aspects. Vol. 2. New York, Raven Press, 1984, pp 301–319. *A detailed study of the clinical characteristics and the biochemistry of male pseudohermaphroditism due to deficiencies in testosterone biosynthesis.*

Disorders of Function at Androgen-Dependent Target Areas

COMPLETE ANDROGEN INSENSITIVITY—TESTICU-LAR FEMINIZATION. *Clinical Presentation.* In this inherited form of male pseudohermaphroditism, genetic and gonadal males have a female phenotype and totally female psychosexual orientation. The testes differentiate normally with adequate secretion of müllerian inhibiting factor, resulting in the absence of fallopian tubes, uterus, and upper portion of the vagina. Despite normal to high-normal plasma levels of testosterone, wolffian structures are absent, and the external genitalia are totally female. Affected subjects are raised as girls, and the condition is rarely suspected prior to puberty. A prepubertal diagnosis is occasionally made when inguinal or labial masses are palpated in a phenotypic female child and are found to be testes.

Adequate breast development occurs at puberty, but pubic and axillary hair is scant to absent. Medical attention is usually sought at this time because of primary amenorrhea. A diagnosis of complete androgen insensitivity or testicular feminization should be considered in a phenotypic female with primary amenorrhea, good breast development, scantness or absence of pubic and axillary hair, a short vagina, and absence of the cervix and uterus. Rarely, patients with 17α-hydroxylase deficiency may have the same phenotypic presentation at puberty.

Pathogenesis. In patients with complete androgen insensitivity, absence of high-affinity dihydrotestosterone binding to the cytosol receptor (receptor-negative) has been demonstrated in cultured fibroblasts from genital skin. Qualitative abnormalities of the androgen receptor have also been described. Finally, postreceptor variants with normal cytosol receptor binding have also been demonstrated. In the latter individuals, the mutation may affect nuclear binding or the steps in the initiation of androgen action subsequent to nuclear binding, i.e., failure of RNA synthesis or an abnormality in its processing (Fig. 234–7).

It has been postulated that the X chromosomes of all mammals, including man, are homologous, and genes X linked in one species are X linked in all. A defect in the receptor-negative form of complete androgen insensitivity has been found to be maternally transmitted with only males expressing the condition, suggesting inheritance as X-linked recessive or autosomal dominant–sex limited (males). Studies of genital skin fibroblasts from mothers of affected subjects demonstrate two clonal populations, one with normal dihydrotestosterone binding and one with absence of binding to the cytosol receptor, confirming X linkage in this form of androgen insensitivity.

Plasma testosterone levels are normal to high with mild to moderately elevated plasma levels of luteinizing hormone (LH). A possible explanation for the increased LH is the relative androgen insensitivity at the level of the hypothalamus resulting in partial negative feedback via conversion of testosterone to estradiol with no direct androgen inhibition. Follicle-stimulating hormone (FSH) levels are normal to elevated. Castration results in further elevation of LH and FSH levels, indicating prior partial feedback control. Urinary estrogens and plasma estradiol levels are generally in the low female range. An increased production rate has been shown for estrone and estradiol, which is mainly testicular in origin. The elevation of plasma estrogens together with the androgen unresponsiveness results in an unopposed estrogen effect that may be the cause of the breast development at puberty.

The histology of the testes cannot be distinguished from that of normal prepubertal males. Postpubertal histologic sections, however, reveal immature tubular development; they contain Sertoli cells and spermatogonia, but no evidence of spermatogenesis. Clumping of tubules with the formation of tubular adenomas is frequently found. The Leydig cells are hyperplastic, correlating with the elevated plasma testosterone levels.

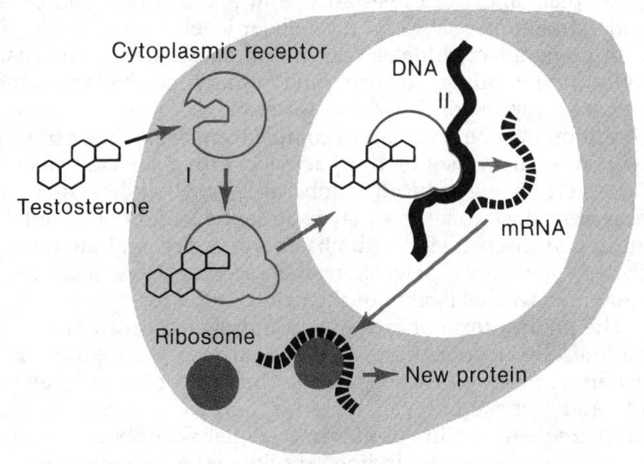

I. Abnormalities affecting binding to the cytosol receptor

   A. Quantitative

      1. Absent binding to cytosol receptor

   B. Qualitative

      1. Thermolability
      2. Failure of stabilization with sodium molybdate
      3. Altered binding affinity
      4. Lability of cytosolic receptor under conditions that normally promote transformation to the DNA–binding state

II. Nuclear or postnuclear receptor binding defect

      1. Impaired nuclear retention
      2. Impaired augmentation of receptor binding following incubation with androgen

FIGURE 234–7. Illustration of the abnormalities of androgen action resulting in androgen insensitivity.

Management and Therapy. The frequency of testicular neoplasms in complete androgen insensitivity is approximately 2 to 5 per cent, tumors rarely occurring before the age of 25 to 30 years. For this reason the testes should be removed following puberty to allow complete breast development. Following castration, intermittent estrogen replacement therapy is necessary to maintain adequate breast turgor. In general, the vagina is adequate for normal coital function. Occasionally it is too shallow, but can frequently be enlarged with vaginal dilators, thereby bypassing the necessity for reconstructive surgery.

PARTIAL ANDROGEN INSENSITIVITY. *Clinical Presentation.* Partial forms of androgen insensitivity have been described. Affected subjects range from XY subjects with genital ambiguity and minimal to moderate pubertal virilization and gynecomastia, to those with a normal male phenotype, normal male secondary sexual development, and infertility. Reifenstein syndrome is a term that is applied to the variety of phenotypic presentations of partial androgen insensitivity. Several pedigrees compatible with X linkage have been reported. Affected subjects within the same pedigree may exhibit the variable phenotypes described. Thus these syndromes may represent variable phenotypic expressions of the same gene mutation.

Pathogenesis. In general, the endocrine profile is similar to that demonstrated in subjects with complete androgen insensitivity. Plasma LH and testosterone levels are generally elevated. The total amount of 17β-estradiol produced and the quantity secreted by the testes can be greater than those found in patients with complete androgen insensitivity. However, despite increased estrogen production, the degree of feminization at puberty is not as marked as in complete androgen insensitivity, which may be a consequence of the incomplete androgen resistance with a less severe androgen and estrogen imbalance at the cellular level.

In many affected males with incomplete androgen insensitivity, the binding capacity and affinity of the androgen cytosol receptor for dihydrotestosterone is normal. Thus this condition may be a variant of complete androgen insensitivity with normal cytosol-binding activity. Other affected males, however, have a reduced number of cytosol-binding sites for dihydrotestosterone; this may represent a variant of complete androgen insensitivity with absence of androgen-binding activity. Qualitative defects in the receptor have also been shown as well as lability of the cytosol receptor.

The mildest form of incomplete androgen insensitivity may be infertility in phenotypically normal men with either azoospermia or severe oligospermia. The mean plasma levels of LH and testosterone can be either normal or elevated. The most frequent finding in cultured genital skin fibroblasts is a decrease in androgen-binding capacity to the androgen cytosol receptor by over 50 per cent in comparison to that found in normal skin samples. A major unknown in this form of androgen resistance is its frequency as a cause of infertility.

Management and Therapy. Incomplete forms of androgen insensitivity can be distinguished biochemically from male pseudohermaphroditism with defects in testosterone biosynthesis. All of these conditions can have the same phenotypic presentation prior to puberty. In the absence of a demonstrable cytosol receptor abnormality, a decrease in the anabolic response to androgen administration, i.e., decreased nitrogen retention, may help clarify the diagnosis. True hermaphrodites most commonly have an XX karyotype and can often be distinguished on that basis. Incomplete androgen insensitivity in puberty commonly results in gynecomastia and varying degrees of virilization. Following puberty, a normal to elevated plasma testosterone level with a normal androstenedione-testosterone ratio as well as normal plasma progesterone and dehydroepiandrosterone levels will distinguish subjects with this condition from subjects with 17β-hydroxysteroid dehydrogenase deficiency, 17α-hydroxylase deficiency, and 3β-hydroxysteroid dehydrogenase deficiency, who can have the same appearance. Those subjects with moderate to severe defects in masculinization of the external genitalia should be raised as females and if possible castrated before puberty because of the possibility of virilization. Estrogen therapy should be added at puberty. Those with mild hypospadias can be raised as males, but will require surgery for correction of both the hypospadias and the gynecomastia.

Wilson JD, Griffin JE: Mutations that impair androgen action. Trends Genet 1:335, 1985. *A comprehensive review of the biochemical abnormalities in complete and partial androgen insensitivity.*

5α-REDUCTASE DEFICIENCY. *Clinical Presentation.* Most patients with this condition have perineal hypospadias with separate urethral and vaginal openings within a urogenital sinus. Rarely a blind vaginal pouch opens into the urethra. The patients have an epididymis, vas deferens, and seminal vesicles. The incidence of cryptorchidism is significantly higher in childhood than adulthood, suggesting that it is not uncommon for the testes to descend during puberty in this condition.

The pubertal events include deepening of the voice, development of a muscular habitus, growth of the phallus, rugation and hyperpigmentation of the scrotum, and testicular descent. The prostate is small or absent, even in elderly subjects. Subjects have erections with ejaculation from the perineal urethra. Facial hair is decreased or absent and body hair is decreased.

Pathogenesis. The enzyme Δ⁴,5α-reductase with NADPH as a cofactor catalyzes the reduction of the double bond at the 4–5 position of both C19 steroids, such as testosterone, and C21 steroids. It is present in high quantities in the liver and peripheral tissues, particularly the sebaceous glands, hair

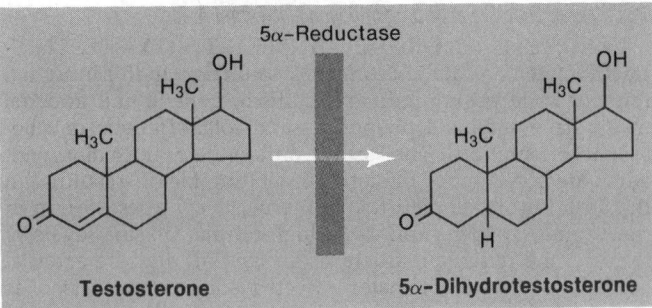

FIGURE 234–8. The conversion of testosterone to dihydrotestosterone by the enzyme 5α-reductase.

follicles, and skin of the external genitalia, where it actively converts testosterone to dihydrotestosterone, a more potent androgen (Fig. 234–8). In subjects with 5α-reductase deficiency, the biochemical abnormality is characterized by normal to elevated levels of plasma testosterone with decreased levels of dihydrotestosterone, resulting in an increased testosterone-dihydrotestosterone ratio. There is decreased production of the urinary 5α-reduced metabolites of testosterone, i.e., androsterone and androstanediol, causing elevated etiocholanolone-androsterone and etiocholanediol-androstanediol ratios. The urinary 5α-reduced metabolites of C21 and C19 steroids other than testosterone, i.e., cortisol, corticosterone, 11β-hydroxyandrostenedione, and androstenedione, are also decreased. Diminished 5α-reductase activity has been demonstrated both in skin slices and in fibroblasts cultured from genital skin. An autosomal recessive inheritance has been demonstrated.

Male pseudohermaphrodites with 5α-reductase deficiency represent a unique clinical model, defining major actions for testosterone and dihydrotestosterone in male sexual differentiation and development. Since the development defect is limited to the external genitalia and prostate, the normal development of these structures appears to be effected through the actions of dihydrotestosterone. In contrast, wolffian differentiation develops normally and appears to be a testosterone-mediated function (Fig. 234–9). At puberty the affected males develop rugation and hyperpigmentation of the scrotum, growth of the phallus, an increase in muscle mass, and deepening of the voice (Fig. 234–10). Their ultimate height is also similar to that of their fathers and normal male sibs. Thus the aforementioned pubertal events are mainly effected through the actions of testosterone. In contrast, prostatic development or enlargement, acne, normal male facial and body hair, and temporal recession of the hairline do not occur in affected males and appear to be effected mainly through the actions of dihydrotestosterone.

Since both androgens share a common cytosol receptor, it is puzzling that the effects of dihydrotestosterone in dihydrotestosterone-dependent areas are not mimicked by testosterone. Two possible explanations can be submitted: (1) the cytosol receptor at certain target sites is modified so that it favors 5α-dihydrotestosterone over testosterone or (2) the 5α-dihydrotestosterone receptor complex has a higher affinity for the acceptor sites in chromatin.

In affected subjects with descended testes, testicular biopsy has demonstrated complete spermatogenesis; thus testosterone may be more important than dihydrotestosterone in the process of spermatogenesis. The question of fertility, however, remains unanswered. The cryptorchid testes of most subjects demonstrate seminiferous tubular damage with either Sertoli cells only or aberrant spermatogenesis. Plasma LH is increased despite normal to high plasma levels of testosterone, suggesting a role for dihydrotestosterone in the negative feedback control of LH. The elevated plasma LH levels correlate with the microscopic findings of Leydig cell hyperplasia. Plasma FSH levels are also elevated, which may be a conse-

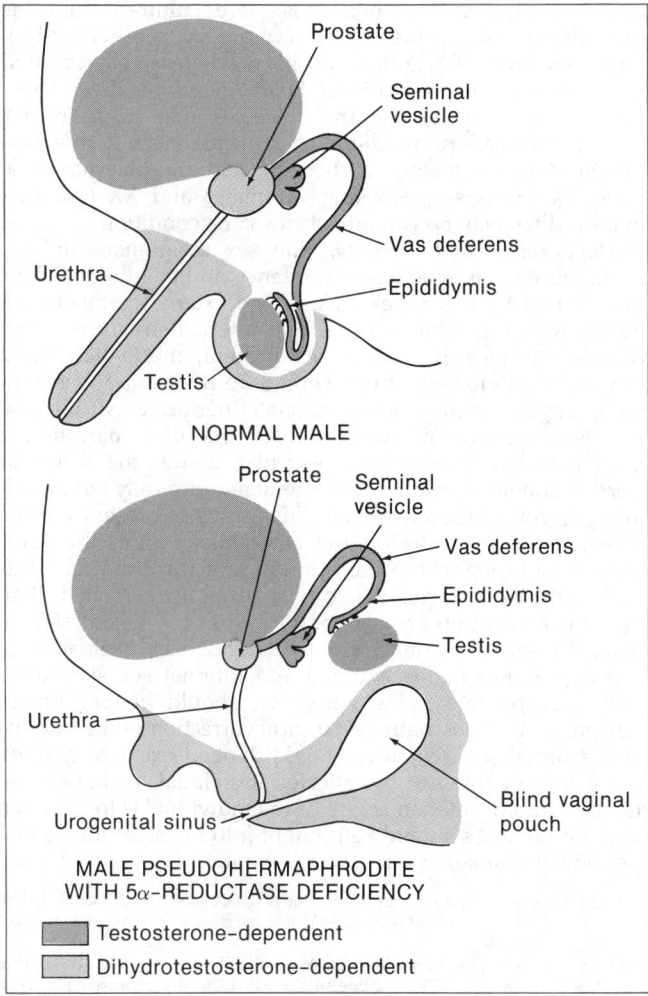

FIGURE 234–9. Illustration of the hypothesis for the specific actions of testosterone and dihydrotestosterone in male sexual differentiation in utero.

quence of the cryptorchidism with its damaging effect on spermatogenesis. Affected males have erections, with ejaculation from the perineal urethra, and thus these male sexual functions appear to be mediated through the actions of testosterone, either directly or via conversion to estradiol in the brain. Conversely, administration of pharmacologic amounts of dihydrotestosterone causes a substantial decrease in plasma testosterone with subsequent loss of libido and impotence.

A documented gender change from female to male in untreated affected subjects in large kindreds underscores the importance of testosterone exposure of the brain in utero, the early postnatal period, and at puberty in the determination of male gender identity. Theoretically, "masculinization" of the brain occurs under the influence of testosterone and, together with activation of testosterone-mediated puberty, a male gender identity develops, overriding the female sex of rearing. It has been proposed that gender identity becomes fixed by 18 months to 4 years of age, around the time of language development. However, from studies with these patients, it appears that the development of gender identity in humans is continually evolving throughout childhood and adolescence, becoming fixed with puberty.

Imperato-McGinley J, Gautier T: Inherited 5α-reductase deficiency. Main Trends Genet 2(5):130, 1986. *A review of the inheritance and clinical and biochemical findings of this unusual experiment of nature.*

Imperato-McGinley J, Peterson RE, Gautier T, et al.: The impact of androgens on the evolution of male gender identity. In Kogan SJ, Hafez ESE (eds.): Clinics in Andrology: Pediatric Andrology. Vol. 7. The Hague, Matinus Nijhoff, 1981, pp 99–105. *A study of gender change from female to male in a large kindred with 5α-reductase deficiency—a comprehensive theory concerning the acquisition of gender identity in males.*

XX Males and True Hermaphroditism

XX Males

Clinical Presentation. Approximately 50 cases of XX males have been reported, including members within the same family. A rare condition, the incidence in newborn males is estimated to be 1 in 20,000. Classically XX adult males have short stature, a normal-sized penis, small firm testes generally less than 2 cm, and infertility. One third have gynecomastia.

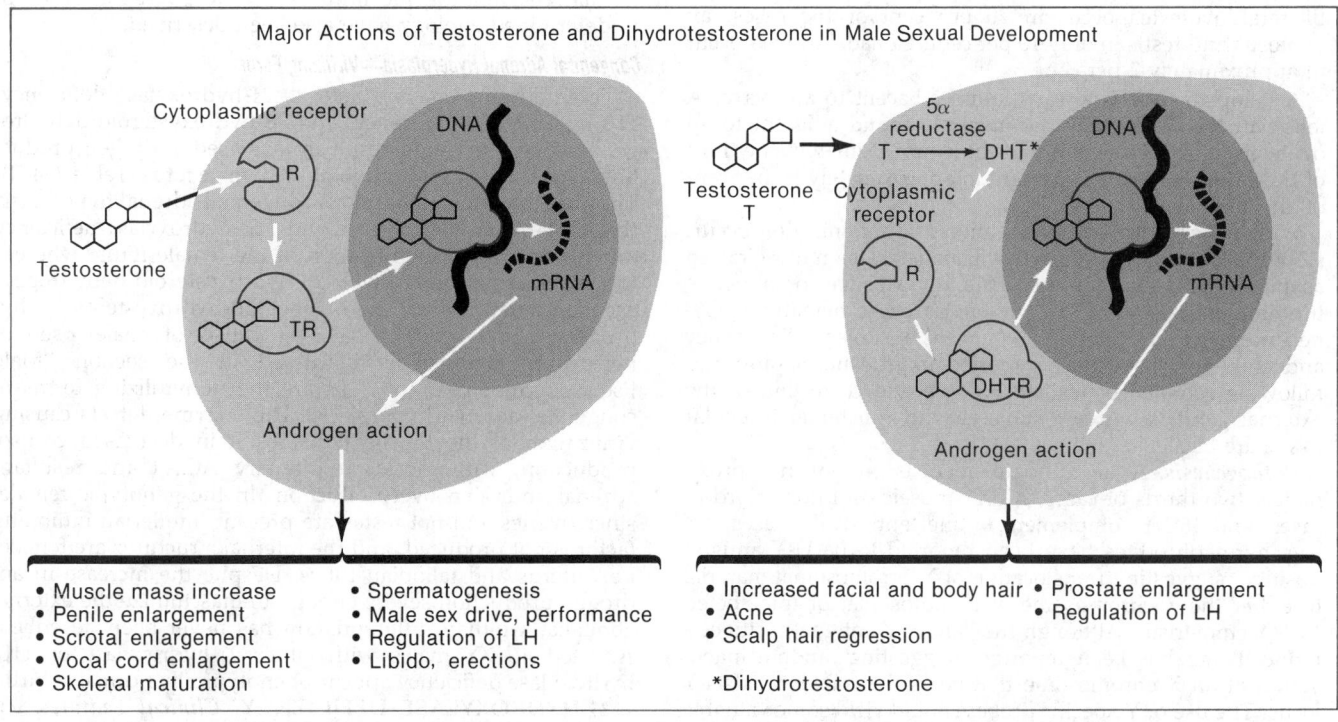

FIGURE 234–10. Illustration of the major actions of testosterone and dihydrotestosterone at puberty.

The phenotypic appearance resembles that of males with Klinefelter's syndrome (XXY) with the notable exception that XX males are shorter in stature, even shorter than the average male. In general, the histologic features of the testes also resemble those of subjects with Klinefelter's syndrome. The seminiferous tubules of the testes are hyalinized and contain only Sertoli cells or occasionally a few immature spermatogonia, correlating clinically with azoospermia or oligospermia. The Leydig cells are hyperplastic. Levels of FSH and LH are elevated, with decreased plasma testosterone and increased plasma estradiol levels. Some XX children with bilateral testes have been reported with ambiguous genitalia, suggesting a phenotypic spectrum of this condition.

Pathogenesis. The etiologic factors for the expression of masculinity in XX individuals have been the subject of much speculation. Three possible mechanisms have been proposed—(1) translocation of part of the Y chromosome to the X chromosome or to an autosome, (2) undetected mosaicism XX/XY or XXY, or (3) a mutant autosomal gene determining maleness in an XX individual. Studies of H-Y antigen in subjects with this condition have revealed a positive titer. Chromosome preparations from 8 to 12 46 XX males were clearly distinguishable from normal 46 XX female preparations secondary to alterations in shape, as well as an increase in the tip of the short arm of the X chromosome. DNA digests from the nuclei of cells from testes of an XX male have demonstrated Y-specific DNA fragments. Studies using Y-specific DNA probes have demonstrated the presence of Y chromosomal material in the genome of some XX males. Thus, the condition in a high percentage of 46 XX males appears to be a consequence of a paternal X-Y interchange affecting the testes-determining area of the Y chromosome.

True Hermaphroditism

Clinical Presentation. The morphologic expression of true hermaphroditism is the presence of both ovarian and testicular tissue, with each gonad containing its corresponding gamete. Most subjects have ambiguous genitalia, although approximately 7 per cent of true hermaphrodites have normal female external genitalia, and 12 per cent have a penile urethra; 75 per cent of affected subjects are raised as males. The most common gonadal associations are an ovary and testis or an ovotestis and ovary, each occurring in 30 per cent of cases. Bilateral ovotestes occur in 20 per cent of the cases; an ovotestis and testis in only 10 per cent. Gonadal tumors occur in approximately 2 per cent.

A fallopian tube is always found adjacent to an ovary. A fallopian tube is also most commonly found adjacent to an ovotestis; an epididymis is present in approximately one third of the cases. A uterus is present in approximately 90 per cent of affected subjects.

With puberty, variable virilization and feminization occur. About half of affected subjects will menstruate; in those raised as males with mild or moderate hypospadias or a penile urethra, menstruation can present as cyclic hematuria. Gynecomastia will develop in 80 per cent of subjects. Pregnancy and childbirth have been reported in true hermaphrodites following removal of testicular tissue and correction of the external genitalia. A few subjects with functional testicular tissue are fertile.

Pathogenesis. A 46 XX complement is present in approximately two thirds of cases, XX/XY mosaicism in one third of cases, and 46 XY complement in one tenth of cases. XX true hermaphrodites have been reported to be H-Y antigen positive, suggesting translocation of Y chromosomal material to either the X chromosome or an autosome, or undetected XX/XY chimerism. Although they are H-Y antigen positive, a reduced titer has been reported, suggesting random inactivation of an X chromosome that bears the translocated H-Y locus. The use of Y-specific probes should yield some valuable information, particularly in those true hermaphrodites with

an XX complement. When cells were cultured from the testicular portion of the ovotestis of an XX true hermaphrodite, they were H-Y antigen positive, whereas cells cultured from the ovarian portion were H-Y antigen negative. These observations suggest that the ovotestes arise from an H-Y +/H-Y− mosaic primordium. A reported case of true hermaphroditism in a subject whose brother and paternal uncle were XX males suggests that XX males and XX true hermaphrodites may be variants of the same condition.

Management and Therapy. The sex assignment in true hermaphroditism diagnosed in infancy and childhood is best determined by the appearance of the external genitalia, together with the gonadal tissue and internal structures. If an ovary-ovotestis and a uterus are present, the ovotestis and any male internal structures should be removed and feminizing surgery of the external genitalia performed. If bilateral ovotestes are present, and if a good line of demarcation is seen between ovarian and testicular tissue, the testicular portion should be removed, the genitalia surgically feminized, and the child raised as female. If a testis is present on one side and an ovotestis on the contralateral side, the testis should be brought into the scrotum and the child raised as male if the external genitalia can be surgically corrected. If an ovary is present on one side and a testis on the contralateral side, the sex of rearing should be decided by evaluation of the appearance of the external and internal sex structures, and appropriate surgical correction should be performed. Peripubertal or postpubertal surgical correction of the internal and external sex structures should depend exclusively upon the gender identity of the affected individual. Although testicular tumor formation is rare, if the individual is to be raised as male the testis should be brought into the scrotum, so that periodic examination can be carried out.

De La Chapelle A: The etiology of maleness in XX men. Hum Genet 58:105, 1981. *A review of clinical characteristics and hypotheses in the occurrence of this unique condition.*

Van Niekerk WA: True hermaphroditism—An analytic review with a report of 3 new cases. Am J Obstet Gynecol 126:890, 1976. *An extensive review of all reported cases to 1976, covering clinical presentation and etiology.*

Female Pseudohermaphroditism

Female pseudohermaphroditism can result from either fetal or maternal androgenic influences (Table 234–3). Cases of undetermined etiology have also been described.

Congenital Adrenal Hyperplasia—Virilizing Forms

Three adrenal enzyme defects, 21-hydroxylase deficiency, 11β-hydroxylase deficiency, and 3β-hydroxysteroid dehydrogenase deficiency, can result in increased androgen production in utero with virilization of the female fetus (Table 234–4). They are the virilizing forms of congenital adrenal hyperplasia (Fig. 234–6). 21-Hydroxylase and 11β-hydroxylase deficiency can result in severe virilization of the female fetus, whereas the virilization reported with 3β-hydroxysteroid dehydrogenase deficiency is very mild. Since 3β-hydroxysteroid dehydrogenase deficiency is also a cause of male pseudohermaphroditism, it is discussed in the section "Male Pseudohermaphroditism," as are the nonvirilizing forms of congenital adrenal hyperplasia. The enzyme defects causing virilization of the female fetus result in decreased cortisol production, with increased pituitary ACTH and resultant adrenal androgen overproduction. In the genotypic female, since ovaries and not testes are present, müllerian inhibiting factor is not produced, and the internal structures are female, i.e., uterus and fallopian tubes. Despite the increase in androgen production severe enough to masculinize the external genitalia, wolffian differentiation has never been described. Affected 46 XY males with either 21-hydroxylase or 11β-hydroxylase deficiency appear phenotypically normal at birth.

21-HYDROXYLASE DEFICIENCY. *Clinical Features.* 21-Hydroxylase deficiency is the most common cause of ambig-

TABLE 234–4. XX FEMALE PSEUDOHERMAPHRODITISM DUE TO CONGENITAL ADRENAL HYPERPLASIA

Enzyme Deficiency	External Genitalia		Salt-wasting	Hypertension	Cortisol	Mineralocorticoids		Androgens	
	Ambiguous	*Postnatal Virilization*							
21-Hydroxylase deficiency	+ + + +	+ + + +	50–80%	−	− ↓	*ALDO ↓		T	↑
						*B ↓		Δ4	↑ ↑
						*DOC ↓		17OHP	↑ ↑ ↑
11β-Hydroxylase deficiency†	+ + +	+ + + +	−	+ +	− ↓	ALDO ↓		T	↑
						B ↓		Δ4	↑ ↑
						DOC ↑		17OHP	↑ ↑
3β-Hydroxysteroid dehydrogenase deficiency	+ +	+ +	±	−	− ↓	ALDO ↓ −		DHEA	↑ ↑ ↑
						B ↓ −		17OH preg	↑
						DOC ↓			

*Mineralocorticoids are significantly decreased in the salt-wasting form of 21 OH deficiency.
†Elevated 11-deoxycortisol and desoxycorticosterone levels are diagnostic of 11β-hydroxylase deficiency.
↑ = elevated, ↓ = decreased, − = normal, + = relative frequency of occurrence; ALDO = aldosterone; B = corticosterone; DOC = desoxycorticosterone; T = testosterone; Δ4 = 4-androstenedione; 17OHP = 17-hydroxyprogesterone; DHEA = dehydroepiandrosterone; 17OH preg = 17α-hydroxypregnenolone.

uous genitalia in 46 XX infants. Its incidence varies from approximately 1 in 300 births in Alaskan Eskimos to 1 in 15,000 births in Caucasians in Wisconsin. The spectrum of masculinization varies from female infants with minimal clitoromegaly and fusion of the labioscrotal folds to infants with a penile urethra and the appearance of a cryptorchid male. Classically, if affected XX children are untreated in infancy, there is rapid acceleration of growth, enlargement of the clitoris, increase in muscle mass, precocious development of pubic, axillary, and body hair, and advancement of bone age. Although they are tall in childhood, premature closure of the epiphyses eventually results in short stature in adulthood. At the time of expected puberty, there is absence of breast development and menstruation. Untreated males with this condition also show precocious maturation and are short in stature in adulthood. The excessive androgen production can inhibit gonadotropin secretion, so that untreated adult males, although strongly virilized, can have small soft testes and azoospermia. However, because of the adrenal androgen excess, they are capable of having erections. Frequently, however, true puberty occurs in untreated males with normal FSH and LH secretion, testicular enlargement, and spermatogenesis. ACTH-dependent testicular "tumors" have been described and can occur either unilaterally or bilaterally; most probably they are of adrenal origin.

Two forms of 21-hydroxylase deficiency have been described, a simple form and a salt-losing form. Infants with the salt-losing form usually have an adrenal crisis within the first two weeks of life. Infants with the simple form do not show signs of adrenal crisis; ambiguity of the external genitalia is the most prominent feature.

Pathogenesis. 21-Hydroxylase deficiency results in decreased synthesis of cortisol with consequent increase in ACTH and increase in plasma progesterone, 17α-hydroxyprogesterone, and C19 androgens (dehydroepiandrosterone, androstenedione, and testosterone; Figure 234–6). In the newborn, determination of plasma 17α-hydroxyprogesterone is the test most diagnostic for this condition. The increased adrenal androgen production in the female fetus in utero results in virilization of the external genitalia. In the salt-losing form, there is a deficiency of aldosterone production. However, an additive factor in the salt loss may be due to increased production of progesterone and 17α-hydroxyprogesterone, which act as aldosterone antagonists.

The gene for 21-hydroxylase deficiency is closely linked to the HLA-B locus of chromosome 6. 21-OH deficiency associated with HLA-Bw47 results from an apparent deletion of a P-450$_{C21}$ structural gene. When 21-hydroxylase deficiency is associated with other HLA-B antigens, there is occasionally deletion of at least part of a gene. Obligate carrier parents and sibs predicted to be heterozygotes by HLA typing frequently demonstrate increased 17α-hydroxyprogesterone lev-

els in response to a one-hour ACTH stimulation test. Although the tests are extremely helpful in heterozygote detection, they are not uniformly conclusive. A late onset or attenuated variant of 21-hydroxylase deficiency has also recently been documented in adult women with hirsutism, or virilization and menstrual irregularities. HLA typing and ACTH testing of affected subjects' parents and sibs with this form also document linkage to HLA-B locus of chromosome 6, as in the classic form of congenital adrenal hyperplasia. It is proposed that they are genetic compounds of two recessive gene defects, 21-OH^{severe}/21-OH^{mild} defect. Family members, both males and females, have also been identified who have biochemical evidence of 21-hydroxylase deficiency but are without signs of virilization, hirsutism, amenorrhea, or infertility. These individuals are designated as having a cryptic form of 21-hydroxylase deficiency. It is proposed that they are genetic compounds, the result of two recessive gene defects, 21-OH^{mild}/21-OH^{mild}.

Management and Therapy. Affected females with 21-hydroxylase deficiency have ovaries and normal internal female structures with potential for fertility. Therefore, diagnosis and treatment should be carried out early and the child appropriately treated and raised as a female. Surgical correction of the masculinized external genitalia should be performed early so that gender confusion does not occur later on in childhood and adolescence. Medical therapy involves adequate glucocorticoid replacement therapy to lower ACTH secretion and to suppress adrenal androgen excess. Overtreatment should be avoided to prevent the signs and symptoms of glucocorticoid excess, which can lead to growth retardation.

Overt salt losers must be given mineralocorticoid as well as glucocorticoid replacement therapy. Many affected subjects without overt signs of adrenal crisis have impaired mineralocorticoid production, characterized by decreased sodium content and plasma volume with resultant increase in plasma renin. The increased plasma renin has been postulated to increase release of ACTH, necessitating more glucocorticoid replacement therapy. Thus mineralocorticoid supplementation should be considered in any subject with increase of plasma renin, despite the absence of signs of adrenal insufficiency.

Assessment of adequate therapy in a child is made on the basis of maintaining normal growth velocity, without signs of excess of either androgen or exogenous glucocorticoid. Monitoring plasma 17α-hydroxyprogesterone and plasma androgens has been helpful in regulating the glucocorticoid dosage; normalization of plasma androstenedione is the most reliable predictor of optimal therapy.

11β-HYDROXYLASE DEFICIENCY. Clinical Features. To date approximately 60 cases of 11β-hydroxylase deficiency have been described. In females with this disorder the enzyme deficiency at birth results in normal female genitalia to varying degrees of masculinization of the external genitalia. Adolescence results in mild hirsutism, clitoral hypertrophy, and irregular menses to severe virilization. Males with this condition show precocious male sexual maturation, but develop gynecomastia at puberty. The cause of the gynecomastia is not known, but it has been postulated to be secondary to elevated plasma desoxycorticosterone levels. Patients usually have hyporeninemic hypertension.

Pathogenesis. 11β-Hydroxylase deficiency results in decreased cortisol production, which causes an increase in ACTH, in C19 androgen secretion, and in desoxycorticosterone production (Fig. 234–6). Elevation of the plasma 11-desoxycortisol level is diagnostic of this enzyme deficiency and distinguishes it from 21-hydroxylase deficiency. Plasma cortisol as well as the urinary cortisol metabolites tetrahydrocortisone and tetrahydrocortisol can be normal to low. Urinary 17-ketosteroids, reflecting adrenal androgen overproduction, and urinary 17-hydroxysteroids, reflecting elevated levels of plasma 11-desoxycortisol, are increased. Excretion of pregnanetriol, a metabolite of 17α-hydroxyprogesterone, is usually normal or slightly increased. Plasma desoxycorticosterone is increased, as is its urinary metabolite tetrahydrodesoxycorticosterone, while corticosterone and aldosterone are decreased. The increased production of desoxycorticosterone results in salt retention, increased plasma volume, hypertension, and decreased plasma renin. Some affected subjects are not hypertensive and have a deficiency of the enzyme that appears to be limited to the 17α-hydroxylated pathway, with normal levels of plasma desoxycorticosterone and its urinary metabolites. This has been explained by postulating the presence of either two 11β-hydroxylase enzyme systems or two different regulatory systems for 17α-hydroxylase steroids and for 17-desoxysteroids.

Management and Therapy. Glucocorticoid replacement therapy will effect biochemical normalization, decrease blood pressure, and arrest precocious development. In females, surgical correction of the external genitalia should be carried out as in females with 21-hydroxylase deficiency.

Virilization of the Female Fetus Secondary to Excess Maternal Androgen Production or Exogenous Maternal Administration of Virilizing Hormones

Masculinization of the female infant has been demonstrated in mothers with ovarian luteomas, virilizing adrenal tumors, and untreated maternal congenital adrenal hyperplasia. Why virilization of the female fetus does not occur in all states of maternal hyperandrogenicity may be related to the onset and the degree of hyperandrogenicity and the potency of the androgens secreted. The placenta may also offer some protection for the fetus by aromatization of the maternal androgens to estrogens.

Administration of testosterone or its derivatives to pregnant women has been associated with virilization of the female fetus. These substances stimulate virilization of the external genitalia with no effect on differentiation of the wolffian ductal system. A causal relationship of the progestational agents progesterone, medroxyprogesterone, and 17α-hydroxyprogesterone has not been definitely proven. Paradoxic masculinization of the female fetus associated with maternal administration of diethylstilbestrol early in pregnancy has been reported rarely. The degree of genital masculinization is correlated with the time of initiation of treatment. The mechanism for the genital masculinization has been postulated to be secondary to inhibition of the enzyme 3β-hydroxysteroid dehydrogenase:Δ^{5-4} isomerase of diethylstilbestrol, with consequent increase of the weak androgen dehydroepiandrosterone and possibly other Δ^{5}-androgenic steroids.

White PC, New MI, Dupont B: Congenital adrenal hyperplasia. N Engl J Med 316:1519, 1580, 1987. *An excellent review and inclusive bibliography of the enzyme deficiencies resulting in adrenal hyperplasia, with particular emphasis on 21-hydroxylase deficiency; 107 references.*

235 THE TESTIS
Alvin M. Matsumoto

The testis has three major physiologic functions: (1) During embryogenesis, the testis plays a vital role in normal male sexual differentiation. Production of testosterone by the fetal testis stimulates the development and growth of male internal and external genitalia. The fetal testis also produces müllerian inhibitory factor, which prevents the differentiation of female internal genitalia (see Ch. 234). (2) Beginning at the time of puberty and continuing into adulthood, testosterone produced by the testis is necessary for the development and maintenance of secondary sexual characteristics (virility) and sexual functioning (libido and potency). (3) Spermatozoa produced by the testis are necessary for fertility.

Disorders of the testis are common and have profound effects on patients. Infertility affects approximately 14 per cent of all married couples in the reproductive age group. Disorders of sperm production cause or contribute to the infertility in 40 per cent of these couples; i.e., 5 to 6 per cent of all men wishing to father children are unable to do so because of a disorder of testicular function. Klinefelter's syndrome, which results in permanent androgen deficiency and infertility, affects approximately one in 400 to 500 males. Impotence and gynecomastia, which may result from testicular dysfunction, are very common complaints for which men seek medical attention. High doses of androgenic steroids are in widespread use by competitive athletes, often with serious side effects. Finally, cancer of the testis remains one of the most common fatal neoplasms of young men.

Disorders of the testis can be treated effectively. Testosterone replacement therapy in androgen-deficient men results in the development or restoration of secondary sexual characteristics and normal sexual functioning. Gonadotropin treatment of gonadotropin-deficient men often stimulates spermatogenesis and induces fertility in addition to restoring secretion of androgens. Finally, seminomas are exquisitely sensitive and responsive to radiation therapy, and the treatment of nonseminomatous testicular cancers with multidrug chemotherapy has markedly improved survival.

TESTICULAR STRUCTURE AND PHYSIOLOGY
Functional Anatomy

The normal adult testis weighs approximately 20 grams and normally measures 3.5 to 5.5 cm in length and 2.0 to 3.0 cm in width. Normal testis volume is between 15 and 30 ml. About 90 per cent of the volume of the testis is composed of seminiferous tubules, where spermatozoa are produced. Therefore, any significant reduction in testicular size is likely to be reflected in a decrease in total sperm production.

During fetal development, the testes descend from an intra-abdominal position into the scrotum. The scrotal location of the testes allows them to function at a temperature approximately 2°C lower than that of the abdomen. The pampiniform plexus of veins that drains the testes surrounds the testicular artery and cools the arterial blood supply to the testes by a countercurrent heat exchange mechanism. The lower testicular temperature is necessary for normal spermatogenesis in man. Failure of the testes to descend into the scrotum (cryptorchidism) impairs sperm production.

The testis is composed of two structurally distinct compartments: the *interstitial* or *Leydig cell compartment* and the *seminiferous tubule compartment* (Fig. 235–1). These compartments are responsible for the two major physiologic roles of the testis, namely production of testosterone and spermatozoa, respectively.

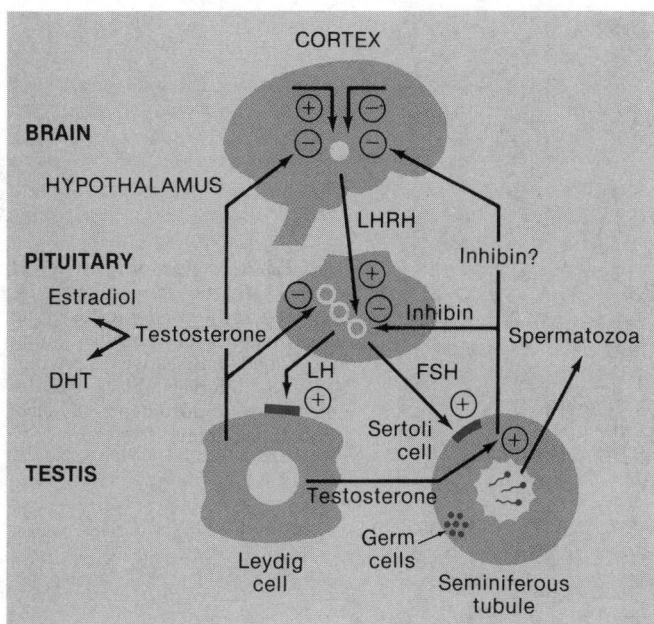

FIGURE 235–1. Diagram of the normal physiology of the hypothalamic-pituitary-testicular axis. (Adapted from Matsumoto AM, Bremner WJ: Bailliere's Clin Endocrinol Metab 1:71, 1987.)

The interstitial compartment is composed of *Leydig cells*, which produce sex steroid hormones, primarily testosterone. Leydig cells are nestled between seminiferous tubules, in close proximity to blood vessels. This location is important, since it facilitates delivery of high concentrations of testosterone to the seminiferous tubule compartment (intratesticular testosterone levels being approximately 100 times those found in peripheral blood) and the diffusion of testosterone into the blood vessels, for delivery to the rest of the body. The high intratesticular concentration of testosterone is important in stimulating normal spermatogenesis.

The seminiferous tubule compartment is composed of developing *germ cells* and *Sertoli cells*. Spermatogenesis involves the differentiation and maturation of spermatogonia, the most primitive germ cell, into spermatozoa. In humans, spermatogenesis takes approximately 74 days. Therefore, processes that adversely affect early spermatogenesis may not be manifest by reduced sperm counts in the ejaculate until 2 to 2½ months after the insult.

Sertoli cells perform many varied functions. By forming tight junctions at the basal portion of the seminiferous tubules, they maintain a barrier to the passage of macromolecules from the blood and interstitial compartment into the seminiferous tubules (the blood-testis barrier). Sertoli cells support spermatogenesis by synthesizing and secreting androgen-binding protein (ABP) and other protein products, by phagocytosing cellular remnants, and by participating in the movement and release of the maturing sperm and the secretion of fluid into the seminiferous tubule lumen. Sertoli cells produce *inhibin*, a glycoprotein that inhibits follicle-stimulating hormone secretion from the pituitary gland, but whose physiologic role remains unclear. They also produce another glycoprotein, *müllerian inhibitory factor (MIF)*, which is responsible, in the fetus, for causing the regression of the müllerian ducts (which normally develop into the female internal genitalia) during male sexual differentiation (see Ch. 234). Finally, Sertoli cells are capable of aromatizing testosterone to estradiol and producing paracrine factors that modulate Leydig cell function.

Central Nervous System Regulation of Gonadotropin Secretion

Normal testicular function depends on adequate stimulation by the gonadotropins, *luteinizing hormone (LH)*, and *follicle-*

stimulating hormone (FSH), which are secreted by the anterior pituitary gland (Fig. 235–1). Like thyroid-stimulating hormone and human chorionic gonadotropin (hCG), both LH and FSH are glycoprotein hormones composed of an alpha and a beta subunit. Alpha and beta subunits are synthesized separately, glycosylated, and noncovalently assembled prior to secretion from the pituitary. The alpha subunits of all four glycoprotein hormones are identical and biologically inactive, whereas the beta subunits are unique for each hormone and determine their biologic activity.

Measurements of serum gonadotropin levels are usually performed by radioimmunoassay (RIA). In normal young men, LH levels range from 5 to 20 mIU per milliliter, and FSH levels range from 5 to 25 mIU per milliliter (normal ranges will vary according to the reference preparations used). Most gonadotropin assays are not sufficiently sensitive to distinguish between low and low-normal gonadotropin levels. Therefore, a hormonal profile of low-normal gonadotropin levels and low testosterone levels is consistent with secondary hypogonadism (see below).

Serum gonadotropin measurements determined by RIA may not always reflect the levels of biologically active hormone present. Free alpha subunit is synthesized in excess and secreted into the circulation by the pituitary. Because it cross-reacts significantly with the RIA for the intact glycoprotein hormones but is biologically inactive, alterations in free alpha subunit production may result in discrepancies between gonadotropin levels determined by RIA and bioassay. Such discrepancies have been found in gonadotropin-secreting pituitary adenomas and alpha subunit–secreting tumors, such as pancreatic islet cell tumors. Discrepancies between the immunoreactivity and bioactivity of gonadotropins may also result from alterations in glycosylation, which can affect both their intrinsic biologic activity and their half-life in the circulation.

Both LH and, to a lesser extent, FSH are secreted into the peripheral circulation from the anterior pituitary in an episodic fashion (Fig. 235–2). Pulsatile gonadotropin secretion begins during sleep in early puberty, and by adulthood it is present throughout the day. Knowledge of the fluctuations of serum gonadotropin levels has influenced blood sampling regimens to determine normal values of these hormones.

The pulsatile secretion of gonadotropins is regulated primarily by the central nervous system through episodic stimulation of the pituitary by *LH releasing hormone (LHRH)*. LHRH, a decapeptide synthesized by hypothalamic neurons, stimulates release of both LH and FSH from the pituitary gland (see Fig. 235–1). Low-dose pulsatile LHRH administration has been used successfully to induce normal testicular function in patients with hypogonadotropic eunuchoidism, who presumably lack endogenous LHRH. By contrast, administration of high-dose, continuous LHRH or potent, long-acting LHRH agonists results in marked suppression of gonadotropin and testicular function. This paradoxic action of superactive LHRH agonists has been used clinically in the treatment of androgen-dependent tumors, such as prostate cancer.

The hypothalamic LHRH neuronal system plays an important integrative role in the regulation of testicular function (see Fig. 235–1). It receives input both from higher neural centers, such as the cerebral cortex and limbic system, through numerous stimulatory and inhibitory neurotransmitter (e.g., catecholamine and serotonin) and neuropeptide (e.g., opioid) systems and from testicular feedback signals, primarily sex steroid hormones. The input from these sources alters LHRH output, which, in turn, regulates pituitary gonadotropin secretion and testicular function. Increasing knowledge of how the central nervous system regulates LHRH secretion has helped increase our understanding of the mechanisms by which stress, malnutrition, and certain pharmacolgic agents (such as catecholaminergic and opiate drugs) affect testicular functon (Ch. 225).

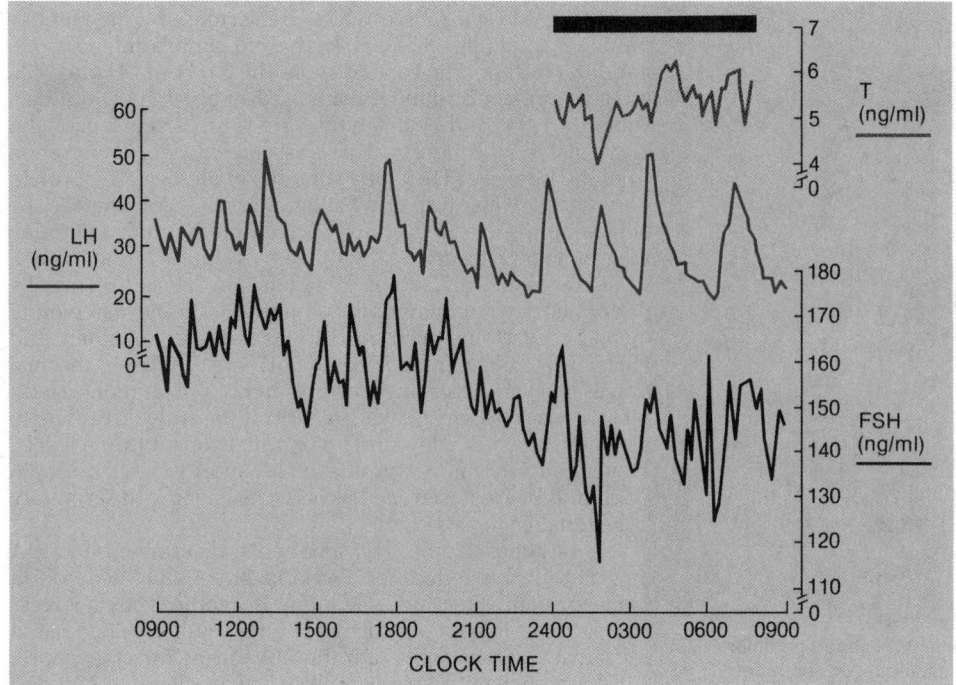

FIGURE 235–2. Example of pulsatile LH and FSH secretion throughout a 24-hour day and episodic testosterone secretion at night in a healthy young man. Blood samples were drawn at 10-minute intervals. Black bar denotes sleep, as documented by electroencephalogram.

Gonadotropin Regulation of Testicular Function

LH REGULATION OF TESTOSTERONE PRODUCTION. LH binds to specific membrane receptors on Leydig cells of the interstitial compartment of the testis and stimulates testicular steroidogenesis and secretion of *testosterone*, the major steroid product of the testis (see Fig. 235–1). LH increases the conversion of cholesterol to pregnenolone by the cholesterol side chain cleavage enzyme complex (20,22 desmolase), the rate-limiting step in testosterone biosynthesis.

Testosterone is secreted both locally within the testes and into the peripheral circulation (see Fig. 235–1). Healthy young men secrete approximately 7 mg of testosterone daily, essentially all from the Leydig cells. Total testosterone concentrations in plasma, as determined by RIA, range from 3 to 10 ng per milliliter (300 to 1000 ng per deciliter). Like gonadotropins, testosterone is secreted in a pulsatile fashion (Fig. 235–2).

In early puberty, testosterone secretion increases from very low to near adult levels during sleep in response to sleep-associated rises in LH levels. In adults, testosterone secretion occurs throughout the entire day. In young healthy men testosterone levels exhibit a circadian variation of about 1.5 ng per milliliter, with maximal levels occurring at 8 A.M. and minimal levels occurring at 9 P.M.

Under the influence of LH stimulation, Leydig cells also convert testosterone to *estradiol*. However, secretion of estradiol by the testis accounts for only about 15 per cent of the daily production of estradiol. The remainder of estradiol in blood is produced from testosterone and androstenedione (an adrenal androgen) by the enzyme aromatase in peripheral tissues (mostly adipose tissue).

TESTOSTERONE TRANSPORT. Like other steroid hormones, the majority of testosterone secreted into the circulation is bound to plasma proteins, primarily albumin and *sex hormone binding globulin (SHBG)*. Approximately 30 per cent of total testosterone is bound to SHBG and is not biologically available. Only 1 to 2 per cent is free (i.e., unbound to plasma proteins) and physiologically active. Albumin-bound testosterone seems also to be available to act on many target organs. Therefore, measurement of non–SHBG-bound testosterone may provide the best estimate of biologically available testosterone. In certain clinical situations (e.g., thyroid dysfunction, hepatic cirrhosis, and obesity), alterations in SHBG levels result in total testosterone measurements that do not reflect bioavailable testosterone levels. In these situations, free or non–SHBG-bound testosterone levels should be obtained.

PERIPHERAL METABOLISM OF TESTOSTERONE. The metabolism of circulating testosterone plays a very important role in its biologic actions on target tissues. Testosterone may be converted in peripheral tissues to either *dihydrotestosterone (DHT)* or *estradiol*, which mediates many of the physiologic actions of testosterone (see Fig. 235–1). These active metabolites of testosterone can be formed and act locally on androgen target tissues or circulate in blood and act on distant target tissues.

In many androgen-dependent target tissues, testosterone is converted intracellularly to a more potent androgen, DHT, by the enzyme 5 alpha-reductase. This conversion is required for normal male sexual differentiation. Males with 5 alpha-reductase deficiency, who cannot form DHT from testosterone in utero, fail to develop normal male external genitalia and as a result are born and raised as phenotypic females (Ch. 234). DHT is also thought to be important in mediating the androgenic effects of testosterone on skin and accessory sexual organs (i.e., prostate, seminal vesicles, and epididymis). In many peripheral tissues, especially in adipose tissue, testosterone is aromatized to estradiol, a potent estrogen. Obesity therefore results in increased peripheral estrogen formation. In men estrogens have diverse physiologic actions that may be agonistic or antagonistic to those of androgens. Therefore, the physiologic effects of testosterone result from the actions of testosterone itself in combination with those of its active metabolites, DHT and estradiol. Finally, 5 beta–reduced metabolites of androgens may be important mediators of androgen action on bone marrow.

Circulating testosterone and its active metabolites are metabolized to inactive metabolites mostly in the liver, and these inactive metabolites are excreted primarily in the urine. In sexual tissue (including skin and prostate), DHT is efficiently metabolized to 3 alpha-androstanediol and then to *3 alpha-androstanediol glucuronide (3 alpha-diol G)*. Blood and urine measurements of 3 alpha-diol G are useful markers of peripheral androgen action. In disorders in which DHT formation is reduced (such as 5 alpha-reductase deficiency), 3 alpha-diol G levels are reduced (Ch. 234).

ANDROGEN ACTION AND FUNCTIONS. At the target cell, testosterone and its active metabolites bind to intracellular androgen (in the case of testosterone and DHT) or estrogen

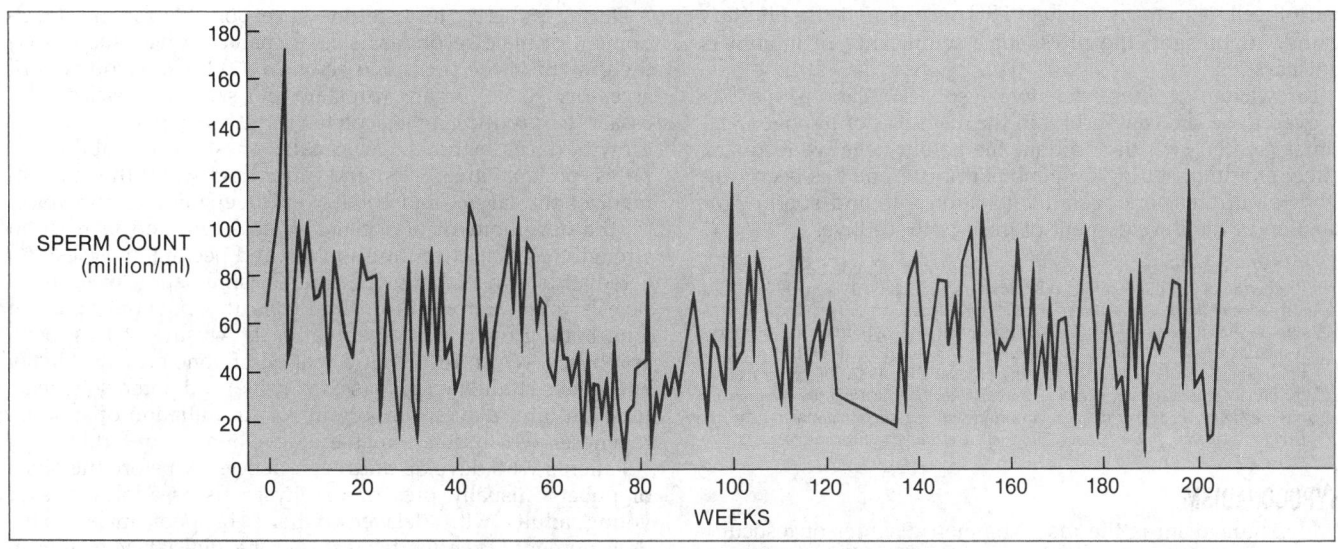

FIGURE 235–3. Example of the normal variations in sperm count in a healthy young man. Normal range of sperm count is generally considered to be between 20 and 200 million per milliliter. Despite good health and no medications, the sperm count may occasionally fall below the normal range, into the oligospermic range. (Adapted from Bardin CW, Paulsen CA: The testes. In Williams RH (ed.): Textbook of Endocrinology. 6th ed. Philadelphia, W.B. Saunders Company, 1981.)

(in the case of estradiol) receptors, which interact with specific chromosomal sites to ultimately alter protein synthesis, resulting in expression of androgen action (Ch. 221). Quantitative or qualitative abnormalities of the androgen receptor, resulting in impaired androgen action, cause varying degrees of male pseudohermaphroditism (Ch. 234).

The major functions of androgens are the differentiation of male internal and external genitalia (primary sexual characteristics) during embryogenesis; the development and maintenance of secondary sexual characteristics, sexual functioning (libido and potency), certain behavioral characteristics (such as aggression), and feedback regulation of gonadotropins; and the initiation and maintenance of spermatogenesis.

FSH REGULATION OF SERTOLI CELL FUNCTION. FSH binds to specific membrane receptors on Sertoli cells of the seminiferous tubule compartment of the testis and stimulates the production of seminiferous tubule fluid and a variety of proteins thought to be important in regulating spermatogenesis (e.g., ABP, transferrin, plasminogen activator), in feedback control of pituitary FSH secretion (inhibin), and possibly in intratesticular paracrine modulation of Leydig cell function (see Fig. 235–1). Testosterone produced by adjacent Leydig cells also regulates these Sertoli cell functions through androgen receptors. The relative roles of FSH and testosterone in the regulation of Sertoli cell function are poorly understood. Developing spermatogenic cells are enveloped in the cytoplasmic processes of the Sertoli cells, which nurture and coordinate the completion of sperm maturation in the seminiferous tubule.

HORMONAL CONTROL OF SPERMATOGENESIS. Both FSH and LH stimulation are required for the initiation of spermatogenesis at the time of puberty. At this time, LH causes the differentiation of Leydig cells from interstitial connective tissue precursors and stimulates them to produce high intratesticular levels of testosterone, which are essential for the initial phases of sperm production. By stimulating Sertoli cell function, FSH plays an important role in the later stages of spermatid maturation (spermiogenesis) during this initial wave of spermatogenesis.

Normal levels of either FSH or LH do not appear to be absolute requirements for the maintenance of spermatogenesis in adult men. Selective gonadotropin replacement in experimentally induced gonadotropin deficiency in adult men results in stimulation of qualitatively normal sperm production with either FSH or LH treatment alone. However, replacement of both LH and FSH is necessary to maintain quantitatively normal spermatogenesis in these hypogonadotropic men.

Clinically, replacement of both FSH and LH activity is generally required to initiate sperm production in prepubertal hypogonadotropic hypogonadal patients. In contrast, initiation and maintenance of spermatogenesis in postpubertal men with acquired hypogonadotropic hypogonadism can usually be achieved with replacement of LH activity alone.

Seminal fluid analysis is used to evaluate the function of the seminiferous tubules. It is performed on seminal fluid samples obtained by masturbation, usually after 48 hours of abstinence from ejaculation. Normal ejaculate volume ranges from 2 to 6 ml. Although the normal range of sperm concentration is generally considered to be 20 to 200 million per milliliter, sperm concentrations below 20 million per milliliter may be sufficient for fertility. In addition to determining sperm count, a careful microscopic examination of the seminal fluid is usually performed to assess sperm motility and morphology. Normally, greater than 60 per cent of sperm examined within one hour after ejaculation are motile, and greater than 60 per cent have a normal oval head morphology.

The minimal levels of sperm concentration, per cent motility, and per cent oval forms compatible with fertility are not clearly defined. In any individual, sperm counts normally exhibit extreme variability (Fig. 235–3) and are often temporarily suppressed by factors such as fever. Therefore, a reasonable estimate of mean sperm production requires at least three seminal fluid analyses over a two-month period. Functional tests of sperm penetration into cervical mucus of various mammalian species or zona pellucida–free hamster ova may be helpful in assessing fertilizing capability of spermatozoa.

Testicular Feedback Regulation of Gonadotropin Secretion

Both steroid and nonsteroidal products of the testis are involved in negative feedback control of pituitary gonadotropin secretion. Increased production of these testicular products results in suppression, whereas decreased production of these factors results in stimulation of gonadotropin secretion (see Fig. 235–1). Testosterone and its active metabolites, DHT and estradiol, exert profound inhibitory effects on both LH and FSH secretion, although the relative roles of these steroids are not clearly defined. Testosterone may affect both the hypothalamic release of LHRH and the pituitary sensitivity to LHRH stimulation. Inhibin, a glycoprotein product of the

Sertoli cell, selectively inhibits FSH secretion at the pituitary gland. At present, the physiologic significance of inhibin is unclear.

Knowledge of these negative feedback relationships has proved to be clinically useful in the diagnosis of hypogonadal states (see below). In addition, the potent negative feedback effect of administering exogenous testosterone has been utilized to suppress endogenous gonadotropin and sperm production in the development of male contraceptives.

Bardin CW: Pituitary-testicular axis. In Yen SSC, Jaffe RB (eds.): Reproductive Endocrinology. Philadelphia, WB Saunders Company, 1986, p 177. *A good discussion of the normal physiology of the reproductive axis.*

Matsumoto AM, Bremner WJ: Endocrinology of the hypothalamic-pituitary-testicular axis with particular reference to the hormonal control of spermatogenesis. Bailiere's Clin Endocrinol Metab 1:71, 1987. *This paper reviews the normal physiologic regulation of testicular function, which forms the basis for understanding the pathophysiology and treatment of testicular disorders. An up-to-date discussion of the hormonal regulation of human spermatogenesis is also provided.*

HYPOGONADISM

Hypogonadism is the most common disorder of testicular function encountered in clinical practice. The clinical manifestations of male hypogonadism differ depending on (1) whether there is *impairment of testosterone production*, which is nearly always accompanied by impairment of sperm production, or *isolated impairment of sperm production*, with normal testosterone production; (2) whether androgen deficiency occurs *during embryogenesis, before puberty,* or *after puberty;* and (3) whether testicular hypofunction is the result of a *primary* defect in the testis or is *secondary* to hypothalamic-pituitary dysfunction.

Androgen Deficiency

The clinical presentation of androgen deficiency depends on the stage of sexual development in which it occurs.

During early fetal development, testosterone and its active metabolite, DHT, mediate the differentiation of male internal and external genitalia from the wolffian duct system and the indifferent anlage of external genitalia, respectively. Androgen deficiency occurring during this period of development results in varying degrees of ambiguous genital development, or *male pseudohermaphroditism.* These disorders are discussed in greater detail in Ch. 234.

During puberty, testosterone is responsible for the development of male secondary sexual characteristics, such as (1) the growth of the penis and scrotum, (2) the development of accessory sexual organs (prostate and seminal vesicles) necessary to produce an ejaculate, (3) a male pattern of hair growth (face, external ear canals, chest, lower abdomen, pubis, perianal area, legs, and inner thighs), (4) the enlargement of the larynx and consequent deepening of the voice, (5) the development of skeletal musculature and increase in strength (especially in the shoulder and pectoral muscles), (6) a redistribution of body fat, and (7) stimulation of erythropoiesis. Testosterone also stimulates the pubertal spurt of long bone growth and, eventually, the closure of long bone epiphyses, which results in cessation of bone growth. Finally androgens stimulate libido (sexual drive) and potency (erectile function) and play an important role in initiation of spermatogenesis, which determines the development of fertility.

Patients who develop androgen deficiency before the onset of puberty usually present to physicians as adolescents or young adults with delayed puberty or poor male sexual development. Prepubertal testosterone deficiency results in *eunuchoidism* (Fig. 235–4), which is characterized by infantile development of genital and accessory sexual organs, failure to develop an ejaculate (aspermia), lack of male hair pattern, high-pitched voice, poor muscular development and strength, lower abdominal–pelvic girdle fat distribution, and excessive long bone growth (due to lack of closure of long bone epiphyses). The testes are small, usually less than 2 cm in length or 2 ml in volume. A eunuchoidal body habitus is characterized by excessively long arms and legs in proportion to height. Although there are racial differences in body proportions, eunuchoidal body measurements consist of an arm span that exceeds height by greater than 4 cm or a distance from the floor to the symphysis pubis that is greater than that from the symphysis to the crown of the head. Patients with prepubertal androgen deficiency fail to develop normal sexual functioning (libido and potency) and are infertile. Testosterone deficiency before puberty may occasionally result in gynecomastia (benign enlargement of breast tissue).

In the adult, testosterone is responsible for the maintenance of libido, potency, and secondary sexual characteristics and participates in the maintenance of spermatogenesis. The major

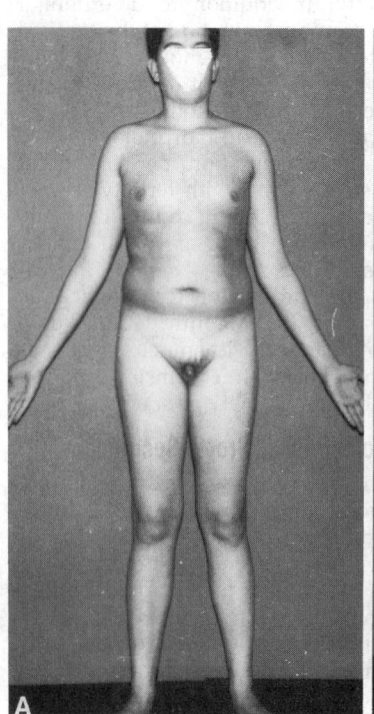
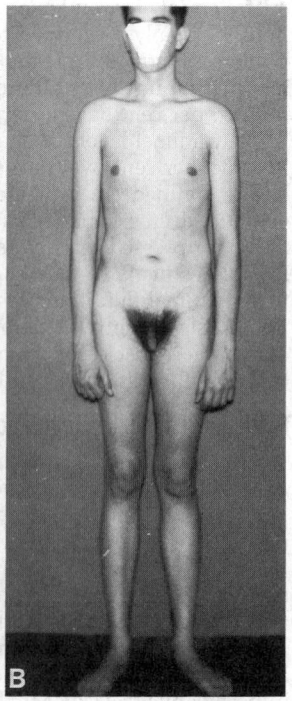
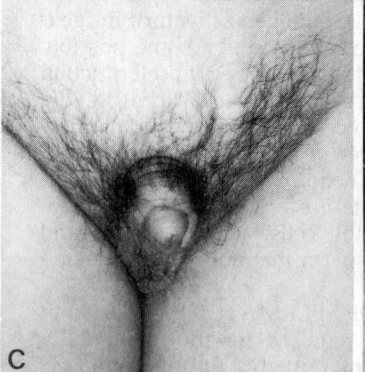
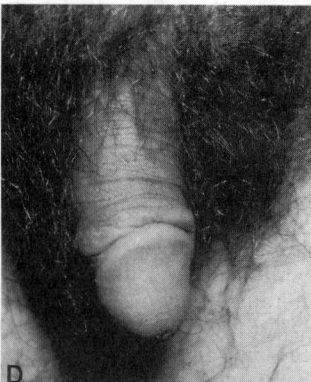

FIGURE 235–4. Example of eunuchoidism as a result of prepubertal androgen deficiency due to functional prepubertal castrate syndrome. *A* and *C,* Before androgen therapy, note the eunuchoidal features of infantile genital development, lack of male hair pattern, poor muscular development, pelvic girdle and abdominal fat distribution, and disproportionately long arms and legs. No testicular tissue was identified at the time of surgical exploration. *B* and *D,* After 18 months of testosterone treatment, scalp hair recession, penile development, and pubic hair growth have occurred. A masculine body habitus has developed, with an increase in pectoral and shoulder muscle development and loss of pelvic girdle and lower abdominal fat. (From Bardin CW, Paulsen CA: The testes. In Williams RH (ed.): Textbook of Endocrinology. 6th ed. Philadelphia, W.B. Saunders Company, 1981.)

complaints of men with adult-onset androgen deficiency are poor sexual performance, as a result of diminished libido and/or impotence; infertility, as a result of impaired spermatogenesis; and gynecomastia. Rapid development of severe androgen deficiency (such as surgical castration) may also result in vasomotor instability or hot flushes, similar to those that many women develop at the time of menopause. Androgen deficiency may also result in behavioral changes, such as passivity, lack of motivation, and irritability.

Secondary sexual characteristics do not regress to the prepubertal state in men who develop testosterone deficiency as adults. However, with long-standing androgen deficiency, there may be significant loss of hair in androgen-dependent areas of the body, fine wrinkling of skin (most noticeable around the eyes and mouth), diminished muscle strength, and altered fat distribution. The amount and distribution of facial and body hair vary considerably, depending on an individual's ethnic and genetic background. The testes are usually small in hypogonadal states that result in androgen deficiency. However, depending on the specific cause and severity of the disorder, testis size may be normal. For example, men with recent onset of gonadotropin deficiency from a destructive pituitary tumor may have normal size testes, despite severe testosterone deficiency.

Serum testosterone levels are low in states of androgen deficiency. Very sensitive and specific RIAs for serum testosterone are generally available and are relatively inexpensive. Routinely available assays measure total testosterone and may give falsely low values in clinical states in which sex hormone binding globulin is reduced (such as protein deficiency states and obesity). In these instances, free serum testosterone levels should be measured.

Testosterone helps to maintain quantitatively normal spermatogenesis in man; androgen deficiency, therefore, almost always results in abnormalities in sperm production. Impaired spermatogenesis is usually confirmed by a low sperm count on seminal fluid analysis. Sperm counts are highly variable in any individual and are often suppressed by illness (e.g., fever). At least three sperm counts should be obtained over a period of two months, while patients are well, before diagnosing low sperm counts (oligospermia).

Isolated Deficiency in Sperm Production

In contrast to patients with androgen deficiency, men with an isolated deficiency of sperm production present postpubertally with infertility as their major complaint, without symptoms of testosterone deficiency. Testis size may be reduced or normal and an undescended testis or *varicocele* (varicose dilatation of the pampiniform venous plexus of the testis) may be found. The remainder of the physical examination is usually unremarkable. Sperm counts are usually low (less than 20 million per milliliter) or zero (*azoospermia*), and there may be isolated or associated abnormalities of sperm motility and/or morphology on seminal fluid analysis. Serum testosterone levels are normal in disorders causing isolated impairment of sperm production.

Differential Diagnosis

The major manifestations of androgen deficiency in adults are impotence, infertility, and gynecomastia. Although hypogonadism resulting in testosterone deficiency is a major cause of these clinical manifestations, there are many other causes.

IMPOTENCE. Impotence is defined as the inability to achieve or maintain penile erection that is adequate for completion of intercourse. It is a commonly encountered complaint in medical practice, occurring in 10 to 35 per cent of adult men with medical problems and increasing in prevalence with advancing age. Impotence is often underdiagnosed because of reluctance of patients and physicians to discuss sexual

TABLE 235–1. CAUSES OF IMPOTENCE

Disorders of Central Nervous System Control	Disorders of Peripheral Erectile Response
Psychiatric Illness	Autonomic Neuropathy
Stress	Pelvic surgery
Performance anxiety	Sympatholytic drugs
Depression	Anticholinergic drugs
Major psychiatric illness	Diabetes
Chronic Illness	Vascular Disease
Cardiac disease	Distal aortoiliac
Respiratory disease	atherosclerosis
Renal disease	Trauma
Liver disease	Venous incompetence
Malignancy	Penile Abnormalities
Central Nervous System–	Peyronie's disease
Active Drugs	Priapism
Sedatives	Chordee
Tranquilizers	Microphallus or
Antidepressants	micropenis
Antihypertensive agents	
Alcohol	
Endocrine Disorders	
Androgen deficiency	
Hyperprolactinemia	
Thyroid disease	
Central Nervous System Disease	
Temporal lobe disorders	
Limbic system disorders	
Spinal Cord Disease	
Trauma	
Multiple sclerosis	
Syphilis	

dysfunction as a medical problem. Although psychogenic impotence is common, the majority of men with impotence who are followed in a general medical clinic have one or more organic causes of erectile dysfunction. Furthermore, organic causes of impotence often result in performance anxiety and secondary psychogenic sexual dysfunction.

Penile erection sufficient to complete intercourse requires (1) normal *central nervous system* and thoracolumbar sympathetic and sacral parasympathetic *spinal cord* outputs to the penis; (2) an intact *arterial supply* and *venous drainage* of the penis; and (3) an *anatomically normal penis*. Dysfunction of any of these components will interfere with normal initiation and maintenance of penile erection (Table 235–1).

Normal central nervous system function is necessary to produce adequate penile erections. *Libido* or sexual desire is mediated by the cerebral cortex and has a profound influence on erectile function. In most central nervous system disorders that cause sexual dysfunction, reduced libido is usually associated with impotence. All degrees of *psychiatric disturbance*, from minor stress and performance anxiety to major psychiatric illness, such as depression and schizophrenia; *chronic debilitating illness*, such as cardiac, respiratory, renal, or liver disease or malignancy; and *drugs* that affect central nervous system function (sedatives, tranquilizers, antidepressants, certain antihypertensive agents, and alcohol), are central nervous system causes of impotence and generally reduce libido as well as erectile function. *Androgen deficiency, hyperprolactinemia*, and *thyroid dysfunction* also impair libido and potency. Elevated prolactin levels may cause impotence by inducing secondary hypogonadism and androgen deficiency. However, impotence may not resolve with androgen replacement therapy alone and may require, in addition, therapy aimed at reducing the elevated prolactin levels. In contrast to these disorders, *destructive or infiltrative diseases* of other parts of the *brain* (such as tumor or infarction of the temporal lobe or limbic system) or *spinal cord* (such as injury, tumor, multiple sclerosis, or syphilis) may cause impotence without associated loss of libido.

In addition to intact central nervous system functioning, normal penile erection requires intact peripheral nervous system functioning, adequate blood flow to the penis, and normal erectile structures within the penis. *Disorders of peripheral autonomic nerve function* which cause impotence include extensive pelvic surgery, such as aortoiliac bypass, pelvic lymph node dissection, abdominoperineal resection of the rectum, lumbar sympathectomy, and prostatectomy; sympatholytic and anticholinergic drugs; and diabetes. Atherosclerotic *peripheral vascular disease* involving the distal aortoiliac arteries and *trauma* to these vessels are the most common causes of vascular impotence. These patients usually have diminished or absent femoral pulses and may present with *Leriche's syndrome*, although claudication may be absent in some cases. Penile venous incompetence is a rare cause of impotence. *Penile abnormalities*, such as Peyronie's disease, chordee, priapism, and microphallus, may also cause erectile dysfunction.

Normal testosterone levels are necessary for maintenance of libido and potency. Hypogonadism resulting in androgen deficiency is a cause of impotence in approximately 15 to 20 per cent of men complaining of sexual dysfunction in a general medical clinic. Therefore, all impotent patients should have serum testosterone and gonadotropin levels measured as part of their diagnostic work-up.

INFERTILITY. Infertility is defined as the inability of a couple to achieve a pregnancy after one year of unprotected intercourse. An estimated 5 to 6 per cent of men in the reproductive age group are infertile. Most causes of male infertility result in abnormal sperm count or semen quality, as reflected by an abnormal seminal fluid analysis. About 90 per cent of male infertility is caused by hypogonadism resulting in impaired spermatogenesis; and 80 to 90 per cent of these men have isolated deficiency of sperm production with normal androgen production of unclear etiology, i.e., *idiopathic oligospermia or azoospermia* (see below). Other causes of male infertility include *coital disorders, ductal obstruction, ejaculatory dysfunction,* and *disorders of accessory sexual organs* (Table 235–2). Even if a cause of male infertility is diagnosed, the female partner should undergo diagnostic evaluation, since a concomitant female factor causing infertility is found in 30 per cent of infertile couples.

Although uncommon, *defects* in the *coital technique*, such as timing of intercourse during menses, rather than at the time of ovulation near mid-cycle, premature withdrawal of the penis, prior ejaculation, and infrequent intercourse are causes of male infertility. They are important to remember because they are potentially reversible with proper patient education. Basal body temperature measurements or rapid RIA kits measuring urinary LH levels are commercially available methods often used to estimate the timing of ovulation in the partner's menstrual cycle. *Erectile dysfunction* from any cause may result in unsuccessful intercourse and infertility.

Impediment of sperm transport from the testis to the urethra results in azoospermia and infertility. Causes of *ductal*

TABLE 235–2. CAUSES OF MALE INFERTILITY

Coital Disorders
  Defects in Technique
    Poor timing with menses
    Premature withdrawal
    Infrequent intercourse
  Impotence

Hypogonadism (Deficiency of Sperm Production)

Ductal Obstruction
  Congenital Defects of Vas Deferens and Seminal Vesicles
  Postinfectious Obstruction
  Cystic Fibrosis/Young's Syndrome
  Vasectomy

Ejaculatory Dysfunction
  Premature Ejaculation
  Retrograde Ejaculation

Disorders of Accessory Glands
  Epididymitis/Seminal Vesiculitis/Prostatitis
  Immunologic

obstruction include congenital absence of the vas deferens or seminal vesicles; congenital defects of the epididymis or vas, e.g., as a consequence of diethylstilbestrol exposure in utero; fibrosis as a complication of genitourinary infection, especially epididymitis; cystic fibrosis or Young's syndrome, in which thickened, inspissated mucous secretions lead to blockage of the epididymis and vas deferens; and vasectomy. Obstructive azoospermia must be differentiated from a severe defect in spermatogenesis. Measurement of a serum FSH level is often helpful, since elevated levels generally indicate disordered seminiferous tubular function. Normal FSH levels may occur in either obstructive azoospermia or seminiferous tubule dysfunction. In obstructive azoospermia, radiologic examination, i.e., a vasogram, will demonstrate the ductal obstruction, and a testicular biopsy will reveal normal spermatogenesis. Evaluation of azoospermia is one of the few indications for performing a testicular biopsy. Vasectomy has been used widely and successfully to induce infertility in men who desire fertility control, without any deleterious effects on the hypothalamic-pituitary-testicular axis or general health.

Ejaculatory dysfunction, such as premature or retrograde ejaculation, can cause infertility by preventing the normal deposition of sperm into the female genital tract. Premature ejaculation is often successfully treated by sex therapy techniques. Retrograde ejaculation most commonly results from diabetic autonomic neuropathy, prostatic resection, pelvic surgery, or administration of sympatholytic drugs. It is suspected if orgasm produces little or no ejaculate and is confirmed by the presence of large numbers of sperm in a postejaculation urine sample. Sympathomimetic drugs, imipramine, and harvesting and concentrating of sperm from the urine for artificial insemination have been used to treat retrograde ejaculation.

Disorders of the *accessory sexual organs* result in infertility by a number of mechanisms. Infections of the epididymis, seminal vesicles, and/or prostate have been reported to cause infertility by affecting sperm maturation or function directly or by inducing antisperm antibodies that, in turn, affect sperm function. Antisperm antibodies present in the semen may cause sperm agglutination and reduce sperm motility. Induction of these antibodies after vasectomy may be responsible for the discrepancy between the success rate for return of sperm in the ejaculate (90 per cent) and restoration of fertility (50 per cent) after vasectomy reversal.

GYNECOMASTIA. Gynecomastia, a benign glandular enlargement of the male breast, is usually asymptomatic, but its rapid development may cause pain and tenderness. It is often very difficult to distinguish between true gynecomastia and an increase in adipose tissue in obese boys or men. Gynecomastia must also be distinguished from other benign chest wall tumors that may occur on or near the breast, such as lipomas, neurofibromas, and lymphomas, and from male breast cancer. Gynecomastia usually results from an increased circulating estrogen level relative to the testosterone level, i.e., an increased estrogen/testosterone ratio. This may result from either an increased estrogen level or from a decreased testosterone level. Unless hyperprolactinemia induces severe androgen deficiency by inhibiting gonadotropin secretion, elevated serum prolactin levels do not usually cause gynecomastia. The clinical causes of gynecomastia are summarized in Table 235–3.

Gynecomastia may sometimes be *physiologic* rather than pathologic. Transient gynecomastia is usually seen in neonatal boys, as a result of exposure in utero to high maternal estrogen concentrations. At the time of puberty, gynecomastia is observed in 60 to 70 per cent of boys. This pubertal gynecomastia usually lasts for months to years and does not persist into adulthood. Although there is a transient rise in the estrogen/testosterone ratio during puberty, the pathogenesis of pubertal gynecomastia is unclear. Finally, small amounts of palpable breast tissue can be detected by careful examination

TABLE 235–3. CAUSES OF GYNECOMASTIA

Physiologic Gynecomastia
  Neonatal
  Pubertal
  Adult
 	
Hypogonadism (Deficiency of Androgen Production)
 	
Androgen Resistance Syndromes
Drug-Induced
  Hormones
    Estrogens
    Aromatizable androgens
    hCG
  Drugs Interacting with Estrogen
  Receptor
    Marijuana
    Digitalis
  Drugs Altering Androgen
  Production or Action
    Spironolactone
    Cimetidine
    Ketoconazole
    Cytotoxic agents
  Central Nervous System–
  Active Drugs
    Antihypertensive agents
    Tranquilizers
    Sedatives
    Antidepressants
    Amphetamines
	Tumors
	  Estrogen-Secreting Tumors
	    Adrenal carcinoma
	    Leydig cell or Sertoli cell
	      tumor of testis
	  Gonadotropin-Secreting
	  Tumors
	    Testicular carcinoma
	    Lung carcinoma
	    Liver carcinoma
	
	Systemic Disorders
	  Hepatic Cirrhosis
	  Renal Failure
	  Thyrotoxicosis
	
	Miscellaneous
	  Refeeding Gynecomastia
	  Familial
	  Increased Peripheral
	    Aromatization
	  Local Chest
	    Trauma

in 40 per cent of healthy normal adult men, increasing in prevalence with advancing age. This mild gynecomastia is always asymptomatic and generally goes unnoticed.

Most of the pathologic causes of gynecomastia are associated with alterations in the hypothalamic-pituitary-testicular axis, resulting in a hypogonadal hormonal profile. Gynecomastia may occur with any of the causes of hypogonadism that result in *androgen deficiency*, including both primary testicular disorders and those secondary to gonadotropin deficiency.

In addition to androgen deficiency or *disorders of androgen action*, gynecomastia may be caused by a number of *drugs*. Gynecomastia may result from exposure to exogenous estrogen, e.g., from administration of diethylstilbestrol for metastatic prostate cancer, ingestion of estrogen-treated animal foodstuffs, use of or contact with estrogen-containing creams, and accidental occupational exposure. Excessive circulating estrogens inhibit endogenous gonadotropin secretion, which results, in turn, in reduced testosterone production. Secondary hypogonadism induced by estrogens may contribute to the development of gynecomastia. Administration of high doses of aromatizable androgens, especially to prepubertal boys or severely hypogonadal men, may induce gynecomastia analogous to that which occurs at puberty. Human chorionic gonadotropin (hCG) binds to the LH receptor on the Leydig cell of the testis and has biologic activities identical to those of LH. By stimulating relatively greater testicular production of estradiol compared to testosterone, hCG treatment of hypogonadotropic hypogonadal men may cause gynecomastia. Certain drugs result in breast enlargement by interacting with the estrogen receptor (marijuana, digitalis) or by interfering with androgen production or action (spironolactone, cimetidine, ketoconazole, certain chemotherapeutic agents). Finally, many central nervous system–active drugs, such as certain antihypertensives, sedatives, tranquilizers, antidepressants, and amphetamines, are associated with gynecomastia.

Although very uncommon, gynecomastia may be the initial manifestation of an *estrogen-secreting tumor* of the adrenal gland or testis. Feminizing adrenal tumors are usually malignant and present with a palpable abdominal mass. In contrast, estrogen-secreting tumors of the testis are often small and benign. Unlike many exogenous estrogen preparations, which do not cross-react with the RIA for estradiol, these tumors secrete large amounts of estradiol, which are detected in blood by clinically available estrogen assays. *hCG-secreting tumors*, such as testicular, lung, and hepatic carcinoma, may cause gynecomastia by stimulating excessive estrogen relative to testosterone secretion by Leydig cells. hCG cross-reacts with most routinely available LH assays; patients with hCG-secreting tumors may therefore have elevated LH levels. Also, since LH cross-reacts with most intact hCG assays, a specific beta-hCG assay should be used to confirm the diagnosis of an hCG-secreting tumor.

Certain *systemic disorders* are associated with gynecomastia. In hepatic cirrhosis, gynecomastia is associated with increased estrogen production, primarily by accelerated peripheral conversion of adrenal androgens (androstenedione) to estrone. In addition, serum SHBG levels are elevated, and total and bioavailable serum testosterone levels are low, which also favor an increased estrogen/testosterone ratio. The gynecomastia observed in patients with renal failure is associated with androgen deficiency resulting from primary testicular failure, and estrogen production is not increased. High estradiol levels and relatively reduced bioavailable testosterone levels (as a result of increased SHBG levels) are commonly found in patients with thyrotoxicosis and contribute to the development of gynecomastia in this condition.

Gynecomastia is often associated with nutritional repletion and weight gain after a period of starvation and weight loss. This *refeeding gynecomastia* was originally described in former prisoners of World War II who developed tender gynecomastia following their liberation and resumption of a normal diet. A similar condition may occur upon recovery from any prolonged, severe illness associated with malnutrition and weight loss. Refeeding gynecomastia may contribute to the gynecomastia associated with hemodialysis in chronic renal failure patients and to that related to isoniazid treatment in men with tuberculosis. Malnutrition results in severe suppression of the hypothalamic-pituitary-testicular axis. Refeeding and restoration of nutrition and body weight result in resumption of normal gonadal function, a dynamic hormonal situation similar to the onset of puberty. The rapid restoration of gonadal function ("second puberty") may explain the gynecomastia associated with refeeding. *Familial gynecomastia* and *idiopathic increase in peripheral aromatase activity* are very rare causes of gynecomastia.

Treatment of gynecomastia should be focused on the correction of the underlying disorder or withdrawal of the offending drug. Prophylactic low-dose irradiation of the breast prior to the institution of diethylstilbestrol treatment in men with prostatic carcinoma will prevent gynecomastia. Testosterone treatment of androgen deficiency may occasionally result in resolution of gynecomastia. However, severe, longstanding gynecomastia of any cause is usually associated with increased fibrous tissue stroma and requires surgical reduction mammoplasty.

Carlson HE: Gynecomastia. N Engl J Med 303:795, 1980. *A review of the causes and treatment of gynecomastia.*

Morley JE: Impotence. Am J Med 80:897, 1986. *This paper reviews the physiology of penile erection and the causes, evaluation, and treatment of impotence.*

Slag MF, Morley JE, Elson MK, et al.: Impotence in medical clinic outpatients. JAMA 249:1736, 1983. *A large study of 1180 men in a medical outpatient clinic who were screened for the presence of impotence. 401 men (34 per cent) were impotent, and evaluation of the causes of impotence in 188 men revealed hypogonadism in 19 per cent.*

Swerdloff RS: Infertility in the male. Ann Intern Med 103:906, 1985. *This is an extensive review of the diagnostic evaluation and treatment of male infertility (over 100 references).*

CAUSES OF MALE HYPOGONADISM

Once the diagnosis of male hypogonadism is suspected from the clinical manifestations described above, the diagnosis is confirmed by measurement of serum testosterone level and sperm count. A low serum testosterone concentration confirms androgen deficiency, and reduced sperm counts confirm a deficiency in sperm production.

The majority of hypogonadal men with *androgen deficiency* also have impairment in sperm production. Once androgen deficiency is diagnosed (low serum testosterone and sperm count), an effort should be made to distinguish between disorders that result from primary testicular disease (*primary hypogonadism*) and those that are secondary to inadequate gonadotropin stimulation of the testis (*secondary hypogonadism*), as a result of either pituitary or hypothalamic disease. In addition to helping to define the specific etiology of androgen deficiency, the distinction between primary and secondary hypogonadism may have practical therapeutic implications. For example, regardless of the specific etiology, primary hypogonadism is usually treated with androgen replacement. In the majority of cases, the infertility in primary hypogonadism is not treatable. However, secondary hypogonadism may result from destruction of pituitary gonadotropin-secreting cells by a pituitary tumor. In this instance, in addition to androgen deficiency, the space-occupying effects of the tumor mass on brain function (such as visual fields and cerebroventricular flow) and alterations (both increase and decrease) in the secretion of other anterior pituitary hormones (such as ACTH, TSH, growth hormone, and prolactin) need to be considered in formulating a therapeutic plan (Ch. 226). Furthermore, since the testes usually function normally in response to adequate gonadotropin stimulation in patients with secondary hypogonadism, gonadotropins or LHRH may be administered in these patients to stimulate spermatogenesis and induce fertility.

The negative feedback relationship between gonadotropin secretion and circulating testosterone levels (see Fig. 235–1) provides the physiologic basis and rationale for the use of serum gonadotropin levels to distinguish between primary and secondary testicular disorders that result in androgen deficiency. Because the negative feedback effect of testosterone on gonadotropin secretion is reduced, men with *primary hypogonadism* have reduced serum testosterone and elevated serum LH and FSH levels; i.e., they have *hypergonadotropic hypogonadism*. Not uncommonly, serum FSH levels may be disproportionately elevated compared to LH levels, especially with severe seminiferous tubule dysfunction. However, selective elevation of serum LH levels is distinctly unusual and suggests the presence of a substance, such as hCG or alpha subunit, that cross-reacts in the RIA for LH. In contrast to primary testicular dysfunction, men with *secondary hypogonadism* are not able to increase gonadotropin secretion appropriately in the presence of reduced testosterone negative feedback and have inadequate gonadotropin stimulation of the testis. These men have a hormonal pattern of reduced serum testosterone and low to low normal serum LH and FSH levels; i.e., they have *hypogonadotropic hypogonadism*. Gonadotropin levels are often in the low normal range in men with secondary hypogonadism because most clinically available gonadotropin assays lack sufficient sensitivity to distinguish low from low normal values.

The majority of hypogonadal patients with *isolated impairment of sperm production* have primary testicular disease. These patients generally present with infertility and have no clinical manifestations of androgen deficiency, and serum testosterone and gonadotropin levels are usually normal. Therefore, hormone determinations are not routinely obtained as part of an infertility work-up unless clinical androgen deficiency is also present. Infertile patients who present with no sperm in their ejaculate, i.e., azoospermia, may have either severe seminiferous tubule failure or obstruction of the genital tract. Measurement of serum FSH level may be helpful in evaluation of an azoospermic patient. A selective elevation of serum FSH levels with normal LH levels in a patient with azoospermia implies severe germ cell dysfunction with loss of negative feedback influences (such as inhibin) on the pituitary gland and poor prognosis for fertility. No further work-up is usually necessary. A normal serum FSH level in an azoospermic

patient leaves open the possibility of a surgically correctable ductal obstruction, and a vasogram and testicular biopsy is usually performed. In addition to severe seminiferous tubule dysfunction, selective elevation in serum FSH levels may be observed in patients with gonadotropin-secreting pituitary adenomas. Uncommonly, isolated deficiency of sperm production results from inadequate gonadotropin stimulation of the testis. In these instances, serum gonadotropin levels are generally reduced, and very rarely selective FSH deficiency may occur.

The vast majority of adults with male hypogonadism have either primary or secondary testicular failure. Very rarely, *disorders of androgen action* may present in adults with a clinical picture of hypogonadism. Unlike the severe androgen resistance syndromes, which present at birth with male pseudohermaphroditism (Ch. 234), these disorders are characterized by mild defects in androgen action, resulting in a nearly normal male phenotype (frequently with varying degrees of hypospadius). Both serum testosterone and gonadotropin levels are usually elevated.

In summary, clinical manifestations combined with measurements of serum testosterone, sperm count, and basal serum gonadotropin levels permit a physiologic classification of the causes of male hypogonadism into *primary* and *secondary hypogonadism* and subclassification into disorders that result in *deficiencies of both sperm and androgen production* and those with *isolated deficiency in sperm production* with normal androgen production (Table 235–4).

Primary Hypogonadism

DEFICIENCY OF SPERM AND ANDROGEN PRODUCTION. *Congenital or Developmental Disorders.* *Klinefelter's syndrome* is the most common cause of primary testicular failure resulting in impairment of both spermatogenesis and testosterone production. The syndrome is characterized by small, firm testes, azoospermia, gynecomastia, varying degrees of eunuchoidism and testosterone deficiency, and elevated gonadotropin levels. Klinefelter's syndrome is a very common disorder, affecting 1 in every 400 to 500 men. The incidence of this syndrome, in particular of its variants, is significantly increased in mentally retarded individuals. The fundamental defect in Klinefelter's syndrome and its variants is the presence of one or a number of extra X chromosomes.

Classically, the karyotype in Klinefelter's syndrome is 47 XXY. Variants of the syndrome demonstrate a variety of karyotypes, including XXYY, more than two X (poly X) plus Y, and mosaicism. The karyotypes in mosaic Klinefelter's syndrome are a combination of the normal, classic, and variant karyotypes and may vary among different tissues within the same individual. In classic Klinefelter's syndrome (47 XXY), the presence of an extra X chromosome is responsible for the presence of a sex chromatin or Barr body in the nucleus of epithelial cells obtained on buccal smear, a normal finding in females, who carry two X chromosomes. Variant syndromes characterized by more than two X chromosomes may exhibit more than one Barr body per nucleus, the number of sex chromatin bodies always being one less than the number of X chromosomes.

Although Klinefelter's disease is a congenital disorder, clinical features are not evident prior to puberty. At the time of puberty, the testes fail to increase in size and become firmer in consistency. This is a result of fibrosis and hyalinization of the seminiferous tubules. The most remarkable clinical feature of Klinefelter's syndrome is the very small size of the testes, rarely exceeding 2 cm in length, in contrast to a lower limit of 3.5 cm in the normal adult. Clinical androgen deficiency is usually present, but the degree of androgen deficiency is variable, resulting in varying degrees of eunuchoidism (Fig. 235–5). In contrast to other conditions that result in prepubertal androgen deficiency and classic eunuchoidism (see above), Klinefelter's syndrome often results in a dispro-

TABLE 235–4. CAUSES OF MALE HYPOGONADISM

Primary Hypogonadism
Deficiency of Sperm and Androgen Production
  Congenital or Developmental Disorders
    Klinefelter's syndrome and variants
    Functional prepubertal castrate syndrome
    Noonan (Bonnevie-Ullrich) syndrome
    Myotonic dystrophy
    Polyglandular autoimmune disease
    Complex genetic disorders
    ? Normal aging
  Acquired Disorders
    Orchitis (mumps, leprosy, etc.)
    Surgical or traumatic castration
    Drugs (spironolactone, ketoconazole, alcohol, digitalis, cytotoxic drugs)
    Irradiation
  Systemic Disorders
    Chronic liver disease
    Chronic renal failure
    Sickle cell disease
    Paraplegia
Isolated Deficiency of Sperm Production
  Congenital or Developmental Disorders
    Germinal cell aplasia (Sertoli cell–only syndrome)
    Cryptorchidism
    Varicocele
    Immotile cilia syndrome (Kartagener's syndrome)
    Myotonic dystrophy
  Acquired Disorders
    Orchitis (mumps, leprosy, etc.)
    Thermal trauma
    Irradiation
    Cytotoxic drugs
    Environmental Toxins
  Systemic Disorders
    Acute febrile illness
    Paraplegia
  Idiopathic Oligospermia or Azoospermia

Secondary Hypogonadism
Deficiency of Sperm and Androgen Production
  Congenital or Developmental Disorders
    Hypogonadotropic eunuchoidism (Kallmann's syndrome)
    Hemochromatosis
    Complex genetic syndromes
  Acquired Disorders
    Hypopituitarism
    Hyperprolactinemia
    Estrogen excess
    Progestins
    Opiate-like drugs
  Systemic Disorders
    Glucocorticoid excess (Cushing's syndrome)
    Acute stress or illness
    Nutritional deficiency (protein-calorie malnutrition, anorexia nervosa)
    Chronic illness
    Massive obesity
Isolated Deficiency of Sperm Production
  Androgen Excess
    Congenital adrenal hyperplasia (21- and 11-hydroxylase deficiency)
    Androgenic anabolic steroids
    Androgen-secreting tumors
  Hyperprolactinemia
  Isolated FSH Deficiency

Androgen Resistance Syndromes
Reifenstein's Syndrome
Idiopathic Oligospermia or Azoospermia

portionate increase in lower extremity compared to upper extremity long bone growth. Careful palpation usually reveals bilateral gynecomastia in about 80 to 90 per cent of patients. Although the incidence of mental retardation is greater, the majority of patients with Klinefelter's syndrome have normal intelligence. Most patients exhibit character and personality disorders, which may be related, in part, to the psychosocial consequences of androgen deficiency. There is a slightly increased incidence of certain systemic diseases in Klinefelter's syndrome. These include diabetes, chronic obstructive pulmonary disease, autoimmune disorders (e.g., systemic lupus erythematosus), and varicose veins.

The clinical manifestations of Klinefelter syndrome variants differ from those of the classic 47 XXY syndrome. In general, the presence of more than two extra X chromosomes results in a much higher incidence of mental retardation and somatic abnormalities, such as hypospadias, cryptorchidism, and bony abnormalities of the radius and ulna. The majority of patients with mosaic Klinefelter's syndrome exhibit less severe clinical manifestations, particularly if a normal XY cell line is present. Indeed, fertility in patients with mosaic Klinefelter's syndrome (XXY/XY) has been documented. Patients with an additional Y chromosome tend to be tall and have extremely aggressive, antisocial behavioral abnormalities. Very rarely, a patient exhibits the classic features of Klinefelter's syndrome with a normal (46 XY) karyotype, a so-called mutant or phenocopy. Finally, phenotypic males with a 46 XX karyotype may demonstrate the typical clinical manifestations of classic Klinefelter's syndrome, except for having shorter stature. The mechanism by which these individuals develop a male phenotype in the apparent absence of a Y chromosome is unclear (Ch. 234).

Azoospermia is present in all patients with classic Klinefelter's syndrome. Serum testosterone levels are usually low but may be in the low normal adult range. However, serum gonadotropin levels, especially serum FSH levels, are uniformly elevated. Occasionally, serum LH levels may fall in the high normal adult range.

Treatment of Klinefelter's syndrome is aimed primarily at correction of the androgen deficiency with testosterone replacement therapy (see below). The infertility is irreversible. Gynecomastia may be a source of great social embarrassment, in which case reduction mammoplasty should be performed.

The *functional prepubertal castrate syndrome (congenital anorchia)* is characterized by bilateral absence of functioning testicular tissue, occasionally associated with absent epididymis, in a genotypic and phenotypic man. The presence of otherwise normal male internal and external genitalia, without müllerian duct derivatives, and descent of the vas and testicular blood vessels into the scrotum imply that a normally functioning testis was present during fetal and prepubertal life. It is hypothesized that testicular damage during the fetal or prepubertal period results in atrophy of the gonads. Pa-

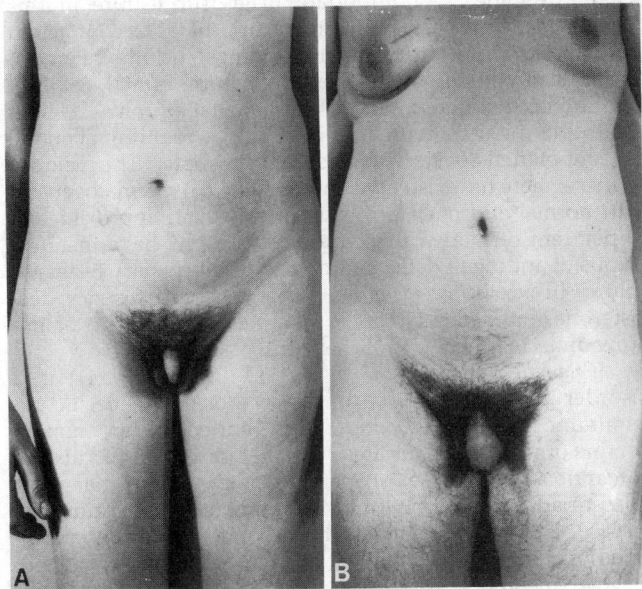

FIGURE 235–5. Two patients with untreated Klinefelter's syndrome, demonstrating the variability in degree of androgenization in this disorder. *A,* The small penis, diminished pubic hair with a female escutcheon, and sparse body hair indicate severe androgen deficiency. *B,* Normal penile development and adequate pubic and body hair indicate nearly normal androgen production by the testes. Gynecomastia is present in both patients, although only visible in the patient shown in *B.* The testes in both subjects were less than 2 cm in length. (From Bardin CW, Paulsen CA: The testes. In Williams RH (ed.): Textbook of Endocrinology. 6th ed. Philadelphia, W.B. Saunders Company, 1981.)

tients with this syndrome usually present with delayed puberty, eunuchoidal features with sexual infantilism, absence of palpable testes ("empty scrotum"), and, unlike other conditions associated with eunuchoidism, short stature (Fig. 235–4). Congenital anorchia must be distinguished from bilateral abdominal cryptorchidism, which also presents with absent scrotal testes. Because of the increased risk of malignancy, intra-abdominal testes require orchiectomy or orchiopexy. The absence of a testosterone response to exogenous hCG (hCG stimulation test) in patients with congenital anorchia may be helpful in distinguishing it from bilateral abdominal testes. However, there have been reports of responses to hCG stimulation in patients with congenital anorchia and absent responses in patients with bilateral cryptorchidism. Surgical exploration is often necessary to confirm the diagnosis. Treatment of this syndrome consists of androgen replacement therapy to induce full sexual maturation. Insertion of a testicular prosthesis may be of psychological value.

Noonan (Bonnevie-Ullrich) syndrome, an autosomal recessive disorder, occurs in karyotypically normal males and females. It is characterized by a number of clinical features similar to those of females with Turner's syndrome. Characteristic findings include short stature, typical facies (hypertelorism, antimongoloid eye slant, ptosis, low-set ears, micrognathia, high-arched palate, and dental malocclusions), webbed neck, shield-like chest, pectus excavatum, cubitus valgus, mental retardation, cardiovascular anomalies, and lymphedema. Males with Noonan syndrome (also called male Turner's syndrome) exhibit primary testicular dysfunction with impairment of both sperm and androgen production and elevated serum gonadotropin levels. Cryptorchidism is frequently present. Treatment of this disorder consists of testosterone replacement to correct the androgen deficiency and orchiopexy for associated cryptorchidism, both for psychological reasons and to monitor the testes for malignancy.

Myotonic dystrophy (see also Ch. 513) is an autosomal dominant disorder characterized by progessive weakness and atrophy of muscles, especially those of the face, neck, and distal extremities. An important diagnostic feature in this disorder is the presence of myotonia, or prolonged contraction of muscles. Other characteristic findings include cataracts, cardiac arrhythmia, dysphagia, premature frontal balding, mild intellectual deterioration, and gonadal atrophy. Testicular atrophy, which occurs in middle age, is found in about 80 per cent of men affected by myotonic dystrophy. The majority of these men have isolated impairment of spermatogenesis with normal androgen production. However, approximately 20 per cent of men with myotonic dystrophy have manifestations of androgen deficiency as a result of primary testicular failure. In addition to treating the androgen deficiency, testosterone replacement therapy may help to maintain or improve muscle function in these men.

Polyglandular autoimmune disease (see also Ch. 241) is a disorder in which there is concurrence of organ-specific autoimmune disease involving several endocrine and nonendocrine organs and associated with the presence of circulating autoantibodies to these organs. Specific conditions that occur in association with each other in this disorder are Addison's disease, hypothyroidism, insulin-dependent diabetes, pernicious anemia, ovarian failure, hypoparathyroidism, vitiligo, mucocutaneous candidiasis, Graves' disease, hypopituitarism, and alopecia. Although much less common than primary ovarian failure, primary testicular failure, associated with antitesticular antibodies and resulting in androgen deficiency, may occur in males with polyglandular autoimmune disease.

Normal aging in healthy men significantly reduces levels of total, free, and non–SHBG-bound testosterone and diminishes spermatogenesis compared to that in young men. In addition, the normal circadian variation in testosterone levels is markedly attenuated in old compared to young men. Both LH and FSH levels are significantly elevated in healthy old men,

suggesting that the reduction in testosterone levels which occurs with normal aging is the result of primary testicular dysfunction. Indeed, elderly men exhibit reduced testosterone responses to stimulation by exogenous hCG administration. The physiologic significance of reduced testosterone levels in aging men is unknown. Normal aging in men is also accompanied by an increased incidence of sexual dysfunction, as well as decreased muscle and bone mass. Whether these changes in body function with aging are related to the reduction in androgen production remains to be investigated.

Complex genetic disorders may be the cause of primary hypogonadism, which is found in the *Alstrom, ataxia telangiectasia, Sohval-Soffer, Weinstein,* and *Werner* syndromes, among others.

Acquired Disorders. In general, seminiferous tubule function and spermatogenesis are much more sensitive to external or environmental influences (such as irradiation, cytotoxic agents, or heat) than is Leydig cell production of testosterone. This greater sensitivity is due, in large part, to the fact that spermatogenesis involves active and coordinated cellular division and differentiation, requiring complex regulation. As a result, most acquired primary testicular disorders causing hypogonadism result more commonly in isolated impairment of spermatogenesis with normal androgen production (see below) than in androgen deficiency.

Viral orchitis, most frequently due to *mumps*, is a very common cause of acquired primary testicular failure. Approximately 15 to 25 per cent of males with mumps develop acute orchitis. The few boys who develop mumps orchitis before puberty usually recover completely without subsequent testicular dysfunction. However, acute mumps infection of pubertal or adult testes usually results in permanent seminiferous tubule damage and, in severe cases, Leydig cell dysfunction with androgen deficiency. Although clinical mumps orchitis is unilateral in the majority of cases, degenerative changes have been observed in the clinically uninvolved testis. During the acute phase of orchitis, which usually develops within a few days of parotitis, there is interstitial edema and sloughing of the germinal epithelium. This may be followed by progressive tubular sclerosis and testicular atrophy over the next several months. Orchitis may complicate infections with viruses such as *echoviruses* and *arboviruses*. Uncommon causes of orchitis include *gonorrhea, leprosy, tuberculosis, brucellosis, glanders, syphilis,* and certain parasitic diseases such as *filariasis* and *bilharziasis*. As in mumps, orchitis complicating these disorders results more commonly in isolated impairment of sperm production, although in severe cases androgen production is also affected.

Bilateral surgical or traumatic castration results in acute androgen deficiency, and castration after puberty often causes hot flushes and irritability, similar to that of women at the time of menopause.

Certain *drugs* may produce androgen deficiency by inhibiting testosterone biosynthesis and/or by blocking androgen action. The aldosterone antagonist *spironolactone* inhibits testosterone synthesis, as well as interfering with androgen action by competitively binding to the adrogen receptor. *Ketoconazole*, an antifungal agent, inhibits testosterone synthesis and in high doses may also inhibit adrenal steroidogenesis. *Alcohol* has direct toxic effects on both spermatogenesis and steroidogenesis in the testis in the absence of alcoholic cirrhosis. *Digitalis* has been reported to elevate serum estradiol levels and reduce serum testosterone levels, perhaps through its interaction with both the estrogen and androgen receptors. A number of *cytotoxic drugs* used in cancer chemotherapy interfere with spermatogenesis and, more rarely, with androgen production. In some malignancies, androgen deficiency may also be present in the absence of exposure to chemotherapeutic agents (e.g., Hodgkin's disease or testicular cancer). Androgen deficiency may be the result of general debilitation and malnutrition associated with some malignancies.

Irradiation of the testes rarely causes permanent androgen deficiency. However, exposure of the testes to very large doses (over 600 to 800 rads) may compromise Leydig cell function.

Systemic Disorders. A number of systemic diseases cause deficiencies in sperm and androgen production, primarily by affecting testicular function directly. In patients with *chronic liver disease* (cirrhosis), gynecomastia and testicular atrophy are commonly present. Total serum testosterone levels are low or low normal. Because SHBG levels are elevated, free or non–SHBG-bound testosterone levels are low. Serum LH levels are usually elevated but may fall in the high normal range. LH secretion may be partially suppressed by the high circulating levels of estrogens found in cirrhotic patients. Increased estrogen concentrations result from impaired hepatic clearance of adrenal androgens (androstendione), leading to an increased substrate for peripheral aromatization to estrone and estradiol. The increased estrogen/testosterone ratio may contribute to the formation of gynecomastia. Treatment of androgen deficiency in patients with cirrhosis with an aromatizable androgen may result in worsening of gynecomastia.

Chronic renal failure usually causes reductions in both sperm and androgen production. LH and FSH levels are elevated, as a result of increased production as well as reduced renal clearance. The response of testosterone levels to hCG stimulation is impaired. Elevated serum prolactin levels may also contribute to testicular dysfunction in uremia. Hemodialysis does not significantly improve testosterone production. However, successful renal transplantation may result in some return of testicular function, which may be tempered by the drugs used for chronic immunosuppressive therapy to prevent graft rejection. In addition to treating androgen deficiency, testosterone replacement therapy may also improve the anemia of renal failure.

Sickle cell disease often results in low serum testosterone and elevated serum gonadotropin levels, implying primary testicular failure. *Paraplegia* may result in a transient reduction in serum testosterone levels that return to normal in the chronic paraplegic state unless chronic malnutrition occurs.

ISOLATED DEFICIENCY OF SPERM PRODUCTION.

Congenital or Developmental Disorders. *Germinal cell aplasia, or Sertoli cell–only syndrome,* is an uncommon condition characterized on testicular biopsy by seminiferous tubules of moderately reduced size, lined with Sertoli cells but devoid of germ cells and having little or no tubular fibrosis. Patients with this syndrome are normally androgenized but infertile. They have slightly smaller than normal testes, azoospermia, and elevated serum FSH levels, indicative of severe seminiferous tubule dysfunction. Serum testosterone levels are normal, and LH levels are normal or slightly elevated. Testosterone response to hCG stimulation may be reduced. These findings suggest that mild, subclinical Leydig cell dysfunction may also be present. It is hypothesized that congenital absence of germ cells is the basis for this syndrome. However, in some familial cases of germinal cell aplasia, germ cells have been found on testicular biopsy prior to puberty but are lost during and after puberty. The karyotype is usually 46 XY, although 47 XYY and 47 XXY karyotypes have also been found. Other gonadal disorders causing severe seminiferous tubule damage (such as mumps orchitis, cryptorchidism, irradiation, or cytotoxic drugs) may result in seminiferous tubules lined only with Sertoli cells. In these acquired causes of Sertoli cell–only syndrome, however, the tubules are usually extensively sclerosed and hyalinized and the testes are much smaller. Infertility in congenital germinal cell aplasia is irreversible but may be reversible with time in acquired cases of severe germ cell damage.

In *cryptorchidism* the testes fail to descend normally into the scrotum. Cryptorchid testes are usually located in the abdomen or inguinal canal. *Ectopic testes* are located outside the normal pathway of testicular descent and may be found in the perineal, femoral, or superficial inguinal areas. To avoid unnecessary treatment, cryptorchid testes must be distinguished from *retractile testes*, which are located in the scrotum, but are withdrawn into the inguinal canal or abdomen with minimal stimulation.

The testes usually descend into the scrotum about the eighth month of fetal life. Undescended testes are found in approximately 3 to 4 per cent of newborn males, but the testes descend during the first year in all but 0.5 per cent. The prevalence of cryptorchidism in adult males is about 0.3 to 0.4 per cent.

Bilateral cryptorchidism may be the presenting complaint in a number of hypogonadal disorders, such as the functional prepubertal castrate, the Noonan syndrome, and Reifenstein's syndrome. It may also be variably associated with many other causes of hypogonadism, such as Klinefelter's syndrome and hypogonadotropic eunuchoidism. In these disorders, cryptorchidism is usually associated with androgen deficiency. In contrast, cryptorchidism, when not associated with other hypogonadal disorders, rarely affects Leydig cell function and usually causes isolated impairment of spermatogenesis.

Even when cryptorchidism is unilateral, testicular dysfunction is very common, suggesting that both testes have altered function. Abnormal testicular function may contribute to the failure of the testes to descend properly. In rare instances, normal testicular descent may be impeded by anatomic abnormalities along the pathway of descent, e.g., external inguinal hernias. In these instances, both testes function normally, and orchiopexy before puberty usually results in preservation of normal testicular function.

Careful physical examination of the scrotum should be performed to distinguish cryptorchidism from retractile testes, which is a more common condition. The diagnosis is particularly difficult in obese patients, and repeated examinations may be necessary. Examination should be performed in the standing, squatting, and recumbent positions, and observation in warm water may be helpful. The Valsalva maneuver and applied pressure to the lower abdomen are useful procedures to detect a mobile testis, which does not require therapy. In patients with retractile testes, elicitation of a cremasteric reflex may result in a localized puckering of the scrotal skin. Failure to palpate a testis after repeated examinations suggests that the testis is intra-abdominal, severely atrophic, or absent.

As a result of exposure of the seminiferous tubules to higher extrascrotal temperatures at the time of puberty, the germinal epithelium of cryptorchid testes shows severe degeneration, eventually resulting in tubular fibrosis. Bilateral cryptorchidism causes infertility. Sperm counts are low, and serum FSH levels are usually elevated. Leydig cell function is usually preserved, and serum testosterone and LH concentrations remain normal. The risk of malignancy in undescended testes is 20 to 40 times greater than in scrotal testes, and the risk remains increased even after orchiopexy.

Therapy for cryptorchidism should be instituted before puberty, when the degenerative changes of the germinal epithelium occur. The exact age at which treatment should be instituted is controversial. Administration of hCG (1000 IU three times weekly) or LHRH to prepubertal boys with cryptorchidism may cause testicular descent in some patients. When such therapy is successful, it is probable that the testis would have descended spontaneously at puberty. Reports of the efficacy of hormonal therapy are widely discrepant, probably as a result of inclusion of variable proportions of patients with retractile testes. If hormonal therapy is unsuccessful in causing testicular descent, orchiopexy is performed in an attempt to preserve testicular function, to allow easier examination of the testis for malignant degeneration, and for cosmetic reasons. Despite orchiopexy, fertility rates in patients with cryptorchidism are usually reduced, particularly in patients with bilateral undescended testes. Often, bilateral testicular biopsies are performed at the time of orchiopexy to determine the degree of testicular abnormality. If a unilateral cryptorchid testis is atrophic and shows extensive tubular fibrosis, an orchiectomy is usually performed, provided that the contralateral testis is in the scrotum.

A *varicocele* is an abnormal dilatation of the pampiniform plexus of veins surrounding the spermatic cord, caused by retrograde blood flow into the internal spermatic vein. Palpable varicocele occurs in about 10 per cent of the general population and in 30 per cent of men with infertility. Varicocele is clearly associated with infertility. However, approximately 50 per cent of men with varicoceles have normal seminal fluid analyses, and some men with varicocele and abnormal seminal fluid parameters are fertile. About 90 per cent of varicoceles occur on the left side, as a result of valvular incompetence between the left internal spermatic vein and the renal vein. Occurrence of a isolated right-sided varicocele may be an early clue to venous obstruction by malignancy or to situs inversus. Varicoceles may affect testicular function by a variety of mechanisms, including increasing testicular temperature and blood flow. Seminal fluid analysis usually shows low sperm concentration with reduced motility and increased numbers of sperm with abnormal morphology (e.g., increased tapered and amorphous forms). Testicular size and serum testosterone, LH, and FSH levels are usually normal. Surgical repair of varicoceles in infertile men has been reported to improve semen quality and fertility, although well-controlled clinical studies have not been performed.

Immotile cilia syndrome, or *Kartagener's syndrome*, is characterized by sinusitis, bronchiectasis, and situs inversus. Patients usually suffer from chronic respiratory infections because of impaired mucociliary clearance in the respiratory tract. In addition, these patients produce nonmotile spermatozoa. Cilia in the respiratory tract and the sperm tail are immotile in Kartagener's syndrome because they lack a specific protein, *dynein*, which is important in microtubular filament movement. Other patients have a *deficiency* in an enzyme, *protein carboxyl methylase*, which is important in sperm motility. Infertility in this disorder is not treatable.

The majority of patients with *myotonic dystrophy* (see above) may have isolated impairment of spermatogenesis with normal androgen production.

Acquired Disorders. The majority of adults who develop mumps *orchitis* and orchitis due to other infectious agents sustain severe germ cell damage and isolated impairment of spermatogenesis with normal Leydig cell function (see above). Seminiferous tubule function is much more sensitive to damage from external or environmental agents than is Leydig cell function. Therefore, exposure of the testis to *thermal trauma, irradiation, cytotoxic drugs,* and *environmental toxins* often results in deficiency of sperm production without androgen deficiency. Even relatively minor thermal trauma, such as that induced by tight underwear or hot tubs, may result in suppression of sperm production.

The human testis is very sensitive to irradiation. Only 15 rads of x-irradiation may suppress spermatogenesis temporarily; more than 700 rads usually produces permanent infertility. Doses of radiation used in therapy of malignant lymphoma have been reported to result in permanent germ cell damage and infertility, despite shielding of the testis. Spermatogenesis is also very sensitive to damage by cytotoxic cancer chemotherapeutic agents, especially to alkylating agents. The likelihood of severe seminiferous tubule damage and permanent infertility is greater with combination chemotherapy regimens, such as MOPP for Hodgkin's disease. Despite being very sensitive to radiation and cytotoxic drugs, the germinal epithelium has great regenerative properties, and recovery of spermatogenesis may occur despite very severe germ cell loss associated with high doses of these cytotoxic agents. Both irradiation and cytotoxic agents occa-

sionally produce androgen deficiency. Sperm banking offers some hope for fertility for patients who will develop permanent infertility as a result of irradiation or chemotherapy for malignant disease.

Damage to the germinal epithelium has been reported in workers exposed to carbon disulfide, a solvent used in production of rayon, and to dibromochloropropane, an insecticide. A number of other chemical agents used in industry and laboratories have been implicated as direct testicular toxins (e.g., deuterium oxide, cadmium, fluoroacetamide, nitrofurans, dinitropyrroles, diamines, alpha-chlorhydrin, other insecticides, and rodenticides).

Systemic Disorders. A number of relatively minor *acute febrile illnesses* may result in temporary suppression of sperm production (e.g., minor viral infections). Over 50 per cent of men with spinal cord lesions resulting in *paraplegia* exhibit diminished testicular function, the majority demonstrating impaired sperm production with normal androgen production. Reduced spermatogenesis may be a result of elevated testicular temperature, caused by increased scrotal skin temperature (from loss of lumbar sympathetic innervation) and loss of the cremasteric reflex.

Idiopathic Oligospermia or Azoospermia. In most men who present with infertility and isolated impairment of spermatogenesis, no apparent cause can be found, leading to the diagnosis of *idiopathic oligospermia or azoospermia.* Because of the high prevalence of male infertility (5 to 6 per cent of reproductive age men), idiopathic oligospermia is the most common cause of male hypogonadism. Since the pathogenesis of impaired sperm production is not known, therapy for this disorder has been largely empiric and unsatisfactory. Trials of treatment with large doses of testosterone, gonadotropins, clomiphene citrate, testolactone, cortisone, thyroid hormone, caffeine, and vitamins have generally been unsuccessful.

Secondary Hypogonadism

Secondary hypogonadism is testicular failure due to inadequate gonadotropin secretion as a result of either hypothalamic or pituitary dysfunction. In the majority of cases, both LH and FSH secretion are diminished, resulting in impairment of both sperm and androgen production. Rarely, there may be isolated deficiency of sperm production.

DEFICIENCY OF SPERM AND ANDROGEN PRODUCTION. *Congenital or Developmental Disorders.* Hypogonadotropic eunuchoidism, or *Kallmann's syndrome,* is a congenital and often familial disorder, characterized by isolated hypogonadotropic hypogonadism (resulting in eunuchoidal features) and anosmia or hyposmia. Gonadotropin deficiency in this disorder is caused by a defect in synthesis and/or release of LHRH from the hypothalamus; chronic exogenous LHRH administration results in stimulation of normal testicular function. A developmental failure of the olfactory lobes is responsible for absent or reduced sense of smell. There is considerable genetic heterogeneity in this disorder. Kallmann's syndrome may be inherited as an autosomal dominant with variable (male-predominant) expression, an autosomal recessive, or an X-linked recessive condition.

Usually, patients with Kallmann's syndrome present with delayed puberty. They exhibit eunuchoidal features and prepubertal size testes. An early prepubertal manifestation of Kallmann's syndrome is micropenis. In addition to anosmia or hyposmia (present in approximately 80 per cent of cases), these patients may also exhibit other mid-line defects (e.g., cleft-lip or -palate, color blindness, renal agenesis, nerve deafness, cryptorchidism, and skeletal abnormalities (e.g., syndactyly, short fourth metacarpals, craniofacial asymmetry). Patients with Kallmann's syndrome are often aspermic (i.e., have no ejaculate). Serum testosterone, LH, and FSH levels are low, while other anterior pituitary functions are normal. A single dose LHRH test may not result in stimulation of gonadotropin secretion, but repeated LHRH administration will increase LH and FSH levels. Clomiphene citrate is an antiestrogen that stimulates hypothalamic release of LHRH and as a result increases gonadotropin secretion. Men with Kallman's syndrome do not respond to clomiphene citrate administration.

The differentiation between Kallmann's syndrome and constitutional delayed puberty is very difficult (especially in the absence of anosmia or hyposmia) and cannot be reliably made in the prepubertal age range. Usually, androgen therapy is initiated to induce sexual maturation in both of these conditions. It is intermittently stopped to determine whether spontaneous onset of puberty occurs. Patients with Kallmann's syndrome will continue to require androgen therapy to achieve and maintain sexual maturation, whereas patients with constitutional delayed puberty will not require treatment after spontaneous endogenous gonadotropin and testosterone secretion begin. When fertility is desired, androgen replacement treatment is discontinued, and spermatogenesis may be induced with gonadotropin or LHRH therapy. Previous androgen therapy does not alter the subsequent testicular response to gonadotropin therapy. However, gonadotropin therapy is much less successful in patients who have associated cryptorchidism, particularly if it is bilateral.

A variant form of Kallmann's syndrome is *isolated LH deficiency*, which is also called the *"fertile" eunuch syndrome*. This syndrome is characterized by a selective deficiency in LH secretion, which results in prepubertal androgen deficiency and eunuchoidism. FSH secretion is preserved, resulting in testes of nearly normal size in which well-advanced spermatogenesis is present. Spermatogenesis is not normal in these patients, however, and they are not fertile, as the name of the syndrome would imply. Treatment with hCG, which contains predominantly LH-like hormonal activity, stimulates Leydig cell production of testosterone, ameliorates androgen deficiency, and increases spermatogenesis.

Hemochromatosis is an autosomal recessive disorder in which there is parenchymal iron deposition in a variety of tissues, most prominently in the liver, skin, pancreas, and heart (Ch. 206). Iron deposition in the pituitary gland selectively inhibits gonadotropin production without significantly affecting other anterior pituitary hormone secretion. The resulting hypogonadotropic hypogonadism and androgen deficiency are responsible for the common complaint of impotence in this disorder. Frequent phlebotomies or treatment with desferioxamine to decrease iron overload may restore gonadotropin secretion in some patients. Even in the presence of significant iron overload, administration of gonadotropins can stimulate testicular function, including induction of spermatogenesis. Parenchymal iron deposition resulting in hypogonadotropic hypogonadism may also occur in patients with conditions that require frequent blood transfusions, such as thalassemia.

Secondary hypogonadism may be present in a number of *complex genetic syndromes*, such as *Prader-Willi, Laurence-Moon-Biedl, Biemond, Carpenter, familial cerebellar ataxia, Fanconi, dyskeratosis congenita, familial ichthyosis, Borjeson, Kraus-Rupert,* and *Richards-Rundle* syndromes.

Acquired Disorders. Hypopituitarism. Any destructive or infiltrative lesion of the hypothalamus and/or pituitary may cause impairment of gonadotropin secretion, either selectively or in conjunction with deficiency of other anterior pituitary hormones (Ch. 226). Specific pathologic conditions include functioning and nonfunctioning pituitary adenomas; suprasellar tumors, such as craniopharyngioma, meningioma, optic glioma, or astrocytoma; surgical ablation or irradiation of the pituitary; infarction; vasculitis; trauma; granulomatous disease, such as tuberculosis, sarcoidosis, and histiocytosis X; and hemochromatosis.

Usually, destructive processes involving the pituitary gland result in progressive loss of anterior pituitary function in the following order: Gonadotropin and growth hormone secretion

are the first to be affected, followed by TSH production, and finally ACTH secretion. The combination of gonadotropin and growth hormone deficiency is most important to recognize in prepubertal children with growth retardation. In adults, clinical secondary hypogonadism, in the absence of other anterior pituitary dysfunction, may be the initial manifestation of a hypothalamic or pituitary process. Because loss of TSH and ACTH secretion is associated with greater degrees of pituitary destruction, secondary hypothyroidism and hypoadrenalism usually do not occur without concurrent secondary hypogonadism.

Patients with prepubertal gonadotropin deficiency present with delayed puberty and have eunuchoidal features and small testes, usually less than 2 cm. Children with associated growth hormone deficiency will also demonstrate short stature (dwarfism). Men with postpubertal gonadotropin deficiency usually present with diminished libido and potency. Initially, testicular size may be normal, but with long-standing gonadotropin deficiency the testes become small. In addition to hypogonadism, patients with hypopituitarism may have findings of deficiency or excess of other anterior pituitary hormones or tumor mass effects.

Serum testosterone levels and sperm counts are low. Serum LH and FSH levels are low or in the low normal adult range. The gonadotropin response to single-dose LHRH administration does not reliably differentiate hypothalamic and pituitary causes of gonadotropin deficiency. In many instances, LHRH administration will fail to stimulate gonadotropin secretion in patients with hypothalamic disease; alternatively, it may stimulate gonadotropin levels in men with pituitary disease. Clinical evaluation of patients with secondary hypogonadism should include anatomic studies (such as CT scan and visual field examination) to determine the presence and effects of a hypothalamic or pituitary tumor and investigation of other anterior pituitary hormone functions.

Treatment is aimed at the process causing hypopituitarism and correction of androgen deficiency with testosterone replacement therapy. If fertility is desired, androgens are discontinued and gonadotropin therapy is instituted.

Hyperprolactinemia. This condition, resulting from either a pituitary adenoma or central nervous system–active drugs (such as phenothiazines), may cause secondary testicular failure (Ch. 239). In men, prolactin-secreting adenomas are usually large (macroadenomas), and gonadotropin deficiency may be caused primarily by destruction of pituitary gonadotrophs. Even in the absence of a tumor, prolactin has an inhibitory effect on gonadotropin secretion, resulting in secondary hypogonadism. In some men with hyperprolactinemia, correction of androgen deficiency with testosterone replacement therapy does not correct impotence. The addition of bromocriptine, a dopamine agonist that decreases pituitary prolactin secretion, may be useful in these situations.

The negative feedback effects of *estrogen excess* in men causes inhibition of gonadotropin secretion and secondary hypogonadism. Estrogen excess may result from either exogenous administration of estrogens or estrogenic substances (e.g., diethylstilbestrol administration in men with prostate cancer) or endogenous secretion from an estrogen-producing neoplasm (e.g., feminizing adrenal carcinoma). Patients with estrogen excess usually manifest varying degrees of gynecomastia. *Progestins* (e.g., medroxyprogesterone acetate) and *opiate-like drugs* (e.g., morphine, methadone, and heroin) also inhibit gonadotropin production and may cause secondary hypogonadism.

Systemic Disorders. Glucocorticoid excess, as a result of either Cushing's syndrome or high-dosage glucocorticoid administration, suppresses gonadotropin secretion, resulting in secondary testicular failure with loss of libido, impotence, and oligospermia. High circulating levels of endogenous glucocorticoids may contribute to the reduction in serum testosterone, LH, and FSH levels observed with a variety of *acute stressful situations or illnesses*, such as emotional stress, vigorous physical exercise, trauma, myocardial infarction, surgery, trauma, burns, sepsis, etc. *Nutritional deficiency*, such as that associated with protein-calorie malnutrition or anorexia nervosa, inhibits gonadotropin production and may cause secondary hypogonadism. Concurrent primary testicular dysfunction may also be associated with inadequate nutrition. Malnutrition may contribute to the secondary testicular failure associated with a number of *chronic illnesses*, such as malignancy and chronic heart, respiratory, liver, and kidney disease. Moderate obesity results in reduction in SHBG and total testosterone levels, with normal free testosterone levels. Some men with *massive obesity* demonstrate clinical androgen deficiency with low free testosterone concentrations and reduced gonadotropin levels.

ISOLATED DEFICIENCY OF SPERM PRODUCTION. *Congenital adrenal hyperplasia* caused by either 21-hydroxylase or 11 beta-hydroxylase deficiency results in excessive production of adrenal androgens. Androgen excess suppresses gonadotropin secretion, resulting in secondary hypogonadism. Testicular androgen and sperm production are suppressed. Excessive adrenal androgen production causes premature virilization and precocious pseudopuberty, rather than androgen deficiency. Secondary hypogonadism is therefore manifested by isolated impairment of spermatogenesis. Glucocorticoid treatment of some patients with congenital adrenal hyperplasia may result in true precocious puberty, with premature activation of the hypothalamic-pituitary-gonadal axis. These patients will demonstrate premature induction of spermatogenesis and normal gonadotropin levels. Androgen excess caused by administration of *testosterone* or *androgenic anabolic steroids* or *androgen-secreting tumors* (e.g., testicular Leydig cell tumors) also result in secondary hypogonadism presenting with isolated deficiency in sperm production with normal androgenization. High doses of testosterone have been used in normal men to suppress sperm production in trials to develop male contraceptives.

Rarely, *hyperprolactinemia* will impair sperm production despite normal gonadotropin and testosterone levels. *Isolated FSH deficiency*, an extremely rare condition, results in normal virilization in males, with normal serum testosterone and LH levels. Spermatogenesis and fertility have not been well characterized in this disorder, although testicular biopsy in one man revealed arrest of sperm maturation at the spermatid stage.

Androgen Resistance Syndromes

Androgen resistance syndromes are caused by defects in androgen action (Ch. 234). The severity of androgen insensitivity determines the clinical presentation of these disorders. Most androgen resistance syndromes result in severely defective androgen action, and patients with these syndromes present at birth as either phenotypic females (testicular feminization) or with ambiguous genitalia (male pseudohermaphroditism). However, some men with mild, incomplete androgen insensitivity or *Reifenstein's syndrome* may present as adults with a clinical picture of mild androgen deficiency with a nearly normal male phenotype. Patients with Reifenstein's syndrome may have hypospadias, gynecomastia, varying degrees of virilization, a small prostate gland, impaired spermatogenesis, and cryptorchidism. They may be distinguished from patients with true hypogonadism by having elevated serum testosterone, LH, and FSH levels. Some men with very mild androgen insensitivity may present with only oligospermia or azoospermia and no other phenotypic abnormalities.

Delayed Puberty

Puberty in boys usually begins at age 11 to 12 years. With the maturation of the central nervous system mechanism that regulates LHRH production, pulsatile gonadotropin and testosterone secretions begin, initially during sleep and then throughout the day. The first clinical indications of the onset of puberty are an increase in the testicular size and a wrinkling and pigmentation of the scrotal skin. Subsequently, there are increase in penile length and appearance of pubic hair, followed by increasing long bone growth and development of other secondary sexual characteristics, such as hair growth in other androgen-dependent areas, increase in muscle mass, enlargement of the larynx, and growth of the prostate. The increase in testicular size precedes the appearance of pubic hair by about two years and the peak velocity in growth of height by three years. The onset and duration of puberty and the degree to which secondary sexual characteristics develop vary considerably, largely attributable to the genetic background of an individual.

Delayed puberty is the lack of sexual maturation before the age of 15 years. A number of the disorders discussed above that cause *hypogonadism*, including those causing primary and secondary testicular failure and androgen resistance, may result in delayed sexual maturation. *Severe systemic illnesses* (such as malabsorption, asthma, diabetes, malignancy) that also cause growth retardation and *thyroid hormone deficiency* may also cause delayed puberty. The great majority of boys with delayed puberty, however, have physiologic or *constitutional delayed puberty*. This is a benign form of delayed adolescence which represents a normal variation in the onset of puberty. It is frequently familial. These boys will eventually undergo a delayed but normal puberty and attain normal sexual maturation and height.

The diagnosis of constitutional delayed puberty can be strongly suspected in a healthy boy with retardation of growth and bone age, normal growth velocity in relation to bone age, a family history of delayed adolescence, a testicular volume above 2 ml, and a bone age between 12 and 13 years. These clinical features are often not present and the diagnosis can be very difficult. Diagnostic evaluation should be undertaken to exclude organic causes of delayed puberty, i.e., hypogonadism, systemic illness, and hypothyroidism. In the absence of anosmia or other morphologic manifestations, constitutional delayed puberty cannot be distinguished from hypogonadotropic eunuchoidism or Kallmann's syndrome (see above).

Delayed sexual maturation often results in severe psychosocial distress to both the patient and his parents. Therefore, after systemic and endocrine disorders are excluded, patients with delayed puberty are usually treated with androgen replacement therapy to induce sexual maturation. It is generally recommended that patients not be treated with androgens until after 15 years of age. The emotional stress and trauma of delayed puberty often results in treatment beginning at about 13 to 14 years of age, however, so that the onset of sexual maturation coincides with those of his contemporaries. Androgen treatment is intermittently stopped to determine if spontaneous onset of puberty has occurred.

TREATMENT OF HYPOGONADISM
Androgen Therapy

Androgens are principally used to treat testosterone deficiency in hypogonadal men; the therapeutic goal of androgen therapy is to restore the normal physiologic effects of testosterone. In prepubertal androgen-deficient boys, the aim of androgen replacement is to stimulate and maintain male secondary sexual characteristics, somatic development, and sexual function without compromising adult height by premature closure of long bone epiphyses. In adult androgen deficiency, the objective of therapy is to restore and maintain libido, potency, and secondary sexual characteristics. Androgen treatment is very successful in accomplishing these goals. However, testosterone cannot be administered in sufficiently high doses to achieve the high intratesticular levels required to stimulate spermatogenesis.

The long-acting 17 beta-hydroxyl esters of testosterone,

testosterone enanthate and *cypionate*, are the most effective, safest, and most practical preparations currently available to treat androgen deficiency. Intramuscular injection of 200 mg of either preparation results in peak serum testosterone levels at the upper limits of the normal adult range in one to two days. Testosterone levels remain in the normal range for about two weeks. Therefore, in adults with androgen deficiency, replacement therapy is usually initiated with either testosterone enanthate or cypionate at a dose of 200 mg intramuscularly every two weeks. In these men, testosterone administration generally results in stimulation of libido and potency, improvement in energy level, increase in physical and social drive, and increase in hemoglobin concentration. In an elderly androgen-deficient man with symptoms of bladder neck obstruction secondary to an enlarged prostate gland, it is wise to begin testosterone therapy gradually with a short-acting testosterone preparation. *Testosterone propionate*, a short-acting 17 beta-hydroxyl ester of testosterone, given in doses of 25 to 50 mg intramuscularly three times weekly, is useful in this situation. The shorter duration of action of this preparation permits rapid withdrawal if androgen stimulation results in prostatic growth or urinary obstruction.

Androgen replacement therapy is much more complicated in prepubertal boys with delayed puberty. Although testosterone is very effective in inducing secondary sexual characteristics and stimulating long bone growth, overly aggressive androgen therapy can result in premature closure of long bone epiphyses and compromise final adult height. Furthermore, it is often not possible to differentiate patients with constitutional delayed puberty, who require only temporary androgen replacement, from those with permanent hypogonadotropic hypogonadism. Therefore, in boys with delayed puberty whose height is far below the expected adult height, androgen therapy is begun with testosterone enanthate or cypionate, 50 to 100 mg intramuscularly every two weeks, and gradually increased to full replacement doses. Androgen therapy is intermittently stopped to determine whether spontaneous pubertal development will occur.

Currently, all oral androgen preparations available in the United States are 17 alpha-alkylated derivatives of testosterone, which have the potential for serious hepatotoxicity. When used for the treatment of androgen deficiency, parenteral 17 beta-hydroxyl esters of testosterone do not cause hepatotoxicity. Because of the greater risk of oral androgen preparations, as well as their increased cost and reduced efficacy, they should be avoided in the treatment of androgen deficiency. In the unusual circumstance of a patient who will not or cannot take parenteral androgens, *methyltestosterone*, 25 to 50 mg orally or 10 to 25 mg buccally, or *fluoxymesterone*, 5 to 10 mg orally daily, may be used.

Androgen therapy is absolutely contraindicated in men with androgen-sensitive cancers, i.e., prostatic carcinoma and male breast carcinoma. Full replacement doses of androgens may be inappropriate for hypogonadal men with mental retardation or severe psychopathology and for elderly androgen-deficient men with severe bladder neck obstruction from prostatic hyperplasia, who are not good surgical candidates.

Excessive stimulation of libido and erections by androgens are very uncommon, usually occurring in prepubertal boys or in men with long-standing androgen deficiency given large doses of testosterone. These symptoms usually resolve with time or reduction in dosage. Androgen administration causing acute urinary retention is very uncommon in the absence of underlying prostatic carcinoma. Patients given testosterone to induce puberty may develop acne or gynecomastia, similar to that observed in normal puberty. Adult hypogonadal men rarely develop gynecomastia, except when a predisposing condition such as hepatic cirrhosis exists. Androgens may cause mild weight gain as a result of sodium retention and protein anabolic effects, and patients with underlying edematous states may develop worsening edema during therapy.

Erythropoiesis is stimulated by androgen administration. Occasionally, significant erythrocytosis requiring phlebotomy and reduced testosterone dosage occurs. Testosterone has also been reported to worsen or induce obstructive sleep apnea. All oral 17 alpha-alkylated androgens have been reported to cause hepatic cholestasis and occasionally clinical jaundice. Although rare, more serious and potentially life-threatening complications of oral androgens are the development of peliosis hepatis (blood-filled cysts in the liver), hepatic adenoma, hepatoma, or hepatic angiosarcoma. Hepatotoxicity does not result from replacement dosages of parenteral 17 beta-hydroxyl esters of testosterone.

Androgens have also been used in the treatment of anemias related to renal and bone marrow failure, micropenis and microphallus, hereditary angioneurotic edema, female breast cancer, lichen sclerosus, and senile osteoporosis. The use of androgenic steroids has not been demonstrated to be of long-term value in promoting protein anabolism in catabolic states associated with a variety of acute and chronic illnesses. However, in many illnesses (such as burns, chronic liver disease, and illnesses requiring chronic glucocorticoid therapy), serum testosterone levels are often low. The efficacy of androgen therapy in this subset of catabolic diseases has not been examined.

Androgenic anabolic steroids are commonly used by competitive athletes with the hope of improving endurance, strength, and performance. Numerous studies have demonstrated that androgens are of dubious value in increasing strength and performance, in the absence of intensive training and high-protein diets. Many athletes often take multiple androgenic anabolic agents (including 17 alpha-alkylated agents) in very high doses, with little regard for potentially serious side effects. Hepatotoxicity (including hepatoma) and impaired spermatogenesis resulting in infertility have been reported in athletes taking these androgenic steroids. Furthermore, the long-term sequelae of taking massive doses of 17 beta-hydroxyl ester preparations are unknown. It is clear that the potential risks of high-dose anabolic steroid use far outweigh the potential benefits to athletic performance, and the use of these agents for this purpose should be strongly discouraged.

Gonadotropin and LHRH Therapy

The aim of gonadotropin therapy is to stimulate spermatogenesis and to establish or restore fertility in gonadotropin-deficient hypogonadal patients. The gonadotropin preparations usually used for this purpose are *human chorionic gonadotropin (hCG)*, which is purified from the urine of pregnant women and contains LH-like biologic activity almost exclusively; and *human menopausal gonadotropin (hMG*, Pergonal), which is purified from the urine of postmenopausal women and contains both FSH and LH activity. Both hCG and hMG are expensive and require multiple injections per week. Therefore, testosterone, rather than gonadotropin therapy, is used to induce and maintain androgenization in patients with hypogonadotropic hypogonadism.

Initiation of spermatogenesis in prepubertal patients with hypogonadotropic hypogonadism usually requires treatment with both hCG and hMG. Because of the relative ineffectiveness of hMG to stimulate the immature testis and the greater expense, treatment is initiated with hCG alone, at a dosage of 2000 IU three times weekly. Clinical evidence of sexual maturation and the increase in serum testosterone levels are monitored to determine the need for adjustments in dose. During hCG treatment, testosterone produced by the Leydig cells causes the Sertoli cells to mature and spermatogenesis to be initiated to varying degrees of completeness. Occasionally, hCG alone will stimulate spermatogenesis sufficiently for sperm to appear in the ejaculate. However, the majority of prepubertal patients with hypogonadotropic hypogonadism require FSH activity, in the form of hMG, in addition to hCG to complete spermatogenesis and induce fertility. Therefore, hMG, at a dosage of 75 IU three times weekly, is usually added to hCG if there is no evidence of sperm in the ejaculate with hCG alone. Gonadotropin induction of sperm production may take as long as one year. Even with combined hCG and hMG treatment, sperm output in the ejaculate may not be normal. Despite very low sperm counts, fertility may be induced, however.

Once initiated, spermatogenesis may be maintained with hCG treatment alone. In adults with acquired hypogonadotropic hypogonadism, sperm production may also be restored with hCG treatment alone. Previous androgen treatment does not alter testicular responsiveness to subsequent gonadotropin therapy. The presence of primary testicular disease, such as cryptorchidism, worsens the prognosis for induction of sperm production and fertility by gonadotropin treatment.

In patients with Kallmann's syndrome, pulsatile administration of low doses of LHRH has been used successfully to stimulate endogenous gonadotropin secretion and to initiate and maintain spermatogenesis to induce fertility. Pulsatile administration more closely mimics the normal physiologic situation; however, a portable infusion pump must be used to deliver small doses of LHRH every few hours throughout the day, making LHRH therapy a much more complex management problem than gonadotropin therapy. LHRH and gonadotropin therapy are probably similar in their ability to stimulate spermatogenesis in men with Kallmann's syndrome.

Bardin CW: Male hypogonadism. In Yen SSC, Jaffe RB (eds.): Reproductive Endocrinology. Philadelphia, WB Saunders Company, 1986, p 614. *A good discussion of disorders causing primary and secondary male hypogonadism.*

Finkel DM, Phillips JL, Synder PJ: Stimulation of spermatogenesis by gonadotropins in men with hypogonadotropic hypogonadism. N Engl J Med 313:651, 1985. *This paper compares the responses of sperm production to gonadotropin therapy in prepubertal and postpubertal hypogonadotropic hypogonadism.*

Handelsman DJ, Swerdloff RS: Male gonadal dysfunction. Clin Endocrinol Metab 14:89, 1985. *A very complete review of clinical and laboratory evaluation of male gonadal disorders.*

Hopwood NJ: Pathogenesis and management of abnormal puberty. Spec Topics Endocrinol Metab 7:175, 1985. *An excellent review of pubertal disorders.*

Lieblich JM, Rogol AD, White BJ, et al.: Syndrome of anosmia with hypogonadotropic hypogonadism (Kallmann syndrome). Clinical and laboratory studies in 23 cases. Am J Med 73:506, 1982. *This paper documents the substantial clinical and endocrine heterogeneity of Kallmann's syndrome.*

Matsumoto AM, Bremner WJ: Hypogonadism: Androgen therapy. In Bayliss TM, Brain MC, Cherniak RM (eds.): Current Therapy in Internal Medicine–2. Philadelphia, BC Decker, Inc, 1987, p 517. *A concise, practical discussion of androgen therapy for male hypogonadism.*

PRECOCIOUS PUBERTY

Isosexual precocity is defined as the development of sexual maturation before the age of 10 years. In boys, premature development of secondary sexual characteristics results in virilization. This is accompanied by accelerated skeletal maturation and linear growth and premature closure of long bone epiphyses, resulting in short stature as an adult. *True precocious puberty* is caused by premature secretion of gonadotropins. Testicular androgen and sperm production are stimulated by gonadotropins and result in virilization and increased testis size. *Precocious pseudopuberty* results from secretion of androgens from the adrenal gland or testis. Androgen excess results in virilization, but sperm production is not stimulated and the testes remain small.

True Precocious Puberty

In the majority of cases of true precocious puberty no identifiable cause for premature activation of gonadotropin secretion is found. This condition is called *idiopathic precocious puberty*. It is often inherited as a male-limited autosomal dominant or X-linked recessive trait. Patients have an increased incidence of seizure disorders and abnormal electroencephalograms. The remaining cases of true precocious puberty are primarily caused by *central nervous system lesions* involving the posterior hypothalamus. Lesions include hypothalamic and pineal tumors, craniopharyngioma, hamartomas, hydrocephalus, postencephalitic lesions, congenital defects, neurofibromatosis, and tuberous sclerosis. Central nervous system lesions may also result in disturbances of other hypothalamic functions, causing diabetes insipidus, eating disorders, somnolence, emotional lability, and altered temperature regulation. Precocious puberty may precede the onset of a clinically detectable neurologic lesion. Therefore, a prolonged period of follow-up observation with repeated neurologic evaluation is necessary to exclude central nervous system lesions. Rarely, an hCG-secreting tumor (e.g., hepatoblastoma) or hCG administration for cryptorchidism (iatrogenic precocious puberty) causes true precocious puberty.

Precocious Pseudopuberty (Ch. 234)

Adrenocortical hyperfunction, either from congenital adrenal hyperplasia (21-hydroxylase or 11-hydroxylase deficiency) or a virilizing adrenocortical tumor, is the most common condition causing precocious pseudopuberty in boys. Patients with congenital adrenal hyperplasia caused by 21-hydroxylase deficiency usually have markedly elevated serum 17-hydroxyprogesterone and urinary pregnanetriol levels. Rarely, *Leydig cell tumor* of the testis, autonomous Leydig cell function (*testotoxicosis*), and administration of *androgenic steroids* may cause precocious pseudopuberty.

Treatment of these conditions is directed at the underlying cause. For idiopathic precocious puberty, drugs to inhibit pituitary gonadotropin secretion (medroxyprogesterone acetate, LHRH analogues) or to block androgen action (cryproterone acetate) have been used with varying success to prevent further sexual maturation. Treatment does not usually prevent premature closure of long bone epiphyses.

Root AW, Shulman DI: Isosexual precocity: Current concepts and recent advances. Fertil Steril 45:749, 1986. *A well-referenced review of the causes and treatment of isosexual precocious puberty.*

TUMORS OF THE TESTIS

Tumors of the testis are uncommon, representing about 1 per cent of all cancers in men. The annual incidence of testicular tumors is 6 per 100,000 males. About 95 per cent of testicular tumors are malignant and derive from the germ cells. The remaining 5 per cent are non–germ-cell tumors derived mostly from Leydig and Sertoli cells of the gonadal stroma and are usually benign. The peak age of incidence of testicular cancer is 20 to 35 years. It is the most common malignancy and the third leading cause of cancer death in this age group. A testicular mass in a patient over 50 years is more likely to be a lymphoma than a germ-cell tumor.

The most significant risk factor for developing testicular cancer is cryptorchidism. In unilateral cryptorchidism, the contralateral, normally descended testis also carries an increased risk of malignant degeneration. Orchiopexy at an early age (two to three years) may reduce the risk of neoplasm.

Germ Cell Tumors

Germ cell cancers may be classified according to their pathologic characteristics into seminoma and nonseminoma. *Nonseminomatous cancers* include *embryonal cell carcinomas, choriocarcinomas,* and *teratomas.* The presence of any nonseminomatous element in a tumor that is predominantly seminoma dictates its classification as a nonseminoma. The distinction between seminoma and nonseminoma is important to plan for staging and subsequent therapy. Seminomas usually metastasize via regional lymph nodes to retroperitoneal, mediastinal, and supraclavicular lymph nodes and are very sensitive to radiation therapy. On the other hand, nonseminomas metastasize by both lymphatic and hematogenous routes (especially to liver and lungs) and are radioresistant.

Most patients with germ cell tumors present with a painless mass in the testis. Rapid onset of a painful testicular mass is usually caused by bleeding into the neoplasm. Back or abdominal pain (from retroperitoneal lymphadenopathy), shortness of breath (from diffuse pulmonary metastases), gynecomastia (from hCG secretion), supraclavicular lymphadenopathy, or ureteral obstruction may also be present.

Germ cell tumors, especially nonseminomatous cancers, often secrete biologic markers (Ch. 172). Embryonal cell cancers may secrete *alpha-fetoprotein*. Pure seminomas never elaborate alpha-fetoprotein, and its presence in serum implies the presence of nonseminomatous elements in the tumor or metastases. *hCG* is most often secreted by choriocarcinomas and embryonal cell carcinomas and, rarely, by pure seminomas. This marker may be detected and differentiated from cross-reacting LH in serum with a specific beta-hCG assay. Both of these tumor markers may be used to monitor response to therapy. They may precede clinically detectable disease by weeks to months.

In seminoma, orchiectomy and radiotherapy to the periaortic and iliac lymph nodes have resulted in cure rates of 80 to 95 per cent. In nonseminomatous testicular cancer, the addition of cisplatin to aggressive, multiple-drug chemotherapeutic regimens has resulted in response rates of 40 to 70 per cent and long-term remission in 40 per cent of patients.

Non—Germ Cell Tumors

Non–germ cell tumors are rare tumors that develop from the two major elements of testicular stroma, the *Leydig* and *Sertoli cells*. They are usually benign, but about 10 per cent are malignant and metastasize via regional lymphatics. Both Leydig and Sertoli cell tumors may secrete a variety of steroid hormones, primarily androgens or estrogens, that may result in virilization or feminization, respectively. Gynecomastia is present in about 30 per cent of patients with non–germ cell tumors. Children may present with either isosexual (virilizing) or heterosexual (feminizing) precocious pseudopuberty.

Einhorn LH: Cancer of the testis: A new paradigm. Hosp Prac 21:165, 1986. *An excellent review of staging, current therapy, and responses to treatment of testicular cancer.*

Einhorn LH, Donohue JP, Reckham MJ, et al.: Cancer of the testes. In DeVita VT, Hellman S, Rosenberg SA (eds.): Cancer: Principles and Practice of Oncology. Philadelphia, JB Lippincott, 1985, p 979. *A comprehensive, well-written discussion of testicular cancer.*

Hainsworth JD, Greco FA: Testicular germ cell neoplasms. Am J Med 75:817, 1983. *The diagnosis and treatment of testicular tumors are well described in this excellent review (121 references).*

236 DISEASES OF THE PROSTATE
Patrick C. Walsh

The adult prostate weighs approximately 20 grams and lies immediately below the base of the bladder surrounding the proximal portion of the urethra. This tubuloalveolar gland secretes a colorless, slightly acidic fluid that contains fibrinolysin, citric acid, acid phosphatase, spermine, potassium, calcium, and zinc. The differentiation, growth, and function of the prostate are under the regulation of testicular androgens. Testosterone, which is secreted by the testes under the control of pituitary luteinizing hormone, is the principal circulating androgen. Testosterone enters the prostatic cell by passive diffusion where it is converted to dihydrotestosterone, the principal intracellular androgen. Dihydrotestosterone then binds to a specific cytosolic receptor protein, translocates to the nucleus, and influences in a complex fashion the expression of genetic information (see Ch. 221 for details).

Unlike most other organ systems, patients with diseases of the prostate do not present with complaints referable to disorders of prostatic function. Indeed, the exact role of prostatic secretion in normal reproduction is unclear. Rather, patients present with inflammatory, congestive, or neoplastic disturbances that most often give rise to difficulties with micturition. For this reason, men are often unaware of the existence of the prostate until one of these disorders develops. Starting at puberty, the prostate increases from approximately 4 grams to 20 grams in weight by age 20. Thereafter, for the next several decades prostatitis is the most common prostatic disorder. Beyond the fifth decade, benign hyperplasia and prostatic carcinoma predominate.

PROSTATITIS

Prostatitis, which refers to any condition associated with prostatic inflammation, is the most imprecise diagnosis in all of medicine. The disease can be acute or chronic and can have either bacterial or nonbacterial causes.

ETIOLOGY AND PATHOGENESIS. Bacterial prostatitis is most commonly caused by gram-negative organisms (predominantly *Escherichia coli*) and more rarely by enterococcus. Possible routes of infection include ascending urethral infection, reflux of infected urine into the prostatic ducts that empty into the posterior urethra, invasion by rectal bacteria via direct extension or lymphogenous spread, and hematogenous infection. Whether infectious prostatitis is a sexually transmitted disease is uncertain. The etiology of nonbacterial prostatitis is unknown. Except in rare instances, the disease does not appear to be caused by fungi, obligate anaerobic bacteria, trichomonads, viral agents, T-mycoplasma, or *Chlamydia*.

CLINICAL MANIFESTATIONS, DIAGNOSIS, AND DIFFERENTIAL DIAGNOSIS. Much of the confusion concerning prostatitis is attributable to imprecise methods of diagnosis. Many male patients have multiple genitourinary complaints centered on the prostate. Often the medical history and physical findings are not helpful in the differential diagnosis. Furthermore, when done as isolated procedures, midstream urinalysis and culture offer little diagnostic assistance. The two most useful tools in forming a differential diagnosis are examination of the expressed prostatic secretions (EPS) and quantitative bacterial localization cultures. Although microscopic examination of the EPS is important, it can be misleading. The clinician should always compare the microscopic appearance of the EPS to smears of the spun sediment of the first voided 10 ml of urine (the urethral specimen) and the midstream urine (bladder specimen) to localize the site of the inflammatory response. The presence of more than 20 white blood cells per high power field in the EPS is abnormal. During prostatic inflammation EPS typically contain leukocytes and abnormal numbers of lipid-laden macrophages (oval fat bodies). The most accurate and useful method of establishing the diagnosis of bacterial prostatitis is the performance of simultaneous quantitative bacterial cultures of the urethral urine, bladder urine, and EPS. Four specimens are collected: the first voided 10 ml (VB1), the midstream aliquot (VB2), the EPS, and the first voided 10 ml immediately after prostatic massage (VB3). All specimens are cultured quantitatively by surface streaking onto blood and MacConkey agar. The diagnosis of bacterial prostatitis is confirmed when the quantitative bacterial colony counts of the prostatic specimens (EPS and VB3) significantly exceed those of the urethral (VB1) and bladder (VB2) specimens by at least one logarithm. Based on these diagnostic maneuvers, the inflammatory diseases of the prostate have been subdivided into four categories: (1) acute bacterial prostatitis, (2) chronic bacterial prostatitis, (3) non-bacterial prostatitis, and (4) prostatodynia.

Acute bacterial prostatitis is a fulminating bacterial infection characterized by fever, chills, low back and perineal pain, and intense irritative voiding symptoms. Rectal examination usually discloses a markedly tender prostate that is swollen, firm, and warm. Prostatic discomfort and the risk of bacteremia generally make prostatic massage unwise. Because bacterial cystitis usually accompanies the disease, the pathogen can be identified by culture of a voided specimen of urine. The disease often responds dramatically to therapy with antibacterial agents.

Chronic bacterial prostatitis is one of the most common causes of relapsing urinary tract infection in men. The majority of patients complain of irritative voiding symptoms (dysuria, urgency, frequency, and nocturia) and pain in various sites (suprapubic, perineal, low back, scrotal, and penile). However, patients are usually asymptomatic until significant bacteriuria develops. Rectal palpation discloses no specific or characteristic finding. The diagnosis is based upon quantitative bacterial localization cultures. Characteristically, these patients have relapsing urinary tract infections caused by the same pathogen. Although the urine may be sterilized and symptoms may disappear during treatment with antimicrobial agents, the organism often persists unaltered in the prostatic fluid; when therapy is discontinued, reinfection of the urine and reappearance of symptoms occur.

Nonbacterial prostatitis, a disease of uncertain cause, is the most common type of prostatitis seen today. The symptoms, physical findings, and microscopic appearance of the EPS in nonbacterial prostatitis and chronic bacterial prostatitis are indistinguishable. However, the patient with nonbacterial prostatitis has no history of documented urinary tract infection, and localization cultures exclude an infectious etiology. The etiology of this disorder is unknown. Finally, some male patients complain of symptoms that mimic prostatitis, especially a painful prostate, but they have negative cultures and no history of documented urinary tract infections. Contrary to the findings in the other categories, the EPS is normal. Since these men do not actually have prostatitis, the diagnostic term *prostatodynia* has been suggested.

All patients with lower urinary tract complaints require a full evaluation. The differential diagnosis of patients with lower urinary tract irritative symptoms should include carcinoma of the bladder, urethral stricture, prostatic obstruction, pericolic abscess, neurogenic bladder, diabetes mellitus, bladder calculus, and detrusor-sphincter dyssynergia. Because the symptoms in men with nonbacterial prostatitis are identical to those of patients with flat in situ carcinoma of the bladder, urinary cytologic studies and cystoscopy should be performed in these patients to exclude the presence of a malignancy.

TREATMENT. In patients with bacterial prostatitis, the use of antibacterial agents is complicated by the fact most of the agents that are useful against gram-negative bacteria diffuse poorly into prostatic fluid. The factors that limit diffusion include lipid solubility, pKa, protein binding, and molecular size and shape. Although trimethoprim fulfills all theoretical criteria and experimentally high levels can be demonstrated in canine prostatic fluid, only one third of patients with chronic prostatitis are cured by treatment with trimethoprim.

In patients with acute bacterial prostatitis, hospitalization may be required. Rest in bed, sexual abstention, increased hydration, analgesics, antipyretics, stool softeners, and suprapubic bladder drainage (the latter for the rare patient who has urinary retention) have been recommended. The diffuse and intense inflammation of acute prostatitis allows many drugs to diffuse readily into the prostatic fluid. Therapy

should be begun with trimethoprim-sulfamethoxazole (160 mg of trimethoprim and 800 mg of sulfamethoxazole), administered twice daily until the results of culture and sensitivity are known. Therapy with the appropriate antibiotic should then be continued for at least 30 days in an effort to prevent the evolution of chronic prostatitis. In patients with chronic bacterial prostatitis, trimethoprim-sulfamethoxazole has the best cure rate that has been documented. Among patients who receive therapy continuously for four to six weeks, the cure rate has been 32 to 71 per cent. If patients fail to respond to this treatment, therapy with erythromycin, minocycline, or oral carbenicillin indanyl sodium may be attempted. In those patients who are not cured by medical therapy, continuous suppressive treatment with low-dose medication can be attempted. The most suitable choices are trimethoprim-sulfamethoxazole, 1 regular tablet daily, or nitrofurantoin, 100 mg by mouth daily. Even though the pathogen persists in the prostatic ducts, suppressive therapy usually prevents bacteriuria and controls the symptoms.

In patients with nonbacterial prostatitis, because the cause of the disease is unknown, definitive therapy is difficult. In these patients treatment is usually directed toward controlling the symptoms. A trial of clinical treatment with a tetracycline preparation or erythromycin in maximal doses is a reasonable approach to initial treatment. Most patients benefit from a frank discussion of the nature of their condition, short-term use of anticholinergic or anti-inflammatory agents, and hot sitz baths. Although prostatic massage is advocated by many, its benefits are questioned by others. The proper management of men with prostatodynia is unclear.

Fair WR (ed.): Managing prostatitis: Practical aspects of antibiotic therapy. Urology 24 (Suppl. to Dec '84), 1, 1984. *A symposium on etiology, diagnosis, and treatment of prostatitis.*

Meares EM Jr: Prostatitis and related disorders. In Walsh PC, Gittes RF, Perlmutter AD, et al. (eds.): Campbell's Urology. 5th ed. Philadelphia, W. B. Saunders Company, 1986, pp 868–887. *A comprehensive review of all aspects dealing with the diagnosis and management of the common forms of prostatitis.*

Meares EM Jr: Prostatitis syndromes: New perspectives about old woes. J Urol 123:141, 1980. *The author has provided an extensive review of the syndromes classified under the term prostatitis. The diagnosis, pathogenesis, and management of each disorder are clearly outlined. It is the most authoritative article published on this subject.*

BENIGN PROSTATIC HYPERPLASIA

INCIDENCE AND PREVALENCE. Benign prostatic hyperplasia (BPH) is probably the most common neoplastic growth in men. The disease characteristically occurs in men older than age 40; few if any patients with true nodular hyperplasia have been observed before this age. In men over the age of 50, the frequency of symptomatic BPH varies from 50 to 75 per cent. The mean age of detection by race is about 65 years for whites and approximately five years earlier for blacks. The probability of a 50-year-old man requiring an operation for BPH if he lives to 80 years of age is approximately 20 to 25 per cent.

ETIOLOGY AND PATHOGENESIS. Although the development of BPH is almost a universal phenomenon in aging men, the cause and pathogenesis of the disorder are not well understood. The two major factors necessary for the onset of BPH are the presence of the testes and aging. Consequently, much interest has been directed at identifying a hormonal etiology. There are several factors that strongly support the possibility that BPH in men is under endocrine control: (1) BPH does not occur in men who are castrated prior to puberty; (2) regression of established BPH has been reported to occur following castration; and (3) in a canine model, BPH can be produced by treatment with hormones. The prostate appears to become more sensitive to androgens as the gland enlarges and as plasma levels of testosterone decline. These observations suggest that other factors, such as induction of increased androgen receptor levels, may sensitize the prostate to adequate levels of dihydrotestosterone and accelerate growth. Medical approaches to the management of BPH must await further elucidation of these factors.

CLINICAL MANIFESTATIONS. Enlargement of the prostate causes no obvious physiologic manifestations. The disturbances that result are entirely secondary to effects on the urethra, the bladder, and the kidneys. In early cases the patient usually has minimal symptoms because the detrusor musculature is capable of compensating for the increased outlet resistance to urine flow. With increasing obstruction, however, the patient develops a constellation of symptoms called "prostatism": diminution in the caliber and force of the urinary stream, hesitancy in initiating voiding, inability to terminate micturition abruptly with postvoid dribbling, a sensation of incomplete emptying of the bladder, and occasionally urinary retention. These are *obstructive symptoms* and they must be carefully distinguished from *irritative* lower urinary tract symptoms such as dysuria, frequency, and urgency. Disastrous results can follow a prostatectomy performed on a patient whose symptoms stemmed from irritation, such as an inflammatory or infectious process, rather than from obstruction. As the amount of residual urine increases, the patient may note nocturia, diurnal frequency, a mass in the lower abdomen, and overflow urinary incontinence. In patients with slowly progressive obstruction, the patient may gradually adjust to the symptoms and present with "silent prostatism." On examination these patients may show the secondary anemia of renal insufficiency, a lower abdominal midline mass representing a distended bladder, and other findings associated with renal insufficiency (see Ch. 83).

DIAGNOSIS AND DIFFERENTIAL DIAGNOSIS. Usually there is no difficulty in establishing the diagnosis of BPH. The patient usually presents with lower urinary tract obstructive symptoms. Prior to examination the physician should observe the patient voiding to completion to document the decrease in size and force of the urinary stream. The prostate is palpated with attention to size, consistency, and shape. Hyperplasia usually produces a smooth, firm, and elastic enlargement of the prostate. However, the size of the prostate on rectal examination does not permit one to estimate the degree of bladder neck obstruction. Patients with marked enlargement of the prostate may have no urinary tract obstruction, and others with a large intravesical median lobe may have marked outflow obstructive symptoms without palpable enlargement of the gland. In addition to revealing the individual characteristics of the prostate, the rectal examination also affords the physician an opportunity to evaluate the intactness of the rectal spincter, which indirectly reflects the state of vesical innervation.

A urinalysis and urine culture are performed to evaluate the presence of infection; a serum creatinine is obtained to evaluate renal function; and a serum acid phosphatase sample is drawn (preferably prior to prostatic examination). In patients whose disease is in an early stage and who have only mild symptoms, no further studies are necessary. However, in men with marked outlet obstructive symptoms, intravenous urography and cystourethroscopy should be performed. The intravenous urogram with a postvoiding film will document the degree of upper tract obstruction, identify the presence of bladder calculi, and estimate the degree of bladder emptying. Cystourethroscopy is valuable in confirming the presence of vesical neck obstruction, in evaluating the degree of detrusor hypertrophy (presence of trabeculation, cellules, and diverticula), and in excluding the presence of a bladder tumor.

Several other conditions produce bladder neck obstruction: carcinoma of the prostate, bladder neck contracture, urethral stricture, bladder calculus, carcinoma of the bladder, chronic prostatitis, and neurogenic bladder. The presence of irritative lower urinary tract symptoms, such as dysuria, urgency, and frequency, should alert the physician to consider conditions

other than obstruction as the cause for the patient's symptoms. In the absence of a large amount of residual urine, frequency and nocturia are not caused by PBH. Bladder neck contracture, urethral stricture, bladder calculi, and bladder neoplasms are best evaluated with endoscopy.

TREATMENT AND PROGNOSIS. At present, there is no effective medical management fo BPH; surgery is the only effective form of therapy. The vast majority of men over the age of 60 have some evidence of BPH, so the mere presence of this disorder is not an indication for its treatment. The general indications for the relief of prostatic obstruction are (1) acute urinary retention, (2) hydronephrosis, (3) recurrent urinary tract infection aggravated by residual urine, (4) severe hematuria from a congestive prostate, and (5) outflow obstructive symptoms that are of sufficient concern to the patient to cause him to desire treatment. When the patient is seen early in the course of the disease, when his symptoms are mild, and before any of these relative indications are present, he is often curious about the natural history of the disease. This question is difficult to answer, because many patients who receive no treatment whatsoever will have no change in their symptoms over many years. Consequently in the group of patients that lack definitive indications for prostatectomy, it appears advisable to examine the patient periodically to observe the natural history of the disease rather than to anticipate its development by advising prophylactic prostatectomy. Simple prostatectomy can be performed in a variety of ways. However, transurethral resection of the prostate is the procedure with the least morbidity.

Walsh PC: Benign prostatic hyperplasia. In Walsh PC, Gittes RF, Perlmutter AD, et al. (eds.): Campbell's Urology. 5th ed. Philadelphia, W. B. Saunders Company, 1986, pp 1248–1265. *A comprehensive review of all aspects relative to the diagnosis and treatment of benign prostatic hyperplasia.*

Wilson JD: The pathogenesis of benign prostate hyperplasia. Am J Med 68:745, 1980. *A concise and lucid discussion of the endocrine factors that may be responsible for the development of benign prostatic hyperplasia. Experimental studies are integrated with clinical findings to formulate a sound understanding of the pathogenesis of this common disease.*

CARCINOMA OF THE PROSTATE

INCIDENCE, PREVALENCE, AND EPIDEMIOLOGY. The prostate is the second leading site of cancer in males, accounting for about 19 per cent of all male cancers. The only female cancer that accounts for more new cancer cases per year is cancer of the breast. Approximately 8.7 per cent of white males and 9.4 per cent of nonwhite males will develop cancer of the prostate. Furthermore, it is calculated that 2.6 per cent of newborn white males and 4.3 per cent of newborn nonwhite males will eventually die of the disease. Although carcinoma of the prostate does not develop in eunuchs, there is no other evidence to suggest that a direct relationship exists between hormone levels and the development of prostatic cancer. Similarly, no relationship between the development of benign prostatic hyperplasia and prostatic cancer has been demonstrated. Furthermore, there is little relationship between prostatic cancer and industrial carcinogens, cigarette smoking, use of alcohol, disease patterns, circumcision, weight, height, blood group, or hair distribution.

PATHOLOGY. More than 95 per cent of all prostatic carcinomas are adenocarcinomas. The tumor is multifocal in 85 per cent of the cases, suggesting a multifocal rather than a single site of origin. Prostatic carcinoma can spread by local extension or by lymphatic or hematogenous dissemination. As carcinoma of the prostate progresses, the tumor extends to the urethra, the bladder neck, the seminal vesicles, and the trigone. The most common sites of lymph node metastases, in descending order of frequency, are the obturator, hypogastric, iliac, presacral, and periaortic nodes. Osseous metastases constitute the most common form of hematogenous spread. The most frequent sites of involvement are, in decreasing order, the pelvis, the lumbar spine, the femora, the thoracic spine, and the ribs. The most common sites for

TABLE 236–1. CARCINOMA OF THE PROSTATE

Stage (Whitmore)	Definition of Stage	Usual Treatment
A	Not palpable; found by histopathology	
A₁	Focal, well differentiated	Observation, except in young men
A₂	Diffuse, poorly differentiated	Radical prostatectomy
B	Palpable, but limited to prostate	
B₁	Solitary nodule < one lobe	Radical prostatectomy
B₂	One lobe or more involved	Megavolt radiation or radical prostatectomy
C	Extension beyond capsule	Megavolt radiation
D	Metastatic disease; acid phosphatase ↑	Hormonal therapy
D₁	Pelvis lymph nodes only	⎫ Rarely chemotherapy
D₂	More widespread metastases	⎭

visceral metastases include the lung and liver. Pulmonary metastases are detected clinically or radiographically in less than 6 per cent of patients.

The prognosis of patients with prostatic cancer correlates well with the grade and stage of the tumor, although grading is somewhat difficult because most tumors exhibit a heterogeneous histologic pattern (Table 236–1): *Stage A* disease is not palpable clinically but is found histopathologically following prostatectomy. It is subdivided into two biologically meaningful subclasses: Stage A1, focal or well-differentiated carcinoma, and Stage A2, diffuse or poorly differentiated carcinoma. *Stage B* tumors are limited to the prostate and on rectal examination can be subdivided into Stage B1, a solitary nodule involving less than one lobe of the prostate, and Stage B2, cancer in which one lobe or more is involved. *Stage C* tumors extend beyond the prostatic capsule but have not metastasized. *Stage D* represents metastatic carcinoma of the prostate and includes any patient with an elevated serum acid phosphatase level. Stage D can be subdivided into Stage D1, the presence of metastatic disease in lymph nodes, and Stage D2, patients with clinical metastatic carcinoma.

CLINICAL MANIFESTATIONS AND DIAGNOSIS. Early in the clinical evolution of prostatic cancer, symptoms may be entirely absent. Later, patients develop symptoms of urinary outflow obstruction or bone pain. Hematuria, lymphadenopathy, and lower extremity edema are uncommon presenting symptoms of prostatic cancer. A careful routine rectal examination is the only means of detecting prostatic cancer at an early stage. Carcinoma of the prostate characteristically has a hard consistency, felt as a region of dense induration within the substance of the prostate. With tumor penetration of the capsule, the margins of the prostate may become obscured and tumor may be palpated extending to the seminal vesicles and regions of the bladder neck. Other causes of prostatic induration include focal regions of benign hyperplasia, prostatic calculi, granulomatous prostatitis, prostatic infarction, and postoperative changes. Approximately 50 per cent of prostatic nodules are malignant.

A clinical suspicion of prostatic cancer requires histologic verification by needle biopsy. If the biopsy is positive, the patient should have a serum acid phosphatase determination, an intravenous urogram, and a bone scan. Because of the lack of specificity of bone scans, skeletal radiographs should be performed of any suspicious areas. Routine lymphangiography or staging pelvic lymphadenectomy is generally unnecessary in the management of patients with prostatic cancer.

Serum acid phosphatase is elevated in most patients with bony metastases and, more rarely, with localized carcinoma. It is not sufficiently sensitive or specific for screening, so it is used mainly to follow the progress of the disease. Acid phosphatase, not inhibited by 1-tartrate, is characteristically elevated in the serum of patients with Gaucher's disease (Ch. 185).

TREATMENT. There is considerable debate concerning the best mode of therapy for each particular stage of carcinoma of the prostate. In selecting treatment there is often the dilemma of attempting both to maintain the quality of life and to increase the duration of survival. Men with carcinoma of the prostate are often old and suffer from other illnesses that may pose a greater threat than the cancer itself. Furthermore, although there are a variety of relatively effective therapeutic modalities from which to choose, there is little information that accurately compares their relative efficacy. Each form of treatment is associated with undesirable side effects. In selecting therapy the physician must determine the long-term threat that the tumor poses to the quality and duration of survival in each individual patient and must select a form of treatment that provides the proper balance between efficacy and morbidity.

In patients over 60 years of age with Stage A1 prostatic cancer, observation but no further treatment is necessary. In younger stage A1 patients active treatment should be considered. Patients with Stage A2 and B1 prostatic cancer who are less than 70 years old are ideal candidates for radical prostatectomy. In these patients, the tumor will be confined to the pathologic specimen in 84 to 95 per cent of the cases, and the long-term survival of these patients is excellent. Although the complications of radical prostatectomy are often emphasized, in the hands of the experienced surgeon the incidence of urinary incontinence should be less than 2 per cent. Previously, most patients were impotent postoperatively. However, with use of a new surgical technique this undesirable side effect can be avoided. In patients with Stage B2 prostatic cancer, 50 to 60 per cent will have involvement of the seminal vesicles. Because only 5 per cent of patients with involvement of the seminal vesicles survive 15 years free of tumor, patients with Stage B2 disease are not ideal candidates for radical surgery. For the treatment of Stage B2 and C disease, megavoltage radiation provides excellent palliation and the possibility of cure. For the treatment of Stage D disease, hormonal therapy is the preferred modality for initial treatment, but there are two major areas of controversy: (1) What are the relative merits of estrogen therapy versus therapy with bilateral orchiectomy or the use of LHRH analogues? (2) What is the preferred timing of endocrine treatment?

The physiologic effects of orchiectomy, treatment with estrogens, and treatment with LHRH analogues are similar; i.e., they produce regression of cancer of the prostate by suppressing plasma testosterone levels. Orchiectomy alone, estrogen, or treatment with an LHRH analogue appears to be equally effective in the treatment of metastatic carcinoma of the prostate. However, because of the untoward cardiovascular side effects associated with estrogen therapy, orchiectomy or treatment with an LHRH analogue is preferred.

The second point of controversy surrounds the proper timing of endocrine therapy: Should it be instituted as soon as the diagnosis is made, or should treatment be delayed until the patient becomes symptomatic? In one study, patients with Stage A and B carcinoma of the prostate who were treated with estrogen had a higher death rate than did patients who were not receiving estrogen. The increase in death rate was caused by cardiovascular complications, suggesting that early treatment with estrogens can be harmful under some circumstances. The survival rate of patients with Stage C and D carcinoma treated with initial hormonal therapy was identical to the survival rate in those patients in whom hormonal therapy was delayed until symptoms appeared. Therefore, delaying hormonal therapy until symptoms occur has no adverse effect on the survival rate in patients with established metastatic disease. Estrogen therapy, treatment with an LHRH analogue, or orchiectomy should probably be delayed until symptoms appear. At that time, treatment with low-dose estrogen (diethylstibestrol, 1 mg per day), therapy with an LHRH analogue, or orchiectomy may be utilized. In patients with a history of cardiovascular disease, bilateral orchiectomy or treatment with an LHRH analogue is preferred. Reactivation of symptoms following an initial response to hormonal therapy usually indicates a tumor no longer under hormonal control. Attempts at further endocrine therapy (adrenalectomy, hypophysectomy, or antiandrogen therapy) are usually disappointing. At present the only hope for treatment of these patients is chemotherapy. Several large-scale clinical studies are currently in progress to evaluate different cytotoxic agents for the treatment of metastatic carcinoma of the prostate.

Catalona WJ, Scott WW: Carcinoma of the prostate. In Walsh PC, Gittes RF, Perlmutter AD, et al.: (eds.): Campbell's Urology. 5th ed. Philadelphia, W. B. Saunders Company, pp 1463–1543. *This article provides a comprehensive review of all aspects relative to the diagnosis and treatment of carcinoma of the prostate.*
Leuprolide Study Group: Leuprolide versus diethylstilbestrol for metastatic prostatic cancer. N Engl J Med 311:1281, 1983. *A randomized controlled study demonstrating that an LHRH analogue is therapeutically equivalent to and causes fewer side effects than diethylstilbestrol.*
Walsh PC, Lepor H: The role of radical prostatectomy in the management of prostatic cancer. Cancer (in press). *This article provides a sound rationale for the use of radical prostatectomy and identifies those patients most likely to benefit from surgical therapy. It outlines the recent advances in preservation of sexual function following radical prostatectomy.*

237 THE OVARIES*

Robert W. Rebar

The ovaries episodically release female gametes (oocytes or eggs) and secrete sex steroid hormones, principally androstenedione, estradiol, and progesterone. Oocytes are released only during the adult reproductive years when sex steroid secretion is also greatest, but the ovaries are physiologically active throughout life.

Sex steroids affect the growth, differentiation, and function of a variety of tissues and organs throughout the body; therefore abnormalities of the ovaries and of sex steroid secretion should be recognized by all physicians. A rational approach to the diagnosis and treatment of reproductive disorders in women requires an understanding of the func-

*Dedicated to the memory of Griff T. Ross.

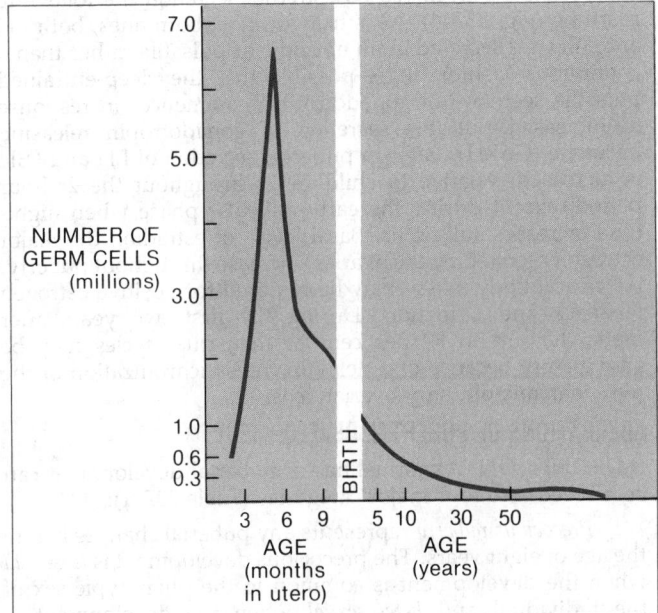

FIGURE 237–1. The number of oocytes present in both ovaries at different ages. (Adapted from Baker TG: In Austin CR, Short RJ (eds.): Reproduction in Mammals. I. Germ Cells and Fertilization. London, Cambridge University Press, 1972, pp 14–45. Reproduced from Rebar RW: Semin Reprod Endocrinol 1:169–176, 1983.)

tions of the ovaries and of their most important unit, the follicle, throughout life.

EMBRYOLOGY AND ANATOMY OF THE OVARIES

EMBRYOGENESIS AND DIFFERENTIATION. Prior to six to seven weeks of fetal age the gonads are paired, undifferentiated gonadal ridges overlying the mesonephros. By the sixth week of gestation, the primordial germ cells have migrated from their site of origin in the yolk sac to the gonadal ridges. Beginning during the sixth to eighth weeks the ovaries rapidly differentiate, and the number of germ cells, now called oogonia, increases by mitosis to 6 to 7 million. The germ cells next undergo meiosis such that all germ cells (now called oocytes) are arrested in meiotic prophase by the seventh month of gestation. From midgestation onward the number of germ cells progressively decreases until the menopause, by which time virtually no oocytes remain (Fig. 237–1). Thus the human female is born with a finite and decreasing number of germ cells. The germ cells are eliminated from ovaries by *ovulation* and by *atresia* (degeneration), which accounts for the elimination of 99.9 per cent of all germ cells. The development of the ovaries is described in greater detail in Ch. 234.

THE ADULT OVARY. The adult ovary consists of two principal parts: a central medulla surrounded by the predominant outer cortex (Fig. 237–2). The entire ovary is limited by a single cell layer termed the germinal epithelium. The medulla contains the blood vessels and nerves as well as nests of steroid-secreting hilus or ovarian Leydig cells. The cortex contains the *follicle complex*, composed of the *oocyte, granulosa cells,* and *theca cells.* Characteristic changes occur in each component during follicle growth and differentiation. Interactions among the follicular components give rise to the gamete (ovum) and to sex steroid hormones necessary for establishing and maintaining early pregnancy following fertilization of the ovum.

Follicles can be divided into two major classes, nongrowing and growing. The nongrowing or *primordial* follicles comprise 90 to 95 per cent of the ovarian follicles throughout reproductive life of the female. The ability of a woman to menstruate and reproduce depends totally upon the pool of primordial follicles. Each primordial follicle contains a small oocyte arrested in meiotic prophase, surrounded by a layer of squamous cells from which granulosa cells originate. These cells are bounded by the basal lamina, which is selectively permeable to solutes in plasma. This complex is surrounded in turn by stroma, which consists of supporting connective tissue cells, contractile cells, and steroid-secreting thecal interstitial cells. Primordial follicles are recruited sequentially to become growing follicles, which then pass through primary, secondary, and tertiary (or graafian) phases. Atresia may occur in any phase.

Baker TG, Sum OW: Development of the ovary and oogenesis. Clin Obstet Gynecol 3:3, 1976. *A detailed summary of ovarian development.*
Erickson GF: Follicular growth and development. In Sciarra JJ (ed.): Gynecology and Obstetrics. Vol. 4. Philadelphia, Harper & Row, 1986 (rev. ed.), pp 1–21. *A treatise on follicular growth and development.*

OVARIAN FUNCTION IN CHILDHOOD AND PUBERTY

PHYSICAL CHANGES AT PUBERTY. Puberty extends from the earliest signs of sexual maturation until the attainment of physical, mental, and emotional maturity. Pubertal changes in girls result directly or indirectly from maturation of the hypothalamic-pituitary-ovarian unit. Hormonally, human puberty is characterized by a resetting of the negative gonadal steroid feedback loop, the establishment of new circadian and ultradian (frequent) gonadotropin rhythms, and the acquisition in the female of a positive estrogen feedback loop controlling the menstrual cycle as interdependent expressions of the gonadotropins and ovarian steroids. In girls, pubertal development generally occurs between eight and fourteen years of age. The age of onset and the rate of progress

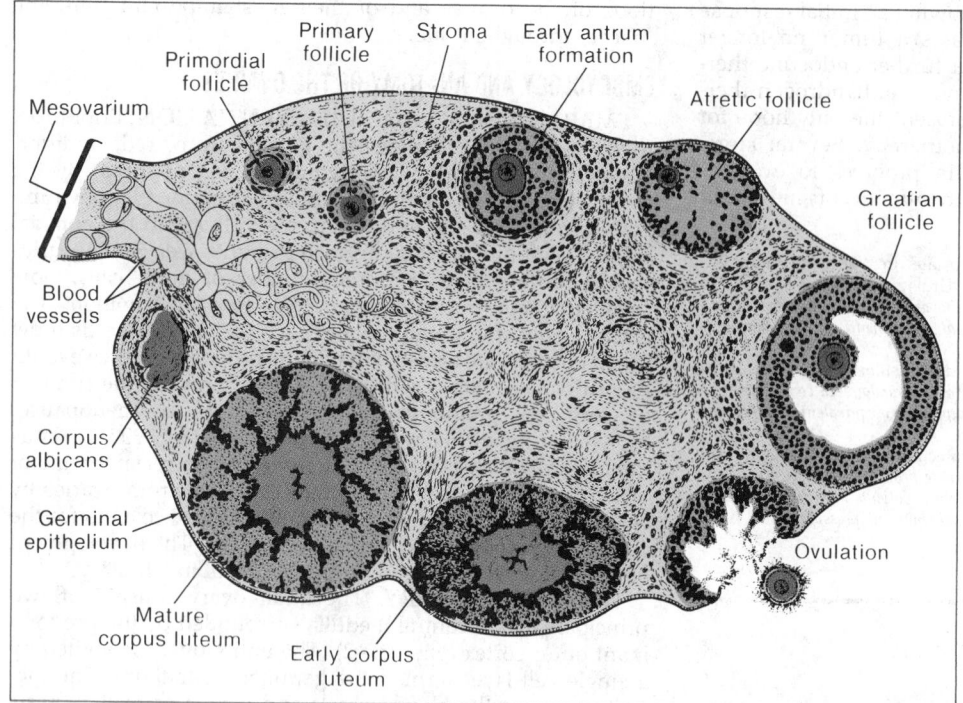

FIGURE 237-2. Diagrammatic illustration of the microscopic anatomy of the ovary. Changes in the components of the follicular complex occurring during atresia and ovulation are shown, progressing clockwise, from a primordial follicle (*upper left*) to a corpus albicans (*lower left*). (Adapted from Ross GT, Schreiber JR: In Yen SSC, Jaffe RB (eds.): Reproductive Endocrinology—Physiology, Pathophysiology and Clinical Management. Philadelphia, W.B. Saunders Company, 1978, pp 63–79.)

through puberty are variable and depend upon genetic, socioeconomic, nutritional, physical, and psychological factors.

Physical changes occur in an orderly sequence over a definite time frame during puberty (Fig. 237–3). Breast budding in girls is usually the first pubertal change, followed shortly by the appearance of pubic hair, with menarche occurring late in pubertal development. The time from breast budding (median age of onset 9.8 years) to menarche approximates two years. Breast development results from increasing ovarian estrogen production; pubic and axillary hair, from increasing ovarian androgen production. Estrogens are required for growth of pubic hair as well.

The ovarian sex steroids join with growth hormone and adrenal androgens to produce the adolescent growth spurt. Peak growth velocity is achieved relatively early with little growth observed following menarche. Lean body mass, skeletal mass, and body fat are equal in prepubertal boys and girls, but by maturity women have twice as much body fat and less lean body mass and skeletal mass as men, as a result of differences in sex steroid secretion beginning at puberty. Estrogens are necessary for normal formation, mineralization, and maturation of bones. Well-established standards exist for determining radiographically, typically by examining radio-

graphs of the bones of the wrist, whether bone age is appropriate for chronologic age. Estrogen deficiencies retard and excesses advance bone age in relation to chronologic age.

HORMONAL CHANGES. The ovaries function even in early childhood. The low levels of luteinizing hormone (LH) and follicle-stimulating hormone (FSH), which are normally present, increase if the ovaries are removed prior to puberty, just as they do later in life, indicating exquisite sensitivity of the hypothalamic-pituitary unit to extremely low circulating sex steroid levels. As puberty nears there is a progressive decrease in sensitivity of the hypothalamic-pituitary unit to sex steroids, leading to increased secretion of pituitary gonadotropins, stimulation of sex steroid output, and the development of secondary sex characteristics. Increased secretion of both LH and FSH initially occurs at night with sleep and is associated with increased estradiol secretion the following morning (Fig. 237–4). As is true for most hormones, both LH and FSH are secreted in an episodic or pulsatile rather than a continuous fashion. It is possible that the sleep-entrained pulsatile secretion of gonadotropins commences in response to increased pulsatile secretion of gonadotropin releasing hormone (GnRH). Later in puberty, secretion of LH and FSH is increased, relative to childhood, throughout the 24-hour period, except during the early follicular phase when nighttime increases still occur. Basal levels of estradiol, the major estrogen secreted by the ovaries, increase throughout puberty. A "critical body mass" may be required for positive estrogen feedback and ovulation. During the first two years after menarche, up to 90 per cent of menstrual cycles may be anovulatory because of a delay in the synchronization of the hypothalamic-pituitary-ovarian axis.

ABERRATIONS OF PUBERTAL DEVELOPMENT

DEFINITION. Abnormalities of pubertal development can be divided into four major categories (Table 237–1):

1. *Precocious puberty* represents any pubertal changes before the age of eight years. The precocious development is *isosexual* when the development is common to the phenotypic sex of the individual and *heterosexual* when the development is characteristic of the opposite sex. *True precocious puberty* is due to premature maturation of the hypothalamic-pituitary axis. In the absence of increased hypothalamic-pituitary activity, *precocious pseudopuberty* exists.

2. *Delayed (or interrupted) puberty* is defined as the absence

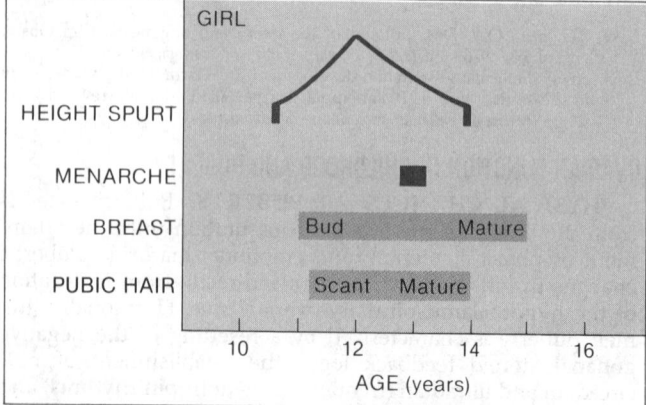

FIGURE 237-3. Temporal sequence of events for the "average" girl during puberty. Reproduced from Rebar RW: In Yen SSC, Jaffe RB (eds.): Reproductive Endocrinology—Physiology, Pathophysiology and Clinical Management. 2nd ed. Philadelphia, W.B. Saunders Company, 1986, pp 683–733.)

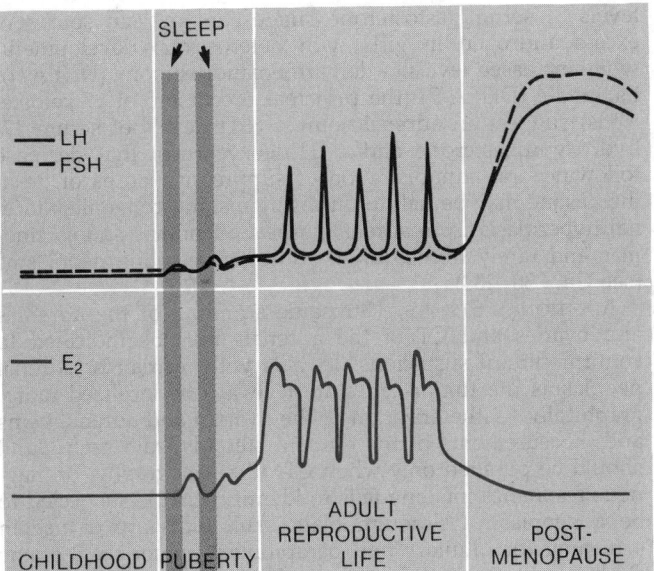

FIGURE 237–4. The changing patterns of LH, FSH, and estradiol (E₂) concentrations in peripheral blood throughout the life of a woman. The elevated levels of LH and FSH present in the first several weeks of life are not shown, nor is the fact that both LH and FSH are secreted in a pulsatile fashion. The pubertal period has been expanded to illustrate the sleep-associated increases in LH and FSH followed by morning increases in E₂ that are observed during puberty. (Reprinted with permission from *Endocrine and Metabolism Continuing Education Quality Control Program*, 1982. Copyright American Association for Clinical Chemistry, Inc.)

of any secondary sex characteristics by the age of 13 years or of menarche by age 16 or by passage of 5 or more years from breast budding to menarche.

3. *Asynchronous pubertal development* occurs when there is deviation from the normal pattern of pubertal development.

4. *Heterosexual pubertal development* is development occurring at the appropriate time, but with some features characteristic of the opposite sex.

PRECOCIOUS PUBERTY. *Differential Diagnosis.* The temporal sequence in which the signs and symptoms of sex steroid hormone excess appeared is most important. *Incomplete isosexual precocious puberty* indicates premature development of only a single pubertal feature. If breast budding occurs prior to the age of eight years in the absence of any other development, the diagnosis may be *premature thelarche*. Premature thelarche is believed due to transient increases in estrogen secretion or increased breast sensitivity to the small quantities of circulating estrogens present prior to puberty. If pubic and/or axillary hair develops alone and persists, *premature pubarche* and *adrenarche* must be considered. These abnormalities are associated with slight increases in adrenal androgen secretion, but not with clitoromegaly or other signs of virilization. These syndromes require no treatment, and affected girls typically begin true puberty at the usual age.

When precocious development is isosexual, the purpose of evaluation is to determine if the cause is central (true precocious puberty) or not. Careful questioning of the patient and her parents may indicate inadvertent ingestion or absorption of sex steroids (iatrogenic or factitious). About 10 per cent of individuals with true precocious puberty have one of several organic brain diseases, including neoplasms, tuberous sclerosis, neurofibromatosis, encephalitis, meningitis, and hydrocephalus. The seriousness of intracranial lesions mandates that girls with precocious puberty have skull films and/or computed tomography (CT) of the brain. In almost 90 per cent of girls with true precocious puberty, however, no cause is identified (idiopathic or constitutional).

The physical examination may also provide critical information about the etiology of the precocious development.

TABLE 237–1. ABERRATIONS OF PUBERTAL DEVELOPMENT

I. Precocious development (before age 8)
  A. Isosexual precocity
    1. Incomplete sexual precocity
      a. Premature thelarche
      b. Premature pubarche
      c. Premature adrenarche
    2. True precocious puberty
      a. Idiopathic (constitutional)
      b. Due to CNS lesions
      c. McCune-Albright syndrome
      d. Primary hypothyroidism
      e. Silver-Russell syndrome
    3. Precocious pseudopuberty
      a. Ovarian neoplasms
      b. Adrenal neoplasms
      c. Iatrogenic (estrogen-containing preparations)
      d. hCG-secreting neoplasms distinct from CNS and ovarian tumors
  B. Heterosexual precocity
    1. Ovarian neoplasms
    2. Adrenal neoplasms
    3. Congenital adrenal hyperplasia
    4. Other rare disorders of sexual differentiation
II. Delayed pubertal development (no development by age 13; absence of menarche by age 16; passage of 5 years or more from breast budding without menarche)
  A. Anatomic abnormalities
    1. Müllerian agenesis or dysgenesis (Rokitansky-Küster-Hauser syndrome)
    2. Distal genital tract obstruction
      a. Transverse vaginal septum
      b. Imperforate hymen
      c. Vaginal agenesis
  B. Hypergonadotropic hypogonadism (FSH > 40 mIU per milliliter)
    1. Gonadal dysgenesis
      a. With stigmata of Turner's syndrome
      b. Pure (46,XX or 46,XY)
      c. Mixed
    2. Ovarian failure with normal ovarian development
      a. Autoimmune disorders
      b. Gonadotropin receptor and/or postreceptor defects (?Resistant ovary or Savage syndrome)
      c. Enzymatic defects (17α-hydroxylase deficiency, galactosemia)
      d. Physical causes
        i. Irradiation
        ii. Chemotherapeutic agents
        iii. Viral agents
      e. Idiopathic
  C. Hypogonadotropic or normogonadotropic hypogonadism (LH and FSH < 10 mIU per milliliter or LH and FSH 6–25 mIU per milliliter with at least one being greater than 10 mIU per milliliter)
    1. Isolated gonadotropin deficiency
      a. In association with midline defects (Kallmann's syndrome)
      b. Independent of associated disorders
    2. Neoplasms of the hypothalamic-pituitary axis
      a. Craniopharyngiomas
      b. Pituitary tumors
      c. Others
    3. Hand-Schüller-Christian disease (eosinophilic granuloma; histiocytosis X)
    4. Idiopathic hypopituitarism
    5. "Hypothalamic" forms of amenorrhea
      a. Psychogenic
      b. Exercise associated
      c. Associated with malnutrition
      d. Anorexia nervosa
    6. Miscellaneous disorders
      a. Práder-Willi syndrome
      b. Lawrence-Moon-Bardet-Biedl syndrome
    7. Constitutional delayed puberty
III. Asynchronous pubertal development
  A. Incomplete forms of androgen insensitivity
  B. Complete forms of androgen insensitivity
IV. Heterosexual pubertal development
  A. Polycystic ovarian syndrome
  B. Congenital adrenal hyperplasia (female pseudohermaphrodism)
    1. 21-Hydroxylase deficiency
    2. 11β-Hydroxylase deficiency
    3. 3β-ol-Hydroxysteroid dehydrogenase deficiency
  C. Male pseudohermaphrodism due to 5α-reductase deficiency
  D. Male pseudohermaphrodism due to partial androgen insensitivity
  E. Mixed gonadal dysgenesis
  F. Androgen-producing neoplasms
    1. Ovarian
    2. Adrenal
  G. Cushing's syndrome

Cutaneous café au lait spots, facial asymmetry, polyostotic fibrous dysplasia, and other skeletal abnormalities and cranial nerve deficits suggest *McCune-Albright syndrome* in a girl with precocious puberty. Precocious development associated with short stature, congenital bodily asymmetry, a triangular facies, and clinodactyly suggests the *Silver-Russell syndrome*. Characteristic signs and symptoms may suggest the coexistence of primary hypothyroidism and precocious puberty, especially if galactorrhea is also present. In these patients, thyroid hormone replacement therapy will halt progression of pubertal development until the expected age of puberty.

Abdominal and rectal examination may reveal a mass and suggest an adrenal or ovarian tumor. Since palpable ovarian cysts may develop rarely prior to ovulation in true precocious puberty, the presence of a mass need not confirm the diagnosis of precocious pseudopuberty.

When vaginal bleeding is the only sign of development, the diagnosis of sexual precocity should be suspect. Common causes of bleeding in this age group include irritation from a vaginal infection or foreign body, sexual assault, prolapse of the urethral meatus, and ingestion of estrogen-containing medications (most commonly oral contraceptive preparations). A vaginal or cervical neoplasm is also a rare possibility. Thus, vaginal bleeding dictates the need for vaginal examination, often best performed under anesthesia, before further evaluation is undertaken.

Heterosexual precocity in an apparent prepubertal female is almost always due to congenital adrenal hyperplasia or to an androgen-secreting adrenal or ovarian neoplasm. Only very rarely must another disorder of sexual differentiation be considered (see Ch. 234). It is important to examine the external genitalia carefully because congenital adrenal hyperplasia is usually associated with some degree of sexual ambiguity.

Excessive androgens produced endogenously by abnormal fetal adrenal glands in utero or diffusing across the placenta to the fetus from the mother can virilize the external genitalia and result in female pseudohermaphroditism. The extent of virilization varies from an enlarged clitoris only to sexual ambiguity sufficient to make gender assignment difficult.

Excessive maternal androgen secretion, typically from an ovarian or adrenal neoplasm, can lead to virilization of a female fetus. This occurs very rarely, because of the great capacity of the placenta to aromatize naturally occurring androgens to estrogens. Virilization of a female fetus is much more apt to occur if a pregnant woman has ingested a synthetic steroid preparation with androgenic properties, because available synthetic compounds generally cannot be aromatized.

Excessive androgen secretion beginning in utero is usually associated with defective cortisol synthesis. As a consequence, ACTH secretion is increased, resulting in congenital adrenal hyperplasia and excessive androgen secretion. The three different enzyme defects in the steroidogenic pathway that can lead to virilization of the female fetus are described in Ch. 234. 21-Hydroxylase deficiency is the most common form of congenital adrenal hyperplasia, accounting for more than 90 per cent of affected individuals. The defect may vary from partial to complete deficiency of the enzyme.

Diagnostic Tests. MEASUREMENT OF PEPTIDE AND STEROID HORMONES. Increased levels of immunoreactive LH may suggest a chorionic gonadotropin (hCG)-secreting neoplasm, most commonly an ovarian teratoma or dysgerminoma. In such cases, the hCG, which is antigenically and biologically similar to LH, stimulates ovarian steroid secretion and pseudopubertal development. Levels and ratios of FSH and LH typical of pubertal as opposed to prepubertal girls help in diagnosing true precocious puberty. Timed urine collections rather than blood samples can be used to measure gonadotropin secretion if necessary. Excessively high circulating levels of estrogen suggest an estrogen-producing neoplasm. High

levels of serum testosterone suggest an ovarian source of excess androgen in girls with heterosexual development, while increased levels of dehydroepiandrosterone (DHEA) or its sulfate (DHEA-S) (the principal precursors of 17-ketosteroids) suggest an adrenal source. High levels of serum 17-hydroxyprogesterone and/or 11-deoxycortisol that decrease following oral administration of suppressive doses of dexamethasone may be helpful in distinguishing congenital adrenal hyperplasia from adrenal cortical adenomas and carcinomas and rarely from ovarian androgen-secreting neoplasms (see Ch. 230, 234).

ADDITIONAL STUDIES. Ultrasonic scanning of the adrenals and ovaries and CT of the adrenals may be indicated to confirm clinical suspicions. In girls with ovarian or adrenal neoplasms the tumor can almost always be localized radiographically. Catheterization of the ovarian and adrenal veins and measurements of the effluent steroids from each gland should be pursued only when CT, ultrasonography, or magnetic resonance imaging fails to identify what is suspected to be a neoplasm. Although plain skull films are of use in screening for pituitary and parapituitary tumors, CT of the skull is indicated in the presence of definite neurologic deficits or if true precocious puberty is suspected. Radiographic estimation of bone age is indicated in all cases and serves as a useful tool to follow the results of treatment.

Treatment. Treatment for precocious puberty should be initiated promptly so that: (1) The patient's ultimate height is not compromised as a result of sex steroid–induced premature epiphyseal closure. (2) Emotional disturbances in the patient and her parents are prevented or attenuated. The usual treatment for constitutional isosexual precocious puberty has been administration of medroxyprogesterone acetate (100 to 200 mg intramuscularly every two to four weeks) to suppress gonadotropin secretion. Medroxyprogesterone acetate, however, does not always prevent premature epiphyseal closure and the resultant short stature. More recently, gonadotropin releasing hormone agonists have been demonstrated to be effective and also may prevent bone maturation. If this is confirmed, use of these analogues may become the preferred therapy.

Individuals with CNS or steroid-secreting neoplasms must undergo therapy appropriate for the particular lesion. Girls with congenital adrenal hyperplasia are appropriately managed with glucocorticoids (plus mineralocorticoids when indicated) as outlined in Ch. 234.

DELAYED PUBERTY. Typically girls with delayed puberty present at the age of 16 years or later because of primary amenorrhea, but younger girls may present because of failure to initiate pubertal development. Because of the anxiety generated by delayed puberty, some evaluation is always indicated regardless of the age of the patient.

When pubertal development progresses normally but menstruation does not begin, an abnormality in the genital tract should be considered. Congenital malformations of the müllerian duct are uncommon, occurring in 0.02 per cent of all women. Most do not cause amenorrhea, and many do not impair reproduction. The anomalies associated with amenorrhea vary in severity from an imperforate hymen to complete aplasia of all müllerian duct derivatives with vaginal atresia. Although aplasia generally involves all of the müllerian duct derivatives, defects may involve only a single part of the distal genital tract.

A müllerian duct anomaly is suggested by (1) normal levels of serum gonadotropins and steroids, (2) an abnormal outflow tract, and (3) a history of cyclic abdominal pain with or without a palpable mass. Normal ovarian function still induces endometrial growth and shedding after menarche if the uterus is normal. In the absence of a normal outflow tract, however, the menstrual effluent is retained and may or may not be able to escape into the abdominal cavity. Free in the abdominal cavity, the effluent may cause endometriosis. Constrained to the uterine cavity, the effluent causes hematometra and a large abdominal mass. In the absence of a mass or cyclic pain, a karyotype is indicated in girls with evidence of an abnormal genital tract to rule out any of several disorders of sexual differentiation (see Ch. 234). Such disorders, however, almost never occur together with completely normal pubertal development. In girls with a normal karyotype and a genital tract anomaly, examination under anesthesia and diagnostic laparoscopy should be undertaken to delineate the extent of the defect. When the abnormality consists of an imperforate hymen or transverse vaginal septum only, surgical restoration can be accomplished relatively simply. Attempts to provide an outflow tract for the uterus should not be undertaken if there is no cervix because of the high risk of recurrent pelvic infection. Even with a functional cervix, the creation of an outflow tract that will permit successful pregnancy is unlikely. A functional vagina can be created surgically or by the daily use of ever larger dilators. To prevent shrinkage and scarring, surgery should be deferred until the patient is willing to use dilators even postoperatively on a daily basis or she is about to become sexually active.

Other causes of delayed puberty and primary amenorrhea are the same as those that may cause amenorrhea in older women (see below). When no apparent cause for delayed development is found, constitutional delayed puberty must be entertained as a diagnosis of exclusion. A strong family history of delayed maturation adds support to this presumption. Small doses of estrogen may be administered to induce some pubertal development, but may obscure a pathologic cause for the delay and may compromise linear growth and ultimate height.

ASYNCHRONOUS PUBERTAL DEVELOPMENT. Asynchronous pubertal development is characteristic of male pseudohermaphroditism due to androgen insensitivity, especially complete testicular feminization. This syndrome of androgen insensitivity is inherited either as an X-linked recessive or as a sex-limited autosomal dominant trait. Despite the presence of intra-abdominal or inguinal testes, there is complete failure of virilization. Affected individuals develop breasts (but only to Tanner stage 3) and a typical female habitus with unambiguous female external genitalia, but with absence of internal female structures, generally having only a foreshortened blind-ending vagina. Little or no pubic and axillary hair develops. The karyotype is obviously 46,XY in these individuals. Circulating testosterone levels are equivalent to or higher than those found in normal men, and LH levels are elevated while FSH levels are normal compared to menstruating women. This syndrome is further discussed in Ch. 234.

HETEROSEXUAL PUBERTAL DEVELOPMENT. *Polycystic ovarian (PCO) syndrome*, by far the most common cause of heterosexual pubertal development, is associated with the development of some secondary sex features characteristic of males at the normal age of puberty. Feminization occurs in affected girls, and they develop normal breasts and a typical female habitus, but masculinization also occurs. (In contrast, girls with congenital adrenal hyperplasia generally show little if any female development at puberty.) A heterogeneous syndrome, PCO syndrome most typically begins at or near puberty with hirsutism and irregular menses from the time of menarche. Menarche may be delayed as well, so that young women may present with primary amenorrhea. Basal LH levels tend to be somewhat elevated in perhaps 80 per cent of cases, and circulating levels of all androgens are elevated moderately.

Congenital adrenal hyperplasia is generally diagnosed prior to puberty, and heterosexual precocious pseudopuberty is typical. However, if the defect is mild and changes to the external genitalia are minimal, masculinization may occur at the expected age of puberty. This attenuated form of 21-hydroxylase deficiency is rare and seems to occur in families with a strong family history of hirsutism. Affected girls generally have some

defeminization with flattening of the breasts, severe hirsutism, relatively short stature, and obesity.

Mixed gonadal dysgenesis designates asymmetric gonadal development with a germ cell tumor or a testis on one side and an undifferentiated streak, rudimentary gonad, or no gonad on the other. The extent of genital virilization prior to puberty is variable in this rare disorder. The vast majority are reared as girls in whom virilization occurs at puberty; some may note breast development as well. Affected individuals generally have a mosaic karyotype, with 45,X/46,XY being most common. Short stature and other stigmata associated with a 45,X karyotype in Turner's syndrome are less common in patients with tumors than in patients with testes. Gonadectomy is indicated in all individuals with a Y chromosome to eliminate the increased neoplastic potential of such dysgenetic gonads and in all patients in whom virilization occurs at puberty to remove the source of androgen. Estrogen replacement therapy is warranted following gonadectomy. Other causes of male pseudohermaphroditism associated with heterosexual pubertal development are described in Ch. 234.

An androgen-producing neoplasm or Cushing's syndrome may occur rarely during the pubertal years and lead to heterosexual development.

Jaffe RB: Disorders of sexual development. In Yen SSC, Jaffe RB (eds.): Reproductive Endocrinology. 2nd ed. Philadelphia, W. B. Saunders Company, 1986, pp 283–312. *A concise but complete discussion of errors in fetal genital differentiation and neonatal gender assignment.*

Marshall WA, Tanner JM: Variations in the pattern of pubertal changes in girls. Arch Dis Child 44:291, 1969. *A classic paper that is required reading for all serious students.*

Styne DM, Grumbach MM: Puberty in the male and female. Its physiology and disorders. In Yen SSC, Jaffe RB (eds.): Reproductive Endocrinology. 2nd ed. Philadelphia, W. B. Saunders Company, 1986, pp 313–384. *A detailed and excellently referenced discussion of normal and abnormal pubertal development.*

THE NORMAL MENSTRUAL CYCLE

CHARACTERISTICS OF THE MENSTRUAL CYCLE. Between menarche at approximately age 12 years and the menopause at about age 51 years, the reproductive organs of normal women undergo a series of closely coordinated changes at approximately monthly intervals that together comprise the normal menstrual cycle. The menstrual cycle is the expression of the coordinated interaction of the hypothalamic-pituitary-ovarian axis with associated changes in the target tissues (endometrium, cervix, vagina) of the reproductive tract.

A menstrual cycle begins with the first day of genital bleeding (day 1; menses) and ends just prior to the next menstrual period. The median menstrual cycle length is 28 days, but normal ovulatory menstrual cycles may range from about 21 to 40 days in length. Menstrual cycles vary most greatly in length in the years immediately following menarche and in the years immediately preceding menopause, largely because of an increased incidence of anovulatory cycles. Irregularities in menstrual cycle length also may be caused by abrupt changes in diet, exercise, or environment; serious emotional disturbances; and following parturition or abortion. The menstrual cycle can be divided into three distinct phases: *follicular, ovulatory,* and *luteal.*

The Follicular or Preovulatory Phase. Variable in length, the follicular phase begins with the first day of menstrual bleeding and extends to the day prior to the preovulatory LH surge. A rise in serum FSH begins in the late luteal phase of the previous menstrual cycle, continues into the early follicular phase, and initiates growth and development of a group of follicles (Fig. 237–5). The preovulatory follicle destined for ovulation will be selected from this cohort in a manner that is not yet understood. Circulating LH levels rise slowly throughout the follicular phase, but FSH levels fall after the early follicular phase increase. Approximately seven to eight days before the preovulatory LH surge, estradiol (E_2) and estrone (E_1) begin to increase, generally reaching a maximum on the day before or the day of the LH surge. The divergence

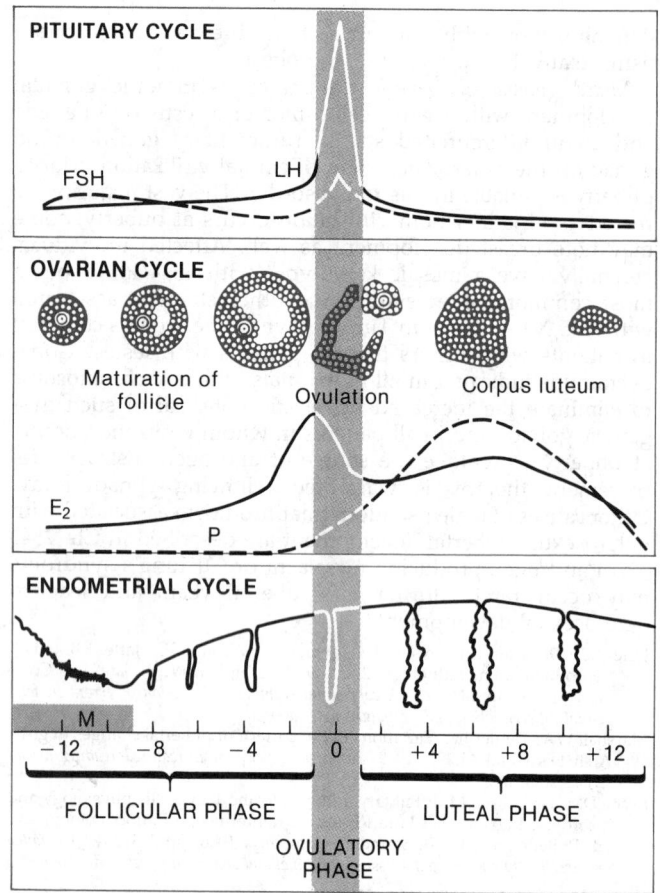

FIGURE 237–5. The idealized cyclic changes observed in gonadotropins, estradiol (E_2), progesterone (P), and uterine endometrium during the normal menstrual cycle. The data are centered about the day of the LH surge (day 0). Days of menstrual bleeding are indicated by M. (Reprinted with permission from *Endocrine and Metabolism Continuing Education Quality Control Program*, 1982. Copyright American Association for Clinical Chemistry, Inc.)

in LH and FSH levels may be related to the follicular secretion of *inhibin* (folliculostatin), a hormone that specifically inhibits the release of FSH. Several days before the LH surge, plasma androgens (androstenedione and testosterone) and some progestins (17α-hydroxyprogesterone and 20α-dihydroprogesterone) begin to increase. They peak on the day of the LH surge. Progesterone itself does not increase until just prior to the onset of the LH surge.

The Ovulatory Phase. During this phase the ovum is released from the mature graafian follicle 16 to 32 hours after the onset of the preovulatory surge of LH by the pituitary gland. The ovulatory phase extends from one day prior to the LH surge to one day following the LH surge. Some women experience brief (a few minutes to few hours in length), dull, unilateral pelvic pain near the time of ovulation, termed mittelschmerz. The association of this pain to ovulation is unknown, but it may be due to leakage of follicular fluid into the abdominal cavity at ovulation. Mittelschmerz may occur before or after actual ovulation or not at all in ovulatory women. During the ovulatory phase a rapid rise in plasma LH results in response to positive estrogen feedback, leading to final maturation of the follicle and to ovulation. As peak LH levels are reached, E_2 levels drop, but progesterone levels continue to increase.

The Luteal or Postovulatory Phase. The more constant half of the menstrual cycle, the luteal phase is approximately 14 days in length and ends with the onset of menses. This phase represents the functional lifespan of the corpus luteum ("yellow body") of the ovary, which supports the released ovum by secreting progesterone. In the luteal phase, progesterone

secretion increases to peak six to eight days after the LH surge. Parallel but smaller increases in 17α-hydroxyprogesterone, E_2, and E_1 levels also occur. Progesterone levels decrease toward menses unless the ovum is fertilized and pregnancy results. The finding of serum progesterone levels greater than 10 ng per milliliter one week prior to menses is probably diagnostic of normal ovulation. Progestins increase basal morning body temperature so that a "thermogenic shift" of more than 0.3°C occurring after a nadir is a presumptive sign of ovulation and progesterone secretion. Unfortunately, taking basal temperatures on a daily basis is tedious, subject to error, and not very reliable.

CYCLIC CHANGES IN TARGET ORGANS. *Endometrium.* During the menstrual cycle the endometrium undergoes remarkable histologic and cytologic changes, which culminate with menstrual bleeding when the corpus luteum ceases to secrete progesterone. The *basal layer of the endometrium*, which is not lost during menses, then regenerates the *superficial layer* of compact epithelial cells lining the uterine cavity and an *intermediate layer of spongiosa*, both of which are shed at each menstruation. Endometrial glands in these layers proliferate under the influence of estrogen in the follicular phase so that the mucosa thickens. In the luteal phase, under the influence of progesterone, the glands become coiled and secretory, with increased vascularity and edema of the stroma. As both E_2 and progesterone decline in the late luteal phase, the stroma becomes increasingly edematous, endometrial and blood vessel necrosis occurs, and endometrial bleeding ensues. Local release of prostaglandins may initiate vasospasm and ischemic necrosis in the endometrium as well as the uterine contractions accompanying menstrual flow. Thus prostaglandin synthetase inhibitors can relieve dysmenorrhea (menstrual cramping). Fibrinolytic activity in the endometrium also peaks at the time of menstruation, accounting for the noncoagulability of menstrual blood. Because the histologic changes during the menstrual cycle are so characteristic, endometrial biopsies are used to date the stage of the cycle and to assess the tissue response to gonadal steroids.

Cervix and Cervical Mucus. During the follicular phase, cervical vascularity, congestion, and edema increase progressively under the influence of estrogen. The external cervical os opens to a diameter of 3 mm at ovulation and then decreases to 1 mm. Cervical mucus increases in quantity (10- to 30-fold) and in elasticity (spinnbarkeit). "Palm leaf" arborization (ferning) becomes prominent just prior to ovulation (if cervical mucus is allowed to dry on a glass slide and examined microscopically). Under the influence of progesterone during the luteal phase, cervical mucus thickens, becomes less watery, and loses its elasticity and ability to fern. The characteristics of cervical mucus are useful clinically to evaluate the stage of the cycle and the amount of estrogen present.

Vagina. When ovarian estrogen secretion is low, as in the early follicular phase, vaginal epithelium is pale and thin. In the follicular phase under the influence of estrogens the epithelium thickens, and the number of mature cornified epithelial cells increases. During the luteal phase, progesterone causes a decrease in the percentage of cornified cells and an increase in the number of precornified intermediate cells and polymorphonuclear leukocytes. There is also increased cellular debris and clumping of shed desquamated cells. Histologic changes in the vaginal epithelium and in the cervical mucus are the most sensitive indicators of estrogen status in the body. However, the reliability of vaginal smears depends upon the absence of infection or exogenously administered steroid hormones that have antiestrogenic effects. Steroid hormones also facilitate progression of spermatozoa toward the ovaries and of ova toward the uterine cavity through effects on the fallopian tubes.

Ovary. A small primordial follicle with a diameter of 50 μm transforms and grows into a mature graafian follicle 1 to 2 cm in diameter in two distinct phases: (1) The oocyte and follicle grow to form a *primary follicle*, apparently independent of gonadotropin control. The oocyte increases tenfold in diameter (from 15 to 150 μm) and becomes surrounded by a zona pellucida, a translucent "shell" of glycoproteins. In addition, the single layer of cells surrounding the oocyte becomes cuboidal and takes on the characteristics of granulosa cells. (2) In a second phase completely dependent upon gonadotropin and steroid hormones, the follicular unit develops into a *mature graafian follicle*, which is capable of being released in response to the midcycle surge of LH and FSH. Under the influence of FSH, granulosa cells acquire specific receptors for FSH, undergo mitosis, multiply to form secondary follicles consisting of several granulosa cell layers, and also acquire the ability to aromatize androgens to estrogens. Simultaneously, thecal interstitial cells begin to develop around the basement membrane surrounding the granulosa cells, develop specific cell membrane receptors for LH, and synthesize and secrete androgens, primarily Δ^4-androstenedione and testosterone, in response to LH. The androgens can diffuse across the basement lamina where they are aromatized to estrogens. The rising E_2 in the follicular phase then feeds back on the hypothalamic-pituitary unit via the systemic circulation (Fig. 237–6). Just described is the so-called *two-cell theory*, which holds that both granulosa and theca are required for estrogen biosynthesis and maturation of the follicle.

A tertiary graafian follicle that contains an antrum or fluid-filled cavity increases from 200 μm to 1 to 2 cm in diameter, primarily because of accumulation of follicular fluid, again under the direct control of FSH. In tertiary follicles, FSH induces the appearance of specific LH receptors on granulosa cell membranes. These LH receptors are responsible for the stimulation of progesterone secretion prior to ovulation (luteinization) and for continued production of progesterone in the luteal phase.

Approximately two weeks are required for the presumptive preovulatory follicle to complete its growth and expel a mature oocyte. The oocyte is inhibited from resuming meiotic maturation by granulosa cell–oocyte interaction and an oocyte maturation inhibitor (OMI) until following the LH-FSH surge. Within 36 hours of the onset of the surge the oocyte completes the first meiotic division (reduction to 22 + X chromosomes) and a first polar body is extruded. The second meiotic division is completed only if the oocyte is fertilized by a spermatozoon. During the LH-FSH surge the preovulatory follicle bulges above the surface of the ovary. A stigma or avascular area develops on the follicle surface. Under the influence of local prostaglandins, plasminogen activator, and other hormones, a cluster of granulosa cells surrounding the oocyte and the oocyte itself (together known as the cumulus oophorus) are extruded.

The corpus luteum is formed from the granulosa and theca cells of the former preovulatory follicle following ovulation and secretes progesterone and E_2 for approximately 14 days. It then degenerates unless fertilization occurs. The lifespan of the corpus luteum may depend in part upon prostaglandins and prolactin as well as upon progestin. If fertilization occurs, chorionic gonadotropin (hCG), which is similar to LH, is secreted by the developing blastocyst and helps to support the corpus luteum until the fetoplacental unit can support itself. Pregnancy tests in common use have been developed utilizing antibodies to the specific β subunit of hCG and have little if any cross-reactivity with LH.

OVARIAN STEROIDOGENESIS. The ovaries and the developing follicles synthesize sex steroid hormones (estrogens, androgens, and progestins), which play important roles in ovulation and in preparing the uterus to accept a fertilized ovum via two separate pathways: (1) the so-called Δ^5 pathway, in which 17α-hydroxypregnenolone and DHEA with double bonds between carbons 5 and 6 are intermediates, and (2) the Δ^4 pathway, in which pregnenolone is converted to progesterone and in which 17α-hydroxyprogesterone and andro-

stenedione with double bonds between carbon 4 and 5 are the alternative intermediates (Fig. 237–7).

Although cholesterol as substrate for steroid synthesis is obtained normally from circulating low-density lipoproteins (LDL), it can be synthesized de novo from two-carbon fragments (acetate). Different structures and cells within the ovary synthesize different steroids, in part because of stimulation by the gonadotropins. Gonadotropin binding to its receptor activates adenylate cyclase and stimulates cyclic AMP production. The cAMP in turn activates protein kinases that catalyze phosphorylation of proteins to mediate the cellular effects of each gonadotropin (see Ch. 221). LH acts primarily to regulate the first step in steroid hormone biosynthesis, that is, the conversion of cholesterol to pregnenolone. FSH acts to aromatize androgens to estrogens. Thus, LH acts to enhance substrate flow and the synthesis of androgens and/or progesterone. In the absence of LH, FSH action is reduced because of diminished substrate for aromatization.

Androgens, primarily androstenedione and testosterone, are secreted by interstitial and theca cells and serve as the substrate for the granulosa cell aromatase enzyme for synthesis of estrogens. Androstenedione, the major ovarian androgen, can also be converted to testosterone and estrogens in peripheral tissues. When ovarian androgen synthesis is excessive, as in ovarian androgen-producing tumors, or when conversion of androgen to estrogen in the ovary is reduced, as in PCO syndrome, hirsutism and even virilism can result. Testosterone, the most biologically potent androgen, is bound tightly to sex hormone–binding globulin (SHBG; also known as testosterone-estradiol binding globulin, TeBG) so that only about 1 per cent of circulating testosterone is biologically free and active. Secretion rates and circulating concentrations in normal adult premenopausal women are given in Table 237–2.

Estrogens are produced predominantly in ovarian follicles by granulosa cell aromatization of the A ring of theca cell androgens. Naturally occurring estrogens are 18-carbon steroids, which by definition stimulate proliferation of the en-

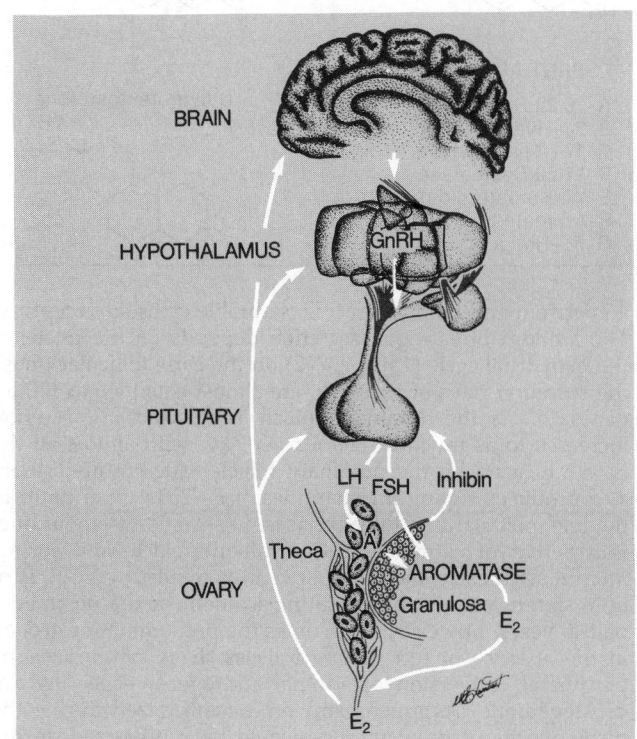

FIGURE 237–6. The hypothalamic-pituitary-ovarian axis in the regulation of follicular maturation and steroidogenesis. A = Androgens; E_2 = estradiol. (Reprinted with permission from *Endocrine and Metabolism Continuing Education Quality Control Program*, 1982. Copyright American Association for Clinical Chemistry, Inc.)

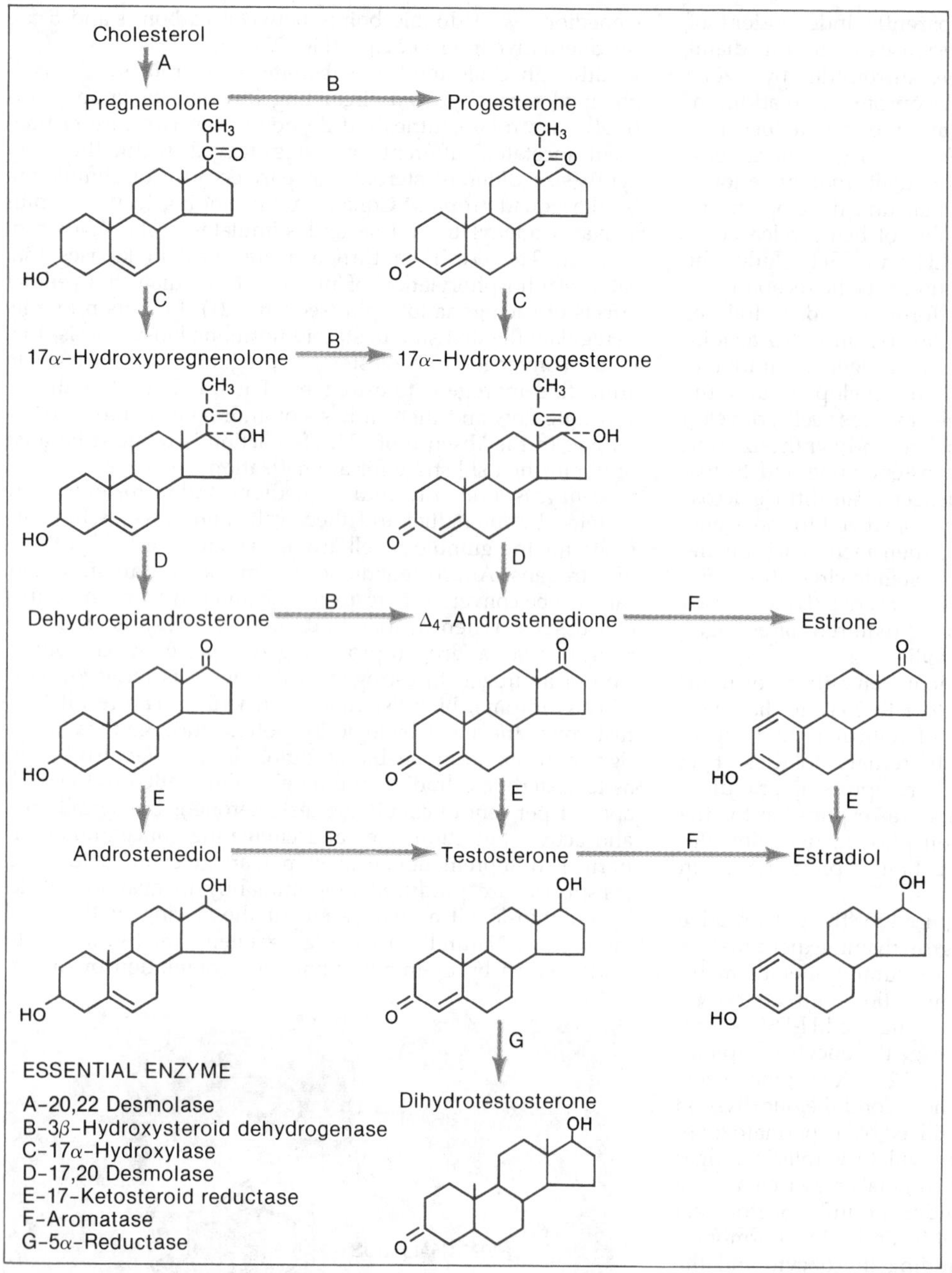

FIGURE 237–7. Steps in ovarian biosynthesis of steroid hormones. (Modified from data of Ross GT: In Rudolph AM (ed.): Pediatrics 16:1726, 1977.)

dometrium and bind to specific, saturable cytosolic receptors. The amount of estrogen secretion depends on the phase of the menstrual cycle (Table 237–2). In the early follicular phase the secretion rates of E_2 and E_1 are almost equal (60 to 170 μg per day). As the dominant follicle is selected, E_2 secretion increases to as much as 800 μg per day, with almost all the E_2 synthesized by the dominant follicle. The corpus luteum also produces significant quantities of E_2 (250 μg per day). In the late follicular and luteal phases, E_1 secretion is about one-fourth that of estradiol. The dominant follicle and corpus luteum synthesize about 95 per cent of circulating E_2; E_1 is of little significance in the ovulating woman. In the postmenopausal years, however, E_1 becomes the predominant estrogen in the absence of functioning follicles. E_1 is synthesized by peripheral conversion of adrenal androgens, especially androstenedione. As much estrogen is synthesized during the nine months of pregnancy as would be synthesized during 100 years of normal menstrual cycles.

Progesterone synthesis is low in the follicular phase, but increases to 10 to 40 mg per day during the luteal phase (Table 237–2). Should pregnancy occur, progesterone production increases to as much as 300 mg per day at term. Why the corpus luteum atrophies at about 14 days is not known, but may be due to the effects of intraovarian estrogen and/or prostaglandins. However, LH stimulation is required for progesterone production by the corpus luteum. Progesterone induces secretory changes in the endometrium in preparation for implantation of the fertilized ovum.

NEUROENDOCRINE REGULATION OF THE OVARIES. Neurons containing various peptide hormones that can release or inhibit secretion of the gonadotropins are found in the hypothalamus (see Ch. 225). Specifically, cells containing gonadotropin releasing hormone (GnRH) occur in the area including the arcuate nucleus and median eminence and the preoptic area. Axons from these neurons run in the tuberoinfundibular tract and terminate on capillaries within the median eminence; this allows for delivery of their products through the portal vascular system to the anterior pituitary gland. It appears that classic neurotransmitters, including norepinephrine, dopamine, and serotonin, as well as neuromodulators, such as endogenous opiates and prostaglandins, influence secretion of GnRH by the hypothalamus. In addition, estrogens and androgens bind to cells in the hypothalamus and the anterior pituitary, and progestins bind to cells

TABLE 237-2. CONCENTRATIONS, METABOLIC CLEARANCE RATES, PRODUCTION RATES, AND OVARIAN SECRETION RATES OF SEX STEROID HORMONES IN BLOOD

Steroid	Plasma MCR (liters/day)	Binding	Phase of Menstrual Cycle or Stage of Life	Plasma Concentration (ng/dl)	Plasma Production Rate (μg/day)	Ovarian Secretion Rate (μg/day)
Androstenedione	2000	Albumin	Premenopausal	40–240	3200	800–1600
			Postmenopausal	30–120	1600	
Testosterone	700	TeBG, albumin	Premenopausal	19–70	260	
			Postmenopausal	15–70	150	
Estradiol	1350	TeBG, albumin	Early follicular	2.5–6	70–200	60–170
			Late follicular	20–40	445–945	400–800
			Midluteal	15–25	270	250
			Postmenopausal	<1.0–2.5		
Estrone	2200	Albumin	Early follicular	2–6	70–200	60–170
			Late follicular	10–20	300–600	250–500
			Midluteal	10–15	240	160
			Postmenopausal	1.5–5.0	55	
Progesterone	2200	CBG, albumin	Follicular	3–10	700–2500	1500
			Luteal	10–25	3000–30,000	24,000

CBG = Cortisol-binding globulin; MCR = metabolic clearing rate; TeBG = testosterone-estradiol binding globulin.

in the hypothalamus to influence hypothalamic-pituitary regulation of ovarian function.

GnRH is secreted in a pulsatile fashion (perhaps because of an inherent oscillator within the arcuate nucleus) and is responsible for pulsatile release of gonadotropins. Pulsatile gonadotropin release in turn appears to account for the pulsatile secretion of sex steroids from the ovaries. The ovarian sex steroids then feed back on the hypothalamic-pituitary unit to modulate both the frequency and amplitude of the gonadotropin pulse (Fig. 237–6). Thus, gonadotropin pulses vary throughout the menstrual cycle. Pulses occur at approximately 60- to 90-minute intervals in the follicular phase and at intervals of greater than 180 minutes in the luteal phase.

Gonadal steroids can exert both negative and positive feedback effects on gonadotropin secretion. Among ovarian steroids, 17β-estradiol is the most potent inhibitor of gonadotropin secretion, acting on both the hypothalamus and pituitary. For women to ovulate, E_2 must also elicit a positive feedback effect on gonadotropin release. The feedback effects are both time and dose dependent. In the normal menstrual cycle the positive feedback action of E_2 leading to the LH surge is preceded by a period when lower E_2 levels are present with their negative feedback effects.

It appears that the ovary is the "clock" for the timing of ovulation, with the hypothalamus stimulating pulsatile release of the gonadotropins. The follicle complex and corpus luteum develop in response to gonadotropin stimulation. For appropriate ovarian regulation of reproductive function in women, three biologic characteristics are necessary: (1) an appropriate balance and sequence of negative and positive feedback actions; (2) differential feedback effects on the release of LH and FSH; (3) local intraovarian controls on follicular growth and maturation, separate from but interrelated to the effects of gonadotropins on the ovaries.

di Zerega GS, Hodgen GD: Folliculogenesis in the primate ovarian cycle. Endocr Rev 2:27, 1981. *A detailed discussion of recruitment and selection of the dominant follicle, summarizing a series of elegant studies.*

Hsueh AJW, Adashi EY, Jones PBC, et al.: Hormonal regulation of the differentiation of cultured ovarian granulosa cells. Endocr Rev 5:76, 1984. *A scholarly review of what is known about the function of granulosa cells.*

Knobil E: The neuroendocrine control of the menstrual cycle. Recent Prog Horm Res 36:53, 1980. *A classic summary of the role of the hypothalamus in the regulation of reproductive function in the primate.*

Richardson GS: Steroidogenesis. In Sciarra JJ (ed.): Gynecology and Obstetrics. Vol. 5. Philadelphia, Harper and Row, 1986 (rev. ed.), pp 1–17. *A detailed summary of the steroidogenic pathway.*

Yen SSC: The human menstrual cycle. In Yen SSC, Jaffe RB (eds.): Reproductive Endocrinology. 2nd ed. Philadelphia, W. B. Saunders Company, 1986, pp 200–236. *A scholarly and well-referenced discussion of the regulation of the human menstrual cycle.*

ABNORMALITIES OF THE REPRODUCTIVE YEARS

DYSMENORRHEA. Dysmenorrhea, perhaps the most common of all gynecologic disorders, affects about 50 per cent of postpubertal women. Dysmenorrhea can be classified as primary or secondary.

Primary dysmenorrhea occurs only in ovulatory cycles. Prostaglandins that are released from the endometrium just prior to and during menstruation cause contraction of uterine smooth muscle and produce dysmenorrhea by initiating painful, exaggerated uterine contractions and myometrial ischemia. Associated systemic symptoms include nausea, diarrhea, headache, and emotional changes. Primary dysmenorrhea is much more common than is secondary amenorrhea.

In *secondary dysmenorrhea* there is a pathologic cause for the dysmenorrhea. Endometriosis, the ectopic occurrence of endometrial tissue generally within the abdominal cavity, is the most common cause in severe cases. Other possible causes include pelvic inflammatory disease, congenital abnormalities such as atresia of a portion of the distal genital tract and cystic duplication of the paramesonephric ducts, and cervical stenosis.

Prostaglandin synthetase inhibitors such as naproxen, ibuprofen, mefenamic acid, and indomethacin are the mainstays of treatment. If the dysmenorrhea is still severe, addition of an oral contraceptive preparation to inhibit ovulation and limit prostaglandin release is generally effective. In cases in which the pelvic pain still remains intractable, additional evaluation is warranted. If thorough evaluation of the gastrointestinal and urinary tracts fails to reveal a definitive cause, examination under anesthesia and diagnostic laparoscopy may be indicated.

If endometriosis is diagnosed at laparoscopy, treatment varies, depending on the severity of the disease and the goals of the patient regarding fertility. It may be possible to fulgurate implants or lyse adhesions through the laparoscope. In general, endometriosis should be treated medically, with additional surgery deferred until infertility (if present) becomes manifest. Medical therapy can consist of continuous suppression with progestins, oral contraceptive agents, or danazol for three to six months. GnRH analogues may be approved soon for suppressive therapy as well. After a course of therapy, use of oral contraceptive agents probably should be continued until fertility is desired. Conservative surgical resection of endometriosis at laparotomy should almost always be deferred until it is established as the cause of infertility. Surgery may be required, however, for continuing severe pain, severe endometriosis, or large ovarian cysts containing endometriosis (endometriomas). If symptoms continue despite adequate treatment or if psychological overlay is suspected, psychiatric evaluation may be indicated. Medical causes of dysmenorrhea, however, should be eliminated first.

PREMENSTRUAL SYNDROME. Premenstrual syndrome (PMS), also known as premenstrual tension (PMT), is a complex of physical and/or emotional symptoms that occur repetitively in a cyclic fashion before menstruation and that

TABLE 237–3. COMMON SYMPTOMS OF CYCLIC PREMENSTRUAL SYNDROME

Somatic Symptoms

Abdominal bloating	Constipation or diarrhea
Acne	Headache
Alcohol intolerance	Peripheral edema
Breast engorgement and tenderness	Weight gain
Clumsiness	

Emotional and Mental Symptoms

Anxiety	Insomnia
Change in libido	Irritability
Depression	Lethargy
Fatigue	Mood swings
Food cravings (especially salt and sugar)	Panic attacks
	Paranoia
Hostility	Violence toward self and others
Inability to concentrate	Withdrawal from others
Increased appetite	

diminish or disappear with menstruation. Typically these cyclic symptoms are sufficiently severe to interfere with some aspects of life. Women with definitive psychiatric disturbances probably should not be included among those with PMS. More than 150 different symptoms are now thought to vary with the menstrual cycle (Table 237–3). Estimates of the prevalence of PMS range from 25 to 100 per cent. For most women the syndrome is merely annoying; it is likely that PMS causes serious difficulties for no more than 5 to 10 per cent. The diagnosis is best established by requiring patients to keep prospective daily records of symptoms over a two- to three-month period. Less than 50 per cent of women presenting with PMS are found to have the syndrome when such records are examined.

Most women seek help for PMS in their 30's after ten or more years of symptoms. Many report that their symptoms began at menarche; approximately half will state that symptoms began following childbirth. Severity and duration of symptoms are often reported to increase following each successive pregnancy, to become more severe with advancing age. Women with severe longstanding PMS almost always experience secondary psychological reactions, including social difficulties, such as marital discord, difficulty relating to their children, difficulty maintaining friendships, and withdrawal from social activities.

The etiology of PMS is unknown, but theories abound: alterations in the ratio of estrogen to progesterone in the luteal phase, alterations in α-melanocyte stimulating hormone (MSH) or β-endorphin activity, alterations in monoamine neurotransmitters, alterations in prolactin activity, increase in vasopressin secretion, alterations in mineralocorticoid secretion, alterations in prostaglandins, endogenous allergies to steroids (especially progesterone), reactive hypoglycemia, and many others.

Patients should be informed that no one therapy has been effective in all women and that none of the currently popular therapies has proved consistently effective. Still, women with mild premenstrual symptoms often benefit from simple changes in lifestyle, including addition of mild aerobic exercise each day; reduction in intake of xanthine-containing beverages, salt, and refined sugar in the day, particularly in the luteal phase; stress reduction; and adequate rest. Women with more severe PMS may benefit from treating predominant complaints symptomatically. Thus bromocriptine* (generally 2.5 mg twice a day) or danazol (100 to 400 mg daily in two divided doses) may be given continuously for relief of mastalgia, with the understanding that both may have unpleasant side effects. Prostaglandin synthetase inhibitors may help reduce dysmenorrhea and may benefit headaches. Mild sedatives and tranquilizers may help reduce insomnia and anxiety. Mild diuretics (especially spironolactone at doses up to 100 mg each morning) may be of benefit if cyclic edema can be documented by the presence of substantial weight gain in

*This use is not listed in the manufacturer's directive.

the luteal phase and by signs of dependent edema. The administration of 50 mg of pyridoxine per day has been urged by many as at least a harmless placebo, since it is a required cofactor in several enzymatic reactions, but, rarely, vitamin toxicity can develop when doses as low as 250 mg per day are given for a protracted time.

Since PMS requires the occurrence of cyclic ovulation, oophorectomy is sometimes considered for patients with particularly intractable symptomatology. Since GnRH analogues that induce a "medical castration" appear to have some effectiveness in PMS, the rationale seems valid. However, oophorectomy may create new problems related to estrogen deficiency for women with PMS treated in this permanent fashion.

Natural progesterone, particularly in the form of vaginal suppositories given at doses of up to 800 mg per day, has been used enthusiastically by many clinicians, but results of double-blind placebo-controlled trials have generally provided no evidence of efficacy. Likewise, the use of large quantities of multiple vitamins or of oil of evening primrose, containing the essential fatty acid gamma-linolenic acid, a precursor of prostaglandins, is unsubstantiated.

Hoffman PG: Primary dysmenorrhea and the premenstrual syndrome. In Glass RH (ed.): Office Gynecology. 2nd ed. Baltimore, Williams & Wilkins Company, 1981. *A rational discussion of difficult clinical problems.*
Reid RL, Yen SSC: The premenstrual syndrome. Clin Obstet Gynecol 26:710, 1983. *A scholarly review about what is and what is not known about this ill-defined disorder.*

ABNORMAL UTERINE BLEEDING. *Differential Diagnosis.* The causes of abnormal uterine bleeding in the reproductive years include complications from the use of oral contraceptive preparations; complications of pregnancy (especially threatened, incomplete, or missed abortion and ectopic pregnancy); coagulation disorders (most commonly idiopathic thrombocytopenic purpura and von Willebrand's disease); and pelvic disease such as intrauterine polyps, leiomyomas, and tumors of the vagina and cervix. Clear-cell adenocarcinoma of the vagina or cervix may occur in women exposed to diethylstilbestrol (DES) during fetal life as a result of maternal ingestion. Affected women also may have congenital abnormalities of the upper vagina, cervix, and uterus. Since a history of DES exposure is not always obtained and since this malignant tumor may be fatal, clinical suspicion should remain high. Women with a history of DES exposure should be reassured, however, that the incidence of malignancy is extremely low. Trauma (postcoital or otherwise), foreign bodies, systemic illnesses including various endocrinopathies (such as diabetes mellitus, hypothyroidism and hyperthyroidism, Cushing's syndrome, and Addison's disease), leukemia, and renal disease may also present with abnormal bleeding.

Dysfunctional uterine bleeding (DUB), abnormal uterine bleeding with no demonstrable organic genital or extragenital cause (75 per cent of cases), is most frequently associated with anovulation. Postmenarchal bleeding in adolescents secondary to immaturity of the hypothalamic-pituitary-ovarian axis accounts for about 20 per cent of all cases, and premenopausal bleeding consequent to incipient ovarian failure constitutes more than half of the cases. Most anovulatory bleeding is due to either estrogen withdrawal or to estrogen breakthrough bleeding. In anovulatory women, estrogen stimulates the endometrium unopposed by progesterone. As a consequence, the endometrium proliferates, becomes thicker, and may shed irregularly, especially if estrogen levels drop. Anovulatory bleeding tends to occur at less frequent intervals, while organic lesions tend to cause bleeding more frequently than cyclic menses.

Evaluation and Treatment. All cases of abnormal bleeding should be evaluated, including obtaining a thorough history with special emphasis on the amount and duration of blood loss. Prospective charting of the days that the patient bleeds may be required to evaluate the bleeding pattern. Complications of pregnancy or a bleeding diathesis must always be ruled out.

The physical examination (including the Papanicolaou smear) is normal in dysfunctional bleeding except for signs of anemia in the more severe cases. Laboratory tests should include a complete blood count, platelet count, coagulation studies, thyroid function tests, and fasting blood glucose. DUB must be a diagnosis of exclusion. Management of DUB depends upon the age of the patient and the extent of the bleeding. A sample of the endometrium should be obtained by biopsy or by dilatation and curettage from all women over age 35 and from those at increased risk of developing endometrial carcinoma because of prolonged anovulatory bleeding.

Even profuse bleeding in anovulatory women can almost always be successfully treated by administering one combination oral contraceptive pill every six hours for five to seven days. Bleeding should cease within 24 hours, but patients should be warned to expect heavy bleeding two to four days after stopping therapy. If anemia and signs of acute blood loss are profound, blood transfusion may be necessary. If the bleeding continues despite therapy, curettage can be carried out. Recurrence can be prevented by giving the patient combination oral contraceptive agents cyclically for three or more months. If spontaneous cyclic menses do not resume and pregnancy is not desired, the patient can be treated with cyclic progestin (medroxyprogesterone acetate 5 to 10 mg for 10 to 14 days each month) or oral contraceptive agents. If pregnancy is desired, ovulation can be induced, as discussed subsequently.

Acute episodes of anovulatory bleeding also can be treated with conjugated estrogens administered intravenously (25 mg every four hours for up to three doses) until bleeding ceases. Progestin therapy (medroxyprogesterone acetate 5 to 10 mg orally for ten days) should be started simultaneously. Withdrawal bleeding will occur after cessation of therapy, and the patient can then be treated with oral contraceptive agents for at least three cycles.

For individuals with anovulatory bleeding without an episode of profuse bleeding, treatment with cyclic oral contraceptive agents or progestin can be provided unless pregnancy is desired, in which case ovulation must be induced.

Speroff L, Glass RH, Kase NG: Dysfunctional uterine bleeding. In Speroff L, Glass RH, Kase NG: Clinical Gynecologic Endocrinology and Infertility, 3rd ed. Baltimore, Williams & Wilkins Company, 1983, pp 225–242. *A detailed and logical approach to the treatment of abnormal uterine bleeding.*

AMENORRHEA. *Definition and Etiology.* Amenorrhea is the absence of menstruation for three or more months in women with past menses (*secondary amenorrhea*) or the absence of menarche by the age of 16 years regardless of the absence or presence of secondary sex characteristics (*primary amenorrhea*). If an intact genital outflow tract exists and there is no primary disease of the uterus, amenorrhea is a sign of failure of the hypothalamic-pituitary-ovarian axis to produce cyclically the hormones necessary for menses. Amenorrhea is a sign of any of several disorders involving different organ systems. Amenorrhea is physiologic in the prepubertal girl, during pregnancy and early in lactation, and after the menopause. At any other time it is pathologic and demands evaluation. Use of the term *post-pill amenorrhea* to refer to women who fail to resume menses within three months of discontinuing oral contraceptives is inappropriate. Such individuals should be evaluated in the same manner as any woman with amenorrhea.

Clinical Evaluation. The patient with amenorrhea should be viewed as a bioassay subject in whom even subtle hormonal abnormalities may be manifested by obvious signs and symptoms. For example, breast development indicates exposure to estrogens, while the presence of pubic and axillary hair indicates androgenic stimulation.

Patients should be questioned especially closely for evidence of psychological disturbances, dietary and exercise habits, lifestyle, environmental stresses, a family history of genetic anomalies, and abnormal growth and development. Patients should also be asked about and examined for the presence of any signs of hyperandrogenism, including hirsutism, temporal balding, deepening of the voice, increased muscle mass, clitoromegaly, and increased libido, as well as for any signs of defeminization, including decreasing breast size and vaginal atrophy. Any history of galactorrhea, the nonpuerperal secretion of milk from the breasts, should be determined (see Ch. 239). A history of symptoms related to thyroid and adrenal dysfunction should also be sought.

The physical examination should focus on evaluating (1) body dimensions and habitus, (2) the extent and distribution of body hair, (3) breast development and secretions, and (4) the genitalia.

In normal adult women the arm span is similar to the height, while in hypogonadal women the span is generally more than 5 cm greater than the height. The general appearance of the patient should be evaluated to determine if the habitus is that of an adult female. The distribution and quantity of body hair should be considered in view of the family history. The extent of any hirsutism (increased sexually stimulated terminal hair; see Ch. 238) should be recorded, preferably by photographs. Other signs of virilization should be sought carefully. Breast development should be graded according to the method of Tanner (Table 237–4). Breast secretion should be sought by applying pressure to the breasts while the patient is seated. Any secretion should be examined microscopically for the presence of perfectly round fat globules of varying size, which are always present in milk and indicate galactorrhea. Finally, the female genitalia should be examined carefully because they are such sensitive indicators of hormonal milieu. The Tanner stage of pubic hair development should be noted (Table 237–4). Since the sensitivity of the genitalia to androgens decreases onward from early in fetal development, the extent of any virilization is important. Fusion of the labia and enlargement of the clitoris with or without formation of a penile urethra are observed in women exposed to androgens during the first three months of fetal development (see Ch. 234). Significant clitoromegaly in the absence of other signs of sexual ambiguity and in the presence of other signs of virilization requires marked androgenic stimulation and strongly implicates an androgen-secreting neoplasm in the absence of a history of ingestion of exogenous steroids. The development of the labia minora in postpubertal women indicates the influence of estrogens. Overt anomalies of the distal genital tract and especially any evidence of obstruction to the escape of menstrual blood should be sought in the remainder of the pelvic examination. The vaginal mucosa and the cervical mucus are exquisitely sensitive to estrogen. Under the influence of estrogen the vaginal mucosa changes during sexual maturation from a tissue with a shiny, bright red appearance with sparse, thin secretions to a dull, gray-pink rugated surface with copious, thick secretions.

The history and physical examination quickly differentiate among several causes of amenorrhea, regardless of the age of the patient (Table 237–5). The various disorders of sexual differentiation and the other peripheral causes are often apparent on inspection. Distal genital tract obstruction should be identified at the time of pelvic examination even if the specific abnormality is not obvious. The physical stigmata of Turner's syndrome, discussed subsequently, generally make the diagnosis simple. Any sexual ambiguity indicates the need for chromosomal analysis and the measurement of 17-α-hydroxyprogesterone to rule out congenital adrenal hyperplasia. Pregnancy and gestational trophoblastic disease may be suspected and confirmed by measuring circulating concentrations of hCG. The possibility of intrauterine synechiae or adhesions (Asherman's syndrome) must be considered in individuals developing amenorrhea following curettage or

TABLE 237–4. CRITERIA FOR DISTINGUISHING TANNER STAGES 1 TO 5 DURING PUBERTAL MATURATION

Tanner Stage	Breast	Pubic Hair
1 (Prepubertal)	No palpable glandular tissue or pigmentation of areola; elevation of areola only	No pubic hair; short, fine vellous hair only
2	Glandular tissue palpable with elevation of breast and areola together as a small mound; areolar diameter increased	Sparse, long, pigmented terminal hair chiefly along the labia majora
3	Further enlargement without separation of breast and areola; although more darkly pigmented, areola still pale and immature; nipple generally at or above midplane of breast tissue when individual is seated upright	Dark, coarse, curly hair extending sparsely over mons
4	Secondary mound of areola and papilla above breast	Adult-type hair, abundant but limited to mons and labia
5 (Adult)	Recession of areola to contour of breast; development of Montgomery's glands and ducts on areola; further pigmentation of areola; nipple generally below midplane of breast tissue when individual is seated upright; maturation independent of breast size	Adult-type hair in quantity and distribution; spread to inner aspects of the thighs in most racial groups

Adapted from Ross GT: Disorders of the ovary and female reproductive tract. In Wilson JD, Foster DW (eds.): Textbook of Endocrinology. 7th ed. Philadelphia, W. B. Saunders Company, 1985, pp 206–258; Speroff L, Glass RH, Kase N: Clinical Gynecologic Endocrinology and Infertility. 3rd ed. Baltimore, Williams & Wilkins Company, 1983, p 377; and Kustin J, Rebar RW: Menstrual disorders in the adolescent age group. Primary Care 14:139–166, 1987.

endometritis. Tuberculous endometritis, especially in younger women, may also lead to this disorder. Without hormonal measurements it may be impossible to distinguish among individuals with chronic anovulation, in whom hypothalamic-pituitary-ovarian function is insufficiently coordinated to produce cyclic ovulation, and those with ovarian failure, in whom in most cases the ovaries are devoid of oocytes. Still, it is generally possible to form some strong clinical impressions about the etiology of the amenorrhea. It can be noted if the patient has absence of, incomplete, or complete development of secondary sex characteristics. The presence of excess body hair or galactorrhea may provide clinical evidence of the pathogenesis of the amenorrhea. Signs and symptoms of adrenal or thyroid dysfunction may be important as well.

To ascertain if the outflow tract is intact and to assess the level of endogenous estrogen, a progestational challenge, consisting of progesterone in oil (100 to 200 mg administered intramuscularly) or medroxyprogesterone acetate (5 to 10 mg orally daily for five to ten days) can be utilized. Any bleeding within ten days of the completion of progestin administration makes the possibility of Asherman's syndrome unlikely and suggests chronic anovulation rather than hypothalamic-pituitary or ovarian failure. If bleeding does not occur, an orally active estrogen, such as 2.5 mg conjugated estrogen daily for

TABLE 237–5. CAUSES OF AMENORRHEA

Disorders of sexual differentiation
Distal genital tract obstruction (müllerian agenesis and dysgenesis)
Gonadal dysgenesis
Ambiguity of external genitalia (male and female pseudohermaphroditism)

Other peripheral causes
Pregnancy
Gestational trophoblastic disease
Amenorrhea traumatica (Asherman's syndrome)

Chronic anovulation or ovarian failure
Degree of absence of sexual development
Galactorrhea
Evidence of androgen excess
Evidence suggestive of adrenal or thyroid dysfunction

21 days with 10 mg of oral medroxyprogesterone acetate for the last five to ten days, should produce bleeding if the endometrium is normal. Still, hysterosalpingography and hysteroscopy may be required to diagnose Asherman's syndrome because some patients do continue to have some withdrawal bleeding.

Laboratory Evaluation. Basal levels of FSH, prolactin, and TSH should be measured in all amenorrheic women to confirm the clinical impression (Fig. 237–8).

Increased TSH levels with or without increased levels of prolactin imply primary hypothyroidism, and further evaluation for this disorder is indicated (see Ch. 229).

If the prolactin concentration is increased (typically greater than 20 to 30 ng per milliliter) and the TSH level is normal (generally less than 5 μU per milliliter), measurement of the prolactin concentration in the basal state should be repeated before more extensive evaluation is undertaken. This is the case because prolactin levels are increased by nonspecific stressful simuli, sleep, and food ingestion. Prolactin levels may be elevated in as many as one third of women with amenorrhea. Evaluation of galactorrhea and hyperprolactinemia is detailed in Ch. 239.

Increased FSH levels (generally greater than 40 milli International Units [mIU] per milliliter) imply ovarian failure and require further evaluation. Chromosomal evaluation is indicated in all individuals with elevated FSH levels who are under the age of 30 years at the time the amenorrhea begins.

If prolactin and TSH concentrations are within normal ranges and FSH levels are low or normal, the measurement of total testosterone levels is indicated whether or not there is any evidence of hirsutism or virilization. Hyperandrogenic women need not be hirsute because some have relative insensitivity of the hair follicles to androgens. Mildly increased levels of testosterone (and perhaps DHEA-S as well) suggest PCO syndrome. However, total circulating androgen levels are rarely not elevated because of the alterations in metabolic clearance rate and SHBG that are present in PCO syndrome. Circulating levels of LH and FSH may aid in differentiating PCO syndrome from hypothalamic-pituitary dysfunction. LH levels are frequently elevated in PCO syndrome such that the ratio of LH to FSH is increased; however, LH levels may be identical to those observed in normal women in the follicular

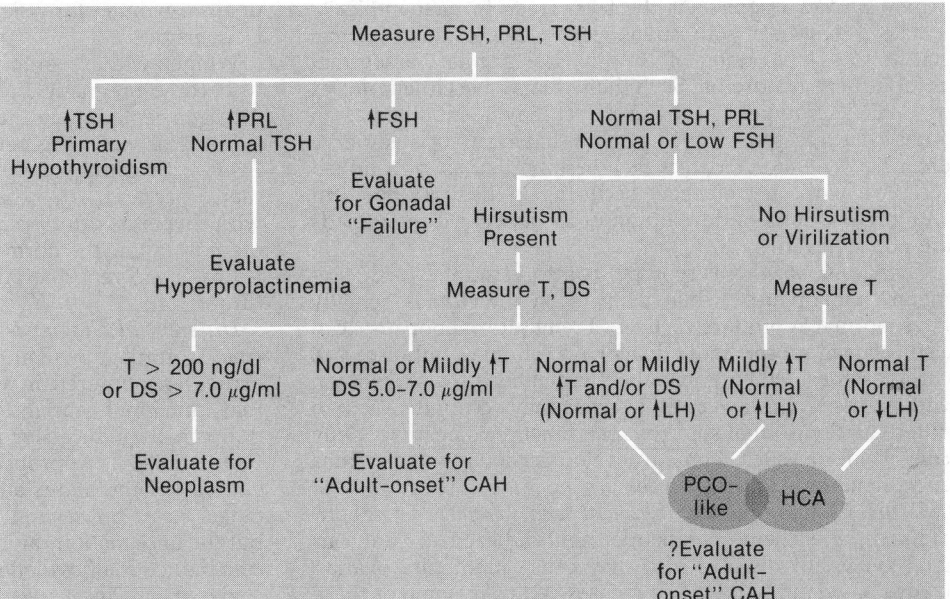

FIGURE 237–8. Biochemical evaluation of amenorrhea. This schema must be considered as an adjunct to the clinical evaluation of the patient. See text for details. **Abbreviations:** FSH = follicle-stimulating hormone; PRL = prolactin; TSH = thyroid-stimulating hormone; T = testosterone; DS = dehydroepiandrosterone sulfate; LH = luteinizing hormone; PCO-like = polycystic ovarian–like; HCA = hypothalamic chronic anovulation; CAH = congenital adrenal hyperplasia.

phase. In contrast, levels of LH and FSH are normal or slightly reduced in hypothalamic-pituitary dysfunction. There is some overlap between women with "PCO-like" disorders and those with hypothalamic-pituitary dysfunction. Radiographic assessment of the sella turcica is indicated in all amenorrheic women in whom both LH and FSH levels are very low to exclude a pituitary or parapituitary neoplasm. Other pituitary functions should be evaluated in any individual with significantly impaired LH and FSH secretion, as detailed subsequently. Both total testosterone and DHEA-S levels should be measured in hirsute or virilized women. Testosterone levels of greater than 200 ng per deciliter should lead to investigation for an androgen-producing neoplasm, most likely of ovarian origin. DHEA-S levels greater than 7.0 µg per milliliter should lead to evaluation for an adrenal neoplasm, and DHEA-S levels between 5.0 and 7.0 µg per milliliter should lead to evaluation for "adult-onset" congenital adrenal hyperplasia (see Ch. 234).

Hypergonadotropic Amenorrhea (Presumptive Ovarian Failure). DIFFERENTIAL DIAGNOSIS. Gonadal failure may begin at any time during embryonic or postnatal development and may result from many causes (Table 237–6). Normally the ovaries fail at menopause when virtually no functioning follicles remain. However, premature loss of oocytes prior to age 40 may occur and lead to premature ovarian failure, possibly from abnormalities in the recruitment and selection of oocytes. Since FSH is the principal regulator of folliculogenesis, it would seem that most causes of premature ovarian failure may somehow involve FSH secretion or action. Circulating gonadotropin levels increase whenever ovarian failure occurs, because of decreased negative estrogen feedback to the hypothalamic-pituitary unit.

Chromosomal Abnormalities. Several pathologic conditions with dysgenetic gonads have elevated gonadotropin levels and amenorrhea. The term *gonadal dysgenesis* refers to individuals with undifferentiated streak gonads without any association with either extragonadal stigmata or sex chromosomal aberrations. Since individuals with gonadal dysgenesis have the normal complement of oocytes at 20 weeks of fetal age but virtually none by birth, this disorder is a form of premature ovarian failure.

Turner's syndrome describes patients with streak gonads composed of fibrous stroma and four cardinal features: (1) a female phenotype, (2) sexual infantilism, (3) short stature, and (4) several physical abnormalities, sometimes including a webbed neck, low-set ears, multiple pigmented nevi, double eyelashes, micrognathia, epicanthal folds, shieldlike chest

with microthelia, short fourth metacarpals, an increased carrying angle to the arms, and certain renal and cardiovascular defects (most commonly coarctation of the aorta and aortic stenosis). The diagnosis can sometimes be made at birth because of unexplained lymphedema of the hands and feet. The syndrome is associated with an abnormality of sex chromosome number, morphology, or both. Most commonly the second sex chromosome is absent (45,X). This is the single most common chromosomal disorder in humans, but more than 95 per cent of such fetuses are aborted so that the incidence in newborns is approximately 1 in 3000 to 5000. Chromosomal breakage and mosaicism occur frequently as well. In mosaic individuals with a normal 46,XX cell line, sufficient follicles may persist postnatally to initiate pubertal changes and to cause ovulation so that pregnancy is possible.

TABLE 237–6. CLASSIFICATION OF HYPERGONADOTROPIC AMENORRHEA (FSH > 40 mIU PER MILLILITER)

I. Menopause
II. Chromosomal abnormalities
  A. Gonadal dysgenesis
    1. With stigmata of Turner's syndrome (45,X)
    2. Pure (46,XX or 46,XY)
    3. Mixed
  B. Trisomy X with or without chromosomal mosaicism
III. Physical causes
  A. Gonadal irradiation
  B. Chemotherapeutic (especially alkylating) agents
  C. Viral agents
  D. Surgical extirpation
IV. Autoimmune disorders
  A. Polyglandular, involving ovarian failure and any combination of thyroiditis, hypoadrenalism, hypoparathyroidism, diabetes mellitus, myasthenia gravis, vitiligo, mucocutaneous candidiasis, and pernicious anemia
  B. Isolated ovarian failure
V. Enzymatic defects
  A. 17α-Hydroxylase deficiency
  B. Galactosemia
VI. Gonadotropin receptor and/or postreceptor defects (resistant ovary or Savage syndrome)
VII. Congenital thymic aplasia
VIII. Inherited tendencies producing premature ovarian failure
  A. Genetically reduced cell endowment
  B. Accelerated atresia
IX. Defects in gonadotropin secretion
  A. Secretion of biologically inactive forms
  B. Alpha or beta subunit defects
X. Circulating gonadotropin antibodies
XI. Idiopathic premature ovarian failure

Pure gonadal dysgenesis is the term given to phenotypically female individuals with streak gonads who are of normal stature and have none of the physical stigmata associated with Turner's syndrome. Such individuals have either a 46,XX or 46,XY karyotype. The 46,XX defect may be inherited as an autosomal recessive with 10 per cent having associated nerve deafness. The 46,XY defect may be inherited as an X-linked recessive with clitoromegaly occurring in 10 to 15 per cent and gonadal tumors developing in 25 per cent if the gonads are not removed.

Trisomy X (46,XXX karyotype) is also associated with premature menopause, while many such individuals actually have normal reproductive lives. Premature menopause can also occur in mosaic individuals with cell lines with excess X chromosomes. When gonadal abnormalities occur in women with excess X chromosomes, it seems they occur after ovarian differentiation so that some ovarian function is possible. Only later in life do such women develop secondary amenorrhea and premature ovarian failure.

OTHER CAUSES. *Physical, Chemical, and Infectious Causes.* Irradiation and chemotherapeutic agents utilized to treat various malignant diseases also may cause premature ovarian failure. Ovulation and cyclic menses return in some of these patients even after prolonged intervals of hypergonadotropic amenorrhea associated with signs and symptoms of profound hypoestrogenism. Rarely, mumps affects the ovaries and causes ovarian failure.

Autoimmune Disorders. Premature ovarian failure may occur in conjunction with a variety of autoimmune disorders. The most common syndrome involves hypoadrenalism, hypoparathyroidism, and mucocutaneous candidiasis together with ovarian failure (see Ch. 241). Antibodies to the FSH receptor have been identified in a very few cases. These associations make it mandatory to rule out other potentially life-threatening endocrinopathies in young women with hypergonadotropic amenorrhea.

Enzymatic Defects. In girls with the rare syndrome of 17α-hydroxylase deficiency who survive until the expected age of puberty, sexual infantilism and primary amenorrhea occur together with elevated levels of gonadotropins. Increased synthesis of desoxycorticosterone leads to hypertension with hypokalemic alkalosis; serum progesterone levels are elevated as well. As with other causes of congenital adrenal hyperplasia, the hypertension is controlled by replacement therapy with glucocorticoids (see Ch. 234). Women with galactosemia also develop ovarian failure early in life, even when a galactose-restricted diet is introduced early in infancy (see Ch. 178).

Gonadotropin Receptor and/or Postreceptor Defects. The resistant ovary (Savage) syndrome occurs in young amenorrheic women who have (1) elevated peripheral gonadotropin concentrations, (2) normal (although immature) follicles present on ovarian biopsy, (3) a 46,XX karyotype with no evidence of mosaicism, (4) fully developed secondary sex characteristics, and (5) ovarian resistance to stimulation with human menopausal or pituitary gonadotropins. There seems to be some block to gonadotropin action within the ovary in this syndrome.

THERAPEUTIC CONSIDERATIONS. Women with hypergonadotropic amenorrhea and ovarian failure should be treated identically whether or not they have signs of hypoestrogenism or desire pregnancy. Ovarian biopsy does not seem indicated to document the existence of follicles because only a small portion of each ovary can be sampled and because pregnancies have resulted in patients who had biopsies devoid of follicles. Estrogen replacement is indicated to prevent the accelerated bone loss known to occur in affected women (see Ch. 250). The estrogen should be given sequentially with a progestin to prevent endometrial hyperplasia. Young women with ovarian failure may require twice as much estrogen as postmenopausal women for relief of signs and symptoms of hypoestrogenism.

Women with hypergonadotropic amenorrhea are rarely able to become pregnant. Pregnancy is more likely to occur with estrogen replacement therapy than with any other therapy. It is not clear why pregnancy is rarely possible in such women. Even with estrogen replacement the pregnancy rate is less than 5 per cent. The experimental treatment of young women with hypergonadotropic amenorrhea by hormone replacement to mimic the normal menstrual cycle and embryo transfer has been reported and will become more common in the future.

Differential Diagnosis and Treatment of Chronic Anovulation. Chronic anovulation, the most frequent form of amenorrhea encountered in women of reproductive age, implies that functional ovarian follicles remain and that cyclic ovulation can be induced or reinitiated with appropriate therapy (Table 237–7). Appropriate management requires that the etiology of the anovulation be determined. The pathophysiologic bases for several forms of anovulation are unknown, but the anovulation can be interrupted transiently by nonspecific induction of ovulation in the majority of affected women.

HYPOTHALAMIC CHRONIC ANOVULATION (HCA). HCA is a heterogeneous group of disorders with similar manifestations. Emotional and physical stress, exercise, diet, weight loss, body composition, malnutrition, environment, and other unrecognized factors may contribute in varying proportions to the anovulation. Abrupt cessation of menses in women under 30 years of age who have no anatomic abnormalities of the hypothalamic-pituitary-ovarian axis and no other endocrine disturbances suggests a diagnosis of HCA. Affected individuals tend to be bright, educated, and engaged in intellectual

TABLE 237–7. CAUSES OF CHRONIC ANOVULATION

I. **Chronic anovulation of hypothalamic-pituitary origin**
  A. Hypothalamic chronic anovulation
    1. Psychogenic
    2. Exercise associated
    3. Associated with diet, weight loss, and/or malnutrition
    4. Anorexia nervosa and bulimia
    5. Pseudocyesis
  B. Forms of isolated gonadotropin deficiency (including Kallmann's syndrome)
  C. Due to hypothalamic-pituitary damage
    1. Pituitary and parapituitary tumors
    2. Empty-sella syndrome
    3. Following surgery
    4. Following radiation
    5. Following trauma
    6. Following infection
    7. Following infarction
  D. Idiopathic hypopituitarism
  E. Hypothalamic-pituitary dysfunction or failure with hyperprolactinemia (multiple causes)
  F. Due to systemic diseases
II. **Chronic anovulation due to inappropriate feedback** (i.e., polycystic ovarian syndrome)
  A. Excessive extraglandular estrogen production (i.e., obesity)
  B. Abnormal buffering involving sex hormone-binding globulin (including liver disease)
  C. Functional androgen excess (adrenal or ovarian)
  D. Neoplasms producing androgens or estrogens
  E. Neoplasms producing chorionic gonadotropin
III. **Chronic anovulation due to other endocrine and metabolic disorders**
  A. Adrenal hyperfunction
    a. Cushing's syndrome
    2. Congenital adrenal hyperplasia (female pseudohermaphroditism)
  B. Thyroid dysfunction
    1. Hyperthyroidism
    2. Hypothyroidism
  C. Prolactin and/or growth hormone excess
    1. Hypothalamic dysfunction
    2. Pituitary dysfunction (microadenomas and macroadenomas)
    3. Drug induced
  D. Malnutrition

Modified from Rebar RW: Chronic anovulation. In Serra GB (ed.): The Ovary. New York, Raven Press, 1983, pp 217–240.

occupations and may well give a history of psychosexual problems and socioenvironmental trauma. HCA is characterized by low to normal levels of gonadotropins and relative hypoestrogenism. Rarely, however, do affected women present with signs and symptoms of estrogen deficiency. Psychological counseling and/or a change in lifestyle, especially for those women engaged in strenuous exercise programs, may be effective in inducing cyclic ovulation and menses. For women desiring pregnancy, ovulation can also be induced with clomiphene citrate (50 to 100 mg per day for five days beginning on the fifth day of withdrawal bleeding). Treatment with human menopausal gonadotropin and human chorionic gonadotropin (hMG-hCG) or with GnRH administered in a pulsatile fashion may be effective in women who do not ovulate in response to clomiphene. Treatment of affected individuals who do not seek pregnancy is controversial. Some physicians advocate the use of exogenous steroids to prevent osteoporosis. A regimen can be used consisting of oral conjugated estrogens (0.625 to 1.25 mg), ethinyl estradiol (20 μg), or micronized estradiol-17β (1 to 2 mg) or of transdermal estradiol-17β (0.05 to 0.10 mg) for the first 25 days of each month with oral medroxyprogesterone acetate (5 to 10 mg) added for days 13 to 25. Sexually active women can be given oral contraceptive agents as an alternative. If steroid therapy is administered, patients must be informed that the amenorrhea probably will be present when therapy is discontinued. Other physicians believe only periodic observation is indicated with barrier methods of contraception recommended for fertility control. Contraception is needed for sexually active women with HCA, because the functional defect is mild in these disorders and may resolve spontaneously at any time with ovulation occurring prior to any episode of menstruation.

Individuals with amenorrhea and significant weight loss should be examined for the possibility of *anorexia nervosa* (see Ch. 215). This disorder may be the most severe form of functional HCA, or it may be a distinct entity.

Kallmann's syndrome (isolated gonadotropin deficiency or familial hypogonadotropic hypogonadism) is a familial disorder consisting of gonadotropin deficiency, anosmia or hyposmia, and color blindness in men or, more rarely, in women. Other midline defects such as cleft lip and palate can occur in the affected individual or in family members. The trait is transmitted as an X-linked recessive or a male-limited autosomal dominant trait, but genetic heterogeneity may occur. Partial or complete agenesis of the olfactory bulb is present on autopsy, accounting for use of the term *olfactogenital dysplasia*. The disorder affects only gonadotropin secretion, and all other pituitary hormones are secreted normally. Isolated gonadotropin deficiency in the absence of anosmia occurs as well, and the syndrome is quite heterogeneous. Sexual infantilism with a eunuchoidal habitus is the clinical hallmark of this disorder, but moderate breast development may occur. Circulating LH and FSH levels are quite low, but almost always detectable. Ovulation induction requires use of hMG-hCG or pulsatile GnRH. Estrogen replacement therapy is indicated in these women until such time as pregnancy is desired. It may not be possible to distinguish between partial isolated gonadotropin deficiency and functional HCA in all cases.

Hypopituitarism may be obvious upon cursory inspection or sufficiently subtle as to require endocrine testing (see Ch. 226). The clinical presentation depends on the age of onset, the etiology, and the nutritional status of the individual. Failure of development of secondary sex characteristics or for development to progress once puberty is initiated must always raise the question of hypopituitarism. Ovulation can be induced successfully with exogenous gonadotropins when pregnancy is desired and after the hypopituitarism is treated appropriately. Replacement therapy with estrogen is indicated to prevent signs and symptoms of estrogen deficiency.

Galactorrhea associated with hyperprolactinemia, whatever the etiology, almost always occurs together with amenorrhea caused by hypothalamic-pituitary dysfunction or failure. Many conditions can cause excess prolactin secretion (see Ch. 239). It is unclear if all individuals with chronic anovulation associated with hyperprolactinemia and no other cause have pituitary microadenomas, even in the absence of identifiable radiographic changes of the sella turcica. Hirsutism may be observed occasionally in association with amenorrhea-galactorrhea and hyperprolactinemia. Elevated levels of the adrenal androgens DHEA and DHEA-S may be observed and may account for the polycystic-like ovaries present in some hyperprolactinemic women.

The hypothalamic-pituitary unit may also fail to function normally in a number of stressful, debilitating, systemic illnesses that interfere with somatic growth and development. Chronic renal failure, liver disease, and diabetes mellitus are the most prominent examples.

CHRONIC ANOVULATION DUE TO INAPPROPRIATE FEEDBACK. PCO syndrome, which causes anovulation because of inappropriate feedback signals to the hypothalamic-pituitary unit, is a heterogeneous disorder in which there is considerable clinical and biochemical variability among affected individuals. Although patients usually present with amenorrhea, hirsutism, and obesity, affected women may instead complain of irregular and profuse uterine bleeding, may not have hirsutism, and may be of normal weight. Excess androgen from any source or increased extraglandular conversion of androgens to estrogens can lead to the typical findings of PCO syndrome. Included are such diverse disorders as Cushing's syndrome, mild congenital adrenal hyperplasia, virilizing tumors of adrenal or ovarian origin, hyperthyroidism and hypothyroidism, obesity, and primary PCO syndrome with no other recognizable etiology. In the primary syndrome the irregular menses, mild obesity, and hirsutism begin during puberty and typically become more severe with time. Obesity alone can lead to a PCO-like syndrome, with the degree of obesity required to cause anovulation varying widely from individual to individual. All such patients are well estrogenized regardless of whether they present with primary or secondary amenorrhea or dysfunctional bleeding. As noted, LH concentrations tend to be elevated, with relatively low and constant FSH levels, but both may be in the normal range compared to levels in women in the follicular phase of the menstrual cycle. Levels of most circulating androgens, especially testosterone, tend to be mildly elevated. The etiology of PCO syndrome is unknown, but current evidence suggests that the hypothalamic-pituitary unit is intact and that a functional derangement results in abnormal gonadotropin secretion.

The aim of the diagnostic evaluation is to rule out any causes (such as neoplasms) that require definitive therapy. Hirsutism should be evaluated as detailed in Ch. 238. PCO syndrome itself is a benign disorder. Patients generally require therapy for hirsutism, for induction of ovulation if pregnancy is desired, and for prevention of estrogen-induced endometrial hyperplasia and cancer. No ideal therapy exists, but rather the therapeutic approach must be individualized to the needs of each patient.

In the anovulatory woman not desiring pregnancy who is not hirsute, therapy with intermittent progestin administration (such as medroxyprogesterone acetate 5 to 10 mg orally for 10 to 14 days each month) or oral contraceptives (if she is under 35 years of age, does not smoke, and has no other significant risk factor) can be provided to reduce the increased risk of endometrial carcinoma that is present in such a woman with unopposed estrogen. All women utilizing intermittent progestin administration should be cautioned about the need for effective contraception if they are sexually active, because these agents will not inhibit ovulation when administered intermittently.

The approach to the hirsute anovulatory woman not desiring pregnancy is detailed in Ch. 238. Oral contraceptive agents are the first line of therapy for such women with mild hirsutism and offer protection from endometrial hyperplasia.

In women with PCO syndrome desiring pregnancy, clomiphene citrate is the first approach to inducing ovulation because of its simplicity and high success rate. Approximately 75 to 80 per cent will conceive with such therapy. Other possible methods of inducing ovulation include use of hMG-hCG, purified FSH, pulsatile GnRH, and wedge resection of the ovaries at laparotomy. Wedge resection should be performed only rarely and only in women in whom all other methods fail, in whom there is a question of an ovarian tumor because of ovarian size or circulating androgen levels, and in whom fertility is not an issue (because of the risk of pelvic adhesions from the surgery leading to infertility).

A particularly severe subset of affected women present with marked obesity, anovulation, mild glucose intolerance and high levels of circulating insulin with insulin resistance, acanthosis nigricans, hyperuricemia, and severe hirsutism with markedly elevated circulating androgen levels. These women have *hyperthecosis of the ovaries* in which the androgen-producing cells in the stromal, hilar, and thecal components of the ovaries are increased greatly in number. Although considered a separate entity by some clinicians, hyperthecosis probably should be viewed as a part of the spectrum comprising PCO syndrome.

Chronic Anovulation Due to Other Endocrine and Metabolic Disorders. Adrenal hyperfunction appears to cause chronic anovulation by inducing a PCO-like syndrome secondary to increased adrenal androgen secretion, but other possible mechanisms also exist.

Both hyperthyroidism and hypothyroidism are associated with a variety of menstrual disturbances, including dysfunctional uterine bleeding and amenorrhea as a result of alterations in the metabolism of androgens and estrogens. These metabolic changes in turn result in inappropriate steroid feedback and chronic anovulation. In hyperthyroidism the increased thyroid hormone levels induce increased SHBG synthesis and reduce clearance of androgens and estrogens from the circulation. Conversion of androgens to estrogens is also increased, leading to increased circulating estrone levels. Estrogen metabolism to 2-hydroxyestrone is increased relative to what occurs in ovulatory women. In hypothyroidism the clearance of testosterone and E_2 from the bloodstream is increased consequent to decreased SHBG. Metabolism of E_2 is altered, with estriol (E_3), a weak estrogen, being formed in increased quantities.

Rebar RW: Effect of exercise on reproductive function in females. In Givens JR (ed.): Hypothalamus in Health and Disease. Chicago, Year Book Medical Publishers, 1984, pp 245–262. *A detailed discussion of the effects of exercise on reproduction in women.*

Rebar RW: Practical evaluation of hormonal status. In Yen SSC, Jaffe RB (eds.): Reproductive Endocrinology. 2nd ed. Philadelphia, W. B. Saunders Company, 1986, pp 683–733. *A clinician describes a systematic approach to assessing ovarian function and clinical diagnosis. Bibliography is exhaustive.*

Rebar RW, Erickson GF, Coulam CB: Premature ovarian failure. In Gondos B, Riddick D (eds.): Pathology of Infertility. New York, Thieme-Stratton (in press). *A detailed discussion of the diagnosis and treatment of premature ovarian failure.*

Yen SSC: Chronic anovulation caused by peripheral endocrine disorders. In Yen SSC, Jaffe RB (eds.): Reproductive Endocrinology. 2nd ed. Philadelphia, W. B. Saunders Company, 1986, pp 441–499. *A detailed discussion of many of the causes of anovulation with an exhaustive bibliography.*

Yen SSC: Chronic anovulation due to CNS-hypothalamic-pituitary dysfunction. In Yen SSC, Jaffe RB (eds.): Reproductive Endocrinology. 2nd ed. Philadelphia, W. B. Saunders Company, 1986, pp 500–545. *A complete discussion of hypothalamic amenorrhea with an extensive bibliography.*

DISORDERS OF FOLLICULOGENESIS. The recognized disorders of folliculogenesis are not identified until at or following ovulation, but they are believed to be manifestations of abnormalities in follicular development.

Luteinized Unruptured Follicle (LUF) Syndrome. The LUF syndrome describes development of a dominant follicle without its subsequent disruption and release of the ovum. The abnormality can be diagnosed by ultrasound or by the absence of evidence of ovulation when the ovary is viewed at laparoscopy. The disorder is believed to occur infrequently and sporadically and is probably not a significant cause of infertility. Menstrual cycles in which no ovum is released are characterized by presumptive evidence of ovulation, including biphasic basal body temperatures, secretory endometrium, a normal LH surge, and normal progesterone production in the luteal phase. In fact, although the syndrome is believed to occur, data to substantiate its existence are only circumstantial (though strongly so) at present.

Luteal Phase Dysfunction. Progesterone secretion in the luteal phase may be reduced in duration (termed luteal phase insufficiency) or in amount (termed luteal phase inadequacy). More rarely the endometrium may be unable to respond to secreted progesterone because of the absence of progesterone receptors. These disorders are believed to represent causes for infertility (because of inability of fertilized ova to implant) in approximately 5 per cent of infertile couples. Abnormalities of the follicular phase, especially in the frequency of gonadotropin pulses, may account for most luteal phase dysfunction. Luteal phase defects also may occur sporadically in normally ovulating women approximately once each year.

Luteal phase dysfunction may be associated with several clinical entities, including hyperprolactinemia (of any etiology), strenuous physical exercise, inadequately treated 21-hydroxylase deficiency, and habitual abortion. Luteal dysfunction occurs more commonly at the extremes of reproductive life and in the first menstrual cycles following full-term delivery, abortion, or discontinuation of oral contraceptives. It also may occur during ovulatory cycles induced with clomiphene citrate or hMG-hCG.

The diagnosis of luteal phase dysfunction can be made either by endometrial biopsy or by serial progesterone determinations. Endometrial biopsies obtained from the uterine fundus in the late luteal phases of two different cycles must be at least two days out of phase from the expected date of bleeding, as judged from the subsequent menstrual cycle, for the diagnosis to be made. The absolute concentration that progesterone must achieve and the length of time progesterone must be increased in the luteal phase to exclude luteal dysfunction are unclear. Luteal dysfunction is extremely rare in women with menstrual cycles greater than 25 days in length in whom a single random progesterone determination is greater than 15 ng per milliliter.

Treatment of luteal dysfunction is controversial. Any underlying defect should be treated. If subsequent luteal function depends on prior follicular development, modification of follicular development with either clomiphene citrate (25 to 100 mg daily by mouth for five days beginning on cycle day 3 to 5) or FSH (75 to 300 IU intramuscularly for three to five days beginning on cycle day 3 to 5) is reasonable. hCG (2500 to 5000 IU intramuscularly at two- to three-day intervals beginning with the shift in basal body temperature) or progesterone (12.5 mg intramuscularly in oil daily or 25 mg twice a day as rectal or vaginal suppositories) can be utilized as well. Synthetic progestational agents should not be used to treat luteal phase defects because of their possible (though unproven) association with congenital anomalies. Furthermore, the synthetic progestins produce an abnormal endometrium. None of these agents has been shown to increase the pregnancy rate.

Wentz AG: Physiologic and clinical considerations in luteal phase defects. Clin Obstet Gynecol 22:169, 1979. *A complete review of what is known about luteal dysfunction.*

INFERTILITY. *Infertility* may be defined as involuntary inability to conceive. *Sterility* is total inability to reproduce. In either case the situation may or may not be correctable, especially for each particular couple. Failure to reproduce thwarts a basic human instinct and causes anger, guilt, and depression. More than 10 per cent of couples in the United States seek medical assistance for infertility.

The requirements for pregnancy to occur are several:

1. The male must produce adequate numbers of normal, motile spermatozoa.

2. The male must be capable of ejaculating the sperm through a patent ductal system.

3. The sperm must be able to traverse an unobstructed female reproductive tract.

4. The female must ovulate and release an ovum.

5. The sperm must be able to fertilize the ovum.

6. The fertilized ovum must be capable of developing and implanting in appropriately prepared endometrium.

Infertility is too frequently viewed primarily as a problem of the female. In fact, in approximately 40 per cent of cases, infertility is caused by the male (Table 237–8). In perhaps one third of couples more than one cause contributes to the infertility.

Peak age of fertility in the female in 25 years. For nulliparous women of this age the average time during which unprotected intercourse occurs until conception is 5.3 months. For parous women the average duration of intercourse until conception is 2.7 months. The reproductive performance of couples is influenced by the ages of the female and male partners, the frequency of intercourse, and the length of time the couple has been attempting to conceive. There is a decline in both female and male reproductive performance after age 25.

TABLE 237–8. CAUSES OF INFERTILITY AND THEIR APPROXIMATE INCIDENCE

I. **Male factors (40%)**
  A. Decreased production of spermatozoa
    1. Varicocele
    2. Testicular failure
    3. Endocrine disorders
    4. Cryptorchidism
    5. Stress, smoking, caffeine, nicotine, recreational drugs
  B. Ductal obstruction
    1. Epididymal (postinfection)
    2. Congenital absence of vas deferens
    3. Ejaculatory duct (postinfection)
    4. Postvasectomy
  C. Inability to deliver sperm into vagina
    1. Ejaculatory disturbances
    2. Hypospadias
    3. Sexual problems (i.e., impotence), medical or psychological
  D. Abnormal semen
    1. Infection
    2. Abnormal volume
    3. Abnormal viscosity
  E. Immunological factors
    1. Sperm-immobilizing antibodies
    2. Sperm-agglutinating antibodies
II. **Female factors**
  A. Fallopian tube pathology (20 to 30%)
    1. Pelvic inflammatory disease or puerperal infection
    2. Congenital anomalies
    3. Endometriosis
    4. Secondary to past peritonitis of nongenital origin
  B. Amenorrhea and anovulation (15%)
  C. Minor ovulatory disturbances (<5%?)
  D. Cervical and uterine factors (10%)
    1. Leiomyomas and polyps
    2. Uterine anomalies
    3. Intrauterine synechiae (Asherman's syndrome)
    4. Destroyed endocervical glands (postsurgery or postinfection)
  E. Vaginal factors (<5%)
    1. Congenital absence of vagina
    2. Imperforate hymen
    3. Vaginismus
    4. Vaginitis
  F. Immunologic factors (<5%)
    1. Sperm-immobilizing antibodies
    2. Sperm-agglutinating antibodies
  G. Nutritional and metabolic factors (5%)
    1. Thyroid disorders
    2. Diabetes mellitus
    3. Severe nutritional disturbances
III. **Idiopathic or unexplained (< 10%)**

Couples who complain of infertility merit evaluation regardless of the length of infertility. If the couple believes there is a problem, it is the physician's responsibility to reassure them by appropriate evaluation and subsequent explanation of all findings and the prognosis.

The evaluation begins with a detailed history obtained from both partners and physical examinations of both individuals. The couple should be seen together for the first visit. Each couple should be questioned together and separately, since separate interviews may uncover information that would not be imparted in the presence of the partner.

Initial evaluation of infertility generally includes (1) assessment of semen, (2) documentation of ovulation by basal body temperature, serum progesterone determination approximately six to eight days before menses, or endometrial biopsy less than three days before onset of menses, and (3) evaluation of the female genital tract by hysterosalpingography. Basal serum levels of prolactin and thyroid hormones should be measured. Diagnostic laparoscopy with tubal dye instillation should be performed if all previous tests are normal, since 30 to 50 per cent of women are found to have endometriosis or tubal disease on surgical evaluation. Treatment must be predicated on the findings of the infertility evaluation.

Glass RH: Infertility. In Yen SSC, Jaffe RB (eds.): Reproductive Endocrinology. 2nd ed. Philadelphia, W. B. Saunders Company, 1986, pp 571–613. *A summary of the approach to the infertile couple.*

SEXUAL FUNCTION AND DYSFUNCTION. Although sexual responses begin following puberty, they can continue for the duration of a woman's life. Sexual responses generally are divided into four phases: excitement, plateau, orgasm, and resolution.

With sexual arousal and excitement, vasocongestion and muscular tension increase progressively, primarily in the genitals, manifested by vaginal lubrication in the female. The lubrication is due to formation of a transudate in the vagina. Sexual excitement is initiated by any of a variety of psychogenic or somatogenic sexual stimuli and must be reinforced to result in orgasm. With continued stimulation, the excitement phase increases in intensity into a plateau phase during which a high state of sexual interest is maintained. The plateau phase may be short or long, and it is from this phase that an individual can shift to orgasm. The orgasmic phase tends to be brief and is characterized by rapid release from the developed vasocongestion and muscular tension. The orgasmic release is also known as the climax because peak psychological and physical intensity is achieved and there is an attendant feeling of satisfaction. Copious secretions and transudate may flow during orgasm in women. While women may resolve toward sleep following orgasm, many remain responsive to sexual stimulation and may return to plateau and subsequent orgasm.

Characteristic genital and extragenital responses occur during these phases. Estrogens magnify the sexual responses, but responses may occur in estrogen-deficient women. For women these changes occur in the breasts and in the pudendal region and are variable from one response cycle to another. For some women, excitement proceeds quickly through plateau to orgasm, and orgasm is explosive and accompanied by vocalization and involuntary contractions of the pelvic skeletal muscles. For other women, the responses are slow in building, controlled in amplitude, and long lasting. For a few women orgasm never occurs; for many it is intermittently absent.

The somatic sensate focus enabling orgasmic release is variable and may include stimulation of the breast, vagina, or clitoris. The psychological aspect of coitus may involve concentration on the current partner or act or fantasies about other times and persons. While orgasms may vary in physiologic intensity, what is important is psychological satisfaction. Satisfaction for both men and women may be had without orgasm.

Women may seek consultation because of disturbances in normal sexual arousal or orgasm. Such sexual dysfunction may be due to either organic or functional disturbances.

A variety of diseases affecting neurologic function, including diabetes mellitus and multiple sclerosis, may prevent sexual arousal. So, too, may local pelvic disorders, such as endometriosis and vaginitis, which cause dyspareunia and lead to sexual avoidance. Estrogen deficiency causing vaginal atrophy and dyspareunia is a relatively common cause of sexual dysfunction. Debilitating systemic diseases such as malignant disease may also affect sexual function indirectly.

In most cases the cause of sexual dysfunction is psychological. For instance, vaginismus involves involuntary contractions of the muscles surrounding the introitus and leads to dyspareunia. It is a conditioned response engendered by a previous imagined or real traumatic sexual experience. Feelings of guilt, caused by incest or rape as examples; of inadequacy, caused by hysterectomy or mastectomy; or of depression or anxiety may lead to failure to be aroused. Failure to achieve orgasm may be viewed as a dysfunction if the woman is frustrated or dissatisfied.

Treatment of sexual dysfunction is best accomplished by eliminating functional causes and providing the patient, often together with her partner, with appropriate psychological counseling. Behavioral modification is effective in treating many women with psychological sexual dysfunction.

Green, R (ed.): Human Sexuality. A Health Practitioner's Guide. 2nd ed. Baltimore, Williams & Wilkins Company, 1979. *A simple and pragmatic approach to dealing with common sexual disorders is provided.*

Kaplan HS: The Evaluation of Sexual Disorders: Psychological and Medical Aspects. New York, Brunner-Mazel, 1983. *A good general text detailing sexual disorders.*

Kolodny RC, Masters WH, Johnson VE: Textbook of Sexual Medicine. Boston, Little, Brown and Company, 1979. *A widely used text detailing sexual problems and their therapy.*

Masters W, Johnson V: Human Sexual Response. Boston, Little, Brown and Company, 1966. *The classic work detailing human sexual response. Required reading for all individuals seriously interested in this field.*

Masters W, Johnson V: Human Sexual Inadequacy. Boston, Little, Brown and Company, 1970. *Identifies the major causes of sexual dysfunction in humans.*

HORMONAL THERAPY DURING THE REPRODUCTIVE YEARS

INDUCTION OF OVULATION. Induction of ovulation should never be attempted until serious disorders precluding pregnancy are ruled out or treated. Furthermore, ovulation induction should be utilized only in women with chronic anovulation, since women with ovarian failure are unresponsive to any form of ovulation induction. In general, the use of pharmaceutical agents does not improve the quality of an ovum, and thus the chance of pregnancy is not improved in women who ovulate regularly.

Clomiphene citrate is the agent that usually induces ovulation most easily. Clomiphene should be utilized in individuals without hyperprolactinemia who have the ability to release LH and FSH. A typical course of clomiphene therapy is begun on the fifth day following either spontaneous or induced uterine bleeding. The initial dosage is 50 mg daily for five days. Clomiphene appears to act as an anti-estrogen and stimulates gonadotropin secretion by the pituitary gland to initiate follicular development. If ovulation is not achieved in the very first cycle of treatment, the daily dosage is increased to 100 mg. If ovulation is still not achieved, dosage is increased in a stepwise fashion by 50 mg increments to a maximum of 200 to 250 mg daily for five days. The highest dose should be continued for three to six months before the patient is regarded as a clomiphene failure. The quantity of drug and the length of time that it can be used, as suggested here, are greater than those recommended by the manufacturers, but conform with published series.

The ovulatory surge of LH may occur five to twelve days (average, seven days) after the completion of the last day of clomiphene treatment in each course. Couples are advised to have intercourse every other day during this time interval.

Ovulation can be documented by monitoring changes in basal body temperature or preferably by measuring serum progesterone approximately 14 days after the last clomiphene tablet is taken. In addition, menses should occur about three weeks after the last day of therapy. Withdrawal bleeding with progestin can be induced if the patient fails to bleed within four weeks of therapy and if a serum hCG level documents that the patient is not pregnant.

Some clinicians give 5000 to 10,000 IU of hCG intramuscularly seven days after the last day of clomiphene therapy to trigger ovulation, but this approach has not been established to increase effectiveness. The administration of hCG, however, does serve to time ovulation and may be helpful in selected couples. Ovulation can be expected to occur approximately 36 hours after hCG administration.

In appropriately selected patients, 75 to 80 per cent will ovulate and 40 to 50 per cent can be expected to become pregnant. About 15 per cent of pregnancies can be expected with each ovulatory cycle. The multiple pregnancy rate is about 8 per cent, with almost all being twins. The incidence of congenital anomalies is not increased.

Side effects of clomiphene are uncommon and very rarely serious. The most serious side effects include vasomotor flushes (10 per cent), abdominal discomfort (5 per cent), breast tenderness (2 per cent), nausea and vomiting (2 per cent), visual symptoms (1.5 per cent), and headache (1 per cent). Significant ovarian enlargement may occur but is rare (5 per cent).

The addition of dexamethasone, 0.5 mg orally at bedtime to blunt the nighttime secretion of ACTH, may be useful in hyperandrogenic women with an adrenal component who fail to ovulate in response to clomiphene. Other individuals failing to respond to clomiphene typically require hMG-hCG or perhaps pulsatile GnRH to induce ovulation.

Bromocriptine, a dopamine agonist, is effective in inducing ovulation in hyperprolactinemic women (see Ch. 239). The drug should be stopped once pregnancy is confirmed. Ovulatory menses and pregnancy are achieved in about 80 per cent of patients with galactorrhea and hyperprolactinemia. The majority of women with prolactin-secreting pituitary tumors remain asymptomatic during pregnancy. It is extremely rare for a patient with either a microadenoma or a macroadenoma to develop a problem related to the tumor that affects either the mother or the fetus during pregnancy. Monitoring during pregnancy need consist only of questioning the patient about the development of visual symptoms and headaches. Formal assessment of visual fields and CT should be carried out in any patient developing suspicious symptoms. Symptoms generally abate with institution of bromocriptine therapy. No adverse effects of bromocriptine on fetuses or pregnancies have been reported.

hMG, a purified preparation of gonadotropins extracted from the urine of postmenopausal women, must be administered intramuscularly. Each vial contains 75 units of FSH and 75 units of LH. Purified FSH has become available for use recently. Biochemically engineered preparations of both products will become available in the future. hMG is administered at doses of two to four vials for five to twelve days to achieve follicular development as monitored by ultrasound and serum or urinary E_2 concentrations. hCG, 5000 to 10,000 IU, is administered as a single intramuscular dose when follicular maturation is apparent. The hCG should be withheld if more than three follicles mature together.

Because of the expense and the complication rate, thorough evaluation should be carried out to exclude other causes of infertility before hMG-hCG is used. Ovulation can be induced in almost 100 per cent of patients, but pregnancy will occur in only 50 to 70 per cent. There is no increased risk of congenital anomalies with hMG-hCG.

The rate of multiple pregnancies with hMG-hCG may approach 30 per cent with 5 per cent being triplets or more.

Ovarian hyperstimulation is the major side effect and may be life threatening. The ovaries enlarge remarkably in this treatment-induced syndrome, and multiple follicle cysts, stromal edema, and multiple corpora lutea are present. There is a shift of fluid from the intravascular space into the abdominal cavity with resultant hypovolemia and hemoconcentration. The cause of the ascites is unknown. Treatment is conservative with monitoring of fluid and electrolyte status. Pelvic examinations should not be performed for fear of rupturing the ovaries. The hyperstimulation generally will resolve slowly over about seven days.

GnRH, administered intravenously or less effectively subcutaneously at doses of 5 to 20 μg every 60 to 120 minutes, also can be used to induce ovulation in women with an intact pituitary gland. hCG can be administered to support the corpus luteum after ovulation at a dose of 1500 IU intramuscularly every three days for three to four doses. The advantage of GnRH rests in the fact that hyperstimulation is extremely unlikely. However, reported pregnancy rates have been no greater than those achieved with hMG-hCG, and this treatment must be considered experimental. Furthermore, some patients do not tolerate wearing the infusion pump that must be utilized.

Speroff L, Glass RH, Kase NG: Induction of ovulation. In Speroff L, Glass RH, Kase NG: Clinical Gynecologic Endocrinology and Infertility. 3rd ed. Baltimore, Williams & Wilkins Company, 1983, pp 523–544. *A detailed and practical survey of how to induce ovulation.*

STEROIDAL CONTRACEPTION. *Physiologic Actions and Metabolic Effects.* Oral contraceptive pills are the most widely used contraceptives worldwide, with more than 50 million users. Combination (estrogen-progestin) and progestin only preparations are available. The estrogen may be either mestranol or ethinyl estradiol, while the progestin is usually one of six derivatives of 19-nor-testosterone: norethindrone, norethindrone acetate, norethynodrel, ethynodiol diacetate, norgestrel, and levonorgestrel. New progestins are under development.

Combination oral contraceptives inhibit the midcycle gonadotropin surge by inhibiting GnRH release from the hypothalamus. Cervical mucus becomes thick, viscid, and scanty in amount, thus retarding sperm penetration. Fallopian tube motility and secretion are altered as well, and the endometrial glands produce less glycogen.

Oral contraceptives decrease maturation of the vaginal epithelium and somehow render the vagina more susceptible to candidiasis. The endometrium becomes atrophic with variable degrees of decidual change, leading to diminished menstrual flow. Follicular development is arrested with low estrogen and progesterone secretion. Both circulating LH and FSH levels are reduced and constant.

The general metabolic effects of oral contraceptives resemble those of pregnancy. Glucose tolerance is impaired with an increase in plasma insulin levels. The "mini-pill" containing progestin only in low dosage may cause no changes in glucose metabolism. Levels of circulating triglycerides and of very low density lipoproteins (VLDL) are often increased, almost entirely because of the estrogenic component (see Ch. 183). Only very high estrogenic formulations will increase mean serum cholesterol levels. Because of a direct effect of estrogens on the endoplasmic reticulum in the liver, alpha$_2$ globulins, including angiotensinogen, and beta globulins are increased, while serum albumin levels are decreased somewhat. A number of blood coagulation factors and carrier proteins (including thyroid-binding globulin, transferrin, ceruloplasmin, SHBG, and corticosteroid-binding globulin) are also increased.

Interactions with Other Drugs. Oral contraceptive steroids interact with several other drugs, leading to reduced effectiveness of the contraceptives or of the other drug. Such interactions occur because of altered drug absorption or metabolism. The majority of these interactions occur only with long-term use of the pharmacologic agent. By inducing hepatic microsomal enzymes, long-term administration of antibiotics may reduce the contraceptive efficacy of the steroids. The short-term use of antibiotics is probably of little concern. Anticonvulsants also sharply reduce the efficacy of contraceptive steroids, as do antacids, which may decrease the absorption of steroids. Conversely, contraceptive steroids oppose the therapeutic effects of anticoagulants, antidiabetic agents, and certain antihypertensive agents, such as guanethidine and alpha-methyldopa, because of their metabolic effects. Because of the impaired elimination of certain drugs, such as phenothiazines, oral contraceptive users may require lower doses.

Complications and Side Effects. The use of oral contraceptives increases the risk of *thromboembolism*, possibly as much as 4- to 13-fold with the doses of estrogens used in early preparations. The estrogen content of oral contraceptives appears to be correlated roughly with the risk of venous thromboembolic disease. Lower dosages of estrogen than were used initially in oral contraceptive preparations may not significantly increase the risk of any cardiovascular complications. Advanced maternal age and smoking seem to be the major risk factors for the use of oral contraceptives. In the absence of smoking and in women under the age of 35 years who do not suffer from obesity, hypertension, diabetes mellitus, or inherited lipoprotein abnormalities, there is little, if any, increased risk to oral contraceptive users for cardiovascular disease, including myocardial infarction.

In the absence of smoking and hypertension, it appears unlikely that there is an increased risk of fatal and nonfatal stroke from the use of low-dose oral contraceptives, in contrast to the enhanced risk of both thrombotic and hemorrhagic stroke reported earlier from the use of preparations containing larger amounts of estrogens. Some but not all women with migraine headaches may note increasingly frequent headaches with oral contraceptive use. Women with migraine headaches do not seem to be at increased risk of stroke.

Women using oral contraceptives are more likely to become hypertensive, especially those over the age of 35 years. Smoking may contribute to the incidence of hypertension. Increases in blood pressure are generally reversible shortly after oral contraceptives are discontinued. Failure of the blood pressure to return to normal when oral contraceptives are discontinued suggests underlying disease.

Contraceptive steroids do not appear to be teratogenic. Derivatives of 19-nor-testosterone can virilize female fetuses when administered in large doses to women early in pregnancy, but the doses required are far in excess of those contained in oral contraceptives.

Use of oral contraceptives reduces the risk of benign breast neoplasia, including fibrocystic disease and fibroadenoma. Since benign breast disease is a significant risk factor for the subsequent development of breast cancer, oral contraceptives may afford protection against breast cancer in this manner. Indeed, the incidence of breast cancer does not seem to be increased by use of oral contraceptives. Furthermore, oral contraceptives protect against the development of both endometrial and ovarian carcinoma.

Use of combined oral contraceptives may result in an increased risk for the development of *hepatocellular adenoma*, and this risk may increase with increased duration of contraceptive use. Rarely in patients with such adenomas the liver may rupture, and death may even occur because of hemorrhage.

The relationships of oral contraceptive use to cervical carcinoma, pituitary tumors, and melanoma are unclear. Some studies show positive relationships between cervical dysplasia and oral contraceptive use, while other studies do not. Cervical dysplasia is increased in women with first coitus at an early age and those who have multiple sexual partners. Since oral contraceptive use may encourage such sexual behavior, any such relationship is difficult to interpret. There is some evidence that the incidence of prolactinomas may be increasing in women, but the use of contraceptive steroids has not been shown to increase this risk.

So-called *post-pill amenorrhea* is sometimes regarded as a side effect of oral contraceptive use. The return to ovulation following discontinuation of contraceptive use is variable, but will occur within four to eight weeks in most patients. Approximately 1 in 500 patients will have amenorrhea for six months or longer, with 15 per cent of these having associated galactorrhea. This prolonged amenorrhea is probably caused by underlying disorders unrelated to oral contraceptive use. In normal women subsequent fertility is unimpaired.

Nausea and vomiting occur occasionally when use begins, but generally abate with continued use. Mastalgia and increased breast size may occur, but also tend to subside in several cycles. Chloasma (hyperpigmentation of the face) is a leading cause of pill discontinuation. Acne is usually improved, but occasionally may be exacerbated. Dizziness, headaches, visual disturbances, depression, and increased or decreased libido have been reported. Easy bruisability due to increased capillary fragility and edema also may occur. Furthermore, uterine leiomyomas may increase in size with use of contraceptive steroids.

Despite these potential side effects, therapeutic benefits exist with oral contraceptive use as well. Decreased menstrual blood loss results in a lower incidence of iron deficiency anemia. Acne frequently improves and dysmenorrhea decreases in the majority of patients. Symptomatic relief of endometriosis occurs in some patients. Women with PCO syndrome treated with oral contraceptives are afforded protection from endometrial carcinoma.

Absolute contraindications to the use of oral contraceptives include thrombophlebitis, thromboembolic disorders, cardiovascular disease, or a history of these conditions; markedly impaired liver function; known or suspected estrogen-dependent neoplasia; undiagnosed abnormal genital bleeding; known or suspected pregnancy; and congenital hyperlipidemia. Oral contraceptives generally should not be administered to women over 35 years of age and only with caution to smokers, women who are obese, and those with varicose veins. If headaches develop or become more frequent with pill use, oral contraceptives should be discontinued. Because of a possible increase in postsurgical thromboembolic complications in women using oral contraceptives, use of oral contraceptives should be discontinued two weeks prior to surgery and begun again two weeks postoperatively.

Henzl MR: Contraceptive hormones and their clinical use. In Yen SSC, Jaffe RB (eds.): Reproductive Endocrinology. 2nd ed. Philadelphia, W. B. Saunders Company, 1986, pp 643–682. *A detailed discussion of steroidal contraception.*

THE MENOPAUSE AND POSTMENOPAUSAL YEARS

DEFINITIONS AND EPIDEMIOLOGY. The *menopause* is the final menstrual period denoting the cessation of cyclic ovarian function as manifested by cyclic menstruation. The *climacteric* is the physiologic period during which regression of ovarian function occurs. Its onset generally is signalled by alterations in the menstrual cycle or vasomotor symptomatology. Menopause occurs at a mean age of approximately 51 years. Today's average woman in the Western world can expect to live one third of her life in the postmenopausal phase.

SYMPTOMATOLOGY AND SIGNS. Most signs and symptoms associated with the postmenopausal years result from decreased circulating estrogen. Common symptoms include hot flushes, paresthesias, palpitations, cold hands and feet, headaches, vertigo, irritability, anxiety, nervousness, depression, fatigue, weight gain, insomnia, night sweats, forgetfulness, and inability to concentrate.

Vasomotor instability is perhaps the most common complaint. Over 75 per cent of women experience hot flushes with decreasing estrogen levels, and these may persist for years.

In a typical hot flush, the skin, especially of the head and neck, becomes red and warm for a few seconds to two minutes with cold chills thereafter. Accompanying physiologic changes include a rise in skin temperature, peripheral vasodilatation, increased heart rate, decreased skin resistance, and concomitant LH pulses. The mechanism for hot flushes is unknown but must involve thermoregulatory centers in the hypothalamus.

During the menopausal years menstrual bleeding usually occurs at more widely spaced intervals. Any increase in bleeding or bleeding after six months of amenorrhea demands examination and sampling of the endometrium to exclude carcinoma. Women note relocation of fat deposits with increased fat in the lower abdomen, hips, and breasts. The genital skin becomes thin and pale with a decrease in the size of the labia minora, clitoris, uterus, and ovaries, and the women often complain of dyspareunia. Decreased elastic tissue of skin is noted, and osteoporosis may occur in about 25 per cent of postmenopausal women (see Ch. 250).

Menopausal signs and symptoms may begin long before menses have ceased. Symptoms may be difficult to diagnose in women with previous hysterectomies. Following bilateral oophorectomy young women develop identical signs and symptoms.

ENDOCRINOLOGIC CHANGES. During the menopausal transition regular menstrual cycles may continue up to the menopause. The cycles may become shorter, due to shortened follicular phases, with increased FSH, normal LH, and decreased E_2 and progesterone levels in comparison to normal ovulatory cycles. Variable cycles also may occur prior to the menopause, with some being ovulatory and others being anovulatory. Waning ovarian follicular activity with decreasing E_2 production must be central to these changes, and yet some follicles have been found on occasion in ovaries of postmenopausal women.

In postmenopausal women, circulating FSH and LH concentrations are greatly increased. Estrogen levels are decreased markedly, but androgen levels are decreased only slightly. The postmenopausal ovaries continue to secrete substantial amounts of androgen (androstenedione and testosterone), which together with adrenal androgens are converted to estrogens by extraglandular conversion in the periphery. The peripheral conversion of androgens accounts for most circulating estrogen in postmenopausal women.

CLINICAL MANAGEMENT. Treatment of postmenopausal women must be individualized and based on a personal dialogue with each patient. Exogenous estrogen replacement will stop or diminish hot flushes, reverse atrophic genital changes, decrease osteoporotic fractures (see Ch. 250), and may decrease the incidence of atherosclerotic coronary artery disease.

Estrogen replacement therapy is absolutely contraindicated in postmenopausal women with estrogen-dependent tumors of the breast, uterus, or kidney; acute liver disease; cerebrovascular disease; deep-vein thrombosis and embolism; malignant melanoma; and undiagnosed genital bleeding. Replacement therapy must be considered carefully and other therapy may require modification in women with estrogen-associated hypertension, diabetes mellitus, cholecystitis and cholelithiasis, pancreatitis, congestive heart failure, past endometriosis, and neuro-ophthalmologic vascular disease. Individual exceptions to these contraindications exist.

Estrogen should be administered together with a progestin in a cyclic fashion to women with a uterus to prevent an increased risk of endometrial hyperplasia and carcinoma. Several different regimens may be utilized. Oral estrone sulfate (0.625 to 1.25 mg), micronized estradiol-17β (1 mg) or transdermal estradiol (0.05 mg) may be given on days 1 to 25 of each month. To this should be added medroxyprogesterone acetate (5 to 10 mg orally for 13 or 14 days each month counting backward from day 25). Menstrual bleeding will occur in more than half of the women given such a regimen. Similar dosages of estrogen alone may be administered continuously to women who have undergone hysterectomy, but this is controversial and some physicians continue to use cyclic therapy with estrogen and a progestin for such women. Younger women may require twice as much estrogen as older women to alleviate symptoms.

Before beginning estrogen replacement therapy, patients should have a complete history and physical examination. A pretreatment mammogram is indicated because estrogens stimulate glandular tissue and may make diagnosis of breast masses more difficult. Periodic Papanicolaou smears should be obtained, and patients should undergo endometrial biopsy for any breakthrough bleeding and perhaps at intervals of one to two years while receiving estrogen replacement therapy.

Side effects of therapy are common and may require modifications of therapy. Breast tenderness occurs frequently if too much estrogen is given. The dose of progestin should be reduced in the woman who complains of depression and/or bloating.

Medroxyprogesterone acetate (20 to 40 mg) or megestrol acetate (40 to 80 mg) orally each day may be utilized to treat hot flushes in women who cannot or will not take estrogens. Vaginal lubricants may be used for symptomatic treatment of dyspareunia in such individuals.

EFFECTS OF ESTROGEN ON LIPIDS AND CARCINOMA. Unlike the effects of oral contraceptives in younger women, estrogen replacement in postmenopausal women does not raise blood pressure. This may be true because some estrogens, particularly those synthetic ones used in oral contraceptives, increase hepatic synthesis of renin substrate (angiotensinogen). The naturally occurring estrogens E_2 and E_1, however, do not increase renin substrate.

Estrogen administration tends to lower total cholesterol levels, although the degree of reduction varies with the dose and potency of the estrogen used. More importantly, estrogen decreases the LDL-cholesterol and increases the HDL-cholesterol fraction. Increased levels of the subfraction HDL_2 are most strongly associated with both estrogen ingestion and diminished cardiovascular risk. Thus the net effect of estrogen administration is to shift the HDL-LDL ratio to one associated with a decreased risk of cardiovascular disease. In fact, most (but not all) studies suggest a protective effect of estrogens on the incidence of heart disease in postmenopausal women. Estrogen administration to postmenopausal women may increase plasma triglycerides slightly, but these increases are generally of no significance except in some individuals with genetic disorders of triglyceride metabolism in whom marked elevations in triglycerides may occur.

Progestins, especially those derived from 19-nor-testosterone, oppose the effects of estrogens on plasma lipid and lipoprotein fractions. Even orally administered medroxyprogesterone, which is relatively neutral when given alone, appears to cancel the favorable changes induced by estrogens when given in combination with estrogen.

Estrogen-containing oral contraceptive preparations have not been linked conclusively to increased risks of endometrial or breast cancer. However, as noted, estrogen given alone to postmenopausal women greatly increases the risk of endometrial cancer over those never given estrogen. The risk of endometrial carcinoma is reduced markedly, if not abolished, by the cyclic addition of a progestin. Whether estrogen therapy increases the risk of breast cancer is not clear, but the majority of studies have not shown such a relationship.

Bush TL, Barrett-Connor E: Noncontraceptive estrogen use and cardiovascular disease. Epidemiol Rev 7:80, 1985. *A thoughtful discussion of the benefits and risks of estrogen replacement therapy.*

Speroff, L: Menopause. Semin Reprod Endocrinol 1:1, 1983. *A review by leading authorities on the physiologic changes and therapeutic approaches to the menopause.*

Wingo PA, Layde PM, Lee NC, et al.: The risk of breast cancer in postmenopausal women who have used estrogen replacement therapy. JAMA 257:209, 1987. *A recently published study which cites the relevant literature and suggests that the risk of breast cancer is not increased appreciably by postmenopausal estrogen use.*

OVARIAN TUMORS

Ovarian tumors may cause ovarian dysfunction, either by secreting hormones or by stimulating adjacent non-neoplastic stromal cells. Only perhaps 5 per cent of ovarian tumors, however, show functional activity. Most nonfunctional tumors are asymptomatic until late in their evolution; more than three fourths are diagnosed only in advanced stages. In contrast, women with functioning neoplasms commonly present with altered sexual development or reproductive abnormalities, and thus diagnosis is made much earlier. Ovarian tumors may occur in all age groups, but are less common in younger women, especially before puberty.

Ovarian tumors generally are classified as (1) common epithelial tumors derived from coelomic epithelial cells; (2) sex cord stromal tumors composed of granulosa cells, theca cells, Sertoli-Leydig cells, or their progenitors; (3) lipid or lipoid cell tumors; (4) germ cell tumors, including teratomas, dysgerminomas, and choriocarcinomas; (5) gonadoblastomas; (6) soft tissue tumors not specific to the ovary; and (7) secondary metastatic tumors. Each of these major classes of

TABLE 237–9. CLINICAL FEATURES OF HORMONE-PRODUCING OVARIAN TUMORS

Tumor	Hormones Produced*	Age in Years Peak	Age in Years Range	Malignancy	Bilaterality	Size Range in cm (per cent Palpable)	Miscellaneous
Androblastoma (arrhenoblastomas)	*Androgens*, estrogens	20–40	4–69	20%	Rare	<5–>25 (85)	Most common virilizing ovarian neoplasm
Dysgerminoma	Androgens, *chorionic gonadotropin*	10–30	6–76	100%	15%	3–50 (60)	May be "mixed" with other tumors originating from germ cells
Gonadoblastoma	*Androgens*, estrogens	10–30	6–38	50%	40%	<1–>30 (?)	Usually occur in genetic males with female external genitalia
Granulosa-theca cell	*Estrogens*, androgens, progestogens	30–70	<1–92	5–20%	10–15%	<1–>30 (80–90)	Most common functioning ovarian neoplasm
Hilar cell	*Androgens*, estrogens	45–75	4–86	Rare	Rare	1–9 (50)	Hypertension in 50%, diabetes in 50%
Lipoid cell (adrenal-like)	*Androgens*, estrogens	20–50	6–78	20%	Rare	0.5–30	Diabetes associated with lesion in 50%
Teratomas, benign	Serotonin, thyroxine	10–40	<1–78	Rare	10%	2–45 (90)	Carcinoid syndrome only in patients with large carcinoid tumors
Teratomas, malignant	Chorionic gonadotropin	6–15	6–42	100%	Rare	>5 (100)	Not all secrete chorionic gonadotropin

Modified from data of Rose GI, Vande Wiele RL; In Williams RH (ed.): Textbook of Endocrinology. 5th ed. Philadelphia, W. B. Saunders Company, 1974, pp 368–422.

*When more than one hormone is secreted, the major one is *italicized*

tumors includes several different histologic types. Sex cord stromal tumors are most apt to be functioning.

Ovarian neoplasms must be distinguished from tumor-like conditions of the ovary, which include luteomas of pregnancy (nodular theca-lutein hyperplasia) that may result in virilization of the mother but regress spontaneously post partum; hyperplasia of ovarian stroma (hyperthecosis), frequently associated with severe hirsutism; functional follicle and corpus luteum cysts; germinal inclusion cysts lined by surface epithelium; simple cysts; paraovarian cysts; inflammatory lesions; and endometrial cysts or endometriomas.

Ovarian neoplasms are diagnosed most commonly at the time of routine pelvic examination. Even most functioning neoplasms are palpable; those that are not may be identified by ultrasound. As an ovarian tumor grows, it distends the abdomen, leading to pressure on the bladder or rectum and a sensation of pelvic fullness and discomfort. Ascites may develop if the neoplasm is malignant or sometimes when it is not (Meigs' syndrome). Abdominal and pelvic pain may occur with torsion, hemorrhage, or rupture of the tumor.

Functioning ovarian tumors can produce other clinical manifestations as well (Table 237–9). Some tumors are associated with clinical manifestations of decreased hormone production. Intervals of amenorrhea caused by steroid suppression of gonadotropins may alternate with excessive vaginal bleeding produced by steroid stimulation of the endometrium during the reproductive years. In some young girls, steroid-secreting ovarian tumors may cause pseudopubertal development. In postmenopausal women, increased estrogens, secreted by the tumor itself or from peripheral aromatization of androgens secreted by the tumor, may stimulate the endometrium and result in bleeding.

Any pelvic mass identified on examination must be investigated. What constitutes such a "mass" and what evaluation is indicated depend on the age of the individual. Adnexal masses less than 5 cm in diameter may well be due to normal follicular development in women of reproductive age and may resolve with observation over two to eight weeks. Even cystic masses greater than 5 cm in diameter, as documented by ultrasound examination, may resolve over a few weeks. Those that do not require surgical removal. Any palpable adnexal mass in a postmenopausal woman, in whom the ovaries normally atrophy and cannot be detected during examination, should be removed.

Scully RE: Ovarian tumors with endocrine manifestations. In De Groot LJ, et al. (ed.): Endocrinology. Vol. 3. New York, Grune & Stratton, 1979, pp 1473–1488. *An excellent discussion of the clinical manifestations of ovarian tumors for any physician who undertakes the medical care of women.*

ACKNOWLEDGMENTS: This chapter is dedicated to the memory of my teacher and friend, Dr. Griff T. Ross, with the hope that it will enable other physicians to learn some of what I learned from Griff. My thanks also to Ms. Claudette Eldridge for assistance with the manuscript.

238 HIRSUTISM

D. Lynn Loriaux

DEFINITIONS. *Normal Hair Growth.* Except for the lips, the palms of the hands, and the soles of the feet, the bodies of men and women are covered with hair follicles. The hairs growing from these follicles are of two types, *vellous* and *terminal.* Vellous hair is the soft, downy hair that is characteristic of the faces of children. Terminal hair (the hairs of the scalp and eyebrows being examples) is usually more deeply pigmented, of greater diameter, and stiffer. Androgens induce follicles to change the nature of the hair produced from vellous

to terminal (or vice versa, as in male pattern baldness) in certain areas of the body, including the mons pubis, axillae, chest, and face (mustache and beard). There is a spectrum of androgen-dependent hair follicle response, the mons pubis being the most sensitive and the beard hairs usually being the least sensitive. In other areas, notably the arms and legs, increased androgen stimulation is not obligatory for the change from vellous to terminal hair. These follicles are considered to be partially androgen dependent.

Hirsutism. In women, excessive growth of body hair is called hirsutism. This is not a disease per se, but it may be a sign of disease. Certain patterns of hair growth can be said to be clearly abnormal in women, e.g., terminal hair on the upper abdomen or shoulders and upper back. Only 3 per cent of women have terminal hair over the sternum. Thus, terminal hair in these locations suggests an underlying disorder. More often, however, women complaining of hirsutism come to the physician not with hair in these abnormal locations, but with the subjective impression that either the rate of hair growth or the distribution of hair, or both seems to be changing. This can be an early indication of serious illness. In the majority of patients, however, no underlying disease can be found.

ETIOLOGY. Etiologically, hirsutism can be divided into two categories: androgen-independent hirsutism and androgen-dependent hirsutism. Ordinarily, the distinction between the two varieties can be made on clinical grounds.

In *androgen-independent hirsutism* the hair is usually vellous and evenly distributed over both androgen-independent areas, such as the forehead, and androgen-dependent areas, such as the chin and upper lip (Fig. 238–1). The more common causes of androgen-independent hirsutism are listed in Table 238–1.

In *androgen-dependent hirsutism,* the hair is of the terminal type and the distribution is restricted to androgen-responsive areas such as the chin, upper lip, and chest. Androgen-dependent hirsutism, caused by androgen excess, may be found in association with other signs of androgen effects, as noted below. The causes of androgen-dependent hirsutism are listed in Table 238–2. Since androgens in women are secreted only by the adrenal glands and by the ovaries, one or the other of these two glands must be the source of the excess androgen, except in cases of factitious hirsutism caused by exogenous androgen administration.

PATHOGENESIS OF ANDROGEN-DEPENDENT HIRSUTISM. Androgen-dependent hirsutism is the result of an elevated plasma protein unbound testosterone concentration. The pathophysiologic mechanism underlying the increased plasma testosterone concentrations found in the adrenal causes of hirsutism, such as adrenal cancer and virilizing adrenal adenomas, and the ovarian causes of hirsutism, including ovarian neoplasms, polycystic ovarian disease, and idiopathic hirsutism, is the excessive secretion of testosterone and/or its immediate precursor, androstenedione. Androstenedione contributes to plasma testosterone by being converted to testosterone in the liver and other peripheral tissues.

The syndromes of congenital adrenal hyperplasia (CAH) also cause hirsutism through increased androgen secretion, but the mechanism is more complex (see Ch. 230). The more common of these virilizing syndromes, 21-hydroxylase deficiency, results in the impaired ability of the adrenal gland to synthesize cortisol. Impaired cortisol production causes increased ACTH stimulation of the adrenal gland with resultant overproduction of 17-hydroxyprogesterone, the substrate for 21-hydroxylase activity, and its metabolic product androstenedione. Androstenedione is partially converted to testosterone, the hormone responsible for hirsutism and virilization. A second and less common form of CAH, 11-hydroxylase deficiency, is also associated with excessive testosterone production. This presumably results from the conversion of 11-deoxycortisol, the cortisol biosynthetic intermediate just be-

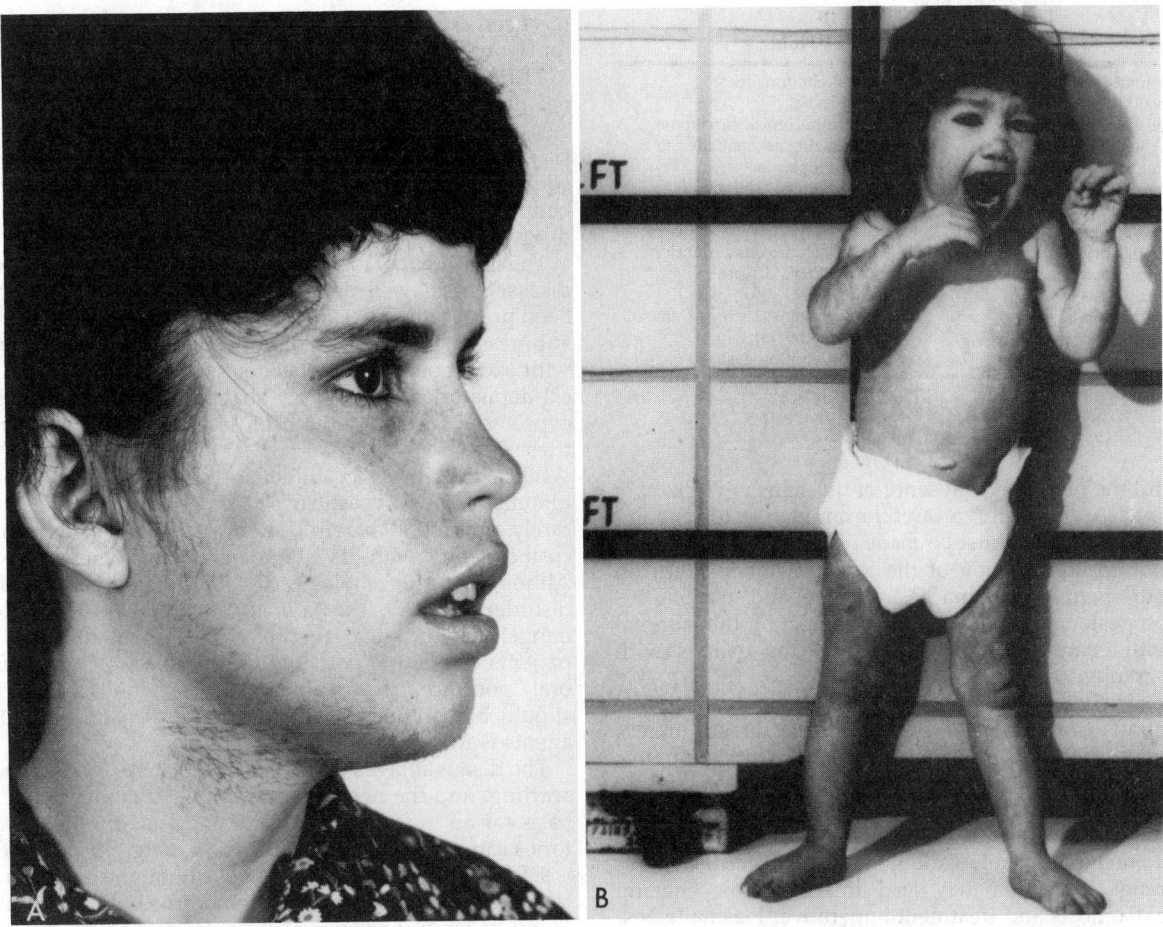

FIGURE 238–1. Examples of androgen-dependent and androgen-independent hirsutism. *A,* Androgen-dependent hirsutism in a woman with the polycystic ovarian syndrome. The terminal hairs are confined to the beard and mustache areas. *B,* A child with androgen-independent hirsutism induced by diazoxide. Note the even distribution of the hair over arms, legs, abdomen, chest, and face.

fore the 11-hydroxylase block, to androstenedione and thence to testosterone.

CLINICAL MANIFESTATIONS. The consequences of elevated plasma testosterone concentrations include hirsutism, acne, temporal balding, increased muscle strength, altered libido, and, in virilized patients, clitoral enlargement and deepening of the voice. There is usually also defeminization with amenorrhea, decrease in the size of the breasts, and change from the female body habitus. The various disorders leading to androgen excess vary primarily in the time of onset of the symptoms and the degree to which they progress.

Idiopathic hirsutism and polycystic ovarian disease tend to present a similar clinical picture, and in fact there may be a continuous spectrum between them. Patients with these disorders rarely become virilized and as such do not have clitoral enlargement or masculinization of the larynx. The hirsutism is usually first noticed in the peripubertal period and tends to stabilize after one to two years of progressive worsening. Menses are often irregular in polycystic ovarian disease and may cease altogether with time. On physical examination

TABLE 238–1. CAUSES OF ANDROGEN-INDEPENDENT HIRSUTISM

1. Medications:	2. Metabolic disorders:
Phenytoin	Starvation (anorexia nervosa)
Diazoxide	Porphyria cutanea tarda
Glucocorticoids	Hypertrichosis lanuginosa
Minoxidil	3. Genetic disorders:
Cyclosporin	Cornelia de Lange syndrome
	Seckel's dwarfism
	Congenital hypertrichosis

hirsutism and the frequent occurrence of enlarged ovaries are usually the only abnormal findings.

Hirsutism that has its onset before or after the pubertal period is suggestive of more serious disease. Adrenal carcinoma can appear at any time in life. These tumors are generally inefficient in producing steroid hormone and hence are large at the time of presentation. Forty per cent are palpable, 90 per cent are detectable by intravenous pyelography, and perhaps all are detectable with computed tomography. The rare virilizing adrenal adenomas, on the other hand, are quite efficient in the synthesis of steroid hormones and are usually only a few centimeters in diameter at the time that symptoms first appear.

Congenital adrenal hyperplasia usually becomes clinically apparent at birth or during childhood. It is characterized, in girls, by rapid growth, by heterosexual precocious puberty, and by hypertension in those having the 11-hydroxylase–deficient variety. Rarely, congenital adrenal hyperplasia may first become clinically apparent at the time of puberty or thereafter. When this occurs, the major clinical manifestations are hirsutism, acne, and menstrual irregularity.

Ovarian neoplasms with manifestations of excessive androgen secretion usually occur in adults (Table 238–2). Most will lead to overt virilization with time, and the majority are palpable on pelvic examination.

DIAGNOSIS. Important historical points include age at onset of hirsutism, rate of progression of hirsutism, the body areas involved, the menstrual history, libidinal changes, changes in appetite and weight, and the family history regarding hirsutism. Important physical findings include the nature of the hair (vellous versus terminal), the hair distri-

**TABLE 238–2. CAUSES OF
ANDROGEN-DEPENDENT HIRSUTISM**

1. Ovarian causes:
   Neoplastic
      Sertoli-Leydig cell tumors
         (arrhenoblastoma)
      Granulosa-stromal cell tumors
      Gynandroblastoma
      Lipid cell tumor
      Gonadoblastoma
   Non-neoplastic
      Polycystic ovarian disease
      Hyperthecosis
      Idiopathic hirsutism
      Insulin resistance

2. Adrenal abnormalities:
   Neoplastic
      Adrenocortical carcinoma
      Virilizing-adrenal adenoma
   Non-neoplastic
      Congenital adrenal
         hyperplasia
      21-Hydroxylase deficiency
      11-Hydroxylase deficiency
      Cushing's disease
3. Medications:
   Androgens (such as Danazol,
      Halotestin)
   "19-Nor" progestins

bution, and the presence or absence of the signs of virilization noted above. Additionally, a careful examination for abdominal and pelvic masses must be made.

The laboratory evaluation of the hirsute woman relies on the measurement of plasma testosterone and plasma 17-hydroxyprogesterone, and on the imaging of the adrenal glands with computed tomography and the ovaries with ultrasonography.

In normal women, the upper limit of plasma testosterone concentrations is about 80 ng per deciliter. Values in excess of 200 ng per deciliter are rarely associated with idiopathic hirsutism or polycystic ovarian disease but are frequently associated with adrenal and ovarian tumors. Hence, values in this range make the diagnosis of an adrenal or ovarian neoplasm much more likely. Additionally, testosterone values in this range will ultimately lead to virilization, making definitive diagnosis and treatment imperative. Plasma testosterone values of less than 200 ng per deciliter are more likely to be associated with a benign process, but periodic re-evaluation (i.e., at three- to six-month intervals) is necessary to ensure that those patients with a progressive disorder will be identified as early as possible.

The measurement of plasma 17-hydroxyprogesterone is the single best test for the diagnosis of congenital adrenal hyperplasia resulting from 21-hydroxylase deficiency. Plasma 17-hydroxyprogesterone values are less than 200 ng per deciliter in normal women. Most patients with 21-hydroxylase deficiency have values at least five times this level. The most reliable diagnostic test for this disorder is determination of the plasma level of 17-hydroxyprogesterone 30 minutes after an intravenous injection of 250 µg synthetic ACTH. In normal subjects the value rarely exceeds 400 ng per deciliter. Patients with 21-hydroxylase deficiency achieve levels of 3000 ng per deciliter or greater. Since 17-hydroxyprogesterone can also be secreted by certain ovarian and adrenal neoplasms, it is essential that plasma 17-hydroxyprogesterone levels be shown to normalize after three days of adrenal suppressive therapy, using 0.5 mg of dexamethasone four times daily to document the adrenal origin of the abnormality.

The diagnosis of 11-hydroxylase deficiency depends, similarly, upon the measurement of plasma 11-deoxycortisol. Because this steroid is also secreted by adrenal neoplasms, distinguishing the 11-hydroxylase type of congenital adrenal hyperplasia from adrenal neoplasms again requires the demonstration that adrenal suppression with dexamethasone lowers the plasma 11-deoxycortisol into the normal range.

Adrenal neoplasms should be sought with computed tomography or ultrasonography, but pelvic ultrasonography is sufficient for diagnosing most virilizing ovarian tumors and does not expose the ovaries to ionizing radiation. If an adrenal or ovarian mass is found and congenital adrenal hyperplasia

has been excluded, surgical exploration should be undertaken for definitive diagnosis and initial treatment.

TREATMENT. The treatments of Cushing's disease, adrenal neoplasms, and congenital adrenal hyperplasia are discussed in Ch. 230. Patients with congenital adrenal hyperplasia should be treated with 12 to 15 mg of hydrocortisone per square meter per day, or its equivalent, given preferably at bedtime, to suppress ACTH secretion and thus adrenal androgen production.

The treatment of idiopathic hirsutism and polycystic ovarian disease is less well defined. Many treatment regimens have been proposed. These include hypothalamic-pituitary-ovarian suppression with oral contraceptives, adrenal suppression with exogenous glucocorticoids, electrolysis, wax and chemical depilatories, and simple shaving. Antiandrogens such as cyproterone acetate have been employed in European countries.

Since the extent of hirsutism in women with idiopathic hirsutism and polycystic ovarian disease is usually stable and rarely progresses to virilization, the problem is primarily a cosmetic one with its attendant psychologic ramifications. Although the psychologic discomfort associated with these disorders may be great, it is difficult to justify potentially dangerous hormonal therapies for the treatment of these patients. Thus, the potential complications of treatment with oral contraceptives, glucocorticoids, and antiandrogens should be carefully considered before treatment with these agents is initiated.

The disadvantages of electrolysis include expense, potential scarring, and the need to continue the treatment on a regular basis for an indefinite period. Using wax or chemical depilatories can be painful and untidy. Shaving, on the other hand is safe, effective, and inexpensive. Although shaving is alleged to exacerbate hirsutism, this is not borne out by clinical study. Many women will reject shaving on the basis that it is unfeminine. They will often relent, however, when it is pointed out that they have no such misgivings about shaving their legs and underarms. On balance then, shaving is the cheapest, safest, and most effective form of treatment for idiopathic hirsutism and should be employed whenever possible.

PROGNOSIS. Since hirsutism is a symptom of many different disorders, prognosis for remission is linked to the efficacy of treatment for these maladies. It should be emphasized again that most patients complaining of hirsutism have no serious underlying disorder. Complete extirpation of an androgen-producing neoplasm can be expected to result in the resolution of hirsutism. However, the recovery period may be as long as two years, and patients should be warned not to expect a dramatic decrease in hair growth immediately following therapeutic intervention.

Hirsutism tends to progress to a given level and to stabilize in idiopathic hirsutism and polycystic ovarian disease. Patients are often aware that the process does not seem to be progressing, but the assurance that it probably will not progress is often helpful in allaying anxiety.

Chrousos GP, Loriaux DL, Mann DL, et al.: Late-onset 21-hydroxylase deficiency mimicking idiopathic hirsutism or polycystic ovarian disease. Ann Intern Med 96:143, 1982. *Clinical and laboratory description of a rare genetic disorder associated with hirsutism with review of the literature and 80 references.*

Ferriman D, Gallway M: Clinical assessment of body hair in women. J Clin Endocrinol Metab 21:1440, 1961. *Delineates normal and abnormal hair growth patterns in women.*

Kirschner MA, Zucker IR, Jespersen D: Idiopathic hirsutism, an ovarian abnormality. N Engl J Med 294:637, 1976. *The best pathogenetic study of idiopathic hirsutism.*

Korobkin M, White EA, Kressel HY, et al.: Computed tomography in the diagnosis of adrenal disease. Am J Roentgenol 132:231, 1979. *An up-to-date discussion of the power of this technique for diagnosing adrenal mass lesions.*

Rittmaster R, Loriaux DL: Hirsutism: A clinical review. Ann Intern Med 106:95, 1987. *A recent review of hirsutism with an extensive (246 references) bibliography.*

239 NONMALIGNANT DISEASES OF THE BREAST*

George Tolis

Diseases of the breast are important in medical practice. In this chapter some of the developmental aspects and the function (lactation) of the breast will be reviewed briefly as a background for more extensive discussions of two clinically important disorders, gynecomastia and galactorrhea. Carcinoma of the breast, by far the most important disease of that organ, will be discussed in Ch. 240.

DEVELOPMENTAL ASPECTS OF THE MAMMARY GLAND. The human breast has a tubuloalveolar structure and consists of 15 to 25 lobes radiating from the nipple. Each lobe is subdivided into lobules from which emerge lactiferous ducts. The mammary line is well developed in the five-week embryo, but it is not until the fifth gestational month that both the nipple and the secondary buds develop. Until puberty the human mammary gland does not develop unless a pathologic condition (e.g., feminizing adrenal carcinoma), or isosexual precocity occurs. With the onset of puberty, the areola enlarges and becomes pigmented, and a significant growth of the tubular duct of the female breast ensues. Estrogens primarily stimulate the development of the mammary duct; progesterone seems to play a major role in alveolar growth. The role of other factors (such as growth hormone, insulin, somatomedins, epidermal growth factor, glucocorticoids, and thyroxine) in the normal growth of the mammary gland is incompletely understood.

INITIATION AND MAINTENANCE OF LACTATION. The hormonal factor absolutely required for lactation is prolactin. In the absence of adequate circulating prolactin, lactation does not occur or ceases if previously established. Furthermore the experimental administration of a specific antiserum to prolactin inhibits galactopoiesis. For prolactin activity to be fully expressed, optimal concentrations of other hormones (such as estrogens, thyroxine, and insulin) are also required. The effects of prolactin upon the female breast are modulated by various factors such as suckling, age, hormones, and medications. The administration of estrogens in the postpartum period will suppress lactation in many women by a mechanism independent of serum prolactin levels. Since serum prolactin concentrations do not decrease, it appears that in this situation estrogens block the action of prolactin. In contrast, the suppression of lactation by bromocriptine, a dopamine agonistic analogue, is due to the inhibition of prolactin release from the pituitary gland. In the breast-feeding mother basal serum prolactin levels fall gradually, yet the amount of milk secreted increases. Although no association exists between the resting serum prolactin levels and the amount of milk produced, there may be a correlation between the amount of lactation and the degree of prolactin increment induced by vigorous suckling.

GALACTORRHEA

Nonpuerperal lactation or galactorrhea is an abnormal physical sign that occurs in both men and women. The amount of milk secreted forms the basis of the grading system used in quantitating the disorder. Grades I and II: Milk can be expressed manually, but the patient may not necessarily be aware of it otherwise. Grades III and IV: Copious milk secretion occurs in an intermittent or continuous manner. The degree of galactorrhea so defined does not correlate with the

---

*The editors acknowledge the assistance of Dr. Robert B. Jaffe in the revision of this chapter.

pathologic significance of the underlying disorder (i.e., pituitary tumors may be associated with Grade II galactorrhea; the use of psychotropic drugs may lead to Grade IV galactorrhea). Galactorrhea often is of benign significance. It becomes an important clinical sign especially when it is associated with disturbances of menstruation, pituitary tumor, or impairment of fertility.

ETIOLOGY AND PATHOGENESIS. The classification of galactorrhea is more meaningful if it takes into account the serum prolactin (PRL) levels (Table 239–1). *Normoprolactinemic galactorrhea* is usually benign as far as hypothalamic-pituitary pathology is concerned. In acromegaly secondary to a growth hormone–secreting tumor, excess milk production may be due to the intrinsic lactogenic activity of growth hormone or to a circulating PRL of different molecular form than that measured by the standard radioimmunoassay. Even when serum PRL is in the normal range, the level may be inappropriately increased for a particular individual, since further lowering of the PRL with bromocriptine may be effective treatment. It has also been speculated that prior to the development of galactorrhea there may have been an increase in PRL that led to an increase in the number of lactogenic receptors and therefore to enhanced sensitivity.

Hyperprolactinemic galactorrhea should prompt a thorough investigation. Increased serum levels of PRL can result either from a decrease in its metabolic clearance (e.g., in liver failure or hypothyroidism) or, more commonly, from an increase in PRL production. The latter can result from conditions decreasing the inhibitory hypothalamic (dopaminergic) control of the pituitary or from the presence of a prolactin-secreting pituitary tumor. A decrease in the hypothalamic suppression of the secretion of PRL by the pituitary can be due either to lesions in the hypothalamus (e.g., gliomas, craniopharyngioma, histiocytosis, infarction) or to disruption of the hypothalamic-pituitary neurovascular connections (e.g., pituitary stalk section, tumoral impingement on the stalk as by suprasellar extension of pituitary tumor). Functional causes of decreased

TABLE 239–1. CAUSES OF NONPUERPERAL GALACTORRHEA

I. **Central origin**
  A. Organic
    1. Suprahypophyseal lesions
      a. Hypothalamic disorders—infiltrative processes (histiocytosis, metastatic diseases); masses (craniopharyngioma, meningioma); infarction; embolism
      b. Pituitary stalk lesions—section; impingement by tumors (all types with suprasellar extension); vascular insult
    2. Hypophyseal tumors
      a. Prolactin secreting* (solitary; part of multiple endocrine adenomatosis syndrome mixed with GH, TSH, ACTH)
  B. Functional
    1. Drug related
      a. Psychotropic (butyrophenones, phenothiazines)*
      b. Antihypertensive (reserpine, alpha-methyldopa)
      c. Cannabinoids (morphine, heroin)
      d. Contraceptives
      e. Antigastroplegics (metoclopramide)*
    2. Unclassified (idiopathic, stress, empty sella syndrome)
II. **Peripheral origin**
  A. Due to pituitary prolactin
    1. Due to primary failure of target endocrine gland
      a. Hypothyroidism
      b. Addison's disease
    2. Due to excess estrogen formation from target endocrine glands
      a. Feminizing adrenal carcinoma
      b. Polycystic ovarian syndrome
    3. Due to decreased metabolic clearance of PRL
      a. Renal failure
      b. Liver failure
      c. Hypothyroidism
    4. Due to local breast conditions
      a. Mechanical stimulation or suckling
      b. Thoracic and/or breast trauma, burn
      c. Inflammation, i.e., mastitis, herpes zoster
  B. Due to ectopic prolactin production
    1. Renal neoplasia
    2. Bronchogenic neoplasia

---

*Most common causes of highest serum PRL levels.

dopaminergic control are mainly due to the intake of drugs that may (1) inhibit dopamine synthesis (e.g., alpha-methyl paratyrosine); (2) deplete the pool of catecholamine (e.g., reserpine); (3) dilute the catecholamine content in the presynaptic neurons (e.g., the false neurotransmitter methyldopa); or (4) occupy the postsynaptic receptor sites (e.g., haloperidol). Other drugs that stimulate the pituitary lactotrope are exogenous opiates and contraceptive steroids, especially those with high estrogen content. In susceptible animals, administration of a large dose of estrogen may induce pituitary prolactin-secreting tumors and result in hyperprolactinemia.

Galactorrhea and hyperprolactinemia may occur in primary myxedema or in Addison's disease. The mechanism whereby hypothyroidism leads to hyperprolactinemia is unknown, but it is believed to be mediated via excessive thyrotropin releasing hormone (TRH) secretion. Whether excess corticotropin releasing factor (CRF) accounts for the hyperprolactinemic galactorrhea of Addison's disease or Cushing's syndrome is unknown. Other conditions associated with excess PRL secretion include the polycystic ovary syndrome and adrenal carcinoma, perhaps because of the excess estrogen production found in the syndromes.

Excess production of PRL has been reported in patients with bronchogenic or renal neoplasms. Ectopic sources of PRL should be considered in the differential diagnosis.

CLINICAL PRESENTATION AND DIFFERENTIAL DIAGNOSIS. The clinical presentation of galactorrhea is highly variable, with milk production anywhere on the scale of I to IV (see above). There may be no other symptoms, or the patient may have the signs or symptoms of any of the disorders listed in Table 239–1. It is particularly important to determine carefully any drugs the patient may be taking.

In humans, the incidence of prolactin-secreting tumors (prolactinomas) is far higher in women then in men. A more general discussion of pituitary tumors has been presented in Ch. 226. Galactorrhea associated with amenorrhea is the most common presentation of a prolactinoma in women. Galactorrhea alone is found in less than one third of patients with prolactinoma. Prolactinomas in men produce galactorrhea much more rarely and, partly because of this, tend to present later as larger, space-occupying tumors with headaches, visual impairment, and impotence.

One should measure serum PRL in every patient with galactorrhea, whether spontaneous or elicited at examination. If the level is elevated and there is no evidence of psychotropic drug intake or primary hypothyroidism, one should exclude the presence of a pituitary tumor. If the tumor is non-prolactin-secreting and impinges upon the stalk, then the administration of TRH (500 µg intravenously) will provoke an increase of at least two-fold in serum PRL in the majority of patients (see Ch. 225 for normal response of PRL to TRH). If the tumor is composed of prolactin-secreting cells, then the diagnosis can be established with a combination of radiologic techniques and hormonal assays. If serum PRL levels exceed 500 ng per milliliter, a macroadenoma of the pituitary will generally be demonstrable by a plain skull film of the sella turcica by both the anteroposterior and lateral views. If the levels are between 100 and 500 ng per milliliter, the plain skull film may be normal, but computed tomography or magnetic resonance imaging will demonstrate a microadenoma in 85 per cent of the patients. In as many as 20 per cent of such patients TRH may elicit a doubling of serum PRL levels. If the levels of PRL are less than 100 ng per milliliter, no sella pathology may be detected even when high-resolution computed tomography is utilized. In these cases a larger proportion of patients may respond to TRH. If PRL is not released by TRH patients with hyperprolactinemia, the diagnosis of an autonomously secreting adenoma is strongly suspected.

TREATMENT. The treatment of the patient with galactorrhea depends on the primary disease. Discontinuation of

medications or treatment of conditions such as hypothyroidism should lessen milk secretion. In persistent hyperprolactinemia without radiologic evidence for prolactinoma, bromocriptine will often be sufficient therapy (see below for treatment schedule). In such patients annual evaluation by sella radiology may be necessary if, upon discontinuation of the medication, hyperprolactinemia again supervenes. If a microadenoma is strongly suspected, the same strategy can be followed even for the woman who desires pregnancy. Small (10 mm or less) noninvasive microadenomas do not usually grow rapidly during the gestational period. If there are signs of tumor growth despite bromocriptine treatment, trans-sphenoidal tumor resection is the preferred treatment. If during bromocriptine treatment there is no radiographic evidence of growth of the tumor, if the serum PRL is maintained within normal limits, and if the clinical abnormality is corrected, the patient can be kept on this regimen indefinitely. Reasons for discontinuation of medical therapy are (1) patient noncompliance, (2) cost of the medication, (3) development of side effects, and (4) failure of the medication to control the clinical and abnormal disorder (e.g., continuation of galactorrhea-amenorrhea and nonsuppression of serum PRL). In these instances, which are not uncommon, trans-sphenoidal resection of the pituitary adenoma could be undertaken in specialized centers. Pituitary tumor irradiation is the alternative to surgery. For those patients with galactorrhea and large adenomas, with or without parasellar and suprasellar extension, a combination of surgery, radiotherapy, and bromocriptine offers the best results. There have been reports of rapid decrease in tumor size with the use of bromocriptine alone, but there have been other reports to the contrary.

The management of patients with idiopathic normoprolactinemic galactorrhea is very difficult. This is more likely to occur in parous than in nulliparous women. Reports of the efficacy of pyridoxine and cyproheptadine in the treatment of these patients are not convincing and may represent only a placebo effect. Bromocriptine has been used to treat normoprolactinemic galactorrhea, but the number of "responders" not unexpectedly is smaller than in hyperprolactinemic patients. A trial of bromocriptine in normoprolactinemic galactorrhea may be warranted, based on the reasoning that (1) the levels of PRL, although within the normal range, may be inappropriately high for a given patient, and (2) there may be a discrepancy between the biologically active versus the immunologically detectable PRL molecule.

Bromocriptine should be administered carefully in the treatment of galactorrhea. Our custom is to begin with 1.25 mg (occasionally even with half that dose) every night for one week, and then to increase it by 1.25 mg every week until a dosage of 2.5 mg twice daily is reached. A total daily dosage of 10 mg is rarely exceeded, although the dosage can be increased to 20 mg per day. Bromocriptine is taken with a meal, and the patient is asked to avoid abrupt postural change to prevent orthostatic hypotensive episodes. Nausea and behavioral changes (of the manic type) are other side effects. Currently there is no evidence for teratogenicity or other defects in the offspring of mothers who conceived while receiving bromocriptine. The drug passes the placental barrier, however, and exposed children have been observed for less than ten years. It is probably prudent, therefore, for women to discontinue the medication during pregnancy.

GYNECOMASTIA

Gynecomastia is defined as a palpable, firm mass, measuring at least 2 cm in diameter in the subareolar region. It represents excessive development of the male breast with a feminine appearance, and is the most common disorder of the male breast; about 85 per cent of male breast masses are due to gynecomastia (Fig. 239–1). Pathologically it may be florid with proliferation of glandular or fibrous elements, characterized by increase of stromal tissue. The florid type may regress or progress to the fibrous type; the fibrous type is typically irreversible.

Gynecomastia usually begins at puberty when it may be unilateral or bilateral. When gynecomastia is unilateral it is more common on the left side for reasons unknown. Approximately 40 per cent of pubescent boys may develop some transient gynecomastia, with the highest incidence being between 14 and 15.5 years of age. Autopsy studies of elderly men have revealed true gynecomastia in as many as 40 per cent of subjects. The development of gynecomastia from late puberty to male senescence may signal a serious underlying disorder, such as adrenal or testicular tumor, and in such cases early diagnosis and treatment may be lifesaving.

ETIOLOGY AND PATHOPHYSIOLOGY. A classification of gynecomastia is contained in Table 239–2. The pathophysiology of gynecomastia has been partly clarified. For the majority of patients it seems to be associated with a disturbance in the balance of estrogenic-androgenic effects on the mammary epithelium. The pathogenesis of gynecomastia may be complex. For example, both increased estrogen production and aromatization of secreted androgens to estrogens may occur in association with adrenal tumors and congenital adrenal hyperplasia. In nonadrenal neoplasms associated with human chorionic gonadotropin (hCG) production, the excess estrogen levels are due to increased secretion of estrogens by the testes. Finally, the estrogen level may be only relatively increased in comparison to the testosterone level, as in Klinefelter's syndrome or in testicular failure, with an increased estrogen-androgen ratio. An increased extraglandular formation of estrogens from androgens is believed to play a significant role in the gynecomastia seen in patients with chronic liver disease, starvation, and thyrotoxicosis. In these conditions, as a result of decreased hepatic extraction, there

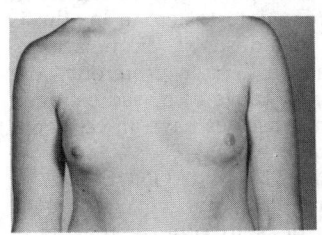
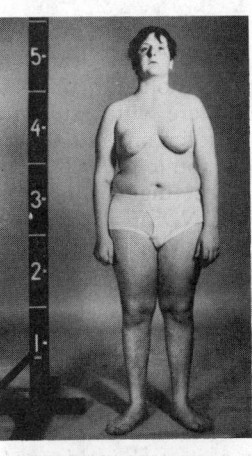
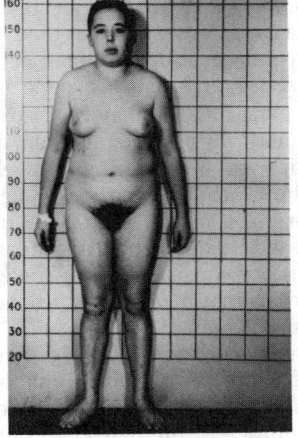
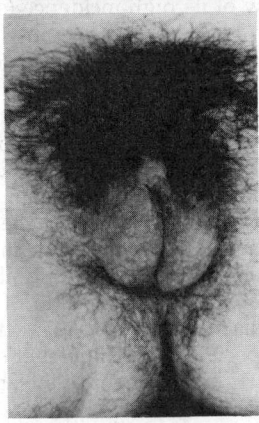

FIGURE 239–1. *Upper left,* Pubertal gynecomastia (physical examination: normal). *Upper right,* Gynecomastia associated with obesity (physical examination: normal except for increased adiposity). *Lower left and right,* Phenotypic appearance of body habitus and external genitalia in a genetically male patient with the syndrome of incomplete testicular feminization (physical examination: female escutcheon, hypospadias, bifid scrotum, normal-sized testes). (Courtesy of Dr. H. Guyda.)

TABLE 239–2. CLASSIFICATION OF THE CAUSES OF GYNECOMASTIA

All true gynecomastia is caused by an estrogenic effect on the male breast. This may result from excessive estrogen or from deficient androgen.

I. **Physiologic—newborn, puberty, senescence**
II. **Pathologic**
   A. Increased estrogen secretion
     1. Hermaphroditism
     2. Klinefelter's syndrome
     3. Congenital adrenal hyperplasia
     4. Neoplastic
       a. Adrenal carcinoma
       b. Testicular tumor (Sertoli cell, Leydig cell, choriocarcinoma)
       c. Paraneoplasms secreting human chorionic gonadotropin (lung, liver, kidney, stomach, lymphopoietic system)
   B. Increased conversion of androgens to estrogens
     1. Adrenal carcinoma
     2. Liver disorders (failure secondary to infectious or nutritional causes, carcinoma)
     3. Nutritional (refeeding after starvation)
     4. Thyrotoxicosis
   C. Decreased androgen secretion
     1. Primary testicular failure (anorchia, Klinefelter's syndrome, enzymatic defects in testosterone synthesis)
     2. Secondary testicular failure (castration; infectious orchitis; mumps and other viruses, lepromatous, tuberculous; neurologic disorders; paraplegia, muscular dystrophy; renal failure; panhypopituitarism; prolactin-secreting tumors)
   D. Decreased androgen activity due to receptor protein abnormalities
     1. Complete testicular feminization
     2. Incomplete testicular feminization
     3. Reifenstein's syndrome
III. **Pharmacologic—a combination of mechanisms**
   A. Cannabinoid—methadone and marijuana
   B. Psychotropics—phenothiazine, butyrophenone, reserpine
   C. Antihypertensives—reserpine, alpha-methyldopa, spironolactone
   D. Cardiac—digitalis
   E. Gastrointestinal—cimetidine, metoclopramide, domperidone
   F. Antituberculous—isoniazid
   G. Hormonal
     1. Sex steroids—estrogens, androgens
     2. Gonadotropins—human chorionic gonadotropin
     3. Antiandrogens
   H. Cytotoxic—cyclophosphamide, mustine, vincristine, mitotane
   I. Miscellaneous—penicillamine
IV. **Idiopathic**

is increased androgen available for peripheral conversion to estrogens. The latter mechanism seems to be operative in some patients with idiopathic gynecomastia, but its significance in that syndrome has not been fully elucidated.

Peptide hormones may contribute to the genesis of gynecomastia directly or indirectly. Human placental lactogen (hPL) is secreted by some testicular tumors, but its role in the proliferation of mammary epithelium is not clear. Some patients with hyperprolactinemia associated with a prolactin-secreting pituitary tumor have gynecomastia. This is probably secondary to a decrease in androgen secretion (suppression of gonadotropins), possibly to a decrease in the peripheral conversion of testosterone to its active metabolite dihydrotestosterone.

In the syndrome of complete testicular feminization, androgen production by the testes is normal but pituitary luteinizing hormone (LH) output is enhanced (because the absence of cytoplasmic androgen receptors in the pituitary impairs feedback control) and leads to testicular estrogen production. The increased estrogen, coupled with a defect in the action of androgen owing to the lack of the receptor in the mammary gland, leads to excessive estrogenic expression and gynecomastia. A similar mechanism has been invoked in incomplete testicular feminization and in Reifenstein's syndrome. Perhaps variations in hormone receptor levels may account for other cases of gynecomastia associated with normal circulating levels of estrogens and androgens.

Gynecomastia occurs in patients receiving various drugs, in particular estrogens (orally, parenterally, or as ointments). Other drugs, however, can also lead to gynecomastia by altering the effective estrogenic-androgenic ratio of activity in the breast. Some lead to decreased testosterone synthesis (e.g., chemotherapeutic agents, high doses of spironolactone) or interfere with testosterone action (e.g., cyproterone, low doses of spironolactone). They may cause increased estrogen production (e.g., hCG) or may themselves have an estrogen-like effect (digitalis, tetrahydrocannabinol).

DIAGNOSIS AND DIFFERENTIAL DIAGNOSIS. It is obviously important to be sure that true gynecomastia is present. The most common error is to confuse the "false gynecomastia" of obesity with true gynecomastia. The obese breast lacks glandular elements on palpation. Palpation will also differentiate gynecomastia from such disorders as carcinoma or neurofibroma. It should be evident that even the presence of true gynecomastia with onset at the time of puberty does not call for a major medical investigation in view of its high incidence (see above) and benign prognosis.

The differential diagnosis of gynecomastia may be accomplished on the basis of history and physical examination. In most instances laboratory studies will be important as well. For example, examination of the head and neck may reveal the presence of signs of compression of the anterior visual pathways consistent with suprasellar extension of a pituitary tumor, or diplopia, lid lag, or goiter consistent with Graves' disease. Examination of the breasts may reveal the presence of galactorrhea, in which case measurement of serum PRL is mandatory. The skin and abdomen may reveal signs of liver failure, and examination of the testes may establish microrchidia, in which case a chromosomal disorder should be suspected (e.g., Klinefelter's syndrome). Alternatively, asymmetric enlargement of a testis raises suspicion of a malignant process.

Laboratory studies will be selected in part based on the clinical circumstances revealed by the history, physical examination, and the age of the patient. A study of liver function is usually indicated. Useful hormone assays include the determination of serum estrogens (estrone and estradiol), androgens (androstenedione and testosterone), and luteinizing hormone (LH), and of urinary 17-ketosteroids or serum dehydroepiandrosterone sulfate (DHAS). Excess serum estrogens are found in patients with Leydig cell tumors and adrenal carcinoma; in such patients serum LH and testosterone levels are low. Elevated serum LH is found in primary testicular failure (in which case testosterone levels are low) and in hCG-secreting tumors (due to cross-reaction of hCG in the assay for LH if a specific hCG assay is not done). If hCG is increased, serum testosterone may be normal, but serum estrogens tend to be increased. Abnormally high LH occurs in the syndrome of peripheral androgen resistance and is accompanied by normal or elevated testosterone levels. Finally, excessive secretion of DHAS or excretion of 17-ketosteroids almost invariably reflects disease of the adrenal cortex. Inability to demonstrate abnormal values in any of the aforementioned measurements does not exclude a metabolic cause of gynecomastia.

Radiologic studies can be of significant help in selected cases. Four radiographic patterns have been identified: (1) the presence of ductlike structures (54 per cent incidence in one series); (2) marked proliferation of the ducts occupying almost the entire breast; (3) homogeneous density occupying either or both subareolar breast areas; and (4) nonhomogeneous density in subareolar or most breast regions. The last appearance was found more often in adults, whereas homogeneity was more prevalent in pubertal gynecomastia. Xeromammography in a patient with a breast mass raises strong suspicions for cancer when the mass is solid, spiculated, and located eccentrically in relation to the nipple; benign gynecomastia, by contrast, is symmetrical in relation to the nipple.

TREATMENT. Regression of gynecomastia can occur in the majority of patients. It is spontaneous in the pubertal cases (up to 90 per cent regress within one to three years). In the rest of the patients, removal of the offending agent or appropriate drug treatment will result in significant improvement when utilized not too late in the course of the abnormality. Thus, impressive improvement occurs with the removal of a sex steroid–producing tumor or treatment of thyrotoxicosis, whereas poor results are obtained in long-standing cases of Klinefelter's or fibrous gynecomastia. In cases of androgen deficiency, androgen administration certainly leads to improvement; however, the active biotransformation of aromatizable androgens to estrogens sustains gynecomastic changes. Attempts to use nonaromatizable androgens or dihydrotestosterone may have promise. As well, independent or combined administration of antiestrogens could theoretically protect the breast tissue from the estrogenic side effects; well-documented series are not as yet reported. A striking reversal of gynecomastia in a child, however, has been demonstrated using a potent aromatase inhibitor. If gynecomastia is long lasting, the ensuing fibrotic changes are irreversible, so that even the removal of the causative agent (e.g., drug withdrawal) may not lead to a return of the breast to normal size. Cosmetic mastectomy may be the preferred mode of "treatment," depending upon the wishes of the patient.

GALACTORRHEA

Friesen HG, Tolis G: The use of bromocriptine in the galactorrhea-amenorrhea syndromes. Clin Endocrinol 6S:91, 1977. *An important document in the North American literature. It is based on the Canadian Comparative Study and should be a standard reference.*

Jaffe RB (ed.): Prolactin. New York, Elsevier, 1981.

Jaffe RB: Pathologic alterations in prolactin secretion. In Yen SSC, Jaffe RB (eds.): Reproductive Endocrinology. Philadelphia, W. B. Saunders Company, 1986, pp 546–570.

Kleinberg DL, Noel GH, Frantz AG: Galactorrhea: A study of 235 cases, including 48 with pituitary tumors. N Engl J Med 296:589, 1977. *This study confirms and extends previous observations. It is among the most comprehensive reports on etiologic entities associated with galactorrhea.*

Koppelman MCS, Jaffe MJ, Rieth KG, et al.: Hyperprolactinemia, amenorrhea and galactorrhea. Ann Intern Med 100:115, 1984. *The authors report on their experiences with 25 patients with this syndrome and emphasize its benign clinical course. Because of this they advocate conservative treatment.*

Tolis G: Galactorrhea. In Krieger DT, Bordin WC (eds.): Current Therapy in Endocrinology 1983–1984. Toronto and St. Louis, B. C. Decker and C. V. Mosby Companies, 1983, pp 427–428. *Report based on the author's data and literature review of normoprolactinemic and hyperprolactinemic galactorrhea.*

Yen SSC: Prolactin in human reproduction. In Yen SSC, Jaffe RB (eds.): Reproductive Endocrinology. Philadelphia, W. B. Saunders Company, 1986, pp 237–263.

GYNECOMASTIA

Chandrakant CK, Parekh NJ: The male breast. Radiol Clin North Am 21:137, 1983. *A thorough review and presentation of the authors' own series of radiologic issues in the evaluation of gynecomastia.*

Large DM, Anderson DC: Twenty-four hour profiles of circulating androgens and estrogens in male puberty with and without gynecomastia. Clin Endocrinol 11:505, 1979. *A significant contribution. It documents the long-held view that there is an estrogen-androgen imbalance associated with pubertal gynecomastia.*

Large DM, Jones JM, Shalet SM, et al.: Gynaecomastia complicating the treatment of myeloma. Br J Cancer 48:69, 1983. *A detailed hormonal study of patients with gynecomastia receiving cytotoxic agents.*

Wilson JD, Aiman J, MacDonald P: The pathogenesis of gynecomastia. Adv Intern Med 25:1, 1980. *This review is based on the authors' longstanding experience in the steroid field and presents a "state of the art" contribution with regard to the pathophysiology of gynecomastia.*

240 BREAST CANCER

Brian J. Lewis

EPIDEMIOLOGY AND PATHOGENESIS

In 1986, 123,000 new cases of female breast cancer and 900 new cases of male breast cancer were projected for the United States. In terms of annual mortality, 40,000 women and 300 men die of breast cancer. These figures and the 1 in 12 lifetime risk that a woman in the United States has for developing breast cancer make this disease a significant health problem.

The cause of breast cancer is unknown, but there are several factors that correlate with its occurrence: age, family history, ethnic influences, and hormonal effects.

AGE. Only about 15 per cent of cases of breast cancer occur before the age of 40. The age-adjusted incidence steadily increases thereafter, with two thirds of cases occurring in postmenopausal women.

FAMILY HISTORY. Daughters or sisters of breast cancer patients have a two- to three-fold greater risk of developing breast cancer than do women without an affected first-degree relative. More specifically, this relative risk can range from 1.5 if the mother or sister was postmenopausal at diagnosis to 8.8 if she was premenopausal and had bilateral disease. Unlike patients in the general population, women with the highest relative risk among those with a positive family history have a greater tendency to have their disease before the age of 40. Careful counseling, screening, and tracking of high-risk patients are essential. Increased monitoring should be given to patients with prior curative treatment for breast cancer, since they have a 10 to 15 per cent lifetime chance of developing a second primary breast cancer.

ETHNIC INFLUENCES. Ninety per cent of breast cancer patients lack a positive family history. While ethnic background has a role, it is necessary to control for the influences of allied cultural and nongenetic factors. Oriental women have a much lower risk of breast cancer than women in western countries. Women of Japanese descent who reside in the United States have a higher risk than women in Japan. Within the United States itself, the probability of developing breast cancer by age 75 shows considerable variation: for white women, it is 8.2 per cent; for black women, 7.0 per cent; for Hispanic women, 4.8 per cent; for native American women, 2.5 per cent; for Japanese-American women, 5.4 per cent; and for Chinese-American women, 6.1 per cent.

HORMONAL EFFECTS. Estrogens have an impact on the development of breast cancer. Early menarche, late menopause, and late or no pregnancy correlate with a higher risk (relative risk of 1.3, 1.5 and 2 to 3, respectively). Conversely, premature loss of ovarian function, late menarche, early menopause, and early or more numerous pregnancies correlate with a decreased risk. The chance for developing breast cancer is increased in men with Klinefelter's syndrome or with other disturbances of estrogen metabolism.

Oral contraceptives seem not to increase the risk of breast cancer, and they may ameliorate the symptoms of fibrocystic disease. There is some concern that the use of exogenous estrogens in postmenopausal patients can increase the risk, but this may correlate with higher doses and more prolonged treatment. There is very little evidence that the replacement doses used for the treatment of osteoporosis increase the risk of carcinoma of the breast (Ch. 250).

Historically, there has been a linkage between fibrocystic disease of the breast and an increased risk for breast cancer. A host of terms has been lumped under "fibrocystic disease" (i.e., macrocysts, microcysts, adenosis, apocrine change, fibrosis, fibroadenoma, and ductal hyperplasia). We now know that the majority of women (70 per cent) who have a biopsy for benign disease are not at increased risk for cancer, but the presence of atypical hyperplasia and a family history of breast cancer greatly increase the probability of developing breast carcinoma (Table 240–1).

OTHER RISK FACTORS. Other risk factors include ionizing radiation and possibly diet. Surprisingly, consumption of even moderate amounts of alcohol appears to increase risk appreciably. Repeated chest fluoroscopy for tuberculosis, therapeutic radiation of mastitis, and exposure of Japanese women to the atomic bomb blast have been linked to increased rates of breast cancer. Animal models and geographic-ethnic differences in incidence suggest that dietary factors, in particular fat (increased in the western diet), may contribute to the development of breast cancer.

TABLE 240–1. RISK FACTORS FOR BREAST CANCER IN WOMEN WITH PROLIFERATIVE BREAST DISEASE

Diagnosis	Relative Risk of Breast Cancer (95% Confidence Interval)
Nonproliferative lesions	1.0
Proliferative disease without atypical hyperplasia	1.9 (1.2 to 2.9)
Atypical hyperplasia	5.3 (3.1 to 8.8)
Atypical hyperplasia + family history of breast cancer	11.0 (5.5 to 24)

Data from DuPont WD, Page DL: Risk factors for breast cancer in women with proliferative breast disease. N Engl J Med 312:146, 1985.

DIAGNOSIS

Clinical Presentation

Breast cancer is usually noted as a painless lump and discovered incidentally by the patient, by routine physical examination, or by mammography. Pain and tenderness are nonspecific findings and herald cancer less than 10 per cent of the time. Physical findings suggestive of a malignancy include a hard, irregular mass and skin dimpling or nipple retraction. Nonbloody nipple discharges are rarely associated with cancer. Bloody discharges correlate with intraductal papillomas in about 30 per cent of cases and with invasive cancer in about one third of cases.

Pertinent history includes a family history of breast cancer on the maternal side, especially in first-degree relatives, prior breast biopsies, whether the lump is new or old, and whether it fluctuates in size, consistency, and tenderness with the menstrual cycle. Such cycling will be more suggestive of a benign process but by no means rules out cancer. Physical examination should include careful inspection and palpation of both breasts and assessment of the axillary, supraclavicular, and infraclavicular node areas.

Evaluation of a Breast Mass

A suspicious breast mass requires systematic evaluation and follow-up. A negative mammogram or needle aspiration does not ensure that a mass is benign, and if it remains of concern, it must be excised. To avoid distortion of breast anatomy, a mammogram should precede any biopsy procedure. Breast imaging rules out contralateral lesions and multiple foci in the ipsilateral breast, and it is sometimes redone after biopsy to confirm that the area of interest was in fact removed.

Formerly, diagnosis and treatment were a one-step procedure. A woman with a suspicious lesion had an excision under general anesthesia with frozen section analysis of the tumor. If cancer was found, mastectomy immediately followed, and the woman awoke to confront both the diagnosis of cancer and the loss of her breast. A two-step procedure is now used. Fine-needle aspiration cytology or excisional biopsy under local anesthesia allows an outpatient diagnosis. If cancer is found, the patient and surgeon can then review treatment options. This approach does not increase the spread of tumor, and the interval of one to two weeks between diagnosis and primary treatment does not represent a significant delay in the therapy of a tumor that has likely been present for years already. It does allow the patient time to make some emotional adjustments and to have a greater sense of involvement in treatment planning.

Screening and Detection

Early detection of a tumor improves the chances for cure. Efforts to screen for and detect early breast cancer have centered on self-examination, physician examination, and techniques for imaging the breast.

Self-examination is simple, without cost, and free of risk. It has been shown to result in earlier detection of tumors, and

TABLE 240–2. GUIDELINES FOR MAMMOGRAPHIC SCREENING OF ASYMPTOMATIC WOMEN (American Cancer Society)

1. Baseline mammogram for all women aged 35 to 40
2. Mammography every one to two years from age 40 to 49
3. Mammography annually for women aged 50 or older

every adult woman should be instructed in its use. Any mass that is new and persists for more than a few weeks, is rapidly enlarging, or changes from a previously stable lump requires a physician's examination.

Examination by a physician as a screening tool is more costly and is applied less frequently than self-examination. Discovery of an unsuspected mass during a periodic examination by a physician leads to detection of tumors at an earlier stage than in patients who do not have periodic breast examinations. The American Cancer Society recommends that every woman have a routine breast examination at least every three years.

Breast imaging techniques include thermography, sonography, and radiographic mammography. Thermography has yet to prove sufficiently sensitive for widespread use, while sonography of the breast remains in a developmental stage. Radiographic mammography is a well-studied and standardized methodology. Annual mammography lowers the mortality from breast cancer in screened populations compared to unscreened control groups. It detects smaller lesions with fewer nodal metastases. Current technology allows a lower dose of radiation per examination. Table 240–2 shows guidelines for screening. Annual examinations are also recommended for women with a prior breast cancer regardless of age.

Breast cancer incidence rose gradually over the first half of the century and turned more sharply upward in the 1960's, concomitant with and possibly as a result of increased attention to education and screening. The mortality (deaths per 100,000), however, has remained constant. It may be that tumors are being found earlier and cured more readily, since more of the tumors found are smaller. Alternatively, a proportion of the early asymptomatic (subclinical) cancers being discovered may have a lower malignant potential than tumors that grow faster and more rapidly become clinically apparent. Thus, screening may appear more efficacious than it really is, since some of the patients discovered to have an "early" cancer may represent a subpopulation with indolent disease who would not otherwise have had clinical expression of the tumor. Nonetheless, there has been a definite reduction in mortality from breast cancer in women who are screened with mammography.

TUMOR BIOLOGY

Breast cancer is more than just a local process; local control of tumor is necessary but not by itself sufficient to address the threat of distant metastases. Breast cancer is also a chronic illness with a potential for recurrence 10 to 15 years after removal of the primary tumor. While one can extirpate apparent disease in the breast and in the axillary nodes in the majority of cases, at least 50 per cent of women found to have tumor in the axillary nodes and 25 per cent of those without axillary node metastases will have metastatic disease.

TABLE 240–3. STAGING OF CARCINOMA OF THE BREAST

Stage I   Tumor < 2 cm without skin involvement and with no clinically suspicious axillary nodes.
Stage II Tumor < 2 cm with clinically suspicious nodes; any tumor 2 to 5 cm with or without clinically suspicious nodes.
Stage III Any tumor > 5 cm; skin involvement or chest wall attachment; any size tumor with clinically fixed axillary nodes; arm edema; supraclavicular nodes.
Stage IV Metastatic disease.

STAGING. The system for clinically staging breast cancer reflects the anatomic extent of tumor (Table 240–3). It allows consistent and comparable description and reporting of cases. The stages correlate with survival and are important in planning treatment, but they do not totally predict the clinical behavior of the tumor. A more complete classification scheme would ideally measure the balance between the inherent virulence of the cancer and the intrinsic antitumor defenses of the host.

METHOD OF SPREAD. Breast cancer spreads directly to the bloodstream as well as to the draining lymphatics. Tumor emboli can traverse the lymph nodes and enter the venous system; and tumor cells can presumably reach lymph nodes by way of the bloodstream. In addition, upon discovery, a breast cancer mass usually contains 10^9 or more cells. Given what is known of doubling times, the cell number at diagnosis implies that the cancer may have been growing for a number of years. It seems logical that there will be shedding of the tumor cells into the venous and lymphatic circulation throughout the life of the tumor, especially early, when tumor growth rate is highest.

Accordingly, it is likely that many more patients with breast cancer have micrometastases than we see with clinical recurrence. Negative axillary nodes may not mean that the tumor was never present in the lymphatic system but rather that it had been there and was unable to flourish. Positive lymph nodes do correlate with subsequent metastases and poor survival. This could reflect simple anatomic spread of cancer past the last "line of defense" imposed by the lymph nodes (Halsted). Alternatively, it could imply that because the tumor persisted in the nodes, however it arrived there, it will also persist and grow in other organs.

In any case, clinical experience has identified important prognostic factors. The size of the primary lesion and particularly the presence or absence of axillary nodal metastases correlate strongly with risk for recurrence. Other features indicating a poor prognosis include an ill-defined tumor border, vascular or lymphatic invasion within the breast, extension of tumor through the axillary node capsule, tumor necrosis, and high-grade histology. The presence of estrogen and progesterone receptor proteins (RP) correlates with a better outcome. A higher proliferative rate of the cancer cells is a strong predictor of recurrence. Patients with locally advanced disease, such as tumor invading the skin or chest wall or those with fixed axillary nodes, are also at high risk for recurrence.

CELL ORIGIN. Most breast tumors derive from mammary epithelium. Eighty per cent of these are infiltrating ductal carcinomas. Less common are infiltrating lobular carcinoma, medullary carcinoma, comedocarcinoma, and colloid carcinoma. Lobular and comedocarcinoma can be bilateral and require increased surveillance of the unaffected breast. Medullary, comedo- and colloid carcinomas are said to have a better prognosis than infiltrating ductal or infiltrating lobular carcinoma. This reflects the lower incidence of nodal metastases with these subtypes. However, when nodes are involved, the five-year survival rate approaches the lower rate seen with node involvement in the ductal or lobular forms. Lobular carcinoma in situ poses a special problem. Although it is not an invasive lesion, it is associated with a 1 per cent annual risk for the development of an invasive lesion in either breast. Some surgeons have therefore advocated prophylactic mastectomy. A more conservative approach is to do a "mirror image" biopsy of the contralateral breast to rule out invasive tumor and then to track the patient closely with periodic examinations and prompt biopsy of any suspicious lesions. Ductal carcinoma in situ carries a higher risk for evolving into invasive cancer and requires surgery. Inflammatory breast cancer represents a highly virulent pathologic variant. Clinically, the patient has a red, swollen, warm breast with a characteristic peau d'orange appearance. Microscopically, this is associated with involvement of dermal lymphatics by tumor. It has proven difficult to achieve long-term survival in patients with this diagnosis.

HORMONE RECEPTOR PROTEINS. Estrogen and progesterone receptor proteins (ERP and PRP) are present in normal mammary epithelium and in a proportion of breast cancers. After binding to the steroid, the activated hormone-receptor complex interacts with specific sites on DNA, and this results in the initiation of steroid-specific protein synthesis. One product of estrogen stimulation is PRP, and the presence of PRP signifies functionally intact ERP. A tumor is considered ERP-positive when it contains more than 10 femtomoles of receptor per milligram of protein, as measured using a radioligand binding assay. Monoclonal antibodies against ERP are now available and permit microscopic visualization and enumeration of ERP-positive tumor cells.

ERP is found more frequently and in higher titer in tumors from postmenopausal patients (60 per cent or more versus 30 to 40 per cent positive in premenopausal women). ERP-positive tumors tend to be less virulent and are more likely to respond to hormonal therapy (see below). Tumors that contain both ERP and PRP have the greatest likelihood of regressing after an endocrine maneuver, and the probability of a response increases directly with the titer of the RP. Given the therapeutic and prognostic implications of hormone receptor levels, it is mandatory that all primary breast cancers be submitted for receptor analysis at the time of removal. There is an 80 per cent concordance between the hormone receptor profile of a primary tumor and its metastases, in the absence of intervening hormone treatment. Breast cancers are heterogeneous in the sense that in RP-positive specimens, the majority but not necessarily all of the cells contain RP. When metastatic disease becomes refractory to hormonal therapy after initially responding, the progression reflects the outgrowth of hormone-independent cells that are usually RP-negative.

PRIMARY MANAGEMENT OF BREAST CANCER
Stage I and Stage II Disease

Since Halsted's time, almost three generations ago, the view of breast cancer as a local or regional process has made radical mastectomy or one of its variants the standard approach to the management of resectable tumor confined to the breast and the axillary lymph nodes. Patients often receive postoperative radiation therapy to the chest wall and the draining lymph node areas. These treatments have produced a local control rate of 95 per cent, but variations in locoregional therapy have not differed significantly in their impact upon distant recurrence or overall survival. Furthermore, more extensive surgery or surgery followed by radiation increases the risk of arm edema.

These approaches entered general use without the testing of alternative approaches, but recently local tumor excision with breast irradiation has been gaining a wider acceptance. Older, largely uncontrolled studies seemed to indicate similar outcomes either with tumor excision and breast irradiation or with traditional mastectomy. While one cannot refer to the decades of observation on local tumor control and side effects that exist for standard surgical approaches, recent and ongoing controlled trials indicate that the techniques are equivalent in terms of tumor recurrence and overall survival.

Public interest in alternatives to mastectomy has increased, and patients are more informed and expect their physicians to provide a comprehensive overview of treatment possibilities, especially ones that would spare them the disfigurement and distress imposed by mastectomy. Likewise, the growing application of plastic surgery for breast reconstruction after mastectomy has lessened the emotional trauma of the operation.

For the present, the most common approach to the primary

TABLE 240–4. REQUIREMENT FOR LIMITED SURGERY AND RADIOTHERAPY FOR EARLY BREAST CANCER

	Comments
Patient Selection	
Adequate resection of tumor without major cosmetic deformity	This requires a single discrete tumor, moderate sized breast, tumor diameter < 4–5 cm.
Surgical Criteria	
Wide resection with specimen orientation	Negative surgical margins are essential—re-resection may be required.
Hormone receptor analysis	
Separate axillary incision	
Radiation Therapy	
4500–5000 rad to entire breast + boost to tumor bed	
Treatment of the Axilla	
Level I *and* Level II axillary dissection* (*not* an informal "sampling")	Permits adequate node sampling, controls local tumor, and obviates the need for axillary radiation. Does not impose a major risk for arm edema.

Sources: Harris, 1985; Danoff, 1985.
*Level I = Complete removal of nodes lateral to the pectoralis minor muscle.
Level II = Removal of nodes beneath the pectoralis minor.

management of a Stage I or Stage II breast cancer remains the modified radical mastectomy. This operation provides important information about the status of axillary nodes and usually allows for breast reconstruction. Postoperative radiotherapy is an individualized rather than "standard" therapy. It is employed when narrow resection margins, extensive nodal disease, the presence of residual tumor, or other high-risk factors for local recurrence are present. With the advent of adjuvant chemotherapy for Stage II disease (see below), there may be even fewer indications for adjuvant radiation therapy, since drug treatment alone may decrease the local failure rate. However, this supposition has yet to be adequately tested in clinical trials.

Table 240–4 lists the requirements for limited surgery and breast irradiation. Mammography is essential to exclude patients with multifocal disease or with diffuse microcalcifications. (Even if the latter prove benign on biopsy, they will interfere with the subsequent mammographic follow-up used to screen for recurrent cancer.) A wide surgical resection of the tumor with negative resection margins is essential and is facilitated by inking the margins of the specimen and orienting it for the pathologist. Axillary node dissection determines whether the patient requires adjuvant systemic treatment because of nodal metastasis.

Clinically suspicious nodes are pathologically negative for tumor 25 to 30 per cent of the time, and, conversely, clinically negative nodes are positive histologically with an equal frequency. With a proper axillary dissection, radiation to the axilla is not necessary (and would significantly augment the risk for arm edema). While positive axillary nodes increase the likelihood of subclinical supraclavicular and internal mammary node metastases, there is no evidence that adjuvant radiation to those areas will improve survival.

Standard pretreatment evaluation for any of these techniques includes a complete blood count, a profile of serum chemistries with particular reference to studies suggestive of liver or bone involvement, and a chest radiograph. Many feel that routine bone scans or liver scans are not indicated in patients with clinical Stage I or II disease, although some advocate a baseline bone scan to be used as a reference if the patient should develop skeletal metastases in the future. The yield of positives is extremely low in the absence of symptoms or signs suggesting visceral disease. On the other hand, with locally advanced tumor (Stage III), the yield of screening bone scans is sufficiently high to warrant their use. Likewise, with abnormal blood chemistries suggestive of liver involvement or with symptoms such as bone pain, scans would be required to avoid inappropriate use of a curative procedure in a patient with advanced, incurable disease.

Stage III Disease and Inflammatory Breast Cancer

If a patient's disease is Stage III solely on the basis of tumor size (tumor > 5 cm), but the tumor appears to be as resectable as that of a Stage I or II patient, mastectomy is the primary treatment. For patients with locally advanced but unresectable disease (i.e., invasion of chest wall, fixation of axillary nodes, or positive supraclavicular nodes), control of persistent or recurrent regional disease as well as latent distant metastases are the dominant problems. Inflammatory breast cancer is aggressive locally as well as metastatically. It is properly considered a systemic disease from the outset, even though it appears to be confined to the breast. The treatment plan for the latter two presentations involves an individualized approach using chemotherapy to reduce the tumor volume, followed by radiation therapy and possibly resection of the breast and draining nodes. This strategy requires close consultation from the outset between surgeons, radiation oncologists, and medical oncologists. Prolonged remissions and perhaps cures can be obtained in a fraction of patients.

Metastatic Breast Cancer

CLINICAL FEATURES. Breast cancer most frequently metastasizes to lymph nodes, skin, lung, pleura, bone, liver, brain, and pericardium. In autopsy series, the adrenals are involved in up to half the patients, but adrenal insufficiency is rarely seen. Likewise, the ovaries contain tumor in up to one quarter of patients at autopsy. Rarely metastatic breast cancer may be found incidentally at oophorectomy in a patient whose first sign of breast cancer is an involved ovary presenting as a pelvic mass. Breast cancer is the most common source of metastases to the eye in women.

PATIENT ASSESSMENT. Once a metastatic focus is found, routine studies to map tumor extent include a complete blood count (which can reflect myelophthisis secondary to marrow metastases) and the measurement of serum levels of liver enzymes, bilirubin, and calcium. The carcinoembryonic antigen titer can be elevated in up to 50 per cent of patients with metastatic disease and can be a useful marker for following response to therapy. A chest radiograph is indicated and can reveal lung nodules, mediastinal or hilar node involvement, or a pleural effusion. A bone scan is also mandatory, and positive areas, especially those that are symptomatic or in weight-bearing bones, require follow-up radiographs to determine whether radiation is needed to prevent collapse or pathologic fracture. If physical findings or laboratory studies suggest hepatic involvement, a radionuclide liver scan, a sonogram of the liver, or a liver CT scan confirms the presence of metastatic disease, gauges its extent, and allows comparison with follow-up studies during treatment. "Routine" liver imaging is widely employed, but its yield and cost-effectiveness in the absence of signs suggesting liver metastasis are open to question. The same statement applies to "routine" studies of the brain, although they are clearly indicated in the presence of neurologic symptoms or signs.

COMPLICATIONS. Certain complications occur with some frequency and require urgent attention in patients with metastatic breast cancer: hypercalcemia, metastases to weight-bearing bones, and metastases to the nervous system (the epidural space, the leptomeninges, or the brain).

Hypercalcemia requires standard methods of therapy, such as saline, furosemide, and mithramycin therapy along with treatment of the breast cancer itself (Ch. 247). A positive bone scan, especially in the femur or vertebral column, or bone pain in these areas requires radiographic analysis of the extent of structural damage. Femoral lesions may necessitate orthopedic stabilization and radiation therapy to prevent pathologic fractures. Vertebral body lesions may require radiation to diminish pain and avoid further collapse.

Patients with persistent back pain are at greater risk for *epidural metastases* and possibly cord compression. Motor or sensory changes in a segmental distribution greatly increase the possibility of an epidural lesion. However, in the presence of back pain, their absence does not exclude an epidural lesion. Pain without a neurologic deficit means that there is still time to treat an epidural lesion with radiation before the cord becomes ischemic and permanently damaged.

Leptomeningeal metastases present with headache and focal sensory or motor changes suggestive of single or multiple nerve root involvement. The diagnosis depends upon the demonstration of breast cancer cells in the cerebrospinal fluid and may require multiple spinal taps to yield a diagnosis (with appropriate studies beforehand, if indicated, to rule out a mass lesion in the brain). Since systemically administered drugs penetrate the blood-brain barrier poorly, intrathecal or intraventricular chemotherapy is necessary.

TREATMENT. The two major types of therapy for disseminated breast cancer are hormonal and cytotoxic. Hormonal therapy is less toxic but can require as long as 8 to 12 weeks to produce maximal benefit. The impact of chemotherapy is more rapid. Responses to all these treatments last a median of 6 to 18 months, and responders have a significantly prolonged survival compared to nonresponders.

The menopausal status of the patient and the hormone receptor profile of the tumor are the major determinants of whether to employ an endocrine maneuver and which particular therapy to use. Other important considerations are the tempo of the disease, the performance status of the patient, and the sites of metastases. A long interval between mastectomy and recurrence suggests indolent disease and would, along with a good performance status, permit the longer observation period needed to gauge response to an endocrine therapy. Bone, soft tissue, and limited pulmonary metastases may respond to hormonal therapy, whereas liver, brain, and extensive lung metastases greatly decrease the probability of a response and therefore require chemotherapy.

Premenopausal Patients. For premenopausal patients with ER-positive tumors, hormonal therapy is first-line treatment in the absence of the contraindications mentioned above. Oophorectomy is the initial choice and causes tumor regression in 30 to 80 per cent of RP-positive patients. If a patient progresses after initial response, then progestins, adrenalectomy (rarely hypophysectomy), and androgens can be used in sequence until there is no longer a response. At that point, the patient should receive chemotherapy.

Some advocate initial endocrine treatment with the antiestrogen tamoxifen, followed later by oophorectomy once the tamoxifen is ineffective. The experience is more limited with this approach. Some women will continue to menstruate while receiving tamoxifen, so its exact mechanism of action and the certainty of adequate estrogen blockade are less well established (in premenopausal women). LHRH agonists are being studied and may become the treatment of choice in the next several years.

Adrenal influences can be removed either by surgical adrenalectomy or by use of medical methods to inhibit adrenal function. Surgical ablation requires permanent replacement therapy in addition to the morbidity of surgery. Medical inhibition with aminoglutethimide, by contrast, is reversible once the drug is stopped. Patients receiving aminoglutethimide experience rash and somnolence 10 to 40 per cent of the time, although these side effects wane after several weeks of treatment. The drug blocks adrenal steroidogenesis by inhibiting conversion of cholesterol to pregnenolone. In peripheral tissue, it also blocks the conversion of androstenedione to estrone, a precursor of estradiol. This latter reaction accounts for the bulk of estrogen production in postmenopausal women. In patients who have RP-positive tumors and responded to prior endocrine therapy, responses to aminoglutethimide occur 30 to 60 per cent of the time. Aminoglutethimide therapy requires replacement corticosteroid treatment with hydrocortisone, which also suppresses the increase in pituitary ACTH secretion produced by aminoglutethimide inhibition of cortisol production, an increase that could otherwise override the blockade. A periodic check of plasma dehydroepiandrosterone levels will confirm the adequacy of adrenal suppression.

Adrenalectomy is usually chosen over hypophysectomy. The two are roughly equal in therapeutic effect. Hypophysectomy requires a neurosurgeon highly skilled in the transsphenoidal approach (less morbid than the transfrontal route), and complications of the surgery range from incomplete pituitary ablation to cerebrospinal fluid leak and infection. Hypophysectomy also requires permanent thyroid *and* adrenal hormone replacement.

Premenopausal patients with RP-negative tumors, or those originally RP-positive who have become refractory to endocrine treatment, require chemotherapy. Drug classes active against breast cancer include alkylating agents (typically cyclophosphamide), antimetabolites (5-fluorouracil, methotrexate), vinca alkaloids (vincristine, vinblastine), anthracyclines (doxorubicin), and mitomycin-C. In various combinations, these agents effect responses in 60 to 70 per cent of patients, with 10 to 15 per cent achieving a complete remission.

Postmenopausal Patients. For RP-positive tumors in postmenopausal patients who are candidates for endocrine therapy, the antiestrogen tamoxifen has replaced estrogen therapy (diethylstilbestrol, DES) as initial treatment. Tamoxifen has few side effects, in contrast to DES, which much more frequently produces nausea, anorexia, and salt retention. Both drugs have been associated with a tumor "flare" consisting of increased bone pain and hypercalcemia. This occurs in patients with skeletal metastases during the initial weeks of treatment, more commonly with DES. These reactions usually herald an antitumor effect and do not necessitate cessation of therapy as long as symptoms and calcium levels are controlled by standard supportive treatments. Withdrawal of DES, once the tumor progresses, produces further regression of tumor in 20 to 30 per cent of patients (withdrawal effect is less common with tamoxifen). Once the disease progresses after this initial therapy, serial endocrine maneuvers are employed, as discussed for premenopausal patients, until the tumor becomes refractory to hormonal therapy. Oophorectomy has no role in the treatment of postmenopausal patients. Again, for RP-negative tumors or for tumors resistant to endocrine treatment, chemotherapy becomes the treatment of choice.

Adjuvant Drug Therapy

The goal of prophylactic chemotherapy after mastectomy is to eliminate the micrometastases likely present in high-risk (e.g., axillary node–positive) patients. Since eradication of tumor cells is more probable when their number is small, the treatment should be applied as soon after mastectomy as possible. Furthermore, because cytotoxic chemotherapy is quite active against metastatic breast cancer in women who have a high tumor burden, it should be all the more effective against microscopic disease.

A number of clinical trials of adjuvant therapy have been carried out: (1) The use of the oral alkylating agent phenylalanine mustard (melphalan) decreased recurrence and improved survival in premenopausal but not postmenopausal patients with Stage II disease. (2) The three-drug combination "CMF" (cyclophosphamide, methotrexate, and 5-fluorouracil) improved outcome, but again, only for premenopausal women. In this Milan trial it appeared that postmenopausal women who had no benefit tended to have received less drug. Those who received 85 per cent or more of standard doses did benefit from adjuvant treatment. (3) A trial of CMFVP (CMF plus vincristine and prednisone) showed an improvement in outcome in those who received the combination compared to women who received melphalan alone, postmenopausal as well as premenopausal patients. (4) A large-scale controlled trial of tamoxifen alone in pre- and

TABLE 240–5. CURRENT RECOMMENDATIONS FOR ADJUVANT TREATMENT (NCI CONCENSUS DEVELOPMENT CONFERENCE, 1985)

Group	Recommendations
Premenopausal, node (+), hormone receptor (+) or (−)	Established combination chemotherapy
Premenopausal, node (−)	No treatment—consider adjuvant chemotherapy for selected high-risk patients (e.g., ERP-negative, adverse pathology)
Postmenopausal, node (+), hormone receptor (+)	Tamoxifen
Postmenopausal, node (+), hormone receptor (−)	Consider chemotherapy but this cannot be recommended as standard practice
Postmenopausal, node (−)	No treatment—possibly consider adjuvant therapy for high-risk patients

From Glick JH, Abeloff MD, Brown BW, et al.: National Institutes of Health Consensus Development Conference Statement; Adjuvant chemotherapy for breast cancer. September 9–11, 1985, CA 36:42, 1986.

postmenopausal women demonstrated an improvement in disease-free and overall survival in treated patients, independent of menopausal status, compared to a group with no treatment.

Based on these and other studies, a National Institutes of Health Consensus Development Conference on adjuvant chemotherapy for breast cancer concluded that: (1) adjuvant chemotherapy and adjuvant hormonal therapy are effective in axillary node–positive patients; (2) *optimal* treatment for any subset of patients has yet to be defined; and (3) physicians should be strongly encouraged to continue to enroll their patients in controlled trials. Interim recommendations for patients outside the context of a formal clinical study are listed in Table 240–5.

Unresolved issues include optimal drug selection, dose, schedule, and duration of adjuvant treatment. Ongoing trials are examining risk factors in the 20 to 25 per cent of Stage I patients who develop metastatic disease. Data suggest that having an RP-negative tumor and a high proliferative rate are major risk factors for recurrence in these patients with negative axillary nodes and that they may also benefit from adjuvant chemotherapy. Long-term sequelae of chemotherapy in patients who have received adjuvant treatment do not appear to be significant, within the limits of the length of observation of the trials.

SPECIAL CONSIDERATIONS
Male Breast Cancer

Carcinoma of the male breast occurs with 1 per cent the frequency of female breast cancer. Its clinical presentation and primary therapy are similar to those in women. Abnormalities of estrogen metabolism are cited as a possible causative factor. The vast majority of tumors that have been examined are estrogen RP-positive. Castration is the treatment of choice for the initial management of metastatic disease. Antiestrogen therapy, adrenalectomy, and hypophysectomy may offer some palliation, and the effects of additive hormonal therapy are less certain than in female breast cancer.

Breast Cancer and Pregnancy

Breast cancer complicates approximately one of every 3,000 pregnancies. It has been held for some time that pregnancy adversely affects the outcome of breast cancer, with studies citing a high frequency of axillary lymph node metastases and shortened survival when the diagnosis is made during pregnancy. To some extent, these poor results may have related to a delay in diagnosis and in the initiation of treatment rather than inherently different biologic factors. The treatment considerations are the same as for the nonpregnant patients, and a standard surgical approach poses a 1 per cent or less risk to the developing fetus. When patients present with disseminated disease in the first or second trimester, cytotoxic drug treatment is a significant risk to the fetus and usually requires termination of pregnancy. If clinical considerations permit, treatment can be delayed to the third trimester to permit delivery of a viable fetus.

Patients who develop cancer during pregnancy tend to present with more advanced stages of disease than nonpregnant patients. However, when compared stage for stage, pregnant women have only a slightly less favorable prognosis than nonpregnant women. In a woman who has had an apparent cure of a breast cancer, subsequent pregnancy is not associated with an excessive risk of recurrence. Patients with early stage breast cancer who bear children appear to have a survival equal to that of women who do not become pregnant. A three-year interval between primary treatment of early breast cancer and a subsequent pregnancy has been advocated.

Brinton LA, Hoover R, Fraumeni JF Jr: Interaction of familial and hormonal risk factors for breast cancer. J Natl Cancer Inst 69:817, 1982. *An evaluation of family history of breast cancer as a risk indicator in relation to hormonal factors. A large, case-controlled study.*

Danoff BF, Haller DG, Glick JH, et al.: Conservative surgery and irradiation in the treatment of early breast cancer. Ann Intern Med 102:634, 1985. *A comprehensive and detailed review of the literature on breast conservation in primary breast cancer management.*

Donegan WL: Cancer and pregnancy. CA 33:194, 1983. *A useful and comprehensive overview of the issues surrounding breast cancer (and other cancers) and pregnancy.*

Dupont WD, Page DL: Risk factors for breast cancer in women with proliferative breast disease. N Engl J Med 312:146, 1985. *A large, retrospective cohort study that advances the understanding of the influence of various types of benign breast disease on cancer risk and their interaction with factors such as family history.*

Fisher B: Laboratory and clinical research in breast cancer—a personal adventure. Cancer Res 40:3863, 1980. *This article, plus the following references by Fisher et al. and the reference by Veronesi et al., detail a shift in thinking about the biology of breast cancer and update clinical trials of primary management designed to test specific hypotheses about the nature of breast cancer.*

Fisher B, Bauer M, Margolese R, et al.: Five year results of a randomized clinical trial comparing total mastectomy and segmental mastectomy with or without radiation in the treatment of breast cancer. N Engl J Med 312:665, 1985.

Fisher B, Redmond C, Fisher ER, et al.: Ten year results of a randomized clinical trial comparing radical mastectomy and total mastectomy with or without radiation. N Engl J Med 312:674, 1985.

Glick JH, Abeloff MD, Brown BW, et al.: National Institutes of Health Consensus Development Conference Statement: Adjuvant chemotherapy for breast cancer. September 9–11, 1985. CA 36:42, 1986. *A summary statement of the conclusions and recommendations reached in the recent national conference on adjuvant therapy.*

Harris JR, Hellman S, Canellos GP, et al.: Cancer of the breast. In De Vita VT, Hellman S, Rosenberg SA (eds.): Cancer. Principles and Practice of Oncology. Philadelphia, J. B. Lippincott, 1985. *A comprehensive treatise detailing areas such as surgical technique, pathology, and chemotherapy.*

Harris JR, Hellman S, Kinne DW: Special Report. Limited surgery and radiotherapy for early breast cancer. N Engl J Med 313:1365, 1985. *Summary statement of a workshop held to define surgical procedures, patient selection criteria, and areas of controversy in the use of more conservative surgery plus radiotherapy for the primary management of breast cancer.*

Kopans, DP, Meyer JE, Sadowsky N: Breast imaging. N Engl J Med 310:960, 1984. *A review of mammography and other breast imaging methods which includes a critique of the utility and limitations of each technique.*

Lippman ME (ed.): Proceedings of the NIH Consensus Development Conference on adjuvant chemotherapy and endocrine therapy for breast cancer. NCI Monographs 1:1, 1986. *This monograph contains articles that update the major trials of adjuvant therapy and review the prognostic significance of breast pathology, cell kinetics, and steroid hormone receptors.*

Petrakis NL, Ernster VL, King M-C: Breast. In Schottenfeld D, Fraumeni JF Jr (eds.): Cancer Epidemiology and Prevention. Philadelphia, WB Saunders Company, 1982. *A detailed review of the range of associated risk factors for breast cancer.*

Schatzkin A, Jones DY, Hoover, RN, et al.: Alcohol consumption and breast cancer in the epidemiologic follow-up study of the first national health and nutrition examination survey. N Engl J Med 316:1169, 1987. *This recent article and its accompanying editorial review the increasing evidence that even modest consumption of alcohol increases the risk of breast cancer by 50 to 100 per cent.*

Veronesi U, Del Vecchio M, Greco M, et al.: Results of quadrantectomy, axillary dissection and radiotherapy (QUART) in T₁N₀ patients. In Harris JR, Hellman S, Silen W (eds.): Conservative Management of Breast Cancer. Philadelphia, J. B. Lippincott Company, 1983.

241 POLYGLANDULAR DISORDERS

John N. Loeb

A number of different syndromes are characterized by autonomous hyperfunction or hypofunction of more than one endocrine gland. Although the majority of these syndromes are clearly of genetic origin, the fundamental mechanisms leading to hyperfunction or hypofunction thus far remain unknown in any instance. The syndromes to be considered in this chapter are those in which dysfunction appears to be autonomous within the affected endocrine glands themselves; multiple glandular abnormalities resulting from primary abnormalities in the hypothalamic-pituitary axis or ascribable to various locally infiltrative processes are discussed elsewhere.

SYNDROMES CHARACTERIZED BY MULTIPLE ENDOCRINE GLAND HYPERFUNCTION OR NEOPLASIA

The major syndromes characterized by multiple endocrine hyperfunction are those of multiple endocrine adenomatosis (MEA) or multiple endocrine neoplasia (MEN). A number of these syndromes are inherited as autosomal dominant traits and are clinically distinct. The term MEN is now generally preferred because it is more inclusive, comprising both hyperplastic and carcinomatous as well as adenomatous abnormalities. Table 241–1 compares the clinical features of some of these syndromes.

MULTIPLE ENDOCRINE NEOPLASIA, TYPE 1 (WERMER'S SYNDROME). In 1954 Wermer reported the familial occurrence of *multiple tumors of the anterior pituitary, parathyroid glands, and pancreatic islet cells* in association with a high incidence of peptic ulcer. This complex of abnormalities is now most commonly referred to as multiple endocrine neoplasia, type 1 (MEN 1). The syndrome may also include tumor or hyperfunction of the adrenal and thyroid glands, but the relation of these latter endocrinopathies to the underlying genetic abnormality is less well defined. Although it has been proposed that the fundamental defect in MEN 1 is an abnormal differentiation of neural crest tissue, current evidence in support of this hypothesis is by no means conclusive (see also below, under MEN 2). In fact, there is now evidence for a circulating growth factor present in excess in the plasma of patients with MEN 1 as the presumed humoral basis for the syndrome.

More than half of patients with MEN 1 have adenomas of two or more different endocrine glands, and involvement of three or more different glands is seen in up to 20 per cent of affected individuals. The approximate frequencies of glandular involvement in patients exhibiting any manifestation of endocrine hyperfunction are, in descending order, parathyroids (90 to 95 per cent), pancreatic islet cells (30 to 35 per cent), and anterior pituitary (15 to 20 per cent). Less commonly there may be hyperfunction (adenomas) of the adrenal cortex and thyroid gland; carcinoid tumors have been reported occasionally. Initial manifestations are most commonly detected in middle age, and many years may elapse between the manifestation of the first endocrine abnormality and ensuing ones. The clinical course is highly variable, depending in part upon which glands are affected and whether the neoplasm results in hypersecretion or instead in compression of surrounding normal glandular tissue with concomitant loss of function. By far the greatest majority of patients (over 90 per cent) have problems related to hypercalcemia, peptic ulcer, hypoglycemia, or pituitary dysfunction. In patients with pituitary neoplasms symptoms are most commonly attribut-

TABLE 241–1. COMPARISON OF THE CLINICAL FEATURES OF THE MAJOR SYNDROMES CHARACTERIZED BY MULTIPLE ENDOCRINE GLAND HYPERFUNCTION

Endocrine Abnormality	MEN 1*	MEN 2 ("2A")*	MEN 3 ("2B")*
Hyperparathyroidism [Hyperplasia or multiple adenomas]	90–95%, with high incidence of hyper-calcemia and nephrolithiasis	20–30%, but only 10% with frank hypercalcemia or nephro-lithiasis	Rare
Pancreatic islet cell hyperfunction [Hyperplasia, adenomas, or carcinoma, with hypersecretion (e.g., of gastrin or insulin)]	30–35%	—†	
Pituitary adenomas ["Nonfunctioning" or with hypersecretion of prolactin (common) or growth hormone (rare)]	15–20%	—	—
Multiple cutaneous lipomas	20%	—	—
Thyroid adenomas, adrenal cortical adenomas, carcinoid tumors	Rare		
Thyroid C-cell hyperplasia with hypersecretion of calcitonin ± medullary carcinoma	—	"100%"‡	"100%"‡
Pheochromocytoma	—	Probably > 20%	Probably > 20%
Multiple mucosal neuromas; marfanoid habitus	—	—	Characteristic
Inheritance	Autosomal dominant	Autosomal dominant	Autosomal dominant, but frequently "sporadic"

*Percentages indicate approximate frequencies among affected individuals manifesting hyperfunction of at least one endocrine gland.

†— = *not* part of the syndrome.

‡Generally taken to be an essential component of the syndrome.

able to pituitary enlargement, with headache or visual-field abnormalities, or to hypopituitarism. Acromegaly, the galactorrhea-amenorrhea syndrome with hyperprolactinemia, and, considerably more rarely, Cushing's syndrome, may also be seen.

Parathyroid gland involvement is by far the most common manifestation of MEN 1 but may be clinically "silent" for many years. Patients may have a history of kidney stones or progressive renal failure as the first manifestation of hyperparathyroidism, or, much more commonly, hypercalcemia may be detected incidentally upon routine screening. All four parathyroid glands are frequently abnormal, and pathologic study may reveal either hyperplasia or multiple adenomas. Parathyroid carcinoma is rare.

Islet cell tumors of the pancreas can be either adenomas (generally multiple) or carcinomas; they may be preceded by diffuse hyperplasia of islet tissue and most typically secrete excess gastrin. Hypersecretion of gastrin may give rise to the *Zollinger-Ellison syndrome* (see Ch. 100) characterized by marked hypersecretion of hydrochloric acid, peptic ulceration (sometimes involving esophageal, distal duodenal, or jejunal sites), and, often, diarrhea. Abdominal pain, bleeding, and perforation are more common than in ordinary instances of peptic ulcer, and radiographic signs consistent with hypersecretion of gastric acid (e.g., hypertrophied gastric rugae) are frequently seen. Many patients in whom the Zollinger-Ellison syndrome initially appears in isolation represent a subset of individuals with MEN 1, and they ultimately develop manifestations of additional endocrine neoplasms.

Hypersecretion of insulin by islet cell neoplasms may produce hypoglycemia as an initial manifestation, whereas the elaboration of other substances may, considerably more rarely, result in a variety of other syndromes. Vasoactive intestinal peptide and prostaglandins have been proposed as agents possibly responsible for the intractable watery diarrhea that can be seen even in the absence of hypersecretion of gastrin and the Zollinger-Ellison syndrome, and hypersecretion of glucagon with hyperglycemia, weight loss, and a characteristic skin rash ("necrotizing migratory erythema") has been reported. Islet cell tumors may also secrete pancreatic polypeptide or, rarely, ACTH, serotonin, or somatostatin.

Symptoms caused by *pituitary adenomas* in MEN 1 are most commonly due to local encroachment of tumor upon other structures, with headache or visual-field abnormalities, or to deficiency of one or more of the tropic hormones. Many of these tumors secrete prolactin and may give rise to the galactorrhea-amenorrhea syndrome. More rarely there is hypersecretion of growth hormone with resulting acromegaly. Hypersecretion of ACTH in MEN 1 is almost always attributable to an ectopic (pancreatic) site.

Adrenocortical hyperfunction may be due to ectopic production of ACTH or to independently functioning adrenal adenomas or carcinomas. Functioning adenomas most commonly elaborate hydrocortisone, giving rise to signs of glucocorticoid excess, but predominant secretion of aldosterone has been reported in rare instances. Hyperfunction of the *thyroid* gland has been reported least frequently of all, and, in part owing to the high incidence of thyroid abnormalities in the population at large, it is possible that sporadic instances of thyroid hyperfunction in MEN 1 represent incidental occurrences unrelated to the underlying genetic abnormality. Adenomas, thyroiditis, and rarely papillary and follicular cell carcinomas have all been reported in association with MEN 1; medullary carcinomas are *not* a part of this syndrome (cf. MEN 2, below). *Other tumors* that can form a part of the clinical picture of MEN 1 include schwannomas, multiple cutaneous lipomas, thymomas, and both bronchial and small intestinal carcinoids.

Management of the various manifestations of MEN 1 is, for the most part, similar to management of the identical manifestations when they occur in sporadic form and hence is considered elsewhere in this textbook. As indicated above, parathyroid involvement, when it occurs, frequently involves more than one gland, and histopathology far more commonly reveals diffuse hyperplasia than a single adenoma. In such instances a number of surgeons now advocate total parathyroidectomy with reimplantation of a glandular fragment in a location conveniently accessible to subsequent exploration if necessary (e.g., the muscle of the forearm). Management of severe peptic ulceration in MEN 1 requires either long-term cimetidine or ranitidine therapy or near-total gastrectomy—rather than an attempt to eliminate the source of excess gastrin—since hypersecretion of gastrin by islet-cell tissue in this syndrome is almost always attributable to either multiple tumors or diffuse hyperplasia.

The sporadic nature of the sequential manifestations of this syndrome makes it important to follow affected individuals with particular attention to the development of new abnormalities. Once the diagnosis has been established in a given patient and baseline films of the sella turcica and prolactin levels have proved to be normal, the major requisite is a careful interval history and a periodic (e.g., yearly) determination of the serum calcium and phosphorus.

Because of the high incidence of the syndrome in first-degree relatives, all such family members should be carefully evaluated, as well as any second-degree relatives with suggestive histories elicited through questioning of the propositus. Determination of fasting blood sugar, serum calcium, and prolactin levels is generally sufficient if menses or sexual potency is present and if the history and physical examination are negative. Films of the sella turcica are usually unrevealing, and CT scanning is too expensive for use as a routine screen.

MULTIPLE ENDOCRINE NEOPLASIA, TYPE 2 (SIPPLE'S SYNDROME). A second and entirely distinct syndrome, multiple endocrine neoplasia, type 2 (MEN 2 or MEN 2A), is characterized by *medullary carcinoma of the thyroid, pheochromocytoma, and parathyroid hyperplasia.* First partially described by Sipple in 1961, this syndrome, like MEN 1, is inherited as an autosomal dominant trait. The pheochromocytomas are frequently bilateral, although rarely extra-adrenal, and the medullary carcinoma of the thyroid generally appears to be multifocal in origin. A particularly convenient and virtually constant feature of the medullary thyroid carcinomas is the hypersecretion of calcitonin, which serves as a useful marker for the presence of this neoplasm. Elevated levels of calcitonin, either under basal conditions or in response to the provocative stimuli of calcium and pentagastrin infusions, are an indication of parafollicular C-cell hyperplasia in the thyroid gland and may herald the presence of the genetic abnormality well before pathologic changes appear that are unequivocally malignant. As in the instance of the pancreatic adenomas in MEN 1, the medullary carcinomas of the thyroid in MEN 2 may secrete a variety of hormones and other biologically active substances that are not secreted by the corresponding normal tissue. These include ACTH, prolactin, histaminase, vasoactive intestinal peptide, serotonin, and a number of prostaglandins. Only rarely does medullary carcinoma of the thyroid present as a palpable mass. Pheochromocytoma is observed in about one half of affected individuals, and hyperparathyroidism in about one quarter. Only about 10 per cent of individuals with MEN 2 exhibit hypercalcemia or nephrolithiasis (cf. the much higher incidence of overt hyperparathyroidism in MEN 1). Glial tumors and meningiomas may also be seen in MEN 2 but occur far less frequently.

It has been suggested that MEN 2 represents a form of neuroectodermal dysplasia in which so-called APUD cells (cells capable of *a*mine *p*recursor *u*ptake and *d*ecarboxylation and possessing rather characteristic histologic staining properties)—following their embryonic migration to the foregut and subsequent localization in a variety of endocrine tissues—later become neoplastic and secrete excessive amounts of hormone in response to a specific genetic defect. Although the evidence for a common APUD cell origin is somewhat better in MEN 2 than it is in MEN 1, it is still by no means wholly convincing. In particular, the high incidence of parathyroid involvement is difficult to reconcile with this theory, since the bulk of present evidence suggests an epithelial rather than a neural crest origin for this tissue.

The pheochromocytomas of MEN 2 are generally benign and are treated surgically. Because they are frequently bilateral, an anterior surgical approach is often recommended; CT scan, multiple-site venous sampling for catecholamines, and angiography can all be helpful in planning surgery. Medullary carcinoma of the thyroid, on the other hand, runs a typically malignant course, and, because of its multifocal nature, requires total thyroidectomy. Elevated levels of calcitonin per se constitute a sufficient indication for total thyroidectomy, even when the tumor is otherwise clinically silent. The tumor is frequently slowly growing, and limited node dissection is thus justified; completeness of tumor removal and the possibility of subsequent recurrence are both conveniently monitored by serum calcitonin levels. The isolated finding of medullary carcinoma of the thyroid should prompt a particularly careful inquiry into the family history, since it is likely that at least 10 per cent of such tumors are familial.

Screening of first-degree relatives of patients with MEN 2 is indicated and should include a 24-hour urine collection for vanillylmandelic acid, metanephrines, and catecholamines (even when the blood pressure is normal) as well as calcium and basal calcitonin determinations. If a thyroid mass is present, a fuller work-up is indicated, including measurement of calcium-pentagastrin–stimulated calcitonin levels.

MULTIPLE ENDOCRINE NEOPLASIA, TYPE 3 (MUCOSAL NEUROMA SYNDROME). This syndrome (MEN 3 or MEN 2B) resembles MEN 2 but differs in four important respects: (1) The medullary carcinoma of the thyroid and the pheochromocytomas may be accompanied by striking and often disfiguring neuromas of the lips, buccal mucosa, and tongue, as well as by ganglioneuromas of the gastrointestinal tract, thickened corneal nerves visible upon slit-lamp examination, and café-au-lait spots, neuromas, or neurofibromas of the skin; (2) the body habitus may somewhat resemble that seen in patients with the Marfan syndrome; (3) parathyroid hyperplasia sufficient to result in frank hypercalcemia is rare; and (4) mean survival time in MEN 3 is considerably shorter than that in MEN 2 (30 versus 60 years). In contrast to MEN 1 and MEN 2, MEN 3 is frequently sporadic, a history of affected family members being obtainable in not more than half of the cases.

McCUNE-ALBRIGHT SYNDROME. In 1937 McCune and Albright and their associates both described a syndrome characterized by a triad of *polyostotic fibrous dysplasia, café-au-lait pigmentation of the skin* (typically over the forehead, nuchal or sacral areas, or buttocks), and *precocious puberty in the female.* The precocious puberty, although predominantly seen in the female, may occur in males as well. This syndrome may be accompanied by a variety of other endocrine abnormalities, including pituitary hyperfunction (with Cushing's syndrome, acromegaly, or gigantism), bilateral pheochromocytomas, hyperthyroidism, and hypercorticism resulting from adrenal adenoma. Frank malignant disease has not been described. Although the sexual precocity appears to be hypothalamic in origin, patients with adrenal adenomas and hyperthyroidism have been found to have low plasma levels of ACTH and TSH, respectively. The cause of the bone lesions is unknown. The disease appears to be sporadic.

SYNDROMES CHARACTERIZED BY MULTIPLE ENDOCRINE GLAND HYPOFUNCTION

Syndromes characterized by hypofunction of multiple endocrine organs will be discussed under the separate headings of Schmidt's syndrome and the syndrome of polyglandular deficiency associated with mucocutaneous candidiasis. As noted below, however, evidence that the two syndromes actually represent different entities is incomplete. Table 241–2 compares the clinical features of these syndromes.

MULTIPLE ENDOCRINE DEFICIENCY SYNDROME (SCHMIDT'S SYNDROME). In 1926 Schmidt described two patients with biglandular failure characterized by *idiopathic Addison's disease and lymphocytic thyroiditis.* This syndrome has subsequently been expanded to include "primary" failure of other endocrine glands, including the gonads, parathyroids, and endocrine pancreas, as well as a number of nonendocrine abnormalities of presumed autoimmune origin (see below). Virtually any combination of the foregoing endocrine deficiencies may appear in a single individual. The order of appearance is extremely variable, and a lag of as much as 17 years has been observed in the manifestation of sequential deficiencies. Hypothyroidism and hypoadrenalism are particularly common; diabetes mellitus, hypoparathyroidism, and gonadal failure are somewhat less so. The frequencies of the different glandular failures probably vary greatly with ascertainment; if one considers juvenile-onset diabetes mellitus as part of the syndrome, the association of this with autoimmune thyroid disease may be the most commonly encountered combination.

TABLE 241–2. COMPARISON OF THE CLINICAL FEATURES OF THE MAJOR SYNDROMES CHARACTERIZED BY MULTIPLE ENDOCRINE GLAND HYPOFUNCTION

	Multiple Endocrine Deficiency Syndrome (Schmidt's Syndrome)	Polyglandular Deficiency with Mucocutaneous Candidiasis
Hypoadrenalism	Common	Common
Hypothyroidism	Common	Less common
Hypoparathyroidism	Less common	Common
Gonadal failure	Less common	Rare
Diabetes mellitus	Less common	Rare
Pituitary insufficiency	Rare	Rare
Autoantibodies to endocrine tissues and gastric parietal cells	Often present	Often present
Sex distribution	Strong female predominance	Female preponderance about 4:1
Inheritance	Usually "sporadic," but susceptibility related to HLA haplotype and may be inherited as autosomal dominant	Generally inherited as autosomal recessive; no apparent HLA association
Time of onset	Usually becomes evident during adult life	Typically becomes evident during childhood preceded by chronic mucocutaneous moniliasis
Other associated "autoimmune" diseases and characteristics	Pernicious anemia; hyperthyroidism; celiac disease; alopecia; vitiligo; myasthenia gravis; isolated red-cell aplasia	Pernicious anemia; malabsorption; alopecia; vitiligo; IgA deficiency; hypergammaglobulinemia; chronic active hepatitis; proliferative glomerulonephritis

Characteristic of this syndrome is the presence of autoantibodies to endocrine tissue and at times to gastric parietal cells as well. Such antibodies are often detectable before the appearance of clinical glandular insufficiency and are a hallmark of syndromes of "idiopathic" endocrine failure. Their presence has been implicated in the pathogenesis of the glandular destruction itself rather than merely as reflecting an immune response to tissue antigens released during antecedent glandular degeneration. Thus, for example, approximately two thirds of patients with idiopathic Addison's disease are reported to have autoantibodies to adrenal tissue, whereas such antibodies are generally absent in patients whose adrenal insufficiency is secondary to tuberculous destruction. About twice as many females are affected with idiopathic adrenal insufficiency as males. Although most cases of multiple deficiency syndromes are sporadic, their occasional appearance in kindreds, as well as the relatively high gene frequency of the HLA-B8 and HLA-DR3 alleles in affected persons, provides strong evidence for a dominantly inherited susceptibility to the development of this type of polyglandular failure. Other "autoimmune" diseases that may accompany the aforementioned endocrine deficiencies include pernicious anemia, celiac disease, myasthenia gravis, alopecia, vitiligo, and isolated red-cell aplasia. Because it occurs in the same families and has the same HLA associations, Graves' disease is considered by many to be another facet of the syndrome.

Although the constellation of adrenal, thyroid, and gonadal failure in a single patient can easily be confused with primary pituitary insufficiency, measurement of the appropriate tropic hormones now permits a ready differentiation of the two syndromes. Occasionally the simultaneous presence of hyperpigmentation in such an individual suggests a diagnosis of primary adrenal failure on "clinical" grounds alone. Because of the sporadic appearance and variable sequence of

subsequent endocrine deficiencies, patients with a proven idiopathic endocrine deficiency should be periodically screened for evidence of additional endocrine involvement.

POLYGLANDULAR DEFICIENCY ASSOCIATED WITH MUCOCUTANEOUS CANDIDIASIS. A clinical picture somewhat different from that of Schmidt's syndrome is presented by patients with the so-called candidiasis-endocrinopathy syndrome. Characteristically this syndrome is dominated by the presence of extensive mucocutaneous candidiasis that appears in early childhood and is followed by the development of idiopathic adrenal insufficiency or hypoparathyroidism or both. Most typically, but not invariably, the appearance of these endocrinopathies postdates the acquisition of chronic monilial infection (mean age of onset, 13 versus 3 years, respectively). As in Schmidt's syndrome, antibodies against endocrine tissues are frequently demonstrable, and pernicious anemia with antibodies against gastric parietal cells may also be present. Diabetes mellitus, in contrast, is relatively rare. Also contrasting with Schmidt's syndrome, which most typically becomes evident in adult life, is the fact that there is no apparent association with the presence of specific HLA alleles, and the apparent inheritance of the syndrome as an autosomal recessive trait within a single generation of siblings. Chronic active hepatitis and proliferative glomerulonephritis have also been reported. The mucocutaneous candidiasis is associated with hypergammaglobulinemia, IgA deficiency, and anergy to *Candida albicans*, and typically is relatively resistant to therapy. No evidence for disseminated candidiasis has been found in autopsied individuals, nor has *Candida* yet been cultured from an affected endocrine gland.

Albright F, Butler AM, Hampton AO, et al.: Syndrome characterized by osteitis fibrosa disseminata, areas of pigmentation and endocrine dysfunction, with precocious puberty in females. N Engl J Med 216:727, 1937. *One of the two classic descriptions of the McCune-Albright syndrome. Excellent figures.*
Brandi ML, Aurbach GD, Fitzpatrick LA, et al.: Parathyroid mitogenic activity in plasma from patients with familial multiple endocrine neoplasia type 1. N Engl J Med 314:1287, 1986. *In a provocative study the plasma of patients with MEN 1 (but not with MEN 2) was found to contain a potent growth factor that stimulated the mitotic activity of parathyroid cells in cell culture. It was concluded that the hyperparathyroidism in MEN 1 may well have a humoral cause.*
Deftos LJ, Catherwood BD, Bone HG III: Multiglandular endocrine disorders. In Felig P, Baxter JD, Broadus AE, et al. (eds.): Endocrinology and Metabolism. 2nd ed. New York, McGraw-Hill Book Company, 1987, pp 1662–1691. *Excellent general review with 198 references.*
Marx SJ, Spiegel AM, Levine MA, et al.: Familial hypocalciuric hypercalcemia: The relation to primary parathyroid hyperplasia. N Engl J Med 307:416, 1982. *Excellent review of hereditary causes of primary parathyroid hyperplasia, including explicit discussion of the different MEN syndromes.*
Neufeld M, Maclaren NK, Blizzard RM: Two types of autoimmune Addison's disease associated with different polyglandular autoimmune (PGA) syndromes. Medicine 60:355, 1981. *A detailed review of a large series of patients with autoimmune Addison's disease, contrasting the different features of the two principal types of autoimmune polyglandular failure.*
Rabinowe SL, Eisenbarth GS: Polyglandular autoimmunity. Adv Intern Med 31:293, 1986. *An excellent review of these syndromes with an up-to-date list of 60 references.*
Schimke RN: Genetic aspects of multiple endocrine neoplasia. Annu Rev Med 35:25, 1984. *A useful review.*
Trence DL, Morley JE, Handwerger BS: Polyglandular autoimmune syndromes. Am J Med 77:107, 1984. *A review of these interesting disorders supplemented by 110 references.*

242 THE ADRENAL MEDULLA AND THE SYMPATHETIC NERVOUS SYSTEM

Philip E. Cryer

The sympathochromaffin system consists of two components: (1) the sympathetic nervous system and (2) the chromaffin tissues, including the adrenal medulla. The primary endocrine, neurotransmitter, and perhaps paracrine products of the sympathochromaffin system are the catecholamines—

epinephrine (adrenaline), norepinephrine (noradrenaline), and dopamine. Cells of the sympathochromaffin system also contain a variety of peptides of potential biologic importance, including enkephalins. Their pathophysiologic roles, if any, are unknown.

Catecholamine excess commonly results in hypertension along with typical symptoms. It has long been suspected, but is still not proven, that increased sympathetic nervous system activity is the cause of primary (essential) hypertension. Catecholamine overproduction from chromaffin cell tumors—pheochromocytomas—is an uncommon, but often curable, cause of hypertension. Deficient sympathetic neuronal norepinephrine release results in postural (orthostatic) hypotension, a sharp decrease in blood pressure when a person stands. Under certain conditions, deficient adrenomedullary epinephrine secretion results in hypoglycemia. These three prominent examples of sympathochromaffin pathophysiology are discussed in the paragraphs that follow. Possible roles of the sympathochromaffin system in the pathophysiology of a variety of human disorders—such as cardiac, hepatic, and renal failure, diabetes, asthma, thyroid disease, myocardial infarction, and cardiac arrhythmias, among others—are emerging but will not be discussed here.

PHYSIOLOGY OF THE SYMPATHOCHROMAFFIN SYSTEM

CATECHOLAMINE BIOSYNTHESIS. The term *catecholamines* is often used to refer to epinephrine and norepinephrine, although dopamine is also a catecholamine, i.e., has the dihydroxyphenyl ("catechol") ring structure and an amine side chain (Fig. 242–1). The catecholamines are synthesized from the amino acid tyrosine, which is derived from the diet or formed by hydroxylation of the essential amino acid phenylalanine. Tyrosine hydroxylase, the enzyme that converts tyrosine to dihydroxyphenylalanine (dopa), is the rate-limiting enzyme in catecholamine biosynthesis. In the presence of a nonspecific decarboxylase, dopa is converted to dopamine, which is the final product in some systems (e.g., interneurons in the sympathetic ganglia). After transport into cytoplasmic vesicles (storage granules), dopamine can be converted to norepinephrine in the presence of dopamine β-hydroxylase. Norepinephrine is the final product in sympathetic postganglionic neurons. Other tissues, such as the adrenal medulla, have cells that also contain phenylethanolamine-N-methyltransferase, the enzyme that converts norepinephrine to epinephrine, the final product of those cells.

Catecholamines are stored in cytoplasmic granules and released from the cell by exocytosis in response to neural stimulation.

CATECHOLAMINE DEGRADATION AND ELIMINATION. Catecholamines are degraded by two principal enzyme systems, catechol-O-methyltransferase (COMT) and monoamine oxidase (MAO) (Fig. 242–1). COMT converts norepinephrine and epinephrine to their respective O-methyl derivatives, the metanephrines (normetanephrine and metanephrine). MAO converts norepinephrine and epinephrine to dihydroxymandelic acid. These intermediates, the metanephrines and dihydroxymandelic acid, can then serve as substrates for MAO and COMT, respectively, resulting in their conversion to the major end product of extra-CNS catechol-

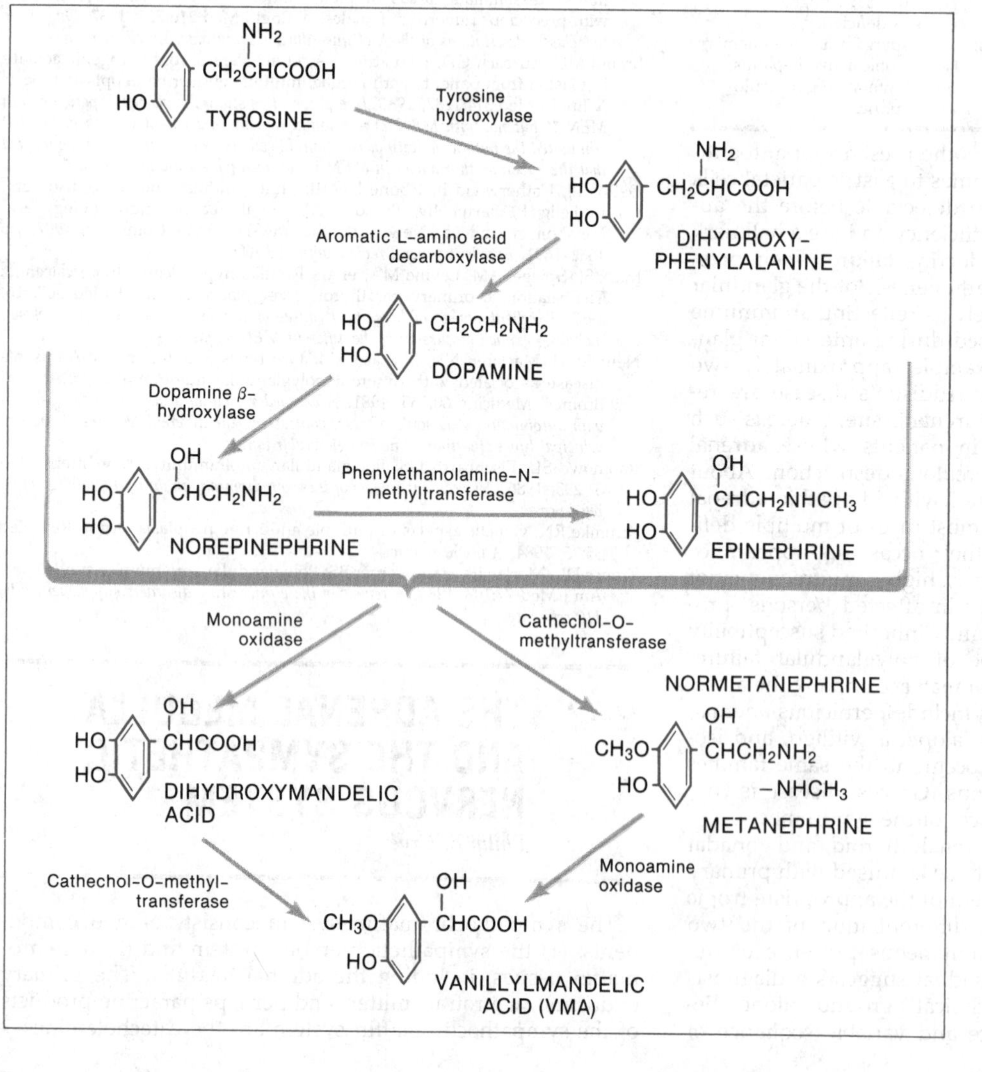

FIGURE 242–1. Catecholamine biosynthesis and metabolic degradation.

amine metabolism, vanillylmandelic acid (VMA). Dopamine metabolism (not shown in Figure 242–1) by MAO and COMT leads to the formation of homovanillic acid (HVA).

In general, catecholamine degradation within the sympathochromaffin cells is via MAO, whereas that of released catecholamines is via COMT. Released catecholamines are also conjugated, largely to sulfate in humans, and this may be another important route of inactivation. Sixty to 80 per cent of plasma epinephrine and norepinephrine and roughly half of the catecholamines excreted in the urine are conjugated.

Catecholamines are cleared rapidly from the circulation. Plasma half-times are 1 to 2 minutes. Clearance is largely extra-renal; less than 5 per cent appears in the urine unaltered.

BIOLOGIC ROLES OF THE CATECHOLAMINES. Epinephrine, norepinephrine, and dopamine are neurotransmitters in the CNS. Outside of the CNS, epinephrine is a hormone of the adrenal medulla, and norepinephrine is primarily the neurotransmitter of sympathetic postganglionic neurons. Dopamine is probably also a neurotransmitter, although its physiologic role has not been defined clearly.

Neurally regulated secretion of epinephrine from extra-adrenal chromaffin tissue (not sympathetic neurons) occurs, but in the absence of the adrenal medulla even stimulated plasma epinephrine levels in adults are not high enough to produce measurable biologic effects. Biologic actions of extra-adrenal epinephrine, if any, must be paracrine/neurotransmitter, not hormonal, in nature, at least in adults. Thus, epinephrine functions primarily as a hormone of the adrenal medulla and its plasma concentration is a valid index of its secretion.

Norepinephrine is released from axon terminals of sympathetic postganglionic neurons in direct relation to adrenergic receptors on innervated target cells. Most released norepinephrine is dissipated locally by reuptake into an axon terminal (uptake$_1$), where it is either stored in vesicles or metabolized, or by uptake into other cells adjacent to the synaptic cleft (uptake$_2$), where it is metabolized. Only a small fraction escapes into the circulation. The plasma norepinephrine concentration is a reasonable index of sympathetic neural activity under common physiologic conditions, at least in the basal state and during upright activity in humans. However, under some conditions, such as hypoglycemia, substantial amounts of norepinephrine (along with large amounts of epinephrine), are released from chromaffin tissues, specifically the adrenal medulla. Under such conditions the plasma norepinephrine concentration is clearly not an index of sympathetic neural activity. During vigorous physical activity and in a variety of pathologic states such as surgery, acute myocardial infarction, and diabetic ketoacidosis, circulating norepinephrine is probably derived from both the sympathetic nerves and the adrenal medulla, and its concentrations can be high enough to produce measurable effects. Under these conditions norepinephrine may function as a hormone as well as a neurotransmitter.

This physiology is relevant to the clinical use of plasma catecholamine measurements. Norepinephrine release from sympathetic neurons in amounts sufficient to produce biologically active norepinephrine concentrations in the synaptic cleft can be associated with very small, even undetectable, increments in its plasma concentration. On the other hand, if norepinephrine is released directly into the circulation (as from a pheochromocytoma) substantial increments in its plasma concentration are required to produce biologically active synaptic cleft concentrations.

BIOLOGIC ACTIONS OF THE CATECHOLAMINES. Catecholamines produce a variety of hemodynamic and metabolic effects. These are the result of catecholamine occupancy of adrenergic receptors (adrenoceptors) on the surface of target cells and a consequent series of intramembrane and intracellular biochemical events. Adrenergic receptors are divided into α- and β-adrenergic receptors, which are subdivided into α$_1$- and α$_2$-adrenergic receptors and β$_1$- and β$_2$-adrenergic receptors on the basis of measurements of the responses to various agonists and antagonists and the binding of a variety of ligands (generally antagonists) and competition for binding of these ligands by agonists and antagonists in vitro. In general, β-adrenergic receptors are linked through a stimulatory guanine nucleotide regulatory protein to adenylate cyclase, and α$_2$- (but not α$_1$-) adrenergic receptors are linked through an inhibitory protein to adenylate cyclase. A discussion of adrenergic receptors is beyond the scope of this chapter, although selected examples are given.

Catecholamines increase the rate and force of myocardial contraction (β$_1$) and produce vasoconstriction (α) in most vascular beds, although vasodilatation (β$_2$) occurs in some vascular beds, e.g., those of skeletal muscle. Norepinephrine produces increased vascular resistance and blood pressure (systolic and diastolic); the increased blood pressure reflexively limits the increase in heart rate. Probably because it has a higher affinity than norepinephrine for β$_2$-adrenergic receptors, epinephrine normally produces a somewhat different pattern: increased systolic, but not diastolic, blood pressure and increased heart rate.

Catecholamines increase the plasma glucose concentration through complex actions. These involve both stimulation of hepatic glucose production and limitation of glucose utilization and are mediated by both direct and indirect mechanisms. Foremost among the indirect mechanisms is limitation of insulin secretion (α). The direct actions are largely β mediated. Catecholamines also stimulate lipolysis, ketogenesis, glycolysis, and mobilization of amino acids such as alanine. They also increase thermogenesis.

Symptoms that occur when the sympathochromaffin system is activated include palpitations, anxiety, headache, and diaphoresis. All but the last are attributable to released catecholamines; diaphoresis has been attributed to a sympathetic cholinergic mechanism.

PHEOCHROMOCYTOMA

Pheochromocytomas are catecholamine-releasing tumors that typically produce hypertension. They are an uncommon cause of hypertension; perhaps 1 in 1000 hypertensive patients harbors a pheochromocytoma. Yet it is important to detect a pheochromocytoma for several reasons: (1) Hypertension due to a pheochromocytoma is usually curable by surgical removal of the tumor. (2) Patients with a pheochromocytoma are at risk for a lethal hypertensive paroxysm. (3) Some pheochromocytomas are malignant; early detection and removal would be expected to reduce the frequency of metastatic disease. Parenthetically, malignancy is established convincingly only by proven metastases; histologic criteria in the primary tumor are not reliable. (4) The presence of pheochromocytomas can be a clue to the presence of associated endocrine and nonendocrine familial disorders (Ch. 241). Pheochromocytomas are components of the multiple endocrine neoplasia, type 2 (MEN 2) and type 3 (MEN 3) syndromes. These familial disorders are inherited as autosomal dominant traits. MEN 2 includes medullary carcinoma of the thyroid, primary hyperparathyroidism, and pheochromocytoma. MEN 3 includes medullary carcinoma of the thyroid, multiple mucosal neuromas, and pheochromocytoma. Pheochromocytomas are not a component of the MEN 1 syndrome (pituitary and pancreatic adenomas and hyperparathyroidism). Familial pheochromocytomas also occur as an isolated disorder, in neurofibromatosis, and in the von Hippel-Lindau syndrome.

PATHOLOGY. Pheochromocytomas arise from chromaffin cells. Chromaffin cells are widespread and associated with sympathetic ganglia during fetal life. Postnatally most chromaffin cells degenerate; the major residual clusters of chromaffin cells comprise the adrenal medulla. Approximately 90 per cent of pheochromocytomas arise from the adrenal medulla. Extra-adrenal pheochromocytomas (paragangliomas) have been found in sites ranging from the carotid body to the pelvic floor. However, the majority are associated with sympathetic ganglia in the abdomen and most of the others with ganglia in the posterior mediastinum. Multiple pheochromocytomas, including bilateral adrenomedullary tumors, occur in up to 10 per cent of apparently sporadic cases. Bilateral adrenomedullary pheochromocytomas, with or without extra-adrenal tumors, are the rule in familial pheochromocytoma. Bilateral adrenomedullary hyperplasia, thought to be a precursor to pheochromocytoma, has been found in members of affected families.

The vast majority of pheochromocytomas release norepinephrine, and most also release some epinephrine. Rarely, a pheochromocytoma releases epinephrine predominantly or even exclusively.

CLINICAL MANIFESTATIONS. The clinical manifestations of pheochromocytomas are commonly due to the effects of released catecholamines and only rarely to the mass effect of the tumor. Common symptoms are *headache, palpitations,* and *diaphoresis.* Less common symptoms include abdominal or chest pain, gastrointestinal symptoms, weakness, or visual symptoms. Symptoms are typically paroxysmal and associated with increments in blood pressure. Hypertension is sometimes truly intermittent. In many cases, hypertension is sustained, but exhibits marked fluctuations with peak values occurring during symptomatic episodes. In general, plasma catecholamine levels are higher during symptomatic, hypertensive episodes than during asymptomatic, less hypertensive, or even normotensive intervals. The event(s) that precipitates episodic catecholamine release is usually not identifiable. However, the relationship between plasma catecholamine concentrations and blood pressure is not tight. This may reflect contrasting effects of norepinephrine and epinephrine but raises the possibility that hypertension in a patient with a pheochromocytoma may not be exclusively the result of direct effects of circulating norepinephrine on the cardiovascular system. Metabolic features of pheochromocytoma include an increased metabolic rate (some patients complain of heat intolerance, weight loss, or both) and an insulin-resistant state. Glucose intolerance and fasting hyperglycemia occur, but overt diabetes is unusual and probably reflects a coexistent defect in insulin secretion, i.e., genetic diabetes mellitus.

The rare epinephrine-releasing pheochromocytomas can produce different paroxysms. These may include hypotension, prominent tachycardia, noncardiac pulmonary edema, and cardiac arrhythmias. It is conceivable that tumor products in addition to epinephrine might contribute to these manifestations.

TABLE 242–1. DIAGNOSIS OF PHEOCHROMOCYTOMA

Clinical Suspicion
1. Paroxysmal symptoms (especially headache, palpitations, and diaphoresis)
2. Intermittent or unusually labile hypertension or hypertension refractory to therapy
3. Incidental adrenal mass (rarely a pheochromocytoma in the absence of one or more of the above)
4. Family history of pheochromocytoma, MEN 2, or MEN 3

Biochemical Confirmation
1. Plasma norepinephrine and epinephrine (± dopamine)
   Patient sampled in the basal state (and supine position) and, if possible, during a paroxysm
   Radioenzymatic or HPLC method
   Note blood pressure, heart rate, and any symptoms
2. Urinary catecholamines or metanephrines (or VMA)
   If plasma values are normal or equivocal but clinical suspicion is high, repeated plasma measurements are an alternative
   Can be used as the initial test

Anatomic Localization
1. Computed tomography
   Of the abdomen, including the adrenals, initially; of the pelvis and thorax if the abdomen is negative
   Indicated in the absence of biochemical evidence only if clinical suspicion is very high (e.g., positive family history)
2. Iodobenzylguanidine scan

DIAGNOSIS. The diagnosis of pheochromocytoma is based upon clinical suspicion and biochemical confirmation (Table 242–1). In general, radiographic studies should be used only to localize pheochromocytomas known to be present on the basis of clinical and biochemical evidence. Fluorometric or high-pressure liquid chromatographic measurement of unconjugated catecholamines or spectrophotometric measurement of total metanephrines or VMA in 24-hour urine collections is the traditional approach to the biochemical diagnosis of pheochromocytoma. The frequency of false-negative findings is slightly higher with VMA determinations. Nonetheless, the excretion of all three is substantially increased in the majority of patients with pheochromocytomas.

With the development of sufficiently sensitive methods, including single isotope derivative (radioenzymatic) or high-pressure liquid chromatographic (HPLC) assays, plasma catecholamine measurements have been effectively introduced into the diagnosis of pheochromocytoma. Plasma catecholamine measurements are probably superior to measurement of 24-hour urinary metanephrine and VMA because of less overlap between affected and unaffected hypertensive patients. However, the two approaches yield somewhat different information. Urinary measurements provide an index of catecholamine release integrated over time. Thus they might reflect intermittent plasma catecholamine elevations that could be missed by plasma measurements that provide information relevant only to a time frame of a few minutes.

Most patients with a pheochromocytoma have markedly elevated plasma catecholamine values (Fig. 242–2). Three points warrant emphasis, however. First, occasional patients with pheochromocytomas and typical histories of paroxysms have normal plasma catecholamine concentrations during an asymptomatic, normotensive interval. Second, some patients, commonly those investigated because of family history of

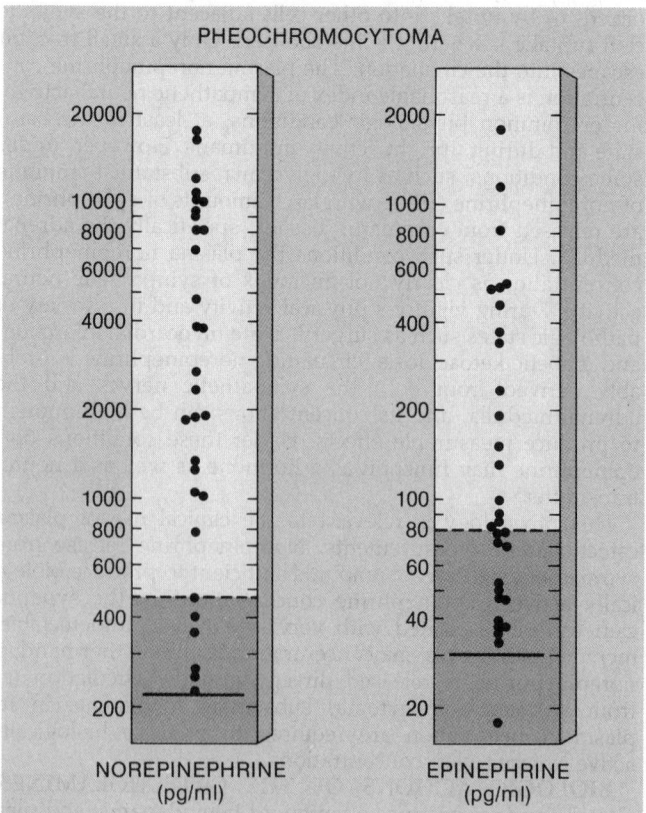

FIGURE 242–2. Plasma norepinephrine and epinephrine concentrations (radioenzymatic method) in 30 patients with pheochromocytomas. Note the semi-logarithmic scales. The interrupted horizontal lines are three standard deviations above the means (solid horizontal lines) of data from 165 normal humans sampled in the supine position.

pheochromocytoma, have no symptoms or signs and have normal plasma catecholamine concentrations but are found to have pheochromocytomas. These are not innocent tumors; lethal hypertensive paroxysms have occurred in such patients. Third, patients thought to have predominant epinephrine-secreting pheochromocytomas on clinical grounds can also have substantial overproduction of norepinephrine.

Strict attention to the details of sample collection, handling and storage, the sources of possible biologic variation, and the effects of drugs is critical if diagnostic error is to be avoided in the biochemical assessment of patients with suspected pheochromocytomas. Patients should be studied in the drug-free state if at all possible. Most antihypertensive drugs (other than clonidine) and many other drugs can elevate plasma and/or urine catecholamine levels. Elevated plasma catecholamine concentrations are to be expected during physical or mental stress and in any acute illness. Elevations, at times marked, have been well documented in patients with acute myocardial infarction, shock, burns, diabetic ketoacidosis, and cerebrovascular accidents, as well as during and immediately after surgery. Stable plasma catecholamine elevations also occur in patients with chronic disorders—for example, hypothyroidism, congestive heart failure, chronic obstructive pulmonary disease, anemia, duodenal ulcer, and depression. Lastly, elevated plasma catecholamine concentrations have been found in some, but certainly not all, patients thought to have essential hypertension.

It is my practice to obtain samples for determination of plasma norepinephrine and epinephrine in the basal state, with the patient supine, when pheochromocytoma is suspected. Substantial elevations over reference values provide strong support for the diagnosis of pheochromocytoma and are commonly found in affected patients. Samples are also obtained during symptomatic paroxysms. However, the interpretation of such values is more judgmental, since reference values cannot be defined precisely. Thus the biochemical diagnosis of pheochromocytoma is more convincingly supported if plasma catecholamine levels are elevated in the basal state and rise further during symptomatic episodes.

It is useful to record the blood pressure and whether or not symptoms are present when plasma samples for catecholamine measurements are drawn from a patient suspected of having a pheochromocytoma. Clearly, normal plasma (or urinary) catecholamine values obtained when the patient is normotensive and free of symptoms do not exclude the presence of a pheochromocytoma. Theoretically, 24-hour urinary catecholamine or metabolite measurements might detect intermittent catecholamine release missed by plasma sampling. These measurements should be obtained if plasma catecholamine levels are normal but clinical suspicion is high.

Substantial plasma norepinephrine elevations are required to produce hypertension in normal humans. Plasma epinephrine elevations within the physiologic range do not raise the diastolic blood pressure. It is reasonable, therefore, to consider normal or even moderately elevated plasma catecholamine levels obtained when the patient is hypertensive to be strong evidence against the diagnosis of pheochromocytoma.

Most patients ultimately found to have pheochromocytomas have distinctly elevated plasma and urinary catecholamine levels. The considerations raised in the preceding paragraphs apply to patients in whom the diagnosis is less clear cut and to the always difficult problem of the degree of certainty of a negative conclusion. Obviously one can never be absolutely certain during life that a given patient does not have a pheochromocytoma. As in many other areas of medicine, clinical judgment must be based upon probability.

Oral clonidine (0.3 mg) suppresses plasma catecholamine levels in hypertensive patients without pheochromocytoma but not in patients with pheochromocytoma. Thus the clonidine suppression test has been suggested to distinguish patients with primary hypertension with elevated basal plasma norepinephrine levels from those with hypertension due to a pheochromocytoma. Definition of the utility of this test awaits further experience. False negatives and false positives have been reported.

LOCALIZATION. Given biochemical confirmation of pheochromocytoma, anatomic localization is desirable. Normal adrenal glands can usually be imaged with modern computed tomography (CT), and the majority of adrenomedullary pheochromocytomas can be seen with this technique. CT is the recommended initial localizing procedure. It is conceivable that ultrasonography of the adrenals might be positive despite negative CT scans in an unusually thin patient. External scanning after the injection of radioactive agents that localize in pheochromocytomas has the conceptual advantage of measuring function rather than anatomy and the practical advantage of permitting scanning of the entire trunk of the body and might, therefore, be expected to localize extra-adrenal pheochromocytomas better than CT scans. The initial experience with $[^{131}I]$-m-iodobenzylguanidine (MIBG) scans has been encouraging in this regard.

TREATMENT. Treatment is surgical removal of the pheochromocytoma. Patients are usually prepared for surgery by administration of an α-adrenergic antagonist, such as phenoxybenzamine or prazosin, in doses sufficient to produce normal blood pressure and to prevent paroxysms. Treatment for 7 to 10 days prior to surgery is often recommended on the premise that this permits expansion of the blood volume. These drugs can also be used to treat chronic catecholamine excess in patients with metastatic tumor, although they do not influence the growth of a malignant pheochromocytoma. A β-adrenergic antagonist, such as propranolol, can be added to the preoperative regimen if arrhythmias are, or become, a problem.

Most patients are cured by surgery. The differential diagnosis of persistent hypertension includes a missed pheochromocytoma, a surgical complication resulting in renal ischemia, and underlying primary hypertension. Long-term follow-up is important, since late recurrences, including metastatic lesions, are being recognized with increasing frequency.

OTHER NEURAL CREST TUMORS. Pheochromocytomas are tumors of differentiated neural crest cells, the chromaffin cells. Tumors of more primitive cells also occur. These include neuroblastoma, a rather common malignant tumor of infancy and early childhood, usually arising in the adrenal medulla, and ganglioneuroma, a generally benign tumor often arising in sympathetic ganglia. These tumors commonly synthesize catecholamines but usually do not release catecholamines in sufficient quantities to produce clinical manifestations. Presumably the catecholamines are largely inactivated within the tumor. Nonetheless, measurements of catecholamine metabolites such as HVA and VMA are useful, particularly in assessing the response to therapy.

AUTONOMIC HYPOFUNCTION

NORMAL PHYSIOLOGY. Assumption of the upright position causes a sharp reduction in venous return to the heart. In the absence of compensatory mechanisms this would result in a corresponding decrease in cardiac output, in arterial pressure, and in blood flow to the brain. Syncope would result from the simple act of standing. Obviously there are effective compensatory mechanisms. The primary compensatory mechanism is a baroreceptor-initiated, CNS-mediated, sympathetic neural reflex that results in a norepinephrine release from axon terminals within the tissues. This results in a sharp increase in systemic vascular resistance (and limitation of the fall in venous return and cardiac output) and, thus, maintenance of the blood pressure in the standing position. Postural activation of this sympathetic reflex is reflected in a rapid, approximately two-fold rise in plasma norepinephrine concentrations. Thus, measurement of the plasma norepinephrine response to standing provides a relatively simple means of assessing the integrity of this sympathetic reflex.

PATHOPHYSIOLOGY. Defective postural adaptation results in a decrement in blood pressure upon standing, termed postural (orthostatic) hypotension. Conceptually, postural hypotension can be caused by one or more of three general mechanisms: (1) absolute or relative intravascular volume contraction; (2) resistance to the cardiovascular actions of norepinephrine; and (3) an afferent, central, or efferent defect in the sympathetic neural reflex arc. Patients with postural hypotension due to intravascular volume contraction or resistance to the action of norepinephrine exhibit an exaggerated plasma norepinephrine response to standing. They have *hyper*adrenergic postural hypotension. In contrast, patients with postural hypotension due to a defect in the sympathetic reflex arc have a blunted plasma norepinephrine response to standing. They have *hypo*adrenergic postural hypotension.

HYPERADRENERGIC POSTURAL HYPOTENSION. The causes of hyperadrenergic postural hypotension (Table 242–2) should be considered in all patients with postural hypotension, including those with overt autonomic disease, because they are commonly treatable. A given patient can have multiple hypotensive mechanisms; correction of one can result in clinical improvement. For example, in a patient with relatively mild autonomic hypofunction, otherwise trivial sodium depletion may result in symptomatic postural hypotension that can be treated by sodium repletion.

HYPOADRENERGIC POSTURAL HYPOTENSION. Hypoadrenergic postural hypotension can result from afferent, central, or efferent lesions in the sympathetic neural arc. Diseases recognized to cause secondary hypoadrenergic postural hypotension produce lesions in the brain, spinal cord, or peripheral nerves (Table 242–2). Diabetes is a common cause. In the absence of such diseases, autonomic hypofunction is considered to be idiopathic or primary. Undoubtedly a heterogeneous group of disorders of unknown etiology, primary autonomic dysfunction can be divided into two clinical and pathophysiologic syndromes. *Primary autonomic dysfunction type 1*, most commonly referred to as idiopathic orthostatic hypotension, is characterized by autonomic hypofunction in the absence of central nervous system disease. In addition to a blunted plasma norepinephrine response to standing, common to both the type 1 and type 2 disorders,

as a group patients with the type 1 disorder have low basal plasma norepinephrine concentrations. They are thought to have lesions of the peripheral autonomic nerves.

Primary autonomic dysfunction type 2 is perhaps best known as the Shy-Drager syndrome; it has also been referred to as multiple system atrophy or idiopathic orthostatic hypotension with somatic neurologic deficit. In addition to autonomic hypofunction, patients with the type 2 disorder have degenerative central nervous system disease most commonly manifested as parkinsonism. Such patients have normal basal plasma norepinephrine concentrations, and their autonomic lesions are thought to be in the central nervous system.

Impairment of both sympathetic and parasympathetic neural functions is the rule in primary autonomic dysfunction. Thus a variety of symptoms, such as diminished sweating and heat intolerance, difficulty in focusing, gastrointestinal symptoms, urinary and fecal incontinence and impotence, in addition to postural symptoms, occur commonly.

Treatment involves correction of the underlying cause of postural hypotension (Table 242–2) when possible. Symptomatic treatment approaches include sodium loading (NaCl tablets plus fludrocortisone [0.1 to 0.3 mg daily], which can produce hypokalemia and might precipitate cardiac failure in a patient with heart disease). Although not approved by the FDA at this writing, the agonist midodrine* (which constricts veins as well as arterioles) appears to be an effective drug.

EPINEPHRINE DEFICIENCY

The prevention or correction of hypoglycemia involves both dissipation of insulin and activation of glucose counter-regulatory systems. Whereas insulin is the dominant glucose-lowering factor, there are redundant glucose counter-regulatory factors, and a hierarchy among these. In defense against decrements in plasma glucose, dissipation of insulin is likely most important. Glucagon plays a primary counter-regulatory role. Epinephrine is not normally critical, but it compensates and becomes critical when glucagon is deficient. Hypoglycemia develops or progresses when both glucagon and epinephrine are deficient and insulin is present. Other hormones, neurotransmitters, or substrate effects may be involved, but they are neither critical nor potent.

Selective deficiency of the glucagon response to decrements in plasma glucose is the rule in patients with insulin-dependent diabetes mellitus (IDDM). To the extent that they have deficient glucagon responses, patients with IDDM are largely dependent upon epinephrine to prevent or correct hypoglycemia. Deficient epinephrine responses, a manifestation of diabetic autonomic neuropathy, to plasma glucose decrements develop in some patients with IDDM, typically later in the course of the disease. Patients with combined deficiencies of the glucagon and epinephrine responses are virtually defenseless against iatrogenic hypoglycemia. They have defective glucose counter-regulation and are at substantially increased risk (25-fold in our experience) for severe hypoglycemia, at least during intensive therapy of IDDM.

Patients with defective glucose counter-regulation often have a history of hypoglycemia unawareness, overt autonomic neuropathy, or both, but some do not. They can be identified prospectively with an insulin infusion test. Clearly, euglycemia is not an appropriate therapeutic goal in patients with IDDM and defective glucose counter-regulation, whether the latter is demonstrated with an insulin infusion test or is apparent from recurrent severe hypoglycemia during an attempt at intensive therapy. Administration of a β-adrenergic antagonist such as propranolol impairs recovery from experimental hypoglycemia in most patients with IDDM. Long-term administration of β-adrenergic antagonists has not been shown to increase the frequency of severe hypoglycemia in

---

TABLE 242–2. DIFFERENTIAL DIAGNOSIS OF POSTURAL HYPOTENSION

I. Hyperadrenergic postural hypotension
  A. Intravascular volume contraction
    1. Hemorrhage
    2. Severe chronic anemia
    3. Sodium (and water) depletion—aldosterone deficiency, diuretics, gastrointestinal or renal diseases
    4. Relative volume contraction—pregnancy
  B. Resistance to released norepinephrine
    1. Sodium depletion (see above)
    2. Glucocorticoid deficiency
    3. Bartter's syndrome
    4. Vasodilator drugs—nitroglycerin; hydralazine and minoxidil; prazosin, bromocriptine, and other α-adrenergic antagonists
II. Hypoadrenergic Postural Hypotension
  A. Secondary
    1. Brain lesions—vascular accidents involving the brainstem, toxic/nutritional encephalopathies, demyelinating and degenerative disorders, neoplasms, trauma, infections, tricyclic antidepressants, and phenothiazines
    2. Spinal cord lesions—cervical transection, mass lesions (tumor, abscess), syringomyelia, combined systems disease, tabes dorsalis
    3. Peripheral nerve lesions—diabetic adrenergic neuropathy, alcoholism, amyloidosis, porphyria, vincristine
  B. Primary
    1. Primary autonomic dysfunction
      a. Type 1: Idiopathic orthostatic hypotension
      b. Type 2: Idiopathic orthostatic hypotension with somatic neurologic deficit (Shy-Drager syndrome, multiple system atrophy)
    2. Familial dysautonomia (Riley-Day syndrome)

---

*This drug is available under the orphan drug program.

patients with IDDM, but this has not been examined in the context of intensive therapy.

Bravo EL, Gifford RW Jr: Pheochromocytoma: Diagnosis, localization and management. N Engl J Med 311:1298, 1984. *An extensive experience, including plasma catecholamine data.*

Cryer PE: Pheochromocytoma. Clin Endocrinol Metab 14:203, 1985. *A more detailed review of the subject, including discussion of the effects of drugs on catecholamine measurements and other details of diagnostic testing.*

Cryer PE: Diseases of the sympathochromaffin system. In Felig P, Baxter JD, Broadus AE, et al. (eds.): Endocrinology and Metabolism. 2nd ed. New York, McGraw-Hill Book Company, 1987, pp 651–692. *A detailed discussion of sympathochromaffin physiology and pathophysiology.*

Cryer PE, White NH, Santiago JV: The relevance of glucose counterregulatory systems to patients with insulin dependent diabetes mellitus. Endocr Rev 7:131, 1986. *A review of the physiology and pathophysiology of glucose counterregulation and its relationship to defective glucose counter-regulation, hypoglycemia unawareness, posthypoglycemic hyperglycemia, and stress hyperglycemia.*

Onrot J, Goldberg MR, Hollister AS, et al.: Management of chronic orthostatic hypotension. Am J Med 80:454, 1986. *Discussion of various supportive measures.*

The French MIBG Study Group: Comparison of iodobenzylguanidine imaging with computed tomography in locating pheochromocytoma. J Clin Endocrinol Metab 61:769, 1985. *A large experience demonstrating the strengths and weakness of the two approaches.*

243 THE CARCINOID SYNDROME

Philip E. Cryer

Carcinoid tumors arise from enterochromaffin (Kulchitsky) cells that are located predominantly in the gastrointestinal mucosa. Enterochromaffin cells have the potential to produce a variety of biologically active amines and peptides, including serotonin, bradykinin, and histamine, as well as prostaglandins. Carcinoid tumors are relatively common. Those that release sufficient quantities of mediators into the systemic circulation to produce the clinical carcinoid syndrome—flushing often with diarrhea and sometimes with wheezing or cardiac failure—are rare. Carcinoid tumors are most commonly found in the appendix or rectum, but these rarely produce the carcinoid syndrome. The tumors that produce the syndrome typically arise in the ileum, although the carcinoid syndrome can also result from tumors of the stomach, bile duct, duodenum, pancreas, lung, or even the ovary. Despite the release of a variety of mediators, the biochemical common denominator of the carcinoid syndrome is the overproduction of serotonin and the excretion of its major metabolite, 5-hydroxyindoleacetic acid (5-HIAA).

A variety of ectopic humoral syndromes have been associated with histologic carcinoid tumors. These include Cushing's syndrome (ACTH) and dilutional hyponatremia (vasopressin) with bronchial carcinoids, gynecomastia (chorionic gonadotropin) with gastric carcinoids, acromegaly (growth hormone–releasing hormone) with foregut carcinoids, and hypoglycemia (insulin) with pancreatic carcinoids. Typically, such patients do not have the carcinoid syndrome.

BIOSYNTHESIS AND DEGRADATION OF SERO-TONIN. Serotonin is synthesized from dietary tryptophan and later is converted to 5-hydroxyindoleacetic acid through the reactions shown in Figure 243–1.

Approximately 90 per cent of serotonin in the body is normally found in the gut. Serotonin synthesis accounts for only 1 per cent of the metabolism of tryptophan in normal individuals. This may be as high as 60 per cent in patients with the carcinoid syndrome. Indeed, a pellagra-like skin rash has been attributed to diversion of tryptophan from nicotinic acid synthesis in such patients. Normal individuals excrete less than 10 mg of 5-HIAA per 24 hours. Patients with the carcinoid syndrome commonly excrete 50 to 100 mg per 24 hours.

CLINICAL MANIFESTATIONS. Clinical carcinoid syndrome is usually associated with an ileal carcinoid tumor that has metastasized to the liver. Although carcinoids in sites, such as the lung or ovary, that do not drain into the portal circulation can rarely produce the carcinoid syndrome without evident hepatic metastases, carcinoid syndrome due to an ileal carcinoid is almost invariably associated with overt hepatic metastases. Presumably the liver clears mediators released from the tumor, and this clearance is impaired by metastatic tumor, resulting in the clinical syndrome.

More than 90 per cent of patients with the carcinoid syndrome have episodes of *cutaneous flushing*. The flush usually begins in the face and may spread to the trunk or even the extremities. It is red initially and then becomes purple; it commonly lasts only a few minutes, but may continue for hours. *Telangiectasias* of the face can result from frequent flushing. The heart rate increases and the blood pressure tends to decrease during a flush. This is in contrast to patients with pheochromocytomas who typically have episodes of pallor with hypertension. Bronchial carcinoids may be associated with more intense and long-lasting flushing episodes. In patients with gastric carcinoids, flushing tends to be patchy initially and may be anywhere on the body. Headache commonly follows the flush.

Flushing can be precipitated by alcohol, food, stress, or palpation of the liver, or it may follow the administration of catecholamines, pentagastrin, or reserpine. A single mediator that causes the carcinoid flush has not been identified. It is not serotonin, since inhibition of serotonin synthesis does not prevent flushing. Candidate mediators include bradykinin, histamine, prostaglandins, and substance P.

More than three quarters of patients with the carcinoid syndrome have *diarrhea*, typically exacerbated during episodes of flushing. Serotonin most likely mediates the diarrhea, since it can be reduced by inhibition of serotonin synthesis in most patients. Intestinal symptoms can also result from mesenteric fibrosis. Pleural, peritoneal, and retroperitoneal fibroses also occur. Serotonin may also cause the fibrotic lesions.

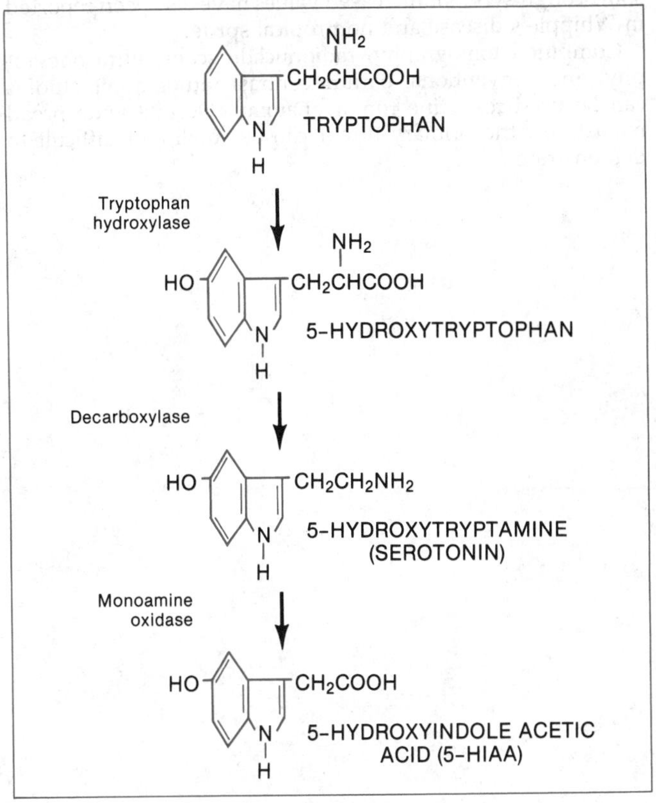

FIGURE 243–1. Synthesis and degradation of serotonin.

Right-sided endocardial fibrosis, perhaps the result of chronic serotonin excess, is found in more than one third of patients with the carcinoid syndrome. Cardiac failure due to pulmonic stenosis or tricuspid insufficiency or both is less common but implies a poor prognosis. Involvement of the left side of the heart is uncommon. It does occur in patients with bronchial carcinoids, which implies that the responsible mediator(s) is ordinarily cleared during passage through pulmonary capillaries.

Bronchoconstriction with wheezing during an episode of flushing is less common, occurring in about 20 per cent of patients. Like flushing, but unlike diarrhea, bronchoconstriction is not prevented by inhibition of serotonin synthesis.

Somatostatin has been reported to decrease flushing, diarrhea, and bronchoconstriction in patients with the carcinoid syndrome. The mechanism(s) of this effect is not known.

DIAGNOSIS. Diagnosis is based upon clinical suspicion—usually a history of flushing and diarrhea—associated with markedly increased urinary 5-hydroxyindoleacetic acid excretion. Metastatic hepatomegaly is common. Since carcinoid tumors produce the carcinoid syndrome rarely, the histologic diagnosis of a carcinoid tumor does not establish the presence of the carcinoid syndrome. Platelet serotonin levels are elevated in most patients with the carcinoid syndrome. Gastric carcinoids appear to have low decarboxylase activity, since 5-hydroxytryptophan, rather than serotonin, is the major product of indole metabolism in some such patients.

Provocative tests, such as the precipitation of episodes with intravenous administration of epinephrine, are seldom necessary and potentially dangerous, since severe hypotension and bronchoconstriction can occur.

False-positive urinary 5-HIAA determinations are common and should be suspected particularly when the values are minimally elevated, e.g., 10 to 20 mg per 24 hours. Increased 5-HIAA excretion can follow the ingestion of chocolate, bananas, tomatoes, pineapples, walnuts, and avocados and the use of drugs, including mephenesin, methocarbamol, reserpine, acetaminophen, and glyceryl guaiacolate (the last in some cough syrups). Increased values have also been reported in Whipple's disease and nontropical sprue.

Computed tomography, radionuclide scans, ultrasonography, and conventional barium-contrast radiographic studies can be used to define tumor anatomy. Despite widespread metastases, the primary tumor can be small and difficult to demonstrate.

TREATMENT. In the presence of documented metastases, resection of a primary ileal carcinoid tumor is not indicated. It may become necessary because of intestinal obstruction or because of intussusception. Rarely, surgical removal of an isolated tumor (e.g., a bronchial or ovarian carcinoid) is curative. Devascularization of metastatic tumor by percutaneous arterial embolization has been reported to produce symptomatic relief in some patients. Resection of localized hepatic metastases and hepatic artery ligation have also been reported to ameliorate symptoms of the carcinoid syndrome temporarily.

Survival of less than five years after the onset of the carcinoid syndrome is the rule, but survival for more than 20 years is well documented. Thus, high-risk attempts at curative therapy are generally not indicated. Carcinoid tumors are not radiosensitive. Low-risk chemotherapy has not been very effective.

Symptomatic therapy includes nutritional support plus the provision of nicotinamide to prevent pellagra. Diarrhea has been treated with serotonin antagonists such as methysergide or cyproheptadine as well as with opiates. The drug parachlorophenylalanine, a tryptophan hydroxylase inhibitor, reduces diarrhea. However, allergic reactions and CNS side effects have occurred, and the drug remains experimental. No drug is consistently effective in preventing flushing; H_1 and H_2 histamine antagonists, including cimetidine, are often tried. Phenothiazines and the α-adrenergic antagonist phenoxybenzamine have also been used, as have glucocorticoids. Treatment with leukocyte interferon was reported to decrease flushing and diarrhea in six of nine patients with the carcinoid syndrome. Symptomatic improvement, reduction of 5-HIAA excretion, and reduction in tumor size were reported in a patient treated with tamoxifen. Long-term symptomatic therapy with somatostatin analogues is promising.

Kvols LK, Moertel CG, O'Connell MJ, et al.: Treatment of the malignant carcinoid syndrome. Evaluation of a long-acting somatostatin analogue. N Engl J Med 315:663, 1986. *Somatostatin analogues represent a potential long-term therapy for carcinoid syndrome.*

Oberg K, Funa K, Alm G: Effects of leukocyte interferon on clinical symptoms and hormone levels in patients with mid-gut carcinoid tumors and carcinoid syndrome. N Engl J Med 309:129, 1983. *Unanticipated clinical and biochemical responses with demonstrable reductions in tumor size.*

Roberts LJ II, Oates JA: Disorders of vasodilator hormones: The carcinoid syndrome and mastocytosis. In Wilson JD, Foster DW (eds.): Williams Textbook of Endocrinology. 7th ed. Philadelphia, W. B. Saunders Company, 1985, pp 1363–1369. *A more detailed discussion of the carcinoid syndrome.*

PART XVII

DISEASES OF BONE AND BONE MINERAL METABOLISM

244 MINERAL AND BONE HOMEOSTASIS

Claude D. Arnaud

THE INTEGRATED CALCIOTROPIC HORMONE SYSTEM

A highly integrated and complex endocrine system maintains calcium, phosphate, and magnesium homeostasis in all vertebrates. It involves an interplay between two polypeptide hormones, parathyroid hormone (PTH) and calcitonin, and a sterol hormone, 1,25-dihydroxycholecalciferol [1,25(OH)$_2$D]. Biosynthesis and secretion of the polypeptide hormones are regulated by a negative feedback mechanism that involves calcium ion activity in the extracellular fluids (Fig. 244–1). Biosynthesis of 1,25(OH)$_2$D from the major circulating metabolite of vitamin D, 25-hydroxycholecalciferol (25OHD) takes place in the kidney and is regulated by PTH and calcitonin as well as by the extracellular fluid concentrations of calcium and phosphate. Other hormones, such as insulin, cortisol, thyroxine, epinephrine, estrogen, and testosterone; inorganic ions, such as calcium, magnesium, and phosphate; growth factors, such as the somatomedins, epidermal growth factor, fibroblast growth factor, platelet-derived growth factor, and the transforming growth factors; the prostaglandins; the lym-phokines; and certain physical factors undoubtedly play roles in the modification and regulation of organ responses to PTH, calcitonin, and 1,25(OH)$_2$D.

Parathyroid hormone, calcitonin, and 1,25(OH)$_2$D regulate the flow of minerals into and out of the extracellular fluid compartment through their actions on intestine, kidney, and bone (Fig. 244–1, Table 244–1). The target cells of these organs function as a barrier between the extracellular fluid compartment and the intestinal lumen, the renal tubular lumen, and the bone fluid compartment (Fig. 244–2). These target cells are highly specialized for solute transport against a concentration gradient and thus are often described as being polarized.

PARATHYROID HORMONE. Under normal circumstances, PTH prevents serum calcium from falling below physiologic concentrations by stimulating calcium movement from the bone fluid compartment and the intestinal and renal tubular lumina into the blood. Whereas its effects on bone and kidney are direct, PTH acts indirectly on the intestine, through the mediation of vitamin D. The hormone stimulates the conversion of 25OHD to 1,25(OH)$_2$D via a 1α-hydroxylase in the mitochondria of the renal tubule (this stimulation works directly and indirectly through a decrease in serum phosphate levels). The 1,25(OH)$_2$D thus formed stimulates intestinal absorption of calcium via a vitamin D–dependent calcium pump.

Parathyroid hormone also prevents serum phosphate levels from rising above normal physiologic concentrations by increasing renal tubular excretion of phosphate. This regulatory

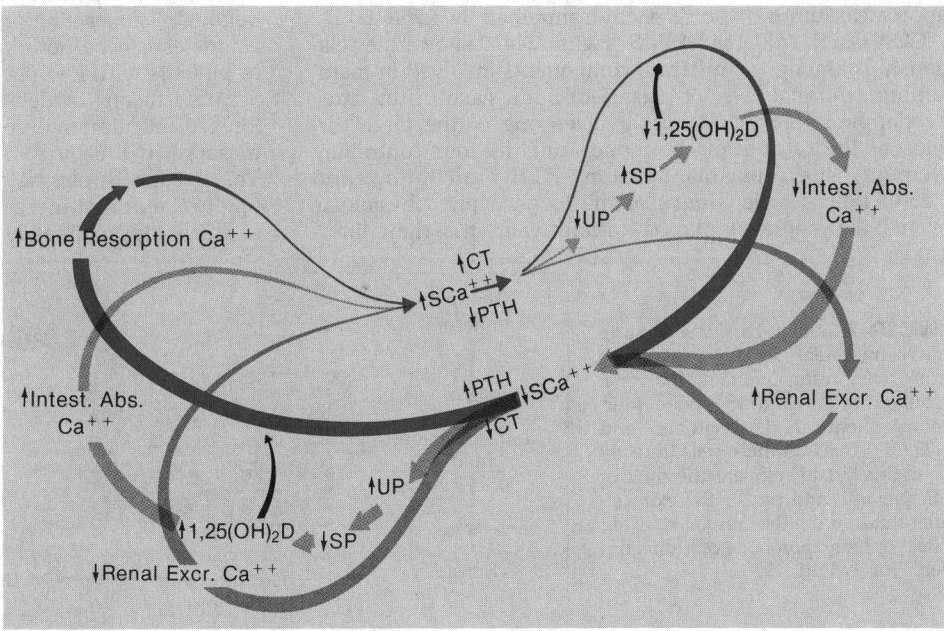

FIGURE 244–1. Schema of calcium homeostasis, consisting of three overlapping control loops that interlock and relate to one another through the level of blood concentrations of ionic calcium, parathyroid hormone, and calcitonin. Each loop involves a calciotropic hormone target organ (bone, intestine, kidney). The loops on the left depict physiologic events that increase the blood concentration of calcium, and the loops on the right, events that decrease this concentration. See text for detailed descriptions. (From Arnaud CD: Calcium homeostasis: Regulatory elements and their integrity. Fed Proc 37:2558, 1978.)

TABLE 244–1. ACTIONS OF MAJOR CALCIUM-REGULATING HORMONES

	Bone	Kidney	Intestine
PTH	Increases resorption of calcium and phosphate.	Increases resorption of calcium; conversion of 25 OHD to 1,25(OH)₂D. Decreases resorption of phosphate and bicarbonate.	No direct effects.
Calcitonin	Decreases resorption of calcium and phosphate.	Decreases resorption of calcium and phosphate. Questionable effect on vitamin D metabolism.	No direct effects.
Vitamin D	Maintains Ca⁺⁺ transport system.	Decreases resorption of calcium.	Increases absorption of calcium and phosphate.

Adapted from Arnaud CD, Kolb FO: The calciotropic hormones and metabolic bone disease. In Greenspan FS, Forsham PH (eds.): Basic and Clinical Endocrinology. Los Altos, CA, Lange Medical Publications, 1983, p 188.

action is important because phosphate, like calcium, is also released into the blood by PTH-induced bone resorption. This function can be particularly appreciated in patients with end-stage renal failure and associated severe hyperparathyroidism. These patients develop hyperphosphatemia because large quantities of phosphate are released from bone and the kidney can no longer excrete it.

CALCITONIN. Calcitonin prevents abnormal increases in both serum calcium and serum phosphate. It decreases the translocation of calcium from the renal tubule and bone fluid compartment into the blood and thus can be considered a counter-regulator of PTH in this regard. The effects of calcitonin on the intestinal absorption of calcium and vitamin D metabolism are uncertain.

VITAMIN D. Vitamin D, as 1,25(OH)₂D, acts primarily to maintain the cellular calcium transport system in the intestine, which causes the active extrusion of calcium against a concentration gradient from the interior of the cell (ionized calcium concentration = 10^{-7} to 10^{-6} M), across the antiluminal membrane, and into the extracellular fluid (ionized calcium concentration = 10^{-3} M) (Fig. 244–3). Thus, PTH and 1,25(OH)₂D are interdependent. The renal production of 1,25(OH)₂D depends upon the prevailing concentration of PTH in the blood, and the ability of PTH to increase plasma calcium depends upon a calcium transport system maintained by 1,25(OH)₂D.

CONTROL MECHANISMS. Figure 244–1 shows the relationships among the different components involved in maintaining a normal level of plasma calcium. Each of the three overlapping feedback loops involves one of the target organs of the calciotropic hormones and the four controlling elements—i.e., plasma calcium, PTH, calcitonin, and 1,25(OH)₂D. The left limbs of the loops depict physiologic events that increase plasma calcium, and the right limbs

events that decrease plasma calcium. Under physiologic conditions, there are small fluctuations in plasma calcium. Decreases in plasma calcium increase PTH secretion and decrease calcitonin secretion. These changes in hormone secretion lead to increased bone resorption, decreased renal excretion of calcium, and increased intestinal calcium absorption (via PTH stimulation of 1,25(OH)₂D production; left side of Fig. 244–1). As a consequence of these events, plasma calcium rises slightly above physiologic levels, inhibiting PTH secretion and stimulating calcitonin secretion. These changes in plasma hormone concentrations decrease bone resorption, increase renal excretion of calcium, and decrease intestinal absorption of calcium (right side of Fig. 244–1), causing plasma calcium to fall below the physiologic level. This sequence of events probably occurs within milliseconds, so that plasma calcium is maintained at physiologic levels with minimal oscillation. The "butterfly" scheme in Figure 244–1 not only shows the relationships among elements that control mineral homeostasis under physiologic conditions but also suggests how potential pathogenetic mechanisms and adaptive responses elicited by disease or treatment would operate in this system.

PLASMA CALCIUM AND PHOSPHATE

CALCIUM. The circulating forms of calcium and phosphorus and their normal ranges are shown in Figure 244–4. Calcium is distributed in three major fractions: ionized, protein-bound, and complexed. The ionized form (Ca⁺⁺), the only biologically active species, constitutes 46 to 50 per cent of total calcium. The protein-bound fraction, roughly equivalent to the ionized fraction in amount, is biologically inert. However, the calcium bound to albumin (80 per cent) and globulin (20 per cent) is important because it provides a readily available reservoir of this important cation. Since the binding of calcium to these proteins obeys the mass-law equation, calcium can dissociate from its binding sites to provide a first-line defense against hypocalcemia. Moreover, hyperproteinemia (e.g., hyperglobulinemia in myelomatosis) can increase and hypoproteinemia (e.g., hypoalbuminemia in cirrhosis of the liver or nephrosis) can decrease total plasma calcium without changing the concentration of ionized calcium. Formulas have been developed to estimate the percentage of calcium bound to the plasma proteins based on the differential binding affinities of albumin and globulin; for example,

Per cent protein-bound Ca⁺⁺ = 8 × albumin (grams per deciliter) + 2 × globulin (grams per deciliter) + 3.

Such formulas permit the calculation of diffusible calcium (see below) by subtracting protein-bound from total calcium. Such estimates can be notoriously inaccurate, however, especially in patients with low plasma protein concentrations. The only accurate means of determining the plasma concentration of ionized calcium in hypo- or hyperproteinemic states is to measure it directly by an ion-selective electrode procedure. The fraction of plasma calcium that is complexed to organic (e.g., citrate) and inorganic (e.g., phosphate or sulfate) acids is small (approximately 8 per cent), and, like the ionized

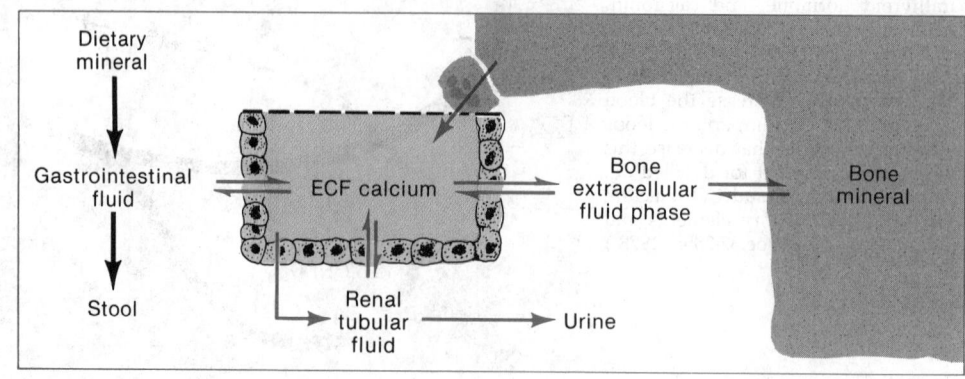

FIGURE 244–2. Cellular barrier separating the extracellular fluid compartment from the intestinal lumen, the renal tubular lumen, and the bone fluid compartment. PTH, calcitonin, and 1,25(OH)₂D act on these cells (directly or indirectly) to regulate the flow of calcium into and out of the extracellular fluid. (From Rasmussen H, et al.: Effect of ions upon bone cell function. Fed Proc 29:1191, 1970.)

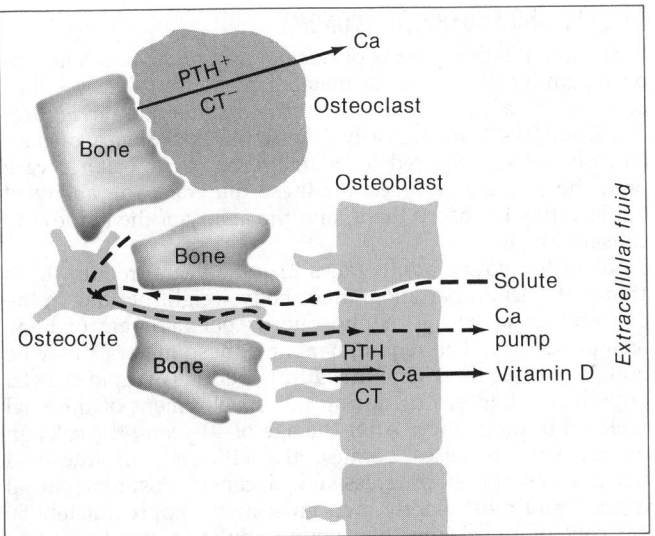

FIGURE 244–3. Relationships between calciotropic hormones, bone cells, and calcium transport. Bone crystal is represented by the shaded areas. The osteoclast, with an active "ruffled border," is shown resorbing bone—a process stimulated by PTH (PTH⁺) and inhibited by calcitonin (CT⁻). The osteoblasts are actively extruding calcium (Ca) from the bone fluid (between cells and crystals) under the influence of hormones. Processes connecting deep osteocytes are shown participating in calcium transport (dashed arrows). (From Arnaud CD, Kolb FO: The calciotropic hormones and metabolic bone disease. In Greenspan FS, Forsham PH (eds): Basic and Clinical Endocrinology. Los Altos, CA, Lange Medical Publications, 1983, p 189.)

fraction, it is ultrafilterable (diffusible). Complexed calcium probably has little importance as a reservoir for ionized calcium, but in states of hyperphosphatemia, such as chronic renal failure, excessive complexing of calcium with phosphate may contribute to the decrease in plasma ionized calcium observed in this condition.

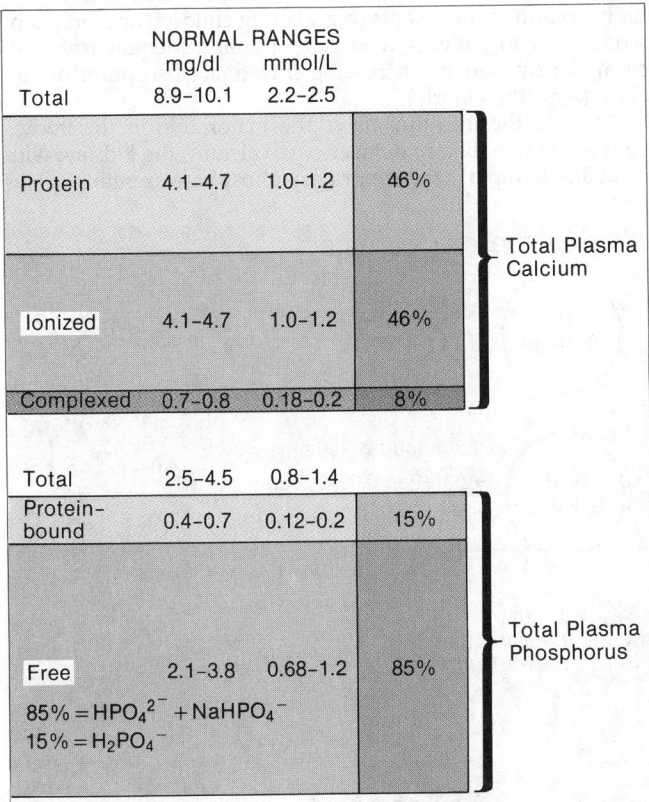

FIGURE 244–4. Distribution and normal ranges of calcium and phosphorus in the plasma.

The normal range for serum calcium (Fig. 244–4) is small (1.2 mg per deciliter) compared to the total concentration of serum calcium (8.9 to 10.1 mg per deciliter), and the same is true for the ionized fraction. Thus, values for total calcium below 8.9 mg per deciliter, assuming that plasma protein concentrations are normal, reflect clinically significant hypocalcemia, and values above 10.1 mg per deciliter reflect hypercalcemia. In recent years, serum calcium has been measured with reasonable accuracy in most clinical laboratories. However, stored plasma samples may yield artifactual decreases in circulating calcium concentrations, and contaminated serum samples may yield artifactual increases. Thus, it is important to use *fresh serum* for calcium measurements and eliminate sources of calcium contamination in order to obtain reliable measurements of calcium.

The plasma calcium concentration varies little in spite of large changes in dietary calcium because of the adaptive alterations in the endocrine system regulating this mineral. Minor diurnal changes (decreases in the afternoon) have been recorded. In addition, plasma calcium decreases with age in men but not in women, probably due to a decrease in the serum albumin concentration in men. Total (but not ionized) serum calcium also decreases during pregnancy, and this change may also be due to the decrease in the serum albumin concentration in this condition.

Hypocalcemia produces a myriad of symptoms, and when severe can result in tetany and possibly convulsions (see Ch. 247 and 493). *Hypercalcemia* can produce functional changes in most organ systems, and these changes may lead to a confusing variety of symptoms and objective findings (see Ch. 247).

PHOSPHORUS. Only 15 per cent of plasma phosphate is bound to proteins in the blood (Fig. 244–4). The rest is ultrafilterable and consists mainly of free HPO_4^{2-} and $NaHPO_4^-$ (85 per cent), with free $H_2PO_4^-$ making up the remainder (15 per cent). By convention, plasma phosphate is expressed in terms of the amount of elemental phosphorus involved.

In comparison to calcium, phosphate has a wider range of normal plasma values (2.5 to 4.5 mg per deciliter) (Fig. 244–4). Moreover, increases or decreases in dietary phosphate are promptly reflected in changes in the same direction in serum phosphorus and urinary phosphorus excretion. There are also marked diurnal variations in serum phosphorus and urinary phosphorus excretion (both may as much as double in the afternoon and evening), even during a fast, which are caused in part by diurnal changes in plasma cortisol. Serum phosphorus concentrations in young children are almost double those in adults, and they increase slightly with age in women. The reason for these differences in children and in aging women is poorly understood but may relate to the increased bone turnover present in both groups.

Serum phosphorus can be measured accurately and precisely in most laboratories. However, spuriously high values may be obtained if (1) serum extracts or dialysates are exposed to acid longer than is prescribed (resulting in hydrolysis of organic compounds containing phosphorus) or (2) hemolyzed serum is used (red blood cells contain phosphorus).

Hyperphosphatemia. Acute, severe hyperphosphatemia, as might be induced by intravenous phosphate infusion, can cause hypocalcemia sufficiently severe to result in tetany and even death. The less severe hyperphosphatemia induced by phosphate ingestion rarely causes symptoms; however, if the patient has an associated disorder in which there is a tendency toward hypocalcemia (e.g., mild hypoparathyroidism or chronic renal failure), frank hypocalcemia may develop.

Hypophosphatemia (see also Ch. 207). Acute respiratory alkalosis, the administration of a large quantity of carbohydrate, and insulin administration all cause a rapid decrease in serum phosphorus. Severe hypophosphatemia may occur during the treatment of diabetic ketoacidosis or forced nutrition of undernourished patients and can cause both skeletal myopathy and cardiomyopathy. These conditions may lead to rhabdomyolysis, as evidenced by increases in serum creatine phosphokinase (Ch. 77). The levels of 2,3-diphosphoglyceric acid and adenosine triphosphate (ATP) in erythrocytes may also decrease; the decrease in 2,3-diphosphoglyceric acid may in turn may decrease oxygen delivery to tissues, and the decrease in ATP may cause hemolytic anemia. Chronic, moderate hypophosphatemia frequently results in osteomalacia or rickets, as in the genetic disorder X-linked hypophosphatemia (Ch. 246). Generally, restoration of serum phosphate concentrations to normal corrects abnormal organ function in hypophosphatemic conditions, except in X-linked hypophosphatemic rickets, which requires regimens specially tailored for individual patients.

INTERRELATION OF PLASMA CALCIUM AND PHOSPHATE

The physiologic importance of the relationship between the circulating concentrations of ionized calcium and diffusible (free) phosphate is poorly understood, especially with regard to the formation and dissolution of amorphous calcium phosphate $(Ca_3(PO_4)_2)$ and hydroxyapatite $(Ca_{10}(PO_4)_6(OH)_2)$ in bone. However, available evidence indicates that the ion product of normal plasma concentrations of calcium and phosphate (the Ca × P ion product) is considerably higher than that necessary to form these two compounds. Thus, in comparison to bone, plasma is supersaturated with calcium and phosphate, and this can be considered an important driving force in bone mineralization. The positive effect of vitamin D on bone mineralization is probably indirect and resides in its ability to maintain the Ca × P ion product in the normal range by increasing calcium and phosphate absorption by the gut and their resorption by bone (Fig. 244–1).

The biologic significance of the Ca × P ion product has been questioned in recent years, but it is important to recognize that products below 20 mg per deciliter (0.7 mmol per liter) usually reflect a mineralization defect in bone, and products above 70 mg per deciliter (2.2 mmol per liter) a propensity toward soft tissue calcification. There are exceptions to these numerical guidelines that will become apparent in future chapters, but, short of directly measuring changes in bone formation in bone biopsy specimens or changes in calcium content in soft tissues, determining the Ca × P ion product may provide the best indication of the presence of these pathologic changes.

CALCIUM AND PHOSPHATE ECONOMY

The quantitative aspects of calcium and phosphorus metabolism, under conditions of metabolic balance (dietary intake equal to urinary and fecal excretion), are illustrated in Figures 244–5 and 244–6, respectively. The amounts of dietary calcium and phosphate required to maintain metabolic balance vary with the physiologic need for these minerals, the ability of the intestine to absorb them, and the ability of the kidneys to conserve them.

Normally, young adults (ages 21 to 35 years) require 12 to 15 mg of calcium per kilogram of body weight per day in the diet and 15 to 20 mg of phosphorus per kilogram of body weight per day. The requirements for these minerals may be double or triple these amounts during periods of rapid skeletal growth (in children) or during the development of the fetal skeleton in pregnancy. After the age of 40 years, the calcium requirement increases because the efficiency of intestinal calcium absorption progressively declines. Postmenopausal women and most elderly men must ingest approximately 50 per cent more calcium than young adults to avoid negative balance.

Dietary deprivation of calcium or phosphorus induces adaptive changes in the production and secretion of the calciotropic hormones that minimize the development of negative balance. In the case of calcium, only 30 to 50 per cent of ingested calcium is normally absorbed (Fig. 244–5). With decreased intake, serum calcium decreases slightly, and the sequence of events depicted in the left limbs of the feedback loops in Figure 244–1 is activated. In severe, chronic dietary deficiency of calcium in normal subjects, PTH stimulates an increase in plasma 1,25(OH)$_2$D levels, which can increase fractional calcium absorption up to 75 per cent; hence, the total body calcium is minimally perturbed. However, this adaptive response requires a chronic increase in plasma concentrations of PTH. The destructive effects of such hyperparathyroidism on bone (see Ch. 247) may be of little consequence to the young adult, in whom the net loss of total body calcium is minimal, but they may be devastating to individuals with high calcium requirements (e.g., young children and pregnant women) or to patients who cannot adapt adequately to calcium deprivation by increasing intestinal absorption of calcium (e.g., the elderly).

Whereas the intestine plays the major role in the body's adaptation to a dietary deficiency of calcium, the kidney, with its ability to rapidly reduce urinary phosphate excretion, plays

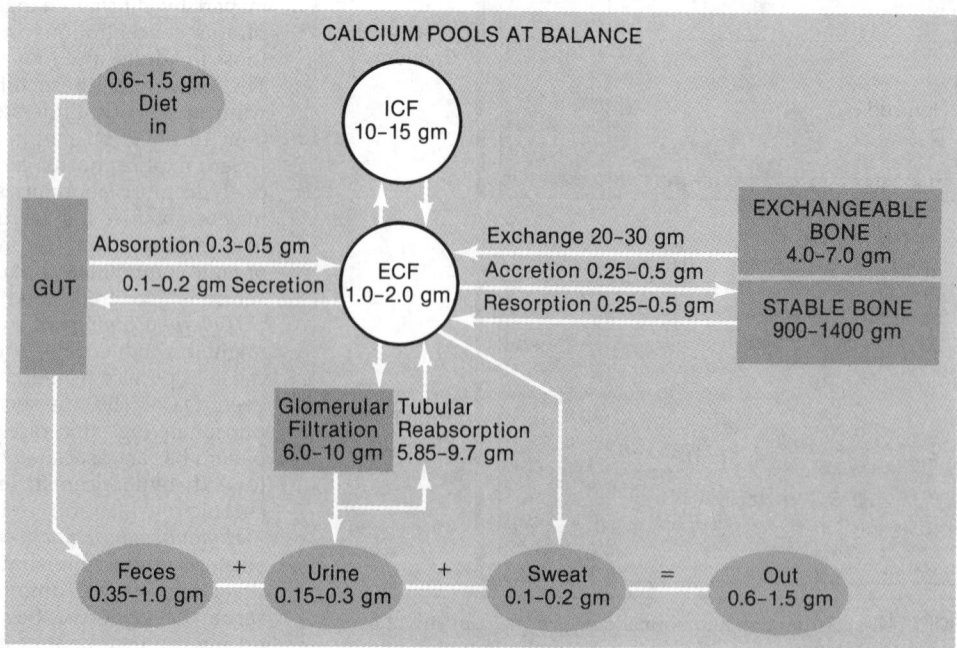

FIGURE 244–5. Normal distribution of calcium in the body. ICF denotes intracellular fluid, and ECF extracellular fluid.

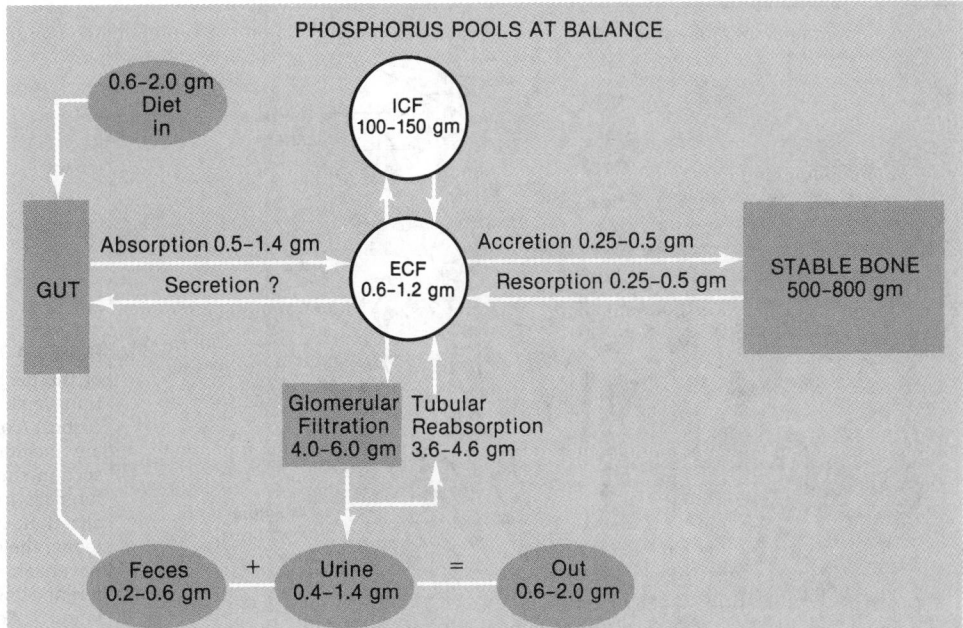

FIGURE 244–6. Normal distribution of phosphorus in the body. ICF denotes intracellular fluid, and ECF extracellular fluid.

the major role in maintaining phosphate balance during a dietary deficiency of this mineral. Normally, 70 to 80 per cent of dietary phosphorus is absorbed, and therefore any increase in its fractional absorption during deprivation would have little influence in preventing the development of negative balance. However, 80 per cent or more of absorbed phosphorus is normally excreted in the urine; thus, decreasing excretion by 50 per cent, for example, would have an effect comparable to that of almost tripling dietary intake.

The mechanism(s) involved in the decrease in urinary excretion of phosphorus in response to dietary deprivation is not entirely understood. Hypophosphatemia in this condition is associated with increased production of 1,25(OH)$_2$D, increased intestinal absorption of calcium, mild hypercalcemia, and decreased PTH secretion (Fig. 244–1, left middle limb). Any one or a combination of these changes could account for part or all of the decrease in urinary excretion of phosphate. However, it is also possible that other, as-yet-undescribed factors may also play a role.

MAGNESIUM HOMEOSTASIS

Magnesium is the major intracellular divalent cation. Its extracellular fluid concentration is normally maintained within a reasonably narrow range (1.5 to 2.2 mg per deciliter), but, in contrast to the inability of low-calcium diets to produce appreciable hypocalcemia, dramatic decreases in the serum magnesium can be observed in humans ingesting diets deficient in this ion for as little as one week (Ch. 208). Thus, even though there are appreciable stores of magnesium in cells and bone, they are not easily mobilized, and serum concentrations of magnesium are heavily dependent upon adequate dietary supplies and its normal intestinal absorption.

Increased renal conservation of magnesium is an almost immediate response to the ingestion of a magnesium-deficient diet. This is thought to be due to an effect of PTH on the renal tubule similar to that which PTH exerts on the renal tubular reabsorption of calcium. Like hypocalcemia, mild to moderate hypomagnesemia stimulates PTH secretion, albeit to a lesser extent, so that at least the rudiments of a negative feedback regulatory system exist which has the potential for maintaining extracellular magnesium homeostasis. Unfortunately, the system is complicated by the fact that severe magnesium deficiency and hypomagnesemia (<1.0 mg per deciliter) inhibit both PTH secretion and action, thus causing functional hypoparathyroidism and hypocalcemia (see Ch. 247).

BONE
Function of Bone

Bone has four major functions: (1) Bones provide rigid support to extremities and to the body cavities that contain vital organs. When bone is weak or defective, erect posture may be impossible and vital organ function may be compromised. (An example is the cardiopulmonary dysfunction that occurs in patients with severe kyphosis due to vertebral collapse.) (2) Bones are crucial to locomotion in that they provide efficient levers and sites of attachment for muscles. With bony deformities, these levers become defective, and severe abnormalities of gait develop. (3) Bone provides a hospitable environment for the dispersed hematopoietic system. (4) Bone provides a large reservoir of ions, such as calcium, phosphorus, magnesium, and sodium, that are crucial for life and can be mobilized when the external environment fails to provide them.

Structure of Bone

Two thirds of the weight of bone is mineral; the remainder is water and collagen. Minor organic components, such as proteoglycans, lipids, noncollagenous proteins, and acidic proteins that contain γ-carboxyglutamic acid, are probably important, but their functions are poorly understood.

There are two types of bone mineral. The major form consists of hydroxyapatite in crystals of varying maturity. The remainder is amorphous calcium phosphate, which lacks a coherent x-ray diffraction pattern, has a lower calcium-to-phosphate ratio than pure hydroxyapatite, occurs in regions of active bone formation, and is present in larger quantities in young bone.

As a living tissue, bone is unique in that it is not only rigid and resists forces that would ordinarily break brittle materials but is also light enough to be moved by coordinated muscle contractions. These characteristics are a function of the strategic location of two major types of bone (Fig. 244–7). Cortical bone, composed of densely packed, mineralized collagen laid down in layers, provides rigidity and is the major component of tubular bones. Trabecular (cancellous) bone is spongy in appearance, provides strength and elasticity, and constitutes the major portion of the axial skeleton. Defective or scanty cortical bone leads to fractures of the long bones, whereas defective or scanty trabecular bone leads to vertebral fractures. Fractures of long bones may also occur because normal reinforcement by trabecular bone is lacking.

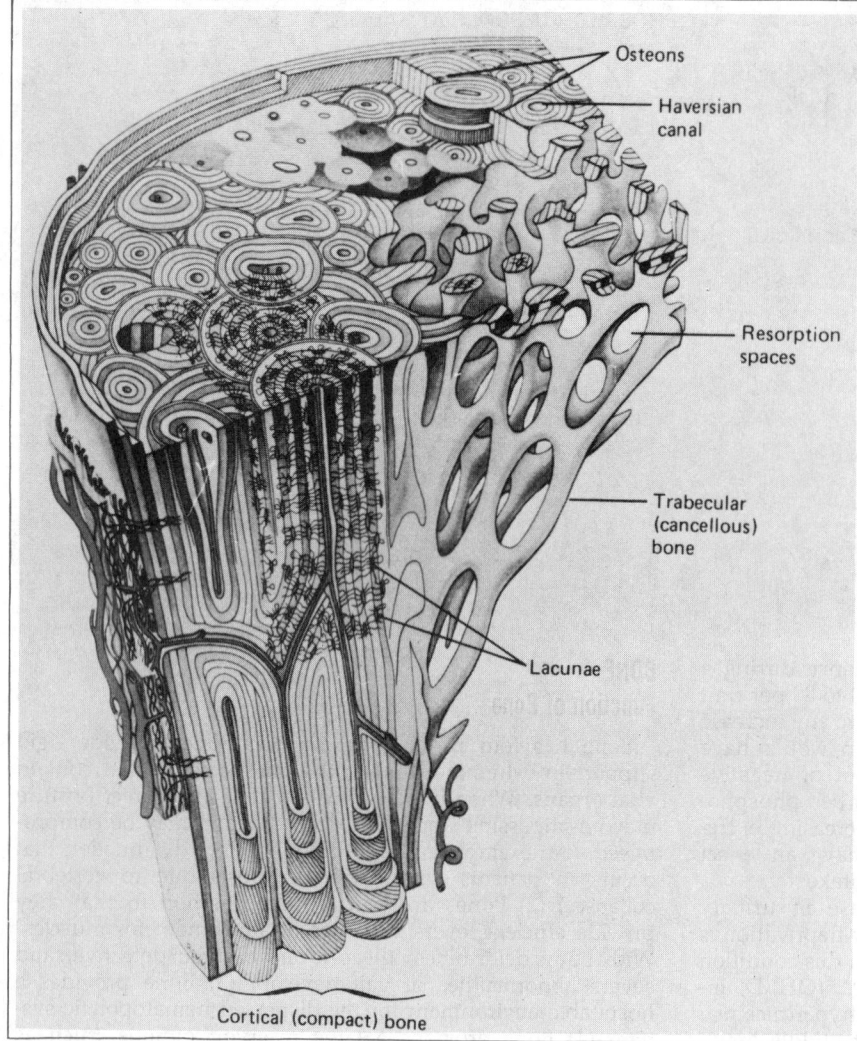

FIGURE 244–7. Diagram of some of the main features of the microstructure of mature bone seen in both transverse (*top*) and longitudinal sections. Areas of cortical (compact) and trabecular (cancellous) bone are included. The central area in the transverse section simulates a microradiograph, with the differences in density reflecting variations in mineralization. Note the general construction of the osteons, the distribution of the osteocyte lacunae, the haversian systems, resorption spaces, and the different views of the structural basis of bone lamellation. (Adapted from Warwick R, Williams PL [eds.]: Gray's Anatomy. 35th ed. Edinburgh. Churchill Livingstone, 1973, p 217.)

Microscopically, there are two types of bone structure: woven and lamellar. Both may be found in either cortical or trabecular bone. Woven bone is a normal constituent of embryonic bone but in adult bone it usually reflects the presence of disease. Lamellar bone is stronger than woven bone and is formed more slowly. It progressively replaces woven bone as the skeleton develops from birth. Whereas woven bone has nonparallel collagen fibers, many osteocytes per unit area of matrix, and mineral that is poorly incorporated into collagen fibrils, lamellar bone has a parallel arrangement of collagen fibers, few osteocytes per unit area of matrix, and mineral that is well incorporated into collagen fibrils. Cortical lamellar bone is present in concentric layers surrounding the vascular channels that compose the haversian systems of cortical bone (osteons) (Fig. 244–7). In contrast, the lamellar bone of trabeculae is present in layers and is laid down in long sheaves and sheets (Fig. 244–8).

Formation and Resorption of Bone

Bone is formed and resorbed continuously throughout life. These important processes depend upon three major types of bone cells, each with different functions.

OSTEOBLASTS. Osteoblasts are thought to be derived from a population of dividing cells, present on bone surfaces, that arise from mesenchymal cells in the connective tissue in bone. These specialized cells form new bone on bone surfaces previously resorbed by osteoclasts and have alkaline phosphatase activity. The exact role of alkaline phosphatase in osteoblast function remains uncertain. Osteoblasts are actively involved in the synthesis of the components of bone matrix (primarily collagen) and probably facilitate the movement of mineral ions between extracellular fluid and the bone surface

(Fig. 244–3). The evidence supporting such ion transport by osteoblasts is sparse, but there is widespread agreement that osteoblast-mediated transport of calcium and phosphate is involved in the mineralization of collagen, which in turn is crucial for formation of bone. In the process of bone formation,

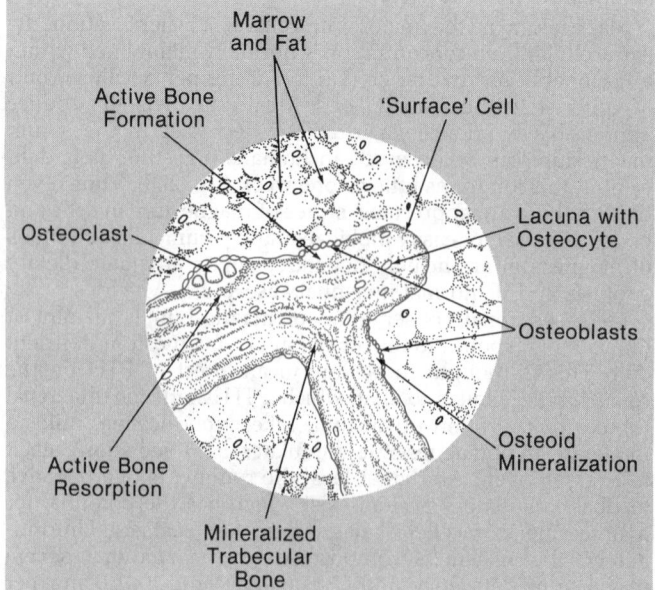

FIGURE 244–8. Schema of typical microscopic appearance of a section of undemineralized trabecular bone showing active bone resorption and formation.

osteoblasts gradually become encased in the bone matrix they have produced.

OSTEOCYTES. Once trapped in the mineralized matrix, the functional and morphologic characteristics of osteoblasts change, and they are then called osteocytes. Protein synthesis decreases markedly, and the cells develop multiple processes that reach out through lacunae (Figs. 244–3, 244–7, and 244–8) in bone tissue to "communicate" with processes of other osteocytes within a unit of bone (osteon) and with the processes of surface osteoblasts (Fig. 244–3). It is believed that osteocytes permit mineral movement in and out of regions of bone that are removed from surfaces.

OSTEOCLASTS. Osteoclasts are multinucleated giant cells that are responsible for the resorption of bone (Figs. 244–3 and 244–8). They are probably derived from circulating monocytic precursor cells, which differentiate into the mature osteoclasts by fusion in the bone environment. These cells contain all of the enzymatic components that, when secreted into their environs, solubilize matrix and release calcium and phosphate. Once released, mineral is transported through the osteoclasts into the extracellular fluid and ultimately into the blood. Opinion has varied over the years concerning the relative importance to extracellular homeostasis of osteoclastic resorption of bone and the translocation of mineral from the surface of bone into the extracellular space by surface osteoblasts. It is likely that the major role of osteoclastic bone resorption is in bone remodeling (see below).

Dynamics of Bone

The term "modeling," as applied to bone, denotes processes involved in the formation of the macroscopic skeleton. Thus, modeling ceases at maturity (age 18 to 20). The term "remodeling" denotes those processes, occurring at bone surfaces before and after adult development, that are required to maintain the structural integrity of bone.

Abnormalities of remodeling are responsible for metabolic bone diseases. These abnormalities involve alterations in the balance between bone formation and resorption, which lead to diminished structural integrity of bone and ultimately compromise its function. Normally, in spite of continuous bone remodeling, there is little net gain or loss of skeletal mass after longitudinal growth has ceased (Figs. 244–5 and 244–6). This has led to the view that bone resorption and formation are closely coupled and that this coupling is the result of the coordinated activity of "packets" of interacting osteoblasts and osteoclasts. These packets have been termed "basic multicellular units." The activity of such a unit is characterized by osteoclastic resorption of a defined quantity of bone (on the surface in trabecular bone and by actual excavation in cortical bone), followed by repair of the defect by osteoblasts. During the repair process, collagen (osteoid) is laid down and subsequently mineralized.

Using timed, sequential labeling of bone with orally administered tetracycline (which binds to recently mineralized collagen) and histomorphometric analysis of transiliac bone biopsies from normal adult humans, it has been possible to time the activities of a basic multicellular unit. Estimates indicate that osteoclastic resorption proceeds for about one month in a normal 30-year-old adult, and osteoblastic repair for about three months. The term "sigma" is used to denote the total duration of activity of a typical basic multicellular unit. The concept of sigma has added a new dimension to the understanding of the pathogenesis of metabolic bone disease. Thus, an imbalance between bone formation and resorption could be due not only to alterations in the relative numbers and activities of osteoblasts and osteoclasts but also to abnormalities in the relative duration of the activities of these two cell types.

General Evaluation of Patients with Metabolic Bone Disease

The early detection and treatment of metabolic bone disease are important because it may be difficult or impossible to restore skeletal mass after bone has been lost. This is particularly true of the bone loss that occurs in postmenopausal women and the elderly. It is insidious but causes symptoms only when skeletal mass has decreased to the point that fractures occur with minimal trauma. Establishing bone loss can be difficult because available techniques cannot always detect a decrease in skeletal mass in individual patients. It is necessary, therefore, to have a high index of suspicion for the presence of metabolic bone disease in patients at risk for its development, so that treatment can be instituted early. Since specific metabolic bone diseases are discussed in other chapters, this section will provide only a broad overview of the evaluation of patients with these disorders.

Any one or a combination of the risk factors listed in Table 244–2, especially if accompanied by symptoms such as back pain and muscular weakness or a history of bone fracture with minimal trauma, should suggest the possibility of metabolic bone disease. The extent and type of investigation done should be determined by the specific metabolic bone disease suspected. More than one pathologic process may be involved in producing skeletal disease in an individual patient. Thus, once metabolic bone disease is discovered, the clinician should evaluate the patient for the presence of all of the diseases and risk factors that could alter skeletal metabolism and aggravate the bone disease. In postmenopausal or elderly patients who have sustained a recent fracture with minimal trauma, the cause of the osseous demineralization underlying the fracture should be investigated. Although a generalized decrease in skeletal mass due to the osteoporosis associated with menopause or aging is the most likely cause, the first diagnostic consideration should be osseous malignancy, and such patients should be investigated for multiple myeloma (using immunoelectrophoresis of serum and urine protein, Ch. 163)

TABLE 244–2. MAJOR RISK FACTORS FOR THE DEVELOPMENT OF METABOLIC BONE DISEASE

A. **Physiologic Factors**
 1. Non-black race
 2. Postmenopausal
 3. Aging
B. **Dietary, Environmental, and Physical Factors**
 1. Decreased calcium intake
 2. Decreased phosphate intake
 3. Decreased vitamin D intake
 4. Sunlight deprivation
 5. Immobilization
C. **Drugs**
 1. Corticosteroids
 2. Thyroid hormone
 3. Anticonvulsants
 4. Alcohol
 5. Antacids containing aluminum
 6. Heparin
 7. Cancer chemotherapy
D. **Diseases**
 1. Endocrinologic
  a. Hyperparathyroidism
  b. Hyperthyroidism
  c. Hyperadrenocorticism
  d. Sex hormone deficiency
 2. Gastrointestinal
  a. Intestinal malabsorption
  b. Malabsorption due to gastric or intestinal resection
  c. Chronic obstructive biliary disease
 3. Renal
  a. Functional impairment of any cause
  b. All tubular disorders resulting in calcium or phosphate loss
  c. Possibly nephrosis

and metastatic malignancy (using radionuclide bone scans). The clinician should also assess vitamin D nutritional status and parathyroid function (serum measurements of calcium, phosphorus, magnesium, alkaline phosphatase, 25OHD, and immunoreactive PTH). Hypercalcemia, if found, should be investigated as described in Ch. 247. Hypocalcemia, especially if it is accompanied by hypophosphatemia, suggests the presence of vitamin D deficiency and osteomalacia. Such a diagnosis is confirmed if serum concentrations of 25OHD are low and serum concentrations of immunoreactive PTH and alkaline phosphatase are increased. These findings should prompt an investigation of possible causes of vitamin D deficiency, such as intestinal malabsorption (e.g., a 72-hour stool fat measurement).

If the noted serum measurements are normal and no evidence for malignancy can be found, the next major objective is to establish the extent and location of the osteopenia so that the effects of treatment can be assessed over time. The only clinical measurement of value is patient height. Decreased height usually reflects the progression of spinal crush fractures and is probably the best indication of disease activity. Although lateral x-rays of the spine, done serially, show only gross decreases in bone mineral, they are the only means of directly assessing new vertebral crush fractures. They should be performed initially and repeated routinely every two years or if there is significant recurrence of back pain. Roentgenograms of the proximal femur yield information about the integrity of the femoral neck and trochanter, which are major sites of osteoporotic fractures that can result in permanent incapacitation and even death (10 to 20 per cent) in the elderly. Disappearance of the superior trabecular pattern that traverses the greater trochanter (arrow in grade 3 sketch, Fig. 244–9) signals that osteoporosis is sufficiently severe to place the patient at increased risk for hip fracture. It is probably wise to obtain x-rays of these areas at the initial evaluation of postmenopausal or elderly patients for two reasons. First, if grade 2 or 3 trabecular patterns are present, patients should be cautioned to eliminate hazards that may cause falls in their home environments. Second, they provide a basis for comparison with similar x-rays obtained during long-term follow-up and treatment.

There are several clinically applicable techniques for measuring bone mass. The first involves careful x-rays of the hands and measurement of the endosteal and periosteal diameters of the second to fourth metacarpal bones with a precision caliper. The combined cortical thickness of bones is then determined by subtracting the internal from the external diameter. The precision of this measurement is about ± 2 per cent, and values obtained are reasonable reflections of appendicular skeletal mass. The second technique, single photon absorptiometry, measures the attenuation by bone (usually the radius) of a gamma-ray beam generated by a ^{125}I or ^{247}Am source. The precision of this measurement is also about ± 2 per cent, and values obtained reflect predominantly appendicular skeletal mass.

Two techniques can directly measure the mineral content in almost any bone in the body, although both have been used mainly to assess the axial skeleton. The first technique, dual photon absorptiometry, measures the combined mineral content of several vertebrae in both cortical and trabecular bone, as well as that present in overlying structures (e.g., in calcified abdominal aorta). It uses equipment that can be modified from equipment available in most nuclear medicine units. The second technique, which uses computer-assisted tomography, is much more selective than the first, measuring the mineral content of only vertebral trabecular bone. Both techniques are reasonably precise and accurate.

The clinical usefulness of techniques that measure bone mineral content is unclear. Unfortunately, they cannot definitely exclude the presence of osteoporosis because there is a large overlap in measurements between patients with proved osteoporotic fractures and age-matched subjects without fractures. However, it may be possible to use single measurements to estimate the fracture risk in individual patients, once data concerning the incidence of fracture are available from long-term, prospective follow-up of such patients.

At present, histomorphometric analysis of transiliac bone biopsies has achieved almost the status of a fine art. The procedure is most useful in establishing a diagnosis of osteomalacia (Ch. 246) and in determining if, in a given patient, diminished bone density is associated with significant changes in the duration of bone formation or resorption. Being an invasive procedure with minimal but definite complications, it should be done after consultation with an expert who can ascertain that both the biopsy and the quantitative histomorphometry will be performed adequately and that an informed interpretation of the results will be made available.

Arnaud CD, Kolb FO: The calciotropic hormones and metabolic bone disease. In Greenspan FS, Forsham PH (eds.): Basic and Clinical Endocrinology. Los Altos, CA, Lange Medical Publications, 1986, pp 202–271. *Brief review of the regulation of bone and mineral metabolism and the disorders affecting them. Heavy emphasis is placed on pathophysiology and treatment.*

Aurbach GD, Marx S, Spiegel AM: Parathyroid hormone calcitonin and the calciferols (Ch. 29). Metabolic bone disease (Ch. 30). In Williams RH (ed.): Textbook of Endocrinology. Philadelphia, W. B. Saunders Company, 1985, pp 1137–1255. *Comprehensive review of the basic science of the mineral-regulating hormones and of bone biology. Full and systematic discussion of metabolic bone diseases and disorders of mineral-regulating hormone secretion, metabolism, and action is provided.*

Avioli L, Raisz L: Bone metabolism and disease. In Bondy PK, Rosenberg LE (eds.): Metabolic Control and Disease. Philadelphia, W. B. Saunders Company, 1980, pp 1709–1786. *Provides an excellent, in-depth description of bone metabolism and disease.*

DeGroot LJ (ed.): Endocrinology. Vol 2. New York, Grune & Stratton, 1979, pp 551–692. *Comprehensive review of the basic science of the mineral-regulating hormones, arranged in 13 chapters written by internationally renowned experts. Topics include parathyroid hormone, calcitonin, and vitamin D chemistry, biosynthesis, secretion, metabolism, and action.*

Singer FR: Metabolic bone disease. In Felig P, Baxter JD, Broadus AE, et al. (eds.): Endocrinology and Metabolism. 2nd ed. New York, McGraw-Hill Book Company, 1987, pp 1454–1499. *Brief but complete review of the metabolic bone diseases with emphasis on diagnosis and treatment.*

Stewart AF, Broadus AE: Mineral metabolism. In Felig P, Baxter JD, Broadus AE, et al. (eds.): Endocrinology and Metabolism. 2nd ed. New York, McGraw-Hill Book Company, 1987, pp 1317–1453. *Incisive review of the basic science of the mineral-regulating hormones and diseases of their secretion, metabolism, and actions.*

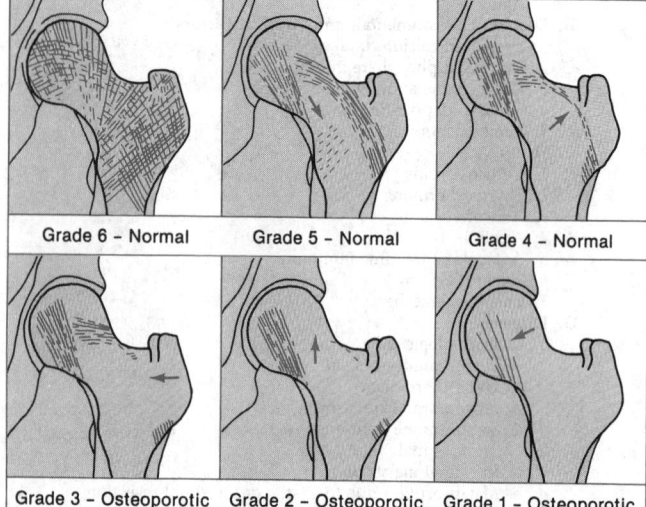

Grade 6 – Normal   Grade 5 – Normal   Grade 4 – Normal

Grade 3 – Osteoporotic   Grade 2 – Osteoporotic   Grade 1 – Osteoporotic

FIGURE 244–9. The effects of increasingly severe osteoporosis on the pattern of trabecular bone in the upper end of the femur. Arrows show progressive radiologic disappearance of trabecular groups. (Adapted from Singh M, et al.: Femoral trabecular-pattern index for evaluation of spinal osteoporosis. Ann Intern Med 77:64, 1972.)

245 VITAMIN D

Daniel D. Bikle

Vitamin D is a steroid hormone with two molecular forms: vitamin D_3 (cholecalciferol), which is produced in the skin, and vitamin D_2 (ergocalciferol), which is derived from the plant sterol ergosterol. Vitamin D_2 is the usual form of vitamin D available for pharmaceutical use, although both vitamin D_2 and D_3 are used as food supplements. Despite subtle differences in physiology and biochemistry, vitamin D_2 and D_3 have equivalent potency and mechanisms of action in humans. In the ensuing discussion, lack of a subscript after the D indicates that both forms of vitamin D are implied.

To achieve biologic potency, vitamin D must be further metabolized. Two of these metabolites, 25-hydroxyvitamin D (25OHD) and 1,25-dihydroxyvitamin D (1,25(OH)$_2$D), are produced by successive hydroxylations; the hepatic enzyme vitamin D 25-hydroxylase catalyzes the formation of 25OHD, and the renal enzyme 25OHD catalyzes the formation of 1-hydroxylase 1,25(OH)$_2$D. Both 25OHD (calcifediol) and 1,25(OH)$_2$D (calcitriol) are available to treat disorders of calcium homeostasis. A third metabolite, 24,25-dihydroxyvitamin D (24,25(OH)$_2$D), also shows promise as a therapeutic agent but as yet is available only for investigational purposes. 24,25(OH)$_2$D, like 1,25(OH)$_2$D, is produced from 25OHD principally in the kidney.

VITAMIN D ENDOCRINE SYSTEM

The vitamin D endocrine system can be divided into three levels (Fig. 245–1): bioavailability of vitamin D from skin and gut, metabolism of vitamin D to its active forms principally by the liver and kidney, and the action of these metabolites on target tissues.

BIOAVAILABILITY. Vitamin D_3 is produced in the skin by a multistep process. Irradiation of 7-dehydrocholesterol by ultraviolet (UV) light converts it to previtamin D_3, which then undergoes thermal isomerization to vitamin D_3. No clear regulation of vitamin D_3 production has been observed other than the amount of UV irradiation that reaches the 7-dehydrocholesterol in the epidermis.

Vitamin D is also available from the diet, as it is commonly used as a food supplement in dairy products. Vitamin D is absorbed principally in the jejunum by a process (chylomicron formation) that is facilitated by bile salts, fatty acids, and monoglycerides. Most of the vitamin D absorbed passes through the lymphatic system before entering the bloodstream. The hydroxylated metabolites of vitamin D (i.e., 25OHD and 1,25(OH)$_2$D) depend less on chylomicron formation for their absorption.

Vitamin D and its metabolites are transported in blood bound mainly to an alpha-globulin called vitamin D–binding protein (DBP). This protein has a higher affinity for 25OHD and 24,25(OH)$_2$D than for vitamin D and 1,25(OH)$_2$D. Since the amount of DBP in blood (5×10^{-6} M) far exceeds that of vitamin D and its metabolites (Table 245–1), 1 per cent or less of the total amount of these metabolites is actually free to diffuse into cells. It is unclear whether DBP serves principally as a circulating reservoir for the vitamin D metabolites in blood or facilitates the transport of these metabolites into target tissues. Changes in DBP levels affect total concentrations of vitamin D metabolites without necessarily affecting the free concentrations. Pregnancy and estrogen increase DBP; liver disease and proteinuria decrease DBP. The relative importance of free versus total concentration of the vitamin D metabolites has not been established.

METABOLISM. *Liver.* The first step in the bioactivation of vitamin D occurs in the liver, where vitamin D 25-hydroxylase converts vitamin D to 25OHD. Since 25OHD production by this cytochrome P450 mixed function oxidase is governed principally by the supply of substrate (i.e., vitamin D), circulating 25OHD levels are a good indicator of vitamin D bioavailability. Hepatic production of 25OHD appears to be well preserved in all but the most severe cases of liver disease unless the vitamin D stores are depleted. Compounds such as phenytoin and phenobarbital, however, which induce drug-metabolizing enzymes in the liver, alter the hepatic metabolism of vitamin D in a manner that may lead to clinical bone disease in subjects with marginal vitamin D stores.

Kidney. The 25OHD produced by the liver is further metabolized to 1,25(OH)$_2$D and 24,25(OH)$_2$D, principally in the kidney. Little if any 1,25(OH)$_2$D is produced outside the kidney (except by the placenta) under normal circumstances, although other tissues, such as bone, cartilage, skin, and

FIGURE 245–1. The vitamin D endocrine system. Vitamin D is made available to the body by photogenesis in the skin and absorption from the intestine. Vitamin D is then hydroxylated in the liver to 25OHD, then in the kidney to 1,25(OH)$_2$D and 24,25(OH)$_2$D. The active vitamin D metabolites act on different tissues to produce a variety of responses. The three target tissues principally responsible for calcium (Ca) and phosphate (Pi) homeostasis are kidney, bone, and intestine. Endocrine tissues such as the parathyroid gland (PTG) and anterior pituitary are also target tissues. Their hormones, parathyroid hormone (PTH), prolactin (PRL), and growth hormone (GH), help regulate vitamin D metabolism in the kidney. In addition, PTH has a direct effect on bone and kidney regulation of calcium and phosphate homeostasis. (Reproduced with permission from Bikle DD: The vitamin D endocrine system. In Stollerman GH, et al. (eds.): Advances in Internal Medicine, Volume 27. Copyright © 1982 by Year Book Medical Publishers, Inc. Chicago.)

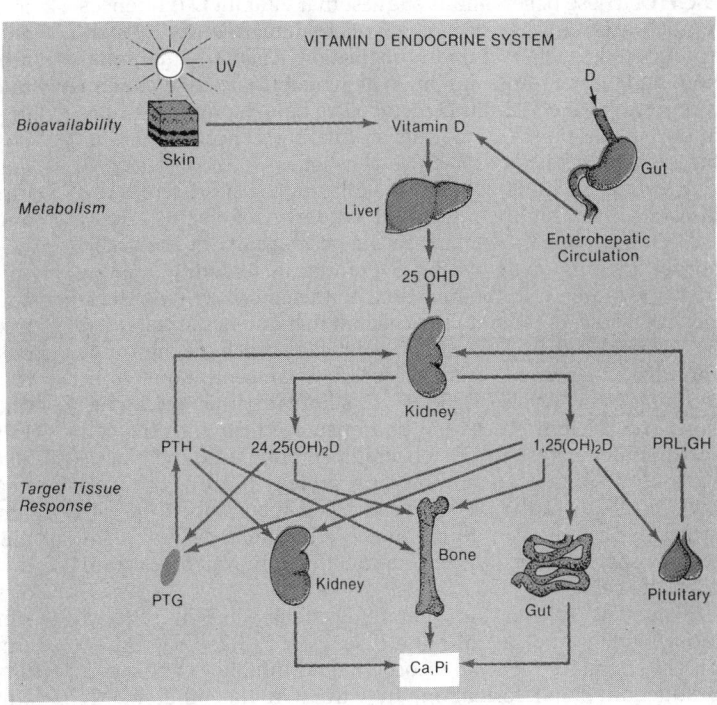

TABLE 245–1. VITAMIN D AND ITS METABOLITES

Name	Abbreviation	Generic Name	Serum Concentration*
Vitamin D	D	Calciferol	1.6 ± 0.4 ng/ml
Vitamin D$_3$	D$_3$	a) Cholecalciferol	
Vitamin D$_2$	D$_2$	b) Ergocalciferol	
25 hydroxy-vitamin D	25OHD	Calcifediol	26.5 ± 5.3 ng/ml
1,25 dihydroxy-vitamin D	1,25(OH)$_2$D	Calcitriol	34.1 ± 9.8 pg/ml
24,25 dihydroxy-vitamin D	24,25(OH)$_2$D		1.3 ± 0.4 ng/ml
25,26 dihydroxy-vitamin D	25,26(OH)$_2$D		0.5 ± 0.1 ng/ml

*Values differ somewhat from laboratory to laboratory, depending on the methodology used and the sunlight exposure and dietary intake of vitamin D in the population studied. Children tend to have higher 1,25(OH)$_2$D levels than adults. Data are derived from Lambert PW, Fu IY, Kaetzel DM, et al.: Assay for multiple vitamin D metabolites. In Bikle DD (ed.): Assay of Calcium Regulating Hormones. New York, Springer-Verlag, 1983, pp 99–124.

intestine, may produce 24,25(OH)$_2$D (and, possibly, 1,25(OH)$_2$D) under some circumstances. Lymphomatous and sarcoid tissue may also contain 1-hydroxylase activity. Both the 1-hydroxylase and the 24-hydroxylase in the kidney are cytochrome P450 mixed function oxidases located exclusively in the mitochondria of the proximal renal tubule. Their activities are closely regulated by a variety of ions and hormones, the most important of which are calcium, phosphate, 1,25(OH)$_2$D itself, and parathyroid hormone (PTH). Low serum calcium and phosphate levels and elevated PTH levels stimulate 1,25(OH)$_2$D production. High 1,25(OH)$_2$D levels inhibit 1,25(OH)$_2$D production but increase 24,25(OH)$_2$D production. Other hormones such as prolactin and growth hormone may also stimulate 1,25(OH)$_2$D production, but whether these hormones are important in the control of 1,25(OH)$_2$D production under normal physiologic conditions is not known.

TARGET TISSUE RESPONSE. Bone, gut, and kidney are the primary target tissues for vitamin D, but many other tissues, including the pituitary, parathyroid glands, pancreas, brain, activated lymphocytes, thymocytes, skin, and a variety of tumors, contain a specific receptor for 1,25(OH)$_2$D and respond to it by a change in function. Muscle contains no receptors for 1,25(OH)$_2$D but appears to be a target tissue for 25OHD. These observations suggest that vitamin D influences a much greater range of biologic phenomena than previously appreciated, such as immunoregulation, cellular differentiation, and neural transmission. Whether all tissues that contain receptors for the vitamin D metabolites have a physiologically important response to normal circulating concentrations of the metabolites has not been established.

Intestine. 1,25(OH)$_2$D regulates calcium transport across the intestine in a highly integrated sequence of events. First, 1,25(OH)$_2$D appears to increase the permeability of the brush border membrane to calcium, permitting calcium to enter from the lumen into the intestinal epithelial cell down a steep electrochemical gradient. The calcium that enters the cell must be accumulated by subcellular organelles, such as the mitochondria, to prevent cytosolic calcium concentrations from reaching toxic levels. 1,25(OH)$_2$D stimulates this accumulation. The calcium must then be transported through the cell and pumped across the basolateral membrane into the bloodstream. A unique calcium-binding protein (CaBP), induced by 1,25(OH)$_2$D in the intestine as well as in a number of other target tissues, appears to modulate intracellular calcium concentrations, perhaps by facilitating the removal of calcium from the cell.

Bone. The role of the vitamin D metabolites in calcium movement in and out of bone is less clear. 1,25(OH)$_2$D is a potent stimulator of bone resorption and inhibitor of collagen production (bone formation) in vitro. On the other hand,

24,25(OH)$_2$D may stimulate bone and cartilage formation without stimulating bone resorption. These results have engendered a controversy as to whether all the effects of vitamin D on bone are mediated by 1,25(OH)$_2$D or whether other metabolites, 24,25(OH)$_2$D in particular, have a unique biologic role.

Kidney. Although the vitamin D metabolites may play a role, independent of PTH, in regulating renal calcium and phosphate excretion, this role has not been well defined.

MEASUREMENT IN SERUM

Most assays for the vitamin D metabolites use naturally occurring binding proteins. Radioimmunoassays employing poly- or monoclonal antibodies and a bioassay evaluating resorption from cultured bone in vitro have also been developed. The principal difficulty in measuring vitamin D metabolites is that chromatographic separation of the metabolites from each other and from other interfering substances is required. Nevertheless, most laboratories generally agree on the measurements of 25OHD and 1,25(OH)$_2$D (Table 245–1). Measurement of vitamin D itself remains difficult because of its poor solubility in aqueous solutions and modest affinity for the binding proteins used in the assays.

HYPOVITAMINOSIS D

Vitamin D deficiency results from insufficient vitamin D in the diet, insufficient production of vitamin D in the skin, inadequate absorption of vitamin D from the diet, or abnormal conversion of vitamin D to its bioactive metabolites. Vitamin D deficiency presents clinically as rickets in children and osteomalacia in adults. This subject is discussed in detail in Ch. 246.

HYPERVITAMINOSIS D

Hypervitaminosis D may occur in three general settings: (1) excessive consumption, usually for therapeutic purposes, of vitamin D, vitamin D analogues (such as dihydrotachysterol), or vitamin D metabolites; (2) the abnormal conversion of vitamin D to its biologically active metabolites, as occurs in sarcoidosis and possibly other granulomatous diseases; or (3) a change in the sensitivity of the target tissue to vitamin D, as can occur with the remission of a variety of gastrointestinal diseases associated with calcium malabsorption. The initial signs and symptoms of vitamin D intoxication include weakness, lethargy, headaches, nausea, and polyuria and are attributable to the hypercalcemia and hypercalciuria. Ectopic calcification may occur, particularly in the kidneys, resulting in nephrolithiasis or nephrocalcinosis; other sites include blood vessels, heart, lungs, and skin. Infants appear to be quite susceptible to vitamin D intoxication and may develop disseminated arteriosclerosis, supravalvular aortic stenosis, and renal acidosis.

The dose of vitamin D required to produce toxicity varies among patients, reflecting differences in absorption, storage, and subsequent metabolism of the vitamin as well as in target tissue response to the active metabolites. For example, an elderly patient with senile osteoporosis and a low turnover rate of bone also tends to have a reduced ability to absorb calcium in the intestine and a reduced ability to produce 1,25(OH)$_2$D in the kidney. Such a patient can usually ingest 50,000 to 100,000 IU of vitamin D per day without developing hypercalcemia or hypercalciuria. In contrast, a patient of similar age with a similar degree of osteoporosis but in whom the osteoporosis develops as a result of primary hyperparathyroidism would almost certainly be harmed by this amount of vitamin D. In the latter patient, the ability of vitamin D to stimulate bone resorption and intestinal calcium absorption is enhanced in part because of the greater rates of 1,25(OH)$_2$D production and bone turnover observed in primary hyperparathyroidism. Patients with sarcoidosis appear to develop vitamin D intoxication because 1,25(OH)$_2$D production in the abnormal tissue is not subject to the normal feedback mechanisms that regulate renal production of 1,25(OH)$_2$D. Analogues of vitamin D, such as dihydrotachysterol, or the renal metabolite of vitamin D, 1,25(OH)$_2$D, which bypass the normal rate-limiting step of vitamin D bioactivation (the renal 1α-hydroxylase), are more likely than vitamin D or 25OHD to result in hypercalcemia if used in excess.

Hypervitaminosis D is treated by stopping the administration of vitamin D or its analogues or metabolites. If the hypercalcemia is severe, the patient should be placed on a low-calcium diet and given glucocorticoids (e.g., 60 mg of prednisone every day) and generous amounts of fluids. Acute hypercalcemia, when symptomatic, can be treated with saline and furosemide diuresis, as described under the general management of hypercalcemia (Ch. 247). Hypercalcemia lasts for only a few days when caused by excess 1,25(OH)$_2$D, but it may persist for weeks or months when caused by excess vitamin D. The hypercalcemia of sarcoidosis tends to respond within days to glucocorticoid therapy.

Adams JS, Singer FR, Gacad MA, et al.: Isolation and structural identification of 1,25-dihydroxyvitamin D$_3$ produced by cultured alveolar macrophages in sarcoidosis. J Clin Endocrinol Metab 60:960, 1985. *Provides direct evidence that sarcoid macrophages make 1,25(OH)$_2$D.*

Bell NH: Vitamin D-endocrine system. J Clin Invest 76:1, 1985. *A short, well-referenced and up-to-date review of the subject.*

Bikle DD, Morrissey RL, Zolock DT, et al.: The intestinal response to vitamin D. Rev Physiol Biochem Pharmacol 89:63, 1981. *A comprehensive discussion of intestinal calcium and phosphate transport and the role of 1,25(OH)$_2$D in this process.*

Bikle DD, Nemanic MK, Gee EA, et al.: 1,25-dihydroxyvitamin D$_3$ production by human keratinocytes. J Clin Invest 78:557, 1986. *Normal skin cells make 1,25(OH)$_2$D and 24,25(OH)$_2$D by a process regulated by parathyroid hormone and 1,25(OH)$_2$D in a manner similar to the renal production of 1,25(OH)$_2$D and 24,25(OH)$_2$D.*

Fraser DR: Regulation of the metabolism of vitamin D. Physiol Rev 60:551, 1980. *A thorough, well-balanced review of vitamin D metabolism in the liver and kidney.*

Lambert PW, Stern PH, Avioli RC, et al.: Evidence for extrarenal production of 1α,25-dihydroxyvitamin D in man. J Clin Invest 69:722, 1982. *The demonstration of 1,25(OH)$_2$D levels in anephric humans and the suggestion that vitamin D treatment increases these levels.*

Lee DBN, Zawada ET, Kleeman CR: The pathophysiology and clinical aspects of hypercalcemic disorders. West J Med 129:278, 1978. *This article discusses all the major hypercalcemic disorders, including the diagnosis and treatment of hypervitaminosis D.*

Norman AW, Roth J, Orci L: The vitamin D endocrine system: Steroid metabolism, hormone receptors and biological response (calcium binding proteins). Endocrine Rev 3:331, 1982. *A thorough compilation of the complexity of vitamin D metabolism and the diversity of vitamin D action.*

246 OSTEOMALACIA AND RICKETS

Daniel D. Bikle

DEFINITIONS

Osteomalacia and rickets are caused by the abnormal mineralization of bone and cartilage. Osteomalacia refers to the defect that occurs in bone in which the epiphyseal plates have closed (i.e., in adults), whereas rickets refers to the defect that occurs in growing bone (i.e., in children). Abnormal mineralization in growing bone affects the transformation of cartilage into bone at the zone of provisional calcification. As a result, an enormous profusion of disorganized, nonmineralized, degenerating cartilage appears in this region, leading to widening of the epiphyseal plate (observed radiologically as a widened radiolucent zone) with flaring or cupping and irregularity of the epiphyseal-metaphyseal junctions. This latter problem gives rise to the clinically obvious beaded swellings along the costochondral junctions (rachitic rosary) and the swelling at the ends of the long bones. Growth is retarded by the failure to make new bone. Once bone growth has ceased (i.e., after closure of the epiphyseal plates), the clinical evidence for defective mineralization becomes more subtle, and special diagnostic procedures may be required for its detection.

PATHOGENESIS

The best known cause of abnormal bone mineralization is vitamin D deficiency. Vitamin D, through its biologically active metabolites, insures that the calcium and phosphate concentrations in the extracellular milieu are adequate for mineralization to occur. Vitamin D also may permit osteoblasts to produce a bone matrix that can be mineralized and then allows them to mineralize that matrix in a normal fashion. Phosphate deficiency can also cause defective mineralization. It may act independently or in conjunction with other predisposing abnormalities, since most hypophosphatemic disorders associated with osteomalacia or rickets also affect the vitamin D endocrine system. Dietary calcium deficiency has been implicated as a cause of rickets and may contribute to the osteomalacia and osteoporosis found in elderly patients. Osteomalacia or rickets may develop despite adequate levels of calcium, phosphate, and vitamin D if the bone matrix cannot undergo normal mineralization. For example, the deficiency in alkaline phosphatase in patients with hypophosphatasia can cause a defect in mineralization. This enzyme cleaves pyrophosphate, an inhibitor of bone mineralization, and a deficiency results in reduced removal of this inhibitor. Finally, drugs such as etidronate and heavy metals such as aluminum can interfere with mineralization and lead to osteomalacia or rickets.

Table 246–1 lists diseases associated with osteomalacia and rickets according to the presumed mechanism responsible for the mineralization defect. Diseases that appear under multiple headings affect bone mineralization via multiple mechanisms. It is important to understand the mechanism by which a particular disease interferes with bone mineralization in order to choose appropriate diagnostic procedures and therapy.

Disorders in the Vitamin D Endocrine System

The exact mechanism(s) by which vitamin D maintains normal bone development is unknown, but disorders in the vitamin D endocrine system are the leading cause of rickets and osteomalacia through decreased bioavailability of vitamin D, abnormal metabolism of vitamin D, and abnormal response of target tissues to the biologically active vitamin D metabolites.

Decreased Bioavailability

REDUCED SUNLIGHT EXPOSURE. The human skin can generate adequate amounts of vitamin D if exposed to sufficient ultraviolet irradiation. In countries with limited sunlight, however, or where the population dresses in a fashion that reduces exposure to sunlight, circulating levels of vitamin D metabolites are often low. These low levels may help explain why the incidence of osteomalacia is higher in Great Britain, the Scandinavian countries, the Middle East, and India than in the United States.

NUTRITIONAL VITAMIN D DEFICIENCY. The fortification of dairy products with vitamin D has made nutritional vitamin D–deficient rickets uncommon in the United States, although it is still prevalent in other parts of the world. Even in the United States vitamin D deficiency may occur in children of vegetarian mothers who avoid milk products (and presumably have reduced vitamin D stores) and in children who are not weaned to vitamin D–supplemented milk by age two. The contribution of nutritional vitamin D deficiency to osteomalacia in elderly people is unknown. Osteomalacia has

TABLE 246–1. THE OSTEOMALACIC SYNDROMES*

A. Disorders in the vitamin D endocrine system
  1. Decreased bioavailability
    Insufficient sunlight exposure
    Nutritional vitamin D deficiency
    Nephrotic syndrome (urinary loss)
    Malabsorption (fecal loss)
      Billroth type II gastrectomy
      Sprue
      Regional enteritis
      Jejunoileal bypass
      Pancreatic insufficiency
      Cholestatic disorders
      Cholestyramine
  2. Abnormal metabolism
    Liver disease
    Chronic renal failure
    Vitamin D–dependent rickets type I
    Tumoral hypophosphatemic osteomalacia
    X-linked hypophosphatemia
    Hypoparathyroidism (?)
    Chronic acidosis (?)
    Anticonvulsants
  3. Abnormal target tissue response
    Vitamin D–dependent rickets type II
    Gastrointestinal disorders
B. Disorders of phosphate homeostasis
  1. Decreased intestinal absorption
    Malnutrition
    Malabsorption
    Antacids containing aluminum hydroxide
  2. Increased renal loss
    X-linked hypophosphatemic rickets
    Tumoral hypophosphatemic osteomalacia
    De Toni-Debré-Fanconi (phosphaturia, aminoaciduria, glycosuria,
      bicarbonaturia)
    Cystinosis
    Oculocerebrorenal syndrome (Lowe's syndrome)
    Paraproteinemias
    Wilson's disease
    Glycogen storage diseases
    Galactosemia
    Tyrosinemia
    Cadmium poisoning
    Neurofibromatosis
C. Calcium deficiency
  1. Dietary insufficiency
  2. Excessive renal loss (?)
  3. Malabsorption of calcium (?)
D. Primary disorders of bone matrix
  1. Hypophosphatasia
  2. Fibrogenesis imperfecta ossium
  3. Axial osteomalacia
E. Inhibitors of mineralization
  1. Aluminum
    Chronic renal failure
    Total parenteral nutrition
  2. Etidronate
  3. Phenytoin (?)
  4. Fluoride (?)

*This table categorizes diseases that produce osteomalacia according to the presumed mechanism(s) by which bone mineralization is inhibited. A question mark indicates that the association of the disease to osteomalacia or the mechanism by which it produces osteomalacia is not established.

been observed in 25 to 30 per cent of bone biopsies from elderly patients who have suffered hip fractures in Scandinavia and Great Britain. Most likely, both reduced vitamin D intake and reduced exposure to sunlight contribute to the development of osteomalacia in the elderly.

NEPHROTIC SYNDROME. Even when vitamin D intake is adequate, vitamin D and its metabolites can be lost in the urine. The vitamin D metabolites in serum are tightly bound to an alpha-globulin called vitamin D–binding protein (DBP). Patients with the nephrotic syndrome may lose substantial amounts of DBP into their urine and consequently have very low circulating levels of the vitamin D metabolites. Although the total concentration of all the vitamin D metabolites is reduced in this situation, the free (or unbound) concentration may be normal. Thus, the measurement of the total concentration may be misleading as to the severity of the vitamin D deficiency. The incidence of osteomalacia in patients with the

nephrotic syndrome is unknown; osteomalacia has only recently been recognized as a complication of this renal disease.

MALABSORPTION. Fecal loss of vitamin D and its metabolites occurs in patients with malabsorption for several reasons. Ingested vitamin D is absorbed primarily in chylomicrons; disorders that involve the biliary tract, pancreas, or mid to distal portions of the small intestine reduce the efficiency of this process (Ch. 104). Endogenous vitamin D and its metabolites undergo enterohepatic circulation; disorders of the distal small bowel disrupt this circulation. In cholestatic disorders, urinary excretion of vitamin D metabolites is increased, and intestinal absorption is decreased. Drugs, such as cholestyramine, that are used in the treatment of cholestatic disorders may compound the problem by binding to the vitamin D metabolites and enhancing their fecal excretion. The resulting bone disease is often a combination of osteomalacia and osteoporosis. The prevalence of osteomalacia in patients with cholestatic and gastrointestinal disorders varies from country to country. It appears to be higher in Great Britain and Northern Europe than in the United States. Fully 25 to 50 per cent of British and European patients who have undergone Billroth type II gastrectomy or jejunoileal bypass or who have cholestatic liver disease or inflammatory bowel disease have osteomalacia when evaluated by bone biopsy.

Abnormal Metabolism

LIVER DISEASE. The hepatic production of 25-hydroxyvitamin D (25OHD) is not tightly controlled. Neither cholestatic nor parenchymal liver disease has much effect on 25OHD production. The low levels of circulating 25OHD found in patients with liver disease can usually be attributed to reduced hepatic synthesis of DBP, poor nutrition, or malabsorption rather than to failure by the liver to metabolize vitamin D. As in patients with the nephrotic syndrome, the low total concentrations of the vitamin D metabolites in patients with liver disease may reflect the low levels of DBP and not a true state of vitamin D deficiency.

CHRONIC RENAL FAILURE (see also Ch. 78). Metabolism of 25OHD to 1,25-dihydroxyvitamin D (1,25(OH)$_2$D) and 24,25-dihydroxyvitamin D (24,25(OH)$_2$D) in the kidney is tightly regulated. Renal disease results in reduced circulating levels of both these metabolites. With the reduction in 1,25(OH)$_2$D levels, intestinal calcium absorption falls, and bone resorption appears to become less sensitive to parathyroid hormone (PTH)—a result that leads to hypocalcemia. Phosphate excretion by the diseased kidney is decreased, resulting in hyperphosphatemia and aggravation of the hypocalcemia. As a consequence, hyperparathyroidism develops, facilitated by the fact that the levels of the vitamin D metabolites are too low to inhibit parathyroid hormone (PTH) secretion. The net effect of deficient 1,25(OH)$_2$D and 24,25(OH)$_2$D and excessive PTH on bone is complex. Patients may have osteitis fibrosa (reflecting excessive PTH), osteomalacia (in part reflecting vitamin D deficiency), or a combination of the two. One particularly debilitating form of renal osteodystrophy is found in a small percentage of patients in whom only osteomalacia occurs. These patients have normal or only modestly elevated levels of PTH and alkaline phosphatase; hypercalcemia, especially after small doses of 1,25(OH)$_2$D, and refractoriness to 1,25(OH)$_2$D therapy are often found. Such patients have increased aluminum content in their bones, particularly in the zone where mineralization is occurring (calcification front).

VITAMIN D–DEPENDENT RICKETS TYPE I. Vitamin D–dependent rickets type I, or pseudo–vitamin D deficiency, is a rare, autosomal recessive disease in which there is a low level of 1,25(OH)$_2$D resulting from a selective deficiency in the renal production of 1,25(OH)$_2$D. Although affected patients do not respond to doses of vitamin D that are adequate to treat vitamin D deficiency (i.e., 400 to 4000 IU per day), they do respond to moderate doses (4000 to 40,000 IU per day) of vitamin D or physiologic doses (0.5 to 1.0 μg per day) of 1,25(OH)$_2$D.

TUMOR-INDUCED HYPOPHOSPHATEMIC OSTEO-MALACIA. Certain unusual tumors (usually mesenchymal) produce osteomalacia associated with low serum levels of phosphorus and 1,25(OH)$_2$D and increased phosphaturia. The cause of this syndrome is unknown, but it is presumed that a humoral product of the tumor suppresses both 1,25(OH)$_2$D production and phosphate reabsorption in the kidney. Removal of the tumor reverses the abnormalities.

X-LINKED HYPOPHOSPHATEMIA. X-linked hypophosphatemia (vitamin D–resistant rickets, or VDRR) is characterized by renal phosphate wasting, hypophosphatemia, and a subtle decrease in 1,25(OH)$_2$D production. Although most cases are diagnosed in childhood and have an X-linked dominant form of inheritance, sporadic adult cases and autosomal transmission occur. Most patients have 1,25(OH)$_2$D levels that are inappropriately low for the degree of hypophosphatemia, which ordinarily increases 1,25(OH)$_2$D production. Treatment with oral phosphate and vitamin D suppresses 1,25(OH)$_2$D to even lower levels. The primary abnormality in these patients is thought to be a defect in renal tubular phosphate transport, resulting in renal phosphate wasting. This defect may secondarily alter vitamin D metabolism. X-linked hypophosphatemia is a fairly common form of metabolic bone disease which should be suspected in all individuals who have low levels of serum phosphorus and evidence of bone disease.

HYPOPARATHYROIDISM. Parathyroid hormone is a major stimulator of 1,25(OH)$_2$D production. One would expect osteomalacia to develop when the hormone is absent, because of the reduction in 1,25(OH)$_2$D production. However, osteomalacia appears to be a rare complication of hypoparathyroidism.

CHRONIC METABOLIC ACIDOSIS. Acute metabolic acidosis results in reduced 1,25(OH)$_2$D production. Although chronic metabolic acidosis is associated with osteomalacia, especially when accompanied by renal loss of phosphate and bicarbonate (as in proximal renal tubular acidosis), it is unclear whether chronic metabolic acidosis has a direct effect on the renal metabolism of vitamin D. Bicarbonate therapy alone is effective in treating the osteomalacia associated with renal tubular acidosis and ureterosigmoidostomy, although the addition of 0.25 to 1 mg of vitamin D per day may facilitate healing.

ANTICONVULSANTS. Phenytoin and phenobarbital induce drug-metabolizing enzymes in the liver that alter the hepatic metabolism of vitamin D. This effect may account for the lower circulating levels of 25OHD found in patients treated with anticonvulsants. Surprisingly, these drugs do not lead to a reduction in 1,25(OH)$_2$D levels. Chronic anticonvulsant therapy does not seem to lead to clinically significant osteomalacia unless accompanied by other predisposing factors such as inadequate sunlight exposure or poor nutrition.

Abnormal Target Tissue Response

VITAMIN D–DEPENDENT RICKETS TYPE II. Vitamin D–dependent rickets type II is a rare condition that occurs in childhood and is not responsive to even huge doses of vitamin D. Unlike patients with vitamin D–dependent rickets type I (see Abnormal Metabolism, above), children with type II disease have high circulating levels of 1,25(OH)$_2$D. Their problem involves an abnormality in the number, affinity, or functions of the intracellular 1,25(OH)$_2$D receptor.

GASTROINTESTINAL DISORDERS. Less exotic examples of abnormal target tissue response include a variety of gastrointestinal diseases, such as sprue, short bowel, and regional enteritis, in which calcium and phosphate malabsorption occurs not only because of vitamin D deficiency but

also because of decreased absorptive surface, steatorrhea, and rapid transit time.

Disorders of Phosphate Homeostasis

Chronic hypophosphatemia may lead to rickets or osteomalacia independently of other predisposing abnormalities. The principal diseases in which hypophosphatemia is associated with osteomalacia or rickets, however, also include other abnormalities that can interfere with bone mineralization. Chronic phosphate depletion is caused by decreased intestinal absorption or increased renal clearance. Acute hypophosphatemia can result from movement of phosphate into cells (e.g., after infusion of insulin and glucose), but this condition is transient and does not result in bone disease (see Ch. 207).

Decreased Intestinal Absorption

MALNUTRITION. Seventy to 90 per cent of dietary phosphate is absorbed, primarily in the jejunum. This process is not tightly regulated, although vitamin D, at least in animal models, stimulates phosphate absorption. Meat and dairy products are the principal dietary sources of phosphate, and vegetarian diets that exclude them can cause phosphate deficiency. The incidence of osteomalacia in vegetarians who avoid all meat and dairy products is unknown. Since these dietary practices also lead to decreased vitamin D intake, such individuals may be predisposed to bone disease.

MALABSORPTION. Intrinsic small bowel disease and surgical rearrangement of the small bowel interfere with phosphate absorption and, if coupled with diarrhea or steatorrhea, can result in phosphate depletion. The hypophosphatemia may contribute to the osteomalacia seen in such patients, especially when vitamin D levels are reduced (see Decreased Bioavailability of Vitamin D, above).

ALUMINUM HYDROXIDE ANTACIDS. A number of widely used antacids (for example, Mylanta, Maalox, Basaljel, and Amphojel) contain aluminum hydroxide, which binds phosphate and prevents its absorption. Patients who ingest large amounts of these antacids may become depleted in phosphate. This mechanism may contribute to the severity of the osteomalacia observed in patients with chronic renal failure and in those who have undergone partial gastrectomy but who continue to ingest large quantities of antacids (see Ch. 249).

Increased Renal Loss

Eighty-five to 90 per cent of the phosphate filtered by the glomerulus is reabsorbed, primarily in the proximal tubule. This process is regulated by PTH, which reduces renal tubular phosphate reabsorption, and probably also by vitamin D, which appears to increase renal tubular phosphate reabsorption. Many diseases that affect renal handling of phosphate are associated with osteomalacia. X-linked hypophosphatemia and tumoral hypophosphatemic osteomalacia have been described above. The de Toni-Debré-Fanconi syndrome is also associated with osteomalacia (Ch. 84). It includes a heterogeneous group of disorders characterized by phosphaturia, aminoaciduria, glycosuria, and bicarbonaturia, and frequently by mild acidosis and hypercalciuria. In general, the osteomalacia or rickets associated with these proximal tubular disorders responds only to large doses of vitamin D with correction of the acidosis and hypophosphatemia as needed. The associated bone disease is most likely the result of a combination of systemic acidosis, hypophosphatemia, and abnormal vitamin D metabolism.

Calcium Deficiency

Calcium deficiency may contribute to the mineralization defect that complicates gastrointestinal disease and proximal tubular disorders, but it is less well established as a cause of osteomalacia than is vitamin D or phosphate deficiency. In one carefully performed study of children who ingested a low-calcium diet, there was clinical, biochemical, and histologic evidence of osteomalacia. The serum phosphorus and 25OHD levels were normal, but the serum calcium levels were low. Since intestinal absorption of calcium decreases with age, the daily requirement for calcium increases from approximately 800 mg in young adults to 1400 mg in the elderly. Calcium deficiency can result not only from inadequate dietary intake but also from excessive fecal and urinary losses.

Primary Disorders of the Bone Matrix

Intrinsic disorders of bone in which matrix is produced but not normally mineralized are rare. Three diseases appear to fit this category, but none is well understood.

Hypophosphatasia

Hypophosphatasia, transmitted in an autosomal recessive pattern, usually presents with a severe form of rickets in children, or merely as a predisposition to fractures in adults. The biochemical hallmarks are low serum (and tissue) levels of alkaline phosphatase and increased urinary levels of phosphoethanolamine. The reason why these patients develop osteomalacia or rickets is unclear, but the following mechanism has been suggested. Skeletal alkaline phosphatase cleaves pyrophosphate, an inhibitor of bone mineralization; patients deficient in alkaline phosphatase may be unable to hydrolyze this inhibitor and so develop a mineralization defect.

Fibrogenesis Imperfecta Ossium

Fibrogenesis imperfecta ossium is a rare, painful disorder that affects middle-aged males in what appears to be a sporadic fashion. Serum alkaline phosphatase is increased. The bones have a dense, amorphous, mottled appearance radiologically and a disorganized arrangement of collagen with decreased birefringence histologically. Presumably, the disorganized collagen matrix retards normal bone mineralization.

Axial Osteomalacia

Unlike fibrogenesis imperfecta ossium, axial osteomalacia is not painful, involves only the axial skeleton, shows no disorganization of collagen on bone biopsy, and is not associated with increased serum alkaline phosphatase. The reason for the mineralization disorder in this rare disease is uncertain.

Inhibitors of Mineralization

Several drugs are known to cause osteomalacia or rickets by inhibiting mineralization, but in no case is the mechanism fully understood.

Aluminum

Patients on hemodialysis are exposed to aluminum in the dialysate if tap water is used and through the antacid preparations used to control serum phosphorus. Most develop bone disease. Bone biopsies show a correlation between the extent of osteomalacia in these patients and the amount of aluminum deposited in bone. It is likely that the aluminum blocks normal mineralization. Severely affected patients respond to a reduction in their exposure to or body stores of the metal.

Many patients who are treated by total parenteral nutrition for extended periods of time develop bone disease characterized by osteomalacia. In some cases the aluminum content of the casein hydrolysate used to provide amino acids is high. Replacement of casein hydrolysate with purified amino acids may correct or prevent this complication.

Etidronate

Etidronate, the only diphosphonate available for clinical use in the United States, produces osteomalacia at doses greater than 5 to 10 mg per kilogram of body weight. Therefore, the dose must be limited. Etidronate affects osteoblast function and inhibits calcium phosphate crystallization. It is unclear why this drug and not other diphosphonates results in osteomalacia.

Phenytoin

As discussed previously (see Anticonvulsants), phenytoin therapy may cause osteomalacia by inducing enzymes that alter the hepatic metabolism of vitamin D. In addition, phenytoin directly and adversely affects bone mineral metabolism in animals. This effect may also contribute to bone disease.

Fluoride

Fluoride stimulates bone formation, but if it is administered in high doses without adequate calcium supplementation, the bone is poorly mineralized. The mechanism(s) by which fluoride alters osteoblast function and bone mineralization is unknown.

DIAGNOSIS

In children, the presentation of rickets is generally obvious from a combination of clinical and radiologic evidence. The diagnostic challenge is to determine the etiology. The most common causes—malabsorption, liver disease, chronic renal failure, X-linked hypophosphatemic rickets, and vitamin D deficiency—are readily distinguished on the basis of history, clinical findings, and routine analyses of blood and urine.

In adults the clinical, radiologic, and biochemical evidence for osteomalacia is often subtle. In situations in which osteomalacia should be suspected (malnutrition, liver disease, malabsorption, renal failure, and unexplained osteopenia), the clinician must decide whether to biopsy the bone for histomorphometric examination. This decision must rest on the availability of resources to perform the biopsy and to evaluate the specimen, the index of suspicion coupled with the lack of certainty from other diagnostic procedures, and the degree to which the therapeutic approach will be altered by the additional information.

Clinical Features

The clinical presentation of rickets depends on the age of the patient and, to some extent, the etiology of the syndrome (Fig. 246–1). The affected infant or young child may be apathetic, listless, weak, hypotonic, and growing poorly. A soft, somewhat misshapen head with widened sutures and frontal bossing may be observed. Eruption of teeth may be delayed, and teeth that do appear may be pitted and poorly mineralized. The enlargement and cupping of the costochondral junctions produce the "rachitic rosary" on the thorax. The tug of the diaphragm against the softened lower ribs may produce an indentation at the point of insertion of the diaphragm (Harrison's groove). Muscle hypotonia can result in a pronounced pot belly and a waddling gait. The limbs may become bowed, and joints may swell because of flaring at the ends of the long bones (including phalanges and metacarpals). Pathologic fractures may occur in patients with florid rickets.

After the epiphyses have closed, the clinical signs of rickets or osteomalacia are subtle and cannot be relied upon to make the diagnosis. Patients with severe osteomalacia, such as occurs with aluminum intoxication, complain of bone pain and muscle weakness. Difficulty climbing stairs or rising from chairs may be reported. Such individuals may have a history of multiple fractures. However, osteomalacia often will be diagnosed by bone histomorphometry in patients who lack obvious symptoms in their musculoskeletal system.

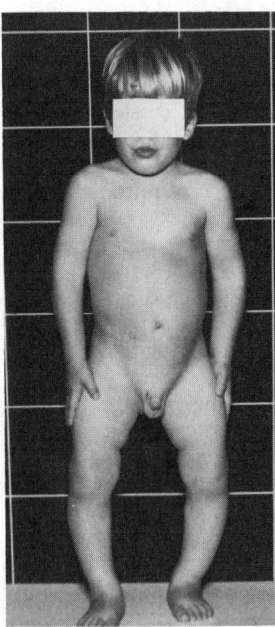 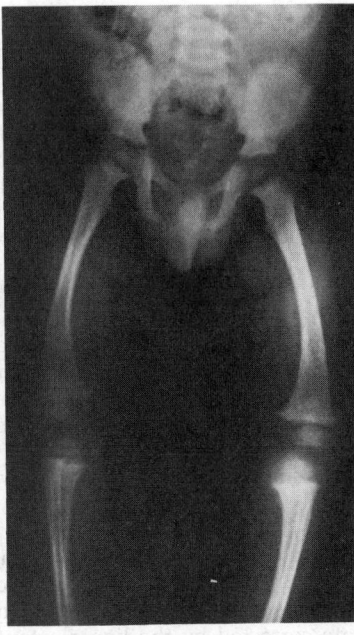

A   **B**

FIGURE 246–1. The clinical (*A*) and radiologic (*B*) appearance of a young boy with X-linked hypophosphatemic rickets. The most striking abnormalities are the bowing of the legs, apparent in both femora and tibiae, with flaring of the ends of these bones at the knee. (Photographs courtesy of Dr. Sara B. Arnaud.)

Radiologic Features

The radiologic features of rickets, like the clinical manifestations, can be quite striking, especially in the young child. In growing bone, the radiolucent epiphyses are wide and flared, with irregular epiphyseal-metaphyseal junctions. Long bones may be bowed. The cortices of the long bones are often indistinct. Occasionally, evidence of secondary hyperparathyroidism—subperiosteal resorption in the phalanges and metacarpals and erosion of the distal ends of the clavicles—is observed.

Pseudofractures (also known as Looser's zones or Milkman's fractures) are an uncommon but nearly pathognomonic feature of rickets and osteomalacia (Fig. 246–2). These radiolucent lines are most often found along the concave side of the femoral neck, the pubic rami, the ribs, the clavicles, and the lateral aspects of the scapulae. Pseudofractures may result from unhealed microfractures at points of stress or at the entry point of blood vessels into bone. They may progress to complete fractures that go unrecognized and thereby lead to

substantial deformity and disability. Bone density is not a reliable indicator of osteomalacia, since bone density can be decreased in patients with vitamin D deficiency or increased in patients with chronic renal failure. In adults with normal renal function, radiologic evidence of a mineralization defect is often subtle and not readily distinguishable from osteoporosis.

Biochemical Features

The multiple etiologies of rickets and osteomalacia do not produce a single pattern of biochemical abnormalities. Furthermore, osteomalacia may be found on bone biopsy with no abnormality in serum or urinary levels of minerals and electrolytes. However, certain general patterns can be recognized.

Vitamin D Deficiency

Vitamin D deficiency, whether it is caused by nutritional deficiency, malabsorption, or abnormal metabolism, results in decreased intestinal absorption of calcium and phosphate. In conjunction with the resulting secondary hyperparathyroidism, vitamin D deficiency leads to an increase in bone resorption, increased excretion of urinary phosphate, and increased renal tubular reabsorption of calcium. The net result tends to be a low normal serum calcium level, low serum phosphorus level (unless chronic renal failure prevents phosphaturia), elevated serum alkaline phosphatase level, increased PTH level, decreased urinary calcium level, and increased urinary phosphate level. Finding a low 25OHD level in combination with these other biochemical alterations strengthens the diagnosis of vitamin D deficiency. The 1,25(OH)$_2$D level may be normal, making this determination less useful for the diagnosis of osteomalacia. Both 25OHD and 1,25(OH)$_2$D levels may be reduced in patients with liver disease or nephrotic syndrome, who nevertheless have normal free concentrations of these metabolites and who may not be vitamin D deficient. Other factors, such as age and diet, must be considered. For example, serum phosphorus values are normally lower in adults than in children. Dietary history is important, since urinary phosphate excretion and, to a lesser degree, urinary calcium excretion reflect dietary phosphate and calcium content. Since phosphate excretion depends on the filtered load (the product of the glomerular filtration rate [GFR] and plasma phosphate), urinary phosphate levels may be normal if either the GFR or plasma phosphate levels are reduced, despite the presence of hyperparathyroidism. Expressions of renal phosphate clearance that account for these variables (e.g., renal threshold for phosphate, or TmP/GFR) are a better indicator of renal phosphate handling than is total phosphate excretion. The TmP/GFR can be calculated from a nomogram using measurements of a fasting serum and urine phosphorus concentration.

Chronic Renal Failure

Most patients with chronic renal failure and renal osteodystrophy have osteitis fibrosa alone or in combination with osteomalacia (see Ch. 249). If not well controlled, these patients will have a low serum level of calcium and high serum levels of phosphorus, alkaline phosphatase, and PTH. A few patients develop severe secondary hyperparathyroidism in which the PTH level increases dramatically, with restoration of the serum calcium to normal or even elevated levels (sometimes called tertiary hyperparathyroidism). Another small subset of patients with renal osteodystrophy presents with normal or low serum levels of PTH and alkaline phosphatase. Their serum calcium levels are often elevated after treatment with small doses of 1,25(OH)$_2$D. These patients have pure osteomalacia on bone biopsy and are thought to suffer from aluminum intoxication (see Ch. 249). Regardless of the type of bone disease, most patients with chronic renal

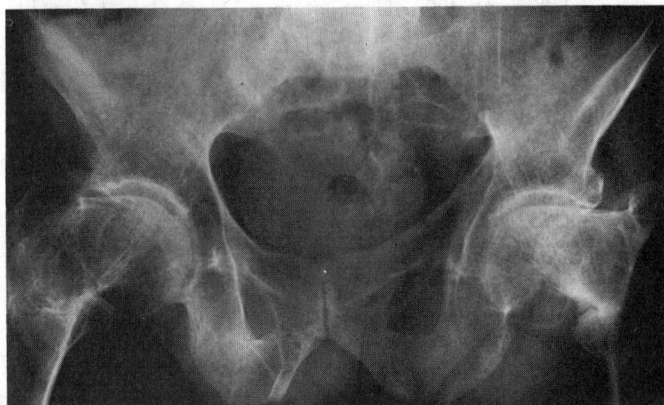

FIGURE 246–2. Roentgenogram of the pelvis of an elderly female with severe osteomalacia. This film reveals marked bowing (varus deformity) of both femoral necks, with pseudofractures of the medial aspect of the femoral necks and the superior aspect of the left pubic ramus. (Photograph courtesy of Dr. Harry K. Genant.)

disease have low $1,25(OH)_2D$ and $24,25(OH)_2D$ levels and, unless treated with vitamin D, tend to have low 25OHD levels as well.

Vitamin D–Dependent Rickets Types I and II

In these rare diseases, serum and urinary levels of calcium and phosphate resemble those in vitamin D–deficient rickets. However, serum 25OHD levels are normal. In type I patients, serum $1,25(OH)_2D$ levels are low in comparison to serum 25OHD levels, whereas in type II patients, serum $1,25(OH)_2D$ levels may be extraordinarily high.

Anticonvulsants

Patients on long-term anticonvulsant therapy tend to have the biochemical findings of mild vitamin D deficiency, including a low serum 25OHD level. Since these patients have normal serum $1,25(OH)_2D$ levels, some investigators have suggested that anticonvulsants may directly inhibit calcium transport in intestine and bone.

Hypophosphatemic Disorders

A low serum phosphorus level combined with its high renal clearance is characteristic of diseases such as X-linked hypophosphatemic rickets, tumoral hypophosphatemic osteomalacia, and the variety of proximal renal tubular disorders that are associated with osteomalacia. Serum calcium is generally normal. In both X-linked hypophosphatemic rickets and tumoral hypophosphatemic osteomalacia, serum $1,25(OH)_2D$ is inappropriately low for the serum phosphorus, although it is often in the low normal range. The proximal tubular diseases that present with the full de Toni-Debré-Fanconi syndrome also result in increased urinary levels of bicarbonate, amino acids, and glucose, as well as metabolic acidosis. Levels of the vitamin D metabolites have not been reported in large series of such patients.

Calcium Deficiency

In one study, children suspected of having rickets on the basis of calcium-deficient diets had normal serum levels of 25OHD and phosphorus, elevated serum levels of alkaline phosphatase, and low serum and urinary levels of calcium. Additional studies of calcium deficiency are necessary to confirm these observations.

Mineralization Disorders

Disorders attributed to an intrinsic defect in mineralization of the bone matrix do not produce the biochemical abnormalities observed in vitamin D deficiency. For example, patients who have developed osteomalacia as a result of long-term hemodialysis or total parenteral nutrition frequently are found to have hypercalcemia and hyperphosphatemia with low or normal levels of PTH. It is possible that the skeleton in these patients is unable to adequately buffer calcium and phosphate from the intestine, total parenteral nutrition solutions, or dialysate, resulting in marked oscillations of serum calcium and phosphorus.

Histologic Features

Because of the difficulty in diagnosing osteomalacia in adults by clinical and radiologic means, transcortical bone biopsy may be necessary. A rib or the iliac crest is the site generally biopsied. To assess osteoid content and mineral appositional rate, the bone biopsy specimen is processed without decalcification. This requires special equipment.

In osteomalacia, bone is mineralized poorly and slowly, resulting in wide osteoid seams (>12 μm) and a large fraction of bone covered by unmineralized osteoid. States of high bone turnover (increased bone formation and resorption), such as hyperparathyroidism, can also cause wide osteoid seams and increased osteoid surface, producing a superficial resemblance to osteomalacia. Therefore, the rate of bone turnover should be determined by labeling bone with tetracycline, which provides a fluorescent marker of the calcification front. When two doses of tetracycline are given at different times, the distance between the two labels divided by the time interval between the two doses equals the mineral appositional rate. The normal appositional rate is approximately 0.74 μm per day. Mineralization lag time, the time required for newly formed osteoid to be mineralized, can be calculated by dividing osteoid seam width by the appositional rate corrected by the linear extent of mineralization or calcification front (a measure of the bone surface that is undergoing active mineralization as measured by tetracycline incorporation). It is normally about 20 to 25 days. Depressed appositional rate, increased mineralization lag time, and reduced calcification front clearly distinguish osteomalacia from high turnover states such as hyperparathyroidism. Low turnover states such as senile osteoporosis can also have low appositional rates and reduced calcification fronts, but these are distinguished from osteomalacia by normal or reduced osteoid surface and volume.

TREATMENT

The goal in treating osteomalacia and rickets is to normalize the clinical, biochemical, and radiologic abnormalities without producing hypercalcemia, hyperphosphatemia, hypercalciuria, nephrolithiasis, or ectopic calcification (especially nephrocalcinosis). To realize this goal, patients must be followed carefully, and as the bone lesions heal or the underlying disease improves, the dose of vitamin D, calcium, or phosphate needs to be adjusted to avoid such complications. Table 246–2 lists the available vitamin D metabolites and analogues, including dose range, duration of action, cost, and clinical applications.

Vitamin D Deficiency

Simple nutritional vitamin D deficiency responds to oral doses of 2000 to 4000 IU of vitamin D per day, taken for several months, followed by replacement doses of 200 to 400 IU per day. Radiologic and biochemical evidence of healing requires several months. If the patient fails to respond to treatment, the physician should consider other possible causes of the bone disease.

TABLE 246–2. AVAILABLE VITAMIN D METABOLITES AND ANALOGUES

	Ergocalciferol	Dihydrotachysterol	Calcifediol	Calcitriol
Abbreviation	D_2	DHT	25OHD$_3$	$1,25(OH)_2D_3$
Physiologic dose	2.5–10 μg (1 μg = 40 units)	25–100 μg	1–5 μg	0.25–0.5 μg
Pharmacologic dose	0.625–5.0 mg	0.2–1.0 mg	20–200 μg	0.25–2.0 μg
Duration of action	1–3 months	1–4 weeks	2–6 weeks	2–5 days
Cost	$0.11/1.25 mg	$0.42/0.4 mg	$0.51/50 μg	$1.50/0.5 μg
Clinical applications	Vitamin D deficiency Vitamin D malabsorption Hypoparathyroidism Hyperphosphatemic rickets Anticonvulsant therapy in institutionalized patients	Chronic renal failure Hypoparathyroidism	Vitamin D malabsorption Chronic renal failure	Chronic renal failure Hyperparathyroidism Hypophosphatemic rickets Acute hypocalcemia Vitamin D–dependent rickets types I and II

Intestinal Malabsorption and Liver Disease

Patients with intestinal malabsorption or liver disease may respond to large doses of oral vitamin D (25,000 to 100,000 IU per day), or they may require parenteral administration of the vitamin. Since patients with steatorrhea absorb 25OHD (calcifediol) better than they do vitamin D, 50 to 100 μg of calcifediol per day or every other day should be tried if large doses of vitamin D fail to raise circulating levels of 25OHD into the high normal range. Vitamin D therapy should be supplemented with 1 to 3 grams of calcium per day. Only the osteomalacic component of the bone disease associated with these conditions responds to vitamin D; the osteoporotic component does not. Consequently, patients must be carefully selected for vitamin D treatment and carefully followed. Histomorphometric evaluation of bone biopsies is particularly useful in this regard.

Chronic Renal Failure

Most patients with renal osteodystrophy respond to 1,25(OH)$_2$D (calcitriol, 0.5 to 1.0 μg per day) or dihydrotachysterol (DHT, 0.25 to 0.5 mg per day), calcium supplementation (1 to 3 grams per day), and phosphate restriction (dietary restriction supplemented with phosphate binders such as aluminum hydroxide). The goal is to achieve and maintain normal serum levels of calcium, phosphorus, PTH, and alkaline phosphatase. This regimen treats osteitis fibrosa more effectively than osteomalacia. Some authorities recommend the use of calcifediol rather than calcitriol or DHT, since calcifediol may treat the osteomalacia more effectively. This issue is unresolved. Patients with only osteomalacia usually fail to respond to 1,25(OH)$_2$D alone, but they have responded to 1,25(OH)$_2$D in combination with 24,25(OH)$_2$D, a metabolite not yet available for clinical use. The osteomalacia in renal osteodystrophy also appears to respond to the removal of aluminum with deferoxamine, a drug approved for the treatment of iron overload. Neither 24,25(OH)$_2$D nor deferoxamine has been approved by the United States Food and Drug Administration for the treatment of renal osteodystrophy, and both must currently be considered investigational drugs for this purpose.

Hypophosphatemia

The bone disease in patients with X–linked hypophosphatemia responds to the combination of phosphate (1 to 3 grams per day) and either large doses (25,000 to 100,000 IU) of vitamin D or more physiologic doses (0.25 to 1.0 μg per day) of 1,25(OH)$_2$D. Neither phosphate nor vitamin D alone is as effective. Unfortunately, oral phosphate preparations also act as laxatives, and tolerance of full doses is sometimes difficult to achieve. Less information is available regarding the efficacy of vitamin D and phosphate in other hypophosphatemic syndromes. When hypophosphatemia is associated with metabolic acidosis, as it often is in the de Toni-Debré-Fanconi syndrome, correction of the acidosis with bicarbonate may improve the associated metabolic bone disease.

Calcium Deficiency

Calcium supplements (1 to 3 grams per day) are useful in the treatment of calcium deficiency resulting from deficient diets, intestinal malabsorption, and aging. The amount of calcium should be adjusted to achieve adequate intestinal absorption, as monitored by urinary calcium excretion and serum levels of calcium and PTH.

Inhibitors of Mineralization

Restricting the use of aluminum-containing antacids in patients with chronic renal failure or peptic ulcer, removing aluminum and other impurities from the water used in hemodialysis, and substituting purified amino acids for the aluminum-containing casein hydrolysate in total parenteral nutrition solutions should reduce the incidence of aluminum intoxication. Chelation and removal of aluminum from the body with deferoxamine shows promise as a remedy of the future.

Patients on long-term anticonvulsant therapy may benefit from the prophylactic use of 2000 to 4000 IU of vitamin D per day and 500 to 1000 mg of calcium per day, especially if their serum 25OHD levels are low.

Etidronate, which is used in the treatment of Paget's disease, should be limited to a dose of 5 mg per kilogram and restricted to therapeutic periods of six months with at least six months between treatment periods.

Fluoride, which is currently under investigation for the treatment of osteoporosis, must be accompanied by 1 to 2 grams of calcium per day.

Bikle DD: Calcium absorption and vitamin D metabolism. Clin Gastroenterol 12:379, 1983. *A review of the effect of vitamin D on the intestine and the gastrointestinal diseases that lead to osteomalacia.*

Bikle DD, Halloran BP, Gee E, et al.: Free 25-hydroxyvitamin D levels are normal in subjects with liver disease and reduced total 25-hydroxyvitamin D levels. J Clin Invest 78:748, 1986. *This article points out that total vitamin D metabolite concentrations may be reduced in patients with reduced DBP levels without a reduction in the free (and, possibly, the more physiologically relevant) vitamin D metabolite concentrations.*

Brenner RJ, Spring DB, Sebastion A, et al.: Incidence of radiologically evident bone disease, nephrocalcinosis, and nephrolithiasis in various types of renal tubular acidosis. N Engl J Med 307:217, 1982. *The authors point out that bone disease (osteomalacia) is much more common in proximal renal tubular acidosis than in distal renal tubular acidosis.*

Chesney RW, Mazess RB, Rose P, et al.: Long-term influence of calcitriol (1,25-dihydroxyvitamin D) and supplemental phosphate in X-linked hypophosphatemic rickets. Pediatrics 71:559, 1983. *This article discusses the modern therapy for this disease.*

Curtis JA, Kooh SW, Fraser D, et al.: Nutritional rickets in vegetarian children. Can Med Assoc J 128:150, 1983. *Nutritional vitamin D deficiency continues to be a problem in those who omit milk and dairy products from their diet.*

Dibble JB, Sheridan P, Losowsky MS: A survey of vitamin D deficiency in gastrointestinal and liver disorders. Q J Med 209:119, 1984. *This article reports the results of a survey of 152 patients with gastrointestinal disease and 104 patients with chronic liver disease in whom 25OHD levels were assessed. Low levels of 25OHD were found in many patients, but osteomalacia was detected almost exclusively in patients with 25OHD levels below 2 ng/ml.*

Goldstein DA, Haldimann B, Sherman D, et al.: Vitamin D metabolites and calcium metabolism in patients with nephrotic syndrome and normal renal function. J Clin Endocrinol Metab 52:116, 1981. *This article describes the pathogenesis of osteomalacia in the nephrotic syndrome.*

Mankin HJ: Rickets, osteomalacia, and renal osteodystrophy. Parts I and II. Am Bone Joint Surg 56A:101, 352, 1974. *A thorough review with an accounting of the history of the subject, a description of the clinical presentation of rickets, and a complete list of the etiologies of bone mineralization disorders.*

Marel GM, McKenna MJ, Frame B: Osteomalacia. Bone Mineral Res 4:335, 1986. *This is an excellent, complete, and up-to-date review of the subject.*

Marie PJ, Pettifor JM, Ross FP, et al.: Histological osteomalacia due to dietary calcium deficiency in children. N Engl J Med 307:584, 1982. *This study indicates that calcium deficiency alone may be sufficient to cause osteomalacia.*

Ott SM, Andress DL, Nebeker HG, et al.: Changes in bone histology after treatment with desferrioxamine. Kidney Int 29:S108, 1986. *This is a preliminary report indicating the potential usefulness of desferrioxamine in the treatment of aluminum-associated osteomalacia.*

Parfitt AM, Gallagher JC, Heaney RP, et al.: Vitamin D and bone health in the elderly. Am J Clin Nutr 36:1014, 1982. *A review of the importance of adequate vitamin D intake in adults, discussing, among other issues, the high incidence of osteomalacia found in patients with hip fractures.*

Voights AL, Felsenfeld AJ, Flach F: The effects of calciferol and its metabolites on patients with chronic renal failure. Arch Intern Med 143:960, 1205, 1983. *In this two-part review, the authors evaluate the data concerning the most appropriate vitamin D metabolite (or analogue) to use in the treatment of the various types of renal osteodystrophy.*

Weider N, Cruz DS: Phosphaturic mesenchymal tumors: A polymorphous group causing osteomalacia or rickets. Cancer 59:1442, 1987. *An excellent review of 17 cases of this syndrome of reversible bone disease caused by tumors.*

247 THE PARATHYROID GLANDS, HYPERCALCEMIA, AND HYPOCALCEMIA

Claude D. Arnaud

PARATHYROID HORMONE

STRUCTURE AND SYNTHESIS. *Parathyroid hormone (PTH),* an 84 amino acid, linear polypeptide with a molecular weight of 9500, is the principal regulator of the concentration of ionic calcium in extracellular fluid. The biosynthesis and intracellular processing of the hormone are complex. The original hormonal gene product of the parathyroid cell is a 115 amino acid precursor termed pre-proparathyroid hormone. In the cisternal space of the endoplasmic reticulum the enzyme "clipase" removes the presequence, leaving the 90 amino acid proparathyroid hormone structure. Proparathyroid hormone is converted to parathyroid hormone in the Golgi apparatus by proteolytic removal ("tryptic clipase") of the remaining 6 amino acids at the amino terminus. Here, the 84 amino acid polypeptide is readied for secretion either in a secretory granule or in its free form. There is no evidence that either of the parathyroid hormone precursor molecules or the "pre" or "pro" peptide sequence normally finds its way into the circulation.

In contrast to the rapid regulation of secretion, hormone biosynthesis is only slowly influenced by changes in concentrations of extracellular ionic calcium. Intracellular stores of parathyroid hormone may be regulated by a degradative pathway that is stimulated by high and inhibited by low extracellular calcium. This degradative pathway may not only provide an important mechanism for regulating parathyroid hormone economy, as noted later, but the fragments of the hormone produced during its intracellular degradation may also provide a major source for the multiple immunoreactive forms of the hormone known to circulate in the blood (see below).

All of the structural information required for full biologic activity of native, 84 amino acid parathyroid hormone lies within the 34 amino acids at the amino terminus. The active fragments of the bovine and human hormones, multiple fragments of the mid and carboxyl regions of the bovine and human hormones, and the full sequence of human parathyroid hormone have been synthesized and are commercially available for investigational use. Limited studies of the mid- and carboxyl-region fragments have shown them to be biologically inert.

CONTROL OF SECRETION. Parathyroid hormone is rapidly released from the parathyroid glands in response to a fall in plasma ionic calcium. It acts on kidney, intestine (indirectly, see below), and bone to restore the concentration of this cation to just above a normal set point, which, in turn, inhibits the secretion of the hormone. This negative feedback cycle is depicted in the "butterfly" diagram shown in Figure 244–1, in which the cycle is dissected into three loops, each involving one of the major target organs of parathyroid hormone. The concentration of extracellular ionic calcium is the major regulator of parathyroid hormone secretion. A more general discussion of calcium metabolism and its homeostasis is provided in Ch. 244. Other factors influence secretion only indirectly. For example, plasma phosphate alters the degree to which calcium is complexed, and blood pH, the degree to which it binds to albumin. The effects of extracellular magnesium concentrations on secretion are qualitatively similar to those of ionic calcium but are physiologically less important. Paradoxically, severe, prolonged hypomagnesemia markedly inhibits secretion of parathyroid hormone and may be associated with hypocalcemia (see below). Known, direct parathyroid hormone secretagogues of questionable physiologic importance include β-adrenergic agonists, prostaglandins, and histamine. These agents, as well as decreased ionic calcium, stimulate the production of cyclic 3'5'-adenosine monophosphate (cyclic AMP) in parathyroid cells in vitro. This compound may be an important mediator of parathyroid cell secretagogues, but the phosphoinositol-diacyl glycerol system may also play an important role in the regulation of PTH secretion.

THE CIRCULATING HORMONE. Circulating parathyroid hormone is heterogeneous. It consists of the intact 84 amino acid polypeptide and multiple fragments of the hormone. These fragments are derived from the mid and carboxyl regions of the hormone molecule and therefore are likely to be biologically inactive. There is no evidence that biologically active fragments are secreted by the parathyroid gland or that they are present in the circulation. It is not possible at present to determine precisely the relative quantities of intact parathyroid hormone and of its fragments in serum, but grossly there are more circulating fragments than intact hormone. This difference is due primarily to the fact that the fragments survive longer in the circulation. The fragments are derived both from the degradative metabolism of intact parathyroid hormone and from glandular secretion, but the quantitative importance of these sources is uncertain.

Biologically active parathyroid hormone normally circulates in the blood at extremely low concentrations (<50 pg per milliliter). It is likely that there are individual, constitutionally derived "set point" values for the plasma ionic calcium above which glandular secretion rates are decreased and below which they are increased. However, steady-state levels of parathyroid hormone are probably determined primarily by the degree to which the parathyroid glands must adapt to individual, chronic, environmentally induced changes in the level of plasma ionic calcium (e.g., dietary calcium and phosphate). There is an inverse relationship between fasting levels of serum calcium and serum immunoreactive parathyroid hormone (iPTH) in normal subjects (Fig. 247–1). Serum iPTH also increases with age (Fig. 247–2).

ACTION OF PARATHYROID HORMONE. The major function of PTH is to defend against hypocalcemia. It carries

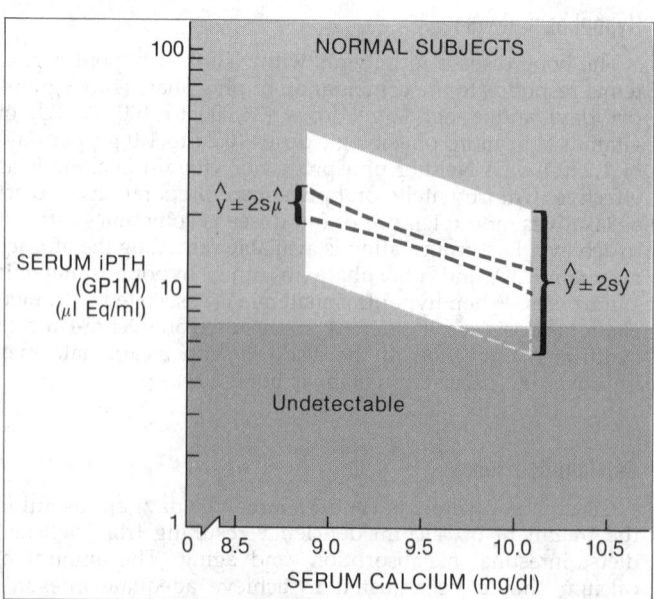

FIGURE 247–1. Serum immunoreactive parathyroid hormone (iPTH) (log scale) as a function of total serum calcium in 150 normal subjects (r = −0.424; p <0.001). (From Purnell D, et al.: Treatment of primary hyperparathyroidism. Am J Med 56:801, 1974.)

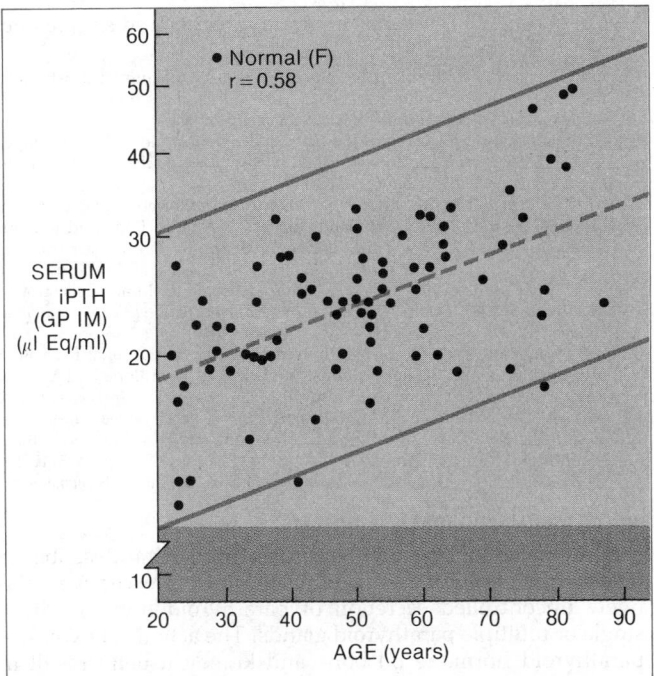

FIGURE 247–2. Serum immunoreactive parathyroid hormone (iPTH) as a function of age in 78 normal Caucasian women. Screened area at bottom represents limit of assay detectability. Mean increase in serum iPTH between age 20 and 90 is 80 per cent and is significant (p <0.001). (From Gallagher JC, et al.: The effect of age on serum immunoreactive parathyroid hormone in normal and osteoporotic women. J Lab Clin Med 95:376, 1980.)

out this function by promoting virtually all of the actions that could be teleologically postulated: (1) release of calcium from bone, (2) conservation of calcium by the kidney, (3) enhanced absorption of calcium from the gut (indirectly via vitamin D), and (4) reduction in plasma phosphate. These physiologic effects of parathyroid hormone will be described after a brief summary of what is known concerning its mechanism of action.

MECHANISM OF ACTION OF PTH. Parathyroid hormone binds to specific plasma membrane receptors of target cells. These occupied receptors interact with a membrane-bound protein that is regulated by guanyl nucleotides; this protein in turn activates membrane-bound adenylate cyclase to convert ATP to cyclic AMP (Fig. 247–3). Cyclic AMP, by virtue of its ability to initiate a cascade of enzyme-activating intracellular phosphorylations, is considered to be one of possibly several intracellular "second messengers" responsible for mediating the final expression of the action of the hormone. The details of these enzyme activations and the manner in which they relate to discrete effects of the hormone are unknown. Other potential second messengers of parathyroid hormone (e.g., calcium itself) that might act in concert with or modulate the actions of cyclic AMP are under investigation. A more general description of the mechanisms by which polypeptide hormones act on target cells is contained in Ch. 221. The region of the molecule essential for receptor binding is the amino acid sequence 25-30, and for receptor activation, the 1-7 sequence.

ACTION OF PTH ON THE KIDNEY. Parathyroid hormone acts most immediately on the kidney (1) to increase renal tubular reabsorption of calcium and magnesium, thus conserving these two divalent cations, and (2) to increase phosphate and bicarbonate excretion by inhibiting their proximal tubular reabsorption. These latter effects have several important, albeit indirect, effects on the homeostasis of extracellular calcium. Hormone-induced bicarbonaturia tends to produce acidosis, which decreases the ability of circulating albumin to bind calcium, thus increasing ionic calcium by physiochemical

means. Hormone-induced phosphaturia assures that the increased release of phosphate from bone, which occurs obligately during hormone-induced calcium mobilization from bone, does not produce hyperphosphatemia. Increased serum phosphate would tend to complex calcium and thereby counteract the physiologic effect of parathyroid hormone to increase plasma ionic calcium.

The most important indirect effect of the phosphaturic action of the hormone is illustrated in the intestinal feedback loop in Figure 244–1. Parathyroid hormone, either directly or by its hypophosphatemic action, stimulates renal tubular 25OH 1α-hydroxylase to convert the major circulating metabolite of vitamin D, 25-hydroxycholecalciferol (25OHD), to its major biologically active metabolite, 1α,25-dihydroxycholecalciferol [1,25(OH)₂D]. This latter metabolite acts directly on the intestinal mucosal cell to increase calcium absorption and on bone to increase resorption (see arrow between the intestinal and bone loop in Fig. 244–1). The metabolism of vitamin D is discussed in detail in Ch. 245.

In the process of stimulating adenylate cyclase in renal tubular cells, parathyroid hormone increases the urinary excretion of cyclic AMP. Presumably, cyclic AMP is simply released into the tubular fluid following its intracellular synthesis, since it has no known extracellular function. Urinary cyclic AMP is increased by the administration of other hormones active in the kidney, including epinephrine and glucagon, but its renal production and excretion are almost entirely due to parathyroid hormone. It can therefore be used as an indirect measure of the action of parathyroid hormone on the kidney, as noted below.

ACTION OF PTH ON BONE. Parathyroid hormone increases the net release of calcium and phosphate from bone into extracellular fluid. Curiously, PTH receptors have been identified on osteoblast-like cells but not on osteoclasts. It is

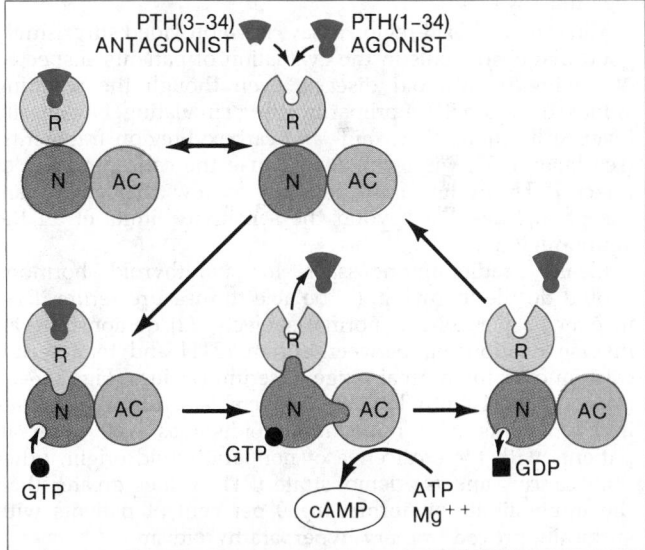

FIGURE 247–3. Mechanism of PTH action on membrane-bound adenylate cyclase. The biologically active PTH agonist ⁸Nle, ¹⁸Nle, ³⁴Tyr bovine PTH(1-34) amide [PTH(1-34)] and the biologically inactive PTH antagonist ⁸Nle, ¹⁸Nle, ³⁴Tyr bovine PTH(3-34) amide [PTH(3-34)] are capable of binding to the PTH receptor (R). However, only PTH(1-34) is capable of converting the receptor to a high-affinity state, so that the guanyl nucleotide regulatory protein (N) can be stimulated to bind guanosine triphosphate (GTP). The binding of GTP to N converts R to a low-affinity state, inducing dissociation of PTH(1-34) *and* the formation of an N-adenylate cyclase (AC) complex, leading to the activation of this enzyme and the increased production of intracellular cAMP. In contrast, the binding of PTH antagonist to R does not change the affinity of R. Consequently, R cannot interact with N or induce activation of AC. (From Arnaud CD, Kolb FO: The calciotropic hormones and metabolic bone disease. In Greenspan FS, Forsham PH (eds.): Basic and Clinical Endocrinology. Los Altos, CA, Lange Medical Publications, 1983, p 193.)

thought, therefore, that PTH exerts its resorptive effect on bone indirectly by stimulating one or more activities of osteoblasts, which in turn facilitate osteoclastic bone resorption and both the recruitment and differentiation of osteoclasts.

ASSAY IN BIOLOGIC FLUIDS. The major tool for measuring parathyroid hormone in biologic fluids is radioimmunoassay. Values for serum iPTH vary from laboratory to laboratory, however, because of the differences in the source (bovine or human) and purity of the parathyroid hormone preparations used as standards and in the specificity of the antisera. Therefore, interpretation of serum iPTH values requires knowledge of the normal range for each assay system. Until recently, most radioimmunoassays of human PTH have used ^{125}I-labeled bovine PTH as the radioligand and cross-reacting antisera directed against porcine or bovine PTH. Use of synthetic human PTH or its fragments may help to minimize some of the inconsistencies in the future. However, variations in the specificities of antisera used in different assays will continue to result in different iPTH values for the same serum sample. Such differences reflect true differences in the concentrations of the various forms of circulating parathyroid hormone.

At present, all available antisera that have a sufficiently high affinity for parathyroid hormone to be useful in radioimmunoassays are multivalent and contain antibodies directed at multiple regions of the PTH molecule. Antisera directed against the mid or carboxyl region of the PTH molecule recognize inactive mid- or carboxyl-region fragments and intact, biologically active PTH, and antisera directed against the amino region recognize amino-region fragments and intact PTH. Because the quantities of mid- and carboxyl-region fragments in the circulation are greater than those of amino-region fragments or intact PTH, values for serum iPTH are higher in mid- and carboxyl-region assays than in amino-region assays.

Mid- and carboxyl-region assays have provided surprisingly good diagnostic tools in the evaluation of patients suspected of having parathyroid disease, even though the resulting values for serum iPTH primarily reflect circulating, biologically inactive hormone (i.e., mid- and carboxyl-region fragments) (see below). This is fortunate because the concentrations of intact PTH in the circulation are so low that, with rare exception, they are beyond the sensitivity limits of all the amino-region assays.

Ideally, radioimmunoassays for parathyroid hormone should do the following: (1) be able to measure serum iPTH in over 95 per cent of normal subjects, (2) demonstrate an inverse relationship between serum iPTH and total serum calcium over the normal range of serum calcium (Fig. 247–1), (3) show consistently low or undetectable serum iPTH values in all patients with hypoparathyroidism as well as in all patients with hypercalcemia of nonparathyroid origin, other than cancer, and (4) demonstrate iPTH values greater than the upper limits of normal in 90 per cent of patients with surgically proved primary hyperparathyroidism.

Until recently, bioassays for parathyroid hormone lacked sufficient sensitivity for the study of circulating parathyroid hormone. This obstacle has now been overcome by two novel approaches. One is a cytochemical bioassay that is based on the PTH-specific stimulation of glucose-6-phosphate dehydrogenase in guinea pig renal slices. This assay is extremely sensitive, measuring femtogram amounts of parathyroid hormone. Its disadvantage is its technical complexity. The other assay, which is more convenient, uses a nonhydrolyzable analogue of guanosine triphosphate, 5' guanyl-imidodiphosphate [Gpp(NH)p], to greatly augment the sensitivity of adenylate cyclase to parathyroid hormone in canine kidneys in vitro. In the presence of Gpp(NH)p, as little as 10 pg per milliliter of intact PTH elicits significant stimulation. However, even with this sensitivity, the measurement of parathyroid hormone in normal serum requires the immunoextraction of

3 ml of serum. This assay is accurate, precise, and simple and can be performed rapidly.

Arnaud C, Tsao HS, Littledike ET: Radioimmunoassay of human parathyroid hormone in serum. J Clin Invest 50:21, 1971. *Detailed description of one of the earliest successful parathyroid hormone radioimmunoassays.*

Bikle DD (ed.): Assay of Calcium-Regulating Hormones. New York, Springer Verlag, 1983. *Detailed descriptions by 21 authors of assay techniques for parathyroid hormone, calcitonin, and the calciferols.*

Cohen DV, Elting JJ: Synthesis and secretion of parathormone and secretory protein I by the parathyroid gland. In Peck WA (ed.): Bone and Mineral Research Annual 2. New York, Elsevier, 1984, pp 67–124. *Incisive review of the physiology and cell biology of parathyroid hormone action on the kidney.*

Draper MW, Nissenson RA (eds.): Parathyroid hormone. Mineral Electrolyte Metab 8:116, 1982. *Extensive review of the basic and clinical science of parathyroid hormone.*

Klahr W, Hruska KA: Effects of parathyroid hormone on the renal resorption of phosphorus and divalent cations. In Peck WA (ed.): Bone and Mineral Research Annual 2. New York, Elsevier, 1984, pp 67–124. *Incisive review of the physiology and cell biology of parathyroid hormone action on the kidney.*

Wong GL: Skeletal effects of parathyroid hormone. In Peck WA (ed.): Bone and Mineral Research Annual 4. New York, Elsevier, 1986, pp 103–129. *A timely and needed review of advances in the study of parathyroid hormone action on bone and in particular on isolated bone cells.*

PRIMARY HYPERPARATHYROIDISM

DEFINITION. Primary hyperparathyroidism describes a disorder or group of disorders resulting from excessive, relatively uncontrolled secretion of parathyroid hormone by a single or multiple parathyroid glands. The actions of excessive parathyroid hormone on bone and kidney usually result in hypercalcemia, the biochemical hallmark of the disorder, but this fails to inhibit PTH secretion normally. Most patients are now detected by routine measurement of the serum calcium while relatively asymptomatic and without other readily demonstrable manifestations of the disease. When present, symptoms can be remarkably varied and vague and are related to hypercalcemia, hypercalciuria (nephrolithiasis), or osteitis fibrosa cystica (bone pain).

ETIOLOGY. The etiology of primary hyperparathyroidism is unknown. In several families the disease has been inherited as an autosomal dominant trait. Patients studied for the detection of thyroid carcinoma following previous neck x-irradiation have incidentally shown a greater than expected number of cases of primary hyperparathyroidism. It is difficult to interpret such studies, however, because information about the general incidence and natural history of primary hyperparathyroidism is incomplete.

Calcium infusions in the hyperparathyroid patients with mild hypercalcemia incompletely suppress serum immunoreactive parathyroid hormone levels. This strongly suggests that increased hormone secretion in these patients is due, at least in part, to a set point error in the level of ionic calcium at which abnormal tissue is suppressed. This defect can be demonstrated in vitro. Higher concentrations of calcium are required in the medium to decrease parathyroid hormone secretion from parathyroid cells isolated from abnormal glands than are required for cells isolated from normal glands.

INCIDENCE. Routine, automated measurement of serum calcium has vastly increased the detection of primary hyperparathyroidism. The incidence of primary hyperparathyroidism increases in both men and women after age 50, but it is two to four times more common in women. The disease is rare in children. In a careful epidemiologic study of cases detected in Rochester, Minnesota, over a 10-year period, the age-adjusted incidence rate was estimated to be 42 per 100,000. Studies of selected populations (mostly older than 40 years of age) have revealed prevalence rates of primary hyperparathyroidism as high as 1 in 1000 to 1 in 200 of those surveyed.

PATHOLOGY. Abnormal parathyroid glands from patients with primary hyperparathyroidism have been characterized as being hyperplastic, adenomatous, or malignant. Unfortunately, it is often difficult, if not impossible, to distinguish between an adenoma and chief cell hyperplasia in a given gland, and, occasionally, abnormal parathyroid tissue that is benign has many of the histologic features of malignant tissue.

Thus, it has generally been necessary to revert to the gross pathology observed at surgery to classify parathyroid lesions. The surgeon determines the number of abnormal glands present on the basis of their size and gross appearance, and the pathologist determines whether the biopsy specimens are parathyroid tissue. Single gland involvement ("adenoma") is observed in about 80 per cent of patients and multiple gland involvement ("hyperplasia") in about 20 per cent. Less than 2 per cent of hyperfunctioning glands are carcinomatous as judged by a combination of gross appearance, histology, and the ultimate biologic behavior of the abnormal tissue. Multiple glands are almost always involved in familial primary hyperparathyroidism and the hyperparathyroidism associated with multiple endocrine neoplasia (MEN) syndromes. Abnormal parathyroid glands usually weigh between 0.2 and 2.0 grams (25 to 75 mg is normal). Occasionally, very large glands (e.g., >10 grams) are observed. The severity of the clinical manifestations, especially the degree of hypercalcemia, is generally proportional to the quantity of hyperfunctioning tissue present and the level of serum immunoreactive PTH (iPTH). The predominant cell type in most abnormal glands is the chief cell, although so-called "water-clear cells" and oxyphilic cells may be admixed, and very occasionally either of these cells may predominate. The secretory capabilities of the "water-clear" and oxyphilic cells are unknown.

Virtually all patients with primary hyperparathyroidism have histomorphometric evidence of excess parathyroid hormone action in bone biopsies from the iliac crest, although most of these patients do not have radiographic evidence of bone disease. An increase in the amount of bone surface undergoing resorption, increased numbers of osteoclasts, osteocytic osteolysis, and, in moderate to severe cases, marrow fibrosis are characteristic of this lesion, which is termed osteitis fibrosa cystica. Only far advanced disease is associated with classic bone cysts and fractures.

Between 20 and 30 per cent of patients have nephrolithiasis, not infrequently complicated by pyelonephritis. Gross nephrocalcinosis or calcification of the renal papillae is unusual, but careful microscopic examinations of kidneys with special calcium stains occasionally reveal peritubular and tubular calcifications at autopsy. The incidence of such soft tissue calcification in patients with mild to moderate disease is unknown; however, it may be relatively frequent because chondrocalcinosis and calcific tendinitis can be demonstrated radiographically in approximately 7.5 to 18 per cent of cases. Calcification of other organs such as stomach, lung, and heart has been observed in patients with hyperparathyroid crisis (serum calcium >15.0 mg per deciliter).

Myopathy is relatively common in primary hyperparathyroidism, and muscle biopsy may show neuropathic atrophy of both type I and type II muscle fibers. These histologic changes parallel clinical, neurologic, and electromyographic dysfunction.

PATHOPHYSIOLOGY. The excessive release of parathyroid hormone from hyperfunctioning parathyroid tissue causes exaggerated physiologic responses of target organs (see Fig. 244–1) and inappropriately raises the concentration of ionized calcium in extracellular fluid. In contrast to other hypercalcemic states, in primary hyperparathyroidism the first lines of defense against hypercalcemia (increased renal and intestinal loss of calcium) are not fully operative, since the kidney and intestine are target organs for PTH and are themselves contributing to the pathogenesis of the hypercalcemia. Early in the course of the disease, when serum calcium values are <11.5 mg per deciliter (normal range, 8.9 to 10.1 mg per deciliter), urinary calcium is often relatively low for the degree of hypercalcemia and may be normal. When serum calcium values exceed 12.0 mg per deciliter, the increased filtered load of calcium overwhelms renal tubular reabsorption and hypercalciuria develops. This assists in limiting the further rise of plasma calcium but at the cost of producing kidney

stone diathesis secondary to continued hypercalciuria, along with other changes in urine composition (e.g., increased pH resulting from bicarbonaturia).

Factors other than urinary loss may tend to limit the degree of hypercalcemia in primary hyperparathyroidism. First, calcium may be "lost" from the extracellular fluid by being deposited in soft tissues. This metastatic calcification may cause symptoms (e.g., joint pain owing to calcific tendinitis and chondrocalcinosis) or compromise function (e.g., nephrocalcinosis leading to renal failure). Secondly, the permissive effect of vitamin D is necessary for the action of parathyroid hormone; in its absence patients with even severe hyperparathyroidism become either eucalcemic or nearly so. In fact, stores of vitamin D may become depleted in a patient who previously was marginally replete because of the increased renal conversion of 25OHD to $1,25(OH)_2D$, which is caused by excessive parathyroid hormone. As a result, such patients may have severe osteomalacia in addition to osteitis fibrosa cystica. Finally, hypercalcemia per se may increase the degradation of biologically active forms of parathyroid hormone peripherally (i.e., in the liver and possibly the kidney) and in the parathyroid tissue itself. In this way plasma calcium not only may regulate parathyroid hormone secretion but also may be an important factor in determining the relative quantities of circulating, biologically active parathyroid hormone and inactive hormone fragments. Increased secretion of calcitonin might be expected to play an important role in correcting the hypercalcemia of primary hyperparathyroidism (see Fig. 244–1), but this seems not to occur in the majority of patients. In fact, the secretory reserve of calcitonin often appears to be depleted.

Parathyroid hormone decreases renal tubular reabsorption of phosphate, and in excess tends to cause hyperphosphaturia and hypophosphatemia. Normally, these effects both support mineral homeostasis (by stimulating $1,25(OH)_2D$ production) and protect it (by clearing from the blood phosphate that is removed from bone during resorption of calcium). In patients with primary hyperparathyroidism, however, hypophosphatemia tends to worsen hypercalcemia by causing increased production of the hypercalcemic compound $1,25(OH)_2D$ and decreased complexing of blood ionic calcium by phosphate.

Patients with primary hyperparathyroidism generally have mild to moderate hyperchloremic acidosis, primarily because excess hormone decreases urinary hydrogen ion excretion and increases urinary bicarbonate excretion. These effects also tend to aggravate existing hypercalcemia by decreasing the ability of blood albumin to bind ionic calcium, and by increasing the dissolution of bone mineral.

Urinary cyclic AMP is increased in as many as 80 per cent of patients with primary hyperparathyroidism. Presumably, increased hormonal occupancy of renal receptors stimulates adenylate cyclase to produce an increase in this intracellular second messenger. Interestingly, the phosphaturic and cyclic AMP responses to exogenously administered parathyroid hormone are blunted in patients with primary hyperparathyroidism, suggesting refractoriness or "desensitization" of one or more of the cellular components responsible for these effects. This desensitization, as well as the increased excretion of nephrogenous cyclic AMP, has been used as a diagnostic test for the presence of hyperparathyroidism.

Patients with radiologic evidence of osteitis fibrosa cystica (a bone lesion caused by excess PTH) almost always have increased serum concentrations of the bone isoenzyme of alkaline phosphatase. This enzyme is produced by osteoblasts and probably constitutes one of several enzymes involved in osseous mineralization. These patients also excrete in their urine greater than normal quantities of small peptides that contain hydroxyproline. This amino acid is unique to collagen, which is the major structural protein in bone. Combined increases in serum alkaline phosphatase and urinary excretion of hydroxyproline reflect grossly increased bone turnover, which can be documented further by studies of the dynamics of intravenously administered, isotopically labeled calcium (^{47}Ca, ^{45}Ca).

SYMPTOMS (Table 247–1). Most patients with primary hyperparathyroidism are relatively asymptomatic when the diagnosis is made, or else they have nonspecific symptoms, especially those of weakness and easy fatigability. When symptoms do occur, they can generally be attributed to either hypercalcemia with associated hypercalciuria or to osteitis fibrosa cystica.

Hypercalcemia. The symptoms attributable to hypercalcemia involve a number of systems: (1) Central nervous system—impaired mentation, loss of memory for recent events, emotional lability, depression, anosmia, somnolence, and even coma. (2) Neuromuscular—weakness (especially of the proximal musculature), arthralgias, severe pruritus (which may be due to metastatic calcification in the skin), and the restless leg syndrome (no comfortable position for legs when attempting to sleep). (3) Rheumatologic—the joint pains may be due to associated gout, intra-articular deposition of calcium pyrophosphate crystals (pseudogout), calcific tendinitis, or chondrocalcinosis. (4) Gastrointestinal—anorexia, nausea, vomiting, dyspepsia, constipation, and possibly an increased incidence of peptic ulcer and acute pancreatitis. (5) Renal—polyuria, nocturia, and increased propensity to form calcium oxalate or calcium phosphate stones, which sometimes leads to renal failure from calcium nephropathy, with associated symptoms of uremia. (6) Cardiovascular—increased frequency of hypertension. In general, all of these abnormalities are related to the degree of increase in ionized calcium in extracellular fluid, but the correlation is a crude one. One patient may be severely incapacitated at a level of serum calcium that produces only moderate symptoms in another.

Osteitis Fibrosa Cystica. Bony abnormalities can be demonstrated by special techniques in biopsy specimens from the iliac crest in most patients with primary hyperparathyroidism. However, symptomatic bone disease is now rare in this disorder. Patients may infrequently complain of diffuse or localized (e.g., to the back) bone pain. Very rarely patients may have a pathologic fracture through a bone cyst. The radiographic changes in osteitis fibrosa cystica are described later.

PHYSICAL SIGNS. Most patients with primary hyperparathyroidism have no abnormal physical signs of the dis-

TABLE 247–1. SYMPTOMS AND SIGNS OF PRIMARY HYPERPARATHYROIDISM

I. **Related to hypercalcemia per se**

Central nervous system	Renal
lethargy	polyuria
drowsiness	calcium nephropathy—
depression	nephrocalcinosis
stupor	Gastrointestinal
coma	nausea
Neuromuscular	vomiting
fatigue	constipation
weakness	dyspepsia
proximal myopathy	possibly increased peptic ulcer
hypotonia	pancreatitis
Cardiovascular	Metastatic calcification (usually
hypertension	requires P to be elevated as
bradycardia	well)
short Q-T interval	band keratopathy
potentiation of digitalis	pruritus
intoxication	

II. **Related to hypercalciuria**
Kidney stone diathesis (10 per cent)

III. **Related to PTH effect on bone and joints**
Bone pain from osteitis fibrosa cystica
Bone cysts—rarely with fracture
Epulis—a brown tumor (osteoclastic) of the jaw
Arthralgias
Increased incidence of gout and pseudogout

From Andreoli TE, Carpenter CCJ, Plum F, et al. (eds.): *Cecil Essentials of Medicine.* Philadelphia, W. B. Saunders Company, 1986, p 511.

order. When present, such signs are usually confined to the neuromuscular system or to organ systems in which soft tissue calcification can be noted. Neurologic abnormalities are nonspecific and include impaired mentation, hyperactive deep tendon reflexes, sensory loss for pain and vibration, proximal muscle weakness (particularly the thighs), abnormal tongue movements (resembling fasciculations), glossal atrophy, and ataxic gait.

Soft tissue calcification can result in arthritis (chondrocalcinosis or calcific tendinitis), conjunctivitis (conjunctival calcium phosphate crystals), and "band keratopathy," which is characterized by deposition of opaque calcium phosphate in vertical lines parallel to and within the ocular limbus, usually laterally in the cornea. These ocular signs, which can be best seen with slit lamp examination, are rare in hyperparathyroidism unless the serum phosphate is elevated, as occurs after the onset of renal failure.

Primary hyperparathyroidism is a prominent component of the rare multiple endocrine neoplasia syndromes (MEN I or IIa), which are described in Ch. 241. The clinician should look for evidence of these abnormalities—e.g., acromegaly, hypopituitarism, pheochromocytoma, and medullary carcinoma of the thyroid—during the physical examination.

Enlarged parathyroid glands are only rarely demonstrable on physical examination. In fact, even in the presence of primary hyperparathyroidism, a nodule in the neck is almost certainly one of the thyroid rather than the parathyroid.

Rarely, patients may exhibit bone tenderness on examination, and even more rarely bone deformities, fractures through an osteoclastic cyst, or the presence of an epulis (brown tumor of the jaw).

RADIOGRAPHIC MANIFESTATIONS. The most specific and frequent radiographic sign of osteitis fibrosa cystica is that of subperiosteal bone resorption. This sign is best demonstrated in magnified, fine-grain, industrial radiographs of the fingers (particularly the index finger) (Fig. 247–4A). Particular attention should be paid to the radial surface of the phalanx, where the cortex is almost completely resorbed, leaving only a lacey edge. Other radiographic manifestations of the disease range from generalized osteopenia to bone cysts ("brown tumors") and erosion of distal phalangeal tufts or of the distal ends of the clavicles. Figure 247–4B provides an example of severe osteitis fibrosa cystica involving the skull.

Soft tissue calcifications (e.g., calcific tendinitis, chondrocalcinosis, nephrocalcinosis, and pulmonary calcifications) may be detected on routine films incidentally. The latter two are demonstrated best with bone scanning techniques, using radioactively labeled diphosphate compounds.

Nephrocalcinosis is rarely seen radiographically, but lithiasis is common. Since the stones are usually radiopaque (i.e., calcium oxalate and calcium phosphate stones), nephrotomograms are helpful in identifying, localizing, and measuring them. This procedure is important in determining the "activity" of the stone disease (see Ch. 90). An increase in stone diameter with time can be taken as objective evidence of "active" stone disease and is probably an additional indication for treatment of hyperparathyroidism (see below). Primary hyperparathyroidism may also be associated, although less commonly, with uric acid stones (not radiopaque). Thus, x-ray examination of the urinary tract with contrast material is also important.

DIFFERENTIAL DIAGNOSIS. In general, the major problem in the differential diagnosis of primary hyperparathyroidism is distinguishing this disease from other conditions associated with hypercalcemia (Table 247–2). Hypercalcemia associated with thiazide diuretic therapy and with nonhematologic malignancy are the most frequently encountered among these. Other important causes of hypercalcemia are (1) hematologic malignancies involving bone (myeloma, lymphoma, and leukemia); (2) granulomatous diseases (sarcoidosis, tuberculosis, and berylliosis); (3) endocrine disorders,

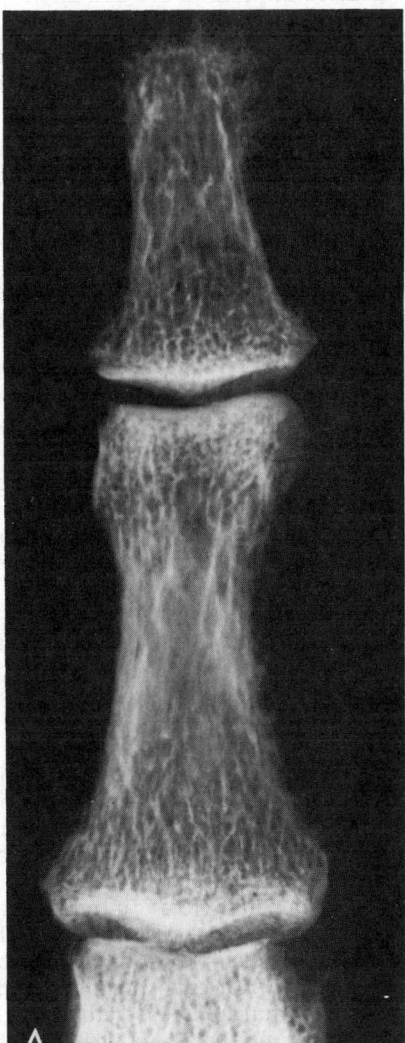

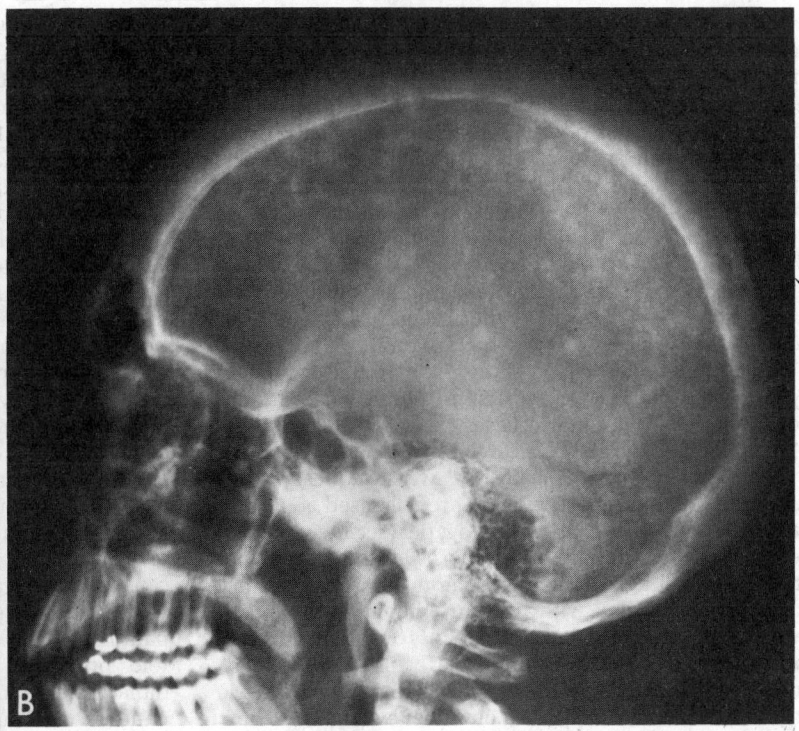

FIGURE 247–4. *A,* Magnified x-ray of index finger on fine-grain industrial film, showing classic subperiosteal resorption in patient with severe primary hyperparathyroidism. *B,* Skull x-ray from a patient with severe secondary hyperparathyroidism resulting from prolonged end-stage renal disease. Extensive areas of demineralization alternate with areas of increased bone density, resulting in an exaggerated picture of the "salt-and-pepper" skull x-ray, which used to be a classic finding in primary hyperparathyroidism. This is rarely seen now and cannot be visualized easily in x-ray reproductions. Although it is difficult to appreciate at this magnification, the dental lamina dura is absent, another classic x-ray finding in severe hyperparathyroidism. (Courtesy of Professor H. Genant, University of California, San Francisco, Department of Radiology.)

including thyrotoxicosis and acute adrenal insufficiency; (4) familial hypocalciuric hypercalcemia (a genetic disorder also called benign familial hypercalcemia); (5) excessive ingestion of calcium, vitamin D, or vitamin A; (6) extensive skeletal immobilization (e.g., spica body cast) in normal young people and prolonged bed rest in patients with osteolytic metabolic bone disease; and (7) idiopathic hypercalcemia of infancy.

Pathophysiologically, hypercalcemic disorders can be segregated into those caused by excess parathyroid hormone and those caused by factors other than parathyroid hormone (see Table 247–2). Only patients with primary hyperparathyroidism and certain patients with malignant diseases have both hypercalcemia and elevated levels of circulating parathyroid

TABLE 247–2. DIFFERENTIAL DIAGNOSIS OF HYPERCALCEMIA

Due to increased serum PTH
Primary and "tertiary" hyperparathyroidism
Some nonhematologic malignant neoplasms
Not due to increased serum PTH
Drug-induced hypercalcemia (thiazides, furosemide, vitamin D, calcium,
vitamin A, lithium)
Granulomatous diseases (sarcoidosis, tuberculosis, berylliosis)
Genetic diseases (familial hypocalciuric hypercalcemia)
Immobilization
"Idiopathic"
Most nonhematologic malignant neoplasms with hypercalcemia
Malignant hematologic diseases
Nonparathyroid endocrine diseases (Addison's disease, hyper- and
hypothyroidism)

From Arnaud CD, Kolb FO: The calciotropic hormones and metabolic bone disease. In Greenspan FS, Forsham PH (eds.): Basic and Clinical Endocrinology. Los Altos, CA, Lange Medical Publications, 1983, p 208.

hormone. In all other patients with hypercalcemia the secretion of parathyroid hormone is suppressed.

The underlying causes of the hypercalcemia in conditions without increased secretion of parathyroid hormone are varied and for the most part uncertain. They are discussed below under "Nonparathyroid Causes of Hypercalcemia." The most important among these, in terms of the differential diagnosis of primary hyperparathyroidism, are the hypercalcemia of malignancy and familial hypocalciuric hypercalcemia.

Hypercalcemia of Malignancy (see "Hypercalcemia and its treatment" below). It is unlikely that metastases to bone produce chronic hypercalcemia simply by physical displacement of bone. Rather, malignant tumors probably produce osteolytic humoral factors that act either systemically or locally in the immediate vicinity of a metastasis. These factors include parathyroid hormone–like substances, prostaglandins, lymphokines such as osteoclast activating factor (OAF), $1,25(OH)_2D_3$, growth factors such as the transforming growth factors, and probably other factors yet to be discovered. Any one or a combination of these factors might be secreted systemically by a tumor or released locally by its bony metastases in sufficient quantities to stimulate osteolysis and produce hypercalcemia.

Benign Familial Hypercalcemia. Benign familial hypercalcemia (or familial hypocalciuric hypercalcemia) is probably the second most important consideration in the differential diagnosis of primary hyperparathyroidism. This rare condition, inherited as an autosomal dominant trait, is characterized by asymptomatic hypercalcemia, hypocalciuria, a tendency toward mild hypermagnesemia, and normal to low levels of serum iPTH. Histologically, the parathyroid glands either are normal or show equivocal "hyperplasia," and subtotal parathyroidectomy has consistently failed to restore eucalcemia. The response of nephrogenous cyclic AMP to exogenous and endogenous parathyroid hormone is greater in patients with familial hypocalciuric hypercalcemia than in normal subjects or in patients with primary hyperparathyroidism. The hypercalcemia in this familial syndrome may be due, at least in part, to renal hypersensitivity to the hypocalciuric effects of parathyroid hormone. In this sense then, familial hypocalciuric hypercalcemia could be considered to be a form of hyperparathyroidism. However, the notable absence of the characteristic sequelae of primary hyperparathyroidism (e.g., renal stones and osteitis fibrosa cystica) in these patients clearly indicates that tissue hypersensitivity to parathyroid hormone is probably not generalized.

DIAGNOSTIC INVESTIGATIONS. *General.* The presence of hypercalcemia is established when at least three measurements of total serum calcium are increased above the normal range, which is 8.9 to 10.1 mg per deciliter. If laboratories use a wider normal range (e.g., 9.0 to 11.0 mg per deciliter), based either on poor selection of normal control subjects or on problems with calcium contamination in the laboratory (Ch. 244), numbers of patients with mild hypercalcemia (i.e., 10.2 to 11.0 mg per deciliter) will go undetected.

Hypercalcemia generally reflects serious underlying disease that may not have been suspected on initial evaluation. Thus, when unsuspected hypercalcemia is found, the history and physical examination should be repeated with specific objectives in mind. These include detailed evaluation of the duration of illness, drug intake, and possible presence of other endocrine diseases, a history of nephrolithiasis with documentation if possible, symptoms of malignancy, a family history of endocrine and mineral disorders, and the possible presence of palpable lymph nodes or masses, unusual skin pigmentation or lesions, and an enlarged thyroid, liver, or spleen.

Illness of long duration associated with kidney stones but no weight loss favors primary hyperparathyroidism; illness of short duration associated with weight loss without nephrolithiasis favors a nonparathyroid cause for hypercalcemia, particularly malignancy. A history of thiazide intake might explain an increase in serum calcium to 11.0 mg per deciliter, but higher values usually indicate that the effects of this drug have augmented the hypercalcemia of another condition (e.g., mild hyperparathyroidism). Patients who are taking thiazides and are hypercalcemic should be re-evaluated one month after discontinuing the drug. Vitamin D in doses exceeding 50,000 units per day can cause hypercalcemia in adults, and its ingestion may not have been elicited in the initial history. Hypercalcemic patients may be abnormally sensitive to vitamin D. Thus, intake of less than 50,000 units per day may aggravate existing hypercalcemia in sarcoidosis or primary hyperparathyroidism. What may appear initially to be a severe form of the primary disorder may prove to be relatively mild when vitamin D intake is curtailed. Excess calcium ingested in the form of antacids containing calcium carbonate (>5 grams per day) can cause severe hypercalcemia in susceptible individuals, especially when coupled with additional intake of alkali (bicarbonate) as in the "milk-alkali syndrome." This condition is rare in the absence of other abnormalities. Many patients actually have underlying primary hyperparathyroidism and are taking calcium carbonate and alkali for associated gastric hyperacidity.

The family history may hold the key to both the correct diagnosis and the correct treatment of a hypercalcemic patient. Systematic inquiry regarding a history of neck exploration and the presence of hypercalcemia, nephrolithiasis, metabolic bone disease, intractable peptic ulcer disease, and endocrine tumors in family members is essential. There is no specific family history in the syndrome of familial hypocalciuric hypercalcemia, although a history of unsuccessful parathyroid surgery in more than one hypercalcemic relative is characteristic of this condition. The diagnosis can be made definitively only by documenting hypercalcemia in the immediate relatives of the patient. If a multiple endocrine neoplasia syndrome or familial hyperparathyroidism is present, the patient will almost certainly have enlargement ("hyperplasia") of all four glands, and subtotal parathyroidectomy (removal of three and one-half glands), as opposed to single gland removal, would be indicated.

Radioimmunoassay of Parathyroid Hormone. The availability of sensitive and specific radioimmunoassays of parathyroid hormone in serum has revolutionized the approach to the diagnosis of primary hyperparathyroidism during the past few years. Previously, patients were first extensively evaluated for nonparathyroid disorders that could cause hypercalcemia, and the diagnosis of hyperparathyroidism was one of exclusion. Now measurements of serum iPTH and calcium allow the assignment of patients either to a group that is very likely to have a surgically resectable parathyroid lesion(s) or to groups that require further diagnostic evaluation for the cause of hypercalcemia (Fig. 247–5).

The author's experience in the diagnosis of primary hyperparathyroidism, using a radioimmunoassay of serum parathyroid hormone that is specific for the mid region of the molecule, is illustrated in Figure 247–6. Ninety per cent of patients with surgically proved disease had values of serum iPTH that exceeded the upper limit of normal, and 10 per cent had values that were in the upper range of normal but inappropriately high for the total calcium concentration. Not shown are serum iPTH values in patients with nonparathyroid hypercalcemia (e.g., sarcoidosis and vitamin D intoxication). These are low or undetectable except in ectopic hyperparathyroidism caused by nonparathyroid cancer (see below). Thus, it is possible, by measuring calcium and iPTH in a single morning fasting serum sample, to categorize correctly 80 to 90 per cent of the hypercalcemic patients who have a potentially resectable hyperfunctioning parathyroid gland(s) and to categorize a similar percentage of the patients who have nonparathyroid hypercalcemia and who therefore require further study to discover the underlying cause of this derangement (see below). The advantages of using the serum iPTH as the principal laboratory probe to "triage" the hypercalcemic patient are clear. In the majority of patients with primary hyperparathyroidism, a correct diagnosis can be made in an outpatient setting, eliminating the costs and inconveniences of hospitalization and the multiple indirect tests required for a similar, less definitive diagnosis by exclusion.

Values of serum iPTH, measured with an assay specific for the mid or carboxyl region, are much lower for a given serum calcium in malignancy-associated hypercalcemia than in primary hyperparathyroidism (Fig. 247–7). This interesting phenomenon is probably due to the fact that patients with the hypercalcemia of malignancy have relatively low serum quantities of carboxyl- and mid-region fragments in comparison to patients with primary hyperparathyroidism. Irrespective of the pathophysiology involved, the relationships shown in Figure 247–7 help greatly in determining the course of action to be followed in some hypercalcemic and hypophosphatemic patients who are suspected of having cancer (e.g., those with weight loss, anemia, or a high erythrocyte sedimentation rate) but in whom proof is lacking (Fig. 247–5). If serum calcium values are greater than 12.5 mg per deciliter and serum iPTH is within the normal range or only slightly increased, more intensive efforts should be made to identify a neoplastic lesion, and the patient should be followed with temporizing medical treatment. If the situation is not clarified after 6 to 12 months, the patient should be re-evaluated for the presence of primary hyperparathyroidism.

Clinical Chemistry. Several serum and urine measurements

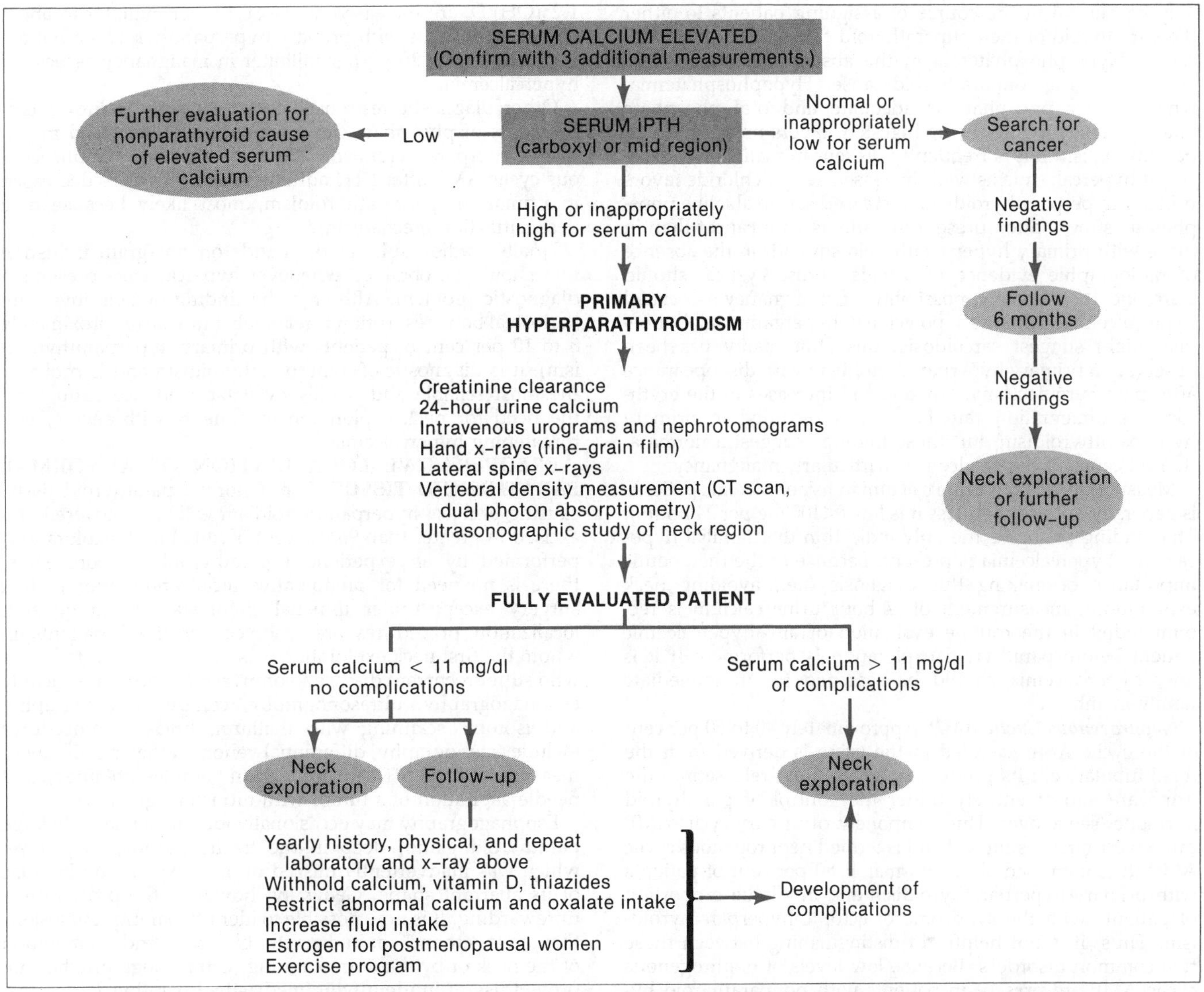

SERUM CALCIUM ELEVATED
(Confirm with 3 additional measurements.)
Further evaluation for nonparathyroid cause of elevated serum calcium
Low
SERUM iPTH
(carboxyl or mid region)
Normal or inappropriately low for serum calcium
Search for cancer
Negative findings
Follow 6 months
Negative findings
Neck exploration or further follow-up
High or inappropriately high for serum calcium
PRIMARY HYPERPARATHYROIDISM
Creatinine clearance
24-hour urine calcium
Intravenous urograms and nephrotomograms
Hand x-rays (fine-grain film)
Lateral spine x-rays
Vertebral density measurement (CT scan, dual photon absorptiometry)
Ultrasonographic study of neck region
FULLY EVALUATED PATIENT
Serum calcium < 11 mg/dl no complications
Serum calcium > 11 mg/dl or complications
Neck exploration
Follow-up
Neck exploration
Yearly history, physical, and repeat laboratory and x-ray above
Withhold calcium, vitamin D, thiazides
Restrict abnormal calcium and oxalate intake
Increase fluid intake
Estrogen for postmenopausal women
Exercise program
Development of complications

FIGURE 247–5. Use of PTH radioimmunoassay in the diagnosis and management of patients with hypercalcemia. (From Arnaud CD, Kolb FO: The calciotropic hormones and metabolic bone disease. In Greenspan FS, Forsham PH (eds.): Basic and Clinical Endocrinology. Los Altos, CA, Lange Medical Publications, 1983, p 211.)

SERUM iPTH (GP1M) (pg Eq hPTH (44–68)/ml)
5000
2000
1000
500
200
100
50
20
10
Primary Hyperparathyroidism (n = 450)
Normal
8.0 9.0 10.0 11.0 12.0 13.0 14.0 15.0 16.0 17.0
SERUM CALCIUM (mg/dl)

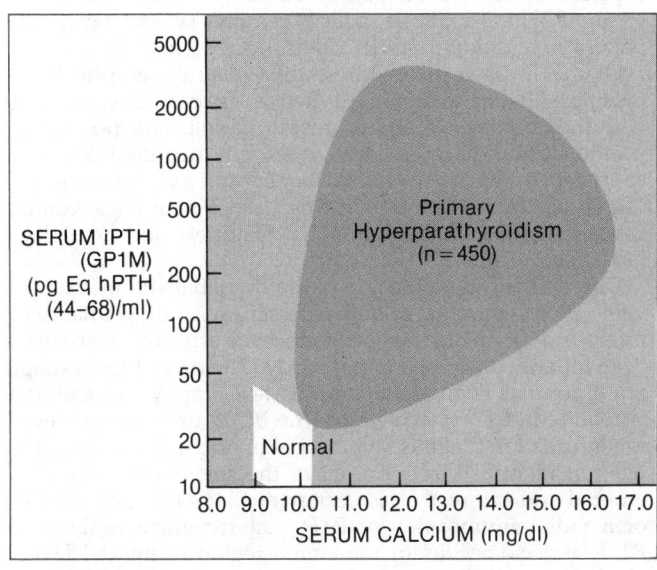

FIGURE 247–6. Serum iPTH in primary hyperparathyroidism.

SERUM iPTH (GP1M) (pg Eq hPTH (44–68)/ml)
1000
300
100
30
10
Primary Hyperparathyroidism
Malignancy-associated Hypercalcemia
Normal
0 9 10 11 12 13 14 15 16 17 18
SERUM CALCIUM (mg/dl)

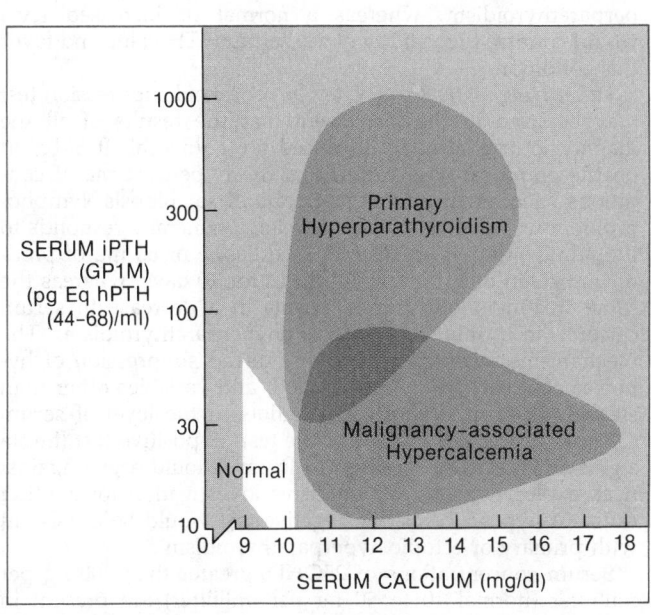

FIGURE 247–7. Serum iPTH in hypercalcemic states.

may be helpful in the course of assigning patients to either the parathyroid or the nonparathyroid categories of hypercalcemia. Hyperphosphatemia in the absence of severe renal failure favors a nonparathyroid cause. Hypophosphatemia, when dietary phosphate is adequate and oral phosphate binding agents are not being ingested, favors primary hyperparathyroidism but is frequently present in malignancy-associated hypercalcemia as well. Increased serum chloride favors primary hyperparathyroidism. Increased serum alkaline phosphatase is more often present in patients with cancer than in those with primary hyperparathyroidism and, in the absence of radiographic evidence of osteitis fibrosa cystica, should alert one to the likely possibility of malignancy-associated hypercalcemia. Although polyclonal hypergammaglobulinemia might suggest sarcoidosis, this abnormality has been observed in primary hyperparathyroidism with disappearance after parathyroidectomy. Anemia and increases in the erythrocyte sedimentation rate have been recorded in primary hyperparathyroidism, but these findings suggest a nonparathyroid cause of hypercalcemia, particularly malignancy.

Measurement of the urine calcium in hypercalcemic patients is generally not useful unless it is low (<100 mg per 24 hours). This finding may give the only indication that familial hypocalciuric hypercalcemia is present. Because of the therapeutic importance of making this diagnosis (i.e., avoiding neck exploration), measurement of 24-hour urine calcium is recommended in the routine evaluation of any hypercalcemic patient before parathyroid exploration is performed. If it is low, hypercalcemia should be searched for in immediate family members.

Nephrogenous Cyclic AMP. Approximately 40 to 50 per cent of the cyclic AMP excreted in the urine is derived from the renal tubular cell. Its production and cellular release into the urine are almost entirely under the control of parathyroid hormone (see above). This component of urinary cyclic AMP can be accurately estimated and is termed nephrogenous cyclic AMP. It is increased above normal in 80 per cent of patients with primary hyperparathyroidism and in a large proportion of patients with the syndrome of ectopic hyperparathyroidism. Thus, it is not helpful in distinguishing between these two common disorders. Because low levels of nephrogenous cyclic AMP are present in patients with nonparathyroid hypercalcemia (excluding malignancy-associated hypercalcemia), the test is useful in those patients whose serum iPTH is equivocally increased. In such patients, a low level of nephrogenous cyclic AMP would suggest that the serum iPTH value was artifactual and would argue against primary hyperparathyroidism, whereas a normal or increased level would confirm the validity of the serum iPTH value and favor this condition.

Other Diagnostic Tests. The glucocorticoid suppression test may be used in the rare event that the results of all the diagnostic tests already discussed are equivocal. It is based on the empirical observation that the hypercalcemia of conditions such as vitamin D intoxication, sarcoidosis, lymphoproliferative syndromes, and myeloma generally responds to the administration of 300 mg of cortisone or 60 mg of prednisone given daily in divided doses for 10 days, whereas the same treatment only rarely results in a decrease in serum calcium in primary or ectopic hyperparathyroidism. The mechanisms involved in steroid-induced suppression of hypercalcemia are poorly understood, and variables other than steroids (e.g., hydration) may influence the level of serum calcium during the 10 days of the test. A positive test (i.e., a significant decrease in serum calcium) should argue against neck exploration and for intensive investigation for another cause of hypercalcemia. A negative test would be consistent with primary or ectopic hyperparathyroidism.

Serum concentrations of $25OHD_3$ greater than 200 ng per milliliter (normal 10 to 50 ng per milliliter) are present in patients with vitamin D intoxication. Serum concentrations of

$1,25(OH)_2D_3$ are increased above 50 pg per milliliter in about half of all patients with primary hyperparathyroidism but are generally below 20 pg per milliliter in malignancy-associated hypercalcemia.

Other diagnostic tests used less frequently include measurements of phosphate clearance (which is increased in primary hyperparathyroidism) and measurement of nephrogenous cyclic AMP after PTH administration (which is decreased in primary hyperparathyroidism, most likely because of a desensitization mechanism).

Finally, radiographs of the hands on fine-grain industrial film should be obtained whenever hypercalcemia presents a diagnostic problem. Although the finding of definitive subperiosteal bone resorption is relatively unusual (approximately 8 to 10 per cent of patients with primary hyperparathyroidism), it is diagnostic of hyperparathyroidism and is probably the most reliable and readily available evidence supporting the need for neck exploration in patients with severe, lifethreatening hypercalcemia.

PREOPERATIVE LOCALIZATION OF ABNORMAL PARATHYROID TISSUE. The abnormal parathyroid tissue causing primary hyperparathyroidism will be discovered and excised in greater than 90 per cent of initial neck explorations performed by an experienced parathyroid surgeon. Thus, there is no need for preoperative localization prior to first surgery except under unusual circumstances. In general, localization procedures are reserved for those patients in whom the first neck exploration was unsuccessful or for those who suffer recurrent disease. Noninvasive procedures include esophagography, ultrasonography, computed tomography, and isotopic scanning with thallium. Invasive procedures include arteriography, differential venous catheterization with measurement of iPTH in the serum samples obtained, and needle aspiration of a tumor with ultrasonic guidance.

Esophagography may occasionally identify a relatively large parathyroid gland, deep in the tracheoesophageal groove, which was inadvertently missed on first exploration because of its aberrant shape. Generally, however, the procedure is unrewarding. It is now possible to identify parathyroid lesions that are less than 1 cm in diameter by ultrasound examination of the neck or by thallium scanning. Ultrasonography has not proved useful in identifying mediastinal parathyroid lesions, but computed tomography has. These noninvasive procedures may also have diagnostic value in the patient with severe hypercalcemia who has not undergone previous neck exploration. When a mass lesion(s) is identified in a location(s) consistent with normal or aberrant parathyroid tissue, the patient probably has primary hyperparathyroidism, and neck exploration should be performed early, before values for serum iPTH are available (usually requires several days) if the patient's condition is sufficiently serious.

Of the invasive procedures, thyroid arteriography is the most useful to the surgeon when a lesion is identified. As with the noninvasive procedures, the results are specific only in the sense that the location of an identified lesion is consistent with that of a normal or aberrant parathyroid gland. This procedure is not without risk, since neurologic complications such as transient occipital blindness and hemiplegia have been recorded.

Differential catheterization of the thyroidal and mediastinal veins for the purpose of obtaining serum for iPTH analysis is rarely indicated but can be performed after the veins have been identified during arteriography. The procedure is simple if a lesion has been identified by arteriography, since all that is required of iPTH analysis of the blood draining the lesion is confirmation that it is parathyroid in origin. If arteriography has not identified a lesion, all of the small veins should be entered and sampled. It is important that a bioassay for PTH or a radioimmunoassay of PTH that recognizes only intact PTH (assays specific for the amino region or intact PTH) be used for measurements of iPTH in sera obtained during differential venous catheterization. Step-up differences in iPTH concentrations between peripheral sera and sera from veins draining parathyroid lesions are greater using such assays because of the relatively low concentrations of intact PTH in the peripheral circulation. By contrast, mid- and carboxyl-region specific assays measure the high concentrations of mid- and carboxyl-region fragments in the peripheral circulation and provide smaller step-up increases.

TREATMENT. The medical treatment of hypercalcemia is described in detail below ("Nonparathyroid Causes of Hypercalcemia"). The discussion here will be confined to the definitive treatment of hyperparathyroidism per se. The surgical removal of abnormal parathyroid tissue should be considered in all patients in whom the diagnosis of primary hyperparathyroidism has been established. Although patients with only biochemical abnormalities do not always develop clinically significant sequelae, they often do. Furthermore, the majority of these patients have histologic evidence of hyperparathyroidism in bone biopsies. This should be kept in mind before a long-term medical follow-up program is embarked upon, especially in older women who may have already suffered considerable bone loss as a result of age-related factors. Age per se should not be a contraindication to neck exploration. In fact, it is better to perform elective parathyroidectomy in an older person than to face hypercalcemia later as a complication of another age-related, serious illness (e.g., MI).

If surgery is withheld and one embarks on following a patient who has hyperparathyroidism with only biochemical abnormalities, there remains a group of compelling indications for neck exploration: (1) radiographic evidence of metabolic bone disease, (2) demonstration of decreasing renal function, (3) active nephrolithiasis, (4) serum calcium concentrations greater than 11.0 mg per deciliter, and (5) the development of one or more "complications" of hyperparathyroidism, such as serious psychiatric disease, peptic ulcer that is resistant to treatment, pancreatitis, and severe hypertension. In any patient proposed for long-term follow-up, certain follow-up studies should be done systematically (Fig. 247–5). At a minimum, these should include a yearly history and physical examination, determinations of serum calcium and creatinine clearance, x-rays of the hand on fine-grain industrial film to detect subperiosteal bone resorption, and a plain film of the abdomen to detect renal calcifications. If inactive nephrolithiasis has been detected on initial examination, nephrotomograms should be done to determine if new stones have developed or old stones have increased in size. By definition, either of these would be interpreted as the recrudescence of active stone disease, which would in turn be an indication for surgery. The cost of such a follow-up program rapidly approaches the cost of parathyroidectomy within several years of the time it is initiated.

The most critical consideration in the surgical treatment of patients with primary hyperparathyroidism is the selection of the surgeon. He should not only have extensive experience in parathyroid surgery but also be able to recognize an abnormal, enlarged parathyroid gland—a difficult skill to attain. The surgeon usually attempts to identify all four parathyroid glands (using biopsy if absolutely necessary), with the plan of removing a single enlarged parathyroid gland or three and one-half parathyroid glands if multiple glands are involved. Less commonly, one side of the neck is explored first and any single enlarged parathyroid gland is removed. If the second parathyroid gland on the same side is normal, the other side of the neck is not explored. If the second parathyroid gland is abnormal, it is removed and the other side of the neck is explored and all the parathyroid tissue removed except for one half of a gland. The second approach has the advantage of leaving the unoperated side without scar tissue and easier to explore at a future time for recurrent hyperparathyroidism, but has the disadvantage of not firmly establishing whether multiple glands are enlarged.

Autotransplantation of parathyroid tissue to the muscles of the forearm may be of considerable value in special circumstances, such as when the last known parathyroid gland is removed because of recurrent primary hyperparathyroidism. Such patients are likely to be rendered hypoparathyroid without successful transplantation. The functioning of such transplants can be easily assessed by determining if there is a step-up in the concentration of parathyroid hormone in venous blood from the ipsilateral forearm in comparison with the other forearm.

Approximately 20 per cent of abnormal parathyroid glands are in the mediastinum, but the great majority of these (~95 per cent) are high enough that they can be readily identified and removed during routine neck exploration. In the remaining cases abnormal parathyroid tissue is located elsewhere in the mediastinum and can be approached for excision only by splitting the sternum. Before the advent of localization procedures (see above), the success rate in removing abnormal parathyroid tissue from the mediastinum was only 50 per cent. The decision to carry out mediastinal exploration depends to a large extent on the accuracy and completeness of the information obtained during initial neck exploration.

Postoperatively, serum calcium concentrations decrease to within the normal range or below within 24 to 48 hours. It is possible to determine if all of the abnormal parathyroid tissue has been removed by measuring urinary cyclic AMP (which should be decreased) within two hours of parathyroidectomy. Patients who have significant bony demineralization may develop significant hypocalcemia postoperatively, presumably owing to the avidity of demineralized bone for extracellular fluid calcium. This "hungry bone syndrome" can be distinguished from hypoparathyroidism by the absence of hyperphosphatemia and the presence of increased concentrations of serum iPTH. Treatment of this syndrome, which may be difficult, requires very large quantities of intravenous calcium given continuously by infusion and administration of calcium carbonate by mouth in doses of 1 to 5 grams per day, depending upon the serum calcium response. Administration of vitamin D (usually 50,000 to 100,000 units daily) is of equivocal value. However, the biologically active metabolite of vitamin D, $1,25(OH)_2D_3$, has proved to be an effective therapeutic agent. It should be given in doses starting at 0.5 μg per day, increasing by 0.25 μg daily until hypocalcemia is controlled. Care should be exerted to avoid overdosage and the development of hypercalcemia. If serum calcium values increase above 10.5 mg per deciliter, $1,25(OH)_2D_3$ treatment should be discontinued and reinstituted only if serum calcium values decrease below 8.0 mg per deciliter.

Most patients who develop hypocalcemia and mild hyperphosphatemia have temporary hypoparathyroidism, as evidenced by low normal values for serum iPTH. A small percentage of these patients will develop permanent hypoparathyroidism requiring treatment (see below).

Worsening of renal function (either temporary or permanent), metabolic acidosis, hypomagnesemia, pancreatitis, and gout or pseudogout may occur in the postoperative period. Deterioration in renal function should be anticipated in patients who have abnormal renal function preoperatively, and prophylactic mannitol infusions should be given early in the postoperative period to initiate an osmotic diuresis. Likewise, a flaring of gout or pseudogout should be anticipated in patients with intra-articular calcification or a history of prior arthritic attacks.

PROGNOSIS. The natural history of primary hyperparathyroidism is not known. This is because the majority of patients, once the diagnosis is established, are subjected to neck exploration and removal of the abnormal parathyroid glands and are cured.

A large proportion of patients have "biochemical" hyperparathyroidism—i.e., only a slightly increased serum calcium (10.1 to 11.0 mg per deciliter) and no clinical manifestations of the disease. In a large prospective study (150 patients), relatively few (10 to 30 per cent) progressed to a more severe form of the disease within five years. In this study, no clinical or biochemical abnormality was found to be predictive of such a progression.

It is presumed that patients with mild to moderately severe manifestations of primary hyperparathyroidism represent progression from a previously "biochemical" form of the disease. Some of these patients appear to attain a degree of disease stability; some patients have been observed for as long as 10 to 15 years without apparent progression. Except for a very small number who progress to severe disease, the remaining patients probably progress slowly in the signs and symptoms of the disease and suffer a gradual deterioration of renal function. Patients with severe primary hyperparathyroidism (serum calcium >15 mg per deciliter) will almost certainly die of their disease unless it is detected and appropriately treated.

Surgical resection of benign parathyroid lesions is generally curative in primary hyperparathyroidism. Recurrences are rare in patients who have single gland disease but relatively common when multiple glands are involved. The calcium nephropathy of hyperparathyroidism may be irreversible; whether improvement in hypertension occurs after successful treatment of hyperparathyroidism has not been established. Active nephrolithiasis generally becomes inactive unless factors other than primary hyperparathyroidism are present to perpetuate this problem. There have been anecdotal reports that severe psychiatric symptoms may disappear after the removal of abnormal parathyroid glands. All but the more severe forms of osteitis fibrosa cystica demonstrate improvement within months of parathyroidectomy and essentially complete resolution within a year. At present it is not known if the surgical treatment of hyperparathyroidism in patients who also have postmenopausal or senile osteoporosis results in improvement of the osteopenic disease. However, this will be important to determine because as many as 8 to 10 per cent of patients with age-related osteopenia have increased circulating levels of immunoreactive parathyroid hormone and may suffer from some form of curable hyperparathyroidism.

Arnaud CD, Clark OH: Primary hyperparathyroidism. In Krieger DT, Bardin CW: Current Therapy in Endocrinology 1983–1984. Philadelphia and St. Louis, BC Decker, Inc, and CV Mosby Company, 1983, pp 277–282. *Review of the medical and surgical treatment of primary hyperparathyroidism.*

Broadus AE, Stewart AF: Humoral mechanisms of hypercalcemia. In Peck WA (ed.): Bone and Mineral Research Annual 2. New York, Elsevier, 1984, pp 311–364. *Broadly based review of the endocrinology of hypercalcemia with emphasis on pathophysiology.*

Christensson T, Hellström K, Wengle B, et al.: Prevalence of hypercalcemia in health screening in Stockholm. Acta Med Scand 200:131, 1976. *In this study at least 3 per cent of 15,903 residents of Stockholm (predominantly middle-aged) had "asymptomatic hypercalcemia" and, most probably, primary hyperparathyroidism.*

Clark OH, Stark DD, Gooding GAW, et al.: Localization procedures in patients requiring reoperation for hyperparathyroidism. World J Surg 8:509, 1986. *Comparison of the efficacy of recently developed techniques for the localization of abnormal parathyroid glands.*

DeGroot LJ (ed.): Endocrinology. Vol 2. New York, Grune & Stratton, 1979, pp 693–737. *Extensive and inclusive review of primary hyperparathyroidism by internationally renowned experts. The subjects discussed include clinical features, differential diagnosis, parathyroid hormone radioimmunoassay, localizing techniques, medical management, and surgical management.*

Foley TP Jr, Harrison HC, Arnaud CD, et al.: Familial benign hypercalcemia. J Pediatr 81:1060, 1972. *First description of the syndrome of familial benign hypercalcemia, or familial hypocalciuric hypercalcemia.*

Heath H III, Hodgson SF, Kennedy MA: Primary hyperparathyroidism: Incidence, morbidity and potential economic impact in a community. N Engl J Med 302:189, 1980. *Only available systematic epidemiologic study of the incidence of primary hyperparathyroidism in a well-characterized general population.*

Strewler GJ, Nissenson RA: Nonparathyroid hypercalcemia. Adv Intern Med 32:235, 1986. *A useful review of the pathophysiology of the disorders that most frequently enter into the differential diagnosis of hyperparathyroidism.*

HYPOPARATHYROIDISM

DEFINITION. Hypoparathyroidism, or deficient secretion of parathyroid hormone, is characterized clinically by symptoms of neuromuscular hyperactivity and biochemically by hypocalcemia, hyperphosphatemia, and diminished to absent levels of circulating immunoreactive parathyroid hormone.

ETIOLOGY. There are three types of hypoparathyroidism: surgically induced, idiopathic, and functional. *Surgically induced hypoparathyroidism,* the most common of these, may occur after any surgical procedure in which the anterior neck is explored, including thyroidectomy, removal of abnormal parathyroid glands, and excision of various malignant lesions in the neck. Parathyroid glands need not actually be removed for hypoparathyroidism to ensue. In such cases it is presumed that the blood supply to the parathyroid glands has been compromised.

Idiopathic hypoparathyroidism occurs spontaneously and can be categorized according to whether it appears early or late in life. Aside from congenital absence of the glands, as in DiGeorge's syndrome (see Ch. 419), the syndromes occurring at an early age are genetic and are transmitted most frequently as an autosomal recessive trait. This type of hypoparathyroidism is called multiple endocrine deficiency–autoimmune–candidiasis (MEDAC) syndrome or juvenile familial endocrinopathy–hypoparathyroidism–Addison's disease–moniliasis (HAM) syndrome. Hypoparathyroidism, Addison's disease, and mucocutaneous candidiasis characterize the disorder. Circulating antibodies specific for parathyroid and adrenal tissues are frequently present, but they correlate poorly with clinical manifestations. Sporadic cases of MEDAC syndrome have been reported, as well as cases that have an autosomal recessive mode of inheritance. The majority of these are generally seen at a later age, and some have hypoparathyroidism only. This syndrome is described in Ch. 241. The late-onset form of idiopathic hypoparathyroidism occurs sporadically and circulating glandular antibodies are absent. The cause of parathyroid gland destruction in these cases is unknown.

Functional hypoparathyroidism occurs in patients with severe and prolonged hypomagnesemia of whatever cause (see Ch. 208). Since magnesium is required for release of parathyroid hormone from the glands, serum iPTH is characteristically low or undetectable in this syndrome. Infusion of magnesium increases serum iPTH rapidly (within minutes), and restoration of magnesium to normal levels ultimately restores eucalcemia. Magnesium is probably also required for the peripheral action of parathyroid hormone; the hypocalcemia in patients with functional hypoparathyroidism may be due, in part, to the failure of PTH to act normally on its target tissues.

Neonatal hypoparathyroidism occurs in infants of mothers who have primary hyperparathyroidism. It is presumed that in utero exposure to maternal hypercalcemia results in prolonged suppression of fetal parathyroid glands and failure of the parathyroid glands to respond to hypocalcemic stimuli after birth.

PATHOLOGY. Patients with MEDAC syndrome may have lymphocytic infiltration and fibrosis of glands. In the few patients with late-onset idiopathic hypoparathyroidism who have been examined, fatty infiltration, fibrosis, and atrophy have been found. Long-standing cases of hypoparathyroidism have characteristic soft tissue calcifications in the lens and basal ganglia of the brain. All types of bone cells are diminished, and both formation and resorption surfaces in bone are decreased.

PATHOPHYSIOLOGY AND CLINICAL CHEMISTRY. The pathophysiology and biochemical consequences of parathyroid gland removal can be appreciated by referring to the "butterfly" diagram (see Fig. 244–1). In hypoparathyroidism the right limbs of the three feedback loops predominate. There is (1) decreased bone resorption; (2) decreased renal phosphate excretion, increased serum phosphate, decreased $1,25(OH)_2D$, and decreased intestinal absorption of calcium; and (3) increased excretion of calcium for the prevailing serum concentration of calcium. Patients have hypocalcemia and generally hyperphosphatemia, provided that dietary phosphate has been normal. Urinary calcium is usually low unless eucalcemia has been restored with treatment. In that case, urinary calcium is generally inappropriately high for the level of serum calcium and occasionally reaches hypercalciuric levels. Nephrogenous cyclic AMP is decreased but increases briskly with the administration of parathyroid hormone.

Hypocalcemia and mild alkalosis (resulting from decreased bicarbonate excretion), if sufficiently severe, cause increased neuromuscular excitability with consequent tetany and, rarely, convulsions.

CLINICAL MANIFESTATIONS (Table 247–3). The clinical manifestations of hypoparathyroidism depend upon the severity of the disease (degree of hypocalcemia) and its chronicity. The rate of decrease in the serum calcium appears to be a major determinant in the development of the neuromuscular complications (see below) of hypocalcemia. Thus, these symptoms are more likely to occur within one to two days after parathyroidectomy, when serum calcium decreases acutely, and at serum calcium values that may be considerably higher (e.g., 8.0 mg per deciliter) than might be found in patients who have had more severe hypocalcemia (e.g., 6.0 mg per deciliter) for a longer time. It is therefore important to observe patients carefully for the development of the clinical signs heralding tetany, immediately and for several days after neck surgery in the region of the parathyroid glands, rather than relying entirely on the absolute concentration of the serum calcium.

Hypocalcemia causes a decreased threshold of excitation, repetitive responses to a single stimulus, reduced accommodation, and, at the extreme, continuous activity of nervous tissues. Such neural activity occurs spontaneously in both sensory and motor fibers in hypocalcemic states and gives rise to neuromuscular symptoms and signs. Symptoms include numbness and tingling around the mouth, in the tips of the fingers, and sometimes in the feet. An attack of tetany usually begins with this prodrome and is followed by muscle spasms in the extremities and face. The hands, forearms, and less commonly, feet become contorted in a characteristic way (Fig. 247–8). First, the thumb is strongly adducted, followed by flexion of the metacarpophalangeal joints, extension of the interphalangeal joints (with fingers together), and flexion of the wrist and elbow joints. This somewhat grotesque spastic condition may be quite painful but is more alarming than dangerous. Because of its alarming quality, patients may hyperventilate and secrete more epinephrine. Hyperventilation causes hypocapnia and alkalosis and worsens hypocalcemia by increasing the binding of ionic calcium to plasma proteins. Increased epinephrine secretion produces further anxiety, tachycardia, sweating, and peripheral and circumoral pallor. Prolonged hyperventilation in normal subjects can lower serum ionic calcium and produce tetany, but great care should be exercised in attributing such findings to hyperventilation alone.

Patients with hypoparathyroidism may have convulsions, especially during childhood. A more generalized form of tetany may be followed by prolonged tonic spasms, or the patient may have a typical epileptiform seizure (grand mal,

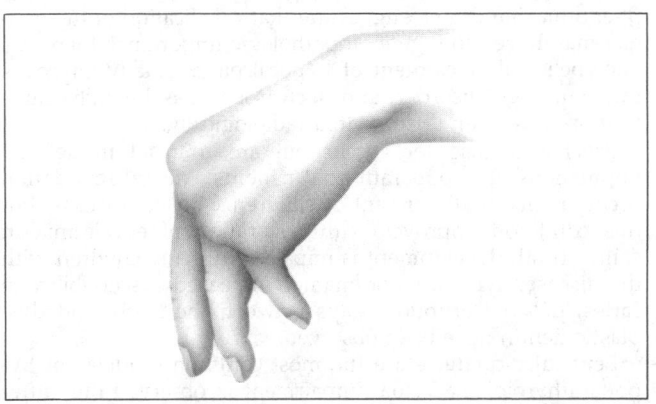

FIGURE 247–8. Position of hand in hypocalcemic tetany (Trousseau's sign). (From Ganong WF: Review of Medical Physiology. 11th ed. Los Altos, CA, Lange Medical Publications, 1983, p 319.)

jacksonian, focal, or petit mal), with characteristic associated electroencephalographic (EEG) findings. Because restoration of eucalcemia results in a decrease in the number of seizures without improvement in the EEG findings associated with seizures, it is thought that hypocalcemia lowers the excitation threshold of pre-existing epilepsy in such patients. The characteristic EEG changes associated with hypocalcemia per se do disappear after restoration of eucalcemia. Laryngeal spasm and stridor may occur during tetany and may precipitate seizures because of hypoxia. The relatively unusual finding of papilledema and increased intracranial pressure resulting from hypocalcemia in association with convulsions may suggest the diagnosis of brain tumor.

Latent tetany can be detected by several relatively specific physical signs. *Chvostek's sign* is elicited by tapping the facial nerve just anterior to the ear lobe, just below the zygomatic arch, or between the zygomatic arch and the corner of the mouth. The response ranges from twitching of the lip at the corner of the mouth to twitching of all of the facial muscles on the stimulated side. Simple twitching at the corner of the mouth occurs in 25 per cent of normal subjects, but more extensive muscle contraction (ala nasi and orbital muscles) is a reliable sign of latent tetany.

Trousseau's sign is demonstrated with a sphygmomanometer cuff inflated about the arm to above the systolic blood pressure for at least two minutes. A positive response consists of the development of typical ipsilateral carpal spasm (Fig. 247–8), with relaxation only occurring five to ten seconds after the cuff is deflated. Apparent spasm disappearing instantly should be regarded with suspicion. Trousseau's sign is the most reliable physical finding of latent tetany, and serial tests for this sign should be done and the results recorded in the immediate postoperative period after anterior neck surgery.

Beyond the neurologic manifestations described above, there are a number of other possible manifestations of hypocalcemia: (1) basal ganglia calcification and occasional extrapyramidal neurologic syndromes; (2) papilledema and increased intracranial pressure; (3) psychiatric disorders; (4) skin, hair, and fingernail abnormalities; (5) susceptibility to *Candida* infections; (6) inhibition of normal dental development; (7) lenticular cataracts; (8) intestinal malabsorption; (9) prolongation of the Q-T$_c$ and S-T intervals of the electrocardiogram, in rare cases 2:1 heart block, and even more rarely heart failure requiring digitalis and diuretics; and (10) increased serum concentrations of creatine phosphokinase and lactic dehydrogenase.

Extrapyramidal neurologic syndromes, including classic parkinsonism, may occur in patients with chronic hypoparathyroidism. Such manifestations are presumably caused by the basal ganglia calcification observed in the majority of such patients. Many untreated patients with extrapyramidal syndromes are unduly sensitive to the dystonic side effects of

TABLE 247–3. SYMPTOMS AND SIGNS OF HYPOCALCEMIA

Enhanced neuromuscular irritability
  Paresthesias (numbness, tingling), especially around mouth and tips of
    fingers
  Tetany—positive Chvostek's and Trousseau's sign
  Grand mal seizures
Lenticular cataracts—decreased vision
Basal ganglia calcification—rarely extrapyramidal abnormalities
Papilledema and increased intracranial pressure
Intestinal malabsorption (which may further exacerbate hypocalcemia)
Trophic changes in skin, fingernails, and developing teeth
Prolonged Q-T interval; rarely heart block and congestive heart failure

From Andreoli TE, Carpenter CCJ, Plum F, et al. (eds.): Cecil Essentials of Medicine. Philadelphia, WB Saunders Company, 1986, p 513.

phenothiazine drugs, suggesting that calcification of the ganglia may have more general pathologic importance than was once believed. Treatment of hypocalcemia usually improves the neurologic disorder, and decreases in basal ganglia calcification have been documented radiologically.

Psychiatric disorders occur but are unusual in defined populations of hypoparathyroid patients. Mental retardation occurs in about 20 per cent of children with the disease, but this condition improves with restoration of eucalcemia in some. Tooth development is impaired in many children with the disease; hypoplasia of enamel, increased susceptibility to caries, delayed eruption, gaps between the teeth, and dysplastic dentin have been observed.

Lenticular cataracts are the most common sequelae of hypoparathyroidism. Visual impairment is observed only after five to ten years of cataract development. Fully mature cataracts in hypoparathyroidism are confluent and produce total opacity of the lens. Such cataracts are different from senile cataracts, which are frequently confined to one segment of the lens. Successful treatment of hypocalcemia generally halts the progress of cataracts, and, rarely, opacities may diminish in size.

The skin of patients with long-standing hypoparathyroidism may be dry and scaling, the nails ridged longitudinally, and the hair coarse, dry, friable, and falling. An occasional patient will suffer exfoliative dermatitis or atopic eczema, and existing psoriasis may be made worse. All of these lesions tend to improve and disappear with restoration of eucalcemia. *Candida* infections can complicate skin, nail, and hair abnormalities. They also improve with treatment of hypocalcemia but may require specific antifungal therapy as well.

Intestinal malabsorption with steatorrhea occurs in rare cases of long-standing untreated hypoparathyroidism. The disorder is presumed to be due to decreased serum calcium because it is reversed by successful treatment of hypocalcemia but not by a gluten-free diet. The problem is particularly difficult to manage because the treatment of hypoparathyroidism largely depends upon the ability to increase calcium transport across a normal gastrointestinal tract with drugs. Conversely, malabsorption may cause functional hypoparathyroidism by producing magnesium deficiency.

Hypocalcemia causes prolongation of the Q-T$_c$ interval in the electrocardiogram, but clinical cardiac abnormalities are rare in hypoparathyroidism. Congestive heart failure, requiring digitalis and diuretics, has been reported, but this condition usually reverses following successful treatment of hypocalcemia.

DIAGNOSIS. The detection of hypoparathyroidism depends upon maintaining a high index of suspicion in certain clinical situations. Serum calcium should be measured yearly in patients who have had anterior neck surgery or who are suspected of having the MEDAC syndrome. Cutaneous candidiasis, cataracts, incidental discovery of basal ganglia calcification, convulsions, numbness and tingling of the fingers, facial muscle spasm (spontaneous or self-induced), delayed dentition, and developmental retardation should all prompt serum calcium measurement.

In the absence of renal failure, the diagnosis of hypoparathyroidism is virtually certain if hypocalcemia and hyperphosphatemia are found. However, some patients may be actually relatively depleted in phosphate because of dietary restriction or the ingestion of aluminum hydroxide gels. In addition, in patients who have undergone parathyroidectomy for primary hyperparathyroidism, bone uptake of minerals may be so great as to produce hypophosphatemia (the "hungry bone syndrome"). The measurement of serum iPTH is crucial for diagnosis. Increased values in a range appropriate to the degree of hypocalcemia would essentially exclude the presence of hypoparathyroidism and suggest the possibility of end-organ resistance to parathyroid hormone (i.e., pseudohypoparathyroidism [see below], vitamin D deficiency, and

vitamin D dependency) or secondary hyperparathyroidism resulting from such disorders as dietary deficiency of calcium, intestinal malabsorption of calcium, or excessive intake of drugs containing absorbable phosphate (Fig. 247–9).

Undetectable serum iPTH confirms the diagnosis of hypoparathyroidism, provided that the assay used is sufficiently sensitive to measure serum iPTH in the large majority of normal subjects. Serum iPTH may be barely detectable in some patients with hypoparathyroidism if the assay employed is very sensitive, but such low values may be due to nonspecific effects of serum per se in radioimmunoassays that do not adequately control for this factor.

Patients with functional hypoparathyroidism resulting from hypomagnesemia also have low to undetectable levels of serum iPTH. Detection of this condition depends upon the measurement of serum magnesium and its diagnosis upon the demonstration that successful treatment with magnesium salts restores eucalcemia and increases serum iPTH (see Ch. 208).

TREATMENT. Theoretically, the most appropriate therapy for hypoparathyroidism would be the physiologic replacement of parathyroid hormone. This approach is impractical at present because the hormone must be administered parenterally and because synthetic human parathyroid hormone is too expensive. Such treatment might become practical in the future for some patients who are poorly controlled on conventional regimens.

Because of the absence of parathyroid hormone and the consequent hyperphosphatemia, the renal enzyme that converts 25OHD to 1,25(OH)$_2$D, 1α-hydroxylase, is relatively inactive in patients with hypoparathyroidism. Conversion of circulating 25OHD to 1,25(OH)$_2$D is poor, and serum levels of this most active vitamin D metabolite are low or undetectable. In fact, hypoparathyroid patients are resistant to pharmacologic quantities of vitamin D for this reason.

The lowering of serum phosphate levels, using diets low in phosphate (i.e., restricting dairy products and meat) and oral aluminum hydroxide gels to bind intestinal phosphate, might be expected to increase the conversion of 25OHD to 1,25(OH)$_2$D, but such treatment has received little attention. Rather, treatment with pharmacologic doses of vitamin D$_2$ or its more potent analogue, dihydrotachysterol, in combination with oral calcium, has been the mainstay regimen for many years. Unfortunately, unpredictable hypercalcemic episodes sometimes occur with this therapeutic regimen unless serum

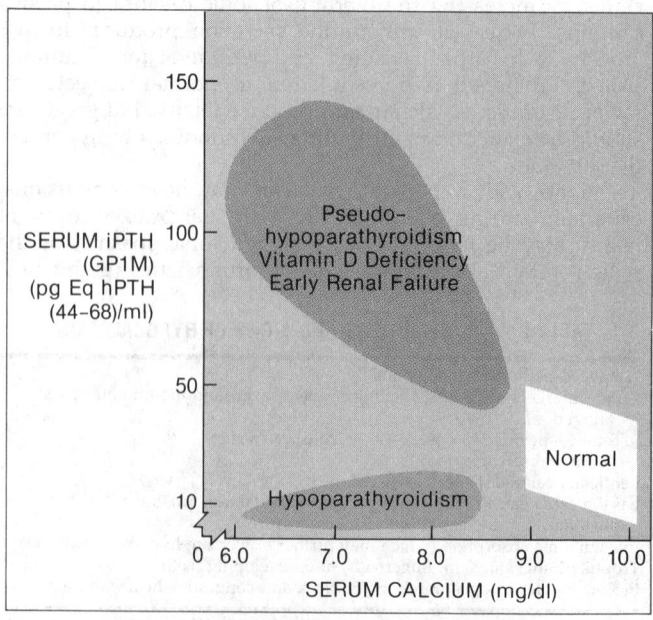

FIGURE 247–9. Serum iPTH in hypocalcemic states.

calcium is monitored at least once per month. A single episode of vitamin D intoxication can irreversibly impair renal function and can last from weeks to months because the body stores vitamin D and its metabolite 25OHD. The treatment of the vitamin D intoxication is similar to that described for severe hypercalcemia (see below), but with the additional use of corticosteroids (60 mg of prednisone or 300 mg of cortisone in four divided doses per day), which appear to antagonize vitamin D action.

Tetany caused by hypoparathyroidism requires emergency treatment with intravenous calcium to prevent laryngeal stridor and convulsions, the occurrence of which cannot be predicted. A 10 per cent solution of calcium gluconate (10 to 20 ml) should be given slowly (not more than 10 ml per minute) intravenously until symptoms are relieved or until serum calcium rises above 7 mg per deciliter. Hypercalcemia should be avoided; maintaining calcium levels between 7.5 and 9.0 mg per deciliter is adequate. Caution should be exercised in patients taking digitalis because calcium potentiates the action of this drug on the heart. Electrocardiographic monitoring during intravenous administration of calcium is prudent. It may be necessary to maintain serum calcium at levels that prevent tetany for several days before treatment with vitamin D or its metabolites or analogues (see below) becomes effective. This is accomplished by combining oral with intravenous calcium administration. Oral calcium is begun as soon as possible, starting with 200 mg of elemental calcium (as the gluconate or chloride salt) every two hours, increasing to 500 mg with each dose. If serum calcium falls below 7.5 mg per deciliter after six hours of the combined intravenous and oral regimen, continuous calcium infusion should be started. Five hundred ml of 5 per cent glucose and water containing 10 ml of 10 per cent calcium gluconate (1 gram) is given over six hours initially, with the quantity of calcium increased in increments of 5 ml (0.5 grams) every six hours until satisfactory control is achieved. In patients with hyperparathyroidism and bone disease who have undergone successful excision of a hyperfunctioning parathyroid gland(s), hypocalcemia may be profound and extremely resistant to treatment. As much as 10 grams of elemental calcium administered intravenously by infusion over 24 hours may be required to increase serum calcium above 7.5 mg per deciliter.

Patients with hypocalcemia due to hypoparathyroidism or postparathyroidectomy "bone hunger" syndrome are resistant to vitamin D, but $1,25(OH)_2D_3$ is highly effective in restoring serum calcium values to normal. It should be used in the acute treatment of symptomatic hypocalcemia concomitantly with oral and intravenous calcium. A dose of 0.5 μg is given initially followed by dose increases of 0.25 μg daily until hypocalcemia is controlled.

Because $1,25(OH)_2D_3$ is expensive, most patients with severe hypoparathyroidism require some form of long-term treatment with vitamin D. The only natural vitamin D preparation currently available for general clinical use is ergocalciferol, or vitamin D_2, which is derived from plant sources (vitamin D_3 is the naturally produced compound in humans). In initiating vitamin D_2 therapy, the development of hypercalcemia can best be avoided by giving small doses initially (0.2 mg [8,000 units] to 0.5 mg [20,000 units]), with gradual increases only after steady-state levels of serum calcium are achieved at each dose level. Most patients can be managed successfully with 1.0 mg (40,000 units) to 3.0 mg (120,000 units) of vitamin D_2 daily. The occasional patient who requires more than 3.0 mg per day is a candidate for the shorter-acting analogues or metabolites of vitamin D.

Dihydrotachysterol, an analogue of vitamin D, is the least expensive of these. An effective regimen is as follows: dihydrotachysterol, 4 mg per day for two days, then 2 mg per day for two days, then 1 mg per day until dose adjustment is required, as judged by serum calcium values. Ideally, serum calcium should be maintained between 8.5 and 9.0 mg per

deciliter, leaving a margin for the calcium to fluctuate upward to levels that are still not dangerous. The major advantage of dihydrotachysterol is its relatively rapid onset of action and short half-life. With regard to the latter, hypercalcemia caused by inadvertent overdosage is relieved within one to three weeks after the drug is discontinued; in comparison, the hypercalcemic effects of overdoses of vitamin D persist for 6 to 18 weeks. Dihydrotachysterol offers another advantage in that parathyroid function can be tested fairly soon after withdrawal of the drug. Hypocalcemia occurring within two weeks of withdrawal proves the persistence of hypoparathyroidism.

Relatively little information is now available concerning the long-term management of hypoparathyroidism with the vitamin D_3 metabolites $25(OH)D_3$ (calcifediol) or $1,25(OH)_2D_3$ (calcitriol). Both appear to be biologically effective and superior to vitamin D_2 with respect to the rapidity of onset and termination of action. Neither seems to have major advantages over dihydrotachysterol, except in patients who are particularly difficult to manage. The initiation and termination of action appear to be faster for $1,25(OH)_2D_3$ than for dihydrotachysterol. Both metabolites are even more expensive than dihydrotachysterol.

Since vitamin D acts primarily to increase intestinal calcium absorption, dietary calcium must be adequate: an approximate total (dietary and supplemental) intake of 1.0 gram daily in patients under 40 and 2 grams in patients over 40. Supplements can be provided by administering calcium as the gluconate, chloride, or carbonate salt. There are disadvantages to each. Calcium gluconate tablets contain relatively small quantities of calcium (9 per cent by weight), so that a large number of tablets must be given. Calcium chloride tablets contain larger quantities of calcium (27 per cent) but tend to produce gastric irritation. Calcium carbonate tablets also contain large quantities of calcium (40 per cent) but tend to produce alkalosis, which may aggravate hypocalcemia.

Patients with milder hypoparathyroidism may require only calcium supplementation (1 to 5 grams daily) and moderate degrees of phosphate restriction (including aluminum hydroxide gels) to maintain serum calcium in a therapeutic range. This treatment should be tried whenever a successful outcome is thought to be possible in order to avoid vitamin D intoxication entirely.

Long-term restoration of serum calcium to normal or nearly normal levels usually results in improvement in most manifestations of surgical and idiopathic hypoparathyroidism, including the skin disorders and associated candidiasis. Unfortunately, the latter appears to persist in the MEDAC syndrome, and resolution usually can be achieved only with iodoquinol or with systemic amphotericin (alone or combined with transfer factor) therapy.

Hypercalciuria can complicate successful restoration of a normal plasma calcium owing to the absence of the influence of parathyroid hormone to maintain normal renal tubular reabsorption of calcium. Accurate measurement of 24-hour urine calcium is therefore mandatory as serum calcium approaches the normal range during calcium and vitamin D treatment in order to avert possible renal stone formation. Thiazide diuretics, which cause increased renal tubular reabsorption of calcium, may be useful in such patients and may have the added advantage of partially restoring eucalcemia as a result of this action.

Anast CS, Mohs JM, Kaplan SL, et al.: Evidence for parathyroid failure in magnesium deficiency. Science 177:606, 1972. *First definitive demonstration of functional hypoparathyroidism in a magnesium-deficient patient with a selective intestinal defect in the absorption of magnesium.*

Attie JM, Kafif RA: Preservation of parathyroid glands during total thyroidectomy. Improved techniques utilizing microsurgery. Am J Surg 130:399, 1975. *Describes techniques in thyroid surgery that should help prevent destruction of the parathyroid glands and consequent hypoparathyroidism.*

Avioli LV: The therapeutic approach to hypoparathyroidism. Am J Med 57:34, 1974. *An important review of the problems encountered in the treatment of hypoparathyroidism.*

Hunt G, Morgan DB: The early effects of dihydrotachysterol on calcium and phosphorus metabolism in patients with hypoparathyroidism. Clin Sci 38:713, 1970. *A careful evaluation of the effects of dihydrotachysterol in patients with hypoparathyroidism.*

Neer RM, Holick MF, DeLuca HF, et al.: Effects of 1α-hydroxyvitamin D₃ and 1,25(OH)₂D₃ on calcium and phosphorus metabolism in hypoparathyroidism. Metabolism 24:1403, 1975. *These authors investigated the acute effects of 1αOHD₃ and 1,25(OH)₂D₃ in five patients with surgical hypoparathyroidism and found that these compounds are rapid acting. Since urinary hydroxyproline levels did not increase, they concluded that these compounds act on the intestine rather than on bone to increase serum calcium.*

Nusynowitz ML, Frame B, Kolb FO: The spectrum of the hypoparathyroid states: A classification based on physiologic principles. Medicine 55:105, 1976. *Broad and in-depth evaluation of all forms of hypoparathyroidism.*

Parfitt AM: The incidence of hypoparathyroid tetany after thyroid operations. Relationship to age, extent of resection and surgical experience. Med J Aust 1:1103, 1971. *Detailed compilation of the factors involved in the production of hypoparathyroidism resulting from thyroidectomy.*

Parfitt AM: The spectrum of hypoparathyroidism. J Clin Endocrinol Metab 34:152, 1972. *This detailed analysis of serum calcium values in hypoparathyroid patients formed the basis for the author's classification of the severity of the disease.*

Parfitt AM: Adult hypoparathyroidism. Treatment with calcifediol. Arch Intern Med 138:874, 1978. *A systematic study of the therapeutic efficacy of 25OHD in hypoparathyroid patients for a total of 19 patient-years.*

Parfitt AM: Surgical, idiopathic, and other varieties of parathyroid hormone–deficient hypoparathyroidism. In DeGroot LJ (ed.): Endocrinology. Vol 2. New York, Grune & Stratton, 1979, pp 755–768. *Comprehensive review of parathyroid hormone–deficient hypoparathyroidism.*

Stewart AF, Broadus AE: Mineral metabolism. In Felig P, Baxter JD, Broadus AE, et al. (eds.): Endocrinology and Metabolism. 2nd ed. New York, McGraw-Hill Book Company, 1987, pp 1317–1453. *This general review of mineral metabolism contains an excellent, succinct summary of hyperparathyroidism and pseudohypoparathyroidism (next section).*

PSEUDOHYPOPARATHYROIDISM AND PSEUDOPSEUDOHYPOPARATHYROIDISM

DEFINITIONS. *Pseudohypoparathyroidism* describes a rare clinical state of hypoparathyroidism that results from target tissue resistance to parathyroid hormone, associated with a secondary, hypocalcemia-induced increase in parathyroid gland function. Patients with pseudohypoparathyroidism classically have a variety of congenital defects in growth and skeletal development including short stature and foreshortened metacarpal and metatarsal bones (Fig. 247–10). Patients with *pseudopseudohypoparathyroidism* have analogous development defects without clinical hypoparathyroidism. Some patients with pseudohypoparathyroidism have target tissue resistance to the hormone but no developmental abnormalities, and others with developmental abnormalities have spontaneous remission of clinical hypoparathyroidism. Very rarely, patients have developmental abnormalities and clinical hypoparathyroidism with typical osteitis fibrosa cystica, a syndrome described by the barbarism "pseudohyperhypoparathyroidism."

ETIOLOGY AND GENETICS. It is difficult to conceive that all these combinations of manifestations could be ascribed to a single underlying biochemical defect. Although abnormal target tissue responses to parathyroid hormone may be the underlying theme, it is likely that an array of separate, rate-limiting steps, from receptor binding of parathyroid hormone to final expression of the cellular actions of the hormone (see Fig. 247–3) could be involved.

In some patients with pseudohypoparathyroidism, the guanyl nucleotide–sensitive regulatory protein (N protein), which couples parathyroid hormone–occupied receptors to adenylate cyclase, is decreased by 50 per cent in the red blood cells (see Fig. 247–3). In such patients this defect appears to produce resistance to several other hormones that apparently exert their actions by stimulating the increased production of cellular cyclic AMP (e.g., vasopressin and glucagon). Other possible mechanisms, as yet largely untested, include the secretion of a biologically inert form of parathyroid hormone, an intrinsic abnormality of parathyroid hormone receptors, autoantibodies to the parathyroid hormone receptor, a defect

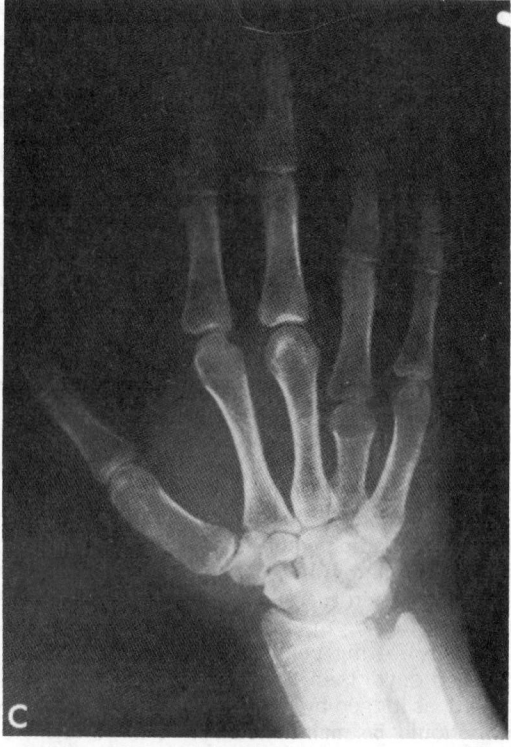

FIGURE 247–10. Hands of patient with pseudohypoparathyroidism. *A,* Note the shortened fourth finger. *B,* Note the "absent" fourth knuckle. *C,* Film shows the foreshortened fourth metacarpal. (From Potts JT Jr: Pseudohypoparathyroidism. In Stanbury JB, Wyngaarden JB, Fredrickson DS [eds.]: The Metabolic Basis of Inherited Disease. 4th ed. New York, McGraw-Hill Book Company, 1978, p 1359.)

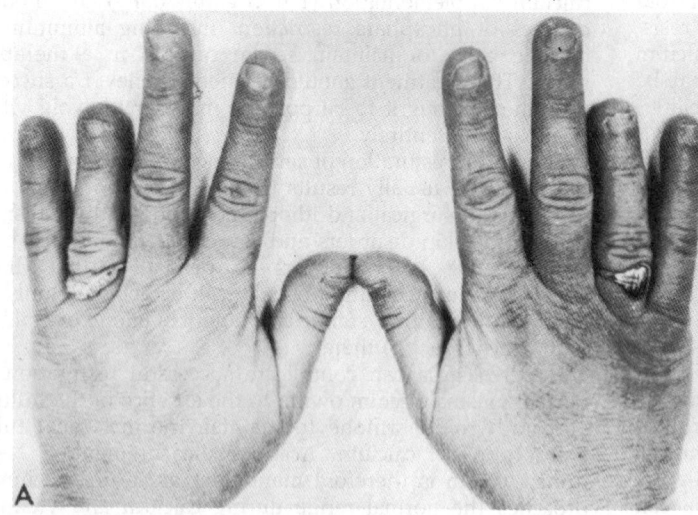

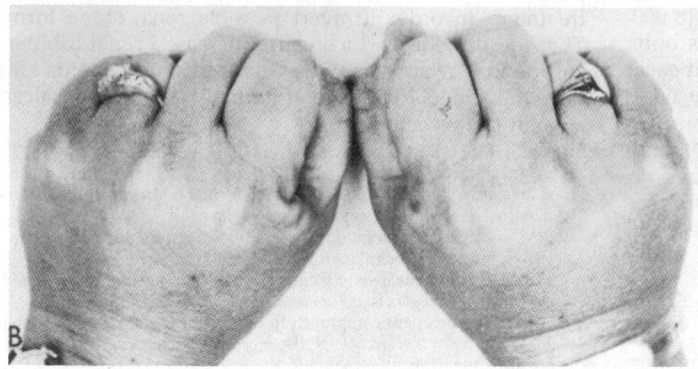

in adenylate cyclase, a disturbance in the process by which parathyroid hormone alters the distribution of ions across membranes, abnormalities of cellular protein kinases or other hormone-dependent enzymes, or gross cellular abnormalities that permit all of the actions of the hormones except the actual transfer of minerals from the cell to the blood.

Patients with pseudohypoparathyroidism generally fail to respond normally to the administration of large doses of parathyroid hormone with an increase in urinary phosphate excretion and nephrogenous cyclic AMP. A few have normal cyclic AMP responses but diminished phosphate responses, whereas others may have the reverse. The implication is that cyclic AMP may not be involved in the biologic actions of PTH. However, these results can be accounted for by several alternative explanations, including the possibility that urinary excretion of cyclic AMP does not accurately reflect all of the cyclic AMP–related cellular events critical to parathyroid hormone action and that only small changes in intracellular cyclic AMP are required for parathyroid hormone action.

Levels of $1,25(OH)_2D$ have been reported to be low in pseudohypoparathyroidism, and, because of this, defective conversion of 25OHD to $1,25(OH)_2D$ has been suggested as the mechanism involved in the abnormal mineral homeostasis in these patients. Support for this argument is derived from the success achieved in restoring serum calcium and urinary phosphate excretion to normal levels with $1,25(OH)_2D$ administration in patients with pseudohypoparathyroidism. Again, alternative explanations for these observations are not only possible but likely. Increased renal tubular cyclic AMP may be involved in the stimulation of 1α hydroxylation of 25OHD. If this is true, normal tissue responsiveness to parathyroid hormone may be necessary for the production of $1,25(OH)_2D$. This would account for the low levels of serum $1,25(OH)_2D$ found in pseudohypoparathyroidism. Likewise, $1,25(OH)_2D$ might be expected to improve the responsiveness of bone to parathyroid hormone in patients with deficient production of $1,25(OH)_2D$ simply because the hypercalcemic action of parathyroid hormone depends upon the presence of biologically active metabolites of vitamin D. Finally, the phosphaturia induced in pseudohypoparathyroidism by $1,25(OH)_2D$ administration could be due to the restoration of eucalcemia; it is well known that phosphaturia occurs when the serum calcium is restored to normal in patients with surgical hypoparathyroidism.

Although pseudohypoparathyroidism is inherited, the mode of its transmission is unclear. A sex-linked dominant mechanism is possible, since there is a female-to-male ratio of 2:1 for the disease. It is difficult to explain how the developmental defects of pseudohypoparathyroidism can be inherited without abnormalities occurring in the adenylate cyclase system. Furthermore, four cases of male-to-male transmission of the developmental defects have been recorded.

PATHOPHYSIOLOGY AND CLINICAL CHEMISTRY. The biochemical findings in patients with pseudohypoparathyroidism are identical to those observed in patients with surgical or idiopathic hypoparathyroidism, except that serum iPTH is increased appropriately for the degree of hypocalcemia. The pathophysiology of the disease can be visualized best by referring to Figure 244–1. Parathyroid hormone action is blocked in all three of the left limbs of the feedback loops. The result in the right limbs is (1) decreased bone resorption caused by decreased bone cell responsiveness to parathyroid hormone; (2) increased serum phosphate caused by decreased renal tubular responsiveness to the phosphaturic action of PTH, which in turn decreases production of $1,25(OH)_2D$ and intestinal calcium absorption; and (3) increased renal excretion of calcium for the degree of hypocalcemia, which is caused again by decreased renal tubular responsiveness to the hypocalciuric effects of parathyroid hormone. The consequent hypocalcemia stimulates parathyroid hormone secretion.

PATHOLOGY. In patients who are hypocalcemic, the parathyroid glands are hyperplastic. Aside from the unique developmental abnormalities noted under Clinical Manifestations, below, the findings are the same as in surgical hypoparathyroidism.

CLINICAL MANIFESTATIONS. Most of the symptoms and signs of pseudohypoparathyroidism are the same as those of surgical and idiopathic hypoparathyroidism and are due almost entirely to hypocalcemia. However, there are certain unique developmental features. Many patients are mentally retarded, have short stocky builds, are obese, have rounded faces, and display one or more short metacarpal or metatarsal bones. A classic sign of the brachymetacarpia, usually most marked in the fourth and fifth metacarpals, is the formation of a dimple over the head of the involved metacarpals when the patient makes a fist (Fig. 247–10). The fingers may be foreshortened. The calvarium is thickened in one third of patients, and there may be delayed dentition, defective enamel, and absence of teeth. There also may be exostoses, coxa vara, coxa valga, and bowing of the radius, tibia, and fibula.

DIAGNOSIS. The diagnosis of pseudohypoparathyroidism or pseudopseudohypoparathyroidism is likely when the described developmental abnormalities are discovered. When normal serum calcium and phosphorus are found in such a patient, the diagnosis of pseudopseudohypoparathyroidism is almost certain, although many of the same developmental abnormalities seen in pseudopseudohypoparathyroidism are present in unusual cases of Turner's, Gardner's, and the basal nevus syndromes. If hypocalcemia and hyperphosphatemia are found, the diagnosis of pseudohypoparathyroidism is highly likely. Increased serum iPTH and markedly diminished phosphaturic and nephrogenous cyclic AMP responses to parathyroid hormone distinguish pseudohypoparathyroidism from surgical, idiopathic, and functional hypoparathyroidism in patients with equivocal signs of the developmental abnormalities (see Fig. 247–9). If serum phosphorus is normal or low in such patients, secondary hyperparathyroidism resulting from vitamin D deficiency, dietary calcium deficiency, or intestinal malabsorption of calcium must be excluded. Measurement of serum 25OHD should help determine the presence of vitamin D deficiency, and dietary history or analysis, the presence of dietary calcium deficiency. The third underlying cause, intestinal malabsorption of calcium, may present difficulties because hypocalcemia per se may produce malabsorption (see above), and, unless magnesium deficiency is present, patients with intrinsic intestinal malabsorption usually have increased levels of serum iPTH. Therapeutic tests may be needed. When treatment of malabsorption with a gluten-free diet restores eucalcemia, the diagnosis is probably gluten-sensitive enteropathy (see Ch. 104). If correction of hypocalcemia with a regimen used in the treatment of hypoparathyroidism cures the malabsorption syndrome, the underlying diagnosis is probably pseudohypoparathyroidism.

Albright F, Burnett CH, Smith PH, et al.: Pseudohypoparathyroidism—an example of "Seabright-Bantam syndrome." Endocrinology 30:922, 1942. *First description of pseudohypoparathyroidism.*

Chase LR, Melson GL, Aurbach GD: Pseudohypoparathyroidism: Defective excretion of 3'5'-AMP in response to parathyroid hormone. J Clin Invest 48:1832, 1969. *First demonstration of renal blockade of parathyroid hormone–stimulated cyclic AMP excretion in pseudohypoparathyroidism.*

Drezner MK, Burch WM: Altered activity of the nucleotide regulatory site in the patient with pseudohypoparathyroidism. J Clin Invest 62:1222, 1978. *Demonstration that the addition of GTP to renal cortical membranes from a patient with pseudohypoparathyroidism restores their sensitivity to parathyroid hormone stimulation of adenylate cyclase in vitro. These results suggest that the molecular defect in some patients with this disease may be an abnormality of the regulatory protein that couples parathyroid hormone to adenylate cyclase.*

Farfel Z, Brickman AS, Kaslow HR, et al.: Defect of receptor-cyclase coupling protein in pseudohypoparathyroidism. N Engl J Med 303:237, 1980. Levine MA, Downs RW Jr, Singer M, et al.: Deficient activity of guanine nucleotide regulatory protein in erythrocytes from patients with pseudohypoparathyroidism. Biochem Biophys Res Commun 94:1319, 1980. *The work described in these two papers was done simultaneously and independently by two different groups. The results are essentially the same: the activity of the guanyl nucleotide regulatory protein in the red blood cell membranes of some patients with pseudohypoparathyroidism was significantly reduced. The work suggests the hypothesis that deficient activity of this protein is the molecular basis for hormone resistance in some patients with this inherited disorder.*

Potts JT Jr.: Pseudohypoparathyroidism. In DeGroot LJ (ed.): Endocrinology. Vol 2. New York, Grune & Stratton, 1979, pp 769–776. *Comprehensive review of pseudohypoparathyroidism.*

Van Dop C, Bourne HR: Pseudohypoparathyroidism. Annu Rev Med 34:259, 1983. *Excellent review of this disease focusing on pathogenesis.*

HYPERCALCEMIA AND ITS TREATMENT

Many diseases and conditions of nonparathyroid origin are associated with hypercalcemia (Table 247–2). Malignancy-associated hypercalcemia and familial hypocalciuric hypercalcemia are discussed above in relation to the differential diagnosis of primary hyperparathyroidism, because these disorders frequently resemble primary hyperparathyroidism in their clinical presentation and biochemical characteristics. This section will describe the spectrum of disorders that can produce hypercalcemia by mechanisms unrelated to parathyroid hormone (these are listed in Table 247–2 under the category of hypercalcemia "not due to increased serum PTH"). This section will also discuss the medical treatment of hypercalcemia, whether of parathyroid or nonparathyroid origin.

Nonparathyroid Causes of Hypercalcemia

Malignancy

The underlying cause of hypercalcemia in patients with nonhematologic malignancies who exhibit the other common biochemical features of primary hyperparathyroidism (i.e., hypophosphatemia and increased nephrogenous cyclic AMP) is probably the secretion of PTH-like substances by malignant tissue. The cancers that are most commonly associated with this syndrome are bronchogenic carcinoma and carcinoma of the kidney. Thus, although not strictly accurate, the term "ectopic hyperparathyroidism" has been used (as well as pseudohyperparathyroidism) to segregate these patients from those with malignancy-associated hypercalcemia who do not have hypophosphatemia and increased nephrogenous cyclic AMP. This segregation appears to be justified on therapeutic grounds because the hypercalcemia in patients with ectopic hyperparathyroidism rarely responds to corticosteroid administration, whereas the hypercalcemia in patients who do not have this syndrome frequently does respond.

Carcinoma of the breast accounts for approximately half of the malignancies associated with hypercalcemia. It is not associated with the biochemical features of ectopic hyperparathyroidism. The cause of the hypercalcemia in patients with breast cancer is uncertain. Many other solid tumors secrete substances that stimulate the cellular elements in bone to increase bone resorption. However, cultured breast cancer cells can increase the release of calcium from devitalized bone in vitro in a manner similar to osteoclasts. Thus, the direct interaction of tumor cells with bone (i.e., metastasis) may be required to produce hypercalcemia in patients with breast cancer.

Serum levels of phosphorus are normal or slightly increased in hypercalcemic patients with breast cancer, and serum levels of iPTH (as measured by mid- or carboxyl-region assays) are low or undetectable. These biochemical findings usually exclude primary hyperparathyroidism as a cause of hypercalcemia, but they cannot differentiate between ectopic hyperparathyroidism and breast cancer associated with hypercalcemia. The measurement of nephrogenous cyclic AMP may be helpful in this regard. It is almost always increased in patients with the syndrome of ectopic hyperparathyroidism and normal or decreased in patients with breast cancer. The hypercalcemia of patients with breast cancer usually responds to corticosteroids.

The finding of increased serum levels of iPTH and hypophosphatemia in hypercalcemic patients with a history of successfully treated breast cancer or with active disease almost certainly reflects associated primary hyperparathyroidism. Successful treatment of the latter (see above) may completely resolve the hypercalcemia. Frankly increased levels of serum iPTH in hypercalcemic patients with nonhematologic malignancies other than breast cancer should be interpreted similarly. As described in Figure 247–7, serum iPTH (as measured by mid- or carboxyl-region assays) is either normal or slightly increased in most patients with the syndrome of ectopic hyperparathyroidism. Thus, values of serum iPTH that are greater than two times the upper limit of normal in such patients indicate the coexistence of malignancy and primary hyperparathyroidism.

Multiple myeloma is the most common of the hematologic malignancies causing hypercalcemia (Ch. 163). Approximately 20 to 30 per cent of patients with this disease have increased serum calcium levels. As in breast cancer, serum phosphorus is normal or slightly increased, and corticosteroid administration frequently resolves the hypercalcemia. Patients with multiple myeloma often present with vertebral compression fractures and can be mistakenly diagnosed as having idiopathic osteoporosis. Roentgenograms of the spine may not distinguish between these two diseases. Interestingly, radionuclide bone scans often do not identify the bony lesions of multiple myeloma; a "positive scan" is more consistent with metastatic malignancy. A definitive diagnosis of multiple myeloma can usually be made if immunoelectrophoresis of serum or urine protein shows immunoglobulin abnormalities or if bone marrow biopsies show increased plasma cells.

The underlying cause of the hypercalcemia in patients with multiple myeloma is probably increased osteoclastic osteolysis induced by the local elaboration by myeloma cells of a lymphokine termed osteoclast-activating factor (OAF) (see Fig. 163–2). However, in some patients with this disease, the hypercalcemia may not be due to osteolysis but to extensive binding of calcium by the high circulating concentrations of myeloma proteins, which results in an increase in the protein-bound, biologically inert fraction of the plasma calcium (Ch. 244).

Hypercalcemia is unusual in other hematologic or lymphoproliferative malignancies, but it can occur in acute lymphocytic leukemia and more rarely in Hodgkin's disease, lymphosarcoma, and reticulum cell sarcoma. Although it has not been proved, the cause of hypercalcemia in these conditions is thought to be osteolysis induced by osteoclast-activating factor (or a similar substance) that is elaborated by tumor deposits (accumulations of malignant cells) in bone. Such lesions are common in patients with acute leukemia (50 to 90 per cent), but the incidence of hypercalcemia is quite low (5 per cent), suggesting that leukemic cells only rarely develop the capacity to produce significant quantities of osteolytic substances. High serum levels of 1,25-dihydroxyvitamin D have been reported in three patients with non-Hodgkin's lymphoma and hypercalcemia; it was speculated that the increased 1,25-dihydroxyvitamin D was synthesized in the neoplastic tissue.

Drugs

Thiazide diuretics regularly cause small increases in the plasma levels of total and ionized calcium in normal subjects by increasing serum protein concentrations (hemoconcentration due to volume depletion) and increasing renal tubular reabsorption of calcium. The widespread use of these agents for hypertension and as diuretics has complicated the diagnosis of hypercalcemia. Two simple rules are valuable in the evaluation of such patients. First, thiazide diuretics rarely increase serum calcium levels above 11.0 mg per deciliter, and therefore patients with higher values probably have a hypercalcemic disorder that is not related to thiazide administration. Secondly, serum calcium should be restored to the normal range (8.9 to 10.1 mg per deciliter) in normal patients within three weeks of discontinuing thiazides. There is no evidence that the mild hypercalcemia causes adverse effects.

Furosemide, a diuretic commonly used in the treatment of severe hypercalcemia (see below), has been reported to cause mild hypercalcemia when administered chronically. There is no explanation for this apparent paradox.

Vitamin D was once used in large doses (>50,000 units per day) to treat rheumatologic conditions; not surprisingly, vitamin D intoxication (see Ch. 245) and consequent hypercalcemia were common complications of that type of therapy. It is relatively rare now but should be considered in the differential diagnosis of hypercalcemia, particularly in those patients treated with large doses of vitamin D or its metabolites (e.g., for hypoparathyroidism and renal osteodystrophy) and in individuals who are prone to self-medication with large doses of vitamins and minerals. The hypercalcemia associated with vitamin D intoxication usually is accompanied by slight to moderate increases in serum phosphorus unless there is some independent reason for phosphate depletion. As with other nonparathyroid disorders, this biochemical feature helps distinguish vitamin D intoxication from primary hyperparathyroidism, but the diagnosis can be confirmed by demonstrating decreased or undetectable serum levels of iPTH and serum levels of 25OHD that are greater than 200 ng per milliliter. Corticosteroids characteristically reverse the hypercalcemia of vitamin D intoxication, as they do the hypercalcemia of breast cancer and hematologic malignancies.

Vitamin A, when ingested in doses of 50,000 to 100,000 units daily (10 to 20 times the recommended daily requirement), may result in hypercalcemia and diffuse bone pain. It is presumed that increased bone resorption underlies these abnormalities, even though skeletal radiographs are generally normal. In some cases these films may show multiple calcifications of the periosteum along the shafts of the phalanges and metacarpals. The diagnosis is confirmed by demonstrating that serum vitamin A levels are two to three times higher than normal. Symptoms, skeletal lesions, and hypercalcemia resolve rapidly after discontinuation of the vitamin.

Lithium, used in doses typical for manic-depressive illness, can cause mild hypercalcemia, which resolves after the drug is discontinued. The mechanism by which lithium induces hypercalcemia is unclear, although increased serum iPTH levels have been demonstrated in patients taking this drug. Further investigation is needed to determine whether increased secretion of PTH plays an important role in the hypercalcemia associated with lithium treatment.

Milk-Alkali Syndrome (Burnett's Syndrome). Ingestion of antacids that contain large amounts of calcium (i.e., >5 grams per day) can produce hypercalcemia in susceptible individuals and should be suspected, particularly in neurotic or psychiatrically ill patients who may be medicating themselves surreptitiously. If excessive calcium intake and the resulting hypercalcemia continue for a long time, the kidney may be damaged and renal failure may occur. This course of events was more frequent many years ago when the treatment of peptic ulcer included the use of large quantities of calcium in the form of milk or calcium cabonate and soluble alkali.

Granulomatous Diseases

Hypercalcemia occurs in 10 to 20 per cent of patients with *sarcoidosis* but is rare in other granulomatous diseases. When hypercalcemia is present, serum levels of phosphorus and alkaline phosphatase are generally increased and hypercalciuria is common. Other manifestations of the sarcoidosis, such as hilar lymphadenopathy, enlarged liver or spleen, peripheral lymphadenopathy, skin lesions, and hyperglobulinemia, are usually present. An increased serum level of angiotensin-converting enzyme in a hypercalcemic patient is highly suggestive of sarcoidosis (see Ch. 69), and the demonstration of noncaseating granulomatous lesions in a biopsied lymph node (e.g., the scalene) is confirmatory.

The presence of low serum levels of phosphorus and increased serum levels of PTH in a hypercalcemic patient with sarcoidosis indicate primary hyperparathyroidism. Diagnosis may be difficult in such patients when sarcoidosis involves the kidneys and compromises renal function.

Patients with sarcoidosis are very sensitive to the hypercalcemic effects of vitamin D. They have an increased ability to convert vitamin D to its biologically active form, 1,25(OH)$_2$D. The site of this increased conversion may be the abnormal granulomatous tissue that these patients harbor. This tissue appears capable of hydroxylating 25OHD to form a compound that has chromatographic properties similar to those of 1,25(OH)$_2$D. It is presumed that the mechanism underlying the hypercalcemia in other granulomatous diseases is similar to that responsible for the hypercalcemia in sarcoidosis. Treatment with corticosteroids lowers serum calcium levels in hypercalcemic patients with sarcoidosis in the same way as in vitamin D intoxication.

Nonparathyroid Endocrine Diseases

Hyperthyroidism frequently (in 20 per cent of patients) causes mild hypercalcemia, which resolves soon after treatment for the hyperthyroidism is instituted. The hypercalcemia is accompanied by normal or slightly increased concentrations of serum phosphorus, decreased concentrations of serum iPTH, and increased excretion of hydroxyproline. As might be expected, bone biopsies from patients with hyperthyroidism are hypercellular and show increases in both formation and resorption surfaces of bone. It is presumed that the hypercalcemia in these patients is due to the uncoupling of bone formation and resorption so that resorption predominates. Serum levels of calcium above 11.5 mg per deciliter are rare in patients with hyperthyroidism; when they occur, they suggest the presence of another hypercalcemic disorder.

Acute adrenal insufficiency may be associated with hypercalcemia. Although the mechanism is poorly understood, increases in serum protein concentrations associated with severe hemoconcentration may be involved. Glucocorticoid replacement restores serum concentrations to normal.

Familial Hypocalciuric Hypercalcemia (See above, p. 1491)
Immobilization

Immobilization of patients in body casts or by quadriplegia frequently causes hypercalcemia as a result of increased dissolution of bone. Hypercalcemia is generally mild in adults but can be severe in children (e.g., >15.0 mg per deciliter). This difference in severity is probably due to the higher turnover rate of bone in children. The mechanism responsible for enhanced dissolution of bone in immobilized patients is unclear, but available evidence from histomorphometric examination of bone biopsies from these patients suggests that bone formation surfaces are decreased and bone resorption surfaces are increased. The hypercalcemia associated with immobilization usually resolves rapidly when patients can bear weight with their lower extremities (as little as one or more hours per day). Treatment of hypercalcemia in adults is rarely needed because it is mild. However, the severe hypercalcemia seen in immobilized children requires prompt treatment using the measures detailed below (i.e., increased fluids, sodium chloride, phosphate, and possibly calcitonin).

Idiopathic Hypercalcemia of Infancy

Idiopathic hypercalcemia of infancy is rare. It is associated with several congenital cardiovascular and facial defects. Hypersensitivity to vitamin D is suspected as the cause of the hypercalcemia because corticosteroids can lower the serum calcium concentrations in these patients. Moreover, there may be increased conversion of vitamin D to 1,25(OH)$_2$D in affected infants.

Neonatal primary hyperparathyroidism, also a rare disease, is easily confused with idiopathic hypercalcemia of infancy. The treatments for these two diseases are different and depend completely upon the correct diagnosis. Measurement of serum iPTH is key in this latter regard; levels are increased in primary hyperparathyroidism and decreased or undetectable in idiopathic hypercalcemia.

Renal Failure and Renal Transplantation

Hypercalcemia may occur during the development of severe secondary hyperparathyroidism caused by chronic renal failure or after renal transplantation. It is also a diagnostic hallmark of the syndrome of aluminum intoxication seen also in patients with chronic renal failure. The pathogenesis and treatment of the hypercalcemia associated with these conditions are described in Ch. 249. Hypercalcemia is a frequent complication of acute renal failure, but its cause is poorly understood. It is usually managed successfully by hemodialysis with dialysis baths that contain low concentrations of calcium.

Medical Treatment of Hypercalcemia

Acute Severe Hypercalcemia

The medical treatment of acute severe hypercalcemia (>13.0 mg per deciliter) should be started immediately, because the condition is life-threatening. Serum levels of calcium, magnesium, sodium, and potassium must be monitored every two to four hours. If possible, patients should remain ambulatory, since immobilization may increase serum calcium in some patients. In patients with heart disease who are in danger of developing heart failure due to volume overload from fluid administration, central venous pressure should be monitored so that appropriate measures can be taken if the pressure increases.

The diagnostic approach to determining the underlying cause of hypercalcemia outlined here should be instituted early so that the cause of hypercalcemia can be specifically identified and treated.

In addition to these measures, dietary calcium should be restricted, and all drugs that might cause hypercalcemia (e.g, thiazides or vitamin D) discontinued. If the patient is taking digitalis, it may be wise to reduce the dose because the hypercalcemic patient may be more sensitive to the toxic effects of this drug. Ideally, the patient should be admitted to an intensive care unit for electrocardiographic monitoring while antihypercalcemic measures are instituted. Beta-adrenergic blockade is useful in protecting the heart against the adverse effects of severe hypercalcemia, especially serious arrhythmias.

The mainstay of therapy is a regimen of hydration, initially with normal saline, plus forced diuresis using furosemide or ethacrynic acid. The objective is to increase the urinary excretion of calcium rapidly, thus decreasing the exchangeable calcium pool and the serum calcium concentration. Saline is given to increase sodium excretion because sodium clearance parallels calcium clearance during water or osmotic diuresis. Furosemide and ethacrynic acid inhibit the tubular reabsorption of calcium and aid in maintaining diuresis. Approximately 4 to 6 liters of isotonic saline (sometimes as much as 12 liters are needed) should be given intravenously each day, along with 20 to 100 mg of furosemide or 10 to 40 mg of ethacrynic acid every 1 to 2 hours (intravenously or orally). Such a regimen usually increases urinary calcium excretion to 500 to 1000 mg per day and lowers serum calcium by 2 to 6 mg per deciliter after 24 to 48 hours. Potassium and magnesium depletion are complications of therapy, and appropriate replacement should be instituted early.

After the serum calcium has decreased to a reasonably safe level (<13.0 mg per deciliter), a chronic regimen may be instituted. At the minimum, this should consist of a daily oral regimen of 40 to 160 mg of furosemide or 50 to 200 mg of ethacrynic acid, 400 to 600 mEq of sodium chloride (in tablet form), and 3 liters of fluid. Serum calcium, magnesium, and potassium should be monitored daily at first, and then weekly when serum calcium has stabilized. Magnesium and potassium should be replaced as necessary. Patient compliance with this excretion can be monitored by measuring 24-hour urinary excretion of sodium (which should exceed 300 mEq per day) and 24-hour urinary volume (minimum required is 2500 ml per day).

Chronic Treatment of Moderately Severe Hypercalcemia

Whereas the acute treatment of severe hypercalcemia (>13.0 mg per deciliter) is nonspecific and relatively straightforward, requiring primarily hydration and saline diuresis (see below), the chronic treatment of moderately severe hypercalcemia (<13.0 mg per deciliter) requires knowledge of the underlying disease and involves trial and error in formulating an effective drug regimen. The problem is less difficult in diseases of nonparathyroid origin because treatment with corticosteroids (e.g., 300 mg of cortisone or 60 mg of prednisone given daily in divided doses for sarcoidosis, multiple myeloma, or vitamin D intoxication) usually results in satisfactory resolution of hypercalcemia. However, the medical treatment of hypercalcemia in those diseases associated with excess circulating levels of PTH or PTH-like substances is considerably more difficult. The drugs that are available may not be completely effective and may have serious side effects.

All patients with moderately severe hypercalcemia should maintain a high fluid intake (3 to 5 liters per day) and, unless contraindicated because of associated diseases, a sodium chloride intake of at least 300 to 400 mEq per day. These measures increase the renal excretion of calcium while maintaining the concentration of urinary calcium below that conducive to renal stone formation. Periodic measurements of serum electrolytes should be made because this regimen can cause magnesium and potassium depletion. These ions should be replaced if their serum concentrations decrease. Except in patients with breast cancer, in whom the administration of estrogens or androgens may induce hypercalcemia for unknown reasons, hypercalcemic postmenopausal women with either primary hyperparathyroidism or the syndrome of ectopic hyperparathyroidism should be given cyclic estrogen-progestin therapy (as described in Ch. 250). Estrogens suppress bone resorption and have been used successfully in the long-term management of mild hypercalcemia in women with primary hyperparathyroidism.

If hypercalcemia is not controlled (10.0 to 11.0 mg per deciliter) using these simple measures, other agents may be tried. Oral phosphate, either as neutral or potassium phosphate, may be given in doses as high as 2 to 4 grams of elemental phosphorus per day. Initial doses should be relatively low (1 to 2 grams per day in divided doses every 6 hours) because gastrointestinal side effects (e.g., nausea and diarrhea) may occur; these should disappear, however, with time. During treatment with phosphate, serum levels of calcium, phosphorus, and creatinine should be monitored to determine whether the serum calcium level has decreased and whether hyperphosphatemia or impaired renal function has developed. Increases in serum phosphorus above 5 mg per deciliter should be avoided because extraskeletal calcification (e.g., in the kidney) may be induced. Phosphate should be discontinued if the serum creatinine level increases significantly.

If phosphate therapy fails, the only effective approach to the treatment of hypercalcemia is to use mithramycin. This cytotoxic antibiotic has been used to treat testicular tumors but also ameliorates hypercalcemia by dramatically inhibiting bone resorption, presumably by killing osteoclasts. However, the drug is associated with renal and hepatic toxicity, thrombocytopenia, nausea, vomiting, stomatitis, and facial swelling.

Therefore, it is usually reserved for hypercalcemic patients with malignancy. The intravenous administration of 15 to 25 μg of mithramycin per kilogram of body weight generally restores serum calcium to nearly normal levels within a few days. The duration of this effect varies, but it can last as long as a month. When hypercalcemia recurs, mithramycin can be administered again, provided that thrombocytopenia has not occurred and renal and hepatic functions have not been impaired. Lower doses (10 to 15 μg per kilogram of body weight) can be tried, with the expectation that there will be fewer side effects. In general, the toxic effects of mithramycin can be reversed by discontinuing the drug.

Whereas intravenous disodium etidronate has been reported to be effective in treating hypercalcemia in patients with malignancy (not yet FDA approved), oral treatment with the same drug is ineffective. This is in contrast to several other bisphosphonate compounds that are extremely effective both orally and intravenously. These latter drug forms are not sold in the United States. However, it is the author's view that they will become the mainstay of medical treatment of hypercalcemia in the future.

The treatment of hypercalcemia with calcitonin, although rational, has been disappointing, and there is no convincing evidence that it is effective in the chronic management of hypercalcemia in these patients.

Indomethacin,* given orally in doses of 25 mg every 6 hours, may be tried, but it is rarely effective. The rationale for its use is that the hypercalcemia may be due to increased bone resorption caused by excess prostaglandins released by the cancer.

Bilezikian JP: Hypercalcemia. In Krieger DT, Bardin CW: Current Therapy in Endocrinology 1983-1984. Philadelphia and St. Louis, BC Decker, Inc, and CV Mosby Company, 1983, pp 272–277. *Brief but incisive review of the treatment of hypercalcemia.*
Rodman JS, Sherwood LM: Disorders of mineral metabolism in malignancy. In Avioli LV, Krane SM (eds.): Metabolic Bone Disease. Vol 2. New York, Academic Press, 1978, pp 577–631. *A systematic assessment of the diagnosis, etiology, and management of patients with malignancy-associated hypercalcemia.*
Suki WN, Yium JJ, Von Minden M, et al.: Acute treatment of hypercalcemia with furosemide. N Engl J Med 283:836, 1970. *Classic paper outlining the acute treatment of hypercalcemia.*

248 THE ULTIMOBRANCHIAL CELLS AND CALCITONIN

Claude D. Arnaud

The ultimobranchial cells develop from neural crest tissue in the ultimobranchial cleft during embryonic life. They form a discrete organ in submammalian vertebrates called the ultimobranchial gland. In the mammal, the anlage of the cells merges with the embryonic thyroid gland, ultimately becoming dispersed in the central region of each lobe (of the thyroid gland), adjacent to the follicular cells.

Calcitonin, a 32 amino acid polypeptide, is biosynthesized and secreted by the ultimobranchial (parafollicular or "C") cells. Calcitonin is rapidly released by the "C" cells in response to small increases in plasma ionic calcium. It acts on kidney and bone to restore the level of this cation to just below a normal set point, which in turn inhibits the secretion of the hormone. Calcitonin is a physiologic antagonist to parathyroid hormone, and these agents presumably act in concert to maintain the normal concentration of ionic calcium in the extracellular fluid (see Fig. 244–1).

The actual importance of calcitonin in the calcium homeostasis of adult humans is not established. An excess or deficiency of parathyroid hormone or vitamin D produces dramatic clinical disorders. In contrast, an excess (medullary carcinoma of the thyroid) or deficiency (post-thyroidectomy) of calcitonin produces few discernible and no serious abnormalities in mineral metabolism. The basal plasma levels of calcitonin and its responsiveness to induced hypercalcemia or pentagastrin injection are lower in women than in men. In adult humans, calcitonin may function primarily to restrain the bone resorptive effects of parathyroid hormone.

Calcitonin exists in multiple molecular forms in ultimobranchial tissue and plasma. In contrast to parathyroid hormone, however, the major circulating species are not hormone fragments but immunoreactive forms with molecular weights larger than 32 amino acid calcitonin. The different antisera used in radioimmunoassays recognize these forms differently, and therefore the normal range for plasma calcitonin must be established for each assay. The concentrations of calcitonin are extremely low (<100 pg per milliliter). Induced hypercalcemia and pentagastrin injection cause an increase in plasma calcitonin in approximately 40 to 50 per cent of normal women and 70 to 80 per cent of normal men. However, it is unlikely that gastrin is a physiologic calcitonin secretagogue. Other calcitonin secretagogues of unproved physiologic significance include glucagon, beta-adrenergic agonists, and alcohol.

When bone turnover rates are high, calcitonin administration produces rapid and profound hypocalcemia and hypophosphatemia. This is largely due to an inhibitory effect on osteoclastic bone resorption. Calcitonin also increases urinary excretion of calcium and phosphate, but its action on the kidney is transient and variable. Calcitonin stimulates adenylate cyclase in bone and kidney, but whether cyclic AMP is the major intracellular mediator of calcitonin action has not been established. It is also unclear whether calcitonin influences intestinal calcium absorption.

HYPOCALCITONINEMIA

No clinical condition has been reported to date in which hypocalcitoninemia plays a definitive role.

MEDULLARY CARCINOMA

DEFINITION. Medullary carcinoma, a malignancy of the parafollicular cells of the thyroid gland, is the only recognized disorder in which calcitonin is inappropriately secreted in excess. It occurs sporadically but also may be inherited as an autosomal dominant trait as part of the multiple endocrine neoplasia (MEN) syndromes, types II and III (Ch. 241). These syndromes include medullary carcinoma of the thyroid gland and pheochromocytoma. Patients with MEN II have a normal appearance but a high incidence of hyperparathyroidism, most frequently resulting from enlargement of multiple parathyroid glands. Patients with MEN III have a striking appearance owing to ganglioneuromas of the labia and mucosae, a marfanoid habitus, and other somatic abnormalities. Hyperparathyroidism is unusual.

INCIDENCE. Medullary carcinoma constitutes between 3.5 and 10 per cent of all thyroid malignancies. The incidence in males and females is almost equal, there being a male-to-female ratio of 1.3:1 in sporadic cases and 1:1 in familial cases. In general, familial cases present at a younger age than do sporadic cases.

PATHOLOGY. Medullary carcinoma manifests as a solid, often hard mass confined to but not encapsulated in the substance of the thyroid gland. In sporadic cases, it is often unilateral, but in familial cases it is frequently bilateral. It is composed of sheets of cells with granular cytoplasms, and usually contains irregular masses of amyloid and fibrous tissue. Most patients who present with a thyroid mass have metastases to cervical lymph nodes. Some lesions spread to the upper mediastinum. Spread beyond the mediastinum, usually delayed until later in the natural history of the disease, is most commonly to lungs, liver, bones, and the adrenal glands.

---

*This use is not listed in the manufacturer's directive.

PATHOPHYSIOLOGY. Medullary carcinomas secrete large quantities of calcitonin and respond to provocative stimuli such as increased serum calcium or intravenous pentagastrin. Although calcitonin produces hypocalcemia and hypophosphatemia in experimental animals, these biochemical findings are unusual in patients with medullary carcinoma in spite of extremely high levels of immunoreactive calcitonin. This paradox is probably due to a combination of factors, including homologous desensitization of tissues that normally respond to calcitonin (i.e., osteoclasts).

Medullary carcinoma may secrete many other bioactive substances in addition to calcitonin, each with the potential of causing clinical symptoms. These substances include biogenic amines, ACTH and corticotropin-releasing hormone, prostaglandins, nerve growth factor, and possibly a prolactin-releasing hormone. Diarrhea is present in 20 per cent of patients. It relents after surgical excision of the tumor and is therefore thought to be humorally mediated. Cushing's syndrome is present in about 5 per cent of cases and is secondary to secretion of excessive ACTH.

CLINICAL MANIFESTATIONS AND DETECTION. The majority of patients with sporadic medullary carcinoma present with an asymptomatic thyroid mass. Patients with MEN III may complain of the neuromas they harbor and their marfanoid habitus. Hypercalcemia may be detected on routine blood screening in patients with MEN II and primary hyperparathyroidism. Most important, hypertension in patients with MEN II and III may lead to the diagnosis of pheochromocytoma, which is more life threatening than is medullary carcinoma.

Paraneoplastic syndromes, such as Cushing's syndrome or intractable diarrhea, should alert the physician to the possible existence of medullary carcinoma. Certainly, a history of more than one family member with thyroid cancer should raise suspicion in a patient with bizarre symptoms.

Other neural manifestations in MEN III include medullated nerves on slit lamp examination of the eye and ganglioneuromas of the gastrointestinal tract. The latter can cause gastrointestinal obstruction as well as megacolon.

Medullary cancers occasionally calcify. The discovery of a calcified thyroidal mass does not indicate that it is benign; rather, it is probably an indication for the measurement of serum immunoreactive calcitonin (see below).

DIAGNOSIS. The cornerstone for the investigation of patients suspected of having medullary carcinoma is the radioimmunoassay of calcitonin in plasma. Although not specific for this tumor, increased levels of immunoreactive calcitonin in patients with a thyroid mass, pheochromocytoma, or a family history of medullary carcinoma virtually assure the diagnosis. Serum immunoreactive calcitonin may be increased in many other conditions, however, including other malignancies that secrete calcitonin ectopically (especially small cell carcinoma of the lung), chronic renal failure, gastrointestinal disorders such as tumors of the pancreas and pernicious anemia, subacute Hashimoto's thyroiditis, and pregnancy. These conditions should be considered in the interpretation of a high value.

The diagnostic power of the calcitonin radioimmunoassay is greatly enhanced when combined with provocative tests. For example, as many as 30 per cent of members of a family with MEN II who actually harbor small medullary carcinomas will have normal unstimulated plasma levels of immunoreactive calcitonin. They can be detected only by intravenous administration of 0.5 µg of pentagastrin* per kilogram of body weight over 5 to 10 seconds, or 150 mg of calcium chloride over 10 minutes. Plasma levels of immunoreactive calcitonin increase abnormally in the majority of these patients, thus establishing the diagnosis; surgery can then be performed before metastatic spread occurs. The calcitonin radioimmuno-

assay should be able to measure normal plasma levels of immunoreactive calcitonin (males, <100 pg per milliliter; females, <70 pg per milliliter). Without such sensitivity it is unlikely that the assay will be able to detect relatively small increases above the stimulated normal range, thus making the test impossible to interpret.

To rule out familial medullary carcinoma, immunoreactive calcitonin should be measured during a provocative test in all primary relatives of all patients with medullary carcinoma, regardless of family history. A significant proportion of these relatives of patients with seemingly "sporadic" medullary carcinoma will turn out to have the familial disease. In a few affected patients with minimal parafollicular cell disease, false-negative results will be obtained with any of the tests outlined. Provocative testing should therefore be performed yearly in primary relatives with previous negative tests, since approximately 50 per cent of the members of a given family with MEN II should eventually develop medullary cancer. Its timely detection will permit definitive surgical treatment.

TREATMENT. After exclusion or treatment of pheochromocytoma, total thyroidectomy is mandatory. This is especially true in patients with MEN II because medullary carcinoma is almost always bilateral and polycentric. Lymph nodes in the midline compartment should be removed and those in both internal jugular chains sampled. If jugular lymph nodes are involved, a modified neck dissection should be performed. Postoperatively, all patients should be studied with a provocative test(s) to determine if residual tumor is present. They should be given thyroid hormone replacement. The overall prevalence of residual medullary cancer after such surgery is about 35 per cent. The majority of these patients are older and have had regional metastases at surgery. Long-term follow-up with provocative tests every year is advised for all patients. Although it is usually difficult to determine the location of metastases responsible for a positive result in a provocative test, local recurrences are likely and can be dealt with surgically. There is no known effective chemotherapeutic, isotopic, or radiologic treatment for medullary carcinoma.

PROGNOSIS. Patients with sporadic medullary carcinoma have the least favorable prognosis. Metastases are usually present, and only 46 per cent of these patients survive for 10 years. Patients with MEN II appear to fare better, with few having been recorded as dying from their disease. Conversely, in the Mayo Clinic series of patients with MEN III, 67 per cent have had residual disease after surgery, and 18 per cent have died of medullary cancer. The reasons for the apparent difference in the prognosis of MEN II and MEN III are unknown.

THERAPEUTIC USE OF CALCITONIN

Calcitonin is used to treat Paget's disease of bone and hypercalcemia of all causes (see Ch. 251). The preparation most frequently employed is synthetic salmon calcitonin because this species is about 30 times more potent in lowering serum calcium than are mammalian calcitonins (porcine, human). The rationale for its use in both Paget's disease and hypercalcemia is its inhibitory effect on bone resorption. In unusual cases, high titers of circulating antibodies are formed against salmon calcitonin. These antibodies may block the action of the hormone and its beneficial effects. In such cases, synthetic human calcitonin may be successfully substituted, but this species of the hormone is not readily available commercially at present.

Austin L, Heath H III: Calcitonin: Physiology and pathophysiology. N Engl J Med 304:269, 1981. *Lively review of advances in calcitonin research in health and disease.*

Deftos LJ, Catherwood BD, Bone HG: Multiglandular endocrine disorders. In Felig P, Baxter JD, Broadus AF, et al. (eds.): Endocrinology and Metabolism. 2nd ed. New York, McGraw-Hill Book Company, 1987, pp 1662–1691. *Comprehensive review of medullary cancer of the thyroid gland.*

Gagel RF, Melvin KEW, Tashjian AH Jr, et al.: Natural history of the familial medullary thyroid carcinoma–pheochromocytoma syndrome and the iden-

*This use is not listed in the manufacturer's directive.

tification of preneoplastic stages by screening studies: A five-year report. Trans Assoc Am Physicians 88:177, 1975. *The first description of the diagnostic power of the calcitonin radioimmunoassay in the diagnosis of familial medullary carcinoma.*

Sizemore GW, Carney JA, Health H III: Epidemiology of medullary carcinoma of the thyroid gland: A five year experience (1971–1976). Surg Clin North Am 57:633, 1977. *Describes this group's extensive experience with both the familial and sporadic forms of medullary carcinoma of the thyroid gland.*

249 RENAL OSTEODYSTROPHY

Eduardo Slatopolsky

Renal osteodystrophy refers to the complex lesions of bone that are present in the majority of patients with advanced renal failure. The main components of renal osteodystrophy are osteitis fibrosa and osteomalacia (Table 249–1). A lesser role is played by osteosclerosis and osteoporosis. Osteitis fibrosa, a consequence of an increased parathyroid hormone, is characterized by an increase in the number of osteoclasts and an increase in bone resorption and marrow fibrosis. Osteomalacia, a condition secondary in part to alterations in vitamin D metabolism, results from a decreased mineralization of osteoid tissue (shown histologically by an abnormal calcification front in bone). Osteosclerosis is due to localized areas of mineralized woven bone which appear as increased bone density on radiographic studies. Osteoporosis, defined as a decrease in the mass of normally mineralized bone, is an infrequent and minor component of renal osteodystrophy.

OSTEITIS FIBROSA

Secondary hyperparathyroidism occurs universally in chronic renal disease. Chief cell hyperplasia of the parathyroid glands and high levels of immunoreactive parathyroid hormone (i-PTH) are among the earliest findings affecting mineral metabolism in patients with chronic renal failure. Several factors contribute to the development of secondary hyperparathyroidism in renal insufficiency (Table 249–1 and Fig. 249–1).

PHOSPHATE RETENTION. An important role of phosphate retention in producing secondary hyperparathyroidism is firmly established. Long-term feeding of a diet high in phosphate to animals with normal renal function can produce secondary hyperparathyroidism. Conversely, restriction of dietary phosphate can prevent the development of secondary hyperparathyroidism in chronic renal failure. The effect of phosphate retention on the parathyroid glands is mediated by lowering the concentration of ionized calcium in extracellular fluid, which in turn results from (1) the complexing of ionized calcium by phosphate, (2) a decreased renal production of calcitriol ($1,25(OH)_2D_3$), the active metabolite of vitamin D, and (3) a direct effect of phosphate on bone, decreasing calcium mobilization from the skeleton. In patients with far-advanced renal failure (GFR less than 20 ml per minute), correction of hyperphosphatemia alone will not completely

TABLE 249–1. FOUR COMPONENTS OF RENAL OSTEODYSTROPHY

1. Osteitis fibrosa (secondary hyperparathyroidism)
   a. Phosphate retention
   b. Altered metabolism of vitamin D
   c. Skeletal resistance to PTH
   d. Unpaired degradation of PTH
   e. Altered feedback regulation of PTH by Ca^{++}
2. Osteomalacia
   a. Altered metabolism of vitamin D
   b. Altered synthesis and maturation of collagen
   c. Acidosis
   d. Increased bone magnesium
   e. Increased pyrophosphate
   f. Retention of aluminum
3. Osteosclerosis } of lesser quantitative importance
4. Osteoporosis

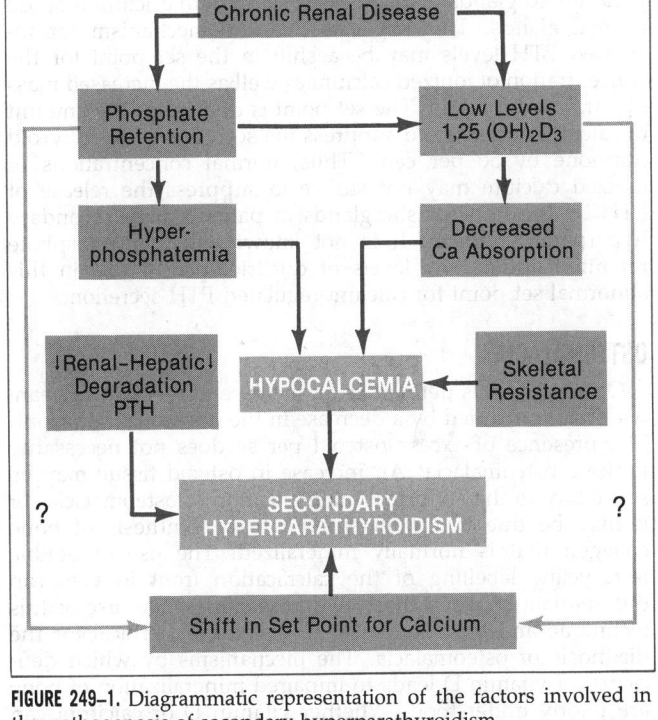

FIGURE 249–1. Diagrammatic representation of the factors involved in the pathogenesis of secondary hyperparathyroidism.

reverse secondary hyperparathyroidism, since many other factors also contribute to the increased PTH levels in blood.

ALTERATIONS IN VITAMIN D METABOLISM (see also Ch. 245). Renal osteodystrophy may arise in part because of defective renal production of the active form of vitamin D in advanced renal failure. The liver hydroxylates vitamin D_3 to 25-hydroxycholecalciferol ($25(OH)D_3$), the predominant form of vitamin D_3 present in plasma. $25(OH)D_3$ is further hydroxylated to $1,25(OH)_2D_3$, also termed calcitriol, by a specific hydroxylase enzyme found in the mitochondrial fraction of the renal proximal tubular cells. Parathyroid hormone and low phosphate diets stimulate the activity of this hydroxylase; lack of parathyroid hormone, hyperphosphatemia, or hypercalcemia decreases the activity of the hydroxylase. Intestinal absorption of calcium is reduced in patients with far-advanced renal insufficiency, and low levels of calcitriol are found in serum as the probable cause. Calcium malabsorption is usually present in patients with GFR's less than 40 ml per minute.

SKELETAL RESISTANCE TO THE ACTION OF PARATHYROID HORMONE. Skeletal resistance to the calcemic action of PTH may also play a role in the development of hypocalcemia seen in patients with renal insufficiency. Higher circulating levels of PTH may be needed for the maintenance of a normal serum calcium in patients with renal failure.

IMPAIRED DEGRADATION OF PTH SECONDARY TO REDUCED RENAL FUNCTION. Parathyroid hormone is metabolized by the liver and the kidney. The liver takes up the intact hormone exclusively; it does not remove either amino terminal or carboxy terminal PTH fragments from the circulation. The kidney, on the other hand, removes both intact PTH and the amino and carboxy terminal fragments from plasma. In chronic renal insufficiency, therefore, the high levels of circulating i-PTH result in part from increased PTH secretion due to chief cell hyperplasia and in part from a decreased catabolism of the hormone secondary to a decreased number of nephrons. There also seems to be decreased hepatic metabolism of intact PTH.

ALTERED FEEDBACK REGULATION BETWEEN IONIZED CALCIUM AND THE SECRETION OF PARATHYROID HORMONE. The control of the secretion of PTH by levels of ionized calcium in extracellular fluid may be blunted in patients with chronic renal insufficiency. Hyperplastic parathyroid glands display less sensitivity to calcium than do normal glands. This suggests that the mechanism for increased PTH levels may be a shift in the set point for the concentration of ionized calcium as well as the increased mass of parathyroid tissue. The set point is defined as the amount of calcium necessary to suppress the secretion of parathyroid hormone by 50 per cent. Thus, normal concentrations of ionized calcium may not suffice to suppress the release of PTH by the hyperplastic glands of patients with secondary hyperparathyroidism. It is not known whether phosphate retention and/or low levels of calcitriol play a role in this abnormal set point for calcium-regulated PTH secretion.

OSTEOMALACIA

Osteomalacia is defined as an increase in the osteoid seam width accompanied by a decrease in the mineralization front. The presence of excess osteoid per se does not necessarily indicate osteomalacia. An increase in osteoid tissue may be secondary to the abnormal mineralization of osteomalacia, or it may be due to an increased rate of synthesis of bone collagen that is normally mineralized. The use of double tetracycline labelling of the calcification front in vivo can differentiate between these two possibilities. The use of this technique and quantitative bone histology is critical for the diagnosis of osteomalacia. The mechanisms by which deficiency of vitamin D leads to impaired mineralization of bone are poorly understood. Whether vitamin D or calcitriol can directly stimulate bone mineralization or whether it leads to mineralization only by increasing the levels of calcium and phosphate in the extracellular fluid surrounding bone is uncertain. Although the plasma levels of calcitriol are reduced in patients with far-advanced renal insufficiency, overt osteomalacia is found in only a small fraction of such patients and may be absent even in anephric patients. Thus, other factors could also participate in the pathogenesis of osteomalacia in uremic patients—for example, the plasma level of phosphate. Hypophosphatemia per se can produce severe osteomalacia even in patients with normal renal function. Additional factors include alterations in collagen synthesis and maturation, defective bone crystal maturation, increased bone magnesium, elevated levels of pyrophosphate, and diminished calcium carbonate. The combination of these factors may influence the maturation of bone and potentially contribute to the development of osteomalacia. Acidosis also contributes to the skeletal disease. In chronic renal insufficiency the skeleton assists in buffering the retained acids. Administration of bicarbonate and correction of the acidosis in azotemic patients can reduce fecal calcium excretion.

Another type of osteomalacia in renal insufficiency, one that is resistant to vitamin D therapy, is caused by an excess of aluminum. Patients with osteomalacia secondary to aluminum have pathologic fractures, complain of severe bone pain, and characteristically have low levels of parathyroid hormone. The source may be a high aluminum content in the water and/or the ingestion of phosphate binders containing aluminum. The aluminum is deposited in the interface between the osteoid tissue and the calcification front and has a toxic effect on the osteoblast.

Finally, after total parathyroidectomy the lack of parathyroid hormone in patients results in low bone turnover and may sometimes precipitate the development of osteomalacia.

CLINICAL MANIFESTATIONS

The symptoms related to renal osteodystrophy usually appear only when renal failure is advanced. On the other hand, certain biochemical alterations may appear early in the course of renal insufficiency. Knowledge of the presence of these alterations may help the physician to introduce treatment early in the course of renal failure and in this way to prevent severe complications in bone and mineral metabolism.

Bone pain can develop and progress slowly to a point where the patient is bedridden, without regard to whether the bone disease is predominantly osteitis fibrosa or osteomalacia. The bone pain is generally vague and commonly located in the lower back, hips, knees, and legs. Low back pain may result from the collapse of a vertebral body, and sharp chest pain may indicate spontaneous rib fracture. Physical findings are frequently lacking.

Muscular weakness, when present, is usually proximal, appears slowly, and progresses with time. Plasma levels of muscle enzymes, creatine phosphokinase, and transaminases are usually normal, and the electron micrographic changes are nonspecific. The pathogenesis of such muscular weakness is uncertain. In patients with myopathy, the myofibrils are disorganized in a patchy fashion and the Z-band material may be dispersed. These changes revert to normal following treatment with $25(OH)D_3$. *Pruritus* due to calcium deposition in skin is a common symptom in uremic patients, particularly with severe secondary hyperparathyroidism.

Vascular calcification and peripheral ischemic necrosis may occur, producing lesions of the tips of the toes and fingers and violaceous discoloration of the skin. Ulcerations and scar formation may occur, with clear demarcation of the lesions from the surrounding skin. Acute pain and swelling around one or more joints may also develop in uremic patients. The syndrome of *calcific periarthritis*, which may be caused by deposition of hydroxyapatite crystals, is accompanied by marked hyperphosphatemia.

Skeletal deformities are common in azotemic children who are growing. Bowing of the tibia and femur and deformities from slipped epiphyses are not uncommon. Children with renal rickets sometimes exhibit typical radiographic findings of vitamin D deficiency. In adults with renal failure, particularly those with osteomalacia, marked skeletal deformities with lumbar scoliosis, thoracic kyphosis, and deformity of the thoracic cage may be observed. Growth retardation is usually seen in young children before and during maintenance hemodialysis. See Chapter 246 for a further discussion of osteomalacia and rickets.

Another clinical manifestation of renal osteodystrophy which occurs in some patients after renal transplant is aseptic necrosis of the head of the femur. This condition is more frequently seen in patients with severe bone disease (osteitis fibrosa) before renal transplant and in those who receive very large doses of glucocorticoids.

BIOCHEMICAL FEATURES

Circulating i-PTH is elevated early in the course of renal insufficiency (GFR 60 to 80 ml per minute). As the disease progresses (GFR less than 40 ml per minute), hypocalcemia and low levels of calcitriol appear. With advanced renal insufficiency, however, the serum calcium may remain close to normal and values below 7.5 mg per deciliter are infrequent. Usually hypocalcemia is more marked in severe osteomalacia or with profound metabolic acidosis. Occasionally, hypercalcemia may be observed in uremic patients, particularly in those undergoing long-term dialysis. This complication can arise from (1) severe hyperparathyroidism, (2) the ingestion of large amounts of calcium and vitamin D, (3) the presence of unrelated diseases such as sarcoidosis or malignancies, or (4) a "pure" mineralizing defect, as may occur in osteomalacia secondary to aluminum retention. Hyperphosphatemia is usually present in patients with GFR less than 25 ml per minute. The degree of hyperphosphatemia depends on the amount of phosphate ingested, the fraction absorbed in the intestine, and that excreted into the urine. If the patient ingests phosphate binders, the serum phosphate may remain normal despite advanced renal insufficiency. Patients with severe hyperparathyroidism and advanced renal insufficiency usually have higher concentrations of serum phosphate in plasma.

Advanced renal insufficiency (GFR less than 15 ml per minute) may be associated with hypermagnesemia and an increased content of magnesium in bone. This may adversely affect crystal formation.

Total serum alkaline phosphatase levels are commonly higher in uremic patients with osteitis fibrosa than in those with osteomalacia. Coexistent liver disease should be excluded as a cause of an elevated alkaline phosphatase.

RADIOGRAPHIC FEATURES

Secondary hyperparathyroidism increases bone resorption, most commonly evident on the subperiosteal surfaces of bone. Erosions that occur in conjunction with formation of new bone may appear as cysts or osteoclastomas (brown tumors). The presence of subperiosteal erosion correlates with serum i-PTH and with the histomorphometric features of osteitis fibrosa on bone biopsy. Subperiosteal resorption of the phalanges may be the most sensitive radiographic sign of secondary hyperparathyroidism (Fig. 247–4). The tuft of the terminal phalanx or the second or third digit commonly shows resorption. With severe tuft erosion there may be a collapse of the soft tissue and change of the contour of the tuft so that the finger appears to show clubbing. Bone erosions may also occur at the upper end of the tibia, the neck of the femur or the humerus, and the lower surface of the medial end of the clavicle. In the skull, resorption leads to the mottled and granular appearance commonly associated with altering areas of osteosclerosis.

Osteosclerosis is thought to be another feature of osteitis fibrosa arising from an increase in the thickness and number of trabecula in spongy bone. Osteosclerosis can lead to a typical "rugger jersey" appearance of the spine.

Osteomalacia is far less distinctive radiographically than is secondary hyperparathyroidism. The Looser zone or pseudofracture is the only pathognomonic radiographic finding of osteomalacia in the adult (Fig. 246–2). Rickets, i.e., widening of the epiphyseal growth plate, cannot develop after epiphyseal closure and hence is limited to children. With mechanical stress following severe prolonged deficiency of vitamin D, a Looser zone may extend across the full width of the bone and produce a true fracture with displacement of fragments. In uremia osteomalacia is commonly associated with secondary hyperparathyroidism with concomitant radiographic features of both. The diagnosis of osteomalacia rests on histologic examinations and can be established with certainty only by bone biopsy.

Soft-tissue calcification is presumed to be influenced by an increase in the calcium phosphate product in plasma, the degree of secondary hyperparathyroidism, the magnitude of alkalosis, and local tissue injury. Three major varieties include (1) calcification of the medium-size arteries, (2) articular or tumoral calcifications, and (3) visceral calcifications affecting the heart, lung, and kidney.

TREATMENT

The objectives of the treatment of patients with renal osteodystrophy are (1) to return the blood levels of calcium and phosphate to normal; (2) to suppress secondary hyperparathyroidism; (3) to reverse the histologic abnormalities in the skeleton; and (4) to prevent and reverse extraskeletal deposits of calcium and phosphate. Guidelines for the management of renal osteodystrophy are summarized in Table 249–2.

CONTROL OF PHOSPHATE AND CALCIUM. To control phosphate, dietary phosphate intake should be reduced to 700 to 800 mg per day (determined as phosphorus) by restricting the ingestion of dairy products and by decreasing the

TABLE 249–2. GUIDELINES FOR MANAGEMENT OF RENAL OSTEODYSTROPHY

Early Treatment
   It is important to begin treatment early, i.e., when the GFR is 30 to 40 ml per min, especially for the control of serum phosphate.
Control of Serum Phosphate (P) (3.5 to 4.5 mg per dl)
   Restrict phosphorus intake in diet to 600 to 800 mg per day
   Phosphate-binding antacids: aluminum carbonate or hydroxide; individualize dosage: Basaljel, Dialume, Alucap, Amphogel, 1–4 capsules with each meal
   Calcium carbonate: 1–3 grams with each meal
   Hypophosphatemia should be avoided
   Predialysis phosphorus: 4.5–5.5 mg per dl
   Minimize the use of aluminum binders
Adequate Calcium Intake
   Oral calcium supplements providing 1–2 grams per day when serum P is controlled: Os-Cal, Titralac
   Dialysate Ca, 6.0–6.5 mg per dl (3.0–3.25 mEq per liter)
Use of Vitamin D Sterols
   Vitamin D₂ or D₃, 50,000 to 250,000 IU (1.25 to 6.25 mg) per day
   Dihydrotachysterol, 0.25–2.0 mg per day
   25-Hydroxyvitamin D₃ (calcifediol), 20–100 μg per day (Calderol)
   1,25-Dihydroxyvitamin D₃ (calcitriol), 0.5–1.0 μg per day (Rocaltrol)
Parathyroidectomy: Severe secondary hyperparathyroidism (bone erosions and increased i-PTH) plus any of the following:
   Persistent hypercalcemia (serum Ca > 11.5 to 12.0 mg per dl)
   Progressive or symptomatic extraskeletal calcification
   Persistently elevated serum calcium × phosphorus product
   Pruritus not responsive to medical treatment
   Calciphylaxis (ischemic ulcers and necrosis)
   Symptomatic hypercalcemia after renal transplantation

amount of protein in the diet. In advanced renal failure, in addition to dietary control, phosphate binders are usually required to reduce its intestinal absorption. Phosphate binders should be ingested along with the meal in order to increase their efficiency. The use of aluminum-containing gels carries the potential of excessive aluminum absorption and accumulation. They should, therefore, be used with caution. If the patient develops symptoms and signs suggesting aluminum-induced osteomalacia, this drug should be discounted. If phosphate is not controlled, the patient will develop severe secondary hyperparathyroidism and extraskeletal calcification. Calcium carbonate (1 to 3 grams with each meal) will help to bind phosphate and thereby reduce the amount of aluminum binders needed for the treatment of hyperphosphatemia. During treatment with oral calcium carbonate, it is important to determinate the total amount of phosphate ingested during 24 hours and during each meal. In this way the relative amount of calcium carbonate given can be adjusted to the phosphate-binding requirements of specific meals. Calcium carbonate also provides a calcium supplement that will help correct the negative calcium balance secondary to the calcium malabsorption of advanced renal insufficiency. The serum phosphorus should be maintained at normal or nearly normal levels, between 3.5 and 4.5 mg per deciliter, if the patient is not yet on dialysis. The serum calcium should be maintained in the upper limits of normal. Severe hyperphosphatemia should be corrected before the administration of calcium in order to reduce the risk of metastatic calcification. Supplemental calcium should be discontinued if the serum calcium increases above 11.0 mg per deciliter. The concentration of calcium in the dialysate affects serum calcium levels during maintenance hemodialysis. The ideal calcium concentration in the dialysate is between 6.0 and 6.5 mg per deciliter.

USE OF VITAMIN D AND ITS METABOLITES. Despite dietary control of phosphate, the use of phosphate binders, an adequate dietary calcium, and appropriate levels of calcium in the dialysate, uremic patients may still develop skeletal disease. Thus, vitamin D and its metabolites are important and effective agents in the treatment of renal osteodystrophy. Calcitriol, the most active metabolite of vitamin D, is the drug of choice in the treatment of hypocalcemia and secondary hyperparathyroidism (see Ch. 247). The usual dose is 0.5 to 1 μg per day. If osteomalacia predominates on bone biopsy, excellent results have been obtained with the use of 25(OH)D$_3$ (20 to 100 μg per day) in addition to calcitriol. With the use of vitamin D or its metabolites, hypercalcemia and, less frequently, hyperphosphatemia may occur as side effects.

PARATHYROIDECTOMY. The regimen outlined above can lead to improved homeostasis of calcium and phosphorus and reverse the symptoms of bone disease and suppression of PTH secretion. Such measures may not be entirely successful, however, and parathyroidectomy may be required. Indications for parathyroid surgery include severe secondary hyperparathyroidism (bone erosions and high levels of i-PTH) in the presence of any of the following: (1) persistent hypercalcemia, particularly when symptomatic; (2) intractable pruritus that does not respond to dialysis or other medical treatment; (3) progressive extraskeletal calcification in conjunction with a high calcium-phosphorus product that is consistently about 75 to 80 despite appropriate phosphate restriction; and (4) the appearance of ischemic lesions of soft tissues. Because of lack of compliance many patients are unable to control their serum phosphorus levels. In these cases neither calcium supplements nor vitamin D or its metabolites can be recommended safely. Such patients are more likely to develop severe secondary hyperparathyroidism and require parathyroidectomy. Postoperative hypocalcemia may pose a problem if the remaining parathyroid tissue is inadequate and if severe osteitis fibrosa is present preoperatively. Preoperative treatment of such patients with calcitriol (1 to 2 μg per day) may obviate such problems. Serum levels of phosphorus and magnesium sometimes decrease after parathyroidectomy. Aluminum-containing phosphate binders should be withheld if the serum phosphorus falls below 3.0 mg per deciliter. Rapid remineralization of the skeleton occurs during this period, but once the "hungry bones" have been mineralized, serum calcium levels will rise. A fall in a previously elevated serum alkaline phosphatase toward normal may indicate that rapid skeletal remineralization is nearly complete and that calcium supplements and vitamin D therapy may be reduced or discontinued. In the past the removal of 3½ parathyroid glands was the procedure of choice. More recently, total parathyroidectomy followed by autotransplantation of some of the parathyroid tissue into the patient's forearm has been utilized. The transplanted tissue is more accessible if subsequent surgical removal is necessary. Total parathyroidectomy without autotransplantation has no place in the management of renal osteodystrophy, since it may predispose to the development of an isolated mineralization defect or osteomalacia in uremic patients. Cryopreservation of removed parathyroid tissue is a useful precaution so that hypoparathyroidism may be treated by reimplantation of parathyroid tissue.

Occasionally after a successful renal transplant the patient may develop hypercalcemia. Usually this is due to persistent hyperparathyroidism and increased renal production of calcitriol. In the majority of cases, the hypercalcemia subsides several months after renal transplantation. In some patients, however, severe hypercalcemia (calcium 12 to 13 mg per deciliter) may persist for several months and may affect renal function. In these patients a subtotal parathyroidectomy is recommended.

Treatment of Aluminum Toxicity. If the patient has aluminum-induced osteomalacia, phosphate binders containing aluminum should be discontinued at once. Phosphate should be controlled by using a more restrictive phosphate diet, and serum phosphorus may be allowed to increase to 6 mg per deciliter. Desferoxamine, a drug used for the treatment of iron excess, also chelates aluminum, and its use may relieve aluminum-induced osteomalacia.

Coburn JW, Slatopolsky E: Vitamin D, parathyroid hormone and renal osteodystrophy. In Brenner BM, Rector FC (eds.): The Kidney. 3rd ed. Philadelphia, W.B. Saunders Company, 1986, pp 1657–1729.
Massry SG: Divalent ion metabolism and renal osteodystrophy. In Massry SG, Glassock RJ (eds.): Textbook of Nephrology. Baltimore, Williams & Wilkins, 1983, pp 7.104–7.148.
Slatopolsky E, Weerts C, Lopez–Hilker S, et al.: Calcium carbonate as a binder in patients with chronic renal failure undergoing dialysis. N Engl J Med 315:157, 1986.

250 OSTEOPOROSIS
B. Lawrence Riggs

GENERAL CONSIDERATIONS

Osteoporosis is defined pathologically as an absolute decrease in the amount of bone, leading to fractures after minimal trauma. The disease is responsible for over 1.2 million fractures in the United States each year. The most common sites are the vertebrae, distal radius (Colles' fracture), and hip. One third of women over age 65 will have vertebral fractures. By extreme old age, one in every three women and one in every six men will have had a hip fracture. This catastrophic fracture is fatal in 12 to 20 per cent of cases and results in the need for long-term nursing home care for half of those who survive. The direct and indirect costs of osteoporosis are estimated at $7 to 10 billion annually in the United States.

After maximal skeletal mass is achieved in young adulthood, there is a period of stability before age-related bone loss begins. Thereafter, women lose about 35 per cent of their cortical bone and 50 per cent of their trabecular bone, and men lose about 25 and 35 per cent, respectively, over their lifetimes. Cortical bone predominates in the appendicular skeleton, whereas trabecular bone is concentrated in the axial skeleton, particularly in the vertebrae and in the ends of the long bones. With its greater surface area, trabecular bone is much more active metabolically than cortical bone and thus is more responsive to changes in mineral status. A biphasic pattern of bone loss has been identified for both cortical and trabecular bone: a protracted slow phase that occurs in both sexes, and a transient accelerated phase that occurs in women after menopause.

In both sexes the slow phase of loss begins about age 40 in cortical bone and possibly earlier in trabecular bone. It continues at a rate of 0.5 to 1 per cent per year in both sexes until it slows or ceases late in life. The proportional losses of cortical and trabecular bone due to this process are similar.

Bone resorption and bone formation occur at discrete foci in the skeleton—bone remodeling units. Osteoclasts appear on a previously inactive surface and create a resorption lacuna. The osteoclasts are then replaced by osteoblasts that fill in the resorption lacuna with new bone. The slow, age-dependent phase of bone loss results mainly from impaired bone formation; the resorption lacunae are of normal depth or even decreased in depth, but the osteoblasts fail to refill them completely.

In postmenopausal women, an accelerated phase of loss is superimposed on this pattern. For cortical bone, the bone loss rate of 2 to 3 per cent per year immediately after menopause decreases exponentially to become asymptotic with the slow phase after eight to ten years. For trabecular bone, there is a similar pattern except that the rate of accelerated loss is about twice as great, so that relatively more trabecular than cortical bone is lost. The accelerated postmenopausal phase of bone loss is associated with a high rate of bone turnover: there is an increase in bone formation but an even greater increase in bone resorption.

ETIOLOGY

GENERAL. The main underlying cause of fractures in osteoporosis is increased bone fragility as a result of bone

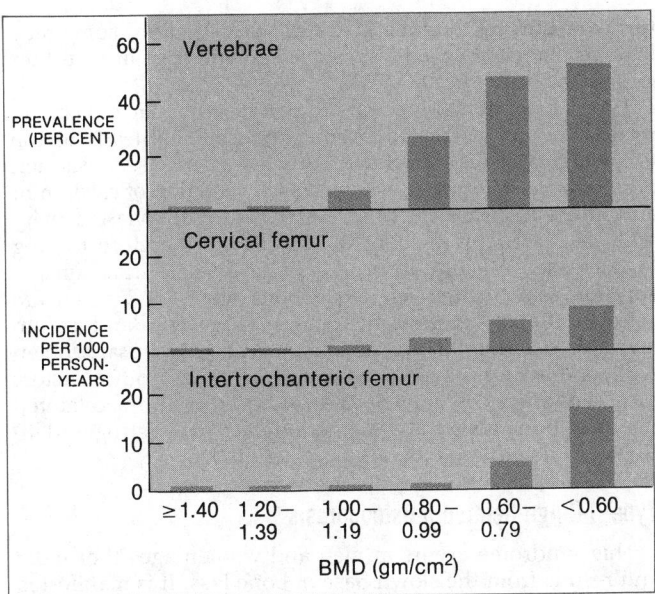

FIGURE 250–1. Occurrence of fractures in vertebrae and proximal femurs at various levels of bone mineral density (BMD). (Adapted from Riggs and Melton. N Engl J Med 314:1676, 1986.)

loss. Fracture risk is determined by absolute bone density, regardless of age. In the absence of severe trauma, fractures do not occur until bone density has fallen below the values found in young adults (about 1.0 gram per square centimeter for both vertebrae and femur). With further decreases in bone density below the fracture threshold, the incidence of fractures increases (Fig. 250–1). In addition, the increased propensity of the elderly to fall is an independent cause of fractures.

The main factors contributing to osteoporosis are shown in Figure 250–2 and are discussed below.

INITIAL BONE DENSITY. Insufficient accumulation of bone mass during skeletal growth predisposes to fractures later in life as age-related bone loss ensues. Differences in bone density at skeletal maturity explain, in part, the racial and sexual differences in the incidence of osteoporosis that have been observed. White women have the lightest skeletons and black men have the heaviest; white men and black women have skeletons of intermediate density. This rank order corresponds to the rank order for the occurrence of fractures. Women of short stature and of northern European extraction tend toward a more gracile skeleton and also have an increased incidence of osteoporosis later in life. Moreover, if the rate of bone loss with age is constant, those white women

with the lowest bone density values at skeletal maturity are at the greatest risk for fracture in later life. The amount of bone present in young adulthood has been shown to have significant genetic determinants, and osteoporotic patients often have affected relatives.

AGE-RELATED FACTORS. These factors are responsible for the slow phase of bone loss. Although they occur universally, variations in their magnitude may account, in part, for individual differences in bone loss. Two age-related factors seem particularly important. First, from the fourth decade onward there is decreased bone formation at the cellular level (each osteoblast does less work), and this abnormality becomes more severe with age. Second, an age-related increase in parathyroid function occurs concomitantly with and probably results from the age-related decrease in calcium absorption. Although serum levels of 25-hydroxyvitamin D (25OHD) are generally normal, serum levels of 1,25-dihydroxyvitamin D [1,25(OH)$_2$D] decrease by about 50 per cent with aging and may be even lower in patients with hip fracture. This decrease appears to be caused by impairment, in the aging kidney, of the activity of 25OHD 1α-hydroxylase, the enzyme that converts 25OHD to 1,25(OH)$_2$D (Ch. 245). The recent observation that serum bone G1a-protein and other biochemical markers increase with aging suggests that secondary hyperparathyroidism may increase overall skeletal turnover (more bone remodeling units are formed). Because of the impairment in osteoblast function, however, increased bone turnover results in increased bone loss.

MENOPAUSE. The accelerated phase of bone loss after menopause is the result of estrogen deficiency and can be prevented by estrogen replacement. The excess loss attributable to menopause may be 10 to 15 per cent for the appendicular skeleton and 15 to 20 per cent for the vertebrae. A form of functional hypogonadism associated with decreased vertebral density has been described in female long-distance runners. Postmenopausal administration of estrogen decreases the occurrence of vertebral fractures and, in most studies, of hip and Colles' fractures as well. Men do not undergo the equivalent of menopause, but gonadal function does decline in some elderly men, and overt hypogonadism is often associated with vertebral fractures.

SPORADIC FACTORS. When present, these sporadic factors increase the rate of bone loss. Smoking and high alcohol consumption increase the risk for developing osteoporosis by twofold. Ethanol is toxic to osteoblasts. Obesity is protective, possibly because of increased loading stress to the spine and, in postmenopausal women, because of increased conversion (in fat tissue) of adrenal androgens to estrogens. Nutritional factors also may be important, although there is considerable controversy regarding this. Some data suggest that premenopausal women require a calcium intake of 1000 mg per day and postmenopausal women require 1500 mg per day to maintain calcium balance. These levels are well above the average intake—550 mg per day—in middle-aged and elderly women. However, other investigators have been unable to demonstrate a relationship between the rate of bone loss assessed densitometrically and the calcium intake. A high protein intake may decrease retention of dietary calcium, possibly because acid radicals increase urinary calcium excretion.

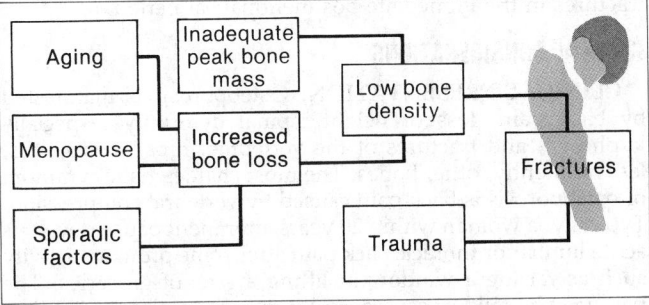

FIGURE 250–2. Model for pathogenesis of osteoporosis. The major cause of fractures in osteoporosis is a decrease in absolute bone density. In the elderly, trauma due to an increased propensity to fall and impaired ability to break the fall further increases the incidence of fractures. Low bone density can occur later in life because the amount of bone formed by the completion of growth in young adulthood was inadequate or the rate of bone loss was increased. The latter is a result of the cumulative effect of factors related to aging (that are universally present), of the menopause (in women), and of various sporadic factors (that are present in some but not in other individuals).

OSTEOPOROSIS SYNDROMES

Osteoporosis can be classified as primary or secondary, depending on the absence or presence of an associated medical condition known to cause bone loss (Table 250–1). Secondary causes of osteoporosis can be identified in 20 per cent of women and 40 per cent of men presenting with vertebral fractures and should always be searched for. Primary osteoporosis may occur, although rarely, in prepubertal boys and girls (juvenile osteoporosis) and characteristically runs an

TABLE 250-1. CLASSIFICATION OF CAUSES OF OSTEOPOROSIS

Primary Osteoporosis
Juvenile
Idiopathic (young adults)
Involutional osteoporosis

Endocrine Diseases
Hypogonadism
Ovarian agenesis
Glucocorticoid excess
Hyperthyroidism
Hyperparathyroidism
Diabetes mellitus (?)

Gastrointestinal Diseases
Subtotal gastrectomy
Malabsorption syndromes
Chronic obstructive jaundice
Primary biliary cirrhosis
Severe malnutrition
Alactasia

Bone Marrow Disorders
Multiple myeloma and related disorders
Systemic mastocytosis
Disseminated carcinoma

Connective Tissue Diseases
Osteogenesis imperfecta
Homocystinuria
Ehlers-Danlos syndrome
Marfan syndrome

Miscellaneous Causes
Immobilization
Chronic obstructive pulmonary disease
Chronic alcoholism
Rheumatoid arthritis (?)
Chronic heparin administration
Chronic administration of anticonvulsant drugs (?)

acute clinical course for two to four years. A spontaneous remission then ensues, followed by resumption of bone growth. An uncommon primary form of osteoporosis occurs in young adults of either sex (idiopathic osteoporosis) and undoubtedly is heterogeneous etiologically. The main manifestation is vertebral fracture, although fractures of the ribs and appendicular skeleton also may occur. The clinical course may be mild but more often is severe, progressive, and relatively refractory to standard therapy.

The common primary form of osteoporosis, termed "involutional osteoporosis," begins in middle life and becomes increasingly more common with advancing age. Involutional osteoporosis can be separated into two major types based on differences in clinical presentation, in densitometric and hormonal changes, and in the relationship of disease patterns to the menopause and age (Table 250-2).

Type I ("Postmenopausal") Osteoporosis

This form of the disease characteristically affects women within 15 to 20 years after menopause. Less commonly, men of the same age are affected with a form of osteoporosis that is indistinguishable from it. Vertebral fractures and Colles' fractures are the main clinical manifestations. The vertebral fractures are often of the "crush type" and are associated with large deformation and pain. The skeletal sites of these manifestations—vertebral body and the ultradistal radius—contain large amounts of trabecular bone. In patients with type I osteoporosis, the rate of trabecular bone loss is usually two to three times normal, but the rate of cortical bone loss is only slightly above normal. During this accelerated phase, trabecular plate perforation with loss of structural trabeculae weakens the vertebrae and predisposes to acute collapse. Iliac crest biopsies have shown bone turnover to be high (in about 25 per cent), normal (in about 45 per cent), or low (in about 30 per cent), but even those with low turnover show evidence of an earlier phase of accelerated bone turnover on stereologic analysis. Thus, all patients with type I osteoporosis may have passed through a phase of high bone

turnover but, by the time of clinical presentation, some may have reached a "burned-out" stage and will have little further loss of trabecular bone.

Type I osteoporosis appears to be caused by factors closely related to or exacerbated by menopause. This leads to the following cascade: accelerated bone loss, decreased secretion of parathyroid hormone and increased secretion of calcitonin, and functional impairment in 25OHD 1α-hydroxylase activity with decreased production of 1,25(OH)$_2$D, therefore leading to decreased calcium absorption. The defect in calcium absorption may further aggravate bone loss. All women are estrogen deficient after menopause, however, and serum levels of sex steroids are similar in postmenopausal women with and without type I osteoporosis. Thus, other factors must augment the rate or the duration of the accelerated phase of bone loss: these factors interact with estrogen deficiency to determine individual susceptibility.

Type II ("Age-Related") Osteoporosis

This syndrome occurs in men and women age 70 or older and results from the slow phase of bone loss. It is manifested mainly by hip and vertebral fractures, although fractures of the proximal humerus, proximal tibia, and pelvis are common. The vertebral fractures are often of the multiple wedge type, leading to dorsal kyphosis ("dowager's hump"). Trabecular thinning associated with the slow phase of bone loss is responsible for gradual and, usually, painless vertebral deformation. In type II osteoporosis, bone density values for the proximal femur, vertebrae, and sites in the appendicular skeleton are usually in the lower part of the normal range (adjusted for age and sex). This suggests proportionate losses of cortical and trabecular bone and a rate of loss that is only slightly higher than the mean for age-matched peers. The age-related processes causing type II osteoporosis affect virtually the entire population of aging men and women and, as the slow phase of bone loss progresses, an increasing number of them will have bone density values below the fracture threshold. The two most important of these age-related factors are decreased osteoblast function and impaired production of 1,25(OH)$_2$D, leading to decreased calcium absorption and secondary hyperparathyroidism. The effects of all risk factors for bone loss encountered over a lifetime, however, are cumulative. Thus, the residual effects of accelerated bone loss after menopause many years before may explain why the incidence of hip fractures is twofold greater in elderly women than in elderly men, although rates of slow bone loss are similar in the two sexes. Conversely, the necessary contribution of age-related slow bone loss accounts for the absence of an acute increase in the incidence of hip fractures in the immediate postmenopausal period.

CLINICAL CONSIDERATIONS

CLINICAL PRESENTATION. Osteoporosis is manifested by back pain, loss of height, spinal deformity (especially kyphosis), and fractures of the vertebrae, hips, wrists, and, less frequently, other bones. The most characteristic symptom of osteoporosis is back pain caused by vertebral compression. Typically, a woman within 20 years after menopause develops acute lumbar or thoracic back pain after some ordinary activity such as raising a window or lifting a sack of groceries. The pain may be mild or severe, and it may be localized or radiate to the flank. It remits in days or weeks but then recurs with the occurrence of new fractures. After several episodes of acute intermittent pain, a chronic mechanical backache may develop as a result of spinal deformity. In untreated or unsuccessfully treated patients, severe kyphosis may develop with a loss of 4 to 8 inches of height. In severe cases, the rib cage comes to rest on the pelvic brim. The frequency of occurrence of vertebral fractures and the number of fractures that eventually occur vary widely among patients, but the

TABLE 250-2. TYPES OF INVOLUTIONAL OSTEOPOROSIS

	Type I	Type II
Age (years)	51–75	>70
Sex ratio, F:M	6:1	2:1
Type of bone loss	Mainly trabecular	Trabecular and cortical
Rate of bone loss	Accelerated	Not accelerated
Fracture sites	Vertebrae (crush) and distal radius	Vertebrae (multiple wedge) and hip
Parathyroid function	Decreased	Increased
Calcium absorption	Decreased	Decreased
Metabolism of 25OHD to 1,25(OH)$_2$D	Secondary decrease	Primary decrease
Main causes	Factors related to menopause	Factors related to aging

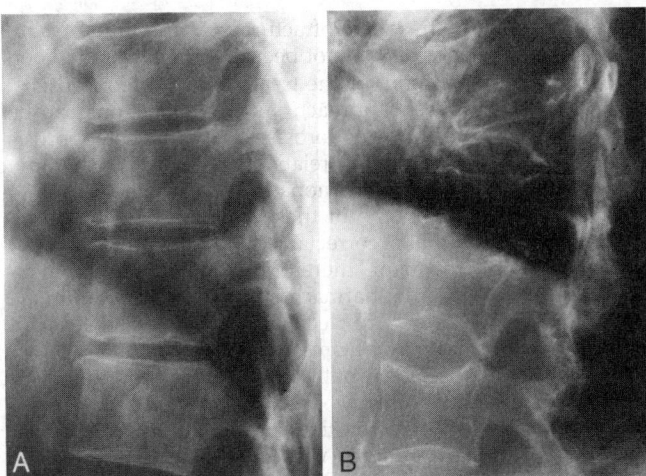

FIGURE 250–3. Radiographs of the spinal column. *A*, Normal bone in a 60-year-old woman. *B*, Vertebral osteoporosis in a 62-year-old woman. There is a decrease in bone density with high-grade collapse fractures of T12 and L1 and ballooning (expansion of the intervertebral discs) of L2 and L3.

average is one per year in the initial phase of the disease. In general, progression is slower in elderly women, and commonly substantial dorsal kyphosis and cervical lordosis—the so-called dowager's hump—develop in the absence of significant pain. Half of the hip fractures in elderly men and women are spontaneous and half are associated with falls.

RADIOLOGIC FINDINGS. Radiographs of the spinal column (Fig. 250–3) show accentuation of the vertebral endplates, prominence of the weight-bearing vertical trabeculae (due to disappearance of the horizontal trabeculae), and loss of contrast in radiodensity between the interior of the vertebral body and the adjacent soft tissue. Vertebral deformity may take the form of collapse (reduction of anterior and posterior height), anterior wedging (reduction in anterior height, usually occurring in the thoracic spinal column), or "ballooning" (biconcave compression of the end-plates by pressure of the intervertebral discs, usually occurring in the lumbar spinal column). Also, the nucleus pulposus may herniate locally into the vertebral body (Schmorl's nodes). Osteoporosis due to glucocorticoid excess should be considered when there is associated osteoporosis of the skull, fractures of the ribs and pelvic rami, and prominent partially mineralized callus at the site of fracture. In the absence of pseudofractures, osteomalacia may be difficult to distinguish from osteoporosis, but it often has a "ground glass" appearance rather than the characteristic "clear glass" appearance of osteoporosis. Posterior wedging of a vertebra suggests a destructive lesion rather than osteoporosis.

DIAGNOSTIC EVALUATION. All patients with newly discovered osteoporosis should have a general medical evaluation to assess severity and exclude secondary diseases that may cause the osteoporosis. Systemic symptoms or abnormal physical findings suggest the presence of an underlying disease. Serum calcium and phosphorus levels are normal in primary osteoporosis. Serum alkaline phosphatase levels also are normal except for transient elevations during healing of vertebral fractures. Sustained elevation of the alkaline phosphatase level, in the absence of liver disease, suggests osteomalacia or skeletal metastasis.

Multiple myeloma may be present without symptoms and with a normal hematogram and erythrocyte sedimentation rate. Although most cases can be diagnosed by serum and urine protein electrophoresis, bone marrow examination may be required to establish its presence (Ch. 163). Sometimes bone marrow examination is also necessary to diagnose disseminated carcinoma.

In the past, severity of osteoporosis has been assessed by

determining the amount of height loss and the number of vertebral fractures. The severity can now be assessed more precisely by direct measurement of vertebral bone density. Two techniques are generally available—dual-photon absorptiometry and quantitative computed tomography using single-energy scanning. Although both methods have advantages and disadvantages, either will provide satisfactory clinical results. Bone density also can be measured at the radius and os calcis by using single-photon absorptiometry. The correlation between bone mineral density (BMD) in the lumbar spine and in the radius, even at an ultradistal site or the os calcis, is too low ($r = 0.5$ to 0.8) for vertebral density to be predicted accurately for individual patients. Bone densitometry also is used to assess whether therapy has been effective in arresting bone loss. BMD should be determined at baseline and at yearly intervals during treatment.

Iliac trephine biopsy may be useful in selected patients to exclude osteomalacia and to assess bone turnover. Biopsy specimens should be obtained after the patient has received tetracycline double labeling (tetracycline is selectively deposited where there is bone formation, and it fluoresces when the bone section is illuminated with ultraviolet light). The biopsy specimen should be processed by an experienced laboratory that will provide quantitative information.

TREATMENT

GENERAL THERAPEUTIC MEASURES. Acute back pain responds to analgesics, heat, and gentle massage to alleviate muscle spasm. Sometimes a brief period of bed rest is required. Chronic back pain often is caused by spinal deformity and thus is difficult to relieve completely. Instruction in posture and gait training and institution of regular back extension exercises to strengthen the flabby paravertebral muscles are usually beneficial. Occasionally, use of an orthopedic back brace is required. All patients with osteoporosis should have a diet adequate in calcium, proteins, and vitamins, should be reasonably active physically, and should take precautions to prevent falls.

DRUG THERAPY. Drugs used in the treatment of osteoporosis can be classified as antiresorptive or formation-stimulating (Fig. 250–4). The drugs currently approved by the Food and Drug Administration for the treatment of osteoporosis—calcium, estrogen, and calcitonin—act by decreasing bone resorption.

Calcium, which may act by decreasing parathyroid hormone

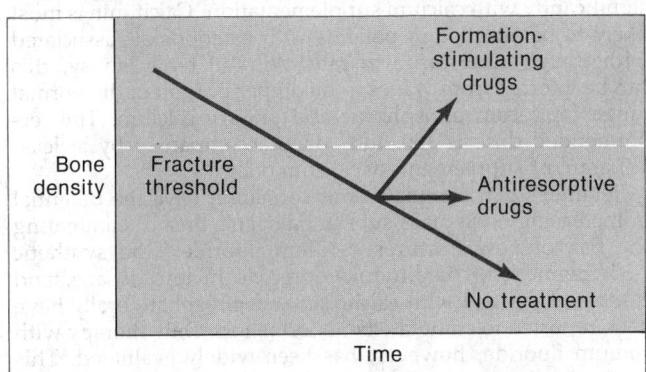

FIGURE 250–4. As bone is lost due to the osteoporotic process, the bone density falls below the fracture threshold. As more bone is lost in the untreated patient, progressively more fractures occur. Antiresorptive drug therapy decreases the bone resorption that is responsible for continued bone loss. When a new steady state is attained, after three to six months of treatment, there also is a decrease in bone formation that approximates the decrease in bone resorption. Thus, the best result that can be obtained with this class of therapeutic agents is maintenance of the existing skeletal mass or slowing of its rate of loss. Regimens that stimulate bone formation have the theoretical potential of increasing bone mass substantially and, thus, of eliminating the risk of new fractures.

secretion, is safe, well-tolerated, and inexpensive. *Vitamin D* and its active metabolites must be used judiciously, if at all, because the dosage that increases calcium absorption is not much smaller than the dosage that increases bone resorption.

Estrogen is more effective than calcium but has significant side effects. These commonly include induction of menstruation, mastodynia, and fluid retention. Less common but more serious side effects are endometrial carcinoma, venous thrombosis and pulmonary embolism, aggravation of hypertension, and cholelithiasis. The effect of estrogen on bone may be mediated by decreasing skeletal responsiveness to circulating parathyroid hormone. The mechanism of action of androgens and synthetic anabolic agents probably is similar to that of estrogen, although some data suggest a weak stimulation of bone formation.

Calcitonin is an effective antiresorption agent, but calcium supplementation must be given concurrently to prevent secondary hyperparathyroidism; disadvantages include the requirement for parenteral administration, a relatively high cost, and the development of neutralizing antibodies in some patients.

Therapy for patients with involutional osteoporosis should be individualized. For patients with mild disease, only calcium supplementation (1.0 to 1.5 grams per day) need be used. For more than minimal disease, especially in women within 15 years of menopause, low-dose estrogen therapy (such as cyclic doses of 0.625 mg of conjugated estrogen or 0.025 mg of ethynyl estradiol daily) may be used. Because the risk of endometrial hyperplasia (and therefore carcinoma) is decreased or eliminated by concomitant progestin therapy, 5 mg of medroxyprogesterone acetate should be given daily during the last 13 days of the cycle. The excessive hepatic production of coagulation factors, renin substrate, and bile cholesterol (accounting for increased risk of venous thrombosis, hypertension, and cholelithiasis) are due to the liver being exposed to increased estrogen concentration in the first pass after oral administration. These problems can be reduced or eliminated by giving the estrogen as a transdermal patch (0.1 mg of 17β-estradiol per day). If bone loss or fractures continue on hormone treatment, the dosage of both estrogen and progestin should be doubled.

Treatment with vitamin D and its active metabolites probably should be reserved for patients with a documented or suspected impairment in calcium absorption. This can be inferred from a relatively low urinary calcium excretion rate (<75 mg per day), especially if this rate does not increase significantly with calcium supplementation. Calcitonin is most likely to be effective in patients with osteoporosis associated with a high bone turnover rate. Without bone biopsy, this can be inferred from values in the upper portion of the normal range for serum phosphorus and urinary calcium. The recommended dose is 100 units daily accompanied by at least 1.0 gram of supplementary calcium daily.

Regimens that stimulate bone formation have the potential of increasing bone mass substantially and thus of eliminating the risk of new fractures. Sodium fluoride,* the synthetic 1-34 fragment of parathyroid hormone in low dosage, and combined therapy with calcitonin and phosphate orally have been reported to stimulate bone formation. Only therapy with sodium fluoride, however, has been widely evaluated. This drug stimulates osteoblasts directly. In doses of 40 to 80 mg per day, sodium fluoride can increase the trabecular bone density of the axial skeleton substantially but does not increase cortical bone density in the appendicular skeleton. Concurrent calcium administration prevents or minimizes the mineralization defect that may occur when fluoride is given alone. Side effects from the drug include symptoms of gastric irritation (in about 30 per cent) and acute lower extremity pain syndrome (in about 10 per cent). The latter may be due to increased bone remodeling in weight-bearing bones and may

be associated with stress microfractures. At the time of publication, sodium fluoride has not been approved by the Food and Drug Administration for the treatment of osteoporosis.

The same therapeutic approach with modifications can be used for other types of osteoporosis. Idiopathic osteoporosis in young adult women often is relatively refractory to therapy. Because the women are premenopausal, there is no reason to prescribe sex steroid. Some of these patients have impaired calcium absorption that is correctable with vitamin D therapy. The mainstay of treatment, therefore, is calcium supplementation with or without pharmacologic doses of vitamin D. Calcitonin can be added to decrease the increased level of bone resorption that may be present.

Men with osteoporosis usually do not have a deficiency of sex steroids and thus have no need for hormonal treatment. But 10 to 20 per cent have partial or complete hypogonadism from various causes. Patients with documented low plasma testosterone levels should receive replacement therapy—for example, with testosterone enanthate in a dose of 200 to 400 mg intramuscularly every four weeks. Calcium supplementation with or without pharmacologic doses of vitamin D should also be given.

The most common cause of secondary osteoporosis is chronic use of pharmacologic dosages of glucocorticoids. The single most effective measure is reduction of dosage or, if possible, complete discontinuation of the glucocorticoid. Administering the glucocorticoid once daily or on alternate days may maintain a more favorable balance between its antiinflammatory and immunosuppressive effects and the osteopenic effect. All patients should be given calcium supplements and postmenopausal women should be given estrogens. Although glucocorticoids inhibit calcium absorption, the use of pharmacologic doses of vitamin D or its metabolites in this circumstance is controversial and may increase the calciuric effect of the glucocorticoid. There is increasing evidence that glucocorticoids do not induce major alterations in vitamin D metabolism.

Patients with type II osteoporosis have already lost most of the bone they ever will lose, their bone differs little in density from that of peers without fractures, and they generally have low bone turnover. There is no evidence that estrogen or calcitonin is beneficial in such patients. Treatment consists primarily of calcium supplementation (because of impaired calcium absorption), a vitamin D supplement (1000 units per day) to correct any deficiency that may be present, and instruction in measures that decrease the risk of falls.

PREVENTION

Considering the magnitude of the problem of osteoporosis, prevention is the only cost-effective approach. Dietary calcium, if low, should be increased at least to the RDA of 1000 mg per day for adults and 1500 mg per day for adolescents. Increased physical activity should be encouraged, and bone toxins, such as cigarettes and heavy alcohol consumption, should be eliminated. The recent NIH Consensus Conference on Osteoporosis recommended a calcium intake of 1000 to 1500 mg per day for all postmenopausal women but left the decision on estrogen replacement therapy to the woman and her physician. Because it is impractical to treat and follow the entire population at risk (all postmenopausal women and all elderly men!), it will be necessary to develop criteria for selecting those at greatest risk for future development of fractures. Prophylactic therapy with agents such as estrogen, which are effective but have potential risks, would be justified in high-risk individuals.

Selection of subjects for prophylactic intervention should follow a two-step process. First, historical risk factors (Table 250–3) should be used to select those who are believed to be at sufficient risk for type I osteoporosis to warrant vertebral bone densitometry. Although it is not yet possible to weigh these quantitatively, the more of them that are present in a

---

*This use is not listed in the manufacturer's directive.

TABLE 250–3. MAJOR RISK FACTORS FOR OSTEOPOROSIS IN WOMEN

Postmenopausal (within 20 years after menopause)
White or Asian
Premature menopause
Positive family history
Short stature and small bones
Leanness
Low calcium intake
Inactivity
Nulliparity
Gastric or small bowel resection
Long-term glucocorticoid therapy
Long-term use of anticonvulsants
Hyperparathyroidism
Thyrotoxicosis
Smoking
Heavy alcohol use

given individual, the greater the likelihood that vertebral bone density values will be low. Persons found to have low, or relatively low, values should be counseled and started on prophylactic therapy. Although longitudinal measurements provide a better estimate of risk than do single measurements, their cost-effectiveness is less because measurements every six months over two to three years are required to estimate individual rates of bone loss. For women over age 75 years, densitometry is less useful because most women already are below the fracture threshold, and those with and without fractures differ only slightly in bone density.

Genant HK, Ettinger B, Cann CE, et al.: Osteoporosis: Assessment by quantitative computed tomography. Orthop Clin North Am 16:557, 1985. *Review of assessment of bone density using quantitative computed tomography.*

Mazess RB: The noninvasive measurement of skeletal mass. In Peck WA (ed.): Bone and Mineral Research, Annual 1. Amsterdam, Excerpta Medica, 1983, pp 223–279. *Review of assessment of bone density using single- and dual-photon absorptiometry.*

Parfitt AM: Morphologic basis of bone mineral measurements: Transient and steady state effects of treatment in osteoporosis. Min Electrolyte Metab 4:273, 1980. *The theoretic basis for differences in early and late effects of therapeutic agents on bone remodeling and bone density in osteoporosis.*

Parfitt AM: Quantum concept of bone remodeling and turnover: Implications for the pathogenesis of osteoporosis. Calcif Tissue Int 28:1, 1979. *A lucid review of the role of abnormalities of bone remodeling in the pathogenesis of osteoporosis.*

Riggs BL, Melton LJ III: Medical progress: Involutional osteoporosis. N Engl J Med 314:1676, 1986. *Review of etiology and treatment of osteoporosis and a summary of the evidence that supports the concept of two distinct syndromes of involutional osteoporosis.*

Riis B, Thomsen K, Christiansen C: Does calcium supplementation prevent postmenopausal bone loss? N Engl J Med 316:173, 1987. *This controlled two-year study in 43 women in the early postmenopausal period found that treatment with estrogen prevented bone loss, whereas treatment with 2000 mg daily of oral calcium was only slightly better than placebo. The data reaffirm that calcium supplementation is not as effective as estrogen therapy in the prevention of early postmenopausal bone loss.*

251 PAGET'S DISEASE OF BONE (Osteitis Deformans)

Frederick R. Singer

INCIDENCE AND EPIDEMIOLOGY

Paget's disease is a common bone disorder second in incidence to osteoporosis. In areas of prevalence it affects approximately 3 per cent of the population over age 40. The disease is commonly diagnosed in the United Kingdom and in the countries to which its inhabitants have migrated, including the United States, Canada, South Africa, Australia, and New Zealand. The disease also is common in France, Germany, and Italy. Patients are rarely found in China, Japan, India, or Scandinavia. There is no major predilection for either sex.

There is evidence of an autosomal dominant transmission that is linked to histocompatibility leukocyte antigens. As high as 25 per cent of patients have been reported to have at least one relative with the disease.

PATHOLOGY

Paget's disease may affect one or many bones, but in the majority of patients most of the skeleton is uninvolved. The earliest phase is characterized by a localized osteolytic process in which proliferation of multinucleated osteoclasts is the dominant lesion. The osteoclasts of Paget's disease are occasionally quite large and may exhibit more than 100 nuclei in a cross-section of one cell. Adjacent to the advancing osteolytic front, the pathology is characterized by a mixed osteolytic and osteoblastic process of great intensity. Numerous plump osteoblasts line bony trabeculae that have previously been partially resorbed by osteoclasts. The marrow spaces may be devoid of hematopoietic cells and instead are filled with fibroblasts, connective tissue, and blood vessels. The resultant architecture of the bone takes on a "mosaic" pattern in which the cement lines are arranged in a haphazard pattern instead of the normal symmetry of parallel collagen fibers in both cortical and trabecular bone. Occasionally this abnormal mosaic pattern is present with little or no cellular activity. Osteolytic, mixed osteolytic and osteoblastic, and "burned out" Paget's disease may be present in a single bone. Paget's disease can usually be readily distinguished from primary hyperparathyroidism, osteomyelitis, and osteomalacia by light microscopy, but electron microscopy studies have provided evidence of a characteristic lesion. The nuclei, and at times the cytoplasm, of the osteoclasts frequently contain abnormal inclusions that resemble the nucleocapsids of viruses of the Paramyxoviridae family. Respiratory syncytial virus and measles virus antigens have been demonstrated in the osteoclasts of Paget's disease by immunohistologic techniques.

ETIOLOGY

Sir James Paget, in his original description of the disease, proposed that the entity was inflammatory in nature. The recent ultrastructural and immunohistologic studies support the concept of a "slow" virus infection, although definitive proof is still to be obtained. No other hypotheses have generated supporting evidence.

CLINICAL FEATURES

In many patients Paget's disease is not appreciated until an abnormal radiograph or laboratory test is encountered either in the course of a routine evaluation or during assessment of an unrelated complaint. The most common complaints of symptomatic patients are *skeletal deformity* and *musculoskeletal pain*. The bones most likely to be abnormal on physical examination are the cranium, the clavicles, and the long bones, particularly of the lower extremities. The complications associated with skull lesions include hearing loss, vertigo, tinnitus and, less commonly, headaches. Severe enlargement of the base of the skull may lead to basilar impression and compression of the spinal cord, the brain stem, the cerebellum, and the basilar and vertebral arteries. Slurred speech, impaired swallowing, diplopia, and urinary incontinence may result. Deformity of the facial bones (leontiasis ossea) is much less common in patients with Paget's disease than in patients with fibrous dysplasia, a disease that usually is diagnosed several decades earlier in life. The spine may be involved at any level, but lumbar and thoracic vertebrae are most commonly affected. One or more vertebrae, consecutive or not, can manifest the disease. Back pain may be severe and of complex origin, since degenerative arthritis is common in this age group, and impingement of skeletal tissue on nerve roots or the spinal cord can occur. The sudden onset of intolerable pain suggests that a compression fracture has occurred. Disease affecting the pelvis and proximal femur produces a common severe pain syndrome, weight-bearing pain from degenerative arthritis of the hip. Ambulation may also be impaired when significant lateral or anterior bowing of the femur or tibia develops. These bones are also prone to pathologic fracture. Evidence of disease activity in long bones is manifested by increased skin temperature over the affected bone. This results from the increased cutaneous blood flow associated with the hypervascular bone beneath.

Defects in Bruch's membrane of the retina, termed angioid streaks, may be observed in about 10 per cent of patients and seldom are associated with impaired vision. Cardiac enlargement and frank congestive heart failure may be manifestations of prior increased cardiac output, which is thought to be a consequence of increased vascularity of affected bones. This usually occurs in patients with more than 20 per cent of the skeleton affected by Paget's disease or when the skull is severely involved. Bone tumors such as osteosarcoma and giant cell tumor may develop in lesions of Paget's disease (Ch. 253). A rapid worsening of bone pain or the relatively sudden development of a mass or both are the common modes of presentation.

RADIOLOGY. The radiologic features of Paget's disease are so characteristic that it is seldom necessary to obtain a bone biopsy for diagnosis. The earliest manifestation is a localized osteolytic lesion most readily detected in the skull and at either end of a long bone. In the skull, the circumscribed radiolucent area has been termed osteoporosis circumscripta (Fig. 251–1). The osteolytic lesion in an extremity bone usually progresses with a sharply defined V-shape at an average rate of progression of 1 cm per year. Linear cortical radiolucencies may develop in the femur or tibia on the convex surface of a curved bone and may be precursors of fractures. An uncommon variant of the osteolytic lesion may occur at the distal end of the tibia, in which a cystlike expansion of the bone is seen. Osteolytic disease of the vertebral bodies is often associated with sclerotic margins, giving a "picture frame" appearance. These vertebrae are prone to compression fractures.

The radiographic manifestations of osteoblastic activity generally appear years or even decades after the onset of osteolysis. In the skull a "honeycomb" appearance of patchy new bone may fill in the underlying osteoporosis circumscripta, and subsequently the classic "cotton-wool" lesions of exuberant chaotic bone formation appear with a strikingly thickened calvarium (Fig. 251–2). In the long bones, the osteolytic lesions evolve into thickened bone with irregular trabeculation. In the pelvis, thickening of the iliopectineal line, the "brim sign,"

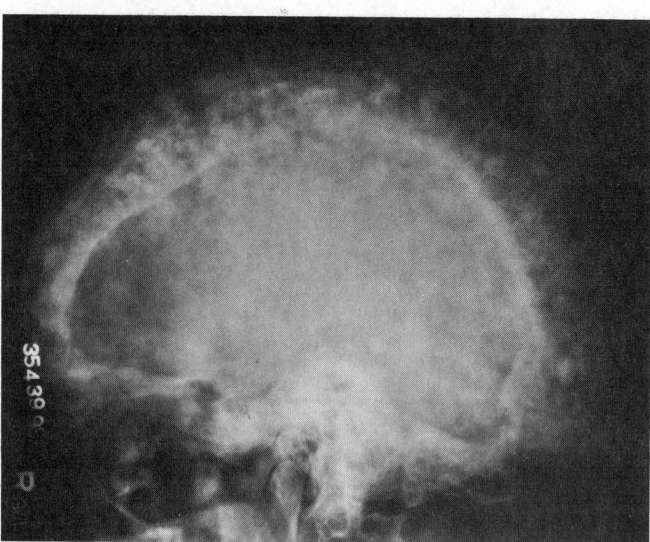

FIGURE 251–2. Advanced involvement of the skull with marked thickening of the entire cranial vault, areas of osteolysis, and patchy new bone formation resulting in a "cotton-wool" appearance.

is nearly pathognomonic of Paget's disease. It is also found in patients with osteopetrosis but rarely in patients with osteoblastic metastases. Enlargement of the ischial and pubic bones is also typical of Paget's disease. Sclerosis of the pagetic vertebral body may be difficult to distinguish from malignant bone involvement, but if the vertebral body is clearly larger than adjacent vertebral bodies, Paget's disease is likely. Computerized tomography of the spine is a useful means of evaluating the detailed anatomy of the spine and is particularly helpful in defining arthritic and neurologic complications in the patient with back pain.

The bone scan is the most sensitive means to detect active lesions of Paget's disease, although it is not a specific diagnostic test. The earliest lesions may not be discernible roentgenographically at the same time an area of increased uptake of the radiolabeled scanning agent is obvious.

BIOCHEMICAL FEATURES

The extent and activity of Paget's disease have been found to correlate reasonably well with serum alkaline phosphatase activity (an index of osteoblastic activity) and urinary hydroxyproline excretion (an index of bone matrix resorption). Patients with very limited active disease have normal biochemical parameters, whereas increases of 50-fold greater than normal sometimes occur in patients with polyostotic disease of greatest extent. The serum calcium concentration is normal except in patients who are immobilized or in whom malignancy or primary hyperparathyroidism develops. Hypercalciuria precedes hypercalcemia in these patients. Hyperuricemia, with or without clinical gout, is sometimes found and may reflect increased turnover of purines.

MEDICAL AND SURGICAL THERAPY

Most patients with Paget's disease do not require any therapy or may only require analgesic agents such as aspirin or indomethacin. The leading indications for medical therapy are bone pain and preparation for orthopedic surgery. Prevention of future complications in patients with osteolytic lesions of the skull and weight-bearing bones may be a reasonable objective.

CALCITONIN. Effective and safe therapy of Paget's disease became possible with the availability of salmon calcitonin. Subcutaneous injections of 50 to 100 MRC units daily or on alternate days produce an average decrease of 50 per cent in biochemical parameters and improve many of the manifestations of the disease. Relief of bone pain, healing of

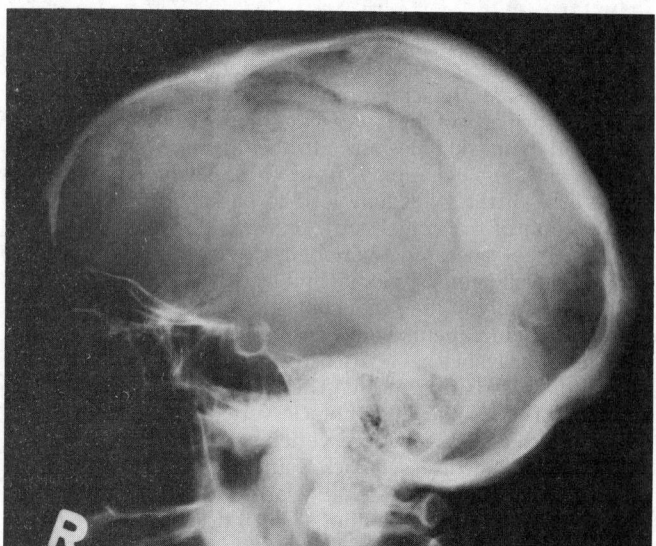

FIGURE 251–1. Osteoporosis circumscripta of the skull involving the frontal, parietal, and temporal bones.

osteolytic lesions, reduction of increased cardiac output and elevated skin temperature, stabilization of auditory acuity, and reversal of various neurologic deficits have all been convincingly documented during chronic therapy. Treatment may be necessary for years in patients with active osteolytic lesions. Side effects include nausea, facial flushing, and polyuria, but they seldom require interruption of therapy. Salmon calcitonin elicits an antibody response in more than 50 per cent of patients, since its amino acid sequence differs considerably from human calcitonin. Approximately 25 per cent of patients acquire high enough antibody titers to become resistant to hormone action. These patients respond to human calcitonin or to other forms of therapy.

DIPHOSPHONATES. An alternate form of therapy is disodium etidronate, whose main advantage is its oral mode of administration. At a dose of 5 mg per kilogram of body weight daily for an initial treatment period of six months, this drug produces benefits similar to calcitonin and can be used in repeated six-month courses after symptoms return. However, healing of osteolytic lesions has seldom been documented. Long-term use of higher doses should be avoided because of impairment of bone mineralization and resulting susceptibility to fracture.

MITHRAMYCIN. Mithramycin is a cytotoxic antibiotic that has not been approved for therapy of Paget's disease by the FDA but has been used in selected patients because of its great potency. Dosage has not been standardized but intravenous infusions of 10 to 15 µg per kilogram daily for 10 days or once weekly have been reported to suppress many of the manifestations of the disease. The platelet, renal, and hepatic toxicity of this agent warrants great caution in its use. It should be reserved for patients with marked symptomatology who fail with other agents.

The effectiveness of medical therapy can usually be objectively assessed by measurement of serum alkaline phosphatase activity alone at intervals of two to four months. Radiographs of osteolytic lesions should be obtained at least annually.

SURGERY. Surgery is an important adjunct to medical therapy in selected patients. Occipital craniectomy may be necessary in patients with basilar impression, and decompression of neurologic structures affected by vertebral lesions is another procedure of critical importance. More commonly orthopedic procedures are required to enable more normal ambulation in patients with pelvic and lower extremity disease. Degenerative arthritis of the hip is a common complication that can produce severe pain and limit ambulation. Results of total hip replacement are excellent. Deformity of the tibia may also limit ambulation because of knee and ankle pain. Tibial osteotomy leading to restoration of a more normal knee-ankle alignment can also markedly alleviate joint pain and restore a near normal gait. If possible, one to three months of medical therapy should be administered prior to surgery in order to reduce the amount of intra- and postoperative bleeding and to prevent immobilization hypercalcemia postoperatively.

Altman RD, Singer FR: Proceedings of the Kroc foundation conference on Paget's disease of bone. Arthritis Rheum 23:1073, 1980. *A comprehensive coverage of etiology, metabolic, and therapeutic aspects of the disease.*

Mills BG, Singer FR, Weiner LP, et al.: Evidence for both respiratory syncytial virus and measles virus antigens in the osteoclasts of patients with Paget's disease of bone. Clin Orth Rel Res 183:303, 1984. *A study documenting antigens of two Paramyxoviridae viruses in osteoclasts of Paget's disease.*

Rebel A: Symposium: Paget's disease. Clin Orthop Rel Res 217:2, 1987.

Singer FR, Krane SM: Paget's disease of bone. In Avioli LV, Krane SM (eds.): Metabolic Bone Disease. New York, Academic Press, 1987. *A comprehensive review of clinical features, pathology, biochemistry, and treatment of Paget's disease.*

252 OSTEONECROSIS, OSTEOSCLEROSIS, AND OTHER DISORDERS OF BONE

Gordon J. Strewler

OSTEONECROSIS

Osteonecrosis is synonymous with aseptic or avascular necrosis of bone; these terms describe infarction of bone, presumably resulting from ischemia. Such infarcts may be asymptomatic or associated with self-limited pain if they occur in the shaft, as in sickle cell disease or hyperbaric injury (caisson disease). Syndromes with greater morbidity occur with infarcts of subarticular bone, especially in the femoral head.

ETIOLOGY. The most common cause of osteonecrosis is fracture or dislocation of the femoral neck. Other bones susceptible to post-traumatic osteonecrosis are the proximal pole of the carpal scaphoid and the body of the talus. Nontraumatic vascular compromise, usually of the femoral head, is the likely cause of osteonecrosis in sickle cell disease (sludging of sickled erythrocytes), caisson disease (gas bubble emboli), Gaucher's disease (obstruction by histiocytes), hemophilia, and polycythemia vera. Other important etiologies are glucocorticoid therapy, cytotoxic chemotherapy, radiation injury, and renal transplantation. The prevalence of osteonecrosis after renal transplantation ranges from 3 to 41 per cent in various reports. In addition to corticosteroid therapy, precedent renal osteodytrophy and persistent secondary hyperparathyroidism may be etiologic factors. Osteonecrosis is associated with alcoholism and diabetes mellitus, but diabetics seem to be relatively protected against its development after renal transplantation. The ossification centers of growing bone in children are susceptible to growth disturbances and sometimes to osteonecrosis; here the relative roles of constitutional factors and trauma are poorly defined. Over 50 eponymic syndromes, collectively called osteochondroses, are associated with growth disturbances at various epiphyseal sites. The most common site of true osteonecrosis is the femoral head (Perthes' disease).

PATHOGENESIS. While in some disorders (e.g., sickle cell disease), osteonecrosis can readily be ascribed to vascular obstruction, in others, such as glucocorticoid excess, its cause is unknown. There is little support for such proposed mechanisms of steroid-induced osteonecrosis as increased intramedullary pressure with obstruction of venous outflow, fat embolization, or osteopenia with nonhealing microfractures. Also poorly understood are the mechanisms by which infarction of bone leads to its eventual collapse. Dead bone does not lose mechanical stability; bone resorption occurring as part of the reparative process may weaken the infarcted area, predisposing the infarcted bone to fractures and fragmentation.

CLINICAL MANIFESTATIONS. Besides the femoral head, common sites of nontraumatic osteonecrosis include the femoral condyles, distal tibia, humeral head, and talus. The presenting symptom is pain, often of acute onset. Radiologic diagnosis may be delayed for weeks or months because dead and living bone are radiologically indistinguishable. Magnetic resonance imaging or radionuclide scanning may be positive earlier than the radiograph. It is mostly slow reparative processes that are visualized radiographically. A linear subchondral lucency, the "crescent sign," indicates collapse of subchondral bone. Patchy lucencies reflect resorption; patchy sclerosis indicates growth of new bone over the scaffolding of dead trabeculae. These reparative processes may lead to healing if fragmentation or collapse of weakened bone does not supervene. Initial therapy consists of avoidance of weight bearing, but surgery, such as transpositional osteotomy, arthrotomy with removal of fragments, or arthroplasty, is frequently required.

Kenzora JE (ed.): Symposium on idiopathic osteonecrosis. Orthop Clin North Am 16:593, 1985. *Articles on pathogenesis, diagnosis, and therapy of osteonecrosis.*

DISORDERS OF INCREASED BONE DENSITY

Radiographic evidence of increased bone density (osteosclerosis) usually reflects increased bone mass per unit volume, rather than increased mineral per unit of bone mass. This increase can result from accelerated synthesis and mineralization of the bone matrix or from decreased bone resorption. The pathogenesis of such disorders is rarely known, and their histologic characteristics are often indistinguishable; hence, they are classified on the basis of their radiographic appearance. Sclerosis of the cortex can produce increased width as the result of new bone formation, and this is sometimes referred to as hyperostosis. Bone shape can also be altered by disorders of modeling, the process by which bones assume their adult shape during development.

Trabecular Osteosclerosis

This form of osteosclerosis is the most frequently encountered. Its causes can be categorized as neoplastic, hematologic, or metabolic.

Neoplastic. Prostatic and breast carcinoma, as well as other neoplasms with osteoblastic metastases, can present on occasion as diffuse osteosclerosis; however, localized blastic or lytic areas are generally also present and permit radiologic diagnosis of malignancy. Generalized osteosclerosis is a rare presentation of myeloma and other hematologic malignancies.

Hematologic. In 40 per cent of cases of agnogenic myeloid metaplasia with myelofibrosis, diffuse skeletal sclerosis is seen. Osteosclerosis is also preceded by myelofibrosis when it occurs in mastocytosis and polycythemia vera. Sickle cell disease is manifested in bone by sclerosis, medullary bone infarcts, and subchondral osteonecrosis.

Metabolic. Renal osteodystrophy characteristically gives rise to sclerosis of the vertebral end-plates—the "rugger-jersey" spine—and to trabecular sclerosis in the metaphyses of long bones and the skull (Ch. 249). Cortical erosions of secondary hyperparathyroidism are also typically present. Diffuse osteosclerosis is an unusual presentation of Paget's disease (Ch. 251) and is rare in primary hyperparathyroidism. Fluorosis occurs endemically in areas of India and Africa where the fluoride content of water is high, following industrial exposure in aluminum and fertilizer plants, and, increasingly, in individuals treated for osteoporosis (see Ch. 250). Uniform sclerosis of bone is accompanied by exostoses and roughened cortical calcifications at muscle and ligamentous insertions, which suggest the diagnosis. Periarticular pain and limitation of motion are common. Histologically, thick trabeculae are covered by wide osteoid seams, which indicate the presence of osteomalacia.

Cortical and Trabecular Osteosclerosis

Osteopetrosis

Osteopetrosis (Albers-Schönberg disease, or marble bone disease), a rare disorder of greatly increased bone density, occurs in several distinct forms. The malignant, autosomal recessive form (osteopetrosis congenita) results in replacement of the marrow space with bone, which causes anemia, infection, and early death. The benign, autosomal dominant form (osteopetrosis tarda) may be asymptomatic and rarely limits

survival. A mild form with autosomal recessive rather than dominant inheritance is characterized by renal tubular acidosis and absence of the isozyme carbonic anhydrase II in erythrocytes. In obligate heterozygotes for this disorder, carbonic anhydrase II activity is half of normal. This is undoubtedly an important clue to the nature of osteoclast dysfunction in these individuals.

PATHOLOGY. Osteosclerosis results from defective osteoclast function with a failure of normal bone resorption. The medullary cavity is occupied by thickened bone trabeculae with central zones of entrapped calcified cartilage, which indicates a failure to resorb the primary spongiosa. Osteoclasts are abundant. In some cases defective osteoclast function is suggested by the absence of a ruffled border, the redundantly invaginated membrane structure normally adjacent to bone in actively resorbing osteoblasts.

MALIGNANT OSTEOPETROSIS. The malignant, autosomal recessive form of osteopetrosis presents in infancy with failure to thrive and delayed development. Proptosis, blindness, and frequently deafness and hydrocephalus ensue before age two, as bone encroaches upon the cranial foramina. Despite its solid appearance, osteopetrotic bone is fragile, and fractures are frequent. Osteomyelitis is common. Obliteration of the marrow space causes extramedullary hematopoiesis, with hepatosplenomegaly and hypersplenism. Leukoerythroblastic anemia and thrombocytopenia are accompanied by elevated acid and alkaline phosphatase levels and, on occasion, hypocalcemia. Radiologically, the bone is everywhere sclerotic, often with metaphyseal bands of increased density. The long bones are poorly modeled and clublike; ragged metaphyseal-epiphyseal junctions may suggest rickets. Untreated, malignant osteopetrosis results in death from infection, bleeding, or anemia.

BENIGN OSTEOPETROSIS. This autosomal dominant variant is asymptomatic in about half of cases and is usually detected in family studies or as an incidental radiologic finding. The remainder of patients present with fractures of brittle osteopetrotic bone (about 40 per cent) or with osteomyelitis, usually of the mandible. Radiographically, the picture resembles that in the malignant form, but bones are well-modeled (Fig. 252–1). The only laboratory abnormality is an increased acid phosphatase level in some patients.

TREATMENT. The observation that osteopetrosis in mice and rats could be cured by transplantation of marrow or spleen cells has led to the successful use of bone marrow transplantation from HLA-identical sibs for treatment of malignant, autosomal recessive osteopetrosis. Establishment of a chimeric state is accompanied by remarkable regression of

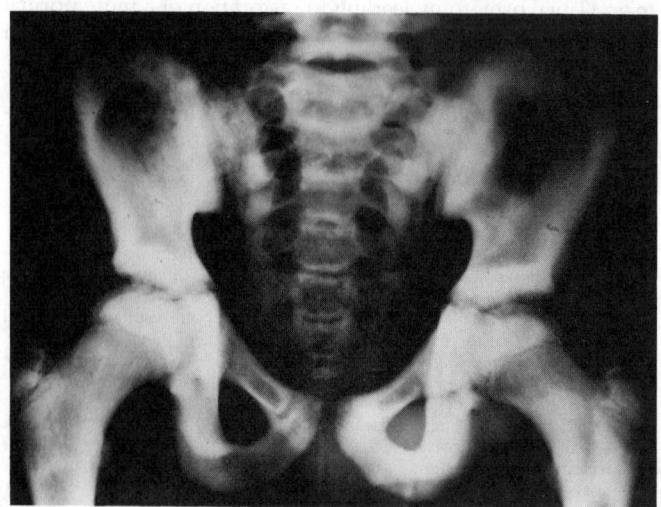

FIGURE 252–1. Roentgenogram of the pelvis of a teenager with the benign, autosomal recessive form of osteopetrosis.

osteosclerosis and the reversal of anemia and incomplete nerve deficits. Defective function of killer T cells, which may predispose to infectious complications, may also be reversed by marrow transplantation. A conceptual by-product of these experiments has been the demonstration that the osteoclast originates from hematopoietic elements.

Pyknodysostosis

This disease has only recently been distinguished from osteopetrosis. Inherited as an autosomal recessive trait, it is characterized by short stature and generalized osteosclerosis and is distinguished from osteopetrosis by several additional features: an obtuse mandibular angle with receding chin, multiple wormian bones with persistently open cranial fontanelles, and hypoplasia of terminal phalanges and clavicles. Fractures are common. Toulouse-Lautrec is thought to have suffered from pyknodysostosis.

Cortical Osteosclerosis

Hypertrophic Osteoarthropathy

This term describes subperiosteal formation of new bone in the long bones, secondary to some other condition. It usually occurs in conjunction with digital clubbing and arthritis (see Ch. 450). The etiologies include pulmonary, hepatic, and intestinal disease. Bronchogenic carcinoma (except small cell carcinoma) is the most common cause of hypertrophic osteoarthropathy and of clubbing; other causes of hypertrophic pulmonary osteoarthropathy are pleural tumors, lung abscesses, and empyema. Hypertrophic osteoarthropathy occurs in as many as 30 per cent of patients with chronic liver disease, often without clubbing. It is occasionally seen in ulcerative colitis and regional enteritis. Hypertrophic osteoarthropathy is unusual in cyanotic congenital heart disease, although clubbing is typically observed.

Hypertrophic osteoarthropathy is usually confined to the distal tibia and fibula and the distal radius and ulna. When advanced, it may involve other bones. However, it rarely involves the distal phalanges, even in the presence of clubbing. Bone pain, tenderness, and soft tissue swelling may be present, but the condition is sometimes asymptomatic. The periosteum is thickened, and subperiosteal formation of new bone is radiographically evident. Initially present as a separate stripe, new bone may eventually fuse with the cortex. The differential diagnosis includes pachydermoperiostosis, thyroid achropachy, hypervitaminosis A, syphilis, and polyarteritis nodosa. The pathogenesis is unknown. However, blood flow to affected extremities is increased, and the condition sometimes responds to vagotomy; these findings suggest that central reflex changes may be operative.

Pachydermoperiostosis

In pachydermoperiostosis, an autosomal dominant condition, periosteal formation of new bone occurs from puberty in the same distribution as in secondary hypertrophic osteoarthropathy. Also classically present are marked clubbing and thickened, oily skin. Facial features are coarse, and the thickened forehead and scalp are often marked by transverse folds (cutis verticis gyrata). The appearance may superficially resemble acromegaly. Pachydermoperiostosis is differentiated from secondary hypertrophic osteoarthropathy by the family history and lack of an antecedent cause.

Vitamin A Intoxication (Ch. 217)

Previously witnessed mostly in abusers of vitamins, this disorder is being seen more often, sometimes with hypercalcemia, in those treated with 13-cis-retinoic acid (isotretinoin) for cystic acne, ichthyosis, or malignancy. The characteristic periosteal new bone is often seen as a fusiform excrescence on the midshaft, or anterior spurs on vertebral bodies.

Progressive Diaphyseal Dysplasia

This rare disorder, also known as Camurati-Engelmann disease, is inherited as an autosomal trait. Classically, it is manifest in childhood by a thin body habitus, muscle wasting and weakness with a waddling gait, and bone pain. Serum biochemistry is usually normal, but the alkaline phosphatase level may be increased; the erythrocyte sedimentation rate is also elevated. X-rays show characteristic hyperostosis of the diaphyseal cortices with symmetric fusiform enlargement of the long bones. The skull is sometimes involved. These changes progress with time, at a pace that slows in adulthood. Bone pain and muscle weakness sometimes respond to corticosteroids, but the bony changes do not. Like other autosomal dominant traits, progressive diaphyseal dysplasia exhibits considerable phenotypic variation; asymptomatic individuals and a mild adult variant (Ribbing disease) are common.

Hereditary Hyperphosphatasia

Hereditary hyperphosphatasia has also been called congenital hyperphosphatasia, osteoectasia with hyperphosphatasia, and juvenile Paget's disease; the last, however, is a poor term, since Paget's disease is probably not heritable. Children affected by this rare, crippling, autosomal recessive condition present before age two with an enlarging skull, bowing of the extremities, bone pain, and fractures. Alkaline and acid phosphatase levels and the urinary hydroxyproline level are greatly increased. The calvaria is thickened, with focal densities that resemble cotton-wool balls. Elsewhere, bones are thickened symmetrically and may be demineralized, sometimes with loss of the normal cortex. Several patients have responded dramatically to calcitonin.

Focal Osteosclerosis

Osteopoikilosis is an asymptomatic, autosomal dominant trait. Pea-sized sclerotic spots, prominent in the metaphyseal area, are accompanied in some kindreds by unique cutaneous lesions (dermatofibrosis lenticularis disseminata). These are yellowish papules or plaques with increased elastin. The combination is known as the Buschke-Ollendorff syndrome. *Osteopathia striata*, another autosomal dominant disorder of the sclerosing type, is usually asymptomatic and is characterized by symmetric, parallel arrays of fine streaks in the long bones and pelvis. *Melorheostosis* is a progressive, painful disorder in which discrete hyperostotic areas appear to flow down the long bones like dripping wax. No hereditary predisposition is evident.

Beighton P, Cremin BJ: Sclerosing Bone Dysplasia. New York, Springer-Verlag, 1980. *A radiographic atlas with useful comments on nosology and a good bibliography.*

Coccia PF, Krivit W, Cervenka J, et al.: Successful bone-marrow transplantation for infantile malignant osteopetrosis. N Engl J Med 302:701, 1980. *The first successful treatment of this disorder.*

Murray RO, Jacobson HG: The Radiology of Skeletal Disorders: Exercises in Diagnosis. 2nd ed. Vol. 4. Edinburgh, Churchill Livingstone, 1977. *The question-answer format and a charming prose style make this an eminently readable book.*

Schneerson JM: Digital clubbing and hypertrophic osteoarthropathy: The underlying mechanisms. Br J Dis Chest 75:113, 1981. *A review of clubbing and hypertrophic osteoarthropathy, with 180 references.*

Sly WS, Whyte MP, Sundaram V, et al.: Carbonic anhydrase II deficiency in 12 families with the autosomal recessive syndrome of osteopetrosis with renal tubular acidosis and cerebral calcification. N Engl J Med 313:139, 1985.

OTHER DISORDERS OF BONE

Fibrous Dysplasia

Fibrous dysplasia occurs in both monostotic and polyostotic forms. The latter is often associated with cutaneous café au lait spots and precocious pseudopuberty in females, and this triad is called the McCune-Albright syndrome.

The etiology of fibrous dysplasia is unknown. It is not

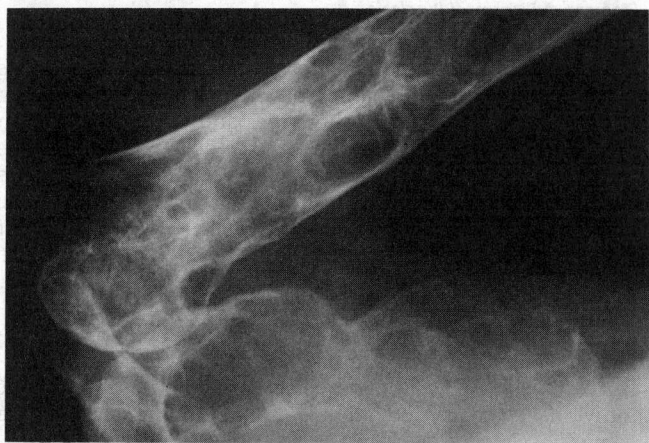

FIGURE 252–2. Roentgenogram of the humerus and scapula of a patient with extensive polyostotic fibrous dysplasia. Both bones are extensively involved with typical lesions.

heritable. Individual lesions are composed of dense fibrous tissue in medullary bone, interspersed with thin bone trabeculae (often covered by wide osteoid seams) and sometimes islands of cartilage. Radiographically, the lesions have a multilocular appearance beneath a thinned cotex (Fig. 252–2). Within, they have the appearance of ground glass, owing to their fine trabeculations. Although monostotic and polyostotic forms are histologically indistinguishable, monostotic lesions are not associated with an endocrinopathy. They commonly involve the proximal femur, tibia, or ribs, may occur at any age, and can cause bone pain, fractures, or deformity. Malignant transformation occurs in about 1 per cent of lesions.

Polyostotic fibrous dysplasia usually presents between the ages of 3 and 10. It may involve over 50 per cent of the skeleton and frequently produces "shepherd's-crook" deformity of the femur and discrepancies in leg length; skull involvement may cause gross facial disfigurement (leontiasis ossea). Fractures are common. Serum biochemistry is frequently normal except for elevation of the alkaline phosphatase level. The café au lait spots sometimes seen in polyostotic fibrous dysplasia have jagged borders that Albright likened to the coast of Maine, to distinguish them from those in neurofibromatosis, which have smooth borders like the coast of California.

About half of girls with polyostotic fibrous dysplasia undergo precocious puberty, which may precede detection of the bony abnormality. Precocious puberty has also been reported in a few boys with this syndrome. Sexual maturation in both sexes is associated with low gonadotropin levels, and fertility does not occur. Histologically, the ovaries display multiple follicle cysts. Several other endocrinopathies have been described in the McCune-Albright syndrome; these include hyperthyroidism (in about 20 per cent), gigantism with acromegaly, and Cushing's syndrome. Levels of thyroid-stimulating hormone (TSH) are suppressed in hyperthyroidism associated with the McCune-Albright syndrome. In these glands, which thus function autonomously, receptors for the respective tropic hormone–luteinizing hormone (LH), follicle-stimulating hormone (FSH), and TSH—are coupled to adenylate cyclase. However, the nature of the regulatory defect remains to be defined and may be unrelated to the receptor–adenylate cyclase system.

Hereditary Multiple Exostoses

This relatively common disorder (also called diaphyseal aclasis) is inherited as an autosomal dominant trait with high penetrance. Irregular bony excrescences protrude from the expanded metaphyses of the long bones. These osteocartila-

ginous exostoses arise from the growth plate and grow as the bone does. They may subsequently become isolated from the epiphysis or remain in continuity, but they reproduce normal structure, with an outer cortex and an inner spongiosa continuous with that of the bone of origin. Growth ceases in adulthood. Disability results principally from limb-length discrepancies: linear bone growth decreases as the bone grows transversely. Less common are syndromes of nerve, spinal cord, and vascular compression. The exostoses undergo sarcomatous degeneration in 3 to 10 per cent of affected individuals, and this must be suspected when a lesion enlarges rapidly, especially during adulthood.

Enchondromatosis (Dyschondroplasia, Ollier's Disease)

A sporadic condition, enchondromatosis becomes symptomatic in childhood as multiple, growing, cartilaginous masses within the trabecular bone, which produce swelling and interfere with linear bone growth. As with cartilaginous exostoses, these arise from the growth plate, growth ceases at puberty, and replacement of cartilage by mature bone may follow. Enchondromas appear radiologically as radiolucent defects in the metaphyseal area of the tubular and flat bones, often with central calcific stippling. The affected area may be expanded, with thinning of the cortex. Enchondromatosis must be distinguished from hereditary exostoses and from fibrous dysplasia. Malignant degeneration is uncommon. When enchondromatosis is associated with multiple hemangiomas (Maffucci's syndrome), the enchondromas or hemangiomas undergo malignant transformation in 15 per cent of cases.

Achondroplasia

Chondrodystrophies are disorders of cartilaginous growth that typically eventuate in disproportionate short stature. The commonest of them is achondroplasia. Affected individuals are easily recognizable: the limbs are short; the trunk is of relatively normal length; and the head is large, with a bulging forehead and scooped-out nose. Achondroplasia is inherited as an autosomal dominant trait. About 80 per cent of cases represent new mutations; the mutation rate increases with paternal age. To account for short bones and a shortened cranial base but a normal cranial vault, the mutation must affect endochondral ossification, as in the limbs and chondrocranium, but not membranous ossification, as in the vault. Surprisingly, the growth plate is not grossly disorganized histologically and chondrocytes are normal ultrastructurally. The pathogenesis of achondroplasia remains an enigma. Radiographically, the cranial base and foramen magnum are small, lumbar lordosis is greatly exaggerated, and the lumbar spinal canal narrows from the upper to lower lumbar spine, as indicated by a decreasing interpeduncular distance. The long bones appear massive, owing to their disproportionately normal width. Complications can include hydrocephalus, presumably related to the small size of the foramen magnum, and spinal cord and root compression, a potential consequence of even minimal impingement by a disk or osteophyte upon the small spinal canal. Reproductive potential is limited by social factors as well as cephalopelvic disproportion. Despite its problems, achondroplasia is compatible with good health and a normal lifespan.

Grabias SL, Campbell CJ: Fibrous dysplasia. Orthop Clin North Am 8:771, 1977. *A review of clinical, radiologic, and orthopedic aspects of monostotic and polyostotic forms of fibrous dysplasia.*

McKusick VA: Heritable Disorders of Connective Tissue. 4th ed. St. Louis, CV Mosby, 1972. *This scholarly, profusely illustrated book remains an excellent source for the inherited diseases of bone.*

Rimoin DL, Lachman RS: The chondrodysplasias. In Rimoin DL, Emory EAH (eds.): Principles and Practice of Medical Genetics. Edinburgh. Vol 2. Churchill Livingstone, 1983, pp 703–735. *Achondroplasia and a host of less common causes of disproportionate short stature are discussed.*

253 BONE TUMORS

Henry J. Mankin

PRIMARY TUMORS OF BONE

Primary bone tumors are uncommon but they are important, since they are most frequent in the young (the second to the fourth decades) and they tend to be extraordinarily malignant. Beyond their random occurrence, bone tumors have been associated with (1) genetic disorders of preosseous cartilage (hereditary multiple osteocartilaginous exostoses and enchondromatosis), (2) radiation injury, (3) Paget's disease, (4) bone infarcts, and (5) chronic osteomyelitis.

CLASSIFICATION AND STAGING

Any connective tissue element that exists in the osseous or preosseous skeleton can be the cell of origin of a neoplastic process; both benign and malignant tumors may be classified according to cell type as osseous, cartilaginous, fibrous, and "other" (including vascular, neural, marrow, lipid, and tumors of unspecified origin). Furthermore, within each broad category, several radiologically, histologically, and biologically distinct types of tumors exist, providing a sometimes puzzling array of diagnoses from which to choose for a patient who presents with an obvious radiographic lesion.

Prior to treatment, all primary bone tumors must be "staged" in order to assess the anatomic extent of the lesion (T), the grade of the tumor (G), and the presence or absence of distant metastases (M). The determination of T is best done by physical examination, radiographs, and special imaging studies, including angiography, computed and planar tomography, magnetic resonance imaging, and ^{99m}Tc bone scanning. The grade of the tumor can be determined only by study of biopsy material using both standard and specialized techniques. Since most bone tumors metastasize to the lungs and occasionally other bones, computed tomography of the chest or with less accuracy, full-lung tomograms, and a bone scan are required to establish "M".

BENIGN BONE TUMORS

Most benign tumors of bone present as a mass or deformity detectable on physical examination, as an incidental finding on a radiograph, or occasionally as a result of a pathologic fracture through a weakened area of the bone. With few exceptions, benign lesions are small and painless. For some, the radiographic features are so characteristic as to be easily recognizable. Benign bone tumors show well-defined cortical margins, absence of a soft-tissue mass, and sclerotic bony margination separating the lesion from the normal tissues. Some lesions may require biopsy for definition, and some, particularly those that threaten the integrity of the skeleton, require treatment, which for most of these lesions is "intralesional" (such as simple excision or curettage and packing of the defect with auto- or allograft bone), although for some benign lesions the recurrence rate may be high and necessitate subsequent surgery. An ultimate "cure" may be anticipated in a high percentage of the cases.

MALIGNANT PRIMARY TUMORS OF BONE

Multiple myeloma, the most common "primary" malignancy of bone, is discussed in Ch. 163. Other primary malignant tumors of bone are considerably less common in frequency than carcinomas or blood element neoplasms. The most frequently encountered bone sarcomas are osteosarcoma and (depending on the age group studied) chondrosarcoma; round cell tumors (Ewing's sarcoma and primary lymphoma of bone), giant cell tumors, and malignant fibrous tumors follow in order of diminishing frequency.

OSTEOSARCOMA. The peak age of incidence for osteosarcoma is in the second decade with a second lesser peak occurring in later years (often in association with Paget's disease). The tumor has a predilection for the distal femur or proximal tibia of the rapidly growing child and occurs more frequently in males. Osteosarcoma in later life usually occurs as a complication of Paget's disease, irradiation injury of bone, or a bone infarct. Pain, limitation of movement, and swelling are the principal complaints, and even at earliest observation, the radiographic findings show obvious destruction and a soft-tissue mass outside the bone. Productive changes within and without the bone suggest the presence of the osteosarcoma. Typically, the serum alkaline phosphatase level is moderately elevated. Fully one fourth of patients have metastases to the lungs at the time of the initial examination or shortly after. If left untreated, the course is fulminant with a rapid progression of the tumor, widespread metastases, and death in less than a year.

Treatment consists of wide excision of the primary tumor, which in some cases will require amputation of the extremity, but in selected instances includes a local resection and limb reconstruction with auto- or allograft or metallic implants. Treatment with chemotherapeutic agents such as doxorubicin, high dose methotrexate with citrovorum rescue and/or cisplatinum may improve the prognosis considerably, with reported survival figures ranging from 50 to 80 per cent, at three years. Even in patients who develop metastases, resection of pulmonary nodules in conjunction with aggressive chemotherapy appears to be successful in effecting cure in over 20 per cent.

ROUND CELL SARCOMA. *Ewing's sarcoma* is a highly malignant tumor of unknown cytogenesis, which primarily affects teenage children and produces a very destructive, lytic tumor often of the pelvis, shaft of the femur, or other long bones. Symptoms and signs include not only local pain, swelling, and a palpable mass, but at times systemic findings such as fever, malaise, chills, and a rapid sedimentation rate. The prognosis for this tumor is particularly poor without treatment, but the lesions, like the lymphomas of bone, are remarkably chemo- and radiosensitive. The combination of local radiation and chemotherapy provides a long survival rate exceeding 60 per cent. *Non-Hodgkin's lymphoma* and less frequently *Hodgkin's lymphoma* may make their appearance as a bony focus difficult to distinguish radiographically and sometimes histologically from Ewing's sarcoma. Staging of these individuals is essential to be certain that the bony tumor is solitary rather than an osseous focus of diffuse disease. The treatment is similar to that of lymphoma of other sites, depending principally on the radiosensitivity of the primary site and the response of the tumor to chemotherapeutic drugs.

CHONDROSARCOMA. The chondrosarcomas are extraordinarily variable in clinical presentation, degree of malignancy, and biologic behavior. Central chondrosarcomas, most prevalent in middle age, occur most frequently in the pelvis and proximal portions of the appendicular skeleton. Neither radiation nor chemotherapy has proved to be very effective in the treatment of chondrosarcomas, particularly for large tumors. With accurate staging, however, surgery with appropriately wide margins may produce a cure in up to 85 per cent of patients, depending on the stage of the disease.

METASTATIC TUMORS OF BONE

Certain of the malignant neoplasms and tumors of the hematopoietic system have a propensity for metastasis to the skeleton. At times, the presenting complaint for a patient with a primary breast, lung, prostatic, renal, or thyroid carcinoma may be pain in the spine, ribs, or long bones or a pathologic fracture through a metastatic focus. In males, the most frequent source of metastatic carcinoma is carcinoma of the prostate, followed closely by carcinoma of the lung and with lesser frequency, tumors originating in the genitourinary or gastrointestinal tracts. In women, carcinoma of the breast is by far the most frequent cause of metastatic bone disease. The frequency of metastatic carcinoma far exceeds that of primary tumors of bone, especially in later life, so that staging of any individual with a bone tumor should include a careful clinical, imaging, and laboratory evaluation of the more frequent sites of origin. Conversely, patients who are under treatment for primary tumors of the organs just cited should have frequent bone scans, which are far more sensitive than radiographs in revealing the presence of distant metastases.

Radiographic findings in metastatic bone disease vary with the type of primary tumor and the bony site involved, but almost always the tumorous deposits are in the axial and proximal appendicular skeleton, are centrally placed within the bone, and are quite destructive in appearance. About 90 per cent of prostatic, 50 per cent of breast, and 25 per cent of lung carcinomatous metastases evoke a sclerotic response in the affected bone, producing a mottled increase in osseous density on the radiograph. The treatment of skeletal metastases from a primary carcinoma depends on the patient's general condition, the radiosensitivity of the lesion, the site and extent of involvement, and the proximity of the tumor to vital structures such as the spinal cord. Most skeletal metastases are radiosensitive and regression and long-term remission can be achieved in some patients with carcinoma of the prostate and breast simply with the use of hormones and radiation (see Ch. 236 and 240). When the integrity of the skeletal system is threatened or a pathologic fracture of a long bone has occurred, prophylactic or therapeutic open reduction and internal fixation are clearly indicated and frequently provide the patient with considerable relief of pain and restoration of function.

Enneking WF: Musculoskeletal Tumor Surgery. New York, Churchill Livingstone, 1983. *A comprehensive text detailing the principles and technical aspects of surgical management of bone tumors.*
Mankin HJ, Gebhardt MC: Advances in the management of bone tumors. Clin Orthop 200:73, 1985. *An extensive review of this general topic.*

PART XVIII

INFECTIOUS DISEASES

SECTION ONE / INTRODUCTION

254 INTRODUCTION TO MICROBIAL DISEASES

Charles C. J. Carpenter

Those diseases for which specific cures are possible and for which immunoprophylaxis is available are caused primarily by infectious agents. Throughout the developing world, acute infections, predominantly acute diarrheal illnesses and acute respiratory disease, are by far the leading causes of mortality. In more circumscribed areas of Asia, Africa, and South America, protozoal diseases (especially malaria) and helminthic infections (notably schistosomiasis and onchocerciasis) continue to affect millions of individuals and cause hundreds of thousands of deaths annually. In the developed world, microbial disease processes remain the most common curable causes of both morbidity and mortality. Pneumococcal pneumonia, although curable by timely antimicrobial therapy and in large part preventable by immunization of susceptible population groups, remains among the 10 leading causes of death in North America. New infectious disease problems have appeared at a rapidly accelerating rate in patients immunocompromised by treatment with cytotoxic or immunosuppressive drugs, and especially by HIV infection. Such patients are susceptible to life-threatening infections caused by a wide range of opportunistic, normally commensal, microorganisms. The great number and variety of unusual infections occurring in immunodeficient patients present rapidly expanding diagnostic and therapeutic challenges.

A new infectious agent, the human immunodeficiency virus (HIV), currently poses the greatest communicable disease challenge of the twentieth century. Efforts to deal effectively with the disease created by this retrovirus have eclipsed other infectious disease problems at the present time. HIV, which was identified as the etiologic agent in the uniformly fatal acquired immunodeficiency syndrome (AIDS) shortly before the publication of the last edition of this textbook, has now infected over 10 million individuals worldwide. Although the prevalence of HIV infection is greatest in central Africa, cases of AIDS have now been identified in over two thirds of the nations of the world, and neither the rate nor the ultimate limits of its spread can be defined at the present time. Current data indicate that 25 to 45 per cent of the individuals infected with HIV will develop AIDS within five to eight years of the initial infection. The response of the biomedical community to the HIV challenge has been swift and, in view of the complexity of the problem, well coordinated. The clinical syndrome was recognized in 1981, and the etiologic retrovirus identified in 1983-1984. In the last two years, the seven viral genes have been isolated. Several of the genes have been cloned and sequenced, a number of the gene products have been identified, and the immune responses to both the whole virus and its products have been intensively studied.

Despite these remarkably rapid accomplishments, neither a curative therapeutic agent nor an effective vaccine has yet been developed. Azidothymidine, an antimetabolite that acts as a DNA-chain terminator, does effectively delay disease progression in a large subset of AIDS patients but does not eliminate HIV; progression of the disease recurs following cessation of therapy. Although a great deal of effort is now directed toward developing more effective antiretroviral agents, the incorporation of the HIV proviral DNA into the genome of the host cell greatly complicates any attempt to eradicate the etiologic retrovirus. The efforts to develop an effective vaccine are also impeded by a number of complex problems. The extraordinarily rapid rate of mutation of certain of the viral genes, especially those coding for the envelope glycoprotein, and the known oncogenic effects of both HIV and related animal retroviruses, make the development of an effective vaccine exceptionally difficult. The biomedical research community has made extraordinary efforts to overcome these many obstacles, but it appears unlikely that an effective vaccine will be available at any time in the next five years. During that time, it can be reasonably predicted that the HIV viral infection will spread inexorably, so that by 1991 there will have been at least 270,000 cases of AIDS and over 30 million individuals will have been infected with HIV worldwide.

Although dwarfed in magnitude and significance by the HIV epidemic, several additional microbial agents have recently been identified as human pathogens, and others have been characterized as probable pathogens. Cryptosporidia, an acid-fast protozoan of the Coccidia order, has been identified as a relatively common cause of acute self-limited diarrheal disease of worldwide distribution, as well as a major cause of severe, protracted diarrhea in immunocompromised individuals, most notably in victims of AIDS. Roughly 4 per cent of AIDS patients have debilitating diarrhea as a result of cryptosporidial infection. There is as yet no therapeutic agent that is effective against this newly identified pathogen.

The human parvovirus, previously known as the cause of a mild febrile exanthem (erythema infectiosum) in children, has been identified as the dominant cause of self-limited aplastic crises in patients with sickle cell anemia. A newly identified (TWAR) strain of *Chlamydia psittaci* has proved to be a frequent cause of acute pneumonia in young adults. New data have pointed to a retroviral etiology for Kawasaki disease (mucocutaneous lymph node syndrome), a serious febrile illness of childhood in which epidemiologic evidence has long pointed to an infectious etiology.

A perplexing challenge has been presented by the recently demonstrated association of small subviral particles, which

1523

contain no detectable nucleic acid and have been called prions, with degenerative central nervous system diseases previously attributed to slow viruses. Should prions ultimately prove to be transmissible agents, they will be unique pathogens that will demand entirely new approaches both to treatment and to possible immunization.

While newly recognized infectious diseases have created unprecedented challenges to the biomedical research community, rapid progress has continued in the development and application of vaccines effective against major life-threatening illnesses; the utilization of recombinant deoxyribonucleic acid (DNA) technology and hybridoma-derived antibodies gives promise of yielding effective means of preventing additional bacterial, protozoal, and helminthic infections. A recombinant hepatitis B vaccine is now available and has proved effective in several field trials. This vaccine, which is free of the potential problem of contamination posed by the original, serum-derived hepatitis B vaccine, is available in adequate quantities to immunize the populations at greatest risk in North America and should soon be available in quantities sufficient to immunize the much larger high-risk populations in the developing world. Recombinant DNA technology also gives promise of the development of an effective antimalarial vaccine in the near future.

In the face of rapid and sometimes bewildering changes, both in the nature of the infectious diseases with which the clinician is confronted and the therapeutic armamentarium at his disposal, two basic principles continue to guide the physicians' approach to patient management. When faced with a sick patient, a physician's primary responsibility is to determine whether or not the illness does indeed represent an acute infectious process—a decision made more complex by such factors as frequent lack of fever in elderly patients with pneumonia and the lack of leukocytosis in many patients on cytotoxic drug therapy. There is probably no situation in clinical medicine in which the thoughtful attention to all relevant details of the patient's medical history and a meticulous physical examination remain more important to the welfare of the patient. Once a physician has made the decision that a patient has an infectious process, his next responsibility must be to determine whether or not the patient has a potentially fulminant, life-threatening illness that could cause death within the next few hours in the absence of prompt and appropriate therapy. These illnesses obviously include such life-threatening diseases as acute bacterial meningitis, falciparum malaria, and gram-negative bacteremia but may also include such generally nonlethal illnesses as acute bacterial pneumonia. Because of the difficulty in determining which infectious processes are potentially death-dealing, it is incumbent upon the physician, when faced with a patient with an acute infectious process, to establish a tentative diagnosis as rapidly as possible (e.g., with the use of Gram-stained preparations in the case of acute bacterial pneumonia or purulent meningitis) and to initiate specific therapy for the presumed pathogen as rapidly as possible. In no other major group of illnesses is the rapid initiation of appropriate therapy so important as in acute infectious diseases.

Despite the prophylactic and therapeutic advances that have resulted from the rapid evolution of cellular and molecular biology, the microbial world continues to present the thoughtful physician with some of the most perplexing, and potentially rewarding, problems in the practice of medicine.

255 THE FEBRILE PATIENT

Sheldon M. Wolff

Fever is one of the most common symptoms that physicians encounter. In the vast majority of patients the fever is secondary to an infectious process, often viral in origin. In such patients, the febrile state is self-limited, and relatively little is needed in terms of diagnostic work-up or therapy. However, when the fever persists for more than a few days or is excessively high, a more thorough evaluation is indicated. Certain aspects of the febrile patient are worth emphasizing. For example, fever is *never* the sole manifestation of an illness. Constitutional symptoms such as headache, myalgias, or malaise almost always accompany fever. In addition, except in rare instances, the type or pattern of fever is of no diagnostic value. When a quotidian fever pattern occurs in the proper setting, then malaria should be considered. Furthermore, a Pel-Ebstein pattern should suggest Hodgkin's disease but is not diagnostic. In fact, viral diseases can cause hectic fevers accompanied by chills and be indistinguishable from the response of patients with bacteremia or fungemia. Thus, when approaching a patient with fever, careful history-taking, thorough physical examination, and close observation are all indicated.

Some patients with febrile illnesses will have persistent symptoms (and fever) for more than two weeks despite a thorough evaluation by history, physical examination, and laboratory tests, including appropriate cultures of blood, sputum, urine, and, if indicated, stools. Such patients can be considered to have a fever of unknown origin (FUO), and they require extensive evaluation.

When attempting to determine the cause of a prolonged fever, the wide spectrum of diseases that cause fever must be considered. Factors such as age, social and economic factors, geography, and recent exposure are all important determinants of the causes of prolonged fevers. In the overwhelming majority of FUO patients, an underlying cause is discovered or the patient recovers spontaneously.

CAUSES OF FEVER OF UNKNOWN ORIGIN. *Infections.* Approximately one third of all FUO patients will have an infectious etiology to explain their illness. Any infectious agent can be the cause of an FUO, although it is rare for a virus to be the cause of such a condition. Although most will be obvious, self-limited, or responsive to therapy, other infectious diseases may still present as an FUO. In particular, certain sites such as bone, sinuses, heart valves, subphrenic area, biliary tract, and the urinary tract may be infected and not provide localizing signs.

Neoplasias. Some tumors are likely to be associated with fever and may present as an FUO. About 25 to 30 per cent of FUO patients will have an underlying tumor as a cause of the FUO. The percentage of such patients is increasing. Examples of such neoplasms include Hodgkin's and other lymphomas, hypernephroma, preleukemia, and atrial myxoma. However, tumors of almost any origin may present as an FUO, and this may occur in the absence of metastases. In addition, the fever may precede the clinical appearance of the underlying disease by weeks or months.

Hypersensitivity Diseases. Although most connective tissue diseases can present as an FUO, systemic lupus erythematosus, Still's disease (in children and adults), and certain of the systemic necrotizing vasculitides such as temporal arteritis are more likely than others. Certain drug reactions may present as an FUO. Scleroderma is one of the collagen vascular diseases that rarely or never presents as an FUO.

Granulomatous Diseases. There are three major granulomatous diseases of unknown etiology that may present as fevers of unknown origin. The most common of these is sarcoidosis. Most, but not all, sarcoid patients who present with an FUO have extrapulmonary disease often involving the liver. In regional enteritis, fever can sometimes be much more prominent than any gastrointestinal signs or symptoms. Many of the well-known causes of granulomatous hepatitis, such as tuberculosis, sarcoidosis, or systemic fungal infections, can present as an FUO. In addition, there is a separate group of patients with granulomatous hepatitis of unknown cause and FUO. Thus, any FUO patient whose symptoms persist despite thorough noninvasive work-up should have a liver biopsy.

Inherited Diseases. There are at least three inherited diseases that present as an FUO. The most common of these is familial Mediterranean fever (FMF). Although FMF is most common in Armenians, Sephardic Jews, and Arabs, it can occur in almost any ethnic group. It is in the latter situation that the diagnosis is most often missed and the patient is considered to have an FUO. Patients with an inherited hyperlipidemia (Type 1) may have fever as a presenting complaint. In patients with Fabry's disease, an X-linked inherited error of glycosphingolipid metabolism characterized by telangiectases and lancinating pain, fever may be a prominent sign. Cyclic neutropenia often presents as an FUO, and a small percentage of patients with this disease seem to have a familial form.

Factitious Diseases. A small number of patients who present with an FUO turn out to have a factitious or self-induced illness. In general, these patients are young female adults who are in the health-related professions. Such patients can be roughly separated into two groups. The first consists of patients who feign illness by manipulating thermometers and often have a bona fide febrile illness prior to the onset of their so-called FUO. The second group is predominantly in the third or fourth decade of life, and these patients have more profound psychiatric problems. They will often induce disease and in fact can do themselves considerable harm.

EVALUATION OF THE PATIENT WITH AN FUO. The approach to the patient with an FUO requires an awareness of the myriad etiologies and a willingness to demonstrate a thoroughness in the workup that few other situations in medicine demand. Careful attention to the history is required. Has there been any exposure to infectious agents? Any unusual travel? These and many other questions must be asked. If the answers are positive, then follow-up laboratory procedures will be required. A thorough and complete physical examination is mandatory. Furthermore, repeated attention must be paid to any changes, such as the appearance of septic phenomena in the skin, fundi, nailbeds, or other areas.

Approximately 10 per cent of FUO patients will defy extensive evaluation and continue to have fevers without a diagnosis forthcoming. Such patients require close observation and follow-up, and workups may have to be repeated. A patient with an ongoing active debilitating illness requires earlier re-evaluation than the patient with a chronic, slowly progressive course. The longer a patient has an FUO, the less likely he is to have an infectious or neoplastic cause for the fever.

The laboratory evaluation of the patient with an FUO should be logical and complete. Knowledge of the causes of fever directs the physician toward appropriate laboratory tests. Certain examinations are mandatory such as skin tests, liver function tests, and complete blood counts. However, tests should not be performed just for the sake of completeness if they have little or no chance of providing useful information. Appropriate cultures must be made, but again reason should prevail regarding the number and sites.

Radiographic studies must include the chest, sinuses (if headache or pain is present), the entire gastrointestinal and biliary tracts, and the urinary tract. Radionuclide scanning should be employed after the appropriate x-rays have been obtained. Finally, CT scans and ultrasonography should be obtained when indicated.

If all of these noninvasive procedures have been performed and a diagnosis still has not been made, then invasive procedures must be employed. Bone marrow and liver biopsies should be done. When indicated, other biopsies will prove of value. For example, biopsy of a skin lesion, biopsy of an enlarged node, or temporal artery biopsy may prove useful in selected patients. The availability of needle biopsy techniques and the use of scanning methods and, when indicated, peritoneoscopy make exploratory laparotomy no longer indicated in the evaluation of FUO patients.

Aduan RP, Fauci AS, Dale DC, et al.: Factitious fever and self-induced infections. Ann Intern Med 90:230, 1979. *A comprehensive review of a large group of patients with factitious and self-induced diseases.*

Dinarello CA, Wolff SM: Approach to the patient with fever of unknown origin. In Mandell G, Bennett JE, Douglas RG (eds.): Principles and Practices of Infectious Diseases, Vol 1. New York, John Wiley & Sons, 1985, pp 347–351. *A detailed discussion of the evaluation and diagnostic procedures to be followed in patients with fevers of unknown origin.*

Dinarello CA, Wolff SM: Fever of unknown origin. In Mandell G, Bennett JE, Douglas RG (eds.): Principles and Practices of Infectious Diseases. New York, John Wiley & Sons, 1985, pp 339–347. *A categorization of the types of diseases that can present in patients with fevers of unknown origin.*

Larson EB, Featherstone HJ, Petersdorf RG: Fever of undetermined origin: Diagnosis and follow-up of 105 cases, 1970–1980. Medicine 61:269, 1982. *A comparison by Dr. Petersdorf's group of their recent experience and the data they published in 1961.*

Petersdorf RG, Beeson PB: Fever of unexplained origin. Medicine 40:1, 1961. *The classic paper on fever of unknown origin.*

Wolff SM, Fauci AS, Dale DC: Unusual etiologies of fever and their evaluation. Ann Rev Med 26:277, 1975. *A summary of a 15-year study of a large group of patients with chronic or recurring fevers.*

256 PATHOGENESIS OF FEVER

Charles A. Dinarello

DEFINITION. Fever is an elevation of temperature above the normal daily variation. Infections are most commonly associated with fever, but several noninfectious diseases may also have fever as their primary clinical presentation. Although the vast majority of patients with elevated body temperature have fever, there are a few instances in which elevated temperature is not fever but hyperthermia. These include heat stroke syndromes, certain metabolic diseases, and the effects of pharmacologic agents that interfere with thermoregulation.

Fever is best understood at the hypothalamic level, and the home thermostat can be used as an analogy for control of body temperature. The thermoregulatory center located in the anterior hypothalamus regulates internal temperature at about 37° C (98.6° F) primarily by its ability to balance heat production and peripheral heat loss. During fever, the thermostat setting in the hypothalamic center shifts upward, e.g., from 37 to 39° C. This results in increased heat production and decreased peripheral heat loss. Heat production from shivering muscles and heat conservation from vasoconstriction continue until the temperature of the blood supplying the hypothalamus matches the higher thermostat setting. In contradistinction to fever, the setting of the thermoregulatory center during hyperthermia remains unchanged at normothermic levels, while, in an uncontrolled fashion, body temperature increases and overrides the ability to lose heat. Exogenous heat exposure and endogenous heat production are two mechanisms by which hyperthermia can result in dangerously high internal temperatures. It is important to make the distinction between fever and hyperthermia. Hyperthermia can be rapidly fatal, and its treatment differs from that of fever.

PATHOGENESIS. In addition to infectious agents, several substances have been recognized to cause fever. These include the lipopolysaccharide of gram-negative bacteria called *endotoxin.* Endotoxin will produce fever in humans when as little as 2 ng per kilogram is injected intravenously. Other substances that produce fever include toxins from gram-positive bacteria, drugs in sensitized individuals, and incompatible blood products. It has become a custom to refer to endotoxin and other substances that produce fever as *exogenous pyrogens.* Exogenous pyrogens share no common physicochemical structure, are derived from varied sources of microbial and nonmicrobial origin, and, in general, do not directly affect the hypothalamus but rather produce fever through the action of mediator molecules, called *endogenous pyrogens.*

ENDOGENOUS PYROGENS. Endogenous pyrogens are polypeptides produced by the host which cause fever by their ability to stimulate hypothalamic prostaglandins. The first endogenous pyrogen was described by Beeson in 1948, and in 1953 Atkins and Wood showed that it circulates during fever. During the next three decades, it was assumed that there was one endogenous pyrogen that caused fever; however, other host-derived polypeptides are produced during infection and injury and are now considered endogenous pyrogens. The first endogenous pyrogen described has now been identified as interleukin-1 (IL-1). There are two IL-1's, alpha and beta, and each has a distinct amino acid sequence. Recombinant human IL-1's produce fever in experimental animals at doses of 50 ng per kilogram. Interferons (alpha and beta), produced as a consequence of viral infection, are also endogenous pyrogens. Recombinant human interferon-alpha produces chills and fever in humans following injections of 1 μg per kilogram. Tumor necrosis factor (also called cachectin) is a polypeptide that is produced during bacterial and parasitic infections and has recently been shown to be an endogenous pyrogen; when injected into human subjects, 100 ng per kilogram produce fever. These substances have widespread biologic effects on many tissues, but it is their ability to initiate fever that identifies them as endogenous pyrogens.

Endogenous pyrogens are potent inducers of prostaglandins in the brain and produce fever as outlined in the following steps: (1) endogenous pyrogens produced as a result of infection or injury reach the anterior hypothalamic area via the arterial circulation; (2) there they stimulate the endothelium of vascular organs to begin synthesizing prostaglandins; (3) the newly synthesized prostaglandins enter the brain substance through large spaces between the endothelial cells; and (4) these prostaglandins activate thermoregulatory neurons via increased cyclic AMP levels. The preoptic area of the hypothalamus is thought to contain the highest concentration of thermosensitive neurons, and the proximity of the vascular organs to these neurons accounts for their responses to the prostaglandins. Lesions near these neurons, in particular hemorrhagic events, may produce prostaglandins that independently activate the thermosensitive neurons. Figure 256–1 illustrates the production of fever.

ACUTE PHASE CHANGES. Although the mechanism above explains how endogenous pyrogens induce fever, endogenous pyrogens can induce similar processes in other tissues. In doing so, prostaglandins, particularly of the E series, are produced in skin, muscle, blood vessels, and other sites and, as a result, account for symptoms such as headache, myalgias, and arthralgias. Laboratory changes in febrile patients include changes in white blood cells, liver proteins, and certain hormones. Endogenous pyrogens are capable of in-

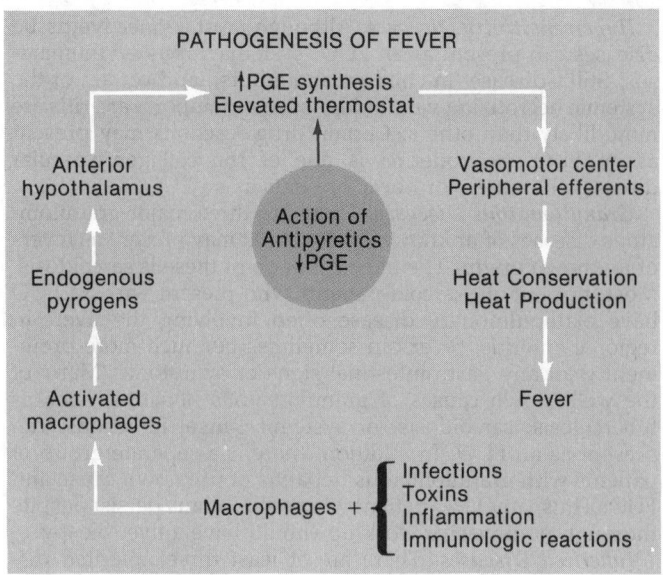

FIGURE 256–1. Steps in the pathogenesis of fever.

ducing these changes, which have been collectively called "acute phase responses" (see Ch. 257).

ACTION OF ANTIPYRETICS. Aspirin and other antipyretics have no effect on the synthesis and release of endogenous pyrogens. Therefore, their role in reducing fever is not directly related to their peripheral anti-inflammatory properties. The potency of an antipyretic in reducing fever is proportionately related to its ability to inhibit prostaglandin synthesis in the hypothalamus. The ability of endogenous pyrogens to raise the hypothalamic thermostat setting is due to its ability to increase the concentration of hypothalamic prostaglandin and hence antipyretics lower fever by preventing pyrogen-induced prostaglandin synthesis. This is corroborated by the clinical observation that antipyretics do not lower normal body temperature. Corticosteroids prevent fever by reducing the synthesis and release of endogenous pyrogens. Therefore, the ability of corticosteroids to reduce fever is related to their peripheral anti-inflammatory properties.

DIAGNOSIS. Individuals maintain body temperature at about 37° C despite wide variations in environmental temperatures. For some individuals, normal body temperature can be below or above 37° C without constituting a pathologic process. During a 24-hour period, body temperature varies from a low point in the early morning to the highest levels at 4 to 6 P.M. The amplitude of this daily variation, also called circadian temperature rhythm, is about 0.6° C (1° F), and individuals retain their circadian rhythm throughout life despite intervening bouts of prolonged illness. During fever, the morning low and evening high temperature pattern can still be observed. In the occasional situation in which elevated temperature is really hyperthermia, this rhythm is absent. A diagnosis of hyperthermia is often made because of a preceding history of heat exposure or use of certain drugs that interfere with normal thermoregulation. In some patients the hypothalamic set-point is elevated owing to local trauma, hemorrhage, tumor invasion, or intrinsic hypothalamic malfunction. The term "hypothalamic fever" is sometimes used to describe elevated temperature caused by abnormal hypothalamic function. However, the majority of patients with hypothalamic damage have hypothermia or do not thermoregulate properly to mild environmental temperature changes. In those few patients in whom hypothalamic fever is suspected, diagnosis depends on demonstrating other abnormal hypothalamic functions, such as production of hypothalamic-releasing factors, abnormal response to cold, and absence of circadian temperature and hormonal rhythms.

MANIFESTATIONS OF FEVER. The subjective symptoms

of fever include sensations of feeling cold or warm, headache, myalgias, arthralgias, and general malaise. The objective signs besides elevated temperature include increased respiratory rate, widened pulse pressure, and rapid heart rate. Laboratory findings may be altered in fever. Elevated erythrocyte sedimentation rate resulting from increased haptoglobin, fibrinogen, ceruloplasmin, and C-reactive protein levels can be present. These are often called "acute phase reactants" and account for the elevation in globulins seen on serum protein electrophoresis. The induction of acute phase changes is discussed in Ch. 257. In some patients the neutrophil count is elevated and young marrow forms appear in the peripheral blood, but these changes may reflect the disease causing the infection rather than the fever itself. Serum iron and zinc levels are decreased during fever, and the low iron may play a role in the anemia that frequently accompanies chronic fever.

Metabolic rate is increased during fever (13 to 15 per cent per degree above 37° C), thus requiring more calories and increased oxygen. For example, tissue breakdown occurs in which the amino acids are inefficiently consumed for energy. Also, fever is accompanied by an increase in urinary calcium, which reflects progressive breakdown of bone. Aminoaciduria and proteinuria reflect the generalized breakdown of tissue during fever.

Fever caused by infectious, toxic, or immunologic diseases rarely exceeds 41.4° C (106° F), and there is clinical as well as animal evidence that the hypothalamic set-point for fever has a ceiling. Extremely high fever (hyperpyrexia), however, can occur in any patient with significant disease, but it is most frequently observed in patients with central nervous system hemorrhage. In general, there are only a few clinical conditions in which moderately elevated temperature is detrimental. These are in patients with central nervous system disease, decreased cardiovascular function, prior history of febrile seizure, and in pregnant women. The increased oxygen demand, cardiac output, and pulse rate associated with fever are particularly dangerous to patients with a compromised myocardium. Fever may also be teratogenic for the developing fetus.

TREATMENT. Most individuals with fever caused by infectious diseases, such as upper respiratory tract infections or flu syndromes, experience unpleasant symptoms and treat their fever with antipyretics. There is no evidence that moderately elevated temperature is harmful to patients who are not in one of the risk groups noted above. It is often desirable to withhold antipyretic therapy so that fever can be used as an index of improvement or worsening of a disease. On the other hand, there are no data on humans to suggest that fever is beneficial, although in some animal models survival from certain bacteremias is increased in febrile as compared with normothermic animals. In most clinical settings, the use of oral antipyretics suffices to reduce fever. In febrile adults, a single oral dose (600 to 900 mg) of acetaminophen or aspirin reduces body temperature to normal levels in three to six hours. Peak plasma levels of the drugs vary and the times of peak drug concentration also vary considerably between one and five hours following oral administration.

Acetaminophen and aspirin in comparable oral doses have approximately equal ability to lower body temperature. The need to repeat the dose of antipyretics may be related to continued synthesis and release of endogenous pyrogens and the short duration of action of antipyretics. In adults, the total daily dose of acetaminophen should not exceed 3 grams under ordinary circumstances and should be lower in patients with impaired hepatic function. The dose limits in children are adjusted on the basis of body surface or weight.

Acetaminophen should be used as an antipyretic in patients who are allergic to salicylates or who have gastrointestinal intolerance to aspirin. In addition, acetaminophen is preferable to aspirin in patients with hemophilia, von Willebrand's disease, or other diseases of blood coagulation or who are being treated with oral anticoagulants. Aspirin is contraindicated in patients with peptic ulcer or asthma or in children with influenza or Reye's syndrome (see Ch. 333). However, with the exceptions cited above, there is no advantage to using acetaminophen rather than aspirin for the reduction of fever.

Several physical methods can also be used to reduce body temperature. The most common is water or alcohol sponging. The use of air-conditioned rooms, fans, and cooling blankets will also reduce core temperature by facilitating air and surface heat conduction from the skin. If physical methods are used to reduce core temperature at a time when the hypothalamic set-point remains elevated, shivering and vasoconstriction will occur as the hypothalamic drive to raise core temperature competes with the peripheral removal of heat. Thus, the ideal circumstance for reducing body temperature during fever combines the use of an antipyretic that lowers the hypothalamic set-point with physical methods that promote heat dissipation. In some circumstances, overzealous methods to reduce fever can lead to hypothermia.

Any patient with fever of 41.4° C (106° F) (hyperpyrexia) requires urgent medical care. For some patients with pre-existing cardiovascular, pulmonary, or central nervous system diseases, or in children who have had a febrile seizure, the temperature at which the individual is at risk may be considerably lower. Efforts to reduce hyperpyrexia should be instituted with rapidity before physiologic changes secondary to prolonged high temperature produce significant morbidity. These may include acidosis, hypovolemia, cardiac arrhythmias, respiratory and contraction alkalosis, and electrolyte abnormalities. It is helpful to use physical methods to reduce body temperature during hyperpyrexia, but core temperature should be carefully monitored.

Atkins E: Fever: Its history, cause and function. Yale J Biol Med 55:283, 1982. *A concise review of the history and function of fever.*

Dinarello CA: Interleukin-1. Rev Inf Dis 6:54, 1984. *A comprehensive review of the interrelationship between fever and the acute phase response.*

Dinarello CA: Interleukin-1: Amino acid sequences, multiple biological properties and comparison with tumor necrosis factor (cachectin). Year Immunol 2:62, 1986. *A comparison between IL-1 and tumor necrosis factor in inducing fever and acute phase changes.*

Dinarello CA, Bernheim HA, Duff GW, et al: Mechanisms of fever induced by recombinant human interferon. J Clin Invest 74:906, 1984. *Identifies interferon as an endogenous pyrogen.*

257 THE ACUTE PHASE RESPONSE

Charles A. Dinarello

ACUTE PHASE CHANGES. Infections, trauma, inflammatory processes, and some malignant diseases induce a constellation of host responses that are collectively referred to as the "acute phase response." The response is associated with characteristic metabolic changes in liver protein synthesis, but, on closer examination, changes also occur in several other systems that include hematologic, endocrinologic, neurologic, and immunologic dysfunctions. These changes are called acute because most are observed within hours or days following the onset of infection or injury, although some acute phase changes also indicate persistent disease. The full spectrum of the response includes dramatic increases in the synthesis of several unique hepatic proteins that are not produced in health. One of these, C-reactive protein, is a marker of the acute phase response and can be used as an indicator of disease. The increased plasma concentrations of acute phase hepatic proteins, glycoproteins, and globulins are responsible for elevated erythrocyte sedimentation rates. Although the liver is producing increasing amounts of a variety of proteins, hepatic albumin synthesis is decreased. Increases in gluconeogenesis, energy expenditure, and muscle proteolysis occur and contribute to weight loss. Fever may be present, and increased sleep and lethargy are frequent clinical complaints. Leukocytosis with increased numbers of circulating immature neutrophils is commmon, and serum iron and zinc levels are depressed while increased ceruloplasmin levels result in elevated serum copper. Thyroid dysfunction can be present and there is often abnormal glucose tolerance and lipid metabolism. In addition, anemia develops despite adequate stores of iron, and hypergammaglobulinemia often occurs.

Although the most florid presentation of the acute phase response is observed in patients with bacterial infections, burns, or multiple injuries, clinicians also encounter acute phase changes in patients with occult infections or chronic illnesses such as rheumatoid arthritis, Crohn's disease, and several autoimmune diseases. The presence of acute phase changes can also serve as an indicator of silent disease and some cancers, particularly renal cell carcinoma and Hodgkin's disease. The acute phase response has the outstanding characteristic of being a generalized host reaction irrespective of the localized or systemic nature of the inciting disease. The various components of the response are remarkably consistent despite the considerable variety of pathologic processes that induce it. For example, plasma levels of several acute phase proteins are elevated following myocardial infarction, fracture of a bone, or bacterial pneumonia.

INDUCTION OF ACUTE PHASE CHANGES. How are infections, injuries, and immunologic and inflammatory reactions able to elicit acute phase changes in the host? Moreover, does the acute phase response serve any purpose, and can its presence be used for diagnosis or monitoring the progression of disease? The initiation of the acute phase response is linked to the production of hormone-like polypeptide mediators. Three substances induce acute phase changes: interleukin-1, cachectin (also called tumor necrosis factor), and interferon. Interleukin-1 and cachectin are produced from phagocytic mononuclear cells, enter the circulation, and affect distant organ systems. Although the primary sources of interleukin-1 and cachectin are blood monocytes, phagocytic lining cells of the liver and spleen, and other tissue macrophages, specialized cells such as keratinocytes, gingival and corneal epithelial cells, renal mesangial cells, and brain microglial and astroglial cells also produce these molecules. Interleukin-1 and cachectin produced by these latter cell types exert their primary effects within these tissues. In fact, the ability of microbial and inflammatory substances to stimulate the production of these mediators in these strategically located, specialized cells appears to be part of local pathologic changes in many diseases.

Interferon is produced primarily during viral infections. Although it shares with interleukin-1 and cachectin the ability to produce fever, sleep, and lethargy, interferon does not induce hepatic acute phase protein synthesis and certain other acute phase changes, and, hence, elevated erythrocyte sedimentation rates and neutrophilia are not commonly observed during viral infections.

The patient with a localized bacterial infection represents an excellent example of the development of the acute phase response. At the onset of the infection, blood monocytes and tissue macrophages become activated either by phagocytosis of the invading microbe or by exposure to its products or toxins; the process results in the synthesis and release of interleukin-1 and cachectin within one to two hours. These mediators enter the circulation and reach the brain where they initiate fever. Fever is the result of prostaglandin E_2 synthesis induced by interleukin-1 or cachectin in the thermoregulatory center of the brain. Whereas fever is clearly one of the most obvious signs of the acute phase response, other components of the response can be present without apparent clinical manifestations. One of the most sensitive measures of the acute phase response is an increase in the number and immaturity of circulating neutrophils. The release of neutrophils is due to the direct action of interleukin-1 on the bone marrow. In human subjects injected with small doses of endotoxin, marked neutrophilia can be measured in the absence of fever. Although not routinely measured, serum zinc and iron levels are depressed. Low serum iron associated with anemia in the face of adequate iron stores is characteristic of the acute phase response. There is a large body of evidence that decreased serum iron probably plays an important role in protecting the host against various bacteria. For example, the reduction in serum iron can suppress the growth rate of several microorganisms and certain tumor cells that have a strict requirement for iron as a growth factor.

Within 8 to 12 hours after the onset of infection or trauma, the liver increases the synthetic rate of the so-called acute phase proteins. The response includes increases in proteins normally found in health as well as the appearance of new proteins that serve as markers of a pathologic event. Several normal plasma proteins increase several-fold during the acute phase response. These include haptoglobin, certain protease inhibitors, complement components, ceruloplasmin, and fibrinogen. However, true acute phase reactants increase several hundredfold. These include serum amyloid A protein, a precursor of the amyloid fibril in secondary amyloidosis, and C-reactive protein. C-reactive protein was named for its ability to interact with the C-polysaccharide of pneumococci and was the first acute phase protein described. Table 257–1 lists the characteristic pattern of increased plasma proteins observed during the acute phase response. Note one exception: the plasma concentration of albumin is decreased.

Of all the acute phase proteins, C-reactive protein and serum amyloid A protein are clinically the most important because their presence serves as an indicator of disease. These proteins are structurally related. C-reactive protein is particularly useful as a marker of the hepatic acute phase protein response and can be measured easily in most hospital clinical laboratories.

Despite the anabolic processes of the liver, the acute phase response is accompanied by a pronounced catabolism of muscle protein associated with loss of body weight and overall negative nitrogen balance. Fever increases oxygen and caloric demands (usually 7 per cent per degree F), and most of the negative nitrogen balance results from oxidation of amino acids from skeletal muscle, which contributes to wasting. These amino acids are largely used for gluconeogenesis. In addition, there can be demineralization of bone. Although the metabolic demands of elevated temperature contribute to the increased need for energy substrates, the host also requires a large supply of amino acids for synthesis of new

Table 257–1. PLASMA PROTEINS THAT INCREASE DURING THE ACUTE PHASE RESPONSE

C-reactive protein
Serum amyloid A protein
Alpha-1-acid glycoprotein
Ceruloplasmin
Alpha-macroglobulins

Complement components (C1-C4, factor B, C9, C11)

Alpha-1-antitrypsin
Alpha-1-antichymotrypsin

Fibrinogen
Prothrombin
Factor VIII
Plasminogen

Haptoglobin
Ferritin

Lipoproteins

protein at a time when food intake may be severely impaired or appetite reduced. Amino acids are required for immunologic and reparative processes such as the clonal expansion of lymphocytes and the proliferation of fibroblasts. Also, they are needed for synthesis of hepatic acute phase proteins, immunoglobulins, and collagen. The mechanism of providing ample amino acids for these cellular functions seems to be well orchestrated during the acute phase response. The catabolism during infection and inflammation differs from that of starvation. Unlike starvation, in which large amounts of ketones are spilled into the urine, a septic individual excretes protein with small amounts of ketones. Interleukin-1 and cachectin, the primary mediators of acute phase changes, inhibit lipoprotein lipase and hence interfere with lipid metabolism.

MEASUREMENT OF ACUTE PHASE CHANGES IN CLINICAL MEDICINE. The acute phase response is nonspecific. However, the presence of certain acute phase changes in an otherwise healthy individual can alert the physician to hidden disease. Measuring the levels of ACTH, cortisol, growth hormone, and vasopressin is not particularly useful, although they are elevated during acute phase responses. Increased peripheral neutrophils and erythrocyte sedimentation rate are often used to detect an acute phase response. Measurement of C-reactive protein can assist the physician in determining the presence of disease in patients with vague, constitutional complaints. C-reactive protein levels are usually less than 100 µg per liter but increase within hours 10- to 1000-fold. In severe bacterial infections, the serum level can rise from undetectable to over 100 mg per liter in 48 hours. The presence of elevated levels of C-reactive protein or serum amyloid A protein, even in the absence of fever or neutrophilia, may indicate occult infection or malignant change. Increases in C-reactive protein and serum amyloid A protein occur in patients of any age and also in immunocompromised patients with opportunistic infections.

Not all inflammatory diseases are associated with elevated C-reactive protein. A refractory state can develop in certain diseases such as scleroderma, ulcerative colitis, and lupus erythematosus. Failure to develop hepatic protein changes and the neutrophilia of the acute phase response seems to be related to the presence of circulating inhibitors of interleukin-1 and cachectin.

TREATMENT OF ACUTE PHASE RESPONSES. Measurements of fever, acute phase plasma proteins, and peripheral leukocyte numbers are well-established procedures for monitoring many disease states. Although nonsteroidal anti-inflammatory agents are used to treat the fever and associated myalgias of acute phase responses, these drugs do not affect other acute phase changes in the liver, various endocrinologic parameters, or the bone marrow response. Antipyretic blood levels of aspirin and therapeutic concentrations of drugs such as indomethacin or ibuprofen do not reduce production of interleukin-1 and cachectin. On the other hand, corticosteroids are highly effective in reducing interleukin-1 and cachectin synthesis as well as the effect of these mediators on various tissue targets. Patients receiving therapeutic doses of corticosteroids have blunted acute phase responses with ongoing infections, inflammatory processes, or immunologic reactions.

Most clinicians would agree that alleviation of fever is indicated in many situations such as in patients with seizure or cardiovascular disorders, in patients with joint destruction, and in patients with debilitating muscle wasting. Treating fever with antipyretics reduces the metabolic and caloric demands of elevated temperature and at the same time ameliorates many of the symptoms of the acute phase response such as headache and myalgias. Yet, some effects of the acute phase response on the host have an important and vital role in defense against infection and malignant transformation, and therefore antipyrexic treatment may be contra-

dicated. For example, elevated temperature has a direct effect on immunologic responses in that temperatures of 38 and 39° C augment T and B cell responses, the generation of cytolytic T cells, B cell activity, and immunoglobulin synthesis. In addition, these febrile temperatures adversely affect the replication of certain viruses, several bacteria, and some tumors. The requirement for iron as a growth factor for microorganisms increases at elevated temperatures. Therefore, the decision to intervene with antipyretics could, in some diseases, increase host comfort at the expense of host defenses.

The role of acute phase proteins in host defense and repair is not entirely clear. Studies suggest that the major role of C-reactive protein is to bind serum lipids or opsonize pneumococci, whereas serum amyloid A is thought to be immunosuppressive. Ceruloplasmin scavenges toxic free oxygen radicals that are injurious to many tissues. What is clear, however, is that the production and physical structure of these acute phase proteins have been conserved through 400 million years of evolution, and therefore they have presumably been useful to the host. The Limulus crab and fish make C-reactive protein that is nearly identical to human C-reactive protein. This argues that the acute phase response plays a role in survival.

Beisel WR: Magnitude of the host nutritional responses to infection. Am J Clin Nutr 30:1236–1247, 1977. *Discussion of the metabolic imbalances seen in patients with infection and injury.*

Dinarello CA: Interleukin-1: Amino acid sequences, multiple biological activities and comparison with tumor necrosis factor (cachectin). Year Immunol. 2:62–89, 1986. *A comprehensive overview of the biologic properties of interleukin-1 and cachectin.*

Kushner I, Gewurz H, Benson MD: C-reactive protein and the acute-phase response. J Lab Clin Med 97:739–749, 1981. *A brief discussion of the usefulness of measuring C-reactive protein levels in clinical practice.*

Pepys MB, Baltz ML: Acute phase proteins with special reference to C-reactive protein and related proteins (pentaxins) and serum amyloid A protein. In Dixon FJ, Kunkel HG (eds.): Advances in Immunology, Vol 34. New York, Academic Press, 1983, pp 141–211. *A comprehensive discussion of the hepatic acute phase protein pattern observed during the acute phase response, with special attention to the acute phase response in various autoimmune diseases.*

Perlmutter DH, Dinarello CA, Punsal PI, et al.: Cachectin/tumor necrosis factor regulates hepatic acute-phase gene expression. J Clin Invest 78:1349–1354, 1986. *Demonstrates the role of cachectin and interleukin-1 as inducers of hepatic acute phase protein synthesis.*

---

258 THE COMPROMISED HOST

Richard K. Root

HOST DEFENSE MECHANISMS

The host defense mechanisms can be divided into three major categories (Table 258–1).

LOCAL DEFENSES. Skin and mucosal defense mechanisms constitute the first line of protection against most microorganisms. Cutaneous defenses include the physical barrier created by keratin and bacteriostatic or bactericidal fatty acids formed by sebaceous glands. On mucosal surfaces cellular integrity provides a mechanical barrier. In addition, lactoperoxidase, lysozyme, and lactoferrin have microbicidal activity in salivary and vaginal secretions and milk. Locally produced immunoglobulin A provides protection on mucosal surfaces, in milk, and in saliva. Gastric acid reduces bacterial counts by 10- to 100,000-fold from those found in the esophagus. Similarly, acidic urine and vaginal secretions may limit bacterial growth at these sites.

Mechanical cleansing of mucous membrane surfaces is accomplished by cough and mucociliary action in the respiratory tract. The anatomic integrity of the biliary tree and the urinary collection system is key to maintaining adequate drainage and prevention of infection of these sites. Diarrhea may serve as a mechanism to expel parasites or enteric bacterial pathogens.

TABLE 258–1. THE HOST DEFENSES

Local
    Mucocutaneous barriers
    Cough
    Mucociliary action
    Patency and function of anatomic drainage tracts
Inflammatory Responses
    Phagocytic cells
        Circulating PMNs, monocytes, eosinophils
        Tissue macrophages
        The reticuloendothelial system
    Complement
    Other humoral mediators
The Specific Immune Response
    Antibodies (B cells)
    Cellular immunity
        T cells
        NK cells
        Lymphokines
        Activated macrophages

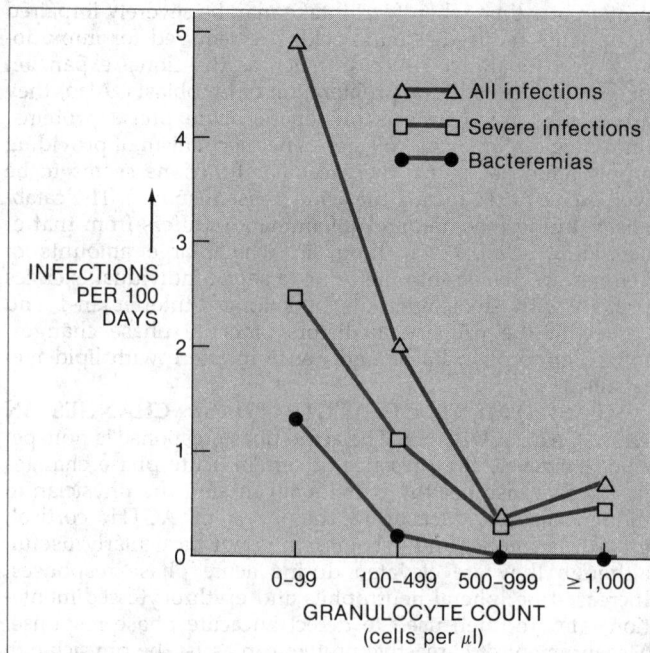

FIGURE 258–1. Incidence of infection in acute nonlymphocytic leukemia during induction therapy. The incidence of infection rises as the absolute granulocyte count is reduced. Graph based on 64 newly diagnosed patients with acute nonlymphocytic leukemia treated with intensive chemotherapy at the University of Maryland Cancer Center between 1974 and 1977. (From Joshi JH, Schimpff SC: Infections in the compromised host. In Mandell GL, Douglas RG Jr, Bennett JE (eds.): Principles and Practices of Infectious Diseases. New York, John Wiley and Sons, 1979, p 1645, with permission.)

Finally, competition between colonizing bacteria can determine the ability of newly acquired organisms to infect the host at mucosal and skin sites. The synthesis of the matrix protein, fibronectin, in the upper respiratory tract promotes selective adherence of gram-positive cocci. Bacteriocins produced by some organisms may be lethal to competing bacteria.

THE INFLAMMATORY RESPONSE. The inflammatory response involves interaction of phagocytes and humoral mediators. The latter can augment regional blood flow, increase capillary permeability, attract and activate phagocytes, and promote microbial killing indirectly (opsonization) or directly (lysis of susceptible organisms). Antibodies developing as part of the specific immune response increase the efficiency of eradicating microbes.

Once local barriers are breached and organisms escape the action of regional tissue macrophages, the acute inflammatory response plays a key role in limiting infections at the entry site.

Phagocytes. Circulating and tissue phagocytes play a central role in eradicating organisms in tissues and on mucosal surfaces. Of these cells polymorphonuclear leukocytes (PMNs) are the most highly motile and rapidly effective. All phagocytes are produced in the bone marrow and after various maturation times (see Ch. 148) enter the circulation in transit to their ultimate sites of operation. The production of PMNs averages 100 billion per day in the normal 70-kg man and can be increased by as much as 10-fold during bacterial infection.

All phagocytes exit the circulation by diapedesis and emigration (Fig. 258–1). Increased surface adherence of phagocytes to each other (aggregation) and to vascular endothelium appears to be essential. A specific group of PMN surface glycoproteins is involved in the adherence/aggregation phenomenon; inflammatory mediators such as C5a or leukotriene B$_4$ increase neutrophil adhesiveness by promoting release of these glycoproteins from an intracellular pool (see Ch. 148). Patients whose cells lack these proteins cannot generate pus.

Besides adherence, diapedesis and emigration are also functions of cellular deformability, of a contractile protein machinery for ameboid motion, the sensing of a chemical signal for attraction (chemotactic factor), and the ability of cells to convert random to directed locomotion (chemotaxis). Actin-myosin interactions are essential to the ameboid movement process. Partial degranulation of PMN-specific granules occurs extracellularly during chemotactic responses and modulates the process by altering the cell surface.

Killing of microorganisms by phagocytes is accomplished by the combined destructive action of oxidative and nonoxidative processes (Table 258–2). Oxidative mechanisms are activated in the plasma membrane during phagocytosis by the assembly of a B-cytochrome with a flavoprotein oxidase. This enzyme complex generates superoxide (O$_2^-$) from molecular oxygen using cytoplasmic pyridine nucleotides as the electron donor. Through a series of reduction reactions, H$_2$O$_2$ as well as the reactive intermediates hydroxyl radical (OH·) and singlet oxygen (^{1}O$_2$) are formed (see Ch. 148). H$_2$O$_2$ also serves as the substrate for the lysosomal enzyme myeloperoxidase (MPO). In the presence of a halide such as Cl$^-$, MPO can utilize H$_2$O$_2$ to form hypochlorous acid (HOCl); this compound then participates in a series of further oxidation reactions that are lethal to many ingested organisms or other cells. Nonoxidative killing is accomplished through the action of proteins located in specific granules (lactoferrin) or primary granules (cationic proteins that alter bacterial permeability, lysozyme and neutral proteases) as well as lowering of intraphagosomal pH.

The mechanisms by which monocytes, macrophages, and eosinophils ingest and kill microorganisms are not so well understood as those for PMNs (see Ch. 148). Monocytes differ importantly from PMNs in their capability to mature further into macrophages in tissue, their resulting long life, and the modulation of their function by lymphokines in the process known as macrophage "activation." Furthermore, during infection or exposure to bacterial lipopolysaccharides, monocytes and macrophages produce and release both interleukin-1 (IL-1) and cachectin. These monokines cause fever, leukocyte mobilization and activation, changes in vascular dynam-

TABLE 258–2. KILLING MECHANISMS OF POLYMORPHONUCLEAR LEUKOCYTES

Oxygen-dependent
    Myeloperoxidase-mediated
    Myeloperoxidase-independent
        H$_2$O$_2$
        Superoxide (O$_2^-$)
        Hydroxyl radical (OH·)
        Singlet oxygen (^{1}O$_2$)
Non–Oxygen-dependent
    Cationic proteins
    Lysozyme
    Neutral proteases
    Acid

ics (cachectin), stimulation of amino acid mobilization from muscle (IL-1), and inhibition of adipocyte metabolism (cachectin). IL-1 activates T-helper lymphocytes to produce the lymphokine IL-2, an important initial step in the clonal proliferation essential to the specific immune response.

The Complement System. The complement system (see Ch. 418) plays a key role in promoting the elimination of organisms from the blood stream as well as in the generation of the acute inflammatory response in tissues. Complement proteins can link the action of specific antibodies to those of phagocytic cells or to lytic destruction of susceptible organisms or infected host cells. The alternative activation pathway can be triggered by microbial products in the absence of antibody; this places the complement system with phagocytic cells in the forefront of the acute inflammatory defenses that precede the development of specific immunity.

A number of intermediate proteins formed by proteolytic cleavage of precursor components of complement have potent biologic effects. These include opsonins (C4b, C3b, C3bi), chemotactic factors (C5a, C5a des arg.), a releaser of PMNs from bone marrow storage pools (C3e), a factor that causes PMN degranulation and oxidative activation (C5a), and factors causing vasodilation and increased capillary permeability (C3a, C5a). The membrane attack complex (C5b6789) lyses the plasma membranes of gram-negative bacteria or other susceptible cells.

Other Humoral Mediators. Bacterial lipopolysaccharides can activate Hageman factor, triggering a series of proteolytic reactions which culminates in the release of kinins from kininogens. Kinins are vasodilatory and increase capillary permeability and stimulate pain fibers.

All inflammatory cells, platelets, endothelial cells, and vascular smooth muscle cells contain arachidonic acid in cell membranes. Phospholipases that release arachidonate are activated by microbial products during phagocytosis. Arachidonate may then be further metabolized to platelet activating factor (PAF), to prostacyclins and thromboxanes, or to leukotrienes and 5-hydroxyeicosotetraenoic acid derivatives (see Ch. 223). PAF has kinin-like activities and can aggregate neutrophils as well as platelets. These actions are mimicked and intensified by leukotriene LTB_4. LTB_4 is also a potent chemoattractant for PMNs.

The Reticuloendothelial System (RES). The fixed macrophages of the RES participate in early removal of organisms by phagocytosis as well as in the specific immune response (see Ch. 148 and 417). The macrophages of the spleen and liver are particularly important in clearing organisms from the blood stream.

SPECIFIC IMMUNE RESPONSES. Specific immunity refers to the capability of the host to recognize unique determinants on proteins or polysaccharides and to develop either antibodies or a cellular response to them. The principal cellular components are B and T lymphocytes and macrophages. B cells are the precursors of plasma cells, which produce antibodies. T cells are involved in antigen recognition and helper or suppressor functions. They may be cytotoxic or may secrete lymphokines that inhibit microbial replication directly or indirectly by activating macrophages. Natural killer (NK) cells are lymphocytes that can kill certain tumors or virally infect cells directly without requiring immune amplification. The details of the mechanisms involved in specific immunity are covered in Ch. 417.

Antibodies in Host Defense (Table 258–3). IgM isotype antibodies are usually the first to be formed in the primary immune response. As high molecular weight pentamers, they are largely retained in the intravascular compartment where they can trigger complement activation by the classic pathway or can neutralize certain viruses. They are formed in easily detectable levels within seven days of contact with a new antigen.

Man makes four subclasses of IgG antibodies. The mono-

TABLE 258–3. ROLE OF ANTIBODIES IN HOST DEFENSE

Inhibit adherence (IgA, IgG)
Opsonization (IgG)
Activate complement (IgM, IgG)
  Opsonization
  Bacteriolysis
Neutralize toxins (IgG)
Neutralize viruses (IgM, IgG, IgA)
Antibody-dependent cellular cytotoxicity (IgG)
Basophil and mast cell granule discharge (IgE)

From Root R: Host defense mechanisms against infection. In Smith LH Jr, Thier SO (eds.): Pathophysiology. Philadelphia, W. B. Saunders Company, 1985, p 157.

meric state and relatively low molecular weight of IgG immunoglobulins (around 150,000) allow free distribution in intravascular and extravascular compartments as well as appearance in low levels in secretions. IgG antibodies have a broad role in antimicrobial defenses; they can activate complement (IgG1, IgG3) and serve as opsonins by binding to Fc receptors on phagocytic cells, neutralize protein toxins or viral invasiveness, inhibit adherence of microbes to cellular surfaces, and participate in antibody-dependent cellular cytotoxicity against virally infected cells (see Ch. 417 for details). Deficiency of IgG leads invariably to infectious complications.

Small amounts of IgA are found in the blood. The role of IgA in host defense is primarily as an inhibitor of bacterial adherence or neutralizer of viruses. IgA antibodies are weak opsonins for alveolar macrophages. IgA antibodies do not fix complement by the classic pathway. The host defense action of IgE antibodies is less clear. No direct role for IgD antibodies in host defense has been documented.

Cellular Immunity and Host Defense (Table 258–4). Cellular immunity refers to the coordinated operation of T lymphocytes and macrophages in the eradication of microorganisms that are often resistant to destruction by phagocytosis or lysis by complement. Such organisms frequently reside in an intracellular location protected from antibodies. Cellular immunity is also important in the destruction of foreign cells introduced into the host or cells transformed by neoplasia. Its functional correlate is the development of a delayed type hypersensitivity reaction to antigens introduced intradermally. It usually takes several weeks for cellular immunity to become established in primary infections.

Details of the development and operation of cellular immunity can be found in Ch. 417. In brief, two primary effector mechanisms are employed: cellular cytotoxicity and modification of host cellular functions by different cytokines, derived from monocytes (monokines) or lymphocytes (lymphokines).

Cellular cytotoxicity mechanisms can involve the direct action of T lymphocytes or NK cells or indirect, lymphokine-enhanced action of macrophages. NK cells can lyse tumor cells, HLA incompatible cells, and some virally infected target host cells. They constitute 10 to 15 per cent of circulating lymphocytes and may provide an immediate defense against some viruses. Their lytic activity can be enhanced by gamma-

TABLE 258–4. CELLULAR IMMUNITY IN HOST DEFENSE

Enhanced Cellular Cytotoxicity
  Natural killer (NK) cells
  T cell cytotoxicity
Enhanced Macrophage Function
  Production
  Chemotaxis
  Phagocytosis and killing of intracellular
    organisms
Enhanced Neutrophil Function
  Production
  Marrow release
  Chemotaxis
  Oxidative metabolism
Eosinophil Function
  Chemotaxis
Inhibition of Viral Replication
  Interferons α and γ

interferon. Cytotoxic T cells undergo clonal proliferation in response to foreign antigens. They are highly specific immunologically and HLA-restricted in their action, which requires cell-to-cell contact.

Lymphokines are glycoproteins produced by antigenically or mitogenically stimulated lymphocytes. T lymphocyte activation and eventual clonal expansion are produced by interleukin-2 (IL-2) following the action of IL-1. B-lymphocyte proliferation and maturation are induced by the lymphokines, interleukin-4, B-cell growth factor, and several differentiation factors. Hematopoietic stem cell proliferation and maturation are induced by the lymphokine IL-3. Granulocyte-myeloid colony stimulating factor (GMCSF) is formed by T lymphocytes and induces myeloid proliferation, release of neutrophils from the marrow, chemotaxis, and activation of neutrophils. Macrophage chemotaxis, inhibition of macrophage movement, activation of macrophage oxidative metabolism, adherence, and increased lysosomal enzyme production can be induced by several other lymphokines. Gamma-interferon is a key factor in promoting killing of intracellular organisms by macrophages. Gamma-interferon also inhibits viral replication in target cells but is not as active as alpha-interferon. Other lymphokines regulate the chemotaxis of polymorphonuclear leukocytes and eosinophils. When fully expressed, the cellular immune response evokes a chronic inflammatory response characterized by granuloma formation and enhanced killing of intracellular and some complex extracellular organisms (see Ch. 417).

ETIOLOGY AND EPIDEMIOLOGY

Single or multiple host defense mechanisms can be altered by inherited disorders or by coexisting disease or therapy. In the United States, the prevalence of host impairment caused by the administration of cytotoxic drugs and/or glucocorticoids for malignancy or autoimmune disorders is much greater than that due to inheritance. Alcoholism and protein-calorie malnutrition are also important modifiers of normal host defenses.

PATHOGENESIS AND PATHOLOGY

The types of infections that complicate discrete inherited defects of host defense have provided great insight into specific pathophysiologic mechanisms (Table 258–5). Patients with altered local defenses are particularly prone to bacterial infections. For example, patients with eczematous dermatitis, skin puncture, or trauma often have complicating local or systemic infection caused by *Staphylococcus aureus* or *Streptococcus pyogenes*. The high incidence of staphylococcal bacter-

emia and endocarditis in intravenous drug addicts and patients with chronic hemodialysis can be directly attributed to heavy colonization with *S. aureus* and entry through the skin.

Recurrent pyogenic infections of the middle ear, sinuses, bronchial tract, and lungs occur in patients with the immotile cilia syndrome (ICS). Caused by the more virulent aerobic flora found in the nasopharynx (*Streptococcus pneumoniae*, *Haemophilus influenzae*), the infections are a consequence of disordered ciliary action. Bacterial respiratory infections in cigarette smokers and heavy ethanol drinkers also reflect impaired ciliary action and in alcoholism, aspiration of oral and nasopharyngeal secretions. Colonic flora cause recurrent, relapsing urinary tract infections in patients with abnormalities of the urinary collecting system, urinary stones, and bladder outlet obstruction. Chronic recurring infections of the apocrine sweat glands with staphylococci and enteric gram-negative rods develop with obstruction of these glands (chronic hidradenitis suppurativa).

Conversely, procedures that violate mucocutaneous barriers induce a defect in local defenses: foreign body insertion can represent a special problem. Plastic intravenous catheters, urinary catheters, sutures, and joint and cardiac valve prostheses all increase susceptibility to infection at their particular sites.

Patients with quantitative or qualitative disorders of polymorphonuclear leukocytes have recurrent or unusually severe systemic infections with bacteria that consititue the normal flora. Skin and soft tissue infections, septicemias, pneumonias, osteomyelitis, and intra-abdominal infections with staphylococci and gram-negative enteric rods predominate. Opportunistic fungi, particularly *Aspergillus* and *Candida*, and *Nocardia* species also cause systemic infection in these patients. The systemic nature of these infections coupled with multiple site involvement distinguishes these patients from those with local defects.

Splenectomized patients have lost an important component of the intravascular phagocytic defense system. Fulminant infections with pneumococci, other streptococci, or unusual organisms such as the bacterium DF-2 or the plasmodium, *Babesia microti*, occur as a consequence of this loss.

Patients with disorders of complement synthesis or metabolism develop recurrent or unusually severe infections only if the alternative activation pathway, C3, or the terminal membrane attack complex is involved. C3-deficient patients are rare and suffer with recurrent bacteremias and pneumonias with encapsulated organisms, highlighting the role of C3 as an opsonin. Deficiency of any of the components of the membrane attack complex (C5-C9) leads to disseminated in-

TABLE 258–5. ABNORMALITIES IN HOST DEFENSE AND THEIR CONSEQUENCES

System	Examples	Consequences
Local	Dermatitis, mucosal ulceration, catheters, foreign bodies, bronchiectasis, urinary stones or strictures, cystic fibrosis, immotile cilia syndrome, hidradenitis suppurativa	Localized infection with regional bacteria
Phagocytic	Neutropenias, PMN adhesion, protein deficiency, Job's syndrome, chronic granulomatous disease, Chédiak-Higashi syndrome, MPO deficiency, myelogenous leukemias, diabetes mellitus, uremia, acidosis, glucocorticosteroid therapy	Localized and systemic infection with *Staphylococcus aureus*, enteric gram negative rods, opportunistic fungi, and *Nocardia*
	Splenectomy	Bacteremias with *Streptococcus pneumoniae*, other streptococci, DF-2. Babesiosis
Complement	C3, C5–C9 deficiency, SLE, immune complex disorders	Disseminated infection with encapsulated bacteria and *Neisseria* species
Antibody	Congenital and acquired hypogammaglobulinemias, multiple myeloma, chronic lymphocytic leukemia, lymphomas, nephrotic syndrome, burns, steroid or cytotoxic therapy	Systemic infections with encapsulated and gram-negative bacteria, prolonged enteroviral infections, intestinal giardiasis
Cellular Immunity	DiGeorge syndrome, mucocutaneous candidiasis, severe protein-calorie malnutrition, steroid therapy, Hodgkin's disease, uremia, cytotoxic therapy	Systemic infection with intracellular bacteria, mycobacteria, DNA viruses, protozoans, invasive fungi, *Strongyloides stercoralis*, and coccidian parasites
Combined Immune Deficiency	SCID, Wiskott-Aldrich syndrome, ataxia telangiectasia, glucocorticosteroid therapy, cytotoxic therapy, AIDS	Systemic infection with bacteria and organisms complicating impaired cellular immunity

MPO = Myeloperoxidase; SLE = systemic lupus erythematosus; SCID = severe combined immune deficiency; AIDS = acquired immune deficiency syndrome due to the human immunodeficiency retrovirus (HIV).

fection with gonococci or meningococci. This demonstrates the importance of the bacteriolytic action of complement.

When production of immunoglobulin G or one of its subclasses is deficient, systemic and sinopulmonary infections with encapsulated organisms predominate and are recurrent. Infection with *S. pneumoniae* is particularly prevalent, highlighting the importance of protective opsonic antibodies against this organism. Once ingested, pneumococci, like other streptococci, are rapidly killed by cellular microbicidal mechanisms. With the exception of prolonged infections with some enteric viruses, viral infections are not usually severe in this group; cellular immunity mechanisms appear to be more important in limiting viral infection.

IgA deficiency occurs with a frequency of 1 per 600 in the United States, yet major infectious complications are comparatively infrequent. Individuals with associated deficiency of IgG$_2$ will have bacterial infections similar to those of other IgG-deficient patients. Some IgA-deficient patients have sinopulmonary infections or malabsorption. Also, some will have persistent intestinal *Giardia lamblia* infections.

Isolated deficiency of IgM is rare and usually of no clinical consequence.

Patients with depressed cellular immunity are subject to recurrent or progressive infections with eukaryotic organisms and/or those that are adapted for intracellular survival. These include mucocutaneous candidiasis and progressive systemic infections with the primary mycoses (in particular, histoplasmosis, coccidioidomycosis, cryptococcosis); disseminated infection with *Listeria monocytogenes*, *Legionella* or mycobacteria; pneumonia caused by the protozoan *Pneumocystis carinii* and toxoplasmosis; disseminated infections with herpesviruses (cytomegalovirus, Ebstein-Barr virus, herpes simplex, and herpes zoster varicellosus viruses); disseminated infection ("hyperinfection syndrome") caused by *Strongyloides stercoralis*, and diarrhea caused by *Cryptosporidium* sp.

Patients with mixed defects develop life-threatening infections with organisms in all of the classes identified above. A prime example is AIDS, in which markedly depressed cellular immunity and disordered production of antibody to new antigens lead to multiple severe infections including bacteremias and pneumonias caused by *S. pneumoniae*.

Administration of glucocorticoids in doses in excess of 0.3 mg per kilogram of prednisone or its equivalent depresses wound healing, impairs the acute inflammatory response by decreasing PMN adherence and diapedesis, reduces humoral antibody production to new antigens, and markedly suppresses cellular immunity. Thus, patients on prolonged high-dose glucocorticoid therapy can develop infection with the complete array of pathogens noted. Cytotoxic chemotherapy has broad effects on neutrophil production and specific humoral and cellular immune responses. Patients who receive heterologous organ transplants are treated with cytotoxic agents (e.g., azathioprine), inhibitors of T helper cell proliferation (cyclosporine), and high-dose glucocorticosteroids. Intense immunosuppressive treatment early in the post-transplant phase and during organ rejection is often complicated by infections with a wide variety of agents, reflecting the broad impairment of host defenses. In bone marrow transplantation, early neutropenia and graft-vs.-host reactions add to the alterations in host defenses.

Severely burned patients have an open portal for infection, reduced immunoglobulins from early leakage into the burn site, and suppressed cellular immune responses.

Malnutrition can be an additive factor in suppressing cellular immunity when other limbs of the host defense system are also impaired.

CLINICAL MANIFESTATIONS

LOCAL DISORDERS IN HOST DEFENSE. A pattern of recurrent bacterial infections in a specific anatomic site iden-

tifies patients who have a disorder of local host defenses at that site. Children and young adults with mucoviscidosis have recurrent bacterial pneumonias, initially with staphylococci and other upper respiratory tract flora and later with *Pseudomonas* species. Most patients with chronic hidradenitis suppurativa are healthy save for the recurrent localized infections that begin with puberty. Approximately one half of patients with the immotile cilia syndrome (ICS) will have *situs inversus* and thus meet the criteria for Kartagener's syndrome (see Ch. 65). Male patients with ICS have immotile spermatozoa and are sterile. Severe recurrent otitis media, sinusitis, and bronchopulmonary infections beginning in early childhood should suggest this diagnosis. Patients with relapsing (same organism) urinary tract infection may have an anatomic defect in the urinary tract (see Ch. 92).

LEUKOCYTE DISORDERS. Patients with inherited disorders of leukocyte production or function will usually present with infectious complications during the first year of life. Skin and soft tissue infections, bacteremias, and pneumonias with pyogenic bacteria are particularly prominent. The heightened susceptibility of low birth weight infants to infections has been ascribed to deficiency in neutrophil production and chemotaxis. These deficiencies usually disappear as these infants mature.

The minimal number of circulating neutrophils necessary to maintain a normal inflammatory response is about 1500 per cubic millimeter. When neutrophil counts fall below 1000 per cubic millimeter and especially below 500 per cubic millimeter, severe bacterial infections almost always result. Invasive opportunistic fungal infection (*Candida* and *Aspergillus* species predominate) is more likely to occur if bacterial flora have been suppressed with antimicrobial therapy. In the case of congenital neutropenias, the infections will become manifest in the first week of life. With the inherited disorder, *cyclic neutropenia*, a characteristic precipitous fall in neutrophil counts occurs at 23- to 28-day intervals. Aphthous ulcers, fever, and bacterial infection can develop. The periodicity of these cycles provides an immediate diagnostic clue.

While some patients with chronic neutropenia suffer relatively few infectious complications, prolonged (more than two weeks) acute neutropenia with counts less than 500 per cubic millimeter is almost invariably complicated by infection. These infections may lack characteristic localizing manifestations (infiltrates on chest x-ray, purulent sputum production, or drainage from soft tissues).

Patients with acute nonlymphocytic leukemia will have disordered neutrophil function either from cellular immaturity (acute myelogenous leukemia) or from abnormalities in cellular development (e.g., myeloperoxidase deficiency in chronic myelogenous leukemia). In the lymphocytic leukemias neutrophils are usually preserved unless the myeloid pool in the marrow becomes totally displaced. Some patients with lymphatic leukemias fail to produce immunoglobulins or have monoclonal gammopathies with suppression of normal antibody responses. Bacterial and opportunistic infections may bring the leukemia to clinical attention. Almost all patients who receive cytotoxic therapy or bone marrow transplantation for leukemias develop infectious complications. The risk of infection can usually be related directly to the degree of neutropenia (Fig. 258–2).

Patients with the sex-linked form of chronic granulomatous disease of childhood will be males with eczematous dermatitis, granulomatous lymphadenopathy, pneumonias that respond poorly to conventional antibiotic therapy, spontaneous liver abscesses (sometimes containing *Nocardia* species), and osteomyelitis in other than the typical hematogenous locations. Neutrophilic leukocytosis develops normally with infection, and hypergammaglobulinemia is frequent. Tissue histopathology discloses necrosis with mixed neutrophilic infiltrates and granuloma formation. Pigment-laden macrophages are sometimes found. Cultures yield *S. aureus*, enteric

PHASES IN NEUTROPHIL FUNCTION

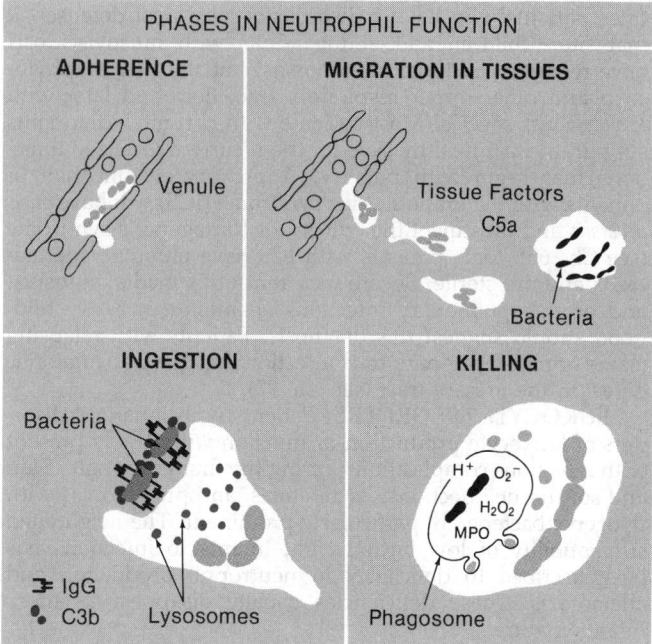

FIGURE 258–2. The four major phases in neutrophil function are adherence to postcapillary venules, migration into tissues in response to chemotactic factors, ingestion of organisms opsonized by IgG and C3B, and, finally, killing of organisms in phagocytic vacuoles by the combined action of lysosomal enzymes (myeloperoxidase), superoxide, H_2O_2, and acidity (H^+). (From Root, R. K.: Host defense factors in infectious diseases. American College of Physicians Medical Knowledge Self Assessment Program V, 1979, p 31, with permission.)

gram-negative rods, opportunistic fungi, or *Nocardia* (all catalase-positive organisms).

Deficiency of the leukocyte adhesion protein complex, CDW18, is inherited as an autosomal disorder. Patients have a characteristic failure of detachment of the umbilicus. They develop necrotizing spreading infections of the skin and soft tissue with common pyogenic organisms but without pus formation. Healing results in very thin scars. Severe periodontal disease occurs with dentition. Chronic circulating neutrophilic leukocytosis sometimes exceeds 100,000 per cubic millimeter with acute infection.

Inherited disorders of chemotaxis lead to severe periodontal disease in juveniles and a triad of eczematous dermatitis, "cold" abscesses caused by *S. aureus*, and eosinophilia in others. The condition is termed "Job's syndrome." Patients have very high circulating levels of IgE and may have skin anergy to a variety of antigens. The chemotactic disorder varies in intensity with time and is the consequence of unregulated production of a normally inhibitory lymphokine that modulates chemotaxis.

The Chédiak-Higashi syndrome is a rare disorder that affects the production of single membrane-bound organelles within a number of different cell types. Patients have partial albinism (giant melanosomes within melanocytes), peripheral neuropathy (abnormalities of Schwann cells), and recurrent sinopulmonary and cutaneous bacterial infections beginning in infancy. They are often moderately neutropenic and have both disordered neutrophil and monocyte chemotaxis as well as intracellular bacterial killing. On Wrights' stain pathognomonic multiple dark inclusions within the neutrophil cytoplasm and single pink inclusions within lymphocytes (giant lysosomes) are seen.

Inherited complete or partial absence of neutrophil and monocyte myeloperoxidase (MPO) is a relatively common occurrence (one in 5,000 to 10,000 of the general American population), yet most people are clinically well unless they develop diabetes mellitus. Visceral candidiasis (pneumonia, hepatic abscesses) may develop in this setting.

The clinical features of other, more rare neutrophil function disorders are described in Ch. 149.

COMPLEMENT DISORDERS. Deficiencies of the first three components of the complement system are rarely complicated by infection unless other disorders coexist. C4 deficiency is most commonly associated with hereditary angioneurotic edema (see Ch. 418). C2 deficiency has sometimes been associated with connective tissue disease. The consequences of C3, alternative complement pathway, or membrane attack complex (C5-C9) deficiencies have been described. A number of these patients have also had connective tissue disorders (Ch. 418).

Acquired complement deficiency severe enough to alter susceptibility to infection may occur in the setting of circulating immune complexes.

CONGENITAL AND ACQUIRED DISORDERS OF IM-MUNOGLOBULINS AND OF CELLULAR IMMUNITY. These lead to life-threatening susceptibilities to infections, which are described in Ch. 419.

DIAGNOSIS

Two major diagnostic problems are posed in considering infections in the immunosuppressed host: the first concerns the detection of host alterations; the second concerns proper approaches to establishing or excluding the possibility of infection in these patients. The latter will be considered in the next section on management.

In considering possible host impairment, the clinician should first note any unusually severe or repetitive infections with specific microbial agents. The location of recurrent bacterial infections will provide a clue to a possible impairment of a local defense mechanism. Repetitive or unusually severe systemic infections with *S. aureus* or gram-negative enteric organisms or visceral infection with opportunistic fungi or *Nocardia* suggests a quantitative or qualitative disorder of neutrophils. Severe or repetitive infections with encapsulated organisms or *Neisseria* should raise the question of a humoral defect involving the complement or antibody systems. Systemic infection with intracellular pathogens, protozoans, primary mycoses, or DNA viruses suggests defective cell-mediated immunity.

If the infections begin in infancy, one should suspect a congenital or inherited defect. A positive family history of similar infections supports the latter and may suggest an inheritance mechanism. Additional clinical features such as eczema, hypocalcemia, and telangiectasias can point the way toward specific etiologic diagnoses (see Ch. 419).

Useful tests in the laboratory evaluation of host defenses are shown in Table 258–6. These tests are divided into those that should be employed as screening assays and those that are generally available only at specialized centers and are used to define the mechanisms of specific defects. Not all screening tests need to be performed in all patients; the selection should be guided by the pattern of infections and the abnormality suggested.

After physical examination radiographic tests can reveal anatomic abnormalities that predispose to localized infections (e.g., intravenous pyelograms for recurrent urinary tract infections). The finding of situs inversus supports a diagnosis of the immotile cilia syndrome, as does a measure of sperm motility in affected postpubertal males. In all patients in whom the diagnosis of ICS is suspected, electron microscopic cross-sections of cilia obtained by nasal scraping may disclose characteristic absence of dynein arms or radial spokes between microtubules. Sweat chlorides should be determined in any child or young adult with recurrent bacterial pneumonias to detect possible cystic fibrosis.

A total and differential white blood cell count and examination of the blood smear will establish a diagnosis of neutropenia, the Chédiak-Higashi syndrome, or various leukemias. Bone marrow aspiration can determine the etiology of neutropenias or leukemias. When megaloblastosis is found, serum B_{12} and folate levels should be measured.

Many major hospital laboratories can perform a nitroblue tetrazolium test to detect chronic granulomatous disease and its variants. Similarly, leukocyte myeloperoxidase activity can easily be evaluated with specific histochemical staining. The increasing commercial availability of monoclonal antibodies makes it possible to evaluate important cell surface antigens by immunofluorescence assay. The OKM_1 and Mac 1 antibodies identify key leukocyte adherence proteins. The remainder of the assays summarized in Table 258–6 are the province of highly specialized laboratories.

Measurement of serum hemolytic complement activity is performed by many commercial and hospital laboratories. Radial immunodiffusion assays are commercially available for C3 and C4 and a number of the other individual components of the complement system.

Quantification of serum immunoglobulins by radial immunodiffusion assay is simple and readily available. The electrophoresis of serum proteins is useful mainly for determining if paraproteins are present. Urinary protein electrophoresis can detect and characterize Bence Jones proteins in patients with suspected myeloma. B cell surface markers can be identified using immunoglobulin-coated erythrocytes (Fc receptors) or specific monoclonal antibodies. Measurements of the production of specific antibodies in vitro and in vivo are generally performed only by specialized research laboratories. A simple screen for the production of any antibodies is the measurement of isohemagglutinins (IgM) by blood banks.

A count of total circulating lymphocytes will document lymphopenia (normally greater than 1000 per cubic millimeter). Administration of intradermal antigens, including those from *Candida albicans* and *Tricophyton* species, the enzyme mixture DNAase and streptokinase from *S. pyogenes*, and purified protein derivative of *Mycobacterium tuberculosis*, will establish the presence of delayed hypersensitivity in over 95 per cent of normal adults. Fluorescence immunoassays with monoclonal antibodies can readily identify T cells (OKT3) and their helper (OKT4) and suppressor/cytotoxic phenotypes (OKT8). Measurements of T-cell mitogenic responses and the production of specific lymphokines are usually performed only by research laboratories or those involved in histocompatibility determinations.

Measurement of antibodies against the human immunodeficiency retrovirus (HIV) is now routinely performed by all blood banks in the United States. The presence of antibodies to HIV documents infection with this organism.

Some patients with repetitive infection may defy a mechanistic diagnosis. No major abnormalities of the inflammatory or specific immune response have been identified in most patients with recurrent viral respiratory infections. A large number of different serotypes of rhinoviruses as well as other organisms can cause the common cold syndrome in normal people (see Ch. 329). Other patients with an unusual sequence of repeated bacterial infections will be found to be purposely inoculating themselves with organisms in a variant of factitious disease. Most such patients profit from confrontation and psychiatric evaluation.

MANAGEMENT

The management of a patient with altered defenses centers on the diagnosis, treatment, and prevention of infection as well as attempts at reconstitution of host defenses (Table 258–7).

LOCAL HOST DEFENSE DISORDERS. Patients with isolated disorders of the local host defenses usually respond with vigorous inflammation acutely; cultures and smears from the relevant local sites will provide an etiologic diagnosis and blood cultures an estimate of dissemination of infection. Treatment with specific antimicrobials will reduce or eliminate the responsible organisms.

The major task of management, however, is treatment of the primary condition as in patients with skin disorders (e.g., eczematous dermatitis, pemphigus vulgaris, burns), which provide a portal of entry for infectious agents. Altered or obstructed drainage tracts may require surgical repair or removal of calculi. Foreign bodies, which provide a focus for relapse or treatment failure, must usually be removed when infected. Patients who have chronic hidradenitis suppurativa may be best managed by excision of the apocrine sweat gland tissue and plastic surgical repair.

LEUKOCYTE DISORDERS. In patients with severe neutropenia or disorders of neutrophil adherence or motility, the inflammatory response at the localized site is often impaired. Some degree of pain, swelling, and tenderness with or without ulceration and nonpurulent discharge typify the soft tissue responses to infection in this group. Pulmonary infiltrates may be scant and sputum production minimal and nonpurulent in bacterial or fungal pneumonias.

TABLE 258–6. DIAGNOSTIC TESTS FOR HOST DEFENSE DEFECTS

System	Test
Local	Radiographs,* sweat chlorides,† sperm motility*
Phagocytic	Leukocyte count,* marrow aspiration,* bone marrow reserve test,† Rebuck skin window,‡ binding of monoclonal antibodies OKM1, Mac1
	Leukocyte functions:
	Adherence‡
	Chemotactic responses‡
	Phagocytosis‡
	Degranulation‡
	Bactericidal activity‡
	Nitroblue tetrazolium (NBT) dye reduction† test
	Chemiluminescence‡
	H_2O_2 and O_2^- production‡
	Myeloperoxidase activity†
Complement	Serum hemolytic complement activity (CH50),* C4,* C3*
	Other complement components†
Antibody Production	Quantitative immunoglobulins*
	Immunoglobulin subclasses†
	Serum protein electrophoresis*
	Isohemagglutinins†
	Antibody response after immunization†
	Quantitation of B cells†
	Lymphocyte mitogenesis to Pokeweed or specific antigens‡
Cellular Immunity	Delayed hypersensitivity skin tests to common antigens*
	Quantitation of T cells†
	Lymphocyte mitogenic responses to phytohemagglutinin‡
	Lymphokine production‡

*Screening tests
†Generally available at major medical centers
‡Available only at specialized laboratories

TABLE 258–7. METHODS TO RESTORE NORMAL HOST DEFENSE MECHANISMS

System	Treatment
Local	Prophylaxis of infection
	Removal of foreign bodies
	Restoration of anatomy
Phagocytic	Antibiotic prophylaxis (selected patients)
	Leukocyte transfusions when infected
	Bone marrow transplantation
Splenectomy	Pneumococcal vaccine
	Antibiotic prophylaxis (selected patients)
Complement	Plasma infusion
	Administration of missing components
Antibodies	Intramuscular or intravenous IgG
Cellular Immunity	Interferon α or γ
	Interleukin-2
	Thymic extracts
	Transfer factor
	Treat underlying conditions
	Bone marrow transplantation
	Reduce glucocorticosteroids

Febrile responses to infection are usually preserved. In most studies over 50 per cent of febrile episodes in subjects with acute nonlymphocytic (myelocytic) leukemia or acute neutropenias from diverse causes are due to infections. A diligent search of skin, mucous membranes, the anorectal area, and chest roentgenograms (even with no pulmonary physical findings) and cultures of the blood, urine, and other secretions are indicated when fever appears or infection is otherwise suspected. Even when there is no sign of inflammation or surrounding soft tissue infection, intravenous catheters (with the exception of Hickman catheters) should be removed or changed.

It may be impossible in the absence of specific localizing findings to differentiate bacteremic illness from other causes for fever in this patient group; prompt treatment with antimicrobials is indicated before culture results are known. The specific choice of antimicrobial should be guided by a knowledge of the patient's previous infections, colonizing flora in the patient's stool or oropharynx, or major flora causing infection in the hospital setting and likely sites of the origin for sepsis based on examination. The initial antibiotic regimen should be composed of at least two antimicrobials with broad-spectrum activity. Table 258–8 lists several such regimens that have been shown to have equivalent efficacy in controlled trials. These antibiotics are bactericidal in their action and must be given intravenously. For precise dosages see Ch. 28.

Once the infecting agent is identified, more selective treatment is indicated. In the severely neutropenic patient therapeutic success has been directly related to treatment of bacteremias or pneumonias with two or more antimicrobials active against the offending organism. These antimicrobials should not be antagonistic in their actions in vitro. (All of the combinations of agents listed in Table 258–8 have been found to be additive or synergistic in their activities against specific bacteria.) Treatment is usually continued until patients have become afebrile and other manifestations of infection have cleared. Some advocate continuation of antibiotics until the neutrophil count rises above 1000 per cubic millimeter.

When patients fail to respond to treatment for bacterial infections, a diligent search for opportunistic fungal or viral infections should be carried out. Early presumptive treatment with amphotericin B has been successful in minimizing or eliminating candidiasis. Control of *Aspergillus* infections complicating neutropenia or neutrophil dysfunction has been more difficult, despite early deployment of antifungals, unless neutropenia resolves.

With improved antimicrobial regimens the indications for leukocyte transfusion therapy have diminished. The number of cells collected by the usual centrifugation procedures (approximately 100 million) is too few to add significantly to the inflammatory response in adults, although it is adequate for children. The administration of neutrophils to sensitized subjects may cause leukagglutination reactions that impact on the lung. Finally, leukocyte transfusions may transmit cytomegalovirus to nonimmune subjects. Because of these risks, this form of treatment is reserved for patients with prolonged neutropenia or selected subjects with disordered neutrophil function (e.g., chronic granulomatous disease) who are failing antimicrobial therapy.

Bone marrow transplantation is the treatment of choice for aplastic anemia and acute myelocytic leukemias and has been successfully accomplished in some patients with chronic granulomatous disease. In patients with active or chronic infections at the time of transplantation, the added broad immunosuppression constitutes a particularly severe risk for mortality.

Pharmacologic augmentation of neutrophil function in vivo is not generally available at the present time. Ascorbic acid administration to patients with the Chédiak-Higashi syndrome has repaired the functional defects in some. Pentoxifylline has some ability to stimulate inflammatory responses in vivo. It apparently works by increasing membrane fluidity and may be useful in augmenting neutrophil function in neonates.

Lithium carbonate administration can lead to expansion of the bone marrow myeloid series and neutrophilic leukocytosis. It has sometimes protected patients during cytotoxic therapy or with Felty's syndrome.

HUMORAL DISORDERS. Replacement therapy with intramuscular or intravenous immunoglobin is reserved for patients with hypogammaglobulinemia (i.e., IgG levels below 200 mg per deciliter). It is without benefit in patients with normal IgG levels or those with IgG paraproteins. It should *not* be used in patients with isolated IgA deficiency because the available preparations do not contain IgA, and anaphylactic reactions may occur owing to anti-IgG antibodies in these subjects. In IgG deficiency the goal is to maintain serum IgG levels above 200 mg per deciliter; at these concentrations serum opsonic activity is returned to normal. Doses of 100 mg per kilogram are administered intramuscularly at monthly intervals. Most adults cannot tolerate more than 40 ml of immune serum globulin given in this manner. Intravenous IgG is more expensive but can be given in higher dosages (200 to 300 mg per kilogram every three to four weeks) with better patient tolerance.

Hyperimmune globulins containing high titers of antibodies against pneumococcal polysaccharides or *Pseudomonas* surface components can be used as an adjunct to antimicrobial management in patients with normal or reduced IgG levels. They can also be given as short-term prophylaxis. Similarly, an antiserum obtained from patients immunized with the core portion of bacterial lipopolysaccharides is additive to antimicrobial therapy in gram-negative bacteremias.

Administration of whole fresh plasma can restore complement defects or replace absent IgG and IgM. The usual dose is 10 to 20 ml per kilogram monthly. The risk of non-A, non-B hepatitis in patients receiving this treatment is substantial. At present, treatment with individual complement components is not generally available.

Some patients with common variable hypogammaglobulinemia have benefited from treatment with cimetidine, which inhibits the action of suppressor T cells containing H$_2$ receptors.

CELLULAR IMMUNE DISORDERS. Attempts at immune reconstitution of AIDS patients have led to the accelerated development of compounds to stimulate cellular immunity. These include recombinant-prepared IL-2, interferons, and thymic extracts. The use of these highly purified substances has largely replaced treatment with cruder preparations such as "transfer factor." In vitro and in experimental animals, the

TABLE 258–8. SUGGESTED REGIMENS FOR INITIAL ANTIMICROBIAL THERAPY IN NEUTROPENIC PATIENTS WITH SUSPECTED SEPSIS

Group 1 β-lactams (a or b) plus an aminoglycoside (c)

a. *Penicillins*	b. *Cephalosporins*	c. *Aminoglycosides*
Carbenicillin	Cefaperazone	Gentamicin
or	*or*	*or*
Ticarcillin	Cefotaxime	Tobramycin
or	*or*	*or*
Piperacillin	Ceftizoxime *PLUS*	Amikacin
or	*or*	
Mezlocillin	Ceftriaxone	
or	*or*	
Azlocillin	Ceftazidime	
or		
Imipenem		

Group 2 "Double" β-lactams
  Combinations of Group 1a and 1b

Vancomycin Substitute for semisynthetic penicillins or cephalosporins in allergy. Use if methicillin-resistant gram-positive infection is suspected (*Staphylococcus aureus*, *S. epidermidis*, JK diphtheroids)

Erythromycin Add if legionellosis suspected.

Trimethoprim-sulfamethoxazole Add if *Pneumocystis* infection is suspected.

interferons and IL-2 can increase macrophage phagocytosis and cytotoxicity, T-cell cytotoxicity, and NK activity. The interferons also have antiviral activity. Interferon-γ, while promoting macrophage activation in vitro, causes fever, neutropenia, and other adverse symptoms in vivo.

Patients given IL-2 may have restoration of cutaneous delayed hypersensitivity and mitogenic responses in vitro. However, profoundly immunosuppressed patients with AIDS have only transient responses, and no overall benefit has been observed in altering morbidity and mortality.

Thymosin fraction 5 has been partially successful in restoring immune defects in the DiGeorge syndrome and ataxia telangiectasia.

In patients with severe combined immunodeficiency, bone marrow transplantation from compatible donors has proven to be life-saving. Patients found to be deficient in adenosine deaminase or purine nucleosidase phosphorylase may benefit from infusion with fresh normal erythrocytes. Adenosine and purine nucleosides will diffuse into the erythrocytes and be deaminated or phosphorylated.

INFECTION PREVENTION. In patients with compromised host defenses, attempts to prevent infection become a particularly important aspect of management. These include protection of mucosal barriers, appropriate antimicrobial prophylaxis, and reconstitution of immune defenses where possible.

Protection of mucosal barriers includes avoiding the use of plastic inlying venous catheters whenever possible, judicious attention to dental hygiene, and reduction of trauma in the rectal area. Inlying Silastic (Hickman) catheters have made it possible to administer blood products and chemotherapy repetitively to cytopenic patients and to draw blood samples at a greatly reduced infection rate.

Gingivitis constitutes a painful and potentially severe complication of neutropenia. Thrombocytopenia leads to hemorrhage and adds to the infectious risk. Saline rinses or irrigation and soft brushes should be used to clean the teeth and gums. The addition of nystatin mouthwash or vaginal troches will reduce the incidence of *Candida* superinfection. Keeping the perirectal area clean and dry, Sitz baths for hemorrhoids, and stool softeners reduce the risk of perirectal infection.

In cytopenic patients who are hospitalized, preceding colonization with nosocomial flora accounts for approximately one half of cases of septicemia. Efforts to reduce colonization must be centered on judicious hand washing by hospital personnel with direct patient contact, the reduction of raw food ingestion, the use of nonaerating faucets to avoid infectious aerosols, minimal use of respiratory therapy and endoscopy equipment, and some type of protective isolation. Strict isolation techniques, including laminar air flow rooms, have not been shown to reduce infection rates impressively and may interfere with patient contact.

Prophylactic antimicrobial administration has been most rewarding when targeted against specific pathogens that frequently cause infection in certain conditions. Daily administration of trimethoprim-sulfamethoxazole to children with lymphocytic leukemias will reduce the incidence of *Pneumocystis carinii* pneumonia. Penicillin prophylaxis in children splenectomized for hemolytic anemias can reduce the incidence of serious pneumococcal infection; however, this practice has largely been supplanted by the administration of pneumococcal vaccine. Isoniazid prophylaxis for patients known to be PPD positive is indicated during immunosuppressive treatment.

Combinations of nonabsorbable antibiotics administered to neutropenic patients are not predictably effective in preventing infection. Oral trimethoprim-sulfamethoxazole with or without nalidixic acid and a quinolone can reduce subsequent sepsis in acutely neutropenic patients and is generally well-tolerated. The success of this approach appears to be related to selective elimination of enteric aerobic flora responsible for sepsis while preserving the anaerobic flora and a resistance to colonization with new organisms.

In patients undergoing bone marrow transplantation, prophylaxis with oral or intravenous acyclovir reduces the incidence and severity of post-transplantation infection with herpesviruses, in particular, those causing herpes simplex and herpes zoster. Administration of zoster immunoglobulin within 24 to 48 hours of exposure to an active case will prevent the development of varicella in immunosuppressed nonimmune children.

Prophylactic therapy with leukocyte transfusions in neutropenic subjects has limited benefit and carries the risk of CMV infection. In patients undergoing marrow transplantation, daily infusion of HLA-matched neutrophils from the marrow donor may reduce the incidence of subsequent infection before engraftment of the myeloid series occurs.

Live virus vaccines should not be given to any subjects suspected of humoral or cellular immune deficiency. The use of inactivated vaccines is acceptable and appropriate in these patients, although immunosuppression may prevent an adequate response. Pneumococcal vaccine should be administered to patients who are splenectomized. In patients about to undergo splenectomy, administration of vaccine approximately two weeks before elective splenectomy will lead to improved antibody responses.

Maintenance of nutritional support of any patient will promote wound healing and persistence or restoration of cellular immunity. It is particularly important to avoid protein malnutrition and zinc deficiency because of the deleterious effect on the cellular-immune system.

Finally, when glucocorticoids and cytotoxic therapy are employed as immunosuppressive treatment, attention should always be directed toward reducing the dosage as soon as clinical responses permit in order to reduce the risk of complicating infections.

GENERAL TEXTS

Mandell GL, Douglas RG Jr, Bennett JH (eds.): Principles and Practice of Infectious Diseases. New York, John E Wiley, 1985. *A complete and comprehensive text of infectious diseases with excellent chapters on host defense mechanisms and host impairment syndromes.*

Root RK: Infectious diseases. Pathogenetic mechanisms and host responses. In Smith LH, Thier SO (eds.): Pathophysiology: The Biologic Principles of Disease. 2nd ed. Philadelphia, WB Saunders Company, 1985. *A more detailed review of many of the points covered in this chapter.*

Stites DP, Stobo JD, Fudenberg HH, et al. (eds.): Basic and Clinical Immunology. 6th ed. Los Altos, CA, Appleton & Lane, 1987. *An excellent basic review of immunologic mechanisms with their clinical application.*

NEUTROPHIL DISORDERS

Gallin JI: Abnormal phagocyte chemotaxis: Pathophysiology, clinical manifestations and management of patients. Rev Infect Dis 3:1196, 1981. *A review of basic mechanisms of phagocytic cell movement and clinical abnormalities.*

Root RK, Cohen MS: The microbicidal mechanisms of human neutrophils and eosinophils. Rev Infect Dis 3:365, 1981. *A comprehensive review of the oxidative killing mechanisms of neutrophils and macrophages.*

Root RK: Genetic disorders of human leukocyte function: What they tell us about normal mechanisms. Bull NY Acad Med 58:669, 1982. *A summary of clinical disorders of neutrophil function, emphasizing insights into normal functional mechanisms of these cells.*

Rubin RH, Young LS, (eds.): The Clinical Approach to Infection in the Compromised Host. New York, Plenum Press, 1981. *A comprehensive series of chapters by authorities in the field. Ideal for residents and specialists.*

Springer TA, Thompson WS, Miller LJ, et al.: Inherited deficiency of the MAC-1, LFA-1, gp 150-95 glycoprotein family and its molecular basis. J Exp Med 160:1901, 1984. *The original description of the mechanisms of leukocyte adhesion protein deficiency.*

Tauber AI, Borregard N, Simons E, et al.: Chronic granulomatous disease: A syndrome of phagocyte oxidase deficiencies. Medicine 62:286, 1983. *A complete review of neutrophil oxidative killing mechanism and an analysis of the clinical variants of their deficiency.*

COMPLEMENT DISORDERS

Ross SC, Denson P: Complement deficiency states and infection. Epidemiology, pathogenesis and consequences of neisserial and other infections in an immune deficiency. Medicine 63:243, 1984. *A review of complement-deficient states, concentrating on terminal component deficiency.*

DISORDERS OF THE SPECIFIC IMMUNE RESPONSE

Cunningham-Rundles C, Siegal FP, Smithwick EM, et al.: Efficacy of intravenous gammaglobulin in primary immunodeficiency disease. Ann Intern Med 101:435, 1984. *Treatment of antibody deficiency states.*

Rosen FS, Cooper MD, Wedgewood RJP: The primary immunodeficiencies. N Engl J Med 311:235, 1984. *A comprehensive review stressing mechanisms and clinical correlations.*

White WB, Ballow M: Modulation of suppressor cell activity by cimetidine in patients with common variable hypogammaglobulinemia. N Engl J Med 312:198, 1985. *Potential role of cimetidine in immune restoration.*

MANAGEMENT

Abraham J: Management of the immunocompromised host. Med Clin North Am 68:617, 1984. *A detailed accounting of management issues in impaired hosts.*

Pizzo PA, Young LS: Limitations of current antimicrobial therapy in the immunosuppressed host: Looking at both sides of the coin. Am J Med 76:78–82, 1984. *A good discussion of the current benefits and limitations of antimicrobial treatment in immunosuppressed patients.*

259 SHOCK SYNDROMES RELATED TO SEPSIS

John N. Sheagren

Sepsis is defined as the presence of various pus-forming and other pathogenic organisms or their toxins in the blood or tissues. A presumptive diagnosis of sepsis is often made on the basis of historical, physical, and laboratory data even in the absence of proof. The most serious complications are produced when infection spreads from the original focus to the bloodstream. Bacteremia can produce two different types of complications: microbiologic and inflammatory. The microbiologic complications result from the local and systemic proliferation and seeding of the causative organism, which cause direct tissue or organ damage. The inflammatory complications are produced locally and can result in tissue or organ destruction independent of toxic factors produced by the causative organism. Bacteremia triggers intravascular activation of the same inflammatory systems that are protective within tissues. These combine with stress-generated endocrine responses to produce a sequence of metabolic events. The end stage of these events is the systemic vascular collapse traditionally termed *septic shock*. The clinical definition of septic shock is a systolic blood pressure less than 90 mm Hg which has become unresponsive to adequate volume replacement.

Morbidity and mortality associated with septic shock are high: approximately two thirds of such patients die, and the cause of death is usually progressive failure of one or more vital organs. Prevention of septic shock should be the primary goal. It is possible to recognize clinically the changes that occur in patients in the early stages of septic shock. Intervention at early stages can reduce morbidity and mortality.

INCIDENCE AND EPIDEMIOLOGY. Infections most commonly occur in the hospital setting. Many infected patients become bacteremic. It is estimated that of 100 randomly chosen patients who appear to be infected (septic) in a hospital setting, approximately 90 per cent will actually be infected. Of these, about 20 per cent will develop some evidence of hemodynamic instability and appear, at least temporarily, "shocky." About half of shocky patients (or about 10 per cent of all septic-appearing patients) will go on to frank septic shock and/or manifest serious end organ malfunction related to the septic episode such as adult respiratory distress syndrome (ARDS), renal failure, or disseminated intravascular coagulation (DIC). Since about 5 per cent of all hospital patients either are admitted with or develop an infection during hospitalization, the number of patients at risk of developing septic shock is large. The clinician must be familiar with the manifestations and differential diagnosis of the septic-appearing patient and have in mind rapid comprehensive diagnostic and therapeutic plans of action.

Shock Related to Gram-Negative as Opposed to Gram-Positive Organisms. Septic shock more commonly follows gram-negative than gram-positive septic episodes, and many textbooks refer to generic septic shock as gram-negative sepsis or endotoxic shock because endotoxin is found only in gram-negative bacterial cell walls. In patients who are bacteremic with gram-negative microbes, the incidence of metabolic complications and shock is high (about 25 per cent). However, about 10 per cent of patients with gram-positive bacteremia, especially those infected with *Staphylococcus aureus*, develop shock. The incidence of suppurative complications (metastatic seeding to bones, joints, viscera, and so on), on the other hand, is much higher with gram-positive microorganisms. Gram-positive bacteria have the capability of adhering to endothelial cells and subendothelial matrix substances (such as fibronectin and laminin) to a much greater degree than do gram-negative organisms, so that seeding to heart valves, to other organs, and especially to foci of trauma and/or preexisting inflammation is much more common.

PATHOGENESIS. Sepsis can cause shock in many ways, either related to the primary focus of infection or to the systemic effects of bacteremia. These mechanisms of shock are listed in Table 259–1.

The classic *septic shock syndrome* results primarily from the sequence of events triggered by bacteremia during which cell wall bacterial substances (endotoxin in gram-negative organisms, the peptidoglycan/teichoic acid complex in gram-positive organisms, and polysaccharide substances in yeast cell walls) activate the complement, coagulation, kinin, and ACTH/endorphin systems. In addition, endotoxin (and probably other toxic microbial cell wall substances) strongly stimulate the production of cachectin (see Ch. 257) by macrophages, which impairs functioning of surrounding cells in multiple ways. Cachectin plays a central role in mediating the toxic effects of endotoxin and other microbial products. These processes initiate a series of metabolic events that ultimately progress to a state of shock. Severe sepsis produces hemodynamic changes in two phases. Septic patients initially have hemodynamic changes primarily reflecting vasodilation. Systemic vascular resistance is decreased and cardiac output is

TABLE 259–1. MECHANISMS OF SHOCK CAUSED BY SEPSIS

1. Shock related to a localized primary focus of infection
   Hypovolemic shock: severe local infection may
   —cause sufficient local fluid accumulation to produce systemic hypovolemia.
   —produce severe diarrhea with gastrointestinal fluid loss.
   —erode into a local vessel with mycotic aneurysm formation and rupture.
   Cardiogenic shock: extension of a pericardiac infection (usually pneumonia) into the pericardium
   —may cause purulent pericarditis and tamponade.
   Toxigenic shock (the toxic shock syndrome): a toxin is produced locally, causing
   —endothelial cell damage with capillary leakage.
   —cardiodepression.
2. Shock related to bacteremic infections
   Cardiogenic shock: seeding of the organism through the bloodstream may cause
   —valvular malfunction (endocarditis).
   —myocarditis secondary to multiple metastatic myocardial abscesses.
   —purulent pericarditis (metastatic).
   Inflammatory-system-mediated shock: bacterial cell wall substances activate the complement, coagulation, kinin, and ACTH/endorphin systems and thus cause
   —vasodilation (roles of endorphins, kinins, and complement).
   —capillary leakage (primarily due to the intracapillary adherence and aggregation of activated polymorphonuclear leukocytes).
   —disseminated intravascular coagulation.
   —cardiodepression (encephalins, vasopressin, possibly other substances).

increased. As this hyperdynamic state develops, complement-mediated leukoagglutination and capillary damage cause a severe capillary leak, intravascular volume decreases, blood pressure falls, and cardiac output declines. Several factors contribute to the decline in cardiac output: peripheral resistance increases in late septic shock and cardiodepressants such as vasopressin and encephalin are demonstrable. Individual organs may be damaged independently of the hypotensive events; for example, direct pulmonary damage by the activated leukocytes may result in ARDS, or the patient may develop renal malfunction. Presumably these end organ manifestations are related to localized direct inflammatory damage. It is in this stage that disseminated intravascular coagulation associated with severe hypoperfusion may occur with extremely high morbidity and mortality.

An important pathophysiologic concept in understanding the damage that occurs during bacteremia or fungemia is that of "multiple organ failure." Septicemia is the most important of a number of precipitating causes. Other causes include severe trauma, burns, pancreatitis, and all other causes of shock. Once the syndrome of multiple organ system failure is triggered, by whatever cause, the patient becomes febrile and hypermetabolic, exhibits hyperactive hemodynamic measurements, and develops progressive failure of one or more organs. It is tempting to speculate that cachectin plays a central role in this syndrome. Mortality exceeds 90 per cent despite all modern therapeutic measures.

Figure 259–1 outlines the sequence of early events initiated from the localized focus of infection. From these events are derived the various complications of bacteremia, which include metastatic abscess formation and the metabolic complications described earlier. Antibiotics limit metastatic abscess formation (the microbiologic complications of bacteremia). However, the other metabolic events, when initiated and independent of bacterial proliferation, still produce substantial morbidity and mortality. Therefore, therapy in addition to antibiotics is recommended to counter these deleterious metabolic sequelae.

The ACTH/Endorphin System. During systemic stress, increased ACTH release occurs. For each molecule of ACTH produced, a molecule of one of the endorphins or encephalins is also produced. The endorphins provide pain relief during severe stress, and high levels of circulating endorphins may contribute to hypotension, changes in vascular permeability, and alterations in mentation.

Coagulation/Kinin System Activation. Bacterial endotoxins and other cell wall materials directly activate the coagulation system both by initiating platelet aggregation and by activating Hageman factor. Subsequently, kinin system activation (see Ch. 431) results in the production of bradykinin, a powerful vasodilator.

Complement System Activation. The complement system is also directly activated by high molecular weight bacterial and fungal polysaccharides primarily by means of the alternative pathway. A sequence of intravascular events ensues, resulting in microvascular instability as well as activation of circulating polymorphonuclear leukocytes (PMNs). The activated PMN has enhanced bactericidal capabilities but also an enhanced capability of damaging host tissues. The activated PMN possesses increased amounts of lysosomal enzymes and produces a variety of toxic metabolites of molecular oxygen, all of which are both bactericidal and cytocidal. Furthermore, the activated PMN produces both inflammatory prostaglandins and several products of the lipoxygenase system, many of which enhance inflammation by also producing vasodilation, capillary leakage, chemotaxis, and PMN activation. The activated PMNs adhere to each other (the *leukopenic phase* of sepsis during which PMN aggregates form in capillaries) and to endothelial cells to cause severe damage and capillary leakage.

CLINICAL MANIFESTATIONS. *The Septic Patient.* The clinical situation in which a patient is considered septic (highly likely to be infected) is common. High fever and a chill strongly indicate that bacterial sepsis is occurring. In this setting, the physician must be alert for signs of septic shock. When a clinical diagnosis of septic shock can be made, the mortality rate is high. Therefore, it is important to develop the concept of a "preshock phase of septic shock" predicated on identifying a subgroup of infected patients more likely than others to develop shock. Treatment before shock develops undoubtedly prevents some of the morbidity and mortality associated with sepsis.

Table 259–2 lists several systemic signs and a variety of physical findings likely to be predictive of septic shock. Extremes of body temperature are often associated with shock. Specifically, fever in excess of 40.6° C and hypothermia associated with sepsis should be alerting signs that hypotension may soon follow. Also, in the febrile patient with a distinct change in mentation the mortality rate is higher. In association with such a finding, primary central nervous system infection may be present, and lumbar puncture is often indicated. Febrile patients who have hemodynamic instability (who are orthostatic with a blood pressure decrease of 30 mm Hg or greater) should be considered on the verge of septic shock.

While it is not possible to distinguish between simple dehydration and early septic shock solely on the basis of orthostatic blood pressure changes, hemodynamic monitoring will show an increase in peripheral vascular resistance in the

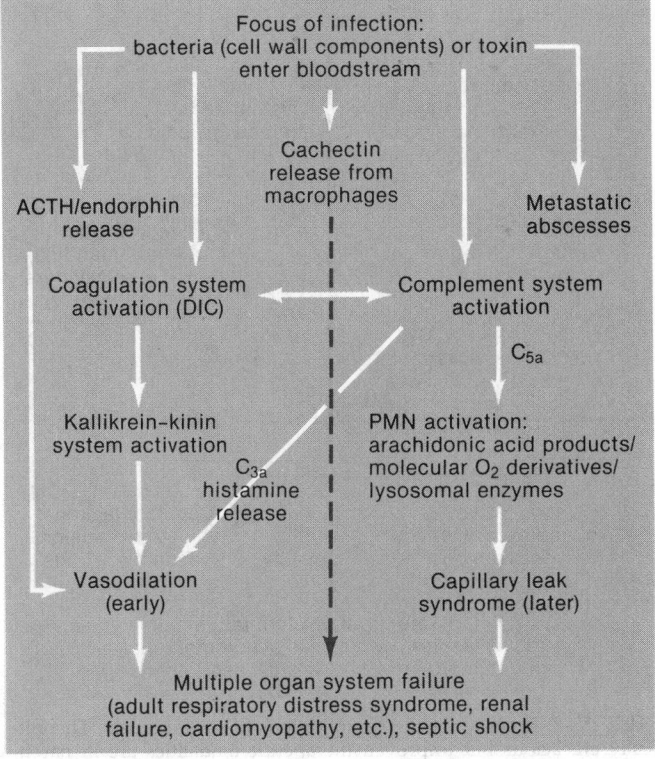

FIGURE 259–1. The complications of severe sepsis.

TABLE 259–2. PHYSICAL SIGNS AND LABORATORY DATA LIKELY TO BE PREDICTIVE OF THE DEVELOPMENT OF SEPTIC SHOCK

1. Extremes of body temperature (fever >40.6°C or hypothermia)
2. Altered mental status
3. Orthostatic blood pressure decrease (>30 mm Hg)
4. Decreasing urine output
5. Unexplained edema, usually associated with a falling serum albumin concentration
6. Tachypnea with hypoxemia and/or the development of a metabolic acidosis
7. Elevated serum lactate concentration
8. Development of leukopenia (predominantly neutropenia)
9. Development of thrombocytopenia with or without petechial skin rash

former case and a reduction in the latter. Also, fluid challenge alone will rapidly stabilize the purely hypovolemic patient. Sepsis is associated in the early stages with a state of "warm shock" in which there is an orthostatic decrease in blood pressure but good perfusion in the extremities (they are warm and pink rather than cool and cyanotic). Tachypnea with hypoxemia or metabolic acidosis or both may be predictive of impending ARDS. The development of peripheral edema, often with a suddenly decreased serum albumin concentration, as in toxigenic shock (see Toxic Shock Syndrome in Ch. 271), is often caused by an unrecognized bacteremic event.

Laboratory Data Suggesting Bacteremia or Toxemia. Several laboratory tests are often helpful in the evaluation of a potentially septic patient (Table 259–2) The blood may show hypoxemia and a metabolic acidosis. Serum lactate elevation is highly predictive of deterioration leading to septic shock. Decreasing urine output, often associated with rising blood urea nitrogen and creatinine, may be seen early in sepsis as renal failure occurs. Serum albumin measurements may show decreases in excess of that calculated by catabolism alone. Often such patients show signs of progressive peripheral edema. In early sepsis, the total white count may be low, with most of the decrease in the PMN count, owing to complement-induced leukoaggregation. As white cells aggregate, platelets become caught up in the process. Thrombocytopenia is predictive of high risk of septic shock and ARDS.

In the future, assistance in clinical decision making will be provided by rapid laboratory measurements of the activation of many of the systems shown in Figure 259–1. For example, the rapid identification of a falling total complement level and elevated levels of C5a, prostaglandins, endorphins, or cachectin might predict subgroups of septic patients at risk of developing shock.

DIAGNOSIS. The presumptive diagnosis of sepsis must be made when the setting and attendant clinical signs are suggestive. In general, patients with fever should be considered septic until proved otherwise. Therapy should always be initiated for high-risk febrile patients in advance of microbiologic confirmation of sepsis.

Evaluation of the Septic Patient. The setting in which the episode is occurring should be evaluated promptly. Crucial to appropriate initial decision making are the background history, which may help to define the type of host defense defect present, and prior cultural data, which might predict the infecting organism. The physical examination should be directed at quickly but thoroughly searching for the septic source as well as signs of end organ failure that might indicate progression to shock such as altered mental status, progressive edema, hypotension, and so on (Table 259–2). All potentially infected foci should be appropriately sampled, and the material obtained should be Gram-stained and cultured.

Differential Diagnosis of Severe Sepsis. Having done a thorough preliminary evaluation and initiated therapy (see below), one can reassess the clinical situation on subsequent days and stop antibiotic therapy if the episode later seems not to be infectious. Many nonseptic events can cause high fever with or without hemodynamic instability. For example, a variety of hypersensitivity reactions (often caused by drugs) may mimic sepsis. Vasculitic disease may present with high fever, unstable blood pressure, and altered mentation. Pulmonary emboli occur frequently in the hospital setting, and especially if the patient develops fever, the embolic event initially may be confused with sepsis. Myocardial infarction may result in hemodynamic instability, and in the subset of patients who develop higher than average fever may lead to initial confusion with sepsis.

There are infectious syndromes against which antimicrobials are of no use in which bacterial sepsis may be suspected. For example, viral syndromes such as those caused by influenza viruses, enteroviruses, adenoviruses, cytomegalovirus, and hepatitis viruses may all have high fever and be difficult

to diagnose. Malaria can be difficult to identify unless the parasite is detected on the peripheral blood smear.

TREATMENT. *Antibacterial Therapy.* Broad coverage is required in patients with severe sepsis. It is best to initiate therapy with a combination of antibiotics when the infecting organism is unknown. An aminoglycoside should always be used, and gentamicin remains the aminoglycoside of choice unless other considerations (such as abnormal renal function and known microbial resistance) dictate the use of tobramycin or amikacin. In the granulocytopenic patient, the aminoglycoside should be combined with high doses of ticarcillin or mezlocillin. In the patient likely to have an anaerobic focus of infection in which *Bacteriodes fragilis* is likely to be present, such as an intra-abdominal or gynecologic infection, or decubitus and lower extremity vascular and neuropathic ulcers, clindamycin is combined with gentamicin. For all other patients, gentamicin plus cefazolin is the combination of choice. When cultures define the causative microbe(s) or other data point to a specific organism, therapy can be tailored to the most appropriate, most specific, least toxic, and least expensive single antibiotic.

Antishock Therapy. The most important component of the therapy of shock associated with sepsis is volume replacement. Sufficient quantities of an appropriate solute (or, where indicated, albumin or whole blood) should be administered in an attempt to provide adequate volume support. Evidence is accumulating, especially in the surgical literature, that colloid-containing solutions are more efficacious than solute solutions once capillary leakage has developed. Hemodynamic monitoring is mandatory and is preferably carried out in the intensive care unit (see Ch. 73). Fluid administration

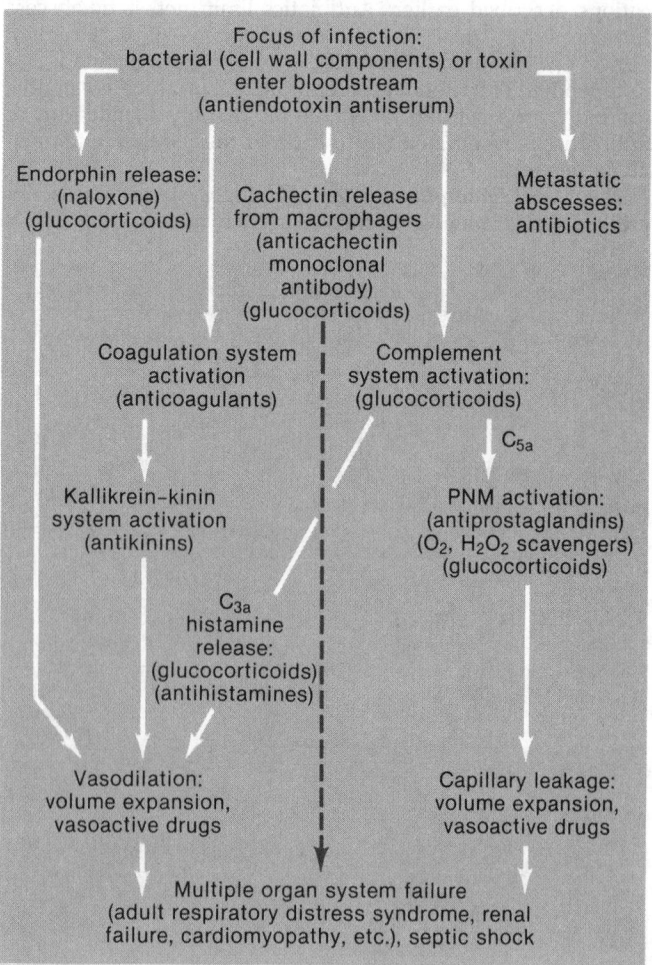

FIGURE 259–2. Therapy for the complications of severe sepsis. Theoretically efficacious but unproven therapeutic modalities are in parentheses.

should be just sufficient to bring the pulmonary capillary wedge pressure to the high normal range.

Recently two multicenter studies prospectively compared high doses of methylprednisolone sodium succinate (MPSS) with placebo in a blinded protocol in over 600 severely septic patients. Glucocorticoids were administered within four hours of recognition of the septic event. Both studies showed *no* efficacy of MPSS and one study showed increased mortality in patients with mild degrees of renal malfunction (creatinines of 2 mg per deciliter or greater). Thus, glucocorticoid therapy seems to have no role in the treatment of human sepsis.

The use of other anti-inflammatory drugs such as the antiprostaglandins is under active investigation. These agents may selectively suppress inflammatory damage caused by the activated PMN without interfering with the antibacterial capabilities of these important host defense cells.

Some clinicians are beginning to use naloxone in severe sepsis on the basis of the contribution of the endorphin system to hemodynamic instability in experimental models of septic shock. However, in primate models naloxone, like alpha agonists (aramine and levophed), appears to increase blood pressure without leading to improved tissue perfusion. Also, some preliminary data from small controlled trials in human sepsis have not documented any long-term benefits from naloxone administration.

In DIC, one should not use anticoagulant therapy when the cause is thought to be sepsis.

The Role of Surgery and Hyperbaric Oxygen. Surgical debridement and drainage of septic foci are especially important. All severe localized infections, especially with gas formation, should be widely debrided and drained. Hyperbaric oxygen has been used in patients with the gangrene syndromes and clostridial myonecrosis. Whether or not it stabilizes patients' conditions or influences the ultimate outcome is unknown.

Antiendotoxin Antiserum. In a prospective randomized study, an antiserum directed against the "core" (common) lipopolysaccharide moiety of an *Escherichia coli* mutant significantly reduced mortality in severely septic patients (Zeigler, 1982). Thus, ultimately the infusion of an antiendotoxin antiserum may be beneficial in patients in the early stages of septic shock.

PROGNOSIS. Most febrile patients lacking other signs of severe sepsis (as described in Table 259–2) will usually do well even when bacteremic. Such patients usually respond quickly to fluid administration, antibacterial therapy, and drainage of the primary focus of infection. However, the presence of shock dramatically increases morbidity and mortality. Even when the inciting infection is localized, shock (with the exception of the toxic shock syndrome) is associated with a 50 per cent mortality. Full-blown, bacteremia-associated septic shock has greater than 70 per cent mortality. A favorable outcome in a patient in frank shock depends on the skill of management in the intensive care unit. Early diagnosis and therapy of severely septic patients will decrease the morbidity and mortality.

PREVENTION. Prevention of infection, especially in the hospital, is the key to reducing morbidity and mortality associated with septic shock. Strict adherence to the hospital infection control program with avoidance of Foley catheters and meticulous attention to the placement and maintenance of intravascular lines dramatically reduces the incidence of bacteremic infections. The concept of the preshock approach to the therapy of septic shock is useful; in all such patients fluids should be administered and broad antibiotic coverage started early. Controlled studies of anti-inflammatory therapy in severe sepsis are under way and better guidelines should be forthcoming.

Abraham E, Shoemaker WC, Bland RD, et al.: Sequential cardiorespiratory patterns in septic shock. Crit Care Med 11:799, 1983. *Describes the hemodynamic patterns occurring in patients as they develop septic shock.*

Beutler B, Cerami A: Cachectin: More than a tumor necrosis factor. N Engl J Med 316:379, 1987. *Excellent review of the role of cachectin in inflammation, sepsis, and septic shock.*

Jacob HS, Craddock PR, Hammerschmidt DE, et al.: Complement-induced granulocyte aggregation: An unsuspected mechanism of disease. N Engl J Med 302:789, 1980. *Describes how complement-induced granulocyte aggregation leads to capillary and organ damage.*

Sande M, Root RR: Septic Shock: Newer Concepts in Pathophysiology and Treatment. New York, Churchill Livingstone, Inc., 1985. *Complete up-to-date review of all aspects of septic shock including papers on the roles of endorphins, complement, prostaglandins, the PMN, and glucocorticoid therapy.*

Sibbald WJ, Sprung CL: New Horizons—Perspectives on Sepsis and Septic Shock. Fullerton, CA, Society of Critical Care Medicine, 1986. *An up-to-date review of all basic and clinical aspects of the sepsis and multiple organ system failure syndromes.*

Spriggs DR: Cachexia and septic shock: What's in a name? J Infect Dis 154:734, 1986. *Describes role of cachectin in sepsis.*

Tracey KJ, Beutler B, Lowry SF, et al.: Shock and tissue injury induced by recombinant human cachectin. Science 234:470, 1986. *Cachectin is capable of producing most of the deleterious effects of endotoxin.*

Weissman G, Smolen JE, Dorchak HM: Release of inflammatory mediators from stimulated neutrophils. N Engl J Med 303:27, 1980. *An excellent description of the events leading to and occurring in the activated PMN.*

Zeigler EJ, McCutchan JA, Fierer J, et al.: Treatment of gram-negative bacteremia and shock with human antiserum to a mutant *Escherichia coli*. N Engl J Med 307:1225, 1982. *Describes therapy of bacteremic patients with human antiserum to endotoxin core resulting in a significant reduction in mortality.*

260 PREVENTION AND TREATMENT OF HOSPITAL-ACQUIRED INFECTIONS

Richard P. Wenzel

HISTORY. The father of infection control is Ignaz Semmelweis (1818–1865), whose observations in Vienna—prior to formulation of the germ theory—laid the foundations for hospital epidemiology. At the Allgemeines Krankenhaus, Semmelweis compiled mortality data on two obstetrics wards: on one ward (I), in which all women were attended by obstetricans and medical students, the mortality was over 8 percent; on the other ward (II), in which all women were attended by midwives, the mortality was 2 per cent. In retrospect the cause of death with puerperal sepsis was the Group A β-hemolytic streptococcus, *S. pyogenes*. Semmelweis made two very important observations: (1) there was a lower mortality on ward I when medical students were on vacation, and (2) the odor of the autopsy room was noted on ward I whenever students were present. Furthermore, a colleague and pathologist, Professor Kolletschka, accidentally cut his own finger while performing a postmortem examination on one of the women who had died of puerperal sepsis, developed a very similar syndrome and died. Semmelweis reasoned that some element was carried on the hands of students and physicians from the autopsy room to the obstetrics ward. Semmelweis introduced the practice of handwashing with an antiseptic (chloride of lime) between the autopsy and delivery room and before examination of each patient. Thereafter, the mortality in ward I fell to less than 2 per cent.

INTRODUCTION. Each year approximately 40 million people are hospitalized in the United States. Between 5 and 10 per cent, or 2 to 4 million patients, develop an infection that was not present or incubating upon admission. Such infections are referred to as hospital acquired or nosocomial.* Nosocomial infections are directly responsible for an estimated 30,000 to 60,000 deaths and lead to excess hospitalization with an economic burden of approximately 5 billion dollars per year.

Approximately half of all hospital infections are caused by gram-positive cocci. In large part, this has resulted from the recent emergence of coagulase-negative staphylococci as true nosocomial pathogens. More hospitals have also witnessed

---

*Nosocomial is derived from the Greek word for hospital.

the presence of methicillin-resistant staphylococci in the mid 1980s and an increased frequency of enterococcal infections. *Candida* species have increased, and there has been a decline in gram-negative rods, especially the more sensitive *Escherichia coli* with the persistence of other Enterobacteriaceae and pseudomonads.

Although urinary tract infections account for the largest proportion (40 per cent) of all nosocomial infections, postoperative wound infections account for the greatest burden (33 per cent) in terms of excess stay in the hospital (Table 260–1).

No matter how effective an infection control program may be, it is impossible to eliminate all infections, in part because many arise endogenously in patients whose immune defense mechanisms are impaired, such as patients with leukemia and those who have received organ transplants. It is important, therefore, to focus on preventable, i.e., device-related and procedure-related, infections. Several priorities can be recognized:

1. Since bloodstream infections account for the greatest mortality and because one third to one half occur in intensive care unit patients, a focus on device-related infections in critical care units is important.

2. Since postoperative wound infections account for most of the morbidity and economic burden, selected surveillance and reporting of common procedures is helpful.

3. Since urinary tract infections are so frequent and almost always catheter-related, continual review of catheter insertion and management and associated infection rates is useful.

Infection or colonization results when a sufficient number of organisms with ability to attach to skin or mucosal surfaces reaches a susceptible host. Colonization implies a peaceful coexistence between organism and host, whereas infection results from an altered balance of power in favor of the organism. Three major routes are recognized by which organisms are transmitted to hospitalized patients: direct contact, the air (via droplet nuclei less than 5 μ in diameter), and common source vehicles such as contaminated equipment. The most likely mode of transmission is direct contact via the hands of medical personnel. Furthermore, the rate of transmission by all mechanisms is highest in patients in close proximity to the reservoir. Simple handwashing is effective in preventing direct contact transmission and remains the most important infection control measure. Optimal technique in managing devices and strict adherence to protocols are helpful. Additionally, infections can be minimized by elimination of the reservoir. If the reservoir is an inanimate object (e.g., a pressure monitor transducer head), infection control is readily accomplished. Unfortunately the reservoirs for most nosocomial infections are patients themselves. Thus, isolation techniques (see below) are utilized to contain certain organisms that cannot be readily eliminated.

HIGH-RISK LOCATIONS. Certain areas of any hospital are likely to foster endemic infections as well as outbreaks or epidemics. High risk areas include critical care areas, burn units, and dialysis units. Critical care areas are usually the birthplace and area of highest prevalence of antibiotic resistance in the hospital, including methicillin-resistant *Staphylococcus aureus* and aminoglycoside-resistant gram-negative rods. The importance of *S. epidermidis* bloodstream infections in patients in intensive care units has been stressed.

Critical Care Areas. Medical, surgical, and neonatal critical care areas provide a concentration of patients at high risk for nosocomial infections. This is a reflection of patients' underlying diseases, the frequent use of invasive monitoring, and alteration of normal flora by antibiotics. Often patients are in close proximity to each other, promoting transmission by busy medical personnel who fail to wash their hands between contacts. Cross-infection is particularly common among burn patients. Furthermore, the widespread use of topical antibiotics may select for colonization and infection with multiply resistant organisms. The major pathogens include *Pseudomonas aeruginosa*, *Providencia stuartii*, or other gram-negative rods, and, in some burn units, methicillin-resistant *S. aureus*.

Proper design of critical care units with regard to separation of patients by partitions and placement of sinks at the entrance to individual cubicles, as well as optimal nursing-to-patient ratios, may minimize the risks of cross-infection. Other suggested infection control measures include (1) the notification of the infection control team of all new procedures or products and (2) use of a clinical flow sheet listing catheters, dates of insertion, and rationale for continued use.

Dialysis Units. Both bacterial and viral infections occur with increased frequency in patients with chronic renal failure. Bacterial infections often affect fistulas and arteriovenous access shunts. With infected fistulas, up to one third of patients may have no objective signs of infection and may complain only of intense pain. With *S. aureus* infections of fistulas or shunts, up to 20 per cent may develop secondary endocarditis. Evidence of viral infection (including both non-A non-B and type B viral hepatitis) is found in virtually all units. Often the virus is introduced by one of the blood products used. Once introduced, transmission to other patients and staff can occur by accidental needle stick exposure, contaminated dialysis equipment, and possibly other contact. Renal patients are more likely to become chronic carriers of hepatitis B surface antigen (HB_sAg) than are patients in the community who become infected with hepatitis B. Staff members working in these units are also at increased risk of infection. Data from the Centers for Disease Control indicate that in 1982 only 0.4 per cent of dialysis personnel and 0.5 per cent of patients acquired hepatitis B. The annual incidence of non-A non-B hepatitis in patients was 1.6 per cent. Thus, there has been a dramatic reduction in hepatitis B relative to the late 1970's and a 3 to 1 ratio of non-A non-B to type B infection in dialysis patients. The infections may result in chronic liver disease, including a susceptibility to delta infection in chronic carriers of HB_sAg, and may expose offspring of pregnant workers to the risk of neonatal hepatitis. Hospital personnel who are exposed to blood products should receive hepatitis B vaccine (see Ch. 121). In addition, the risk to the staff can be minimized and epidemics identified early or prevented with proper control practices: (1) Strict handwashing procedures should be observed. (2) Serologic surveillance of patients and dialysis staff for hepatitis at three- to six-month intervals is recommended unless anti-HB_s antibody is present. (3) Protective clothing should be worn in the area. (4) Eating, drinking, smoking, and mouth pipetting should be prohibited in the unit. (5) Contaminated materials should be autoclaved or incinerated. (6) Contaminated surfaces should be washed with 0.5 to 1.0 per cent sodium hypochlorite

TABLE 260–1. IMPACT OF HOSPITAL-ACQUIRED INFECTIONS IN ACUTE CARE INSTITUTIONS

Anatomic Site	Number of Infections per 100 Admissions	Proportion of All Hospital-Acquired Infections	Estimated Direct Mortality	Estimated Number of Excess Hospital Days per Infection	Proportion of All Excess Hospital Days
Urinary tract	2.5	40%	<1%	2	19%
Postoperative wound	1.5	20%	<1%	7	33%
Pulmonary	1	10%	5–10%*	8	21%
Bloodstream	0.5–1	5–10%	25%	14	16%
Others	1	20–25%	Varies with site	2	12%

*Crude mortality was 35 and 30 per cent, respectively, in two uncontrolled studies at two university hospitals.

prior to routine cleanup. (7) Needles used to draw blood should not be recapped or clipped and they should be discarded into large impenetrable containers. (8) Pregnant staff members might consider transferring to another area of the hospital in order to avoid acquiring viral hepatitis and transmitting the infection to the baby.

SURVEILLANCE. Surveillance refers to the routine and orderly collection of information regarding the occurrence of a disease. In the hospital it is primarily used to define endemic rates and to identify high and low risk areas. Data from surveillance identify clusters and epidemics when certain threshold rates are exceeded and form the basis for alteration of existing procedures and practices. Results of the SENIC study (study of the efficacy of nosocomial infection control) by the Centers for Disease Control showed lower infection rates in hospitals routinely performing surveillance. A minimal data base is necessary to satisfy the requirements of the Joint Commission for Accreditation of Hospitals (JCAH).

In general, surveillance is performed by infection control practitioners, most of whom are nurses. While gathering data, they reinforce isolation procedures and identify new problems. The starting point for data collection varies; review of nursing care plans or bacteriology reports is useful to identify patients at high risk. Once they are identified, trained practitioners can then review their charts, seeking evidence for infection. Practitioners who wish to compare infection rates among similar categories of hospitals should use identical definitions for infection (Table 260–2). Infection rates for a defined period are later compiled by identifying the number of infections (numerator) and the total number of patient-days or patients at risk (denominator). By convention, the number of patients admitted or discharged is often substituted for the number of patients at risk. Infection rates by site, service, organism, and procedure are tallied. In hospitals with sophisticated surveillance, infection rates by underlying diagnosis are also reported. In addition, a summary of antibiotic sensitivity patterns for hospital pathogens may help clinicians select proper initial antimicrobial therapy of nosocomial infections.

Analysis of data collected by surveillance requires knowledge of basic epidemiologic measurements. These include the following: (1) Incidence—the number of new cases of a disease in a population at risk over a specified unit of time. An example is the number of new cases of bloodstream infection per 100 patient-days of risk. (2) Prevalence—the number of persons with a disease (newly acquired or not) at a given time. An example is the number of patients on January 1 with an obvious wound infection per 100 patients on the ward. (3) Attack rate—the number of new cases of a disease in a particular population exposed to a particular risk. No defined unit of time is implied, although the period of risk is assumed to be limited. An example is the number of patients with a wound infection per 100 undergoing appendectomies.

Surveillance data should be summarized in a report for distribution throughout the hospital. This enables the various services to review their performance routinely and to become aware of potential problems. If a change in the infection rate appears to be significant, it is necessary to use statistical testing to be sure.

URINARY TRACT INFECTIONS. The upper and lower urinary tracts are the source of approximately 40 per cent of all nosocomial infections. Almost all occur in patients who have undergone some form of instrumentation, usually catheterization.

A simple in-and-out catheterization is frequently used to obtain urine samples from patients who cannot give a clean voided sample. Although this procedure carries a relatively low risk of significant bacteriuria in healthy ambulatory men and women (2 to 3 per cent), the risk is 6 per cent in hospitalized women, 9 per cent in postpartum women, and 23 per cent in postpartum women who have had complicated labors. Although the risk may be justified in postoperative patients with transient retention, routine catheterization should be discouraged in healthy obstetric patients at the time of delivery.

Indwelling Foley catheters are used in 10 to 20 per cent of hospitalized patients. They are the major predisposing agents of nosocomially induced urinary tract infection. Bacteriuria occurs at a rate of 5 per cent per day that the indwelling catheter is left in place. Evidence of upper tract involvement by antibody coating tests and the presence of circulating endotoxins is not infrequent in patients with catheter-related infection. In addition, urinary infections serve as the most common predisposing source for secondary gram-negative rod bacteremia, which occurs in 3 per cent of bacteriuric patients. Since the rate of secondary bacteremia with *Serrata marcescens* bacteriuria is very high (16 per cent), all bacteriuric patients with the organism should be given appropriate therapy regardless of symptoms.

The principal organisms involved in nosocomial urinary tract infections are as follows: *E. coli* (33 per cent), enterococci (15 per cent), *Proteus* (15 per cent), *Klebsiella* (10 per cent), and *Pseudomonas* (10 per cent). Unlike community-acquired urinary tract infections, these organisms are usually resistant to sulfonamides and ampicillin. Newer β-lactam antibiotics and aminoglycosides are effective in most cases, but outbreaks of multiply resistant organisms have occurred.

Hematogenous spread of bacteria to the urinary tract is uncommon. In approximately 80 per cent of infections, organisms migrate from the perineum, then gain entrance to the bladder along the external catheter surface. However, in 20 per cent of infections, the organisms travel intraluminally from the collection bag or from the connection site of catheter and drainage tubing after the system is broken.

All patients requiring indwelling catheters should have closed drainage systems. Proper care is important in minimizing the risk of infection. Basic practices include the following: (1) Aseptic insertion by trained personnel, e.g., specially instructed physicians. (Catheter care teams have not been shown to be cost effective or efficacious.) (2) Drainage bags should be hung and kept upright below the level of the patient's bladder to prevent retrograde flow. They should never be allowed to rest on the floor or to be inverted. (3) Drainage bags should be emptied frequently to avoid distention and contamination. All vessels used to measure urine output should be disinfected between patients to avoid cross-infection. (4) The system should not be irrigated unless absolutely necessary and then under strict asepsis. Small specimens of urine can be aspirated from the proximal lumen of the catheter with a sterile syringe after proper disinfection. (5) Routine changing of the catheters is probably unnecessary unless they become obstructed or encrusted.

Perineal care and use of antimicrobial lubricants either around the catheter or impregnated within the catheter are not of proven efficacy. Similarly, the use of disinfectants in the drainage bag has not reduced infections in patients catheterized one week or less. Furthermore, the practice of cul-

TABLE 260–2. DEFINITIONS OF NOSOCOMIAL INFECTIONS*
USED IN SURVEILLANCE

Anatomic Site	Criteria
Urine	≥100,000 colonies of bacteria per milliliter of urine
Postoperative wound	Pus at the incision site
Blood	Positive culture (exclude contaminant)
Pulmonary	New infiltrate on chest film associated with purulent sputum (exclude atelectasis and pulmonary embolus with infarction) Sputum production is not required for immunosuppressed patients
Burns	≥10^6 organisms per gram of biopsy tissue

*Infections that are not incubating or present upon admission.

turing the tip of catheters at the time of removal has been shown not to be a valuable monitor of infection.

Several authors have suggested the use of prophylactic irrigation of closed drainage systems with acetic acid or polymyxin-neomycin solutions. Their use should probably be reserved for those who require irrigation to relieve obstruction by clots. The efficacy of prophylactic antibiotics appears to be limited to the first four days of catheterization. Although this may be of value in selected patients such as those undergoing prostate surgery, prolonged or widespread use should be discouraged, since it will most likely select for resistant organisms. In addition, the efficacy of prophylactic antibiotics has not been critically evaluated in closed drainage systems.

NOSOCOMIAL PNEUMONIAS. Approximately 1 per cent of hospitalized patients will develop a nosocomial pneumonia. Hospital-acquired pneumonias tend to be more common in university than community hospitals owing to differences in patient populations. Although crude mortality for nosocomial pneumonias in university patients has been reported to be 30 to 35 per cent, a recent case control study suggested that the attributable mortality (direct mortality after controlling for the underlying disease) was low (approximately 7 per cent) and not statistically significant. The infections do, however, contribute significantly to hospital stay. *Pseudomonas* pneumonia appears to carry a particularly high mortality (70 per cent), as do pneumonias in compromised hosts and those that are superinfections. A survey by the Centers for Disease Control's National Nosocomial Infectious Study suggested that 7 per cent of nosocomial pneumonias led to secondary bacteremias.

The most common causes of nosocomial pneumonias are the gram-negative bacilli, accounting for over 50 per cent of cases. No study has employed transtracheal aspirates or lung aspirates to confirm the etiology of nosocomial pneumonias in a large series of patients. *Klebsiella, S. aureus, Pseudomonas aeruginosa*, and *E. coli* are frequently isolated from sputum. These organisms colonize the upper airways of up to 50 per cent of critically ill hospitalized patients, usually within four to five days of admission. Once colonized, a patient is at higher risk for the development of pneumonia; in one study of intensive care unit patients, pneumonia occurred in 23 per cent of colonized, in contrast to 3 per cent of noncolonized, patients. Factors influencing colonization are multiple and poorly understood. Organisms appear to come from exogenous sources (especially *Pseudomonas)* via respiratory care equipment or the hands of medical personnel; organisms (especially Enterobacteriaceae) may also come from the patient's own gastrointestinal tract. Encouraging work in Europe suggests that reducing the number of organisms in the stomach and mouth might reduce the incidence of nosocomial pneumonia. The use of local oral and gastric antibiotics is not generally recommended, however.

Aspiration of gastric contents with subsequent pneumonitis is common in the patient with cerebrovascular disease, seizures, drug overdose, cardiopulmonary arrests, and any condition which alters the patient's respiratory clearing mechanisms. Similarly, postoperative patients are at higher risk of developing pneumonia. Chemical pneumonitis from aspiration of gastric contents generally develops immediately and may be associated with respiratory failure. The pneumonia may result in death or resolve over a five-day period. Chemical pneumonitis does not require antimicrobial therapy, nor is steroid therapy helpful. Bacterial pneumonia, however, may develop as a complication of aspiration. Bacterial infection is characterized by deterioration after a transient period of recovery.

Frequently, postoperative and seriously ill patients have endotracheal or nasotracheal tubes or tracheostomies. Although these protect the patient from aspiration, they also bypass normal defense mechanisms and predispose to tracheal injury from suctioning. Uncommonly, secretions and gastric contents may be aspirated around the tube. There are occasionally serious problems associated with respiratory therapy. Outbreaks of pharyngeal colonization and pneumonia have been associated with the use of contaminated anesthesia equipment, ventilators, and IPPB machines with medication nebulizers. Usually, the gases from oxygen and air compressors, and internal parts of the machines, do not become contaminated or promote bacterial growth. The changeable tubing and masks can become contaminated if not disinfected or sterilized between patients. The greatest source of contamination is large volume Venturi nebulizers. Nebulizers produce liquid in aerosol (droplet) form by either ultrasonic or centrifugal means. These droplets can emit aerosols containing large numbers of gram-negative rods that may be delivered to terminal bronchi, resulting in pneumonia. Contamination of the large volume cascade humidifier may occur during cleaning or replenishing water. Organisms capable of growing under these conditions include *P. aeruginosa, P. cepacia, Serratia marcescens, Acinetobacter calcoaceticus*, and *Flavobacterium meningosepticum*. Pneumonia caused by any of these suggests the possibility of exogenous contamination. The risk of contamination appears to be minimal with small volume medication nebulizers as long as the medications used are sterile. Humidifiers uncommonly may serve as a potential risk to patients, but it unusual because bacteria are not transported by molecules of water in vapor form.

The immunocompromised host with pulmonary infiltrates represents a particularly difficult diagnostic and therapeutic problem. These patients are generally being treated with steroids or cytotoxic agents or both. Although the most common causes for their pneumonias are aerobic gram-negative rods, up to 25 per cent may become infected with fungi, herpesviruses, *Legionella pneumophila, Legionella (Tatlockia) micdadei, Nocardia*, acid-fast bacilli, and combinations of these. Optimal therapy generally requires a tissue diagnosis, often an open lung biopsy of diffuse infiltrates, or needle aspirate of solitary nodules. Hospitals with clusters of patients with *Legionella pneumophila* have usually identified water as the significant vehicle, and control of contamination has been followed by a reduction in number of cases.

A great deal of attention has been focused on the infection control practices necessary to minimize the risk of pneumonias from respiratory care equipment. Although the data are incomplete, important points include the following: (1) Large volume reservoir nebulizers should be replaced by humidifiers if possible. Water used for humidification should be sterile. (2) All medication used for respiratory therapy should be sterile and preferably administered as a single unit dose. (3) Equipment such as tubing that comes into direct contact with patients should be changed between patients and every 24 to 48 hours when in continuous use.

BLOODSTREAM INFECTIONS. Hospital-acquired bloodstream infections may be primary (without an apparent source) or secondary to infection at a distal site. The distinction is important for both epidemiologic and clinical reasons. Secondary bloodstream infections complicate 3 per cent of urinary tract infections, 5 to 7 per cent of postoperative wound and pulmonary infections, and 7 per cent of cutaneous infections. *E. coli, S. aureus, K. pneumoniae, S. marcescens*, and *P. aeruginosa* are the usual pathogens. Identification of the source allows one to treat both the underlying condition and the complicating bacteremia. For example, bacteremia developing in patients with a urinary tract infection should suggest the possibility of obstruction, which may require surgery as well as antibiotics.

When true primary bacteremias occur, even in the compromised host, one must always consider the possibility of an infusion- or instrument-related infection. Twenty-five per cent of all patients hospitalized receive intravenous infusions, and the use of hyperalimentation, arterial, Swan-Ganz and the subcutaneously tunneled Hickman and Broviac catheters has increased greatly in recent years.

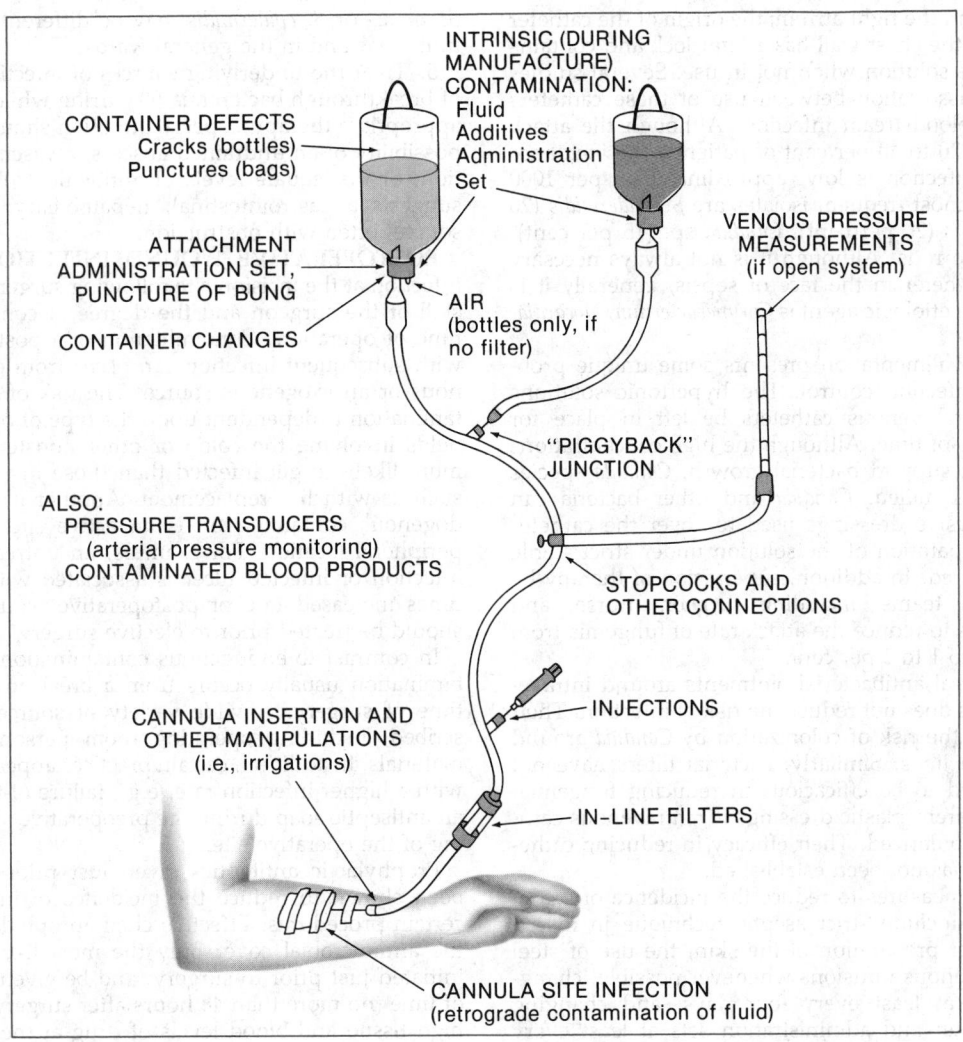

FIGURE 260–1. Sites at which contamination of intravenous fluids or intravascular devices may occur.

Infections related to intravenous fluids or intravascular devices may occur from either intrinsic or extrinsic contamination of the system (Fig. 260–1). Contamination of the infusion or administration set at the site of manufacture (intrinsic) may be extremely difficult to detect. In the early 1970's, at least 400 cases of *Enterobacter* sepsis occurred secondary to contaminated dextrose infusions. A similar outbreak was reported in 1984 in Greece. Because only 0.7 to 0.9 per cent of all manufactured bottles were contaminated and because these were shipped to many different hospitals, the association was difficult to detect. Certain clues, however, should serve as a flag for such a possibility: (1) sepsis occurring in an otherwise low risk patient receiving an intravenous solution, or (2) a cluster of primary bloodstream infections with an unusual pathogen. Only certain organisms are capable of growing well in intravenous solutions. *Klebsiella*, *Enterobacter*, and *Serratia* can readily grow in 5 per cent dextrose in water, exceeding 10^5 colonies per milliliter within 24 hours at room temperature. Thus, careful examination of intravenous infusion bags or bottles may be useful, but even when the infusion contains 10^6 organisms per milliliter, cloudiness may be difficult to detect with the unaided eye. *Pseudomonas cepacia*, *Citrobacter freundii*, and *Flavobacterium* species are also likely to contaminate intravenous infusions. In contrast, *Proteus* species, *Pseudomonas aeruginosa*, *S. aureus*, *E. coli*, *Acinetobacter* species, and *Candida* species are unable to survive in significant numbers under these conditions.

Extrinsic contamination, usually at the catheter site, is the most likely source of infusion-related infections. Steel needles carry a lower risk than plastic catheters. The incidence of a catheter-related infection rises with the length of time the catheter is left in place. Inflammation at the catheter site (a "cord," redness, swelling, pain) strongly suggests catheter-associated sepsis. Catheters introduced via surgical cutdowns, femoral catheters, and devices left in place for more than 48 hours are particularly at risk. In contrast to contamination of the infusion, cannula-related sepsis is likely to be caused by gram-positive organisms, predominantly by *S. aureus* (50 per cent), *S. epidermidis*, and enterococci, although some are caused by gram-negative rods. Preliminary data suggest that intra-arterial catheters should not remain in place longer than four days. *S. epidermidis* bloodstream infections are primarily catheter related, occur in critical care units 70 per cent of the time, and, in one study, had a crude mortality rate of 36 per cent. It is thought that the organism's relative resistance to commonly used antibiotics and its ability to attach to catheter surfaces with an extracellular glycocalyx (slime) have been important selective factors.

An unusual complication of catheters is suppurative thrombophlebitis, a purulent infection involving the entire vein, often occurring in the burn patient. Although local evidence of infection may be absent, the patients have unremitting sepsis. Therapy often requires surgical excision of the vein, beginning proximal to the involved section, as well as antimicrobial therapy.

Hickman-Broviac intravenous catheters are currently popular, both for infusing fluids and for withdrawing blood from selected patients. The catheters are tunneled under the skin of the chest wall midway between the nipple and sternum and enter the subclavian vein superiorly. The tip of the catheter is placed in the right atrium; the origin of the catheter on the outside of the chest wall has a Luer lock and contains heparinized saline solution when not in use. Several studies have shown an association between use of these catheters and subsequent bloodstream infection. Although the attack rate is as high as 20 to 40 per cent of patients, the incidence of bloodstream infection is low, approximately 3 per 1000 days of use. The most frequent isolates are *S. epidermidis* (20 per cent), *S. aureus* (20 per cent), *Candida* sp. (15 per cent), and gram-negative rods. Although it is not always necesary to remove the catheter in the face of sepsis, generally it is wise to do so if the etiologic agent is *Corynebacterium, Nocardia,* or a fungus.

Parenteral hyperalimentation presents some unique problems regarding infection control. The hypertonic solutions require that central venous catheters be left in place for prolonged periods of time. Although the high concentrations of glucose do not support bacterial growth, *Candida* species grow well in this milieu. *Candida* and other bacteria can colonize the occlusive dressings used to cover the catheter insertion site. Preparation of the solution under strict sterile technique is required. In addition, supervision of therapy by hyperalimentation teams, including surgeon, nurse, and pharmacist, seems to reduce the attack rate of fungemia from 10 to 20 per cent to 1 to 2 per cent.

The use of topical antibacterial ointments around intravenous catheter sites does not reduce the risk of infection. Their use may increase the risk of colonization by *Candida* around hyperalimentation lines. Similarly, bacterial filters have not been demonstrated to be efficacious in reducing fungemia. The use of transparent plastic dressings for intravenous catheters has been popularized. Their efficacy in reducing catheter-related sepsis has not been established.

Recommended measures to reduce the incidence of catheter-related sepsis include strict aseptic technique in inserting a cannula after preparation of the skin, the use of steel needles for intravenous infusions whenever possible, changing arterial lines at least every four days, and changing intravenous catheter and administration sets at least every 48 hours. The use of flow sheets to keep track of the multiple monitoring devices used in intensive care areas should be encouraged.

Despite control measures, bloodstream infections related to infusion therapy will occur. The following is offered as a general guide in the approach to the hospitalized patient with sepsis:

1. Determine the most likely source of infection (is it primary or secondary?). If secondary, where is the other infection site: urinary tract, lung, wound, or elsewhere?

2. What intravenous and intra-arterial devices are in place? How long have they been there? Is there any evidence of local inflammation? If the bacteremia is primary or caused by an unusual pathogen, or occurs while the patient is receiving appropriate antimicrobial therapy, the following measures should be undertaken: (a) Discontinue the intravenous device immediately. (b) After iodine prep of the latex injection port at the distal end of the intravenous tubing (allow iodine to remain at least two minutes and then remove with 70 per cent isopropyl alcohol), aspirate 10 ml of the intravenous contents. Place 5 ml into each of two blood culture bottles (one set), and send to the bacteriology laboratory. (c) Remove the indwelling catheter aseptically, and send it to the laboratory for semiquantitative culture. (d) Record the lot number of all intravenous products the patient was receiving.

3. Draw blood cultures and obtain appropriate cultures at distal sites.

4. Initiate intravenous antimicrobial therapy. Until sensitivities are available, initial antibiotic selection should be based on the surveillance data for the hospital ward(s) in which the patient has resided. The probability of specific aminoglycoside-resistant gram-negative rods and of methicillin-resistant

S. aureus or *S. epidermidis* may be different in intensive care unit areas and in the general wards.

5. Treat the underlying sources of infection. In the setting of breakthrough bacteremia (occurring while the patient is on appropriate therapy), special attention should be given to the possibility of an undrained abscess, a vascular focus of infection, or inadequate levels of antibiotic. Polymicrobial sepsis suggests a gastrointestinal, hepatobiliary, or genitourinary source, often with obstruction.

POSTOPERATIVE WOUND INFECTIONS. The rate of infection at the incision site following surgery depends on the skill of the surgeon and the degree of contamination at the time of operation. Contamination of a postoperative wound with subsequent infection can occur from either an endogenous or an exogenous source. The risk of endogenous contamination is dependent upon the type of operation. Surgical fields involving the colon or other nonsterile structures are more likely to get infected than those involving clean areas such as with hip replacement. Another likely source of endogenous contamination is an active site of infection at a peripheral location. For example, an untreated urinary tract infection or infected ulcer is associated with a two to three times increased rate of postoperative wound infection and should be treated prior to elective surgery.

In contrast to endogenous contamination, exogenous contamination usually occurs from a break in technique at the time of surgery. A wide variety of sources have been described, including operating room personnel and surgical materials. In addition, certain practices appear to be associated with a higher infection rate, e.g., failure of the patient to use an antiseptic soap during the preoperative shower, and shaving of the operative site.

Prophylactic antibiotics given just prior to surgery have been shown to reduce the incidence of infection following certain procedures. Effective chemoprophylaxis requires that the antimicrobial cover only the most likely pathogens, be initiated just prior to surgery, and be given for brief periods of time (no more than 48 hours after surgery). There must be high tissue and blood levels of drug at the time of surgery. When wound infections do occur, they are generally caused by *S. aureus, S. epidermis,* or gram-negative rods. Patients with *S. aureus* infections should be placed on "contact" or "drainage/secretion" precautions to minimize the risk of cross-contamination. Treatment usually requires drainage followed by antibiotic therapy for approximately seven days.

If pus is found after surgery and no organisms are recovered from routine cultures, then a possibility exists that infection is caused by anaerobic bacteria, rapid-growing atypical mycobacteria, or a saprophytic fungus. The latter two situations are distinctly unusual and should be considered only if there are clinical or laboratory features suggesting nonvegetative bacterial infection.

Wound infections occurring unusually early (within 24 to 48 hours of surgery) should suggest the possibility of infection with β-hemolytic Group A streptococci (*S. pyogenes*), *Clostridium* species (gas gangrene) or organisms causing necrotizing fasciitis. These are especially serious and life-threatening infections requiring immediate evaluation and therapy. Their management is discussed elsewhere in this text.

OTHER INFECTION SITES. A wide variety of infections occurs in hospitalized patients in addition to those previously discussed. Nosocomial meningitis usually occurs following neurosurgical shunting procedures and is usually caused by *S. aureus, S. epidermidis,* or gram-negative rods, rarely by *Candida* as a late infection. In the compromised host, nosocomial meningitis may occur without prior surgery. *Listeria, Cryptococcus,* and gram-negative rods are the likely pathogens. Group B streptococci are a common cause of meningitis in the neonate, and there have been reports of *Citrobacter* and *Campylobacter* bloodstream infections and meningitis in a few neonatal units.

Infections following the insertion of artificial joints are particularly difficult to treat. Those occurring in the hospitalized patient usually are "early onset" infections. *S. epidermidis*, *S. aureus*, and gram-negative rods are involved. In a large study of infections following total knee arthroplasty at the Mayo Clinic, the significance of anaerobes was stressed. Unless the infection is of a superficial wound, salvage of the prosthesis is infrequent. Infections with a late onset (beyond eight weeks) account for at least 50 per cent of infections involving prosthetic joints.

In the last 10 years, the percentage of infants delivered by cesarean section has risen. Currently, up to 25 per cent of all deliveries are performed in this manner. In contrast to the incidence of endometritis following vaginal deliveries (1 per cent or less), that following cesarean section ranges from 20 to 30 per cent. The specific contribution to the increased infection risk by the cesarean section, underlying disease, or use of fetal monitoring is unclear.

INFECTION CONTROL COMMITTEE. In order to be accredited by the Joint Commission for Accreditation of Hospitals (JCAH), all hospitals in the United States are required to have an infection control committee that meets at least six times a year. The committee formulates and reviews hospital policies with regard to infection control practices. Usually, its members are diverse, representing the medicine, surgery, microbiology laboratory, nursing, and pharmacy departments. One member of the committee serves as the hospital epidemiologist, usually someone with training in infectious diseases or clinical microbiology who has a strong interest in infection control.

An important task of the committee is to adopt and enforce proper isolation practices to prevent the transmission of communicable diseases within the hospital. Most hospitals utilize a limited number of types of isolation based upon the route of transmission of the disease. The Centers for Disease Control (CDC) released a new set of isolation guidelines in 1983 (Table 260–3). Hospitals may utilize the CDC guidelines verbatim or modify them for local use. An isolation manual listing the precautions and the type of isolation a specific disease requires should be distributed to each ward. Infection control practitioners then review on-ward practices to assure compliance and to prevent unnecessary isolation, which is costly and inefficient. "Isolation" is used to imply that a private room is necessary, and "precaution" is used when a private room is optional or not indicated.

INANIMATE OBJECTS. The inanimate environment of a hospital may serve as a potential reservoir for microorganisms. Water in flower vases may contain up to 10^9 organisms per milliliter (usually *Pseudomonas*), and stethoscopes are capable of being colonized. The risks associated with toilets and laundry chutes appear minimal. In one cancer hospital, fireproofing materials were shown to be a reservoir for *Aspergillus*, which caused deep tissue infections in patients. In all outbreaks of nosocomial *Aspergillus* pulmonary infections, the mode of transmission was airborne.

Based on the limited amount of information available, several recommendations can be made: (1) Flower vases probably do not belong in burn units or intensive care areas. (2) Patients on isolation should be issued a single stethoscope to be used by all physicians entering the room. In addition, alcohol swabs will kill most bacteria on the stethoscope to be used on high risk patients (those with severe dermatitis or burns). (3) Prior to construction or installation of waste disposal chutes, fire-proofing material, or other environment changes, an infection control specialist should be consulted. (4) In general, routine culturing of the inanimate environment should be discouraged. Only in working up an outbreak might this be essential.

STERILIZATION AND DISINFECTION. In order to reduce the number of organisms that come in contact with patients, sterilization, disinfection, and antiseptics are employed. Sterilization refers to the killing of all forms of microbiologic life, including spores. The term disinfection implies that there is a marked reduction of the number of microorganisms but that spores are not killed. Antiseptics are degerming agents which can be used on the skin.

Sterilization. Two types of sterilization are generally employed in hospitals: autoclaving and gas. The former, use of moist heat under pressure, is the more effective and less expensive method. Boiling at normal atmospheric pressure is not sufficient to sterilize (kill spores). Gaseous sterilization, using ethylene oxide, is an acceptable alternative for use on items that cannot withstand heat. The gas is effective at lower temperatures and can penerate plastics and other materials. However, ethylene oxide is an explosive and a skin irritant and is potentially mutagenic and carcinogenic. The Occupational Safety and Health Administration has proposed to reduce the current permissible exposure limit for ethylene oxide from 50 parts per million to 1 part per million as an eight-hour time-weighted average. Therefore, external ex-

TABLE 260–3. NEW ISOLATION PROCEDURES RECOMMENDED BY THE CENTERS FOR DISEASE CONTROL IN 1983

Isolation Category	Private Room Necessary	Masks	Gowns	Gloves	Handwashing	Examples of Diseases for Which It is Recommended
Strict	+	+	+	+	+	Pharyngeal diphtheria; varicella; zoster (localized in immunocompromised patient or disseminated)
Contact	+	For those in close contact	If soiling likely	If contact with infective material	+	Staphylococcal furunculosis in newborns; herpes simplex disseminated, severe primary, or neonatal; methicillin-resistant *S. aureus*
Respiratory	+	For those in close contact	—	—	+	Measles; meningococcal pneumonia, meningitis, or meningococcemia; *H. influenzae*, pneumonia, or meningitis
Tuberculosis (AFB)	+	If patient is coughing	Only to prevent gross contamination	—	+	Tuberculosis
Enteric precautions	Only if patient's hygiene is poor	—	If soiling likely	If contact with infective material	+	Viral hepatitis A; *Salmonella*, *Shigella*, or *C. difficile* enterocolitis
Drainage/secretion precautions	—	—	If soiling likely	If contact with infective material	+	Minor or limited skin infections including those caused by *S. aureus*
Blood/body fluid precautions	Only if patient's hygiene is poor	—	If soiling with blood or body fluids likely	If contact with blood or body fluid	+	AIDS; Creutzfeldt-Jakob disease; viral hepatitis B

haust systems are recommended. Regardless of the method of sterilization used, biologic sterility testing with spore strips must be used to document adequacy of the sterilization process. *Bacillus stearothermophilus* spores are very heat resistant and are used to monitor sterilization processes using moist heat. *Bacillus subtilis* spores are used to monitor the efficacy of gas sterilization processes.

Disinfection. Several different classes of chemical disinfectants exist. Commonly used agents include chlorine, iodine, phenols, hexachlorophenes, alcohols, and second generation quaternary ammonium compounds. They vary in their ability to kill microorganisms, and the type of agent utilized depends upon the likely pathogens and the properties of the object to be disinfected. Two epidemics of idiopathic neonatal hyperbilirubinemia have been linked to excessive use of a phenolic disinfectant plus detergent. Thus, alternatives are recommended for use in the newborn area. Particular care must be taken with hepatitis B virus and the Jakob-Creutzfeldt agent. Both are resistant to killing by most disinfectants, but they are thought to be susceptible to high concentrations of hypochlorite. For the Jakob-Creutzfeldt agent, the preferred method is autoclave sterilization for unusually long times (one hour at 121° C). It has been suggested that if autoclave sterilization is not possible, a one-hour exposure to 1 N sodium hydroxide inactivates Jakob-Creutzfeldt agent. Furthermore, it is less corrosive than hypochlorite for all materials except aluminum.

Bloodstream infections and pseudoinfections and peritonitis have been traced to contaminated povidone iodine and polyximer iodine antiseptic compounds. The organisms were *Ps. cepacia* and *Ps. aeruginosa*, respectively, species that are naturally resistant to many antibiotics, have minimal growth requirements, and are ubiquitous. Their ability to survive in an iodine-containing product has stimulated research into the chemistry of these agents and an increased awareness of infectious complications with antiseptics.

Following isolation of *Legionella pneumophila* from cooling towers, the Centers for Disease Control recommended that cooling towers undergo periodic maintenance to ensure low levels of slime bacteria and algae in accordance with the American Society of Heating, Refrigeration and Air Conditioning Engineers and the Environmental Protection Agency. Field trials are being planned to evaluate the efficacy of various water additives to eliminate *L. pneumophila*.

With respect to the acquired immunodeficiency syndrome (AIDS), the Centers for Disease Control (CDC) have recommended that the same precautions be used as when caring for patients with viral hepatitis B, in whom blood and body fluids likely to have become contaminated with blood are considered infective. The same guidelines also hold for reusable instruments. Specifically, the CDC stated that lensed instruments should be sterilized after use on AIDS patients. A similar statement regarding endoscopes was made by the American Hospital Association's Advisory Committee on Infections Within Hospitals.

HANDWASHING. Proper and frequent handwashing is the most important control measure available in preventing the transmission of infectious diseases in hospitalized patients. The role of antiseptics is secondary in importance to standard handwashing with plain soap and water before and after routine patient contact.

The normal flora of the skin consists of a transient and permanent group of organisms. Transiently present organisms are more often the gram-negative rods and at times *S. aureus.* Permanent flora include the micrococci *S. epidermidis* and *Propionibacterium acnes.* Certain gram-negative rods appear to be persistent after standard handwashing efforts and thus may be part of the permanent flora. *S. aureus* can also become part of the permanent flora of the anterior nares and thereby repeatedly colonize the hands. Soap and water are generally effective in removing the transient flora. Various antiseptics,

including isopropyl and ethyl alcohol, are more effective in reducing, but not eliminating, the permanent flora. Hexachlorophene is highly effective against *S. aureus*, but has little or no activity against gram-negative rods and fungi. In addition, absorption of hexachlorophene through the skin has been shown to cause vacuolization of brain tissue in some infants and experimental laboratory animals, and therefore its routine use for washing babies in the newborn and premature units is discouraged. Aqueous benzalkonium chloride (aqueous Zephiran) is relatively ineffective and will sustain the growth of gram-negative rods. Its use as an antiseptic should be discouraged. Iodine remains an excellent antiseptic with a wide range of action but causes local irritation. Chlorhexidine is also an effective antiseptic but may cause dermatitis with excessive use.

EMPLOYEE HEALTH. The employee health division should be concerned with protecting both patients and employees from the transmission of infectious diseases. Problems most frequently arise regarding the transmission of tuberculosis, viral hepatitis, herpesvirus infections, and meningococcal infections.

Tuberculosis. The risk of tuberculosis is related to exposure to unsuspected cases among patients. After patients have been placed in respiratory isolation, the risk becomes minimal. Unfortunately, routine chest x-rays are not specific or sensitive enough to screen for suspected cases. The addition of a tuberculin skin test for all patients who have respiratory symptoms or radiographic abnormalities may lead to earlier diagnosis and may prevent early transmission.

All employees should receive a tuberculin skin test (intermediate strength or 5 tuberculin units PPD-S) prior to beginning work. These are repeated yearly or three months after exposure to an initially unsuspected case. Employees who convert their PPD skin test result from negative to positive (10 mm induration or greater) should be considered for therapy with isoniazid (INH), 300 mg per day for one year.

Viral Hepatitis. Transmission of hepatitis A to employees or other patients is very unusual. Unlike hepatitis B and non-A non-B viral hepatitis, hepatitis A is transmitted almost exclusively by the fecal-oral route. In addition, peak viral excretion occurs prior to development of symptoms. Enteric precautions are probably effective in protecting medical personnel from acquiring hepatitis A from hospitalized patients with the disease.

Hepatitis B is transmitted by parenteral or mucous membrane exposure to infected blood or body fluids. Because of their frequent exposure to blood from accidental needle sticks and blood spills, medical personnel are at increased risk. The prevalence of both HB_sAg and anti-HB_s has been shown to be higher in medical personnel than in control populations: approximately 15 per cent of physicians are positive for anti-HB_s, and 1 per cent carry HB_sAg. Dentists and oral surgeons appear to be at even higher risk.

With the availability of a safe and effective vaccine for viral hepatitis B, the protection of employees at risk by vaccination should be a high priority. Despite the institution of proper isolation of infected patients, needle stick accidents will occur. Currently it seems reasonable to draw blood from both the donor (source) and the recipient in order to clarify the risk of transmitting hepatitis B to a susceptible hospital employee. If the donor shows evidence of infection with hepatitis B and the recipient is susceptible, then both high titered anti-hepatitis B immunoglobulin (HBIG) and the first dose of vaccine should be offered to the hospital worker. At one month and six months, the second and third doses of vaccine should be given. A second dose of high titered globulin is *not* necessary. If there is concern about the transmission of either hepatitis A or non-A non-B hepatitis, standard immune serum globulin could be given, although its efficacy in preventing non-A non-B disease is uncertain. This virus has replaced hepatitis B as the most common cause (80 per cent) of post-transfusion-related hepatitis. Its exact role in needle stick–associated disease, however, is unknown.

Herpes Infections. Nonimmune personnel having direct contact with the oral secretions of patients are at risk for developing herpes skin infections. Usually a nurse involved in suctioning a tracheostomy comes in contact with virus-contaminated secretions at the site of a locally traumatized or minimally lacerated finger. This exposure is followed by the development of a localized, painful, herpes simplex infection referred to as "whitlow." These infections are often misdiagnosed as bacterial infections and may get secondarily infected if incised and drained. The use of gloves will probably prevent the transmission of herpes, although personnel with vesicles should avoid contact with immunosuppressed patients, including neonates.

Meningococcal Disease. Few events produce more panic among hospital employees than exposure to a patient suspected of having meningococcal disease. Nevertheless, cases among exposed medical personnel are very rare. Secondary attack rates are significantly higher in household contacts. Close contact with the index case appears to be required. Guidelines recommended by the Centers for Disease Control include the following: (1) Suspected cases of meningococcal disease should be placed in respiratory isolation immediately. (2) A contact list of those who have had *close* (possible secretion) contact with the case should be compiled. The Public Health Department should be notified immediately to supervise the identification of contact exposures made in the community prior to admission. (3) Personnel who have known close contact should be given antimicrobial prophylaxis as soon as possible and should not await cultural confirmation of the diagnosis or susceptibility testing. Recommended prophylaxis for adults is rifampin, 600 mg orally daily for four days. If rifampin is not tolerated, minocycline, 100 to 200 mg orally every 12 hours, can be given for three days. Sulfonamides may be used only if the organism has been shown to be sensitive. Penicillin is not effective for prophylaxis for elimination of the carrier state. (4) Routine nasopharyngeal cultures of employees are not useful. (5) Indiscriminate use of prophylactic therapy should be discouraged (in those who have had fleeting or casual contact). (6) In the setting of an epidemic, the use of vaccines an adjunct to antimicrobial prophylaxis should be considered if the offending organism is in the serogroup A or C.

AIDS. With the increasing numbers of patients with AIDS being hospitalized, there has been a parallel increase in hospital workers' concern for their health risks. The extremely low risk has been recently stressed by the Infectious Disease Society of America. There is no evidence for transmission of this disease by casual contact. As of late 1986, only two instances of seropositivity have been recognized in hospital employees who were in no apparent risk group. Furthermore, only three of over 1500 employees who have sustained a needle-stick injury or direct exposure to potentially infectious secretions from patients with AIDS have developed antibody to HTLV-III. The Centers for Disease Control have developed numerous guidelines for hospitals.

American Hospital Association: A hospitalized approach to AIDS. Recommendations of the Advisory Committee on Infections Within Hospitals. Infect Control 5:242, 1984.

Bennett J, Brachman S: Hospital Infections. Boston, Little Brown & Company, 1986. Wenzel RP: Prevention and Control of Nosocomial Infections. Baltimore, Williams and Wilkins, 1987. *Recently published, scholarly texts on nosocomial infections.*

Centers for Disease Control: Recommendation for preventing possible transmission of human T-cell lymphotrophic virus Type III/lymphadenopathy-associated virus from tears. MMWR 34:533, 1985; Recommendation for preventing transmission of infection with human T-lymphotrophic virus type III/lymphadenopathy-associated virus in the workplace. MMWR 34:681, 1985; Update: Revised Public Health Service definition of persons who should refrain from donating blood and plasma—United States. MMWR 34:547, 1985.

Garner JS, Simmons BP: CDC guidelines for isolation precautions in hospitals. Infect Control 4 (Special Suppl):245, 1983.

Infectious Diseases Society of America: Acquired immunodeficiency syndrome. J Infect Dis 154:1–9, 1986. *Statement of the Infectious Diseases Society of America regarding the very low risk of transmission of AIDS to hospital workers from infected patients.*

Kunin CM: Detection, Prevention and Management of Urinary Tract Infections. 4th ed. Philadelphia, Lea & Febiger, 1986. *A readable reference that provides both basic and advanced knowledge regarding all aspects of urinary tract infections.*

Russell AD, Hugo WB, Ayliffe GAJ: Principles and Practice of Disinfection, Preservation and Sterilization. Boston, Blackwell Scientific Publications, 1982. *Provide detailed discussion of the chemical agents and modes of action, as well as tests of sterility. Two chapters are devoted specifically to issues in the hospital.*

The SENIC Project: The study on the efficacy of nosocomial infection control by the Centers for Disease Control. Methods published as a special issue of the American Journal of Epidemiology 111 (May) 1980. *The final report in the same journal 116 (February) 1985.*

Simmons RL, Howard RJ: Surgical Infectious Diseases. New York, Appleton-Century-Crofts, 1982. *Comprehensive review of infections in surgical patients.*

261 ADVICE TO TRAVELERS
Jeffrey A. Gelfand

Travelers frequently make precise arrangements with connecting flights, hotels, theater tickets, and tours—yet give little or no advance consideration to their health while traveling. This can result in disrupted plans, physical misery, serious illness, and considerable expense. Vaccination requirements for entering different countries vary and depend on where the traveler stopped en route. There are several publications that address these issues. The most useful of these is published annually by the Centers for Disease Control (CDC): *Health Information for International Travel*. It contains a compendium of the vaccination requirements for entry into other countries, epidemiologic information, current CDC recommendations for vaccinations, chemoprophylaxis, and other helpful information. It can be obtained for $5.00 by writing to the Superintendent of Documents, U.S. Government Printing Office, Washington, D.C. 20402; telephone (202) 783-3238. The HHS publication number is the year followed by "8280" (e.g., 88-8280). Finally, local health departments and "Traveler's Clinics" (now available in a number of hospitals) can provide up-to-the-minute information about changing epidemiologic and vaccination requirements.

Travel to Europe, Australia, and New Zealand poses no greater health hazard than travel in the United States or Canada. The risks of travel to other areas vary greatly from country to country and depend on the traveler's local living conditions and length of stay. In general, brief visits to large cities, with accommodations in good tourist hotels and meals in reputable restaurants, carry little risk of exotic infection. Travel to rural areas may greatly increase such risks.

GENERAL MEASURES

Gastronomic curiosity should be restrained by prudence. Meat and fish should be well cooked. Smoking, salting, and drying are not sufficient to kill tapeworm cysts. Peelable raw fruits and vegetables with unbroken skins are safe if peeled by the diner and the skin discarded. Lettuce is especially to be avoided, as it is virtually impossible to cleanse it of protozoal cysts. In general, dairy foods, including local cheeses, should be avoided. Milk can be safely consumed after boiling. Untreated water should be avoided, as should ice. Alcohol does not confer "sterility" to local water, and many pathogens can tolerate alcohol better than can the traveler. Very hot tap water is safer but not risk-free. Bottled water is not necessarily safe, although carbonated bottled water and beverages usually are. Tea and coffee made with boiled water are safe. Beer and wine present few hazards (save for the next morning). While recent evidence suggests that following such rules will not help the traveler evade the ever-present threat of uncomplicated traveler's diarrhea (see Ch. 289), these measures are likely to reduce the probability of developing more serious food-borne bacterial and parasitic diseases. Swimming in fresh water in tropical areas where schistosomiasis is found should be avoided; salt water and chlorinated pools are safe. Walking barefoot could lead to infection with hookworm or *Strongyloides*. Measures to prevent insect bites (clothing, netting, repellents) should be strongly considered where appropriate. There is no other preventive measure for dengue, for example. Patients should be cautioned against taking over-the-counter medications proffered by pharmacists and physicians abroad. These medications, as well as prescription drugs, may contain agents of dubious efficacy and significant toxicity. For example, chloramphenicol may be present in cold remedies. Finally, lists of English-speaking physicians can be supplied by the American and other consulates general.

IMMUNIZATIONS

There are two immunizations occasionally required for entry into other countries—yellow fever and cholera. In general, these vaccinations are not required for travel from the United States, to Canada, Mexico, Europe, or Caribbean countries, nor for re-entry to the United States. Measles, mumps, and rubella are still widespread in many countries. Approximately 50 per cent of imported measles cases reported for 1980 to 1983 were in citizens returning to the United States. Those born before 1957 are presumed to be immune. All persons born in 1957 or later should have been immunized. If one lacks documentation of prior live-measles vaccination, evidence of immunity, or physician-diagnosed measles, vaccination is indicated. Persons who received killed virus vaccine during 1963 to 1967 should be revaccinated. Female travelers of childbearing age should be immune before leaving the United States. All travelers should receive a tetanus-diphtheria toxoid booster if the tetanus immunization status is uncertain, or if 10 or more years have passed since the last vaccination. Polio is a real threat in developing nations, and all travelers to such areas should receive a booster dose of trivalent oral polio vaccine (TOPV). Adults not previously immunized should receive the primary series of inactivated polio vaccine (IPV). Those with depressed immune function should receive IPV, as should the family members of those who are immunosuppressed.

CHOLERA. The risk of cholera to most tourists is low, and cholera vaccines are of limited effectiveness in protecting against clinical cholera. Vaccination is not recommended unless the traveler will be visiting an area experiencing an outbreak or living in an endemic area with poor sanitation. Travel to other countries from such areas may require vaccination as a condition of entry.

HEPATITIS A. Antibody for hepatitis A can be measured to determine susceptibility. Immune serum globulin is effective in reducing the risk of hepatitis A in those without pre-existent antibody. A dose of 5 ml is recommended for adults traveling in the developing world or areas with poor sanitation for periods of over three months, and is repeated every four to six months. For those staying in endemic areas for a briefer period, a dose of 2 ml can be used.*

HEPATITIS B. Hepatitis B vaccine (HBV) is not generally recommended for travelers, save for medical personnel who might handle blood or blood-derived fluids, persons residing for long term, or those expecting to have sexual contact in areas of high endemicity for hepatitis B, such as Southeast Asia, sub-Saharan Africa, and Haiti. Antibody titers should be measured prior to immunization, as immunity may already

---

*These dosages differ from the manufacturer's recommendations.

be present. Deltoid vaccination is preferred, to ensure intramuscular vaccination. Six months are required to complete the primary immunization series before travel.

JAPANESE ENCEPHALITIS. Japanese encephalitis vaccine (JEV) should be considered for those residing (for more than one month) in endemic rural areas of India, Bangladesh, China, Korea, Thailand, and elsewhere in Southeast Asia. It is readily available in Japan but is available in the United States only from the CDC Vector-Born Viral Disease Branch (telephone [303]-221-6429).

MEASLES. For those born after 1956 without prior physician-documented history of the disease or immunization, vaccination is advised.

PLAGUE. Plague vaccine is recommended only for those traveling to enzootic rural areas of Asia, South America, and Africa.

RABIES. Anyone anticipating exposure to animals in an enzootic or epizootic area ought to receive pre-exposure prophylaxis. Simple residence for several months in such an area is sufficient for some to advocate vaccination. A new human diploid cell vaccine is now available in the United States.

SMALLPOX. Smallpox vaccine should not be given for international travel.

TYPHOID. Typhoid vaccination is only partially effective, and the protective effect may be overcome by large inocula. It is recommended for travelers to endemic areas experiencing an outbreak. Highly susceptible travelers (patients with achlorhydria, immunosuppression, sickle cell disease) should be immunized.

YELLOW FEVER. Yellow fever vaccination is recommended for travel to endemic areas of South America and Africa. Vaccination is also required for travel to and between such areas. It can be given only at designated Yellow Fever Vaccination Centers (travelers should check with the local board of health).

MALARIA CHEMOPROPHYLAXIS

Travelers to areas where malaria is endemic should receive prophylaxis. Malaria chemoprophylaxis is not recommended for those visiting only urban centers of Asia (China, Indonesia, Malaysia, the Philippines, Thailand) or South America (except the Amazon River basin areas and the Ecuadoran coast), or those with only daytime exposure in rural areas. Travelers to malaria-endemic areas of Africa, India, Bangladesh, and Pakistan, including urban areas, are at considerable risk. All such travelers should receive one dose of chloroquine phosphate (300 mg base or 500 mg salt) weekly (on the same day of the week), beginning one to two weeks before entering and continuing six weeks after leaving malarious areas. Considerable change and controversy have developed with regard to additional recommendations for preventing malaria in travelers to areas with chloroquine-resistant *Plasmodium falciparum* (CRPF) and reflect both the severity of reactions to prophylactic therapy and changing resistance patterns. Regardless of the prophylactic regimen employed, malaria may still develop. This further emphasizes the fact that general protection measures (netting, screens, repellants, etc.) and prompt recognition and treatment of possible malaria are imperative.

In areas where CRPF is infrequent, only weekly chloroquine is recommended. In areas where CRPF is endemic, but travel will be less than three weeks, weekly chloroquine should continue, but travelers should be provided with a single-treatment dose (three tablets) of Fansidar (pyrimethamine-sulfadoxine) to be kept in their possession during travel. They should be advised to take the Fansidar promptly in the event of a febrile illness during or after their travel, if professional medical care is not available. As considerable *combined* chloroquine and Fansidar resistance now occurs in *P. falciparum* in East Africa and Thailand, an alternative regimen (although not officially recommended by the CDC) for presumptive therapy would be quinine sulfate 650 mg every eight hours for three days, plus tetracycline 250 mg every six hours for seven days. Fansidar should not be used by anyone with a history of sulfa allergy. An alternative regimen for short-term prophylaxis of CRPF is doxycycline 100 mg *daily*, taken with weekly chloroquine prophylaxis. There are considerably fewer data to confirm the efficacy of this regimen, however, and photosensitivity with sun exposure and contraindications in children and pregnant women limit its usefulness.

For longer-term travel in CRPF areas, or very intense exposure, consideration should be given to the addition of Fansidar, one tablet weekly, to the weekly dose of chloroquine. The individual risk of developing CRPF malaria must be balanced against both the risk of potentially serious side effects of Fansidar and the risk of failure of prophylaxis. Fansidar has been associated with 24 episodes of erythema multiforme, Stevens-Johnson syndrome, or toxic epidermal necrolysis in American travelers, seven of these fatal. The incidence of fatal reactions in Americans has been estimated at between 1 in 11,000 and 1 in 25,000 users. In addition, serum-sickness, hepatitis, and exfoliative dermatitis have been described with Fansidar. Obviously, anyone with sulfa sensitivity should avoid the drug, and any ill effects should terminate its use. An alternative to weekly prophylaxis with chloroquine and Fansidar for the long-term traveler is weekly chloroquine plus daily doxycycline (100 mg), with the same limitations as previously noted. Finally, there is the alternative of presumptive therapy, as previously outlined. Travelers returning from prolonged, heavy exposure in areas where *P. vivax* and *P. ovale* are endemic can be given a course of primaquine phosphate during the last two weeks of post-exposure chloroquine prophylaxis to prevent relapse from extraerythrocytic infection, although such therapy is not recommended for the average traveler. In such persons, glucose-6-phosphate dehydrogenase deficiency should be ruled out prior to primaquine therapy.

TRAVELER'S DIARRHEA

This frequent problem is discussed in Ch. 289.

ADVICE ON RETURNING HOME

The most important single piece of advice is to remind the traveler to include the history of travel when seeking medical attention. Delay in the diagnosis of falciparum malaria can be fatal. Febrile illnesses should never be assumed to be "the flu." Vague gastrointestinal symptoms may be due to giardiasis, frequently overlooked. The clinical onset of certain diseases may occur months or even years after the traveler returns home, and the traveler should be reminded of this possibility.

Centers for Disease Control: Health information for international travel. U. S. Public Health Service, Dept. of Health and Human Services (publication no. [CDC] 87-8280), 1987. *This is a thorough and helpful guide with information on a country-by-country basis. It is the best single reference, and every physician dealing with travelers should have access to a copy.*

Centers for Disease Control: Revised recommendations for preventing malaria in travelers to areas with chloroquine-resistant *Plasmodium falciparum*. MMWR 34:185, 1985. *This bulletin contains critical information regarding the risk of developing chloroquine-resistant falciparum malaria in various areas and outlines the official CDC recommendations for prophylaxis.*

Miller KD, Lobel HO, Pappaioanou M, et al.: Failures of combined chloroquine and Fansidar prophylaxis in American travelers to East Africa. J Inf Dis 154:689, 1986. *Documents P. falciparum infection in American travelers (one fatal) in whom compliance with prophylactic therapy was proven by adequate serum levels of both chloroquine and sulfadoxine.*

Wyler DJ: Malaria-resurgence, resistance, and research. N Engl J Med 308:875, 1983. *A comprehensive review. Includes such problems as Fansidar-resistant P. falciparum, and other topics beyond the scope of this chapter.*

SECTION TWO / BACTERIAL DISEASES
Pneumonia

262 INTRODUCTION TO PNEUMONIA

Waldemar G. Johanson, Jr.

Pneumonia is a term used to indicate inflammation of the distal lung—terminal airways, alveolar spaces, and interstitium. To improve the precision of communication, the term "pneumonia" is usually further qualified with words that imply an etiology, mechanism, anatomic site, or clinical course. Thus, descriptors such as "viral bronchopneumonia," "aspiration pneumonia," "chronic interstitial pneumonia," or "acute bacterial pneumonia" serve to identify patients with clinical illnesses characterized by signs and symptoms of lung inflammation in a variety of clinical situations. This chapter will provide the background for the ensuing chapters that deal with specific forms of bacterial pneumonia.

PATHOPHYSIOLOGY. Bacterial pneumonia can be simply defined as a condition that results when host defense mechanisms are insufficient to meet a bacterial challenge presented to the lungs. This definition emphasizes the two key aspects of bacterial pneumonia—host defenses and the type and route of bacterial challenge.

Bacterial Challenges to the Lungs. Bacteria may be introduced into the lungs by any of four routes (Table 262–1). The most common routes are aspiration of contaminated oropharyngeal secretions and inhalation of airborne bacteria. Organisms arriving in the lungs via the bloodstream may produce pneumonia, but the originating site of infection and the severe systemic effects of sepsis usually outweigh the importance of the resulting pneumonia. Direct extension from a focus of infection adjacent to the lungs is uncommon, and the initial site of infection is always more important.

Aspiration of contaminated oropharyngeal secretions is by far the most common route of lung inoculation leading to pneumonia. Organisms transmitted from person to person are usually deposited in the nose or mouth by one means or another, including the inhalation of large droplets generated by cough, sneeze, or even talking. These organisms initially establish themselves in the nasopharynx or oropharynx, where they join the plethora of organisms already present and multiply to achieve high local concentrations. They gain entry into the lungs in a bolus of secretions in the company of other organisms. Aspiration of large amounts of oropha-

TABLE 262–1. ROUTES OF BACTERIAL INOCULATION OF THE LUNGS

Aspiration of contaminated oropharyngeal secretions
Inhalation of airborne bacteria
Bacteremia
Direct extension into the lungs

ryngeal secretions occurs regularly in individuals with impaired levels of consciousness, but aspiration of small volumes of secretions occurs regularly, at least during sleep, in normal people as well. The concentration of aerobic bacteria in upper respiratory tract secretions is about 10^8 organisms per milliliter, while that of anaerobic organisms is about 10 times greater. Thus, aspiration of even small quantities of oropharyngeal secretions causes inoculation of the lung with an enormous bacterial challenge.

The number of bacteria present in ambient air is small, although some are available for inhalation with each breath. The organisms present are highly selected by environmental conditions, as they must have survived aerosolization, drying, temperature changes, and ultraviolet irradiation. Further, since only a few bacteria will be inhaled with each breath, those that arrive in the lungs must be capable of causing infection with a very small inoculum; this is not true for most pathogenic bacteria. In fact, the inability of investigators in the early twentieth century to produce pneumonia in experimental animals by exposing them to massive numbers of aerosolized bacteria nearly halted research on the airborne transmission of disease. Subsequently it was learned that a few organisms meet all of the criteria listed above and are often transmitted by the airborne route. *Mycobacterium tuberculosis* was one of the first to be identified. The infective dose may be as low as a single organism, most often resulting in only a positive skin test as the evidence of infection. Many viruses are transmitted by this route as well. However, the list of bacteria capable of transmission by this route is short and includes only organisms that are unusually invasive, such as the plague bacillus, and organisms particularly adapted to certain environments, such as *Legionella*, so that they are present in large numbers in the air in confined spaces such as buildings served by contaminated air conditioning systems. Organisms capable of airborne transmission often produce outbreaks of infection when groups of susceptible people are exposed, a striking characteristic of *Legionella* infections, for example.

Host Defenses. A variety of mechanisms defends the host against bacterial invasion of the respiratory tract. Some of them should be evident from the discussion above. The anatomy of the upper air passages is an important aspect of defense against inhaled particulates, including bacteria. Droplets that exceed 10 μ in diameter are deposited by inertial impaction in the upper airways, a process that is promoted by the angulations of these structures. About 90 per cent of particles 5 to 10 μ in diameter are deposited along the tracheobronchial tree, while only those particles of 0.5 to 3 μ diameter tend to be deposited in the alveoli. Smaller particles tend to behave like gas molecules and are exhaled to a large extent. "Droplet nuclei" is the term applied to particles about 1 to 3 μ in diameter containing a single bacterium, the likely infecting unit for organisms transmitted by the airborne route.

Organisms that are deposited in the upper air passages are immediately exposed to local secretions. The antibacterial capacity of normal respiratory secretions has been investigated for many years without a firm conclusion. There is little doubt that an antibacterial effect can be demonstrated under various experimental conditions or in vitro. These effects have been attributed to a variety of factors, including lysozyme, complement, immunoglobulins, and products of resident bacteria. The biologic significance of these factors remains uncertain, however. Of much greater significance is the process of physical removal effected by the movement of secretions toward the esophagus and ultimate swallowing.

To avoid physical removal, newly arrived bacteria must persist in the upper air passages. This is facilitated by adherence of bacteria to the regional epithelium. Normal mucosal cells of the upper respiratory tract contain cell-surface receptors for a variety of bacteria. The chemical nature of receptors for different species of bacteria is highly variable, and the site

of the receptor may be either an integral part of the cell surface or contained in proteins attached to the cell. For example, *Streptococcus hemolyticus* binds to fibronectin, a protein that is not an integral constituent of the cell membrane but is acquired normally by respiratory mucosal cells following exposure to respiratory secretions. By contrast, gram-negative bacilli such as *E. coli* or *P. aeruginosa* adhere in large numbers to respiratory cells only after the surface fibronectin is removed. While many details of bacteria–host cell adherence remain to be defined, it is clear that this phenomenon is a major determinant of the composition of the normal bacterial flora of the oropharynx and that changes in adherence are important in promoting or inhibiting colonization of this region by exogenous bacteria.

Under ideal conditions aspiration of oropharyngeal secretions is prevented by the normal swallowing mechanisms and the presence of reflexes that close the vocal cords when foreign materials enter the larynx. The latter are highly effective in preventing the aspiration of large volumes of fluid in normal persons but apparently do not prevent the aspiration of small volumes, at least during sleep. In view of the high concentration of bacteria in oropharyngeal secretions, aspiration of even 0.0001 ml may be important in initiating pneumonia, depending upon the nature of the bacteria aspirated and the state of lung defenses. Aspiration of such volumes may be an everyday occurrence in normal people and the infrequence of pneumonia due principally to lung defenses.

The first line of defense against bacteria that have gained entry into the lungs is physical removal from the airways. This is accomplished by the mucociliary escalator, an integrated multifaceted system consisting of the ciliated cells lining the airways, the secretory cells (goblet cells and submucosal glands), and the secretions. Propulsion of secretions toward the mouth is provided by cilia beating at the incredible rate of 1200 times per minute. However, the effectiveness of this activity depends on the perpendicular depth and the viscosity of secretions. The perpendicular depth of secretions within the airways appears to be relatively constant. This is somewhat puzzling when one considers the total cross-sectional area of the airways, which becomes markedly smaller as the large number of peripheral airways converge on the fewer central bronchi and ultimately on the trachea alone. Mucus moves twice as rapidly in the trachea as in small bronchi but the difference in area is much greater, a finding that has led to speculation that fluid in secretions must be resorbed in proximal airways to maintain the perpendicular depth of the mucous layer in a range compatible with the length of the cilia. Obviously, processes that impair ciliary movement, cause excessive secretion of respiratory mucus, or change the viscosity of secretions may each impair the effectiveness of this transport system.

Bacteria that penetrate to the distal airways or alveoli are killed in situ prior to physical transport out of the lung. The principal mechanism of bacterial killing is ingestion and killing by phagocytic cells. The quantitative aspects of this phenomenon have been extensively investigated in experimental animals, using a variety of bacterial species. The initial experiments were performed with relatively nonpathogenic staphylococci, and the results indicated that the antibacterial capacity of the lung is enormous and that phagocytosis and killing are accomplished almost solely by resident alveolar macrophages. This finding fits nicely with the concept that the lung is normally sterile and that polymorphonuclear leukocytes comprise a very small proportion of the total phagocytic cells on the alveolar surface. Further, these experiments indicated that neither antibody nor other humoral components are required for phagocytosis of bacteria on the alveolar surface. Subsequent experiments with more highly pathogenic bacteria showed that the situation is more complicated; some species cause a prompt recruitment of neutrophils, and in fact bacterial killing appears to depend much more upon the availability of neutrophils than on the presence of alveolar macrophages. Further, clearance of viable bacteria from the lung is enhanced by the presence of specific antibody and is delayed in the absence of complement, findings that indicate an important role for circulating factors.

In general, bacterial killing is more efficient following aerosol deposition than following deposition of a fluid bolus containing equal numbers of bacteria. The reasons for this difference are not entirely clear but probably have to do with the local concentration of bacteria, changes induced in the organisms by the process of aerosolization, e.g., loss of capsular material, and the antiphagocytic effects of the fluid bolus in which the bacteria are suspended.

If bacteria on the alveolar surface are not promptly engulfed and killed, an inflammatory response swiftly develops that is characterized by interstitial and alveolar edema and an influx of neutrophils from the vascular space. The chemoattractants responsible for the latter may include bacterial products, activation of complement proteins that are present in small concentration in alveolar lining fluid, and the elaboration of neutrophil chemotactic factors by alveolar macrophages. In any case, once alveolar edema and inflammation are initiated, the process of bacterial ingestion and killing is remarkably retarded. As neutrophils and bacteria accumulate, the local milieu becomes acidic and hypoxic, since ventilation is impaired by alveolar filling. These conditions further impair phagocyte function so that a population of viable organisms persists, albeit with a reduced rate of multiplication.

In the preantibiotic era, patients with pneumonia often improved dramatically on about the seventh day of illness with a sudden loss of fever, a process that was termed the "crisis" or "breaking of the fever." This event correlated with the development of antibody, which interrupted the standoff between bacteria and phagocytes in the consolidated regions of lung. This clinical phenomenon rarely occurs with antibiotic treatment because the drugs assist in bacterial killing. However, many antibiotics penetrate poorly into lung tissue and treatment must be relatively prolonged.

Community-acquired pneumonias are usually due to a single organism, an observation that appears to contradict the aspiration mechanism that necessarily includes multiple species. The susceptibility of individual bacterial species to lung defenses varies widely. While mucociliary transport is presumably equally effective for all bacteria, phagocytosis by the resident alveolar macrophages clearly is not. Further, previous exposure or immunization may have led to the development of antibody against some species, a factor that promotes phagocytosis and killing by neutrophils. The result of these differences is that the lung's defenses select the organism(s) that will go on to cause pneumonia—the species most capable of evading phagocytosis and killing.

A number of conditions are clinically associated with increased risk of bacterial pneumonia. Many of these have been confirmed in studies of experimental animals in attempts to relate susceptibility to pneumonia to specific defects in one or another of the lung's defenses (Table 262–2).

CLINICAL MANIFESTATIONS. The signs and symptoms associated with bacterial pneumonia vary widely depending on several factors, most importantly the nature of the offend-

ing pathogen and the state of the host. Extremes in presentation can be easily described, although most patients will fall somewhere in between. At one extreme is the previously healthy person with pneumococcal pneumonia. Such patients complain of a brief prodromal upper respiratory illness followed by fever, a single shaking chill, pleuritic chest pain, and a cough productive of purulent or "rusty" sputum. Physical examination reveals signs of consolidation which are readily confirmed by chest radiography. Gram's stain of the sputum reveals numerous neutrophils and abundant pneumococci. In such a patient there is no doubt that a lower respiratory tract infection is present, and the stain of the sputum strongly suggests the etiology. At the other extreme might be an elderly, confused patient who presents only with deterioration in mental function. Physical examination reveals only rhonchi without signs of consolidation, and the chest radiograph shows only bilateral lower lobe interstitial infiltrates that might represent acute or chronic changes. Gram's stain of the sputum (obtained with difficulty) shows many squamous epithelial cells, a few neutrophils, and a pleomorphic bacterial flora that includes both gram-positive and gram-negative organisms. In such patients it may not be clear whether or not the patient has pneumonia, and the information at hand offers few clues as to etiology.

The history-taker should explore the presence of risk factors, including chronic illnesses, recent acute illnesses, illness in family members, use of alcohol or other drugs, and possible exposures to infectious agents. A thorough physical examination, posteroanterior and lateral chest radiographs, and blood leukocyte count with differential should be performed. Based on the data available from these steps, it is usually possible to conclude that pneumonia is present and the remaining task is to determine its etiology.

Controversy exists over the proper microbiologic evaluation of the patient with pneumonia because of questions of sensitivity, specificity, cost, and benefit. These problems are created basically by the presence of abundant organisms in the upper tract and the resultant contamination of expectorated specimens. Further, since most patients with pneumonia respond satisfactorily to simple, relatively nontoxic antibiotic regimens, the need to document the etiology of the process is uncertain. It is impossible to define rules that apply to all patients, and knowledgeable physicians will differ in their approach to an individual patient.

There is little disagreement that sputum should be examined microscopically. The portion chosen should be purulent and contain fewer than 10 squamous cells and more than 25 leukocytes per low power field. A well-done Gram's stain will disclose whether or not one species of organism predominates. Often, such specimens contain a vast preponderance of a single species and if these are encapsulated gram-positive diplococci (pneumococci), clumps of large gram-positive cocci (staphylococci), or small pleomorphic gram-negative coccobacilli (*Haemophilus*), a presumptive diagnosis can be made. Problems arise when a predominant organism is less apparent, when enteric gram-negative bacilli are present, or when an adequate specimen cannot be obtained. Special stains for acid-fast organisms, fungi, *Legionella*, *Pneumocystic carinii*, and others should be used selectively when the clinical situation suggests infection with one of these organisms.

Aerobic culture of expectorated sputum suffers from a lack of sensitivity (organisms causing pneumonia are not detected) and specificity (organisms are present which are not the cause of pneumonia); both have been estimated to occur in up to 50 per cent of cases. The results may be improved by microscopic screening of the specimen prior to culture. Other approaches have included washing the specimen repeatedly to remove contamination by oral secretions, and quantitative culture techniques on the assumption that the organism causing pneumonia will be present in the greatest concentration. While both of these techniques have merit, the time and

TABLE 262–2. CONDITIONS ASSOCIATED WITH INCREASED RISK OF BACTERIAL PNEUMONIA

Condition	Impaired Defense Mechanism
Chronic airway obstruction	Reduced mucociliary transport
	Alveolar hypoxia
Pulmonary edema	Reduced phagocyte function
Unconsciousness	Increased aspiration
Immunoglobulin deficiency	Impaired phagocytosis
Neutropenia	Impaired phagocytosis
Viral infection	Altered mucosal adherence
	Reduced mucociliary transport
	Impaired phagocytosis

effort required to perform them preclude their use as a routine part of the evaluation of a sputum specimen.

Contamination of sputum by oral secretions may be avoided by collecting the specimen proximal to the mouth. The most direct approach involves puncture of the trachea with a large-bore needle and insertion of a plastic cannula into the trachea, a technique called transtracheal aspiration. If secretions cannot be harvested by suction, a small amount of sterile saline is injected through the cannula and suction reapplied. In the hands of experienced operators this technique provides better results than sputum examination in some situations. It is most useful in documenting the absence of bacteria in the secretions of individuals with nonbacterial (e.g., viral, mycoplasmal, etc.) pneumonias, but these pneumonias can usually be strongly suspected on clinical grounds alone. In patients in whom an accurate bacteriologic diagnosis is urgently required, such as elderly or immunocompromised patients, contamination of tracheal secretions by aspirated oropharyngeal secretions renders the technique of less value. Absolute contraindications to the performance of transtracheal aspiration include abnormal bleeding/clotting values and an uncooperative patient. The major complications are bleeding and the occurrence of barotrauma, usually manifested as subcutaneous emphysema in the neck only. Because of the risk of bleeding, the procedure should not be performed in patients with a small trachea (children) or in those with a markedly impaired cough who may not be able to expectorate blood effectively. Transtracheal aspiration remains an excellent method for identifying anaerobic bacteria as responsible for pleuropulmonary infections, if this diagnosis cannot be made by other means.

Another method for bypassing the mouth in the collection of specimens is to aspirate directly from the area of lung consolidation, using either physical findings or fluoroscopy to guide the approach. This technique, called transthoracic lung aspiration, has proved to be an excellent technique in children with complicated pneumonias, since sputum samples may be impossible to obtain. In adults, especially those with underlying lung disease, the rate of complications, especially pneumothorax and bleeding, limits its usefulness. This direct approach is further compromised by the fact that the false-negative rate may be as high as 30 per cent.

Fiberoptic bronchoscopy provides a relatively safe way to collect specimens from the periphery of the lung. Specially designed protected brushes are available which permit the operator to obtain endobronchial specimens that have not been contaminated by proximal airway secretions, even though the instrument has traversed the upper airways. Complications of the procedure are infrequent, and the major limiting factors are expense and time. In addition to the small specimens collected by brushing of the peripheral airways, sterile fluid can be instilled and aspirated to obtain material from a larger area of the lung (bronchoalveolar lavage).

In addition to improving the site of specimen collection, increased diagnostic accuracy may accrue from the application of new diagnostic techniques applied to the specimens obtained. A variety of immunologic procedures have been evaluated as alternatives or adjunctives to Gram's stain and culture. Since these procedures usually provide prompt results, they have been referred to as "rapid diagnostic techniques." They depend upon the demonstration of microbial antigens, either capsular or somatic, in the specimen. While pneumococcal capsular material can be readily demonstrated in the sputum of patients with pneumococcal pneumonia by any of several immunologic techniques, it has not been conclusively shown that this approach provides any greater diagnostic accuracy than conventional techniques. It is likely that these newer techniques will find their greatest usefulness in the identification of organisms that are difficult to identify microscopically and/or difficult to recover in culture, such as *Legionella* or *Chlamydia*. As a general rule, it appears that the more distally the specimen is obtained, the more reliable the rapid tests become. Thus, the value of subjecting expectorated sputum to these procedures is uncertain, whereas their use in evaluating bronchoscopically obtained specimens appears to be more fruitful. These immunologic techniques are highly specific. While culture of respiratory secretions casts a broad net, restricted only by the variety of culture media chosen, immunologic techniques can demonstrate the presence of only a narrow spectrum of related organisms. This difference can be either an advantage or a disadvantage depending on clinical considerations. For example, immunologic demonstration of influenza virus in respiratory secretions would unequivocally prove the presence of this infection, whereas proof of the etiology of a complicating bacterial process would require immunologic studies for a variety of bacteria or the presence of a single organism on culture.

Lastly, it must be remembered that cultures of the blood and pleural fluid, if present, provide results that are highly specific if positive. However, only about 30 per cent of patients with bacterial pneumonia are bacteremic. About the same percentage of pleural fluid aspirates are positive in the absence of antibiotic therapy, but since only 10 to 15 per cent of patients with pneumonia have a pleural effusion, the applicability of this approach is limited. Nevertheless, blood cultures should be obtained in patients with serious illness due to pneumonia, and a diagnostic thoracentesis should be performed in patients with effusions large enough to be aspirated safely.

Proper utilization of these techniques must be individually determined for each patient with pneumonia. In many patients, the history, physical examination, radiographic studies, and evaluation of the sputum by Gram's stain provide all the data that might be reasonably required. Invasive procedures should be reserved for those patients in whom a delay in making an accurate diagnosis will have serious consequences or those in whom the diagnosis cannot be reasonably suspected on the basis of simpler approaches.

Dal Nogare AR, Toews GB, Pierce AK: Increased salivary elastase precedes gram-negative bacillary colonization in postoperative patients. Am Rev Respir Dis 135:671, 1987. *Evidence that acute changes in the enzymatic activity of oral secretions mediate bacterial adherence and colonization of the respiratory tract.*

Green GM, Jakab GJ, Low RB, et al.: Defense mechanisms of the respiratory membrane. Am Rev Respir Dis 115:479, 1977. *Still the best, most comprehensive review of lung defense mechanisms.*

Onofrio JM, Toews GB, Lipscomb MF, et al.: Granulocyte-alveolar-macrophage interaction in the pulmonary clearance of *Staphylococcus aureus*. Am Rev Respir Dis 127:335, 1983. *Illustrates how the lung defenses vary in response to differing bacterial challenges.*

van Uffelen R, van Saene HKF, Fidler V, et al.: Oropharyngeal flora as a source of bacteria colonizing the lower airways in patients on artificial ventilation. Intensive Care Med 10:233, 1984. *Demonstrates the progression from oropharyngeal colonization to colonization of distal airways to bacterial pneumonia.*

Wanner A: Clinical aspects of mucociliary transport. Am Rev Respir Dis 116:78, 1977. *An excellent, complete review of the mucociliary system.*

Woods DE, Straus DC, Johanson WG Jr, et al.: Role of salivary protease activity in adherence of gram-negative bacilli to mammalian buccal epithelial cells in vivo. J Clin Invest 68:1435, 1981. *Describes the phenomenon of bacterial adherence to buccal epithelial cells and its acute alteration following surgery leading to gram-negative colonization of the oropharynx.*

263 PNEUMOCOCCAL PNEUMONIA

David T. Durack

DEFINITION. Pneumococcal pneumonia is a common bacterial infection of the lungs caused by *Streptococcus pneumoniae*. This illness is usually characterized by sudden onset, high fever, shaking chills, pleuritic chest pain, and a racking cough that raises thick, blood-stained sputum.

MICROBIOLOGY. Pneumococci are gram-positive streptococci, each organism measuring about 0.8 μ in diameter.

They associate in pairs much more often than in chains. They are not quite spherical, so that on a Gram-stained slide these diplococci look like two short, fat bullets pointing away from each other, with bases touching.

Pneumococci are facultative anaerobes. They flourish in nutrient media containing 5 to 10 per cent blood or serum, and their growth is encouraged by carbon dioxide. On blood agar plates they form circular colonies 0.5 to 1.5 mm in diameter. These are dome shaped at first but often become umbilicated as time passes owing to autolysis of the cocci in the older, central part of the colony. Autolysis is a characteristic attribute of pneumococci; for example, a broth culture full of living pneumococci sometimes spontaneously becomes sterile, containing nothing but bacterial debris, within a day. This self-destruction is caused by a pneumococcal enzyme, L-alanine muramyl amidase. Pneumococci also elaborate a hyaluronidase, but unlike other common pathogens such as staphylococci, clostridia, and pseudomonas, they produce no known toxins. Colonies of pneumococci growing on blood agar are surrounded by a zone of green (alpha) hemolysis caused by a hemolysin, which under anaerobic conditions causes clear (beta) hemolysis. Pneumococci undergo rapid autolysis when exposed to bile or sodium deoxycholate and are highly sensitive to optochin. These characteristics are exploited in the laboratory to distinguish pneumococci from other alpha-hemolytic streptococci.

Possession of a capsule is an important attribute of pneumococci. Each capsule consists of a high molecular weight polysaccharide polymer that forms a glutinous coat around each bacterium. Variations in the composition of these capsular carbohydrates allow serologic differentiation of at least 83 antigenically distinct types of pneumococci. The capsule is also a crucial virulence factor. It confers resistance to ingestion by phagocytes; this can be partially or completely overcome if type-specific antibody and complement are available to opsonize the pneumococci. Encapsulated, virulent strains form smooth, glistening, mucoid colonies, whereas noncapsulated, nonvirulent strains form rough, dry, granular colonies. The Type 3 pneumococcus is a particularly virulent strain that is noted for producing an abundance of capsular polysaccharide; its colonies are therefore unusually large and mucoid. Admixture of pneumococci with homologous anticapsular serum causes the capsule to become refractile, hence readily visible under the microscope. This is the quellung reaction, which can be used for rapid confirmation of presence of pneumococci in clinical specimens as well as for typing.

Because the lungs in pneumococcal pneumonia can contain as much as 1 to 2 grams of polysaccharide, it is not surprising that this substance can be found in patients' blood and urine by special techniques such as counterimmunoelectrophoresis (CIE). CIE will be positive on blood from one half or more of patients with bacteremia. High levels indicate severe disease and a worse prognosis. Although more valuable in evaluation of meningitis than of pneumonia, CIE occasionally confirms a diagnosis missed by blood and sputum cultures and provides another means to type the pneumococcus. Polysaccharide can sometimes be detected in the urine of a patient with pneumococcal infection for days or even weeks after eradication of living pneumococci.

Pneumococci are ordinarily highly sensitive to a broad range of antibiotics, including the penicillins, cephalosporins, chloramphenicol, erythromycin, tetracyclines, clindamycin, and vancomycin. They are relatively resistant to aminoglycosides. For penicillin, the minimal inhibitory concentration (MIC) is usually 0.01 μg per milliliter or less, but intermediate (MIC 0.1 to 1.0 μg per milliliter) or high-level resistance (MIC 1.0 μg per milliliter or more) can occur. Penicillin resistance in pneumococci, in contrast to gonococci, is mediated by chromosomal mutations, not by plasmids. High-level resistance was extremely rare until 1977, when many resistant strains appeared among pneumococci isolated from children in Dur-

ban and Johannesburg, South Africa. Subsequently, a large number of strains that were resistant to many other antibiotics as well as to penicillin were isolated from patients and carriers in these cities. Currently intermediate resistance can be expected in 2 to 5 per cent of clinical isolates in the United States, and high-level resistance in less than 0.1 per cent. Isolates from blood or cerebrospinal fluid should be screened for penicillin resistance when practicable. Routine sensitivity testing of isolates from sputum is not necessary. The prevalence of antibiotic resistance seems to be stable at present, but clinicians should be alert to the possibility of treatment failures due to antibiotic resistance in the future.

EPIDEMIOLOGY. Pneumococci are commonly present in the upper respiratory tract as part of the normal microbial flora. From 10 to 60 per cent of healthy people carry one or more types of pneumococci at any one time. These are most often the higher-numbered, less pathogenic types, with the exception that Type 3 is carried quite commonly by healthy people. Lower-numbered, more pathogenic types are found less frequently in the oropharynx but presumably must have been acquired transiently by patients who develop pneumococcal pneumonia.

Pneumococci cause about 50 per cent of *all* bacterial pneumonias and 90 per cent of all cases of *lobar* pneumonia. In children, Types 6, 14, 18, 19, and 23 predominate. In adults, Types 1, 3, 4, 6, 7, 8, 9, 12, 14, 18, 19, and 23 cause about four fifths of pneumococcal infections. Typing is not merely of academic interest, because polyvalent vaccines must include antigens from the predominant types.

The ratio of males to females among patients with pneumococcal pneumonia is about 3:2. Most cases occur during winter and early spring, when viral respiratory infections are prevalent. Pneumococcal pneumonia is generally a sporadic rather than epidemic disease; it should not be regarded as highly contagious. Rarely, epidemics of pneumonia have occurred in closed communities when the carriage rate of a pathogenic pneumococcus has become unusually high, and a viral respiratory infection passes through the group. This observation demonstrates that pneumococci carried in the nasopharyngeal flora of healthy persons can cause infection under suitable circumstances. When bacterial pneumonia complicates influenza, the pneumococcus is the most common etiologic agent, followed in frequency by *Staphylococcus aureus*. Therefore, epidemiologists are able to monitor the advent and progress of influenza epidemics by watching the monthly death rate from pneumonias.

PATHOGENESIS. Microorganisms enter the lower airways every day in everyone. The likelihood that pneumonia will result is directly proportional to the *inoculum size* and *virulence* of the organisms, and inversely related to the adequacy of pulmonary *host defenses*. These include the epiglottal and cough reflexes, the carpet of mucus lining the large airways (which is kept moving away from the alveoli at a rate of 1 to 3 cm per hour by the cilia of the respiratory epithelium), lymphatic drainage of alveoli, alveolar macrophages, opsonins, antibodies, and neutrophil leukocytes. Partial or complete obstruction of a bronchus interferes with local defenses and strongly predisposes to infection.

Pneumonia occurs when defenses are impaired and a sufficient number of pneumococci is aspirated (Table 263–1). The central importance of aspiration in pathogenesis is supported by experiments in laboratory animals. Other experiments have shown that fluid-containing alveoli are far more susceptible to infection than are dry alveoli; hence the increased risk of pneumonia in patients with heart failure. Like any aspiration pneumonia, pneumococcal pneumonia shows a predilection for dependent portions of the lung: the lower lobes and the posterior segments of the upper lobes. However, the right middle lobe is involved more often in pneumococcal pneumonia than in other forms of aspiration pneumonia.

The mouse provides a useful model for study of the patho-

TABLE 263–1. CONDITIONS THAT PREDISPOSE TO PNEUMOCOCCAL PNEUMONIA AND OTHER LOWER RESPIRATORY TRACT INFECTIONS BY INTERFERING WITH THE NORMAL DEFENSE MECHANISMS

Impairment of Defenses	Causes
Depressed epiglottal and cough reflexes	Unconsciousness, seizures, alcohol, anesthesia, CNS depressants, neuromuscular diseases
Decreased activity of cilia	Smoking, inhaled pollutants and toxic gases, upper respiratory infections, pertussis, chronic bronchitis, intubation, cilial dysmotility syndromes
Increased secretions	Common cold, other viral respiratory infections, anesthesia, bronchiectasis
Decreased lymphatic flow	Congestive heart failure, tumor
Atelectasis	Tumor or foreign body in bronchi, anesthesia, trauma
Fluid in the alveoli	Congestive heart failure, aspiration, hypoproteinemia, trauma
Abnormality of phagocytes	Neutropenia, sickle cell disease, influenza, asplenia
Abnormality of humoral immunity	Hypogammaglobulinemia, congenital or acquired, e.g., multiple myeloma; starvation; sickle cell disease; hypocomplementemia

genicity of pneumococci. Most encapsulated strains are "mouse virulent"; i.e., injection of only one to ten pneumococci into the peritoneal cavity of a mouse will result in its death from overwhelming pneumococcal bacteremia. If the capsule is removed by treatment with a polysaccharidase before inoculation, more than 1 million of the same pneumococci are needed to kill a mouse. Similarly, a rough (unencapsulated) mutant is far less virulent than its smooth parent. These observations indicate the crucial importance of the capsule as a virulence factor.

Opsonizing antibodies to the capsule are vitally important in host defense against pneumococci. This is evident from the clinical observation that patients with immunoglobulin deficiency are at increased risk for pneumococcal infections. For example, pneumococcal pneumonia occasionally provides the presenting evidence of multiple myeloma. During the first few days of an infection, only nonspecific antibodies possessing relatively weak opsonizing capacity are present in serum. If the patient survives, monospecific anticapsular antibody usually appears after five to ten days, promoting efficient phagocytosis and thus assisting in recovery. Because the issue of death or recovery is often decided before this, great efforts have been made to provide a patient with specific antibodies early enough to influence the course of illness. In the preantibiotic era, passive immunity was provided by administration of specific horse or rabbit antisera, resulting in significant improvement in outcome. Today, a degree of active humoral immunity can be provided by administering polyvalent pneumococcal vaccine to selected high-risk patients.

PATHOLOGY. Once enough inoculum of sufficiently virulent pneumococci has reached the alveoli, pneumonia develops and evolves in a stereotyped fashion. First, fluid pours out from capillaries to fill the alveoli, spreading concentrically outward via the pores of Kohn and the smallest airways to fill adjacent alveoli and acini. This infected tide carries pneumococci into contiguous areas until its flow is stopped by an anatomic barrier, usually the visceral pleura investing a segment or lobe of the lung. Edema fluid containing pneumococci also enters the bronchi, by way of which it can bypass segmental anatomic divisions to involve nearby segments or other lobes. The normally smooth, slippery surface of the pleura overlying an affected segment or lobe becomes roughened as dilated vessels leak plasma and inflammatory cells, forming a patch of fibrinous pleurisy. The movements of breathing then give rise to pleuritic chest pain and a friction rub at the site. Often there is an associated exudative pleural effusion.

Next, the interaction of pneumococci with serum opsonins and complement in the alveolar exudate generates chemotactic factors, which stimulate an outpouring of neutrophils into the alveoli. These phagocytes, together with many red cells that spill out from damaged capillaries, pack the alveoli to cause *consolidation*. Although neutrophils do not phagocytose bacteria efficiently when suspended in fluid, they can ingest pneumococci that are trapped against cell surfaces such as the alveolar wall (surface phagocytosis) or immobilized in consolidated exudate. Thus a finely balanced contest develops between the spreading pneumococcal infection and pursuing phagocytes brought to the site by the host's inflammatory reaction. Even without treatment, polymorphonuclear phagocytes will eventually contain the acute infection in a majority of patients. Therefore, antibiotic treatment should be regarded as only one of many antibacterial mechanisms working together to overcome pneumococcal infection. Antibiotics need not *kill* pneumococci to be effective; bacteriostatic agents work as well as bactericidal drugs in this infection because treatment need only tip the balance slightly in favor of the host, whose phagocytes will then effect cure. Unfavorable factors for the host include a high inoculum, a virulent infecting strain, a wide area of involved lung, lack of specific opsonizing antibody, and anatomic abnormalities such as bronchial obstruction, especially when the patient is elderly and debilitated by other diseases.

Finally, macrophages migrate into the consolidated alveoli and ingest the debris left behind as the acute infection resolves. This, together with expectoration of alveolar contents by coughing, results in ultimate resolution of the exudate. Because the alveolar wall is not destroyed when consolidation occurs, recovery is complete in most cases, with restoration of normal pulmonary anatomy.

In a fully developed case of pneumonia, all of the three main stages of the inflammatory reaction described above may be present at once. At the periphery is a spreading zone of serous edema fluid containing bacteria but few cells. Within is a zone of early consolidation, marked by hemorrhage and migration of neutrophils into alveoli, causing the pathologic appearance graphically described as "red hepatization" by pathologists. In the oldest part of the lesion is found a zone of advanced consolidation in which leukocytes predominate; this is termed "gray hepatization." Here the process of resolution begins.

Pneumococcal pneumonia can develop in a patchy, multifocal, and peribronchial rather than segmental or lobar distribution. This form of the disease may be termed *bronchopneumonia*. It is more common in infants and young children, and in elderly, immobile, or debilitated patients, especially those with cardiac failure, and is often a preterminal complication contributing to, or causing, death.

Spread of Infection. The most common and most important form of spread from the lungs is *bacteremia*. Pneumococci travel via pulmonary lymphatics through hilar lymph nodes to the thoracic duct, thence to the blood. Pneumococci can infect contiguous pleural or pericardial spaces by direct spread from the lung. The organisms may travel via lymphatics, spread across anatomic barriers breached by inflammation, or pass through new communications such as bronchopleural fistulas. Hematogenous seeding of distant susceptible sites can lead to pneumococcal meningitis, endocarditis, pericarditis, peritonitis, arthritis, or ophthalmitis. Metastatic infections have become less common in the antibiotic era.

CLINICAL FINDINGS. The bedside examiner finds a patient suffering from a serious febrile illness, intermittently sweating, breathing fast, distressed by frequent bouts of coughing, and preoccupied with pleuritic pain. The patient may be too ill to cooperate fully with history or examination until these symptoms are relieved.

Many patients have had an upper respiratory infection for several days before the onset of pneumonia. This may be as mild as a common cold or as severe as influenza. Then they experience an abrupt chill, followed quickly by fever, cough, and chest pain, often with rapid progression over 12 to 24 hours. Patients may vomit once or twice early in the course.

The *chill* is often severe, being accompanied by a teeth-chattering, bed-rattling rigor lasting from 10 to 30 minutes. Chills may continue intermittently, but frequently only a single episode of true rigor occurs; repeated rigors over several days are unusual unless a complication has developed. The *fever* is usually high and continuous, with temperatures ranging between 39.5 and 40°C. This contributes to the patient's striking malaise, weakness, myalgia, and prostration. Temperature should be measured rectally, because the patient is usually breathing rapidly through his or her mouth. Anxiety, restlessness, and delirium are common.

Cough occurs in more than 90 per cent of patients; it may be dry at first, but soon the patient begins to raise sputum. This is blood tinged or bloody in about three fourths of cases. The blood is usually well mixed through the sputum rather than streaked on the surface, because bleeding occurs directly into the exudate in the alveoli. This gives the sputum a characteristic "rusty" or "prune-juice" appearance. The pneumococcal capsular polysaccharide itself may be present in the sputum in such abundance as to lend it a sticky, tenacious mucoid character, especially in Type 3 infections. In some cases the sputum is simply mucopurulent.

Chest pain is common and frequently severe. It is stabbing in nature, localized over the involved lobe, and sharply exacerbated by deep breathing or coughing. The patient often carefully adjusts his position in bed in order to "splint" the ribs, reducing chest wall movement over the area of pleurisy. Diaphragmatic pleurisy may cause upper abdominal pain or pain referred to the supraclavicular fossa or shoulder.

On examination, the patient's brow is usually beaded with sweat and his skin is hot. Fresh "fever blisters" of reactivated herpes simplex virus infection are commonly present around the lips. Rapid pulse and wide pulse pressure accompany the fever. Respiratory distress is evident, with tachypnea, dyspnea, and use of the accessory muscles. Breathing may be so restricted by pleuritic pain that each shallow breath is followed by an audible, grunting expiration. Mild central cyanosis may be present owing to alveolar hypoventilation as a consequence of shallow breathing, and to shunting of venous blood through consolidated lung. Shock may supervene.

On inspection, chest wall movements may be diminished on the affected side owing to the combined effect of consolidation of the underlying lung and splinting of voluntary muscles. Palpation confirms decreased respiratory movement and will occasionally reveal a palpable pleural rub. The trachea is usually central but occasionally deviates toward the affected side if there is associated atelectasis, or away from it if there is a large pleural effusion. Vocal fremitus is increased owing to conduction of vibrations from patent bronchi through solid lung.

Percussion reveals dullness over the affected lung, unless the area of consolidation is too small or too deep to be detectable. Even light percussion may cause local pain at the site of underlying pleurisy.

Auscultation over consolidated lung reveals suppressed breath sounds at first, soon followed after 24 to 48 hours by bronchial breath sounds, increased vocal resonance, whispered pectoriloquy, egophony ("*e to a* change"), and crackling rales. A localized pleural friction rub is often present.

Other findings that may be present include *jaundice*, which occurs in a few severe cases and indicates a worse prognosis, and *abdominal distention*, which can be due to gastrectasia (acute gastric dilatation) or generalized ileus. *Neck stiffness* could be due to concomitant meningitis, and the neurologic examination should be at least complete enough to exclude this complication and to detect any focal neurologic signs. Signs of shock or heart failure can be present in severe cases. *Systolic murmurs* in the aortic area are common, most often signifying no more than a high cardiac output. Murmurs caused by aortic or mitral regurgitation should raise the possibility of pneumococcal endocarditis.

Many patients with pneumococcal pneumonia have milder symptoms and less striking physical signs. Not all need admission to hospital.

LABORATORY FINDINGS. The leukocyte count is usually elevated to 15,000 to 30,000 cells per cubic millimeter, with an increased percentage of mature and immature neutrophils. These often show toxic granulation. Painstaking examination of a Gram-stained smear of the buffy coat (if time is available) will show intraleukocytic pneumococci in a few cases, especially in patients who are asplenic. Leukopenia occurs in some severe cases and is associated with a worse prognosis. The infection is usually too short lived to cause anemia; if present, anemia probably reflects a pre-existing condition. Moderate free-water depletion caused by fever and sweating is reflected by raised serum sodium concentration in many patients. Hypovolemia may occur owing to the combined effects of vomiting, vasodilatation, and ileus.

Examination of *Gram-stained sputum* is an important step in evaluation of a patient with pneumonia. Smears containing many epithelial cells associated with normal flora should be discarded, because they are heavily contaminated with saliva and can only be misleading. Presence of many polymorphonuclear leukocytes indicates that the specimen is sputum. A smear showing predominant gram-positive bullet-shaped diplococci associated with pus cells together with a positive *sputum culture* for pneumococci provides good evidence (but not proof) of pneumococcal infection in a patient with pneumonia. Interpretation of the sputum Gram stain should be tempered by the knowledge that false positives are common because pneumococci are part of the normal flora, and that the Gram stain may not correlate with the results of sputum culture. Sputa from many patients with pneumococcal pneumonia show only mixed flora. In practice, the sputum Gram stain is sometimes more useful to help rule out staphylococcal or gram-negative pneumonia than to rule in pneumococcal disease.

In seriously ill patients with pneumonia, further measures to identify the causative organism may be considered necessary. Transtracheal aspiration provides a more reliable specimen for Gram stain and culture than sputum, but about one third of transtracheal specimens will yield one or more contaminating organisms from the upper airways. Direct needle aspiration of the lung will not yield contaminants, but a false-negative result is obtained in about one third of cases. Bronchoscopy is of limited value in diagnosis of acute pneumonia, except when endobronchial obstruction must be excluded. Fortunately, these techniques are not necessary for diagnosis and management of most cases of pneumococcal pneumonia.

Two *blood cultures* should be taken prior to treatment from all patients with pneumonia who are ill enough to be hospitalized. Fifteen to 25 per cent of patients with pneumococcal pneumonia have positive blood cultures. Unlike a positive sputum culture, a positive blood culture proves the diagnosis and also indicates that the patient has a higher risk of complications and death than patients with negative blood cultures.

ROENTGENOGRAPHY. The chest x-ray usually shows a homogeneous opacity in one or more segments or lobes of the lung (Fig. 263–1). An air bronchogram is almost always present, and volume loss is slight or nonexistent. Patients with bronchopneumonia have diffuse, patchy infiltrates on x-ray rather than consolidation. In a patient with emphysema, pneumonia causes poorly defined opacities that are honeycombed with small holes, presumably emphysematous spaces that escape consolidation (Fig. 263–2). Rarely, pneumococcal pneumonia may produce a spherical opacity on the chest film.

Resolution after treatment may be rapid, progressing to completion in two weeks or less, but in some cases the radiologic appearance of consolidation persists for several weeks despite successful treatment. This may cause unjusti-

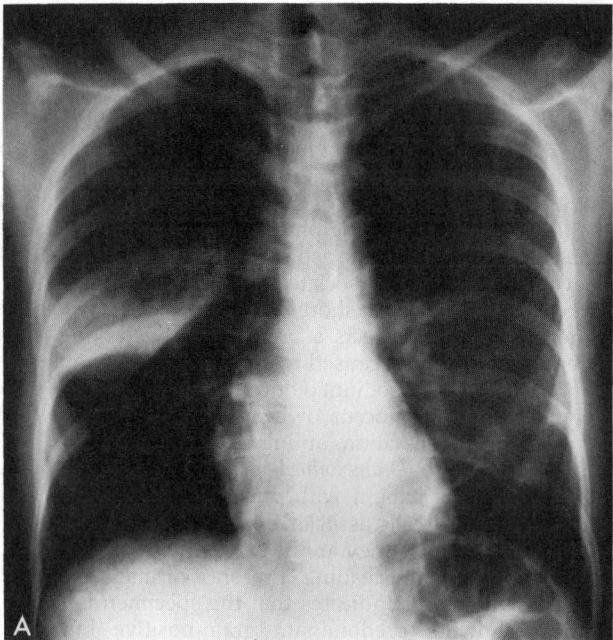

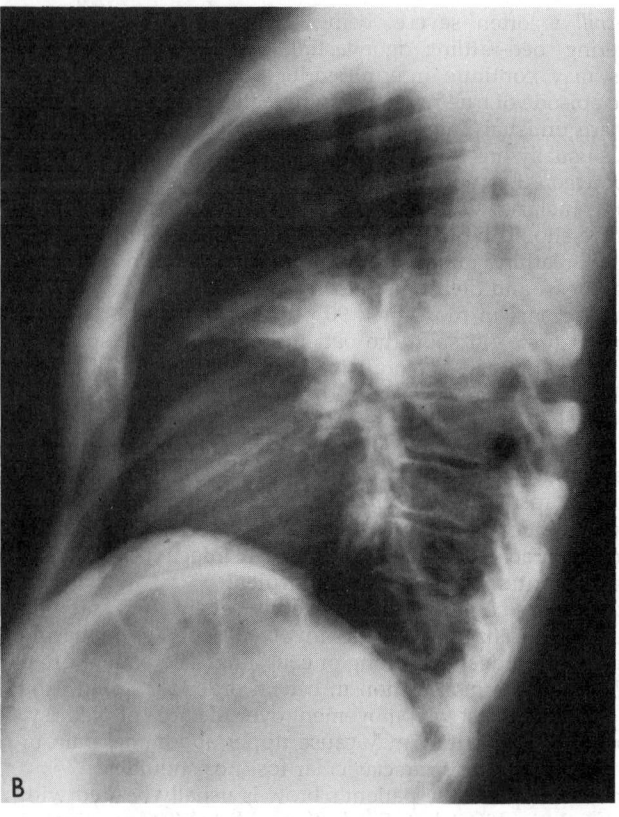

FIGURE 263–1. Chest radiograph from a typical case of pneumococcal pneumonia showing segmental consolidation in the anterior and posterior segments of the right upper lobe, bounded by pleural surfaces. *A*, Posteroanterior view. *B*, Lateral view.

fied alarm and despondency on the part of the physician; therefore, frequent follow-up x-rays should be avoided in patients who are clinically cured. On the other hand, follow-up x-rays are mandatory for patients who do not recover promptly. They may reveal various causes of treatment failure, including tumor, lung abscess, empyema, or bronchopleural fistula.

DIFFERENTIAL DIAGNOSIS. Many other infections can simulate pneumococcal pneumonia. *Klebsiella pneumoniae* causes a form of lobar pneumonia that may be radiologically indistinguishable. Some cases show a bulging interlobar fis-

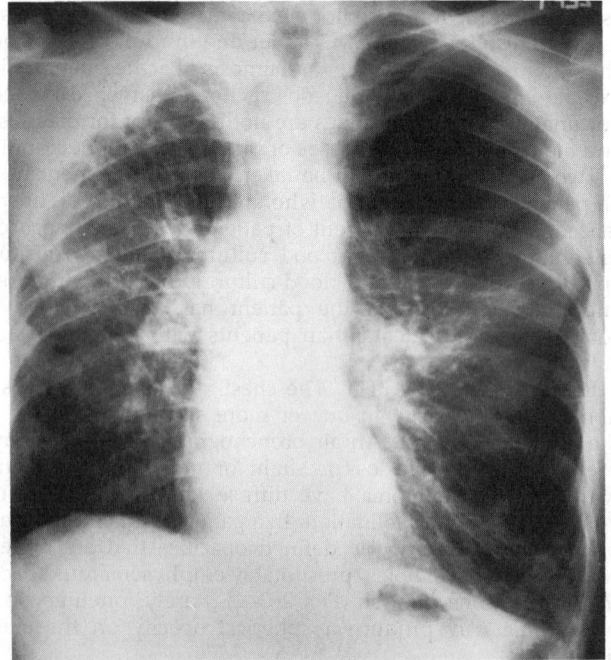

FIGURE 263–2. Chest radiograph showing pneumococcal pneumonia in the right upper lobe of a patient with severe emphysema. Instead of homogeneous consolidation there is diffuse, patchy ("Swiss-cheese") opacification.

sure on x-ray, but this sign is not specific. *Klebsiella* pneumonia shows some predilection for the upper lobes and frequently causes necrosis of pulmonary parenchyma. Patients often produce sputum likened to red currant jelly, composed of necrotic tissue and blood mixed with gelatinous capsular polysaccharide. Staphylococcal pneumonia occurs as a complication of influenza or as part of disseminated staphylococcal infections; it often causes multiple patchy infiltrates that may progress to form pneumatoceles or abscesses. *Haemophilus influenzae* type b pneumonia may be clinically indistinguishable from pneumococcal infection but is much more common in children under five years of age than in adults. *Streptococcus pyogenes* and *Neisseria meningitidis* (usually group Y) are other rare causes of pneumonia that can be distinguished with certainty only by the results of culture.

Mycoplasma and chlamydial pneumonias are usually less acute in onset and less likely to cause lobar consolidation. Patients with tuberculous pneumonia show less acute prostration and are less likely to have neutrophil leukocytosis. Legionnaires' disease usually does not evolve as rapidly as pneumococcal pneumonia, is less likely to show lobar distribution, and more likely to be associated with gastrointestinal upset.

The differential diagnosis between pulmonary infarction and pneumonia is frequently difficult but must be made in order to treat these conditions correctly. Misdirected treatment of pulmonary embolus as pneumonia (or vice versa) can have serious consequences. Careful consideration of the differential features (Table 263–2) may be sufficient to clarify the diagnosis, but in some cases only pulmonary angiography can resolve the issue.

Infections below the diaphragm such as subphrenic or hepatic abscesses can cause fever, cough, low chest pain, referred pain to the shoulder, atelectasis, and pleural effusion, thus closely simulating lower lobe pneumonia. Gonococcal perihepatitis can mimic right lower lobe pneumonia.

TREATMENT. *Supportive measures* are important for the comfort and safety of patients with pneumococcal pneumonia. They should be put at bed rest, without undue disturbances except for regular checks of respiratory rate, blood pressure,

TABLE 263–2. COMPARATIVE FEATURES OF PNEUMOCOCCAL PNEUMONIA AND PULMONARY INFARCTION*

	Pneumococcal Pneumonia	Pulmonary Infarction
Predisposing factors	Alcoholism, measles, debility	Recent trauma or operation; immobility
Previous upper respiratory infection	Frequent	No
Fever, sweating	Yes, usually >39.5°C	Yes, usually <39.5°C
Rigors	Yes	No
Cough	Severe, in paroxysms	Slight or none
Purulent sputum	Yes	No
Hemoptysis	Yes; rusty color, well mixed with sputum	Yes; bright red blood
Pleuritic chest pain, pleural rub	Yes	Yes
Dyspnea, cyanosis	Yes	Yes
Sputum Gram stain	Gram-positive diplococci or mixed flora; leukocytes present	Mixed flora from saliva; few leukocytes
Leukocytosis	Yes, usually >15,000/cu mm	Yes, usually <15,000/cu mm
Shift to the left, toxic granulations	Yes	No
Bilirubin	May be elevated	May be elevated
Arterial oxygen	Moderate reduction	Moderate reduction
Chest roentgenogram	Lobar or segmental opacity	Pleural-based, segmental, wedge-shaped opacity
Radionuclide scan	Matched ventilation and perfusion defect	Matched ventilation and perfusion defect
Pulmonary angiogram	Normal	Obstruction of pulmonary arteries

*In practice, exceptions to these guidelines are common, making this a difficult differential diagnosis.

and urine output until there is clearly no danger that shock will develop.

Adequate *analgesia* is needed, both to relieve distress and to allow deeper breathing and coughing to help raise secretions. Codeine tablets may suffice but will not be adequate for some patients with severe pleurisy or those not absorbing oral drugs because of ileus. These patients should receive parenteral meperidine, 50 to 100 mg every three to six hours until relief is provided, unless there is *real* danger of harming the patient by depressing the respiratory center. In many patients with pneumonia, the benefits of parenteral narcotic treatment for pleuritic pain far outweigh any risks, so they should not be allowed to suffer because of excessive reluctance to use a respiratory depressant. An intracostal nerve block can relieve pleuritic pain without depressing respiratory drive. Aspirin should be avoided because it interferes with evaluation of progress by means of the temperature chart. Moreover, haphazard use of antipyretics can actually increase the patient's discomfort by subjecting him to intermittent swings in temperature with associated heavy sweats. If antipyretic therapy seems truly necessary, it should be given on a round-the-clock dosage schedule.

Because pneumococcal pneumonia is common in alcoholics, delirium tremens often develops during treatment, requiring additional nursing care, sedation, and fluid replacement. Its manifestations must be distinguished from those of unsuspected bacterial meningitis.

Oxygen should be administered to moderately or severely ill patients until improvement begins, preferably by a mask with humidification to avoid desiccation of the mucosae of the upper airways. Intubation and mechanical ventilation may be necessary if respiratory failure develops.

Significant fluid and electrolyte depletion should be treated, with the aim of keeping up a good urine flow with specific gravity less than 1.020 and maintaining the serum sodium below 145 mEq per liter. Because the degree of free-water depletion caused by fever is usually greater than the degree of salt depletion, half-normal saline or quarter-normal saline plus 5 per cent dextrose will usually provide correct replacement therapy. Intravenous fluid therapy is not always needed, because some patients with mild disease have no disturbance of fluid balance.

If the patient has significant distention and discomfort from ileus or gastrectasia, oral treatment should be avoided and nasogastric suction should be instituted until peristalsis returns. Otherwise, patients may be given clear liquids until improvement begins, after which a light diet can be given when the patient requests it. Because the illness is usually brief, tube feeding or intravenous alimentation should not be necessary.

Even though many patients would recover completely without treatment, *antibiotics* reduce mortality, shorten the duration of illness, and prevent development of complications, especially bacteremia and metastatic infections. Therefore all patients should be treated as soon as a clinical diagnosis of pneumococcal pneumonia is made, without waiting for results of cultures.

Penicillin is the drug of choice. The selection of one of several well-tried regimens employing one of the various forms of penicillin (Table 263–3) should be based upon the severity of the illness and convenience for the patient. Neither oral nor intramuscular therapy should be used for patients in shock. For most patients the course of penicillin need not be prolonged beyond five to seven days.

For patients who give a history of penicillin allergy, a cephalosporin often can be substituted, because the cross-reaction rate is low. Care should be taken, however, to administer the first dose in a setting in which an immediate allergic reaction can be treated adequately. For added safety a simple scratch test through a drop of the cephalosporin solution placed on the skin, to look for wheal and flare reaction, may be performed. All beta-lactam drugs should be avoided if the patient has a convincing history of immediate (Type 1) hypersensitivity. These patients, who may not tolerate either penicillins or cephalosporins, may be treated with erythromycin. This antibiotic is also active against *Mycoplasma pneumoniae*. Therefore, it is particularly useful for patients with mild symptoms who could have either mycoplasmal or pneumococcal pneumonia and who could be treated as outpatients.

Response to treatment is usually rapid, gratifying both patient and physician. Temperature often falls to normal by crisis within 24 hours, but persistence of fever with resolution by lysis over several days is *not* uncommon and need not be interpreted as treatment failure. Fever recurring or persisting after three days may be due to a focus of extrapulmonary pneumococcal infection that is more resistant to treatment,

TABLE 263–3. STANDARD ANTIBIOTIC REGIMENS FOR TREATMENT OF PNEUMOCOCCAL PNEUMONIA

For patients with mild symptoms, treated outside hospital	Penicillin V, 500 mg PO four times daily for seven days *or* Erythromycin, 250 mg PO four times daily for seven days*
For inpatients with uncomplicated pneumonia	Crystalline penicillin G, 1.0 million units (600 mg) IV every six hours for five to seven days *or* Procaine penicillin G, 300,000–600,000 units IM every 12 hours for five to seven days
If the patient is allergic to penicillin	Cefazolin, 0.5 gram IM or IV every eight hours for five to seven days
If the patient is allergic to penicillins and cephalosporins	Erythromycin, 250 mg IV every eight hours for five to seven days
For inpatients with pneumonia plus meningitis, pericarditis, arthritis, or endocarditis	Crystalline penicillin G, 3.0–4.0 million units IV every four hours for seven to ten days (meningitis) or two to four weeks (pericarditis, endocarditis)

*If etiology is uncertain, erythromycin is a good first choice because it also treats *Mycoplasma pneumoniae* and *Legionella pneumophila*.

such as empyema, pericarditis, or arthritis. Other causes of fever during treatment include polymicrobial infection, drug fever, or another underlying disease that was overlooked or misdiagnosed. Failure of the pneumonia to resolve may be due to obstruction of a bronchus by tumor or foreign body, or to infection with more than one organism.

COMPLICATIONS. At least 10 to 20 per cent of patients with pneumococcal pneumonia develop a concomitant *pleural effusion*. The true incidence is considerably higher, but the effusions pass unnoticed because patients are not routinely radiographed in the lateral decubitus position. Small effusions usually resolve spontaneously after successful treatment, and pleural aspiration is not mandatory. Pleural fluid should be obtained, cultured, and tested for pH, cell count, protein, and lactic dehydrogenase concentration in severely ill patients, in those with large effusions, in those who do not recover smoothly, and whenever empyema is suspected.

Most parapneumonic effusions resolve after treatment, but a few progress to *empyema*. This complication is more likely to develop in untreated cases, or in patients whose treatment was delayed or inadequate. Empyema occurs in less than 5 per cent of adequately treated patients. The clinical distinction between simple effusions and empyemas is important, because most empyemas require drainage. Small or moderate effusions noted early in the course of treatment often do not require drainage, even though the fluid has the biochemical characteristics of an exudate and occasionally is infected with pneumococci. Later, if the fluid turns to thick pus composed of fibrin, serum, organisms, and disintegrating leukocytes releasing enzymes and nucleic acids, spontaneous resolution is unlikely to occur. At this stage the effusion has evolved into a true empyema; loculations that cannot be drained by simple needle aspiration have usually formed. Drainage via a chest tube should be instituted. Because a thick, infected exudate often cannot move freely with changes in position, radiographic diagnosis of empyemas can be difficult. Loculated empyemas can be misinterpreted on x-ray as unresolved pneumonia, or tumor. Ultrasonography and needle aspiration can help to make the diagnosis.

The possibility that pneumococcal *meningitis* is present in a patient with pneumonia must be carefully considered (even though this complication is uncommon), because meningitis requires a much higher dosage of penicillin than pneumonia for cure (Table 263–3). If there is any doubt about this issue, a spinal tap should be performed. A small subgroup of patients, usually alcoholics, develops the triad of pneumonia, meningitis, and endocarditis (Austrian's syndrome). These patients are always bacteremic, and their prognosis is very grave; about 80 per cent will die despite treatment. First- or second-generation cephalosporins or erythromycin must not be used in a patient with pneumococcal meningitis; if a patient with this complication is allergic to penicillin, a third-generation cephalosporin that provides good concentrations in cerebrospinal fluid (such as cefotaxime 2.0 grams intravenously every four hours or ceftriaxone 2.0 grams intravenously every 12 hours) should be used.

Pneumococcal pericarditis, peritonitis, endocarditis, and arthritis all may occur in association with pneumonia. These conditions are discussed in Ch. 54, 270, and 435, respectively.

PROGNOSIS. The overall case fatality rate for untreated pneumococcal pneumonia is about 25 per cent. This varies widely among subgroups: In young people without pre-existing diseases and without bacteremia, mortality would be only 5 per cent even without treatment, whereas in bacteremic, elderly patients with chronic heart or lung disease, mortality would be about *10 times* higher.

Recognized adverse prognostic factors include pneumonia occurring in old age or in infancy; chronic heart, lung, or liver disease; malnutrition; debilitation; bacteremia; shock; meningitis, endocarditis, or pericarditis; alcoholism or delirium

tremens; advanced pregnancy; involvement of more than one lobe; infection with virulent serotypes, e.g., Type 3; leukopenia; jaundice; and delayed treatment.

In the pre-penicillin era, both serotherapy and sulfonamide treatment improved the prognosis significantly. Penicillin further improved these figures, so that overall mortality is now about 5 per cent. However, for those patients with several major adverse prognostic factors, mortality remains higher than 20 to 30 per cent, even with penicillin treatment and modern intensive care.

PREVENTION. Even though the sputum of a patient with pneumococcal pneumonia contains the etiologic organism, there is negligible risk that medical staff and other patients who come in contact with him will "catch pneumonia." Isolation during treatment is therefore not necessary.

Antibiotic treatment given empirically for viral upper respiratory infections undoubtedly prevents or aborts some cases of pneumococcal pneumonia. However, because upper respiratory infections are hundreds of times more common than pneumonia, the cost and risks of treating all of them with antibiotics outweigh the benefit of preventing an occasional case of pneumonia. In young children with absent or hypofunctioning spleens, long-term, low-dose penicillin prophylaxis may be appropriate, but in this setting the primary aim is to prevent fulminant pneumococcal *bacteremia* rather than pneumonia.

The currently available polyvalent pneumococcal vaccine contains purified polysaccharide antigens derived from the 23 types most commonly recovered from infected patients. These 23 types cause about 90 per cent of pneumococcal infections, and the vaccine is estimated to be about 80 per cent effective. This means that theoretically the vaccine could prevent about two thirds of pneumococcal pneumonias, and possibly some other pneumococcal infections. Not all vaccinated persons will produce protective levels of antibody, and infections caused by types contained in the vaccine have occurred after vaccination. It does not seem to be effective in prevention of pneumococcal otitis. Children less than two years of age should not receive this vaccine, because their antibody response is inadequate. This is unfortunate because among asplenic patients, very young children are at the greatest risk for severe pneumococcal infection.

Present recommendations call for vaccination of high-risk patients over two years of age, including those with sickle cell disease; patients with splenic hypofunction or asplenia; the elderly; and patients with chronic cardiac or respiratory disease. Apart from children with asplenia, this is essentially the same population that should receive influenza vaccine.

Because the vaccine consists of purified polysaccharide, there is no risk of inadvertently causing infection if an immunosuppressed patient is vaccinated. Even though such patients' antibody responses are unpredictable, it is reasonable to vaccinate them in the hope that partial protection will result. Side effects are limited to local tenderness. Immunity appears to be long lasting; patients should not be revaccinated in less than five years, lest a more severe local reaction occur.

Austrian R: Life with the Pneumococcus. Notes from the Bedside, Laboratory, and Library. Philadelphia, University of Pennsylvania Press, 1985. *A potpourri of interesting observations on pneumococci, by a true authority.*

Austrian R, Douglas RM, Schiffman G, et al.: Prevention of pneumococcal pneumonia by vaccination. Trans Assoc Am Physicians 89:184, 1976. *This paper summarizes the rationale for vaccination against pneumococcal infection and gives the results of clinical studies proving efficacy of a vaccine.*

Coonrod JD, Kunz LJ, Ferraro MJ (eds.): Direct Detection of Microorganisms in Clinical Samples. New York, Academic Press, 1983. *The title of this comprehensive volume is self-explanatory. It provides numerous references to detection of pneumococci in body fluids, including notes on counterimmunoelectrophoresis and coagglutination.*

Heffron R: Pneumonia, with Special Reference to Pneumococcus Lobar Pneumonia. New York, Commonwealth Fund, 1939. *This is a classic description of large numbers of patients studied in the preantibiotic era. Valuable today for its superb detail on clinical findings and the natural history of pneumonia.*

Hook EW, Horton CA, Schaberg DR: Failure of intensive care unit support to influence mortality from pneumococcal bacteremia. JAMA 249:1055, 1983. *This clinical brief shows that even the most intensive modern medical care cannot save 30 to 76 per cent of patients with pneumococcal bacteremia and thus emphasizes the need for vaccines.*

Istre GR, Humphreys JT, Albrecht KD, et al.: Chloramphenicol and penicillin resistance in pneumococci isolated from blood and cerebrospinal fluid: A prevalence study in metropolitan Denver. J Clin Microbiol 17:472, 1983. *A short recent paper with current information on the prevalence of antibiotic resistance among clinical isolates of pneumococci in the United States.*

Jacobs MR, Koornhof HJ, Robins-Browne RM, et al.: Emergence of multiply resistant pneumococci. N Engl J Med 299:735, 1978. *An important report describing the emergence of a large number of strains of antibiotic-resistant pneumococci in South Africa. Emphasizes the potential for worldwide spread of resistant strains, and supports the need for an effective vaccine.*

Robbins JB, Austrian R, Lee C-J, et al.: Considerations for formulating the second-generation pneumococcal capsular polysaccharide vaccine with emphasis on the cross-reactive types within groups. J Infect Dis 148:1136, 1983. *An extensive review of pneumococcal serotypes, related specifically to human infection and vaccines.*

Ward J: Antibiotic-resistant *Streptococcus pneumoniae*: Clinical and epidemiologic aspects. Rev Infect Dis 3:254, 1981. *A broad review of the advent and clinical implications of antibiotic resistance among pneumococci.*

264 MYCOPLASMAL INFECTIONS

Stephen G. Baum

In the late 1930's, a group of pneumonias was delineated that did not resemble typical bacterial lobar pneumonia. Because the cause of the pneumonias was unknown, and because the radiographic appearance and low mortality distinguished these cases from pneumococcal and other bacterial respiratory infections, these were called *primary atypical pneumonias*. In the 1950's, the organism responsible for many cases of so-called atypical pneumonia was isolated by Eaton and was shown to be similar to one causing pleuropneumonia in cattle; hence the names Eaton agent and pleuropneumonia-like organisms (PPLO). In 1962, this agent was reclassified as *Mycoplasma pneumoniae*.

The most significant human infections caused by mycoplasmas are diseases of the respiratory tract, including pharyngitis, tracheobronchitis, and pneumonia. Also, one species of mycoplasmas, *Mycoplasma hominis*, and a closely related organism, *Ureaplasma*, have been etiologically implicated in some diseases of the human urogenital tract.

The high incidence of mycoplasmal infection is not generally appreciated. Factors responsible for this include lack of familiarity with mycoplasmal syndromes; the absence of specific, rapid tests for diagnosis in the early phases of these diseases; and the relative difficulty of growing the organisms in the diagnostic laboratory.

Accurate etiologic diagnosis of mycoplasmal diseases, however, is of considerable clinical importance. Mycoplasmal infections do not respond to the antimicrobial therapies usually used for respiratory or genital infections, but treatment with erythromycins or tetracyclines leads to amelioration of symptoms, decrease in the likelihood of spread, and eventually, true microbiologic cure.

DESCRIPTION OF THE ORGANISM AND RELATIONSHIP TO PATHOGENESIS. The mycoplasmas, members of the class Mollicutes, represent the smallest free-living forms, i.e., they do not require host cells for replication. For many years the question of whether these organisms were viruses or bacteria was debated. However, it appears that they are neither, and there is no significant deoxyribonucleic acid similarity between mycoplasmas and any known bacterium or virus.

The average diameter of mycoplasmas (125 to 150 nm) is in the size range of large viruses. They have no cell wall but are bounded by a limiting membrane containing lipid. Absence of a cell wall renders them susceptible to lysis by hypotonic solutions but insensitive to cell-wall active antibiotics such as the penicillins. Mycoplasmas and *Ureaplasma* can be grown on agar supplemented with serum proteins and sterols. Most *Mycoplasma* species form 200- to 300-μm colonies, which look much like a fried egg. They have a peripheral halo and a thicker central portion lying just below the surface of the agar. *M. pneumoniae* colonies, however, lack the halo and resemble a mulberry. *Ureaplasma* was previously called "T-strain" *Mycoplasma* because it formed tiny colonies on agar. When *M. pneumoniae* is grown on agar containing mammalian erythrocytes, it rapidly produces a clear zone of hemolysis similar to β-hemolysis of some bacteria. *M. pneumoniae* also differs from many other mycoplasmas in that it grows more slowly, ferments glucose to produce acid, adsorbs red cells to growing colonies, and reduces the dye tetrazolium under aerobic conditions. All of these characteristics have been exploited to establish a rapid microbiologic diagnosis.

When mycoplasmas contaminate tissue culture systems, as they often do, they are found intracellularly. This fact has led to speculation as to the mechanisms of persistence of these organisms in vivo. However, electron microscopic studies using tracheal organ culture systems have demonstrated most of the infecting organisms extracellularly at the base of the cilia of epithelial cells.

Two properties of *M. pneumoniae* seem to correlate extremely well with its pathogenicity in humans. *M. pneumoniae* has a selective affinity for respiratory epithelial cells and produces hydrogen peroxide. The H_2O_2 is thought to be responsible for much of the initial cell disruption in the respiratory tract. H_2O_2 also causes damage to erythrocyte membranes. In the laboratory, this damage results in hemolysis, and, in the patient, may alter erythrocyte antigens, thereby stimulating cold agglutinins. These agglutinins appear in the serum of over 50 per cent of patients who develop mycoplasmal pneumonia and are capable of clumping red blood cells in vitro at 4° C. They are different from cold precipitins or cryoglobulins occurring in other diseases. Cold agglutinins are IgM antibodies directed at the I antigen on the surface of normal erythrocytes. There is increasing evidence that cold agglutinins are antibodies to a glycolipid in the membrane of *M. pneumoniae*, which happens to cross-react with a similar erythrocyte antigen. Cold agglutinins occur rarely in other diseases, including influenza and adenoviral pneumonia.

RESPIRATORY DISEASES CAUSED BY *M. pneumoniae*

DEFINITION. Respiratory infection by *M. pneumoniae* may be asymptomatic or may lead to inflammation of the upper airways (pharyngitis or tracheitis) or lower respiratory tract (bronchitis or pneumonia). In the vast majority of cases, disease is self-limited, but proper antibiotic therapy can shorten the duration of symptoms.

EPIDEMIOLOGY. Each year about one out of every thousand people in the United States will experience mycoplasmal pneumonia. The incidence of all other mycoplasmal upper and lower respiratory infections is probably 10 times that of mycoplasmal pneumonia. From one quarter to three quarters of all pneumonias occurring in "closed" populations (military recruit camps, boarding schools, and colleges) are caused by *M. pneumoniae*.

Mycoplasmal respiratory infection is most common in children and young adults, with a peak incidence in the age range of 5 to 20 years; however, infants and elderly patients are also infected. Distribution is worldwide. Although documented epidemics have occurred primarily in the fall months, this disease does not have the marked seasonal predominance that is found with influenza.

Infection is spread from person to person by respiratory secretions expelled during bouts of coughing. The organism is present in these secretions for several days prior to the onset of symptoms and peaks in titer in the sputum during the first week of clinical illness. *M. pneumoniae* organisms persist in the sputum, albeit in reduced numbers, for weeks after the cessation of appropriate antimicrobial therapy.

In open populations under nonepidemic conditions, the infection seems to be spread most easily among playmates and within the household. The index case is usually a child. The majority of households having an index case will experience secondary infections, and the majority of susceptible family members will become infected, with resultant symptomatic disease or asymptomatic seroconversion.

In comparison with viral respiratory disease, the incubation period for mycoplasmal infection is relatively long, averaging two to three weeks. Therefore, unless two or more people from a household are simultaneously infected from an index case, it is unusual for several family members to be ill at the same time, and the disease may take several months to run its course through a household.

CLINICAL PRESENTATIONS. Mycoplasmal infection of the upper airways is impossible to distinguish clinically from infection by other agents. On the other hand, mycoplasmal pneumonia has several characteristics that may help the physician to diagnose this disease (see Fig. 264–1). The onset of mycoplasmal pneumonia is usually insidious in contrast to the abrupt onset of adenoviral or influenzal pneumonia. Mild fever is usually the first sign of infection. The hallmark of the disease is severe, disabling, paroxysmal cough, which usually becomes prominent two or three days after the onset of fever and often requires narcotic medication for suppression. Although usually nonproductive, the cough may yield small amounts of whitish sputum. Occasionally the sputum may contain flecks of blood, but grossly purulent sputum and marked hemoptysis are rare. Production of purulent or bloody sputum is actually more prevalent in tracheobronchitis than in pneumonia.

Headache occurs commonly in conjunction with the cough. During the first week of illness, many patients complain of burning soreness in the chest, though true pleuritic pain is uncommon. Fever rarely exceeds 39.5° C (102 to 103° F), and mild myalgias and malaise occur early in the disease. A history of shaking chills, severe myalgias, or gastrointestinal complaints is unusual.

On physical examination, the pharynx may be slightly injected or inflamed. Much diagnostic emphasis has been placed on the presence of bullous myringitis in patients with mycoplasmal respiratory disease. This finding was noted in less than 25 per cent of volunteers experimentally infected with *M. pneumoniae* and is very rare in naturally occurring mycoplasmal infection. Bacteria are much more commonly cultured than are *M. pneumoniae* from patients with bullous myringitis, and the relationship between *M. pneumoniae* infection and bullous myringitis or otitis remains tenuous.

Examination of the chest usually fails to show signs of dense consolidation or fluid accumulation. Auscultation reveals fine rales either unilaterally or bilaterally, which are often not very impressive. Findings from the remainder of the physical examination are usually normal.

The radiographic appearance of the lungs frequently presents a surprise. There is marked patchy infiltration of the lungs consistent with extensive interstitial pneumonia; bilateral involvement is evident in about one quarter of the patients. Infiltration is most prominent at the base of the lungs, although mycoplasmal pneumonia can be seen in any pulmonary segment. There may be slight blunting of the costovertebral angle on the affected side(s) in 10 to 20 per cent of patients, but large pleural effusions are rare. If thoracentesis is performed, it yields a serous or serosanguineous transudative fluid.

COMPLICATIONS. Spread of infection within the lung and pleural effusions are the most common pulmonary complications. Involvement of a number of extrapulmonary sites has been attributed to infection with *M. pneumoniae*, usually occurring as complications of pulmonary disease. Occasionally, they have been seen without pneumonia, and mycoplasmal causation has been substantiated on the basis of culture of the organism from involved organs, four-fold or greater rises in mycoplasma-specific antibodies, or demonstration (described later) of less specific cold hemagglutinins.

Three extrapulmonary complications are relatively common (occurring in 2 to 10 per cent of patients). These deserve comment because, when present, they help to confirm the diagnosis of mycoplasmal pneumonia.

Erythema Multiforme Major (Stevens-Johnson Syndrome). Some patients with mycoplasmal pneumonia develop blistering lesions involving the mouth, eyes, and skin. Usually, although the lesions look quite severe, they heal with minimal scarring. However, when the cornea is involved, blindness

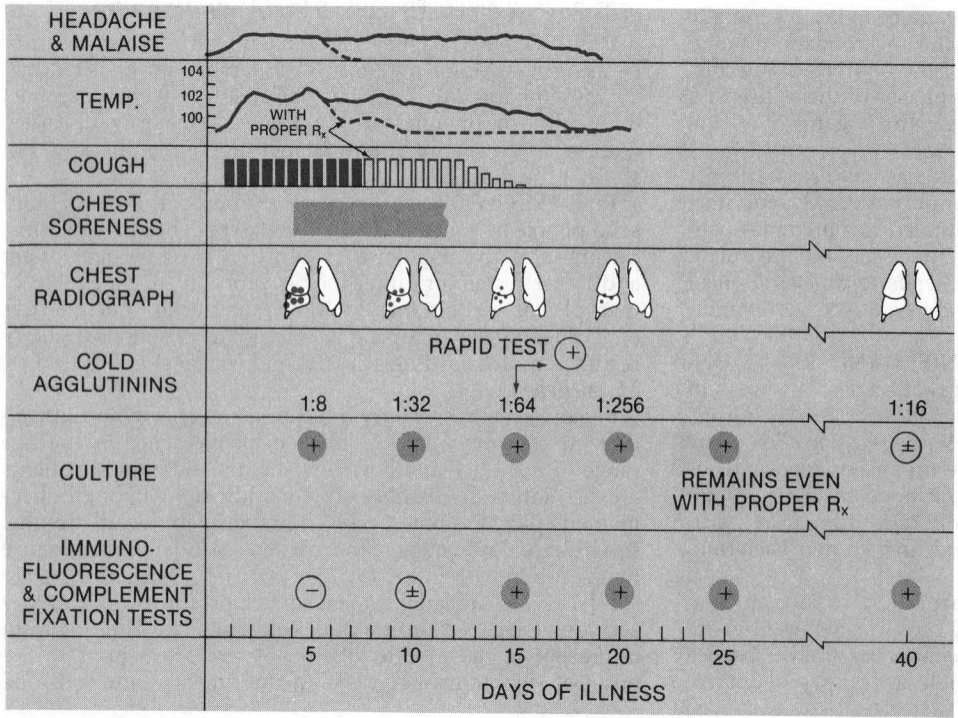

FIGURE 264–1. Major clinical manifestations of mycoplasmal pneumonia.

may ensue, and local and systemic steroid therapy is often recommended in these instances. This dermatologic syndrome has many causes, including adverse reaction to drugs. When, however, it occurs in conjunction with interstitial pneumonia in a child or young adult, its presence helps confirm the clinical diagnosis of mycoplasmal pneumonia.

The pathogenesis of this syndrome is unknown. There is one report of isolation of *M. pneumoniae* from skin lesions, but most authorities consider Stevens-Johnson syndrome an allergic reaction. A great variety of other skin rashes in mycoplasmal pneumonia has been described, but these are not diagnostically helpful.

Raynaud's Phenomenon. A second syndrome, occurring in fewer than 5 per cent of mycoplasmal pneumonia patients, is Raynaud's phenomenon. This consists of painful blanching of the distal parts of fingers and toes upon exposure to cold and may occur whether or not the patient has a history of Raynaud's phenomenon unrelated to mycoplasmal infection. The pathogenesis of this complication in *M. pneumoniae* infection is unknown. However, it is tempting to hypothesize that high titers of cold hemagglutinins could play a role by creating minute thrombi in the microcirculation of the distal extremities when exposed to cold. Patients with sickle cell disease may have particularly severe symptoms when they contract mycoplasmal pneumonia. In the presence of extremely high titers of cold agglutinins (1:20,000), gangrene of the distal parts of fingers and toes in these patients has been reported.

Hemolysis. Patients with cold agglutinin titers of greater than 1:500 may experience rapid and severe hemolysis with decreases of 50 per cent in hematocrit. This complication occurs in less than 5 per cent of patients in the second or third week of illness.

LESS COMMON COMPLICATIONS. Among the organ systems reported to be rarely involved in mycoplasmal infection are the cardiovascular, skeletal, and central nervous systems. In a very few cases involving each of these systems, the organism has been cultured directly from the affected organ.

NEUROLOGIC COMPLICATIONS. Aseptic meningitis, meningoencephalitis, cranial nerve neuritis, peripheral neuritis, Guillain-Barré syndrome, transverse myelitis, and psychosis all have been reported as complications of *M. pneumoniae* infection. Most often, etiologic diagnosis is made on the basis of exclusion of other agents and antibody response to *M. pneumoniae*. Spinal fluid cell counts and glucose and protein levels are extremely variable in these cases, ranging from normal to patterns consistent with aseptic meningitis. In some cases, elevated cerebrospinal fluid proteins were found to contain antibodies to *M. pneumoniae*, but these often paralleled serum antibody levels, and it was unclear whether or not cerebrospinal fluid antibody represented diffusion from the serum. There are only two or three reports of isolation of *M. pneumoniae* from cerebrospinal fluid or neural tissue, and the prevailing hypothesis is that mycoplasmal central nervous system disease occurs on the basis of allergic reaction.

Patients with neurologic complications seem to have greater mortality than is commonly associated with mycoplasmal disease. This could signify either a group of patients at increased risk of death from mycoplasmal infection or alternatively, support the hypothesis that these patients had a second (concurrent) undiagnosed disease with greater inherent mortality.

CARDIOVASCULAR COMPLICATIONS. Pericarditis and myocarditis are the most commonly reported cardiovascular complications of mycoplasmal infection. In general, the major criteria of heart disease have been congestive failure and abnormal electrocardiographic results. Large pericardial effusions have not occurred. There have been a few deaths during the acute phase of the disease, but recovery without sequelae is the rule. In most cases documentation of *M. pneumoniae* infection has been made by noting seroconversion. In one

retrospective study based on seroconversion, 8 per cent of patients with *M. pneumoniae* infection had evidence of pericarditis or myocarditis. The average age of these patients was 46 years, considerably older than the mean for patients with *M. pneumoniae* infection.

MUSCULOSKELETAL COMPLICATIONS. Arthralgias are common in association with mycoplasmal pneumonia, but frank arthritis is rare. When it does occur, arthritis may continue long after the other manifestations of mycoplasmal infection are gone. Large joints seem to be preferentially affected, and the arthritis may be migratory. *Mycoplasma* has not been cultured from joint fluid of immunocompetent patients.

M. pneumoniae and other mycoplasmas have been implicated as the causative agents of a number of other connective tissue diseases, including rheumatoid arthritis, juvenile rheumatoid arthritis, and Reiter's syndrome. Nonhuman mycoplasmas have been shown to cause arthritis in the animals they infect, and *M. pneumoniae* has been cultured on several occasions from the joints of immunocompromised patients. To date, however, there is no evidence that human mycoplasmas cause joint disease, except perhaps as an acute manifestation of pneumonia.

CLINICAL COURSE. Mycoplasmal respiratory disease is almost invariably self-limited and very rarely results in death. In the absence of treatment, upper respiratory infection usually lasts one to three weeks, and pneumonia may persist from four to six weeks. Recovery is gradual, with clinical improvement preceding roentgenographic clearing. Development of any of the severe cardiovascular, dermatologic, hematologic, or neurologic complications described earlier may prolong resolution. Proper treatment, which is often not begun until other antibiotics have failed, would appear to shorten the duration of symptoms by about one half. Results might be even better if treatment were begun earlier. Relapse occurs in 5 to 10 per cent of patients. In most cases these patients receive courses of therapy less than two weeks in duration.

Two groups of patients commonly appear to develop severe disease. The first group consists of infants who, until recently, were thought not to be particularly susceptible to *M. pneumoniae* infection. Many infants develop severe respiratory distress requiring intubation and supported respiration. Fortunately, despite severe illness the prognosis for these children is excellent. The second group contains patients with sickle cell disease. In addition to digital gangrene, these patients are prone to develop large multilobar pneumonias and pleural effusions. The possibility of mycoplasmal infection should be considered in a patient with sickle cell crisis and interstitial pneumonia.

PATHOLOGY. Since death is rare in patients with mycoplasmal pneumonia, descriptions of pathologic changes in this disease rest on a very small number of specimens. The tracheobronchial tree and lungs are generally hyperemic. There is evidence of interstitial pneumonia with engorged lungs consistent with the findings on x-ray. Cellular infiltrate, usually minimal, consists mostly of mononuclear elements. Tracheal organ culture systems have been used to demonstrate that infection with *M. pneumoniae* causes a marked decrease of ciliary action, followed by complete loss of cilia and sloughing of epithelial cells.

IMMUNITY. There are varied antibody responses to infection with *M. pneumoniae*. It is unclear what role these immune responses play in the pathogenesis of, and recovery from, infection. Secretory IgA antibody is thought to be the most protective immunoglobulin in this disease. Individual immunity may be relatively short-lived, and there are well-documented instances of recurrent disease within 2 to 10 years following primary infection.

DIAGNOSIS. A clinical diagnosis of mycoplasmal pneumonia should be seriously entertained whenever interstitial pneumonia occurs in a young adult. Examination of the Gram-stained sputum is helpful in that it reveals inflammation but no bacterial organisms. The peripheral leukocyte count may be normal or slightly elevated. There is minimal shift toward immature forms, and mild lymphopenia may exist. The diagnosis is substantiated by finding a cold agglutinin titer greater than 1:32 in the serum.

Hospital bacteriology or serology laboratories titrate cold agglutinins in the patient's serum using Rh-positive, type O erythrocytes to avoid reactions due to major blood-group isoantibodies present in the patient's serum. However, a simple, rapid bedside procedure for finding cold agglutinins can be performed using only the patient's blood. One milliliter of freshly drawn blood is placed in a tube containing anticoagulant. The tube used for prothrombin determinations is suitable. The tube is chilled on ice for two or three minutes and then gently rotated in a horizontal position. Development of small clumps of erythrocytes, similar to those seen when typing blood, which disappear on warming the tube between the hands, indicates the presence of cold agglutinins. The agglutination-dissociation cycle can be repeated many times with the same blood sample. This differentiates the reaction from direct hemagglutination by viruses—a process that generally cannot be recycled. A positive test result correlates with a cold agglutinin titer of 1:64 or greater. When the cold agglutinin titer is extremely high, an easily dissociable clot may form in the tube. Blood from a patient with an unrelated disease should be used as a control. Cold agglutinins are usually found during the second and third weeks of illness and may peak one month or more after the onset of symptoms.

Diagnosis of mycoplasmal pneumonia should be further supported by finding rising titers of specific antibodies to the *Mycoplasma* organism. These can be measured by complement fixation, inhibition of metabolism, indirect hemagglutination, or immunofluorescence techniques. In addition, patients with mycoplasmal pneumonia may develop a false-positive test result for syphilis.

Definitive diagnosis of mycoplasmal pneumonia rests, however, on coupling an antibody rise with culturing *M. pneumoniae* from sputum. Although growth on agar may take two to three weeks, rendering results useless for initiating drug therapy, a more rapid (three to four days) presumptive diagnosis can be based on the use of a diphasic medium available in some diagnostic laboratories.

DIFFERENTIAL DIAGNOSIS. The most common respiratory infections mimicking mycoplasmal pneumonia are influenza and adenoviral and *Legionella* pneumonia. These tend to be more fulminant in onset and are associated with more severe systemic symptoms and greater respiratory insufficiency. Patients with legionnaires' disease are likely to be older males with histories of smoking. Confusion and gastrointestinal disturbance are common in *Legionella* pneumonia. Often one cannot definitively distinguish between these diseases, and a therapeutic trial with erythromycin (which will also treat *Legionella pneumophila*) may be warranted. Psittacosis and ornithosis (chlamydial diseases) and Q fever (a rickettsial disease) should also be considered in the diagnosis. In such cases, history of exposure to birds on the one hand and to cattle on the other may prove diagnostically helpful.

THERAPY. Treatment with appropriate antibiotics can terminate symptoms abruptly and usually must be begun on the basis of clinical diagnosis. Penicillins, cephalosporins, and aminoglycosides, such as streptomycin, kanamycin, and gentamicin, have little or no effect against these organisms.

M. pneumoniae is sensitive in vitro and in vivo to erythromycin and to the tetracyclines. These agents appear to be equally effective in diminishing the symptoms of the disease. Because there are fewer adverse effects, especially in children under age 10 years, erythromycin is preferred. The dosage

for either drug is 250 to 500 mg four times daily for two weeks. Although erythromycin and the tetracyclines are effective in ending symptoms, *M. pneumoniae* can be isolated from the sputum of patients for several weeks after the onset of therapy. The mechanism of persistence is unknown but does not depend on the emergence of drug-resistant organisms.

PREVENTION. The frequency of mycoplasmal infection makes the development of a vaccine an attractive objective. Inactivated vaccines, while producing rises in serum antibody levels, give little protection.

The possible role of IgA antibodies in combating disease has prompted the trial of intranasally administered vaccines using live temperature-sensitive (ts) mutants of *M. pneumoniae*. The rationale was that these mutants would induce a localized nasopharyngeal immune response but would not replicate in the warmer lower respiratory tree and cause disease. The results of initial trials of these vaccines have been variable.

GENITAL INFECTION BY MYCOPLASMA AND UREAPLASMA

INTRODUCTION. One strain of human mycoplasmas, *M. hominis*, and a closely related organism, *Ureaplasma urealyticum*, frequently colonize the male and female genital tracts. During the past decade, there has been increasing interest in discovering the role these organisms might play in causing disease of the genitourinary system.

EPIDEMIOLOGY. *M. hominis* and ureaplasmas can be included in the group of venereally transmitted infectious agents. Infants are colonized during birth, but carriage of the organism is lost during the first year of life. After this, the prevalence of colonization increases with age and sexual experience, as it does for other sexually transmitted organisms. At all ages, females seem to be more readily colonized than males, and colonization is found most frequently in patients from lower socioeconomic groups. *U. urealyticum* carriage may decrease with increasing age over 40 and with hypoestrogenism.

CLINICAL PRESENTATIONS. *M. hominis, U. urealyticum,* or both organisms have been implicated in nongonococcal urethritis (NGU) and inflammatory disease of the prostate, vagina, cervix, upper urinary tract, and female pelvic organs. In addition, colonization by one or both of these organisms has been associated with male and female infertility, habitual abortion, and recurrent production of premature and underweight infants.

INFECTION OF THE LOWER URINARY TRACT. Chlamydia are responsible for a large percentage of cases of NGU. *U. urealyticum* is probably the cause of many of the remaining cases of NGU. Evidence for this stems from the many patients with NGU from whom ureaplasmas are cultured and from these patients' poor clinical response to treatment with sulfa drugs, to which chlamydia are susceptible and to which *Ureaplasma* is not. *M. hominis* probably does not cause urethritis.

INFECTION OF THE UPPER URINARY TRACT. *M. hominis* has been isolated from the kidneys and ureters of patients with clinical pyelonephritis. Antibody to the organism was detected in serum and urine from some of these patients, providing moderately strong evidence that *M. hominis* causes some cases of pyelonephritis. *U. urealyticum* infection may infrequently play a role in urinary calculus formation.

INFECTION OF THE FEMALE GENITAL TRACT. *M. hominis* probably causes a small proportion of the cases of vaginitis and cervicitis. Infection of the uterus and fallopian tubes with this organism has also been documented. *Ureaplasma* rarely, if ever, causes infection in the female pelvis.

MYCOPLASMAS AND REPRODUCTIVE ABNORMALITIES. *U. urealyticum* has been cultured from the sperm of males with fertility disorders. Treatment to eradicate *Urea-*

plasma has resulted in increased motility and number of sperm as well as improved morphology. However, recent studies do not indicate a causal role for ureaplasmas in infertility.

Ureaplasma has also been isolated from internal organs of the products of conception of patients with repeated spontaneous abortions. In addition, in some studies *U. urealyticum* was more often isolated from the genital tracts of women with this syndrome than from control populations. Finally, treatment with tetracycline prior to conception in women with histories of habitual abortion has been reported to increase fetal salvage rate. Unfortunately, few if any of these studies took into account the presence of chlamydia, which might have been responsible for the reproductive disorders.

LOW BIRTH WEIGHT. Prior to the realization that tetracycline is contraindicated in pregnancy, it was shown that tetracycline treatment of mothers who habitually gave birth to underweight fetuses would increase birth weight. In addition, vaginal colonization by ureaplasmas was correlated with decreased birth weight. However, these studies did not take into account the presence or absence of chlamydia.

PUERPERAL INFECTION. *M. hominis* infection and septicemia have been associated with some cases of postpartum fever. This organism has been found in the blood of up to 10 per cent of women with fever after delivery, and antibody response indicating true infection has been noted in many cases.

THERAPY. Mycoplasmas and *Ureaplasma* are all susceptible to the tetracyclines. *U. urealyticum* is sensitive to erythromycin, but *M. hominis* is not. Spectinomycin, an antimicrobial agent used in cases of penicillin-resistant gonococcal disease, appears to be effective against both *M. hominis* and *U. urealyticum*. Since both *U. urealyticum* and *C. trachomatis* are sensitive to tetracycline, it is recommended that patients with NGU be treated with a tetracycline at a dose of 1 to 2 grams daily for one to two weeks. The patient should abstain from sexual intercourse during this period, and sexual partners should be evaluated for therapy.

In addition, tetracycline therapy prior to conception and erythromycin therapy during pregnancy should be considered for couples with gestational problems who are shown to harbor *U. urealyticum* in the genitourinary tract.

Episodes of postabortal and puerperal fever are usually self-limited and do not require antimicrobial therapy directed at mycoplasmas. Should such therapy be deemed necessary, tetracycline is the drug of choice.

Couch RB: Mycoplasma diseases. In Mandell G, Douglas RG, Bennett JE (eds.): Principles and Practice of Infectious Diseases. 2nd ed. New York, John Wiley & Sons, 1985, pp 1064–1080. *An up-to-date chapter dealing with both clinical and microbiologic aspects.*

Roberts DB: The etiology of bullous myringitis and the role of mycoplasmas in ear disease. A review. Pediatrics 65:761, 1980. *A definitive review of several studies indicating no significant relationship between this organism and ear disease.*

Taylor-Robinson D, McCormack WM: The genital mycoplasmas. N Engl J Med 302:1003, 1980; 302:1063, 1980. *A comprehensive two-part article on epidemiology, microbiology, clinical presentation, and therapy.*

265 PNEUMONIA CAUSED BY AEROBIC GRAM-NEGATIVE BACILLI

Waldemar G. Johanson, Jr.

Over the past 30 years the group of organisms known collectively as aerobic gram-negative bacilli (GNB) has assumed an increasing importance in clinical respiratory infections. There is no evidence that this phenomenon is due to a change in the virulence of these organisms. Rather, it is due to changes in the human hosts they infect and, to some degree, to changes in the environment induced by antibiotics and other factors, especially in hospitals. Each of the GNB has its place (or places) in nature. Many are regular inhabitants of the human gastrointestinal tract while others are found in water or other sites in the environment. None is especially virulent for the respiratory tract of healthy mammalian hosts; all are distinctly inferior to the pneumococcus, for example, in that regard. A careful review of the preantibiotic literature reveals that the presence of these organisms in the respiratory tracts of seriously ill patients is not a recent occurrence; rather, the presence of these organisms was disregarded for many years, an approach that was not unjustified considering the pre-eminence of the pneumococcus as a cause of fatal pneumonia prior to the availability of highly efficacious antibiotics. The emergence of GNB as respiratory pathogens in recent years is the result of suppression of more aggressive organisms by effective therapy and the long-term survival of people who would have succumbed to other infections or other processes in an earlier era.

PATHOGENESIS. Pneumonias due to GNB are caused by one of three mechanisms: inhalation of contaminated aerosols, hematogenous infection of the lungs from another primary source of infection, or aspiration of oropharyngeal secretions that are colonized by these organisms.

Inhalation therapy became a popular mode of treatment in the mid-1960's. Shortly thereafter it was recognized that up to 80 per cent of aerosol treatments contained viable bacteria, most often *P. aeruginosa*. The cause of this phenomenon was traced to contaminated water in nebulization equipment that was allowed to remain in service for a number of days without decontamination. In one hospital 12 per cent of randomly selected patients at autopsy showed evidence of necrotizing gram-negative bacillary pneumonia. Following recognition of this problem and institution of effective control strategies that decreased the frequency of contaminated inhalation therapy equipment from 80 per cent to essentially zero, the incidence of necrotizing pneumonia at autopsy decreased to 1 to 2 per cent. The data obtained during this period are extremely important in that they indicate the magnitude of the potential problem that contamination of inhalation therapy equipment can create. However, with the current use of disposable nebulizers the frequency of contaminated equipment remains very low. Outbreaks of pneumonia caused by contaminated respiratory medications, resuscitation equipment, and even devices used to measure vital capacities have been reported, findings that indicate that continued vigilance is required to prevent such sources from becoming important causes of infections. However, as a practical matter, pneumonias due to GNB are rarely caused by inhalation of contaminated aerosols today.

The incidence of pneumonia caused by bacteremic spread to the lungs has probably been overestimated in the literature. *P. aeruginosa* causes a distinctive vasculitis involving pulmonary arteries and veins, and pneumonia in adjacent lung units associated with bacteremia, but this is uncommon with other organisms. It is likely that most instances of bacteremia from a nonpulmonary source such as the gastrointestinal or urinary tract, associated with pulmonary infiltrates, fever, and hypoxemia, represent noncardiogenic pulmonary edema, or the "adult respiratory distress syndrome," and not actual pneumonia. In fact, pneumonia due to this cause is sufficiently uncommon that the presence of bacteremia in association with new pulmonary infiltrates should initiate a vigorous search for a primary site of infection outside the lungs before it is concluded that pneumonia is responsible.

Aspiration of oropharyngeal secretions that contain GNB is the usual event leading to pneumonia caused by these organisms. Colonization of the upper respiratory tract with GNB occurs in 10 per cent or less of normal people, but the prevalence of such colonization is markedly increased among patients with acute or chronic diseases. Colonization rates are similar among populations with chronic disease such as alcoholics and residents of skilled nursing facilities and previously healthy individuals with acute but severe illnesses or trauma; in both types of patient groups colonization rates approach 50 per cent. Similarly, colonization of the oropharynx by GNB among healthy persons undergoing elective surgical procedures rises from essentially zero to 35 to 50 per cent within 24 hours following surgery. The organisms responsible for colonization vary from one study to another but only rarely can this sudden acquisition of GNB be attributed to demonstrable environmental sources. Instead, colonization appears to be caused by a translocation of the patient's fecal flora or the transfer of organisms from one patient to another on the hands of personnel. However, the root cause of this colonization is the great susceptibility of ill patients to the acquisition of GNB from the immediate environment.

Healthy people are resistant to the implantation of GNB in the oropharynx; even gargling a broth culture of GNB fails to produce colonization. This difference between healthy and ill people is related to the ability of GNB to adhere to epithelial cells of the oropharynx. Buccal epithelial cells obtained from healthy subjects adhere few GNB during incubation in vitro while cells obtained from either acutely or chronically ill patients adhere large numbers. The ability of cells to resist adherence by GNB is directly related to the concentration of fibronectin on the cell surface; loss of cell surface fibronectin, whether removed by proteolytic enzymes experimentally in vitro or by endogenous enzymes in vivo, appears to expose binding sites on the cells to which GNB can adhere and thus achieve colonization.

Once established in the oropharynx GNB multiply, achieve high concentrations in secretions, and are aspirated in small liquid boluses into the lungs (see Ch. 262). Since lung defenses are often impaired by the same underlying conditions that promote changes in cell resistance to adherence and colonization, the ability of the lungs to handle this bacterial inoculum is insufficient and pneumonia results. The specific lung defense mechanism that might be impaired in a given patient varies with the nature of underlying illness. For example, patients with chronic airway obstruction have impaired mucociliary transport and alveolar hypoxia that impairs the effectiveness of phagocytic cells. Some data suggest that the bronchial abnormalities in these patients allow persistent colonization of the distal airways by potentially pathogenic bacteria, a factor that affords the bacteria the advantage of access to the distal lung. Patients who are neutropenic are remarkably predisposed to develop pneumonias with GNB, a clinical observation that correlates nicely with the experimental finding that swift recruitment of circulating neutrophils into the lungs is a crucial aspect of host defense against *Pseudomonas* infection. Alcoholism seems to predispose to GNB pneumonias in several ways. Malnutrition promotes colonization of the upper tract by GNB, aspiration is facilitated by episodes of impaired consciousness, and acute alcohol intoxication impairs the ability of phagocytes to migrate to the site of inflammation.

Of the many species of gram-negative aerobic bacilli that colonize human hosts, only *Hemophilus influenzae* can be classified as a true respiratory pathogen, if the ability of the organism to produce infections in previously normal individuals is accepted as a reasonable criterion of pathogenicity. All of the others together, including Enterobacteriaceae (*E. coli, Klebsiella, Enterobacter, Serratia,* and *Proteus*), *Pseudomonas,* and *Acinetobacter* account for 10 to 20 per cent of community-acquired pneumonias and these occur almost exclusively in patients with serious underlying disease. The genus *Klebsiella* contains four species of which only *K. pneumoniae* and *K. oxytoca* cause pneumonia; infections due to *K. pneumoniae* are by far the most common.

Pneumonia due to *Klebsiella* has been held separate from

that caused by other gram-negative bacilli largely for historical reasons. It was the first such organism to be recognized as a pulmonary pathogen and the pneumonia it caused was distinctive from that caused by the pneumococcus, especially in its lack of response to early forms of treatment and its predilection to cause upper lobe pneumonias in alcoholic males. However, the classic features of *Klebsiella* pneumonia as described in the earlier literature, such as "currant jelly" sputum (a mixture of blood and mucus), the bulging fissure associated with upper lobe consolidation, and the syndrome of "chronic cavitary pneumonia," are rarely observed today. While *Klebsiella* remains an important pulmonary pathogen, the illness it causes cannot be clinically differentiated from those caused by other aerobic gram-negative bacilli, and its treatment is similar.

CLINICAL MANIFESTATIONS. Pneumonias caused by GNB may be community-acquired or hospital-acquired (nosocomial). Virtually all patients with community-acquired pneumonias caused by GNB have serious underlying chronic illnesses, especially chronic obstructive lung disease, alcoholism, or malignancy. Nosocomial pneumonias resulting from GNB occur principally in patients with severe, acute illnesses whether or not they have underlying chronic disease as well. Thus, these infections are most likely to be found in postoperative patients or patients who require intensive care for other reasons. The clinical manifestations of infection are influenced by the nature of the associated processes.

Community-acquired gram-negative bacillary pneumonias share the common features of all bacterial pneumonias—fever, cough productive of purulent sputum, chest pain, and shortness of breath. The illness tends to be abrupt and associated with prominent systemic signs and symptoms such as mental confusion, vomiting, and hypotension. Physical examination reveals rales in most patients, but the classic findings of dense consolidation are uncommon. Pleural effusion is present in 15 to 20 per cent of patients. Radiographic infiltrates may involve any lobe and are bilateral in about one third of patients. Although cavitation is most likely to occur in pneumonia caused by *Klebsiella,* it also occurs commonly with *Pseudomonas* infections and occasionally with other organisms. Laboratory features include leukocytosis or leukopenia, either of which is characteristically associated with a marked left shift. Leukopenia is a poor prognostic sign.

Nosocomial pneumonia produced by GNB can be an explosive illness similar to the community-acquired form but frequently proceeds with a more indolent but seemingly inexorable course. Often the patient is in respiratory failure, intubated, and receiving mechanical ventilation. GNB are initially found colonizing the oropharynx, and over the subsequent few days appear in tracheal secretions followed by increasing numbers of neutrophils. Finally, the patient becomes febrile and develops new radiographic infiltrates and worsening hypoxemia. Another common presentation is fever on the second or third postoperative day. Postoperative pneumonias are most common after lateral thoracotomies (especially combined thoracoabdominal procedures) and upper abdominal incisions. When nosocomial GNB pneumonia complicates the course of an already seriously ill patient, it is frequently associated with evidence of impaired function of other organs, commonly the liver, kidneys, hematopoietic system, and central nervous system. Upper gastrointestinal bleeding and impaired coagulation are also common. This phenomenon is referred to as the syndrome of multiple organ failure and is the most common cause of death in patients with protracted serious illness. The occurrence of any of these complications should alert the clinician to the probable presence of bacterial infection. If no apparent site is found elsewhere in the patient, the lungs must be highly suspect even in the absence of strong clinical signs since such pulmonary infections are often difficult to detect in the setting of serious disease.

DIAGNOSIS. Confirming the role of GNB as the etiologic agent in the patient with pneumonia is a major clinical problem that is created largely by the propensity to colonization of proximal airways by these organisms in patients subject to such pneumonias. Thus, GNB will be present in the secretions of these patients whether they have pneumonia or not, and whether or not the GNB are the cause of pneumonia. Blood cultures are positive in 20 to 30 per cent of patients with community-acquired infections but in as few as 8 per cent of nosocomial pneumonias. Nevertheless, because the information gained from a positive blood culture as to the causative organism and its antimicrobial susceptiblity is so important in patient management, blood cultures should always be obtained when GNB pneumonia is suspected. Similarly, while pleural effusion is usually not present, the yield of positive cultures from such fluid when it is present is about 30 per cent, and a diagnostic thoracentesis should be performed if a sufficient volume of fluid is identified radiographically.

A variety of approaches have been utilized to improve the accuracy of cultures of respiratory secretions (see Ch. 262). Gram staining a portion of purulent sputum is always important; the presence of numerous gram-negative bacilli in a patient at risk of pneumonia caused by these organisms certainly supports the diagnosis. However, GNB do not demonstrate sufficiently distinct morphological characteristics to permit accurate identification, and culture with determination of antibiotic sensitivities is important. Some authorities recommend that sputum specimens be screened microscopically prior to culture and only those that contain more than 25 neutrophils and fewer than 10 squamous cells per low-power field be studied further. These criteria obviously cannot be applied to markedly neutropenic patients. Whether or not to employ one of the invasive techniques for sampling respiratory secretions must be decided in each patient on an individual basis (Ch. 262).

TREATMENT. Recommendations for the antimicrobial treatment of pneumonia due to GNB are changing rapidly as new drugs aimed at this group of organisms are entering clinical practice. However, certain principles apply whichever drugs are selected. First, remember that GNB are relatively poor respiratory pathogens and patients susceptible to infection by them are at even greater risk of pulmonary infection by more virulent organisms such as the pneumococcus, *Hemophilus*, and *S. aureus*. Thus, despite the presence of GNB in sputum, initial treatment of these pneumonias—particularly those acquired outside the hospital or in the absence of concomitant antibiotic therapy—should include coverage of usual respiratory pathogens. Penicillin, a first- or second-generation cephalosporin, and even erythromycin or clindamycin are good choices. Second, the use of multiple agents is advisable for initial therapy for several reasons. The susceptibility of the infecting organisms is not known and two agents provide broader coverage; emergence of antibiotic resistance may be retarded by the use of multiple agents; and antibacterial synergism may result from the use of multiple agents. Bacteriologic cure rates of experimental GNB pneumonias are increased when two agents are used in contrast to those for single-agent therapy. Agents with good coverage of the common GNB include the aminoglycosides (gentamicin, tobramycin, amikacin), second- and particularly third-generation cephalosporins (cefamandole, cefoxitin, cefotaxime, ceftriaxone), and the monolactams (aztreonam). The third principle is that the agents chosen must be given parenterally and in adequate dosage. Metabolic clearance rates of the aminoglycosides in particular vary widely, and standard dosages based on body weight and renal function may result in either excessively high or low plasma concentrations in the individual patient. Improved clinical outcomes in the treatment of pneumonia produced by GNB have been associated with peak plasma levels of gentamicin or tobramycin of 6 μg per milliliter and 28 μg per milliliter for amikacin.

On the basis of the foregoing, a reasonable therapeutic approach to the patient with a community-acquired pneumonia suspected to be of gram-negative bacillary etiology would be to initiate treatment with a beta-lactam agent plus an aminoglycoside, for example penicillin, ampicillin, or cephalothin plus gentamicin or tobramycin. This combination will provide coverage for the usual respiratory pathogens as well as the most common GNB (*K. pneumoniae* and *E. coli*) in this setting. If the patient has recently received antimicrobial therapy or has been recently hospitalized, a third-generation cephalosporin such as cefotaxime can be substituted for the other beta-lactam agents, although such a regimen provides poor coverage for gram-positive organisms.

Treatment of nosocomial infection is often made more difficult by previous antimicrobial therapy, and drug susceptibility studies are critically important. However, empiric therapy must usually be initiated before the results of such studies are available. Agents should be chosen on the basis of several factors including knowledge of local resistance patterns, previous cultures, and prior treatment. For example, resistance of *P. aeruginosa* to gentamicin varies from 5 to 50 per cent in different hospitals and knowledge of resistance patterns in one's hospital can be very helpful in selecting empiric therapy. Most clinicians choose an aminoglycoside, usually amikacin because of the less frequent resistance to this agent, and a third-generation cephalosporin such as cefotaxime. If *P. aeruginosa* is strongly suspected on the basis of previous cultures or the clinical setting (respiratory failure, neutropenia) an agent with greater antipseudomonas activity such as piperacillin or ticarcillin can be substituted for the cephalosporin. Because new beta-lactam agents with good activity against gram-negative bacilli are less active than earlier generations against a number of important respiratory pathogens, great care needs to be given to the spectrum of organisms covered until the results of cultures are available.

PROGNOSIS. The mortality of GNB pneumonias remains high—in the range of 30 to 50 per cent. It has been argued that this is the result of the underlying disease usually present in patients who develop these pneumonias. This notion could lead to therapeutic nihilism. Other data clearly indicate that GNB pneumonias increase hospital mortality among patients who have nonlethal disease processes, a finding that would support an aggressive diagnostic and treatment approach. It is probable that both conclusions could be correct, depending on the population of patients studied. There is little doubt that GNB pneumonias represent the terminal event for a number of patients with irreversible and lethal diseases and that such patients form a large fraction of all hospital patients. On the other hand, there is reason to expect recovery rates of 80 per cent or more among patients who develop GNB pneumonias in the context of acute, severe, but nonlethal disease processes and in these patients aggressive diagnostic maneuvers and intensive therapy are clearly indicated.

COMPLICATIONS. Pneumonias caused by GNB are more likely than other pneumonias to be complicated by one or another adverse event. Important complications include empyema, lung necrosis, superinfections, and multiple organ failure; metastatic seeding of infection to other sites is an uncommon complication.

Empyema occurs in perhaps as many as 30 per cent of patients with GNB pneumonias. Criteria for the diagnosis of empyema vary among clinicians, but all agree that empyema is present if the pleural space contains gross pus. Other criteria accepted by many are the presence of bacteria on Gram stain, a pleural fluid pH of 7.2 or less, and a pleural fluid white cell count exceeding 30,000 per deciliter. Each of these criteria is important because it indicates a condition unlikely to respond to antimicrobials alone but that will usually require drainage of the pleural space as well. Thus, the term "complicated effusion" has gained favor over the use of "empyema" to identify pleural fluid collections for which drainage needs to be considered. The occurrence of a complicated effusion generally prevents the recovery of the patient until it is recognized and effectively treated. Signs and symptoms of continuing illness such as fever, persistent leukocytosis, and the onset of multiple organ failure in a patient undergoing treatment for a GNB pneumonia should raise suspicion of a complicated effusion. If pleural fluid is identified on upright PA and lateral chest radiographs, thoracentesis should be performed; useful studies of the fluid obtained include measurements of pH and glucose, white cell count, Gram stain, and cultures for aerobic and anaerobic organisms.

If the fluid qualifies as a complicated effusion, most authorities recommend prompt placement of a thoracostomy tube and drainage. Alternative approaches, principally repeated thoracentesis, are less successful owing to loculation of the pleural space. Surgical drainage of the pleural space, using localized resection of an overlying rib with creation of a larger drainage tract, is reserved for patients who do not respond to tube drainage. Decortication of the pleura may be necessary if the clinical signs of uncontrolled infection are not ameliorated by simple drainage plus antimicrobial therapy. In such patients radiographic evidence of effusion persists along with continued fever and leukocytosis. At surgery, the pleural space is found to contain numerous loculated pockets of pus. The timing of intervention with these techniques requires excellent clinical judgment, because the patients are usually seriously ill and poor candidates for surgical treatment of any kind; on the other hand, they will not recover unless the pleural space is adequately drained.

Extensive lung necrosis has been termed "lung gangrene" because of the rapid occurrence of pulmonary cavitation associated with marked systemic toxicity and the appearance of extensive devitalization of lung tissue at necropsy. Occasionally, an entire lung will appear to dissolve within a few days, leaving multiple cavities with air-fluid levels. This complication occurs with all of the common GNB, although perhaps more commonly in infections produced by *K. pneumoniae* and *P. aeruginosa*. Lung necrosis may be caused by the extracellular products of these organisms. *P. aeruginosa* makes a number of "virulence factors" including exotoxin A, exoenzyme S, elastase, and a neutral protease. However, *K. pneumoniae* makes none of these and the propensity of this organism to cause lung necrosis remains unexplained.

Extensive lung necrosis may be followed by massive hemoptysis, continued suppuration because of inadequate drainage of the massively disrupted lung parenchyma, or bronchopleural fistula owing to extension of the necrotizing process through the pleura. The latter must be promptly treated with placement of a chest tube because of the attendant pneumothorax. However, definitive treatment of extensive lung necrosis is surgical resection of the involved lobe or lobes. As with management of complicated effusion, the timing of such an intervention must be carefully considered in light of the control of the underlying infection, severity of complicating problems (hemoptysis, air leak, and so on) and the patient's general condition.

Assessment of the patient with multiple organ failure in the context of a serious illness complicated by a GNB pneumonia is always difficult. The major question is usually whether a new complication such as oliguria is due to the underlying disease, to the current treatment, or to the infection. Each of the common manifestations of multiple organ dysfunction—altered liver function, acute renal failure, hematopoietic abnormalities, upper gastrointestinal bleeding, and altered mental state—may be multifactorial in etiology, and the antimicrobial agents used to treat GNB pneumonia may cause most of them. The guiding principles are to treat

the infection aggressively and to correct life-threatening complications as they occur.

Superinfections may develop during treatment of GNB pneumonia, just as GNB pneumonia may occur as a superinfection of a previous pneumonia. Unfortunately, treatment of the patient's pneumonia does not prevent colonization of the oropharynx and tracheobronchial tree by additional GNB or fungi. Thus, the clinician is often faced with evaluating a new set of microorganisms recovered from the patient's secretions. The guiding principle here is to treat patients, not culture results. If the patient is responding well and appears to be improving, the new cultures can be disregarded for the time being. On the other hand, if the new cultural data correspond to a worsening clinical course, the process of evaluation and revision of treatment must be begun again.

Bell RC, Coalson JJ, Smith JD, et al.: Multiple organ failure and infection in adult respiratory distress syndrome. Ann Intern Med 99:293, 1983. *A detailed analysis of 84 patients with ARDS with autopsy confirmation of sites of infection in those who succumbed.*

Karnad A, Alvarez S, Berk SL: Pneumonia caused by gram-negative bacilli. Am J Med 79(Suppl 1A):61, 1985. *Many well-documented cases are described which indicate clearly the variable clinical presentation of these infections and the generally poor response to treatment.*

Levison ME, Kaye D: Pneumonia caused by gram-negative bacilli: An overview. Rev Infect Dis 7(Suppl 4):S656, 1985. *A thorough review from the standpoint of microbiology and antimicrobial therapy.*

Moore RD, Smith CR, Lietman PS: Association of aminoglycoside plasma levels with therapeutic outcome in gram-negative pneumonia. Am J Med 77:657, 1984. *Emphasizes the importance of adequate aminoglycoside dosing and monitoring of blood levels in improving the outcome of treatment.*

266 RECURRENT ASPIRATION PNEUMONIA

Waldemar G. Johanson, Jr.

Categorization of the various syndromes associated with aspiration of liquids into the tracheobronchial tree is not an area distinguished by precise terminology or even consistency in the use of terms. Most of the important syndromes are dealt with elsewhere in the volume: gastric acid aspiration (Ch. 537), anaerobic pneumonias and lung abscess (Ch. 64), lipoid pneumonia (Ch. 68), and hydrocarbon aspiration (Ch. 537). In this chapter, we will concentrate on an infrequent but difficult problem: that of recurrent bacterial pneumonias associated with aspiration. Such pneumonias are defined as recurring clinical illnesses characterized by fever, purulent sputum, and new radiographic infiltrates in the lungs in a patient with known or suspected chronic aspiration of oropharyngeal contents.

ETIOLOGY. Most patients afflicted with this problem have serious problems with swallowing for one or another reason. Common predisposing conditions are carcinoma of the esophagus with obstruction, tracheobronchial fistula (usually following treatment for cancer), and neurologic diseases affecting deglutition. Strokes are certainly the most common cause of the latter but amyotrophic lateral sclerosis (including bulbar palsy), multiple sclerosis, and the myopathies may be responsible. Recurrent nocturnal aspiration of gastric contents by patients with esophageal reflux represents the one situation in which the swallowing mechanism may be intact in this syndrome.

Impaired swallowing having neural or myopathic causes is most pronounced when the patient attempts to swallow liquids. By contrast, dysphagia caused by obstruction is always worst with solid foods. Thus, it is not surprising that the patient with myoneural deficits of the pharyngeal musculature repeatedly aspirates oropharyngeal secretions. In patients with esophageal obstruction, secretions accumulate proximal to the obstruction, especially at night, and are aspirated. Gastric contents are normally sterile. However, as the patient with reflux aspirates gastric contents a certain volume of oropharyngeal secretions is necessarily carried along.

Oropharyngeal secretions are massively contaminated containing 10^6 to 10^8 aerobic bacteria per milliliter and about 10 times as many anaerobic organisms. Although the majority of organisms comprising the normal flora of this region have little invasiveness for the normal host, highly pathogenic organisms including *Streptococcus pneumoniae*, *Staphylococcus aureus*, and *Hemophilus influenzae* may be present in the secretions of normal people. Since most of the patients susceptible to recurrent aspiration have serious underlying diseases, their upper respiratory tracts are likely to be colonized by enteric gram-negative bacilli and *Pseudomonas* as well. The presence of oropharyngeal mucus is probably important in promoting infection in these patients, since it tends to retard bacterial ingestion by phagocytic cells.

Normal individuals aspirate small volumes of oropharyngeal secretions during sleep but do not develop recurrent pneumonias. The difference between normal people and those who do develop recurrent pneumonias is probably the volume of material aspirated and the underlying chronic illnesses of the latter patients; differences in the bacterial composition in secretions may play a role as well.

CLINICAL MANIFESTATIONS. Episodes of recurrent pneumonia associated with aspiration tend not to be acute, fulminant illnesses but rather are characterized by progressive fever, purulent sputum production, shortness of breath, and systemic symptoms (such as loss of appetite and malaise) over a period of days. The frequency of such episodes in an individual prone to recurrent aspiration varies widely. In patients with tracheobronchial fistulas the episodes are essentially continuous until an effective preventive measure can be implemented or the patient dies. By contrast, patients with esophageal reflux may go years between episodes. The frequency of episodes is usually directly related to the frequency and volume of material aspirated and thus is increased in conditions in which aspiration is a daily event, especially if coupled with a decreased level of awareness as occurs in some patients following strokes.

Physical findings include those related to the underlying illness and the presence of coarse rhonchi over dependent lung zones. Rales and signs of consolidation may or may not be present. Fever and leukocytosis are regularly present. Radiographs of the chest reveal infiltrates of varying intensity with a preponderance of change in the dependent zones, i.e., posterior aspects of the lower lobes and posterior segments of the upper lobes. Pleural effusion is uncommon unless anaerobic infection is present.

DIAGNOSIS. Examination of expectorated sputum is helpful in confirming the suspicion of aspiration pneumonia but of little help in defining a specific bacterial etiology. Typically, the sputum of such patients is intensely purulent with a wide spectrum of bacterial forms present on Gram stain. Cultures of this material yields the same flora as in upper respiratory secretions and the clinical problem consists of trying to discern which of several pathogenic organisms should be treated. Cultures should be obtained, however, since knowledge of the sensitivity of the organisms present may be needed to guide therapy. Blood cultures are rarely positive. The presence of food particles in tracheal secretions is clear evidence of aspiration. In patients receiving enteral feedings, the presence of glucose in secretions may be demonstrable by bedside tests. Since normal secretions contain an undetectable level of glucose, a positive result is highly specific for aspiration. Dietary lipids form large intracellular deposits when ingested by phagocytic cells, and examination of sputum with a lipid stain may confirm the clinical impression of chronic aspiration. The microscopic appearance of the large lipid deposits is important in differentiating this type of lipid inclusion from the foamy deposit which occurs in macrophages due to the accumulation of endogenous lipid distal to an obstructing lesion in the airways.

When the diagnosis of recurrent aspiration is in doubt, cineradiographic studies of the patient swallowing a thin, water-soluble contrast material is usually definitive. Thick barium should be avoided as aspiration of this material compounds the patient's problems and the use of a thick solution is less likely to identify the swallowing difficulty. The procedure may need to be repeated with the patient in the supine position in questionable cases. Follow-up films of the chest reveal the presence of contrast material in the airways.

Patients with infrequent episodes of recurrent pneumonia caused by esophageal reflux and nocturnal aspiration represent a somewhat different problem. The presence of a hiatal hernia or the demonstration of reflux during an upper gastrointestinal contrast study does not necessarily prove that pneumonia was caused by this mechanism, although that would be a reasonable presumption if other aspects of the patient's presentation were compatible with the diagnosis. Probably the best diagnostic test in uncertain circumstances is to monitor the pH in the upper esophagus during sleep. Reflux into the upper esophagus is marked by a sudden fall in pH, an event which is easily captured on a long-term strip chart recorder for review the next morning. Attempts to document aspiration by placing contrast material or radioisotopes in the stomach prior to sleep are of limited value since such patients do not aspirate every night.

TREATMENT. Initial antibiotic therapy should provide broad coverage. Pending the results of culture and sensitivity studies, therapy with intravenous penicillin and an aminoglycoside is reasonable. Alternatively, a second- or third-generation cephalosporin can be used as long as coverage for gram-positive, gram-negative, and anaerobic organisms is provided. Supportive care, including aggressive tracheobronchial toilet, is required. Nutrition must not be overlooked despite the difficulties encountered in many of these patients. If swallowing is impossible and a small feeding tube cannot be placed in the intestinal tract via the nose or mouth, parenteral nutrition should be provided while a long-term solution to the patient's problem is sought. Failure to address the nutritional deficits of these patients is a common cause of protracted and often lethal complications.

Surgical intervention to prevent esophageal reflux is indicated for the patient in whom recurrent pneumonia can be reasonably attributed to this mechanism. Long-term solutions for the other patients with this syndrome often involve difficult choices. Bypassing the mouth to facilitate feeding can be accomplished with a feeding gastrostomy or enterostomy. The former can be performed noninvasively via fiberoptic gastroscopy with the feeding tube being passed percutaneously into the stomach. In some patients, cessation of swallowing food diminishes the frequency and severity of aspiration and successfully ameliorates the clinical problem. However, in many it does not because patients must still handle their own secretions. Drug therapy aimed at reducing the volume of secretions in this situation is usually not successful. The only certain preventive measure is tracheostomy with all of the complications attendant to this procedure. Even tracheostomy does not negate the possibility of aspiration around the tube unless the larynx is removed or the vocal cords are sewn together. The latter can be undone at a later date if the patient's condition improves. These procedures should not be contemplated in all patients with the syndrome of recurrent aspiration since many patients have underlying conditions that will be lethal in a short period of time. However, if the patient has a reasonable chance of long-term survival in the absence of recurrent episodes of pneumonia, these steps should be considered.

Bartlett JG: The triple threat of aspiration pneumonia. Chest 68:560, 1975. *A useful classification and review of the bacteriology of aspiration pneumonias.*

Lorber B, Swenson RM: Bacteriology of aspiration pneumonia. A prospective study of community and hospitalized cases. Ann Intern Med 81:329, 1974. *Emphasizes the differences in bacteriology among these two groups of patients.*

Winterbauer R, Durning R Jr, Baron E, et al.: Aspirated nasogastric feeding solution detected by glucose strips. Ann Intern Med 95:67, 1981. *Provides insight into the problem and a simple approach to diagnosis.*

267 LEGIONELLOSIS

David W. Fraser

DEFINITION. Legionellosis refers to acute bacterial infections of humans caused by *Legionella pneumophila, L. micdadei, L. bozemanii, L. dumoffii, L. gormanii, L. longbeachae, L. jordanis, L. wadsworthii, L. feeleii, L. hackeliae, L. maceachernii, L. oakridgensis, L. sainthelensi, L. anisa, L. jamestowniensis, L. rubrilucens, L. erythra, L. spiritensis, L. parisiensis, L. cherrii, L. steigerwaltii, L. santicrucis,* and *L. israelensis.* The first 11 have been implicated in human disease. Previous experience with *Legionella* suggests that upon further investigation others may be expected to be implicated. Infections caused by *Legionella* spp. have occurred in two distinct forms: legionnaires' disease, which is characterized by pneumonia, involvement of other organ systems, and (at least for *L. pneumophila*) a two- to ten-day incubation period; and Pontiac fever, which is characterized by fever without pneumonia or involvement of other organ systems and an incubation period of 5 to 66 hours.

ETIOLOGY. Members of the genus *Legionella* are aerobic, weakly staining, gram-negative bacilli that will not grow on most commonly used bacteriologic media but will grow on media containing supplementary L-cysteine, ferric salts, and activated charcoal. Growth is best at 35° C, but colonies may take up to 12 days to appear on primary culture, especially if the inocula are small. All except *L. erythra* have cellular fatty acids with a large proportion of branched chains. They are catalase-positive but do not ferment sugars. *Legionella* species can be distinguished most readily by direct immunofluorescence but phenotypic differences are seen in regard to the presence and color of colonial autofluorescence in ultraviolet light, the pattern of fatty acids in gas liquid chromatography, browning of yeast extract agar medium supplemented with L-tyrosine, ability to hydrolyze hippurate, and gelatinase and oxidase activity. Eleven serogroups of *L. pneumophila* and two each of *L. longbeachae, L. feeleii, L. hackeliae,* and *L. bozemanii* have been identified that can be distinguished by direct immunofluorescence or slide agglutination. In addition, antigens are shared among the serogroups of *L. pneumophila,* the species of *Legionella,* and other genera of gram-negative bacilli. Legionellae are found in a wide variety of watery environments. *L. pneumophila* can survive more than one year in tap water, apparently by associating with protozoa (including amoebae and *Tetrahymena*), cyanobacteria, and other bacteria. Variations in the virulence of strains of *L. pneumophila* have been related to the presence or absence of plasmids and particular surface antigens.

EPIDEMIOLOGY. Although only recently recognized to cause human disease, the three species of *Legionella* that cause most *Legionella* pneumonia were first isolated decades ago (*L. micdadei,* 1943; *L. pneumophila,* 1947; *L. bozemanii,* 1959). Legionellae cause outbreaks of both pneumonic and nonpneumonic disease, as well as sporadic cases of pneumonia. The incidence of sporadic *L. pneumophila* pneumonia caused by serogroups 1 or 2 has been estimated from a prospective serologic study to be 12 cases per 100,000 population per year. Those serogroups cause 57 per cent of cases of *Legionella* pneumonia diagnosed at the Centers for Disease Control, whereas *L. micdadei* and *L. bozemanii* cause 6 per cent and 3

per cent, respectively. Five per cent of recognized pneumonia cases caused by *L. pneumophila* and most so far recognized as being caused by *L. micdadei* are nosocomial. Cases of *Legionella* pneumonia have been documented in six continents. Cases occur throughout the year but primarily in the summer. Epidemiologic factors associated with increased risk of *L. pneumophila* pneumonia include male sex, middle or old age, cigarette smoking, excessive consumption of alcohol, travel, work in construction, residence near excavation or construction, and underlying medical conditions or therapy commonly associated with immunosuppression. Immunosuppression is also common in those with *L. micdadei* and *L. bozemanii* pneumonia.

The only proven mode of spread of *Legionella* is the airborne route. Outbreaks have been traced to airborne spread of bacteria released in aerosols by air-conditioning cooling towers, evaporative condensers, humidifiers, and industrial grinding machinery and inhaled by people downwind. *L. pneumophila* infections have been traced to contamination of the hot water in potable water systems, but whether spread in these cases is by aerosolization, drinking, or mucous membrane contact is unknown. Person-to-person spread has not been documented.

Clusters of *Legionella* infections have occurred in one of two epidemiologic patterns. Outbreaks of legionnaires' disease (named for the group most affected in the 1976 Philadelphia outbreak) are characterized by attack rates of 0.1 to 5.0 per cent for people presumed to be exposed. All documented point-source outbreaks have been caused by *L. pneumophila,* and the usual incubation period has been two to ten days (mean = 5.5 days). Continuing common-source outbreaks of *L. micdadei* and *L. bozemanii* pneumonia have not permitted estimation of incubation periods. Pontiac fever outbreaks (named for the city in which an outbreak occurred in 1968) are characterized by attack rates of 95 to 100 per cent for people intensively exposed and by incubation periods of 5 to 66 hours (mean = 36 hours). They have been caused by *L. pneumophila* and *L. feeleii.* No differences in the source or mode of spread of the organism appear to explain the epidemiologic (or clinical—see later discussion) differences between legionnaires' disease and Pontiac fever.

PATHOGENESIS. Legionnaires' disease appears to occur two to ten days after inhalation of *L. pneumophila.* About half of those infected develop clinical illness. The only consistent pathologic condition found is in the lung and includes areas of acute fibrinopurulent pneumonia bounded by lobular septa. The infiltrate comprises polymorphonuclear leukocytes and macrophages, many of which are necrotic, mixed with proliferating type II pneumocytes and fibrin. Large numbers of bacteria can be demonstrated by Dieterle silver stain or direct immunofluorescence in areas of pneumonia and commonly clustered in macrophages. Bacteria can also be seen in areas of pleuritis. The lung architecture is usually intact, although focal septal necrosis is sometimes seen, and frank lung abscess may occur in immunosuppressed people. Respiratory bronchioles are affected, but larger bronchioles and bronchi (and their cilia) are spared, perhaps explaining in part the usual paucity of sputum and rarity of person-to-person spread. Healing is commonly complete, but in some patients residual fibrosis can be detected by diminished capacity to diffuse carbon monoxide.

The degree to which involvement of organs other than the lungs is due to direct invasion by *L. pneumophila* or to remote effects of the organism in lung tissue is uncertain. Rarely, *L. pneumophila* has been visualized in mediastinal lymph nodes, blood vessels, liver, spleen, bone marrow, and kidneys and has been recovered from blood. *L. pneumophila* has some of the properties of endotoxins and produces proteases and a lymphocytotoxin, but the role of these or other toxins in the pathogenesis of disease is unclear.

L. pneumophila organisms are ingested by monocytes, including human alveolar macrophages. In unactivated macrophages, the bacteria multiply freely—apparently helped by their ability to inhibit phagosome-lysozyme fusion. In macrophages that are activated, as by incubation with lymphocytes stimulated by concanavalin A, *L. pneumophila* multiply more slowly and may indeed be killed. The intracellular location of *Legionella* may help explain the poor agreement between antibiotic sensitivities observed in vitro and in vivo. Although complement-mediated opsonization and killing of *L. pneumophila*, by the classic pathway, are accelerated by specific antibody in vitro, a protective effect of antibody has not been shown in humans. The possibility that opsonic activity of serogroup-specific antibody is more protective of bacterium than host has been suggested.

Little is known about the pathophysiology of the Pontiac fever syndrome of *L. pneumophila* or *L. feeleii* infection or of the cases of pneumonia caused by legionellae other than *L. pneumophila*. Pathologically, the latter cases resemble *L. pneumophila* pneumonia. No differences have been found in *L. pneumophila* strains that cause legionnaires' disease and Pontiac fever.

CLINICAL MANIFESTATIONS. *Legionella* infections occur in at least two distinct syndromes: legionnaires' disease and Pontiac fever. Pontiac fever is an acute influenza-like illness characterized by fever, headache, and myalgia. Cough, sore throat, diarrhea, confusion, and chest pain occur but are not usually prominent. Pneumonia does not occur, although one patient had a pleural friction rub during convalescence. The illness is debilitating for two to seven days, but all patients recover completely.

Legionnaires' disease varies in severity from a mild grippe to a severe multisystem disease affecting lungs, liver, kidney, gastrointestinal tract, and central nervous system. Typically, patients have the subacute onset of malaise, weakness, anorexia, dry cough, and fever, without accompanying upper respiratory symptoms. Illness progresses over the next day or two, commonly with repeated rigors, pleuritic chest pain, headache, watery diarrhea, generalized abdominal pain, and confusion. Sputum may be expectorated but is often scant and nonpurulent and may be streaked with blood. Patients appear acutely ill, usually with temperatures of 38.9 to 40.4° C. The degree of tachypnea reflects the severity of the pneumonia, but the pulse rate is often slower than would be expected from the temperature. Pulmonary rales are common early, and signs of consolidation may appear later. Nonfocal neurologic disturbances (confusion, clumsiness, ataxia, slurred speech, and apparent hallucinations) occur and often are of a severity disproportionate to the degree of fever or metabolic derangements.

Laboratory testing shows normal or moderately elevated leukocyte counts with an excess of juvenile neutrophils. Erythrocyte sedimentation rate is greatly elevated. Modest elevations of serum concentrations of transaminases are common. Microscopic hematuria is seen in one third of patients and is often accompanied by cylindruria and proteinuria. Azotemia is found at some time during the illness in about 15 per cent of patients and occasionally necessitates dialysis. Chest radiographs may show patchy infiltrates early in the disease, which later progress to dense consolidation, often in a lobar or segmental pattern and commonly bilaterally. Cavitation is sometimes seen in the immunocompromised host. Pleural effusions are seen in up to one third of patients but are small except in occasional immunosuppressed patients. Gram staining of transtracheally aspirated material usually shows moderate numbers of neutrophils, but large numbers of bacilli are rarely seen. The protein and cellular composition of pleural fluid suggests an exudate in half and a transudate in the other half of the cases in which it is examined. Cerebrospinal fluid is usually normal, although small numbers of lymphocytes have been seen. Without specific therapy fever, pneumonia, and accompanying hypoxemia may pro-

gress for five to seven days and be complicated by the syndrome of inappropriate secretion of antidiuretic hormone. Death occurs in 15 to 20 per cent of patients (up to 60 per cent in nosocomial cases) and is usually the result of progressive pneumonia; however, in a few cases a syndrome resembling septic shock precedes death. With specific therapy temperature generally begins to decrease within 24 hours and may be normal within two days, although radiographically the pneumonia may continue to progress for two to five days. Radiographic resolution of *L. pneumophila* pneumonia may take many weeks, longer than for pneumococcal or *Mycoplasma* pneumonia. Residual scarring can be seen histologically and radiographically. In rare cases patients with severe neurologic involvement show mild residual aphasia and impaired memory. Amnesia for the acute illness is common.

Rare cases of *Legionella* infection localized outside the lungs have involved perirectal abscess, focal myocarditis, pericarditis, cutaneous abscess, hemodialysis fistula infection, or pyelonephritis. Coinfection with other bacteria may occur in such sites.

DIAGNOSIS. *Legionella* pneumonia must be distinguished from pneumonia caused by other bacteria or infections caused by *Mycoplasma pneumoniae*, *Chlamydia psittaci*, *Coxiella burnetii*, influenza virus, or several other respiratory viruses. Clinical clues that may be of differential value for *L. pneumophila* pneumonia include very high fever with repeated rigors, lack of preceding upper respiratory symptoms, diarrhea, unexplained impairment of mental function, hematuria, abnormal liver function, negative routine bacteriologic cultures, and failure to respond to therapy with penicillins, cephalosporins, or aminoglycosides. Epidemiologic clues (see above) may also be helpful in suggesting the diagnosis. With *Legionella* pneumonia, staining well-collected lower respiratory secretions by the Gram method reveals neutrophils accompanied by no bacteria or by weakly staining gram-negative bacilli.

Specific diagnosis is made by isolation of *Legionella* from lung tissue, respiratory secretions, pleural fluid, or blood; detection of specific antigens in lung tissue, respiratory secretions, extrapulmonary tissue, or urine; or demonstration of a significant rise in serum antibody titer during convalescence. Buffered charcoal yeast extract (CYE) agar supports growth of all species, but isolation of *L. pneumophila* from sputum is aided by the incorporation of cefamandole (or vancomycin), polymixin B, and anisomycin in the agar to inhibit other organisms. A biphasic medium with CYE agar as the solid phase has been successful for culture of *L. pneumophila* from blood. Direct immunofluorescence using species- and serogroup-specific conjugated antisera is useful in detecting *Legionella* in tissues and secretions. For *L. pneumophila*, about two thirds of infected patients have organisms detectable in lower respiratory tract secretions, and they remain detectable for an average of four days after specific therapy is started. *L. pneumophila* serogroup 1 antigen can be detected in the urine of most infected patients by latex agglutination, enzyme-linked immunoassay, or radioimmunoassay and may persist for many weeks. The procedure used for serologic detection of infection is usually indirect immunofluorescence, but this procedure is not well standardized for strains other than *L. pneumophila* serogroup 1. About 80 per cent of patients with *L. pneumophila* pneumonia have a four-fold or greater rise in antibody titer to 1:128 or greater within two to six weeks after onset of symptoms. Rises in titer are not always serogroup specific and may involve IgM, IgG, or IgA. Because rises in titers to *L. pneumophila* have been found in patients with culture-confirmed plague, tularemia, or *Bacteroides fragilis* bacteremia and in patients with simultaneous rises in antibody titers to *M. pneumoniae* or *Leptospira interrogans*, it is likely that serologic diagnosis is not always specific.

THERAPY. Patients with severe *Legionella* pneumonia require supportive respiratory therapy, including supplemental oxygen and mechanical ventilation with or without positive end-expiratory pressure. Careful management of fluid and electrolytes may be necessary in cases of renal insufficiency and inappropriate secretion of antidiuretic hormone. Dialysis may be needed as a temporary measure in frank renal failure.

Experimental studies suggest that erythromycin and rifampin are effective specific therapy against all *Legionella* species, although information about other antimicrobials is conflicting. Retrospective studies of epidemic cases show that therapy of *L. pneumophila* pneumonia with erythromycin is associated with a decrease in case-fatality rate from 24 to 5 per cent.

Recommended initial therapy for pneumonia suspected to be caused by any of the *Legionella* species is erythromycin, 2 grams per day (50 mg per kilogram per day for children) given in four divided doses orally, or in seriously ill patients, intravenously. The dose for adults can be doubled if clinical response is not prompt. Patients with confirmed disease who do not respond to high-dose erythromycin given intravenously may be given rifampin, 600 mg daily, in addition. Because of concern about development of resistance to the drug, rifampin should not be given alone. Therapy should continue for 14 days, although pulmonary cavitation may require therapy to be prolonged. The possibility of relapse after specific therapy is stopped should be remembered. In cases of relapse, erythromycin therapy should be resumed promptly. The potential value of sulfamethoxazole-trimethoprim and tetracyclines in treating *Legionella* pneumonia deserves further study.

Initial treatment of adults with pneumonias of uncertain cause but suspected to be of bacterial origin can usefully include erythromycin—with or without an aminoglycoside—because of the relative safety of erythromycin and its broad spectrum of activity against the most common bacterial agents of pneumonia in this group. Doses are as recommended for *Legionella* pneumonia.

No specific therapy is needed for Pontiac fever.

PREVENTION. Outbreaks caused by organisms from contaminated cooling towers, evaporative condensers, humidifiers, or industrial grinding coolants can be stopped by turning off this equipment or perhaps by treating it with chemicals effective against *L. pneumophila*, such as calcium hypochlorite, quaternary ammonium compounds, and dibromonitrilopropionamide. Whether these chemicals would be helpful in preventive maintenance of these units is unknown. Outbreaks traced to potable water have been controlled by raising the temperature of the hot water to ≥55° C or by hyperchlorination (to ≥2 mg free residual chlorine per liter). Secretion precautions in hospitalized cases may be helpful in decreasing the theoretical possibility of person-to-person spread. In the laboratory caution should be exercised to prevent generation of aerosols to live organisms or to contain them in a biologic safety cabinet.

Brenner DJ, Steigerwalt AG, Gorman GW, et al.: Ten new species of *Legionella*. Int J System Bacteriol 35:50, 1985. *A clear guide to the species of Legionella.*

Fraser DW, Tsai TR, Orenstein W, et al.: Legionnaires' disease. Description of an epidemic of pneumonia. N Engl J Med 297:1189, 1977. *The 1976 Philadelphia outbreak.*

Helms CM, Viner JP, Weisenburger DD, et al.: Sporadic Legionnaires' disease: Clinical observations in 87 nosocomial and community-acquired cases. Am J Med Sci 288:2, 1984. *Good clinical summary with illustrative case reports and extensive references.*

Horwitz MA: Phagocytosis of the Legionnaires' disease bacterium (*Legionella pneumophila*) occurs by a novel mechanism: Engulfment within a pseudopod coil. Cell 36:27, 1984. *One of a series of papers that emphasize the role of cell-mediated immunity in legionellosis.*

Johnson JT, Yu VL, Best MG, et al.: Nosocomial legionellosis in surgical patients with head-and-neck cancer: Implications for epidemiological reservoir and mode of transmission. Lancet 2:298, 1985. *Impressive evidence that legionellosis may be overlooked.*

Kohler RB, Winn WC Jr, Wheat LJ: Onset and duration of urinary antigen excretion in Legionnaires' disease. J Clin Microbiol 20:605, 1984. *Utility of urinary antigen detection in diagnosis of legionellosis.*

Parry MF, Stampleman L, Hutchinson JH, et al.: Waterborne *Legionella bozemanii* and nosocomial pneumonia in immunosuppressed patients. Ann Intern Med 103:205, 1985. *Concise review of problems of diagnosis and control of legionellosis.*

Winn WC, Myerowitz R: The pathology of *Legionella* pneumonias: A review of 74 cases and the literature. Hum Pathol 12:401, 1981. *Documents the similarity of pneumonias caused by the various Legionellae.*

Zuravleff JJ, Yu VL, Shonnard JW, et al.: Diagnosis of legionnaires' disease. JAMA 250:1981, 1983. *A summary of laboratory methods, emphasizing value of culture.*

Streptococcal Diseases

268 STREPTOCOCCAL DISEASES

Richard M. Krause

Streptococci are ubiquitous, gram-positive globular bacteria that grow in chains. They were first described by Billroth in 1874 in purulent exudates from erysipelas lesions and infected wounds. Subsequently they were shown to cause different forms of streptococcal disease, including streptococcal sore throat, scarlet fever, streptococcal skin infections (impetigo or pyoderma), suppurative infections including abscesses and pneumonia, food poisoning, septicemia, bacterial endocarditis, and urinary tract infections. A single streptococcal species may be responsible for a variety of diseases, and many different kinds of streptococci may be cultured from humans and animals.

The first classification of these organisms was based on their capacity to lyse red blood cells. When streptococci are cultured on blood agar plates, three types of hemolytic reactions are observed. Streptococcal colonies surrounded by a clear zone of hemolysis are termed beta, colonies surrounded by green partial hemolysis are termed alpha, and the nonhemolytic colonies are termed gamma.

Primarily through the efforts of Lancefield, the beta-hemolytic streptococci were further differentiated into a number of immunologic categories, designated groups A to H and K to T, on the basis of specific polysaccharide antigens. Most streptococci causing pharyngitis and impetigo belong to group A. Rheumatic fever occurs only after group A pharyngitis. Streptococci belonging to certain other Lancefield groups are now recognized as important causes of infection. Alpha-hemolytic and gamma streptococci can cause sepsis with systemic illness.

Group A streptococcal pharyngitis has been intensely studied over the years because it may give rise to the delayed, nonsuppurative sequelae acute rheumatic fever (ARF) and acute glomerulonephritis (AGN). While ARF is less common in the United States today than 30 years ago, it still persists as a common cause of heart disease in the developing world. Pyoderma due to group A streptococci may lead to AGN but not to ARF.

CLASSIFICATION OF STREPTOCOCCI OF CLINICAL IMPORTANCE

The classification of streptococci on the basis of hemolysis patterns on blood agar plates and antigenic composition was a major advance. Nevertheless, it is frequently necessary to employ a combination of features, including growth charac-

TABLE 268–1. CLINICAL CLASSES OF STREPTOCOCCAL INFECTIONS

Lancefield Groups	Hemolysis on Blood Agar	Representative Species	Major Clinical Syndromes	Colonization (Carriage)
A	Beta	S. pyogenes	Pharyngitis (scarlet fever), pyoderma, wound infection, sepsis, rheumatic fever, acute glomerulonephritis	Pharynx
B	Beta	S. agalactiae	Perinatal sepsis, newborn meningitis, subacute bacterial endocarditis, urinary tract infection, adult sepsis	Adult urogenital tract, gastrointestinal tract, throat, rectum, pharynx
C and G	Beta	—	Mild pharyngitis	Pharynx
D	Variable (usually nonhemolytic)	Enterococci (S. faecalis)	Subacute bacterial endocarditis, urinary tract infection	Bowel
		Nonenterococci (S. bovis)	Subacute bacterial endocarditis	
Nongroupable: viridans streptococci	Alpha (green)	S. salivarius, S. sanguis, S. mutans	Subacute bacterial endocarditis, caries	Oropharynx, saliva
Anaerobic (microaerophilic streptococci)	Gamma (nonhemolytic) or variable	Peptostreptococcus	Abscesses, gangrene, necrotizing fasciitis, peritonsillar abscess	Mouth, intestine, vagina

teristics and biochemical reactions, to fully characterize these organisms because they are such a heterogeneous group. A classification of streptococci with a clinical orientation for the most important streptococcal infections is presented in Table 268–1. While group A streptococci remain important human pathogens, beta-hemolytic non–group A, alpha-hemolytic, and nonhemolytic streptococci are of increasing importance as the cause of suppurative infections in all regions of the body.

GROUP A INFECTIONS. Group A streptococci are the most common cause of streptococcal pharyngitis. They are recognized by the characteristic group A carbohydrate cell wall antigen, which is identified by serologic reactions to specific rabbit antiserum. In this way they can be distinguished from other beta-hemolytic streptococci that are also frequently isolated from the human pharynx, vagina, or skin.

GROUP B INFECTIONS. Group B streptococci are identified serologically by their characteristic cell wall polysaccharide. Group B streptococci were first recognized as a cause of bovine mastitis, but since the 1960's they have emerged as a major cause of neonatal sepsis with or without meningitis. Carriage of group B streptococci in the female genital tract is a major source of these infections.

GROUP D INFECTIONS. Group D streptococci consist of two major categories: enterococci (such as S. faecalis) and nonenterococci (such as S. bovis). Strains isolated from clinical cultures are usually nonhemolytic or alpha-hemolytic, but beta-hemolytic strains are seen.

Enterococci are present in the normal intestinal flora and are a significant cause of community-acquired and hospital-acquired sepsis, as demonstrated by the cultivation of these organisms from the blood. Enterococci are a frequent cause of urinary tract infections, particularly in patients with structural abnormalities of the urinary tract. They are also a frequent cause of endocarditis. Enterococci are frequently resistant to many antibiotics, which complicates treatment. For the treatment of enterococcal endocarditis, combined therapy should be employed, including intravenously administered penicillin in high doses plus an aminoglycoside antibiotic. In combination, these drugs have a synergistic killing effect on enterococci.

In contrast to enterococci, nonenterococcal group D streptococci isolated from patients with endocarditis are extremely sensitive to penicillin. Because of these differences in antibiotic sensitivity, it may be necessary to perform additional biochemical tests to differentiate enterococci from nonenterococcal group D organisms. One simple procedure that may be

useful is to attempt growth in a broth containing 6.5 per cent sodium chloride. Enterococci will usually grow under these conditions, whereas other streptococci will not.

OTHER STREPTOCOCCAL INFECTIONS. Not infrequently, the beta-hemolytic streptococci cultured from the throat or other sites are identified as group C or G organisms. Most commonly when they colonize the pharynx, these organisms produce no symptoms or illness. But on occasion pharyngitis occurs, which may be exudative. A rise in the convalescent antistreptolysin O titer indicates that these groups actually can cause an infection of the pharynx and other sites and are not just passively carried. An unexpected event was the occurrence of ten cases of group C streptococcal sepsis, including meningitis, in New Mexico in the summer of 1983. In addition to groups C and G, case reports indicate that streptococci belonging to most of the other groups can cause sporadic infections, including meningitis, infected heart valves, visceral abscesses, and soft tissue infections following surgical procedures. Furthermore, these less common organisms are now known to cause opportunistic infections in individuals whose resistance has been compromised by other diseases or treatments.

The predominant aerobic flora of the oral pharynx normally consists of a large variety of streptococci. These are classified as viridans, alpha-hemolytic, or green streptococci. It is probable that they might play some useful role by maintaining a favorable ecologic balance. However, they can produce disease in abnormal circumstances. They are a common cause of subacute bacterial endocarditis and enter the bloodstream most often from diseased teeth and gums.

Special interest has now centered on a species of these organisms identified as S. mutans. These bacteria colonize the oral cavity and have been implicated in the development of dental caries. They produce a mucoid substance that becomes part of the plaque adhering to the tooth enamel. The bacteria remain embedded in the plaque and excrete metabolic products that are a factor in the production of caries. Currently there is evidence that dental caries can be prevented by decreasing sugar in the diet to diminish the growth of these bacteria as well as by practicing proper oral hygiene to remove the plaque containing the S. mutans organisms.

Anaerobic streptococci are also a prominent part of the normal flora in the mouth, intestine, and vagina. It is suspected that they maintain an ecologic balance on the surface of these tissues, but the mechanism is unknown. The presence of this normal flora appears to be important, however, because when the ecologic balance is disturbed by the use of antibiotics, pathogens such as *Candida albicans* may cause infections of these sites.

Anaerobic streptococci may cause abscesses in many different regions of the body, including retropharyngeal spaces, paranasal sinuses, dental structures, and the brain. Visceral infections include lung abscesses and empyema fluids, abscesses of the liver and other intra-abdominal viscera, and perirectal and pelvic abscesses. Anaerobic streptococci are especially prone to thrive in dead or devitalized muscle, skin, or subcutaneous tissue. A rapidly progressing necrotizing fasciitis or *progressive synergistic gangrene* is usually produced by these anaerobic streptococci along with *Staphylococcus aureus*. While these anaerobic organisms are frequently sensitive to penicillin, debridement and drainage of abscesses is an important aspect of treatment.

GROUP A STREPTOCOCCAL INFECTIONS

BACKGROUND AND PATHOGENESIS. Although streptococci were identified as the cause of scarlet fever and tonsillitis in 1895, determination of the origin and epidemiology of streptococcal infections stems from the serologic classification of the organisms into groups by Lancefield and into types by Lancefield and Griffith. With these developments it was possible to identify group A streptococci as the most common cause of streptococcal pharyngitis. The ability to measure serologic responses was another important advance. Most widely used has been the antistreptolysin O (ASO) test developed by Todd in 1932. This was a major achievement because a rise in an ASO titer or a markedly elevated titer was indicative of a prior streptococcal infection. These immunologic and bacteriologic developments led to the firm conclusion that ARF and AGN were nonsuppurative sequelae to group A streptococcal infections and that infections by *any* of the other streptococcal groups did not result in such sequelae. The rare exception to this rule is that, on occasion, group C streptococcal infections appear to cause AGN. ARF is *only* observed after group A pharyngitis, but AGN is seen after pharyngitis and pyoderma.

Epidemics of streptococcal disease in the armed forces have been known since the Civil War. The epidemics in World War I, World War II, and the Korean War were studied in detail, and much of the current knowledge concerning the epidemiology of group A streptococcal disease rests on this research. A major advance was the prevention of rheumatic fever by penicillin treatment of streptococcal pharyngitis and the use of penicillin prophylaxis to prevent recurrences of ARF in patients who had had prior ARF. Epidemics have not been confined to the armed forces, however. Epidemics of streptococcal sore throat and scarlet fever were once commonly observed among school children, and this resulted in extensive programs for the early detection and treatment of pharyngitis and the subsequent prevention of rheumatic fever. While epidemics of streptococcal pharyngitis are now less common, sporadic outbreaks in schools or other closed populations still occur as minor epidemics. As a result, occasional cases of ARF and AGN are still seen in civilian populations.

Group A streptococci are subdivided into M types on the basis of an antigen known as *M protein*. More than 70 antigenically distinct M types have been identified. This substance plays a very important role in the pathogenesis of group A streptococcal infections. The M protein is a surface component of the streptococcus and is correlated with its ability to resist phagocytosis. Streptococci that have large amounts of M protein are highly resistant to phagocytosis, whereas those with no, or small, amounts of M protein are susceptible to phagocytosis. Following an infection with streptococci of a particular M type, homologous type-specific immunity develops, so that the individual is resistant to infection by organisms of the same M type. Because this type-specific antibody can persist for many years, reinfection with the same M type is rare. Penicillin or other antibiotic therapy can suppress the type-specific immune response, however; for this reason reinfection with the same M type has been seen in recent years. Because immunity is M-type–specific and because there are numerous M types of streptococci, repeated streptococcal infections caused by different M types are common, particularly in childhood and early adult life.

Because of the importance of M-type–specific immunity in resistance to group A streptococcal infections, intensive research has centered on the immunochemistry of the M protein and the immune response to it. The complete chemical structure of several different M proteins is now known, and with the use of recombinant deoxyribonucleic acid technology, pure type 6 M protein has been produced by *Escherichia coli*. It should now be possible to examine at the molecular level the chemical basis for the antiphagocytic properties of M protein and to explore the molecular interactions that occur when specific antibody promotes phagocytosis of group A streptococci. While these recent developments on the chemistry of M protein again have raised the possibility of a multivalent streptococcal vaccine for use in regions where streptococcal disease still flourishes, a number of theoretical and practical impediments to the development of such a vaccine have to be overcome.

The T antigen is another streptococcal surface protein that has assisted in the classification of streptococci isolated from clinical material. As with M proteins, there are multiple serotypes of T antigens. While T antigens (unlike M proteins) play no part in virulence, they have become very useful antigenic markers, particularly in the recognition of less virulent strains that have lost their M protein. The T antigen classification also has been useful in identifying strains isolated from patients with pyoderma for which an M protein has not yet been identified.

Group A streptococci grown in vivo and in vitro produce a great variety of antigenic extracellular products such as the two hemolysins—streptolysin O and streptolysin S—streptokinase, hyaluronidase, nicotinamide adenine dinucleotidase (NADase), and several deoxyribonucleases (DNAses). The antibody responses to several of these substances are useful in clinical diagnosis. Streptolysin O is reversibly inhibited by oxygen. Because anaerobic conditions prevail beneath the surface of the blood agar, hemolysis in this region is due to streptolysin O. Streptolysin O is produced by almost all group A strains as well as by many group C and G organisms. Since streptolysin O is a good antigen, titration of ASO antibodies in human sera is the most widely used serologic procedure in clinical practice to detect a prior group A streptococcal infection. In recent years, a test to measure anti-DNAse B antibodies has been used in the evaluation of streptococcal pyoderma as well as upper respiratory tract infections.

The erythrogenic toxins cause the typical erythema of scarlet fever. There are three serologically distinct toxins, each neutralized by its respective antibody. For this reason scarlet fever may occur more than once. Not all strains of streptococci produce an erythrogenic toxin.

Group A streptococci most commonly infect the tonsils, nasopharynx, and skin. A number of features of streptococcal skin infections set them apart from streptococcal tonsillitis and, for this reason, the clinical features of skin infections will be considered separately.

EPIDEMIOLOGY. Streptococcal pharyngitis and tonsillitis are the most common group A streptococcal infections. Their most frequent occurrence is in children between 5 and 15 years of age, but both younger and older persons are still highly susceptible to infection. This is particularly true when special environmental circumstances enhance transmission. For example, mobilization of troops during wartime results in an increased incidence of streptococcal infections in individuals 18 to 25 years of age. The high attack rate in children and military recruits is related to the mode of transmission of group A streptococcal infections. Transmission occurs as a result of close contact between susceptible individuals and either infected persons or healthy individuals who carry contagious streptococci in the pharynx. Organisms are transmitted from one person to another on saliva droplets produced by sneezing or coughing. For this reason, transmission of this disease requires close association with an individual who harbors infectious streptococci in the pharynx.

Untreated patients are the primary source of the spread of streptococcal disease, especially during the period of acute pharyngitis and for the first several weeks of convalescence. Studies of kindergarten and school-age children indicate that an untreated child is often the source of the disease in the classroom as well as in the home. It is therefore important to identify and treat patients as soon as possible to prevent secondary spread of the disease.

Throat cultures of untreated patients obtained during the illness and early convalescence (one to three weeks) usually reveal large numbers of streptococci, and therefore the source of spread. Small numbers of streptococci may be detected in the throat cultures for many weeks or months after an untreated infection. However, individuals in whom small amounts of streptococci persist for long periods are an unusual source of secondary spread.

Nasal or throat carriage (or both) of virulent streptococci is also a source of infection of open wounds and skin abrasions as well as of puerperal sepsis. Secondary infection of the lungs may occur, particularly after a respiratory infection such as influenza. Indeed, streptococcal pneumonia may be seen with greater frequency during an influenza epidemic.

A confusing aspect of streptococcal pharyngitis is that a significant number of individuals have "silent" infections that are detected by positive throat cultures *and* a rise in the ASO titer. In early studies it was learned that at least 25 to 30 per cent of all patients who developed ARF had had a preceding silent throat infection. Such silent infections complicate the control of spread of streptococcal disease in a family or community. Epidemiologic studies have shown that patients with subclinical or silent infection are capable of disseminating the streptococci to other individuals who then may develop overt disease.

Currently there is debate concerning reasons for the declining frequency of severe acute pharyngitis with exudate. Certainly the number of such patients with severe disease is much smaller than it was 30 years ago, while the mild form appears more common. It is unknown whether this change in the clinical picture is due to a decline in the virulence of the streptococci, to host factors, or to the widespread use of antibiotics to treat patients who have been infected with the more virulent forms of streptococci, thus eliminating these organisms from the reservoir of potential pathogens.

A number of epidemiologic factors influence the spread of streptococcal disease. Clearly, socioeconomic factors that promote crowding will result in close contact between individuals and therefore in the spread of streptococci. Climate, season, and geography also can enhance the spread of streptococci because of their influence in bringing people into close contact. It has already been mentioned that military recruits are susceptible because they are clustered in large camps under crowded conditions. Similarly, streptococcal disease is common in civilian populations where poverty and poor housing promote crowding and therefore the spread from one individual to another. It is probable that these factors continue to influence the widespread occurrence of streptococcal disease, and therefore ARF and rheumatic heart disease, in developing countries.

Scarlet fever is now uncommon in the United States. The reasons for this are not clear, because the decline began before the widespread use of antibiotics. Streptococcal strains that produce scarlet fever are the same as those that produce group A infections except that they are lysogenized by a bacteriophage that induces the production of erythrogenic toxin.

Although streptococcal pharyngitis is most common in the winter months when close contact between individuals is greatest, streptococcal pyoderma occurs in the late summer and early fall. Presumably this is due to exposure of uncovered skin, during the warmer months, to minor trauma and insect bites, which favor skin infections. Although streptococcal pharyngitis and streptococcal pyoderma occur worldwide, geography clearly influences the occurrence of these diseases. Pharyngitis is most common in temperate and cold climates, and pyoderma is more frequent in hot or tropical climates.

The attack rate of ARF after streptococcal infections may vary widely. During the major epidemics of World War II and the Korean War, the attack rate was 3 per cent or more in military recruits with untreated group A streptococcal infections. Since that time, studies of children and other civilian populations, particularly those experiencing the sporadic infections that occur today, have suggested that the attack rate may be as low as 0.3 per cent or less.

The epidemiology and bacteriology of the streptococcal infections that precede ARF differ in important respects from those of the streptococcal infections that precede AGN. In the early years of streptococcal bacteriology, ARF was seen as a complication of epidemic pharyngitis due to nearly all of the different types of group A streptococci. For example, certain M types such as 1, 3, 5, 6, 14, 18, 19, and 24 have all produced epidemics of pharyngitis in the United States that have resulted in ARF. In contrast, AGN was not a constant complication of these epidemics. The occurrence of AGN has been associated with epidemics of pharyngitis caused by a limited number of M types, such as type 12. Such differences in the bacteriology of ARF and AGN have raised speculation concerning "rheumatogenic" and "nephritogenic" strains of streptococci. However, such designations become blurred on the basis of epidemiologic information. Sporadic outbreaks of AGN caused by types 1, 3, and 6 have been seen, all of which have been associated with ARF. There is no doubt that certain outbreaks of type 12 pharyngitis have resulted in an unusually high incidence of AGN, but type 12 strains in the general population have not consistently resulted in outbreaks of AGN. Therefore, no single M type can be arbitrarily designated "nephritogenic." Clearly the *antecedent* streptococcal infection that results in AGN must be due to an organism that has acquired some special characteristic other than a particular M protein. Despite intensive study, there is no certainty as to the nature of this special characteristic. Efforts are under way to identify streptococcal antigens in the immune complexes of patients with AGN that are associated with "nephritogenic" streptococci. It is tempting to speculate that strains acquire the "nephritogenic" property by some form of gene transfer from those streptococci that already possess the capacity to produce AGN.

As attention was focused on the epidemiology of streptococcal infections and AGN, additional M serotypes that had not been associated with pharyngitis were identified, primarily from skin infections. Nearly 20 new M serotypes have been identified from skin cultures as the cause of impetigo. AGN has been associated with skin infections due to several of these types, such as M types 2, 49, 55, and 57.

Streptococcal Sore Throat

The usual incubation period of streptococcal pharyngitis is between two and four days. Typically, in both children and adults there is a rather abrupt onset of sore throat. A particular characteristic is pain on swallowing. Hoarseness is rare. Other symptoms include headache, malaise, feverishness, and anorexia. Chilliness is common, but not rigor. Nausea, vomiting, and abdominal pain are common in children. The patient appears mildly to moderately ill, but signs and symptoms depend upon the severity of the illness. Temperature frequently exceeds 38.5° C. In the moderately severe case, examination of the throat reveals diffuse erythema, edema, and lymphoid hyperplasia of the posterior pharynx. The uvula may be edematous. The tonsils are enlarged and reddened, with either a punctate or a confluent yellow-gray exudate. There may be discrete areas of exudate about 1 to 2 mm in diameter on the posterior pharynx. The anterior cervical nodes are usually enlarged and tender. The white blood cell count is usually greater than 12,000 per cu mm. When properly taken, the throat culture usually reveals large numbers of group A beta-hemolytic streptococci. Not uncommonly, group A streptococci are the predominant organisms observed on the culture plate. The course of streptococcal pharyngitis is usually self-limited and the fever and other symptoms abate within a week.

A pharyngitis of the severity just described is typical of the infections seen in earlier years in civilian populations and during military epidemics, but such infections occur less commonly today. Many patients do not have all of the signs and symptoms just described. For example, in mild pharyngitis, there may be no exudate and the throat culture may reveal modest numbers of group A streptococci.

If antimicrobial therapy has not been used, group A streptococci may persist in the pharynx for weeks or months following acute pharyngitis. Some patients who are treated with penicillin will carry the streptococci for several weeks. If the course of antibiotics has been adequate, these patients need not be retreated, since they are unlikely to be a source of spread to other individuals.

The diagnosis of streptococcal pharyngitis in infants and small children presents a special challenge. The disease lacks a well-defined onset. Often there is rhinorrhea as a dominant manifestation. Fever is low grade. Usually the physical signs in the throat are not helpful in the differential diagnosis. A throat culture is positive when properly taken, as is the culture of the anterior nares. Despite the mildness of the pharyngitis in infants, suppurative complications such as otitis media can occur.

Scarlet Fever

Scarlet fever occurs in those patients with streptococcal pharyngitis in whom the infected organism produces an erythrogenic toxin and who are not immune to the toxin because they have had no prior exposure. The enanthem of scarlet fever includes a tongue that may be bright red with large papillae (raspberry tongue) or coated, with the red papillae protruding (strawberry tongue). These manifestations of the disease are rarely seen in adults. The rash appears shortly after the onset of the sore throat, usually within two days, and involves the neck, upper chest, and back and then spreads to the remainder of the trunk and the extremities. The palms and the soles are spared. The rash consists of a diffuse erythema that blanches on pressure, with numerous 1-mm punctate elevations that give a sandpaper texture to the skin. There is a generalized facial flush with a pale area often seen around the mouth, the *circumoral pallor*. The distribution of the rash is variable. The trunk and inner aspects of the arms and thighs are most often affected, but in milder cases the rash is seen only in the axilla or groin. Linear striations of confluent petechiae are known as *Pastia's lines*. A tourniquet applied to the arm for five minutes results in large numbers of petechiae distal to the obstruction in nearly all cases (the *Rumpel-Leede sign*). The erythema usually disappears by the sixth to ninth day after the onset of infection. Desquamation of the skin is a characteristic of scarlet fever. It begins with a fine scaling of the face and body and is usually completed during the second week. There then occurs an extensive and characteristic desquamation of the palms and soles. Eosinophilia has been observed, particularly during the period of desquamation.

SUPPURATIVE COMPLICATIONS. The most frequent suppurative complications of streptococcal pharyngitis are perinasal sinusitis, otitis media, and mastoiditis. Suppurative cervical adenitis may occur. Bacteremia was seen more commonly in earlier times prior to the use of antibiotics; this resulted in metastatic lesions in joints, bones, and other sites. Group A streptococcal meningitis is now uncommon.

An unusual and infrequent complication of streptococcal tonsillitis is *peritonsillar abscess*, or *quinsy*. While it is probable that the streptococcal infection leads to the formation of the abscess, the abscesses themselves do not contain group A streptococci but a variety of oropharyngeal flora, including anaerobic bacteria. This complication should be suspected if there is an abrupt increase in (1) soreness in the throat, (2) swelling in the neck, and (3) fever during or shortly after streptococcal pharyngitis. Inspection of the throat will reveal the displacement of the tonsil on the affected side toward the midline. A fluctuant mass may be felt in the affected area with a gloved finger; it should be treated promptly because complications arise when the infection extends further into the neck and surrounding tissues.

NONSUPPURATIVE COMPLICATIONS. The nonsuppurative complications of streptococcal disease are ARF and AGN. These are discussed in Ch. 269 and 81.

DIAGNOSIS. Group A streptococcal pharyngitis must be differentiated from pharyngitis due to other bacterial and viral agents. Gonococcal tonsillopharyngitis should be suspected if there is a history of homosexuality or fellatio. *Vincent's angina* usually has an insidious onset without the constitutional symptoms characteristic of a streptococcal sore throat. Signs of this infection, including an exudate, are commonly unilateral, whereas streptococcal pharyngitis is not. *Diphtheria* is now rare, although it should be recognized by the presence of the characteristic diphtheritic membrane as well as the other signs and symptoms of the disease.

The major confusion in the differential diagnosis will stem from viral respiratory infections, which not only occur more frequently than do streptococcal infections but which also may cause pharyngeal and tonsillar exudate. While many upper respiratory infections have a "common cold–like" quality, the symptoms may overlap considerably with those of streptococcal disease. Adenoviruses can cause an exudative pharyngitis clinically indistinguishable from that due to group A streptococci. A severe exudative pharyngitis with fever and toxicity is seen in infectious mononucleosis. The generalized symptoms and signs associated with infectious mononucleosis, however, should assist in the differential diagnosis. Pharyngitis due to group A coxsackieviruses (herpangina) or to herpes simplex will result in formation of vesicles. When these rupture they may leave shallow ulcers that can often be differentiated by inspection from streptococcal disease. Because it is frequently not possible to distinguish streptococcal from nonstreptococcal sore throat on clinical grounds, precise diagnosis requires a throat culture.

Before any antimicrobial therapy is administered, swabs should be passed through the mouth under direct vision and a good light and rubbed over the tonsils and posterior pharynx. The swabs should be streaked directly, with a minimum of delay, on a sheep blood agar plate of low dextrose content. After incubation overnight, the number of hemolytic streptococci present should be recorded in a roughly quantitative manner. The organisms will be very numerous in most cases if they are the cause of the infection. The presence of a few colonies does not provide convincing evidence that they are responsible for the illness, because 5 to 10 per cent of the general population (and a higher percentage of children) may be nasopharyngeal carriers of these organisms. Serologic grouping and typing of the isolated organisms are usually not necessary for routine clinical diagnosis. Because the growth of group A streptococci is inhibited in vitro by paper discs containing less than 0.02 unit of bacitracin, some laboratories routinely determine the bacitracin susceptibility of hemolytic streptococci. Hemolytic bacteria resistant to such low concentrations of bacitracin are unlikely to be group A streptococci. On the other hand, approximately 5 per cent of nongroup A hemolytic streptococci are also susceptible to this low concentration. New rapid antigen detection systems have been developed to identify group A streptococci directly from the cotton swab, including latex agglutination of throat swab extracts. The specificity of these tests is reasonably good, but when small numbers of streptococci are present, the test is less sensitive than the culture methods.

If the pharyngitis persists with adequate penicillin therapy, it is unlikely to be due to group A streptococci. However, viral pharyngitis is often of brief duration, and if such patients are treated with penicillin, it may appear that there has been a therapeutic response when in fact the disease has abated spontaneously.

The ASO test is not useful in the diagnosis of streptococcal pharyngitis. An elevation in titer is evidence of a recent infection and is employed in the diagnosis of patients with rheumatic fever and rheumatic heart disease.

TREATMENT. There are four reasons for treating streptococcal pharyngitis: (1) the prevention of suppurative complications, (2) the prevention of the nonsuppurative complications ARF and AGN, (3) the prevention of spread of the disease to family contacts or to persons in small social units such as school rooms and army barracks, and (4) the relief of symptoms. Prevention of ARF depends upon the eradication of the organism from the pharynx, and this requires treatment for at least ten days. Because signs and symptoms frequently subside in a few days, there is a tendency to shorten the time antibiotics are given. Brief periods of antibiotic therapy do not eliminate the streptococci from the pharynx. Patients treated briefly have a greater risk of developing ARF than do those who are adequately treated for at least ten days.

Penicillin is the drug of choice. Group A streptococci are highly susceptible to the action of penicillin. Despite its use for over 40 years, no penicillin-resistant strains have developed. A single intramuscular injection of 1.2 million units of benzathine penicillin G provides a sufficiently prolonged level of penicillin in the blood to eradicate the organism. For children weighing less than 60 pounds, the dose is 600,000 units. If oral therapy is used, 250,000 units of penicillin G or 250 mg of penicillin V, three or four times daily, is the treatment of choice. If penicillin allergy is suspected or known to exist, erythromycin is the drug of choice, 20 mg per pound per day (not to exceed 1 gram per day) for a period of ten days. Erythromycin resistance is not yet a serious problem in the United States. Many group A streptococci have developed resistance to tetracycline, and it is no longer recommended for treatment of group A infections. Sulfonamides, when used to treat streptococcal pharyngitis, are ineffective in preventing rheumatic fever. They do not suppress the immune response, do not terminate pharyngeal carriage of streptococci, and thus do not reduce the attack rate of subsequent rheumatic fever. They may be used, however, as continuous prophylaxis to prevent new infections in patients who have had an initial attack of rheumatic fever.

Treatment of streptococcal sore throat should be started as soon as a definite diagnosis of streptococcal infection is made. It has been shown, however, that a short delay while awaiting throat culture results (even for several days) in initiating antimicrobial therapy does not significantly interfere with rheumatic fever prevention. One exception to this statement involves the patient with a history of rheumatic fever. In such a patient, the prevention of rheumatic occurrence is not always possible unless treatment is instituted at the first clinical sign of streptococcal infection. For such a patient, any delay of therapy entails the risk of reactivation of the disease.

If severe suppurative streptococcal infections such as mastoiditis, pneumonia, wound infections, or other forms of sepsis are present, patients should receive 600,000 units of procaine penicillin G twice a day intramuscularly for several days until the illness is under control. Then a shift can be made to benzathine penicillin or oral penicillin. It may be necessary to prolong therapy for several weeks whenever pus or necrosis is present, particularly when adequate debridement is not possible.

STREPTOCOCCAL PNEUMONIA

Streptococcal pneumonia is now uncommon. It can be seen, however, as a complication of influenza, measles, pertussis, or varicella. It is characterized by abrupt onset of fever, chills, myalgia, dyspnea, cough, pleuritic chest pain, and hemoptysis. Patients are severely ill. Radiologically, there is usually bronchopneumonia. Lobar consolidation is less common. One characteristic feature of streptococcal pneumonia is the early and rapid accumulation of a large volume of thin empyema fluid. The pneumonic infection can extend to the mediastinum and pericardium. Bacteremia occurs in 10 to 15 per cent of the cases. Bacteriologic diagnosis depends on recovering group A streptococci from the sputum, empyema fluid, and blood. Because the patient is very ill, treatment should be started promptly. Therapy consists of 4 to 6 million units of parenteral procaine penicillin G given daily; this total daily dose is given in two to four intramuscular injections. There must also be adequate drainage of the empyema fluid. This may require insertion of a chest tube.

STREPTOCOCCAL SKIN INFECTIONS

PYODERMA. Group A streptococci can produce localized purulent skin infections known as pyoderma. While some of the lesions represent secondary infections of wounds or burns, most commonly the infection is primary and is usually referred to as *streptococcal impetigo* or *impetigo contagiosa*. Intensive studies over the past 20 years have revealed a number of important bacteriologic and epidemiologic differences between streptococcal impetigo and streptococcal pharyngitis (Table 268–2). Impetigo occurs in the summer and fall, but

TABLE 268–2. COMPARISON OF THE FEATURES OF STREPTOCOCCAL PHARYNGITIS AND PYODERMA*

Features	Pharyngitis	Pyoderma
Clinical illness	Acute	Indolent
Laboratory		
Leukocytosis	Usually present	Often absent
Antistreptolysin O response	Common	Uncommon
Epidemiology		
Seasonal occurrence	Winter and spring	Late summer and early fall
Geographic distribution	More common in temperate or cold climates	Common in hot or tropical climates
Age	School-aged children	Children of preschool age
Transmission	Direct spread from human reservoirs	Unknown; insects may be mechanical vectors
Carrier state	Common in pharynx of many populations	Unusual on skin
Preceding trauma	Not present	May predispose to infection
Complications		
Acute nephritis	Occurs; partially preventable (50%)	Occurs; preventability unknown
Acute rheumatic fever	Occurs; preventable	Does not occur
Treatment		
Local	Not important	Removal of crusts and scrubbing with hexachlorophene soap
Systemic	Single intramuscular injection of benzathine penicillin or oral penicillin for 10 days	May not be necessary; extensive lesions may require intramuscular benzathine penicillin

*Modified from Wannamaker LW: N Engl J Med 282:23, 78, 1970.

pharyngitis is seen in the winter and spring. Children between the ages of two and five years are more commonly infected. They are usually from underprivileged families residing in the southern United States or the tropics. Nevertheless, outbreaks can be seen among children of similar circumstances in other areas of the United States, such as those in American Indian reservations.

Epidemiologic studies have not clarified the mode of spread of streptococcal pyoderma, but it is reasonable to assume that personal contact with those infected, and perhaps insect vectors, may be important. Despite the uncertainty about the mode of spread, a number of important epidemiologic and clinical facts have emerged from recent studies. In general, the streptococci that cause pyoderma are the higher numbered M types, whereas pharyngitis is usually due to M types 1 through 40. Children who develop streptococcal impetigo and who carry the higher types on the skin may then develop pharyngeal carriage of these skin strains, which are unlikely to cause pharyngitis. Such pharyngeal carriage must be taken into consideration in the diagnosis of respiratory disease in these children, because carriage of these strains alone is not indicative of streptococcal pharyngitis.

Differences have been seen also in the immune response, depending on the site of the streptococcal infection. While the ASO response is usually brisk following streptococcal pharyngitis, it is weak or absent in patients with impetigo. It has been suggested that inactivation of streptolysin O by the lipids present in the skin accounts for this feeble antibody response. Brisk antibody responses do occur, however, to DNAse B in patients with impetigo. M type-specific protective antibodies are almost always produced after streptococcal pharyngitis, but the response to the M type-specific antigens is variable in the case of impetigo. It is not surprising, therefore, that lesions due to the same serotype may persist for months if untreated.

The lesions of streptococcal impetigo occur over the exposed areas of the body. They are more common on the lower extremities, undoubtedly because abrasions of the skin are more common in these areas. The lesions begin as papules but rapidly evolve into vesicles surrounded by erythema. They may be localized but are often multiple. As the papules enlarge, they break down over five or six days to form a thick crust. The lesions heal slowly, leaving a depigmented area. While there may be some regional lymphadenitis, systemic symptoms are not usually present.

While streptococcal impetigo can be suspected from the history as well as the examination, definite diagnosis requires bacteriologic culture. The crust must be removed to obtain specimens from the base of the lesion after washing the infected area of the skin with sterile water. Soap or other detergents can kill or reduce the number of group A streptococci. Culturing the surface of the lesion itself will usually give a negative result. Culture results may show both group A streptococci and *Staphylococcus aureus*, but it is generally believed that the streptococcus is the primary pathogen. In many instances mild impetigo responds to local treatment. The crusts should be removed and the skin washed with soap and water. Topical antibiotics and other antiseptics have little or no value in treatment or prevention. When the lesions are more extensive, parenteral use of benzathine penicillin is indicated. The lesions respond well to penicillin therapy. The antibiotic regimen is the same as used for the treatment of pharyngitis. Even though the *S. aureus* present may produce penicillinase, this does not interfere with penicillin treatment. Prevention of impetigo is achieved with good personal hygiene and liberal use of soap and water.

The importance of streptococcal impetigo beyond the inconvenience and some disfiguration of the skin relates to its association with AGN. Not all strains of group A streptococci that cause impetigo and other forms of pyoderma result in AGN; nevertheless, certain M types such as 49, 55, and 57

have been associated with sporadic cases as well as large epidemics of pyoderma-associated AGN. These have occurred in many different geographic regions. Although there is evidence to suggest that treatment of streptococcal pharyngitis will prevent AGN 50 per cent of the time, there is no conclusive evidence that treatment of an individual case of pyoderma will prevent subsequent occurrence of AGN. Nevertheless, treatment of the individual is important, particularly in a setting in which AGN is occurring or has occurred in the past, because this eradicates the streptococcus from the environment. The individual is therefore less of a risk to siblings and other school children.

A more severe ulcerated form of pyoderma is known as *ecthyma*. During the Vietnam conflict, this was seen in combat troops serving in the jungle. The ulcers, located on the ankle or dorsum of the foot, are circular, have a punched-out appearance, and are 0.5 to 3 cm in diameter. They contain purulent material and may be covered with a yellowish-gray crust. They are surrounded by a zone of erythema, and in more severe cases there may be cellulitis and lymphadenitis.

ERYSIPELAS. Erysipelas (St. Anthony's fire) is an acute infection of the skin and subcutaneous tissues caused by group A streptococci. The disease is more common in infants, young children, and elderly people. It is most commonly seen on the face and has a "butterfly" distribution when the bridge of the nose and the cheeks are involved. Eyelids are edematous and often swollen shut. The source of the infection is the patient's nasopharynx. Erysipelas may also develop from streptococcal infections elsewhere on the body, including surgical incisions and wounds. In some cases the disease has been seen in association with dermatophytosis.

As with streptococcal pharyngitis, the onset is usually abrupt, and similar systemic symptoms are frequently present. The lesion initially begins with an area of mild discomfort at the site of infection. Erythema follows and enlarges rapidly, reaching a maximum in three to six days. The lesion, pink to deep red in color, has an advancing irregular margin. It is warm to the touch. Vesicles and bullae may appear, which then rupture and become crusted. As the margin advances, the central area begins to clear and the skin returns to a normal appearance, usually with some residual pigmentation.

While recovery is usually seen in a week or ten days, this varies with the severity of the infection. High fever and bacteremia were often present before antibiotics were available, and mortality was not uncommon, particularly in patients who had bacteremia. Death is rare when the disease is adequately treated with penicillin or another appropriate antibiotic. Early diagnosis and treatment are important in infants and in elderly, debilitated, or immunosuppressed individuals. Death can occur in these cases if treatment is not prompt. Not uncommonly the disease will recur in the same site, particularly if there are areas of lymphatic obstruction.

Large numbers of group A streptococci can usually be cultured from the nasopharynx of patients with early erysipelas. Efforts to culture the streptococci from the edema fluid of the lesion are not always successful. Diagnosis is primarily made on the basis of clinical findings.

PREVENTION AND PROPHYLAXIS OF GROUP A STREPTOCOCCAL DISEASES AND THEIR NONSUPPURATIVE SEQUELAE

Views on the antibiotic treatment of streptococcal pharyngitis to prevent ARF and AGN are undergoing re-evaluation because of the decrease in the severity of streptococcal pharyngitis in recent years and the dramatic decline in the occurrence of ARF. Do the low attack rates of ARF (1 to 2 per 100,000 people per year for the age group 5 to 17 years) justify intensive efforts to detect streptococcal infections by bacteriologic cultures? Do they justify a prolonged course of antibiotic therapy for all patients in whom streptococcal infection is suspected, however mild it may be? Views are currently changing on these matters, and there is now discussion of some relaxation of the vigorous efforts used in the past to diagnose and treat streptococcal pharyngitis.

From this debate several principles are emerging. While direct proof is lacking, it is probable that the decline in the incidence of ARF and the clinical severity of streptococcal pharyngitis is due at least in part to the widespread use of penicillin to treat this infection during the past 25 years. It is difficult to believe that this decline in disease has occurred as a result of genetic changes in the streptococci. This would have required the simultaneous occurrence of similar genetic events in a large number of different streptococci during this interval, which seems unlikely. Certainly the decline in both diseases has been too precipitous to have been the result of changes in the genetic background of the population that would have enhanced natural immunity. These considerations suggest that the treatment of pharyngitis with penicillin has been a major factor in reducing the incidence of this infection; it follows that penicillin treatment has also influenced the decline in ARF. It seems likely that continuation of treatment in the future will maintain this low incidence. It is known that virulent group A streptococci lurk in the shadows and are the cause of occasional outbreaks of streptococcal pharyngitis and ARF. It is certainly conceivable that such outbreaks would become more common if penicillin treatment were no longer used. Therefore, arguments to discontinue the use of penicillin to treat streptococcal pharyngitis, even though the disease is less virulent today than in previous times, are reminiscent of the arguments to discontinue the use of pertussis or poliomyelitis vaccines now that these diseases are rare. We know that failure to vaccinate will result in the re-emergence of these diseases.

Until there is more evidence concerning the benign nature of the streptococcal diseases that are occurring today, it will be prudent to maintain vigilance concerning streptococcal infections. Nevertheless, a consensus is emerging that the milder forms of pharyngitis need not be treated until the diagnosis is confirmed by throat culture. Furthermore, many specialists question the value of a throat culture in all cases of upper respiratory tract disease. These authors would reserve the throat culture for laboratory confirmation of streptococcal disease that is suspected on clinical grounds. Throat cultures of family members in contact with the usual case of streptococcal pharyngitis seem unnecessary.

The occurrence of an index case of either ARF or AGN should alert the physician to the possibility that an outbreak of streptococcal disease is occurring in a family or school.

It is apparent from this discussion concerning the infrequency of ARF and the milder nature of streptococcal disease that there is probably much less risk today of the recurrence of rheumatic fever in patients with prior history of the disease following an untreated streptococcal infection. Continuous antibiotic prophylaxis has been employed in the past to prevent recurrences of rheumatic fever in such patients, and while discussions are under way concerning modification of the recommendations, the three regimens listed below are still recommended at this time.

1. Benzathine penicillin G given in a single injection of 1.2 million units every four weeks usually will provide protection for about 30 days. The disadvantages and discomfort of this regimen should be weighed against the individual patient's susceptibility to rheumatic occurrences. Those with rheumatic heart disease, those who have had a recent attack of rheumatic fever, and those exposed to an environment in which the incidence of streptococcal infection is frequent deserve the most effective protection. For such patients, benzathine penicillin by monthly injection is recommended.

2. Sulfonamide given daily by mouth in the form of 1.0 gram of sulfadiazine or one of the other sulfapyramidines provides satisfactory prophylaxis, but failures will occur. Toxic reactions may be observed during the first 60 days of continuous treatment. These have been rare, however, with the small doses of sulfadiazine that have been employed extensively.

3. Oral penicillin V is the preferred form because it is relatively resistant to gastric acid. The dose is 125 or 150 mg twice a day. This regimen has not been any more effective, however, than the daily dose of 1.0 gram of sulfadiazine. Indeed, 200,000 units of penicillin twice daily has not proved as yet to be clearly superior to the single dose. It is possible that the oral dose of penicillin may have to be increased to nearly therapeutic proportions to be more effective than sulfonamides, and this would increase further its expense and impracticability.

GROUP B STREPTOCOCCAL INFECTIONS

In the past, group B streptococci were primarily of interest to veterinarians because they were the cause of bovine mastitis. However, in recent years human strains of group B streptococci that appear to be distinct from the bovine strains have received considerable attention because they frequently produce neonatal sepsis. Group B streptococci are subdivided by means of surface polysaccharides into five serotypes: Ia, Ib, Ic, II, and III. Recent evidence suggests that group B streptococci normally colonize the intestine, and it is speculated that there is then secondary spread from the rectum to the vagina. This raises the possibility of sexual transmission of these organisms. Vaginal carriage is asymptomatic in post-pubertal women. The incidence of carriage and of neonatal infection varies widely depending on socioeconomic status and geographic residence.

Infections due to group B streptococci are associated with perinatal events. Maternal infections include chorioamnionitis, septic abortion, and puerperal sepsis. Group B streptococci are now recognized as one of the most frequent causes of neonatal sepsis and meningitis. Extensive clinical and epidemiologic studies have delineated two forms of the disease. "Early-onset disease" primarily involves infection of the lungs. The disease usually occurs within the first ten days of life, but cases after this period have been reported. The organisms are usually acquired from the maternal genital tract. This may be secondary to aspiration of infected amniotic fluid. Septicemia usually is present. Early-onset disease occurs as frequently as in 5 of every 1000 live births, although this varies depending upon the region of the country and the specific hospital reporting. Early-onset disease tends to occur in infants of certain high-risk pregnancies, such as those involving prematurity, prolonged rupture of membranes, and maternal infection. The other form of group B streptococcal neonatal infection has been referred to as "late-onset disease." Affected infants develop meningitis and bacteremia. The infant is usually over ten days old, but cases have occurred at four or five days of age. Infection may be due to nosocomial transmission. The disease has a much lower mortality rate than early-onset disease. Type III organisms predominate as the cause of early- and late-onset disease.

Because all the evidence suggests that early-onset disease in the newborn infant is acquired by vertical transmission from the mother who has vaginal colonization by group B streptococci, intravenous administration of ampicillin sodium has been used to treat such women during labor in an effort to prevent transmission. While recent reports suggest that the disease in newborns is prevented by selective chemoprophylaxis of the mother, more research remains to be done in this important area. One reason for some uncertainty is that not all newborns who acquire group B carriage in the ear, nose, umbilicus, and rectum develop early-onset disease. Nevertheless, prevention of vertical transmission of carriage is a promising development, particularly if further documented.

While group B streptococci frequently may be cultured from the throat, they rarely, if ever, cause pharyngitis. Group B streptococcal infection can, however, cause urinary tract infections in both sexes. Infected men are likely to be elderly. Group B streptococci may produce suppurative gangrenous lesions in adults with insulin-dependent diabetes mellitus who have peripheral vascular insufficiency. Any large series of infectious diseases will reveal group B streptococci as a cause of endocarditis, pneumonia, empyema, meningitis, peritonitis, and terminal bacteremia in patients with malignancy.

All group B streptococci are susceptible to penicillin. It is the drug of choice for these infections. Thus far, most strains are susceptible to erythromycin. Tetracycline should not be used because the organisms have developed resistance to this antibiotic.

Baker CJ: Group B streptococcal infections. Adv Intern Med 25:475, 1980. *A brief but comprehensive review of the clinical features, epidemiology, and clinical microbiology of this most important cause of sepsis and meningitis in the newborn. Approximately 100 references are annotated.*

Bass JW: Treatment of streptococcal pharyngitis revisited. JAMA 256:740, 1986. *An excellent recent review of current indications for treatment and the choice of therapy.*

Boyer KM, Gotoff SP: Prevention of early-onset neonatal group B streptococcal disease with selective intrapartum chemoprophylaxis. N Engl J Med 314:1665, 1986. *The most recent paper that suggests intrapartum ampicillin prophylaxis in women with positive prenatal cultures for group B streptococci who have certain risk factors can prevent early-onset disease in the newborn.*

Johnston KH, Zabriskie JB: Purification and partial characterization of the nephritis strain-associated protein from Streptococcus pyogenes, Group A. J Exp Med 163:697, 1986. *The most recent evidence suggesting a possible role for a streptococcal extracellular product in the pathogenesis of AGN.*

Kimura Y, Kotami S, Shiokawa Y (eds.): Recent Advances in Streptococci and Streptococcal Diseases. Berkshire, England, Readbooks Ltd., 1985. *The proceedings of the recent ninth symposium consisting of over 100 short research papers on all aspects of streptococcal bacteriology, immunology, and pathogenesis.*

McCarty M: Streptococci. In Davis BD, Dulbecco R, Eisen HN, Ginsberg HS (eds.): Microbiology. New York, Harper & Row, 1980, pp 607–622. *A good brief review of all aspects of streptococcal bacteriology and streptococcal disease.*

Read SE, Zabriskie JB (eds.): Streptococcal Diseases and the Immune Response. New York, Academic Press, 1980. *An exhaustive symposium of immunology in general and streptococcal diseases in particular by leading American and British investigators.*

Rheumatic Fever Committee, American Heart Association: Prevention of rheumatic fever. Circulation 70:1118A–1122A, 1984. *Standard recommendations for the prevention of rheumatic fever, which should be basic knowledge for all physicians.*

Shulman ST (ed.): Management of Pharyngitis in an Era of Declining Rheumatic Fever. Columbus, Ohio, Ross Laboratories, 1984. *A collection of papers that thoroughly reviews the changing patterns of streptococcal diseases and the implications of these changes for treatment and management.*

Wannamaker LW: Immunology of streptococci. In Nahmias AJ, O'Reilly RJ (eds.): Immunology of Human Infection. Part I: Bacteria, Mycoplasmae, Chlamydiae, and Fungi. New York, Plenum Medical Book Company, 1981, pp 47–92. *An excellent review of the humoral and cellular immune responses to many different streptococcal products and antigens. Includes 400 references.*

Wood HF, Feinstein AR, Taranta A, et al.: Rheumatic fever in children and adolescents. III. Comparative effectiveness of three prophylaxis regimens in preventing streptococcal infections and rheumatic recurrences. Ann Intern Med 60 (S5):31, 1964. *A classic controlled long-term study of the prevention of rheumatic recurrences and the relative effectiveness of the three regimens commonly in use for secondary prophylaxis.*

269 RHEUMATIC FEVER

Alan L. Bisno

DEFINITION. Rheumatic fever is a delayed, nonsuppurative sequel of upper respiratory infection with group A streptococci. The disease is characterized by inflammatory lesions involving primarily the joints, heart, and subcutaneous tissues; its pathogenesis remains obscure. The clinical manifestations include polyarthritis, carditis, subcutaneous nodules, erythema marginatum, and chorea in varying combinations. In its classic form, the disorder is acute, febrile, and largely self-limited. However, damage to heart valves may be chronic and progressive, causing cardiac disability or death many years after the initial episode.

ETIOLOGY. The development of acute rheumatic fever (ARF) requires antecedent infection with a specific organism, the group A *Streptococcus*, at a specific body site, the upper respiratory tract. Cutaneous streptococcal infection, a frequent precursor of poststreptococcal acute glomerulonephritis, has never been shown to cause rheumatic fever.

Strains representing a number of the more than 80 M protein serotypes of group A streptococci are capable of eliciting ARF. Whether *all* clinically virulent strains of *S. pyogenes* are equally "rheumatogenic" remains a matter of controversy. There is evidence to suggest, however, that group A streptococci vary in their rheumatogenic potential. Analysis of epidemics of ARF caused by a variety of serotypes shows a striking absence of certain highly prevalent types (e.g., type 12) and an over-representation of others, particularly type 5. Reports from the preantibiotic era document epidemics of streptococcal tonsillitis, even among rheumatic subjects, in which ARF failed to appear. Prospective studies from Trinidad, where poststreptococcal acute glomerulonephritis and ARF occur simultaneously in the same indigent population, indicate that the streptococcal strains responsible for each sequel are serotypically distinct.

PATHOGENESIS. The mechanism by which group A streptococci elicit the connective tissue inflammatory response that constitutes ARF remains unknown. Various theories have been advanced, including (1) toxic effects of streptococcal products, particularly streptolysins S and O, both of which are capable of initiating tissue injury; (2) a serum sickness–like reaction mediated by antigen-antibody complexes, perhaps localized to sites of tissue injury; and (3) "autoimmune" phenomena induced by the similarity of certain streptococcal and human tissue antigens.

Efforts to discriminate among these potential pathogenetic mechanisms have been hampered by the lack of an animal model of rheumatic fever. Many authorities currently favor the theory that ARF is an "autoimmune" disorder, in which tissue damage is mediated by the host's own immunologic responses to the antecedent streptococcal infection. This theory is rendered more credible by the relatively long latent period between the onset of pharyngitis and ARF and by the demonstration of numerous examples of antigenic similarity between somatic constituents of the group A *Streptococcus* and human tissues. The most intensively studied of these antigenic cross-reactions is that between streptococci and human heart. Many patients with ARF (as well as patients with uncomplicated streptococcal infections) have in their sera antistreptococcal antibodies that cross-react with heart tissue in a variety of test systems. Moreover, both the group A streptococcal M-protein molecule (located in the cell wall) and the cell membrane contain epitopes that share antigenic determinants with certain constituents of the human heart.

Another intriguing cross-reaction is that between the group A carbohydrate in cell walls of *S. pyogenes* and a glycoprotein in bovine heart valves. This cross-reaction is of special interest because serum levels of antibodies to group A carbohydrate remain elevated for years in patients with rheumatic valvulitis (but not in rheumatic patients without valvulitis) and decline remarkably if valve resection is performed.

Patients with ARF have, on the average, higher titers of antibodies to streptococcal extracellular and somatic antigens than do patients with uncomplicated streptococcal infections. Data relating to cellular immunity are more limited. ARF patients exhibit an exaggerated cellular reactivity to streptococcal cell membrane antigens, as demonstrated by inhibition in vitro of migration of peripheral blood lymphocytes.

Chronic remittent nodular lesions have been produced in dermal connective tissue following injection into experimental animals of a streptococcal mucopeptide-polysaccharide cell wall complex. Antibodies to the cytoplasm of neurons located in the caudate and subthalamic nuclei of the brain have been identified in sera of patients with Sydenham's chorea, and such antibodies cross-react with group A streptococcal membranes. Streptococcal extracellular products appear to be present in immune complexes circulating in the blood of ARF patients. Taken together, these and other reported immunologic cross-reactions and toxic phenomena could theoretically account for most of the manifestations of ARF. As yet, however, there is no direct evidence that any of them is of pathogenetic significance.

Several observations suggest that development of rheumatic fever may be modulated, at least in part, by the specific genetic constitution of the host. These include (1) the tendency of rheumatic fever to affect more than one member of a given family; (2) the fact that only a small percentage of all individuals experiencing an immunologically significant streptococcal infection develop ARF; (3) the tendency of rheumatic individuals to experience recurrent attacks; and (4) the propensity of rheumatic subjects to exhibit exaggerated immunologic responses to streptococcal antigens. Analyses of the relative frequencies of histocompatibility antigens in rheumatic subjects and controls have been inconclusive. Recently, however, certain B cell alloantigen(s) have been found to be present in three fourths or more of ARF patients but in less than 20 per cent of controls.

EPIDEMIOLOGY. The epidemiology of ARF mirrors that of streptococcal pharyngitis. The peak age incidence is 5 to 15 years, but both primary and recurrent cases occur in adults. ARF is rare in children less than four years of age, a fact that has led some observers to speculate that repetitive streptococcal infections are necessary to "prime" the host for the disease. There is no clear-cut sex predilection, although females are more likely to develop certain manifestations such as Sydenham's chorea and mitral stenosis.

Rheumatic fever occurs in all parts of the world; there is no known racial predisposition. In temperate climates, ARF peaks in the cooler months of the year, in the winter and early spring or shortly after schools open in the fall. The major environmental factor favoring occurrence appears to be crowding, as in military barracks or similar closed institutions and in large households. Crowding favors interpersonal spread of group A streptococci and perhaps enhances streptococcal virulence by frequent human passage. At present, ARF is primarily a disease of lower socioeconomic groups, particularly those massed in the densely populated core areas of major urban metropolitan centers. The disease remains rampant in developing areas such as the Middle East, the Indian subcontinent, and many nations of Africa and South America. It has been estimated that rheumatic heart disease causes 25 to 40 per cent of all cardiovascular disease in the third world.

The precise incidence of ARF in the United States is difficult to ascertain. In many localities the disease is not reportable. Cases manifested by carditis alone may not come to medical attention during the acute phase, and instances of polyarthritis or cardiac disease of other etiologies are frequently confused with ARF. All observers agree, however, that the incidence of ARF and the prevalence of rheumatic heart disease have declined dramatically both in America and in Western Europe over the past four to five decades. Studies of the incidence of ARF (hospitalized and nonhospitalized cases) among children aged 5 to 19 years in Baltimore and Nashville during the 1960's indicated rates in the range of 24 to 34 per 100,000 population. The rate for blacks was about twice that for whites, a fact thought to be related to socioeconomic rather than to genetic factors. At present, rates of less than 2 per 100,000 school children have been reported from several centers. In the affluent suburbs of many United States cities, ARF is now rare. Surprisingly, however, a sizable outbreak of ARF occurred in 1985-1986 among middle-class families in Salt Lake City, Utah, and environs.

The frequency with which ARF develops following untreated group A streptococcal upper respiratory infection differs with the epidemiologic circumstances. In the years

following World War II, careful prospective studies were conducted among personnel in military recruit camps suffering from exudative tonsillitis or pharyngitis caused by M typable group A streptococci. Under such circumstances, in which cases of streptococcal pharyngitis tend to be clinically severe and to appear in epidemics, approximately 3 per cent of untreated patients developed ARF. Studies of endemically occurring streptococcal infection among open populations of children are complicated by the difficulties of differentiating cases of streptococcal pharyngitis from viral pharyngitis occurring in streptococcal carriers; nevertheless, the ARF attack rate in such circumstances is clearly lower than in the military experience, with an overall attack rate of less than 1 per cent.

Certain features of the antecedent streptococcal infection are associated with an increased risk of ARF. Among these are the magnitude of the ASO titer rise and the persistence of the infecting organism in the pharynx. Prospective civilian studies indicate that ARF is more likely to occur following clinically severe exudative pharyngitis than following mild, nonexudative illness. On the other hand, one third or more of cases of ARF occur after streptococcal infections that are asymptomatic or so mild as to have been forgotten by the patient.

Patients with a history of ARF are at greatly increased risk of recurrent disease following an immunologically significant streptococcal infection. In long-term prospective studies of rheumatic subjects carried out at Irvington House, a rheumatic fever sanitarium outside New York City, one of every five documented streptococcal infections gave rise to a recurrence of ARF. The risk of recurrence is greater in patients with pre-existing rheumatic heart disease and in those experiencing symptomatic throat infections; the risk declines with advancing age and with increasing interval since the most recent rheumatic attack. Nevertheless, rheumatic patients remain at increased risk well into adult life, perhaps indefinitely.

PATHOLOGY. ARF is characterized by exudative and proliferative inflammatory lesions in the connective tissues, especially those of heart, joints, and subcutaneous tissues. The early lesions consist of edema of the ground substance, fragmentation of collagen fibers, cellular infiltration, and fibrinoid degeneration. In the heart, diffuse degeneration and even necrosis of muscle cells may be observed. At a slightly later stage, focal perivascular inflammatory lesions develop. These so-called *Aschoff nodules* (Fig. 269–1), considered pathognomonic of rheumatic fever, consist of a central area of fibrinoid surrounded by lymphocytes, plasma cells, and large

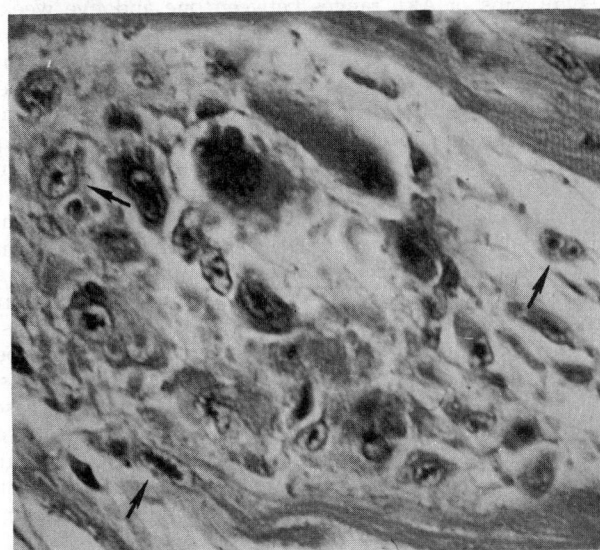

FIGURE 269–1. Myocardial Aschoff nodule demonstrates areas of fibrinoid degeneration and numerous large cells with polymorphous nuclei; several of the nuclei have "owl eye" or "caterpillar" configurations (*arrows*). × 630. (Courtesy of Robert Peace, M.D.)

basophilic cells, some of them multinucleate. Many of these cells have elongated nuclei with a distinctive chromatin pattern, sometimes called "caterpillar" or "owl-eye" nuclei, depending on their orientation in microscopic cross-section. Cells containing these nuclei are called "Anitschkow myocytes," despite the fact that most authorities believe them to be of mesenchymal origin.

Cardiac findings may include pericarditis, myocarditis, and endocarditis. Foci of coronary arteritis may also be observed. A thickened and roughened area ("MacCallum's patch") is frequently present in the left atrium above the posterior leaflet of the mitral valve. Valvular lesions appear early as small verrucae along the line of closure. Later, as healing occurs, the valves may become thickened and deformed, the chordae shortened, and the commissures fused. These changes result in valvular stenosis or insufficiency. The mitral valve is most commonly involved, followed by the aortic, the tricuspid, and, rarely, the pulmonic.

Pathologically, the *arthritis* of ARF is characterized by a fibrinous exudate and sterile effusion without erosion of the joint surfaces or pannus formation. *Subcutaneous nodules* have many histologic features in common with the Aschoff nodules. These consist of central zones of fibrinoid necrosis surrounded by histiocytes, fibroblasts, occasional lymphocytes, and rare polymorphonuclear cells. Inflammation of the smaller arteries and arterioles may occur throughout the body. Despite pathologic evidence of diffuse vasculitis, aneurysms and thrombosis are not typical features of ARF.

CLINICAL MANIFESTATIONS. Rheumatic fever may involve a number of different organ systems, most notably the heart, joints, skin, and central nervous system. The clinical picture of the disease may thus be quite variable, depending upon which systems are attacked, whether they are involved singly or in combination, the order in which they are affected, and the severity of the involvement. Five clinical features of the disease are so characteristic that they are recognized as "major manifestations" according to the revised Jones criteria (see below) for diagnosis of ARF: carditis, polyarthritis, chorea, subcutaneous nodules, and erythema marginatum. Certain other findings, frequently present but nonspecific, have been designated "minor manifestations." These include arthralgia, fever, history of previous rheumatic fever or evidence of pre-existing rheumatic heart disease, and certain laboratory findings (see below).

In cases in which it can be determined, the *latent period* between the antecedent streptococcal infection and the onset of symptoms of ARF ranges between one and five weeks. The average latent period is 19 days for both primary and recurrent attacks. When acute polyarthritis is the presenting complaint, the onset is often rather abrupt and may be marked by high fever and toxicity. If isolated carditis is the initial manifestation, the onset may be insidious or even subclinical. Between these two extremes, a wide variety of gradations exists in the initial presentation of ARF. In most attacks, fever and joint involvement are the earliest clinical manifestations, although they may occasionally be preceded by abdominal pain localized to the periumbilical or infraumbilical areas. At times the location and severity of the pain, as well as fleeting signs of peritoneal inflammation, may lead to a misdiagnosis of acute appendicitis. Carditis, if it is to appear, usually does so within the first three weeks of the illness. In contrast, chorea tends to occur later in the course of the disease, sometimes after all other manifestations have subsided. Fortunately, chorea and polyarthritis almost never occur simultaneously. Epistaxis may be a feature of ARF, occurring both at the onset and throughout the acute phase of the illness; it may be quite severe.

Overall, arthritis occurs in approximately 75 per cent of first attacks of ARF, carditis in 40 to 50 per cent, chorea in 15 per cent, and subcutaneous nodules and erythema marginatum in fewer than 10 per cent. The incidence of individual manifestations, however, varies with age. Carditis is more frequent in the youngest age groups and is relatively rare in first attacks occurring in adults. Chorea occurs primarily in persons between age five years and puberty. It is seen more frequently in females and virtually never occurs in adult males. Thus, most attacks of ARF occurring in adults are manifested primarily by arthritis.

Arthritis. Joint involvement ranges from arthralgia alone to acute, disabling arthritis characterized by swelling, warmth, erythema, severe limitation of motion, and exquisite tenderness to pressure. The larger joints of the extremities are usually involved—most frequently the knees and ankles, but also the wrists and elbows. The hips and small joints of the hands and feet are affected occasionally. Involvement of shoulders and lumbosacral, cervical, sternoclavicular, and temporomandibular joints occurs in a relatively small percentage of cases. The synovial fluid contains thousands of white blood cells with a marked preponderance of polymorphonuclear leukocytes; bacterial cultures are sterile.

Characteristically, the articular involvement in ARF assumes a pattern of *migratory polyarthritis*. This does not mean that inflammation in one joint disappears before the next is attacked. Rather, a number of joints are affected in succession and the periods of involvement overlap. Inflammation in one joint may subside while another is becoming symptomatic so that the process seems to migrate from joint to joint. In untreated cases, as many as 16 joints may be affected, and about half the patients develop arthritis in more than six joints. When effective anti-inflammatory therapy is administered early in the course of the disease, the involvement not infrequently remains monoarticular or pauciarticular.

In most instances, inflammation in any one joint begins to subside spontaneously within a week and the total duration of involvement is no more than two or three weeks. The entire bout of polyarthritis rarely lasts more than four weeks and resolves completely, leaving no residual joint damage. Some authors have described the rare occurrence of *Jaccoud's arthritis,* so-called chronic post-rheumatic fever arthropathy of the metacarpophalangeal joints, following repetitive bouts of rheumatic polyarthritis. This entity is not a true arthritis but a form of periarticular fibrosis; its relationship to rheumatic fever remains unresolved.

Carditis. Rheumatic fever may involve the endocardium, myocardium, and pericardium (Table 269–1), and thus the disease is capable of inducing a true *pancarditis.* Carditis is the most important manifestation of ARF because it is the only one capable of causing significant permanent organ damage or death. Although the clinical picture may at times be fulminant, it is more frequently mild or even asymptomatic and may escape notice in the absence of more obvious associated findings such as arthritis or chorea. The diagnosis of carditis requires the presence of one of the following four manifestations: (1) organic cardiac murmurs not previously present, (2) cardiomegaly, (3) pericarditis, or (4) congestive heart failure. In practice, the characteristic murmurs of ARF are almost always present in cases of rheumatic carditis, unless the ability to hear them is obscured (e.g., loud pericardial friction rub, large pericardial effusion, low cardiac output, severe tachycardia). The diagnosis of carditis should be made with caution in the absence of one of the following

TABLE 269–1. CLINICAL MANIFESTATIONS OF CARDITIS IN ACUTE RHEUMATIC FEVER

Murmurs*
   Apical systolic
   Apical mid-diastolic (Carey-Coombs murmur)
   Basal diastolic
Pericarditis
Cardiomegaly
Congestive heart failure

*At least one of the characteristic murmurs is almost always present in acute rheumatic carditis (see text for details).

three murmurs: apical systolic, apical mid-diastolic, and basal diastolic. Such murmurs, if they are destined to develop, do so usually within the first week and almost always within the first three weeks of illness. (An exception to this rule may occur in the patient with "pure" chorea; see later discussion.) The *apical systolic murmur* of relative or actual mitral regurgitation encompasses most of systole. It is blowing, relatively high pitched, and heard best at the apex; it radiates to the axilla and at times to the base of the heart or the back. It must be distinguished carefully by quality, location, and radiation from a variety of functional precordial systolic murmurs heard in normal individuals, especially in children. The *apical mid-diastolic* (Carey-Coombs) murmur is a low-pitched sound replacing or immediately following the third heart sound and ending distinctly before the first heart sound. It may be heard in a variety of conditions associated with increased flow across the mitral valve and is thus not pathognomonic of ARF. It may be differentiated from the diastolic rumble of mitral stenosis by the absence of an opening snap, presystolic accentuation, or accentuated first sound at the mitral area. The high-pitched, descrescendo *basal diastolic murmur* of aortic regurgitation is best heard along the upper left sternal border or over the aortic area. It may be brief and faint, best heard after expiration with the patient leaning forward.

Other prominent auscultatory findings in patients with active rheumatic carditis include tachycardia, which persists during sleep; protodiastolic, presystolic, or summation gallops; an indistinct or "mushy" quality to the first heart sound (resulting in some cases from first-degree heart block); pericardial friction rub; or muffing of heart tones caused by pericardial effusion. In the early stages of congestive heart failure, rapid distention of the hepatic capsule may lead to right upper quadrant aching and tenderness over the liver. All the usual clinical findings of pericarditis or congestive failure may be observed.

A number of different rhythm disturbances may occur during the course of ARF. By far the most common is first-degree atrioventricular block. Second- and third-degree heart block, nodal rhythm, and premature contractions may also be observed; atrial fibrillation, on the other hand, is usually a feature of chronic rather than acute rheumatic involvement. Conduction disturbances do not in themselves indicate acute carditis, and their presence or absence is unrelated to the subsequent development of rheumatic heart disease.

In cases of ARF with severe carditis, areas of patchy pneumonitis are sometimes seen. Many observers feel that these pulmonary infiltrates represent a specific *rheumatic pneumonia.* The case is difficult to prove, however, because of the confusion induced by such confounding clinical entities as pulmonary edema, pulmonary embolization, superimposed bacterial pneumonia, and the acute respiratory distress syndrome in these severely ill and toxic patients.

Sydenham's Chorea (Chorea Minor, "St. Vitus' Dance"). This neurologic syndrome occurs after a latent period which is variable but on the average longer than that associated with the other manifestations of ARF. It frequently occurs in "pure" form, either unaccompanied by other major manifestations or, after a latent period of several months, at a time when all other evidence of acute rheumatic activity has subsided. Chorea is characterized by rapid, purposeless, involuntary movements, most noticeable in the extremities and face. The arms and legs flail about in erratic, jerky, incoordinated movements that may sometimes be unilateral (hemichorea). Facial tics, grimaces, grins, and contortions are evident. The speech is usually slurred or jerky. The tongue, when protruded, retracts involuntarily, while asynchronous contractions of lingual muscles produce a "bag of worms" appearance. The involuntary motions disappear during sleep and may be partially suppressed by rest, sedation, or volition. Patients with chorea display generalized muscle weakness

and an inability to maintain a tetanic muscle contraction. Thus, when the patient is asked to squeeze the examiner's fingers, a squeezing and relaxing motion occurs which has been described as "milkmaid's grip." The knee jerk may have a pendular quality. There is no cranial nerve or pyramidal involvement, and sensory modalities are unaffected. The electroencephalogram may display abnormal slow wave activity.

Emotional lability is characteristic of Sydenham's chorea and often may precede other neurologic manifestations, leaving teachers and parents puzzled over apparently inexplicable personality changes.

Subcutaneous Nodules. These are firm, painless subcutaneous lesions that vary in size from a few millimeters to approximately 2 cm. The skin overlying them is freely movable and is not inflamed. The lesions tend to occur in crops over bony surfaces or prominences and over tendons. Sites of predilection include the extensor surfaces of elbows, knees, and wrists; the occiput; and spinous processes of the thoracic and lumbar vertebrae (Fig. 269–2). Nodules are virtually never the sole major manifestation of ARF; they almost always appear in association with carditis, and the cardiac involvement in such cases tends to be clinically severe. Nodules ordinarily do not appear until at least three weeks after the onset of an attack, usually lasting one to two weeks. They may appear in repeated crops in patients with protracted carditis. Similar nodules may be seen in systemic lupus erythematosus and in rheumatoid arthritis. Subcutaneous nodules in the latter disease are larger and more persistent than those in rheumatic fever.

Erythema Marginatum. The rash begins as an erythematous macule or papule, which then extends outward, while the skin in the center returns to normal. Adjacent lesions coalesce, forming circinate or serpiginous patterns (see Color plate 9). The lesions are neither pruritic nor indurated, and they blanch on pressure. They vary greatly in size, and appear mostly upon the trunk and proximal extremities, sparing the face. Erythema marginatum may be raised or flat; the latter was termed *erythema annulare* in the older literature. The lesions

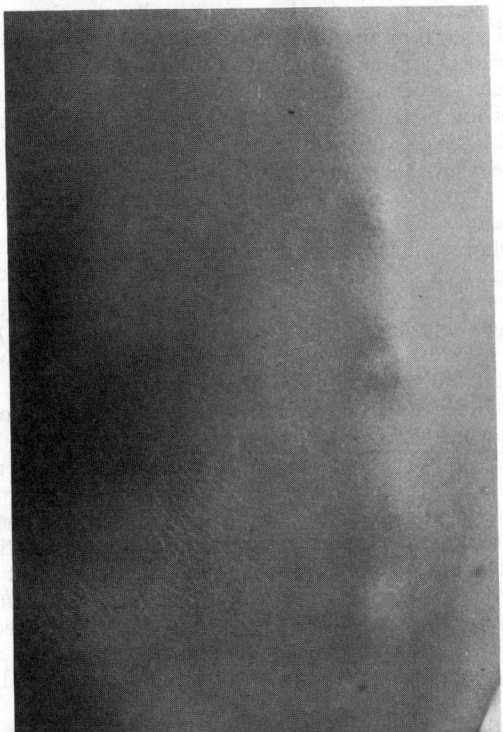

FIGURE 269–2. Subcutaneous nodules over spinous processes on the back of a patient with acute rheumatic carditis. (Courtesy of S. Levine, M.D.)

are evanescent, migrating from place to place, at times changing before the observer's eyes, and leaving no residual scarring. The erythema may be brought out by the application of heat. Individual lesions may come and go in minutes to hours, but the process may go on intermittently for weeks to months uninfluenced by anti-inflammatory therapy; its persistence is not necessarily an adverse prognostic sign. In the great majority of cases, erythema marginatum is accompanied by carditis; it also tends to be associated with subcutaneous nodules.

LABORATORY FINDINGS. No specific laboratory test is diagnostic of ARF. Usually there is a leukocytosis with an increase in the proportion of polymorphonuclear leukocytes. A mild to moderate normocytic normochromic anemia is the rule. In some patients the serum glutamic oxaloacetic transaminase level is elevated. Evidences of acute inflammation are prominent, including readily detectable quantities of C-reactive protein in the blood and elevation of the erythrocyte sedimentation rate. An exception is "pure" chorea, which may appear long after indices of inflammation have returned to normal. The urine may contain protein, white cells, and red cells. Biopsy studies have revealed a variety of renal abnormalities, but the classic proliferative glomerular abnormalities that characterize post-streptococcal acute glomerulonephritis occur quite rarely in ARF. Electrocardiographic and radiographic studies may reveal evidence of rhythm disturbances, pericarditis, or congestive heart failure. Echocardiography may document myocardial and valvular dysfunction and pericardial effusion.

The major laboratory contribution to the work-up of ARF is the documentation of recent group A streptococcal infection. Throat culture should always be performed but is positive in only a minority of cases. This is perhaps due to the time lapse of several weeks between the onset of the pharyngeal infection and the throat culture. The serum titer of antistreptolysin O (ASO) is elevated in 80 per cent or more of ARF patients. If two streptococcal antibody tests, e.g., ASO plus either anti-DNAse B or antihyaluronidase, are performed, an elevated titer of at least one will be found in 90 per cent of ARF patients. A battery of three tests will establish the presence of recent, immunologically significant streptococcal infection in more than 95 per cent of individuals experiencing an acute rheumatic attack. The definition of an "elevated" titer varies, depending upon the test employed, age of the patient, and geographic locale. ASO titers greater than 200 to 250 Todd units per milliliter are generally considered elevated. At times, serial sampling may detect a rising titer of streptococcal antibodies in patients seen early in the course of a rheumatic attack.

A simple slide agglutination test (Streptozyme) is positive in high titer in over 90 per cent of ARF patients. However, the test must be performed by a technician skilled in interpreting hemagglutination reactions, and values of 1:100 to 1:200 should be considered equivocal. Care should be taken to test simultaneously controls of known titer.

COURSE AND PROGNOSIS. The average duration of an untreated attack of ARF is approximately three months. The duration tends to be longer, up to six months, in patients with severe carditis. Less than 5 per cent of patients have continuing rheumatic activity for longer than six months. In a few of these the disease is limited to chorea and is otherwise benign. Other patients exhibit evidence of persistent inflammatory activity, including arthritis, carditis, and subcutaneous nodules. "Chronic rheumatic fever" occurs more frequently in patients who have had one or more previous attacks; cardiac involvement in chronic rheumatic fever tends to be frequent and severe.

Death from intractable myocarditis during the acute phase of ARF is now very rare. Once the acute attack has subsided, the only long-term sequel is that of rheumatic heart disease, manifested primarily by insufficiency and/or stenosis of the mitral and aortic valves. The prognosis from a cardiac standpoint is very much dependent upon the clinical findings at the time the patient is first seen. In one large study, for example, 347 patients were examined during an acute rheumatic attack and again 10 years later. Among patients who had been free of carditis during their acute attack, only 6 per cent had residual heart disease on follow-up. Patients with no pre-existing heart disease and with mild carditis during their acute attack (i.e., apical systolic murmur without pericarditis or heart failure) had a relatively good prognosis in that only approximately 30 per cent had heart murmurs 10 years later. About 40 per cent of subjects with apical or basal diastolic murmurs and 70 per cent of subjects with failure and/or pericarditis during their acute attacks had residual rheumatic heart disease. The prognosis was worse in patients with pre-existing heart disease and in those who had experienced recurrent attacks of ARF in the 10-year interval.

The data cited above indicate that patients who do not develop carditis during an acute attack and are protected from ARF recurrences are most unlikely to suffer from rheumatic heart disease. The patient with "pure" chorea represents an exception to this rule. A significant proportion of such patients who have no evidence of carditis when first examined may develop rheumatic valvular disease on prolonged follow-up. Although the explanation for this phenomenon is unknown, it is conceivable that, in view of the long latent period associated with chorea, signs of carditis might have been present earlier but subsided by the time the neurologic abnormality became evident.

DIAGNOSIS. Although ARF is readily recognized in the individual who presents with multiple major manifestations or in epidemic circumstances, at other times the disease may be extraordinarily difficult to diagnose with confidence. This is because of the variability of its clinical presentation, the frequency with which only a single major manifestation is detected, and the fact that there is no definitive diagnostic laboratory test. Nevertheless, precise diagnosis is especially important in this disease because of the necessity to advise the patient regarding prolonged antimicrobial prophylaxis (see below).

The diagnostic criteria of T. Duckett Jones, as subsequently modified by a committee of the American Heart Association, attempt to minimize over- and underdiagnosis (Table 269–2). Two major manifestations, or one major and two minor manifestations, indicate a high probability of ARF, *provided that there is supporting evidence of recent streptococcal infection.* Although a positive throat culture for group A streptococci

TABLE 269–2. JONES CRITERIA (REVISED) FOR GUIDANCE IN THE DIAGNOSIS OF RHEUMATIC FEVER*

Major Manifestations	Minor Manifestations
Carditis	*Clinical*
Polyarthritis	Previous rheumatic fever or rheumatic heart
Chorea	disease
Erythema marginatum	Arthralgia
Subcutaneous nodules	Fever
	Laboratory
	Acute phase reactions
	Erythrocyte sedimentation rate, C-reactive
	protein, leukocytosis
	Prolonged P-R interval
	Plus

Supporting evidence of preceding streptococcal infection (increased ASO or other streptococcal antibodies; positive throat culture for group A *Streptococcus*; recent scarlet fever).

The presence of two major criteria, or of one major and two minor criteria, indicates a high probability of the presence of rheumatic fever if supported by evidence of a preceding streptococcal infection. The absence of such evidence should make the diagnosis doubtful, except in situations in which rheumatic fever is first discovered after a long latent period from the antecedent infection (e.g., Sydenham's chorea or low-grade carditis).

*Modified from Jones criteria (revised) for guidance in the diagnosis of rheumatic fever. Circulation 69:204A, 1984, by permission of the American Heart Association, Inc.

technically satisfies this requirement, streptococcal carriage rates of 15 per cent are not uncommon among school-aged children during the fall and winter. Elevated titers of antibodies to streptococcal extracellular products, although not diagnostic of ARF, do indicate a recent, *immunologically significant* streptococcal infection. Conversely, if a battery of streptococcal antibody tests fails to reveal any evidence of recent infection, the diagnosis of ARF must be considered unlikely. This statement does *not* necessarily hold true in patients whose only rheumatic manifestation is Sydenham's chorea. Because of the long latent period associated with chorea, previously elevated antibody titers may have declined to normal.

The modified Jones criteria are of course only guidelines. They are most difficult to apply confidently when polyarthritis is the single major manifestation present. Under such circumstances, serious consideration must be given to various other entities, including rheumatoid arthritis, Still's disease, viral arthritides (e.g., rubella, hepatitis B), the early prepurpuric phase of Henoch-Schönlein purpura, and septic arthritis. The last-named entity has come to the fore with the resurgence of gonococcal arthritis as a relatively common cause of febrile polyarthralgia and polyarthritis in adolescent females in certain population groups.

Serum sickness is frequently a serious consideration, particularly if the patient has received penicillin or other antibiotics for a preceding respiratory infection. Systemic lupus erythematosus, sickle cell hemoglobinopathies, and infective endocarditis may involve the joints and the heart. Other differential diagnostic considerations include congenital heart lesions, viral and idiopathic forms of myocarditis and pericarditis, and functional heart murmurs. Nonfamilial forms of chorea have been described in systemic lupus erythematosus, and rarely in association with the use of birth control pills. It remains uncertain how often episodes of chorea occurring during pregnancy ("chorea gravidarum") represent attacks of rheumatic fever. Other disorders that may at times be confused with ARF are gout, sarcoidosis, Hodgkin's disease, and acute leukemia.

Following an episode of acute streptococcal pharyngitis, a small proportion of patients may experience persistent symptoms of malaise, arthralgia, low grade fever, and lymphadenopathy plus laboratory evidences of mild inflammation. It is difficult to classify such cases, but the affected individuals do not meet the criteria for diagnosis of ARF and, moreover, do not appear to be at risk for the delayed cardiac sequelae of ARF.

TREATMENT. Antibiotics neither modify the course of a rheumatic attack nor influence the subsequent development of carditis. Nevertheless, it is conventional to give a course of antibiotics designed to eradicate any group A streptococci remaining in the tonsils and pharynx, at least in part to prevent spread of the organism to close contacts. The recommended regimens are as follows: intramuscular benzathine penicillin G, 600,000 units for children less than 60 pounds and 1,200,000 units for heavier individuals; or penicillin V orally, 125 to 250 mg four times daily for 10 days. Penicillin-allergic individuals may receive erythromycin. The specific dosage of erythromycin varies somewhat with the preparation selected but is in the range of 20 to 40 mg per kilogram of body weight per day divided in two to four equal doses. The maximum dose is 1 gram per day. Following completion of this therapy, continuous antistreptococcal prophylaxis should commence (see below).

Treatment with anti-inflammatory agents is effective in suppressing many of the signs and symptoms of ARF. These agents do not "cure" the disease, nor do they prevent the subsequent evolution of rheumatic heart disease. They should be avoided in very mild or equivocal cases, because, by suppressing the clinical manifestations, they may obscure the diagnosis. The two drugs most widely used are aspirin and

corticosteroids. The former is used in patients with acute polyarthritis, provided that carditis is either absent or mild and there is no evidence of congestive heart failure. Aspirin is very effective in decreasing fever, toxicity, and joint inflammation. It should be given in a dosage of 90 to 100 mg per kilogram per day. This is administered in equally divided doses, every four hours for the first 24 to 36 hours; thereafter it may be given in four doses during waking hours. A salicylate level of 25 mg per deciliter is usually satisfactory. The incidence of nausea and vomiting may be minimized by starting somewhat below the optimal dosage level and gradually increasing over a few days. The patient should be observed for evidence of significant gastrointestinal bleeding and for signs and symptoms of salicylism. After two weeks, the dosage is reduced to 60 to 70 mg per kilogram per day for an additional six weeks. These dosage schedules represent general guidelines only. The precise aspirin dose must be determined by the patient's clinical response, blood salicylate levels, and tolerance of the drug.

Corticosteroids are generally reserved for patients who have severe carditis manifested by congestive heart failure, who are unable to tolerate large doses of salicylates, or whose signs and symptoms are inadequately suppressed by aspirin. As with aspirin, the dosage must be individualized. Prednisone, 40 to 60 mg per day in divided doses, may be used initially; after two to three weeks it should be withdrawn slowly over an additional three-week period. In cases of fulminating carditis with profound heart failure, intravenous corticosteroids may be employed. Aspirin should be administered for a month after discontinuation of prednisone. As is the case for other patients receiving corticosteroids, the physician should be alert to problems such as gastrointestinal bleeding, sodium and water retention, potassium depletion, and impairment of glucose tolerance. Suppression of the pituitary-adrenal axis or of the host immune system is a potential problem but not ordinarily a major one during this relatively short course of treatment. The role of nonsteroidal anti-inflammatory agents in management of ARF remains to be defined.

Following cessation of anti-inflammatory therapy, clinical or laboratory evidence of ARF may reappear. Such therapeutic "rebounds" occur more frequently after corticosteroid therapy than after treatment with aspirin. They may be minimized by prolonging salicylate therapy for 9 to 12 weeks and, when corticosteroids have been required, by continuing aspirin use for a month after corticosteroids have been discontinued.

Congestive heart failure is managed by the usual measures of bed rest, sodium restriction, diuretics, and, if necessary, oxygen and digitalis. The potential risk of digitalis-induced arrhythmias in the patient with active myocarditis must be borne in mind.

All patients should be kept at bed-chair rest for the first three weeks of illness, during which time carditis will usually manifest itself if it is destined to appear. Bathroom privileges may be allowed unless arthritis or chorea make this infeasible or unless frank heart failure supervenes. Subsequently the level of physical activity should be guided by the patient's clinical status, primarily by the presence and activity of rheumatic carditis. Patients with congestive heart failure should be kept at bed rest until compensation has been achieved. Patients with Sydenham's chorea require a quiet environment, and sedatives such as phenobarbital may be helpful.

Once the acute attack has subsided completely, the patient's subsequent level of physical activity is dependent upon his cardiac status. Patients without residual heart disease may resume full and unrestricted activity. It is important that the patient not be subjected to unwarranted invalidism, either because of his own inaccurate perceptions of the nature of the rheumatic process or because of those of his parents, teachers, or employers.

PREVENTION. "Primary prevention" of ARF consists of accurate diagnosis and appropriate treatment of streptococcal sore throat (Ch. 268). Although straightforward in theory, primary prevention is often frustratingly difficult to achieve. In many of the densely populated, indigent communities in which the risk of ARF is greatest, children with self-limited illnesses such as sore throats may never come to medical attention, and throat culture services are usually unavailable to aid in diagnosis. Moreover, in one third or more of cases, ARF may arise after a clinically inapparent streptococcal infection.

Perhaps the most effective strategy for avoiding the mortality and chronic cardiac disability associated with ARF is that of "secondary prevention." This strategy focuses upon the group of persons who have already suffered a rheumatic attack and who are inordinately susceptible to a recurrence following an immunologically significant streptococcal upper respiratory infection. Recurrent attacks tend to be mimetic in nature so that patients who have suffered carditis with their previous attack are likely to have repetitive cardiac involvement and progressive cardiac damage. Because even patients who experienced only arthritis or chorea may develop carditis with recurrent attacks of ARF, *all* patients who have experienced a documented attack of ARF should receive continuous antimicrobial prophylaxis to prevent either symptomatic or asymptomatic streptococcal infections. The specific regimens to be used are indicated in Ch. 268. By far the most effective of these is monthly benzathine penicillin G. Rheumatic recurrences are very unusual in patients faithfully adhering to this regimen.

The total duration of rheumatic prophylaxis remains unresolved. Some authorities recommend lifelong prophylaxis. On the other hand, the risk of rheumatic recurrence is known to diminish with increasing age and increasing interval since the most recent rheumatic attack. Patients who escape carditis during their initial attack are less likely to experience rheumatic recurrences and less likely to develop carditis if a recurrence does ensue. These facts, coupled with the relative rarity of ARF itself in most parts of the United States at present, suggest that prophylaxis need not be perpetual for all rheumatic subjects. Continuous prophylaxis should be maintained indefinitely for those with clinically significant rheumatic heart disease. Other rheumatic subjects should be protected until reaching adulthood, for at least five years after their most recent attack, and if they are in an epidemiologic circumstance that places them at high risk of streptococcal acquisition (e.g., parents of small children, school teachers, military recruits, nurses, pediatricians). The decision to remove a rheumatic subject from continuous prophylaxis should be an individualized one, based upon the physician's assessment of the risk and likely consequences of recurrence, and taken with the patient's informed consent. Patients taken off prophylaxis must be instructed to return immediately for medical follow-up whenever symptoms of pharyngitis occur.

Patients with rheumatic valvular heart disease must receive prophylaxis designed to avoid bacterial endocarditis whenever they undergo dental or surgical procedures likely to evoke bacteremia. This is not necessary in the rheumatic subject who is free of residual heart disease. The regimens for prevention of endocarditis (see Ch. 270) are entirely different from those prescribed for prevention of ARF, and the fact that a patient is receiving rheumatic fever prophylaxis in no way exempts him from endocarditis prophylaxis. This is a frequent point of confusion not only among patients but among physicians and dentists as well.

Ben-Dov I, Berry E: Acute rheumatic fever in adults over the age of 45 years: An analysis of 23 patients together with a review of the literature. Sem Arth Rheum 10:100, 1980. *A detailed review of clinical data relating to nearly 500 published cases of ARF in adults over 45.*

Bisno AL: Acute rheumatic fever: Current concepts and controversies. In Swartz MN, Remington JS (eds.): Current Clinical Topics in Infectious Diseases. New York, McGraw-Hill Book Company, 1984, pp 316:341. *A review of the epidemiology, theories of pathogenesis, and clinical aspects of acute rheumatic fever.*

Bisno AL: The concept of rheumatogenic and non-rheumatogenic group A streptococci. In Read SE, Zabriskie JB (eds.): Streptococcal Diseases and the Immune Response. New York, Academic Press, 1980, pp 789-803. *Summarizes data supporting the hypothesis that group A streptococci vary in rheumatogenic potential.*

Committee on Rheumatic Fever and Infective Endocarditis, American Heart Association: Prevention of rheumatic fever. Circulation 70:1118A-1122A, 1984. *Official recommendations of the American Heart Association for primary and secondary prevention of rheumatic fever. Includes specific antibiotic regimens.*

Feinstein AR, Spagnuola M: The clinical pattern of acute rheumatic fever. A reappraisal. Medicine 41:279, 1962. *An extremely careful and comprehensive analysis of the clinical patterns observed in 374 episodes of ARF admitted to the Irvington House rheumatic fever sanitarium.*

Stollerman GH: Rheumatic Fever and Streptococcal Infection. New York, Grune & Stratton, 1975. *A comprehensive, extremely readable summary of all aspects of rheumatic fever.*

United Kingdom and United States Joint Report: The natural history of rheumatic fever and rheumatic heart disease: Ten year report of a cooperative clinical trial of ACTH, cortisone and aspirin. Circulation 32:457, 1965. *This definitive international study of the natural history of rheumatic fever relates the risk of developing rheumatic heart disease to the cardiac status during the acute attack. Long-term prognosis was not improved by the use of corticosteroids or ACTH.*

Veasey LG, Wiedmeier SE, Orsmond GS, et al.: Resurgence of acute rheumatic fever in the intermountain area of the United States. N Engl J Med 316:421, 1987. *A detailed description of a recent major epidemic of ARF in the United States.*

Zabriskie JB: Rheumatic fever: The interplay between host, genetics and microbe. Circulation 71:1077, 1985. *A useful summary of immunologic data relating to the pathogenesis of ARF, with newer data on a possible genetic marker of susceptibility to this disease.*

Endocarditis

270 INFECTIVE ENDOCARDITIS
David T. Durack

When microbes colonize the endocardium, they cause the disease termed *infective endocarditis*. The organism is usually a common bacterium, the site affected is usually one of the heart valves, and the characteristic lesion is a vegetation. For general use, the term infective endocarditis is more appropriate than *bacterial endocarditis,* because this disease also can be caused by fungi and chlamydia. Serviceable terms in general use include *subacute* and *acute bacterial endocarditis* (SBE and ABE), *native valve endocarditis* (NVE), *prosthetic valve endocarditis* (PVE), and *nonbacterial thrombotic endocarditis* (NBTE).

MICROBIOLOGY. Most of the species of bacteria that have been isolated from humans have been reported to cause endocarditis. However, a few common gram-positive species account for the great majority of infections. Streptococci and staphylococci dominate the list: together these organisms cause more than 80 per cent of infections on native valves. Table 270–1 shows representative figures for the reported frequency of the main etiologic microbes on native valves, on prosthetic valves, and in drug addicts. Individual and local experience may differ widely.

The Gram-Positive Cocci. The various alpha-hemolytic (viridans) streptococci together cause more cases of endocarditis than any other bacteria. These relatively avirulent streptococci

TABLE 270–1. APPROXIMATE FREQUENCY OF VARIOUS ORGANISMS CAUSING INFECTIVE ENDOCARDITIS ON NATIVE VALVES, IN DRUG ABUSERS, AND ON PROSTHETIC VALVES*

	NVE (%)	Intravenous Drug Abusers (%)	Early PVE (%)	Late PVE (%)
Streptococci	65	15	10	35
Viridans, alpha-hemolytic	35	5	<5	25
S. bovis (group D)	15	<5	<5	<5
S. faecalis (group D)	10	8	<5	<5
Other streptococci	<5	<5	<5	<5
Staphylococci	25	50	50	30
Coagulase-positive	23	50	20	10
Coagulase-negative	<5	<5	30	20
Gram-negative aerobic bacilli	<5	15	20	15
Fungi	<5	5	10	5
Miscellaneous bacteria	<5	5	5	5
Diphtheroids, propionibacteria	<1	<5	5	<5
Other anaerobes	<1	<1	<1	<1
Rickettsia	<1	<1	<1	<1
Chlamydia	<1	<1	<1	<1
Polymicrobial infection	<1	5	5	5
Culture-negative endocarditis	5–10	5	<5	<5

*These are representative figures collated from the literature; wide local variations in frequency are to be expected.

Adapted from Durack DT: Infective and non-infective endocarditis. In Hurst JW (ed.): The Heart. 6th ed. New York, McGraw-Hill Book Company, 1986, pp 1130–1157.

are found in large numbers in the oropharyngeal and gastrointestinal flora. In order of frequency, the species that cause SBE most often are *Streptococcus sanguis, S. mutans, S. intermedius,* and *S. mitis.* Next in frequency among the streptococci causing endocarditis are the Group D streptococci, *S. bovis* and *S. faecalis. S. bovis* bacteremia and endocarditis are strongly associated with the presence of lower gastrointestinal lesions, including polyps and colonic cancer. Therefore, recovery of this species from blood cultures should be followed up by investigation for colonic tumors, whether or not the patient has any symptoms. *S. faecalis* (enterococcus) causes endocarditis in association with infections of the genital and urinary tract in women of childbearing age and of the urinary tract in elderly men with prostatic disease.

S. pneumoniae occasionally causes acute endocarditis. The triad of coexisting pneumococcal pneumonia, meningitis, and endocarditis is known as *Austrian's syndrome.* It is found in debilitated alcoholics and carries a very poor prognosis.

A few cases of endocarditis are caused by nutritionally dependent streptococci that require media supplemented with L-cysteine or pyridoxine for growth. These fastidious organisms can be difficult to isolate from blood cultures, and the infections they cause are more difficult to cure than infections caused by other streptococci.

Staphylococcus aureus is (1) the leading cause of acute bacterial endocarditis, (2) the predominant species in narcotic addicts with endocarditis, and (3) an important cause of PVE (Table 270–1). *Staphylococcus epidermidis* rarely causes NVE, but it is a leading cause of PVE.

Other Etiologic Organisms. Gram-negative and fungal infections are described later. Endocarditis caused by *Haemophilus* species is usually associated with *H. aphrophilus, H. paraphrophilus,* or *H. parainfluenzae,* rarely with *H. influenzae. Neisseria gonorrhoeae* causes acute endocarditis; this complication of gonorrhea has become rare since the introduction of penicillin. Endocarditis caused by anaerobic bacteria is also rare, accounting for less than 1 per cent of cases.

PATHOGENESIS AND PATHOLOGY. Figure 270–1 illustrates the sequence of events in pathogenesis of SBE, which usually develops on previously abnormal heart valves. Thirty years ago, the underlying cardiac condition was most often chronic rheumatic valvular heart disease. Today, the leading pre-existing condition for SBE in the United States is congenital heart disease in its various forms, including mitral valve prolapse. The number of cases engrafted upon rheumatic valvular disease will decline even further in the United States and other developed countries as the prevalence of chronic rheumatic heart disease in the general population continues to fall. Other important predisposing conditions are cardiac surgery (especially if a prosthetic valve has been implanted) and previous episodes of infective endocarditis. ABE can attack previously normal as well as damaged valves. Estimates of the frequency of the main underlying heart conditions for patients of various ages with acute or subacute endocarditis are shown in Table 270–2. Table 270–3 ranks the relative risks for endocarditis posed by various cardiac lesions.

The pathogenetic sequence leading to SBE begins with endothelial damage. When subendothelial connective tissue containing collagen fibers is denuded of endothelium, platelets aggregate at the site. These aggregates have been found occasionally on normal valves, but they occur more frequently on the surfaces of valves damaged by congenital or rheumatic disease or by a previous episode of infective endocarditis. These microscopic platelet thrombi may form and resolve harmlessly, but sometimes they are stabilized by deposition of fibrin and grow to form nodular sterile vegetations that are referred to as NBTE. Microscopic examination shows bundles of degenerating platelets held together by strands of fibrin, with few other cells present. This process can be induced in experimental animals by passing a catheter into the heart; NBTE forms at sites where the catheter damages the endothelium. Intracardiac pressure-monitoring catheters produce NBTE in humans in the same way. For unknown reasons, patients with cachexia caused by advanced malignancy or other wasting diseases are prone to form NBTE, which in this setting is usually termed *marantic endocarditis.* The sterile vegetations found in a few patients with systemic lupus erythematosus (Libman-Sacks endocarditis) are another form of NBTE.

The vegetations of NBTE are irregular friable white or tan masses of variable size that are usually found along the lines where valves touch upon closing. They may be so small as to be easily missed on inspection but are frequently rather large.

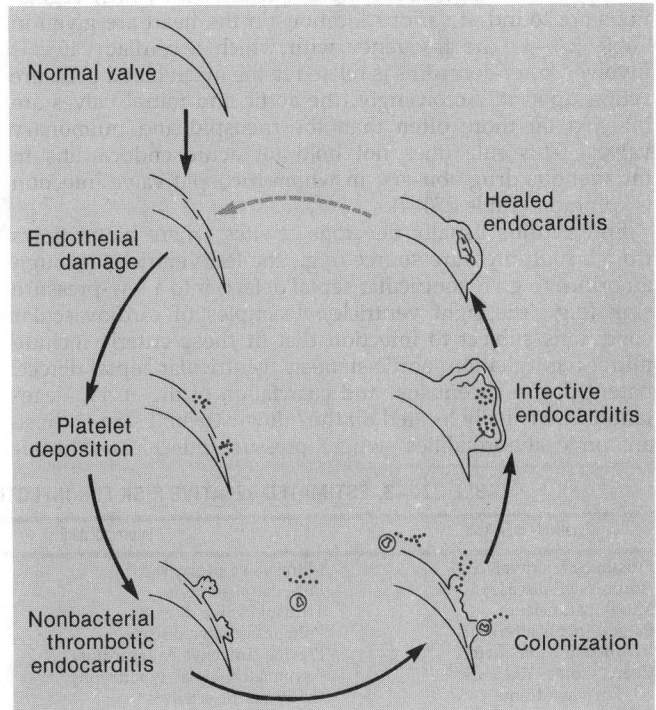

FIGURE 270–1. A diagram to illustrate the main events in pathogenesis of subacute bacterial endocarditis. (Adapted from Durack DT: Infective and non-infective endocarditis. *In* Hurst JW (ed.): The Heart. 5th ed. New York, McGraw-Hill Book Company, 1982.)

**TABLE 270–2. APPROXIMATE FREQUENCY OF THE MAJOR CATEGORIES
OF PRE-EXISTING CARDIAC LESIONS IN PATIENTS WITH INFECTIVE ENDOCARDITIS**

	Children Under 2 Years Old (%)	Children 2 to 15 Years Old (%)	Adults 15 to 50 Years Old (%)	Adults > 50 Years Old (%)	Adults, Intravenous Drug Abusers
No known heart disease	50–70	10–15	10–20	10	50–60
Congenital heart disease	30–50	70–80	20–30	10–20	10
Rheumatic heart disease	Rare	10	20–30	20–30	10
Degenerative heart disease	0	0	Rare	10–20	Rare
Previous cardiac surgery	5	10–20	10–20	10–20	10–20
Previous endocarditis	Rare	5	5	5–10	10–20

Adapted from Durack DT: Infective and non-infective endocarditis. In Hurst JW (ed.): The Heart. 6th ed. New York, McGraw-Hill Book Company, 1986, pp 1130–1157.

Because there is no inflammatory reaction at the site of attachment, the vegetations of NBTE can often be picked off easily with forceps at necropsy, leaving a normal-looking valve surface. These easily dislodged vegetations embolize frequently, often blocking peripheral arteries and causing infarction in myocardium, spleen, kidney, brain, gut, or extremities.

When NBTE is colonized by circulating bacteria, infective endocarditis results. Two important factors that determine which organisms will be most likely to cause endocarditis are (1) the frequency with which they are found in the blood and (2) their ability to adhere to fibrin and platelet thrombi. Viridans streptococci enter the blood from the oral cavity frequently (probably daily) and adhere well. Therefore, it is not surprising that they are the leading cause of SBE (Table 270–1). In contrast, *Escherichia coli* adheres poorly and rarely causes infective endocarditis even though it is a very frequent cause of bacteremia.

Once lodged upon the surface of NBTE, bacteria multiply rapidly and attain high numbers within the vegetation, after which many enter the stationary or resting phase. The presence of bacteria is a powerful stimulus for further localized thrombosis, which causes vegetations to enlarge by accretion of new layers of fibrin. Because these layers protect bacteria from phagocytes, the vegetation provides a sanctuary in which even avirulent bacteria can flourish.

Approximate figures for the frequency with which vegetations are found at various locations in the heart are given in Table 270–4. The frequency with which a cardiac valve is involved by endocarditis is related to the mean blood pressure acting upon it. Accordingly, the aortic and mitral valves are infected far more often than the tricuspid and pulmonary valves. This rule does not hold for acute endocarditis in intravenous drug abusers, in whom tricuspid valve infection is common (Table 270–4).

Endocarditis usually develops at sites where blood flows from a high-pressure source (e.g., the left ventricle) through an orifice (e.g., a ventricular septal defect) into a low-pressure sink (e.g., the right ventricle). Examples of cardiovascular conditions subject to infection that fit these criteria include mitral regurgitation, aortic stenosis, ventricular septal defect, patent ductus arteriosus, and coarctation of the aorta. Vegetations are usually located on the "downstream" side of these anatomic abnormalities, where pressure effects and turbu-

lence favor deposition of bacteria from the swift stream of blood. Vegetations also may develop at sites where a turbulent regurgitant jet of blood strikes the wall of a cardiac chamber, causing endothelial roughening and reactive endocardial fibrosis. These are called *jet lesions*.

The vegetations of infective endocarditis are variable in appearance. Some are small warty nodules, while others have the cauliflower-like polypoid appearance that gave rise to the descriptive term *vegetation*. Some are less than 1 sq mm in size, while others are so large as to block valve orifices and cause functional stenosis. They may be white, red, tan, or gray. Vegetations in patients with ABE or fungal endocarditis are often larger than those of SBE. Microscopic examination shows colonies of bacteria or masses of fungal hyphae embedded in fibrin and platelets. Infected vegetations usually contain surprisingly few leukocytes. Inflammatory cells may accumulate at the base of the vegetation, where it attaches to the valve. This distorts the valve, superimposing new damage on any pre-existing pathology. If this reaction is severe, the valve may perforate, or an abscess may develop in adjacent tissues. Abscess formation is common in ABE and PVE but not in SBE.

Antibodies to many of the commensal organisms that cause SBE are present in low titer before infection occurs, increase in number during the course of SBE, and decrease after successful treatment. These antibodies do not arrest the progress of SBE and do not provide immunity to future endocardial infection.

The healing process begins even in untreated endocarditis but only reaches completion if antibiotic treatment kills the bacteria. Host cells move in to organize the vegetation; macrophages ingest bacterial and cellular debris; and fibroblasts lay down new collagen. The vegetations gradually shrink over a period of weeks or months and become endothelialized. Recognizable but nonviable bacteria can sometimes be found in sections of valves resected at operation or necropsy, months after infection has been eradicated. The healed valve is often scarred, thickened by fibrosis, and calcified. It may be perforated, and the supporting structures may be damaged. Residual hemodynamic dysfunction, mild or severe, is therefore likely. This condition may worsen over time, even though the bacteria had been eradicated long before by antibiotic treatment. The scarred valve remains susceptible to reinfection for life.

TABLE 270–3. ESTIMATED RELATIVE RISK FOR INFECTIVE ENDOCARDITIS POSED BY VARIOUS CARDIAC LESIONS

Relatively High Risk	Intermediate Risk	Very Low or Negligible Risk
Prosthetic heart valves	Mitral valve prolapse	Atrial septal defects
Aortic valve disease	Pure mitral stenosis	Arteriosclerotic plaques
Mitral insufficiency	Tricuspid valve disease	Coronary artery disease
Patent ductus arteriosus	Pulmonary valve disease	Syphilitic aortitis
Ventricular septal defect	Previous infective endocarditis	Cardiac pacemakers
Coarctation of the aorta	Asymmetric septal hypertrophy	Surgically corrected cardiac lesions (without prosthetic
Marfan's syndrome	Calcific aortic sclerosis	implants, more than 6 months after operation)
	Hyperalimentation or pressure-monitoring lines that reach the right atrium	
	Nonvalvular intracardiac prosthetic implants	

Adapted from Durack DT: Infective and non-infective endocarditis. In Hurst JW (ed.): The Heart. 6th ed. New York, McGraw-Hill Book Company, 1986, pp 1130–1157.

TABLE 270–4. FREQUENCY WITH WHICH ANATOMIC SITES ARE INVOLVED IN SUBACUTE ENDOCARDITIS, ACUTE ENDOCARDITIS, AND ENDOCARDITIS IN DRUG ADDICTS

	SBE (%)	ABE (%)	Endocarditis in Intravenous Drug Abusers (%)
Left-sided valves	85	65	40
Aortic	15–26	18–25	25–30
Mitral	38–45	30–35	15–20
Aortic *and* Mitral	23–30	15–20	13–20
Right-sided valves	5	20	50
Tricuspid	1–5	15	45–55
Pulmonary	1	Rare	2
Tricuspid *and* pulmonary	Rare	Rare	3
Left- *and* right-sided sites	Rare	5–10	5–10
Other sites (patent ductus, VSD, coarctation, jet lesions)	10	5	5

Adapted from Durack DT: Infective and non-infective endocarditis. In Hurst JW (ed.): The Heart. 6th ed. New York, McGraw-Hill Book Company, 1986, pp 1130–1157.

CLINICAL FEATURES. All the clinical and laboratory manifestations of infective endocarditis reflect the effects of a systemic intravascular infection and the patient's physiologic and immunologic reaction to it.

History. The onset of subacute endocarditis is usually insidious, with nonspecific complaints, general malaise, anorexia, weakness, and fatigue. This nonspecific syndrome is often described as a "flu-like illness." Low grade intermittent fevers with chills and night sweats are usual. Headaches, myalgias, arthralgias, and back pain are common. A history of heart murmur, congenital heart disease, rheumatic fever, or cardiac surgery may help identify the underlying lesion. The patient may conceal intravenous drug abuse, which should be kept in mind during both interview and examination as a possible mode of infection.

Symptoms of heart failure must be carefully sought because their presence is of great prognostic significance. Embolization and infarction can cause sudden onset of neurologic syndromes such as hemiparesis, or abdominal pain due to infarction of spleen, kidney, or gut. Embolization of a coronary artery can cause silent or symptomatic myocardial infarction.

Perforation of a valve or rupture of chordae tendineae can cause sudden onset of severe heart failure.

Physical Examination. Patients with subacute endocarditis may have nonspecific symptoms of subacute systemic infection including pallor, asthenia, and sweating. A variety of interesting peripheral signs may be found on further examination, including petechiae, splinter hemorrhages, Roth's spots, Osler's nodes, Janeway lesions, and clubbing of the fingers. Some of the characteristics of these signs are summarized in Table 270–5.

Examination of the spleen often shows moderate enlargement, usually without notable tenderness unless there is a splenic abscess or recent embolic infarction.

On examination of the cardiovascular system, the peripheral pulse is usually rapid because of fever, heart failure, or both. A collapsing pulse may be present, indicating aortic incompetence associated with pre-existing aortic valve disease, or new aortic insufficiency associated with endocarditis. Individual peripheral arteries may be occluded by emboli, or they may be the site of a mycotic aneurysm.

One or more cardiac murmurs are present in virtually all patients with endocarditis. Murmurs may be caused by preexisting heart disease, by endocarditis itself, or by both. Up to 15 per cent of patients do not have a heart murmur when first examined, but nearly all will develop a murmur before the disease has run its course. New murmurs and changing murmurs are more likely to occur in acute endocarditis than in subacute disease. Development of a new murmur of aortic insufficiency during a febrile illness of unknown origin strongly suggests the diagnosis of infective endocarditis.

COMPLICATIONS. Heart failure is by far the most important complication of infective endocarditis; it exerts more influence on prognosis and treatment than any other. In one representative series, some degree of heart failure was present in 75 per cent of patients with aortic valve disease and endocarditis, in 50 per cent with mitral valve involvement, and in 19 per cent with tricuspid disease.

Arterial embolization is diagnosed in about one third of patients with subacute endocarditis and in up to two thirds of patients with acute endocarditis. Many small or large arterial emboli go undetected. Any artery may be affected. In

TABLE 270–5. CHARACTERISTICS OF SOME PERIPHERAL SIGNS OF INFECTIVE ENDOCARDITIS

	Petechiae	Splinter Hemorrhages	Roth's Spots	Osler's Nodes	Janeway's Lesions	Clubbing
Appearance	Tiny red hemorrhagic spots	"Splinters" under nails; red when fresh, then brown or black	Small bright red patches with white centers	Pea-sized red or purplish nodules	Red macules	Curvature of the nails in two planes, with swelling of the terminal phalanges
Distribution	Anywhere, especially above clavicles, in mouth and in conjunctivae	Distal third of nails	Retinae	Fingers and toes; occasionally hands and feet	Palms and soles; occasionally on flanks, forearms, ankles, feet, ears	Fingers and/or toes
Incidence	Common, in both SBE and ABE	Common, in both SBE and ABE	Infrequent; usually in SBE	Infrequent; usually in SBE	Infrequent; usually in ABE	Rare; in SBE only
Pathology	Increased capillary permeability; microemboli	Blood in avascular squamous epithelium under nail; due to microemboli or increased capillary fragility	Inflammation and hemorrhage	Intracutaneous local vasculitis; bacteria rarely found; occasional abscess formation; probably embolic in origin	Origin uncertain; possibly embolic or allergic in origin	Soft tissue proliferation, occasionally periosteal new bone formation
Pain	None	None	None	Mild to moderately severe	None	Usually none; sometimes painful
Duration	Days	Weeks	Days	Days	Several hours to days	Weeks to months
Diagnostic significance	Nonspecific; also found in septicemia, after cardiac surgery, and in many other disorders	Nonspecific; found in up to 10% of normal people and up to 40% of patients with mitral stenosis	Strongly suggestive of endocarditis but not diagnostic	Almost pathognomonic for endocarditis	Unusual in bacteremia without endocarditis	Nonspecific; found in many cardiopulmonary disorders; can be congenital

Adapted from Durack DT: Infective and non-infective endocarditis. In Hurst JW (ed.): The Heart. 5th ed. New York, McGraw-Hill Book Company, 1982, pp 1250–1277.

order of frequency, arteries supplying the brain, lung, myocardium, spleen, and extremities are involved.

Neurologic manifestations of endocarditis are common and clinically important. These include toxic confusional states, stroke, meningoencephalitis, cranial or peripheral nerve lesions, and psychiatric symptoms. About 10 per cent of patients with endocarditis have complaints involving the central nervous system, while 30 to 50 per cent have nervous system involvement at some point during the course of the disease. Cerebral infarction is usually caused by embolism, while cerebral hemorrhage, which is less common than infarction, may be associated with emboli or rupture of a mycotic aneurysm. Heparin therapy increases the risk that an intracranial hemorrhage will occur during the course of infective endocarditis.

Cerebritis secondary to impaction of infected emboli or hematogenous spread of bacteria is quite common, especially in acute bacterial endocarditis caused by S. aureus. Cerebritis may progress to form a frank cerebral abscess, which is found in 1 to 5 per cent of cases of acute endocarditis. However, brain abscesses rarely complicate subacute endocarditis.

In up to 15 per cent of patients, examination of the cerebrospinal fluid may show reactive changes consisting of the presence of polymorphonuclear leukocytes and moderately elevated protein concentration. Such reactions are particularly common in acute staphylococcal endocarditis. In most cases cerebrospinal glucose concentrations do not decrease, cultures are negative, and true bacterial meningitis does not develop, except in a few patients with acute pneumococcal or staphylococcal endocarditis.

Mycotic aneurysm is an unusual but important complication that is diagnosed in 3 to 5 per cent of patients. The true incidence is probably higher, but a number pass undetected, especially small aneurysms in the brain. Mycotic aneurysms are caused by an inflammatory reaction in the arterial wall associated with septic microemboli to vasa vasorum, or to impaction of an infected embolus in the arterial lumen. The site most often involved is the proximal aorta, including the sinuses of Valsalva, followed by arteries to the viscera, extremities, and brain. Living organisms are seldom found in the wall of these aneurysms, even when the underlying endocardial infection is still active. Presumably, the damage that weakens the arterial wall was done by an earlier inflammatory reaction to infected emboli. If an aneurysm enlarges to a certain critical size (probably about 1 cm in diameter), it is likely to continue to enlarge and eventually rupture as a result of the physical force exerted by the arterial pressure, despite eradication of the infecting organisms by antimicrobial therapy.

Most patients with subacute endocarditis show abnormalities in the urinary sediment. In some cases this is due to glomerulonephritis, a relatively common complication that is usually not severe enough to cause significant renal failure. Glomerulonephritis is caused by deposition of immune complexes on the glomerular basement membrane. Other inflammatory manifestations of subacute infective endocarditis that may be mediated by immune complexes include arthritis, tenosynovitis, and possibly pericarditis, Osler's nodes, and Roth's spots. In a few patients with long-term SBE, glomerulonephritis is severe enough to necessitate dialysis. Renal function usually recovers steadily within a few weeks after the start of effective treatment.

SPECIAL FORMS OF INFECTIVE ENDOCARDITIS

ACUTE BACTERIAL ENDOCARDITIS. Several important features distinguish acute from subacute bacterial endocarditis. The diagnosis is usually made within seven days from onset of symptoms. The clinical course is usually measured in days rather than in weeks or months. The associated systemic illness is more severe, and early mortality is higher than in subacute endocarditis.

Acute endocardial infection is usually caused by primary pathogens capable of producing invasive infection at other sites. S. aureus is the most common cause of acute endocarditis. This species alone accounts for 50 to 70 per cent of cases. The patient is more likely to suffer rapid destruction of the valve, including perforation, so the likelihood that valve replacement will be required is greater. Patients with acute bacterial endocarditis are also more likely to have one or more focal infections outside the heart—in brain, bone, lungs, or other sites. Such foci could be either primary (that is, the portal of entry for the organism causing endocarditis) or secondary hematogenous infections. In contrast, the organisms that cause subacute bacterial endocarditis rarely cause localized hematogenous infection elsewhere in the body.

Abscesses in the fibrous cardiac skeleton or myocardium are much more likely to form in acute than in subacute endocarditis. If such abscesses are adjacent to the fibers of the conduction system, they may cause conduction defects. Abscesses may be responsible for antibiotic treatment failure.

Because acute bacterial endocarditis is caused by invasive organisms and progresses rapidly, treatment should not be delayed until blood culture results are available. It is important to clear the bloodstream of circulating organisms as soon as possible, both to reduce the risk of death from septicemia and to lessen the chances that metastatic infection will develop elsewhere. When acute endocarditis is strongly suspected, empiric antibiotic therapy should be started immediately after three blood samples have been drawn for culture.

ENDOCARDITIS IN DRUG ADDICTS. Endocarditis is the most important of the many infective complications experienced by intravenous drug abusers. Salient features that distinguish endocarditis in this subgroup from the disease in general include a younger age of onset, a higher proportion of acute cases, a correspondingly higher proportion of cases involving normal cardiac valves, and a high frequency of tricuspid valve infection. The etiologic organisms can gain entry into the bloodstream in various ways: directly, by injection of contaminated materials; or indirectly, from the patient's skin flora, from cellulitis caused by subcutaneous injection of drugs, or from suppurative thrombophlebitis or drug-related infections in other sites such as the lungs. S. aureus is the leading etiologic organism. Addicts also have an increased incidence of endocardial infection with gram-negative bacilli, especially Pseudomonas species, and fungi.

Drug addicts with acute endocarditis usually experience a brief severe illness, with heavily positive blood cultures. Because the etiologic organisms are often primary pathogens, hematogenous infection elsewhere in the body is common. A common finding on admission is multiple patches of pneumonitis visible on chest x-ray. These are caused by small septic pulmonary emboli arising from vegetations on the tricuspid or occasionally the pulmonary valve. Although acute disease is typical, subacute endocarditis in addicts is not rare, especially in those who have had previous episodes of endocarditis.

The prognosis for young drug addicts with right-sided S. aureus infection is good, with mortality rates being less than 5 per cent. Factors that worsen the prognosis include left-sided involvement, particularly aortic, and infection with gram-negative bacilli or fungi. Recurrent episodes of endocarditis are common in addicts who continue to use drugs after their first episode of endocarditis, especially if a prosthetic valve has been inserted.

PROSTHETIC VALVE INFECTION. Prosthetic valve endocarditis should be regarded as a special category, because it differs in many ways from other forms of endocarditis. By arbitrary definition, early PVE occurs within 60 days of valve placement and late PVE more than 60 days postoperatively. Early PVE occurs at a rate of about 1 per cent, although this figure varies between hospitals. Late PVE is estimated to occur at an overall rate of about 1 per cent per year. The rate for infection of aortic valve prostheses is four to five times higher than for mitral prostheses.

The progress of PVE may be either acute or subacute, but this cannot be predicted reliably from the infecting organism. For example, even *S. epidermidis*, a nonpathogen that causes indolent chronic disease on native valves, can cause an acute syndrome in early PVE.

The spectrum of organisms causing PVE is quite distinct. *S. epidermidis*, which rarely infects native valves, is a leading cause of both early and late prosthetic valve infection. Gram-negative bacilli and fungi infect prosthetic valves notably more often than they do native valves, especially in early onset cases. The later the onset of PVE after operation, the more nearly the spectrum of etiologic organisms resembles that of native valve endocarditis.

In addition to forming vegetations, infection may spread around the circumference of the sewing ring of the prosthesis, often causing partial dehiscence and paravalvular leaks. Abscess formation in fibrous tissue or myocardium adjacent to the sewing ring is common. Despite these adverse factors, when a prosthetic valve is replaced for infection, early reinfection with the same organism is uncommon.

In general, PVE is harder to cure than most other forms of endocarditis (Table 270–6). This is due partly to the increased frequency of antibiotic-resistant organisms in PVE, and partly to the fact that a foreign body is present at the site of infection. Not surprisingly, the risk of relapse after antibiotic therapy is much higher for PVE than for native valve infection. Valve replacement is often necessary to achieve cure. Antibiotic treatment usually must be continued for a minimum of four to six weeks, sometimes for many months. In some cases in which repeated valve replacement is contraindicated, cure cannot be achieved but suppressive antibiotic therapy is continued indefinitely.

GRAM-NEGATIVE BACTERIAL ENDOCARDITIS. This term usually refers to infection with enteric or environmental gram-negative aerobic bacilli such as *Klebsiella*, *Pseudomonas*, *Serratia*, *Enterobacter*, and *E. coli*. (*Haemophilus* species usually cause subacute endocarditis and are not considered in this group.) Gram-negative endocarditis is a rare disease except

in two settings: early prosthetic valve infection and intravenous drug addiction. In these two groups, gram-negative bacilli can account for up to 15 to 20 per cent of cases.

Gram-negative endocarditis often progresses acutely. Patients may develop septic shock. The mortality rate is higher than for gram-positive infections, approaching that of fungal endocarditis. Antibiotic treatment alone is often unsuccessful, so valve replacement is frequently necessary. Treatment with combinations of two or more antibiotics for six weeks or more is often necessary. Relapse after antibiotic treatment is much more common than for gram-positive infection.

FUNGAL ENDOCARDITIS. Like gram-negative endocarditis, fungal infection of the endocardium is rare except in two groups of patients: those with prosthetic valves and intravenous drug addicts. Although a wide variety of fungal species have been recovered from patients with endocarditis over the years, only two predominate: *Candida* and *Aspergillus* spp. *C. albicans* endocarditis occurs in patients with central intravascular lines, especially hyperalimentation lines that are allowed to reach the level of the tricuspid valve. Therefore, these infections often involve the right side. *C. parapsilosis* and *C. tropicalis* are more likely to occur in drug addicts and can infect valves on either side of the heart. Fungal vegetations tend to be bulky and often cause infarctions as a result of embolization of peripheral arteries. Because blood cultures are commonly negative in fungal endocarditis (see earlier discussion), surgical removal of a large embolus from an artery to one of the limbs may be diagnostic as well as therapeutic. Histologic examination may show hyphae of the infecting fungus in tissue sections.

Few drugs are available for treatment of fungal endocarditis. Amphotericin B is generally used, but the chances of achieving cure with drug therapy alone is extremely low. Cure rates can be increased by surgical removal of vegetations and valve replacement, but mortality remains relatively high compared with that for other forms of endocarditis (Table 270–6).

ENDOCARDITIS IN INFANTS AND CHILDREN. Infective endocarditis is an unusual occurrence in infants. When it does occur, it is most often only one component of systemic bacterial infection caused by an invasive organism such as *S. aureus*. The endocardial infection is likely to follow an acute course, being discovered unexpectedly at necropsy in an infant who has died with bacterial infection. Often a normal cardiac valve is involved, as in other forms of acute endocarditis. The remaining cases are associated with congenital cardiac defects. Because the diagnosis is often delayed or missed, endocarditis in infants has a higher mortality than in other age groups.

In children more than one year old, infective endocarditis is not rare. Most affected children have subacute disease involving congenital cardiac defects. The spectrum of etiologic organisms and the approach to diagnosis and treatment are similar to those in adults with infective endocarditis. However, the age and physical size of children must be carefully considered when choosing the best time for cardiac surgery, especially when prostheses must be implanted.

ENDOCARDITIS IN OBSTETRIC AND GYNECOLOGIC PRACTICE. Pregnancy itself poses little increased risk for infective endocarditis. Septic abortion or pelvic infection related to intrauterine contraceptive devices can lead to endocarditis in susceptible patients. Occasionally, infective endocarditis develops during delivery or in the puerperium. If the mother has pre-existing valvular disease, bacteremias associated with perinatal infective complications such as amnionitis, endometritis, parametritis, septic thrombophlebitis, or urinary tract infection can seed the endocardium. The leading etiologic organisms in this setting are *S. faecalis*, *S. agalactiae* (Group B), *S. aureus*, and occasionally *Bacteroides* or gram-negative enteric bacilli.

NOSOCOMIAL ENDOCARDITIS. Intensive medical care

TABLE 270–6. ESTIMATED BACTERIOLOGIC CURE RATES FOR ETIOLOGIC ORGANISMS TREATED WITH ANTIMICROBIAL THERAPY ALONE OR ANTIMICROBIALS PLUS SURGERY*

Native Valve Endocarditis	Antimicrobial Therapy Alone	Antimicrobial Therapy Plus Surgery
Viridans streptococci, group A streptococci, *S. bovis*, pneumococci, gonococci	98	98
S. faecalis	90	>90
S. aureus (in young drug addicts)	90	>90
S. aureus (in elderly patients with chronic underlying diseases)	50	70
Gram-negative aerobic bacilli†	40	65
Fungi	<5	50

Prosthetic Valve Endocarditis	Early PVE	Late PVE	Early PVE	Late PVE
Viridans streptococci, group A streptococci, *S. bovis*, pneumococci, gonococci	‡	80	‡	90
S. faecalis	‡	60	‡	75
S. aureus	25	40	50	60
S. epidermidis	20	40	60	70
Gram-negative aerobic bacilli†	<10	20	40	50
Fungi	<1	<1	30	40

*Morbidity and mortality will be significantly greater than these figures for *bacteriologic* cure indicate.

†Excluding *Haemophilus* species, which carry a better prognosis.

‡Insufficient data to estimate rate.

Adapted from Durack DT: Infective and non-infective endocarditis. In Hurst JW (ed.): The Heart. 5th ed. New York, McGraw-Hill Book Company, 1982, pp 1250–1277.

can predispose to endocarditis in many ways. Endothelial damage can be caused by intracardiac surgery, pressure-monitoring catheters, ventriculoatrial shunts, and hyperalimentation lines if they reach into the right atrium. Portals of entry for microorganisms are provided by wounds, burns, biopsy sites, intravenous and arterial catheters and pacemakers, hemodialysis access sites, urinary catheters, and intratracheal airways. Nosocomial bacteremias are common in seriously ill patients. Therefore, it is not surprising that hospital-acquired infective endocarditis has become increasingly common in the past two decades, as intensive care units have proliferated. Perhaps the highest risk is found in severely burned patients, who may sustain repeated episodes of bacteremia while pressure-monitoring catheters are kept in the right side of the heart for long periods. In contrast, diagnostic right heart catheterization over brief periods in patients in a coronary care unit, who seldom develop bacteremia, presents a very low risk for infective endocarditis.

The microbes likely to cause nosocomial endocarditis are staphylococci, *Candida* species, and gram-negative bacilli. The prognosis is worse than for most other forms of infective endocarditis. This is because the patients have serious pre-existing diseases that may obscure the symptoms and signs, thus delaying diagnosis. Also, nosocomially acquired organisms are more likely to be resistant to antibiotics.

CULTURE-NEGATIVE ENDOCARDITIS. This term refers to the situation in which the endocardium is infected, but blood cultures remain persistently negative. Possible causes include antibiotic therapy, and infection by slow-growing or fastidious microorganisms that are missed because of suboptimal blood culture technique. Culture-negative endocarditis is an uncommon disease. Therefore, when blood cultures from a patient not receiving antibiotics remain *persistently* negative, that patient probably does not have endocarditis. Fungal endocarditis is an exception. Blood cultures are positive in only about half of patients with *Candida* endocarditis and in less than one fifth of those with *Aspergillus* infection. When culture-negative disease does occur, it is much more likely to follow a subacute than an acute course.

If the clinical findings strongly support the diagnosis of culture-negative endocarditis, a therapeutic trial of antibiotic therapy may be given. This usually consists of a penicillin plus an aminoglycoside for subacute infection, a combination that will cover viridans streptococci, enterococci, *Haemophilus* species, and diphtheroids. If the disease is acute, treatment for *Staphylococcus aureus* must be included. To be of diagnostic value, a proper therapeutic trial must be continued for at least two weeks unless new information changes the situation.

INFECTIVE ENDARTERITIS. An infection located within an artery can mimic infective endocarditis. Possible sites of vegetations include patent ductus arteriosus, coarctation of the aorta, arteriovenous fistulas, and prosthetic vascular grafts. In the past, about one quarter of all patients with an uncorrected patent ductus arteriosus eventually developed bacterial endarteritis. Because many of the underlying lesions are surgically correctable, infective endarteritis is now uncommon in developed countries, with the exception of infections in arteriovenous shunts constructed for the purpose of hemodialysis. When bacterial endarteritis occurs in an aneurysm, the etiologic organisms are usually found within a multilayered thrombus in the lumen of the aneurysm rather than in vegetations.

RECURRENT ENDOCARDITIS. The term *recurrent endocarditis* includes both *relapses* and *reinfections*. Recurrent endocarditis has been reported in 2 to 30 per cent of cases. This wide variation is partly explained by variable duration of follow-up. Intravenous drug abusers are at higher risk than any other group for recurrent endocarditis. A few patients with more than four separate episodes of infective endocarditis have been reported.

The likelihood of relapse after treatment of different forms of infective endocarditis can be predicted from published experience (Table 270–6). Because occasional relapses occur even after optimal treatment, careful follow-up for several months after treatment is mandatory. Most relapses occur within a few days or weeks of ending treatment, but occasional late relapses occur as a result of a few organisms surviving in a metabolically inactive state deep within vegetations.

Reinfection means a new episode of endocarditis has developed after cure of a previous episode. Usually a different species or strain of etiologic organism is involved, but if the second organism is a common viridans streptococcus that appears identical to the first, one cannot be certain whether an episode of recurrent endocarditis represents reinfection or relapse.

DIFFERENTIAL DIAGNOSIS. The differential diagnosis of endocarditis is very wide because its manifestations are numerous and often nonspecific. SBE must be considered in the evaluation of every patient with fever of unknown origin. It can be confused with rheumatic fever, osteomyelitis, tuberculosis, meningitis, intra-abdominal infections, salmonellosis, brucellosis, glomerulonephritis, myocardial infarction, stroke, endocardial thrombi, atrial myxoma, connective tissue diseases, vasculitis, occult malignancy (especially lymphomas), congestive heart failure, pericarditis, and even psychoneurosis. ABE shares many manifestations with septicemias caused by *S. aureus*, *Neisseria*, pneumococci, and gram-negative bacilli in patients who do not have endocarditis. ABE may mimic pneumonia, meningitis, brain abscess, stroke, malaria, acute pericarditis, vasculitis, and disseminated intravascular coagulation.

INVESTIGATIONS. *Routine Tests.* Results of urinalysis are abnormal in about 50 per cent of cases, showing microscopic hematuria or slight proteinuria or both. Gross hematuria suggests that renal infarction may have occurred. Red cell casts and heavy proteinuria indicate that immune complex glomerulonephritis may be present.

The automated blood count shows only nonspecific abnormalities. Anemia is usual in SBE and fairly common in ABE. Anemia is most often of the hypoproliferative type, with a normochromic normocytic smear. ABE may cause acute hemolysis. A prosthetic valve may cause chronic low grade hemolysis in the absence of infection.

A moderate leukocytosis with some immature forms apparent on smear is often found in SBE, but in many cases the leukocyte count is normal. Patients with ABE usually show a striking neutrophilia with band forms, vacuoles, Döhle bodies, and toxic granulation. In a few cases, careful examination of a Gram-stained smear of the buffy coat will reveal organisms within neutrophils.

The erythrocyte sedimentation rate is almost always elevated, except in a few acute cases of very brief duration.

Blood Culture. This is the single most important investigation in diagnosis of endocarditis. Blood cultures should be drawn from all patients with fever and heart murmur unless their illness is clearly due to another diagnosed disease or the fever resolves quickly without recurrence. Blood cultures should also be taken if a patient with a heart lesion susceptible to endocarditis has other symptoms or signs consistent with infection.

The bacteremia of infective endocarditis is usually continuous, with between 1 and 100 organisms per milliliter of blood in subacute cases. Therefore, it is seldom necessary to draw a large number of blood cultures. The causative organism can be recovered from culture samples taken on the first day of admission in over 90 per cent of patients with culture-positive endocarditis. No more than three separate venous blood cultures should be drawn on the first day. If these show no growth by the second day, two or three further culture samples may be drawn. If the patient has received prior antibiotic therapy, further blood samples may be taken over the following week in a search for recrudescence of bacteremia after antibiotic effect has passed. Otherwise, repeated blood cultures are likely to be uninformative and wasteful.

After careful skin cleansing, 10 to 20 ml of blood should be drawn for each culture. Skin preparation is especially important because common skin flora (*S. epidermidis* and diphtheroids) can cause endocarditis, and their isolation from blood cultures can cause diagnostic confusion. Pour plates can help to distinguish contaminants from true positive cultures. The culture medium should be adequately supplemented to allow growth of fastidious, nutritionally variant bacteria. When endocarditis is suspected, cultures should be incubated for at least three weeks and stains made at intervals even if no growth is apparent on inspection.

Subacute endocarditis stimulates the humoral immune system to produce both nonspecific and specific antibodies. A positive test for rheumatoid factor is found in 40 to 50 per cent of subacute cases, but rarely in ABE. This can provide a useful diagnostic clue in culture-negative cases. A polyclonal increase in gamma globulins is characteristic. Occasional false-positive serologic test results for syphilis occur. Hemolytic complement levels may be moderately elevated, normal, or low. The lowest levels are found in patients with immune complex glomerulonephritis. Circulating immune complexes are present in more than 80 per cent of patients with either ABE or SBE. All these immunologic findings revert to normal after eradication of the organisms.

Electrocardiography. Electrocardiography may reveal evidence of myocardial infarction due to embolization of a vegetation to a coronary artery. When a disturbance of conduction develops during the course of endocarditis, extension of infection into the myocardium may have occurred. This could be focal myocarditis, or an abscess located close to the conduction system.

Echocardiography. Echocardiography may detect valvular vegetations or help in evaluation of underlying heart disease and cardiac function. This tool can be very helpful, but its sensitivity and specificity for diagnosis of endocarditis are limited. Negative echocardiographic study results do not rule out endocarditis. Very small vegetations cannot be detected, and all the leaflets of the valves cannot be visualized in every patient. Occasional false-positive readings for vegetations occur, particularly in patients with myxomatous degeneration of a valve.

The larger vegetations typical of acute infection in narcotic addicts and of fungal endocarditis are easier to demonstrate than the smaller lesions found in some patients with SBE. Vegetations on prosthetic valves are difficult to visualize. Sequential echocardiographic studies of vegetations during and after treatment are unreliable as a criterion for success or failure of antibiotic therapy.

Radiography. The chest x-ray is most useful as a means of providing evidence of congestive heart failure. Multiple small patchy infiltrates in the lungs of an intravenous drug abuser with fever strongly suggest the diagnosis of septic emboli arising from right-sided infective endocarditis. Valvular calcification may identify a valve affected by chronic rheumatic or congenital disease. A mycotic aneurysm could cause widening of the aorta.

Abnormal motion of a prosthetic valve can be detected by fluoroscopy, indicating presence of a vegetation or partial dehiscence of the valve from the aortic root. This information can indicate that valve replacement is needed during management of PVE.

Computerized axial tomography can be very useful to define the cause of focal neurologic lesions in patients with endocarditis. Such lesions could be caused by various complications, including cerebritis, infarction, hemorrhage from a mycotic aneurysm, or brain abscess. Angiography is occasionally necessary to demonstrate mycotic aneurysms in the brain or elsewhere.

Cardiac catheterization and cineangiography are not necessary for most patients who respond well to antimicrobial therapy without developing cardiac failure. When treatment seems to be failing and/or operation is considered, cardiac catheterization can provide vital information. In one study of 35 patients who underwent cardiac catheterization during active endocarditis, the precatheterization assessment was significantly modified for 23, the diagnosis of site of valve involvement was altered for 14, and six valve ring abscesses were revealed. Surgery was postponed or cancelled for six patients when catheterization indicated only mild hemodynamic abnormalities. There were no serious complications. This study suggests that catheterization for selected patients with endocarditis provides such important information that it should not be avoided for fear of dislodging emboli.

TREATMENT. *General Measures.* The patient should be informed of the diagnosis and treatment plan and comforted. Heart failure, if present, should be managed with bed rest, salt restriction, and drug treatment as necessary. High temperatures and headaches can be treated symptomatically.

Antibiotic Therapy. For optimal antibiotic therapy, certain microbiologic information on the infecting organism is necessary. For most bacteria, both the minimal inhibitory concentration (MIC) and minimal bactericidal concentration (MBC) of the antibiotics likely to be used should be determined. This will form the basis for choice of curative therapy.

The serum bactericidal titer (SBT or Schlichter test) is frequently used and sometimes useful in the management of endocarditis. The infecting organism is exposed in vitro to the patient's serum, which is drawn while antibiotic therapy is being administered, to determine the maximum dilution of serum that will inhibit and kill the organism. The SBT provides assurance that the antibiotic(s) present in the patient's serum is actually capable of killing the infecting organism. Clinical experience indicates that the SBT should be 1:8 or higher at intervals during each day of treatment. For gram-positive organisms the serum usually can kill the organism without difficulty, and SBT's are often very high (1:128 to 1:1024). In such cases, SBT's need not be measured repeatedly. SBT's for gram-negative bacilli are usually rather low (1:2 to 1:16). The SBT is most likely to be clinically helpful when the physician is treating an unusual organism, using unusual antibiotics, using an unusual regimen (such as oral treatment), or encountering treatment failure. If treatment with unusual combinations of antibiotics is needed, further laboratory tests should be performed to find out whether they are synergistic, indifferent, or antagonistic in combination.

Bactericidal antibiotics should be used for treatment of endocarditis whenever possible. Some patients have been cured with bacteriostatic drugs, but results of treatment with these agents are usually poor, presumably because host defense mechanisms are inadequate in the vegetations. With respect to treatment, the vegetations of infective endocarditis provide a contrast to bacterial pneumonia, in which phagocytes are plentiful and bacteriostatic antibiotics are usually effective. Curative antibiotic therapy for endocarditis must eradicate organisms completely, without the help of phagocytes to eliminate microbes that are relatively resistant to antibiotics because they are in the resting phase.

Clinical experience with treatment of the common forms of bacterial endocarditis caused by gram-positive cocci is so extensive that specific therapeutic regimens can be recommended with confidence. Standard regimens for streptococcal and staphylococcal endocarditis are listed in Table 270–7. Regimens for treatment of endocarditis caused by less common organisms are not listed. For these, treatment must be chosen on the basis of more limited published experience, together with the results of tests performed upon the infecting organism in the microbiology laboratory. One of the beta-

TABLE 270–7. TREATMENT REGIMENS FOR INFECTIVE ENDOCARDITIS CAUSED BY GRAM-POSITIVE COCCI

Organism	Antibiotic Regimen	Duration (Weeks)	Comments
Alpha-hemolytic (viridans) streptococci, S. bovis	1. Penicillin G 2 million units every 6 hours IV plus streptomycin 7.5 mg per kilogram every 12 hours IM, or	2	For patients <65 years old without renal failure, eighth-nerve defects, or serious complications
	2. Penicillin G 2 million units every 6 hours IV plus streptomycin 7.5 mg per kilogram every 12 hours IM (for first 2 weeks only), or	4	For patients with complicated disease, e.g., CNS involvement, shock, moderately penicillin-resistant organism, failed previous treatment
	3. Penicillin G 4 million units every 6 hours IV, or	4	For patients >65 years old or with renal failure or eighth-nerve defect
	4. Cefazolin 2 grams every 8 hours IV, or	4	For patients allergic to penicillin
	5. Vancomycin 15 mg per kilogram (not to exceed 1 gram) every 12 hours IV	4	For patients allergic to penicillin
Group A streptococci, S. pneumoniae	1. Penicillin G 2 million units every 6 hours IV, or	2–4	These organisms are usually highly sensitive to pencillin; 2–3 weeks will be adequate for most cases
	2. Cefazolin 2 grams every 8 hours IV	2–4	
S. faecalis, other penicillin-resistant streptococci	1. Ampicillin 2 grams every 4 hours IV plus gentamicin 1.5 mg per kilogram every 8 hours IV, or	4–6	Four weeks will be adequate for most cases. Serum levels must be checked and dose adjusted accordingly.
	2. Vancomycin 15 mg per kilogram (not to exceed 1 gram) every 12 hours IV plus streptomycin 15 mg per kilogram (not to exceed 1 gram) every 12 hours IM	4–6	Four weeks will be adequate for most cases The dose of streptomycin may have to be reduced as treatment progresses, to avoid toxicity
S. aureus	1. Nafcillin 2 grams every 4 hours IV, or	4 or longer	Standard regimen
	2. Nafcillin as above plus gentamicin 1.5 mg per kilogram every 8 hours IV for the first 3–5 days, or	4 or longer	For patients with severe disseminated staphylococcal disease, gentamicin synergy may be advantageous during early stages of treatment
	3. Cephalothin 2 grams every 4 hours IV, or	4 or longer	For patients allergic to penicillin
	4. Vancomycin 15 mg per kilogram (not to exceed 1 gram) every 12 hours IV	4 or longer	For patients allergic to penicillin and cephalosporin; for resistant organisms

lactam antibiotics should be included in the regimen whenever possible.

Empiric Therapy. When the causative organism is unknown, the choice of empiric therapy depends upon whether the patient has acute or subacute disease. For ABE, broad-spectrum therapy that will cover *S. aureus* as well as many species of streptococci and gram-negative bacilli is required. For SBE, a regimen that will treat most streptococci including *S. faecalis* is appropriate. To meet these requirements, the following regimens are suggested:

1. For ABE, a combination of nafcillin, 2 grams intravenously every four hours plus ampicillin, 2 grams intravenously every four hours plus gentamicin, 1.5 mg per kilogram intravenously every eight hours.

2. For SBE, a combination of ampicillin, 2 grams intravenously every four hours plus gentamicin, 1.5 mg per kilogram intravenously every eight hours.

These regimens should be adjusted if and when the causative organism is identified.

Duration of Therapy. Because infective endocarditis carries significant mortality even when well managed, it is important that treatment be continued long enough to ensure that relapse will not occur. On the other hand, patients with the most easily treated forms of endocarditis should not be subjected to unnecessarily long and expensive treatment in hospital. Extensive experience with treatment of the streptococci provides sufficient grounds for firm recommendations on duration of therapy for these organisms (Table 270–7).

In contrast, the natural history of *S. aureus* endocarditis is more variable. Some patients recover swiftly without complications, whereas others remain febrile for several weeks, sometimes owing to manifestations of disseminated staphylococcal disease such as osteomyelitis. While four weeks of therapy will be adequate for most cases, this must not be regarded as a rigid rule because some patients require treatment for six to eight weeks or longer to achieve cure. In general, the less extensive the published experience with a particular infective agent, the more one should lean toward prolonging treatment in order to provide a reasonable margin of safety. Guidelines on duration of treatment for other organisms are not listed in Table 270–7 because the duration required varies greatly according to individual circumstances.

Anticoagulants. Although the infected vegetation is essentially a thrombotic lesion, there is no evidence that anticoagulants provide any useful therapeutic effect in endocarditis. In fact, simultaneous treatment with antibiotics plus heparin carries a higher risk of serious or fatal intracerebral hemorrhage from mycotic aneurysm or infarction than treatment with penicillin alone. However, Coumadin can be given to most patients with endocarditis without excessive risk.

It is therefore best to avoid use of heparin entirely in endocarditis and to discontinue or avoid anticoagulation therapy if possible. However, Coumadin may be given if there is a clear-cut indication, taking care not to allow the prothrombin time to rise above 1.5 times normal values. An antibiotic treatment regimen that does not require intramuscular injections should be used if the patient is receiving anticoagulants.

Surgical Treatment. Modern operative treatment constitutes the greatest advance in management of endocarditis since the advent of antibiotics. Because surgery may be needed for any patient during the course of endocarditis, they should be treated close to a thoracic surgical unit. Consultation should be obtained early, so that immediate operation can be performed if necessary.

Aortic or mitral valvular incompetence with consequent acute left ventricular failure can occur without warning, even in the most favorable forms of endocarditis. These patients need valve replacement in order to reverse cardiac failure resulting from new or worsening valvular dysfunction. Replacement of an infected prosthesis is often necessary for cure because prosthetic valve infection is more difficult to eradicate with antibiotics than is native valve infection. Repeated major emboli constitute a relative indication for valve replacement. Occasionally, a patient remains septic despite antibiotic therapy. Operation may then be required for infection control rather than for the hemodynamic consequences of infection. Operation to close a patent ductus arteriosus or septal defect, to excise a coarctation of the aorta, or to relieve asymmetric septal hypertrophy may be required as part of treatment of endocarditis engrafted upon these lesions.

Good surgical management for endocarditis depends on correct timing for valve replacement. If operation is undertaken too soon, unnecessary operative mortality and early and late morbidity of valve replacement may result. Some patients will respond quickly to medical therapy, so that operation can be postponed indefinitely. If time is available for treatment of septicemia, renal failure, pneumonia, myocarditis, conduction defects, or other complications before valve replacement, ventricular function will improve and operative risk will be correspondingly lower. Given for a few days, antibiotic therapy should eradicate or at least greatly reduce the population of organisms on the valve, thus increasing the chance that an artificial valve can be inserted without itself becoming infected. However, if surgery is delayed too long patients may die suddenly, or their hemodynamic status may deteriorate so that operation is no longer feasible. This is a tragic error, because some of these patients could have been saved by earlier operation.

Frequent re-examination of the patient, together with echocardiography and/or cardiac catheterization to extend the clinical findings, is indicated in every case in which operation may be needed. The natural history of the type of endocarditis being treated should be taken into account. Penicillin-sensitive streptococcal endocarditis can almost always be bacteriologically cured (see Table 270–6), and the prognosis is good if cardiac failure does not occur. Thus, operation should usually be considered only for patients with cardiac failure who do not respond to medical treatment. Similarly, narcotic addicts with acute staphylococcal endocarditis have a relatively good prognosis, so operation should be reserved for those who develop serious heart failure. At the other end of the spectrum, the likelihood that fungal prosthetic valve endocarditis can be eradicated with antifungal drugs alone is negligible, even in the absence of heart failure (see Table 270–6). Such patients usually should undergo valve replacement early, without waiting to test the remote possibility that antifungal treatment could eradicate the infection. Aortic valve involvement, staphylococcal infection in patients other than drug addicts, gram-negative infection, prosthetic valve infection, and extension of infection into the myocardium should be regarded as other relative indications favoring early valve replacement.

PROGNOSIS. Infective endocarditis is unusual among infectious diseases in that it is always fatal if untreated. Most of the rare cases of apparent recovery reported in the preantibiotic era probably did not have infective endocarditis, which can be diagnosed with absolute certainty only at operation or necropsy. The median interval between onset of symptoms and death in patients with untreated subacute endocarditis was about six months, with wide individual variation. Almost all patients with acute infective endocarditis died in less than four weeks.

Favorable prognostic factors include infection with penicillin-sensitive streptococci, a youthful patient, absence of serious pre-existing diseases, and early diagnosis and treatment. The rate of recovery for many young drug addicts with *S. aureus* infection of the tricuspid valve is excellent—greater than 95 per cent.

Heart failure is by far the most important adverse prognostic factor. Other adverse factors include aortic valve involvement, renal failure, culture-negative disease, gram-negative or fungal infection, prosthetic valve infection, and presence of an abscess in the valve ring or myocardium.

Today, bacteriologic cure can be achieved in most patients with bacterial endocarditis (see Table 270–6). This is not true for infection with resistant gram-negative bacilli and fungi, but fortunately these are uncommon. Despite the ability to eradicate most organisms, both early and long-term mortality and morbidity of infective endocarditis remain significant because of damage already done before treatment. Follow-up of patients cured of infective endocarditis shows a five-year survival of only 60 to 70 per cent.

PREVENTION. Because endocarditis is a serious disease, antibiotics are usually given to susceptible patients during medical and dental procedures known to cause bacteremia, in an attempt to prevent this infection. Unfortunately, there is no proof that this practice is effective. Meaningful cost-benefit ratios cannot be calculated, and any recommendations are therefore necessarily empiric.

One approach is to consider two factors in each situation: (1) the relative risk for endocarditis posed by the patient's

heart condition and (2) the relative risk for endocarditis posed by the procedure. If both risks are judged to be significant, prophylactic antibiotics should be given. If one or both of these risk factors is judged to be negligible, prophylaxis should be omitted. The first of these two questions can be approached by using a ranking like that shown in Table 270–3. The second can be approached by knowing something of the frequency of bacteremia after the procedure in question and the number of cases of endocarditis attributed to it. For example, if a patient with aortic stenosis were to have dental extraction or urologic surgery, attempted prevention with antibiotics would be appropriate. If the same patient were to undergo gastroscopy, antibiotics would not be indicated because that procedure poses very little risk for endocarditis.

Prophylaxis for endocarditis is probably not required to cover most gastrointestinal diagnostic procedures such as endoscopy or radiocontrast studies, nor for normal delivery, therapeutic abortion, dilation and curettage, insertion or removal of intrauterine contraceptive devices in the absence of local infection, cardiac catheterization, insertion of pacemakers, endotracheal intubation, or bronchoscopy. However, some physicians choose to cover even these low-risk procedures in patients with prosthetic valves because they are at higher risk for endocarditis.

The indication for prophylactic antibiotics in patients with mitral valve prolapse remains controversial. MVP increases an individual's risk for endocarditis by five to eight times and

TABLE 270–8. AUTHOR'S RECOMMENDATIONS FOR PROPHYLAXIS OF ENDOCARDITIS *

	Indications	Drug and Dosage
Standard regimen	For dental procedures and oral or upper respiratory tract surgery	Penicillin V 2 grams orally 1 hour before, then 1 gram 6 hours later†
Special regimens	Parenteral regimen for high-risk patients; also for gastrointestinal or genitourinary tract procedures	Ampicillin 2 grams IM or IV *plus* gentamicin 1.5 mg per kilogram IM or IV, 0.5 hours before†
	Parenteral regimen for penicillin-allergic patients	Vancomycin 1 gram IV *slowly* over 1 hour, starting 1 hour before; *add* gentamicin 1.5 mg per kilogram IM or IV if gastrointestinal or genitourinary tract is involved†
	Oral regimen for penicillin-allergic patients (oral and respiratory tract procedures)	Erythromycin 1 gram orally 1 hour before, then 0.5 gram 6 hours later†
	Oral regimen for minor gastrointestinal or genitourinary tract procedures	Amoxicillin 3 grams orally 1 hour before, then 1.5 grams 6 hours later†
	Parenteral regimen for cardiac surgery including prosthetic valve placement	Cefazolin 2 grams IV on induction of anesthesia, repeated 8 and 16 hours later,‡ *or* Vancomycin 1 gram IV *slowly* over 1 hour, starting on induction of anesthesia, then 0.5 gram IV 8 and 16 hours later‡

*These are empiric suggestions. No regimen has been proven effective, and prevention failures may occur with any regimen. These recommendations are not intended to cover all clinical situations; practitioners should use their own judgment on safety and cost-benefit issues in each individual case. Several additional doses may be given if the period of risk for bacteremia is prolonged, but prophylaxis should not be extended for days.

†Pediatric dosages: ampicillin 50 mg per kilogram; erythromycin 20 mg per kilogram for first dose, then 10 mg per kilogram; gentamicin 2 mg per kilogram; vancomycin 20 mg per kilogram; penicillin V, cefazolin, and amoxicillin for children weighing more than 60 pounds, use same dose as for adults; for children weighing less than 60 pounds, use half the adult dose.

‡Gentamicin 1.5 mg per kilogram IV may be given with each dose only if postoperative gram-negative infections have occurred with significant frequency.

Adapted from Durack DT: Nine controversies in the management of endocarditis. In Petersdorf RG, et al. (eds.): Update V. Harrison's Principles of Internal Medicine. New York, McGraw-Hill Book Company, 1984, pp 35–46.

underlies a significant proportion of cases of subacute bacterial endocarditis. However, mitral valve prolapse is very common in the general population, while endocarditis is relatively uncommon, so prolapse should be regarded as a low-risk lesion for endocarditis. Many authorities currently recommend prophylaxis for patients with prolapse, especially those with mitral regurgitation, but an estimate of benefits in relation to costs has indicated that parenteral prophylaxis for prolapse is probably not cost-effective. In the author's opinion, it is reasonable to give oral antibiotic prophylaxis to MVP patients undergoing procedures that cause significant bacteremia because the costs and risks of oral penicillin therapy for an individual are very low, and a serious disease may occasionally be prevented. However, use of antibiotics in this setting should be considered optional rather than mandatory. Parenteral prophylaxis for MVP patients probably should be avoided to reduce the risk of anaphylaxis.

Specific recommendations for prophylaxis of endocarditis are listed in Table 270–8.

AHA Committee Report: Treatment of infective endocarditis due to viridans streptococci. Circulation 63:730A, 1981. *A brief, authoritative statement on treatment options for endocarditis caused by streptococci.*

Bisno AL: Treatment of Infective Endocarditis. New York, Grune & Stratton, 1982. *This book deals with many aspects of endocarditis besides treatment. It provides a good source for references.*

Durack DT: Infective and non-infective endocarditis. In Hurst JW (ed.): The Heart. 6th ed. New York, McGraw Hill Book Company, 1986, pp 1130–1157. *A general review of infective and noninfective endocarditis in a leading cardiology textbook (181 references).*

Durack DT: Prophylaxis of endocarditis. In Mandell GL, Douglas RG, Bennett JE (eds.): Principles and Practice of Infectious Diseases. New York, John Wiley & Sons, 1984. *This chapter analyzes the problems of endocarditis prophylaxis in detail and reviews current recommendations (52 references).*

Karchmer AW, Dismukes WE, Buckley MJ, et al.: Late prosthetic valve endocarditis: Clinical features influencing therapy. Am J Med 64:199, 1978. *This paper reports on patients with late prosthetic valve endocarditis, comparing survival according to etiologic organisms and medical as opposed to surgical treatment. Various features that carry a poor prognosis are identified, and relative indications for surgery are discussed.*

Rahimtoola SH: Infective Endocarditis. New York, Grune & Stratton, 1978. *A heavily referenced book, with good material on pathogenesis, pathology, and endocarditis in addicts and fungal endocarditis.*

Reisberg BE: Infective endocarditis in the narcotic addict. Prog Cardiovasc Dis 22:193, 1979. *A useful review of infective endocarditis in narcotic addicts. The importance of tricuspid valve infection and the effect of different infecting organisms and the sites involved on prognosis are analyzed.*

Reller LB: The serum bactericidal test. Rev Infect Dis 8:803, 1986. *A concise analysis of the strengths and weaknesses of the SBT as a means to monitor therapy.*

Weinstein L: Infective endocarditis. In Braunwald E (ed.): Heart Disease. A Textbook of Cardiovascular Medicine. Philadelphia, W. B. Saunders Company, 1988. *A long, detailed chapter in a major cardiology textbook (approximately 400 references).*

Staphylococcal Infections

271 STAPHYLOCOCCAL INFECTIONS

John N. Sheagren

Staphylococci are ubiquitous in nature. All humans are colonized by "nonpathogenic" staphylococci. In addition the "pathogenic" coagulase-producing *Staphylococcus aureus* is present transiently in a high percentage of people and is chronically carried by about 15 per cent of the normal population.

S. aureus itself is one of the most important bacterial pathogens of man. It can be aggressively invasive, spreading rapidly through soft tissues, directly invading bones and other support structures and ultimately, under conducive circumstances, seeding the bloodstream to produce septic shock and disseminated intravascular coagulation. Conversely, *S. aureus* can lie dormant deep within tissues for years without causing disease. The balance between host and parasite that results in infection with a given strain of staphylococci is not known and continues to be the subject of active research. Staphylococci rank only behind *Escherichia coli* in overall incidence of infections in the hospital setting. In the community, staphylococci, particularly *S. aureus*, are the leading cause of acute, serious, and progressive skin, soft tissue, and post-traumatic infections. A thorough understanding of the pathogenetic mechanisms and clinical manifestations of staphylococcal infections is crucial to the care of septic patients in every medical environment.

BACTERIOLOGY. Staphylococci are members of the family Micrococcaceae, of which there are two genera of major clinical importance, the micrococci and the staphylococci. These two genera are both catalase positive, but only staphylococci can anaerobically ferment glucose to produce acid. The staphylococci in turn have three clinically important species: *S. aureus*, *S. epidermidis*, and *S. saprophyticus*. *S. aureus* alone has the capacity to produce coagulase. Almost all laboratories label all coagulase-negative organisms as "*S. epidermidis*," which results in the failure to differentiate at least one clinically important subspecies, *S. saprophyticus*. *S. saprophyticus* ferments mannitol and can also be identified by resistance to novobiocin. *S. saprophyticus* is a frequent cause of urinary tract infections, almost always in young women; these organisms are sensitive to all generally prescribed urinary tract antibiotics.

The word *aureus* comes from the Latin word meaning gold and refers to the fact that most *S. aureus* colonies develop a bright golden-yellow color on blood agar media. However, *S. aureus* speciation is now assigned to all strains producing coagulase, whether or not they are golden in color. In addition, almost all strains of *S. aureus* ferment mannitol and contain deoxyribonuclease (DNAase). Staphylococci grow well both anaerobically and aerobically: thus, both aerobic and anaerobic bottles in a blood culture set from a truly bacteremic patient are usually positive.

The name staphylococcus comes from the fact that these organisms grow in clusters in liquid or semisolid media or within tissues when causing infection. However, in material obtained from abscesses, the organisms can sometimes be confusing in morphology, being quite variable in size, shape, and tendency toward clustering. Occasionally the organisms may grow in pairs or even chains, and confusion with streptococci is possible. Nonetheless, to the trained eye the size and general characteristics of the organism usually permit an accurate diagnosis of a pure staphylococcal lesion when the stained smear is carefully examined.

No reproducible serologic typing schemes are available to classify staphylococci. However, bacteriophage typing has been extremely useful in identifying strain characteristics of *S. aureus* and in providing epidemiologic data. Recently, bacteriophage typing has begun to be applied to *S. epidermidis*, and over 50 per cent of recovered strains can now be typed by this system. Bacteriophages are viruses that attach to the mucopeptide–teichoic acid complex of the cell wall. Over 100 different phages are now available for use in typing *S. aureus*, and five major groups of organisms having generally similar characteristics have been designated (phage groups I through V). For example, some phage groups of staphylococci are more likely to produce certain toxins than are others. Coagulase-negative *S. epidermidis* has also been divided into subgroups, known as biotypes, based on biochemical testing.

EPIDEMIOLOGY. Staphylococci may colonize almost all animal species, and *S. epidermidis* is universally present on the human skin. The carrier state of *S. aureus* is clinically important. Humans carry *S. aureus* predominantly in the nasopharynx, although some individuals can be heavily colonized in the axillae, groin, and perirectal region. The heavily colonized individual may become a source of recurrrent infections both to himself and to surrounding contacts. Most humans probably carry a few *S. aureus* organisms among the normal flora of every body site but at such a low level that routine cultures rarely reveal the organism. About 15 per cent of normal, non–hospital-associated persons more or less chronically carry a heavy growth of *S. aureus* in their noses.

The definition of the carrier state is a simple one: from swab culture of the anterior nares of a carrier, multiple colonies of *S. aureus* are visually identified on a blood agar culture plate. Clearly this definition is imprecise, because the more intensely one focuses attention on the organism the higher will be the percentage of normal individuals found to carry it. Nonetheless, colony counts of the nasopharyngeal flora consistently indicate a small group of persons who harbor relatively large numbers of the organism.

The factors that result in high growth rates and numbers of *S. aureus* in the nares of certain individuals and not in others are unknown. There is no evidence that the immune response to the organism (for example, secretory immunoglobulins or other inhibitory substances) plays a major role in the acquisition and loss of the organism from the nose and throat, as is the case for the meningococcus. Data indicate that the teichoic acid moiety in the cell wall of *S. aureus* mediates the adherence of the organism to nasal mucosal cells, a phenomenon of major import in mucous membrane colonization. Also, it is highly probable that the carrier state is influenced by the ability of other members of the normal bacterial flora of the nose, throat, and skin to suppress growth of a given strain of *Staphylococcus*. Most probably, other staphylococci or micrococci (or both) will turn out to be instrumental in controlling the growth of a newly introduced staphylococcal strain. In fact, clinical use of this concept has already been attempted via the process termed *bacterial interference*. Bacterial interference is the concept that a nonpathogenic strain of *Staphylococcus*, once established, seems to reduce the likelihood of acquisition of another, more pathogenic strain (see later section).

There is an interesting association between the nasal carriage of *S. aureus* and any condition associated with small breaks in the skin and mucous membranes. It has been known for a long time that patients with a variety of dermatoses, especially atopic dermatitis, are very likely to be heavily colonized with *S. aureus*. In fact, patients with eczematous skin diseases may be heavily colonized in the lesions but have few organisms on the intervening normal skin. Possibly related to these observations is the fact that patients who regularly use needles have an increased rate of carriage of *S. aureus*. Drug addicts, diabetics injecting insulin, patients on hemodialysis, and even patients receiving brief courses of allergy shots all have an increased rate of nasal carriage of *S. aureus*. This phenomenon is clinically important, because the organism carried in the nose and throat is often identical to that in the bloodstream of drug-abusing patients with endocarditis. Similarly, studies done years ago demonstrated that patients who entered hospitals for surgical procedures and who were carriers of *S. aureus* had increased rates of wound infections with the carried organism. The same phenomenon has recently been shown for hemodialysis patients, 60 to 80 per cent of whom are colonized in the nose with *S. aureus*. The colonizing organism often causes recurrent infections. Prophylaxis of the nasal carrier state with rifampin significantly reduces the subsequent incidence of infections (see later section on Treatment of Chronic Carriers).

Thus, the sequence of events leading to infection with *S.*

aureus seems to be the following: persons who for whatever reason begin to carry the organism in the nose are at risk of seeding the organism to other bodily sites and to breaks in the skin (for example, wounds or points of insertion of intravascular catheters). From such colonized peripheral sites, the organism may invade and cause destructive and rapidly progressive local and systemic septic complications.

Carriage of staphylococci within the gastrointestinal tract has not been extensively studied. However, normally a few staphylococci can usually be isolated. *S. epidermidis* is not uncommonly isolated from the stool but probably represents contamination from the perianal skin. Staphylococci, especially *S. aureus*, may grow to very high titers in the gastrointestinal tract in the presence of antibiotic therapy and cause gastrointestinal symptoms; the presumption is that antibiotics suppress the more sensitive normal floral components that are responsible for inhibiting the growth of *S. aureus*. This rationale is similar to that for the emergence of *C. difficile* in the syndrome of antibiotic-associated colitis (see Ch. 279).

Newborn infants rapidly experience an increasing rate of colonization following birth. It is not uncommon within nurseries to note infant colonization rates of 25 to 30 per cent. Most infants remain asymptomatic; on occasion, however, outbreaks of disease within nurseries may occur, sometimes traceable to a common carrier. Adult patients become increasingly colonized with *S. aureus* the longer they remain in the hospital. Once a hospitalized individual becomes a carrier (especially individuals with open, actively infected lesions), the nasally carried organisms may spread to other anatomic sites, to clothing and other items within the room, and to individuals with whom the patient has contact. The most effective technique for stopping transmission of staphylococci from person to person, especially in a hospital setting, is to wash one's hands meticulously immediately before and after examining each patient. This process is particularly important when examining a patient with a gross, obviously staphylococcal lesion or with a chronic exudative dermatosis. Such patients should always be managed by appropriate isolation procedures while they are hospitalized.

PATHOGENESIS. Whether or not an infection develops with any microorganism depends on the balance between the aggressiveness of the organism and the level of defense provided by the host. Thus, organisms that are highly virulent may regularly infect normal hosts and, conversely, nonpathogenic (saprophytic) organisms usually only cause infection in the face of a significant impairment of host defense. The following paragraphs will first describe those microbial characteristics that lead to the presence or absence of virulence and then the primary mechanisms by which the host attempts containment.

Microbial Virulence. The factor that makes certain strains of staphylococci virulent and others nonpathogenic is unknown. Several extracellular enzymes are produced by *S. aureus*, many probably participating in the pathogenic capabilities of the organism. For example, as in the case of streptococci, hyaluronidase probably assists the organism in its rapid spread through tissues. A variety of other enzymes may also degrade other tissue elements, may lyse inflammation-associated coagulation (coagulase), and may be directly toxic to either white cells (leukocidins) or platelets. Studies in experimental models have shown a high correlation between coagulase production and organism virulence.

The ability of *S. aureus* to adhere to damaged endothelial surfaces explains why the organism has a high likelihood of seeding to traumatized or inflamed tissues. Adherence is mediated by receptors on the surface of *S. aureus* for laminin and fibronectin, components of the subendothelial matrix.

Numerous toxins are produced by *S. aureus*. Some have endotoxic capabilities when injected into tissues (for example, the alpha and beta toxins). *S. aureus* frequently produces an enterotoxin, and at present six enterotoxins (A through F) have been described. Enterotoxin F is identical to pyrogenic exotoxin C, the toxin involved in the toxic shock syndrome. Another well-described toxin is the exfoliative toxin responsible for the staphylococcal scalded skin syndrome.

The capsular and cell wall components of *S. aureus* clearly participate in the pathogenesis of certain clinical syndromes produced by the organism. Many *S. aureus* strains have a polysaccharide capsule covering the complex rigid cell wall matrix that consists of peptidoglycan and teichoic acid (ribitol in *S. aureus* and predominantly glycerol in *S. epidermidis*). In most strains of *S. aureus*, a unique substance, *protein A*, is also part of the cell wall. Protein A is an immunologically active substance having high affinity for the Fc fragment of immunoglobulins, particularly subgroups of IgG. Thus, protein A binds to and aggregates IgG molecules and, interestingly, fixes complement in the process. Protein A has emerged as an extremely useful immunochemical substance for extraction and quantitation of IgG molecules from biologic specimens. Whether protein A plays a role in any of the clinical syndromes produced by *S. aureus* is unknown.

The presence of a capsule varies greatly from strain to strain and may explain some of the biologic differences between organisms as they invade tissues or the bloodstream. The capsule inhibits phagocytosis by interfering with the interaction between the underlying teichoic acid-peptidoglycan complex and complement, which is activated primarily via the alternative pathway. Thus, encapsulated strains are protected in tissues from the complement-mediated attack by polymorphonuclear leukocytes (PMNs). Along with the enzymes described above, the capsule undoubtedly increases the ability of *S. aureus* to protect itself as it spreads through tissues and therefore is an important virulence factor for tissue infections. Paradoxically, while unencapsulated organisms are more likely to be contained in tissues, should the bloodstream be reached (for example in a narcotics addict directly injecting carried organisms into the blood stream), the syndrome of septic shock and disseminated intravascular coagulation (DIC) may result. The syndrome of septic shock follows massive intravascular activation of cachectin and the complement, coagulation, and kinin systems (see Ch. 257). In such a situation, unencapsulated strains of *S. aureus* produce septic shock exactly like gram-negative bacteria wherein the cell wall lipopolysaccharide (endotoxin) activates the responsible inflammatory systems.

Host Defense Aspects. The primary mechanism by which the host defends against staphylococci, especially *S. aureus*, is via the nonspecific defense system. The specific antibody and T cell-mediated host defenses appear to participate very little, if at all, in defense against *S. aureus*. Thus, while antibodies are of theoretical value against encapsulated strains of *S. aureus*, no data exist to show that antibody (commonly present in the sera of most individuals against a variety of cell wall antigens and toxins of *S. aureus*) is of any clinical value. Previous attempts to develop vaccines against the organism have not yielded documented clinical benefits.

The nonspecific host defense system consists of the barrier systems (skin and mucous membranes) plus the complement-mediated polymorphonuclear (PMN) leukocyte assault on invading organisms. Patients with defects in intracellular killing of bacteria by the PMN (for example, as in the chronic granulomatous disease of childhood or the Chédiak-Higashi syndrome) are particularly prone to develop serious infections with *S. aureus*.

Certain pathologic states with highly elevated levels of IgE predispose the patient to recurrent, chronic infections with *S. aureus*. *Job's syndrome* is a condition wherein an elevated IgE level associated with eczematous skin changes somehow predisposes the patient to recurrent soft tissue infections. No one knows how or why staphylococcal infections are enhanced by highly elevated levels of IgE. The theory is that mast cell activation in the neighborhood of a focus of *S. aureus*

infection somehow impairs normal PMN-mediated defense mechanisms. Some recent studies have shown that antihistamines may at least partially correct the defect demonstrated in these patients.

The presence of a foreign body has a dramatic effect on the development of staphylococcal infections. For example, infections with *S. epidermidis* strains are particularly common in patients harboring foreign bodies such as prosthetic heart valves, cerebrospinal fluid shunts, and artificial joints. As for *S. aureus*, the inoculum required experimentally to produce a skin infection in a healthy individual is very large (10^6 to 10^7 organisms); however, the presence of even a small foreign body such as a suture reduces the dose required to produce an infection to less than 100 organisms. Thus, foreign bodies must provide a nidus of chronic inflammation in which leukocyte accumulation and function are impaired.

CLINICAL MANIFESTATIONS

This section will review two broad categories of human diseases produced by staphylococci: first, diseases related to the production of toxins by staphylococci (exclusively *S. aureus*) and, second, diseases related to direct organism invasion.

TOXIN-PRODUCED DISEASES. Clinically, the most important toxins produced by *S. aureus* are the enterotoxins and exfoliative toxin. The distinction between the different types of toxins is becoming less clear: for example, the toxin involved in the toxic shock syndrome (pyrogenic exotoxin C) has recently been shown to be identical to enterotoxin F; furthermore, that toxin clearly has exfoliative properties.

Staphylococcal Gastroenteritis. Most cases of gastroenteritis caused by *S. aureus* follow the ingestion of foods containing a preformed toxin. The toxin itself is not produced within the gastrointestinal tract. A number of extracellular toxins are produced in large amounts when the culture media contain high amounts of carbohydrate (as in sugary and starchy foods contaminated by *S. aureus*) and when such a mixture is incubated at appropriate conditions of temperature and acidity. Toxin ingestion results in increased intestinal peristalsis, profuse nausea, vomiting, diarrhea, and in some cases fever. The organism and its preformed toxin can usually be identified in point source outbreaks from the epidemiologically implicated foodstuff. Toxin-mediated staphylococcal gastroenteritis is usually self-limited, lasting anywhere from 12 to 24 hours; however, supportive therapy (fluid and electrolyte maintenance) may on occasion be required. Antibiotics are not useful.

The Toxic Shock Syndrome (TSS). TSS is almost certainly caused by the production of a toxin at the site of a localized, often relatively asymptomatic or unnoticed infection with any strain of *S. aureus* capable of toxin production. The most common site of infection is the vagina, almost invariably in association with tampon usage. The few (less than 10 per cent) TSS cases that have not been associated with infection of the female genital tract have usually been associated with infected foreign bodies (such as sutures) in surgical wounds. Both enterotoxin F and pyrogenic exotoxin C were described by independent investigators as putative toxins responsible for the syndrome. Recent studies have confirmed the two substances to be identical. The new name for the toxin responsible for TSS is "toxic shock syndrome toxin-1" (abbreviated TSST-1). The unit "1" designation was chosen in case other such toxins are ultimately discovered. TSST-1 production by strains of *S. aureus* isolated from cases of TSS have been shown to be related to lysogeny, the presence of a temperate bacteriophage. Presumably, the clinical manifestations of the syndrome are produced when the toxin is absorbed either through mucous membranes or from a subcutaneous tissue site of colonization or infection. TSST-1 production by toxigenic strains of *S. aureus* is markedly enhanced in Mg^{++}-depleted media; further, superabsorbent tampon materials chelate Mg^{++}, resulting in ideal conditions for toxin production, explaining the relationship between superabsorbent tampon introduction and the TSS. The toxin probably produces its systemic effects by directly damaging cell membranes in peripheral tissues.

The clinical syndrome that results is dramatic. The patient, almost always unaware of the focus of toxin production, experiences the abrupt onset of high fever, myalgias, and profuse nausea, vomiting and watery diarrhea. Within the first several days, a sunburn-like rash appears, and the conjunctivae become injected. On biopsy of the skin lesions, the epidermis exhibits cleavage in the basilar layers, differentiating it from the staphylococcal scalded skin syndrome (discussed later) and from viral and drug eruptions. The patient often becomes progressively more ill and is frequently in frank shock when presenting for care. A diffuse capillary leak syndrome rapidly develops, and the serum albumin concentration often plummets to less than 2 grams per 100 ml. Hypotension and frank shock are common and are often associated with the adult respiratory distress syndrome (ARDS), acute renal failure, and abnormalities in literally every organ system evaluated. For example, almost all patients exhibit an altered state of mentation, hepatocellular malfunction, elevated levels of muscle enzymes, thrombocytopenia, and a low serum calcium concentration (far out of proportion to the hypoalbuminemia). Highly elevated levels of calcitonin are present for which no explanation currently exists.

Therapy is both supportive and specific. Identification of site of infection, drainage thereof (most frequently consisting of removal of contaminated tampons), and antibiotic therapy with beta-lactamase–resistant antistaphylococcal agents are all indicated. Antibiotics do not change the course of the initial illness but seem to prevent relapse, at least in tampon-associated cases. Patients with TSS are rarely bacteremic, and therefore this type of shock syndrome is different from bacteremic, inflammatory system-mediated shock (see Ch. 257), wherein complement, coagulation, and kinin system activation seem to be primary events.

The prognosis in TSS is favorable despite the fact that most patients are critically ill for a period of time in the hospital. However, between 5 and 10 per cent of patients studied so far succumb to the illness. Since recurrences, generally milder, are relatively common following tampon associated TSS (up to 10 per cent over the subsequent three menstrual cycles), women who have recovered from TSS should avoid tampon use for at least six months following the illness.

The Staphylococcal Scalded Skin Syndrome (SSSS). SSSS is another toxin-mediated disease produced by certain strains of *S. aureus*, usually of phage group II. These organisms produce an exfoliative toxin that when injected experimentally into infant mice produces dramatic skin desquamation and mimics in every way the clinical syndrome seen in human infants. The human disease is produced by a toxin originating in a distant focus of infection. The exfoliative toxin is absorbed and disseminated systemically and causes cleavage of the middle layers of the epidermis, bulla formation, and ultimately slippage of the superficial layer of the epithelium on gentle pressure (a positive *Nikolsky's sign*). The skin is often tender and very erythematous, producing a sunburn-like rash during the initial phase. Infants are most commonly involved, and outbreaks of this syndrome have occurred in nurseries after introduction of a toxin-producing strain. Often mild or asymptomatic omphalitis is the source. In older children, the portal of infection can be any minor skin abrasion, furuncle, or some other infected local site. The conjunctival sac may be the source as a result of mild conjunctivitis, and this source often goes undetected. The syndrome has occasionally been reported in adults. The rash proceeds rapidly to desquamation, but healing is rapid and is related to how promptly the

peripheral site has been treated. Mortality of SSSS is very low.

Differentiation of SSSS from viral exanthems and drug allergies is very important. The most important disease with which SSSS can be confused is *toxic epidermal necrolysis (TEN)*, an often fatal variant of erythema multiforme usually caused by a drug allergy (see Ch. 534). The two illnesses can be differentiated on skin biopsy, and therapy is very different for each: local care and antibiotics suffice to cure SSSS, whereas high-dose systemic glucocorticoids are indicated in TEN, with mortality still remaining high.

DISEASES RELATED TO DIRECT INVASION AND SYSTEMIC SPREAD OF STAPHYLOCOCCI. In the following subsections, the classic clinical manifestations of invasive staphylococcal infection, bacteremia, and endocarditis are described.

Dermal Infections. Most minor skin infections in man are caused by either *S. aureus* or group A beta-hemolytic streptococci. There is no way clinically to differentiate between diseases produced by the penicillin-sensitive streptococci and *S. aureus*; obviously, this is an important point, for all skin infections in which antibiotic therapy seems indicated therefore require the use of a beta-lactamase–resistant antibiotic (see Ch. 28). Direct invasion through minor breaks in skin and mucous membranes is the hallmark of disease produced by *S. aureus*. A wide variety of dermal and soft tissue infections may result, including cellulitis, local abscess formation (furuncles and carbuncles), lymphangiitis, and lymphadenitis. Direct extension can occur to deep support structures such as bones and joints and result in primary osteomyelitis and septic arthritis. Even dermal staphylococcal infections that appear minor are important to recognize because they may become a source of bacteremia. When a patient with a localized *S. aureus* skin infection manifests fever and chills, bacteremia must be assumed to be present, and prompt diagnostic and therapeutic intervention should be initiated.

Diagnosis of dermal infections is usually relatively easy. The aspirate of a large, well-developed abscess (furuncle or carbuncle) almost always reveals typical creamy pus, and on Gram's stain the clustered organisms are mixed with inflammatory debris. One should perform Gram's stains of materials from every dermal infection because occasionally gram-negative organisms may cause a clinical picture similar to that of gram-positive infections, especially in immunocompromised hosts, and obviously the initial therapeutic approach will be very different.

Therapy must always be initiated with a beta-lactamase–resistant antibiotic if antimicrobial therapy is indicated at all. In fact, the backbone of therapy of dermal staphylococcal infections continues to be debridement and drainage. Only large lesions associated with signs of surrounding cutaneous spread or systemic clinical symptoms need be treated with antibiotics. It is usually wise, however, before incising a large staphylococcal abscess (even when localized) to treat the patient with an oral dose of a penicillinase-resistant antibiotic (250 mg of dicloxacillin). Such a dose should be administered 30 minutes to one hour before incision and drainage are carried out.

The prognosis for most localized infections is excellent, but infections due to *S. aureus* often recur. Population surveys have found that each year most persons develop one to several isolated local lesions, most probably caused by *S. aureus*. However, not infrequently an individual may suffer from recurrent crops of extremely debilitating local skin lesions. In this situation the patient is usually found to be carrying the causative organism in the anterior nares, axilla, groin, or perirectal region. Most such individuals are nasal carriers, and an attempt to eradicate nasal carriage is worth making (see later section on Treatment of Chronic Carriers).

Bone and Joint Infections. Through a variety of mechanisms

S. aureus commonly involves bone (osteomyelitis, see Ch. 275) and joints (see Ch. 435 on Septic Arthritis). Direct inoculation by *S. aureus* can occur in trauma or penetrating wounds. Bone and joint infections can also result from bacteremia. In children and young adults it is assumed that bacteremia originates from a minor dermal source (such as folliculitis) or from heavily colonized mucous membranes. Seeding of *S. aureus* from the blood tends to occur to areas previously traumatized or harboring foreign bodies. In young children, the organism tends to seed into the diaphyseal plates of the long bone, areas of greatest vascularity. The affected area (usually on the ankle, knee, or shin) becomes acutely warm and swollen and may appear at first to be a primary cellulitis. Fever and shaking chills are common. Blood cultures are usually positive. In adults, the syndrome of hematogenous osteomyelitis is usually less acute, often involving the lumbar vertebrae. The individual will begin to develop low-grade fever, night sweats, and back pain that gradually becomes localized to an area of point tenderness. In such cases, *S. aureus* may be grown from the blood, but more commonly the organism is isolated from an aspirate of the bone or intervertebral space obtained by an orthopedic surgical consultant.

Staphylococcal septic arthritis usually involves a joint afflicted by pre-existing chronic arthritis (such as rheumatoid arthritis or osteoarthritis). Again, an episode of bacteremia causes seeding to a previously inflamed joint. The only indication in some patients is the development of increasing symptoms in one joint, usually accompanied by fever. Joint aspiration reveals a purulent effusion; Gram's stains may be negative, but the organism can usually be cultured. *S. epidermidis* increasingly is being described as a cause of chronic osteomyelitis, especially in debilitated patients such as those on hemodialysis or with underlying neoplastic diseases.

The diagnosis of staphylococcal bone and joint infections depends on recovering the organism from an aspirate of the involved site; every effort should be made, with the assistance of orthopedic surgeons, to aspirate or biopsy the involved area *before* antibiotics are started. Newer techniques permit core biopsies to be obtained from deep tissues and may in future permit more frequent definitive bacteriologic diagnosis of low-grade, chronic bone and joint infections. The diagnosis becomes especially difficult if patients have been treated with antibiotics before appropriate culture material has been obtained. In such cases a rising or significantly elevated teichoic acid antibody titer may assist in diagnosing deep infections due to *S. aureus* (see later section on The Teichoic Acid Antibody Assay).

Treatment of osteomyelitis in adults must be prolonged. While it is becoming customary to treat children with a brief course of parenteral antibiotics, adults on oral antibiotics tend to relapse if a prolonged parenteral course of antibiotics is not administered. Four weeks of parenteral therapy is the minimum acceptable course, and most clinicians prefer to treat for six weeks. An oral antistaphylococcal agent (for example, dicloxacillin 2 grams daily) should be continued for several weeks following discharge. Gradual reduction of the dose of oral antibiotic over a three- to six-month period may leave the patient symptom-free for an extended period of time. Some clinicians treat isolated septic arthritis for only two weeks. However, it is extremely difficult to differentiate septic arthritis *without* bone involvement from that with osteomyelitis. Therefore, a four-week course of therapy with appropriate parenteral antibiotics is recommended. Staphylococcal osteomyelitis tends to relapse even after years of quiescence, and one can never be sure of complete eradication of the disease. Once a relapse has occurred, chronic recurrence will be the rule. In such situations carefully planned surgical debridement and drainage under the cover of a prolonged parenteral and oral course of antibiotics may result in ex-tended quiescence or even apparent cure. Some of the newer beta-lactam antibiotics have favorable pharmacokinetics, permitting once-daily parenteral therapy to be administered long term to outpatients. The most widely used new antibiotic is ceftriaxone.

Staphylococcal Pneumonia and Empyema. Although most cases of *S. aureus* pneumonia follow acute viral infections of the lower respiratory tract (especially influenza), the disease occasionally occurs de novo in elderly and debilitated individuals. *S. aureus* pneumonia is most often acquired in the hospital. Primary staphylococcal pneumonia is most common in children and usually evolves radiologically from patchy pulmonary infiltrates into harder nodules and then pneumatoceles. Rapid development of pleural effusions and empyema often accompanied by pneumothorax may occur. Staphylococcal bronchitis and recurrent pneumonias are also seen in children and young adults with cystic fibrosis, and a young adult suffering from recurrent bronchitis from which *S. aureus* and/or *Pseudomonas aeruginosa* (usually with mucoid colonial morphology) are isolated should have a sweat test evaluation.

Adult patients with influenza have an increased incidence of *S. aureus* pneumonia. The patient is usually recovering from typical symptoms of influenza when the rapid onset of fever, chills, and chest pain supervenes. Gram's stain of the sputum in such cases reveals large clumps of gram-positive cocci. Therapy must be intense with appropriate antibiotics. Nonetheless, such patients often do poorly and frequently develop secondary infections with gram-negative organisms, chronic respiratory failure, and progressive debility. Mortality rates remain high. Even in young people, morbidity is substantial, related to serious, rapidly progressive pulmonary disease often with empyema as well as the sequelae of the accompanying bacteremia.

In particular, pleural effusions accompanying *S. aureus* pneumonia require early drainage to prevent empyema formation. If thorough drainage cannot be accomplished by needle aspiration, a chest tube must be inserted. Every effort should be made to avoid the debilitating, prolonged sequelae that result from an extensive, multiloculated *S. aureus* infection of the pleural space.

Staphylococcal Meningitis, Cerebritis, and Brain Abscess. Meningitis due to *S. aureus* most commonly develops as a complication of a central nervous system diagnostic or neurosurgical procedure. Occasionally, however, meningitis may develop during an episode of bacteremia from a peripheral site. Many patients with staphylococcal bacteremia, with or without endocarditis, develop transient but sometimes focal central nervous system symptoms. On lumbar puncture, such patients commonly have a PMN pleocytosis with elevated protein but a normal to low normal glucose concentration and a *negative* Gram's stain. These individuals probably have begun to develop multiple perimeningeal foci or areas of cerebritis (or both) and not yet frank meningitis. Almost certainly, if left untreated such patients would develop frank brain abscesses or fulminant staphylococcal meningitis. On occasion, such a patient may also exhibit purpura, disseminated intravascular coagulation, and shock in which the differentiation from *meningococcal meningitis* (see Ch. 273) is difficult. Treatment of such patients is particularly difficult, for the initial inclination is to use penicillin, an inappropriate antibiotic choice. Thus, for any patient whose Gram's stain of the spinal fluid does not reveal identifiable organisms (such as meningococci or pneumococci), a beta-lactamase–resistant antibiotic must be included in the initial antibiotic coverage.

Brain abscesses in general are usually caused by anaerobes, but not infrequently *S. aureus* is found to accompany them. Therefore, antistaphylococcal drugs should be included with antianaerobic antibiotics in the initial coverage of such individuals. For example, nafcillin plus chloramphenicol is a combination frequently used for the patient who has a brain abscess with the source and causative organisms not yet defined. Surgical drainage is required only if the abscess is large and encapsulated.

Therapy of staphylococcal meningitis and cerebritis is usually that of the underlying syndrome (for example, endocarditis). However, even in the rare patient with an uncomplicated case of pure meningitis, therapy should be prolonged, at least four weeks parenterally, in contrast to the customary 10 to 14 days of therapy for patients with uncomplicated meningitis caused by *S. pneumoniae* or *N. meningitides*.

Staphylococcus epidermidis may cause meningeal signs and symptoms, almost always in a patient with a central nervous system shunt in place. In such instances, the infection has originated in the shunt, and the organism has proliferated and seeded back into the spinal fluid. In many such cases, the individual known to have a shunt in place simply has fever with few if any central nervous system signs. Only an aspirate of the shunt itself will reveal the organism. Therapy may result in quiescence of symptoms, but removal of the infected shunt is almost always required before cure can be accomplished.

Staphylococcal Urinary Tract Infections. Here the species spectrum changes, and coagulase-negative staphylococci become the more common infecting organisms. *S. epidermidis* may occasionally cause urinary tract infections, especially in elderly hospitalized men with obstructive urinary tract pathology or indwelling Foley catheters.

Staphylococcus saprophyticus accounts for between 5 and 10 per cent of urinary tract infections in otherwise healthy young women. Presumably the organism colonizes the genitalia and for reasons not yet ascertained may ascend the urethra to involve the bladder and cause symptomatic cystitis. *S. saprophyticus* is easily treated, being sensitive to essentially all commonly used antibiotics, including penicillin, ampicillin, sulfonamides, and cephalosporins.

S. aureus may involve the urinary tract by either of two mechanisms: first, the organism may seed to the renal cortex during an episode of staphylococcal bacteremia; second, usually in patients with lower urinary tract pathology or indwelling Foley catheters, the organism may ascend to cause a primary lower urinary tract infection. Approximately 10 per cent of patients with staphylococcal bacteremia eventually excrete the organism in the urine; other studies have found that about 25 per cent of patients with a defined urinary tract infection caused by *S. aureus* had had a preceding bacteremic episode. Thus, small cortical abscesses must occur frequently during bacteremia and ultimately rupture in some patients into the tubules and the urine. Most such patients respond promptly to therapy for the underlying disease, and renal carbuncles are now rare.

Conversely, about 5 per cent of patients with a primary staphylococcal urinary tract infection may develop secondary bacteremia. In some patients, the renal infection may seed to the perinephric and retroperitoneal structures, with resultant chronic infection and fibrosis. Frank perinephric abscess is a complication associated with high morbidity and mortality. This condition occurs most frequently in patients with chronic underlying renal diseases who are also often diabetic. Aggressive drainage along with prolonged antibiotic therapy is required for cure.

Staphylococcal Endocarditis. This condition follows staphylococcal bacteremia during which a nidus of infection becomes established on one or more heart valves. Endocarditis consists of two clinical syndromes (see Ch. 270): the first is "subacute" bacterial endocarditis, and the second is "acute" bacterial endocarditis.

SUBACUTE BACTERIAL ENDOCARDITIS. The patient presents with a history of days to weeks of low-grade fever with or without chills, myalgias, night sweats, and weight loss. The word subacute refers to the clinical manifestations: the clinical course is one of a chronic, febrile illness. The patient almost always has a history of pre-existing organic valvular heart disease, and the species of *Staphylococcus* involved is usually *S. epidermidis*. *S. epidermidis* accounts for approximately 5 per cent of all cases of subacute endocarditis, the vast majority being caused by streptococcal species. *S. epidermidis* is the most common cause, however, of endocarditis occurring in association with prosthetic heart valves (see Ch. 270). The organism, being a contaminant from the patient's or surgeon's skin flora, is inoculated at the time of the surgical valve replacement. Most such infections occur within the initial two months after surgery. In such instances, the outlook for therapy with antibiotics alone is poor, and reoperation with removal of the infected valve or valve ring is often required. More than half of such patients die.

ACUTE BACTERIAL ENDOCARDITIS. The word acute refers to the clinical presentation of the patient who experiences the rapid onset of fever, chills, and myalgias, often with back pain or some gastrointestinal symptoms. The fever is often quite high (103 to 105° F), and the individual at first has the feeling of developing a very bad case of the flu. In the majority of cases, the individual has not had a history of pre-existing valvular heart disease, although it is assumed that many of these individuals have had asymptomatic organic valvular lesions (such as a fenestrated or bicuspid aortic valve, mitral valve prolapse, and so forth). Frequently, therapy for such individuals, who previously had been well, is delayed because the patient and the physician do not realize the gravity of the situation.

S. aureus is almost always the cause of the syndrome of acute endocarditis. At the time of presentation, the patient may not have an obvious heart murmur or show evidence of embolic phenomenon. Thus, the differentiation between primary staphylococcal bacteremia, which may remain uncomplicated, and acute staphylococcal bacterial endocarditis is clinically difficult. The physician must closely follow every patient whose blood samples grow *S. aureus* and must examine carefully each day for the presence of a new murmur, the signs of embolic phenomena, or the observable development of vegetation(s) by echocardiography. Valve destruction, especially of the aortic valve, may progress quite rapidly, and surgery may be necessary even within the first few days of presentation.

S. aureus endocarditis in the drug addict is almost always on one of the right-sided heart valves, usually the tricuspid valve. Therefore, pleuritic chest pain and pulmonary infiltrates are common occurrences due to embolization. In drug-abusing patients who have surreptitiously taken antibiotics, the syndrome may be of a much lower grade and may mimic that of subacute bacterial endocarditis.

The treatment of bacterial endocarditis must be prolonged (see Ch. 270). Four weeks of parenteral therapy is the minimum for staphylococcal endocarditis, although some authors have reported that two weeks may suffice for the drug addict, usually a young, otherwise healthy individual with right-sided endocarditis. All staphylococcal infections should be treated with a "cidal" antibiotic, and serum bactericidal levels must be monitored to guide effective therapy. For infections caused by beta-lactam antibiotic-resistant staphylococci, whether *aureus* or *epidermidis* species, a cephalosporin is not adequate therapy (see later discussion of treatment), although data may indicate sensitivity to the cephalosporins in vitro. As noted earlier, patients with prosthetic valve endocarditis often require surgery to eradicate the infection. Even those patients with prosthetic valve infections who respond to antibiotics alone probably should be treated with a prolonged course of an appropriate oral antistaphylococcal drug following the six-week course of parenteral therapy in the hospital.

The prognosis for patients with staphylococcal endocarditis is guarded. Patients with prosthetic valve endocarditis have about a 50 per cent mortality rate. Patients with acute bacterial endocarditis caused by *S. aureus* will do well if they are young and otherwise healthy and especially if the vegetations are on the right-sided valves. The older the patient with left-sided valvular involvement, the higher the mortality (approaching 60 to 80 per cent). Pre-existing symptomatic heart disease is a particularly ominous prognostic sign. The patients who have the subacute syndrome due to *S. epidermidis* not on prosthetic valves, in which the organism is susceptible to the usual antibiotics, usually do quite well: survival rates are comparable to those of patients with streptococcal endocarditis (in the range of 80 to 90 per cent).

Staphylococcal Bacteremia. Sustained bacteremia due to *S. epidermidis* is uncommon. Although blood cultures frequently yield the organism, 80 to 90 per cent of the time it is a contaminant. The occasional case of true, sustained *S. epidermidis* bacteremia is usually caused by infection of an intravascular line or a prosthetic valve. The commonest species causing true bacteremia, especially in the hospital, is *S. aureus*.

There are two varieties of *S. aureus* bacteremia: primary and secondary. Primary bacteremia exists when a patient presenting with fever and chills grows *S. aureus* out of multiple blood cultures but does *not* have an identifiable primary focus of infection. In this situation, the patient may have unrecognized endocarditis and should be treated accordingly. Secondary bacteremia is that associated with an obvious, peripheral focus of infection, for example, an intravascular line. Many such patients have a benign clinical course after line removal and a brief course of antibiotic treatment. The problem is to select from the overall group of such patients those who have not developed metastatic septic complications. Patients without metastatic sequelae require only a short (14-day) course of therapy. The typical patient who develops *S. aureus* bacteremia has usually been hospitalized for some other medical problem and has had a neglected peripheral or central venous or arterial access line in place. The patient suddenly develops fever and chills with or without signs of local infection at the site of the line. Other common sources are hemodialysis access shunts, postsurgical or traumatic wounds, and decubitus ulcers. The diagnosis of staphylococcal bacteremia is made when *S. aureus* grows from several blood cultures obtained before an empiric course of antibiotics is begun. Some patients already will have an obvious metastatic complication of the bacteremic episode when first examined.

The complications of an episode of *S. aureus* bacteremia are of two varieties: the first type is nonsuppurative, involving patients who develop the septic shock syndrome, including, in some, disseminated intravascular coagulation; the second type is suppurative, involving the metastatic spread of the organism via the bloodstream to heart valves or other organs. The development of endocarditis in this setting is distinctly uncommon; most suppurative spread occurs to bones, joints, and kidneys, occasionally to other deep viscera, and rarely to the meninges. Following the episode of bacteremia, the patient is placed first on broad, empiric and later on specific antistaphylococcal antibiotic therapy. Throughout this period, the patient must be examined carefully each day for metastatic suppurative sites. Laboratory evaluation may also be helpful, yielding pyuria and the organism from the urine, abnormalities of liver function, and other data. Vegetations may become demonstrable by echocardiography. Radionuclide scans may reveal infectious foci within bones, joints, or soft tissues.

Those patients who develop a clinically evident metastatic focus are treated as dictated by the type of complication that has evolved. Approximately 20 per cent of previously healthy persons who acquire *S. aureus* bacteremia develop some type of complication. In the absence of clinical findings after two weeks of observation, some experts now recommend discontinuation of antibiotics. At that point the results of a teichoic acid antibody (TA-AB) analysis reassure the clinician that no metastatic seeding had occurred. While most positive TA-AB titers will be from patients who already have developed obvious metastatic sequelae, a small subgroup of clinically

well patients will also develop a positive TA-AB test, probably representing response to subclinical suppuration. Administration of an oral antistaphylococcal drug (dicloxacillin) should be continued for several weeks if there is any doubt about the possibility of residual metastatic abscesses.

If the following criteria are present, such patients qualify for a short course (14 days) of antibiotic therapy following an episode of *S. aureus* bacteremia:

1. Host defenses are normal.
2. The patient should have no seedable sites (pre-existing valvular heart lesions, implanted prostheses, chronic arthritis).
3. The primary focus of infection should be obvious and easily managed.
4. There should be a prompt, complete response to the initial course of antimicrobial therapy.
5. The *S. aureus* recovered should be fully sensitive to the antibiotics initially chosen.
6. No clinical evidence of a metastatic, suppurative complication should be found.
7. No rise in the titer of teichoic acid antibodies should occur over a 14-day period of observation.

Septic Shock Syndromes Due to Staphylococci. Staphylococci can produce shock by five mechanisms:

1. The local infection can generate a massive inflammatory reaction resulting in sufficient "third spacing" (i.e., fluid accumulation into the area of infection) to lead to hypovolemic shock.
2. Enterotoxin-producing *S. aureus* occasionally causes diarrhea severe enough to cause hypovolemia and shock.
3. Cardiogenic shock can be produced by staphylococci by causing either valve malfunction (usually aortic), multiple myocardial abscesses, or purulent pericarditis.
4. Endotoxic-like shock can be produced via intravascular complement activation (see Ch. 259).
5. Toxigenic shock—the toxic shock syndrome—can produce shock, probably by direct capillary endothelial and end-organ damage.

Massive local infection due to staphylococci is uncommon, and such infections usually involve several organisms, usually anaerobes coinfecting with *S. aureus*. *S. epidermidis* may be a part of the flora in these infections but is probably not pathogenic. Specifically, patients with one of the gangrene syndromes (for example, necrotizing fasciitis or synergistic gangrene) may develop shock not caused by bacteremia but by fluid accumulation in the infected area. Such individuals require massive fluid and albumin replacement, extensive local debridement, and broad antibiotic coverage.

Diarrhea, nausea, and vomiting may be so severe in some patients with staphylococcal food poisoning that shock may develop from hypovolemia secondary to gastrointestinal fluid loss. Hospitalization with fluid replacement may be required and will usually suffice because the disease is self-limiting.

Cardiogenic shock is self-explanatory (see Ch. 44).

During acute sepsis *S. aureus* may produce shock that mimics that produced by endotoxin during gram-negative organism septicemia (see Ch. 259). Briefly, the primary event in endotoxic shock is the following: on entering the bloodstream, endotoxin activates a sequence of endocrine and inflammatory events leading first to vasodilation and subsequently to a primarily complement- and PMN-mediated capillary leak syndrome resulting in full-blown septic shock. The coagulation and kinin systems also become activated, and such patients may suffer frank DIC. The presence or absence of a capsule seems to be a major factor determining whether or not a particular strain of *S. aureus* in the bloodstream will cause an endotoxic shock–like syndrome. Encapsulated organisms are virulent in tissues and are *more* likely to reach the bloodstream in the course of a peripheral infection. However, once there they are *less* likely to produce the septic shock syndrome. Unencapsulated strains activate complement readily in tissues and therefore are *more* likely to be contained and are least likely to reach the bloodstream and to cause bacteremia. Yet, these are the organisms that can cause shock when directly inoculated into the bloodstream, as by a parenteral drug user or when having colonized an intravascular line.

For a discussion of the toxigenic shock caused by *S. aureus*, refer to the earlier section on the toxic shock syndrome.

Miscellaneous Staphylococcal Infections. This section focuses on several relatively unusual infections that require special diagnostic and therapeutic considerations.

STAPHYLOCOCCAL PYOMYOSITIS. This malady is primarily a tropical disease, rare enough to be reportable in the United States. The patient develops pain, warmth, and swelling over a muscle region, usually of the lower extremities and buttocks. The overlying skin may appear quite normal or may look like a mild cellulitis; however, when drainage is attempted, the surgeon discovers that the infection extends into muscle, often with extensive destruction. In the tropics, the disease afflicts malnourished individuals.

S. AUREUS EPIDURAL ABSCESS. This infection is often related to the presence of vertebral osteomyelitis wherein periosseus inflammation extends into the epidural space. The inflammation causes localized tenderness over the spine at point of infection followed by weakness and progressive neurologic signs of paraplegia. Effective therapy depends on early diagnosis and *prompt* surgical intervention and drainage.

DIAGNOSIS. Knowledgeable interpretation of the Gram's stain of an adequately obtained specimen will usually suggest the presence of staphylococci. Culture of such a specimen almost always will yield the responsible staphylococcus, and confirmation is provided by positive blood cultures. Some judgment is required in deciding whether *S. epidermidis* in blood cultures is a contaminant or a true infection. The presence of the organism *in more than two* consecutive blood cultures and associated with proper clinical circumstances (the presence of an indwelling intravascular catheter or a prosthetic device) strongly suggests true bacteremia. The vast majority (80 to 85 per cent) of *S. epidermidis* isolated from blood culture bottles are single organisms, usually in only one of the two bottles in a set, and are contaminants. While *S. aureus* may on occasion contaminate blood cultures, the clinician must determine the significance of the isolation of *S. aureus* from the blood under any condition. In most cases multiple blood cultures will be positive, and there is no question about the diagnosis of the true bacteremic state. If there is any doubt as to the origin of *S. aureus* either in blood, urine, or other fluid specimens, appropriate therapy should be continued.

The Teichoic Acid Antibody (TA-AB) Assay. This assay measures the presence (and titer) or absence of antibodies to staphylococcal cell wall teichoic acids. It is of no use in diagnosing infections with *S. epidermidis* because it only identifies antibodies to the ribitol teichoic acid moiety in the wall of *S. aureus*. Approximately 90 per cent of patients with *S. aureus* endocarditis develop a significant titer of teichoic acid antibodies. The test is fairly sensitive but only moderately specific for other types of serious, deep-seated *S. aureus* infections. The major role of the TA-AB assay is not primarily to diagnose *S. aureus* infections, most of which are diagnosed on clinical grounds, but to assist the clinician in deciding how long to treat bacteremic patients. Patients with *S. aureus* bacteremia who develop disseminated or metastatic abscesses will usually develop an increase in the titer of TA-AB acid antibodies as opposed to those with benign, self-limited bacteremias. The predictive value of a negative assay in someone who has experienced an episode of *S. aureus* bacteremia is high; therefore, the test is useful in *ruling out* metastatic infections in such patients. Other situations in which the teichoic acid antibody may be of some use in clinical decision making are the following:

1. For patients with endocarditis and negative blood cultures, usually because of prior antibiotic therapy (in a drug addict). A rise in TA-AB titers to a positive level confirms the diagnosis.

2. For deep tissue infections thought likely to be due to *S. aureus* but inaccessible to culturing (osteomyelitis or visceral abscesses). Again, a rising TA-AB titer is confirmatory, but a negative result does *not* rule out the involvement of *S. aureus*.

3. To determine the response to therapy of patients with endocarditis. Patients responding to therapy will have a prompt (two- to four-weeks) decrease in the titer of antibodies. A titer that remains elevated suggests an undrained focus of residual infection.

4. To detect relapse. Relapse is associated with a rapidly rising antibody titer; thus, sequential titers may help the clinician analyze febrile episodes occurring late in the course of treatment of an episode of endocarditis.

TREATMENT. Effective therapy of staphylococcal infections depends on early, effective debridement and drainage of the primary focus of infection along with the selection of antibiotics to which the organisms are susceptible. At present, more than 90 per cent of all organisms, whether nosocomial or community-acquired, are resistant to penicillin. Therefore, no patient suspected of having an infection with *S. aureus* should be started on a penicillinase-susceptible penicillin. Most staphylococci are still susceptible to nafcillin and oxacillin; methicillin is an antiquated drug, more toxic than either of the aforementioned parenteral alternatives. Usual doses of nafcillin and oxacillin are in the range of 6 to 12 grams daily, and patients with endocarditis should receive between 9 and 12 grams daily. In the penicillin-allergic individual, the cephalosporins can be used in the absence of a history of an anaphylactic type of penicillin hypersenstivity; however, the most effective alternative continues to be vancomycin. Vancomycin is used in a dose of 2 to 4 grams per day parenterally and should be equal to the penicillins and cephalosporins in terms of therapeutic outcome.

Beta-Lactam Antibiotic-Resistant Staphylococci (BLARS). These organisms are usually referred to as "methicillin-resistant staphylococci." However, methicillin is simply the drug used to determine resistance of these organisms and many methicillin-resistant organisms remain sensitive to the cephalosporins in vitro. However, the clinical responses to the cephalosporins of cephalosporin-sensitive but methicillin-resistant organisms have not been good. Thus, when any species of staphylococcus has been identified as being methicillin-resistant (or, therefore, nafcillin- or oxacillin-resistant) it should be considered resistant to *all* beta-lactam antibiotics regardless of contrary data in vitro. The drug of choice in the treatment of BLARS is vancomycin. Alternative drugs include rifampin and trimethoprim/sulfamethoxazole (TMS). Some BLARS remain sensitive to the aminogloycosides, and aminogloycosides may provide a synergistic effect with whatever other antibiotic is used. Newer antibiotics that will be very effective against BLARS are teichoplanin* and the quinolones. A new beta-lactam-like antibiotic, imipenem (a carbapenem), should probably not be used against BLARS, despite sensitivity in vitro. These recommendations hold true both for *S. aureus* and *S. epidermidis*.

Treatment of Chronic Carriers. Certain individuals may suffer recurrent staphylococcal infections of the skin (furunculosis), and eradication of the nasal carrier state may be required to terminate the series of infections. Nasal carriage termination may be difficult by local means. Traditionally, individuals so afflicted have been advised to observe meticulous personal hygienic measures such as frequent bathing or showering, using pHisoHex or other bactericidal soap preparations, and the application of an antibacterial ointment such as bacitracin to the anterior nares. While such a treatment

---

*Investigational drug.

program will clear a portion of chronic carriers, many will relapse and develop recurrent crops of boils. The drug most helpful in this situation is rifampin, known to be excreted in bactericidal concentrations in external secretions. Rifampin should always be used with another oral antistaphylococcal drug that, even though present in low concentrations, will delay the emergence of rifampin resistance. Thus, a five-day course of rifampin* (600 mg twice daily) plus, for example, dicloxacillin (125 mg four times a day) or in the penicillin-allergic patient cephalexin or TMS is very effective in eliminating nasal carriage of S. aureus and the associated dermal infections. A percentage of individuals will reacquire the organism and the course of therapy may have to be repeated; the physician should be sure to ascertain that the carried organism is still sensitive to rifampin. As discussed earlier, five days of rifampin treatment administered every three months to colonized hemodialysis patients significantly reduced the incidence of subsequent infections with S. aureus.

Bacterial Interference. Bacterial interference is the process of recolonizing an individual with an organism in order to displace a more pathogenic microbe. Initially, investigators found that patients heavily colonized with an aggressive strain of S. aureus that was associated with recurrent infections (boils, omphalitis, or conjunctivitis) could be helped by being recolonized with a nonpathogenic strain (designated strain 502A) of the organism. Reports in the 1960's and 1970's attested to the efficacy of bacterial interference. However, from time to time, there were reports of a serious infection caused by the 502A strain of S. aureus. The use of bacterial interference to treat recurrent infections due to a carried strain of S. aureus therefore has declined. The potential usefulness of this process should be kept in mind as one considers therapeutic approaches to patients with recurrent furunculosis recalcitrant to repeated courses of therapy.

PREVENTION. Prevention of nosocomial staphylococcal infections depends on breaking the chain of transmission between a carrier and a susceptible noncarrier. Transmission

from person to person is interrupted by thorough handwashing before and after examination of each patient. Certain other hospital infection control recommendations and procedures apply in particular to staphylococcal infections. For example, hospitals are required to have specific recommendations about the placement and maintenance of intravascular catheters; such instructions should be followed *meticulously.* Staphylococci are among the leading causes of infection of indwelling intravascular catheters, and proper catheter maintenance substantially reduces the incidence of nosocomial infections with these organisms.

While in theory vaccines containing capsular polysaccharides might enhance host defenses against the encapsulated strains of staphylococci, vaccines developed in the past were not shown to be of major clinical benefit. It is probable that some acquired immunity does develop against staphylococci, since the incidence of S. aureus infections decreases with increasing age. However, firm evidence is lacking that enhancement of humoral or cellular immunity against staphylococci significantly assists the host in its struggle with the organism.

Aldridge KE: Methicillin-resistant *Staphylococcus aureus*: Clinical and laboratory features. Infect Control 6:461–465, 1985. *Describes all aspects of infections with beta-lactam antibiotic resistant staphylococci.*

Chambers HF, Korzeniowski OM, Sande MA: *Staphylococcus aureus* endocarditis. Clinical manifestations in addicts and nonaddicts. Medicine 62:170–177, 1983. *Data from a prospective, multicenter study will describe and contrast the clinical presentation of the syndromes in addicts and nonaddicts.*

Esperson F, Frimodt-Møller N: *Staphylococcus aureus* endocarditis: A review of 119 cases. Arch Intern Med 146:1118–1121, 1986. *Excellent review of the syndrome of acute bacterial endocarditis with emphasis on community-acquired cases.*

Kaplan MH, Tenenbaum MJ: *Staphylococcus aureus*: Cellular biology and clinical application. Am J Med 72:248–257, 1982. *Reviews the clinically relevant molecular biologic aspects of* S. aureus.

Musher DM, McKenzie SO: Infections due to *Staphylococcus aureus*. Medicine 56:383-409, 1977. *A nice review of most clinical aspects of* S. aureus *infections.*

Sheagren JN: *Staphylococcus aureus*—the persistent pathogen. N Engl J Med 310:1368-1372, 1437-1442, 1984. *A complete review of all aspects of infections with* S. aureus.

Yu VL, Goetz A, Wagener M, et al.: *Staphylococcus aureus* nasal carriage and infection in patients on hemodialysis. Efficacy of antibiotic prophylaxis. N Engl J Med 315:91–96, 1986. *The incidence of infection in hemodialysis patients can be decreased by treating the nasal carrier state.*

---

*This use of rifampin is not listed in the manufacturer's directive.

Bacterial Meningitis

Morton N. Swartz

272 BACTERIAL MENINGITIS

Meningitis is an inflammation of the arachnoid, the pia mater, and the intervening cerebrospinal fluid. The inflammatory process extends throughout the subarachnoid space about the brain and spinal cord and regularly involves the ventricles. Pyogenic meningitis, considered in this chapter, is usually an acute infection with bacteria that evoke a polymorphonuclear response in the cerebrospinal fluid (CSF). One of its major forms, that caused by meningococci, is considered in Ch. 273; less acute forms of bacterial meningitis, characterized by a mononuclear cell response in the CSF, are discussed in Ch. 302 and 467.

ETIOLOGY AND INCIDENCE. Approximately 20,000 to 25,000 cases of bacterial meningitis occur annually in the United States. If all cases are included regardless of the age of patients, data from the Centers for Disease Control indicate that *Hemophilus influenzae* type b is the most frequent bacterial cause (46 per cent), followed by *Neisseria meningitidis* (27 per cent) and *Streptococcus pneumoniae* (11 per cent). About 70 per

cent of all cases occur in children under 5 years of age. The relative frequencies with which the different bacterial species cause meningitis are age related (Table 272–1). In the newborn, gram-negative bacilli (most frequently E. coli, but also other enteric bacilli and Pseudomonas) and group B streptococci are the principal causes. In the past 20 years the group B

TABLE 272–1. BACTERIAL CAUSES OF MENINGITIS

	Neonates (≤ 1 month) (%)	Children (1 month–15 years) (%)	Adults (> 15 years) (%)
S. pneumoniae	0–5	10–20	30–50
N. meningitidis	0–1	25–40	10–35
H. influenzae	0–3	40–60	1–3
Streptococci	20–40 *	2–4	5
Staphylococci	5	1–2	5–15
Listeria	2–10	1–2	5
Gram-negative bacilli	50–60 †	1–2	1–10

*Almost all isolates from neonatal meningitis are group B streptococci.
†Of all cases of neonatal meningitis, E. coli accounts for about 40 per cent and Klebsiella-Enterobacter for about 8 per cent.

Streptococcus has increased in importance in neonatal meningitis; in some hospitals it is the single most frequent etiology, surpassing *E. coli*. Beyond the first month of life and extending through childhood, *H. influenzae* and *N. meningitidis* are the most frequent causes of bacterial meningitis. In adults *S. pneumoniae* and *N. meningitidis* are responsible for most cases. Meningococcal meningitis is the only type that occurs in outbreaks; its relative frequency among the meningitides will depend on whether statistics have been gathered during an epidemic period. In about 10 per cent of patients with pyogenic meningitis the bacterial cause cannot be defined. Simultaneous mixed meningitis is rare, occurring in the setting of neurosurgical procedures, penetrating head injury, or intraventricular rupture of a cerebral abscess; the isolation of anaerobes should strongly suggest the last of these.

Important changes have occurred in the frequencies of several types of bacterial meningitis over the past 25 years. Gram-negative bacillary meningitis has almost doubled in frequency, probably reflecting more frequent and extensive neurosurgical procedures as well as other nosocomial factors. *Listeria monocytogenes* has increased eight- to tenfold as a cause of bacterial meningitis in urban general hospitals, reflecting the enlarging immunosuppressed population at particular risk. *Listeria* infections appear to be food borne (dairy products, uncooked vegetables) and involve particularly organ transplant recipients, other patients receiving corticosteroids and cytotoxic drugs, patients with liver disease, pregnant women, and neonates. Meningitis due to *Staphylococcus epidermidis*, essentially unheard of 30 years ago, now represents about 2 per cent of cases in large urban hospitals. It occurs as a complication of neurosurgical procedures and may present a particular therapeutic problem due to methicillin resistance of many of the *S. epidermidis* strains.

CLINICAL SETTINGS. The clinical setting in which meningitis develops may provide a clue to the specific bacterial cause. Meningococcal disease, including meningitis, may occur sporadically and in cyclic outbreaks; military recruits are particularly susceptible, but large urban outbreaks also occur.

Certain predisposing factors are frequently associated with the development of *pneumococcal meningitis*. Acute otitis media (± mastoiditis) occurs in about 30 per cent of patients. Pneumonia is present in about 15 per cent of patients with pneumococcal meningitis, a much higher frequency than in meningitis caused by *H. influenzae* or *N. meningitidis*. Acute pneumococcal sinusitis is occasionally the initial focus from which infection spreads to the meninges. A significant head injury (recent or remote) has occurred in about 10 per cent of patients with pneumococcal meningitis. CSF rhinorrhea (usually caused by a defect or fracture in the cribriform plate) is present in about 5 per cent of patients with pneumococcal meningitis. Meningitis occurring in young children with sickle cell anemia is most likely to be caused by *S. pneumoniae*. A variety of defects in host defenses (primary or acquired immunoglobulin deficiencies, the asplenic state) may predispose to pneumococcal disease, particularly meningitis. Alcoholism is an underlying problem in 10 to 25 per cent of adults with pneumococcal meningitis in urban hospitals.

S. aureus meningitis is seen most commonly as a complication of a neurosurgical procedure, following penetrating skull trauma, or secondary to staphylococcal bacteremia and endocarditis. Meningitis caused by *gram-negative bacilli* takes one of three forms: neonatal meningitis, meningitis following trauma or neurosurgery, or spontaneous meningitis in adults (e.g., bacteremic *Klebsiella* meningitis in a patient with diabetes mellitus). The most common causes of gram-negative bacillary meningitis in the adult are *E. coli* (about 30 per cent) and *Klebsiella-Enterobacter* (about 40 per cent). The most frequent causes of bacterial meningitis in patients with neoplastic disease are gram-negative bacilli (particularly *Pseudomonas aeruginosa* and *E. coli*), *Listeria monocytogenes*, *S. pneumoniae*,

and *S. aureus*. Meningitis caused by *group A streptococci* is uncommon, but occasionally occurs following acute otitis media.

The age-related incidence (children under five years) of *H. influenzae* type b meningitis is so striking that the occurrence of this disease in an adult should raise the question of the presence of an underlying anatomic or immunologic defect, circumventing the usual barrier interposed by serum bactericidal mechanisms.

Neonatal Meningitis. The incidence of meningitis is higher in the first month of life than in any other single month. The principal cause, *E. coli* strains containing the K1 capsular antigen, is usually acquired by the neonates from their mothers who carry the organism in their stool. In the newborn the group B *Streptococcus* can produce either an "early onset" (occurring within eight days of delivery and characterized by a fulminant illness with septicemia, severe respiratory distress, and sometimes meningitis) or a "late onset" (occurring ten days to two months after delivery and presenting a more insidious, slowly progressive illness which usually includes meningitis) infection.

The clinical signs in neonatal meningitis suggest sepsis but not necessarily central nervous system involvement: fever (in only 60 per cent), jaundice, diarrhea, lethargy, poor feeding or vomiting, respiratory distress (including apnea), seizures, irritability, bulging fontanel (in only 30 per cent), and nuchal rigidity (15 per cent). Frequently, only by examination of the CSF can the presence of meningitis be ruled in or out.

PATHOLOGY. The purulent exudate is distributed widely in the subarachnoid space, most abundant in the basal cisterns and about the cerebellum initially, but also extending into the sulci over the cerebrum. There is no direct invasion of cerebral tissue by the infecting organism or the inflammatory exudate, but the subjacent brain becomes congested and edematous. The effectiveness of the pial barrier accounts for the fact that cerebral abscess does not complicate bacterial meningitis. Indeed, when these two processes coexist, the sequence usually has been that of an initial abscess subsequently leaking its contents into the ventricular system, producing meningitis. There are two possible exceptions to the aforementioned generalization: (1) neonatal meningitis due to *Citrobacter*, where the organisms appear to invade the brain after producing a necrotizing vasculitis of small penetrating blood vessels; (2) *Listeria* rhombencephalitis, a very rare process where brain stem infection can occur simultaneously with *Listeria* meningitis (or alone). Structures adjacent to the meninges may show a variety of pathologic changes secondary to bacterial meningitis. *Cortical thrombophlebitis* results from venous stasis and adjacent meningeal inflammation. Infarction of cerebral tissue may follow. *Involvement of cortical and pial arteries* with peripheral aneurysm formation and vascular occlusion occurs occasionally in bacterial meningitis. Rarely, narrowing of the supraclinoid portion of the internal carotid artery at the base of the brain occurs as a result of arteritis and arterial spasm. In fulminating cases (particularly meningococcal meningitis), *cerebral edema* may be marked even though the CSF pleocytosis is only moderate. Rarely such patients develop temporal lobe and cerebellar herniation, resulting in compression of the midbrain and medulla. *Damage to cranial nerves* occurs in areas where dense exudate accumulates; the third and sixth cranial nerves are also vulnerable to damage by increased intracranial pressure. *Ventriculitis* probably occurs in most cases of bacterial meningitis; rarely this progresses to the accumulation of pus, *ventricular empyema*. *Hydrocephalus* can develop during meningitis from obstruction to CSF flow within the ventricular system (obstructive hydrocephalus) or extraventricularly (communicating hydrocephalus). *Subdural effusions* are sterile transudates which develop over the cerebral cortex in about 15 per cent of infants with bacterial meningitis. Rarely such effusions become infected, producing a subdural empyema.

In the past the diagnosis has been made almost exclusively in infants, in whom abnormal transillumination or increasing head size can be detected. Now, sterile or infected (showing peripheral contrast enhancement) subdural collections can be demonstrated readily by CT scan as low-density areas about the cerebrum.

PATHOGENESIS. Bacteria may reach the meninges by several routes: (1) systemic bacteremia, (2) direct ingress from the upper respiratory tract or skin through an anatomic defect (e.g., skull fracture, eroding sequestrum, meningocele), (3) passage intracranially via venules in the nasopharynx, or (4) spread from a contiguous focus of infection (infection of the paranasal sinuses, leakage of a brain abscess). Bacteremic spread to the meninges is probably the most frequent path of infection. However, not all bacteremic organisms have the same likelihood of causing meningitis. Most bacterial species causing meningitis (*H. influenzae b, N. meningitidis, S. pneumoniae, E. coli* K1, group B *Streptococcus*) have definable capsules which are antiphagocytic. Whether the capsular polysaccharide confers some special meningeal tropism, possibly through surface receptors, is not known. The primary focus initiating the bacteremia is usually in the upper respiratory tract or lung (pneumonia) but may be in the heart (endocarditis) or the gastrointestinal or urinary tracts. Once established in any part of the meninges, infection quickly extends throughout the subarachnoid space. Bacterial replication proceeds relatively unhindered, since CSF levels of complement are low early in meningeal inflammation, resulting in minimal opsonic and bactericidal activity (or none), and since surface phagocytosis of unopsonized organisms is meager in such a fluid environment. A secondary bacteremia may follow meningeal infection and itself contribute to continuing further inoculation of the cerebrospinal fluid.

CLINICAL MANIFESTATIONS. *History.* An acute onset of fever, generalized headache, vomiting, and stiff neck are common to many types of meningitis. The majority of patients with pyogenic meningitis of the three common causes have had an antecedent or accompanying upper respiratory tract infection, acute otitis (or mastoiditis), or pneumonia. Myalgias (particularly in meningococcal disease), backache, and generalized weakness are common symptoms. The illness usually progresses rapidly with development of confusion, obtundation, and loss of consciousness. Occasionally the onset may be less acute, with meningeal signs present for several days to a week.

General Physical Findings. Evidences of meningeal irritation (drowsiness and decreased mentation, stiff neck, Kernig's and Brudzinski's signs) are usually present. In certain patients the findings of meningitis may be easily overlooked; infants, obtunded patients, or elderly patients with congestive failure or pneumonia may develop meningitis without prominent meningeal signs. Their lethargy should be investigated carefully and meningeal signs should be sought; if any doubt exists, examination of the CSF is indicated.

The presence of a petechial, purpuric, or ecchymotic rash in a patient with meningeal findings almost always indicates meningococcal infection and requires prompt treatment because of the rapidity with which this infection can progress (see Ch. 273). Rarely, extensive petechial and purpuric lesions occur in meningitis caused by *S. pneumoniae* or *H. influenzae*. Very rarely skin lesions almost indistinguishable from those of meningococcal bacteremia occur in patients with acute *S. aureus* endocarditis who also have meningeal signs and a CSF pleocytosis (secondary either to staphylococcal meningitis or to embolic cerebral infarction). Usually one or two of the lesions in such a patient are those of purulent purpura; aspiration of material reveals staphylococci on Gram stain. In the summer months viral aseptic meningitis may produce meningeal signs, macular and petechial skin lesions, and a CSF pleocytosis of several hundred cells, with neutrophils predominating initially.

Neurologic Findings and Complications. Cranial nerve abnormalities, involving principally the third, fourth, sixth, or seventh nerves, occur in 10 to 20 per cent of patients with bacterial meningitis. These usually disappear shortly after recovery. Persistent sensorineural hearing loss occurs in 10 per cent of children with bacterial meningitis. In another 16 per cent a transient conductive hearing loss develops. The most likely sites of involvement in persistent sensorineural deafness appear to be the inner ear (infection possibly spreading from the subarachnoid space along the cochlear aqueduct) and the acoustic nerve. In children permanent hearing impairment is more common following meningitis due to *S. pneumoniae* than to *H. influenzae* or *N. meningitidis*.

Seizures (focal or generalized) occur in 20 to 30 per cent of patients and may result from readily reversible causes (high fever in infants; penicillin neurotoxicity when large doses are administered intravenously in the presence of renal failure) or to focal cerebral injury. Seizures can occur during the first few days, or can appear with associated focal neurologic deficits caused by cortical vein phlebitis seven to ten days after the onset of the meningitis.

Brain swelling and increased CSF pressure are associated with seizures, third nerve dysfunction, abnormal reflexes, coma, hypertension, and bradycardia. Two anatomic features of brain capillaries account for the functioning of the blood–brain barrier in controlling the concentration of substances in brain interstitium. They are the presence of tight junctions fusing brain capillary endothelial cells together and the paucity of pinocytotic vacuoles in the same cells. With bacterial meningitis, separation of intercellular junctions occurs, and pinocytotic vacuoles increase, probably accounting for the development of complicating cerebral edema.

Papilledema is rare in bacterial meningitis even with high CSF pressures. Its presence should indicate the possibility of some other associated or independent suppurative intracranial process (subdural empyema, brain abscess). Marked central hyperpnea sometimes occurs in patients with severe bacterial meningitis; CSF acidosis (principally caused by increased lactic acid levels) provides much of the respiratory stimulus.

Focal cerebral signs (hemiparesis, dysphasia, visual field defects) occur in about 15 per cent of patients with bacterial meningitis. They may develop during early meningitis secondary to occlusive vascular processes or some days later. It is important to distinguish lateralizing findings resulting from postictal changes (Todd's paralysis), which usually persist for no more than several hours.

Prompt treatment of bacterial meningitis usually results in rapid recovery of neurologic function. Persistent or late onset obtundation and coma without focal findings suggests development of brain swelling, subdural effusion (in the infant), hydrocephalus, loculated ventriculitis, cortical thrombophlebitis, or sagittal sinus thrombosis. The last three are commonly associated with fever and continuing CSF pleocytosis.

Residual neurologic damage remains in 10 to 20 per cent of patients who recover from bacterial meningitis. Developmental delay and speech defects are each observed in about 5 per cent of children. In infants surviving neonatal meningitis, significant sequelae are much more frequent (30 to 50 per cent).

LABORATORY DIAGNOSIS. *Cerebrospinal Fluid Examination.* Initial CSF pressure is usually moderately elevated (200 to 300 mm H_2O). Striking elevations (over 400 mm) occur in occasional patients with acute brain swelling complicating meningitis in the absence of an associated mass lesion.

GRAM-STAINED SMEAR. By the time of hospitalization, most patients with pyogenic meningitis have large numbers (at least 10^5 per milliliter) of bacteria in the cerebrospinal fluid. Careful examination of the Gram-stained smear of the spun sediment of CSF reveals the etiologic agent in 70 to 80 per cent of cases. In most instances when gram-positive diplococci (or short chaining cocci) are observed on stained CSF smear they are pneumococci. In certain clinical settings it is important to distinguish this organism from the relatively penicillin-resistant enterococcus, which would require the addition of an aminoglycoside to penicillin in treatment. This can be done by employing the quellung reaction or by identifying pneumococcal polysaccharide in the CSF by latex particle agglutination. Culture of the cerebrospinal fluid reveals the etiologic agent in 80 to 90 per cent of patients with bacterial meningitis.

SPECIAL IMMUNOLOGIC AND SEROLOGIC PROCEDURES. In patients in whom the etiologic agent is not identified on Gram-stained smear of the CSF, rapid diagnosis may often be made by detection of specific bacterial antigens by latex agglutination (LA) or countercurrent immunoelectrophoresis (CIE). These techniques have been employed most extensively in the rapid diagnosis of meningitis caused by *H. influenzae* type b, but have also been used in the diagnosis of meningococcal (groups A,B,C, and Y) and pneumococcal meningitis. Antigen detection by LA is more sensitive and provides results more rapidly than CIE. Since *E. coli* K1 and *N. meningitidis* serogroup B share a common antigenic determinant, immunologic cross-reactivity may cause a false-positive reaction with the group B meningococcal reagent. Since the bacterial cause can be found on Gram-stained smear in most cases of bacterial meningitis, the role of latex agglutination appears to be as an adjunct in rapid diagnosis when no organisms are observed or in providing a specific rather than a morphologic (Gram stain) diagnosis.

The limulus gelation assay for endotoxin is positive in the CSF of patients with meningitis caused by gram-negative but not by gram-positive bacteria.

CELL COUNT. The cell count in untreated meningitis usually ranges between 100 and 10,000 per cubic millimeter, with polymorphonuclear leukocytes predominating initially (80 per cent or more) and lymphocytes appearing subsequently. Extremely high cell counts (>50,000 per cubic millimeter) may occur rarely in primary bacterial meningitis, but should also raise the possibility of intraventricular rupture of a cerebral abscess. Cell counts as low as 10 to 20 may be observed early in bacterial meningitis (particularly that caused by *N. meningitidis* and *H. influenzae*). Occasionally, in granulocytopenic patients or in the elderly with overwhelming pneumococcal meningitis, the CSF may contain very few leukocytes and yet may appear grossly turbid because of the presence of myriads of organisms. Meningitis caused by several bacterial species (*M. tuberculosis, T. pallidum*) characteristically produces a lymphocytic pleocytosis. *Listeria monocytogenes* meningitis in infants may produce a primarily lymphocytic response in the CSF; in the adult there is usually a polymorphonuclear response, but rarely lymphocytes predominate.

GLUCOSE. The CSF glucose is reduced to values of 40 mg per deciliter or below (or less than 50 to 60 per cent of the simultaneous blood level) in over 50 per cent of patients with bacterial meningitis; this finding can be very valuable in distinguishing bacterial meningitis from most viral meningitides or parameningeal infections. A normal CSF glucose does not exclude the diagnosis of bacterial meningitis. The simultaneous blood glucose level should be determined, because patients with diabetes mellitus (or who are receiving intravenous glucose infusions) will have an elevated level of glucose in the CSF, and its significance can be appreciated only on comparison with the simultaneous blood level. However, it may take 90 to 120 minutes for equilibration to occur after major shifts in the level of glucose in the circulation. The hypoglycorrhachia characteristic of pyogenic meningitis appears to be due to interference with normal carrier-facilitated diffusion of glucose.

PROTEIN. The level of protein in the CSF is usually elevated above 100 mg per deciliter, and the higher values are more commonly observed in pneumococcal meningitis. Extreme elevations, 1000 mg per deciliter or more, indicate subarachnoid block secondary to the meningitis.

OTHER ABNORMALITIES IN THE CSF. Elevated levels of lactic acid occur in pyogenic meningitis. Although lactic dehydrogenase levels are higher in patients with bacterial meningitis than in those with viral infections of the central nervous system, these alterations are not of help in determining the specific etiologic agent involved. C-reactive protein is increased in about 95 per cent of patients with bacterial meningitis and is not increased in most patients with viral meningitis. However, it does not seem to provide more information than the CSF cell count, is not helpful in diagnosing bacterial meningitis in newborns, and does not provide clues to the bacterial species involved.

Other Laboratory Tests. BLOOD and RESPIRATORY TRACT CULTURES. Bacteremia is demonstrable in about 80 per cent of patients with *H. influenzae* meningitis, 50 per cent of those with pneumococcal meningitis, and 30 to 40 per cent of those with meningococcal meningitis. Cultures of the upper respiratory tract are not helpful in establishing an etiologic diagnosis. Determination of serum creatinine and electrolytes is important in view of the gravity of the illness, the occurrence of specific abnormalities secondary to the meningitis (syndrome of inappropriate secretion of antidiuretic hormone), and problems in therapy in the presence of renal dysfunction (seizures and hyperkalemia with high-dose penicillin therapy). In patients with extensive petechial and purpuric skin lesions, evaluation for coagulopathy is indicated.

RADIOLOGIC STUDIES. In view of the frequency with which pyogenic meningitis is associated with primary foci of infection in the chest, nasal sinuses, or mastoid, roentgenograms of these areas should be taken at the appropriate time after institution of antimicrobial therapy. Computerized tomography (CT) scans are not indicated in most patients with bacterial meningitis. If a mass lesion (cerebral abscess, subdural empyema) is suspected by history, clinical setting, or physical findings (papilledema), then CT scans should be performed. *Bacterial meningitis is a medical emergency requiring immediate diagnosis and rapid institution of antimicrobial therapy.* Delay in performing a diagnostic lumbar puncture in order to obtain a CT scan should be avoided except on the basis of findings indicative of a parameningeal collection or other intracranial mass lesion. Changes may be observed on CT scan during meningitis itself: enlargement of the subarachnoid spaces; contrast enhancement of the leptomeninges and the ependyma; or patchy areas of diminished density owing to associated cerebritis and necrosis. In the patient with meningitis whose clinical status deteriorates or fails to improve, the CT scan may be helpful in demonstrating suspected complications: sterile subdural collections or empyema; ventricular enlargement secondary to communicating or obstructive hydrocephalus; prominent persisting basilar meningitis; extensive areas of cerebral infarction resulting from occlusion of major cerebral arteries or veins; or marked ventricular wall enhancement, suggesting ventriculitis or ventricular empyema.

DIAGNOSIS. Diagnosis of bacterial meningitis is not difficult in a febrile patient with meningeal symptoms and signs developing in the setting of a predisposing illness. The diagnosis may be less obvious in the elderly, obtunded patient with pneumonia or the confused alcoholic patient in impending delirium tremens. Examination of the CSF should be carried out promptly whenever there is any question of meningitis.

Headache, fever, vomiting, stiff neck, and CSF pleocytosis are features of meningeal inflammation and are common to many types of meningitis (e.g., bacterial, fungal, viral) and also to some parameningeal processes. The CSF findings are most helpful in distinguishing among these processes (see Ch. 481). In the patient with meningitis whose CSF does not reveal the etiologic agent on examination of Gram-stained smear, particularly when the CSF glucose is normal and the polymorphonuclear pleocytosis is atypical, certain treatable processes which can mimic bacterial meningitis should be considered in differential diagnosis: (1) *Parameningeal infections*. The presence of infections (chronic ear or nasal accessory sinus infections, lung abscess) predisposing to brain abscess, epidural (cerebral or spinal) abscess, subdural empyema, or pyogenic venous sinus phlebitis should be sought. Neurologic findings may appear in the course of primary bacterial meningitis, but their presence should alert the physician to the need for close scrutiny for the presence of a space-occupying infectious process in the central nervous system. Neurologic symptoms or findings antedating the onset of meningeal symptoms should suggest the possibility of a parameningeal infection. The isolation of an anaerobic organism should suggest the possibility of intraventricular leakage of a cerebral abscess. (2) *Bacterial endocarditis*. Bacterial meningitis may occur during bacterial endocarditis caused by pyogenic organisms such as *S. aureus* and enterococci. In subacute bacterial endocarditis sterile embolic infarctions of the brain may occur and produce meningeal signs and a CSF pleocytosis containing several hundred cells, including polymorphonuclear leukocytes. A history of dental manipulation, fever, and anorexia antedating the meningitis should be sought; careful examination for heart murmurs and peripheral stigmata of endocarditis is indicated. (3) *"Chemical" meningitis*. The clinical and CSF findings (polymorphonuclear pleocytosis and even reduced glucose level) of bacterial meningitis may be produced by chemically induced inflammation. Acute meningitis following a diagnostic lumbar puncture or spinal anesthesia may be due to bacterial or chemical contamination of equipment or anesthetic agent. Endogenous chemical meningitis resulting from leakage into the subarachnoid space of material from an epidermoid tumor or a craniopharyngioma can produce a polymorphonuclear pleocytosis and hypoglycorrhachia. Birefringent material may be seen on polarizing microscopy of the CSF sediment.

Rarely, a patient develops meningitis characterized by subacute onset and persistent neutrophilic CSF pleocytosis lasting weeks or months without ready bacteriologic diagnosis. The etiologic agent in such cases of *chronic neutrophilic meningitis* has usually been either a fungus (*Aspergillus, Candida, Blastomyces*, etc.) or a bacterium such as *Nocardia* or *Actinomyces* species.

NON-NEUROLOGIC COMPLICATIONS. Shock. When shock occurs in pyogenic meningitis it is usually a manifestation of an accompanying intense bacteremia, as in fulminant meningococcemia, rather than of the meningitis itself. Management is guided by the principles of septic shock therapy with appropriate modifications for myocardial failure (see Ch. 273).

Coagulation Disorders. Coagulopathies are frequently associated with the intense bacteremias (usually meningococcal, occasionally pneumococcal) and hypotension which can accompany meningitis. The changes may be mild such as thrombocytopenia (with or without prolongation of prothrombin and partial thromboplastin times) or more marked with clinical evidences of disseminated intravascular coagulation (see Ch. 273).

Septic Complications. ENDOCARDITIS. Previously, 5 to 10 per cent of patients with pneumococcal meningitis, particularly those with bacteremia and pneumonia as well, developed acute endocarditis, most commonly on the aortic valve. The incidence is currently much lower, as a result of earlier treatment of the initiating infection. In such patients, febrile relapse and a new murmur may appear shortly after completion of antimicrobial therapy for meningitis.

PYOGENIC ARTHRITIS. Septic arthritis may result from the bacteremia associated with meningitis caused by *S. pneumoniae, N. meningitidis*, or *H. influenzae*.

Prolonged Fever. With appropriate antimicrobial treatment of meningitis of the three most common bacterial causes, patients become afebrile within two to five days. Sometimes fever persists beyond this or recurs after an afebrile period. In the patient with persisting headache, obtundation, and cerebral findings, inadequate drug therapy or neurologic sequelae (cortical venous thrombophlebitis, ventriculitis, subdural collections) are important considerations. Re-evaluation of the CSF, particularly Gram-stained smear and culture, is essential under these circumstances. Drug fever may be responsible in the patient who continues to show clinical improvement in all other respects. Metastatic infection (septic arthritis, purulent pericarditis, thoracic empyema, endocarditis) may be the cause of continuing or recurrent fever.

A syndrome consisting of fever, arthritis, and pericarditis three to six days after initiation of effective antimicrobial therapy of meningococcal meningitis occurs in about 10 per cent of patients (see Ch. 273).

RECURRENT MENINGITIS. Repeated episodes of bacterial meningitis generally indicate a host defect, either in local anatomy or in antibacterial and immunologic defenses (e.g., recurrent *N. meningitidis* infections in patients with congenital or acquired deficiencies of complement, particularly late-acting components). *S. pneumoniae* is by far the most frequent cause of recurrent meningitis. Eleven per cent of patients with pneumococcal meningitis have had more than one episode, whereas 0.5 per cent of patients with meningitis caused by other organisms have had recurrent attacks. A history of head trauma is much more frequent in patients with recurrent meningitis. Organisms may directly enter the subarachnoid space, through a defect in the cribriform plate (the most common site), in association with the empty sella syndrome, via a basilar skull fracture, through an erosive sequestrum of the mastoid, through congenital dermal defects along the craniospinal axis (usually evident before adult life), or as a consequence of penetrating cranial trauma or neurosurgical procedures. The anatomic defect may produce a frank CSF leak (rhinorrhea or, less commonly, otorrhea) or may entrap a vascular cuff of meninges which might subsequently serve as a direct route for organisms to reach the meninges. CSF rhinorrhea may be intermittent, and meningitis may occur months or years after head injury.

Any patient with bacterial meningitis, particularly if meningitis is recurrent, should be evaluated carefully for any congenital or post-traumatic defects. The presence of CSF rhinorrhea should be sought at admission and subsequently (rhinorrhea may clear during active meningitis only to recur when inflammation has resolved). Clinical clues suggesting the presence of a CSF fistula through the cribriform plate, pericranial air sinuses, or temporal bone include (1) salty taste in the throat, (2) positionally dependent rhinorrhea (rhinorrhea only in the lateral recumbent or prone position suggests an otic or sphenoid origin), (3) anosmia (cribriform plate leak), (4) hearing loss or full feeling in the ear, often with a finding of fluid or bubbles behind the tympanic membrane (leakage into the middle ear). Demonstration of glucose in nasal secretions with glucose oxidase "sticks" (Dextrostix) suggests the presence of CSF. Quantitative determination of glucose and chloride content of nasal secretions can definitively establish the presence of CSF rhinorrhea.

Recurrent pneumococcal meningitis may occur without apparent predisposing circumstances, and cryptic CSF leaks should be sought actively in such patients by polytomography of the frontal and mastoid regions and by radioisotope techniques. (Radioiodine-labeled albumin is introduced intrathecally, and pledgets of cotton placed in the nares are subsequently examined for the radionuclide. Radioisotopic cisternography has been used successfully recently.) Intrathecal introduction of fluorescein as a visual tracer (under ultraviolet light) can be employed similarly in detecting active leaks. Surgical closure of CSF fistulas should be carried out to prevent further episodes of meningitis. Newer extracranial approaches via the ethmoid sinuses for repair of cribriform plate or sphenoid sinus dural defects are successful and avoid the higher morbidity associated with craniotomy.

In most patients with CSF otorrhea and rhinorrhea following an acute head injury, the leak ceases in one or two weeks. *Persistent rhinorrhea for more than four to six weeks is an indication for surgical repair.* Prolonged administration of penicillin will not prevent pneumococcal meningitis and may encourage infection with more drug-resistant species.

Rarely, recurrent meningitis of nonbacterial etiology may mimic bacterial meningitis. *Mollaret's meningitis* consists of repeated febrile episodes of mild meningeal symptomatology, usually without neurologic abnormalities. Initially, large "endothelial" cells may be seen in the CSF along with polymorphonuclear leukocytes, which subsequently are replaced by lymphocytes. *Behçet's syndrome,* characterized by relapsing oral and genital ulcers and ocular lesions (hypopyon), may exhibit a variety of neurologic abnormalities, including recurrent meningitis.

PROGNOSIS. The introduction of antimicrobial agents has converted bacterial meningitis from a disease that was almost always fatal to one in which the majority of patients survive without significant neurologic residua. The mortality rate for bacterial meningitis varies with the etiologic agent and the clinical circumstances. With current antimicrobial therapy the mortality rate for *H. influenzae* meningitis is below 5 per cent and that for meningococcal meningitis is about 10 per cent. The highest mortality is with pneumococcal meningitis, in which the rate is about 25 per cent. Poor prognostic factors include advanced age, presence of other foci of infection, underlying diseases (leukemia, alcoholism), coma, and delay in instituting appropriate therapy.

TREATMENT. *Antimicrobial Agents. Antimicrobial therapy should be begun promptly in this life-threatening emergency.* Treatment should be aimed at the most likely causes based on clinical clues (age of the patient, presence of a purpuric rash, a recent neurosurgical procedure, CSF rhinorrhea). If the infecting organism is observed on examination of the Gram-stained smear of the CSF sediment, specific therapy is initiated. If the etiologic agent is not seen on smear (or not detected by latex agglutination), treatment for bacterial meningitis of unknown etiology should be carried out (see below).

With the exception of chloramphenicol, the commonly employed antimicrobial agents do not readily penetrate the normal blood-brain barrier; but the passage of penicillin and other antimicrobials is enhanced in the presence of meningeal inflammation. Antimicrobial drugs should be administered intravenously throughout the treatment period; reduction in dosage as the patient improves should be avoided, because normalization of the blood-brain barrier during recovery reduces the CSF levels of drug that are achievable. Bactericidal drugs (penicillin, ampicillin, third-generation cephalosporins) are preferred whenever possible in the treatment of meningitis caused by susceptible bacteria. In animal models of bacterial meningitis CSF levels of antibiotics at least 10 to 20 times the minimal bactericidal concentration appear to be needed for optimal therapy. Several antimicrobial drugs (first or second generation cephalosporins, clindamycin) which do not provide effective levels in the cerebrospinal fluid should not be used.

MENINGITIS OF SPECIFIC BACTERIAL CAUSE. The treatment of choice for pneumococcal meningitis in the adult is penicillin (24 million units daily in divided doses every two hours) or ampicillin (12 grams daily in divided doses every two to three hours). In the patient with a major penicillin allergy, chloramphenicol (4 to 6 grams intravenously daily in the adult) is a reasonable alternative. However, several points of caution should be made: (1) resistance to chloramphenicol has been reported from Spain in 45 per cent of pneumococcal strains, (2) the response to chloramphenicol of granulocytopenic pa-

tients may be suboptimal, and (3) recently, isolates of *S. pneumoniae* that are relatively resistant (minimum inhibitory concentration [MIC] of 0.1 to 1.0 μg per milliliter) or highly resistant (South African strains with MIC of 4 to 8 μg per milliliter) to penicillin have been identified. In the United States, relative pneumococcal resistance to penicillin occurs in 1 to 2 per cent of clinical isolates (in a few geographic areas the figures are as high as 6 to 8 per cent). (In one area of Spain 50 per cent of pneumococcal isolates have been reported to be penicillin resistant). In addition to cases of meningitis due to highly penicillin-resistant *S. pneumoniae* that occurred during the outbreak in South Africa in the late 1970s, seven cases of meningitis due to moderately penicillin-resistant strains (including two that were multiply-resistant) have been described in the United States and abroad. Thus, antimicrobial susceptibilities should be determined for all pneumococcal isolates from cerebrospinal fluid and blood. Chloramphenicol is a reasonable alternative to penicillin G in treatment of pneumococcal meningitis due to strains that are penicillin-resistant, provided they are not multiply-resistant. The multiply and highly penicillin-resistant strains in South Africa were susceptible only to vancomycin among the commonly employed antimicrobials. The third-generation cephalosporins cefotaxime and ceftriaxone have good in vitro activity against moderately penicillin-resistant *S. pneumoniae* and achieve adequate CSF levels in meningitis, but their effectiveness in meningitis due to such strains requires clinical evaluation.

The treatment of meningococcal meningitis is the same as for pneumococcal meningitis (see Ch. 273).

At present 30 per cent of isolates of *H. influenzae* b in the United States are ampicillin resistant. Thus, chloramphenicol (100 mg per kilogram intravenously daily for a child; 4 grams intravenously daily for an adult), either alone or in combination with ampicillin (300 to 400 mg per kilogram intravenously per day for a child; 12 grams intravenously per day for an adult), has been the preferred treatment until drug susceptibilities are determined. If the organism proves susceptible to ampicillin, then this drug can be used alone in treatment. In the rare instance of *H. influenzae* meningitis caused by a strain resistant to both ampicillin and chloramphenicol or occurring in a patient who cannot tolerate chloramphenicol, cefotaxime (180 mg per kilogram intravenously daily in divided doses every 4 to 6 hours for children) or ceftriaxone (loading dose of 75 mg per kilogram intravenously followed by 50 mg per kilogram every 12 hours intravenously in children; not to exceed a total of 4 grams daily) are alternatives. Although experience is not yet extensive, available results indicate ceftriaxone to be as effective as conventional chloramphenicol plus ampicillin therapy of *H. influenzae* meningitis. Thus, it may soon supplant this combination as routine primary therapy.

Adult meningitis caused by methicillin-sensitive *S. aureus* should be treated with a penicillinase-resistant penicillin (nafcillin 10 to 12 grams intravenously per day). Rifampin (600 mg orally daily), because adequate CSF levels can be achieved and because of its capacity to penetrate leukocytes and kill intracellular organisms, may be added as a second antimicrobial in difficult cases. In the penicillin-allergic patient, vancomycin (2.0 grams intravenously in divided doses every 6 hours) is the alternative of choice. Since penetration of vancomycin into the CSF is limited, adjunctive intrathecal therapy (5,000 to 10,000 units of bacitracin slowly in 10 ml of CSF in the adult; or 5 to 20 mg of vancomycin in 10 ml of 5 per cent dextrose–0.85 per cent NaCl slowly in the adult)* has been used when CSF cultures have remained positive after 48 hours of intravenous therapy alone. For adult meningitis due

---

*Intrathecal use is not mentioned in the manufacturer's package insert approved by the U.S. Food and Drug Administration. Therefore its use in these circumstances must be considered investigational.

to methicillin-resistant *S. aureus*, intravenous vancomycin (with adjunctive intrathecal bacitracin or vancomycin) is the treatment of choice. In refractory cases the addition of another drug for systemic therapy (rifampin or gentamicin) may be warranted.

Treatment of enterococcal meningitis in the adult involves the use of intravenous penicillin (24 million units daily) or ampicillin (12 grams daily), supplemented with parenterally administered gentamicin (3 to 5 mg per kilogram daily in divided doses every eight hours). In the patient who fails to respond promptly to parenteral therapy, adjunctive intrathecal therapy with gentamicin (3 to 5 mg per day) should be considered.

Cefotaxime (12 grams daily intravenously in divided doses every 4 hours in adults) is now being used extensively in the treatment of meningitis known to be due to susceptible gram-negative bacilli (*E. coli, Klebsiella, Proteus,* etc.). It should not be used in the treatment of meningitis due to less susceptible species such as *Pseudomonas aeruginosa* and *Acinetobacter*. Initial treatment (on the basis only of findings on Gram-stained smear of CSF) of adults with gram-negative bacillary meningitis involves the combination of cefotaxime (or ceftazidime) with an aminoglycoside (e.g., gentamicin 5 mg per kilogram daily intravenously in divided doses every 8 hours). Adjunctive intrathecal therapy with gentamicin (3 to 5 mg administered at intervals of 24 hours for the first few days) may be indicated as well. Following identification of the specific pathogen and determination of its drug susceptibilities, alterations in antimicrobial therapy may be indicated. If the organism is *Pseudomonas aeruginosa*, a third-generation cephalosporin with antipseudomonal activity, ceftazidime (2 grams intravenously every 6 or 8 hours in an adult), or an antipseudomonal penicillin, ticarcillin (3 grams intravenously every 4 hours in an adult), is combined with parenteral (and intrathecal, if needed) tobramycin in treatment. Although ceftazidime has been used alone successfully in a few patients, the addition of a parenteral aminoglycoside is aimed at preventing emergence of resistant organisms either in the subarachnoid space or at the initiating site of infection.

BACTERIAL MENINGITIS OF UNKNOWN ETIOLOGY. Initial treatment of meningitis when the etiologic agent cannot be identified on Gram-stained smear of cerebrospinal fluid is based on available clinical clues. *In the neonate,* a wide range of gram-positive (group B streptococci, *Listeria*) and gram-negative organisms (*E. coli, Klebsiella, H. influenzae*) may be the cause, indicating the intravenous use of combined therapy with drugs such as ampicillin with gentamicin (or amikacin), or ampicillin with cefotaxime (or ceftriaxone), until results of cultures become available. *In children,* therapy is directed at the three most frequent pathogens: *H. influenzae, S. pneumoniae,* and *N. meningitidis*. The appearance of ampicillin resistance among strains of *H. influenzae* necessitated the shift from single drug therapy (ampicillin) to a two-drug approach (ampicillin-chloramphenicol) in the treatment of meningitis of unknown cause in this age group, pending results of culture. Currently, equally effective alternatives, cefuroxime (240 mg per kilogram intravenously daily in divided doses every 6 hours) and ceftriaxone (same dosage as for *H. influenzae* meningitis), are being employed increasingly. *In adults,* therapy with ampicillin or penicillin is directed at the most common community-acquired pathogens (*S. pneumoniae* and *N. meningitidis*). However, because *H. influenzae* type b infections appear to be increasing in adults, and because of the increased incidence of gram-negative bacillary and staphylococcal meningitis in certain clinical settings, broader initial therapy may be indicated if clinical features suggest unusual organisms.

Duration of Therapy. The frequency of cerebrospinal fluid examinations depends on the clinical course, but a repeat examination should be done in 24 to 48 hours if there has not

been satisfactory improvement. Routine "end-of-treatment" CSF examination is unnecessary in most patients with the common types of community-acquired bacterial meningitis. Meningococci are rapidly eliminated from the circulation and CSF with appropriate antimicrobial therapy, which should be continued for five to seven days after the patient becomes afebrile. If the patient has responded well, a follow-up lumbar puncture is not necessary. *H. influenzae* meningitis should be treated for ten days (at least for seven days after the patient becomes afebrile). Follow-up CSF examination may be omitted in those patients who have responded with rapid clinical resolution of the meningitis. In pneumococcal meningitis antimicrobial treatment should be continued for 10 to 14 days and follow-up examination of the CSF should be done. More prolonged therapy is indicated with concomitant parameningeal infection. Treatment of gram-negative bacillary meningitis with parenteral antimicrobials is prolonged, usually for a minimum of three weeks (particularly in patients with a recent neurosurgical procedure) in order to prevent relapse. Repeated examinations of the CSF are necessary both during and at the conclusion of treatment to determine whether bacteriologic cure has been achieved.

Other Aspects of Treatment. Occasional patients with acute bacterial meningitis develop marked brain swelling (CSF pressure exceeding 450 mm H_2O), which may lead to temporal lobe or cerebellar herniation following lumbar puncture. To reduce this increased pressure, an intravenous infusion of 20 per cent mannitol solution (0.25 to 0.5 gram per kilogram) is administered over 20 to 30 minutes. Continued control of increased intracranial pressure, if needed thereafter, may be effected with mannitol, dexamethasone (10 mg intravenously, followed by 4 mg every six hours), or both. Brain swelling is about the only indication for the use of corticosteroids in the treatment of pyogenic meningitis; they should be employed only when the appropriate antimicrobial drugs are administered. Fluid restriction (1200 to 1500 ml daily in adults) is advisable during the first 24 to 48 hours to minimize brain swelling.

Patients with acute bacterial meningitis should receive constant nursing attention to ensure prompt recognition of seizures and to prevent aspiration. If seizures occur, they should be treated acutely with diazepam (Valium) administered slowly intravenously in a dose of 5 to 10 mg in the adult. Maintenance anticonvulsant therapy can be continued thereafter with intravenous phenytoin (Dilantin) until the medication can be administered orally. Sedation should be avoided because of the danger of respiratory depression and aspiration.

Surgical treatment of an accompanying pyogenic focus such as mastoiditis should be carried out when complete recovery from the meningitis has occurred, but under continuing antibiotic administration. Rarely, the mastoid infection (e.g., Bezold abscess) is so hyperacute that early drainage may be required after 48 hours or so of antibiotic therapy when the acute meningeal process will have subsided somewhat.

Berk SL, McCabe WR: Meningitis caused by gram-negative bacilli. Ann Intern Med 93:253, 1980. *Good descriptions of gram-negative bacillary meningitis occurring spontaneously and after surgery.*

Cherubin CE, Corrado ML, Nair SR, et al.: Treatment of gram-negative bacillary meningitis: Role of the new cephalosporin antibiotics. Rev Infect Dis 4:S453, 1982. *Summary of results of cefotaxime treatment of 137 patients with various types of bacterial meningitis.*

Del Rio M, Skelton S, Chrane D, et al.: Ceftriaxone versus ampicillin and chloramphenicol for treatment of bacterial meningitis in children. Lancet 1:1241, 1983. *A clinical and bacteriological study of meningitis in 78 children showing the equivalence of ceftriaxone treatment to that of the heretofore conventional regimen.*

Dodge PR, Davis H, Feigin RD, et al.: Prospective evaluation of hearing impairment as a sequela of acute bacterial meningitis. N Engl J Med 311:869, 1984. *An excellent detailed prospective study of deafness as a complication of childhood meningitis. A model study of this sort..*

Durack DT, Spanos A: End-of-treatment spinal tap in bacterial meningitis. Is it worthwhile? JAMA 248:75, 1982. *Places in perspective the role of end-of-treatment CSF examination.*

Geiseler PJ, Nelson KE, Levin S, et al.: Community-acquired purulent meningitis: A review of 1316 cases during the antibiotic era, 1954–1976. Rev Infect Dis 2:725, 1980. *Extensive experience at one of the last contagious disease hospitals in the United States is recounted. Effects of prior antibiotic therapy on culture results are particularly well studied.*

Hyslop NE Jr, Montgomery WW: Diagnosis and management of meningitis associated with cerebrospinal leaks. In Remington JS, Swartz MN (eds.): Current Clinical Topics in Infectious Diseases, 3. New York, McGraw-Hill Book Company, 1982, pp 254–285. *Most complete review of the bacteriology, anatomy, diagnostic approach, and surgical repair of CSF leaks associated with meningitis.*

Marks WA, Stutman HR, Marks MI, et al.: Cefuroxime versus ampicillin plus chloramphenicol in childhood bacterial meningitis. J Pediatr 109:123, 1986. *Results from a multicenter randomized trial involving 107 children with bacterial meningitis indicate similar clinical cure and relapse rates in those receiving ampicillin plus chloramphenicol and those receiving cefuroxime.*

New PFJ, Davis KR: The role of CT scanning in diagnosis of infections of the central nervous system. In Remington JS, Swartz MN (eds.): Current Clinical Topics in Infectious Diseases, 1. New York, McGraw-Hill Book Company, 1980, pp 1–33. *Comprehensive review of the changes on CT scan in a wide variety of CNS infections. Large number of illustrative scans with good descriptions.*

Overturf GD: Treatment of the child with bacterial meningitis. In Remington JS, Swartz MN (eds.): Current Clinical Topics in Infectious Diseases, 3. New York, McGraw-Hill Book Company, 1982, pp 218–253. *Excellent review of management of childhood meningitis.*

Sande MA, Smith AL, Root RL (eds.): Bacterial Meningitis. New York. Churchill–Livingstone, 1985. *A collection of articles reviewing current issues and recent progress in understanding bacterial meningitis. Provides valuable insights in pathogenesis and pathophysiology.*

Swartz MN, Dodge PR: Bacterial meningitis—a review of selected aspects. N Engl J Med 272:725, 779, 842, 898, 954, 1003, 1965. *Detailed account of experience at the Massachusetts General Hospital. Particularly good on clinical aspects, neurologic complications, and differential diagnosis.*

273 MENINGOCOCCAL DISEASE

DEFINITION. Meningococcal infections are caused by *Neisseria meningitidis*. The best known syndromes are *meningococcal meningitis* ("epidemic cerebrospinal meningitis") and *fulminant meningococcemia*. Infections also occur in the upper and lower respiratory tracts, joints, pericardium, eyes, and genitourinary tract.

ETIOLOGY. *N. meningitidis* is a gram-negative coccus which appears on smears of infected fluids as biscuit-shaped diplococci, located either extracellularly or within polymorphonuclear leukocytes. Colonies are best isolated on blood, "chocolate," or enriched Mueller-Hinton agar in an atmosphere of 3 to 10 per cent CO_2. Modified Thayer-Martin selective medium is useful in detection of meningococcal carriers or in initial isolation of *N. meningitidis* from areas with an extensive indigenous flora. The organism is susceptible to drying or chilling, and specimens should be inoculated and incubated promptly. Sodium polyetholesulfonate, frequently included in commercial blood culture media as an anticoagulant and to neutralize inhibitory factors in human blood, may inhibit isolation of occasional strains of *Neisseria* species.

Since other *Neisseria* species and related organisms (*Branhamella catarrhalis*), as well as morphologically similar gram-negative coccobacilli (e.g., *Moraxella*), may be isolated from clinical specimens, biochemical and immunologic methods are needed for identification. *Neisseria* species are oxidase positive. Whereas *N. gonorrhoeae* ferments only glucose (but not maltose or lactose) to acid, *N. meningitidis* ferments both glucose and maltose (but not lactose). *N. lactamica*, a species sometimes present in throat cultures, may be mistaken for the meningococcus, since it too ferments both glucose and maltose; however, it also utilizes lactose. Occasional maltose-negative strains of *N. meningitidis* have been noted; fluorescent antibody or coagglutination tests or electrophoretic analysis of hexokinase isoenzymes may be helpful in distinguishing such strains from *N. gonorrhoeae*, particularly when isolated from atypical locations.

N. meningitidis are classified by serogroup and further defined by serotype. There are 13 serogroups, including groups A, B, C, D, X, Y, Z, 29E, and W135: they differ in the structures of their capsular polysaccharides and can be identified by agglutination reactions with specific antisera. Most meningococcal disease is due to strains belonging to groups A, B, C, and Y. Twenty to 50 per cent of isolates from carriers are nongroupable (unencapsulated). Subcapsular protein antigens located in the outer bacterial membrane have been used to identify 20 serotypes among the various serogroups, providing a classification useful in epidemiologic studies. Serotype 2 (2a, 2b) strains are responsible for most cases of meningococcal disease due to group B (50 per cent) and group C (80 per cent) organisms (and also are associated with groups Y and W135), but they are rarely isolated from carriers not in direct contact with clinical cases. In contrast, other serotypes are commonly isolated, but primarily from carriers. More detailed differentiation between strains can be carried out by including lipopolysaccharide typing in addition. Group A meningococcal strains show no variation in their outer membrane proteins and are unrelated serologically to the serotypes of other groups.

Strains of *N. meningitidis* produce extracellular proteases that cleave the IgA1 heavy chain in the hinge region. Although the role of this protease in infection is unknown, its elaboration also by the other principal causes of bacterial meningitis (*H. influenzae*, *S. pneumoniae*) and the importance of IgA in mucosal immunity at the pharyngeal portal for these organisms suggests a possible role in pathogenicity.

Fresh isolates of *N. meningitidis* from the pharynx of carriers and from patients with meningococcal disease contain pili, which appear to have an important role in attachment to nonciliated columnar human nasopharyngeal cells.

Meningococci contain endotoxins, and these lipopolysaccharides may play a role in the purpura and other clinical features of meningococcemia.

INCIDENCE. *N. meningitidis* is second only to *H. influenzae* as a cause of bacterial meningitis in this country. In the period 1984 to 1986, 2,400 to 2,700 cases of meningococcal infection were reported annually in the United States.

EPIDEMIOLOGY. The natural reservoir of *N. meningitidis* is the human nasopharynx, and transmission occurs principally through airborne droplets or close contact. Infection may occur as the *asymptomatic carrier state* (the most common form), *endemic disease* (sporadic cases occurring at a relatively stable rate), *hyperendemic disease* (cyclic waves of increased incidence), or *epidemic disease* (major outbreaks involving large portions of the population or focal outbreaks involving particularly lower socioeconomic groups).

Carrier State. Nasopharyngeal carrier rates may fluctuate widely. The rate varies with age: 0.5 to 1.0 per cent in children 3 to 48 months of age, 5 per cent in those 14 to 17 years of age, and 20 to 40 per cent in young adults. In the nonepidemic setting carriage usually lasts weeks to months. The carrier rate in close family contacts of a case of meningococcal disease is increased and may reach 40 per cent. In crowded populations (e.g., military training camps) the carrier rate ranges between 20 and 60 per cent and may reach 90 per cent during epidemics. Although it has often been stated that meningococcal outbreaks occur when the rate of nasopharyngeal carriage exceeds 20 per cent in a military camp, there is in reality no clear relation between the overall carriage rate in a community and the occurrence of meningococcal disease. The strain (serotype)-specific acquisition rate appears to be a more reliable indicator of an outbreak than the group-specific carriage rate.

Spread of disease appears to be mediated by carriers rather than by direct case-to-case transmission. An adult family member generally is the one who brings *N. meningitidis* into a household, where it spreads to others and often colonizes younger children and infants last. As yet unknown host and environmental factors are of decisive importance in determining whether the organism will be confined to the nasopharynx or whether dissemination will take place.

Meningococcal Disease. The annual attack rate for meningococcal disease in the United States in recent years has been about 1.2 cases per 100,000 population. The highest incidence is in the first year of life (17.1 per 100,000), declining in the one- to four-year age group (5.2 per 100,000), and ultimately reaching the level of 0.3 per 100,000 in adults. During epidemics of meningococcal disease, overall annual attack rates of 5 to 24 cases per 100,000 are observed (as high as 370 per 100,000 in Sao Paulo, Brazil, in 1974). The peak incidence is in the winter and early spring.

During a nonepidemic period the risk of meningococcal illness for household contacts of an initial case is about 3 per 1000 (500- to 1000-fold higher than the overall endemic rate for meningococcal disease) and stems from the higher carriage rate in this setting. The secondary attack rate appears to be age related, with most cases occurring in younger children.

Major meningococcal epidemics, caused primarily by group A strains, tend to recur at 20- to 30-year intervals. More circumscribed outbreaks have taken place in interepidemic periods, as in Detroit in 1929, when about 750 cases occurred. Aside from several minor urban outbreaks, particularly among alcoholics, group A strains have only rarely been implicated in meningococcal disease in North America during the past decade. However, serious epidemics caused by group A meningococci have occurred in Finland in 1973, in Brazil in 1974, and in northern Nigeria in 1977. The outbreak in Nigeria is but one of many that have occurred about once every ten years in the "meningitis belt" in sub-Saharan Africa. In the 1948–49 epidemic, about 93,000 cases were reported, with over 14,000 deaths. Although group A meningococci had been susceptible to sulfonamides in the past, resistant strains first appeared in the epidemics in Africa in the late 1960's and subsequently in Brazil and Finland.

Although group A meningococci have been involved in the most extensive epidemics of meningococcal disease, groups B and C have been responsible for focal outbreaks and for *endemic disease* both in this country and abroad. In the United States in 1963 and 1964, outbreaks caused by group B meningococci (noteworthy for their frequent resistance to sulfonamides) occurred in military camps. By 1967 serogroup B was responsible for the majority of infections occurring in military and civilian populations. By the early 1970's serogroup C strains were those most frequently isolated, only to be supplanted by group B in the mid 1970's. Currently, serogroup B accounts for 50 to 55 per cent of cases; serogroup C, for 20 to 25 per cent; serogroup W135, for 15 per cent; serogroup Y, for 10 per cent; and serogroup A, for 1 to 2 per cent.

Just as serogrouping of meningococcal strains has been invaluable in the study of major epidemics and in the development and use of polysaccharide vaccines, serotyping can be helpful in evaluating changes in ambient strains. Between epidemics sporadic cases are caused by heterogeneous strains belonging to many serogroups and a variety of serotypes. In military recruit populations, the serogroup carried is not a valid indicator of epidemic potential. At intervals of 5 to 10 years a single serotype (e.g., serotype 2, present in most disease-related strains of groups B and C and in some strains of groups Y and W135 during this past decade) becomes preeminent, producing *hyperendemic disease*, sometimes accompanied by scattered small outbreaks.

Nosocomial transmission of infection occasionally occurs. Meningococcal meningitis has developed in several physicians who gave mouth-to-mouth resuscitation to infected patients. Group Y meningococci particularly have been implicated in meningococcal pneumonia, and such patients, if not isolated, may be responsible for nosocomial spread of infection.

Immunity. The age-specific incidence of meningococcal disease is inversely proportional to the prevalence of antimeningococcal bactericidal antibodies (against serogroups A, B, C). At birth, over 50 per cent of infants have bactericidal antibody as a result of transplacental transfer. Group B organisms present a special problem that accounts for the occurrence of group B meningococcal disease in neonates. Because the capsular polysaccharide of group B meningococci is a polymer of α 2–8–linked sialic acid and is immunologically identical to oligosaccharides of several human glycoproteins (including brain gangliosides), immunologic tolerance for this molecule exists in humans. IgM antibody can be induced but without the usual switch to IgG. As a result, maternal antibody to group B capsular antigen is entirely IgM and cannot be passed transplacentally. All infants are born lacking antibody to group B (but not to other common serogroup) capsular antigens. Because the capsular polysaccharide of *E. coli* K1 is the same, infants are born also lacking antibody to this organism, the major cause of neonatal sepsis and meningitis.

From six to 24 months of age, the prevalence of antibodies is lowest, and thereafter it increases to early adulthood, when over 70 per cent of individuals have bactericidal activity. The protective role of bactericidal antibodies against *N. meningitidis* was demonstrated during an outbreak of group C meningitis among army recruits in 1968. Eleven per cent of recruits lacked serum antibody against the outbreak-associated strain, and one quarter of these susceptibles acquired this strain during their training period. Of the susceptibles exposed, 38 per cent developed systemic meningococcal disease; in contrast, only 1 per cent of the entire trainee group developed disease.

IgA antibody to meningococcal polysaccharide may have a paradoxic effect. When a large part of an individual's antibodies to a meningococcal serogroup is of this class, serum complement-mediated immune lysis by IgM is blocked, enhancing susceptibility to meningococcal disease. This was demonstrated in several outbreaks. Sera drawn from susceptibles at the time of acute meningococcal infection lacked bactericidal activity for the infecting strain; removal of IgA restored this activity which was in the IgM class. This odd phenomenon is observed for a short time following the induction of IgA by asymptomatic carriage of *N. meningitidis* or an immunologically related organism.

Following meningococcal meningitis serum bactericidal antibody develops, and the patient is immune to clinical reinfection with the same serogroup. However, this is not the usual means of acquiring immunity. Nasopharyngeal carriage of *N. meningitidis* is an effective immunizing process, producing rises in bactericidal antibody within five to twelve days of acquisition of the organism. About 90 per cent of carriers of group B, C, or Y meningococci develop increased serum bactericidal titers, primarily to the colonizing strain but also to heterologous strains. Similarly, nasopharyngeal carriage of nongroupable meningococci, strains rarely causing human disease, can induce antibodies against various groupable pathogenic isolates.

The group-specific capsular polysaccharides of group A and group C meningococci are good immunogens and have been used in successful vaccines. The capsular polysaccharide of group B meningococci is a very poor immunogen because of its immunologic identity with oligosaccharides of several human glycoproteins, and this likely contributes to the failure to develop an effective group B vaccine.

In young children, colonization with *N. lactamica* may induce cross-reactive antibodies to *N. meningitidis* and thus contribute to natural immunity. *N. lactamica* is relatively avirulent and has only rarely been involved in systemic infections. During the first eight years of life the age-related prevalence of meningococcal carriage is between 0.5 and 2 per cent, whereas that of *N. lactamica* is considerably higher (4 to 20 per cent).

In addition to antibody, complement is an important component of serum bactericidal activity. Isolated congenital deficiency of one of the late complement components (C5, C6, C7, or C8) is rare and has been associated with recurrent or chronic (chronic meningococcemia) infections with *N. meningitidis* or *N. gonorrhoeae*. Repeated episodes of meningococcal meningitis have occurred in patients with late complement component deficiencies in the absence of enhanced susceptibility to organisms other than *N. meningitidis*. Measurement of total hemolytic complement is helpful for screening purposes in a patient with recurrent systemic *Neisseria* infections. The course of infection, whether meningitis or meningococcemia, is not unusual, and the response to antimicrobial treatment is satisfactory. Complement deficiency, either congenital (late-acting components) or due to a complement-depleting (C1, C3, C4) underlying disease (systemic lupus, multiple myeloma, C3 nephritic factor, hepatic failure) also may be an important risk factor for the occurrence of first episodes of endemic meningococcal disease: among 20 patients presenting with invasive infection 30 per cent had decreased complement function. Fulminant meningococcal disease has also occurred in several members of a family with properdin deficiency.

PATHOGENESIS AND PATHOLOGY. The factors that determine whether initial exposure to *N. meningitidis* will result in benign nasopharyngeal carriage or serious invasive infection are unclear. About one third of patients with invasive infection have had antecedent symptoms referable to the upper respiratory tract. Whether these prodromal symptoms are produced by *N. meningitidis* or a predisposing viral respiratory infection is difficult to determine, particularly since many cases of meningococcal disease occur in winter when viral respiratory infections are frequent. A simultaneous outbreak of meningococcal disease and influenza A2 infection has occurred in a closed institutional setting. The predisposing role of influenza for meningococcal lower respiratory infections may be clearer (e.g., numerous cases of meningococcal pneumonia complicating influenza during the 1918–19 pandemic).

The incubation period from initiation of nasopharyngeal infection to bloodstream dissemination is probably under 10 days. The incubation period may be quite short, judging by the fact that the interval between primary and secondary cases in the same household is often only one to four days. Also, among prospectively studied military recruits cultured within seven days preceding hospitalization for meningococcal disease, only about 20 per cent were carriers of the implicated strain. Once the organism has entered the circulation, the predominant (over 90 per cent) clinical expression is as meningitis or meningococcemia.

The pathologic findings in acute meningococcemia are observed when shock and disseminated intravascular coagulation have occurred. The skin lesions show evidence of fibrin thrombi and vasculitis in small blood vessels. *N. meningitidis* can be seen in endothelial cells and in neutrophils surrounding damaged vessels. The prominent purpura has been attributed to the enhanced capacity to elicit the dermal Shwartzman reaction of its endotoxin compared to endotoxin from enteric gram-negative bacilli. Hemorrhagic adrenal infarction is often observed in patients with fulminant meningococcemia (Waterhouse-Friderichsen syndrome). Shock in this disease is a consequence of bacteremia and not of adrenal failure, since (1) fulminant meningococcemia can occur without adrenal hemorrhage, (2) serum cortisol levels are normal or elevated, and (3) patients who have recovered have not developed Addison's disease. It has been suggested that the shock, purpura, and widespread microvascular thrombi are consequences of an endotoxin-initiated generalized Shwartzman-like reaction or endotoxin-activated disseminated intravascular coagulation. Depressed levels of complement components

are found in some patients with acute meningococcemia and may reflect complement activation by circulating endotoxin. Interstitial myocarditis is observed in about 70 per cent of cases of fatal meningococcal disease.

CLINICAL MANIFESTATIONS. Overt illness develops when the initial, often minimally symptomatic nasopharyngeal infection has progressed to bloodstream invasion. The subsequent clinical picture may be mild, or sudden in onset and fulminant, and may reflect principally the bacteremia or features referable to metastatic localization of infection. The most common clinical syndromes are acute meningococcemia, acute purulent meningitis, and a combination of the two (meningococcemia-meningitis).

Meningitis. Most cases occur in children between three months of age and adolescence. Isolated meningitis is less common than meningococcemia-meningitis. The clinical picture may be dominated by manifestations of either meningococcemia or meningitis. In the latter instance the findings are similar to those of meningitis caused by any of the common pyogens (see Ch. 272). Predisposing acute otitis media or pneumonia is unusual in contrast to *H. influenzae* or pneumococcal meningitis. The onset of meningeal symptomatology (1) may be rapid (less than 24 hours) without premonitory symptomatology, (2) may follow an upper respiratory infection of one or two weeks' duration, or (3) may evolve gradually over several days of upper respiratory or nonlocalizing symptoms. Rarely, the clinical course with fever and meningismus may be indolent and persist unchanged for a week or longer, suggesting the diagnosis of "aseptic" meningitis. In the last-named instance CSF examination during this period may reveal minimal or no increase in cell count and no organisms on Gram-stained smear, but *N. meningitidis* may be isolated, indicating early meningeal involvement. A "clear" CSF in this setting should *not* preclude careful culture. The rapid onset of delirium is seen occasionally in bacterial meningitis (more frequently meningococcal), but it also may occur with a temporal lobe abscess or encephalitis. The neurologic features and complications of meningococcal meningitis are generally the same as for other bacterial meningitides.

The course of meningococcal meningitis may differ from that of other pyogenic meningitides in the occasional occurrence during convalescence of a nonseptic arthritis-pericarditis syndrome.

Meningococcemia. About 20 per cent of patients with meningococcal disease have meningococcemia without meningitis. The clinical expression of meningococcemia varies from an acute process (mild systemic illness or rapidly lethal course) to a chronic, indolent, relapsing disease that may go on for months.

MILD ACUTE MENINGOCOCCEMIA. This is the most common form of meningococcemia, characterized by the rapid development of malaise, fever, chills, myalgias, and arthralgias, often following a minor upper respiratory infection. In a few patients diarrhea has been an early symptom. The subsequent course may follow one of several paths: (1) Symptoms may abate in two or three days, and the diagnosis is made in retrospect when *N. meningitidis* is isolated from a blood culture. (2) Initial symptomatology is followed over 24 to 48 hours by recurrent chills and the appearance of erythematous macular lesions, particularly on the extremities, often accompanied by petechiae. In more severe infections, purpura and ecchymotic areas with gunmetal gray necrotic centers appear. Tachycardia and tachypnea are prominent. Mild hypotension may be present, and shock is a feature if fulminant meningococcemia ensues. In some patients headache may appear and confusion and stiff neck develop; the syndrome then becomes one of combined *meningococcemia-meningitis*. A meningoencephalopathic picture has been described in up to 15 per cent of patients. This probably represents a heterogeneous group (some with meningitis and others with fulminant meningococcemia and central nervous system changes secondary to shock), in whom confusion, delirium, or coma is striking. (3) Occasionally, initial malaise, fever, and arthralgias (accompanied by a few macular and petechial skin lesions) may persist for about a week, during which one or more joint effusions may develop. Blood cultures reveal *N. meningitidis*, and all manifestations promptly subside on treatment with penicillin.

FULMINANT MENINGOCOCCEMIA. This is the most dramatic form of infection, with an abrupt onset and extraordinarily rapid progression (occasionally less than 10 hours from onset to fatal termination). It occurs in about 10 per cent of patients with meningococcal disease. Violent chills, high fever, dizziness, headache, and profound weakness develop over a few hours. Petechiae appear initially on the extremities; they rapidly increase in number and coalesce as new ones appear in the conjunctivae and buccal mucosa. Hypotension with peripheral vasoconstriction quickly appears. Purpura soon develops (Fig. 273–1). At this point the patient may still be febrile or may have become hypothermic. As shock supervenes, restlessness, mental obtundation, and coma may follow in rapid succession. Disseminated intravascular coagulation (DIC) is commonly present, with enlarging hemorrhagic areas in the skin and sometimes mucosal and gastrointestinal bleeding. Cardiac (myocarditis) and respiratory ("shock lung") failure may be terminal events. *The relentless course, once shock develops, makes mandatory early diagnosis and immediate institution of antibiotic treatment even while parts of the initial examination are being performed.*

CHRONIC MENINGOCOCCEMIA. This uncommon form of meningococcemia is characterized by intermittent febrile episodes lasting one to six days, or, rarely, by sustained fevers for several weeks. It begins with chills, migratory arthralgias (or occasionally mild arthritis), and headache, but minimal toxicity. A transient polymorphous (erythematous macules and papules, rare petechiae, and purpuric nodules) nonpruritic rash appears with each febrile episode. The total number of skin lesions is small, and Gram stain and culture only rarely reveal the etiologic agent. Biopsy reveals a leukocytoclastic angiitis, which may be mistaken for a collagen disease or allergic vasculitis. Splenomegaly is observed in 20 per cent of patients. Blood cultures are not positive during apyrexial periods and may not yield the organism until the second or third febrile episode.

Untreated, about 20 per cent of patients ultimately develop meningitis. Rarer complications include endocarditis and epididymitis.

Where the organism resides between episodes is unclear. Throat cultures frequently have not revealed meningococci. The occurrence of chronic meningococcemia in several patients with congenital late complement component deficiencies suggests a possible factor in pathogenesis.

Upper Respiratory Tract Infection. How frequently nasopharyngeal infection is symptomatic is unclear. Nasopharyngeal symptoms preceding some systemic meningococcal infections may be due to this organism or to ambient viral respiratory infections.

Pneumonia. Meningococcal pneumonia is much more often of bronchogenic than of hematogenous origin. Other than during the 1918 influenza pandemic, it has been reported only rarely until this past decade. Primary meningococcal pneumonia is most often due to group Y; in recent years among recruits pneumonia caused by group Y has become the most common form of meningococcal disease. Primary meningococcal pneumonia may be segmental, lobar, or bronchopneumonic in pattern. It sometimes follows antecedent influenza or adenoviral infection. Clinical features are similar to those of community-acquired pneumonias. The onset may be gradual or abrupt. Lower lobes are usually involved. Bacteremia occurs in about 15 per cent of cases. In some patients purulent sputum is produced, containing numerous gram-negative diplococci; in others sputum is scanty, and diagnosis is made on a transtracheal aspirate or by blood culture. Response to treatment with penicillin is prompt.

Meningococcal pneumonia occasionally develops in the course of clinical meningococcemia or meningitis, but the clinical picture is dominated by the extrapulmonary aspects.

To be distinguished from meningococcal pneumonia are pulmonary infections due to *Branhamella catarrhalis* (gram-negative biscuit-shaped diplococci) or rarely to other usually noninvasive *Neisseria* species (e.g., *N. sicca*). Such infections usually take the form of acute exacerbations of chronic bronchitis or of pneumonia, occurring particularly in immunodeficient individuals, patients with chronic pulmonary disease, or as a nosocomial infection. *B. catarrhalis* can also be the etiology of acute sinusitis, bacteremia, and, rarely, meningitis. In children this organism, after *S. pneumoniae* and *H. influenzae*, is the third commonest cause of acute otitis media. Beta-lactamase production occurs in 75 per cent of strains isolated

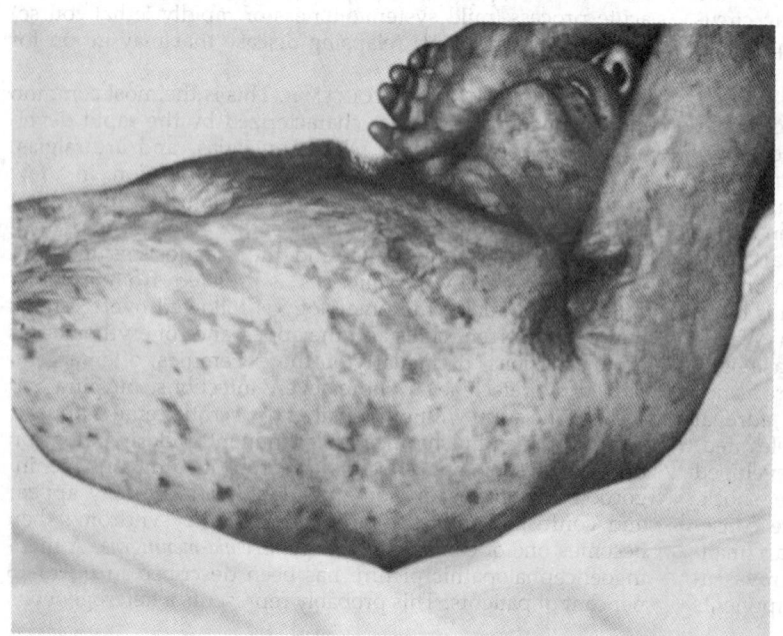

FIGURE 273–1. Skin lesions in fulminating meningococcemia. (Courtesy of Dr. Worth B. Daniels.)

currently from children. Alternatives to ampicillin or penicillin for therapy, based on in vitro susceptibilities, include erythromycin, trimethoprim-sulfamethoxazole, chloramphenicol, amoxicillin-clavulanic acid, tetracycline, and cefuroxime.

Arthritis. Arthritis complicates 2 to 16 per cent of acute meningococcal illness and may take several forms: (1) *Isolated, acute suppurative meningococcal arthritis,* a rare type occurring in the absence of meningitis or clinical meningococcemia. The joint fluid has the characteristics of septic arthritis. (2) *Early onset (first two to three days) arthritis* during meningococcal meningitis or meningococcemia, the most common form. It is a polyarthritis with acutely inflamed joints; effusions are small or absent. It responds promptly to penicillin. (3) *Late onset (fourth to tenth day, when meningitis is subsiding) arthritis.* This is commonly a subacute mono- or oligoarthritis accompanied by joint effusions. It is associated with recrudescence of fever, pleuropericarditis, and, occasionally, new papulobullous skin lesions. Synovial and pericardial fluids are characteristically serosanguineous (but sometimes purulent) and sterile. Immunopathologic study of synovial lesions implicates immune complex formation in their genesis. Treatment involves joint aspiration and the use of anti-inflammatory agents.

Pericarditis. Pericarditis complicates 2 to 20 per cent of meningococcal disease. It may take several forms: (1) *Early onset pericarditis,* appearing in the first several days of clinical meningococcemia or meningitis, may be purulent and may be due to invasion by *N. meningitidis.* (2) *Late onset pericarditis,* developing four to ten days after onset of meningitis, may cause large sterile, serosanguineous effusions. The favorable response to anti-inflammatory agents and adrenal corticosteroids supports the proposed role of hypersensitivity in pathogenesis. (3) *Isolated purulent pericarditis,* occurring in the absence of meningitis or clinical meningococcemia, is the least common form of meningococcal pericarditis and usually presents with a purulent effusion and tamponade requiring surgical intervention.

Other Meningococcal Infections. Ocular involvement (panophthalmitis, conjunctivitis) occurs in less than 1 per cent of patients with meningococcal disease. Primary conjunctivitis, an acute purulent process, is even less common. Since dissemination develops in 10 per cent of children with primary meningococcal conjunctivitis, systemic therapy with penicillin should be employed along with topical antimicrobials.

Genital tract and anal infections with *N. meningitidis* occasionally occur, the latter in homosexual males. In the female symptomatic or asymptomatic infections of the cervix and vagina may be associated with salpingitis or subsequent clinical meningococcemia. Urethral infection is less common than anal infection but is usually symptomatic. Treatment, as for gonococcal infection, is warranted to eliminate symptomatic disease and to prevent the rare instance of disseminated infection.

COURSE AND COMPLICATIONS. Acute meningococcemia may run a varied course, from that of mild disease to that of fulminant illness with death in a day or less. Certain features (particularly if present simultaneously) indicate a poor prognosis: (1) petechiae for less than 12 hours prior to hospitalization (rapid development of crops of new petechiae and purpura from one hour to the next is ominous); (2) shock; (3) fever above 40° C; (4) absence of meningitis; (5) leukopenia; (6) thrombocytopenia or evidence of DIC; and (7) extremes of age.

Extensive purpura, acral cyanosis, hemorrhagic bullae, and peripheral gangrene are features of fulminant meningococcemia, usually occurring in the presence of shock and DIC. DIC may be evident on hospitalization or may develop precipitously in some patients who are stable initially. In acute DIC platelets, fibrinogen, prothrombin, and factors V, VII, and VIII are reduced. Abnormalities in three screening tests (prothrombin time prolongation, platelet count reduction, hypofibrinogenemia) aid in detection of DIC, which occurs to

some extent in about one quarter of patients with meningococcemia. The partial thromboplastin time may also be prolonged. Confirmation is provided by demonstration of circulating fibrin degradation products in concentrations greater than 40 μg per milliliter. These coagulation defects can result in upper gastrointestinal bleeding, hematuria, and bleeding from the respiratory tract. Despite all therapeutic interventions, some patients show progressive deterioration with marked tachycardia, hyperventilation, refractory shock, metabolic acidosis, deepening coma, and "shock lung." Myocardial involvement may be manifest as either transient electrocardiographic changes or left ventricular failure.

In those who recover, resolution of the hemorrhagic or gangrenous lesions is slow and may require skin grafting. Areas of the hands and feet may remain edematous, cold, and cyanotic and may show demarcation after some weeks.

DIAGNOSIS. *Laboratory Findings.* Bacteriologic diagnosis is established by the finding of organisms on stained smears from an infected area (in an appropriate clinical setting), by isolation of *N. meningitidis* from blood or infected body fluids, or by demonstration by latex agglutination or counterimmunoelectrophoresis of group A, B, C, or Y polysaccharide antigen in blood or CSF. Blood cultures reveal *N. meningitidis* in about one third of patients with meningococcal meningitis and in 50 to 75 per cent with clinical meningococcemia or meningococcemia-meningitis. In rare patients with fulminant meningococcemia, diplococci can be seen on Gram-stained smears of blood or buffy coat. Demonstration of organisms on scrapings from skin lesions in acute meningococcemia has been variable: 70 per cent in one study, but much lower in more recent experience.

Since *N. gonorrhoeae* can be isolated from the pharynx and *N. meningitidis* can occasionally be found in the anogenital area, since both species may invade the bloodstream, and since gonococci and *N. lactamica* have on rare occasions been implicated in meningitis, accurate bacteriologic identification is important. However, 0.5 to 5 per cent of meningococci are maltose negative and may thus resemble gonococci and cause confusion.

Meningococcal polysaccharide antigen is demonstrated in the CSF of about 70 per cent of patients with meningococcal meningitis. Antigen is detected in the blood of 10 to 25 per cent of patients with meningococcemia, and its presence is associated with a poorer prognosis and higher incidence of late onset arthritis.

The CSF findings in meningococcal meningitis are those of pyogenic meningitis.

Differential Diagnosis. The differential diagnosis of meningococcal meningitis in the absence of clinical meningococcemia is that of acute meningitis with a purulent CSF formula. With the meningococcemia-meningitis syndrome it should be remembered that very rare instances of meningitis caused by *H. influenzae* and *S. pneumoniae* may be accompanied by petechial skin lesions. Occasional patients with enteroviral meningitis may have a brisk CSF pleocytosis (up to several thousand cells, with as many as 50 to 80 per cent neutrophils and a maculopetechial rash). Rarely, acute bacterial endocarditis caused by *Staphylococcus aureus* can produce a clinical picture almost indistinguishable from that of meningococcemia-meningitis, with a polymorphonuclear CSF pleocytosis and petechial and purpuric skin lesions. In *S. aureus* endocarditis there are a few skin lesions of purulent purpura which show the etiologic agent on Gram-stained smear. Occasionally measles or other viral exanthems may resemble early meningococcemia. Rocky Mountain spotted fever may mimic meningococcemia, but the absence of meningitis in the former, epidemiologic considerations, and demonstration of the etiologic agent aid in distinguishing between these processes.

Chronic meningococcemia, because of its protean manifestations, may be mistaken for Henoch-Schönlein purpura, acute vasculitis, gonococcemia, rheumatic fever, and subacute bacterial endocarditis.

TREATMENT. *Antibiotic Management.* As soon as the diagnosis is made, the patient should be put on respiratory isolation to minimize nosocomial spread of infection. Whereas practically all meningococci isolated prior to 1963 were susceptible to sulfadiazine (formerly the treatment of choice), since that time isolates resistant to sulfonamides have become common. Sulfonamide resistance in this country peaked in 1970, when 67 per cent of strains were resistant, and has since decreased (1980) to 12 per cent (8 per cent of group B, 30 per cent of group C, 4 per cent of group W135; all group Y strains susceptible). Should resistance to sulfonamides decline to less than 10 per cent, sulfonamides may again become appropriate drugs for prophylaxis.

Antimicrobial therapy should be initiated *immediately* in patients with suspected meningococcal meningitis or clinical meningococcemia because of the rapidity with which the illness may progress. Clinical isolates have been uniformly susceptible to penicillin and ampicillin (one penicillin-resistant genitourinary tract isolate, a strain with an R-factor–mediated β-lactamase, has recently been described). Intravenous penicillin G is the drug of choice (24 million units daily in the adult in divided doses every two hours) for meningococcal meningitis. Alternatively, intravenous ampicillin can be employed in the adult (12 grams daily in divided doses every two to three hours). In patients allergic to penicillin, intravenous chloramphenicol (4 to 6 grams daily in the adult) is the recommended alternative, with appropriate monitoring of the hematopoietic system. Third-generation cephalosporins such as cefotaxime and ceftriaxone are active in vitro against *N. meningitidis* and have been used successfully in treatment of meningococcal meningitis. They may now provide an alternative when the use of chloramphenicol is considered. The duration of treatment of meningococcal meningitis and the management of complications are considered in Ch. 272.

Intravenous penicillin G is the treatment for acute clinical meningococcemia without meningitis. Although 8 to 10 million units daily is usually adequate to sterilize the blood and most areas of metastatic infection, it may not provide therapeutic CSF levels in the patient with incipient meningitis. For this reason, initial therapy with "meningitis" doses is often employed. Treatment is continued until the patient has been afebrile for five days. Penicillin (5 to 8 million units daily intravenously in the adult) is effective treatment for chronic meningococcemia.

Other Aspects of Treatment. Treatment of severe meningococcemia requires supportive measures to deal with shock and other complications (DIC, congestive failure, metabolic acidosis, "shock lung"). These include cardiovascular monitoring in an intensive care setting, initial volume expansion, use of vasoactive agents, attention to fluid balances, maintenance of adequate oxygenation, and possible use of digoxin. A central venous pressure (CVP) catheter is placed (a flow-directed pulmonary catheter for evaluation of left atrial and ventricular filling pressures may be necessary if cardiac decompensation develops). Volume expansion (dextrose-saline infused rapidly) is necessary initially to assure that intravascular volume is optimal. If there is no sudden or progressive rise in CVP, then volume expansion (utilizing both crystalloid and colloid) is continued until shock is corrected or fluid overload (increased CVP, rales) develops. Urine output should be monitored and maintained at 40 to 50 ml per hour.

If rapid improvement does not follow volume expansion or if the CVP exceeds appropriate limits, a catecholamine should be added to enhance cardiac output and raise arterial pressure to the range of 90 to 100 mm Hg. Dopamine has been widely used because of its ability to increase renal blood flow (at dosage below 6 μg per kilogram per minute) while increasing cardiac contractility. It is administered by continuous intravenous (initial rate of 2 to 5 μg per kilogram per minute) infusion at a rate sufficient to maintain an adequate arterial pressure and urine volume.

Evidence as to whether adrenal corticosteroids have a beneficial effect in bacteremic shock is still conflicting. One or two pharmacologic doses (3 mg per kilogram of dexamethasone or 30 mg per kilogram of methylprednisolone intravenously) have been used in patients not responding to the aforementioned initial measures. Smaller maintenance doses do not appear beneficial, and continued administration predisposes to superinfection.

Adequate oxygenation is essential in a patient with shock, particularly if meningitis is also a feature (in which hypoxia can aggravate cerebral edema). Oxygen administration, and intubation with ventilatory assistance if needed, should be an integral part of therapy aiming at restoring the arterial P_{O_2} to appropriate levels (80 to 120 mm Hg). Acidosis should be corrected by intravenous administration of sodium bicarbonate (45 mEq) as needed. Digoxin is not of value in meningococcemic shock but may have a role if fluid overload complicates volume expansion or secondary myocarditis. Generally, diuretics such as furosemide have been of more value in this acute situation.

The initial enthusiasm for heparin treatment of DIC in meningococcemia and septic shock has waned, since evidence of efficacy in reducing mortality has been conflicting despite improvement in coagulation factors. Heparin treatment on the basis of laboratory abnormalities alone is inadvisable. Reversal of hypotension is often associated with improvement in laboratory evidences of DIC and a halt in further clinical progression of the coagulopathy. Only if bleeding into deep tissues or from mucosal surfaces develops or thrombotic manifestations occur in the presence of DIC might heparinization be considered. After initiation of heparin therapy coagulation factor deficiencies can be repaired by administration of fresh frozen plasma. Once heparin is started, prothrombin time and partial thromboplastin time determinations are no longer helpful in following laboratory evidences of DIC; levels of fibrin degradation products, fibrinogen, and platelets are of greatest assistance.

PREVENTION. *Chemoprophylaxis.* Close contacts (e.g., same household or daycare center, medical personnel exposed by intimate contact such as mouth-to-mouth resuscitation) of a patient with meningococcal disease are at increased risk of developing systemic disease and should receive chemoprophylaxis. Since secondary (or coprimary) cases usually occur within four days of the initial case, prophylactic treatment should begin as soon as the initial case is identified. Rifampin has been shown to be 80 to 90 per cent effective in eliminating meningococci from the nasopharynx of asymptomatic carriers, and minocycline has been almost as effective. Because of reports of vestibular side effects with minocycline, rifampin is the recommended drug for chemoprophylaxis. It is administered for two days: to adults at a dosage of 600 mg orally every 12 hours; to children (one month of age or older) at a dosage of 10 mg per kilogram every 12 hours; and to children under one month of age, at a dosage of 5 mg per kilogram every 12 hours. Since even the high doses of penicillin used to treat meningococcal meningitis or meningococcemia may not eradicate nasopharyngeal carriage, rifampin should be administered also to the index patient prior to discharge from hospital. Rifampin-resistant strains appear readily and would be selected if use of the drug for prophylaxis were widespread.

Meningococcal Vaccine. A quadrivalent (groups A, C, Y, W135) vaccine is now commercially available. A previous serogroup A vaccine showed efficacy of 85 to 95 per cent and was helpful in controlling epidemics; similar clinical efficacy has been demonstrated for a serogroup C vaccine in military recruits and in an epidemic. The polysaccharide vaccines are immunogenic in adults but do not induce a good antibody response in children under two years of age. A vaccine against serogroup B, the major cause of meningococcal disease in the United States, is not available.

The principal indication for use of meningococcal vaccines is the presence of outbreaks of meningococcal disease caused by *N. meningitidis* belonging to serogroup A or C (or more recently Y and W135).

The routine immunization of individuals against meningococcal disease is not recommended because of the low risk of disease in the absence of outbreaks. However, immunization would be advisable for high-risk groups such as those with complement deficiencies or with anatomic or functional asplenia. Also, vaccination should be considered for travelers to countries in which there is epidemic meningococcal disease. Since about 50 per cent of secondary cases among close contacts occur more than five days following the primary case, consideration should be given to the use of immunization as an adjunct to chemoprophylaxis to extend protection if the latter has been unsuccessful.

PROGNOSIS. The mortality from meningococcal meningitis before any treatment was available was about 75 per cent, and residual neurologic damage in the survivors was extensive. The advent of the sulfonamides brought a dramatic reduction in mortality to 5 to 15 per cent. Despite the emergence of sulfonamide-resistant *N. meningitidis*, mortality has been kept at the same low level through the use of high doses of penicillin G or ampicillin. The case-fatality ratio for patients with meningococcemia without accompanying meningitis is higher (25 per cent) than for meningococcal meningitis and reflects the fulminant course in some patients. The case-fatality ratio is highest in children under two years of age and in adults over 50.

Band JD, Chamberland ME, Platt T, et al.: Trends in meningococcal disease in the United States, 1975–1980. J Infect Dis 148:754, 1983. *Most current review of incidence of meningococcal disease in the United States, with emphasis on the role of various serogroups and the prevalence of sulfonamide resistance.*

Benoit FL: Chronic meningococcemia. Case report and review of the literature. Am J Med 35:103, 1963. *The best review of the clinical features of this fascinating entity.*

DeVoe IW: The meningococcus and mechanisms of pathogenicity. Microbiol Rev 46:162, 1982. *Comprehensive review of the biologic properties of N. meningitidis and of the epidemiologic and immunologic aspects of meningococcal disease.*

Feldman HA: Meningococcal infections. Adv Intern Med 18:117, 1972. *The best overview of the major aspects of meningococcal disease, including epidemiology, clinical aspects, treatment, and prevention. Authoritative; very well referenced.*

Goldschneider I, Gotschlich EC, Artenstein MS: Human immunity to the meningococcus. I. The role of humoral antibodies. J Exper Med 129:1307, 1969. *A most important paper, relating susceptibility to meningococcal infection to the lack of serum bactericidal activity against N. meningitidis. A lucid presentation of the basic facts necessary to understand the epidemiology of meningococcal disease.*

Goldschneider I, Gotschlich EC, Artenstein MS: Human immunity to the meningococcus. II. Development of natural immunity. J Exper Med 129:1327, 1969. *A second landmark paper by these authors on immunity to meningococcal infection. The role of the carrier state as an immunizing process is clearly demonstrated.*

Griffiss JM, Brandt BL: Nonepidemic (endemic) meningococcal disease: Pathogenetic factors and clinical features. In Remington JS, Swartz MN (eds.): Current Clinical Topics in Infectious Disease, 7. New York, McGraw-Hill Book Company, 1986, pp 27–50. *Provides important new insights into the endemic and hyperendemic forms of meningococcal disease in the U.S. The role of host:parasite interactions is emphasized.*

Koppes GM, Ellenbogen C, Gebhart RJ: Group Y meningococcal disease in United States Air Force recruits. Am J Med 62:661, 1977. *A very good description of the spectrum of disease produced by group Y meningococci. The importance of pneumonia in a recruit population is emphasized.*

McGowan JE Jr: Respiratory tract infections due to Branhamella catarrhalis and Neisseria species. In Remington JS, Swartz MN (eds.): Current Clinical Topics in Infectious Disease, 8. New York, McGraw-Hill Book Company, 1987. *Comprehensive appraisal of Branhamella catarrhalis as a cause of human disease. Neisseria species (other than N. meningitidis) are also evaluated as pathogens.*

Peltola H: Meningococcal disease: Still with us. Rev Infect Dis 5:71, 1983. *Authoritative evaluation of the current status of meningococcal disease around the world.*

274 INFECTIONS CAUSED BY *HEMOPHILUS* SPECIES

DEFINITION. *Hemophilus* infections involve primarily the upper respiratory tract and the bronchopulmonary system. Invasive infections (bacteremia, meningitis, pericarditis, septic arthritis, cellulitis) may sometimes ensue; they occur predominantly in young children and are almost always due to one species, *Hemophilus influenzae* type b. Endocarditis is occasionally caused by *Hemophilus* species other than *H. influenzae* b. One *Hemophilus* species (*H. ducreyi*) is the cause of chancroid (see Ch. 309), and another (*H. vaginalis*—more recently designated *Gardnerella vaginalis*) is implicated in "nonspecific vaginitis." With the exception of these last two species, the normal habitat of the *Hemophilus* species is the upper respiratory tract.

GENERAL MICROBIOLOGIC FEATURES. The various *Hemophilus* species (Table 274–1) are similar in morphology (small, pleomorphic, gram-negative bacilli) and growth requirements (facultatively aerobic, media supplemented with blood). *H. influenzae* requires for aerobic growth both the X factor (hematin) and the V factor (NAD, NADP, or nicotinamide nucleoside) present in erythrocytes. Since some strains of *H. influenzae* grow best in 5 to 10 per cent carbon dioxide and other *Hemophilus* species have a CO_2 dependence, clinical specimens should be incubated in a CO_2 incubator. Media for isolation of *Hemophilus* species include chocolate agar, agar containing horse (*not* sheep) blood, or enrichment agar (Levinthal).

H. hemolyticus rarely is isolated from sites outside the upper respiratory tract and is of dubious pathogenicity.

INFECTIONS DUE TO *HEMOPHILUS INFLUENZAE*. *Etiology.* *H. influenzae* strains are either encapsulated (typable) or unencapsulated (nontypable). The former consist of six distinguishable types, designated a to f. Nearly all strains causing invasive infection belong to type b, and the capsular polysaccharide contains both ribose and ribitol phosphate (PRP). However, encapsulated strains make up only a small percentage of clinical isolates of *H. influenzae*. Nontypable strains are more likely to be implicated in localized infections and rarely are associated with bacteremia. Encapsulated strains can be identified by a variety of methods employing antisera to their capsular antigens (immunofluorescence; production of immunoprecipitin halos ringing colonies on agar plates containing antiserum; demonstration by counterimmunoelectrophoresis or latex particle agglutination of capsular antigen in culture supernatants). The outer membrane of *H. influenzae* strains contains a lipopolysaccharide with the properties of endotoxin. A classification of *H. influenzae* b into 21 subtypes based on differences in outer membrane proteins has been developed and is of use in epidemiologic studies.

Smears of clinical specimens usually show pleomorphic gram-negative coccobacilli. Occasionally, in underdecolorized

TABLE 274–1. DIFFERENTIAL PROPERTIES OF *HEMOPHILUS* SPECIES

Species	Growth Factor Requirement		CO_2 Dependence	Hemolysis
	X	V		
H. influenzae	+	+	−	−
H. parainfluenzae	−	+	−	−
H. aphrophilus	−, +	−	+	−
H. paraphrophilus	−	+	+	−
H. hemolyticus	+	+	−	+
H. ducreyi	+	−	−	−

gram-stained smears of spinal fluid, bipolar concentration of stain may incorrectly suggest gram-positive diplococci.

Incidence and Prevalence. Nontypable *H. influenzae* are commonly carried in the nasopharynx of asymptomatic individuals. Rates of carriage for encapsulated strains (usually type b) are much lower (less than 5 per cent of children and less than 1 per cent of adults). However, the carriage rate of household contacts, at the time of hospitalization of a child with invasive *H. influenzae* b, is much higher, 20 to 25 per cent (50 per cent in children under five years). Nasopharyngeal carriage of *H. influenzae* b may develop in some persons in the presence of circulating antibody to PRP, and successful antibiotic treatment of *H. influenzae* meningitis may not eliminate it from the upper respiratory tract. The carrier state may persist for weeks to months.

H. influenzae b is the principal (estimated 8000 to 11,000 cases annually) cause of bacterial meningitis in the United States. It is estimated to cause an additional 6000 cases per year of other invasive diseases such as bacteremia, epiglottitis, pneumonia, and cellulitis. By five years of age, one in every 200 children has had a systemic infection from *H. influenzae* b. In the past decade many clinicians have had the impression that systemic disease caused by *H. influenzae* b has become more frequent in adults. Systemic infection with *H. influenzae* probably should be considered in the adult in the proper setting more frequently than was formerly the case.

Epidemiology. Infections in the first two months of life are rare, probably because of transplacental transfer of maternal antibody. Most cases (about 80 per cent) of meningitis and invasive infections caused by *H. influenzae* in the United States occur in children under two years of age. The mean age of children with epiglottitis is three to five years. Host factors appearing to contribute to increased susceptibility include immune globulin deficiencies, sickle cell disease, CSF fistulas, splenectomized states, and chronic pulmonary infections. Alcoholism appears to be a risk factor in adults. In certain racial groups (Eskimos, American Indians, blacks) children are at higher risk of invasive *H. influenzae* infection; socioeconomic factors undoubtedly play a role.

Unlike *Neisseria meningitidis*, *H. influenzae* b does not cause epidemics in the community, but it is responsible for an increased incidence of secondary cases among susceptibles in families or possibly in daycare centers exposed to an index case. The risk of serious *H. influenzae* illness among exposed household contacts of a child with *H. influenzae* meningitis is age dependent: 4 per cent among children under two years of age, 2 per cent among children two to three years of age, and 0.1 per cent among children four to five years of age. The risk of infection in household contacts represents a 600-fold increase over the age-adjusted risk in the population at large.

Pathogenesis and Immunity. Most nasopharyngeal infections with *H. influenzae* are unrecognized and occur by age five years. Type b strains may occasionally invade locally, producing epiglottitis, pneumonia, or buccal cellulitis, or may be disseminated directly from the nasopharynx via the bloodstream, producing meningitis. Intense ($> 10^3$ organisms/ml of blood) sustained bacteremia resulting from intravascular bacterial replication (rather than growth at a focal site of initial infection) appears to be a prerequisite for the development of meningitis. Pathogenicity of type b strains owes principally to the antiphagocytic activity of its PRP capsule. Nonencapsulated strains rarely produce bacteremic infection but can produce disease involving the upper (otitis media, sinusitis) and lower (pneumonia, exacerbations of chronic bronchitis) respiratory tracts.

In Finland, studies of anti-PRP antibodies by radioimmunoassay indicate an inverse correlation between age-related antibody levels and incidence of bacteremic *H. influenzae* disease (confirming Fothergill and Wright); 90 per cent of children (3 to 12 months of age) had antibody levels below 150 ng per milliliter, whereas all adults had higher levels. In the presence of complement, IgG class antibodies to PRP are not only bactericidal (bacteriolytic) but are also opsonic. Such antibodies are protective in vivo. Antibodies to outer membrane proteins also play a role in immunity, but they appear to be protective primarily against strains of the same subtype.

The antibody response to *H. influenzae* b meningitis is age related (infants responding poorly and older children and adults developing high titers) and related to PRP load and clearance rate. Antigenemia may persist for as long as several weeks in younger children; an antibody response may be delayed until antigenemia has cleared. Anti-PRP antibody responses are observed within about three months in about 80 per cent of children with meningitis.

Failure of specific anti-PRP antibody response occurs in individuals with agammaglobulinemia and with IgG_2 subclass deficiency. In addition, during the first one or two years of life polysaccharide antigens such as PRP vaccine are not efficient immunogens. The rare recurrence of *H. influenzae* b meningitis in the first 24 months of life may reflect failure even of invasive infection to elicit a protective antibody response.

It has been suggested that the age-related acquisition of anti-PRP antibodies is too rapid and extensive to be accounted for by the low incidence of *H. influenzae* b carriage or disease, and that cross-reacting *E. coli* strains in the intestine may serve as the primary immunogen.

Clinical Manifestations. In one survey of children with serious *H. influenzae* infections, meningitis was the most common manifestation (about 50 per cent), followed by pneumonia (15 per cent), bacteremia without definable portal (10 per cent), cellulitis (10 per cent), epiglottitis (10 per cent), and pericarditis (4 per cent).

Among adults with *H. influenzae* bacteremia, pneumonia is the commonest cause. About one half of isolates are nontypable, and most of the typable strains belong to type b. Other sources of *H. influenzae* bacteremia in adults include obstetric infections (nontypable strains), meningitis, occult bacteremias, cellulitis, acute sinusitis, and epiglottitis. Metastatic *H. influenzae* infections in the adult include septic arthritis and purulent pericarditis.

MENINGITIS (See Ch. 272). *H. influenzae* type b is the pre-eminent cause of bacterial meningitis in childhood, most cases occurring between ages four months and two years. The clinical features are not distinctive except as they relate to pyogenic meningitis occurring at that age. The manifestations may be nonspecific (fever, irritability, listlessness, poor feeding, vomiting) initially, especially in the younger child, and there may be only minimal nuchal rigidity. If the fontanel is still open, it may not be tense, particularly if the infant is dehydrated. Subdural effusions occur more frequently (20 to 30 per cent) with *H. influenzae* meningitis, but this is related to age and ease of detection by transillumination.

Anemia is more frequent in patients with *H. influenzae* b meningitis and invasive infections than in those with comparable meningococcal or pneumococcal illnesses. It appears, in patients with prolonged antigenemia coinciding with production of antibody to PRP, to be a consequence of splenic removal of PRP-coated erythrocytes to which antibody and complement have been bound, or of intravascular hemolysis.

EPIGLOTTITIS. This pediatric otolaryngologic emergency begins abruptly with a severe sore throat, fever, and dysphagia; progression is swift, usually requiring hospitalization (and intubation) within 12 hours of onset. In the adult the onset of epiglottitis may be more prolonged and respiratory difficulty less pronounced initially despite severe pharyngitis and dysphagia; occasionally, the clinical picture may be mistaken for that of asthma. Airway obstruction in the child develops early with a sensation of choking, inspiratory (but not expiratory) distress, drooling, and anxiety. Speech is muffled, but the barking cough observed in croup is uncommon. The patient sits leaning forward with arms, back, and neck hyperextended to provide maximal airway. Pneumonia occurs in 15 to 25 per cent of patients, but simultaneous meningitis is uncommon. *Intraoral examination of the child (particularly in the supine position) may precipitate a cardiorespiratory arrest and should be performed only with the means of establishing an airway immediately at hand.* The pharynx is reddened; the epiglottis is bright red and markedly swollen. Lateral radiographs of the neck can demonstrate swelling of the epiglottis, but are of less value in acute cases (the procedure may delay establishment of an adequate airway) than in subacute ones.

Viral croup may resemble epiglottitis but occurs in younger children (3 to 36 months), has a more gradual onset, and frequently is preceded by an upper respiratory infection; the airway obstruction is subglottic.

PNEUMONIA. Most cases occur in children, are caused by type b, and are accompanied by bacteremia. Lobar consolidation occurs more commonly than bronchopneumonia, and pleural effusions (or empyema) are present in 75 per cent of cases. Lung abscess is rare. Meningitis occurs in about 15 per cent of patients.

In the adult, *H. influenzae* pneumonia occurs more frequently in the setting of chronic lung disease, alcoholism, immunologic deficiency, or following viral respiratory tract infection, but it may develop in previously healthy individuals. The majority of sputum isolates are nontypable, as are most blood isolates from the approximately 20 per cent of patients in whom bacteremia occurs. The radiologic pattern is usually that of bronchopneumonia. Small sterile parapneumonic effusions are common. The diagnosis can be suspected on the basis of findings on Gram-stained smears of sputum, but confirmation requires isolation of the organism from blood, pleural fluid, or lower respiratory tract.

BRONCHITIS. *H. influenzae* (nontypable) has been associated with purulent sputum and clinical exacerbations (dyspnea, wheezing, low-grade fever) of chronic bronchitis. A direct etiologic role is difficult to establish because of the frequent (20 to 80 per cent) carriage of these organisms in the upper respiratory tract of normal adults.

CELLULITIS. *H. influenzae* b causes cellulitis in children below two years of age, but may also cause cellulitis on rare occasions in older adults. The cheek, periorbital area, head, and neck are the most common sites. An associated ipsilateral otitis media or upper respiratory infection is a frequent precursor. It begins with fever, local pain, and increasing toxicity. The lesion develops within a few hours and progresses rapidly; it is poorly demarcated, tender, and edematous. Although usually described as having a distinctive bluish purple color, the lesion is commonly erythematous like other types of cellulitis. Bacteremia occurs in 80 per cent of cases. Diagnosis is made on the basis of the appearance and location of the lesion, the patient's age, Gram-stained smears and culture of an aspirate, and blood cultures.

BACTEREMIA WITHOUT OBVIOUS PORTAL. *H. influenzae* b is responsible for about 20 per cent of cryptogenic bacteremias occurring in febrile children with mild nonspecific illnesses. Such patients are at considerable risk for subsequent serious localized infection (meningitis, pneumonia, epiglottitis). Unsuspected *H. influenzae* bacteremia also occurs in patients with neoplastic disease undergoing chemotherapy. Fulminant *H. influenzae* bacteremia with fatal shock and disseminated intravascular coagulation can develop in splenectomized patients.

SKELETAL INFECTIONS. Septic arthritis accounts for 1 to 8 per cent of cases of invasive *H. influenzae* b infection in children. It is the cause of pyogenic arthritis in about one half of cases in children under two years of age. Weight-bearing joints are most often involved. Most commonly pyarthrosis is secondary to bacteremic spread from an upper respiratory tract infection, but joint involvement may result from direct spread of adjacent osteomyelitis in the first year of life.

A "reactive" arthritis has recently been described in children in association with *H. influenzae* b meningitis. Whereas the articular manifestations of pyogenic arthritis are usually present within the first day of admission with meningitis, the joint findings in the "reactive" form usually appear about a week following institution of appropriate antimicrobial therapy. Gram-stains and cultures of repeated synovial fluid aspirates are negative. Whether this process is comparable to the reactive arthritis of meningococcal meningitis, in which immune complexes are present in blood and synovial fluid, is not known. Joint effusions with a neutrophilic pleocytosis occurring in this setting should be considered to be those of pyogenic arthritis until results of repeated bacteriologic studies are available.

H. influenzae is a rare cause of osteomyelitis in children, usually occurring in the first year of life.

PERICARDITIS. *H. influenza* b is the cause of 10 to 15 per cent of cases of purulent pericarditis in children. It is a rare cause of pericarditis in adults. Over one half of the children have an associated pneumonia. The hemodynamic manifestations of cardiac tamponade are commonly present. Treatment involves pericardiocentesis for diagnosis followed by surgical drainage (closed catheter drainage or anterior pericardectomy), along with antimicrobial therapy. With treatment 85 to 95 per cent of patients recover.

OTITIS MEDIA AND SINUSITIS. *H. influenzae* is second in frequency to *Streptococcus pneumoniae* as the cause of acute otitis media in children. In most instances the *H. influenzae* strains are not typable, but type b stains can be isolated in 10 per cent of cases. Serous middle ear fluid in children with chronic low-grade otitis media with effusion may be colonized by *H. influenzae*, which may contribute to its persistence. *H. influenzae* also appears to be a significant cause of otitis media in older children and adults. The manifestations of acute otitis media caused by *H. influenzae* are indistinguishable from those caused by other pyogens: otalgia, fever, hyperemia of the tympanic membrane, and middle ear fluid. Tinnitus, vertigo, and nystagmus may develop.

Acute sinusitis is more common in adults than in children. In about 25 per cent of cases *H. influenzae* (nontypable) is the cause. Facial pain, frontal headache, purulent nasal discharge or nasal obstruction, anosmia, and nasal speech are common features. Sinus tenderness and opacity on transillumination are helpful findings.

CONJUNCTIVITIS. Most strains of *Hemophilus* isolated from conjunctivae are unencapsulated and formerly were designated as *H. aegyptius* (Koch-Weeks bacillus). Currently these strains are considered as biotypes of *H. influenzae*. *H. influenzae* mucopurulent conjunctivitis occurs principally in children, particularly in the summer. The findings of acute catarrhal conjunctivitis are present, but petechial hemorrhages on the tarsal and epibulbar conjunctivae are suggestive of *H. influenzae* or a pneumococcal cause. Diagnosis is made on the basis of Gram-stained smears of conjunctival scrapings and culture of the outer eye.

H. influenzae conjunctivitis is often self-limited, clearing in 7 to 14 days. Treatment consists of moist soaks to keep the eyelids clean and topical antimicrobials (e.g., 10 to 30 per cent sulfacetamide eyedrops).

OTHER INFECTIONS. *H. influenzae* is a very rare cause of endocarditis and brain abscess. *H. influenzae* may occasionally be the cause of nonexudative pharyngitis (with prominent pain and dysphagia), but its presence in the pharynx often merely represents colonization. Rare cases of genital tract infections (salpingitis, endometritis, puerperal sepsis) and urinary infections have occurred.

Diagnosis. Certain serious infections (purulent meningitis, epiglottitis, facial and orbital cellulitis) in young children should suggest the possibility of *H. influenzae* b as the cause. In meningitis the presence of gram-negative pleomorphic coccobacillary forms in smears of CSF is highly suggestive of *H. influenzae*, but other organisms (*Pasteurella multocida, Aci-*

netobacter) which only rarely cause meningitis may have a similar appearance. Rapid and sensitive methods of antigen (PRP) detection such as latex particle agglutination (LPA), coagglutination (CoA), countercurrent immunoelectrophoresis (CIE), and enzyme-linked immunosorbent assay (ELISA) have detected *H. influenzae* b antigen in initial CSF specimens of 60 to 90 per cent of cases of *H. influenzae* meningitis; they are particularly helpful in early diagnosis and in the diagnosis of patients whose cultures may be negative because of prior antibiotic therapy. LPA is positive in 90 to 95 per cent of culture-confirmed cases of *H. influenzae* b meningitis and has the advantages over CIE and ELISA of being easier to perform and more rapid. Antigenemia can be demonstrated in 60 to 100 per cent of patients with *H. influenzae* b meningitis but much less frequently in children with epiglottitis and cellulitis. False-positive reactions may occur owing to cross-reactive antigens in other bacteria such as *E. coli*, but these are infrequent.

Bacteremia is commonly demonstrable in patients with invasive infections (at least 80 per cent of children with meningitis, epiglottitis, or cellulitis) caused by *H. influenzae* b. *H. influenzae* is generally isolated on cultures of the epiglottis, joint fluid, and empyema fluid when it is the cause of infection in those areas.

Treatment. Currently, about 30 per cent of strains of *H. influenzae* b isolated in this country from systemic infections are ampicillin-resistant. Resistance to chloramphenicol is found in less than 1 per cent of strains. Regional variations in resistance patterns exist. In Barcelona, Spain, 50 per cent of strains are ampicillin resistant, 52 per cent are resistant to chloramphenicol, and 18 per cent are resistant to both drugs. Most ampicillin-resistant *H. influenzae* strains are resistant by virtue of plasmid-encoded β-lactamase production. Detection of β-lactamase production is commonly employed to determine ampicillin resistance. Recently a few isolates of ampicillin-resistant *H. influenzae* that are resistant because of alterations in penicillin-binding proteins rather than β-lactamase production have been detected. Since routine testing for β-lactamase would indicate incorrectly such strains to be ampicillin susceptible, special disc or agar-dilution testing would be required if this were suspected. About 15 per cent of strains (usually nontypable) associated with childhood otitis media are ampicillin resistant, as are 2 to 8 per cent of strains (mostly nontypable) isolated from adults with invasive infections or chronic bronchitis.

Because of the prevalence of ampicillin resistance, ampicillin should not be used as single-drug therapy of systemic illnesses caused by *H. influenzae* b unless it has been established that the organism is ampicillin susceptible. Several forms of initial therapy are currently being employed (see Ch. 272). These include: a third-generation cephalosporin such as ceftriaxone or cefotaxime; chloramphenicol (alone, or in combination with ampicillin until testing for ampicillin resistance has been performed); and cefuroxime (a second-generation cephalosporin resistant to many β-lactamases). Ceftriaxone or cefotaxime would be the drug of choice in areas where resistance to both chloramphenicol and ampicillin exists or when such resistance is suspected on the basis of clinical response to other therapy.

Ampicillin (50 to 100 mg per kilogram per day in four divided doses) or amoxicillin (50 mg per kilogram per day in four divided doses), because each is active against *S. pneumoniae* and most strains of *H. influenzae*, is still the drug of choice for initial treatment of otitis media in children. Alternatives include trimethoprim (TMP)-sulfamethoxazole (SMX) (40 mg TMP-200 mg SMX twice daily per 20 pounds), the combination of penicillin (or erythromycin) with a sulfonamide, or cefaclor. Treatment should be continued for 10 to 14 days. Initial treatment of *H. influenzae* pneumonia in the adult should be with ampicillin, since these infections are infrequently caused by ampicillin-resistant strains, and there is sufficient time to shift therapy (chloramphenicol, cefuroxime)

if the response is unsatisfactory. Based on the bacteriology (*S. pneumoniae* and *H. influenzae* are frequently identified) of acute sinusitis, ampicillin is a reasonable initial antibiotic choice. (In the patient with rapidly progressive frontal sinusitis, *S. aureus* must be considered as a cause as well, and a penicillinase-resistant penicillin should be included in the initial therapeutic program.)

Prevention. A vaccine (*Hemophilus b polysaccharide vaccine*) against invasive infection with *H. influenzae* b has recently been licensed. This vaccine was demonstrated in Finland to have 90 per cent efficacy among children 18 to 71 months of age. It was not possible statistically to demonstrate efficacy in children immunized at 18 to 23 months of age. The vaccine was ineffective in children under 18 months of age. Children should be immunized at two years of age. Consideration may be given to immunization of children in high-risk groups (sickle cell disease, asplenic states, malignancies associated with immunosuppression) at 18 months of age even though efficacy has not been established in this age group. If this is done, a booster dose within 18 months may be necessary.

Since the majority of cases of *H. influenzae* meningitis occur in the first 18 to 24 months of life when the current polysaccharide vaccine is not efficacious, other vaccines have been developed. Since there appears to be an age-specific defect in the response of infants to polysaccharide antigen (thymus-independent), attempts have been made to overcome this limitation by linking the PRP antigen to a protein (e.g., diphtheria toxoid) thus invoking T cell participation and establishing immunologic memory. In infants 9 to 15 months of age such a PRP-protein conjugate vaccine is more immunogenic than the current PRP vaccine, with antibody levels for the former of 0.15 μg per milliliter or higher (considered protective) in all recipients one year after immunization. Large-scale trials of such conjugate vaccines in young infants are currently under way in Alaska and Finland.

The rate of secondary cases among young children who are close household contacts of a patient with invasive *H. influenzae* b infection indicates the need for an effective prophylactic antibiotic program. Since rifampin has efficacy in eliminating nasopharyngeal carriage of *H. influenzae* b, the following management of household contacts has been recommended: (1) if another child less than four years of age resides in the household of an index case, all household members (including adults) should receive rifampin (20 mg per kilogram orally once daily for four days, with a maximal daily dose of 600 mg); (2) rifampin in the same dosage should also be administered to the index patient prior to discharge from the hospital, since nasopharyngeal carriage may reappear after discontinuation of ampicillin or chloramphenicol therapy for systemic infection; (3) rifampin prophylaxis is probably not indicated if over two weeks have elapsed since illness began in the index patient or if the youngest child in the household is four years of age or older.

Whether the risk of subsequent invasive *H. influenzae* infection is increased in contacts of patients in daycare facilities is controversial; the risk may vary from region to region. If two or more cases occur in a daycare center within 60 days, rifampin prophylaxis should be given to all contacts in the facility, including adults. Whether to do likewise if only one case has occurred is controversial. However, if any of the exposed classroom contacts is under two years of age, institution of chemoprophylaxis seems warranted.

INFECTIONS CAUSED BY OTHER *HEMOPHILUS* SPECIES. *Hemophilus parainfluenzae*. This *Hemophilus* species is part of the normal flora of the nasopharynx and is found in dental plaque. It is very uncommonly responsible for human disease. It has been a rare cause of meningitis, epiglottitis, otitis media, puerperal bacteremia, brain abscess, and pneumonia in adults. Ampicillin is the drug of choice, except when ampicillin resistance is present (6 per cent of isolates), in which case chloramphenicol should be used. The most common association of *H. parainfluenzae* with disease has been with infective endocarditis. It may take as long as 14 to 18 days to grow out of blood cultures. The only distinctive clinical feature (also observed with *H. aphrophilus* endocarditis) appears to be the frequent occurrence of embolic occlusion of large arteries. For endocarditis in the adult, treatment with ampicillin (12 grams daily intravenously) alone or in combination with gentamicin (4 mg per kilogram per day in divided doses every eight hours intravenously) for four to six weeks has been employed successfully.

Hemophilus aphrophilus. This organism is part of the normal gingival flora and is a rare cause of disease, generally acting as an "opportunist." The infections it produces, often following oropharyngeal foci of infection or trauma, include abscesses (particularly brain abscess), bacteremia, and endocarditis. Most strains are susceptible to penicillin, ampicillin, cephalothin, chloramphenicol, and gentamicin. Successful treatment of endocarditis has involved the use of ampicillin or penicillin, alone or in combination with streptomycin for four to six weeks.

Hemophilus ducreyi. See Ch. 309.

Hemophilus vaginalis. *Hemophilus vaginalis* is now designated as a new species, *Gardnerella vaginalis*. *G. vaginalis* is found in the vaginal flora of 40 per cent of normal women but in large numbers in the vaginal fluid of over 95 per cent of patients with nonspecific vaginitis. It appears that this organism, acting in concert with certain anaerobes, causes this type of vaginal infection. Oral metronidazole, which is active against both anaerobes and *G. vaginalis*, suppresses both organisms and produces clinical improvement. Such improvement does not occur on treatment with oral ampicillin or doxycycline. Findings suggesting the diagnosis of nonspecific vaginitis include the presence of "clue" cells (vaginal epithelial cells with numerous adherent small gram-negative bacilli) in a vaginal discharge with pH 5.0 (exhibiting a "fishy" amine-like odor upon addition of potassium hydroxide). Treatment with metronidazole is effective, but its possible toxicity must be considered in view of the mildness of the disease and the possibility of reinfection.

G. vaginalis has also been a cause of puerperal fever with bacteremia, septic abortion, and neonatal bacteremia.

HEMOPHILUS INFLUENZAE

Campos J, Garcia-Tornel S, Sanfeliu I: Susceptibility studies of multiply resistant *Haemophilus influenzae* isolated from pediatric patients and contacts. Antimicrob Agents Chemother 25:706, 1985. *Summarizes the extent of a major endemic problem in Spain of resistance to ampicillin and chloramphenicol in H. influenzae strains. Alternative therapeutic approaches are suggested.*

Cherry JD: Acute epiglottitis, laryngitis, and croup. In Remington JS, Swartz MN (eds.): Current Clinical Topics in Infectious Disease, 2. New York, McGraw-Hill Book Company, 1981, pp 1–30. *Provides a particularly vivid clinical picture of acute H. influenzae epiglottitis. Valuable points on differential diagnosis and treatment are emphasized. A very well organised and thoroughly referenced presentation.*

Dajani AS, Asmar BI, Thirumoorthi MC: Systemic *Haemophilus influenzae* disease. J Pediatr 94:355, 1979. *This is a thorough review of an extensive pediatric experience with systemic H. influenzae b infections. It provides helpful data on the relative frequencies of the various clinical syndromes and an extensive bibliography.*

Fothergill LD, Wright J: Influenzal meningitis: Relation of age incidence to bactericidal power of blood against causal organism. J Immunol 24:273, 1933. *This is the original and "classic" study demonstrating an inverse relationship between the presence of serum bactericidal antibody and the incidence of H. influenzae meningitis at various ages.*

Granoff DM, Ward JI: Current status of prophylaxis for *Hemophilus influenzae* infections. In Remington JS, Swartz MN (eds.): Current Clinical Topics in Infectious Disease, 5. New York, McGraw-Hill Book Company, 1984. *Provides excellent background regarding secondary spread of H. influenzae infections and concrete recommendations for chemoprophylaxis of close family and daycare center contacts.*

Mayo-Smith MF, Hirsch PJ, Wodzinski SF, et al.: Acute epiglottitis in adults. An eight year experience in the state of Rhode Island. N Engl J Med 314:1133, 1986. *A clinical and bacteriologic review of 56 cases of acute epiglottitis (supraglottitis) in adults, indicating that H. influenzae is an important etiology in this age group (28 per cent of published cases in which blood cultures were obtained). Practical management issues are considered.*

Peltola H, Kayhty H, Virtanen M, et al.: Prevention of *Hemophilus influenzae* type B bacteremic infections with the capsular polysaccharide vaccine. N Engl J Med 310:1561, 1984. *This article describes a long-term follow-up of a very well conducted, large scale trial of the type b capsular polysaccharide vaccine, which protected against bacteremic H. influenzae b disease in children older than 24 months of age.*

Shurin SB, Anderson P, Zollinger J, et al.: Pathophysiology of hemolysis in infections with *Hemophilus influenzae* type b. J Clin Invest 77:1340, 1986. *In a careful laboratory study the authors demonstrate that the anemia observed in invasive H. influenzae b infections is hemolytic in origin and may be due to coating of PRP on erythrocytes and their subsequent immune destruction.*

Spagnuolo PJ, Ellner JJ, Lerner PL, et al.: *Haemophilus influenzae* meningitis: The spectrum of disease in adults. Medicine 61:74, 1982. *These 15 cases represent the largest series of cases of H. influenzae meningitis reported in the past 20 years. Particular emphasis is on predisposing factors in this unusual form of meningitis in adults.*

Wallace RJ Jr, Musher DM, Septimus EJ, et al.: *Haemophilus influenzae* infections in adults: Characterization of strains by serotypes, biotypes, and β-lactamase production. J Infect Dis 144:101, 1981. *This is a detailed review of 103 cases of H. influenzae bacteremia or meningitis. Noteworthy is the frequency of nontypable strains among blood isolates in adults and the infrequency of ampicillin resistance in the same group.*

HEMOPHILUS PARAINFLUENZAE AND HEMOPHILUS APHROPHILUS

Bieger RC, Brewer NS, Washington JA II: *Haemophilus aphrophilus*: A microbiologic and clinical review and report of 42 cases. Medicine 57:345, 1978. *A comprehensive review of the bacteriologic features, ecologic niche, and clinical impact of this uncommon cause of human disease.*

Oill PA, Chow AW, Guze LB: Adult bacteremic *Haemophilus parainfluenzae* infections: Seven reports of cases and a review of the literature. Arch Intern Med 139:985, 1979. *The type of infection (exclusive of endocarditis) caused by H. parainfluenzae and the antibiotic susceptibilities of this organism are summarized concisely.*

GARDNERELLA VAGINALIS (HEMOPHILUS VAGINALIS)

Spiegel CA, Amsel R, Eschenbach D, et al.: Anaerobic bacteria in nonspecific vaginitis. N Engl J Med 303:601, 1980. *Strong circumstantial evidence implicating both anaerobic bacteria and Gardnerella vaginalis (Hemophilus vaginalis) in the production of "nonspecific vaginitis" is presented. Good references for those uninformed about this entity.*

Osteomyelitis

275 OSTEOMYELITIS

Francis A. Waldvogel

DEFINITIONS. Osteomyelitis is an infection of bacterial, exceptionally of fungal, or viral origin that invades and destroys bone. Osteomyelitis is a well known, albeit rare, consequence of bacteremia. In other situations, such as open fractures, wounds, and orthopedic procedures, the microorganism gains access to bone from a contaminated or infected contiguous structure. Finally, peripheral bones can also be invaded by contiguity in case of severe vascular insufficiency. In the latter case, other metabolic and neurologic factors play an important contributory role.

ETIOLOGY. Most cases of osteomyelitis are of bacterial origin. Of all pathogenic organisms, *Staphylococcus aureus* is still the most common offending agent, whatever the mechanism of the infection. However, *S. epidermidis* has emerged in recent years as a frequent offender as well, for instance in hematogenous spread to the sternoclavicular joint or to a vertebral body from an infected intravenous line. *S. epidermidis* is also responsible for many bone infections secondary to implantation of prosthetic material, such as total hip prosthesis, where it can account for up to 30 per cent of the cases.

Other etiologic agents include gram-negative enteric organisms, which are often responsible for hematogenous vertebral osteomyelitis, certain *Salmonella* species that cause hematogenous disease in patients with sickle cell anemia, and rarely *Pseudomonas aeruginosa*, which can involve the spine in heroin addicts. Anaerobic organisms, either in pure or mixed cultures, have been isolated from infected bone in the vicinity of an anaerobic reservoir (maxilla, sinuses, sacrum), after human or animal bites, or from infected extremities in diabetic patients, where it may be associated or not with anaerobic cellulitis. *Mycobacterium tuberculosis* remains a diagnostic possibility in osteomyelitis of the spine with limited periosteal reaction, and in nonhealing bone infections. Various fungi can cause osteomyelitis under exceptional conditions, such as hematogenous spread from a chronically infected intravenous device or in connection with prosthetic material. Finally, exceptional cases of viral osteomyelitis have been described after chickenpox or smallpox.

All causes of osteomyelitis have not been discovered yet. Thus, multifocal hematogenous osteomyelitis is a syndrome occurring in children and young adults characterized by multiple, lytic inflammatory bone lesions in patients with various skin conditions such as pustulosis palmoplantaris and acne fulminans. Conventional bacterial cultures of biopsy specimens are negative, and the disease usually evolves toward cure without specific antibacterial therapy.

INCIDENCE, PREVALENCE, AND EPIDEMIOLOGY. Hematogenous osteomyelitis has a biphasic incidence, occurring mainly in children, in whom it shows a predilection for the metaphysis of long bones, and in adults beyond the age of 50 years, in whom it most often involves the spine. Blunt trauma is considered by many to be a favoring factor in children. In adults, any factor favoring bacteremia (urinary tract infection, prostatitis, various skin infections, prolonged intravenous therapy, or repeated injections) can occasionally lead to hematogenous osteomyelitis of the spine. The prevalence of osteomyelitis secondary to a contiguous focus varies according to the primary trauma, the invasive procedure performed, the type of material inserted, the underlying disease, and the degree of contamination of the wound. For instance, in well-planned aseptic interventions such as total hip replacement, the risk of infection is usually less than 1 per cent; insertions of total knee prostheses, on the other hand, are associated with a higher risk of infection, particularly in patients with rheumatoid arthritis; at the other end of the spectrum, the prevalence of postoperative osteomyelitis can reach 15 per cent after comminuted fracture.

PATHOGENESIS AND PATHOLOGY. The development of experimental models and the collection of better morphologic data have shed some new light on the mechanisms leading to bone destruction in osteomyelitis. The porous structure of bone, its canaliculi filled with capillaries and/or osteoblast cytoplasmic extensions, and the space between these organic structures and the mineral constituents, account for a nonnegligible fluid volume in bone, in the range of 5 per cent. In hematogenous osteomyelitis, microorganisms settle probably first in this fluid phase, where they will stimulate an active inflammatory reaction. Whether microorganisms have to adhere on the hydroxyapatite surface to escape host defense mechanisms, as suggested by other infection models, is uncertain at the present time. Since, however, microorganisms per se are unable to destroy bone tissue, one has to postulate that the inflammatory reaction, the metabolic alterations, and the vascular changes triggered by the bacterial invasion play a preponderant role in the development of an osteomyelitic focus, i.e., in bone destruction and regeneration. From a morphologic point of view, the following major changes can be identified: (1) bone necrosis, with death of the cellular constituents and disappearance of bone mass. Sometimes devitalized bone persists as a dead fragment called a sequestrum; (2) a heavy inflammatory reaction, in which granulocytes predominate initially but are replaced over time by a mononuclear infiltrate; (3) new bone apposition, originating from periosteal activation; this periosteal reaction is often the first sign of osteomyelitis identified on x-rays. In some cases, this bone apposition can be exuberant and lead to bridging of two adjacent bone structures, as in vertebral osteomyelitis. In other cases, bone apposition is very modest, and x-ray examination may show only an intraosseous, punched-out radiolucent lesion, as in subacute hematogenous osteomyelitis (Brodie's abscess) (Fig. 275–1).

CLINICAL MANIFESTATIONS. Acute hematogenous osteomyelitis involving long bones usually does not pose any major diagnostic problems: it starts as an acute episode with chills and fever, the young patient usually complaining of severe pain in the affected bone, most often the tibia or femur, more rarely the humerus. Clinical examination of the affected limb is usually unremarkable, except for pain on palpation of the affected area, usually the metaphysis. Characteristically, the adjacent joint is freely mobile and painless. If the infection is caused by an organism less virulent than *S. aureus*, however, the onset can be protracted, the pain less severe, and the fever moderate.

In hematogenous osteomyelitis of the spine, the clinical presentation is often characterized by progressive, ill-defined pain with low fever, following, for instance, an episode of urinary tract infection, bacteremia, or skin infection. The dull pain is usually located in the lower dorsal or lumbar segments of the spine ("febrile lumbago"). Any vertebral body can occasionally become involved by the disease, even the cervical spine ("febrile torticollis"). On physical examination, the mildly febrile patient usually has vertebral and paravertebral tenderness, but the overlying skin is normal. At this stage, there is usually no radicular pain and no sign of pyramidal tract involvement. Either of the two latter findings should suggest a paraspinal abscess, a dreaded complication of vertebral osteomyelitis calling for immediate neuroradiologic evaluation, surgical decompression, and appropriate antibiotic therapy (see Spinal Epidural Abscess in Ch. 481).

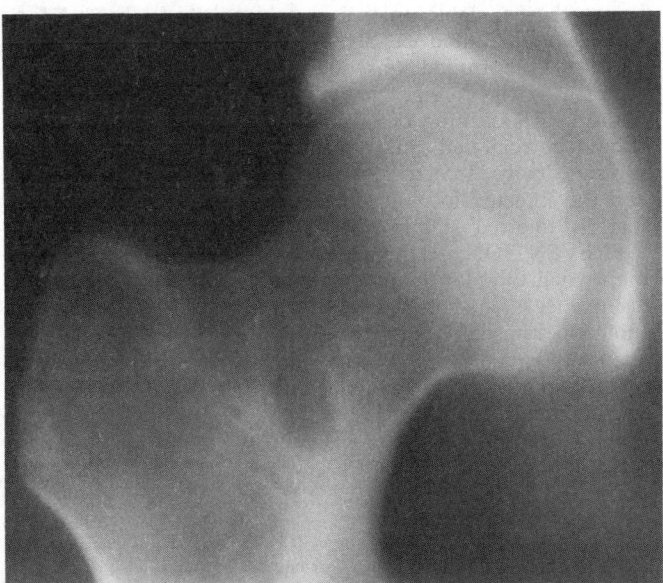

FIGURE 275–1. Subacute osteomyelitis (Brodie's abscess), hematogenous, in the right femur of a 31-year-old male.

Under exceptional circumstances, a patient with hematogenous osteomyelitis—usually of long bones—will present only with pain in the affected area, without fever. X-rays show a punched-out lesion, without expansion beyond cortical bone. Without biopsy, it is difficult to differentiate such a lesion (Brodie's abscess) from benign tumors.

Osteomyelitis secondary to a contiguous focus of infection after open trauma or secondary to orthopedic reconstructive surgery is a diagnostic challenge, since pain, low-grade fever, local signs of low-grade inflammation, and x-ray findings are all compatible with postoperative repair and infection. Recurrence of mild fever one week after surgery or trauma, increasing pain on weight bearing after total joint prosthetic replacement (Fig. 275–2), poor healing of the incision, and drainage of increased amounts of serosanguineous fluid should alert the physician to the possibility of ongoing infection.

DIAGNOSIS AND DIFFERENTIAL DIAGNOSIS. Positive cultures for *S. epidermidis* should not be discarded as contaminants, but the organism should be further characterized as to sensitivity patterns, biotypes, even plasmid fingerprinting, since this organism has become a common pathogen in bone infection. If the blood cultures remain negative, a direct aspiration and/or bone biopsy should be performed for full microbiologic diagnosis. This is particularly true for vertebral osteomyelitis, which can be due to a great variety of microorganisms.

In osteomyelitis secondary to a focus of infection, the clinician is often tempted to perform a local superficial aspiration or to culture the fistulous tract for microbiologic diagnosis. Such cultures often yield multiple organisms, and it is often difficult to differentiate the pathogenic organisms from contaminants. Deep bone aspiration and/or biopsy is of greater value under these circumstances, and usually yields the offending organism in pure culture. For all cases of osteomyelitis, other laboratory tests are noncontributory: erythrocyte sedimentation rate is usually increased; the white blood cell count is normal or high; and blood chemical values, including alkaline phosphatases, are normal.

Radiologic changes are delayed, appearing several weeks after the onset of the disease. In hematogenous osteomyelitis of long bones, periosteal elevation and subsequent bone destruction are the first changes to be observed. In veretebral osteomyelitis, progressive piecemeal destruction of two adjacent vertebral plateaus, narrowing of the intervertebral space, and progressive anterior periosteal bridging are the hallmarks of the disease, bone sclerosis being a late event. In tuberculous

osteomyelitis of the spine, the changes just mentioned are delayed and occur over several months, periosteal reaction usually being absent.

In most cases of hematogenous osteomyelitis, ^{99m}Tc-polyphosphate uptake, although nonspecific, can be of great diagnostic help by identifying the suspected areas of infection for appropriate tomograms at a stage when conventional x-ray results are still normal. In osteomyelitis secondary to a contiguous focus of infection, radiologic techniques and bone scanning are less helpful, since they cannot distinguish between normal bone reaction and infection. When detailed radiologic information is mandatory, such as in identifying an abscess in acute osteomyelitis, demonstrating sequestra in chronic osteomyelitis, or searching for a possible paraspinal abscess in vertebral body infection, CT scanning can offer additional diagnostic help. However, besides identifying such complications, this procedure has not been helpful in decreasing the delay in early diagnosis of osteomyelitis.

Acute hematogenous osteomyelitis of long bones has to be differentiated clinically from septic arthritis, bursitis, and cellulitis. These more superficial infections are accompanied by local skin changes, and x-ray results remain normal. Osteomyelitis of the spine is a diagnostic challenge and has to be differentiated from bone tumors such as myeloma and metastases, which usually do not involve two adjacent vertebral plateaus. In case of doubt, bone biopsy may be indicated.

TREATMENT. The therapeutic approach to osteomyelitis is both surgical and medical: For instance, although acute hematogenous osteomyelitis is usually treated medically, an orthopedic surgeon should be ready to intervene in case of abscess or sequestrum formation, pathologic fracture, etc.

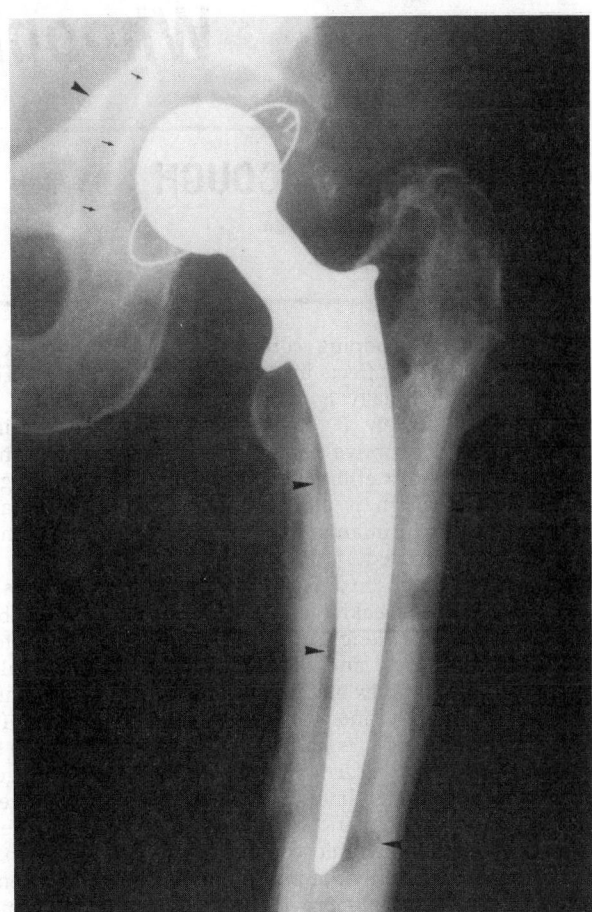

FIGURE 275–2. Osteomyelitis secondary to a contiguous focus of infection: infection after placement of a total hip prosthesis in a 63-year-old patient.

Conversely, osteomyelitis after total hip replacement will need prompt surgical intervention for debridement, and possibly for hip replacement, under coverage of appropriate antibiotic therapy.

Appropriate medical treatment of osteomyelitis implies isolation of the offending organism and a complete assessment of its antibiotic sensitivities. In case of *S. aureus* sensitive to cloxacillin, this drug should be used at a dosage of 8 grams per day parenterally. In case of an *S. aureus* or *S. epidermidis* resistant to cloxacillin, vancomycin at a dosage of 2 grams per day given every 12 hours as a slow infusion is the treatment of choice. For all other organisms, the following rule can be applied: Those parenteral antibiotics usually effective for the treatment of septicemia due to a particular organism will also be appropriate for osteomyelitis, provided that they are administered over a four- to six-week period. Thus, osteomyelitis of the spine caused by a gram-negative organism will be cured by a four- to six-week course of ampicillin, a first or second generation cephalosporin, or an aminoglycoside, depending on the sensitivity pattern. Although some investigators have advocated oral therapy in uncomplicated pediatric cases, no comparable studies, with adequate follow-up, are currently available in adults. Bed rest is usually recommended until all signs of inflammation have abated, pain has subsided, and x-rays show signs of improvement. This is particularly true for osteomyelitis of the spine. Surgery is generally unnecessary in hematogenous infection, except for drainage of intramedullary abscesses, removal of sequestra, and decompression if neurologic signs supervene in vertebral osteomyelitis. In osteomyelitis secondary to a contiguous focus of infection, however, careful evaluation of the situation by a skilled orthopedic surgeon is mandatory. In case of infected fractures or prostheses, stable union is a prerequisite for bacteriologic cure. Union should be achieved first despite sepsis, and infection is controlled subsequently by antibiotic therapy after removal of the foreign material. In case of nonunion of a fracture or loosening of the prosthesis, the foreign material should be removed, and if possible replaced by an external fixation device. Infected prostheses should also be removed and the infected focus cleaned out, with reinsertion of new material in a one-step or two-step procedure.

PREVENTION. At present, there is no preventive treatment available for hematogenous osteomyelitis, since the occurrence of the disease after bacteremia is unpredictable. Infection rates after insertion of hip prostheses have been shown to be markedly decreased by short-term coverage (two to three days) with parenteral antistaphylococcal antibiotics. Such coverage should also be considered in high-risk operations, such as reduction of comminuted fractures, open fractures, and insertion of joint prostheses in high risk patients.

Kido D, Bryan D, Halpern M: Hematogenous osteomyelitis in drug addicts. Ther Nucl Med 118:356, 1973. *A concise study of 32 cases, most of them due to* Pseudomonas *species. Discusses their clinical and radiologic manifestations.*

Larde D, Mathieu D, Frija J, et al.: Vertebral osteomyelitis: Disk hypodensity on CT. AJR 139:963, 1982. *Thirty-six cases of vertebral osteomyelitis, investigated by CT scan for early diagnosis of complications.*

Waldvogel FA, Medoff G, Swartz MN: Osteomyelitis: A review of clinical features, therapeutic considerations and unusual aspects I. II. III. N Engl J Med 282:198, 260, 316, 1970. *A retrospective review of 247 cases of osteomyelitis, their clinical and radiologic presentations, and their treatment.*

Waldvogel FA, Vasey H: Osteomyelitis: The past decade. N Engl J Med 303:360, 1980. *A review update of newer approaches in diagnosis and treatment of osteomyelitis, with emphasis on a combined surgical and medical approach.*

Wing VW, Jeffrey RB, Federle MP, et al.: Chronic osteomyelitis examined by CT. Radiology 154:171, 1985. *The additional information obtained by CT scanning in case of sequestra is well illustrated in 14 out of 25 patients with chronic osteomyelitis.*

Whooping Cough

276 WHOOPING COUGH (Pertussis)

Samuel L. Katz

DEFINITION. Whooping cough is an acute respiratory illness that classically affects infants and young children. The etiologic agent is usually *Bordetella pertussis;* occasionally *B. parapertussis* and rarely *B. bronchiseptica* produce a similar syndrome. The descriptive name derives from a distressing, prolonged inspiratory effort that follows paroxysmal coughing. Whooping cough is still responsible for a significant number of deaths in infants in areas where pertussis immunization is not practiced.

ETIOLOGY. When first isolated, *Bordetella pertussis* is a minute, nonmotile, weakly staining, gram-negative coccobacillus, 0.5 to 1.0 μ in length. Capsules can be demonstrated by special procedures, and bipolar metachromatic granules are present. The complex medium containing blood originally employed by Bordet and Gengou is still often used for cultivation. *Primary isolates, phase I organisms, will not grow on conventional laboratory media,* but will do so after prolonged passage. At the same time colonial morphology changes, marked pleomorphism of individual cells is evident, and there is an alteration in antigenic composition. This occurs in a series of phases, but only the phase I organisms are virulent, and *only phase I organisms* provide effective immunizing material.

The addition of blood to Bordet-Gengou medium is required for the growth of phase I organisms, but charcoal, starch, or ion exchange resins can be substituted for blood.

A single protein exotoxin ("pertussis toxin") purified from the organism's envelope is antigenic and responsible for the induction of histamine sensitization (HSF), activation of pancreatic islet cells (IAP), and lymphocytosis (LPF). Other toxins of *B. pertussis* include a heat-labile toxin and a heat-stable toxin (lipopolysaccharide). There are an extracytoplasmic adenylate cyclase, two hemagglutinins (the filamentous protein from fimbria, FHA, and the HSF-LPF-IAP hemagglutinin) as well as O and K surface and capsular antigens. The roles of these constituents in disease production and in the development of protective immunity are under investigation. The fimbrial hemagglutinin is apparently responsible for attachment of *B. pertussis* to ciliated respiratory epithelial cells. The systemic disease manifestations are likely caused by circulating pertussis toxin.

Approximately 5 to 10 per cent of clinical whooping cough may be caused by *B. parapertussis.* The animal pathogen *B. bronchiseptica* is responsible for a very minor percentage of cases. These organisms can be differentiated from *B. pertussis* by growth requirements, enzyme production, and presence of species-specific antigens. It has been suggested that adenoviruses, alone or in concert with *B. pertussis,* may play an etiologic role in some cases of whooping cough.

EPIDEMIOLOGY. In communities of susceptibles the family attack rate is 80 to 90 per cent. Transmission is by droplet infection. Carriers of *B. pertussis* are found infrequently, but persons previously immunized have been shown during outbreaks of disease to excrete the organism in the absence of clinical illness.

The mortality rate from whooping cough has fallen since

the turn of this century owing to improved supportive therapy. The incidence of whooping cough, however, did not change until after the 1940's, when immunization of young children became standard practice. In the 1940's, approximately 200,000 cases of pertussis were reported annually in the United States; in 1986, 4100 cases were reported. At the same time, the fatality rate has dropped from 20 per 1000 patients to 3. The majority of deaths, over 70 per cent, occur in children under one year of age, with the preponderance in infants under the age of six months.

Neither immunization against pertussis nor natural disease provides lifelong protection. In the case of artificial immunization, an attack rate greater than 50 per cent has been reported when the interval after immunization exceeds 12 years.

PATHOLOGY. Interpretation of pathologic material obtained at autopsy is difficult because of the common presence of complicating respiratory infections. Lesions caused by *B. pertussis* are found principally in the bronchi and bronchioles, but changes are also seen in the nasopharynx, larynx, and trachea. Masses of bacteria are intertwined with the cilia of the columnar epithelium together with mucopurulent exudate. Adherence of organisms to ciliated respiratory epithelial cells is the crucial element in pathogenesis of disease. There is also necrosis of the midzonal and basilar epithelium with infiltration of polymorphonuclear leukocytes and macrophages. Peribronchial accumulation of lymphocytes and granulocytes produces the picture of interstitial pneumonitis. Secondary atelectasis and localized emphysema are common.

CLINICAL MANIFESTATIONS. After an incubation period of 7 to 16 days, symptoms appear. It is customary to divide the clinical course into three stages, each of two weeks' duration, but variation is frequent.

Catarrhal Stage. Whooping cough begins with symptoms indistinguishable from those of a mild viral upper respiratory infection or common cold. Sneezing is frequent, the conjunctivae are injected, and a nocturnal cough appears. The temperature may be slightly elevated at this time. Infectivity is greatest at this stage.

Paroxysmal Stage. Seven to 14 days after onset, the cough becomes more frequent, diurnal, and then paroxysmal. In a typical paroxysm there is a series of 15 to 20 short coughs of increasing intensity, and then with a deep inspiration the air is drawn into the lungs, making the "whoop." A tenacious mucous plug is usually expelled, and vomiting frequently follows. Paroxysms may occur as often as every half hour and are accompanied by signs of increased venous pressure. The conjunctivae are deeply engorged; there is periorbital edema; and petechial hemorrhages, particularly about the forehead, as well as epistaxis are common. During the attack the infant may be cyanotic until the crowing whoop occurs. In between paroxysms the child usually feels well, although justifiably apprehensive. This phase lasts two to four weeks.

Physical examination of the chest is often unremarkable, although scattered rhonchi may be heard. The chest roentgenogram sometimes reveals hilar and mediastinal nodal enlargement. The presence of fever immediately suggests the development of a secondary infectious process.

Convalescent Stage. Gradually the paroxysms become less frequent and less intense; vomiting ceases, and slow recovery ensues. Convalescence requires 4 to 12 weeks. Often for many months even a mild, unrelated respiratory infection will induce a return of paroxysmal cough and whoop.

In very young infants the paroxysms and the whoop are often absent; instead, choking spells and apneic episodes may be the major manifestations. Second attacks of whooping cough as well as disease occurring in previously immunized individuals often present simply as an upper respiratory illness or bronchitis.

Complications. Complications may be related to the primary disease or to secondary events. Alterations in acid-base bal-

ance occur as a result of metabolic alkalosis when vomiting is severe. Recurrent vomiting can also lead to malnutrition. Anoxemic manifestations are seen when ventilation is markedly impaired. Central nervous system changes can result from cerebral anoxia or hemorrhages consequent to the elevated venous pressure. Rarely, cortical degeneration occurs, but the exact pathogenesis of the encephalopathy is unknown. A serous meningitis with lymphocytosis of the cerebrospinal fluid has been described. Localized areas of emphysema and atelectasis generally return to normal after the disease has run its course, and pneumothorax and interstitial emphysema are infrequently seen.

The major cause of death in whooping cough is complicating pneumonia or bronchopneumonia caused by other bacteria or viruses. In addition, secondary bacterial otitis media occurs frequently.

DIAGNOSIS. There is little difficulty in making the clinical diagnosis of whooping cough in a patient who, after a variable period of coryzal symptoms, develops paroxysmal coughing with a terminal inspiratory whoop. Toward the end of the catarrhal stage, or early in the spasmodic phase, leukocytosis often occurs. In contrast to the leukocytosis found in most bacterial diseases, the predominating cell type is the mature small lymphocyte. Characteristically the leukocyte count ranges from 15,000 to 30,000 per cubic millimeter or higher, and 80 per cent of the cells are small lymphocytes. Polymorphonuclear leukocytosis suggests a secondary bacterial complication.

Difficulty in recognizing whooping cough occurs in the catarrhal stage, in abortive or mild cases, and in young infants. Epidemiologic awareness may suggest the possibility, but microbiologic identification of the organisms is required. During the early stages *B. pertussis* can be isolated from approximately 90 per cent of patients. By the third or fourth week the organism can be recovered in only 50 per cent of cases, and in the convalescent stage it is unusual to obtain a positive culture.

Adequate specimens and appropriate media are essential if bacteriologic diagnosis is to be efficient. *Specimens are best obtained by pernasal swab rather than by the cough plate method.* A sterile cotton swab wrapped about a flexible copper wire is passed through the nares, and mucus is obtained from the posterior pharynx. The swab must not be allowed to dry out because *B. pertussis* is readily killed by desiccation. As quickly as possible the specimen is plated onto fresh medium, to which penicillin has been added to prevent overgrowth of adventitious organisms.

A fluorescent antibody staining procedure that can be applied directly to clinical specimens as well as to organisms grown in culture has been utilized by many state diagnostic laboratories and the Centers for Disease Control. It greatly accelerates the identification of organisms after isolation, but is less reliable in its direct application to nasopharyngeal swabs or other clinical material.

Serologic procedures are of little help in the diagnosis of whooping cough because a rise in titer of most antibodies does not occur until at least the third week of illness. Tests are not well standardized, and few laboratories perform them.

It is difficult to distinguish abortive or mild cases of pertussis from tracheobronchitis caused by other agents.

TREATMENT. Mild cases of pertussis require only supportive treatment. Specific therapy of severe whooping cough has been disappointing despite the in vitro susceptibility of *B. pertussis* to various antimicrobial agents and the protective effect of passively administered antibody in experimental disease.

Antimicrobials. A number of antimicrobial drugs have significant activity against *B. pertussis* in vitro. In the established paroxysmal stage the organisms can be readily eliminated by antimicrobials, but the course of the illness is unaltered.

Antibiotics may be justified in order to render the patient noninfectious.

Erythromycin, oxytetracycline, and several other drugs are effective in eliminating organisms. Erythromycin is the drug of choice. The daily dose is 50 mg per kilogram of body weight given in four divided doses. The organism is eliminated after a few days of therapy, but because bacteriologic relapse may occur, treatment should be continued for 14 to 21 days.

Immunotherapy. Hyperimmune human gamma globulin has previously been used in therapy of unimmunized patients, particularly small infants, with no efficacy demonstrated in controlled trials.

Supportive Therapy. Particularly in the young infant, supportive measures combined with careful nursing care are of paramount importance. Specific attention must be devoted to the maintenance of proper water and electrolyte balance, adequate nutrition, and sufficient oxygenation. Constant alertness for the presence of secondary infectious complications such as pneumonia is required.

PREVENTION. Unfortunately, the diagnosis is usually not made until the end of the catarrhal stage, and by then spread of the disease has already occurred. Exposed susceptibles should receive erythromycin prophylaxis, and close (household, day care classroom) contacts under seven years of age who have been previously immunized should receive a booster dose of vaccine in addition to erythromycin. Booster doses of vaccine have been used to protect adults, such as hospital staff, but side effects tend to be frequent, and erythromycin chemoprophylaxis may be preferable.

Active Immunization. The fall in incidence of whooping cough in the very young is directly related to widespread immunization. The highest risk of serious morbidity and mortality is in the young infant. Women of childbearing age generally do not have significant levels of protective antibody in their sera, and these antibodies do not cross the placenta. Consequently, newborns are not protected by maternal antibodies. Therefore active immunization is begun as early as is commensurate with the production of a satisfactory immune response. At present, it is recommended that the infant receive three injections of pertussis vaccine at eight-week intervals commencing at age two months. The pertussis suspension is incorporated into a triple vaccine with alum-precipitated diphtheria and tetanus toxoids (DTP). Booster injections are given one and five years after completion of the initial course. Administration of pertussis vaccine to those over six years of age is not generally recommended because of an apparent increased incidence of untoward reactions and the diminished risk of the illness itself in the older child. However, low doses have been administered to adults without incident.

As previously noted, immunization does not confer lifelong protection. Approximately 80 per cent of those vaccinated within four years of exposure will be protected, whereas 80 to 90 per cent of a matched unimmunized group with similar exposure will contract pertussis. The prophylactic efficacy of pertussis vaccine was clearly demonstrated when epidemics occurred in the United Kingdom in 1977–1979 and 1982 following a three- to five-year period during which vaccine acceptance had declined to very low levels. More than 170,000 cases of whooping cough were reported, including 42 deaths, principally among children under five years of age. Similar outbreaks have followed diminished vaccine utilization in Japan and Sweden.

Local reactions as well as fever, hyperirritability, or seizures may occur after injection of pertussis vaccine. The exact incidence of the more severe complication of encephalopathy is uncertain. A recent British study suggests a risk of 1 in 100,000 immunizations for previously normal infants, with residual neurologic damage in 30 per cent of those affected. Despite the small, but real, incidence of neurologic complications of pertussis immunization, the risk is far less than the hazards of whooping cough in the young child. Nevertheless, in infants with a personal history of convulsions or other neurologic disorders, pertussis immunization should be deferred until the condition has stabilized and is under medical control. A Japanese vaccine containing only the two *B. pertussis* hemagglutinins (pertussis toxin and the filamentous hemagglutinin), extracted, purified, and formalin-treated, is far less reactogenic than the whole bacterial cell vaccine. If tests currently under way in Sweden and the United States of its immunogenicity and prophylactic efficacy are convincing in field use, it should replace the killed whole cell vaccine. An inactivated pertussis toxin vaccine is also under investigation.

Aoyama T, Murase Y, Kato T, et al.: Efficacy of an acellular pertussis vaccine in Japan. J Pediatr 107:180, 1985. *Seventy-nine per cent prophylactic efficacy of the Japanese acellular vaccine in prevention of secondary household cases.*

Geller RJ: The pertussis syndrome: A persistent problem. Pediatr Infect Dis J 3:182, 1984. *A succinct "state-of-the-art" presentation of diagnosis, clinical picture, and management today.*

Lewis K, Cherry JD, Holroyd HJ, et al.: A double-blind study comparing an acellular pertussis-component DTP vaccine with a whole-cell pertussis-component DTP vaccine in 18-month-old children. Am J Dis Child 140:872, 1986. *The first study in this country of the cellular vaccine, demonstrating diminished reactogenicity but intact immunogenicity.*

Manclark CR, Hill JC: International Symposium on Pertussis. Washington, D.C., US Dept HEW NIH, 1979. *This 387-page volume contains informative papers on research dealing with the organism, its components, infection, disease control, and vaccine development.*

Miller DL, Alderslade R, Ross EM: Whooping cough and whooping cough vaccine: The risks and benefits debate. Epidem Rev 4:1, 1982. *Particularly cogent at this time when public confidence in pertussis vaccine has been eroded by media presentations.*

Sato Y, Kimura M, Fukumi H: Development of a pertussis component vaccine in Japan. Lancet 1:122, 1984. *The great hope for an improved less reactive vaccine in the 1980's.*

Diphtheria

277 DIPHTHERIA

Erik L. Hewlett

Diphtheria is an acute infectious disease caused by toxigenic *Corynebacterium diphtheriae.* The infection usually localizes in the pharynx, larynx, nostrils, and occasionally the skin. Severe systemic disease and mortality occur most frequently in patients with pharyngeal infection and are largely attributable to an exotoxin released by the bacteria at the site of localized infection. The disease, but not necessarily the local infection, is preventable by immunization with diphtheria toxoid.

ETIOLOGY. *Corynebacterium diphtheriae* is a pleomorphic, non–spore-forming, non–acid-fast, non-motile gram-positive rod that on smears is often seen in palisades or configurations resembling Chinese characters. Its club-end appearance is the origin of the name *Corynebacterium,* from the Greek *korynee,* meaning club. The heterogeneous morphology of corynebacteria makes diagnosis on the basis of stained smear unreliable. *C. diphtheriae* grows well on tellurite agar or Loeffler's serum slants under aerobic conditions and is distinguished from related corynebacteria by fermentation of glucose and maltose, but not sucrose. Although the organisms are killed by mild heating (56° C for 10 minutes), they are strikingly resistant to damage from drying and can be cultured from floor dust for five weeks or longer.

The species is divided into three stable biotypes, named *gravis*, *intermedius*, and *mitis*, to indicate their relative virulence in epidemics during the early twentieth century. Although there is not now a direct correlation between biotypes and severity of disease, their identification on the basis of cell and colony morphology, fermentation patterns, and hemolytic activity remains useful for epidemiologic purposes. Recent data from the United States indicate that the *intermedius* type is the most commonly isolated, with *mitis* second and *gravis* least. Similarly, among all isolates, the *intermedius* biotype was most frequently toxigenic (98.9 per cent) followed by *gravis* (84.0 per cent) and *mitis* (34.1 per cent). *Gravis* is frequently associated with epidemics of clinical diphtheria, whereas *mitis* is more often isolated from endemic cases or asymptomatic carriers.

The major virulence determinant is an exotoxin that is produced by organisms infected by a lysogenic β-phage. The toxin structural gene is carried in the genome of the phage, and toxin is produced by lysogenized *C. diphtheriae* only after exhaustion of the iron in the medium. Toxigenicity of an isolate can be determined in vitro by the Elek test, in which the clinical isolate is streaked at right angles to an antitoxin-impregnated strip of filter paper on a plate. If the strain is toxigenic, a precipitin line of toxin-antitoxin complex forms during culture. Toxigenicity testing in vivo involves intraperitoneal injection of a suspension of organisms into naive and antitoxin-treated guinea pigs. Death of the test animal, but not the antitoxin recipient, in one to four days indicates toxin production.

EPIDEMIOLOGY. Diphtheria is a highly contagious infection that is spread most easily under socioeconomic conditions in which there is poor personal hygiene, crowding, and limited access to medical care. The primary route of transmission has been by aerosol or other transfer of respiratory secretions from an infected individual. As illustrated by several outbreaks among adults in the United States, however, direct spread from cutaneous lesions of subjects with little or no systemic disease is of increasing importance epidemiologically. The skin infections of these carriers may occur in many different forms, such as purulent, punched-out ulcers, impetiginous lesions, and wound infections, and, as a consequence, are frequently difficult to identify in the absence of classic cases of diphtheria in contacts. Furthermore, the diagnosis may be missed because of the presence of a mixed infection with staphylococci or streptococci. Such localized infections with limited toxin absorption are postulated to be the source of acquired immunity among unimmunized children in the tropics. Less frequently, transmission may occur by contact with fomites (such as unclean blankets) or by ingestion of infected milk. While infections of animals, especially cattle, can be the source of human disease, this is an uncommon mechanism of transmission and there are no known reservoirs in nature. Molecular epidemiologic studies indicate that strains of *C. diphtheriae* are stable in a population and that changes in disease rates may occur by introduction and transmission of the β-phage among previously nontoxigenic strains.

Immunization status influences severity of disease in the individual patient. When disease does occur in immunized or partially immunized patients, mortality (1.3 per cent) is 10-fold lower than in unimmunized individuals (13.4 per cent). Herd immunity has a major impact on patterns of transmission and carriage of *C. diphtheriae*. Although it was expected by some that immunization with diphtheria toxoid would increase the rate of carriage of *C. diphtheriae* in a population, the opposite is true. The selective advantage of toxigenicity is

lost, and fewer toxigenic strains are found in an immunized population. Although some serologic surveys indicate a high proportion of susceptible adults in the population, clinical diphtheria is at its lowest level ever, with no cases reported in the United States in 1986.

PATHOGENESIS. Following arrival of *C. diphtheriae* at the site of infection, organisms proliferate and elaborate toxin. As with other bacterial diseases that are mediated in large part by exotoxins, the rapidity of onset, severity of disease, and ultimate outcome are determined by the rate of production, absorption, and dissemination of the toxin. The determinants of these variables include the site of infection, the virulence of the strain (quantity of toxin produced and availability of ancillary factors to facilitate toxin absorption), and the status of host immunity. For example, individuals with *C. diphtheriae* infection of the skin, middle ear, or anterior nares, sites from which toxin absorption is less than across the pharyngeal mucosa, may have little or no systemic disease. Prior immunity, by virtue of immunization or prior infection, may prevent systemic manifestations of disease without affecting the localized carriage of the organism.

Diphtheria toxin, probably the best studied of all bacterial toxins, is synthesized as an inactive single polypeptide of MW = 61,000. It is activated by proteolytic cleavage and reduction of the interchain disulfide bonds, yielding two subunits (A or active subunit and B or binding subunit). Upon reaching the host cell, the B subunit attaches to a specific glycoprotein receptor, a step that is required for internalization of the A subunit by receptor-mediated endocytosis. Within mammalian cells, the A subunit catalyzes the transfer of the adenosine diphosphate ribose (ADPR) portion of nicotinamide adenine dinucleotide (NAD) to a novel and specific target amino acid (modified histidine named diphthamide because of this reaction) on a single protein, elongation factor 2, which is required for protein synthesis. The consequence to the cell is interruption of protein synthesis, disruption of cell processes requiring new proteins, and, ultimately, cell death. The consequences to the infected host depend upon the type of cells intoxicated and the extent of intoxication. The toxin and other ancillary factors probably contribute to the formation of the characteristic membrane, which is composed of necrotic epithelial cells, leukocytes, bacteria, and fibrin. It is hypothesized that the cardiomyopathy, the cardiac conduction abnormalities, and the neuropathy are attributable to action of the toxin on cardiac and nerve cells. Other products of the organism must be involved in the establishment of the infection and the development of local pathology, however, since nontoxigenic strains can produce localized infection.

CLINICAL MANIFESTATIONS. The manifestations of infection with *C. diphtheriae* can range from a single, localized lesion without systemic signs or symptoms to a rapidly progressive, fatal illness. In general, the severity of the disease is correlated with the magnitude and site of the local lesion, and, in fact, the different clinical presentations have been classified on the basis of the primary site of infection.

Symptoms begin after an incubation period of less than one week. Patients with anterior nasal or middle ear infection with *C. diphtheriae* are generally well, with little or no local pain and often only purulent drainage from the involved site. Occasionally, a thin membrane with associated crusting can be seen. Because of the infrequent occurrence of systemic toxicity, these lesions can become chronic, providing a source for transmission to contacts.

Tonsillar or faucial diphtheria, while not frequently life-threatening, can be associated with severe complications. At the time of presentation, patients are moderately ill, with complaints of low grade fever, fatigue, headache, and sore throat. The typical adherent, grayish-green membrane may be localized to one tonsil or may extend across the midline and anteriorly. Such patients have the potential for abrupt deterioration and warrant close observation.

Pharyngeal diphtheria, especially associated with laryngeal and bronchial extension, represents an extreme in the spectrum of clinical presentations. The patient is gravely ill with weak pulse, restlessness, and confusion, but at the same time may be afebrile. The diphtheritic membrane may be extensive, covering the posterior pharynx and extending upward into the nasopharynx, forward onto the hard palate, and downward through the larynx. The thick, partially necrotic membrane is difficult to remove and is the source of the classic, but not diagnostic, foul odor associated with this disease. Development of anterior cervical warmth and edema resulting in the "bull neck" appearance is not uncommon in extensive pharyngeal disease. Patients in whom the membrane extends to the larynx and beyond experience airway obstruction with stridor and cyanosis.

Clinical diphtheria may be associated with dysfunction of a variety of tissues, especially heart and nerve, and these complications are the major cause of morbidity and mortality. Myocarditis, for example, occurs in 50 per cent of patients with moderately severe disease, apparently as a result of direct toxin action on myocardial cells and perhaps subsequent inflammation and fibrosis. The onset may be slow, with manifestations after the local pharyngeal lesion is improving. There are concurrent abnormalities of the cardiac conducting system, as indicated by ECG abnormalities such as ST-T wave changes, arrhythmias, and heart block. The rapid onset of ECG changes, circulatory collapse, and congestive failure indicates a high level of systemic intoxication and a very poor prognosis.

Functionally significant intoxication of neural tissue occurs in 10 to 20 per cent of patients and is manifested by cranial nerve palsies, peripheral neuropathies, and frank paralysis. Patients may experience difficulty swallowing with regurgitation and aspiration of liquids, extremity weakness, and even respiratory failure. These deficits may be first recognized four or more weeks after onset of the illness, but, if the patient survives, are generally slowly reversible.

DIAGNOSIS. Although bacteriologic identification is a critical feature of diphtheria diagnosis, therapy for this life-threatening illness must not await culture confirmation. Gram-stained or fluorescent antibody–stained material can be used to increase the index of suspicion but is not adequate for definitive diagnosis. Swabs from nose and pharynx or other sites should be cultured on Loeffler's slants and the more selective tellurite agar, as well as blood agar. All clinical isolates of *C. diphtheriae* should be tested for toxigenicity by the Elek test. Since coinfection with staphylococci and streptococci can occur, the presence of these organisms does not rule out diphtheria.

In milder cases, the diphtheritic membrane may not be striking and other physical findings are not distinguishing. Although the sore throat is generally less than with a streptococcal infection, the differential diagnosis should include streptococcal pharyngitis, oral candidiasis, infectious mononucleosis, and Vincent's angina.

TREATMENT AND PREVENTION. The goals of therapy in a patient with presumed or documented diphtheria are neutralization of free toxin, elimination of further toxin production, control of the local infection, support during the course of the systemic intoxication phase, and prevention of transmission. The mainstays of treatment, therefore, are (1) equine diphtheria antitoxin (human diphtheria immune globulin is not available in the United States), (2) antibiotics, (3) supportive intervention directed at complications such as respiratory compromise, congestive heart failure, cardiac arrhythmias, neuropathies, renal failure, and bleeding diatheses, and (4) strict isolation.

Presumptive diagnosis of diphtheria is adequate justification for use of diphtheria antitoxin, since the severe life-threatening complications are the result of toxin action at distal sites and immediate neutralization of circulating toxin is essential. The dose of antitoxin is based upon the site and extent of the local infection and the severity and duration of symptoms at the time of presentation. Patients with cutaneous infection generally do not experience toxicity, but a low dose of antitoxin (20,000 units) is sometimes given. A dose of 20,000 to 40,000 units of antitoxin is recommended for patients with limited pharyngeal disease of two days or less duration. Patients with more extensive nasopharyngeal involvement, especially of greater than three days duration and associated with bull neck and other complications, require 80,000 to 100,000 units of antitoxin. The antitoxin is most effective when given intravenously, but because it is of equine origin, patients must be tested for hypersensitivity before administration and desensitized as necessary.

Antibiotics are required for prevention of further toxin production, control of local infection, and reduction of transmission, as untreated convalescent carriage can persist for weeks. Treatment with penicillin or erythromycin should be followed by repeat culture to document elimination of the organism. Since the consequences of toxin action within target cells cannot be reversed pharmacologically, patients with life-threatening complications need intensive monitoring and specific supportive therapy as indicated. For example, myocarditis with arrhythmias and congestive heart failure may necessitate salt restriction, digitalis, antiarrhythmics, and even temporary pacing during the height of the illness. As with other toxin-mediated diseases, there may not be a sufficient immune response to provide future protection, and convalescent individuals should receive diphtheria toxoid immunization.

All contacts should be cultured. Those immunized five or more years previously should receive a booster and those never immunized should be treated prophylactically with antibiotics. All asymptomatic carriers detected should be treated with antibiotics to eliminate the organism and immunized with either a primary series or booster as indicated.

The only effective measure for prevention of clinical diphtheria is immunization with diphtheria toxoid. The primary series is three doses given in conjunction with tetanus toxoid and pertussis vaccine during the first six months of life. Boosters are given at 15 months and 4 to 6 years of age. In order to maintain immunity during adolescence and adulthood, boosters are needed at 10-year intervals using a preparation containing a reduced amount of the diphtheria toxoid, owing to adverse reactions related to some prior immunity. The reduced dose for adults is available alone or in combination with tetanus toxoid (Td).

Although not commonly determined at the present time except as an epidemiologic research tool, susceptibility of an individual to clinical diphtheria can be assessed by quantitation in vitro of toxin-neutralizing antibody in the serum or by the Schick test, which involves injection of a low dose of native diphtheria toxin intradermally and observation for evidence of local toxin damage (redness, edema at 48 to 96 hours). A positive reaction indicates lack of neutralizing antibody and susceptibility to disease.

Chen RT, Broome CV, Weinstein RA, et al.: Diphtheria in the United States, 1971–1981. Am J Public Health 75:1393, 1985. *Summary of recent trends in diphtheria epidemiology.*

Hewlett EL: Selective primary health care: Strategies for control of disease in the developing world. XVIII. Pertussis and diphtheria. Rev Infect Dis 7:426, 1985. *Review of approaches to control of diphtheria, compared and contrasted with pertussis.*

McCloskey RV, Ellner JJ, Green M, et al.: The 1970 epidemic of diphtheria in San Antonio. Ann Intern Med 75:495, 1971. *Complete and careful evaluation of an epidemic.*

Pappenheimer AM: Diphtheria: Studies on the biology of an infectious disease. The Harvey Lectures, Academic Press, 1982. Series 76, pp 45–73. *Detailed description of the cellular and molecular biology of toxin structure and function.*

Wilson G: Corynebacteriae and other coryneform organisms. Chapter 25, vol. 1, pp 94–110, and Wilson G, Smith G: Diphtheria and other diseases due to corynebacteria. Chapter 53, vol. 2, pp 73–97. In Wilson GS (ed.): Topley and Wilson's Principles of Bacteriology, Virology and Immunity. 7th ed. Baltimore, Williams & Wilkins, 1983. *Useful compilation of microbiologic and epidemiologic data.*

Clostridial Diseases

John G. Bartlett

278 CLOSTRIDIAL MYONECROSIS AND OTHER CLOSTRIDIAL DISEASES

Clostridia are gram-positive, spore-forming anaerobic bacteria that are widely distributed in soil and in the normal intestinal microflora of humans and animals. Sporulation permits survival in adverse conditions so that these organisms can be isolated with ease from almost any environmental source. Concentrations vary considerably, but any fertile loam is expected to contain at least 10^3 clostridia per gram. Clostridia have been found in the intestinal tract of almost all animals examined. Most humans harbor 10^9 to 10^{10} clostridia per gram of stool; these organisms are less commonly found in the normal flora of the skin, oral cavity, and female genital tract. *Clostridium perfringens*, the most frequent clinical isolate, is found in virtually all soil samples and, along with *C. ramosum*, is the most frequent clostridial species found in the intestinal flora of humans. Nevertheless, there are over 60 recognized species, and about 30 species have been found in human infections. Most clinical laboratories do not perform the extensive biochemical testing necessary to speciate clostridial isolates, and even when this is done, many organisms do not fit current taxonomic schema.

Clostridia cause diverse disease processes including bacteremia, localized infections at various anatomic sites, and the histotoxic clostridial syndromes. The latter refers to well-characterized syndromes caused by toxins elaborated under appropriate cultural conditions by various clostridial species (Table 278–1). The most commonly encountered histotoxic species is *C. perfringens*, which is divided into five types designated A to E on the basis of the production of the four major lethal toxins designated alpha, beta, epsilon, and iota. All *C. perfringens*, and many other species of clostridia (Table 278–1), produce alpha toxin, a phospholipase that splits lecithin to phosphoryl choline and a diglyceride. Intravenous administration of alpha toxin in experimental animals causes massive hemolysis, platelet destruction, and widespread capillary damage. Other clostridial toxins cause diseases of the intestine (enteric toxins) or of the nervous system (neurotoxins). The toxins of *C. botulinum* and *C. tetanus* are lethal to mice in doses of 1 ng. By extrapolation, the lethal dose in the bloodstream of humans is approximately 10^{-9} mg per kilogram body weight, making these toxins the most potent microbial poisons known. The toxins of *C. difficile* and the alpha toxin

of *C. perfringens* are about 100 to 1,000 times less potent in mouse lethality testing.

Smith LDS: The Pathogenic Anaerobic Bacteria. 2nd ed. Springfield, Charles C Thomas, 1975, pp 109–324. *The author, a noted authority in the field, provides a scholarly review of clostridia, including a description of the species, their natural habitat, their toxins, and their role in disease.*

CLOSTRIDIAL MYONECROSIS

DEFINITION. Clostridial myonecrosis, or gas gangrene, is a life-threatening infection involving muscle caused by toxins produced by clostridia, usually *C. perfringens*.

ETIOLOGY. Clostridial myonecrosis usually follows wounding from trauma or surgery, contamination with histotoxic clostridia, and toxin elaboration. It is estimated that 30 to 80 per cent of serious traumatic open wounds are contaminated by clostridia, although gas gangrene remains a relatively rare infection. This experience emphasizes the decisive role of local conditions that promote toxin production primarily by decreasing the oxidation-reduction potential. Contributing factors to tissue hypoxia include vascular insufficiency, the presence of foreign bodies, tissue necrosis, and concurrent infection involving other microbes.

The most frequent pathogen, *C. perfringens*, is found in approximately 80 per cent of cases with positive cultures. Other clostridial species implicated include *C. novyi, C. septicum, C. histolyticum, C. bifermentans,* and *C. fallax.* In many instances, there are several clostridial species isolated from the infected site. Species causing gas gangrene produce over 20 exotoxins, including seven that are lethal to experimental animals. Perhaps the most important toxin is *alpha toxin*, a lecithinase that destroys cell membranes, alters capillary permeability, destroys platelets, and causes severe hemolysis. In appropriate environmental conditions, vegetative forms of the histotoxic clostridia replicate and elaborate toxins that diffuse into adjacent soft tissue to promote local spread as well as extensive systemic effects.

CLINICAL MANIFESTATIONS. Gas gangrene is a devastating infection characterized by prominent findings at the site of injury and profound systemic toxicity. Most cases occur in association with wounding from trauma or surgery. The usual clinical settings are (1) traumatic injury or penetrating wound; (2) surgery, especially intestinal or biliary tract operations; (3) uterine gas gangrene, which most frequently follows delivery or septic abortions; (4) soft tissue lesions associated with vascular insufficiency; (5) intestinal gas gangrene, which is most commonly found in compromised hosts, especially patients with leukemia or colonic carcinoma; and (6) "spontaneous gas gangrene," a rare form of the disease in which there is no readily identifiable predisposing condition. During peacetime in the United States approximately 50 per cent of cases follow severe traumatic injury and 40 per cent follow surgery. The most frequent traumatic injuries are car accidents, crush injuries, industrial accidents, and gunshot wounds. The most frequent antecedent surgical procedures are colon resection and biliary tract surgery. About two thirds of cases involve extremities, and one third involve the abdominal wall.

The usual incubation period from the time of wounding to the onset of symptoms is one to four days, with a range of eight hours to several weeks. The first symptom is usually sudden and severe pain at the site of injury. Observations at this time typically show tense edema and tenderness. Gas may be noted in the soft tissues by palpation, x-ray, computed tomography, or ultrasound studies. The skin is initially pale and then progresses to a magenta or bronze discoloration,

TABLE 278–1. HISTOTOXIC CLOSTRIDIAL SYNDROMES

Disease	Agent	Toxin
Enteric diseases		
Food poisoning	*C. perfringens*, type A	Enterotoxin
Antibiotic-induced diarrhea or colitis	*C. difficile*	Toxins A and B
Enteritis necroticans	*C. perfringens*, type C	Beta toxin
Neurologic syndromes		
Botulism	*C. botulinum*	Botulinal toxins A, B, E, and F
Tetanus	*C. tetanus*	Tetanospasmin
Myonecrosis (gas gangrene)	*C. perfringens, C. novyi, C. septicum, C. histolyticum, C. bifermentans, C. fallax*	Multiple toxins, especially alpha toxin

and there is often cutaneous necrosis with hemorrhagic bullae. As the lesion evolves, there may be a thin, serosanguineous discharge with characteristic sweet odor. The systemic findings that accompany the evolving changes at the wound are profound. These include diaphoresis, low grade fever, and tachycardia. Common complications include hemolytic anemia, hypotension, and renal failure. The patient is typically anxious throughout the disease but remains alert despite profound systemic toxicity.

DIAGNOSIS. The diagnosis of clostridial myonecrosis is based on a constellation of clinical findings, observations at the site of injury, and supporting microbiologic data. X-rays or computed tomography studies often show gas bubbles distributed in and around muscle, and Gram stains of discharge typically show large, gram-positive bacilli with blunt ends and a paucity of polymorphonuclear leukocytes. Approximately 15 per cent of patients have clostridial bacteremia. Nevertheless, the findings of Gram stain and the detection of gas in the soft tissue cannot be considered specific. Moreover, most patients with clostridial bacteremia do not have myonecrosis. The definitive diagnostic procedure is surgical incision to expose muscle that may appear pale and edematous, beefyred, or, in the most advanced stages, black and friable. The muscle is nonviable, it fails to contract with stimulation, and the cut surface does not bleed.

The differential diagnosis includes a number of soft tissue infections that may also involve clostridia, or occur in association with severe systemic toxicity, tissue necrosis, a fulminant course, or gas formation. Important findings in the differential diagnosis are summarized in Table 278–2. This classification includes two anatomic patterns: infections involving the enveloping fascia and infections within the fascial compartment. The latter category includes infections associated with myonecrosis which are classified by microbiologic pattern as streptococcal myonecrosis, synergistic necrotizing cellulitis due to mixtures of aerobic and anaerobic bacteria, and gas gangrene. None of these infections is common, but all require aggressive treatment including early surgical intervention. Clinical clues suggesting these devastating conditions include severe systemic toxicity, severe pain that is sponta-

neous (tenderness suggests a more superficial infection such as cellulitis), bullae, gas in the soft tissue, and rapid extension. Computed tomography or magnetic resonance imaging will often demonstrate the tissue plane of involvement, and deep aspirates and blood cultures may reveal microbiologic patterns. However, surgery provides a definitive diagnosis.

TREATMENT. The most important facet of treatment is extensive surgical debridement with wide excision of involved muscle, amputation when an extremity is involved, or hysterectomy with uterine gas gangrene. The preferred antibiotic is aqueous penicillin G given intravenously in doses of 10 to 40 million units daily for adults or chloramphenicol in doses of 1 gram intravenously every six hours. Cephalosporins and clindamycin are less active against clostridia. The therapeutic value of hyperbaric oxygen is controversial. Advocates claim that this will clearly demarcate the necrotic tissue to simplify surgery and improve survival rates. Nevertheless, controlled studies to document efficacy are not available, and there may be major problems in transferring critically ill patients to centers with this type of facility. Surgery should not be delayed. Supportive measures include fluid and electrolyte replacement, control of acidosis, transfusions for severe anemia, and appropriate measures for renal failure.

PROGNOSIS. Clostridial myonecrosis is a devastating infection that often requires mutilating surgery and prolonged hospital courses. The overall mortality rate in 116 reports summarizing over 1200 cases is 25 per cent. However, many reported cases actually represent other types of soft tissue infections involving clostridial species, and the mortality rate for true gas gangrene is probably far higher.

PREVENTION. The inoculum of *C. perfringens* required to produce gas gangrene is reduced by 10^6 organisms in experimental animals if the organism is delivered into devitalized muscle containing dirt instead of normal tissue. As noted earlier, contamination of wounds by clostridia either from soil sources or from the endogenous fecal flora is common with both traumatic injuries and surgical incisions. The incidence of clostridial myonecrosis following battlefield injury was 10 per cent in World War I, 1 per cent in World War II, and 0.01 per cent (22 cases in 139,000 battle injuries) in the Vietnam

TABLE 278–2. DEEP AND SERIOUS SOFT TISSUE INFECTIONS

	Gas-Forming Cellulitis	Synergistic Necrotizing Cellulitis	Gas Gangrene	"Streptococcal" Myonecrosis	Necrotizing Fasciitis	Infected Vascular Gangrene	Streptococcal Gangrene
Predisposing conditions	Traumatic	Diabetes, prior local lesion, perirectal lesion	Traumatic or surgical wound	Trauma, surgery	Diabetes, trauma, surgery, perineal infection	Arterial insufficiency	Traumatic or surgical wound
Incubation period	>3 days	3–14 days	1–4 days	3–4 days	1–4 days	>5 days	6 hours—2 days
Etiologic organism(s)	Clostridia, others	Mixed aerobic-anaerobic flora	Clostridia, esp. *C. perfringens*	Anaerobic streptococci	Mixed aerobic-anaerobic flora	Mixed aerobic-anaerobic flora	*S. pyogenes*
Systemic toxicity	Minimal	Moderate to severe	Severe	Minimal until late in course	Moderate to severe	Minimal	Severe
Course	Gradual	Acute	Acute	Subacute	Acute or subacute	Subacute	Acute
Wound findings							
Local pain	Minimal	Moderate to severe	Severe	Late only	Minimal to moderate	Variable	Severe
Skin appearance	Swollen, minimal discoloration	Erythematous or gangrene	Tense and blanched, yellow-bronze, necrosis with hemorrhagic bullae	Erythema or yellow-bronze	Blanched, erythema, necrosis with hemorrhagic bullae	Erythema or necrosis	Erythema, necrosis
Gas	Abundant	Variable	Usually present	Variable	Variable	Variable	No
Muscle involvement	No	Variable	Myonecrosis	Myonecrosis	No	Myonecrosis limited to area of vascular insufficiency	No
Discharge	Thin, dark, sweetish or foul odor	Dark pus or "dishwater," putrid	Serosanguineous, sweet or foul odor	Seropurulent	Seropurulent or "dishwater," putrid	Minimal	None or serosanguineous, no odor
Gram stain	PMNs, grampositive bacilli	PMNs, mixed flora	Sparse PMNs, grampositive bacilli	PMNs, grampositive cocci	PMNs, mixed flora	PMNs, mixed flora	PMNs, grampositive cocci in chains
Surgical therapy	Debridement	Wide filleting incisions	Extensive excision, amputation	Excision of necrotic muscle	Wide filleting incisions	Amputation	Debridement of necrotic tissue

War. These figures reflect improvements in the management of battlefield injuries with major emphasis on prompt and thorough debridement. There should also be care in preserving the vascular supply, particularly with the use of tourniquets and casts. Judicious decisions regarding closure of traumatic wounds and the prophylactic use of antibiotics are also important. There is no effective means of active immunization.

Baxter CR: Surgical management of soft tissue infections. Surg Clin North Am 52:1483, 1972. *Soft tissue infections are reviewed using three categories: infections requiring incision and drainage, infections requiring excision of tissue, and infections not requiring extensive surgery.*

Dellinger EP: Severe necrotizing soft tissue infections. JAMA 246:1717–1721, 1981. *The author reviews management principles for severe soft tissue infections and emphasizes the differential diagnosis based on clinical presentation, Gram stain, and operative inspection.*

Heimbach RD: Gas gangrene: Review and update. HBO Review 1:41, 1980. *The author reviews gas gangrene and presents an endorsement for hyperbaric oxygen treatment which may be overly enthusiastic.*

Weinstein L, Barza M: Gas gangrene. N Engl J Med 289:1129, 1972. *A review of clinical features and management recommendations for gas gangrene.*

OTHER CLOSTRIDIAL DISEASES

SEPTICEMIA. Clostridia account for up to 3 per cent of all positive blood cultures in most clinical microbiologic laboratories. The most frequent species is *C. perfringens*, which accounts for 50 to 60 per cent. Most patients have other conditions and the significance of the clostridia is enigmatic. Less frequently there is an associated mixed infection, such as an intra-abdominal abscess, that represents the presumed portal of entry. Gas gangrene is rare and this diagnosis should be based on compatible clinical features. Special notation must be made for bacteremia with *C. septicum*. Many of these patients have a hematologic malignancy, neutropenia, or colonic carcinoma. The usual portal of entry in these cases is the distal ileum or cecum, most patients are acutely ill, and aggressive antibiotic therapy with penicillin is indicated.

MISCELLANEOUS INFECTIONS. Clostridia are frequently isolated from infections involving the host's normal flora. This situation especially applies to cases in which the infecting flora originates in the colon, such as in intra-abdominal sepsis, wound infections after intestinal surgery, and wounds, ischemic ulcers, diabetic ulcers, or decubitus ulcers located on the lower trunk or lower extremities. These organisms are also found in 5 to 10 per cent of anaerobic pulmonary infections and with similar frequency in nonvenereal infections of the female genital tract. Such infections usually involve a mixture of aerobic and anaerobic bacteria so that the role of clostridia is uncertain. The major concern is often gas gangrene and, as already emphasized, this diagnosis is best established by supporting clinical findings. Other considerations in the differential diagnosis include soft tissue infections associated with gas formation, such as gas-forming cellulitis, necrotizing fasciitis, infected vascular gangrene, and synergistic necrotizing cellulitis. All of these may involve clostridia as well as other microbes, but they are quite different in terms of prognosis, clinical findings, and type of surgery required (Table 278–2). Penicillin G is the preferred antibiotic for clostridial infections; chloramphenicol or metronidazole is also appropriate; clindamycin and cephalosporins are somewhat inferior.

CLOSTRIDIA ENTEROTOXEMIAS. Clostridia cause three different types of enteric disease, each of which is ascribed to a unique toxin (Table 278–1). *C. difficile*, the major cause of antibiotic-associated colitis, is discussed in Ch. 279.

C. perfringens is commonly responsible for foodborne outbreaks of a self-limited enteric disease. The cause is an enterotoxin produced by some type A strains during sporulation. Requirements for infections are (1) ingestion of at least

10^8 viable vegetative cells; (2) enterotoxigenic potential of the ingested strain; and (3) sporulation with toxin production in the alkaline medium of the small bowel. The usual symptoms are diarrhea and abdominal cramps ascribed to fluid secretion, morphologic damage to the intestinal mucosa, and altered motility in the small bowel. Less frequent symptoms are nausea, vomiting, and fever. The usual vehicle is meat or food made with meat, such as stews, meat pies, gravies, or casseroles. The attack rate among exposed persons is usually 30 to 60 per cent, and the incubation period ranges from 7 to 15 hours. The diagnosis is suspected in any outbreak of gastrointestinal disease associated with typical symptoms and incubation period among persons sharing a common and likely food source. Confirmation requires the recovery of *C. perfringens* in concentrations of at least 10^5 per gram of epidemiologically implicated food and recovery of at least 10^6 spores per gram of stool obtained within 48 hours after onset of symptoms from victims. Nearly all patients have spontaneous resolution of symptoms within 6 to 24 hours and do not require any specific form of therapy.

Enteritis necroticans is a serious gastrointestinal disease caused by the beta toxin of *C. perfringens*, type C. This disease, once called "darmbrand," occurred in epidemic form in malnourished individuals from Norway and Germany at the end of World War II. More recently, the same condition, known locally as "pigbel," has been found to be endemic in the highlands of New Guinea. Most victims are children who have participated in pig feasts. The toxin is susceptible to proteolytic enzymes including trypsin. However, toxin inactivation in the small bowel fails because of enzyme deficiency ascribed to protein malnutrition, excessive consumption of sweet potatoes, which contain trypsin inhibitors, or colonization with *Ascaris lumbricoides*, which secretes trypsin inhibitors. The predilection for children presumably reflects antigenic naiveté. Pathologically, enteritis necroticans is a segmental disease of the small bowel which is characterized by mucosal infarction, edema, hemorrhage, and infiltration with polymorphonuclear cells. In advanced stages the bowel is thinned, friable, and subject to perforation. Medical therapy consists of intestinal decompression, penicillin or chloramphenicol, and intravenous fluid support. About half of the patients require resectional surgery, and the overall mortality rate is 15 to 40 per cent. Prevention is achieved with a beta-toxoid vaccine that is currently recommended for children in the endemic area.

Gorbach SL, Thadepalli H: Isolation of *Clostridia* in human infections: Evaluation of 114 cases. J Infect Dis 131:S81–S85, 1975. *The authors review their experience with 152 strains of clostridia recovered from 144 patients at Cook County Hospital. Sixty-five patients had soft tissue infections or intra-abdominal sepsis, and 84 per cent of these had polymicrobial infections. Clostridia bacteremia in 49 patients usually occurred with no apparent relation to the clinical setting.*

Lawrence G, Walker PD: Pathogenesis of enteritis necroticans in Papua New Guinea. Lancet 1:125–126, 1976. *The authors, noted authorities in the field, provide a postulate for the pathophysiology of pigbel.*

Lawrence G, Shann F, Freestone DS, et al.: Prevention of necrotising enteritis in Papua New Guinea by active immunization. Lancet 1:227–230, 1979. *The authors provide data from a controlled trial showing success of vaccination with beta toxin toxoid.*

Koransky JR, Stargel MD, Dowell VR Jr.: Clostridium septicum bacteremia. Am J Med 66:63–66, 1979. *A review of 59 patients with* C. septicum *bacteremia which showed 71 per cent had malignancy, most presented with a fulminant clinical course, and most died unless appropriate antibiotics were given soon after admission.*

Ramsay AM: The significance of *Clostridium welchii* in the cervical swab and blood stream in postpartum and postabortum sepsis. J Obstet Gynecol Br Commonwealth 56:247–258, 1949. *The author refers to* C. perfringens *(welchii) as a "harmless saprophyte" in a discussion of 28 women with bacteremia, since most had minimal clinical disturbance despite the fact that the majority were studied before antibiotics were available.*

Shaudera WX, Tacket CO, Blake PA: Food poisoning due to *Clostridium perfringens* in the US. J Infect Dis 147:167–170, 1983. *The authors review the Centers for Disease Control's experience with* C. perfringens *food poisoning.*

279 PSEUDOMEMBRANOUS COLITIS

DESCRIPTION. Pseudomembranous colitis is a severe gastrointestinal disease characterized by exudative plaques on the intestinal mucosa.

ETIOLOGY. Pseudomembranous colitis is usually found in association with other conditions, although occasional cases occur in healthy persons with no identifiable risk factors. This condition was initially described in the preantibiotic era when it most frequently followed intestinal surgery, and the predominant site of involvement was the small bowel, hence the term "pseudomembranous colitis." Additional recognized risk factors include intestinal obstruction, uremia, the hemolytic-uremic syndrome, Hirschsprung's disease, inflammatory bowel disease, shigellosis, intestinal ischemia, and neonatal necrotizing enterocolitis. During the past three decades, the great majority of cases represent a complication of antimicrobial use, and the pathologic changes are restricted to the colon. The etiologic agent in nearly all cases of antibiotic-associated pseudomembranous colitis is *Clostridium difficile*. The pathophysiologic mechanism is elaboration of toxins designated toxin A and toxin B during replication of vegetative forms of *C. difficile*, a process that is presumably promoted by suppression of the competitive flora.

INCIDENCE. Most patients with pseudomembranous colitis have recent antibiotic exposure, and the other risk factors noted appear to account for less than 10 per cent of all cases. The incidence of antibiotic-associated pseudomembranous colitis depends on the frequency with which endoscopy is performed to establish the diagnosis, antimicrobial use patterns, and epidemiologic patterns. Nearly all antimicrobials with an antibacterial spectrum of activity have been implicated. The most frequent are ampicillin, clindamycin, and cephalosporins. Less frequent are penicillins other than ampicillin, erythromycin, and sulfamethoxazole-trimethoprim. Drugs rarely implicated include tetracyclines, chloramphenicol, sulfonamides, and parenterally administered aminoglycosides. *C. difficile*–induced diarrhea or colitis may occur sporadically or in clusters within institutions. Epidemiologic studies indicate that *C. difficile* may be found in the colonic flora of about 3 per cent of healthy adults, is widely distributed in the environment, and is especially common in areas subject to fecal contamination from patients who have *C. difficile*–induced diarrheal complications. This last observation provides an explanation for focal outbreaks of the disease in hospitals and nursing homes where there is clustering of vulnerable patients, mainly the elderly and antibiotic recipients.

MECHANISM. *C. difficile*–induced colitis is a toxin-mediated enteric disease in which there is no microbial invasion of the intestinal mucosa.

CLINICAL MANIFESTATIONS. Virtually all patients are at risk for antibiotic-associated pseudomembranous colitis, although there appears to be an increased risk with increasing age. The most common symptom is diarrhea consisting of watery or semiliquid stools without visible blood. Stool examination may show fecal leukocytes, but this is inconsistent and nonspecific. Many patients also have fever, which is usually moderate but may reach 40° C. Other common findings are abdominal cramps, lower quadrant tenderness, leukocytosis, and hypoalbuminemia. Systemic symptoms and abdominal findings are not invariably present, and some patients simply have annoying diarrhea. Complications in severe cases include dehydration, hypoalbuminemia with anasarca, electrolyte disturbances, toxic megacolon, and colonic perforation. Symptoms may begin at any time during the course of antimicrobial treatment or up to six weeks after antimicrobials have been discontinued. The differential diagnosis includes acute and chronic diarrhea caused by enteric pathogens other than *C. difficile*, intra-abdominal sepsis, and idiopathic inflammatory bowel disease.

DIAGNOSIS. The preferred method to establish the anatomic diagnosis is endoscopy. Gross inspection of the colon typically reveals punctate, raised, yellowish-white plaques with "skip areas" of a normal mucosa or a mucosa showing erythema or edema. The plaques are usually 2 to 10 mm wide but may enlarge and coalesce over extensive segments of the colon in the late stages. Pseudomembranes are often located throughout the colon, but up to 20 per cent of patients have segmental involvement of the right side of the colon, necessitating colonoscopy. Recognition of typical lesions on gross inspection often requires an experienced endoscopist using care to wipe away mucus to detect adherent plaques. Some cases are recognized only with histologic studies of biopsy specimens. Microscopic examination shows epithelial necrosis, goblet cells distended with mucus, and infiltration of the lamina propria with polymorphonuclear cells and eosinophilic exudate. The pseudomembrane is attached to the surface epithelium and is composed of fibrin, mucin, and polymorphonuclear cells.

The preferred diagnostic test to implicate *C. difficile* is a tissue culture assay of stool to demonstrate a cytopathic toxin that is neutralized by antitoxin to *C. difficile* or *C. sordellii*. Antitoxin neutralization with antisera to *C. sordellii* reflects antigenic cross-reactivity. Toxin titers may also be performed using serial dilutions of stool specimens, although there is little correlation between the toxin titer and the severity of the disease.

Anatomic changes in the colonic mucosa noted in patients with the diarrheal complications of antibiotic use include an entirely normal colonic mucosa; erythema or edema; colitis with friability, ulceration, or hemorrhage; and pseudomembranous colitis. The toxin of *C. difficile* has been implicated in the entire spectrum of anatomic changes, but the frequency of this toxin correlates to a large extent with the severity of the disease process. Tissue culture assays for *C. difficile* toxin are positive in over 90 per cent of patients with pseudomembranous colitis and in approximately 20 per cent of those with antibiotic-associated diarrhea and an entirely normal colonic mucosa. Thus, the tissue culture assay defines the etiologic agent and does not establish the anatomic diagnosis. There is no identifiable pathogen in most patients with antibiotic-associated diarrhea or colitis in whom the assay for *C. difficile* toxin is negative, except for occasional cases that may involve *S. aureus* or *C. perfringens*.

TREATMENT. The most important therapeutic decision with antibiotic-associated diarrhea or colitis is discontinuation of the implicated agent. This often results in resolution of symptoms with no necessity for further diagnostic tests or therapy. Patients with severe or persistent symptoms should undergo endoscopy to define anatomic changes and stool examination to detect *C. difficile* cytotoxin. Patients with severe fluid, albumin, or electrolyte depletion often require intravenous replacement and may require hyperalimentation. The role of corticosteroids and attempts to manipulate the flora, as with oral lactobacilli or fecal enemas, is uncertain. Antiperistaltic drugs are contraindicated.

Specific therapy is available for diarrhea caused by *C. difficile*, using cholestyramine to bind the toxin or antibiotics to inhibit the pathogen. The preferred agent for seriously ill patients is orally administered vancomycin, 125 to 500 mg four times daily for 7 to 14 days. Vancomycin is active against virtually all strains of *C. difficile*, the levels in the colon with oral administration are extremely high, and systemic toxicity is nil owing to poor absorption with oral administration even in the presence of an inflamed bowel. The major problems with vancomycin are high cost, noxious taste, and relapses in about 20 per cent of patients when vancomycin is discontinued. Relapses are characterized by the recurrence of typical symptoms, positive tissue culture assays for *C. difficile* cytotoxin, and stool cultures that yield vancomycin-sensitive strains of *C. difficile*.

Alternative and less expensive treatments are anion exchange resins that bind *C. difficile* toxins, such as cholestyramine (4 gm packet orally three times daily for 5 to 10 days) and metronidazole (500 mg orally 3 or 4 times daily for 7 to 14 days). These drugs should be reserved for less seriously ill patients or those who have suffered a relapse with vancomycin therapy.

PROGNOSIS. *C. difficile* causes a disease spectrum ranging from asymptomatic carriers of the toxin to patients with life-threatening pseudomembranous colitis. The most common clinical expression is "simple diarrhea" that resolves when the implicated antibiotic is discontinued. Even patients with PMC usually recover without specific forms of therapy. However, symptoms may be prolonged and debilitating, with persistent diarrhea for several weeks or months. Reports that focus on more seriously ill patients indicate mortality rates of 10 to 30 per cent. With early institution of vancomycin therapy there is a prompt symptomatic response, and virtually all patients recover. Following recovery, there are no recurrences except with the previously noted relapses following treatment with antimicrobial agents. The incidence of relapse following vancomycin or metronidazole treatment is 15 to 35 per cent, and some patients suffer multiple relapses following each course of treatment. Recurrence following a subsequent course of antibiotics for other purposes appears to be unusual.

PREVENTION. The most important preventive measure is judicious use of antimicrobial agents. Patients with *C. difficile*–induced diarrhea or colitis should be isolated and placed on enteric precautions to limit spread to susceptible hosts within institutions.

Bartlett JG, Gorbach SL: Pseudomembranous colitis. Adv Intern Med 22:455, 1977. *Review of the topic with extensive reference list for publications prior to evidence implicating* C. difficile.

Bartlett JG: Treatment of *Clostridium difficile* colitis. Gastroenterology 89:1192, 1985. *Editorial review of treatment strategies.*

Bartlett JG: Antibiotic-associated colitis. DM 30:1–54, 1984. *A review of the clinical findings, laboratory findings, and management recommendations in patients with antibiotic-associated diarrhea and colitis.*

Fekety R, Kim K-H, Brown D, et al.: Epidemiology of antibiotic-associated colitis. Am J Med 70:906, 1981. *A survey of the epidemiology of* C. difficile.

Price AB, Davis DR: Pseudomembranous colitis. J Clin Pathol 30:1, 1977. *A review of histopathologic changes.*

280 BOTULISM

DEFINITION. Botulism is a severe neuroparalytic disease caused by botulinal toxin produced by clostridial species, usually *C. botulinum*. There are four recognized disease categories: (1) foodborne botulism, (2) infant botulism, (3) wound botulism, and (4) unclassified cases.

ETIOLOGY. At least six different types of clostridia produce botulinal neurotoxin, but the four types referred to as *C. botulinum* are the most common. *C. botulinum* is a gram-positive, spore-forming obligate anaerobe that is widely distributed in nature and frequently found in soil, marine environments, and agricultural products. Adults regularly ingest *C. botulinum* spores from fresh agricultural products without deleterious consequences, and this organism is not recognized as a component of the normal fecal flora. Each strain produces one of seven antigenically distinct toxins of approximately 150,000 daltons, designated A through G. Human disease is caused by types A, B, E, and rarely F. These toxins are hematogenously disseminated to peripheral cholinergic synapses where they bind irreversibly and block acetylcholine release. The result is hypotonia with a descending symmetric flaccid paralysis. Botulinal toxin is the most potent poison of man; it has an estimated lethal dose in the bloodstream of 10^{-9} mg per kilogram.

FOOD POISONING. Foodborne botulism results from the ingestion of preformed toxin in inadequately prepared food. There are an average of 15 "outbreaks" annually in the United States, most of which involve a single case. The most frequently implicated vehicle in the United States is home-canned foods, which usually have a putrefactive odor. Meat and meat products are more commonly responsible in Europe, and preserved fish is most frequent in Japan, Scandinavia, and Russia. Type A and B organisms predominate in the United States. Type E organisms are usually, but not exclusively, associated with an aquatic source in northern latitudes, where they are found in coastal waters, lakes, and intestines of fish that inhabit these areas.

CLINICAL MANIFESTATIONS. The incubation period is usually 18 to 36 hours but may be as short as two hours or as long as eight days. Persons with the shortest incubation period usually have the most severe disease. The bulbar musculature is affected first, with resultant diplopia, difficulty in focusing to a near point, dry mouth, and dysphagia. Common gastrointestinal symptoms include nausea, vomiting, and abdominal pain. Neurologic examination shows lateral rectus muscle weakness (cranial nerve VI), ptosis, dilated pupils with sluggish reaction, decreased gag reflex, or medial rectus paresis. This is followed by descending involvement of the motor neurons to peripheral muscles, including the muscles of respiration. Some patients have only mild illness, whereas others have severe paralysis that may require intensive supportive care for weeks. Mentation remains clear, there is no fever, and neurologic dysfunction is bilateral but not necessarily symmetric. The principal causes of death are respiratory or bulbar paralysis and infectious complications during the period of supportive care.

DIAGNOSIS. The usual laboratory test in suspected cases is analysis of serum, stool, and food suspected of harboring botulinum toxin. The classic test is a mouse assay in which specimens are injected intraperitoneally to demonstrate a lethal toxin that is neutralized by type-specific antitoxin. Alternative antigen assays, such as the enzyme-linked immunoassay, have been developed, but are not widely available. Contaminated foods and patient stool may also be cultured for *C. botulinum*. Among patients with clinical evidence of botulism, the toxin is detected in sera from one third, the toxin is found in the stool from one third, and the organism is recovered in stool from 60 per cent.

Botulism should be suspected in patients with acute flaccid paralysis, especially when there is bilateral sixth cranial nerve dysfunction, associated gastrointestinal symptoms, prior ingestion of possibly contaminated food, and typical symptoms in other persons who shared this food. The differential diagnosis includes myasthenia gravis, Guillain-Barré syndrome, tick paralysis, cerebrovascular accident involving branches of the basilar artery, trichinosis, the Eaton-Lambert syndrome, hypocalcemia, hypermagnesemia, organophosphate poisoning, atropine poisoning, paralytic poisoning caused by shellfish or puffer fish, and psychiatric syndromes. Electromyography using repetitive stimulation at 40 Hz or greater is useful in differentiating botulism from other neurologic syndromes. This shows a diminished amplitude of muscle action potentials with a single supramaximal stimulus and facilitation of action potentials using paired or repetitive stimuli. These findings do not appear until the patient develops peripheral muscle weakness and are most likely to be positive in an affected limb.

TREATMENT. The patient's vital capacity should be monitored, and ventilatory support is most important. Elimination of the toxin from the gastrointestinal tract may be facilitated using gastric lavage, cathartics, and enemas early in the course. Antitoxin is usually given irrespective of the duration of illness, since the toxin may persist in the blood for extended periods. Treatment is initiated using two vials of the trivalent antitoxin, each containing 7500 IU type A, 5500 IU type B, and 8500 IU type E antitoxin; this is given intravenously and repeated at two to four hours. The antitoxin is horse serum and is associated with a 20 per cent incidence of hypersensitivity reactions, the most serious being anaphylaxis in 3 to 5 per cent. Efficacy of the antitoxin is most clearly established with type E botulism. Other therapeutic considerations include guanidine hydrochloride (15 to 50 mg per kilogram daily) to enhance acetylcholine release, but efficacy has not been established. Antimicrobial agents are advocated only for infectious complications.

PROGNOSIS. The case fatality rate for foodborne botulism was formerly 60 to 70 per cent. Improved methods of management, especially support of respiratory function, have reduced the fatality rate to less than 10 per cent. Patients who survive generally have complete recovery.

PREVENTION. Foodborne botulism is caused by germination of spores in food with toxin produced by vegetative forms, although the toxin may also be produced in vivo by simultaneous ingestion of spores. The disease may be prevented by destruction of spores in the original food source, inhibition of germination, or destruction of preformed toxin. Specific measures are as follows:

1. Destruction of spores with heat or irradiation. Spores of types A and B may survive boiling for several hours, especially at high altitudes (such as in Colorado) where the boiling point may be substantially lower. These spores may be destroyed if kept at 120° C for 30 minutes using pressure cookers. Spores of type E are most heat-labile and are killed with heating at 80° C for 30 minutes.

2. Germination may be inhibited by a reduction in pH, refrigeration, freezing, drying, or addition of salt, sugar, or other inhibitory substances such as sodium nitrite.

3. Inactivation of preformed toxin is accomplished by terminal heating for 20 minutes at 80° C or 10 minutes at 90° C.

INFANT BOTULISM. Infant botulism results from production of botulinal neurotoxin in vivo following colonization of the gastrointestinal tract in children ages one to nine months. This is the most common form of botulism in the United States, where 30 to 80 cases are documented annually. Spores of *C. botulinum* (but not the toxin) have been found in about 10 per cent of honey supplies, which presumably account for one third of cases. The disease spectrum varies considerably, ranging from "failure to thrive" or mild changes in bowel habits to the sudden infant death syndrome or "crib death." The most commonly recognized form of the disease is the "floppy baby syndrome." Initial symptoms are lethargy, diminished suck, weakness, feeble cry, and diminished spontaneous activity with loss of head control. This is followed by extensive flaccid paralysis. The diagnosis is established with the recovery of *C. botulinum* or its toxin in stool. The toxin has rarely been detected in the serum. Fecal carriage of the organism and the toxin may persist for weeks to months following clinical improvement and hospital discharge. The major therapeutic need is supportive care with special attention to nutrition and maintenance of respiratory function. The role of antitoxin, guanidine, and antibiotics in this form of botulism has not been established, and generally their use is not advised. The mortality rate for hospitalized patients given supportive care is only 2 per cent.

WOUND BOTULISM. This is a rare form of botulism in which a traumatic wound is infected by *C. botulinum* with toxin production in vivo. Clinical features are identical to those of foodborne botulism except that the incubation period is 4 to 14 days and there is a paucity of gastrointestinal symptoms. The diagnosis is established by recovering *C.*

botulinum from the wound or by detection of the toxin in serum.

UNCLASSIFIED BOTULISM. This category includes persons over the age of 12 months who have typical symptoms and signs of botulism with no identifiable vehicle. It is possible that some cases result from production of toxin in vivo by organisms colonizing the intestine in a fashion comparable to the mechanism described for infant botulism.

SPECIAL NOTE. Physicians who suspect foodborne botulism or wish to receive botulinal antitoxin should contact the state health department (daytime and 24-hour numbers listed in JAMA 256:1105, 1986) or contact the CDC 24-hour number (404-329-2888).

Arnon SS: Infant botulism. Ann Rev Med 31:541, 1980. *A review of infant botulism.*

Chia JK, Clark JB, Ryan CA, et al.: Botulism in an adult associated with foodborne intestinal infection with *Clostridium botulinum*. N Engl J Med 315:239, 1986. *This is a case report of an adult with the infant form of botulism and an accompanying editorial that places this observation in perspective.*

Dowell VR Jr, McCroskey LM, Hathaway CL, et al.: Coproexamination for botulinal toxin and *Clostridium botulinum*. JAMA 238:1829, 1977. *Reviews methods to establish the diagnosis in foodborne botulism.*

Merson MH, Hughes JM, Dowell VR, et al.: Current trends in botulism in the United States. JAMA 229:1305, 1974. *Summary of the CDC experience with foodborne botulism.*

281 TETANUS

DEFINITION. Tetanus is a neurologic syndrome caused by a neurotoxin elaborated at the site of injury by *Clostridium tetani*.

ETIOLOGY. *C. tetani* is an anaerobic, gram-positive, slender, motile bacillus. The sporulated form has a characteristic drumstick or tennis racket shape with a terminal spore. The vegetative form produces tetanospasmin, a protein neurotoxin with a molecular weight of approximately 150,000. Tetanospasmin ranks with botulism toxin as the most potent known microbial toxin; 1 mg is capable of killing 50 to 70 million mice. The vegetative forms of *C. tetani* are highly susceptible to heat, disinfectants, and other adverse environmental conditions, but the spores are highly resistant and can survive in soil for months to years. Killing of spores requires boiling for at least four hours or autoclaving for 12 minutes at 121° C.

EPIDEMIOLOGY. *C. tetani* can be found in 20 to 65 per cent of soil samples, the highest yields being in cultivated land and the lowest yields, in virgin soil. The organism can also be found in stool from a variety of animals, house dust, operating rooms, and contaminated heroin. Approximately 10 per cent of humans harbor *C. tetani* in the colon.

Tetanus is most common in warm climates and in highly cultivated rural areas. The greatest problem is in economically deprived countries, owing to poor immunization standards and unhygienic practices. An example is the practice of dressing the umbilical stump with animal dung or "dusting powder," a local dried clay sold for cosmetic purposes, after childbirth by unimmunized mothers. It is estimated that the annual toll from neonatal tetanus in developing countries is one half to one million. In the United States, there are 70 to 100 reported cases annually, and almost all occur in unimmunized or inadequately immunized persons. Over 70 per cent of these patients are 50 years of age or older, and less than 4 per cent are under 20 years; there is only about one case of neonatal tetanus per year. This predilection for the disease in the elderly appears to reflect waning immunity associated with aging. Another risk group in industrialized countries is comprised of drug addicts, primarily "skin poppers," who inject illicit drugs at multiple subcutaneous sites.

PATHOGENESIS. Clinical tetanus requires a source of the organism, local tissue conditions that promote toxin production, and immunologic naiveté. The usual portals of entry are traumatic wounds, surgical wounds, subcutaneous injection sites, burns, skin ulcers, infected umbilical cords, and otitis media with tympanic membrane perforation. Most cases in the United States occur with a puncture wound or cut incurred while gardening, working, or handling animals. In approximately 10 per cent of cases no likely portal of entry is identified. The spores are ubiquitous in the environment, and most cases reflect contamination from exogenous sources, although endogenous infection is conceivable in occasional cases that follow intestinal surgery. Important factors at the site of injury are necrotic tissue, suppuration, and the presence of a foreign body. These are responsible for a reduction in the local oxidation-reduction potential (Eh), thus promoting reversion of spores to the vegetative forms that produce tetanospasmin. Tetanospasmin is taken up by the peripheral nerve terminals and carried intra-axonally within membrane-bound vesicles to spinal neurons at a transport rate of approximately 250 mm per day. Upon reaching the perikarya of the motor neurons the toxin passes to the presynaptic terminals where it blocks release of neurotransmitters including glycine which is the neurotransmitter used by group 1A inhibitory afferent motor neurons. Loss of the inhibitory influence results in unrestrained firing with sustained muscular contraction. The result with spinal cord neurons is rigidity. In severe cases there is also involvement of the sympathetic chain causing autonomic dysfunction.

CLINICAL FEATURES. Forms of tetanus include generalized, localized, cephalic, and neonatal.

Generalized tetanus is the most common. The extent of the associated trauma varies from a rather trivial injury that may be forgotten by the patient to a severe, contaminated crush injury. The usual incubation period is seven to 21 days, depending largely on the distance of the site of injury from the central nervous system. The "onset period" refers to the time from the first clinical symptoms of tetanus to the first generalized spasm. An incubation period of less than nine days and an onset period of less than 48 hours appear to be associated with more severe symptomatology. Trismus is the presenting complaint in 75 per cent of cases, so the patient is often initially seen by a dentist or oral surgeon. Other early features include irritability, restlessness, diaphoresis, and dysphagia with hydrophobia and drooling. Sustained trismus may result in a characterisic sardonic smile, or "risus sardonicus," and persistent spasm of the back musculature may cause opisthotonos. These early manifestations reflect involvement of the bulbar muscles and paraspinous muscles, possibly because they are innervated by the shortest axons. Waves of opisthotonos are highly characteristic of the disease. With progression, the extremities become involved in episodes that may be extremely painful. Noise or tactile stimuli may precipitate spasms and generalized convulsions, although they occur spontaneously as well. Involvement of the autonomic nervous system may result in severe arrhythmias, oscillation in the blood pressure, profound diaphoresis, hyperthermia, rhabdomyolysis, laryngeal spasm, and urinary retention. In most cases the patient remains lucid. Complications include fractures from sustained contractions and convulsions, pulmonary emboli, bacterial infections, and dehydration.

Localized tetanus refers to involvement of the extremity with a contaminated wound and shows considerable variation and severity. In the more severe cases there are intense, painful spasms that usually progress to generalized tetanus. Cases that remain localized tend to be less severe. This is a relatively unusual form of tetanus, and the prognosis for survival is excellent.

Cephalic tetanus generally follows a head injury or occurs with C. *tetani* infection of the middle ear. The clinical symptoms consist of isolated or combined dysfunction of the cranial motor nerves, most frequently the seventh cranial nerve. This

may remain localized or progress to generalized tetanus. Again, this is a relatively unusual form of tetanus, but the incubation period is only one or two days, and the prognosis for survival is extremely poor.

Tetanus neonatorum refers to generalized tetanus resulting from C. *tetani* infection in neonates. This occurs primarily in underdeveloped countries where various contamined materials are used to sever or dress the umbilical cord in newborn infants of unimmunized mothers. The usual incubation period following birth is three to ten days, and it is sometimes referred to as "the disease of the seventh day," reflecting the average incubation period. The child typically shows irritability, facial grimacing, and severe spasms with touch. The mortality rate usually exceeds 70 per cent.

DIAGNOSIS. The diagnosis of tetanus is usually made on the basis of clinical observations. The putative agent, C. *tetani*, can be recovered with cultures of the wound in only about 30 per cent of cases at best. Spinal fluid analysis is entirely normal, and the electroencephalogram generally shows a sleep pattern. The differential diagnosis includes oculogyric crisis secondary to phenothiazine toxicity, meningitis, subarachnoid hemorrhage, hypocalcemic or alkalotic tetany, and strychnine poisoning. Strychnine poisoning produces very similar symptoms, but differs from tetanus in that patients usually recover rapidly following supportive care.

TREATMENT. *Surgery.* Debridement of any associated wound. (This may pose a problem in "skin poppers," who often have multiple possibly infected sites.)

Antibiotics. Penicillin G should be given parenterally in doses of 1 to 10 million units daily for ten days; tetracycline, erythromycin, and chloramphenicol are alternative agents for penicillin-allergic patients.

Antitoxin. Human tetanus immunoglobulin (TIG) should be given as soon as possible in a dose of 3,000 to 6,000 units intramuscularly or in split doses intramuscularly and by infiltration into the wound. The high dose is recommended to maintain high circulating levels. The serum half-life is four weeks, and substantial levels are noted for up to 16 weeks. Equine tetanus immune globulin (50,000 to 100,000 units in split doses intramuscularly) is equally effective, but the rate of reactions is high owing to the equine source. Epinephrine 1:1000 should be readily available for severe reactions. This preparation is far less expensive and is consequently used most extensively in underdeveloped countries.

ACTIVE IMMUNIZATION. Natural infection does not result in detectable levels of circulating antibody, so a full course of immunization with tetanus toxoic in three doses should be given.

Muscle Spasms. Chlorpromazine (50 to 150 mg every four to eight hours in adults), meprobamate (400 mg every three to four hours in adults*), or diazepam (2 to 20 mg intravenously every two to eight hours) are given to control spasms and convulsions, and short-acting barbiturates are useful for sedation. Overuse of these agents may lead to hypoventilation. When muscle spasms are severe or interfere with ventilation, therapeutic paralysis should be introduced using pancuronium bromide or metocurine combined with mechanical ventilation.

SUPPORTIVE CARE. Trismus, dysphagia, laryngeal spasm, respiratory muscle spasm, and sedatives all contribute to the high frequency of pulmonary complications. Maintenance of a patent airway is imperative, often with intubation followed by a tracheostomy. The patient may then be maintained with mechanical ventilation in conjunction with sedation, usually with diazepam.

Patients with dysphagia should be fed via a nasogastric tube. Fluid balance needs to be followed assiduously since large losses may occur and may be difficult to measure owing to profuse sweating and unswallowed saliva. Autonomic

---

*May exceed manufacturer's recommended dosage.

nervous system involvement may result in tachycardia and hypertension with high cardiac output and cardiac arrhythmias. Alpha- and beta-adrenergic blocking agents were used formerly, but beta blockade was sometimes complicated by cardiac arrest. Additional concerns are pulmonary emboli requiring anticoagulation, gastrointestinal bleeding that may be prevented with proper maintenance of the gastric pH, renal failure that may require dialysis, superimposed infections requiring judicious use of antibiotics, hyperthermia requiring a cooling blanket, and hypertension requiring pressor agents.

PROGNOSIS. The overall mortality rate for generalized tetanus is 25 to 50 per cent even in modern medical facilities with extensive resources. Important prognostic features are the form of tetanus, as described above, the incubation period, the onset period, patient's age, and severity of symptoms. Patients with mild disease have only trismus with or without minor and brief muscle spasms. Moderate disease is characterized by trismus, dysphagia, rigidity, and intermittent muscle spasms. With severe tetanus there are generalized convulsions. The most important therapeutic maneuvers are to insure airway patency and to provide mechanical ventilation to counter the tendency for respiratory arrest. Other therapeutic principles include antimicrobial drugs, active and passive immunization, wound debridement, and supportive care. Patients with moderate or severe generalized tetanus generally require three to six weeks for recovery. They may require intensive care during most of this time, but if they survive their recovery is usually complete. Specific recommendations follow. The highest mortality rates are at the extremes of age, in neonatal tetanus and in persons over 60 years of age. The most frequent cause of death is pneumonia, but many patients have no obvious findings at autopsy, suggesting that death was directly due to the neurotoxin.

PREVENTION. Nearly all cases of tetanus occur in unimmunized or inadequately immunized individuals. The Immunization Practices Advisory Committee recommends active immunization of infants and children with DPT (diphtheria and tetanus toxoids and pertussis adsorbed) at two months, four months, six months, 15 months, and four to six years. Tetanus toxoid is a highly effective antigen and protective levels of serum antitoxin in persons who complete the primary series persist for at least ten years. Td (tetanus and diphtheria toxoids adsorbed for adult use) is recommended every ten years at mid-decade ages (15 years, 25 years, 35 years, etc.). This is commonly neglected as disclosed by serosurveys showing that 40 per cent of persons over 60 years in the U.S. lack protective levels of tetanus antitoxin. The recommended primary immunization series for unimmunized persons over seven years is Td at time 0, four to eight weeks, six to twelve months after the second dose, and then every ten years. Nearly all states now require DPT immunization for school enrollment. About 95 per cent of cases in the United States occur in persons who have not received the primary series of tetanus toxoid. Immunized childbearing women confer protection on their infants through transplacental maternal antibody.

Prevention of tetanus after injury requires appropriate wound management, assurance of adequate immunity, and consideration of antibiotic prophylaxis. The aim of surgery is to eliminate necrotic tissue, purulent collections, and foreign bodies that promote the environmental conditions necessary for spore germination. Guidelines for wound management based on immunization status and wound characteristics are summarized in Table 281–1. Passive immunization is recommended only for "tetanus prone" wounds, preferably with TIG consisting of globulins prepared from plasma of adults hyperimmunized with tetanus toxoid. The alternative is tetanus antitoxin equine prepared from hyperimmunized horses. The horse serum is associated with a high reaction rate including pain at the injection site, serum sickness, and anaphylactic shock. Equine antitoxin also generates immune complexes that are rapidly excreted so that larger doses are required to produce sustained blood levels. The definition of *tetanus-prone* depends on the interval between injury and treatment, the degree of contamination, the extent of devitalized tissue or foreign bodies within the site of injury, and the depth of the injury. Antimicrobial agents such as penicillin or erythromycin may be given to inhibit replication of the vegetative forms of *C. tetani*, but immunization and wound cleansing are more important and therefore the use of antibiotics is generally dictated by other considerations.

TABLE 281–1. GUIDELINES FOR TETANUS PROPHYLAXIS IN WOUND MANAGEMENT

History of Adsorbed Tetanus Toxoid	Clean and Minor Wounds		Other Wounds*	
Number of Doses	*Td†*	*TIG‡*	*Td†*	*TIG‡*
Unknown or less than three	Yes§	No	Yes§	Yes
Three or more	Yes if over 10 years since last dose	No	Yes if over 5 years since last dose	No

*Included but not limited to wounds contaminated with dirt, feces, soil, saliva, puncture wounds; avulsions; and wounds resulting from missiles, crushing, burns, and frostbite.

†Td: Tetanus and diphtheria toxoids adsorbed. Children under seven should receive DPT (diphtheria and tetanus toxoids and pertussis vaccine adsorbed). Too frequent booster doses of tetanus toxoid have been associated with hypersensitivity reactions.

‡TIG: Tetanus immune globulin in a dose of 250 to 500 units intramuscularly. The usual dose is 250 units. The usual prophylactic dose of equine tetanus immune globulin is 1,500 to 5,000 units intramuscularly. When tetanus toxoid is given concurrently there should be separate syringes and injection sites.

§Unimmunized or incompletely immunized persons (1 or 2 doses of toxoid) should receive complete immunization with Td at time 0, 4–8 weeks later, and 6–12 months later.

Armitage P, Clifford R: Prognosis in tetanus: Use of data from therapeutic trials. J Infect Dis 138:1–8, 1978. *Data for 1385 patients with tetanus in India are reviewed to propose a prognostic classification.*

Bizzini B: Tetanus toxin. Microbiol Rev 43:224, 1979. *An extensive discussion of tetanus toxin.*

Centers for Disease Control: Diphtheria, tetanus and pertussis: Guidelines for vaccine prophylaxis and other preventative measures. Ann Intern Med 103:896–905, 1985. *The recommendations of the Immunization Practices Advisory Committee are summarized for wound management to prevent tetanus.*

Communicable Disease Center: New recommended schedule for active immunization of normal infants and children. JAMA 256:2311–2312, 1986. *The revised recommendations of the Immunization Practices Advisory Committee for childhood immunizations are summarized.*

Faust RA, Vickers OR, Cohn L Jr: Tetanus: 2,449 cases in 68 years at Charity Hospital. J Trauma 16:704–712, 1976. *The authors review a large clinical experience with tetanus in a United States hospital.*

Griffin JW: Local tetanus. Johns Hopkins Med J 149:84–88, 1981. *A good review of local tetanus and the pathophysiology of tetanospasmin.*

Anaerobic Bacteria

282 DISEASES CAUSED BY NON–SPORE-FORMING ANAEROBIC BACTERIA

Sherwood L. Gorbach

DEFINITIONS. Anaerobic bacteria are the major constituents of the microflora that colonizes the gastrointestinal tract, upper respiratory tract, skin, and vagina. Under normal circumstances these organisms exist in a *commensal* (literal meaning "dining at the same table") relationship with their host. Anaerobic bacteria require reduced oxygen tension for growth; the more fastidious strains cannot survive exposure to atmospheric oxygen for more than five minutes. As a general rule, anaerobes associated with infectious processes are relatively aerotolerant. Teleologically, aerotolerance provides anaerobic bacteria with a survival advantage in mammalian tissues, since the extremely oxygen-sensitive forms perish almost immediately upon escape from their natural ecologic niche, whereas aerotolerant forms can establish a septic focus.

Regardless of the organ site, anaerobic infections have three characteristics in common. First, such infections are truly endogenous, since the pathogens originate from the normal flora of the host. Second, certain pathogenic conditions predispose to anaerobic infections by initiating spread of the normal flora beyond the confines of mucosal barriers. These inciting events also produce a low *oxidation-reduction potential* (Eh) in the tissues, thereby favoring the growth of anaerobic organisms. Compromised vascular supply, trauma, tissue destruction, and antecedent infections caused by aerobic bacteria or viruses that result in necrosis are among the situations that precede anaerobic infection. Third, the infecting flora is highly complex. Abdominal infections, for example, harbor an average of five different bacterial species, usually three anaerobes and two aerobic or facultative strains.

ANAEROBIC GRAM-NEGATIVE BACILLI. *Bacteroides.* *B. fragilis* is the preeminent anaerobic pathogen in humans. This distinction is based on its virulence, its ubiquity in various organ sites, and its resistance to many conventional antimicrobial drugs. The organism frequently produces abscesses and causes tissue destruction. The *B. fragilis* group has been divided into five distinct species, based on biochemical differences and DNA homology: *B. fragilis, B. distasonis, B. vulgatus, B. ovatus,* and *B. thetaiotaomicron.* Although these organisms are recognized pathogens, they all lack one of the prime virulence factors of other gram-negative organisms, endotoxin. While *Bacteroides* strains do possess a surface lipopolysaccharide (LPS), this substance differs in chemical composition from LPS of other gram-negative organisms. In addition, *B. fragilis* LPS lacks the biologic activities of classic endotoxin, such as production of septic shock and vascular collapse in experimental animals. On the other hand, *B. fragilis* contains on its outer cell membrane a specific, large molecular weight capsule composed of polysaccharide. In a purified form the capsular material is highly antigenic, and it can produce abscesses when it is injected into experimental animals.

B. fragilis causes infections in the abdominal cavity that are associated with contamination by the intestinal flora. These organisms also are found in female pelvic infections and in mixed infections of skin and soft tissue such as decubitus ulcer, diabetic foot ulcer, and gangrene of the perineum.

B. bivius and *B. disieus* are frequent isolates in female pelvic infections. These organisms often are resistant to conventional penicillins and cephalosporins.

The *Bacteroides melaninogenicus-asaccharolyticus* group is found in the normal flora and in association with various infections. The major distinguishing feature of *B. melaninogenicus* is the production of a brown-black pigment, formed in the colony after five to seven days of growth on blood agar. Many strains require blood and vitamin K or its analogues for growth. Infections caused by *B. melaninogenicus* are most commonly found in the respiratory tract, head and neck region, and female pelvic area.

Fusobacterium. The major species found in clinical specimens are *F. nucleatum* and *F. necrophorum.* In Gram-stained preparations, these organisms take up stain poorly and appear as slender spear-shaped bacilli with parallel sides and tapered ends. The LPS of *F. nucleatum* causes septic shock and vascular collapse when injected intravenously into rabbits, in contrast to the material found in *B. fragilis,* which is biologically inactive in this model. *Fusobacterium* species are regular constituents of the normal flora of the oral cavity, gastrointestinal tract, and female genital tract. Among the infectious processes, these organisms are major causes of pleuropulmonary infections and various abscesses of the head and neck region. They are also responsible for bacteremia. The most common sites of origin are the female genital tract, orofacial region, and lower respiratory tract.

ANAEROBIC GRAM-POSITIVE COCCI. This diverse group of organisms ranks second in importance to *Bacteroides* in frequency of isolation from infected sites. The two genera are *Peptostreptococcus* and *Peptococcus.* (There are also gram-negative cocci known as *Veillonella,* that are only rarely involved as pathogens.) Peptostreptococci form long chains of cocci in culture. Peptococci occur as irregular clumps of gram-positive cocci that resemble *Staphylococcus aureus* in morphologic appearance.

Anaerobic gram-positive cocci are important components of the normal flora of humans. Within the oral cavity peptostreptococci represent a significant percentage of the anaerobic isolates in saliva and dental plaque. They are also among the leading components of the fecal flora and the vaginal flora. As pathogenic organisms these anaerobic cocci are found in virtually all sites where anaerobes have been identified. Approximately 50 per cent of such isolates in a clinical bacteriology laboratory are from surgical wounds, mostly associated with abdominal operations and hysterectomies. The gram-positive cocci are also found in skin and soft tissue infections and in blood cultures. About one third of anaerobic pleuropulmonary infections are associated with these gram-positive cocci. In the female genital tract they are probably the most important cause of salpingitis and are frequently isolated in cases of pelvic abscess.

GRAM-POSITIVE NON–SPORE-FORMING BACILLI. The two leading isolates are *Propionibacterium acnes* and various species of *Eubacterium. P. acnes* is the most frequent anaerobe found on normal skin. Many laboratories incorrectly identify it as a diphtheroid. This organism is commonly recovered from blood cultures, most often as a contaminant. It is also isolated from wound infections as part of a mixed flora. Although these organisms have little intrinsic pathogenicity, they are important causes of infection in patients with artificial heart valves, vascular grafts, orthopedic prostheses, or ventricular shunts. *Eubacterium* is isolated from wound infections, particularly in association with *Bacteroides.* Insofar as can be determined, *Eubacterium* plays no pathogenic role in the infective process.

PATHOGENESIS OF ANAEROBIC INFECTIONS. *Unitarian Compared with Synergistic Infections.* Our theoretical models of infections are based on concepts of microbial monoetiology. Pasteur established that certain microorganisms are responsible for a specific disease state. His theory was formalized by Robert Koch in his famous postulates. Finally, Ehrlich created the concept of a single drug, the "magic bullet," designed for a specific infection. Thus, the principle states: one microbe, one disease, one drug. This concept applies to classic infections such as typhoid fever, diphtheria, and cholera. However, the classic design does not fit most infections associated with anaerobic bacteria, since these processes harbor multiple strains of organisms with varying oxygen sensitivities and undefined pathogenic potentials. Anaerobic infections follow the model of bacterial synergy, in which several bacteria behave in a cooperative fashion to produce infection. In experimental model systems of mixed infection, various microbial components contribute virulence factors or growth substances that permit other more pathogenic forms to invade the tissues. Most clinical anaerobic infections are mixed, containing several species of bacteria. Because it is not clear which are the primary pathogens and which are the symbionts and commensals, it is often necessary to treat all of the potential pathogens.

Virulence Factors. The microenvironment of an anaerobic abscess has features that insure its own survival. An abscess has an Eh of -250 mv, with an extremely low concentration of oxygen. Anaerobiosis is a hostile condition for host-defense mechanisms. Within this oxygen-free zone, neutrophils are unable to kill bacteria by their oxidative metabolic pathway. Low oxygen tension also inhibits the activity of aminoglycoside antibiotics, since they require an oxidative transport system to cross the bacterial cell envelope. The abscess itself contains a large concentration of microorganisms, approximately 10^8 to 10^9 per milliliter. A high inoculum and a relatively low growth rate are adverse conditions for the activity of beta-lactam antibiotics. Thus, host defenses and antibiotic interventions are hindered in an anaerobic abscess.

Individual anaerobic microorganisms possess virulence factors that promote their survival in the host's tissues. *B. fragilis* elaborates a polysaccharide capsule that provides protection against phagocytosis by neutrophils. Membrane-associated enzymes are found in many virulent anaerobes, including beta-lactamases and superoxide dismutase (SOD). The beta-lactamases destroy antibiotics such as penicillin and cephalosporin. SOD, an enzyme present in virtually all pathogenic anaerobes studied thus far, seems to protect the organism in its initial exposure to oxygenated tissues.

Immunologic factors are affected by anaerobic bacteria. Several species of anaerobes are more resistant to phagocytosis than coliforms and other facultative organisms. Anaerobic bacteria can also interfere with phagocytosis of aerobes when both organisms are present in a mixed infection. *B. fragilis* appears to influence the alternative pathway of serum complement. Cell-mediated immunity also plays a role in anaerobic infections, at least in abscess formation by *B. fragilis.*

Role of Facultative Organisms. Facultative or aerobic organisms are frequent partners in anaerobic infections. In some settings these organisms seem to initiate the infective process, perhaps by promoting early tissue necrosis or by consuming oxygen in the tissues. In abdominal infections coliforms and *Bacteroides* are often isolated together.

An animal model of intra-abdominal infection has delineated the role of these pathogens in the septic process. Following intestinal perforation, the initial phase consists of peritonitis, bacteremia, and septic shock. This phase is caused, at least in the animal model, by coliforms such as *E. coli* and *Proteus.* The later abscess formation, is associated with anaerobes, particularly *Bacteroides.* Antimicrobial drugs active only against coliforms suppress the initial septicemic and shock phase but have no effect on abscess formation. Similarly, antianaerobic drugs do not protect against coliform bacteremia, but they do suppress formation of abscess. The clinical picture is complex, with overlapping of the septic shock stage

and the abscess stage. However, the therapeutic implications are clear: both components of abdominal sepsis should receive appropriate antimicrobial attention.

ANAEROBIC BACTERIA IN VARIOUS INFECTIONS. Aerobic and facultative microorganisms have been traditionally considered the major pathogens in infectious diseases. Recent improvements in laboratory techniques have facilitated the identification of anaerobic bacteria, and it has become clear that these oxygen-sensitive organisms share responsibility for a significant number of infections seen in clinical practice. Certain types of infection, such as those appearing in the abdomen, chest, female genital tract, and head and neck, characteristically are caused by anaerobes. Other infections such as lobar pneumonia, acute pharyngitis, and pyogenic meningitis are rarely associated with anaerobic bacteria.

Intra-abdominal Infections. Infections within the peritoneal cavity usually are related to contamination by the intestinal flora. The microflora of the upper intestine, from the stomach to the upper ileum, consists of sparse numbers of facultative gram-positive organisms derived from the oropharynx. Relatively few coliforms and obligate anaerobes are encountered. The lower bowel, on the other hand, harbors a luxuriant flora in which anaerobes outnumber facultative organisms such as coliforms by a factor of 1000 to 1. Hence, injuries to the upper intestinal tract, such as perforated ulcer or trauma, result in a small inoculum of microorganisms and a low risk of infection. But colonic perforations release a large inoculum of bacteria, causing a high rate of infection.

Peritonitis and intra-abdominal abscess are associated with anaerobic bacteria in 95 per cent of cases. The most frequent finding is a mixture of aerobes and anaerobes. (Infection by a single facultative organism such as *E. coli* is uncommon and usually is seen in *primary peritonitis* associated with cirrhosis of the liver.) In a large series of intra-abdominal infections, an average of five different organisms were isolated from each patient, including three types of anaerobes and two aerobes. Of the anaerobes, *Bacteroides, Clostridium,* anaerobic cocci, and *Fusobacterium* are the major pathogens. The specific site of infection does not determine the flora, since the same pathogens are found in peritonitis, appendicitis, subphrenic abscess, and diverticular abscess.

Anaerobic Pleuropulmonary Infections. Anaerobic infections of the lower respiratory tract produce four clinical conditions: *aspiration pneumonia, lung abscess, necrotizing pneumonia,* and *empyema.* The pathogenesis of these conditions is aspiration of oropharyngeal contents, a situation associated with compromised state of consciousness, obstruction of the esophagus, and neurologic deficits. The oral flora is permitted admission to normally sterile regions of the lower respiratory tract. Approximately 90 per cent of patients with aspiration pneumonia have anaerobes as the major infecting flora. The situation applies to patients who have aspirated outside the hospital or shortly after admission, since they harbor normal oral flora. When the aspiration event occurs after hospitalization or after treatment with antibiotics, at which time the oral flora becomes colonized by gram-negative facultative organisms, the aspirated flora assumes a different character. Coliforms and *Pseudomonas* account for most cases of hospital-acquired aspiration pneumonia. Lung abscess is associated with anaerobic bacteria in over 90 per cent of cases. The aerobes that occasionally cause a solitary lung abscess include *Klebsiella* and *S. aureus.* Necrotizing pneumonia is actually an earlier stage of lung abscess in which a specific segment or lobe of the lung is extensively damaged with multiple small abscesses. In the more advanced stage these abscesses coalesce to form a single large cavity, leaving in its wake a large area of destroyed lung. Necrotizing pneumonia is a more aggressive condition than lung abscess, with higher mortality. Anaerobes are responsible for the vast majority of cases. Empyema is an infection usually associated with underlying pneumonitis or lung abscess. Nearly 75 per cent of the cases of empyema are associated with anaerobes, most frequently in patients with chronic infection. The remaining cases are caused by the classic aerobic pathogens such as staphylococci, group A streptococci, and pneumococci; these organisms produce an acute onset and a more virulent course. Formerly, most cases of empyema were caused by these aerobic gram-positive organisms, but the situation has been reversed with the advent of antimicrobial agents.

Anaerobic pleuropulmonary infections involve multiple bacterial species including *B. melaninogenicus, F. nucleatum,* and anaerobic gram-positive cocci. *B. fragilis* is found in 15 per cent of cases. The fact that these organisms are found in the same relative concentrations in the various clinical cases suggests that the inoculum of oral contents is similar in each setting. Corroboration for this hypothesis is provided by animal studies in which a spectrum of pulmonary infection is produced by the same inoculum of mixed bacteria derived from gingival scrapings.

Obstetric and Gynecologic Infections. The source of infections of the female upper genital tract is the vaginal flora, which has aerobic and anaerobic bacteria as normal constituents. The clinical conditions in which anaerobes are frequently encountered include tubo-ovarian abscess, pelvic abscess, septic abortion, endomyometritis, and postoperative wound infection (following hysterectomy). Polymicrobic bacteremia is a frequent occurrence in patients with severe pelvic infections. One important difference between pelvic abscesses derived from the female genital tract and those in the abdomen is that pure anaerobic infections—those without coliforms or other facultative forms—occur with a higher frequency in the pelvic location. The major anaerobic pathogens are *Bacteroides* gram-positive cocci (especially *Peptostreptococcus*), *Fusobacterium,* and *Clostridium.* Pelvic inflammatory disease, also known as salpingitis, is a milder condition that is caused by an array of organisms, including gonococci, *Chlamydia,* and anaerobes, particularly *Peptostreptococcus.*

Head and Neck Infections. Because the anaerobic bacteria in the normal flora of the upper airways have limited invasive properties, they require an antecedent event that permits their movement into deeper structures. Dental manipulation, trauma, prior bacterial or viral infections, and operative interventions can provide the initiating circumstance. Necrotizing infections of the gingiva are usually associated with *B. melaninogenicus,* as well as other anaerobes. This organism is also present in endodontal infections. Spirochetes have been found at the advancing border of inflammation in histologic sections of acute ulcerative gingivitis, noma, and lung abscess. Since these organisms cannot be grown in subculture, their role in pathogenesis cannot be assessed. In patients with *sinusitis,* anaerobes are recovered from 50 per cent of patients with chronic processes. However, acute or subacute sinusitis, lasting three months or less, is rarely associated with anaerobes. *Otitis media* may be either acute or chronic. As in sinusitis, anaerobes may be present in the chronic forms but are rarely present in the more acute cases. *Space infections,* occurring in the potential spaces formed by fascial planes of the head and neck, are usually associated with three types of organisms: either *S. aureus, Streptococcus pyogenes,* or anaerobic bacteria. The first two organisms occur in space infections related to overlying skin processes such as boils or impetigo. Anaerobes are associated with space infections that arise from diseases of the mucous membrane, dental manipulations, or in those cases that occur spontaneously. *Ludwig's angina* is an example of a space infection associated with anaerobes.

Of the central nervous system infections, *brain abscess* is the one most frequently associated with anaerobic bacteria. These organisms are isolated from 85 per cent of suppurative brain abscesses unrelated to trauma or operative procedures. Gram-positive cocci, followed in frequency by *Fusobacterium* and *Bacteroides,* are the most common strains, often in association with facultative streptococci and coliforms. *Subdural empyema* may also be caused by anaerobes, particularly when it occurs in association with a parameningeal focus in an ear or nasal sinus. Classic pyogenic meningitis, however, is rarely caused by anaerobes.

Skin, Bone, and Soft Tissue Infections. The predisposing factors in anaerobic skin and soft tissue infections are trauma, ischemia, and surgery. The organisms often derive from the fecal or oral flora, particularly in wounds associated with intestinal surgery, decubitus ulcer, and human bites. The clinical presentations are *crepitant cellulitis, synergistic gangrene or cellulitis,* and *necrotizing fasciitis.* Anaerobes are also regularly encountered in *diabetic foot ulcers;* 75 per cent of such lesions are associated with *Bacteroides,* anaerobic cocci, and *Clostridium,* usually in mixed culture. Anaerobic *osteomyelitis* is associated with trauma or prior surgery, although some cases arise from hematogenous spread.

CLUES TO PRESUMPTIVE DIAGNOSIS OF ANAEROBIC INFECTION. Clinicians should suspect the diagnosis of an anaerobic infection before the bacteriologic results are available on the basis of the following features: (1) Any infection that is contiguous or in proximity to a mucosal surface normally harboring an anaerobic flora—the gastrointestinal tract, female genital tract, and oropharynx. (2) A foul-smelling discharge; this odor is pathognomonic evidence of anaerobic infection. The absence of odor, however, is not helpful, because 50 per cent of anaerobic infections lack the characteristic odor. (3) The presence of severe tissue necrosis, abscess formation, fasciitis, or gangrene. (4) Gas in the tissue, which is highly suggestive, although not absolutely diagnostic. (5) A mixed infection, indicated by a Gram's stain of exudate showing a polymorphic array of organisms. Certain anaerobes have a characteristic appearance under the microscope, especially *Clostridium, Fusobacterium, Actinomyces,* and certain strains of *Bacteroides.* (6) The failure to recover organisms by conventional aerobic culture in the presence of clinical infection. (7) Failure to respond to antibiotics that have poor anaerobic activity, such as aminoglycosides and certain penicillins and cephalosporins.

TREATMENT STRATEGIES FOR ANAEROBIC INFECTIONS. Successful therapy for anaerobic infections involves rational antibiotic selection in conjunction with judicious surgical resection and drainage. The operative approach may be ultimately decisive, but it should be emphasized that surgical intervention alone may be inadequate. Anaerobic infection can continue to simmer with intermittent sepsis and insidious extension of the process unless appropriate antimicrobial agents are employed. Selection of initial antibiotic therapy should be based on knowledge of the pathogens likely to be present in a specific clinical setting. Because many anaerobic infections tend to be mixed with coliforms and other facultative organisms, it is advisable to use antimicrobial drugs active against both components. With regard to the anaerobic components, important differences are seen in infections above and below the diaphragm. Anaerobic infections above the diaphragm, including those in the central nervous system, head and neck region, and pleuropulmonary area, tend to involve organisms sensitive to penicillin. This observation is not invariably true, since certain organisms, especially *B. melaninogenicus,* can elaborate beta-lactamases, which inactivate penicillins and cephalosporins. Anaerobic infections below the diaphragm, such as those in the abdominal cavity and female genital tract, commonly involve *B. fragilis* as a major pathogen. Because this organism is commonly resistant to several antimicrobial agents, infections in these sites require special consideration for choice of antimicrobial drugs.

TREATMENT. The range of choice among antimicrobial drugs is somewhat limited with regard to anaerobic bacteria in general and even more so with *B. fragilis.* A United States survey of antibiotic susceptibility among strains of *B. fragilis* from eight medical centers was conducted during 1983.

Among the 550 isolates, piperacillin was the most active beta-lactam antibiotic, with resistance rates running from 3 to 16 per cent in various centers. Cefoxitin and moxalactam were the next most active beta-lactam antibiotics. Since high blood levels can be achieved with these drugs, they can be used to treat clinical infections caused by this organism. Disappointing results were seen with penicillin, carbenicillin, ticarcillin, cephalothin, cefamandole, and certain third-generation cephalosporins such as cefotaxime and cefoperazone. The drugs in this grouping are not considered good choices for infections associated with *B. fragilis*. Clostridia, fusobacteria, and gram-positive cocci are usually sensitive to several drugs, including penicillins, cephalosporins, clindamycin, and metronidazole.

The explanation for variations in activity of the beta-lactam drugs against anaerobes is the presence in certain strains of constitutive beta-lactamases. This enzyme is found in most strains of *B. fragilis* isolated from clinical sources. It is also found in 20 to 40 per cent of strains of *B. melaninogenicus* and in occasional strains of *Fusobacterium*. The increased activity of cefoxitin, imipenem, and cefotetan against *B. fragilis* is based on their resistance to hydrolysis by beta-lactamase elaborated by anaerobic organisms.

Metronidazole, a bacteriocidal drug, has excellent activity against *Bacteroides*, *Fusobacterium*, *Clostridium*, and most strains of anaerobic cocci. Resistance to metronidazole among *Bacteroides* is extremely rare. Since the drug has a spectrum limited almost exclusively to anaerobes, another agent such as an aminoglycoside should be included for facultative organisms. In clinical trials metronidazole has produced excellent results in intra-abdominal infections, female pelvic infections, brain abscess, and anaerobic osteomyelitis. Many failures, however, have been noted in anaerobic pleuropulmonary infections. Such failures are probably related to the relatively poor activity against microaerophilic organisms that may accompany this infectious process.

Clindamycin is highly active against most anaerobic isolates with resistance rates among *Bacteroides* running at about 5 per cent. Some resistant isolates of *Clostridium* and *Fusobacterium* have been encountered, but they have been relatively uncommon in clinical practice. The drug is also active against streptococci, both aerobic and anaerobic, and most strains of *S. aureus*. Because it has very little activity against coliforms and other facultative gram-negative organisms, a second drug is used in mixed anaerobic infections. Clindamycin has produced excellent results in intra-abdominal infections, female pelvic infections, and skin and soft tissue infections. Some authorities consider it the drug of choice for anaerobic pleuropulmonary infections, preferring it to penicillin because of apparent failures associated with penicillin treatment. Erythromycin is less active than clindamycin, although resistance patterns commonly overlap. The problem with erythromycin is the difficulty in administering it parenterally. By the oral route only low serum levels of erythromycin are obtained, often below the amount needed to inhibit many anaerobic bacteria.

Tetracyclines were once touted as drugs of choice for anaerobic infections, but their performance against *Bacteroides* and many gram-negative cocci has considerably altered this view. Widespread tetracycline resistance has been noted. As a result, this class of compounds is not recommended for treatment of anaerobic infections. Chloramphenicol shows excellent activity in vitro against *Bacteroides* and most other anaerobic pathogens. It also has activity against coliforms, staphylococci, and streptococci. Whereas some clinical trials have shown good results with chloramphenicol, others have encountered therapeutic failures. In addition, animal models

of anaerobic infection have shown poor results with chloramphenicol treatment. Anaerobic organisms can inactivate chloramphenicol by at least two mechanisms, acetylation and nitroreduction. It is possible that one or both of these mechanisms are responsible for the occasional clinical failures with this drug.

Aminoglycoside and quinilone antimicrobial drugs, as well as aztreonam and ceftazidime, are inactive against most anaerobic bacteria. These drugs are included in antimicrobial regimens for therapy of mixed infections, although their role is clearly to suppress the facultative gram-negative components.

PROGNOSIS. Prognosis of anaerobic infections is related to the site of infection, the type of pathogen, the underlying condition of the patient, and the choice of antimicrobial therapy. In general, anaerobic pleuropulmonary infections have a good outcome, especially when adequate drainage can be achieved. Penicillin G has been successful in treating these infections in the past, curing up to 95 per cent of patients with aspiration pneumonia or lung abscess, for example. Some failures have been noted with penicillin, and in such instances clindamycin has been used to advantage. Metronidazole treatment has been associated with failures in lung abscess. In certain series poor outcomes are noted in 25 to 50 per cent of treated patients.

Severe intra-abdominal infections have a failure rate of 10 to 20 per cent even with optimal surgery and antimicrobial therapy. Higher failure rates in controlled clinical trials have been associated with treatment regimens using antimicrobial agents with poor activity against *B. fragilis* such as cephalothin, doxycycline, cefamandole, and cefoperazone. Infections of the female genital tract generally have a good prognosis, since most patients tend to be rather healthy prior to the onset of the septic process. Good results have been reported with cefoxitin, clindamycin, and metronidazole, usually in association with another antibiotic. In one clinical trial penicillin combined with gentamicin produced a poor result in endomyometritis when compared with the alternative regimen of clindamycin and gentamicin.

In general, clinical trials with new antimicrobial agents have corroborated the findings in animal models and susceptibility testing in vitro. Because of the vast array of anaerobic organisms and their varying patterns of susceptibility, it is best to base empiric therapy on known sensitivity patterns and performance of the specific drugs in controlled clinical trials.

Bartlett JG, Louie TJ, Gorbach SL, et al.: Therapeutic efficacy of 29 antimicrobial regimens in experimental intra-abdominal sepsis. Rev Infect Dis 3:535, 1981. *An experimental model of intra-abdominal infections that explains the pathophysiologic events and the rationale for antimicrobial treatments.*

Finegold SM (ed.): International Symposium on Anaerobic Bacteria and Their Role in Disease. Rev Infect Dis 6:S1, 1984. *Complete clinical and laboratory aspects, presented by foremost experts in the field.*

Finegold SM, George WL, Mulligan ME: Anaerobic infections: Parts I and II. DM 31:Oct, Nov, 1985. *A fine treatise, mostly clinical, which provides 279 references.*

Gorbach SL, Bartlett JG: Medical progress: Anaerobic infections. N Engl J Med 290:1177, 1974. *The clinical and microbiologic features of anaerobic infections in many organ sites.*

Tally FP, Cuchural GJ Jr, Jacobus NV, et al.: Nationwide study of the susceptibility of the *Bacteroides fragilis* group in the United States. Antimicrob Agents Chemother 28:675, 1985. *The antimicrobial susceptibilities of 555 strains of this important pathogen, collected in eight medical centers.*

Wasserheit JN, Bill TA, Kiviat NB, et al.: Microbial causes of proven pelvic inflammatory disease and efficacy of clindamycin and tobramycin. Ann Intern Med 104:187, 1986. *Isolations of the important pathogens from the fallopian tubes and endocervix, studied by good microbiologic techniques.*

Zaleznik DF, Kasper DL: The role of anaerobic bacteria in abscess formation. Ann Rev Med 33:217, 1982. *Discussion of pathophysiology of abscess supported by observations in microbiology, experimental animals, and patients.*

Enteric Infections

283 TYPHOID FEVER

Thomas Butler

DEFINITION. Typhoid fever is a bacterial disease caused by *Salmonella typhi*. It is characterized by prolonged fever, abdominal pain, diarrhea, delirium, rose spots, and splenomegaly and complicated sometimes by intestinal bleeding and perforation. Enteric fever is synonymous with typhoid fever, which is occasionally caused also by *S. enteritidis* bioserotype paratyphi A or B.

ETIOLOGY. The typhoid bacillus is a motile gram-negative rod in the family Enterobacteriaceae. It possesses a flagellar (H) antigen, a cell wall (O) lipopolysaccharide antigen, and a polysaccharide virulence (Vi) antigen located in the cell capsule. The polysaccharide side chain of the O antigen confers serologic specificity to the organism and is essential in virulence because salmonellae other than *S. typhi* and *S. enteritidis* bioserotype paratyphi A or B do not produce enteric fever in humans. These antigens play critical roles in permitting the organisms to invade lymphoid tissue from the gut lumen and to multiply within macrophages.

INCIDENCE AND PREVALENCE. Typhoid fever has been almost eliminated from developed countries because of sewage and water treatment facilities but remains a common disease in developing countries. In 1980, the number of cases occurring yearly was estimated as about seven million in Asia, over four million in Africa, and half a million in Latin America. About 500 cases are diagnosed each year in the United States, and over half of these are in recently arrived travelers who contracted their infections abroad.

EPIDEMIOLOGY. Adults and children of all ages and both sexes appear equally susceptible to infection. In developing countries, most cases occur in school-age children and young adults. Although acquired immunity provides some protection, reinfections have been documented. Typhoid fever occurs during all seasons.

Transmission is by the fecal-oral route through contaminated water or food. The main human sources of infection in the community are asymptomatic fecal carriers and cases during either disease or convalescence. Females and older males are prone to become chronic fecal carriers because underlying cholecystitis enables them to harbor chronic infection in the gallbladder. *S. typhi* is resistant to drying and cooling, thus allowing bacteria to survive prolonged periods in dried sewage, water, food, and ice.

Vi-phage typing of *S. typhi* is a useful epidemiologic tool to trace cases of typhoid fever to a carrier or food source. Single-source outbreaks of typhoid fever are rare. In endemic situations, multiple phage types are present, and several phage types may be responsible for an epidemic.

PATHOGENESIS AND PATHOLOGY. After ingestion of *S. typhi*, the part of the inoculum that survives the acidity of the stomach enters the small intestine, where bacteria penetrate the mucosa and enter mononuclear phagocytes of ileal Peyer's patches and mesenteric lymph nodes. Inocula of at least 10^5 bacteria are necessary to initiate disease, and inocula of 10^7 and more will cause disease regularly. The incubation period ranges from 8 to 28 days, depending on inoculum size and immune status of the host. Bacteria proliferate in mononuclear phagocytes and spread by way of the blood to the spleen, liver, and bone marrow, where further proliferation in macrophages occurs. The earliest symptoms of fever and chills (Table 283–1) are associated with bacteremia. Inflammatory reactions occur in the spleen, liver, bone marrow, Peyer's patches mainly in the terminal ileum, and skin,

consisting of mononuclear cell infiltration, hyperplasia, and focal necrosis. Focal collections of mononuclear leukocytes are called "typhoid nodules." Fever and other constitutional symptoms are probably caused by the release of interleukin-1 (endogenous pyrogen) from infected mononuclear phagocytes. Endotoxemia does not occur in typhoid fever. Intestinal manifestations are caused by hyperplasia of Peyer's patches with ulcerations of overlying mucosa, resulting in pain, diarrhea, bleeding, or perforation.

CLINICAL MANIFESTATIONS. In the first days of illness the nonspecific symptoms of fever, chills, and headache are mild and in the typical case build up in intensity during the first week, resulting in prostration. The evolution of disease syndromes occurs stepwise over one to three weeks (Table 283–1) but may be variable in the time of appearance. The early symptoms of fever, abdominal pain, and prostration tend to persist throughout the illness, which in untreated cases lasts a month or longer. Abdominal pain occurs in more than half of patients and is frequently diffuse or located in the right lower quadrant over the terminal ileum. Diarrhea occurs in about a third of patients and consists of either watery stools or semisolid stools described as "pea soup." Melena occurs less commonly. Rose spots occur in more than half of light-skinned individuals but are often not visible in dark-skinned patients. The rash is seen most commonly on the shoulders, thorax, and abdomen and rarely affects the extremities. The lesions are erythematous macules or papules about 1 to 5 mm in diameter which typically blanch with pressure but may become hemorrhagic. They fade quickly after a few days of treatment. Many patients display abnormal behavior or altered mental status that may be out of proportion to the severity of the systemic illness. Among the common presentations are "toxic" staring, delirium, aphonia, and coma. Seizures are common in children. Patients are rarely jaundiced.

In about 5 per cent of patients, intestinal bleeding or intestinal perforation will occur, usually after the second week of illness. Bleeding occurs from ileal ulcers and may present as melena or bright red blood in stools. Brisk bleeding develops rarely but is an occasional cause of death. Intestinal perforation presents as the sudden onset of more severe abdominal pain, distention, and tenderness. Bowel sounds are diminished and the abdominal radiograph usually reveals free air. Perforation most often occurs unexpectedly after a few days of treatment when a patient has started to improve. Other complications of typhoid fever include pneumonia, which develops as a superinfection due to other bacteria, myocarditis, acute cholecystitis, and acute meningitis.

Relapses occur in about 10 to 20 per cent of patients treated with chloramphenicol. Patients with relapses experience the reappearance of typical symptoms about 7 to 14 days after the end of treatment. Relapses tend to be less severe than the initial episode.

DIAGNOSIS. The preferred method of diagnosis is isolation of *S. typhi* from a blood culture, which is positive in most patients during the first two weeks of illness. Urine and stool cultures are positive less frequently but should be taken to increase the diagnostic yield. The bone marrow culture is the most sensitive test, positive in nearly 90 per cent of cases, and can be used when a bacteriologic diagnosis is crucially needed or in patients who have been pretreated with antibiotics. The duodenal string test to culture bile has also been used with success in typhoid fever.

The Widal test for agglutinating antibodies against the somatic (O) and flagellar (H) antigens of *S. typhi* is widely used for serodiagnosis. An O agglutinin titer of ≥1:80 or a fourfold rise supports a diagnosis of typhoid fever, whereas the H agglutinins are more often nonspecifically elevated by immunization or previous infections with other bacteria. Sero-

TABLE 283–1. EVOLUTION OF TYPICAL SYMPTOMS AND SIGNS OF TYPHOID FEVER

Disease Period	Symptoms	Signs	Pathology
First week	Fever, chills gradually increasing and persisting; headache	Abdominal tenderness	Bacteremia
Second week	Rash, abdominal pain, diarrhea or constipation, delirium, prostration	Rose spots, splenomegaly, hepatomegaly	Mononuclear cell vasculitis of skin, hyperplasia of ileal Peyer's patches, typhoid nodules in spleen and liver
Third week	Complications of intestinal bleeding and perforation, shock	Melena, ileus, rigid abdomen, coma	Ulcerations over Peyer's patches, perforation with peritonitis
Fourth week and later	Resolution of symptoms, relapse, weight loss	Reappearance of acute disease, cachexia	Cholecystitis, chronic fecal carriage of bacteria

diagnosis is of limited value because false-positive results are often obtained in endemic areas and false-negative results occur in some cases of bacteriologically proven typhoid fever.

Other laboratory findings are anemia of variable severity and a white blood cell count that is normal or decreased with an increased percentage of band forms. Platelets are often diminished, and signs of disseminated intravascular coagulation are present. Liver function tests frequently show elevated aminotransferases and bilirubin concentrations. Renal failure is an infrequent complication. In patients with diarrhea, the stool shows fecal leukocytes.

The differential diagnosis depends on infections that are endemic in the area where an individual contracted his infection. For returned travelers from developing countries, the common possibilities are malaria, hepatitis, typhus, amebic liver abscess, shigellosis, nontyphoid salmonellosis, and leptospirosis. In the United States one must consider septicemias originating from the urinary tract, GI tract, or gallbladder as well as influenza, infectious mononucleosis, meningococcemia, miliary tuberculosis, and bacterial endocarditis.

TREATMENT. Chloramphenicol has remained the drug of choice since its introduction in 1948 because no other drug has been demonstrated to cause more rapid or consistent improvement of disease. Resistance to chloramphenicol mediated by plasmid R factors has been reported only occasionally in patients who acquired infections in Mexico, India, and Thailand. Chloramphenicol is given orally in a dose of 50 to 60 mg per kilogram of body weight per day in four equal portions every six hours. After defervescence and clinical improvement the dosage can be reduced to 30 mg per kilogram per day to complete a 14-day course. In patients unable to take oral medication the same dosage should be given intravenously until the patient can take capsules.

Alternative drugs should be considered when *S. typhi* resistant to chloramphenicol is isolated or strongly suspected. Several are nearly equal to chloramphenicol in efficacy. Trimethoprim-sulfamethoxazole is effective in a standard adult dose of 160 mg trimethoprim and 800 mg sulfamethoxazole given orally or intravenously twice a day for 14 days. Other drugs that are effective include ampicillin (intravenously), amoxicillin, cefoperazone, and ceftriaxone.

Patients who are dehydrated, anorectic, or suffering from diarrhea should receive intravenous saline with attention to electrolyte and acid-base disturbances. Patients with brisk intestinal bleeding will require blood transfusion. Patients with suspected perforation should have an abdominal radiograph to look for free air and peritoneal fluid. Laparotomy should be undertaken as early as possible to suture the perforation, and gentamicin should be added to broaden coverage for polymicrobial peritonitis.

In some high-risk patients with delirium, coma, or shock, high-dose dexamethasone in addition to antibiotics reduces mortality. The dose should be 3 mg per kilogram initially, followed by 1 mg per kilogram every 6 hours for 48 hours. One must be cautious with this therapy because signs and symptoms of perforation will be masked by steroids. Antipyretic drugs such as aspirin should be administered with

caution because they occasionally cause marked reductions in blood pressure.

Patients with relapses of typhoid fever should be treated the same as patients with a first attack. Chronic fecal carriers (asymptomatic excretion for a year or longer) should be given high doses of ampicillin or amoxicillin, 100 mg per kilogram per day, plus probenecid 30 mg per kilogram per day for four to six weeks. Trimethoprim-sulfamethoxazole is also effective. Patients with gallstones or cholecystitis may require cholecystectomy for eradication of the carrier state. Chloramphenicol neither prevents nor effectively treats the chronic carrier state.

PROGNOSIS. Typhoid fever carried a case fatality rate of about 12 per cent in the preantibiotic era which was reduced to about 4 per cent after chloramphenicol became available. Case fatality rates over 10 per cent continue to be reported in developing countries despite availability of antibiotics, whereas developed countries show case fatality rates less than 1 per cent. After treatment with chloramphenicol or other effective drug, most patients become afebrile in four to seven days. In the preantibiotic era about 10 per cent of recovered patients had relapses, and chloramphenicol treatment has not reduced this rate. Intestinal bleeding or perforation occurs in about 5 per cent of patients and may not be prevented by antibiotic treatment. Thus, bleeding or perforation is occasionally detected after patients have defervesced during treatment. About 1 to 3 per cent of patients become chronic fecal carriers after recovery.

PREVENTION. Travelers to developing countries should avoid drinking untreated water, drinks served with ice, peeled fruits, and other food that is not served hot. American international travelers face an overall risk of developing typhoid fever of less than 1 case in 10,000 trips, but travelers to high-risk countries like India and Pakistan have a probability of about 4 in 10,000 trips of getting typhoid fever. Travelers wishing protection should receive typhoid vaccine, U.S.P., administered as two subcutaneous injections of 0.5 ml each at intervals of four weeks, with booster doses given every three years if needed. The live oral vaccine Ty21a has been field tested and is available commercially in Europe. These vaccines give only partial protection, and thus vaccinated persons should still exercise dietary precautions. The traditional method of controlling typhoid is to follow stool cultures of convalescent cases and report positive cultures to the Health Department. The Health Department investigates nonimported typhoid cases to identify possible food sources or contact with a chronic carrier.

Butler T, Knight J, Nath SK, et al.: Typhoid fever complicated by intestinal perforation: A persisting fatal disease requiring surgical management. Rev Infect Dis 7:244, 1985. *A useful summary of 76 papers, advancing the argument that surgical intervention for intestinal perforation gives better results than medical treatment alone.*

Edelman R, Levine MM: Summary of an international workshop on typhoid fever. Rev Infect Dis 8:329, 1986. *An overview of a workshop presenting current research on epidemiology and vaccine development.*

Hoffmann SL, Punjabi NH, Kumala S, et al.: Reduction of mortality in chloramphenicol-treated typhoid fever by high dose dexamethasone. N Engl J Med 310:82, 1984. *In typhoid patients with delirium, obtundation, stupor, coma, or shock, dexamethasone therapy was highly efficacious.*

Hoffmann TA, Ruiz CJ, Counts GW, et al.: Waterborne typhoid fever in Dade County, Florida: Clinical and therapeutic evaluation in 105 bacteremic patients. Am J Med 59:481, 1975. *Good account of an epidemic. The illness was generally mild. Chloramphenicol seemed to be superior to ampicillin for therapy.*

Hornick RB, Greisman SE, Woodward TE, et al.: Typhoid fever: Pathogenesis and immunologic control. N Engl J Med 283:686, 739, 1970. *A good account of pathophysiology, including a discussion of the role of endotoxin. Human volunteer studies are reviewed.*

Wahdan MH, Serie C, Cerisier Y, et al.: A controlled field trial of live *Salmonella typhi* strain Ty21a oral vaccine against typhoid: Three-year results. J Infect Dis 145:292, 1982. *An important vaccine, not only for excellent activity against an ancient enemy, typhoid fever, but also because this is the first effective oral bacterial vaccine.*

284 SALMONELLA INFECTIONS OTHER THAN TYPHOID FEVER

Richard B. Hornick

DEFINITION. Salmonellae comprise a large group of gram-negative bacilli that cause a broad spectrum of disease in humans and animals. The most common disorder in humans is gastroenteritis or salmonellosis, usually a mild, self-limited diarrheal illness. Systemic spread from the gut is unusual. Other patients may develop septicemia, a stubborn infection for the host to eradicate, even with antimicrobial therapy. Localized infections may present in the form of osteomyelitis, mycotic aneurysms, or abscesses. The unique human pathogen *S. typhi* produces enteric fever, an illness also caused by several other select *Salmonella* species. A prolonged carrier state, which mimics that seen following infection with *S. typhi*, may result from *Salmonella* infections.

Many animals suffer fatal diarrheal disease caused by species of salmonellae that infect only animals. Some animals have an asymptomatic infection caused by strains that infect both humans and animals. Meat and eggs and other animal-derived food products serve as the most important source of infections in humans.

ETIOLOGY. Salmonellae are motile, gram-negative bacilli that do not ferment lactose or sucrose but metabolize glucose, maltose, and mannitol. They grow readily on many media.

Salmonellae contain a thick, complex lipopolysaccharide cell wall that is the O antigen, made up of several specific O antigen types. The specificity of each of the O antigens is determined by the sequence of sugars that constitute the outer layer of the cell wall. Strains lacking the outer layer are characterized as "rough" because of the wrinkled surface of the colonies. Such strains appear to be nonpathogenic. Antibodies directed at the R core protect against infections caused by many gram-negative bacilli. The inner or basal layer is the lipid moiety, a bridging structure between the outer two layers and the foundation of the cell wall. This whole substance is the endotoxin, the ubiquitous lipopolysaccharide material of all gram-negative bacilli that causes fever plus other severe host reactions during active disease.

There are at least 60 specific O-antigen complexes. Group-specific antibodies can be used to classify salmonellae into many serotypes. The H antigens are the flagellae of the organisms. Serotyping, using O and H antisera plus biochemical tests, has established at least 2200 species. A simplified characterization has been suggested based on host preferences and adaptations: (1) *Salmonella* serotypes highly adapted to man. These include *S. typhi*, *S. paratyphi A*, *S. schottmülleri* (paratyphi B), *S. hirschfeldii* (paratyphi C), and *S. sendai*. There is no animal reservoir for these strains, animal infection is rare, and accidental and human-to-human transmission is critical in the epidemiology of the disease they produce.

(2) *Salmonella* serotypes highly adapted to specific nonhuman hosts. Most strains cause only illness in animals. *S. dublin* from cattle and *S. choleraesuis* from swine are two exceptions that often cause human disease. (3) *Salmonella* serotypes unadapted to specific hosts. This is a large group (>1400 strains), ubiquitous in nature, that usually causes gastroenteritis, rarely invades the bloodstream, and is responsible for about 85 per cent of all *Salmonella* infections in the United States. The strains of this last group will be mainly discussed in this chapter. The most common serotypes involved in human disease are *S. typhimurium* (accounts for about 25 to 30 per cent of all cases), *S. enteritidis*, *S. heidelberg*, *S. newport*, *S. infantis*, *S. agona*, *S. montevideo*, *S. saint-paul*, and *S. javiana*. *Salmonella* infections are reportable diseases, and the ranking listed comes from the annual compilation published by the Centers for Disease Control.

EPIDEMIOLOGY. Humans ingest salmonellae primarily in contaminated food, less frequently in water, and in rare instances from exotic sources. Salmonellae can infect many species of animals. Those of greatest hazard to human health are meat-producing animals and poultry. Eggs and egg products have been a consistent source of salmonellae. The organisms can be incorporated into the egg before the shell is completely calcified in the chicken, or the egg becomes contaminated during laying. Cracked or dirty eggs should raise a suspicion of contamination with salmonellae. An egg containing salmonellae requires at least three minutes of boiling to ensure complete bacterial killing. Poultry may become infected, have no significant disease, and yet be fecal shedders. During the processing of poultry, the carcasses may become surface contaminated from water baths or conveyer belts that were colonized by microorganisms from previously processed birds. Consumers handling such poultry products are at risk of infection. The organisms persist on the fingers for several hours and can be transferred to other foods that permit further multiplication. The meat of animals usually does not contain abscesses, nor are the salmonellae isolated from mesenteric lymph nodes of meat-producing animals. Thus, most salmonellae represent skin colonization from the contaminated surfaces of the processing plant. Raw milk is a persistent source of *S. dublin* for consumers. Up to 10 per cent of healthy cattle may carry this species.

Pet turtles have been an important source of salmonella infections in this country. Chickens and cattle can deposit salmonellae into the soil upon which the turtles feed. The legs of the common housefly can also carry salmonellae. Transmission to human food is possible but not likely. Contaminated carmine red dye, derived from female scale insects and larvae, has caused hospital epidemics of salmonellosis when given to determine intestinal transit time. Recently, an outbreak of salmonellosis occurred among teenagers and young adults using marijuana contaminated with *S. muenchen*, an organism isolated from poultry, swine, and cattle.

Human-to-human spread via contaminated food or water is the second most common means of transmitting salmonellae. Transient or convalescent carriers have frequently been the source of large foodborne outbreaks of gastroenteritis. Improper hand washing, inadequate refrigeration of prepared foods prior to serving, and insufficient cooking of poultry products have been common epidemiologic features of outbreaks occurring after large public feasts.

Most cases of salmonellosis occurring in healthy adults are of little medical significance. However, outbreaks in nursing homes or nurseries cause severe morbidity and unnecessary mortality. Epidemics may arise owing to contaminated hospital food; cross-infections have been documented in pediatric wards resulting from contaminated fingers or clothes of attending personnel or via aerosols from sick infants. A rare source of infection has been *S. kottbus* excreted by the donor of breast milk. Faulty refrigeration allowed for multiplication of this species in the milk.

The most common form of illness is the diarrheal disease salmonellosis. Children have the greatest incidence (median age, 10 years), and the highest rate is in infants. In the United States, this disease occurs most frequently in the summer and early fall.

The epidemiologic characteristics of other strains causing systemic infection are also varied. *S. choleraesuis*, which is associated with swine and pork products, is an unusual isolate in the United States but is the predominant cause of localized or enteric fever syndromes. Children with this strain may develop a moderately severe form of enteric fever. Infected adults are more likely to present with bacteremia or localized infectious conditions such as abscesses in deep muscle groups, osteomyelitis, or mycotic aneurysms. This difference may reflect a partial immunity developed in adults and resulting from previous subclinical infections.

Enteric fever may also be produced by *S. paratyphi* A and B. These infections are unusual in this country but are common in late-developing countries where typhoid fever is also prevalent. Patients with enteric fever induced by *S. paratyphi* B frequently respond less promptly to antibiotic treatment than do patients with typhoid fever.

PATHOLOGY. *Salmonella*-induced gastroenteritis rarely causes death. Infants and the aged are at the greatest risk. Death usually occurs as a result of dehydration caused by the diarrhea. Intestinal mucosa is red and swollen and often shows petechial hemorrhages. Salmonellae induce a polymorphonuclear leukocyte infiltration in the lamina propria region. The organisms reach that area by penetrating through the epithelial cell layer. Those patients suffering from bacteremia or localized disease have collections of neutrophils in the areas of bacterial localizations. By contrast, *S. typhi* induces mononuclear cell responses in the liver or in the lamina propria and at sites of intestinal perforation. These differences in cellular responses may be due to small concentrations of endotoxin present at the sites of *S. typhi* multiplication.

PATHOGENESIS. Ingested salmonellae must penetrate through the epithelial cell layer in order to produce disease. Stomach acid is an effective barrier to large inocula reaching the small and large intestine, where disease is initiated. Persons who are taking antacids, or who have achlorhydria because of drugs, marijuana use, surgery, or age, are at increased risk of acquiring salmonellae or other enteric pathogens. Passage through the stomach appears to be facilitated by ingestion of the bacilli in a small volume of fluid (50 ml or less). This small volume is not retained in the stomach. Nonspecific defense mechanisms in the small and large bowel such as rapid transit time, inactivation by enzymes or lysozymes, and nosocomial bacteria may decrease the number of bacteria able to penetrate through the epithelial cells.

In order to invade, salmonellae and other enteric pathogens must first adhere to the surface of the cells. Two virulence factors are involved in this process, one in the large bowel and the other in the small intestine. Colonization factors (pili) on the surface of the salmonellae are needed to allow adherence to epithelial cells in the small intestine. Specific receptor sites on the epithelial cell surface, glycosides, are involved. The lipopolysaccharide (LPS) of the bacteria appears to be critical in the colon. In experimental animals, organisms lacking the complete LPS are unable to adhere to colonic mucosa. Penetration through the cell is associated with a plasmid that also provides the organism with other virulence functions. Similar plasmids are found in other enteric pathogens.

Once the bacteria reach the lamina propria area, further penetration into the lymphatics or capillaries is impeded by the inflammatory response. Presumably the polymorphonuclear leukocytes effectively phagocytize and eliminate these salmonellae. However, certain species of *Salmonella* have a predilection for extraintestinal spread. *S. heidelberg* and *S. dublin* are responsible for small numbers of cases of diarrhea

but of those infected, about 15 per cent may develop bacteremia. As many as 79 per cent of patients who are infected with *S. dublin* and who have compromised immune systems develop bacteremia and infections in extraintestinal sites. This species is frequently isolated from raw milk.

The watery stools elicited by salmonellae probably originate in the upper small intestine, a section that has a great secretory capacity. An enterotoxin stimulates the secretion of electrolytes and fluid into the lumen. This process is similar to that induced by enterotoxigenic *E. coli*. No penetration occurs; the toxin is released on the surface of the cells and activates adenylate cyclase; secretion of chloride and sodium ions results. The inflammatory process associated with penetration in the ileum may cause diarrheal disease characterized by stools of smaller volume. These presumably result from the lesser capacity of the ileum to secrete fluid and perhaps from failure to absorb all the fluid presented to the inflamed ileum. The secretion in the ileum may be stimulated by the enterotoxins, by prostaglandins released from the inflammatory exudate, or by both. This latter mediator also activates the adenylate cyclase energy system. A smear of a small specimen of stool stained with methylene blue will reveal large numbers of neutrophils. These are indicative of involvement of the large bowel in the inflammatory process initiated by salmonellae.

The number of organisms necessary to induce gastroenteritis in humans is unknown. Limited studies in volunteers have suggested that large doses of *S. typhimurium*, e.g., 10 million to 1 billion cells, are required to cause disease. The incubation period falls within a relatively narrow range—12 to 24 hours. An inverse relationship between the size of the inoculum and the length of the incubation period probably exists. The short incubation period of salmonellosis suggests that this infection is superficial in the gut and causes disease through quick-acting substances such as enterotoxins. The self-limiting nature is consistent with rapid clearing mechanisms, e.g., short life span of the epithelial cells and efficient cellular clearing systems in the lamina propria.

Patients with certain chronic diseases are prone to *Salmonella* infections. Patients with sickle cell disease develop septicemia or localized *Salmonella* infection. Osteomyelitis caused by one of the *Salmonella* strains is especially common. These patients are deficient in opsonizing capabilities, have reduced numbers of phagocytes in the spleen and elsewhere, and sustain bone and gut infarcts. Taken together, these changes permit easy access of salmonellae through the gut, survival in the circulation, and infection in the bone. Patients with acute hemolytic processes caused by bartonellosis and malaria have an increased incidence of salmonellosis. Diseases that impair cellular immune mechanisms, e.g., AIDS, leukemias and lymphomas, are associated with a high incidence of salmonellal septicemic infections. Patients with chronic *Schistosoma haematobium* infections of the genitourinary tract are prone to chronic bacteriuria and bacteremia caused by *S. typhi* and *S. paratyphi* strains. These strains have pili that permit attachment to surface receptors on the schistosomes. Treatment of the schistosomiasis as well as the bacterial infection can be curative.

The pathogenesis of the chronic asymptomatic carrier state caused by salmonellae other than *S. typhi* is not clearly understood. A few persons will have chronic low grade infection in a diseased gallbladder identical to the typhoid carrier state. The paratyphi strains are involved in this manner. However, for those strains causing salmonellosis, carriage may persist for many months without evidence of biliary tract dysfunction. Some of those patients have received unnecessary antibiotic therapy for their diarrhea, and this can prolong the carrier state. In mice, the antibiotic eliminates part of the nosocomial flora that normally inhibits the colonization and multiplication of salmonellae. The mechanism involves the acid environment associated with the production of short chain fatty acids by the normal flora. This explanation, if applicable to the human situation, suggests that chronic carriage occurs primarily in the intestinal tract. Rarely will these patients shed salmonellae for more than eight months.

CLINICAL MANIFESTATIONS. *Gastroenteritis.* Gastroenteritis begins abruptly with nausea and crampy abdominal pain followed by diarrhea. The stools are watery, initially in large volume, and occasionally will contain mucus and a trace of blood. A smaller number of patients will have paste-like or semisolid stools that are associated with cramps in the lower quadrants. These stools are likely to contain mucus and blood, and white cells are seen on a methylene blue–stained specimen. Vomiting is not frequent and, if present, does not persist throughout the period of the diarrhea. Fever of 38.5 to 39° C is seen in 50 to 70 per cent of patients. Chills are noted in about 30 per cent of patients. Physical findings are few and relate to the inflammatory process in the gastrointestinal tract. Palpation tenderness resulting from contraction of loops of bowel is present in variable locations of the abdomen. Symptoms in otherwise healthy adults last about two to five days. The disease persists for a longer period in patients debilitated by extremes of age, malignancy, or antibiotic or steroid therapy.

The symptoms and signs of enteric fever have been described for typhoid fever. An identical presentation is associated with disease produced by paratyphi strains.

Bacteremia. Patients with this form of salmonellal disease have a history of fever, chills, sweats, malaise, anorexia, and weight loss for several days to a week or more. Stool cultures may not reveal salmonellae, but blood cultures will be positive. A search for the source of bacteremia is mandatory but often unrewarding. Osteomyelitis, mycotic aneurysm or infection of a pre-existing aneurysm (abdominal aorta and femoral artery are common sites), pericarditis (minimal amount of exudate present), abscesses, arthritis, meningitis, pneumonia, and hepatitis are all representative of localized infections with bacteremia. Patients with solid tumors may have abscesses in these lesions that serve as a source of *Salmonella* bacteremia. Pheochromocytoma, ovarian cyst, renal cell carcinoma, uterine myomas, and metastatic tumors to bone or skin are common examples of such tumors.

The isolation of *S. choleraesuis* from the blood of an adult is usually indicative of an abscess.

DIAGNOSIS. The diagnosis of any form of *Salmonella* infection is confirmed by isolation of the organism from blood or stool or both. Other isolations can be made from liver, abscesses, or localized infections when systemic disease is present. Fresh diarrheal stool specimens should be cultured. Serologic information is not helpful for salmonellosis but is useful for the systemic infections, especially enteric fever. About 65 to 70 per cent of patients with enteric fever will have a four-fold or greater increase in O and/or H antibody titers over a two- to three-week span.

Patients with gastroenteritis will have a normal white blood cell count. Hemoconcentration may occur with significant fluid loss. A smear of the diarrheal stool stained with methylene blue will often reveal numerous leukocytes, indicating colitis. Similar findings are noted with other bacteria that invade epithelial cells, e.g., *Shigella, Campylobacter, Yersinia.*

The differential diagnosis of *Salmonella* gastroenteritis includes a broad spectrum of enteric pathogens: enterotoxigenic *E. coli* (heat-stable and heat-labile toxins), *Campylobacter fetus* subspecies *jejuni, Vibrio parahaemolyticus, Shigella* species, *Yersinia enterocolitica,* and other bacteria associated with food-induced diarrhea. The diarrheal syndromes produced by these organisms can mimic that caused by salmonellae. Historical facts may suggest a cause (seafood—*Vibrio parahaemolyticus;* refried rice—*B. cereus*), but confirmation requires cultural proof. Viral agents such as the parvoviruses and rotovirus can also cause the same illness; however, the highest attack rate is in infants and children. Isolation techniques for these

viruses are not readily available. Most patients with infectious diarrhea have almost recovered from their illness when culture results are available. In certain patients, e.g., those with persistent diarrhea or those debilitated by other illness, specific cultural information is necessary to prescribe appropriate therapy. More rapid culture techniques are needed.

TREATMENT. Fluid replacement is the uniform approach to treatment of any patient with a diarrheal illness. It is especially critical in the management of patients who cannot readily tolerate a reduction in plasma volume. In most adults with salmonellosis, self-treatment with tolerated liquids is satisfactory. Fruit juices, broths, tea, and water are useful. In children an acquired lactase deficiency during the diarrhea is common, and milk can therefore prolong the diarrheal state because of the osmotic effect of undigested lactose. Intravenous fluids are necessary only for severely dehydrated patients unable to take oral replacement fluid because of nausea and vomiting.

Antibiotic treatment is not usually required to treat salmonellosis although selected patients may benefit. Infants and elderly nursing-home patients who are known to be at greatest risk of mortality from this infection should be treated. A short course (three to five days) of ampicillin (4 to 6 grams per day) or amoxicillin (2 to 4 grams per day) may be used in adults. Sensitivity of the isolate to various antibiotics should be ascertained, since ampicillin-resistant strains are becoming increasingly common. Trimethoprim-sulfamethoxazole or chloramphenicol is an effective alternative. Antibiotic treatment will prolong the excretion of salmonellae in the stools and may not shorten the clinical course of the patient's illness. Adults usually recover without antibiotic therapy in two to five days.

The uncomfortable abdominal cramps may be relieved with atropine or drugs with a similar smooth muscle relaxing effect. However, such drugs have an antiperistaltic effect that can prolong the diarrhea. Thus, these drugs should be used intermittently for relief of pain only.

The treatment of the systemic forms of *Salmonella* infection requires appropriate antibiotic therapy. The approach is similar to that for typhoid fever. Three drugs have been generally effective: chloramphenicol, trimethoprim-sulfamethoxazole, and ampicillin or amoxicillin. Drainage of abscesses is mandatory. Resection of infected aneurysms is indicated, but the surgical results have been poor. Antibiotic coverage is required before, during, and after surgery.

PROGNOSIS. Gastroenteritis is a mild self-limiting infection, and recovery is complete in several days. Complications are mainly related to consequences of dehydration, e.g., azotemia, stroke, or myocardial infarction, occurring in those patients with significant arteriosclerosis or tenuous fluid balance. Mortality occurs in infants and the elderly. In some epidemics in nurseries or nursing homes, the rate has been 3 to 5 per cent. Immunity to reinfection is incomplete and repeated episodes of salmonellosis will occur following reexposure.

The prognosis for patients with bacteremic forms of salmonellae may be poor, since many of these patients have underlying diseases. The mortality with *S. choleraesuis* infections has been reported to be as high as 20 per cent. Infants with meningitis have a mortality of 40 per cent, and residual neurologic defects are common.

PREVENTION. There is no vaccine to prevent gastroenteritis or the systemic forms of *Salmonella* infection. Typhoid fever prevention is possible with a new oral attenuated vaccine strain. Careful attention to handwashing, refrigeration of prepared foods, and proper cooking of poultry and their products can help reduce the opportunities to acquire salmonellosis.

Aserhoff B, Bennett JV: Effect of antibiotic therapy in acute salmonellosis on the fecal excretion of salmonellae. N Engl J Med 281:636, 1969. *This paper* presents evidence that suggested antibiotic treatment prolongs the fecal secretion of salmonellae in patients with salmonellosis.

Black PH, King LJ, Swartz MN: Salmonellosis: A review of some unusual aspects. N Engl J Med 262:811, 1960. *A classic paper that highlights many of the epidemiologic and clinical curiosities of* Salmonella-*induced disease.*

Giannella RA, Broitman SA, Zamcheck N: Influence of gastric acidity on bacterial and parasitic enteric infections: A perspective. Ann Intern Med 78:271, 1973. *A good review of the topic dealing with the gastric acid barrier.*

Huang CT, Lo CB: Human infection with *Salmonella choleraesuis* in Hong Kong. J Hyg 65:149, 1967. *The authors present a complete summary of the clinical manifestations of infection with this important Salmonella strain.*

Riley LW, DiFerdinando GT Jr, DeMelfi TM, et al.: Evaluation of isolated cases of salmonellosis by plasmid profile analysis: Introduction and transmission of a bacterial clone by precooked roast beef. J Infect Dis 148:12, 1983. *A new epidemiologic tool for identifying* Salmonella *isolated from patients in scattered locations as coming from a common source.*

285 SHIGELLOSIS

Thomas Butler

DEFINITION. Shigellosis is an acute bacterial infection caused by the genus *Shigella* resulting in colitis affecting predominantly the rectosigmoid colon. Bacillary dysentery is synonymous with shigellosis. The disease is characterized by diarrhea, dysentery, fever, abdominal pain, and tenesmus. Shigellosis is usually limited to a few days. Early treatment with antimicrobial drugs results in more rapid recovery.

ETIOLOGY. Shigellae are nonmotile gram-negative bacilli belonging to the family Enterobacteriaceae. Four species of shigellae are recognized on the basis of antigenic and biochemical properties: *S. dysenteriae* (group A), *S. flexneri* (group B), *S. boydii* (group C), and *S. sonnei* (group D). Among these species there are over 40 serotypes, each of which is designated by the species name followed by a specific Arabic number. *S. dysenteriae* 1 is called the Shiga bacillus and causes epidemics with higher mortality than other serotypes. With the exception of *S. flexneri* 6, they do not ferment lactose.

Serotypes are determined by the O polysaccharide side chain of the lipopolysaccharide (endotoxin) in the cell wall. Endotoxin is detectable in the blood of severely ill patients and may be responsible for the complication of the hemolytic-uremic syndrome. To be virulent, shigellae must be able to invade epithelial cells, as tested in the laboratory by kerato-conjunctivitis in the guinea pig (Sereney test) or HeLa cell invasion. Bacterial invasion of cells is genetically governed by three chromosomal regions and a 140 Mdal plasmid. Shiga toxin is produced by *S. dysenteriae* 1 and in lesser amounts by other serotypes. It inhibits protein synthesis and has entero-toxic activity in animal models, but its role in human disease is uncertain.

INCIDENCE AND PREVALENCE. In the United States in 1984, there were about 13,000 reported cases of shigellosis. The predominant species was *S. sonnei* (64 per cent), followed by *S. flexneri* (31 per cent), *S. boydii* (3 per cent), and *S. dysenteriae* (2 per cent). Most cases were in young children, and a large proportion occurred in population groups living in homes for the mentally ill or in nursing homes. Among cases occurring on Indian reservations, 64 per cent were due to *S. flexneri*.

Worldwide most cases of shigellosis occur in children of developing countries, where *S. flexneri* is the predominant species. During the past 15 years, major epidemics due to *S. dysenteriae* 1 have occurred in Central America, Central Africa, India, and Bangladesh.

EPIDEMIOLOGY. Shigellosis is transmitted by the fecal-oral route. Crowded living conditions, low standards of personal hygiene, poor water supply, and inadequate sewage facilities all contribute to an increased risk of infection. Transmission most often occurs by close person-to-person contact through contaminated hands. During clinical illness and for up to six weeks after recovery, organisms are excreted in the feces. Although the organisms are sensitive to desiccation, they may survive several months in food or water, which are occasional vehicles of transmission.

Children between one and four years of age have the greatest risk of developing shigellosis. Inhabitants of custodial institutions, such as homes for retarded children, are at highest risk. Intrafamilial spread follows often when the initial case has occurred in a pre-school child. In young adults the incidence is higher in women than men, which probably reflects closer contact of women with children. The male homosexual population in the United States is at increased risk for shigellosis, which is one of the causes of the "gay bowel syndrome."

Humans and higher primates are the only known natural reservoirs of shigellosis. Transmission shows variable seasonal patterns in different regions. In the United States, the peak incidence is in late summer and early autumn.

PATHOGENESIS AND PATHOLOGY. Since the micro-organisms are relatively resistant to acid, shigellae pass the gastric barrier more readily than other enteric pathogens. In volunteer studies, as few as 200 ingested bacilli regularly initiate disease in 25 per cent of healthy adults. This contrasts strikingly with the much larger numbers of typhoid or cholera bacilli required to produce disease in normal individuals. During the incubation period, usually 12 to 72 hours, the organisms traverse the small bowel, penetrate colonic epithelial cells, and multiply intracellularly. An acute inflammatory response ensues in the colonic mucosa attended by prodromal symptoms (Table 285–1). Epithelial cells containing bacteria are lysed, resulting in superficial ulcerations and shedding of shigella organisms into stools. The mucosa is friable and covered with a layer of polymorphonuclear leukocytes. Advancing inflammation causes the formation of crypt abscesses. Initially the inflammation is confined to the rectosigmoid colon but after about four days of illness may advance to involve the proximal colon also. In severe cases, there may be pan-colitis with extension of inflammation into the terminal ileum; a pseudomembranous type of colitis may develop. Diarrhea results because of impaired absorption of water and electrolytes by the inflamed colon.

Although the colonic inflammation is superficial, bacteremia occurs occasionally, especially in *S. dysenteriae* 1 infections. Susceptibility of organisms to serum complement–mediated bacteriolysis may explain the infrequency of bacteremia and disseminated infection. Colonic perforation is a rare complication during toxic megacolon. Children with severe colitis due to *S. dysenteriae* 1 are prone to develop the hemolytic-uremic syndrome. In this complication fibrin thrombi are deposited in the renal glomeruli, causing cortical necrosis and fragmentation of red cells.

CLINICAL MANIFESTATIONS. Most patients with shigellosis begin their illness with a nonspecific prodrome (Table 285–1). The height of the temperature varies, and children may have febrile convulsions. The initial intestinal symptoms soon follow as cramps, loose stools, and watery diarrhea, which usually precede the onset of dysentery by one or more days. The average fecal output is about 600 grams a day for adults. The dysentery consists typically of flecks and small clots of bright red blood and mucus in stools that are small in volume. Frequency of passage is often as high as 20 to 40 times a day, with excruciating rectal pain and tenesmus during defecation. Some patients develop rectal prolapse during severe straining. The amount of blood in stools varies widely but usually is small because of the superficial colonic ulcerations. Abdominal tenderness is often most marked in the left lower quadrant over the sigmoid colon but may also be generalized. The fever is likely to abate after a few days of dysentery, making afebrile bloody diarrhea an occasional clinical presentation. After one to two weeks of untreated disease, spontaneous improvement occurs in most patients.

TABLE 285–1. EVOLUTION OF CLINICAL SYNDROMES IN SHIGELLOSIS

Stage	Time of Appearance After Onset of Illness	Symptoms and Signs	Pathology
Prodrome	Earliest	Fever, chills, myalgias, anorexia, nausea, vomiting	None or early colitis
Nonspecific diarrhea	0–3 days	Abdominal cramps, loose stools, watery diarrhea	Rectosigmoid colitis with superficial ulceration, fecal leukocytes
Dysentery	1–8 days	Frequent passage of blood and mucus, tenesmus, rectal prolapse, abdominal tenderness	Colitis extending sometimes to proximal colon, crypt abscesses, inflammation in lamina propria
Complications	3–10 days	Dehydration, seizures, septicemia, leukemoid reaction, hemolytic-uremic syndrome, ileus, peritonitis	Severe colitis, terminal ileitis, endotoxemia, intravascular coagulation, toxic megacolon, colonic perforation
Postdysenteric syndromes	1–3 weeks	Arthritis, Reiter's syndrome	Reactive inflammation in HLA-B27 haplotype

Some patients with mild disease develop only the prodrome or experience only watery diarrhea without dysentery.

Complications include dehydration, which can be a cause of death, especially in children and the elderly. Shigella septicemia occurs mainly in malnourished children with *S. dysenteriae* 1 infections. The leukemoid reaction and hemolytic-uremic syndrome may develop in children late in the course when the dysentery has started to improve. Neurologic manifestations can be striking and include delirium, seizures, and nuchal rigidity.

The important postdysenteric syndromes are arthritis and Reiter's triad of arthritis, urethritis, and conjunctivitis (see Ch. 434). These are nonsuppurative phenomena that occur in the absence of viable *Shigella* organisms about one to three weeks after resolution of dysentery.

DIAGNOSIS. Shigellosis should be considered in any patient with acute onset of fever and diarrhea. Examination of the stool is essential. Blood and pus are grossly apparent in severe bacillary dysentery; even in milder forms of the disease, microscopic examination of the stool often reveals numerous leukocytes and erythrocytes. The fecal leukocyte examination should be performed with a portion of liquid stool, preferably containing mucus. A drop of stool is placed on a microscopic slide, mixed thoroughly with two drops of methylene blue, and overlaid with a coverslip. The presence of abundant polymorphonuclear leukocytes helps in distinguishing shigellosis from diarrheal syndromes caused by viruses and enterotoxigenic bacteria. The fecal leukocyte examination is not helpful in distinguishing shigellosis from diarrheal illnesses caused by other invasive enteric pathogens (nontyphoidal *Salmonella, Campylobacter,* and *Yersina*). Amebic dysentery is excluded by the absence of trophozoites on a microscopic examination of fresh stool under a cover slip. The peripheral white cell count is of little diagnostic value, since it may range from less than 3,000 to more than 30,000. Sigmoidoscopic examination reveals diffuse erythema with a mucopurulent layer and friable areas of mucosa with shallow ulcers 3 to 7 mm in diameter.

Definitive diagnosis depends upon isolating shigellae by selective media. A rectal swab, a swab of a colonic ulcer obtained by sigmoidoscopic examination, or a freshly passed stool specimen should be inoculated immediately on culture plates or into carrying media. Since isolation rates of shigellae from freshly passed stools of patients with shigellosis may be as low as 67 per cent, culturing for three successive days is recommended. Stool cultures are generally positive within 24 hours after onset of symptoms and may remain positive for several weeks in the absence of antimicrobial therapy. Appropriate culture media include blood, desoxycholate, and Salmonella-Shigella (S-S) agars. Selected colonies should be diagnosed by agglutination with polyvalent *Shigella* antisera. S-S agar is inhibitory for *S dysenteriae* 1.

Definitive bacteriologic diagnosis becomes of critical importance in distinguishing the more severe and prolonged cases of shigellosis from ulcerative colitis, with which it may be confused both clinically and on sigmoidoscopic examination. Patients with shigellosis have been subjected to colectomy because of a mistaken diagnosis of ulcerative colitis; a positive culture should prevent such a misadventure.

TREATMENT. The effectiveness of antimicrobial agents in treating shigellosis has been well established. Appropriate antimicrobial therapy instituted early may decrease the duration of symptoms by 50 per cent and decrease the duration of excretion of shigellae (an important epidemiologic factor) by a far greater percentage. Ampicillin is currently the drug of choice for sensitive strains in the United States. It should be administered orally in four divided doses for a total of 2 grams a day to adults and 100 mg per kilogram per day to children for a five-day period. Single-dose therapy of 100 mg per kilogram of ampicillin orally for adults and children older than four years is also effective. Because of the increasing frequency of plasmid-mediated antimicrobial resistance in *Shigella* infections, drug susceptibility testing is important. Trimethoprim-sulfamethoxazole administered in standard doses twice daily for five days is now the treatment of choice for *Shigella* strains of unknown antibiotic sensitivity in both adults and children. Certain drugs that appear effective in vitro, including amoxicillin and nonabsorbable antimicrobials such as neomycin or kanamycin, are not effective in vivo. Sulfonamide resistance is so widespread as to nullify the value of these agents.

Fluid losses in shigellosis are qualitatively similar to those in other infectious diarrheal diseases, and the patient should be treated with appropriate intravenous or oral electrolyte repletion fluids in quantities adequate to correct clinical signs of saline depletion. The requirement for fluids is generally small, but fluid repletion will be lifesaving in exceptional cases.

Agents that decrease intestinal motility should not be used. Such preparations as diphenoxylate and paregoric may exacerbate symptoms, presumably by retarding intestinal clearance of the microorganisms. There is no convincing evidence that pectin- or bismuth-containing preparations are helpful.

PROGNOSIS. The mortality rate in untreated shigellosis is dependent upon the infectious strain and ranges from 10 to 30 per cent in certain outbreaks caused by *S. dysenteriae* 1 to less than 1 per cent in most *S. sonnei* infections. Even with infection caused by *S. dysenteriae* 1, mortality rates should approach zero if appropriate fluid replacement and antimicrobial therapy are initiated early.

About 2 per cent of patients may develop arthritis or Reiter's syndrome weeks or months after recovery from shigellosis.

PREVENTION. Individuals excreting shigellae should be excluded from all phases of food handling until negative cultures have been obtained from three successive stool specimens collected after completion of antimicrobial therapy. In institutional outbreaks, strict and early isolation of infected individuals is mandatory. Targeted antimicrobial chemoprophylaxis has been disappointing. The most important control measure is scrupulous handwashing by all individuals involved in handling of food. Reporting of shigellosis cases to health authorities should be mandatory.

For the traveler to countries with major *Shigella* problems, no chemoprophylactic agent is an adequate substitute for good personal hygiene and the avoidance of contaminated food and water. A variety of vaccines has been developed and tested, but no vaccine is now commercially available.

Butler T, Speelman P, Kabir I, et al.: Colonic dysfunction during shigellosis. J Infect Dis 154:817, 1986. *Studies perfusing the human colon showed diminished colonic water absorption, increased potassium secretion, and normal ileocecal flow rates.*

Haltalin KC, Kusmiesz HT, Hinton LV, et al.: Treatment of acute diarrhea in outpatients. Am J Dis Child 124:554, 1972. *An unequivocal demonstration of the value of appropriate antimicrobial therapy in the management of shigellosis.*

Keusch GT: Shigella infections. Clin Gastroenterol 8:645, 1979. *A review of clinical features and pathogenesis which highlights controversies.*

Koster F, Levin J, Walker L, et al.: Hemolytic-uremic syndrome after shigellosis. Relation to endotoxemia and circulating immune complexes. N Engl J Med 298:927, 1978. *New light on the pathogenesis of this frequently lethal complication of shigellosis in children.*

Levine MM: Bacillary dysentery. Mechanisms and treatment. Med Clin North Am 66:623, 1982. *A good review of microbiologic and clinical aspects of shigellosis.*

Struelens MJ, Patte D, Kabir I, et al.: Shigella septicemia: Prevalence, presentation, risk factors, and outcome. J Infect Dis 152:784, 1985. *A report of this complication from Bangladesh and the high case fatality rate in malnourished children.*

286 CAMPYLOBACTER ENTERITIS

Richard L. Guerrant

Enteric infection with a member of the genus *Campylobacter* usually results in an inflammatory, occasionally bloody diarrhea or dysentery syndrome. In industrialized, temperate areas, *Campylobacter jejuni* is often the most commonly recognized cause of inflammatory enteritis. The diarrhea may also be watery, especially in developing, tropical areas. An enterocolitis or protocolitis syndrome similar to that seen with *C. jejuni* is also increasingly appreciated in homosexual males with several "*Campylobacter*-like organisms." The other major *Campylobacter* species that infects humans is *Campylobacter fetus*, a relatively uncommon cause of bacteremia and occasional intravascular infection in immunocompromised hosts. Finally, gastric *Campylobacter* isolates have recently been associated with histologic gastritis.

ETIOLOGY. *Campylobacter* (meaning curved rod) is a curved or spiral, motile, non–spore-forming, gram-negative rod measuring 1.5 by 3.5 microns which is distinguished from Enterobacteriaceae by its inability to ferment or oxidize carbohydrates. It was formerly called a vibrio, but is now recognized as a separate genus, on the basis of its distinctive DNA content. It is both oxidase- and catalase-positive and is a microaerophilic organism that requires reduced oxygen (5 to 10 per cent) and increased carbon dioxide (3 to 10 per cent). The organism will not grow at either aerobic or strictly anaerobic conditions. Perhaps reflecting its avian reservoir, *C. jejuni* also requires an increased temperature to 42° C for optimal growth. *C. jejuni* is distinguished from *C. fetus* by its higher growth temperatures, cephalothin resistance, and nalidixic acid sensitivity. As shown in Table 286–1, the additional *Campylobacter* species that infect humans include *C. laridis*, a thermophilic organism commonly found in healthy sea gulls which has been reported in children with mild recurrent diarrhea and in an elderly patient with sepsis and terminal multiple myeloma. Additional "*Campylobacter*-like organisms" are now being increasingly appreciated in at least two clinical settings. Up to three distinct species (including proposed species names *C. fennelliae* and *C. cinaedi*) are associated with protocolitis in homosexual males and the *Campylobacter*-like organisms (proposed name *C. pyloridis*) now being found in patients with varying symptoms and histologic evidence of gastritis. Like *C. fetus*, these *Campylobacter*-like organisms will not grow at 42° C or in the presence of cephalosporin anti-

TABLE 286–1. HUMAN *CAMPYLOBACTER* INFECTIONS

Species	Growth Temperature	Reservoir	Clinical Manifestations
C. jejuni/coli	37–43° C	Poultry, mammals	Common cause of dysentery/diarrhea
C. fetus (sub sp. *fetus*, old sub sp. *intestinalis*)	25–37° C	Cattle, sheep	Uncommon, bacteremia; intravascular infections in debilitated hosts
C. laridis	30–43° C	Sea gulls	Uncommon, childhood diarrhea, one case of sepsis
"*Campylobacter*-like organisms":			
"Gay CLO's" (*C. cinaedi*, *C. fennelliae*)	37° C	?	Proctocolitis, rarely sepsis, in homosexual males
"Antral CLO" (*C. pylorids*)	37° C	?	Histologic gastritis ? ulcer or gastritis symptoms

biotics and may require several days to a week or more to grow in culture. *C. jejuni* is further subdivided into over 60 serotypes on the basis of heat-stable O antigens or over 50 serotypes on the basis of heat-labile capsular and flagellar antigens, markers that are helpful in tracing the epidemiology of this common enteric pathogen.

EPIDEMIOLOGY. Although the frequency of other *Campylobacter* infections is either low or unclear, *C. jejuni* infections are extremely common throughout the world. In many studies, the frequency of *Campylobacter* enteritis exceeds that of *Salmonella* or *Shigella* infections, and it has been estimated that as many as two million *Campylobacter* enteritis cases occur annually in the United States. The reservoirs of *C. jejuni/coli* include a wide range of mammalian species. Thirty to 100 per cent of chickens, turkeys, and water fowl may be infected asymptomatically in their intestinal tracts, and commercially prepared poultry in supermarkets can often be shown to be culture positive. In addition, swine, cattle, sheep, horses, and even household pets and rodents may carry *Campylobacter jejuni*, *C. coli*, or *C. fetus*. Enteric symptoms may be found, particularly in puppies, kittens, calves, or lambs, which may have diarrhea when infected. Furthermore, the organisms survive days to weeks in fresh or salt water and in milk and are killed most effectively by pasteurization, chlorination, drying, or freezing.

The transmission of *Campylobacter* infections is likely via the fecal-oral route. Fecal-oral spread may occur by contact among animals, homosexual males, and those in day care centers. However, secondary transmission is relatively infrequent and the infectious dose appears to vary from 500 to over one million organisms. The majority of infections, however, are probably acquired via ingestion of contaminated food, water, or milk vehicles. Many cases and outbreaks are associated with ingestion of inadequately cooked poultry, unpasteurized milk, inadequately treated water, and even cake icing, salads, beef, and clams.

The majority of those infected in well-described outbreaks are symptomatic. Asymptomatic infection appears to be relatively infrequent in temperate climates and in adults. An exception is among young children in certain tropical developing areas such as Bangladesh, where as many as 39 per cent of children under the age of two years may be infected asymptomatically (Table 286–2). These frequent asymptomatic infections in tropical areas raise important questions about possible strain differences in virulence, host susceptibility, and protective immunity against disease that might be acquired very early in developing areas.

Throughout the world, *Campylobacter* infections appear to predominate during the warmer or wet season. As with diarrheal illnesses in general, the highest age-specific attack rate is in young children. However, the greatest proportion of positive fecal cultures occurs in older children and young adults. There is little if any sexual predominance of recognized *C. jejuni* infections.

TABLE 286–2. CLINICAL PRESENTATIONS OF *CAMPYLOBACTER JEJUNI* INFECTION

	Industrialized Countries	Developing Countries
Per cent of all diarrhea with *C. jejuni*	5–13	2–35
Per cent of *C. jejuni* diarrhea with:		
Fecal PMN	78–93	22–46
Blood in stool	60–65	5–17
Asymptomatic infection rates (%)	< 2	0–39*

*Depending on age—39% if less than two years old.

PATHOGENESIS AND PATHOLOGY. *Campylobacter jejuni* and *C. coli* are reasonably susceptible to gastric acidity. However, the reported variation in infectious dose suggests considerable host or strain variability. After an incubation period of one to seven (median four) days, symptoms of the enteric infection begin. *C. jejuni* organisms are attracted toward mucus and fucose in bile, and the flagellae may be important in both chemotaxis and adherence to epithelial cells or mucus. Adherence may also involve lipopolysaccharide or other outer membrane components. Several laboratories around the world have documented the production by *C. jejuni* of a cholera-like, heat-labile enterotoxin that binds to ganglioside and is neutralized by anticholera toxin antiserum. However, the genetic code and role of this toxin in disease remain elusive to date. Studies from Mexico have shown that antitoxic immunity develops after infection, often with watery diarrhea, suggesting that this toxin is significant in those infections.

However, more characteristic in temperate areas is a diffuse, often bloody exudative enteritis involving the ileum and colon. These pathologic changes may include nonspecific crypt abscesses that on colonoscopy and histopathology may mimic the changes seen with inflammatory bowel disease. Such invasive pathology is also seen in rabbit, chick, mouse, dog, and monkey models of infection. Although *C. jejuni* is negative in the Sereny test for guinea pig conjunctivitis, some have reported the production of cytotoxins by certain strains of *C. jejuni* that may be involved in the pathogenesis of the invasive colitis. The relative infrequency of bloodstream invasion by *C. jejuni*, compared to *C. fetus*, likely relates to the relative serum sensitivity of most *C. jejuni* strains and to the rapid development of bactericidal antibody with infection in normal individuals. Volunteer studies suggest that effective immunity develops to rechallenge with the homologous strain, and animal studies suggest that protective immunity may be transferred in immune milk to suckling offspring. Additional evidence of effective immunity comes with the decreasing illness:infection ratio among children in endemic areas as well as among regular consumers of raw milk.

Once patients are infected, they shed 10^7 to 10^9 organisms per gram of stool for a median duration of two to three weeks, if not treated with effective antibiotics. While some may continue to excrete the organism for two to three months, chronic asymptomatic intestinal carriage is rare.

CLINICAL MANIFESTATIONS. As noted in Table 286–1, the major recognized disease with human *Campylobacter* infections is the characteristic diarrheal illness seen with *C. jejuni* or *C. coli* infections. Although asymptomatic infections and watery, noninflammatory diarrhea are seen with *C. jejuni* infections in tropical, developing areas as shown in Table 286–2, *C. jejuni* is characteristically associated with an inflammatory, febrile enteritis in industrialized countries throughout the world. After an incubation period of one to seven days, a brief prodrome of fever, headache, and myalgias lasting for 12 to 24 hours is promptly followed in a case of *C. jejuni* enteritis in a child or young adult with the symptoms of acute enteritis. These characteristically include crampy abdominal pain, fever to 39 or 40° C, and diarrhea with up to 10 or more loose, often bloody bowel movements per day. Occasionally

the crampy abdominal pain may predominate as an appendicitis-like syndrome with mesenteric adenitis or terminal ileitis being the predominant pathology. On physical examination the abdomen is diffusely tender and again may mimic appendicitis. Although the acute febrile enteritis is usually self-limited to five to seven days, 10 to 20 per cent of cases may last longer than one week and 5 to 20 per cent of untreated cases may relapse with a similar illness.

Complications, particularly if antimotility agents are used, include toxic megacolon, pseudomembranous colitis, and colonic hemorrhage. In addition hemolytic-uremic syndrome, postinfectious polyneuritis, or Guillain-Barré syndrome may follow *C. jejuni* enteritis. As with many inflammatory colitis syndromes, reactive arthritis and full-blown Reiter's syndrome may follow weeks after *Campylobacter* enteritis. Bacteremia may occur relatively rarely (< 1 per cent of cases), particularly in the very young or the elderly, in whom meningitis, endocarditis, cholecystitis, urinary tract infections, and pancreatitis have been described.

In striking contrast to *C. jejuni*, the slow-growing *C. fetus* is primarily an uncommon cause of bacteremia, often in immunocompromised hosts. Although *C. fetus* would be missed on most routine stool cultures for *C. jejuni*, studies with filtration methods suggest that it is a relatively infrequent cause of diarrhea. Instead, *C. fetus* tends to cause intravascular, meningeal, or localized infections such as arthritis, cellulitis, abscesses, cholecystitis, and urinary, placental, or pleural infections, often in elderly or debilitated hosts. As it does in animals, *C. fetus* may cause stillbirth or septic abortions more often than generally recognized in humans. *C. fetus* infections are often recognized only by astute clinical microbiology technicians who methodically examine or subculture specimens of blood or other body fluids after one week in the laboratory. The clinical course of *C. fetus* bacteremia is often related to its recognition and appropriate treatment as well as to the underlying disease.

DIAGNOSIS. The diagnosis of *Campylobacter* infections is related to a careful history for exposure or characteristic clinical syndromes, direct stool examination, and selective culture methods. *C. jejuni* enteritis should be suspected in anyone presenting with a febrile enteritis, especially if there is a history of recent ingestion of inadequately cooked poultry, unpasteurized milk, or untreated water. As suggested in Figure 286–1, such a history should prompt the obtaining of a fecal specimen in a cup if at all possible and direct microscopic examination using methylene blue or Gram stain for leukocytes as well as gross and/or occult blood. In many industrialized areas, the presence of blood or fecal leukocytes with fever strongly suggests the presence of a cultivable enteric pathogen such as *C. jejuni*, *Salmonella*, or *Shigella*, with *C. jejuni* being most common. Additional immediate clues to *C. jejuni* infection may be seen on darkfield or phase microscopy for characteristic darting motility or on a carbol-fuchsin Gram stain of stool for characteristic curved rods or sea gull morphology. However, darkfield and Gram stains, while reasonably specific with trained observers, are each only 50 to 66 per cent sensitive. Patients with febrile enteritis, particularly with blood and leukocytes in the stool, should be cultured for *C. jejuni*.

Additional differential diagnostic possibilities for febrile inflammatory enteritis include *Salmonella* and *Shigella* infections, for which one should seek a history of an outbreak or contact exposure (such as in day care centers or among homosexual males, respectively). If the patient has recently taken antibiotics, *C. difficile* colitis or *Salmonella* enteritis should be considered. Recent ingestion of raw seafood should prompt investigation for *Vibrio* infection that may present with either inflammatory or noninflammatory diarrhea. A history of sick pet exposure, persisting abdominal pain, or unexplained inflammatory diarrhea should also prompt consideration of *Yersinia enterocolitica* infections, and travel exposure to tropical

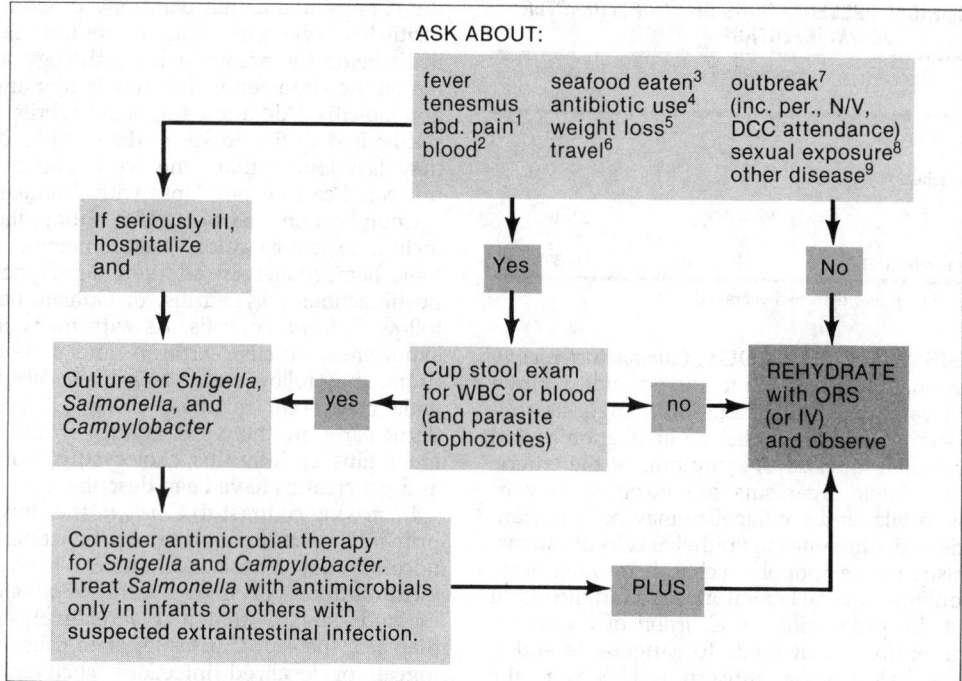

FIGURE 286–1. Approach to the diagnosis and management of acute infectious diarrhea.

1. If unexplained abdominal pain and fever persist or suggest an appendicitis-like syndrome, culture for *Yersinia enterocolitica.*

2. Bloody diarrhea especially if without fecal leukocytes, suggests enterrohemorrhagic (Shiga toxin–producing) *E. coli* 0157 or amebiasis (where leukocytes are destroyed by the parasite).

3. Ingestion of inadequately cooked seafood should prompt consideration of *Vibrio* infections or Norwalk-like viruses.

4. Associated antibiotics should be stopped if possible and cytotoxigenic *C. difficile* considered.

5. Persistence (> 10 days) with weight loss should prompt consideration of giardiasis or cryptosporidiosis.

6. Travel to tropical areas increases the chance of enterotoxigenic *E. coli* as well as viral (ex. Norwalk-like or rotaviral), parasitic (ex. *Giardia; Entamoeba, Strongyloides, Cryptosporidium*), and, if fecal leukocytes are present, invasive bacterial pathogens as noted in the algorithm.

7. Outbreaks should prompt consideration of *S. aureus, B. cereus, Anisakis* (incubation period < 6 hour), *C. perfringens, ETEC, Vibrio, Salmonella, Campylobacter, Shigella* or EIEC infection. If unexplained, consider saving *E. coli* for LT, ST, invasiveness, adherence testing, and serotyping, and save stool for rotavirus and stool + paired sera for Norwalk-like virus testing

8. Sigmoidoscopy in symptomatic homosexual males should distinguish proctitis in the distal 15 cm only (caused by herpesvirus, gonococcal, chlamydial, or syphilitic infection) from colitis [*Campylobacter, Shigella, C. difficile,* or chlamydial (LGV serotypes) infections] or noninflammatory diarrhea (due to giardiasis).

9. Immunocompromised hosts should have a wide range of viral (ex. CMV, HSV, coxsackie, rotavirus), bacterial (ex. *Salmonella, Mycobacterium avium-intracellulare, Listeria*), fungal (ex. *Candida*), and parasitic (ex. *Cryptosporidium, Strongyloides, Entamoeba,* and *Giardia*) agents considered.

(Adapted from Guerrant RL, Shields DS, Thorson SM, et al.: Evaluation and diagnosis of acute infectious diarrhea. *Am. J. Med.* 78:91–98, 1985.)

areas should prompt an examination of stool and possibly rectal biopsy specimens for *E. histolytica* (which often destroys fecal leukocytes). Another frequent diagnosis that is considered, especially if *Campylobacter* enteritis has relapsed once or twice, is inflammatory bowel disease. However, it is imperative that anyone who is being considered for that diagnosis have treatable causes such as *Campylobacter* enteritis or amebiasis excluded by appropriate cultures or stains, as treatment with steroids may worsen *Campylobacter* or amebic enteritis with potentially devastating consequences. Additional noninfectious causes of bloody diarrhea with abdominal pain include intussusception and vascular insufficiency.

THERAPY. The most important treatment for *Campylobacter* enteritis, as with all diarrheal illnesses, is adequate rehydration and maintenance fluid therapy, which can often be accomplished with oral glucose-electrolyte solutions. The effectiveness of specific antimicrobial therapy remains debated. Although most *C. jejuni* strains are sensitive to erythromycin as well as to tetracyclines, chloramphenicol, clindamycin, and aminoglycosides, they are characteristically resistant to penicillin, ampicillin, cephalosporins, and sulfamethoxazole-trimethroprim. Indications for antibiotic treatment remain controversial. Several studies have failed to show a significant reduction in the duration of illness with erythromycin treatment despite its prompt eradication of the organism from the stool. Some reserve antimicrobial treatment for those with particularly severe symptoms of high fever, bloody or severe diarrhea, young children in day care centers, or prolonged or relapsing illnesses. Antimotility agents should be avoided in *Campylobacter* enteritis, as with any inflammatory diarrhea.

It should be remembered that erythromycin orally may not be adequate for systemic *C. jejuni* or *C. fetus* endovascular infections, which probably warrant two to four weeks of parenteral bactericidal antimicrobial therapy.

PROGNOSIS. The prognosis of *C. jejuni* enteritis is generally quite good, and the disease is usually self-limited with or without specific therapy.

PREVENTION. As most *Campylobacter* infections arise from fecal contamination, often from animal reservoirs, many if not most *Campylobacter* infections are potentially preventable by education. The most common recognized vehicles of spread are inadequately cooked food, unpasteurized milk, and inadequately treated water. Consequently, thorough cooking of meats, careful hand washing after food preparation, pasteurization of milk, and adequate chlorination of drinking water should greatly reduce the frequency of *Campylobacter* infections. Parents should be warned that sick pet kittens or puppies may harbor potential human pathogens such as *C. jejuni* and keep them away from small children and practice careful hygienic measures in their care.

Blaser MJ, Reller LB: Campylobacter enteritis. N Engl J Med 305:1444–1451, 1981. *Excellent overall review of the epidemiology and manifestations of C. jejuni in tropical and industrialized areas.*

Blaser MJ, Wells JG, Feldman RA, et al.: Campylobacter enteritis in the United States. Ann Intern Med 98:360–365, 1983. *Critical analysis of the presentation of C. jejuni and other enteritides in the United States.*

Butzler JP, Skirrow MB: Campylobacter enteritis. Clin Gastroenterol 8:737–765, 1979. *Good review of cultivation methods, epidemiology, clinical presentation, and models of C. jejuni infections.*

Guerrant RL, Lahita RG, Winn WC, et al.: Campylobacteriosis in man: Pathogenic mechanisms and review of 16 bloodstream infections. Am J Med 65:584–592, 1978. *Review of both C. fetus and C. jejuni infections and their presentations as bacteremic illnesses.*

Guerrant RL, Shields DS, Thorson SM, et al.: Evaluation and diagnosis of acute infectious diarrhea. Am J Med 78:91–98, 1985. *Review of a more cost-effective approach to selecting patients for stool culture who are likely to have an identifiable bacterial pathogen, such as C. jejuni.*

Quinn TC, Corey L, Chaffee RG, et al.: The etiology of anorectal infections in homosexual men. Am J Med 71:395–406, 1981. *Review of the clinical manifestations and diagnostic approach to the wide range of enteric infections commonly seen in promiscuous homosexual males.*

Ruiz Palacios GM, Torres J, Torres NI, et al.: Cholera-like enterotoxin produced by Campylobacter jejuni. Lancet 2:250–252, 1982. *Original report of evidence for production of a cholera-like enterotoxin by C. jejuni in a developing area.*

Walker RI, Caldwell MB, Lee EC, et al.: Pathophysiology of Campylobacter enteritis. Microbiol Rev 50:81–94, 1986. *Excellent recent review of the virulence traits, pathogenic mechanisms, and animal models of C. jejuni infections.*

287 CHOLERA (Asiatic Cholera)

Nathaniel F. Pierce

DEFINITION. Cholera is an acute, sometimes fulminant, diarrheal disease during which *Vibrio cholerae*, serogroup 1, is abundant in liquid stool. It occurs only in humans and varies in severity from a mild diarrheal illness to a dramatically severe disease that causes death from hypovolemic shock in a few hours owing to the passage of voluminous, watery, electrolyte-rich stools. Cholera often occurs in epidemic form; it has caused seven pandemics in the past two centuries.

ETIOLOGY. *Vibrio cholerae* organisms are short, slightly curved, motile gram-negative rods that grow aerobically at 37° C. There are more than 60 O serogroups of *Vibrio cholerae*, but only serogroup 1 causes epidemic cholera. Some of the others sporadically cause acute diarrhea, which is occasionally severe. *Vibrio cholerae*, serogroup 1, occurs as two serotypes, *Ogawa* and *Inaba*, which reflect differences in the somatic antigen; there are also two biotypes: the *classic* and the *eltor*. The eltor biotype is recognized by its resistance to polymyxin B and by characteristic patterns of susceptibility to vibriophage. Distinction between the two biotypes has epidemiologic importance; the eltor biotype causes a higher proportion of mild or asymptomatic infections and survives better outside the human host.

EPIDEMIOLOGY. The Seventh Pandemic. The traditional "home" of cholera is the delta region of the Ganges and Brahmaputra rivers, where thousands of cases occur during annual epidemics. During pandemics the disease has spread in Asia, Africa, Europe, and North America. The current pandemic is due to the eltor biotype; it involves Southeast Asia, the Indian subcontinent, the Middle East, Africa, and the Gulf Coast of North America. Cholera now appears to be endemic in many of these recently involved areas and has been imported to Japan, Israel, Spain, Italy, and Portugal, where it has caused isolated outbreaks. Individual cases have also occurred among travelers returning from affected areas. In North America, cholera has occurred sporadically along the Gulf Coast since 1973. All cases were caused by the same unusual strain of *Vibrio cholerae*, which suggests that Gulf Coast waters may have been contaminated since 1973.

Mode of Spread. Cholera is largely waterborne, usually by means of fecal contamination of drinking water. However, food exposed to contaminated water may also be the vehicle for infection. Examples of the latter include fresh vegetables washed in contaminated water and shellfish or other seafood harvested from contaminated water. Evidence that *Vibrio cholerae* adheres to shellfish suggests that these may be an especially important means of spread.

Secondary cases of cholera in affected households are common because of direct contamination of water or food with infected excreta. Persons with self-limited, mild, or asymptomatic infections outnumber those with serious illness and are probably the major means by which cholera is spread from affected to nearby nonaffected communities. Prolonged biliary infection with *V. cholerae* also occurs in about 3 per cent of older adults convalescent from cholera; however, their role in transmission of cholera is uncertain.

Susceptibility to Cholera. The age distribution of cholera cases reflects the level of naturally acquired immunity in the population. In endemic areas, accidental ingestion of the organism occurs periodically and substantial immunity develops by early adulthood; in such areas, cholera is largely a disease of children. In Bangladesh, for example, attack rates among children under five years old are 10 times those of adults. By contrast, attack rates in newly affected areas, where there is no naturally acquired immunity, are nearly equal among adults and children.

Vibrio cholerae is quickly killed by pH levels below 5.5. Thus, normal gastric acidity is an important barrier to infection. Impairment of gastric acidity by mucosal atrophy, the use of antacids, or subtotal gastrectomy increases susceptibility to cholera. Cholera also occurs with greater severity in persons with blood group O and is least severe with blood group AB.

PATHOGENESIS. The incubation period for cholera is usually one to two days but may vary from 12 hours to six days. Cholera occurs when *Vibrio cholerae* organisms are ingested, survive passage through the stomach, colonize and multiply in the small bowel, and release the cholera enterotoxin. Colonization is promoted by adherence of the vibrios to the small bowel mucosa. The enterotoxin is a protein (molecular weight 84,000) composed of A and B subunits. The B subunit binds irreversibly to its receptor, GM_1 ganglioside, on the brush border of small bowel epithelial cells. This assists entry of the A subunit into epithelial cells, which causes activation of adenylate cyclase, an increase in intracellular content of 3′,5′-cyclic adenosine monophosphate, and the secretion of electrolytes into the bowel lumen. Cholera enterotoxin does not cause morphologic damage to the bowel mucosa, does not alter its permeability to serum proteins, and does not affect the active absorption of monosaccharides (e.g., glucose) or amino acids. The secreted electrolyte solution passes through the gut and emerges as watery stool, which rapidly becomes free of fecal material. Flecks of mucus give the stool its characteristic "rice-water" appearance. The stool is isotonic with plasma but has concentrations of bicarbonate and potassium greater than plasma (see Table 287–1). All of the signs, symptoms, and metabolic disorders of cholera are related to the rapid loss of this electrolyte-rich liquid stool. This loss causes hypovolemia, base-deficit acidosis, and potassium depletion.

CLINICAL MANIFESTATIONS. Cholera begins with the

TABLE 287–1. TYPICAL CHEMICAL VALUES IN STOOL AND PLASMA FROM PATIENTS WITH SEVERE CHOLERA

	Stool	Plasma	
		Untreated	Treated†
Sodium*	138 (105)	141	142
Chloride*	102 (90)	107	106
Potassium*	18 (25)	4.5	3.6
Bicarbonate*	45 (30)	9	21
Arterial pH	—	7.21	7.43
Plasma specific gravity	—	1.040	1.026

*Milliequivalents per liter. Stool values in parentheses are for children less than 10 years old.

†Four hours after water and electrolyte replacement.

abrupt onset of watery diarrhea. Many cases are mild, cause little morbidity, and cannot be distinguished clinically from other types of gastroenteritis. In severe cases, however, stool loss is dramatic, sometimes exceeding 1 liter per hour. Collapse from shock occurs when unreplaced fluid losses equal about 10 per cent of body weight. This may happen within 6 hours but usually requires 18 to 24 hours. Greater fluid losses are rapidly lethal. Vomiting, painful cramps of the gastrocnemius muscles, and severe thirst are other prominent features of severe cholera.

The outstanding physical findings in severe untreated cholera are the result of marked isotonic fluid deficit. These include collapse, poor skin turgor, weak or absent peripheral pulses, hypotension, tachycardia, and cyanosis. Eyes are sunken, the voice is faint and high-pitched, heart sounds are faint, and bowel sounds are hypoactive. Adults are usually normally oriented but apathetic. Features that occur only in children under seven years are fever and occasionally coma or convulsions.

Initial laboratory findings reflect the loss of isotonic bicarbonate-rich stool (Table 287–1). These include increased plasma protein concentration, increased plasma-specific gravity, low arterial pH, and low plasma bicarbonate concentration. Plasma sodium concentration is normal. Small children occasionally have severe hypoglycemia.

DIAGNOSIS. Cholera should be suspected in any acute case of watery, shock-producing diarrhea, especially in an adult. Travel to or residence in a cholera-affected area makes the diagnosis more likely. A diagnosis of cholera should also be considered in exposed persons who develop mild, painless, nonbloody diarrhea.

After treatment has begun, a direct stool examination should be performed. A fecal smear stained with methylene blue usually reveals neither erythrocytes nor leukocytes, which is a feature also characteristic of infections with enterotoxigenic *Escherichia coli* and rotavirus. Darkfield microscopy of dilute feces reveals numerous bacilli with the rapid, darting movement characteristic of vibrios. Immobilization of these organisms by addition of group-specific antisera confirms that they are *Vibrio cholerae*, serogroup 1.

Stool should also be obtained for diagnostic culture. The simplest method involves direct plating of feces on thiosulfate-citrate-bile salt-sucrose (TCBS) agar, a medium highly selective for vibrios. Opaque flat yellow colonies form on TCBS agar within 18 hours at 37° C. Confirmation of serogroup and serotype is made by direct bacterial agglutination in specific antiserum. The eltor biotype is identified by its resistance to polymyxin B.

The diagnosis can be confirmed by showing significant rises during convalescence in the serum titers of *Vibrio cholerae* agglutinating antibody or of complement-dependent vibriocidal antibodies. Serodiagnostic techniques are used mostly for epidemiologic studies.

TREATMENT. The mainstay of cholera therapy is prompt, complete replacement of lost water and electrolytes. In severe cases, this should be done immediately, before diagnostic studies. Fluid replacement therapy for cholera is fully effective for cholera-like diseases sometimes caused by other bacterial or viral agents.

Water and electrolytes can be replaced intravenously or in many cases orally. The choice depends upon the patient's condition and the treatment materials available. Intravenous rehydration is required for severely hypovolemic patients and is acceptable for those less seriously ill. Oral replacement of water and electrolytes can be used throughout the course of mild cases and in severe cases after hypovolemia has been corrected by rapid intravenous replacement. Oral therapy is especially useful in rural or underdeveloped areas where intravenous fluids are in short supply.

Lactated Ringer's solution is satisfactory for intravenous rehydration. Initial treatment should aim to restore an effective blood volume as rapidly as possible. Fluid should be given through a large bore needle at 50 to 100 ml per minute until a strong radial pulse is restored. The remainder of the intial deficit is then replaced within two hours. For example, a 50-kg patient with severe dehydration has a fluid deficit of about 5 liters (10 per cent of body weight); 1 to 2 liters is replaced within 20 minutes, and the remainder (3 to 4 liters) by the end of two hours. The response to rapid rehydration is usually dramatic, patients becoming alert, comfortable, and fully cooperative within an hour. After initial rehydration, if administration of intravenous fluids is continued, the infusion should be given at a rate equal to the rate of ongoing measured stool loss until diarrhea subsides. If stool loss cannot be measured, the rate should be sufficient to maintain a strong pulse and normal skin turgor. In severe cases, stool losses may average 10 to 25 ml per kilogram per hour for the first 24 hours. Overhydration can be detected by frequent examination of the neck veins and auscultation of the lungs.

Oral therapy is effective because enteric glucose absorption and glucose-facilitated sodium absorption are intact in patients with cholera. A suitable glucose-electrolyte solution is made by adding the following (in grams per liter) to drinking water: sodium chloride, 3.5; trisodium citrate, 2.9 (or sodium bicarbonate, 2.5); potassium chloride, 1.5; and glucose, 20. If glucose is unavailable, sucrose (40 grams per liter) is nearly as effective. An effective solution can also be prepared by boiling 50 grams rice starch per liter of water, allowing the solution to cool, and adding the salts. Oral rehydration requires 50 to 100 ml per kilogram, depending upon the degree of dehydration. Replacement of ongoing stool losses requires 5 to 15 ml per kilogram per hour. Thirst is a valuable guide to oral fluid requirements; however, patients may need encouragement to drink the large amounts required for rehydration (up to 1000 ml per hour for adults). Vomiting may occur but does not affect the success of oral therapy unless it is severe.

The treatment of small children with cholera resembles that of adults. The same solutions may be used for oral or intravenous replacement. If lactated Ringer's solution is given, oral supplementation with glucose and potassium is needed to prevent symptomatic hypoglycemia and hypokalemia. The rate of intravenous rehydration should be slower to minimize the risk of coma or seizures caused by cerebral edema. After rapid restoration of a strong radial pulse, by infusing up to 30 ml per kilogram in 30 minutes, the remainder of the initial deficit is replaced in about six hours. Thereafter, ongoing stool losses are replaced as they occur.

Adjunctive therapy with oral antibiotics markedly reduces the duration and volume of stool loss and shortens the period of vibrio excretion. Oral tetracycline (50 mg per kilogram per day in six-hourly doses for two days, maximum daily dose 2 grams) is usually most effective. Recently, resistance of *Vibrio cholerae* to tetracycline has been encountered. Trimethoprim-sulfamethoxazole, furazolidone, or chlorampheniocol may be used in such instances. A normal diet should be given as soon as appetite returns. Drinking water should be freely available and frequently offered to small children.

The complications of cholera depend largely upon the adequacy of treatment. Uncorrected hypovolemia is the major cause of death. Transient oliguria occurs in many patients, but renal failure with acute tubular necrosis occurs only when hypovolemia is poorly corrected. Inadequate potassium replacement causes cardiac arrhythmias in adults and serious paralytic ileus in children. Water and electrolyte replacement without correction of acidosis can cause pulmonary edema. Uncorrected hypoglycemia can contribute to coma or seizures in children. Severe cholera during the third trimester of pregnancy carries a high risk of fetal death.

PROGNOSIS. Mortality from serious cholera, if untreated, reaches 50 per cent. With adequate replacement therapy, however, mortality approaches zero. Despite adequate therapy, a mortality of about 1 per cent persists among small children, owing largely to complicating coma and seizures.

PREVENTION. Safe sewage disposal and pure water supply are the only certain means of preventing cholera. There is no satisfactory cholera vaccine. However, results of trials with experimental vaccines given orally strongly suggest that one can be developed. Tetracycline taken prophylactically by household contacts of proven cases prevents secondary cases, but community-wide prophylaxis is not recommended. Infants breast fed by mothers whose milk contains antibodies to *V. cholerae* antigens are significantly protected against cholera.

Barua D, Burrows W: Cholera. Philadelphia, W. B. Saunders Company, 1974. *A broad review of bacteriologic, epidemiologic, immunologic, and clinical aspects of cholera written by a variety of experts.*

Carpenter CCJ, Mitra PP, Sack RB: Clinical studies in Asiatic cholera. Parts I–VI. Bull Johns Hopkins Hosp 118:165, 1966. *This is an excellent series of reports concerning the pathophysiology of cholera, rational fluid replacement, and the value of antibiotic therapy.*

Glass RI, Becker S, Hug MI, et al.: Endemic cholera in rural Bangladesh, 1966–1980. Am J Epidemiol 116:959, 1982. *This is a comprehensive review of the epidemiology of cholera in a highly endemic area.*

Hirschhorn N: The treatment of acute diarrhea in children. An historical and physiologic perspective. Am J Clin Nutr 33:637, 1980. *A thorough review of the special concerns that surround treatment of acute diarrhea, including cholera, in children. The review serves to "bridge" the traditional pediatric literature and the recent literature on cholera and related diarrheal diseases.*

Johnston JM, Martin DL, Perdue J, et al.: Cholera on a Gulf Coast oil rig. N Engl J Med 309:523, 1983. *This is the most recent in a series of articles since 1974 describing outbreaks of cholera along the coast of the Gulf of Mexico.*

Recent advances in cholera research: Memorandum from a WHO meeting. Bull WHO 63:851, 1985. *A recent summary of research on the epidemiology and pathogenesis of cholera, and on progress toward vaccine development.*

World Health Organization. Programme for Control of Diarrhoeal Diseases: A manual for treatment of acute diarrhoea. WHO/CDD/SER/80.2 REV. 1, 1984. *A practical guide designed especially for workers in developing countries. It includes valuable guidelines on using oral rehydration solutions for all types of acute dehydrating diarrhea.*

288 ENTERIC *ESCHERICHIA COLI* INFECTIONS

Richard L. Guerrant

Escherichia coli is the predominant aerobic, coliform species in the normal colon. However, *E. coli* can also be an enteric pathogen and cause intestinal disease, usually diarrhea. Diarrhea caused by *E. coli* may be watery, inflammatory, or bloody, depending on which genetic codes for virulence traits the organism happens to possess. Consequently, diarrheogenic *E. coli* must be defined more specifically according to its virulence traits. Specific virulence traits determine the type of disease the organism causes, such as enterotoxigenic, enteroinvasive, or enteropathogenic (enteroadherent or enterohemorrhagic) *E. coli* diarrhea. Each of these categories is being further resolved by the type of enterotoxin (such as the cholera-like, heat-labile toxin, LT, or the heat-stable toxin, ST)

or adherence (such as close, focal, epithelial cell effacing, or diffuse) it causes. Taken separately, organisms such as enterotoxigenic *E. coli* constitute major bacterial causes of diarrhea morbidity and mortality on a global scale, particularly among children in tropical, developing areas and in travelers. Taken together, the varied types of *E. coli* diarrhea not only constitute the major category of bacterial enteric pathogens, but illustrate the wide array of ways that enteric pathogens can cause disease.

As noted in Table 288–1, at least three different types of *E. coli* enterotoxins may cause intestinal secretion (ETEC), others are enteroinvasive (EIEC), while the classically recognized enteropathogenic *E. coli* (EPEC) serotypes are neither enterotoxic nor invasive but are often tightly enteroadherent (EAEC), and still others cause food-borne hemorrhagic colitis (EHEC) and produce large amounts of Shiga-like toxin (EHEC).

ETIOLOGY. *Escherichia coli* is a small, catalase-positive, oxidase-negative, gram-negative bacillus in the family Enterobacteriaceae. It characteristically reduces nitrates, ferments glucose and usually lactose, and is either motile (with peritrichate flagella) or nonmotile. It gives a positive methyl red reaction and negative reactions with Voges-Proskauer, urease, phenylalanine deaminase, and citrate agents. *E. coli* constitutes the predominant facultative gram-negative bacillus in the intestinal tract of humans and other mammals. As with other gram-negative organisms, the lipopolysaccharide cell wall contains lipid A and 2-keto-3-deoxyoctanate (KDO), a core glycolipid that has been used in vaccine development to provide cross-protection against systemic infections with other gram-negative organisms. Smooth (S) forms of *E. coli* have O specific carbohydrate chains attached to this core glycolipid to provide 169 O serogroups as well as at least 60 heat-labile protein flagellar (H) antigens by which strains are currently serotyped. Historically some 80 variably heat-labile capsular (K) antigens have also been described (L, B, and A), not to mention the more recently appreciated numerous adherence, enterotoxin, cytotoxin, and invasiveness factors that may be gained or lost by a particular serotype, as they are characteristically encoded on transmissible genetic elements such as plasmids or bacteriophages. Consequently, this common inhabitant of the normal human intestinal tract becomes a pathogen when it houses one or more specific traits that contribute to its virulence in the intestinal tract. Other traits such as O and H serogroup appear also to be important for certain enteropathogenic and enteroinvasive organisms. For reasons that remain obscure, only a few O serogroups tend to predominate in the normal human colon (O groups 1, 2, 4, 6, 7, 8, 18, 25, 45, 75, and 81), while others noted in Table 288–1 tend (albeit not absolutely) to be associated with specific virulence traits and thus different types of pathogenesis in the intestine. The O antigens of invasive *E. coli* often cross-react with various *Shigella* species, suggesting further that, in addition to the 140 Mdal plasmid, serotype also has a role in pathogenesis.

EPIDEMIOLOGY. Enteric *E. coli* infections are essentially acquired by the fecal-oral route, reflecting primarily a human reservoir for most recognized types of *E. coli* enteropathogens. Enterotoxigenic *E. coli* is also an important veterinary pathogen, especially in calves and piglets. However, the attachment traits of animal strains are different from those that infect humans and likely substantially influence their epidemiology.

The infectious doses of enterotoxigenic *E. coli* and enteroinvasive *E. coli* have been determined in volunteers to be 10^6 to 10^8, numbers that usually require multiplication in contaminated food or water vehicles for their transmission. Heavy contamination with enterotoxigenic *E. coli* has been documented in foods prepared in homes, restaurants, and at street vendors as well as in drinking water in many tropical areas, and contaminated water and foods likely represent the major sources of their acquisition, primarily in the warm or wet

TABLE 288–1. DIFFERENT TYPES OF ENTERIC *E. COLI* INFECTIONS

Type	Mechanism	Predominant O Serogroups	Genetic Code	Detection	Clinical Syndromes
Enterotoxigenic E. coli (ETEC)					
1. Cholera-like, heat-labile toxin (LT)	Activates intestinal adenylate cyclase	6, 8, 15, 20, 25, 78, 115 (LT, ST)	Plasmid	ELISA, RIA, PIH, CHO, Y1 cells, 18 h loops, gene probe	Watery diarrhea, Travelers' diarrhea
2. Heat-stable toxin (STa: STh or STp)	Activates intestinal guanylate cyclase	20, 27, 63, 148, 159	Plasmid (transposon)	ELISA, RIA, suckling mice, 6 h loops, gene probes	Watery diarrhea, Travelers' diarrhea
3. Heat-stable toxin (STb)	?; Not cAMP or cGMP		Plasmid	Piglet loops, gene probe	?
Enteroinvasive E. coli (EIEC)					
4. Enteroinvasive E. coli (EIEC)	Invasive	28ac, 29, 42, 112ac, 124, 136, 143, 144, 147, 152, 164, 167	Plasmid (140 Mdal, pWR110)	Sereny test, gene probe, (lys⁻, NM, oft. lactose⁻)	Inflammatory dysentery
Enterohemorrhagic E. coli (EHEC)					
5. Enterohemorrhagic (EHEC)	Shiga-like toxin(s)	26, 39, 145, 157, occ 55, 111	Phage(s)	Serotype, HeLa, Vero cells, sorbitol	Bloody noninflammatory diarrhea; hemolytic-uremic syndrome
Enteropathogenic E. coli (EPEC)					
6. Enteroadherent (EAEC)	Attach, efface the mucosa	55, 111, 119, 125, 126, 127, 128, 142	Plasmid (50 Mdal, pMAR2)	Serotype, local HEp2 adhesion, gene probe	Infantile diarrhea
7. Other EPEC	?	44, 86, 114	?	Serotype	?

season. In the United States, major outbreaks of water- or food-borne *E. coli* diarrhea of different types have been documented in the last 10 to 15 years. A large water-borne outbreak of diarrhea at a popular national park was found to be caused by enterotoxigenic *E. coli* (ETEC), and a widespread outbreak of enteroinvasive *E. coli* (EIEC) enteritis was traced to consumption of French Camembert cheese. More recently, bloody, noninflammatory diarrhea was noted in two states in association with enterohemorrhagic *E. coli* (O157) in specialty hamburgers in a fast-food chain. Occasional nosocomial outbreaks of enterotoxigenic *E. coli* and enteropathogenic *E. coli* serotypes have also occurred in hospitalized infants in the United States or other industrialized countries in the last 10 to 20 years.

As with most diarrheal illnesses, the highest age-specific attack rates of enterotoxigenic *E. coli* infections are in young children, especially at the time of weaning, when enterotoxigenic *E. coli* account for 15 to 50 per cent of illnesses. Like immunologically inexperienced young children, the traveler visiting tropical areas has a 30 to 50 per cent chance of acquiring travelers' diarrhea over a two- to three-week stay unless untreated water or ice and uncooked foods such as salads are strictly avoided. The most commonly recognized pathogen associated with travelers' diarrhea around the world is enterotoxigenic *E. coli* that produces either the STa, LT, or both enterotoxins (see Ch. 289).

Of potential immunologic significance is the continued occurrence of symptomatic infections with *E. coli* which produce the less immunogenic STa in adult residents of tropical or other areas endemic for enterotoxigenic *E. coli* infections. In contrast, adult residents in endemic areas often carry LT-producing *E. coli* asymptomatically, suggesting that they may be protected from symptoms, if not from colonization.

Limited data on invasive *E. coli* suggest that the infectious doses are relatively high. As with enterotoxigenic *E. coli* infections, such large numbers have been readily spread in food with high attack rates. Enteropathogenic *E. coli* have been recognized primarily in urban areas, especially among hospitalized infants in their first year of life, with apparent cross-infection in hospital nurseries. While sporadic cases still occur, nosocomial outbreaks of EPEC diarrhea during summer months appear to have become less common and less severe in industrialized countries in the last decade or two.

PATHOGENESIS AND PATHOLOGY. The pathogenesis of enteric *E. coli* infections begins with the ingestion of the organism in contaminated food or water, which then faces the normal gastric acid barrier. Both enterotoxigenic *E. coli* and enteroinvasive *E. coli* appear to be sensitive to gastric acid; neutralization by gastric acid will reduce the infectious dose by 100- to 1000-fold. This is followed by an incubation period of two to seven days, during which colonization of the involved part of the intestinal tract and enterotoxin production or invasion takes place. Best characterized is the colonization by enterotoxigenic *E. coli* in the upper small bowel which involves one of at least three major colonization factor antigen groups (which are fimbriate or fibrillar protein structures on the surface of the organism). The colonization fimbriae bind the organism to cell surface receptors in the upper small bowel where the enterotoxin is delivered to reduce normal absorption and cause net electrolyte and water secretion. The heat-labile toxin (LT) with a molecular weight of about 86,000 has a binding and active subunit that, like choleratoxin, binds to a monosialoganglioside (Gml) receptor. Also like choleratoxin, the active subunit ADP-ribosylates the regulatory subunit of adenylate cyclase to activate adenylate cyclase. The consequently increased chloride secretion and reduced sodium absorption combine to cause net isotonic electrolyte loss that must be replaced to prevent severe dehydration and hypotension and its potential consequences. Other strains produce the heat-stable toxin (STa), a much smaller molecule of 18-19 amino acids (molecular weight less than 2000) which activates intestinal particulate guanylate cyclase. Like cyclic AMP, the cyclic GMP thus formed also causes net secretion. A third type of *E. coli* enterotoxin (STb) causes secretion in porcine intestine without activating adenylate or guanylate cyclase; STb has no known role in human disease. Both the colonization traits and enterotoxin production are encoded on transmissible plasmids. Besides the complications of dehydration, the only significant pathologic change is depletion of mucus from intestinal goblet cells.

Other *E. coli*, often of certain serogroups noted in Table 288–1, have the capacity, analogous to *Shigella*, to invade and multiply in epithelial cells, cause conjunctivitis in guinea pigs (Sereny test), and cause inflammatory colitis and dysenteric or bloody diarrhea. As seen with shigellosis, there is a striking inflammatory response with sheets of polymorphonuclear leukocytes in the stool. The colon shows patchy, acute inflammation in the mucosa and submucosa with focal denuding of the surface epithelium but usually without deeper invasion or systemic spread. While epithelial cell invasiveness in both enteroinvasive *E. coli* and *Shigella* appears to be encoded on a large 120-140 Mdal plasmid, several chromosomal determinants, including the O antigen, are critical for full invasive virulence.

Classically recognized enteropathogenic *E. coli* serotypes often fail to produce known enterotoxins or to be invasive. Nevertheless, they are well established causes of infantile diarrhea. Recent studies document at least two separate mechanisms by which different EPEC serotypes may cause diarrhea. The first, demonstrable with the majority of classically recognized EPEC serotypes such as O55 and O111, is a plasmid-encoded adherence to epithelial cells. This close adherence is associated with dissolution of the glycocalyx, disruption and effacement of the microvilli, villus atrophy, mucosal thinning, inflammation in the lamina propria, and variable crypt cell hyperplasia. These morphologic changes are associated with a reduction in the mucosal brush border enzymes and may contribute to the impaired absorptive function and diarrhea.

Other *E. coli*, notably of serogroups O26, 39, and 157, have been associated with food-borne outbreaks of bloody, noninflammatory diarrhea and with the hemolytic-uremic syndrome. These organisms produce large amounts of Shiga-like toxin that may be responsible for the characteristic colonic mucosal inflammation, edema, and hemorrhage. Sigmoidoscopy usually reveals only moderately hyperemic mucosa, and barium enema may reveal a thumb-print pattern of submucosal edema in the ascending and transverse colon. Some patients have superficial ulceration with mild neutrophil infiltration in the edematous submucosa.

Still other EPEC serotypes have historically been associated with diarrhea and have caused diarrhea in volunteers without recognized attachment, enteroadherence, enterotoxin, or enteroinvasiveness traits to date, suggesting that still other mechanisms remain to be unraveled for *E. coli* strains that cause diarrhea. The roles of a recently recognized LT-like toxin (which activates adenylate cyclase but is immunologically distinct from LT), of STb (a unique large heat-stable toxin that causes secretion without altering cyclic AMP or cyclic GMP in porcine intestine), or of colonization alone offer three additional potential types of enteric *E. coli* infections for which roles in human disease remain unclear at present.

CLINICAL MANIFESTATIONS. The most common clinical manifestation of enteric *E. coli* infections is the watery diarrhea that characterizes enterotoxigenic *E. coli* infections, particularly in young children and travelers to tropical or developing areas. This may range from mild to severe, cholera-like diarrhea that may be life-threatening, especially in small children and elderly patients who are particularly prone to suffer the severest consequences of dehydration, undernutrition, and electrolyte imbalance (especially hypokalemia and acidosis).

The incubation period (two to seven days) varies with the size of the inoculum. Characteristic symptoms include malaise, abdominal cramping, anorexia, and watery diarrhea, occasionally associated with nausea, vomiting, or low-grade fever. The illness is usually self-limited to one to five days and rarely extends beyond 10 days or two weeks. Infections with *E. coli* which produce both ST and LT or ST alone may be more severe than those with only LT-producing *E. coli*. The persistence of impaired mucosal absorptive capacity for one to three weeks may further compound the cycle of malnutrition that complicates diarrheal illnesses in children in developing, tropical areas.

Infection with enteroinvasive *E. coli* is characterized by inflammatory colitis, often with abdominal pain, high fever, tenesmus, and bloody or dysenteric diarrhea essentially like that seen with *Shigella*, to which this organism is closely related. The incubation period is usually one to three days with the duration usually self-limited to seven to ten days.

Outbreaks of enteropathogenic *E. coli* infections in newborn nurseries have ranged from mild transient diarrhea to severe and rapidly fatal diarrheal illnesses, especially in premature or otherwise compromised infants. The more severe illnesses appear to have been more common in industrialized countries prior to 1950. However, more recent outbreaks and sporadic cases are well documented.

Recently recognized outbreaks of hemorrhagic colitis associated with the Shiga-like toxin producing *E. coli* (EHEC) O157:H7 and O26:H11 have been characterized by grossly bloody diarrhea with remarkably little fever or inflammatory exudate in the stool. Although the diarrheal illnesses have been self-limited, a significant number of children have subsequently developed a hemolytic-uremic syndrome. The incubation period in two outbreaks has been three to four days (range one to seven days), and the illness is characteristically self-limited to 5 to 12 days (mean 7.8).

DIAGNOSIS. A definitive etiologic diagnosis of *E. coli* diarrhea requires the documentation of a specific virulence trait such as enterotoxin, invasiveness, enteroadherence, or serotype which usually requires specialized immunologic, tissue culture, animal bioassay, or gene probes that are available only in research and reference laboratories. Such tests are rarely cost effective or clinically indicated, except in outbreak or research situations. Fortunately, a likely diagnosis can often be suspected by the clinical and epidemiologic setting. For example, self-limited, noninflammatory diarrhea in tropical, developing areas is most likely due to enterotoxigenic *E. coli*, rotaviruses (young children), or Norwalk-like viruses (older children and adults). Noninflammatory diarrhea in winter months in temperate areas in older children or younger adults is more likely to be due to Norwalk-like viruses. Specific tests for the respective virulence traits of different types of *E. coli* are noted in Table 288–1. One should also consider *Vibrio* infections in areas endemic for cholera or in any coastal area where inadequately cooked seafood may be eaten. If noninflammatory diarrhea persists, especially with weight loss, one should also consider *Giardia lamblia* or *Cryptosporidium* infection. In outbreaks of food poisoning, *S. aureus*, *Clostridium perfringens*, and *Bacillus cereus* should be considered.

Inflammatory colitis with high fever, tenesmus, and leukocytes, mucus, and blood in the stool may well be due to enteroinvasive *E. coli* but should prompt a stool culture for more common invasive pathogens such as *Campylobacter jejuni*, *Shigella*, and *Salmonella* or even *Clostridium difficile*, *Yersina enterocolitica*, or non-cholera *Vibrio* (see Ch. 286). On the other hand, bloody diarrhea without high fever or fecal leukocytes should prompt consideration of the Shiga-like toxin producing enterohemorrhagic *E. coli* (EHEC) such as strain O157:H7. This organism is often suspected as a sorbitol-negative *E. coli*, which may require further study for serotype or Shiga-like toxin production.

THERAPY. As with all diarrheal illnesses, the primary treatment is replacement and maintenance of water and electrolytes. Losses of water and electrolytes may be particularly severe and even life-threatening with enterotoxigenic *E. coli* and can usually be replaced with a simple oral rehydration solution that employs the intact, sodium-coupled glucose, and/or amino acid absorption to replace fluid losses, as described in Ch. 287. This oral rehydration solution should be given ad libitum with free water and, in breast-fed infants, continued breast feeding and early refeeding to compensate for the nutritional losses.

Because most *E. coli* diarrhea is self-limited, the role of antimicrobial agents is debated and remains of secondary importance to rehydration. In areas where the enterotoxigenic *E. coli* remains sensitive, early initiation of sulfamethoxazole-trimethoprim, tetracycline, or new quinolone derivatives may reduce a three- to five-day illness to a one- to two-day illness if started with the first loose stool in travelers to endemic, tropical areas. The use of antimotility agents should be tempered by the potential added risk of worsening or prolonging inflammatory diarrheas and by their lack of effectiveness in reducing fluid loss even though abdominal cramping and overt diarrhea may be temporarily reduced. Because of the potential severity of the disease in infants, some pediatricians use neomycin, 100 mg per kilogram per day P.O., divided into three daily doses for five days, for documented enteropathogenic *E. coli* infections in neonates. Bismuth subsalicylate may reduce symptoms in travelers' diarrhea but should be used with caution to avoid toxic doses of salicylate. A number of pharmacologic agents have been shown to enhance absorption or reduce secretion with experimental diarrhea but remain inadequately studied or too toxic for recommended use to date.

PROGNOSIS. The overall prognosis in *E. coli* diarrheas of the various types noted, if fully and adequately treated, is generally excellent. However, the impact of *E. coli* and other common diarrheas on mortality and morbidity (particularly with repeated infections compounding malnutrition in developing young children) remains one of the major health problems on a global scale; this problem may actually be worsening in some transitional areas.

PREVENTION. The prevention of *E. coli* enteric infections is ultimately related to basic economic development and adequate sanitary facilities and wide availability of sufficient quality and quantity of water. In the interim, especially in areas where adequate water supplies and sanitary facilities are not available, such measures as breast feeding for at least 6 to 12 months and hygienic measures like hand washing should reduce the likelihood of acquiring *E. coli* enteric infections. Travelers to developing or tropical areas should avoid drinking untreated or unboiled water or ice and eating uncooked fruits or vegetables that may have been "freshened" with highly contaminated water. Although a number of antimicrobial agents have been documented to be effective over short periods of time when taken prophylactically, their effectiveness is sharply limited by the rapidly emerging resistance to antimicrobial drugs as well as by the potential side effects of their indiscriminate, widespread use. For example, tetracycline resistance among enterotoxigenic *E. coli* is common, and combined sulfamethoxazole-trimethroprim resistance is rapidly emerging around the world. Finally, currently developing toxoid or colonization factor vaccines hold considerable promise for the prevention of enterotoxigenic *E. coli* diarrhea.

Black RE, Merson MH, Hug I, et al.: Incidence and severity of rotavirus and *Escherichia coli* diarrhoea in rural Bangladesh. Implications for vaccine development. Lancet 1:141–143, 1981. *Concise report of community-based studies of enterotoxigenic E. coli and rotaviral diarrhea in a rural area of Bangladesh.*

DuPont HL, Formal SB, Hornick RB, et al.: Pathogenesis of *Escherichia coli* diarrhea. N Engl J Med 285:1–9, 1971. *Classic early clinical, pathologic, and pathogenetic studies of enterotoxigenic and enteroinvasive E. coli diarrhea in human volunteers.*

Guerrant RL, Kirchhoff LV, Shields DS, et al.: Prospective study of diarrheal illnesses in northeastern Brazil: Patterns of disease, nutritional impact, etiologies and risk factors. J Infect Dis 148:986–997, 1983. *A detailed study of endemic diarrhea in a tropical area, including seasonality, risk after weaning, and nutritional impact, as well as relationship of enterotoxigenic E. coli to other pathogens.*

Levine MM, Edelman R: Enteropathogenic *Escherichia coli* of classic serotypes associated with infant diarrhea: Epidemiology and pathogenesis. Epidemiol Rev 6:31–51, 1984. *A thorough historical review of classic enteropathogenic E. coli diarrhea as well as an update on recent volunteer studies and pathogenesis.*

Levine MM, Kaper JB, Black RE, et al.: New knowledge on pathogenesis of bacterial enteric infections as applied to vaccine development. Microbiol Rev 47:510–550, 1983. *A detailed analysis of current work on vaccines against E. coli as well as V. cholerae, Shigella, Salmonella, and other enteric infections.*

Microbial Toxins and Diarrheal Diseases. CIBA Foundation Symposium No. 112, 1985. *Thorough review of the mechanisms of enterotoxin action, relating the pharmacology of E. coli toxins (LT, STa, STb, Shiga) to those of other enteric pathogens like V. cholerae, Shigella, and C. difficile.*

NIH Consensus Development Conference on Traveler's Diarrhea. JAMA 253:2700–2704, 1985. *A balanced critical appraisal of the epidemiology, etiologies, presentation, and treatment of concise travelers' diarrhea.*

Remis RS, MacDonald KL, Riley LW, et al.: Sporadic cases of hemorrhagic colitis associated with *Escherichia coli* O157:H7. Ann Intern Med 101:624–626, 1984. *Review of clinical and pathologic presentations of enterohemorrhagic E. coli (EHEC) O157:H7 infections in adults and children, since the first report of outbreaks in two states related to fast-food hamburger consumption.*

Sansonetti PJ, Hale TL, Oaks EV: Genetics of virulence in enteroinvasive *Escherichia coli*. Microbiology, 1985, pp 67–82. *One of a series of three brief reviews that offer a considerable amount of new information on the pathogenesis of the major types of E. coli enteric infection including ETEC, EIEC, EPEC, and EHEC.*

289 THE DIARRHEA OF TRAVELERS

R. Bradley Sack

Travelers from the developed world who visit the developing world are highly susceptible to an acute diarrheal illness known as "travelers' diarrhea" or by more colorful names that fit the locale in which the travelers find themselves incapacitated. Although at one time this condition was blamed on a change in diet, minerals in the water, and travel fatigue, it is now known to be an acute infection, caused by enteric pathogens that are endemic throughout the areas of the world where sanitation is less than optimal. In those areas the diarrhea produced by these pathogens is primarily a childhood disease that decreases markedly in incidence after the first few years of life, because of the development of protective immunity. Travelers are, in a sense, immunologically naive "children" who are suddenly placed in an endemic area of infection and therefore are highly susceptible to the disease. The predictable, high attack rates of diarrhea in travelers make this syndrome one that can be conveniently and intensively studied by investigators attempting to prevent and treat it. Perhaps other than a common source outbreak of diarrheal disease, the attack rates among travelers are the highest known in any identifiable population. Among travelers from the United States to the developing world, attack rates vary from about 25 to 75 per cent during the first three weeks of stay, with rates decreasing markedly as immunity develops.

By way of contrast, travelers from developing countries who visit other developing countries usually have a considerably lower attack rate, based on their prior exposure to these organisms. However, they are still susceptible to "new" agents that they may not have encountered previously. Visitors from the developing countries who visit the developed world, on the other hand, have a very low attack rate of diarrhea, as would be expected.

ETIOLOGY. Multiple studies have now been done on the etiology of this syndrome throughout the world, and it is clear that enterotoxigenic *Escherichia coli* (Ch. 288) is the predominant organism. Other bacteria, viruses, and protozoa are also involved, but with lesser frequency (Table 289–1). In different geographic areas, the rank order of these pathogens varies, but *E. coli* heads the list; because of this observation, studies of treatment and prophylaxis have been possible by focusing on this single group of organisms. However, a considerable percentage of episodes is undiagnosed etiologically, in spite of the best available laboratory techniques; evidence from studies employing antimicrobials suggests that a large number of these are also bacterial in origin. Contrary to "popular" notions about travelers' diarrhea, relatively few cases are caused by protozoa, particularly *Entameba histolytica*.

PATHOGENESIS AND CLINICAL PICTURE. The clinical syndrome of travelers' diarrhea is typically that of a secretory watery diarrhea caused by the enterotoxins of *E. coli* (see Ch. 288). The entire process is analogous to the pathogenesis of cholera (Ch. 287). The watery diarrhea usually lasts three to four days, and when most severe, may result in watery stools as frequent as 15 to 20 times per day, with significant water and electrolyte loss, leading to clinical signs of dehydration.

TABLE 289–1. ETIOLOGIC AGENTS OF TRAVELERS' DIARRHEA*

Agent	Percentage
Enterotoxigenic *E. coli*	30–70
Shigella	5–10
Salmonella	<5
Campylobacter	<5
Enteroadherent *E. coli*	
Rotavirus	
Norwalk-like virus	
Giardia lamblia	
Entameba histolytica	
Cryptosporidium	
Unknown agents	30–40

*Agents listed without percentages are usually found infrequently, or studies have not been sufficient to establish a frequency.

Although deaths due to this illness are extremely rare, definitive replacement of fluid and electrolytes lost in the stool may be necessary, and hospitalization may be required. The vast majority of illnesses are much milder, however, consisting of only three to five diarrheal stools per day, and are of importance primarily because of limitation of activities.

Those episodes due to *Shigella* organisms are usually typical of a dysentery-like illness, with abdominal pain, fever, and blood and inflammatory cells in the stool.

Nearly all episodes are self-limited, but a few (less than 1 per cent) may become persistent and require evaluation following return home.

Although the clinical syndrome in children traveling to the developing world has been less well studied, there are a number of reports of severe, persistent diarrhea and marked nutritional wasting following visits to high-risk areas.

TRANSMISSION. The transmission of the enteric pathogens occurs almost exclusively through fecally contaminated food and water. Of highest risk to the traveler are foods that are not cooked or peeled and are consumed raw. Foods obtained from road-side vendors or foods kept unrefrigerated for long periods of time are also in the highest risk category.

PREVENTION. Since the mode of transmission is known, prudent attention to the ingestion of uncontaminated food and water should entirely prevent the disease. This has been shown in the military and on board cruise ships, where all food is hygienically prepared and packaged. For the usual traveler, however, food must be obtained from local sources, and contamination cannot be entirely prevented. Even the "best" hotels in the developing world may have unsanitary kitchens, and "first class" travelers are therefore not exempt.

A number of studies have been carried out in an attempt to prevent the disease with drugs, and many agents have been shown to be highly protective. The most protective are antimicrobials directed against the most common etiologic agents, the enterotoxigenic *E. coli*. Both doxycycline (100 mg, once daily with food) and trimethoprim-sulfamethoxazole (160 + 800 mg, once daily), taken for a period of up to three weeks, have provided a high degree of protection against travelers' diarrhea, in the neighborhood of 75 to 90 per cent. A nonantimicrobial drug, bismuth subsalicylate taken four times a day has also given a significant degree of protection (approximately 60 per cent). Other antimicrobial drugs have also been used successfully (erythromycin, mecillinam, trimethoprim alone) but have not been tested as extensively. Drugs that have been tested and found to be of little or no benefit include neomycin, streptotriad, hydroxyquinolines, and *Lactobacillus* preparations.

The main questions relating to the use of prophylactic medications are not the efficacy, but rather the side effects; this issue will be further discussed later.

THERAPY. Therapy is based on recognition of clinical disease and a general knowledge of the causative organisms, since identity of specific etiologic agents will usually not be known (Table 289–1). The therapy of travelers' diarrhea falls under three general categories: (1) replacement of fluid and electrolytes lost to prevent and treat the resulting dehydration, (2) symptomatic therapy directed at relieving the frequency of stooling or the attendant abdominal cramps, and (3) specific antimicrobial therapy directed at the causative agent, in order to decrease the severity and shorten the duration of the illness.

Replacement therapy is done best with the oral glucose-electrolyte solutions developed for therapy of all dehydrating diarrheas, regardless of etiologic agent or age of the patient. These are now available commercially in packets, which can be carried by the traveler and used as required by mixing the contents with the appropriate volumes of potable water.

Symptomatic therapy may be useful for travelers with a typical secretory diarrhea who need to participate in certain vital events, such as long bus rides or important business or social occasions. The drugs used (loperamide, diphenoxylate) primarily interfere with intestinal motility and therefore can decrease the rate of stooling in persons with mild disease. However, because of this action, there is the possibility of actually intensifying the clinical illness due to invasive bacteria, since they will be more slowly cleared from the bowel.

Preparations of bismuth subsalicylate have also been shown to give mild symptomatic relief, although the mechanism of action is unknown. Kaolin/pectin preparations are of no significant effect in treatment.

Specific antimicrobial therapy has been shown to be highly effective for this illness. The same three drugs used for prophylaxis—trimethoprim (160 mg)-sulfamethoxazole (800 mg) twice daily; trimethoprim, 200 mg twice daily; and doxycycline, 100 mg twice daily—are also effective in shortening the duration of the disease to 24 to 36 hours. A three-day course of therapy is sufficient.

THE STRATEGY OF MANAGING THE PROBLEM OF TRAVELERS' DIARRHEA. The questions relating to the prevention and treatment of travelers' diarrhea have recently been reviewed at an NIH Consensus Conference, which should be consulted for further details. The most difficult issue is who, if anyone, should receive prophylactic antimicrobials. Since antimicrobials are widely available as over-the-counter medications throughout the developing world, the small addition to the antimicrobial pool by tourists is thought to be inconsequential to the larger issue of antibiotic pressure on a worldwide basis. Of more importance is the issue of adverse reactions to the drugs being taken for prophylaxis. Although none of the published controlled studies demonstrated any significant side effects, all were done using primarily young healthy adults. Since these drugs have significant side effects, although at low frequency, they are not recommended for routine prophylaxis. For the short-term individual traveler, however, who is advised of the possible side effects and who wishes to avail him/herself of the protection, these drugs can be considered for use.

Since the same drugs can be taken as treatment the preferred strategy in most cases would be to have the traveler carry along sufficient medication, so that he or she can administer appropriate treatment when indicated. Oral rehydration therapy should be given simultaneously for the prevention of dehydration. For milder episodes of diarrhea, drugs like bismuth subsalicylate or antimotility drugs can be taken for symptomatic relief.

The problem of travelers' diarrhea will continue until the general sanitation of the developing world approaches that of the industrialized countries or until effective vaccines against the major diarrheal pathogens are available. Neither of these occurrences is expected soon, and therefore this common syndrome will need to be addressed for some time; this can now be done rationally and effectively based on our knowledge of etiologies and modes of transmission.

Consensus Conference: Travelers' Diarrhea. JAMA 253:2700, 1985. *A summary of the NIH conference in which all aspects of the problem were reviewed; a complete publication of the conference is given in Rev Infect Dis 8:(Suppl 2), 1986.*

DuPont HL, Reves RR, Galindo E, et al.: Treatment of travelers' diarrhea with trimethoprim/sulfamethoxazole and with trimethoprim alone. N Engl J Med 307:841, 1982. *A controlled therapeutic study showing marked efficacy of these drugs.*

Sack RB: Treatment and prevention of travelers' diarrhea. In Holmgren J, Lindberg A, Mollby R (eds.): Development of Vaccines against Diarrhea, 11th Nobel Conf., Stockholm 1985, pp 289–301. Lund, Sweden, Studentlitteratur, 1986. *A comprehensive review of all controlled studies of prophylaxis and treatment.*

Other Bacterial Infections

290 EXTRAINTESTINAL INFECTIONS CAUSED BY ENTERIC BACTERIA

Elizabeth J. Ziegler

Bacteria comprise over half the dry weight of stool. *Bacteroides* species far outnumber other genera, at 10^{12} organisms per gram. Other anaerobes such as *Fusobacteria, Clostridia,* and peptostreptococci also are abundant. Among the facultative bacteria, members of the family Enterobacteriaciae predominate, at about 10^9 organisms per gram. Pseudomonads, enterococci, other nonhemolytic streptococci, and yeasts are present as well.

These bacteria that normally inhabit the human gastrointestinal tract perform important functions beneficial to the host. *Bacteroides fragilis, Clostridia,* and enterococci deconjugate bile acids for participation in fat metabolism. Some intestinal bacteria synthesize menaquinone, or vitamin K, a cofactor for blood coagulation. The normal gut flora discourage colonization of bowel with primary pathogens and overgrowth of bacteria usually present in small numbers. Colonization resistance is not understood completely, but it must involve bacteriocins, regulation of local oxidation-reduction potential, and balance of nutrients as well as unknown factors. Breakdown of colonization resistance can be observed in the increase in susceptibility of antibiotic-treated animals to *Salmonella* and in the emergence of fecal *Pseudomonas aeruginosa* and *Candida* in patients receiving antimicrobial agents.

PATHOGENESIS OF INFECTIONS

Enteric bacteria are not primary pathogens but cause disease when they escape from their usual gastrointestinal habitat. Direct penetration of the bowel wall by surgical, traumatic, or spontaneous rupture spills fecal contents into the peritoneal cavity and into open wounds. Gut bacteria on the perineal skin gain access to the urinary tract and proliferate there, especially when the flushing action of urine flow is disrupted by mechanical obstruction or neurologic dysfunction. When the biliary tract is obstructed by gallstones or tumor, the upper small bowel, which normally is sterile, becomes colonized with facultative bacteria (*E. coli, Klebsiella,* enterococci) or, less often, with *Bacteroides* and *Clostridia,* which then infect the gallbladder and bile ducts. Intestinal flora can be introduced into the respiratory tract from contaminated skin or the environment; they proliferate there under the influence of antibiotics and in the presence of underlying pulmonary disease and tracheal instrumentation. Penetrating foreign bodies such as intravenous catheters and intraventricular cerebral pressure monitors become colonized by gut flora on the skin and in respiratory secretions and then induce infection in adjacent tissues. In burns, destruction of the skin barrier, the rich culture medium of oozing tissue fluid, and a shift of surface flora by application of local and systemic antibacterial agents result in local necrotizing infection of the burn wound with gut flora and frequent secondary gram-negative bacteremia.

In the absence of mechanical and surface abnormalities such as those outlined above, systemic resistance to enteric bacteria is very strong. The mainstay of this resistance is the polymorphonuclear neutrophil, destruction or malfunction of which leads almost inevitably to blood stream invasion by bowel bacteria. Serum complement must be protective against invasion of some organisms, since very few of the gram-negative bacilli isolated from blood are sensitive to complement-mediated bacteriolysis, whereas many enteric rods in feces are susceptible. Newborn infants, whose neutrophils and complement activity have not fully matured, are at high risk of disseminated infections with facultative enteric rods. Microbial factors are important, too. Although anaerobes predominate over facultative bacteria and aerobes in the gut, these anaerobes rarely cause bacteremia or metastatic infection even in neutropenia. The presence of certain bacterial polysaccharide capsules (e.g., *E. coli* K1) or production of large amounts of capsule (e.g., by *Klebsiella pneumoniae* in hyperglycemic or glycosuric diabetics) predisposes to systemic invasion by these organisms.

Infections with enteric bacteria have increased dramatically during the past four decades. The reasons should be apparent from the discussion above. Advances in surgical and intensive care, trauma and burn management, blood transfusion, antimicrobial and cancer chemotherapy, transplantation, and immunosuppression all create opportunities for these infections. The average life span has lengthened so that those receiving medical attention carry the added risks of advanced age. The majority of extraintestinal infections with enteric bacteria now arise in the hospital, and they exact a high toll in mortality and increased hospital costs. Furthermore, they jeopardize the success of the advanced treatments we have worked so hard to develop. For these reasons, physicians should understand the pathogenesis of each infection so that they can effect a cure and prevent recurrence if possible.

SPECIFIC LOCAL INFECTIONS WITH ENTERIC BACTERIA

The diagnosis and management of each of the following gram-negative infections are discussed in depth in the appropriate section elsewhere in the textbook. A few points are emphasized here.

PERITONITIS (see Ch. 112). It can be difficult to recover bacteria from cases of spontaneous bacterial peritonitis; large volumes of fluid should be submitted for culture. Patients undergoing chronic peritoneal dialysis frequently develop peritonitis. If the same organism is isolated from repeated episodes and especially if it is an enteric rod or *Pseudomonas,* infection of the subcutaneous catheter tunnel should be suspected. A radiolabelled white blood cell scan can be helpful in detecting such infections so that the infected catheter can be removed.

PYELONEPHRITIS (see Ch. 86). Localizing urinary tract infections to bladder or kidneys can have important implications for therapy. Symptoms may be misleading, selective ureteral catheterization carries considerable risk, and examination of urine for antibody-coated bacteria is not practical in routine laboratories. A simple culture technique can differentiate between upper and lower urinary tract infections in difficult cases in which parenteral antibiotics would be required for kidney infection. In brief, the test (Fairley et al., 1967) employs a newly placed three-way bladder catheter through which a combination of antibiotic and enzyme mixture (fibrinolysin and DNAase) is instilled to sterilize the bladder. Neomycin is employed for most organisms; polymyxin can be used for *Pseudomonas* and amphotericin for yeast. Bladder instillation is followed by a large-volume sterile water wash. Then the catheter is clamped and three 10-minute specimens are collected. Increasing bacterial counts after the wash point to pyelonephritis. If infection is limited to the bladder, the Fairley procedure can cure it. The test is unreliable in patients with low urinary output and it should not be performed in patients with neutropenia.

PROSTATITIS (see Ch. 236). Most antibiotics available for treatment of enteric bacilli do not penetrate the prostate well. For this reason, chronic prostatitis rarely is cured. However, the role of chronic prostatitis as a nidus of recurrent acute urinary tract infection in males can be curbed by low levels of suppressive antibiotics in bladder urine, achieved by a single daily tablet of an oral antibiotic.

MENINGITIS (see Ch. 272). Enteric rods, especially *E. coli* and *Klebsiella,* are a frequent cause of neonatal meningitis. In adults, meningitis with enteric bacilli is exceedingly rare except in cases of head trauma or neurosurgery. Bacteria may be infrequent and difficult to see on stained smears of spinal or ventricular fluid. Treatment with a third-generation cephalosporin that penetrates the blood-brain barrier at high dose may be sufficient, but infections with organisms resistant to such drugs may require chloramphenicol or a combination of intravenous and intrathecal aminoglycosides. Infected foreign bodies must be removed.

PNEUMONIA (see Ch. 262, 265, 266). Seeing or growing gram-negative rods from respiratory secretions does not necessarily imply infection. Susceptible patients often have severe chronic lung disease with abnormal chest radiographs. Many are on respirators with inflammation around endotracheal tubes and have abnormal gram-negative nasopharyngeal flora. Evidence of increasing infiltrates, fever, increasing leukocytosis, and/or worsening respiratory function should be sought before the diagnosis of gram-negative pneumonia is made in such cases.

INFECTIONS OF INTRAVENOUS CATHETERS. Patients who are critically ill may have limited numbers of sites for placement of intravenous catheters. If catheter infection is suspected, it may be impractical or impossible to remove all the lines. Comparison of quantitative blood cultures drawn through each catheter and from one peripheral vein can identify the infected site and preserve the uninfected catheters in place.

INFECTIONS IN NEUTROPENIA (see Ch. 258). The most common bowel infection in neutropenia is perirectal abscess. Inflammation may be modest, but patients complain of severe pain. Examination can cause bacteremia. Surgical drainage may not be required unless neutropenia resolves and fluctuance develops. A less common but much more serious condition is typhlitis, an infection of the cecum associated with gas in the bowel wall, peritonitis, perforation, and bacteremia. This condition can be fatal within hours. Surgical resection has been helpful in a few cases, but surgical mortality is very high. Aggressive antibiotic therapy should be directed against *E. coli* and *P. aeruginosa,* the most common etiologic agents.

Necrotic skin lesions can accompany gram-negative bacteremia in neutropenic patients. These lesions are called ecthyma gangrenosum, and they are seen most frequently in *Pseudomonas* bacteremia. Cases have been reported with other gram-negative rods and with *Candida* and *Aspergillus* septicemia as well. The lesions can be scraped to search for the organism on smear. If nothing is seen, a punch biopsy for culture and histologic section can be done safely even in severe thrombocytopenia. In fungemia, the histologic section may be the only premortem diagnostic specimen obtained.

GRAM-NEGATIVE BACTEREMIA AND ENDOTOXIC SHOCK

Gram-negative bacteria gain access to the bloodstream from foci of tissue infection or, when host resistance is depressed, from sites of heavy colonization and minor trauma. Although bacteremia creates the opportunity for metastatic infections, a more immediate and serious consequence of gram-negative bacteremia is bacteremic shock. The incidence of gram-negative bacteremia has risen steadily during the past three decades. Now there are at least 140,000 episodes in the United States each year, of which 50,000 are fatal. Death is caused by either irreversible hypotension or damage to vital organs such as lung or kidney, which cannot be salvaged despite recovery from circulatory collapse.

Rates of shock vary in different series from less than 20 per cent to more than 50 per cent. In comparable groups shock is somewhat more frequent in gram-negative bacteremia than in gram-positive bacteremia or fungemia. However, gram-negative bacteremia is distinguished from the other septicemias by the fact that very small numbers of circulating bacteria are capable of causing hypotension. It is generally agreed that the principal instigator of gram-negative shock is endotoxin, a major structural component of the gram-negative bacterial cell wall, for the abnormalities seen in endotoxic shock can be duplicated with intravenous infusions of pure endotoxin in experimental animals. Endotoxin is a lipopolysaccharide (LPS) consisting of a long chain of strain-specific repeating sugar subunits at one end, some connecting core sugars in the middle, and lipid A, a fatty acid– and phosphate-substituted diglucosamine, at the other end, embedded in the cell wall. Lipid A, the biologically active portion of the molecule, is highly conserved with little variation among gram-negative bacteria. An exception is *Bacteroides fragilis*, which makes an unusual lipid A; its LPS is virtually nontoxic and *B. fragilis* bacteremia is rarely associated with shock. In gram-negative bacteremia, endotoxin is available on the bacterial surface and free in the circulation to stimulate mediators of shock. There is evidence that antibiotics, especially those directed at the cell wall, release substantial amounts of LPS from bacteria while killing them; this may explain the transient worsening of hypotension occasionally seen after the first dose of antibiotics.

Man is one of the species most sensitive to endotoxin. Subnanogram quantities of LPS stimulate beneficial host responses such as lymphocyte activation and fever (interleukin 1). However, even a few nanograms given intravenously elicit a panoply of toxic reactions including complement activation, production of procoagulant factors with disseminated intravascular coagulation (DIC), neutrophil aggregation, lung capillary damage, and perturbation of circulatory control with splanchnic pooling of blood, hypotension, and metabolic acidosis. Many mediators are involved in these reactions; recent work suggests that tumor necrosis factor, a small protein produced by endotoxin-stimulated macrophages, may be responsible for most of the phenomena leading to death from endotoxin (see Ch. 256, 257).

CLINICAL MANIFESTATIONS (see also Ch. 259). Since focal infections usually precede bloodstream invasion, patients are likely to have had fever and leukocytosis for several days before the sudden deterioration that marks the onset of gram-negative bacteremia. The temperature may suddenly increase or it may fall to subnormal levels, especially in elderly patients or those who are debilitated. Rarely, fever is obliterated by chronically administered high-dose steroids. There may be frank shaking chills. Patients may exhibit new anxiety, agitation, or confusion. For some reason, patients with burns often develop unexplained ileus as one of the few clues to bacteremia on a background of fever, leukocytosis, and vascular instability associated with the burn itself. Even though blood pressure still may be normal, orthostatic pulse and blood pressure changes may be seen. Resting tachycardia and/or increased respiratory rate is helpful (unless the patient has a pacemaker, is on drugs that affect heart rate, or is on a respirator at controlled rate). In patients under less strict surveillance, the first symptom of hypotension may be a significant decrease in urine output. When the blood pressure is obtained, it is important to consult the medical record for the patient's normal reading. Formerly hypertensive patients will suffer poor perfusion at levels of blood pressure which are normal for most individuals. In general, the traditional distinction between "warm" and "cold" shock has not been helpful in separating gram-positive from gram-negative shock, and no reliance should be placed on it. When measured, cardiac output is high and systemic resistance is low in cases of endotoxic shock uncomplicated by other diseases. In late stages of untreated or irreversible shock, patients will exhibit intense vasoconstriction, then cyanosis. Symptoms of shock-induced organ failure—bleeding, adult respiratory distress syndrome, azotemia, and infarcts of brain, heart, and bowel—will appear and may dominate the picture.

DIAGNOSIS. For therapeutic purposes the diagnosis of gram-negative bacteremia cannot await the results of blood cultures but must be made on clinical grounds alone. The clinical setting is very helpful. A diagnosis of gram-negative bacteremia should be entertained when acute deterioration occurs in patients with focal infections usually caused by gram-negative bacteria (e.g., pyelonephritis, cholecystitis), patients with significant focal infections from which gram-negative bacteria already have been isolated, and patients with compromise in host defenses (e.g., neutropenia, burn) rendering them susceptible to their own bacterial flora. Neutropenic patients rarely have physical signs to localize the source of their bacteremia, but a careful conversation often reveals a history of minor trauma, slight pain, or diarrhea.

When gram-negative bacteria grow in blood cultured at the time of clinical deterioration, the diagnosis of gram-negative bacteremia is certain. With increased use of prophylactic and empiric antibiotics, negative blood cultures are being obtained more frequently in series of cases with the typical presentation and outcome of endotoxic shock. When shock is coupled with a single, major, culture-proven gram-negative focal infection in patients on antibiotics appropriate for the isolates, the diagnosis of endotoxic shock can be made even with negative blood cultures. Some authorities accept the entity of "endotoxemia with bacteremia" when blood cultures are negative in the absence of antibiotics. Confirmation of this syndrome awaits development of a sensitive test for LPS in plasma; the Limulus lysate assay, which is excellent in CSF and intravenous fluids, is still not reliable enough in plasma to be applied diagnostically.

Gram-negative bacteremia and endotoxin infusion both cause transient neutropenia followed by neutrophilic leukocytosis. Large "toxic" vacuoles are seen. The first leukocyte count often is obtained after the leukopenic phase, but patients recovering from chemotherapy may have limited leukocyte reserves and thus will exhibit only an apparent reversal of marrow recovery. Isolated thrombocytopenia or full-blown disseminated intravascular coagulopathy is not diagnostic of gram-negative bacteremia but, if present, is good supporting evidence. Arterial blood gas determinations reveal unexplained respiratory alkalosis, then metabolic acidosis.

The differential diagnosis of gram-negative shock includes septicemias caused by gram-positive bacteria and fungi, staphylococcal toxic shock syndrome, clostridial shock, pulmonary embolus, acute allergic reactions, myocardial infarction, and a long list of less common conditions.

TREATMENT. There are three essential elements in the management of gram-negative bacteremia: physiologic support, antibiotics, and identification of the source so that it can be eradicated. These are listed in the order in which they should be addressed but all three should be considered urgently, generally within one hour. If the patient is in shock or impending shock, physiologic monitoring in an intensive care unit should be applied if available. Good intravenous access should be obtained and a bladder catheter placed for hourly measurement of urine flow.

The aim of physiologic support is to restore adequate tissue perfusion. This is judged most easily by urine flow and mental status; perfusion of vital organs may be adequate when systolic blood pressure remains low and there is marked peripheral vasoconstriction. The principles of management of septic shock are the same as those used for other kinds of shock. If urine flow is less than 30 ml per hour, fluids should be infused at the maximum rate tolerated by the patient. The composition, infusion rate, and total amount of fluid must be tailored to individual cardiac capacity. If urine flow is not restored with the pulmonary wedge pressure at upper limits of normal or if the wedge pressure cannot be raised by fluids, a sympathetic amine such as dopamine or dobutamine should be administered without delay. If excessive quantities of fluid are used, severe pulmonary edema may develop just as the patient is recovering from septic shock. Dopamine is diluted to a concentration of 0.8 to 1.6 mg per milliliter and is given intravenously at an initial rate of 2 to 5 μg per kilogram per minute. The rate may be increased gradually up to 20 to 50 μg per kilogram per minute as needed. Dobutamine may be preferable in patients with congestive heart failure because it does not increase the pulmonary wedge pressure; however, in contrast to dopamine, it does not produce renal vasodilation. Therefore, dopamine is preferable in profound, prolonged shock. If pressors are used for many days, patients may require very slow weaning; continued hypotension does not necessarily imply continuing infection. Supplemental oxygen is commonly used in endotoxic shock, but its value has not been assessed rigorously. It does little harm.

The correct choice of antibiotics is crucial to successful treatment of gram-negative bacteremia. When inappropriate drugs are used or the doses are too low, outcome is poor. It is never wise to give a single antibiotic to a patient at the onset of a bacteremic episode, even if the diagnosis and etiology seem certain. Many other infections can mimic gram-negative bacteremia, as discussed. Sometimes more than one bacterial species is involved. In neutropenia, the outcome of *Pseudomonas* bacteremia is much better if more than one effective antibiotic is used. The choice of empiric antibiotics should be made on the basis of the site of the focal infection(s) present, the known antimicrobial sensitivities of previous isolates from the patient and of agents of recent nosocomial infections in the hospital, and the patient's underlying diseases. At the present time the best regimen seems to be a combination of an aminoglycoside with a third-generation cephalosporin. An antistaphylococcal drug should be added if *S. aureus* infection is likely. If bowel perforation or infarction has occurred, *Bacteroides fragilis* must be covered. If *Clostridium perfringens* is suspected to be part of a mixed infection, concomitant high-dose penicillin should be used. (*C. perfringens* decolorizes easily in the Gram's stain and may be distinguishable from gram-negative rods only by its boxlike rectangular shape.) A common mistake in the use of aminoglycosides is to tailor the initial regimen to the first renal function tests. If azotemia is acute and attributable to poor perfusion, initial low doses will give inadequate levels as soon as hypotension is reversed. Renal toxicity from these drugs rarely occurs early; it is far more important to treat infection effectively in the first 24 hours than to avoid aminoglycoside toxicity.

Gram-negative bacteremia cannot be cured without eradication of the source of bacteremia. In cases of infection associated with ureteral or biliary obstruction, bacteremia and shock may persist in the face of adequate antibiotics until the obstruction is relieved. All likely sites of infection should be cultured, if possible, before antibiotics are given. However, antibiotic treatment should not be delayed for this reason. Wound cultures often remain positive after blood and urine have been sterilized. The physician should not be content until he has found a satisfactory explanation for bacteremia. New fever or clinical deterioration can signal a new infection in a susceptible patient, the emergence of resistant bacteria, spread of the original focal infection, inadequate antibiotic levels, or a drug reaction. Such an episode requires complete re-evaluation with physical examination and repeat cultures.

Several modes of adjunctive treatment for endotoxic shock are being evaluated at the present time. High-dose corticosteroids have been used empirically for many years because of beneficial effects seen in experimental animal models of septic shock. Their value has not yet been established in patients despite several large clinical trials. Nonsteroidal anti-inflammatory drugs also are being studied in endotoxic shock. Because endotoxin seems to play a central role in the evolution of gram-negative shock, several groups have raised antibodies to LPS determinants common to most gram-negative bacteria and have found these anti-endotoxin antisera effective in preventing LPS toxicity and bacteremic death in experimental gram-negative infections. A controlled clinical trial of human anti-LPS antiserum to treat established bacteremia showed a lower bacteremic death rate in patients given antiserum than in those given preimmunization control serum; the protective effect extended to patients in profound endotoxic shock. Several murine and human monoclonal antibodies to lipid A are being evaluated for their protective capacity in experimental infection and their safety in man, but none has yet been subjected to controlled clinical trials.

Bryan CS, Reynolds KL, Brenner ER: Analysis of 1,186 episodes of gram-negative bacteremia in non-university hospitals: The effects of antimicrobial therapy. Rev Infect Dis 5:629, 1983. *A thorough study of gram-negative bacteremia in community hospitals from 1977 to 1981, this article discusses the factors that are most important in determining outcome. An interesting contrast to series from academic centers.*

DuPont HL, Spink WW: Infections due to gram-negative organisms: An analysis of 860 patients with bacteremia at the University of Minnesota Medical Center, 1958–1966. Medicine 48:307, 1969. *This article is a classic in the field; it describes the early years when gram-negative bacteremia first was flourishing.*

Fairley KF, Bond AG, Brown RB, et al.: Simple test to determine the site of urinary tract infection. Lancet 1:427, 1967. *A brief description of the details of the Fairley test.*

Kreger BE, Craven DE, Carling PC, et al.: Gram-negative bacteremia: III. Reassessment of etiology, epidemiology and ecology in 612 patients. Am J Med 68:332, 1980. *A recent classic clinical description of gram-negative bacteremia in an academic hospital setting, with emphasis on the pathogenesis and the influence of underlying condition on outcome.*

Tracey KJ, Beutler B, Lowry SF, et al.: Shock and tissue injury induced by recombinant human cachetin. Science 234:470, 1986. *An excellent review of tumor necrosis factor and experimental evidence of its role in endotoxic shock.*

Ziegler EJ, McCutchan JA, Fierer J, et al.: Treatment of gram-negative bacteremia and shock with human antiserum to a mutant *Escherichia coli*. N Engl J Med 307:1225, 1982. *Description of the clinical trial of antiserum against LPS core in treatment of endotoxic shock, with a review of the antecedent animal experiments.*

291 YERSINIA INFECTIONS

Thomas Butler

PLAGUE

DEFINITION. Plague is a bacterial infection of animals and humans caused by *Yersinia pestis*. The most common clinical form is *acute regional lymphadenitis*, called *bubonic plague*. Less common forms include *septicemic, pneumonic, cutaneous,* and *meningeal plague*. Mortality is high in untreated cases, but antibiotic treatment administered early in the course of the disease markedly reduces fatalities.

HISTORY. *Y. pestis* has caused devastating pandemics with high mortality rates throughout history. The fourth great pandemic in the world is currently under way. The first three are believed to have occurred in the following times: the first originated in Egypt in 542 A.D. and spread to Turkey and Europe. The second started in the 14th century in Asia Minor and Africa; after spreading to Europe the black death killed about a fourth of the continent's people. The third occurred in Europe during the 15th to 18th centuries. The present fourth pandemic began around 1860 in the Chinese province of Yunnan. It spread to the southern coast of China, reaching Hong Kong in 1894. Subsequently plague was carried by ship to India, other countries of Asia, Brazil, and California. An estimated 10 million deaths were caused by this disease in India during this century. The plague bacillus was discovered by Alexandre Yersin in 1894 in Hong Kong and was called *Pasteurella pestis* until 1970. Transmission by flea bites was suggested by Ogata in 1897.

ETIOLOGY. The causative agent, *Y. pestis*, belongs to the family of bacteria Enterobacteriaceae. It is virulent by virtue of plasmid-mediated V and W antigens, which confer calcium dependency and are believed to enable the plague bacillus to proliferate inside mammalian mononuclear phagocytic cells. In the capsular envelope there is an antiphagocytic protein called Fraction 1 antigen. In the cell walls there is a potent lipopolysaccharide endotoxin, which like endotoxins of other gram-negative bacteria produces fever, disseminated intravascular coagulation, complement activation, B lymphocyte activation, and many kinds of tissue damage. Additionally, *Y. pestis* elaborates *murine toxin*, which produces beta-adrenergic blockade, but the role of this exotoxin in human disease is unclear.

PATHOLOGY. The pathology of bubonic plague is unmistakable. The capsules of the lymph nodes are obliterated by an inflammatory process that involves the periglandular tissues as much as the lymph nodes themselves. The normal architecture that separates cortex from medulla is destroyed. The lymphoid cells of the medulla are necrotic. There are large phagocytic cells, polymorphonuclear leukocytes, hemorrhage, and a granular material that is a pure culture of plague bacilli. Blood vessels are thrombosed.

DISTRIBUTION AND EPIDEMIOLOGY. During the five years from 1980 to 1984, 3036 cases of human plague were reported to the World Health Organization. Countries reporting the most cases were Vietnam, 654 cases; Brazil, 508 cases; Peru, 468 cases; Tanzania, 441 cases; Burma, 335 cases; Madagascar, 156 cases; and United States, 121 cases. In the United States, plague is limited almost entirely to the Southwestern states of New Mexico, Arizona, Colorado, Nevada, and California.

Plague is primarily a zoonotic infection. It is transmitted among the natural animal reservoirs by flea bites or by ingestion of contaminated animal tissues. Throughout the world domestic and urban rats are the most important reservoirs of the plague bacillus. In sylvatic foci of plague, however, as occur in the United States, the important reservoirs are the ground squirrel, rock squirrel, and prairie dog. Humans are an accidental host in the natural cycle of plague, when rodent fleas bite people, and appear to play no role in the maintenance of plague in nature. Only rarely, during epidemics of pneumonic plague, is the infection passed directly from person to person. Occasionally the infection develops in humans by the direct handling of contaminated animal tissues, as when hunters skin dead rabbits.

The incidence of plague in humans for any particular locality is a function of both the frequency of infection in local rodent populations and the intimacy with which the people live with the infected rodents and their fleas. In the United States, the season for plague is April to September, when people are out of doors. Off-season cases are often hunters who handle their prey. Although humans develop acquired immunity after plague infection, the role of immunity in determining host susceptibility to infection of individuals in a population appears to be small.

PATHOGENESIS AND CLINICAL FEATURES. The most common clinical form is bubonic plague, which presents a distinctive clinical picture (Table 291–1). During an incubation period of two to eight days following a bite by an infected flea, bacteria proliferate in the regional lymph nodes. Patients are typically affected by the sudden onset of fever, chills, weakness, and headache. Usually at the same time, or after a few hours or the next day, patients notice the *bubo*, which is signaled by intense pain in one anatomic region of lymph nodes, usually the groin, axilla, or neck. A swelling evolves that is so tender that the patient typically avoids any motion that would provoke tenderness of the affected nodes.

The buboes of patients with plague are oval swellings varying from about 1 to 10 cm in length and elevating the overlying skin, which may appear stretched or erythematous. They appear either as a smooth uniform egg-shaped mass or an irregular cluster of several nodes. Palpation will typically elicit extreme tenderness. There is warmth of the overlying skin and an underlying, firm nonfluctuant mass. Usually around the lymph nodes there is considerable edema, which can be gelatinous or pitting in nature. Occasionally edema extends into the skin region drained by the affected lymph nodes. Although infections other than plague can produce acute lymphadenitis, plague is unique for the suddenness of onset of the fever and the bubo, the rapid development of intense inflammation in the bubo, and the fulminant clinical course that can produce death as quickly as two to four days after the onset of symptoms. The bubo of plague is also distinctive for the usual absence of a detectable skin lesion and likewise for the absence of an ascending lymphangitis nearby.

In uncomplicated *bubonic plague*, the patients are typically prostrate and lethargic and often exhibit restlessness or agitation. Occasionally they are delirious with high fever, and seizures are common in children. Temperature is usually in the range of 38.5 to 40.0° C, and the pulse rate is increased to 110 to 140 beats per minute. Blood pressure is characteristically low, in the range of 100/60 mm Hg, owing to extreme vasodilation. Pressure determinations may be unobtainable if shock ensues. The liver and spleen are often palpable and tender. Abdominal pain, vomiting, and diarrhea are common.

The majority of patients with bubonic plague do not have skin lesions. About a fourth of patients in Vietnam, however, did show varied skin findings. The most common were pustules, vesicles, eschars, or papules near the bubo or in the anatomic region of skin that is lymphatically drained by the affected lymph nodes. These presumably represent sites of flea bite inoculations. When these lesions are opened, they usually contain white cells and plague bacilli. These skin lesions rarely progress to extensive cellulitis or abscesses. Ulceration may lead, however, to a larger plague carbuncle. Another kind of skin lesion in plague is purpura, which may become necrotic, resulting in gangrene of distal extremities that is the probable basis of the term black death. These purpuric lesions result from vasculitis and occlusion by fibrin thrombi, resulting in hemorrhage and necrosis.

A distinctive feature of plague is the propensity for massive growth of bacteria in the blood. In the early acute stages of bubonic plague, all patients probably have intermittent bacteremia. Single blood cultures obtained at the time of hospital admission from Vietnamese patients were positive in 27 per cent of cases. A hallmark of moribund patients with plague is high-density bacteremia, so that a blood smear revealing characteristic bacilli has been used as a prognostic indicator in this disease. Occasionally in the pathogenesis of plague infection bacteria are inoculated and proliferate in the body, producing bacteremia without a bubo. This syndrome has been termed *septicemic plague.*

One of the feared complications of bubonic plague is secondary pneumonia. The infection reaches the lungs by hematogenous spread from the bubo. In addition to the high mortality, plague pneumonia is highly contagious by airborne transmission. It is characterized by fever and lymphadenopathy with cough, chest pain, and often hemoptysis. Radiographically there is patchy bronchopneumonia or confluent consolidation. The sputum is usually purulent and contains plague bacilli.

Primary inhalation pneumonia is rare now but is a potential threat to the individual exposed to a patient with plague who has a cough. Plague pneumonia is often fatal when antibiotic therapy is delayed more than a day after the onset of illness.

Plague meningitis is a rarer complication and typically occurs more than a week after inadequately treated bubonic plague. Less commonly, plague meningitis appears as a primary infection without antecedent lymphadenitis. Bacteria are frequently demonstrable with a Gram's stain of spinal fluid sediment, and endotoxin has been demonstrated in spinal fluid by the limulus gelation assay.

LABORATORY FEATURES. The white blood cell count is typically elevated in the range of 10,000 to 20,000 cells per cubic millimeter, with a predominance of immature and mature neutrophils. Patients who are most severely ill tend to have higher counts. Occasionally some patients, especially children, may develop myelocytic leukemoid reactions with white cell counts as high as 100,000 per cubic millimeter. The white blood cells in the peripheral blood typically show cytoplasmic vacuolations, toxic granulations, and Döhle bodies that are characteristic of acute bacterial infections. Blood platelet counts may be normal or low in the early stages of bubonic plague. Although a generalized bleeding tendency from profound thrombocytopenia is rare, disseminated intravascular coagulation (DIC) is common. Fibrinogen-fibrin degradation products in the serum that are indicative of DIC were detected in elevated titers in most patients tested in Vietnam.

DIAGNOSIS. Plague should be suspected in febrile patients who have been in known endemic areas. A bacteriologic diagnosis is readily made in most patients by smear and culture of a bubo aspirate. The aspirate is obtained by inserting a 20-gauge needle on a 10-ml syringe containing 1 ml of sterile saline solution into the bubo and aspirating several times until the saline solution has become blood-tinged. Because the bubo does not contain liquid pus, it may be necessary to inject some of the saline solution and to immediately reaspirate it. Drops of the aspirate should be placed on microscope slides. The Gram's stain will reveal polymorphonuclear leukocytes and gram-negative coccobacilli and bacilli ranging from 1 to 2 μm in length. Smears of blood, sputum, or spinal fluid can be handled similarly.

The aspirate, blood, and other appropriate fluids should be inoculated onto blood and MacConkey's agar plates and into infusion broth. For definitive identification, cultures can be mailed in double containers to the Centers for Disease Control, Plague Branch, P.O. Box 2087, Fort Collins, Colorado 80422 (telephone no.: 303–482–0213). At this same laboratory, a serologic test, the passive hemagglutination test utilizing Fraction 1 of *Y. pestis*, can be performed on acute- and convalescent-phase serum. For patients with negative cultures, a four-fold or greater increase in titer or a single titer of greater than or equal to 1:16 is presumptive evidence for plague infection.

TABLE 291–1. PLAGUE SYNDROMES

Syndrome	Features
Bubonic	Fever, painful lymphadenopathy (bubo)
Septicemic	Fever, hypotension without bubo
Pneumonic	Cough, hemoptysis with or without bubo
Cutaneous	Pustule, eschar, carbuncle, or ecthyma gangrenosum usually with bubo
Meningitis	Fever, nuchal rigidity usually with bubo

The differential diagnosis of bubonic plague includes tularemia, streptococcal and staphylococcal lymphadenitis, secondary syphilis, and lymphogranuloma venereum. For pneumonia, the physician also should consider common forms of bacterial and viral pneumonia. For meningitis and septicemia, the common bacterial causes need to be assessed by age groups.

TREATMENT AND PROGNOSIS. Untreated plague has an estimated mortality rate of greater than 50 per cent and can evolve into a fulminant illness complicated by septic shock. Therefore the early institution of effective antibiotic therapy is mandatory. In 1948, streptomycin was identified as the drug of choice for the treatment of plague by reducing mortality to less than 5 per cent. No other drug has been demonstrated to be more efficacious or less toxic. Streptomycin should be administered intramuscularly in two divided doses daily, totaling 30 mg per kilogram of body weight per day for ten days. Most patients improve rapidly and become afebrile in about three days. The ten-day course is recommended to prevent relapses because viable bacteria have been isolated from buboes of patients with plague during convalescence. The risk of vestibular damage and hearing loss caused by streptomycin is minimal during a ten-day course. This antibiotic should be used cautiously, however, during pregnancy, in older patients who would have trouble adapting to vestibular damage, and in patients with previous hearing difficulty. In such patients, the course of streptomycin can be shortened to three days after the patient becomes afebrile. Renal injury as a result of streptomycin therapy is rare with this regimen; however, renal function should be monitored. If the serum creatinine concentration rises significantly, the dose of streptomycin should be reduced. In mild renal failure the recommended dose is about 20 mg per kilogram per day and in advanced renal failure 8 mg per kilogram every three days.

For patients allergic to streptomycin or for whom an oral drug is strongly preferred, tetracycline is a satisfactory alternative. It is administered orally in a dose of 2 to 4 grams per day in four divided doses for ten days. Tetracycline is contraindicated in children under seven years of age and in pregnant women in order to avoid staining of developing teeth. It is also contraindicated in patients with renal failure.

For patients with meningitis who will require a drug that penetrates well into the cerebrospinal fluid and for patients with profound hypotension in whom an intramuscular injection may not be well absorbed, chloramphenicol should be administered intravenously with a loading dose of 25 mg per kilogram of body weight followed by 60 mg per kilogram per day in four divided doses. After clinical improvement oral chloramphenicol administration should be continued to complete a total course of 10 days; the dosage may be reduced to 30 mg per kilogram per day to reduce the magnitude of bone marrow suppression, which is reversible after completion of therapy.

Antibiotic resistance in human isolates of *Y. pestis* has never been reported, nor has resistance emerged during antibiotic therapy. The three antibiotics streptomycin, tetracycline, and chloramphenicol given alone are clinically very effective and relapses are exceedingly rare. Therefore, there is no rationale for using multiple antibiotics to treat plague.

Because patients are febrile and often have nausea or vomiting, hypotension, and dehydration, intravenous 0.9 per cent saline solution should be given to most patients for the first few days of the illness or until improvement occurs. Patients in shock will require additional quantities of fluid with hemodynamic monitoring and the judicious use of epinephrine or dopamine. There is no evidence that corticosteroids are beneficial in plague. Although disseminated intravascular coagulation is commonly present and purpura occasionally develops in severely ill patients, therapy with heparin has no proven benefit in plague infections.

The buboes usually recede without need of local therapy. Occasionally, however, they may enlarge or become fluctuant during the first week of treatment and require incision and drainage. The aspirated fluid should be cultured for evidence of superinfection, but this material is usually sterile.

PREVENTION. All patients with suspected plague should be reported to the local health department. Patients with uncomplicated infections who are promptly treated present no health hazards to other persons. Those with cough or other signs of pneumonia must be placed in strict respiratory isolation for at least 48 hours after the start of antibiotic therapy or until the sputum culture is negative. The bubo aspirate and blood must be handled with gloves. Standard bacteriologic techniques that safeguard against skin contact with and aerosolization of infected fluids and cultures should be adequate to protect laboratory personnel.

A formalin-killed vaccine, plague vaccine U.S.P. (Cutter Laboratories, Berkeley, California 94710) is available for travelers to epidemic areas, for individuals who must live and work in close contact with wild rodents, and for laboratory workers who must handle live *Y. pestis* cultures. A primary series of two injections is recommended with a one- to three-month interval between them. Booster injections are given every six months for as long as exposure continues. In addition, persons living in endemic areas should protect themselves against rodents and fleas. Measures include living in ratproof houses, reducing opportunities for rodent harborage near homes, wearing shoes and garments to cover the legs, and application of insecticide dusts to houses and household pets.

Butler T: A clinical study of bubonic plague. Observations of the 1970 Vietnam epidemic with emphasis on coagulation studies, skin histology, and electrocardiograms. Am J Med 53:268, 1972. *This paper describes clinical features of serious cases in Vietnam.*

Butler T: Plague and other *Yersinia* infections. New York, Plenum Publishing Corp., 1983. *This monograph gives full clinical description and contemporary literature citations.*

Hull HF, Montes JM, Mann JM: Septicemic plague in New Mexico. J Infect Dis 155:113, 1987. *One fourth of 71 recent cases of plague in New Mexico were septicemic without a bubo. To prevent the observed 33 per cent mortality rate, earlier empiric antibiotic treatment is advised.*

Welty TK, Grabman J, Kompare E, et al.: Nineteen cases of plague in Arizona. West J Med 142:641, 1985. *This paper describes clinical features of recent cases in Arizona.*

OTHER YERSINIA INFECTIONS

DEFINITION. The non-plague yersinioses are caused by *Yersinia enterocolitica* and *Y. pseudotuberculosis*. These gram-negative rod bacteria produce fever, diarrhea, and abdominal pain that can mimic acute appendicitis. The common pathologic lesions in yersiniosis are acute enteritis and mesenteric lymphadenitis. Extraintestinal disease may result from septicemia or appear as arthritis and erythema nodosum.

ETIOLOGY. Of the 34 different O serotypes of *Y. enterocolitica* that have been identified, the ones most commonly associated with human disease are types 3, 8, and 9. All virulent strains possess a plasmid that encodes the V and W antigens, which confer calcium dependency on the bacteria. Like other gram-negative bacteria, the yersiniae contain a lipopolysaccharide endotoxin in the cell wall that may be responsible, in part, for the fever and inflammation.

EPIDEMIOLOGY. The yersinioses are distributed worldwide. Large numbers of confirmed cases have been reported in Europe, Canada, the United States, and Japan. This infection has also been reported from Africa and Asia. In the United States, infection with *Y. enterocolitica* appears to be rare when compared with infection with *Salmonella* and *Shigella* species, but in other countries such as Finland and Sweden the incidence of infection is higher. Both adults and children are susceptible to infection. Males acquire the infection more commonly than females. The natural reservoirs of *Y. enterocolitica* are farm animals, especially pigs and goats, and other domestic animals, including dogs and cats. The natural reservoirs of *Y. pseudotuberculosis* include birds and other diverse domestic and farm animals. These animals harbor the bacteria in their intestines and excrete them in feces. Humans become infected by ingesting food or water contaminated by animal feces or directly by the ingestion of certain fomites. Person-to-person transmission seems to be rare. Well-defined outbreaks of *Y. enterocolitica* infection have occurred in a North Carolina family with a sick dog, in a New York school at which chocolate milk was the source of infection, in members of a Brownie scout troop in Pennsylvania who ate infected bean sprouts, and in persons who drank milk from a dairy in Tennessee. There are no clear seasonal patterns of infection.

PATHOGENESIS OF CLINICAL SYNDROMES. An inoculum with as many as 10^9 organisms may be required to produce infection. During the incubation period, estimated at 4 to 10 days, bacteria proliferate in the small bowel; invade the mucosa, especially that of the ileum; and elicit an acute inflammatory response. Ulcerations may occur and polymorphonuclear leukocytes appear in the stool. Some bacteria migrate via the lymphatics to the mesenteric lymph nodes, where inflammation occurs. The initial symptoms include fever and either diarrhea or abdominal pain. In these instances, the corresponding pathologic finding is terminal ileitis or mesenteric lymphadenitis or both. The colon is less frequently affected, but aphthoid ulcers and hemorrhagic colitis have been described in yersiniosis. The tissues are affected by acute inflammation, thrombosis of blood vessels, hemorrhage, and necrosis. The diarrhea results from the mucosal invasion by bacteria or the action of an enterotoxin. Diarrhea varies from semisolid or watery to grossly bloody. In some patients the abdominal pain is severe and located in the right lower quadrant and may be mistaken for appendicitis; the appendix is usually normal. A few days later, some patients may develop extraintestinal complications of arthralgias, arthritis, and erythema nodosum. Since the synovial and cutaneous tissues in these syndromes are sterile, an immunologic reaction has been postulated to explain their pathogenesis. Arthritis, including sacroiliitis, is more likely to occur in individuals of haplotype HLA-B27, and erythema nodosum occurs more commonly in women. Septicemia is a rare complication that occurs in the setting of prior liver disease, malignancies, or immunosuppressive therapy. Rarer clinical forms of yersiniosis include pneumonia, pharyngitis, and meningitis. Antibodies appear in the blood against the O and other antigens of *Y. enterocolitica*, and nearly all infections are self-limited. However, fatalities have occurred from extensive ulceration and necrosis of the intestine and from septicemia.

DIAGNOSIS. The diagnosis requires the isolation of yersiniae from stool, blood, or surgical specimens. The number of bacteria in stool may be small, and a cold-enrichment technique may be required. A rectal swab or piece of stool is placed into 0.067 M phosphate-buffered saline solution at a pH of 7.6 and incubated at 4° C for four weeks. Most other stool bacteria die, whereas *Y. enterocolitica* will grow. At weekly intervals, subcultures should be made on MacConkey agar. A presumptive diagnosis can be made from serologic test results by showing a rise in agglutinin titer in paired serum specimens. The existence of cross-reacting antigens in the genera *Brucella*, *Vibrio*, and *Salmonella* indicates that false-positive serologic results sometimes occur.

TREATMENT AND PROGNOSIS. Yersiniosis is usually self-limited and so rarely diagnosed that it is impossible to assess the possible benefits of antibiotic treatment. Most isolates of *Y. enterocolitica* are susceptible to streptomycin, gentamicin, tetracycline, chloramphenicol, and sulfamethoxazole-trimethoprim and resistant to the penicillins and cephalosporin antibiotics. *Y. pseudotuberculosis* isolates usually have been susceptible to penicillin. It is important to suspect the diagnosis in patients with severe abdominal pain to avoid unnecessary surgery for appendicitis. The recognition that

early fever accompanies yersiniosis may be helpful, as is epidemiologic information pertaining to outbreaks in the community.

PREVENTION AND CONTROL. The presumed origin of *Y. enterocolitica* infection in farm and domestic animals suggests that transmission may be similar to that of *Salmonella*. Meat and dairy products and other farm produce should periodically be examined for *Y. enterocolitica* content. During outbreaks, public health authorities should identify sources of infection in food (especially milk), water, or persons.

Bottone EJ: *Yersinia enterocolitica*: A panoramic view of a charismatic organism. CRC Crit Rev Microbiol 5:211, 1977. *A useful review of microbiologic aspects of these infections.*

Hoogkamp-Korstanje JAA, de Koning J, Samsom JP: Incidence of human infection with *Yersinia enterocolitica* serotypes 03, 08, and 09 and the use of indirect immunofluorescence in diagnosis. J Infect Dis 153:138, 1986. *This report from Holland showed that awareness of this disease by physicians and laboratories will increase its diagnosis and that serotype 08 was associated with extraintestinal features.*

Kohl S: *Yersinia enterocolitica* infections. Pediatr Clin North Am 26:433, 1979. *This clinical discussion emphasizes disease syndromes in children.*

Vantrappen G, Agg HO, Geboes K, et al.: *Yersinia* enteritis. Med Clin North Am 66:639, 1982. *This article contains a good clinical description of gastroenterologic features of the disease.*

292   TULAREMIA

Richard B. Hornick

DEFINITION. Tularemia is a rare infectious disease caused by a small gram-negative pleomorphic rod, *Francisella tularensis*. This organism is acquired from an animal reservoir, frequently cottontail rabbits, by direct contact with diseased animal tissues, the bite of an infected tick or deer fly, ingestion of contaminated food or water, and inhalation of aerosolized bacteria. Clinical manifestations usually include a cutaneous ulcer with enlargement of regional lymph nodes. Rarely, a pneumonitis will result from inhalation of *F. tularensis* or secondary spread from the skin ulcer and lymph nodes. Confirmation of the diagnosis by cultural technique is not advocated because of the high contagion risk to personnel handling this organism. The therapeutic response to effective antibiotic therapy is rapid.

The typhoidal form of tularemia was first described in Japan in 1818. A clear description of the organism occurred in 1906 when McCoy uncovered a "plague-like" disease among ground squirrels in Tulare County, California. In Japan, tularemia may be referred to as Ohara's disease, or Yato-byo (wild hare disease).

ETIOLOGY, SPECIFIC LABORATORY DIAGNOSIS, AND EPIDEMIOLOGY. *F. tularensis* is a small gram-negative pleomorphic rod-shaped bacterium. Organisms are not seen in smears of infected tissue unless special staining techniques are used. Fluorescent antibody conjugate staining and modified Dieterle staining are the best methods for demonstrating them. All tularemia strains are serologically identical, but there are biochemical and virulence differences for mammals that have allowed differentiation of two strains. These are called Jellison A and B; the former, found only in North America, is lethal for domestic rabbits (*Oryctolagus*) and causes severe disease in man. The unique biochemical capabilities of this strain—e.g., it ferments glycerol and contains citrulline ureidase—do not explain its increased virulence. Strain B lacks these biochemical features, is not lethal for cottontails, causes milder disease in man, usually is isolated from rodents or from water, and is distributed over Europe, Asia, and North America. Reasons for the differences in virulence are unknown.

Culture Methods. The direct isolation of *F. tularensis* from blood (rarely), pus from ulcers or buboes, sputum, or pharyngeal or gastric aspirations in a patient with pneumonitis can be achieved by two methods. This is a class 4 organism requiring an effective hood or an adequate isolation laboratory to prevent human disease or epizootics. The two methods for isolation are intraperitoneal inoculation of guinea pigs and direct plating of a specimen onto glucose cysteine blood agar, cystine heart agar, or eugon agar. As few as one to five viable organisms will cause death of guinea pigs in five to ten days. Appropriate facilities are needed to prevent spread of the disease to other animals. The media employed to isolate the organism usually contain drugs to suppress other flora and allow the tularemia colonies to be visible. Useful additions are 0.1 mg of cycloheximide and 20 units of penicillin per milliliter of media. The colonies are small on these media; they appear in 48 to 72 hours of incubation at 37° C.

Serologic Diagnosis. The measurement of serum agglutinating antibodies is a useful and safer method of diagnosing tularemia. Titers begin to rise in about seven to ten days and peak in three to four weeks. Paired serum specimens obtained two weeks apart and demonstrating a four-fold or greater rise are diagnostic of tularemia. However, a single specimen with a titer of 1:160 or greater in a patient thought to have tularemia on clinical grounds is diagnostic. Antibiotic therapy does not appear to dampen the antibody response. Titers remain elevated for six to eight months and then decline in the subsequent one to one and a half years to low or undetectable levels. There is a cross-reaction with brucella antigen during the early phase of the antibody response. The brucella titer falls off faster than and is never so high as the tularemia titer.

Skin Testing. A skin test antigen has proved to be reliable for diagnostic and epidemiologic purposes. A positive test result, similar in appearance to a tuberculin test response, is present during the first week of illness, frequently before the agglutinins are detectable, and remains positive for years. There is no known cross-reacting skin test antigen. The antigen is derived from *F. tularensis* by ether extraction; however, it is not commonly available. It can be obtained from the Centers for Disease Control, Atlanta. In 10 per cent of patients, the skin test antigen may boost pre-existing agglutinating antibody titers. Skin test reactivity can be shown to be associated with sensitized lymphocytes.

Epidemiology. Tularemia is a sporadic disease; humans acquire it when bitten by an infected tick or deer fly or when handling an infected animal. In the process of dressing a rabbit or skinning a muskrat, the hands may become contaminated with infected blood, subcutaneous abscesses, or liver and spleen that contain millions of organisms. The act of eviscerating the animal can create an aerosol that can be inhaled. The ingestion of contaminated water or food is the least likely method of acquiring tularemia. Many carnivores such as dogs, cats, bull snakes, and others may feed on diseased rabbits. This results in contamination of the teeth and saliva. These animals are relatively resistant to tularemia. Contact with the teeth of a pet dog or cat has resulted in ulceroglandular tularemia. Studies in volunteers have quantified the susceptibility of humans to infection and disease and the virulence of *F. tularensis* for humans. As few as 50 type A organisms injected subcutaneously will cause ulceroglandular disease. Pneumonic tularemia can be induced by a similar inoculum size if the aerosolized and inhaled particles are small (less than 5 microns). Type B organisms require an inoculum about 1000 times larger to induce ulceroglandular or respiratory disease in humans.

The incidence of tularemia is low, 200 to 300 cases a year having been reported in each of the past 10 years. The peak incidence was in 1939, when almost 2300 cases were reported. Laws passed at that time prohibited the sale of wild rabbits, especially cottontails, and this legislation plus increased public awareness of the danger of handling sick or dying wild animals has contributed to the decline. Most cases occur in the Midwest, but the disease is not restricted to any one geographic location in the United States. Cottontail rabbits in urban and suburban areas throughout the country provide the reservoir from which tularemia can occur. Epizootics among these or other animals can cause epidemics in man. Tularemia has been reported only north of the thirtieth parallel. The cottontail rabbit is not found in Europe; various rodents such as voles, muskrats, and hares carry *F. tularensis* (Jellison B type) in that part of the world. Diseased jack rabbits, found west of the Mississippi River, may be an important source of contamination of ticks and deer flies.

In the summer months, most cases of tularemia are caused by tick or deer fly bites. Ulceroglandular disease begins with an ulcer at the site of the bite, e.g., groin, axilla, or scalp. In the fall, during hunting season, sporadic cases, usually ulceroglandular, occur among hunters and trappers. In the Scandinavian countries, epidemics have occurred in the winter months when farmers handling stored hay contaminated by diseased voles inhaled *F. tularensis* and developed pneumonic tularemia.

MECHANISMS OF INFECTION AND PATHOLOGY. The most common form of tularemia results from the penetration of *F. tularensis* into the skin. This penetration may be through hair follicles or minute areas of trauma. The development of the subsequent disease takes two to six days, depending upon the number of bacteria and their virulence. The organisms multiply in the dermis and induce a marked inflammatory process consisting primarily of mononuclear cells with a perivascular distribution. This process produces an erythematous tender papule. The inflamed area continues to swell until the induced ischemia causes the skin to ulcerate. The base of the ulcer becomes black and depressed. The edges are sharply demarcated. At the time of penetration some organisms may be phagocytized and transported in the lymph to regional nodes. There is no clinically apparent lymphangitis. The nodes enlarge and become painful when caseation occurs. Histologic sections reveal geographic necrosis and disruption of the capsule. Fluctuation of the node is a late and rare event. It may then rupture. The necrotic, purulent, painful lymph node is termed a bubo. Healing of a bubo takes months even with appropriate antibiotic treatment. Aspiration of an unruptured node may lead to an indolent draining sinus tract. *F. tularensis* may remain in the necrotic tissue and purulent drainage for many weeks. The ulcer heals slowly and usually leaves a depigmented, rounded area in the skin.

Oculoglandular tularemia may occur when the conjunctival sac is infected from an ulcer or contaminated finger. Small yellowish granulomatous lesions develop on the palpebral conjunctivae, accompanied by enlargement of the preauricular lymph nodes. In untreated patients the cornea may perforate.

Inhaled small particle aerosols (<5 microns in diameter) containing *F. tularensis* (usually type A) are ultimately deposited in the terminal bronchioles and alveoli, although infection of the trachea and large bronchi also occurs. A peribronchial inflammation develops with infiltration by neutrophils and mononuclear cells. This produces necrosis of alveolar walls and results in localized pneumonitis. In man, small areas of pneumonitis represent the most common findings on chest roentgenograms. Often these are ill defined and difficult to interpret. Lobar consolidation or lung abscesses represent extensive spread and necrosis. These are infrequent in man. Mediastinal and peritracheal lymph nodes enlarge and may be apparent on chest x-ray films. They may be partially responsible, along with the bronchitis, for the substernal burning that is common in patients with tularemic pneumonia. The incubation period for this form of tularemia varies inversely with the size and virulence of the inhaled inoculum. Following an inoculum of 10 to 50 organisms, disease appears in about four to seven days in volunteers.

Typhoidal tularemia follows systemic spread of *F. tularensis* from the oropharynx and probably the gastrointestinal tract when a huge inoculum is swallowed. Enlargement of cervical lymph nodes, and presumably nodes in the mesentery, occurs. This latter process causes abdominal pain and is associated with an ileus. This is the most unusual form of tularemia in this country.

CLINICAL MANIFESTATIONS. Disease initiated by a tick bite is manifested by an ulcer at the site or adjacent to it. The tick defecates after feeding, and the infected feces may be scratched into the epidermis. Usually the lesion will be in the inguinal, axillary, or scalp skin. If contact with tularemia organisms results from the handling of an infected animal, an ulcerative lesion evolves in the skin of the hands, frequently around a fingernail. This lesion may be so trivial that it is ignored by the patient. The ulcer is depressed into the dermis, has sharply demarcated edges, and gradually develops a black base. In the initial stage of development the lesion produces a thick, yellowish exudate. Regional lymph nodes enlarge and are tender to palpation. Fever and chills are common. The temperature curve is usually remittent or continuous in character. Without antibiotic therapy, most patients remain febrile for several weeks, the ulcer heals slowly over weeks to months, and the enlarged lymph nodes persist for months. Untreated patients may occasionally develop a secondary necrotizing pneumonia as a consequence of bacteremia. These patients may be acutely ill.

Primary tularemia pneumonia presents with the sudden development of substernal burning and a nonproductive paroxysmal cough associated with fever and chills. Headache, myalgia, photophobia, malaise, and prostration are common findings. The temperature elevates quickly to 39.4 to 40° C and remains at that level (continuous fever curve) until antibiotic treatment is given. Sixty to 70 per cent of patients will survive without specific therapy, and in these a slow defervescence occurs over several months. X-ray of the lungs may reveal ill-defined, scattered oval areas of infiltration, with enlarged peritracheal lymph nodes. Pleural effusions, lobar consolidation, and lung abscess are other manifestations of this form of tularemia. Cervical lymph nodes are palpable and tender.

DIAGNOSIS AND DIFFERENTIAL DIAGNOSIS. The diagnosis of ulceroglandular tularemia is made by the clinical manifestations and serologic studies. Paired serum specimens collected over a two- to three-week period are required to demonstrate a fourfold rise in titer. A baseline agglutinin titer of 1:160 in a patient with a history of an indolent ulcer for two or more weeks is diagnostic of tularemia. Culture of an ulcer and blood should be performed only if the hospital laboratory has appropriate protective isolation hoods. Patients with sporotrichosis or *Mycobacterium marinum* infections may have ulcers suggestive of tularemia but are usually afebrile. Enlarged lymph nodes extending centripetally as a beaded chain are a characteristic finding in sporotrichosis. Lesions of the fingers infected with staphylococci or beta streptococci usually produce more pus and may be associated with lymphangitis. *B. anthracis* can produce an ulcer (anthrax) with black-based, sharply demarcated edges similar to that initiated by *F. tularensis*. A careful history and serologic data will help in the differential diagnosis. In patients in whom any form of tularemia is suspected, the use of the skin test antigen will be helpful. The test result is usually positive prior to the development of agglutinating antibodies.

Tularemia pneumonia must be differentiated from the more common bacterial, viral, and mycoplasmal pneumonias. The history and the presence of ulceroglandular disease are helpful. Skin testing and serologic studies are diagnostic. The chest x-ray may yield suggestive findings consisting of ill-defined, small, oval, multiple infiltrates but is not diagnostic.

Patients infected with *F. tularensis* usually have a normal leukocyte count with an elevation of the sedimentation rate and a positive C-reactive protein (CRP) determination. The white count is elevated when a bubo or a lung abscess is present.

COMPLICATIONS. Pericarditis and meningitis are rare events that usually occur in patients who have been misdiagnosed and have received inappropriate treatment. Pericarditis results from direct extension of the infection from the purulent, necrotic mediastinal lymph nodes or the involved lung. Constrictive pericarditis has been reported. Meningitis develops rarely, represents a seeding of the meninges during bacteremia, and is characterized by a lymphocytic pleocytosis in the cerebrospinal fluid.

TREATMENT. Patients with all forms of tularemia respond to the following antibiotics: streptomycin, gentamicin, tetracycline, and chloramphenicol. The aminoglycoside antibiotics are recommended, since they produce a prompt cure of patients with the most severe form of tularemia. Patients with pneumonitis are afebrile within 24 to 48 hours and do not relapse. Ulcers and tender lymph nodes heal in seven to ten days. Gentamicin, 5 mg per kilogram per day in divided doses, is given for ten days. Streptomycin was the principal drug for treating tularemia before gentamicin; 1 gram is given every 12 hours for ten days. Treatment with tetracycline or chloramphenicol may produce an equally rapid response, but relapses occur in 15 to 20 per cent of the patients. These drugs are not recommended unless gentamicin and streptomycin are contraindicated. Doses of 3 to 4 grams of tetracycline or 3 grams of chloramphenicol daily for ten days can be employed. Naturally acquired resistance to any of these antibiotics has not been found.

Patients with ulceroglandular tularemia respond well to these antibiotics. Fluctuant lymph nodes should not be aspirated until the patient has finished the course of the antibiotic treatment. Isolation of patients with any form of tularemia is not required; there is no evidence of person-to-person spread.

PROGNOSIS. The mortality rate for untreated ulceroglandular disease is about 5 per cent. Patients infected with type B strains and untreated probably have a mortality rate less than 1 per cent. Many of these patients probably go undiagnosed, as the disease is mild and self-limiting. Treatment with antibiotics prevents death and promotes healing in a week to ten days.

The mortality rate for pneumonic tularemia in the preantibiotic period was 30 to 60 per cent. Treatment with streptomycin or tetracycline has lowered this figure to less than 1 per cent. Healing occurs without residual lung damage or deficits in pulmonary function.

PREVENTION. Patients who recover from tularemia have a high degree of resistance to reinfection. If *F. tularensis* is reintroduced into the skin, a positive skin test reaction ensues without ulceration. Resistance to pulmonary disease may be associated with sensitized lymphocytes and alveolar macrophages.

A live attenuated strain of *F. tularensis* has been prepared as a vaccine. This can be administered by the acupuncture route, and it produces excellent immunity. The vaccine can be obtained from the Commander, U.S. Army Medical Research Institute of Infectious Diseases, Frederick, Maryland 21701. Its use is limited to persons considered at high risk such as selected laboratory workers, forest rangers, game wardens, and perhaps others known to be exposed during an outbreak. The vaccine exerts its effect through the stimulation of cellular immune mechanisms. Circulating agglutinins are not associated with resistance to disease.

Buchanan TM, Brooks GF, Brachman PS: The tularemia skin test; 325 skin tests in 210 persons: Serologic correlation and review of the literature. Ann Intern Med 74:336, 1971. *This study is an extension of the study reported by Young et al. (see below). It clearly presents proof of the efficacy of the skin test as a diagnostic test for tularemia. In addition it shows the amount of antigen stimulation needed to cause a conversion to a positive reactor.*

Tärnvik A, Sandström G, Löfgren S: Time of lymphocyte response after onset of tularemia and after tularemia vaccination. J Clin Microbiol 10:854, 1979. *Presents evidence on the development of cellular immunity in patients with tularemia or who have received the attenuated vaccine.*

Teutsch SM, Marone WJ, Brink EW, et al.: Pneumonic tularemia on Martha's Vineyard. N Engl J Med 301:826, 1979. *This study illustrates the suddenness with which tularemia may appear in a geographic area. Furthermore it indicates a unique mechanism by which man can acquire pneumonic tularemia.*

Young LS, Bicknell DS, Archer BG, et al.: Tularemia epidemic: Vermont, 1968. Forty-seven cases linked to contact with muskrats. N Engl J Med 280:1253, 1969. *This represents one of the largest outbreaks occurring in the United States in the past 20 years. It is one of the best described epidemiologic studies of infection caused by the Jellison type B organism.*

293 ANTHRAX

Philip S. Brachman

DEFINITION. Anthrax is a zoonotic disease transmitted to humans through contact with animals or animal products. Its primary forms are cutaneous, inhalational, and gastrointestinal. Occasionally, meningitis and septicemia occur, almost always secondary to one of the primary forms. In the United States, the most common form of the disease is the cutaneous lesion; inhalation anthrax occurs rarely; gastrointestinal anthrax has never been reported in the United States. Synonyms for anthrax include charbon, malignant pustule, Siberian ulcer, malignant edema, splenic fever, milzbrand, woolsorter's disease, and ragpicker's disease.

ETIOLOGY. *Bacillus anthracis* is a gram-positive, nonmotile, spore-forming bacillus (1 to 1.3 mμ × 3 to 10 mμ) that on ordinary laboratory media at 35 to 37°C produces round, grayish white, ground-glass-appearing, convex, tenacious colonies 2 to 5 mm in diameter with comma-shaped projections. Microscopic examination of artificial media growth shows long parallel chains of organisms, referred to as "boxcars." Material from a fresh lesion reveals shorter chains with individual organisms having slightly rounded ends. Fluorescent antibody staining and a specific gamma bacteriophage can be used to identify *B. anthracis*. Parenteral inoculation of mice, guinea pigs, or rabbits with agar-grown cells or washed liquid growth will result in death in 24 to 72 hours. Growth on bicarbonate agar under CO_2 produces capsular material.

B. anthracis spores may persist for years in the industrial or agricultural environment.

INCIDENCE AND PREVALENCE. The true worldwide incidence of anthrax is unknown owing to the lack of diagnosis and poor reporting of cases to health authorities. Estimates have been made that range from 2,000 to 100,000 cases annually. Cutaneous anthrax is reported to be endemic in Haiti, South Africa, and several Asiatic countries. There are undoubtedly other countries that have similar endemic disease but do not report their data. Occasionally, epidemics occur; one of the largest was reported in Zimbabwe from 1978 to 1980, when almost 10,000 cases of cutaneous and a few cases of gastrointestinal anthrax occurred related to an extensive epizootic infection among cattle.

In the United States, the average annual occurrence from 1916 to 1925 was 127 cases, and from 1977 to 1986, 0.8 case. Ninety-five per cent of the cases in the United States are cutaneous; the other 5 per cent are inhalational. Twenty of the 232 cases reported from 1955 through 1986 were fatal, for a case-fatality rate (CFR) of 8.6 per cent. Two hundred and twenty-one cases with 11 deaths were cutaneous (CFR, 5 per cent); 11 cases with 9 deaths were inhalational (CFR, 82 per cent). Anthrax meningitis occurred in less than 5 per cent of the cases.

EPIDEMIOLOGY. Cases are classified as either industrial (80 per cent) or agricultural (20 per cent). Industrial anthrax results from contact with animal products, usually from Asia or Africa, including goat hair, wool, hides and skin, and animal bones. Transmission is by direct contact with contaminated animal products, or by indirect contact with a contaminated environment, or with airborne particles created during the processing of animal products. Occasional laboratory-acquired infections are reported.

Agricultural anthrax results from contact with infected animals (cattle, horses, sheep, goats, or swine) or their discharges. Animal vaccine inadvertently injected into the injector's hand has also caused disease.

In the United States, the majority of cases are sporadic, although there are occasional epidemics. The largest epidemic occurred during 10 weeks in 1957, when nine of 600 employees in a processing plant acquired anthrax; four cutaneous and five inhalation (four fatalities) cases were associated with one batch of contaminated goat hair imported from Asia.

Human-to-human transmission has not been reported.

PATHOGENESIS. Cutaneous anthrax results from the introduction of *B. anthracis* through a wound or by means of an infected animal fiber penetrating the skin. Organisms in the subcutaneous tissue germinate, multiply, and produce toxin with tissue necrosis. Organisms and toxin may be distributed by the vascular or lymphatic system, resulting in involvement of regional lymph nodes, septicemia, and toxemia.

Inhalation anthrax results from the inhalation of airborne droplet nuclei less than 5 μ in size, with subsequent deposition in the terminal alveoli, where they are phagocytized by macrophages, carried through the alveolar membranes, and deposited in the regional lymph nodes; there they germinate, multiply, and produce toxin. The resulting reaction causes necrosis of the mediastinal tissue, leading to hemorrhagic, edematous mediastinitis, a unique pathologic finding. There may be a direct toxic effect on the pulmonary capillary endothelium, causing pulmonary capillary thrombosis and respiratory failure. Primary anthrax pneumonia is not seen, although there may be secondary pneumonic involvement.

Gastrointestinal anthrax results from ingestion of contaminated meat and deposition of spores in the submucosa of the intestinal tract (commonly ileum or cecum), where they germinate, multiply, and produce toxin, with resultant edema, hemorrhage, and necrosis. A mucosal lesion may develop with hemorrhage; there may be regional lymph node involvement. Occasionally organisms are introduced through the oral mucosa (oropharyngeal anthrax) and deposited in the regional lymph nodes, where they germinate, multiply, and produce toxin.

Anthrax meningitis results from hematogenous spread of bacteria from a primary focus.

B. anthracis produces a toxin consisting of three components: edema factor, lethal factor, and protective antigen. The virulence of *B. anthracis* is characterized by the presence of two factors, capsular material and toxin, which are mediated by different plasmids. In human disease antibiotic therapy may sterilize the tissue (usually within 24 hours of initiation), but the persistence of the toxin results in continued development of clinical disease until it is metabolized.

Clinical disease probably imparts permanent immunity; purported second cases have not been confirmed.

CLINICAL MANIFESTATIONS. Cutaneous anthrax usually occurs on the upper extremities or face. There may be mild fever, malaise, and headache. After an incubation period of three to ten days (usually five to seven days), a small pruritic, painless papule (approximately 1.0 cm) develops at the site of inoculation. Several days later a small vesicle or ring of vesicles is noted; this may be surrounded by erythema and slight nonpitting edema. The lesion may enlarge to approximately 4 cm. Within several days a dark hemorrhagic area develops beneath the center of the vesicular tissue. Disruption of the tissue releases a clear or slightly serous liquid teeming with organisms. Beneath this tissue will be a well-demarcated depressed ulcer crater in the center of which a black eschar is developing. The eschar dries and separates from the tissue within one to three weeks, leaving a scar. There may be lymphangitis and regional lymphadenopathy.

The lesion is not painful except when secondarily infected. Rarely the lesion is large and irregularly shaped. Significant edema may develop, particularly with lesions near the eye. Malignant edema refers to an especially serious form with spreading edema, induration, formation of bullae, high fever, and severe toxemia. Rarely, multiple simultaneous lesions have been reported, probably resulting from simultaneous coprimary infections.

Antibiotic therapy will not alter the progression of the lesion, although it may influence the development of secondary infection and of septicemia.

Inhalation anthrax has an incubation period of one to five days (commonly three to four days). This form of the disease is biphasic, with an initial phase similar to a mild upper respiratory tract infection, with mild fever, malaise, fatigue, myalgia, nonproductive cough, and occasionally a sensation of precordial oppression. The only physical finding may be rhonchi on auscultation of the chest. Within several days there may be clinical improvement, but then the second or acute phase develops with severe respiratory distress as manifested by dyspnea, cyanosis, respiratory stridor, and profuse diaphoresis. Subcutaneous edema of the chest and neck may develop. The vital signs are elevated; moist, crepitant rales may be heard; minimal pleural effusion may be evident; shock may develop. On chest x-ray, the typical finding is that of an enlarged mediastinum and possible pleural effusion. The patient usually dies within 24 hours.

Gastrointestinal anthrax has an incubation period of two to five days. In the abdominal form of the disease, the initial symptoms are nausea, vomiting, anorexia, and fever. With progression of the disease, significant abdominal pain, hematemesis, and bloody diarrhea may develop. In some instances the findings simulate an acute surgical abdomen. Ascites may be present. Further progression leads to toxemia, cyanosis, shock, and death. In the oropharyngeal form, patients develop fever, anorexia, cervical or submandibular lymphadenopathy, and edema. A primary anthrax lesion of the pharynx has also been reported.

Anthrax meningitis resembles typical hemorrhagic meningitis.

DIAGNOSIS. In cutaneous anthrax, the typical lesion is a painless, pruritic papule that progresses into a vesicle, beneath which a depressed black eschar develops. Microscopic and bacteriologic examination of fluid from a vesicle or exudate from beneath the eschar should reveal organisms. The differential diagnosis includes staphylococcal skin infections, tularemia, plague, contagious pustular dermatitis (ecthyma contagiosum or orf), and milker's nodule.

The initial phase of inhalation anthrax is indistinguishable from a mild upper respiratory tract infection, and the acute phase of severe respiratory distress will resemble other diseases that cause respiratory insufficiency. The classic physical finding of inhalation anthrax is widening of the mediastinum. Sputum cultures are not generally positive for *B. anthracis*.

Gastrointestinal anthrax has no characteristic signs and symptoms, but organisms may be demonstrable in feces or vomitus. The clinical course may resemble shigellosis or *Yersinia* gastroenteritis. Severe involvement may lead to surgery of the abdomen. Involvement of the upper gastrointestinal tract is not distinctive of infection with *B. anthracis*.

Anthrax meningitis resembles hemorrhagic meningitis or possibly a cerebrovascular accident, but there should be evidence of a primary site of infection. The organism should be demonstrable in the cerebrospinal fluid.

In any of these forms of the disease, appropriate serum specimens may demonstrate a significant titer by the ELISA or a new test, the electrophoretic immunotransblot test.

TREATMENT. The drug of choice in anthrax is penicillin;

B. anthracis organisms resistant to penicillin have not been identified from clinical specimens. In mild cutaneous anthrax, oral potassium penicillin, 2 grams per day for five to seven days, is recommended. With extensive lesions or with significant systemic illness, intramuscular procaine penicillin, 4 to 6 million units per day for five to seven days, should be given. Tetracycline or erythromycin may also be used in oral doses of 2 grams per day for five to seven days. In malignant edema, additional therapy with intravenous hydrocortisone, 100 to 200 mg per day, has been reported to be effective.

The lesion in cutaneous anthrax should be covered with a clean dressing. Hospitalized patients should be on Drainage/Secretion Precautions. No ointments have been shown to be effective; excision of the lesion has been reported to increase the severity of symptoms.

Therapy of inhalation anthrax is based primarily on empirical knowledge and extrapolation from animal experiments. Penicillin G should be administered intravenously in doses of 18 to 24 million units per day. Streptomycin, 1 to 2 grams per day intravenously, may also be used. Supportive therapy such as volume expanders and vasopressor agents should be used as necessary. There may be a need to ensure an adequate airway if edema results in compression of the trachea.

For gastrointestinal anthrax, the therapeutic regimen for inhalation anthrax should be initiated. Tetracycline, 1 gram per day intravenously, has also been reported to be effective.

Anthrax meningitis should be treated in the same way as inhalation anthrax.

PROGNOSIS. The case-fatality ratio for cutaneous anthrax is 20 per cent without treatment and less than 5 per cent with appropriate treatment. Inhalation anthrax is almost always fatal. Gastrointestinal anthrax has a case fatality rate of 25 to 75 per cent.

PREVENTION. Formaldehyde has been successfully used to decontaminate raw hair and wool; gamma irradiation, steam under pressure, and ethylene oxide sterilization have been used with less effectiveness. Currently, prevention is directed toward protecting the employee by use of an effective, cell-free vaccine; education; good personal hygiene; and use of protective clothing, including respirators if aerosols are created. Gastrointestinal anthrax can be prevented by education concerning the ingestion of potentially contaminated meat. Prophylactic antibiotics or hyperimmune serum have not been shown to be effective.

Agricultural cases can be prevented by practicing good animal husbandry, including annual immunization of animals.

Brachman PS: Anthrax. In Evans A, Feldman H (eds.): Bacterial Infections of Humans: Epidemiology and Control. New York, Ms. Hilary Evans Publishing Company, 1982, pp 63–74. *Comprehensive summary of all aspects of anthrax, with emphasis on the epidemiology.*

Brachman PS: Inhalation anthrax, New York Academy of Science, Conference on Airborne Contagion, November 8, 1979. Ann NY Acad Sci 353:83, 1980. *A review of all aspects of inhalation anthrax.*

Doyle PJ, Keller KF, Ezzell JW: *Bacillus anthracis.* In Lenette EH, Balows A, Hausler Jr WJ, Shadomy HJ (eds.): Manual of Clinical Microbiology. 4th ed. Washington, D.C., American Society for Microbiology, 1985, pp 211–215. *A thorough review of the laboratory identification of anthrax.*

Harrison LH, Ezzell JW, Abshire T, et al.: Application of an electrophoretic immunotransblot method for the serologic diagnosis of anthrax. Abstract number 877, Interscience conference on antibiotics and chemotherapy, p 258, 1986. *Discusses a new and sensitive serologic test for anthrax.*

Knudson GB: Treatment of anthrax in man: History and current concepts. Military Med 151:71, 1986. *Reviews the history of anthrax with emphasis on treatment.*

Little SF, Knudson GB: Comparative efficacy of *Bacillus anthracis* live spore vaccine against anthrax in guinea pigs. Infect Immun 52:509, 1986. *Compares two different anthrax vaccines and discusses ELISA testing.*

Plotkin SA, Brachman PS, Utell M, et al.: An epidemic of inhalation anthrax. The first in the twentieth century. I. Clinical features. Am J Med 29:992, 1960. *Summarizes the clinical features of an epidemic of inhalation anthrax in the United States.*

294 DISEASES CAUSED BY PSEUDOMONADS

Michael Barza

Melioidosis and glanders are caused by closely related bacteria of the genus *Pseudomonas*. Like other pseudomonads, these are strictly aerobic, nonfermentative, gram-negative bacilli. Both species show distinctive bipolar staining with various dyes.

MELIOIDOSIS

DEFINITION. Melioidosis, caused by *P. pseudomallei*, is a rare disease acquired in equatorial areas. It may produce fulminant septicemia with widespread suppurative lesions or a chronic, tuberculosis-like illness with lung cavitation. Infection occurs through contact with contaminated soil or water.

ETIOLOGY. In 1912, Whitmore and Krishnaswami, while performing autopsies on derelicts in Rangoon who had died of a glanders-like illness, recovered a unique bacillus. Because of the resemblance to glanders, this bacterium came to be called *P. pseudomallei* and the disease, melioidosis.

EPIDEMIOLOGY. *P. pseudomallei* is found in a narrow belt ranging 20 degrees on either side of the equator. Most cases have been acquired in Southeast Asia, but some have been reported from the Philippines, Guam, Australia, and, rarely, Central or South America. Over 300 cases of melioidosis with 36 deaths were recorded among United States troops stationed in Vietnam.

The organism is widespread in soil and stagnant water, particularly in paddy fields. Epizootic infection occurs among sheep, goats, swine, and horses, but, in contrast to glanders, animals do not seem to be a reservoir of human disease. Most infections in humans are believed to arise by contamination of skin abrasions by soil or water. This may explain the marked predilection for males. Ingestion and inhalation and aspiration of contaminated water are occasional routes of entry. Rarely, laboratory workers have been infected while working with this organism. Only one instance of human-to-human transmission has been reported.

Inapparent infection in the form of seroreactivity is common in endemic areas. Significant titers have been found in as many as 15 to 30 per cent of healthy Malaysians, Thais, and Vietnamese and in 1 to 2 per cent of United States soldiers who spent at least six months in Vietnam. Seropositivity has been reported in up to 32 per cent of soldiers severely wounded or burned in Vietnam. This is important because of the remarkable ability of melioidosis, like tuberculosis, to become clinically manifest many years after exposure. A population of veterans in the United States is now at risk for this disease.

PATHOGENESIS AND PATHOLOGY. In acute septicemic melioidosis, organisms are disseminated widely throughout the body, particularly the lungs, liver, spleen, and lymph nodes. Lung lesions usually result from hematogenous spread, but sometimes arise from aspiration or inhalation of bacteria. Multiple small abscesses are formed, containing necrotic material, neutrophils, and abundant bacteria. With time, the lesions coalesce and may cavitate. A rim of hemorrhage may be evident in pulmonary abscesses.

Chronic melioidosis most commonly affects the lungs and lymph nodes. The lesions show central necrosis containing polymorphonuclear leukocytes, and peripheral granulomas. Giant cells may be seen. Organisms are sparse in these lesions.

CLINICAL MANIFESTATIONS. The most common manifestation of infection with *P. pseudomallei* is simply a positive serologic test result. Clinical disease ranges from an acute septicemic form to a subacute or chronic localized form. At both extremes, the lung is commonly involved. The incubation period is usually a few days, but may be as long as 20 years or more. In late-onset cases, the illness often seems to be triggered by intercurrent trauma or other disease such as diabetes mellitus, alcoholism, cancer, or malnutrition.

Acute septicemic melioidosis, which often seems to strike diabetic individuals, causes fever, chills, tachypnea, and muscle pain, as well as signs and symptoms attributable to local abscess formation. Macroscopic abscesses are common in the liver, spleen, and lymph nodes. They are especially prominent in the lungs, chiefly in the upper lobes. Radiographic changes range from bronchopneumonia through lobar consolidation to nodular lesions that coalesce and may cavitate. There may be pleuritic chest pain and a pleural rub. Rales and rhonchi are often heard. Pustular skin lesions are sometimes seen. Routine laboratory tests show anemia and a variable polymorphonuclear leukocytosis.

Subacute or chronic melioidosis may follow the acute infection or may arise indolently. The typical presentation is cavitary disease of the upper lobes of the lungs, resembling tuberculosis. The liver, skin, bones, and soft tissues may be affected, and sinus tracts may be formed. The general picture is of a chronic, wasting, usually febrile illness with occasional periods of remission.

Variations upon these themes may be encountered. A nodular abscess with regional lymphadenitis may occur at the site of the original infection, usually the skin. Focal and diffuse encephalitis and meningitis, as well as pleural mass and effusion, have been described.

DIAGNOSIS. Melioidosis should be suspected in subjects from an endemic area who manifest either an acute, febrile illness with widespread suppurative lesions, especially in the lungs and skin, or who exhibit progressive cavitary lung disease without a clear cause. *A high level of suspicion in individuals who have resided in endemic areas may be lifesaving, especially in the septicemic form of the illness, because the organisms are usually resistant to agents such as various first- and second-generation cephalosporins, gentamicin, and tobramycin, which might be used for empiric treatment.* Gram's stain of infected material may show the organisms poorly, but Wright's, Giemsa, and other techniques usually demonstrate the bacteria and reveal the bipolar accentuation.

The laboratory should be alerted to the suspected diagnosis. The organisms usually grow well in ordinary media, but they may be sparse in chronic infections and may be overgrown by normal flora. The use of selective media may increase the yield. After several days of incubation, the colonies usually assume a typical "wrinkled" appearance on agar media. *P. pseudomallei* can be differentiated from other pseudomonads by a variety of biologic features. Fluorescent-antibody staining, one of the most definitive tests, cross-reacts with *P. mallei*, but the two organisms can be distinguished by the lack of motility of the latter. A rapid slide-agglutination test using commercially available antiserum also distinguishes *P. pseudomallei* from other pseudomonads but cross-reacts with *P. mallei*.

Serologic studies may be helpful. The complement fixation test is suggestive at titers above 1:8 and the hemagglutination test at titers above 1:80. A four-fold rise in titer is essentially diagnostic. Serologic tests are occasionally negative in patients with active disease. Elevated titers may persist despite successful treatment of melioidosis. Tests for specific IgM antibody appear to be more sensitive and specific than other serologic tests in detecting patients with active infection.

TREATMENT. There is no general agreement upon an optimal regimen for the treatment of melioidosis. The choice of drugs must, to some extent, be based upon sensitivity tests. Most active in vitro are the tetracyclines, chloramphenicol, novobiocin, kanamycin, amikacin, sulfonamides, and trimethoprim-sulfamethoxazole. Recently, the third-generation cephalosporin ceftazidime was reported to be active against an isolate resistant to most other drugs.

For *acute septicemic melioidosis*, high intravenous doses of trimethoprim-sulfamethoxazole (9 and 45 mg per kilogram per day), ceftazidime (2 grams every 6 to 8 hours), kanamycin (30 mg per kilogram per day*), or amikacin are recommended. Other potentially useful agents include tetracycline (4 to 6 grams or 80 mg per kilogram per day), chloramphenicol (80 mg per kilogram per day), sulfisoxazole (140 mg per kilogram per day), and novobiocin (60 mg per kilogram per day). In general, at least two drugs should be used simultaneously for the first 30 days, and the dosages of the more toxic agents should be reduced as the infection comes under control. Thereafter, a single agent such as trimethoprim-sulfamethoxazole may be given for two to six months.

For *chronic melioidosis*, tetracycline, chloramphenicol, sulfisoxazole, or trimethoprim-sulfamethoxazole should be given in about half the dosage recommended for acute disease. One drug to which the organism is sensitive usually suffices, but two drugs may be recommended initially if the patient is very sick. Because the bacteria are difficult to eradicate, treatment should be continued for at least three months for chronic pulmonary melioidosis and for at least six months for chronic extrapulmonary melioidosis. Abscesses should be drained according to usual principles; however, surgical intervention without adequate antibiotic coverage can be dangerous. The indications for operation on patients with active lung disease are not settled.

PROGNOSIS. The mortality rate of untreated septicemic melioidosis exceeds 90 per cent, but with treatment this is reduced to about 50 per cent. Subacute or chronic infection carries a lower mortality which, with treatment, may be diminished to 10 per cent or less.

PREVENTION. No vaccine is available. It seems reasonable to recommend thorough cleansing of abrasions sustained in endemic areas. Despite the rarity of person-to-person transmission, patients with active infection, especially pulmonary infection, should probably be isolated.

Everett ED, Nelson RA: Pulmonary melioidosis. Observations in thirty-nine cases. Am Rev Respir Dis 112:331, 1975. *A thorough account of the clinical presentation of a large group of United States soldiers, most of whom had subacute or chronic pulmonary infection. Therapeutic recommendations, including the role of surgery, are discussed at length.*

Howe C, Sampath A, Spotnitz M: The pseudomallei group: A review. J Infect Dis 124:598, 1971. *An excellent review of the bacteriology and epidemiology of the disease and of what little is known about the pathogenetic factors involved.*

John JF Jr: Trimethoprim-sulfamethoxazole therapy of pulmonary melioidosis. Am Rev Respir Dis 114:1021, 1976. *Presentation of a case and brief review of the limited information available regarding therapy of cavitary lung disease.*

Puthucheary SD, Lin HP, Yap PK: Acute septicemic melioidosis. Trop Geog Med 33:19, 1981. *A good account of the fulminant septicemic form of acute melioidosis; four of the seven patients had diabetes mellitus.*

So SY, Chau PY, Leung YK, et al.: Successful treatment of melioidosis caused by a multiresistant strain in an immunocompromised host with third generation cephalosporins. Am Rev Resp Dis 127:650, 1983. *This strain was resistant to most other drugs and was only moderately susceptible to cefoperazone and moxalactam but was highly susceptible to ceftazidime.*

GLANDERS

DEFINITION. Glanders is primarily an infection of horses, mules, or donkeys, but can produce an acute septicemic illness in humans or a more chronic one involving principally the skin and lungs.

ETIOLOGY. The causative organism, *Pseudomonas mallei*, derives its species name from the Latin *malleus*, connoting "severe disease." It is a strictly aerobic, nonfermentative, gram-negative rod that closely resembles *Pseudomonas pseudomallei*, the agent of melioidosis, but is nonmotile.

EPIDEMIOLOGY. Glanders occurs almost exclusively in people handling horses, mules, or donkeys. In horses, there may be pulmonary involvement ("glanders") or subcutaneous nodules, especially about the head and neck ("farcy"). The

---

*Dosage exceeds manufacturer's recommendations.

infection is occasionally transmitted to domestic animals. In the rare instances of infection in humans, transmission appears to be via broken skin or mucous membranes or possibly aerosol inhalation. Glanders has been eradicated from the United States, but cases still occur in Asia and South America. Laboratory personnel working with the organism may become infected. In contrast to melioidosis, glanders can be transmitted fairly readily from person to person.

PATHOLOGY AND PATHOGENESIS. The lesions of glanders range from acute cellulitis with necrosis and abscess formation to a chronic necrotizing process with granuloma formation.

CLINICAL MANIFESTATIONS. Within a few days of cutaneous inoculation, subcutaneous nodules appear with regional lymphadenitis. When the portal of entry is the upper respiratory tract, draining mucosal ulcers occur. Lower respiratory infection following inhalation may have a longer incubation period, 10 to 14 days, and results in a necrotizing lobar pneumonia or bronchopneumonia, nodular lung infiltrates, or lung abscess; accompanying features include chills, myalgias, headache, and pleuritic chest pain. Systemic spread may complicate infection in any of these sites, producing a rapidly fatal illness with a generalized pustular rash.

Physical findings may include local suppuration, generalized adenopathy, and splenomegaly. The white blood cell count may be mildly elevated. Occasionally there is severe leukopenia.

In some patients, a chronic form of disease occurs with subcutaneous or intramuscular abscesses. There may be lymphadenitis and ulceration of the nasal mucosa. Involvement of the liver, spleen, lung, eye, and central nervous system has been reported.

DIAGNOSIS. Glanders should be considered when persons handling potentially infected animals or laboratory material develop acute or chronic nodular, suppurative infections of the skin or respiratory tract or an acute, septicemic illness. Bacteria are sparse even in abscesses and may not be well seen with Gram's stain. Giemsa, Wright's, or methylene blue stain, however, may reveal organisms with irregular staining. *P. mallei* grows slowly on various standard laboratory media. The bacteria can be identified presumptively by their biochemical characteristics and lack of motility, as well as by fluorescent-antibody staining. Serologic tests (agglutination, complement fixation) may be useful.

TREATMENT. The mortality of untreated glanders is high. Experience with therapy is limited. Sulfadiazine appears to be effective. It should be administered in a dosage of 100 mg per kilogram per day for three weeks or more. By analogy with melioidosis, other drugs such as tetracycline, chloramphenicol, or an aminoglycoside might be administered concomitantly.

Infected animals should be destroyed, and infected humans should be isolated to prevent spread of the disease.

Howe C, Miller WR: Human glanders: Report of six cases. Ann Intern Med 26:93, 1947. *A review of cases that occurred among workers in a single laboratory. The diagnoses were made serologically, and all patients survived.*

295 LISTERIOSIS

Michael Barza

DEFINITION. Infection caused by *Listeria monocytogenes*, a distinctive gram-positive bacillus, occurs worldwide. The organism has a propensity to afflict people with underlying diseases but also affects previously healthy individuals. Meningitis, bacteremia, and focal infections, as well as devastating neonatal sepsis, can occur.

ETIOLOGY. In 1926, Murray, Webb, and Swann isolated a new bacterium from sick rabbits and guinea pigs. Because it produced a monocytosis in these animals, they suggested the species name *monocytogenes*. The first human isolation, in 1929, was from a patient with an illness resembling infectious mononucleosis.

EPIDEMIOLOGY. *L. monocytogenes* is widespread in soil, water, and sewage, and can survive in moist environments for months. A large variety of healthy mammals, fowl, and fish are sporadically colonized. Listeriosis is a well-recognized cause of abortion, septicemia, and encephalitis in various animal species. As many as 5 per cent of well individuals and a higher proportion of household contacts of patients with listeriosis carry the organism in the feces. Fecal carriage is common in individuals who are heavily exposed to animals. The organisms can occasionally be recovered from the nose, throat, or genitalia of healthy persons.

Most sporadic listerial infections in humans are of uncertain origin. Patients are usually urban dwellers with no obvious contact with animals, unpasteurized milk, or contaminated food or water. However, a number of outbreaks of listeriosis have been attributed to the ingestion of contaminated foods, including pasteurized and unpasteurized milk, cheese, and coleslaw. The dairy products in these instances were presumably contaminated by milk from cows with subclinical listerial mastitis and the coleslaw by cabbage fertilized with manure from infected sheep. In one survey from the northeastern United States, 12 per cent of raw milk samples contained *L. monocytogenes*. Patients taking medications to reduce gastric acidity may be at increased risk of infection because of loss of the antibacterial effect of stomach acid.

The frequency of listeriosis appears to be increasing. This may be due in part to heightened awareness, but probably also reflects the increasing population of patients with immunosuppressive disorders who now constitute the majority of patients with *Listeria* infection. Males are more often affected than females. In Europe two thirds of cases occur in neonates, whereas in the United States most infections occur in later life. The reasons for these differences in sex, age, and geographic distribution are not known.

L. monocytogenes can be grouped into 11 serotypes, of which type 1 (especially 1b) and type 4 (especially 4b) are the most common in the United States. Clusters of cases caused by a single serotype have occasionally been described in the community and in the hospital, suggesting that either person-to-person or common-source spread has occurred. Nursery outbreaks are well recognized.

PATHOLOGY AND PATHOGENESIS. The usual portal of entry of *L. monocytogenes*, except for fetal infections, is the gastrointestinal tract. In animals, the organisms are taken up by the epithelial cells of the gut. Bacteremia may ensue with seeding of various sites. The usual histologic response in humans is a polymorphonuclear leukocytosis with formation of microabscesses. Occasionally, there is a monocytic reaction.

L. monocytogenes shares with mycobacteria, fungi, *Salmonella*, and *Brucella* the ability to survive within macrophages of the nonimmune host. Resistance to infection appears to depend mainly on the acquisition of cell-mediated immunity; humoral immunity probably plays a lesser role. Thus, patients who have diseases that depress cellular immunity or who are taking immunosuppressive drugs or are pregnant are especially susceptible to infection.

The pathogenetic properties of the organism are beginning to be understood. A high molecular weight component of the cell wall is immunosuppressive. A low molecular weight component of the cell membrane produces a monocytosis in animals. There is some evidence that various hemolysins, termed lysteriolysins, are produced by pathogenic isolates of *L. monocytogenes*, and that these hemolysins are virulence factors.

L. monocytogenes shows striking tropism for the fetus and placenta of most animals and for the central nervous system of monkeys and humans. Meningitis results in a dense, purulent reaction, especially over the base of the brain. The infection sometimes extends more deeply to produce "cerebritis" or bacterial encephalitis. Brain abscess may supervene. In perinatal infection, miliary necrotizing granulomas are found in the liver, spleen, lungs, and central nervous system.

CLINICAL MANIFESTATIONS. Listeriosis most commonly affects elderly patients, especially males. The major presentations are meningitis (55 per cent), bacteremia (25 per cent), endocarditis (7 per cent), and nonmeningitic parenchymal infection of the central nervous system (6 per cent). More than one half of patients have an underlying disorder such as malignancy, cirrhosis, alcoholism, diabetes, or vasculitis, or are undergoing chronic hemodialysis or are receiving immunosuppressive drugs such as corticosteroids. Gastrointestinal symptoms sometimes occur at the onset of the systemic illness, further suggesting that the intestinal tract is the likely portal of entry.

L. monocytogenes accounts for about 2 per cent of cases of meningitis in the population at large. However, it is a leading cause of bacterial *meningitis* among people with cancer, especially lymphoma and leukemia, and among recipients of renal transplants. About 30 per cent of patients with *Listeria* meningitis have no preceding disease. The onset of illness is usually fairly sudden with headache and fever. Nuchal rigidity is present in 85 per cent of patients. Although the signs and symptoms generally resemble those of other pyogenic meningitides, coarse tremors or cerebellar ataxia may be striking. The cerebrospinal fluid in most patients (70 per cent) shows a polymorphonuclear leukocytosis and increased protein concentration; in fewer than one half is the glucose decreased below 40 mg per deciliter. Occasionally, the course of *Listeria* meningitis is indolent and the spinal fluid contains a predominance of lymphocytes, leading to suspicion of tuberculous or cryptococcal infection.

Focal cerebritis or one or more *brain abscesses* may complicate the course of *Listeria* meningitis, especially in renal transplant recipients. In some patients, these focal lesions may appear without other evidence of meningitis. They usually affect the cerebral hemispheres, causing hemiplegia, or the brain stem or cerebellum, causing vomiting, headache, vertigo, and cranial nerve palsies ("listerial rhombencephalitis"). In the absence of meningitis, there is no nuchal rigidity and the spinal fluid abnormalities are relatively mild. Radionuclide scan and computed tomographic (CT) scan may be helpful in delineating the lesions.

Bacteremia caused by *L. monocytogenes* usually affects patients under 50 years of age. About 90 per cent of patients have an underlying illness or are pregnant. There are no specific features to distinguish this from other forms of bacteremia. Fever, chills, and tachycardia are usual; hypotension and confusion may occur. Peripheral leukocytosis is the rule, but monocytosis has been reported. The major complications are meningitis and endocarditis.

Endocarditis caused by *L. monocytogenes* is rare. In contrast to other forms of listeriosis in adults, most patients have not had an immunosuppressive illness, but pre-existing valvular disease has been noted in over one half of cases. In several instances, infection occurred on a prosthetic valve.

Other *localized infections*, all rare, include pneumonia, hepatitis, pericarditis, infected aortic aneurysm, osteomyelitis, conjunctivitis, intraocular infection, and primary skin infection.

L. monocytogenes has occasionally been recovered from lymph nodes, blood, or spinal fluid of patients with a syndrome resembling infectious mononucleosis. However, this presentation is exceedingly rare and is unrelated to EB-virus infection.

Listerial infection occurring during *pregnancy* may have devastating consequences for the fetus, including abortion or stillbirth. If the infant is born alive, the distinctive syndrome known as *granulomatosis infantiseptica* may supervene with signs of septicemia, fetal distress, pneumonia, diarrhea, seizures, and rash; this syndrome, which has a high mortality, develops within hours or a day or two after birth and is referred to as "early-onset" infection. Microabscesses, sometimes with a granulomatous component, are found in various organs of the newborn. In most instances of fetal listeriosis, the mother sustains a mild influenza-like illness with fever, myalgias, diarrhea, sore throat, or urinary symptoms. Infection of the fetus is assumed to occur through the hematogenous route, but some infections may occur through ascent from the lower genital tract of the mother.

The second form of neonatal listeriosis, known as "late-onset" infection, occurs after the first five to seven days of life. Infection is believed to be acquired during passage through the colonized birth canal. Meningitis is the usual presentation; sequelae include hydrocephalus and mental retardation. Overall, about 10 to 20 per cent of neonatal meningitis is caused by *L. monocytogenes.*

The overall importance of listeriosis in the causation of spontaneous abortion is controversial. In one study, the organism was cultured from the cervix of 25 of 34 women who had had repeated abortions, but in none of 87 control patients. In another study, antibiotic treatment of three couples in which the wives had suffered repeated abortions resulted in successful pregnancies. However, a large body of data suggests that this sequence of events is unusual and that *Listeria* is not implicated in most instances of spontaneous abortion.

DIAGNOSIS. Beyond the neonatal period, there is little that is specific about the syndrome of listeriosis. Clearly, this organism must be suspected when meningitis occurs in a setting of diminished host defenses. However, the diagnosis rests upon bacteriologic grounds, and the key to diagnosis is awareness. Laboratories frequently misinterpret *L. monocytogenes* as diphtheroids, which are discarded as "contaminants." Gram's stain of infected material may reveal the typical, pleomorphic, palisading, gram-positive bacilli. However, organisms are not seen in Gram's stain of the spinal fluid in 60 to 75 per cent of patients with *Listeria* meningitis. Moreover, the organisms sometimes resemble streptococci, or in other instances, stain irregularly so that they are mistaken for *Haemophilus influenzae.* If the clinical setting is suggestive, the physician should alert the laboratory to the possibility of listeriosis. Cultures can then be examined for β-hemolysis, catalase positivity, and tumbling motility of organisms at room temperature, which distinguish *L. monocytogenes* from other agents.

Listeria is generally not difficult to grow from infected material unless the patient has received antibiotics. The use of selective media may be helpful with samples such as sputum and vaginal secretions that contain other bacteria. In addition to blood cultures, spinal fluid should be obtained if there is any suggestion of meningitis, for nuchal rigidity may be absent. In the newborn, material from the eye, ear, nose, throat, amniotic fluid, and meconium should be examined in addition to blood cultures.

TREATMENT. Ampicillin or penicillin G is the mainstay of therapy for listeriosis. The organisms are generally susceptible to these antibiotics as well as to trimethoprim-sulfamethoxazole, chloramphenicol, clindamycin, erythromycin, gentamicin, vancomycin, and tetracyclines, but individual strains may depart from the usual pattern. Penicillins are slowly bactericidal against *L. monocytogenes* in vitro; by contrast, erythromycin, chloramphenicol, the tetracyclines, and rifampin are only bacteriostatic, a distinction that may be important in the treatment of meningitis. Trimethoprim-sulfamethoxazole is

rapidly bactericidal in vitro and penetrates the meninges well, whereas imipenem may be less satisfactory in these respects. Cephalosporins should be avoided because of their limited meningeal penetration and generally poor activity against the organisms. In one retrospective study, ampicillin appeared somewhat better than penicillin G. There is some evidence that ampicillin or penicillin G, given alone, is more effective than chloramphenicol given alone or in combination with ampicillin or penicillin G.

For initial therapy in adults, pending the results of sensitivity tests, ampicillin is recommended in a dosage of 200 mg per kilogram per day in six divided doses; alternatively, penicillin G, 300,000 units per kilogram per day in six or eight divided doses, may be used. Higher dosages may occasionally be required. There is synergy between these drugs and gentamicin or streptomycin in vitro. Thus, concomitant administration of an aminoglycoside, intrathecally for meningitis, might be considered in seriously ill patients or those who relapse. Therapy may have to be given for several weeks to prevent relapse. On the basis of activity in vitro and a limited experience in vivo, trimethoprim-sulfamethoxazole appears to be a useful alternative in the penicillin-allergic patient.

PROGNOSIS. The overall mortality of untreated listeriosis exceeds 70 per cent for meningitis or bacteremia. The outcome with treatment is influenced by coexisting diseases. In adults with meningitis, the mortality rate was 13 per cent in those without other disorders, 28 per cent in immunosuppressed patients without malignancy, and 60 per cent in those with malignancy. A low glucose concentration and high protein concentration in the cerebrospinal fluid appear to herald an unfavorable outcome of meningitis. Brain abscess or cerebritis carries a mortality rate of about 50 per cent, and residual defects are common.

Among patients treated appropriately for bacteremia with ampicillin or penicillin G, 90 per cent survive. Fatalities occur primarily among those with immunosuppressive illnesses in whom there is undiagnosed central nervous system infection. Patients being treated for bacteremia should be carefully watched for signs of meningitis, especially if they are being given antibiotics that penetrate the meninges poorly. Well-demarcated brain abscesses require surgical drainage. About one third of patients with endocarditis die, primarily of myocardial infarction, congestive heart failure, or subarachnoid hemorrhage.

Antibiotics have reduced the mortality rate of perinatal infection from almost 100 per cent to about 50 per cent.

PREVENTION. There is no vaccine available to prevent listeriosis. On occasion, clusters of cases have occurred in hospitalized patients, suggesting possible cross-infection. Although such events are rare, it seems prudent to use isolation precautions for patients with listeriosis, especially if there are transplant recipients or patients with immunosuppressive disorders nearby.

It may be worthwhile to culture the cervix of women who have repeated abortions or whose infants die early in life and the blood of women who are febrile during pregnancy for the possibility of treatable *Listeria* infection.

Fleming DW, Cochi SL, MacDonald KL, et al.: Pasteurized milk as a vehicle of infection in an outbreak of listeriosis. N Engl J Med 312:404, 1985. *Forty-nine patients in Massachusetts developed listeriosis following ingestion of properly pasteurized milk. L. monocytogenes may be uniquely suited to survive pasteurization, as is discussed in the article and an accompanying editorial.*

Galsworthy SB: Immunomodulation by surface components of Listeria monocytogenes: A review. Clin Invest Med (Can) 7:223, 1984. *A readable review of some of the newer investigations of the effects of various components of the cell wall and cell membrane of this species on host defense mechanisms.*

Lavetter A, Leedom JM, Mathies AW, et al.: Meningitis due to Listeria monocytogenes. N Engl J Med 285:598, 1971. *A retrospective comparison of the outcome of disease in 25 patients treated mainly with ampicillin or penicillin G. Although concomitant antibiotics may have skewed the results somewhat, the data suggest some advantage for ampicillin.*

Nieman RE, Lorber B: Listeriosis in adults: A changing pattern. Report of eight cases and review of the literature, 1968–1978. Rev Infect Dis 2:207, 1980. *A thorough review of the clinical aspects of listeriosis in the postnatal period, with a detailed analysis of risk factors and prognostic features.*

Perinatal listeriosis. Lancet 1:911, 1980. *A concise account of the current status of the diagnosis, treatment, and prevention of this highly fatal disease.*

Stamm AM, Dismukes WE, Simmons BP, et al.: Listeriosis in renal transplant recipients: Report of an outbreak and review of 102 cases. Rev Infect Dis 4:665, 1982. *An excellent review of this continuing problem. Has 110 references.*

Tuazon CU, Shamsuddin D, Miller H: Antibiotic susceptibility and synergy of clinical isolates of *Listeria monocytogenes*. Antimicrob Agents Chemother 21:525, 1982. *Stresses the lack of bactericidal activity of the penicillins (the drugs of choice) and of chloramphenicol and the excellent activity of trimethoprim-sulfamethoxazole in vitro.*

296 ERYSIPELOID

Michael Barza

DEFINITION. *Erysipelothrix rhusiopathiae* is an important cause of disease in animals. In humans, it produces a characteristic violaceous erythema of the fingers and hands known as erysipeloid (of Rosenbach). Disseminated infection and endocarditis rarely occur.

ETIOLOGY. *E. rhusiopathiae* is a slender, pleomorphic, non–spore-forming gram-positive rod that grows well on ordinary laboratory media. Its lack of motility or catalase production and its ability to form hydrogen sulfide on TSI slants help distinguish it from *Listeria monocytogenes* and *Corynebacteria* (diphtheroids).

EPIDEMIOLOGY. Erysipeloid is contracted through exposure to infected tissue. *E. rhusiopathiae* is found in various *animals*, including sheep, lambs, cattle, horses, dogs, and mice; *fish* and *shellfish*; and *fowl*, including turkeys, chickens, and ducks. It is carried by 50 per cent of healthy swine and is an economically significant cause of disease in swine and turkeys. Swine develop septicemia, chronic arthritis, endocarditis, and a rhomboid urticarial skin reaction ("diamond skin"). *E. rhusiopathiae* appears to colonize the slime of fish. It survives in decaying organic matter. Although resistant to salting, pickling, and smoking, the bacteria are killed at 55° C for 15 minutes.

Humans are quite resistant to infection by ingestion, but are readily infected through superficial abrasions. The disease is most common in abattoir workers, butchers, fish-handlers, and the like. There is often no definite recollection of trauma.

CLINICAL MANIFESTATIONS. Within a few days of inoculation, a purplish erythema develops, usually on the finger or hand. Pain or itching, tingling, and throbbing usually accompany the skin lesions. The rash slowly spreads to involve other fingers, but rarely the fingertips or the skin above the wrist. It is sharply demarcated, and there is central clearing. Vesicles and even bullae are sometimes seen. Lymphangitis or regional lymphadenitis occurs in about 20 per cent of patients and constitutional symptoms such as fever occur in about 10 per cent. The joints in the affected extremity may be stiff and swollen. Untreated, the lesions usually resolve spontaneously over a period of weeks, but persistent sterile arthritis has been reported in up to 10 per cent of patients. In rare instances, a more diffuse skin eruption occurs.

Occasionally, *E. rhusiopathiae* causes septicemia. This almost always signifies endocarditis. About one half of patients with endocarditis have no antecedent history of valvular disease; some have evidence of recent erysipeloid. The endocarditis may be very destructive, with a high mortality rate. Septic shock has been reported in one patient with *E. rhusiopathiae* bacteremia.

DIAGNOSIS. The characteristic skin lesion and history of animal contact point to the diagnosis. The violaceous hue, burning or painful sensation, and absence of suppuration or constitutional symptoms distinguish this from ordinary pyogenic infections. The organisms can rarely be grown from aspirates of infected material but can often (7 of 20 cases in one series) be cultured from full-thickness skin biopsy of the advancing edge. Septicemia is diagnosed by blood culture.

TREATMENT. The organisms are generally sensitive to penicillins, cephalosporins, erythromycin, clindamycin, tetracyclines, and chloramphenicol, but not to vancomycin or aminoglycosides. However, strains resistant to erythromycin and tetracycline have been recovered from antibiotic-fed swine in Japan. Uncomplicated cutaneous lesions generally respond well to oral penicillin G, although parenteral therapy is occasionally necessary. Relapse sometimes occurs after treatment. Surgical incision offers no benefit and may lead to secondary infection. A suggested regimen for endocarditis is intravenous penicillin G, 12 to 20 million units daily for four to six weeks. Valve excision may be required. With early and aggressive therapy of endocarditis, the survival rate is about 85 per cent.

There is no vaccine available to prevent the disease. Highly exposed persons should wear gloves and wash their hands frequently at work.

Barnett JH, Estes SA, Wirman JA, et al.: Erysipeloid. J Am Acad Dermatol 9:116, 1983. *A good review of the clinical features and appearance of the lesions on electron microscopy and enunciation of the hypothesis that L-forms may play a role in the pathogenesis of the infection.*

Grieco MH, Sheldon C: Erysipelothrix rhusiopathiae. Ann NY Acad Sci 174:523, 1970. *A concise and detailed review of the bacteriology, epidemiology, and clinical features of this disease. Many references.*

Klauder JV: Erysipeloid as an occupational disease. JAMA 111:1345, 1938. *An account of the epidemiology of the infection in 100 patients, together with a vivid, illustrated, clinical description.*

Kramer MR, Gombert ME, Corrado ML, et al.: Erysipelothrix rhusiopathiae endocarditis. South Med J 75:892, 1982. *The first reported case in a drug addict. Points out the improved survival with current treatment, including valve replacement.*

297 ACTINOMYCOSIS

David J. Drutz

DEFINITION. Actinomycosis is a chronic suppurative and granulomatous bacterial infection characterized by contiguous spread, abscess formation, and sinuses that discharge grains ("sulfur granules"). There are four clinical forms: cervicofacial ("lumpy jaw"), thoracic, abdominal, and disseminated.

ETIOLOGY. Etiologic agents include *Actinomyces israelii*, *A. naeslundii*, *A. viscosus*, *A. odontolyticus*, *A. meyeri*, and *Arachnia propionica*. *Actinomyces bovis* produces lumpy jaw in cattle but is virtually never a human pathogen. These filamentous bacteria are anaerobic or facultative, capnophilic, gram-positive, and non–acid-fast. Filaments may break up into coccobacilli. All are normal oral flora; none is recoverable from the environment. Sulfur granules may be found in normal tonsillar crypts in the absence of an inflammatory reaction.

Actinomycosis is characterized by "associate" bacteria (e.g., *Actinobacillus actinomycetemcomitans* or various streptococci in cervicofacial actinomycosis; *E. coli* and diverse enteric organisms in abdominal actinomycosis). Given the disruption of mucous membranes necessary for initiation of actinomycosis, the presence of these bacteria is not surprising. These aerobes may play a synergistic role by helping maintain the low oxygen tension necessary for growth of the actinomycetes.

EPIDEMIOLOGY. Actinomycosis occurs worldwide and is unrelated to climate, occupation, race, or age. It may be more common in men than in women. Accurate data on incidence and prevalence are not available, but the disease is not rare. Actinomycosis occurs in many animal species but is not transmissible to man.

PATHOGENESIS AND PATHOLOGY. The etiologic agents are poorly invasive, generally requiring a break in the mucous membrane and the presence of devitalized tissue suitable to their anaerobic growth requirements. Unlike *Nocardia* species, they are not usually opportunistic in a setting of depressed cell-mediated immunity.

In animal studies mycelia and grains are more difficult to eliminate than coccobacilli. When the suppurative response fails to eradicate the bacteria, a granulomatous reaction ensues, accompanied by intense fibrosis. Contiguous spread of infection characteristically ignores tissue boundaries and ultimately produces draining sinus tracts and invasion of surrounding tissues.

The histopathologic picture is characterized by a mixed suppurative, granulomatous, and fibrotic process in which grains are a major distinguishing feature. When stained with hematoxylin-eosin, grains are centrally basophilic with eosinophilic rays (*Actinomyces* = "ray fungus"), terminating in pear-shaped "clubs." The clubs consist of an immune complex–derived sheath enclosing a single central filament that represents the organism itself. The grains stain well with methenamine silver, but Gram's stain is needed to identify the actinomycetes.

CLINICAL MANIFESTATIONS. Cervicofacial actinomycosis accounts for 60 per cent of infections and generally occurs in a setting of tooth decay, gingival disease, dental extraction, or serious injury sufficient to disrupt mucosal integrity. Manifestations include pain (some are painless); woody-hard swelling, often in the parotid or mandibular region (attributable to fibrosis); discoloration; trismus; and multiple sinuses that discharge odorless pus containing yellow-white granules. Fever and leukocytosis may occur. The disease spreads by direct extension and may involve tongue, salivary glands, pharynx, and larynx. Periostitis is followed by osteomyelitis. Cervical spine or cranial bone disease may lead to subdural empyema and central nervous system invasion. Cervicofacial actinomycosis may be confused with tuberculosis, nocardiosis, mycotic infections, osteomyelitis caused by other microorganisms, or neoplasm.

Thoracic actinomycosis accounts for 15 per cent of cases and may result from the aspiration of pharyngeal contents, dental plaque, or tonsillar grains; from organisms carried to the lung by a foreign body; by direct extension from cervicofacial or abdominal (especially hepatic) infection; or by hematogenous spread. There is often a history of underlying lung disease. Thoracic actinomycosis resembles other chronic inflammatory processes and malignancies. The tendency for the infection to cross pulmonary fissures and to form draining chest wall sinuses suggests the correct diagnosis. The pericardium and mediastinum may be invaded. Sulfur granules are rarely present in the sputum.

Abdominal actinomycosis accounts for about 20 per cent of cases and usually arises weeks to months following a perforation of the gastrointestinal tract. Most cases present in the right iliac fossa, reflecting a frequent association with appendicitis. Abdominal actinomycosis may spread by contiguity to other intra-abdominal structures (especially the liver), the lung, pelvis, spine, or abdominal wall. The eventual development of draining fistulas offers an important clue, and the diagnosis should be considered even in cases of perirectal abscess or fistula in ano. Abdominal actinomycosis may be confused with Crohn's disease, ulcerative colitis, tuberculosis, or malignancy. Colonization of the uterine cervix with *A. israelii* and other actinomycetes has become common with the use of intrauterine contraceptive devices (IUD's). Cases of pelvic actinomycosis have originated in this fashion.

Disseminated actinomycosis may result from the hematogenous spread of bacteria from any of the sites mentioned above but most frequently follows thoracic disease. Hematogenous dissemination is rare. Tissues most commonly involved include the skin and subcutaneous tissues, bone, brain, liver, and kidneys.

DIAGNOSIS. The diagnosis of actinomycosis should be made by direct isolation of the infecting organism from clinical specimens or from washed, crushed sulfur granules. Bacteriologic confirmation is achieved in less than 50 per cent of cases because of failure to obtain anaerobic cultures or overgrowth by the "associate" bacteria. Examination of Gram-stained tissue for filamentous, branching, non–acid-fast, gram-positive organisms often provides the clue to diagnosis. The organisms can also be seen in Gram's stains of crushed granules but must be differentiated from those seen in the grains of botryomycosis, eumycetomas, or actinomycetomas (see Ch. 378). The diagnosis of pelvic actinomycosis is usually first suspected when organisms are seen on cytologic preparations from the cervix.

Transtracheal aspiration has been complicated by formation of actinomycotic neck abscess at the site of needle introduction.

There are no reliable serologic tests for actinomycosis and no skin tests. Fluorescent antibody staining techniques have been used to identify actinomycetes in tissue sections, to identify their presence in mixed cultures, and to verify their final identity after isolation. However, these tests are not generally available.

TREATMENT. Actinomycosis has a strong tendency to recur, at least partially because of inaccessibility of the disease process to antibiotic penetration. Therefore, prolonged treatment courses may be necessary. There is no generally agreed upon formula for antibiotic dose or duration, and treatment should be tailored to disease severity. Cervicofacial actinomycosis may be easier to cure than the other forms. Penicillin is the drug of choice. In severe cases, 10 to 20 million units are given intravenously daily for four to six weeks, followed by 2 to 5 million units of oral phenoxymethyl penicillin (or its equivalent) for a total of 12 to 18 months of treatment. Alternative antibiotics (given in full dosage) include tetracycline, erythromycin, lincomycin, and clindamycin. *A. israelii* is exquisitely sensitive to rifampin, but no data are available on therapy with this drug. Although *Actinobacillus actinomycetemcomitans* is not particularly susceptible to penicillin or ampicillin, patients with actinomycosis improve on these regimens. Therefore, it is not necessary to tailor therapy to the drug susceptibilities of "associate" bacteria. Adjunctive therapeutic measures for actinomycosis include surgery.

PROGNOSIS. The advent of antibiotics has greatly improved the prognosis for all forms of actinomycosis, and neither deformity nor death is common.

Bennhoff DF: Actinomycosis: Diagnostic and therapeutic considerations and a review of 32 cases. Laryngoscope 94:1198, 1984. *A recent general review.*
Bernardi RS: Abdominal actinomycosis. Surg Gynecol Obstet 149:257, 1979. *A thorough and up-to-date review of all aspects of actinomycosis, with particular emphasis on the abdominal form.*
Flynn MW, Felson B: The roentgen manifestations of thoracic actinomycosis. Am J Roentgenol 110:707, 1970. *An outstanding guide to the roentgenographic diagnosis of pulmonary actinomycosis.*
Nayar M, Chandra M, Chitraratha K, et al.: Incidence of actinomycetes infection in women using intrauterine contraceptive devices. Acta Cytol 29:111, 1985. *Ten of 350 women using intrauterine contraceptive devices (IUD's) had actinomyces-like organisms in Papanicolaou-stained smears; 8 of the 10 were symptomatic. Seven of the 10 patients had been using an IUD for more than two years.*
Richtsmeier WJ, Johns ME: Actinomycosis of the head and neck. CRC Crit Rev Clin Lab Sci 11:175, 1979. *An excellent review, with an emphasis on infection of the head and neck.*

298 NOCARDIOSIS

David J. Drutz

DEFINITION. Nocardiosis is a subacute or chronic suppurative bacterial infection characterized by pneumonia and hematogenous dissemination, especially to the central nervous system. In immunosuppressed patients, the disease pursues a more acute, aggressive course.

ETIOLOGY. The etiologic agent is *Nocardia asteroides*, a gram-positive, aerobic actinomycete that is partially, and weakly, acid fast. Filamentous branching cells occur during logarithmic phase growth but later fragment to small coccobacillary forms. There are also numerous other *Nocardia* species, and some aspects of classification are unsettled. All nocardiae contain mycolic acid and are similar to mycobacteria in this regard. All are commonly found in soil and on straw, grasses, and rotting vegetation. Nocardiae are resistant to rifampin, a useful point in taxonomy. *N. caviae*, *N. farcinica*, and *N. brasiliensis* can produce pulmonary and disseminated infection in man, but only rarely. *N. brasiliensis* is, however, a common cause of actinomycetoma (see Ch. 378).

INCIDENCE AND PREVALENCE. Nocardiosis occurs worldwide, in all ages, races, and climates. It is two to three times as common in men as in women, but there is no occupation-related susceptibility. Five hundred to 1000 clinical cases occur yearly in the United States, but because of underreporting the true incidence and prevalence of nocardiosis are unknown.

EPIDEMIOLOGY. Nocardiosis is presumed to result from inhalation of airborne bacteria. At least one common-source outbreak in immunocompromised patients has been reported. *N. asteroides* has been recovered from the sputum and other body sites in patients without apparent clinical disease.

Nocardiosis can occur in apparently normal persons or in those with chronic obstructive pulmonary disease but is encountered more commonly in patients with impaired cell-mediated immunity (including AIDS). The recovery of *N. asteroides* from any immunocompromised person must be considered evidence of infection, not colonization, and must be appropriately treated.

Nocardiosis can occur as a primary cutaneous infection, usually following a local injury. Dissemination may occur.

PATHOGENESIS AND PATHOLOGY. In congenitally athymic nude mice, *N. asteroides* produces a fatal disseminated infection, but in their syngeneic thymus-bearing littermates, the disease is limited in extent and animals survive. *N. asteroides* growing in log phase prevents the phagolysosomal fusion necessary for alveolar macrophages to kill the ingested bacteria. These observations suggest that macrophages, T lymphocytes, and cell-mediated immunity play a crucial role in host defense against nocardiosis. The roles that serum factors and polymorphonuclear leukoyctes fulfill are poorly defined.

Nocardiosis disseminates hematogenously, with a tendency to involve the central nervous system, kidneys, and skin. However, no organ is exempt. The histologic picture is dominated by suppuration, mimicking pyogenic bacterial infection. *N. asteroides* is usually overlooked in hematoxylin-eosin-stained tissue, but is seen with tissue Gram's stain or Gomori methenamine silver (if staining time is extended). Acid-fast stains (appropriately modified to prevent overdecolorization) will demonstrate the organism, but its tendency to fragment into coccobacillary forms may cause it to be confused with *Mycobacterium tuberculosis* or atypical mycobacteria.

CLINICAL MANIFESTATIONS. Nocardiosis presents as a pneumonic process in about 75 per cent of cases; in others, the pulmonary involvement may be transient or inapparent.

Fever and cough are common. The radiographic picture is characterized by segmental or lobar infiltrates, often with rapidly developing thick-walled cavities. Masses, nodules, empyema, bulging fissures, and even chest wall extension reminiscent of actinomycosis may be encountered. Other radiographic presentations include chronic solitary lung abscess or indolent progressive fibrosis. Hilar involvement and calcification are uncommon. The radiographic picture has no pathognomonic features and is often complicated by pre-existing lung disease.

In 25 to 40 per cent of patients there is dissemination to the central nervous system. Occasionally, there is meningitis, but more frequently there are one or more space-occupying lesions, with headache and focal neurologic findings. Other common sites of dissemination include the skin and subcutaneous tissues, pleura and chest wall, kidneys, eyes, liver, and lymph nodes. Fifty-five per cent of patients have no identifiable foci of secondary infection. However, dissemination is more common in the immunosuppressed and must be aggressively sought. A negative chest film does not exclude disseminated nocardiosis.

DIAGNOSIS. In a patient with a generally intact immune system and a chronic disease course, nocardiosis may be confused with tuberculosis, mycoses, a variety of bacterial infections, or a malignancy. Repeated sputum cultures or more invasive diagnostic procedures may be required to reach the diagnosis. In the immunosuppressed patient, the disease may be confused or may coexist with other opportunists. In such patients, an aggressive diagnostic evaluation is indicated. Diagnostic flexibility is limited by the unavailability of reliable skin or serologic tests. Specimens of sputum, pleural fluid, tracheostomy secretions, transtracheal aspirates, bronchial washings and brushings, and transbronchial biopsy specimens should be stained and cultured. With failure of these methods, percutaneous lung aspiration or open lung biopsy should be carried out. Skin abscesses should be aspirated and smears examined for organisms. In addition, skin lesions should be biopsied, with portions submitted for histology and for culture. Computed tomographic (CT) scans of the brain should be obtained, as otherwise silent cerebral abscesses or foci of cerebritis have been identified in this manner.

N. asteroides will grow on most standard media. However, unless the organism is suspected, its recognition poses a practical problem because culture plates tend to be overgrown by microbial contaminants (especially in sputum) and are often discarded after 48 hours, whereas *N. asteroides* may require three to seven days for growth. As a result, the organism is more likely to be identified on media used for mycobacteria or fungi, which are observed for longer periods of time. Although chances for recovery of *N. asteroides* from the blood, urine, bone marrow, and spinal fluid are slim, cultures should nevertheless be obtained in difficult diagnostic situations.

TREATMENT. Most *N. asteroides* strains are sensitive to sulfonamides in vitro, and sulfonamides are the treatment of choice. Therapy should be initiated with 6 to 10* grams of sulfadiazine or sulfisoxazole daily. These regimens produce peak serum levels of 12 to 15 mg per deciliter. Subsequent dosage can be modified according to measured serum concentrations and clinical response. The duration of therapy is poorly standardized but should be prolonged, since relapse is common. In patients with intact host defenses, treatment should be continued for at least six weeks following clinical recovery. In the immunosuppressed, therapy should be given for at least one year. In patients with cerebral involvement, the progress of treatment should be monitored with serial CT scans. Surgery is usually required for brain abscesses and may also be necessary for subcutaneous abscesses or empyema.

*This dose exceeds the manufacturer's recommendations.

Not all patients respond to sulfonamide therapy, especially those who are profoundly immunosuppressed. In these patients it may be necessary to reduce dosage of immunosuppressive drugs. It has also been common to employ supplemental drugs (cycloserine, ampicillin, amoxicillin, tetracycline, erythromycin, aminoglycosides, or imipenem), but proof of efficacy of combined drug regimens is lacking. This statement also applies to co-trimoxazole, a fixed combination of one part trimethoprim to five parts sulfamethoxazole. Nevertheless, trimethoprim-sulfamethoxazole has come to be widely used, especially in immunocompromised patients or those with central nervous system involvement.

In patients unable to tolerate or not responding to sulfonamides, therapeutic alternatives include amikacin, minocycline, and chloramphenicol, and possibly imipenem, or amoxicillin plus clavulanic acid.

PROGNOSIS. Nocardiosis is not restricted to the immunosuppressed. However, those who are immunosuppressed have the most acute process, the greatest propensity to hematogenous dissemination, and the poorest prognosis. Prior to the sulfonamide era, only 25 per cent of patients recovered; in patients treated with a sulfonamide, the recovery rate is 54 per cent. However, Palmer et al. have recorded 75 per cent survival, even in immunosuppressed patients, when the diagnosis was established promptly and sulfonamide therapy begun. Thus, the chances for cure are directly related to the aggressiveness of management. Patients with cerebral involvement generally have a poorer prognosis.

Holtz HA, Lavery DP, Kapila R: Actinomycetales infection in the acquired immunodeficiency syndrome. Ann Intern Med 102:203, 1985. *Four parenteral drug abusers with AIDS had nonmycobacterial Actinomycetales infection (three with nocardiosis; one with Streptomyces lymphadenitis). Three of eight nocardiosis cases reported to the Centers for Disease Control have had concomitant mycobacterial disease, including one of the three cases described here.*

Palmer DL, Harvey RL, Wheeler JK: Diagnostic and therapeutic considerations in Nocardia asteroides infection. Medicine 53:391, 1974. *A comprehensive literature review of 243 cases of nocardiosis (including 13 patients in their own experience) occurring between 1961 and 1972. Still the best single review on the subject.*

Simpson GL, Stinson EB, Egger MJ, et al.: Nocardial infections in the immunocompromised host: A detailed study in a defined population. Rev Infect Dis 3:492, 1981. *Twenty-one of 160 patients undergoing cardiac transplantation at Stanford developed nocardiosis. Percutaneous lung aspiration was of particular value in reaching the diagnosis; sputum survey cultures were rarely positive. Patients responded surprisingly well to sulfisoxazole, despite the fact that immunosuppressive therapy was not altered.*

Smego RA Jr, Moeller MB, Gallis HA: Trimethoprim-sulfamethoxazole therapy for Nocardia infections. Arch Intern Med 143:711, 1983. *This article provides an extensive literature review and argues that trimethoprim-sulfamethoxazole is likely to be superior to sulfonamides alone for patients with all forms of nocardiosis. The authors acknowledge that no direct comparative data exist but offer pharmacokinetic evidence and discussion of synergy in vitro to support the use of the combination.*

Stevens DA: Clinical and clinical laboratory aspects of nocardial infection. J Hygiene 91:377, 1983. *A current review, including discussion of epidemiology, diagnosis, clinical manifestations, and treatment. Additional papers found in the same issue include: (1) Stanford JL: A simple view of nocardial taxonomy. p 369; and (2) Hay RJ: Nocardial infection of the skin. p 385.*

299 BRUCELLOSIS

Robert A. Salata

DEFINITION. Bacteria of the genus *Brucella* cause disease with protean manifestations. Transmission of infection to man from animals occurs as a consequence of occupational exposure or ingestion of contaminated milk products. Despite the attempt to institute effective control measures, brucellosis remains a significant health and economic burden in many countries.

ETIOLOGY. Brucellae are slow growing, small, aerobic, nonmotile, nonencapsulated, non–spore-forming gram-negative coccobacilli. *B. abortus*, *B. suis*, *B. melitensis*, and *B. canis*

are known to infect man and are typed on the basis of biochemical, metabolic, and immunologic criteria. There are differences in virulence among these four species. *B. abortus*, with a reservoir in cattle, usually is associated with mild sporadic disease; suppurative or disabling complications are rare. *B. suis* infection, resulting from swine contact, is often associated with destructive, suppurative lesions and may have a prolonged course. *B. melitensis*, with a reservoir in sheep and goats, may cause severe acute disease and disabling complications. *B. canis*, spread to man from infected dogs, causes disease with an insidious onset, frequent relapse, and a chronic course that is indistinguishable from infection related to *B. abortus*.

EPIDEMIOLOGY. Over 500,000 cases of brucellosis are reported yearly to the World Health Organization. *B. melitensis* infection, distributed primarily in the Mediterranean, Latin America, and Asia, accounts for the majority of cases. *B. abortus* infection occurs worldwide but has been effectively eradicated in several European countries, Japan, and Israel. *B. suis* occurs mainly in the midwestern United States, South America, and Southeast Asia, whereas *B. canis* infection is most common in North and South America, Japan, and Central Europe.

In association with effective control programs in animals, human brucellosis has decreased dramatically in the United States, from over 6000 cases in 1947 to 130 cases in 1985 (Fig. 299–1). States reporting the greatest number of cases include Texas, California, Florida, Virginia, and Iowa. In North America, brucellosis occurs mostly in spring and summer and is most common in adult males. Most occupationally related infection occurs in young workers as a primary infection, suggesting that immunity to brucellosis is acquired.

Brucella infection in the United States most frequently occurs in high-risk groups, including slaughterhouse workers, farmers and dairymen, veterinarians, travelers to endemic areas, and laboratory workers handling the organisms. Over one half of reported cases occur in the meat processing industry, particularly in the kill areas where infection is spread through abraded or lacerated skin and the conjunctiva, possibly by aerosolization, and rarely by ingestion of infected tissue. Many cases of *B. abortus* infection in veterinarians have accidentally occurred from the strain 19 vaccine used to immunize cattle. In American travelers or immigrants, Mexico has been the most frequent source of *B. melitensis* infection, transmitted through the ingestion of goat's milk cheese.

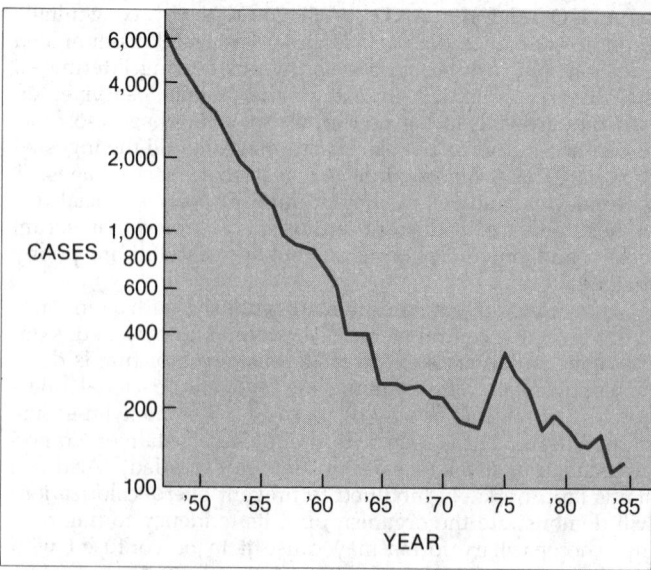

FIGURE 299–1. Incidence of human brucellosis, United States, 1947 to 1985. Following the implementation of eradication programs in cattle, the incidence of human brucellosis in the United States has steadily declined from 6321 cases in 1947 to 133 cases in 1985.

Brucellosis in children accounts for only 3 to 10 per cent of all reported cases, is most common in endemic areas, and is often a mild, self-limited process. There is no convincing evidence to associate *Brucella* infection with abortion in humans.

PATHOGENESIS AND IMMUNITY. After penetrating the epithelial cells of human skin, conjunctiva, pharynx, or lung, *Brucella* organisms initially induce an exuberant polymorphonuclear neutrophil response in the submucosa. Following ingestion of organisms by neutrophilis and tissue macrophages, spread to regional lymph nodes occurs. If host defenses within the lymph nodes are overwhelmed, bacteremia follows. The usual incubation period between infection and bacteremia is 1½ to 3 weeks. Bacteremia is accompanied by phagocytosis of free *Brucella* organisms by neutrophils and localization of bacteria primarily to the spleen, liver, and bone marrow with the formation of granulomas.

If the inoculum is large and the patient is untreated, large granulomas may form, suppurate, and serve as a source of persistent bacteremia with the potential for multiorgan spread.

Both virulent and attenuated strains of *Brucella* are readily phagocytized by neutrophils after opsonization with normal human serum. However, whole bacteria and extracts of *Brucella* species may inhibit neutrophil oxidative burst activity and degranulation. Intracellular killing of ingested bacteria has been demonstrated with *B. abortus* but not *B. melitensis*; this may explain differences in pathogenicity between these species.

Humoral factors may be important in the host defense against *Brucella*. Even in the absence of specific agglutinating antibody, normal human serum is bactericidal for *Brucella* organisms; *B. abortus* is more susceptible to serum lysis than *B. melitensis*. The intracellular location of the organism may provide a means for the bacteria to escape the lethal effects of serum. Specific serum agglutinating antibody has opsonic activity but does not correlate with the development of protective immunity.

A vital role for mononuclear phagocytes and cell-mediated immunity in brucellosis has been demonstrated. Protection against *Brucella* infection in animals is associated with preceding infection with *Listeria monocytogenes* or *Mycobacterium tuberculosis*, both of which stimulate cell-mediated immune mechanisms. Skin testing with *Brucella* proteins elicits a typical delayed hypersensitivity response in infected individuals. Activated macrophages kill *Brucella* in vitro. In some cases of chronic brucellosis, depressed proliferative responses to classic T-cell mitogens or to *Brucella* antigen occur. An increased incidence of *Brucella* infections occurs in patients with Hodgkin's disease and other lymphomas.

CLINICAL MANIFESTATIONS. Clinically, human brucellosis may be conveniently divided into subclinical illness, acute/subacute disease, localized disease and complications, relapsing infection, and chronic disease (Table 299–1).

Subclinical Illness. Detected only with serologic testing, asymptomatic or clinically unrecognized human brucellosis often occurs in high-risk groups including slaughterhouse workers, farmers, and veterinarians. Greater than 50 per cent of abattoir workers and up to 33 per cent of veterinarians have high anti-*Brucella* antibody titers but no history of recognized clinical infection. Children in endemic areas frequently have subclinical illness. Subclinical cases outnumber clinically evident cases of brucellosis by 12 to 1.

Acute and Subacute Disease. After an incubation period of several weeks or months, acute brucellosis may occur as a mild, transient illness (with *B. abortus* or *B. canis*) or as an explosive, toxic illness with the potential for multiple complications (with *B. melitensis*). Approximately 50 per cent of patients have an abrupt onset over days, while the remainder have an insidious onset over weeks. Symptoms in brucellosis are protean and nonspecific. Over 90 per cent of patients experience malaise, chills, sweats, fatigue, and weakness. More than 50 per cent of patients have myalgias, anorexia, and weight loss. Fewer patients complain of arthralgias, cough, testicular pain, dysuria, ocular pain, or visual blurring. Likewise, few localizing physical signs are apparent. Fever, often greater than 103° F, occurs in 95 per cent. An undulating or intermittent fever pattern is unusual. Because *Brucella* organisms are intracellular pathogens, a relative pulse-temperature deficit may occur. Splenomegaly is present in 10 to 15 per cent, lymphadenopathy occurs in up to 14 per cent (axillary, cervical, and supraclavicular locations are most frequent, related to hand-wound or oropharyngeal routes of infection); hepatomegaly is less frequent. Acute/subacute disease is usually associated with a significant serologic response by the standard tube agglutination assay. Other laboratory findings in acute or subacute disease may include mild anemia, lymphopenia or neutropenia (especially with bacteremia), lymphocytosis, thrombocytopenia, or (rarely) pancytopenia. The majority of infected individuals recover completely without sequelae if the diagnosis is appropriately made and prompt therapy is initiated.

Localized Disease and Complications. *Brucella* organisms may localize in almost any organ, most commonly in bone, CNS, heart, lung, spleen, testes, liver, gallbladder, or prostate. Localized disease may occur simultaneously at multiple sites. Localized complications most often appear in association with a more chronic course of illness, although complications may occur with acute disease due to *B. melitensis* or *B. suis*.

TABLE 299–1. CLINICAL CLASSIFICATION OF HUMAN BRUCELLOSIS

	Duration of Symptoms Before Diagnosis	Major Symptoms and Signs	Diagnosis	Comments
Subclinical	—	Asymptomatic	Positive (low titer) serology, negative cultures	Occurs in abattoir workers, farmers, and veterinarians
Acute and Subacute	Up to 2–3 months and 3 months to 1 year	Malaise, chills, sweats, fatigue, headache, anorexia, arthralgias, fever, splenomegaly, lymphadenopathy, hepatomegaly	Positive serology, positive blood or bone marrow cultures	Presentation can be mild, self-limited (*B. abortus*), or fulminant with severe complications (*B. melitensis*)
Localized	Occurs with acute or chronic untreated disease	Related to involved organs	Positive serology, positive cultures in specific tissues	Bone/joints, genitourinary hepatosplenic involvement most common
Relapsing	2–3 months after initial episode	Same as acute illness but may have higher fever, more fatigue, weakness, chills, and sweats	Positive serology, positive cultures	May be extremely difficult to distinguish relapse from reinfection
Chronic	Greater than 1 year	Nonspecific presentation but neuropsychiatric symptoms and low-grade fever most common	Low titer or negative serology, cultures negative	Most controversial classification, localized disease may be associated

In the United States, localized disease is most frequently related to *B. suis*.

Relapsing Infection. Up to 10 per cent of patients with brucellosis relapse after antimicrobial therapy. This probably results from the intracellular location of the organisms, which protects the bacteria from certain antibiotics and host defense mechanisms. Relapses occur most frequently within months after initial infection but may occur as long as two years after apparently successful treatment. Relapsing infection is difficult to distinguish from reinfection in high-risk groups with continued exposure. Nearly all relapsed cases respond to a repeated course of antimicrobial agents.

Chronic Disease. Disease with a duration greater than one year is called chronic brucellosis. Chronic brucellosis may be manifested in four ways: an insidious onset of disease, acute disease followed by repetitive relapses, localized disease, or persistent fatigue and weakness unresponsive to multiple antibiotic courses but with no focal signs of disease. Much controversy surrounds the inclusion of this last presentation as chronic brucellosis. Fever is seen in less than 50 per cent. Physical signs (e.g., splenomegaly, hepatomegaly, or joint involvement) are evident in only the 15 per cent of patients in whom localization of infection has occurred. Standard serology may be positive, normal, or negative. Blood cultures are typically negative.

DIAGNOSIS. Many more common illnesses mimic the clinical presentation of brucellosis. The most conclusive means of establishing the diagnosis of brucellosis is by positive cultures from normally sterile body fluids or tissues. Special media are necessary because of the unusual metabolic requirements and slow growth of *Brucella*. The culture of *Brucella* organisms is potentially hazardous to laboratory personnel; a laboratory should not undertake isolation and identification of *Brucella* unless Biosafety Level 3 facilities are available. Therefore, most cases of brucellosis are diagnosed by serologic testing.

In acute brucellosis, positive blood cultures are obtained in 10 to 30 per cent of cases (as high as 85 per cent with *B. melitensis*). Blood culture positivity decreases with increasing duration of illness. With *B. melitensis* infection, bone marrow cultures are of higher yield than blood cultures. With localized brucellosis (e.g., lymph nodes, spleen, liver, or skeletal system) cultures of purulent material or tissues usually yield *Brucella* organisms. Culture of cerebrospinal fluid is positive in 45 per cent of patients with meningitis. Antibody against *Brucella* may be demonstrated in CSF.

Most patients mount significant serologic responses to *Brucella* infections. The most frequently utilized test is the standard tube agglutination (STA) test, measuring antibody to *B. abortus* antigen. A fourfold or greater rise in titer to 1:160 or higher is considered significant. A presumptive case is one in which the agglutination titer is positive (≥ 1:160) in single or serial specimens, with symptoms consistent with brucellosis. By three weeks of illness over 97 per cent of patients demonstrate serologic evidence of infection. Several problems exist, however, with the STA test. This test equally detects antibodies to *B. abortus*, *B. suis*, and *B. melitensis*, but not to *B. canis*. Serologic confirmation of *B. canis* infection requires *B. canis* or *B. ovis* antigen. Despite adequate antibiotic treatment, significant STA titers persist for up to two years in 5 to 7 per cent of cases. As the STA titer may remain elevated, it is not useful in differentiating relapsing infection from other febrile illnesses in patients with past *Brucella* infections. Individuals with subclinical infection may demonstrate significant STA titers. In chronic localized brucellosis, STA titers may appear absent or low owing to a prozone phenomenon. This prozone effect appears to be related to the presence of IgG or IgA blocking antibodies; it can be eliminated if dilutions are carried out to at least 1:1280. False-positive STA titers due to immunologic cross-reactivity have been associated with *Bru-cella* skin testing, cholera vaccination, or infections due to *V. cholerae*, *F. tularensis*, or *Y. enterocolitica*.

IgM is the major agglutinating antibody formed in the first few weeks following infection with *Brucella* organisms. Thereafter IgG levels also rise. The STA test measures both IgM and IgG. With prompt and adequate therapy, IgG antibody levels usually become undetectable after 6 to 12 months. If therapy is given, those patients who develop persistent *Brucella* infection usually maintain elevated IgG agglutinins. The addition of 2-mercaptoethanol (2-ME) to the STA test results in the detection of only IgG antibodies. In the absence of rising STA titers, a single elevated 2-ME *Brucella* agglutination titer (≥ 1:160) suggests either current or recent infection. Since a substantial number of patients maintain elevated IgM antibodies for years after treatment, the 2-ME agglutination test helps to identify those patients who have been cured. as IgG titers usually disappear within six months of adequate treatment. Certain newer antibody tests, including an ELISA and RIA, are more sensitive than the STA; these methods have not been widely employed, and agglutination tests remain the standard for serologic diagnosis.

TREATMENT. Antibiotic treatment of *Brucella* infections is complicated by a number of complex issues. These include the requirements for antibiotic that penetrate intracellularly, for prolonged therapy to prevent relapse, and for bactericidal antibiotics in treating CNS infection and endocarditis, as well as the lack of controlled, randomized, double-blind studies comparing different antimicrobial regimens.

Tetracyclines remain the drugs of choice for brucellosis. Because of high relapse rates with short-term therapy, tetracycline at 2 grams per day in adults should be administered for four to six weeks. Tetracyclines are less effective in children. *B. canis* has also demonstrated resistance to tetracycline in vitro. The addition of streptomycin at 1 gram IM per day for the first 14 days of tetracycline therapy decreases the incidence of both relapse and localized complications; this antibiotic combination is recommended in seriously ill patients. The effectiveness of other aminoglycosides has not been evaluated in controlled studies.

Rifampin, at 600 mg daily, is brucellacidal and penetrates well both into cells and into the CSF; it should be used in cases that are refractory to tetracycline and streptomycin and should be employed in combination therapy for endocarditis and meningitis. As an alternative to tetracycline regimens, trimethoprim-sulfamethoxazole at high doses (480 mg/2400 mg per day) for at least four weeks has been generally effective; relapse rates of 40 per cent have occurred with lower doses and/or shorter duration of therapy. In limited studies, trimethoprim-sulfamethoxazole has been moderately effective in patients who have relapsed after tetracycline plus streptomycin therapy and in cases of chronic brucellosis.

In localized brucellosis, following surgical drainage of abscesses, antimicrobial agents should be administered for at least six weeks. *Brucella* endocarditis, which accounts for the highest mortality rates among *Brucella* infections, requires bactericidal drugs; early valve replacement is often necessary because of aortic valve destruction and/or major arterial emboli.

PROGNOSIS. Brucellosis appropriately treated within the first month of symptom onset is curable. Acute brucellosis often produces severe weakness and fatigue, and patients are frequently unable to work for up to two months. Immunity to reinfection follows initial *Brucella* infection in the majority of individuals.

With early antimicrobial therapy, cases of chronic brucellosis or localized disease and complications are rare. Of patients who die of brucellosis, 84 per cent have endocarditis involving a previously abnormal aortic valve, often associated with severe congestive heart failure.

PREVENTION. The control of human brucellosis relates

directly to prevention programs in domestic animals and avoidance of unpasteurized milk and milk products. In North America, the control of brucellosis in cattle involves identification and elimination of infected animals as well as vaccination of young, seronegative animals. Application of this program to swine has been much more limited to date. With control in animals and the resultant marked decrease in human cases, the need for a vaccination program in humans has been less pressing. In other countries, the experience with human vaccination has showed a narrow range between efficacy and toxicity. In slaughterhouses, important means of prevention include careful wound dressing, protective glasses and clothing, prohibition of raw meat ingestion, and the use of previously infected (immune) individuals in high-risk areas. Eradication of human cases will require elimination of disease in animals and a greater physician awareness of the epidemiology, nuances of clinical presentation, and available diagnostic and treatment strategies in *Brucella* infections.

Ariza J, et al.: Brucella spondylitis: A detailed analysis based on current findings. Rev Infect Dis 7:656, 1985. *The epidemiologic, clinical, diagnostic, and therapeutic features of spondylitis due to B. melitensis are detailed in 20 patients included in a 10-year prospective study from Barcelona, Spain.*

Arnow PM, Smaron M, Ormiste V: Brucellosis in a group of travelers to Spain. JAMA 251:505, 1984. *Describes the risk of brucellosis in travelers to endemic areas and the value of epidemiologic investigation to detect unrecognized cases.*

Buchanan TM, Faber LC, Feldman RA: Brucellosis in the United States, 1960–1972: An abattoir-associated disease. I. Clinical features and therapy. Buchanan TM, Sulzer CR, Frix MK, et al.: II. Diagnostic aspects. Buchanan TM, Hendricks SL, Patton CM, et al.: III. Epidemiology and evidence for acquired immunity. Medicine 53:403, 415, 427, 1974. *A very complete description of all aspects of brucellosis derived from a study of 160 patients in a large Iowa slaughterhouse.*

Crosby E, et al.: Hematologic changes in brucellosis. J Infect Dis 150:419, 1984. *An excellent prospective study of hematologic abnormalities in 38 patients with B. melitensis infection.*

Gotuzzo E, Carrillo C, Guerra J, et al.: An evaluation of diagnostic methods for brucellosis—The value of bone marrow culture. J Infect Dis 153:122, 1986. *The high yield of bone marrow culture in patients with B. melitensis infection is emphasized.*

Young EJ, Borchert M, Kretzer FL, et al.: Phagocytosis and killing of *Brucella* by human polymorphonuclear neutrophils. J Infect Dis 151:682, 1985. *This study provides a possible explanation for the differences in pathogenicity between B. abortus and B. melitensis based upon their susceptibility to killing by neutrophils.*

300 CAT SCRATCH DISEASE

Andrew M. Margileth

DEFINITION. Cat scratch disease is characterized by tender regional chronic lymphadenopathy that is frequently preceded by a primary skin lesion related to cat contact or scratches. The disease is usually benign, and the adenopathy resolves spontaneously in three weeks to several months.

ETIOLOGY. Since 1983, studies by Wear et al. have continued to identify a pleomorphic gram-negative rod-shaped bacterium in tissue from patients with clinical and histopathologic criteria of cat scratch disease. These specimens include 400 lymph nodes, 10 primary inoculation skin lesions, and over 12 from patients with ocular granulomas. Recently, a gram-negative pleomorphic bacillus was cultured from eight patients with subacute cat scratch disease. Further identification of this organism is pending.

EPIDEMIOLOGY. Since the initial description by Debré (1950), about 3000 patients with cat scratch disease have been reported. Cat scratch disease may occur in preschool children and in adults, but about 60 per cent present between ages 5 and 21 years. An estimated 2000 unreported cases occur annually in the United States. The disease is worldwide, occurring in all races with a predominance in males (57 per cent). In temperate zones, most cases have occurred during fall and winter. Seasonal variation is minimal in warmer climates.

TRANSMISSION AND COMMUNICABILITY. The mode of transmission is presumably by direct contact, since the bubo usually follows a scratch, bite, or lick from a young cat. Cat contact occurs in 93 per cent of patients. The disease has also developed after a dog bite or scratch and rarely after a scratch from a thorn, wood splinter, or fish bone. Person-to-person transmission has not been reported. Attempts to isolate an infectious agent from cat saliva or claws have been unsuccessful. The healthy cat—often a kitten—apparently acts as a mechanical vector for the infective agent, for skin tests with CS antigen on the implicated cats have been nonreactive. Studies in family outbreaks have shown that the family cat usually transmits the causative agent no longer than two to three weeks.

PATHOGENESIS AND PATHOLOGY. No serologic test is available to measure antibodies to the causative agent. Fortunately, the cat scratch skin test is reliable and has a high degree of specificity; the reaction is a delayed hypersensitivity type. A positive reaction is usually detected at the time the clinical diagnosis is suspected; however, conversion may be delayed up to four weeks thereafter. Cutaneous reactivity lasts up to 10 years. Recurrent lymphadenopathy has been reported recently in three adults.

Histopathologic findings of biopsied lymph nodes may show a broad spectrum of reactions: arteriolar proliferation and widening of arteriolar walls, reticulum cell hyperplasia, multiple microabscesses, frank abscess formation, and round or stellate granulomas. Other than the vascular changes, similar histopathologic findings may be found in tularemia, brucellosis, tuberculosis, lymphogranuloma venereum, and the solid granulomas in sarcoidosis. One presentation, reticulum cell hyperplasia and granulomas, is suggestive of Hodgkin's disease. Cat scratch bacilli were best demonstrated by the Warthin-Starry silver impregnation stain in nodes removed during the first three to four weeks of the illness. In early lesions these bacteria were abundant in clumps or filaments, and most readily found in vessel walls, collagen fibers, and microabscesses. The bacilli ranged in size from 0.2 to 0.3 μm in diameter, and 0.5 to 1.5 μm in length.

CLINICAL MANIFESTATIONS. The patient usually is not ill in spite of impressive lymphadenopathy; however, malaise, fever, sore throat, headache, and anorexia may be present. Three to 10 days elapse from the time of the scratch or contact until a primary skin papule or pustule forms. It may exhibit one or more erythematous papules. Unilateral conjunctival granuloma or conjunctivitis occurred in 9 per cent of the author's 832 patients. An inoculation site (a scratch or a

TABLE 300–1. CLINICAL FEATURES IN 832 PATIENTS WITH CAT SCRATCH ADENOPATHY AND A POSITIVE SKIN TEST (April 1975 to July 1986)

Category	Percentage of Patients
Animal contact	
Cat	93
Dog	6
None	1
Animal scratch	
Cat	73
Dog	2
None	25
Primary lesion	
Skin papule or pustule	49
Eye granuloma	7
Mucous membrane	5
Symptoms and signs	
None except adenopathy	51
Fever (38.3–42.1° C)	31
Malaise/fatigue	28
Headache	13
Anorexia/emesis/weight loss	13
Splenomegaly	12
Sore throat	9
Exanthem	4.4
Parotid swelling	2

primary lesion, or both) may be detected in 61 to 96 per cent of patients, depending on the thoroughness of the examination and the duration of the bubo. Most primary lesions persist for one to three weeks, rarely for months, and heal without scar formation. Regional lymphadenopathy usually develops about two weeks after the scratch (range, 3 to 50 days). Lymphangitis has not been observed. Tender nodes, present in 80 per cent of patients for the first one or two weeks, are commonly found in the head, neck, or axilla. Epitrochlear, inguinal, femoral, or occipital areas are involved less frequently. Multiple site involvement occurred in one third of the author's cases. Node size varies from 1 to 8 cm. Enlargement persists for two to four months, rarely for 6 to 24 months. Suppuration occurs in about 10 per cent of patients seen in office practice and in about 25 per cent of those admitted to hospitals.

About one half of patients have no clinical signs other than lymphadenopathy. About one third have fever (38.3 to 41.2° C) lasting for 5 to 9 (1 to 42) days; one fourth have malaise or an influenza-like syndrome lasting about 4 (1 to 21) days. Less common manifestations include splenomegaly (12 per cent), the oculoglandular syndrome of Parinaud (6 per cent), central nervous system involvement (2 per cent), and severe chronic systemic disease (2 per cent) (see Tables 300–1 and 300–2).

Children with central nervous system involvement may develop encephalopathy, meningitis, radiculitis, polyneuritis, or myelitis with paraplegia. Onset of neurologic symptoms is sudden, usually with fever, and occurs within one to six weeks of the onset of adenopathy. There may be cerebrospinal fluid pleocytosis, elevated protein, or both. Electroencephalograms are abnormal in most patients. Severe manifestations last for one to two weeks, with gradual recovery to normal status in one to six months in 90 per cent of patients.

DIAGNOSIS. Regional lymphadenopathy developing two weeks after cat contact, and especially if a primary inoculation papule or pustule followed a scratch, suggests cat scratch disease. Three of the four following manifestations would confirm the diagnosis in a typical case, whereas all four would be necessary in an atypical case: (1) a history of animal (usually cat) contact with presence of a scratch or a primary dermal or eye lesion; (2) negative laboratory studies (serology, cultures of aspirated pus or lymph node, PPD-T, and PPD-Battey) for other causes of lymphadenopathy; (3) a positive skin test result to one or two cat scratch antigens; (4) node biopsy

revealing typical histopathology, especially if pleomorphic rod-shaped bacilli can be demonstrated with the Warthin-Starry silver stain.

If a negative skin test result is found to one or two different cat scratch antigens applied simultaneously and again four weeks later, and if results of other sudies are negative, a biopsy must be considered to rule out a benign tumor or lymphoma. The presence of tenderness favors cat scratch or a pyogenic or mycobacterial adenopathy rather than a neoplasm. Ultrasonography has been very useful in deciding whether or not to aspirate nontender or nonfluctuant cervical masses. It may also aid needle placement for cyst or abscess aspiration.

Skin Tests. A skin test using cat scratch antigen is positive in 98 per cent of patients who are clinically suspected of CSD. A negative result often occurs if the duration of illness is less than three or four weeks, and 1 to 2 per cent of patients with typical cat scratch disease will have negative test results with one or two different antigens. The positive reaction consists of a wheal or papule with 5 mm or more of induration, with or without erythema, occurring 48 to 72 hours after intradermal inoculation of 0.1 ml of antigen. Induration may persist for five to six days or longer. A positive test result may be obtained for years (10 to 28) after the initial episode.

Positive reactions have been reported in veterinarians (12 to 29 per cent), healthy persons (5 per cent), and family contacts (18 per cent); the overall incidence is 5 per cent. Thus the limit of confidence for a positive reaction in a person suspected of having CSD is about 95 per cent. If the reaction is negative at four-week intervals, the disease can be excluded with reasonable certainty, especially if two different antigens are used. Repeated skin testing with CS antigen in the same patients has not produced positive reactions.

Since CS antigen is not available commercially, all aspirated pus from affected nodes should be saved to prepare test antigen. CS antigen for medical diagnosis is usually available from the author upon written request.

Laboratory Data. Laboratory tests are not diagnostic. Eosinophilia has been reported. At the onset there may be a mild leukocytosis. The erythrocyte sedimentation rate is usually elevated during the first few weeks of adenopathy.

DIFFERENTIAL DIAGNOSIS. Cat scratch disease should be considered in all patients with persistent lymphadenopathy (over three weeks), because it is the most common cause of chronic regional lymphadenitis in children or adolescents.

**TABLE 300–2. CAT SCRATCH LYMPHADENOPATHY IN 832 PATIENTS—
CLINICAL CHARACTERISTICS OF INVOLVED NODES AND DURATION OF ADENOPATHY
(April 1975 to July 1986)**

Adenopathy (N = 832)	Per Cent	Size (cm) (N = 832)	Per Cent
Single node	39	1.0 to < 3.0	43
Multiple nodes	26	3.0 to < 5.0	39
Multiple sites	35	≥ 5.0	18
Tender nodes	78		
Suppuration	16		

Location (N = 1106*)	Per Cent	Duration (N = 702)	Per Cent
Head: total (N = 196†)	18	Prior to diagnosis‡	
Submandibular	12	2 to < 4 weeks	44
Preauricular	5	1 to < 2 months	32
Neck: total (N = 437)	40	2 to < 4 months	15
Posterior	16	4 to < 6 months	3
Anterior	20	6 to < 12 months	3
Supraclavicular	3	Regression (months, < 1.0 cm)§ (N = 832)	
Extremities: total (N = 470)	42	1 to < 2	15
Axillary	25	2 to < 6	61
Epitrochlear	5.6	6 to < 12	15
Inguinal	7	12 to < 24	6
Femoral	5	≥ 24	0.7

*Mediastinal = 2, breast = 2: N = 4 (0.3%).
†Occipital = 10 (0.9%).
‡Duration ≥ 12 months = 20 (3%).
§2 to 4 weeks = 19 (2.3%)

The presence of an inoculation (dermal or ocular) lesion strongly suggests cat scratch disease. Other less common causes are sporotrichosis, primary syphilis, lymphogranuloma venereum, typical or atypical tuberculosis, other bacterial adenitis, tularemia, brucellosis, histoplasmosis, coccidioidomycosis, sarcoidosis, toxoplasmosis, infectious mononucleosis, and benign or malignant tumors. In atypical forms of cat scratch disease, one may observe benign parotid lymphosialadenopathy, Parinaud's oculoglandular disease, encephalitis, pneumonia, thrombocytopenic purpura, erythema nodosum, and osteomyelitis, as well as fluctuant lymphadenopathy simulating cystic hygroma or a thyroglossal duct cyst. If CS skin test reactions, appropriate cultures, and serologic and PPD-T and PPD-Battey skin tests are negative, a node biopsy will usually determine the cause.

TREATMENT. The best therapy is reassurance that the adenopathy is benign and in most cases will subside spontaneously within two or three months. Management consists of appropriate follow-up examination, analgesics for pain, and aspiration if suppuration occurs. The efficacy of antimicrobial therapy is unproven. In the child whose node suppurates, needle aspiration on an ambulatory basis is preferred to incision and drainage. After washing with Betadine cleanser, a needle (18 or 20 gauge) is inserted through normal unanesthetized skin at the base of the mass in order to avoid a chronic sinus tract in the event that a tuberculous lesion is present. Aspiration provides material for skin test antigen, relieves painful adenopathy, and usually allows the patient to become symptom free within 24 to 48 hours. If fluid recurs, reaspiration may be necessary. Application of moist soaks to the primary lesion may facilitate drainage and shorten the duration of lymphadenopathy. The efficacy of steroid therapy is questionable, and it is not recommended. Excisional biopsy of the node may be necessary in selected patients because of persistent pain or for diagnostic purposes.

PROGNOSIS. The prognosis is excellent; lymphadenopathy usually regresses spontaneously in two to four months. One attack appears to confer lifelong immunity. Complications and sequelae are almost nonexistent. Rarely, patients have been observed to have had chronic adenopathy for two years.

PREVENTION. Because of the number of household pets (50 million cats in the United States), cat scratch disease will be difficult to prevent. Disposal of the suspect cat is not recommended, because the cat involved is invariably well. Four to 9 per cent of family members scratched by the same cat may develop cat scratch disease. The patient with the disease does not require isolation or quarantine. Active or passive protection is not available.

Carithers HA: Cat scratch disease: An overview based on a study of 1200 patients. AM J Dis Child 139:1124, 1985. *A review of the clinical features of cat scratch disease in 1200 patients during 30 years by one author. Cat contact occurred in 99 per cent of cases, an inoculation site was detected in 93 per cent, and the cat scratch antigen test was positive in 99 per cent of patients. Unusual manifestations of CSD were observed in 60 patients: 48 had the oculoglandular syndrome of Parinaud. The remainder had osteolytic lesions, encephalopathy, erythema nodosum, and/or thrombocytopenic purpura.*

Lewis DW, Tucker SH: Central nervous system involvement in cat scratch disease. Pediatrics 77:714, 1986. *Thirty-four children had cat scratch disease associated with alterations of mental status and convulsions. The spectrum of CNS involvement is reviewed for this usually benign disease. Prognosis is generally excellent.*

Margileth AM, Wear DJ: Systemic Cat Scratch Disease: Report of 23 patients with prolonged or recurrent severe, bacterial infection. J Infect Dis 155:390, 1987. *The clinical features were evaluated in 23 patients with prolonged or recurrent severe systemic cat scratch disease. Seven patients with systemic disease had either splenic abscesses, pleurisy, hepatosplenomegaly, or enlarged lymph nodes involving the mediastinum or head of the pancreas. Compared to the usual benign course of CSD, these 23 patients had prolonged morbidity (fever, malaise, fatigue, weight loss, arthralgia, myalgia, and/or recurrent lymphadenopathy). Cat scratch bacilli were found in 15 lymph nodes and/or 4 skin biopsies of 18 of the 23 patients. All patients recovered within 21 months.*

Margileth AM, Wear DJ, Hadfield TL, et al.: Cat scratch disease: Bacteria in skin at the primary inoculation site. JAMA 252:928, 1984. *Five patients with CSD had biopsy or aspiration of adenopathy and biopsy of the primary inoculation*

skin lesion. In three patients gram-negative pleomorphic bacilli were demonstrated in the skin lesion by the Warthin-Starry silver stain, and identical bacteria were also seen in the regional lymph nodes of two of these patients.

Wear DJ, Malaty RH, Zimmerman LE, et al.: Cat scratch disease bacilli in the conjunctivae of patients with Parinaud's oculoglandular syndrome. Ophthalmology 92:1282, 1986. *Unilateral conjunctivitis with regional lymphadenitis has been designated Parinaud's oculoglandular syndrome. In 1983–84 the cause of CSD in lymph nodes and skin was established as small pleomorphic gram-negative bacilli. In this report, identical bacteria were found in the conjunctival lesions in 9 of 24 patients with Parinaud's syndrome.*

301 BARTONELLOSIS

Theodore C. Eickhoff

DEFINITION. Synonyms for bartonellosis include Carrión's disease, Oroya fever, and verruga peruana. Bartonellosis is an insect-borne bacterial disease found only in South America and characterized by two distinct stages. The first, Oroya fever, is an acute febrile hemolytic anemia with an appreciable mortality; the second, verruga peruana, is a benign cutaneous eruption of hemangiomatous papules and nodules.

ETIOLOGY. The disease is caused by *Bartonella bacilliformis*, a small gram-negative pleomorphic bacillus that may be cultivated readily in enriched bacteriologic media. The disease is transmitted to man by the bite of phlebotamine sandflies.

EPIDEMIOLOGY. Although a number of epidemics have been reported, Oroya fever is more commonly seen as sporadic cases among populations of Peru, Colombia, and Ecuador, where occurrence of the disease is restricted to those who live at or visit altitudes of 1500 to 9000 feet on both slopes of the Andes. This coincides in general with the ecologic zones supporting populations of the phlebotamine vector.

The disease is transmitted by *Lutzomyia verrucarum*, a night-biting sandfly, and possibly by other unidentified species of sandfly. The principal reservoir of the disease appears to be man; no additional animal reservoirs have been implicated. Reports of cultivation of the agent from apparently healthy persons suggest that as much as 10 per cent of infection may be subclinical.

PATHOLOGY. In Oroya fever, the causative organism may be found in peripheral blood smears stained with Giemsa's or Wright's stain, as well as in the reticuloendothelial cells. In the blood the parasite is found both free in the plasma and adherent to erythrocytes. Parasitization of the erythrocytes causes increased mechanical fragility and also increased sequestration of the cells in the spleen and liver. Because as many as 90 per cent of erythrocytes may be parasitized, a severe hemolytic anemia develops rapidly during the febrile period, erythrocyte counts decreasing within only a few days to levels of 1 to 2 million cells per cubic millimeter. Coombs' tests and tests for red cell agglutinins and hemolysins give negative results, and the mechanism of hemolysis remains poorly understood.

CLINICAL MANIFESTATIONS. Characteristic symptoms of Oroya fever follow an incubation period of two to six weeks. The presenting symptoms are intermittent high fever, painful muscles and joints, tender enlarged lymph nodes, and the systemic symptoms and prostration of a severe anemia. The patient's skin color may reflect the presence of both jaundice caused by hemolysis and marked pallor caused by profound anemia. Peripheral blood films show macrocytosis, hypochromasia, poikilocytosis, Howell-Jolly bodies, and nucleated erythrocytes. Muscle and joint pain and headache may be severe. After three to six weeks, survivors begin a slow convalescence marked by disappearance of bartonellae from the blood and gradual normalization of temperature and red cell mass.

After a variable length of time, survivors may develop the second (verruga peruana) stage of the disease, characterized by cutaneous nodules that develop over one to two months. The "verrugas" are nodular hemangiomatous lesions, 0.5 to 2 cm in diameter, that most frequently involve exposed skin but occasionally may appear on mucous membranes or in viscera. The verrugas may persist for several months to several years in untreated persons, but mortality is infrequent. The cutaneous verrugas may at times resemble the lesions of Kaposi's sarcoma. Occasional patients may experience only the fever and anemia without the skin manifestations or only the cutaneous lesions without the initial fever. Although these two aspects of the infection were once thought to be different diseases, there is ample evidence that both syndromes are manifestations of infection with the same organism. The skin lesions are believed to be an expression of incomplete immunity in the patient.

DIAGNOSIS. In the acute stage of Oroya fever both blood smears and blood culture usually reveal the presence of the agent. As the patient progresses toward the verruga stage of infection, the organism becomes more difficult to demonstrate in blood but can be regularly cultured from the cutaneous lesions.

TREATMENT AND PROGNOSIS. Mortality in the Oroya fever phase of the disease may approach 50 per cent, partic-ularly when the infection is complicated by concurrent attacks of malaria, amebiasis, tuberculosis, or salmonellosis. The disease responds well to treatment with penicillin, tetracyclines, streptomycin, or chloramphenicol. Because of the high frequency of intercurrent *Salmonella* infections, chloramphenicol is widely used for seven or more days in a dose of 2.0 to 3.0 grams daily. Patients become afebrile in 24 to 48 hours, and, if they receive transfusions, recover strength rapidly. The mortality of the verruga stage of infection is less than 5 per cent, and the lesions respond variably to chemotherapy.

PREVENTION. Prevention requires control of the sandfly vector. Spraying of interior and exterior dwellings with residual insecticide has been helpful. Personal protection may be augmented by insect repellents and bed nets.

Archer GL, Coleman PH, Cole RM, et al.: Human infection from an unidentified erythrocyte-associated bacterium. N Engl J Med 301:897, 1979. *Although bartonellae are the only well-characterized hemotrophic bacteria known, this case report suggests the possibility that there may be others. See also the accompanying editorial by Ristic M, Kreier JP: Hemotropic bacteria, pp 937–939.*

Dooley JR: Haemotropic bacteria in man. Lancet 2:1237, 1980. Kreier JP, Ristic M: The biology of hemotrophic bacteria. Ann Rev Microbiol 35:325, 1981. *These two reviews are an excellent introduction to the broad topic of hemotrophic bacteria.*

Schultz MG: Daniel Carrión's experiment. N Engl J Med 278:1323, 1968. *A fascinating account of the young Peruvian medical student, Daniel Carrión, who demonstrated by his death that verruga peruana and Oroya fever were caused by the same etiologic agent.*

Diseases Due to Mycobacteria

302 TUBERCULOSIS

Emanuel Wolinsky

DEFINITION. Tuberculosis is a chronic infectious disease caused by mycobacteria of the "tuberculosis complex," mainly *Mycobacterium tuberculosis*.

INCIDENCE. During the Industrial Revolution of the eighteenth and ninteenth centuries, the disease was known as the *white plague*. It was the leading cause of death in young people all over the world. Today, despite great progress in its treatment and control, it is still an important medical problem in many developing countries. There are still 4 to 10 million new cases and about 1 million deaths each year from tuberculosis. In the United States tuberculosis mortality has decreased from a rate of 202 per 100,000 in 1900 to less than 1 in 1982. The new case rate has also declined from about 60 per 100,000 in 1950 to 9 in 1985. During the last few years, however, there has been little decline, and even an upsurge in 1986, in the number of new cases reported, thought to be partially related to the association of tuberculosis with the acquired immunodeficiency syndrome (AIDS).

The rate of infection as determined by skin test surveys remains high in many developing countries. In the United States the rate has become increasingly difficult to estimate because of the abandonment of large-scale testing in cities. Information obtained in 1977 from selected urban areas of the country indicated that the rate of infection varied from less than 3 per cent in young children to 14 to 40 per cent in adults over the age of 65. Tuberculosis is becoming more and more a disease of middle-aged and older nonwhite men in residual urban pockets of disease associated with poverty and overcrowding.

ETIOLOGY. The microorganism that causes tuberculosis belongs to the genus *Mycobacterium*, which is classified in the family Mycobacteriaceae of the order Actinomycetales. Other families in this order are the Actinomycetaceae, with genera *Actinomyces* and *Nocardia*, and the Streptomycetaceae, which includes the genus *Streptomyces*. Taxonomists do not agree on the further classification of the genus *Mycobacterium*, but a useful concept is that of the tuberculosis complex to include *M. tuberculosis*, *M. bovis*, and probably *M. africanum*. Some taxonomists would subdivide *M. bovis* into European, Afro-Asian, and African variants. A few suggest that there should be just one species, *M. tuberculosis*, with subclassifications of bovine type, African type, and so forth.

M. tuberculosis is an obligate intracellular parasite that shares with other mycobacteria a characteristic staining quality. The popular abbreviation *AFB* for *acid-fast bacilli* is based on this quality. Acid-fastness is the result of retention of carbol fuchsin (or certain fluorochrome dyes) after washing with acid, alcohol, or both. It is not unique to mycobacteria, since *Nocardia* and certain *Corynebacterium* strains may also be acid fast. Mycobacterial cell walls are rich in lipids, existing mainly as complexes with peptides and polysaccharides. Certain stains can form a stable complex with one of these lipid compounds, mycolic acid, provided the latter is contained within an intact cell wall structure.

In addition to the members of the tuberculosis complex, the genus *Mycobacterium* may be divided into about 30 species. Again, there is disagreement among the taxonomists on the definition of many of these species (see Ch. 303).

PATHOLOGY AND PATHOGENESIS. Tuberculosis is derived from the word tubercle, meaning a small lump or nodule. Histopathologically, the tubercle is a more or less discrete focus of granulomatous inflammation consisting of lymphocytes, epithelioid cells, macrophages, and giant cells. The granulomas seen in tuberculosis are characterized by a form of tissue necrosis known as *caseation*, so called because the caseum has the consistency of soft cheese. Prior to the time of necrosis the lesion may heal completely by resolution, but once necrosis and caseation have occurred it heals by fibrosis, encapsulation, calcification, and scar formation. Breakdown of the lesion occurs when the caseum softens and liquefies and is expelled through the bronchial system. This process results in the formation of a cavity in the lung. Spread of disease may occur by local extension, by an intrabronchial route, or through the lymphohematogenous pathway. Early in the primary infection the organisms are transported to the draining lymph nodes and may be widely disseminated throughout the body. In the apical posterior areas of the upper lobes the seeded organisms may remain dormant in inactive lesions for many years only to reactivate during a period of lowered host immunity. The processes of healing and breakdown may occur sequentially and repeatedly so that various stages of the inflammatory reaction are seen in different areas.

The primary lesion in a nonsensitized individual consists of an area of nonspecific pneumonitis in a middle or lower lung zone at the site of deposition of the inhaled droplet nuclei. The initial inflammatory response is the same as that seen in any bacterial pneumonia and consists mainly of fibrin, edema, and polymorphonuclear leukocytes. The extent of this primary exudative response varies with the number and virulence of the bacilli inhaled, the native resistance of the host, and the effectiveness of the immune response. The change to a granulomatous type of reaction occurs coincidentally with the development of delayed hypersensitivity after two or three weeks. The mechanisms of cellular immunity may allow the host to wall off the lesion and to halt the lymphohematogenous spread. It is the softening and liquefaction of the caseous focus that leads to further trouble and the provision of a favorable environment for the rapid multiplication of the mycobacteria. In the encapsulated lesion that does not soften, the bacilli slowly lose their viability.

Stages in the natural history of untreated pulmonary tuberculosis, especially as it occurs in childhood, may be described as follows:

1. During the primary phase and throughout the development of the lesions there are usually no symptoms. Even in the so-called manifest primary stage, symptoms may be mild or absent despite parenchymal lesions and enlarged hilar or mediastinal lymph nodes. Pleurisy with effusion may occur. Life-threatening complications at this stage are meningitis and miliary disease.

2. The primary disease usually heals, leaving evidence of its presence in the form of a calcified pulmonary scar along with calcifications in the draining lymph nodes, which together are known as a *Ghon's complex.*

3. The third stage is one of latency, during which the bacilli remain dormant but still viable within inactive lesions. This situation may exist for the remainder of the patient's life.

4. Reactivation may occur in a relatively small proportion of infected individuals. This is the mechanism by which tuberculosis in the adult usually develops, either in the lung or in an extrapulmonary site.

5. Exogenous reinfection occasionally may be documented by the demonstration of bacilli with a different phage type or drug sensitivity pattern from those of the primary infection.

EPIDEMIOLOGY. Infection is usually transmitted from person to person by the inhalation of infective droplet nuclei that result from the aerosolization of respiratory secretions. The source of the infected material usually is an adult with cavitary pulmonary tuberculosis. The most important determinants of infectivity are the concentration of organisms in the sputum and the closeness and duration of contact with the index case. Other factors of importance are the cough frequency and the personal habits of the index case, the efficiency with which aerosols are produced by such activities as singing, loud talking, and laughing, and the air circulation and ventilation in the area of contact. A situation favorable to acquisition of infection would be an overcrowded and poorly ventilated house in which there were several young children and an adult with highly positive sputum.

Ingestion is no longer a common pathway for infection, although in the days of unpasteurized milk and widespread tuberculosis in cattle this was a common route of infection for *M. bovis,* especially for the production of tuberculosis of the tonsils and subsequent involvement of the submandibular lymph nodes. Another route of infection that still may be observed, however, is primary inoculation through the skin. Laboratory workers may inoculate themselves with actively growing cultures via needle puncture or broken glass, and pathologists may sustain a penetrating injury while doing a postmortem examination.

Many localized outbreaks or miniepidemics have been reported in the past and continue to be observed today (Lincoln, 1967; Stead, 1979). The pattern of airborne transmission in a closed environment is well described in these accounts of infections aboard ships, in day care centers, nursing homes, prisons, industrial school dormitories, school buses, and among members of a choir.

Tuberculosis Control. Tuberculosis is perpetuated by the repeated cycle of new infections that result from the inhalation of infected droplet nuclei coughed into the air by adults with cavitary pulmonary disease. This cycle may be attacked at several points. Case-finding efforts are needed to recognize individuals with active disease so that they may be placed under treatment to terminate the infectivity. Large-scale roentgenographic surveys have been abandoned in favor of contact investigation, recognition of symptomatic cases at entry points to the medical care system, and surveillance of high-risk groups such as hospital personnel, prisoners, and nursing home patients.

Protection from the complications of primary disease may be afforded by vaccination with bacille Calmette-Guérin (BCG). This was a strain of *M. bovis* attenuated by many passages on artificial media. There are now many different strains, each unique, maintained in laboratories across the world. Vaccination has been utilized mainly in areas of the world that have a high rate of tuberculosis infection. Although vaccination may protect the individual, it does not reduce the overall rate of infection in the community, since it does not prevent the transmission of infection. Its effectiveness depends on an enhancement of the immune response, which enables the host to eliminate most of the bacilli before tissue destruction and dissemination occur. The efficacy of BCG is controversial. It has not been used extensively in the United States because it interferes with the subsequent use of the tuberculin test in recognizing tuberculosis infection and because the major source of morbidity is people already infected. Nevertheless, a case could be made for BCG in certain special circumstances such as to protect the infant whose mother has active disease and to prevent infection in close contacts of an index case with drug-resistant bacilli.

Chemoprophylaxis may prevent infection in close contacts with negative skin tests, prevent disease in those already infected, and prevent subsequent recurrences in individuals with inactive pulmonary disease. The recommended drug for prophylaxis is isoniazid, once daily, in a dosage of 300 mg for adults and 10 mg per kilogram (not to exceed 300 mg) for children. When taken for one year, such treatment results in a reduction of at least 70 per cent in the appearance of primary disease in household contacts. Protection is about 90 per cent in those who actually take the drug as prescribed. The effectiveness of shorter courses of therapy has not been adequately investigated. Six months of chemoprophylaxis, while not completely ineffective, protects less well than 12 months. The two principal drawbacks to this method of control are isoniazid-related hepatitis and the failure of about 30 per cent of patients to take the prescribed medication.

The risk of developing active disease in recent tuberculin converters of any age is about 3.3 per cent in the first year after infection. From 5 to 15 per cent may progress to active disease within five years. The risk is greater in infants. Chemoprophylaxis is recommended for close contacts of patients with recently diagnosed active disease; for persons with recent infection documented by skin test conversion within the past two years; for individuals with positive skin test results, radiographic findings consistent with inactive tuberculous disease, and neither positive bacteriologic findings nor a history of adequate chemotherapy; and for individuals with positive skin test results who have additional risk factors (such as malignancy or severe diabetes) or who are undergoing prolonged immunosuppressive or corticosteroid therapy. Although chemoprophylaxis is one of the important methods of tuberculosis control in this country, it has not been accepted in many other parts of the world. Isoniazid will not prevent disease resulting from infection with isoniazid-resistant bacilli. Rifampin has been suggested as a substitute, although no good studies of its efficacy have been published.

IMMUNOLOGY. Tuberculosis is the classic example of disease caused by an intracellular parasite. Protection is afforded by the mechanisms of cell-mediated immunity rather than by those associated with antibodies. Immunity may be natural or acquired, but in either case it is the macrophage that assumes the major burden of protection. Polymorphonuclear leukocytes have the ability to phagocytize but not to destroy mycobacteria. Although the results of some experiments are contradictory, most researchers have been able to demonstrate that macrophages from an immunized animal kill the bacilli more efficiently and at a more rapid rate than do control cells. Macrophages may be activated by immunologically specific mechanisms as well as by nonspecific stimulation. Specific stimulation occurs when sensitized T lymphocytes contact mycobacterial antigens that have been properly processed by macrophages. The lymphocytes then release a number of active chemical substances known as *lymphokines*, one variety of which activates macrophages.

Native immunity certainly has played a role in the global aspects of tuberculosis. Good examples exist in the animal kingdom; the rat and the cat are quite resistant to infection with *M. tuberculosis*, in contrast to the guinea pig and the monkey, which are highly susceptible. Lurie was able to breed two races of rabbits, one susceptible and one resistant to infection. Although it is difficult to separate the factors of social and economic conditions from those of race, the Eskimo peoples and blacks are considered by some researchers to be more susceptible. The forces of natural selection probably contributed to the decline of tuberculosis prior to the introduction of chemotherapy, although improved socioeconomic conditions played an important role. Acquired immunity may occur as a result of natural infection or by vaccination. Recovery from tuberculosis confers protection against reinfection with a new inoculum, even though the original bacilli may remain latent for many years and be capable of producing recrudescent disease. Whether acquired by natural infection or vaccination, the protection is only relative and may be overwhelmed by a sufficiently large infecting dose.

The relationship between delayed hypersensitivity and immunity is still controversial. The two functions appear at about the same time after infection and are intimately related thereafter. Nevertheless, it has been shown in experimental animals that immunity may remain despite abolition of a positive skin test result by desensitization and that immunity may be induced by ribosome preparations that do not induce a positive skin reaction.

The balance between the reactions of delayed hypersensitivity and those of the humoral antibody response is very important in determining the clinical presentation and prognosis in leprosy. A similar but less dramatic situation exists in tuberculosis. A more favorable prognosis may be expected for patients who have strong reactivity in their cell-mediated immune functions than for those who are hypoergic and have abundant antibody production. Patients with nonreactive tuberculosis tend to have disseminated disease with almost unopposed multiplication of the organisms in reticuloendothelial cells and a lack of granulomatous response. The question

of whether the anergic state is the cause or the result of severe tuberculosis is moot. Recovery of the compromised cell-mediated immune functions, including delayed hypersensitivity, usually accompanies clinical improvement. A patient's location in the immune spectrum usually is dynamic and changeable rather than fixed.

The Tuberculin Skin Test. The biologically active material in the liquid medium after growth of *M. tuberculosis* was named *tuberculin* by Robert Koch. This crude material was later called *Old Tuberculin (OT)*. A purified protein derivative of tuberculin *(PPD)* was made by Siebert in 1924 by precipitation with saturated ammonium sulfate. The World Health Organization adopted a large batch, designated *PPD-S*, as the international standard tuberculin. Five tuberculin units *(TU)* was defined as the biologic activity contained in a specified weight of PPD-S. Solutions with much greater stability were achieved by the addition of a wetting agent. All preparations of PPD commercially available in this country must be bioequivalent to 5 TU of PPD-S as demonstrated by comparative testing in humans.

The intracutaneous, or Mantoux, test is performed by injecting 5 TU contained in 0.1 ml of solution intracutaneously with needle and syringe. This is known as the intermediate-strength test. It corresponds to 0.1 µg of the standard preparation. A more dilute solution containing 1 TU is available to test those who may be expected to have a very strong reaction, especially children. This preparation is known as first-strength PPD and is essentially a fivefold dilution of the 5 TU material. Second-strength PPD contains what is calculated to be 250 TU.

In the sensitized individual a reaction of redness, swelling, and induration will begin at about 6 hours, reach a maximum intensity at 36 to 60 hours, and then fade over the next several days. A positive result usually is defined as 10 mm or more of induration at 48 hours. This arbitrary definition is based on results of large-scale testing that showed that a reaction of 10 mm best separated those with from those without tuberculosis. The reading of the test is a subjective evaluation, with wide observer variation. It is only by averaging multiple readings made blindly by at least two expert readers that an accuracy within 3 mm may be approached.

It is unwise to have an arbitrary definition of a positive reaction in the diagnostic evaluation of a sick patient. Many factors may diminish the response in a nonspecific manner. They include virus infections or live virus vaccination; immunosuppression by disease, drugs, or steroids; malnutrition; overwhelming infection of any kind; and old age. It is best to measure the induration as accurately as possible and, in addition, to describe the intensity of both the erythema and the induration. Erythema that persists for 72 hours is usually indicative of a positive reaction. In case of doubt, it is often useful to repeat the test using 250 TU. If there is no reaction to the second-strength material, the odds against the diagnosis of nondisseminated tuberculosis are approximately 50 to 1. It is helpful to determine the reaction to other antigens utilizing the so-called *anergy panel*. The most useful are mumps, *Candida*, trichophytin, tetanus toxoid, and a streptococcal antigen such as streptokinase. Failure to react to the panel indicates a generalized state of cutaneous anergy, which may be expected to include tuberculin. Several multiple puncture devices are available for performing a tuberculin test. They should all be regarded as screening tests, and any doubtful or positive reactions should be tested with the Mantoux technique.

Intradermal administration of tuberculin in the recommended dosage does not induce an immunologic response even after repeated injections. However, a second injection from 2 weeks to 12 months after an original negative reaction may produce a booster response from recall of waning delayed hypersensitivity. To avoid the assumption that the positive reaction represents a new infection, it has been suggested that negative reactors be retested up to a week later in surveillance programs such as those for hospital personnel. Infection with any mycobacterium and probably with organisms of related genera, such as *Nocardia* and *Corynebacterium*, may give cross-reactions with the tuberculin test materials available today. Tuberculin reactivity is a quantitative function that may vary in intensity from time to time in a given person.

Factors Modifying the Course of Tuberculosis. Before chemotherapy, tuberculosis patients were considered to be at risk for recrudescent disease for the rest of their lives. Mitchell was able to follow over 2000 patients for 15 to 25 years after their moderately or far advanced disease had become inactive. He found a relapse rate of 28 per cent. Even with modern drug therapy relapse occasionally may occur, depending mainly on whether or not the patient was cooperative in taking medication. A study of 20,000 cases reported to the Centers for Disease Control in 1980 revealed that 7 to 8 per cent represented recurrent disease.

Many conditions are known to increase the risk for the recurrence of tuberculosis. Among these are emotional stress, malnutrition, drug addiction, alcoholism, immunosuppression by diseases that interfere with cell-mediated immunity, and the use of drugs such as corticosteroids. Gastric resection is a risk factor, presumably in relation to malnutrition. A risk over ten times that of suitable controls has been documented for patients with chronic renal failure on maintenance dialysis or for those with renal transplants. Influenza, pneumonia, and cancer of the lung may cause local reactivation of dormant lesions. Another local factor is pneumoconiosis, especially silicosis and coal worker's pneumoconiosis.

CLINICAL DESCRIPTION. *Pulmonary Tuberculosis.* Tuberculosis may involve any organ system, but the lung is the usual site of the primary lesion and the principal organ involved. In roughly one half of patients with extrapulmonary disease, however, the original pulmonary lesions may not be discernible clinically or radiographically.

PRIMARY TUBERCULOSIS. Primary tuberculosis refers to disease in a person not previously infected with a virulent mycobacterium of the tuberculosis complex. This definition excludes persons who have had BCG vaccination or infection with other mycobacteria. Primary tuberculosis formerly was seen almost exclusively in children and was known as the childhood type. At present it is not uncommon in adults of all ages. Most primary infections are subclinical and not detectable by ordinary radiographic procedures. They may be recognized, however, by a documented tuberculin skin test conversion. When accompanied by symptoms or radiographic evidence, or both, the disease is called manifest or overt primary tuberculosis. Enlarged hilar lymph nodes are almost always seen. Complications of the primary infection include pleurisy with effusion, miliary disease, meningitis, bone and joint disease, and progressive primary infection. In progressive primary disease the lesions enlarge, caseate, liquefy, and cavitate. Primary disease in adults is especially prone to progression and cavity formation.

The morbidity and mortality associated with primary infection are related to age. Although usually benign in older children and adults, it is life threatening when it occurs in infants. In a New York City study before the development of chemotherapy, tuberculosis in children less than six months of age had a mortality rate of 50 per cent. Congenital tuberculosis, often fatal, may be acquired from a mother with active disease by the hematogenous route or by the aspiration or ingestion of contaminated amniotic fluid. A unique finding in primary tuberculosis of young children is the development of consolidated and collapsed segmental lesions resulting from a combination of bronchial compression from enlarged hilar lymph nodes and extrusion of caseous contents into the bronchial lumen. This situation usually is clinically benign despite the alarmingly unhealthy appearance of the chest

roentgenogram. The spectrum of primary tuberculosis in adults was documented by Stead and colleagues in 1968. In almost half of 37 adults the disease progressed without interruption into chronic pulmonary tuberculosis.

REACTIVATION TUBERCULOSIS. This term refers to the pattern of disease in adults. It usually results from the reactivation of dormant foci in the posterior portions of the upper lobes that had been seeded by the bloodstream during the early primary infection. Occasionally adult disease is the result of a new inoculum of tubercle bacilli in a person already sensitized by a previous infection *(exogenous reinfection)*. Adult disease is characterized by chronicity, caseation, sloughing of liquefied caseous material, cavity formation, and the simultaneous occurrence of healing and progression in different areas of the lung. Lymph node involvement is usually minimal or absent, at least in those nodes that directly drain the pulmonary foci. Phage typing of strains recovered from different areas of the body and correlation between antimicrobial susceptibility patterns and the history of drug intake have been used to document both recrudescence of an old infection and exogenous reinfection.

The onset of disease may be *insidious, catarrhal, hemoptoic,* or *acute.* With insidious onset there is gradual development of fatigue, anorexia, weight loss, and other vague complaints. Later, a low-grade intermittent fever may develop that is commonly associated with excessive sweating at night. The temperature elevation tends to occur in the late afternoon. The catarrhal onset is characterized by an increasingly productive cough and occasional blood streaking of the sputum. Fever and night sweats may also be noted. In the hemoptoic variety, the presenting symptom is hemoptysis either with or without other symptoms already mentioned. Occasionally, the onset is acute and influenza-like with high fever, chills, myalgia, and productive cough. Pleuritic pain may be the presenting complaint, often without pleural fluid but sometimes ushering in the appearance of an effusion. Many cases of adult-type pulmonary tuberculosis in the past were discovered by routine chest films in asymptomatic persons. Some individuals might recall minor symptoms, such as slight pleurisy, night sweats, or tiredness, but others would deny all warning signs despite the presence of advanced disease. Before the advent of chemotherapy it was not unusual for the patient to have hoarseness or perirectal abscess—both conditions being secondary to the long-term presence of highly positive sputum.

DIAGNOSIS. A careful history and physical examination often suggest the diagnosis of pulmonary tuberculosis before any laboratory test is ordered. The most characteristic physical findings of adult-type disease are rales heard posteriorly near the apex of one or both lungs. The chest radiographs will then confirm the presence of disease in the posterior portion of the upper lobes. Visualization of one or more cavities strengthens the diagnosis. In primary tuberculosis the initial pneumonic area may be anywhere in the lung, especially in the middle or lower lobes, with enlargement of the draining lymph nodes in the mediastinum. These characteristic patterns are not always seen, however. In a recent report from a large teaching hospital, the diagnosis of tuberculosis was not suggested by the radiologist in 26 per cent of 100 consecutive cases. A wide variety of unusual patterns may be encountered, from mass lesions resembling malignancy to widespread interstitial disease of a nonspecific nature. Diabetics are more likely than nondiabetics to have lower lobe disease, which may also be noted as a bronchogenic spread from apical cavities.

Confirmation of the diagnosis should be sought by bacteriologic examination of the sputum. It may be necessary to obtain specimens by the inhalation of nebulized distilled water or saline solution or by gastric lavage. In addition to properly stained smears and cultures for acid-fast bacilli, it is useful to search for elastic fibers by unstained potassium hydroxide wet mounts. The presence of these fibers indicates destruction of lung tissue and should be accompanied by smears positive for AFB. Occasionally, it may be necessary to resort to bronchoscopy and even to lung biopsy to establish the diagnosis.

The tuberculin skin test is very useful in diagnosis, despite the fact that 5 to 20 per cent of those with newly diagnosed cases may have a negative response to the initial test. Transient depression of cell-mediated immune reactions either may be specific for tuberculin or may take the form of a generalized anergy to all skin test antigens. For immediate diagnostic purposes in such cases, it is useful to apply a second-strength PPD containing 250 TU, which will give a false-negative reaction in no more than 1 to 2 per cent of patients without disseminated disease or severe debility.

Recent innovations in laboratory tests include automated radiometric culture methods that allow for more rapid results and simultaneous differentiation of *M. tuberculosis* from other mycobacteria; enzyme immunoassay recognition of mycobacterial antigens in the sputum; and serodiagnosis by enzyme-linked immunosorbent assay to detect antibodies against specific *M. tuberculosis* antigens.

DIFFERENTIAL DIAGNOSIS. Many subacute and chronic pulmonary conditions, both infectious and noninfectious, may be confused with tuberculosis. Some pulmonary mycoses, especially histoplasmosis, may present with a similar clinical and radiologic picture. Pyogenic lung abscess as well as pneumonia with a delayed resolution may be confused with tuberculosis. A pyogenic lung abscess is likely to have more fluid within it, hence a higher air-fluid level, and more dense consolidation around it. When repeated examinations of the sputum are negative for AFB, one should increase efforts at establishing another diagnosis. Tuberculomas may be confused with similar lesions arising from several different fungal infections and with pulmonary neoplasms. Sarcoidosis and tuberculosis may have similar manifestations. One third of cases of fever of unknown origin are due to infection, and extrapulmonary tuberculosis is still prominent among these cases.

TREATMENT. *Historical Perspective.* For many decades the physician relied upon nonspecific measures to treat tuberculosis. These measures included fresh air, good food, bed rest, and graded exercise, among others. The idea of the cottage sanatorium was started in this country in 1884 to accommodate these feeble attempts at treatment. Measures designated to collapse cavities and to put diseased portions of the lungs "at rest" included artificial pneumothorax, pneumoperitoneum, phrenic nerve crush, and various forms of thoracoplasty. Resectional surgery became popular after the introduction of effective drug therapy.

The era of chemotherapy began in 1945 with Waksman's discovery of streptomycin. In 1949 it was shown that treatment with the combination of streptomycin and para-aminosalicylic acid (PAS) delayed the emergence of streptomycin-resistant tubercle bacilli. With the introduction of isoniazid in 1952 it became possible to treat the disease with two drugs given by mouth. A course of 18 to 24 months was recommended by studies of relapse rates and the bacteriology of lesions removed at lung resection as related to duration of treatment. Ethambutol, marketed in 1961, replaced PAS because of its relative lack of annoying side effects. These drugs rendered all previous modes of therapy obsolete, and most sanatoriums in this country were closed by 1960. A study done in India in 1960 demonstrated that home treatment was not risky for the patient or his or her family. It was documented in 1973 that supervised intermittent treatment twice a week was just as beneficial as daily treatment, especially for the ambulatory continuation phase after a period of daily drug therapy. Such intermittent treatment is especially suited for uncooperative patients. The introduction of rifampin in 1966 provided not only another very powerful antituberculosis agent, but also the opportunity to shorten the duration of therapy by at least one half. Published reports on short-course chemotherapy began to appear in 1972. With proper combinations and rhythm of administration it is now possible to achieve excellent results with six months of treatment, provided that all doses are consumed as prescribed.

The Antituberculosis Drugs. Isoniazid (INH) is the most important drug in original treatment regimens. It is easily synthesized, highly stable, inexpensive, and well tolerated. The drug is well absorbed when given by mouth and also may be administered parenterally. It is widely distributed throughout the body, including the central nervous system, and it reaches bacilli within cells. The drug exerts a bactericidal effect on actively multiplying bacilli. Adverse reactions may occur in approximately 5 per cent of cases with a daily dose of 5 mg per kilogram per day, usually given as 300 mg once daily for adults. A common toxicity is peripheral neuropathy, based on interference with the metabolism of pyridoxine. It is directly related to the dose and blood level and is more likely to be seen in genetically constituted slow acetylators and in malnourished individuals. Neuropathy can be prevented by the administration of 25 mg of pyridoxine daily and is not likely to occur when ordinary doses of INH are used in nonalcoholic, nondiabetic, well-nourished, and relatively young patients. The most important adverse reaction is hepatitis of the hepatocellular variety. Although approximately 10 per cent of healthy individuals may have asymptomatic elevations of aminotransferases within the first two months of treatment, the enzyme levels usually return to normal despite the continued administration of the drug. The risk of hepatitis is related to age, being less than 1 per cent in those under 35 and increasing with age to 2.3 per cent at age 60. Hepatitis usually occurs within the first few months of treatment but occasionally appears in later stages. Heavy alcohol intake is associated with a greater risk of hepatitis. Several fatalities from INH hepatitis have been reported, mainly in patients whose reaction occurred late and in those who continued to take the drug despite progressive symptoms.

Some rare untoward effects include encephalopathy, loss of memory, optic atrophy, convulsions, hemolytic anemia, and purpura. The usual hypersensitivity reactions such as drug fever and skin rash occasionally may be seen. Isoniazid is one of several drugs that can produce a lupus-like syndrome. Although INH is excreted promptly and mainly by the kidneys, the half-life is prolonged only slightly in patients with renal failure.

Rifampin (RMP) is comparable to INH in its bactericidal effect on metabolically active bacilli. It is an antibiotic of the rifamycin family and is much more expensive than INH. Well absorbed when taken orally in a fasting state, the drug is widely distributed and penetrates well into cells and into the central nervous system when the meninges are inflamed. It differs from most of the antituberculosis drugs in that it has good activity against a variety of gram-positive and gram-negative bacteria. Its activity depends upon inhibition of DNA-dependent RNA polymerase activity. Rifampin is well tolerated by most patients in a dosage of 10 mg per kilogram per day, usually given to adults as 600 mg once daily by mouth. A parenteral preparation is not yet generally available, although it may be obtained from the manufacturer in emergency situations. Hepatitis is the most important adverse effect, occurring in about 1 per cent of patients. There are conflicting reports on the risk of hepatitis when INH and RMP are given together. Most studies now indicate no excessive risk. An exception occurs in the treatment of children, for whom a dosage of greater than 10 mg per kilogram per day of INH given with RMP is associated with a high risk of hepatitis.

Allergic reactions occasionally occur, especially in those individuals who take the drug irregularly or in those who are given intermittent treatment twice weekly in a dosage greater than 600 mg. These reactions include chills and fever and more rarely acute renal failure, thrombocytopenia, and massive hemolysis. Rifampin may induce enzymes in the liver that increase metabolic degradation of several other drugs, such as oral contraceptive agents and anticoagulants. The drug is excreted mainly by the liver and biliary tract and therefore must be given with caution to patients with liver failure.

Ethambutol (EMB) is a synthetic chemical compound that is well absorbed when given by mouth and is excreted mainly in the urine. Thus, the drug should be given with great care to patients with poor renal function, for whom dosage must be reduced and blood levels followed carefully. Aside from its principal toxicity, optic neuritis, there are very few adverse effects. Optic nerve toxicity is directly related to dosage and blood levels. At the recommended dosage of 15 mg per kilogram per day, optic neuritis is very rare, but some physicians administer 25 mg per kilogram per day for the first two or three months, at which dosage approximately 3 per cent of patients may have impaired visual acuity. When the higher dose is used, periodic examinations for visual acuity are indicated. The toxicity usually is reversible if administration of the drug is discontinued promptly.

Pyrazinamide (PZA) is an important drug because of its excellent tissue-sterilizing ability when used in combination with other bactericidal drugs. It is well absorbed from the gastrointestinal tract, is widely distributed throughout the body water, and penetrates well into the central nervous system. The drug is active against only one species of *Mycobacterium*, *M. tuberculosis*, and then only at the low pH of 5.0 to 5.5. It is especially useful to kill tubercle bacilli within macrophages, into whose acidic environment it penetrates well. It is excreted mainly by way of the kidneys. Allergic reactions are rare, but joint pains and occasionally gout may occur as the result of a hyperuricemic effect. Hepatitis may occur in about 1 per cent of patients receiving the recommended daily dose of 20 to 30 mg per kilogram, usually 1.5 grams for small and 2.0 grams for large adults, given by mouth once daily.

Streptomycin (SM) is an aminoglycoside antibiotic that has been chemically defined and synthesized. It is not absorbed when given by mouth. The principal method of elimination is through the kidneys, so that dosage adjustment is necessary when renal function is reduced. It is distributed largely in the extracellular fluid and does not enter appreciably into the central nervous system or into macrophages. The dosage is 10 to 15 mg per kilogram per day, given intramuscularly, usually as 0.75 to 1.0 gram once daily in adults with normal renal function. As with other aminoglycosides, damage to the renal tubules is common, as manifested by cylindruria, but renal function is not compromised unless blood levels of the drug are excessive. The major toxicity is exerted against the eighth nerve, of which the vestibular division is more likely to be affected, although deafness may also be produced. The seriousness of these reactions makes periodic testing of renal and eighth nerve function advisable, especially in the elderly. Measurements of blood levels should be obtained whenever renal function is in question. Allergic reactions are fairly common, as are paresthesias of the lips and extremities immediately after injection. The drug is bactericidal against tubercle bacilli. The maximum effect is exerted at a pH of 7.7.

Kanamycin and *capreomycin* are used as substitutes for SM when the organisms are resistant to that drug or on the rare occasions when the patient cannot tolerate SM. Dosages, methods of administration, and adverse reactions are similar to those of SM. More care is needed with kanamycin, since it is slightly more ototoxic and nephrotoxic than SM, especially on the cochlear division of the eighth nerve.

Ethionamide and *cycloserine* are not used for initial therapy but are reserved for retreatment cases and for special situa-

tions of drug intolerance and bacillary resistance. Both drugs are given by mouth in dosages of 10 to 15 mg per kilogram per day. The administration of ethionamide is accompanied by rather severe gastrointestinal upset and occasionally by hepatitis, and allergic reactions are common. Allergic reactions with cycloserine are rare, but aberrations of mental function and seizures are quite common.

Drug Regimens. Until the landmark short-course chemotherapy studies of the British Medical Research Council and its cooperative investigators, the conventional drug regimens for initial treatment consisted mainly of INH and EMB for one and one half to two years, supplemented by RMP or SM for the first month or two in patients with far advanced disease. An intermittent regimen consisting of supervised twice-weekly drug administration can be used after the initial two or three months of daily treatment. Dosages in milligrams per kilogram recommended for intermittent treatment are as follows: INH 15, SM 25 to 30, EMB 50, and RMP 10 to 15 (usually no more than 600 mg total). With a fully compliant patient and drug-sensitive bacilli, the success rate is well over 95 per cent with long-term treatment. The main problems are related to the long-term administration of a drug regimen and include ensuring compliance with recommended treatment and the cost of supervision and follow-up to the local health department. The conventional regimen has been all but abandoned in favor of short-course treatment.

SHORT-COURSE TREATMENT. The first report of successful short-course treatment was published in 1968 and involved experience in East Africa. From the results of many other trials conducted since then, it appears that the minimum requirements include therapy with INH and RMP for at least nine months. The addition of a third drug—EMB, SM, or PZA—for the first one to three months of intensive treatment guards against the eventuality of infection with INH- or RMP-resistant bacilli. To shorten the course to six months, a third drug is necessary. That drug should be PZA for the initial two months. Treatment may then be continued with daily INH plus RMP for the remaining four months. When the patient is in a high-risk group for infection with INH-resistant or RMP-resistant organisms, use of a four-drug regimen has been suggested for the first two months (INH/RMP/PZA/SM), followed by administration of two or three drugs, depending on drug susceptibility, for four months. A modification of the 6-month treatment involving only 62 doses, fully supervised, is as follows: INH/RMP/PZA/SM daily for 2 weeks, then twice weekly for 6 weeks, then INH/RMP twice weekly for 18 weeks. These intensive regimens should be considered for patients who are likely to resist treatment, such as prisoners and urban homeless alcoholics. Even shorter regimens consisting of INH/RMP/PZA/SM daily for four months may be advisable for problem patients for whom ambulatory treatment of any kind is unsuitable. Success rates of 70 to 80 per cent have been reported.

Short-course treatment has the obvious advantages of smaller amounts of drugs used and less time needed at the ambulatory health facility for supervision of treatment. Another benefit is more rapid sputum conversion. In addition, if relapse occurs following short-course treatment, it is usually caused by drug-susceptible organisms. The main disadvantage of intensive three- and four-drug regimens, drug toxicity, has proved to be less troublesome than was predicted.

The remarkable success of short-course treatment has been attributed to special characteristics of certain drugs, e.g., the ability of INH, RMP, and PZA to penetrate macrophages and to kill rapidly growing bacilli; the effectiveness of PZA in the acid environment of the phagolysosome; and the more rapid bactericidal activity of RMP during periods of intermittent growth of otherwise dormant bacilli.

Results of Treatment. The success of treatment may be judged by clinical assessment, decreased bacillary count of the sputum, and clearing of the lungs as shown on radiographs. The temperature usually returns to normal within a week or two, but in some patients who are highly febrile, defervescence may not occur for many weeks. The speed of radiographic improvement depends upon the nature and extent of pulmonary disease and the age of the patient. Chronic, cavitary, and fibrotic lesions do not clear rapidly. The sputum should be examined at frequent intervals during the first few months of treatment, since a decreasing number of acid-fast bacilli is the surest indication of successful treatment. The best of regimens in patients with far advanced disease will take four to six weeks to convert sputum cultures to negative in 50 per cent of cases; to convert 75 per cent of cases usually requires about ten weeks. The rate of conversion depends on the same factors that determine the rate of radiographic clearing. Failure of the sputum to convert to negative or a rise in the bacillary count after an initial decrease represents a treatment failure. Such failures are usually the result of poor compliance on the part of the patient but occasionally are related to bacillary drug resistance or an inappropriate drug regimen. The aim of chemotherapy is an initial success rate of 100 per cent without relapses. When relapse occurs, it is usually within a year of the completion of therapy. Rarely, relapses may occur with decreasing frequency up to five to ten years after completion of therapy. This is so infrequent after adequate drug therapy that it is no longer necessary for the local health department to carry out periodic follow-up examinations.

Corticosteroids. Corticosteroids may be a useful adjunct to chemotherapy for selected patients. They usually produce a dramatic reversal of overwhelming sepsis. Absorption of the fluid may be hastened in tuberculous pleurisy and pericarditis, although there is no evidence that late complications in the pleural and pericardial spaces are prevented. In tuberculous meningitis it was often the custom to give steroids routinely, but there is no good evidence that this is necessary. Steroids should be given for as short a time as possible, preferably for no longer than three or four weeks. A more controversial issue is whether or not to use INH prophylaxis to cover the administration of steroids in the patient with a history of tuberculosis or with a positive tuberculin skin test result. This situation is most likely to occur in patients receiving steroids to prevent rejection of transplanted organs, to help control lymphoma or leukemia, or to control severe asthma. One year of INH preventive therapy is recommended when steroids will be used on a long-term basis.

Reversal of Infectiousness. Some experts believe that it takes only about two weeks of effective chemotherapy to render patients noninfectious to others, even when large numbers of viable acid-fast bacilli are still present in the sputum. The evidence for this is inconclusive, and it is more reasonable to consider a patient with smear-positive sputum to represent a gradually diminishing risk until the smears are negative.

Drug Resistance. The phenomenon of clinical bacillary resistance was recognized soon after SM was tried as single drug therapy. The emergence of drug-resistant strains was at least delayed, if not prevented, by the use of two or more drugs in combination. Resistant populations emerge by a selective process in which resistant cells are favored that have arisen by spontaneous random mutation at the rate of about 1×10^{-8} to 1×10^{-10} per bacterium per generation.

Modern drug regimens are designed to prevent the emergence of drug resistance unless the patient is noncompliant or infection occurs with strains already resistant to one or more drugs—a situation known as *primary drug resistance*. The rate of primary drug resistance in a community will influence the choice of drug regimens for initial treatment. In this country the overall rate is 7 per cent and varies in different locations from 3 to 15 per cent, depending mainly on the relative numbers of Asian and Hispanic individuals in the population. Age is another important factor; the highest rate is seen in young children. The highest single drug rate is for INH, with SM second. In another study from the Centers for Disease Control, 41 per cent of unsuccessfully treated patients harbored strains resistant to at least one drug. The known contacts of an index case excreting INH-resistant tubercle bacilli should receive careful follow-up, and appropriate treatment should be given if active disease develops. Alternatively, prophylaxis may be attempted with RMP either alone or with another drug such as EMB or PZA, although it has not yet been proved that RMP alone is effective in prophylaxis.

Retreatment. The choice of proper therapy for initial treatment failures and disease that relapses after apparently successful treatment requires special expertise. Accurate drug susceptibility testing is a prerequisite for devising the best drug regimen, but while awaiting test results the following guidelines may be followed: A single new drug should not be added to a regimen that has failed, since rapid emergence of resistance to the new drug may occur. Instead, the new regimen should contain at least two drugs that the patient has never received previously. In selecting the proper drugs, all available information should be gathered from the patient, the patient's family and former physicians, and health departments. The chosen regimen should be adjusted according to any newly available information. It may be necessary to use combinations of four or more drugs, some of which have high rates of adverse reactions. After two or three relapses, especially when the infecting strain is resistant to INH, RMP, and SM, the chances of success are slim. The best approach to retreatment of patients with multiply resistant strains is to prevent this unfortunate turn of events by proper supervision of the initial course of drug therapy.

Patients with Impaired Renal and Hepatic Function. Isoniazid is excreted mainly in the urine, and it has been reported that the drug will accumulate in patients with markedly impaired renal function. However, the drug is dialyzable, and others have reported that the half-life is prolonged only slightly in patients with renal failure. It is probably not necessary to reduce the dosage, but pyridoxine supplementation should be given and patients should be monitored for hepatitis and peripheral neuropathy. It may also be advisable to assay INH serum concentrations from time to time. Rifampin is metabolized in the liver and excreted mainly in the bile. When hepatic function is impaired, the drug may accumulate to toxic levels. It is only slightly, if at all, dialyzable. Both EMB and SM are cleared by dialysis and are excreted mainly through the urine. The dosage of SM must be reduced in proportion to the renal function; serum levels should be checked frequently, and the patient should be monitored for signs of eighth nerve toxicity. In a similar fashion, the dosage of EMB must be reduced, serum levels checked, and the visual acuity monitored. Since about 20 per cent of EMB is metabolized in the liver, it would be wise to check serum levels when there is hepatic failure. There is insufficient information upon which to base recommendations for use of PZA, ethionamide, and cycloserine in patients with impaired renal or hepatic function. Since PZA and cycloserine are excreted mainly by the kidneys, the dosage should be reduced and blood levels monitored when these drugs are used in patients with poor kidney function. It is not known how ethionamide is metabolized; only a very small amount may be found unchanged in the urine. Drug levels should be monitored to avoid accumulation.

Treatment of Pregnant Women. Ethionamide and SM should be avoided, the first because of teratogenic potential and the second because eighth nerve damage has been reported in the offspring. Cycloserine and PZA should also be avoided because of a lack of information on possible adverse effects. Rifampin crosses the placental barrier readily and inhibits ribonucleic acid (RNA) polymerase. It should be used with caution and only with a very strong indication, perhaps only for the first few weeks of treatment. The combination of INH and EMB is most suitable for pregnant women.

Treatment of Children. There are conflicting recommendations for drug regimens and dosages of individual drugs for treatment of children with tuberculosis. The most suitable combination is INH 10 mg per kilogram daily (maximum of 300 mg daily) and RMP 15 mg per kilogram daily (maximum of 600 mg daily). A third drug should be added if there is risk of infection with drug-resistant organisms. The third drug, given for the first two or three months of therapy, may be SM, EMB,* or PAS. All three drugs have drawbacks: SM has a high rate of adverse effects and must be given by injection; PAS is difficult to administer to children because of stomach irritation, and the drug is no longer available in the liquid form; young children cannot be monitored for the major toxicity of EMB, optic neuritis. Ethambutol* is probably the best choice of therapy. It has been used successfully in other countries in a dosage of 15 mg per kilogram daily. The duration of treatment should be one year, although some reports indicate that nine months may be sufficient.

Surgical and Collapse Procedures. The need for collapse procedures such as pneumothorax, pneumoperitoneum, and phrenic nerve crush and for excisional surgery with or without thoracoplasty has been virtually eliminated by the success of chemotherapy. The surgeon may still be called upon to correct late complications of previous attempts at treatment such as bronchopleural fistula or persistent empyema.

EXTRAPULMONARY DISEASE. In contrast to the declining incidence of pulmonary tuberculosis, there has been little change in the number of extrapulmonary cases reported in the United States since 1964, about 4000 per year (Alvarez and McCabe, Weir and Thornton). This may be partially explained by the higher rate of infection in the immunocompromised states associated with old age, renal failure (including dialysis and transplant patients), cirrhosis, malnutrition, hematologic malignancies, and AIDS. In England, extrapulmonary disease is reported mainly in recent immigrants from the Asian subcontinent.

Thoracic Cavity and Chest Wall. Tuberculosis of the pleura is almost always associated with disease of the lung, arising by contiguous spread or rupture of a subpleural tubercle. It usually begins as a localized fibrinous inflammation, which produces pleuritic chest pain. Pleurisy with effusion is often associated with primary infection. When this occurs in young adults who are untreated, approximately 75 per cent may be expected to develop overt pulmonary tuberculosis within five years. The onset may be either abrupt or insidious, with cough and fever accompanying the chest pain. Pain and friction rub often disappear as pleural fluid accumulates. Most primary tuberculous pleural effusions will resorb spontaneously, sometimes within a week or two, but the diagnosis can be made on the basis of a positive tuberculin skin test result, the exudative characteristics of the fluid, and the preponderance of lymphocytes. Tubercle bacilli are usually very scarce in the fluid so that stained smears may be negative and cultures only weakly positive. Imprints and cultures made from pleural tissue removed by closed needle biopsy are more likely than the fluid to be positive. Histologic examination also may be helpful. Pleural effusions in young adults who have positive tuberculin skin test results are best treated as tuberculosis unless some other cause can be identified. The fluid should be aspirated for diagnosis and perhaps once or twice more if it accumulates rapidly. Chest tube drainage should be avoided. Corticosteroids should not be used routinely but may be given in selected cases to hasten symptomatic improvement and absorption of the fluid. Pleural effusion may also occur in disseminated tuberculosis with multiple organ and serous membrane involvement. Tuberculous empyema may be secondary to involvement of the vertebral column or result from a bronchopleural fistula.

Endobronchial tuberculosis commonly accompanies pulmonary disease but now rarely results in identifiable symptoms and signs. In primary tuberculosis of children it is the pressure of enlarged lymph nodes together with ulceration and rupture through the bronchial wall that produce endobronchial disease. Endobronchial disease in adults usually starts as inflammatory lesions from repeated implantations of tubercle bacilli originating in lung parenchyma. These lesions may progress to ulceration and narrowing of the bronchi and eventually to cicatricial stenosis. Secondary changes include atelectasis and obstructive pneumonitis, tension cavity from involvement of the distal small bronchi or bronchioles, and accumulation of fluid within cavities. The symptoms of endobronchial disease are spasmodic coughing and a localized wheeze. Bronchial ulceration or erosion of a caseating lymph node may cause positive sputum in the absence of recognizable pulmonary disease. Bronchoscopy usually serves to identify the lesions.

Although tuberculosis of the endocardium and myocardium has been described, the most common involvement of the heart is *pericarditis*. Rupture into the pericardium of nearby caseous lymph nodes is the common route of infection, although lymphohematogenous dissemination may occur. The serofibrinous pericardial effusion usually is associated with substernal pain, fever, pericardial friction rub, and left-sided pleural effusion. Cardiac tamponade occasionally develops in the acute stage. A search for tuberculosis elsewhere and a tuberculin skin test should be performed. A thorough examination of the pericardial fluid obtained by needle aspiration or surgical drainage also may be helpful. Obtaining a pericardial biopsy sample in the operating room may be justified in obscure cases because of the importance of early drug treatment. The differential diagnosis includes benign or viral pericarditis, pyogenic infection, other granulomatous inflammations, and malignant effusion. The diagnosis is made more difficult by the facts that the skin test reaction is negative in a sizable minority; the fluid rarely contains enough organisms to be positive by smear and often not even by culture; the characteristics of the fluid are nonspecific; and about half of the individuals have no other obvious sites of tuberculosis. The administration of corticosteroids may be beneficial, but antituberculosis drugs should be used in addition even when tuberculosis is only suspected.

The most important sequela is constrictive pericarditis, which usually occurs two to four years after the acute disease. At this stage the heart is small and relatively immobile and there is a paradoxical pulse and obstruction of venous return to the heart, with congestion of the liver, peripheral edema, and later ascites. Calcification of the pericardium may be seen on x-ray films. Treatment consists of removal of the pericardium, although it is preferable to perform the operation at an earlier stage.

The chest wall may be the site of one or more subcutaneous abscesses as a result of hematogenous dissemination or sometimes as the peripheral manifestation of an empyema necessitatis as it burrows through the chest wall. Chest wall abscesses may also result from drainage of underlying caseous lymph nodes along the intercostal lymphatics.

Extrathoracic. LYMPHATIC. Tuberculous lymphadenitis is the most common manifestation of extrathoracic disease throughout the world, and the most frequently involved nodes are cervical. The disease in this location was known as *scrofula*, or the *King's Evil*. The latter name was used because the condition was supposedly amenable to cure by the royal touch. Although it was once thought that infection with *M. bovis* was responsible for most cases of scrofula, a recent study from England emphasized that *M. tuberculosis* accounted for more cases than did the bovine organism, although the latter is relatively more common in lymphatic tuberculosis than in other forms of the disease. Infection of the tonsils through the ingestion of contaminated milk was the usual route of infection for the tonsillar node high in the neck, near the angle of the jaw. At present, scrofula in young children is

---

*Not recommended for use in children under 13 years of age.

mainly due to infection with mycobacteria other than *M. tuberculosis* and *M. bovis* (see Ch. 303). Supraclavicular node involvement usually arises by lymphatic spread from mediastinal disease. Affected nodes elsewhere in the neck, as well as those in the axilla and inguinal area, the other common sites of involvement, may be the result of drainage from a primary site or from hematogenous spread.

The infected nodes are usually detectable by sight and palpation. Although the nodes usually are not painful, they may be tender during the phase of rapid enlargement early in the infection. Later they become matted together and eventually soften, slough, and drain. Draining sinuses may persist for many months, sometimes for years, with intermittent healing and breakdown. The diagnosis may be made by bacteriologic study of the pus from draining sinuses or by biopsy together with bacteriologic studies. The presence of calcific densities in the neck and axilla as seen in the chest radiograph may provide evidence of healed tuberculous adenitis.

Lymphatic tuberculosis tends to heal but often not completely, so that relapse is common even many years after the primary infection. Treatment with antituberculosis drugs is usually successful, although the tendency to late relapse may still be seen. Good results have been reported with short-course regimens. Excision of large caseous nodes in accessible sites sometimes is advisable.

GENITOURINARY. The second most common site of infection is the genitourinary tract. Disease is usually centered in the kidney, which becomes seeded either during the primary infection or later. These foci may remain dormant for many years. When reactivation occurs, one or more renal abscesses are produced, followed by spread to the remainder of the urinary tract. Extensive scarring of the ureters eventually occurs. This scarring produces obstructive hydronephrosis, which together with renal caseation may destroy the kidney completely. Specific symptoms may be lacking until the hydronephrotic kidney becomes secondarily infected or until the development of tuberculous cystitis manifested by frequency and dysuria. Long before the onset of symptoms, the examination of the urine may show hematuria, pyuria, and albuminuria, along with cultures negative for pyogens. The diagnosis is made by radiographic examination of the urinary tract, cystoscopy, and demonstration of tubercle bacilli by cultures of first morning voided urines. It was found that approximately 10 per cent of a general tuberculosis patient population had positive urine cultures, and in 7 per cent of these patients the urinary tract disease was completely unanticipated. Renal tuberculosis responds well to drug treatment. According to recent recommendations, conventional long-term regimens may be replaced by six- to nine-month courses of INH, RMP, and a third drug (either EMB or PZA). The role of surgery remains controversial. Some urologists would remove destroyed kidneys and repair strictures of the ureter, while others claim that surgery is almost never indicated.

Genital tuberculosis in the male may involve the prostate, seminal vesicles, and epididymis. The acute inflammation is later replaced by induration and hard nodules, sometimes followed by obstruction, calcification, and chronic draining sinuses of the scrotum. The diagnosis is made by finding tubercle bacilli in the urine, sinus drainage, or biopsied tissues. In the female, tuberculous salpingitis is the common manifestation, followed by disease of the uterus and ovaries. Sterility almost always results, and peritonitis may occur secondarily. The symptoms are those of chronic pelvic inflammatory disease. Diagnosis should be based on examination of tissue from the endometrium and from lesions visible through the laparoscope and cultures of the menstrual fluid or vaginal discharge. As with renal tuberculosis, drug therapy usually is successful, but excisional surgery may be indicated for residual lesions or persistently draining sinuses.

SKELETAL TUBERCULOSIS. The presence of a gibbus or hunchback deformity of the thoracic spine (Pott's disease) has served as a marker of tuberculosis since prehistoric times. *Tuberculous spondylitis* is still the most common manifestation of bone and joint infection. At present, it is mainly a disease of adults that arises by reactivation of dormant foci. The common areas of involvement are thoracic and lumbar; the cervical spine may be involved in 2 to 3 per cent of cases. The destructive process usually begins in the intervertebral discs, where it first produces narrowing of the disc space, then destruction of the two adjacent vertebral bodies through the bony end-plates. Sometimes, however, the anterior portion of the vertebral body is destroyed first. Inflammation often extends into the soft tissues surrounding the spine, either in the form of a spreading, phlegmonous reaction or as a cold abscess that may be paravertebral, in and around the psoas muscle, or retropharyngeal, depending upon the site of disease. The symptoms are usually dominated by back pain, sometimes followed by the neurologic manifestations of compression of the spinal cord and nerve roots. There may be fever. Active tuberculosis of the lungs may be absent, although some evidence of past disease usually is seen.

Radiographic examination of the spine shows destructive lesions in the commonly involved sites. The paraspinal involvement appears as widening of the mediastinum or an oval-shaped density behind the heart. It may be manifested as a psoas abscess, a retropharyngeal abscess, or a mass in the groin or in the supraclavicular area. A similar radiographic appearance may occur in pyogenic infection of the spine. A needle biopsy sample usually is necessary to establish the proper diagnosis. Even when a pyogenic organism such as *Staphylococcus aureus* is isolated, caseating granulomas and a culture positive for *M. tuberculosis* sometimes can be found by biopsy. Occasionally open biopsy of the vertebral body may be necessary.

The disease has a natural tendency to heal by spontaneous fusion of the vertebral bodies. Treatment consists of antituberculosis chemotherapy according to the modern regimens described under Treatment. Preliminary results with short-course treatment are encouraging, but they cannot be recommended for routine use until further experience has accumulated. Prolonged bed rest, immobilization of the spine, and spinal fusion operations are no longer necessary, although some indications still exist for surgical procedures: decompression of the spinal cord if there has been no neurologic improvement after several weeks of drug treatment and debridement and anterior spinal fusion for dangerous instability of the spine. The inflammatory reaction with or without pus around the spine often improves with drug treatment so that drainage is not always necessary.

Tuberculous arthritis occurs mainly in hips and knees but also may involve many other joints, including elbows, shoulders, and the joints of the hands and feet. The patient usually has chronic monoarticular arthritis. Diagnosis is made by synovial biopsy and bacteriologic study of tissues and pus. The process usually responds to antituberculosis chemotherapy without the necessity for operative procedures, but occasionally excision of extensively destroyed synovium and temporary immobilization may be beneficial.

Tuberculous tenosynovitis is usually secondary to involvement of adjacent bone. At least two distinctive processes may result from involvement of the hand: carpal tunnel syndrome, and compound palmar ganglion, a distinctive bilobed swelling on either side of the volar carpal ligament. Chemotherapy often needs to be supplemented by debridement and evacuation of fibrinous material.

ABDOMINAL TUBERCULOSIS. *Intestinal tuberculosis* secondary to chronic pulmonary disease once was so common that patients were routinely screened by radiography of the small bowel upon admission to the sanatorium. This situation continued long after the ingestion of *M. bovis* was brought under control by the pasteurization of milk. Lately, the emphasis has been on primary intestinal disease in the absence of recognizable pulmonary lesions. The route of infection in these cases remains unknown. Tuberculosis may involve all parts of the alimentary canal from top to bottom, but by far the most common location is in the ileocecal area. The predominant tissue reaction may be either ulcerative or hyperplastic, with accompanying bleeding, perforation, fistula formation, obstruction, or combinations of two or more of these processes. The early symptoms are nonspecific, consisting mainly of anorexia, loss of weight, abdominal pain, and alternating periods of diarrhea and constipation. The clinical picture is not unlike that of Crohn's disease. Indeed, the differential diagnosis of these two conditions may not be possible, even on the basis of intestinal radiography. Tuberculosis of the colon also may occur and needs to be distinguished from carcinoma, diverticulitis, and inflammatory bowel disease of nonspecific nature. Perirectal abscess and fistula formation may result from lower colon lesions. The disease usually responds well to antituberculosis chemotherapy, but surgical correction may be necessary for the complications described earlier. The diagnosis often is made unexpectedly at surgery or autopsy.

Tuberculous peritonitis may result from bloodborne infection or by extension of disease from the intestine, mesenteric lymph nodes, or fallopian tubes. The classic form is that of a chronic adhesive peritonitis that produces a doughy, tender abdomen, abdominal masses, low-grade fever, anorexia, and weight loss. A much more common manifestation is painless ascites. When this occurs in adults with alcoholic cirrhosis and ascites, it makes for a difficult differential diagnosis. Tuberculosis should be suspected when the combination of fever, ascites, and a positive tuberculin skin test reaction are found. Examination of the fluid is helpful. A high total protein concentration with a moderate number of leukocytes, mostly lymphocytes, is suggestive of tuberculosis. A more definitive diagnosis may be obtained by laparoscopy or laparotomy. Usually the entire peritoneal surface is studded with tubercles that are easily differentiated from carcinomatosis histologically. The fluid is rarely positive for AFB by stained smear and even by culture is positive in somewhat less than 50 per cent of cases. Response to antituberculosis chemotherapy is good.

Isolated tuberculosis of the liver or spleen occasionally has been described. These organs are usually involved in disseminated or miliary tuberculosis, but occasionally a liver biopsy done in an attempt to explain enlargement of the liver, jaundice, or abnormal liver function studies leads to a diagnosis of tuberculosis when there is apparently no disease elsewhere.

CENTRAL NERVOUS SYSTEM. In the past, *tuberculous meningitis* was one of the most dreaded complications of primary tuberculosis in young children, appearing in about one in a thousand cases and almost always resulting in fatality. It usually occurred two to six months after the primary infection in infants and was commonly associated with miliary tuberculosis. In this country it is now more likely to be seen in adults than in children. Invasion of the meninges occurs by direct extension from subjacent caseous foci in the cerebral cortex, cerebellum, choroid plexus, middle ear, or spine. Brain infarcts secondary to tuberculous arteritis sometimes occur. The syndrome of inappropriate secretion of antidiuretic hormone may accompany the meningitis.

The inflammatory reaction is concentrated around the base of the brain, where the thick exudate may eventually obstruct the basal foramina to produce hydrocephalus. Examination of the spinal fluid reveals a characteristic pattern of high protein, low sugar, and a moderate number (up to a few hundred) of leukocytes, most of which are lymphocytes. However, early in the course of the disease neutrophils may predominate; rarely the shift to a lymphocytic exudate does not occur; the sugar level may be normal or only slightly decreased; and the number of leukocytes may reach several thousand. Occasionally the protein content is high enough that a thin web or pellicle appears in undisturbed refrigerated fluid. Acid-fast bacilli may be seen in this web, although they are not visible in the sedimented fluid. Stained smears of the fluid are usually positive in no more than 25 per cent of samples, but there are a few colonies of tubercle bacilli in cultures in about 75 per cent of cases. The larger the sample of spinal fluid submitted, the greater the chance of finding the organism. The tuberculin skin test should be positive in approximately 75 per cent of cases, provided that those nonreactive to 5 TU are retested with 250 TU. A careful search reveals evidence of tuberculosis elsewhere in the majority of cases, although the disease in the lungs may appear to be inactive.

The onset is usually insidious, extending over a period of many weeks. Occasionally, however, there is a much more acute onset that resembles pyogenic or aseptic meningitis. The most common symptoms are headache, fever, lethargy, and confusion. Later, focal neurologic signs appear in the form of ocular palsies, other cranial nerve palsies, and increasing stupor progressing to coma. Stiffness of the neck is common. The outcome of therapy depends mainly on the stage of disease at the time treatment is instituted. Treatment should start immediately when tuberculous meningitis is suspected, without waiting for confirmation of diagnosis. A triple-drug regimen including INH and RMP is recommended. Ethionamide and PZA achieve therapeutic concentrations in spinal fluid even in the absence of an inflammatory reaction. Ethambutol penetrates reasonably well through inflamed meninges. It should be remembered that SM does not appear in therapeutic concentrations and that infections with INH-resistant organisms occur more often in children than in adults. Treatment should be continued for at least one year, although administration of the third drug may be discontinued after two or three months once it has been determined that drug resistance is not a problem. The use of corticosteroids is controversial. Intrathecal treatment is usually not necessary.

Tuberculomas of the brain may be seen at any age. Cases involving children still predominate in the developing countries, while in the United States they occur mainly in adults. The clinical presentation is that of a brain tumor with signs and symptoms of increased intracranial pressure, focal seizures, and focal neurologic defects. Indications of infection, such as fever, often are absent. Lesions may be single or multiple and must be differentiated from tumor and abscess. The spinal fluid may show slight lymphocytosis and elevated protein concentration, but often it is normal. The correct diagnois may be suggested by radiographic scanning techniques, a positive tuberculin skin test reaction, and the presence of tuberculosis elsewhere, but the definitive procedures are needle aspiration through a burr hole and craniotomy for open biopsy. Drug treatment similar to that used for tuberculous meningitis should be used.

MISCELLANEOUS. Almost every organ and tissue of the body can be involved in tuberculosis. In the upper respiratory tract and oral cavity, the larynx and the middle ear are most prone to infection. *Tuberculous laryngitis* used to be a rather common complication that was considered to be secondary to long-standing highly positive sputum associated with chronic cavitary disease. It was extremely painful and resulted in such difficulty in swallowing that severe inanition resulted. Response to drug treatment, even to administration of SM alone, was rapid and dramatic. The new face of tuberculous laryngitis is that of a primary laryngeal lesion that must be distinguished from carcinoma. Tuberculous middle ear disease, formerly common, is now rare. It was usually associated with advanced pulmonary or disseminated disease. Involvement of the eye is in the form of chronic uveitis, such as chorioretinitis, iridocyclitis, or iritis. Phlyctenular conjunctivitis produces small, yellowish vesicles. Direct inoculation into the eye may produce conjunctivitis or keratitis. The specific origin of eye disease is difficult to prove. Cutaneous tuberculosis has all but disappeared, except for lesions associated with direct inoculation in laboratory workers and pathologists. Other manifestations include lesions like lupus vulgaris, in which tubercle bacilli may be located, and the tuberculids that are considered to be hypersensitivity reactions, in which the organisms usually are not found. The larger blood vessels may harbor infections in their walls. Tuberculosis is a rare cause of aortic aneurysm. At one time tuberculosis of the adrenal gland was a common cause of adrenal insufficiency. Occasional cases of tuberculosis of the thyroid, breast, and soft tissues elsewhere than in the chest wall are still being reported.

DISSEMINATED AND MILIARY TUBERCULOSIS. These terms are used synonymously, although miliary tuberculosis is but one form of disseminated tuberculosis in which the widely dispersed small tubercles resemble millet seeds. During life these lesions usually are first recognized in the chest roentgenogram as very small nodules of uniform size that are evenly distributed throughout both lungs. The acute form was predominantly an early complication of untreated primary tuberculosis, occurring mainly in young children and often associated with meningitis. During the past three decades the predominant age group has changed to the elderly, and the disease has become more subacute in its progression.

The diagnosis often is missed because it is difficult to distinguish the tuberculosis symptoms from those of the many underlying conditions that could be responsible for the weight loss, increasing fatigue, and low-grade fever. Skin test anergy and frequent absence of chronic pulmonary tuberculosis may compound the difficulty. This sort of subacute disseminated tuberculosis has been called *cryptic* or *nonreactive tuberculosis.* In a series of autopsied cases analyzed by Slavin and colleagues in 1980, only 15 per cent of patients admitted during the antibiotic era had the correct diagnosis made ante mortem. A composite of such a case would be an elderly anergic patient without previously recognized tuberculosis who presented to the hospital with malignancy, renal failure, a renal transplant, or chronic alcoholism. Constitutional symptoms would be nonspecific, mainly fever, loss of weight, and increasing fatigue. Examinations would reveal no obvious tuberculosis in lungs or other organs, no hepatosplenomegaly, and no enlarged peripheral lymph nodes. There would be moderate anemia, a slight elevation of alkaline phosphatase, and a negative initial bacteriologic workup. The correct diagnosis depends upon a high index of suspicion and the demonstration of characteristic microscopic lesions and mycobacteria by biopsy. The most productive tissue is the liver, usually sampled by needle biopsy, with bone marrow next in line. Blood cultures should be obtained, since they are sometimes positive at this stage of disease. At a later stage choroidal tubercles may be seen and radiographs of the lungs may show the typical miliary pattern.

Miliary tuberculosis almost always results from the discharge of infected caseous material into the bloodstream, usually from a well-hidden lymph node in the mediastinum or the abdomen. When multiple bacteremic episodes occur, the process may be protracted. The patient may have serositis manifested by pleural effusion, pericardial effusion, or ascites. Hematologic abnormalities may be so prominent that a primary blood disease is suspected. The most common abnormality is a leukemoid reaction, although leukopenia, thrombocytopenia, and hemolytic anemia may occur. More commonly the primary disease is hematologic, complicated by a secondary tuberculosis dissemination, especially when large doses of corticosteroids have been given.

Treatment should consist of an intensive antituberculosis drug regimen using three drugs, including INH and RMP, plus EMB or PZA. After a few months, when a good response

has occurred and after the drug susceptibility pattern of the infecting strain is known, the third drug can be discontinued. The total duration of therapy has not been established, but it probably should be at least one year. Disseminated mycobacteriosis is one of the common opportunistic infections in immunosuppressed and debilitated patients, including those with AIDS. Nontuberculous mycobacteria are the causative agents in these cases even more often than *M. tuberculosis*—a fact that should be considered in the choice of proper treatment.

Alvarez S, McCabe WR: Extrapulmonary tuberculosis revisited: A review of experience at Boston City and other hospitals. Medicine 63:25, 1984. *This paper, along with that of Weir and Thornton, provides the information needed to understand why extrapulmonary disease is still common throughout the world.*

Andrew OT, Schoenfeld PY, Hopewell PC, et al.: Tuberculosis in patients with end-stage renal disease. Am J Med 68:59, 1980. *A study of 10 patients with tuberculosis from a group of 172 undergoing dialysis in San Francisco gave a risk ratio of 12:1. The problems of diagnosis and treatment are admirably discussed.*

Anonymous: Is BCG vaccination effective? Tubercle 62:219, 1981. *The failure of the most recent large-scale trial in South India to demonstrate protection is brought into focus by this concise article.*

Centers for Disease Control: Primary resistance to antituberculosis drugs—United States. MMWR 32:521, 1983. *The final report of a seven-year study in which 20 selected laboratories throughout the country submitted over 12,000 cultures to the CDC laboratory to be tested for drug susceptibility in a uniform manner.*

Chaparas SD: Immunologic tests for the diagnosis of tuberculosis. Indian J Tuberc 32:2, 1985. *The possible applications of new monoclonal antibody, molecular biology, and immunoassay techniques are discussed.*

Chaparas SD: The immunology of mycobacterial infections. CRC Crit Rev Microbiol 9:139, 1982. *A good recent and thorough summary of a subject important for the understanding of the immune system's role in all infections.*

Chow AW, Jewesson PJ: Pharmacokinetics and safety of antimicrobial agents during pregnancy. Rev Infect Dis 7:287, 1985. *This paper includes a discussion of the antituberculosis drugs.*

Costello HD, Caras GJ, Snider DE Jr: Drug resistance among previously treated tuberculosis patients: A brief report. Am Rev Respir Dis 121:313, 1980. *Among 4000 unsuccessfully treated patients in the United States, 41 per cent harbored drug-resistant strains.*

Daniel TM, Debanne SM, van der Kuyp F: Enzyme linked immunosorbent assay using *Mycobacterium tuberculosis* antigen 5 and PPD for the serodiagnosis of tuberculosis. Chest 88:388, 1985. *Potentially a long-awaited, clinically useful serodiagnostic test for tuberculosis.*

Dannenberg AM Jr: Macrophages in inflammation and infection. N Engl J Med 293:489, 1975. *This study utilizing skin lesions in rabbits demonstrates the dynamic nature of mycobacterial lesions. Macrophages enter the arena as novices, become activated locally by interaction with immune lymphocytes, ingest bacilli, die, and are replaced by fresh cells recruited from the circulation.*

Fox W: The chemotherapy of tuberculosis: A review. Chest 76S:785, 1979. *An excellent review of antituberculosis drug treatment up to 1979.*

Gorse GJ, Pais MJ, Kusske JA, et al.: Tuberculous spondylitis: A report of six cases and a review of the literature. Medicine 62:178, 1983. *This review from the University of California, Irvine, presents a thorough and unbiased account of spinal tuberculosis as it exists today.*

Laszlo A, Handzel V: Radiometric diagnosis of mycobacteria. Eur J Clin Microbiol 5:152, 1986. *An automated, more rapid method for the culture of mycobacteria from clinical specimens.*

Lichtenstein IH, MacGregor RR: Mycobacterial infections in renal transplant recipients: Report of 5 cases and review of the literature. Rev Infect Dis 5:216, 1983. *Among the cases were two that probably represented reactivation tuberculosis in the transplanted kidney. A survey of 26 transplantation centers revealed a tuberculosis rate of 480 cases per 100,000.*

Lincoln EM: Epidemics of tuberculosis. Arch Environ Health 14:473, 1967. *A review of 109 epidemics in 12 countries, the majority of them occurring in schools.*

Lorin MI, Hsu KHK, Jacob SC: Treatment of tuberculosis in children. Pediatr Clin North Am 30:333, 1983. *The latest recommendations for treatment of children, from a Houston group with longstanding interest in pediatric tuberculosis.*

Mackay AD, Cole RB: The problems of tuberculosis in the elderly. Q J Med 53:497, 1984. *The case rate of tuberculosis is increasing among the elderly, and physicians should understand the special problems of diagnosis and management so well presented in this report.*

Sahn SA, Lakshminarayan S: Tuberculosis after corticosteroid therapy. Br J Dis Chest 70:195, 1976. *This review emphasizes the usefulness of preventive therapy with isoniazid in patients already infected with M. tuberculosis.*

Schofield PF: Abdominal tuberculosis (leading article). Gut 26:1275, 1985. *The author gives a good discussion of all aspects of abdominal disease as it is seen today.*

Singapore Tuberculosis Service/British Medical Research Council: Long-term follow-up of a clinical trial of six-month and four-month regimens of chemotherapy in the treatment of pulmonary tuberculosis. Am Rev Respir Dis 133:779, 1986. *A good example of the efficacy of ultra-short regimens from experts in cooperative chemotherapy studies.*

Slavin RE, Walsh TJ, Pollack AD: Late generalized tuberculosis: A clinical pathologic analysis and comparison of 100 cases in the preantibiotic and antibiotic eras. Medicine 59:352, 1980. *This study, from the Department of*

Pathology at Johns Hopkins University, consists of an analysis of 200 autopsied cases. It contains a wealth of useful information on one form of disseminated tuberculosis.

Snider DE Jr, Cohn DL, Davidson PT, et al.: Standard therapy for tuberculosis. Chest 87 (Suppl 2):117S, 1985. A consensus of an expert group of clinicians and public health officials.

Stead WW: Control of tuberculosis in institutions. Chest 76 (suppl):797, 1979. Reviews recent outbreaks in nursing homes, prisons, schools, and hospitals and suggests common-sense methods of control.

Stead WW, Kerby GR, Schlueter DP, et al.: The clinical spectrum of primary tuberculosis in adults. Ann Intern Med 68:333, 1968. Primary pulmonary disease was documented in 37 adults, of whom 9 had only minor symptoms, 11 developed pleural effusion, and 16 showed progression to adult-type chronic pulmonary disease.

Weir MR, Thornton GF: Extrapulmonary tuberculosis: Experience of a community hospital and review of the literature. Am J Med 79:467, 1985. See Alvarez and McCabe, above.

303 OTHER MYCOBACTERIOSES

Emanuel Wolinsky

Organisms of the tuberculosis complex are not the only mycobacteria associated with human disease. The most popular label at present for these other mycobacteria is "nontuberculous." They have become more prominent in the total picture of mycobacterial disease because of the declining incidence of tuberculosis and a greater awareness and recognition of the other mycobacterioses. Indeed, there is evidence that the frequency of nontuberculous pulmonary disease may be increasing in certain areas of the country. In addition, disseminated mycobacterial infection is now recognized much more frequently as an opportunistic infection in immunosuppressed individuals, especially in those with the acquired immunodeficiency syndrome (AIDS). Infection with other mycobacteria has been blamed, perhaps unfairly, for the apparent failure of bacille Calmette-Guérin (BCG) vaccination to protect adults in South India from subsequent tuberculosis. Leprosy, also a mycobacterial disease, is discussed in Ch. 304.

Although the existence of nontuberculous mycobacteria was recognized in the late 1800's, they were first identified as causes of human disease in the mid 1950's.

MYCOBACTERIA. *Mycobacterium avium-intracellulare (MAI).* Mycobacteria of this species or complex constitute the most important agents of nontuberculous mycobacteriosis throughout the world. The organism known as the avian tubercle bacillus was described in 1890, although tuberculosis of chickens had been recognized for 22 years before that time. Supposedly quite resistant to infection with *M. avium*, people with documented *M. avium* disease were the subjects of occasional literature reports. Recognition of the expanded role of these mycobacteria in pulmonary and disseminated disease occurred in the 1950's, when the organism was misnamed *Nocardia intracellularis* and given the common name of Battey bacillus. The official name of *Mycobacterium intracellulare* was assigned in the 1960's. The realization that *M. intracellulare* could not be distinguished from *M. avium* in most laboratories dictated another change to the presently used term MAI or *M. avium* complex. In this complex one can recognize 28 types by seroagglutination, of which types 1 to 3 represent the classic *M. avium* strains. Strains of MAI grow slowly; usually are nonpigmented or slightly yellow, becoming more highly pigmented with age but independently of light; are resistant to most antituberculosis drugs; and often produce colony variants of two or three types, including smooth translucent, smooth domed, and rough opaque. Of the three variants, the translucent colonies are usually most drug resistant and most virulent for experimental animals. Strains of MAI may be associated with all varieties of mycobacterial disease, especially pulmonary disease, childhood lymphadenitis, and opportunistic infection in patients who have AIDS. AIDS-asso-

ciated strains tend to be deeply pigmented and are mainly serotypes 1, 4, and 8.

Mycobacterium scrofulaceum. This is a scotochromogenic mycobacterium similar in many ways to MAI. The pigmentation varies from light yellow to dark orange. In some publications these organisms are lumped together with MAI, and the combination is called the *MAIS complex.* The name derives from the fact that the organism was recognized as the cause of scrofula in young children. Rarely, *M. scrofulaceum* may be associated with pulmonary disease in adults. Most of the disease-associated strains belong to one of three seroagglutination types, but it is not uncommon to see a strain of *M. scrofulaceum* agglutinate in one of the MAI serotypes.

Mycobacterium kansasii. The "yellow bacillus" was described in 1953 in Kansas City and was later given the official name of *M. kansasii.* It is responsible for a large number of pulmonary mycobacteriosis cases in some areas of the world. The organisms may be recognized in the initial sputum smears as large cross-barred acid-fast bacilli. Positive cultures may be identified by their distinctive photochromogenicity. The yellow color is light dependent, developing within hours after the colonies have been exposed to light. Most strains are fully susceptible to rifampin and only slightly resistant to isoniazid, ethambutol, and streptomycin. *M. kansasii* is not found in nature except occasionally in samples of water.

Mycobacterium fortuitum-chelonae. Strains of this group grow rapidly, even on ordinary laboratory media. They are sometimes spoken of as the *M. fortuitum complex,* but it is better to retain at least two separate species because they can be distinguished from each other readily in the laboratory, and *M. chelonae* tends to be much more drug resistant than *M. fortuitum.* Both species are pathogenic for mice and resistant to the usual antituberculosis drugs. Long known for their ability to produce injection site abscesses and severe infections of traumatic wounds, strains of this group recently have become prominent as the cause of sternal osteomyelitis after cardiac surgery, of wound infection after implantation of silicone breast prostheses, of disseminated and localized infection in dialysis patients, of prosthetic valve endocarditis, and of disseminated infections with skin lesions in the immunosuppressed host.

Mycobacterium marinum. This organism is distinctive by virtue of its photochromogenicity and an optimal growth temperature of 30 to 33° C. It was named and recognized as a pathogen of fish in 1926. It is a common contaminant in fresh and salt water, accounting for the frequent occurrence of skin infection in individuals who work or play in a marine environment. Deep infections of the hand may also occur. Almost all strains are resistant to isoniazid but susceptible to rifampin and ethambutol. The organisms are also susceptible to tetracycline and sulfonamides.

Other Slow-Growing Species. *Mycobacterium xenopi* has an optimal growth temperature of 43° C and has been found as a contaminant in hot water generators and storage tanks. From these sites several outbreaks have occurred of respiratory tract colonization and pulmonary disease in the hospital environment. Other species that may cause disease are *M. simiae,* *M. szulgai,* and *M. malmoense.* Two species that may be associated with superficial soft tissue disease but not with pulmonary disease are *M. ulcerans* and *M. hemophilum.*

Species of Low Pathogenic Potential. A few cases have been reported in which strains of the *M. terrae* complex (including *M. triviale*) were the cause of pulmonary disease, arthritis, or tenosynovitis. Strains of this complex may be found in the soil. An organism long associated with water and considered to be saprophytic is *M. gordonae.* Documented infections with this organism now range from bursitis to widely disseminated disease. Cases of pulmonary disease and synovitis also have been ascribed to *M. flavescens,* an organism with an intermediate growth rate that was previously considered to be nonpathogenic for humans.

EPIDEMIOLOGY. In contrast to tuberculosis, the other mycobacterioses are not transmitted from person to person but are acquired from the environment by mechanisms that are not well understood. For *M. xenopi* and *M. kansasii* the evidence points to aerosols of infected water. Strains of MAI may be found in domestic animals, soil, dust, and water. There is evidence that infected droplet nuclei may be produced along coastlines. Still largely unexplained is the geographic variability in the incidence of other mycobacterioses and the relative proportion of these infections attributable to each of the two most important agents of disease, MAI and *M. kansasii.* In this country the highest rates of *M. kansasii* disease have been reported from New Orleans, Dallas, Houston, Kansas City, and Chicago, while Milwaukee and the states of Georgia and Florida have reported a predominance of MAI disease. From one institution in St. Louis, 27 per cent of newly diagnosed cases of mycobacterial pulmonary disease were associated with an equal proportion of MAI and *M. kansasii.* Australia, Israel, and Japan have reported an overwhelming predominance of MAI infections over those caused by *M. kansasii.* In the Scandinavian countries, southeast England, and the Canadian province of Ontario, *M. xenopi* is an important pathogen. These figures refer to pulmonary disease; they do not reflect the distribution of disseminated infections. A recent increase in MAI and a concomitant decrease in *M. kansasii* pulmonary disease have been reported from Virginia and have been noted elsewhere, as well.

PATHOGENESIS. The localization of disease in the lungs suggests that the inhalation of infectious aerosols represents the primary route of infection. In many cases infection occurs by inoculation as a result of puncture wounds, lacerations, and foreign bodies. The question of whether the disease in adults usually represents primary infection or recrudescence of dormant foci cannot be answered at this time. The alimentary tract may be the route of infection in AIDS, since the intestinal tract is so often involved.

CLINICAL DESCRIPTION. *Pulmonary Disease.* The classic description is that of chronic cavitary disease resembling tuberculosis that occurs in a middle-aged rural man who has one or more of the following predisposing conditions: pneumoconiosis, healed tuberculosis, chronic bronchitis and emphysema, bullous disease, bronchiectasis, and malignant disease. However, there are many exceptions: The disease may be seen in all age groups except rarely in children, in either sex, and in some individuals without any apparent predisposing factor. It sometimes appears as an acute condition in which there is an infected bulla or cyst or in a case resembling pneumonia. Solitary pulmonary nodules also have been described.

The diagnosis may be suspected from the clinical appearance and the x-ray film, but it is the laboratory that must supply the correct identification of the mycobacterial agent. Skin tests are not helpful owing to a lack of adequately standardized antigens and the poor specificity of the presently available reagents. Pulmonary changes are characterized by one or more thin-walled cavities with little or no pleural disease or spread to the basal segments of the lungs. The sputum usually contains many acid-fast bacilli visible on smear and yields a heavy growth of the infecting agent. It may be possible to recognize the large banded forms of *M. kansasii* in the direct smear. A single positive culture result in which there are only a few colonies usually represents environmental contamination. Repeatedly positive specimens may be indicative of transient or long-term colonization of the respiratory tract when they are not associated with new or enlarging cavities and a compatible clinical picture.

Treatment for *M. kansasii* disease usually is highly successful, provided that rifampin is included in the regimen. It is recommended that isoniazid, rifampin, and ethambutol be given for one year after the sputum becomes negative for the organism. Results of preliminary trials of short-course treatment have not been encouraging.

Therapy for MAI disease, on the other hand, has proved to be difficult. Most strains are resistant to the available antituberculosis drugs as well as the other anti-infectives, and the drug regimens recommended up to now have been chosen empirically. The necessity for treatment must first be established by an observation period to determine the stability of disease and the rate of progression if it is advancing. During this period the sputum should be examined at frequent intervals, and the patient should receive a comprehensive course of bronchial hygiene, including cessation of smoking, bronchodilator therapy, chest physiotherapy, and antibiotics if there are purulent secretions. These maneuvers have served to eliminate the organism from the sputum of some patients with chronic pulmonary disease. It may be necessary to initiate therapy immediately in certain cases of severe acute disease with a new cavitary lesion and no other apparent cause. Drug treatment may be considered at three levels. Level 1 is a triple-drug regimen consisting of isoniazid, rifampin, and ethambutol for a duration of at least two years provided there is some response within the first few months. This level would be suitable for a patient who had chronic stable disease with consistently positive sputum test results and in whom the mycobacterial infection was adding to the burden of pulmonary disease. Level 2 treatment consists of the same three drugs plus daily streptomycin administration for at least two years. Administration of streptomycin may be reduced to two or three times a week after an initial response has been demonstrated. This treatment level would be suitable for a patient who had slowly progressive disease, who had a poor response to level 1 treatment, or who had a relapse after discontinuation of level 1 drug therapy. Drug treatment at level 3 may be empiric combinations of five or six drugs or, more reasonably, a regimen consisting of isoniazid, ethambutol, streptomycin, and rifabutin.* Most strains of MAI are susceptible to rifabutin in vitro.

The response to drug treatment depends to a large extent on the underlying chronic lung disease and on the rate of progression of the mycobacterial infection. For those patients who have rapidly progressive infection in lungs that are already severely damaged, the prognosis is poor even with level 3 treatment. Some of these individuals have defects in cellular immune functions, especially those associated with T cells. Resectional surgery should be considered after a few months of treatment for those patients who have adequate pulmonary function and sufficiently localized mycobacterial disease. Treatment is not necessary for solitary pulmonary nodules that result from MAI infection, usually recognized after resection.

Disease caused by *M. xenopi* and *M. szulgai* usually is amenable to drug therapy. The exact combinations of drugs to be used depend on the drug susceptibility patterns in vitro. Suggested for *M. xenopi* disease is a regimen consisting of isoniazid, rifampin, and streptomycin and for *M. szulgai,* rifampin, ethambutol, and either ethionamide or streptomycin.

Infections associated with *M. scrofulaceum, M. simiae,* and *M. fortuitum-chelonae* are more difficult to control because of natural drug resistance. Strains of *M. simiae* usually are resistant to all of the antituberculosis drugs except cycloserine and ethionamide. Limited information on susceptibility of *M. scrofulaceum* suggests that ethionamide, rifampin, and ethambutol are most likely to be active in vitro. The same considerations as those described for MAI infection are applicable to these resistant infections. Although pulmonary infections with *M. fortuitum-chelonae* are quite rare, there is some infor-

---

*Investigational drug made by Farmitalia Carlo Erba in Italy, represented by Adria Laboratories of Dublin, Ohio.

mation about the response to drug treatment from cases of extrapulmonary disease. Before sensitivity test results are available, full doses of amikacin should be given intramuscularly, together with one or more of the following drugs: doxycycline, erythromycin, cefoxitin, and a sulfonamide.

Lymphadenitis. Mycobacterial lymphadenitis is almost exclusively a disease of children of preschool age. Data from British Columbia published in 1974 indicated that the case rate for this new kind of scrofula was 0.37 per 100,000 persons per year, about ten times higher than for that caused by *M. tuberculosis.* Involved nodes may be found in the femoral, inguinal, epitrochlear, and axillary areas, although the most common location is around the angle of the jaw. The route of infection to the groin area is a penetrating injury or splinter entry into an extremity. The cervical nodes probably become infected by mucous membrane penetration in the mouth or pharynx. Examination shows a child who has had a painless localized swelling for several weeks and who is otherwise healthy. An unknown proportion of cases goes on to suppuration and breakdown. Draining sinuses, whether spontaneous or following incision and drainage, may persist for many months. *M. scrofulaceum* was the most common cause of this infection, with MAI the second. However, there has been a recent reversal of this ratio so that strains of MAI now are the most common isolates from these infected nodes. Rare cases caused by several other species have been reported.

Correct diagnosis depends on the physician's familiarity with the disease, a positive tuberculin skin test result (sometimes requiring the use of second-strength purified protein derivative), the absence of a history of contact with tuberculosis, absence of thoracic disease, and the location as well as the appearance of the involved nodes. Other conditions that need to be differentiated are tuberculosis, pyogenic lymphadenitis, cat scratch disease, congenital cyst, and lymphoma. The treatment of choice is excision of the involved nodes. In about 10 per cent of cases there is a recurrence of the infection in another group of nodes near the original site, occasionally on the other side. Rarely there may be a third episode. Recurrences should be treated in the same manner as the original infection. There is no convincing evidence that drug treatment is beneficial. It should be remembered that as a result of this infection a child may have a positive tuberculin skin test reaction for many years.

Skin and Soft Tissue Infections. CUTANEOUS GRANULOMA. Localized groups of papules have been called swimming pool granuloma or fish tank granuloma, depending on the source of infection. In another form of the disease there is a local abscess at the inoculation site, usually on the hand, followed by a series of secondary nodules that progress centrally along the lymphatics in a manner not unlike that seen in sporotrichosis. A few deep hand infections have also been described. The infection is not uncommon as an occupational or recreational illness in people who work or play in a marine environment. With few exceptions, the etiologic agent is *M. marinum.* Most superficial infections are self-limited. When treatment is deemed necessary, the physician may use a combination of rifampin and ethambutol, rifampin alone, one of the tetracyclines, or trimethoprim-sulfamethoxazole. All of these regimens have been reported to be successful.

LOCAL ABSCESS. Many cases of local abscess following subcutaneous or intramuscular injection have been reported, some in outbreaks. The trouble usually is traced to a contaminated multiple injection vial, and the etiologic agent usually is *M. fortuitum-chelonae.* Incision and drainage usually will suffice to control the infection.

LOCAL TRAUMA. Most of these infections caused by *M. fortuitum-chelonae* occur as a result of penetrating or lacerating wounds contaminated with soil. Expert surgical handling is necessary, along with appropriate drug therapy as outlined under Pulmonary Disease.

DISSEMINATED NODULES. Multiple nodules and abscesses may be associated with widely disseminated mycobacterial disease, almost always in an immunocompromised host. The species most often isolated is *M. fortuitum-chelonae.* In addition, such nodules have been described in renal transplant patients as a result of infection with *M. hemophilum.*

BURULI ULCER. This deeply penetrating ulcer caused by *M. ulcerans* is confined mainly to Africa, Papua New Guinea, Malaysia, and Australia. The treatment is difficult and controversial.

Skeletal Infections. The synovia, tendon sheaths, and bursae are involved more often than other parts of the skeletal system in nontuberculous mycobacterial infections. A wide variety of species may be associated, including environmental strains with little pathogenicity for humans, such as *M. terrae, M. gordonae,* and *M. flavescens.* Leading the list of etiologic agents is *M. kansasii,* with *M. fortuitum-chelonae* and MAI following in that order. Many of these infections follow trauma in which the wound is contaminated with soil or water. Others have occurred after injections of corticosteroids into arthritic joints; in these cases it is difficult to determine which condition was primary. The most common site is the hand, where the infection produces an indolent but persistent tenosynovitis, including the carpal tunnel syndrome. Osteomyelitis may occur in the form of multifocal lesions from hematogenous dissemination, often as a slowly progressive rather than a fulminant infection. The principal etiologic agent in these cases is MAI.

Treatment for skeletal infection usually demands close cooperation between a skilled surgeon and a physician specializing in infectious disease. Drug therapy depends on the etiologic agent (refer to earlier discussion).

Postsurgical Infections. Infections following surgery mainly are caused by *M. fortuitum-chelonae.* They include prosthetic valve endocarditis, sternal wound infection and osteomyelitis after open heart surgery, wound infection after augmentation mammoplasty, and infections associated with hemodialysis and peritoneal dialysis.

Disseminated Disease. Patients who develop disseminated disease usually are severely immunocompromised from the standpoint of cellular immune functions. The recently recognized AIDS has been associated with a dramatic increase in disseminated mycobacterial infections, since up to 50 per cent of such patients coming to autopsy in several cities have been found to have disseminated MAI infections. Prior to 1980 there were relatively few cases of disseminated mycobacterial disease reported throughout the world. Such cases usually involved patients who had underlying hematologic malignancies or who were under treatment with corticosteroids, or both. Both children and adults were affected, and the most common etiologic agents were *M. kansasii* and MAI. The case fatality rate was very high, even with the most intensive multiple-drug treatment. Diagnosis is most commonly made by biopsy and culture of liver, bone marrow, or lymph nodes. Cultures of the blood are often positive. Skin lesions or subcutaneous nodules or abscesses should be biopsied and examined for acid-fast bacilli. Strains of *M. fortuitum-chelonae* often are associated with these superficial lesions. The tissues may show a nonspecific necrotizing reaction in which macrophages are loaded with acid-fast bacilli, rather than a granulomatous reaction.

Treatment for disseminated disease is based on the same principles as those outlined for pulmonary disease. Infections caused by drug-sensitive organisms such as *M. kansasii* can usually be brought under at least temporary control provided that the human host is able to provide an adequate immune response. For infections related to MAI a multiple-drug regimen is usually chosen empirically, with a core of ansamycin* LM 427 (rifabutin) and clofazimine.*

---

*Investigational drugs available from Adria Laboratories, Dublin, OH, and Ciba-Geigy, Summit, NJ, respectively.

Beyt BE Jr, Ortbals DW, Santa Cruz DJ, et al.: Cutaneous mycobacteriosis: Analysis of 34 cases with a new classification of the disease. Medicine 60:95, 1980. *In 8 of these 34 patients from St. Louis, positive cultures for 3 different species other than M. tuberculosis were obtained.*

Chapman JS: The Atypical Mycobacteria and Human Mycobacteriosis. New York, Plenum Medical Book Company, 1977. *A very informative monograph from one of the leaders in the field.*

Good RC: Opportunistic pathogens in the genus *Mycobacterium*. Ann Rev Microbiol 39:347, 1985. *The reports of Good and of Wayne (see below) provide a thorough review of the microbiology and classification of the mycobacterial pathogens.*

Granger JM, Yates MD: Infections caused by opportunist mycobacteria: A review. J R Soc Med 79:226, 1986. *A succinct, informative account of mycobacteriosis as seen in England.*

Hawkins CC, Gold JWM, Whimbey E, et al.: *Mycobacterium avium* complex infections in patients with the acquired immunodeficiency syndrome. Ann Intern Med 105:184, 1986. *A report of 67 patients from New York, emphasizing the unsatisfactory result of treatment; mycobacteremia persisted in 24 of 26 treated patients. Previous reports are reviewed.*

Horsburgh CR Jr, Mason UG III, Farhi DC, et al.: Disseminated infection with *Mycobacterium avium-intracellulare*: A report of 13 cases and a review of the literature. Medicine 64:36, 1985. *A thorough analysis of 13 cases from the National Jewish Hospital and 24 cases from the literature, with emphasis on response to treatment.*

Iseman MD, Corpe RF, O'Brien RJ, et al.: Disease due to *Mycobacterium avium-intracellulare*. Chest 87 (Suppl 2): 139, 1985. *A consensus conference hammered out these concepts of diagnosis, pathogenesis, and treatment.*

Lichtenstein IH, MacGregor RR: Mycobacterial infections in renal transplant recipients: Report of five cases and review of the literature. Rev Infect Dis 5:216, 1983. *Renal transplant recipients have a high risk of disseminated mycobacteriosis, and 34 per cent of reported cases have been attributed to nontuberculous species.*

Marchevsky AM, Damsker B, Green S, et al.: The clinicopathological spectrum of nontuberculous mycobacterial osteoarticular infections. J Bone Joint Surg 67A:925, 1985. *A report of eight cases, attributed to five different species, with a good literature review. Infection of bone, synovium, and tendon sheaths may be seen.*

Marchevsky A, Damsker B, Gribetz A, et al.: The spectrum of pathology of nontuberculous mycobacterial infections in open-lung biopsy specimens. Am J Clin Pathol 78:695, 1982. *From 1969 to 1980 at New York's Mt. Sinai Medical Center, biopsy material from 40 patients revealed AFB. M. avium-intracellulare accounted for 24 cases and M. tuberculosis for 6. A variety of histopathologic reactions are described in addition to the classic granulomas.*

Margileth AM, Chandra R, Altman RP: Chronic lymphadenopathy due to mycobacterial infection: Clinical features, diagnosis, histopathology, and management. Am J Dis Child 138:917, 1984. *From Washington and New York comes this informative report of 153 cases, of which 86 per cent were due to nontuberculous mycobacteria. Unfortunately, no speciation of the positive cultures is presented.*

Moran JF, Alexander LG, Staub EW, et al.: Long-term results of pulmonary resection for atypical mycobacterial disease. Ann Thorac Surg 35:597, 1983. *This report documents the good results of resectional surgery in 37 patients seen by the surgical group at Duke University from 1967 to 1981. All disease was attributed to M. avium-intracellulare.*

Roth RI, Owen RL, Keren DF, et al.: Intestinal infection with *Mycobacterium avium* in AIDS: Histological and clinical comparison with Whipple's disease. Dig Dis Sci 30:497, 1985. *A good account of the fascinating similarity of some MAI intestinal infections to Whipple's disease.*

Wayne LG: The "atypical" mycobacteria: Recognition and disease association. CRC Crit Rev Microbiol 12:185, 1985. *See Good, above.*

Wolinsky E: Nontuberculous mycobacteria and associated diseases. Am Rev Respir Dis 119:107, 1979. *A "state of the art" review of the entire subject.*

304 LEPROSY (Hansen's Disease)

Ward E. Bullock

DEFINITION. Leprosy is a chronic granulomatous disease of humans that is caused by *Mycobacterium leprae*. The spectrum of its clinical manifestations is broad. At one end is tuberculoid (TT) leprosy, in which the clinical manifestations are localized to a single area of skin and the associated nerve supply. At the opposite end is lepromatous (LL) leprosy, in which there is massive infection of the dermis by *M. leprae* as well as involvement of the nerves, nasopharynx, testes, and lymphoreticular system. The intermediate forms of leprosy display mixtures of the clinical, histopathologic, and immunologic features typical of TT or LL disease. The intermediate

forms are less stable clinically and often progress toward the lepromatous type; spontaneous improvement with a shift toward the tuberculoid spectrum occurs less frequently unless antimicrobial therapy has been instituted. These "upward" or "downward" shifts, as defined by gain or loss of host resistance, may be marked by inflammatory reactions within infected tissues, the immunologic mechanisms of which are poorly understood. Such reactions produce considerable functional impairment when they involve the peripheral nerve trunks. Reactions of this type occur in individuals with intermediate forms of leprosy but not in those with TT or LL disease. LL leprosy is associated with a different type of tissue reaction, erythema nodosum leprosum (ENL), that likewise may precipitate acute nerve dysfunction, possibly as a result of the humoral response to antigens of *M. leprae*.

EPIDEMIOLOGY. *Incidence and Prevalence.* The World Health Organization has estimated the number of leprosy cases in the world to be approximately 11 million. However, valid statistics are not available from several countries with a high prevalence of leprosy, including China. The actual number probably exceeds 15 million. The highest prevalence rates are in Asia and Africa, followed by Central and South America and Oceania. Overall, the prevalence rate does not exceed 25 to 55 per 1000 in these areas, although it may be greater than 200 per 1000 within particular villages and surrounding areas.

The proportion of cases with lepromatous leprosy varies considerably from region to region; in Asia and the Americas it ranges from 25 to 65 per cent. In Africa the lepromatous forms of disease are distinctly less common, constituting from 6 to 20 per cent of the leprosy population. Roughly 20 per cent of the known cases in India are of the lepromatous type. Although most cases of leprosy are found in the tropics, leprosy can flourish in colder climates, as for example in Korea, northern China, and Siberia. Within the United States, leprosy is endemic in Hawaii and in small areas of Texas, Louisiana, and Florida. Nevertheless, of the 1923 new cases reported to the United States Public Health Service from 1981 through 1985, 90 per cent occurred in foreign-born patients. This percentage represents a significant shift since the period from 1947 to 1966, when only 55 per cent of patients were foreign born. The largest number of patients with leprosy from 1981 through 1985 have come from the Philippines, Mexico, Vietnam, and Kampuchea.

TRANSMISSION. The incubation period of leprosy is generally three to five years but may range from six months to decades. The precise modes of transmission have not been established. Traditionally, it had been thought that transmission involved prolonged close exposure of susceptible persons to the skin of an index case, especially one with lepromatous infection. In an endemic area, the risk of acquiring leprosy among household contacts of lepromatous cases is about eight times that in normal households; the risk of acquisition in households with tuberculoid leprosy is approximately four times normal. In fact, very few leprosy bacilli are shed from the intact skin of lepromatous patients; large numbers of organisms may be shed from skin ulcers, but these are relatively uncommon. By contrast, the nasal secretions of those with lepromatous disease contain up to 2×10^8 *M. leprae* in a single nose blow. Thus, a major portal of entry may be the respiratory tract. To date, however, there is little evidence to document primary respiratory tract infection *prior* to the onset of skin lesions. The granulomatous inflammation of leprosy does not caseate except occasionally within nerves. Since lesions heal without calcification, there are no residual tissue markers of primary infection equivalent to the Ghon complex of tuberculosis that might suggest the initial site of infection.

The gastrointestinal tract is a possible route for primary infection, since breast milk contains large numbers of *M. leprae*, but primary lesions have not been recognized within the gastrointestinal tract. Biting insects may provide still another means of transmission, since viable *M. leprae* can be isolated from the midguts of laboratory-bred arthropods for at least 48 hours after they have fed on lepromatous cases.

Although humans have been thought to be the only natural hosts of *M. leprae*, a disease resembling lepromatous leprosy has been recognized in up to 10 per cent of feral armadillos from certain regions of Louisiana. The organism recovered from these animals is indistinguishable from *M. leprae* by available techniques. Leprosy has also been discovered in the sooty mangabey, a New World monkey. Thus, there may exist reservoirs of *M. leprae* other than the human.

Susceptibility to Leprosy. The host factors that determine susceptibility to disease once an individual has been infected with *M. leprae* are poorly understood. The incidence of new cases usually is highest among older children and young adults. Although the cell-mediated immune responses of younger children may be relatively immature at the time of initial exposure to *M. leprae* and thereby predispose to increased disease incidence, environmental factors undoubtedly play a major role as well. The index case in childhood leprosy frequently is a parent with untreated disease with whom the child will have had prolonged and close contact.

Leprosy is diagnosed more frequently in males than in females, the ratio being 3:1 in some areas. The apparent predominance of leprosy in males probably is specious, since census figures in many regions are uncontrolled for sex selection.

Genetic factors long have been held to be important in determining susceptibility to leprosy, especially to the lepromatous type. Strong support for this concept is lacking. In a large study of monozygotic twins, 37 of 62 (60 per cent) of monozygotic twin pairs were concordant for leprosy of similar type, whereas in 25 pairs (40 per cent) only 1 member had leprosy. Others have failed to detect differences from normal in the segregation patterns of multiple genetic polymorphic systems among leprosy cases. Likewise, no consistent associations have been found between leprosy and HLA-A, B, or C antigens.

ETIOLOGY. The causative agent of leprosy is a bacillus measuring 0.3 to 0.4 μm × 4 to 7 μm that is acid-alcohol fast when stained by the Ziehl-Neelsen method. Although the lepra bacillus was the first to be identified as the cause of human disease by Hansen in 1874, successful cultivation of this organism in vitro has not yet been achieved conclusively, and hence relatively little is known of its biology. A significant advance was made in 1960, when Shephard observed that a small inoculum (10^4) of *M. leprae* prepared from infected human tissues will multiply in the footpads of mice to a plateau level of 10^6. During multiplication, the doubling time of *M. leprae* is extraordinarily long, ranging from 10 to 13 days. The mouse footpad model has also made it possible to study the efficacy of many compounds against *M. leprae* in vivo.

Systemic infections with *M. leprae* can be achieved in mice and rats that are congenitally athymic or have been neonatally thymectomized. It is difficult to maintain immunodeficient animals for prolonged periods, and thus the utility of these models has been limited. Nine-banded armadillos and some species of monkeys are susceptible to infection with *M. leprae*. The former tend to develop an overwhelming infection that is analogous to lepromatous leprosy.

PATHOGENESIS AND HISTOPATHOLOGY. Whatever the portal of entry for *M. leprae* may be, the first clinical manifestations of leprosy appear in the skin. The histopathology of an early lesion may be indeterminate, revealing only nonspecific inflammation composed of a scanty lymphocytic infiltrate around the dermal appendages and neurovascular bundles. Rarely, an acid-fast bacillus can be seen within small nerves of the dermis. In untreated cases, indeterminate lesions may resolve spontaneously or evolve until the histopathology becomes more characteristic of leprosy. It is then possible to

TABLE 304–1. IMMUNOLOGIC MANIFESTATIONS WITHIN THE LEPROSY SPECTRUM*

Manifestation	TT	BT	BB	BL	LL
Lepromin reaction	3+	1+	±	–	–
ENL	–	–	–	±	2+
Bacilli in nose	–	–	–	1+	2+
Bacilli in granuloma	0	1–3+	3–4+	4–5+	5–6+
Epithelioid cells	1+	1+	1+	–	–
Langhans giant cells	1+	2+	–	–	–
Foam cells	–	–	–	1+	3+
Lymphocytes	3+	2+	1+	1+	±
Nerve destruction (skin)	2+	2+	1+	±	–

*Modified from Ridley DS: Int J Leprosy 40:102, 1972.

classify a lesion within the leprosy spectrum based on the cell types and the number of bacilli observed within the areas of granulomatous inflammation. The best standardized classification of leprosy is that developed by Ridley and Jopling, in which the leprosy spectrum is divided into five groups as outlined in Table 304–1.

Tuberculoid (TT) Leprosy. The lesion of TT leprosy is characterized by well-developed granulomas composed of epithelioid cells with a uniform appearance and giant cells of the Langhans or foreign-body type. Lymphocytes are abundant at the periphery of the granuloma, and acid-fast bacilli usually cannot be identified. Dermal nerves involved by the granulomatous inflammation are destroyed.

Borderline Tuberculoid (BT) Leprosy. The pathology of TT and BT leprosy is similar except that acid-fast bacilli are more readily seen in the latter, especially in dermal nerves, although the number is small.

Borderline (BB) Leprosy. In BB leprosy, the histologic picture may vary considerably from lesion to lesion or even within the same lesion. Typically, the granuloma formation is less well developed. Epithelioid cells are spread more diffusely throughout the granuloma, giant cells are not present, and there are fewer lymphocytes within the infiltrate. The dermal nerves are less damaged, and therefore more easily visible. Acid-fast bacilli are numerous.

Borderline Lepromatous (BL) Leprosy. In this form, histiocytes are the predominant cell type with relatively few lymphocytes scattered among them, sometimes in aggregates. Epithelioid cells are absent. The damage within dermal nerves is less than that observed in BB disease, but there is increased perineural inflammation. This produces lamination of the perineurium that imparts an "onion skin" appearance to the nerve. Large numbers of acid-fast bacilli are present.

Lepromatous Leprosy (LL). The inflammatory infiltrate is composed almost exclusively of histiocytic cells that have a foamy appearance. Masses of bacilli are present intracellularly, many in large clumps called globi. Lymphocytes are very sparse. Characteristically, there is a "clear zone" beneath the epidermal basement membrane in which there is no inflammatory infiltrate, as contrasted with the tuberculoid forms of leprosy, in which the granulomas extend to the dermal-epidermal junction.

Granulomas can be identified in the lymphoreticular organs of persons with tuberculoid leprosy. However, granulomatous pathology is far more extensive in BL and LL disease. For example, the paracortical regions of lymph nodes are heavily infiltrated by masses of histiocytes and literally are "choked" with acid-fast bacilli; T lymphocytes, normally abundant in this area, are largely displaced. The germinal centers, containing a predominance of B lymphocytes, are spared; they tend to be increased in both size and number. In the spleen, the white pulp is especially prone to invasion by histiocytic cells, although the red pulp also may be infiltrated. Aggregates of foamy histiocytes are present in the liver, most frequently around the portal tracts and scattered within the lobules. Patients suffering from LL disease manifest a continuous bacteremia with up to 1×10^5 bacilli per milliliter of blood, and the total body burden of *M. leprae* may approach 10^{12}.

IMMUNOPATHOLOGIC CONSIDERATIONS. Intracutaneous injection of healthy individuals and of patients with TT or BT leprosy with a heat-killed suspension of *M. leprae* (integral lepromin) prepared from skin lepromas will induce local granuloma formation within a three- to four-week period. Conversely, patients with LL disease are completely anergic to lepromin. Thus, the lepromin test provides a crude indication of an individual's capacity to mount a cell-mediated immune response against *M. leprae*. If more purified preparations of *M. leprae* are employed to skin test for delayed-type hypersensitivity or to measure the proliferative responses of lymphocytes in vitro, the response to these antigens decreases progressively across the leprosy spectrum, i.e., they are greatest in TT leprosy and least in LL cases. Moreover, in a high percentage of the latter group, there is a generalized impairment of the delayed-type hypersensitivity response to a variety of "recall" antigens as measured by skin testing and lymphocyte proliferative responses. The anergy to antigens of *M. leprae* is very persistent despite long-term treatment, whereas the anergy to other antigens tends to be reversible.

Serum levels of the immunoglobulins generally are normal in tuberculoid patients, whereas polyclonal hypergammaglobulinemia is a common feature of lepromatous leprosy. More than 90 per cent of lepromatous sera contain antibodies to antigens of *M. leprae*, many of which are cross-reactive with other mycobacteria; as antimicrobial therapy is continued, titers of these antibodies decline over a period of years. Ten per cent or more of patients with LL disease will have biologic false-positive reactions in tests for syphilis employing cardiolipin-type antigens, and more than 30 per cent will have cryoglobulinemia. Circulating immune complexes are present in a substantial but variable percentage of lepromatous cases, and in more than 50 per cent the serum contains elevated levels of amyloid-related serum protein component (SAA), an acute phase reactant. Although the relationship of SAA to tissue amyloid is unclear, secondary amyloidosis is not an uncommon complication of longstanding lepromatous leprosy. At least 50 per cent of cases have greatly elevated serum levels of C-reactive protein. Less frequently, antinuclear antibodies and rheumatoid factor are present, as well as low titers of antibody to thyroglobulin. In tuberculoid forms of leprosy, the prevalence of these serologic abnormalities is very low, presumably because the host immunoregulatory control mechanisms are less disordered.

CLINICAL MANIFESTATIONS. The variations of histopathology within the skin and peripheral nerves are reflected clinically by a wide range of skin lesions and peripheral neuropathies. The typical indeterminate lesion is usually, but not always, seen in children. It is a hypopigmented macule, of which there are rarely more than three or four. The macule measures 2 to 5 cm in diameter, and sensation may be impaired slightly within the macular area. In many cases the macules resolve spontaneously, whereas in others they evolve to become lesions more typical of tuberculoid or lepromatous disease.

TT leprosy generally presents as a single large plaque or macule that is very well defined. Occasionally, up to two or three lesions are present. Plaques are erythematous with sharply elevated outer borders that slope toward a flattened center, which is rough, dry, hairless, and anesthetic. Macules may be either erythematous or hypopigmented in the center. Enlarged dermal nerve twigs and related peripheral nerve trunks may be palpable or visible within the involved skin area. The most frequently enlarged nerves are the greater auricular, the ulnar above the elbow, the peroneal as it curves around the head of the fibula, and the posterior tibial. As with skin lesions, nerve damage is localized. Any area of the body may be affected, although the axillae, inguinal region, and perineal areas are spared, presumably because of the proclivity of *M. leprae* to grow in cooler areas of the body.

BT leprosy closely resembles TT disease; however, the plaques or macules tend to be more numerous, and satellite lesions sometimes are present near the larger lesions. The peripheral nerve trunks frequently are enlarged by granulomatous infiltrates. Some of the more common complications are (1) traumatic plantar ulcerations of the feet, (2) footdrop, (3) loss of hand function as a result of flexion contracture and repeated trauma to anesthetic digits, and (4) corneal abrasions if there is corneal nerve dysfunction.

The lesions of BB leprosy are polymorphic in appearance. Generally they are numerous and vary considerably in size. Unlike the tuberculoid forms of disease, in which lesions are localized to one side of the body, the lesions of BB leprosy are more symmetric. In some cases they appear as large, erythematous bands with sharply demarcated centers and outer edges. Others appear as irregular erythematous plaques with poorly defined outer margins and hypopigmented centers that have a characteristic "punched-out" appearance. Not infrequently, both types are present simultaneously, and satellite lesions are common. The lesions tend not to be as anesthetic as those in TT or BT disease.

Skin manifestations of BL leprosy are perhaps the most heterogeneous of all. They are numerous, are distributed bilaterally, and can present as macules, plaques, papules, or nodules. BL skin lesions tend to include some nodules with "dimpled" appearance in the center, and some plaques have centers that appear hypopigmented and "punched out." As a rule, the nasal structures are not involved, although the ear lobes may be thickened. Nerve thickening can be quite prominent near the site of cutaneous lesions, but anesthesia is less evident than in the forms described above.

During early stages of LL leprosy, the extensive inflammatory response within the dermis gives rise to widely distributed erythematous macules or papules. In dark-skinned individuals these are difficult to see unless viewed obliquely in good light. With progression, plaques and nodules become evident. In later stages they are the predominant types of lesions. The skin becomes progressively thickened with infiltrate to produce the classic leonine facies in association with thinning and loss of eyebrows. Occasionally, cases of LL leprosy can present without obvious localized lesions but instead have diffuse lepromatous infiltrates in the skin. This type of disease is observed most frequently in Central America. Those who suffer from it are prone to develop a distinctive vasculitis (the so-called "Lucio's phenomenon") involving the dermal vessels that results in ischemic necrosis of the epidermis. The lesions are stellate in appearance and heal with atrophic scar formation.

In LL leprosy, the eyes frequently are involved by keratitis and iritis; there is progressive destruction of the nasal cartilage and anterior maxillary spinous process, resulting in saddle nose deformity. Incisor teeth may be lost, and chronic inflammation of the larynx can lead to life-threatening stenosis. Extensive infection of the testes is common, leading to fibrosis and hyalinization of the seminiferous tubules and azoospermia; the testicular damage is reflected by elevated gonadotropin levels, reduced plasma testosterone levels, and gynecomastia. The ovaries are infected only rarely. Nerve involvement is more extensive in LL leprosy than in other forms, although functional deficits are less severe because the intensity of the intraneuronal inflammation is reduced consequent to poor cell-mediated immunity to *M. leprae*. The neurologic damage usually manifests as mononeuritis multiplex, i.e., an asymmetric sensory polyneuropathy.

Reactional States. Although leprosy itself is an extremely torpid infection, the clinical course all too frequently is punctuated by acute and subacute reactional states that produce serious morbidity and even death. The most common of these reactional states is erythema nodosum leprosum (ENL), which occurs only in patients with high bacterial loads—namely, those with BL or LL disease. Occasionally, untreated patients experience ENL. Much more frequently, effective antileprosy treatment triggers the onset of ENL, which occurs in more than 50 per cent of patients within the first year. The onset of ENL is sudden over a 24- to 48-hour period with eruption of painful red papules or nodules over the face, trunk, arms, and thighs. Nodules may proceed to frank suppuration, requiring several weeks to heal, generally without scarring. Occasionally, ENL is chronic lasting several months. Histologically, early ENL nodules reveal polymorphonuclear infiltration within the lepromatous granulomas, and frequently there is panniculitis; a panvasculitis may involve both arteries and veins in the dermis. It is widely believed that ENL activated by antimycobacterial therapy is precipitated by degradation of *M. leprae* with release of antigenic material. Antibodies to *M. leprae* are presumed to complex with these antigens, thereby inducing a number of serious constitutional distrubances, including severe pyrexia, iridocyclitis, neuritis, orchitis, lymphadenitis, and polyarthritis. In addition, there is a high prevalence of glomerulonephritis in ENL. Acute proliferative glomerulonephritis and focal mesangial hypercellularity with thickening of the glomerular capillary loops are the most consistent findings. Deposits of subendothelial or subepithelial electron-dense material are seen by electron microscopy, and discontinuous linear deposits of IgG, IgM, and C3 have been demonstrated along the capillary membranes by fluorescence microscopy. To date, it has not been established that antigenic material derived from *M. leprae* is actually present within the glomeruli. Notwithstanding the severity of the inflammatory response in many cases of ENL, hypocomplementemia is unusual.

Reversal Reactions. Patients with BT, BB, or BL disease may experience a quite different type of tissue reaction after several months of treatment. As patients improve, typically from a BL to a BB classification, some will develop induration and erythema within infected areas of the skin. Histologic examination reveals an influx of lymphocytes into areas of granulomatous inflammation, with concomitant reduction in the number of bacilli. Reversal reactions generally develop over days or weeks and last for weeks or months. Although these reactions are regarded as an "upgrading" of the host's cellular immune responses, the clinical consequences can be serious. For example, augmentation of the inflammatory response within peripheral nerves can irreversibly damage the already compromised fascicles. Reactions quite similar in appearance to reversal reactions but that signal a deterioration in the immune response may be experienced by patients whose compliance with therapy is poor or in whom the *M. leprae* has become drug resistant. These so-called "downgrading" reactions are associated with worsening of the clinical condition and an increased bacillary index.

DIAGNOSIS AND DIFFERENTIAL DIAGNOSIS. Isolation of a phenolic glycolipid I that appears unique to *M. leprae* offers promise that serologic tests may aid in the early diagnosis of leprosy. At present, however, the diagnosis must be established by clinical examination and histopathologic study. An anesthetic or hypoesthetic skin lesion immediately suggests leprosy; associated nerve thickening further supports the diagnosis. A skin biopsy is essential for confirmation and accurate classification of the disease. An adequate biopsy specimen must include both central and peripheral areas of a lesion and should be deep enough to remove subcutaneous fatty tissue en bloc. Elliptical excision biopsy 12 to 15 mm long is preferred to punch biopsy. When lesions of varying types are present, it is advisable to obtain biopsies from two different sites.

M. leprae in paraffinized tissues is poorly stained by the Ziehl-Neelsen method. A much better stain is obtained by the Wade-Fite method, or its equivalent, which restores the acid-fast property of *M. leprae* by impregnating the tissue section with an oily substance such as turpentine or peanut oil. Control sections known to contain acid-fast staining organisms should be prepared simultaneously. In patients with paucibacillary disease (i.e., TT or BT), serial histologic sections may have to be searched for hours to identify one or two bacilli, most frequently within dermal nerve twigs. The Ziehl-Neelsen stain is adequate for smear preparations as from nasal scrapings and the buffy coat of blood. Acid-fast staining bacilli are readily visualized in both types of smears in BL or LL disease. In buffy coat smears, mononuclear cells contain bacilli, as do occasional polymorphonuclear leukocytes.

Clinical signs and symptoms that may be helpful in establishing the diagnosis of lepromatous leprosy include the following: (1) The ear lobes are thickened and have a "succulent" appearance. (2) The patient complains of a chronically stuffy nose with discharge that sometimes is bloody; frequently the examiner will note a fetid odor. (3) There may be ENL lesions scattered widely over the body, including the face. Erythema nodosum that is associated with other conditions usually is localized to the pretibial regions of the lower extremities. ENL is not seen in tuberculoid leprosy. (4) Not infrequently there is brawny edema involving the lower extremities and hands. Fusiform swelling of the digits that extends to the dorsum of the hands is seen, mimicking scleroderma.

Certain types of nerve deficits or deformities should suggest the possibility of leprosy in any form. These include (1) plantar ulcerations in a person who is neither diabetic nor tabetic; (2) footdrop without a history of poliomyelitis or heavy metal exposure; and (3) a characteristic claw deformity of the hands, with digital damage resulting from motor and sensory dysfunction of the ulnar nerve and other nerve supply to the hand. Occasionally, leprosy will be misdiagnosed as lupus erythematosus; fluorescent antibody staining of a skin biopsy may reveal immunoglobulin deposits resembling those of lupus within the epidermal basement membrane. A Wade-Fite stain is most helpful in such situations.

TREATMENT—PRINCIPAL DRUGS. *Dapsone.* A major drug for leprosy is 4,4'-diaminodiphenylsulfone (dapsone, DDS). DDS is thought to block the *p*-aminobenzoic acid condensation reaction necessary for folate synthesis. The minimal inhibitory concentration (MIC) of DDS for *M. leprae* that are susceptible to the drug ranges between 0.01 and 0.001 μg per milliliter as determined by the mouse footpad assay. DDS is inexpensive, a factor of great economic significance in countries with high prevalence rates of leprosy. Its toxicity is low; however, adverse reactions to DDS occasionally occur. The most serious are hemolysis, agranulocytosis, hepatitis, exfoliative dermatitis, and, very rarely, severe hypoalbuminemia. A devastating combination of exfoliative dermatitis and hepatitis, known as the "DDS syndrome," has been observed in perhaps 1 per 5000 cases in the early stages of treatment (less than seven weeks). Immediate cessation of DDS, intensive care, and massive corticosteroid therapy (in excess of 100 mg per day of prednisone or its equivalent) may be lifesaving.

Twenty-four hours after ingestion of DDS, 100 mg, the plasma concentration in a 60-kg person ranges from approximately 0.12 to 0.4 μg per milliliter. This rather wide range is explained by large individual differences in rates of clearance from the body, resulting in part from genetic polymorphism in acetylation of the drug. Thus, the half-life in plasma varies from 10 to 50 hours, with an average of 28 hours. Regardless of an individual's acetylation status, the plasma levels of DDS under daily therapy with 50 to 100 mg will remain well in excess of the MIC for susceptible *M. leprae*.

*Rifampin.** The MIC of rifampin against *M. leprae* is less than 1 μg per milliliter, and it provides a rapid bactericidal effect against organisms in tissues and nasal secretions. As little as four weeks of therapy with rifampin prevent multiplication in the mouse footpad of acid-fast bacilli harvested from tissue specimens or nasal secretions of patients with lepromatous leprosy. A comparable loss of infectivity cannot

---

*This use is not listed in the manufacturer's directive.

be achieved with DDS until 10 to 12 weeks of treatment. Rifampin therapy also rapidly reduces the morphologic index (MI) of *M. leprae*. The MI expresses a ratio of the number of bacilli, within tissues or secretions, that stain uniformly by acid-fast methods and that therefore are considered viable, to the number of bacilli that strain irregularly and are considered to be nonviable. The MI of *M. leprae* in lepromatous patients falls to nearly zero within four weeks after the start of rifampin therapy. By contrast, three to six months of DDS therapy may be required for comparable reduction of the MI.

Clofazimine. Clofazimine (B663) is a phenazine iminoquinone derivative that is effective in the treatment of leprosy, although its mechanism of action is not well understood. There is some evidence that it may act by inhibiting template formation of deoxyribonucleic acid. The compound is highly lipophilic and is deposited within fatty tissues, the skin, and the reticuloendothelial system, where it is taken up by macrophages. Clofazimine is a dye and causes skin pigmentation over time, with a coloration varying from a reddish hue to a deep purple. After discontinuation of clofazimine therapy, the pigmentation clears gradually over a period of months to years. Clofazimine is eliminated very slowly, with a half-life following oral administration of 70 days or more. Urinary excretion is negligible, whereas approximately 50 per cent of an administered dose may be recovered unchanged from the feces, possibly as a result of incomplete absorption from the gut and excretion via the bile, in which high concentrations have been found. Given in high concentrations (200 to 300* mg per day) for extended periods of time, the drug is deposited in the small intestinal wall and causes segmental thickening that may be associated with midabdominal burning or cramping pain, diarrhea, and rarely partial small bowel obstruction.

TREATMENT—CURRENT RECOMMENDATIONS. Of great concern has been the emergence of both primary and secondary resistance to DDS. Worldwide, the prevalence of secondary resistance currently ranges from 20 to 190 per 1000, depending on locale. Primary resistance to DDS of varying prevalence and degree also has been reported worldwide. In view of these findings, it is essential that multiple antibiotics be administered to all patients with leprosy.

For treatment of multibacillary forms of leprosy (BB, BL, and LL types), the following triple-drug combination is suggested by the World Health Organization (WHO): (1) a self-administered oral dose of DDS, 50 to 100 mg daily; (2) a self-administered oral dose of clofazimine, 50 mg daily plus a 300-mg* dose given once monthly under supervision; and (3) an oral dose of rifampin, 600 mg once monthly under supervision. When clofazimine is unacceptable, ethionamide† or prothionamide‡ should be considered in a self-administered oral dose of 250 to 375 mg daily. The case for use of the latter antibiotics is more compelling in patients harboring *M. leprae* that is resistant to DDS. Proof of resistance requires special procedures that are available at centers for the treatment of leprosy.

Combined therapy should be given for a minimum of two years. If possible, such therapy should be continued until all skin scrapings and biopsies become negative for acid-fast bacilli, a process that may require several years.

The WHO recommendation for intermittent rifampin† treatment is made in part because of the heavy economic burden that the drug places upon nations with a high prevalence of leprosy. The scientific rationale is based on clinical trials and studies of intermittent chemotherapy in the mouse footpad infection model. Despite the early promise of intermittent rifampin therapy and the low incidence of reactions to the drug when it is given in this manner (influenza-like syndrome, thrombocytopenic purpura, and shock), the WHO recommendation is based on limited data. Many experienced physicians prefer to give 450 or 600 mg of rifampin* daily for two to three years when possible.

For treatment of paucibacillary disease (indeterminant, TT, and BT types), the WHO recommends administration of rifampin,* 600 mg orally once per month under supervision for a six-month period, plus DDS, 100 mg orally daily for six months, self-administered. If relapse occurs, the treatment regimen should be repeated. The number of *M. leprae* in patients with paucibacillary disease rarely exceeds 10^6. Therefore, the risk of selecting drug-resistant mutants by treatment appears to be quite low. Moreover, the cell-mediated immune defense mechanisms of these patients are better able to deal with the leprosy bacillus than are those of patients with multibacillary disease. However, the long-term efficacy of intermittent rifampin therapy for paucibacillary disease has not been established. Thus some leprologists prefer to treat such cases with DDS, 50 to 100 mg daily, plus rifampin, 450 to 600 mg daily for six months, with DDS therapy continued for two to five years.

In patients with multibacillary disease who are treated appropriately, clinical improvement generally can be detected after the third month of treatment and clearly is evident by the sixth month. Disappearance of recognizable bacillary forms usually requires three to five years even though viable bacilli rapidly become undetectable by currently available assay methods. Thus patients with lepromatous leprosy have difficulty not only in disposing of viable *M. leprae* but also in clearing nonviable organisms.

Patients with lepromatous leprosy who are under treatment with a drug regimen that includes rifampin can be regarded as noncontagious after a two- to three-week period. However, even the untreated patient represents only a very low risk of contagion and can be admitted to any general hospital in which ordinary procedures of barrier nursing are observed. Tuberculoid leprosy should be viewed as noncontagious.

Treatment of Reactions. ENL is by far the most common reaction in lepromatous leprosy. When mild, it can be managed with aspirin. Severe episodes are controlled rapidly by high dosages of prednisone (60 to 80 mg per day). However, as the dosage is tapered, a flare-up of ENL is encountered frequently. Thalidomide† is very effective in treating severe ENL. The initial dosage is usually 200 mg given twice daily with gradual tapering over several weeks to maintenance levels of 50 to 100 mg per day. This dosage can be continued for several months. Administration of both prednisone and thalidomide brings about prompt improvement and permits rapid steroid withdrawal within a few days as the thalidomide takes full effect. The use of thalidomide in women of childbearing age is hazardous because of its teratogenicity. Clofazimine is also effective in the management of ENL, although it requires from four to six weeks to exert its effect. ENL reactions in patients with BL leprosy are poorly controlled by thalidomide and are best managed by judicious use of steroids and/or clofazimine.

Reversal reactions associated with severe neuritis or in which there is a risk of skin ulceration should be treated with steroids in high dosage, followed by gradual tapering. Alternatively, steroids plus clofazimine can be employed to attempt more rapid withdrawal of the steroid. Reversal reactions are far more chronic than the usual episodes of ENL and may require anti-inflammatory therapy for several months. Thalidomide is ineffective in treating these reactions.

Treatment of Other Complications. A cold abscess within a peripheral nerve requires surgical drainage. A sudden in-

---

*Manufacturer does not recommend doses above 200 mg/day.
†This use is not listed in the manufacturer's directive.
‡Investigational drug.

---

*This use is not listed in the manufacturer's directive.
†Investigational drug in leprosy.

crease in the intensity of nerve pain and/or increase in the functional deficit of a nerve under full medical therapy may be helped in some cases by surgical decompression to relieve the intraneural edema. Excellent corrective surgical procedures are available for deformity of the hands secondary to permanent loss of motor innervation. The common problem of footdrop can be greatly improved by transfer of the tibialis posterior muscle so that it becomes a dorsiflexor. Plantar ulceration secondary to sensory loss responds well to appropriate medical and surgical management. Subsequently the patient should be fitted carefully with special footwear that will increase the area of loadbearing and reduce pressure at the ulcer-prone site. Madarosis (complete loss of eyebrows) can be corrected by swinging scalp flaps to the eyebrow area after infection has been arrested. This cosmetic procedure can make the difference between social acceptance or nonacceptance, since laymen in regions endemic for leprosy are well aware of the cause of eyebrow loss. Leprotic iridocyclitis is an insidious complication in lepromatous patients that may progress without pain. Treatment with mydriatrics and steroids is essential to prevent destruction of the ciliary body. Lagophthalmos secondary to involvement of the seventh cranial nerve also must be corrected to prevent exposure keratitis.

PROGNOSIS. Most cases of TT leprosy are self-curing, as are many of those with indeterminate disease. Some individuals with BT leprosy may self-cure with or without permanent nerve damage; however, there is a tendency for others to lose cell-mediated immune responsiveness to *M. leprae* and to drift toward the lepromatous end of the disease spectrum. Notwithstanding the more favorable prognosis in tuberculoid leprosy, all patients should be treated as detailed above.

Most cases of lepromatous leprosy can be brought to a state of arrest if not cure, provided that compliance is good and that appropriate therapy is continued for a prolonged period.

Death caused by amyloidosis or inadequately treated ENL is infrequent.

PREVENTION AND PROPHYLAXIS. The household contacts of leprosy patients, especially children, should be examined carefully for signs of leprosy, and suspicious skin lesions must be biopsied. Generally, household contacts of TT and BT patients should not be given prophylaxis, although they should be examined annually. Children who have had extensive household contact with BL or LL patients who have been untreated should be considered for DDS prophylaxis; DDS has been shown to be of prophylactic value in children under the age of 16 when given according to recommended dosage schedules (Filice and Fraser). Adults appear to be less susceptible to leprosy; since the efficacy of DDS prophylaxis in this group has not been established, preventive treatment of older age groups usually is not recommended.

Three major trials to determine the preventive role of bacille Calmette-Guérin (BCG) vaccine against leprosy have yielded different results. At this time BCG is not recommended for prevention of leprosy. *M. leprae* vaccine trials currently are in progress worldwide.

Bullock WE: Immunology of leprosy. In Nahmias A, O'Reilly R (eds.): Immunology of Human Infection, Part I. New York, Plenum Publishing Corporation, 1981, p 369. *A thorough discussion of the immunologic disturbances associated with leprosy.*

Filice GA, Fraser DW: Management of household contacts of leprosy patients. Ann Intern Med 88:538, 1978. *Detailed recommendations.*

Ridley DS, Jopling WH: Classification of leprosy according to immunity. A five-group system. Int J Leprosy 34:255, 1966. *Most helpful for comprehending the spectrum of leprosy. Good illustrations.*

Serjeantson SW: HLA and susceptibility to leprosy. Immunol Rev 70:89, 1983. *A good review of the genetic aspects of leprosy.*

WHO Study Group Report: Chemotherapy of leprosy for control programmes. WHO Technical Report Series No. 675. Geneva, WHO, 1982. *A new report containing important recommendations for changes in the treatment of leprosy.*

Yawalkar SJ, Vischer W: Lamprene (Clofazimine) in Leprosy. Basel, Ciba-Geigy Limited, 1984, pp 1–19. *A concise summary of what is known about this important drug.*

Sexually Transmitted Diseases

P. Frederick Sparling

305 INTRODUCTION AND COMMON SYNDROMES

Sexually transmitted diseases (STD's) are a diverse group of infections, caused by biologically dissimilar microbial agents, which are grouped together because of certain common clinical and epidemiologic features. In recent years there has been a remarkable accumulation of information about venereal infections. Advent of the acquired immunodeficiency syndrome (AIDS) has heightened public awareness of the importance of STD's and the dangers of unsafe sexual practices. New knowledge has accumulated rapidly about old diseases; for instance, it is now clear that cervical carcinoma is a complication of certain human papillomavirus (genital wart virus) infections. Some relatively less severe infections, such as chlamydial ones, are known to be alarmingly prevalent in young persons. This chapter will discuss certain common features of some of these infections, as well as the differential diagnosis and management of several of the common syndromes of genital infections.

DEFINITIONS. Those infectious agents that are frequently transmitted by sexual contact, and for which sexual transmission is epidemiologically important, are considered sexually transmitted diseases. In some cases, such as gonorrhea and genital herpes simplex virus infection, sexual transmission is the only important mode of transmission, at least between adults. In others, such as the hepatitis viruses, giardiasis, shigellosis, and amebiasis, there are also important nonsexual means of acquiring infection. Table 305–1 lists the important infectious agents that are commonly transmitted sexually, as well as their known or probable disease syndromes. "Sexual" includes the full range of heterosexual or homosexual behavior, including genital, oral-genital, oral-anal, and genital-anal contact.

EPIDEMIOLOGIC CONSIDERATIONS. Sexually transmitted infections are prevalent in many segments of society, but, for obvious reasons, are most prevalent in the groups with the most promiscuous sexual activity. It is not sexual activity per se, but the number and type of different sexual partners that determine the risk of acquiring STD. The highest rates of gonorrhea are found in the young (15 to 30) and unmarried and in groups of low educational and socioeconomic status. Rates of gonococcal infection may be 50-fold higher in young, single inner-city persons than in married middle to upper-middle-class persons. Decisions regarding the cost-effectiveness of screening for STD should be governed by these considerations; screening is most effective in high-risk groups.

Multiple infections are frequent in patients with sexually transmitted infection. In venereal disease clinics, about 20 per cent of men with gonorrhea also have urethral chlamydial

TABLE 305–1. SEXUALLY TRANSMITTED AGENTS AND THEIR SYNDROMES*

Microorganism	Syndromes
Bacteria	
Neisseria gonorrhoeae	Urethritis, cervicitis, bartholinitis, proctitis, pharyngitis, salpingitis, epididymitis, conjunctivitis, perihepatitis, arthritis, dermatitis, endocarditis, meningitis, amniotic infection syndrome
Mobiluncus species and *Gardnerella vaginalis*	"Nonspecific" vaginosis
Treponema pallidum	Syphilis (multiple clinical syndromes)
Hemophilus ducreyi	Chancroid
Calymmatobacterium granulomatis	Granuloma inguinale
Shigella species	Enteritis in homosexual men
Campylobacter species	Enteritis in homosexual men
Group B *Streptococcus*	Neonatal sepsis and meningitis
Chlamydiae	
Chlamydia trachomatis	Nongonococcal urethritis, purulent hypertrophic cervicitis, epididymitis, salpingitis, conjunctivitis, trachoma, pneumonia, perihepatitis, lymphogranuloma venereum, Reiter's syndrome
Mycoplasmas	
Ureaplasma urealyticum	Nongonococcal urethritis, ? premature rupture of membranes and abortion
Mycoplasma hominis	Postpartum fever, pelvic inflammatory disease
Viruses	
Herpes simplex virus	Genital herpes, proctitis, meningitis, disseminated infection in neonates
Hepatitis A virus	Hepatitis in homosexual men
Hepatitis B virus	Hepatitis, ? periarteritis nodosa, hepatoma; especially prevalent in homosexual men
Cytomegalovirus	Congenital infection (birth defects, infant mortality, mental deficiency, hearing loss); mononucleosis syndrome
Human papillomavirus	Condyloma acuminatum; cervical carcinoma
Molluscum contagiosum virus	Molluscum contagiosum
Human immunodeficiency virus	Acquired immunodeficiency syndrome and related illnesses
Protozoa	
Trichomonas vaginalis	Trichomonal vaginitis, occasional urethritis
Entamoeba histolytica	Enteritis in homosexual men
Giardia lamblia	Enteritis in homosexual men
Fungi	
Candida albicans	Vaginitis, balanitis
Ectoparasites	
Phthirus pubis	Pubic lice infestation
Sarcoptes scabei	Scabies

*The relative importance of sexual transmission in the epidemiology of several of these agents remains to be defined; these include Group B streptococci, hepatitis A virus, cytomegalovirus, *Candida albicans*, and others.

infection, and 30 to 50 per cent of women with gonorrhea also have cervical chlamydial infection. In women with vaginitis, one study showed that 16 per cent of cases were caused by mixed infection with various combinations of *Candida*, *Trichomonas*, and *Gardnerella vaginalis*. However, there is no convincing evidence that one sexually transmitted infection directly increases the risk of acquiring others. Rather, the frequent coexistence of multiple sexually acquired infections probably reflects the frequency of these organisms and the multiplicity of sexual partners among patients who were the subjects of these studies.

Control of sexually transmitted infections is complicated by the frequent lack of significant symptoms. The majority of gonococcal and chlamydial infections in women probably are associated with few symptoms. From 10 to 50 per cent of urethral gonococcal infections in men are oligo- or asymptomatic. Urethral chlamydial infections of men are more common than gonococcal infections and frequently are asymp-

tomatic. The importance of the asymptomatic male is underscored by the repeated observation that women with gonococcal pelvic inflammatory disease have male partners whose infection is asymptomatic. Thus, one of the crucial issues in management is proper diagnosis and treatment of the asymptomatically infected partner.

STD IN HOMOSEXUAL MALES. Homosexual males are recognized as a group at particularly high risk of acquiring sexually transmitted disease. The current epidemic of AIDS in homosexual or bisexual men is a major concern. This subject is discussed in Ch. 346. AIDS is but one of many STD-related problems in homosexual males, however. Currently, over one half of all male patients in the United States with infectious (primary and secondary) syphilis name other males as their contacts. Some homosexual males are exceptionally promiscuous and are at high risk of acquiring not only syphilis but also gonococcal urethritis, proctitis, and pharyngitis; herpes genitalis and proctitis; hepatitis A and B; and a variety of enteric infections that are rarely transmitted in heterosexual sex, including giardiasis, amebiasis, and shigellosis. These enteric infections are probably transmitted by oral-anal or anal-penile-oral contact. In recent years, however, the incidence of some STD's, such as gonorrhea, has declined in homosexual males owing to adoption of changed and safer sex practices (fewer partners, condoms) resulting from the fear of acquiring AIDS. Homosexual women apparently do not have increased rates of STD.

INCIDENCE OF STD's. The true incidence of the STD's is not known in the United States because of serious problems of under-reporting. Gonorrhea is the most common of the reported infectious diseases in the United States, with over 1,000,000 reported infections annually. Although genital chlamydial infections generally are not reported, their prevalence certainly exceeds gonorrhea. The relative incidence of STD is quite variable in different areas of the world. For instance, chancroid is currently quite uncommon in the United States but is about as common as gonorrhea in certain areas of the Far East.

COMMON SYNDROMES. *Urethritis in Males.* Urethritis in males is a very common syndrome. It is ordinarily classified as either gonococcal or nongonococcal urethritis (NGU), depending on whether the presence of gonococci can be demonstrated by Gram's stain or culture. In venereal disease clinics, the prevalence of gonococcal and nongonococcal urethritis is similar, but NGU is considerably more common in private practice and in college infirmaries. Several recent studies of asymptomatic sexually active young persons found a prevalence of up to 15 per cent of genital chlamydial infection.

A large number of studies have established *Chlamydia trachomatis* as a cause of approximately 40 per cent of cases of NGU. Case-control studies have provided suggestive evidence that *Ureaplasma urealyticum* (formerly "T-strain" mycoplasma) is a significant factor in chlamydia-negative NGU. In addition, urethral inoculation of volunteers with pure cultures of *U. urealyticum* produced rather typical NGU. In practice, however, it is difficult to define the importance of *Ureaplasma* infection in patients with urethritis, because up to 70 per cent of asymptomatic sexually active persons are colonized by these organisms. A very small proportion of cases of NGU in men is due to *Trichomonas vaginalis* or herpes simplex virus infection.

Diagnosis of urethritis requires demonstration of an inflammatory urethral exudate. A discharge may not be evident if the patient has recently voided, and patients preferably should be examined several hours after their last urination. The discharge may be present only in the morning, prior to urination. Demonstration of discharge often requires urethral "milking" and may require insertion of a small calcium alginate or similar swab into the anterior urethra, with examination of a direct Gram-stained smear of the swab for leukocytes. Presence of an average of at least five polymorphonuclear leukocytes per high power (100×) field suggests the diagnosis of urethritis.

The patient should be questioned for past history of urethritis and for symptoms suggestive of systemic diseases such as Reiter's syndrome or disseminated gonococcal infection. Examination should be made for signs of conjunctivitis, arthritis, dermatitis, and epididymitis. Prostatitis is rarely present unless there are symptoms of perineal, suprapubic, or rectal discomfort, and rectal examination is not routinely indicated. Rectal examination and urine culture are indicated in men with dysuria but without signs of anterior urethral discharge.

Laboratory studies are ordinarily limited to a Gram's stain of urethral exudate. Demonstration of typical gram-negative diplococci, many of which are inside neutrophils, establishes the diagnosis of gonococcal urethritis. At least 90 per cent of men with symptomatic culture-proven urethral gonorrhea have a positive Gram's stain. In occasional patients, especially those with equivocal Gram's stain, it may be necessary to culture the anterior urethra or freshly voided urine sediment for gonococci. This is particularly important in asymptomatic male contacts of patients with disseminated gonococcal infection or gonococcal salpingitis, since Gram's stain of urethral contents is positive in only about 60 per cent of men with asymptomatic urethral gonorrhea.

Diagnosis of NGU usually is made by exclusion of gonorrhea. Monoclonal antibodies recently were made available for diagnosis of chlamydiae in secretions; results indicate a sensitivity of over 90 per cent compared with culture, with nearly 100 per cent specificity. This test requires use of a fluorescence microscope, and cost considerations (about $20 per test) preclude widespread use. Other immunoassays are being developed, and cultures for *Chlamydia* (even more expensive) are now more widely available than in the past. There is no serologic test that is clinically useful. Tests for *Ureaplasma* are not readily available and rarely are indicated. Examination of a saline suspension of urethral exudate occasionally may reveal motile trichomonads in patients with recurrent urethritis who fail to respond to appropriate therapy. A serologic test for syphilis should be obtained, but the diagnostic yield is low.

Management is outlined in Figure 305–1 and is discussed further in Ch. 306. Sexual partners of men with gonococcal or nongonococcal urethritis should be treated both to prevent reinfection of the patient and to prevent development of complications in the partners.

The syndrome of *postgonococcal urethritis* (persistence or crudescence of urethritis after administration of therapy that has eradicated gonococcal infection) is usually due to concomitant urethral chlamydial infection that was not eradicated by the original treatment. This syndrome is more common after therapy with intramuscular procaine penicillin or a single oral dose of ampicillin than after a five-day regimen of tetracycline, undoubtedly because of the greater efficacy of tetracycline for treating chlamydial infections. Accordingly, there is considerable merit to use of oral tetracycline to follow up penicillin or ampicillin therapy for genital gonorrhea.

Genital Ulcer Syndrome. Genital skin lesions may be either ulcerative or nonulcerative. In patients seen in a venereal disease clinic, the most common sexually transmitted nonulcerative genital lesions are due to scabies, genital warts, molluscum contagiosum, or *Candida* species, but differential diagnosis includes a long list of dermatologic conditions.

The most common cause of ulcerative genital lesions in patients in the United States is herpes simplex virus, but differential diagnosis includes syphilis, chancroid, lymphogranuloma venereum (LGV), granuloma inguinale (GI), and trauma. Chancroid is uncommon in Western nations, and LGV and GI are rare. The most important distinction is between syphilis and genital herpes. Sometimes, the appearance is virtually diagnostic: Grouped, painful, superficial vesicles are nearly diagnostic of herpes, whereas a single, clean-based, nonpainful ulcer with indurated margins suggests primary syphilis. In recent studies, only about 60 per cent of penile syphilitic chancres had this classic appearance. Painful ulcers suggest herpes, or possibly chancroid. Genital herpes may present as a single ulcer, particularly in patients with recurrent herpes, and syphilis may present with multiple ulcers. Secondarily infected lesions of primary syphilis may be painful.

It is a useful rule to obtain a serologic test for syphilis on all patients with genital ulcers, and, if the initial serology is negative and if the diagnosis remains uncertain, to obtain a second serology about two weeks later. A darkfield examination for syphilis should also be done, and it should be repeated twice on successive days if syphilis is seriously suspected and the initial examination is negative.

Infection by herpes simplex virus may be efficiently diagnosed by viral culture or by immunofluorescent methods, but these are frequently unavailable in practice. Papanicolaou's smear is suggestive of herpes in about two thirds of culture-positive cases. Giemsa's or Wright's stain of cells scraped from the base of a vesicle may reveal multinucleate giant cells

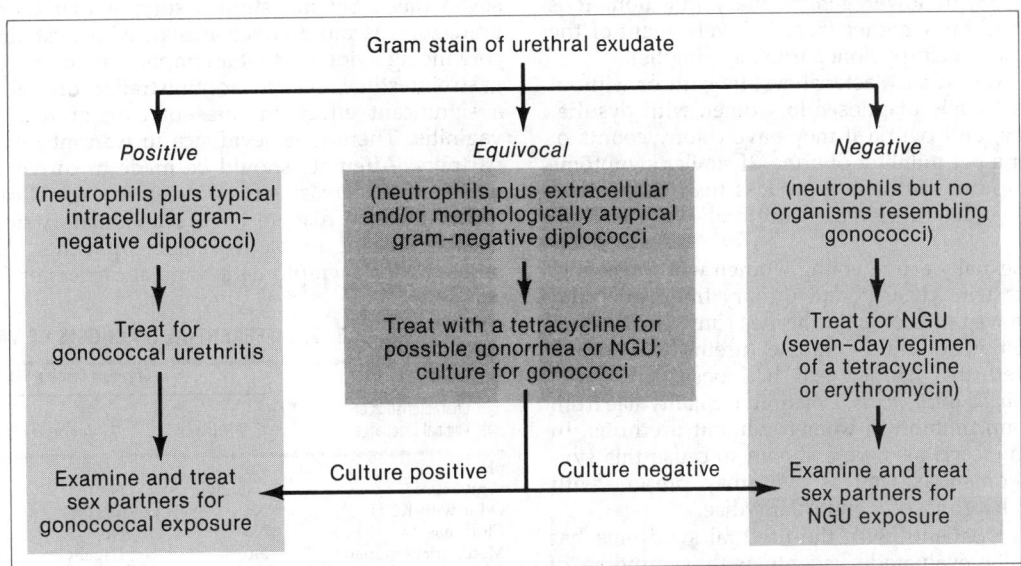

FIGURE 305–1. Management of male patients with urethritis.

(Tzanck's test), but this test is particularly insensitive in herpetic lesions that have become ulcerated. Serologic tests for herpesvirus are not helpful. Referral of patients to centers with capability of viral culture may be indicated in diagnostically difficult patients.

In addition to herpesvirus infection, chancroid should be suspected in patients with painful genital ulcers. Chancroid is more likely if there has been recent sexual contact in Africa or the Far East. Attempts should be made to isolate the causative agent, *Hemophilus ducreyi;* selective culture media are an improvement over previously available methods. No serologic tests are available.

Therapy clearly depends on the correct diagnosis. Topical antibiotics are never indicated. Initial genital herpes (first infection) is best treated with topical or oral administration of acyclovir or intravenous administration for severe infections (see Ch. 29). Therapy of chancroid is with co-trimoxazole or erythromycin. Occasional empiric trials of oral co-trimoxazole or erythromycin are warranted in patients with persistent genital ulcers not readily attributable to herpesvirus or syphilis, but repeated attempts to isolate *H. ducreyi* should be made in such instances. It is not possible to arrive at an unequivocal diagnosis of the cause of genital ulcers in all patients.

Lower Genital Tract Infections in Women. Infections of the female genitourinary tract produce a variety of syndromes, often with overlapping symptoms (dysuria, vaginal discharge, vulvar irritation). These infections are very common, relatively poorly understood by most physicians, sometimes difficult to treat, and often frustrating for both doctor and patient. However, the various syndromes usually can be distinguished on relatively simple clinical and laboratory grounds, and a precise microbial etiology often can be established.

It is most helpful first to determine the primary anatomic site of infection: urethra or bladder, endocervix, or vagina. This can sometimes be accomplished by history; women with urinary tract infection (UTI) usually experience "internal" dysuria, whereas women with dysuria associated with vaginitis usually experience "external" dysuria owing to passage of urine over inflamed labia. Cervicitis is diagnosed by physical examination; there are mucopurulent secretions emanating from the endocervical canal, and there is often a hypertrophic, mucoid, reddened "cobblestone" appearance to the cervical mucosa. Patients with cervicitis may also have urethritis or vaginitis. Vaginitis is associated with increased vaginal discharge of several types, as discussed below, and frequently there are associated signs and symptoms of vaginal, vulvar, and perineal irritation (dyspareunia, external dysuria, itching, pain). In patients with lower genitourinary infection, it is important to determine whether there is involvement of the upper genitourinary tract (pyelonephritis, salpingitis).

THE URETHRAL SYNDROME. Bacterial cystitis with or without pyelonephritis is usually diagnosed in women with dysuria, urinary frequency, and pyuria if they have colony counts of at least 10^5 bacteria per milliliter of urine. If similar symptoms are present but routine cultures grow less than 10^4 bacteria per milliliter of voided urine, the "urethral syndrome" is likely.

In a study of sexually active young women who presented to walk-in clinics with dysuria and urinary frequency, and who did not have vaginitis or active herpes simplex infection, 43 per cent had the urethral syndrome (urethritis). Among women with urethritis, 25 per cent had positive urethral cultures for *Chlamydia trachomatis.* Isolation of chlamydiae from the urethra was uncommon in women without urethritis. In other studies, gonococci also were shown to cause this syndrome. Thus, women as well as men may present with urethritis caused by gonococci and chlamydiae.

Management of patients with the urethral syndrome has not been carefully evaluated. Patients with symptoms of urinary tract infection who do not have bacteriuria should

have urethral and cervical cultures for *Neisseria gonorrhoeae.* If these cultures are also negative, a therapeutic trial may be made with a tetracycline or a sulfonamide for approximately seven days. There are no controlled trials of such therapy or of the management of sexual partners of women with the urethral syndrome.

VAGINITIS. In a large study of women in a primary care clinic who presented with lower genitourinary complaints, vaginitis was more than five times as common as urinary tract infections. In this and similar studies, there were three predominant types of vaginitis: yeast infection (*Candida albicans*), trichomonas (*T. vaginalis*) infection, and "nonspecific" vaginitis caused by organisms other than *Candida* and *T. vaginalis.* The incidence of these types of vaginitis varies in different patient populations, but in general *Candida* and nonspecific vaginitis are more common than *T. vaginalis* vaginitis.

Symptoms of vaginitis include increased volume of vaginal discharge, which is often abnormally yellow or green in appearance, and may be malodorous. Vaginal and vulvar itching may be troublesome, especially in *Candida* infection. There may be vaginal tenderness and pain, dyspareunia, or dysuria.

The most common sign of vaginitis is an increased vaginal discharge. In *T. vaginalis* infections, there is often a profuse and frothy discharge. A curdlike, white discharge is common in *Candida* infections, and many patients with nonspecific vaginitis have an adherent, often gray, and frequently malodorous discharge. Microscopic examination shows many polymorphonuclear leukocytes in the discharge in all but nonspecific vaginitis. Speculum examination may show signs of endocervicitis as well, with purulent discharge issuing from the cervical os. In occasional patients, no objective signs of vaginal inflammation are found despite the presence of troublesome symptoms. See Table 305–2.

Candida Vaginitis. Most vaginal yeast infections are due to *C. albicans.* Diagnosis is usually made by visualizing yeasts or pseudohyphae by microscopic examination of vaginal secretions suspended in normal saline or 10 per cent KOH. Microscopic examination is less sensitive than culture. However, many asymptomatic women have positive vaginal cultures for *C. albicans,* and therefore some authorities advocate using microscopy in preference to culture. The discharge in *Candida* vaginitis is not malodorous and has a pH of less than 4.5 when a drop is applied to pH paper with a range of 4.0 to 5.5.

Therapy of *Candida* vaginitis is with intravaginal nystatin twice daily for seven days, or with one of the imidazole compounds (clotrimazole or miconazole) once each night for seven days. Several studies suggest that therapy with the imidazoles is more effective than with nystatin. There is no convincing evidence that attempts to eradicate yeast from the gastrointestinal tract by administration of oral nystatin have a significant effect on rates of cure or relapse of *Candida* vaginitis. There is no evidence to warrant therapy of sexual partners. Attempts should be made to correct ancillary conditions that increase susceptibility to vaginal candidiasis: antibiotic therapy, diabetes, or oral anovulatory steroids. Relapse is a significant problem in some patients. No therapy is indicated for asymptomatic vaginal carriers of *C. albicans.*

TABLE 305–2. DIFFERENTIAL DIAGNOSIS OF VAGINITIS

Characteristics of Vaginal Discharge	Organism Causing Vaginitis		
	C. albicans	*T. vaginalis*	*Mobiluncus, G. vaginalis*
pH	4.5	>5.0	>5.0
White curd	Usually	No	No
Odor with KOH	No	Yes	Yes
Clue cells	No	No	Usually
Motile trichomonads	No	Usually	No
Yeast cells	Yes	No	No

T. vaginale Vaginitis. Diagnosis is made ordinarily by visualizing motile trichomonads in a normal saline suspension of vaginal secretions. The organisms are easily seen at high-dry ($100\times$) magnification, and may usually be seen under low-power magnification. The saline suspension should be examined promptly. Culture is more sensitive, but about 80 to 90 per cent of culture-positive cases are detected by microscopy. Addition of a drop of 10 per cent KOH to vaginal secretions usually results in liberation of a detectable fish-like odor, attributed to release of volatile amines. The pH of vaginal secretions is usually greater than 5.0. In these latter two respects, *T. vaginale* vaginitis is similar to nonspecific vaginitis.

Therapy of trichomoniasis is with one of the nitroimidazoles, either metronidazole or newer compounds such as tinidazole. The latter is extensively used in Europe but is not approved in the United States. A single 2.0-gram oral dose of metronidazole is as effective as multiple-day regimens. Metronidazole is mutagenic, and there is evidence that it is a weak carcinogen in certain animal systems (but, so far, not in humans). Accordingly, it should be used with caution; it has been advocated for women with asymptomatic trichomoniasis, but others would reserve its use for women with symptomatic infections because of possible adverse effects. Metronidazole should not be used in the first trimester of pregnancy. Since over one third of male sexual partners of women with trichomoniasis are asymptomatic urethral carriers of *T. vaginale*, the male partners should also be treated with a single 2.0-gram dose of metronidazole.

Although *T. vaginale* can be transmitted sexually, it probably is transmitted by other means as well. This conclusion is based on prevalence studies that show one peak in young, sexually active women and a second peak in older women who have no other evidence for sexually transmitted infection.

Nonspecific Vaginosis. This syndrome is probably due to infection by an organism formerly called either *Corynebacterium vaginale* or *Hemophilus vaginalis*, but now termed *Gardnerella vaginalis*, in association with anaerobic bacteria, including the curved or comma-shaped rods now known as *Mobiluncus* species. *G. vaginalis* is a small, gram-variable coccobacillus, which can be grown quite successfully on partially selective enriched media. Among women with abnormal vaginal discharge who do not have yeast infection or trichomoniasis, over 90 per cent will grow *G. vaginalis*, whereas fewer than 10 per cent of matched controls grow the same organism. There usually are increased numbers of anaerobic vaginal bacteria as well, and decreased numbers of the normal vaginal lactobacilli. Development of full symptoms may require both *G. vaginalis* and vaginal anaerobes, although the precise pathophysiology of this syndrome is still under investigation.

Diagnosis of nonspecific vaginosis is by exclusion of trichomoniasis, candidiasis, and purulent cervicitis. Abnormal cells termed "clue cells" are often seen in a wet mount of vaginal secretions in normal saline; these are stippled, granular-appearing vaginal epithelial cells that contain large numbers of adherent *G. vaginalis*. Few polymorphonuclear leukocytes are present. Addition of a drop of 10 per cent KOH usually results in production of an unpleasant fishy odor. The pH of the vaginal secretions is nearly always greater than 5.0.

Optimal therapy is being investigated. Some, but not all, studies show that oral ampicillin (500 mg four times daily for seven days) is effective. Metronidazole has only borderline activity in vitro against *G. vaginalis*, but in a dose of 500 mg by mouth twice daily for seven days it was effective in eradicating both *G. vaginalis* and the symptoms of vaginitis from 80 of 81 patients in one trial; similar results have been obtained in other trials. This suggests that the principal cause of this syndrome is an anaerobe, since metronidazole is principally effective against anaerobes. Oral tetracycline and topical vaginal creams containing sulfonamides are usually ineffective. Over 90 per cent of male partners are urethral carriers of *G. vaginalis* and therefore probably should be treated with the same regimen as the patient.

Mixed Vaginitis. In 2 to 16 per cent of patients, vaginitis may be due to polymicrobial infection with two or three organisms. Such mixed infection may account for some instances of treatment failure. Particular care should be given to identification of all causative organisms in patients who have recurrent or relapsing vaginitis.

CERVICITIS. Two organisms are recognized as probable causes of mucopurulent endocervicitis: *N. gonorrhoeae* and *C. trachomatis*. Women who are sexual partners of men with chlamydia-positive NGU have a much higher rate of isolation of chlamydiae from the cervix than do women who are partners of men with chlamydia-negative NGU, and they also have significantly higher rates of mucopurulent cervicitis. Herpes simplex virus can also cause cervicitis, especially in primary infection. However, the clinical appearance in herpetic cervicitis is different, with cervical vesicles and ulcers rather than mucopurulent cervicitis.

True cervicitis should not be confused with cervical ectopy, which is merely the appearance of endocervical columnar epithelium on the exposed, visible exocervix. This results in a red-appearing cervix and may result in increased production of a mucoid vaginal discharge but does not require therapy.

Diagnosis of mucopurulent endocervicitis requires visualization of purulent discharge from the cervical os. There often is a roughened "cobblestone" appearance to the cervix. Gram's stain is about 60 per cent sensitive and over 90 per cent specific for gonorrhea if typical intracellular gonococci are seen, but cultures for *N. gonorrhoeae* should be taken. Tissue culture for isolation of *C. trachomatis* may be employed if available. Cytology is not sufficiently sensitive to warrant widespread use. New monoclonal antibodies against *C. trachomatis* allow rapid, sensitive, specific immunofluorescent diagnosis from patient secretions and undoubtedly should be more widely employed to document etiology and to initiate proper treatment for cervicitis due to chlamydiae.

Antibiotic therapy appears to result in clinical improvement in mucopurulent cervicitis. Patients with negative cultures for the gonococcus probably should be treated with tetracycline or erythromycin in a dose of 500 mg four times daily for at least seven days; their sexual partners probably should be treated similarly. One should recognize that only modest data support these recommendations. No other form of cervicitis has been shown to respond to antimicrobial therapy.

Upper Genital Tract Disease in Women: Salpingitis. Full coverage of this important topic is precluded by space considerations. This is a very important clinical problem, resulting in considerable morbidity in the estimated 250,000 to 500,000 women who are affected yearly in the United States.

ETIOLOGY. The gonococcus may account for as much as 50 per cent of cases in the United States, particularly among women with relatively severe and first-episode salpingitis. About 15 to 20 per cent of women with gonococcal cervicitis probably subsequently develop salpingitis. Strong evidence now implicates genital chlamydial infections as another significant cause of salpingitis; in Sweden, more cases of salpingitis are due to *C. trachomatis* than to *N. gonorrhoeae*. Salpingitis due to genital chlamydial infections may be mild, and patients may not seek medical care. Nevertheless, complications may follow, particularly tubal scarring and infertility. There is less convincing evidence that *Mycoplasma hominis* may occasionally cause a similar syndrome. Many cases of salpingitis are caused by mixed infection with microaerophilic streptococci and enteric bacilli, often including *Bacteroides* species. These polymicrobial infections appear to be more common in recurrent attacks of salpingitis.

DIAGNOSIS. Clinical diagnosis of salpingitis is inexact. Perhaps only 20 per cent of patients have the classic syndrome of lower abdominal pain and tenderness, cervical tenderness, fever, leukocytosis, and elevated sedimentation rate. The most common findings are lower abdominal tenderness. which is usually bilateral, and adnexal and cervical tenderness. Patients with gonococcal salpingitis are more likely to present with fever, and more commonly have onset near the menses, whereas patients with nongonococcal salpingitis more commonly present with adnexal masses. Laparoscopy is commonly used to diagnose salpingitis in certain countries, but is invasive and requires general anesthesia. In the United States, laparoscopy is usually used only in selected patients whose differential diagnosis includes ectopic pregnancy, appendicitis, ruptured abscess, or other potential emergencies.

COMPLICATIONS. Complications are primarily infertility and ectopic pregnancies. Rates of involuntary infertility are about 15 per cent after one attack of salpingitis and about 75 per cent after three or more attacks. Total hysterectomy may eventually be necessitated by symptoms of chronic salpingitis.

THERAPY. A controlled trial of outpatient therapy showed that ten-day regimens of either oral tetracycline or ampicillin were equally effective in both gonococcal and nongonococcal salpingitis. Recommendations from the Centers for Disease Control suggest initial therapy with cefoxitin 2.0 grams intramuscularly, or ampicillin 3.5 grams orally, or aqueous procaine penicillin G 4.8 mU intramuscularly, each along with probenecid 1.0 gram orally, followed by doxycycline 100 mg orally twice daily for 10 to 14 days. There are no controlled data on efficacy of various regimens used for hospitalized patients. Current recommendations call for doxycycline 100 mg intravenously twice daily plus cefoxitin 2.0 grams intravenously four times daily; or clindamycin 600 mg intravenously four times daily plus gentamicin or tobramycin 1.5 mg per kilogram intravenously three times daily; or doxycycline 100 mg intravenously twice daily plus metronidazole 1.0 gram intravenously twice daily in patients with normal renal function. Patients should usually be hospitalized if they are very ill, are pregnant, have significant adnexal masses, or have failed previous therapy, or if the differential diagnosis includes surgical emergencies such as appendicitis or ectopic pregnancy.

PREVENTION. Sexual partners of women with gonococcal salpingitis must be identified, examined, and treated to prevent subsequent reinfection of the patient. About one half of the infected male partners of women with gonococcal salpingitis are asymptomatic. Treatment of women with tetracycline (as compared with penicillin) to eradicate chlamydiae from the cervix reduces the incidence of post-therapy salpingitis (Rees, 1980), which suggests that increased emphasis on treatment of chlamydiae in the male and female genital tract might reduce the incidence of salpingitis.

Baldson MJ, Pead L, Taylor GE, et al.: *Corynebacterium vaginale* and vaginitis: A controlled trial of treatment. Lancet 1:501, 1980. *A randomized trial of the therapy of nonspecific vaginitis. Tetracycline was ineffective, but metronidazole was effective.*

Bowie WR, Wang S-P, Alexander ER, et al.: Etiology of nongonococcal urethritis: Evidence for *Chlamydia trachomatis* and *Ureplasma urealyticum*. J Clin Invest 59:735, 1977. *An excellent epidemiologic and clinical study of the etiology and therapy of nongonococcal urethritis in males.*

Brunham RC, Paavonen J, Stevens CE, et al.: Mucopurulent cervicitis—the ignored counterpart in women of urethritis in men. N Engl J Med 311:1, 1984. *Genital chlamydial infection causes mucopurulent cervicitis, and proper diagnosis leads to effective treatment.*

Mårdh P-A, Møller BR, Paavonen J: Chlamydial infection of the female genital tract with emphasis on pelvic inflammatory disease. A review of Scandinavian studies. Sex Transm Dis 8(Suppl):140, 1981. *Review of the role of chlamydiae in pelvic inflammatory disease.*

McCue JD, Komaroff AL, Pass TM, et al.: Strategies for diagnosing vaginitis. J Fam Pract 9:395, 1979. *A study in a primary care clinic of simple methods for diagnosing the etiology of genitourinary symptoms in women.*

Nettleman MD, Jones RB, Roberts SD, et al.: Cost-effectiveness of culturing for *Chlamydia trachomatis*: A study in a clinic for sexually transmitted diseases. Ann Intern Med 105:189, 1986. *Cultures were most cost effective in low-risk women. In high-risk groups, empiric therapy is suggested.*

Pheifer TA, Forsyth PS, Durfee MA, et al.: Nonspecific vaginitis: Role of *Haemophilus vaginalis* and treatment with metronidazole. N Engl J Med 298:1429, 1978. *A clinical and therapeutic study of nonspecific vaginitis, showing that both G. vaginalis and vaginal anaerobes are probably important in causation of the syndrome and also that metronidazole is effective therapy.*

Rees E: The treatment of pelvic inflammatory disease. Am J Obstet Gynecol 138:1042, 1980. *Treatment of women with chlamydial infection of the cervix with tetracycline compared with penicillin reduced the incidence of subsequent salpingitis.*

Stamm WE, Harrison HR, Alexander ER, et al.: Diagnosis of *Chlamydia trachomatis* infections by direct immunofluorescence staining of genital secretions: A multicenter trial. Ann Intern Med 101:638, 1984. *Immunofluorescence was reasonably sensitive (89 to 92 per cent) and specific (96 to 99 per cent) in the diagnosis of genital chlamydial infection in symptomatic men and women, compared with culture. Other reports show less sensitivity in asymptomatic screening.*

Stamm WE, Koutsky LA, Benedetti JK, et al.: *Chlamydia trachomatis* urethral infections in men: Prevalence, risk factors, and clinical manifestations. Ann Intern Med 100:47, 1984. *Asymptomatic male urethral carriers of chlamydiae are very common.*

Stamm WE, Wagner KF, Amsel R, et al.: Causes of the acute urethral syndrome in women. N Engl J Med 303:409, 1980. *Females may also develop a form of nongonococcal urethritis resulting from infection with Chlamydia trachomatis.*

Tait IA, Rees E, Hobson D, et al.: Chlamydial infection of the cervix in contacts of men with nongonococcal urethritis. Br J Vener Dis 56:37, 1980. *Chlamydia trachomatis is shown to cause mucopurulent cervicitis, and appropriate antibiotic therapy results in clinical improvement.*

Taylor-Robinson D, Csonka GW, Prentice MJ: Human intraurethral inoculation of ureaplasmas. Q J Med 46:309, 1977. *Inoculation of the investigator's urethra with ureaplasmas resulted in nonspecific urethritis.*

306 GONOCOCCAL INFECTIONS

INTRODUCTION. *Neisseria gonorrhoeae* is a common sexually transmitted organism that causes anterior urethritis in males and endocervicitis and urethritis in females. Other types of primary infection include pharyngitis, proctitis, conjunctivitis, and vulvovaginitis; the last-named disorder occurs principally in prepubescent females. Complications may occur by direct extension of infection, including epididymitis, prostatitis, Bartholin gland abscess, salpingitis, and perihepatitis. Bacteremia may occur, with production of characteristic cutaneous lesions, arthritis, and tenosynovitis; rare complications include endocarditis and meningitis. Conjunctival infection formerly was a common cause of blindness in neonates.

Gonorrhea is the most common reportable infectious disease in the United States, with about 1 million reported cases annually. The true incidence is probably at least 2 million cases annually.

EPIDEMIOLOGY. The only natural hosts for *N. gonorrhoeae* are humans. The organism normally resides on the columnar epithelium of mucosal surfaces and is usually transmitted by intimate sexual contact.

The prevalence of gonorrhea varies greatly in different groups. As many as 5 per cent of persons in high-risk populations may be infected at any time. Surveys of private practices in the United States in the 1970's showed that about 2 per cent of sexually active young women had positive endocervical cultures for the gonococcus. Highest prevalence was found in young (15 to 30) single persons of low socioeconomic and educational status, probably because these factors correlate positively with sexual promiscuity.

The risk of acquiring infection depends on the type of contact with an infected person. About 60 to 80 per cent of females in contact with a male with urethral gonorrhea will develop gonococcal cervicitis. By contrast, it is estimated that only 20 to 30 per cent of males having sex with an infected female will develop gonorrhea. This difference may be due to exposure of females to a larger inoculum of gonococci. A person having oral sex with a male with gonococcal urethritis has considerable risk of acquiring pharyngeal gonorrhea. Transmission of infection by oral contact with the genitals of an infected female is rare. Infection is apparently efficiently spread by penile-rectal contact.

Gonococci die rapidly upon drying, and transmission by fomites is rare. Epidemics were reported in prepubertal females living in close proximity in orphanages, but such episodes are now very uncommon.

Control of gonorrhea is difficult because of the frequency of asymptomatic infection. Perhaps 50 per cent of infections in females are asymptomatic or only minimally symptomatic, and at least 10 per cent of infected males are asymptomatic.

In past years there was considerable emphasis on case finding by endocervical culture of young, sexually active females. The merit of this strategy depends on the prevalence of infection in the community and the lifestyle of the patient. A more cost-effective method for finding infected patients is to culture patients about six weeks after treatment for gonorrhea; as many as 15 to 20 per cent of such persons will be culture positive, usually because of reinfection.

THE ORGANISM. *N. gonorrhoeae* is a gram-negative, aerobic diplococcus. Many strains require 3 to 10 per cent CO_2 for optimal growth. They are highly autolytic and die rapidly when outside their normal human environment. They are sensitive to fatty acids and grow best on media with added starch to inhibit fatty acids present in agar. Several partially selective media are available; most employ antibiotics such as trimethoprim, vancomycin, colistin, and nystatin to inhibit growth of other microorganisms. Replacement of vancomycin with lincomycin seems to improve the rate of isolation of gonococci.

Presumptive identification in vitro is made by colonial morphology, Gram's stain, and a positive oxidase test. Differentiation from the closely related meningococcus and the various nonpathogenic *Neisseria* is ordinarily by patterns of utilization of various simple carbohydrates; gonococci use glucose but not maltose or sucrose.

Gonococci are highly variable and occur in a number of different colonial forms. Small colonial types are piliated and more virulent in humans than the larger, nonpiliated variants. Variation is also found in certain outer membrane proteins. Gonococci undergo rapid variation in the antigenic type of pilus expressed, which probably contributes to prolonged infections without treatment and to the ability of persons to acquire repeat infections after treatment. The importance of surface components of the gonococcus in the pathogenesis of infection is under intense investigation.

Gonococci can be serotyped on the basis of antigenic differences in pili, outer membrane proteins, and other antigens. They also can be reliably biotyped by definition of their nutritional requirements on defined agar media ("auxotypes"). These tests are not routinely available at present.

PATHOGENESIS. The minimal infective dose of gonococci for establishment of urethritis in male volunteers is between 100 and 1000 colony-forming units. Surface pili undoubtedly help to attach the bacteria to the mucosal surface, and they also help prevent ingestion and killing by polymorphonuclear leukocytes. Typical urethral infections result in a moderately severe inflammatory response, which is probably due to release of toxic lipopolysaccharide from gonococci and to production of chemotactic factors that attract neutrophilic leukocytes. Certain strains are likely to cause asymptomatic urethral infection for reasons not completely understood. These strains are usually penicillin sensitive, resistant to the bactericidal effects of normal human serum, and particularly likely to cause bacteremia and septic arthritis.

In the preantibiotic era, symptoms usually persisted for two to three months before host defenses finally succeeded in eradicating the infection. Host defenses include serum opsonic and bactericidal antibodies, as well as local (mucosal) antibodies of the IgG and IgA classes. All gonococci produce an enzyme, IgA protease, which cleaves the major class of secretory IgA, perhaps contributing to persistence of local gonococcal infections.

Serum bactericidal antibodies are undoubtedly important in prevention of bacteremic infection. The best evidence for this has been provided by patients who suffer from homozygous deficiency of one of the complement components C6, C7, C8, or C9. This results in deficiency of serum bactericidal activity but no alteration of serum opsonic activity. Such individuals are particularly prone to recurrent bacteremic gonococcal infection or to recurrent meningococcal meningitis or meningococcemia.

CLINICAL PATTERNS OF DISEASE. *Gonorrhea in Males.* Gonococcal urethritis in males ("the clap," or "the strain") is characterized by a yellowish, purulent urethral discharge and dysuria. The usual incubation period is two to six days. The discharge of gonorrhea is slightly more copious and purulent than in nongonococcal urethritis (NGU). Symptoms are probably produced by 90 per cent of infections, although asymptomatic infections do occur and may persist for many months. Males with asymptomatic infection do not seek treatment, whereas those with symptomatic infection are usually promptly treated and cured. This is the probable explanation for prevalence studies that show that up to 50 per cent of infected males are asymptomatic. Asymptomatic infection in males and females is of great epidemiologic importance, since such carriers may continue to spread infection to new sexual partners for months if they are not properly diagnosed and treated.

Complications of gonococcal urethritis in males are now rare. Urethral stricture was formerly a common complication, but was probably due in part to the use of caustic treatment regimens. Epididymitis and prostatitis, relatively common complications in the past, are seen only occasionally today. The principal complication is disseminated gonococcal infection, which is estimated to affect about 1 per cent of men with gonorrhea. This entity is discussed below.

The differential diagnosis of gonococcal urethritis is discussed in Ch. 305.

Gonococcal infections of the pharynx and rectum are common problems in homosexual males. Most patients with pharyngeal infection are asymptomatic, but occasional patients have exudative pharyngitis with cervical adenopathy. Gonococcal infection of the rectum causes a wide spectrum of symptoms, ranging from asymptomatic carriers to severe proctitis with tenesmus and bloody, mucopurulent discharge. Although approximately 40 per cent of females with cervical gonorrhea also have positive rectal cultures, symptoms of proctitis in females are unusual. This has suggested that the trauma of rectal intercourse may contribute to the proctitis observed in males. Sigmoidoscopy may be indicated to exclude ulcerative colitis, Crohn's colitis, rectal lacerations, or other infections such as shigellosis, amebiasis, or syphilis, all of which are common in male homosexuals.

Gonococcal epididymitis is usually unilateral. Both *Chlamydia trachomatis* and the gonococcus are significant causes of epididymitis in men under 35 years, whereas coliform bacteria are the usual cause in older males. The differential diagnosis includes trauma, tumor, and torsion of the testicle, the last of which is suggested by sudden onset and elevation of the testicle. If there is question of testicular torsion, consultation with a urologist is necessary. In epididymitis there is often a urethral exudate, which should be cultured for gonococci and other bacteria. Treatment of gonococcal epididymitis includes scrotal elevation and seven to ten days of appropriate antibiotics, as indicated in Table 306–1.

Gonorrhea in Females. In prevalence studies, approximately one half of women infected with the gonococcus are asymptomatic or have so few symptoms that they do not seek medical care. The most commonly involved site is the endocervix (80 to 90 per cent), followed by the urethra (80 per cent), rectum (40 per cent), and pharynx (10 to 20 per cent). Most pharyngeal, urethral, and rectal infections cause few or no symptoms. Cervical infection may result in vaginal discharge or abnormal menstrual bleeding. Neither of these symptoms is specific for gonococcal infection. Gonococcal urethritis may mimic cystitis caused by enteric bacilli, although standard urine cultures are negative because gonococci do not grow on culture media ordinarily used to diagnose urinary tract infection. Culture methods are discussed below under Laboratory Diagnosis. The differential diagnosis of cervicitis, vaginitis, and the urethral syndrome is discussed in Ch. 305.

The most important complication of gonorrhea is salpingitis. The less precise term "pelvic inflammatory disease" (PID) is often used synonymously. Although many other organisms can cause a similar syndrome, the gonococcus accounts for about half of the estimated 500,000 annual cases of PID in the United States. About 15 per cent of women with gonococcal cervicitis develop PID, often in close proximity to a menstrual period. Symptoms usually include abdominal pain, and often there is fever. Physical examination usually discloses cervical motion tenderness and bilateral adnexal tenderness; in a small proportion of cases the disease may be unilateral, causing confusion with appendicitis or ectopic pregnancy. There may be signs of generalized peritonitis. Laboratory studies often show an elevation of the white blood cell count and sedimentation rate. The diagnosis of PID is inexact, as shown by laparoscopic examination; many patients with PID will be missed if undue reliance is placed on presence of fever or elevation of white blood cell count or sedimentation rate.

Although PID is uncommon in pregnancy, it may be particularly severe, and pregnant patients with PID should probably be hospitalized. The incidence of gonococcal PID is increased about threefold in women using an intrauterine device (IUD) for contraception.

A single attack of gonococcal PID seems to increase twofold the risk of developing another bout of PID with subsequent gonococcal cervicitis. About half of the male sexual partners of women with gonococcal PID are infected, and half of these infections are asymptomatic. Failure to diagnose and treat properly the male partners exposes the patient to the risk of further attacks of PID. After the patient has been effectively treated, it often is wise to refer her and her sexual partners to a public health clinic for follow-up.

The major complication of gonococcal PID is tubal scarring and infertility. The incidence of involuntary infertility is estimated as 15 per cent after one attack of PID and about 50 per cent after three attacks. The incidence of ectopic pregnancy is increased from seven- to tenfold in women with previous salpingitis, with resultant increased fetal and maternal mortality. Treatment is indicated in Table 306–1.

Gonococci may spread upward to the liver, causing perihepatitis (Fitz-Hugh-Curtis syndrome). Gonococcal perihepatitis causes tenderness and pain in the region of the liver, mimicking acute cholecystitis. However, it resolves promptly with appropriate antibiotic therapy. Peritoneoscopy may be indicated rarely for diagnostic purposes; "violin-string" adhesions between the liver capsule and the peritoneum are seen.

Gonorrhea in Children. Infants born to a mother with cervicovaginal gonorrhea may develop a gonococcal conjunctivitis, although routine use of prophylactic 1 per cent silver nitrate eye drops (or, in some hospitals, topical erythromycin or tetracycline) has markedly reduced the incidence of this problem. Neonates may also acquire pharyngeal, respiratory, or rectal infection, and may develop gonococcal sepsis. Older children up to one year of age usually acquire conjunctival or vaginal infection by accidental contamination from an adult, whereas from one year to puberty most childhood gonorrhea is the result of purposeful sexual abuse by an adult.

Gonococcal Bacteremia. Approximately 1 per cent of adults with gonorrhea develop the syndrome of gonococcal bacteremia, dermatitis, and arthritis, or disseminated gonococcal infection (DGI). In most series, the majority of patients with DGI are women. The regional incidence of DGI probably varies because of geographic differences in prevalence of the usually antibiotic-sensitive, serum-bactericidal-resistant strains of N. gonorrhoeae that cause this syndrome. The severity of the syndrome is variable, from a slowly evolving mild illness with little or no fever, mild arthralgias, and few skin

TABLE 306–1. ANTIBIOTIC REGIMENS RECOMMENDED FOR GONOCOCCAL INFECTIONS

Diagnosis	Treatment
Uncomplicated genital infection, men and women	Aqueous procaine penicillin G (APPG), 4.8 million units IM in two divided doses, plus 1.0 gram of probenecid PO *or* Tetracycline, 0.5 gram PO four times daily for seven days *or* Ampicillin, 3.5 grams (or amoxicillin, 3.0 grams), in a single PO dose, plus 1.0 gram of probenecid PO *or* Spectinomycin, 2.0 grams IM
Anorectal infections in men	APPG, 4.8 million units IM, plus 1.0 gram of probenecid PO *or* Spectinomycin, 2.0 grams IM
Pharyngeal infection	APPG, 4.8 million units IM, plus 1.0 gram of probenecid PO *or* Tetracycline, 0.5 gram PO four times daily for seven days
Treatment failure (patients should be recultured and isolates tested for production of β-lactamase)	Spectinomycin, 2.0 grams IM *or* Ceftriaxone, 125 mg IM
Penicillinase-producing N. gonorrhoeae or infection acquired in Africa or the Far East where PPNG are common	Spectinomycin, 2.0 grams IM *or* Ceftriaxone, 125 mg IM
Gonorrhea in pregnancy	APPG, 4.8 million units IM, plus 1.0 gram of probenecid *or* Spectinomycin, 2.0 grams IM
Salpingitis—outpatient	APPG, 4.8 million units IM, plus 1.0 gram of probenecid, or cefoxitin, 2.0 grams IM, followed by doxycycline, 100 mg PO two times daily for ten days *or* Doxycycline, 100 mg PO two times daily for ten days
Salpingitis—inpatient	Doxycycline, 100 mg IV twice daily plus cefoxitin, 2.0 grams IV four times daily until improved, followed by doxycycline, 100 mg PO twice daily to complete 14 days of therapy; alternative regimens include clindamycin plus an aminoglycoside, cefoxitin, or doxycycline, 100 mg IV twice daily plus metronidazole, 1.0 gram IV twice daily until improved, followed by same drugs, same dose PO to complete 14 days of therapy
Disseminated gonococcal infection	Penicillin G, 10 million units IV daily until improvement, followed by ampicillin, 0.5 gram PO four times daily to complete a minimum of seven days of therapy *or* Ampicillin, 3.5 grams PO, plus 1.0 gram of probenecid, followed by ampicillin, 0.5 gram PO four times daily for seven days *or* Tetracycline, 0.5 gram PO four times daily for seven days

lesions to a fulminant illness with high fever and prostration. Most episodes of DGI are relatively mild in comparison with meningococcemia.

Many patients with DGI have no local symptoms of gonococcal infection. Initial manifestations are usually migratory asymmetric polyarthralgias and skin lesions that are often accompanied by fever. Many patients have tenosynovitis, typically involving the flexor tendon sheaths of the wrist or the Achilles tendon (colloquially known as "lover's heels"). Skin lesions are few in number (less than 30 usually), are acral in distribution (fingers, toes, extremities), and may be painful before they are visible. The individual lesions may be papules, pustules, or bullae on an erythematous base; less commonly seen are petechiae or necrotic lesions. The rash is not pathognomonic, but is sufficiently typical that it should strongly suggest DGI when seen in young patients with polyarthralgias. Blood cultures are often positive at this stage, and circulating immune complexes may be present. Gram's stain of the skin lesions is positive in only about 5 per cent of patients, but gonococcal antigens can be detected in these lesions in about two thirds of patients by use of immunofluorescent-labeled antigonococcal antibody.

The early stage of gonococcemia may subside spontaneously, or may merge indistinctly after one week into a second stage of septic arthritis. Skin lesions have usually disappeared by this time, and blood cultures are nearly always negative. Septic arthritis may occur without preceding skin lesions or polyarthralgia. One large joint (elbow, wrist, hip, knee, ankle) is usually involved, although some series report involvement of two joints in a significant minority of patients. On infrequent occasions symmetric involvement of the fingers may mimic acute rheumatoid arthritis. Physical examination typically discloses a swollen, warm joint with evident intra-articular fluid. Aspiration of the joint often reveals a marked neutrophilic leukocytosis (50,000 to 100,000 leukocytes per cubic millimeter), although early in the development of the septic joint the synovial leukocyte count may be much lower. Cultures of joint fluid are usually positive if the leukocyte count is 80,000 or greater, but are often negative when leukocyte counts are 20,000 or less.

Other complications of gonococcal bacteremia include mild hepatitis, myocarditis, the Fitz-Hugh-Curtis syndrome, meningitis, and endocarditis. In the preantibiotic era gonococcal infection accounted for up to 10 per cent of all endocarditis, but it is now rare. Gonococcal endocarditis is often a rapidly progressive infection with severe valvular damage; it should be suspected in patients with a new murmur, severe prostrating illness, severe myocarditis, or evidence of renal failure, or in the presence of stigmata of peripheral embolization.

The differential diagnosis of the gonococcal bacteremia arthritis syndrome includes Reiter's syndrome, rheumatic fever, rheumatoid arthritis, systemic lupus erythematosus, other infectious or postinfectious arthritis, subacute bacterial endocarditis, meningococcemia, and viral hepatitis. In young males, Reiter's syndrome is the principal consideration. Conjunctivitis is rarely seen in gonococcemia, but is common in Reiter's syndrome. In the absence of typical skin lesions, DGI may not be suspected until culture results are known.

Diagnosis of DGI is secure when gonococci are recovered from the blood, skin lesions, or synovial fluid. The diagnosis of DGI is probably correct in patients in whom the only positive cultures are from local mucosal surfaces, but in whom there are both typical skin lesions and a prompt response to antigonococcal therapy.

LABORATORY DIAGNOSIS. Gram's stain of urethral exudate in symptomatic males has a sensitivity of 90 to 98 per cent and a specificity of 95 to 98 per cent. Accordingly, urethral cultures are not ordinarily indicated in untreated symptomatic males. Since the sensitivity of the Gram stain is only about 60 per cent in asymptomatic male urethral infection, cultures of the anterior urethra or fresh urine sediment are recommended when epidemiologic evidence suggests possible asymptomatic urethral infection. Gram's stain of the endocervix is about 50 to 60 per cent sensitive and about 82 to 97 per cent specific in women with positive cervical cultures for *N. gonorrhoeae*. Care must be taken to avoid mistaking normal endocervical flora and neutrophils for gonorrhea; only smears showing several neutrophils with multiple, typical intracellular gram-negative diplococci should be read as presumptively positive for gonorrhea. All women should be cultured for *N. gonorrhoeae*, even if the Gram's stain appears positive.

Cultures should be plated immediately if possible onto chocolate agar or chocolate agar containing selective antibiotics (e.g., modified Thayer-Martin medium, MTM). Holding media such as Amies' or Stuart's transport media may be used if necessary, but viability of gonococci drops after 12 to 24 hours in such media. In infected women, a single endocervical culture on MTM is about 80 to 90 per cent sensitive, as judged by yields obtained with multiple cultures from multiple sites. About 3 to 5 per cent of women will have their only positive culture at the pharyngeal, urethral, or rectal site. The yield from these sites is too low to warrant routine pharyngeal, urethral, or rectal cultures. Urethral cultures are indicated in women with the urethral syndrome. Both cervical and rectal cultures should be obtained as part of the test of cure in women after treatment, since inclusion of the rectal culture increases the diagnostic yield of treatment failures by as much as 50 per cent. Pharyngeal cultures should be obtained from patients with symptomatic pharyngitis or from persons exposed by fellatio to infected males. Patients with possible disseminated gonococcal infection should have culture samples taken from all possible mucosal sites (pharynx, urethra, cervix, rectum), as well as blood and synovial fluid.

Cultures of the cervix should be taken under direct visualization during speculum examination, using a cotton-tipped swab. Lubricant jellies may be deleterious to gonococci and should be avoided. Cultures of tampons can be used if speculum examination is not possible. Cultures of the anterior urethra of males should be taken with calcium alginate swabs or a sterile wire loop.

Positive cultures from the pharynx or rectum should be carefully evaluated by the microbiology laboratory to avoid confusion between gonococci and meningococci. Meningococci are more common than gonococci in throat cultures. Male homosexuals apparently transmit meningococci sexually, and positive rectal cultures for meningococci are relatively common in this group.

A variety of inexpensive office kits is available for culturing gonococci. These offer the advantages of media with long shelf life. They are approximately equal to standard cultures when their use is limited to urethral or cervical samples; the currently available systems should not be used for pharyngeal or rectal cultures.

A variety of serologic tests for gonorrhea has been developed in the past, and more are being tested currently. No test available in 1987 is sufficiently sensitive and specific to merit use for screening purposes. Patients with complications of gonorrhea usually have detectable serum antibodies against crude or purified gonococcal antigens, but none of the tests is routinely available at present.

TREATMENT. Gonococci frequently have chromosomal mutations that result in relative resistance to penicillin, tetracycline, and other antibiotics. The resistance in these strains is usually low level and can be overcome by appropriate doses of penicillin or tetracycline. Recently, strains with slightly higher levels of chromosomally mediated resistance (CMRNG strains) have become prevalent in certain areas of the United States and are more common in parts of Asia. These strains do not respond to penicillin but do respond to spectinomycin or ceftriaxone.

Gonococci that carry a β-lactamase (penicillinase) plasmid recently emerged in the Far East and elsewhere and have spread to much of the world. Penicillinase-producing gonococci (PPNG) account for about 30 per cent of all gonorrhea in certain cities in the Philippines but are quite uncommon (less than 0.5 per cent) in the United States. The prevalence of PPNG is only about 1 per cent in northern Europe but seems to be rising. There are two closely related gonococcal penicillinase plasmids of either 3.2 or 4.4 × 10⁶ daltons; each encodes a typical enteric-type TEM β-lactamase. The gonococcal plasmids are similar to penicillinase plasmids found in *Hemophilus* species. PPNG are resistant to clinically attainable doses of penicillins but are sensitive to spectinomycin and to certain cephalosporins (cefuroxime, cefoxitin, ceftriaxone). PPNG are known to cause DGI and salpingitis.

Quite recently, a new problem has arisen: plasmid-encoded tetracycline resistance. These strains do not respond to tetracycline but do respond to spectinomycin or ceftriaxone and may respond to penicillin.

The antibiotic regimens recommended for gonorrhea in the United States are summarized in Table 306-1. Because gonococcal infections commonly are associated with genital chlamydial infection, most authorities now recommend a seven-day course of a tetracycline for all patients with gonorrhea as follow-up to initial penicillin or ampicillin therapy.

Although the risk of anaphylaxis after penicillin is low (0.05 per cent if there is no history of penicillin allergy), up to 1 per cent of patients treated with 4.8 million units of procaine penicillin develop an acute neurotoxic syndrome caused by inadvertent intravenous administration of procaine, and up to 5 to 15 per cent develop rash caused by penicillin. The procaine penicillin regimen has the advantages of proven efficacy for incubating syphilis and single-dose administration.

In pharyngeal gonorrhea, the single-dose ampicillin and spectinomycin regimens result in about 50 per cent treatment failures. Consideration should be given to use of a pretreatment pharyngeal culture in patients treated with either of these regimens.

Each of the recommended regimens is highly effective for genital gonorrhea. If patients fail to respond to therapy, they should be cultured so that their isolates can be tested for production of penicillinase, and spectinomycin should be used for retreatment. However, most apparent failures are really reinfections. Some studies show that 15 per cent of patients are reinfected within six weeks of successful therapy. On this basis, many authorities recommend that patients should be recultured six weeks after treatment.

In the absence of an effective vaccine, control of this disease depends on proper diagnosis and treatment of patients' sexual contacts. If patients are given simple instructions, many will bring their contacts to the physician for examination. There are sound epidemiologic reasons for treating contacts immediately. Local health departments are not utilized sufficiently for help in examination and treatment of contacts.

Treatment of salpingitis (PID) has not been studied adequately. Two studies comparing ten-day oral ampicillin and tetracycline regimens found that they were equally effective in gonococcal and nongonococcal PID. Little is known about the relative merits of various regimens for hospitalized patients. Most authorities recommend removal of intrauterine devices in women with PID. It is crucial to examine and treat all sexual partners of women with gonococcal PID.

Therapy of gonococcal arthritis is ordinarily highly successful with each of the recommended regimens (Table 306-1). Failure to improve in three days suggests that the patient does not have DGI. Septic joints should be aspirated, both to make the initial diagnosis and to remove inflammatory exudate. Open drainage is rarely indicated, except in infection of the hip in childhood. Repeat closed aspiration may be necessary if joint fluid rapidly reaccumulates, but most patients require only one or a few joint aspirations. Antibiotics should not be injected into the joint space. Most patients with DGI should be hospitalized initially, but outpatient therapy may be used occasionally in carefully selected, compliant patients with a definite diagnosis and only mild infection.

Gonococcal conjunctivitis should be treated by immediate saline irrigation and intravenous penicillin G.

PREVENTION. Although vaccines are presently under intense study, an effective gonococcal vaccine is still only a hope. Condoms will prevent most infection, but those who need them most will often not use them. Certain contraceptive foams have antigonococcal activity but are of unproven effi-

cacy clinically. Prophylaxis with a single dose of a tetracycline antibiotic was partially protective in a recent study but failed in patients exposed to relatively resistant strains and therefore cannot be recommended.

Barlow D, Phillips I: Gonorrhoea in women: Diagnostic, clinical, and laboratory aspects. Lancet 1:761, 1978. *A concise description of the clinical and laboratory findings in a large group of women.*
Collier AC, Judson FN, Murphy VL, et al.: Comparative study of ceftriaxone and spectinomycin in the treatment of uncomplicated gonorrhea in women. Am J Med 77:68, 1984. *Ceftriaxone was effective in a single dose of 125 mg intramuscularly without probenecid for oropharyngeal and genital infections. Spectinomycin resulted in a 50 per cent failure rate in oropharyngeal infection, in agreement with earlier reports.*
Dans PE, Judson F: The establishment of a venereal disease clinic. II. An appraisal of current diagnostic methods in uncomplicated urogenital and rectal gonorrhea. J Am Vener Dis Assoc 1:107, 1975. *A critical examination of the utility of various diagnostic methods, including multiple cultures and Gram's stains.*
Eisenstein BI, Sox T, Biswas G, et al.: Conjugal transfer of the gonococcal penicillinase plasmid. Science 195:998, 1977. *Gonococci contain a conjugal plasmid that enables them to transfer sexually their penicillinase plasmid with efficiency.*
Faruki H, Kohmescher RN, McKinney WP, et al.: A community-based outbreak of infection with penicillin-resistant Neisseria gonorrhoeae not producing penicillinase (chromosomally mediated resistance). N Engl J Med 313:607, 1985. *Drug resistance among gonococci is an increasing problem everywhere.*
Handsfield HH, Lipman TO, Harnisch JP, et al.: Asymptomatic gonorrhea in men: Diagnosis, natural course, prevalence and significance. N Engl J Med 290:117, 1974. *Asymptomatic infection of the male urethra by gonococci is carefully described and is shown to be much more common than previously recognized.*
Handsfield HH, Murphy VL: Comparative study of ceftriaxone and spectinomycin for treatment of uncomplicated gonorrhoea in men. Lancet 2:67, 1983. *Among newer antibiotics, ceftriaxone appears most promising for single-dose therapy of penicillin-resistant gonorrhea.*
Handsfield HH, Wiesner PJ, Holmes KK: Treatment of the gonococcal arthritis-dermatitis syndrome. Ann Intern Med 84:661, 1976. *This is probably the best evaluation of the efficacy of various regimens for therapy of disseminated gonococcal infection.*
Hook EW, Holmes KK: Gonococcal infections. Ann Intern Med 102:229, 1985. *An excellent, clinically relevant review.*
Lebedeff DA, Hochman EB: Rectal gonorrhea in men: Diagnosis and treatment. Ann Intern Med 92:463, 1980. *This paper briefly reviews the clinical findings, diagnostic methods, and efficacy of various methods of treatment for gonococcal proctitis in men.*
Luciano AA, Grubin L: Gonorrhea screening: Comparison of three techniques. JAMA 243:680, 1980. *Culture of the first-voided urine in asymptomatic males is shown to be a highly reliable method for diagnosis.*

307 LYMPHOGRANULOMA VENEREUM

Lymphogranuloma venereum (LGV) is an acute to chronic sexually transmitted disease caused by strains of *Chlamydia trachomatis*. LGV typically produces transient genital lesions followed by significant regional lymphadenopathy, which may progress to late fibrosis and tissue destruction in untreated cases.

ETIOLOGY. The organisms causing LGV are closely related to the *C. trachomatis* strains that cause trachoma (serotypes A–C) or nongonococcal urethritis (serotypes D–K). By use of a microimmunofluorescent procedure the LGV strains have been grouped into three serotypes (L1, L2, and L3), of which L2 is apparently the most common. On one occasion the related organism *Chlamydia psittaci* caused a similar syndrome. All chlamydiae contain a common group antigen, but an LGV-specific protein antigen has been partially characterized. As is the case with all chlamydiae, the LGV strains can be isolated only in tissue culture or in yolk sac culture.

EPIDEMIOLOGY. LGV is more common in tropical and subtropical climates but does occur in relatively low incidence throughout the western world. The true incidence is unknown. Screening of patients in venereal disease clinics with the LGV complement fixation test has sometimes shown 10 per cent with positive serologies; however, this may merely reflect cross-reactions between antibodies directed against the *Chlamydia trachomatis* serotypes D–K (the causes of nongonococcal urethritis and related syndromes) and the LGV serotypes L1, L2, and L3.

The disease is almost always transmitted by sexual contact. The site of primary infection is usually around the genitals but may be anal or oral, depending on the mode of sexual practice.

PATHOGENESIS AND PATHOLOGY. The incubation period is uncertain but has been estimated to be anywhere from a few days to several weeks. In approximately one fourth of patients a small, evanescent primary lesion develops at the site of inoculation, but in the other three fourths of patients no primary lesion is clinically evident. Occasional patients may have symptoms of nonspecific urethritis, presumably owing to intraurethral infection. Approximately two to six weeks after sexual contact most patients develop significant regional lymphadenopathy. Primary infection of the anterior vulva or penis results in inguinal adenopathy, whereas primary infection of the vagina or posterior vulva or rectum results in primary perirectal or pelvic adenopathy. Most patients seen in venereal disease clinics are males with inguinal adenopathy. In about one third of patients the adenopathy is bilateral. Involvement of lymphatic tissue may result in significant lymphedema and, if untreated, may lead to elephantiasis of the external genitalia. Chronic infection of the perirectal tissues may lead to rectal strictures. The histologic appearance of involved tissues is nonspecific with acute and chronic inflammation.

CLINICAL MANIFESTATIONS. The transient primary lesion usually appears as an infiltrated papule or small erosion. It may mimic herpes but is frequently unnoticed or not present. In its earlier stages the adenopathy syndrome is manifested by discrete, tender, movable nodes. After several days the nodes become matted, with an ovoid, firm, lobulated swelling with adherent, erythematous overlying skin. In about 10 to 20 per cent of patients, nodes are involved above and below the inguinal ligament, and fibrosis may result in the so-called "groove sign" (linear depressions parallel to the inguinal ligament). The nodes may undergo necrosis, and, if not aspirated, spontaneous fistula tracts may develop. Lymphatic obstruction may result in vulvar edema or polypoid masses around the anal orifice. In early stages anal masses may resemble hemorrhoids. There may be fever, chills, and headache, associated with other nonspecific systemic symptoms such as nausea and weight loss. Infrequently, there is generalized rash, polyarthralgia, splenomegaly, generalized lymphadenopathy, or meningismus. Cutaneous manifestations may include erythema nodosum, erythema multiforme, urticaria, or a scarlatiniform eruption.

Late complications are usually limited to strictures or scarring of the rectum. This complication is more common in women, but is now fortunately rare. There is often no preceding adenopathy syndrome. The strictures may be bandlike or may involve extensive areas of the lower large bowel.

DIAGNOSIS. LGV must be considered in patients with enlarged inguinal lymph nodes, draining inguinal fistulas, and rectal strictures. Differential diagnosis includes reactive nodes secondary to distal sites of pyogenic infection on the extremities (which may be small and not noticed unless careful examination is performed), chancroid, granuloma inguinale, syphilis, and a variety of other diseases associated with adenopathy or adenitis. Diagnosis is made by one of two methods: either by direct demonstration of LGV organisms in lesion material or by appropriate serologic tests. Material may be obtained for culture from affected lymph nodes by inserting a needle into the area of fluctuance, being careful to insert the needle through normal skin. The aspirated pus is characteristically extremely viscous. Organisms may sometimes be directly demonstrated in this material by immunofluorescence, although this test is not routinely available. Culture

may be performed in yolk sacs or in tissue cell culture. A complement fixation test, using group-specific antigen, is widely available for serologic diagnosis. In the presence of a compatible clinical syndrome, a titer greater than or equal to 1:16 is strongly suggestive of LGV. Serial samples frequently show a fourfold or greater rise in titer in the acute stage of the disease. Most patients with LGV develop peak titers of at least 1:64. Other serologic tests are under development, including indirect immunofluorescence and counterimmunoelectrophoresis; each of these tests uses antigens specific for LGV, but neither is widely available at present. A direct immunofluorescence test employing monoclonal antibodies against *C. trachomatis* serotypes L1, L2, and L3 offers promise for rapid specific diagnosis, but it is not yet widely available.

Other laboratory tests are of little help. Many patients have a modest elevation in total leukocyte count with predominance of lymphocytes. There may be a reversal of the albumin globulin ratio, and some patients have elevated cryoglobulins or rheumatoid factor.

TREATMENT. Both tetracycline and sulfonamide drugs are effective. Usual therapy for adults is tetracycline, 500 mg four times daily for at least three weeks. When tetracycline is contraindicated as in pregnancy, sulfisoxazole may be given in a dose of 500 mg four times daily for at least three weeks. Tense nodes should be aspirated through normal skin to prevent formation of fistulous tracts. Patients with early stages of the disease respond well to therapy, but those with late complications, including chronic lymphatic obstruction and rectal stricture, respond poorly or not at all to antibiotic therapy. Surgery may be needed to correct rectal stricture. After an initial course of treatment, patients should be seen at least every three months for one year, and the titer of the LGV complement fixation test should be followed. Retreatment should be given if there is a fourfold increase in serologic titer or if there is clinical evidence of relapse. Sexual contacts should be treated similarly.

PREVENTION. There are no specific data regarding modes of prevention. Presumably, use of condoms would help to prevent transmission. An effective vaccine is not available.

Klotz SA, Drutz DJ, Tam MR, et al.: Hemorrhagic proctitis due to lymphogranuloma venereum serogroup L2: Diagnosis by fluorescent monoclonal antibody. N Engl J Med 308:1563, 1983. *LGV may cause hemorrhagic proctitis that mimics ulcerative colitis in homosexual males; monoclonal antibodies provide rapid diagnosis.*

Schachter J: Lymphogranuloma venereum and other nonocular *Chlamydia trachomatis* infections. In Hobson D, Holmes KK (eds.): Nongonococcal Urethritis and Related Infections. Washington, D.C., American Society for Microbiology, 1977, pp 91–97. *An excellent short review of the biology of the organism and the clinical manifestations of the disease.*

Sowmini CN, Gopalan KN, Chandrasekhara RG: Minocycline in the treatment of lymphogranuloma venereum. J Am Vener Dis Assoc 2:19, 1976. *Tetracyclines were effective in infected military personnel in Vietnam.*

308 GRANULOMA INGUINALE (Donovanosis)

Granuloma inguinale, also known as donovanosis, is a slowly progressive ulcerative disease involving principally the skin and subcutaneous tissues of the genital, inguinal, and anal regions. It is primarily transmitted sexually, but probably can be transmitted by nonsexual contact as well. Multiple sexual contacts with an infected partner seem necessary for transmission of infection. The disease is uncommon in the United States, with less than 100 recorded cases annually. It is quite common, however, in certain other areas of the world, especially Papua New Guinea.

ETIOLOGY. The causative organism is *Calymmatobacterium granulomatis*, a gram-negative bacterium which is immunologically related to certain *Klebsiella* strains. Current evidence suggests that *C. granulomatis* is not a member of the *Klebsiella-Enterobacter-Serratia* family; its exact taxonomic status is uncertain. The organism can be grown in yolk sacs, but only with great difficulty on artificial medium. It is apparently a facultative intracellular parasite, since in infected lesions it is found primarily in histiocytes or other mononuclear cells.

CLINICAL MANIFESTATIONS. The initial lesion usually appears as a subcutaneous nodule which erodes through the surface and develops into a beefy, elevated granulomatous lesion. This usually is painless and unassociated with systemic symptoms. Secondary bacterial infection may cause a necrotic painful ulcerative lesion which may be rapidly destructive. A cicatricial form may also occur with a depigmented elevated area of keloid-like scar containing scattered islands of granulomatous tissue. Lesions in the genital area are commonly associated with pseudobuboes in the inguinal region; these swellings are usually not due to involvement of the inguinal lymph nodes but rather to granulomatous involvement of the subcutaneous tissues. Metastatic infection of bones or other viscera is occasionally seen. Clinical experience suggests that secondary carcinomas may be a complication of granuloma inguinale.

DIFFERENTIAL DIAGNOSIS. The differential diagnosis includes tumor, lymphogranuloma venereum, chancroid, syphilis, and other ulcerative granulomatous diseases. Chancroid is usually differentiated by its irregular undermined borders, which are not seen in the usual cases of granuloma inguinale. Darkfield examination and serologic tests should help to distinguish syphilis. Biopsies may be necessary to distinguish granuloma inguinale from certain tumors.

DIAGNOSIS. Diagnosis is made by demonstrating intracellular "Donovan bodies" in histiocytes or other mononuclear cells from lesion scrapings or biopsies. Wright's stain or Giemsa stain of fresh impression smears or unfixed biopsies will usually demonstrate the bacilli relatively easily, although multiple biopsies may be necessary in chronic cases. Culture is not practical at present. A serologic test has been devised but is not clinically available. Histologic examination of biopsies shows mononuclear cells with some infiltration by polymorphonuclear leukocytes but no giant cells.

TREATMENT. Treatment consists of tetracycline or sulfisoxazole in a dose of 0.5 gram four times daily for at least three weeks. Other regimens which have proved effective include ampicillin, chloramphenicol, gentamicin, or co-trimoxazole. Limited experience suggests that lincomycin may be used successfully. Patients should be followed for at least several weeks after discontinuation of treatment because of the possibility of relapse. Although the risk of communicability appears to be low, sexual contacts should also be examined; at present, treatment of contacts is not indicated in the absence of clinically evident disease.

PREVENTION. No effective prevention is known.

Breschi LC, Goldman G, Shapiro SR: Granuloma inguinale in Vietnam: Successful therapy with ampicillin and lincomycin. J Am Vener Dis Assoc 1:118, 1975. *Ampicillin was frequently effective in patients previously unresponsive to tetracycline.*

Garg BR, Lal S, Sivamani S: Efficacy of co-trimoxazole in donovanosis. A preliminary report. Br J Vener Dis 54:348, 1978. *Trimethoprim and sulfamethoxazole were effective.*

Kuberski T: Granuloma inguinale (donovanosis). Sex Trans Dis 7:29, 1980. *An excellent short review.*

Maddocks I, Anders EM, Dennis E: Donovanosis in Papua New Guinea. Br J Vener Dis 52:190, 1976. *A description of the epidemiology and clinical manifestations in an endemic area of granuloma inguinale.*

Rosen T, Tschen JA, Ramsdell W, et al.: Granuloma inguinale. J Am Acad Dermatol 11:433, 1984. *An American epidemic of this relatively rare disease is described.*

309 CHANCROID

Chancroid is a sexually transmitted infection caused by the gram-negative bacillus *Hemophilus ducreyi*.

EPIDEMIOLOGY. On a worldwide basis chancroid is considerably more common than syphilis, and in parts of Africa and in Southeast Asia is nearly as great a problem as gonorrhea. In the United States it is an uncommon disease, but the incidence is rising. Epidemics have been documented in several cities in North America in recent years. The majority of reported cases occur in males. An outbreak in Greenland was exceptional in that about 40 per cent of cases were noted in women. It is quite likely that there has been significant underdiagnosis in women in the past.

CLINICAL MANIFESTATIONS. The usual incubation period is 2 to 5 days but may be up to 14 days. In the Greenland outbreak the incubation period averaged nearly two weeks in women. The initial clinical manifestation is an inflammatory macule that then becomes a vesicle-pustule and finally a sharply circumscribed, somewhat ragged, and undermined painful ulcer. The base is moist and may be covered with a grayish necrotic exudate. Removal of the exudate reveals purulent granulation tissue. There is usually surrounding cutaneous erythema. Lesions typically are single but may be multiple, possibly owing to autoinoculation of nearby tissues. There are rarely systemic symptoms. Inguinal adenopathy is noted in one half of patients, approximately two thirds of whom have unilateral adenopathy. Lesions are usually noted on the shaft or glans of the penis or around the anal orifice in males. In females lesions may occur on the cervix, vagina, vulva, or perianal area. Lesions may occasionally occur primarily on or spread to the abdomen, thigh, breast, fingers, or lips. Intraoral lesions are uncommon.

There are reports of a transient genital ulcer, followed by significant inguinal adenopathy. This may be difficult to distinguish from lymphogranuloma venereum. Other uncommon clinical variants include the *phagedenic type* of ulcer with secondary suprainfection and rapid tissue destruction; *giant chancroid*, which is characterized by a very large single ulcer; *serpiginous ulcer*, which is characterized by rapidly spreading, indolent, shallow ulcers on the groin or the thigh; and a *follicular* type with multiple small ulcers in a perifollicular distribution.

DIFFERENTIAL DIAGNOSIS. The differential diagnosis includes syphilis, herpes genitalis, lymphogranuloma venereum, traumatic ulcers, and granuloma inguinale. Of these the most commonly confused are syphilis and herpes genitalis. Multiple infections are relatively common. Outpatients with suspected chancroid should have a serologic test for syphilis and preferably a darkfield examination as well.

DIAGNOSIS. The diagnosis of chancroid is made on the basis of the clinical appearance of the lesions plus either morphologic demonstration of typical organisms in the lesions or recovery of *H. ducreyi* by culture. Culture is the preferred method. Positive cultures can be obtained in over 80 per cent of cases. Best culture results seem to be obtained with a chocolate agar medium containing 3 μg per milliliter of vancomycin. Necrotic debris should be removed from the ulcer with physiologic saline. The base and edges of the ulcer should be swabbed with a cotton-tipped swab and inoculated directly onto the culture plate if possible; swabs may be put into Amies transport medium if culture plates are not immediately available. Smears obtained from the undermined edges should be gently rolled onto a slide. *H. ducreyi* is a small gram-negative bacillus with rounded ends, which typically forms chains or parallel aggregates in lesions. Typical organisms are seen in 50 to 80 per cent of cases. Organisms may also be obtained by aspiration of inguinal nodes. Nodes should be aspirated by placing the needle through normal skin to avoid formation of fistulous tracts. Nodes should not be incised. There is no serologic test for chancroid.

TREATMENT. The drug of choice is probably erythromycin, in a dose of 500 mg orally four times daily for ten days. Combinations of trimethoprim and sulfamethoxazole (co-trimoxazole) usually are effective. Ampicillin should not be used, since some strains of *H. ducreyi* produce a typical TEM-type β-lactamase and are quite ampicillin resistant. Interestingly, the plasmids containing the gene for production of β-lactamase are very closely related to the penicillinase plasmids found recently in *H. influenzae* and *Neisseria gonorrhoeae*. Tetracycline resistance is common. All regular sexual partners should be examined and epidemiologically treated with a similar regimen.

PREVENTION. No vaccine is available. Use of a condom is presumably helpful. There are no data regarding efficacy of antibiotic prophylaxis.

Blackmore CA, Limpakarnjanarat K, Rigau-Perez JG, et al.: An outbreak of chancroid in Orange County, California: Descriptive epidemiology and disease-control measures. J Infect Dis 151:840, 1985. *A very large continental United States outbreak is described. Sulfa and tetracycline resistance was common, but erythromycin and co-trimoxazole were effective.*

Hammond GW, Slutchuk M, Scatliff J, et al.: Epidemiologic, clinical, laboratory, and therapeutic features of an urban outbreak of chancroid in North America. Rev Infect Dis 2:867, 1980. *An excellent summary of a recent epidemic in Winnipeg.*

Lykke-Olesen L, Larsen L, Pedersen TG, et al.: Epidemic of chancroid in Greenland 1977–78. Lancet 1:654, 1979. *A remarkable epidemic, affecting 3 per cent of the adult population. Tropical climates are not necessary for disease transmission or expression.*

Plummer FA, D'Costa LJ, Nsanze H, et al.: Antimicrobial therapy of chancroid: Effectiveness of erythromycin. J Infect Dis 148:726, 1983. *Documents the efficacy of erythromycin.*

Taylor DN, Pitarangsi C, Echeverria P, et al.: Comparative study of ceftriaxone and trimethoprim-sulfamethoxazole for the treatment of chancroid in Thailand. J Infect Dis 152:1002, 1985. *Ceftriaxone appears to be effective for this infection as well, in a single intramuscularly administered dose of 250 mg.*

310 SYPHILIS

DEFINITION. Syphilis is a subacute to chronic infectious disease caused by the bacterium *Treponema pallidum*. It is usually acquired by sexual contact with another infected individual. Syphilis is remarkable among infectious diseases in its large variety of clinical presentations. It progresses, if untreated, through primary, secondary, and tertiary stages. The early stages (primary and secondary) are infectious. Spontaneous healing of early lesions occurs, followed by a long latent period. In about 30 per cent of untreated patients, late disease of the heart, central nervous system, or other organs ultimately develops. At one time this disease was termed "the great imitator." Although the disease is less common now than previously, it remains a great challenge to the clinician because of its protean manifestations and is of great interest to biologists as well because of the long and tenuous balance between the host and the invading spirochete.

ETIOLOGY. The etiology of syphilis was discovered in 1905 by Schaudinn and Hoffman when they visualized spirochetal organisms in early infectious lesions. The causative agent of syphilis, *Treponema pallidum*, is closely related to

other pathogenic spirochetes, including those causing yaws (*Treponema pertenue*) and pinta (*Treponema carateum*).

T. pallidum is a thin, helical cell approximately 0.15 μ wide and 6 to 50 μ long. Ordinarily there are approximately 6 to 14 spirals. The organism is tapered on either end. It is too thin to be seen by ordinary Gram's stain but can be visualized in wet mounts by darkfield microscopy (see below) or by silver stains or fluorescent antibody methods.

The organism bears considerable structural resemblance to gram-negative bacteria. A superficial hyaluronic acid slime layer is formed around the organism and may contribute to virulence. Beneath the slime layer is the outer membrane, or outer envelope, which is structurally similar to the outer membrane of gram-negative bacteria. Between the outer membrane and the peptidoglycan cell wall are six axial fibrils. The axial fibrils are attached three at each end and overlap in the center of the organism. They are structurally and biochemically similar to flagella and may be in part responsible for the motility of the organism.

It is possible to culture *T. pallidum* in vitro, but yields are very low; culture is of limited use in research but of no use in clinical practice. *T. pallidum* can be maintained by serial passage in rabbits without loss of virulence. Only a few strains have been isolated in rabbits and carefully studied, and little evidence is available regarding the genetic diversity of the organism. All studied isolates have been susceptible to penicillin and are similar antigenically. Immunity to the homologous strain develops after prolonged infection in rabbits. The only known natural hosts for *T. pallidum* are humans and certain monkeys and higher apes.

PATHOGENESIS AND HOST RESPONSE. *T. pallidum* may penetrate through normal mucosal membranes and also through minor abrasions of epithelial surfaces. In experimental rabbit syphilis, spirochetes can be found in the lymphatic system within 30 minutes of inoculation and are found in blood shortly thereafter. There have been occasional instances in humans of transfusion syphilis resulting from use of blood from a donor who was in the incubation stage of the disease. Therefore it seems clear that syphilis is a systemic disease from the onset in humans as well. However, the first lesions appear at the site of primary inoculation, presumably because of the large numbers of treponemes implanted at this site. In laboratory animals, there is an inverse relationship between numbers of treponemes inoculated and time required for development of the primary cutaneous lesion. The minimal number of treponemes required to establish infection is not known but may be as low as one treponeme. Multiplication of organisms is very slow, with a division time in rabbits of approximately 33 hours. Similarly slow growth of treponemes in humans probably accounts in part for the protracted nature of the illness and for the relatively long incubation period.

T. pallidum is not known to produce any toxins. Although the outer membrane structurally resembles those of gram-negative bacteria, there is no biologically active endotoxin in *T. pallidum*. Treponemes are capable of specific attachment to host cells, but it is not known whether attachment results in damage to host cells. Most treponemes are found in intercellular spaces, but occasional treponemes can be seen within phagocytic cells. However, there is no evidence for intracellular survival of treponemes.

The primary pathologic lesion of syphilis is a focal endarteritis. There is an increase in adventitial cells, endothelial proliferation, and presence of an inflammatory cuff around affected vessels. Lymphocytes, plasma cells, and monocytes predominate in the inflammatory lesion, and in some cases polymorphonuclear cells are seen as well. The vessel lumen is frequently obliterated. With healing there is considerable fibrosis. Treponemes may be seen in most early lesions of syphilis and in some of the late lesions such as the meningoencephalitis of general paresis.

Granulomatous reaction is also frequent in secondary syphilis and in late syphilis. The granuloma is histologically nonspecific, and cases of syphilis have been incorrectly diagnosed as sarcoidosis or other granulomatous diseases. Human inoculation studies suggest that the pathogenesis of the gumma, which is a granulomatous lesion, involves hypersensitivity to small numbers of virulent treponemes introduced into a previously sensitized host.

Intracutaneous inoculation of patients with syphilis in various stages with partially purified antigens of *T. pallidum* showed that delayed cellular hypersensitivity developed only in late secondary syphilis but was uniformly present in latent syphilis. There may be temporary hyporesponsiveness of lymphocytes from patients with primary and secondary syphilis to treponemal antigens. It is possible but not proved that the unusual waxing and waning of lesions in early syphilis depend on the balance between development of effective cellular immunity and suppression of thymus-derived lymphocyte function.

The host also responds to infection with production of numerous antibodies, and in some instances circulating immune complexes may be formed. The nephrotic syndrome has been recognized occasionally in secondary syphilis, and renal biopsies from such cases have shown membranous glomerulonephritis characterized by focal subepithelial basement membrane deposits. The deposits contain both IgG and C3, and treponemal antibody.

Rarely patients may develop paroxysmal cold hemoglobinuria. This is due to production of an IgG antibody that binds to the red cell at 4° C and, upon rewarming of the blood in the presence of complement, results in hemolysis. Thus patients may develop massive hemolysis and hemoglobinuria after cold exposure. This was formerly usually due to congenital syphilis but is now almost always due to other infections. Treatment with penicillin usually stops the attacks.

Antibodies useful in diagnosis are discussed under Serologic Tests, below.

EPIDEMIOLOGY. Syphilis, with the exception of congenital syphilis, is acquired almost exclusively by intimate contact with the infectious lesions of primary or secondary syphilis (chancre, mucous patches, condylomata lata). This is usually through sexual intercourse, including anogenital and orogenital intercourse. Health workers have sometimes been infected during unsuspecting examination of patients with infectious lesions. Infection by contact with fomites is extremely uncommon.

Syphilis is most common in large cities and in young, sexually active individuals. The highest rate in both men and women occurs at ages 20 to 24, followed by ages 25 to 29 and 15 to 19 years. Among predominantly rural areas in the United States the disease is most prevalent in the southeast.

Syphilis spares no class, race, or group but is more prevalent in the United States among the poorly educated and economically deprived than among more prosperous groups. Increased numbers of different sexual partners and perhaps indiscriminate choice of partner increase the risk of acquiring sexually transmitted disease. Patients with primary and secondary syphilis name on the average nearly three different sexual contacts within the previous 90 days. A cornerstone of syphilis control is epidemiologic investigation of sexual contacts of patients with primary or secondary lesions, and of patients with early latent disease.

In recent years male homosexuals have accounted for an increasing proportion of the total cases of infectious syphilis. The ratio of male:female cases of primary and seondary syphilis in the United States rose from 1.6:1.0 in 1965 to 2.5:1.0 in 1975 and is now about 3:1. In many large cities over 50 per cent of all infectious syphilis occurs in male homosexuals. Currently, more than half of all white males with infectious syphilis name at least one male sexual partner during the recent past. In contrast, only 2 per cent of primary and secondary syphilis in females occurs in women who name a female sexual contact. Similar trends have been noted in other countries.

The annual incidence of syphilis has generally declined worldwide for approximately 100 years with the exception of periods of extensive war. With introduction of penicillin there was a rapid decline in primary and secondary syphilis after World War II, to annual rates of approximately 4 cases per 100,000 in 1957. This resulted in declining federal expenditure for syphilis control, however, and there was a subsequent resurgence in infectious primary and secondary syphilis in the United States, reaching peaks of over 12 cases per 100,000 several times in the period 1965–1983. Total reported cases of primary and secondary syphilis in 1983 were 33,613. Since many cases of syphilis are not reported, the true incidence is much higher, perhaps 75,000 to 100,000 annually.

Reported deaths from syphilis declined from 2434 in 1965 to 200 in 1976. Infant deaths from syphilis and first admissions for syphilitic psychoses have fallen by 98 to 99 per cent since 1940. Patients with clinically manifest late syphilis, particularly gummas, are becoming less common, perhaps as a result of the effectiveness of penicillin therapy for early syphilis. However, surveys indicate that there still are significant numbers of patients with untreated cardiovascular and neurologic syphilis, especially among older age groups. There is suggestive evidence that neurosyphilis may be presenting with atypical clinical manifestations and therefore may not be easily recognized.

NATURAL COURSE OF UNTREATED SYPHILIS. The incubation period from time of exposure to development of the primary lesion at the place of initial inoculation of treponemes averages approximately 21 days but ranges from 10 to 90 days. A painless papule develops and gradually breaks down to form a clean-based ulcer with raised, indurated margins. This persists for two to six weeks and then heals spontaneously. Several weeks later the patient characteristically develops a secondary stage characterized by low-grade fever, headache, malaise, generalized lymphadenopathy, and a mucocutaneous rash. There may be involvement of visceral organs. The secondary eruption may occur while the primary chancre is still healing or several months after the disappearance of the chancre. The secondary lesions heal spontaneously within two to six weeks, and the infection then enters latency. Some patients may later develop relapsing lesions similar to those of the secondary stage; rarely the relapse will take the form of recurrence of the primary chancre. About one third of untreated patients eventually develop late destructive tertiary lesions involving one or more of the eyes, central nervous system, heart, or other organs, including skin. These may occur at any time from a few years to as late as 25 years following infection.

The incidence of late complications of untreated syphilis is currently unknown but seems less than noted previously. Cases of gumma are at present so rare as to be reportable.

CLINICAL MANIFESTATIONS. *Primary Syphilis.* The typical lesion of primary syphilis is the chancre, a painless, clean-based, indurated ulcer. The chancre starts as a papule, but then superficial erosion occurs, resulting in the typical ulcer. The borders of the ulcer are raised, firm, and indurated. Occasionally, secondary infections change the appearance, resulting in a painful lesion. Most chancres are single, but multiple ulcers are sometimes seen, particularly when skin folds are opposed ("kissing chancres"). The untreated chancre heals in several weeks, leaving a faint scar. The chancre is usually associated with regional adenopathy, which may be either unilateral or bilateral. The regional nodes are movable, discrete, and rubbery. If the chancre occurs in the cervix or in the rectum, the affected regional iliac nodes are not palpable. See Figure 310–1.

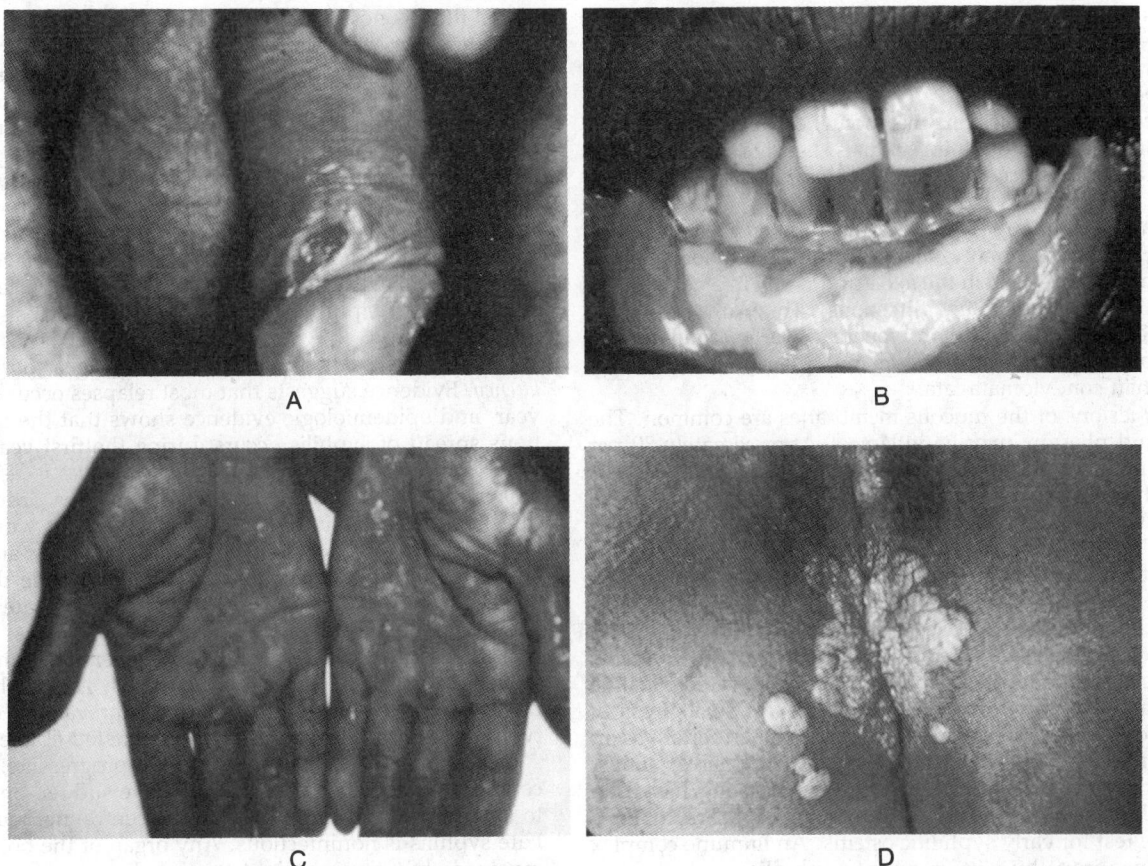

FIGURE 310–1. *A*, Primary syphilis, chancre. *B*, Secondary syphilis, mucous patch. *C*, Secondary syphilis, papulosquamous rash. *D*, Secondary syphilis, condylomata lata.

It was formerly taught that 90 per cent of chancres occurred in the genital region. Currently, a much higher proportion of nongenital chancres is observed, particularly among male homosexuals, in whom chancres in or near the rectum are common. Rectal chancres may have an atypical appearance, mimicking rectal fissures or other more benign lesions, and are frequently overlooked. Conversely, they have also been mistaken for malignant disease. In general it is reasonable to assume that any ulcer occurring in the genital area or, in male homosexuals, around the rectum is syphilitic until proved otherwise. Chancres may also be seen in the pharynx, on the tongue, around the lips, on the fingers, on the nipples, or in diverse other areas. The morphology depends in part on the area of the body in which they occur and also on the host immune response. Chancres in previously infected individuals may be small and may remain papular. Chancres of the finger may appear more erosive and may be quite painful.

The *differential diagnosis* of a genital ulcer should include genital herpes. Herpetic ulcers can usually be distinguished because they are multiple, superficial, and, if seen early, vesicular. They are often painful. Herpetic ulcers, unlike syphilitic ulcers, may yield positive findings on Tzanck's test—multinucleated giant cells in the base of the ulcer. The ulcers of chancroid are usually painful, often multiple, and frequently exudative and nonindurated. Lymphogranuloma venereum may produce a small papular lesion associated wtih a regional adenopathy. Other conditions that must be distinguished include granuloma inguinale, drug eruptions, carcinoma, superficial fungal infections, traumatic lesions, and lichen planus. Final distinction in most cases is made on the basis of darkfield examination, which is positive only in syphilis.

Secondary Syphilis. Approximately four to eight weeks following the appearance of the primary chancre, patients typically develop lesions of secondary syphilis. They may complain of *malaise, fever, headache, sore throat,* and other systemic symptoms. Most patients have generalized lymphadenopathy, including the epitrochlear nodes. Approximately 30 per cent of patients will have evidence of the healing chancre, although many patients, including male homosexuals and women, give no history of a primary lesion.

At least 80 per cent of patients with secondary syphilis have cutaneous lesions or lesions of the mucocutaneous junctions at some point in their illness. The diagnosis is usually first suspected on the basis of the cutaneous eruption. The rash is often minimally symptomatic, however, and many patients with late syphilis do not recall either primary or secondary lesions. The rashes are quite varied in their appearance but have certain characterisitc features. The lesions are usually widespread and are symmetric in distribution. They often are pink, coppery, or dusky red, particularly the earliest macular lesions. They usually are nonpruritic, although occasional exceptions have been noted, and are almost never vesicular or bullous in adults. They are indurated except for the very earliest macular lesions and frequently have a superficial scale (papulosquamous lesions). They tend to be polymorphic and rounded, and on healing they may leave residual pigmentation or depigmentation. The lesions may be quite faint and difficult to visualize, particularly on dark-skinned individuals.

The earliest pink macular lesions are frequently seen on the margins of the ribs or the sides of the trunk with later spread to the rest of the body. The face is often spared except around the mouth. Subsequently a papular rash appears, which is usually generalized but is *quite marked on the palms and soles.* These frequently are associated with a superficial scale and may be hyperpigmented. When the rash occurs on the face, it may be pustular, resembling acne vulgaris. On occasion the scale may be so great as to resemble psoriasis. Deep nodular lesions may cause confusion. Ulceration may occur, producing lesions resembling ecthyma. In malnourished or debilitated patients extensive destructive ulcerative lesions with a heaped-up crust may occur, the so-called rupial lesion. Lesions around the hair follicles may result in patchy alopecia of the beard or of the scalp.

Ringed or annular lesions may occur, especially around the face, particularly on black individuals. Lesions at the angle of the mouth or the corner of the nose may have a central linear erosion (the so-called "split papule").

In warm, moist areas such as the perineum, large, pale, flat-topped papules may coalesce to form condylomata lata. These may also be seen in the axilla and rarely in a generalized form. They are extremely infectious. They are not to be confused with the common venereal warts (condylomata acuminata), which are small, often multiple, and more sharply raised than condylomata lata.

Other lesions of the mucous membranes are common. The palate and pharynx may be inflamed. Approximately 30 per cent of patients develop the so-called mucous patch. This is a slightly raised oval area covered by a grayish-white membrane, which when raised reveals a pink base that does not bleed. These may be seen on the genitalia, in the mouth, or on the tongue and, like condylomata lata, are highly infectious.

Other manifestations of secondary syphilis include hepatitis, which has been reported in up to 10 per cent of patients in some series. Jaundice is rare, but an elevated alkaline phosphatase is common. Liver biopsy reveals small areas of focal necrosis and mononuclear infiltrate or periportal vasculitis. Spirochetes can often be visualized with silver stains. Periostitis with widespread lytic lesions of bone has been reported occasionally; use of bone scans appears to be a sensitive test for early syphilitic osteitis. An immune complex type of nephropathy with transient nephrotic syndrome has been rarely documented. There may be iritis or an anterior uveitis. From 10 to 30 per cent of patients have pleocytosis in the cerebrospinal fluid, but symptomatic meningitis is seen in less than 1 per cent of patients. Symptomatic gastritis may be present.

Differential diagnosis of secondary syphilis includes a large number of diseases. The cutaneous eruptions may be mimicked by pityriasis rosea, which can be differentiated by the occurrence of lesions along lines of skin cleavage and frequently by the presence of a herald patch. Drug eruptions, acute febrile exanthems, psoriasis, lichen planus, scabies, and other diseases must also be considered in some cases. The mucous patch may superficially resemble oral candidiasis (thrush). Infectious mononucleosis may appear very similar to secondary syphilis, with sore throat, generalized adenopathy, hepatitis, and a generalized rash. Infectious hepatitis may also cause confusion. A high index of suspicion is required to make the diagnosis of syphilis in some cases. Unfortunately even classic cases with widespread, hyperpigmented, papulosquamous lesions involving the palms and the soles are not infrequently misdiagnosed in the current era. Fortunately, if the serologic tests for syphilis are obtained, they will be positive in 99 per cent of patients. The condylomata lata and mucous patches contain large numbers of treponemes on darkfield examination. Aspiration of lymph nodes may occasionally reveal motile *T. pallidum*.

Relapsing Syphilis. Condylomata lata are likely to recur. The skin manifestations tend to be unilateral, the eruptions more dense, marked, with fewer lesions, and sometimes solitary. They are also more infiltrated and of somewhat longer standing and have some characteristics that resemble the skin lesions in late syphilis. This reflects the increasing immunity with the duration of the early disease. Neurorecurrences, as well as ophthalmic and other relapsing manifestations, may occur. If the patient has been inadequately treated, relapses may be delayed.

Latent Syphilis. By definition latent syphilis is that stage in which there are no clinical signs of syphilis and the cerebro-

spinal fluid is normal. Latency begins with the passing of the first attack of secondary syphilis and may last for a lifetime thereafter. It is usually detected by positive specific treponemal antibody tests for syphilis. The test must be shown to be reactive on more than one occasion to rule out technical errors. Diseases known to cause occasional false-positive treponemal reactions for syphilis, such as systemic lupus erythematosus, must be excluded. In addition, congenital syphilis must be excluded before the diagnosis of latent syphilis can be made. Patients may or may not have a history of earlier primary or secondary syphilis, although such history is obviously helpful in making a firm diagnosis of latent syphilis.

Latency has been divided into two stages: *early* and *late latency.* Evidence suggests that most relapses occur in the first year, and epidemiologic evidence shows that the most infectious spread of syphilis occurs during the first year of infection. *Therefore early latency in the United States is defined as the first year after infection.* Late latent syphilis is ordinarily not infectious except for the case of the pregnant woman, who may transmit infection to her fetus after many years.

Late Syphilis. Late, or tertiary, syphilis is the destructive stage of the disease and can be crippling. Late syphilitic complications are still important medical problems, but newly recognized cases of late syphilis have been declining steadily in the United States since World War II. Although the incidence of late syphilis is unknown, the prevalence of various types of late syphilis has been approximated (Table 310–1).

Late syphilis is usually very slowly progressive, although certain neurologic syndromes may have sudden onset owing to endarteritis and thrombosis in the central nervous system. Late syphilis is noninfectious. Any organ of the body may be involved, but three main types of disease may be distinguished: late benign (gummatous), cardiovascular, and neurosyphilis.

LATE BENIGN SYPHILIS. Late benign syphilis, or gumma, was the most common complication of late syphilis in the Oslo Study of untreated patients (1891–1951). In the penicillin era gummas are rare. They typically develop from one to ten years after the initial infection and may involve any part of the body. Although they may be very destructive, they respond rapidly to treatment and therefore are relatively benign. Histologically the gumma is a granuloma. The histologic findings are nonspecific and may be associated with central necrosis surrounded by epithelioid and fibroblastic cells and occasionally giant cells. There is sometimes vasculitis. *T. pallidum* is ordinarily not demonstrable by silver stains but can sometimes be recovered by inoculation of rabbits.

Gummas may be solitary or multiple. They are usually asymmetric and are often grouped. They may start as a superficial nodule or as a deeper lesion that breaks down to form punched-out ulcers. They are ordinarily indolent and slowly progressive with curving or polycyclic borders. They are indurated on palpation. There often is central healing with an atrophic scar surrounded by hyperpigmented borders.

TABLE 310–1. NEWLY DIAGNOSED TERTIARY SYPHILIS IN 105 PATIENTS IN DENMARK, 1961–1970

Type of Tertiary Syphilis	Number Observed*
Neurosyphilis	72
Asymptomatic	45
Tabes dorsalis	11
General paralysis	13
Meningovascular	1
Optic atrophy	2
Cardiovascular syphilis	44
Aortic insufficiency	16
Aortic aneurysm	13
Uncomplicated aortitis†	15
Late benign syphilis (gumma)	4

*Some patients had more than one form of late syphilis.
†Autopsy diagnoses only.

Cutaneous gummas may resemble other chronic granulomatous ulcerative lesions caused by tuberculosis, sarcoidosis, leprosy, and other deep fungal infections. Precise histologic diagnosis may not be possible. However, the syphilitic gumma is the only such lesion to heal dramatically with penicillin therapy. Another form of gumma is papulosquamous and may mimic psoriasis.

Gummas may also involve deep visceral organs, of which the most common are the respiratory tract, the gastrointestinal tract, and bones. In earlier centuries gummas of the nose and palate commonly resulted in septal perforations and disfiguring facial lesions. Gummas may also involve the larynx or the pulmonary parenchyma. Gumma of the stomach may masquerade as carcinoma of the stomach or lymphoma. Gummas of the liver were once the most common form of visceral syphilis, presenting often with hepatosplenomegaly and anemia, occasionally with fever and jaundice. Skeletal gummas typically produce lesions in the long bones, skull, and clavicle. A characteristic symptom is nocturnal pain. Radiologic abnormalities, when present, include periostitis and either lytic or sclerotic destructive osteitis.

CARDIOVASCULAR SYPHILIS. The primary cardiovascular complications of syphilis are aortic insufficiency and aortic aneurysm, usually of the ascending aorta. Less commonly other large arteries may be involved, and rarely involvement of the coronary ostia results in coronary insufficiency. These complications in all cases are due to obliterative endarteritis of the vasa vasorum with resultant damage to the intima and media of the great vessels. This results in dilatation of the ascending aorta and eventually in stretching of the ring of the aortic valve, producing aortic insufficiency. The valve cusps remain normal. Death may eventually result from congestive heart failure. There has been some success with placing prosthetic heart valves in patients with syphilitic aortic insufficiency. Aneurysms occasionally present as a pulsating mass bulging through the anterior chest wall. Syphilitic aortitis may involve the descending aorta, but this is almost always proximal to the renal arteries, unlike atherosclerotic aneurysms, which typically involve the descending aorta below the renal arteries.

The disease usually begins within 5 to 10 years after initial infection but may not become clinically manifest until 20 to 30 years after infection. Cardiovascular syphilis is thought to be more common in men than in women and possibly in blacks than in whites. Cardiovascular syphilis does not occur after congenital infection—a phenomenon that remains unexplained.

Asymptomatic aortitis is best diagnosed by visualizing linear calcifications in the wall of the ascending aorta by radiography. The signs of syphilitic aortic insufficiency are the same as for aortic insufficiency of other causes. In aortic insufficiency resulting from dilatation of the aortic ring, the decrescendo murmur is often loudest along the *right* sternal margin. Syphilitic aneurysms may be fusiform but are more typically saccular and do not lead to aortic dissection. Approximately 10 to 25 per cent of patients with cardiovascular syphilis have coexistent neurosyphilis, and it is therefore mandatory to do a lumbar puncture in all patients with cardiovascular syphilis.

At present, syphilis is a relatively more common cause of aortic insufficiency among the elderly than among younger patients; this is due to the progressively decreasing incidence of new cases of late cardiovascular syphilis.

NEUROSYPHILIS. Neurosyphilis may be divided into four groups: asymptomatic, meningovascular, tabes dorsalis, and general paresis. These are more fully described in Ch. 482. Division is not absolute, and there may be considerable overlap between syndromes. Current cases of neurosyphilis are more likely than heretofore to be variants of the classic syndromes, possibly as a result of use of antimicrobials for other diseases.

Asymptomatic Neurosyphilis. Asymptomatic neurosyphilis is

diagnosed when there is a positive VDRL* in the cerebrospinal fluid (CSF) in the absence of signs and symptoms of neurologic disease. False-positive VDRL test results are very rare in CSF in the absence of a traumatic tap. The CSF usually shows an increased total protein and a lymphocytic pleocytosis. If the CSF is normal two or more years after the initial infection, the patient is not likely to develop a positive CSF later. Although up to 30 per cent of patients with untreated secondary syphilis have an abnormal CSF, penicillin therapy apparently prevents progression to late symptomatic neurosyphilis. Because of this, routine lumbar punctures for examination of CSF are not indicated in early syphilis. Unfortunately, it has become common practice to avoid lumbar punctures in later stages of syphilis as well. Instead, patients are treated with doses of penicillin thought to be effective for neurosyphilis, if present. As a result, there are few data on the present frequency and course of asymptomatic neurosyphilis.

Some laboratories perform an FTA-ABS* test on spinal fluid. Interest in tests such as this has been prompted by good evidence that patients with untreated neurosyphilis may have a negative CSF-VDRL. There are published reports of positive FTA-ABS test results in the CSF of patients with otherwise normal spinal fluid, in whom there were clinical signs and symptoms compatible with neurosyphilis. However, the CSF FTA-ABS test has not been standardized, and there is some evidence that positive CSF test results are caused by passive transfer of serum antibody into spinal fluid. At present no diagnosis of asymptomatic (or symptomatic) neurosyphilis should be based solely on the CSF FTA-ABS* test.

Meningovascular Syphilis. An acute to subacute aseptic meningitis may occur at any time after the primary stage but usually within the first year of infection. It frequently involves the base of the brain and may result in unilateral or bilateral cranial nerve palsies. In about 10 per cent of cases, the onset of meningitis coincides with the rash of secondary syphilis. The spinal fluid shows a lymphocytic pleocytosis with increased protein and usually normal glucose concentration. The CSF-VDRL is nearly always positive. Rarely CSF glucose concentration is decreased. This syndrome can mimic tuberculous or fungal meningitis or nonpurulent meningitis of various causes.

In other patients, the meningeal involvement may be less prominent, but there is sufficient endarteritis and perivascular inflammation to result in cerebrovascular thrombosis and infarction. This usually occurs five to ten years after the initial infection and is more common in males. There often is an associated aseptic meningitis as well. Most cerebrovascular accidents are not due to syphilitic arteritis even in patients with a positive serologic test for syphilis. However, syphilis should be considered as the cause in young patients with a history of syphilis and without other causes for cerebrovascular accidents.

Tabes Dorsalis. Tabes dorsalis is a slowly progressive degenerative disease involving the posterior columns and posterior roots of the spinal cord, resulting in progressive loss of peripheral reflexes, impairment of vibration and position sense, and progressive ataxia. There may be chronic destructive changes in the large joints of the affected limbs in far advanced cases (Charcot's joints). Incontinence of the bladder and impotence are common. Sudden and severe painful crises of uncertain cause are a characteristic part of the syndrome. These may involve the larynx, vagina, rectum, or other organs. Not infrequently severe, sharp abdominal pains lead to exploratory surgery. Lightning pains in the extremities may require opiates for relief. These may be triggered by exposure to cold or other stresses or may arise with no obvious precipitating cause.

Optic atrophy is seen in 20 per cent of cases. The pupils

---

*See Serologic Tests, below. Also refer to Table 310–2.

are abnormal in 90 per cent of cases, with bilaterally small pupils that fail to constrict further in response to light but that do constrict normally to accommodation (Argyll Robertson pupils).

The cause of tabes dorsalis is unclear. Spirochetes cannot be demonstrated in the posterior column or dorsal root.

Onset of the disease is usually delayed, often 20 to 30 years after initial onset of infection. It is thought to be more common in whites and in males. Typical cases of patients presenting with lightning pains, ataxia, Argyll Robertson pupils, absent deep tendon reflexes, and loss of posterior column function are easy to diagnose. Atypical cases may be more troublesome, particularly because the VDRL test result in the serum is normal in as many as 30 to 40 per cent of patients, and 10 to 20 per cent of patients (even before the advent of penicillin) have normal CSF-VDRL results as well. The FTA-ABS test in serum is nearly always positive.

Treatment is unsatisfactory. Penicillin does not reverse the symptoms, although it does usually result in clearing of the abnormal spinal fluid. Carbamazepine in doses of 400 to 800 mg per day has been reported to be effective in treatment of the lightning pains.

Tabes dorsalis is now thought to be uncommon, although a survey of newly diagnosed late syphilis in Denmark in the decade 1961 to 1970 showed that in approximately 10 per cent of all persons with late syphilis and 40 per cent of all with clinical neurosyphilis there was evidence of tabes dorsalis.

General Paresis. This form of neurosyphilis is a chronic meningoencephalitis resulting in gradually progressive loss of cortical function. It typically occurs 10 to 20 years after the initial infection. Pathologically there is a perivascular and meningeal chronic inflammatory reaction with thickening of the meninges, a granular ependymitis, degeneration of the cortical parenchyma, and abundant spirochetes in the tissues.

The most devastating effect of general paresis is on the mind. With effective penicillin therapy this disease has become much less common; in the United States, first admissions to mental hospitals because of syphilitic psychosis declined from 7694 in 1940 to 154 in 1968, the last year for which definite figures are available.

In its early stages general paresis results in nonspecific symptoms such as irritability, fatigability, headaches, forgetfulness, and personality changes. Later there is impaired memory, defective judgment, lack of insight, confusion, and often depression or marked elation. The patients may be delusional, and seizures are sometimes seen. There may also be loss of other cortical functions, including paralysis or aphasia.

Physical signs are primarily those of the altered mental status. Cranial nerve palsies are uncommon. Optic atrophy is rare. The complete Argyll Robertson pupil is also uncommon, but irregular or otherwise abnormal pupils are not infrequent. Peripheral reflexes are often somewhat increased.

The CSF is nearly always abnormal with lymphocytic pleocytosis and increased total protein. The VDRL is usually reactive in both spinal fluid and serum. The disease responds well to penicillin therapy if administered early, although as many as a third of treated patients may develop progressive neurologic decline in later years. Fever therapy induced with malaria was formerly an effective adjunct to treatment with arsenicals but has now been abandoned.

Even though classic general paresis is now infrequent, it remains reasonable to suspect syphilis as the cause of undiagnosed neurologic illness. Since the VDRL may be negative in patients with late neurologic syphilis, the FTA-ABS test on serum must be performed before syphilis can be excluded.

Congenital Syphilis. Congenital syphilis results from transplacental hematogenous spread of syphilis from the mother to the fetus. The incidence of congenital syphilis among newborns or infants under one year of age in the United States rose from 180 cases in 1957 to 422 cases in 1972 but has

since declined to about 100 cases annually. Each case of congenital syphilis represents a tragedy that could have been prevented by better case reporting and by proper prenatal care. A VDRL should be obtained in all expectant mothers at the beginning and near the end of pregnancy.

Spirochetes can be found in abortuses of as little as nine to ten weeks' gestation. The risk of fetal infection is greatest in the early stages of untreated maternal syphilis and declines slowly thereafter, but the mother may infect her fetus during at least the first five years of her infection. Adequate treatment of the mother prior to the sixteenth week will usually prevent manifest clinical illness in the neonate. Later treatment may not prevent late sequelae of the disease in the child. Untreated maternal infection may result in stillbirth, neonatal death, prematurity, or syndromes of early or late congenital syphilis among surviving infants.

Manifestations of early congenital syphilis are often seen in the perinatal period but may not develop until the infant has been discharged from the hospital. The disease resembles secondary syphilis of the adult except that the rash may be vesicular or bullous, which is extremely rare in adults. There often is rhinitis, hepatosplenomegaly, hemolytic anemia, jaundice, and pseudoparalysis (immobility of one or more extremities) resulting from painful osteochondritis. There may be thrombocytopenia and leukocytosis. The early stages of congenital syphilis must be differentiated from rubella, cytomegalovirus infection, toxoplasmosis, bacterial sepsis, and other diseases.

Late congenital syphilis is defined as congenital syphilis of more than two years' duration. The disease may remain latent with no manifest late damage. Cardiovascular alterations have not been observed in congenital syphilis. Neurologic manifestations are common, and there may be eighth cranial nerve deafness and interstitial keratitis. The latter occurs in over 10 per cent of patients but may not be manifest until the tenth year of life or later. Periostitis may result in prominent frontal bones, depression of the bridge of the nose ("saddle nose"), poor development of the maxilla, and anterior bowing of the tibias ("saber shins"). There may be late-onset arthritis of the knees (Clutton's joints). The permanent dentition may show characteristic abnormalities known as Hutchinson's teeth; the upper central incisors are widely spaced, centrally notched, and tapered in the manner of a screwdriver. The molars may show multiple poorly developed cusps (mulberry molars). Some of the late manifestations such as interstitial keratitis and Clutton's joints may be due to hypersensitivity responses and are benefited by corticosteroids in some cases.

DIAGNOSIS. *Darkfield Examination.* The most definitive means of making a diagnosis is finding spirochetes of typical morphology and motility in lesions of early acquired or congenital syphilis. The darkfield examination is almost always positive in primary syphilis and in the moist mucosal lesions of secondary and congenital syphilis. It may occasionally be positive in aspirates of lymph nodes in secondary syphilis. Problems arise, however, because of false-negative results in primary syphilis owing to application by the patient of soaps or other toxic compounds to the lesions. A single negative result is therefore insufficient to exclude syphilis. Patients with suspicious lesions but with an initially negative darkfield examination should be instructed to avoid washing the lesion and to return daily for two successive examinations. Confusion may also arise because of the presence of spirochetes that are morphologically indistinguishable from *T. pallidum* in the mouth, particularly around the gingival margins. For lesions in these areas, therefore, diagnosis often depends upon clinical appearance, history, and serologic testing.

To perform the darkfield examination, the surface of the suspected ulcerative lesion should be cleaned with saline solution and gauze without production of bleeding. The presence of red cells in the specimen makes it difficult to visualize small numbers of *T. pallidum*. Squeezing of the lesion (with gloves on) may help produce serous fluid, which is picked up on a glass slide, covered with a coverslip, and examined with the darkfield microscope. Living *T. pallidum* organisms demonstrate gradual motion to and fro, rotational movement around the long axis, and rather sudden 90-degree bending near the center of the organism. Since most physicians do not have the proper equipment and are not familiar with the techniques of darkfield microscopy, the state public health authorities can be called for assistance.

T. pallidum may also be demonstrated in biopsies or pathologic specimens by fluorescent antibody stains or by silver stains.

Serologic Tests. Two basic types of humoral antibody are stimulated by infection with *T. pallidum*: nonspecific antibody directed against diphosphatidylglycerol (cardiolipin), which is a normal component of many tissues; and specific treponemal antibodies. Nonspecific antibodies against cardiolipin were formerly designated "reagin," a term that should be discarded to avoid confusion with another "reagin," IgE. The kinds of tests used in syphilis are summarized in Table 310–2.

NONSPECIFIC TESTS. Anticardiolipin antibodies were first discovered by Wassermann in 1907, using extracts of congenitally syphilitic livers as the antigen for a complement fixation test. Subsequently it was shown that normal livers contained the same antigen as do many other tissues; the antigen for this class of test is now extracted from beef heart. As yet there is no convincing explanation for why patients infected with *T. pallidum* develop increasing titers of antibody against a normal tissue component.

The Wassermann test has now been replaced by related tests. The standard test in use today for detection of anticardiolipin antibody is the Venereal Disease Research Laboratories (VDRL) test, which is an easily quantified slide flocculation test. Many similar tests, including the rapid plasma reagin (RPR) test and the unheated serum reagin (USR) test, are frequently used for screening for syphilis.

The VDRL and related tests are simple, well standardized, cheap, and the screening tests of choice. The VDRL is the test of choice for following the response of patients to treatment. Since the VDRL detects antibody against a normal tissue component, it may be falsely positive in a significant number of patients. The relative proportion of patients with a false-positive VDRL depends on the prevalence of syphilis in the community; the lower the prevalence of syphilis, the higher the proportion of positive VDRL tests that are due to nonsyphilitic causes.

The VDRL test begins to turn positive a week or two after the onset of the chancre. In large series of patients with primary syphilis, approximately two thirds have had a positive VDRL test result. Obviously, then, a negative VDRL test does not exclude primary syphilis, particularly if the lesion is less than two weeks old. The VDRL is positive in 99 per cent of patients with secondary syphilis, the only exceptions being patients with such high titers of antibody that they are in

antibody excess; dilution of the serum will then paradoxically result in conversion of a negative test to positive. VDRL reactivity tends to diminish in later stages of the disease, and only about 70 per cent of patients with cardiovascular or neurosyphilis have a positive VDRL test result.

The *quantitative titer* of the VDRL test is somewhat useful in diagnosis and quite useful in following therapeutic response. The titer is reported as the highest dilution that gives a positive response. Most patients with secondary syphilis have titers of at least 1:16. Most patients with false-positive VDRL tests have titers of less than 1:8. No single titer is in itself diagnostic. Significant rises (fourfold or greater) in paired sera, however, are strongly indicative of acute syphilis.

TREPONEMAL TESTS. There are many varieties of specific treponemal antibody tests. The most widely used is the fluorescent treponemal antibody absorption (FTA-ABS) test. Patient serum is absorbed with extracts of nonpathogenic cultivable treponemes to remove cross-reacting group treponemal antibody. Agglutination of red cells to which *T. pallidum* antigens have been fixed is the basis of the microhemagglutination assay for *T. pallidum* (MHA-TP).

The precise nature of the antigens involved in these tests is not known. Characterization of the antigens of *T. pallidum* has been greatly hindered by inability to grow the organism in cell-free culture. Recent success in cloning *T. pallidum* antigens into *Escherichia coli* may circumvent this problem. Antibodies reactive in the various tests are found in all major immunoglobulin classes (IgG, IgM, IgA). A modification of the FTA-ABS test has been developed using fluorescein-labeled anti–human IgM (IgM FTA-ABS). The IgM FTA-ABS test is of some use in the diagnosis of early congenital syphilis but is of no use in distinguishing acute disease from old infections in adults.

The FTA-ABS test is best used as a confirmatory test. It is somewhat more difficult to perform than the VDRL test and cannot be easily quantified. It is sensitive and has a high degree of specificity, being positive in only approximately 1 per cent of normal individuals. It is positive in 85 per cent of patients with primary syphilis, 99 per cent with secondary syphilis, and at least 95 per cent with late syphilis. It may therefore be the only test positive in patients with cardiovascular or neurologic syphilis. In late syphilis the FTA-ABS test usually remains positive for life despite adequate therapy. It (as well as the MHA-TP) is positive in other treponemal diseases, such as pinta, yaws, and bejel.

The FTA-ABS test is reported in terms of relative brilliance of fluorescence, from borderline to 4+. Borderline reactivity has the same meaning as nonreactive for clinical purposes. Most laboratories report 1+ positive tests as reactive, but some studies have shown that such tests may be difficult to reproduce. Occasional laboratories therefore only report as positive tests with 2+ or greater reactivity. In patients lacking historical or clinical evidence of syphilis but with a reactive FTA-ABS test, one should repeat the FTA-ABS test. Use of another treponemal test such as the MHA-TP may be helpful in problem cases.

The MHA-TP test is less sensitive than either the VDRL or the FTA-ABS test in primary syphilis. Its sensitivity and specificity otherwise are nearly identical to those of the FTA-ABS test, being positive in nearly all patients with secondary syphilis and in 95 per cent or more of patients with late syphilis. The reactivity of serologic tests for syphilis in various stages of disease is shown in Table 310–3.

False-Positive Serologic Test Results for Syphilis. The VDRL or RPR test may be positive in a variety of diseases other than syphilis. A false-positive result is defined as a reproducible positive test in a patient with no clinical or historical evidence of syphilis and whose serum FTA-ABS or MHA-TP test is negative.

"Acute" (less than six months) false-positive VDRL test results occur with low frequency in atypical pneumonia, malaria,

TABLE 310–2. SEROLOGIC TESTS FOR SYPHILIS

Type	Use
Nonspecific (anticardiolipin) antibodies:	
VDRL (slide flocculation)	Screening, quantitation, following response to treatment
RPR (circle-card) (agglutination)	Screening
Specific treponemal antibodies:	
FTA-ABS (immunofluorescence with absorbed serum)	Confirmatory, diagnostic, not for routine screening
MHA-TP (microhemagglutination)	Similar to FTA-ABS but can be quantified and automated

VDRL = Venereal Disease Research Laboratories test.
RPR = Rapid plasma reagin test.
FTA-ABS = Fluorescent treponemal antibody absorption test.
MHA-TP = Microhemagglutination assay for *T. pallidum*.

TABLE 310–3. FREQUENCY OF POSITIVE SEROLOGIC TESTS IN UNTREATED SYPHILIS

Stage	VDRL (%)	FTA-ABS (%)	MHA-TP (%)
Primary	70	85	50–60
Secondary	99	100	100
Latent or late	70	98	98

and other bacterial or viral infections and may occur after smallpox or other vaccinations as well. *Chronic false-positive VDRL tests* (lasting longer than six months) are relatively common in autoimmune disorders such as systemic lupus erythematosus (SLE), in narcotic addicts, in leprosy, and in aged persons. From 8 to 20 per cent of patients with SLE have been reported as having a false-positive VDRL test, and the false-positive result may develop many years prior to the onset of other manifestations of the disease. A chronic false-positive VDRL test in females age 20 or younger carries a significant risk of future development of SLE, thyroiditis, or other autoimmune disorders, and such patients should be followed carefully for a considerable period of time. As many as one third of patients with narcotic addiction have a false-positive VDRL test. Over 1 per cent of patients aged 70 and 10 per cent of patients over age 80 have a low-titer false-positive VDRL test. Most false-positive VDRL tests have a titer of 1:8 or less, although occasional patients with lymphoma and other diseases have been described with very high-titer false-positive VDRL tests.

A positive FTA-ABS result is usually indicative of recent or past syphilis. However, there is an increased incidence of false-positive FTA-ABS results in SLE and in other chronic diseases associated with hyperglobulinemia, including rheumatoid arthritis, biliary cirrhosis, and others. False-positive results are of two kinds in SLE: The most common is one with a beaded pattern of fluorescence, which has been shown to be due to anti-DNA antibodies; there also may be homogeneous fluorescence of the treponeme indistinguishable from a true positive result in syphilis. Patients with SLE who have a false-positive FTA-ABS result almost always have a negative VDRL result (and conversely, patients with SLE with a positive VDRL usually have a negative FTA-ABS).

Occasionally one encounters reproducible positive FTA-ABS results in patients with no clinical or historical evidence of syphilis and in whom there is no evidence of diseases associated with false-positive FTA-ABS results. It may be wise to obtain CSF for examination of total protein, cells, and VDRL reactivity in order to rule out neurosyphilis. If in doubt and if the patient is not allergic to penicillin, it is often wisest to treat such patients for possible syphilis.

IgM FTA-ABS Test for Congenital Syphilis. Mothers with a positive VDRL or FTA-ABS will deliver infants with a positive VDRL and FTA-ABS because of passive transfer of the IgG antibodies reactive in these tests. Since many infants with congenital syphilis are clinically normal at birth but develop serious symptomatic disease some weeks later, it is important to determine whether a newborn with a positive VDRL or FTA-ABS test has passively transferred maternal antibody or is actively infected. Since maternal IgM antibodies are not passively transferred to the fetus, an IgM FTA-ABS test has been developed to detect syphilis in the newborn. Unfortunately there is approximately a 35 per cent incidence of false-negative IgM FTA-ABS test results in delayed-onset congenital syphilis. There also is a false-positive rate of approximately 10 per cent. For these reasons the IgM FTA-ABS test is of limited use in the diagnosis of neonatal syphilis.

If the mother has been adequately treated for syphilis during pregnancy and the infant is clinically normal at birth, one may elect to follow the infant carefully by serial examination and VDRL titers. If the positive VDRL in the infant is due to passively transferred maternal antibody, the titer of reactivity will fall markedly in the first two months of life. A

rising titer indicates active disease and the need for treatment. Many physicians are unwilling to risk failure of proper follow-up of VDRL-positive but clinically normal neonates and instead administer effective therapy immediately. The risk of penicillin allergy in neonates is very low.

TREATMENT. *T. pallidum* is highly susceptible to penicillin, being inhibited by less than 0.01 μg of penicillin G. Since treponemes divide slowly, and since penicillin acts only on dividing cells, it is necessary to maintain serum levels of penicillin for many days. Studies in animals and in humans show that more therapy is required as the length of infection increases. Current recommendations for treatment of syphilis are summarized in Table 310–4.

Early (Less Than One Year) Infectious Syphilis. Early syphilis may be treated with a single injection of 2.4 million units of *benzathine penicillin G,* which provides low but effective serum levels for over two weeks. Extensive studies in the 1940's and 1950's with regimens that provided similar serum levels and duration of therapy showed that approximately 95 per cent of patients were cured by such treatment. Many of the remaining 5 per cent who had clinical or serologic evidence of relapse may actually have been reinfected. It is not necessary to examine the CSF at this stage because penicillin prevents development of later neurosyphilis. Motile treponemes disappear from primary lesions in 24 hours.

A single injection of 2.4 million units of *aqueous procaine penicillin,* which provides relatively high serum levels for a brief period, is ineffective in established early syphilis but is curative if the disease is still in the incubating stage (e.g., in a patient who is being treated for gonorrhea and who happened to acquire syphilis simultaneously). Other regimens currently useful for gonorrhea have uncertain effects on

TABLE 310–4. PENICILLIN TREATMENT PRACTICE IN SYPHILIS AS RECOMMENDED BY UNITED STATES PUBLIC HEALTH SERVICE

Indications for Syphilis Therapy†	Dosage and Administration*	
	Benzathine Penicillin G	Aqueous Benzyl Penicillin G or Procaine Penicillin G
Primary, secondary, and early latent syphilis (<1 year); epidemiologic treatment	Total of 2.4 million units; single IM dose of two injections of 1.2 million units in one session	Total of 4.8 million units IM in doses of 600,000 units daily for 8 consecutive days
Late latent (>1 year) or when CSF was not examined in "latency"; asymptomatic neurosyphilis, symptomatic neurosyphilis, cardiovascular syphilis, late benign (cutaneous, osseous, visceral gumma)	Total of 7.2 million units IM in doses of 2.4 million units at 7-day intervals, over 21 days	Total of 9 million units IM in doses of 600,000 units daily over 15 days; in selected cases of symptomatic central nervous system syphilis, 2 to 4 million units of aqueous (crystalline) penicillin G intravenously every 4 hours for at least 10 days
Congenital Early Up to 2 years of age	If CSF is normal: Total of 50,000 units per kilogram IM in a single or divided dose at one session	If CSF is abnormal: Total of 50,000 units per kilogram IM per day for 10 consecutive days‡
Late Two to 12 years, weight 32 kg (71 lb) or less	Same as for early congenital syphilis	Same as for early congenital syphilis
Over 12 years, or over 32 kg	Same as for adult late latent syphilis	Same as for adult late latent syphilis

*Individual doses can be divided for injection in each buttock to minimize discomfort.

†In *pregnancy,* treatment is dependent on the stage of syphilis.

‡For aqueous penicillin, give in two divided doses per day; for procaine penicillin, give as one daily dose.

incubating syphilis, and careful follow-up for syphilis is indicated in gonorrhea patients treated with regimens other than procaine penicillin. The incidence of incubating syphilis in gonorrhea patients is 2 per cent or more in several series.

For patients allergic to penicillin, tetracycline hydrochloride or erythromycin base may be given in a total dose of either agent of 30 grams over 15 days. Particularly careful follow-up is necessary in patients treated with drugs other than penicillin, because patients may not be fully compliant with these prolonged courses of oral therapy and these regimens have been less fully evaluated clinically. Cephaloridine or other cephalosporins may be effective but have not been well studied. Chloramphenicol is of equivocal efficacy and for this reason, as well as because of the risk of toxicity, should not be used. Spectinomycin has essentially no effect on syphilis.

Syphilis of More Than One Year's Duration. Larger doses of penicillin are needed for *neurosyphilis* (see Ch. 482) than for syphilis of less than one year's duration. In general, patients with general paresis respond better to treatment than do patients with tabes dorsalis, although patients with paresis should be expected to show residual effects of the infection. This is particularly true in advanced cases. Meningovascular syphilis usually responds well, except for residual damage to cranial nerves or cortical function resulting from ischemic infarcts. Published studies show that a total of 6.0 to 9.0 million units of penicillin G results in a satisfactory clinical response in approximately 90 per cent of patients with neurosyphilis.

Currently used benzathine penicillin regimens have received relatively little study in neurosyphilis. Benzathine penicillin G in a total dose of 7.2 million units given as 2.4 million units weekly for three successive weeks is effective in most patients. However, there are reports of patients who have failed standard penicillin therapy for neurosyphilis but who responded to intensive intravenous therapy that provided high serum levels of penicillin. Benzathine penicillin does not provide measurable levels of penicillin in the spinal fluid or aqueous humor of the eye. *Therefore in cases of symptomatic central nervous system syphilis, which is a serious disease, there is considerable rationale to treatment with intravenous penicillin G (20 million units per day for at least ten days in hospital).* Therapy of neurosyphilis not infrequently results in increased CSF pleocytosis for seven to ten days after starting treatment and may transiently convert a normal CSF to abnormal.

Limited evidence suggests that treating *latent syphilis* with 7.2 million units total dose of benzathine penicillin is curative even if the patient has asymptomatic neurosyphilis. However, because of the possible lack of the efficacy of benzathine penicillin in some patients with central nervous system syphilis, it is desirable to examine CSF in all patients with latent syphilis to exclude asymptomatic neurosyphilis. Alternatively, one may reasonably elect to perform a lumbar puncture at the conclusion of the follow-up period (two years); if the CSF is normal, the patient can be reassured that neurosyphilis will not develop.

There is no evidence that therapy with antimicrobial drugs is clinically beneficial to patients with *cardiovascular syphilis.* Nevertheless, treatment of cardiovascular syphilis is recommended in order to prevent further progression of disease and because approximately 15 per cent of patients with cardiovascular syphilis have associated neurosyphilis.

There is no evidence regarding the efficacy of other antimicrobials in the treatment of later syphilis. Therefore if patients are allergic to penicillin, it is mandatory that the CSF be examined before therapy is undertaken. Either tetracycline or erythromycin, 2 grams daily for 30 days, is probably effective.

Syphilis in Pregnancy. All pregnant women should be examined with a VDRL or RPR test during pregnancy; if they are at high risk for syphilis, a second test should be obtained before delivery. Because of the risk to the fetus, evaluation and treatment of the VDRL-positive patient should be done as rapidly as possible, particularly for patients first seen in the later stages of pregnancy. If a confirmatory FTA-ABS is positive and the patient has not been treated, penicillin (or erythromycin for patients who are allergic to penicillin) should be administered in doses appropriate for early or late syphilis as outlined above. For patients who are VDRL positive but FTA-ABS negative and who have no clinical signs of syphilis, treatment may be withheld. In such patients a quantitative VDRL test and another FTA-ABS test should be repeated in four weeks. If the VDRL titer has risen by fourfold or more, or if clinical signs of syphilis have developed, the patient should be treated. If after repeat examination the diagnosis remains equivocal, the patient should be treated to prevent possible disease in the neonate. After treatment a quantitative VDRL titer should be followed monthly; if it rises fourfold, the patient should be treated a second time.

Congenital Syphilis. Proper treatment of the mother usually prevents active congenital syphilis in the neonate. However, infected infants may be clinically normal at birth, and the infant may be seronegative if the mother's infection was acquired late in pregnancy. The infant should be treated at birth if the mother has received no or inadequate treatment, or has been treated with drugs other than penicillin, or if the infant cannot be carefully followed up for several months after birth. The CSF should be examined before treatment of the infant. If the CSF is normal, treatment may be with a single injection of 50,000 units per kilogram of benzathine penicillin G. If the CSF is abnormal, treatment should be with aqueous penicillin G, 50,000 units per kilogram intramuscularly or intravenously daily, given in two divided doses, for a minimum of ten days. Alternatively, a single daily intramuscular injection of procaine penicillin G, 50,000 units per kilogram, may be given for ten days. These recommendations are based upon the failure of benzathine penicillin to provide adequate treponemicidal levels in spinal fluid and on evidence that aqueous or procaine penicillin does provide adequate CSF levels of penicillin.

Tetracycline should not be used to treat children of less than eight years of age. Antimicrobial agents other than penicillin are not recommended for treatment of congenital syphilis.

Follow-up Examinations. All patients with early syphilis or congenital syphilis should return for quantitative VDRL titers and clinical examination 3, 6, and 12 months after treatment. Patients with late latent syphilis should be examined also at 24 months after therapy; if CSF was not examined prior to therapy, a lumbar puncture should be done prior to discharge to rule out inadequately treated asymptomatic neurosyphilis.

The quantitative VDRL titer should return to normal within 12 months after therapy of primary syphilis or 24 months after therapy of secondary syphilis. In a small percentage of patients with early syphilis, the VDRL will remain reactive in low titer for long periods of time. Chronic low-titer VDRL reactivity after therapy is much more common in late syphilis and should not be viewed with alarm. The FTA-ABS test usually remains positive for years, despite adequate therapy. The influence of therapy on serologic tests is shown in Table 310–5. A fourfold or greater rise of VDRL titer after therapy is sufficient evidence for retreatment. Patients with treated early syphilis are fully susceptible to reinfection, and many clinical and serologic relapses after therapy are probably reinfections. As such they represent failures of proper epidemiologic case finding and preventive therapy of the patient's sexual contacts.

Patients with neurosyphilis should be followed with serologic tests for at least three years and with repeat examination of CSF at six-month intervals. The CSF pleocytosis is the first abnormality to disappear, but cell counts may not be normal for one to two years. The elevated CSF protein level falls

TABLE 310–5. EFFECT OF RECOMMENDED TREATMENT SCHEDULES ON SEROLOGIC TESTS FOR SYPHILIS

Stage of Disease When Treated	Time to Follow-up (years)	Frequency of Positive Serologic Tests (%)	
		VDRL†	FTA-ABS
Primary (seropositive)*	2	0–3‡	>80
Secondary	2	0–24	>80
Late latent or tertiary	5–13	56–70	98

*Patients with primary syphilis and a positive VDRL test.

†Positive VDRL tests after treatment are almost always *low titer* unless reinfection or relapse has occurred.

‡The range of results reflects inclusion of data from several series, using different patient selection and treatment regimens.

more slowly, followed by the positive CSF-VDRL test, which may take years to become negative. It is not known whether use of high-dose intravenous penicillin therapy will accelerate the return of CSF to normal. Rising CSF cell counts, protein, and VDRL titer obtained at follow-up are an indication for retreatment.

Epidemiologic Investigation and Treatment. All patients with syphilis should be reported to public health authorities. In the absence of an effective vaccine, control of syphilis depends on finding and treating persons with infectious lesions of primary and secondary syphilis before they can further transmit the disease and on finding and treating persons with incubating syphilis before they develop infectious lesions. All patients with early syphilis (less than one year) should be carefully interviewed by qualified persons to determine the nature of their recent sex contacts. Approximately 16 per cent of the named recent contacts of patients with early syphilis will be found to have active untreated syphilis on examination, and a similar proportion of individuals named as suspects or associates will also have active syphilis.

Most authorities, particularly in the United States, recommend treatment of sexual contacts of patients with early syphilis even if the contacts are clinically and serologically normal on examination. This is justifiable, because 30 per cent of clinically normal individuals named as contacts of persons with infectious lesions of syphilis within the previous 30 days will go on to develop syphilis if untreated. In general, preventive treatment is given to all sexual contacts of the past 90 days, although nearly all cases of syphilis in contacts will have developed within 60 days of exposure.

Jarisch-Herxheimer Reactions. Up to 60 per cent of patients with early syphilis, and a significant proportion of patients with later stages of syphilis, experience a transient febrile reaction after therapy for syphilis. This usually occurs in the first few hours after therapy, peaks at 6 to 8 hours, and disappears within 12 to 24 hours of therapy. Temperature elevation is usually low grade, and there is often associated myalgia, headache, and malaise. The skin lesions of secondary syphilis are often exacerbated during the Herxheimer reaction, and cutaneous lesions that were not visible may become visible. It is usually of no clinical significance and may be treated with salicylates in most cases. In patients with syphilis of the coronary ostia or of the optic nerve, there is a theoretic risk that local inflammation coincident with the Herxheimer reaction could precipitate serious damage. This is the subject of much discussion in the old literature, but there is little current evidence that "local Herxheimer rections" constitute a significant risk to the patient. Corticosteroids have been used to prevent adverse effects of the Herxheimer reaction, but there is no evidence that they are clinically beneficial (other than reducing fever) or necessary. Institution of treatment with small doses of penicillin does not prevent the Herxheimer reaction.

The pathogenesis of the Herxheimer reaction is unclear. It may be due to liberation of antigens from the spirochetes.

There is evidence of activation of the complement cascade, including transient consumption of C3, C4, C6, and C7, and of transient decrease in treponemal antibodies coincident with the Herxheimer reaction. There is also evidence for endotoxemia, obtained by positive limulus amebocyte gelatin tests, at the time of the Herxheimer reaction, although *T. pallidum* does not contain biologically active endotoxin. These seemingly contradictory observations could be explained if the reaction resulted in release of endogenous endotoxin from the gut.

Persistence of Treponemes After Treatment. Studies in humans and in rabbits have shown that spiral forms may be visualized by silver stains in lymph nodes after effective treatment. Living virulent treponemes have occasionally been recovered by rabbit inoculation from lymph nodes, CSF, or ocular fluids after effective treatment has been given. These documented cases of treponemal persistence are very rare, however. At present there is little reason to worry about persistence of virulent treponemes after therapy with penicillin, with the possible exception of central nervous system syphilis, which needs further evaluation. There is no evidence for selection of penicillin-resistant mutants of *T. pallidum* to date.

PROSPECTS FOR PREVENTION. Solid immunity develops in rabbits following prolonged infection with virulent *T. pallidum*. It has not yet been possible to transfer immunity passively in laboratory animals by either immune serum or immune lymphocytes alone, suggesting that both cellular and humoral systems are necessary for immunity. Rabbits have been effectively immunized with multiple injections of treponemes that have been rendered avirulent by irradiation or by exposure to cold. However, a very large number of injections and a large mass of treponemes are necessary to effect immunity in the laboratory animal. For this reason and since *T. pallidum* cannot yet be grown in a virulent state in cell-free medium, there is no immediate prospect for a vaccine. However, significant immunity does develop in humans after prolonged infection. For the present, control depends entirely on clinical awareness on the part of physicians, adequate reporting to public health authorities, and vigorous application of epidemiologic investigation and preventive treatment of sexual contacts.

Drusin LM, Singer C, Valenti AJ, et al.: Infectious syphilis mimicking neoplastic disease. Arch Intern Med 137:156, 1977. *A fascinating and frightening account of diagnostic problems caused by oral, rectal, or lymphatic syphilis, nearly leading to cancer surgery.*

Feher J, Somogyi T, Timmer M, et al.: Early syphilitic hepatitis. Lancet 2:896, 1975. *A description of the frequency and histology of early syphilitic hepatitis.*

Fischer A, Kristensen JK, Husfelt V: Tertiary syphilis in Denmark 1961–1970. A description of 105 cases not previously diagnosed or specifically treated. Acta Dermatovener 56:485, 1975. *One of few studies of the prevalence of newly diagnosed late syphilis in the antibiotic era.*

Gamble CN, Reardan JB: Immunopathogenesis of syphilitic glomerulonephritis: Elution of antitreponemal antibody from glomerular immune-complex deposits. N Engl J Med 292:449, 1975. *Clear evidence for an immune-complex etiology of syphilitic nephrosis.*

Gjestland T: The Oslo study of untreated syphilis: An epidemiologic investigation of the natural course of the syphilitic infection based upon a restudy of the Boeck-Bruusgaard material. Acta Derm Venereol 35:Suppl 34, 1955. *A medical classic, in which the long-term course of untreated syphilis is evaluated.*

Holmes KK, Märdh P-A, Sparling PF, et al.: Sexually Transmitted Diseases. New York, McGraw-Hill Book Company, 1984. *The definitive text on sexually transmitted diseases.*

Lee TJ, Sparling PF: Syphilis. An algorithm. JAMA 242:1187, 1979. *An algorithm for management of patients who present with a positive VDRL or similar test.*

Lugar A, Schmidt B, Spendlingwimmer I, et al.: Recent observations on the serology of syphilis. Br J Vener Dis 56:12, 1980. *A current evaluation of the merits of serologic tests for syphilis.*

Magnuson HJ, Thomas EW, Olansky S, et al.: Inoculation syphilis in human volunteers. Medicine 35:33, 1956. *A classic paper, in which prison volunteers were inoculated with virulent* T. pallidum. *Immunity to inoculation syphilis was observed only in individuals who had congenital or late syphilis.*

Prewitt TA: Syphilitic aortic insufficiency. JAMA 211:637, 1970. *Observations on the epidemiology, serology, and clinical manifestations of syphilitic aortitis in the United States.*

Raskind MA, Eisdorfer C: Screening for syphilis in an aged psychiatrically impaired population. West J Med 125:361, 1976. *Syphilitic disease of the central nervous system may be more prevalent than hospital surveys suggest.*

Schroeter AL, Turner RH, Lucas JB, et al.: Therapy for incubating syphilis: Effectiveness of gonorrhea treatment. JAMA 218:711, 1971. *A controlled study showing that single-dose procaine penicillin eradicates incubating syphilis.*

Tramont EC: Persistence of *Treponema pallidum* following penicillin G therapy: Report of two cases. JAMA 236:2206. *At least one of the cases of neurosyphilis probably was a true penicillin treatment failure.*

Wilner E, Brody JA: Prognosis of general paresis after treatment. Lancet 2:1370, 1968. *Neurosyphilus frequently shows clinical progression despite what is probably adequate therapy.*

Spirochetal Diseases Other Than Syphilis

311 NONSYPHILITIC TREPONEMATOSES*

Thomas Butler

DEFINITION. The nonsyphilitic treponematoses are the skin diseases called *yaws*, *bejel*, and *pinta*. They occur predominantly in tropical regions and are transmitted by skin contact with infected persons. Disfiguring ulcerations of the skin may be produced, and invasion of bone and other tissues has been described. Treatment with benzathine penicillin G is effective, and the World Health Organization has carried out extensive treatment campaigns in endemic areas.

ETIOLOGY. Yaws is caused by *Treponema pertenue*; pinta is caused by *T. carateum*; and bejel is caused by a treponeme that is indistinguishable from other species. Like *T. pallidum*, these treponemes are spirochetal bacteria with helical structures and measure about 0.2 μ in diameter and 10 μ in length. They are visible by darkfield microscopy but cannot be cultivated in vitro.

DISTRIBUTION AND EPIDEMIOLOGY. Yaws is prevalent in rural areas of tropical Africa, the Americas, Southeast Asia, and Oceania. The highest incidence is in children between ages two and five years. Bejel occurs in Africa, in Eastern Mediterranean countries, on the Arabian peninsula, in Central Asia, and in Australia. It is most prevalent in arid regions. Pinta occurs in rural areas of tropical Central and South America. Pinta affects mostly older children and adolescents. Humans are the only known carriers of the nonsyphilitic treponematoses. The portal of entry is the skin, which must be broken, as by a scratch or insect bite, before the spirochete can enter. Transmission is believed to be by direct skin contact or indirectly by contaminated hands or fomites and is facilitated by conditions of poor personal hygiene and crowding.

CLINICAL FEATURES. *Yaws* produces a skin papule at the site of inoculation after an incubation period of three to four weeks. The most common sites are the legs and buttocks. The papule enlarges, ulcerates, and develops a serous crust from which treponemes can be recovered. Regional lymphadenitis may accompany the papule, which will heal spontaneously within six months. A generalized secondary rash will occur before or after healing of the initial lesion, and these rashes are also papular and often covered with brown crusts. Relapsing crops of lesions can occur. Papillomas may result, and the plantar surfaces of the feet are involved with hyperkeratotic lesions. Periostitis of long bones leads to tender

bones, and fever may be present. Relapsing lesions may occur over several years, resulting in chronic ulcerations and destructive gummatous lesions affecting the skin and bones.

Bejel produces patches on the mucous membranes of the oral cavity and pharynx and can cause split papules at the mucocutaneous junction of the oral angles. Anal, genital, and other intertriginous skin areas can be affected by lesions that resemble secondary syphilis. Regional lymphadenitis is common, and generalized rashes are rare. Healing of these early lesions is followed by latency manifested by seropositivity or by late lesions that resemble tertiary syphilis. These include nodular ulcers of skin, deformities of bones, and gummatous lesions that can perforate the palate.

Pinta starts similarly as a cutaneous papule with regional lymphadenitis that is followed by a generalized maculopapular eruption. One to three years after healing of the initial lesion, large hyperpigmented macules that are brown or blue develop and subsequently lose their pigment and become white. The time required for lesions to pass through these stages varies, so that the same patient may have coexisting areas of increased pigment and loss of pigment.

DIAGNOSIS. By darkfield microscopy, the causative spirochetes from early skin lesions can be observed directly. Spirochetes have been demonstrated also in lymph node aspirates. Serologic tests for syphilis will detect cross-reacting antibodies in these diseases. The VDRL test, the serologic test for syphilis, and the fluorescent treponemal antibody absorption test will all give positive results if serum is taken at least two weeks after the appearance of initial lesions.

TREATMENT AND PROGNOSIS. Long-acting benzathine penicillin G given as 1.2 million units intramuscularly is the preferred treatment for patients with early lesions. For patients with late manifestations, this therapy should be repeated twice at approximately seven-day intervals. The early lesions will heal rapidly, and most seropositive patients will convert to seronegative status. Late destructive lesions take longer to show improvement.

PREVENTION. The prevalence of these diseases has been reduced in several areas of the world by mass treatment campaigns using penicillin. The World Health Organization has treated about 53 million cases of yaws and 350,000 cases of pinta in the field with good results. These campaigns, however, are not adequate to eradicate the disease. It has been suggested that reduction in transmission requires improvements in the sanitation and economic standards of people living in endemic areas.

Guthe T: Clinical serological and epidemiological features of framboesia tropica (yaws) and its control in rural communities. Acta Dermatovener 49:343, 1969.

Hackett CJ, Lowenthal LJA: Differential Diagnosis of Yaws. WHO Monograph Series No. 45. Geneva, WHO, 1960.

Kantor I, Wilentz JM, Berger BB: Yaws. Arch Dermatol 103:546, 1971.

Vorst FA: Clinical diagnosis and changing manifestations of treponemal infection. Rev Infect Dis 7(Suppl 2):S327, 1985. *This paper shows that yaws in populations after mass treatment with penicillin assumes attenuated forms characterized by shorter duration of papillomas and lower antibody titers.*

*The author acknowledges the contribution of Dr. Thorstein Guthe on this subject in the 16th edition of the *Cecil Textbook of Medicine*, pages 1584–1589, and refers the interested reader to this more complete treatment of the subject, which includes photographs of skin lesions.

312 RELAPSING FEVER

Thomas Butler

DEFINITION. Relapsing fever is an acute febrile illness caused by blood spirochetes belonging to *Borrelia* species. The two major kinds of relapsing fever are *louse-borne relapsing fever*, for which the human is the reservoir and the body louse is the vector, and *tick-borne relapsing fever*, for which rodents and other animals are the predominant reservoirs and ticks are the vectors. The clinical course consists of one or more phases of fever and spirochetemia, which last for several days and are separated by afebrile intervals of several days without spirochetemia. The relapsing fevers are effectively treated with antibiotics, but after treatment patients will often experience a Jarisch-Herxheimer-like reaction.

ETIOLOGY. Relapsing fevers are caused by blood spirochetes of *Borrelia* species, which belong to the order of bacteria called Spirochaetales. *Borrelia* species differ from the other two genera of pathogenic spirochetes, *Leptospira* and *Treponema*, by structure, biochemical characteristics, and antigenic determinants. *Borrelia* spirochetes are spiral organisms that measure 5 to 40 μ in length and about 0.5 μ in diameter. They are too thin to be seen reliably by light microscopy of wet preparations, but they are easily visible when viewed by darkfield or phase contrast microscopy. They are stainable with aniline dyes, such as Wright's or Giemsa's stains, and can be visualized well in tissue by the application of silver stains. Between the cell wall and the cytoplasmic membrane there are 15 to 20 flagella, which are anchored to the ends of the spirochete and wrap around its body until they meet at the middle region. Under darkfield or phase contrast microscopy, *Borrelia* spirochetes display an active corkscrew-like motility consisting of rotation and motion in helical waves to produce translational movement. *Borrelia* spirochetes are microaerophilic and fermentative in their growth characteristics. They require long-chain fatty acids for growth and are cultivable in Kelly's medium.

The species names of the tick-borne *Borrelia* are derived from the species names of *Ornithodorus* tick vectors that carry them. The more common ones in North America are *B. turicatae*, *B. hermsii*, and *B. parkeri* and in Africa *B. duttonii*. Louse-borne disease is caused solely by *B. recurrentis*. *Borrelia* spirochetes produce fever when injected into rabbits but do not possess endotoxin.

The relapsing feature of *Borrelia* infection has been attributed to antigenic variation in the infecting population of spirochetes. In experimental infections of rats with *B. hermsii*, three separate serotypes emerged sequentially during relapses, and specific antibody appeared in response to each of the antigenic variants.

DISTRIBUTION AND EPIDEMIOLOGY. Between 1910 and 1945, there have been at least seven epidemics of relapsing fever in North Africa, Sudan, Ethiopia, West Africa, Central Africa, Eastern Europe, and Russia. An estimated 15 million cases occurred with over 5 million deaths and case fatality rates as high as 73 per cent. Louse-borne relapsing fever has disappeared from the United States but still occurs in parts of South America, Europe, Africa, and Asia. From 1960 to 1979 louse-borne relapsing fever was documented in Ethiopia and Sudan. Although accurate statistics on the incidence of this disease are not available, Ethiopia appears to be the country with the highest incidence, estimated at approximately 10,000 or more cases a year.

The two types of relapsing fever, louse-borne and tick-borne, differ so much in their epidemiology that they must be considered separately. *Epidemic relapsing fever* refers to the louse-borne kind and *endemic* or *sporadic relapsing fever* to the tick-borne variety. For louse-borne relapsing fever, the cycle of infection is from person to person via the louse. Body lice acquire the infection by feeding on a spirochetemic person, and they remain infected for their entire lifespan, which is 10 to 61 days under laboratory conditions. Spirochetes do not reach the salivary glands or ovaries of the lice. Therefore, infection is not transmitted to humans by bites of lice. Infection is believed to be transmitted to humans by the crushing of lice on the skin, which allows liberated spirochetes to penetrate through a bite site or through intact skin.

The persons at greatest risk for acquiring louse-borne relapsing fever are those living under crowded, unhygienic conditions that favor infestation with body lice. Migrant workers and soldiers in war are particularly prone to develop this infection. Males are at much greater risk than females. A strain-specific, short-lived acquired immunity develops following infection. This immunity helps to explain why migrant workers coming into an endemic area are more susceptible to infection than are the permanent inhabitants. In some endemic areas, such as Addis Ababa, Ethiopia, there is an increased incidence during the cool winter season when people wear heavier clothing that becomes louse infested.

The vectors for tick-borne relapsing fever are argasid soft ticks of the genus *Ornithodorus*. The major reservoirs of tick-borne relapsing fever are wild rodents, including squirrels, deer mice, rats, chipmunks, and rabbits, and occasionally lizards, toads, turtles, and owls. The infection is passed between the reservoir animals by tick bites, and humans are accidental hosts when they come into contact with infected animal ticks.

Ticks acquire the infection by biting and sucking blood from a spirochetemic animal. Transmission of the infection to animals or to humans follows injection of infected saliva through the bite site or intact skin. Ticks are more durable vectors than body lice, being able to survive as long as 15 years between blood meals and to harbor viable spirochetes for years. In addition, female ticks can pass *Borrelia* spirochetes transovarially to their offspring, thus permitting ticks to be infective without having previously bitten an infected host.

Persons at greatest risk of infection are those who come in contact with infected ticks from wild rodents. The largest outbreak of tick-borne relapsing fever occurred in 62 campers and employees in the National Park at the Northern Rim of the Grand Canyon, Arizona, in 1973. They had all slept in log cabins that were inhabited by wild rodents. Another outbreak in Washington State affected 42 boy scouts who also camped in a log cabin.

PATHOGENESIS AND PATHOLOGY. After exposure to an infected louse or tick, spirochetes enter through the skin, and in the subcutaneous tissue they have access to the blood and lymphatic circulations. After an incubation period of 4 to 18 days, during which the spirochetes build up to a concentration of 10^6 to 10^8 per milliliter of blood, the symptoms of shaking chills and fever begin. A decrease in blood platelets leads to diffuse petechial skin rashes. There also is disseminated intravascular coagulation, which contributes to the decrease in platelets and produces prolonged prothrombin and partial thromboplastin times and elevated titers of fibrinogen-fibrin degradation products. During acute relapsing fever, there are decreased levels of serum complement, the Hageman factor, and prekallikrein, suggesting that activation of certain plasma proteins contributes to the pathogenesis of features such as hypotension and disseminated intravascular coagulation.

In the hours after antibiotic treatment, most patients undergo a Jarisch-Herxheimer reaction characterized by rigor, rising temperature, and falling blood pressure. Disseminated intravascular coagulation is accelerated, and spirochetes are phagocytosed at increased rates while being cleared from the plasma. Some patients not receiving antibiotic treatment undergo a similar spontaneous crisis. It is during this crisis of Jarisch-Herxheimer reaction that patients are at the greatest risk of dying.

Autopsies performed in Ethiopia and Sudan in fatal cases of louse-borne relapsing fever show characteristic disease most regularly in the spleen, liver, heart, and brain. The spleen is enlarged to as much as 900 grams, and the cut surface shows white microabscesses, which consist of necrosis and hemorrhage in the white pulp. Occasionally there are splenic infarcts and splenic rupture. The liver is also enlarged, often to over 2000 grams. The midzonal region shows scattered necrosis and hemorhage, and Kupffer's cells are enlarged and numerous. The heart is normal in size but frequently shows evidence of myocarditis, consisting of interstitial edema and a cellular infiltrate of lymphocytes and plasma cells. Examination of the brain usually indicates cerebral edema, and in some cases there is hemorrhage into the subarachnoid space or cerebrum. Thus, the immediate causes of death in relapsing fever are varied and in any particular case may be liver failure, cerebral hemorrhage, or acute cardiac arrhythmia caused by myocarditis.

The majority of patients with relapsing fever recover from illness either with or without antibiotic treatment. Patients develop antiborrelial antibodies that agglutinate, kill, and opsonize the spirochetes. These antibodies participate also in rendering patients immune to future infection with the same serotype of *Borrelia*.

CLINICAL SYNDROMES. The illness begins abruptly with shaking chills, fever, headache, and fatigue. Most patients have these symptoms almost continuously throughout the day, whereas some patients report intermittent symptoms several times a day. Patients complain frequently of myalgias, arthralgia, anorexia, dry cough, and abdominal pains. These symptoms are usually mild on the first day of illness and increase in intensity over a few days, until they result in prostration and a visit to a physician. The nonspecific nature of the symptoms leads the patient or the physician to believe the illness is flulike.

The temperature is elevated in the range of 38.5° to 40°C, and the pulse rate is increased to about 115 beats per minute. The blood pressure is lowered to about 105/70 mm Hg. Patients appear lethargic or may be delirious. Common physical signs are conjunctival injection, petechial skin rash that is more apparent on the trunk than on the extremities, and palpable liver and spleen. Jaundice is occasionally present. Generalized muscle weakness is common. Some patients have nuchal rigidity.

The white blood cell count is usually normal, with increased band forms and decreased eosinophils. The platelet counts are often less than 50,000 per cubic millimeter, and there may be prolongation of prothrombin and partial thromboplastin times. Liver function test results are frequently abnormal, with elevations in concentrations of serum alanine aminotransferase and bilirubin that are evenly divided between the conjugated and unconjugated fractions. Renal function studies often show mild abnormalities of the serum urea nitrogen and creatinine values, and patients may have proteinuria and microscopic hematuria.

DIAGNOSIS. The diagnosis of relapsing fever depends on the demonstration of spirochetemia. In most patients, this is readily accomplished by obtaining peripheral blood by either fingerstick or venipuncture methods and preparing a thin film on a microscope slide. *Borrelia* spirochetes are stained blue by aniline dyes. Thus a routine blood smear stained with Wright's or Giemsa's stain is adequate. Blood smears, thin or thick, prepared for examination for malaria parasites, are also satisfactory. The spirochetes are 5 to 20 µ in length and lie in the plasma spaces between blood cells or may overlie the blood cells. Febrile patients with relapsing fever typically have large numbers of spirochetes in the blood, approximately 10^6 to 10^8 per milliliter, or several per high-power field. Patients

who are afebrile in the interval between relapses will have smears negative for *Borrelia* and should be re-examined when the fever reappears. Spirochetemia also may be detected by darkfield or phase contrast microscopy. A drop of fresh blood is diluted with another drop of 0.9 per cent NaCl and overlaid with a coverslip. Spirochetes are readily identified by their characteristic rotational motility.

TREATMENT AND PROGNOSIS. The relapsing fevers are effectively treated with tetracycline and erythromycin. Tetracycline is the treatment of choice except in children less than seven years old and in pregnant women, in whom tetracycline may stain developing fetal teeth. Recent studies in Ethiopia indicate that a single oral dose of tetracycline, 500 mg, is as effective in clearing spirochetemia and preventing relapse as a longer course of treatment. Eythromycin, 500 mg given orally as a single dose, is equally effective and is a satisfactory alternative to tetracycline. For patients unable to take oral medication, intravenous injections of 250 mg of tetracycline or erythromycin are curative. For children weighing less than 30 kg, the dosage of tetracycline or erythromycin should be reduced to approximately 10 mg per kilogram. Penicillin G has been used to treat relapsing fever, but its use has been associated with slow clearance of spirochetes and relapses following treatment.

In most patients with louse-borne relapsing fever and in some with tick-borne relapsing fever, a distressing Jarisch-Herxheimer–like reaction occurs within four hours after antibiotic treatment. During the reaction, the patient is extremely uncomfortable, feeling very cold with severe headache and myalgia. The blood leukocyte and platelet counts sharply decrease, and spirochetes disappear from the plasma. The patient may require intravenous infusions of 0.9 per cent NaCl to maintain adequate blood pressure. Over several hours, the temperature declines and the patient's condition improves. Attempts to ameliorate the severity of the reaction by giving antipyretic or anti-inflammatory drugs have not been entirely successful. The best approach is to anticipate the reaction and to provide intensive nursing care and intravenous fluid support during the first day of treatment.

The prognosis is favorable for complete recovery in 95 per cent or more of treated cases of relapsing fever. Bad prognostic signs are the presence of jaundice, high spirochete counts in the blood, and hypotension. The prognosis of untreated disease is grave in the case of louse-borne relapsing fever, for which mortality rates of 40 per cent have been reported during recent epidemics. Untreated patients will also experience relapses. In louse-borne relapsing fever, the first attack lasts about six days and is followed by an afebrile period of about nine days. There usually is one relapse, which will last only about two days. In tick-borne relapsing fever, the first attack lasts about three days and is followed by an interval of about seven days, after which an average of three relapses occur, each lasting about two days. Relapses are usually milder in intensity than the first attacks.

PREVENTION. Available approaches for the control of relapsing fevers include the detection and treatment of human cases, vector control, rodent control, and public health education. Vaccines are not available for the prevention of relapsing fever. Delousing of clothing and bodies with insecticides such as DDT (chlorophenothane) can be employed, as can the application of insect repellents. In known epidemic situations, prophylactic antibiotics are a temporary measure to contain spread of infection to persons at high risk. For tick-borne relapsing fever, campers and hikers going into endemic areas should be advised to avoid cabins that are inhabited by rodents and ticks and to apply topical tick repellents to the skin.

Butler T, Hazen P, Wallace CK, et al.: *Borrelia recurrentis* infection: Pathogenesis of fever and petechiae. J Infect Dis 140:665, 1979. *Demonstration of a nonendotoxic pyrogen in spirochetes.*

Butler T, Jones PK, Wallace CK: *Borrelia recurrentis* infection: Single dose antibiotic regimens and management of Jarisch-Herxheimer reaction. J Infect Dis 137:573, 1978. *Clinical trials in Ethiopia showed that single-dose regimens of tetracycline and erythromycin were effective.*

Fihn S, Larson EB: Tick-borne relapsing fever in the Pacific Northwest: An underdiagnosed illness? West J Med 133:203, 1980. *This article advises physicians to suspect relapsing fever in nonspecific febrile illnesses of exposed persons.*

Horton JM, Blaser MJ: The spectrum of relapsing fever in the Rocky Mountains. Arch Intern Med 145:871, 1985. *This report of 23 recent cases indicated an increased incidence of the disease in Colorado. Severe Jarisch-Herxheimer reactions occurred in four patients.*

313 LYME DISEASE

Stephen E. Malawista

Lyme disease is a tick-borne inflammatory disorder caused by a newly recognized spirochete, *Borrelia burgdorferi*. Its clinical hallmark is an early expanding skin lesion, *erythema chronicum migrans* (ECM), which may be followed weeks to months later by neurologic, cardiac, or joint abnormalities. Symptoms may refer to any one of these four systems alone or in combination. Foci of Lyme disease are widely distributed within the United States and Europe.

"Lyme arthritis" was recognized in November 1975 because of unusual geographic clustering of children with inflammatory arthropathy in the region of Lyme, Connecticut. It soon became clear that this was a multisystem disorder (Lyme *disease*) occurring at any age, in both sexes, and often preceded by a characteristic expanding skin lesion, *erythema chronicum migrans* (ECM). In Europe ECM had been associated with the bite of the sheep tick, *Ixodes ricinus*, and with tick-borne meningopolyneuritis. In the Lyme region, a closely related deer tick, *Ixodes dammini*, was implicated as the principal disease vector on epidemiologic grounds. In 1982, Burgdorfer and associates isolated a spirochete from *Ixodes dammini* and linked it serologically to patients with Lyme disease. It was soon recovered from patient specimens.

DISTRIBUTION AND EPIDEMIOLOGY. Lyme disease is widespread. In the United States there are three distinct foci: the Northeast from Massachusetts to Maryland, the Midwest in Wisconsin and Minnesota, and the West in California, southern Oregon, and western Nevada. However, the illness has been reported in over one half of the states, as well as throughout Europe and in Australia. The earliest known cases in the United States occurred on Cape Cod in 1962 and in Lyme, Connecticut, in 1965; cases now number in the thousands. Disease can occur at any age and in either sex. Onset of illness is generally between May 1 and November 30, with the peak in June and July.

The primary vectors of Lyme disease are tiny ixodid ticks. Major foci of disease correspond to the distribution of *I. dammini* (Northeast and Midwest), *I. pacificus* (West), and *I. ricinus* (Europe), but other vectors, including the Lone Star tick, *Amblyomma americanum*, are likely in some areas. In one United States study, 31 per cent of 314 patients recalled a tick bite at the skin site where ECM developed days to weeks later. The six ticks that were saved were invariably nymphal *I. dammini*, whose peak questing period is May through July and which seems to be the stage primarily responsible for transmission of disease. Preferred hosts for *I. dammini* nymphs are white-footed mice and, for adults, white-tailed deer, in whose fur they may survive the winter.

B. burgdorferi has been recovered from all three major ixodid tick vectors; in some areas, its prevalence in *I. dammini* is as high as 60 per cent (compared with *I. pacificus*, ≈ 1 per cent). The organism has been isolated, or specific antibody found, in blood and tissues of a wide variety of large and small animals, including domestic dogs and birds. Indiscriminate feeding on a variety of animals by immature *I. dammini* may favor the spread of infection.

PATHOGENESIS. Recovery of *B. burgdorferi* is straightforward from the tick (see above) but difficult from patients, perhaps because of a relative paucity of organisms in specimens of tissue and fluids from the latter. Nevertheless, rare positive cultures are reported at all stages of the illness—from blood (early), *erythema chronicum migrans*, meningitic cerebrospinal fluid, joint fluid, and even a late skin lesion, *acrodermatitis chronica atrophicans*, that had been present for 10 years. Spirochetes have been identified by silver stain or by immunofluorescence in some histologic sections of ECM and rarely of secondary annular lesions, synovium, brain, eye, and heart.

From these data, combined with clinical (see below) and epidemiologic features of Lyme disease, the following pathogenetic sequence is likely. *B. burgdorferi* is transmitted to the skin of the host via the tick vector. After an incubation period of 3 to 32 days, the organism migrates outward in the skin (ECM), spreads in lymph (regional adenopathy), or disseminates in blood to organs (e.g., central nervous system and presumably liver and spleen) or other skin sites (secondary annular lesions; see below). Although organisms are hard to find in later stages of Lyme disease, it is likely that persistent live spirochetes are driving the illness throughout its course. Evidence for this interpretation includes the responsiveness of many patients to antibiotics, the rare sightings of spirochetes in affected tissues, and an expansion of the antibody response to additional spirochetal antigens over time.

Lyme disease is associated with characteristic immune abnormalities. At disease onset (ECM), almost all patients have evidence of circulating immune complexes. At that time, the findings of elevated serum immunoglobulin M (IgM) levels and cryoglobulins containing IgM predict subsequent nervous system, heart, or joint involvement—i.e., early humoral findings have prognostic significance. Serial determinations of serum IgM are often the single most helpful laboratory indicator of disease activity. These abnormalities tend to persist during neurologic or cardiac involvement. Later in the illness, when arthritis is present, serum IgM levels are more often normal. By then, immune complexes are usually lacking in serum but are present uniformly in joint fluid. Mononuclear cells from peripheral blood increase their antigen-specific proliferative response as the disease progresses, but the greatest reactivity to antigen is seen in cells from inflamed joints. Adjacent to that joint fluid, one sees on biopsy a proliferative synovium often replete with lymphocytes and plasma cells that are presumably capable of producing immunoglobulin locally. Thus, an initially disseminated, immune-mediated inflammatory disorder becomes localized in some patients and propagated in joints.

CLINICAL CHARACTERISTICS. Lyme disease is conveniently divided into three clinical stages, but the stages may overlap and most patients do not exhibit all of them. The illness usually begins with ECM and associated symptoms (stage 1), sometimes followed weeks to months later by neurologic or cardiac abnormalities (stage 2) and weeks to years later by arthritis (stage 3). Chronic neurologic and skin involvement may also occur years after onset.

Early Manifestations. *Erythema chronicum migrans*, the unique clinical marker for Lyme disease, begins as a red macule or papule at the site where the tick vector, usually long gone, had engorged. As the area of redness expands to 15 cm or so (range, 3 to 68 cm), there is usually partial central clearing (see color plate). The outer borders are red, generally flat, and without scaling. The centers are occasionally red and indurated, even vesicular or necrotic. Variations may occur—multiple rings, for example. The thigh, groin, and axilla are particularly common sites. The lesion is warm to touch, but not often sore, and is easily missed if out of sight. Routine histologic findings are nonspecific: a heavy dermal infiltrate

TABLE 313–1. EARLY SIGNS OF LYME DISEASE

Signs	No. of Patients N = 314	(%)
Erythema chronicum migrans	314	(100)*
Multiple annular lesions	150	(48)
Lymphadenopathy		
Regional	128	(41)
Generalized	63	(20)
Pain on neck flexion	52	(17)
Malar rash	41	(13)
Erythematous throat	38	(12)
Conjunctivitis	35	(11)
Right upper quadrant tenderness	24	(8)
Splenomegaly	18	(6)
Hepatomegaly	16	(5)
Muscle tenderness	12	(4)
Periorbital edema	10	(3)
Evanescent skin lesions	8	(3)
Abdominal tenderness	6	(2)
Testicular swelling	2	(1)

*Erythema chronicum migrans was required for inclusion in this study.
From Steere AC, Bartenhagen NH, Craft JE, et al.: The early clinical manifestations of Lyme disease. Ann Intern Med 99:76, 1983.

of mononuclear cells, without epidermal change except at the site of the tick bite.

Within days of onset of ECM, one half of United States patients develop multiple annular secondary lesions (see color plate; Table 313–1). They resemble ECM itself but are generally smaller, migrate less, and lack indurated centers; they are not associated with the sites of previous tick bites. Individual lesions may come and go, and their borders sometimes merge. Other occasional skin lesions are noted in Table 313–1. In addition, benign lymphocytoma cutis has been reported in Europe. *Erythema chronicum migrans* and secondary lesions fade in three to four weeks (range, 1 day to 14 months). They may recur.

Skin involvement is often accompanied by flulike symptoms—malaise and fatigue, headache, fever and chills, myalgia, and arthralgia (Table 313–2). Some patients have evidence of meningeal irritation or mild encephalopathy—for example, episodic attacks of excruciating headache and neck pain, stiffness, or pressure—but typically lasting only for hours at this stage of the illness, and without spinal fluid pleocytosis or objective neurologic deficit. Except for fatigue and lethargy, which are often constant, the early signs and symptoms are typically intermittent and changing. For example, a patient may have meningitic attacks for several days, a few days of improvement, and then the onset of migratory musculoskeletal pain. This last may involve joints (generally without

TABLE 313–2. EARLY SYMPTOMS OF LYME DISEASE

Symptoms	No. of Patients N = 314	(%)
Malaise, fatigue, and lethargy	251	(80)
Headache	200	(64)
Fever and chills	185	(59)
Stiff neck	151	(48)
Arthralgias	150	(48)
Myalgias	135	(43)
Backache	81	(26)
Anorexia	73	(23)
Sore thorat	53	(17)
Nausea	53	(17)
Dysesthesia	35	(11)
Vomiting	32	(10)
Abdominal pain	24	(8)
Photophobia	19	(6)
Hand stiffness	16	(5)
Dizziness	15	(5)
Cough	15	(5)
Chest pain	12	(4)
Ear pain	12	(4)
Diarrhea	6	(2)

From Steere AC, Bartenhagen NH, Craft JE, et al.: The early clinical manifestations of Lyme disease. Ann Intern Med 99:76, 1983.

swelling), tendons, bursa, muscle, and bone. The pain tends to affect only one or two sites at a time and to last a few hours to several days in a given location. The various associated symptoms may occur several days before ECM (or without it) and last for months (especially fatigue and lethargy) after the skin lesions have disappeared.

Later Manifestations. NEUROLOGIC INVOLVEMENT. Within several weeks to months of the onset of illness, about 15 per cent of patients develop frank neurologic abnormalities, including meningitis, encephalitis, chorea, cranial neuritis (including bilateral facial palsy), motor and sensory radiculoneuritis, or mononeuritis multiplex, in various combinations. The usual pattern is fluctuating meningoencephalitis with superimposed cranial nerve (particularly facial) palsy and peripheral radiculoneuropathy, but Bell's palsy may occur *alone*. By now, patients with meningitic symptoms have a lymphocytic pleocytosis (about 100 cells per cubic millimeter) in cerebrospinal fluid and sometimes diffuse slowing on electroencephalogram. However, the neck is rarely stiff except on extreme flexion; Kernig's and Brudzinski's signs are absent. Neurologic abnormalities typically last for months but usually resolve completely (late neurologic complications are noted below).

CARDIAC INVOLVEMENT. Also within weeks to months of onset, about 8 per cent of patients develop cardiac involvement. The commonest abnormality is fluctuating degrees of atrioventricular block (first-degree, Wenckebach, or complete heart block). Some patients have evidence of more diffuse cardiac involvement, including electrocardiographic changes compatible with acute myopericarditis, radionuclide evidence of mild left ventricular dysfunction, or, rarely, cardiomegaly, None has had heart murmurs. Cardiac involvement is usually brief (three days to six weeks), but it may recur.

ARTHRITIS. From weeks to as long as two years after the onset of illness, about 60 per cent of patients develop frank arthritis, usually characterized by intermittent attacks of asymmetric joint swelling and pain primarily in large joints, especially the knee, one or two joints at a time. Affected knees are commonly more swollen than painful, often hot, and rarely red; Baker's cysts may form and rupture early. However, both large and small joints may be affected, and a few patients have had symmetric polyarthritis. Attacks of arthritis, which generally last from weeks to months, typically recur for several years. Fatigue is common with active joint involvement, but fever or other systemic symptoms at this stage are unusual. Joint fluid white cell counts vary from 500 to 110,000 cells per cubic millimeter, with an average of about 25,000 cells per cubic millimeter, mostly polymorphonuclear leukocytes. Total protein ranges from 3 to 8 grams per deciliter. The C3 and C4 levels are generally greater than one-third, and glucose levels usually greater than two-thirds, that of serum. Rheumatoid factor and antinuclear antibody are absent.

In about 10 per cent of patients with arthritis, involvement in large joints may become chronic, with pannus formation and erosion of cartilage and bone. Synovial biopsy findings may mimic those of rheumatoid arthritis: surface deposits of fibrin, villous hypertrophy, vascular proliferation, and a heavy infiltration of mononuclear cells. In addition, there may be an obliterative endarteritis and (rarely) demonstrable spirochetes. In one patient with chronic Lyme arthritis, synovium grown in tissue culture produced large amounts of collagenase and prostaglandin E$_2$. Thus, in Lyme disease the joint fluid cell counts, the immune reactants (except for rheumatoid factor), the synovial histology, the amounts of synovial enzymes released, and the resulting destruction of cartilage and bone may be similar to those in rheumatoid arthritis.

Other late findings (years) associated with this infection include a chronic skin lesion—*acrodermatitis chronica atrophicans*—well known in Europe but still rare in the United States. One sees violaceous infiltrated plaques or nodules, especially on extensor surfaces, that eventually become atrophic. Late chronic neurologic disease includes transverse myelitis and demyelinating lesions of the central nervous system.

LABORATORY TEST RESULTS. Determination of specific antibody titers is currently the most helpful diagnostic test for Lyme disease. Culture of *B. burgdorferi* from patients permits definitive diagnosis but is rarely successful. Similarly, spirochetes are not often seen by direct examination of blood, plasma, plasma pellets, or skin transudate specimens of ECM, and special tissue-staining techniques are low in yield and not readily available.

In serum, specific IgM antibody titers against *B. burgdorferi* usually reach a peak between the third and sixth weeks after the onset of disease; specific immunoglobulin G (IgG) antibody titers rise more slowly and are generally highest months later when arthritis is present (Fig. 313–1). To date, no one with established Lyme arthritis has failed to have an elevated titer of specific IgG antibody. This finding makes antibody titers against *B. burgdorferi* particularly useful in differentiating Lyme disease from other rheumatic syndromes, especially when ECM is missed, forgotten, or absent. This antibody cross-reacts with other spirochetes, including *Treponema pallidum*, but patients with Lyme disease do not have positive VDRL test results.

The most common nonspecific laboratory abnormalities, particularly early in the illness, are a high erythrocyte sedimentation rate, an elevated serum IgM level, or an increased serum glutamic-oxaloacetic transaminase (SGOT) level. The enzyme levels generally return to normal within several weeks. Patients may be mildly anemic early in the illness and occasionally have elevated white cell counts with shifts to the left in the differential count. A few patients have had microscopic hematuria, sometimes with mild proteinuria (dipstick); values for creatinine and blood urea nitrogen have been normal. Throughout the illness, serum C3 and C4 levels are generally normal or elevated. Rheumatoid factor and antinuclear antibodies are usually absent.

DIFFERENTIAL DIAGNOSIS. *Erythema chronicum migrans* is the unique herald lesion of Lyme disease (color plate). When present in its classic form, there is little else that might be confused with it. However, some patients are not aware of having had ECM, and in others, its appearance is not always characteristic. Secondary lesions might suggest *erythema multiforme*, but blistering, mucosal lesions, and involvement of the palms and soles are not features of Lyme disease. Malar rash may suggest systemic lupus erythematosus; an urticarial rash, hepatitis B infection or serum sickness. Evanescent blotches and circles may resemble *erythema marginatum*, but those of Lyme disease do not expand.

Early flulike symptoms may be misleading, especially when *erythema chronicum migrans* is absent or missed or is not the first manifestation. Severe headache and stiff neck may resemble aseptic meningitis; abdominal symptoms, hepatitis; and generalized tender lymphadenopathy and splenomegaly, infectious mononucleosis. As in the last infection, profound fatigue in Lyme disease may be a major and persistent complaint.

In later stages, Lyme disease may mimic other immune-mediated disorders. Like rheumatic fever, Lyme disease may be associated with sore throat followed by migratory polyarthritis and carditis, but without evidence of valvular involvement or of a preceding streptococcal infection. Migratory pain in tendons and joints may also suggest disseminated gonococcal disease. An isolated facial weakness may mimic Bell's palsy of other causes. Late neurologic involvement may suggest multiple sclerosis (transverse myelitis), Guillain-Barré syndrome (symmetric peripheral neuropathy), primary psychosis, or brain tumor. In adults with Lyme arthritis, the large knee effusions can resemble those in Reiter's syndrome, and the occasional symmetric polyarthritis, that of rheumatoid arthritis. In children, the attacks of arthritis, although generally shorter, may be identical to those seen in the oligoarticular form of juvenile rheumatoid arthritis, but without iridocyclitis.

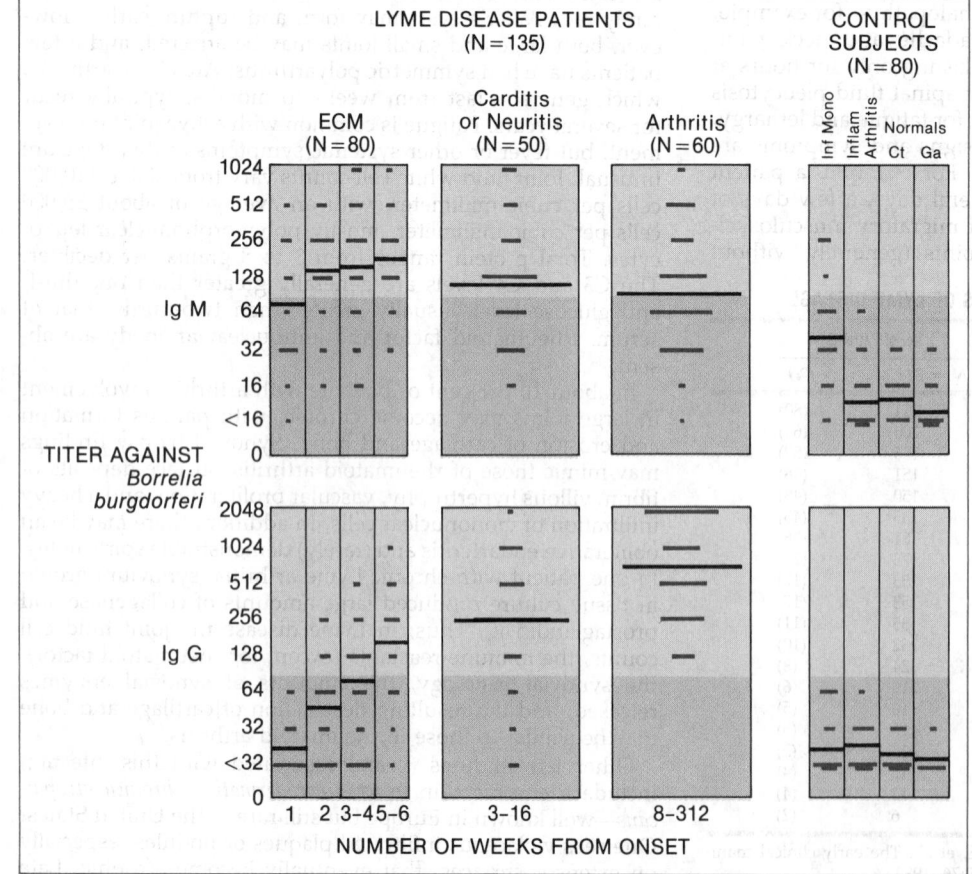

FIGURE 313–1. Antibody titers against *Borrelia burgdorferi* are shown in serum samples from 135 patients with different clinical manifestations of Lyme disease, and from 80 control subjects with infectious mononucleosis, inflammatory arthritis, or no disease (titers determined by indirect immunofluorescence). The black bar shows the geometric mean titer for each group; the pink shaded areas indicate the range of values generally observed in control subjects. Note that all patients with Lyme arthritis have elevated IgG antibody titers. (Adapted from Steere AC, Grodzicki RL, Kornblatt AN, et al: The spirochetal etiology of Lyme disease. N Engl J Med 308:733–740, 1983.)

TREATMENT. *Stage 1.* In patients treated early with anti-biotics, *erythema chronicum migrans* and its associated symptoms resolve in days, and subsequent major sequelae (myocarditis, meningoencephalitis, or recurrent arthritis) usually do not occur. For adults, therapy, in order of preference, includes oral tetracycline, 250 mg four times a day, phenoxymethyl penicillin, 500 mg four times a day, or erythromycin, 250 mg four times a day, each for 10 to 20 days, depending on the response. In children, phenoxymethyl penicillin, 50 mg per kilogram per day (not less than 1 gram or more than 2 grams per day), is given in divided doses for the same period, or, in cases of penicillin allergy, erythromycin, 30 mg per kilogram per day, in divided doses for 15 or 20 days. About 10 per cent of patients experience a Jarisch-Herxheimer–like reaction (higher fever, redder rash, or greater pain) during the first 24 hours of therapy.

Whichever drug is given, nearly half of patients have brief (hours to days) recurrent episodes of headache or pain in joints, tendons, bursae, or muscle, often with lethargy, which may continue for extended periods. Such symptoms may represent undegraded antigen rather than persistent live spirochetes.

Stage 2. For meningitis and cranial or peripheral neuropathies, intravenous penicillin G, 20 million units a day in six divided doses for ten days, is effective therapy. Headache, stiff neck, and radicular pain usually begin to subside by the second day of therapy and disappear by seven to ten days; motor deficits frequently require seven to eight weeks for complete recovery. Carditis also responds rapidly (in days) to this regimen. Prednisone, 40 to 60 mg a day in divided doses, may be added when a strong anti-inflammatory effect is important (e.g., persistent complete heart block).

Stage 3. For established Lyme arthritis, even with unremitting involvement, parenteral penicillin is curative in some patients. During treatment, the affected joint should be at rest, and accumulated fluid removed by needle aspirations. In a double-blind, placebo-controlled trial, 7 of 20 patients given intramuscular benzathine penicillin, 2.4 million units weekly for three weeks, were cured (mean follow-up of 33 months), versus none of 20 control patients. This regimen provides low serum levels of penicillin for about six weeks. The high-dose intravenous regimen of penicillin G (above), which yields much higher serum levels over its ten-day course, cured 11 of 20 patients, including 2 in whom benzathine penicillin had failed. Optimal therapy for this problem and for the later neurologic complications of Lyme disease is not yet clear. Synovectomy may be useful for treatment failures. The infiltrative lesions of *acrodermatitis chronica atrophicans* are usually cured by three weeks of oral phenoxymethyl penicillin, 2 to 3 grams daily in divided doses.

Malawista SE, Steere AC: Lyme disease: Infectious in origin, rheumatic in expression. Adv Int Med 31:147, 1986. *Review of the first ten years of Lyme disease, with a discussion of its importance as a unique human model for an infectious etiology of rheumatic disease.*

Pachner AR: Spirochetal diseases of the CNS. Neurol Clin 4:207, 1986. *Central nervous system complications of Lyme disease in the context of other spirochetal infections: neurosyphilis, leptospirosis, and relapsing fever.*

Schmid GP: The global distribution of Lyme disease. Rev Infect Dis 7:41, 1985. *Where the disease is and where the known vectors are, with maps.*

Steere AC, Green J, Schoen RT, et al.: Successful parenteral penicillin therapy of established Lyme arthritis. N Engl J Med 312:869, 1985. *Cure by antibiotics of a rheumatoid "look-alike."*

Steere AC, Grodzicki RL, Kornblatt AN, et al.: The spirochetal etiology of Lyme disease. N Engl J Med 308:733, 1983. *Borrelia recovered from blood, ECM, and cerebrospinal fluid of patients.*

Steere AC, Malawista SE, Fischer DK, et al. (eds.): Lyme Disease: First International Symposium. Yale J Biol Med 57:445, 1984. *The international experience, as the scope of this illness began to become clear.*

Steere AC, Malawista SE, Syndman DR, et al.: Lyme arthritis: An epidemic of oligoarticular arthritis in children and adults in three Connecticut communities. Arthritis Rheum 20:7, 1977. *The first description of a new nosologic entity, recognized because it clusters geographically; rheumatoid arthritis does not.*

Steere AC, Pachner AR, Malawista SE: Neurologic abnormalities of Lyme disease: Successful treatment with high-dose intravenous penicillin. Ann Intern Med 99:767, 1983. *Meningitis, formerly treated with high-dose prednisone tapered over months, responds to penicillin in days.*

314   RAT-BITE FEVERS

J. Bruce McClain

The term *rat-bite fevers* refers to illnesses caused by *Streptobacillus moniliformis* or *Spirillum minus.*

S. moniliformis previously has been called *Actinomyces muris*, *Streptothrix muris ratti*, or *Haverhillia multiformis*. It is an aerobic, gram-negative, branching rod in the same family as mycobacteria, 2 to 15 μ in length, and an inhabitant of the respiratory tracts of mice and rats.

Spirillum minus, sometimes called *Spirillum minor*, is a twisted, gram-negative, aerobic rod with bipolar tufts of flagella, which has not been grown on artificial media but which has been passed to animals. It is 2 to 5 μ in length and has been identified in the drainage from interstitial keratitis in rats.

EPIDEMIOLOGY. Neither streptobacillary nor spirillary rat-bite fevers are reportable diseases. The Centers for Disease Control receive two to three isolates annually. A survey from the 1940's of 400 rat bites reported 16 cases of clinical rat-bite fever, 8 of which had organisms identified. The highest reported rate of post–rat-bite fevers is 10 per cent. Many factors make the current prevalence in the United States difficult to determine: innate antibiotic responsiveness, the difficulty with which the causative organisms are isolated, and the lack of widely available serologic tests. The majority of recently reported cases are in laboratory workers with definite bite exposure, and these individuals constitute the population at highest risk. Other animals have been reported to transmit the disease, including weasels, dogs, cats, pigs, and mice. Streptobacillary fever may be transmitted by non-bite mechanisms, as demonstrated by an outbreak associated with consumption of unpasteurized milk in Haverhill, Massachusetts, and case reports of illness associated with trauma.

CLINICAL MANIFESTATIONS. *Streptobacillary Fever (Haverhill Fever).* The initial injury heals promptly in most cases. The incubation period from bite exposure is usually 3 to 4 days, with a range of 1 to 22 days. In the Haverhill outbreak most cases occurred within three days of exposure to contaminated milk. Ninety-five percent of patients will complain of fever, frequently in the 38.8° to 40° C range, usually with a sudden onset and a toxic effect on the patient. Bifrontal headache, nausea, vomiting, and myalgias usually accompany the fever initially. Occasionally there is a lessening of fever after a few days, with subsequent return of higher temperatures. A maculopapular rash develops within the first five days of illness in almost all patients. The rash is distributed distally and may involve the palms and soles of the feet. Occasionally the centers of the 0.3- to 1-cm lesions develop pustules. A fine desquamation occurs on healing in 20 per cent of patients. Arthritis occurs in 70 per cent of patients on the second through fourteenth days of illness and almost always involves more than one joint, especially the wrists and elbows. The arthritis is nondeforming, although in untreated cases it may persist for months and has been known to damage joints. Less frequently reported complications of streptobacillary fever are endocarditis, pericarditis, soft tissue abscesses, and amnionitis.

Spirillary Fever (Sodoku). The initial injury heals promptly in most cases, although induration, ulceration, or eschar may develop at the site of injury with the onset of illness. Regional adenopathy is frequently present. The incubation period is generally greater than 7 days, with a range of 1 to 36 days. The onset of sodoku is less abrupt than in streptobacillary fever, and temperatures are in the 38.8° C range. Fevers are recurrent with several days between episodes. Headaches, nausea, and vomiting are common, and a roseolar-urticarial rash is seen in one half of patients. Arthritis is rare.

Spirilla are poorly characterized organisms. It seems that on occasion nonsodoku spirilla may cause illness in humans. These illnesses tend to be prolonged and to resemble endocarditis.

LABORATORY MANIFESTATIONS. Most patients with spirillary fever and fewer than 20 per cent with streptobacillary fever have false-positive results of serologic tests for syphilis. Leukocyte counts in both illnesses range from normal to 30,000 per cubic millimeter. Results of urinalysis usually are normal, although nephritic sediments have been seen in sodoku.

DIAGNOSIS. The diagnosis of streptobacillary rat-bite fever is made by culturing the organism from blood, joint fluid, or tissue or by demonstrating a fourfold rise in titer by an agglutination test that is available through the Centers for Disease Control. Titers may persist for two to four years. Streptobacilli from blood cultures will usually grow within a week. Their cultivation is complicated by requirements for animal serum in the medium and a CO_2 atmosphere as well as sensitivity to sodium polyanethol sulfonate (Liquoid, SPS), which is found in most automated blood culture systems at levels that are inhibitory (over 0.01 per cent). Specific measures to cultivate the organisms must be arranged with the laboratory.

Spirillary fever may be diagnosed by inoculation of mice with infected tissues or fluids and demonstration of morphologically compatible organisms in the peripheral blood by darkfield examination. Occasionally the diagnosis has been established by darkfield examination of peripheral blood or eschars in humans.

The differential diagnosis of rat-bite fever includes Still's disease, arthritis associated with hepatitis B, rubella, gonococcemia, meningococcemia, rickettsial disease, hypersensitivity vasculitis, and leptospirosis.

TREATMENT AND PROGNOSIS. Penicillin G, 1.2 million units per day in divided doses, is the treatment of choice for both types of rat-bite fever. Ampicillin or penicillin V, 2 grams per day, is effective oral therapy. The duration of therapy should total ten days, and parenteral therapy may be followed with oral therapy. Higher doses have been used in endocarditis. The streptobacillary illness has responded to parenteral cephalosporin therapy. Oral cephalosporin therapy should not be substituted until more information is available. In the patient allergic to penicillin, both forms of the illness may be treated with tetracyclines, chloramphenicol, or streptomycin.

About 12 per cent of untreated patients with streptobacillary disease die, although in most cases the disease will run a course of 25 days with spontaneous resolution. Treatment with penicillin G will resolve most symptoms in one to four days, although patients who receive less than 400,000 units per day of penicillin have had illnesses persisting for several weeks. Penicillin resistance has been reported and should be kept in mind if treatment failure is suspected.

The mortality in untreated spirillary fever is 7 per cent. Without therapy the disease will last an average of 35 days. Spontaneous resolution is the rule. Penicillin therapy will cause resolution of symptoms in one or two days. A Herxheimer reaction is common.

Anderson LC, Leary SL, Manning PJ: Rat-bite fever in animal research laboratory personnel. Lab Anim Sci 33:292, 1983. *A case report and review of the clinical and epidemiologic characteristics of the group at risk for disease.*

Kowal J: Spirillum fever, report of a case and review of the literature. N Engl J Med 264:123, 1961. *An interesting review of nonsodoku spirillary illness.*

Roughgarden JW: Antimicrobial therapy of rat-bite fever. Arch Intern Med 116:39, 1965. *A comprehensive review of therapeutic results with various antimicrobials.*

Watkins CG: Ratbite fever. J Pediatr 28:429, 1946. *The best review of the clinical syndromes of rat-bite fever.*

315 LEPTOSPIROSIS

J. Bruce McClain

The term *leptospirosis* describes an infection with any serovar of *Leptospira interrogans*, regardless of the syndrome. Old names such as *canicola fever*, *Fort Bragg fever*, *Weil's disease*, or *peapicker's disease* are potentially confusing and should be avoided.

ETIOLOGY. *Leptospira* consists of two species: *interrogans*, which is pathogenic, and *biflexa*, which is saprophytic. Serotyping and serogrouping have established over 170 serovars in the species *L. interrogans*. The proper designation of a serovar is *L. interrogans* serovar pomona not *L. pomona*. The latter usage, although widespread, represents serovars as species and is incorrect.

The organism is a tightly coiled spirochete with one axial filament. With a diameter of about 0.15 μm, it is invisible on light microscopy and must be visualized by phase contrast or darkfield microscopy. It is easily cultured on Fletcher's medium and is an obligate aerobe.

EPIDEMIOLOGY. Leptospirosis is a ubiquitous enzootic disease. Reservoirs of infection include rodents, skunks, foxes, domestic livestock, and dogs. Many animals exhibit a prolonged urinary shedding of the organism without clinical illness. When humans contact infected tissues, fluids, or contaminated waters, they contract the illness. Transmission may occur through cuts, mucous membranes, and possibly unabraded skin. In earlier series illness was reported associated with occupational exposure, such as among sanitation, dairy, slaughterhouse, or fishing workers. The epidemiology has changed over the last 15 years, owing to the advent of multiuse land development with farmlands draining into recreational bodies of water. More recent reports indicate that at least one half of cases result from nonvocational exposure. There has been a corresponding decrease in the age of persons infected, although males still comprise 80 per cent of cases. In the United States between 50 and 150 cases are reported annually. The national attack rate is 0.05 per 100,000, although rates as high as 1 per 100,000 occur in Hawaii. The disease is probably substantially under-reported. Leptospirosis shows an annual peak in the summer months and has had a 4- to 5-year periodicity in attack rates over the last 25 years.

PATHOLOGY AND PATHOGENESIS. Gross anatomic findings in patients dying from leptospirosis are (1) widespread hemorrhage in skin, mucosa, serosa, heart, lungs, spleen, liver, and kidneys; (2) hepatomegaly without prominent splenomegaly; (3) bile staining; and (4) enlargement of the heart and kidneys.

Histologic examination of the liver in autopsy material shows nonspecific inflammatory changes, bile stasis, and disruption of the limiting plate. Biopsy materials under light and electron microscopic examination show similar features with less destruction of architecture.

Kidneys in autopsy series show a spectrum of changes that reflect an initial tubular injury that is acellular. As the disease progresses and antibodies appear, inflammatory changes occur that result in an overt interstitial nephritis with disruption of the tubular architecture. Biopsy series show similar changes to a lesser degree. The glomeruli have foot-process fusion and mesangial hypertrophy but are otherwise spared. Leptospires are seen in most of the renal material.

Hemorrhagic manifestations are associated with areas of capillary wall damage and necrosis with perivascular round cell infiltration.

Striated muscle is frequently involved with degeneration of

individual fibrils and loss of architecture associated with inflammation. This pattern is considered specific for leptospirosis. The myocardium is affected with similar changes. In one fourth of autopsy cases, myocarditis is listed as serious enough to be a contributing cause of death.

The mechanism by which *Leptospira* organisms cause damage to tissues is obscure. Toxic factors have been identified in culture supernatants, but organisms that do not produce some of these factors may cause serious disease. Early in the illness the evidence favors a direct leptospiral toxicity to certain tissues, while later in the illness damage secondary to inflammation is more pronounced.

CLINICAL FEATURES. Most natural infections appear 7 to 14 days after exposure, although the incubation period ranges from 2 to 20 days. The length of the incubation period has no prognostic significance. Clinical findings vary among reported series, but a general description includes fever and headache, 95 per cent; myalgia and conjunctival suffusion, 80 per cent (in nonmilitary series suffusion is reported less often); gastrointestinal symptoms (nausea, vomiting, or abdominal pain), 60 per cent; cough or pharyngitis, 40 per cent; lymphadenopathy, 25 per cent; hepatomegaly, 15 per cent; rash, 10 per cent; and jaundice and gastrointestinal hemorrhage, 5 per cent each. Less commonly reported symptoms are splenomegaly, uveitis, and diarrhea. About one half of patients exhibit a "brutal beginning" with an abrupt onset of symptoms over a one- to two-hour period. The clinical picture that should bring leptospirosis to mind is a febrile patient with severe muscle aches and pain who is nauseated or vomiting. The presence of conjunctival suffusion may be very helpful in detecting the illness in military populations. It is not conjunctivitis as seen in allergic or viral conjunctivitis, but rather a *pericorneal reddening* or *hyperemia.*

The fever is high, usually above 38° C and frequently up to 40° C, and is accompanied by chills. Headache is severe and is characterized as retro-orbital or occipital. The presence of headache, high fever, and neck stiffness or pain due to profound myalgias suggests meningitis and may necessitate a lumbar puncture. Spinal fluid is usually acellular in the first five to seven days of illness, although leptospires may be seen. With the onset of antibody in the serum, an aseptic meningitis may occur in up to 90 per cent of patients, but only one half will have meningeal symptoms. When a cutaneous hypesthesia is also present, patients may not tolerate the touch of a sheet. Other neurologic manifestations, such as changes in the level of consciousness, encephalitis, and cranial nerve palsies, have been reported less often. The muscle pains and tenderness are truly remarkable. The severity of myalgias may even prevent the patient from standing. The presence of nausea, vomiting, and anorexia with abdominal tenderness caused by muscle involvement can mimic pancreatitis. Acute dilatation of the gallbladder and cholecystitis can occur in leptospirosis and make the clinical evaluation of an ill patient very difficult, especially since there is already laboratory evidence of inflammation.

The illness usually lasts four to nine days. During that period all clinical findings resolve simultaneously, and both doctor and patients are surprised at how quickly the recovery has taken place and at how well the patient feels. In about 15 per cent of patients the illness persists beyond the ninth day. It rarely may last six to seven weeks.

Leptospirosis is generally a monophasic illness. In a minority of patients after an initial illness there will be a period of apparent recovery, after which symptoms worsen. This second phase is termed the *immune phase.* It lasts two to four days in most patients. It differs from initial illness in being more variable. Fever is not so high, myalgias and gastrointestinal symptoms are not so severe, but meningitis and abnormal spinal fluids and iridocyclitis are more common. The immune phase is so named because of its correlation with the onset of antibodies to leptospirosis in the blood, the disap-

pearance of leptospiremia, and the onset of urine cultures positive for the germ.

The term *Weil's syndrome* is applied to one pole of a continuum of illness. It is not a specific subgroup of leptospirosis; it is simply severe leptospirosis. Any of the several manifestations of Weil's syndrome may occur alone. The clinical findings of intense jaundice, mental status changes, hemorrhage, purpura or petechiae, and renal insufficiency occurring in a previously normal patient are so memorable that it is not surprising that this was the syndrome that stimulated the search for leptospires. The first manifestation of severe illness is usually jaundice that develops between the fifth and ninth days. The intensity of jaundice has no prognostic significance. Renal insufficiency may develop concomitantly with jaundice. Oliguria is a grave prognostic sign. Hemorrhagic manifestations may develop: Purpura and petechiae may appear on the oral, vaginal, or conjunctival mucosa. A biphasic pattern frequently may be seen, although the "stages" tend to merge into a single severe illness. Convalescence is rapid in most patients but may be delayed for up to ten weeks.

Childhood Disease. A recent report of nine pediatric cases reiterated the close contact of children to common reservoirs such as dogs. The pediatric syndrome shares many features of adult disease but is more intense, with several atypical features such as shock, hydrops of the gallbladder, skin desquamation, and chest radiograph abnormality.

LABORATORY FEATURES. Leukocyte counts are usually below 15,000 per cubic millimeter but may be as high as 50,000 per cubic millimeter. There is almost always neutrophilia. Hematocrit is normal in anicteric illness, but in prolonged illness anemia is common. The causes of anemia are many, with blood loss, microangiopathy, and leptospiral hemolysin all implicated in clinical cases. Thrombocytopenia is seen in severe cases. Coagulation studies occasionally demonstrate a vitamin K reversible prolongation of prothrombin time. However, this is not responsible for the hemorrhagic diathesis of severe leptospirosis. The sedimentation rate is elevated in one half of cases.

Liver function tests reveal a mean serum glutamic-oxaloacetic transaminase/serum glutamic-pyruvic transaminase (SGOT/SGPT) elevation of 5 times normal, with occasional patients having elevations up to 20 times normal. The direct bilirubin concentration may rise as a manifestation of severe disease and may reach 64 mg per deciliter, but in most icteric cases it is below 20 mg per deciliter. The pattern is one of intrahepatic cholestasis.

Early in the illness 80 per cent of patients have abnormal urine findings. The most common abnormalities are microscopic hematuria, pyuria, and "2+" proteinuria. Gross hematuria rarely has been reported. One fourth of patients demonstrate elevations of the blood urea nitrogen between 20 and 100 mg per deciliter. The most common electrolyte abnormality is hyperkalemia, primarily in patients with renal failure.

The chest radiograph appears abnormal in one fourth of patients, including anicteric cases. The most common abnormality is patchy bronchopneumonia. A small pleural effusion is seen in 10 per cent of patients.

Electrocardiographic abnormalities occur in 10 to 40 per cent of patients, with bradycardia and low voltage accounting for one half of abnormalities. The remainder consists of nonspecific ST-T wave changes.

Cerebrospinal fluid may be abnormal in up to 90 per cent of patients. In 70 per cent of specimens the total cell count is below 500 per cubic millimeter, with frequent presence of neutrophils. Protein ranges from 50 to 110 mg per deciliter in 80 per cent of cases. The glucose concentration is usually normal.

IgM antibodies may be detected in blood by day four or five of illness in most patients.

DIAGNOSIS. A diagnosis of leptospirosis must be suspected in any patient with fever, myalgias, headache, and nausea or vomiting. The presence of conjunctival suffusion is an early and helpful sign. The most common misdiagnosis of a patient with leptospirosis is aseptic meningitis followed by viral hepatitis, viral syndrome, fever of unknown origin, bronchitis, influenza, nephritis, and rickettsiosis. The following differential points aid the clinician: (1) The myalgias of leptospirosis are not a prominent feature of viral hepatitis; (2) creatine kinase is frequently elevated in leptospirosis, and this seldom occurs in viral hepatitis; (3) liver enzyme values in viral hepatitis may average 10 to 15 times higher than normal, but the average is 5 times higher in leptospirosis; (4) a conjunctival suffusion is very helpful in separating leptospirosis from other processes.

The diagnosis may be confirmed by culture (on Fletcher's semisolid medium) of the blood in the first week of illness or of the urine thereafter. Cultures may take up to eight weeks to become positive. Since leptospires may be excreted in the urine for prolonged periods, the diagnosis may be established by urine culture in untreated patients even after clinical illness is over. Direct examination of the urine and blood is not sufficient to establish the diagnosis. There are many artifacts that may be mistaken for leptospires, especially by the inexperienced laboratory worker. When cultures are performed three to four times, organisms are recovered with regularity. The diagnosis may be established serologically by two methods. The macroagglutination is a screening test that uses pooled antigens from all of the serogroups of leptospirosis. Diagnosis is made by a fourfold rise in titer. This test is broadly available but will not detect infecting serovars that are not included in the pooled test antigens. The microagglutination requires a live pathogenic leptospiral culture and therefore is performed mainly in reference laboratories. Techniques for detecting genus-specific antibody or antigen using hemolytic assays and counterimmunoelectrophoresis have been published and are available as research tools. The most promising test for early diagnosis is a genus-specific antibody detection system.

PROGNOSIS. In most untreated cases this is a nonfatal, self-limited illness. The reported mortality of leptospirosis varies greatly among series. In military populations it is around 0.1 per cent. In civilian series it ranges from 5 to 10 per cent. In both military and civilian series mortality is related to age and presence of jaundice. Thirty per cent of patients over age 60 die. Jaundiced patients have a 15 per cent mortality. The differences in mortality may have to do with the underlying health of the host and the bias toward reporting of more serious cases. In the military series, involving large groups of well men, high attack rates have been documented and physicians are sensitive to the diagnosis. If the patient lives, sequelae are uncommon even in severe cases. When sequelae occur, they consist of focal cerebral or peripheral nerve deficits or ocular problems caused by persistent uveitis. Several patients have been reported with persistent renal abnormalities.

THERAPY AND PREVENTION. Tetracycline and doxycycline (in controlled trials) are both effective in shortening the course of anicteric leptospirosis when they are given in the first two to four days of illness. Their efficacy in reducing symptoms if given later has not been established. Therapeutic trials were done in populations with no mortality in the placebo group, so the effect of these drugs on mortality is unknown. Doxycycline therapy prevents leptospiruria in infected patients. If leptospiruria is necessary for the mediation of renal damage, as some investigators have speculated, then doxycycline may affect the development of renal failure or Weil's syndrome. Although activities in vitro have been demonstrated for penicillins, aminoglycosides, and erythromycin, they have not been studied in a controlled trial. Uncontrolled experience suggests that penicillin is effective. The balance of therapy in leptospirosis consists of careful attention to the details of care in patients with renal, hepatic, hematologic, and central nervous system complications.

Doxycycline, 100 mg once a week, will prevent leptospirosis in high-risk groups for three weeks. Efficacy in longer periods of exposure has not been evaluated. There are no leptospiral vaccines for humans in use, although effective vaccines for animals are available.

Edwards GA, Domm BM: Human leptospirosis. Medicine 39:117, 1960. *An extensive analysis of the clinical and laboratory features of leptospirosis with a review of early papers.*

Feigin RD, Anderson DC: Human leptospirosis. CRC Crit Rev Clin Lab Sci 5:413, 1975. *The most comprehensive review of leptospirosis, including history, microbiology, pathogenesis, clinical findings, and therapy.*

McClain JBL, Ballou WR, Harrison SH, et al.: Doxycycline therapy of leptospirosis. Ann Intern Med 100:696, 1984. *A description of therapeutic effects of doxycycline in therapy of leptospirosis.*

Schmid GP, Steere AC, Kornblatt AN, et al.: Newly recognized *Leptospira* species ("*Leptospira inadai*" serovar lyme) isolated from human skin. J Clin Microbiol 24:484, 1986. *What may be a third species of leptospire with pathogenic potential.*

Takafuji ET, Kirkpatrick JW, Miller RN, et al.: An efficacy trial of doxycycline chemoprophylaxis against leptospirosis. N Engl J Med 310:497, 1984. *Demonstrates efficacy in American soldiers with placebo controls.*

Diseases Caused by Chlamydiae

Walter E. Stamm

316 INTRODUCTION

Because of their obligate intracellular growth cycle, chlamydiae were originally considered large viruses and were variously called *Bedsonia* or *TRIC* (for *trachoma-inclusion conjunctivitis*) agents. These terms have been discarded, and chlamydiae now constitute a separate order (Chlamydiales), family (Chlamydiaceae), and genus (*Chlamydia*). All members of the genus are obligate intracellular pathogens, but they more closely resemble bacteria than viruses in that they possess both deoxyribonucleic acid (DNA) and ribonucleic acid (RNA), divide by binary fission, have bacterial ribosomes and a cell wall not unlike that of Enterobacteriaceae, and can be inhibited by antibiotics. Compared with other bacteria, they have a small genome of 6 to 8 $\times$ 10^5 base pairs. They also lack adenosine triphosphate (ATP)–generating enzymes and hence depend entirely upon host cell metabolism for energy production.

The genus *Chlamydia* contains two species, *C. psittaci* and *C. trachomatis*. The former is a ubiquitous cause of infection in birds and lower mammals, with humans being occasional accidental hosts, while *C. trachomatis* infects humans and has no apparent natural animal hosts. Characteristically, *C. psittaci* produces long-lived, persistent infections of birds and mammals. Transmission to humans occurs via exposure to infected animal tissues or secretions. Persistent infections caused by *C. trachomatis* in humans may also be common but have been less well documented. In the United States, *C. trachomatis* is transmitted sexually and from mother to infant at the time of birth. Trachoma, still endemic in arid parts of the Third World, spreads within families via close nonsexual contact. Recently, Grayston and colleagues have described a fastidious *C. psittaci*–like strain, termed the TWAR agent, which may be a common cause of human upper respiratory infection and pneumonia. No animal reservoirs have as yet been identified, and the mode of transmission is unknown (see Ch. 319).

All chlamydiae possess a genus-specific, heat-stable lipopolysaccharide antigen that serves as the basis for the widely available complement fixation serologic test. Species- and immunotype-specific antigens have also been described and serve as the basis for subdividing *C. trachomatis* into 15 immunotypes using the microimmunofluorescence test of Wang and Grayston. Specific immunotypes tend to cause particular clinical syndromes. Types A, B, Ba, and C produce endemic trachoma (see Ch. 317). Types D, E, F, G, H, I, J, and K cause oculogenital infections in adults (see Ch. 305) and ocular, respiratory, and genital infections in infants. Types L1, L2, and L3 produce lymphogranuloma venereum (LGV) (see Ch. 307) and proctocolitis (see Ch. 105). LGV strains of *C. trachomatis* possess properties that distinguish them from non-LGV strains biologically, including more efficient cell entry and cell-to-cell infectivity in tissue culture, as well as mouse lethality upon intracerebral injection.

Chlamydiae replicate by means of a unique life cycle unlike that of other bacteria. The 300-nm elementary body (the infective and extracellular form of a chlamydia) initiates infection by attachment to specific receptors in the susceptible host cell's outer membrane. Subsequently, the elementary body enters the host cell by endocytosis. Within the resulting phagosome, the elementary body reorganizes within six hours into the larger 800- to 1000-nm and more metabolically active reticulate body. These reticulate bodies undergo repeated binary division until a large inclusion occupying much of the cell's cytoplasm and containing many reticulate bodies is formed. Reticulate bodies possess many ribosomes and synthesize deoxyribonucleic acid (DNA), ribonucleic acid (RNA), proteins, and other molecules but cannot generate ATP. After 24 hours, some of the reticulate bodies condense to form compact elementary bodies in the mature inclusion, and the latter are released into the extracellular environment to begin the cycle anew.

C. trachomatis preferentially infects columnar epithelial cells, while *C. psittaci* has a broader host cell range, including macrophages. In most patients, *C. trachomatis* infections remain superficial, involving mucosal surfaces of the eye, nasopharynx, cervix, urethra, and rectum (Table 316–1). Many of these infections produce few or no symptoms and tend to be subacute in nature and mild in terms of the signs they produce. Ascending infections of the endometrium, fallopian tube, liver capsule, epididymis, or lung produce more severe symptoms and signs and can be regarded as more extensive or invasive infections. Infection of the upper genital tract in women is of particular importance, often leading to tubal scarring with resultant complications of infertility and ectopic pregnancy. LGV strains of *C. trachomatis* cause the most invasive disease, manifested either by proctocolitis or by painful inguinal adenopathy and fever. *C. trachomatis* occasionally causes nongenital systemic infection, including culture-negative endocarditis, peritonitis, and pneumonia in adults.

Since many chlamydial infections produce either no symptoms or nonspecific symptoms and signs, laboratory confirmation of infection should be sought. Available techniques include direct microscopic examination of tissue scrapings or secretions for typical inclusions or for elementary bodies; isolation of the organism in cell culture; and assessment of antichlamydial antibody in serum or secretions. Widespread adoption of cell culture techniques for isolation of *C. trachomatis* from patients' secretions or biopsies (replacing the more cumbersome embryonated yolk sac method) has been a major factor contributing to recognition of the wide spectrum of infections caused by *C. trachomatis*. Inclusions formed in cell culture monolayers can be visualized using iodine, Giemsa's, or immunofluorescent staining procedures. Despite widespread use in research laboratories, cell culture procedures for isolation of *C. trachomatis* have not been generally available to clinicians because of their expense and technical difficulty. Lack of an available confirmatory diagnostic test and the inability to screen high-risk populations for infection have been major factors contributing to the increasing incidence of genital and neonatal *C. trachomatis* infections in this country. Newer immunodiagnostic procedures that detect chlamydial antigen in patients' secretions have recently been developed and can be used for diagnostic confirmation and for screening where cultures are not available. These tests utilize monoclonal or polyclonal antichlamydial antibodies to demonstrate the presence of chlamydial antigens in infected secretions by either enzyme-linked immunosorbent assay (ELISA) or immunofluorescence techniques. These methods have approximate sensitivities of 80 to 90 per cent and specificities of 95 to 99 per cent compared with culture in high-risk populations.

Chlamydial infection stimulates both a humoral and a cellular immune response, but neither appears to be completely protective against subsequent infection with either homologous or heterologous strains. Both local and systemic antibody can be demonstrated after acute infection, and immunoglobulin G (IgG) antibody neutralizes infective elementary bodies. Some have advocated that the immune response actually participates in the disease process by producing continued inflammation. Serodiagnosis of chlamydial infections has limited applicability except in specific circumstances. The complement fixation test, available in most health department laboratories, should be used for confirmation of suspected psittacosis or LGV. The microimmunofluorescence test may be useful in the diagnosis of infant pneumonia, pelvic inflammatory disease, or Fitz-Hugh-Curtis syndrome but is available only in research laboratories. Uncomplicated genital infections evoke only low titer-antibody responses, and acute infections cannot be easily distinguished from preexisting antibody in many patients.

C. trachomatis infections can be treated with a variety of antimicrobial agents. Those with greatest activity in cell culture assays and in clinical studies include the tetracyclines (tetracycline HCl, doxycycline, and minocycline), erythromycin, sulfonamides, sulfamethoxazole-trimethoprim, and rifampin. The beta-lactam antibiotics produce abnormal inclusions in cell culture and inhibit replication but have been largely ineffective in clinical treatment trials. The aminogly-

TABLE 316–1. CLINICAL SPECTRUM OF *C. TRACHOMATIS* INFECTIONS*

Males	Females	Infants
Uncomplicated Infections		
Urethritis (NGU, PGU)	Cervicitis	Conjunctivitis
Proctitis	Urethritis	Pharyngitis
Conjunctivitis	Proctitis	Asymptomatic rectal
Pharyngitis	Conjunctivitis	and vaginal carriage
	Pharyngitis	
	Bartholinitis	
Invasive Infections		
Proctocolitis	Endometritis	Pneumonia
Lymphogranuloma venereum	Salpingitis	? Otitis media
Epididymitis	Perihepatitis	
? Prostatitis	Postpartum endometritis	
Complications		
Reiter's syndrome	Infertility	? Chronic pulmonary impairment
Rectal strictures	Ectopic pregnancy	
? Urethral strictures	Chronic salpingitis	
? Sterility	Complications of pregnancy (? prematurity, stillbirth)	

*Excludes trachoma.
NGU = nongonococcal urethritis; PGU = postgonococcal urethritis.

cosides, vancomycin, and spectinomycin have no activity against chlamydiae. In general, chlamydial infections require 7 to 21 days of antibiotic treatment; single-day regimens have been largely ineffective. Treatment failure usually indicates noncompliance, reinfection, or inadequate duration of drug therapy. Resistance to tetracycline or erythromycin has not been described.

Chlamydia trachomatis infections: Policy guidelines for prevention and control. MMWR 34(Suppl):53s, 1985. *Excellent overview of* C. trachomatis *infections (including clinical aspects) with current bibliography.*

Stamm WE, Harrison HR, Alexander ER, et al.: Diagnosis of *Chlamydia trachomatis* infections by direct immunofluorescence staining of genital secretions: A multicenter trial. Ann Intern Med 101:638, 1984. *Illustrates the potential value of a noncultural diagnostic test for* Chlamydia.

Thompson SE, Washington AE: Epidemiology of sexually transmitted *Chlamydia trachomatis* infections. Epidemiol Rev 5:96, 1983. *Reviews current view of the epidemic of sexually transmitted* C. trachomatis *infections in the United States.*

317 TRACHOMA

Chlamydia trachomatis causes two epidemiologically distinct patterns of ocular infection. In endemic parts of the world, *C. trachomatis* immunotypes A, B, Ba, and C cause trachoma, a chronic eye disease that may lead to severe visual impairment or blindness. In nonendemic areas, immunotypes D through K produce a milder, self-limited conjunctivitis in infants born to mothers with cervical infection or in adults who acquire ocular infection after secondary spread from genital sites.

Since antiquity, trachomatous infection has been recognized in the Mediterranean basin and in the Orient, and it remains prevalent in Africa and Asia. Although the incidence has been decreasing over the last 30 years, more than 500 million persons have eye infections with chlamydiae, with millions blinded as a result. Trachoma flourishes in hot, dry areas that have a shortage of available water and poor hygienic customs. Initial infection usually occurs in early childhood, and in certain parts of the world virtually the entire population is infected with chlamydiae before reaching adulthood. Repeated exposure to chlamydiae and the high prevalence of bacterial superinfection with *Hemophilus* spp., pneumococci, staphylococci, and Enterobacteriaceae in these populations contribute to the severity of the resulting eye disease. In the United States, trachoma is occasionally seen on Indian reservations in the southwestern United States, in Mexican-Americans, and in immigrants from endemic areas, but such cases rarely result in major visual impairment, perhaps because bacterial superinfection is infrequent.

Persons with active trachoma shed chlamydiae in desquamated conjunctival cells, in conjunctival exudate, and in tears, which then may be transmitted by fingers, fomites, and perhaps flies. In endemic areas, transmission by these routes occurs through close personal contact, especially within family units and in groups of young children. Patients with early active infection shed more infective chlamydiae than those with chronic infection. However, even patients with long-term eye disease unaccompanied by signs of current activity may shed chlamydiae and thus serve as a source of infection.

Typical trachoma in children begins insidiously at about age two as a follicular conjunctivitis, most noticeable in the conjunctiva of the upper lid and the tarsal plate. Histologically, inclusion bodies appear within the conjunctival epithelial cells, polymorphonuclear leukocytes infiltrate the epithelium, and subepithelial lymphoid follicles develop. Reinfection is common during this period. Next the cornea becomes involved, with epithelial keratitis and subepithelial corneal infiltration resulting in opacities. Blood vessels from the limbus, accompanied by fibroblasts, invade the cornea to form a pannus. Progression of the inflammatory response leads to necrosis and scarring of the conjunctiva and gradual corneal vascularization from the upper limbus downward. Eventually a dense fibrovascular pannus extends over part or all of the cornea to impair vision grossly. Linear or stellate scars appear on the conjunctiva. Progressive scarring of the subepithelial tissues leads to deformation of the tarsal plate that results in entropion, trichiasis, and further corneal damage. Destruction of the conjunctival goblet cells and lacrimal ducts and gland produces xerosis. The latter changes often follow secondary bacterial infection, which may also produce corneal ulceration and accelerate loss of vision. Typically there are no systemic symptoms or signs of infection. The disease process evolves over about ten years in endemic areas but may be milder and more slowly progressive in other cases.

The traditional diagnostic criteria for trachoma include lymphoid follicles on the upper tarsal plate, limbal follicles, typical conjunctival scars, and vascular pannus. Early in the disease the last two can be detected only by slit-lamp examination. The presence of any two of these features confirms the diagnosis. Laboratory confirmation of trachoma is based on (1) identification of typical inclusions in epithelial cells from a conjunctival swab or scraping (usually done by Giemsa's or immunofluorescence staining); (2) cultivation of chlamydiae from a conjunctival specimen in cell culture; or (3) microimmunofluorescent antibody in high titer in tears. Approximately 20 to 60 per cent of children with early inflammatory trachoma have Giemsa-positive scrapings; higher yields result from cultures of chlamydiae.

In the differential diagnosis of ocular chlamydial infection, epidemic keratoconjunctivitis (usually caused by adenovirus type 8 or type 19), herpetic keratoconjunctivitis, Newcastle disease virus conjunctivitis, acute hemorrhagic conjunctivitis caused by enterovirus type 70 or coxsackievirus, reactions to allergens and irritating chemicals, and other bacterial causes of conjunctivitis must be considered. Some of these entities may coexist with chlamydial infections, and repeated ophthalmologic examinations and extensive laboratory evaluation may be required to establish a correct diagnosis.

Adult inclusion conjunctivitis caused by *C. trachomatis* usually presents as an acute follicular conjunctivitis with preauricular lymphadenopathy. Untreated, it regresses slowly, but keratitis with marginal infiltrates, subepithelial opacities, and corneal neovascularization may develop in the conjunctiva. Unlike trachoma, adult inclusion conjunctivitis rarely impairs vision permanently.

Control of chronic trachoma in endemic areas has been attempted using tetracycline or erythromycin ointment in the eyes of all affected children in the community for 21 to 60 days. Oral administration of erythromycin has been used as an alternative. Antibiotic therapy usually suppresses clinical activity and chlamydial as well as bacterial growth but may not eradicate chlamydiae permanently. However, in endemic areas, repeated courses of drug treatment are beneficial because they reduce severity of eye disease and thus avoid progression toward blindness. Even one dose per month of doxycycline, 300 mg (2.5 to 4 mg per kilogram), can provide clinical benefit by converting severe to mild eye disease. Drug therapy has no influence on scars or pannus. Surgical correction is required in serious entropion or trichiasis. Topical corticosteroids and caustic substances have no place in therapy. For acute adult inclusion conjunctivitis, tetracycline HCl, 1.0 to 2.0 grams given orally daily in divided doses, or erythromycin, 1.0 to 2.0 grams given daily for two weeks, will successfully treat genital tract as well as ocular involvement. Sulfisoxazole, 4 grams daily, may also be effective. Sexual partners must be treated simultaneously in order to avoid reinfection.

The potential measures to prevent trachoma include efforts to increase the supply of water; practices to maintain cleanliness, such as frequent handwashing and avoidance of use of common towels; and measures to reduce flies. It is also important to detect mild early infection in young children in endemic areas and to apply effective drug treatment repeatedly to prevent the blinding progression of the disease. Detection and treatment of adults who already have visual impairment probably can reduce the source of infection for children. Entire family groups or communities should be treated simultaneously. Efforts to prevent trachoma with a vaccine have been unsuccessful.

Dawson CR: Eye disease with chlamydial infection. In Oriel D, Ridgway G, Schachter J, et al. (eds.): Chlamydial Infections. Cambridge, Cambridge University Press, 1986, pp 135–144. *Excellent recent overview of all aspects of trachoma.*

318 NEONATAL CHLAMYDIAL INFECTIONS

Between 5 and 22 per cent of pregnant women have *Chlamydia trachomatis* infection of the cervix, with neonatal infection occurring when the infant passes through the infected birth canal. Ascending intrauterine infection of the fetus has not been demonstrated. After birth, 30 to 50 per cent of infants born to infected mothers have cultural evidence of infection, 25 per cent manifest clinically apparent conjunctivitis, and 10 to 15 per cent acquire nasopharyngeal infection, which in some cases progresses to chlamydial neonatal pneumonitis. Otitis media and symptomatic nasopharyngitis may be caused by *C. trachomatis* in some infants.

Neonatal *C. trachomatis* inclusion conjunctivitis begins 5 to 14 days after birth. The infection must be differentiated from gonococcal ophthalmia (which has a shorter incubation period of one to three days) and from other common causes of neonatal conjunctivitis (*Streptococcus pneumoniae*, *Hemophilus influenzae*, *Staphylococcus aureus*, and group D streptococci). Typical manifestations include lid and conjunctival swelling, mucopurulent ocular discharge, conjunctival hyperemia, and membrane formation. Untreated, the disease persists 3 to 12 months but usually heals without sequelae. Rarely, conjunctival scarring and corneal neovascularization occur. Neonates with inclusion conjunctivitis frequently have concomitant chlamydial infection of the nasopharynx, rectum, urethra, and vagina, usually without associated clinical manifestations at these sites.

The diagnosis can be rapidly established by demonstration of chlamydial inclusions or elementary bodies in conjunctival scrapings stained by Giemsa's stain or immunofluorescence. Cultures for *C. trachomatis* can also be used if available and will be positive in some smear-negative cases. Tear antibody to *C. trachomatis* can be demonstrated in most cases, but the test is not readily available.

Silver nitrate drops instilled at birth do not prevent chlamydial inclusion conjunctivitis and in some instances cause chemical conjunctivitis. For this reason, many health departments now recommend prophylactic use of erythromycin ointment at birth. However, topical erythromycin prophylaxis does not cure concomitant nasopharyngeal or rectal infection. Perhaps a better preventive approach would be screening and treatment of pregnant women for *C. trachomatis* infection before term. This approach essentially eliminates *C. trachomatis* infections in neonates and should be the strategy of choice in high risk women.

Since many infants with inclusion conjunctivitis have concomitant nasopharyngeal, rectal, and vaginal *C. trachomatis* infection, systemic rather than topical therapy should be used. In addition, relapses often follow topical therapy. Erythro-

mycin, 40 to 50 mg per kilogram per day in four divided doses for 14 to 21 days, cures more than 80 per cent of cases. Both parents should be examined for *C. trachomatis* infection and should be treated with tetracycline or erythromycin (for nursing mothers) if cultures or immunodiagnostic tests are not available.

Approximately 10 per cent of infants born to infected mothers develop a distinctive subacute chlamydial pneumonia between the first and fourth months of life. Typically, tachypnea, a staccato cough, inspiratory rales, elevated serum globulin concentrations, and eosinophilia are seen, but fever is absent. Hyperinflated lungs with scattered interstitial infiltrates are evident on chest radiographic examination. The disease lasts for weeks to months but is mild in most infants and will resolve without specific therapy. However, marked hypoxemia and apnea have been reported in some cases. Lung biopsies have demonstrated chlamydial inclusions, alveoli with inflammatory exudate, and a lymphocytic interstitial infiltration of the bronchial submucosa. In some cases, *C. trachomatis* has been recovered from lung tissue. Diagnosis in most instances can be suspected on clinical grounds and confirmed by the demonstration of chlamydial inclusions or elementary bodies on Giemsa- or immunofluorescent-stained smears of the conjunctivae or nasopharynx. If available, *C. trachomatis* should be sought by cell culture of eye scrapings, nasopharyngeal swabs, or rectal swabs. Rising high-titer immunoglobuin M (IgM) microimmunofluorescent antibody to *C. trachomatis* can be demonstrated in the majority of infants with pneumonia. Erythromycin, 50 mg per kilogram per day in four divided doses for 14 to 21 days, has been recommended for treatment of pneumonia in infants, although there are no control trials demonstrating the benefits of this regimen. Chronic respiratory impairment and persistent pulmonary symptoms may develop in some patients.

Alexander ER, Harrison HR: Role of *Chlamydia trachomatis* in perinatal infection. Rev Infect Dis 5:713, 1983.
Harrison HR: Chlamydial infection in neonates and children. In Oriel D, Ridgway G, Schachter J, et al. (eds.): Chlamydial Infections. Cambridge, Cambridge University Press, 1986, pp 283–292.

319 PSITTACOSIS AND RELATED INFECTIONS*

DEFINITION. Psittacosis (ornithosis), an infection of birds caused by *Chlamydia psittaci*, can produce asymptomatic infection, a transient influenza-like illness, or serious pneumonic disease when transmitted to humans.

ETIOLOGY. *C. psittaci*, an obligate intracellular bacterium, is one of two species within the genus *Chlamydia* (see Ch. 316). Parrots and parakeets are common carriers and until recently represented the major source of human infection. With better control of psittacine disease in aviaries, other birds now contribute more human infections. Cases have resulted from contact with turkeys, pigeons, ducks, and other fowl. Persons working with birds are at greatest risk, notably pet shop employees, pigeon handlers, and poultry workers. There is no risk associated with eating poultry products.

The agent is present in the blood, tissue, feathers, and discharges of infected birds. Although the avian disease can be fatal, infected birds frequently show only minimal evidence of illness, such as ruffled feathers, lethargy, diarrhea, and failure to eat. Birds having active infections are most likely to transmit the disease, but asymptomatic carriers are common, and birds can transmit the agent for months.

---

*This chapter is based upon "Psittacosis (Ornithosis, Parrot Fever)" by William Schaffner, in the 17th edition of the *Cecil Textbook of Medicine.*

Psittacosis is generally acquired by the respiratory route through inhalation of infected dried bird excreta or by handling of infected birds. Cases have been reported after only brief exposure to birds, and 20 per cent of patients can show no history of exposure to birds. Person-to-person transmission of psittacosis is rare.

Recently, Grayston and colleagues have described a fastidious *C. psittaci*–like strain, termed the TWAR agent, which may be a frequent cause of human respiratory tract infection. Serologic evidence of prior infection has been demonstrated in 20 to 40 per cent of adult populations in many parts of the world. Seroprevalence is low among children and increases in adolescence and young adulthood. Reservoirs and modes of transmission for the organism have not been defined, but epidemics of pneumonitis have been demonstrated. Isolation of the TWAR strain in association with rising antibody titers in young adults with idiopathic pneumonitis, nasopharyngitis, and bronchitis suggests that the agent causes these syndromes. Specific diagnostic tests are not yet available; erythromycin or tetracycline should be used for presumptive therapy.

PATHOLOGY. In birds, the principal sites of disease are the liver, spleen, and pericardium. In humans, the lung is most commonly involved. *C. psittaci* gains access to the human body via the respiratory route, rapidly enters the blood, and reaches the reticuloendothelial cells of the liver and spleen. After replication in these sites, invasion of the lung occurs via hematogenous spread. The mature pulmonary lesion, a lobular pneumonitis, results from inflammation and progressive edema of the alveoli, often accompanied by small hemorrhages. Thick, gelatinous plugs of mucus may fill major and minor bronchi and account for the severe cyanosis and progressive anoxia seen in fatal cases. Foci of necrosis may occur in more severely affected parts of the lung and are sometimes associated with capillary thrombi. The process is generally most severe in dependent bronchopulmonary segments. Monocytes and macrophages containing cytoplasmic inclusion bodies, which represent the agent (LCL bodies), are characteristic. Hyperplasia and monocytic infiltration of pulmonary and hilar lymph nodes and splenic enlargement with occasional areas of focal necrosis occur. Rarely the liver shows intralobular focal necrosis and swollen Kupffer's cells containing psittacosis elementary bodies. Changes in the myocardium, heart valves, pericardium, meninges, brain, adrenal glands, pancreas, and kidneys have been reported.

CLINICAL MANIFESTATIONS. Wide variations can occur in the clinical picture. The incubation period ranges from 7 to 15 days but may be longer. Asymptomatic or mild influenza-like infections probably are the rule. Moderate or severe infections, although less frequent, are more commonly diagnosed. The onset of illness may be insidious, but it often starts with chills and a fever that rises slowly to 39 to 40.5°C during the first week of illness. The pulse may be slow relative to the level of the fever. Headache is severe. Malaise, anorexia, nausea, vomiting, severe myalgias, particularly in the neck and back, and arthralgias are common. Cough is generally prominent but may be delayed until late in the first week. Small amounts of mucoid sputum with occasional blood streaking are the rule. Changes in mentation are often seen. Delirium or stupor may occur in severe cases toward the end of the first week and usually are associated with severe pulmonary involvement, cyanosis, and anoxia. Other neurologic manifestations are uncommon. A macular rash (Horder's spots) resembling that seen in typhoid has occasionally been described. Jaundice and progressive nitrogen retention have been reported in severe cases. Severe dyspnea, tachypnea, tachycardia, cyanosis, jaundice, delirium, and stupor are all poor prognostic signs.

The physical findings of pneumonia are usually sparse. Chest roentgenograms often reveal infiltrates not detected at the bedside. Examination may reveal only fever, painful muscle groups, an elevated respiratory rate, and a relative bradycardia. Fine, crepitant rales may be heard in localized areas over the lungs, but true consolidation is less common. Pleurisy with effusion occurs but is unusual. Mild hepatomegaly is frequent. A palpable spleen has been noted in a substantial number of patients. Splenomegaly in a patient with undiagnosed acute pneumonitis should raise the consideration of psittacosis. An erythematous pharynx may be noted. In rare instances there may be signs of pericarditis or myocarditis. In prolonged, severe illness, thrombophlebitis and pulmonary infarction have been reported as late complications.

Patients with mild cases may recover in seven days. More severe infections may last 12 to 21 days without specific treatment. Defervescence is generally slow, and a prolonged convalescence is common. Relapses have been reported even after appropriate treatment. Reinfections have been described. Occasional cases of endocarditis caused by *C. psittaci* in patients with sterile blood cultures have been described.

LABORATORY FINDINGS. Simple laboratory studies are not helpful in establishing a diagnosis . The leukocyte count is usually normal or slightly elevated. The erythrocyte sedimentation rate is generally elevated. Chest roentgenograms show soft, patchy infiltrates radiating outward from the hilum, which tend to be more prominent in dependent lobes or segments. Occasionally diffuse miliary, nodular, or frank lobar distribution of infiltrates is seen.

A specific diagnosis can be made only by isolation of the agent or by serologic studies. The agent is present in the blood and sputum during the first two to three weeks, but owing to the high risk of laboratory-acquired infection, isolation is hazardous and should not be attempted except in special laboratories. Diagnosis is generally made by a fourfold rise in complement-fixing antibodies. A significant change in antibody titers is generally present by the twelfth to fourteenth day of disease; the titers are usually maximal by 30 days, then slowly wane. Treatment can delay or suppress antibody response. A serum complement-fixation titer of 1:32 during the acute illness is presumptive evidence of psittacosis. There is considerable cross-reaction between antigens prepared from psittacosis and lymphogranuloma venereum agents. False-positive complement-fixation tests may occur with Q fever, brucellosis, or legionnaires' disease.

DIFFERENTIAL DIAGNOSIS. Specific diagnosis of psittacosis is of extreme importance because of its potential severity, its response to antimicrobials, and the public health significance of psittacosis infection. All cases should be reported to the local health department. The syndrome of idiopathic pneumonia accompanied by protracted high fever, usually severe headache, and relative bradycardia should suggest psittacosis. Often a history of contact with birds is the only clue to diagnosis and may be elicited only by repeated questioning of the patient and family. When pneumonic symptoms are prominent, psittacosis must be differentiated from legionnaires' disease, viral pneumonias, mycoplasmal pneumonia, influenza, Q fever, tularemia, tuberculosis, fungal infection, and bacterial pneumonia distal to an obstructed bronchus. If pneumonic symptoms are not prominent, psittacosis can be confused with other systemic febrile illnesses such as typhoid fever, brucellosis, infectious mononucleosis, infectious hepatitis, miliary tuberculosis, or the viral meningoencephalitides.

TREATMENT. The tetracyclines are the drugs of choice, and early diagnosis and initiation of treatment may be lifesaving. After institution of therapy with 2 to 3 grams daily, both fever and symptoms are generally controlled within 48 to 72 hours, although the response may be indolent. Although the disease apparently responds to penicillin in doses above 2 million units daily and to erythromycin, tetracycline remains the drug of choice. Treatment should be continued for at least ten days after defervescence to prevent relapse. With treatment, mortality rates as low as 1 to 5 per cent can be achieved.

Byrom NP, Walls J, Mair HJ: Fulminant psittacosis. Lancet 1:353, 1979. *The difficulty in differentiating psittacosis and legionnaires' disease at the bedside is emphasized.*

Grayston JT, Kuo CC, Wang SP, et al.: A new *Chlamydia psittaci* strain, TWAR, isolated in acute respiratory tract infections. N Engl J Med 315:161, 1986. *Description of this new agent and the infections it appears to cause.*

Jariwalla AG, Davies BH, White J: Infective endocarditis complicating psittacosis: Response to rifampicin. Br Med J 1:155, 1980. *Endocarditis caused by psittacosis is reviewed concisely.*

Macfarlane JT, Macrae AD: Psittacosis. Br Med Bull 39:163, 1983. *A well-written review.*

Schaffner W, Drutz DJ, Duncan GW, et al.: The clinical spectrum of endemic psittacosis. Arch Intern Med 119:433, 1967. *Good descriptions of clinical presentations.*

Rickettsial Diseases

320 INTRODUCTION

Richard B. Hornick

The rickettsiae are small obligate intracellular, gram-negative pathogens. They do not have a symbiotic relationship with human host cells and therefore cause metabolic derangements that result in cell death. Infections with the typhus and spotted fever groups of rickettsiae involve endothelial cells. This host-pathogen interaction results in a perivasculitis. Q fever induces granulomas in the liver plus interstitial pneumonia. Fortunately, these small, gram-negative organisms are susceptible to tetracycline and chloramphenicol antibiotics so that patients recover quickly once the drugs are administered.

Each of the rickettsiae is transmitted to humans by ticks, mites, lice, fleas, or aerosols originating from animal products (placentas, Q fever) or from feces of the aforementioned insects. In the United States, there are relatively few cases of rickettsial infections. Rocky Mountain spotted fever is the most prevalent, 800 to 900 cases having been reported annually from 1983 to 1985. Fewer cases of Q fever and murine typhus are identified each year. Certain other rickettsial infections are major public health problems in developing coun-

TABLE 320–1. SUMMARY OF SOME EPIDEMIOLOGIC FEATURES OF SELECTED RICKETTSIAL DISEASES OF HUMANS

| Disease | Organism | Natural Cycle | | Usual Mode of Transmission to Humans | Common Occupational or Environmental Association | Geographic Distribution |
		Arthropod Vector	Reservoir/ Mammalian Host			
Typhus group						
Murine typhus	*Rickettsia mooseri* (*R. typhi*)	Flea	Rodents	Infected flea feces into broken skin or aerosol to mucous membranes	Rat-infected premises (shops, warehouses, grain elevators)	Scattered foci, worldwide
Epidemic typhus	*R. prowazekii*	Body louse	Humans*	Infected crushed louse or feces into broken skin or aerosol to mucous membranes	Lousy human population with louse transfer	Worldwide
Brill-Zinsser disease	*R. prowazekii*	Recrudescence months to years after primary attack of louse-borne typhus			Unknown; ?stress	Worldwide
Spotted fever group (selected examples)						
Rocky Mountain spotted fever	*R. rickettsii*	Ixodid ticks	Ticks/small mammals	Tick bite, mechanical transfer to mucous membranes, ?airborne	Tick-infested terrain, houses, dogs	Western hemisphere
Boutonneuse fever	*R. conorii*	Ixodid ticks	Ticks/rodents, dogs	Tick bite	Tick-infested terrain, houses, dogs	Mediterranean littoral, Africa, ?Indian subcontinent
Rickettsialpox	*R. akari*	Mouse mite	Mite/mice	Mouse mite bite	Unique mouse- and mite-infested premises (incinerators)	United States, U.S.S.R., Korea, ?Central Africa
Scrub typhus						
Tsutsugamushi disease	*R. tsutsugamushi* (multiple serotypes)	Chigger	Chigger/?rodents	Chigger bite	Chigger-infested terrain; secondary scrub, grass airfields, golf courses	Asia, Australia, New Guinea, Pacific islands
Q fever	*Coxiella burnetii*	?Ticks	Ticks/mammals	Inhalation of dried airborne infective material; ?tick bite	Domestic animals or products, dairies, lambing pens, slaughterhouses	Worldwide
Trench fever	*Rochalimaea quintana*	Body louse	Humans	Infected crushed louse or feces into broken skin; ?aerosol to mucous membranes	Lousy human population with louse transfer	Africa, Mexico, ?South America, ?Eastern Europe

*Recent isolations of putative *R. prowazekii* from flying squirrels in the eastern United States have not been evaluated as reservoirs for human infection. Previous claims of involvement of domestic animals are now largely discounted.

TABLE 320–2. RICKETTSIA TARGET CELL RELATIONSHIPS, PATHOLOGIC LESIONS, AND CLINICAL MANIFESTATIONS OF HUMAN RICKETTSIOSES*

Disease	Target Cell	Host-Cell Association	Basic Lesion	Clinical Manifestations
Typhus-like fevers				
Typhus group	Endothelial	Free intracytoplasmic	Vasculitis	Acute self-limited fever
Scrub typhus	Endothelial	Free intracytoplasmic	Vasculitis	Acute self-limited fever
Spotted fever group	Endothelial, smooth muscle	Free intracytoplasmic and intranuclear	Vasculitis	Acute self-limited fever
Q fever	Reticuloendothelial	Intracytoplasmic vacuole	Granulomas	Acute self-limited fever, "atypical pneumonia," subacute hepatitis, subacute endocarditis
Trench fever	Unknown	Pericellular (in louse and cell culture)	Unknown	Recurring febrile episodes

*Adapted from Strickland (ed.): Hunter's Tropical Medicine. Philadelphia, W. B. Saunders Company, 1984.

TABLE 320–3. SOME CLINICAL FEATURES OF SELECTED RICKETTSIAL DISEASES

Disease	Usual Incubation Period (Days)	Eschar	Rash — Onset, Day of Disease	Rash — Distribution	Rash — Type	Usual Duration of Disease* (Days)	Usual Severity†	Fever After Chemotherapy (Hours)
Typhus group								
Murine typhus	12 (8–16)	None	5–7	Trunk → extremities	Macular, maculopapular	12 (8–16)	Moderate	48–72
Epidemic typhus	12 (10–14)	None	5–7	Trunk → extremities	Macular, maculopapular, petechial	14 (10–18)	Severe	48–72
Brill-Zinsser disease	—	None		Trunk → extremities	Macular	7–11	Relatively mild	48–72
Spotted fever group								
Rocky Mountain spotted fever	7 (3–12)	None	3–5	Extremities → trunk, face	Macular, maculopapular, petechial	16 (10–20)	Severe	72
Boutonneuse fever	5–7	Often present	3–4	Trunk, extremities, face, palms, soles	Macular, maculopapular, petechial	10 (7–14) 7	Moderate	—
Rickettsialpox	?9–17	Often present	1–3	Trunk → face, extremities	Papulovesicular	7 (3–11)	Relatively mild	—
Scrub typhus (tsutsugamushi disease)	1–12 (9–18)	Often present	4–6	Trunk → extremities	Macular, maculopapular	14 (10–20)	Mild to severe	24–36
Q fever	10–19	None		None		6 (2–21)	Relatively‡ mild	48 (occasionally slow)

*Untreated disease.
†Severity can vary greatly.
‡Occasional subacute infections occur (e.g., hepatitis, endocarditis).

tries but are not found in the United States, e.g., scrub typhus. The potential for tourists to return to the United States with an emerging rickettsial infection is increasing. Because of the rarity of rickettsial infections in the United States, diagnosis may be delayed. Delays in diagnosing these illnesses can adversely affect the potential for recovery.

In this introductory chapter, three tables* are included that summarize, first, the epidemiologic features of rickettsial infections; second, the host cells involved in the pathogenesis of the clinical manifestations of the disease; and third, those clinical features that will assist in differentiating the various forms of rickettsial infections. The following chapters provide additional details on the major rickettsial infections that are found in this country or that represent potential threats to persons traveling abroad.

*The author is indebted to Dr. Charles L. Wisseman, Jr., for permission to reprint these tables from the 17th edition of the *Cecil Textbook of Medicine.*

321 THE TYPHUS GROUP

Richard B. Hornick

This group of conditions includes three established clinical and epidemiologic entitis: epidemic louse-borne typhus fever, the oldest disease known to be caused by rickettsiae; Brill-Zinsser disease, a classic example of reactivation of a latent infection; and flea-borne murine typhus. The first two conditions are induced by *Rickettsia prowazekii*, a pathogen transferred from person to person by the bite of body lice. Persons who have recovered from epidemic typhus have persistent rickettsiae in various host cells, presumably in the reticuloendothelial cells; stresses that cause a defect in the suppressive lymphocytes will, years later, permit these rickettsiae to be

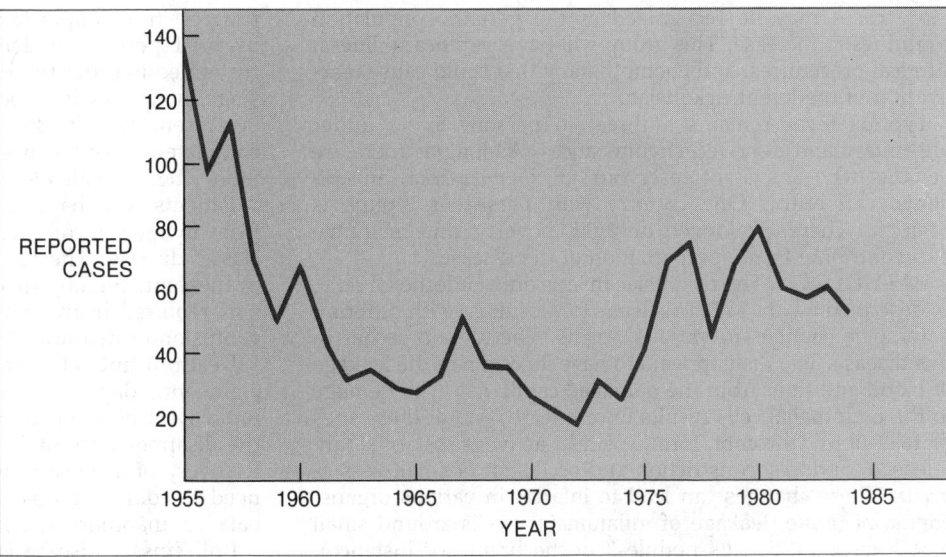

FIGURE 321–1. Flea-borne (endemic, murine) typhus fever: cases, by year in the United States, from 1955 to 1984. For 1984, 53 cases of murine typhus were reported from six states. Thirty-seven of the cases were reported from Texas, eight from California, and five from Hawaii.

reactivated, resulting in a mild typhus-like illness, called Brill-Zinsser disease. In 1975, *R. prowazekii* was isolated from flying squirrels in the southeastern United States. A number of persons acquired typhus fever from squirrels living in their attics and probably harboring infected fleas or lice or both.

Flea-borne murine typhus, caused by *R. typhi*, is a mild form of typhus fever occurring in this country and elsewhere. It is transmitted by fleas from rodents (Fig. 321–1). Finally a new species in this group, *R. canada*, has been isolated. It is transmitted by a tick, but it has serologic cross-reactions with *R. prowazekii*. Additional clinical information is needed to determine what role *R. canada* plays in inducing human rickettsial disease.

EPIDEMIC LOUSE-BORNE TYPHUS

INTRODUCTION. Synonyms include classic, historic, and European typhus; jail, war, camp, and ship fever; *Flichfieber* (German); *typhus exanthematique* (French); and *tifus exantematico* and *tabardillo* (Spanish). Many of these names indicate the location of the outbreaks—military and concentration camps, crowded ships with poor and starved immigrants, outbreaks in persons living in occupied countries during wartime, and so forth. Each implies crowded, unsanitary living conditions where bathing and laundry facilities are inadequate. These conditions allow for the breeding and propagation of body lice. The impact of typhus fever on military campaigns and immigration patterns is a fascinating and provocative story. The reader is referred to Woodward for an introduction to the effects of this disease on history.

DEFINITION. Classic typhus fever is manifested by the sudden onset of headache, fever, rash, and an altered mental state. (Typhus is derived from the Greek word meaning cloudy or misty. Applied to typhus, it describes the obtunded, lethargic state of mind.) *R. prowazekii* is transmitted by human body lice (*Pediculus humanus humanus*).

ETIOLOGY. *R. prowazekii* is a small obligate intracellular, gram-negative bacillus. In cells it stains red when exposed to Gimenez's stain. Viable rickettsiae stimulate the endothelial cell to act like a phagocyte to engulf the rickettsiae in a phagosome and internalize it. If rickettsiae do not break out of the phagosome promptly, they begin to disintegrate, perhaps owing to enzymatic activities. The rickettsiae have an enzyme, phospholipase A, that enables them to lyse the phagosome wall and to multiply freely in the cytoplasm. *R. prowazekii* escape from the cell by destroying it. The necrotic cell stimulates an inflammatory response that leads to the vasculitis and subsequent clotting abnormalities.

TRANSMISSION AND EPIDEMIOLOGY. The unique feature of infection with *R. prowazekii* is that no animal reservoir has been implicated at least until its isolation from the flying squirrel (*Glaucomys volans*). It is still uncertain how significant the flying squirrel will be in amplifying the incidence of this disease. Very few, if any, cases of classic typhus occur each year in this country (Centers for Disease Control does not have an active surveillance for it). Fifteen cases were reported in 1980 and 1981, all in persons having contact with flying squirrels.

Classic typhus is a disease of humans. An individual with rickettsemia can infect body lice. The lice acquire the organisms in their blood meal. These ectoparasites may then find another person to whom they transmit the rickettsiae via infected feces. Body lice do not survive the ingestion of rickettsiae. The organisms multiply in the gut of the louse, destroy the epithelial cells, and the louse dies (usually in one to three weeks). However, during the period of infection, the louse will pass feces heavily laden with rickettsiae. Either the human host will scratch the site of the bite and thereby self-inoculate the rickettsiae, or the feces and rickettsiae can contaminate minute apertures in the epidermis, allowing the organisms to find cells in which to multiply. Dried, contaminated feces can also become airborne, e.g., by shaking out one's clothes loaded with lice and feces and thereby creating an infectious aerosol. When inhaled, the rickettsiae can penetrate the mucosal cells and enter endothelial cells. Laboratory accidents frequently generate aerosols that induce infection in technicians. Nurses and other medical personnel are at risk of inhaling airborne particles when they remove the clothing from a patient.

When the body louse obtains a blood meal containing antibody-coated rickettsiae, the louse may modify the infectivity of the rickettsiae-antibody combination by partially digesting the antibody coating of the organism in its gut. This digestion destroys the Fc portion of the antibody that would have permitted attachment to macrophages. The rickettsia is then free of the inhibiting action of the antibody when it infects the next person.

The louse does not transmit *R. prowazekii* transovarially to offspring and is not an amplifier for further propagation. Patients who recover from classic typhus have the opportunity to develop Brill-Zinsser disease and at that time will have rickettsemia and be able again to infect body lice. However, this happens rarely, for few cases of Brill-Zinsser disease have been detected among the many hundreds of thousands of soldiers who acquired typhus in World War II; one estimate suggested a rate of 10 per 100,000 cases of primary typhus.

More cases may be recognized as the geriatric population continues to increase. This group will have significant illness, surgical procedures, and chemotherapy that could cause reactivation of the latent rickettsiae.

Typhus fever remains a threat to persons living under unsanitary and deprived circumstances. As long as there are persons who are latent reservoirs for *R. prowazekii*, an epidemic can erupt. One country with persistent typhus is Ethiopia. There, prolonged drought, poverty, and malnutrition contribute to the perpetuation of the disease.

PATHOLOGY. The rickettsiae invade only endothelial cells, as described in Ch. 322. This leads to vasculitis, with differing pathologic changes in various organs. There is no eschar in this disease. The rash appears to have its origin in the leakage of blood and fluid from the damaged capillaries. The damage to the endothelial cells results in cell death, and at these sites platelet-fibrin thrombi form, platelet-active substances are released, and vasoconstriction and occlusion of small vessels occur. These changes can lead to infarcts in various organs, edema of tissue, leakage of inflammatory cells around small blood vessels ("typhus nodules" of the brain, for instance), stimulation of clotting mechanisms, and the development of shock. Almost all organs are involved in patients with untreated disease. The inflammatory exudate consists of mononuclear cells, plasma cells, histiocytes, and polymorphonuclear leukocytes. Gangrene of skin and limbs occurs in the presence of extensive thrombotic activity.

CLINICAL MANIFESTATIONS AND COURSE. The incubation period is about 7 days on the average but can range from 6 to 15 days. The onset is abrupt with intense headache, chills, fever, and myalgia. There is back or leg pain—presumably due to the muscle damage secondary to the vasculitis. Bites of lice may cause pruritus, and persons infested with lice may have numerous scratches in the skin. Sometimes the skin will have a yellow-gold hue because of frequent lice bites. The headache is described as the "worst ever," and the pain is unremitting unless treated with narcotic analgesics. The temperature rises quickly during the first two days and persists for about two weeks, maintaining a continuous fever pattern if not altered by antibiotics or antipyretic medications. During the first week, there is a bradycardia relative to the temperature elevations of 39° to 41°C. Conjunctivae are injected, and photophobia is present. Deafness, tinnitus, and sometimes vertigo are prominent features. The patient appears to be in a toxic state, with a flushed face, obtundation, and profound weakness. There may be a cough, but no rales are apparent on auscultation of the lungs. The pharyngeal mucous lining is dry and inflamed.

The rash, characteristic of the typhus group, appears on the fourth to seventh day of disease. The lesions appear first on the trunk and axillary folds (areas of skin stress) and spread to the extremities but spare the palms and soles of the feet. The lesions are reddish-pink macules that fade on pressure. With treatment or in mild cases, the rash disappears within several days. In untreated patients, it can spread and coalesce, leading to gangrene of portions of the skin, especially over regions of bony prominences. In 5 to 10 per cent of patients, the rash may not be present.

These and other manifestations of the disease occur because of the initial unchecked multiplication and spread of the rickettsiae, involving ever-enlarging segments of the endothelial surface. The resulting damage to the organs evolves because of the compromised circulation and the associated acute inflammatory responses. Whether rickettsial toxin or endotoxin contributes to the pathologic changes is still a debated point. Whatever processes are involved, certain organs are regularly involved: the skin, heart, kidneys, and skeletal muscle. In patients with severe disease, hypotension and renal failure portend a fatal outcome.

The altered mental status that occurs as the disease progresses (in untreated patients) is striking. The patient may progress from stupor to coma. The stupor may be interrupted by brief periods of delirium. The patient may have to be restrained in order to protect him or her from trauma. At this stage, lymphocytic pleocytosis of the cerebrospinal fluid may be present. Despite the seriousness of the patient's condition, complete recovery can ensue. Cranial nerve lesions are common. There are also temporary mental aberrations.

Patients who have acquired typhus fever in this country from flying squirrels have had signs and symptoms of the classic disease. The rash was noted in 8 of 15, and it was evanescent. Significant central nervous system involvement was reported in five patients; two had coma and three had confusion or delirium.

Death in untreated patients occurs between the ninth and eighteenth days. Recovery from the disease begins with a rapid lysis of fever after about two weeks of disease. With the disappearance of fever, mental function returns quickly. Recovery of a sense of well-being is protracted owing to the need to counter the stresses of prolonged negative nitrogen balance, inanition, and loss of muscle mass.

Brill-Zinsser disease is manifested in a manner similar to classic typhus. All signs and symptoms are milder, presumably because the host has well-developed immune mechanisms that can regain control in a short time. Serologic studies in these patients demonstrate immunoglobulin G (IgG) rather than immunoglobulin M (IgM) antibodies. Occasionally, patients with unrecognized Brill-Zinsser disease will die. An underlying disease or procedure may permit activation of the latent rickettsiae, and this combination can culminate in death. Reactivation has been noted following surgical procedures and the use of immunosuppressive drugs. In experimental animals that have recovered from the primary disease, isolation of rickettsiae at a future date is facilitated by the administration of steroids.

PROGNOSIS. The fatality rate in untreated groups of patients with classic typhus is 10 to 60 per cent. Children usually have a mild illness with minimal risk of death. Patients over 60 years of age have the highest mortality rate. Recovery is the rule with appropriate antibiotic treatment.

TREATMENT. *R. prowazekii* responds well to tetracycline and chloramphenicol antibiotics. Doxycycline, 200 mg as a single oral dose, is the treatment of choice. Tetracycline, 25 mg per kilogram daily in four doses, is chloramphenicol, 50 mg per kilogram daily in four doses, is an effective alternative. Therapy should be continued for two to three days after the fever has defervesced. Most patients are afebrile within 48 to 72 hours and improve quickly from the debilitating headache or mental aberrations or both. Relapses occur in persons who are treated early, on day 1 or 2 of illness. Such patients do not develop the required immune mechanisms to contain the proliferation of the residual rickettsiae. Furthermore, both antibiotics are rickettsiostatic and do not eradicate all of these intracellular parasites even with the introduction of specific immune mechanisms. Recovery from disease without the assistance of antibiotic therapy also allows rickettsiae to remain in cells, later to be activated and cause Brill-Zinsser disease. In the severely ill patient, fluid therapy and proper nutrition are mandatory. Fortunately, antibiotic therapy has simplified the need for supportive care.

PREVENTION AND CONTROL. To prevent and control the spread of classic typhus, the body lice (and feces) associated with patients and their clothes must be destroyed. The clothing should be carefully placed in plastic bags and sealed and carefully removed only in the area where they are to be treated. Clothes that can sustain boiling are boiled, and the rest should be subjected to steam and dry heat. It is also possible to kill the lice (also the eggs present in seams and elsewhere—these eggs will hatch in a week) with insecticides. Formerly, 10 per cent DDT (chlorophenothane) was used, but lice are now generally resistant to it. Resistance has also become a problem with 1 per cent lindane dust. Malathion

(1 per cent) and 2 per cent temefos (Abate) are effective in most areas. These dusts are applied to the fully clothed individual. This approach will control the acute outbreaks of disease when applied to all persons in the community. Long-time use of insecticides is not effective because of the development of resistance, because long-term compliance is difficult, and because the insecticides may have a deleterious effect on the ecology of the region. Control requires improvement of sanitary conditions and standards of living as well as health education.

Health personnel who encounter patients with classic typhus are at risk for acquiring the disease from lice picked up from the patient or his or her clothes. There is no risk of direct human-to-human transfer of the rickettsiae other than by aerosolized, dried, contaminated feces. Once the patient has been deloused, no isolation barriers are required.

No vaccine is currently available for preventing classic typhus.

Travelers to endemic areas are rarely at risk unless, for example, they work in camps for displaced persons or carry out relief work that brings them in contact with persons with lice. Decontaminating the clothing overnight with insecticides or wearing insect repellent–treated clothes will provide some protection. Prophylactic doxycycline has been effective when given weekly to prevent scrub typhus and would be expected to be effective in preventing *R. prowazekii* infections. This drug should be used only for short periods, two to four weeks. It is important under these circumstances to monitor the temperature for two weeks at least, as the drug may have masked the initial infection and delayed the onset of symptoms. Retreatment with doxycycline at the onset of the fever is curative.

MURINE TYPHUS

DEFINITION. Murine typhus, a milder form of classic typhus, is caused by *Rickettsia typhi* and is transmitted from rodents to humans by means of the rat flea (*Xenopsylla cheopis*). It is the only disease of the typhus group that occurs regularly in the United States, albeit in small numbers.

ETIOLOGY. *R. typhi* is a small, gram-negative, obligate, intracellular pathogen. Like *R. prowazekii*, it can penetrate into endothelial cells by induced phagocytosis. Its disease potential resides in its ability to multiply in these cells, destroy them, and initiate a vasculitis. *R. typhi* is catalogued with the typhus group because it shares common antigens with *R. prowazekii* and *R. canada*. In addition, there is cross-immunity between *R. prowazekii* and *R. typhi* induced by infections. Despite these similarities, it is clear from deoxyribonucleic acid (DNA) homology studies that the two are not closely related.

TRANSMISSION AND EPIDEMIOLOGY. *R. typhi* causes disease worldwide. Wherever there are large rodent populations, there is the potential for outbreaks. The rat and other small animals serve as reservoirs of this disease. *Rattus rattus* and *Rattus norvegicus* are two species of rats that can sustain the *R. typhi*, serve as a source of rickettsiae for the rat flea, and have no obvious illness from carrying this human pathogen. The rat flea disseminates the infection not through its bite but by placing contaminated feces on the skin. These may be rubbed or scratched into the skin; they can be carried to the conjunctival sac or mucous membranes on the fingers, where the rickettsiae can invade; or they can be aerosolized after drying and cause infection if inhaled. In the flea, the rickettsiae multiply in the enterocytes in the gut, do not kill the flea, and continue to be shed in the feces for the life of the flea. The rickettsiae are not transmitted by fleas to their offspring.

The numbers of cases reported to the Centers for Disease Control (CDC) from 1955 to 1984 are shown in Figure 321–1. Fifty-three cases were reported in 1984, most from Texas and California. These numbers probably represent an under-reporting of the true incidence. There was a dramatic drop in the number of reported cases after the mid 1940's. In 1944 there were over 5400 cases. By 1954 there were 163. This decline was due to intensive efforts at rodent control. Most of the cases occur in the warmer months, when rat fleas are plentiful.

PATHOLOGY. Descriptions of the pathologic lesions in this disease are few because of the rarity of fatal cases. Since the rickettsiae are known to invade endothelial cells, the pathologic consequences should mimic those seen in other rickettsial infections. The reasons for the differences in virulence of these rickettsiae and the varying severity of illnesses produced are unknown.

CLINICAL MANIFESTATIONS AND COURSE. Headache, fever, and myalgia are the principal symptoms and signs associated with illness produced by *R. typhi*. These appear after an incubation period of about one to two weeks. A faint macular-papular pink-colored rash appears in about 80 per cent of patients after four to five days of illness. It may be difficult to see in poor light. When present, it may be visible for four to eight days before it gradually fades.

Rarely are there any significant complications of this infection, but as it is an infection of the endothelial cells, there is a vasculitis that can cause widespread organ derangement. The patients, especially if older, are debilitated by the infection when not treated. They may remain febrile, with a temperature of 39 to 40°C for two weeks. This metabolic stress necessitates prolonged convalescence. Antibiotic therapy brings about a prompt recovery.

DIAGNOSIS. This disease has no distinguishing characteristics during the early days of symptoms. The rash appearing on the fourth or fifth day of illness should alert the physician to the possibility of a rickettsial infection. The history of a possible exposure to areas where rats are known to exist, e.g., grain elevators, port facilities, and farm buildings, will provide useful information. Flea bites, if seen early, are discrete and may have a central hemorrhagic punctum. The location and grouping of flea bites are important diagnostic features. They occur in covered parts of the body, in irregular groups of several to a dozen or more. They may be in the region of the belt, shoulders, and hips or on the legs.

Differentiating this disease from Rocky Mountain spotted fever (RMSF) may be difficult. The rash of RMSF usually begins on the wrists and palms and on the soles of the feet and then extends to the skin of the thorax and abdomen. In murine typhus the lesions are on the skin of the chest and abdomen and rarely on the extremities. The history of a tick bite or exposure provides evidence for a clinical diagnosis of RMSF.

Serologic studies will confirm the rickettsial infection. Weil-Felix OX-19 reaction is positive in most patients who have not received antibiotic treatment. This test, however, will not distinguish murine typhus from the spotted fever group of infections. The indirect immunofluorescent test can be used to identify *R. typhi* infections. However, because of the common antigens shared with *R. prowazekii*, the serum requires cross-absorption with special antigens from these two rickettsia strains. Isolation of the organism is possible but should be done only in special laboratories where containment facilities are available.

PROGNOSIS. The mortality rate is less than 5 per cent in untreated patients. Appropriate antibiotic treatment results in prompt cure, and the mortality rate is reduced almost to zero.

TREATMENT. Tetracycline and chloramphenicol are effective drugs for treating this rickettsial infection. A five- to seven-day course of either is effective. The usual dosage of 25 mg per kilogram of tetracycline per day in four doses or chloramphenicol, 50 mg per kilogram per day in four doses, will effect a prompt cure. The organisms are sensitive to these antibiotics. No resistant strains have been identified. Relapses do occur when antibiotics are administered early in the course of the illness. Retreatment with the antibiotic of choice provides prompt response.

PREVENTION AND CONTROL. There is no vaccine to prevent this disease. Control of rats has been shown to be very effective. When rat control programs are instituted, appropriate insecticides should be simultaneously used to prevent the fleas from seeking humans for feeding as the rat population is decreased.

Bozeman FM, Maisello SA, Williams MG, et al.: Epidemic typhus rickettsia isolated from flying squirrels. Nature 225:545, 1975. Duma RJ, Sonenshine DE, Bozeman FM, et al.: Epidemic typhus in the United States associated with flying squirrels. JAMA 245:2318, 1981. *These two papers provide a good background on the discovery of the flying squirrel as a reservoir of R. prowazekii and the disease associated with exposure to these animals and their ectoparasites.*

Gaon JA, Murray ES: The natural history of recrudescent typhus (Brill-Zinsser disease) in Bosnia. Bull WHO 35:133, 1966. *Classic paper describing the studies conducted to prove that Brill-Zinsser disease is truly a recrudescence of classic typhus fever.*

Rollivagen FM, Bakun AJ, Dorsey CN, et al.: Mechanisms of immunity to infection with typhus rickettsiae: Infected fibroblasts bear rickettsial antigens on their surfaces. Infect Immun 50:911, 1985.

Walker TS: Rickettsial interactions with human endothelial cells in vitro: Adherence and entry. Infect Immun 44:205, 1984.

Wohlbach SB, Todd JI, Palfrey FW: The Etiology and Pathology of Typhus. Cambridge, Mass., Harvard Press, 1922. *This book will provide the reader with an excellent description of the natural course of classic typhus fever.*

Woodward TE: A historical account of the rickettsial diseases with a discussion of unsolved problems. J Infect Dis 127:5, 1973.

322 ROCKY MOUNTAIN SPOTTED FEVER

Richard B. Hornick

SYNONYMS. Rocky Mountain spotted fever (RMSF) is also known as typhus fever, tick-borne, by the Centers for Disease Control (CDC), *fiebre manchada* (Mexico), *fiebre petequial* (Colombia), and *febre maculosa* or Sao Paulo typhus (Brazil).

DEFINITION. Rocky Mountain spotted fever is a sometimes fatal systemic infection manifested by fever, severe headache, rash, and other organ disease caused by the vasculitis induced by *Rickettsia rickettsii*. The organism is usually transmitted to humans from animal reservoirs by a tick bite.

ETIOLOGY. *R. rickettsii* organisms are small, gram-negative, coccobacillary bacteria that can grow only inside eukaryotic host cells. They cannot be isolated on cell-free culture media. In human infections the rickettsiae invade and multiply within endothelial cells of arteries and veins. Different strains of *R. rickettsii* vary in virulence in human as well as animal hosts. Mortality rates appear to be higher in Montana than on the Eastern seaboard. Attempts to correlate virulence with structural components in the polysaccharide portion of the cell wall have been unsuccessful. However, two surface proteins, with molecular weights of 120,000 and 155,000, have been identified as possible virulence factors (protective antigens), and the latter has been produced from cloned genes in *Escherichia coli*. The antigenic material protects mice from lethal infection and will be studied as a potential vaccine.

DISTRIBUTION AND INCIDENCE. This disease was named for the geographic site of its original discovery; the causative agent was named for the discoverer, Howard T. Ricketts. By the 1940's the disease had become more common on the East Coast than in the West. The incidence rose sharply beginning in 1971, peaked at 1.91/100,000 population in 1980 in the eight South Atlantic states. Subsequently, it has fallen to a value similar to that of 1970 (Fig. 322–1). In other parts of the United States, the incidence increased slightly from 1970 to 1977 but has remained stable at that level in the past eight years. A total of 847 cases of RMSF were reported in 1984 in the United States.

Serologic surveys in children and adults in North Carolina, the state with the highest number of reported cases, demonstrate that subclinical infections occur. Almost 20 per cent of the children had OX-19 agglutination titers in the diagnostic range, and a smaller number had positive indirect fluorescent antibody titers, a more specific test. None of these children was previously diagnosed as having had Rocky Mountain spotted fever.

TRANSMISSION AND EPIDEMIOLOGY. Ninety-five per cent of reported cases occur between April 1 and September 30, with two thirds in May, June, and July. Children and young adults account for about 40 per cent of cases. Ninety per cent of patients will give a history of a tick bite or attachment or of having been in a tick-infested area 14 days prior to onset of illness.

Rocky Mountain spotted fever occurs in humans when an infected tick bites and injects *R. rickettsii* into the skin. Probably fewer than ten organisms injected intradermally are sufficient to induce disease.

Several species of ticks are commonly involved in transmission of disease: *Dermacentor andersoni*, the wood tick, in the Rocky Mountain states; *Dermacentor variabilis*, the dog tick, in the East and Oklahoma; *Amblyomma americanum* in Texas and Oklahoma; and *Rhipicephalus sanguineus* in Texas and Mexico. These ticks feed on small mammals such as ground squirrels and rabbits as well as on larger animals such as bear and deer. Dogs serve as a reservoir to infect ticks and then other animals or humans. Figure 322–2 shows the distribution of cases of Rocky Mountain spotted fever by county in the United States in 1984.

Laboratory-acquired infections have occurred in persons exposed to droplets from accidental generation of aerosols from solutions of the organism. However, even in circumstances conducive to airborne transmission, person-to-person transmission does not occur. Rocky Mountain spotted fever can also be acquired by the transfusion of contaminated blood.

PATHOLOGY. The basis of the pathologic changes in this disease, as in other rickettsial infections, is the inflammatory response stimulated by the irreparable damage of the endothelial cells. In patients dying within three to five days of onset of disease, significant coagulation abnormalities are present. Causes may include damage to the endothelial cells with release of factor VIII; and stimulation of the release of platelet factors by damage to the endothelium or by activation of the kallikrein-kinin system by the Hageman factor. Microinfarcts result from occlusions of small vessels, and edema and hemorrhages occur secondary to increased permeability of the vasculature. Such lesions can be found in the heart, kidneys, adrenals, lungs, brain, skin, spleen, and subcutaneous tissues.

The rash is thought to result from the vasculitis and the associated permeability changes. Petechial lesions are caused by microhemorrhages secondary to the vasculitis and thrombocytopenia.

Patients with glucose-6-phosphate dehydrogenase (G6PD) deficiency appear to be prone to severe infections caused by *R. rickettsii* and other rickettsial agents. These patients have severe hemolytic reactions and significant thrombotic lesions in the glomeruli, resulting in oliguria.

CLINICAL MANIFESTATIONS. The incubation period of naturally acquired disease has a range of 2 to 14 days with an average of 7 days. The onset of disease in the typical case is sudden, with a severe headache, often retrobulbar in location, chills, fever, myalgia, malaise, nausea and vomiting, conjunctival injection, and photophobia. Tenderness may be present in large muscle groups. The duration of fever in untreated cases is about two weeks, but recovery from the debilitating effects of the disease requires several additional weeks.

Rash appears in 80 to 90 per cent of patients—usually on the third or fourth day of fever, rarely after five or more days. It consists of pink macules, 2 to 5 mm, often noted first about

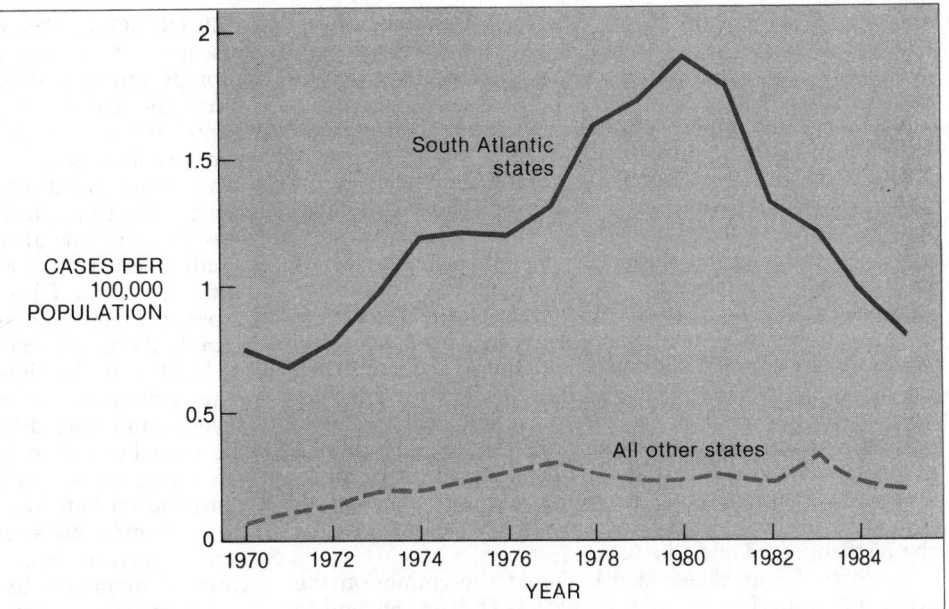

FIGURE 322–1. Rates of reported Rocky Mountain spotted fever cases, by year, in the South Atlantic states and all other states, from 1970 to 1985. The South Atlantic states comprise Delaware, Maryland, Virginia, West Virginia, North Carolina, South Carolina, Georgia, Florida, and the District of Columbia.

the wrists and ankles. Lesions then spread to arms, chest, face, feet, and abdomen. Rarely does the rash involve the mucous membranes. Initially, these lesions will blanch with pressure, but after two to three days they become fixed and turn dark red or purple and then slowly disappear during convalescence. The latter lesions represent microhemorrhages. Lesions on the palms and soles of the feet, in conjunction with the rash elsewhere, and petechial lesions in the skin folds of the axillae and around the ankles, constitute the classic distribution of the rash. Biopsy of the rash will reveal perivascular round cell infiltration. Staining of the specimens of skin with fluorescent tagged antibodies to *R. rickettsii* will reveal the intracellular organisms.

In patients with unrecognized and inappropriately treated disease, the rash will coalesce as the spread of the infectious process involves additional and larger vessels. This can result in large ischemic and gangrenous lesions. Especially susceptible is the skin of the tip of the nose, ear lobes, digits, and scrotum. Involvement of the cooler portions of the body may reflect the optimal temperature for growth of *R. rickettsii* (32°C). Thrombosis of larger arteries can cause gangrene of a limb or hemiplegia. Patients with untreated disease may die of myocarditis and pulmonary edema.

The reported incidence of pulmonary abnormalities varies from 10 to 40 per cent in large series of patients. Respiratory symptoms and signs as part of this illness have not been

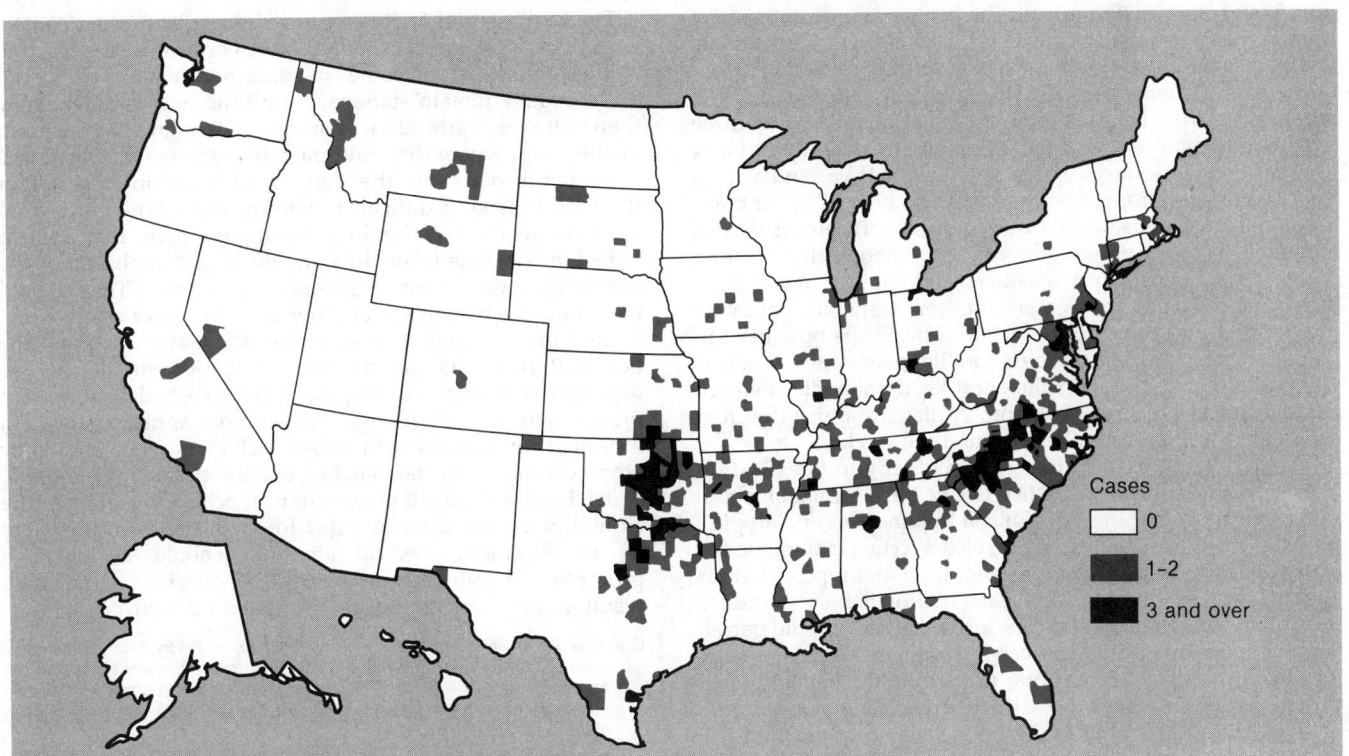

FIGURE 322–2. Tick-borne typhus fever (Rocky Mountain spotted fever): Cases, by county, in the United States in 1984.

emphasized sufficiently. In fact, after the spleen, the heaviest concentrations of rickettsiae can be demonstrated by fluorescent antibody staining in the endothelial cells of the pulmonary vasculature.

Edema of the brain and ring hemorrhages may cause delirium and stupor and ultimately lead to death.

DIAGNOSIS. The diagnosis of RMSF is difficult in the patient presenting with nonspecific complaints such as sudden onset of fever, headache, myalgia, and malaise. A history of travel, camping, or outdoor recreational activities where tick exposure could occur and of recent tick bites is an especially important part of any workup of a febrile patient during the warmer months of the year. The patient will complain of a severe headache, photophobia, and pain when moving the eyes. There is no meningismus. Lumbar puncture will usually reveal normal cerebrospinal fluid (CSF). Patients with stupor or coma may demonstrate elevated CSF protein and a few mononuclear cells. The presence of a faint, pink-colored rash on wrists and ankles should raise a suspicion of RMSF. Helpful in making the diagnosis is the knowledge that the rash appeared after the fever.

A search for an attached tick should concentrate on the scalp and groin. Hard body ticks such as *D. andersoni* tend to remain attached for long periods. The finding of an engorged tick should provide the needed information for a clinical diagnosis. There will usually be no ulceration or scar from the tick bite.

Most patients will have thrombocytopenia but not significant clotting abnormalities. In severe cases, disseminated intravascular coagulopathy (DIC) occurs with hypofibrinogenemia and prolonged prothrombin and partial thromboplastin times. Other laboratory studies are not helpful in making a diagnosis. The white blood cell count is usually normal.

Confirmation of RMSF is achieved by immunofluorescence staining of tissue specimens and by serologic analyses. The detection by immunofluorescence of rickettsiae in tissues, such as skin or rash biopsies, is the one test that can provide the most rapid (four to six hours) and early (day three to four) diagnosis. The state health department should be contacted about the availability of this test.

Serologic tests do not provide rapid diagnostic confirmation. The Weil-Felix reaction utilizes the polysaccharide antigens of three *Proteus* strains (OX-19, OX-2, and OX-K) to agglutinate antibodies produced by a rickettsial infection. Serum specimens from patients with RMSF agglutinate OX-19 and OX-2, but not OX-K. The peak titer occurs at about two to three weeks and then falls rapidly. Antibiotic treatment will blunt the antibody response. The test is inexpensive, and with a fourfold or greater increase in titer of OX-19 or OX-2, or both, in paired specimens (drawn two weeks apart) confirmation is obtained. Indirect immunofluorescent antibody (IFA) testing is the most specific and sensitive serologic test available. It has replaced the complement fixation test and, in many laboratories, the Weil-Felix reaction. The IFA is now used in epidemiologic surveys because of the persistence of these antibodies compared with the short-lived antibodies demonstrated in the Weil-Felix reaction. A diagnostic rise (fourfold or greater) in titer also takes two to three weeks.

Differentiation of this disease from other infections is difficult without the history of a tick bite or the information about the fever preceding the rash. In children measles and atypical measles (in those who received killed vaccine) can mimic the early phase of RMSF illness. The location and type of lesions making up the rash, the presence of Koplik's spots, and a history of measles-like illness in close associates should permit a differentiation. Meningococcemia with meningitis usually produces petechiae or purpura, or both, in the patient earlier in the course of the disease than expected in all but rare patients with RMSF. Furthermore, the cerebrospinal fluid will indicate the septic nature of the meningitis caused by the meningococci.

PROGNOSIS. Patients with RMSF have a serious infectious disease that involves endothelial cells throughout the host. Prompt antibiotic therapy is necessary to assist cellular immune mechanisms to eliminate the pathogen. In some patients, the pathologic processes spread rapidly and cause irreversible damage, and death ensues within three to five days (fulminant disease). Certain risk factors correlate with severe diseases: presence of G6PD/A−, time of onset of specific antibiotic therapy, and black males living in the southeastern United States during the tick season. Patients with the classic form of RMSF who are untreated have a prolonged febrile illness lasting two to three weeks with many complications. The mortality rate in such patients is 20 to 30 per cent, with the highest rate occurring in the elderly. Death may occur from the ninth to the fifteenth day, often from severe pulmonary disease. Antibiotic treatment has lowered the mortality rate to 3 to 10 per cent. The 1985 case fatality rates were greater for blacks (16 per cent) than whites (3 per cent) and for individuals 40 years of age or older (9 per cent) than for individuals under 40 years (2 per cent). This is a serious disease requiring that patients be hospitalized and carefully monitored to detect changes in pulmonary findings and evidence of hypotension, oliguria, myocarditis, or increasing intracranial pressure.

TREATMENT. Prompt initiation of tetracycline or chloramphenicol therapy is mandatory to insure optimal chances for recovery. Tetracycline (25 to 50 mg per kilogram per day), doxycycline (100 mg every 12 hours in adults), and chloramphenicol (50 mg per kilogram per day) are the drugs of choice. Usually the fever abates in two to three days, and concurrently a sense of well-being is restored. Antibiotic treatment can be discontinued two to three days thereafter. No reported instances of strains resistant to the tetracyclines or chloramphenicol have been reported. The newer third-generation cephalosporins, 4-amino-quinolones, or the aminoglycoside antibiotics have not been evaluated in RMSF. Relapses after tetracycline or chloramphenicol treatment are uncommon.

PREVENTION AND CONTROL. Immunity to reinfection after recovery from RMSF appears to be complete. No naturally acquired second cases have been reported. There is no effective vaccine.

The best method for preventing disease is to avoid contact with ticks. Ticks are brushed off leaves or blades of grass onto clothes or skin as one comes in contact with such vegetation. Ticks usually remain stationary until the host is quiet. They then will seek warm, dark areas and will migrate to the groin or the scalp, where they can grasp hair shafts while inserting their mouth parts into the skin. Small barbs on each side of the mouth make it difficult to withdraw the whole tick from the skin while it is feeding; the mouth parts may remain imbedded. A search for ticks should be accomplished at the end of each day spent in tick-infested country. They should be removed with forceps or tweezers. A drop of acetone or a lighted match brought close to the tick may insure that the tick withdraws its mouth parts. The tick should not be removed with exposed fingers. A tick crushed between the fingers may induce disease. Prophylactic antibiotics are not indicated for persons with known tick bites. They should be advised concerning the usual incubation period and urged to watch for development of fever or headache. Oral temperature should be recorded twice a day for two weeks. In the event of an elevation, medical attention should be obtained promptly. Therapy begun before the onset of fever could result in a prolongation of the incubation period.

Donohue JF: Lower respiratory tract involvement in Rocky Mountain spotted fever. Arch Intern Med 140:223, 1980. *This retrospective review of pulmonary findings in patients with RMSF points out the delays that occurred in making the correct diagnosis because the respiratory symptoms were not considered to be a part of the clinical picture of RMSF.*

DuPont HL, Hornick RB, Dawkins AT, et al.: Rocky Mountain spotted fever: A comparative study of the active immunity induced by inactivated and viable pathogenic *Rickettsia rickettsii*. J Infect Dis 128:340, 1973. *A study of* induced disease in volunteers that demonstrated the minimal effectiveness of killed vaccines in preventing RMSF. In addition, new information about the number of rickettsiae required to cause diseases was obtained.

Kaplowitz LG, Lange JV, Fischer JJ, et al.: Correlation of rickettsial titers, circulating endotoxin, and clinical features in Rocky Mountain spotted fever. Arch Intern Med 143:1149, 1983.

Marx RS, McCall CE, Abramson JS, et al.: Rocky Mountain spotted fever: Serological evidence of previous subclinical infection in children. Am J Dis Child 136:16, 1982. Wilfert CM, MacCormack JN, Kleeman K, et al.: The prevalence of antibodies to *Rickettsia rickettsii* in an area endemic for Rocky Mountain spotted fever. J Infect Dis 151:823, 1985. *Two good studies attempting to assess the specificity and sensitivity of various serologic tests in measuring antibodies as an indicator of subclinical infections.*

Silverman D: *Rickettsia rickettsii*—induced cellular injury of human vascular endothelium in vitro. Infect Immun 44:545, 1984. *Electron microscopic study of cellular derangements caused by* R. rickettsii.

Yamada T, Harber P, Pettit GW, et al.: Activation of the kallikrein-kinin system in Rocky Mountain spotted fever. Ann Intern Med 88:764, 1978. *This article presents a thorough discussion of the pathogenesis of the vasculitis and associated coagulopathies that occur in this disease.*

323 OTHER TICK-BORNE RICKETTSIOSES

Richard B. Hornick

DEFINITIONS. *Mediterranean spotted fever*, also known as North African tick typhus, Kenya tick-bite fever, Indian tick typhus, and boutonneuse fever, is caused by *Rickettsia conorii*. A second disease, called North Asian tick-borne rickettsiosis, is induced by *Rickettsia siberica*. A third tick-borne rickettsial infection, called Queensland tick typhus, is caused by *Rickettsia australis*. The disease produced by these agents consists of headache, fever, rash, myalgia, and malaise. The rickettsiae induce disease by invading endothelial cells and producing a vasculitis. The outcome of disease is usually favorable. The illnesses are mild compared with Rocky Mountain spotted fever (RMSF). One other difference is the usual presence of a depressed, black ulcer—the site of the tick bite. This is the *tache noire*, or eschar, and has been likened to a cigarette burn.

ETIOLOGY, DISTRIBUTION, AND EPIDEMIOLOGY. Mediterranean spotted fever (MSF) occurs in countries bordering the Mediterranean Sea, but also in the Middle East, India, and Pakistan. Several species of ticks are involved. The brown dog tick, *Rhipicephalus sanguineus*, is the main vector, but ticks common to wild animals transmit *R. conorii* in African countries. Italian epidemiologists have demonstrated a dramatic increase in the incidence of this disease in Italy, Spain, and Israel. The assumption is that the suburbanization of cities and towns resulted in increased opportunities for humans to contact ticks.

The distribution of *R. siberica* extends from European Russia through Siberia to the Soviet Far East and south into the Indo-Pakistan subcontinent. Several species of hard, or ixodid, body ticks appear to be the vectors: *Haemaphysalis concinna*, *Dermacentor sylvarum*, and *Dermacentor nuttallii*. Transovarian transmission occurs in these three naturally infected ticks.

Queensland tick typhus is one of several rickettsial infections found in Australia. The *R. australis* is carried by the tick *Ixodes holocyclus*, and marsupial animals are among known animal reservoirs.

PATHOLOGY. These three rickettsiae are very similar to *R. rickettsii*. There is greater than 90 per cent homology by DNA hybridization between the latter strain and *R. conorii*. All share group-specific antigens but have species-specific antigens as well that allow for their identification. These strains will invade endothelial cells and cause cell death, resulting in a vasculitis (see Ch. 322). Each of these three strains produces an eschar (*tache noire*) at the site of the tick bite.

SYMPTOMS, LABORATORY FINDINGS, AND DIAGNOSIS. The onset of disease caused by each of these three rickettsiae is sudden and characterized by fever, headache, malaise, myalgia, and conjunctival injection. These symptoms and signs appear about five to seven days after the tick bite. The eschar is the distinguishing sign that confirms the diagnosis. It should be looked for in the scalp, axillae, and groin area, regions of the body favored by ticks. Because of the necrotic nature of the eschar, lymph nodes draining the region of the eschar will be enlarged. The lesion has been appropriately likened to a cigarette burn, about 2 to 5 mm in diameter with a black center and a raised, erythematous rim. The lesion is only mildly tender.

As with RMSF, a rash appears on the fourth to fifth day. The faint pink macular-papular lesions represent small hemorrhages into the skin. The rash is generalized, including the palms and soles of the feet. The duration of the disease is about two weeks. Mortality is unusual.

The Weil-Felix reaction will demonstrate agglutinating antibodies to OX-19 antigen is most patients; these appear in the second to third week of disease. The microimmunofluorescence test for detection of antibodies to *R. conorii* is the serologic test of choice, if available.

A skin biopsy stained with immunofluorescent antibody stain is the most rapid and earliest diagnostic procedure. This approach is indicated only when the diagnosis of spotted fever is suspected and a *tache noire* eschar is not present.

TREATMENT. Tetracycline and chloramphenicol are the drugs of choice. Defervescence occurs within two days. Therapy (see Ch. 322) should be continued for at least two days after the patient becomes afebrile.

PROPHYLAXIS. Prevention of human disease requires avoidance of tick bites. Travelers into wild game country of Africa should check their clothes and skin carefully for ticks. Tourists traveling to southern European countries should search for ticks if they go on hiking tours through suburban and rural areas during the spring and summer months.

Recovery from these rickettsial infections imparts solid immunity. In experimental animals *R. conorii* is relatively avirulent compared with most strains of *R. rickettsii*. However, animals recovered from infections with the former strain are protected against challenge with virulent *R. rickettsii*. This protection is mediated by T lymphocytes that recognize antigens on other species of rickettsial agents of the spotted fever group.

De Micco C, Raoult D, Toga M: Diagnosis of Mediterranean spotted fever by using an immunofluorescence technique. J Infect Dis 153:137, 1986; Raoult D, De Micco C, Gallais H, et al.: Laboratory diagnosis of Mediterranean spotted fever by immunofluorescent demonstration of *Rickettsia conorii* in cutaneous lesions. J Infect Dis 150:145, 1984. *These investigators studied two groups of patients to demonstrate the usefulness of the technique and then to establish the sensitivity and specificity of the procedure.*

Harris RL, Kaplan SL, Bradshaw MW, et al.: Boutonneuse fever in American travelers. J Infect Dis 153:126, 1986. *Excellent color print of eschar. Provides warning to American physicians to be alert to the tick-borne rickettsial disease that tourists can acquire overseas.*

Mansueto S, Tringali G, Walker DH: Widespread simultaneous increase in the incidence of spotted fever group rickettsiosis. J Infect Dis 154:539, 1986.

Vicente V, Alegre A, Ruiz R, et al.: Kinin-prekallikrein system in Mediterranean spotted fever. J Infect Dis 154:541, 1986. *These authors carefully studied the kinin system and found that it, unlike in RMSF, was not activated in MSF; additional laboratory evidence confirmed the lesser virulence of* R. conorii.

324 RICKETTSIALPOX

Richard B. Hornick

DEFINITION. Rickettsialpox is a rare mite-borne infectious disease caused by *Rickettsia akari*. This mild, self-limited illness consists of headache, fever, an eschar at the site of the mite bite, and a papulovesicular rash.

ETIOLOGY. *R. akari* is classified with the spotted fever group of rickettsia. It is a small, gram-negative, coccobacillus-shaped, obligate intracellular organism.

DISTRIBUTION AND INCIDENCE. Rickettsialpox was first described in 1946. In the subsequent few years, more than 500 cases were diagnosed, primarily in New York City. Since the early 1950's, only one outbreak has occurred, again in New York City. The disease is virtually unknown throughout the rest of the United States.

TRANSMISSION AND EPIDEMIOLOGY. The original description of this disease included the isolation of *R. akari* from persons with the disease, from mites (*Allodermanyssus sanguineus*) that feed on rodents, and from house mice (*Mus musculus*). Engorged mites were occasionally found on the mice; attachment was usually around the rump. The mites remain in the nest, where access to mice is readily available. Intrusion into this animal-ectoparasite cycle by humans can result in an infected mite's biting and inducing disease. The ecologic range of *A. sanguineus* covers most of the United States, and mice are ubiquitous animals. Thus the elements for potential epidemics exist. Isolated cases may develop from unusual exposure to mice, as in persons working in land fills or in homeless persons sleeping in abandoned buildings.

Rickettsialpox is fairly common in some urban areas of the Ukraine, where rats appear to be the animal reservoir. In Korea small field mice are infected.

PATHOLOGY. The known pathologic changes are limited to the skin, since this is a nonfatal infection. Histologic examination of the eschar (site of mite bite) reveals intense inflammation with necrosis. Other findings are similar to those in Rocky Mountain spotted fever: thrombosis and necrosis of capillaries, edema, and a monocytic perivascular infiltrate. The characteristic rash in this disease is papulovesicular. The lesions contain fluid that may yield *R. akari* on culture.

CLINICAL MANIFESTATIONS AND COURSE. The bite of the mite is not painful and will go unnoticed. This site will undergo a localized inflammatory reaction over the next week to ten days. During this time the edema and cellular components of the reaction create a slowly enlarging, firm, erythematous papule, which may reach 1 to 1.5 cm in diameter. The involved skin separates gradually, creating a vesicle that finally breaks down to form an ulcer. The base of the ulcer is usually black and is surrounded by a rim of erythematous skin. This progression occurs over a three- to seven-day period, at the end of which there is the sudden onset of fever, chills, sweats, headache, backache, and malaise. The lymph nodes draining the area of the eschar enlarge but are nontender. These symptoms and signs may be present for a week if no specific antibiotic treatment is administered.

As with other members of the spotted fever group, a rash appears after two to three days of illness. Initially the lesions are maculopapular, few in number, and distributed mostly on the trunk and abdomen, rarely involving the palms or soles. The lesions evolve quickly and uniformly into vesicular lesions; the vesicle appears to sit on top of an erythematous papule. These lesions persist for about a week; the fluid in the vesicle is slowly absorbed, and a scab forms, which leaves a brownish discoloration in the skin after it falls off. This gradually clears without leaving a scar. There is no significant internal organ involvement.

DIAGNOSIS. The diagnosis is made by clinical observation; the unique lesions of the rash, the presence of the eschar, and a history that suggests contact with rodents in the past two weeks provide sufficient evidence to make the diagnosis. Serologic studies confirm the diagnosis; complement-fixing antibody titers have been the standard, but indirect immunofluorescent antibodies are more specific, when available. Confusion exists regarding whether the Weil-Felix reaction can be used to diagnose rickettsialpox. In about 10 per cent of patients in small series, significant titer rises to OX-19 and OX-2 have been observed. The test lacks sensitivity for con-

firming the diagnosis. The organism can be isolated from the vesicular fluid or from clotted blood specimens. These materials must be injected into animals or embryonated eggs. Laboratory tests are of no diagnostic help, although leukopenia is common.

The rash may be confused with the lesions of chickenpox, but no eschar will be present in chickenpox. In addition, the lesions of chickenpox are usually in various stages of maturity, whereas the character of those in rickettsialpox is more uniform. Finally, the vesicle of rickettsialpox appears to sit on a papule, whereas those of chickenpox lack such a base.

PROGNOSIS. Rickettsialpox is a benign illness, and recovery occurs without therapy.

TREATMENT. Treatment with tetracycline or doxycycline will shorten the febrile period and hasten recovery. Antibiotic treatment need only be administered for three to four days to insure a cure. No relapse will occur.

PREVENTION AND CONTROL. Rickettsialpox is a zoonosis involving a common house pest, the mouse. Control of this reservoir through elimination of mouse harborages and the application of residual acaricides to walls adjacent to mice-infested areas should control mite populations. There is no available vaccine.

Brettman LR, Lewin S, Holzman RS: Rickettsialpox: Report of an outbreak and a contemporary review. Medicine 60:363, 1981. *Good summary of clinical features of recent outbreak.*

Dolgopol VB: Histologic changes in rickettsialpox. Am J Pathol 24:119, 1948.

Greenberg M, Pelliteri O, Klein IF, et al.: Rickettsialpox—a newly recognized rickettsial disease. II. Clinical observations. JAMA 133:901, 1947. *Original clinical description of a newly recognized spotted fever group infection.*

Huebner RJ, Stamps P, Armstrong C: Rickettsialpox—a newly recognized rickettsial disease. I. Isolation of the etiological agent. Public Health Rep 61:1605, 1946. *Excellent description of the discovery of rickettsialpox.*

Lackman DH: A review of information on rickettsialpox in the United States. Clin Pediatr 2:296, 1963. *A resource for information on rickettsialpox in the United States.*

325 SCRUB TYPHUS

Richard B. Hornick

DEFINITION. Scrub typhus is an acute febrile illness caused by *Rickettsia tsutsugamushi* (from the Japanese: *tsutsuga*, "dangerous"; *mushi*, "bug"). This rickettsia is inoculated into humans during the bite by a chigger. The site of the bite develops into an eschar.

ETIOLOGY. *R. tsutsugamushi* (*R. orientalis*) is a small, gram-negative, obligate intracellular organism. Unlike other rickettsial infections, infection with *R. tsutsugamushi* does not induce solid protection against additional bouts of scrub typhus. This results from the variable antigenic compositions of the strains.

This is the only rickettsia whose polysaccharides bear an antigenic relationship to *Proteus* OX-K. This *Proteus* strain is used in serologic tests to confirm scrub typhus.

DISTRIBUTION. This disease occurs almost exclusively in the large triangular region extending from the northern islands of Japan southwest to Australia and southeast to the South Pacific Islands. This region contains the larval form of mites that are both vector and reservoir of rickettsiae.

TRANSMISSION AND EPIDEMIOLOGY. *R. tsutsugamushi* is transmitted to humans by the bite of the larva of trombiculid mites (chiggers). Chiggers are the only stage in the life cycle of these mites (*Leptotrombidium deliensis* and others) that can feed on humans. Chiggers are almost microscopic, often brilliantly colored (red bugs). The chiggers feed on rats and other small rodents. The word "scrub" was applied because of the type of vegetation—transitional between forests and clearings—that maintains the chigger-mammal relationship. But other regions (semiarid, sandy beaches, and so on) also support rodents and mites. Humans encounter scrub typhus when they enter such areas to build roads, to clear fields or forests, or on military expeditions. Circumscribed regions are highly endemic, a reflection of the lack of mobility of the chiggers and their rodent hosts. Mites transmit the rickettsiae to their offspring via the ova. In this fashion they can serve as vector and reservoir of the etiologic agent.

This disease has been called river or flood fever because of the increased incidence during the rainy seasons. Chiggers and mites proliferate in warm, wet environments.

PATHOLOGY. *R. tsutsugamushi* invades endothelial cells to produce a vasculitis (see Ch. 322). The serious pathologic manifestations in untreated patients are predominantly myocarditis, meningoencephalitis, and pneumonitis. Coagulopathy develops but is less severe than in Rocky Mountain spotted fever or typhus.

The site of the chigger bite develops into a papular lesion that ulcerates to form an eschar. This is associated with regional and later generalized lymphadenopathy.

CLINICAL MANIFESTATIONS AND COURSE. The incubation period for development of the primary papular lesion ranges from 6 to 18 days. This lesion can occur anywhere on the body. It enlarges, undergoes central necrosis, and crusts to form the eschar. As the eschar matures, the patient has the sudden onset of headache, fever, chills, and malaise. Over the next several days, these symptoms increase in severity with further elevation of the temperature. The patient, if untreated, may become stuporous as meningoencephalitis develops. Signs of cardiac dysfunction, including minor electrocardiographic abnormalities such as first-degree heart block and inverted T waves, can appear. The rash of scrub typhus appears at the end of the first week of disease. This is a faint, pink maculopapular rash appearing first on the trunk and spreading to the extremities.

Physical findings late in the first week of illness include generalized lymphadenopathy and palpable spleen and occasionally liver. Pulmonary findings are often absent despite radiographic evidence of interstitial pneumonia. In those patients with myocarditis, there may be a gallop rhythm, poor-quality heart sounds, and systolic murmurs.

Various cranial nerve deficits have been noted in untreated patients. Deafness, dysarthria, and dysphagia may occur but are usually transient, although deafness can last for several months.

All of 87 (nonimmune) soldiers in Vietnam who developed scrub typhus had fever and headache, 46 per cent had an eschar, and 35 per cent had a rash. Eighty-five per cent had generalized lymph node enlargement. It is not surprising that many were misdiagnosed as having infectious mononucleosis.

Laboratory studies reveal leukopenia early in the disease with subsequent increase of white blood cell counts to normal levels. Coagulopathies can be demonstrated, but only rare patients develop the disseminated intravascular clotting syndrome. Liver enzyme values may be elevated, indicating hepatocellular damage. Proteinuria is common.

Patients with untreated disease remain febrile for about two weeks and have a long convalescence of four to six weeks thereafter.

DIAGNOSIS. The variable presentations in this disease make the clinical diagnosis difficult. The eschar and rash should suggest a rickettsial infection, but these may be found in fewer than one half of patients. Furthermore, the eschar and rash may suggest other rickettsial infections, such as tick-borne typhus. A knowledge of the endemic foci of scrub typhus and determination of whether the patient has traveled or worked in such areas constitute important epidemiologic information. A therapeutic trial of tetracycline or chloramphenicol is indicated in patients in whom the diagnosis of scrub typhus is suspected. Defervescence should occur within 24 hours.

The specific serologic test is the detection of significant increases (> fourfold) of indirect immunofluorescent antibodies in paired serum specimens obtained two weeks apart. The *Proteus* OX-K antigen test is readily available and inexpensive, so that it is frequently employed in endemic areas. About 50 per cent of patients will have diagnostic titers. In Malaya, the sensitivity and specificity of both tests were found to be about the same, but their usefulness was enhanced when they were used concurrently.

R. tsutsugamushi can be isolated from a patient's blood by inoculating it, intraperitoneally, into white mice. The rickettsiae can be demonstrated in the tissues of the mice.

PROGNOSIS. Without treatment, the mortality rate ranges from 0 to 30 per cent depending upon virulence and resistance factors; with treatment, survival is the expected outcome. Second or third attacks of scrub typhus, caused by different serotypes, usually result in a mild illness, usually with no eschar or rash.

Persistence of *R. tsutsugamushi* in lymph node tissues has been demonstrated one year after recovery. This finding raises the possibility of reactivation of disease during immunosuppression.

TREATMENT. Tetracycline, doxycycline, and chloramphenicol are all effective. The drug should be continued for at least two days after the patient has become afebrile.

PREVENTION AND CONTROL. Vaccines were developed and tested during and after World War II. Some were effective against homologous strains. However, no single antigen has been identified that induces protection against all of the antigenically diverse strains of *R. tsutsugamushi*. In military populations in endemic areas, weekly doses of doxycycline protect against scrub typhus.

Avoidance of chigger attachment can be accomplished by insect repellents applied to the skin and by wearing protective clothing impregnated with benzyl benzoate. Diethyltoluamide preparations such as OFF and DEET are also effective if sprayed on clothing and exposed skin but are removed rapidly by water. Application of this chemical to socks is especially important in preventing chigger bites.

Berman SJ, Kunidin WD: Scrub typhus in South Vietnam: A study of 87 cases. Ann Intern Med 79:26, 1973. *A good analysis of the clinical features of scrub typhus appearing in United States troops. Helpful in assessing potential for disease in tourists returning from endemic areas.*

Brown GW, Saunders JP, Singh S: Single dose doxycycline therapy for scrub typhus. Trans R Soc Trop Med Hyg 72:412, 1978. *Clinical investigation on the feasibility of a single dose of drug to treat scrub typhus.*

Traub R, Wisseman CL Jr: The ecology of chigger-borne rickettsiosis (scrub typhus) (review article). J Med Entomol 11:237, 1974. *Excellent summary by two experts who have clarified much of what is now known about the ecology of this disease.*

326 TRENCH FEVER

Theodore C. Eickhoff

DEFINITION. Trench fever is also called *five-day* or *quintan fever*, *shin-bone fever*, and *Volhynia fever*. It is a self-limited febrile disease transmitted by the body louse, *Pediculus humanus corporis*, and characterized by headache, fever, and severe pain in the bones, joints, and muscles. Fatalities are rare, but the disease is characterized in most patients by a relapsing course.

ETIOLOGY AND EPIDEMIOLOGY. The etiologic agent, *Rochalimaea quintana*, is a rickettsia-like agent that grows extracellularly in the louse gut and is excreted in louse feces. Human infection follows accidental inoculation of contaminated feces into abraded skin or conjunctivae. The etiologic agent is differentiated from other rickettsiae by its ability to grow on artificial media, true rickettsiae being obligate intracellular parasites.

The disease was a major military problem during World Wars I and II in Europe and occurs in endemic form in Mexico, parts of North Africa, and eastern Europe and Asia. Humans are generally considered to be the prinicipal reservoir, since the agent has been isolated from asymptomatic patients years after their initial infection. The louse then acquires its infection by ingesting the blood of an infected human. The recent finding that the so-called "vole agent" is in fact a strain of *Rochalimaea quintana* suggests that reservoirs may also exist in certain rodent populations.

PATHOLOGY AND CLINICAL MANIFESTATIONS. Histopathologic data are limited to skin biopsy studies that have revealed only nonspecific perivascular inflammation. Following an incubation period of 10 to 30 days, the presenting symptoms are fever, of either gradual or abrupt onset, severe weakness, headache, dizziness, and bone and body pain, frequently most dramatically severe in the shins. Physical and laboratory examination generally reveals only slight enlargement of the liver and spleen, pain and soreness in the muscles, and erythematous macules or papules, which occur transiently in 70 to 80 per cent of patients. There may be a moderate leukocytosis. The initial febrile episode generally lasts three to five days but frequently recurs after a symptom-free interval of four to five days. Up to eight relapses of fever and symptoms similar to the initial episode have been described, but most patients fortunately experience only a few such relapses. In some patients, the fever and symptoms are continuous for two to three weeks. In still others, the initial fever may decline, only to relapse without a true afebrile period, producing a typical "saddle-back" fever curve. Persistent rickettsemia is present during the initial attack and continues during the relapses as well as the intervening asymptomatic periods; it may persist for months or sometimes years after apparent recovery.

DIAGNOSIS. A history of contact with lice within the appropriate incubation period is helpful. *R. quintana* can be cultivated on agar containing 10 per cent fresh defibrinated horse blood. Both a passive hemagglutination and an enzyme-linked immunosorbent assay test have proved useful in serologic diagnosis. During epidemics, typical cases may be diagnosed on clinical grounds alone. The differential diagnosis should include typhoid fever, typhus, dengue, relapsing fever, and leptospirosis.

TREATMENT AND PROGNOSIS. *Rochalimaea quintana* is highly sensitive in vitro to the tetracyclines and other broad-spectrum antimicrobials, and these may be expected to be as effective in the treatment of trench fever as in the treatment of other rickettsial diseases; there is, however, no direct information supporting their efficacy. Mortality is negligible, and the long-term prognosis is excellent. Approximately 85 per cent of patients recover fully within two months of onset; a few, however, continue to experience recurrences for months or years.

PREVENTION. Elimination of the louse vector by dusting clothing with residual insecticides should be as effective in controlling trench fever as in controlling epidemic typhus. Ten per cent DDT (chlorophenothane) powders proved highly effective for louse control during World War II, but development of DDT resistance may require the use of lindane or malathion as a dusting powder.

Hurst A: Trench fever. Br Med J 2:318, 1942. *This is a lucid account of the clinical characteristics of trench fever in British troops in World War I.*

Myers WF, Grossman DM, Wisseman CL Jr: Antibiotic susceptibility patterns in *Rochalimaea quintana*, the agent of trench fever. Antimicrob Agents Chemother 25:690, 1984. *This study documents the broad susceptibility of the organism to antimicrobial agents, with resistance found only to vancomycin and aminoglycosides.*

Weis E, Dasch GA, Woodman DR, et al.: Vole agent identified as a strain of the trench fever rickettsia, *Rochalimaea quintana*. Infect Immun 19:1013, 1978. *One of the few recent studies of trench fever, providing interesting, but speculative, epidemiologic insights.*

327 Q FEVER

Theodore C. Eickhoff

DEFINITION. Q fever is a self-limited rickettsial infection characterized by fever, chills, headache, and constitutional symptoms. In less than one half of patients, there may be an associated pneumonitis. It is unique among the rickettsial diseases of humans in that infection is acquired by inhalation rather than by contact with an arthropod vector.

ETIOLOGY. The disease is caused by *Coxiella burnetii*, a rickettsial agent possessing a unique resistance to desiccation and to exposure in dusts and soils. The organism may be propagated in embryonated eggs and in mice, hamsters, and guinea pigs. Both patients and animals develop agglutinating and complement-fixing antibodies to the agents. *C. burnetii*, unlike other rickettsiae, does not stimulate the production of agglutinins to the X strain of *Proteus vulgaris*. There is recent evidence from examination of plasmid DNA profiles of strain differences that may be associated with different virulence characteristics.

EPIDEMIOLOGY. *Incidence and Distribution.* The true incidence of the disease in humans is impossible to determine because the majority of infections are undiagnosed. In the United States the disease, first found in Montana and California, is now recognized as prevalent in most of the states in which sheep and cattle are produced. Small numbers of cases have been reported from most of the remaining states. Serologic surveys have revealed that many persons exposed to infection in sheep and cattle ranches, abattoirs, meat packing plants, or wool processing plants have serologic evidence of past infection. *C. burnetii* is now known to be distributed on a worldwide basis, but is still rare in Scandinavian countries.

TRANSMISSION. The epidemiology of Q fever is complex, involving two major patterns of transmission. The first pattern, described in Australia, is a disease cycle in wild animals with transmission of the agent from animal to animal by a tick vector. Such cycles involve up to 40 species of tick vectors. The agent can be transmitted indefinitely as an inapparent infection in the wild reservoir, such as kangaroos, by ticks, but it may also be transmitted laterally by arthropod vectors to a domestic animal in close contact with humans. In these and similar cycles recognized in other parts of the world, *C. burnetii*, like the other rickettsial agents of human disease, is vector transmitted.

However, Q fever patients rarely give a history of tick bite. Human infection is now known to result almost exclusively from a second transmission cycle capable of sustaining itself independently of the wild animal cycle. The reservoirs of infection in the second pattern are domestic animals, principally cattle, sheep, and goats, in which *C. burnetii* produces an inapparent or at most mild infection. The organisms do, however, localize in placental tissue and mammary glands of pregnant animals. In sheep, *C. burnetii* is present in up to 10^{12} organisms per gram of placental tissue and to a lesser degree in amniotic fluid, milk, and feces. In the cow, and probably the goat, excretion occurs mainly through the placenta and milk. With all infected animals, the period of parturition is associated with the formation of a highly infectious aerosol. Such aerosols infect other cattle in the herd and also the human population in close contact with the animals. Further, because contaminated clothing, wool, hide, bedding, and soil may be the source of secondary aerosols, the infection may be transmitted by these vehicles at considerable distances from the infected cattle. The unique resistance of *C. burnetii* to prolonged exposure in nature contributes to the spread of the agent by such infectious microenvironments.

The domestic animal cycle has also resulted in several outbreaks of Q fever in personnel in United States medical schools carrying out research studies with pregnant ewes. In addition, Q fever is a recognized laboratory hazard; 50 cases were reported among personnel in one laboratory over a 15-year period. Only 21 of these personnel had been working directly with the organism. Rare reports of nosocomial transmission of Q fever suggest person-to-person transmission; this must be considered infrequent and unlikely.

C. burnetii is easily found in unpasteurized milk from infected cows. Several studies have reported serologic evidence of infection in raw milk drinkers, but there is no clear evidence of disease transmission via raw milk.

PATHOLOGY. Because the mortality rate is quite low, postmortem studies have been few. In patients with pneumonitis, the histopathology is similar to that seen in the viral pneumonias and psittacosis. During the acute phase of the disease, the systemic nature of Q fever is demonstrable both in biochemical abnormalities of liver function and in focal inflammation and noncaseating granulomas in hepatic biopsy specimens. Q fever endocarditis is the major serious complication of the disease, producing valvular vegetations from which rickettsiae may be isolated.

CLINICAL MANIFESTATIONS. After an incubation period of 10 to 28 days following exposure, most patients complain of an abrupt onset of high fever, rigors, headache, muscle pains, and profound malaise. The temperature may rise as high as 40° C and remain elevated, with considerable fluctuation, for one to two weeks. In older patients, three weeks of fever is not unusual. In contrast to all other rickettsial infections, there is generally no rash.

In up to one half of patients, there is roentgenographic evidence of pneumonitis, manifested clinically as a nonproductive cough developing usually in the second week of fever; significant respiratory distress is unusual. Q fever is more properly considered a severe systemic infection that frequently causes an associated pneumonitis, rather than a primary pneumonia. Convalescence tends to be prolonged, lasting up to several months even in uncomplicated cases.

Hepatic involvement is common, manifested by hepatic enlargement, tenderness, and biochemical evidence of hepatitis; significant jaundice is infrequent. Other complications of acute illness reported include myocarditis, pericarditis, and encephalitis. The most serious late sequela, fortunately infrequent, is Q fever endocarditis, which may or may not be preceded by an illness compatible with the acute form of Q fever. Q fever endocarditis should be considered in any patient with culture-negative endocarditis who has resided in an endemic area.

DIAGNOSIS. Q fever should always be suspected in a patient having a severe febrile illness for which no obvious cause can be found. If the patient's vocation or avocation brings him or her into contact with sheep, cattle, or goats, or by-products such as wool or hides, it should be particularly suspected.

The differential diagnosis of the acute systemic febrile illness includes influenza, infectious mononucleosis, brucellosis, typhoid fever, cytomegalovirus infection, leptospirosis, and toxoplasmosis. If pneumonitis is prominent, viral pneumonia, mycoplasma, psittacosis, and *Legionella pneumophila* must be considered as well. Evidence of hepatic involvement should suggest viral hepatitis or other intrahepatic processes in addition to those mentioned previously.

Diagnostic studies are usually limited to serologic studies. The complement-fixation test is the most generally available. Recent reports have emphasized the importance of phase variation in the selection of antigens for diagnostic use. Sixty-five per cent of patients will develop elevated titers against phase II antigen by the end of the second week of illness, and 90 per cent of patients will do so after four weeks. Elevated ($\geq 1:200$) antibody to phase I antigen is seen in patients with Q fever endocarditis, and the finding of such an elevated titer to phase I antigen during convalescence should raise a strong suggestion of subacute or chronic infection.

TREATMENT AND PROGNOSIS. The tetracyclines and chloramphenicol are both effective in treatment of acute infections with *C. burnetii*, but owing to potential chloramphenicol toxicity, tetracycline is preferred, in a dose of 500 mg four times daily. The mortality is low (1 per cent or less) in untreated patients and is lower still in those treated with antimicrobial drugs. Therapy should be continued for approximately 1 week, even though patients usually become afebrile within 48 to 72 hours. Patients occasionally may experience relapse after treatment, and when this occurs additional drug therapy should be administered.

Prognosis is less favorable for the rare patient in whom Q fever endocarditis develops. In some of these patients the disease has been reported to be unresponsive to antimicrobial therapy; long-term tetracycline therapy with valve replacement as necessary is reported to reduce mortality in such patients to about 30 per cent.

PREVENTION. Experimental lots of inactivated yolk-sac vaccines have been effective in preventing clinical disease in volunteers experimentally infected via the respiratory route, and active immunization has proven effective in abattoir workers. Although not yet generally available, immunization should be considered for workers in research or diagnostic laboratories and for others who are occupationally heavily exposed.

Other control measures are limited to minimizing exposure to the organism insofar as possible. Milk from cattle, sheep, and goats in endemic areas should be pasteurized before use.

Ascher MS, Berman MA, Ruppanner R: Initial clinical and immunologic evaluation of a new phase I Q fever vaccine and skin test in humans. J Infect Dis 148:214, 1983. *Description of a promising vaccine.*

Clark WH, Lenette EH, Railsback OC, et al.: Q fever in California. VII. Clinical features in one hundred eighty cases. Arch Intern Med 88:155, 1951. *Well over 30 years old, but still among the best clinical studies of Q fever to be found.*

Marmion BP, Ormsbee RA, Kyrkou M, et al.: Vaccine prophylaxis of abattoir-associated Q fever. Lancet 2:1411, 1984. *This field trial documents the efficacy of the formalin-inactivated vaccine for up to two years in a high-risk population.*

Meiklejohn G, Reimer EG, Graves PS, et al.: Cryptic epidemic of Q fever in a medical school. J Infect Dis 144:107, 1981. *Provides an insight into the potential Q fever problem in research settings.*

Tobin MJ, Cahill N, Gearty G, et al.: Q Fever endocarditis. Am J Med 72:396, 1982. *Good discussion of the management of Q fever endocarditis.*

328 INTRODUCTION TO VIRAL DISEASES

R. Gordon Douglas, Jr.

Viruses are among the simplest and smallest of all forms of life. They are obligate intracellular parasites that require host cell structural and metabolic components for replication. They infect bacteria as well as plants and animals. More than 400 distinct viruses infect humans. They produce diseases ranging from subclinical infections and mild, self-limited, localized infections to common systemic infections and overwhelming, highly lethal infections such as meningoencephalitis or hemorrhagic fever with shock.

CHARACTERISTICS OF VIRUSES

Virus particles, or virions, consist of one type of nucleic acid, either deoxyribonucleic acid (DNA) or ribonucleic acid (RNA). They lack metabolic activity and do not possess ribosomes or most enzymes necessary for replication. Essentially, virions consist of nucleic acid enclosed in a protein coat. In addition, some possess a lipid envelope. Both the lipid and the protein coats protect the nucleic acid from enzymatic degradation. The nucleic acid may code for only a few or, in some cases, nearly 50 proteins. The protein coat, or capsid, consists of repeating, identical subunits called capsomeres. The capsid and nucleic acid together are called the nucleocapsid. The smallest (parvoviruses) are only 18 nm in diameter, whereas some poxviruses may be as large as 450 nm in diameter.

There are two major types of structure of virus particles. In the first type, capsomeres are arranged as a regular polyhedron with 20 triangular faces and 12 corners. Such a virus exhibits icosahedral symmetry. Many nonenveloped viruses are of this type. Other viruses exhibit helical symmetry in which a helix is formed of ribonucleoprotein and nucleic acid. Helical viruses are always enveloped, whereas icosahedral viruses may be enveloped or nonenveloped. The envelope is derived from host cell membranes and modified by insertion of one or more spike-like glycoproteins. These and other proteins on the surface of enveloped or nonenveloped viruses are important for two reasons: they provide specific interaction with receptors on host cells, and they serve as the major antigens of the virus.

Figure 328–1 demonstrates schematically the marked variety in size, shape, and structure of human viruses. In addition, there is great diversity in the structure of the viral genome: either RNA or DNA may be single stranded or double stranded. The genome may be linear or circular and may exist as single or multiple segments.

Viruses are classified by the International Committee on Taxonomy of Viruses according to the scheme presented in Table 328–1. The following order of virion characteristics is used: nucleic acid type, presence or absence of envelope, genome replication strategy, positive- or negative-sense genome, and genome segmentation.

As a result of the variety of structures of viruses and the complexities of genomes, mechanisms of replication are diverse and dependent upon the structure of the virus and its genome. Attachment to a host cell occurs by binding of a surface protein of a virus to a host cell virus receptor. Entry occurs by fusion of the virus envelope to the host cell

membrane, a mechanism operative for many enveloped viruses, or by endocytosis, a process similar to phagocytosis, with formation of an endosome. Following acidification, fusion of the viral membrane with that of the vesicle occurs, releasing the nucleocapsid. After uncoating of the viral nucleic acid, macromolecular synthesis of nucleic acid and protein occurs. Genome replication resembles RNA synthesis. Assembly of virus components then occurs, with release of mature viruses by budding, in the case of enveloped viruses, or by lysis of the cell, in the case of some nonenveloped viruses. Such released viruses are infectious for other cells.

Viruses cause cell injury by a number of mechanisms: directly by lysis resulting from viral replication, by lysis induced by antiviral antibody and complement, or by cell-mediated immune mechanisms recognizing infected host cells. As virus infection spreads and sufficient numbers of cells are injured, disease results. A role for viral toxins has

TABLE 328–1. CLASSIFICATION OF HUMAN VIRUSES

Dividing Characteristics	Virus Families	Important Human Viruses
DNA Viruses		
dsDNA, enveloped	Poxviridae	Variola (smallpox) virus
		Vaccinia virus
	Herpesviridae	Herpes simplex virus types 1 and 2
		Varicella-zoster virus
		Human cytomegalovirus
		EB virus
dsDNA, nonenveloped	Adenoviridae	Human adenovirus
	Papovaviridae	Papillomavirus
	Hepadnaviridae	Hepatitis B virus
ssDNA, nonenveloped	Parvoviridae	Parvovirus B19
RNA Viruses		
dsRNA, nonenveloped	Reoviridae	Colorado tick fever virus
		Human rotaviruses
ssRNA, enveloped		
No DNA step in replication		
Positive-sense genome	Togaviridae	Alphavirus: Eastern equine encephalitis, Western equine encephalitis
		Rubivirus: Rubella virus
	Flaviviridae	Yellow fever virus
		Dengue viruses
		St. Louis encephalitis
	Coronaviridae	Human coronaviruses
Negative-sense genome		
Nonsegmented genome	Paramyxoviridae	Parainfluenza virus
		Measles virus
		Respiratory syncytial virus
	Rhabdoviridae	Rabies virus
	Filoviridae	Marburg and Ebola viruses
Segmented genome	Orthomyxoviridae	Influenza A and B virus
	Bunyaviridae	California encephalitis virus
	Arenaviridae	LCM virus
		Lassa virus
DNA step in replication	Retroviridae	HTLV I, II, III (HIV)
ssRNA, nonenveloped	Picornaviridae	Polioviruses, coxsackieviruses, echoviruses, rhinoviruses
	Caliciviridae	? Norwalk virus

EB = Epstein-Barr; LCM = lymphocytic choriomeningitis; SS = single stranded; ds = double stranded.
From Murphy FA: Virus taxonomy. In Fields BN: Virology. New York, Raven Press, 1985. With permission.

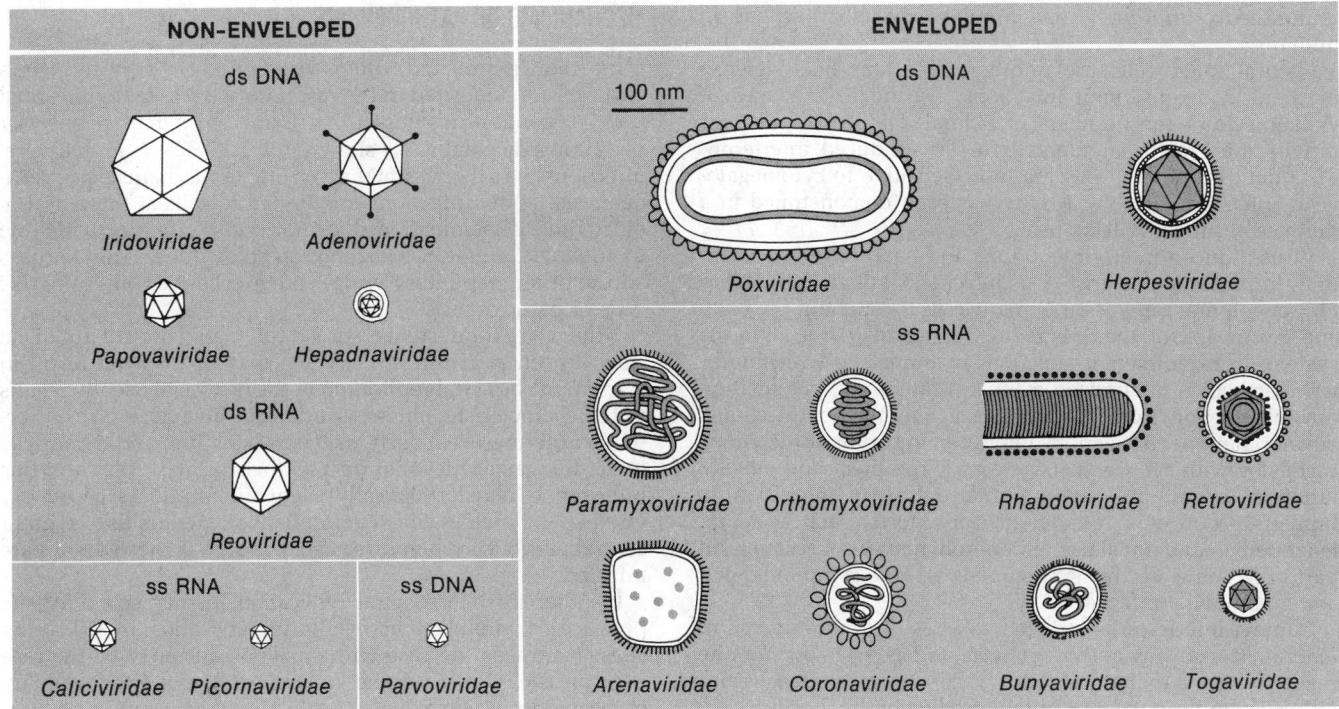

FIGURE 328–1. Structure and relative size of human virus families. (Modified from Matthews, REF: Intervirology 12:158, 1979.)

never been established, and such enzymes as are virus coded have a role in viral replication, but not directly in cellular injury, and they do not affect host tissues at distant sites. However, release of products of inflammation from sites of cell injury and circulating interferon may contribute to the signs and symptoms of viral infection.

In addition to lytic effects on cells, viral infection may transform cells so that they will proliferate continuously, and in vertebrates, mammals, and humans, may produce tumors, sometimes as a result of the occurrence of viral oncogenes in such viruses.

HOST DEFENSE MECHANISMS

In addition to nonspecific barriers such as skin, respiratory epithelium, gastric acidity, and so on, three main host defense mechanisms against viral infections have been described: (1) production of specific antiviral antibody; (2) development of specific cell-mediated immunity involving cytotoxic T cells and nonspecific effector cells such as natural killer (NK) cells; and (3) proliferation of macrophages that restrict virus replication and dissemination and can also destroy infected cells.

Antiviral antibodies develop in response to viral infection and to immunization with attenuated or inactivated virus or viral components. In the serum, antibodies of all classes and subclasses of immunoglobulins are found; in addition, secretory antibodies consisting predominantly of immunoglobulin A (IgA) molecules develop on mucosal surfaces in response to infection of their surfaces. They are of critical importance in diseases in which the primary site of inoculation is a mucosal surface.

The immune system may interact with extracellular (free) virus or cell-associated virus. Specific antibody will inactivate (neutralize) extracellular virus, and this activity may be enhanced by complement. Thus, it can prevent initial infection or restrict cell-to-cell spread of virus through extracellular fluids. It cannot, however, penetrate into cells and neutralize intracellular virus. Thus, virus may escape the effects of antibody by direct cell-to-cell transfer. Virus-infected cells possess viral antigens on their surface and may be lysed by specific antibody and complement, by specific cytotoxic T

cells, or by nonspecific cells such as NK cells or macrophages. Virus released in the process may be neutralized by antiviral antibody.

Cytotoxic T cells (Tc), which are HLA class I antigen restricted, also develop in response to infection or immunization (Ch. 417). They are important in limiting the growth of certain viruses in the infected host. This has been most clearly shown for influenza infections in mice, and Tc are

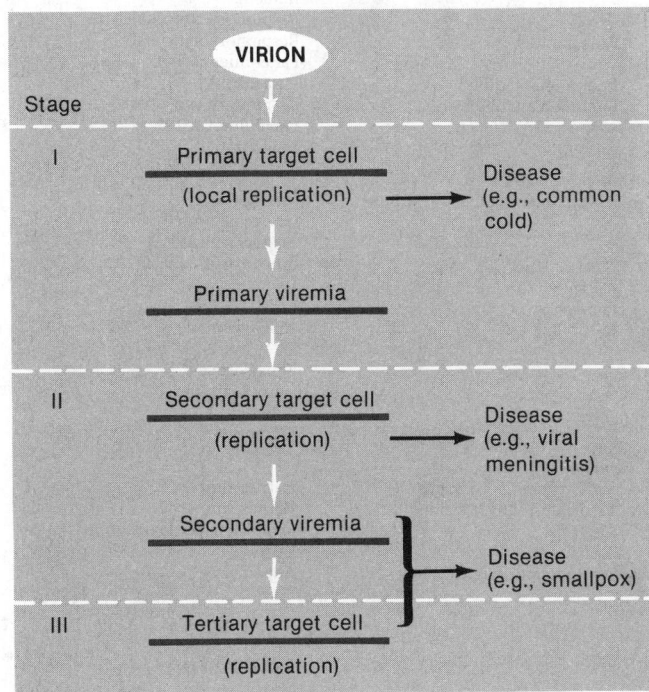

FIGURE 328–2. Stages of viral pathogenesis. Initial invasion may involve only primary target cells or may lead to secondary or tertiary target cell invasion, which results in the characteristic disease. (Courtesy of ED Kilbourne.)

undoubtedly important in a number of viral infections in humans.

Natural killer cells are another important host defense mechanism against viral infections. During early stages of viral infection, the numbers of natural killer cells and their activity are greatly augmented by virus-induced interferon. Mice deficient in NK cells are more sensitive to cytomegalovirus infection, and NK activity has been demonstrated in a number of human infections.

Virus-induced interferons (alpha and beta) have important roles in protection against virus infection through their ability to prevent viral replication in many cells throughout the body and by means of their regulatory function in the immune system. In experimental infections in animals in which interferon activity is neutralized by specific antibody, potentiation of viral infection occurs. In humans, in a number of infections, development of endogenous interferon in serum or secretions correlates with recovery: decreasing virus titers and amelioration of symptoms. Since administration of interferon to humans produces a number of side effects, such as fever, leukopenia, and myalgias, interferon may also account, in part, for some of the systemic signs and symptoms that accompany viral infections.

Gamma interferon is induced as a result of immune stimulation. It also has antiviral effects and is a major immune regulatory protein that induces Tc, activates macrophages and NK cells, and regulates antibody production by B cells.

MECHANISMS OF PATHOGENESIS

Infection is initiated, often when one or a very few virus particles are deposited in the respiratory tract, gastrointestinal tract, or genitourinary tract or are injected percutaneously or pass transplacentally. As shown in Figure 328–2, human viral infections may be classified according to mechanisms of pathogenesis. Many infections are limited to cells at the portal of entry, and dissemination does not occur. Conjunctivitis due to adenovirus type 8 and common colds due to rhinoviruses and to other respiratory viruses are excellent examples of this type of pathogenesis.

Other virus infections spread hematogenously to distal sites. Infection at the primary site may or may not result in symptoms, but viral replication in the distal site usually results in the characteristic illness associated with such a virus infection. Enteroviruses such as coxsackievirus and echovirus infect the gastrointestinal tract as their primary site, and this infection is usually clinically silent but produces a primary viremia, following which encephalitis, meningitis, or other central nervous system disease may occur as these tissues are infected.

In other infections, viral replication in the secondary site produces a viremia that results in replication in still other sites. Such was the case with smallpox and may be the case with measles. Rash may be a manifestation of either primary or secondary viremia.

TABLE 328–2. VIRUSES COMMONLY ASSOCIATED WITH DIFFERENT SYNDROMES

Disease Category	Common Associated Virus	Disease Category	Common Associated Virus
Respiratory Tract		*Immune System*	
Upper respiratory infection (including common cold and pharyngitis)	Rhinoviruses	Acquired immunodeficiency syndrome	Human immunodeficiency virus
	Coronaviruses	*Gastrointestinal Tract*	
	Parainfluenza 1–3	Gastroenteritis	Rotavirus
	Influenza A, B		Norwalk-like agents
	Herpes simplex	Hepatitis	Hepatitis A
	Adenoviruses		Hepatitis B
	Echoviruses		Delta virus
	Coxsackieviruses		Epstein-Barr virus
	Epstein-Barr virus		Cytomegalovirus
	Respiratory syncytial	*Skin*	
Croup	Parainfluenza 1–3	Maculopapular rash	Measles
	Influenza A, B		Rubella
	Respiratory syncytial		Echoviruses
Bronchiolitis	Respiratory syncytial		Coxsackievirus A16
	Parainfluenza 1–3		Enterovirus 71
Pneumonia (adults)	Influenza A	Hemorrhagic rash	Alphavirus
Pneumonia (children)	Respiratory syncytial		Bunyavirus
	Parainfluenza 1–3		Flaviviruses
	Influenza A	Localized lesions	Herpes simplex
Central Nervous System			Warts
Aseptic meningitis	Mumps		Molluscum contagiosum
	Coxsackievirus B1–5	*Neonatal*	
	Coxsackievirus A9	Teratogenic effects	Rubella
	Echovirus 4, 6, 9, 11, 14, 18, 30, 31		Cytomegalovirus
Paralysis	Polio 1–3	Disseminated disease	Coxsackievirus B1–5
Encephalitis	Alphaviruses		Echoviruses
	Flaviviruses		Hepatitis B
	Bunyaviruses		Cytomegalovirus
	Herpes simplex 1		Herpes simplex
	Enterovirus 71	Lower respiratory disease	Respiratory syncytial
	Mumps		Influenza
Genitourinary Tract		Enteritis	Rotavirus
Vulvovaginitis, cervicitis	Herpes simplex 2	*Other*	
Penile and vulvar lesions	Herpes simplex 2	Arthritis	Rubella
	Molluscum contagiosum		Hepatitis B
	Warts	Myositis	Togaviruses
Acute hemorrhagic cystitis	Adenovirus 11		Influenza B
Ocular		Carditis	Coxsackievirus B
Conjunctivitis	Adenovirus 3, 4, 7, 8, 19	Parotitis, pancreatitis, and orchitis	Mumps
	Herpes simplex		
	Varicella-zoster		
	Measles		
Acute Hemorrhagic Conjunctivitis	Enterovirus 70		
	Coxsackievirus A 24		

Modified from Menegus MA, Douglas RG Jr: The clinician and the microbiology laboratory: Viruses, rickettsia, chlamydiae, and mycoplasmas. In Mandell GL, Douglas RG, Jr, Bennett JE: Principles and Practice of Infectious Diseases. 2nd ed. New York, John Wiley & Sons, 1985.

Many virus infections have clinical characteristics that permit diagnosis: measles, mumps, chicken pox, and poliomyelitis. However, many others do not, and many syndromes have multiple etiologies, as is shown in Table 328–2. In fact, as many as 200 serologically distinct viruses may cause the common cold and related disorders. In the case of some syndromes—for example, atypical pneumonia—the etiology may be shared with other infectious organisms: *Mycoplasma pneumoniae*, *Chlamydia trachomatis*, and *Legionella pneumophila*. Others, however, are exclusively viral in etiology.

PREVENTION AND CONTROL

Recent advances in antiviral chemotherapy have produced a number of specific antivirals that are available and effective for prophylaxis or treatment, or both, of certain viral diseases. Drugs such as idoxuridine, amantadine, ribavirin, acyclovir, vidarabine, and azidothymidine (see Ch. 29) are available in the United States. For many other viral infections, however, no specific therapy exists. Proper use of antivirals requires specific viral diagnosis. Fortunately, in the case of herpes zoster, the diagnosis can usually be made clinically, and in influenza, the diagnosis can often be made on clinical and epidemiologic grounds; however, for many infections, viral diagnosis is required. Viral diagnostic laboratories are more common than in the past, and rapid techniques are gaining acceptance.

Vaccines are available for a number of viral infections, and many have greatly affected morbidity and mortality due to specific infections. Antibodies induced by vaccination may block initiation of infection in a primary site, as is the case in influenza. Others, such as inactivated poliomyelitis vaccine, are designed to prevent primary viremia after initial infection has occurred.

Belshe RB (ed.): Textbook of Human Virology. Littleton, MA, PSG Publishing Company, 1984. *A shorter text with clinical emphasis.*

Dolin R: Antiviral chemotherapy and chemoprophylaxis. Science 227-1296, 1985. *An excellent review of approved and promising antivirals.*

Fields BN (ed.): Virology. New York, Raven Press, 1985. *Excellent recent definitive textbook of basic virology.*

Mandell GL, Douglas RG Jr, Bennett JE (eds.): Principles and Practice of Infectious Diseases. 2nd ed. New York, John Wiley & Sons, 1985. *Excellent reference work about clinical aspects of viral infections; both syndromes and specific viruses are discussed.*

McGeoch DJ, Halliburton IW, Meulen VT, et al.: Some highlights of animal virus research in 1985. J. Gen Virol 67:813, 1986. *Up-to-date and well-referenced review of most recent advances in basic virology, some of which have clinical relevance.*

Mills EL: Viral infections predisposing to bacterial infections. In Creger WP, Coggins CH, Hancock EW (eds.): Annual Review of Medicine: Selected Topics in the Clinical Sciences. Palo Alto, CA, Annual Reviews, Inc., 1984. *Describes effects of viruses on neutrophils, lymphocytes, and macrophages.*

Viral Infections of the Respiratory Tract

329 THE COMMON COLD

Albert Z. Kapikian

DEFINITION. Although the term "common cold" does not denote a precisely defined disease, it has an almost universally comprehended meaning of an acute, self-limited, common illness of all age groups, in which the major clinical manifestations involve the upper respiratory tract, with nasal discharge (coryza) or nasal obstruction as the predominant symptom.

ETIOLOGY. Although it was known since 1914 that bacteria-free filtrates of nasal secretions from patients with a common cold could induce similar illnesses in volunteers inoculated intranasally, the discovery of etiologic agents from common colds eluded scientists for many years. Despite the isolation of numerous viruses that were associated etiologically with acute respiratory illnesses, such as influenza virus in 1933, and the adeno-, parainfluenza, and respiratory syncytial viruses in the 1950's, it was clear that the major etiologic agent or agents of the common cold had not yet been discovered. However, beginning gradually in the 1950's and escalating rapidly in the 1960's, about 100 distinct common cold viruses were discovered and shown to be the major causative agents of the common cold. These heretofore fastidious agents were named rhinoviruses (rhin- is Greek for nose), since they caused predominantly nasal symptoms. Shortly thereafter, another group of fastidious viruses, the coronaviruses, were discovered and shown to be the second most important etiologic agents of the common cold and related diseases.

Rhinoviruses have emerged as the major known causative agents of adult upper respiratory illnesses such as common colds. They have been isolated from approximately 15 to 40 per cent of adults with these illnesses (Table 329–1). The isolation rate is lower in children with upper respiratory tract illness, as only 4 to 5 per cent are rhinovirus positive. Rhinoviruses are classified as a genus in the picornavirus family and possess certain common characteristics, including small size (approximately 27 nm), ribonucleic acid (RNA) core, ether resistance, and complete or almost complete inactivation at pH 3. The last property is a major characteristic distinguishing rhinoviruses from another genus of the picornaviruses, the enteroviruses (poliovirus, coxsackievirus, and echovirus), which are stable at pH 3. There are now 100 officially designated rhinovirus serotypes, and it appears that this number includes most circulating strains.

The second most important etiologic agents of common colds are the coronaviruses, which are associated with 10 to 20 per cent of common colds in adults. Their importance as etiologic agents of common colds in infants and young children has not been determined. The human coronaviruses possess certain common characteristics, including (1) a unique electron microscopic appearance characterized by pleomorphic 100- to 150-nm enveloped particles possessing relatively widely spaced club- or pear-shaped surface projections

TABLE 329–1. PERCENTAGE OF COMMON COLDS ASSOCIATED WITH SPECIFIC ETIOLOGIC AGENTS IN ADULTS*

Rhinoviruses (100 serotypes)	15–40%
Coronaviruses (at least 3 serotypes)	10–20%
Influenza viruses A, B, C Parainfluenza viruses (4 serotypes) Respiratory syncytial virus (1 serotype) Adenoviruses (various serotypes)	5–10%
Coxsackieviruses (various serotypes) Echoviruses (various serotypes)	1–2%
Group A beta-hemolytic streptococci	2–10%
No specific agent known but presumed to be viral	30–50%

*Each of these agents can also cause common colds in the pediatric age group, but their relative roles are not clearly defined. Viruses associated with specific syndromes such as rubeola, rubella, and varicella have also been associated with common cold–like symptoms in children.

(reminiscent of the solar corona, from which the name coronavirus is derived); (2) an RNA genome; and (3) ether and acid lability. There are at least three distinct human coronavirus serotypes, designated B814, 229E, and OC43. As a result of difficulties in propagating these fastidious agents, fewer than 50 isolates have been recovered since their discovery; most epidemiologic studies have thus relied on serologic studies with the 229E and OC43 viruses, for which suitable antigens could be prepared. As shown in Table 329–1, many other viruses, such as influenza, parainfluenza, respiratory syncytial, adeno-, echo-, and coxsackieviruses, can also cause common cold-like symptoms. These other agents are described in other sections of this text. A determination of the etiology of a common cold cannot be made clinically, since the agents causing the syndrome are so numerous. In addition, about one third to one half of common colds have yet to be associated with an etiologic agent.

INCIDENCE AND PREVALENCE. The common cold is probably the most frequently occurring illness in humans worldwide. The National Center for Health Statistics estimated that in the United States in 1981 the population experienced more than 93 million common colds for an incidence of 41.4 per 100 persons per year. Common colds represented 19.5 per cent of all acute conditions and were estimated to cause over 261 million days of restricted activity.

In the Cleveland Family Study, which spanned a period of about 10 years and included over 25,000 illnesses, common respiratory diseases accounted for 60 per cent of all illnesses. The overall incidence of common respiratory diseases (which included illnesses diagnosed as the common cold, rhinitis, laryngitis, bronchitis, and other undifferentiated acute respiratory illnesses) was 5.6 per person per year. Children under one year of age experienced about seven respiratory illnesses per year; the highest incidence occurred in the one-year age group (8.3 cases per year) and the incidence remained rather high through age five (7.4 cases per year). A progressive decrease was observed beginning at age six. As expected, adults had relatively fewer common respiratory illnesses than children (adults averaged over four per year). The average incidence was slightly greater in boys than in girls, whereas in adults, mothers experienced higher rates than fathers. In addition, the incidence of common respiratory diseases was greater in young children attending school than in those of the same age who were not in school; also, preschool siblings of school children had more respiratory illnesses than preschool siblings without brothers or sisters attending school. The incidence of common respiratory diseases increased progressively as family size increased from three to seven members. Such illnesses were introduced into the home most frequently by school children under six years of age, followed in order of decreasing frequency by preschool children, school children six years of age and over, mothers, and fathers. Analysis of secondary attack rates in families revealed that on the average 25 per cent of all exposures in the home were followed by illness; one- and two-year-olds experienced the highest secondary attack rates (about twice the average).

In a more recent survey of acute respiratory illnesses over a six-year period in Tecumseh, Michigan, the mean incidence of respiratory illnesses per person per year was 3. The highest incidence was in the one-year age group (6.1) and the next highest in the one- to two-year age group (5.7). A viral or potentially pathogenic bacterial agent was isolated from about 25 per cent of the specimens collected, with rhinoviruses accounting for 38.5 per cent of the total number of isolates, a figure representing more than twice the number of isolates of the next most frequently detected group, the parainfluenza viruses.

Studies of the prevalence of neutralizing antibodies in serum against various rhinovirus serotypes have revealed a gradual acquisition of antibody beginning early in childhood and reaching a maximum of at least 50 per cent in the fifth decade. The prevalence of serum antibody to specific serotypes was not consistent. Although all individuals studied had neutralizing antibodies to each of the 55 serotypes tested, the prevalence of antibody to each serotype varied from about 10 to 80 per cent. Limited surveys of the prevalence of neutralizing antibody to rhinoviruses in various developed and developing countries, including several tropical areas, indicated a generally worldwide presence of rhinovirus antibody.

The prevalence of coronavirus serum antibody has been difficult to ascertain, since only two serotypes, 229E and OC43, can be cultivated with consistency in cell cultures and, in addition, results have been variable in different locations with these two viruses. For example, in one study in the United States, 29 per cent of children and 69 per cent of adults had serum complement-fixing (CF) antibody to OC43 virus. Such antibody to 229E virus was present very infrequently in children, whereas about one third of adults were antibody positive. However, in the United Kingdom, about 25 per cent of children and 41 per cent of adults had neutralizing antibody to 229E virus. In United States marine recruits, over 80 per cent had serum hemagglutination inhibition antibody to OC43 virus and 12 per cent had CF antibody to 229E virus. By recently developed enzyme- or radio-immunoassays, the prevalence of serum antibody to 229E and OC43 or related coronaviruses was over 80 per cent in adults in different geographic areas. A true evaluation of the prevalence of antibody to the coronavirus group must await the development of serologic assays for other members of this fastidious group of agents.

EPIDEMIOLOGY. In the temperate climates common colds occur most frequently in the colder months of the year. For example, in the Cleveland Family Study a consistent pattern of a low summer and high winter incidence of common respiratory diseases was documented. In September, a rise in respiratory illnesses to about six cases per person-year from a summer low of three cases per person-year was observed. After a slight dip in October an average rate of about seven cases per person-year was observed for each month from November through March.

Rhinoviruses are spread from person to person by direct contact, usually with transmission by infected droplets. In early volunteer studies, rhinoviruses induced common colds when administered in nasal drops or by swabbing the nasal mucosa or conjunctiva but not by swabbing the throat. More recent volunteer studies have highlighted a heretofore unrecognized mode of transmission that involves self-inoculation of the conjunctival or nasal mucosa with a rhinovirus-contaminated finger. Virus was recovered in 15 of 16 trials from fingers that were rubbed on plastic surfaces contaminated with rhinovirus one to three hours previously. In addition, rhinovirus dried on volunteers' fingers could be transferred to uncontaminated fingers of other volunteers following skin contact, in three of five trials. The efficiency of transmission of infection from experimentally infected volunteers to susceptible volunteers by hand-to-hand contact followed by self-inoculation was compared with that of transmission by large- and small-particle aerosols. It was striking that 11 of 15 hand-to-hand exposures initiated infection, whereas only 1 of 12 large-particle exposures (donor and contact in social setting) and none of 10 small-particle exposures (donor and contact separated by double mesh barrier) induced such infection.

Rhinovirus communicability was evaluated in childless married couples in a study in which both lacked serum neutralizing antibody to the challenge viruses. The overall transmission of a rhinovirus-related cold between partners was 38 per cent, which is similar to the secondary attack rate in the Cleveland Family Study or to those in epidemiologic studies of naturally occurring rhinovirus infections. Transmission rarely occurred unless (1) at least 1000 TCID$_{50}$ (50 per cent tissue culture infective doses) of virus were present in the donor's nasal washing, (2) the donor's hands and anterior nares were rhinovirus positive, (3) the donor had at least moderate symptoms, and (4) the partners spent many hours together (at least 122 hours during a seven-day period). Virus in saliva was not strongly associated with transmission.

The effect of exposure to cold temperatures on the course of common colds was evaluated in volunteers who were challenged with rhinovirus by small-particle aerosol or intranasal instillation. Exposure to the cold environment did not have a significant effect on host resistance to rhinovirus infection and illness. Exposure to cold temperature did not induce a common cold in uninoculated volunteers. This finding is consistent with results of early studies on the epidemiology of common colds on the island of Spitzbergen. These studies demonstrated that very few colds occurred during the bitter Arctic winter, but sharp outbreaks began shortly after the first ship arrived at the end of May. Thus, cold weather by itself did not induce common colds; the ingredient needed to initiate the outbreak was exposure to infected individuals. In early volunteer studies using common cold virus-like agents for challenge, fatigue and sleep deprivation caused an insignificant increase in the frequency with which colds occurred; however, in females, susceptibility was related to the menstrual cycle, with attempts to induce colds during menstruation being relatively unsuccessful.

The incubation period of rhinovirus-related common colds is quite short, ranging from one to five days with a mean of two days. Virus shedding generally begins with the onset of symptoms and continues for one week or even longer. Although there are 100 distinct rhinovirus serotypes, no one serotype has assumed special importance because numerous serotypes usually circulate at the same time. Rhinoviruses can be detected during most months of the year but reach peak prevalence during the fall and spring seasons. They are least prevalent during the cold winter months of December, January, and February, when common colds still occur frequently. However, coronavirus infections have been found to be prevalent during the late fall, winter, and early spring, when rhinovirus infections occur less frequently. Thus, coronaviruses can be considered to be the major known etiologic agents of the common cold in the winter.

A cyclic pattern in infection rates of coronaviruses 229E and OC43 has been described. With the 229E virus, infections appear to occur in the same years in various locations, including Chicago, Maryland, Virginia, and Michigan; a two-year cycle of activity has been suggested. For OC43 virus, a two- to four-year cycle was found that did not coincide in all locations. The 229E virus was shed in nasal washings of volunteers for one to at least four days after challenge; the peak frequency of virus excretion generally coincided with the peak of clinical symptoms. Virus shedding was also detected in certain volunteers who did not develop colds after challenge. Reinfections have also been observed frequently with coronaviruses under natural conditions; however, volunteers inoculated with the same coronavirus strain 8 to 12 months after initial challenge failed to develop illness on rechallenge.

It appears that serum antibody to a specific rhinovirus serotype correlates with protection against natural or experimental challenge with that serotype. However, serum antibody may not in itself be responsible for protection but may be a reflection of the level of specific nasal secretory antibodies. In one volunteer study in which the protective effects of neutralizing antibody in serum and in nasal secretions were compared, it was found that only nasal secretory antibody was associated with resistance to rhinovirus infection and illness.

PATHOLOGY. The pathologic mechanisms whereby a common cold is induced by a virus are not known. However, the pathology of viral rhinitis in general has been described. In the initial acute period of viral rhinitis the nasal mucosa is thickened and edematous and, depending on the degree of hyperemia, is pale gray to red in color and covered by a thin, watery mucoid discharge. The nasal cavities are narrowed by the enlargement of the turbinates. Histologically, there is extreme edema of the mucosal tissue, which is also infiltrated sparsely with neutrophils, lymphocytes, plasma cells, and eosinophils. Secretory hyperactivity of the mucus-secreting submucosal glands is also observed. The edematous nasal mucosa can cause obstruction of the orifices of the accessory air sinuses and lead to sinusitis. Extension of bacterial superinfections can result in serious sequelae, including osteomyelitis, cavernous sinus thrombophlebitis, epidural or subdural abscess, meningitis, or brain abscess. However, such complications are exceedingly rare.

Information on the pathologic findings in acute rhinovirus infections is extremely limited. Biopsies of nasal epithelium obtained from volunteers with experimentally induced rhinovirus colds failed to demonstrate consistent histologic changes. However, sloughed ciliated epithelial cells are found in nasal secretions.

CLINICAL MANIFESTATIONS. The major clinical manifestation of common colds occurring under natural or experimental conditions is coryza or nasal congestion. The most common complaints in rhinovirus-positive respiratory illnesses in 139 civilian adults were rhinorrhea and sneezing, which were recorded in one half to two thirds of the cases. The next most frequent complaint was sore throat, which occurred in nearly one half, while hoarseness and cough were less common, being present in one quarter to one half of the cases. Temperature elevation was unusual. An oral temperature of 99.6° F (37.6° C) or greater at the time of study was documented in less than 1 per cent of the cases. Nonrespiratory complaints were not common except for headache, which occurred in approximately one quarter of the cases. The mean duration of symptoms was about 9 days with a median of 7.4 days and a mode of 4 days.

The clinical manifestations of coronavirus-229E–like infections under natural conditions in adults are quite similar. Of nine patients who shed this agent, all had coryza, eight had nasal congestion, seven had sneezing, and five had sore throat at the time of study. Less common manifestations were headache (in four), cough (in three), muscular or general aches (in three), and chills and fever (in two). Coryza or nasal congestion was the chief complaint in eight of the nine patients.

Administration of rhinoviruses or coronaviruses to volunteers has provided an opportunity to define the clinical manifestations associated with these agents under carefully controlled conditions (Table 329–2). The mean incubation period of colds induced by coronaviruses was significantly longer (about one day), the duration of the illness somewhat shorter, and the mean maximum number of paper tissues used per day (for nasal discharge) greater than in rhinovirus-induced illnesses. In later studies, each of six other coronavirus strains was also administered by the nasal route to volunteers: cumulatively, 35 of 49 volunteers developed common cold-like illnesses. Thus, the ability to induce common colds in adults under experimental conditions is now as firmly established for the coronaviruses as for the rhinoviruses.

Rhinoviruses also cause common colds in children. The role of rhinoviruses as etiologic agents of bronchitis, bronchiolitis, bronchopneumonia, pneumonia, and croup in the pediatric age group is unclear. However, it appears certain that rhinoviruses are not important causes of these syndromes, even though nasal inhalation of a rhinovirus by small-particle aerosol induces a tracheobronchitis in volunteers. Rhinoviral respiratory illness has also been implicated as an important precipitant of asthmatic attacks in children with a history of asthma. Rhinoviruses have been recovered from certain hospitalized pediatric patients with lower respiratory tract disease; most of these patients had significant underlying disease

**TABLE 329–2. COMPARISON OF THE CLINICAL FEATURES OF COLDS
PRODUCED BY INTRANASAL ADMINISTRATION OF CORONAVIRUSES OR RHINOVIRUSES**

	Coronaviruses		Rhinoviruses	
	229E	B814	Type 2 (HGP or PK)	DC
Number of volunteers inoculated	26	75	213	251
Number getting colds	13 (50%)	34 (45%)	78 (37%)	77 (31%)
Incubation period (days)				
Mean	3.3	3.2	2.1	2.1
Range	2–4	2–5	1–5	1–4
Duration (days)				
Mean	7	6	9	10
Range	3–18	2–17	3–19	2–26
Maximum number of tissues used daily				
Mean	23	21	14	18
Range	8–105	8–120	3–38	3–60
Malaise	46%	47%	28%	25%
Headache	85%	53%	56%	56%
Chill	31%	18%	28%	15%
Pyrexia	23%*	21%	14%	18%
Mucopurulent nasal discharge	0	62%	83%	80%
Sore throat	54%	79%	87%	73%
Cough	31%	44%	68%	56%
Number of volunteers with colds of indicated severity				
Mild	10 (77%)	24 (71%)	63 (80%)	36 (47%)
Moderate	2 (15%)	7 (20%)	12 (15%)	28 (36%)
Severe	1 (8%)	3 (9%)	4 (5%)	13 (17%)

*Between 99.2° F (37.3° C) and 100.4° F (38° C) (oral). After Bradburne, Bynoe, Tyrrell: Br Med J 3:767, 1967.

involving the immune or cardiopulmonary system. In addition, rhinoviruses were recovered from patients with cyanosis and apnea in an intensive care nursery. Coronaviruses can also cause common cold–like illnesses in children. In one study, coronavirus 229E was recovered from two infants with pneumonia, and serologic evidence of coronavirus infection was demonstrated in 8.2 per cent of pediatric patients hospitalized with lower respiratory tract disease. However, in other studies such an association was not found. Coronavirus infection has been associated with exacerbations of wheezing in young children with asthma. Coronavirus OC43 and rhinovirus infections also were observed in several military trainees with pneumonia with pleural reaction and with atypical pneumonia, respectively. The etiologic significance of such associations is not known. Rhinovirus and coronavirus infections have been associated with exacerbations of chronic bronchitis in adults. A transient decrease in pulmonary function has also been observed in volunteers infected with rhinovirus. Rhinovirus has also been recovered from the lung of an adult patient with a fatal pulmonary infection and other underlying disease involving the immune system. Other complications of common colds include sinusitis, otitis media, and extensions of infections into the central nervous or cardiovascular systems, as noted in the pathology section. Rhinovirus has been recovered from sinus and middle ear fluids. The role of bacteria acting in concert with the virus infection in certain of these complications must be kept in mind in establishing therapeutic regimens.

DIAGNOSIS. Since most respiratory viruses can induce common colds, an etiologic diagnosis cannot be made on clinical grounds. Specific viral diagnosis of the common cold is essentially a research procedure that requires tissue or organ cultures for virus isolation or antigens for certain serologic studies. Complement fixation (229E, OC43), hemagglutination-inhibition (OC43), enzyme-linked immunosorbent assay (229E), or radioimmunoassay (OC43) can be performed in order to detect serologic evidence of infection with certain coronaviruses. However, antigens for such tests are not generally available. The most important test for a patient with a common cold-like illness is a throat culture for group A beta-hemolytic streptococci because symptoms of illnesses associated with the common cold viruses and the streptococcus may overlap. Appropriate antibiotic therapy is available for treatment of this bacterial infection.

TREATMENT AND PREVENTION. There is no specific treatment for patients with the common cold. Only symptomatic treatment measures should be employed. At this time, it appears that acetylsalicylic acid (aspirin) should not be used in children with colds because of the epidemiologic association of this drug with Reye's syndrome (see Ch. 490) when the drug is administered during a viral illness, usually influenza or varicella, both of which can cause symptoms resembling those of the common cold (Table 329–1).

Antibiotics have no value in the therapy of the uncomplicated common cold. Previous tonsillectomy did not significantly affect the number of common respiratory illnesses or the induction of experimental colds in volunteers in the Cleveland Family Study. Available evidence indicates that vitamin C does not reduce the number of episodes of respiratory illness but does decrease somewhat the total number of days of disability. The routine use of large doses of vitamin C for preventive treatment of common colds does not appear to be warranted from evidence available at this time.

Currently 100 serotypes of rhinovirus are known to exist, and no one serotype or group of serotypes appears to be consistently more important than others. Experimental rhinovirus vaccines against single serotypes have been made and shown to be effective in preventing or modifying illnesses induced by the serotype present in the vaccine. Although some heterotypic antibody responses have been observed with decavalent rhinovirus vaccines, the production of a rhinovirus vaccine appears to be impractical because of the multiplicity of serotypes. Until the number of serotypes of coronaviruses can be elucidated and the role of antibody in preventing or modifying illnesses can be established, consideration of a coronavirus vaccine is premature.

Since the three-dimensional structure and the cellular receptors of rhinovirus have been determined recently, it may be possible to design effective and practical antiviral compounds based on these findings. In addition, there has been renewed interest in the use of interferon to prevent common colds, since interferon can now be produced by recombinant deoxyribonucleic acid (DNA) techniques. Interferon applied topically by nasal spray was effective in reducing the number of symptomatic illnesses when given prophylactically to volunteers challenged with rhinovirus or following natural exposure to a rhinovirus cold in a family setting. Nasal irritation from interferon was minimized by short-term application.

Interferon nasal sprays are not effective as treatment for common colds caused by rhinovirus after symptoms have begun. Prophylactic interferon nasal spray has also been shown to shorten the duration and reduce the severity of coronavirus (229E)–induced cold symptoms. The use of interferon for prophylaxis of common colds does not appear practical for general usage but may be beneficial under special circumstances.

One method available for preventing rhinovirus-induced colds may be the application of rigid personal hygienic measures when a family member has a common cold. This would entail hand washing and avoidance of finger-eye and finger-nose contact.

Recently, the use of virucidal paper handkerchiefs has been shown to interrupt the transmission of rhinovirus-induced colds. This intervention awaits further evaluation in various settings.

Committee on Infectious Diseases of the American Academy of Pediatrics (Fulginiti VA, Brunell PA, Cherry JD, Ector WL, Gershon AA, Gotoff SP, Hughes WT, Mortimer EA Jr, Peter G): Special Report: Aspirin and Reye syndrome. Pediatrics 69:810, 1982. *After weighing the available evidence, this Committee has made a strong recommendation against the use of aspirin under usual circumstances in children with varicella or influenza (both of which can cause common cold-like symptoms).*

Couch RB: Rhinoviruses. In Fields BN, et al. (eds.): Virology. New York, Raven Press, 1985, pp 795–816. *An up-to-date review of the rhinoviruses (154 references).*

Dick EC, Hossain SU, Mink KA, et al.: Interruption of transmission of rhinovirus colds among human volunteers using virucidal paper handkerchiefs. J Infect Dis 153:352, 1986. *An imaginative study in which the spread of rhinovirus-induced colds is prevented by the use of paper handkerchiefs treated with virucidal ingredients.*

Fox JP, Cooney MK, Hall EC, et al.: Rhinoviruses in Seattle families, 1975–1979. Am J Epidemiol 122:830, 1985. *A comprehensive epidemiologic study of rhinovirus infections in families in Seattle, Washington.*

Hayden FG, Albrecht JK, Kaiser PL, et al.: Prevention of natural colds by contact prophylaxis with intranasal alpha$_2$-interferon. N Engl J Med 314:71, 1986. *Describes how interferon sprayed intranasally, following contact with a family member with a common cold, significantly reduced the number of rhinovirus colds in the contacts.*

Lowenstein SR, Parrino TA: Management of the common cold. Adu Intern Med 32:207–234, 1987. *A review of the management of common colds (121 references).*

McIntosh K: Coronaviruses. In Fields BN, et al. (eds.): Virology. New York, Raven Press, 1985, pp 1323–1330. *An up-to-date review of the coronaviruses (62 references).*

Remington PL, Rowley D, McGee H, et al.: Decreasing trends in Reye syndrome and aspirin use in Michigan, 1979 to 1984. Pediatrics 77:93, 1986. *The decreasing use of aspirin in children with colds or influenza and the decrease in Reye syndrome in Tecumseh is evaluated.*

Scott G: Interfering with the real cold. Br Med J 292:1413, 1986. *In this editorial the use of interferon for preventing common colds is reviewed.*

Smith TJ, Kremer MJ, Luo M, et al.: The site of attachment in human rhinovirus 14 for antiviral agents that inhibit uncoating. Science 233:1286, 1986. *A basic paper describing the three-dimensional structure of a rhinovirus and the application of this information to the development of antiviral compounds.*

Tomassini JE, Colonna RJ: Isolation of a receptor protein involved in attachment of human rhinoviruses. J Virol 58:290, 1986. *The discovery of cellular receptors for rhinoviruses may lead to the development of antiviral compounds.*

Turner RB, Felton A, Kosak K, et al.: Prevention of experimental coronavirus colds with intranasal α-2b interferon. J Infect Dis 154:443, 1986. *Describes how interferon administered prophylactically under experimental conditions shortened the duration and decreased the severity of cold symptoms due to a coronavirus in volunteers.*

Tyrrell DAJ: Common colds. Intervirology 25:177–189, 1986. *A review of common colds from a historical perspective by a pioneer in this field.*

330 VIRAL PHARYNGITIS, LARYNGITIS, CROUP, AND BRONCHITIS

Maurice A. Mufson

DEFINITION. Viral infections that localize to the upper and middle respiratory passages produce an acute inflammatory response and, depending upon the anatomic site involved, evoke the clinical manifestations of pharyngitis, laryngitis, croup (laryngotracheobronchitis), and bronchitis. These infections do not ordinarily involve the pulmonary alveoli. Pharyngitis, laryngitis, and bronchitis can occur in persons of any age. Croup occurs exclusively in children and mainly during the second year of life. These illnesses usually begin abruptly with predominant upper respiratory tract signs and symptoms and limited systemic findings, and the uncomplicated illness abates after five to ten days. Croup can be a life-threatening illness; the most common complications include respiratory failure and pneumonia.

ETIOLOGY. The main viral pathogens of pharyngitis and laryngitis include rhinoviruses, coronaviruses, influenza A and B viruses, adenoviruses, parainfluenza viruses, enteroviruses, and respiratory syncytial virus (see Table 330–1). The principal viral pathogens of croup are the parainfluenza viruses types 1, 3, and 2 (in decreasing frequency). Acute viral bronchitis has been associated with influenza A and B virus, coronavirus, adenovirus, respiratory syncytial virus, and rhinovirus infections. In any individual case, the etiology of pharyngitis, laryngitis, croup, and bronchitis cannot be determined on the basis of the clinical characteristics of the illness. A definitive etiologic diagnosis can be made only by application of diagnostic virology tests, either virus isolation or one of the newer rapid diagnostic procedures using respiratory secretions.

Pharyngitis also can occur as part of systemic viral illnesses associated with *Epstein-Barr virus* (see Ch. 342) or *cytomegalovirus* (see Ch. 341) infection, and laryngitis and bronchitis occur in *measles* virus infection (see Ch. 336). When coryza represents the main feature of an upper respiratory infection, the term *common cold* (see Ch. 329) prevails. When the infecting virus is an influenza virus, the designation *influenza* describes an acute respiratory tract infection with fever and prostration (see Ch. 333).

INCIDENCE AND PREVALENCE. Viral pharyngitis, laryngitis, and bronchitis occur commonly. Most children and adults experience three to five viral infections of the upper respiratory tract each year. Croup is a serious illness of infants and children immediately recognizable by a distinctive complex of symptoms and signs (see later discussion); the incidence of croup peaks in the second year of life, as high as 47 cases per 1000 children per year, and by age four to five it declines to under 15 cases per 1000 children per year (Denny, 1983).

EPIDEMIOLOGY. Viral pharyngitis, laryngitis, croup, and bronchitis occur during all months of the year, with peaks of occurrence paralleling epidemics of individual viruses. Respiratory syncytial virus, influenza A and B viruses, coronaviruses, parainfluenza virus type 1, and to a lesser extent type 2, occur in epidemics, mainly in the late fall, winter, and spring (see Table 330–1). The other viral pathogens occur endemically, although they may exhibit some seasonal variation from year to year. Virus infections of the respiratory tract spread by direct person-to-person contact, by infectious aerosols, or by fomites.

CLINICAL MANIFESTATIONS. *Viral Pharyngitis.* Acute viral pharyngitis is characterized by a scratchy and sore throat, but pain upon swallowing is not a prominent or constant feature. When dysphagia is present, it suggests a streptococcal infection. Cough is not a feature of acute viral pharyngitis. Fever and malaise accompany influenza and adenovirus infections, but these findings are infrequent with the other respiratory viral pathogens. Pharyngeal erythema and edema and enlarged and tender lymph nodes may be the only physical findings. Adenovirus pharyngitis may be associated with conjunctivitis. Exudative tonsillitis occurs in adenovirus infections, infectious mononucleosis associated with Epstein-Barr virus infection, herpetic pharyngitis (with or without vesicles or small ulcers), as well as streptococcal pharyngitis. Exudative tonsillitis alone does not distinguish these infections.

TABLE 330–1. EPIDEMIOLOGY AND ETIOLOGY OF VIRAL PHARYNGITIS, LARYNGITIS, CROUP, AND BRONCHITIS

Virus	Serotype	Epidemiology	Occurrence in Indicated Illness			
			Pharyngitis	*Laryngitis*	*Croup*	*Bronchitis*
Respiratory syncytial	Two subgroups: A and B	Annual epidemics	+		+	+ + +
Parainfluenza	Type 1	Epidemic alternate years	+ +	+ +	+ + + +	+ +
	Type 2	Sporadic	+	+	+ + +	+
	Type 3	Endemic	+ +	+ +	+ + + +	+ +
Influenza	Type A	Epidemic	+ + +	+ + +	+	+ + +
	Type B	Epidemic; less common than influenza A	+ +	+		+
Adenovirus	Types 1, 2, 3, 4, 5, 6, and 7	Endemic	+ + + +	+ +		+ +
Coronavirus	Several	Endemic	+ +	+		+ + +
Rhinovirus	More than 100 serotypes	Endemic	+ + + +	+ + +		+ +
Enterovirus	Many	Endemic	+ +			
Herpes simplex	Type 1	Endemic	+ +			

Frequency and importance of virus occurrence are graded from minimal importance (+) to major importance (+ + + +). Blank = uncommon occurrence.

Viral Laryngitis. In acute viral laryngitis, hoarseness predominates, associated with difficulty in talking, pain on clearing respiratory secretions, and often fever, depending upon the infecting virus. Cough and pharyngitis may be present. The larynx is erythematous and edematous, and the regional lymph nodes are slightly enlarged and tender. Wheezes may be audible upon auscultation.

Viral Croup. The clinical picture of croup characteristically includes inspiratory stridor, hoarseness, and a brassy cough. This distinctive triad of symptoms reflects the acute and intense edema and mucoid exudative secretions of the larynx and associated obstruction of the subglottic portion of the upper airway. These symptoms develop acutely, accompanied by fever, cough, tachypnea, and wheezing. Retractions of the chest wall occur. Hemoptysis does not occur. Rhonchi, rales, or wheezes, alone or in combination, may be audible upon auscultation of the lungs. Radiographic examination of the neck can demonstrate subglottic narrowing, and a chest roentgenogram may show hyperinflation of the lungs. In the uncomplicated case, the findings resolve in several days, but some children develop respiratory failure and pneumonia. Children who previously experienced multiple episodes of croup manifest hyper-reactive airways several years later.

Viral Bronchitis. In acute viral bronchitis, cough, with or without sputum production, and fever are the main features. The sputum is slightly mucoid or watery and white. Other common symptoms include hoarseness, nonpleuritic substernal chest pain, and malaise. Rhonchi or rales may be heard upon auscultation of the chest. The chest roentgenogram may show increased intensity of the vascular pattern, but pulmonary infiltrates do not occur. Acute bronchitis associated with influenza or coronavirus infection occurs often as an exacerbation of chronic bronchitis.

TREATMENT AND PROGNOSIS. The treatment of pharyngitis, laryngitis, and bronchitis associated with virus infections of the upper respiratory tract aims at the relief of distressing local and systemic symptoms. These illnesses are self-limited and not severe. Antibiotics are not indicated, except when secondary bacterial infection occurs; it is likely to develop mainly with influenza virus infections. In pharyngitis, pharyngeal pain or dysphagia should be treated with analgesics and fluids. The treatment of laryngitis and bronchitis also requires analgesics, fluids, and rest. Cough in adults and older children that is relentless and causes fatigue should be treated with cough suppressant preparations. Influenza virus vaccine must be administered to persons in the high-risk group (unless contraindicated) to diminish the chance of infection (see Ch. 17).

The less serious cases of croup can be managed by having the child rest in bed at home. Vaporizers that produce a mist of moist air may be beneficial. Children with severe croup require hospitalization, supportive treatment, and constant monitoring for the development of respiratory distress. If hypoxemia develops, oxygen therapy is essential; hypoxemia requiring oxygen can develop even before cyanosis becomes evident. Subglottic edema may be reduced by the administration of racemic epinephrine. Administration of corticosteroids in the treatment of croup may have limited benefit.

Denny FW, Murphy TF, Clyde WA Jr, et al.: Croup: An 11-year study in a pediatric practice. Pediatrics 71:871, 1983. *A comprehensive investigation of the viral etiology and epidemiology of croup among a large population of ambulatory children. Viral infections were identified by virus isolation attempts on oropharyngeal cultures.*

Gwaltney JM Jr, Hendley JO: Transmission of experimental rhinovirus infection by contaminated surfaces. Am J Epidemiol 116:828, 1982. *The first demonstration that environmental surfaces contaminated with rhinovirus-containing secretions could serve as a reservoir for the spread of these viruses to susceptible persons.*

Koren G, Frand M, Barzilay Z, et al.: Corticosteroid treatment of laryngotracheitis v spasmodic croup in children. Am J Dis Child 137:941, 1983. *Recent re-evaluation of the effectiveness of corticosteroid therapy for croup. Double-blind random design was employed in the treatment of two categories of croup using a single high dose of dexamethasone. Six hours after the start of corticosteroid therapy, the respiratory rate of patients classified as having spasmodic croup had decreased significantly compared with the placebo group, but no change in respiratory rate was detected among patients classified as having laryngotracheitis.*

Mufson MA, Örvell C, Rafnar B, et al.: Two distinct subtypes of human respiratory syncytial virus. J Gen Virol 66:2111, 1985. *New description of two subtypes (or subgroups) of respiratory syncytial virus recognized by their pattern of reaction with monoclonal antibodies generated against the major proteins of the virus.*

Ruuskanen O, Sarkkinen H, Meurman O, et al.: Rapid diagnosis of adenoviral tonsillitis: A prospective clinical study. J Pediatr 104:725, 1984. *Description of a radioimmunoassay for the detection of adenovirus antigen in nasopharyngeal secretions of persons with adenovirus pharyngitis with exudative tonsillitis.*

331 RESPIRATORY SYNCYTIAL VIRUS

Robert M. Chanock

DEFINITION. Respiratory syncytial virus (RSV) is the most important cause of viral lower respiratory tract disease in infants and children. This ubiquitous virus causes an extensive epidemic every year during fall, winter, or early spring. During these epidemics there is a dramatic increase in admission to hospitals of infants and young children with severe lower respiratory tract disease. Older children and adults commonly undergo reinfection, but disease is usually milder than that experienced during infancy and early childhood.

ETIOLOGY. RSV, an enveloped virus that belongs to the family Paramyxoviridae, genus *Pneumovirus*, resembles the parainfluenza viruses of the genus *Paramyxovirus* but differs from them in morphology of its nucleocapsid, in failure to agglutinate erythrocytes (hemagglutination), and in absence of a neuraminidase enzyme. The RSV negative (−) strand RNA genome, approximately 15,000 bases in length, is transcribed as a series of 10 separate messenger ribonucleic acids (mRNAs), each of which is translated into a separate viral protein. One of these proteins, nucleocapsid protein, coats the viral RNA to form a helical nucleocapsid. This structure is enclosed within a bilayer lipid membrane that is studded with two different viral glycoproteins. One of these, the fusion protein, lyses the host cell membrane, permitting entry of virus into the cell. This protein is also responsible for fusion of infected cells to neighboring cells, a process that results in syncytium formation, a prominent feature of the virus during its growth in tissue culture.

Although antigenic variation among strains has been noted, it does not appear to have major epidemiologic significance. A related RSV is a common cause of respiratory disease in calves, but this virus does not appear to infect humans.

EPIDEMIOLOGY. Whenever appropriate studies have been performed, RSV has been found to be the major pediatric respiratory tract viral pathogen. The highest incidence of severe lower respiratory tract disease is observed in infants between one and six months of age, with a peak incidence at two months. Serious lower respiratory tract disease occurs more commonly in males than in females and in nonblack than in black infants. Approximately 50 per cent of infants who live through a single RSV epidemic become infected. In certain settings, such as day-care centers, the attack rate approaches 100 per cent during an outbreak.

Reinfection occurs with high frequency during childhood. Adults are also reinfected frequently, particularly when there is exposure to a large amount of virus. For example, in families into which virus is introduced, spread of RSV among older siblings occurs with high frequency (40 per cent). In individuals of all ages, reinfection is usually symptomatic, and adults exposed to a large amount of virus may develop an influenza-like disease.

Most individuals infected with RSV have upper respiratory illness. However, a surprisingly large proportion of infants (25 to 40 per cent) also develop lower respiratory tract disease. Hospitalization of infants for RSV disease varies with environmental and socioeconomic conditions. Overall, 1 in 120 to 1 in 200 infants requires hospital care for RSV pneumonia or bronchiolitis during the first year of life. RSV is responsible for approximately 50 to 75 per cent of bronchiolitis and for 20 to 25 per cent of pneumonias that necessitate admission of infants and young children to hospital.

In developed countries, severe RSV lower respiratory tract disease is rarely fatal (0.5 to 2.5 per cent). Fatal RSV disease occurs most often in infants with other underlying illnesses, particularly congenital heart disease (37 per cent), bronchopulmonary dysplasia, serious renal disease, and diseases such as cancer that are treated with immunosuppressive drugs. In a British study of 46 infants and children who died with lower respiratory tract disease, 13 were infected with RSV. In addition, a number of babies dying of sudden infant death syndrome are infected with RSV.

RSV has a clear seasonality in temperate zones of the world. In urban centers, epidemics occur yearly in the late fall, winter, or spring but not during the summer. In the northern hemisphere, the virus is rarely isolated during August or September. Each RSV epidemic lasts approximately five months, with 40 per cent of infections occurring during the peak month in the temporal center of the outbreak. In the northern hemisphere, most outbreaks peak in February or March, but the peak may occur as early as December or as late as June. RSV is spread by infected respiratory secretions in the form of large droplets or through fomite contamination.

During epidemic intervals, RSV is one of the most common causes of hospital-acquired infection on pediatric wards. The risk of infection increases as the hospital stay is extended beyond one week. The mortality in such hospital-acquired infections is considerably higher than in community-acquired infections because the patients involved are frequently at high risk from other diseases, malnourishment, or immunosuppressive drugs.

Since reinfection with RSV is common and often associated with disease, it is clear that immunity is neither permanent nor complete. However, multiple reinfections induce temporary immunity to infection and a more long-term resistance to severe RSV lower respiratory tract disease. Studies in adult volunteers indicate that immunity to induced upper respiratory tract infection correlates better with the level of nasal neutralizing immunoglobulin A (IgA) antibody than with serum antibody. On the other hand, there is some epidemiological evidence that the high levels of maternally derived RSV antibodies possessed by many small infants provide protection from serious lower respiratory tract disease. However, lower levels of such antibodies present in the serum of older infants are not protective.

CLINICAL MANIFESTATIONS. During infancy, RSV infection usually causes upper respiratory symptoms. In 25 to 40 per cent of infections the respiratory tract below the larynx is also involved. Lower respiratory tract signs are preceded by a prodromal phase of rhinorrhea that is sometimes accompanied by a decrease in appetite. Low-grade fever is common. Cough is often accompanied by wheezing, and if disease is mild, symptoms may not progress beyond this stage. Examination usually reveals moderate tachypnea, diffuse rhonchi, fine rales and wheezes, as well as profuse rhinorrhea and intermittent fever. Otitis media is also common. The chest radiograph usually appears normal. In most instances, uneventful recovery occurs after 7 to 12 days.

In more severe cases, coughing and wheezing progress and the child becomes dyspneic and refuses feedings. Hyperexpansion of the chest is evident, and there may be intercostal and subcostal retractions. Severe tachypnea is common even in the absence of visible cyanosis, and in advanced disease, as the child tires and hypoxia becomes more extreme, listlessness and apnea occur. The chest may appear normal on radiographic examination, but often there is a combination of air trapping (hyperexpansion) and peribronchial thickening or interstitial pneumonia. Segmental or lobar consolidation is also occasionally seen, usually involving the right upper lobe. Pleural effusion is rare. In infants with underlying cardiac or respiratory disease, the progression of symptoms may be rapid. In these instances, respiratory failure requiring intubation and ventilation may appear on the second or third day of illness.

Almost all infants who require hospitalization are hypoxemic on admission and remain so for a prolonged period—up to several weeks—although recovery has ensued. The hypoxemia reflects an abnormally low ventilation-perfusion ratio. Hypercarbia may also be present.

In infants who were born prematurely, and sometimes in normal infants under six weeks of age, apneic spells may develop during RSV infection. These often occur in the absence of significant respiratory signs and may be the predominant symptom bringing the infant to medical attention. Such apneic spells, while often recurrent during acute infection, are usually self-limited and rarely cause neurologic or systemic damage. However, exceptions to this pattern occur, and such episodes are an indication for hospitalization and careful medical supervision. Apnea at the peak of severe illness is a poor prognostic sign.

In the newborn infant, most RSV infections produce only

upper respiratory symptoms. Bronchiolitis is rare, and severe infection is more often characterized by lethargy, irritability, and fever or unstable body temperature than by specific respiratory signs.

Children who have apparently recovered completely from RSV bronchiolitis or pneumonia may still retain both measurable and symptomatic respiratory abnormalities for many years. A study of 23 children examined ten years after an episode of bronchiolitis found that although all were symptom free (a criterion for admission to the study), 20 had some measurable physiologic abnormality of lung function or arterial blood gases.

Acute RSV infections are common in adults, particularly in medical personnel or in those caring for small children. These reinfections are occasionally asymptomatic but usually are associated with rhinorrhea, pharyngitis, cough, constitutional symptoms of headache and fatigue, and fever. Disease usually lasts about five days but may be more prolonged, particularly in hospital staff. Alterations in pulmonary function, such as elevated total respiratory resistance and increased airway reactivity, often last for eight weeks. There is some evidence that RSV infection in the elderly is a cause of febrile bronchitis and severe or even fatal pneumonia.

DIAGNOSIS. Presumptive diagnosis of RSV infection can often be made on the basis of the clinical syndrome in relation to the time of year and other epidemiologic features. Definitive diagnosis depends upon the laboratory. In older children and adults, an increase in serum RSV antibody concentration, either complement fixing (CF) or neutralizing, is a fairly sensitive index of reinfection with RSV. Serologic tests in infants are less sensitive, particularly in patients under four months of age. In young infants, only 2 to 15 per cent of RSV infections are detectable by CF and 2 to 20 per cent by neutralization assay. Antibody measurement by solid-phase immunoassay (enzyme-linked immunosorbent assay, or ELISA) recently has been shown to be a more sensitive indicator of infection in small infants than CF or neutralization. At all ages, however, isolation of virus or detection of antigen in respiratory secretions is the procedure of choice. Specimens are best obtained by aspiration or gentle washing out of nasopharyngeal secretions. These may be examined by inoculation of tissue culture, immunofluorescence, or ELISA. Infectivity of RSV in secretions is labile; hence samples should be placed on wet ice while being transported to a tissue culture laboratory.

TREATMENT AND PREVENTION. Treatment of RSV infections of the lower respiratory tract consists primarily of supportive care: mechanical removal of secretions, proper positioning of the infant, administration of humidified oxygen, and in severe cases respiratory assistance. When wheezing is an important symptom, some patients, particularly those over a year of age, will benefit from the use of theophylline or adrenergic drugs.

Ribavirin (1β D-ribofuranosyl-1,2,4-triazole-3-carboxamide), delivered by small-particle aerosol, is now licensed for treatment of severe RSV disease in young infants. The drug hastens recovery and diminishes virus shedding.

Because immunity to RSV is neither permanent nor complete, the goal of immunoprophylaxis is prevention of severe lower respiratory tract disease. It should be possible to achieve this through the cumulative effect of repeated vaccination. Efforts to develop an effective vaccine have been frustrated by the ineffectiveness of formalin-inactivated virus and by the genetic instability of satisfactorily attenuated temperature-sensitive mutants that initially showed promise as live virus vaccine strains. Perhaps recent success in constructing recombinant vaccinia viruses that express RSV surface glycoproteins and induce resistance in experimental animals to RSV infection may open the way to effective immunoprophylaxis for this virus.

Hall CBH, Geiman JM, Biggar R, et al.: Respiratory syncytial virus infections within families. N Engl J Med 294:414, 1976. *Longitudinal surveillance of RSV infections in families. During an epidemic, infection occurred in 44 per cent of families; within these families the infection rate was 62 per cent in infants and 43 per cent in adults, the latter rate representing reinfection.*

Hall CBH, McBride JT, Walsh EE, et al.: Aerosolized ribavirin treatment of infants with respiratory syncytial viral infection. N Engl J Med 308:1443, 1983. *Administration of ribavirin by small-particle aerosol hastened recovery of infants with severe RSV lower respiratory tract disease.*

Henderson FW, Collier AM, Clyde WA Jr, et al.: Respiratory-syncytial-virus infections, reinfections and immunity. N Engl J Med 300:530, 1979. *Longitudinal surveillance of children in a day care center demonstrated high frequency of reinfection; also, after several reinfections partial immunity developed to RSV.*

McIntosh K, Chanock RM: Respiratory syncytial virus. In Fields B (ed.): Virology. New York, Raven Press, 1985, pp 1285–1304. *A summary of biologic properties of RSV as well as its epidemiology and the pathogenesis of the disease.*

Olmsted RA, Elango N, Prince GA, et al.: Expression of the F glycoprotein of respiratory syncytial virus by a recombinant vaccinia virus: Comparison of the individual contributions of the F and G glycoproteins to host immunity. Proceed Nat Acad Sci USA 83:7462, 1986. *Immunization of cotton rats with a vaccinia virus—RSV surface glycoprotein gene recombinant induces resistance to RSV infection in the lungs.*

332 PARAINFLUENZA VIRAL DISEASES

Robert M. Chanock

DEFINITION. Infection with parainfluenza viruses occurs early in life and is an important cause of *pediatric respiratory tract disease.* The spectrum of illness varies from mild upper respiratory disease to severe croup, pneumonia, or bronchiolitis. Reinfection is common in later life and is associated with mild respiratory tract disease.

ETIOLOGY. The parainfluenza viruses are enveloped viruses that belong to the family Paramyxoviridae, genus *Paramyxovirus.* The single-stranded ribonucleic acid (RNA) viral genome has negative polarity (antimessenger sense) and is approximately 15,000 bases in length. Its genetic information is expressed as a series of messenger RNAs (mRNAs) transcribed from the viral genome that codes for seven viral-specific proteins. One of these proteins, nucleocapsid protein, coats the viral RNA to form a helical nucleocapsid. This structure is enclosed within a lipid bilayer envelope that is studded with the two viral glycoprotein surface antigens, the hemagglutinin-neuraminidase, and the fusion protein. Parainfluenza viruses share many properties with the influenza viruses, but they differ from these agents in their wider RNA nucleocapsid (18 nm as compared with 9 nm) and in the distribution of hemagglutination and neuraminidase functions on their surface glycoproteins. Both parainfluenza hemagglutinin and neuraminidase are located on the same surface glycoprotein, whereas these functions reside on separate surface glycoproteins of the influenza viruses. The parainfluenza viruses have common antigens that are not shared by the influenza viruses. Mumps virus shares the foregoing properties, as well as related antigens, with the parainfluenza viruses.

There are four antigenically distinct serotypes of human parainfluenza virus. Related parainfluenza viruses cause respiratory disease in mice (Sendai virus, a subtype of type 1), dogs (SV5, a subtype of type 2), calves (bovine shipping fever virus, a subtype of type 3), and birds (seven distinct serotypes not closely related to human parainfluenza viruses). Animal and avian parainfluenza viruses are distinct antigenically from human parainfluenza viruses and do not appear to infect humans.

EPIDEMIOLOGY. The four parainfluenza virus types have wide geographic distribution. The first three types have been identified in most areas where appropriate tissue culture and hemadsorption techniques have been applied to the study of childhood respiratory tract diseases. So far, type 4 viruses (subtypes 4A and 4B), which are more difficult to recover in tissue culture, have been isolated in fewer areas, but serologic studies suggest that they are also relatively ubiquitous.

The parainfluenza viruses are exceeded only by *respiratory syncytial virus (RSV)* as an important cause of lower respiratory tract disease in young children. These viruses, particularly type 3, commonly reinfect older children and adults to produce upper respiratory tract disease. Illness usually occurs less often and is less severe during reinfection than during primary infection.

There is considerable diversity in both epidemiologic and clinical manifestations of infections caused by the parainfluenza viruses. Parainfluenza virus type 1 is the principal cause of croup (laryngotracheobronchitis) in children, and parainfluenza virus type 3 is second only to RSV as a cause of pneumonia and bronchiolitis in infants less than six months of age. Parainfluenza virus type 2 resembles type 1 virus in clinical manifestations but causes serious illness less frequently. Infections with parainfluenza virus type 4 are detected infrequently, and associated illnesses are usually mild.

The parainfluenza viruses are most important as respiratory tract pathogens during infancy and childhood, when they (types 1 through 3) cause a spectrum of effects ranging from inapparent infection to life-threatening lower respiratory tract disease. Studies in different parts of the world indicate that types 1, 2, and 3 are associated with approximately 40 to 70 per cent of severe croup. In addition to croup, these three viruses are also responsible for a smaller but appreciable percentage of other acute respiratory tract diseases of infancy and early childhood. Eighty per cent of individuals undergoing primary infection with type 3 virus develop a febrile illness, and in one third there is involvement of the lower respiratory tract. Approximately one half of initial type 1 virus infections and two thirds of initial type 2 virus infections produce a febrile illness. Severe croup, although the most dramatic and serious manifestation of initial parainfluenza virus infection, is noted in only 2 to 3 per cent of primary type 1 or type 2 virus infections.

Primary parainfluenza virus infection generally occurs early in life. Type 3 virus often causes illness during the first months of life while infants still possess circulating neutralizing antibody derived from their mothers. In contrast, in young infants, maternally derived antibody appears to prevent both infection and severe disease caused by type 1 and type 2 viruses. After age four months, there is an increase in the incidence of croup and other lower respiratory tract diseases caused by type 1 and type 2 viruses. This high incidence continues until approximately six years of age, after which there is a much lower incidence. It is unusual for type 1 or type 2 virus to cause lower respiratory tract illness during adolescence or adult life, although this does occur on occasion.

At present, type 1 and type 2 virus epidemics are synchronous, occurring during the autumn of odd-numbered years. For many years, type 3 virus exhibited an endemic pattern, with infection occurring during all seasons of the year. Within this endemic pattern, small outbreaks occurred, but there was no predictable periodicity. Within the past seven years, there has been a shift toward yearly spring epidemics of type 3 virus infection. Nosocomial infection with the parainfluenza viruses, particularly type 3 virus, is common and often leads to serious lower respiratory tract disease.

Transmission of parainfluenza viruses is by direct person-to-person contact or large droplet spread. The high rate of infection early in life, coupled with the high frequency of reinfection, suggests that these viruses spread readily from person to person. Reinfected individuals appear to be infectious, and a relatively small inoculum is able to initiate infection. Type 3 virus appears to be the most transmissible of the parainfluenza viruses.

In experimental infection of adult volunteers, the interval between administration of type 1, 2, or 3 virus and onset of upper respiratory tract symptoms ranged from three to six days. The incubation period in pediatric infections has not been defined; however, the interval between exposure to type 3 virus and the subsequent initial shedding of this virus is two to four days. Resistance to type 1 or type 2 parainfluenza virus infection and associated upper respiratory disease appears to be a function of local respiratory tract, secretory, immunoglobulin A (IgA)–neutralizing antibodies. Infants may also be partially protected from infection and lower respiratory tract disease by serum antibodies. This protective relationship is suggested by the relative sparing of young infants from type 1 and type 2 virus infection and associated disease at a time when they possess serum antibodies passively acquired from their mother. Also, the risk of infection with type 3 virus during the first four months of life is inversely related to the level of neutralizing antibody present in cord serum at birth. However, the protective effect of passive immunity is less than that observed for type 1 and type 2 viruses, since a significant number of infants with moderately high levels of maternally derived serum antibody become infected with type 3 virus and develop severe illness.

CLINICAL MANIFESTATIONS. In children, the most common type of illness consists of rhinitis, pharyngitis, and bronchitis, usually with fever. The most common initial symptoms are cough, hoarseness, and fever. The cough may be croupy, but respiratory distress is not present. Approximately three fourths of such ill children have temperatures above 37.8° C; fever usually lasts two to three days. Coarse breath sounds, rhonchi, erythema of the pharyngeal mucous membranes, and rhinitis are characteristic physical findings. Cervical adenopathy is uncommon.

When croup develops, the initial symptoms of rhinitis, pharyngitis, fever, and cough progress. After several days, the cough worsens and becomes brassy, seal-like, or barking, and stridor ensues. At this stage, most children recover uneventfully after 24 to 48 hours, but in some air hunger develops, with cyanosis, sternal and intercostal retractions, and progressive airway obstruction. The lateral x-ray of the neck (which should be obtained only under carefully controlled medical supervision, if at all) shows glottic and subglottic narrowing (the "steeple sign") and differentiates this disease from epiglottitis.

When bronchiolitis or pneumonia develops, fever persists and the cough progresses and becomes somewhat productive. It is accompanied by wheezing, tachypnea, and retractions and in severe cases by cyanosis. The x-ray film shows interstitial or perihilar infiltrates and air trapping. In some patients a combined bronchopneumonia-croup syndrome occurs.

DIAGNOSIS. Presumptive diagnosis of parainfluenza virus infection can be made on the basis of age, history, clinical findings, and relation to known or characteristic prevalence of virus in the community. Definitive diagnosis, however, requires recovery of the virus from appropriate specimens taken from the respiratory tract or identification of viral antigens in respiratory tract secretions by immunofluorescence or another form of immunoassay. Serodiagnosis by hemagglutination inhibition, complement fixation, or neutralization can establish that infection with a member of the parainfluenza virus group has occurred, but frequent heterotypic responses make type-specific diagnosis by serology extremely difficult.

TREATMENT. Symptomatic treatment of croup usually includes humidification of air by ultrasonic nebulizer and periodic inhalation of racemic epinephrine. Antibiotics are usually contraindicated. The use of corticosteroids is controversial, but many physicians prescribe high doses of dexamethasone if croup is severe. Specific antiviral treatment or effective vaccines for prevention of parainfluenza virus disease are not available.

Chanock RM, McIntosh K: Parainfluenza viruses. In Fields B (ed.): Virology. New York, Raven Press, 1985, pp 1241–1253. *Summary of natural history of parainfluenza virus infection and pathogenesis of disease.*

Chanock RM, Parrott RH, Johnson KM, et al.: Myxoviruses: Parainfluenza. Am Rev Respir Dis 88:152, 1963. *A discussion of the importance of parainfluenza viruses in pediatric respiratory tract disease and the first description of pattern of spread and reinfection.*

Denny FW, Murphy TF, Clyde WA, Jr, et al.: Croup: An 11-year study in a pediatric practice. Pediatrics 71:871, 1983. *Eleven-year evaluation of the role of parainfluenza viruses in croup. These viruses accounted for 74 per cent of all virus isolates from croup patients.*

Fox JP, Hall CE: Infections with other respiratory pathogens: Influenza, mumps, and respiratory syncytial viruses; Mycoplasma pneumoniae. In Fox JP (ed.): Viruses in Families. Littleton, MA, John Wright/PSG Inc, 1980, pp 335–381. *Longitudinal surveillance of families for parainfluenza virus infection and illness. Infection rate was 44 per 100 person-years for all ages, while attack rate for illness associated with parainfluenza virus infection was 76 per cent for babies under age 2 years and 25 per cent for adults.*

Glenzen WP, Denny FW: Epidemiology of acute lower respiratory disease in children. N Engl J Med 288:498, 1973. *Excellent summary of contribution of parainfluenza viruses to pediatric respiratory disease.*

333 INFLUENZA

R. Gordon Douglas, Jr.

DEFINITION. Influenza is an acute, usually self-limited febrile illness that occurs in outbreaks of varying severity almost evey winter. The causative virus is transmitted by the respiratory route; however, systemic symptoms are out of proportion to those in the respiratory tract. Infection with influenza virus can produce several other clinical syndromes common with infection with respiratory viruses, such as common colds, pharyngitis, croup, tracheobronchitis, bronchiolitis, or pneumonia. Conversely, infections with other respiratory viruses, such as respiratory syncytial virus, rhinovirus, or adenovirus, may produce sporadic cases indistinguishable from those of typical influenza. In addition to enormous morbidity and loss of time from school and work, influenza epidemics are associated with substantial mortality caused in large part by pulmonary complications

Since the year 1510, 31 pandemics of respiratory disease similar to modern influenza have been described, 5 of which have occurred in the twentieth century (1900, 1918, 1957, 1968, and 1977). Of these, the pandemic of 1918 was the most severe, accounting for at least 21 million deaths. Over 500,000 deaths have occurred in the United States from epidemic influenza in the past 20 years.

ETIOLOGY. Influenza viruses belong to the family Orthomyxoviridae. Influenza A virus constitutes one genus and influenza B virus another. The virion is a medium-sized (80 to 100 nm in diameter) enveloped spherical or elongated particle covered with surface projections that are glycoproteins possessing either hemagglutinin (H) or neuraminidase (N) activity (Fig. 333–1). The envelope is composed of a lipid bilayer, on the inner surface of which is the matrix (M) protein. Within the envelope are eight segmented pieces of nucleocapsid, formed by a single species of protein, the nucleoprotein (NP), and by pieces of segmented, single-stranded ribonucleic acid (RNA). Three polymerase (P) proteins and two nonstructural (NS) proteins of unknown function are found within the envelope. The H is responsible for binding of the virus to the cell. Antibody to this protein neutralizes viral infectivity and thus is the major determinant of immunity. The viral N is instrumental in release of virus from cells. Antineuraminidase antibody is not neutralizing but limits viral replication and therefore the severity of infection. The M protein plays a role in stability of the membrane and in organization of the virion during assembly. The three polymerases are important in viral replication. The internal M, NP, and P proteins are antigenically indistinguishable in all influenza A viruses but

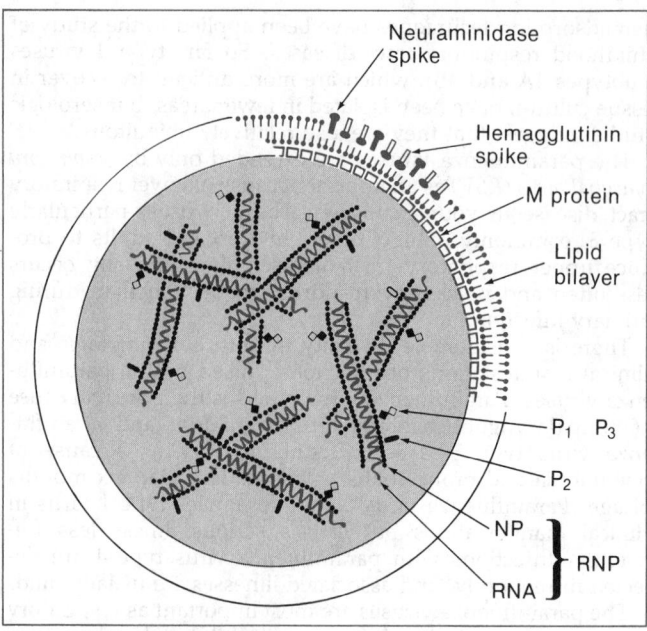

FIGURE 333–1. Schematic model for influenza virus virions. (Modified from Ginsberg HS: Orthomyxoviruses. In Davis BD, Dulbecco R, Eisen HN, Ginsburg HS [eds.]: Microbiology. 3rd ed. Hagerstown, MD, Harper & Row, Publishers, 1980, p. 1119.)

vary for influenza B and C viruses. Thus, type-specific (A, B, or C) distinction of influenza viruses depends on serologic reactions mediated by these internal antigens. However, the surface proteins (H and N) do vary, not only among influenza virus types but also among subtypes of influenza A.

The viral genome comprises eight segments of RNA, seven of which code for a single viral protein each. The eighth codes for the two nonstructural proteins. Reassortment of gene segments occurs frequently during coinfection of cells with two influenza A viruses. Influenza B and C viruses have been studied much less but appear to be structurally similar to influenza A virus. Antigenic variation is much less frequent with influenza B, and it may not occur with influenza C.

EPIDEMIOLOGY. *Antigenic Variation.* One of the unique and most remarkable features of influenza virus is the frequency with which changes in antigenicity occur. Such changes help explain why influenza continues to be a major epidemic disease in humans. As noted previously, antigenic variation involves only the H and N proteins among the proteins of influenza virus. The H is the more important, since it is more frequently involved in antigenic variation than the N protein and since antibody to this protein neutralizes infection. Antigenic variation is referred to as *antigenic drift or antigenic shift*, depending on whether the variation is small or great.

Antigenic Drift. Antigenic drift refers to relatively minor changes that occur frequently (every year or every few years) within an influenza A subtype. Each subtype is named by its hemagglutinin and neuraminidase. To date, three hemagglutinins (H1, H2, and H3) and two neuraminidases (N1 and N2) have been recognized in humans. The former designations, HO and HSW, are now classified as variants of H1. Each strain within the subtype is identified by site and year of isolation. Thus, influenza A/Bangkok/79/H3N2 indicates an influenza virus of type A and subtype H3N2 that was isolated in 1979 in Bangkok. The original H3N2 variant, A/Aichi/68/H3N2, was isolated in Aichi, Japan, in 1968. All isolates worldwide for the next three years were serologically identical. Subsequent antigenic drifts resulted in recovery of variants possessing minor differences: A/England/72/H3N2, A/Port Chalmers/73/H3N2, A/Scotland/74/H3N2, A/Georgia/74/H3N2, A/Victoria/75/H3N2, A/Texas/77/H3N2, A/Bangkok/79/H3N2, A/Philippines/2/82/H3N2, A/Mississippi/1/85/H3N2, and so on. Antigenic drift results from point mutations that usually affect the RNA segment coding for the hemagglutinin, resulting in an alteration in protein structure that involves one or a few amino acids. Complete nucleotide sequencing of hemagglutinins of several H3 strains has been determined, in support of this hypothesis. There is immunologic selection in which a new virus is favored over the old for person-to-person transmission because of the less frequent presence of antibody in the population to the new virus.

Antigenic Shift. Major antigenic shifts result from genetic reassortment when two influenza viruses simultaneously infect a single cell. Such an event results in a hemagglutinin or neuraminidase, or both, that is completely new in comparison with the previously circulating strain. Because of the high level of immunity to the old strain and lack of immunity to the new strain within the human population, the new strain, provided that it possesses intrinsic viral properties such as virulence and transmissibility, can readily cause a major outbreak of influenza.

Epidemic Influenza. An epidemic is an outbreak of influenza

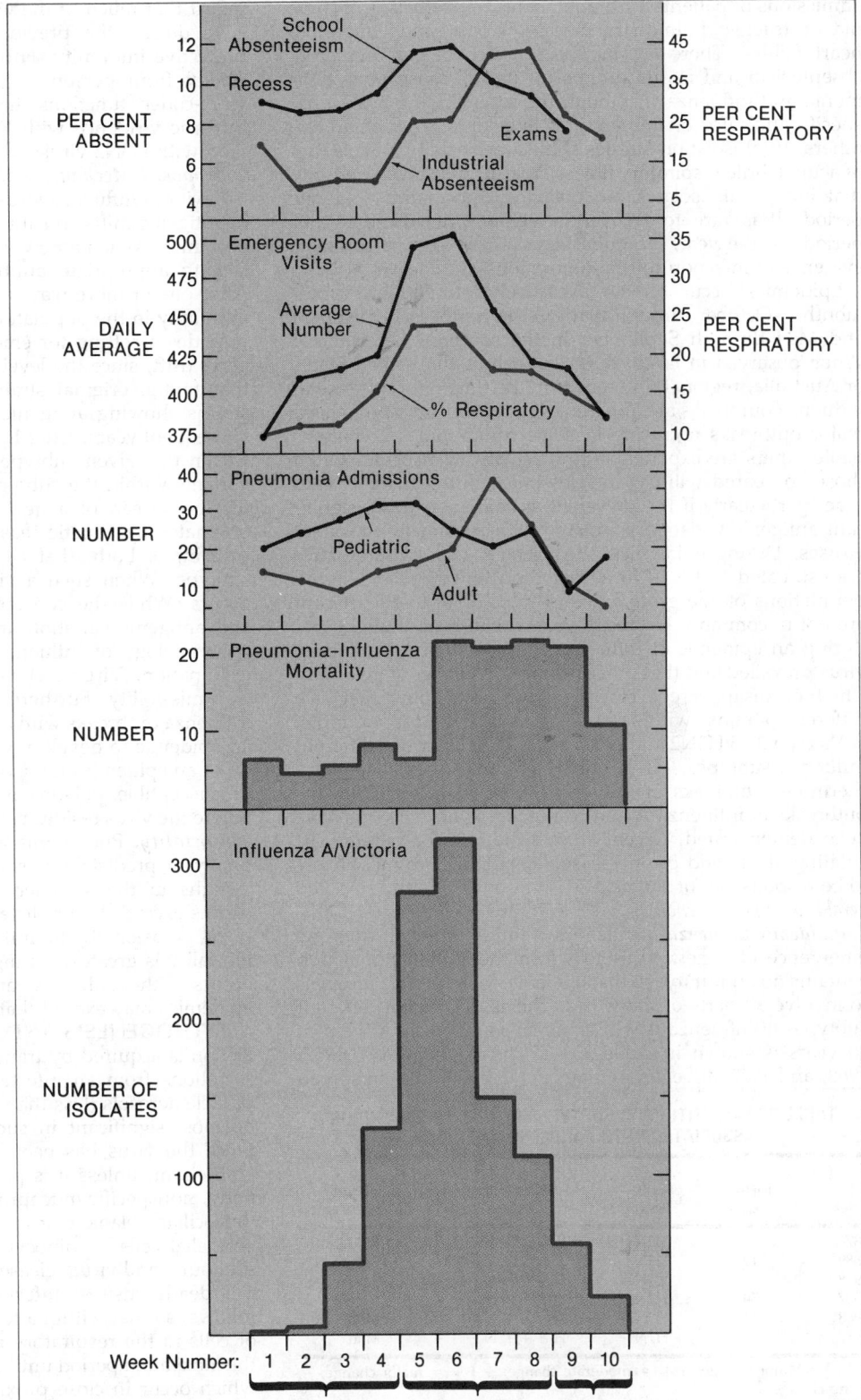

FIGURE 333–2. Correlation of the nonvirologic indexes of epidemiologic influenza with the number of isolates of influenza A/Victoria virus according to week, Houston, 1976 (industrial absenteeism is indicated by percentage with respiratory complaints). (Modified from Glezen WP, Couch RB, Six HR: N Engl J Med 298:589, 1978.)

confined to one location such as a city, town, or country. In a given community, epidemics of influenza A virus infection have a characteristic pattern. A graphic description of an epidemic due to an A/Victoria/75/H3N2–like virus, which occurred in 1976 in Houston, Texas, is shown in Figure 333–2. Such localized epidemics begin rather abruptly, reach a sharp peak in two to three weeks, and last five to six weeks. Reports of increased numbers of children with febrile respiratory illness are often the first indication of influenza in a community. This is soon followed by the occurrence of influenza-like illnesses among adults. The next event is increased hospital admissions of patients with pneumonia, exacerbation of chronic obstructive pulmonary disease, croup, and congestive heart failure. There are increases in school and industrial absenteeism and in the number of deaths caused by pneumonia and influenza. Although the latter finding is a highly specific indicator of influenza, it invariably lags behind the others. Viral isolation studies show a peak that parallels that of acute febrile respiratory illness. Year-round studies indicate that almost all isolates are obtained during the epidemic period. It is rare to recover influenza virus during other periods of the year, although occasionally there is serologic evidence of infection during other months.

Epidemics occur almost exclusively during the winter months—October through April in the northern hemisphere and May through September in the southern hemisphere. When observed in large countries such as the United States or Australia, regional differences in the time of occurrence of influenza outbreaks are apparent. It is not uncommon to have major outbreaks occurring in some communities or regions while others are experiencing no activity whatsoever. Often those so spared will experience similar outbreaks at a later time, particularly if the prevalent virus demonstrates significant antigenic variation compared with previously prevalent viruses. During epidemics, the average overall attack rates are estimated to be 10 to 20 per cent; however, in selected populations of age groups, attack rates of 40 to 50 per cent are not uncommon. For many years it had been thought that during an epidemic of influenza a single strain of influenza virus prevailed and that other respiratory viruses were diminished or disappeared. However, we now know that two different strains within a single subtype, for example, A/Victoria/3/75/H3N2 and A/Texas/1/77/H3N2, or two different influenza subtypes, H1N1 and H3N2, may cocirculate. Furthermore, outbreaks of influenza A and B or simultaneous outbreaks of influenza A and respiratory syncytial virus have been demonstrated. Recent studies indicate that strains circulating at the end of one season's epidemic are most likely to be responsible for the next season's outbreak (the so-called *herald wave phenomenon*).

Pandemic Influenza. Pandemics of influenza result from the emergence of a new virus to which the overall population contains no immunity, so that epidemics of influenza progress to involve all parts of the world. The association of different subtypes of influenza A with pandemic influenza for the past 80 years is shown in Table 333–1. The pandemics of 1957, 1968, and 1977 all began in mainland China and then spread east and west, but primarily to the USSR and Western Europe before reaching the American continent. The interval between pandemics is variable and unpredictable, and this fact, in part, led to the national immunization program against swine influenza, when a small outbreak of A/New Jersey/76/H1N1 infection was detected at Fort Dix, New Jersey. The most severe pandemics have resulted when there were major antigenic alterations in both of the major surface antigens. A striking exception to this occurred when A/USSR/77/H1N1 did not cause a severe pandemic in 1977 to 1978, despite major shifts in both surface glycoproteins. This discrepancy may reflect that much of the world's population in 1977 had been alive during the previous H1N1 era and thus possessed protective immunity. Furthermore, it appears that transmissibility from person to person and intrinsic virulence are virus-coded functions that vary much as does antigenicity. Intrinsic virulence with H1N1 viruses appears to be milder than with H3N2 viruses.

Proposed Mechanism of Epidemic Behavior. The epidemic behavior of influenza virus is partly explained by the concepts of antigenic shifts and antigenic drifts in relation to population immunity. When a new virus is introduced into a population lacking appropriate antibody, pandemic influenza results. After one or more waves of pandemic influenza, the level of immunity in the population increases. Such a chain of events provides a setting for emergence of a variant showing antigenic drift, since the level of immunity to it will be less than that to the original strain. Repeated epidemics caused by strains showing antigenic drift within the subtype occur in subsequent years. After 10 to 40 years of circulation of variants within this given subtype, the population's immunity to all variants within the subtype is very high, and the conditions for the spread of a new virus are favorable. Such a virus originates by genetic reassortment. It possesses an H or N protein, or both, that is markedly different from the prior subtype. When such a virus circulates, the next pandemic occurs. While the concepts of immunity of the population and antigenic variation are important in understanding the epidemiology of influenza, they do not provide the entire explanation. Virus factors also contribute to virulence and transmissibility. Furthermore, other than the association of influenza outbreaks with colder seasons, the factors that allow an epidemic to develop or those responsible for the tapering off of an epidemic after five or six weeks, when only a portion of susceptible persons is infected, are unknown. Finally, where the virus resides between epidemics is not understood.

Mortality. Pneumonia and influenza deaths fluctuate annually in predictable fashion, with peaks in the winter and troughs in the summer. When pneumonia and influenza deaths exceed the predicted number, this is due to influenza A or occasionally to influenza B virus activity. Although mortality is greatest during pandemics, substantial mortality occurs with epidemics, and the cumulative mortality from epidemics may exceed that of pandemics (Fig. 333–3).

PATHOGENESIS AND PATHOLOGY. Influenza virus infection is acquired by transfer of virus-containing respiratory secretions from an infected to a susceptible person. Small-particle aerosols (less than 10 μ mass medium diameter) may be most significant in such person-to-person transmission. Once the virus has been deposited in the respiratory tract epithelium, unless it is prevented by specific secretory antibody, nonspecific mucoproteins, or mechanical actions of the mucociliary blanket, it attaches to and penetrates columnar epithelial cells by pinocytosis. Viral replication lasts four to six hours, and virus release continues for several hours before cell death ensues. Infection of adjacent and nearby cells follows, so that within a few replication cycles large numbers of cells in the respiratory tract are infected. The duration of the incubation period until onset of illness and virus shedding, which occur in close proximity, varies from 18 to 72 hours, depending in part on the inoculum size. Quantitation of virus

TABLE 333–1. ANTIGENIC SUBTYPES OF INFLUENZA A VIRUS ASSOCIATED WITH PANDEMIC INFLUENZA

Year	Interval (Years)	Designation	Extent of Antigenic Change in Indicated Surface Protein*	Severity of Pandemic
1870	—	H2N?	?	Moderate
1889	19	H3N8	H + + +N?	Severe
1918	29	H1N1†	H + + + N + + +	Severe
1957	39	H2N2	H + + + N + + +	Severe
1968	11	H3N2	H + + + N −	Moderate
1977	9	H1N1	H + + + N + + +	Mild

*+ = Minor change; + + = moderate change; + + + = major change; − = no change.
†Former designation was Hsw1N1 (35).

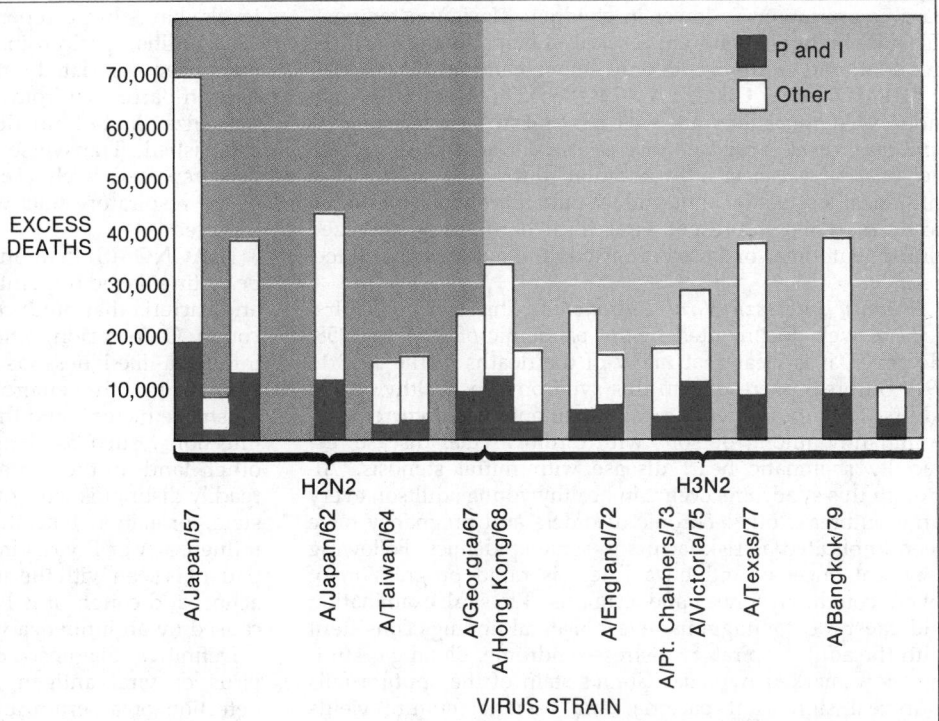

FIGURE 333–3. Excess mortality associated with influenza A epidemics in the United States 1957–58 to 1983–84. P and I = Pneumonia and Influenza. (Modified from Kendal AP, Lui KJ, Cox JN, et al.: The Effect of Influenza Virus Genetic Alteration on Disease in Man and Animals. Banbury Report 22: Genetically Altered Viruses and the Environment. Cold Spring Harbor Laboratory, 1985, pp. 119–143.)

in respiratory tract specimens reveals a characteristic pattern that correlates with severity of illness, suggesting that a major mechanism in the production of illness is cell death resulting from viral replication. Serum or secretory antibody or cell-mediated immune mechanisms are not detectable at this time, indicating that immunologic mechanisms are probably not involved in production of illness, with the possible exception of circulating interferon, which may contribute to systemic symptoms and fever. Such symptoms suggest hematogenous dissemination of virus or release of cellular products into the blood, but infectious virus only rarely has been detected in the blood.

Interferon is frequently detected in respiratory tract and serum specimens. Shedding of virus precedes by one to two days the appearance of interferon, which is correlated with improvements of signs and symptoms and decrease of virus titer, suggesting that interferon is active in the recovery process.

Neutralizing, hemagglutination-inhibiting (HAI), antineuraminidase, complement-fixing, enzyme-linked immunosorbent assay (ELISA), and immunofluorescent antibodies begin to develop in the sera of persons with primary influenza virus infection during the second week after exposure to antigen and reach a peak by four weeks. Secretory antibodies develop in the respiratory tract after influenza infection and consist predominantly of immunoglobulin A (IgA) antibodies that reach peak titers in 14 days. Protection against infection is afforded by serum HAI titers of 1:40 or greater, serum-neutralizing titers of 1:8 or greater, or nasal-neutralizing antibody titers of 1:4 or greater.

Nasal and bronchial biopsy specimens from persons with uncomplicated influenza reveal desquamation of the ciliated columnar epithelium. Individual cells show shrinkage, pyknotic nuclei, and loss of cilia. In addition, the lungs in fatal influenza show extensive hemorrhage, hyaline membrane formation, and paucity of polymorphonuclear cell infiltration. Patients with secondary bacterial pneumonia have the changes characteristic of bacterial pneumonia in addition to the tracheobronchial findings of influenza in the tracheobronchial tree.

CLINICAL FINDINGS. Many patients can pinpoint the hour of onset. Initially, systemic systems predominate, and symptoms include feverishness, chilliness or frank shaking chills, headache, myalgias, malaise, and anorexia. In more severe cases, prostration is observed. Usually myalgias or headaches are the most troublesome symptoms, and their severity is related to the level of the fever. Arthralgias are commonly observed. Ocular symptoms, although less commonly present, are helpful diagnostically and include photophobia, tearing, burning, and pain on moving the eyes. Respiratory symptoms, particularly dry cough and nasal discharge, are usually also present at the onset but are overshadowed by the systemic symptoms. Nasal obstruction, hoarseness, and dry sore throat may also be present.

Fever is the most important physical finding. The temperature usually rises rapidly to a peak of 38 to 40° C and occasionally to 41° C within 12 hours of onset, concurrently with the development of systemic symptoms. Fever is usually continuous but may be intermittent, especially if antipyretics are administered. On the second and third days of illness, the temperature elevation is usually less than on the first day. As fever subsides, the systemic symptoms diminish. Typically, the duration of fever is three days, but it may last from one to five or more days. In a few cases, a second fluctuation in fever occurs on the third or fourth day, resulting in a biphasic fever curve. Early in the course of illness, the patient appears toxic, the face is flushed, and the skin is hot and moist. The eyes are watery and reddened. Clear nasal discharge is common, but nasal obstruction is uncommon. The mucous membranes of the nose and throat are hyperemic, but exudate is not observed. Small, tender cervical lymph nodes are often present, and transient, scattered rhonchi or localized areas of rales are found in less than 20 per cent of cases.

As systemic signs and symptoms diminish, respiratory complaints and findings become more apparent. Cough is the most frequent and troublesome of these symptoms and may be accompanied by substernal discomfort or burning. Nasal obstruction, discharge, pharyngeal pain, and injection are also common. Such symptoms and signs usually persist three to four days after fever subsides; however, cough, lassitude, and malaise may persist for one, two, or more weeks before full recovery.

This pattern of illness just described occurs with any type or subtype of influenza A or B virus. Attack rates are higher in children than in adults, although the incidence of pulmonary complications is lower in children. Maximum temperatures are higher in children, cervical adenopathy may be more frequent, and croup occurs only among children.

PULMONARY COMPLICATIONS. Three kinds of pulmonary complications are well recognized: *primary influenza viral pneumonia, secondary bacterial pneumonia,* and *mixed viral and bacterial pneumonia.* In addition, during an outbreak of influenza, less distinct and milder pulmonic syndromes often occur that may represent viral tracheobronchitis, localized viral pneumonia, or possibly mixed viral and bacterial infection.

Primary Influenza Viral Pneumonia. This syndrome first became well documented in the pandemic of 1957 to 1958. However, it is clear that many of the deaths in the 1918 to 1919 outbreak were due to this syndrome in healthy young adults. Primary influenza viral pneumonia has occurred predominantly among persons with cardiovascular disease, especially rheumatic heart disease with mitral stenosis. Although this syndrome occurs in healthy young adults in every large outbreak, other chronic disorders and pregnancy have been implicated as risk factors in some epidemics. Following a typical onset of influenza, there is rapid progression of fever, cough, dyspnea, and cyanosis. Physical examination and chest roentgenograms reveal bilateral findings consistent with the adult respiratory distress syndrome. Blood gas studies show marked hypoxia. Gram's stain of the sputum fails to reveal significant bacteria, and bacterial culture yields sparse growth of normal flora. Viral cultures of sputum or tracheal aspirates yield high titers of influenza virus. Such patients do not respond to antibiotics, and mortality is high.

Secondary Bacterial Pneumonia. Bacterial superinfection is often clinically distinguishable from primary viral pneumonia. The patients are most often elderly or have chronic pulmonary, cardiac, metabolic, or other diseases. Following a typical influenza illness, a period of improvement lasting from one to four days may occur. Recrudescence of fever is associated with symptoms and signs of bacterial pneumonia, such as cough, sputum production, and a localized area of consolidation apparent on physical and chest roentgenogram examination. Gram's stain and culture sputum reveal predominance of a bacterial pathogen, most often *Streptococcus pneumoniae, Staphylococcus aureus,* or *Hemophilus influenzae.* Such patients will usually respond to specific antibiotic therapy.

Mixed Viral and Bacterial Pneumonia. During an outbreak of influenza, many cases are observed that do not clearly fit into either of the categories just described. The disease is not relentlessly progressive, and yet the fever pattern may be persistent and not biphasic. These patients may have a milder form of primary viral, secondary bacterial, or mixed viral and bacterial infection. Many will respond to antibiotics. Milder forms of primary viral pneumonia involving only one lobe or segment have been described that do not invariably lead to death. Such cases are more likely to be confused with a pneumonia due to *Mycoplasma pneumoniae* than to that produced by bacterial infection. Pneumonia may occur in children, but it is less common than in adults. In addition, bronchiolitis and croup may be caused by influenza A or B virus infection.

Exacerbation of Chronic Obstructive Pulmonary Disease. In adults with chronic obstructive pulmonary disease, influenza A or B virus infection may lead not only to pneumonia but also to acute exacerbation of chronic bronchitis, a syndrome that is associated with other respiratory viruses and bacteria as well.

NONPULMONIC COMPLICATIONS. *Reye's Syndrome.* Reye's syndrome is a frequently recognized hepatic and central nervous system complication of influenza A and B infection. Reye's syndrome is discussed in Ch. 490.

Other Complications. Myositis and myoglobinuria with tender leg muscles and elevated serum creatine kinase (CK)

levels have been reported, mostly occurring in children. Myocarditis, pericarditis, and myocardial infarction rarely have been associated with influenza A and B virus infection. Gullain-Barré syndrome has been reported to occur after influenza A, but no definite causal relationship has been established. Transverse myelitis and encephalitis have also been reported rarely. Toxic shock syndrome due to infection of the respiratory tract with toxin-bearing *S. aureus* has been reported.

DIAGNOSIS. In an individual case, influenza often cannot be distinguished from infection with a number of other viruses and bacteria that produce headache, muscle aches, fever, and cough. On occasion, other respiratory viruses can produce an influenza-like illness, as can streptococcal pharyngitis. In the summer months, enteroviruses produce a clinically indistinguishable picture, and the acute manifestations of many other infections, such as dengue, may mimic influenza. On the other hand, in the context of an epidemic, influenza may be readily distinguished from other acute infections. When local, state, or national health authorities report an epidemic of influenza A or B virus infection in a given community, and a patient is seen with the acute onset of fever, headache, muscle aches, and cough, it is highly likely that these symptoms are caused by an influenza virus infection.

Definitive diagnosis depends on detection of infectious virus or viral antigen in secretions from patients or the detection of a serum antibody response. Influenza virus is readily isolated from throat or nasal specimens, sputum, or tracheal secretion specimens in the first two or three days of illness. Usually infectivity is detected within 48 to 72 hours in cell cultures. Viral antigen may be detected more rapidly in such specimens by use of immunofluorescence or ELISA. Serologic methods are less useful clinically because they require a convalescent serum obtained 10 to 14 days after the onset of infection. However, they are of great use in epidemiologic studies and to document the occurrence of an outbreak. A fourfold increase in antibody titer, comparing an acute with a convalescent phase, is diagnostic. The complement fixation antibody test is most useful for diagnosis because it is not dependent on strain or subtype variation, as is hemagglutination inhibition.

TREATMENT. Amantadine shortens the duration of fever and of systemic and respiratory symptoms by about 50 per cent. The dose is 100 to 200 mg per day orally for three to five days. Rimantadine, although not yet licensed, has a similar effect and reduces the likelihood of the mild, transient central nervous system side effects that occur with amantadine. Other symptomatic measures include antipyretics and cough suppressants. Many authorities consider that aspirin should not be used, especially for persons under 16 years of age, because of its possible association with the occurrence of Reye's syndrome. There is no evidence that amantadine or rimantadine is effective in treatment of pulmonary complications of influenza.

Currently, primary influenza viral pneumonia in its severe stages is best managed in an intensive care unit with supportive measures such as respiratory therapy, supplemental oxygen, and fluids. Secondary bacterial pneumonia should be treated with appropriate antibiotics. When studies of the sputum do not clearly indicate which bacterium may be infecting the patient, coverage should include antibiotics that are effective against *S. aureus, S. pneumoniae, and H. influenzae.*

PREVENTION. The mainstay of prevention is the use of inactivated influenza virus vaccines. These vaccines provide about 80 per cent protective efficacy. The antigenic composition is reviewed annually so that the vaccine contains the most recently circulating strains. Usually the vaccine is a trivalent product containing one or more subtypes of influenza A and influenza B. The recent vaccines have been purified by density gradient centrifugation or chromatography and have very low reaction rates. One to two per cent of persons vaccinated will have fever and systemic symptoms peaking at 8 to 12 hours after vaccination, and up to 25 per cent may have mild local reactions at the site of vaccination. "Split" virus (subvirion) vaccines contain antigens with disrupted virus and may be less reactigenic than "whole" virus vaccines. The highest priority for vaccination should be given to persons with cardiac or pulmonary conditions requiring ongoing medical care and to residents of nursing homes and other chronic care facilities. Physicians, nurses, and other personnel who have extensive contact with high-risk patients constitute the next priority for vaccination. Finally, persons over age 65 and persons with other chronic disease of any age should be vaccinated. Vaccine may also be given to well persons under age 65 who wish to reduce the likelihood of acquiring influenza. Vaccine should be administered each year in the fall prior to the influenza season.

Amantadine and rimantadine are also effective in preventing influenza A and should be used to supplement vaccine programs. Persons who are not vaccinated in the fall should be placed on amantadine when an outbreak occurs or throughout the influenza season for the highest risk group. If vaccine is available, persons may be vaccinated simultaneously, and amantadine therapy should be stopped after 14 days. Alternatively, if vaccine is not available, amantadine administration may be continued for the duration of the outbreak, the dose being 100 to 200 mg per day orally. Amantadine, administered to patients and staff alike, is very helpful in managing nosocomial outbreaks.

A Consensus Development Conference: Diagnosis and treatment of Reye's syndrome. JAMA 246:21, 1982. *Up-to-date summary of Reye's syndrome with description of staging.*

Centers for Disease Control: Prevention and Control of Influenza. Morbidity and Mortality Weekly Report 35:317, 331, 1986. *Details of extensive revisions of recommendations for use of influenza vaccine.*

Dolin R, Reichman RC, Madore HP, et al.: A controlled trial of amantadine and rimantadine in the prophylaxis of influenza A infection. N Engl J Med 307:580, 1982. *Definitive study comparing prophylactic efficacy of amantadine and rimantadine.*

Glezen WP, Couch RB, Six HR: The influenza herald wave. Am J Epidemiol 116:4, 1982. *Prediction of epidemic influenza from previous year's outbreak.*

Hauptmann R, Clarke LD, Mountford RC, et al.: Nucleotide sequence of the hemagglutinin gene of influenza virus A/England/321/77. J Gen Virol 64:215, 1983. *Studies on the molecular mechanism of antigenic drift.*

Kendel AP, Patriarca PA (eds.): Options for the Control of Influenza. New York, Alan R. Liss, 1986. *Excellent recent review of rationale for vaccine and amantadine use. In addition, an up-to-date summary of epidemiology.*

Younkin SW, Betts RF, Roth FK, et al.: Reduction in fever and symptoms in young adults with aspirin or amantadine. Antimicrob Agents Chemother 23:577, 1983. *Recent study comparing therapeutic effects of amantadine and aspirin.*

334 ADENOVIRUS DISEASES

Stephen G. Baum

The most clinically significant diseases caused by adenoviruses are infections of the respiratory system and the eye. Recently, adenoviruses have been shown to play a significant role in causing diarrheal disease in children and respiratory infections in immunocompromised patients. Adenoviruses are the object of intensive research efforts because they possess several fascinating and important biologic capabilities, including oncogenesis and latency. Today they are perhaps the best characterized human virus group.

ETIOLOGIC AGENT. Adenoviruses are double-stranded DNA viruses that average 70 nm in diameter and have a unique outer structure, which permits their morphologic identification by electron microscopic examination. The virus is icosahedral with 20 equilateral triangular faces and 12 vertices. The faces are made up of hexon subunits, and the vertices each contain a penton subunit. From each vertex, an antenna-like structure, the fiber, projects with a knob at the end. Each class of these surface subunits differs antigenically from the others. The hexon contains group-specific and type-specific antigens. Forty-one serotypes of human adenovirus have been identified (types 1 to 41). Many of the serotypes have been associated with specific syndromes, but over half the adenovirus types have not been shown to cause disease. The 41 serotypes have been divided into six groups by DNA homology and four groups according to ability to agglutinate different erythrocytes. The latter grouping correlates well with the ability of different serotypes to cause specific syndromes and to induce tumors in animals.

In acute infections, adenoviruses cause cell death and lysis with release of new progeny virions. The mechanisms of latency and animal oncogenesis are not completely understood, although many of the functions of adenovirus have been accurately mapped on the deoxyribonucleic acid (DNA) genome. Adenoviruses can form a family of hybrid viruses with an unrelated DNA virus, SV40. Portions of the DNA of adenovirus and SV40 are covalently linked within an adenovirus outer coat. The hybrid virus has unique biologic and oncogenic capabilities in vitro and in animals in vivo. Neither adenovirus alone nor the hybrid viruses have been shown to cause cancer in humans.

A small defective DNA parvovirus has been isolated from some adenovirus preparations and from some patients with adenovirus infection. This *adeno-associated virus (AAV)* requires adenovirus for its replication. It is not known to cause disease by itself and does not appear to contribute to adenovirus pathogenesis. A related parvovirus (B19) has recently been implicated as the cause of erythema infectiosum (fifth disease) and of aplastic crisis in patients with hemoglobinopathies.

EPIDEMIOLOGY. Most people experience an adenovirus infection during the first decade of life. The initial infecting serotype and the syndrome it causes are a function of the age of the patient and the route of infection. Studies of large populations show that adenoviruses cause 3 to 5 per cent of all clinically apparent infections in children. Adenoviruses are the most common viral isolates in this age group, and at least half of these isolations are associated with subclinical infections. Respiratory infection is transmitted by person-to-person contact or through contaminated swimming water.

Conjunctival infection may be transmitted directly, through water, or by fomites such as towels or ophthalmologic equipment and solutions. Pneumonia and urinary tract infection in immunocompromised patients may be acquired exogenously or may represent reactivation of latent infection. There are many adenoviruses that infect other animals and birds, but these play no known role in human disease.

CLINICAL PRESENTATIONS OCCURRING MOSTLY IN CHILDREN. *Respiratory Infection.* Infants most commonly manifest adenovirus infections as coryzal symptoms, but occasionally adenovirus type 7 causes fulminant bronchiolitis and pneumonia in this age group. Recently, Reye's syndrome has been reported as a complication of severe adenovirus infection in infants. In older children, pharyngitis and tracheobronchitis are most prevalent. Adenoviruses are the most common viral isolate from children with the whooping cough syndrome. It is not known whether this virus contributes to the pathogenesis of *Bordetella pertussis* infection or whether adenovirus alone can cause the syndrome.

Pharyngoconjunctival Fever. This syndrome occurs in small epidemics in summer camps where it is probably spread in swimming water. Adenovirus type 3 has been the most common isolate. The incubation period is three to five days, and symptoms, which are acute, include pharyngitis, rhinitis, conjunctivitis, cervical adenitis, and elevation in temperature to about 38°C. The bulbar and palpebral conjunctivae have a granular appearance. The symptoms last one to two weeks. Permanent sequelae are rare, and there is no specific therapy.

Intestinal Disease. Immunoelectron microscopy has revealed viruses in the stool in many cases of infantile diarrhea. The most common viruses visualized are rotaviruses and adenoviruses. These adenoviruses appear to be defective in their replication and require special cells for isolation in tissue culture. Serotypes 40 and 41 have been found most often in this situation. Intussusception in children has also been linked to adenovirus types 1, 2, 3, and 5, although a causal role is unproven. Many of the children with this syndrome have intercurrent adenoviral respiratory infection.

Hemorrhagic Cystitis. Adenovirus types 11 and 21 have been associated with hemorrhagic cystitis in American and Japanese children. Boys are affected more often than girls, in contrast to the situation with bacterial cystitis. Gross hematuria may persist for one to two weeks.

CLINICAL PRESENTATIONS OCCURRING MOSTLY IN ADULTS. *Respiratory Infection.* The first isolation of adenoviruses directly from sick patients occurred during an epidemic of acute respiratory disease in military recruits. This population seems extremely susceptible to infection with types 4 and 7, as it is to infection with *Mycoplasma pneumoniae* and the meningococci. In general, the manifestations are those of atypical pneumonia, of which up to 40 per cent of cases are caused by adenovirus. Fever to 39°C, cough, pharyngitis, rhinorrhea, and pulmonary rales are the most common signs and symptoms. Radiographic examination of the chest shows patchy interstitial infiltrates that are unilateral in most cases. Small pleural effusions can occur.

In nonepidemic situations, it is impossible to make a definitive clinical diagnosis of adenoviral pneumonia. Some factors useful in comparing adenoviral with mycoplasmal pneumonia are lower incidence of cold agglutinins, shorter incubation period, and better correlation of x-ray and physical findings in the chest in adenovirus infection. Influenza and parainfluenza viruses produce similar syndromes. Adenoviral pneumonia usually lasts one to two weeks. There is no specific therapy, and bacterial superinfection and death are rare.

Adenoviruses have been isolated from the lungs of immunocompromised patients with pneumonia and from the urine of renal transplant recipients and patients with acquired immunodeficiency syndrome (AIDS). Several of the higher serotypes were first isolated from such patients. In these instances, adenovirus operates as an opportunistic agent.

Neurologic disease, most often appearing as meningoencephalitis, has been attributed to adenovirus. It sometimes occurs in minor epidemic form and is frequently associated with recent respiratory infection. The clinical presentation is that of encephalitis or aseptic meningitis. There are no pathognomonic findings.

Epidemic Keratoconjunctivitis. The initial epidemic of adenoviral keratoconjunctivitis involved shipyard workers who sustained minor eye trauma from paint and rust fragments. Adenovirus type 8 was isolated in this and many other epidemics. Serotypes 19 and 37 have caused keratoconjunctivitis that was spread by fomites such as roller towels. The incubation period is from 3 to 24 days. The onset is insidious, and both eyes often are affected. Eye irritation and exudation may last one to four weeks. Preauricular adenopathy often occurs early. Corneal involvement is a late complication and may persist for a month or more with blurring of vision. Residual blindness is unusual. There is no specific antiviral therapy as there is for herpes keratitis. Secondary spread to household contacts occurs in about 10 per cent of cases, varying with the duration of the index case.

TREATMENT AND PREVENTION. There is no effective antiviral chemotherapy for human adenoviral infections. Live, enteric-coated oral adenovirus vaccines of types 4 and 7 have been effective in immunizing military populations. In epidemic situations, mass immunization with the live virus vaccine promptly interrupts the epidemic. The vaccine is not recommended or available for civilians because of the low incidence and sporadic occurrence of infection with adenovirus types 4 and 7.

Baum SG: Adenovirus. In Mandell A, Douglas RA, Bennet JE (eds.): Principles and Practice of Infectious Diseases. 2nd ed. New York, John Wiley & Sons, 1985, pp 988–993. *An expanded version of the material in this chapter, containing correlative tables, fully referenced.*
Horwitz MS: Adenoviruses. In Fields BN, Melnick JL, Chanock R, et al. (eds.): Human Viral Diseases. New York, Raven Press, 1985, pp 433–476. *An encyclopedic chapter on the molecular biology of the adenoviruses.*

Viral Diseases of the Gastrointestinal Tract

335 VIRAL GASTROENTERITIS

Albert Z. Kapikian

DEFINITION

Viral gastroenteritis (acute infectious nonbacterial gastroenteritis, epidemic diarrhea, winter vomiting disease, sporadic infantile gastroenteritis) is a common acute infectious disease of all age groups, characterized by vomiting or watery diarrhea, or both, that may be accompanied by fever, nausea, anorexia, and malaise. It ranges from a mild, self-limited illness of short duration to life-threatening dehydration, especially in infants and young children.

The importance of this disease in a developed country was highlighted in the Cleveland Family Study, in which infectious gastroenteritis, presumably nonbacterial, was the second most common disease experience, accounting for 16 per cent of some 25,000 illnesses in a period of almost 10 years. In developing countries the impact of diarrheal illnesses is staggering: in Asia, Africa, and Latin America, 3 to 5 billion cases of diarrhea and 5 to 10 million diarrhea-associated deaths occur annually, with the major impact in infants and young children. In addition, diarrheal illness was ranked first in disease incidence and mortality in these developing areas.

In spite of major discoveries in bacteriology and parasitology in the past century, the etiology of most acute diarrheal illnesses remained elusive for many years. In the 1940's and 1950's, oral administration of bacteria-free stool filtrates from patients with acute diarrhea induced illness in volunteers, but the suspected viral etiologic agent could not be identified. In 1972, Kapikian and colleagues, employing immune electron microscopy (IEM), discovered virus-like particles in a stool suspension derived from a gastroenteritis outbreak in Norwalk, Ohio. In 1973, Bishop and associates, employing electron microscopy (EM), discovered rotavirus particles in duodenal biopsies from infants and young children hospitalized with acute gastroenteritis.

ETIOLOGY

NORWALK VIRUS GROUP. The Norwalk virus is the prototype strain of a group of fastidious, nonenveloped particles usually named after the geographic location of the gastroenteritis outbreak from which they are recovered. They share these common characteristics: (1) a diameter of approximately 27 nm; (2) indistinct morphology; (3) presence in feces; (4) noncultivable in vitro; (5) unknown nucleic acid content; and (6) a buoyant density of 1.36 to 1.41 grams per cubic centimeter in cesium chloride. The group includes at least four serotypes—Norwalk, Hawaii, Ditchling, and Snow Mountain agents—and several other strains (Montgomery County, "W", cockle, Taunton, and Parramatta) that share an antigenic relationship with one of the known serotypes or have not been characterized. Classification of these fastidious viruses into a virus family has not been feasible. However, the protein composition of Norwalk and Snow Mountain viruses resembles that of the caliciviruses, since they each possess a single primary virion-associated protein with an approximate molecular weight of 60,000.

ROTAVIRUS. Rotaviruses are classified as a new genus in the family Reoviridae and are etiologic agents of diarrhea in humans and in numerous animal and avian species. They are 70 nm in diameter, with a genome consisting of 11 segments of double-stranded ribonucleic acid (RNA), and possess a distinctive double-layered capsid. The name rotavirus (rota = wheel) was adopted because the sharply defined circular outline of the outer capsid was reminiscent of the rim of a wheel placed on short spokes radiating from a wide hub (the inner capsid). The virions have a density of 1.36 grams per cubic centimeter in cesium chloride and are antigenically distinct from the three reovirus serotypes. Rotaviruses possess three important antigenic specificities—group, subgroup, and serotype—which are mediated by different proteins: group and subgroup by VP6 (encoded by RNA segment 6), and serotype by VP7 and VP3 (encoded by RNA segment 8 or 9, and 4, respectively) (Fig. 335–1). Most animal and human rotaviruses share the common group antigen and are thus classified as group A rotaviruses. In addition, certain group A rotaviruses also share neutralization and subgroup specificities. Five human rotavirus serotypes are recognized, and these are further divided into two subgroups. The human rotaviruses have only recently been grown efficiently in cell culture. Several human and animal rotavirus strains have been discovered that do not share the common group antigen. These are referred to as "pararotaviruses," or non–group A rotaviruses (groups B to F). In this chapter, when the term rotavirus is used, it is meant to describe only those rotaviruses belonging to group A, unless specified otherwise.

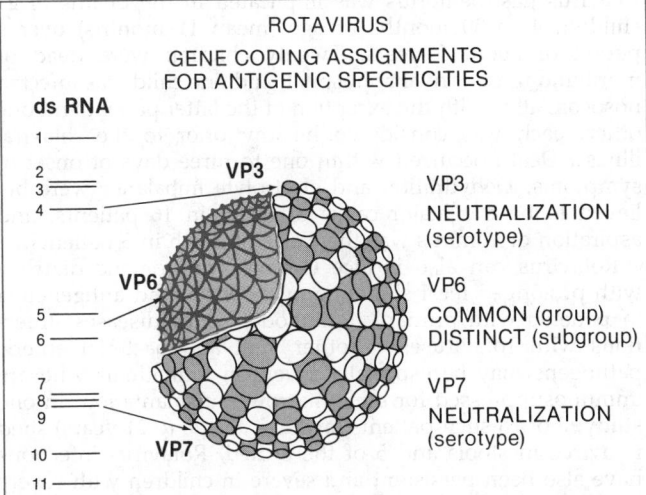

FIGURE 335–1. Gene coding assignments for various antigenic specificities of rotaviruses. (From Kapikian AZ, Flores J, Hoshino Y, et al.: Rotavirus: The major etiologic agent of severe infantile diarrhea may be controllable by a "Jennerian" approach to vaccination. J Infect Dis 153:815, 1986.)

OTHER AGENTS. Other viral agents have been associated with gastroenteritis and include enteric adenoviruses belonging to types 40 and 41 (70 to 80 nm in diameter); caliciviruses (30 to 40 nm); astroviruses (28 to 30 nm); small, round viruses other than the Norwalk virus group (20 to 30 nm); putative coronavirus–like particles (100 to 150 nm); the Otofuke and Sapporo agents (33 to 40 nm); the minireoviruses (30 to 40 nm); and the pleomorphic, fringed, Breda or Berne virus-like particles (100 to 140 nm). The role of these viruses as etiologic agents of severe infantile diarrhea appears to be minor, with the exception of the enteric adenoviruses, which are associated with approximately 5 per cent of the diarrheal illnesses of infants and young children requiring hospitalization. In addition, the role of these other agents in epidemic viral gastroenteritis appears to be minor with the exception of the caliciviruses. However, about one third to one half of gastroenteritis episodes have yet to be associated with an etiologic agent.

EPIDEMIOLOGY

NORWALK VIRUS GROUP. The Norwalk group of viruses comprises major etiologic agents of acute nonbacterial gastroenteritis, which typically occurs as a sharp outbreak affecting adults, school-age children, and family contacts. The location or source of contamination responsible for these outbreaks include various settings such as schools, camps and recreational areas, nursing homes, swimming facilities, cruise ships, and restaurants. For example, the Norwalk virus was derived from an outbreak in an elementary school in Norwalk, Ohio, in which 50 per cent of the students and teachers developed gastroenteritis within a two-day period. Norwalk virus has been linked with 42 per cent of 74 nonbacterial gastroenteritis outbreaks investigated from 1976 to 1980 and approximately 10 per cent of all acute gastroenteritis outbreaks. In the United States, antibody to the Norwalk virus is usually acquired gradually in childhood and somewhat more rapidly in the adult years, so that by age 40 at least 50 per cent of individuals have serum antibody. In developing countries, infants and young children acquire Norwalk antibody at an earlier age, and the virus is associated with mild gastroenteritis in this age group.

Norwalk virus is most likely transmitted via the fecal-oral route; however, it has also been detected in vomitus. Although sporadic cases attributed to person-to-person transmission may occur, the explosive nature of outbreaks associated with the Norwalk virus group often suggests a common source of infection, such as water or food. Common-source outbreaks have been attributed to contamination of community and noncommunity public water systems, stored water on cruise ships, or recreational swimming water and to ingestion of tainted oysters, cockles, lettuce, or cake frosting. Secondary person-to-person transmission to contacts is relatively common. The incubation period ranges from 10 to 51 hours, with a mean of 24 hours, and symptoms usually last 24 to 60 hours. Norwalk virus outbreaks occur throughout the year without a peak season.

Norwalk virus infections have been detected in individuals with travelers' diarrhea. However, this agent is not considered to be an important cause of this disease.

ROTAVIRUS. Rotaviruses are the major known etiologic agents of severe diarrhea in infants and young children in most areas of the world and are usually associated with sporadic infantile gastroenteritis, which differs from epidemic viral gastroenteritis associated with the Norwalk virus group in the following characteristics: (1) it usually does not occur in sharp outbreaks; (2) it is associated with a severe diarrheal illness in infants and young children; (3) it does not usually cause illness in adults; and (4) the attack rate among family contacts of index cases is low, although subclinical infections occur frequently in contacts.

The most compelling evidence for the importance of rotaviruses in severe infantile gastroenteritis has emerged from numerous cross-sectional studies in developed and developing countries. In developed countries, including the United States, rotaviruses are associated with approximately 35 to 52 per cent of acute diarrheal illness requiring hospitalization of infants and young children. The contribution of other enteric pathogens is consistently relatively minor. A similar pattern is also usually observed in developing countries, where rotaviruses are the most frequently detected pathogens in children less than two years of age who have severe gastroenteritis; however, bacterial agents also play an important role in such areas. In addition, during longitudinal studies in a community setting where all diarrheal episodes are monitored, the incidence of rotavirus diarrhea is lower than that of diarrhea caused by other pathogens, but dehydration is more often associated with rotavirus disease than with illness caused by other agents.

In temperate climates, rotavirus gastroenteritis has a characteristic seasonal occurrence during the cooler months of the year with peak prevalence in the winter months. In tropical countries it occurs throughout the year, with less pronounced peaks. Rotavirus diarrhea occurs most frequently in children between 6 months and 24 months of age. Infants less than six months of age have the next highest frequency, although in certain studies the highest frequency is observed in this age group. The low frequency of clinical illness in neonates who undergo rotavirus infection is an unusual paradox that has not been explained. Rotavirus gastroenteritis occurs infrequently in adults, but subclinical infections are common.

Rotaviruses are likely transmitted by the fecal-oral route, although respiratory transmission remains a possibility, since there is such a rapid acquisition of serum antibody during the first two years of life regardless of hygienic conditions. Nosocomial rotavirus infections occur frequently. The incubation period of rotavirus illness is approximately two to four days. There are five recognized human rotavirus serotypes, but the relative importance of each serotype has not been studied thoroughly. Serotype 1 strains have been detected most frequently, but these viruses are not necessarily more virulent. Although a group B rotavirus is responsible for widespread outbreaks of gastroenteritis in adults in China, the role of the non–group A rotaviruses in other regions of the world appears to be minor.

Rotavirus infections have been observed in individuals with travelers' diarrhea. However, rotaviruses are not considered to be an important cause of this illness.

PATHOLOGY AND PATHOGENESIS

NORWALK VIRUS GROUP. Histopathologic lesions following Norwalk or Hawaii virus infections are characterized by a reversible involvement of the upper jejunum. The jejunal mucosa remains intact with marked broadening and blunting of the villi and shortening of the microvilli, along with mononuclear cell infiltration and cytoplasmic vacuolization. Functional alterations may include a transient malabsorption of fat, D-xylose, and lactose and a significant decrease in levels of small intestinal brush border enzymes (alkaline phosphatase and trehalase). Adenylate cyclase activity in the jejunum is not elevated. Delay in gastric emptying may be responsible for the nausea and vomiting associated with these agents.

The nature of immunity to Norwalk virus is perplexing, since a high percentage (~50 per cent) of adults are susceptible to both natural and experimental illness. In addition, although immunity has been observed in approximately 50 per cent of adults, it appears to correlate inversely with the level of serum or local jejunal antibody.

ROTAVIRUS. The major histopathologic lesions are characterized by reversible involvement of the proximal small intestine. The mucosa remains intact, with shortening of the villi, mononuclear cell infiltration in the lamina propria, dis-

tended cisternae of the endoplasmic reticulum, mitochondrial swelling, and sparse, irregular microvilli. Functional alterations may include impaired D-xylose absorption and depressed levels of disaccharidases (maltase, sucrase, and lactase).

The mechanism of immunity to human rotaviruses is not completely clear. Although serum antibodies correlate with resistance to illness (but not infection), the role of local intestinal immunity has not been elucidated. Animal studies indicate that antibody in the small intestine is the major determinant of resistance to illness. A high rate of subclinical infection in neonates is well documented and may be related to passively acquired maternal antibody, host factors, or naturally attenuated rotaviruses that are able to persist in newborn nurseries.

CLINICAL MANIFESTATIONS

NORWALK VIRUS GROUP. Clinical characteristics of illness induced by the Norwalk group of viruses include nausea, vomiting, diarrhea, anorexia, or abdominal discomfort, or any combination. Accompanying clinical manifestations may also include myalgias, low-grade fever, headache, and chills. In children, vomiting occurs more often than diarrhea, whereas in adults the opposite is observed. The onset of illness may be abrupt, marked by vomiting, diarrhea, or both. The illness is usually mild and lasts about 24 to 60 hours. However, severe gastroenteritis has been observed in middle-aged patients and has contributed to the death of elderly, debilitated individuals. The stools are characteristically loose and watery; blood, mucus, and leukocytes are not typically present. A transient decrease in the T, B, and null cell lymphocyte subpopulations has been observed.

ROTAVIRUS. Rotavirus infection can produce a variety of responses in infants and young children, ranging from subclinical infection and mild diarrhea to a severe and occasionally fatal dehydrating illness. Clinical characteristics include vomiting, diarrhea, abdominal discomfort, or fever, or any combination. Fever and vomiting often develop before the diarrhea. Accompanying clinical manifestations may include dehydration, irritability, and pharyngeal or tympanic membrane erythema. In hospitalized patients, the mean duration of confinement is 4 days, with a range of 2 to 14 days. The stools are characteristically loose and watery and only infrequently contain blood or leukocytes.

Although rotaviruses can cause severe or fatal dehydrating illnesses in developing countries, deaths have also been documented in developed countries. In a study in Canada, rotavirus gastroenteritis was implicated in the deaths of 21 children 4 to 30 months of age (mean 11 months) over a period of about 5 years. Twenty children were dead or moribund upon arrival at hospital, and one child was infected nosocomially. With the exception of the latter patient and one other, each was considered healthy prior to the rotaviral illness. Death occurred within one to three days of onset of symptoms. Dehydration and electrolyte imbalance were believed to be the major cause of death in 16 patients, and aspiration of vomitus was the cause of death in 3 patients.

Rotavirus can also induce chronic symptomatic diarrhea with prolonged fecal shedding of the virus and antigenemia in patients with primary immunodeficiency diseases. Infections with rotaviruses or other viral and bacterial enteric pathogens may be especially severe in individuals who are immunosuppressed for bone marrow transplantation. In one study, 8 of 78 such patients (average age 20 to 21 years) shed rotavirus in stools and 5 of the 8 died. Rotavirus infections have also been persistent and severe in children with severe combined immunodeficiency.

DIAGNOSIS

NORWALK VIRUS GROUP. Since a specific diagnosis of infection with this group cannot be made by clinical observation, the diagnosis must be made in the laboratory and relies on the detection of virus in the stool or a serologic response to a viral-specific antigen. These tests include IEM (for the entire group), radioimmunoassay (Norwalk and Snow Mountain agents), and enzyme-linked immunosorbent assay (ELISA) (Norwalk virus). These are still research procedures, since reagents are not generally available. Virus shedding is maximal at or shortly after onset of illness and minimal at 72 hours following onset. The characteristic absence of fecal leukocytes in Norwalk infection may be helpful for differentiation from *Shigella* or *Salmonella* enteritis.

Although a specific clinical diagnosis of infection with Norwalk virus cannot be made in the individual patient, a tentative diagnosis of infection can be made during an outbreak if certain criteria are met: (1) bacterial or parasitic pathogens are not detected; (2) vomiting is present in at least 50 per cent of cases; (3) incubation period is 24 to 48 hours; and (4) mean or median duration of illness is 12 to 60 hours.

ROTAVIRUS. The clinical manifestations of rotavirus gastroenteritis are not distinctive enough to enable diagnosis. Thus, diagnosis requires either detection of the virus or demonstration of a significant serologic response to rotavirus in paired acute and convalescent sera. The epidemiologic pattern relating to the age of the patient, the temporal occurrence of illness, and the signs and symptoms of illness, however, may suggest the diagnosis. In addition, the usual absence of fecal leukocytes in rotavirus diarrhea may help in early differentiation from *Shigella* or *Salmonella* enteritis.

Stools obtained from the first to fourth day of illness are optimal for rotavirus detection, but virus shedding may continue up to 21 days. Virus is characteristically present in stools during the early phase of diarrhea, but diarrhea may continue for two to three days after the cessation of virus shedding.

Over 25 assays have been developed for the detection of rotavirus in stools. The most rapid method is still direct EM because in negatively stained preparations these agents have a distinctive morphologic appearance and are present in large amounts. The non–group A rotaviruses, which do not share the common group antigen, can also be detected by EM. However, an electron microscope may not be readily available, and its use may be impractical when evaluating a large number of specimens. Thus, other rapid and highly effective methods for virus detection have been developed, including ELISA, counterimmunoelectro-osmophoresis (CIEOP), radioimmunoassay (RIA), reverse passive hemagglutination assay (RPHA), latex agglutination (LA), RNA electrophoresis, and dot hybridization. Commercial kits are now available for the ELISA, LA, RPHA, and RNA electrophoresis assays. A popular method is the confirmatory ELISA because it is simple to perform, is sensitive, does not require specialized equipment, and has a negative control for excluding nonspecific reactions. The non–group A rotaviruses cannot be detected by these assays, since they lack the common group antigen; however, an ELISA for group B rotaviruses has recently been developed. Diagnosis of group A rotavirus infection by growth in cell cultures is not practical.

There are many methods for measuring a serologic response to rotavirus infection, including IEM, complement fixation (CF), immunofluorescence, immune adherence hemagglutination assay, ELISA, neutralization, hemagglutination-inhibition (HI), and inhibition of RPHA. Complement fixation is an efficient assay for detecting a serologic response to rotavirus in patients 6 to 24 months of age but is not as effective in adults or infants below 6 months of age.

Detection of rotavirus or demonstration of a serologic response does not necessarily establish an etiologic association with the patient's illness, especially in newborns and adults, who frequently undergo subclinical infection.

TREATMENT

NORWALK VIRUS GROUP. Since the Norwalk group of viruses characteristically causes a mild, self-limited gastroenteritis, replacement of fluid and electrolyte loss with orally administered isotonic fluids is usually sufficient. However, if severe vomiting or diarrhea occurs, parenteral fluid replacement may be necessary. Oral administration of bismuth subsalicylate significantly reduces the severity of abdominal cramps, with a decrease in the median duration of gastrointestinal symptoms from 20 hours to 14 hours. However, the number, weight, and water content of stools and the level of virus excretion are not affected significantly.

ROTAVIRUS. Since rotavirus gastroenteritis may lead to severe dehydration in infants and young children, the early replacement of fluids and electrolytes is essential. Intravenous fluids have been used effectively in the treatment of dehydration. However, in many parts of the world where such treatment is not feasible, efforts have been made to evaluate the effectiveness of an oral rehydration salts (ORS) solution. In a double-blind study comparing ORS with intravenous fluids in children with rotavirus gastroenteritis, ORS solution containing either glucose (20 grams per liter) or sucrose (40 grams per liter) plus electrolytes was found to be as effective as intravenous therapy for rehydration. Glucose electrolyte solutions are recommended for optimal results. The recommended World Health Organization (WHO) ORS solution is made by adding the following to 1 liter of water: sodium chloride, 3.5 grams; trisodium citrate, dihydrate, 2.9 grams; potassium chloride, 1.5 grams; and glucose, anhydrous, 20 grams. Sodium bicarbonate, 2.5 grams, may be substituted for the trisodium citrate, dihydrate. The efficacy of oral glucose-electrolyte solutions that contained either 90 mmol of sodium per liter (as in the WHO formula above) or 50 mmol of sodium per liter, plus additional electrolytes, was examined in well-nourished ambulatory or hospitalized children with mild or moderate dehydrating diarrheal illnesses of varied etiology (including rotavirus but excluding cholera), and each was found to be safe and effective. After the initial calculated fluid deficit is corrected by the ORS, water or fluids without added electrolytes, such as breast milk or some other form of low-solute feeding, should be given orally in addition to the ORS solution, to replace both continued diarrheal fluid and electrolyte losses and to provide normal daily fluid requirements. If oral rehydration fails to correct the fluid and electrolyte loss or if the patient is severely dehydrated or in shock, intravenous therapy must be given.

Chronic rotavirus illness in immunodeficient children has been treated effectively by oral feeding of human milk that contained rotavirus antibody. However, oral administration of preparations containing rotavirus antibody is not effective for treatment of normal children during episodes of rotavirus gastroenteritis.

PREVENTION

NORWALK VIRUS GROUP. There are no specific methods for the prevention of illness by the Norwalk virus group. However, because of the extremely infectious nature of these agents, careful handwashing and proper disposal of contaminated material should minimize transmission. In addition, hygienic preparation of food and measures to decrease contamination of drinking water or swimming facilities should limit the frequency of Norwalk virus outbreaks. Active immunization against this group of viruses is not yet feasible.

ROTAVIRUS. Epidemiologic studies indicate the global need for a rotavirus vaccine to prevent rotavirus diarrhea in the first two years of life, when illness is most severe. Current efforts are focused on developing a live, attenuated oral vaccine that is effective against all serotypes. A promising method involves the "Jennerian" approach, in which a related rotavirus from a nonhuman host is used as the immunizing agent. Efficacy trials of several candidate rotavirus vaccines are currently under way.

Breast milk is generally considered to confer some degree of protection against clinically significant rotavirus diarrhea during infancy. The prophylactic oral administration of human serum globulin containing rotavirus antibody to low birth weight neonates provides significant protection against rotavirus diarrhea.

Chiba S, Yokohama T, Nakata S, et al.: Protective effect of naturally acquired homotypic and heterotypic rotavirus antibodies. Lancet 2:417, 1986. *An important study that examines the relationship of serotype-specific and heterotypic rotavirus neutralizing antibodies to immunity against rotavirus gastroenteritis.*

Ciba Foundation Symposium 128: Novel Diarrhea Viruses. Chichester, John Wiley and Sons, 1987. *An entire volume by various contributors, with special emphasis on non–group A rotaviruses, enteric adenoviruses, caliciviruses, astroviruses, Berne and Breda or Breda-like viruses, the Norwalk virus and rotavirus vaccines.*

Kapikian AZ, Chanock RM: Norwalk group of viruses. In Fields BN, et al. (ed.): Virology. New York, Raven Press, 1985, pp 1495–1517. *A detailed current review of the Norwalk group of viruses from a virologic, epidemiologic, and clinical point of view. Has extensive bibliography with 167 references.*

Kapikian AZ, Chanock RM: Rotaviruses. In Fields BN, et al. (ed.): Virology. New York, Raven Press, 1985, pp 863–906. *A detailed current review of rotaviruses from a virologic, epidemiologic, and clinical point of view. Has extensive bibliography with 513 references.*

Kapikian AZ, Flores J, Hoshino Y, et al.: Rotavirus: The major etiologic agent of severe infantile diarrhea may be controllable by a "Jennerian" approach to vaccination. J Infect Dis 153:815, 1986. *A perspective on various approaches to rotavirus vaccination.*

Kaplan JE, Gary WG, Barron RC, et al.: Epidemiology of Norwalk gastroenteritis and the role of Norwalk virus in outbreaks of acute nonbacterial gastroenteritis. Ann Intern Med 96:756, 1982. *A review of outbreaks of viral gastroenteritis associated with the Norwalk virus from 1976 to 1980.*

Rodriguez WJ, Kim HW, Arrobio JO, et al.: Clinical features of acute gastroenteritis associated with human reovirus-like agent in infants and young children. J Pediatr 91:188, 1977. *A comprehensive description of the clinical features of rotavirus gastroenteritis from a clinical, epidemiologic, and laboratory point of view.*

Santosham M, Burns B, Nadkarni V, et al.: Oral rehydration therapy for acute diarrhea in ambulatory children in the United States: A double-blind comparison of four different solutions. Pediatrics 76:159, 1985. *A recent update on the evaluation of various oral rehydration solutions in infants and young children with diarrhea and mild dehydration. Of special interest to the clinician.*

Santosham M, Daum RS, Dillman L, et al.: Oral rehydration therapy of infantile diarrhea. A controlled study of well-nourished children hospitalized in the United States and Panama. N Engl J Med 306:1070, 1982. *An evaluation of oral glucose-electrolyte rehydration solutions containing different sodium concentrations in children hospitalized with diarrhea. An important study for the clinician.*

Tyrrell DAJ, Kapikian AZ (eds.): Virus Infections of the Gastrointestinal Tract. New York, Marcel Dekker, Inc., 1982. *An entire volume on viral infections of the gastrointestinal tract by numerous contributors. Includes relevant data on virtually all viral agents associated with gastroenteritis with extensive references.*

Viral Infections Characterized by Cutaneous Lesions

336 MEASLES (Morbilli, Rubeola)

Samuel L. Katz

DEFINITION. Measles is an acute, highly contagious disease characterized by fever, coryza, cough, conjunctivitis, enanthem, and exanthem. Its morbidity and mortality vary greatly with host and environmental factors, and its epidemiology has been altered strikingly in the past 25 years in those nations where vaccine has been utilized widely.

ETIOLOGY. The virus is an enveloped, single-stranded RNA paramyxovirus (genus *Morbillivirus*) measuring 120 to 250 nm in diameter, similar to other members of the paramyxovirus family but lacking a neuraminidase. Its single antigenic serotype has been remarkably stable throughout the world for many years with no variation noted. Related animal morbilliviruses are canine distemper and bovine rinderpest, which show some cross-reactivity with measles. The virus contains six major polypeptides, which are responsible for a number of structural and functional properties, including hemagglutination (of primate erythrocytes), hemolysis, cell fusion, viral assembly, and virus penetration. Isolation of virus from clinical specimens is most successful with primary kidney cell cultures of human or simian origin. Laboratory passage has selected variants which grow well in other primary and continuous cell lines of mammalian and avian origin.

Certain simian species provide a reliable animal model of measles after respiratory tract or parenteral inoculation of human isolates. Some virus strains have been adapted to produce central nervous system infection in rodents.

EPIDEMIOLOGY. Classic descriptions of measles epidemiology are no longer applicable to those many areas of the world where measles vaccination is widely practiced. Instead of an inevitable childhood illness, the disease has become an unusual one. The age pattern has shifted to a greater proportion of cases among adolescents and young adults who remain susceptible because of lack of either childhood immunization or exposure to natural infection. In contrast, the epidemiology has been unaltered in developing nations where vaccine programs have been sporadic, incomplete, or totally lacking. Isolated communities such as the Faröe Islands (Panum) are infrequently attacked by measles, at which time manifest illness appears in virtually all persons not previously infected.

Throughout most of the world, measles was a disease of children; most adults acquired active immunity in childhood. Beyond the age of ten more than 90 per cent of the population had specific antibody. Although the peak attack rate coincided with the beginning of school (age six) in technologically advanced societies, it occurs much younger in most developing countries. Morbidity and mortality rates do not appear to be influenced by sex or race. Case fatality rates are highest in children less than five years of age, and are also relatively high in the aged. Congenital infection has occurred but intrauterine infection is more apt to produce a stillborn or premature infant.

There is no evidence that the virus varies significantly in virulence in nature. The excess morbidity and mortality of the disease in developing, isolated, or crowded populations may be explained as a corollary of (1) more prevalent infection of infants under one year of age, (2) poor environmental conditions, (3) inadequate medical care, and (4) secondary bacterial infections. A strikingly increased mortality rate is observed in areas where protein-calorie malnutrition is prevalent.

Communicability. Measles is one of the most highly contagious infections. Demonstration of virus in nasopharyngeal secretions during the prodromal, pre-eruptive phase and in the first days of rash is in accord with epidemiologic evidence that infection is disseminated and acquired by the respiratory tract. Close physical proximity or direct person-to-person respiratory droplet contact is the usual requisite for infection, although uncommon examples of airborne transmission have been reported.

Immunity. An unmodified attack of measles is usually followed by lifelong immunity. This observation is in accord with the observed enduring persistence of antibodies after infection. The mechanism of lifelong immunity after measles is undefined.

Careful studies of isolated or closed populations after administration of live virus vaccine have demonstrated lower titer of antibody than in populations in which measles virus is circulating. Anamnestic antibody response in the absence of disease has been shown in immune contacts of patients with measles. However, studies of children in protected environments have demonstrated that re-exposure or reinfection is not necessary for maintenance of enduring immunity. Passively transferred maternal antibody protects the young infant for the first four to eight months of life.

PATHOLOGY AND PHYSIOLOGIC RESPONSES. Pathologic changes in fatal measles usually represent the compound effect of viral and secondary bacterial infection. Pneumonia is almost invariably present; it is most frequently interstitial. More representative are changes of the uncomplicated viral disease within the tonsillar, nasopharyngeal, and appendiceal tissue removed during the prodrome. These changes consist of round cell infiltration and the presence of multinucleated giant cells. Similar cells are commonly observed in tissue cultures infected with measles virus. Cytoplasmic and nuclear inclusions may be seen in epithelial cells. Koplik's spots show inflammatory mononuclear cell infiltration of buccal submucous glands and necrosis of focal vesicular lesions of the mucosa. Rash is the result of proliferation of capillary endothelial cells in the corium and the coincident exudation of serum, and occasionally erythrocytes, into the epidermis. Viral microtubular aggregates are found in the endothelium of dermal capillaries, but not in the epidermal layer. Simultaneous with the onset of rash, measles-specific antibodies are detectable in serum and, by immunofluorescence, in areas of rash. A marked leukopenia is frequently observed throughout the febrile period. Initially, the leukopenia is occasioned by a decline in lymphocytes on the first day of fever; subsequently, granulocytopenia ensues as well. Measles virus replicates in lymphoid tissues (spleen, thymus, lymph nodes), can multiply in vitro in peripheral blood T and B lymphocytes and monocytes, and can be isolated from blood leukocytes during the course of the disease. The virus is propagable in suspensions of leukocytes in vitro.

Immunosuppressive Effects of Measles. It has long been known that cell-mediated immunity is impaired during measles. There is transient suppression of the tuberculin reaction (observed also with measles vaccines), improvement in eczema and allergic asthma, delay in wound healing, and the induction of remissions in nephrosis. Infection of activated lymphocytes may explain the depression of cell-mediated immunity during the acute disease. In severe disease, the magnitude of depression of the total lymphocytes has been positively correlated with a lessened chance of recovery.

CLINICAL MANIFESTATIONS. After an incubation period that averages 11 days, measles becomes clinically manifest with symptoms of fever, malaise, myalgia, and headache. Within hours *ocular symptoms* of photophobia and burning pain are manifested by conjunctival injection, tearing, and exudate in the conjunctival sac. Concomitantly, or soon thereafter, *catarrhal inflammation of the respiratory tract* leads to sneezing, coughing, and nasal discharge. Less commonly, hoarseness and aphonia may reflect laryngeal involvement. In this prodromal stage of one to four days' duration, petechial lesions of the palate and pharynx or tiny white spots on the buccal mucosa *(Koplik's spots)* may herald the appearance of skin rash. The white lesions described by Koplik characteristically occur lateral to the molar teeth, and typically are mounted on red areolae of injected mucosa, which may

coalesce to form a diffuse red background. They constitute a pathognomonic diagnostic sign. The enanthem may involve other mucous membranes such as the palpebral conjunctiva and vaginal lining. It may "overlap" the subsequent appearance of the cutaneous rash by one to three days. See Figure 336–1.

The *rash* of measles follows the prodromal symptoms by two to four days, occasionally as late as seven days. It first appears behind the ears or on the face and neck as a blotchy erythema, spreads downward to cover the trunk, and finally is manifest on the extremities. The hands and feet may escape involvement. Initially, the eruption consists of discrete, red macules that blanch with pressure. Subsequently, these lesions become papular, tend to coalesce, and may develop a hemorrhagic, nonblanching component. Rash is sometimes very extensive in children with protein-calorie malnutrition, and skin lesions associated with kwashiorkor may develop at the site of the exanthem. The rash fades in the order of its appearance; its disappearance about five days after onset is attended by a fine, powdery desquamation that spares the hands and feet. At its maximum the exanthem usually marks

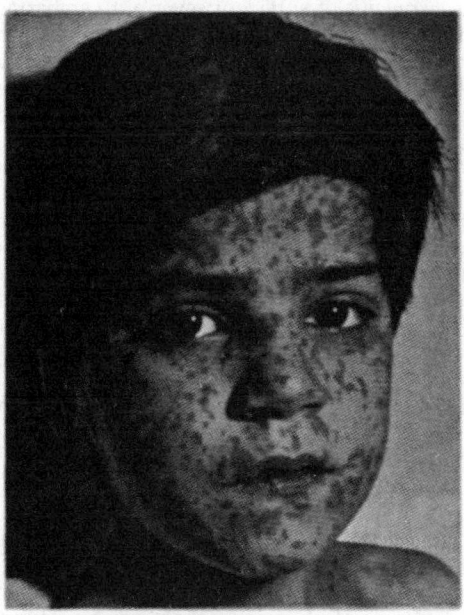

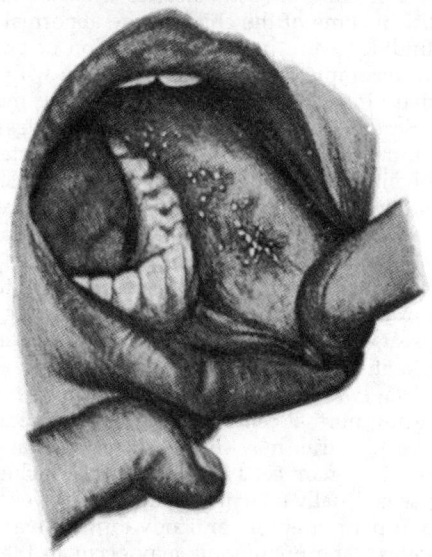

FIGURE 336–1. *Upper*: Early measles eruption. (Reproduction from Therapeutic Notes, by courtesy of Parke, Davis & Company.) *Lower*: Koplik's spots in measles (Hecker, Trumpp, and Abt).

the termination of malaise and fever in the uncomplicated illness.

The *fever* of measles is commonly of the typhoidal, progressively rising type, and falls by lysis. It persists for about six days, and frequently reaches 40 or 41° C. Throughout the febrile period, productive *cough* and auscultatory evidence of bronchiolitis may be evident. These manifestations may persist after defervescence, and cough is often the last symptom to disappear. Bronchopulmonary symptomatology is an integral part of the primary viral infection; roentgenographic evidence of pulmonary involvement is frequently seen in the uncomplicated disease in the absence of leukocytosis and obvious bacterial infection. Generalized lymphadenopathy accompanies the acute febrile illness and may persist for several weeks thereafter.

COMPLICATIONS. The persistence or recurrence of fever and the development of leukocytosis are presumptive evidence of the common bacterial sequelae of *otitis media* or *pneumonia*. Pneumococcus, *Streptococcus hemolyticus, Staphylococcus aureus*, and *Hemophilus influenzae* are the usual secondary invaders.

Serious complications directly related to the measles virus are rare. *Laryngitis* of sufficient severity to embarrass respiration has been observed, and may warrant tracheostomy. Keratoconjunctivitis is part of the acute phase but rarely progresses to actual corneal ulceration. *Electrocardiographic abnormalities* may be found in as many as 30 per cent of children, but clinical evidence of cardiac disease is absent. *Abdominal pain* or *diarrhea* may be related to invasion of lymphoid tissue of the appendix or Peyer's patches. These symptoms may lead to unnecessary surgery before the appearance of the typical rash. The frequency of stomatitis and gastrointestinal symptoms is greater in malnourished children in tropical areas and may reflect coincident bacterial and parasitic infection. They may result in severe dehydration and acidosis as fluid and electrolyte losses rise in the face of diminished oral intake.

Encephalomyelitis. A rare (0.1 per cent) but serious consequence of measles is a demyelinating encephalomyelitis that may appear from 1 to 14 days after the onset of infection. This complication is associated with a recurrence of fever, and headache, vomiting, and stiff neck. Stupor and convulsions usually follow. Localizing neurologic symptoms may be present. Death ensues in about 10 per cent of patients; more than half of survivors suffer permanent residuals of varying severity. Abnormal electroencephalograms were recorded in 51 per cent of children with measles *without clinical signs of encephalitis*. In some of the children the abnormal encephalographic findings were persistent. Infection of brain cells results in an incomplete viral replicative cycle with production of defective virions lacking one ("M") of the measles virus proteins. Studies of patients with acute measles encephalomyelitis and of those with late onset subacute sclerosing panencephalitis show high titers in serum and cerebrospinal fluid of antibodies to all the measles virus proteins except M. This protein is an internal membrane protein crucial to viral assembly.

Other late sequelae of measles are thrombocytopenic purpura and exacerbation or activation of pre-existing pulmonary tuberculosis. The late complication of subacute sclerosing panencephalitis is discussed in Ch. 488.3.

Giant-Cell Pneumonia. In children with severe disease compromising normal cellular and humoral immune mechanisms, measles virus may induce an interstitial pneumonia characterized by giant cells and intracellular inclusion bodies. The disease is usually fatal; if the patient survives, persistence of virus and poor or absent antibody formation are evident in convalescence. The pneumonia may occur in the absence of rash so that its etiologic relation to measles may be unsuspected.

Measles Modified by Antibody Administration. Attenuation of the natural disease by antibody prophylaxis may result in an illness of lessened severity comparable with the milder infection of the maternally immunized newborn. Fever alone may be observed, but some degree of exanthem is usually apparent. Koplik's spots may not appear. In general, the course is truncated and relatively uncomplicated. Lasting immunity is uncertain and serologic studies should be obtained to check for measles-specific antibodies after modified illness.

Atypical Measles—A New Disease. From 1963 to 1967, two types of measles vaccine, one live attenuated, the other inactivated or "killed," were available in the United States. The live attenuated vaccine has since 1967 been the sole product licensed and utilized in this country. From 1965 to 1968 a series of reports was published describing a severe, atypical form of disease occurring after exposure to natural measles of children who had previously received the inactivated vaccine. These patients had high fever, pneumonia, pleural effusion, obtundation, and an unusual rash. The exanthem frequently was initially urticarial and rapidly progressive to maculopapular, petechial, and sometimes vesicular lesions. It was most striking, and often began, on the extremities and was sometimes accompanied by edema of hands and feet. Concomitantly these patients' sera revealed extraordinarily high titers of measles-specific antibodies (25,000 to 200,000 by hemagglutination-inhibition testing).

Subsequent investigations showed that patients who had received inactivated measles vaccines failed to develop antibodies to the "F" protein of the virus. This polypeptide is responsible for cell fusion, viral penetration, and hemolysis. Lack of antibodies to the cell fusion factor permitted these patients to support measles infection in superficial respiratory mucosal cells by cell-to-cell spread. The other measles virus antigens released by these infected cells stimulated a hyperimmune response to those polypeptides that had been present in the inactivated vaccines. Thus the atypical measles syndrome is an imbalance of immune response.

In addition to the rash and pulmonary findings, these patients may have elevated liver enzymes, disseminated intravascular coagulation, and marked myalgia. The pulmonary changes have persisted for longer than 18 months in patients followed with serial chest films. Initial diagnoses on presentation have included Rocky Mountain spotted fever and meningococcemia because of the similarities of rash and toxicity. Since inactivated vaccines were available only from 1963 through 1967, the past recipients are now young adults. This atypical measles syndrome is of increasing importance to the internist.

DIAGNOSIS. The experienced layman can diagnose typical measles. The querulous, bleary-eyed child, his face blotched and his nose crusted with exudate, presents a characteristic, if miserable, picture as he breathes open-mouthed between paroxysms of sneezing and coughing. The severity of the catarrhal symptoms distinguishes the disease from other eruptive fevers. In the prodromal period the diagnosis should be suggested by (1) fever higher than that of the usual respiratory virus infection, (2) known measles in the community, and (3) Koplik's spots on the buccal mucosa.

Differential diagnosis (see Table 336–1) includes consideration of rubella, scarlet fever, exanthem subitum, infectious mononucleosis, secondary syphilis, drug eruptions, and infection with certain adenoviruses, coxsackieviruses, and echoviruses. Of value in excluding these possibilities are the milder course, postauricular nodes, and pinker rash of rubella; the sore throat, eventual desquamation, strawberry tongue, and leukocytosis of scarlet fever; and serologic tests for infectious mononucleosis and syphilis. The rash of exanthem subitum does not appear until the termination of fever. Fever, enanthem, and catarrh are uncommon with the cutaneous mani-

TABLE 336–1. A GUIDE TO THE DIFFERENTIAL DIAGNOSIS OF MEASLES

	Conjunctivitis	Rhinitis	Sore Throat	Enanthem	Leukocytosis	Specific Laboratory Tests Available
Measles	+ +	+ +	0	+	0	+
Rubella	±	±	±	±	0	+
Exanthem subitum	±	±	0	0	0	0
Enterovirus infection	0	±	±	0	0	+
Adenovirus infection	+	+	+	0	0	+
Scarlet fever	±	±	+ +	0	+	+
Infectious mononucleosis	0	0	+ +	±	±	+
Drug rash	0	0	0	0	0	0

0 Not usually present; no test available.
± Variable in occurrence.
+ Present; test available (virus or bacterial culture, serology).
+ + Present and severe.

festations of drug hypersensitivity. Erythema infectiosum is usually an afebrile illness with rash on the cheeks, arms, and legs. There is no prodrome or accompanying respiratory tract involvement.

Specific Diagnosis. Specific diagnosis depends on the isolation of measles virus from throat washings, blood, or urine by inoculation of tissue culture with materials obtained optimally during the prodrome or first days of rash. Increase in specific antibody may be detected as early as the first or second day of rash by the complement fixation test. Antibody is also demonstrated by neutralization, ELISA, or hemagglutination-inhibition procedures. The HI test is generally employed because of rapidity and reliability.

Presumptive diagnosis may be made if giant cells are detected in stained smears of nasal exudate in the pre-eruptive period.

PROGNOSIS. Uncomplicated measles is rarely fatal, and complete recovery is the rule. Fatalities are almost always the result of pneumonia, occurring principally in children below the age of two years. Mortality in economically underdeveloped countries may be 250 times that observed in the United States or northern Europe. Case fatality rates are also high in elderly and tuberculous patients. Congestive cardiac failure is a common cause of death in patients over 50 years old.

Antimicrobial drugs effective against the usual secondary invaders have reduced the case fatality rate of measles sharply. They have proved effective in therapy of bacterial complications, but not in prophylaxis.

Encephalitis occurs as frequently in mild as in severe measles (i.e., about one in a thousand cases); subacute sclerosing panencephalitis follows 1 in 100,000 cases.

TREATMENT. There is no specific antiviral therapy for measles.

Symptomatic Therapy. In the absence of complications, bed rest is the essence of treatment in this usually benign, self-limited disease. Codeine sulfate may be useful in the amelioration of headache and myalgia and is effective in the management of cough. Aspirin or acetaminophen may be employed for its analgesic and antipyretic actions. Fluids should be encouraged. Bright light is not an ocular hazard, but photophobia may require darkening of the patient's room.

Antimicrobial Prophylaxis. The course of uncomplicated measles is not influenced by antimicrobial drugs, and their use during the acute illness has resulted in no decrease of secondary bacterial complications (otitis, sinusitis, pneumonia). Instead, the same rates of complications (about 10 to 15 per cent) have been observed, but with organisms resistant to the antibiotics used during the viral illness. If careful observation of the patient is possible, rational therapy is based on the prompt recognition and etiologic definition of complications, followed by initiation of the appropriate antimicrobial drug in proper dosage.

PREVENTION. *Vaccination.* A highly effective vaccine available for the prevention of measles is derived from the Edmonston strain of virus isolated originally in the laboratory of Dr. John Enders. This live virus vaccine produces immunity by infection and therefore needs to be given only as a single injection. It induces antibody response of somewhat lesser magnitude than that following natural infection. In children over one year of age, seroconversion after vaccination is 90 to 97 per cent. Although a gradual fall in antibody titer occurs in the absence of exposure to wild type virus (see Epidemiology: Immunity), serum antibody is demonstrable in most individuals more than 15 years after a single administration of vaccine. The occasional failure of live virus vaccine to protect has recently been related to vaccination at less than 12 months of age, at which time maternal antibody may inhibit replication of the vaccine virus. It is now recommended that measles immunization be deferred until 15 months of age in technologically advanced countries in which infantile infection is uncommon. Reimmunization is not harmful and is recommended for those who have received vaccine before age one year. The current vaccine is fully effective and safe in susceptible adults also.

Contraindications to live virus vaccine include pregnancy, immunodeficiency, leukemia and other systemic malignant diseases, active tuberculosis, and administration of resistance-depressing drugs such as corticosteroids and antimetabolites.

The introduction of immunization in the United States in 1963 and the subsequent use of more than 150 million doses of vaccine have led to a decrease in incidence from about 500,000 cases annually to a nadir of fewer than 1500 cases in 1983. Although it may be possible to eliminate indigenous measles in the United States, the problem of "imported infection" has arisen with the influx of susceptible children from Southeast Asia and certain Latin American nations where vaccine is not widely employed.

Annunziato D, Kaplan MH, Hall WW, et al.: Atypical measles syndrome: Pathologic and serologic findings. Pediatrics 70:203, 1982. *Excellent clinical description and explanation of a syndrome now seen in young adults.*

Arbeter AM, Baker L, Starr SE, et al.: Combination measles, mumps, rubella and varicella vaccine. Pediatrics 78(Suppl):742, 1986. *The next(?) childhood vaccine, adding varicella to the current MMR.*

Bloch AB, Orenstein WA, Ewing WM, et al.: Measles outbreak in a pediatric practice: Airborne transmission in an office setting. Pediatrics 75:676, 1985. *Although respiratory droplets still form the primary mode of transmission, this study defines epidemiologically the possibility of occasional airborne spread of measles without face-to-face contact of patients and susceptibles.*

Johnson RT, Griffin DE, Hirsch RL, et al.: Measles encephalomyelitis—clinical and immunologic studies. N Engl J Med 310:137, 1984. *Pathogenesis of central nervous system complications studied by modern immunologic approaches.*

Katz SL, Krugman S, Quinn TC (eds.): International symposium on measles immunization. Rev Infect Dis 5:389, 1983. *An all-inclusive presentation of measles and its prevention throughout the world.*

Khanum S, Uddin N, Garelick H, et al.: Comparison of Edmonston-Zagreb and Schwartz strains of measles vaccine given by aerosol or subcutaneous injection. Lancet 1:150, 1987. *A most encouraging demonstration of successful measles immunization of four- to six-month-old infants in a setting where epidemic disease occurs at six to nine months of age.*

Panum PL: Observations Made During the Epidemic of Measles on the Faröe Islands. Delta Omega Society, 1940. *A classic clinical epidemiologic description of measles introduced into an isolated population with disease among all susceptibles born since the previous epidemic 65 years earlier.*

337 RUBELLA (German Measles)

Samuel L. Katz

DEFINITION. Rubella is an acute, usually benign infectious disease characterized by a three-day rash, generalized lymphadenopathy, and minimal or absent prodromal symptoms. Since 1941, it has been known to cause congenital malformations when infection occurs during the early months of pregnancy.

Rubella was recognized as a distinct clinical entity by German physicians in the mid-eighteenth century; it continued to be the subject of moderate interest through the next two centuries until 1941, when the Australian ophthalmologist Gregg called attention to its role as a teratogen. Over the next 20 years the association of rubella in early pregnancy with fetal defects (cataracts, heart disease, and deafness) was corroborated by a number of clinical epidemiologic studies. In 1962, techniques for viral culture and serologic confirmation became available.

ETIOLOGY. Rubella virus is a pleomorphic agent when viewed by electron microscopy, usually spherical, with a central nucleoid 30 nm in diameter contained within an outer envelope 60 to 70 nm wide. Its genome is single-stranded RNA, and the virus is classified as a special member (genus *Rubivirus*) of the togavirus group on the basis of its biochemical, biophysical, and ultrastructural properties. Unlike most of the togaviruses it does not utilize an arthropod vector in its natural cycle. In the human, its only natural host, the virus behaves like a paramyxovirus, and many of its laboratory characteristics are like those of that group. It will multiply in a variety of primary cell culture systems and in some continuous cell lines, usually without detectable cytopathic effects. Hemagglutination of avian (chicken, goose, pigeon) erythrocytes provides a convenient method for virus assay, and by inhibition of this hemagglutination the presence and titer of antibody are readily measured. By polyacrylamide-gel electrophoresis eight distinct viral polypeptides have been identified.

EPIDEMIOLOGY. Prior to the availability of rubella vaccines, the disease was worldwide in distribution, produced major epidemics at six- to nine-year intervals, and occurred mainly in school-age children, but also produced outbreaks in settings such as military recruit bases and college campuses where large numbers of susceptible young adults gathered in relatively crowded conditions. The use, since licensure in 1969, of more than 130 million doses of rubella vaccine in the United States has strikingly altered the epidemiology. There has been no major epidemic since 1964–1965, and the age-specific attack rate has altered with a significant increase in the proportion of cases reported in adolescents and young adults who failed to be immunized in childhood. In other nations, where rubella vaccine has not been widely utilized, the epidemiology has remained unchanged and epidemics were observed in 1971–1972, 1978–1979, and 1982–1983. Because the usual disease may be quite nonspecific clinically, with evidence that nearly one third of adults may undergo infection without rash, epidemiologic reporting has been variable. Since 1966, congenital rubella has been a reportable disease. It is probable that rubella is spread by the respiratory route by close and sustained personal contact. The usual infection is contagious throughout the period of prodromal symptoms and for as long as seven days after the appearance of rash. However, the infant with congenitally acquired infection may excrete virus in respiratory secretions and in urine for months after birth and is contagious during this time. In hospital environments, especially in nurseries, the congenital rubella baby has been a source of nosocomial infection of personnel involved in his care.

Immunity is lifelong in duration after initial infection. Au-thenticated second attacks are exceedingly rare, and require serologic documentation because of the nonspecific nature of the clinical syndrome. *Subclinical* reinfection demonstrated by increase in IgG serum antibody has been documented with increasing frequency as better serologic methods and increased surveillance have become available. Reinfection occurs most commonly in crowded populations in which the density of infection and probability of spread are high. Such reinfections are not associated with viremia and thus pose little threat in pregnant women. IgM response serves to distinguish primary infection from reinfection. Immunity that follows artificial immunization with live virus vaccine is apparently of equal duration even though the antibody titers induced may be somewhat lower. (See Prevention, below.)

PATHOLOGY. Death from postnatal rubella is an almost unheard-of event, so the histology has not been studied. Since 1962, it has been possible to investigate the pathogenesis and to correlate clinical findings with virologic events. After initial invasion of the upper respiratory tract, virus spreads to local lymphoid tissue where it multiplies and initiates a viremia of approximately seven days' duration. Respiratory tract shedding of virus and the viremia rise to peak levels until the onset of rash, at which time the latter becomes undetectable, whereas respiratory secretions contain diminishing quantities of virus over the succeeding 5 to 15 days. Specific serum antibodies can be demonstrated with the onset of rash, and circulating immune complexes are detectable soon thereafter.

Congenital Rubella. Necropsies of fetal and neonatal victims of intrauterine infection have shown a variety of embryonal defects related to developmental arrest involving all three germ layers.

The virus establishes chronic persistent infection of many tissues, with inhibition of mitosis and a resultant intrauterine growth retardation. Delayed and disordered organogenesis produces embryopathic structural defects (eye, brain, heart, large arteries), and continued viral infection in fetal and postnatal cells causes organ and tissue damage (hepatitis, nephritis, myocarditis, pneumonia, osteitis, meningitis, cochlear degeneration, pancreatitis).

CLINICAL MANIFESTATIONS. *Postnatally Acquired Rubella.* Fourteen to 21 days after exposure, the onset of rubella is manifested by the appearance of a rash with mild accompanying constitutional symptoms of malaise and occasional sore throat. Palpable, tender, and occasionally visible lymphadenopathy involves postauricular and suboccipital nodes. Moderate fever, coryza, and faint conjunctivitis may accompany the rash. Generalized peripheral lymphadenopathy and, more rarely, splenomegaly may occur.

The exanthem of rubella is usually apparent within 24 hours of the first symptoms as a faint macular erythema that first involves the face and neck. Characterized by its brevity and evanescence, it spreads rapidly to the trunk and extremities, sometimes leaving one site even as it appears at the next. The pink macules that constitute the rash blanch with pressure and rarely stain the skin. Rubella virus has been isolated from the skin lesions as well as from uninvolved sites. The truncal rash may coalesce, but the lesions on the extremities remain discrete. The eruption vanishes by the third day. Rubella may occur without rash. An enanthem has been described that is inconstant in form and occurrence. The lesions consist of red macules that usually involve the soft palate. Infections with adenoviruses, enteroviruses, and Epstein-Barr virus can mimic rubella with rash, fever, and lymphadenopathy. In the absence of an epidemic and of serologic (or virologic) confirmation, the clinical diagnosis of rubella is not reliable.

COMPLICATIONS. Recovery is almost always prompt and uneventful. In contrast to measles, secondary bacterial infections are not encountered in rubella. Transient polyarthralgia and polyarthritis are more common among adolescents and adults with rubella, particularly females. They appear three or more days after onset of rash and may last five to ten days. Large joints (knees, elbows, ankles) are most often involved, but small and medium-sized joints may also be affected. Surveys during urban epidemics have revealed rates of 5 to 15 per cent in males and 10 to 35 per cent in females. A relationship to later-onset rheumatoid arthritis is a subject of continuing investigation (Chantler).

Thrombocytopenia, when sought by serial platelet counts, is a common complication but rarely of clinical significance. The unusual patient who develops purpuric manifestations may also have evidence of increased capillary fragility and a prolonged bleeding time. A meningoencephalitis of short duration may occur one to six days after the appearance of rash. Its incidence is estimated at 1 in 6000 cases, and it is fatal in approximately 20 per cent of those afflicted. Rubella encephalopathy is not associated with demyelinization (in contrast to other postviral encephalitides). Survivors may have electroencephalographic abnormalities, but intellectual function seems to be preserved.

Congenital Rubella. Congenital transplacental infection of the fetus occurs as a consequence of maternal infection (which may or may not be clinically evident), usually in the first four months of pregnancy. Virus is demonstrable in placental and fetal tissues obtained by therapeutic abortion at that time. If pregnancy is not interrupted, fetal infection persists, and upon delivery of the infant, virus is recoverable from the throat, urine, conjunctivae, bone marrow, and cerebrospinal fluid of the living infant and from most organs at autopsy. From 20 to 80 per cent of infants born to mothers infected in the first trimester of pregnancy have stigmata of infection readily recognizable in the first year of life. These include *cardiac lesions* and *eye defects* (cataracts, glaucoma, retinitis, microphthalmia). Most infants in whom virus is detectable do not have evidence of disease at birth or may simply have intrauterine growth retardation. In others, disease of intermediate severity occurs. Most prominent of these manifestations is *thrombocytopenic purpura*, which disappears soon after birth. *Hepatosplenomegaly* with active hepatitis may persist for months. Other involvement includes *interstitial pneumonia, meningoencephalitis, hearing loss* of varying extent, and *lesions of the long bones.* A chronic recurrent erythematous rash associated with the presence of rubella virus in the skin has been reported in some patients. Recently, a progressive panencephalitis simulating subacute sclerosing panencephalitis has been observed in the second decade following congenital infection. The long-term sequelae for most congenital rubella infants include psychomotor retardation, hearing loss, and retinopathy.

A striking finding has been the persistence of virus in the pharynx, urine, and cerebrospinal fluid for as long as one year after birth (9 per cent). Infective virus was present in a congenital cataract after three years, and in the urine of a victim of congenital rubella 29 years after her birth. This evidence of continuing viral synthesis occurs coincidentally with circulating antibody (initially of maternal origin). The character of the antibody changes during the first months from IgG (presumably maternal) to IgM, indicating a primary response of the infant to the persisting viral antigen. Studies of older infants and children with stigmata of congenital rubella show them to be free of demonstrable virus and to possess the IgG immunoglobulins that characteristically persist after other viral infections. The defect in host response that is responsible for viral persistence has not yet been defined fully, but there is depressed T cell response to rubella virus antigens in some congenitally infected infants.

DIAGNOSIS. Rubella may be diagnosed clinically with assurance only during an epidemic. Distinction from measles may be made on the basis of fainter, nonstaining rash, the milder course, and the minimal or absent systemic complaints. Sore throat is a more prominent complaint in scarlet fever; the course of infectious mononucleosis is often more pro-

tracted, and splenomegaly is more frequent than in rubella. Specific diagnosis of rubella is made by isolation of the virus in any of several cell culture systems, or by demonstration of neutralizing, hemagglutination-inhibiting (HI), ELISA, or complement-fixing antibody response during infection. HI antibodies are most rapidly and reproducibly available in diagnostic laboratories throughout the nation.

PROGNOSIS. Complete recovery from postnatally acquired rubella is almost invariable. The rare deaths attributable to rubella follow the infrequent complication of meningoencephalitis. Infection in pregnancy constitutes a grave hazard to the fetus but not to the mother.

TREATMENT. There is no specific antiviral therapy. Few patients suffer discomfort severe enough to warrant symptomatic medication. Headache and myalgia may be controlled by aspirin.

PREVENTION. *Passive Immunization. Administration of gamma globulin to the pregnant woman may only mask her symptoms of infection and not protect the fetus from viral invasion. Its use may thus only obscure the picture and confound decision about the need for therapeutic abortion.*

Active Immunization. Rubella may be prevented in children and adults by the parenteral administration of attenuated live virus vaccines produced in cell cultures. Seroconversion rates after immunization are at least 95 per cent. As with other live virus vaccines, serum antibody titers are somewhat lower than those that follow natural infection. However, antibody persists for at least 15 years after vaccination. Natural reinfection of individuals immunized with vaccine is not uncommon, although such infection is asymptomatic and without viremia. In children, vaccination is attended by little or no reaction; but in women, malaise, arthralgia, and mild, acute arthritis occur frequently, the incidence being directly related to age. It was initially recommended in the United States that immunization be carried out principally in childhood. The success of these efforts, with reduction of rubella cases to fewer than 600 reported in 1986, has encouraged a more aggressive attempt to immunize those remaining susceptible women and adolescent girls. Current policy recommends vaccination of all such persons who have no history of previous rubella immunization. Of this population, only nonpregnant individuals should be immunized, and contraception (when appropriate) should be carried out for at least three months after vaccination. The inadvertent administration of vaccine to pregnant women, however, has demonstrated that attenuated vaccine viruses can reach the products of conception; but in more than 500 such cases studied, no infant has been observed with congenital malformations as a result. The use of vaccine in the United States prevented a large epidemic of rubella expected in the early 1970's and has reduced the reported annual occurrence from more than 50,000 cases annually (with epidemic peaks of 200,000 to 500,000) to an all-time low in 1986 (500 to 600 cases) with only 11 infants with congenital rubella.

Burke JP, Hinman AR, Krugman S (eds.): International symposium on prevention of congenital rubella infection. Rev Infect Dis 7(Suppl)1, 1985. *Fifteen years of vaccine use summarized by investigators from the developed nations.*

Centers for Disease Control: Elimination of rubella and congenital rebella syndrome—United States. MMWR 34:65, 1985. *A summary report of progress in rubella "eradication" in the United States; points out the need to target "at-risk" groups.*

Chantler JK, Tingle AJ, Petty RE: Persistent rubella virus infection associated with chronic arthritis in children. N Engl J Med 313:1117, 1985. *Continuing provocative investigations of the possible etiologic role of rubella virus in some cases of juvenile rheumatoid arthritis.*

Clarke M, Schild GC, Miller C, et al.: Surveys of rubella antibodies in young adults and children. Lancet 1:667, 1983. *The English approach to prevention of congenital rubella, very different from that in the United States and with persistence of congenital rubella 13 years after its initiation.*

Gregg NM: Congenital cataract following German measles in the mother. Trans Ophthal Soc Aust 3:35, 1941. *The original "classic" associating rubella in pregnancy with congenital malformations.*

Hanshaw JB, Dudgeon JA: Rubella. In Viral Diseases of the Fetus and Newborn. Philadelphia, W. B. Saunders Company, 1978. *For the interested scholar, an all-inclusive presentation with nine pages of references.*

338 FOOT AND MOUTH DISEASE
Catherine M. Wilfert

Foot and mouth disease (FMD) (aphthous fever, epizootic stomatitis) is a highly contagious illness of cloven-hoofed animals, especially cattle, sheep, goats, and pigs. The causative agent is a member of the picornavirus family. It belongs to the *Aphthovirus* genus, which is composed of small (diameter of 25 to 30 nm) acid-labile RNA viruses containing naked icosahedral nucleocapsids. The disease in animals is characterized by fever and increased salivation, with the appearance of vesicular lesions on the mucous membranes of the mouth, tongue, and lips, between the paws, and on the teats and udder. Vesicular fluid is highly infectious. Persistent asymptomatic infection with detectable excretion of infectious virus from the epithelial cells of the pharynx occurs for several years in cattle, sheep, and goats. There are seven different serotypes of FMD, which tend to be found in localized geographic areas. This virus is highly communicable among animals, and the epidemic spread of this agent among domestic animals can result in tremendous loss of livestock. The rigid quarantine regulations of the Bureau of Animal Diseases, United States Department of Agriculture, in the United States has freed this country of FMD. Indeed, public law prevents importation of the virus into the mainland of the United States even for experimental purposes. An inactivated vaccine for use in animals utilized polyvalent, cell culture–grown FMD virus. More recently, DNA recombinant technology and chemically synthesized peptides corresponding to specific regions of a capsid polypeptide (VP1) coupled to a carrier molecule have been successfully used as immunogens in animals.

FMD in its natural hosts is clinically indistinguishable from two other diseases that do occur in the United States. These are vesicular stomatitis virus of horses, cattle, and occasionally humans, and vesicular exanthema of swine. The rapid diagnosis of FMD in cattle is important to allow its differentiation from the other two diseases. This is accomplished by a qualified laboratory with the use of differential inoculations of infectious material into appropriate hosts.

The human is an extremely rare incidental host of FMD. The illness is usually self-limited, febrile, and characterized by excessive salivation and vesicular lesions on the buccal or lingual epithelium, and possibly the skin of the hands, feet, and other parts of the body. Humans apparently carry the virus for at least 24 hours in their nasopharynx and can transmit it to other humans or susceptible animals via infectious droplets. For diagnostic purposes vesicular fluid can be used as antigen in a serotype-specific complement fixation test. Antibody assessment can be accomplished by hemagglutination inhibition assays and tissue culture neutralization assays. This illness has no relationship to hand-foot-and-mouth disease caused by coxsackieviruses.

Bittle JL, Houghten RA, Alexander H, et al.: Protection against foot-and-mouth disease by immunization with a chemically synthesized peptide predicted from the viral nucleotide sequence. Nature 298:30, 1982.

Brooksby JB: Portraits of viruses: Foot-and-mouth disease virus. Intervirology 18:1, 1982. *Historical review of these viruses, illustrating their economic importance and advances in investigative methodology.*

Kleid DG, Yansura D, Small B, et al.: Cloned viral protein vaccine for foot and mouth disease: Responses in cattle and swine. Science 214:1125, 1981. *Description of recombinant DNA technology applied to development of specific polypeptide antigen.*

339 MUMPS
Catherine M. Wilfert

DEFINITION. Mumps, or epidemic parotitis, is an acute communicable viral infection. The characteristic clinical manifestations were described in the fifth century B.C. by Hippocrates.

ETIOLOGY. Mumps virus is placed in the *Paramyxovirus* genus of the Paramyxoviridae family. The diameter of the virus particle is approximately 150 nm, and it has enveloped helical nucleocapsids. It is a ribonucleic acid (RNA) virus with a nonsegmented, single-stranded genome that apparently codes for six polypeptides, three of which are nucleocapsid proteins and three of which are envelope proteins. One of the surface glycoproteins is the spike containing the hemagglutinin and neuraminidase (HN). The hemagglutinin causes the agglutination of erythrocytes of several species. The second surface glycoprotein spike (F) is responsible for the cell fusing and hemolyzing activities of the virus. The remarkable feature of the two paramyxovirus glycoproteins F and HN is that they must be cleaved once by a cellular protease for the virus particles to become infectious. If the cells lack protease, only noninfectious virus particles are produced. The paramyxoviruses enter cells by fusing with cell membranes and liberating their nucleocapsids into the cytoplasm of the host cell. Mumps virus replication occurs in a variety of cell cultures and is infective for monkeys and chick embryos. It is relatively heat labile, with loss of infectivity resulting from heating to 55 to 60°C for 20 minutes.

EPIDEMIOLOGY. Mumps virus infection is endemic in all areas of the world and occurs throughout the year. Mumps is predominantly a disease of childhood, and prior to the advent of vaccine the majority of clinically evident infections were seen in children between the ages of five and ten years. Serologic evidence suggested that approximately 85 per cent of mumps infections occurred in those under 15 years of age. In the United States, immunization has now increased the age-specific attack rate in 10- to 14-year-old children because they were not required to be immunized at school entry.

Infection is transmitted via respiratory droplets, but mumps virus is less communicable than measles or varicella. Epidemiologic evidence suggests that the period of infectivity is from several days before onset of symptoms until the subsidence of the salivary gland swelling. Prolonged or recurrent excretion of virus has not been observed. As many as 25 to 40 per cent of mumps infections are entirely asymptomatic. For these reasons attempts to control the spread of mumps infection by isolation of a patient are usually futile. The asymptomatic patients excrete virus, may transmit infection, and have a self-limited infection. The resulting immunity is comparable to that following symptomatic infection. There are no known animal reservoirs for mumps.

PATHOGENESIS AND PATHOLOGY. The portal of entry of the virus is thought to be the upper respiratory tract. The time interval after exposure to virus before the appearance of the clinical symptoms ranges from 14 to 21 days, with the usual incubation period being 16 to 18 days. After entering the host, the virus replicates and viremia occurs, which may result in secondary invasion of several organ systems. Tissues such as the salivary glands (predominantly the parotids), meninges, testes, pancreas, ovaries, thyroid, and heart may show evidence of infection. Virus is also excreted in the urine, and transient abnormalities in renal function have been found.

Pathologic examination of involved tissues has been infrequent because of the usually benign nature of the illness. Available studies of salivary glands indicate that there is no disruption of the general architecture of the gland. The involved salivary ducts may demonstrate changes in the epithelial lining cells, ranging from edema to complete desquamation. The ducts are dilated, and the lumen may be filled with cellular debris and polymorphonuclear cells. There may be a moderate amount of periductal edema around the involved ducts. Mononuclear inflammatory cells predominate in the interstitium. The pathology of other involved tissues is similar, and no specific hallmarks allow the diagnosis of mumps infection to be made solely on the basis of the observed pathology.

CLINICAL MANIFESTATIONS. Salivary gland involvement usually precedes other clinical symptoms, lasts for two to seven days, and may be unilateral or bilateral. Infection of the salivary glands is manifested by pain, and the characteristic swelling of the parotid gland provides the diagnosis of mumps. The infection less frequently involves the submandibular or sublingual salivary glands. Although other manifestations of mumps most often coincide with the parotid swelling, they may precede or occur in the absence of salivary gland involvement.

Meningitis. Central nervous system involvement with mumps virus occurs frequently. Viral meningitis has been said to occur in 65 per cent of hospitalized persons with parotid swelling when lumbar puncture is done. The cerebrospinal fluid (CSF) shows a predominantly lymphocytic pleocytosis in affected individuals, although only one half of them will display clinical signs of meningitis. The signs of meningeal involvement are most often manifest two to ten days after the onset of parotitis and last three to five days. Illness is characterized by fever, headache, nausea, vomiting, and nuchal rigidity and is self limited and clears with minimal (if any) sequelae.

Encephalitis. A more serious and much less frequent central nervous system manifestation is encephalitis or encephalomyelitis. The onset is usually later than the transient meningitis and occurs 10 to 14 days after the clinical salivary gland involvement. The patient appears severely ill, is deeply obtunded, and may have seizures or die. Although occurring much less often than the encephalitis associated with measles or varicella, mumps encephalitis is clinically and pathologically indistinguishable from them.

Epididymo-orchitis. The complication of mumps infection best known by nonmedical persons is the involvement of the testes. This manifestation occurs predominantly in postpubertal males with 20 to 30 per cent manifesting orchitis during the course of mumps infection. Bilateral testicular involvement occurs in 2 to 6 per cent of patients with orchitis. Orchitis usually begins abruptly with fever, chills, headache, and lower abdominal pain. The systemic reaction ordinarily parallels the extent of gonadal involvement. The testis swells rapidly and becomes very painful and tender. The pain and swelling disappear as fever subsides, usually within five days of onset. Testicular tenderness may persist for a longer period. There is no theoretic or factual basis for the fear of sexual impotence following mumps orchitis. In the vast majority of instances the disease is unilateral. At least one half of those patients who have unilateral disease have completely normal testes after the acute infection; the remainder may have some degree of unilateral testicular atrophy that does not result in sterility.

Pancreatitis. Pancreatitis may occur in association with mumps infection, with typical symptoms of abdominal pain, fever, and vomiting. Symptoms gradually subside over a period of three to seven days, and the patient usually recovers completely. Studies in vitro have demonstrated that mumps virus can replicate in human pancreatic beta cells and pancreatic epithelial cells. There is no firm epidemiologic or

clinical evidence linking mumps virus infection to the subsequent development of diabetes mellitus.

Other Clinical Manifestations. Especially in adults, infection of other tissues may rarely occur. Oophoritis has been described in adult females. The characteristic lower quadrant or back pain suggests the clinical diagnosis, but involvement of the ovaries may occur in the absence of recognizable symptoms. Sterility is not a known consequence of mumps oophoritis. Arthritis may occur alone or in concert with other manifestations. It may be mono- or polyarticular, is self-limited, and affects young adult males most often. Extremely rare manifestations of infection include mastitis, myocarditis, thyroiditis, dacryoadenitis, and bartholinitis.

HOST RESPONSE. In the normal individual a single infection with mumps virus confers permanent immunity against clinically evident infection. It is probable that reinfection, defined as an antibody rise after exposure to the virus, may occur, but neither virus shedding nor clinical illness has been demonstrated with such reinfection. Although second attacks of parotitis have been observed, there are other possible causes, including coxsackievirus or lymphocytic choriomeningitis virus infections, starch ingestion, sarcoidosis, iodine sensitivity, and thiazide therapy. At present there is no documentation by culture or serology of two clinical attacks of mumps virus infection in the same individual.

Mumps virus infection induces the formation of specific humoral antibodies. Initially antibody of the IgM class and subsequently antibody of the IgG class are formed. Neutralization of infectivity, inhibition of hemagglutination, and the inhibition of neuraminidase activity are functions attributable to antibody to the HN protein. Specific neutralizing antibodies can be detected during the first week of symptoms and ordinarily persist for a lifetime. Hemagglutinating-inhibiting and complement-fixing antibodies become detectable from one to three weeks after onset and usually reach peak titers within three to six weeks.

In vitro, mumps virus replicates in human lymphoblastoid cell lines with T cell characteristics and in peripheral blood mononuclear cells. Pokeweed mitogen enhances replication that occurs primarily in T lymphocytes, suggesting that these cells might be infected during natural infection.

DIAGNOSIS. The clinical diagnosis is strongly suggested when a known exposure to mumps is followed in two to three weeks by an illness with compatible clinical findings, such as parotitis. In the absence of parotitis or if parotitis has occurred previously, specific laboratory studies are necessary to confirm the diagnosis.

Virus has been isolated from such varied sources as blood, cerebrospinal fluid (CSF), urine, saliva, salivary gland tissue, and human milk. Viral diagnostic laboratories are available in many academic and large hospital settings for unusual or complicated situations.

Many diagnostic laboratories are better able to offer serologic diagnosis than viral isolation. Evaluation of sera for antibodies to mumps virus is readily accomplished. With acute serum one can determine if a person has ever had mumps infection. An increase in antibody titer in convalescent serum is indicative of recent mumps virus infection. Complement-fixation (CF) tests have been most commonly employed by diagnostic laboratories for this purpose. Occasionally it is useful to obtain additional information about the temporal relationship of an illness to the antibody response. Two complement-fixing antigens, the nucleoprotein or soluble (S) antigen and the viral surface antigen (V), have been recognized for years. CF antibodies against the S antigen are detectable within two to three days of onset, peak at about ten days, and disappear in eight to nine months. CF antibodies against the V antigen, which includes the HN and F proteins, are not detectable until approximately the tenth day of infection and persist for years. Comparison of the transient nature of the S antibodies with the delayed appearance of the

V antibodies may assist in defining recent infection. Although tedious to perform, neutralization assays have traditionally been used as the most accurate assessment of immunity. Enzyme-linked immunoassays (ELISA) have been developed, are sensitive and specific, and will become generally available.

PROGNOSIS. In general the prognosis of infection with mumps virus is excellent. Fatalities have been associated with encephalitis, myocarditis, and nephritis but are extremely rare. An occasional sequel to mumps virus infection is deafness, which may occur even in the absence of other evidence of central nervous system involvement. The loss of hearing may be preceded by tinnitus and a sense of fullness of the ear. Deafness is relatively uncommon but occurs suddenly during the period of parotid swelling. It is usually unilateral, but an estimated 20 per cent of those affected may have bilateral disease. Once deafness has occurred, the damage is irreversible.

TREATMENT. Mumps is a self-limited infection, and there is no specific therapy available.

PREVENTIVE MEASURES. *Passive Protection.* A common question concerns what to do when a susceptible person is exposed to mumps infection. Administration of hyperimmune globulin or pooled serum IgG after such exposure has not decreased the number of patients acquiring illness nor has it lessened the severity of illness. There is a single controlled study reporting that administration of hyperimmune globulin after the appearance of parotitis can decrease the incidence and severity of orchitis. Other studies under epidemic conditions failed to demonstrate any alteration in the attack rate or in the subsequent development of orchitis or meningoencephalitis. Therefore, the use of hyperimmune globulin is of dubious value.

Immunization. Live attenuated mumps virus vaccine is available for prophylactic use. The attenuated virus vaccine is produced in tissue cultures of chick embryo fibroblasts and is administered parenterally. Virus is not shed by the vaccinee, and immunization rarely causes any side effects. Transient, mild parotitis in the several weeks following immunization has been observed in a very few children. The vaccine produces 95 to 100 per cent serologic conversion from antibody negative to positive in vaccinated susceptibles. Although the antibody levels are considerably lower, they parallel those produced by natural infection and have persisted for the 19 to 20 years that the vaccine has been available for study. The presence of detectable mumps antibody correlates with protection against clinical illness. Immunized children in contact with naturally occurring mumps have been protected against clinical illness. It is recommended for administration to children more than one year of age and to adolescents and adults for induction of immunity. Live attenuated mumps vaccine has been combined with measles and rubella virus vaccines. This vaccine (MMR) is routinely administered to children at 15 months of age, and 31 states require immunity to enter school. Vaccine can be given without adverse consequences to adults whose immune status is unknown with regard to the other antigens. That is, inadvertent immunization of a person already immune (either from vaccine or disease) to any of the three viruses is safe.

There is only a single serologic strain of mumps virus; hence a single infection with either natural or attenuated virus confers immunity. More than 59 million doses of mumps vaccine have been distributed since 1967, and this increasing use of mumps vaccination has resulted in a marked decline in the incidence of reported disease in the United States. In 1967, 185,691 cases were reported, compared with 3021 in 1984 for the entire United States.

The vaccine will not offer protection against mumps if someone has already been exposed to natural infection and is in the incubation period of illness. On the other hand, no harmful effects have been noted after administration of vaccine to an exposed susceptible person. If the original exposure is not followed by mumps infection, the vaccine would then induce protection against subsequent exposures.

Fleischer B, Kneth HW: Mumps virus replication in human lymphoid cell lines and in peripheral blood lymphocytes: Preference for T cells. Infect Immun 35:25, 1982. *In vitro studies suggesting that activated T lymphocytes are the major site of replication of mumps virus in peripheral white blood cells.*

Jensik SC, Silver S: Polypeptides of mumps virus. J Virol 17:363, 1976. *Viral glycoprotein containing neuraminidase and hemagglutinating activity corresponds to V antigen of mumps virus.*

Kilham L, Margolis G: Induction of congenital hydrocephalus in hamsters with attenuated and natural strains of mumps virus. J Infect Dis 132:462, 1975. *Experimental induction of intrauterine infection with attenuated and wild-type mumps virus resulting in central nervous system infection.*

Orvel C: Structural polypeptides of mumps virus. J Gen Virol 41:527, 1978. *The experimental definition of mumps virus polypeptides is described.*

Prince GA, Jenson AB, Billups LC, et al.: Infection of human pancreatic beta cell cultures with mumps virus. Nature 271:158, 1978. *The demonstration by immunofluorescence of mumps antigen in human beta cells.*

Shehab ZM, Brunnell PA, Cobb E: Epidemiological standardization of a test for susceptibility to mumps. J Infect Dis 149:810, 1984. *Utilization of an ELISA for antibody measurement.*

Sullivan KM, Halpin TJ, Kim-Farley R, et al.: Mumps disease and its health impact: An outbreak–based report. Pediatrics 76:533, 1985. *Impact on children of mumps illness and the costs of this disease in the 1980's.*

Westmore GA, Pickard BH, Stern H: Isolation of mumps virus from the inner ear after sudden deafness. Br Med J 1:14, 1979. *A case report documenting mumps virus in the inner ear in association with subsequent deafness.*

Diseases Caused By Herpes-Type Viruses

340 HERPES SIMPLEX VIRUS INFECTIONS

R. Gordon Douglas, Jr.

Herpes simplex virus produces diseases ranging from inapparent infections and fever blisters to fatal encephalitis. The word herpes is derived from the Greek work "herpein," meaning "to creep," in reference to the skin manifestations.

ETIOLOGY. Herpes simplex virus (HSV) is a member of the Herpetoviridae family. Herpes simplex virus has an internal core containing linear double-stranded deoxyribonucleic acid (DNA) large enough to encode 60 to 70 gene products. It is surrounded by an electron-dense capsid, an icosahedron of 162 hollow capsomeres surrounded by a lipid-containing laminated envelope studded with five or six glycoproteins. Between the capsid and the envelope is the tegument composed of several proteins. Because of the variable size of the envelope, the overall diameter of the virus ranges from 150 to 200 nm.

Viral replication occurs primarily within the cell nucleus, and viral envelopes are derived from the nuclear membrane. Complete replication is associated with lysis of the infected cell due to inhibition of cell macromolecular synthesis.

Herpes simplex virus grows well in a variety of human and

animal cell lines, in embryonated hens' eggs, and in laboratory animals.

HSV types 1 and 2 share common antigens so that cross-reacting antibodies are induced following infection with either virus. They can be differentiated by monoclonal antibody and restriction enzyme techniques. They differ also by route of transmission, usual site of disease, type of complications, and a few differences in physical properties and characteristics in cell cultures.

EPIDEMIOLOGY. Herpes simplex viruses are distributed worldwide. There are no known seasonal patterns of infection. Since infection with virus is followed by development of antibody that persists for life, incidence of infection can be determined by antibody studies. The prevalence of antibody is inversely related to socioeconomic status. In underdeveloped areas, almost 100 per cent of adults have antibody to HSV, whereas in higher socioeconomic groups, this proportion falls to 30 to 50 per cent. The time of maximal acquisition of infection varies with the two types. The prevalence of antibody to HSV type 1 rises during childhood, whereas the major period of infection with HSV type 2 follows puberty.

Transmission apparently occurs by direct contact from person to person, and there is no animal reservoir. HSV type 1 is transmitted primarily by contact with oral secretions, and HSV type 2 by contact with genital secretions. A small percentage of adults may be excreting HSV type 1 or type 2 at any time, and this may occur in the absence of active lesions. Apparently, transmission can occur both from overtly infected persons and from asymptomatic excretors, but the efficiency of transmission is greater from symptomatic persons. The portal of entry is most commonly the oral cavity for HSV type 1 and the genital tract for HSV type 2. However, either type of HSV may be introduced directly into the eye, a skin site, or the oral cavity or genital area. Transmission of HSV type 2 can occur in infants born to mothers with genital infections. Also, anal and perianal infections of HSV type 2 are common among male homosexuals. Autoinoculation from either oral or genital sites to hands, thighs, or buttocks is not unusual. Extraoral acquisition of HSV is a hazard in certain occupations, and persons such as dentists, respiratory care unit personnel, and wrestlers are at risk. Laboratory-acquired infection and nosocomial outbreaks in hospital personnel or in neonatal nurseries have been reported.

Recurrent infections are one of the hallmarks of the Herpetoviridae family, and they occur frequently with both HSV type 1 and type 2. Recurrent infections of the lips or perioral area with HSV type 1 occur in 20 to 40 per cent of the population. Recurrences may occur as frequently as once every several weeks or as infrequently as once or twice per year. They usually occur at the same site and despite the presence of circulating or local antibodies. They may be triggered by sunlight, fever, local trauma, menstruation, emotional stress, or other factors.

Recurrent HSV type 2 usually presents as lesions on the external genitalia, and with either type recurrences may appear at other sites, e.g., the eye. Genital recurrences occur in up to 80 per cent of those with initial episodes. Although most recurrences are due to reactivation of latent virus, exogenous reinfection accounts for some cases.

PATHOGENESIS AND PATHOLOGY. Following spread of virus from one person to another, the virus replicates locally in peribasal and intermediate epithelial cells, resulting in lysis of cells and initiation of a local inflammatory response. This results in a characteristic thin-walled vesicle on an inflammatory base. Histologic study reveals multinucleated cells with ballooning degeneration, marked edema, and the characteristic Cowdry type A intranuclear inclusions, which are indistinguishable from those caused by varicella-zoster virus. Sensory or autonomic nerve endings are also infected, and virus is transported intra-axonally to the nerve cell bodies in ganglia (Fig. 340–1). Lymphatics and regional lymph nodes

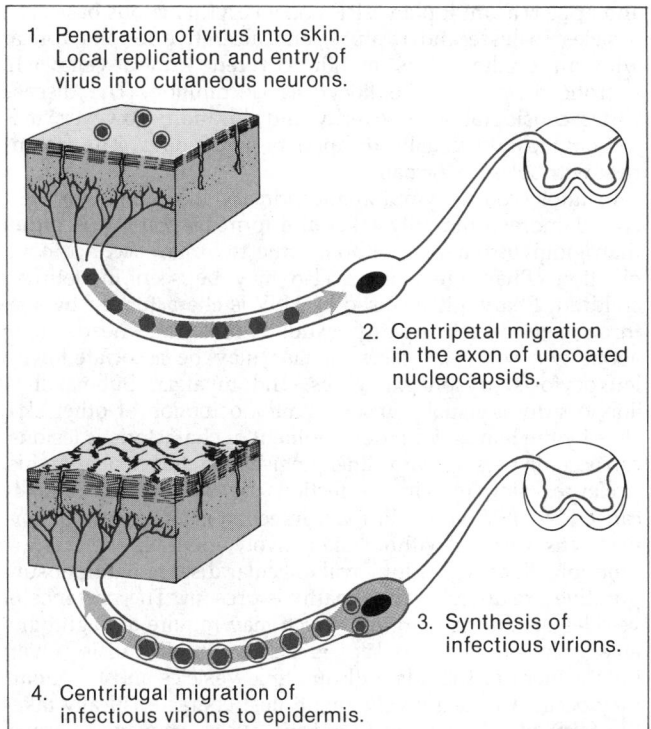

1. Penetration of virus into skin. Local replication and entry of virus into cutaneous neurons.

2. Centripetal migration in the axon of uncoated nucleocapsids.

3. Synthesis of infectious virions.

4. Centrifugal migration of infectious virions to epidermis.

FIGURE 340–1. Schematic diagram of the pathogenesis of primary mucocutaneous HSV infection. (Modified from Corey L, Spear PG: Infections with herpes simplex viruses. N Engl J Med 344:686, 1986.)

may become infected, and in neonates or compromised hosts viremia and visceral dissemination may occur. In most persons, however, infection is controlled at the local site by host defense mechanisms. Although neutralizing antibody may contribute, cellular immune mechanisms, such as the production of interferon and other lymphokines and induction of T cell reactivity, natural killer cells, macrophages, and antibody-dependent lymphocyte cytotoxicity, are thought to have the major function in controlling HSV infections. Adults and children with depressed cell-mediated immune mechanisms appear to be more susceptible to severe, disseminated HSV infections than those with depressed humoral immunity. Disease resulting from primary infection with HSV type 2 is more severe in those who have not experienced HSV type 1 infection previously than in those who have, suggesting that heterotypic protective immunity is present.

Following primary infection, HSV becomes latent in the ganglia of the nerves supplying the infected areas; for HSV type 1 the trigeminal ganglion and for HSV type 2 the lumbosacral ganglia are most frequently involved. The virus does not remain latent at the skin or mucous membrane site. While the virus is latent, infectious virus is no longer detectable in specimens from patients and lesions do not occur. Viral DNA is present as circular episomes or concatemers or is integrated into the cell genome. With reactivation, infectious virus is transported to the body surface along sensory nerves to skin sites where productive infection leads to cell lysis, an inflammatory response, and development of the characteristic lesions.

CLINICAL MANIFESTATIONS. *Primary Infection.* Most commonly, primary infection with HSV type 1 is asymptomatic, but *gingivostomatitis* will occur in a small number, usually children one to three years of age. It can also occur in older children and adults. Following an incubation period of 2 to 12 days, prodromal symptoms of low-grade fever and cervical adenopathy may occur. As the oral lesions appear, the temperature rises to 38.3 to 38.9° C, and there is intense oral pain, increased salivation, and foul breath. The oral lesions begin on the buccal and gingival mucosa and tongue and appear as multiple vesicles on an erythematous base. The vesicles coalesce and rupture, and ulcerative lesions appear with an erythematous margin covered with a yellowish, necrotic membrane. Leukocytosis is common. The disease varies considerably in severity and duration; however, it is self-limited and usually disappears by 14 days. The lesions heal without scar formation.

In adolescents, symptomatic primary infection with HSV type 1 more commonly takes the form of *pharyngitis* rather than gingivostomatitis, although the two may occur in combination. Pharyngitis alone also may be seen in younger children. Pharyngitis caused by HSV is characterized by sore throat, cervical adenopathy, exudate, fever, and headache in about two thirds of cases. It also may be associated with leukocytosis, dysphagia, chills, and myalgia. Submaxillary adenopathy is usually absent. Autoinoculation of other skin sites by the hands, with development of characteristic lesions, can occur in persons with either gingivostomatitis or pharyngitis.

Herpes simplex virus infections of the eye are usually caused by HSV type 1. Primary infection is an acute *keratoconjunctivitis* with or without skin involvement. If the lids are uninvolved, acute conjunctival follicular disease with nonsuppurative preauricular adenopathy is present. The presence of vesicles on the lid margins, which may require a magnifying lens or a slit lamp to see, is helpful in diagnosis. Overt involvement of the lids with multiple vesicles and lid edema may occur. Corneal involvement most characteristically takes the form of a branching (dendritic) ulcer. However, corneal manifestations may be atypical, especially early in illness, and consist of diffuse punctate lesions or wandering serpiginous ulcers without clear-cut branching. The disease is self-limited and resolves entirely without scarring in many cases. However, corneal involvement may lead to permanent scarring.

Primary *genital infection* is most common in adolescents and in young adults and is usually caused by HSV type 2. In the male, characteristic vesicular lesions on an erythematous base usually appear on the glans penis or the penile shaft. In the female, lesions may involve the vulva, perineum, buttocks, cervix, and vagina and are frequently accompanied by vaginal discharge. Primary infection in both sexes may be associated with fever, malaise, anorexia, and tender bilateral inguinal adenopathy. Although vesicular lesions may persist for several days, they usually ulcerate rapidly and become covered with a grayish-white exudate. These lesions are often exquisitely tender, and in the female urethral involvement may result in dysuria or urinary retention. Lesions of primary genital herpes may persist for several weeks before healing is complete. Herpetic sacral radiculomyelitis may rarely accompany genital infection.

Although manifestations of primary infection are generally oral or genital with either type of HSV, primary infection may involve other skin sites. When it involves the fingers, it is referred to as herpetic whitlow.

Primary perianal and rectal HSV infections are being recognized more frequently, particularly in male homosexuals. Pain, tenesmus, discharge, difficulty in urinating, and sacral paresthesias, as well as fever, chills, malaise, and headache occur commonly. Examination reveals vesicles and ulcerations. The disease is usually self-limited except in the setting of acquired immunodeficiency syndrome (AIDS), in which proctitis may be progressive.

Recurrent Infections. The most common manifestation of recurrent infection with HSV type 1 is herpes labialis (fever blister, herpes simplex). The lesions of recurrent labial herpes are localized to the mucocutaneous junction of the lips or adjacent skin. The lower lip is more frequently involved than the upper lip, and in an individual patient lesions tend to occur at the same site. It is notable that although primary infections commonly occur within the mouth, recurrent oral herpes infections rarely involve mucous membranes. They are frequently heralded by prodromal symptoms, such as

tingling or itching, which last for a few hours, and facial hyperesthesia and pain, which may last one to two days. Vesicles then appear and are often associated with considerable pain. The lesions progress from vesicle to ulcer to crust within 48 hours. Pain is most severe in the first 24 hours, and healing is complete within 8 to 10 days.

Recurrent ocular infection may take the form of epithelial infections or trophic ulcers, stromal disease (interstitial or disciform keratitis), iridocyclitis, or combinations of these. It is usually unilateral. Often the characteristic branching (dendritic) ulcers that stain with fluorescein are observed, and these are virtually diagnostic of HSV infection. Stromal disease is manifested by various forms of infiltrates underlying the ulcers, which result in opacification. Superficial keratitis usually heals, but recurrent infection with deep stromal involvement and uveitis may persist. Gradual diminution in visual acuity takes place with recurrent attacks, and permanent visual loss may result.

Recurrent genital lesions in both sexes are associated with less severe systemic symptoms and less extensive local involvement than primary attacks. They are often preceded by a prodrome of tenderness, itching, burning, or tingling. However, in occasional individuals, severe recurrent attacks may occur over a period of one or more years.

Other Manifestations. ENCEPHALITIS. Herpes simplex encephalitis is a rare complication of herpesvirus infection. It is thought to be the most common sporadic viral encephalitis in the United States and is fully described in Ch. 484.

ASEPTIC MENINGITIS. Infrequently, in association with HSV type 2 genital infection, the clinical syndrome of aseptic meningitis, including fever, headache, stiff neck, and cerebrospinal fluid (CSF) pleocytosis, may occur (see Ch. 485.1).

CONGENITAL INFECTIONS. Congenital infection is very rare and probably results from retrograde spread of HSV type 2 from maternal genital infection to the placenta. Such infection may be recognized at birth by central nervous system manifestations such as microcephaly, intracranial calcifications, microphthalmia, seizures, and chorioretinitis, which are common to a number of chronic intrauterine infections.

NEONATAL INFECTIONS. Neonatal infections result from passage of the infant through an infected maternal genital tract or retrograde ascending infection if the membranes have ruptured. The overall risk of neonatal infection is low in women with primary or recurrent HSV type 2 infection after 32 weeks' gestation, but is higher if lesions are present at delivery. Infants born to mothers with primary infection during pregnancy are at greater risk of developing severe infection than are those whose mothers have recurrent genital herpes. Disease may range from mild, self-limited skin infection to fatal, disseminated infection with or without encephalitis. Localized skin disease occurs in 10 per cent of cases and is self-limited. Isolated involvement of the central nervous system (encephalitis) and eye (chorioretinitis) may lead to death or serious sequelae.

Disseminated neonatal infection usually appears a few days after birth, and vesicles may or may not be present. Vesicles eventually occur in 50 per cent of the infants, but may be absent early in infection. Patients may show constitutional signs and symptoms, irritability, seizures, respiratory distress, jaundice, petechiae, ecchymosis, and shock-like syndrome. Neurologic signs occur in 50 per cent of cases and include seizures, cranial nerve palsies, lethargy, and coma. CSF pleocytosis with increased protein and normal glucose also is commonly observed. Many of these patients will develop destructive encephalitis, disseminated intravascular coagulation, or hepatic and adrenal necrosis. About 75 per cent of patients die, and few recover without sequelae.

COMPROMISED HOSTS. Patients compromised by immunodeficiency or immunosuppression, by malnutrition, or by disorders of skin integrity such as burns or eczema are at greater risk of developing severe herpes simplex viral infections. Frequently the cardiac or bone marrow transplant recipient, and less so the renal transplant recipient, excretes HSV in throat washings for the first few months following grafting. Although some such patients may not have overt disease, some develop lesions that can be severe and persist for many weeks to months. Lesions may spread down the respiratory or gastrointestinal tracts and result in tracheobronchitis, pneumonia, or esophagitis. Patients with hematologic and lymphoreticular neoplasms and children with congenital thymic disorders may develop severe, chronic, progressive mucocutaneous HSV infection or disseminated disease. Disseminated disease has also been observed in pregnancy and in geriatric populations. Herpetic esophagitis may be related to nasogastric intubation and results in dysphasia and substernal pain. Burn wound infections with HSV are becoming increasingly well recognized, as are HSV infections in patients with a variety of other skin disorders.

Severe herpes infections, particularly progressive perianal ulcers, colitis, esophagitis, and pneumonia, are prominent features of AIDS.

ERYTHEMA MULTIFORME. About 5 to 15 per cent of all cases of erythema multiforme are regularly preceded by an attack of herpes simplex. Either HSV type 1 or HSV type 2 infections may be involved, and the cutaneous manifestations may range from mild to severe (Stevens-Johnson syndrome) and may be recurrent.

OTHER SYNDROMES. Hepatitis, monoarticular arthritis, adrenal necrosis, idiopathic thrombocytopenia, and glomerulonephritis have been reported. Attempts have been made to relate HSV infections to a variety of neurologic syndromes such as multiple sclerosis, Bell's palsy, some atypical pain syndromes, ascending myelitis, trigeminal neuralgia, temporal lobe epilepsy, and others, but there is no definitive proof of a causal relationship for any of these associations.

DIAGNOSIS. In most minor infections, diagnosis is dependent on clinical recognition. Gingivostomatitis must be differentiated from aphthous stomatitis, Stevens-Johnson syndrome, Vincent's infection, infectious mononucleosis, herpangina, and streptococcal or diphtheritic pharyngitis. Pharyngitis caused by HSV infection must be differentiated from that caused by streptococci, Epstein-Barr (EB) virus, and other viruses. Cervical adenopathy, exudate, and fever are common in HSV infection. If dendritic ulcers are present in patients with keratitis, they are virtually diagnostic of HSV infection; however, these ulcers have also been observed in varicella-zoster virus infections, and corneal abrasions are occasionally mistaken for HSV infection. The presence of multiple vesicular genital lesions or ulcerative lesions associated with pain helps differentiate herpes simplex genital infections from other forms of venereal disease such as syphilis and chancroid. Infections of other skin sites, particularly if they have a dermatomal distribution, must be distinguished from varicella-zoster virus infection. Severe anorectal pain, difficulty in urination, and sacral paresthesias are more common in HSV perianal and rectal disease than in other forms of proctitis. Recurrent herpes labialis is easily recognized clinically. Recurrent intraoral lesions are usually not herpes simplex but rather aphthous stomatitis or some other malady, but intraoral lesions may occur with HSV infections in the immunocompromised or immunosuppressed patient. Recurrent eye and genital infections commonly can be recognized by their characteristic clinical manifestations. Congenital infections may be difficult to distinguish from similar syndromes caused by rubella virus, cytomegalovirus, or *Toxoplasma gondii*. Neonatal infection with HSV may be mistaken for neonatal sepsis, erythema toxicum, streptococcal infection, and enteroviral infection. In more severe infections viral isolation attempts are helpful. Severe skin infection in older patients and disseminated infection in immunocompromised patients may also be diagnosed by recovery of virus. Burn wound infections, unless

there are typical vesicular areas, usually must be diagnosed by viral isolation or biopsy for intranuclear inclusions.

Definitive diagnosis can be made by isolation of HSV from lesions. However, 1 to 15 per cent of asymptomatic normal persons will shed HSV in oral secretions and a similar number in genital secretions. Therefore, isolation of virus from these sites may not be related to active disease. HSV types 1 and 2 replicate in a variety of cell lines, and cytopathic effects appear rapidly, usually within 24 to 48 hours. Specimens should be collected early by aspiration of vesicles or swabbing the open lesions, and promptly inoculated into cell cultures. If transportation to the laboratory must be delayed, specimens can be stored at 4°C for a few hours, or, if storage is longer than 24 hours, they should be stored at −70°C. Rapid detection of antigen by monoclonal antibodies or DNA hybridization is becoming more widely available.

Histologic diagnosis is based on the presence of giant cells, intranuclear inclusions, or both in scrapings of lesions or biopsies of tissue. Scrapings may be smeared, fixed with ethanol or methanol, and stained with Giemsa, Wright, or Papanicolaou (preferred) stain. Usually only giant cells are seen on scrapings and smears, and intranuclear inclusions in HSV infection cannot be distinguished from those of varicella-zoster virus infection.

Development of serum antibodies when none existed previously is often helpful in recognizing primary infection but is of little value in recurrent infections. Measurement of IgM antibodies of HSV may be helpful in the diagnosis of neonatal infection. Such antibodies usually appear within the first four weeks of life in infected infants and persist for many months. Unfortunately, measurement of IgM antibodies in older persons has not proved useful in separating primary from recurrent infection.

TREATMENT. Specific antiviral chemotherapy is now available for some HSV infections.

Idoxuridine (IDU or 2'-deoxy-5-iodouridine) and trifluridine have been shown to be effective in the treatment of HSV keratitis, and are licensed for this purpose in the United States. Trifluridine is the drug of choice.

Vidarabine (adenine arabinoside, ara-A), has been shown to be effective and is licensed in the United States. Ophthalmic ointment is effective in keratoconjunctivitis. Intravenous vidarabine is effective in patients with HSV encephalitis in a dose of 15 mg per kilogram per day for ten days. Intravenous vidarabine has also been shown to be effective in neonatal disseminated herpes simplex infections. It is not effective topically against herpes labialis or other skin or genital infections.

Acyclovir is effective for treatment of herpes genitalis, mucocutaneous disease in immunosuppressed patients, herpes keratitis, herpes encephalitis, and neonatal herpes. It is available in a topical, oral, and intravenous form. Topical therapy is effective in primary but not in recurrent genital infections. Intravenous and oral acyclovir are more effective in primary and are effective in recurrent genital infections. Topical acyclovir therapy is not effective for recurrent herpes labialis. Except for ophthalmic infections, acyclovir has largely replaced vidarabine. Acyclovir is the drug of choice for herpes simplex encephalitis, mucocutaneous HSV infections in immunocompromised patients, and first-episode genital herpes in immunocompetent patients. Oral acyclovir is effective in preventing recurrence of herpes genitalis, and oral or intravenous acyclovir may prevent reactivation of HSV in patients undergong induction chemotherapy or transplantation. Acyclovir is not recommended for routine use in treatment of recurrent HSV genital infections. In recurrent genital disease, prophylaxis with oral acyclovir does not eliminate ganglionic latency, and recurrences occur after therapy is discontinued.

PROPHYLAXIS. Medical and dental personnel should be strongly encouraged to avoid direct contact with potential infectious lesions by wearing gloves. Patients with extensive herpetic lesions should be isolated. Either temporary abstinence or at least the use of condoms has been recommended to prevent genital spread when one sexual partner has active lesions. Continued use of condoms may be useful if there is a history of recurrent genital infections.

Prevention of neonatal disease in offspring of mothers with genital infection presents special problems. If there is clinically apparent cervical infection or genital virus excretion is detected at parturition before membranes rupture, a cesarean section is recommended. If rupture of the membranes has occurred, it is uncertain whether cesarean section will be effective in preventing infection, although rapid delivery by either route is clearly indicated to lessen exposure to the infant. If no lesions are obvious at delivery, only rarely is virus recoverable and vaginal delivery appears safe.

Corey L, Adams HG, Brown ZA, et al.: Genital herpes simplex virus infections: Clinical manifestations, course and complications. Ann Intern Med 98:958, 1983. *Recent, well-referenced review of genital HSV.*
Corey L, Spear PG: Infections with herpes simplex viruses. N Engl J Med 314:686, 1986. *Recent, well-referenced summary of virology, pathogenesis, immunology, epidemiology, and clinical manifestations.*
Goodell SE, Quinn TC, Mkrtichian E, et al.: Herpes simplex virus proctitis in homosexual men. Clinical, sigmoidoscopic and histopathological features. N Engl J Med 308:868, 1983.
Hirsch MS, Schooley RT: Treatment of herpes virus infections. N Engl J Med 309:963, 1983. *An up-to-date, well-referenced review of acyclovir, vidarabine, and other therapeutic agents in HSV infections.*
Whitley RJ, Alford CA, Hirsch MS, et al., and the National Institute of Allergy and Infectious Diseases (NIAID) Collaborative Antiviral Study Group: Vidarabine versus acyclovir therapy in herpes simplex encephalitis. N Engl J Med 314:144, 1986. *Documentation of superiority of acyclovir to vidarabine in HSV encephalitis.*
Wong KK, Hirsch MS: Herpes virus infections in patients with neoplastic disease. Ann Intern Med 76:464, 1984. *Well-referenced summary of diagnosis and therapy with vidarabine, acyclovir, and alpha interferon.*

341 CYTOMEGALOVIRUS INFECTION

David J. Lang

DEFINITION. Infections caused by cytomegalovirus (CMV) may be asymptomatic or may cause disseminated and even fatal multisystem disease, depending upon the mode and timing of virus acquisition and the immunocompetence of the host. CMV infections occur commonly, although with variable severity, in the fetus and in immunocompromised individuals.

ETIOLOGY. CMV is a species-specific member of the herpes virus group. Like other herpesviruses, CMV has the capacity to replicate persistently in the face of normal host immunity and to establish latent infections subject to reactivation. CMV cytopathology is focal in vitro, and replication of the virus is largely limited to cell cultures of species-specific fibroblasts. In vivo, however, CMV replicates in epithelial as well as fibroblastic elements. Subtypes of CMV can be distinguished, although the variants are without apparent clinical significance.

EPIDEMIOLOGY. CMV is worldwide in distribution, and infection shows no seasonal preference. Persistence, latency, and reactivation of CMV make it difficult to interpret the etiologic significance of the recovery of the virus.

The age of acquisition of CMV is variable. In less developed parts of the world, CMV infection is acquired universally in infancy, probably at or shortly after parturition. Where interpersonal contact is reduced and sanitation is more advanced, acquisition of CMV infection is delayed and occurs gradually through infancy, childhood, and even adulthood. Transmission of CMV is associated with close interpersonal (including sexual) contact or with direct introduction of cells or body fluids. CMV has been recovered from virtually all organs and tissues and can be found in urine, saliva, blood, semen, milk, secretions of the uterine cervix, and stool. CMV is opportunistic; it reactivates in, is transmitted to, and spreads from hosts whose defenses are compromised. Since these patients are often found in hospital settings, this virus poses a theoretic risk for nosocomial spread. However, no substantial evidence has been found of patient-to-patient or patient-to-staff transmission.

Transmission of CMV occurs with blood (estimated 5 per cent of whole-blood units) and with a proportion of organ transplants. Horizontal interpersonal transmission of CMV occurs, but not in epidemics. Young children, infected as neonates from blood or as toddlers by contact in daycare centers, can serve as a source of family infection.

Prenatal CMV infection is the most common known congenital infection of humans. It occurs in about 1 per cent of infants born in the United States (0.5 to 8 per cent depending upon the population studied). Most of these infections reflect prenatal transmission of CMV reactivated during pregnancy in otherwise healthy immune women. As many as 30 per cent of pregnant women may shed CMV at some time and from some site during pregnancy.

PATHOGENESIS AND PATHOLOGY. CMV replicates slowly in vitro. Infected cells swell and develop characteristic intranuclear and paranuclear inclusions. CMV infections in vitro are accompanied by some changes associated with morphologic transformation. It has been possible to transform cells permanently by infecting with irradiated virus and in this way interfering selectively with the full cycle of virus replication and cytopathology. These CMV-transformed cells have malignant potential in certain animals. Whether CMV plays a role in the pathogenesis of malignancy in humans is unresolved.

CMV can and frequently does reactivate in immune hosts. When immune function is immature or compromised, reactivated virus can spread, causing significant injury and functional impairment. The pathogenesis of transplacental spread in the presence of intact maternal immunity remains unclear.

That CMV is carried in circulating cells of healthy individuals appears certain on the basis of epidemiologic observations. Nevertheless, it has been difficult to recover this virus from the circulating cells of healthy individuals. The use of CMV antibody–negative blood units has been recommended for transfusion in high-risk groups such as selected newborns or allograft recipients.

CLINICAL MANIFESTATIONS. *Postnatal CMV Infection in Normal Hosts.* In healthy individuals CMV infection is usually asymptomatic or unrecognized. Occasionally primary CMV infection is accompanied by a self-limited, mononucleosis-like syndrome characterized by fever, splenomegaly; mild hepatocellular dysfunction; lymphoid hyperplasia, including the presence of atypical lymphocytes; occasional thrombocytopenia; hemolysis; and inconsistent skin rash. Pharyngitis is not prominent. The fever may range from 39° to over 40° C and in some instances is accompanied by night sweats and chills. Between febrile episodes the patient, although tired, does not feel very ill.

Some cases of mild-to-moderate hepatitis have been associated with CMV infection, and infrequently a normal host will experience an interstitial pneumonitis caused by this virus. There have been reports associating prior CMV infection with the Guillain-Barré syndrome. CMV infections have also been associated with isolated thrombocytopenia, hemolytic anemia, and ulcerative gastrointestinal disease.

Postnatal CMV Infection in Abnormal Hosts. Individuals undergoing open heart surgery requiring perfusion and others receiving multiple units of blood may experience a mononucleosis-like illness about three to six weeks later. The illness can be mistaken for bacterial sepsis or endocarditis, a particularly important distinction in recipients of cardiac prostheses.

CMV infections have been a major problem for allograft recipients. Latent virus may be reactivated by immunosuppression. Alternatively, the response to the allograft or, in the case of marrow transplantation, a graft versus host (GVH) reaction, may stimulate virus reactivation. Immunosuppression limits the ability of the host to restrict virus spread. To complicate matters further, CMV infections also seem to enhance graft rejection, though the mechanism mediating this process remains uncertain. In any case, infection with CMV in allograft recipients can be associated with significant and even fatal interstitial pneumonitis, hepatitis, encephalitis, retinitis, and diffuse cytomegalic inclusion disease.

CMV infections have been found prominently in the acquired immunodeficiency syndrome (AIDS), which occurs in response to infection with human immunodeficiency virus (HIV). Evidence suggests that reciprocal interaction may exist between CMV and HIV infections. On the basis of seroepidemiologic as well as molecular evidence, it is suspected that CMV may play a role in the etiology of Kaposi's sarcoma. Overall, CMV infections associated with AIDS are likely to be opportunistic, although since CMV infections are often associated with some depression of the helper-suppressor T cell ratio, as well as suppression of natural killer (NK) cell activity and T cell proliferation, the precise distinction between cause and effect, opportunism and pathogenesis, remains to be elucidated.

Significant and even fatal CMV infections are prominent in recipients of bone marrow transplants, and this virus remains the most common cause of serious post-transplant infection. Both newly acquired (from transplant or blood cell components or both) and endogenous (reactivated in host) CMV infections occur. The progress and effect of these infections may be mediated by direct cytopathology or by immunopathologic mechanisms. Some controversy exists concerning the role of CMV in the progress of GVH reactions in marrow graft recipients.

CMV infections are very common among male homosexuals, and disseminated symptomatic CMV infections are prominent in patients with AIDS. Indeed, much of the morbidity and some mortality associated with AIDS has been ascribed to CMV infections of the liver, brain (associated with glial nodules), gastrointestinal tract (ulcerative lesions), lungs (diffuse interstitial pneumonitis often coexisting with *Pneumocystis carinii* infection), and eyes (retinitis).

Prenatal and Perinatal CMV Infection. Prenatal CMV infections were first appreciated through retrospective pathologic studies. Since the recognition of the infection depended on postmortem examinations, it was initially concluded that prenatal CMV infection was rare and always fatal. The severe, disseminated infection was termed *cytomegalic inclusion disease.* Subsequently, cytologic techniques identified CMV infection in living infants by the presence of large, intranuclear-inclusion-bearing cells in urinary sediment. The isolation of virus in vitro proved to be an even more sensitive technique. It became apparent that infants congenitally infected with CMV could survive and that manifestations of these infections resembled those associated with other prenatal infections. The CMV-infected infants were often small for gestational age and microcephalic. In some cases they exhibited intracerebral calcifications, hepatosplenomegaly, chorioretinitis, thrombocytopenia with purpura, macular rash, hemolytic anemia, and a variety of structural and functional organ impairments.

Prospective studies determined that congenital infections with CMV were not rare. Overall, about 1 per cent of babies were found to be prenatally infected with CMV. Prenatal CMV infection is particularly prevalent among infants of primiparous, young, unmarried, and promiscuous women. Most CMV-infected infants appear normal at birth, but as many as 10 to 20 per cent ultimately display learning disabilities, hearing impairment, or evidence of cognitive dysfunction.

Women who are immune prior to conception may give birth to CMV-infected infants. The birth to a woman of more than one CMV-infected infant with identical viral strains has been documented. It seems certain that many prenatal CMV infections are acquired from previously latent maternal virus reactivated during gestation.

Perinatal acquisition of CMV infection (from infected cervix, breast milk, or saliva) is usually asymptomatic. However, an infant born to a CMV-seronegative woman may develop significant postnatal pneumonia or hepatitis if infected with CMV via transfusions.

DIAGNOSIS. The laboratory isolation of CMV is accomplished in tissue culture and requires the prompt transportation of refrigerated specimens to a prepared virus laboratory. Up to five weeks can be required for recovery and identification of virus. Although the evolution of cytopathology may be slow, some viral antigens appear rapidly (hours) in inoculated cells. Furthermore, CMV replication in cell culture can be enhanced by centrifugation of specimens on monolayers in shell vials. The use of monoclonal antibodies to early CMV antigens, coupled with labeled antiglobulin preparations, can provide rapid and specific virus detection. The recovery of cloned subgenomic fragments of CMV deoxyribonucleic acid (DNA) has permitted detection of CMV directly and specifically by hybridization procedures.

Regardless of the technique used, occasional prolonged shedding of virus and the intermittent reactivation of latent CMV may confuse the interpretation of virus recovery. The isolation of CMV at certain times (from urine taken during the first days of life) or from unusual sites (blood, spinal fluid, or tissues specifically involved in the disease process) makes the etiologic association of virus and clinical condition more likely. Demonstration of simultaneous seroconversion or significant (fourfold or greater) serologic change further strengthens the association. CMV serology may be assessed by complement fixation, immunofluorescence, and enzyme-linked immunosorbent assay (ELISA) procedures. The use of CMV-specific IgM serology to identify recent infections may be rendered less useful by the presence of rheumatoid factor (false-positives) and by the tendency of CMV IgM to persist in some instances and to reappear when latent virus is reactivated.

DIFFERENTIAL DIAGNOSIS. Postnatally acquired CMV infections in normal hosts may be difficult to distinguish from those caused by Epstein-Barr virus (EBV). However, EBV mononucleosis is often associated with a positive heterophil-agglutination reaction, whereas CMV mononucleosis is always heterophil-negative. CMV mononucleosis tends to occur in older individuals, and is associated with more prominent fever and night sweats and less adenopathy than EBV mononucleosis. Hepatitis associated with CMV infection is generally milder than that associated with hepatitis A, B, or non-A non-B viruses. The ultimate distinction between these conditions is dependent upon the results of virus-specific tests.

CMV interstitial pneumonitis, similar to that caused by *Pneumocystis carinii*, cannot be identified on clinical grounds alone but requires the use of virologic studies applied to clinical samples, especially those from lung biopsies and needle aspirations, bronchoscopy, and bronchoalveolar lavage. Accurate and rapid identification of CMV infections may be made in these specimens by application of histologic and cytologic techniques as well as by specific procedures employing monoclonal antibodies, immunofluorescence, and DNA hybridization.

Congenital infections caused by toxoplasmosis, rubella, syphilis, and herpes simplex virus may be difficult to distinguish from those caused by CMV. All may be associated with intrauterine growth retardation, hepatic and splenic enlargement, purpura, thrombocytopenia, and hemolysis. Congenital toxoplasmosis can be associated as well with chorioretinitis and intracerebral calcifications.

Congenital rubella is associated with glaucoma, microphthalmia, cataracts, and cardiac malformations more frequently than is congenital CMV infection. The retinitis of congenital rubella, unlike that of CMV, is often marked by punctate retinal pigmentation.

Herpes simplex virus can be transmitted transplacentally, although usually neonatal herpes simplex infection reflects the perinatal acquisition of the virus. Herpes simplex infections are often associated with vesicular skin lesions, although systemic visceral and central nervous system infection may occur without rash.

In all of these instances the distinctions are made ultimately by laboratory studies. Specific IgM determinations are available for CMV, toxoplasmosis, rubella, and herpes simplex. The presence of a positive test for specific IgM to only one of these agents is usually diagnostic. The recovery of the specific agent in the case of CMV, rubella, or herpes simplex is also a rigorous means of identification. Differentiation of all of these conditions is important, since specific treatment is available for herpes simplex and for toxoplasmosis. The distinction of congenital syphilis or of bacterial sepsis, other potentially confusing entities in the neonate, is also important to facilitate specific therapy.

PROGNOSIS. Among individuals with acquired CMV infections, the prognosis is dependent upon the immune status of the host. In otherwise healthy persons, acquired CMV infections are self-limited and generally not associated with late complications. Among immunocompromised individuals, including patients with AIDS, those with disseminated neoplasms, and transplant recipients, the outlook may vary from those who recover, maintain (allograft) function, and are without sequelae, to those who die with progressive interstitial pneumonitis. Disseminated CMV may also predispose to significant life-threatening bacterial infections.

The outlook for normal development is variable in infants who are infected prenatally with CMV. Even among those with the apparently symptomless congenital CMV infections, by school age as many as 20 per cent may manifest significant sensorineural dysfunction.

TREATMENT. Until recently, a variety of nucleoside analogues, other antiviral drugs, transfer factor, antiserum, and steroids have been administered in an effort to treat CMV infections without any conclusive success. The most that has been achieved was the transient depression of virus titer without alteration of the clinical condition or ultimate course of the virus infection. The intensive use of interferon in renal transplant recipients has reduced the shedding of virus and apparently improved the associated clinical conditions. Withdrawal of immunosuppression has been used as a means to control CMV infections in allograft recipients. Recent preliminary studies have shown improvement in some immunodeficient patients with severe CMV infections when treated with 9-(1,3 dihydroxy-2-propoxymethyl) guanine (DHPG). Those who received DHPG for retinitis or gastrointestinal disease fared better than did patients with CMV pneumonitis.

PREVENTION. CMV infections have been prevented in seronegative at-risk patients (newborns, allograft recipients) by the use of only CMV-seronegative blood products and allografts. The administration of specific CMV immune globulin has not definitely been shown to prevent or to reduce the occurrence of CMV infection and disease in at-risk individuals. Attenuated CMV vaccine strains have been produced in England and the United States. These candidate vaccine strains have been administered to volunteers, including health care workers, and to some individuals awaiting an allograft. The vaccines are immunogenic and have not been associated with detectable virus shedding or reactivation. Inoculated

individuals who later received transplants and were immunosuppressed nevertheless did experience CMV reinfection and associated virus shedding.

Because of the questions associated with the production and use of attenuated CMV strains, coupled with the evidence that immunity does ameliorate, if not prevent, prenatal and postnatal CMV infections, attention is also being directed to the development of subunit and peptide immunogens.

Adler SP: Transfusion-associated cytomegalovirus infections. Rev Infect Dis 5:977, 1983. *Comprehensive review of transfusion-associated CMV infections with discussion of mechanisms as well as straightforward clinical issues.*

Betts SP: Cytomegalovirus infection in transplant patients. Prog Med Virol 23:44, 1982. *A very good discussion of the reciprocal impact of CMV upon all varieties of allograft. Contains an excellent summary of epidemiologic factors.*

Ho M: Cytomegalovirus: Biology and Infection. New York, Plenum Publishing Corporation, 1982. *Treatise covering all aspects of CMV infection in humans. Small but thorough section pertinent to murine CMV. Very comprehensive bibliography.*

Onorato IM, Morens DM, Martone WJ, et al.: Epidemiology of cytomegaloviral infections: Recommendations for prevention and control. Rev Infect Dis 7:479, 1985. *A thorough review of epidemiologic aspects of CMV infection with concise descriptions of the current status of control measures.*

Zaia JA: The biology of human cytomegalovirus infection after bone marrow transplantation. Int J Cell Cloning 4(Suppl.):135, 1986. *Excellent review of the experience with CMV infections as complications of bone marrow transplantation. Some relevant data are presented, and an hypothesis is proposed to explain the occurrence of CMV interstitial pneumonia.*

Zaia JA, Lang DJ: Cytomegalovirus infection of the fetus and neonate. Neurol Clin 2:387, 1984. *Covers all aspects of pre- and perinatal CMV infection with discussion of some current hypotheses as well as comprehensive data review.*

342 INFECTIOUS MONONUCLEOSIS (Epstein-Barr Virus Infection)

Elliott Kieff

DEFINITION. Infectious mononucleosis is a clinical syndrome characterized by malaise, fever, pharyngitis, pharyngeal lymphatic hyperplasia, lymphadenopathy, lymphocytosis, and IgM heterophile antibodies production. The syndrome occurs most commonly in adolescents and young adults.

ETIOLOGY. Primary Epstein-Barr virus (EBV) infection is the cause of almost all typical infectious mononucleosis syndromes. EBV is a herpes virus. In vitro, it infects only human B lymphocytes. Virus infection results in cell proliferation and immunoglobulin secretion. EBV usually remains latent in the infected B cell.

EPIDEMIOLOGY. The usual mode of EBV infection is by inoculation of the oropharynx of susceptible (nonimmune) persons with saliva from infected persons. Infection may result from an infant eating food premasticated by an infected mother or from salivary exchange during kissing. Virus survival in expectorated saliva is probably brief, since infection does not spread to susceptible roommates. The virus replicates in oropharyngeal epithelial cells. Although the amount of virus in saliva is highest in the months following primary infection, virus replication in the oropharynx persists indefinitely. EBV has also been found in cervical secretions suggesting hematogenous dissemination to other epithelial surfaces. In the course of primary oropharyngeal infection, EBV infects tonsillar and peripheral B lymphocytes. Virus persists indefinitely in a small fraction of the peripheral B lymphocytes. Transfusion of whole blood or fractions containing viable B lymphocytes to susceptible (nonimmune) persons may result in symptomatic primary infection. Previously infected persons are immune to the development of infectious mononucleosis. Among lower socioeconomic groups, most children experience primary infection in the first decade of life. Among middle and higher socioeconomic groups, primary infection usually occurs as a consequence of adolescent or postadolescent kissing. More than 90 per cent of adults in all human populations have been infected with EBV and are carriers. EBV infection is limited to humans, although each Old World primate species has a related virus.

CLINICAL MANIFESTATIONS. The syndrome of infectious mononucleosis was a distinctive clinical entity for at least 40 years before the discovery of its etiologic agent. The syndrome has been intensively studied by university health physicians, particularly at military service academies where exposure to infection was limited to brief and infrequent vacation periods. After an incubation period of two to five weeks, most infected adolescents or young adults develop malaise, fever, lymphadenopathy, and pharyngitis lasting from one to several weeks. Temperatures may reach 40°C. Tonsillar or cervical lymph nodes may be quite enlarged, painful, and tender. Laboratory findings include a relative or absolute lymphocytosis and high titers of IgM heterophile antibody to horse or ox red blood cells. A substantial fraction of the peripheral lymphocytes are atypical large cells with unusually abundant cytoplasm and variable nuclear shape. Other common manifestations include splenomegaly (50 per cent), mild hepatitis or hepatomegaly (20 per cent), headache (20 per cent), vomiting (20 per cent), jaundice (5 per cent), palatal petechiae, skin rash (4 per cent), and albuminuria (10 per cent). Less frequent (0.5 to 1 per cent) manifestations include cough, pneumonitis, neck stiffness, cerebritis, cerebellar dysfunction, mono- or polyneuritis, Guillain-Barré syndrome, subcapsular splenic hemorrhage or rupture, myocarditis, pericarditis, cardiac conduction abnormalities, hemolytic anemia with anti-I antibody, thrombocytopenia, or agranulocytosis. Malaise or weakness may recur over several months. Rashes are significantly more common in patients with primary EBV infection receiving penicillin or ampicillin treatment than in untreated patients or patients with other diseases who are treated with penicillin. Persistence of illness beyond several months is unusual.

Outside of the adolescent and young adult populations, primary EBV infection frequently does not result in the full infectious mononucleosis syndrome. In younger children, fever and pharyngitis from primary EBV infection may be clinically indistinguishable from upper respiratory tract infections caused by other viruses, mycoplasma, or streptococci. In children or adults, cerebritis, neuritis, pneumonitis, hepatitis, carditis, or autoimmune hemolytic anemia or thrombocytopenia may be the predominant clinical manifestation. Atypical lymphocytosis or heterophile antibody may be less prominent or absent.

Severe, chronically progressive, and sometimes fatal, primary EBV infections occur in children with X-linked lymphoproliferative disease or Duncan's syndrome. Non–X-linked, sporadic cases have also been reported. Although these children have no obvious pre-existing immune deficiency, primary EBV infection leads to massive lymphoproliferation, fever, anemia, hepatitis, or fulminant hepatic necrosis. Some recover except for persistent anemia or pancytopenia. Uniclonal or oligoclonal EBV–infected B cell lymphomas may occur during primary infection or after recovery. Similar illnesses occur in other immunosuppressed patients with primary EBV infection. Children with AIDS associated with human immunodeficiency virus infection (HIV) are particularly at risk for severe EBV infection and lymphoproliferative disease. Pneumonitis may be prominent in such patients. EBV has also been found in hairy leukoplakia of the tongue in AIDS patients.

Rare cases of chronic progressive primary EBV infection in young adults have been well documented. These patients have severe acute mononucleosis and persistent clinical manifestations that include lymphadenopathy or intermittent visceral organ involvement and markedly abnormally high titers to EBV replicative cycle or nuclear antigens. Most patients eventually recover without specific treatment. Persistent active EBV infection has also been proposed to be the cause of a syndrome called *chronic mononucleosis*. This is a syndrome of adult neurasthenia characterized by recurrent episodes of weakness, fatigue, myalgia, arthralgia, pharyngitis, or fever. Careful documentation of clinical findings helps to distinguish these patients from those without objective manifestations of illness. The role of EBV infection in this illness can be established only when the antibody titers to EBV-specific antigens differ significantly from those of normal infected adults (see below).

After primary infection, EBV persistently replicates in the oropharynx and is found in peripheral B lymphocytes. EBV is associated with B cell lymphomas in immunosuppressed patients, with Burkitt-type lymphoma in African children, and with anaplastic nasopharyngeal carcinoma. In B cell lymphomas in which the virus is latent in all of the tumor cells, the virus probably provided an initial stimulus for cell proliferation. Malignant conversion required at least one additional factor since the cells also have a translocated c-myc oncogene. In a prospective study of African children, a correlation was noted between the EBV antibody response and Burkitt tumor incidence, suggesting that the extent of EBV replication was important in tumor induction. EBV has also been found in each of the tumor cells of the anaplastic nasopharyngeal carcinomas that have been analyzed. The virus is, therefore, likely to be necessary for oncogenic conversion. Chinese populations have a high incidence of nasopharyngeal carcinoma. Tumors occur only among patients with high antibody titers to EBV.

PATHOLOGY AND PATHOGENESIS. EBV first infects pharyngeal epithelial cells and then spreads to subepithelial and circulating B lymphocytes. Infection may be confined to epithelial and B lymphocyte tissues because only these cells have EBV receptors. The EBV receptor is also the complement (C3d) receptor. Tonsils and regional and systemic lymph nodes enlarge because of follicular hyperplasia and infiltration of sinuses and paracortex with atypical lymphocytes. Loss of normal architecture and the presence of Reed-Sternberg–like cells may make it difficult to distinguish EBV infection from Hodgkin's disease. Similar changes occur in the spleen. In patients with significant hepatitis, hepatic lobules or portal areas may be infiltrated with mononuclear cells. The bone marrow is usually unaffected. Early in the illness up to 1 per cent of the circulating leukocytes may be EBV-infected B cells. Those cells can be detected by their expression of EBV nuclear proteins (EBNAs) or by their ability to proliferate continuously in vitro, a property that normal B cells lack. The predominant atypical lymphocyte in the peripheral blood, however, is a reactive T cell.

EBV infection of B cells stimulates both B cell proliferation and Ig secretion, particularly IgM. In vivo, this results in transient hypergammaglobulinemia. The induction of IgM antibodies that react with heterologous erythrocyte glycoprotein antigen is the basis for the heterophile test. The preexistence of B cells with heterophile antibody specificity remains an enigma perhaps explainable by cross-reactivity of some of these antibodies with bacterial glycoproteins. The T cell response (atypical lymphocyte) is multifunctional. Some T cells suppress both B cell proliferation and Ig secretion. Other peripheral blood T lymphocytes and natural killer cells from patients with infectious mononucleosis are cytotoxic to autologous EBV-infected B cells.

After recovery from acute infectious mononucleosis, the proportion of circulating B cells infected with EBV is one in 10^5–10^6. There are also circulating T cells that suppress or kill only HLA-related EBV-infected cells. EBV-infected B cells and reactive T cells circulate in the peripheral blood indefinitely after primary infection. Cyclosporin A is a potent inhibitor of those T cells that suppress or kill autologous EBV-infected cells, and its use enables such cells to overgrow in patients receiving high doses of cyclosporin and other immunosuppressive drugs. EBV-associated lymphoproliferative diseases have been a significant, albeit unusual, problem in organ transplant recipients.

DIAGNOSIS. In normal adolescents, the diagnosis of acute infectious mononucleosis can usually be made on clinical grounds and confirmed by the laboratory findings of atypical lymphocytosis and heterophile antibodies to ox or horse erythrocytes. Bacterial throat culture should be done in patients with significant pharyngitis to exclude concomitant beta-hemolytic streptoccoccal infection. The rapid heterophile tests are more than 95 per cent sensitive and more than 95 per cent specific. Titers are substantially diminished by three months after primary infection and not detectable by six months. In patients with equivocal or absent heterophile antibodies, specific serologic testing for EBV infection should be done. The differential diagnosis may include streptococcal or gonococcal (pharyngeal) infection, cytomegalovirus, hepatitis A or B, HIV or toxoplasma infection, leukemia, or lymphoma. Most heterophile-negative infectious mononucleosis with pharyngitis is also caused by EBV. In the absence of pharyngitis, however, cytomegalovirus, toxoplasma, or hepatitis virus infections are likely causes of heterophile-negative infectious mononucleosis.

Specific serologic testing for EBV infection involves determining antibody titers to latently infected (anti-EBNA), early replication cycle (anti-EA), or late replication cycle (anti-VCA) viral proteins. This is usually done by indirect immunofluorescence microscopy or by enzyme-linked immunoassay. With acute primary infection, EA and IgM VCA titers are high; and IgG VCA and EBNA titers are low. Convalescent patients have lower EA or IgM VCA titers, higher IgG VCA titer, and low EBNA titer. After several months, EA and IgM VCA titers are negative, whereas IgG VCA and EBNA titers are high. The high IgG VCA and EBNA titers frequently persist for many years. Those rare patients with chronically progressive EBV infection tend to have very high titers of antibodies to all of the EBV antigens. Serologic diagnosis may be misleading in immunosuppressed patients, including children with X-linked immunodeficiency. These infected children may have high or low antibody titers. EBV serologies are helpful in following patients with anaplastic nasopharyngeal carcinoma or in screening for early detection of this malignancy in high-risk populations. Patients at risk for primary tumors or for recurrences have high IgG or IgA EA antibody titers.

TREATMENT. No treatment is necessary for most EBV infections. Rest during the period of acute symptoms and slow return to normal activity are commonly advised, although therapeutic efficacy has not been firmly established. Patients with splenomegaly should restrict their involvement in sports to avoid traumatic rupture. Acetaminophen or aspirin may be used to reduce temperature and pharyngeal pain. Very brief courses of glucocorticoid treatment (e.g., 60 mg prednisone per day for four days followed by rapidly decreasing doses) have been effective in shrinking obstructing tonsils. Autoimmune hemolytic anemia, granulocytopenia, and thrombocytopenia usually respond to longer courses of glucocorticoid therapy. Use of glucocorticoids for other manifestations of EBV infection is less certain to be beneficial. Glucocorticoids have no antiviral activity and are contraindicated in most herpes virus infections. Acycloguanosine and its derivatives have activity against EBV in vitro but are not approved for use against EBV. These drugs should not be used in normal patients with EBV infections.

Buchwald D, Sullivan J, Kamaroff A: Frequency of chronic active Epstein-Barr virus infection in a general medical practice. JAMA, 1987 (in press). *The relationship of EBV infection to chronic mononucleosis-like illnesses. See also Jones et al., Straus et al.*

Epstein MA, Achong BG: The Epstein-Barr Virus: Recent Advances. London, William Heinemann Medical Books Ltd, 1986. *Review of the biology and biochemistry of EBV.*

Ho RW, Miller G, Atchison RW, et al.: Epstein-Barr virus infections and DNA hydridization studies in post-transplantation lymphoma and lymphoproliferative lesions: The role of primary infection. J Infect Dis 152:876–886,

1985. *The relationship of primary EBV infection to lymphoproliferative syndromes in organ transplant recipients.*

Jones JF, Ray CG, Minnich LL, et al.: Evidence for active Epstein-Barr virus infection in patients with persistent unexplained illnesses: Elevated anti-early antigen antibodies. Ann Intern Med 102:1–6, 1985.

Straus SE, Tosato G, Armstrong G, et al.: Persisting illness and fatigue in adults with evidence of Epstein-Barr virus infection. Ann Intern Med 102:7–16, 1985.

Tosato G, Blaese R: Epstein-Barr virus infection and immunoregulation in man. Adv Immunol 37:99–147, 1985. *Review of the pathophysiology of EBV infection.*

---

343 VARICELLA

Philip A. Brunell

DEFINITION. Varicella, or chickenpox, is an acute communicable disease characterized by a generalized vesicular rash with relatively mild systemic symptoms. Because it is highly contagious, most individuals will contract it in childhood.

ETIOLOGY. Varicella is caused by varicella zoster (VZ) virus, sometimes referred to as human herpesvirus type III. This enveloped herpesvirus contains five glycoproteins, some of which bear some homology to those of other members of the human herpesvirus group. The double-stranded DNA has a molecular weight of approximately 80 million. There is some diversity in the restriction enzyme patterns among wild isolates; there is only a single serotype. Although the human is the only known natural host, a closely related virus has been identified in a simian species.

EPIDEMIOLOGY. Varicella is a highly contagious disease. After continuing household exposure, as would occur in a family, almost all susceptibles are infected. The subclinical attack rate is believed to be no more than 4 per cent. The results of nonhousehold exposure are less certain. Although chickenpox may be contagious prior to the onset of rash, this has been difficult to prove. Virus has been virtually impossible to isolate from respiratory secretions either prior to or following the onset of rash. Chickenpox is contagious for as long as five days after the appearance of the first lesion. Patients are customarily isolated for a week. The incubation period is usually about 14 days. Ninety-nine per cent of the cases will occur 10 to 20 days following exposure. The disease is known to be spread by direct contact. Airborne spread also has been demonstrated, most notably in hospitals.

Nosocomial spread of varicella has been well documented. This has occurred room to room by airborne spread as well as by patient-to-patient or staff-to-patient contact. Adults with herpes zoster who are hospitalized are less likely to cause secondary cases of chickenpox among adult contacts than among children. The reason is that hospitalized children are more likely to be susceptible to chickenpox than hospitalized adults. Strict isolation is recommended for hospitalized patients with varicella and for children or immunocompromised adults with herpes zoster. Adults with localized herpes zoster require less stringent isolation procedures.

Most cases of chickenpox occur in childhood. Most children will contract chickenpox either in daycare situations or shortly after they enter school. Fewer than 2 per cent of the cases occur following the second decade. Approximately 2.5 per cent of entering professional students at our institution are seronegative; of those with a negative history for chickenpox, only about 15 per cent are seronegative. Approximately 10 per cent of hospital workers with a negative history are seronegative. Almost all individuals with a positive history are seropositive. A single attack of chickenpox usually confers lifetime immunity.

There appears to be more efficient transmission of disease in temperate than in tropical climates. The reason for this is uncertain but may be due to temperature rather than urbanization. Varicella occurs most commonly during the late winter and spring months, the peak being about in March. Sporadic cases occur into the early summer and start in late fall.

Varicella is more common than other childhood diseases during the early months of life. In this situation the disease is generally mild. Maternal antibody transferred across the placenta may not be as effective in protecting infants against this disease as are antibodies against other viruses. However, nursery outbreaks have been rare. Children who develop varicella during the early months of life, or are exposed in utero, have a greater risk of developing herpes zoster in childhood.

PATHOGENESIS. Varicella zoster virus produces a disseminated rash, which indicates that bloodstream distribution must have occurred. Virus has been isolated from white blood cells just prior to and during the first one or two days following the appearance of rash. After clinical recovery, the virus infection continues in the absence of clinical symptoms in a latent phase. During this time, virus deoxyribonucleic acid (DNA) or messenger ribonucleic acid (RNA) can be demonstrated in dorsal root ganglion cells. The segmental distribution of herpes zoster (see Ch. 485.3), which usually occurs decades after the initial VZ infection, is consistent with a dorsal root ganglion site for the latent virus. In uncomplicated chickenpox, rises in serum transaminase levels have been demonstrated. This suggests that there is visceral involvement in the normal course of this disease.

The vesicular lesions of varicella contain a predominance of polymorphonuclear leukocytes even during the early phase of vesicle formation. Multinuclear giant cells are occasionally found in the base of the lesions, often containing eosinophilic intranuclear inclusions. Large amounts of virus can be demonstrated in vesicular fluid by electron microscopy.

Postmortem descriptions of patients with varicella have usually involved immunocompromised subjects. In these cases inflammatory changes are usually found in multiple organs, including the lung, liver, spleen, and skin, together with anoxic changes in the brain. Similar involvement is found in the newborn. Focal areas of necrosis and intranuclear eosinophilic inclusions in mononuclear cells are common. Changes in otherwise normal individuals usually include myocardial and pulmonary lesions. On microscopic examination, the brain has demonstrated edema with some lymphocyte cuffing around the cerebral vessels.

CLINICAL MANIFESTATIONS. Varicella is characterized by a generalized eruption that is centripetal in distribution; erythematous macules, papules, vesicles, and scabbed lesions may be present at the same time. The vesicles are superficial, with varying amounts of erythema at their bases. Adults tend to have considerably more erythema than children. During the early phase of the eruption, lesions are found on the face, scalp, and trunk. By running the fingers through the hair, one will often detect lesions that were not visible. Later, new lesions will appear on the extremities. By this time, the earlier lesions will have dried and crusted. Excoriations are common, attesting to the pruritic nature of the lesions. Mucous membranes of the conjunctiva and oropharynx are more frequently involved in adults than in children. New lesions will continue to appear over a three- or four-day period, after which the rate of their appearance decelerates markedly.

There is a striking variation in the extent of systemic symptoms associated with varicella. Most children have a mild illness with few systemic complaints and an average maximal temperature of about 38.3°C. It is more common for adults to have considerable malaise, muscle ache, arthralgia, and headache. These may precede the first skin lesions by 24 to 48 hours.

In the immunocompromised subject, the disease often is very severe. Approximately 30 per cent of children with leukemia or lymphoma who get varicella will develop "progressive varicella." Vesicles will continue to erupt into the second week of illness, accompanied by high fever. Lesions tend to be deep seated rather than superficial. Toward the end of the first week and the beginning of the second week, the lesions are more common on the extremities than on the trunk. Indeed, the distribution and lesions may resemble those with smallpox. Visceral involvement occurs in about 30 per cent of these patients. The lung, liver, pancreas, and brain may be involved. Death occurs in about 7 per cent of immunocompromised patients who develop varicella. The death usually is due to pulmonary involvement.

Varicella in pregnant women is believed to be more serious than in nongravid females; fatalities have been reported. The rate of fetal wastage is not increased. Zero to 9 per cent of infants born to mothers who have had varicella early in pregnancy, however, have occasionally been found at birth to have "varicella embryopathy." The infants are born with cerebral damage and a variety of ocular findings, and characteristically they have a scarred, atrophic limb. The children are generally small for gestational age and may have other abnormalities as well. When mothers develop chickenpox within a few days of delivery, "varicella of the newborn" may occur. If the onset of varicella is between five and ten days after birth, it is associated with a high risk of serious disease and even death.

Bacterial infections of the skin are the most common complication of chickenpox in childhood. The rate of complications is much higher in adults than in children. Although fewer than 2 per cent of the reported cases occur after the second decade, almost a quarter of the deaths occur in this group. A disproportionate rate of hospitalization also is found in adults. The major complications of varicella in adults are encephalitis and pneumonia.

Approximately 1 in 400 adults with chickenpox will be hospitalized for pneumonia. In a prospective study, however, it was found that only 6 per cent of young adults with chickenpox had respiratory symptoms, whereas 16 per cent had roentgenographic evidence of pulmonary involvement.

Infection produces a diffuse interstitial type of pneumonia with hypoxia resulting from poor diffusion of gases. Diffuse calcification of the lung parenchyma may be found years after recovery.

Encephalitis in childhood is most commonly manifested by a cerebellitis, which usually occurs at the end of the first week or during the second week following onset of rash. This complication is almost always self limited. In contrast, an acute form of encephalitis usually occurring soon after the onset of rash often has a fulminating course; it is characterized by severe brain swelling. It has been estimated that as many as 20 per cent of cases of Reye's syndrome may be preceded by chickenpox. A variety of other neurologic complications, including optic neuritis, transverse myelitis, and Guillain-Barré syndrome, may be associated with chickenpox. Hemorrhagic complications of chickenpox include thrombocytopenic purpura and purpura fulminans. Nephritis, myocarditis, and arthritis also have been described.

DIAGNOSIS. There is usually little difficulty in recognizing typical forms of chickenpox, particularly if there has been a history of exposure. The disease is seen more commonly by pediatricians than internists. The latter may not consider the diagnosis or may be less familiar with its clinical characteristics. The diagnosis may be more difficult in immunocompromised hosts, as they may have features of progressive varicella with visceral involvement. Modified cases of chickenpox may occur following passive or active immunization. These cases may require laboratory confirmation. The most comon sources of confusion are insect bites; generalized herpes in the immunocompromised host; rickettsialpox; or "hand, foot, and mouth disease" caused by an enterovirus. The differentiation of disseminated herpes zoster from chickenpox may be difficult. The former will have dermatomal involvement initially. Generalization usually does not occur until three to five days after onset of the zosteriform rash. In severely immunocompromised patients the clinical differentiation may be difficult.

The Tzanck smear is a frequently used laboratory aid for diagnosis. Multinucleated giant cells identify the lesions as being caused by one of the herpesviruses, but this is not specific for varicella. A properly stained smear will also contain eosinophilic intranuclear inclusions. Virus can usually be isolated during the first three or four days after the onset of lesions. The virus is quite labile; it must be stored at −70°C if cultures cannot be inoculated immediately. Our preference is to collect vesicular fluid in unheparinized capillary tubes and put the specimen directly into human embryonic lung fibroblasts at the bedside. Specimens from throat, urine, or stool are of no value for isolation of virus.

Serologic confirmation of diagnosis can be made using a variety of techniques. The enzyme-linked immunosorbent assay (ELISA) and complement fixation are the most generally available. The laboratory director should be consulted regarding appropriate time of collection of specimens as well as interpretation of data. Because complement-fixing antibody generally does not persist, a single high titer often is confirmatory evidence of recent infection.

Determining the immune status of contacts can be done with the ELISA or fluorescent antibody against membrane antigen (FAMA). The ELISA is a much simpler and technically less demanding test. Because complement-fixing antibody is lost rapidly after infection, it cannot be used for determining susceptibility. A number of laboratories have developed tests for VZ immunoglobulin M (IgM). It was hoped that these might differentiate varicella from herpes zoster in cases where this was unclear. Unfortunately, these tests have not been very useful, as VZ IgM is present in the sera of many patients with acute herpes zoster.

TREATMENT. Major therapeutic objectives are the prevention of superinfection and relief of pruritus. The latter can be accomplished frequently by application of calamine lotion. Occasionally this will not suffice, and a systemic antipruritic agent such as trimeprazine may be necessary. It is advisable to trim and file nails to reduce the damage from scratching. Bacterial superinfection can best be prevented by encouraging daily bathing with soap or hexachlorophene. Following this with a colloidal starch bath may also be useful in relief of pruritus.

Relief of systemic symptoms may require additional medication such as acetaminophen. Salicylates are contraindicated, as there is an association between their use and development of Reye's syndrome in children. Special care should be taken to be certain that over-the-counter medications containing salicylates are avoided.

Some patients, particularly those who are immunocompromised, may require antiviral therapy. Acyclovir has been shown to be effective in immunocompromised children with varicella. A dose of 500 mg per square meter repeated every eight hours has been used. Varicella zoster virus is generally less sensitive to acyclovir than herpes simplex. For this reason, larger doses are probably required. There are no controlled studies on the use of oral antiviral drugs in the treatment of varicella. Patients who are sick enough to require antiviral therapy probably should be treated with parenteral rather than oral medication. In comparative studies, acyclovir appears to be somewhat safer and probably more effective than vidarabine.

Patients on high doses of steroids or other immunosuppressive drugs who have been exposed to chickenpox are at high risk of developing progressive varicella. Whenever possible, the dose of these drugs should be reduced or the medications discontinued at the time of exposure. Steroids appear to be most deleterious when given during the incubation period. They have been used in the treatment of pneumonia after the eruption has occurred without any obvious deleterious effects.

PREVENTION. Immune serum globulin will not prevent varicella. Massive doses are required to produce measurable modification. If prevention or modification is indicated, varicella zoster immune globulin (VZIG) should be given. Candidates are those who (1) are susceptible, (2) are at high risk of developing complicated varicella, and (3) have had an adequate exposure to the disease. Any individuals fulfilling the first two criteria who have had a household exposure should receive prophylaxis. It is often difficult to judge the degree of intimacy in other types of exposure. Reference to guidelines published by the Academy of Pediatrics or Centers for Disease Control (CDC) may be helpful.

Patients considered at high risk are (1) those who are immunocompromised by virtue of either disease or immunosuppressive therapy, (2) infants born to mothers who have had varicella less than five days prior to or two days following delivery, (3) bone marrow transplantation recipients regardless of susceptibility, and (4) certain adults.

A history of varicella is usually reliable in both adults and children. Children who have a negative history are usually susceptible. In children who are at high risk, such as those with leukemia, it is advisable to do serologic testing. The majority of adults who have a negative history will be found to be seropositive on testing. Often a detailed history will disclose the occurrence of varicella in siblings.

Nosocomial infection following herpes zoster or varicella has been well documented. These outbreaks may result in significant morbidity and cause disruption of hospital routine. These situations are best managed by serologic screening of personnel and by permitting only those who are seropositive to care for patients with varicella or herpes zoster. Patients who are hospitalized with varicella should be isolated until all lesions are crusted. Susceptible persons who are exposed to active cases should be isolated from the tenth to the twenty-first day after the last exposure if they cannot be discharged. Whenever possible, patients with chickenpox should be isolated in a room with negative pressure in order to prevent dissemination of infectious virus to other patients. Airborne spread in hospitals has been documented.

An attenuated live vaccine has been licensed for use abroad and is being considered for licensure in the United States. Susceptible adults who receive the vaccine have some local reactions and occasionally develop a varicelliform rash. Protection against infection is less complete than in children. In normal children, the vaccine is virtually benign and appears to offer very good protection. Initial data suggest that herpes zoster would be no more frequent and perhaps less common following immunization than following natural infection. Live varicella vaccine also has been used to protect children with acute lymphocytic leukemia. Protection is less complete than in normal children. Some of these vaccinated children develop a varicelliform illness from the vaccine.

Advisory Committee on Immunization Practice: Varicella-zoster immune globulin for the prevention of chickenpox. MMWR 33:84, 95, 1984. *Guidelines for passive immunization against chickenpox.*

Brunell PA: Fetal and neonatal varicella-zoster infections. Semin Perinatol 7:47, 1983. *A critical review of fetal, neonatal, and maternal varicella.*

Brunell PA: Varicella vaccine—where are we? Pediatrics 78:721, 1986. *A symposium on the epidemiology, cost burden, and complications of varicella and on varicella vaccine.*

Committee on Infectious Diseases, American Academy of Pediatrics: Expanded guidelines for use of varicella zoster immune globulin. Pediatrics 72:886, 1983. *A useful guide to management of patients exposed to varicella, including control of nosocomial infection.*

Prober CG, Kirk LE, Keeney RE: Acyclovir therapy of chickenpox in immunosuppressed children—a collaborative study. J Pediatr 101:622, 1982. *A controlled study of acyclovir use in children.*

Shehab ZM, Brunell PA: Varicella-zoster virus. In Rose NR, Friedman H, Fahey JL (eds.): Manual of Clinical Laboratory Immunity. 3rd ed. Washington, DC, American Society for Microbiology, 1986, pp 502–503. *A review of serologic tests for varicella-zoster antibody.*

Takahashi M: Chickenpox virus. Adv Virus Res 28:285, 1983. *A comprehensive review of both basic science and information on the vaccine.*

Weller TH: Varicella and herpes zoster. N Engl J Med 309:1362, 1983. *A review of immunology, immunization, and therapy.*

344 VARIOLA AND VACCINIA

Donald A. Henderson

The Thirty-third World Health Assembly "declares solemnly that the world and all its peoples have won freedom from smallpox. . . an unprecedented achievement in the history of public health. . . ." (Resolution 33.3, May 8, 1980, Geneva, Switzerland).

This announcement was made some 30 months after the last known endemic case, in Somalia, on October 26, 1977. In 1978, two additional cases of smallpox occurred in Birmingham, England, as a result of a laboratory infection, but except for these cases no others have been found.

To confirm that eradication had been achieved, each country where smallpox had been endemic since 1967 and those at risk of importations conducted a search for cases for at least two years after the last known case. At the end of this period, World Health Organization (WHO)–appointed International Commissions reviewed the records of work and conducted extensive field visits to confirm the results. Between 1973 and 1979, 21 different commissions visited and certified eradication in 49 countries.

Finally, a Global Commission for the Certification of Smallpox Eradication reviewed the findings and made special field visits. After satisfying itself that eradication had been achieved, the commission reported its findings to the World Health Assembly. The assembly members concurred and recommended that "smallpox vaccination be discontinued in every country except for investigators at special risk," and advised that "an international certificate of vaccination against smallpox should no longer be required of any traveller."

Thus concluded the first successful global program to eradicate a disease—one that had proved to be one of the most devastating known to man.

HISTORY. Because of the need for variola virus to spread continually from person to person to survive, historians speculate that it emerged after the first agricultural settlements, about 10,000 B.C. A distinctive smallpox rash has been identified on the mummy of Pharaoh Ramses V (1160 B.C.). In ancient times, only a few populated areas, probably in India, could have sustained its transmission. In the early Christian era descriptions suggestive of smallpox appear in historical accounts of western Asia, and by the eighth century it had established itself in Europe. Central and southern Africa were probably infected sometime later. In 1520, Spanish conquistadors brought the disease to the Americas.

Case-fatality rates of 20 per cent and greater were characteristic, and where population densities permitted the disease to become endemic virtually all persons eventually contracted smallpox. At the end of the eighteenth century, it was killing an estimated 400,000 Europeans each year and was responsible for one third of all cases of blindness.

VACCINATION. Edward Jenner discovered in 1796 that smallpox could be prevented by "vaccination" with material from a cowpox lesion. Before his discovery, the only defense against smallpox was deliberately to inoculate (variolate) scabs or pustular material from smallpox patients into the skin of susceptible persons. The resulting infection was usually less severe than infection acquired naturally by inhalation. Although case-fatality rates among those with induced infection were sometimes as low as 1 per cent, they readily transmitted infection to others. Within three years after Jenner first published his findings, more than 100,000 had been vaccinated in England. By 1803, the new vaccine had been transported to the Americas, Asia, and Africa.

During the nineteenth century, vaccination was increasingly widely practiced in temperate-climate countries, but the difficulties of sustaining the virus through arm-to-arm inoculation resulted in an uncertain supply. The discovery, late in the nineteenth century, that vaccinia virus could be propagated on the flank of a calf was an important advance. However, such vaccine remained viable for only a few days at ambient temperature. Finally, in the 1950's a commer-

cially feasible technique was developed for producing a dried, heat-resistant vaccine.

In the industrialized countries, smallpox incidence declined steadily, and Europe and North America succeeded in interrupting smallpox transmission after World War II. In these areas, the impetus for vaccination had diminished early in the century when a less virulent strain, variola minor, with a case-fatality rate of about 1 per cent, replaced variola major. In most of Africa, however, 5 to 15 per cent died of smallpox, and in Asia the virulent variola major prevailed. Neither in Africa nor in Asia was vaccination widely practiced.

ERADICATION OF SMALLPOX. Smallpox was a problem to all countries. Even those without disease feared importations and conducted vaccination programs. Although the global control of smallpox was in everyone's best interests, progress was slow. Finally, in 1959, the World Health Assembly decided that a global eradication program should be undertaken. During the succeeding seven years, a number of countries undertook campaigns, but few succeeded in interrupting smallpox transmission.

In 1966, the assembly decided that one further effort should be made. A 10-year goal was proposed. The program commenced on January 1, 1967 (Fenner and colleagues). In 1967, smallpox was endemic in 31 countries, and 13 additional countries reported importations. Although 131,768 cases were officially reported, the true number was about 10 to 15 million. Four geographic reservoirs of smallpox were identified: (1) Africa south of the Sahara; (2) a group of Southeast Asian countries, extending from Bangladesh through India, Nepal, Pakistan, and Afghanistan; (3) Indonesia; and (4) Brazil. The estimated population of these countries was more than 1 billion persons.

WHO's strategy called for each country to undertake a program of vaccination with the objective of reaching at least 80 per cent of the population during a two- to three-year period. During this time, a reliable reporting system was to be developed to identify foci of smallpox that would be eliminated by isolation of patients and vaccination of contacts. Extensive vaccination was believed necessary to increase population immunity and so reduce the number of cases to permit disease surveillance and containment activities to be effective.

Experience soon showed that the surveillance-containment strategy was more effective than had been thought, and this proved to be a key to success. In part, this was due to the unique characteristics of smallpox. An infected patient was able to transmit infection only from the time of first appearance of rash until the last scabs had separated. There were no chronic carriers or individuals with latent infection and no animal reservoir. The rash was sufficiently characteristic to be diagnosed with a high degree of accuracy. The presence or absence of smallpox in an area could thus be reliably determined without laboratory studies. Moreover, approximately two thirds of recovered patients had characteristic residual facial scars. Thus, it was possible to determine both the present status of smallpox and its past history in an area.

To persist, smallpox virus had to be transmitted from patient to susceptible contact. By isolation of the patient and by vaccination of contacts, a barrier to transmission was created. In small villages and in scattered populations, chains of transmission often terminated without intervention. Because smallpox did not spread rapidly, and then only to those in contact, secondary cases usually were found among neighbors and relatives. A patient rarely infected more than two to three others. Because of these factors, early detection of outbreaks and their containment proved effective in stopping transmission.

Smallpox vaccine that conferred excellent and durable immunity was an important factor in the program's success. Studies revealed vaccine efficacy ratios of more than 90 per cent after 20 years. Because the lyophilized vaccine retained its potency after incubation at 37° C for at least one month, the logistics of vaccine storage and distribution were greatly simplified. Vaccination was greatly facilitated by the inexpensive, newly developed bifurcated needle. Vaccine was held between the tines by capillarity. Fifteen rapid punctures were made with the needle held perpendicular to the skin. The technique was learned quickly and produced a high proportion of successful vaccinations.

PROGRESS IN THE PROGRAM. By 1969, eradication programs were in progress in all of the infected and immediately adjacent countries except for Ethiopia, whose program began in 1971. By 1970, the number of endemic countries had decreased from 31 to 18. Brazil registered its last case in 1971 and Indonesia and Afghanistan in 1972. By 1973, all of Africa had become smallpox free except for Ethiopia and Botswana. In Asia, there remained only four smallpox-endemic countries: India, Pakistan, Nepal, and Bangladesh. However, the population of these four was over 700 million, and the techniques of surveillance and containment that had been applied in other areas proved to be less successful.

A new strategy in India began in the autumn of 1973 (Basu and colleagues). Far more rapid case detection and more effective containment of outbreaks were required. Accordingly, for one week each month more than 100,000 health workers were mobilized to search house by house to detect cases. Hundreds of special teams contained the outbreaks that were found. Between searches, the teams asked questions at markets and in schools to uncover rumors of cases. By the summer of 1974, new cases began to decline, and a cash reward was offered to anyone who reported a case. In May 1975 the last case was detected in India, and on October 16, 1975, the last case in Asia.

The only remaining endemic country was Ethiopia. More than half of its population of 25 million lived more than a day's walk from any road, and its health structure was all but nonexistent. With the end of smallpox in Asia, resources were shifted to Ethiopia. In August 1976, the last case was isolated. Unfortunately, Somalian guerrilla forces had meanwhile introduced the disease into neighboring Somalia, and yet another year was to elapse before finally, on October 26, 1977, the last case occurred.

POSSIBLE SOURCES FOR A RETURN OF SMALLPOX. As of September 1987, variola virus was known to exist in only two laboratories, where it was kept under high-security conditions.

Extensive studies has been conducted since 1967 to discover a possible animal or other natural reservoir of the virus. None was found. However, some 400 cases of a newly recognized disease that is clinically indistinguishable from smallpox but caused by the related monkeypox virus occurred in seven central and west African countries between 1970 and 1987. Genome maps of this and other animal poxviruses reveal many differences between them and variola, suggesting that mutation to variola would be highly unlikely.

The recurrence of smallpox resulting from a deliberate release of variola virus cannot be ruled out. However, the potential damage of such an act should not be exaggerated. Smallpox does not spread rapidly, and an outbreak caused in this manner should be able to be contained within three to four weeks.

As insurance against unforeseen events, WHO has established vaccine storage reserves of some 200 million doses of vaccine. Additional stocks are being retained by a number of governments.

Barring improbable circumstances, a human case of smallpox will never again be seen. However, the problem of mistaken diagnosis is a real one. For this reason, WHO medical officers with expertise in diagnosis remain on call to investigate rumors, and an expertise in laboratory diagnosis will be maintained by WHO Diagnostic Reference Laboratories (Centers for Disease Control, Atlanta, and the Institute for Virus Preparations, Moscow).

VARIOLA (Smallpox)

ETIOLOGY. Variola virus is one of a group of orthopoxviruses that includes vaccinia, monkeypox, rabbitpox, cowpox, camelpox, buffalopox, and ectromelia. The poxviruses are the largest viruses so recognized. The virions are brick-shaped structures with a diameter of about 200 mμ. The genome consists of a single molecule of a double-stranded DNA.

INCIDENCE AND PREVALENCE. The disease was declared to be eradicated on May 8, 1980.

PATHOLOGY AND PATHOGENESIS. The site of entry of the smallpox virus was probably the respiratory tract. In the 12-day incubation period the virus multiplied in the regional lymphoid tissues. Viremia occurred at the onset of fever and continued during the first two or three days of the pre-eruptive phase. During this time, the virus localized in mucous membranes, skin, and internal tissues. Virus multiplication in the epithelial cells of the skin and mucous membranes caused pustulation. Antibodies appeared as early as the fourth day of disease.

CLINICAL MANIFESTATIONS. The incubation period of smallpox was about 12 days with a range of 7 to 17 days. The illness began with severe malaise, prostration, head- and backache, and high fever lasting two to five days (Rao). Following the initial febrile period, a macular rash developed, which quickly became papular, and within two days the papules developed into vesicles and then pustules. On the eighth or ninth day of rash, crusting began. The scabs separated over the succeeding two to three weeks, leaving pigment-free skin. Subsequently, scarring or pitting developed. The eruption was characteristically more severe on the face and the distal parts of the arms and legs, and less severe over the trunk and abdomen. Lesions were often found on the palms of the hands and the soles of the feet.

VARIOLA MINOR AND INTERMEDIATE FORMS. In the early twentieth century, a milder clinical form of smallpox (variola minor, or alastrim) became prevalent in the Americas, Europe, and parts of southern and eastern Africa. Case-fatality rates were 1 per cent or less. Variola major and minor were distinct although at times coexisting. Each of the two types gave rise to illnesses with a wide spectrum of severity. There was cross-protection between each of these forms and vaccinia.

DIFFERENTIAL DIAGNOSIS. Most cases of smallpox could readily be identified by the typical deep-seated rash, the centrifugal distribution of lesions, and the fact that in any area on the body all lesions were at the same stage of development. The infrequent severe hemorrhagic cases were frequently mistakenly diagnosed as meningococcemia, acute leukemia, or drug toxicity. Mild cases with few lesions were confused with varicella. Most problematic were severe cases of chickenpox in adults. Of help in diagnosis, however, was the fact that in any outbreak 80 per cent or more of the cases were clinically typical.

LABORATORY TESTS. Diagnosis of a poxvirus infection can be rapidly established by electron microscopic identification of virus particles in vesicular or pustular fluid or scabs. Differentiation among poxviruses requires that the virus be isolated on chick chorioallantoic membrane and its properties characterized by specific biologic tests. WHO Reference Laboratories are prepared to undertake necessary diagnostic studies. For patients who have recovered, neutralizing antibody in serum specimens serves to identify which poxvirus was responsible for the illness.

TREATMENT. No specific treatment is available.

IDENTIFICATION OF A SUSPECT CASE OF SMALLPOX. Because smallpox has been eradicated, the occurrence of a single case has profound international implications. Should a suspect case be identified, *immediate notification of local, state, and national health officials is essential.* Most suspected cases in recent years have been cases of varicella in adults. Should a case prove to be smallpox, the source of virus must be assumed to be inadvertent or deliberate release from a laboratory. A suspect patient should be placed under strict isolation. Additional measures will be dictated by epidemiologic circumstances.

VACCINIA (Vaccination)

No countries now require international certificates of vaccination, and none conducts civilian vaccination programs. Several countries, including the United States, continue to vaccinate military personnel. Vaccination is recommended only for investigators who are working with poxviruses in the laboratory.

THE VACCINE. Vaccinia virus is grown in tissue culture or on the scarified flank of a calf. After purification and the addition of stabilizing agents, the suspension is freeze dried. Inoculated intradermally, vaccinia virus induces a mild infection and confers protection against all orthopoxviruses known to infect man—monkeypox, variola, and cowpox.

VACCINE PROTECTION. Following successful vaccination, protection against variola is virtually complete for five years, but effectiveness wanes over time. In poxvirus laboratories, vaccination at least every three years has been customary.

RISKS OF VACCINATION. Those who are candidates for vaccination are adults, a diminishing proportion of whom have received primary vaccinations as children. Although the risk of complications following revaccination is very low, primary vaccination of adults has been thought to be associated with a higher incidence of serious complications. However, a special study of vaccination complications among military recruits failed to document any cases of the most important, postvaccinal encephalitis, among an estimated 2 million primary vaccinees.

FIRST VACCINATION (PRIMARY TAKE). Three days after vaccination a papule appears at the vaccination site; the papule changes to a vesicle and by the seventh day is a fully developed pustule. It is whitish, umbilicated, and multilocular and contains clear lymph. An erythematous areola expands to reach a maximal diameter about nine days after vaccination. A crust forms and falls off about three weeks after vaccination, leaving a scar.

REVACCINATION. When persons are vaccinated a second time, a gradation of cutaneous responses is observed. Individuals who have not been vaccinated for several decades may develop what appears to be a primary take. In persons with an intermediate level of immunity, development of the lesion is more rapid, and the maximal diameter of erythema is reached in three to seven days. In the highly immune person, virus multiplication may not occur. In such persons, a hypersensitivity response to vaccinial protein may occur. A papule and sometimes a vesicle with erythema may develop, reaching its peak in 48 hours.

To distinguish the hypersensitivity type of reaction, which may be caused by heat-inactivated vaccine, from one in which virus multiplication has taken place, the site of inoculation is examined between the sixth and eighth days. If there is evidence of induration or congestion, virus multiplication may be assumed.

CONTRAINDICATIONS. Four groups of persons are at special risk of complications: (1) persons with eczema or other forms of chronic dermatitis; (2) pregnant women; (3) patients with leukemia, lymphoma, and other reticuloendothelial malignancies; and (4) those receiving immunosuppressive drugs,

especially glucocorticosteroids. Vaccinees in close contact with persons with eczema may infect them, sometimes with serious consequences. If vaccination is required for persons at special risk, vaccinia immune globulin (0.3 ml per kilogram intramuscularly) should be administered simultaneously.

COMPLICATIONS. *Postvaccinal Encephalitis.* Encephalitis following vaccination is a rare event and occurs between the eighth and fifteenth days. Paralysis, when it occurs, is generally spastic in type. Residual paralysis and other central nervous system symptoms may persist. There is no treatment. Studies conducted in the United States in 1963 and 1968 (Neff and colleagues, Lane and associates) revealed 28 cases, 9 fatal, among 11.3 million primary vaccinees. No cases occurred among 16.3 million revaccinees.

Progressive Vaccinia (Vaccinia Gangrenosa). Progressive vaccinia is an exceedingly rare but often fatal complication among vaccinated persons who have deficient immune responses. The initial vaccinial lesion fails to heal and progresses to involve adjacent skin with necrosis of tissue. Dissemination may result in metastatic vaccinial lesions in other parts of the skin, bones, or viscera. Treatment with vaccinia immune globulin is beneficial.

Eczema Vaccinatum. Eczema vaccinatum is sometimes a serious complication, which may occur in vaccinated persons with active or healed eczema, or in subjects in contact with recent vaccinees. The disease tends to localize at sites where eczematous lesions are or have been present. A few cases continue to appear in the United States in children of vaccinated military personnel. Vaccinia immune globulin is of help in therapy.

Generalized Vaccinia. Generalized vaccinia represents a secondary eruption resulting from bloodborne dissemination of vaccinia virus. Almost all cases occur after primary vaccination. The lesions become evident between six and nine days after vaccination. The number of lesions may range from a few to a generalized involvement of the skin. It is a self-limited illness, and complete recovery occurs without specific therapy.

Fetal Vaccinia. Fetal vaccinia results from a bloodborne dissemination of vaccinia virus in the pregnant woman given primary vaccination. It may occur during any trimester of pregnancy and frequently results in death of the fetus.

Miscellaneous Complications. A great variety of rashes has been reported to be caused by vaccination. Most common are erythema multiforme and variously distributed urticarial, maculopapular, blotchy erythematous eruptions.

Basu RN, Jerek Z, Ward NA: The Eradication of Smallpox from India. New Delhi, India, World Health Organization, 1979. *A well-written, detailed, profusely illustrated book describing the epidemiologic and operational aspects of the program in India.*

Fenner F, Henderson DA, Jerek Z, et al.: Smallpox and its Eradication. Geneva, Switzerland, World Health Organization, 1988. *This 1400-page, extensively illustrated and referenced book is the definitive text, providing a historical account of smallpox control and eradication as well as a summary of current knowledge regarding the epidemiology, virology, and pathogenesis of the disease.*

Hopkins DR: Princes and Peasants: Smallpox in History. Chicago, University of Chicago Press, 1983. *The only comprehensive history of smallpox prepared in this century, this interesting and readable book complements the book by Fenner and associates.*

Lane JM, Ruben FL, Neff JM, et al.: Complications of smallpox vaccination, 1968. N Engl J Med 281:138, 1969. *With the paper by Neff and co-workers, one of the few detailed studies of the frequency of complications following smallpox vaccination.*

Neff J, Lane JM, Pert JH, et al.: Complications of smallpox vaccination. N Engl J Med 276:1, 1967. *With the paper by Lane and associates, one of the few detailed studies of the frequency of complications following smallpox vaccination.*

Rao AR: Smallpox. Bombay, India, Kothari Book Depot, 1972. *Written by a clinician who treated more than 3000 cases, this book is an excellent reference on the clinical aspects of variola major.*

Diseases Caused by Retroviruses

345 RETROVIRUSES THAT CAUSE HUMAN DISEASE*

Robert C. Gallo

The history of retroviruses encompasses three eras: (1) *Animal retrovirology:* This era began with the discovery of retroviruses in chickens at the beginning of this century and extended into the decades from 1950 to 1970, when they were established as important causes of lethal infections of poultry as well as many mammals, including monkeys. (2) *Molecular retrovirology:* This period ranged from 1970 to 1980 and established the details of their replication cycle, the nature and function of their genes, the characteristics of their proteins, and some aspects of their biologic effects. (3) *Human retrovirology:* Human retroviruses were discovered at the end of the 1970's. Within a few years, four types were defined; systems for their study in vitro were developed; their modes of transmission and geographic prevalence were determined; their genomes were analyzed and some novel genes were found; the mechanism of their effects on cells was partly unraveled; and, most importantly, some were causally linked to fatal human diseases, including the emerging pandemic of acquired immunodeficiency syndrome (AIDS). In this chapter, some of the general properties of this remarkable virus class are considered.

DEFINITION, GENERAL FEATURES, AND CLASSIFICATION

Retroviruses are 100-nm ribonucleic acid (RNA) viruses consisting of an outer envelope and an inner core that contains two molecules of a single-stranded, relatively small (8.0 to 9.5 Kb), and simple (three to eight genes) RNA genome. The envelope and core are made from viral coded proteins, but as the virus is about to be released from the cell the envelope also acquires a lipid bilayer from the cell membrane. The hallmark of retroviruses is the replication of viral RNA through a deoxyribonucleic acid (DNA) intermediate called a provirus (Fig. 345–1). The DNA arises from transcription of the viral RNA genome soon after the virus enters the cell. This unique mechanism is catalyzed by *reverse transcriptase*, a special RNA-dependent DNA polymerase that is also encoded by a viral gene and is complexed to the RNA in the core. Retroviruses are unique among microorganisms because of this mechanism and enzyme. Another salient feature of retroviruses is the integration of the DNA intermediate into the host cell DNA. Consequently, infections can be lifelong, and the virus may remain "hidden" (unexpressed or nonreplicative) in cells for very long periods. This may contribute to the long interval (sometimes many years) between the time of infection and disease induction. When the DNA provirus is expressed (transcribed by a cellular RNA polymerase), viral genomic and messenger RNA and subsequently viral proteins are made. These assemble at the cell membrane to be packaged and released, thereby completing the replication cycle.

Retroviruses are found in many different vertebrates. Their principal target cells in most animals are those of the hematopoietic and immune systems. Consequently, they induce a wide range of diseases, including malignancies, which chiefly consist of leukemias and lymphomas. Yet retrovirus infection can produce quite the opposite effect. Sometimes they interfere with cell growth, leading to aplasias of various cell types (e.g., aplastic anemia). Some retroviruses alter cell function (e.g., immune impairment), whereas others may be cytopathic, killing the infected cell (AIDS). The kind of disease

*The author acknowledges the assistance of Dr. Howard Z. Streicher in the preparation of this chapter.

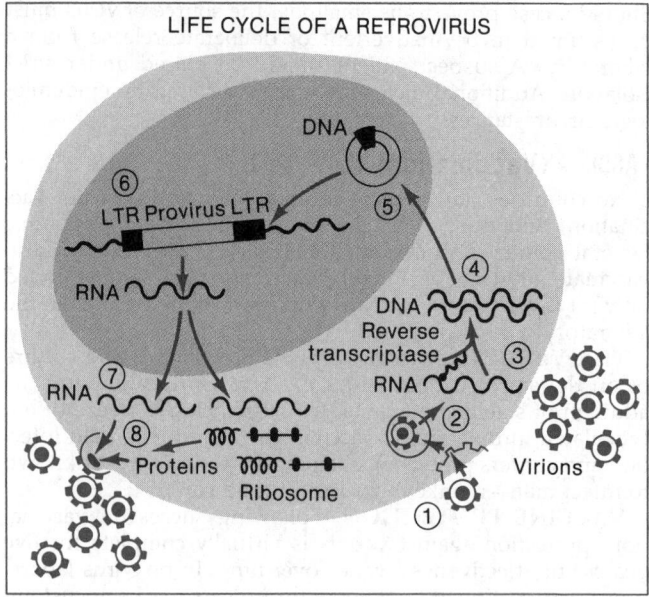

LIFE CYCLE OF A RETROVIRUS

FIGURE 345–1. Viral life cycle: (1) Retrovirus enters the cell by a specific receptor; (2) virus is uncoated in an endosome; and (3) viral RNA is transcribed to double-stranded viral DNA (4) and is transported to the nucleus (5) and integrates into the cellular genome (6). Viral DNA is transcribed as genomic RNA and viral messenger RNA (7), which is translated into new viral protein and assembled at the cell membrane to complete the viral life cycle by budding (8).

induced by a retrovirus partly depends upon its major target cell, which in turn depends upon the viral envelope and sometimes upon the proviral regulatory elements known as long terminal repeat sequences, or LTR's. Depending on the specific retrovirus, the LTR's are sequences of 300 to 900 nucleotides that flank both ends of the double-stranded DNA form of the viral genome. They form the sites of covalent attachment of the provirus to cellular DNA. Other special genes peculiar to a few retroviruses (and especially the human retroviruses) may also contribute to virus effects, as will be illustrated below.

Retroviruses are named and classified according to their species, their mode of transmission (endogenous, exogenous), the type of disease produced (e.g., leukemia viruses, sarcoma viruses), their morphology and mode of maturation (types C, D, B, foamy, and lenti), the organization of their genome, and the genetic relatedness of one to another. Many of these terms and descriptions are no longer useful and will not be considered here. For example, most of the ubiquitous endogenous retroviruses are transmitted in the germ line as genetic elements and have no known role in the origin of disease except in a few highly inbred strains of laboratory mice. These retroviruses will not be considered any further. By contrast, exogenous viruses are transmitted by infection of a somatic cell like any other virus and frequently cause disease.

It is useful to consider retroviruses according to the organization of their genome and the degree to which they share nucleotide sequence homology and biologic properties. In this respect, there are three general groups: (1) those with the three genes necessary for virus replication (*gag* gene for core proteins, *pol* gene for reverse transcriptase, and *env* gene for envelope); (2) those carrying a cellular *onc* gene that codes for a protein that transforms each infected cell; viruses belonging to this second type are rare and usually defective and have never been found in humans; and (3) retroviruses that contain the three requisite genes for viral replication plus one or more additional genes that encode protein or proteins that may regulate virus expression and also may directly or indirectly alter cell function. The majority of known animal retroviruses are of the first type. The mechanisms by which they induce disease often involve extensive replication of the virus and random integration of transcribed DNA into the target cell DNA with occasional chance integration in a region in which the viral LTR may promote altered expression of one or more nearby cellular genes important to cell growth or differentiation or both. This process is sometimes called cis-activation. The third type includes all of the known human retroviruses.

HUMAN RETROVIRUSES: COMMON AND DISTINGUISHING FEATURES

The human retroviruses include two groups, leukemia viruses and the AIDS or AIDS-related viruses (Table 345–1). Their major common characteristics are as follows. The major target cell of each is the T4 cell, and the diseases they cause chiefly involve this cell (hence we call them human T lymphotropic retroviruses, or HTLV's) or cells present in the central nervous system. All the human retroviruses are transmitted by intimate contact, blood contamination (intravenous drug abuse, blood transfusions, and so forth), and infection in utero or after birth by milk. A role for mosquitoes in transmission has also been suggested for HTLV-I. It is likely that all of the human retroviruses originated in Africa and that they might have first entered humans through interspecies infection, perhaps from African green monkeys or a related species. They all contain one or more extra genes that encode proteins involved in the regulation of viral expression. Finally, all of the known human T lymphotropic retroviruses actively replicate after immune stimulation of the infected T cell.

We now distinguish two groups of human retroviruses: leukemia viruses and AIDS viruses. The human retroviruses first discovered, HTLV-I and HTLV-II (human T cell leukemia or lymphotropic viruses), can immortalize (transform) some infected human T cells in vitro and have a preferential tropism for T4+ cells. They can also infect some T8+ cells. They have a spherical core; contain at least one extra gene (*tat* gene) in addition to the *gag*, *pol*, and *env* genes necessary for viral replication; cross-react immunologically with each other; share significant sequence homology; and are chiefly associated with a T cell proliferative disease (leukemias and lymphomas) (Fig. 345–2). The second group includes the more recently discovered AIDS virus—variously termed the third human T lymphotropic retrovirus (HTLV-III) or lymphadenopathy-associated virus (LAV), and now generically called human immunodeficiency virus (HIV-1)—and three very closely and recently isolated related retroviruses now known as HTLV-IV, SBL-6669, and LAV-2 (or collectively as HTLV-IV/HIV-2), whose role in immunodeficiency is under study. Among T cells these viruses infect only T4 cells. When the T4 cell is immune activated and the virus is expressed, HTLV-III kills the T4 cell. The T4 molecule is, itself, part of the receptor for the virus, and since some monocytes and macrophages also express T4, HTLV-III and IV also infect these cells. HTLV-III

TABLE 345–1. HUMAN T LYMPHOTROPIC RETROVIRUSES

Group A (Leukemia Viruses)	Group B (AIDS-related Viruses)
subgroup 1: HTLV-I [STLV-I]	subgroup 1: HTLV-III (HIV-1)
subgroup 2: HTLV-II	subgroup 2: HTLV-IV (HIV-2)
	[STLV-III]
	LAV-2
	SBL virus

HIV-1 and HIV-2 are generic designations corresponding to subgroup 1 and subgroup 2 of the AIDS-related viruses.

STLV-I means simian T-lymphotropic virus I. It has been isolated from several old-world monkeys and from chimpanzees. It is very closely related to HTLV-I.

STLV-III means simian T-lymphotropic virus III. It has been isolated from African green monkeys and other cercopithicenes. It is very closely related to the group B human retroviruses, especially those of subgroup 2 (the West African human retroviruses), and among these it is almost identical to some isolates of HTLV-IV.

All of these different strain isolates from West African patients or healthy people are sometimes collectively called HIV-2.

and IV are immunologically related and share significant nucleotide sequence homology, but cross-react only weakly with the leukemia viruses HTLV-I and II and appear to be more closely related to animal lentiviruses. Compared with HTLV-I and II, they have a smaller cylindrically shaped core and contain at least five genes in addition to the *gag*, *pol*, and *env* genes necessary for viral replication. There are two other major differences between the two human retrovirus groups: (1) There is substantial variation in the genome of HTLV-III (HIV-1) from one isolate to another, especially in the envelope gene, whereas the genomes of the leukemia viruses are remarkably stable; and (2) HTLV-II (HIV-1) (but, as yet, unknown for HTLV-IV (HIV-2)) has entered human populations very recently, whereas human infections caused by HTLV-I and II are much older.

HTLV-I—ASSOCIATED T CELL LEUKEMIAS AND LYMPHOMAS

HTLV-I is chiefly associated with lymphoproliferative diseases of the T cell (Fig. 345–3A). The most common malignancy caused by HTLV-I is adult T cell leukemia (ATL). Clusters of this malignancy were first described in southern Japan at about the same time HTLV-I was isolated from sporadic cases of adult T cell malignancies in the United States. Later, the cluster in Japan was linked to HTLV-I infection. Clear epidemiologic, virologic, and biologic evidence was soon obtained that the virus was causally associated with this malignancy in many parts of the world. The type of transformed T cell may determine the clinical presentation, and the virus-associated malignancy may be occasionally a T cell chronic lymphocytic leukemia, Sézary's syndrome, mycosis fungoides, or a histiocytic or mixed cell lymphoma. The worldwide prevalence of these HTLV-I–associated leukemias is unknown; the incidence in any population depends on the prevalence of viral infection. In endemic areas such as southern Japan and the Caribbean islands, the prevalence of virus-associated leukemia is approximately 3/100,000 and may acount for one half of adult lymphoid malignancies. The chance of an infected individual's developing malignancy over a lifetime is 0.2 to 1 per cent. The prevalence of infection and, therefore, of virus-associated malignancies, is on the increase owing to travel, changes in sexual habits, and spread by intravenous drug abuse and possibly by blood products.

MECHANISM, PATHOGENESIS, AND PATHOLOGY. Perhaps more is known about the pathogenesis of HTLV-I–associated leukemia than any other human malignancy. Early in infection, HTLV-I infects only a small number of T cells. (No other cell types are known to be infected except a very small number of B cells.) The DNA provirus randomly integrates into the DNA of infected cells. At some point, a clone of transformed, but not yet malignant, cells emerges, probably from a polyclonal transformed population. After a long latency period (a few years to several decades), a monoclonal malignancy may develop. The reasons why only a small percentage of infected individuals develop malignancy, the disease takes so long to develop, and T4 cells are selectively involved (although T8 cells can also be infected) remain unknown. When malignancy develops, the HTLV-I provirus is found integrated in the DNA of the leukemic cells in a clonal fashion. The tumor contains one (or occasionally two) copies of the provirus integrated in the same chromosomal location in each cell. This means that the tumor was derived from a single transformed cell and that the virus infection occurred before transformation and clonal expansion, rather than later as a passenger virus. Tumors from different patients, however, have the provirus in different locations. This means that the mechanism cannot be a *cis*-activation of a nearby cellular gene by the LTR of the virus, as occurs with some animal leukemia viruses. Transformation involves the *tat* protein encoded by the extra gene of HTLV-I. The *tat* protein induces expression of cellular genes critical for T cell

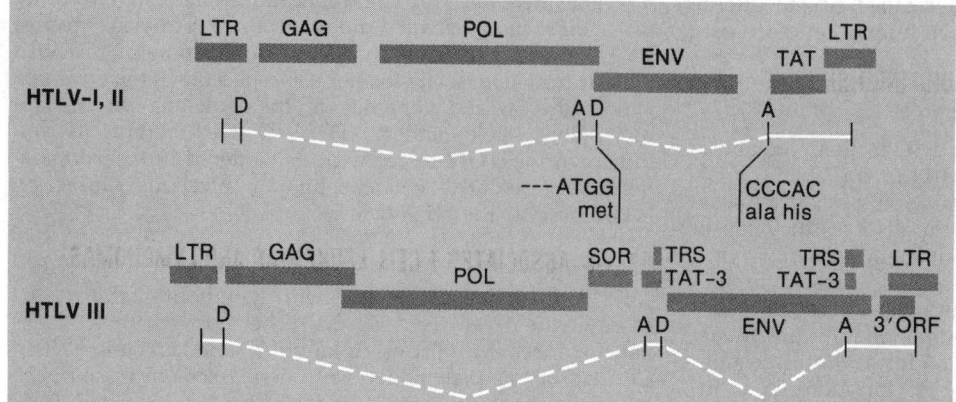

FIGURE 345–2. Genomic organization and splicing of human retrovirus (proviral form); LTR = long terminal repeat; GAG = gene for core proteins; POL = gene for reverse transcriptase; ENV = envelope gene; TAT = transacting gene; TRS, SOR, 3'ORF = genes important for viral regulation whose function has not been determined; D = donor site; A = acceptor site for splicing of mRNA.

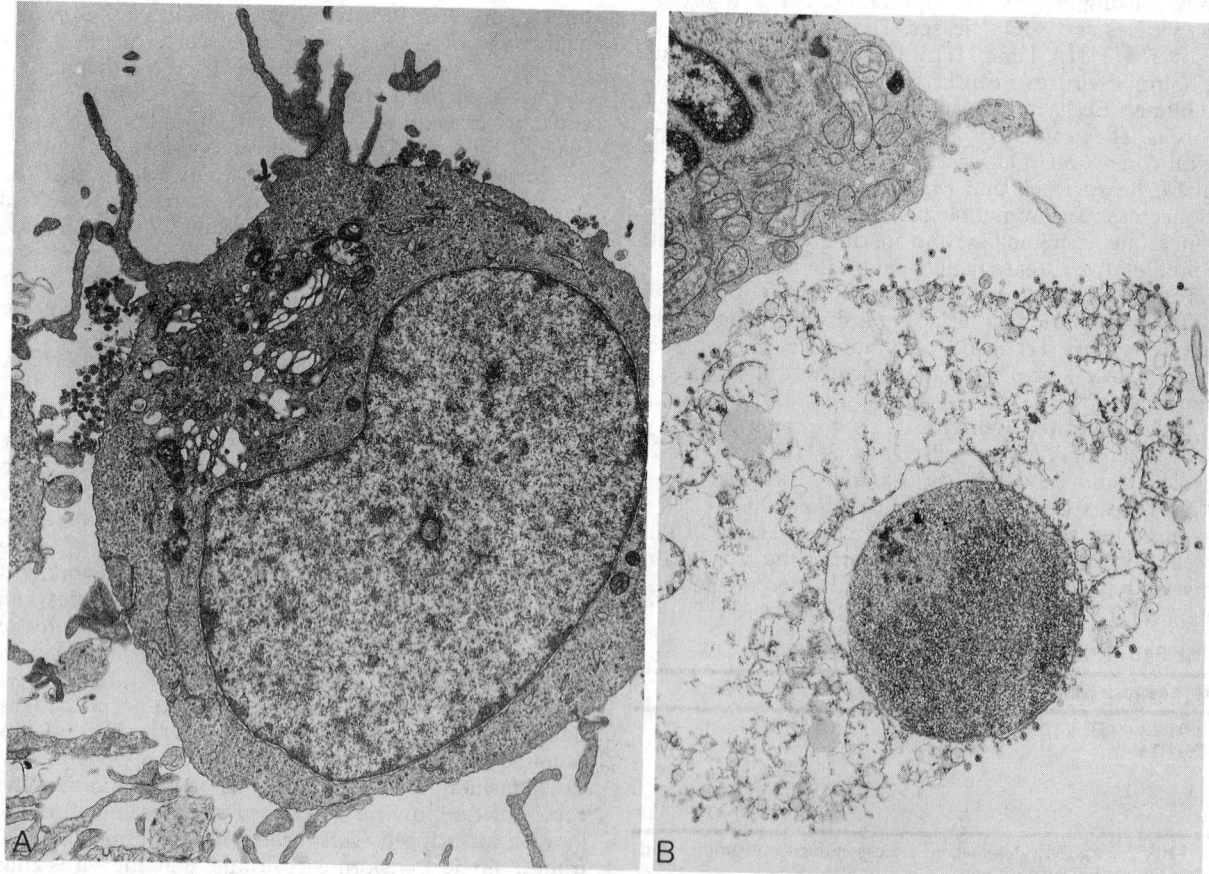

FIGURE 345–3. *A*, T cell infected by HTLV-I is transformed in culture. *B*, T cell infected by HTLV-III shows evidence of viral production and cellular death.

proliferation: T cell growth factor (interleukin-2, or IL-2) and its receptor (IL-2R). The cells apparently both produce and respond to their growth factor (autocrine or autostimulation). This is probably the first step in leukemogenesis, and it leads to polyclonal T cell proliferation. For the development of malignancy, one or more additional genetic changes are probably required because these cells become independent of IL-2 requirements for growth, even though the leukemic cells usually do not express any viral genes (including the *tat* gene). The nature and cause of the additional genetic changes are unknown, but these changes do not appear to require additional specific environmental factors, since the incidence of ATL remains similar wherever the infected individuals may live and since they do not involve any of the so-called known cellular *onc* genes. However, we do know that the malignant cells continue to express the receptor for IL-2 constitutively and in large amounts. Normal T cells do not express IL-2 receptors unless they are activated and then only transiently. Thus, the continued expression of these growth factor receptors is likely to be a major abnormality in this leukemia.

PATHOLOGY OF HTLV-I–ASSOCIATED LEUKEMIA. The pathology reflects infiltration of tissues with leukemic cells. The leukemic cells are usually T4 cells that exhibit extensive nuclear convolution. However, the histopathology varies. Some virus-associated tumors appear similar to lymphomas of various histologic types. The leukemic cells usually infiltrate the viscera and often the dermis, appearing as papules or larger lesions that can become necrotic. Infiltration of the lung can be easily confused with pneumonitis in radiographic analysis. Lytic lesions of the bones are common. Their mechanism is not understood, but they are usually associated with hypercalcemia.

CLINICAL MANIFESTATIONS AND DIAGNOSIS. By far the most common form of malignancy is the acute T cell leukemia or lymphoma mentioned above and known as adult T cell leukemia (ATL). The chief clinical manifestation of ATL is an extremely rapid course. Most patients die within six months of diagnosis. The cause of death is usually an explosive growth of tumor cells but can also be hypercalcemia and infection. In over 80 per cent of cases, HTLV-I malignancy is one of the most acute cancers of humans. Other cases have a more protracted course. Some are indistinguishable from T cell lymphomas of many types. Hallmarks of ATL include elevated white blood cell counts (in close to 100 per cent of cases at some period of the disease); skin abnormalities, e.g., erythema, exfoliative dermatitis, and papules due to infiltration with leukemic cells (in about 50 per cent of cases); and hypercalcemia (in about 75 per cent). The age group includes young to middle-aged adults. The diagnosis should be suspected in any adult with malignancy of T4 cells and in people with unexplained hypercalcemia or unexplained skin abnormalities, particularly if the individual is from a known risk group or known endemic region. The diagnosis is established by testing serum for HTLV-I antibodies and finding leukemic T cells with the provirus in the blood or in biopsy specimens.

TREATMENT AND PREVENTION. There is no proven effective therapy, but exciting experimental approaches now include the use of monoclonal antibodies to the IL-2 receptor. These antibodies can be linked with cell toxins, and the combination can be selectively targeted to the leukemic cells because most normal cells do not express these receptors. Treatment of the complicating hypercalcemia, infections, and skin lesions is a major part of care of these patients. Prevention is achieved by avoiding infection: testing blood prior to transfusion, care in sexual practices, and avoidance of conception by virus positive women. No vaccine is available.

OTHER HTLV-I–ASSOCIATED DISEASES. An association between HTLV-I and B cell leukemias and lymphomas is now recognized. In this case, the role of the virus appears to be indirect. No viral sequences are found in the tumor. It may be that chronic stimulation of B cell proliferation by viral

antigens, coupled with virus-induced impairment of T4 cell function, leads to an increase in the probability of an abnormal genetic change in B cells. T cells infected with HTLV-I have altered functional capacity. This alteration may be responsible for increased rates of infection in HTLV-I–positive people even in the absence of malignancy.

Recently, HTLV-I has been linked to a central nervous system disease called HTLV-I–associated myelopathy, or HAM. This disease is similar to the chronic, progressive form of multiple sclerosis and has been called tropical spastic paraparesis. The incidence, prevalence, and mechanisms of this disease are unknown. The clinical manifestations are usually those of a progressive, bilateral, symmetric loss of pyramidal tract function mainly at the lumbar level. There may also be involvement of the posterior columns. The clinical signs include difficulty in walking, spasticity, hyperreflexia, spastic bladder, constipation, impotence in males, extensor plantar responses, and loss of vibratory perception. The diagnosis is suspected in unexplained central nervous system disease with loss of pyramidal tract functions and is confirmed by testing sera for HTLV-I antibodies. There is no known treatment.

HTLV-II AND LEUKEMIA

This virus has been found in several cases of T cell variants of hairy cell leukemia. Although molecular biologic studies of the leukemic cells strongly suggest that HTLV-II is causally involved in these virus-positive cases, there are insufficient epidemiologic results to draw firm conclusions.

THE THIRD HUMAN RETROVIRUS (HTLV-III/HIV-1) AND AIDS

APPEARANCE AND NATURE OF AIDS. Acquired immunodeficiency syndrome was recognized as a new disease among United States homosexual males in 1981. The disease was associated with a loss of T4 cells, progressive immunodeficiency manifesting with opportunistic infections, frequent development of certain tumors (particularly the peculiar multifocal proliferation known as Kaposi's sarcoma), and frequent impairment of the central nervous system. It was soon learned that the causal agent could also be transmitted by blood, plasma, and factor VIII, and additional risk groups were identified (hemophiliacs, other recipients of blood, and intravenous drug abusers). The same disease was reported in central Africa, first among promiscuous heterosexuals, and further studies showed that this disease was present there even earlier than in other regions of the world. Haitians were also identified as a risk group. By 1983 there were many theories on the cause of AIDS. One of these, the hypothesis that AIDS was caused by a new human T4 lymphotropic retrovirus, was proposed in 1982 and turned out to be correct. This idea was based on information derived from experiences with HTLV-I (and II) and from the feline leukemia virus. The latter virus causes a T cell leukemia of cats, but a minor variant (of the envelope gene) causes an AIDS-like disease in cats. With the use of the same basic technology that had been employed for the isolation of HTLV-I, a new retrovirus was identified in a patient with lymphadenopathy in 1983. In early 1984, numerous isolates of a new human retrovirus (called HTLV-III) were described, and the virus was characterized, produced in permanent cell lines, used for development of a successful test to screen blood prior to transfusion, and unambiguously shown to be the cause of AIDS. In addition, reagents specific for this virus were developed and the virus was shown to be the same as the isolate obtained in 1983. The virus could now properly be called the AIDS virus or the human immunodeficiency virus. Furthermore, as a result of these developments, remarkable progress was made in our understanding of the epidemiology of the disease; the spectrum of disease the virus induces; its latency, target cells, and replication cycle; and some aspects of its mechanism of disease induction—within the span of only a few years. A blood test was developed which can now protect against blood transfusion–induced AIDS.

ETIOLOGY, EPIDEMIOLOGY AND PREVALENCE. HTLV-III was convincingly demonstrated to be the cause of AIDS by showing that the same virus could be isolated from numerous AIDS patients and from people in known risk groups but not from healthy heterosexuals by the study of antibodies to HTLV-III in the sera of hundreds of patients and many control subjects along with the demonstration that the virus infected and killed T4 cells (Fig. 345–3B). This conclusion was supported by studies of recipients of blood transfusions and blood products contaminated with HTLV-III.

The origin of HTLV-III is unknown, but it is likely to have infected humans first in central Africa as a nonpathogenic retrovirus derived from the African green monkey or related monkeys. Genetic change in the virus may have resulted in its striking capacity to cause disease. HTLV-III is transmitted by blood, by sexual contact (semen and cervical fluids), by congenital infection (in utero), and possibly by breast milk. The virus can also be found in tears, urine, and saliva, but there is no proof that these fluids are sources of infection. The virus appears to have spread rapidly in central Africa among sexually promiscuous heterosexuals beginning in the 1960's or 1970's. By the mid 1980's it has become the most serious worldwide infection of this century. In 1987, an estimated 1.5 million Americans were infected, about 35,000 had AIDS, and many thousands of others had developed less severe disease.

PATHOGENESIS AND MECHANISMS. HTLV-III may be transmitted either as free extracellular virus or by virus-infected cells. When transmitted by an infected cell, this "donor" cell may contact a target cell, the viral genes may then become activated, and virus is transmitted directly to the recipient cell. This route could avoid immune detection or exposure of the virus to antibodies. Several weeks after infection, a humoral immune response develops. High titers of antibodies are often made against every viral protein. This includes antibodies to the envelope of the virus, but the critical neutralizing antibodies (against one or more epitopes of the envelope) made after infection do not appear to prevent disease, presumably because the titers are too low or the response is too late, or both. Cellular immunity (T cell cytotoxicity against infected cells) has been difficult to demonstrate. The major target cells of HTLV-III are the T4 cell and the monocyte-macrophage. Cells of the reticuloendothelial system, such as the Langerhans cells of the skin and follicular dendritic cells of the lymph node germinal centers, may also be infected. It appears that all target cells have T4 on the cell surface. Usually, the early response is a lymphocytic proliferation in the lymph nodes, but in time an involution of the lymph nodes occurs.

When the T4 cell containing integrated HTLV-III DNA is immune stimulated, the HTLV-III provirus is activated, the virus forms, the T4 cell dies, and the virus spreads to reinitiate the process, which in time leads to a progressive depletion of the T4 cells. Infected macrophages may bring the virus to the brain, or free virus may cross the blood-brain barrier and infect microglial and possibly other non-neuronal cells. These cells may release factors that cause the major pathologic changes in the brain.

The average period between infection and disease is about four years, but shorter and longer periods are frequent. About 30 per cent of infected people are known to develop serious disease (AIDS), but other studies portend a more ominous future. For example, the Walter Reed Army Institute Study indicates that 90 per cent of infected people progress from their presenting stage to a more advanced disease stage within 1½ to 3 years. Since retroviral infections are lifelong, these statistics predict that the virus may eventually produce serious disease in most infected people. Although the question of

cofactors is constantly raised, there is no evidence that *specific* cofactors are necessary. However, malnutrition and other infections (especially those that provide chronic stimulation of T cells) obviously may accelerate the disease process.

How do the T4 cells become depleted? It seems that the major mechanism is direct killing by the virus as it is expressed following immune activation of infected cells. Since only a minority of T4 cells are infected at any one time, indirect mechanisms may also play a role. Suppressor-like factors have been found in AIDS sera and could be involved. When the T4 cells become depleted, opportunistic infections develop. The mechanism by which HTLV-III kills T4 cells is not completely understood, but we know T4 cell death follows immune activation and virus expression. We also know the killing effect involves the T4 molecule, not only for virus entry but also for the final events of cell killing, since transfection of the viral genes into T4-negative cells does not necessarily lead to their death even after virus is made. Preparation of deletion mutants of the various genes of HTLV-III, followed by transfection of the mutant viral DNA into human T4 cells, shows that in addition to the basic retroviral genes (*gag, pol, env*) some of the regulatory genes, such as *tat*$_{iii}$ and *trs*, are also essential for virus replication. Related studies also suggest that the viral envelope is probably critical to the cell killing. Exactly how T4 molecule and virus envelope interaction leads to cell death is unknown, but it is more complicated than simple induction of cell fusion (giant multinucleated cell formation).

Certain malignancies such as Kaposi's sarcoma (KS), B cell lymphomas, and some carcinomas are more common in HTLV-III–infected people (with or without immune impairment). We know that these malignancies are not directly due to HTLV-III as a transforming virus, since viral genes are not present in the DNA of the cells of any of these tumors. Kaposi's sarcoma associated with HTLV-III is composed of endothelial cells, fibroblasts, and other infiltrating cells and may be a polyclonal, multicentric tumor rather than a true malignancy. Since KS is very common in HTLV-III–infected homosexuals, but much less so in other HTLV-III–infected individuals, another still unknown environmental factor may be involved. The B cell lymphomas are of several types. Recently, a new virus called HBLV (human B lymphotropic virus) was isolated from some, but it is not yet known whether it is involved in causing these tumors. Rearranged *c-myc* genes have been found in some of these tumors, but even in these cases the initiating event is unknown.

PREVENTION. The variation in latency, clinical course, and outcome of HTLV-III/HIV-1 infection may, in part, be dependent upon the variation in the viral genome among various isolates of HTLV-III/HIV-1, especially in the envelope gene. It appears that different individuals are infected with different strain variants and that immune mechanisms protect an infected individual against a second infection by another strain. If this is the case, it may mean that infected people are effectively immunized against infection with another strain. The goal of vaccine development is to do precisely that: to generate an immune response that will be broadly reactive against all variants of the AIDS virus. Because of the theoretic hazards of deliberately introducing retroviral nucleic acids into humans, the approach has been to develop subunit vaccines based on viral envelope proteins. Although type-specific neutralizing antibodies can be induced in many species, including primates, using native envelope glycoprotein, no broadly reactive immunity has yet been achieved in animal studies, but such studies are in their early stages.

The variations in the viral genome may confer advantages on the virus, but since these variations may be generated by an error-prone DNA polymerase (reverse transcriptase), this property may also be exploited to the advantage of the patient. Nucleotide analogues can be used as antimetabolites that are utilized more indiscriminately by the viral enzyme than by cellular DNA polymerases. In fact, this is the rationale for the use of the DNA chain terminator azidothymidine (AZT) in therapy of AIDS. To date, AZT is the only antiviral treatment with documented objective efficacy in vitro and benefits to the patient.

A final point to be emphasized is the recognition of double retrovirus infection (I or II plus III). In this situation, T4 cell depletion increases the probability that HTLV-I will infect (directly) T8+ rather than T4+ cells, leading to unusual clinical presentations. Since the prevalence of HTLV-I infection is increasing in some of the same risk groups exposed to HTLV-III, we can expect more of the unexpected.

The story of human retrovirology is in its infancy, but it is already one of the most fascinating and important chapters in contemporary medicine. These viruses seem destined to open up many doorways to our knowledge of disease causation and provide conceptual advances in our understanding of disease pathogenesis. The human retroviruses—or viruses with similar properties of long latency, minimal replication, lymphotropism, and neurotropism–may be at the heart of some of our important unexplained autoimmune and immunodeficiency diseases. Some may be involved in other human malignancies.

Broder S. (ed.): AIDS: Modern Concepts and Therapeutic Challenges. New York, Marcel Dekker, 1986, pp 1–21. *Detailed articles describing the biology, molecular biology, clinical features, and treatment of HTLV-III (HIV-1) infection.*

Broder S, Bunn PA Jr, Jaffe ES, et al.: T-cell lymphoproliferative syndrome associated with human T-cell leukemia/lymphoma virus. Ann Intern Med 100:543, 1984. Gallo RC, Blattner WA: Human T cell leukemia/lymphoma viruses ATL and AIDS. In DeVita VT, Hellman S, Rosenberg SA (eds.). Important Advances in Oncology, 1985. Philadelphia, J. B. Lippincott Company, 1985, pp 104–138. *These two articles present the clinical description and epidemiology of HTLV-I–associated leukemia.*

Gallo RC: The AIDS virus. Sci Am 256:46, 1987. *Recent summary with clearly illustrated concepts of human retrovirology.*

Gallo RC: The first human retrovirus. Sci Am 255:88, 1986.

Gallo RC: The Henry Kaplan Memorial Lecture: The family of human lymphotropic retroviruses called HTLV: HTLV-I in adult T cell leukemia (ATL), HTLV-II in hairy cell leukemias, and HTLV-III in AIDS. In Miwa M, et al. (eds.): Retroviruses in Human Lymphoma/Leukemia. Utrecht, Japanese Science Society Press, 1985, pp 13–38. *An account of the concepts leading to the isolation of the first human retroviruses with details of the first ones and questions for the future.*

Wong-Staal F, Gallo RC: Human T-lymphotropic retroviruses. Nature 317:395, 1985. *A complete review of the biology of the known human retroviruses (HTLV-I, II, III) up to 1985, with emphasis on the molecular biology.*

Yarchoan R, Broder S: Development of anti-retroviral therapy for the acquired immunodeficiency syndrome and related disorders: A progress report. N Engl J Med 316:557, 1987. *A review of strategies and current status of development of antiviral agents in AIDS.*

346 THE ACQUIRED IMMUNODEFICIENCY SYNDROME

Jerome E. Groopman

INTRODUCTION. The first recognized cases of the disorder now known as acquired immunodeficiency syndrome, or AIDS, were reported in 1981. Soon many new cases were diagnosed among male homosexuals and intravenous drug abusers, and then among hemophiliac patients, recipients of contaminated blood transfusions, and persons from Haiti. For a time the number of new cases doubled about every six months. The largest numbers of cases appeared in the great urban centers, especially the New York City area, San Francisco, and Los Angeles. Over 90 per cent were males.

By 1984 the etiologic agent, a new retrovirus, had been identified, and a blood test for antibodies to the virus had been introduced to assure a virtually safe blood supply. By May, 1987, epidemiologic studies had disclosed an alarming worldwide distribution of the disease. Over 35,000 cases had been reported in the United States, with 20,000 known deaths.

Although the doubling time of new cases has lengthened to 13 months, reflecting behavioral changes among high-risk groups and the success of control measures based on the blood test, prospects for the next few years are staggering. In the United States alone there are an estimated 1 to 1.5 million individuals infected with the AIDS virus, and by the end of 1991 a total of 270,000 cases will have been reported, with 179,000 deaths—80 per cent of them outside New York and San Francisco.

The wave of AIDS in the United States, the Caribbean, and Latin America appears to be running behind that of central Africa and ahead of that of Europe and Asia. Estimates of the number of infected individuals worldwide range as high as 5 to 10 million and of AIDS deaths in Africa in the hundreds of thousands. In Africa the sex ratio of patients with AIDS is 1:1, and heterosexual transmission predominates.

A few drugs have been identified that will block viral replication. One, azidothymidine, has shown beneficial clinical effects in early studies. A few viral proteins, especially one termed gp 120, have shown antigenic properties that have encouraged vaccine development studies and preliminary tests in animals. Intensive, ongoing research centers on the properties of the virus, the pathogenesis of the disease, its epidemiology worldwide, drug discovery and evaluation, and vaccine development. Public education about risk avoidance needs to be intensified, and developing countries need to institute controls to assure safety of their blood supplies.

DEFINITION. The acquired immunodeficiency syndrome (AIDS) was originally defined for purposes of epidemiologic surveillance as a life-threatening opportunistic infection or as Kaposi's sarcoma, or both, developing in a previously healthy individual with cellular immunodeficiency of unknown cause (Table 346–1). Although this case definition still serves some use in tracking the spread of the epidemic, we now know that a variety of clinical disorders, beyond those in this initial surveillance definition, result from infection with the human immunodeficiency virus, HIV, the etiologic agent of the syndrome. The clinical outcomes of HIV infection range from the asymptomatic carrier state to a generalized lymphadenopathy, which may be symptomatic (AIDS-related complex or ARC), to a rapidly progressive disease with high mortality from opportunistic infections or neoplasm (AIDS). Neurologic involvement is common. Because the full clinical spectrum of HIV infection is not yet known, new disorders related to HIV will likely continue to be identified.

ETIOLOGY AND PATHOPHYSIOLOGY. The etiologic agent of AIDS and related human immunodeficiency virus disorders is a cytopathic retrovirus—variously termed human T cell leukemic-lymphoma virus–III (HTLV-III), lymphadenopathy virus (LAV), and now human immunodeficiency virus (HIV)—that has been discussed in detail in the preceding chapter. A small number of patients with AIDS in West Africa have been found to be infected with a related retrovirus, HIV-2, rather than with HIV. The biology of human retroviruses is such that once the host has been infected, there is permanent integration of viral material in the form of proviral genome in the deoxyribonucleic acid (DNA) of the host target cells. This provirus is capable of replication and production of new virions. From an epidemiologic point of view, therefore, a person with evidence of prior infection, such as specific serum antibodies to HIV proteins, must be considered permanently infected and potentially infectious to others. The presence of antibodies to HIV is taken to signify sustained infection that will probably persist for the life of the person.

There are four major apparent target cells of the retrovirus in humans. These are the T4 lymphocyte, the monocyte-macrophage, certain cell populations in brain and spinal cord (possibly microglia), and colorectal epithelial cells. The clinical manifestations of HIV infection may result, at least in part, from progressive dysfunction of the first three of these target cell populations. Colorectal cell infection may be important in

TABLE 346–1. CENTERS FOR DISEASE CONTROL SURVEILLANCE DEFINITION OF AIDS

1. Diagnosed disease process that is at least moderately predictive of a defect in cell-mediated immunity occurring in a person with no known cause for diminished resistance
2. Diseases diagnostic for AIDS include the following:
   Kaposi's sarcoma
   Pneumocystis carinii pneumonia
   Serious opportunistic infections

   Pneumonia
   Meningitis
   Encephalitis
   {
     Aspergillosis
     Candidiasis
     Cryptococcosis
     Cytomegalovirus infection
     Nocardiosis
     Strongyloidosis
     Toxoplasmosis
     Zygomycosis
     Atypical mycobacteriosis
   }

   Esophagitis
   {
     Candida, cytomegalovirus, herpes simplex virus, progressive multifocal leukoencephalopathy
     Chronic (>4 weeks) cryptosporidiosis
     Severe, chronic (>5 weeks) mucocutaneous herpes simplex
   }

3. Diagnostic only if HIV-positive antibody or culture:
   a. Disseminated histoplasmosis
   b. Isosporiasis with chronic (>1 month) diarrhea
   c. Bronchial or pulmonary candidiasis
   d. Non-Hodgkin's lymphoma of high-grade, B lymphocyte type
   e. Kaposi's sarcoma in patients older than 60 years
4. Miscellaneous changes:
   a. Chronic lymphoid interstitial pneumonitis in child (<13 years of age) unless proven HIV negative
   b. Lymphoreticular malignancy occurring greater than 3 months after other disease diagnostic of AIDS will not alter patient's AIDS diagnosis
   c. Patients with any disease processes that are HIV antibody–negative and who have normal immune studies will not be diagnosed as having AIDS irrespective of disease process

Data from MMWR 31:507, 1982; 34:373, 1985.

transmission among homosexuals. The T4 lymphocyte and monocyte-macrophage serve as pivotal cells in the armada of the cellular immune system, critical components of the network for recognition and processing of antigen and production of soluble cytokines such as interferons, interleukins, and hematopoietic colony-stimulating factors. They effectively mobilize immune defense against certain pathogens. Dysfunction or loss of these cell types results in cellular immune impairment. The effects of HIV on cell populations in the brain are less well understood.

The major receptor for HIV on the surface of target cells is the CD4 (T4) antigen. Whether HIV can by itself infect, impair, and destroy target cells is controversial. Target cells, such as T4 lymphocytes, display increased efficiency of infection following stimulation with a variety of mitogens or antigens. These observations, as well as frequent co-infection of high-risk subjects with other viruses, such as cytomegalovirus, Epstein-Barr virus, herpes simplex virus, and exposure to alloantigens in the form of concentrated blood products or semen, suggest that "cofactors" may be important in the pathogenesis of AIDS. This hypothesis holds that HIV infection and replication are relatively inefficient without coexisting stimulation of the immune system. Furthermore, should infection occur, reduction of clinical antigenic stimulation, mainly by reduced exposure to sexually or parenterally transmitted DNA viruses or antigens, may maintain a dormancy of the virus and reduce its cytopathic effects. This hypothesis lacks a firm scientific basis. Data do not support the contention that exposure to cofactors, or lack thereof, will modulate the clinical outcome of HIV infection.

DETECTION OF HIV INFECTION. The most frequently employed test to detect HIV-infected individuals assays serum antibodies to the retrovirus. HIV antibodies can be detected by several techniques, including enzyme-linked immunosorbent assay (ELISA), immunofluorescent assays (IFA), Western blot, and radioimmunoprecipitation (RIP). When performed by an experienced laboratory, each is quite accurate in de-

tecting antibody to HIV. The ELISA is the most frequently used owing to its relatively low cost, simplicity, and capacity to be done on a large scale. The "first generation" of the ELISA has employed whole virus antigens harvested from cultures of lymphocytes infected with HIV. The sensitivity and specificity of such whole virus ELISA tests are 95 to 99 per cent. In a population with a high prevalence of HIV infection, such as homosexual men, the ELISA has a positive predictive value approaching 100 per cent. In populations with a low estimated prevalence of HIV infection, such as volunteer blood donors, the positive predictive value is much lower. Infected individuals in the 8- to 12-week period following exposure may test negative by the ELISA method. Such individuals have been found to be infected with the retrovirus by direct culture of their blood. The major limitation of the current ELISA is a relatively high rate of false-positive reactions. Nearly 1 per cent of healthy, uninfected blood donors will initially show a generally weak but apparently positive result. This appears to be a nonspecific reaction of serum antibodies with contaminating cell debris from the lymphocyte culture. Because of the importance of accurately determining infection by antibody detection, a second or "confirmatory" test is frequently performed. The combination of ELISA with other methods increases the positive predictive value of the test. The algorithm currently used in testing donated blood requires that an ELISA be reactive on two or more determinations with the serum specimen for the test to be considered positive. All ELISA-positive sera are then evaluated by Western blot analysis. The subject is not considered seropositive, and is not notified of the result, unless the results are positive by both techniques.

The indications for HIV testing are controversial. Because of the social stigma associated with a positive result, as well as concerns regarding discrimination and insurability, the application of the test to different social and clinical situations is still debated. It is clear that for blood donation, semen donation for artificial insemination, and organ donation all potential donors should be tested. The United States military currently tests all prospective members and recruits. Future applications of the test may include premarital screening, prenatal screening, and testing of individuals with professions involving high risk to themselves or others, such as airplane pilots or heavy machine operators. It is likely that the insurance industry will attempt to employ HIV testing. Given the increasing use of the test, and its psychologic and clinical impact, accuracy is paramount. A "second-generation" ELISA test using genetically engineered recombinant HIV antigens will likely replace the current whole virus ELISA test, providing a higher degree of accuracy.

EPIDEMIOLOGY. *Transmission.* Transmission of an infectious agent is accomplished via three basic elements: an infectious source, a vector of spread, and a susceptible host. The transmission of HIV has been well defined in the United States by serologic testing. The mechanisms of spread of HIV appear to be limited to sexual, parenteral, and maternal-infant routes. Because the etiologic agent of AIDS was not identified for several years following the initial recognition of the syndrome, considerable public anxiety and misconception have developed regarding transmission. Similarly, because AIDS was first described in homosexual and bisexual men, it was presumed that the virus would not pose a risk to the larger heterosexual population. About 75 per cent of AIDS cases in the United States occur among homosexual men. It appears that receptive anal intercourse is an important and efficient route of HIV spread in this population. This may be related to the relatively high concentration of virus in semen that encounters target colorectal cells bearing CD4 (T4) antigen. Some male sexual partners of AIDS patients, however, have had considerable exposure to the retrovirus and yet not become infected. Such observations raise questions concerning different degrees of infectiousness and host susceptibility.

HIV has been isolated from blood, urine, semen, vaginal fluid, cerebrospinal fluid, tears, and saliva. Identification of the retrovirus in a particular body fluid does not necessarily mean that such a fluid transmits the virus. Epidemiological studies do not support the transmission of HIV by "casual" contact in the home or workplace. Such casual contact includes handshaking, sharing of bathroom facilities, eating or preparing meals, and airborne transmission. Kissing does not appear to transmit the virus efficiently, if at all.

HIV is transmitted during heterosexual contact. Male-to-female transmission occurs in 15 to 30 per cent of regular female sexual partners of infected men. Either vaginal intercourse or rectal intercourse between men and women can transmit the virus. This has been dramatically demonstrated by an unfortunate situation in which several women were artificially inseminated with semen from an HIV-infected donor and nearly half of the exposed women became infected. HIV can also be transmitted from women to men, although the efficiency of such transmission appears to be much lower than from men to women. Female-to-male transmission may occur with greater frequency outside the United States, particularly in central Africa. The presence of HIV in vaginal fluid may allow for infection during vaginal intercourse or oral-genital contact with women. No information exists concerning transmission by oral sex with men.

Parenteral transmission occurs in three major populations: intravenous drug abusers, hemophiliacs who have received clotting factor concentrates, and random blood transfusion recipients. Intravenous drug abusers account for the second largest number of AIDS cases in the United States, constituting 15 to 20 per cent. HIV seropositivity is high among intravenous drug abusers on the East Coast of the United States, and the virus is spreading in this population throughout the country. It is estimated that in New York City 40 to 60 per cent of intravenous drug addicts in 1986 carried the retrovirus. Hemophiliacs are exposed to thousands of different donors per year, since factor VIII concentrate is prepared from pooled plasma. In most hemophilia centers, there is a seroprevalence for HIV ranging from 60 to 90 per cent. As of May, 1987, about 350 cases of AIDS had been reported in patients with hemophilia or other coagulation disorders. Between 5 and 15 per cent of the spouses of hemophiliacs have been infected primarily through vaginal intercourse with their husbands. Factor VIII concentrate is now heat-treated to inactivate HIV. Fortunately, there have been no recorded seroconversions of hemophiliacs who have received only the newer preparations. Over 775 cases of AIDS have been reported in the United States among recipients of random blood component transfusions. Study of the blood donors implicated in AIDS cases resulting from transfusion has nearly always identified at least one donor who was a member of a high-risk group and who was serologically positive for the virus antibody. Recipients of blood products from HIV-seropositive donors appear to be at extraordinarily high risk for infection with the virus. It is estimated that 90 to 100 per cent of transfusion recipients of blood from a seropositive donor will become infected. Serologic testing for HIV has been offered to all individuals transfused in the United States between 1978 and 1985, the year blood products began to be tested for the retrovirus. In spite of the institution of screening, transmission of HIV via blood products may still happen if blood is donated during the period of HIV viremia prior to antibody seroconversion or if infected individuals fail to develop antibody detectable by current methods. Such events are expected to be extraordinarily rare, so that the current risk of HIV transmission by blood transfusion is estimated to be less than 5 to 10 per million units transfused.

Infection through accidental needle sticks is rare, occurring at a frequency of less than 1 in 1000 needle sticks. The difference in risk of transmission between transfusion and needle stick exposure may be attributable to the dose of virus.

Presumably, a relatively large inoculum of virus is transmitted via transfusion of contaminated blood or during intravenous drug abuse. This does not appear to occur during a needle stick. By contrast, hepatitis B, caused by a less fragile virus than HIV, is often transmitted through needle stick accidents.

Parenteral exposure to HIV is a potential risk in the hemodialysis setting, as with hepatitis B virus infection, but current evidence is that HIV is not transmitted among dialysis patients. Similarly, HIV has not been transmitted by the hepatitis B vaccine derived from plasma donors or by immunoglobulin preparations.

Infants born to HIV-seropositive mothers become infected with the retrovirus in a significant number of cases. It is still unclear whether transmission occurs in utero, during delivery, or in the postnatal period. Isolation of HIV from breast milk suggests that the retrovirus could be transmitted orally to infants. This issue is of special importance in central Africa, where breast feeding is encouraged for nutritional reasons and high infant mortality is associated with inappropriately prepared bottled milk.

Definition of these transmission vectors of HIV led to recognition of epidemiologically "high-risk groups." These include homosexual and bisexual men, hemophiliacs, intravenous drug abusers, persons from Haiti and central Africa, and infants born to infected mothers. At much lower risk, although higher than the general population, are recipients of blood products between 1978 and 1985. Heterosexual transmission of HIV appears to be occurring at an increasing rate, particularly in large urban settings. This mainly results from exposure of women to men who have used intravenous drugs or are bisexual, or both. Data derived from screening of military recruits in the Northeast demonstrate a ratio of seropositive men to women of 2:1. This contrasts with a ratio of men to women among AIDS cases of 16:1. This worrisome statistic emphasizes the need for public awareness of the magnitude of the problem and for broad education regarding sexual practices and intravenous drug abuse.

Dimensions of the Epidemic. Over 35,000 cases of AIDS have been reported in the United States, with almost 20,000 deaths, but since only AIDS is reportable, it is difficult to determine accurately the number of people with subclinical HIV infection. Estimates range from 1 to 1.5 million HIV-seropositive, and thus infected, individuals in the United States and 5 to 10 million worldwide. Although people in this group are generally asymptomatic, laboratory abnormalities related to HIV infection of target cells are frequent. Two major subsets of peripheral blood T lymphocytes have been defined through the use of monoclonal antibodies that recognize specific cell surface antigens. These are the T4-bearing helper-inducer and T8-bearing cytotoxic-suppressor lymphocytes. T4 lymphocytes appear to be one major target of HIV. Asymptomatic HIV-seropositive individuals often show a decrease in the absolute numbers of circulating T4 lymphocytes and a consequent decrease in the ratio of T4 to T8 lymphocytes. The majority of HIV-seropositive subjects who are asymptomatic at baseline demonstrate progressive depletion of the T4 helper-inducer lymphocyte population and further laboratory evidence of immune deterioration. Asymptomatic HIV-seropositive individuals have an uncertain prognosis, with 10 to 30 per cent progressing to AIDS and 30 to 50 per cent developing other clinical disorders such as ARC within five years of infection with the virus. Periodic clinical evaluation with attention to signs and symptoms of AIDS or related disorders is the best approach for monitoring asymptomatic HIV-seropositive persons.

IMMUNOLOGY. Although AIDS was initially defined for epidemiologic surveillance purposes as manifesting infectious and/or neoplastic disorders indicative of cellular immune dysfunction, it is now clear that there are changes in the humoral (B lymphocyte) immune system as well. HIV infects not only T4 lymphocytes but also monocyte-macrophages and therefore might be able to interfere with normal processing and/or presentation of antigen by these effector cells to immunoglobulin-producing B lymphocytes. Indeed, in the spectrum of infectious diseases associated with AIDS, pathogens handled in large part by the B lymphocyte system, such as *Salmonella, Hemophilus influenzae,* and *Staphylococcus* species, appear with increased frequency. Nonetheless, AIDS should still be thought of as most commonly manifesting infection with organisms associated with cellular immune dysfunction, such as protozoa, fungi, mycobacteria, and herpesviruses.

Quantitative abnormalities in circulating cell populations are frequent in AIDS. Lymphopenia often follows HIV infection, generally owing to an absolute decrease in the number of the helper-inducer subset of T lymphocytes, which express the T4 (OKT4/Leu3/CD4) surface antigen. In more advanced cases, lymphopenia may also include a decrease in the cytotoxic-suppressor (T8/Leu2/CD8) population. These alterations in helper-inducer and cytotoxic-suppressor T-lymphocyte subsets generally lead to reversal of the T4-T8 ratio. This ratio may also be reversed following infection in normal individuals with herpesviruses such as cytomegalovirus or Epstein-Barr virus, but this reversal occurs on the basis of an absolute increase in the T8 cytotoxic-suppressor population. Some individuals, following HIV infection, may also manifest a minor or no decrease in helper-inducer lymphocytes associated with an apparent increase in the T8 cytotoxic-suppressor population.

The pathophysiology of the decrease in the helper-inducer population is not clear. Although HIV is tropic for T4-bearing lymphocytes, HIV viral sequences can be detected in only a small number of circulating cells, generally less than 1 in 10,000. How are the T4 lymphocytes lost if so few cells are infected? Several hypotheses have been advanced to address this apparent paradox. Cell fusion with formation of syncytia or multinucleated giant cells is frequently observed in vitro in lymphocyte cell lines following HIV infection. It has been suggested that expression of the major HIV envelope glycoprotein, gp120, on the surface of the infected T4 lymphocyte leads to binding with the T4 antigen on the surface of an uninfected lymphocyte and then to fusion. Cell death may follow formation of such multinucleated cells. However, multinucleated cells are rarely observed in lymphoid tissues such as spleen or lymph nodes. They are seen in the central nervous system but are of unclear origin and significance. An alternative hypothesis holds that the helper-inducer T lymphocyte is an important source of regulatory growth factors for lymphoid stem cells, which could fail to grow and differentiate owing to lack of these regulatory growth factors. Furthermore, infected lymphocytes or monocytes may produce suppressor factors that inhibit lymphoid development. In the more advanced stages of AIDS, panlymphopenia may reflect poor production of T lymphocytes from stem cell populations following organ invasion by opportunistic pathogens or the toxic effects of antibiotics and chemotherapy, or both.

Leukopenia is frequent in patients with HIV infection. Its etiology is unknown. It is mainly due to granulocytopenia, but occasionally monocytopenia as well. The bone marrow morphology often reveals dysplasia, hypercellularity, and maturational abnormalities. Monocyte-macrophages can easily be infected by HIV in vitro but show relatively few cytopathic changes. They appear to be infected in vivo as well. Initial studies of bone marrow progenitor cells demonstrate that growth of both granulocyte and macrophage progenitors (CFU-GM) is suppressed in vitro by HIV antibodies. Suppression of hematopoiesis by a serum antibody suggests that an acquired antigen, possibly a viral protein encoded by HIV, is expressed on the surface of the progenitor cell.

Thrombocytopenia frequently follows HIV infection. Indeed, it may be a presenting abnormality suggesting infection with this retrovirus. The possible pathogenesis of thrombocytopenia following HIV infection includes production of an autoantibody to a 25,000-dalton protein found in the membrane of the platelet and nonspecific binding of circulating immune complexes to the F_c receptor of the platelet. The former mechanism is still under study, and the nature and acquisition of the antigen by the circulating platelet are unexplained. The latter "innocent bystander" hypothesis is suggested by elevated circulating immune complexes in AIDS and ARC patients and immunoglobulin on the surface of the platelet.

Anemia is also frequent in AIDS patients. Only occasionally is the direct Coombs' test result positive. The anemia is probably multifactorial, since patients are often infected with one or several pathogens and are receiving myelosuppressive antibiotics or chemotherapy. Studies of bone marrow erythroid progenitors suggest impaired development. Other processes that may contribute include splenomegaly with sequestration and hemolysis (which are frequent with mycobacterial or cytomegalovirus infection) and direct bone marrow invasion by fungi, mycobacteria, or lymphoma.

Functional cell defects have been well described following HIV infection. Decreased lymphocyte proliferation in response to lectins such as phytohemagglutinin (PHA) or concanavalin A (Con A) is frequently observed. Similarly, response to soluble antigens is impaired and may reflect abnormalities in vivo that lead to opportunistic infections and possibly neoplasms. Impaired production of immunoregulatory mediators (lymphokines) such as gamma-interferon and interleukin-2 has also been observed. In consequence, there is decreased cytotoxic cellular response, decreased reactivity to allogeneic cells, and decreased T lymphocyte helper function for production of immunoglobulins by B lymphocytes. There is debate whether these abnormalities are qualitative, reflecting intrinsic dysfunction of different immune effector cells, or quantitative, reflecting absolute decreases in T4 lymphocyte number or increases in T8 suppressor lymphocytes. In highly enriched preparations of helper T lymphocyte subpopulations, the response to lectins appears normal, whereas the response to soluble antigens is still impaired. This observation implies that the T helper-inducer lymphocytes responding to specific soluble antigen are dysfunctional.

T lymphocyte helper function, defined by "help" to B lymphocytes in production of immunoglobulin, appears to be abnormal following HIV infection. By contrast, immunoglobulin production is suppressed in vitro by T8 cytotoxic-suppressor lymphocytes from patients with AIDS. These observations in vitro appear paradoxical in that HIV-infected patients show polyclonal hypergammaglobulinemia, rather than hypogammaglobulinemia. Levels of all classes of immunoglobulin (IgG, IgA, IgM, IgD) are elevated. Thus, there may be a stimulus to B lymphocyte production of immunoglobulins independent of T lymphocytes following HIV infection. Preliminary studies indicate that HIV antigens and reactivated Epstein-Barr virus serve as potent direct stimuli to B lymphocyte immunoglobulin production.

The number of circulating B lymphocytes is generally normal in HIV-infected patients, but the number of circulating immunoglobulin-secreting cells (plasma cells) appears to be increased. Nevertheless, the capacity of B lymphocytes from AIDS patients to respond to stimuli such as pokeweed mitogen or *Staphylococcus aureus* Cowan I is often decreased. Such abnormalities indicate an intrinsic functional abnormality of B lymphocytes following HIV infection. Patients with AIDS and ARC do not develop a normal antibody response upon immunization with pneumococcal vaccine. This abnormal response to a new antigen may explain in part the blunted serologic response to certain infectious pathogens in patients with AIDS, such as *Toxoplasma.* Infection of transformed B lymphocytes by HIV can be accomplished in vitro, but it is unclear whether B lymphocytes are infected in vivo.

Defects in monocyte-macrophage function have also been

observed with respect to both chemotaxis and microbicidal function. Some of these defects can be reversed in vitro by addition of lymphokines such as gamma-interferon and colony-stimulating factor. There appears to be an abnormality in secretion of important regulatory cytokines, such as interleukin-1, by monocytes from AIDS patients. This dysfunction may reflect direct HIV infection of this cell or abnormalities in the induction of macrophage function by regulatory lymphokines from the T4 lymphocyte, or both. Many of the opportunistic pathogens of AIDS patients, such as atypical mycobacteria, *Toxoplasma*, and fungi, are normally eliminated by the monocyte-macrophage system. The frequent pulmonary infections in AIDS patients may represent dysfunction of the pulmonary alveolar macrophage, a primary cell in host lung defense. The monocyte-macrophage may also act as an important reservoir for HIV. The nature of HIV infection of monocyte-macrophages differs substantially from that of the T4 lymphocyte, at least in vitro. HIV is not particularly cytopathic for monocyte-macrophages and appears capable of persistence in a relatively dormant "reservoir" state in this cell type. Cells resembling monocyte-macrophages in the central nervous system may act as a reservoir of HIV in brain and spinal cord. It is still unclear whether the monocyte-macrophage is an important vector for spread of HIV.

Other cellular defects of immune function have also been reported in AIDS patients. Decreased number and function of natural killer (NK) cells have been observed. Although in some animal models decreased NK cell function is correlated with development of certain neoplasms, the significance of this observation following HIV infection is unclear.

Serologic abnormalities have been extensively studied following infection. Nonspecific markers of lymphocyte injury, such as serum beta$_2$-microglobulin, are frequently elevated. A species of acid-labile alpha-interferon has also been reported in the serum of AIDS patients. The immunopathologic significance of these findings is not known.

CLINICAL SPECTRUM OF HIV INFECTION. The clinical spectrum of HIV infection ranges from the asymptomatic carrier state to overt AIDS. The disease may progress through an influenza-like illness, generalized adenopathy, and AIDS-related complex, to AIDS with its opportunistic infections, Kaposi's sarcoma, and dementia, but not all AIDS patients experience all earlier stages. In many, the first indication of AIDS is the development of Kaposi's sarcoma or *Pneumocystis carinii* pneumonia.

Primary HIV Infection: The "Acute Syndrome." Primary HIV infection may present as acute febrile illness resembling influenza or infectious mononucleosis. Incubation time from infection to onset of symptoms varies from 6 days to 7 weeks. Symptoms last 2 to 4 weeks. The most common clinical features are fever, sweats, myalgias, arthralgias, and malaise. One half or more of symptomatic subjects report sore throat, adenopathy, anorexia, nausea, vomiting, and/or a maculopapular rash. Less common complaints include diarrhea, stiff neck, severe shooting pains, urticaria, sacral hyperesthesia, major weight loss, abdominal cramps, and desquamation of the palms and soles. Laboratory abnormalities include mild leukopenia and lymphopenia, with a few cases of T4:T8 inversion following the acute illness. Cerebrospinal fluid changes consistent with a lymphocytic meningitis may be found in rare patients presenting with headaches and stiff neck. Seroconversion for antibodies to the virus follows the presumed exposure by 3 to 12 weeks. Antibodies to gp120, gp160, and p24 develop first. Antibodies to -41 (transmembrane protein) and other antigens develop approximately 4 weeks later. Viral isolation has been reported prior to seroconversion in a number of subjects. The acute viral illness may occur in one third or more of subjects infected by contaminated needles or transfused blood but is much less common in those infected by homosexual contacts.

Persistent Generalized Lymphadenopathy. Persistent generalized lymphadenopathy is frequent after HIV infection. It is operationally defined as involvement of at least two extrainguinal lymph node groups with other causes of diffuse lymphadenopathy investigated and excluded. A staging system from the Centers for Disease Control distinguishes between individuals with only persistent generalized lymphadenopathy and those who are clinically symptomatic with enlarged lymph nodes. This distinction is probably an accurate one in that progression to AIDS appears to be correlated with clinical symptoms among persons with generalized lymphadenopathy. The utility of lymph node biopsy in an asymptomatic individual with persistent generalized lymphadenopathy is controversial. Although occasionally occult Kaposi's sarcoma or B lymphocyte lymphoma may be detected in the enlarged nodes, this is rather rare in the absence of constitutional symptoms. Furthermore, detection of an opportunistic infection by lymph node biopsy is very unusual in the asymptomatic patient. Pathologically, the lymph nodes usually demonstrate follicular hyperplasia with enlargement of the germinal centers. Immunohistochemical stains demonstrate depletion of the T4 population in the node similar to that in peripheral blood. Indications for lymph node biopsy include rapid enlargement of nodes and development of symptoms such as fevers, night sweats, or weight loss, suggesting an infectious or malignant process. In such cases, the highest yield is generally obtained by biopsy of a cervical or axillary lymph node.

AIDS-Related Complex (ARC). The definition of the AIDS-related complex (ARC) is not precise. Several working definitions have been developed, but there is no consensus, and the distinction between generalized lymphadenopathy and ARC is often unclear. However, ARC can be diagnosed when an individual infected with HIV demonstrates persistent clinical abnormalities that do not satisfy the epidemiologic surveillance definition of AIDS (see Table 346–1). Laboratory abnormalities without clinical symptoms or signs are not sufficient to establish the diagnosis of ARC. Nonetheless, laboratory abnormalities are frequent in ARC and help support the diagnosis. These include hematologic, immunologic, and chemical imbalances. The clinical and laboratory abnormalities associated with ARC are listed in Table 346–2. Certain findings, particularly constitutional symptoms of persistent unexplained fever, weight loss, unexplained diarrhea, and

TABLE 346–2. CLINICAL AND LABORATORY FEATURES OF AIDS-RELATED COMPLEX

Clinical

Fever: >100° F (37.7° C), intermittent or continuous ≥3 months, in the absence of other identifiable cause

Weight loss: 10 per cent of normal body weight or ≥15 lb

Lymphadenopathy: persistent ≥3 months, involving two or more extrainguinal node-bearing areas

Diarrhea: intermittent or continuous ≥3 months, in the absence of other identifiable cause

Fatigue: to the point of decreased physical or mental function

Night sweats: intermittent or continuous ≥3 months, in the absence of other identifiable cause

Laboratory

Depressed helper T lymphocytes (≥2 SD below the mean)

Depressed helper suppressor ratio (≥SD below the mean)

At least one of the following: leukopenia, thrombocytopenia, absolute lymphopenia, or anemia

Elevated serum globulins

Depressed blastogenesis (pokeweed, phytohemagglutinin [PHA] mitogens)

Abnormal intradermal tests for delayed cutaneous hypersensitivity (using multitest or equivalent)

Working Definition of Persistent Generalized Lymphadenopathy

1. Lymphadenopathy of a least 3 months' duration involving two or more extrainguinal sites and confirmed on physical examination by patient's physician

2. Absence of any current illness or drug use known to cause lymphadenopathy

3. Presence of reactive hyperplasia in a lymph node if a biopsy was performed.

Data from Adv Host Defense Mech 5:5, 1985; MMWR 31:249, 1982.

oral candidiasis, are particularly ominous with respect to progression from ARC to AIDS. Such symptoms and signs are indicative of severe immunologic damage resulting from HIV infection. Although there is considerable variability, most patients with ARC demonstrate severely depleted numbers of circulating T4 lymphocytes, a marked reversal of the T4:T8 ratio, and occasionally anergy on skin testing. Leukopenia, thrombocytopenia, and anemia with polyclonal hypergammaglobulinemia are frequent in ARC.

Management of thrombocytopenia associated with HIV infection is controversial. Many patients do not develop significant clinical bleeding. Corticosteroids, often used in immune-related thrombocytopenia, have the potential risk of accelerating immunosuppression and precipitating an opportunistic infection. Danazol has rarely been effective. Splenectomy may improve the number of circulating platelets but is a procedure of last resort in such individuals. Transient increases in circulating platelet count and in white blood cell count may be achieved by the use of high-dose intravenous gamma globulin preparations. This appears to reduce the destruction of antibody-coated platelets or leukocytes by the monocyte-macrophage system.

Opportunistic Infections in AIDS. Progressive immunologic deterioration following HIV infection may ultimately result in life-threatening opportunistic infection or neoplasm or both. The list of infections and cancers accepted as diagnostic of AIDS by the Centers for Disease Control is shown in Table 346–1. The opportunistic infections seen in AIDS patients are characterized by an aggressive clinical course, frequent resistance to standard therapy, and a high rate of relapse. Diagnosis of these infections requires a high index of suspicion, an expert microbiologic laboratory, and a familiarity with the clinical presentation of a specific pathogen in AIDS patients. Generally, duration of therapy is more prolonged than for most infections, and drug toxicities may occur at increased frequency compared with other patient populations.

PROTOZOAL INFECTIONS. Protozoal infections, particularly *Pneumocystis carinii pneumonia*, are the most common AIDS-related opportunistic infections in patients in the United States. *Pneumocystis carinii* pneumonia (see Ch. 386) accounts for over one half of all initial AIDS diagnoses. Symptoms at presentation generally include fever, nonproductive cough, dyspnea at rest or on exertion, and chest tightness. The time course of symptoms may range from several days to months, and the onset may be insidious or rapidly progressive. Although the chest radiograph in *Pneumocystis carinii* pneumonia generally shows increased bronchovascular and interstitial markings typical of a bilateral diffuse infiltrate, about 5 to 10 per cent of patients will have an apparently normal chest radiograph. Noninvasive studies that are helpful in the presence of a normal chest radiograph include pulmonary function testing and gallium scanning. There is generally a severely restrictive profile, an increased alveolar arterial oxygen gradient, and a decreased diffusion capacity of carbon monoxide in infected patients. The pulmonary gallium scan reveals diffusely increased uptake of the isotope in more than 95 per cent of cases. Pleural effusion or mediastinal adenopathy should suggest a secondary process, since they are rarely associated with *Pneumocystis carinii* infection alone.

Although a microbiologic diagnosis of *Pneumocystis carinii* infection can be made on a transbronchial biopsy specimen, bronchoalveolar lavage is as sensitive and less invasive than transbronchial biopsy. In some cases, *Pneumocystis* infection can be diagnosed in expectorated sputum. Serologic testing is not sufficient for the diagnosis, and empiric therapy for *Pneumocystis* infection should be avoided because of frequent drug toxicity. Two antibiotics, trimethoprim-sulfamethoxazole and pentamidine isethionate, are the mainstays of therapy (see Table 346–3 and Ch. 386). A 21-day course of therapy with either drug is recommended for AIDS-related *Pneumocystis* pneumonia, but a shorter course of 10 to 14 days may be effective in some cases. Both drugs have appreciable

TABLE 346–3. TREATMENT OF FREQUENTLY ENCOUNTERED INFECTIONS IN AIDS

Infection	Treatment	Toxicity	Comment
Candida	Clotrimazole, oral troche 5 times/day for 10 days to indefinite time	Negligible	Chronic suppression with 1–3 troches per day
Thrush	Nystatin vaginal suppository melted orally t.i.d.–q.i.d.	Negligible	Unpleasant taste, poor compliance
	Nystatin suspension, 100,000 units/ml–5 ml swish and swallow q.i.d.		
	Nystatin powder (to dentures)		May be used in conjunction with other therapies
	Ketoconazole, 200 mg p.o. b.i.d.	Hepatitis, endocrine dysfunction	For refractory cases, maintain at 200 mg q.d. or t.i.w.
Esophagitis	Ketoconazole, 200 mg p.o. b.i.d. *or*	As above	
	Amphotericin 0.3 mg/kg day × 3–10 days	As for cryptococcus	
Disseminated	Amphotericin 0.3–0.6 mg/kg/day	As for cryptococcus	
Cryptococcus	Amphotericin (AMB) 0.3–0.5 mg/kg/day IV *plus*	AMB: Azotemia Hypokalemia	Poor cerebrospinal fluid penetration Intrathecal therapy not established for routine use
Meningitis Fungemia Pneumonia	5-Fluorocytosine (5FC), p.o. 150 mg/kg/day in 4 doses Treat for at least 6 weeks	Marrow suppression Hypomagnesemia Fever and chills Thrombophlebitis 5FC: Rash Marrow suppression Hepatitis	Maintenance therapy advised but specific treatment programs not studied
Cryptosporidium	None established Supportive care: Fluids Antispasmodics Analgesics		No effective therapy in clinical or animal studies Spiramycin possibly effective in some cases
Cytomegalovirus (CMV) Pneumonia Encephalitis Esophagitis Colitis Adrenalitis Retinitis	None established; BW759 (DHPG) experimental	Neutropenia Rash Testicular atrophy	Experimental No effective therapy commercially available Acyclovir is not effective for CMV infection

TABLE 346–3. TREATMENT OF FREQUENTLY ENCOUNTERED INFECTIONS IN AIDS *Continued*

Infection	Treatment	Toxicity	Comment
Herpes simplex			
Severe cutaneous disease	Acyclovir, 200 mg p.o. 5 times/day for 10 days	Negligible	Response to therapy may be dramatic No treatment trials in AIDS
Esophagitis or disseminated (non-[CNS] central nervous system)	Acyclovir, intravenous 5–7.5 mg/kg t.i.d. for 7–14 days	Crystalluria rare Occasional CNS changes	
Encephalitis	Acyclovir, 10 mg/kg q. 8 hr IV*	Rash Chemical hepatitis Azotemia (mild) Crystalluria CNS changes Herpes zoster (rare)	Vidabarine, 15 mg/kg/day over 12 hours for 10 days Less effective and more toxic
Disseminated	Acyclovir, 10 mg/kg t.i.d. IV for 7 days	As above	Role of acyclovir for cutaneous disease or prevention of dissemination not established in this population
Isospora belli	Furazolidone, 100 mg q.i.d. × 4 weeks Trimethoprim-sulfamethoxazide	Gastrointestinal (GI) upset As for *pneumocystis*	Effective in 5–15% of patients treated
Mycobacterium tuberculosis Pulmonary Disseminated	Choose from isoniazid (INH), rifampin, ethambutol, pyrazinamide, streptomycin, depending on sensitivity	Toxicities as established in conventional cases	Treatment in AIDS patients same as in other hosts—see Ch. 302 Use pyridoxine, 50 mg q.d., in patients on INH
Mycobacterium avium complex Disseminated (bone marrow, lung, blood, lymph node)	Five drugs from among INH, rifampin, ethambutol, cycloserine, ethionamide, amikacin	As established in other populations	Not enough cumulative data to establish any unique frequency of adverse effects in AIDS patients; prognosis poor even with aggressive therapy
	Ansamycin (experimental), 150–300 mg p.o. daily	Similar to rifampin	Available to specific investigators through Centers for Disease Control, Atlanta, Georgia
	Clofazimine (experimental), 100–200 mg/day p.o.	Abdominal pain, blue discoloration of skin	Experimental Used in treatment of leprosy Often used in conjunction with ansamycin Efficacy not established
Pneumocystis carinii	Trimethoprim-sulfamethoxazole, 20/100 mg/kg/day in 4 doses IV or p.o. Treat for 2–3 weeks	Rash Neutropenia Thrombocytopenia Hepatitis Azotemia	Mean time to toxicity is 10 days Switch to alternative drug required in 50–60% Monitor: CBC, platelets, liver function tests, creatinine
	Pentamidine isethionate, 4 mg/kg/day or IV infusion, 1–2 hours daily; IM may be used Treat for at least 2 weeks	Neutropenia Thrombocytopenia Hepatitis Azotemia Hypoglycemia Diabetes (rare) Hypotension Pain at IM injection site	Mean toxicity in 10 days Switch to other drug often necessary Monitor: CBC, platelets, liver function tests, creatinine, glucose, blood pressure
Salmonella Septicemia	Ampicillin Trimethoprim-sulfamethoxazole Chloramphenicol, depending on sensitivity	Trimethoprim-sulfamethoxazole, as in *Pneumocystis* infection	Relapse common even on suppressive antibiotics
Toxoplasma gondii	Pyrimethamine, 25 mg per day p.o. with 50–100 mg loading if WBC normal *plus*	Thrombocytopenia Neutropenia Rash	Rapid resolution of CNS lesions in those who recover; relapse common; sustained treatment required; dose may be modified for chronic treatment; only oral therapy available
	Sulfadiazine, 1–1.5 gm p.o. q.i.d. with 2–4 gm load if white blood cells (WBC) normal *with* Folinic acid, 10 mg q.d. Treatment for at least 6–10 wk suppressive therapy indefinite	Thrombocytopenia Neutropenia Rash (may be severe)	

*May exceed manufacturer's recommended dosage.

toxicity (see Ch. 386). The use of these drugs prophylactically is controversial and under investigation. Other antibiotics, including dapsone and difluoromethornithine (DFMO), are being studied for their efficacy.

Toxoplasma gondii (see Ch. 385) is one of the most common causes of central nervous system infection in AIDS patients. Clinical presentation often includes focal or diffuse seizures, mental status change, or focal neurologic deficits resembling stroke. Serologic testing for toxoplasmosis is insensitive and nonspecific, so that microbiologic confirmation is required. Brain biopsy should be performed if the patient is able to undergo the procedure, although some patients, particularly those with lesions deep in the cortex, are empirically treated. Computed tomographic (CT) scans of the brain generally show multiple lesions with ring enhancement deep in brain tissue. Although such lesions are highly suggestive of toxoplasmosis in this population, a similar radiologic picture may be seen with central nervous system lymphoma. Therapy for toxoplasmosis is discussed in Ch. 385.

Another less common protozoa in AIDS patients is *Cryptosporidium* (See Ch. 387). This parasite may produce a self-limited diarrheal illness in animals and immunocompetent persons. In AIDS patients, *Cryptosporidium* infection generally results in a sustained, profuse diarrhea that leads to malabsorption and inanition. Occasionally, the parasite may be found in the lungs or gallbladder and can produce a picture of biliary tract obstruction. Identification of *Cryptosporidium* requires careful analysis of stools and a sugar flotation test. No effective therapy has been found to date. Spiramycin,* a macrolide antibiotic not yet commercially available, has been used experimentally but with limited efficacy. Therapy is generally supportive, with fluid replacement and control of bowel motility with antidiarrheal agents. Another coccidian parasite, *Isospora belli*, may also be seen in AIDS. It is generally invasive and produces a severe diarrhea clinically indistinguishable from that caused by *Cryptosporidium*. Therapy is also supportive, without specific effective antibiotics.

FUNGAL INFECTIONS. *Oral candidiasis* (thrush) (see Ch. 375) is a frequent manifestation in AIDS and ARC. In patients at risk for AIDS, oral candidiasis is strongly indicative of subsequent development of overt AIDS. However, only invasive esophageal candidiasis, not simply thrush, fulfills the current surveillance definition of AIDS. Disseminated candidiasis, particularly candidemia, is unusual in AIDS patients. Several therapeutic approaches have been taken to oral candidiasis, including administration of clotrimazole, nystatin, and ketoconazole. Maintenance therapy is frequently required to suppress oral candidiasis. Esophageal candidiasis is often suspected clinically, if dysphagia is present. Nearly all patients with esophageal candidiasis have oral thrush. Therapy with low doses of amphotericin B or high doses of ketoconazole has been effective for esophageal candidiasis.

Cryptococcal meningitis (see Ch. 373) is not infrequent in AIDS patients, generally presenting with fever, severe headache, and mental status changes. The meninges are the sole site of the cryptococcal infection in nearly 75 per cent of such cases, although concurrent or isolated cryptococcal infection of blood, lungs, or other sites may occur. Diagnosis is greatly assisted by positive cryptococcal antigen response or positive culture results, or both. In nearly one half of cases of meningitis, the cerebrospinal fluid may not show marked pleocytosis or elevation of protein. Therapy has generally involved amphotericin B with or without 5-fluorocytosine for at least six weeks. Because of the high rate of relapse, many patients are maintained on weekly amphotericin B.

Other fungal infections, such as *histoplasmosis* (Ch. 369), *coccidioidomycosis* (Ch. 370), and *aspergillosis* (Ch. 376), have been reported in AIDS patients. The number of cases is too small to evaluate therapeutic outcome, although there appears to be a high rate of relapse, particularly with histoplasmosis, following amphotericin B therapy.

MYCOBACTERIA INFECTIONS. *Mycobacterium avium-intracellulare* (see Ch. 303) is a frequent isolate in sputum, blood, urine, and feces of AIDS patients. It is found in multiple sites in nearly one half of AIDS patients at autopsy. Its clinical significance is controversial. Because it may occur with other opportunistic infections and neoplasms, it may be difficult to attribute fever, anorexia, weight loss, and gastrointestinal dysfunction directly to it. Nonetheless, in some patients it does appear to account for these symptoms as well as hepatosplenomegaly and bone marrow failure. *Mycobacterium avium-intracellulare* is generally resistant to standard antituberculous therapy. Although there is sensitivity in vitro to experimental agents such as ansamycin and clofazimine, they rarely suppress blood culture positivity for the organism or eliminate organ invasion.

Mycobacterium tuberculosis (see Ch. 302) is being seen with increased frequency in HIV-infected individuals. This is particularly true among persons from endemic areas such as Haiti. In patients with AIDS, *Mycobacterium* tuberculosis is often disseminated, and the organism may even be recovered from blood. Response to standard antituberculous therapy is

generally good. Some AIDS patients may present with extrapulmonary tuberculosis, particularly cervical lymphadenopathy reminiscent of scrofula. Such involvement is generally easily treated with standard antituberculous therapy despite the underlying cellular immunodeficiency.

BACTERIAL INFECTIONS. *Salmonella infections* with bacteremia or sustained bowel carriage with diarrhea, or both, are frequent in AIDS patients. The rate of recurrence of *Salmonella* infections after standard antibiotic therapy is high. Recurrence may occur despite maintenance antibiotic therapy.

Pyogenic infections, although relatively uncommon in AIDS patients, may occur with frequent relapses. This is particularly true for *Hemophilus influenzae* and severe *pneumococcal* infections. Patients with AIDS are not immunologically competent to respond to pneumococcal vaccine, and it is unlikely that attempts at vaccination are indicated. Some patients require maintenance antibiotics for prophylaxis against relapse. Such infections illustrate the humoral (B lymphocyte) dysfunction in AIDS in addition to the cellular (T lymphocyte and monocyte-macrophage) immunodeficiency.

VIRAL INFECTIONS. *Herpes simplex* (see Ch. 340) is frequent in patients with AIDS and ARC. Severe cutaneous herpes simplex persisting for greater than four weeks satisfies the diagnostic criterion for AIDS. This infection may be the initial presentation only or may be an ongoing problem throughout the course of the illness. Herpes simplex may also involve the oral mucosa and face and occasionally results in encephalitis, myelitis, and pneumonia. Acyclovir, given either intravenously or orally, may reduce viral shedding, facilitate healing of lesions, and occasionally serve as prophylaxis for patients with severe, recurrent, invasive herpes simplex. *Herpes zoster* infection is also frequent in patients with AIDS or ARC. There are few data on frequency of dissemination or on incidence of postherpetic neuralgia.

Cytomegalovirus (CMV) (see Ch. 341) is a very frequent pathogen in patients with AIDS. It is often difficult to distinguish between colonization and invasive disease. At bronchoscopy, more than one third of patients with interstitial pneumonia have CMV cultured from the lavage fluid; a much smaller proportion have histologic evidence of tissue invasion. In preliminary studies, the presence of CMV at bronchoscopy had no clear effect on survival in patients with *Pneumocystis carinii* pneumonia. Cytomegalovirus is significantly associated with symptomatic retinitis, adrenalitis, colitis, and encephalitis in AIDS. An experimental nucleoside analogue, dihydroxymethyl propoxymethylguanine (DHPG) has been generally successful in suppressing progression of CMV retinitis and colitis but shows less clear benefit in CMV pneumonitis and encephalitis. Bone marrow suppression is the major toxicity seen with DHPG. There is a very high rate of relapse of cytomegalovirus retinitis following discontinuation of the drug. Many patients require sustained intravenous therapy.

Other viral infections, such as *hepatitis B, hepatitis A, non-A, non-B hepatitis*, and *Epstein-Barr* infection, are all frequent in populations at high risk for HIV. The clinical outcome is similar to that in individuals not infected with HIV.

Neoplasms Associated with HIV Infection. *Kaposi's sarcoma* (see Ch. 534), one of the initial manifestations of AIDS, remains a component of the syndrome. In general, patients with Kaposi's sarcoma who have not had an opportunistic infection are less severely immunocompromised than those who have had such infections. Prior to the AIDS epidemic, there was considerable speculation that classic Kaposi's sarcoma in the West might be associated with underlying cellular immunodeficiency, as was seen in immunocompromised individuals who had undergone renal transplantation or who had received therapy for lymphoma. Anecdotal reports of resolution of Kaposi's sarcoma in renal allograft recipients following discontinuation of immunosuppressive therapy further supported the suspected relationship.

Kaposi's sarcoma occurs in nearly one half of homosexual

---

*Available from the National Information Center for Orphan Drugs and Rare Diseases, Washington, DC.

males with AIDS but in only about 10 per cent of heterosexual patients. Although there has been considerable speculation that CMV or environmental toxins, such as recreational nitrites popular in the male homosexual community, could contribute to the development of the neoplasm, there are few compelling data to identify a factor with the sarcoma.

The clinical spectrum and natural history of Kaposi's sarcoma in AIDS are quite wide ranging, probably reflecting a variable degree of immune dysfunction. Patients usually present with mucocutaneous lesions or lymph node involvement. Lesions on the face and in the oral cavity are particularly common. Visceral lesions, particularly in the gastrointestinal tract, occur in nearly one half of patients but are usually clinically silent. The skin or mucous membrane lesions are usually red or purple, do not blanch on pressure, and may appear as round or elliptical papules, plaques, or nodules. Occasionally lesions are linear and follow cutaneous lymphatics. The lesions are generally painless in the early stages of the disease, but pain may occur, particularly in the lower extremities, with extensive lesions and development of lymphedema. Pulmonary Kaposi's sarcoma is usually very aggressive and may be confused with *Pneumocystis carinii* pneumonia, since both present with interstitial infiltrates and fever. The pulmonary gallium scan is generally negative in Kaposi's sarcoma in the absence of concurrent infection. Furthermore, pleural effusions are more common with pulmonary Kaposi's sarcoma than with *Pneumocystis carinii* infection. The prognosis is extremely poor, with survival generally measured in several weeks to a few months.

Most striking is the variable natural history of Kaposi's sarcoma in AIDS patients. Some have remarkably indolent lesions without disease progression for months to years. Other patients have rapidly advancing lesions that may extend over the integument and involve viscera. At the time of initial diagnosis, prediction of clinical course may be difficult, but factors that indicate disease progression and short survival include a history of prior opportunistic infection, constitutional symptoms, absolute T helper lymphocyte count below 100 per cubic millimeter, and pulmonary involvement.

Therapy in AIDS-related Kaposi's sarcoma is controversial because of the variable natural history of the illness and the concern that treatment could exacerbate the underlying immunodeficiency. Alpha-interferon therapy has resulted in an objective response rate of between 30 and 40 per cent; single-agent chemotherapy with vinblastine or doxorubicin achieves similar results. A subset of patients with Kaposi's sarcoma treated with recombinant alpha-interferon has not developed opportunistic infections and has survived nearly three years. It is unclear whether this course represents the natural history of disease in these individuals or is a direct benefit of interferon therapy. In some patients with large erosive or painful lesions, particularly those on the lower extremities causing lymphedema, or on the face, radiation therapy with doses between 1800 and 3000 rads affords effective palliation.

Non-Hodgkin's lymphoma of B lymphocyte origin associated with HIV infection is now a diagnostic criterion for AIDS. It appears that Epstein-Barr virus may have a role in the pathogenesis of these lymphomas. There are no data to support HIV infection of B lymphocytes in these cases. Aggressive B lymphocyte lymphomas had been previously observed in association with abnormal cellular immunity, in patients with liver and kidney transplantation, and in congenital immunodeficiency disorders. Many patients with AIDS and non-Hodgkin's lymphoma have a history of generalized lymphadenopathy. Lymph node biopsies in these patients frequently initially demonstrated follicular hyperplasia. Extranodal sites of lymphoma are frequent in AIDS patients. Central nervous system lymphoma, again previously reported in immunocompromised patients without AIDS, is frequent in AIDS patients. There is often involvement of bone marrow, gastrointestinal tract, and liver. Histopathologically, B lymphocyte lymphoma in AIDS is often large cell, undifferentiated, or immunoblastic sarcoma. The growth rate of these lymphomas may be quite rapid, with clinical doubling occurring in weeks, reminiscent of African Burkitt's lymphoma. Although patients have been treated with combination regimens that have benefited those with aggressive B lymphocyte lymphoma in other settings, death occurs in greater than 90 per cent of AIDS patients.

There is accumulating evidence linking HIV infection with *Hodgkin's disease* in homosexual men. Although not yet accepted as a diagnostic criterion for AIDS, Hodgkin's disease may occur at an increased frequency in HIV-infected men and presents with a clinical picture different from that of classic Hodgkin's disease. The major histopathologic types are nodular sclerosing and mixed cellularity. The disease is often advanced with stage IIIB and IVB presentations and extralymphatic involvement of skin, liver, and bone marrow. In contrast to classic Hodgkin's disease, involvement of mesenteric nodes is common. Although Hodgkin's disease in HIV-infected homosexual men responds well to conventional combination chemotherapy, there are often prolonged pancytopenia and complications with secondary opportunistic infections are frequent. Often these opportunistic infections limit achievement of complete remission and result in death.

Neurologic Disorders. Neuropsychiatric abnormalities, particularly cognitive dysfunction, memory loss, and mild dementia, have a high incidence in patients with AIDS and ARC. The encephalopathy may progress to severe cortical dysfunction. Chronic meningitis has been described, characterized by cerebrospinal fluid with a mild lymphocytic pleocytosis and elevated protein and normal glucose levels. HIV meningitis is diagnosed by ruling out other causes of meningitis and, if available, by direct culture of the retrovirus from CSF. Spinal cord abnormalities with vacuolar myelopathy, as well as peripheral neuropathy, are also frequent complications of HIV. Therapy in these cases is supportive. Progressive, multifocal leukoencephalopathy, perhaps due to the Creutzfeldt-Jakob virus, has also been reported in AIDS patients.

THERAPY AND PUBLIC HEALTH RECOMMENDATIONS REGARDING HIV. The care of patients with AIDS is at present largely symptomatic and supportive, with specific therapy for opportunistic infections and Kaposi's sarcoma, as discussed earlier in this chapter. Therapy for HIV infection itself is experimental. The life cycle of HIV reveals several potential targets for therapeutic agents. The most prominent initial success has been achieved with azidothymidine, which is an inhibitor of HIV reverse transcriptase. Azidothymidine increases survival and prevents development of recurrent opportunistic infections when compared with placebo in patients with AIDS who had recently recovered from their first episode of *Pneumocystis carinii* pneumonia. Approximately 50 per cent of those receiving AZT for 6 months or longer require frequent transfusions. Current clinical trials include testing of azidothymidine in patients with other manifestations of AIDS, as well as in earlier stages of HIV infection, such as ARC. Recombinant alpha$_{2a}$ interferon has a direct antiviral effect in vitro, probably via disruption of assembly of the virion. Immunomodulatory agents, such as interleukin-2 and colony-stimulating factor, are being tested as single agents and, in the near future, in combination with reverse transcriptase inhibitors such as azidothymidine. The feasibility of immune reconstitution in AIDS patients may be assessed in syngeneic (identical twin) bone marrow transplantation with antiretroviral therapy of the AIDS patient, who then receives normal, but genetically identical, marrow stem cells from his or her sibling. Ultimate therapy of AIDS will probably require several agents that act on different parts of the life cycle of HIV as well as drugs that foster immune reconstitution. To date, no treatment has been identified as a "cure" for AIDS. It is likely that beneficial therapy would be chronic, involving suppression of HIV for sufficiently long periods of time to allow immune reconstitution to occur.

Persons who are infected with HIV and are asymptomatic should be vigorously counseled with respect to restricting sexual behavior that could transmit the virus, avoidance of donation of blood products, deferral of pregnancy, and cessation of intravenous drug abuse.

Barre-Sinoussi F, Chermann JC, Rey F, et al.: Isolation of a T-lymphotropic retrovirus from a patient at risk for acquired immune deficiency syndrome (AIDS). Science 220:868, 1983. Levy JA, Hoffman AD, Karmer SM, et al.: Isolation of lymphocytotropic retroviruses from San Francisco patients with AIDS. Science 225:840, 1984. Popovic M, Sarngadharan MG, Reed E, et al.: Detection, isolation, and continuous production of cytopathic retroviruses (HTLV-III) from patients with AIDS and pre-AIDS. Science 224:497, 1984. *These three papers contain the initial descriptions of the etiologic agent of AIDS, now termed human immunodeficiency virus.*

Classification system for human T-lymphotropic virus type III/lymphadenopathy associated virus infections. MMWR 35:334, 1986. *The most useful current classification of HIV disorders.*

Clavel F, Mansinhok K, Chamaret S, et al.: Human immunodeficiency virus type 2 infection associated with AIDS in West Africa. N Engl J Med 316:1180, 1987. *First report that some cases of AIDS in West Africa are associated with HIV-2 rather than HIV-1.*

Cooper DA, MacLean P, Finlayson R, et al.: Acute AIDS retrovirus infection: Definition of a clinical illness associated with seroconversion. Lancet 1:537, 1985. Ho DD, Sarngadharan MG, Resnick L, et al.: Primary human T-lymphotropic virus type III infection. Ann Intern Med 103:880, 1985. *Clinical descriptions of acute HIV infection; important for clinicians to recognize this entity.*

De Vita VT, Broder S, Fauci AS, et al.: Developmental therapeutics and the acquired immunodeficiency syndrome. Ann Intern Med 106:568, 1987. *An NIH conference on antiviral drugs, immune modulators, and opportunistic infections in AIDS.*

Fauci AS, Masur H, Gelmann EP, et al.: The acquired immunodeficiency syndrome: An update. Ann Intern Med 102:800, 1985. International Conference on AIDS: Ann Intern Med 103:653, 1985. *These two publications present excellent comprehensive reviews of etiology, pathogenesis, and clinical manifestations of AIDS and related disorders.*

Francis D, Pettricianni J: The prospects for and pathways toward a vaccine for AIDS. N Engl J Med 313:1586, 1985. *These two articles present the scientific basis for ultimate development of an AIDS vaccine.*

Groopman JE, Salahuddin SZ, Sarngadharan MG, et al.: Virologic studies in a case of transfusion-associated AIDS. N Engl J Med 311:1419, 1984. *Detailed case report demonstrating HIV as necessary and sufficient for the development of AIDS.*

Lasky LA, Groopman JE, Fennie CW, et al.: Neutralization of the AIDS retrovirus by antibodies to a recombinant envelope glycoprotein. Science 233:209, 1986.

Enteroviral Diseases

Raphael Dolin

347 INTRODUCTION

Enteroviruses cause a wide variety of diseases in humans and other mammals. These viral agents compose a separate genus (enterovirus) within the picornavirus (*pico*, small; *rna*, ribonucleic acid) family and share the following common properties: (1) size of 17 to 30 nm, (2) capsids with cubic symmetry, (3) RNA genome, and (4) four major structural polypeptides. The virion lacks a lipid envelope; hence the viruses are resistant to lipid solvents.

Enteroviruses have been historically subdivided into *polioviruses, groups A* and *B coxsackieviruses,* and *echoviruses.* These divisions were based on antigenic relationships and differences in host range. Sixty-seven distinct immunotypes (species) were originally identified, although these have been reduced to 63 because of reclassification and redundancy in numbering. However, this classification is not entirely satisfactory, since several enteroviruses have properties that overlap groups defined by the criteria cited above. Therefore, newly recognized enteroviruses are no longer classified as echoviruses or coxsackieviruses but are simply designated "enterovirus" and are numbered sequentially beginning with enterovirus 68. To avoid confusion within the older literature, the previous classification (coxsackievirus groups A and B, and echovirus) have been retained for the 63 original immunotypes (Table 347–1).

Since infections with polioviruses are presented in Ch. 486, this discussion will be limited to consideration of nonpolio enteroviruses.

CHARACTERISTICS OF NONPOLIO ENTEROVIRUSES

COXSACKIEVIRUSES. Coxsackieviruses were originally isolated from stools of children who were suffering from paralytic poliomyelitis in Coxsackie, New York. Unlike polioviruses, these viruses caused disease in suckling mice and were therefore presumed to be distinct from polioviruses (see Table 347–1). Subsequently, additional coxsackievirus immunotypes have been isolated from widespread geographic locations. These viruses are divided into two groups, A and B, depending on the histopathology of lesions induced in mice. Group A coxsackieviruses produce a generalized myositis of skeletal muscle, which results in flaccid paralysis. Group B coxsackieviruses produce a focal myositis and a generalized infection of brown fat, myocardium, pancreas, and central nervous system, which results in spastic paralysis. Group B coxsackieviruses can be readily cultivated in primate tissue culture, whereas group A coxsackieviruses grow inconsistently or not at all in tissue culture. Twenty-three immunotypes of group A and six of group B have been identified.

ECHOVIRUSES. Echoviruses were first isolated from the stools of healthy children but were not pathogenic for primates or suckling mice. They were given the acronym echo (*e*nteric *c*ytopathic *h*uman *o*rphan), indicating that they were not associated with disease. Subsequently, a variety of diseases have been associated with echoviruses, and 31 immunotypes have been recognized. Most echoviruses can be readily cultivated in tissue culture (see Table 347–1).

NEWLY RECOGNIZED ENTEROVIRUSES. Four newly recognized enteroviruses, immunotypes 68 to 71, have been reported since the adoption of the new classification schema. Illnesses produced by enteroviruses 68 and 71 are similar to those produced by coxsackieviruses and echoviruses (Table 347–2). Enterovirus 70 causes acute hemorrhagic conjunctivitis and is discussed in Ch. 351. Enterovirus 69 has not as yet been associated with illness. In addition, hepatitis A virus has now been demonstrated to have the biophysical properties of enteroviruses and has been designated as enterovirus 72. Hepatitis A infections are discussed in Ch. 121.

GENERAL FEATURES OF NONPOLIO ENTEROVIRAL INFECTIONS

EPIDEMIOLOGY. Enteroviruses have a worldwide distribution. In temperate climates, the incidence of infection and illness is markedly increased in the summer and early fall, although enterovirus-associated disease has been reported at other times as well. In tropical climates, enterovirus infections occur throughout the year. The prevalence of individual immunotypes varies widely according to geographic locale and year. Generally, one or two immunotypes account for the bulk of enterovirus-induced disease during any given season, but occasionally multiple immunotypes may be equally prevalent. Because of the prolonged shedding of virus from the gastrointestinal tract (see below), the presence of enteroviruses in surface waters and in sewage is a good indicator of the prevalence of infection in the community.

Transmission of enteroviruses is primarily by the fecal-oral route, and the frequency of infection is increased by factors that promote such transmission, e.g., poor hygiene and low socioeconomic status. Young children have the highest attack rates and serve as the vehicles for spread within communities. Once infection occurs within a family, susceptible (nonim-

TABLE 347–1. CHARACTERISTICS OF HUMAN ENTEROVIRUSES

Virus	Number of Immunotypes	Numerical Designation	Isolated in Tissue Culture	Pathogenic for Suckling Mice	Pathogenic for Primates
Polioviruses	3	1–3	Yes	No	Yes
Coxsackieviruses A	23	A1–A24*	Occasionally†	Yes	No‡
Coxsackieviruses B	6	B1–B6	Yes	Yes	No
Echoviruses	31	1–34§	Yes	No	No
Enteroviruses	5	68–72¶	Yes	Variable	Variable

*A23 has been reclassified as echovirus 9.
†Primary isolation in tissue culture is difficult for most immunotypes except A7, 11, 13, 15, 16, 18, 20, and 21.
‡Coxsackie A7 is neuropathogenic for monkeys.
§Echovirus 10 is reovirus 1; echovirus 28 is rhinovirus 1A; echovirus 34 is a variant of coxsackievirus A24.
¶Enteroviruses 70 and 71 are neuropathogenic for monkeys; enterovirus 72 (hepatitis A virus) is pathogenic for monkeys.

mune) family members are rapidly infected. Coxsackievirus infections appear to be somewhat more communicable than echovirus infections.

PATHOGENESIS AND CLINICAL MANIFESTATIONS. Models of the pathogenesis of enteroviral infection are based largely on studies with polioviruses. However, the pathogenesis of nonpolio enteroviral infection appears to be similar, except for the major organs that are affected. Initial replication of the virus takes place in the oropharynx or in the gastrointestinal tract. Viral infection may be limited to the mucosa or may proceed deeper into lymphoid tissue. The latter may be followed by viremia and dissemination of virus to distant organs, such as the heart or the central nervous system. The marked variation in clinical manifestations associated with nonpolio enteroviral infection reflects the relative involvement of different target organs (Table 347–2).

The bulk of enteroviral infections (50 to 80 per cent) are asymptomatic, and many of the remainder consist of "undifferentiated febrile illnesses," often with respiratory symptoms. The latter illnesses are generally mild and last a few days. The enterovirus infections most frequently coming to the attention of a physician are those resulting in central nervous system, heart, or skin involvement. Enteroviruses have been associated with a wide variety of clinical syndromes referable to those organ systems (Table 347–2), the most important of which are discussed below. As with "undifferentiated febrile illnesses," these syndromes are rarely sufficiently distinct to permit diagnosis of infection with a particular immunotype. Immunotypes from different groups can produce similar syndromes, and alternatively a single immunotype can produce clinically diverse illnesses. Thus, coxsackievirus B1 can induce aseptic meningitis in one patient and pericarditis in another, even during the same outbreak. The factors that determine which clinical manifestation will be expressed in any individual infection are poorly understood.

LABORATORY DIAGNOSIS. Laboratory diagnosis is based on virus isolation and/or immunotype-specific antibody rises in acute and convalescent serum specimens. Enteroviruses can frequently be isolated from throat secretions and stools obtained from patients with enteroviral infections. Such isolations are most frequent in young children, particularly in lower socioeconomic groups. However, interpretation of the significance of such isolates in individual cases is difficult. Intercurrent subclinical infections or prolonged fecal shedding of virus (up to three months) may occur, so that an etiologic association between an isolate and a current disease episode cannot be made with certainty. A rising titer of immunotype-specific antibodies in acute and convalescent sera indicates that a recent infection has taken place but similarly does not assign an etiologic role to the virus in question. The strongest evidence for enteroviruses as etiologic agents of a variety of diseases originates from two sources: (1) large-scale studies in which isolation rates from cases are matched with controls and (2) isolation of virus from sites from which asymptomatic shedding of virus does not occur, e.g., cerebrospinal fluid, myocardium, or pericardial fluid. In this regard, virus culture of blood has been reported to be useful in infants with enterovirus-related illness.

Serologic diagnosis of enteroviral infections is particularly difficult because group-specific tests, such as complement fixation, do not exist, and thus immunotype-specific neutralization tests must be carried out. Since there are 68 currently recognized immunotypes, neutralization tests against all potential agents cannot be performed. Of necessity, neutralization tests must be limited to those directed against the patient's isolate (if one is present) or perhaps against isolates prevalent in the community. A possible exception is the case in which only a few immunotypes are likely to be present (e.g., hand-foot-and-mouth disease—coxsackievirus A16; myocarditis—coxsackieviruses B1 to 6). In addition, patients may be seen late in the course of illness, at which time high, stable antibody titers are present, which further reduces the utility of serologic tests.

PREVENTION AND TREATMENT. Highly successful live and inactivated virus vaccines directed against poliovirus infections have been developed (see Ch. 486). Immunity to nonpolio enteroviruses has been less well studied but appears to be similarly dependent on the presence of immunotype-specific local and humoral antibodies. Thus, the development of vaccines against these agents is theoretically possible. However, the large number of immunotypes among nonpolio enteroviruses (68), compared with polioviruses (3), and the

TABLE 347–2. ILLNESSES ASSOCIATED WITH NONPOLIO ENTEROVIRUSES*

Coxsackieviruses Group A	Coxsackieviruses Group B	Echoviruses	Enteroviruses
Asymptomatic infection	Asymptomatic infection	Asymptomatic infection	Asymptomatic infection
Undifferentiated febrile illness with or without respiratory symptoms; common cold (21, 24); pneumonitis of infants (9, 16)	Undifferentiated febrile illness with or without respiratory symptoms; upper respiratory tract infection and pneumonia (4, 5)	Undifferentiated febrile illness with or without respiratory symptoms (4, 9, 11, 20, 25)	Undifferentiated febrile illness with or without respiratory symptoms; pneumonia, bronchiolitis (68)
Aseptic meningitis (1-14, 16, 17, 21, 22, 24); rare paralysis or encephalitis (4-7, 9, 10, 16)	Aseptic meningitis (1-6); rare paralysis or encephalitis (2-5)	Aseptic meningitis (all); rare paralysis or encephalitis (all except 23, 26, 28, 29, 32)	Aseptic meningitis (70, 71); paralysis (70, 71)
Mucocutaneous infection: herpangina (2-6, 8, 10, 22); lymphonodular pharyngitis (10); hand-foot-and-mouth disease (5, 9, 10, 16); exanthem (4, 5, 6, 9, 16)	Myocarditis (1-5)†	Exanthem (2, 4, 6, 9, 11, 16, 18)	Acute hemorrhagic conjunctivitis (70)
	Pericarditis (1-5)†	Neonatal diarrhea (18)	Hand-foot-and-mouth disease (71)
	Pleurodynia (1-6)		Exanthem (71)
	Generalized disease of newborn (1-5)		Hepatitis A (72)
Acute hemorrhagic conjunctivitis (24)	Exanthem (1-5)		

*Immunotypes with strongest association are in parentheses.
†Myopericarditis has less frequently been associated with coxsackieviruses A1, 4, 9, and 16 and echoviruses 1, 3, 6 to 9, 11, 14, 19, 22, and 30.

benign nature of most enterovirus-induced disease have precluded the development of such vaccines.

Specific antiviral chemotherapy or chemoprophylaxis directed at enteroviral infection is not currently available. Treatment consists of symptomatic or supportive therapy for severe illness, particularly that involving the central nervous system or the heart (see below). However, the vast majority of enteroviral illnesses are self-limited and require no therapy. Appropriate control measures include maintenance of good hygienic practices, such as handwashing, and proper disposal of potentially infectious stools. Isolation of patients is impractical and rarely indicated.

Huang AS, Modlin JF: Picornaviridae. In Mandell GL, Douglas RG, Bennett JE (eds.): Principles and Practice of Infectious Diseases. New York, John Wiley & Sons, 1985, p 800. *An extensive review that covers the molecular biology, epidemiology, and clinical manifestations of enteroviral diseases. Contains an excellent bibliography.*

Melnick JL: Enteroviruses: Polioviruses, coxsackieviruses, echoviruses, and newer enteroviruses. In Fields BN (ed.): Virology. New York, Raven Press, 1985, p 739. *An up-to-date review with a comprehensive bibliography.*

Moore M: Enteroviral disease in the United States, 1970–1979. J Infect Dis 146:103, 1982. *A summary of the most recent ten-year experience of surveillance data from the Centers for Disease Control. Provides an excellent epidemiologic overview.*

NEUROLOGIC AND OTHER COMPLICATIONS OF NONPOLIO ENTEROVIRUSES

Paralysis has been rarely associated with nonpolio enteroviral infections. The majority of reported cases have been diagnosed on the basis of isolation of echoviruses and coxsackieviruses from stool, with relatively few isolations from central nervous system tissue or cerebrospinal fluid. Generally, muscle weakness rather than paralysis has been observed in these patients. When present, paralysis and weakness are generally less extensive than in poliomyelitis and tend to resolve with time. Cranial nerve and severe bulbar involvement have also been reported. Coxsackievirus A7 has been the immunotype most commonly implicated in paralytic disease, and small outbreaks have been recognized in the USSR and Scotland. A poliomyelitis-like syndrome has also been reported to accompany acute hemorrhagic conjunctivitis caused by enterovirus 70 (see Ch. 351). Enterovirus 71 has been recently associated with both small outbreaks and epidemics of central nervous system disease, including a substantial proportion of cases with paralysis and encephalitis. Other neurologic complications include transverse myelitis and the Guillain-Barré syndrome, although the precise relationship of these illnesses to enteroviral infection is unclear. Aseptic meningitis caused by coxsackieviruses and other enteroviruses is discussed in Ch. 484.

Infants, children, and occasionally young adults infected with nonpolio enteroviruses have developed encephalitis as manifested by seizures, coma, cerebellar ataxia, hemiplegia, or extrapyramidal movements. Up to 10 per cent of children who acquired enteroviral meningitis during the first year of life have developed mild mental retardation and spasticity, suggesting that involvement of central nervous system parenchyma may be more frequent than has previously been suspected. Echovirus infection of the central nervous system in agammaglobulinemic patients has resulted in a chronic meningoencephalitis associated with a dermatomyositis-like syndrome.

Enteroviruses have been associated with upper respiratory tract illness, primarily the "common cold syndrome," in both children and adults. Lower respiratory tract illness, including bronchitis, tracheitis, bronchiolitis, croup, and pneumonia, has been induced by enteroviruses in children, but infrequently in adults. The majority of respiratory tract symptoms have presented as part of the "undifferentiated febrile illness" or "summer grippe" associated with enteroviral infections (see Table 347–2). Coxsackievirus A21 has caused outbreaks of pharyngitis in military recruits and has induced respiratory tract disease in normal adult volunteers. Group B coxsackie-

viruses, enterovirus 68, and several echoviruses (chiefly echovirus 11) have also been implicated as causes of respiratory tract illness. Respiratory illness induced by enteroviruses cannot be differentiated on clinical grounds from that caused by respiratory tract viruses, such as rhinoviruses, parainfluenza viruses, respiratory syncytial virus, or adenoviruses. However, infection with the latter groups of viruses occurs most frequently during the winter months, whereas enterovirus infection is seen most frequently in the summer and early fall. Viral respiratory tract infections are discussed in Ch. 329 to 334.

Grist NR, Bell EJ: Enteroviral etiology of the paralytic poliomyelitis syndrome. Arch Environ Health 21:382, 1970. *A good review of the uncommon association of nonpolio enteroviruses with paralytic disease.*

Melnick JL: Enterovirus 71 infections: A varied clinical pattern sometimes mimicking paralytic poliomyelitis. Rev Infect Dis 6(Suppl):387, 1984. *A review of recent information associating enterovirus with central nervous system disease.*

Wilbert CM, Buckley RH, Mohanakumarz T, et al.: Persistent and fatal central nervous system echovirus infections in patients with agammaglobulinemia. N Engl J Med 296:1485, 1977. *A description of the syndrome of chronic echovirus central nervous system infection and dermatomyositis in patients with abnormal B cell function.*

348 EPIDEMIC PLEURODYNIA

DEFINITION. Epidemic pleurodynia (*pleura,* side; *odyne,* pain) (Bornholm disease, epidemic myalgia, devil's grip, Sylvest's Disease) is an acute febrile disease characterized by sudden, sharp chest (intercostal) or abdominal pain. Pain is paroxysmal in nature, and relapses frequently occur after periods of well-being.

ETIOLOGY. Group B coxsackieviruses (1 to 6) are the major causes of pleurodynia. Outbreaks have also been associated with echovirus 1, and sporadic cases with coxsackieviruses A4, A6, and A10 and echoviruses 1, 6, 9, and 19.

EPIDEMIOLOGY. Epidemic pleurodynia was first described in the mid-nineteenth century in Iceland and Norway. In 1933, Sylvest published a classic monograph describing the illness on the Danish island of Bornholm. Subsequently, outbreaks and sporadic cases have been described in many parts of the world. In contrast to the annual occurrence of aseptic meningitis, epidemics of pleurodynia occur much less frequently, often 10 to 20 years apart. As with other enteroviral infections, illness is most common in summer and early fall. Person-to-person transmission occurs, particularly within families, with incubation periods of two to five days. Attack rates are highest in children, but the peak incidence is at a somewhat older age (5 to 15 years) than with other enteroviral infections.

PATHOGENESIS. Although detailed studies of the histopathology of pleurodynia are not available, the infection appears to involve skeletal muscle rather than pleura or peritoneum. Often muscle tenderness and occasionally swelling can be noted at the site of pain. Hyperesthesia can be elicited over affected muscles as well. In contrast, pleural rubs have been infrequently and inconstantly noted, and peritonitis has not been present in cases that have come to laparotomy. However, coxsackievirus B has not been unequivocally isolated from affected muscle.

CLINICAL MANIFESTATIONS. Characteristically, pleurodynia begins as an abrupt paroxysm of pain, located over the lateral chest (ribs) or upper abdomen. The pain is of variable intensity, but can be severe, and is often described as "catching," "stabbing," "crushing," or "viselike." Acute shortness of breath is also frequently present. Adults most commonly have chest pain, whereas children more frequently have abdominal pain, generally in the epigastrium and upper abdomen. Patients have been described with pain primarily in the lower abdomen, as well as in the extremities. Prodromal symptoms are not present in the majority of cases, although up to 25 per cent of individuals report headache, malaise, myalgia, and sore throat prior to the onset of pain. Fever of 37.8 to 40.0°C is present at the onset of pain but resolves between paroxysms. Multiple paroxysms of pain occur and last from two to ten hours, during which time the patient may appear diaphoretic and acutely ill. The initial paroxysm of pain is most severe, and subsequent ones are generally milder. Splinting of the chest or guarding of the abdomen is usually observed, so that in one outbreak 9 of 49 patients underwent laparotomy before the disease was recognized. Tenderness or swelling of the affected muscles or both have been noted in up to 25 per cent of cases. During paroxysms, patients tend to lie quietly in bed and avoid any motion that may aggravate the pain. The patient may appear relatively well between bouts of pain.

Acute illness generally lasts one to six days, but a range of up to three weeks has been reported. Approximately 10 per cent of the patients experience at least one recurrence of pain within one or more months after the last paroxysm. Such recurrences often develop at the same site as the initial paroxysm of pain.

LABORATORY DIAGNOSIS. Specific diagnosis is made by isolation of coxsackievirus B from the throat or stools of acutely ill patients, along with rises in immunotype-specific neutralizing antibody titers in acute and convalescent sera. Detection of virus is most frequent in samples taken early in illness. Other laboratory tests are not helpful in making the diagnosis. White blood cell and differential counts are generally normal, although mild leukopenia has been reported in approximately 25 per cent of cases.

DIFFERENTIAL DIAGNOSIS. Because of the location of the pain, Bornholm disease can be confused with a variety of acute chest diseases, including pneumonia, pulmonary infarction, and myocardial ischemia. The absence of physical and roentgenographic signs of pulmonary infiltrates, the lack of sputum production, and a normal electrocardiogram help exclude these diagnoses. When the pain is primarily abdominal, differentiation from other causes of an acute abdominal pain can be difficult. The absence of signs of peritonitis and a normal white cell count may be helpful. The most useful distinguishing clinical feature of Bornholm disease is the paroxysmal nature of the pain. Epidemiologic information, such as the occurrence of a cluster of cases in the late summer, may also suggest the diagnosis.

PROGNOSIS AND TREATMENT. Patients with epidemic pleurodynia will eventually recover fully, although relapses are common. Occasionally, malaise or asthenia may persist for months after the acute illness. Complications may include a septic meningitis (3 to 7 per cent of cases), orchitis (fewer than 5 per cent), and rarely pericarditis.

Treatment is supportive and symptomatic. Episodes of acute pain can usually be controlled by salicylates or other mild analgesics. Occasionally, narcotics may be required for relief.

Finn JJ Jr, Weller TH, Morgan HR: Epidemic pleurodynia: Clinical and etiologic studies based on one hundred and fourteen cases. Arch Intern Med 83:305, 1949. *An excellent clinical review of the subject.*

Huebner RJ, Risser JA, Bell JA, et al.: Epidemic pleurodynia in Texas: A study of 22 cases. N Engl J Med 248:267, 1953. *Demonstration of the viral etiology of an outbreak of pleurodynia.*

Pickles NW: Sylvest's disease (Bornholm disease). N Engl J Med 250:1033, 1954. *A vivid and dramatic discussion of the clinical presentation.*

Sylvest E: Epidemic Myalgia: Bornholm Disease. London, Oxford University Press, 1934, pp 1–155. *The classic monograph in the field.*

349 MYOCARDITIS AND PERICARDITIS CAUSED BY ENTEROVIRUSES

Enteroviruses are well-recognized causes of myocarditis and pericarditis, with clinical manifestations that appear to be age dependent. Neonatal infection is a severe illness in which extensive involvement of the myocardium, widespread dissemination to other organs, and high fatality rates are seen. In older children and adults, pericarditis is most prominent, and the disease is generally self limited.

ETIOLOGY. The group B coxsackieviruses, immunotypes 1 to 5, are the enteroviruses most frequently implicated in pericarditis and myocarditis. Depending on the study, group B coxsackieviruses have been reported to cause from 3 to 44 per cent of cases of acute pericarditis and approximately 33 per cent of cases of acute myocarditis. Group A coxsackieviruses (1, 4, 9, and 16) and echoviruses (1, 3, 6 to 9, 19, and 22) have also been implicated, but considerably less frequently. Since routine serologic testing is available for group B, but not for group A coxsackieviruses or echoviruses, it is conceivable that the proportion of cases caused by the latter groups may be higher. The etiology of the majority of cases of "idiopathic" pericarditis and myocarditis remains unknown (see Ch. 53).

EPIDEMIOLOGY. Enteroviral myopericarditis occurs most frequently during the summer and early fall, and both epidemics and sporadic cases are seen. Neonatal myocarditis was first recognized in outbreaks in nurseries for the newborn in South Africa, Rhodesia, and the Netherlands in the mid 1950's. Subsequent reports have been largely confined to sporadic cases. Illness in nursery outbreaks appears to be postnatally acquired, presumably by the fecal-oral route. However, cases in which infection was acquired at birth and even in utero have been described. In the latter cases, infection of mothers appeared to take place within two weeks of delivery.

Among older children and adults, myopericardial involvement with enteroviral infection is sporadic, and even in the presence of outbreaks of enteroviral infection, myopericardial involvement in this age group is uncommon. Despite the likely over-reporting of serious infections, only 3 per cent of group B coxsackievirus infections reported to the World Health Organization involved the myocardium predominantly.

PATHOGENESIS. Infection of the heart by enteroviruses is most likely a result of viremia after initial replication of virus in the gastrointestinal tract. Histopathology of acute enteroviral myocarditis consists of a mixed polymorphonuclear leukocytic and lymphocytic infiltrate, which can be either diffuse or focal. Focal myocardial muscle degeneration and necrosis are also seen. The histopathology of enterovirus-induced pericarditis is similar and is frequently accompanied by focal areas of subepicardial myocarditis. For this reason, some authors prefer the term "myopericarditis" rather than simply "pericarditis."

During acute illness, virus may be isolated from myocardium, pericardium, or pericardial fluid, and therefore the pathogenesis appears to be direct viral invasion of myopericardium. However, chronic inflammatory lesions from which infectious virus cannot be isolated have been described in humans and in experimental myocarditis. Chronic lesions, and perhaps clinically apparent relapses, may have an immunopathologic basis. Direct evidence is lacking in humans, but in weanling mice the severity of coxsackie B3 myocarditis is increased by intact T lymphocyte functions.

CLINICAL MANIFESTATIONS. *Neonatal Myocarditis.* Myocarditis of the newborn presents from two days to three weeks after birth (mean of seven days) with the acute onset of fever and listlessness, often accompanied by coryza or diarrhea or both. When congestive heart failure is present, respiratory distress and tachycardia are prominent. In approximately one third of patients, a biphasic illness is seen. The first phase consists of a febrile prodrome followed by a period of well-being lasting one to seven days, after which the phase of clinically evident cardiac involvement appears. The latter is predominantly myocarditis with little or no pericarditis. Circulatory failure can develop rapidly and be profound, as manifested by cyanosis, abdominal distention, and edema. In addition, viral infection may be disseminated widely, with involvement of the central nervous system, lungs, liver, pancreas, spleen, and kidney. In cases of fulminant disease, death may ensue within 24 hours, although the majority of fatalities occur two to seven days after the onset of illness. Among survivors, cardiac function and general well-being improve rapidly once the fever and acute illness have resolved.

Myopericarditis of Older Children and Adults. In older children and adults, the clinical features of enteroviral infection of the heart are those of acute pericarditis as discussed in Ch. 53. Sixty to 90 per cent of patients present with fever and chest pain, preceded by an upper respiratory tract illness in approximately two thirds of cases. Dyspnea, malaise, myalgias, and arthralgias are frequently seen. Physical examination reveals a pericardial friction rub, often transient, in 35 to 75 per cent of cases. Pericardial effusions have been reported in 0 to 45 per cent of cases, but acute cardiac tamponade is rare. Increased areas of cardiac dullness and gallop rhythms have been reported in up to 25 per cent of patients in some series. Despite histopathologic evidence of subepicardial myocarditis accompanying pericarditis, clinically apparent congestive heart failure is unusual. When present, the latter indicates widespread myocardial involvement. Serologic evidence of enteroviral infection in cases clinically diagnosed as acute myocardial infarctions has been reported, but the etiologic role, if any, of viruses in that setting is unknown. Pleural effusions, particularly left-sided, have been reported in 20 to 50 per cent of cases of enterovirus-associated myopericarditis.

LABORATORY DIAGNOSIS. The etiology of illness is established by isolation of enterovirus from the myocardium, pericardium, or pericardial fluid. Isolation of virus from throat or stool cultures, along with rises in immunotype-specific serum antibodies, provides circumstantial evidence for the diagnosis of enteroviral myopericarditis. Diagnosis is difficult because patients often present late in the course of illness, when virus shedding has ceased, and when high, stable titers of antibodies are already present. In the last case, detection of immunotype-specific IgM antibodies indicates recent infection.

In myopericarditis an abnormal electrocardiogram (ECG) is seen in virtually all cases. Changes in pericarditis or mild myopericarditis are ST segment elevation and T wave flattening or inversion. In severe myocarditis, Q waves, conduction disturbances, and arrhythmias can be seen. In the latter cases, elevations of myocardial enzymes have been noted. Analyses of pericardial fluid in documented viral myopericarditis have been infrequent, but the characteristics of the fluid are gen-

erally those of an exudate, with a predominantly polymorphonuclear leukocytic content. Considerable overlap exists between the cell counts, differentials, and protein content of pericardial fluid in cases of viral pericarditis and these same values of fluid in cases of pericarditis of other etiologies.

Other laboratory tests are generally not helpful in establishing the diagnosis. A moderate polymorphonuclear leukocytosis may be present, and elevated erythrocyte sedimentation rates have been reported in 70 to 90 per cent of patients.

DIFFERENTIAL DIAGNOSIS. Neonatal myocarditis can mimic pneumonia, bacterial sepsis, or other disseminated viral infections such as those caused by herpes simplex and cytomegalovirus. The prominent ECG changes, evidence of congestive heart failure, and absence of skin lesions may be helpful in suggesting the diagnosis of neonatal myocarditis. The differential diagnosis of myopericarditis in older patients is discussed in Ch. 53 and 54.

PROGNOSIS. Neonatal myocarditis was initially reported to have an extremely high case-fatality rate; however, recent experience suggests that with aggressive supportive therapy, mortality is less than 50 per cent. Long-term follow-up of survivors is not available.

The majority of older children and adults with enteroviral myopericarditis recover without clinically apparent sequelae. The duration of illness is highly variable (days to weeks), and up to 20 per cent of patients experience one or more episodes of recurrent myopericarditis within one year of the initial illness. Electrocardiographic abnormalities may persist in 10 to 20 per cent of patients, and long-term cardiomegaly has been described in 5 to 10 per cent. Constrictive pericarditis is a rare complication. Chronic congestive heart failure also appears to be an unusual sequel of illness, although it occurred in 5 of 22 patients in one series. The role of enterovirus-induced myocarditis in chronic cardiomyopathies of unknown etiology remains controversial.

TREATMENT. Specific antiviral chemotherapy for enteroviral infections is not available. Management of patients with enteroviral myopericarditis consists primarily of control of pain with analgesics and treatment of arrhythmias or congestive heart failure as they appear. In experimentally induced myocarditis in mice, vigorous exercise is deleterious, and therefore bed rest or restriction of activity is frequently recommended to patients. Corticosteroids also increase the severity of infection in the same animal model, but anecdotal reports of corticosteroid treatment of cases in humans have claimed either benefit or lack of harm. Controlled studies of corticosteroid therapy of enteroviral myopericarditis are not available.

PREVENTION. Specific preventive measures have not been developed. In neonatal myocarditis, patients and mothers should be isolated as a unit, and women at term should subsequently be admitted to a separate facility. Isolation of cases of myopericarditis in older children and adults is not indicated.

Grist NR, Bell EJ: A six-year study of coxsackievirus B infections in heart disease. J Hyg 73:165, 1974. *A solid, laboratory-based investigation of the problem.*

Lansdown ABG: Viral infections and diseases of the heart. Prog Med Virol 24:70, 1978. *A comprehensive review of infections with all known virus groups, as well as with enteroviruses.*

Lerner MA: Myocarditis and pericarditis. In Mandell GL, Douglas RG, Bennett DE (eds.): Principles and Practice of Infectious Diseases. New York, John Wiley & Sons, 1985, p 544. *A thoughtful review of the subject, with a good presentation of the evidence for a viral etiology. Mechanisms of pathogenesis are also discussed.*

Sainani GS, Krompotic E, Slodki SJ: Adult heart disease due to coxsackievirus B infection. Medicine 47:133, 1968. *A study of 22 adult patients that illustrates the clinical presentations and difficulty in establishing an etiologic diagnosis.*

Woodruff J: Viral myocarditis: A review. Am J Pathol 101:425, 1980. *A good general review of the subject.*

350 MUCOCUTANEOUS INFECTIONS CAUSED BY ENTEROVIRUSES

ENANTHEMS

Herpangina (*herpes,* vesicular eruption; *angina,* inflammation of the throat) is a vesicular eruption of the posterior pharynx that is most frequently caused by coxsackievirus A (1 to 6, 8, 10, 16, and 22), although other enteroviruses have also been implicated. Lesions most commonly occur on the soft palate and anterior pillars of the tonsils and less commonly on the posterior pharyngeal wall or buccal mucosa. Illness begins abruptly with fever ranging from 37.8 to 40.5°C, sore throat, and dysphagia. The pharynx appears mildly injected, with little or no tonsillar exudate. Discrete oropharyngeal lesions can be seen, which begin as macules, progress to gray papules, and eventually become erythema-based vesicles, 2 to 5 mm in diameter. Lesions progress from macules to papules over a period of one to two days and may evolve into ulcers that can last up to one week. The lesions are usually less than 6 in number, occasionally up to 12, and are only moderately painful. Malaise, myalgia, and headache frequently accompany the fever at the onset of illness but resolve over two to four days as the fever abates. Abdominal pain and vomiting have also been noted during acute illness.

Acute lymphonodular pharyngitis is a syndrome in which lesions occur with a distribution similar to that seen in herpangina. However, the lesions consist of small nodules of lymphocytes on an erythematous base, rather than vesicles or ulcers. Mild-to-moderate fever, headache, and sore throat are present as in herpangina, and symptoms last 4 to 14 days. Coxsackievirus A10 has been isolated from patients with this syndrome.

Hand-foot-and-mouth disease (vesicular stomatitis with exanthem) is a mucocutaneous infection with both an enanthem and an exanthem. The enanthem consists of vesicles or ulcers, or both, in the anterior pharynx, most commonly on the anterior buccal mucosa, tongue, lips, and hard palate. The oral lesions are accompanied in 75 per cent of cases by vesicular or papulovesicular lesions on the palms, soles, or extensor surfaces of the hands and feet. Occasionally, lesions are seen on the buttocks or genitalia. Lesions are surrounded by erythema and are usually tender. Initially, patients complain of sore throat or refuse to eat, and manifest a low-grade fever (38 to 39°C) for 24 to 48 hours. Illness is generally mild and lasts less than one week. This syndrome is caused most frequently by coxsackievirus A16, less frequently by A5, A9, and A10, and occasionally by B2 or B5 or enterovirus 71.

EPIDEMIOLOGY. As with other enteroviral infections, the enanthems are seen most frequently during the summer and early fall. Attack rates are highest in younger children, but cases occur in adolescents and young adults as well. Both sporadic cases and outbreaks have been described. Several children within a family unit can become infected sequentially, with an incubation period of two to ten days. Less frequently, illness can spread to adults. Asymptomatic infection of contacts is common.

DIFFERENTIAL DIAGNOSIS. Herpangina and acute lymphonodular pharyngitis involve the posterior pharynx, whereas hand-foot-and-mouth disease involves the anterior pharynx. The latter is associated with cutaneous lesions, which are absent in herpangina. Primary herpes simplex stomatitis is also an anterior stomatitis, but it often has gingivitis and more prominent systemic signs and symptoms, including cervical lymphadenitis. Chickenpox occasionally has

an enanthem, but cutaneous lesions are more numerous and widely distributed than in hand-foot-and-mouth disease. Bacterial pharyngitis or tonsillitis is generally manifested by more systemic signs of illness, as well as by the presence of more extensive pharyngeal exudate. However, individual cases of bacterial infection may be difficult to distinguish from those caused by enteroviruses. Bacterial pharyngitis, as well as pharyngitis caused by viruses other than enteroviruses, generally does not produce vesicular lesions.

LABORATORY DIAGNOSIS. Virus is frequently isolated from throat, stool, or vesicular lesions.

TREATMENT. The enteroviral enanthems are benign, self-limited illnesses that ordinarily require only symptomatic therapy for sore throat and headache.

EXANTHEMS

Nonpolio enteroviruses cause a variety of exanthems that accompany "undifferentiated febrile illness" or specific disease syndromes such as aseptic meningitis or that occur independently. The rate of exanthems associated with enteroviral infection is highest in young children, and the pathogenesis of the majority of these exanthems has not been clearly established. Virus has been isolated from the vesicular exanthem associated with hand-foot-and-mouth disease, and it is likely that these lesions are the result of viremia. Virus isolation has not been reported from enteroviral maculopapular exanthems, and some authors have suggested that an immunopathologic component may be present.

The characteristics of the enterovirus exanthems are not sufficiently distinctive for establishment of an etiologic diagnosis on clinical grounds alone. Multiple immunotypes of echoviruses, coxsackieviruses, and enterovirus 71 cause exanthems. The most common clinical presentation is that of a *morbilliform* exanthem caused most frequently by echovirus 9. The rash consists of fine, discrete macules or papules, or both, and occurs primarily on the face, neck, and, to a lesser extent, chest and extremities. It is most commonly confused with rubella, although posterior cervical and auricular lymphadenopathy is generally not present. Occasionally, rashes may have petechial components and even frank purpura, which may lead to confusion with meningococcemia. Fever is generally low grade and is present at the time that the rash develops. The rash and fever last for three to seven days. Both outbreaks and sporadic cases have been described.

Roseoliform exanthems have been caused most commonly by echovirus 16 ("the Boston exanthem"). Typically, fever (38 to 39.5°C) appears first, and the rash develops as the fever subsides. The rash consists of salmon pink macules and papules on the face and chest but may involve the extremities on occasion. Fever lasts for 24 to 36 hours, and the rash persists for 1 to 5 days. The rashes in roseoliform as well as rubelliform exanthems are usually not pruritic or painful, and complete resolution is the rule. Exanthems are seen most frequently in the summer and early fall. Attack rates are highest in very young children, and both epidemic and sporadic cases are seen.

Diagnosis of enteroviral exanthems depends on laboratory demonstration of viral infection. In general, patients with enteroviral exanthems are only mildly ill, although occasionally infants may be more severely affected. Since little morbidity is associated with enteroviral exanthems, supportive or symptomatic therapy is rarely required. However, the presence of enteroviral exanthems should alert physicians to the potential development of other types of enteroviral illness in the community.

Adler JL, Mostow SR, Mellin H, et al.: Epidemiologic investigation of hand-foot-and-mouth disease. Am J Dis Child 120:309, 1970. *A detailed investigation of an outbreak due to coxsackievirus A16.*

Horstmann DM: Viral exanthems and enanthems. Pediatrics 41:867, 1968. *A concise review of the subject.*

Huebner RJ, Cole RM, Beeman EA, et al.: Herpangina. Etiologic studies of a specific infectious disease. JAMA 145:628, 1951. *Demonstration of association of herpangina with coxsackievirus A infection.*

Neva FA, Feemster RF, Gorbach IJ: Clinical and epidemiological features of an unusual epidemic exanthem. JAMA 155:544, 1954. *The original description of the Boston exanthem.*

Sabin AB, Krumbiegel ER, Wigand R: ECHO type 9 virus disease. J Dis Child 96:197, 1958. *A detailed review of the spectrum of disease associated with an epidemic of this immunotype and the types of rashes that were present.*

351 ACUTE HEMORRHAGIC CONJUNCTIVITIS

DEFINITION. Acute hemorrhagic conjunctivitis (AHC) is an acute viral infection of the eye characterized by painful conjunctival inflammation, subconjunctival hemorrhages, and swelling of the eyelids. AHC has occurred in explosive epidemics in Africa, India, and Asia.

ETIOLOGY. Epidemic AHC has been caused primarily by enterovirus 70. A smaller number of cases have been caused by coxsackievirus A24 and by adenovirus 11.

EPIDEMIOLOGY. Epidemics of AHC caused by enterovirus 70 first appeared in Ghana and Indonesia in 1969. Extensive outbreaks were subsequently observed in northern and southeastern Africa, as well as in India, Southeast Asia, and other areas of the Far East. Localized outbreaks have occurred in the United Kingdom, continental Europe, and the USSR. The USSR outbreaks have been most often related to index cases in travelers and subsequent spread at eye clinics. Cases in the United States had been reported only in Southeast Asian refugees until 1981, when cases originating in the Western hemisphere with subsequent spread to the southern United States were first noted.

Patterns of antibody prevalence to enterovirus 70 suggest that AHC has emerged as a relatively new disease. In endemic areas, antibody studies of serum specimens obtained prior to 1969 revealed low or absent levels of neutralizing antibody to enterovirus 70 in the population. After the occurrence of epidemics in 1969 to 1972, antibody prevalence rates of 40 to 50 per cent were noted, indicating that widespread subclinical as well as clinical infection had taken place. Attack rates for clinical illness are highest among young adults, but infection is most common in young children. It is estimated that tens of millions of cases of AHC caused by enterovirus 70 have occurred since 1969. Simultaneously, a variant of coxsackievirus A24 has been implicated in several hundred thousand cases of AHC, including cases in mixed outbreaks.

PATHOGENESIS. In contrast to other enteroviral infections, AHC is spread by fomites and by direct inoculation of conjunctiva from contaminated fingers. Incubation periods are relatively short (12 to 72 hours) and likely reflect the large inoculum transmitted by these means. Transmission rates are increased by crowding and by poor hygiene. Enterovirus 70 appears to replicate preferentially at 33 to 35°C, which may represent an adaptation to conjunctival temperatures.

CLINICAL MANIFESTATIONS. AHC begins abruptly with pain, photophobia, swelling of the eyelids, and serous or seromucous conjunctival discharge. Involvement is initially unilateral but rapidly spreads to the other eye. Subconjunctival hemorrhages are present in up to 90 per cent of patients with disease caused by enterovirus 70 but are less frequent in disease caused by coxsackievirus A24. Lesions vary in size from petechiae to hemorrhages that cover the entire bulbar conjunctiva. Conjunctival folliculitis and periauricular lymphadenopathy are also frequently present. Slit-lamp examination often reveals corneal erosions or punctate epithelial keratitis. Low-grade fever, headache, coryza, and malaise may be present in up to 20 per cent of cases.

LABORATORY DIAGNOSIS. Virus can be recovered from conjunctival scrapings in a high proportion of cases. Unlike other enteroviral infections, virus is rarely isolated from the throat or stool. The diagnosis is supported by immunotype-specific antibody rises in acute and convalescent sera.

PROGNOSIS. Signs and symptoms peak on the first day of illness, abate over the next 48 hours, and resolve within 10 days. Permanent sequelae are rare, although discoloration from hemorrhages can persist for days. Keratitis rarely leads to permanent corneal damage. Occasionally, secondary bacterial infection may follow the acute viral conjunctivitis. In adults, a rare aseptic meningitis accompanied by a poliomyelitis-like motor paralysis has been reported, usually in association with enterovirus 70 infection. Paralysis develops 5 to 42 days after acute illness and has been observed almost exclusively in adults with an increased prevalence in men. The pathogenesis of the neurologic syndrome is unclear, although enterovirus 70 has been reported to be neuropathogenic in monkeys.

TREATMENT AND PREVENTION. Treatment is symptomatic. If bacterial conjunctivitis develops, topical application of antibacterial ophthalmic ointment is indicated. Prevention of spread of AHC depends on careful handwashing, avoidance of contaminated towels or clothing, and sterilization of ophthalmologic instruments.

Arnow JC, Hierholzer JC, Higbee J, et al.: Acute hemorrhagic conjunctivitis: A mixed virus outbreak among Vietnamese refugees on Guam. Am J Epidemiol 105:68, 1977. *Description of an outbreak caused by enterovirus 70 and adenovirus 11.*

Christopher S, Theogaraj S, Godbole S, et al.: An epidemic of acute hemorrhagic conjunctivitis due to coxsackievirus A24. J Infect Dis 146:16, 1982. *Report of a large outbreak of AHC in India with good clinical descriptions and virologic studies.*

Hierholzer JC, Hilliard KA, Esposito JJ: Serosurvey for "acute hemorrhagic conjunctivitis" virus (enterovirus 70) antibodies in the southeastern United States, with review of the literature and some epidemiologic implications. Am J Epidemiol 102:533, 1975. *A detailed review of the seroepidemiology and spread of this agent.*

Arthropod-Borne Viral Diseases

352 INTRODUCTION

Robert E. Shope

Arthropod-borne viruses (arboviruses) are transmitted biologically by an arthropod to a vertebrate host, either a human or a lower animal. The viruses replicate during an extrinsic incubation period in the arthropod, which may be a mosquito, tick, phlebotomine sandfly, or culicoid midge. The viruses are then transmitted by bite to the vertebrate, which becomes viremic and is in turn capable of infecting another biting arthropod. Some arboviruses also are transmitted vertically through the egg of the arthropod and may be maintained this way between seasons.

There are nearly 500 arthropod-borne viruses and at least 90 of these infect humans. These viruses contain RNA and all except the Reoviridae have lipid-containing envelopes. They are classified by biologic, physical, and chemical properties. Most fit into five families—Togaviridae, Flaviviridae,

TABLE 352–1. SOME PROPERTIES OF RNA VIRUSES CAUSING FEVER, ARTHRITIS, ENCEPHALITIS OR HEMORRHAGIC FEVER

Family (*Genus*) Virus	Human Disease	Distribution	Vector
Togaviridae (*Alphavirus*)			
Mayaro	Fever, arthritis, rash	South America	Mosquito
Ross River	Arthritis, rash, sometimes fever	Australia, S. Pacific	Mosquito
Chikungunya	Fever, arthritis, hemorrhagic fever	Africa, Asia, Philippines	Mosquito
Eastern encephalitis	Fever, encephalitis	Americas	Mosquito
Western encephalitis	Fever, encephalitis	Americas	Mosquito
Venezuelan encephalitis	Fever, sometimes encephalitis	Americas	Mosquito
Flaviviridae (*Flavivirus*)			
Dengue (4 types)	Fever, rash, hemorrhagic fever	Worldwide (tropics)	Mosquito
Yellow fever	Fever, hemorrhagic fever	Tropical Americas, Africa	Mosquito
St. Louis encephalitis	Encephalitis, hepatitis (rare)	Americas	Mosquito
Japanese encephalitis	Encephalitis	Asia, Pacific	Mosquito
West Nile	Fever, rash, hepatitis, encephalitis	Asia, Europe, Africa	Mosquito
Bunyaviridae (*Bunyavirus*)			
LaCrosse encephalitis	Encephalitis	North America	Mosquito
Bunyaviridae (*Phlebovirus*)			
Sandfly fever viruses	Fever	Asia, Africa, tropical Americas	Sand fly, mosquito
Rift Valley fever	Fever, hemorrhagic fever, encephalitis, retinitis	Africa	Mosquito
Bunyaviridae (*Nairovirus*)			
Crimean–Congo hemorrhagic fever	Hemorrhagic fever	Asia, Europe, Africa	Tick
Bunyaviridae (*Hantavirus*)			
Hantaan	Hemorrhagic fever, renal syndrome	Asia	Rodent-borne
Puumala	Hemorrhagic fever, renal syndrome	Europe	Rodent-borne
Arenaviridae (*Arenavirus*)			
Junin	Hemorrhagic fever	Argentina	Rodent-borne
Machupo	Hemorrhagic fever	Bolivia	Rodent-borne
Lassa	Hemorrhagic fever	West Africa	Rodent-borne
Reoviridae (*Orbivirus*)			
Colorado tick fever	Fever	Western U.S.A.	Tick
Filoviridae (*Filovirus*)			
Marburg	Hemorrhagic fever	Africa	Unknown
Ebola	Hemorrhagic fever	Africa	Unknown

Bunyaviridae, Rhabdoviridae, and Reoviridae. Within each family are one or more genera, the genus usually corresponding to an antigenic group. These groups are important, because the clinician must rely heavily on the laboratory for a serologic diagnosis or identification of an isolate.

Table 352–1 lists some of the arboviruses that cause disease in humans. The viruses described in this section were selected as a few of the more important of approximately 90 that are known to infect people.

Most infections are inapparent. The remainder are associated with one or more of four major syndromes: (1) undifferentiated fever, (2) fever with rash and/or arthritis, (3) encephalitis, and (4) hemorrhagic fever (Ch. 360).

The diseases described in this section are nearly all zoonoses (i.e., diseases caused by viruses transmitted from animals to man). The diseases are more prevalent in the tropics and subtropics and are usually focal because of ecologic restrictions on their transmission (Table 352–1). Diagnosis depends on a careful history encompassing exposure to vertebrate animals and arthropod vectors, season, and travel, including geographic site of exposure. The physician must have a high index of suspicion. Fevers may often be diagnosed erroneously as malaria; indeed, in malaria-endemic regions the patient will frequently have malaria concomitantly with an arboviral infection.

Laboratory confirmation of infection is essential. Classically the virus was isolated from acute phase serum or whole blood in laboratory animals such as the mouse or in tissue culture. The neutralization, complement fixation, and hemagglutination-inhibition tests of acute and three-week convalescent sera also led to the correct diagnosis. Now the fluorescent antibody and enzyme-linked immunosorbent assays (ELISA) are supplanting the classic techniques. Antigen detection and IgM capture ELISA permit diagnosis on the initial visit to the physician in many cases, and at least within a week of onset of the illness in most cases.

Control can be achieved by interrupting the cycle, including vaccination of reservoir animals, vector control, and education on methods to avoid the vector. Vaccines are available or under development for some of the agents such as Rift Valley fever, Venezuelan encephalitis, yellow fever, and dengue.

Karabatsos N (ed.): International Catalogue of Arboviruses Including Certain Other Viruses of Vertebrates. 3rd ed. San Antonio, TX, American Society of Tropical Medicine and Hygiene, 1985. *Encyclopedic listing of 504 arboviruses and rodent-borne viruses with detailed description of epidemiologic, serologic, biochemical, and physical properties.*

Shope RE, Sather GE: Arboviruses. In Lennette EH, Schmidt NJ (eds.): Diagnostic Procedures for Viral, Rickettsial and Chlamydial Infections. 5th ed. Washington, D.C., American Public Health Association, 1979, pp 767–814. *Detailed description of classic diagnostic technology with clearly defined explanation of indications and limitations of procedures.*

Undifferentiated Fevers

353 DENGUE

Robert B. Tesh

DEFINITION. "Classic" dengue is an acute, self-limited illness characterized by fever, prostration, headache, myalgia, rash, lymphadenopathy, and leukopenia. It is caused by a mosquito-borne flavivirus. Typically the disease lasts five to seven days and is followed by one or more weeks of depression and weakness.

ETIOLOGY. Four antigenically related but distinct subtypes of dengue virus have been recovered from patients. Infection with each of these agents results in long-lasting immunity against the homologous virus and partial immunity, which persists only for about six months, against the other three heterologous subtypes. This is important, since in many areas of the world endemic for dengue, two or three subtypes may be active simultaneously.

EPIDEMIOLOGY. Dengue fever affects millions of people annually; in terms of human morbidity, it is by far the most important arthropod-transmitted viral illness. Dengue is mainly a disease of the tropics and subtropics, although it can also occur in temperate areas during warm weather. In fact, the first accurate clinical description of the disease was provided by Benjamin Rush during an epidemic in Philadelphia in the summer of 1780. However, the inability of *Aedes aegypti*, the principal mosquito vector, to survive prolonged winter weather has prevented the disease from becoming permanently established in temperate regions of the world.

The basic cycle of dengue virus involves humans and certain *Aedes* mosquitoes. The character of dengue outbreaks often varies from one locality to another, depending on climatic conditions, the size and age of the susceptible human population, and the abundance and vector competence of the local mosquitoes. Thus dengue may appear as a nearly silent, continuously endemic infection, as repeated seasonal epidemics, or as massive outbreaks affecting populations previously free of the disease for many years. Classic dengue is generally a much milder disease in children than in adults.

When a dengue-infected mosquito feeds or probes, it usually introduces virus-contaminated saliva into its host. If the person is susceptible (nonimmune), the virus multiplies, and within five to seven days viremia follows. This viremic period usually corresponds with the acute phase of the illness and lasts about six days. During this time, the patient is infectious to mosquitoes. After ingestion of infected human blood by a susceptible mosquito, eight to ten days is required at warm temperatures for the virus to multiply in the insect's body and to infect its salivary glands. The mosquito is then able to transmit the virus by bite and remains infectious for life.

Aedes aegypti is by far the most important vector. It breeds, rests, and feeds in or near human habitations. It is strongly attracted to humans, biting in daylight or twilight. These attributes make it an ideal virus vector and explain why dengue is principally an urban disease. In rural areas of Africa and Asia, other *Aedes* species also serve as dengue vectors. The recent infestation of the southeastern United States with one of these species, *Aedes albopictus*, raises the possibility that it may soon become an important vector of dengue virus in the Americas.

PATHOLOGY. Dengue virus infection occasionally produces hemorrhagic fever and shock. This syndrome is discussed in Ch. 362. Since classic dengue is rarely fatal, the only information available about its pathology is from biopsies of the skin rash. Such lesions consist of endothelial swelling, perivascular edema, and mononuclear infiltration of small vessels. Petechiae are characterized by extravasation of blood without significant inflammatory reaction.

CLINICAL MANIFESTATIONS. The incubation period of dengue fever is five to eight days. The onset in adults is sudden; during the first 12 to 24 hours the patient develops progressively severe malaise, fever, chills, headache, backache, and generalized myalgia. By the second day the patient is usually acutely ill and prostrate with fever up to 40°C, severe headache, retro-orbital pain, photophobia, generalized muscle aches, and joint stiffness. Other frequent symptoms include anorexia, altered taste sensations, nausea, vomiting, abdominal tenderness, sore throat, and depression. During this early phase, a flush or fleeting erythematous eruption may appear on the face, neck, and chest. The lymph nodes usually become enlarged and palpable, but the liver and spleen do not. The fever generally lasts five to seven days.

About the third or fourth day of illness, a maculopapular or scarlatiniform rash appears, beginning on the trunk and spreading in centripetal fashion. This lasts several days, becomes itchy as it fades, but rarely desquamates. Initially, the leukocyte count may be normal; but by the third or fourth day of illness, a generalized leukopenia develops. Toward the end of the febrile period, small clusters of petechiae may appear, especially on the lower extremities, but the thrombocyte count and clotting time are normal in classic dengue. Convalescence begins on the sixth or seventh day when the fever ends, but full recovery often takes several weeks because of lingering weakness and depression.

DIAGNOSIS. During epidemics of dengue fever, when a large number of cases occur within a short time, the diagnosis is relatively easy. Isolated cases of the disease are more difficult to recognize, because influenza, rubella, and a number of other arbovirus diseases may be mistaken for dengue. Thus laboratory confirmation of a *few* cases during an epidemic and of *every* case when the pattern is sporadic is important. Dengue is endemic in a number of countries in the Caribbean, South and Central America, Africa, and Southern Asia; thus a history of travel during the previous ten days is essential whenever dealing with a suspect case in areas where the disease is rare.

Isolation of the virus is the preferred method of diagnosis. Dengue virus can frequently be recovered from the blood or serum of patients during the febrile stage of their illness. Inoculation of specimens into live mosquitoes or mosquito cell cultures is the most sensitive culture technique. Serologic diagnosis, using acute and convalescent specimens drawn 14 to 21 days apart, is the alternative. However, interpretation of serologic results may be difficult if the patient has been previously infected with another flavivirus. An anamnestic immune response generally develops after a second flavivirus infection, making identification of the specific infecting agent difficult or impossible.

TREATMENT AND PROGNOSIS. There is no specific therapy. Bed rest is indicated, as well as the usual supportive measures to maintain fluid and electrolyte balance, particularly if repeated vomiting occurs. Secondary bacterial infection is uncommon but should be anticipated and treated appropriately. Aspirin should be avoided in dengue patients to prevent exacerbation of the hemorrhagic manifestations that occasionally develop. The prognosis in patients with classic dengue is excellent, although convalescence may be prolonged.

PREVENTION. No vaccines for dengue viruses are yet available. Individual protection is difficult, because the mosquito vectors bite during the day, and continuous use of repellents is not practical. Community protection is possible through effective control or eradication of the *Aedes* vectors.

Dengue patients should be protected from mosquitoes during the first five or six days of their illness in order to prevent further virus transmission, and buildings frequented by patients should be sprayed to eliminate mosquitoes possibly infected prior to the diagnosis of the disease.

Centers for Disease Control: Control of Dengue: Vector Topics No. 2. Atlanta, U.S. Dept Health, Education and Welfare, July 1977. *This short publication (39 pages) provides useful and current information on dengue vectors and their control.*

Guard RW, Stallman ND, Wieners MA: Dengue in the northern region of Queensland, 1981–82. Med J Aust 140:765, 1984. *This paper summarizes the clinical, laboratory, and epidemiologic findings during a dengue outbreak in Australia in 1981 and 1982.*

Pang T: Delayed-type hypersensitivity: Probable role in the pathogenesis of dengue hemorrhagic fever/dengue shock syndrome. Rev Infect Dis 5:346, 1983. *This article reviews the current and most widely accepted hypothesis on the etiology of dengue hemorrhagic fever.*

354 WEST NILE FEVER

Robert B. Tesh

DEFINITION. West Nile fever is an acute, febrile, mosquito-borne viral illness marked by headache, myalgia, lymphadenopathy, and rash. It is generally self limited, although occasional deaths resulting from encephalitis occur in aged persons.

ETIOLOGY. The disease is caused by a flavivirus that is closely related antigenically to Japanese B, Murray Valley, St. Louis, and Rocio encephalitis viruses. West Nile virus also is related to dengue and yellow fever viruses.

EPIDEMIOLOGY. Millions of people have been infected with West Nile virus, which occurs in many rural areas of Africa, the Middle East, southwest Asia, and southern Europe. The disease occurs in both endemic and epidemic forms. In areas where the virus is highly endemic, infection occurs early in childhood and most adults are immune. In regions where the virus is less active, sporadic epidemics of West Nile fever occur at all ages. Epidemics usually occur during the summer months and are correlated with seasonal peaks in populations of culicine mosquitoes. The virus is thought to be maintained in nature by a cycle involving *Culex* mosquitoes and birds, with the human serving as only an incidental host.

CLINICAL MANIFESTATIONS. The disease begins suddenly after an incubation period of three to six days. The character of clinical illness produced by West Nile virus infection is largely age dependent. Infants and young children generally experience a mild, nonspecific febrile illness. Adolescents and adults usually develop a dengue-like disease, characterized by fever, rash, severe frontal headache, orbital pain, backache, generalized myalgia, anorexia, lymphadenopathy, and leukopenia. The rash is nonpruritic and maculopapular, occurs mainly on the trunk, and clears without desquamation. Less frequent symptoms include sore throat, nausea, vomiting, and diarrhea. A few patients in this age group also have meningeal involvement (stiff neck, Kernig's sign) during the acute phase of their illness. The cerebrospinal fluid in these cases usually shows a slight increase in cells and protein. In elderly and debilitated patients, West Nile virus infection sometimes produces meningoencephalitis and occasionally causes death. Neurologic symptoms in the last group of patients may include depressed sensorium, somnolence, involuntary twitches, and coma.

West Nile fever is generally a self-limited disease, lasting three to six days, although general weakness and fatigue may persist for one or two weeks. In patients who develop neurologic involvement, the encephalitic signs usually appear on the fourth or fifth day of illness, after the temperature has returned to normal.

DIAGNOSIS. Clinically this disease is so similar to dengue and phlebotomus fever that laboratory diagnosis is essential in all cases. Virus isolation is by far the best method, and blood specimens obtained as late as the fourth symptomatic day yield a reasonably high percentage of strains when inoculated into newborn mice or a variety of cell cultures. Serologic diagnosis may also be attempted with acute and convalescent serum samples, but previous infection with related flaviviruses, such as the 17D yellow fever vaccine strain, may render interpretation of results difficult owing to the heterologous immune response that develops after a second flavivirus infection.

TREATMENT AND PREVENTION. Management of patients is symptomatic. Complications are uncommon. Since there is no vaccine available, the only effective prevention of West Nile fever is to avoid mosquito bites. Mosquito control programs can reduce the vector population and thus the incidence of the disease. Visitors to areas where West Nile virus is endemic should use mosquito netting, screens, and insect repellent.

Goldblum N: West Nile fever in the Middle East. Proc 6th Int Congr Trop Med Malar 5:112, 1959. *A review of the clinical picture and epidemiology of West Nile fever in Israel.*

Southam CM, Moore AE: Induced virus infections in man by the Egypt isolates of West Nile virus. Am J Trop Med Hyg 3:19, 1954. *This paper reports in great detail the clinical course of terminal cancer patients inoculated with West Nile virus. Encephalitic symptoms were common in this group of patients.*

355 PHLEBOTOMUS FEVER

Robert B. Tesh

DEFINITION. Phlebotomus fever, also referred to as sandfly or pappataci fever, is an acute, self-limited, flulike illness of two to four days' duration, which is transmitted by the bite of infected phlebotomine sandflies. The disease occurs annually during the warm season in the Mediterranean littoral and central Asia. Sporadic cases also occur in tropical America.

ETIOLOGY. The phlebotomus fever group of arboviruses (family Bunyaviridae, genus *Phlebovirus*) currently consists of 40 antigenically distinct and geographically dispersed virus serotypes. Although many of these agents are capable of producing "classic" phlebotomus fever, most cases are due to the Naples and Sicilian serotypes.

EPIDEMIOLOGY. Phlebotomus fever is a public health problem mainly in the Old World, where it occurs in both endemic and epidemic forms. The disease closely parallels the geographic distribution and abundance of *Phlebotomus papatasi*, its principal vector. In areas where the disease is endemic, most of the indigenous population is infected and thereby acquires immunity early in life. The disease in children is a relatively benign, nonspecific febrile illness. However, when nonimmune adults enter an endemic area and are bitten by infected sandflies, they develop "classic" phlebotomus fever. Historically the disease has been of some military importance.

The principal vector, *Phlebotomus papatasi*, is a tiny (2 to 3 mm) sand-colored midge that can readily pass through ordinary screens and mosquito netting. Sandflies usually move in short hops and rarely travel more than a few hundred meters from their resting and breeding sites. The larvae develop in loose soil and organic debris in stone walls, wells, gardens, animal shelters, and privies, usually near human dwellings. *P. papatasi* is active mainly at night and readily feeds on humans. Available evidence suggests that many viruses in the phlebotomus fever group are maintained in the sandfly population by transovarial (hereditary) transmission. This mechanism ensures survival of the viruses during winter months when the vector is inactive and during periods when susceptible vertebrate hosts are not available.

Phlebotomus fever also occurs in tropical America; however, in this region the important vectors are sylvan species belonging to the genus *Lutzomyia*. Therefore cases of the disease in the New World are sporadic and found mainly in persons who enter the tropical forests for work and recreation.

PATHOGENESIS. Since there are no fatalities, the pathology of this disease in humans is unknown. Experimental studies in humans, however, indicate that after intracutaneous inoculation the incubation period is three to six days. Viremia is brief and lasts only one or two days. Postinfection immunity is type specific and probably lifelong; but because of the large number of virus serotypes, a person can have phlebotomus fever more than once.

CLINICAL MANIFESTATIONS. The onset is sudden and is characterized by fever, headache, myalgia, photophobia, retro-orbital pain, and marked conjunctival injection. The face is often flushed, but a true rash is absent. Nausea and vomiting sometimes occur, but other gastrointestinal and respiratory symptoms are uncommon. Most patients with phlebotomus fever develop a marked leukopenia, consisting of an initial lymphopenia followed by a protracted neutropenia. The acute symptoms last only two to four days; however, a general feeling of weakness and depression often persists for a week or more.

DIAGNOSIS AND TREATMENT. Epidemiologic or travel history represents the best clue to diagnosis. Virus isolation is difficult. Serologic procedures serve principally to exclude other possible causes such as dengue, West Nile fever, and influenza. Management of patients is symptomatic. No vaccine is available, but insecticides are effective in controlling the sandfly vectors.

Bartelloni PJ, Tesh RB: Clinical and serologic responses of volunteers infected with phlebotomus fever virus (Sicilian type). Am J Trop Med Hyg 25:456, 1976. *A description of the clinical, hematologic, and serologic responses of volunteers infected with sandfly fever. References are given to other similar studies.*

Sabin AB, Philip CB, Paul JR: Phlebotomus (pappataci or sandfly) fever. JAMA 125:693, 1944. *A report of research on sandfly fever among American troops during World War II. It presents a detailed clinical description of the disease.*

Tesh RB, Saidi S, Gajdamovic SJ, et al.: Serological studies on the epidemiology of sandfly fever in the Old World. Bull WHO 54:663, 1976. *A review of the epidemiology of phlebotomus fever in the Old World. It includes a map showing the geographic distribution of the principal vector,* Phlebotomus papatasi.

356 RIFT VALLEY FEVER
Robert B. Tesh

DEFINITION. Rift Valley fever is an acute viral illness, usually of short duration, which is characterized by high fever, headache, retro-orbital pain, myalgia, prostration, photophobia, and conjunctival injection. A small percentage of patients develop hemorrhagic and encephalitic complications that are sometimes fatal. Humans generally acquire the disease by contact with infected domestic animals, although the virus may also be mosquito borne.

ETIOLOGY. The causative agent is a 90-nm, ribonucleic acid–containing virus that is antigenically related to a number of viruses in the phlebotomus fever serogroup (family Bunyaviridae, genus *Phlebovirus*). However, because of the virulence of Rift Valley fever virus for animals and humans, the disease that it causes is considered separately.

EPIDEMIOLOGY. The known geographic distribution of the virus includes most of sub-Saharan Africa. Rift Valley fever is primarily a disease of domestic ruminants. Epizootics produce heavy mortality among lambs and calves and cause increased rates of abortion among ewes and cows. Outbreaks

of the disease in domestic animals are sporadic; the virus is presumed to be transmitted from animal to animal by infected mosquitoes. The maintenance mechanism of the virus between epizootics is unclear, although there is some evidence that it may survive dry periods by vertical transmission in mosquito vectors.

Humans usually acquire the virus by aerosol transmission or by direct contact with blood or tissues of infected animals. Veterinarians, ranchers, herdsmen, slaughterhouse employees, and persons working in animal disease diagnostic laboratories are all at special risk during epizootics. Rift Valley fever virus is highly infectious to humans; cases of the disease have occurred in persons who have only been present in a room where a sick animal has been slaughtered or autopsied. It is uncertain what role, if any, mosquitoes play in the transmission of Rift Valley fever to humans. Because of the value of domestic animals in many economically depressed regions of Africa, animals are often housed within family compounds. Furthermore, sick or dying animals are usually killed to salvage their meat. Both of these practices greatly increase the risk of virus transmission to humans.

CLINICAL MANIFESTATIONS. The incubation period is three to six days. Uncomplicated Rift Valley fever in humans is similar to phlebotomus fever. The disease begins suddenly with fever up to 40°C, chills, severe headache, retro-orbital pain, photophobia, generalized myalgia, and prostration. Patients with this disease appear acutely ill, with flushed faces and marked conjunctival injection. Occasionally nausea, vomiting, and diarrhea occur. Physical examination early in the disease is unremarkable. The white blood count may be decreased, normal, or elevated. In most cases the illness lasts two to four days, although sometimes a brief recrudescence of fever occurs, giving a biphasic temperature curve. Recovery in uncomplicated cases is complete.

A few patients with Rift Valley fever develop serious complications. One is *loss of central visual acuity* and occasionally blindness. The eye symptoms do not usually become apparent until several days or weeks after the febrile illness has ended. Funduscopic examination in these cases shows white macular exudates and occasionally retinal hemorrhages. In some patients, vision gradually improves; in others, it does not.

A second complication is *hemorrhagic manifestations*. These usually appear between the second and fourth days of illness, about the time that the patient becomes afebrile. The patient becomes progressively jaundiced and drowsy and manifests petechiae, purpura, bleeding gums, hematemesis, and melena. Liver function test results, including bilirubin, serum transaminases, alkaline phosphatase, and prothrombin time, are abnormal. The prognosis in these cases is poor; death often occurs within a week and is due to shock and hepatic failure.

A third complication is *meningoencephalitis*. Neurologic symptoms appear several days after the febrile period ends and may include mental confusion, hallucinations, vertigo, meningismus, paresis, convulsions, and coma. The cerebrospinal fluid shows increased protein and pleocytosis. The outcome is gradual recovery or death.

PATHOGENESIS. At autopsy, patients with hemorrhagic complications have petechiae and hemorrhages throughout the gastrointestinal tract. The most characteristic lesion is in the liver and consists of diffuse central necrosis and hemorrhage. Affected hepatic cells show eosinophilic cytoplasmic degeneration similar to that seen in yellow fever. The brain in fatal cases of encephalitis shows focal necrosis and perivascular infiltration with macrophages and lymphocytes.

DIAGNOSIS. Rift Valley fever is primarily a disease of place and particular human activity. A history is more valuable than any other procedure. Blood obtained during a febrile period almost always contains virus. Serologic diagnosis is also fairly specific, although low-level cross-reactions may occur with some heterologous antigens in the phlebotomus fever group.

TREATMENT AND PREVENTION. Management of patients with this disease is entirely symptomatic. Those with hemorrhage and shock obviously need blood replacement.

Live attenuated and formalin-killed vaccines are available in limited quantities for certain high-risk groups such as veterinarians and laboratory workers. These are protective for at least two years. Individual antimosquito measures would also seem prudent during epizootics.

Peters CJ, Meegan JM: Rift Valley fever. In Steele JH (ed.): CRC Handbook Series in Zoonoses, Section B: Viral Zoonoses. Vol. 1. Boca Raton, Fla., CRC Press, 1981, pp 403–420. *A complete review of all aspects of the disease.*

357 FEVERS CAUSED BY ALPHAVIRUSES: CHIKUNGUNYA, O'NYONG-NYONG, MAYARO, ROSS RIVER, AND OCKELBO

Robert B. Tesh

DEFINITION. Chikungunya, o'nyong-nyong, Mayaro, Ross River, and Ockelbo virus infections are acute nonfatal illnesses that usually include fever, arthralgia, and rash. They are caused by a group of antigenically related, geographically diverse, mosquito-borne viruses.

EPIDEMIOLOGY. These five diseases affect persons of all ages, although they are generally milder in children. Clinically, they are practically indistinguishable, but their epidemiology is quite different. Chikungunya is the most widely distributed of the five diseases and occurs in sub-Saharan Africa, India, Southeast Asia, and the Philippines. Epidemics are sporadic in occurrence and usually appear during warm, rainy months. In rural Africa, the virus is maintained in a cycle involving wild primates and forest mosquitoes (*Aedes africanus* and *Ae. furcifer*). Urban outbreaks of chikungunya are usually associated with *Aedes aegypti*. In this situation the virus is probably transmitted from human to mosquito to human.

Little is known about the epidemiology of o'nyong-nyong fever. It has occurred in Uganda, Kenya, Tanzania, Malawi, and Senegal. Between 1959 and 1962, a major epidemic swept across East Africa, affecting millions of people. The suspected vectors are *Anopheles funestus* and *An. gambiae*.

Mayaro virus has been isolated in Trinidad, Surinam, Brazil, Colombia, and Bolivia. Cases of this disease have been associated mainly with persons who live or work in tropical forests, mostly males. Sylvan mosquitoes of the genus *Haemagogus* are thought to be the principal vectors. Wild animals probably serve as the virus reservoir.

Ross River fever, also known as "epidemic polyarthritis," has occurred in Australia, New Guinea, the Solomon Islands, Fiji, American Samoa, and a number of other South Pacific islands. In southern Australia, sporadic cases of the disease usually occur during warm weather among vacationers traveling in rural areas. There the virus is thought to be maintained in a wild vertebrate-mosquito cycle, with *Culex annulirostris* and *Aedes vigilax* serving as principal vectors. However, explosive epidemics of this disease have also occurred on several South Pacific islands, where the virus appeared to be transmitted from human to mosquito to

human, analogous to urban outbreaks of chikungunya. In the latter epidemics, *Aedes polynesiensis* was the presumed vector.

Ockelbo fever was first recognized in Sweden. A similar illness has also been reported in Finland and adjacent regions of the Soviet Union, where it is referred to as "Pogasta disease" and "Karelian fever," respectively. In all three countries, the disease typically occurs in late summer among picnickers, berry collectors, and other persons entering wooded areas. A single recovery of the virus from *Culiseta* mosquitoes suggests that these insects serve as vectors.

CLINICAL MANIFESTATIONS. The usual incubation period for this group of illnesses is three to five days. Typically, the onset is abrupt with fever, headache, myalgia, and weakness. In Mayaro and chikungunya infections, the fever may reach 39 to 40°C. A saddleback or biphasic temperature curve sometimes occurs with chikungunya. In Ross River, Ockelbo, and o'nyong-nyong infections, the fever is generally lower and constitutional symptoms are milder. Arthralgia and rash may appear with the initial symptoms or develop several days later. Arthralgia is the most striking feature of these illnesses. It is usually bilateral and mainly affects joints in the extremities. Symptoms vary from excruciating pain to vague joint stiffness. Affected joints are often swollen and tender, but other signs of inflammation are absent. Previously injured joints are particularly susceptible. The rash is maculopapular and occurs mainly on the trunk and extremities. It clears in four or five days without desquamation, leaving a brownish stain to the skin. Lymphadenopathy is also common. Many patients have a leukopenia with relative lymphocytosis during the first week of illness. One serious but rare complication of chikungunya virus infection is hemorrhagic manifestations. Epistaxis, hematemesis, melena, petechiae, and purpura have all been reported.

DIAGNOSIS. These viruses can usually be recovered from the blood or serum of patients during the first few days of illness by inoculation of newborn mice or various cell cultures. Standard serologic techniques are also highly reliable in making a specific diagnosis, provided that a first serum specimen is collected early in the disease and a second is obtained 10 to 14 days later. Diagnosis during epidemics is relatively easy; the isolated case is more difficult to recognize. The differential diagnosis includes other diseases producing fever, arthralgia, and rash.

TREATMENT AND PROGNOSIS. Treatment is symptomatic, and the prognosis is excellent. In general, these illnesses last only about one week, although the arthralgia sometimes persists for several weeks or months. In such a case, recurrent attacks of joint pain and swelling are common. The pathogenesis of the joint disease is unknown.

Espmark A, Niklasson B: Ockelbo disease in Sweden: Epidemiological, clinical, and virological data from the 1982 outbreak. Am J Trop Med Hyg 33:1203, 1984. *Good clinical description of Ockelbo outbreak.*
Tesh RB: Arthritides caused by mosquito-borne viruses. Ann Rev Med 33:31, 1982. *A review of the clinical manifestations and epidemiology of diseases caused by five alphaviruses. Many references are given.*

358 COLORADO TICK FEVER

Theodore C. Eickhoff

DEFINITION. Colorado tick fever (CTF) is an acute, benign, tick-transmitted viral infection that occurs throughout the Rocky Mountain area and is characterized by headache, back pain, a biphasic febrile course lasting about one week, and leukopenia.

ETIOLOGY. CTF virus is an RNA virus in the orbivirus genus of the reoviruses. Although unrelated to other major arbovirus groups, it is an arbovirus because it replicates in ticks. The virus is transmitted to humans by the bite of the hard-shelled wood tick, *Dermacentor andersoni*. Human cases appear to be limited to the combined geographic distribution of the tick vector and to the major mammalian reservoirs, ground squirrels and chipmunks.

EPIDEMIOLOGY. The disease occurs during the spring and summer months, when tick exposure in the mountains is common. Disease activity appears to follow springtime in the mountains, for cases occur at lower altitudes during April and May, and at higher altitudes during June and July, presumably reflecting the slower emergence of ticks at higher altitudes. Most patients give a history of having found attached ticks, but others will not be aware of the tick attachment and bite, even though they may have seen ticks on their body or clothing. Cases may occasionally be encountered in other areas of the country as a result of travel outside the endemic area during the incubation period or accidental transportation of infected adult ticks in clothing or bedding.

CTF virus has been recovered from as many as 14 per cent of *Dermacentor andersoni* collected in endemic areas. The virus is passed transovarially within the vector species. The reservoir of the virus probably resides in numerous small mammals, particularly golden mantled ground squirrels and chipmunks, which have a prolonged viremia and infect nymphal ticks. Overwintering may thus occur in either nymphal ticks or hibernating small mammals. Adult ticks then transmit the virus to other small animals, with humans being accidental hosts.

INCIDENCE AND PREVALENCE. The disease has been reported from most states in the Rocky Mountain area and from western Canadian provinces, but the largest number of cases has generally been reported in Colorado. Several hundred cases are diagnosed annually in the endemic area, but it is likely that this represents only a fraction of the total. Mild or wholly subclinical infections do occur, but their frequency has not been systematically evaluated.

The virus has been isolated from other species of ticks and from numerous species of small mammals, suggesting that the disease may occur over a wider geographic area than is currently appreciated.

PATHOGENESIS. There is no unusual local reaction at the site of the tick bite inoculation, and the site of initial localization and replication of the virus is unknown. Symptoms begin three to seven days after tick exposure. Viremia can be demonstrated at the time of onset of fever, not only persisting during the febrile illness itself, but remarkably persisting in red blood cells long after the virus has disappeared from serum and neutralizing antibody has appeared. The virus can be demonstrated within erythrocytes by fluorescent antibody staining for up to 120 days and has been grown from washed erythrocytes 100 days after the original infection. Transfusion-transmitted CTF has been documented.

Few pathologic data in humans are available, since only one fatal case has been recorded. In experimental animals, the heart, lungs, spleen, bone marrow, and lymph nodes are important sites of viral replication. Occasional patients have clinical evidence of central nervous system or meningeal involvement, and CTF virus has been recovered from cerebrospinal fluid.

CLINICAL MANIFESTATIONS. The disease begins abruptly, with chilly sensations, fever of 38 to 40°C, myalgias most prominent in the back and legs, headache, retro-orbital pain, and photophobia. Malaise and nausea may occur, but vomiting is uncommon. Physical findings during the first two to three days of illness are nonspecific. The patient may be flushed, with conjunctival and pharyngeal erythema. Lymphadenopathy is not prominent, although mild splenomegaly is sometimes present. Rashes have been reported in up to 12 per cent of patients, commonly macular or maculopapular

and distributed over the entire body, sometimes petechial and involving primarily the extremities. Tachycardia is in proportion to the temperature elevation.

In approximately one half of cases, a distinctly biphasic illness occurs, the so-called "saddleback" fever. Symptoms abate after two to three days, temperature becomes normal or nearly so, and the patient feels relatively well for one or two days, following which there is an abrupt return of fever, headache, and back pain, often more intense than in the first phase. The second phase lasts two to four days and then subsides, leaving the patient with weakness and lassitude that disappear entirely during the succeeding week or two. Convalescence may be prolonged in patients over 30 years of age to three weeks or more. Some patients do not exhibit the typical biphasic course and experience only one bout of fever or have a typical illness but with a third phase of fever or have a single prolonged febrile illness lasting five to eight days.

Central nervous system involvement has occurred in a few patients, usually children. The presenting findings have been those of aseptic meningitis with nuchal rigidity and mononuclear pleocytosis or of encephalitis with a depressed sensorium or stupor. Hemorrhagic manifestations have been described in a few children with encephalitis.

Laboratory findings very early in the illness are generally not helpful, but leukopenia is usually present by the third day of illness and becomes even more pronounced during the second phase, reaching levels as low as 2000 per cubic millimeter. The most striking decrease is in the granulocyte series, with a relative lymphocytosis, and there is frequently an accompanying thrombocytopenia. Atypical, vacuolated lymphocytes are frequently observed. Bone marrow examination reveals a maturation arrest in the granulocyte series. The white blood count returns to normal during convalescence.

DIAGNOSIS. The diagnosis should be suspected in any person with a history of tick exposure in the endemic area three to seven days prior to the onset of a febrile illness. Findings during the first phase, however, cannot be differentiated from many other acute febrile illnesses. A brief symptom-free interval followed by a second febrile illness should strongly suggest CTF. Profound leukopenia is usually present by that time and lends support to the diagnosis.

The diagnosis is confirmed by isolation of the virus from serum or whole blood, via inoculation of suckling mice. More rapid diagnosis is possible by direct immunofluorescent staining of virus in the patient's erythrocytes. A diagnostic rise in both neutralizing and complement-fixing antibodies can generally be detected by examination of acute and convalescent sera. An enzyme-linked immunoassay has been developed.

The differential diagnosis can be troublesome, inasmuch as Rocky Mountain spotted fever is transmitted in the tick fever endemic area by the same vector, *Dermacentor andersoni*. Paradoxically, Rocky Mountain spotted fever has become an unusual disease in the state of Colorado and is outnumbered by CTF in Colorado by at least 20-fold. Nevertheless, differential diagnosis may be impossible early in the course of disease, before the characteristic rash of Rocky Mountain spotted fever appears. A relatively symptom-free interval after two or three days would be most unusual in Rocky Mountain spotted fever and strongly favors the diagnosis of CTF.

TREATMENT. Therapy is entirely supportive, there being no specific therapy. Salicylates or acetaminophen may be necessary to minimize headache and myalgias but are neither required nor advisable in most patients.

PROGNOSIS. The disease is almost invariably benign, and the prognosis is excellent. Severe illness, complicated by central nervous system involvement, is seen infrequently and only in children.

PREVENTION. Both inactivated and live attenuated vaccines have been studied, but the modest number of cases and the benign nature of the disease suggest little need for active immunization.

The most effective means of preventing the disease is the use of protective clothing or repellents by people outdoors in endemic areas during the spring and summer months, together with frequent body inspection and prompt removal of ticks. Transfusion-associated disease can be prevented by exclusion of convalescent donors for a minimum of six months.

Anderson RD, Entringer MA, Robinson WA: Virus-induced leukopenia: Colorado tick fever as a human model. J Infect Dis 151:449, 1985. *An interesting exploration of the pathogenesis of the profound leukopenia observed in CTF.*

Goodpasture HC, Poland JD, Francy DB, et al.: Colorado tick fever: Clinical, epidemiologic and laboratory aspects of 228 cases in Colorado in 1973–1974. Ann Intern Med 88:303, 1978. *A recent, thorough clinical study.*

Oshiro LS, Dondero DV, Emmons RW, et al.: The development of Colorado tick fever virus within cells of the haematopoietic system. J Gen Virol 39:73, 1978. *Recommended for those interested in the unusual host-parasite relationship in CTF.*

Encephalitides

359 ARTHROPOD-BORNE VIRAL ENCEPHALITIDES

Thomas P. Monath

Of the more than 500 arboviruses currently registered, 13 are important causes of encephalitis, some responsible for intermittent epidemics, and 14 are occasionally associated with encephalitis (see Table 359–1). Arboviral encephalitis is a significant health problem in Europe and the Soviet Union (tick-borne encephalitis), in parts of Asia (Japanese encephalitis), and in the New World, where the disease assumes great importance, owing to a proliferation of etiologic agents, widespread occurrence, potential for epidemic spread, and concurrent affliction of domestic animals and humans. Only the African continent is spared from epidemiologically important arboviral encephalitides. The physician faced with a case should attempt to establish an early specific diagnosis, because it provides information about the occurrence of a potentially epidemic disease and directs investigative, preventive, and control measures by the responsible public health authority.

The viruses under consideration are transmitted between wild or domestic animals by the agency of blood-feeding mosquitoes or ticks (see Fig. 359–1). Vertebrate hosts circulate virus in their blood at titers sufficiently high to infect a specific arthropod vector or vectors. After ingestion of an infectious blood meal, a temperature-dependent delay (extrinsic incubation period) of a week or more is required for replication in salivary gland tissue before transmission by bite can occur;

thereafter arthropods remain infective for life. The human is not an essential host in the transmission cycles of the arboviral encephalitides. Human infection is most often abortive or subclinical, and the severe manifestations of central nervous system inflammation occur in only a small fraction of persons infected. The ratio of inapparent to clinically overt infections is a distinctive, age-dependent quality of each disease.

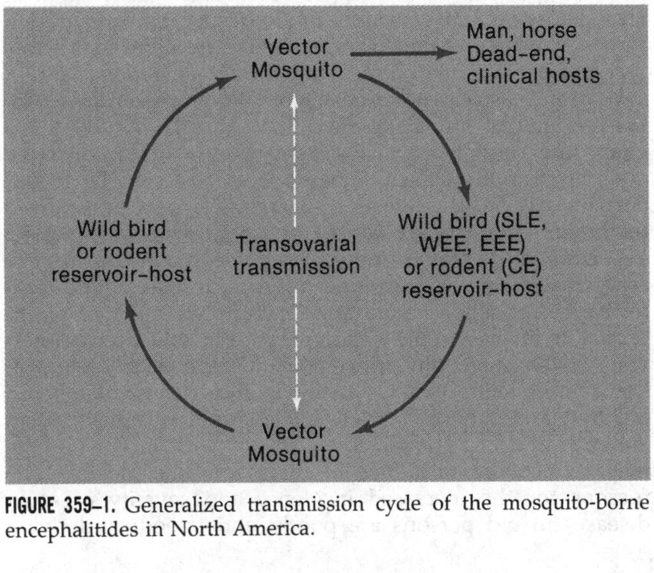

CLINICAL FEATURES. In encephalitis, the brain parenchyma itself is affected, resulting in diffuse or localizing signs of cerebral dysfunction. Signs of meningeal irritation are also nearly always present (*meningoencephalitis*) but may be masked in the very young, the elderly, or the comatose patient. In some patients, inflammation of the leptomeninges may occur without evidence for disturbance of brain function (aseptic meningitis). A still milder form of arboviral central nervous system infection is manifested by fever and headache only; in such cases, however, cerebrospinal fluid pleocytosis may be present, indicating a forme fruste of meningitis.

The neurologic disease usually begins after a variable period of nonspecific, grippelike symptoms. The clinical features and rate of evolution of encephalitis are quite variable. A degree of alteration of the state of consciousness is a universal finding in encephalitis. Convulsions, more often generalized than focal, may occur. Paresis, paralyses, hyperactive reflexes, and plantar extensor responses reflect damage to corticospinal tracts. A prominent feature of some infections (especially St. Louis and Japanese encephalitis) is involvement of extrapyramidal structures, with tremor and muscular rigidity. Cerebellar dysfunction is manifested by muscular incoordination, dysmetria, and ataxic speech. Cranial nerve palsies are not uncommon and reflect damage to brain stem nuclei or supranuclear tracts. Autonomic disturbances (sialorrhea, cardiovascular irregularity, urinary retention) may be present. Infection of the cerebral cortex or hypothalamic-thalamic-temporal lobe regions produces confusion; defective memory; changes in speech, personality, and behavior; and the appearance of pathologic reflexes (e.g., suck, snout). Hyperthermia and the syndrome of inappropriate antidiuretic hormone secretion indicate disturbance of the pituitary-hypothalamic axis. Spinal cord involvement may be manifested by lower motor neuron and sensory deficits, hyperreflexia, and bladder paralysis. Interference with respiratory function, laryngeal paralysis, cardiac arrhythmia, and cerebral edema are potentially life-threatening complications. Surviving patients may be left with permanent neuropsychiatric sequelae. In the pregnant female, infection of the developing fetus may result in central nervous system damage or fetal death.

Clinical laboratory findings are relatively nonspecific. A modest peripheral leukocytosis is usual. The cerebrospinal fluid is under increased pressure and contains white blood cells (predominantly polymorphonuclear cells early and lymphocytes later). The cell count is generally less than 500 per cubic millimeter. Cerebrospinal fluid protein may be moderately elevated; glucose and lactate concentrations are generally

FIGURE 359–1. Generalized transmission cycle of the mosquito-borne encephalitides in North America.

TABLE 359-1. ARTHROPOD-BORNE VIRUSES THAT CAUSE ACUTE CENTRAL NERVOUS SYSTEM INFECTION AND ENCEPHALITIS

Virus	Taxonomic Group	Mode of Transmission	Geographic Distribution	Disease in Domestic Livestock
I. Viruses Principally Associated with the Encephalitis Syndrome; Epidemic and Endemic				
Eastern equine encephalitis	Togaviridae, alphavirus	Mosquito	Eastern North America, Caribbean, South America	Equines, penned pheasants
Western equine encephalitis	Togaviridae, alphavirus	Mosquito	Western North America, South America	Equines
Venezuelan equine encephalitis	Togaviridae, alphavirus	Mosquito, possibly other modes (see text)	Florida, Central and South America	Equines
St. Louis encephalitis	Flaviviridae, flavivirus	Mosquito	North America, Caribbean, Central and South America	None
Japanese encephalitis	Flaviviridae, flavivirus	Mosquito	East, Southeast Asia; India	Equines, swine
Rocio encephalitis	Flaviviridae, flavivirus	Mosquito	Brazil	None
Murray Valley encephalitis	Flaviviridae, flavivirus	Mosquito	Australia	(Equines)*
California encephalitis, La Crosse, Jamestown Canyon	Bunyaviridae, California serogroup	Mosquito	North America	None
Tick-borne encephalitides: Russian spring-summer and Central European encephalitis	Flaviviridae, flavivirus	Tick, ingestion of milk	Europe, USSR	None
Louping ill	Flaviviridae, flavivirus	Tick	British Isles	Sheep, equines, cows
Powassan	Flaviviridae, flavivirus	Tick	North America	None
II. Viruses Principally Associated with Other Syndromes, but Occasionally Causing Encephalitis; Epidemic and Endemic				
Sindbis (febrile illness with rash)	Togaviridae, alphavirus	Mosquito	Africa, Europe	None
West Nile (febrile illness with rash)	Flaviviridae, flavivirus	Mosquito	Africa, Middle East	(Equines)*
Yellow fever (hemorrhagic fever)	Flaviviridae, flavivirus	Mosquito	Africa, tropical America	None
Rift Valley fever (febrile illness, hemorrhagic fever, retinitis)	Bunyaviridae, phlebotomus fever group	Mosquito, direct contact	Africa	Sheep, cows, goats
Colorado tick fever (febrile illness)	Reoviridae, orbivirus	Tick	Western North America	None
Tick-borne hemorrhagic fevers:				
Kyasanur Forest disease	Flaviviridae, flavivirus	Tick	India	None
Omsk hemorrhagic fever	Flaviviridae, flavivirus	Tick	Central Asia	None
Crimean hemorrhagic fever—Congo	Bunyaviridae, nairovirus	Tick	Eastern Europe, USSR, Africa	None
III. Rare and Sporadic Infections Associated with Encephalitis				
Semliki Forest†	Togaviridae, alphavirus	Mosquito	Africa, Southeast Asia	(Equines)*
Ilheus	Flaviviridae, flavivirus	Mosquito	South America	None
Negishi	Flaviviridae, flavivirus	Tick	Japan	None
Langat†	Flaviviridae, flavivirus	Tick	Asia	None
Thogoto	Orthomyxovirus	Tick	Africa	None

*Disease rare or suspected but not well documented.
†Encephalitis recorded in laboratory infections or experimental infections of cancer patients only; significance in naturally acquired infections unknown.

normal. Changes in serum enzyme levels have been reported, reflecting myocarditis or damage to skeletal muscle or liver.

PATHOLOGY AND PATHOGENESIS. Two basic pathologic processes are common to the arboviral encephalitides: (1) neuronal and glial damage mediated by intracellular viral infection, and (2) an inflammatory response involving migration of immunologically active cells (T and B lymphocytes, macrophages) into the perivascular space and brain parenchyma. Endothelial cell swelling and proliferation, vasculitic changes, and destruction of myelin sheaths in deep white matter areas are present in some of the arboviral encephalitides. Since the immune mechanism is responsible for the inflammatory response, an immunopathologic component has been postulated to occur in arboviral encephalitis. A balance apparently occurs between dual roles of the immune response in (1) viral clearance and recovery from infection and (2) enhancement of pathologic processes and acceleration of death.

After inoculation of virus by the bite of an infected arthropod, primary replication occurs in local tissues and in regional lymph nodes. Virus is carried by efferent lymphatics to the thoracic duct and into the bloodstream. This primary viremia seeds extraneural tissues, which in turn support further replication and release into the circulation. Viremia is modulated by replication in extraneural sites, by the rate of viral clearance by the reticuloendothelial system, and by the appearance of humoral antibodies. If viremia is prolonged and intense enough, the neural parenchyma is invaded, with or without ensuing clinical disease. The sites of extraneural infection vary from virus to virus. In the case of many alpha- and flaviviruses, experimental studies have shown that striated muscle and vascular endothelium are important sites of replication; in the case of Venezuelan encephalitis virus, myeloid and lymphoid tissue tropism has been emphasized. The mode of penetration of virus across the blood-brain junction is incompletely understood. Passive movement of virus across cerebral capillaries or virus replication and growth across capillary endothelium are possible mechanisms. Factors that increase vascular permeability (heavy metal poisons, CO_2 inhalation, vasoactive amines) promote viral neuroinvasion. In experimental animals infected with some flaviviruses, virus enters the central nervous system by way of the olfactory neuroepithelium. Olfactory neurons are infected by bloodborne virus, and the infection spreads by axonal transport to the brain.

The immature brain is more susceptible to damage by some arboviruses (e.g., western and Venezuelan equine and California encephalitis), accounting for the predominance of encephalitis in the younger age groups. But other central nervous system infections principally affect the elderly (e.g., St. Louis encephalitis) or have a bimodal incidence, striking both children and the very old (e.g., Japanese encephalitis). In endemic areas, accumulated immunity with increasing age may reduce the incidence of disease in the elderly. The reasons for the increased incidence and severity of some diseases in old persons are poorly understood; underlying hypertensive and arteriosclerotic cerebrovascular disease is suspected to play a role in viral neuroinvasion.

DIFFERENTIAL DIAGNOSIS. The primary task is to differentiate viral encephalitis from acute central nervous system infection by organisms that may respond to antibiotic therapy. Early clinical manifestations of bacterial meningitis (especially if partially treated), brain abscess, subdural empyema, and cerebral thrombophlebitis may mimic viral encephalitis, and cerebrospinal fluid changes are sometimes similar. Culture and repeated examination of the cerebrospinal fluid will help clarify the etiology in cases of bacterial meningitis. Diagnostic tests (computed tomography [CT], electroencephalography, brain scan) help define localized lesions, such as abscess. Subacute bacterial endocarditis may present with meningoencephalitis. Tuberculosis and fungal meningitis cause a mononuclear pleocytosis but reduced glucose values in the cerebrospinal fluid. Other infections that occasionally cause meningoencephalitis include Rocky Mountain spotted fever, leptospirosis, falciparum malaria, trichinosis, *Naegleria*, typhoid, Lyme disease, and *Mycoplasma pneumoniae*.

Acute infection with viral agents other than arboviruses is associated with meningoencephalitis, including herpesviruses, mumps virus, enteroviruses, lymphocytic choriomeningitis virus, rabies, influenza, adenoviruses, respiratory syncytial virus, and encephalomyocarditis virus. Principal clues to an arboviral etiology are the history, presence of an outbreak of similar disease in the community, summer-fall occurrence, and the probable geographic locality in which infection was acquired. Echo- and coxsackieviruses cause summer-fall outbreaks in arbovirus epidemic areas, but the predominant syndrome produced is aseptic meningitis, and there may be clinical clues to the diagnosis (e.g., presence of rash, pleurodynia). In the individual case, herpes encephalitis presents the most important diagnostic challenge, since chemotherapy may be indicated. The presence of localizing neurologic signs, other clinical features (previous herpetic infection, subacute onset, predominant behavioral or confusional disturbance), and tests (e.g., CT scan) to detect a masslike lesion are clues to the clinical diagnosis of herpes encephalitis. If brain biopsy is performed, fluorescent antibody tests and virus isolation attempts may be performed for both herpes and, if suspected, the arthropod-borne encephalitides.

Acute encephalitis may occur following exanthematous viral infections of childhood or administration of rabies or smallpox vaccines. The history of antecedent illness or vaccination and the prominence of myelitis in many cases are clues to the diagnosis.

Cerebrovascular accident may be confused with viral encephalitis. St. Louis encephalitis, a disease of the elderly, has been misdiagnosed as stroke. Subarachnoid hemorrhage produces meningismus, fever, headache, and neurologic signs that mimic an infectious etiology; CT scanning and lumbar puncture clearly distinguish these etiologies.

Metabolic (toxic) encephalopathies (caused by hypoxia, hypoglycemia, diabetic ketoacidosis, hepatic and renal failure, remote carcinoma, intoxications, and addisonian crisis) may present features suggesting infectious encephalitis. Careful history and physical, neurologic, and cerebrospinal fluid examination usually differentiate these conditions.

Neoplastic or *granulomatous diseases* involving the central nervous system and a variety of diseases of uncertain etiology (cat scratch disease, Behçet's disease, Reye's syndrome, acute multiple sclerosis, and systemic lupus erythematosus) must occasionally be considered in the differential diagnosis.

WESTERN EQUINE ENCEPHALITIS (WEE)

ETIOLOGIC AGENT. WEE virus, a member of the family Togaviridae, alphavirus genus, was first isolated in 1930 from a horse with encephalitis in California. A relative of WEE virus (Highlands J virus) present in the eastern United States is very rarely associated with human and equine disease.

WEE virus is pathogenic for a wide range of laboratory animals, embryonated eggs, and cell cultures. Isolation and viral assays are generally performed in infant mice inoculated intracranially or by plaque formation in primary avian cell cultures.

EPIDEMIOLOGY. *Incidence and Prevalence.* Between 1955 and 1985, 982 cases of WEE were reported in the United States. The annual incidence has varied from fewer than 10 cases to over 170 cases in epidemic years. Although classically an important disease on the West Coast, the area most affected in recent years has been the central tier of states from the Mississippi River west to the Rocky Mountains, including adjacent parts of Canada. In Argentina and Uruguay, equine epizootics ocur with little involvement of humans.

Epidemics generally occur in early or midsummer and may be precipitated by heavy snow melt or flooding, which produces conditions favorable for breeding of mosquito vectors. Cases of encephalitis in equines frequently precede the appearance of human disease by several weeks. The disease principally affects residents of rural agricultural communities. The incidence is higher in males than in females because of increased exposure to the vector during farming and recreational pursuits. WEE is most severe in infants and young children; these age groups also represent the immunologically most susceptible population in endemic areas. The case-fatality rate is between 3 and 7 per cent. The ratio of inapparent to apparent infection is age dependent, ranging from about 1:1 in infants under 1 year to 58:1 in children 1 to 4 years old to over 1000:1 in persons over 14 years of age. In the western United States, mixed outbreaks of WEE and St. Louis encephalitis are the rule.

Transmission. The virus circulates between wild birds and *Culex tarsalis* mosquitoes. *Culex tarsalis*, an abundant breeder in irrigated areas and flooded pastures, is responsible for infection of humans and equines, which develop low or undetectable viremias and do not perpetuate the chain of transmission. In temperate areas, transmission ceases during the winter months; the mechanism or mechanisms whereby WEE virus persists in local winter reservoirs or is reintroduced in the spring are unknown.

CLINICAL FEATURES AND PATHOLOGY. The disease usually begins with generalized and nonspecific symptoms of fever, headache, malaise, and aches, lasting one to four days. Somnolence and lethargy, photophobia, vomiting, and neck stiffness signal the neurologic infection and progress, often quite rapidly, to stupor, coma, and, in a high proportion of children, convulsions. Paresis, cranial nerve deficits, tremors, and abnormal reflexes may be present. In fatal cases patients die one to two days after development of coma. Recovery often begins suddenly and progresses rapidly. About one third of surviving infants suffer retardation, cerebellar damage, choreoathetosis, and spastic paralysis. Young age at onset, duration of illness, and convulsions during the acute phase are harbingers of permanent sequelae. Adults may have a prolonged convalescent syndrome of asthenia and neuropsychiatric complaints, but objective residua are rare and parkinsonism is extremely uncommon. Congenital infections are documented and result in severe and progressive neurologic deterioration.

A moderate leukocytosis and left shift are usual. The cerebrospinal fluid contains white cells (at first polymorphonuclear, then mononuclear), rarely in excess of 500 per cubic millimeter, and elevated protein concentration (usually 90 to 110 mg per deciliter).

Pathologic examination of the brains of infants reveals massive neuroparenchymal destruction; children dying months or years after the acute insult often have large cystic lesions in many areas of the brain. In older children and adults, acute WEE is characterized by focal necrosis and perivascular cuffing, predominantly in the basal ganglia and thalamic nuclei, but also in deep cerebral white matter. The highest titers of virus and interferon have also been found in basal ganglia and thalamus.

DIAGNOSIS. Viral isolation from blood or cerebrospinal fluid is almost never successful; a diagnosis may sometimes be achieved by isolation of the virus from brain tissue, obtained by biopsy or at autopsy. Diagnosis is usually achieved by demonstration of a rise in hemagglutination-inhibiting (HI), fluorescent, complement-fixing (CF), enzyme-linked immunosorbent assay (ELISA), or neutralizing (N) antibody titers in appropriately timed paired sera. An acute phase serum is obtained as early as possible in the illness, and a second serum a minimum of 10 to 14 days later. Demonstration of immunoglobulin M (IgM) antibodies in cerebrospinal fluid by ELISA provides a presumptive diagnosis.

TREATMENT. No specific chemotherapeutic agent is known. Supportive nursing care is essential and may reduce mortality. Control of high fever by sponging or ice packs and administration of antipyretics orally or rectally are recommended. Prompt administration of anticonvulsants (intravenous diazepam for acute control and phenytoin for more prolonged control) should be used to prevent protracted seizures and attendant hypoxia. Dehydration caused by fever, vomiting, and insufficient oral intake may be prominent, especially in children, and fluid and electrolyte balance must be restored and maintained by intravenous infusions. Management of airways in semicomatose and comatose patients is essential. Arterial blood gases should be monitored and respiratory assistance provided if hypoxia occurs. Prevention and treatment of secondary bacterial infections may be required; good pulmonary toilet and care of urinary catheters are essential. If clinical signs suggest cerebral edema or if the cerebrospinal fluid pressure is very high (>400 mm H$_2$O), measures to reduce brain swelling are indicated. Clinical signs that suggest progressive intracranial hypertension include deepening obtundation; prolonged delirium; respiratory, ocular, and motor signs of diencephalic deterioration; and loss of brain stem reflexes. Treatment consists of intracranial pressure monitoring, osmotic agents (mannitol), neuromuscular blocking agents, and/or hyperventilation.

PREVENTION AND CONTROL. An experimental formalin-inactivated vaccine grown in chick embryo cell cultures has been used exclusively for protection of laboratory workers. A commercial vaccine is available for horses; since equines are dead-end hosts, vaccination plays no role in preventing human disease. A high level of vaccine immunity in equines reduces their value as sentinels of WEE activity (see Epidemiology). In threatened or ongoing epidemics, residents should be advised to avoid mosquito bite by use of protective clothing, repellents, window screens, and restricted outdoor activity in the early morning, late afternoon, and evening. Public health measures include spray application of insecticides aimed at the adult *Culex tarsalis* vector.

EASTERN EQUINE ENCEPHALITIS (EEE)

ETIOLOGIC AGENT. EEE virus, first isolated in 1933, is an alphavirus. Two antigenic subtypes (North and South American) are distinguishable by special serologic tests. Methods for viral isolation and assay are as described for WEE.

EPIDEMIOLOGY. *Incidence and Prevalence.* The disease in humans is relatively rare; 178 recognized cases were reported in the United States between 1955 and 1985. The largest outbreak occurred in 1959 in New Jersey (32 cases), but the usual pattern is one of a predominant equine epizootic involving 100 to 300 animals and associated with several human cases. The Atlantic and Gulf coastal areas are prone to recrudescent viral activity. Enzootic transmission and sporadic cases occur in inland freshwater swamp areas of the United States east of the Mississippi River. Outbreaks also occur in eastern Canada and in the Caribbean area (Jamaica,

Hispaniola, Cuba) caused by the North American viral subtype. Equine epizootics have appeared in Panama, Brazil, Guyana, Venezuela, and Argentina, but human disease is rare or unrecognized.

Despite the small size of EEE epidemics, their cost in terms of severity is high. The case-fatality rate is 60 to 70 per cent. The incidence and mortality are highest in children under 15 and in persons over 55 years, with no sex predilection. A risk of human disease may be predicted by the occurrence of equine cases or outbreaks of fatal encephalitis in penned exotic birds (pheasants, chukar partridges), which precede the appearance of human cases by several weeks or more. Vaccination of horses and birds or inadequate surveillance may abrogate their usefulness as sentinels. Outbreaks occur during the late summer and early fall.

Transmission. In temperate areas, EEE virus circulates between wild birds and *Culiseta melanura* mosquitoes in freshwater swamp habitat. Sporadic infections may be acquired by the bite of the primary enzootic vector, which is principally attracted to birds and rarely feeds on horses and humans. Other species—in particular, *Aedes sollicitans* and *Coquillettidia perturbans*—are implicated in epidemic-epizootic spread and extension of viral activity from swamp to salt marsh and woodland habitat. Transmission between penned pheasants and chukars is by contact, through pecking and cannibalism. The overwintering cycle is at present unknown.

CLINICAL FEATURES AND PATHOLOGY. The disease is more acute and rapidly progressive than the other arboviral encephalitides. The onset is abrupt, with high fever, vomiting, somnolence, stupor, coma, myoclonus, and generalized convulsions appearing within 24 to 48 hours. Autonomic disturbances (sialorrhea) may be prominent, and respiratory difficulty and cyanosis are frequent. A curious feature of the disease in children is facial, periorbital, or generalized edema. Death usually occurs during the first week; in surviving patients, recovery begins during the second week and may progress rapidly. Residual damage, in 30 to 50 per cent of the patients, is often severe, especially in children, and is characterized by retardation, spastic paralyses, and atrophy of brain substance.

Examination of the cerebrospinal fluid provides a clue to the diagnosis. Early in infection, EEE is characterized by high cell counts (500 to 2000 per cubic millimeter) and a predominance of polymorphonuclear cells. The total cell count falls after day three or four, but polymorphonuclear cells persist as a significant fraction. Red blood cells may be present, the protein elevated, and glucose normal. A striking peripheral leukocytosis and left shift are frequent findings.

In contrast to St. Louis and western equine encephalitis, the brain is grossly edematous and congested, and the inflammatory response is predominantly polymorphonuclear. Focal vasculitic lesions, endothelial cell swelling, and intravenous and arteriolar thrombus formation are present. Demyelination, necrosis, neuronolysis, and neuronophagia are prominent. The areas most affected are basal ganglia, thalamus, hippocampus, and frontal and occipital cortex.

SPECIFIC DIAGNOSIS. Isolation of virus from blood and spinal fluid is rarely successful. A postmortem diagnosis can be achieved by virus isolation from brain in approximately 75 per cent of fatal cases. Serologic diagnosis is as described for WEE virus; because of the rapid course of the clinical disease, sera should be obtained at two- to three-day intervals during the acute phase of illness. An early serologic diagnosis can often be made by this means.

TREATMENT. Treatment is supportive (see previous discussion of WEE).

PREVENTION AND CONTROL. An experimental formalin-inactivated chick embryo cell culture vaccine is used to protect laboratory and field workers. Vaccination prevents disease in equines but does not interrupt transmission or prevent human infection. Reduction of mosquito populations by appropriate use of insecticides may be effective in threatened or established outbreaks.

VENEZUELAN EQUINE ENCEPHALITIS (VEE)

ETIOLOGY. The causative agent is an alphavirus first isolated in 1938 from a sick horse in Venezuela. Six antigenic subtypes (I to VI) are separable by serologic tests; multiple antigenic variants of subtypes I and III are also recognized. Subtypes IAB and IC are responsible for epidemics involving humans and equines. In Florida, subtype II is enzootic and produces sporadic human disease. Definition of the antigenic subtype and variant responsible for infection requires isolation of the virus and characterization by a specialty laboratory.

EPIDEMIOLOGY. *Incidence and Prevalence.* Large equine epizootics occur at five- to ten-year intervals in Venezuela, Colombia, Ecuador, and Peru. The capacity of VEE virus to invade new territory was demonstrated in 1969, when subtype IAB virus appeared in Guatemala and spread in waves throughout Central America, Mexico, and south Texas. Individual epizootics have involved many thousands (sometimes more than 100,000) of animals, with up to 40 per cent mortality rates. Associated human morbidity has also been great (up to 30,000 clinical cases). Truly subclinical infections are rare. The predominant syndrome is a self-limited grippelike illness, and only about 4 per cent of infected persons, principally children under 15 years, develop encephalitis. The case-fatality rate in children up to five years old with encephalitis is approximately 35 per cent, but in older persons it is less than 10 per cent. Laboratory infections are common in unvaccinated persons working with the virus or infected animals.

Transmission. Transmission of subtypes IAB and IC viruses during epizootic-epidemics is effected by a large variety of mosquito vectors, including species of the genera *Aedes*, *Psorophora*, and *Mansonia*; equines are the principal viremic hosts. Viremia in humans is of sufficient magnitude to infect mosquitoes, but human-mosquito-human transmission is of minor importance in the generation and maintenance of an outbreak. Virus may be present in pharyngeal excretions of human patients; contact or aerosol person-to-person spread, although possible, is not epidemiologically important. Aerosol transmission in the laboratory is nevertheless well documented. The interepidemic maintenance transmission cycle of these viral subtypes is unknown.

The other members of the VEE viral complex, including subtype II in Florida, have enzootic transmission cycles involving *Culex (Melanoconion)* species mosquitoes and small forest rodents and marsupials. Equines are not involved in transmission; human disease is sporadic and relatively uncommon but may be clinically severe.

CLINICAL FEATURES AND PATHOLOGY. The incubation period is two to five days. Onset is sudden, with fever, chills, generalized malaise, and headache; these symptoms are followed by myalgia (especially in the lumbar region), nausea, vomiting, and occasionally diarrhea. Physical examination reveals fever, tachycardia, conjunctival injection, and, in some cases, nonexudative pharyngitis. Acute symptoms generally subside in four to six days; a convalescent fatigue syndrome may follow, lasting up to three weeks. A biphasic course has sometimes been noted; acute symptoms reappear after a brief remission, within a week after the initial onset.

Evidence of mild central nervous system involvement (photophobia, somnolence, confusion) may be present in cases of the typical grippelike illness described above. Severe encephalitis develops in a small proportion of those infected, principally children, and is characterized by meningeal signs, convulsions, tremor, stupor, coma, spastic paralysis, abnormal reflexes, cranial nerve palsies, and central respiratory failure. Residual neurologic damage occurs in severe cases. Infections of pregnant women acquired during the first and second trimesters may result in fetal encephalitis and death,

but the risk of congenital infection has not been quantitatively defined.

In the first few days of illness, the peripheral leukocyte count may be depressed, with decrease in both lymphocytes and neutrophils, or normal, with a relative lymphopenia. Eosinopenia and vacuolization of monocytes have been described. In patients with central nervous system signs, the cerebrospinal fluid contains up to 500 cells per cubic millimeter, predominantly lymphocytes. The serum lactic dehydrogenase and glutamic-oxaloacetic transaminase levels may be elevated.

Pathologic changes in the central nervous system include edema, congestion, meningeal and perivascular inflammation, intracerebral hemorrhages, neuronal degeneration, and vasculitis. In addition, hepatocellular degeneration and individual cell necrosis, widespread lymphoid depletion and follicular necrosis, and interstitial pneumonitis are frequent findings. In the congenitally infected fetus, there is massive and widespread necrosis of brain tissue, hemorrhages, and resorption of brain material, resulting in hydranencephaly.

DIAGNOSIS. Virus can be isolated from the blood during the first three or four days after onset, with peak titers on day two. Isolation from throat swabs or washings may also be successful. HI and N antibodies appear in the first week and CF antibodies in the second week after onset; serodiagnosis is achieved by testing appropriately timed paired sera.

TREATMENT. No specific therapy is available, and treatment of encephalitis cases is supportive (see earlier discussion of WEE).

PREVENTION AND CONTROL. An experimental live, attenuated vaccine (TC-83) is used in adult laboratory personnel and provides solid immunity to the immunizing subtype (IAB) and its closest relative (IC), but incomplete protection against infection with some heterologous VEE viruses. Epidemics and epizootics can be prevented by effective vaccination of equines (the principal viremic hosts), using live, attenuated, or inactivated vaccines. In the face of an ongoing epidemic, spraying of insecticides to reduce the adult (infective) mosquito populations is the only means of immediate control; vaccination of equines at the periphery of the outbreak prevents spread.

ST. LOUIS ENCEPHALITIS (SLE)

ETIOLOGY. St. Louis encephalitis virus, a member of the family Flaviviridae, shares close antigenic relationships with Japanese encephalitis, Murray Valley encephalitis, and West Nile viruses. The virus is pathogenic for infant and adult mice inoculated intracerebrally and may also be assayed in a variety of avian and mammalian cell cultures. Strain differences in pathogenicity and genome composition are recognized and provide a geographic and epidemiologic classification. Strains associated with *Culex pipiens*-borne epidemics in the eastern United States are distinct from endemic strains transmitted by *Culex tarsalis* in the western states.

EPIDEMIOLOGY. *Incidence and Prevalence.* The virus is present in all parts of the Western Hemisphere, but causes epidemics only in North America and some Caribbean islands. During epidemic years, the virus has been responsible for up to 80 per cent of all reported cases of encephalitis of known etiology in the United States. A total of 5073 cases were reported between 1955 and 1985. In recent years, epidemics have occurred mainly in urban-suburban localities of the Ohio–Mississippi River basin, in eastern and central Texas, and in Florida. Small outbreaks have also occurred in the western United States. Epidemics generally occur between July and September, with a peak in August, but may arise later in the year in warm areas such as Florida. No racial difference in disease susceptibility exists. Prior exposure and immunity to dengue may provide a degree of cross-protection against clinical SLE.

The overall case-fatality rate is approximately 9 per cent; mortality is negligible in persons under 20 years, and it rises steeply after age 55 to approximately 30 per cent in patients over 65 years of age. The inapparent:apparent infection ratio is 800:1 in children up to nine years, 400:1 in persons 10 to 49 years, and 85:1 in persons over 60 years.

In tropical America, a high prevalence of antibody in many areas indicates widespread transmission; disease is sporadic and rarely recognized.

Transmission. In most of the eastern United States, SLE virus circulates between wild birds and *Culex pipiens* mosquitoes. *Culex pipiens* breeds in polluted water and achieves high densities in urban-suburban areas with poor sanitation. In Florida and in parts of the Caribbean, *Culex nigripalpus* is the principal vector. The cycle in the western United States also involves wild birds, but the vector is *Culex tarsalis.* The ecology of SLE and WEE viruses in the west is thus similar, and transmission occurs predominantly in rural, agricultural areas. Horses develop antibodies but not overt disease or significant viremia. The primary vectors (*C. pipiens, nigripalpus, tarsalis*) are responsible for transmission to humans.

Above-average summer temperatures and deficient rainfall (which creates stagnant pools suitable for *Culex pipiens* breeding) are associated with epidemics in the eastern United States. *Culex tarsalis*–borne SLE in the western states is favored by warm spring temperatures, heavy winter-spring precipitation, high river runoff, and flood conditions.

During the winter, the virus is probably maintained locally in infected hibernating adult female *Culex.*

CLINICAL FEATURES AND PATHOLOGY. Three clinical syndromes are recognized: febrile headache, aseptic meningitis, and encephalitis. As discussed above, encephalitis is a more frequent presentation in the elderly and the milder syndromes in young patients. The incubation period is 4 to 21 days. Onset is characterized by a variable period of non-specific symptoms, including fever, headache, generalized malaise, drowsiness, myalgias, and sore throat, followed by the acute or subacute onset of meningeal or encephalitic signs or both. Fever ranges from 38.3 to 41°C; poor prognosis is associated with persistent high temperatures of 40 to 41°C. Nausea and vomiting and photophobia are common. Neurologic abnormalities include altered sensorium, meningismus, cranial nerve deficits (principally lower motor neuron N. VII), abnormal reflexes, and tremors. Signs of thalamic, brain stem, and cerebellar dysfunction include myoclonic twitching, nystagmus, and ataxia in up to 25 per cent of patients. Motor abnormalities are infrequent and sensory changes extremely uncommon. Convulsions occur in 10 per cent of patients and are a poor prognostic sign. In general, extrapyramidal abnormalities (tremor of tongue, face, and limbs) and the altered state of consciousness are the most significant findings. Signs of markedly increased intracranial pressure are very unusual. Acute inflammatory polyradiculoneuropathy (Guillain-Barré syndrome) has occasionally been associated with SLE, both as an acute presentation and during the convalescent period. Approximately half of the patients with fatal outcome succumb during the first week and 80 per cent within two weeks after onset. Complications of the neurologic disease include pneumonia, bacterial septicemia, pulmonary embolism, and gastrointestinal hemorrhage. Underlying conditions, especially hypertensive and arteriosclerotic disease, chronic brain syndromes, diabetes mellitus, and chronic bronchopulmonary disease, appear to play a role in determining severity and outcome.

In uncomplicated cases of SLE, there is a moderate peripheral neutrophilic leukocytosis and left shift. Cerebrospinal fluid is under increased pressure and contains up to 500 cells per cubic millimeter, with polymorphonuclear predominance early, changing to lymphocyte predominance within several days. Spinal fluid protein is mildly elevated and glucose usually normal. Elevations of serum enzymes (creatine phos-

phokinase and glutamic-oxaloacetic transaminase) are frequently found. Serum aldolase levels may be elevated, but muscle biopsies have shown no changes. The electroencephalogram typically shows amorphous delta wave activity and diffuse generalized slowing most prominent in the frontal and temporal regions. The brain scan is normal. Disproportionately high cerebral blood flow in relation to metabolic demands has been documented, indicating a disturbance in cerebrovascular autoregulation. The syndrome of inappropriate secretion of antidiuretic hormone is present in about one third of patients.

Genitourinary tract symptoms (urgency, frequency, incontinence, and retention), microscopic hematuria, pyuria, and proteinuria, and elevated blood urea nitrogen are frequent. SLE viral antigen in cells of the urinary sediment has been detected by fluorescent techniques and virus-like particles in urine by immunoelectronmicroscopy.

A convalescent fatigue syndrome characterized by weakness, fatigue, nervousness, tremulousness, sleeplessness, irritability, depression, difficulty in concentrating, and headaches occurs in 30 to 50 per cent of older persons and clears in 80 per cent of these within three years.

Pathologic changes in fatal cases are limited to microscopic findings. Leptomeningitis is characterized by lymphocytic inflammation. Parenchymal changes consist of lymphocytic perivascular cuffing, cellular nodule formation, and neuronal degeneration. Changes are most pronounced in substantia nigra, thalamus and hypothalamus, cerebellar cortex, cerebral cortex, and basal ganglia.

DIAGNOSIS. In approximately half of the fatal cases, a diagnosis may be made by virus isolation from brain tissue or immunofluorescent staining of frozen sections of brain. The virus is rarely isolated from blood or spinal fluid obtained during the acute phase of illness. Serologic diagnosis is achieved by demonstration of changing antibody titers; the HI, fluorescent antibody (FA), ELISA, and N tests demonstrate antibody within the first week after onset, and titers rise during the ensuing two weeks. CF antibodies appear 10 to 20 days after onset. Rapid, early diagnosis is possible by measurement of IgM antibodies by ELISA in serum and cerebrospinal fluid. Specific serologic diagnosis may be complicated by cross-reactions in persons with prior exposures to dengue and other related flaviviruses.

TREATMENT. Treatment is supportive (see earlier discussion of WEE). Hyponatremia and clinical signs of water intoxication are managed by restricting fluid intake.

PREVENTION AND CONTROL. No vaccine is available. Surveillance of vectors, antibody prevalence in wild birds, or serologic conversions in sentinel fowl are used to detect viral transmission before the occurrence of human infections. The information may be used to initiate vector control efforts. Source reduction and larviciding of vector breeding sites are useful preventive measures. In the case of an established outbreak, avoidance of mosquito bites and spraying to reduce infected adult mosquitoes are the only effective means of control.

CALIFORNIA ENCEPHALITIS

ETIOLOGY. At least four members of the California serogroup of the *Bunyavirus* genus—LaCrosse, California encephalitis, Jamestown Canyon, and snowshoe hare viruses—cause encephalitis. A fifth virus (Trivittatus) has also been implicated as a pathogen, but on the basis of meager evidence. California encephalitis virus occurs in the western United States (California, New Mexico, Utah, Texas) and has been implicated in only three human cases. In contrast, LaCrosse virus, distributed more widely in the eastern half of the United States and southern Canada, is a major human pathogen. Recently Jamestown Canyon and snowshoe hare viruses have been implicated in sporadic human encephalitis cases in the north central United States and in Canada.

EPIDEMIOLOGY. *Incidence and Prevalence.* Between its recognition as a nosologic entity in 1964 and 1985, a total of 1661 cases of California encephalitis have been reported in the United States, with an annual incidence of 50 to 150 cases. The vast majority of these cases is probably due to LaCrosse virus; a total of 39 cases have been associated with the Jamestown Canyon virus. Undoubtedly far under-reported, California encephalitis occurs as an endemic rather than an epidemic disease, with individual or small clusters of cases scattered across the affected areas. It is most prevalent in the north central states, where it is responsible for as many as 20 per cent of cases of acute central nervous system infection in children. It primarily affects persons less than 15 years of age living in rural and suburban areas characterized by deciduous hardwood forests. Focal "hot spots" (communities, even backyards) of recurrent summertime viral activity are recognized. Cases occur between July and September, with peak incidence in August. The case-fatality rate is low (less than 1 per cent). The inapparent:apparent infection ratio has been variably estimated at between 26:1 and 1571:1.

Transmission. The vectors of LaCrosse virus are *Aedes* mosquitoes (principally *Ae. triseriatus*), which breed both in forest tree-holes and in peridomestic artificial containers. The vector serves as a reservoir of LaCrosse virus, which is efficiently passed transovarially from female mosquitoes to progeny. The virus survives the winter months in infected eggs of *Aedes triseriatus*. In the summer months, wild rodents (squirrels, chipmunks) contribute to a cycle of transmission as viremic hosts. Humans become infected by the bite of an infected mosquito but do not play a role in transmission.

Aedes communis, Ae. stimulans, Ae. triseriatus, and possibly anopheline mosquitoes are involved in transmission of Jamestown Canyon virus, and deer are the principal vertebrate hosts.

CLINICAL FEATURES. The true clinical spectrum of California virus infection is not known but undoubtedly includes nonspecific febrile illness, aseptic meningitis, and meningoencephalitis. Repiratory symptoms have been a prominent feature of Jamestown Canyon virus infections. Encephalitis may be quite severe in the acute stage, but the disease is almost always self limited and death is extremely uncommon. The disease begins with a nonspecific syndrome of fever, headache, sore throat, and gastrointestinal symptoms, with appearance of the neurotropic disorder within one to three days. In mild cases of encephalitis, central nervous system signs appear on the third day after onset and subside within seven to eight days. In the more severe form, neurologic signs appear earlier (within 24 to 48 hours of onset), usually in the form of generalized seizures and altered consciousness, and are more prolonged. Papilledema or abnormal optic disc margins have been noted, but signs of progressive intracranial hypertension are rare. Intensive care and respiratory support are frequently required in severe cases. The question of permanent sequelae is unsettled. Many workers believe LaCrosse virus infection is responsible for residual psychologic problems, emotional lability, hyperkinesis, infantilism, compulsive behavior, and auditory and visual perceptual problems. There are case reports of hemiparesis and persistent seizure disorders.

The peripheral white cell count is often moderately elevated, with a predominance of granulocytes and band forms. The cerebrospinal fluid shows up to 500 lymphocytes per cubic millimeter, normal or mildly elevated protein, and normal glucose concentrations. The abnormalities on the electroencephalogram include generalized slowing in the delta and theta range, indicating diffuse cortical dysfunction. Focal delta wave activity related to cortical destruction or focal seizures is also a common finding.

Histopathologic features in the central nervous system are qualitatively similar to those of other viral encephalitides; however, absence of inflammatory lesions in cerebellum, medulla, and spinal cord has been postulated to be a distinguishing feature of LaCrosse infection.

DIAGNOSIS. The virus has been recovered from the brain in fatal cases, but not from blood or spinal fluid obtained during the acute phase. Diagnosis is best achieved by tests for antibody in paired acute and convalescent sera. The counterimmunoelectrophoresis, HI, CF, FA, ELISA, and N test are applicable. However, the most practical, sensitive, and reliable methods are the HI test using the LaCrosse viral antigen and the IgM antibody capture ELISA.

TREATMENT. Treatment is supportive.

PREVENTION AND CONTROL. There is no vaccine. Vector control methods are of uncertain usefulness in this disease because of the multifocal, endemic pattern of disease incidence and the inherited nature of infection in mosquito vectors. In defined "hot spots" of recurrent viral activity, efforts to eliminate breeding sites for *Aedes triseriatus* should be made. Avoidance of mosquito bites and protection of children by limiting exposure and use of repellents are reasonable suggestions to parents.

JAPANESE ENCEPHALITIS (JE)

ETIOLOGY. Japanese encephalitis is caused by a flavivirus first isolated in 1934 from the brain of a person who died of encephalitis in Japan. Unlike SLE, it causes epizootics of clinical encephalitis in equines. The virus also produces abortion and stillbirth in swine, an important economic problem in parts of Asia. Serologic cross-reactivity with other flaviviruses may lead to confusion in diagnostic tests.

EPIDEMIOLOGY. *Prevalence and Incidence.* The disease is endemic and epidemic in Asia, including Japan, Korea, Taiwan, China, Okinawa, Vietnam, the Philippines, Burma, Malaysia, Bangladesh, east and south India, Sri Lanka, Thailand, and Indonesia. Over 10,000 cases occur annually in Asia, and morbidity in some individual epidemics is high; case-fatality rates of 50 per cent or more have been reported but reflect under-recognition of nonfatal cases. In hyperendemic areas, over 70 per cent of adult populations surveyed have antibodies, and children under 15 years old are principally affected by the disease. In areas without a high prevalence of background immunity (e.g., northern India), however, all age groups are affected; and in Japan, where school children have been protected by vaccination campaigns targeted at this age group, occurrence of encephalitis in the elderly has become evident. The inapparent:apparent infection ratio is over 500:1 in children and decreases with age; in Korea, the ratio among American servicemen was estimated at 25:1. In temperate areas, JE is a summertime disease; in the tropics, it occurs year-round as a sporadic infection. Epidemics have been most frequent at the northern fringe of the tropical zone. JE is predominantly a rural disease, and the incidence in males is often higher than in females.

Transmission. The natural cycle involves *Culex* mosquito vectors and vertebrates susceptible to viremic infection, including wild birds and swine. Humans and equines are incidental (dead-end) hosts. The vector species varies with geographic area; *Culex tritaeniorhyncus*, a rice-paddy breeder, is the most widespread and important. Overwinter survival and springtime recrudescence in temperate areas are unexplained, but evidence suggests that transovarial viral transmission in mosquitoes may play a role.

CLINICAL FEATURES AND PATHOLOGY. The spectrum of illness includes febrile headache, aseptic meningitis, and meningoencephalitis. The disease is more severe than St. Louis encephalitis. Onset is abrupt, with fever, headache, and gastrointestinal symptoms. Meningeal irritation develops within 24 hours and is followed on the second or third day by the appearance of irritability, impaired consciousness, convulsions (especially in children), muscular rigidity, mask-like facies, ataxia, coarse tremor, involuntary movements, cranial nerve deficits, paresis, hyperactive deep tendon reflexes, and pathologic reflexes. Weight loss and dehydration are often striking findings. In patients with mild involvement, fever subsides on the sixth or seventh day and neurologic signs resolve by the end of the second week after onset. In severe cases, hyperpyrexia and progressive neurologic dysfunction and coma result in death between the seventh and tenth days, or the patient undergoes a prolonged recovery, often leaving permanent sequelae. Cardiorespiratory complications are frequent during the acute stage in these patients. Atypical forms with predominance of bulbar or myelitic signs have been described. A poor prognosis is associated with prolonged high fever, frequent or prolonged seizures, high protein content in the cerebrospinal fluid, Babinski signs, and early appearance of respiratory depression.

The occurrence of sequelae correlates with severity of the acute stage of illness; young children are most susceptible, and sequelae, including mental impairment, emotional lability, choreoathetosis, tremor, parkinsonism, autonomic disturbances, motor paralysis, and pathopsychologic syndromes, including schizophrenia, have been reported in up to 75 per cent of patients.

Transplacental infection, resulting in fetal death and abortion, has been reported.

Clinical laboratory tests show a moderate peripheral leukocytosis early in the disease (usually characterized by neutrophilia) and cerebrospinal fluid pleocytosis, polymorphonuclear early but predominantly mononuclear later in the disease. Spinal fluid protein is mildly elevated, and glucose concentration is normal.

Neuropathologic changes and distribution of lesions are similar to those described for St. Louis encephalitis (see earlier discussion of SLE).

DIAGNOSIS. In many patients dying during the first week after onset, the virus may be isolated from brain or viral antigen demonstrated by immunofluorescence. Isolation from blood is uncommon; virus is cultivatable from cerebrospinal fluid from about one third of patients who progress to a fatal outcome, but rarely from patients with nonfatal cases. HI and N antibodies appear during the first and CF antibodies during the second week after onset. In areas where other flaviviral infections are common, cross-reactions make serodiagnosis difficult; increased precision may be obtained by measuring early, specific IgM antibodies by immunoassays on serum or cerebrospinal fluid. Diagnostic levels of IgM antibody are detectable in cerebrospinal fluid in over three fourths of patients at the time of hospital admission.

TREATMENT. Treatment is supportive (see earlier discussion of WEE).

PREVENTION AND CONTROL. Inactivated, partially purified mouse brain vaccines produced in Japan are used principally in preschool- and school-age children. This vaccine has been found safe and extremely effective in a controlled field trial. Although not yet licensed for use in the United States, a vaccine produced in Japan is available on a limited scale to United States citizens traveling to high-risk areas. Information should be sought from state health departments or the Centers for Disease Control. Since three doses of the inactivated vaccine are used, and approximately one month is required to confer protection, vaccination is not a practical measure in the face of an ongoing epidemic. Reduction of vector mosquito populations by application of insecticides may be used to abort outbreaks.

MURRAY VALLEY ENCEPHALITIS AND ROCIO ENCEPHALITIS

Murray Valley encephalitis and Rocio encephalitis are similar to Japanese encephalitis in pathogenesis and clinical features and are caused by closely related flaviviruses.

Murray Valley encephalitis has occurred in small epidemics in the Murray and Darling River valleys of Victoria and New

South Wales, Australia. The virus is endemic in Northern Australia and New Guinea, where it is maintained in a bird-mosquito cycle. It has been postulated that the virus is intermittently brought south by migratory birds; in southern Australia, transmission involves water birds, domestic fowl, and *Culex annulirostris* mosquitoes. Diagnosis requires laboratory studies similar to those for other flaviviruses. No vaccine is available.

Rocio encephalitis was first described in 1975, when a new flavivirus by the same name was isolated from the brains of patients with fatal encephalitis during an epidemic in São Paulo State, Brazil. In several discrete outbreaks in 1975 and 1976, over 1000 cases occurred in this region, but the disease has not been recognized elsewhere. The transmission cycle is poorly understood but probably involves wild birds and mosquitoes. An inactivated suckling mouse brain vaccine has been prepared but has been found to be of low potency.

TICK-BORNE ENCEPHALITIS (TBE)

ETIOLOGIC AGENTS. A complex of six antigenically related tick-borne flaviviruses consists of Powassan, tick-borne encephalitis virus (TBE), louping ill, Kyasanur Forest disease (KFD), Omsk hemorrhagic fever (OHF), and Langat viruses. The predominant syndrome in KFD and OHF is hemorrhagic fever (see Ch. 363), but meningoencephalitis may be a component of the disease spectrum. Two subtypes of TBE virus (Central European encephalitis and Russian spring-summer encephalitis) are distinguished by special serologic tests, are ecologically distinct, and differ in virulence for humans. Powassan and louping ill viruses are rare causes of encephalitis in North America and the British Isles, respectively. These viruses are serologically easily distinguished from mosquito-borne flaviviruses but induce cross-reactions within the complex. The viruses may be isolated and assayed in infant mice and a variety of cell cultures.

EPIDEMIOLOGY. *Incidence and Prevalence.* TBE occurs in Europe (including European Russia), southern Scandinavia, and the far eastern USSR. Several hundred to 2000 cases are reported annually, with morbidity rates of up to 20 per 100,000 inhabitants. Inapparent infections are common. The disease is seasonal, corresponding to peak summertime tick vector populations. Adults over 20 years are principally affected, and persons frequenting tick-infested foci (e.g., forestry workers, shepherds, campers) are at highest risk. Family outbreaks are caused by drinking infected milk (see Transmission, below). In Europe, the disease is relatively mild (case-fatality rate 1 to 2 per cent); but in the Far East, it is severe (20 to 25 per cent). In the United States, the disease should be considered in persons with a history of travel to endemic areas.

Louping ill causes encephalitis in sheep and cattle in Scotland and in northern England and Ireland. Sporadic human cases have been recognized in veterinarians, butchers, and laboratory workers. Serologic surveys indicate that natural infections are uncommon. Powassan virus encephalitis has been documented in a total of 15 cases in the northeastern United States and eastern Canada. The case-fatality rate is 50 per cent. The virus is not associated with animal disease. Serosurveys indicate that human infections in the endemic area are rare (prevalence rates less than 1 per cent).

Transmission. In Europe, the vector of TBE is *Ixodes ricinus*, and in the Far East, *I. persulcatus*. The tick vector also serves as a reservoir of the virus, which is transmitted both transovarially and from one stage (instar) to the next. Larval ticks parasitize small rodents, which serve as amplifying viremic hosts during the spring and summer; hibernating rodents may also harbor the virus during the winter. The human is a dead-end host, incidental to the transmission cycle. Large vertebrates (goats, sheep, cattle) are hosts for nymphal and adult ticks and may become infected and shed virus in the milk. Outbreaks have occurred in families or groups of individuals ingesting unpasteurized goat or sheep milk or cheese.

Louping ill virus is maintained in nature by *Ixodes ricinus* ticks and a variety of hosts, including small mammals, ground-dwelling birds (grouse), and probably sheep. Humans become infected by direct contact with infected sheep or by tick bite. The transmission cycle of Powassan virus involves *Ixodes cookei, I. marxi* (and possibly other tick species), and mammals, particularly rodents and carnivores. Human infection is acquired by tick bite; because of the small size of the vector, a history of bite is infrequently obtained.

CLINICAL FEATURES. TBE in Europe typically (but not invariably) has a diphasic course, beginning 7 to 14 days after exposure with an influenza-like syndrome lasting one week, followed by a period of clinical remission for several days, and then abrupt onset of aseptic meningitis or meningoencephalitis. The latter is usually benign, although severe paralytic illness, myelitis, myeloradiculitis, and bulbar forms may occur. Convalescence is often prolonged, and residual paralysis may follow in severe cases. In the Far East, TBE begins suddenly with fever, headache, and gastrointestinal symptoms, followed rapidly by appearance of depressed sensorium, coma, convulsions, and paralysis. Bulbar paralysis and cervical myelitis are frequent findings. In fatal cases, death occurs in the first week after onset. Survivors have a high incidence of residual paralyses, especially lower motor neuron paralysis of upper extremities or shoulder girdle. Aseptic meningitis and milder forms of encephalitis also occur. Chronic forms of TBE have been described, with active clinical and pathologic abnormalities a year or more after onset.

The clinical features of louping ill resemble the European form of TBE. Powassan encephalitis is characterized by a variable period of fever and nonspecific symptoms, followed by the development of encephalitic signs, which are frequently severe. Residual paralysis may occur.

Peripheral blood and cerebrospinal fluid changes are similar to those described in other forms of flaviviral encephalitis.

DIAGNOSIS. The virus may be isolated from brain tissue. In TBE, virus isolation from blood is also possible during the early phase of illness. Serologic diagnosis is achieved by the HI, CF, N, or ELISA techniques.

TREATMENT. Treatment is supportive (see earlier discussion of WEE).

CONTROL. In eastern Europe and the USSR, TBE vaccines are used in high-risk groups (forestry and agricultural workers, military personnel). Avoidance of tick exposure by use of protective clothing and repellents may be recommended in areas of high TBE activity. In years of high rodent population density, rodent control in natural foci has also been recommended.

Blaškovič D, Nosek J: The ecological approach to the study of tick-borne encephalitis. Prog Med Virol 14:275, 1972. *Comprehensive review of the ecology, epidemiology, prevention, and control of tick-borne encephalitis; exhaustively referenced.*

Calisher CH, Thompson WH (eds.): California Serogroup Viruses. New York, Alan R. Liss, Inc., 1983. *Symposium covering all aspects of this virus group.*

Grabow JD, Matthews CG, Chun RWM, et al.: The electroencephalogram and clinical sequelae of California arbovirus encephalitis. Neurology 19:394, 1969. *Clear descriptions of clinical course and residual damage in children with California encephalitis; should be consulted together with reference by Matthews et al.*

Johnson KM, Martin DH: Venezuelan equine encephalitis. Adv Vet Sci Comp Med 18:79, 1974. *A superbly written, detailed, and well-referenced review of the clinical, virologic, and epidemiologic aspects of this disease.*

Leon CA, Jaramillo R, Martinez S, et al.: Sequelae of Venezuelan equine encephalitis in humans: A four-year follow-up. Int J Epidemiol 4:131, 1975. *The only well-documented study of neurologic residua of this infection.*

Lincoln AF, Sivertson SE: Acute phase of Japanese B encephalitis. Two hundred and one cases in American soldiers, Korea, 1950. JAMA 150:268, 1952. *The leading reference in English to the clinical features of Japanese encephalitis.*

Lopes O de S, Sachetta L de A, Coimbra TLM, et al.: Emergence of a new arbovirus disease in Brazil [Rocio]. II. Epidemiologic studies on 1975 epidemic. Am J Epidemiol 108:394, 1978. *First description of this newly recognized disease; contains only epidemiologic information.*

Matthews CG, Chun RWM, Grabow JD, et al.: Psychological sequelae in children following California arbovirus encephalitis. Neurology 18:1023, 1968. *Useful to the physician facing questions from patients about sequelae in children recovering from this infection.*

Monath TP (ed.): Saint Louis Encephalitis. Washington, D.C., American Public Health Association, 1980. *Encyclopedic coverage of all aspects of St. Louis encephalitis, including clinical features and differential and definitive laboratory diagnosis. Contains references to all previously published studies.*

Viral Hemorrhagic Fevers

Robert E. Shope

360 INTRODUCTION

The viral hemorrhagic fevers encompass syndromes that vary from febrile hemorrhagic disease with capillary fragility to acute severe shock leading rapidly to death. The causative agents include arthropod-borne and rodent-borne viruses. The rodent-borne viruses do not require an arthropod vector, but are transmitted directly to vertebrates by aerosol spread or contact with infected excreta or body secretions of the rodent. The reservoir and natural mode of transmission for the African hemorrhagic fever viruses, Marburg and Ebola, are not known.

There are at least 15 viruses that cause human hemorrhagic fevers (see Table 352–1). They are in the families Flaviviridae, Bunyaviridae, Arenaviridae, and Filoviridae (proposed family name). All contain RNA and all are zoonoses.

The hemorrhagic fevers form a special group of diseases characterized by viral replication in lymphoid cells, followed by fever and myalgia and leading to hemorrhagic manifestations and hypovolemic shock. The basic physiologic defect in most is capillary leakage. In some, such as yellow fever, hepatocellular damage is prominent. In others, such as hemorrhagic fever with renal syndrome, renal lesions are striking. The mortality rates may be high and the pathogenesis is poorly understood. Disseminated intravascular coagulopathy (DIC) is a feature in some cases, but probably not all. Antigen-antibody complexes may lead to release of mediators of shock in some cases, and direct effects of viral replication on capillary permeability in some have not been ruled out. It is important to understand the pathogenetic mechanism in order to manage the patient, but our knowledge is sparse at present.

Control can be achieved by interrupting the cycle, including peridomestic rodent control (Bolivian hemorrhagic fever) and, in those that are arboviruses, by vaccination of reservoir animals (Rift Valley fever), vector control, and education on methods to avoid the vector (dengue). Vaccines are available or under development for some of the agents such as Rift Valley fever, yellow fever, dengue, and Junin viruses. For others such as Lassa virus, we now have an antiviral drug, and for still another (Junin) pre- and postexposure protection is afforded by human immune plasma.

361 YELLOW FEVER

DEFINITION. Yellow fever is an acute viral disease caused by infection with yellow fever virus. The disease is exemplary of the viral hemorrhagic fevers described in the following sections (Table 361–1). The infection is often subclinical but may lead to disease whose severity varies from mild and self-limited to a fulminant fatal outcome. Classic yellow fever is characterized by sudden onset, moderately high fever, nausea, bradycardia, prostration, vomiting of altered blood, jaundice, oliguria, and albuminuria. Natural cycles of the infection occur periodically in mosquitoes and primates of tropical South America as far north as Panama and in tropical west, central, and east Africa.

ETIOLOGY. Yellow fever virus is in the genus *Flavivirus* of the family Flaviviridae. Members of the family are single-stranded, negative-sense, RNA viruses, spherical, and approximately 40 nm in diameter. Particles form in the cytoplasm in close association with endoplasmic reticulum. They contain a lipid envelope and replicate in both arthropod and vertebrate cells. Other members of the Flaviviridae, including dengue, West Nile, and St. Louis encephalitis, cross-react with yellow fever virus in serologic tests and may confound the diagnosis. Minor antigenic differences exist between strains of yellow fever virus from Africa and South America, and among strains from different regions of Africa; however the 17D yellow fever vaccine protects against all strains. The virus can be isolated in mosquitoes, arthropod and vertebrate tissue cultures, baby mice, and several monkey species. Rhesus monkeys regularly succumb following experimental inoculation and mimic severe human disease.

EPIDEMIOLOGY. Two epidemiologic types of yellow fever are distinguished: the urban and the sylvan (jungle) forms. Urban yellow fever is transmitted by *Aedes aegypti* mosquitoes from person to person, whereas yellow fever is maintained in a forest cycle of monkeys and forest-canopy mosquitoes; humans are infected when they enter the forest. The two types do not differ clinically.

A. aegypti is a peridomestic mosquito that breeds in abandoned tires, jars, cans, water storage containers, roof catchments, and drains in and around houses. Urban yellow fever was a major killer until the early 1900s when mosquito control in Havana, Rio de Janeiro, Guayaquil, and the other large urban centers eliminated the disease. The last recorded urban case in the Americas was in Trinidad in 1954. *A. aegypti* continues to be prevalent in African cities, and *A. aegypti*–

transmitted outbreaks still occur there. Major epidemics were recorded in Ethiopia, 1960–1962; Nigeria, 1969; Senegal, 1965 and 1979; Gambia, 1978; and Ghana and Burkina Faso, 1983. In 1986, an epidemic involving at least 3000 persons occurred in Nigeria, in Benue and Cross River States. Yellow fever virus in Africa is transmitted by *A. aegypti* not only in the cities, but also in semirural areas. In addition, some African epidemics are maintained by other *Aedes* species, such as *simpsoni* and the tree-hole breeding *Africanus, leuteocephalus,* and *furcifer-taylori,* which transmit the virus in savannah and the transition forest-savannah zones of west Africa.

Sylvan yellow fever was recognized initially in Brazil in 1932. After urban yellow fever had been controlled in the Americas, sporadic cases continued to occur in persons exposed to mosquitoes in the jungles of South America and Africa. This sylvan form is maintained in tropical America by *Haemagogus* mosquitoes and forest primates, and sometimes by other sylvan animals. Evidence favors the hypothesis that the virus moves through the forest, cycling in one place until the monkeys are immune, then dying out and moving to areas where there are susceptible monkeys. People entering the forest are at risk. Sylvan yellow fever extends periodically outside the enzootic zone into forests such as those in Panama and Central America. The virus can be maintained over dry periods by transovarial transmission in mosquitoes, although it remains to be shown whether maintenance in mosquito eggs is more than a temporary mechanism.

The sylvan cycle in Africa is more complicated than in the Americas; in tropical Africa the virus cycles between *A. africanus* and monkeys. Another African mosquito, *A. simpsoni,* which feeds on both humans and monkeys, serves in some areas as a link between primates in the deep forest and people in the African villages.

A. aegypti was once carried on sailing ships between tropical ports and into temperate-zone cities. Modern ocean-going ships no longer harbor mosquito breeding sites, but the mosquito continues to travel by small boats, airplanes, cars, and especially in the form of dried eggs transported by used tires. Cities such as Rio de Janeiro, which were once freed of the mosquito, are now reinfested. Dengue fever reappeared there in 1985. To control the mosquito again in this area will be difficult because of insecticide resistance and the high price of labor and materials. Jungle yellow fever continues to cycle, reappearing in the same locale every 5 to 40 years. The scene is thus set again for emergence of the virus from the jungle to reinitiate the urban cycle in the Americas.

A. aegypti is easily identified. It has white thoracic scales in the shape of a lyre and black legs with white bands. Mosquitoes that have fed on a viremic vertebrate become infective after an extrinsic incubation period of 9 to 30 days, the shorter

TABLE 361–1. CLINICAL PARAMETERS OF VIRAL HEMORRHAGIC FEVERS

| Disease | Viral Agent | Incubation Period (Days) | Clinical Syndromes | | | | Case-Fatality Rate (%) |
			Hemorrhage	*Hepatitis*	*Encephalitis*	*Nephropathy*	
Yellow fever	Yellow fever	3–6	major	major	absent	moderate	2–20
Dengue hemorrhagic fever	Dengue 1–4	5–8	moderate	moderate	absent	absent	2–5
Rift Valley fever	Rift Valley fever	3–6	major	major	moderate	absent	30–50
Crimean-Congo hemorrhagic fever	Crimean-Congo hemorrhagic fever	2–9	major	major	minor	absent	30–50
Kyasanur Forest disease	Kyasanur Forest disease	3–8	minor	minor	moderate	absent	5–10
Omsk hemorrhagic fever	Omsk hemorrhagic fever	3–8	minor	minor	moderate	absent	0.4–2.5
Hemorrhagic fever with renal syndrome	Hantaan	2–42	moderate	rare	minor	major	2–5
Argentine hemorrhagic fever	Junin	10–14	minor	rare	moderate	minor	1–15
Bolivian hemorrhagic fever	Machupo	7–14	moderate	rare	moderate	minor	15–30
Lassa fever	Lassa	3–16	minor	major	minor	minor	10–25
African hemorrhagic fever	Marburg	3–9	major	major	minor	absent	20–30
	Ebola	3–18	major	major	minor	absent	60–90

periods correlating with higher ambient temperatures. This extrinsic incubation period in the mosquito accounts for the delay from the first human infection in an urban outbreak to subsequent clusters of infection.

Yellow fever is not found in Asia, although large areas harbor *A. aegypti* that are capable of transmitting the virus should it be introduced. India and other Asian nations require vaccination of travelers from yellow fever–endemic regions.

All age groups and races are susceptible. However, sylvan yellow fever is found almost always in young males because they are the individuals who venture into the forest. Immunity following vaccination or infection is long-lasting. During an epidemic the population at risk, therefore, may be limited to age groups not covered by prior immunization or those born since a prior outbreak. There is also some evidence that persons may be protected by antibody to heterologous flaviviruses.

During the 20-year period from 1965 to 1984, there were 2475 cases of sylvan yellow fever reported in the Americas, and 2885 in Africa. The numbers of cases are greatly underestimated, probably by a factor of at least 10. Case-fatality rates are usually about 20 per cent, but are higher in some epidemics. Apparent to inapparent infection ratios, estimated at 1:10, may vary greatly.

PATHOLOGY AND PATHOGENESIS. The lesions of yellow fever involve primarily the liver, heart, kidneys, and lymphoid tissues. Grossly, the skin is icteric, and there may be multiple hemorrhages or petechiae of the skin, mucous membranes, and of multiple organs. The liver is normal in size, icteric, and fatty. The heart is soft and flabby, and the kidneys are swollen and a pink-grey color. Small peritoneal and pleural effusions are sometimes observed.

Histology is often characteristic in patients who die before the ninth day of illness, but the lesions are not always pathognomonic. The most striking lesion is the eosinophilic degeneration and coagulation of hepatocytes (Councilman bodies). Hepatocyte destruction is most marked in the midzone of the lobule, with relative sparing of the central vein and portal areas. Intranuclear eosinophilic granular inclusions or enlarged nucleoli (Torre's bodies) are also described. Both micro- and multivacuolar fatty changes are prominent, especially after the first week of illness. Inflammation is uncommon, and the reticulum framework is unaffected, probably accounting for the absence of postnecrotic fibrosis in convalescence and the regeneration of hepatocytes in recovered cases. The kidneys show cloudy swelling of tubular epithelium leading to acute tubular necrosis. The glomeruli are not obviously affected, but special stains indicate Schiff-positive alterations in the basal membranes, and proteinaceous material accumulates in the capsular spaces and lumina of the proximal tubules. The myocardium is characterized by granular or fatty infiltration of muscle fibers and of the A-V conduction system and cloudy swelling and degeneration of myocytes without inflammation. Large monocytes replace lymphocytic cells in the splenic follicles and lymph nodes. Encephalitis is rare, although petechial hemorrhage in the brain stem and cerebral edema are observed.

Knowledge of the pathogenesis of yellow fever is sparse. Yellow fever cases occur in remote areas, and pathophysiologic studies of yellow fever patients are usually done with only rudimentary laboratory facilities. The virus replicates in the hepatocytes and myocytes, and it is presumed that lesions in these target cells are a direct effect of the virus. Jaundice and prolonged prothrombin time can be explained by hepatocellular damage; bradycardia and arrhythmias, by myocyte and A-V node perturbation.The etiology of renal tubular necrosis is not clear but it may be secondary to hepatic changes. Some, but not all, fatal cases are associated with thrombocytopenia, increased prothrombin, partial thromboplastin, and thrombin times, diminished factor VIII and fibrinogen, and the presence of fibrin split products. The

bleeding in these cases may be secondary to disseminated intravascular coagulopathy, but this is not generally accepted by all investigators. Hypoglycemia, metabolic acidosis, and hyperkalemia characterize the terminal stage and are probably the result of multiple organ system failure.

CLINICAL MANIFESTATIONS. Severe yellow fever is a fulminant febrile illness with 50 per cent or greater mortality. There is a great deal of variation, however; most cases are mild with a better prognosis, and only about 10 to 20 per cent are in the severe category. The intrinsic incubation period is three to six days, exceptionally as long as ten days.

The clinical syndrome is classified as very mild, mild, moderately severe, or malignant. Very mild cases have fever and headache, and the patient recovers in 48 hours or less. Mild cases have sudden fever and headache with nausea, sometimes bleeding of the gums or epistaxis, bradycardia, or albuminuria. The patient recovers in two or three days. Moderately severe cases have more marked manifestations of bleeding, definite bradycardia in relation to the fever, nausea and vomiting, jaundice, and striking albuminuria. The illness may be aborted after three to four days or may develop serious hemorrhagic manifestations such as black vomit, melena, and metrorrhagia. Moderately severe yellow fever may last one week or even longer.

Classic yellow fever is characterized as malignant and is divided into three periods. The period of infection has sudden onset of fever and headache, with initial rapid pulse, but by day two, the pulse slows in spite of continued fever (Faget's sign). Headache, back, and muscle pain may be severe, blood oozes from the gums, and other signs of bleeding become prominent. The face is flushed, the tongue reddened (strawberry tongue), and the conjunctivae injected; the patient is irritable, unable to sleep, and frequently constipated. The temperature is often 40°C or higher. On the third day of illness, there is nausea, vomiting of coffee-ground material, and notable albuminuria. The bleeding is usually gastric, not lower intestinal. In the period of remission, often on day four, the patient feels better, the fever drops, and headache and nausea subside. Remission lasts a few hours to two days. It is followed by the period of intoxication in which the classic signs of fever, epigastric tenderness with vomiting of altered blood, nosebleeds, and albuminuria leading to oliguria or anuria occur. Dehydration may predispose to suppurative parotitis; the lungs are usually normal, but bacterial pneumonia may complicate the disease. Intoxication lasts from three days up to two weeks and may be accompanied by heart failure with drop in blood pressure, hiccough, coma, and death. Sometimes the patient is lucid until the end.

The clinical syndrome may be predominantly one of hepatic, renal, or cardiac failure. Meningoencephalitis has also been recorded. Death usually occurs between the seventh and the tenth day of illness. Patients who survive generally recover completely, although the convalescence may be prolonged, and late death from cardiac failure or arrhythmias is a rare complication.

CLINICAL LABORATORY FINDINGS. Early in the course there may be leukopenia with relative neutropenia (but sometimes with normal or elevated leukocyte count), decreased prothrombin time, and elevation of serum bilirubin. After the third day of illness, full-blown yellow fever is associated with abnormalities referable to the liver, kidneys, and heart. The total and conjugated bilirubin concentration values are elevated and rise together. The mean bilirubin is 9 to 10 mg per deciliter, but averages 15 to 20 mg per deciliter in severe cases and may be much higher. There are increased prothrombin and partial thromboplastin times; decreased platelets, blood glucose, and clotting factors II, V, VII, IX, and X. Alkaline phosphatase levels are normal. Aminotransferase levels are of prognostic value; serum glutamic oxaloacetic and glutamic pyruvic transaminase levels are consistently elevated in jaundiced patients.

Albuminuria usually appears on the fourth day reaching levels of 3 to 5 mg per liter (in severe cases much higher). Blood urea averages 109 mg per deciliter, and creatinine averages 5.9 mg per deciliter in fatal cases; the averages are 5.9 and 2.6 mg per deciliter, respectively, in nonfatal yellow fever. The urine may contain bile and casts. Electrocardiogram abnormalities are sometimes present including abnormal ST–T waves and prolonged P–R and Q–T intervals. The CSF is under increased pressure and may contain increased protein with normal cell counts.

DIAGNOSIS. Diagnosis can be made by histopathologic examination of the liver, by isolation of yellow fever virus from blood during life and from liver and other tissues post mortem, by demonstration of specific nucleic acid, or by serologic tests. Yellow fever should be suspected in any febrile patient from endemic zones of Africa and the Americas and in areas of high *A. aegypti* prevalence where yellow fever may be introduced. Diagnosis post mortem by examination of liver taken by a viscerotome was successfully used in South America routinely for many years. Liver biopsy should not be attempted because of danger of uncontrolled bleeding.

Yellow fever virus can be isolated from serum and blood during the first four days of fever by inoculation intracerebrally into baby mice or onto mammalian or mosquito cell cultures. Mice are observed for death; the virus causes cytopathic effect in Vero cells and is detected by immunofluorescence tests in mosquito cells three to six days after inoculation. The most rapid method of diagnosis is detection of antigen in acute-phase blood by the antigen-capture ELISA. The test can be completed in a few hours, although detection of antigen by ELISA is less sensitive than virus isolation.

Serologic diagnosis is made by demonstrating IgM by the antibody-capture ELISA. Since IgM is relatively specific and is detectable for only a short time after infection, this technique is reliable using a single convalescent serum specimen. Alternatively, tests of sera collected during the acute and convalescent phases are diagnostic if they show a fourfold or greater rise (or fall) of yellow fever antibody. The neutralization test is highly specific, but the complement fixation, hemagglutination-inhibition, and ELISA methods are usually used because they are quicker and lend themselves to field laboratory use. The laboratory must also rule out cross-reacting antibody by related viruses such as dengue. Probes to detect yellow fever nucleic acid are being developed but are not available yet.

DIFFERENTIAL DIAGNOSIS. The mild form of yellow fever is not clinically distinguishable from other tropical fevers. Severe yellow fever simulates viral hepatitis including delta hepatitis; other hemorrhagic fevers, leptospirosis, rickettsial fevers, malignant malaria, and drug- and toxin-related conditions.

PROGNOSIS. Two to 20 per cent of patients with clinically evident yellow fever will die, although as many as 50 per cent of severely ill patients succumb. It is not clear whether these patients would survive if they received the most modern supportive treatment, because most cases are treated in primitive clinics in Africa and South America. Patients who enter the period of intoxication have a guarded prognosis, especially if they develop anuria, high levels of albuminuria and bilirubinemia, a prothrombin time prolonged beyond 25 per cent of normal, a rapid weak pulse, uncontrolled bleeding, persistent hiccough, delirium, hypotension, or coma.

TREATMENT. The treatment consists of complete bed rest, fluid and blood replacement, and supportive care, including monitoring of vital signs. Analgesics and antiemetics may be useful, but aspirin is contraindicated because it may exacerbate bleeding. Patients are placed under bed nets to prevent possible mosquito transmission to other patients and to hospital personnel. Malaria and bacterial complications should be treated if diagnosed. Electrolyte imbalance should be corrected. Dialysis has not been used in cases of renal tubular

damage, but on theoretical grounds may benefit patients in renal failure. If disseminated intravascular coagulopathy is evident by laboratory tests, heparin may be used cautiously, although there is insufficient experience to date to predict its efficacy. Interferon and other antiviral substances have not been tried in patients with yellow fever.

PREVENTION AND CONTROL. Yellow fever can be prevented by inoculation of 17D attenuated vaccine. This vaccine is safe and in over 90 per cent of vaccinees induces antibody that persists at least 10 years, and usually for life. The vaccine is produced in eggs and should not be given to persons with egg allergies. Travellers should be vaccinated at least 10 days before arrival in yellow fever–endemic areas. Since the presence of yellow fever often goes undetected and unreported in tropical Africa and South America, the vaccine should be given to travellers whether or not there is known active transmission. Unless the risk of exposure to yellow fever is great, vaccine is not recommended during pregnancy; however, it is not known to have caused fetal damage. In an epidemic, mosquito control measures and use of bed nets and repellents are recommended until vaccine can be obtained.

362 HEMORRHAGIC FEVER CAUSED BY DENGUE VIRUSES

DEFINITION. Dengue hemorrhagic fever (DHF) is an acute febrile illness characterized by decreased platelet counts and hemoconcentration in patients infected with any one of the four serotypes of dengue virus. The disease affects children mainly and, sometimes, adults. Capillary permeability and coagulation defects lead to hemorrhagic manifestations, and in the more severe cases to hypovolemic shock (dengue shock syndrome) with death in 40 to 50 per cent of untreated shock syndrome patients. The disease has been endoepidemic in Southeast Asia since 1953. It was restricted to Asia and the Pacific until 1981 when epidemic DHF appeared in Cuba.

ETIOLOGY. DHF is caused by infection with dengue viruses, but it is not yet established why one patient develops hemorrhagic fever and another develops classic dengue fever. Initially it was hypothesized that strains of dengue virus that caused DHF were more virulent than others; another current theory holds that infection is enhanced and the disease is more severe when the host has been sensitized by a prior dengue infection of a different serotype.

EPIDEMIOLOGY. The epidemiology of DHF is that described for dengue fever with some added features. Epidemics of DHF are limited to Southeast Asia, the Pacific Islands, and, since 1981, the Caribbean. It is estimated that less than 5 per cent of dengue cases develop DHF. The attack rate in Thailand is highest in children, with a minor peak in infants when maternal antibody is waning and a major peak at four to seven years of age, when second dengue infections are most common; adults as well as children develop DHF in some outbreaks such as that in Cuba in 1981. Well-nourished children in Southeast Asia appeared to be at higher risk than the undernourished, and blacks in the Cuban epidemic had milder illness than whites; well-controlled studies are needed to substantiate these observations.

PATHOLOGY. Post mortem there are focal hemorrhages, vascular congestion, and edema in multiple organs. The spleen and lymphoid tissues show marked lymphocytolysis and phagocytosis of lymphocytes, primarily in the T cell–dependent zones. There is also proliferation of lymphoblasts and young plasma cells. Monocytic and lymphocytic non-necrotizing perivascular infiltration is found in skin lesions resembling an antibody-dependent Arthus reaction.

PATHOGENESIS. Dengue virus infects the macrophages, lymphocytes, and endothelial cells. On rare occasions DHF occurs in primary dengue, indicating that direct infection of these cells with the virus can lead to the syndrome; however, the vast majority of cases are secondary infections. In these cases there is a rapid anamnestic antibody response with formation of antigen-antibody complexes. Experimentally, formation of complexes enhances infectivity of the virus for monocytes through attachment of complexes at the FC receptor site and entry of virus into the cell. Between 0.05 and 0.1 per cent of monocytes in the peripheral blood can be visualized carrying dengue antigen. The replication of dengue virus in the monocyte is postulated to be the effector pathway leading to vascular permeability. Monocyte infection is presumably responsible for the observed complement activation and consumption via the classic and perhaps the alternate pathway. This process may result in formation of C3a and C5a which are anaphylatoxins, or some other as yet unknown mediator of vascular permeability may be activated. Another effector pathway leads to coagulation defects including thrombocytopenia and abnormal clotting. The entire process is rapid. It may evolve in a few hours to shock and death or, if managed effectively, to complete recovery. Although the pathogenesis is not understood, the pathophysiologic events are known and can be treated rationally.

CLINICAL MANIFESTATIONS. DHF usually starts with sudden onset of high fever and the signs and symptoms of dengue fever which include facial flush, anorexia, headache, nausea, and pains in the muscles and joints. Hepatic tenderness, epigastric or generalized abdominal pain, and sore throat are frequent. The liver is usually palpable, and the spleen is characteristically prominent on x-ray. The temperature continues high for two days to a week. A positive tourniquet test result, easy bruising, and fine petechiae on the face, soft palate, and extremities indicate a hemorrhagic disorder. Sometimes gum bleeding and epistaxis are noted. The majority of cases are moderately severe or mild and recover after lysis of fever. The lysis may be associated with sweating, coolness of extremities, and transient lowering of blood pressure.

More severe cases are associated with shock. The fall in blood pressure occurs suddenly on the third to the seventh day of illness and is accompanied by cool, blotchy skin, circumoral cyanosis, and tachycardia. The patient becomes restless and may complain of acute abdominal pain. The pulse pressure drops to 20 mm Hg or less, and in severe cases the blood pressure and pulse may not be detectable. Uncorrected shock may lead to metabolic acidosis and severe bleeding from the gastrointestinal tract and other sites. Death or recovery usually occurs in 12 to 24 hours. Surviving patients do not usually have sequelae. The white blood cell count is normal or slightly elevated with lymphocytosis and atypical lymphocytes commonly seen. There is hemoconcentration and elevated serum aspartate aminotransferase and blood urea nitrogen levels.

DIAGNOSIS. The laboratory diagnosis is that of dengue fever, which is usually made retrospectively. DHF with shock syndrome is a medical emergency and therefore early clinical diagnosis is essential. DHF presents with (1) acute onset of fever which is high, continuous, and lasts two days or more; (2) positive tourniquet test result, with spontaneous petechiae or ecchymoses; bleeding from gums or nose; hematemesis or melena; (3) hepatomegaly, observed in >90 per cent of Asian patients; (4) hypotension with cold, clammy skin, restlessness, and pulse pressure <20 mm Hg; (5) thrombocytopenia; (6) hematocrit increased 20 per cent over convalescent value. Fever, hemorrhagic phenomena, thrombocytopenia, and hemoconcentration are the hallmarks of DHF, and, with hypotension or narrow pulse pressure, of dengue shock

syndrome (DSS). Bacterial endotoxic shock and meningococcemia can mimic DHF/DSS.

TREATMENT. There is no specific treatment. The object of therapy is to maintain hydration, to combat acidosis, and to correct coagulation abnormalities. Salicylates may contribute to bleeding and acidosis and are contraindicated. Paracetamol may be used. Hematocrit should be determined frequently, at least daily, to measure the degree of plasma loss and the need for intravenous fluid. Fluid should be started at 20 ml per kilogram body weight. One third to one half of fluid should be physiological saline and the remainder, 5 per cent glucose in water. If acidosis is present, one quarter of fluid should be 0.167 mol per liter sodium bicarbonate. In shock cases one should use Ringer's lactate, 5 per cent glucose in physiological saline, 5 per cent glucose in one-half physiological saline, 5 per cent glucose in one-half Ringer's lactate, or 5 per cent glucose in one third physiological saline (depending on degree of dehydration and age). One should monitor for signs of cardiac failure during rapid fluid administration.

In case of shock, one should administer fluid rapidly and under pressure if necessary. One should give plasma or another volume expander if shock persists, and follow the vital signs and hematocrit. The hematocrit should decline with fluid therapy, which is continued until the hematocrit is under 40 per cent, urine output is adequate, and the appetite returns. If electrolytes and blood gases indicate acidosis, sodium bicarbonate should be administered. Heparin for intravascular coagulopathy (prolonged prothrombin and partial thromboplastin times) is usually not needed, but may be used cautiously in refractory cases. Chloral hydrate for sedation, oxygen for shock, and blood should be administered as needed.

PROGNOSIS. Case fatality from DHF is 2 to 5 per cent; deaths occur in shock cases. Most patients will survive when treated early by experienced health care workers. Recovery is rapid and without sequelae.

PREVENTION. Prevention is as described for dengue fever.

363 TICK-BORNE FLAVIVIRUS DISEASES: KYASANUR FOREST DISEASE AND OMSK HEMORRHAGIC FEVER

DEFINITION. Kyasanur Forest disease (KFD) of India and Omsk hemorrhagic fever (OHF) of western Siberia are tick-transmitted flavivirus fevers characterized by hemorrhage or encephalitis. Some patients manifest both syndromes.

ETIOLOGY. KFD and OHF viruses belong to the tick-borne complex of flaviviruses which also encompasses the closely related viruses of central European tick-borne encephalitis, Russian spring-summer encephalitis, and Powassan encephalitis of North America.

EPIDEMIOLOGY. KFD was originally limited to the forests of Shimoga District of Karnataka State, India, but since its discovery in 1957 it has spread in an unpredictable fashion to three other neighboring forested districts. The largest and most recent outbreak occurred during 1982–83 in a new focus in Nidle Forest. Many tick species are involved in transmission, especially nymphal *Haemaphysalis spinigera*. Small terrestrial mammals as well as birds and bats are infected in nature. When the forest is felled for plantations, the ecology is upset. Cattle brought in to graze at the forest fringe are not infected but serve as hosts that greatly increase the numbers of ticks. Infected ticks feed on black-faced langur monkeys and South Indian bonnet macaques which become viremic, serve as amplifiers of infection, and often die. At the same time epidemics occur in persons involved in forest occupations. People are infected incidentally and do not form part of the transmission cycle.

OHF occurs in the forest-steppe areas of the lake region of western Siberia. Epidemics of as many as 600 cases were recorded in the 1940's, but in recent years the disease has virtually disappeared. Numbers of cases peak in May and again in August and September. The virus is transmitted by *Dermacentor pictus* ticks and is maintained in small mammal populations. Muskrats, which were introduced for hunting in the 1920s, are susceptible and apparently transmit OHF virus to other muskrats and to hunters by direct contact. Lake water contaminated by dead muskrats is said to be responsible for water-borne disease. Both KFD and OHF are transmitted transovarially and trans-stadially in ticks.

CLINICAL MANIFESTATIONS AND PATHOLOGY. The incubation period is three to eight days. Onset is sudden with fever up to 40°C, headache, myalgia, and prostration lasting one to two weeks. In more severe cases there may be nasal, enteric, uterine, or pulmonary hemorrhage. Leukopenia, thrombocytopenia, and albuminuria are found. Some patients have a diphasic course with a more severe illness and meningoencephalitis after a one- or two-week afebrile period. The second phase is characterized by fever, severe headache, meningismus, mental disturbances, and tremors. Hemorrhagic manifestations or pneumonia may also be prominent in the second phase. The case fatality rate of KFD is 5 to 10 per cent; that of OHF is 0.4 to 2.5 per cent. There are no sequelae. Infections in laboratory workers are common, but are usually mild. Histopathology is minor in comparison to the gravity of the clinical disease. Findings include extravasation of red blood cells, edema, and thrombi in the small vessels.

DIAGNOSIS AND TREATMENT. Diagnosis is by isolation of virus from the blood during the first 10 days of illness and by demonstration of antibody rise during convalescence. There is no specific treatment, but fluid and electrolyte balance should be maintained and blood transfused if needed. Analgesics other than aspirin may be indicated.

PREVENTION. Tick repellents, protective clothing, and spraying of forest tracks with acaricides are the only measures available for prevention.

364 CRIMEAN-CONGO HEMORRHAGIC FEVER

DEFINITION. Crimean-Congo hemorrhagic fever (CCHF) is an acute febrile hemorrhagic tick-borne disease of Asia, Europe, and Africa. Mortality is high and hospital-based outbreaks are common.

ETIOLOGY. The disease is caused by CCHF virus of the *Nairovirus* genus, family Bunyaviridae. The virus kills baby mice and replicates in CER cells and several other cell culture systems.

EPIDEMIOLOGY. CCHF virus is transmitted in nature principally by hard ticks of the genus *Hyalomma*, but also by ticks in the genera *Rhipicephalus, Boophilus,* and *Amblyomma.* Virus is maintained by transovarial and trans-stadial passage in the tick and is amplified by hares and possibly hedgehogs, sheep, and cattle. Giraffe, rhinoceros, eland, buffalo, kudu, zebra, and dogs in southern Africa have antibody to CCHF virus.

The virus or its antibody is found in the distribution of *Hyalomma* ticks. Foci occur in the Soviet Union, the Balkan nations, Iraq, Iran, Pakistan, Afghanistan, western China, the Middle East, and most of sub-Saharan Africa including South Africa. Outbreaks occur in military personnel, campers, and in persons tending sheep and cattle. Medical workers are at high risk because of frequent spread in hospitals from infected human blood and tissues.

CLINICAL MANIFESTATIONS. The incubation period is usually between two and nine days. Onset is sudden with severe headache, fever, chills, myalgia especially in the back and legs, sore throat, abdominal pain, nausea, vomiting, diarrhea, photophobia, and conjunctival infection. The fever is constant but may be remitting. The patient is often confused or aggressive with a marked mood change. Leukopenia and thrombocytopenia are usually observed. On days three to six hemorrhagic manifestations and a petechial rash on the trunk, limbs, and oral cavity appear. Epistaxis, hematemesis, melena, and uterine bleeding may be severe and require transfusion. The liver is sometimes enlarged and tender. In severe cases, hepatorenal failure or multiple organ system failure leads to death, usually on days 6 to 14 of illness. Death may also result from blood loss, cerebral hemorrhage, dehydration after diarrhea, or pulmonary edema. Patients recover gradually starting on day 10 when the rash fades. Asthenia may last for a month or more. Recovery is usually complete, although neuritis may persist for months. Liver function tests are abnormal, especially the aspartate aminotransferase, and serum bilirubin levels are often elevated late in the illness.

DIAGNOSIS. Virus is easily isolated during the first eight days of illness. Antibodies are detectable by the immunofluorescence and enzyme-linked immunosorbent assays. Specific IgM and IgG are present by days seven to nine of illness.

TREATMENT AND PROGNOSIS. Patients suspected of having CCHF should be housed in an isolation facility with needle and blood precautions. Health care personnel should use respirators and protective clothing. Treatment is supportive including monitoring and correction of fluid and electrolyte imbalance. The vital signs and hematocrit should be tested frequently and blood should be replaced by transfusion. Case-fatality rates range from 30 to 50 per cent.

PREVENTION. Protection from tick bites and care in handling blood and tissues of sick sheep and cattle are the only preventive measures available in the case of exposure in natural foci.

365 HEMORRHAGIC DISEASES CAUSED BY ARENAVIRUSES (Argentine and Bolivian Hemorrhagic Fevers and Lassa Fever)

DEFINITION. Argentine and Bolivian hemorrhagic fevers and Lassa fever are acute febrile diseases characterized by hemorrhagic diatheses, marked myalgia, and, in severe cases, shock. Case-fatality rates are between 5 and 30 per cent.

ETIOLOGY. The diseases are caused by the viruses Junin (Argentina), Machupo (Bolivia), and Lassa (West Africa) of the family Arenaviridae.

EPIDEMIOLOGY. The reservoirs are rodents which excrete virus in urine and possibly other body fluids. The rodents involved are: Junin virus, *Calomys musculinus, Calomys laucha,* and *Akodon arenicola*; Machupo virus, *Calomys callosus*; and Lassa virus, *Mastomys natalensis.* People are believed to be infected by inhaling or eating contaminated excreta or by passage of virus through abraded skin or mucous membranes. In Argentina, exposure to Junin virus is primarily in workers harvesting corn in Cordoba and Buenos Aires provinces in the north. In Bolivia, domestic and peridomestic exposure to Machupo virus occurs in Beni province. Lassa virus is endemic in west and central Africa, especially in Liberia, Sierra Leone, and parts of Nigeria, where it is transmitted in and around homes that have an abundance of domestic rats.

Argentine hemorrhagic fever epidemics are recorded annually involving hundreds to thousands of farm workers. Bolivian hemorrhagic fever epidemics were common in the 1960's, but after institution of rodent control measures, the disease has not been reported since 1974. Lassa fever was recognized first in 1969 in a nosocomial outbreak in Nigeria. Several other nosocomial outbreaks were subsequently diagnosed, but studies in Sierra Leone established the basic endemic nature of the disease. In the eastern province, 8 to 52 per cent of the population have antibody, and the annual seroconversion rate in susceptible subjects ranges between 5 and 22 per cent. It is estimated that 5 to 14 per cent of the fevers are Lassa virus infections and that Lassa fever accounts for 10 to 16 per cent of the adult hospital admissions.

PATHOGENESIS AND PATHOLOGY. The diseases are characterized by multiple organ impairment, yet specific lesions are absent. The prominent findings are focal diapedesis and capillary hemorrhage, but there is minimal inflammation. Focal areas of liver necrosis in Lassa fever are not sufficient to account for the profound shock and death. It is postulated that the virus infects cells of the reticuloendothelial system, including the B and T cells. It causes temporary inhibition of immune cell function leading to prolonged and high-titered viremia. It is not known whether subsequent capillary damage and parenchymal edema are direct or indirect effects of the virus.

CLINICAL MANIFESTATIONS. The three diseases have many similarities. The incubation period of Lassa fever is 3 to 16 days; of Argentine hemorrhagic fever, 10 to 14 days; and of Bolivian hemorrhagic fever, 7 to 14 days. Onset is insidious, initially with fever, chills, malaise, asthenia, headache, retro-ocular pain, anorexia, nausea, vomiting, and muscle pain, (especially at the costovertebral angle in the South American forms and the legs in Lassa fever). Fever is nonremitting between 39° and 40.5°C. Sore throat is not prominent in the Argentine and Bolivian diseases, but purulent pharyngitis and aphthous ulcers are common in Lassa fever.

Signs include conjunctivitis, facial edema, exanthem with pharyngeal vesicles, exanthem of the face, neck, and upper thorax, tenderness of thighs, laterocervical and other polyadenopathy, and petechiae, especially in the axillae. There is no jaundice or hepatosplenomegaly. Leukopenia, thrombocytopenia, and albuminuria with casts are characteristic.

Late in the first week of illness, the signs and symptoms become more pronounced. Signs of dehydration, decreased blood pressure, and relative bradycardia are prominent. Hemorrhage from the gums, nose, stomach, intestines, uterus, and urinary tract indicates a severe hemorrhagic diathesis. Bleeding was observed commonly in the South American forms, but in only 17 per cent of Lassa fever cases. Blood loss is not massive enough to account for the shock. The acute phase usually lasts 7 to 15 days. Death is the result of uremia or hypovolemic shock, usually in the second week of illness. Recovery is heralded by lysis of fever; there is usually a prolonged convalescence marked by periods of sweating, flush, and postural hypotension, but patients suffer no permanent sequelae.

Neurologic signs are prominent in Bolivian hemorrhagic fever; nearly 50 per cent of patients have an intention tremor of the tongue and hands at about the fifth day of illness, and 25 per cent of these progress to more serious encephalopathy with delirium and convulsions. The cerebrospinal fluid is normal in these patients. A similar syndrome is occasionally seen in Lassa fever, and about 5 per cent of patients develop unilateral or bilateral eighth cranial nerve damage which may

be permanent. Other transient complications are loss of hair and Beau's lines of the nails.

Most patients have leukopenia with depression of both lymphocytes and neutrophils; however, some Lassa fever patients have markedly elevated white counts. Thrombocytopenia is present during the first week of illness.

DIAGNOSIS. The diagnosis can be made definitively only with laboratory tests. Fever, muscle pain, and diminished white cell count in the endemic areas should alert the physician to the diagnosis. Virus can be isolated in Vero cells from blood, cerebrospinal fluid, and throat washings during life and from most tissues at necropsy. Virus is recoverable even in the presence of antibody. Isolation of virus from Bolivian hemorrhagic fever cases is more difficult than from the Argentine or West African form. Virus isolation should be attempted only in laboratories with high biosecurity containment equipment because of the risk of infection of laboratory workers. Serologic diagnosis is made by the immunofluorescence test. Immunoglobulin G is present in 53 per cent of Lassa fever patients on admission to hospital and IgM, in 67 per cent. The IgM test is useful for early and rapid diagnosis.

TREATMENT. Supportive therapy including attention to electrolyte and fluid balance is essential. Hematocrit and urine protein measurements aid in detection of hypovolemic shock. Plasma expanders are effective if used early but may precipitate pulmonary edema late in the clinical course.

Specific Junin virus–immune human plasma given during the first eight days of Argentine hemorrhagic fever reduced the case-fatality rate from 16 to 1 per cent. A neurologic illness was observed about three weeks after the acute attack in some patients receiving this therapy. Most of these persons recovered completely.

Ribavirin given to Lassa fever patients early in the illness significantly reduced mortality. The drug was administered intravenously 60 mg per kilogram per day for the first four days, then orally 30 mg per kilogram per day for six days more. Immune plasma was not effective in Lassa fever patients in controlled trials.

PROGNOSIS. In Lassa fever, high levels of circulating virus in the blood and elevated aspartate aminotransferase in serum are predictive of death. There are no such predictors for the South American arenavirus hemorrhagic fevers. Shock or abnormal neurologic findings indicate a poor prognosis.

PREVENTION AND CONTROL. Environmental sanitation including rodent-proofing of homes and proper storage of grains and other foods to diminish rodent populations are the only community control measures now available. An experimental vaccine for Junin virus has been developed but is not yet available. Barrier nursing with use of gloves and gowns should be instituted in suspected cases of arenaviral hemorrhagic fevers. Blood and other tissues are infective and should be decontaminated.

366 AFRICAN HEMORRHAGIC FEVER (Marburg-Ebola Disease)

DEFINITION. African hemorrhagic fever is an acute, often fatal, hemorrhagic disease. Fever, rash, hemorrhage, hepatic and pancreatic inflammation, and prostration are hallmarks of the illness.

ETIOLOGY. The disease is caused by Marburg and Ebola viruses, which are distinct antigenically but of very similar morphology. The name Filoviridae has been proposed for this new family of viruses.

EPIDEMIOLOGY. Marburg disease was described in 1967 in Germany and Yugoslavia, where workers in vaccine manufacturing facilities sickened and died after they were exposed to infected tissues of African green monkeys from Uganda. Where the monkeys became infected is not known, although Marburg virus is indigenous to Africa. (Additional isolated cases in South Africa and Kenya are recorded.) Ebola virus epidemics in Sudan and Zaire in 1976 were traced to contact with infected patients and, in Zaire, to spread by needle. The disease recurred in Sudan in 1979, and there was an isolated case in Kenya in 1980. The source of the outbreaks is unknown, and the natural history remains a mystery.

PATHOLOGY. African hemorrhagic fever is a systemic disease with multiple organ involvement, most prominently the lymphatic system, testes, ovaries, and liver. Liver cell necrosis with eosinophilic inclusions, unlike that in yellow fever, is random and focal. Fibrin deposits are found in the renal glomeruli consistent with disseminated intravascular coagulopathy. There is edema and diffuse inflammation in the brain.

CLINICAL MANIFESTATIONS. The incubation period is 3 to 9 days for Marburg virus infection and 3 to 18 days for Ebola. Onset is abrupt, with severe headache, backache, muscle pains, and sometimes abdominal pain. At this stage the disease is not readily differentiated from malaria, typhoid fever, and other bacterial, rickettsial, or viral illnesses. On about the third day, nausea, vomiting, and profuse watery diarrhea with mucus and blood commence. Diarrhea may continue for several days. A maculopapular rash appears on the trunk and spreads to the rest of the body. On day 4 or 5 the patient's status becomes critical, with high unremitting fever and an altered mental state including confusion, aggression, or lethargy. There is spontaneous bleeding from injection sites, hematemesis, melena, hemoptysis, and, in pregnant patients, abortion, often with massive blood loss. Renal failure may be a terminal event. Death occurs from day 8 to 17, often on day 8 or 9. Recovery is marked by fatigue, anorexia, weight loss, hair loss, and, sometimes, psychological problems.

The pathophysiology is characterized by leukopenia, thrombocytopenia, increased prothrombin time, and other abnormalities in the liver function tests, increased serum amylase, proteinuria, and electrocardiographic changes indicative of myocardial disease. Disseminated intravascular coagulopathy has been documented in some cases.

DIAGNOSIS. Virus is isolated from acute-phase blood, liver, and other organs by inoculation into guinea pigs or cell culture. The immunofluorescence assay becomes positive during the second week of illness.

TREATMENT AND PROGNOSIS. There is no specific treatment. Supportive therapy consists of maintenance of fluid and electrolyte balance and administration of blood, platelets, or fresh frozen plasma to control bleeding. Peritoneal dialysis for renal failure and heparin for disseminated intravascular coagulopathy have been recommended, but their value in African hemorrhagic fever is not established. The case-fatality rate under relatively sophisticated hospital conditions in Marburg, Germany, was 22 per cent in 1967, and under Third World rural conditions in Zaire during 1976, was 90 per cent.

PREVENTION. Control activities are not carried out because the natural reservoir is unknown. Nosocomial spread can be minimized by barrier nursing and handling of blood and tissues in isolator laboratory units with proper decontamination.

367 HEMORRHAGIC FEVER WITH RENAL SYNDROME

DEFINITION. Hemorrhagic fever with renal syndrome (HFRS) is a disease of Europe and Asia characterized by fevers, capillary dilatation, and leakage of blood leading to hemorrhagic manifestations, and in severe cases, shock and renal tubular disease.

ETIOLOGY. HFRS is caused by any one of several closely related viruses of the genus *Hantavirus*, family Bunyaviridae. The prototype is Hantaan virus, originally isolated from *Apodemus agrarius* field mice in the endemic region of Korea.

EPIDEMIOLOGY. The virus is transmitted from rodents. *Apodemus agrarius* in Korea and other parts of Asia, *Clethrionomys glareolus* in Finland and west of the Ural Mountains, and *Rattus rattus* and *R. norwegicus* in cities of Japan, Korea, and Belgium serve as reservoirs. The rodent excretes virus in urine, saliva, and feces for weeks, and sometimes for months, after infection. Transmission is presumably by respiratory spread or direct contact with fomites contaminated by rodent excretions. Persons at risk include soldiers in field operations, campers, farmers, woodsmen, and, especially in the winter, family groups in houses harboring field rodents that seek shelter from the cold. Outbreaks have also occurred in laboratories housing field rodents or housing laboratory rats that carry the virus as an inapparent infection. Nosocomial infections are not reported. Viruses of the genus *Hantavirus* have been isolated from rodents in the Americas, but HFRS is absent.

PATHOLOGY. Patients who die of shock in the early stages demonstrate retroperitoneal gelatinous edema. There are macroscopic hemorrhages in the pituitary and right auricle. The renal medulla is congested and hyperemic, and patients who die later in the course of the disease have marked renal tubular necrosis. Petechial hemorrhages found in the skin and in multiple organs indicate widespread capillary fragility.

CLINICAL MANIFESTATIONS AND PATHOLOGIC PHYSIOLOGY. The incubation period ranges from two to 42 days but is usually about two weeks. Eighty per cent of cases are mild (demonstrating only fever, facial flush, back and muscle aches) or moderate (fever plus proteinuria, and petechial hemorrhages). The remaining 20 per cent are severe. They progress through five characteristic phases: febrile, hypotensive, oliguric, diuretic, and convalescent. The febrile phase lasts about five days, during which fever, facial flush, conjunctival injection, and backache precede appearance of petechial hemorrhages and albuminuria. In the hypotensive phase, the temperature returns to baseline, and the patient manifests nausea, vomiting, abdominal pain, and about three days of capillary leakage with a rising hematocrit, heavy proteinuria, leukocytosis, thrombocytopenia, and decreased renal clearance. This is followed for about four days with the oliguric phase when extravascular fluid is resorbed leading to relative hypervolemia, hypertension, metabolic acidosis, and sometimes pulmonary edema and/or acute renal failure. The diuretic phase is accompanied by return of renal clearance to normal, but with marked electrolyte and fluid imbalance which may lead to death if not adequately managed. The convalescent phase may last one to three months with slowly recovering renal function. The clinical diagnosis may be reliable during an outbreak with classic severe cases but not with mild infections; serologic confirmation is obtained by the immunofluorescence and neutralization tests, which become positive at the end of the first week of illness. Antibody titers peak at two weeks and last for many years.

TREATMENT AND PROGNOSIS. There is no specific treatment. Management includes careful monitoring of electrolytes and fluid intake and output with correction, especially during the oliguric and diuretic phases. Plasma expanders can be used for shock, and hemodialysis in cases of renal failure with hyperkalemia. The case fatality in Korea is about 5 per cent with hospital management; the disease in northern Europe is milder with a more favorable prognosis.

PREVENTION. Rodent control should be practiced where feasible, especially in urban settings.

Halstead SB: In vivo enhancement of dengue virus infection in rhesus monkeys by passively transferred antibody. J Infect Dis 140:527, 1979. *The definitive experimental evidence conferring credibility to the secondary infection hypothesis of dengue hemorrhagic fever.*

Hoogstraal H: The epidemiology of tick-borne Crimean-Congo hemorrhagic fever in Asia, Europe, and Africa. J Med Entomol 15:307, 1979. *Extensive description and bibliography of natural history of CCHF.*

Maiztegui JI, Fernandez NJ, deDamilano AJ: Efficacy of immune plasma in treatment of Argentine hemorrhagic fever and association between treatment and a late neurological syndrome. Lancet 2:1216, 1979. *Definitive study showing that immune plasma is efficacious for treatment of Argentine hemorrhagic fever.*

Monath TP: Lassa fever—New issues raised by field studies in West Africa. J Infect Dis 155:433, 1987. *An up-to-day perspective on Lassa fever surveillance, treatment, and research.*

Monath TP: Yellow fever: A medically neglected disease. Report on a seminar. Rev Infect Dis 90:165, 1987. *Excellent summary of state-of-the-art yellow fever case management and diagnosis.*

Pattyn SR (ed.): Ebola Virus Haemorrhagic Fever. New York, Elsevier/North-Holland, 1978. *Descriptions of the outbreaks of African hemorrhagic fever in 1976 in Zaire and Sudan.*

Rosen L: The pathogenesis of dengue haemorrhagic fever: A critical appraisal of current hypotheses. S Afr Med J (Suppl) 11 Oct:40, 1986. *An animated attack on the secondary infection hypothesis of dengue hemorrhagic fever.*

Sangkawibha N, Rojanasuphot S, Ahandrik S, et al.: Risk factors in dengue shock syndrome: A prospective epidemiologic study in Rayong, Thailand: I. The 1980 outbreak. Am J Epidemiol 120:653, 1984. *Strong field evidence favoring the secondary infection hypothesis of dengue hemorrhagic fever.*

Strode GK (ed.): Yellow Fever. New York, McGraw-Hill Book Company, 1951. *Classic description of history, epidemiology, and clinical details of yellow fever cases.*

Swanepoel R, Shepherd AJ, Leman PA, et al.: Epidemiologic and clinical features of Crimean Congo hemorrhagic fever in Southern Africa. Am J Trop Med Hyg 36:120, 1987. *Current clinical description and review of recent CCHF literature.*

Symposium on epidemic hemorrhagic fever. Am J Med 16:617, 1954. *Detailed information on the pathophysiology of HFRS.*

WHO Expert Committee Report: Viral Haemorrhagic Fevers. WHO Tech Rep Ser No 721, 1985. *Excellent review of hemorrhagic fevers by an international group of experts with detailed guide to management of patients, investigation of outbreaks, and vector control.*

WHO Scientific Group Report: Arthropod-borne and rodent-borne viral diseases. WHO Tech Rep Ser No. 719, 1985. *Authoritative discussion of epidemiologic principles, laboratory safety, vector control, and epidemic preparedness.*

WHO Technical Advisory Group Report: Dengue haemorrhagic fever: Diagnosis, treatment and control. World Health Organization, Geneva, 1986. *A most comprehensive manual for the physician faced with management of DHF patients.*

SECTION FOUR / THE MYCOSES

David J. Drutz

368 INTRODUCTION

Fungi differ from bacteria in four major respects:

1. Like mammalian cells, they are *eukaryotes*; that is, they possess a discrete nucleus bounded by a membrane containing several chromosomes. Bacteria are *prokaryotes*, possessing a single continuous chromosome and no true nucleus or nuclear membrane.

2. Fungi may reproduce sexually or asexually. When mating has taken place, the *"perfect state"* is said to be present. Spores formed by the perfect state are of major importance in taxonomy. When the perfect form of fungi has not been identified, they are referred to as *fungi imperfecti* (e.g., *Coccidioides immitis, Candida albicans*).

3. Fungi may be *dimorphic (biphasic)*, with one form in nature and a different form in the infected host. For example, *C. immitis, Histoplasma capsulatum, Blastomyces dermatitidis,* and *Sporothrix schenckii* are mycelia (filamentous forms; molds) in the environment, but yeasts (*H. capsulatum, B. dermatitidis, S. schenckii*) or endosporulating spherules (*C. immitis*) in humans. Because these fungi are basically soil saprobes (saprophytes) and do not appear to require mammalian hosts, it is not clear what benefit accrues to them by attacking humans.

4. Fungal infections may be initiated by specialized structures (propagules), rather than by the filamentous forms of a fungus, per se. In general, asexual propagules are called conidia; those formed sexually are called spores (*exception:* zygomycosis, in which the term spore is used to describe sexual or asexual propagules). Conidia are numerically more common than spores and are the more likely vehicles of infection. Conidia are generally of a size appropriate to be inhaled into the distal airways.

Fungal diseases are referred to as *mycoses*. Some mycoses are *endemic;* that is, susceptibility is conferred by living in a geographic area constituting the natural habitat of that fungus. Most endemic mycoses (coccidioidomycosis, paracoccidioidomycosis, histoplasmosis, blastomycosis) are acquired by the inhalation of conidia, are minimally symptomatic, and are recognized in retrospect by skin tests or serology. Occasionally pulmonary disease may be progressive, or systemic infection may occur.

Some mycoses are chiefly opportunistic. Granulocyte dysfunction (quantitative or qualitative) predisposes to disseminated candidiasis, aspergillosis, and zygomycosis. Depressed cell-mediated immunity (CMI), including that in patients with acquired immunodeficiency syndrome (AIDS), predisposes to disseminated coccidioidomycosis, cryptococcosis, histoplasmosis, and mucosal candidiasis (thrush, esophagitis). Diabetic ketoacidosis is associated with invasive sinusitis due to mucormycosis.

A separate phenomenon is the occurrence of anergy and depressed correlates of CMI in vitro that are seen in some patients with disseminated histoplasmosis, coccidioidomycosis, sporotrichosis, and paracoccidioidomycosis. Such defects may be associated with excessive suppressor T cell activity and are reversible with elimination of the pathogen.

Diagnosis of the mycoses is usually dependent on morphologic and cultural criteria. *Serologic tests* show cross-reactions and are often more confusing than helpful. However, there are outstanding exceptions: Coccidioidomycosis complement-fixing (CF) antibody in the cerebrospinal fluid (CSF) is diagnostic of coccidioidal meningitis; detection of cryptococcal polysaccharide antigen in the blood or CSF is virtually diagnostic of systemic cryptococcosis; antibody to the A antigen may be specific for blastomycosis. *Skin tests* are more useful in epidemiologic surveys than in diagnosis of individual infections. A positive skin test result indicates merely that infection has taken place in the past. Many skin tests are poorly standardized; some (e.g., blastomycin) are valueless for any purpose. The histoplasmin skin test stimulates antibody formation, thereby canceling the limited capabilities of histoplasma serology.

Effective antifungal therapy is limited. Amphotericin B has been in use for nearly three decades and remains the treatment of choice for most mycoses. Only *Pseudallescheria boydii* and *Candida lusitaniae* are considered routinely resistant to amphotericin B. Dosage regimens are based more on clinical experience than on objective criteria, and therapy is limited by toxic side effects, principally azotemia. Flucytosine is an orally absorbed drug with value in the therapy of candidiasis, cryptococcosis, and chromoblastomycosis. Its therapeutic efficacy is limited by rapid development of resistance by fungi, and by bone marrow toxicity that appears at least partially related to its conversion to 5-fluorouracil in vivo. Miconazole is a parenteral imidazole with efficacy in coccidioidomycosis and several other mycoses. Its side effects include hyperlipidemia, hyponatremia, and pruritus. It is currently secondary in importance to amphotericin B, except in the treatment of *Pseudallescheria* infection. Ketoconazole, an orally administered, broad-spectrum antifungal azole, has shown benefit in the gamut of nonfilamentous mycoses. However, its efficacy does not generally extend to patients with aspergillosis, mucormycosis, or severe immunodeficiency, and its poor penetration of the blood-brain barrier precludes its routine use in central nervous system disease. It can be administered on a long-term basis with minimal side effects (gastrointestinal distress; hepatitis; and interference with endogenous steroid synthesis, especially testosterone and cortisol). Antifungal azoles currently in clinical trials (especially itraconazole and fluconazole) may offer improved pharmacokinetics and reduced toxicity.

Drutz DJ: Newer antifungal agents and their use, including an update on amphotericin B and flucytosine. In Remington JS, Swartz MN (eds.): Current Clinical Topics in Infectious Diseases, 3. New York, McGraw-Hill Book Company, 1982, pp 97–135. *The clinical roles of amphotericin B, flucytosine, and miconazole are discussed in detail.*

Hawkins Van Tyle J: Ketoconazole: Mechanism of action, spectrum of activity, pharmacokinetics, adverse reactions and therapeutic use. Pharmacotherapy 4:343, 1984. *A broad general review of this important new antifungal agent.*

Jorgensen JH, Rinaldi MG: A Clinician's Dictionary of Bacteria and Fungi. Indianapolis, IN, Eli Lilly and Company, 1986. *Designed as a "quick reference" to bacterial and fungal isolates from the clinical laboratory, this 130-page booklet offers a great deal more. It is an excellent "painless introduction" to medical mycology and is especially valuable for extensive, up-to-date references and simple definitions of complicated terms.*

369 HISTOPLASMOSIS

DEFINITION. Histoplasmosis is the most common endemic respiratory mycosis in the United States. The disease is noncommunicable and ordinarily self limited, but reinfection, chronic pulmonary infection, and disseminated infection all may occur.

ETIOLOGY. *Histoplasma capsulatum* (perfect form: *Emmonsiella capsulata*) is a dimorphic fungus, occurring in the mycelial phase in the environment, and in the yeast phase at 37°C and in infected hosts. The mycelial form produces two types of conidia: tuberculate macroconidia (8 to 16 μm), and microconidia of a size (2 to 5 μm) more appropriate to be inhaled. The yeasts are ovoid (2 to 3 × 3 to 4 μm) and unencapsulated, bud singly from a narrow neck, and occur intracellularly in macrophages.

INCIDENCE AND PREVALENCE. Histoplasmosis occurs worldwide. Over 40 million people have been infected in the United States, and about 500,000 develop skin test positivity each year. Eighty to 95 per cent of persons in the Mississippi, Missouri, and Ohio River valleys are histoplasmin positive. *H. capsulatum var. duboisii* produces a disease restricted largely to central Africa ("African histoplasmosis") with slightly different clinical and histopathologic features.

EPIDEMIOLOGY. *H. capsulatum* is a soil saprobe that prefers moderate temperatures and moist environments. Droppings from chickens, pigeons, starlings, blackbirds, and bats support its growth. Birds are not infected but carry the fungi on their feathers. Bats are infected and excrete yeasts from an ulcerated intestinal mucosa. Histoplasmosis ("cave disease") may follow exploration of bat-infested caves. Although the fungus is found in greatest abundance in bat- or bird-related microenvironments, microconidia are commonly present as "air pollutants" in endemic areas and probably account for the majority of sporadic infections. Focal outbreaks occur with disturbances that raise dust (e.g., demolition of old buildings where birds or bats have roosted). Because histoplasmin reactivity may wane, persons who live in highly endemic areas are subject to reinfection.

PATHOGENESIS AND PATHOLOGY. Following the inhalation of microconidia, fungi replicate locally and disseminate hematogenously to the mononuclear phagocyte system. With the development of cell-mediated immunity, granuloma formation occurs, often with caseation necrosis, and the histoplasmin skin test becomes positive. Healing may be marked by exuberant calcification at pulmonary parenchymal and hilar loci (Ghon's complex) and in the spleen. An exaggerated fibrotic response may lead to *fibrosing mediastinitis* with bronchial or vascular occlusion (e.g., superior vena caval obstruction). Layers of collagen may be deposited at the site of pulmonary coin lesions *histoplasmomas)*, their growth leading to thoracotomy for suspected malignancy.

H. capsulatum stains poorly with hematoxylin-eosin, but well with periodic acid–Schiff, Giemsa's, or Gomori's methenamine silver stains. Organisms are ordinarily found in macrophages, but large, bizarre extracellular forms or mycelia may be seen in endocarditis lesions or necrotic loci. The spectrum of host response is related directly to the effectiveness of cell-mediated immune mechanisms. With optimal immunity, fungi are rare, granuloma formation is well developed, and the disease is restricted in extent. With deficient immunity, macrophages, including those in circulating blood, are packed with intracellular yeasts, granuloma formation is poor, and disease is extensive.

In patients with centrilobular or bullous emphysema, histoplasmosis is opportunistic. Subintimal arterial proliferation leads to infarct-like pulmonary necrosis. In infants and older adults without obvious host defense defects, and in patients with chronic lymphocytic leukemia, Hodgkin's disease, steroid therapy, or other defects of cell-mediated immunity, progressive hematogenous dissemination may occur. Some of the manifestations (meningitis, adrenal insufficiency, intestinal ulceration) are attributable to an accompanying perivasculitis.

CLINICAL MANIFESTATIONS. *Primary Histoplasmosis.* At least 90 per cent of all respiratory encounters with *H. capsulatum* pass unnoticed or are attributed to "the flu." Manifestations include cough, fever, headache, myalgias, stomach cramps, and pleuritic pain. With heavier exposure, there may be dyspnea, cyanosis, deep chest pain, and pericarditis. Occasionally, there may be erythema nodosum, erythema multiforme, diffuse rash, or arthralgias—especially in white women. The chest roentgenogram may show patchy infiltrates; mediastinal and hilar lymphadenopathy is common, especially in children. Cavitation and pleural effusion may occur. Ghon's complexes tend to be more highly calcified than in tuberculosis. Multifocal pulmonary lesions may heal with diffuse "buckshot" calcifications. These may erode into bronchi and be expectorated later as broncholiths.

Reinfection Histoplasmosis. The potential for re-exposure to microconidia is constantly present in endemic areas. Reinfection is characterized by a shorter incubation period (3 to 7 versus 10 to 18 days), miliary nodulation (rather than patchy bronchopneumonia), lack of hilar adenopathy, and a shorter and less severe disease course. However, very severe pulmonary disease with cyanosis and respiratory distress may also be seen.

Chronic Pulmonary Histoplasmosis. This disease occurs most commonly in middle-aged white men with pre-existing chronic obstructive pulmonary disease and centrilobular or bullous emphysema. Multiplication of inhaled *H. capsulatum* in an emphysematous bleb (characteristically in an apical-posterior location) results in antigenic spillage to contiguous lung areas and an acute segmental interstitial pneumonitis. Symptoms include cough, fever, and malaise. Microorganisms are sparse, and in 80 per cent of cases the disease resolves over two to three months with infarct-like necrosis, contraction of damaged tissue, and a fibrous residual. There may be later recurrences. In 20 per cent of patients, persistent infection leads to chronic cavitary disease. Thick-walled cavities expand by contiguity into the surrounding lung ("marching cavity"), and bronchogenic spread of their contents results in pneumonitis and fibrosis in dependent lung areas. Patients may have fever and a productive cough; one third have hemoptysis. Sputum cultures are positive in only 50 to 70 per cent. The patients usually pursue a declining course, less from actual infection than from progressive loss of functioning lung.

Disseminated Histoplasmosis. One third of cases occur in infants, the remainder predominantly in men over age 40. A clinically apparent pulmonary infection may precede dissemination in infants but is less likely to do so in adults. Dissemination in adults may follow immunosuppression, with arousal of disease from latency. Patients with acquired immunodeficiency syndrome (AIDS) are at increased risk of dissemination from primary or reactivated disease. Infants and patients with AIDS have the poorest host response to infection and the most fulminating course; disease in otherwise normal adults is usually subacute or chronic.

Clinical manifestations include weight loss, fever, weakness and malaise, hepatosplenomegaly, lymphadenopathy, and impaired bone marrow function (anemia, leukopenia, and thrombocytopenia). Oropharyngeal, nasopharyngeal, and laryngeal ulcerations, usually painful and often associated with dysphagia or hoarseness, constitute a major clue to the diagnosis. Gastrointestinal tract ulcerations (especially common in the ileocecal area) may present with bleeding, obstruction, perforation, or malabsorption. Adrenal insufficiency is common and may occur years after successful eradication of fungi. Chest roentgenograms may show evidence of primary or hematogenous infection. Endocarditis (predominantly aortic valve) may present with emboli to large blood vessels. Central nervous system histoplasmosis may present with focal cerebritis or diffuse chronic meningitis with hypoglycorrhachia. The kidneys, prostate, and skin may also be involved, but osteomyelitis and arthritis are rare.

Ocular Histoplasmosis. Presumed ocular histoplasmosis syndrome (POHS) refers to a focal chorioretinitis in the macular area that is thought to be related to a hypersensitivity response to products of *H. capsulatum*. No direct relationship to fungal infection has been proved.

DIAGNOSIS. Histoplasmosis is as clinically diverse as tuberculosis. Particularly suggestive features include mucous

membrane ulcerations, leukopenia, thrombocytopenia, adrenal insufficiency, buckshot pulmonary calcifications, and splenic calcifications. The diagnosis depends on demonstrating or culturing *H. capsulatum* from involved tissues, seldom a simple task. The roles of skin and serologic tests are limited. The histoplasmin skin test (mycelial phase) is seldom useful diagnostically because positive results are common in the endemic area. Conversely, disseminated disease is not necessarily associated with a negative result (unlike the situation with coccidioidomycosis). A positive histoplasmin skin test result also elevates titers of serum antibodies. This skin test should therefore be restricted to use in epidemiologic investigations. The Histolyn CYL skin test (yeast phase) has many of the limitations of histoplasmin. However, it has a minimal tendency to elevate antibody titers.

The *complement fixation test* (using mycelial or yeast phase antigen) may show cross-reactions with blastomycosis or coccidioidomycosis. Low-level antibody titers may persist for years following primary histoplasmosis. A titer $\geq$1:32, or a fourfold titer rise, suggests but does not prove active histoplasmosis; nor does a negative titer rule out the disease. Titers do not parallel disease activity and are of little value in following therapy or estimating prognosis. Tests for antibody by the *immunodiffusion* method produce two bands (m, h) of potential diagnostic value. The occurrence of both bands in the serum of a patient who has not been skin tested with histoplasmin is highly suggestive of histoplasmosis. If only an m band is observed, early histoplasmosis may be present because the m band usually precedes the h band. The *latex agglutination test* with histoplasmin-sensitized latex particles is a potential aid to diagnosis of acute histoplasmosis, especially in titers $\geq$1:16. False-positive and false-negative results may occur, and confirmatory diagnostic tests are required. A recently described radioimmunoassay for antigenuria and antigenemia may add to the diagnostic armamentarium.

Primary pulmonary histoplasmosis is rarely diagnosed in the absence of a suggestive epidemiologic history or the investigation of a common-source outbreak. Most cases are probably overlooked or misdiagnosed as bacterial or viral processes. Sputum cultures are positive in only 20 per cent of cases. Skin test conversion is diagnostic, but seldom documented. Serologic tests may be helpful in diagnosis, as noted above.

Chronic pulmonary histoplasmosis is diagnosed on the basis of suggestive roentgenographic changes and positive sputum smears or cultures. Fewer than one third of cultures are positive in early, self-limited disease, whereas 70 per cent are positive in patients with marching cavities. Multiple cultures may be required before the fungus is found.

Disseminated histoplasmosis in one large series demonstrated positive cultures in the following distribution: oral lesions (91 per cent), lymph node (72 per cent), bone marrow (70 per cent), sputum (60 per cent), liver biopsy (57 per cent), blood (54 per cent), CSF (45 per cent), and urine (43 per cent). Organisms have also been cultured from the stool, prostatic secretions, and skin lesions. Fungi may be demonstrated directly by Wright's, Giemsa's, or methenamine silver stains of the buffy coat of blood, ulcer swabs or scrapings, sputum, or other infected materials.

TREATMENT. Primary pulmonary infection rarely requires treatment. Those with acute respiratory insufficiency following massive fungal exposure may require a brief course of corticosteroid therapy, with or without accompanying antifungal therapy. Chronic pulmonary histoplasmosis resolves spontaneously in 80 per cent of cases, but resolution may be assisted by restriction of activity or bed rest. Amphotericin B (2 grams over ten weeks for adults; 1 mg per kilogram per day for six weeks in infants) is the drug of choice in patients with disseminated histoplasmosis, especially those with immunodeficiency. Ketoconazole (200 to 400 mg daily for six months) may be ameliorative or curative in adults with chronic cavitary pulmonary histoplasmosis and allows outpatient therapy. Surgical resection of marching cavities should also be considered. Treatment of either pulmonary or disseminated histoplasmosis may be initiated with amphotericin B, but completed with ketoconazole. Chronic ketoconazole administration may prevent histoplasmosis relapse in patients with AIDS.

Adrenal function of patients with disseminated histoplasmosis (especially those receiving ketoconazole) should be evaluated at the time of diagnosis and monitored indefinitely thereafter. Adrenal insufficiency may occur years later, and patients should be warned of this possibility. Fibrosing mediastinitis is a manifestation of excessive host response rather than progressive infection. Antifungal chemotherapy is not necessarily indicated.

PROGNOSIS. Chronic cavitary pulmonary histoplasmosis usually results in death from respiratory insufficiency. Progressive disseminated histoplasmosis (once uniformly fatal in those with poor host defenses) is curable, although relapses may occur.

PREVENTION. A 3 per cent solution of formalin sprayed on *H. capsulatum*–containing soil will destroy the fungi and control common-source outbreaks.

Goodwin RA Jr, Loyd JE, Des Prez RM: Histoplasmosis in normal hosts. Medicine 60:231, 1981. *When learning about histoplasmosis, this is the paper with which to begin.*

Goodwin RA Jr, Shapiro JL, Thurman GH, et al.: Disseminated histoplasmosis: Clinical and pathologic correlations. Medicine 59:1, 1980. *An extensive review of experience with this disease in middle Tennessee. Immunopathogenesis is emphasized, but this paper is also an outstanding clinical contribution. Amphotericin B was usually curative.*

Sathapatayavongs B, Batteiger BE, Wheat J, et al.: Clinical and laboratory features of disseminated histoplasmosis during two large urban outbreaks. Medicine 62:263, 1983. *Although the diagnosis was proved by culture in approximately 88 per cent of the 66 cases documented, serologic tests were of additional diagnostic value. Amphotericin B was the drug of choice, but ketoconazole appeared effective in patients who were not immunosuppressed.*

Wheat LJ, Small CB: Disseminated histoplasmosis in the acquired immune deficiency syndrome (editorial). Arch Intern Med 144:2147, 1984. *This editorial calls attention to the ways in which histoplasmosis presentation differs in patients with AIDS. Amphotericin B was suppressive, but not curative. The authors speculate that ketoconazole may have a role in perpetuating remissions induced by amphotericin B.*

Wheat LJ, Kohler RB, Tewari RP: Diagnosis of disseminated histoplasmosis by detection of *Histoplasma capsulatum* antigen in serum and urine specimens. N Engl J Med 314:83, 1986. *Antigenuria was documented in 20 and antigenemia in 11 of 22 episodes of disseminated histoplasmosis occurring in 16 patients. Antigenuria alone was found in 6 of 32 patients with self-limited infection, 2 of 32 with cavitary histoplasmosis, and 4 of 8 with a sarcoidosis-like presentation. Antigenuria and antigenemia decreased after initiation of antifungal therapy and recurred in patients who had a relapse.*

Wheat LJ, Wass J, Norton J, et al.: Cavitary histoplasmosis occurring during two large urban outbreaks: Analysis of clinical, epidemiologic, roentgenographic, and laboratory features. Medicine 63:201, 1984. *Chronic obstructive pulmonary disease, advanced age, male sex, white race, and immunosuppression were important risk factors for cavitary histoplasmosis. The diagnosis was proved by culture in only approximately 60 per cent of cases; serologic tests provided useful clues to diagnosis.*

370 COCCIDIOIDOMYCOSIS

DEFINITION. Coccidioidomycosis is a noncontagious respiratory mycosis of the Southwest and the second most common endemic mycosis in the United States, after histoplasmosis. It is usually self limited but may lead to chronic pulmonary infection or hematogenous dissemination.

ETIOLOGY. *Coccidioides immitis* is a dimorphic fungus. The mycelial phase, a soil saprobe of semiarid regions, fragments to release boxlike arthroconidia of a size suitable to be inhaled (2 to 5 μm). In the infected host, the fungus grows as large spherules, 10 to 80 μm in diameter, the cytoplasm of which segments to produce hundreds of endospores (2 to 5 μm diameter). Spherule rupture results in dispersal of endospores

to surrounding tissues, where they mature to spherules, repeating the growth cycle.

INCIDENCE AND PREVALENCE. Coccidioidomycosis occurs in the southwestern United States and neighboring Mexico (the "Lower Sonoran life zone") and in parts of Central and South America. Approximately 100,000 cases occur yearly. The *spherulin* (spherule-endospore) and coccidioidin (mycelial) skin tests detect approximately equal numbers of *C. immitis*–exposed patients. Each test misses about 5 per cent of patients that the other test detects. Eighty to 95 per cent of the population is skin test positive in parts of California and Arizona. Infection is more common in those with outdoor activities. Extrapulmonary dissemination occurs in 1 of 2000 to 3500 white women, 1 of 500 white men, and 1 of 50 black men. The risk may be even greater in Filipinos. Pregnancy, depressed cell-mediated immunity, and corticosteroid therapy increase the risk of dissemination.

EPIDEMIOLOGY. *C. immitis* is distributed sporadically within the endemic zone. Arthroconidia are spread on the wind by any activity that raises dust; fomites may carry the conidia outside the endemic area. Risk of infectivity drops dramatically once land is cultivated. Animals are commonly infected but pose no hazard for humans. Newcomers to the Southwest are at high risk for infection. A World War II study documented a 50 per cent skin test conversion rate within six months in airmen stationed in the Phoenix area. Skin test reactivity is associated with solid immunity; reinfection is almost unknown.

PATHOGENESIS AND PATHOLOGY. Coccidioidomycosis is characterized by suppuration (endospore response) and granuloma formation (spherule response). Cell-mediated immunity is the major host defense mechanism, and patients with AIDS are at increased risk of coccidioidal dissemination. In patients with extrapulmonary dissemination or chronic progressive pulmonary coccidioidomycosis, *C. immitis* skin test reactivity may never develop or may wane, and there is nonspecific suppression of reactivity to recall-type skin tests and tests of cell-mediated immunity in vitro. Most defects are reversible with therapy. Granuloma formation may be deficient, and suppuration may dominate.

CLINICAL MANIFESTATIONS. *Primary Coccidioidomycosis.* Sixty per cent of primary infections are asymptomatic. Symptoms in the other 40 per cent include cough, fever, headache, and pleuritic pain. Up to 5 per cent (predominantly white women) present with erythema nodosum or erythema multiforme and arthralgias ("valley fever"). Others may have "toxic erythema" resembling measles. Eosinophilia is common. The chest roentgenogram may show segmental or lobar infiltrates, often with hilar adenopathy. Pleural fluid is present in 5 to 20 per cent of cases, and fungi may be demonstrable by pleural biopsy. Cavitation may occur, usually without specific symptoms. Thin-walled cavities may persist and be discovered later on a routine roentgenogram. They are usually single, less than 4 cm in diameter, and seldom symptomatic, although the sputum may contain *C. immitis*. Up to one half of cavities will close spontaneously in two to four years. Rarely, they may lead to hemoptysis, become secondarily infected, or enlarge to encroach on normal surrounding lung.

Persistent coccidioidal pneumonia is manifested by persistence of the primary infection for six to eight weeks, with worsening pulmonary infiltrates, fever, chest pain, prostration, and productive cough. Resolution is slow; healing may result in fibrosis, bronchiectasis, and calcification. Fatality is especially common in immunosuppressed patients.

Chronic progressive coccidioidal pneumonia is an indolent disease process with weight loss, fever, hemoptysis, chest pain, and dyspnea. It is characterized by chronicity and biapical fibronodular lesions and cavities that resemble tuberculosis or histoplasmosis.

Pulmonary nodules (coccidioidomas) result from resolution of earlier infiltrative disease. Most are 1 to 4 cm in size and have semisolid centers that contain *C. immitis.* The lesions may cavitate, resulting in an "abscessing nodule."

Disseminated Coccidioidomycosis. Extrapulmonary dissemination usually occurs soon after primary infection, but diagnosis may be delayed, depending on the pace and sites of dissemination. The chest roentgenogram may or may not be abnormal. Dissemination may be unifocal or multifocal. The *skin and subcutaneous tissues* are the most common sites involved. Lesions are papular, verrucous, or ulcerative; subcutaneous abscesses may occur. *Osteomyelitis* occurs in 10 to 50 per cent of cases, involves single or multiple bones, and is most common in the vertebrae, tibia, skull, metatarsals, and metacarpals, especially at sites of tendon or ligament insertion. Complications include muscle abscesses or draining cutaneous fistulas. *Joints* may be involved by penetration from contiguous osteomyelitis or by hematogenous infection of the synovium. Large weight-bearing joints such as the knee and ankle are most commonly involved. There may be rapid joint destruction or chronic nonerosive synovitis with progressive villous hypertrophy and pannus formation resembling rheumatoid arthritis. *Meningitis* occurs in 30 to 50 per cent of patients, often as the sole site of involvement. Most cases are hematogenous in origin; some reflect direct spread from skull or vertebral osteomyelitis. The disease process is subtle, with headache, lethargy, personality changes, and diverse neurologic abnormalities. The meningitis is predominantly basilar in location; intracerebral infection may be demonstrable by computed tomographic scan; hydrocephalus is common. Liver, spleen, lymph node, and kidney involvement is common but often clinically silent. Adrenal insufficiency may occur. Gastrointestinal tract involvement is rare.

DIAGNOSIS. Coccidioidomycosis may be confused with a variety of infections, including tuberculosis and other mycoses. Joint involvement may mimic primary rheumatologic disorders. Diagnosis is readily achieved by demonstrating endosporulating spherules in 10 per cent KOH wet mounts of sputum or inflammatory exudates. Biopsy specimens stained with hematoxylin-eosin, Gridley's, periodic acid–Schiff, or Gomori's methenamine silver stains may demonstrate the fungi in diverse tissues. Cerebrospinal fluid (CSF) findings include pleocytosis, elevated protein, and hypoglycorrhachia; when present, eosinophils are a valuable clue to the diagnosis. *C. immitis* is not fastidious and can be recovered on most standard media. However, the mycelial phase is biohazardous and demands great care in laboratory handling. Fungi can be cultured from the CSF in only 20 to 40 per cent of instances. Urine cultures may disclose *C. immitis* in the absence of an abnormality of renal function or urinalysis. Blood cultures may be positive in patients with severe disseminated infection, especially those with AIDS. Bone marrow cultures may also be positive.

Serologic tests are extremely important in diagnosis and prognosis and are uninfluenced by skin testing. Patients with symptomatic disease generally manifest an immunoglobulin M (IgM) antibody response that peaks by the second to third week of illness and is replaced by an immunoglobulin G (IgG) response. The IgM antibody is demonstrable by tube precipitin, latex particle agglutination, or immunodiffusion (ID) techniques. The IgG response is detectable by complement fixation (CF) or ID methods. CF titers seldom exceed 1:8 to 1:16 in uncomplicated primary infection. Persistent elevations at 1:16 to 1:32 or more raise the likelihood of dissemination, particularly if associated with loss or absence of skin test reactivity. Minimal workup for suspected dissemination includes wet mounts, biopsies and cultures from any suspicious lesions, lumbar puncture, bone scans, and cultures of concentrated morning urine. Patients with unifocal dissemination (particularly meningitis) may not show elevated CF titers in the serum or loss of skin test reactivity. CF antibody is present in the CSF in 75 to 95 per cent of patients with meningitis, however, and is diagnostic.

TREATMENT. Primary pulmonary infection seldom requires treatment, although a "prophylactic" course of 1 gram of amphotericin B may be given to patients at particular risk of dissemination (blacks, immunosuppressed patients). Isolated thin-walled cavities are usually asymptomatic, although surgical resection may be required for life-threatening hemoptysis or threatened rupture into the pleural space. Progressive pulmonary infection may benefit from a total course of 1 to 2 grams of amphotericin B; fungi are difficult to eradicate once significant destruction of pulmonary parenchyma has occurred. Disseminated coccidioidomycosis is characterized by spontaneous exacerbations and remissions, making therapeutic response difficult to interpret. Amphotericin B is often more likely to be ameliorative than curative. A total dose of 2 grams constitutes a minimal course of therapy; the goal is to produce clear clinical improvement and a persistent fourfold fall in the serum CF titer. Relapse is typical and necessitates retreatment. Meningitis must be treated by the intrathecal or intraventricular route; cure is elusive and may require the use of high intrathecal dosages of amphotericin B. Synovitis may require synovectomy or arthrodesis for cure.

Miconazole lacks nephrotoxicity but is not clearly superior to amphotericin B in any other sense and must also be given intrathecally for meningitis. Ketoconazole (400 to 800 mg daily* for six months) has shown benefit in pulmonary coccidioidomycosis and in disseminated infection limited to the skin and soft tissues. It is not curative for bone, joint, or central nervous system disease but may have a role in maintaining remissions induced by amphotericin B.

PROGNOSIS. Meningitis is usually fatal within two years without therapy. Even with therapy, mental deterioration or fatality may occur from hydrocephalus unless the complication is anticipated and managed by CSF shunting. Other forms of coccidioidomycosis tend to be more debilitating than lethal, although fulminating pulmonary infection may be fatal in the severely immunosuppressed.

PREVENTION. A killed *C. immitis* spherule vaccine is currently being evaluated in the southwest United States. Partial control of *C. immitis* at dusty sites can be achieved by saturating the soil with 1-chloro-2-nitropropane. Patients from nonendemic areas who have risk factors for coccidioidal dissemination should be warned of the danger in working or residing in highly endemic areas.

Ampel NM, Ryan KJ, Carry PJ, et al.: Fungemia due to *Coccidioides immitis*: An analysis of 16 episodes in 15 patients and a review of the literature. Medicine 65:312, 1986. *Coccidioidal fungemia is a marker for an acute, severe form of disseminated coccidioidomycosis that occurs principally in immunocompromised patients, is associated with a miliary pattern on chest roentgenogram, and carries a mortality approaching 70 per cent within one month of the positive blood culture. Fungemia is common in patients with AIDS.*

Bouza E, Dreyer JS, Hewitt WL, et al.: Coccidioidal meningitis: An analysis of thirty-one cases and review of the literature. Medicine 60:139, 1981. *Coccidioidal meningitis is difficult to diagnose, harder to manage, and refractory to cure. This paper recounts the experience of ULCA-affiliated hospitals with coccidioidal meningitis between 1964 and 1976 and provides a valuable literature review.*

DeFelice R, Galgiani JN, Campbell SC, et al.: Ketoconazole treatment of nonprimary coccidioidomycosis: Evaluation of 60 patients during three years of study. Am J Med 72:681, 1982. *Although ketoconazole may produce clinical improvement in patients with various forms of coccidioidomycosis, relapse is not uncommon. Similar results are reported in a series of 29 patients (Catanzaro A, Einstein H, Levine B, et al.: Ketoconazole for treatment of disseminated coccidioidomycosis. Ann Intern Med 96:436, 1982).*

Drutz DJ, Catanzaro A: Coccidioidomycosis. State of the art. Am Rev Respir Dis 117:559, 727, 1978. *A review of all aspects of coccidioidomycosis and its treatment.*

Kabadue EK, Hamilton RH: Survival improvement in coccidioidal meningitis by high-dose intrathecal amphotericin B. Arch Intern Med 146:2013, 1986. *Cure of coccidioidal meningitis may require higher doses of intrathecal amphotericin B than have been recommended heretofore. This study suggests that intrathecal amphotericin (plus hydrocortisone) administered at a high-dose rate of 0.75 mg or more, three times per week, promptly reaching 20 mg, with a total dose surpassing 40 mg, is associated with significantly enhanced survival rates. The study lacks internal controls, but the findings are impressive nonetheless.*

---

*May exceed manufacturer's recommended dosage.

371 BLASTOMYCOSIS

DEFINITION. Blastomycosis (North American blastomycosis, Gilchrist's disease) is a noncontagious, subacute or chronic endemic mycosis that follows inhalation of the conidia of *Blastomyces dermatitidis*. The organs most commonly affected are the lungs, skin, bones, and male genitourinary system.

ETIOLOGY. *B. dermatitidis* (perfect form: *Ajellomyces dermatitidis*) is a dimorphic fungus, occurring in the mycelial phase at ambient temperatures and as yeasts at 37°C. The yeast phase is characterized by cells of 8 to 15 (or more) μm in diameter that reproduce by single budding. Daughter cells are attached at a very broad (4 to 5 μm) base.

INCIDENCE AND PREVALENCE. Blastomycosis is encountered far less commonly than histoplasmosis and coccidioidomycosis. There is no diagnostic skin test. Hence, the extent to which subclinical disease occurs is largely unknown, and endemic areas are defined in terms of clinical cases.

EPIDEMIOLOGY. Blastomycosis occurs most commonly in the southeastern United States and in areas surrounding the Great Lakes. However, the disease is also encountered in Africa, Mexico, and Central and South America, so that "North American blastomycosis" is a misnomer. The ecologic niche for the fungus appears to be the soil, particularly riverbanks, but its recovery has been sporadic, and the factors governing its distribution are unknown. Persons at risk often have outdoor vocations or avocations. Clinical illness is most common in middle-aged men. However, studies during common-source outbreaks indicate that self-limited infection is independent of sex, age, or race. Dogs and horses are highly susceptible to blastomycosis, and the occurrence of veterinary cases helps to define endemic areas. In some instances hunters and their dogs have acquired blastomycosis simultaneously. Percutaneous inoculation of fungi has been documented in laboratory accidents, but in virtually all other circumstances cutaneous lesions result from hematogenous spread of apparent or inapparent pulmonary disease.

PATHOGENESIS AND PATHOLOGY. Blastomycosis is marked histopathologically by the simultaneous presence of suppuration (microabscesses) and granulomas. In fulminating infections, suppuration may dominate. Caseation necrosis is uncommon. Cutaneous and mucous membrane lesions are characterized by the presence of pseudoepitheliomatous hyperplasia.

Studies in vitro indicate that macrophages kill *B. dermatitidis* yeasts with far greater efficiency than granulocytes, especially when sensitized lymphocytes are present. Animal studies indicate that cell-mediated immunity is central to host defense. Clinical data suggest a greater frequency of disseminated infection in patients with defective cell-mediated immunity.

CLINICAL MANIFESTATIONS. *Pulmonary Blastomycosis.* In most cases, respiratory infection is probably asymptomatic. In some cases, pleuritic chest pain, nonspecific "flu-like" symptoms, or arthralgias and erythema nodosum may mark the occurrence of acute infection. The correct diagnosis is probably seldom made in the absence of a specific search for a fungal etiology, as during a suspected common-source outbreak. Clinically apparent pulmonary blastomycosis has no distinguishing clinical or radiographic characteristics. Bronchitis is present in up to one third of cases and may contribute to rapid endobronchial spread. Cavitation, hilar adenopathy, and pleural involvement are all well documented. Fibrosis is common, but residual calcification is rare. Expanding masslike lesions may be confused with malignancies. Acute respiratory distress syndrome and miliary pulmonary lesions may be present in cases with fulminating hematogenous dissemination.

Disseminated Blastomycosis. Extrapulmonary disease may occur in the presence or absence of obvious lung disease, either during or after the initial pulmonary infection. Some cases may reflect late endogenous reactivation. The frequency of multisystem involvement is directly related to the thoroughness of diagnostic studies. The most common site of extrapulmonary dissemination is the skin, and skin lesions are often the presenting feature of blastomycosis. Lesions begin as papules, pustules, or subcutaneous nodules and may involve exposed or unexposed areas. Some become verrucous and progress over weeks or months to produce an elevated, warty, crusted lesion with a serpiginous, indurated, dusky red or violaceous, abruptly sloping outer border. Prominent "black dots" at the surface mark the location of necrotic papillary blood vessels. Removal of crusts reveals a granulomatous base with numerous ulcers exuding bloody purulent material. Central healing and scarring may occur, with disease activity most prominent at the advancing borders. In some patients superficial ulcerative lesions may predominate. Disseminated papulopustular skin lesions have followed incision of pulmonary blastomycotic mass lesions at exploratory thoracotomy for suspected malignancy.

Bone lesions are encountered in 25 to 60 per cent of cases. They are most common in the axial skeleton (especially the vertebrae) and long bones but may be detectable only by bone scan or radiographic bone survey. Lytic lesions with or without sclerotic margins may be seen. Draining sinuses without a verrucous appearance may mark underlying osteomyelitic foci. An acute arthritis, usually monarticular, occurs in 3 to 5 per cent of cases, either hematogenously or by direct bony spread. Involvement of the prostate, testis, and epididymis may be signaled by dysuria, pyuria, hematuria, urinary hesitancy, and tender intrascrotal mass lesions. Renal, hepatic, and splenic infections are common but are usually clinically inapparent. Adrenal involvement may rarely cause Addison's disease. Central nervous system invasion occurs in about 5 per cent of cases and may present as an intracranial mass, isolated meningitis, or spinal epidural granulomas or abscesses. Gastrointestinal involvement is rare.

DIAGNOSIS. Pulmonary blastomycosis may be confused with tuberculosis, other mycoses, bacterial pneumonia, or malignancy. Cutaneous blastomycosis is highly characteristic in appearance but may be confused with chromoblastomycosis, coccidioidomycosis, or some cutaneous malignancies. Diagnosis may be reached most quickly by direct microscopic examination of biologic specimens digested in 10 per cent KOH. Under these circumstances, characteristic single-budding yeasts may be seen in sputum, prostatic fluid, and other biologic specimens. Stains are not necessary. *B dermatitidis* will grow on most standard culture media, but specimens should be held for at least one month. In fixed-tissue specimens, hematoxylin-eosin staining reveals characteristic yeast cells with a doubly refractile cell wall, often accentuated by retraction of the protoplast from the outer cell wall. The periodic acid–Schiff stain preserves intracellular detail and helps differentiate *B. dermatitidis* (multinucleated) from *C. neoformans* and *H. capsulatum* (single nuclei). Fungi are easily seen with Gomori's methenamine silver stain, but internal detail is lost.

Patients with blastomycosis should have complete evaluation for skin, bone, and genitourinary lesions, as the response to therapy may be monitored by observing the progress of disease in these sites. Adrenal function should also be evaluated, as a few patients may go on to develop adrenal insufficiency.

The blastomycin skin test is valueless as a diagnostic or prognostic tool and should not be used. The blastomycin complement fixation test shows extensive cross-reactivity and is also without value. Detection of the A antigen of *B. dermatitidis* by immunodiffusion or enzyme immunoassay shows promise for specific diagnosis of blastomycosis.

TREATMENT. Amphotericin B (given in a total dose of 2 grams) has been the traditional drug of choice for all forms of blastomycosis. 2-Hydroxystilbamidine* (225 mg daily, to a total dose of 4 to 15 grams) is less efficacious in cavitary pulmonary disease or multifocal extrapulmonary dissemination and is associated with a higher relapse rate and substantial drug toxicity. Ketoconazole (400 to 800 mg daily† for six months) shows great promise in both pulmonary and disseminated blastomycosis. This drug may become preferable to amphotericin B except in situations of severe illness or profound immunosuppression, in which therapeutic failures have been reported.

PROGNOSIS. The natural history of extrapulmonary blastomycosis is that of a slowly progressive disease with a 20 to 90 per cent mortality and severe disfigurement, depending upon the series reported. Case mortality with either amphotercin B or 2-hydroxystilbamidine is about 8 per cent. Most relapses occur within one year of treatment but have been documented after as long as nine years. All patients with untreated pulmonary disease should be carefully observed for later evidence of disease activity.

Klein BS, Kuritsky JN, Chappell A, et al.: Comparison of enzyme immunoassay, immunodiffusion and complement fixation tests in detecting antibody in human serum to the A antigen of *Blastomyces dermatitidis*. Am Rev Respir Dis 133:144, 1986. *Detection of antibody to the A antigen of* B. dermatitidis *is useful for serologic screening (enzyme immunoassay) and serologic confirmation (immunodiffusion) of suspected blastomycosis, especially in disseminated disease.*

National Institute of Allergy and Infectious Diseases Mycoses Study Group: Treatment of blastomycosis and histoplasmosis with ketoconazole. Results of a prospective randomized clinical trial. Ann Intern Med 103:861, 1985. *This study demonstrates that ketoconazole in a dose of 400 or 800 mg daily for at least six months is effective for patients with non–life-threatening, nonmeningeal forms of blastomycosis. The higher dose gave better results. However, a companion paper published in the same issue recorded excellent results with the lower dose (Bradsher RW, Rice DC, Abernathy RS: Ketoconazole therapy for endemic blastomycosis. Ann Intern Med 103:872, 1985).*

Sarosi GA, Davies SF: Blastomycosis. State of the art. Am Rev Respir Dis 120:911, 1979. *A valuable review paper with a particular emphasis on pulmonary blastomycosis. An excellent companion piece to the Witorsch and Utz reference.*

Witorsch P, Utz JP: North American blastomycosis: A study of 40 patients. Medicine 47:169, 1968. *This paper contains a wealth of information concerning both pulmonary and systemic blastomycosis.*

372 **PARACOCCIDIOIDOMYCOSIS**

DEFINITION. Paracoccidioidomycosis (South American blastomycosis) is a noncontagious respiratory mycosis that may be acute and self limited or may produce progressive pulmonary disease or extrapulmonary dissemination. It is the most common systemic mycosis in South America.

ETIOLOGY. *Paracoccidioides brasiliensis* is a dimorphic fungus that in its mycelial phase is probably a soil saprobe that favors humid or aquatic environments. In tissues or at 37°C the fungus is a spherical yeast, 6 to 60 μm in diameter, that has multiple buds on narrow necks, producing the appearance of "ship's wheels," "crown of buds," or "Mickey Mouse" figures.

INCIDENCE AND PREVALENCE. Paracoccidioidomycosis is limited to an area 20° N in Mexico to 34° S in Argentina. Brazil accounts for 70 per cent of the 5000 to 6000 reported cases, followed by Venezuela and Colombia. Natural infection in armadillos has been recently documented. Common-source outbreaks in humans have not been reported.

EPIDEMIOLOGY. Equal numbers of men and women have positive paracoccidioidin skin tests, but clinical disease is 15 times more prevalent in men. Only 4 per cent of cases have been reported in children. Asian and European immigrants often have more severe illness than patients who are native born. Whether this indicates a racial predisposition or merely exposure of a population with a lack of prior disease experience is uncertain.

Virtually all cases are acquired by the respiratory route. The vast majority of cases are probably self limited, manifesting themselves by positive skin tests and minimal abnormalities of the chest roentgenogram.

PATHOGENESIS AND PATHOLOGY. The spectrum of disease encountered clinically is a function of the integrity of cell-mediated host defense responses. The host response consists of a combination of suppuration and granulomas. In patients with impaired cell-mediated immunity, the suppurative response may dominate. The disease process is limited to the lungs in most cases, but lymphohematogenous dissemination may occur, especially in males beyond puberty and in immunosuppressed patients.

CLINICAL MANIFESTATIONS. Pulmonary paracoccidioidomycosis may be symptomatic or asymptomatic and may or may not be apparent when extrapulmonary disease is discovered. There is nothing distinctive about the acute pulmonary process. Progressive pulmonary lesions may be unilateral or bilateral, with or without hilar adenopathy. Chest roentgenograms may reveal cavitation (20 to 33 per cent of cases), infiltration, nodules, tumor-like masses, or fibrosis.

Extrapulmonary dissemination may occur acutely, especially in young persons, under which circumstance the disease process is dominated by lymphadenopathy, hepatosplenomegaly, and a miliary pattern on the chest roentgenogram. The disease may also disseminate after a period of years to decades. Many cases have been documented in persons who have long since emigrated from endemic areas so that continued exposure to the fungus is not an important predisposing factor. The clinical presentation is variable, depending on the sites of involvement. Oropharyngeal mucosal invasion is characteristic. Ulcerating lesions involve the gums, lips, tongue, palate, uvula, pharynx, tonsillar areas, or floor of the mouth. Lesions eventually become so painful that eating is extremely difficult. Gingival destruction may result in loss of teeth. Involvement of the epiglottis and larynx results in dysphonia. Ulcers of the nasal, conjunctival, and perianal mucous membranes may be encountered. There may be massive cervical and abdominal lymphadenopathy. Lymph nodes may break down to produce draining fistulas. A wide variety of crusted ulcerative, verrucous, and granulomatous skin lesions have been described, often on the face or at mucocutaneous borders. Ulcerating lesions of the intestinal tract may be encountered; the stomach is usually spared. Complications include malabsorption, protein-losing enteropathy, and intestinal perforation. There may be signs of adrenal insufficiency and involvement of the bones, testes, epididymis, heart, and pancreas. Central nervous system disease may present as a space-occupying lesion or meningitis. Hepatic, splenic, and renal involvement is common but usually clinically silent.

DIAGNOSIS. Paracoccidioidomycosis must be differentiated from tuberculosis, histoplasmosis, sporotrichosis, leishmaniasis, yaws, and syphilis.

Multiple-budding *P. brasiliensis* can usually be demonstrated in wet mounts or 10 per cent KOH preparations from sputum or infective foci. Characteristic fungus cells can also be seen in hematoxylin-eosin–stained slides from biopsy material, but special stains (e.g., periodic acid–Schiff, Gridley's, and Gomori's methenamine silver) demonstrate the cells much more effectively. Fungi can be recovered in two to four weeks on blood agar at 37°C (tissue phase) or on Sabouraud's agar at 30°C (saprobic phase). Cultures of blood, urine, bone marrow, spinal fluid, and biopsy specimens (liver, lymph node, intestine) may be helpful in appropriate instances. In one study of

---

*Discontinued by the manufacturer.
†May exceed manufacturer's recommended dosage.

39 cases, diagnosis could be made from direct examination of biopsy material in 95 per cent and by culture of these materials or sputum in 85 per cent.

Serologic tests are useful in following the course of established disease. Precipitins are the first antibodies to appear and the first to disappear with successful therapy. Complement-fixing (CF) antibodies appear later in a titer proportional to the severity of infection. Sera from 85 to 95 per cent of patients with active disease demonstrate CF titers $\geq$1:32. Numbers of precipitin bands formed in the immunodiffusion (ID) test indicate the degree of disease activity. (ID and CF tests are available at the Centers for Disease Control in Atlanta.) There is still a need for a specific paracoccidioidin skin test. The present preparations appear to share antigens with *Histoplasma capsulatum* and *Sporothrix schenckii*. There is no commercially available paracoccidioidin skin test reagent in the United States.

TREATMENT. The largest therapeutic experience is with sulfonamides. Their low cost, relatively low toxicity, and good gastrointestinal absorption are partially offset by slow response, a 40 per cent failure and relapse rate, and the occurrence of sulfonamide resistance. The recommended dose of sulfadiazine for adults is 4 to 6 grams per day. Once clinical improvement has occurred (a matter of weeks to months), dosage is reduced by one half and continued for three to five years. Amphotericin B produces a higher response rate and has been considered the drug of choice for disseminated disease. However, relapses occcur even after total doses of 2 grams, whether or not sulfonamides are added to the regimen. Recent studies indicate that ketoconazole (200 to 400 mg daily for 18 months) is equivalent in therapeutic efficacy to amphotericin B plus sulfonamides. Given the problems with the latter medications, it is likely that ketoconazole will soon be considered the therapy of choice for patients who can take medication orally. Miconazole can be substituted in patients who must receive parenteral therapy.

Regardless of the regimen chosen, therapy should be continued until CF and immunodiffusion antibody are undetectable or until titers become stabilized at a low level. A decrease in the number of immunoprecipitin bands is also desirable.

PROGNOSIS. Disseminated paracoccidioidomycosis is generally fatal in the absence of therapy, with death occurring from extensive pulmonary disease, central nervous system lesions, intestinal perforation, or adrenal insufficiency.

Ajello L, Polonelli L: Imported paracoccidioidomycosis: A public health problem in non-endemic areas. Eur J Epidemiol 1:160, 1985. *Cases of paracoccidioidomycosis acquired in the endemic area, but presenting in Europe, resulted in major diagnostic confusion. Incorrect diagnoses included tuberculosis, blastomycosis, Wegener's granulomatosis, syphilis, and cancer. Patients had been away from endemic areas for 4 months to 60 years (mean 14 years). It is important to appreciate the prolonged potential dormant period of this mycosis.*

Londero AT, Ramos CF, Lopes JOS: Progressive pulmonary paracoccidioidomycosis. A study of 34 cases observed in Rio Grande do Sul (Brazil). Mycopathologia 63:53, 1978. *Emphasizes the pulmonary aspects of this respiratory mycosis.*

Marques SA, Dillon NL, Franco MF, et al.: Paracoccidioidomycosis: A comprehensive study of the evolutionary serologic, clinical, and radiologic results for patients treated with ketoconazole or amphotericin B plus sulfonamides. Mycopathologia 89:19, 1985. *Thirty-two patients received ketoconazole (400 mg for 30 days; 200 mg for 18 months); 32 received amphotericin B plus sulfonamides. Antibody titers dropped more sharply in the ketoconazole-treated patients, and there was excellent response to therapy.*

Restrepo A, Greer DL, Vasconcellos M: Paracoccidioidomycosis: A review. Rev Med Vet Mycol 8:97, 1973. *A thorough review of the disease; a classic article.*

Restrepo A, Robledo M, Giraldo R, et al.: The gamut of paracoccidioidomycosis. Am J Med 61:33, 1976. *An excellent review with an emphasis on pulmonary and extrapulmonary clinical manifestations, and helpful photographs.*

373 CRYPTOCOCCOSIS

DEFINITION. Cryptococcosis is a noncontagious, often opportunistic mycosis characterized by acute or chronic pulmonary infection, or hematogenous dissemination, usually with meningitis.

ETIOLOGY. Pathogenic cryptococci are budding yeasts, 4 to 20 μm in diameter with a characteristic polysaccharide capsule. Buds are usually single and narrow necked. There are four serotypes. Nomenclature is currently in a state of turmoil because of the discovery that there are no mating barriers among the serotypes. Until recently, however, serotypes A and D (*Cryptococcus neoformans var. neoformans*) and B and C (*C. neoformans var. gattii*) were considered to show exclusive mating compatibility, leading to the names *Filobasidiella neoformans* and *F. bacillispora* for their respective perfect states. For now, all four serotypes should be considered *C. neoformans* without variety definition. *C. neoformans* is not found as a laboratory contaminant.

INCIDENCE AND PREVALENCE. Because there is no skin test or epidemiologically useful serologic test, the incidence and prevalence of cryptococcosis are unknown. However, the disease occurs worldwide, with several hundred new cases yearly in the United States. Most pulmonary infections are probably overlooked. Cryptococcal meningitis, which accounts for some 90 per cent of reported disease, is dramatic and seldom overlooked. Cryptococcosis has increased in incidence as immunosuppression has become more common and diagnostic techniques have improved and has emerged as a particular problem in patients with acquired immunodeficiency syndrome (AIDS).

EPIDEMIOLOGY. Serotype A causes most disease worldwide; serotype D is common only in Europe. Disease caused by serotypes B and C is found predominantly in the tropics and subtropics. Although most disease in the United States is attributable to serotype A, there is a focus of serotypes B and C in southern California. All cases of cryptococcosis in AIDS patients have involved serotype A or D, regardless of country of AIDS acquisition.

Serotypes A and D are most commonly found in avian habitats, especially in pigeon dung. Up to 5×10^7 viable *C. neoformans* per gram of pigeon feces has been recovered from urban environments. Although the feet, beaks, crops, and gut contents of pigeons may harbor cryptococci, the birds are not infected. High humidity and protection from weathering or soil contact promote survival of *C. neoformans* in the environment. Indoor sites may harbor cryptococci more frequently than outdoor sites. Serotypes B and C are rarely recoverable from the environment, suggesting that these serotypes occupy a unique ecologic niche.

Because most patients give no history of contact with pigeons, infection probably results from inhalation of airborne organisms. Ocular cryptococcosis has been transmitted by corneal transplantation. Many animals are infected with cryptococci but pose no threat to humans.

PATHOGENESIS AND PATHOLOGY. Cryptococci in the environment are unencapsulated. Either these forms or the basidiospores of *Filobasidiella* are small enough to be inhaled. Encapsulation takes place in the lung, and virulence is related to capsule formation and the capacity to synthesize melanin (phenoloxidase activity). Occasional infections with unencapsulated cryptococci occur. Activation of C3 by the alternative complement pathway is sufficient to support phagocytosis of cryptococci by neutrophils; however, immune serum is required for optimal phagocytosis by macrophages. Cell-mediated immunity appears to play the major role in host defense against *C. neoformans*, as exemplified by the greatly increased susceptibility of patients with AIDS.

The histopathology of cryptococcosis varies from a foamy, gelatinous process to a more granulomatous response. Caseation, calcification, and fibrosis are rare. Cryptococci are fragile and may collapse during fixation, leading to a crescentic appearance. They stain poorly with hematoxylin-eosin, but well with methenamine silver and periodic acid-Schiff. Mucicarmine specifically stains capsular mucopolysaccharide.

CLINICAL MANIFESTATIONS. Respiratory tract colonization usually occurs in patients with underlying lung disease and may be transient or persistent.

Pulmonary Cryptococcosis. Manifestations include fever, malaise, pleuritic pain, cough, scanty sputum, and hemoptysis. A pleural effusion or friction rub may be present. Solitary or multiple nodules or nodular-confluent infiltrates, tumor-like masses, or miliary densities may be found on chest roentgenograms; any lobe may be involved. Cavitation is present in 10 to 16 per cent of cases. Hilar adenopathy may occur with advanced disease. Chronic infection is common; slowly progressive pulmonary involvement over 4 to 19 years has been documented. Many such cases are diagnosed at thoracotomy for suspected malignancy. Although some cases are associated with alveolar proteinosis, only 10 per cent of all patients with pulmonary cryptococcosis have evidence of immunologic deficiency.

Disseminated Cryptococcosis. Clinical manifestations relate in part to host defense status; patients with AIDS may have few symptoms or signs despite far-advanced infection. Manifestations of central nervous system cryptococcosis reflect exudate over the base of the brain (meningitis and hydrocephalus), extension of infection along perivascular spaces with involvement of the gray matter (encephalitis), direct invasion of the optic pathways (visual impairment), focal ischemic damage related to brain stem vasculitis, and cryptococcomas in the brain or spinal cord. Meningitis is the most common manifestation of systemic cryptococcosis, and its principal symptom is headache. Associated findings include mental changes (confusion, lethargy, personality alteration, defective memory, agitation, or frank psychosis); ocular symptoms (blurred vision, retrobulbar pain, diplopia, and photophobia); stiffness of the neck and back; nausea and vomiting; and fever, nystagmus, ataxia, aphasia, hearing deficits, cranial nerve palsies, seizures, and paresthesias. Up to 50 per cent of patients have papilledema or optic neuritis. Deterioration of mentation may reflect the development of hydrocephalus. Cryptococcal meningitis may be quite chronic, with disease presenting over weeks to months, or very rarely even years. *Skin and mucous membrane* involvement is seen in 10 to 15 per cent of cases and can take the form of papules, pustules, abscesses, chancres, nodules, or cellulitis followed by vesiculation and ulceration. *Bone* involvement occurs in 5 to 10 per cent of cases and may be mistaken for malignancy. Joint involvement is extremely rare. Other sites of invasion may include the *liver* (hepatitis, hepatic necrosis, cholangitis), *kidneys* (pyelonephritis, papillary necrosis), *prostate* (prostatism), *adrenals* (adrenal insufficiency), spleen, lymph nodes, and testes.

DIAGNOSIS. The differential diagnosis of pulmonary cryptococcosis includes diverse infections and malignancies. Cryptococcal meningitis may be confused with various hypoglycorrhachic syndromes, including tuberculosis and coccidioidomycosis. A primary psychiatric disorder is often suspected.

Sputum cultures are positive in only 20 per cent of pulmonary infections. Sixty per cent of cases have been diagnosed by exploratory thoracotomy for suspected malignancy in older series. Patients with positive sputum cultures should be evaluated for systemic infection, with cultures of blood and urine; biopsy and culture of skin lesions; and a lumbar puncture, whether or not central nervous system disease is apparent. Bone marrow aspiration, liver biopsy, and prostatic massage may also be indicated. Positive blood cultures do not routinely predict a poor therapeutic outcome.

In patients presenting with meningitis, the chest roentgenogram may or may not be abnormal. Sputum cultures should be obtained along with a careful baseline evaluation for other foci of infection. Characteristic cerebrospinal fluid (CSF) findings include elevated pressure (90 per cent of cases); pleocytosis (usually lymphocytic, sometimes polymorphonuclear) with a total white blood cell concentration generally below 500 per cubic millimeter; and hypoglycorrhachia (CSF glucose level less than 50 per cent of a simultaneously obtained blood glucose) (55 per cent of cases). When spun CSF sediment (or other body fluid) is mixed with a drop of India ink or nigrosin and examined under high dry magnification, cryptococci stand out against the darkened background by their halo-like capsules. The India ink preparation is positive in only about 50 per cent of cases of cryptococcal meningitis, whereas CSF cultures are eventually positive in about 95 per cent. Diagnostic yield is improved by examining CSF by cytologic techniques, looking carefully for extracranial sites of infection, obtaining large volumes of CSF exclusively for culture (~10 ml, provided that there are no contraindications to removal of this volume), repeated lumbar punctures, and, in particularly refractory diagnostic situations, tapping the cisterna magna or lateral ventricles. In patients with AIDS, fungi are more abundant, but the CSF shows fewer other abnormalities.

Tests for cryptococcal antibody lack diagnostic value, but serologic testing for cryptococcal polysaccharide antigen by agglutination of antibody-coated latex spheres is an extremely important adjunct to diagnosis. Cryptococcal antigen is found in the CSF in up to 93 per cent of proven cases of cryptococcal meningitis and may also be found in the blood. Titers are particularly high in patients with AIDS. In some patients, serology is positive when all other tests of CSF are nondiagnostic. Serum or pleural fluid polysaccharide determinations may be helpful in the differential diagnosis of pneumonia in immunocompromised patients. Recently, patients infected with *Trichosporon beigelii*, an unencapsulated opportunistic yeast, have been shown to have positive serologic test results for cryptococcal antigen. The basis for this cross-reactivity is unknown.

TREATMENT. Patients with respiratory tract colonization or resolving pulmonary infection and intact immunity seldom require therapy. Patients whose pulmonary cryptococcosis is diagnosed at thoracotomy should have careful postoperative evaluation for extrapulmonary disease, including a lumbar puncture. If none is found, therapy may be safely withheld in those with intact host defenses, provided that there is careful follow-up evaluation. If long-term follow-up is unlikely, antifungal therapy should be administered because there may be a 3 to 10 per cent risk of meningitis occurring up to three years following surgery. Patients with progressive pulmonary infection, especially if immunosuppressed, and all patients with extrapulmonary infection require systemic antifungal therapy.

Therapy for pulmonary cryptococcosis is poorly defined, but an arbitrary total dose of 1 gram of amphotericin B delivered intravenously over five to six weeks (up to 50 mg on alternate days), or ketoconazole in a dose of 200 to 400 mg daily for six months, would be expected to control most cases. The use of ketoconazole in this setting, however, must be considered experimental; few data exist regarding the efficacy of this approach. Immunosuppressed patients should not receive ketoconazole as primary therapy; amphotericin B therapy may have to be more aggressive as well.

Therapeutic guidelines for cryptococcal meningitis are more clearly defined. Combination therapy with amphotericin B and flucytosine is currently favored on three bases: (1) The two drugs are synergistic against cryptococci in vitro; (2) flucytosine reliably crosses the blood-brain barrier, whereas amphotericin B does not; and (3) a national cooperative study has demonstrated that a six-week treatment course with intravenous amphotericin B (0.3 mg per kilogram per day) plus oral flucytosine (150 mg per kilogram per day) cured or improved more patients, produced fewer failures or relapses, and was associated with less nephrotoxicity than amphotericin B given alone for ten weeks in a dose of 0.4 mg per kilogram per day. Potential problems relate to the added toxicity of flucytosine (bone marrow suppression, liver function abnormalities, diarrhea, and rash), particularly in patients with AIDS. Treatment of cryptococcosis in AIDS patients may require deletion of flucytosine and more aggressive use of amphotericin B. Long-term suppressive therapy with amphotericin B is required to prevent relapse; ketoconazole may also prove to be beneficial for this purpose.

In patients who fail to show clinical improvement with combination chemotherapy, or in those whose CSF cultures remain persistently positive, consideration must be given to delivery of amphotericin B into the lumbar sac, cisterna magna, or a lateral ventricle via an Ommaya reservoir or similar device. Complications related to amphotericin B irritability or catheter placement are common. Patients must also be carefully evaluated for hydrocephalus, since therapeutic CSF shunting may be required.

PROGNOSIS. Prior to the amphotericin B era, 80 per cent of patients with cryptococcal meningitis died within two years. With current therapeutic regimens, 80 to 90 per cent of patients can be cured, although more than one treatment course may be required. Patients with AIDS cannot be cured, but cryptococcosis can be suppressed. Additional adverse prognostic factors include lymphoreticular malignancy or corticosteroid therapy; cerebrospinal fluid with high opening pressure, a low glucose level, less than 20 leukocytes per cubic millimeter, and positive India ink preparations; cryptococci isolated from the blood or extraneural sites; and high titers of cryptococcal antigen in CSF and serum. Treated patients with persistently elevated titers of cryptococcal antigen have a tendency to relapse. Elevated CSF protein concentrations and positive India ink preparations may persist for years following curative therapy and have no apparent prognostic significance.

PREVENTION. Hydrated lime and sodium hydroxide may be used to control cryptococcal growth in droppings of pet pigeons but are otherwise impractical. Control of pigeon populations in urban areas might be expected to reduce the risk of acquiring cryptococcosis in this setting.

Bennett JE, Dismukes WE, Duma RJ, et al.: A comparison of amphotericin B alone and combined with flucytosine in the treatment of cryptococcal meningitis. N Engl J Med 301:126, 1979. *This important paper provides the rationale for the combined therapeutic approach to cryptococcal meningitis used in the United States at this time.*

Hermann KJ, Powell KE, Christianson CS, et al.: Pulmonary cryptococcosis: Clinical forms and treatment. A Center for Disease Control Cooperative Mycoses Study. Am Rev Respir Dis 108:1116, 1973. *This interesting paper compares the presentation of pulmonary cryptococcosis in patients in chronic chest hospitals with that of patients in other settings. Colonization, infection, and treatment are discussed.*

Kovacs JA, Kovacs AA, Polis M, et al.: Cryptococcosis in the acquired immunodeficiency syndrome. Ann Intern Med 103:533, 1985. *In patients with meningitis, leukocyte count, protein level, and glucose level in the CSF were frequently normal, but blood and CSF cultures and antigen tests were usually positive. Response to treatment with amphotericin B with and without flucytosine was poor, and relapses were frequent. A similarly grim picture emerges in a subsequent paper: Zuger A, Louie E, Holzman RS, et al.: Cryptococcal disease in patients with acquired immunodeficiency syndrome: Diagnostic features and outcome of treatment. Ann Intern Med 104:234, 1986.*

Perfect JR, Durack DT, Gallis HA: Cryptococcemia. Medicine 62:98, 1983. *Cryptococcemia identifies patients with poor prognoses, largely because of underlying disease. However, some patients will respond to aggressive therapy with amphotericin B and flucytosine.*

374 SPOROTRICHOSIS

DEFINITION. Sporotrichosis is a subacute or chronic mycosis of the skin and regional lymphatics that results from the percutaneous introduction of *Sporothrix schenckii*. In some cases, pulmonary disease results from inhalation of conidia. Rarely, there is lymphohematogenous dissemination to joints, bones, and skin.

ETIOLOGY. *Sporothrix schenckii* is a dimorphic fungus. In tissues and at 37°C it is yeastlike, appearing as spherical or cigar-shaped budding cells. In nature (25°C), the fungus exists as hyphae that produce conidia of a size (2 to 3 μm) suitable to be inhaled. *S. schenckii* is commonly found on vegetation or wood, or in the soil.

INCIDENCE AND PREVALENCE. Sporotrichosis occurs worldwide. Susceptibility is less related to sex, age, or race than to opportunities for environmental exposure. Skin test data suggest that sporotrichosis may occur as a subclinical infection, especially in nursery workers.

EPIDEMIOLOGY. *S. schenckii* is a potential cause of infection in anyone who has frequent contact with vegetation (e.g., sphagnum moss, timber, hay, thorn bushes). Thus, it is an occupational hazard for farmers, gardeners, florists, greenhouse workers, timber cutters, hay mulchers, and others. Some cases may be transmitted by insects or animal bites or scratches. The source of infection may be obscure in those with pulmonary or visceral involvement. In the most famous outbreak of sporotrichosis, nearly 3000 otherwise healthy South African gold miners acquired lymphocutaneous sporotrichosis from brushing past contaminated mine timbers. Spread from patient to patient, pulmonary disease and disseminated disease did not occur. Epidemiologic proof that alcoholism predisposes to sporotrichosis ("syndrome of the alcoholic rose gardener") is lacking.

PATHOGENESIS AND PATHOLOGY. *S. schenckii* enters the skin through apparent or inapparent trauma. Strains that multiply well at 35°C but poorly at 37°C can produce cutaneous lesions, but not lymphatic spread or systemic involvement. Strains that multiply well at 35°C or 37°C are capable of producing lymphocutaneous or visceral disease. Cell-mediated immunity is important in determining the extent of disease, and immunosuppressed patients appear more likely to develop multifocal systemic spread of infection.

The basic histopathologic pattern is a combination of suppuration and granulomas, occasionally with caseation necrosis. Chronic cutaneous lesions demonstrate prominent pseudoepitheliomatous hyperplasia and may be confused with malignancies.

CLINICAL MANIFESTATIONS. In lymphocutaneous sporotrichosis, which accounts for 75 per cent of cases, a single lesion usually develops on an exposed skin surface, commonly following trauma. The pimple, wart, pustule, ulcer, abscess, or chancre fails to heal and typically spreads up the extremity over days to weeks, evoking a series of subcutaneous nontender nodular lesions along the thickened lymphatics. The nodules may ulcerate, releasing thin pus. Systemic signs and symptoms of infection are notably absent. Incision and drainage and antibacterial drugs are without benefit. The disease may slowly progress over months or even years; a few cases heal spontaneously.

In 20 per cent of cases, the process is strictly limited to the site of introduction in the skin ("fixed"). It is likely that this disease pattern is produced by *S. schenckii* strains that grow poorly at 37°C. Lacking the diagnostic appearance of nodules following lymphatics, this form of sporotrichosis may be quite difficult to diagnose.

About 70 cases of pulmonary sporotrichosis have been reported. Disease may occur acutely but more frequently presents as a chronic cavitary process involving upper lobes and apices. Chronic sinusitis has also been reported. Extracutaneous sporotrichosis is very rare. It may result from direct, deep implantation of fungi; from direct contiguous spread of lymphocutaneous disease; or by hematogenous spread from apparent or inapparent cutaneous or pulmonary loci. Common sites of dissemination include joints (especially knees, ankles, wrists, and small joints of the hands and feet) and bones (especially the tibia), sometimes with pathologic fractures. When joint disease occurs in the absence of a primary lymphocutaneous focus (as it does in more than 80 per cent of cases), it is classically confused with rheumatoid arthritis, sarcoidosis, villonodular synovitis, or gout. In immunocompromised patients with multifocal disease, there is often abrupt development of widespread subcutaneous nodules in a hematogenous distribution. Multiarticular joint disease may be present, and multifocal osteolytic foci may be visible roentgenographically. Cultures of the urine, bone marrow, and rarely even the blood may be positive. There are a few recorded cases of central nervous system sporotrichosis; chronic meningitis may be present.

DIAGNOSIS. The differential diagnosis of lymphocutaneous sporotrichosis includes "sporotrichoid granulomas" caused by atypical mycobacterial infections, other cutaneous mycoses, leishmaniasis, syphilis, anthrax, tularemia, cat-scratch disease, and even furunculosis. Pulmonary sporotrichosis resembles pulmonary tuberculosis; sometimes the diseases coexist.

The diagnosis of lymphocutaneous sporotrichosis on histopathologic grounds is very difficult, as the fungi may not be easily demonstrable. Direct immunofluorescence or immunoperoxidase staining may be helpful but is not generally available. *S. schenckii* is also difficult to identify directly in the sputum. In deep lesions, fungi may be demonstrable with special stains (e.g., methenamine silver, PAS). Regardless of the locus of infection, diagnosis is made most accurately by recovering *S. schenckii* in culture. These fungi grow well on most standard media; cultures should be held at least four weeks before being discarded as negative. Conversion to yeast form in vitro or animal inoculation may assist in identification. Rarely, *S. schenckii* may be recovered from the sputum in the absence of any demonstrable disease process, thus reflecting the possibility of asymptomatic colonization.

Serologic tests are useful in establishing the diagnosis of extracutaneous or systemic forms of sporotrichosis when distinct clinical features are lacking. The yeast cell and latex particle agglutination tests are more sensitive than immunodiffusion or complement fixation techniques. In general, patients with extracutaneous disease have higher titers than those with lymphocutaneous involvement. A slide latex agglutination titer of 1.8 or above is considered presumptive evidence of sporotrichosis by the Centers for Disease Control, Atlanta. The test has limited prognostic value, since antibody levels may show little change during or after convalescence.

A sporotrichosis skin test is not commercially available.

TREATMENT. The treatment of choice for lymphocutaneous sporotrichosis is saturated solution of potassium iodide (SSKI). Its mechanism of action is unclear. Daily dosage is increased in dropwise fashion (usually 50 mg per drop) in a palatable vehicle until 3 to 5 grams or more is being administered each day. If signs of toxicity ensue (e.g., indigestion, rash, lacrimation, parotid swelling), dosage may have to be reduced. Ketoconazole (200 to 600* mg daily for three to six

months) has been beneficial in many cases but has failed inexplicably in others. Success may be related to the use of higher dosages (400 to 600* mg daily). Amphotericin B is indicated when SSKI and ketoconazole fail. Disseminated sporotrichosis is generally treated with intravenous amphotericin B (minimal dose, 2 grams), together with local intralesional therapy, arthrotomy, and other indicated drainage procedures.

SSKI and ketoconazole may deserve evaluation in cases of noncavitary pulmonary sporotrichosis, but even amphotericin B is of limited value in cavitary infection. Resectional surgery may offer the only real possibility of cure. Amphotericin B is superior to SSKI, miconazole, or ketoconazole in disseminated infection.

PROGNOSIS. Cutaneous, lymphocutaneous, and mucocutaneous sporotrichosis commonly remit and relapse for years without therapy. Spontaneous cures are unknown in disseminated disease. The natural history and, indeed, the incidence and prevalence of pulmonary sporotrichosis are unknown. Cavitary pulmonary disease may be curable medically but more often requires surgery. Untreated chronic pulmonary sporotrichosis is usually fatal.

Lavelle P, Mariat F: Sporotrichosis. Bull Institute Pasteur 81:295, 1983. *A complete and current literature review.*

Pluss JL, Opal SM: Pulmonary sporotrichosis: Review of treatment and outcome. Medicine 65:143, 1986. *A review of 68 cases. Ketoconazole was without benefit in the two patients who received it.*

Urabe H, Honbo S: Sporotrichosis. Int J Dermatol 25:255, 1986. *A more limited review, but perhaps more easily accessible than the Lavelle-Mariat reference.*

Wilson DE, Mann JJ, Bennett JE, et al.: Clinical features of extracutaneous sporotrichosis. Medicine 46:265, 1967. *Still the best reference concerning extracutaneous sporotrichosis.*

375 CANDIDIASIS (Candidosis)

DEFINITION. Candidiasis is a general term for diseases produced by *Candida* species and encompasses colonization; superficial infection (e.g., thrush, vaginitis, cystitis, intertrigo); deep local invasion (e.g., esophagitis); and hematogenous dissemination (e.g., endophthalmitis, hepatic abscesses). "Systemic candidiasis" is a term without clear meaning and will be avoided.

ETIOLOGY. The most common etiologic agent is *Candida albicans* (closely related to *C. stellatoidea*). Others include *C. tropicalis, guilliermondii, krusei, lusitaniae, parapsilosis,* and *pseudotropicalis. C. albicans* and *C. tropicalis* are fungi imperfecti, whereas the others have identifiable perfect states, representing diverse genera. Thus "candidiasis" is actually produced by a variety of fungi that happen to share two morphologic features: (1) yeasts ("blastospores"; more properly, blastoconidia)—these forms reproduce by budding and constitute the principal colonizing form; (2) pseudomycelia (pseudohyphae)—these are chains of elongated yeasts separated by constrictions (like chains of sausages); they often form under suboptimal growth conditions. Since *Torulopsis glabrata* has only a yeastlike form, it cannot be considered a species of *Candida. C. albicans* is capable of producing true mycelia (hyphae with cross walls, but no constrictions). Mycelia begin as "germ tubes." The ability of *C. albicans* to form germ tubes in serum is an important presumptive laboratory test for this fungus.

INCIDENCE AND PREVALENCE. Candidiasis occurs worldwide. Superficial infections such as thrush, paronychia, and intertrigo are universal. Invasive candidiasis has become a problem with the advent of antibiotics (destruction of normal inhibitory bacterial flora) and the use of myelotoxic or immunosuppressive agents, especially corticosteroids. Mucosal

*May exceed manufacturer's recommended dosage.

*May exceed manufacturer's recommended dosage.

candidiasis is a characteristic early manifestation of acquired immunodeficiency syndrome (AIDS).

EPIDEMIOLOGY. *Candida* species can be found in nature but more commonly originate with humans. *C. albicans* is found in the oropharynx, gastrointestinal tract, and vagina of a variable proportion of normal persons, but only rarely on the skin. Non-*albicans* species more frequently colonize the skin. Vaginal colonization is increased by diabetes, pregnancy, and oral contraceptive agents. Carriage at all sites is increased by antibiotics. Unlike most other fungi, *C. albicans* is transmissible (e.g., from colonized birth canal to neonatal oropharynx; between sexual partners; by hands of medical attendants). Cutaneous infection generally requires skin trauma, maceration, and persistent moisture. Invasive or disseminated candidiasis occurs most frequently in a hospital setting, among severely ill, antibiotic-treated patients with breaches of normal mucocutaneous barriers (e.g., indwelling intravascular lines or Foley catheters; gastrointestinal ulceration from chemotherapeutic agents; burns). Abdominal surgery is one of the most important settings for hematogenously disseminated candidiasis. Chronic ambulatory peritoneal dialysis (CAPD) may be complicated by *Candida* peritonitis. Endocarditis may follow intravenous drug abuse, prolonged intravenous therapy, or placement of a prosthetic heart valve.

PATHOGENESIS AND PATHOLOGY. The pathogenic capability of *Candida* species is a function of their ability to adhere to tissues (e.g., mucosal or endothelial cells). *C. albicans* and *C. tropicalis* are more adherent than other species, perhaps explaining their dominance as pathogens. Mechanisms of adherence vary widely under experimental conditions. The most important fungal "adhesin" may be a mannoprotein surface glycocalix; pseudomycelia may be more adherent than yeasts. When deep tissue invasion occurs, yeasts have generally converted to pseudomycelia. However, this does not imply that yeasts themselves lack invasive potential. Putative virulence factors include phospholipases, proteinases, and toxins (e.g., "canditoxin"). Disruption of mucosal integrity by underlying disease processes is probably of greatest importance in explaining *Candida* invasion.

Both neutrophils and cell-mediated immunity (CMI) are important in host defense against candidiasis. Neutropenia is a major risk factor for hematogenous *Candida* dissemination, whereas defective CMI is associated with an increased incidence of mucosal disease (e.g., AIDS; the syndrome of chronic mucocutaneous candidiasis).

CLINICAL MANIFESTATIONS. *Mucocutaneous Infection.* *Thrush* is characterized by a creamy to gray pseudomembrane, patchy or confluent, that covers the tongue, buccal mucosa, or other oropharyngeal surfaces. Ulceration and necrosis may be present. Membrane removal leaves a red, oozing base. Laryngeal involvement results in hoarseness. *Esophagitis* is often an extension of oropharyngeal disease, may be manifested by retrosternal pain and dysphagia, and may be complicated by hemorrhage or stricture. *Gastritis* or gastroduodenal ulcer invasion may occur in patients receiving H$_2$ blockers. *Intestinal candidiasis* is commonly asymptomatic but is a major source of hematogenous invasion in the immunosuppressed. *Perianal* candidal overgrowth may follow antibiotic therapy and produces or aggravates pruritus ani. *Intertrigo* involves the axillae, groins, inframammary folds, and other warm, moist areas. Lesions may be red and oozing or dry and scaly, with sharp, scalloped borders and satellite vesicles, pustules, or bullae. *Paronychia* often follows chronic exposure of the hands or feet to moisture. The nails may become hardened, thickened, grooved, and discolored (*onychomycosis*). *Vulvovaginitis* is characterized by a variable discharge and pruritus. *Balanitis* is manifested by superficial penile erosions and pustules. *Cystitis* looks identical to thrush under the cystoscope.

Chronic mucocutaneous candidiasis is a rare syndrome based upon limited T cell immunodeficiency. One fifth of patients show a familial tendency. In about one half of cases, there is associated endocrinopathy (especially hypoparathyroidism, hypoadrenalism, hypothyroidism, or diabetes mellitus). Clinical features include persistent superficial *Candida* infection of the skin, scalp, nails, and mucous membranes, often in association with a dermatophyte infection. Disease may begin at any age and be extensive or very limited. Associated findings include alopecia, depigmentation, cheilosis, blepharitis, keratoconjunctivitis, and corneal ulcers. In the most severe cases, there is horn formation with thick, plaque-like, hyperkeratotic scales (*Candida* granuloma) involving the skin or nails. Immunologic abnormalities include decreased or absent response to *Candida* antigens by skin test or by tests of cell-mediated immunity in vitro.

Hematogenously Disseminated Candidiasis. Most cases of disseminated candidiasis are due to *C. albicans* and *C. tropicalis*, with an increasing number attributable to *T. glabrata*. Clinical manifestations of *C. albicans* and *C. tropicalis* infection tend to be apparent in specific "target organs":

Eyes: A variable proportion of patients have *Candida* endophthalmitis, with single or multiple raised, white, fluffy chorioretinal lesions, in the presence or absence of overlying vitreous haze. Lesions are usually in the macular area within easy range of the ophthalmoscope and extend forward into the vitreous. They serve as a major clue to diagnosis and are a potential cause of blindness.

Kidneys: Renal involvement is attributable to the ability of bloodborne *Candida* to invade the renal tubules directly. Manifestations include diffuse cortical and medullary abscesses, papillary necrosis, obstruction of the ureters by sloughed papillae or *Candida* balls (bezoars), and progressive renal insufficiency with flank pain and dysuria. *Candida* pyelonephritis must be differentiated from *Candida* cystitis, a benign infection often associated with prolonged catheterization or vaginitis.

Skin: Macronodular skin lesions may mark the occurrence of hematogenous *Candida* infection, sometimes with accompanying arthralgias or myalgias. Subcutaneous nodules and folliculitis may occur, especially in users of "brown" heroin. *Candida* folliculitis must be differentiated from that produced by *Pityrosporum* (*Malassezia*) species. The latter are lipophilic fungi, normally resident on skin. (They may invade the pulmonary vasculature in patients who receive intravenous lipid supplement.)

Liver: "Focal hepatic candidiasis" occurs characteristically during the remission phase of hematologic malignancies, in patients who have been on broad-spectrum antibiotic therapy and who have reversed their neutropenia. It is manifested by persistent fever, abdominal signs and symptoms, alkaline phosphatase elevation, and mass lesions in the liver (or spleen). Presumably, the hepatosplenic focus of infection, often without evidence of disease in other organs, reflects an intense portal fungemia from a heavily infected gastrointestinal tract that has been damaged by cytoreductive therapy.

Lung: *Candida* pneumonia is rare, despite the prominence of oral thrush and the likelihood for aspiration in seriously ill patients. Although hematogenous involvement of the lungs is common, the miliary pulmonary lesions are usually too small to be seen on a chest roentgenogram.

Other manifestations include meningitis and cerebral abscesses (up to 10 per cent of cases), myocardial invasion, osteomyelitis (especially vertebral), arthritis, and thyroid abscesses.

Endocarditis. *C. albicans* endocarditis is most common in a setting of prolonged intravenous therapy, hyperalimentation, or a cardiac valve prosthesis. Non-*albicans* species are most frequent with intravenous narcotic abuse. Fungal valvular lesions are large and friable. Embolization and occlusion of large blood vessels are more common than in bacterial endocarditis; intracerebral lesions are common.

DIAGNOSIS. Superficial infections are diagnosed by examination of scrapings or swabs of infected lesions in the presence of 10 per cent KOH. *Candida* organisms can also be demonstrated by Gram's stain. Endocarditis is diagnosed by blood cultures, echocardiographic demonstration of bulky valvular vegetations, or demonstration of fungi in an excised embolus. Hematogenously disseminated candidiasis may be difficult to diagnose. The presence of heavy colonization at usual carriage sites sets the stage for bloodstream invasion but does not prove that dissemination has occurred. The most reliable evidence of disseminated candidiasis is biopsy demonstration of tissue invasion or recovery of fungi from fluid in a closed body cavity (e.g., cerebrospinal fluid [CSF], pleural or peritoneal fluid). Blood cultures are most likely to be positive when biphasic media or lysis-centrifugation (Isolator) methods are used. However, positive blood cultures or cultures from the tips of an intravenous line do not necessarily establish the diagnosis of disseminated candidiasis, because fungemia may clear spontaneously with the removal of an intravascular focus of infection. Positive urine cultures may indicate lower tract or invasive upper urinary tract disease. The differentiation is not assisted by quantitative urine cultures (even 10^3 *Candida* per milliliter may be associated with pyelonephritis), fluorescent antibody coating studies, or the presence of pseudomycelia in the urine. Declining renal function and evidence of renal destruction (papillary necrosis), *Candida* entrapped in tubular casts, urinary tract fungal bezoars, and fungi from catheterized renal pelvis urine suggest that invasive disease is present. Positive sputum cultures usually indicate respiratory tract colonization; pneumonia is relatively rare and must be documented by invasive means. Meningitis is usually manifested by polymorphonuclear neutrophil (PMN) pleocytosis, hypoglycorrhachia, and a positive CSF culture in 40 to 45 per cent of cases. Hepatosplenic disease is diagnosed by scanning procedures followed by open biopsy. Although easily seen on tissue sections, the fungi may be difficult to culture.

Skin testing is not helpful in diagnosing candidiasis, because delayed type hypersensitivity to *Candida* antigens is so common among normal persons that the test is used to screen for cutaneous anergy. *Serologic* studies based upon detection of antibodies (precipitins or agglutinins) may be falsely positive or negative and do not clearly differentiate heavy colonization from systemic infection, although rising titers must be considered compatible with dissemination. Tests for unique antigens (e.g., mannan) or fungal metabolites (e.g., mannose; arabitol) are not of proven diagnostic efficacy, but they do show promise.

TREATMENT. Topical preparations (nystatin, clotrimazole, econazole, miconazole, or haloprogin) may be useful in the treatment of superficial mucocutaneous infections. Chronic mucocutaneous candidiasis syndrome responds to chronic therapy with ketoconazole (200 to 400 mg daily); relapse occurs if treatment is discontinued. Ketoconazole is also beneficial in patients with esophagitis.

Deeply invasive candidiasis (e.g., severe esophagitis, peritonitis) or hematogenously disseminated candidiasis should be treated with amphotericin B. The removal of precipitating factors (especially intravenous lines) is very important. Because removal of an intravascular focus does not guarantee that fungemia will be self-limited, treatment should be instituted in immunocompromised patients. In acutely ill patients, dosage should be raised quickly to 0.5 to 1.0 mg per kilogram of body weight per day, as tolerated. Alternate-day therapy can be employed and the dosage lowered once clinical improvement is apparent. The usual total dosage recommendation is 1.5 to 2.0 grams, but higher dosage or prolonged therapy may be required in refractory cases. Flucytosine may be added, using the same rationale as that employed for cryptococcosis (see Ch. 373). There are too few clinical data

with either miconazole or ketoconazole to judge their value in disseminated candidiasis; thus, amphotericin B remains the drug of choice.

Candida cystitis is often cured by Foley catheter removal and the substitution of intermittent ("straight") catheterization. Eradication of infection in those who must have an indwelling catheter, or those with non–catheter-related infection, may be attempted with amphotericin B bladder rinses; with low-dose short-course intravenous therapy (amphotericin is excreted in the urine at a therapeutic level for days following intravenous dosing); or even with oral flucytosine, provided no catheter is in place. This is one of the few situations in which flucytosine may be used alone. Ketoconazole is largely metabolized by the liver; therefore, little active ketoconazole reaches the kidneys. There is an approximate 50 per cent failure rate when ketoconazole is used to treat candiduria.

Endocarditis is essentially incurable without valve replacement. Surgical treatment should be accompanied by a six- to ten-week course of amphotericin B and flucytosine, but cure is elusive. Endophthalmitis generally responds to amphotericin B and flucytosine. Local (sub-Tenon) treatment is employed in addition by many ophthalmologists.

PROGNOSIS. Chronic mucocutaneous candidiasis can be ameliorated, but rarely cured. Endocarditis patients often show evidence of disease activity after having been declared cured. Systemic candidiasis is curable, especially in those with intact immune mechanisms. Disseminated candidiasis is common but difficult to document in febrile neutropenic patients. Empiric therapy with amphotericin B has led to an improved prognosis for recovery in these patients.

PREVENTION. Deeply invasive or hematogenously disseminated candidiasis is avoided by adherence to sound principles of antibiotic use (avoidance of excessive dosage, duration, or breadth of antimicrobial spectrum) and avoidance of indwelling intravascular devices in favor of steel needles. If plastic cannulas are used, they must be changed at least every three days. In immunosuppressed patients, lowering colonization of the gastrointestinal tract with nystatin or ketoconazole is widely practiced, although its efficacy in preventing systemic spread is questionable. Foley catheters should be avoided whenever possible.

Bodey GP, Fainstein V (eds.): Candidiasis. New York, Raven Press, 1985. *This book provides an excellent introduction to candidiasis. It is particularly valuable in describing the manifestations of infections in immunocompromised patients but covers all relevant topics in a comprehensive manner.*

DeRepentigny L, Reiss E: Current trends in immunodiagnosis of candidiasis and aspergillosis. Rev Infect Dis 6:301, 1984. *The best current review of serologic tests for antibody, antigen, and fungal metabolites of the two principal opportunistic mycoses.*

Dupont B, Drouhet E: Cutaneous, ocular and osteoarticular candidiasis in heroin addicts: New clinical and therapeutic aspects in 38 patients. J Infect Dis 152:577, 1985. *Users of brown heroin, which is often solubilized in lemon juice, developed a peculiar form of disseminated candidiasis in which folliculitis and subcutaneous nodules were the dominant clinical manifestations. Many of these patients responded to ketoconazole, but other authors have reported less satisfactory results. Thus amphotericin B remains, when possible, the drug of choice. Studies by others suggest that the patients' skin, and not the lemon juice, is the source of the C. albicans.*

Horn R, Wong B, Kiehn TE, et al.: Fungemia in a cancer hospital: Changing frequency, earlier onset, and results of therapy. Rev Infect Dis 7:646, 1985. *A review of 200 episodes of fungemia in cancer patients at Memorial Sloan-Kettering between 1978 and 1982.*

Solomkin JS, Flohr AB, Quie PG, et al.: The role of *Candida* in intraperitoneal infections. Surgery 88:524, 1980. Solomkin JS, Flohr AB, Simmons RL: *Candida* infections in surgical patients: Dose requirements and toxicity of amphotericin B. Ann Surg 195:177, 1982. *Abdominal surgery is one of the most common settings for hematogenously disseminated candidiasis. These two papers enumerate clearly the diagnostic and therapeutic problems encountered in surgical patients who develop invasive infection.*

Tashjian LS, Abramson JS, Peacock JE Jr: Focal hepatic candidiasis: A distinct clinical variant of candidiasis in immunocompromised patients. Rev Infect Dis 6:689, 1984. *This is a newly recognized manifestation of candidiasis but is not rare. It is not clear why fungi that are easily visible in tissue specimens from biopsied material are so difficult to culture.*

376 ASPERGILLOSIS

DEFINITION. Aspergillosis is a poorly descriptive term encompassing a variety of disease processes that share an etiologic relationship with *Aspergillus* species. The dominant element may be any of the following:

1. *Colonization* of previously damaged respiratory tissues (aspergillary bronchitis, aspergilloma).
2. *Allergy* to inhaled conidia or to fungi colonizing the bronchial tree (atopic asthma, allergic bronchopulmonary aspergillosis, extrinsic allergic alveolitis).
3. *Invasion* of (a) the lung, especially in immunocompromised hosts, with or without systemic spread, or (b) other loci, e.g., eyes, external ear canals, paranasal sinuses, burn wounds, prosthetic heart valves.
4. *Intoxication and/or neoplasm,* especially with ingestion of aflatoxin.

ETIOLOGY. *Aspergillus* species are ubiquitous and can be isolated from numerous sources (e.g., grains, leaves, grasses, soil, refrigerator walls, wet paint, construction and fireproofing materials). Their conidia are frequently isolated from the air and are constantly being inhaled. The rarity of disease attests to the potency of normal host defenses. Although hundreds of *Aspergillus* species are known, only a few thermotolerant species are ordinarily pathogenic for humans: *A. fumigatus* (the most common overall), *A. flavus* (especially in upper airway disease and sinusitis), *A. niger* (especially in external otitis), *A. nidulans, A. terreus, A. sydowi, A. clavatus,* and *A. glaucus.* In the tissues, *Aspergillus* hyphae are uniform, 2 to 7 μm in diameter, septate, and dichotomously branched with angles of ~ 45 degrees. These features are not diagnostic. *Aspergillus* species grow rapidly on most media and can be differentiated by their pattern of conidiation or sporulation.

INCIDENCE AND PREVALENCE. Aspergillosis is increasing in prevalence, particularly in patients with chronic respiratory disease or immunosuppression. Among the immunosuppressed, aspergillosis is second only to candidiasis as an opportunistic mycosis, and both are increasing in frequency because of better methods of controlling bacterial infection.

EPIDEMIOLOGY. *Aspergillus* infections occur worldwide, with no regard to age, sex, race, or occupation. Outbreaks of invasive aspergillosis in burned or immunosuppressed patients have followed exposure to conidia released by hospital construction, contaminated air-conditioning ducts and filters, and fireproofing materials above false ceilings. Aflatoxin-related hepatotoxicity and malignancies have been documented in African tribes among whom spoiled peanuts are a major dietary component. *Aspergillus* infections are not considered transmissible from animals to humans or from humans to humans.

SPECIFIC SYNDROMES. *Colonization. Aspergillary bronchitis* is characterized by the growth of mycelia on the surface of the bronchial mucosa, without tissue invasion. The mucosa shows only a mild inflammatory response. Bronchial casts containing mucus and mycelia may be expectorated.

Aspergillomas are fungal balls composed of tangled, degenerating hyphae and amorphous debris that lie free in pulmonary cavities lined partially by modified bronchial epithelium. There is little surrounding inflammation. The cavities have generally been produced by other disease processes (tuberculosis, sarcoidosis, bronchiectasis, bullae, infarcts, necrotic neoplasms) and are particularly common in the upper lobes. The typical radiographic appearance is that of a freely movable intracavitary mass surrounded on its superior surface by a crescent of air (crescent sign, Monod's sign). This sign is not pathognomonic and may be mimicked by necrotizing tumors or pulmonary infarcts, echinococcal cysts, or other fungal balls. The natural history of aspergillomas is quite variable. Lesions may remain stable for long periods, grow or shrink along with the surrounding cavity, or undergo spontaneous lysis (about 10 per cent of cases). Invasiveness is extremely rare. Hemoptysis is encountered in 60 to 75 per cent of cases and is sometimes life threatening. Sputum cultures are positive in 60 per cent and *Aspergillus* precipitins in 90 per cent of patients. Diagnosis requires a suggestive chest radiograph combined with either positive serum precipitins or a positive culture obtained directly from the cavitary lesion. Sputum cultures are not diagnostic. Systemic antifungal therapy has been valueless. Intrabronchial amphotericin B therapy may occasionally be successful. Treatment is probably not indicated except with life-threatening hemoptysis, for which segmental resection or lobectomy is the treatment of choice. Selective bronchial artery embolization has been used in nonsurgical candidates.

Allergy. Allergic bronchopulmonary aspergillosis (ABPA) occurs in up to 20 per cent of patients with asthma and is related to the development of tissue hypersensitivity to antigens of *Aspergillus* species (usually *A. fumigatus*) that colonize the bronchial mucous membranes. Its immunopathogenesis includes type I hypersensitivity (IgE-mediated) with bronchospasm, and type III (immune complex) and perhaps type IV (cell-mediated) hypersensitivity with permanent bronchial damage. Manifestations in the paranasal sinuses may include sinusitis and nasal polyps.

Any patient with asthma may have ABPA. Diagnostic features include episodic bronchial obstruction; peripheral blood eosinophilia; elevated total serum immunoglobulin E (IgE) levels (above 1000 ng per milliliter); and immediate (type I) skin sensitivity, precipitating serum antibodies, and elevated serum IgE and immunoglobulin G (IgG) antibody levels against *Aspergillus* antigens. Chest radiographs reflect the bronchial location of the disease process and the intermittent occurrence of bronchial obstruction attributable to mucous impactions: central saccular bronchiectasis; bronchial wall thickening ("gloved fingers"); fluctuating bronchial dilation; (upper) lobar shrinkage; perihilar consolidation; collapse of a segment, lobe, or entire lung. These findings may be transient or permanent; the chest radiograph may be normal between episodes.

Additional, less constant features include *Aspergillus* species in smears or cultures of sputum, eosinophils in the sputum, history of expectoration of brown plugs or flecks, and fever. Irreversible complications of ABPA include pulmonary fibrosis, lung retraction, and bronchiectasis. In rare instances, aspergillomas may mimic some of the immunologic features of ABPA. Also, aspergilloma is a rare complication of the saccular bronchiectasis of ABPA.

Patients with a history of asthma and pulmonary infiltrates should be skin tested with *Aspergillus* antigen. If positive, serum should be obtained for determination of IgE and *Aspergillus* precipitins. The treatment of choice is prednisone in a dose of 0.5 mg per kilogram of body weight per day for two weeks, followed by the same dose on alternate days for three months. Steroids are reinitiated during exacerbations of ABPA, as defined by a greater than twofold rise in serum IgE level and an unexplained pulmonary infiltrate. The goal of this regimen is the prevention of progression to fibrotic lung disease in patients with ABPA who do not have corticosteroid-dependent asthma.

In patients with *atopic asthma,* the inhalation of *Aspergillus conidia* results in immediate bronchospasm based upon a type I immune response. There is no conidial germination in bronchial passageways.

Extrinsic allergic alveolitis occurs predominantly in nonatopic patients who inhale *Aspergillus* conidia and is characterized by dyspnea, dry cough, malaise, myalgias, rales, diffuse micronodular infiltrates, and serum precipitins to *Aspergillus.*

The skin test shows an Arthus' response, with or without the preceding wheal and flare reaction. Similar processes include farmer's lung, maple bark stripper's disease, pigeon breeder's disease, and bagassosis.

Invasion. Chronic necrotizing pulmonary aspergillosis is an indolent cavitary process, often with mycetoma formation, that occurs predominantly in middle-aged patients with underlying pulmonary parenchymal disease. It is distinct from aspergilloma in that invasion of pulmonary tissue is clearly present. However, it is only semi-invasive when compared with the invasive form of infection described later. Patients have fever, productive cough, and pulmonary infiltrates with cavities. Demonstration of lung invasion by *Aspergillus* species and response to amphotericin B support the diagnosis, as does an elevated *Aspergillus* precipitin titer.

Invasive pulmonary aspergillosis occurs characteristically in patients with hematologic and lymphoreticular malignancy or organ transplants, generally in the face of intense immunosuppression and often following the use of various antibacterial drug regimens for septic episodes. Macrophages are responsible primarily for the killing of conidia, whereas neutrophils attack mycelia. Invasive disease generally occurs in settings in which there is damage to both arms of the immune system. However, even isolated neutrophil defects such as chronic granulomatous disease are characterized by an increased incidence of pulmonary infection and osteomyelitis caused by *Aspergillus* species. Occasional cases have been described in chronic alcoholics or influenza patients.

Invasive pulmonary aspergillosis is characterized by widespread bronchial erosion and ulceration, followed by invasion of the pulmonary vasculature with thrombosis, embolization, and infarction. Clinical manifestations include a necrotizing, patchy bronchopneumonia with or without hemorrhagic pulmonary infarction. The disease process may evolve slowly or rapidly, and abscesses may appear at the site of an apparently resolving pneumonia. In many instances, the abscesses have "crescent signs" and have been referred to as aspergillomas. However, they contain sequestra of infarcted lung tissue and invasive *Aspergillus* infection and are thus distinct from the benign aspergillomas described earlier. In about 60 per cent of cases, the disease process remains confined to the lungs. In the others, there is hematogenous spread to the brain, liver, kidneys, gastrointestinal tract, thyroid, heart, skin, and other sites. Sometimes the pulmonary process itself is inapparent. In all infected loci, the disease is characterized by vascular invasion and tissue infarction and necrosis. Massive gastrointestinal bleeding and cerebral infarcts and abscesses may occur. Suppuration predominates; granulomatous response is rare. The differential diagnosis includes mucormycosis, nocardiosis, and necrotizing bacterial pneumonia.

Invasive aspergillosis is commonly fatal. For survival, an aggressive approach to diagnosis and treatment is required, and return of bone marrow function (reversal of neutropenia) is essential. Patients whose therapy begins more than three to four days after the initiation of the infection seldom survive. Invasive aspergillosis must be strongly considered in high-risk patients with persistent fever and pulmonary infiltrates despite broad-spectrum antibacterial therapy. Antemortem diagnosis is difficult and often requires invasive biopsy procedures. The diagnostic value of cultures of nasal swabs or sputum specimens is undefined. Whereas a negative culture does not rule out the diagnosis, a positive culture in high-risk patient supports the diagnosis of invasive aspergillosis. Blood, urine, and CSF cultures are rarely positive. Skin tests and precipitin tests are of no value in diagnosis. Experiences with detection of *Aspergillus* antigen in blood, urine, and lung washings provide hope that serologic methods may play a more useful role in diagnosis.

Because delays in therapy are associated with reduced survival, empiric therapy has been advocated in neutropenia patients who have unexplained fever despite seven days of broad-spectrum antibacterial therapy. The treatment of choice is amphotericin B. The dosage should be raised rapidly to 0.5 to 1.0 mg per kilogram of body weight per day, as tolerated. Treatment may be given on alternate days once improvement is under way. Total dosage should be no less than 2 grams. The efficacy of granulocyte transfusions, flucytosine, and rifampin is unproven. Miconazole and ketoconazole are not useful in the management of aspergillosis.

Laminar airflow facilities provide the only known means of preventing invasive aspergillosis. Prophylactic antifungal drugs lack proven efficacy. At construction sites, 8-copper quinolinate may control fungal growth on inanimate surfaces.

Other loci: Aspergillosis is the most common fungal infection of the paranasal sinuses in otherwise healthy patients. Roentgenograms show opacification, with or without bony erosion. Surgery is usually sufficient for cure. Immunosuppressed patients may exhibit facial cellulitis and palatal necrosis reminiscent of mucormycosis. Aspergillosis is a rare but devastating complication of burn wounds. Antibiotics and local debridement are seldom effective. Amputation is often required for cure. *Aspergillus* infection of prosthetic cardiac valves is a rare but devastating complication of cardiac surgery. Blood cultures are virtually never positive. Antifungal antibiotics are ineffective, and valve replacement is necessary if there is to be any possibility of cure. Invasive cutaneous aspergillosis has occurred at the site of taping of extremities to boards used to stabilize intravenous infusions. Invasive eye disease may follow local trauma, surgery, or hematogenous spread of infection from other sites.

Dupont B, Huber M, Kim SJ, et al.: Galactomannan antigenemia and antigenuria in aspergillosis: Studies in patients and experimentally infected rabbits. J Infect Dis 155:1, 1987. Talbot GH, Weiner MH, Gerson SL, et al.: Serodiagnosis of invasive aspergillosis in patients with hematologic malignancy: Validation of the *Aspergillus fumigatus* antigen radioimmunoassay. J Infect Dis 155:12, 1987. *These two papers provide the latest information concerning the potential diagnostic utility of tests for* Aspergillus *antigen. At this time, there is no commercial source for these tests.*

Gerson SL, Talbot GH, Hurwitz S, et al.: A discriminant scoreboard for diagnosis of invasive pulmonary aspergillosis in patients with acute leukemia. Am J Med 79:57, 1985. *Eleven parameters are identified that assist in determining the presence or absence of invasive aspergillosis. Among these are total febrile days without an apparent source, total febrile days while receiving antibiotics, rales, nasal or sinus abnormalities, pleuritic or back pain, hospital day upon which pulmonary changes were noted, distribution of the pulmonary infiltrate, and the appearance of nodules or cavities.*

Another study from this group has shown that pulmonary cavitation is a late phenomenon, reflecting bone marrow recovery and the return of circulating granulocytes (Albeda SM, Talbot GH, Gerson SL, et al.: Pulmonary cavitation and massive hemoptysis in invasive pulmonary aspergillosis: Influence of bone marrow recovery in patients with acute leukemia. Am Rev Respir Dis 131:115, 1985).

Levitz SM, Diamond RD: Changing patterns of aspergillosis infections. In Stollerman GH (ed.): Advances in Internal Medicine. Vol. 30. Chicago, Year Book Medical Publishers, 1984, pp 153–174. *An excellent review of aspergilloma, ABPA, chronic necrotizing pulmonary aspergillosis, and invasive aspergillosis. A good place to begin when reading about these diseases.*

Patterson R, Greenberger PA, Halwig JM, et al.: Allergic bronchopulmonary aspergillosis: Natural history and classification of early disease by serologic and roentgenographic studies. Arch Intern Med 146:916, 1986. *This paper makes the point that ABPA may be diagnosable before central saccular bronchiectasis develops. Current recommendations for exclusion or diagnosis of ABPA in patients with asthma are provided, as are guidelines for treatment of ABPA patients with and without central bronchiectasis.*

Weiland D, Ferguson FM, Peterson PK, et al.: Aspergillosis in 25 renal transplant patients: Epidemiology, clinical presentation, diagnosis, and management. Ann Surg 198:622, 1983. *During a nosocomial outbreak of aspergillosis at the University of Minnesota Hospitals, 25 renal transplant patients developed invasive aspergillosis manifested as cavitary lung disease, diffuse lung disease, or central nervous system disease. Diagnosis was aided by the presence of two positive sputum cultures, positive transbronchial lung biopsy, or covered brush biopsy culture. A more recent study also suggests that two or more positive cultures from respiratory secretions may assist in diagnosis, especially if heavy growth occurs and only one* Aspergillus *species is isolated (Treger TR, Visscher DW, Bartlett MS, et al.: Diagnosis of pulmonary infection caused by* Aspergillus: *Usefulness of respiratory cultures. J Infect Dis 152:572, 1985).*

377 ZYGOMYCOSIS (Mucormycosis)

DEFINITION. Zygomycosis includes diseases produced by fungi in the order Entomophthorales and order Mucorales (both in the class Zygomycetes). Mucormycosis is an acute suppurative opportunistic mycosis that produces predominantly rhinocerebral disease in patients with diabetic ketoacidosis; rhinocerebral, pulmonary, or disseminated disease in immunosuppressed patients; local or disseminated disease in patients with burns or open wounds; and gastrointestinal disease in patients with malnutrition or pre-existing intestinal disorders. Although correct mycologic usage dictates that diseases produced by Mucorales be referred to as "zygomycosis," the more clinically familiar term "mucormycosis" will be retained in this chapter.

ETIOLOGY. Mucorales known to produce mucormycosis include *Rhizopus, Mucor, Absidia, Mortierella, Cunninghamella,* and *Saksenaea* species. In the tissues, all these fungi appear as broad (6 to 50 μm), wavy, nonseptate (coenocytic), thick-walled hyphae with right-angle branching at haphazard intervals. They can be distinguished from one another only in vitro.

INCIDENCE AND PREVALENCE. Mucorales occur worldwide in soil and on decaying organic debris and are economically important as food spoilage agents, Airborne spores may contaminate bacteriologic media. Colonization and infection are uncommon in normal persons. Mucormycosis is increasing in incidence because of expanding numbers of susceptible, immunosuppressed patients.

EPIDEMIOLOGY. Mucormycosis is acquired sporadically, by inhalation, by ingestion, or by contamination of wounds with spores. It is not communicable. Infection is unrelated to age, sex, race, or climate. One outbreak of *Rhizopus* wound infections was related to the use of elasticized adhesive tape (Elastoplast, a nonsterile product), in direct contiguity with open wounds. The tape was found to be contaminated with spores of *R. oryzae* and *R. rhizopodoformis*. Mucormycosis of burn wounds may follow the use of topical mafenide, which suppresses other etiologic agents of burn wound infection. Mucormycotic abscesses of the central nervous system have been described in intravenous narcotic addicts.

PATHOGENESIS AND PATHOLOGY. Mechanisms of immunity are poorly understood. Acidosis appears more important than hyperglycemia in the susceptibility of experimental animals to rhinocerebral disease. This may relate to the acidic growth optima of the causative fungi and to the delay in polymorphonuclear leukocyte chemotaxis engendered by diabetic ketoacidosis. Diabetic serum also promotes spore germination while impairing attachment of alveolar macrophages to the fungi.

The pathologic process in humans is characterized by suppuration with little granulomatous response. Invasion of blood vessels is characteristic, resulting in thrombosis, infarction, and embolization. Disease spreads by both direct and hematogenous extension, but the fungi are almost never recovered from the blood. Agents of mucormycosis stain readily with hematoxylin-eosin (eosinophilic hyphae). The Gomori methenamine silver stain is also useful, but results with the periodic acid–Schiff and Gridley stains are poor. Hyphae are generally surrounded by an acute inflammatory cell infiltrate, but sections with marked hyphal invasion sometimes show little or no cellular response.

CLINICAL MANIFESTATIONS. *Rhinocerebral mucormycosis* accounts for about half of all cases of mucormycosis. More than 75 per cent of cases of rhinocerebral mucormycosis occur in patients with acidosis, especially diabetic ketoacidosis.

However, increasing numbers of cases are being seen in neutropenic patients with hematologic malignancies. It is one of the most rapidly fatal fungus diseases of humans, death occurring within two to ten days of onset in untreated patients. Infection is presumably initiated by the germination of spores deposited on the nasopharyngeal mucous membranes. Early clinical manifestations include nasal stuffiness, blood-tinged nasal discharge, facial swelling, and facial or orbital pain. Examination of the nasal mucosa reveals dirty red or black necrotic turbinates—an appearance commonly mistaken for dried blood and a major clue to the diagnosis. Facial cellulitis, palatal or nasal septal perforation, and signs of sinusitis may be present. Radiographs of the sinuses reveal nodular thickening of the mucous membranes, spotty destruction of the bony walls, and the absence of air-fluid levels. Spread of infection to the orbit results in orbital cellulitis, proptosis, and failing vision. Ultimately, there is a full-blown orbital apex syndrome reflecting the destruction of cranial nerves (III, IV, VI, and the ophthalmic branch of V) and blood vessels traversing the optic foramen and superior orbital fissure. Manifestations include complete ophthalmoplegia; a fixed dilated pupil; corneal and upper facial anesthesia; chemosis and conjunctival hemorrhage; and blindness resulting from obstruction of the central artery of the retina. The disease commonly spreads to involve the internal carotid artery and sometimes the cavernous sinus, cribriform plate, meninges, brain, and bones of the skull. Cerebral infarction caused by vascular compromise is common. The cerebrospinal fluid may disclose pleocytosis (≥50 per cent polymorphonuclear leukocytes) and elevated protein concentration, but hypoglycorrhachia is rare, and fungi are virtually never seen or cultured.

Pulmonary mucormycosis is nearly as common as rhinocerebral disease and typically occurs as a complication of hematologic malignancy and cytotoxic or immunosuppressive therapy. Infection presumably follows inhalation of fungal spores. There are no characteristic clinical or roentgenographic findings, but the pattern of infarction and cavitation may resemble that of invasive pulmonary aspergillosis. Sputum cultures are rarely positive, and successful diagnosis usually requires invasive techniques such as open lung biopsy.

Gastrointestinal mucormycosis may result from the ingestion of fungal spores in patients with pre-existing gastrointestinal abnormalities or malnutrition. It is seldom suspected prior to laparotomy or autopsy.

Cutaneous mucormycosis: Local cutaneous infection may follow deep burns, application of contaminated wound dressings, or injections at contaminated skin sites.

Disseminated mucormycosis may follow pulmonary or burn wound infection. Cerebral involvement is common, but no organ is spared.

DIAGNOSIS. Rhinocerebral mucormycosis may be confused with midline granuloma, rhinoscleroma, thyroid disease, syphilis, tuberculosis, or nasal and orbital tumors. Pulmonary mucormycosis may be confused with a variety of opportunistic pulmonary infections in the immunosuppressed host or with bland pulmonary embolization and infarction. The diagnosis of all forms of mucormycosis depends upon the *direct demonstration* of the characteristic hyphae in the tissues. Diagnosis is urgent and may be achieved by crushing fresh biopsy material between two slides, clearing with 10 to 20 per cent KOH, and examining for hyphae. Smears and swabs of sputum or wound exudate rarely disclose the fungus. Cultures are positive in fewer than 20 per cent of cases, and even positive cultures from superficial tissues might reflect the presence of fungal contaminants. No skin test is available, and there are no reliable serologic tests. Neither a negative tissue examination nor a negative culture rules out mucormycosis in the presence of a suggestive clinical picture, and collection of additional tissue specimens is indicated along with appropriate, aggressive therapy.

TREATMENT. Amphotericin B is the only drug with

proven efficacy, and results of therapy do not necessarily correlate with results of tests of susceptibility to the drug in vitro. Successful therapy requires early diagnosis, control of the underlying disease process, aggressive debridement, and aggressive use of amphotericin B. Control of burn infection may necessitate amputation. The dose of amphotericin B should be rapidly increased to 0.5 to 1.0 mg per kilogram per day, in accordance with the patient's ability to tolerate the drug. Consideration should be given to local administration of drug into infected paranasal sinuses. With clinical improvement, amphotericin B can be given in an alternate-day regimen. A total dose of 2 to 4 grams is commonly suggested.

PROGNOSIS. The prognosis of mucormycosis is directly related to the rapidity of diagnosis and the aggressiveness of therapy. Prior to the advent of amphotericin B, rhinocerebral disease was fatal in 80 to 90 per cent of instances. Current data indicate that 75 per cent of patients with no systemic disease, 60 per cent of diabetics, and 20 per cent of patients with other underlying disorders survive rhinocerebral disease. Prognosis is poor in patients with hemiplegia, facial necrosis, or nasal deformity. Only about 15 patients have been reported to have recovered from pulmonary infection.

Blitzer A, Lawson W, Meyers BR et al.: Patient survival factors in paranasal sinus mucormycosis. Laryngoscope 90:635, 1980. *An analysis of 179 cases of rhinocerebral infection with emphasis on significant prognostic factors.*

Morduchowicz G, Schmueli D, Shapira Z, et al.: Rhinocerebral mucormycosis in renal transplant recipients: Report of three cases and review of the literature. Rev Infect Dis 8:441, 1986. *A restricted review of rhinocerebral mucormycosis occurring in predominantly nondiabetic renal transplant recipients. Of 14 patients discussed, 6 had symptoms during or immediately following a rejection episode.*

Parfrey NA: Improved diagnosis and prognosis of mucormycosis: A clinicopathologic study of 33 cases. Medicine 65:113, 1986. *This review covers all cases of mucormycosis encountered at Johns Hopkins Hospital since 1941. There has been a dramatic improvement in clinical outcome, with a major shift from postmortem to premortem diagnosis. Premortem diagnosis gives the opportunity for metabolic stabilization, surgical excision, and amphotericin B therapy appropriate to this disease.*

378 MYCETOMA (Maduromycosis)

DEFINITION. A mycetoma is a localized lesion, usually of an exposed area such as the unshod foot (Madura foot), characterized by swelling and deep sinuses that discharge pus and grains (microbial colonies embedded in a host-derived proteinaceous matrix).

ETIOLOGY. One half of all mycetomas are produced by fungi (eumycetoma); the other one half by actinomycetes (actinomycetoma). The etiologic agents originate in plant debris and soil and are introduced by trauma. Etiologic agents of eumycetoma include (1) white to yellow grains—*Pseudallescheria boydii* and *Acremonium (Cephalosporium)*, *Trichophyton*, and *Microsporum* species; (2) yellow to brown grains—*Neotestudina (Zophia) rosatii*, and (3) black grains—*Madurella mycetomatis* and *grisea (Pyrenochaeta romeroi)*, *Exophiala jeanselmei*, and *Leptosphaeria senegalensis* and *thompkinsii*. Etiologic agents of actinomycetoma include (1) white to yellow grains—*Nocardia asteroides*, *brasiliensis*, and *cavae* (tiny grains) and *Actinomadura madurae* (extremely large grains); (2) yellow to brown grains—*Streptomyces somaliensis*; (3) red grains—*Actinomadura pelletierii*, and (4) black grains—*Streptomyces paraguayensis*.

EPIDEMIOLOGY. Mycetomas are encountered worldwide, but especially in semitropical zones such as Sudan and Mexico. *P. boydii* is the most common cause of mycetoma in Europe and the United States, *N. brasiliensis* in Mexico.

The mycetomas occur most frequently in adult males from rural areas who work out of doors, experience repeated trauma, and care poorly for local wounds. The disease is not contagious, occurs in sporadic fashion, and is unrelated to animal contact. Mycetomas usually involve the feet or legs but may involve the back, neck, or shoulders (in bearers of burdens) or the head (where *Trichophyton* and *Microsporum* eumycetomas are especially likely to occur).

PATHOGENESIS AND PATHOLOGY. The host-parasite interactions that foster the development of grains instead of free filaments by the weakly pathogenic organisms responsible for mycetomas are unknown.

Typical mycetomas consist of large granulomatous areas with a purulent center surrounded by a thick, fibrous capsule. Fistulous tracts that contain grains pass deep into underlying tissues, usually along fascial planes, and also drain at the skin surface. Focal areas of subcutaneous necrosis and intense fibrosis result in typical tumefaction. Tracts open and close over long periods of time. In actinomycetomas, the suppurative response tends to persist indefinitely, and there is a tendency to invade bones and muscles. Eumycetomas take on the character of foreign body granulomas.

CLINICAL MANIFESTATIONS. Mycetomas usually begin as a painless draining nodule at a site of trauma. Multiple secondary nodules develop over years and drain through sinus tracts. Lesions extend deeply into subcutaneous tissues, under the cover of thick, fibrosclerous tissue. A common complaint is a sensation of deep itching. Disease may spread to bone (including medullary canal and epiphyses), joints, muscles, tendons, and nerves. When extensive bony remodeling occurs, the process becomes painful. Blood and lymphatic vessels are damaged or interrupted, but regional lymphadenopathy is rare. In the typical "Madura foot," the destruction of tarsal bones, nonimpairment of the tendons, and widespread plantar fibrosis give the foot a characteristic shortened and raised appearance. The sole is typically convex. The general health of the patient remains little affected. Rapid local or lymphohematogenous spread may occur when mycetomas involve the buttocks, chest, or trunk.

DIAGNOSIS. Mycetomas can be diagnosed by the presence of characteristic sinuses and grains. Collection of grains may be facilitated by gentle abrasion of lesions or overnight occlusion with saline-saturated gauze. Grains should be crushed, and wet mounts prepared in 10 to 20 per cent KOH. Examination of grains permits the broad differentiation of actinomycetoma (fine filaments), eumycetoma (broad hyphae), and botryomycosis (cocci or rods without filaments). Culture is necessary for etiologic diagnosis. Serologic tests are not routinely available.

TREATMENT. Treatment for actinomycetomas depends upon identification of the infecting agent and determination of its in vitro antibiotic susceptibility. Therapeutic responses have followed high-dose penicillin regimens (e.g., 10 million units per day), with or without probenecid, 1 gram per day; sulfadiazine, 3 to 10 grams per day; or minocycline, 150 mg twice daily. *Nocardia brasiliensis* infections are especially likely to respond. Other useful drugs include diaminodiphenylsulfone (dapsone), 50 to 200 mg daily by mouth; co-trimoxazole (160 mg trimethoprim plus 800 mg sulfamethoxazole daily, by mouth); or streptomycin (3 grams intramuscularly per day for three weeks, then 2 grams daily for three weeks, then 1 gram daily). Prolonged streptomycin regimens carry the danger of vestibulotoxicity. Limb perfusion therapy and topical antimicrobial agents have also been used, together with judicious resectional surgery. Eumycetoma is considerably more difficult to treat. Amphotericin B given intravenously or locally has produced equivocal results. *P. boydii* may respond to miconazole, ketoconazole, or even thiabendazole. Unfortunately, eumycetoma often requires amputation.

PROGNOSIS. The mycetomas are often brought to medical attention late in the course of illness. Reasons include the absence of pain, the remote living conditions of patients, and the fear of amputation. In general, the prognosis for life is good, but the disease may be incapacitating.

Magana M: Mycetoma. Int J Dermatol 23:221, 1984. *A complete review of clinical aspects of mycetoma, including therapy.*

Mariat F, Destombes P, Segretain G: The mycetomas: Clinical features, pathology, etiology and epidemiology. In Contributions to Microbiology, Vol. 4, Host-Parasite Relationships in Systemic Mycoses; Part II, Specific Diseases and Therapy. Basel, Karger, 1977, pp 1-39. *A masterful, easily readable, and up-to-date review article with an emphasis on pathophysiology.*

Smego RA Jr, Gallis HA: The clinical spectrum of *Nocardia brasiliensis* infection in the United States. Rev Infect Dis 6:164, 1984. *Nocardia brasiliensis is a common cause of mycetomas throughout the world. It can also produce a variety of other skin, soft tissue, and systemic manifestations. This is an important review of the pathogenesis, diagnosis, and therapy of the gamut of N. brasiliensis infections.*

Tight RR, Bartlett MS: Actinomycetoma in the United States. Rev Infect Dis 3:1139, 1981. *A case report and review of 28 cases of actinomycetoma in the United States that emphasizes the importance of etiologic diagnosis, antibiotic susceptibility testing in vitro, identification of osteomyelitis, and protracted therapy in disease management.*

379 INFECTIONS DUE TO DEMATIACEOUS FUNGI

"Dematiaceous" is the term applied to fungi that produce intrinsic melanin-like pigmentation. Such fungi are widely distributed environmental saprobes. They produce two principal syndromes: chromoblastomycosis and phaeohyphomycosis.

CHROMOBLASTOMYCOSIS

DEFINITION. Chromoblastomycosis (chromomycosis; verrucous dermatitis) is a noncontagious chronic granulomatous infection, usually of exposed areas such as the extremities, characterized by warty plaques, nodules, and cauliflower-like excrescences.

ETIOLOGY. Chromoblastomycosis is produced by several brown-pigmented saprobic soil fungi that are macroscopically identical, but distinguishable in vitro. They include principally members of the genera *Acrotheca, Cladosporium, Fonsecaea, Phialophora,* and *Rhinocladiella. Fonsecaea pedrosoi* is the most common etiologic agent.

INCIDENCE AND PREVALENCE. Chromoblastomycosis occurs worldwide but is most common in the tropics and subtropics. Numerous cases have been documented in Louisiana and Texas.

EPIDEMIOLOGY. The etiologic agents reside in soil, decaying wood, or rotting vegetation. They are usually introduced by trauma, especially in barefoot persons. Chromoblastomycosis is most common in adult males who work out of doors, especially those with suboptimal nutritional or hygienic status.

PATHOGENESIS AND PATHOLOGY. There is pseudoepitheliomatous hyperplasia of the surface epithelium, and microabscesses with epithelioid and giant cell granulomas in the underlying dermis. Eventually, a chronic fibrosing inflammatory reaction supervenes. The characteristic tissue fungi develop as large, thick-walled, chestnut-brown, rounded cells (4 to 12 μm in diameter), the so-called "sclerotic bodies" ("copper pennies"; "sclerotia"). Sclerotic bodies represent a form intermediate between yeasts and hyphae. They can be produced in vitro under acidic conditions (pH approximately 2.5). Sclerotic bodies are muriform, i.e., they multiply by horizontal and vertical septation, and not by budding. They may remain attached to one another in clusters of two or more.

CLINICAL MANIFESTATIONS. Chromoblastomycosis starts as a small, pink, scaly papule and slowly enlarges to a warty tumor that may spread to form a plaque. Mucous membranes are not involved. Plaques may be verrucous with central scarring, extensively scarred with a serpiginous border, scaly, or indurated with fistulas. Some patients develop a papillomatous tumor reminiscent of a cauliflower. Ulceration may follow trauma or secondary infection, and local spread may occur by direct or lymphatic extension, or by autoinoculation through scratching. Regional lymphadenopathy is not common. It may take 10 to 15 years for a whole limb to be involved. Lymphedema and elephantiasis may result. Rarely the disease may be complicated by an epithelioid carcinoma. In some patients, widespread hematogenous dissemination occurs. Lesions have been documented in the pancreas, liver, bowel, lymph nodes, brain, and meninges. The organs may contain sclerotic bodies and/or hyphae.

DIAGNOSIS. Early lesions may be confused with malignancy, mycetoma, other mycoses, cutaneous tuberculosis, leishmaniasis, yaws, and "mossy foot" (lymphostatis verrucosis). Laboratory diagnosis is relatively easy. Although superficial crusts digested in 10 to 20 per cent KOH may contain long, brown, branching hyphae, the diagnostic sclerotic bodies are more likely to be found intracellularly or extracellularly in pus, in granulation tissue obtained by curettage, or in biopsy specimens. The brown pigmentation of the fungi serves to identify them; special stains are seldom needed. Cultures may grow slowly and should be kept at least eight weeks. Serologic or skin tests are not available.

TREATMENT. Treatment is successful in inverse relation to the duration and extent of infection. Except when the lesions are small and early, surgery is nearly always followed by recurrence. Systemic amphotericin B may not produce fungicidal concentrations at the lesions. Intralesional amphotericin B has been tried with variable success but is painful. Flucytosine* (150 mg per kilogram of body weight per day by mouth) cured 16 to 23 patients in a recent series. The other seven developed flucytosine-resistant fungi. Amphotericin B given simultaneously with flucytosine might retard emergence of flucytosine-resistant fungi. Thiabendazole (2 grams per day, orally), an anthelmintic, has given promising results but is not approved for this use in the United States. Unpublished results suggest that ketoconazole, an orally administered imidazole, may be efficacious.

Response to therapy may be monitored by serial biopsies and cultures.

PROGNOSIS. Chromoblastomycosis usually remains localized and will not debilitate the patient if left untreated. Secondary infection resulting in lymphostasis and elephantiasis is disabling. There is a slight risk of hematogenous dissemination, probably increased by immunosuppression.

PHAEOHYPHOMYCOSIS

DEFINITION. Phaeohyphomycosis is a general term referring to an infection with dematiaceous fungi, but one differing from chromoblastomycosis in three major respects: (1) clinical appearance; (2) absence of sclerotic bodies; and (3) scores of potential etiologic agents. At least six clinical forms of phaeohyphomycosis can be recognized.

Superficial Phaeohyphomycosis

These infections are confined to the stratum corneum, with little or no tissue response. Fungi may grow around the hair shaft, but the hair is not damaged. Examples include black piedra (*Piedraia hortae*) and tinea nigra (*Exophiala werneckii, Stenella araguata*).

Cutaneous and Corneal Phaeohyphomycosis

These infections generally involve nonliving layers of keratinized tissues; extensive tissue destruction may occur. Examples include dermatomycosis (*Alternaria, Scytalidium, Taeniolella* species); mycotic keratitis (*Bipolaris, Botryodiplodia, Curvularia, Exophiala, Exserohilum, Rhizoctonia, Tetraploa* spe-

---

*Investigational drug for this purpose.

cies); and onychomycosis (*Botryodiplodia, Phylosticta, Scytalidium* species).

Subcutaneous Phaeohyphomycosis

Subcutaneous infections generally result from the traumatic implantation of fungi, resulting in a cystlike lesion with well-developed fibrous walls. There may be central abscess formation, but spontaneous drainage is uncommon. Histologic examination sometimes discloses an initiating splinter. Etiologic agents include *Alternaria, Bipolaris, Cladosporium, Exophiala, Exserohilum, Phialophora, Phoma, Scytalidium, Wangiella,* or *Xylohypha* species. The treatment of choice is simple excision.

Sinusitis

Alternaria, Bipolaris, Cladosporium, Curvularia Exserohilum, or *Xylohypha* species are capable, like nondematiaceous fungi (*Aspergillus, Pseudallescheria,* Zygomycetes), of producing localized infection of the paranasal sinuses. Most patients respond to surgical debridement, although amphotericin B may also be required in the presence of bony invasion or immunosuppression.

Peritonitis

Chronic ambulatory peritoneal dialysis (CAPD) is often complicated by peritonitis; fungi may be responsible for up to 8 per cent of episodes. In addition to *Candida* species, infections have also been attributable to dematiaceous fungi such as *Bipolaris, Exophiala, Exserohilum,* and *Fusarium* species. Cure usually requires removal of the dialysis catheter and systemic amphotericin B therapy.

Systemic Phaeohyphomycosis

These infections are often initiated in the lungs, with subsequent dissemination to other organs. Blood vessel invasion and tissue infarction are characteristic. Etiologic agents include *Bipolaris, Cladosporium, Curvularia, Exophiala, Exserohilum, Mycocentrospora, Wangiella,* and *Xylohypha* species.

"Cerebral cladosporiosis" is the term most often used for cerebral mycoses caused by dematiaceous fungi. The most important form, caused by *Xylohypha bantiana* (formerly *Cladosporium bantianum* or *Cladosporium trichoides*) is characterized by the formation of abscesses containing pus, giant cells, and pigmented hyphae. Meningitis is present in about one half of the cases, sometimes as an isolated occurrence. The cerebrospinal fluid usually shows a polymorphonuclear leukocyte response; hypoglycorrhachia has not been reported. The site of primary infection may be the lung, but there is seldom evidence of pulmonary involvement. Cerebral cladosporiosis is rarely diagnosed early enough to permit the evaluation of the therapeutic regimens. Optimal management would seem to require surgical debridement and the use of flucytosine* or an imidazole, with or without amphotericin B.

---

*Investigational drug for this purpose.

Adam RD, Paquin ML, Petersen EA, et al.: Phaeohyphomycosis caused by the fungal genera *Bipolaris* and *Exserohilum.* Medicine 65:203, 1986. *These fungi have been previously misclassified as* Helminthosporium *or* Drechslera *species, but the latter fungi appear not to produce human disease. This paper serves as an excellent update to the McGinnis paper (see below). Another review of merit, albeit using* Drechslera *terminology, is Rolston KVI, Hopfer RL, Larson DL: Infections caused by* Drechslera *species: Case report and review of the literature. Rev Infec Dis 7:525, 1985.*

Bennett JE, Bonner H, Jennings AE, et al.: Chronic meningitis caused by *Cladosporium trichoides.* Am J Clin Pathol 59:398, 1973. *Comprehensive discussion of cerebral infection with dematiaceous fungi.*

Eisenberg ES, Leviton I, Soeiro R: Fungal peritonitis in patients receiving peritoneal dialysis: Experience with 11 patients and review of the literature. Rev Infect Dis 8:309, 1986. *Ten per cent of cases of fungal peritonitis in patients receiving CAPD are attributable to dematiaceous fungi. This paper summarizes general principles of diagnosis and management.*

McGinnis MR: Chromoblastomycosis and phaeohyphomycosis: New concepts, diagnosis and mycology. J Am Acad Dermatol 8:1, 1983. *Essential reading for the understanding of these mycoses. Contains a clear-cut exposition of clinical and mycologic criteria for these diagnoses.*

PART XIX

DISEASES CAUSED BY PROTOZOA AND METAZOA

380 INTRODUCTION TO PROTOZOAN AND HELMINTHIC DISEASES

Adel A. F. Mahmoud

Human infections with parasitic protozoa and helminths account for a major proportion of the diseases caused by infectious agents. The magnitude of these infections is staggering; malaria infects 600 million, and ascariasis and trichuriasis 1 billion each, and 600 million are estimated to be infected with either schistosomiasis or filariasis. Other infectious protozoa and helminths such as *Toxoplasma gondii, Entamoeba histolytica, Giardia lamblia, Pneumocystis carinii*, and *Strongyloides stercoralis* occur worldwide. In spite of some worldwide efforts to control the spread and consequences of these infections, the associated morbidity and mortality have not been appreciably reduced. Furthermore, in the developed countries infection with protozoa and helminths is being seen with increasing frequency in immigrants and is also among the more important causes of disease in the growing number of patients with depressed immune responses.

The biology of the interaction between protozoa and helminths and their host is less well understood than that of other infectious agents. Most of these infections are prevalent in the developing countries in which limited attention has been paid to studies on pathogenesis, chemotherapy, or control. An additional dimension of the problem of protozoan and helminthic infections concerns the lack of effective chemotherapeutic agents in some instances and the excessive toxicity of these agents or the development of resistance to them in other instances.

BIOLOGY OF PARASITIC PROTOZOA AND HELMINTHS

This group of infectious agents belongs to the animal kingdom, unlike bacteria, viruses, or fungi. Such distinction led to restricting the term "parasite" to include only protozoa and helminths and may have hampered our clinical as well as basic understanding of the mechanisms by which they cause disease and how to enhance host resistance effectively. The host-parasite relationship in protozoan and helminthic infections is complex because of the distinctive biologic features of the organisms. Although protozoa are unicellular pathogens and are mainly microscopic in size, they are far larger than viruses and bacteria. A major biologic feature of protozoa is their ability to multiply within mammalian hosts as do viruses, bacteria, and fungi. Protozoan infection, therefore, can be initiated by a relatively small inoculum of organisms, which then multiply within the host and reach the numbers that cause disease.

In contrast, helminths are multicellular organisms with well developed organ system structures. They vary in size from 1 cm to approximately 10 meters. Unlike other infectious agents, helminths do not multiply within mammalian hosts. Reexposure is, therefore, necessary to increase the number of helminths in a host. This distinguishing feature has important clinical significance, as disease in most helminthiasis is closely related to intensity of infection. For example, anemia results from hookworm infection only if the individual is harboring a significant worm load or there are other reasons for nutritional deficiencies. In rare circumstances such as strongyloidiasis in the immunosuppressed, the worm can increase its population through an autoinfection cycle. This leads to life-threatening infection that necessitates aggressive medical attention.

Eosinophilia, when present, is a useful clinical manifestation of worm infections that migrate in host tissues. Worms that reside exclusively in body cavities such as adult cestodes in the lumen of small intestines are not associated with eosinophilia. Increased eosinophil counts may be observed in peripheral blood or affected tissues of infected individuals. Specific chemotherapy is usually followed by an increase of cell count before it subsides to normal levels. Eosinophilia in helminthic infections results from a combination of specific worm components that are chemotactic or that induce other host cells to release chemotactic, eosinophilopoietic, or activating factors. The cells obtained from individuals with helminthiases and eosinophilia exhibit more Fc and complement receptors on their surface, are metabolically activated, and may be more efficient than those from uninfected subjects in killing invading stages of worms. Because of the large size of most invading stages of worms, killing of these targets by eosinophils occurs extracellularly and is mediated by a combination of oxidative and nonoxidative mechanisms.

Parasitic protozoa and helminths have developed elaborate mechanisms for evasion of host protective responses. One of the best studied is antigenic variation noted in African trypanosomiasis. Parasitemia in infected individuals declines with the development of a protective antibody response but is followed by the emergence of a new parasite variable antigen and an increase in their numbers. These organisms are capable of expressing at least 100 different variable antigens allowing a long chronic course of infection. The phenomenon of antigenic variation in trypanosomiasis is expressed through a surface glycoprotein of a molecular weight 65,000. The trypanosomes contain individual genes for all the different variable glycoproteins but only one is expressed at a time. The multiplicity of trypanosome variable glycoprotein genes and mechanisms for introducing mutations into them illustrate the degree of complexity and sophistication of these human pathogens.

The constantly changing nature of infectious disease is best illustrated in some parasitic protozoan and helminthic infections. For example, relatively unsuspected pathogens such as *Giardia lamblia* are now being recognized as the major identifiable cause of water-borne diarrhea in North America and several parts of the world. New human pathogens such as *Isospora* and *Cryptosporidium* species have been appreciated only recently as causes of diarrheal illness, particularly in the immunosuppressed. This group of patients, including those with acquired immune deficiency syndrome (AIDS), is particularly susceptible to several opportunistic protozoan organisms such as *Pneumocystis carinii*, *Toxoplasma gondii*, and the coccidia. These new developments add to the difficulties experienced in the treatment and control of parasitic protozoa and helminths. For several, effective and safe chemotherapeutic agents are lacking (e.g., onchocerciasis and South American trypanosomiasis). In some circumstances the pathogen (e.g., *Plasmodium falciparum*) is rapidly developing resistance to the available drug; insecticide resistance is also complicating vector control attempts. On the other hand, malaria vaccine may be a reality soon, and new chemotherapeutic agents for onchocerciasis are to be introduced in the near future.

APPROACH TO THE PATIENT WITH PROTOZOAN OR HELMINTHIC INFECTION

Since most of the clinical manifestations of protozoan and helminthic diseases are not specific or pathognomonic, a high degree of suspicion is essential. The simple question "Where have you been?" and knowledge of the general geographic distribution of parasitic protozoa and helminths will often save exhaustive and costly diagnostic workups and may spare human lives. Furthermore, inquiry of the immune status of individual patients, other drug therapies, or diseases may be helpful in establishing the diagnosis of an opportunistic protozoan or helminth infection.

The next phase in attempting to reach correct diagnosis involves interpretation of the presenting symptoms and signs. Definitive diagnosis in most cases requires isolation and identification of the specific pathogen. Since the number of cases seen by any single laboratory in North America is limited, certain expertise is required for correct identification that may not be available to many practicing physicians. Consultations with the Centers for Disease Control are therefore helpful.

Schmidt GD, Roberts LS (eds.): Foundations of Parasitology. 2nd ed. St. Louis, C. V. Mosby Company, 1981. *A concise text for basic information on morphology and biology of protozoa and helminths.*

Warren KS, Mahmoud AAF, (eds.): Tropical and Geographical Medicine. New York, McGraw-Hill Book Company, 1984. *Detailed description of the biology and molecular understanding of protozoa and helminths and the diseases they cause in individuals and in populations.*

Warren KS, Mahmoud AAF (eds.): Geographic Medicine for the Practitioner. 2nd ed. New York, Springer-Verlag, 1985. *A concise description of the major imported diseases. Step-by-step diagnostic algorithms are included.*

SECTION ONE / PROTOZOAN DISEASES

381 MALARIA
Louis H. Miller

DEFINITION. Malaria remains today one of the major health problems in the tropics. It is caused by four species of *Plasmodium*: *P. falciparum*, *P. vivax*, *P. ovale*, and *P. malariae*. Each species has its own morphology and produces disease with its own clinical characteristics (Table 381–1). The asexual erythrocytic parasite is the stage in the life cycle that causes disease, including the characteristic malarial paroxysm (fever, chills, and sweats). *P. falciparum* malaria causes the most morbidity and mortality and presents the therapeutic problem of chloroquine resistance. Since effective therapy is available for *P. falciparum* malaria, high mortality usually results from failure of the physician to include malaria in the differential diagnosis of a febrile patient who has traveled in the tropics or received a blood transfusion.

ETIOLOGY. Malaria parasites undergo a developmental cycle in the female anopheline mosquito, the vector, and in humans. Mosquitoes, during a blood meal, inoculate *sporozoites* that rapidly enter liver parenchymal cells. Sporozoites may develop immediately in liver cells into thousands of individual merozoites (all types of malaria) or remain dormant as uninucleate hypnozoites for months to years before undergoing proliferation (the relapsing malarias, caused by *P. vivax* and *P. ovale*). Different strains of *P. vivax* produce their own characteristic timing patterns of relapse in patients who contract the disease. Some strains (e.g., from New

TABLE 381–1. CLINICAL AND DIAGNOSTIC DIFFERENCES AMONG THE FOUR SPECIES OF MALARIA

	P. falciparum	*P. vivax*	*P. ovale*	*P. malariae*
Clinical features	High parasitemia, severe anemia, renal failure, cerebral malaria, pulmonary edema, death	Splenic rupture, anemia		RBC infection persists for years; nephritis
Chloroquine resistance	Yes	No	No	No
Asexual cycle	48 hours	48 hours	48 hours	72 hours
Relapse	No	Yes	Yes	No
Characteristic on thin blood film	Rings predominate; multiply infected RBCs, rings with thread-like cytoplasm, double nuclei, crescent shaped gametocytes	Enlarged RBCs with Schüffner's dots; trophozoite cytoplasm amoeboid; 12 to 24 merozoites in mature schizont	Oval RBCs with fringed edges; Schüffner's dots; trophozoite cytoplasm compact; 6 to 16 merozoites in mature schizont	Trophozoite cytoplasm compact (band forms); 6 to 12 merozoites in mature schizont; RBCs unchanged

Guinea) cause relapse monthly after the primary attack. Others cause relapse six months or longer after the primary attack or may not produce a primary attack.

Merozoites rupture from liver cells and pour into the bloodstream to invade erythrocytes. Development of the intraerythrocytic parasite follows one of two pathways: asexual proliferation or differentiation into sexual parasites, the gametocytes, which await ingestion by the mosquito. In the mosquito they ultimately develop into infectious *sporozoites*. Asexual erythrocytic parasites develop from young ring forms through *trophozoites* to the dividing form, the *schizont*. Each mature schizont contains 6 to 24 merozoites, the number varying with the particular species. Merozoites, on rupture of infected erythrocytes, are released to invade other erythrocytes and thus continue the cycle.

Merozoites attach to erythrocytes by specific receptors. Erythrocytic determinants required for *P. vivax* and *P. falciparum* invasion are the Duffy blood group system and glycophorin, respectively. Blacks who are Duffy-blood-group–negative (*FyFy*) are completely refractory to erythrocytic infection by *P. vivax*. En(a-) erythrocytes that completely lack glycophorin A have reduced susceptibility to invasion by *P. falciparum*.

The agents producing the three types of malaria, *P. vivax*, *P. ovale*, and *P. falciparum*, invade reticulocytes preferentially. *P. falciparum*, however, can infect erythrocytes of all ages and produces high-level parasitemias with resultant morbidity and mortality. *P. malariae* infects mature erythrocytes.

Each type of malaria induces characteristic morphologic changes on the infected erythrocyte membrane: knob protrusions by asexual parasites of *P. falciparum*; knobs by sexual and asexual parasites of *P. malariae*; and *Schüffner's dots*, pink stippling of the infected erythrocyte, by sexual and asexual parasites of *P. vivax* and *P. ovale*. Knob protrusions on the membranes of *P. falciparum*-infected erythrocytes mediate attachment to venular endothelium (sequestration), which explains the predominance of young parasites, ring forms, in the peripheral blood.

The asexual erythrocytic parasitic has a haploid genome. Cloned populations of asexual parasites can change their expression of antigens on the erythrocyte surface (antigenic variation) to evade the host immune response.

EPIDEMIOLOGY. Most malaria patients seen in Europe and in the United States are infected in Africa, Asia, and Latin America (imported cases). Mosquito vectors capable of transmitting malaria still exist in countries where malaria has been eradicated (e.g., *Anopheles freeborni* in the western United States). In these areas, rare episodes of transmission have occurred following infection of local mosquitoes by individuals infected in the tropics (introduced cases). Congenital infections occur; the clinical symptoms are not evident until weeks to months after delivery. Other causes of infection in nonendemic areas include blood transfusion and communal use of syringes by drug addicts. The single most important factor in preventing transfusion malaria is the exclusion of donors who have lived or traveled in endemic areas until their risk of infection is negligible, because chronic infections are often asymptomatic. Most *P. falciparum*-infected individuals undergo self-cure in three years; a rare case may persist for four years. Diseases caused by *P. vivax* and *P. ovale* may last for three to five years. That from *P. malariae* may persist as an asymptomatic, erythrocytic infection for decades. Since infection by *P. falciparum* is most serious, blood donation should be excluded for three years after the traveler's return from the tropics.

INNATE RESISTANCE. Genetically determined host factors influence susceptibility to malaria. Certain polymorphisms have been associated with the distribution of *P. falciparum* in the world (e.g., hemoglobin S, thalassemia, and glucose-6-phosphate dehydrogenase [G6PD] deficiency). The evidence for a selective advantage of polymorphisms in malarious areas is most convincing for sickle trait (HB SA). Children who die of malaria in West Africa rarely have sickle trait, although the frequency of this phenotype is high in this region. In areas where the heterozygote has an advantage over either homozygote, a balanced polymorphism results.

Black Africans who have the Duffy-blood-group–negative genotype (*FyFy*) are resistant to infection by *P. vivax*. Elliptocytosis, a skeletal abnormality of erythrocytes, occurs throughout lowland tropical areas of Southeast Asia and Melanesia that are endemic for malaria; the erythrocytes are partially resistant to invasion by all types of malaria.

IMMUNITY. Immunity to malaria is primarily directed against the asexual erythrocytic parasite and develops only after prolonged or repeated infection. Immunity usually does not prevent reinfection but reduces the severity of the disease or leads to an asymptomatic infection. The asymptomatic person, however, can infect mosquitoes and can transmit the infection directly to others through blood transfusion. Immunity wanes in a few years when the person is unexposed to reinfection. Disease may recur in an immune person immediately after surgery or during pregnancy.

Immunity is species-specific (e.g., immunity to *P. falciparum* does not protect against *P. vivax*). Further, the immunity against *P. falciparum* is strain-specific, indicating variant antigens among strains. Passive transfer of antibody from hyperimmune adult West Africans to East or West African children reduced parasitemia. In addition to providing antibody, immunity may function through several other nonantibody mechanisms dependent on T cells, macrophages, and the spleen. After splenectomy even previously immune humans die of severe *P. falciparum* infections.

PATHOGENESIS AND PATHOLOGY. The asexual erythrocytic cycle causes the symptoms and pathology. Fever and the associated symptoms of headache, nausea, and muscular pain occur at the time that schizont-infected erythrocytes rupture and new ring forms appear. Although pyrogens and other toxins may be released from ruptured schizonts to cause fever and symptoms of malaria, none has been identified to date.

Anemia is caused by hemolysis of infected erythrocytes and dyserythropoiesis. Coombs-positive hemolytic anemia occurs rarely and usually results from quinine sensitivity. Severe acute hemolytic anemia results in patients who are heavily infected with *P. falciparum*. African children with chronic low-grade *P. falciparum* parasitemia have severe anemia associated with dyserythropoiesis and a low reticulocyte count. Primaquine administered to patients with G6PD deficiency may cause severe hemolysis. Thrombocytopenia results from binding of malaria-specific IgG to malaria antigen adsorbed on platelets.

Renal failure occurs in *P. falciparum* malaria. Mechanisms for renal failure include severe hemolytic anemia, hemoglobinuria, hypovolemia, and possibly vasoconstriction. *Blackwater fever* is severe hemolytic anemia and hemoglobinuria in a falciparum malaria patient; it may cause renal failure. Prior to the introduction of chloroquine in the 1940's, quinine was used for prevention and treatment of malaria. Because of this, Coombs-positive hemolytic anemia following quinine administration was the most common cause of blackwater fever. Today, blackwater fever results from high-level parasitemia.

P. falciparum malaria causes diffuse cerebral disease (cerebral malaria). The cerebral capillaries and venules are plugged by infected erythrocytes that obstruct because of their decreased deformability and their adherence to endothelium by knob protrusions. Ring hemorrhages develop around obstructed capillaries. Cerebral edema is unusual except in severe, advanced cerebral malaria.

Unusual complications of severe falciparum malaria include centrilobular necrosis of the liver and noncardiac pulmonary edema. The lungs have microvascular congestion, interstitial edema, and hyaline membrane formation as evidence of increased capillary permeability.

P. malariae produces chronic progressive nephritis. Immune complexes are deposited in the glomerular capillary wall. Antibody in the complexes is specific for *P. malariae*. The majority of kidneys with immune complexes contain the C3 component of complement; 25 per cent have *P. malariae* antigen.

CLINICAL MANIFESTATIONS. No sign or symptom is pathognomonic of malaria. *Fever* need not be accompanied by the characteristic *malarial paroxysm*. The paroxysm begins with a chilly feeling, bed-shaking chills, and a rise in temperature. The skin appears pale, with cyanosis of the lips and nail beds. The patient experiences *headache* and *nausea* and may vomit. Within one to two hours the temperature rises toward 39 to 40.5°C, the patient feels hot, and the skin is warm and dry. As the temperature falls, *sweating* begins and drenches clothing. The patient feels fatigued and weak and often sleeps. This description is most typical of benign malarias; fever may persist and symptoms are prolonged in *malignant falciparum malaria*. Fever is usually not periodic in malignant falciparum malaria, and during the initial attack of *P. vivax* malaria, when the infection is asynchronous. Periodicity of fever occurs only in synchronized infections when the majority of infected erythrocytes containing mature schizonts rupture at the same time. This occurs at intervals determined by the length of the asexual erythrocytic cycle. The cycle in *P. vivax* and *P. ovale* malaria takes 48 hours, and thus the fever occurs every other day. *P. malariae* matures in 72 hours and causes fever every third day.

The pulse rate is elevated but not commensurate with the fever. A nonproductive cough may occur during fever. Orthostatic hypotension is common in falciparum malaria, and weakness may persist for weeks. Splenomegaly occurs frequently and hepatomegaly less frequently. Tenderness on palpation of liver and spleen may be due to sudden stretching of their capsules; splenic rupture, a potentially fatal complication, should be considered. The absence of hepatosplenomegaly does not exclude the diagnosis of malaria. Labial herpes simplex lesions are often present. Rashes, pharyngitis, and lymphadenopathy are uncommon and point to a diagnosis other than malaria.

Abnormalities in routine laboratory test results in uncomplicated malaria may include evidence of a hemolytic anemia, leukopenia caused by a decrease in granulocytes and lymphocytes, thrombocytopenia, and minimal albuminuria. The thrombocyte count returns rapidly to normal on treatment. Hyponatremia, which is seen frequently in *P. falciparum* malaria, is caused by salt depletion and water retention.

Asymptomatic Infection and Recrudescence. Partial therapy or immunity reduces parasitemia and symptoms may disappear. Despite persistent erythrocytic infection during these asymptomatic periods, parasites are difficult to locate on blood films. Periodic increases in parasitemia cause recurrent clinical attacks (recrudescence). The total duration of erythrocytic infection varies for each type of malaria. Most falciparum infections are eliminated in one year; a few persist for up to three years. *P. malariae* infection may persist as an asymptomatic infection for the life of the patient. How *P. malariae* evades the immune response for years while infecting new erythrocytes every 72 hours remains a mystery. The asymptomatic erythrocytic infection poses two potential risks to other individuals: First, donated blood induces malaria in the recipient; second, the asymptomatic patient can infect vector mosquitoes.

Relapse differs from recrudescence in that the infection that induces the relapse persists as a latent form in hepatic parenchymal cells. Relapses occur only in *P. vivax* and *P. ovale* malaria.

COMPLICATIONS. High-level parasitemia in *P. falciparum* infection accounts for the severe morbidity and mortality. When the number of infected erythrocytes rises above 100,000 per cubic millimeter and the hematocrit falls below 30 per cent, the patient may develop serious complications, which most commonly include severe hemolytic anemia, renal failure, and coma. Acute renal failure can be associated with hemolytic anemia and hemoglobinuria (blackwater fever). The hemolytic anemia may be caused by the high number of parasites in the blood, quinine sensitivity, or oxidant drugs in patients with G6PD deficiency. Renal failure may occur in the absence of severe hemolysis and may be associated with hypovolemia. It may occur with normal urine volume. Blood urea nitrogen may increase rapidly in renal failure because of an increased catabolic rate.

Cerebral malaria presents as disturbances in consciousness ranging from somnolence to coma, major motor seizures, and organic psychosis. Since the signs and symptoms are not pathognomonic of malaria, other diseases should be excluded, even in patients with circulating malaria parasites. Marked hypoglycemia, especially during infusion of quinine and in pregnancy, may cause lapses in consciousness. Febrile seizures in young children are impossible to distinguish from seizures of malaria. Neurologic examination may reveal hyperreflexion and bilateral Babinski's signs. Focal neurologic findings occur rarely. The cerebrospinal fluid pressure is usually normal. The concentration of protein may be increased. Pleocytosis is rare.

Greatly increased bilirubin and transaminase occur rarely. Another unusual complication, pulmonary edema, may be associated with fluid overload. Since it is caused by increased capillary permeability, it is difficult to reverse, and the outcome is often fatal.

Although splenic tenderness is common in acute malaria, evidence of peritoneal and diaphragmatic irritation may indicate splenic rupture. This life-threatening complication is more common in *P. vivax* malaria.

Chronic infection with *P. malariae* in children may produce progressive nephritis that responds poorly to treatment with antimalarials or steroids.

Falciparum Malaria During Pregnancy in the Semi-immune. Parasites sequester in the vascular beds of the placenta. The primigravida, although previously immune, may have severe attacks of malaria and marked anemia. Consequently, chemoprophylaxis is indicated throughout the first pregnancy in the semi-immune. Malaria causes stillbirths and underweight newborns, especially in the primigravida.

Tropical Splenomegaly Syndrome. Patients living in regions of Africa and New Guinea endemic for falciparum malaria develop massive splenic enlargement, hepatic sinusoidal lymphocytic infiltrates, and elevated levels of serum IgM. They respond to chronic antimalarial chemoprophylaxis with decrease in spleen size and reversal of liver pathology. Mortality is high in patients who do not receive antimalarial therapy. Splenectomy is contraindicated because severe malaria may occur following splenectomy, even in a previously immune individual.

Burkitt's Lymphoma. This tumor occurs in areas of Africa hyperendemic for *P. falciparum* and is believed to be an atypical response to Epstein-Barr virus infection.

DIAGNOSIS. The high mortality from falciparum malaria in nonendemic areas results from the failure of clinicians to consider the diagnosis and to obtain malaria blood films. The diagnosis of malaria should be suspected in any febrile patient who has traveled in the tropics, despite a history of antimalarial chemoprophylaxis, or who has received a blood transfusion. The incubation period—the time from inoculation of sporozoites by mosquito to the first symptoms—is about 10 to 16 days. Drug prophylaxis may suppress the initial attack of *P. falciparum* malaria for weeks to months and of the relapsing malarias caused by *P. vivax* and *P. ovale* for months to years. The definitive diagnosis is made from identification of malarial parasites on a Giemsa-stained thick and thin blood film. Blood should be examined immediately and at 12-hour intervals, because the parasitemia may fluctuate. Parasites may be undetectable during the first few days of the initial attack and in asymptomatic, semi-immune persons. The clinician should not wait for a paroxysm to obtain a blood film, since delay in diagnosis and treatment of *P. falciparum* malaria increases the risk to the patient. If malaria is strongly suspected on clinical grounds in a patient with repeatedly normal blood films, a therapeutic trial may be instituted.

Well-prepared and properly stained thick and thin blood films simplify diagnosis. Both should be stained with Giemsa at pH 7.0 to 7.2. (See Color plate 5.)

Once malaria parasites are identified on the blood film, the most important distinction is whether the patient has *P. falciparum* malaria, because this will influence the initial therapy. Criteria suggestive of *P. falciparum* include predominant small ring forms and multiply infected erythrocytes, rings with double nuclei, rings that appear to lie along the circumference of the erythrocyte, and the diagnostic crescent-shaped gametocytes (Table 381–1). Except during high-level parasitemia, trophozoites and schizonts are rarely seen; infected erythrocytes adhere to venular endothelium. *P. falciparum* does not cause enlargement or pink stippling (Schüffner's dots) of infected erythrocytes. If more than 5 per cent of the erythrocytes are infected, *P. falciparum* should be suspected. Diagnosis of a malaria other than that caused by *P. falciparum* does not exclude the diagnosis of *P. falciparum* malaria, since mixed infections may occur. Slides should be saved for evaluation by an expert. Inclusions in erythrocytes (e.g., Howell-Jolly bodies and siderocytes) and artifacts (e.g., platelets on erythrocytes, precipitated stain and dirt) may be confused with malarial parasites. *Babesia microti* resembles *P. falciparum* rings but can be differentiated by an experienced microscopist.

In the future, probes for parasite DNA in the blood may be a useful adjunct to blood films. Serologic tests have no place in the diagnosis of the acutely ill patient. The indirect fluorescent antibody test is useful in identifying infected donors in cases of transfusion malaria.

THERAPY. *P. falciparum.* Prompt diagnosis and early treatment are essential. Delay in chemotherapy increases morbidity and mortality. All patients should be hospitalized and the case treated as a medical emergency. Patients whose condition appears stable on admission may have rapid worsening.

The decision on drug regimen will depend on the origin of the infection. Chloroquine resistance is widespread and will continue to appear in new areas. Therefore, every falciparum malaria case should be considered potentially chloroquine resistant. Resistance extends today from Pakistan and India through Southeast Asia to New Guinea and Vanuatu in the Pacific, from Panama to South America, and from East Africa to Zambia, Madagascar, and the Comoros, and westward to Zaire, the Congo, Central African Republic, and the Cameroons. Because partial resistance to quinine (i.e., response followed by recrudescence) occurs in Southeast Asia and other areas, quinine is usually not used alone in treatment. Resistance to Fansidar, a fixed-drug combination of pyrimethamine and sulfadoxine, has been reported in Southeast Asia, South America, and East Africa.

Since treatment failure may occur with any drug regimen, the course of parasitemia must be followed at 12-hour intervals. Failure to reduce parasitemia in the first 24 to 48 hours of treatment should raise the possibility of parasite resistance to that treatment. No asexual parasites should be detectable on smears four to five days after a course of chloroquine is completed; persistence after the fifth day indicates drug failure.

Gametocytes may persist in the blood for weeks after asexual forms have been successfully eliminated. Gametocytes do not cause disease and their presence does not indicate treatment failure.

Partially resistant parasites recrudesce up to two months after treatment in the nonimmune. The patient should be warned that any febrile episode weeks to months after treatment may indicate drug failure and requires evaluation for malaria.

SYMPTOMATIC AND SUPPORTIVE MEASURES. Treatment includes aspirin, sponging with tepid water, and fanning to increase evaporation. Orthostatic hypotension, usually observed early in infection, is an indication for complete bed rest.

Packed erythrocytes or whole blood should be infused slowly in severe anemia. Platelet transfusions are generally not indicated for thrombocytopenia, as the platelets rapidly return toward normal during specific chemotherapy. Uremia may progress rapidly because of the high catabolic rate and is an indication for early hemodialysis. Administration of excessive fluids may aggravate cerebral symptoms or precipitate pulmonary edema. Pulmonary edema is usually not associated with a rise in central venous pressure during intravenous fluid administration and often results in death despite treatment.

TREATMENT OF CHLOROQUINE-SENSITIVE *P. falciparum.* The majority of infections contracted in western India, Pakistan, West Africa, Central America (except Panama), and Haiti are chloroquine sensitive. These patients should be treated with chloroquine unless infection occurs while the patient is undergoing chloroquine prophylaxis or if the parasite count is greater than 1 per cent, in which case treatment should be as described in the sections on chloroquine-resistant *P. falciparum* and severe and complicated malaria. The recommended therapy for adults is chloroquine phosphate, 1000 mg initially, 500 mg six hours later, and 500 mg on each of two succeeding days. The major acute toxicity occurs in Africans who experience severe itching of the palms of the hands and soles of the feet without any obvious skin abnormalities, but this is not an indication for discontinuing chloroquine unless the symptoms are severe.

Because of the possibility of chloroquine resistance, the parasitemia should be followed closely during treatment (see above) and alternative drugs instituted if indicated. Fever occurring weeks after therapy may indicate a recrudescence.

TREATMENT OF CHLOROQUINE-RESISTANT *P. falciparum.* The regimen combines quinine sulfate, 650 mg every eight hours for seven days, and Fansidar (pyrimethamine, 25 mg, and sulfadoxine, 500 mg), three tablets immediately. Occasionally after treatment with this regimen, the patient may suffer a recrudescence. Recrudescent attacks may be treated with the following regimen: quinine sulfate, 650 mg every eight hours for three days, plus tetracycline hydrochloride, 250 mg every six hours for ten days.

Cinchonism (nausea, vomiting, tinnitus, and vertigo) commonly results from treatment with quinine and is not an indication to alter or discontinue therapy. A rare complication of quinine therapy, Coombs-positive hemolytic anemia, is an indication for immediate withdrawal of the drug.

Mefloquine, an experimental antimalarial drug, is highly effective against chloroquine-resistant *P. falciparum.* As more data become available on its relative safety, it may become the treatment of choice for *P. falciparum* malaria. Mefloquine alone or in combination with pyrimethamine and sulfadoxine is now undergoing extensive clinical trials. Rarely, mefloquine causes disorientation, hallucinations, and lapses of consciousness two to three weeks after drug administration.

TREATMENT OF SEVERE AND COMPLICATED MALARIA. Patients with *P. falciparum* malaria who have a parasite count greater than 100,000 per microliter, marked anemia, cerebral complications, or are vomiting repeatedly should be treated with intravenous quinine dihydrochloride as follows: quinine dihydrochloride,* 20 mg per kilogram, in 250 ml of 0.15 M

---

*Available from the Centers for Disease Control, Atlanta, GA.

sodium chloride infused over four hours, followed at eight-hour intervals for a total of 72 hours with quinine dihydrochloride, 10 mg per kilogram, infused over four hours. When oral medication is tolerated the patient should receive Fansidar or tetracycline (see Treatment of Chloroquine-Resistant *P. falciparum*) in addition to the quinine. Since quinine is excreted by the kidneys and metabolized by the liver, the dosage in patients with renal failure and hepatic disease should be monitored by determination of blood quinine levels.

Hypoglycemia is a life-threatening complication of severe malaria and occurs most commonly during intravenous quinine therapy and in pregnant women. Blood glucose should be monitored, especially in patients who have a change in the level of consciousness.

If quinine is not immediately available, the Centers for Disease Control may be contacted any time of the day or night for advice on therapy. Intravenous quinidine appears to be as effective as intravenous quinine for the treatment of severe malaria. Quinidine does not have FDA approval for use in malaria; therefore the physician should obtain informed consent. Quinidine gluconate (10 mg per kilogram) should be infused slowly over a period of 60 minutes, followed by a continuous infusion of quinidine gluconate (0.02 mg per kilogram per minute) for three days and then by Fansidar or tetracycline (see Treatment of Chloroquine-Resistant *P. falciparum*). The infusion rate of quinidine will be lowered if the serum quinidine level is greater than 6 μg per milliliter, the uncorrected Q-T interval is greater than 0.6 second, QRS widening is more than 25 per cent of baseline, or hypotension is unresponsive to saline infusion. The quinidine infusion should be discontinued if there is severe persistent hypotension or a severe cardiac arrhythmia.

Exchange transfusions may improve survival in patients who have parasitemia greater than 15 per cent ring-infected erythrocytes, although controlled studies have not been performed. Glucosteroids are contraindicated because they increase morbidity and mortality. Heparin is contraindicated even in patients with disseminated intravascular coagulation because of the risk of hemorrhage.

P. vivax, P. ovale, and P. malariae. Acute attacks with any of these species should be treated with chloroquine (see regimen under Treatment of Chloroquine-Sensitive *P. falciparum*).

P. vivax and *P. ovale* infections acquired by mosquito bites may have persistent hepatic forms, and these must be eliminated to prevent relapses. After completion of chloroquine treatment, primaquine phosphate, 26.6 mg daily for 14 days, is administered. Primaquine causes hemolysis in patients with G6PD deficiency. Patients who have a mild G6PD deficiency may be treated under close supervision because the hemolysis is self-limited. Severe G6PD deficiency is a contraindication to the use of primaquine, each relapse requiring retreatment with chloroquine. Primaquine is not indicated in the treatment of transfusion malaria because erythrocytic parasites of blood-induced infections do not infect the liver.

PREVENTION. *Protection for the Individual.* Ideal chemoprophylaxis is not available because of multi-drug-resistant *P. falciparum* in many areas of the world. In addition, chloroquine eliminates only the primary attack of *P. vivax* and *P. ovale* but has no effect on relapses that may occur months to years later. Therefore the patient should be warned that fever during or after travel in endemic areas may be caused by malaria, even though the patient was undergoing drug suppression.

Because drug prophylaxis is not ideal, the traveler should be advised to prevent contact with night-biting *Anopheles*. The traveler should use netting over the bed, insecticides, and mosquito repellents such as Off (N,N-diethyltoluamide).

All adult travelers to malarious areas should take chloroquine phosphate, 500 mg orally once weekly. Long-term use of chloroquine at recommended doses for malaria prophylaxis

does not cause eye disease. The drug should be continued for six weeks after leaving an endemic area. Travelers who were heavily exposed to malaria and are not G6PD deficient should receive primaquine phosphate, 26.6 mg daily for 14 days, on return from an endemic area to eliminate hepatic forms of *P. vivax* and *P. ovale*.

Fansidar, one tablet weekly, should be used together with weekly chloroquine in East and Central Africa where transmission of chloroquine-resistant *P. falciparum* is intense. Fansidar causes serious mucocutaneous reactions (Stevens-Johnson syndrome and toxic epidermal necrolysis) in one of 20,000 people. Because of this toxicity, Fansidar is not recommended for most travelers to Asia and Latin America except in those localities of heavy transmission. Travelers should be warned to discontinue Fansidar if any mucocutaneous symptoms develop. As an alternative to weekly Fansidar in countries outside of Africa, the traveler may carry a single-treatment dose of Fansidar (three tablets) for self-medication of a febrile illness if medical care is not available. Fansidar resistance occurs in Southeast Asia, Brazil, and Africa.

Chemoprophylaxis in Pregnancy and for Nursing Mothers. Drugs in pregnancy always present a potential risk to the fetus, especially for prolonged use as in chemoprophylaxis. Chloroquine is considered generally safe when used at the recommended dosage. Chemoprophylaxis in areas of chloroquine-resistant *P. falciparum* where Fansidar is recommended (see above) presents a more difficult problem. Although Fansidar has not been proven to be teratogenic in humans, it should be avoided if possible for malaria prophylaxis in pregnant women. In addition, sulfonamides may increase the risk of kernicterus in hyperbilirubinemic neonates, because sulfonamides displace unconjugated bilirubin from albumin. Therefore, short-acting sulfonamides should be used close to term, should be discontinued as soon as labor begins, and should not be given to a mother nursing a newborn.

Acute malaria because of its risk to mother and child should be treated according to the regimens outlined under Therapy. Primaquine is contraindicated during pregnancy for treatment or prevention of relapsing malaria (*P. vivax* or *P. ovale*) because of the risk of inducing a fatal hemolytic crisis in the fetus who has G6PD deficiency.

Eradication and Control in Endemic Areas. The major tools for the control of malaria have been directed against the vector. Antimalarial drugs, especially chloroquine, are used primarily to reduce morbidity and mortality. When malaria eradication was first instituted as a program of WHO in the 1950's, the program mainly emphasized spraying walls with residual insecticides, detecting malaria cases, and treating patients with antimalarial drugs. Insecticide resistance, avoidance by mosquitoes of sprayed surfaces, and outdoor feeding of mosquitoes have created major problems and have led to the failure of malaria eradication in many areas. In addition, the spread of multi-drug-resistant *P. falciparum* will probably increase morbidity and mortality in regions of resurgent malaria. There is no question that new tools such as vaccines and novel approaches to vector control will be sorely needed in the decades ahead.

Boyd MF (ed.): Malariology. Philadelphia, W. B. Saunders Company, 1949. *The best description of the course of each of the four human malarias in the nonimmune.*

Brown HW, Neva FA: Basic Clinical Parasitology. 5th ed. Norwalk, Appleton-Century-Crofts, 1983. *Color plates of malaria parasites for the inexperienced microscopist.*

Miller LH: Malaria. In Warren KW, Mahmoud AAF (eds.): Tropical and Geographical Medicine. New York, McGraw-Hill Book Company, 1983. *A general review of malariology with references.*

Miller LH, Howard RJ, Carter R, et al.: Research towards malarial vaccines. Science 234:1349, 1986. *Review of the status of malaria vaccine research.*

Udeinya IJ, Miller LH, McGregor IA, et al.: *Plasmodium falciparum* strain-specific antibody blocks binding of infected erythrocytes to amelanotic melanoma cells. Nature 303:429, 1983. *An example of variant antigens in falciparum malaria.*

White NJ, Warrell DA, Chanthavanich P, et al.: Severe hypoglycemia and hyperinsulinemia in falciparum malaria. N Engl J Med 309:61, 1983. *A new complication of falciparum malaria.*

World Health Organization Malaria Action Programme. Severe and complicated Malaria. Trans Roy Soc Trop Med Hyg 80 (Suppl):1, 1986. *A review of malaria chemotherapy.*

382 AFRICAN TRYPANOSOMIASIS (Sleeping Sickness)

Thomas C. Quinn

DEFINITION. Known widely as sleeping sickness, African trypanosomiasis is an acute and chronic disease caused by *Trypanosoma brucei*. The parasites are transmitted to humans through the bite of tsetse flies located in regions of Africa between 15 degrees north and 15 degrees south latitude. In humans, there are two distinct forms of the disease, East African trypanosomiasis caused by *T. brucei rhodesiense* and West African trypanosomiasis caused by *T. brucei gambiense*. Although there is some clinical overlap, East African trypanosomiasis primarily causes an acute febrile illness with myocarditis and meningoencephalitis that is rapidly fatal if not treated, while West African trypanosomiasis is characterized as a chronic debilitating disease with mental deterioration and physical wasting (Table 382–1). A closely related variant, *T. brucei brucei*, is noninfectious for man, but causes a chronic wasting illness in cattle, called nagana, which has a considerable indirect effect on human nutrition in sub-Saharan Africa.

ETIOLOGY AND LIFE CYCLE. Trypanosomes are motile hemoflagellates with a single undulating membrane that passes along the length of the parasite, terminating in an anterior flagellum (Fig. 382–1). Located anteriorly is a kinetoplast, an organelle containing topologically interlocked circular DNA molecules and mitochondria. In the peripheral blood of humans trypanosomes vary in length from 10 to 40 μ. Both short stumpy and long slender forms can be present in a patient at the same time. The different variants of *T. brucei* cannot be distinguished morphologically, but can be identified by differences in pathogenicity for certain animals, and in biochemical requirements, electrophoretic pattern of component enzymes, and DNA hybridization.

T. brucei is transmitted by the tsetse fly *Glossina*, within which it undergoes several developmental changes. During the bite of an infected host, trypanosomes are ingested, and within the insect midgut rapidly differentiate into procyclic forms with loss of their dense surface coat, composed of variant surface glycoprotein. After two to three weeks of multiplication within the midgut the procyclic trypanosomes migrate to the insect's salivary glands, where they change morphologically into epimastigotes. These forms further undergo multiplication and ultimately differentiate into meta-

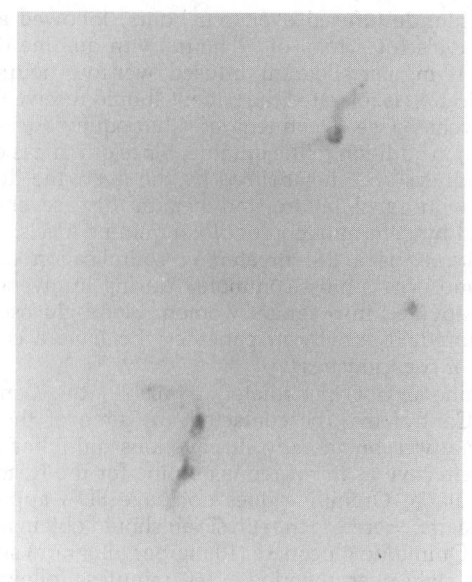

FIGURE 382–1. *Trypanosoma brucei rhodesiense* in a peripheral blood smear from an American safari hunter with African trypanosomiasis. (Giemsa, original magnification, ×1000).

cyclic trypanosomes that are coated with characteristic variant surface glycoprotein and are infectious to mammalian hosts. When a new host is bitten by the tsetse fly the trypanosomes present in the salivary glands are injected into the connective tissue and blood. Within the human host they divide by binary fission and undergo antigen variation, a process by which they continually change their surface glycoproteins and evade the immune system of the host. With the bite of another tsetse fly, ingestion of the parasite occurs, and the life cycle of the organism is completed (Fig. 382–2). Mechanical transmission can theoretically also occur via blood transfusion or by interrupted biting of a tsetse fly feeding on an infectious person, and directly thereafter biting an uninfected individual.

EPIDEMIOLOGY. It is estimated that African trypanosomiasis infects more than 10,000 Africans annually and that approximately 45 million people live at risk of acquiring trypanosomiasis because of the presence of the disease and its vector. Approximately 4 million square miles in Africa remain unpopulated because of the presence of *T. brucei brucei* infection, which results in the loss of domestic and wild animals, including cattle, waterbuck, bushbuck, and buffalo.

T. b. gambiense occurs primarily in the west and central regions of sub-Saharan Africa. Although it primarily infects humans, there may be animal reservoirs, such as pigs, dogs, and sheep. Gambian sleeping sickness is spread mainly by three species of tsetse fly, *Glossina palpalis*, *G. tachinoides*, and *G. fuscipes*. Distribution of these flies includes shaded areas along rivers and streams where the conditions of temperature, darkness, and moisture are optimum. Contact between humans and tsetse flies is often very close and as a result of the chronic course of *T. b. gambiense* infection, many of these

TABLE 382–1. A COMPARISON OF GAMBIAN AND RHODESIAN SLEEPING SICKNESS

	Gambian (West African)	Rhodesian (East African)
Etiologic agent	*Trypanosoma brucei gambiense*	*Trypanosoma brucei rhodesiense*
Vector	*Glossina palpalis* or *tachinoides* (riverine tsetse)	*Glossina morsitans* (savanna tsetse)
Distribution	West and Central Africa	East Africa
Reservoir	Humans (domestic animals)	Wild game
Course of infection	Slow (months–years)	Rapid (<1 year)
Clinical features		
Lymphadenopathy	+ + (Winterbottom's sign)	±
Myocarditis, heart failure	—	+ +
Neurologic symptoms	+ +	+
Disseminated intravascular coagulation	—	+
Parasitemia	Low	High

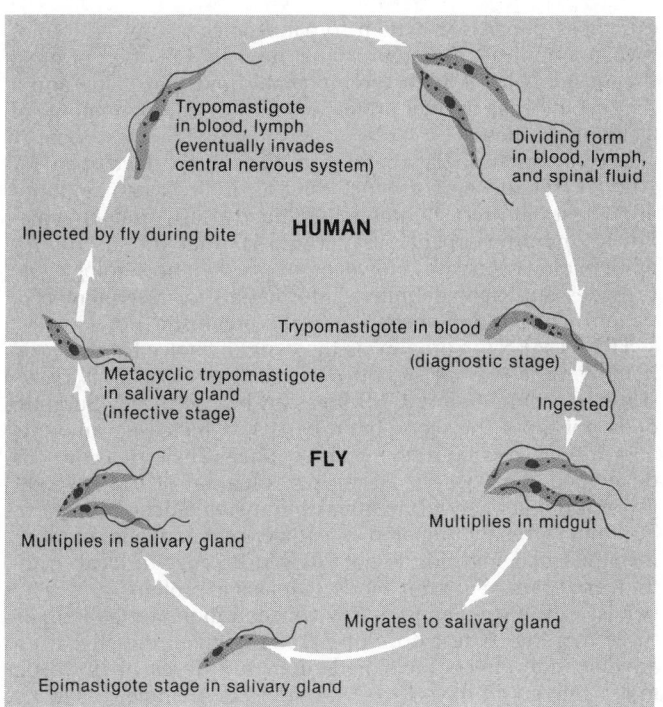

FIGURE 382–2. Life cycle of *Trypanosoma* (*Trypanozoon*) *brucei*, T. (T.) b. *gambiense*, and T. (T.) b. *rhodesiense*.

infected patients remain exposed to flies over a long period, providing ideal conditions for continued transmission of infection.

T. b. rhodesiense differs from *T. b. gambiense* in that it is primarily a parasite of wild game, with man serving only as an occasional host. The geographic distribution of *T. b. rhodesiense* is primarily East Africa from Ethiopia and eastern Uganda south to Zambia and Botswana. Rhodesian sleeping sickness is spread by tsetse flies of the *G. morsitans* group, including *G. pallidipes* and *G. swynnertoni*. These flies can survive in the open savanna, and Rhodesian sleeping sickness usually occurs among individuals visiting or traveling through an endemic area. Consequently, hunters, fishermen, and tourists are at risk, exposing themselves to vectors that usually feed on wild animals. This form of trypanosomiasis is usually sporadic, but epidemics have been reported.

Imported African trypanosomiasis is a rare disease with only 11 cases diagnosed in Americans since 1967. Seven of these cases were among Americans who had been on safari in east Africa for a very brief period. Nearly all of these cases were initially misdiagnosed because of the unfamiliarity of American physicians with this disease. With an increase in international travel, 20,000 Americans are now estimated to visit endemic areas yearly, and approximately 10,000 aliens enter the United States each year from countries in Africa where the infection is endemic.

PATHOGENESIS AND PATHOLOGY. Following the bite of the tsetse fly, trypanosomes accumulate in the connective tissue where they multiply to produce a local chancre (trypanoma). The organisms subsequently spread through the lymphatics, resulting in enlargement of lymph nodes secondary to reactive plasma cell and macrophage infiltration. Later the lymph nodes shrink, and patchy fibrosis occurs. The trypanosomes eventually disseminate to the circulatory system where the parasitemia usually remains at low intensity and the organisms multiply by binary fission.

The host immune response plays an integral role in the pathogenesis of African sleeping sickness, although the exact nature of the immunopathogenic reactions have not been clearly defined. African trypanosomes possess surface antigens that induce an antibody response. Trypanosomes survive by periodically altering their surface antigenic coat, avoiding

successful eradication by the host. One organism can produce multiple antigenic variants (100 or more), each genetically determined and selected by the host antibody response. Consequently trypanosomes occur in the peripheral blood of infected individuals in waves, with each parasite wave consisting of a serologically distinct organism. These specific biologic features of African trypanosomes with their consequent immunologic sequelae in the host may be directly related to the pathogenesis of the disease.

Tissue damage is induced by either toxin production or immune complex reaction with release of proteolytic enzymes. Immune complexes consisting of variant antigens of the organism and complement-fixing antibodies have been demonstrated in both the circulation and target organs of infected patients. The production of autoantibodies is a prominent feature, and they are frequently directed against antigen components of red cells, brain, and heart. Anemia secondary to autoimmune hemolysis can be severe, resulting in anoxia and further tissue destruction. Thus the host-parasite interaction can result in generalized febrile episodes, lymphadenopathy, myocardial and pericardial inflammation along with anemia, thrombocytopenia, disseminated intravascular coagulation, and renal disease primarily during the acute stage of the disease.

During this period of circulatory dissemination, trypanosomes localize in the small vessels of the CNS. Pathologic changes in the CNS are most prominent in chronic cases of gambian sleeping sickness. The meninges are thickened and infiltrated with lymphocytes, plasma cells, and morular cells. Morular cells are modified plasma cells (up to 20 mm in diameter) with large granular inclusions that have been shown to consist of immunoglobulin. These cells may play an important role in the local production of IgM in the cerebrospinal fluid. Chronic inflammatory changes result in perivascular infiltration associated with prominent neuroglial proliferation in the pia-arachnoid of the brain and spinal cord. Edema, hemorrhages, and granulomatous lesions are frequently present, along with thrombosis as a result of endoarteritis and with neuronal degeneration.

African trypanosomes appear to induce a state of B cell polyclonal activation caused either by interference with host T cell lymphocyte control of antibody production or by a B cell mitogen released by the parasite. Polyclonal hypergammaglobulinemia, with very high levels of IgM, is commonly seen. High levels of nonspecific heterophile antibody, rheumatoid factor, and autoantibodies are also produced. In addition, several other immunologic impairments have also been demonstrated in patients with African trypanosomiasis, including impairment of both cellular and humoral immunity with decreased skin reactivity to recall antigens, and reduced antibody response to bacterial and viral vaccines.

CLINICAL FEATURES. The signs and symptoms of sleeping sickness differ according to infecting organism (Table 382–1). Rhodesian sleeping sickness, due to *T. b. rhodesiense*, causes a rapid progressive disease often resulting in cardiac failure and acute neurologic manifestations. Gambian sleeping sickness, caused by *T. b. gambiense*, is typically a more chronic illness with primarily neurologic features. However, this difference is not absolute, and in some cases Gambian sleeping sickness can progress rapidly, and occasionally Rhodesian sleeping sickness may follow a more chronic course.

Gambian Sleeping Sickness. Within several days following the bite by an infected tsetse fly, a trypanosomal nodule or chancre develops, typically on the exposed parts of the body. Within a week the lesion becomes a hard, painful nodule surrounded by erythema and swelling, which persists for about one to two weeks. Following this incubation period, clinical features develop following systemic lymphatic and circulatory invasion of the trypanosomes. Fever, headache, dizziness, and weakness occur in the majority of these patients. Febrile episodes may last one to six days, alternating with afebrile periods. Lymphadenopathy with prominent supraclavicular and posterior cervical enlargement is seen in more than 80 per cent of infected individuals. Known as Winterbottom's sign, these enlarged lymph nodes are usually discrete, rubbery, and painless. Moderate splenomegaly may occur, and urticaria and erythematous rashes have also been observed. Electrocardiograms are often abnormal, but clinical signs of heart disease are unusual.

Six months to several years after the first appearance of symptoms the clinical features of this early hemolymphatic stage progress to a late meningoencephalitic stage. Behavioral and personality changes are often the first signs of CNS involvement. Later, more florid psychologic changes may occur, with hallucinations and delusions. Reversion of sleep rhythm is characteristic, with drowsiness during the day, a feature from which the disease derives its name. Other nervous symptoms include tremor, most characteristically of the face and lips, and hyperesthesia, causing some patients to avoid common practices such as closing (Kerandel's sign) or locking doors (key sign). Without treatment, the patient's level of consciousness progressively deteriorates until he or she finally lapses into stupor. Alterations in thermoregulation may lead to hypothermia or hyperthermia, and progressive neurologic alterations lead to convulsions, chorea, and athetosis. The cerebrospinal fluid shows an increase in cells and protein, much of which is IgM. Free immunoglobulin light chains may be present. Most of the cells are lymphocytes, but a few are plasma cells and morula cells. Trypanosomes may also be evident within the cerebrospinal fluid.

Rhodesian Sleeping Sickness. This disease is more acute than Gambian sleeping sickness, and symptoms usually occur a few days after the victim has been bitten by the tsetse fly. Alternating periods of high fever, malaise, and headache, followed by several days of well-being, are often misinterpreted as acute malaria infection. Lymphadenopathy is not prominent in this variety of the disease, and Winterbottom's sign is usually absent. Tachycardia with arrhythmias and extrasystoles is common. Anemia, thrombocytopenia, and disseminated intravascular coagulation are usually evident within the first several weeks of infection. Liver enzyme values are often elevated, and electrocardiograms are abnormal, usually reflecting underlying myocarditis. Neurologic features are similar to those described for Gambian sleeping sickness, but occur much earlier and with more rapid deterioration. Without treatment the disease may result in death within a matter of weeks to months, without clear distinction into an early and late phase as described for Gambian trypanosomiasis.

DIAGNOSIS. Although a presumptive diagnosis of trypanosomiasis is based on clinical suspicion, history of travel to areas where this disease is endemic, and tsetse fly exposure, confirmation of the diagnosis is based solely on the demonstration of trypanosomes. These organisms may be found in the blood (Color plate 5E), bone marrow, centrifuged cerebrospinal fluid, lymph node aspirates, and scrapings from the chancre. Giemsa or Wright's stain of the buffy coat of centrifuged heparinized blood make identification easier, since the trypanosomes are often concentrated in the buffy coat. In patients with Gambian sleeping sickness, in which trypanosomes are found less frequently in the blood, concentration methods such as ion-exchange chromatography, DEAE filtration, culture, or animal inoculation should be used.

All patients should have a lumbar puncture prior to and following therapy to determine whether there is CNS involvement. Documentation of CNS involvement is imperative since suramin, a drug effective against the hemolymphatic stage of *T. brucei*, does not penetrate into the spinal fluid. CNS disease is manifested by pleocytosis and elevation of spinal fluid total protein and IgM levels. Trypanosomes can be found in most patients, provided that the cerebrospinal fluid is examined immediately after collection and that clean glassware is used.

For those patients in whom trypanosomes cannot be found, measurement of the cerebrospinal fluid IgM is often of great diagnostic help. A high cerebrospinal fluid IgM value and a modest increase in total protein are almost pathognomonic of sleeping sickness.

Several immunodiagnostic tests have been developed for African trypanosomiasis, including an indirect hemagglutination test, indirect fluorescent antibody test, and enzyme-linked immunosorbent assay (ELISA), that are useful for epidemiologic surveys. However, at present, no serologic test provides sufficient definitive information for treatment of a patient without demonstration of the organism.

TREATMENT. Suramin* is the drug of choice for the early hemolymphatic stage of both *T. b. gambiense* and *T. b. rhodesiense* infections before CNS invasion has occurred. Suramin does not cross the blood-brain barrier in increased amounts and it will not cure the disease once CNS invasion has developed. The dose is 20 mg per kilogram of body weight given intravenously up to a maximum single dose of 1 gram. Suramin is freshly prepared as a 10 per cent aqueous solution. Intramuscular injection is not advised because of local irritation and pain. Suramin binds to plasma proteins and may persist in the circulation at low concentrations for as long as three months. A test dose of 200 mg is given initially; if no adverse side effects are noted, then full doses of the drug may be given on days 1, 3, 7, 14, and 21. A single course for an adult is usually 5 grams; it should not exceed 7 grams.

Suramin is a toxic drug that may result in idiosyncratic reactions in some individuals (one of 20,000). The drug is excreted entirely by the kidneys; renal damage may result because of deposition of the drug in the renal tubules. The urine should be examined prior to administration of each dose of suramin, and if proteinuria or casts are present, treatment should be stopped. Other side effects include a papular eruption, photophobia, peripheral neuritis, and agranulocytosis.

Pentamidine isethionate* is an alternative drug for the treatment of early hemolymphatic African trypanosomiasis, but it is much less active against *T. rhodesiense* than is suramin. The dose is 4 mg per kilogram body weight; it is given every other day by intramuscular injection for a total of ten injections. Pentamidine is also ineffective in the treatment of CNS trypanosomiasis.

Melarsoprol* (Mel B) is the treatment of choice for both Gambian and Rhodesian sleeping sickness once involvement of the CNS has occurred, even though the drug is very toxic. It is possible that toxicity is reduced by prior treatment with one or two injections of suramin, but melarsoprol should be started immediately in patients who are very ill with CNS disease. Mel B, an arsenic derivative of British antilewisite (BAL), is given intravenously in a 3.6-per cent solution in propylene glycol. This is very irritating and may produce thrombophlebitis. Initially melarsoprol is administered slowly intravenously in doses of 1.5, 2.0, and 2.2 mg per kilogram of body weight at 48-hour intervals. One week later, doses of 2.5, 3.0, and 3.6 mg per kilogram are injected on a similar schedule; finally, after another week, there is a third course of three injections, each of 3.6 mg per kilogram of body weight. If signs of arsenical toxicity occur, the drug should be discontinued.

A reactive encephalopathy, probably due to release of trypanosomal antigens, may occur early in the course of treatment. A hemorrhagic encephalopathy may also occur at the time of the third or fourth injection. It may develop very rapidly, and its mortality is about 50 per cent. It is uncertain whether it is due to arsenical poisoning or to an immunopathogenic reaction. Dimercaprol (BAL) has been used to treat this complication, but its value has not been clearly established. It has been suggested that corticosteriods protect

---

*Available from the Centers for Disease Control, Atlanta, GA.

patients from Mel B encephalopathy, but this assertion has not been clearly documented. Alternative drugs for CNS involvement include tryparsamide, melarsonyl potassium (Mel W), and nitrofurazone. These drugs appear either to be more toxic than Mel B or less effective in the treatment of CNS disease. Difluoromethylornithine (DFMO), a specific, irreversible inhibitor of polyamine biosynthesis, has been shown to be curative in animal models inoculated with *Trypanosoma* species. In a preliminary open field trial, 20 patients, 18 of whom had central nervous system infection with *T. b. gambiense*, had a clinical response with parasitic clearance of the CSF at doses of 400 mg per kg per day for six weeks with minimal toxicity. Further studies are under way to define optimal treatment regimens. Regular follow-up with clinical examination and lumbar puncture is necessary for all patients for at least one year after treatment.

Patients with neurologic disease require frequent follow-up examinations for treatment failures, and relapses occasionally occur. Patients with a relapse of CNS disease should receive another course of Mel B together with nitrofurazone. Despite the toxicity of the latter drug, there is an impression that in patients with relapse, treatment with melarsoprol and nitrofurazone is more effective than melarsoprol alone. The adult dosage of nitrofurazone is 0.5 gram given orally every six hours for five days, this course being repeated on three occasions with one week between each course. A peripheral neuropathy and hemolytic anemia in patients with G6PD deficiency are the most frequent side effects of nitrofurazone.

PROGNOSIS. Untreated, African sleeping sickness is almost invariably fatal. Many patients with early Gambian sleeping sickness may remain relatively well for months to years without treatment, but once CNS involvement has occurred, death is inevitable unless treatment is given. Death frequently results from pneumonia in Gambian sleeping sickness and from heart failure in Rhodesian sleeping sickness. Treatment with suramin in the early phase of sleeping sickness results in a cure rate of over 90 per cent. A few patients may subsequently develop CNS involvement and require further treatment. Mel B achieves a parasitologic cure in at least 90 per cent of cases of advanced disease, and many patients may recover completely. Unfortunately, some patients are left with irreversible neurologic damage. Approximately 5 per cent of patients may die during the course of Mel B therapy.

CONTROL AND PROPHYLAXIS. Measures to prevent and control African trypanosomiasis can be instituted at three different levels: surveillance and treatment, chemoprophylaxis, and vector control. Surveillance with treatment is necessary to reduce the human reservoir of infection, particularly in areas where epidemics have occurred in the past. Pentamidine has been successfully used as a chemoprophylactic in Gambian sleeping sickness when given as a single intramuscular injection of 4 mg per kilogram every three to six months. However, the drug is generally not recommended for mass use, since it has toxic side effects and carries the risk of producing cryptic infections. It also appears to be ineffective against Rhodesian trypanosomiasis.

Vector control requires destruction of tsetse fly habitats by selective clearing of vegetation and spraying with insecticides, which are effective only temporarily. Because of the wide range of the tsetse fly, these vector control measures are not economically feasible except when it is necessary to break transmission in epidemics. For individual protection, avoidance of contact with infected tsetse flies is best achieved by the use of repellents and protective clothing.

A vaccine is not presently available because of the occurrence of antigenic variation. However, the potential for development of a vaccine has increased with the progress in cultivation of *T. brucei* in vitro and analysis of the chemical structure of its variant antigens.

Englund PT, Hajduk SL, Marini JC: The molecular biology of trypanosomes. Ann Rev Biochem 51:695, 1982. *An excellent analysis of the biology of trypanosomes.*

Greenwood BM, Whittle HC: The pathogenesis of sleeping sickness. Trans R Soc Trop Med Hyg 74:716, 1980. *A review of the interactions of the host immune response to trypanosomes and their contributions to the pathology and clinical features of sleeping sickness.*

Hajduk SL, Englund PT, Mahmoud AAF, et al.: African trypanosomiasis. In Mandel GL, Douglas RJ, Bennett JE (eds.): Principles and Practice of Infectious Disease. New York, J. Wiley & Sons, 1985, pp 244–252. *An excellent chapter on the biology and clinical features of African trypanosomes.*

Lambert PH, Berney M, Kazyumba G: Immune complexes in serum and in cerebrospinal fluid in African trypanosomiasis. Correlation with polyclonal B cell activation and with intracerebral immunoglobulin synthesis. J Clin Invest 67:77, 1981. *A study of the possible role of immune complexes in the pathogenesis of sleeping sickness.*

Molyneux DH: Selective primary health care: Strategies for control of disease in the developing world: VIII. African trypanosomiasis. Rev Infect Dis 5:945, 1983. *A review of the various chemotherapeutic, vector, and environmental control measures for sleeping sickness.*

Turner M: Antigenic variation in the trypanosome. Nature 298:606, 1982. *A review of this very interesting biologic phenomenon.*

Van Nieuwenhove S, Schechter PJ, DeClercq J, et al.: Treatment of gambiense sleeping sickness in the Sudan with oral DFMO, an inhibitor of ornithine decarboxylase; first field trial. Trans R Soc Trop Med Hygiene 79:692, 1985. *A successful clinical treatment trial of 20 patients with chronic Gambian trypanosomiasis with DFMO, a new nontoxic trypanosomocidal drug.*

Wery M, Mulumba PM, Lambert PH, et al.: Hematologic manifestations, diagnosis and immunopathology of African trypanosomiasis. Semin Hematol 19:83, 1982. *A concise review of the complex immunopathogenesis of African trypanosomiasis and its consequences within the hematopoietic system.*

383 AMERICAN TRYPANOSOMIASIS (Chagas' Disease)

Franklin A. Neva

DEFINITION. Chagas' disease, resulting from infection with the protozoan parasite, *Trypanosoma cruzi*, is named after the Brazilian physician Carlos Chagas, who discovered the parasite. Distinction should be made between infection caused by the parasite, as manifested by positive serologic findings, and clinical disease. Chronic disease manifestations develop years after initial infection in the form of chronic cardiomyopathy with conduction defects or with dysfunction of the esophagus or colon (mega syndromes).

LIFE CYCLE OF ETIOLOGIC AGENT. The causative agent, *T. cruzi*, is usually transmitted as a zoonosis. Various species of blood-sucking reduviids become infected when they take a blood meal from animals or humans who have circulating parasites, trypomastigotes, in the blood. The ingested parasites transform into epimastigotes and multiply in the midgut of the insect vector, where they later transform once again into metacyclic trypomastigotes in the hindgut of the bug. When the infected bug takes a subsequent blood meal, it frequently defecates during or after feeding so that the infective metacyclic forms are deposited on the skin. Transmission to a second vertebrate host occurs when the feeding puncture site or a mucous membrane is inadvertently contaminated with infective bug feces. The parasites can penetrate a variety of host cell types within which they transform into intracellular amastigote forms. In contrast to certain other intracellular organisms, amastigotes of *T. cruzi* are not enclosed in phagolysosomes. They multiply in the cytoplasm, elongate, transform into motile trypomastigotes, and rupture out of the cells. Liberated organisms penetrate new cells or are carried into the bloodstream to initiate further cycles of multiplication, preferentially in muscle cells, or are ingested by new vectors to maintain the cycle (Fig. 383–1).

Asymptomatic infected individuals with low-level parasi-

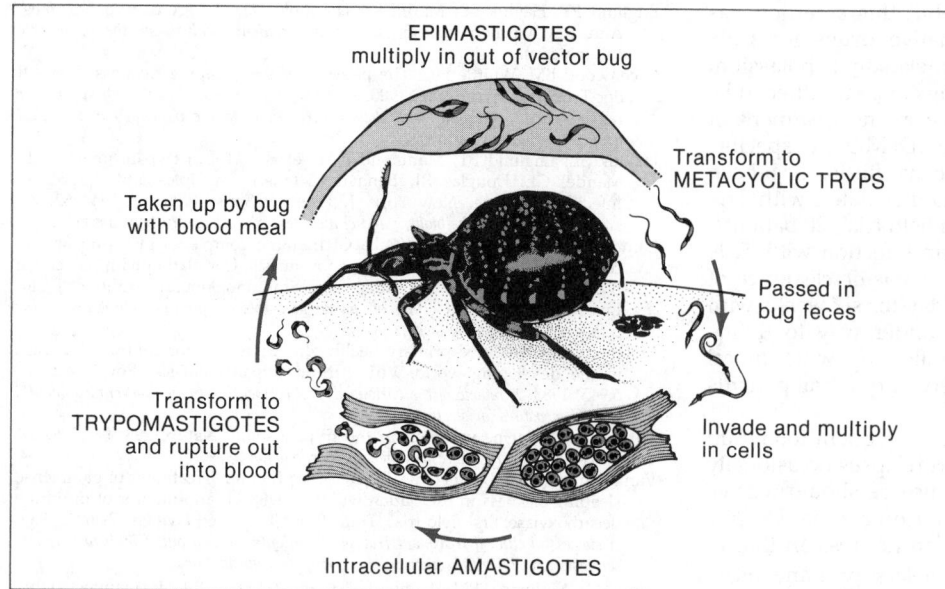

FIGURE 383–1. Life cycle of *Trypanosoma cruzi*.

temia can transmit *T. cruzi* via blood transfusion. Another route of transmission of the parasite is congenital infection.

EPIDEMIOLOGY. *T. cruzi* and its arthropod vectors are widely distributed from the southern United States through Mexico and Central America into South America down to central Argentina and Chile. The parasite is restricted to the Western hemisphere. In most countries where it occurs the parasite cycle is sylvatic, i.e., it takes place in wild animals and vector bugs that associate with them. Human contact with sylvatic vectors is sporadic and accidental. A peridomestic cycle occurs under conditions in which infected animals, such as opposums and rats, live close to human habitations, and vector bugs may invade houses to seek a blood meal. Certain species of triatomine bugs such as *Triatoma infestans*, *Rhodnius prolixus*, and *Panstrongylus megistus* have a great propensity to invade, live, and breed in houses if suitable microenvironments are present. Cracks and holes in adobe mud huts or in crude wooden walls, thatched roofs, and household rubble provide ideal hiding and breeding places for the bugs, which venture out at night to feed upon sleeping inhabitants. Under these conditions *T. cruzi* is transmitted from person to person—a domiciliary cycle—and Chagas' disease becomes a public health problem. Thus, human trypanosomiasis in Latin America is primarily an infection of poor people living in substandard housing in rural areas.

The prevalence of antibodies to the parasite in human populations varies widely in different countries, as well as within regions of a country. A recent nationwide survey in Brazil found about 10 percent of the rural population to be infected. It is not unusual for up to half of all inhabitants in selected villages to have positive serologic findings. Countries with the highest incidence of both infection and disease due to *T. cruzi* include Brazil, Argentina, Chile, Bolivia, and Venezuela. It is estimated that in all of the Americas a total of 15 million people are infected. In many Latin American countries positive serologic findings for *T. cruzi* constitute a social stigma; a lower socioeconomic background is implied, and employers are reluctant to hire someone who may later develop chronic Chagas' disease.

Considerable geographic variation exists in both the prevalence and the type of chronic disease manifestations. In Brazil, for example, cardiomyopathy and megadisease are common, and often a patient has both types of involvement. However, chagasic megaesophagus and megacolon are virtually unknown in Venezuela, Colombia, and Panama, whereas cardiomyopathy is relatively high, moderate and low in prevalence, respectively. In general, the frequency of cardiac disease in Central America and Mexico in seropositive persons

is low, even though rates of seropositivity may be substantial. Also in these countries heart disease tends to develop later in life than in Brazil.

The situation regarding Chagas' disease in the United States is interesting because only four autochthonous acute cases have been recognized despite the presence of *T. cruzi* in vector bugs as well as in animal reservoirs. The lack of transmission of *T. cruzi* to humans in this country is probably due to preference of the vectors for sylvatic habitats and their tendency to defecate late after feeding. Yet in some areas of the West, bites from aggressive and abundant reduviid bugs can be a source of annoyance and allergic reactions to suburbanites and outdoorspeople.

PATHOLOGY AND PATHOGENESIS. In *acute Chagas' disease* a local inflammatory lesion called a chagoma may develop at the site of entry of the parasite. Histologically the chagoma shows mononuclear cell infiltration, interstitial edema, and intracellular aggregates of amastigotes in cells of the subcutaneous tissue and muscle. Other pathologic changes in the acute disease are known only for the severe cases that come to autopsy, since the great majority of cases are subclinical and self-limiting. Biopsy specimens from enlarged lymph nodes show hyperplasia, and amastigotes may be present in reticular cells. Skeletal muscle tissue from muscle biopsies have shown organisms and focal inflammation. In acute cases that have a fatal outcome there is invariably myocarditis with an enlarged heart. Microscopically there is degeneration of cardiac muscle fibers and prominent but patchy areas of inflammation with nests of amastigotes in the muscles. One striking feature of heavily parasitized tissue is the presence of inflammatory foci around infected cells that have ruptured and released parasites, but not around intact infected cells. The brain and meninges may also be parasitized in acute Chagas' disease. Virtually all organs and cell types can be invaded by *T. cruzi*.

The organs primarily affected in *chronic Chagas' disease* are the heart and certain hollow viscera, such as the esophagus and colon. Surprisingly the intracellular *T. cruzi* usually cannot be found in the affected organs, or a few may be demonstrable after protracted search of many tissue sections. The heart in those patients with chronic disease who die suddenly, presumably of ventricular arrhythmias or heart block, may be normal in size or only moderately enlarged. The presence of a prominent lymph node between atria and ventricles in some of these cases has been described. Other patients with chronic chagasic cardiomyopathy develop cardiomegaly and die of intractable failure. The hearts are both hypertrophied and dilated, with thinning, especially at the apex to form a characteristic apical aneurysm. Mural thrombi, with subsequent embolization of the lungs and peripheral organs, are frequently seen. The coronary arteries are generally normal.

Microscopic findings in the heart are not specific, consisting of focal mononuclear cell infiltrates, hypertrophy of cardiac fibers with patchy areas of necrosis, variable fibrosis, and edema. The conduction system of the heart is frequently involved by the inflammatory changes, especially the sinoatrial and atrioventricular nodes and the right branch and left anterior branches of the bundle of His. Andrade's detailed studies of the pathology of the conducting system showed that they correlated well with electrocardiographic changes during life.

When either the esophagus or colon is affected in chronic Chagas' disease, the gross appearance is of dilatation and hypertrophy of the affected organ. As with the heart, the microscopic pathologic changes are disappointing, since they consist of mononuclear inflammatory foci, hypertrophied muscle fibers, patchy fibrosis, and, again, no or very rare organisms. However, myenteric ganglion cells are strikingly reduced in number. This type of parasympathetic denervation may also be found in other hollow viscera, such as duodenum, ureters, or biliary tree.

The significant pathology of *congenital Chagas' disease* is chronic placentitis, with inflammatory changes and focal necrosis in the chorionic villi. Amastigotes of *T. cruzi* are present in the lesions. Presence of lesions and organisms in the placenta may be associated with abortion, stillbirth, or acute disease in the fetus. However, pregnancy may result in a normal fetus even though placental lesions are present.

The extent and clinical significance of pathologic changes in those individuals with antibodies to *T. cruzi* but without evidence of disease, i.e., *the indeterminate form*, is not yet clear. Such indeterminate cases may have significantly reduced numbers of esophageal or colonic ganglion cells. It has been claimed that endocardial biopsy specimens from indeterminate cases have recognizable pathologic changes. In addition, in some indeterminate cases there is a chronic low level of parasitemia. Therefore, one point of view is that everyone with positive serologic findings has a continuing subclinical disease process that will become manifested with time. On the other hand, even in those areas where chronic Chagas' disease is common, one half or more of those with a positive serologic findings will die of causes other than Chagas' disease. In most Latin American countries, where endemicity is much lower, a positive serologic finding constitutes a relatively small risk factor for later chronic disease. Until better information on this issue becomes available, and more importantly, until the pathogenesis of chronic Chagas' disease is unraveled, the distinction between infection and disease caused by *T. cruzi* appears to be valid.

Pathogenesis of acute Chagas' disease is straightforward, but the sequence of events leading to the late manifestations of chronic cardiomyopathy or megadisease is still poorly understood. Key features of the chronic disease that must be explained include the following: (1) a latent period of up to 20 years from presumed initial infection with *T. cruzi* before manifestations of cardiomyopathy or megadisease appear, (2) no or very few intracellular parasites in the affected organs, in contrast to abundant parasites in tissues in acute cases, (3) destruction of autonomic parasympathetic ganglia (Auerbach's plexus) of the esophagus and colon, and (4) great geographic variation in the frequency and type of chronic Chagas' disease. Support for the latter point can be found in recent evidence that different clones of *T. cruzi* have a wide spectrum of biologic characteristics, including virulence for mice. Köberle argued that damage to the autonomic ganglia occurred during the acute disease, but this theory does not readily explain the long interval before chronic disease develops. Some type of autoimmune process affecting the conduction system of the heart and autonomic ganglia of the gut was a popular hypothesis to explain the chronic disease. The demonstration of antibodies in infected patients that reacted with tissue elements gave strong support to the autoimmune concept, but it has been set back by the finding that the autoimmune antibody is heterophile in nature. Direct cell-mediated cytotoxicity to heart muscle has also been proposed as a mechanism for the chronic disease. Exaggerated immune responses to *T. cruzi* are not present in patients with chronic Chagas' disease as compared to those with the indeterminate form, at least as judged by humoral antibody levels and lymphocyte proliferative responses. However, this does not rule out some other autoimmune or immunologic mechanism. In summary, the fundamental mechanism for pathogenesis of chronic Chagas disease remains to be determined.

CLINICAL PRESENTATION. In endemic areas, first exposure to *T. cruzi* generally is subclinical and goes unnoticed. When those initially exposed do develop clinical manifestations the disease is an acute systemic infection. Chronic Chagas' disease, in contrast, evolves as a later sequel with specific organ involvement and no systemic features.

Acute Chagas' Disease. Although acute Chagas' disease is most commonly seen in children, it can occur at any age, depending upon the nature of exposure to the causative organism. The incubation period under natural conditions cannot be established accurately, but is probably at least a week. A local area of erythema and induration (chagoma) may develop in the skin at the site of parasite entry. When infection takes place via the conjunctival route, as it frequently does, the local periorbital swelling is referred to as Romaña's sign. The chagoma is often accompanied by regional adenopathy and persists for several weeks. Other signs of acute Chagas' disease include fever, generalized lymphadenopathy, and hepatosplenomegaly.

Myocarditis, accompanied by tachycardia and nonspecific electrocardiographic changes, can occur in the acute stage. Meningoencephalitis is another serious complication, particularly in very young patients. Fatal outcome in acute Chagas' disease is rare, but when it does occur, it is due to myocarditis and congestive failure or to meningoencephalitis.

Signs and symptoms of acute disease gradually subside within a few weeks to several months even without treatment. Trypanosomes, which have been demonstrable by direct microscopy in the peripheral blood during the acute phase, become more difficult to find and then disappear. The patient then enters the *indeterminate phase*, which is characterized by the presence of antibodies to *T. cruzi*, and often also by the presence of low-level parasitemia in the blood demonstrable only by special sensitive methods. This state of apparent complete recovery with positive serologic findings may continue indefinitely without further evidence of disease or sequelae. However, a variable proportion of indeterminate cases, years to a decade or more later, will develop signs and symptoms of chronic Chagas' disease. Except for epidemiologic experience from a particular geographic region, there are no laboratory or clinical indicators to predict likelihood of future chronic disease.

Chronic Chagas' Disease. Cardiac signs and symptoms are the most common manifestations of chronic disease and are apt to begin with palpitations, dizziness, precordial discomfort, and even syncope. These reflect a variety of arrhythmias, including ventricular extrasystoles, bouts of tachycardia, and various degrees of heart block. Sudden death due to ventricular tachycardia in an otherwise healthy young adult is not at all unusual. Symptoms due to arrhythmias may be present for a long time before cardiomegaly or evidence of cardiac failure appears. When congestive failure develops, it is predominantly right sided and is likely to lead to a fatal outcome within a few years. Peripheral emboli to the brain or other organs are frequent.

Physical examination reveals only an irregular pulse, distant heart sounds, and perhaps a gallop rhythm. With failure, the heart can be very large, functional regurgitant murmurs may be heard, and there is often congestive hepatomegaly and peripheral edema.

The second most common chronic manifestation is megadisease of the esophagus or colon, most frequently the former. The symptoms are indistinguishable from idiopathic achalasia and include dysphagia, feeling of fullness after eating or drinking only small amounts, chest pain, and regurgitation. Aspiration with secondary pneumonia is a common complication in advanced cases, as are weight loss and cachexia. Salivary gland hypertrophy secondary to hypersalivation is sometimes seen. Esophageal cancer is reported to be more frequent in patients with chagasic megaesophagus, as with idiopathic achalasia.

Patients with chagasic megacolon suffer from chronic constipation and abdominal pain. Volvulus, obstruction, and perforation of the bowel may occur. An astonishing history of going several weeks between bowel movements can be obtained from some patients with severe megacolon. Megaesophagus and megacolon may both be present in the same patient, and cardiomyopathy can occur with either form of megadisease.

DIAGNOSIS. For both acute and chronic Chagas' disease a history of possible exposure to *T. cruzi* should be sought. Usual tourist travel to endemic areas is not likely to provide sufficient exposure to infected vectors. Blood transfusion from a chronically infected donor can be a source of infection.

For *acute Chagas' disease* direct microscopic examination of anticoagulated blood or a buffy coat preparation for motile trypanosomes is the most important procedure. Organisms are more difficult to find on stained thin or thick blood films, but the morphology of organisms seen on direct microscopy should be confirmed in a stained preparation. Red cells may be lysed, using 0.083 per cent NH_4Cl to concentrate parasites by centrifugation. If parasites cannot be found in the peripheral blood and acute disease is still suspected, blood can be cultured on NNN or other suitable media. Inoculation of mice with patient's blood may sometimes result in recovery of the parasite. Biopsy of an enlarged lymph node or of skeletal muscle for culture and/or histologic examination is another possibility.

The most sensitive technique for recovery of trypanosomes from the blood is a procedure referred to as xenodiagnosis. It is basically a form of blood culture using the insect vector, by allowing up to 40 normal, laboratory-reared reduviid bugs to feed directly upon the patient, or on the patient's blood through a membrane. Circulating parasites ingested by the bugs multiply in the gut and can be detected when the intestinal contents are examined 30 days later.

Serologic testing is generally not needed for diagnosis of acute disease. Parasite-specific IgM antibodies detected by immunofluorescence or direct agglutination do not become positive until 20 to 40 days after onset of symptoms. In certain situations this delayed antibody response will permit demonstration of seroconversion. Other laboratory tests often show nonspecific changes, such as a lymphocytic leukocytosis, elevated sedimentation rate, or transient electrocardiographic abnormalities. Reversible cardiomegaly and even pericardial effusion may occur.

The diagnosis of *chronic Chagas' disease* requires demonstration of antibodies to *T. cruzi* in the presence of the characteristic cardiac abnormalities and/or megadisease. Thus, except for the positive serologic findings, the diagnosis relies heavily upon clinical judgment in excluding other causes of heart disease or gastrointestinal dysfunction. A positive xenodiagnosis is strongly supportive, but not in itself diagnostic of chronic disease, since patients in the indeterminate phase may have low-level parasitemia. A variety of assays for specific antibody are available, and generally the results of different tests are comparable. However, there are crossreactions in some tests with sera from patients with leishmaniasis or syphilis, for example. Therefore, in individual cases it may be very helpful to confirm the presence of antibody to specific antigens of *T. cruzi* with more sophisticated tests, such as immunoblots.

Symptomatic heart involvement in the chronic disease is manifested by characteristic electrocardiographic abnormalities, often without cardiomegaly. The most common of these is complete right bundle-branch block. Other frequent electrocardiographic findings are left anterior hemiblock, ventricular extrasystoles, and even complete heart block. If heart failure is present, radiographs and echocardiograms will show generalized cardiomegaly with a reduced ejection fraction (Fig. 383–2).

Chagasic megaesophagus in the early stages will show only delayed emptying and minimal dilatation on studies after a barium swallow. With more advanced disease, retention of swallowed material and eosophageal dilatation are progressively increased. Manometric studies will show spasm of the esophageal sphincter and uncoordinated peristaltic movements. Endoscopy should be performed to rule out malignant disease. However, all of these findings are indistinguishable from idiopathic achalasia. Barium enema with air contrast will show the dilated colon with impaired peristalsis, but other causes of colonic obstruction must be ruled out.

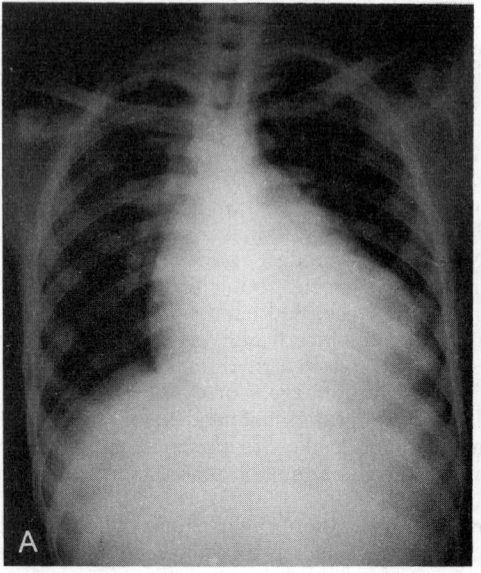
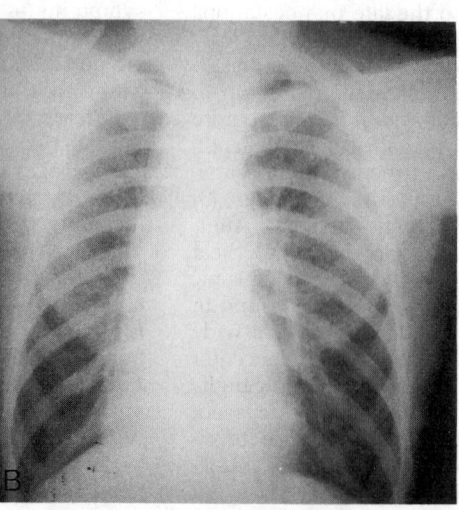

FIGURE 383–2. *A*, Cardiac silhouette in a patient with chronic chagasic cardiomyopathy and heart failure. *B*, Chest x-ray showing a widened mediastinum due to a greatly dilated megaesophagus of chronic Chagas' disease.

DIFFERENTIAL DIAGNOSIS. When acute Chagas' disease is symptomatic and severe, it can resemble a variety of acute systemic infections. Romaña's sign must be distinguished from other causes of unilateral orbital edema, such as the reaction to an insect bite, trauma, or orbital cellulitis.

Congenital infections are virtually indistinguishable from congenital toxoplasmosis, cytomegalic inclusion disease, and syphilis.

Various cardiomyopathies, such as postpartum, alcoholic, and endomyocardial fibrosis can resemble chronic Chagas' heart disease. The characteristic heart murmurs of rheumatic valvular disease are helpful in differentiating this entity from chagasic cardiomyopathy. The value of positive serologic findings for *T. cruzi* in differential diagnosis of both heart and megadisease will depend upon the background prevalence of antibodies in the general population.

TREATMENT. Two drugs with reasonable antitrypanosomal activity are currently in use for treatment of Chagas' disease. One of these is a nitrofuran derivative, nifurtimox (Lampit, Bayer 2502), which has been extensively evaluated. Nifurtimox* is the only drug available in the United States for treatment of Chagas' disease; it is used in a dose of 8 to 12 mg per kilogram per day. The second drug, benznidazole (Radinil, Roche 7-1051), is a nitroimidazole derivative that appears to be equal to nifurtimox in efficacy, although there is less experience with its use. The exact mechanism of antitrypanosomal action of both of these drugs is not known.

There is now considerable evidence that if patients with acute Chagas' disease are treated with either nifurtimox or benznidazole the course of disease and parasitemia usually are reduced. But more importantly, many patients treated in the acute phase never develop antibodies to *T. cruzi*, or do so only transiently. From this observation, plus the fact that xenodiagnosis in such treated patients often does not indicate parasites, it is assumed that parasites can be eliminated and the patient cured if treated in the acute stage. However, nifurtimox is not uniformly effective in producing these results, and parasite strains from certain geographic areas (Brazil) appear to be less responsive to treatment than strains from other countries (Argentina and Chile).

The frequency of side effects from both nifurtimox and benznidazole is high, and since they are administered for 60 to 90 days, drug toxicity is a serious problem. The most common adverse effect with nifurtimox is gastrointestinal intolerance with anorexia, nausea, vomiting, and abdominal pain. Neurologic symptoms include restlessness, insomnia, disorientation, paresthesias, polyneuritis, and even seizures. Skin rashes can also occur. Peripheral neuropathy and bone marrow suppression have been reported with benznidazole. These side effects subside when dosage of the drugs is reduced or treatment is stopped.

Since these drugs have shown effectiveness in treatment of acute Chagas' disease, some Latin American physicians are also treating chronic and indeterminate cases. There is no evidence that established pathologic changes of chronic Chagas' disease can be reversed by nifurtimox or benznidazole therapy. The question whether drug treatment in the indeterminate case, i.e., the asymptomatic patient with positive serologic findings, would prevent development of later chronic disease is controversial. Although it would not be easy, the issue ideally could be settled by a controlled, long-term prospective study. There are some data suggesting that low-level parasitemia, as assessed by xenodiagnosis, can be reduced or eliminated after a course of treatment, but the duration of this effect and the ultimate influence on chronic disease have not been determined. The morbidity, or risks of such treatment versus benefits to be expected, should also be evaluated.

The treatment of patients with established chronic heart disease is supportive. Patients with frequent ventricular premature beats can benefit from antiarrhythmic drugs such as amiodarone. Cardiac pacemakers may prolong survival of those with complete heart block. The congestive failure of chagasic cardiomyopathy is disappointingly refractory to the usual cardiotropic drugs.

More options are open for the management and treatment of megadisease. In the early stages of megaesophagus, pneumatic dilatation of the sphincter is probably more effective than bougienage. For more advanced cases, various surgical procedures involving myotomy of the sphincter or partial resection are necessary. Early stages of megacolon can be managed by manipulation of diet and use of laxatives and occasional enemas. Sometimes resection of an aperistaltic section of the colon can be done in more severe cases.

PREVENTION. Chagas' disease could be eliminated as a serious health problem for the rural poor of Latin America by adequate housing and education. But stark socioeconomic realities dictate another approach to control. This consists mainly of the use of residual insecticides directed at domiciliary vectors. The use of benzene hexachloride (BHC), sprayed once or twice a year, has been very effective when used systematically.

Serologic testing in blood banks to avoid use of seropositive donors is carried out in endemic areas. Another precaution is to add 1:4000 gentian violet to blood 24 hours before use to kill trypanosomes that may be present. Development of vaccines is still in the research stage.

American Trypanosomiasis Research. PAHO Scientific Publication 318, 1975. *Proceedings of an international symposium with useful reviews on all aspects of the subject, including the vector bugs and control of the disease.*

Dvorak J, Gibson C, Maekelt A: A bibliography on Chagas' disease (1968–1984). Washington, D.C., National Institutes of Health, Pan American Health Organization and World Health Organization, 1985. *This Medlars-based computer-processed bibliography is a complete listing of references on an annual basis, by author and subject for the period indicated. For real students of the subject!*

Kirchhoff LV, Neva FA: Trypanosoma species (Chagas' Disease). In Mandel GL, Douglas RG Jr, Bennett JE (eds.): Principles and Practice of Infectious Diseases. 2nd ed. New York, John Wiley & Sons, 1985, pp 1531–1537. *This account has additional details on the parasite, epidemiology, and treatment, as well as many references.*

Laranja FS, Dias E, Nobrega G, et al.: Chagas disease—A clinical, epidemiologic and pathologic study. Circulation 14:1035, 1956. *Even though an old paper, it is an excellent presentation by experienced authors of the clinical epidemiology of heart disease in Brazil.*

Recent advances in Chagas' disease. Papers by various authors. Memorias do Instituto Oswaldo Cruz. Special issue. Supplement to vol. 79, 1984. *This special issue, with all articles in English but by Brazilian authors, consists of papers presented at a symposium held on the 50th anniversary of the death of Carlos Chagas. Articles are largely research oriented, but many are clinical as well.*

384 LEISHMANIASIS

Franklin A. Neva

DEFINITION. Leishmaniasis is a protozoan infection caused by various species of the genus *Leishmania*. Paradoxically the host cells for these intracellular parasites are macrophages, cells that normally help destroy microorganisms. In nature the infection is usually a zoonosis, with transmission of the parasite by sandflies among wild or domestic animals, especially rodents and canines, with humans as incidental hosts.

Human leishmanial infections can result in three main forms of disease, sometimes with dual manifestations in the same patient. The *visceral* form (kala-azar) is a systemic disease with parasites in the reticuloendothelial system, characterized by hepatosplenomegaly, fever, weight loss, leukopenia, and ultimately death if untreated. The *cutaneous* disease is generally

---

*An investigational drug that must be obtained from the Centers for Disease Control Drug Service (404-329-3670).

manifested by one or more indolent ulcers, but a wide spectrum of skin involvement can occur. When parasites from skin lesions sometimes metastasize to produce later destructive lesions of the oronasopharynx, the result is *mucocutaneous leishmaniasis.* Although parasite species is the main determinant for the form of disease, clinical manifestations and outcome are also dependent upon the immune response of the host.

ETIOLOGY. *Leishmania* exist in two morphologic forms, a motile flagellate, or *promastigote,* and a smaller, nonmotile intracellular form, the *amastigote.* Promastigotes are found in the sandfly vector as well as in cultures, both habitats requiring temperatures of about 22 to 26°C. Also called *Leishman-Donovan* or *LD bodies* after their describers, amastigotes are the form of parasite found in humans or other vertebrate hosts. In addition to a nucleus, these 2 by 5 μ round or oval bodies contain a characteristic rodlike structure of extranuclear DNA, the *kinetoplast,* a useful structure in morphologic identification and differentiation from other intracellular organisms.

In the infected animal, leishmania are found only in macrophages, where they multiply by binary fission. An appropriate sandfly vector becomes infected by ingesting infected cells from the skin or blood during a blood meal. In the gut of the sandfly the parasites transform to promastigotes and multiply as spindle-shaped flagellates 15 to 26 μ long and 2 to 3 μ wide. In vectors ultimately capable of transmitting the parasite, promastigotes tend to migrate into the pharynx and buccal cavity. At least seven days are needed before the sandfly becomes infective. The actual mechanism by which infective promastigotes are transferred to a new vertebrate host is not clear—possibly by regurgitation into the bite wound during a blood meal or perhaps even by being rubbed into abrasions after a successful swat. Once inoculated, the promastigotes are taken up by macrophages; they transform into amastigotes and begin to multiply. Amastigotes that rupture from infected macrophages are taken up by adjacent cells; some infected cells may be transported to distant sites via the blood or lymphatics.

Classification of *Leishmania* is based primarily upon patterns of parasite isoenzymes separated by electrophoresis and immunologic reactions of surface and parasite-soluble (EF factors) antigens with monoclonal and polyclonal antisera. Additional taxonomic criteria include hybridization of kinetoplast DNA after treatment with restriction endonucleases and the type of disease produced in experimental animals. For example, *L. donovani* produces a progressive disease in hamsters similar to human visceral disease, and strains of *L. major* produce cutaneous ulcers in BALB/c mice with later visceralization and death. The most meaningful classification of *Leishmania* will probably come from correlating biochemical and immunologic results with biologic characteristics of the organisms. Table 384–1 summarizes geographic distribution and usual clinical features of the main species of *Leishmania.*

PARASITE-HOST INTERACTION. Some of the early events in parasite-macrophage interaction are easier to understand since the recent finding with *L. major* that only organisms in the stationary growth phase, both in culture and in the sandfly vector, are infective. Log phase promastigotes are readily lysed by activation of the classic complement pathway in fresh serum and are susceptible to the oxygen burst of macrophages when ingested. Stationary, or infective, stages are more resistant to both of these host defenses. With *L. donovani,* certain macrophage membrane receptors appear to be required for binding and ingestion of the parasite. After ingestion by macrophages, leishmania are enclosed in a phagocytic vacuole. In contrast to some other intracellular organisms, leishmania not only survive but multiply within phagolysosomes into which lysosomal enzymes are discharged. The parasite is probably protected from this enzyme assault by presence of abundant membrane-bound acid phosphatase. Most, but not all, species of leishmania within infected macrophages can be destroyed by activating the cells or exposing them to specific or nonspecific lymphokines.

Variation in temperature sensitivity of various species of leishmania is a critical factor that determines clinical expression of the disease. For example, *L. donovani* can survive and multiply in macrophages at higher temperatures than cutaneous strains. Among isolates causing cutaneous disease in the Americas, most members of the *L. mexicana* complex are inhibited to a greater extent at 37°C than are strains of the *L. braziliensis* complex. These differences in temperature tolerance probably explain why some varieties of cutaneous leishmaniasis can be treated successfully by local heat.

IMMUNOLOGY. The pattern of humoral and cell-mediated immune responses that normally develops during or after leishmanial infection varies with the clinical form of disease. Serum antibody can be demonstrated by a variety of tests, usually indirect immunofluorescence (IFA) or enzyme-linked immunosorbent assay (ELISA), in patients with established

TABLE 384–1. GEOGRAPHIC DISTRIBUTION AND CLINICAL DISEASE CAUSED BY DIFFERENT SPECIES OF *LEISHMANIA*

Species	Geographic Distribution	Clinical Manifestations
L. mexicana complex (L. m. mexicana, L. m. amazonensis, L. m. venezuelensis, ? others)	New World—from southern U.S. through Central America, northern and central South America, Dominican Republic	Cutaneous ulcers; small proportion of cases may develop diffuse cutaneous (DCL) or mucocutaneous (MCL) leishmaniasis
L. braziliensis complex (L. b. braziliensis, L. b. panamensis, L. b. guyanesis, L. b. peruviana)	New World—from Central America through various parts of South America, including Brazil, Venezuela, Bolivia, Peru to northern Argentina	Cutaneous ulcers; some cases may later develop MCL (probably more likely if cutaneous lesion not treated adequately)
L. major	Northern Africa, Middle East, Central Africa, and southern Asia	Cutaneous ulcers
L. tropica	Middle East and south Asia	Cutaneous ulcers and chronic relapsing cutaneous disease (recidivans form)
L. aethiopica	Ethiopia	Cutaneous ulcers, rarely DCL
L. donovani	Old World—East Africa and south of Sahara, south Asia, including India and Iran	Visceral leishmaniasis; small proportion may develop post-kala-azar dermal leishmaniasis
L. infantum (? separate species)	Old World—North Africa and southern Europe	Visceral leishmaniasis
L. chagasi (? separate species)	New World—Foci in several areas of Brazil, Venezuela, and Colombia, and isolated cases in Central and South America	Visceral leishmaniasis

*DCL = diffuse cutaneous leishmaniasis; MCL = mucocutaneous leishmaniasis.

visceral or cutaneous leishmaniasis. Cell-mediated immunity in leishmaniasis can be evaluated by a delayed hypersensitivity skin test (leishmanin or Montenegro test) or by lymphocyte proliferation to leishmanial antigen. Positive skin test results and lymphocyte proliferation are normally present in patients with cutaneous disease, but only after recovery or effective treatment in patients with visceral disease. Cell-mediated immunity is absent or suppressed during active visceral infections.

Resistance to leishmaniasis is best correlated with presence of cell-mediated immunity. Its absence in visceral disease has already been noted, and it is dramatically demonstrated in a rare form of disease called *diffuse cutaneous leishmaniasis* (DCL). In patients with DCL, not only is there specific anergy to the skin test but parasites are very abundant in lesions, lymphocytes are scanty, lesions do not ulcerate, and response to chemotherapy is poor. Antigen-specific suppressor cells have been demonstrated in DCL. In contrast, a normal immune response in cutaneous leishmaniasis is generally associated with lesions that ulcerate and show relatively few parasites but abundant lymphocytes and even giant cells, plus a positive skin test. This relationship of immune response to clinical forms of disease in leishmaniasis is similar to that in leprosy (see Ch. 304).

Neva FA: Recent advances in the diagnosis and management of leishmaniasis and American trypanosomiasis. In Sande MA, Leech JH, Root RK (eds.): Contemporary Issues in Infectious Diseases. Vol. 7, Parasitic Infections. New York, Churchill Livingstone, (in press). *A recent review that covers details of diagnosis and management of leishmaniasis.*

Sacks DL, Hieny S, Sher A: Identification of cell surface carbohydrate and antigenic changes between noninfective and infective developmental stages of *Leishmania major* promastigotes. J Immunol 134:564, 1985. *This paper provides further evidence of biochemical and immunologic differences between the log phase and stationary infective form of the parasite.*

Turk JL, Bryceson ADM: Immunological phenomena in leprosy and related diseases. Adv Immunol 13:209, 1971. *Provides the clinical and experimental bases for regarding leishmaniasis as a disease spectrum.*

VISCERAL LEISHMANIASIS (Kala-Azar)

EPIDEMIOLOGY. The visceral form of leishmaniasis, caused by *L. donovani* and related organisms, has worldwide distribution. Certain regions continue to be endemic areas of this disease. These include the following: northeastern India, especially Assam and Bihar states; Kenya, Sudan, and Ethiopia in eastern Africa; northeastern China, the shores of the Caspian Sea and Iran in southern Asia; the countries of Europe, North Africa, and the Middle East surrounding the Mediterranean; and northeastern Brazil. In addition to these macrofoci, smaller foci occur outside these areas. In the western hemisphere, for example, visceral leishmaniasis is sporadically seen in southern Brazil, Paraguay, and northern Argentina, as well as in the vicinity of Belem at the mouth of the Amazon. Additionally, there are foci of transmission in Venezuela and Columbia and extending north into Central America with isolated cases reported from El Salvador, Guatemala, Honduras, and even from Mexico.

With such a wide geographic distribution of the disease, it is not surprising that different species of phlebotomine flies are involved in the various regions. What is surprising is that the causative organisms from these widely separated regions are relatively uniform in their properties. Yet some investigators prefer to assign separate species designations to the parasites from certain geographic foci, such as *L. infantum* for the Mediterranean variety and *L. chagasi* for that from Brazil. Although up to now such species designations have been based partly upon epidemiologic grounds, they are likely to be upheld by more discriminating analyses of isoenzyme patterns and DNA characteristics.

FACTORS AFFECTING TRANSMISSION. A common transmission cycle for *L. donovani* that takes place close to people involves dogs as reservoir hosts and sandfly vectors that will also feed on humans. The domestic dog, as well as

wild canines such as the fox, develop a chronic systemic disease very similar to that of humans when infected with *L. donovani*. But an additional unique feature of leishmanial infection in canines is the frequent presence of organisms in the skin, including the nose and ears, which are favorite feeding sites of sandflies. An epidemiologic cycle of the parasite involving wild foxes, domestic dogs, and humans via the vector *Lutzomyia longipalpis* has been documented in northeastern Brazil. The domestic dog has also been incriminated as an important reservoir host for visceral leishmaniasis of the Mediterranean region and in certain areas of China.

Rodents are the likely reservoir in the Sudan, and the activity of the vector, *Phlebotomus orientalis*, is high in clumps of acacia woodland near villages. In Kenya, transmission of disease is associated with termite hills, which serve as resting places for the vector, *P. martini*, and around which village men gather in the evening. However, the animal reservoir in Kenya has not been identified. In some regions such as northeastern India, humans appear to be their own reservoir, and several factors serve to facilitate person-to-person transmission. The vector, *P. argentipes*, has a preference for human blood. The parasite is found in circulating monocytes in Indian cases of kala-azar more frequently than usual. Dermal lesions that develop after the initial disease in Indian patients may be an additional source of parasites for the vector.

The last few decades have seen a resurgence of visceral leishmaniasis in regions where it had disappeared after the widespread use of DDT for malaria control. Phlebotomine populations were greatly reduced around houses, but zoonotic transmission was not affected. When use of residual insecticides was discontinued, transmission to people was reestablished. This has occurred in the countries around the Mediterranean, with an epidemic reported in western Italy.

Outbreak of visceral leishmaniasis have often followed famine, wars, and civil or political disturbances resulting in malnutrition and mass migration of people. It is not known whether this is due to greater exposure to infected vectors, defective immune response, reactivation of latent infection, or a combination of these and other factors.

PATHOLOGY. The organs mainly affected are the liver, spleen, bone marrow, and elements of the reticuloendothelial system in diverse sites. These organs and tissues hypertrophy, with the increased cells made up of parasitized macrophages and histiocytes, but with little or no lymphocytic response. Generalized enlargement of lymph nodes is not a consistent finding (see below), but hyperplasia of lymphoid tissue in the nasopharynx and in the Peyer's patches of the gut is common. Endothelial proliferation occurs in certain organs as within septa of pulmonary alveoli and in renal glomeruli.

The spleen is enlarged, sometimes to tremendous size, but is firm and has a thick capsule. Although the splenic pulp is friable and there may be infarcts, the nature and chronic course of the enlargement make the spleen relatively resistant to tears from an aspirating needle. Enlargement of the liver is due to hyperplasia of the Kupffer cells, which are packed with amastigotes. Only rarely are parenchymal cells of the liver parasitized. There may be focal granulomas and some fibrosis in the liver in chronic untreated cases.

The bone marrow is infiltrated with parasitized macrophages, a process that may later impair red and white cell production. The enlarged spleen undoubtedly also contributes to the anemia and leukopenia. There is a striking polyclonal B cell activation that results in high IgG and total serum protein values. Some organs, most notably the kidneys, may show pathologic changes secondary to deposition of immune complexes.

In the early stages of visceral leishmaniasis, small nodules in the skin containing parasites have been described at or near the site of inoculation. There are scattered reports of parasites being demonstrated even in apparently normal skin. A more obvious type of skin involvement, although variable

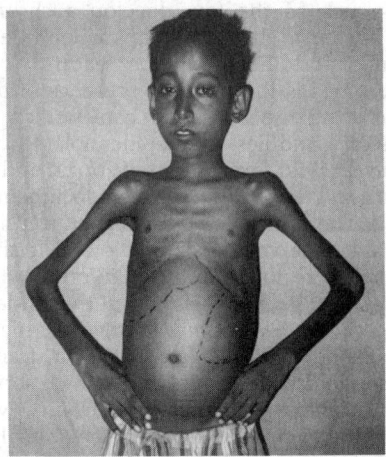

FIGURE 384–1. Indian patient with kala-azar. Note wasting of thorax and shoulder girdle and hepatosplenomegaly as outlined.

by geographic location, is post–kala-azar dermal leishmaniasis (PKDL). This is the development in some patients after recovery from disease of a variety of skin lesions, some of which may contain large numbers of parasites (see below).

CLINICAL FEATURES. The incubation period is long, generally one to three months, but it may be as short as 10 to 14 days. There are well documented instances of activation of latent infection several years after exposure to the parasite, under conditions of immunosuppression. The onset is usually insidious and difficult to date, especially among people who regard intermittent fevers and lassitude as normal. Fever, accompanied by sweating, weakness, and weight loss, gradually becomes noticeable. These symptoms, perhaps including nonproductive cough and abdominal discomfort produced by an enlarging liver and spleen, may continue for months with the patient still up and about. In some patients the course of disease is more rapid, with high temperature and chills, simulating typhoid fever or acute brucellosis. The most prominent physical findings are fever, splenomegaly, and cachexia, which is especially evident in the thorax and shoulder girdle (Fig. 384–1). Although the fever pattern can be variable, ultimately it often exhibits characteristic twice-daily elevations to 38 to 40°C for some time. Generalized adenopathy is common in patients from some geographic areas, but it is seldom striking. In light-skinned patients hyperpigmentation of the skin may be noted; the term *kala-azar* is Hindi for black sickness. Splenic enlargement can be extreme in this disease, often reaching the iliac fossa, and the organ is firm and nontender. Some otherwise typical cases may involve only modest hepatosplenomegaly.

COURSE AND COMPLICATIONS. Although there is strong indirect evidence from skin tests and serologic results that spontaneous recovery from visceral leishmaniasis can occur, it probably happens only early in the course of infection. As the disease progresses, weight loss, anemia, and other signs become clinically more apparent. Subcutaneous edema, ascites, and other evidence of hypoalbuminemia may develop. Bleeding from the nose or gums can occur. Finally, after an illness that may be as short as a few months or as long as a year, the patient becomes emaciated and exhausted. In the great majority of instances death is due to intercurrent infections such as pneumonia, tuberculosis, dysentery, and gangrenous stomatitis. Advanced cases are particularly susceptible because of leukopenia and undoubted impairment of cell-mediated immunologic function, although specific mechanisms have not been defined. Another cause of death is massive gastrointestinal bleeding.

POST–KALA-AZAR DERMAL LESIONS OR PKDL. As noted earlier, a wide spectrum of skin lesions has been described after recovery from kala-azar. They have been reported more often in India than elsewhere and are often

located on the face. Papular or nodular lesions may resemble DCL and contain many parasites, but macular and depigmented lesions without parasites have also been noted. No consistent immunologic abnormality has been demonstrated in patients with PKDL, and they have no systemic evidence of disease.

SPECIFIC LABORATORY DIAGNOSIS. Since other clinical states may mimic certain features of visceral leishmaniasis, demonstration of the parasite, preferably by culture, is essential before treatment is undertaken. In addition, presence or absence of the parasite can be used to monitor response to treatment. Organisms are most readily recovered by aspiration from bone marrow, spleen (Color plate 5F), liver, lymph nodes, or blood. Material obtained is:

1. Used to make smears and slides stained with Giemsa or other Romanovsky stains for examination under oil immersion for amastigotes. Although bone marrow aspiration is usually the method of choice, splenic aspiration can be done if the spleen is readily palpable, if prothrombin and bleeding times are normal, and if proper technique is used. For this, a 21-gauge needle on a 10-ml syringe, with insertion and withdrawal in one second or less, is recommended (see Chulay and Bryceson for details).

2. Inoculated into one or more NNN slants and overlaid with a liquid phase of balanced salt solution containing antibiotics (not antifungal agents!). Other liquid media containing 30 per cent fetal bovine serum (FBS) can be used, but efficacy may vary, depending upon strain or species of *Leishmania* and lots of FBS used. Cultures are incubated at 22 to 26°C (not 37°C); if cultures are positive, organisms are usually seen within 10 to 14 days, but up to 30 days may be required.

3. Inoculated into hamsters, since they are usually quite susceptible to *L. donovani*. However, three to four months may be required before organisms are found in their liver or spleen, so this method is not very practical.

Immunologic Tests. By the time patients with visceral leishmaniasis come to clinical attention, they invariably have readily demonstrable antileishmanial serum antibodies. For this, the ELISA test using promastigotes as antigen, is probably the most practical; it can be read visually if necessary and is applicable for testing large numbers of sera, including specimens eluted from filter paper. The IFA test employing either amastigotes or promastigotes as antigen has been used, as has direct agglutination of fixed promastigotes. In certain areas of Latin America, there may be cross-reactions with sera from people infected with *Trypanosoma cruzi*. The leishmanin skin test for delayed hypersensitivity is negative in cases of active visceral leishmaniasis, but becomes positive after recovery. A low frequency of positive leishmanin reactors among certain populations residing in endemic areas but without a history of visceral leishmaniasis is generally interpreted as evidence for inapparent or subclinical infections.

Laboratory Findings. Most of the laboratory abnormalities involve the hematopoietic system. Leukopenia, with absolute reductions in neutrophils and eosinophils and a relative increase in lymphocytes and monocytes, is characteristic. In one series the total white cell count was below 4000 in 90 per cent of cases by one month after onset of symptoms, and it frequently may be around 2000. Thrombocytopenia is also present, and the erythrocyte sedimentation rate is increased. A moderately severe normocytic and normochromic anemia, unless complicated by blood loss or deficiency states, is very common, caused by increased red cell destruction. In late stages of the disease prothrombin, bleeding, and clotting times are prolonged.

Total serum proteins are increased to levels of 9 to 10 grams per deciliter, virtually all IgG, because of polyclonal B cell activation. Serum albumin levels, especially in advanced cases, are normal or low. The striking hyperglobulinemia is the basis for the old recommended diagnostic tests, such as the formol-gel test and Chopra reaction, before specific serodiagnosis was available. Evidence for circulating immune complexes, based upon C1q binding in the serum, is readily demonstrable. Liver function tests show only mild abnormalities, if any.

DIFFERENTIAL DIAGNOSIS. Chronic malaria in endemic regions may present some problems in differential diagnosis. In malaria-immune individuals the presence of malaria parasites in the blood does not rule out the additional diagnosis of leishmaniasis. Conversely, an enlarged spleen is hardly enough on which to base the diagnosis. Tropical splenomegaly syndrome (an exaggerated immune response to malaria) easily could be confused with the clinical picture of visceral leishmaniasis. Several different forms of schistosomiasis may also mimic visceral leishmaniasis: the acute disease with fever and hepatosplenomegaly, the severe chronic variety with Symmers' fibrosis and portal hypertension, and chronic relapsing enteric fever that can be a complication of schistosomiasis. Other diseases that may resemble kala-azar include lymphoma, cirrhosis of the liver with hypersplenism, miliary tuberculosis, brucellosis, typhoid fever, and subacute bacterial endocarditis.

TREATMENT. The drug of choice for treatment has been and remains pentavalent antimony, even with novel approaches to possible use of other drugs. The antimony preparation available in the United States* and some European countries is sodium stibogluconate (Pentostam), a preparation containing 100 mg antimony (Sb) per milliliter. The dose is 0.2 ml per kilogram of body weight, given daily by intramuscular or intravenous injection, not exceeding 1000 mg Sb per day. Another pentavalent antimony preparation used in Latin America, meglumine antimonate (Glucantime), is virtually identical, but contains 85 mg Sb per milliliter. The total dosage required for cure varies in different parts of the world; Mediterranean kala-azar generally responds to 10 or 15 doses, whereas the disease in Kenya requires 30 injections, and up to 30 per cent of cases may still relapse within six months. Pentavalent antimony is relatively nontoxic in comparison to trivalent Sb, except for local pain at the injection site when given intramuscularly. Other side effects are cumulative with dose and include arthralgias, weakness, nausea, vomiting, slight elevation of liver enzyme values, and nonspecific T wave changes if electrocardiograms are obtained.

Response to treatment is not dramatic and may not be apparent for several weeks. Useful indicators to follow are temperature, spleen size, hemoglobin, and white blood count. Weekly splenic aspirates were used by one group, with "cure" defined as two successively negative aspirates a week apart. Since relapse may occur up to a year after apparent cure, monthly follow-up for six months and then follow-up after a year are recommended.

Primary unresponsiveness to Sb, that is, little or no improvement during or after the first course, occurs in up to 10 per cent of cases. Actual resistance of the parasite to Sb has been difficult to document in man; therefore, lack of response may reflect ineffective immune mechanisms of the host. Allopurinol, in a dosage of 15 mg per kilogram per day combined with Sb, is reported of benefit in some unresponsive cases. Pentamidine is a second-line drug. The dosage of pentamidine† is 4 mg per kilogram given intramuscularly three times weekly for ten doses, but severe pain at the injection site is common, and sterile abscess formation can occur. Additional systemic side effects of anorexia, nausea, abdominal pain, hypotension, and development of diabetes in 10 per cent of patients make the decision to use pentamidine a difficult one. Another second-line drug, amphotericin B, must be given intravenously on alternate days at 1 mg per kilogram each time over many weeks to achieve the recom-

mended total dosage of 1.5 to 2.0 grams. This drug regularly produces chills, fever, and nausea with each dose and a cumulative reduction of hemoglobin and renal function. New approaches to treatment include use of allopurinol derivatives and incorporation of drugs in liposomes for more efficient and prolonged uptake by macrophages.

Supportive treatment can be very important, especially in the malnourished and debilitated. These patients are prone to develop complicating bacterial infections for which proper treatment must be instituted. Fluid and electrolyte imbalance must be corrected, and hemorrhagic complications may require blood transfusion. Good nursing care, attention to oral hygiene, adequate diet, and correction of nutritional deficiencies are, of course, desirable.

PREVENTION. Since the epidemiology of kala-azar varies between different geographic areas, the local conditions responsible for transmission must be understood to implement preventive measures. Where sandflies are in or around houses, vector control with insecticides is appropriate. If an animal reservoir such as the domestic dog is involved, destruction of infected dogs, especially strays, can be instituted. If focal sites of infected flies are known, they can be destroyed or avoided. Personal protection by wearing protective clothing in the evenings, use of insect repellents, and sleeping under fine mesh netting is applicable under some circumstances.

Badaro R, Jones TC, Carvalho EM, et al.: New perspectives on a subclinical form of visceral leishmaniasis. J Infect Dis 154:1003, 1986. *A prospective epidemiologic study in Brazil that documents a feature of kala-azar long suspected, namely, that subclinical infection is common and some infected individuals recover spontaneously.*

Chulay JD, Bryceson ADM: Quantitation of amastigotes of *Leishmania donovani* in smears of splenic aspirates from patients with visceral leishmaniasis. Am J Trop Med Hyg 32:475, 1983. *This reference describes the way to observe patients under treatment, including details of their technique for splenic aspiration.*

CUTANEOUS LEISHMANIASIS OF THE OLD WORLD (ORIENTAL SORE) AND NEW WORLD (INCLUDING MUCOCUTANEOUS OR ESPUNDIA)

EPIDEMIOLOGY. Although basically the same disease, there are differences in epidemiology and clinical course in cutaneous leishmaniasis of the Old and New Worlds. In the Mediterranean basin, Middle East, and southern Asia the disease tends to be clinically more benign and occurs in semiarid and desert climates; transmission can become established in villages and cities. Cutaneous leishmaniasis in the Americas is acquired by workers in the jungle or by farmers and their families living at its edges. The New World disease sometimes produces later metastatic and destructive lesions of the mucous membranes.

The epidemiology of cutaneous leishmaniasis is best understood in southern Russia, Iran, and Middle Eastern countries where infected desert rodents (*Rhombomys opimus* and *Psammomys obesus*) live in burrows with phlebotomine vectors (often *Phlebotomus papatasii*). People are infected with *L. major* when they invade this environment to establish settlements or excavate archaeologic ruins. If settlements are established, the parasite may adapt to a new transmission cycle with dogs and humans as reservoirs and an urban sandfly such as *P. sergenti* as vector. Parasite species from such locations are often identified as *L. tropica*. The commonness of typical face scars in adults in Iran, Afghanistan, Syria, and Iraq indicates the high frequency of cutaneous leishmaniasis in these countries.

The epidemiology of cutaneous leishmaniasis in West Africa and the sub-Sahara belt is less clear. Human cases are sporadic, with a rural transmission cycle, and the parasite species is often *L. major*. In Ethiopia and Kenya, however, the animal reservoir is often the hyrax (*Procavia*), the vector is *Phlebotomus longipes*, and the parasite species is *L. aethiopica*.

In the Americas, cutaneous leishmaniasis occurs from Texas to northern Argentina, with only Chile free of the disease. Except for some areas of Peru, where the domestic dog is a

---

*From Centers for Disease Control, 404-329-3670, 8:00 A.M. to 4:39 P.M. EST Monday through Friday; 404-329-2888, evenings, weekends, and holidays.

†Available from Centers for Disease Control, Atlanta.

reservoir, New World cutaneous leishmaniasis is a forest or jungle zoonosis with forest rodents or sloths serving as animal reservoirs. Western hemisphere sandfly vectors are now classified as members of the genus *Lutzomyia*.

The organism in Texas (ten human cases), Mexico, and northern Central America is mainly *Leishmania m. mexicana*. Members of the *L. braziliensis* complex are predominant in the remainder of Central America, Panama, and northern South America. This species complex also extends into Brazil, Bolivia, and tropical regions of Peru, with complex ecologic combinations of jungle animal reservoirs and sandfly vectors. Yet within the major distribution of a group, there may be isolated pockets of a second species complex, such as *L. b. braziliensis* from Belize where *L. mexicana* predominates, or *L. mexicana* from the Atlantic coast of Panama, and *L. m. amazonensis* from many sites of central Brazil. Additional members of the two major complexes, or even new species, are likely to be described as newer methods of taxonomy are applied.

PATHOLOGY. The earliest changes at the site of inoculation have not been described. Established lesions show a large accumulation of macrophages containing amastigotes, with variable numbers of lymphocytes and plasma cells. There may be focal accumulations of polymorphonuclear cells, especially in areas of necrosis, but the exact mechanism for ulceration of the epithelium is not clear. With time, numbers of parasites diminish and the lesion heals. In other instances the lesion persists and a granulomatous histologic reaction is seen, including multinucleated giant cells. This is the type of pathology seen in *chronic relapsing cutaneous leishmaniasis*, also known as the *lupoid* or *recidivans* form. Delayed skin test reactivity to leishmanial antigen is present in normally healing and recidivans leishmaniasis.

The unusual complication known as diffuse cutaneous leishmaniasis (DCL), associated with anergy to leishmanial antigen, has a different histologic picture. DCL lesions show a heavy infiltrate of foamy or vacuolated macrophages containing large numbers of amastigotes with only scant numbers of lymphocytes. Moreover, the overlying epithelium is not ulcerated.

The lesions of mucocutaneous leishmaniasis (espundia) represent metastatic spread of organisms via the bloodstream to mucuous membranes of the nose, mouth, and upper pharyngeal tissues. The histology is a confusing mixture of granulomatous inflammatory cell reaction with necrosis, fibrosis, and often response to secondary bacterial infection. Organisms are usually scanty. Tissue destruction can involve cartilage with perforation of the nasal septum, loss of much of the nose and palate, and even involvement of the larynx.

CLINICAL MANIFESTATIONS. The lesion begins as a small erythematous papule on exposed areas, often the face or extremities, within two to eight weeks after infection. The papule develops a tiny vesicle that opens and oozes some serous fluid and enlarges to form an ulcer with firm, raised, and reddened edges. The ulcer can remain relatively dry with a central crust (dry form) or may ooze (wet form). Lesions can be single or multiple; small satellite papules may occur at the edge of a larger lesion. Subcutaneous nodules in a centripetal alignment from an ulcer may develop (sporotrichoid form). Cutaneous leishmanial lesions will generally heal spontaneously, but the process can take a few months to a year or more. The result is a depressed, depigmented scar. *Recidivans* or *lupoid leishmaniasis* may sometimes develop, persisting for years. This lesion exhibits central healing with papules developing in the periphery or center of the scar. Regional adenopathy may or may not occur with cutaneous leishmaniasis; this finding is not helpful in differential diagnosis.

COMPLICATIONS. Metastatic spread of parasites and development of destructive naso-oropharyngeal lesions is a serious later sequel to cutaneous disease. This mucuos membrane involvement occurs almost exclusively in the western hemisphere and is said to be associated primarily with *L. braziliensis* infections. Mucocutaneous disease due to *L. mexicana amazonensis* does occur, so until more data correlating parasite type with clinical disease are available, this complication is best related to geographic region rather than parasite species. Thus, mucocutaneous leishmaniasis is most common in central Brazil and adjacent portions of Bolivia, Peru, and Ecuador, and relatively uncommon in Panama and Central America. Mucosal involvement generally does not become manifested until the initial skin lesion has healed, even many years later, and presumably is more likely to occur if there has been no or inadequate treatment of the original ulcer.

Earliest signs and symptoms of mucosal disease commonly involve the nose, with epistaxis and obstruction. Perforation of the nasal septum is common, or the upper lip may be involved. The process can destroy cartilaginous structures of the nose and palate and extend to the larynx. Death may result from aspiration pneumonia or suffocation. Distinction should be made between the mucuous membrane involvement that occurs as direct extension from a facial lesion, as in Ethiopia, and the late metastatic form seen in South America.

DCL is a rare complication that offers insight into immunity to leishmaniasis because it features antigen-specific anergy and cell-mediated imunosuppression. DCL seems to occur more commonly in certain countries (Dominican Republic, Venezuela, and Ethiopia) and in the Americas is caused by organisms belonging to the *L. mexicana* complex. The disease begins with one or only a few nodular lesions that do not ulcerate but go on to metastasize to other cutaneous sites, primarily the face and extensor surfaces of the limbs. The subcutaneous nonulcerative nodular lesions are not associated with fever or other systemic symptoms and do not involve visceral organs. The appearance, distribution, and chronic nature of DCL have often led to the erroneous diagnosis of lepromatous leprosy (Fig. 384–2). There is no mortality associated with DCL, but disfigurement and ulceration secondary to trauma at pressure points lead to morbidity, since this disease is notoriously unresponsive to the usual antileishmanial drugs.

DIAGNOSIS. Leishmaniasis can be suspected in anyone who develops one or more chronic ulcers on exposed areas of skin after recently visiting or working at archaeologic sites in the Middle East, at Mayan ruins, or in jungle or rural areas of Latin America. Ideally, diagnosis should be confirmed by culture of the organism in NNN or other appropriate media

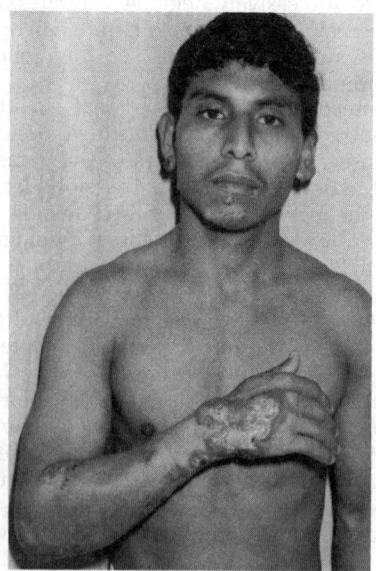

FIGURE 384–2. Patient with diffuse cutaneous leishmaniasis of five years duration. Note nonulcerative lesions of chin, earlobes, right arm, and hand.

from a biopsy or aspirated specimen obtained from the edge of the lesion. Culture is the most sensitive method for detection of organisms. Excisional or punch biopsy offers an additional advantage of providing a portion of the specimen for histopathologic examination and routine bacteriologic, fungal, and acid-fast cultures in cases in which a wider differential diagnosis is required. Appropriate impression smears can also be made and stained from biopsy material, whether culture is possible or not. If biopsy is not possible because of circumstances or location of the lesion, scrapings from a slit made in involved skin or from the debrided base of an ulcer can be cultured or stained for organisms. The characteristic amastigotes in lesions appear larger and are more easily recognized in smears than in tissue sections. A recent technique that may permit direct and rapid diagnosis, as well as species differentiation of leishmania, is blotting with radiolabeled DNA probes. The numbers of parasites present and ease of culture vary with the strain, but the concentration of parasites in lesions tends to diminish with time as healing occurs, and they are also reduced if the ulcer is secondarily infected with bacteria. It is usually more difficult to culture or demonstrate organisms in lesions of mucocutaneous disease.

A positive leishmanin skin test and serum antibody can usually be demonstrated in patients by the time a cutaneous lesion has ulcerated. These tests remain positive in mucocutaneous disease. Serologic tests are not very useful in diagnosis because antibody levels are low. It must also be remembered that positive skin and serologic tests can reflect a previous rather than a current leishmanial infection.

Cutaneous leishmaniasis must be differentiated from the following conditions, with decreasing likelihood of occurrence: nonspecific tropical or traumatic ulcers due to bacterial infection or stasis; fungal infections, especially sporotrichosis and blastomycosis; mycobacterial infections such as *Mycobacterium marinum* and *tuberculosis*; syphilis and other treponematoses of the skin; sarcoidosis and neoplastic ulcers. Mucocutaneous leishmaniasis is especially likely to mimic infection with *Paracoccidiodes brasiliensis*, histoplasmosis, Wegener's disease, midline granuloma, or rhinoscleroma.

TREATMENT. As described earlier for visceral leishmaniasis, the standard and recommended treatment for cutaneous leishmaniasis is pentavalent antimony, available in the United States as Pentostam.* The dose is 0.15 to 0.2 ml per kilogram by intramuscular or slow intravenous injection, not exceeding 10 ml per dose. The drug is given daily for 10 to 20 days. Modest elevation of liver enzymes and/or mild nonspecific ST or T wave electrocardiographic changes may occur during therapy, especially after six or eight doses. These changes are generally not associated with symptoms, but it may be prudent to monitor them.

Old World cutaneous leishmaniasis, especially in patients from the Middle East, will often heal spontaneously within six months. Since leishmaniasis in this region does not metastasize to mucosal tissues, treatment may justifiably be withheld if the lesion is not extensive and appears to be healing.

In contrast, if the infection is known or suspected to originate from an endemic area of mucocutaneous disease, some authorities recommend prolonged (15 to 20 days) or multiple-course therapy. However, healing of the lesion is the ultimate clinical criterion for successful treatment.

Regardless of the infecting species of parasite, it is not unusual for cutaneous leishmanial lesions to require a second course of antimony treatment. Two weeks of rest and clinical observation are generally allowed between courses of treatment. Although different strains of leishmania can vary in their susceptibility to antimony, there is no evidence of drug resistance. Yet the circumstances required to eliminate the

organisms from a lesion are not fully understood, and probably a normal immunologic response on the part of the host is required.

Amphotericin B is indicated in cases in which antimonials have failed to control the disease. Side effects are common and can be severe. The effective total dose is lower than for many systemic mycoses, with a total dose of 1.5 to 2.0 grams for a 60-kg adult often being sufficient.

A number of other drugs with varying degrees of antileishmanial activity may be useful in treatment under certain circumstances. Ketoconazole* in a daily dose of 400 or 600† mg may be effective, but must be given for four weeks. Other orally administered drugs such as rifampin or metronidazole have been touted on the basis of limited or uncontrolled trials, but they are clearly inferior to antimony. Innovative approaches to therapy are under way with allopurinol analogues, liposome-encapsulated compounds, and even topically applied drugs; their ultimate usefulness remains to be established. The application of local heat (40° to 41°C) for 25 hours or more over a period of four or five days may be effective for lesions caused by the *L. mexicana* complex organisms.

PREVENTION. Transmission of leishmaniasis in cities can be prevented by control of sandfly populations with insecticides or destruction of breeding sites. Where reservoirs and vectors are sylvatic, other measures must be employed, such as insect repellents and use of protective clothing over exposed part of the body. Vaccines should theoretically be effective, since there is immunity to second episodes of cutaneous disease. However, the effectiveness of immunization with either viable or killed organisms has been difficult to evaluate.

---

*This use is not listed in the manufacturer's directive.
†Exceeds the dose recommended by the manufacturer.

Neva FA: Diagnosis and treatment of cutaneous leishmaniasis. In Remington JS, Swartz MN (eds.): Current Clinical Topics in Infectious Diseases. New York, McGraw-Hill Book Company, 1982, Vol 3, p 364. *More detailed account of these aspects of the subject.*

Petersen EA, Neva FA, Barral A, et al.: Monocyte suppression of antigen-specific lymphocyte responses in diffuse cutaneous leishmaniasis patients from the Dominican Republic. J Immunol 132:2603, 1984. *Further characterization of the immune defect in DCL patients, including restoration of cell-mediated response by HLA-matched monocytes from skin test–positive relatives.*

---

385 TOXOPLASMOSIS
Henry Masur

Toxoplasmosis is a common disease of birds and mammals caused by the protozoon *Toxoplasma gondii*. The name *T. gondii* is descriptive of this arc-shaped protozoon, being derived from the Greek word *toxon*, meaning arc, and from the name of the North African rodent *gondi*. in which the organism was first recognized. *T. gondii* currently infects over 500 million humans around the world. This obligate intracellar organism can proliferate readily and cause clinically important disease in individuals with normal or abnormal immune function. A clear distinction must be kept in mind between *T. gondii* infection, which is defined by the presence of viable organisms in a patient, and toxoplasmosis, a relatively uncommon occurrence that indicates an active disease process.

THE PROTOZOAN. Three forms exist in the life cycle of *T. gondii*: the *cyst*, the *trophozoite*, and the *oocyst*. The trophozoite has an arc or oval form and is about 3 to 4 μ in diameter and 6 to 7 μ in length. It is an obligate intracellular form that proliferates in acute infection. Trophozoites can enter vacuoles in any nucleated mammalian cell. They divide by endodyogeny, an asexual process whereby two daughter cells are formed within one parent cell. Division continues until the cell ruptures, releasing trophozoites to infect adjacent cells. As the host develops immunity, trophozoite proliferation slows.

Toxoplasma cysts are 10 to 200 μ forms that contain several thousand very slowly dividing organisms; these appear to develop within host cells. Cysts can be seen in any tissue, but they are most commonly found in brain, skeletal muscle, and cardiac muscle. Cysts are more resistant to environmental conditions than are trophozoites, and are able to remain viable after exposure to digestive enzymes.

Oocysts are 10 to 12 μ oval forms that exist uniquely in the intestinal mucosa of cats. Toxoplasma released from cysts or oocysts in the cat intestine enter epithelial cells where they proliferate and then mature by gametogony into microgametocytes or macrogametocytes. A zygote is formed by the union of the gametocytes; this zygote matures in one to four days into an oocyst. Large quantities of oocytes (up to 10 million per day) are excreted by the cat for one to three weeks beginning three to five days after ingestion of the *Toxoplasma*-containing tissue. Cats also get a concurrent systemic infection. Oocysts are not infectious until they undergo sporogony outside the body, a process that requires 1 to 21 days, depending on environmental conditions. Oocysts are quite hardy: they can exist outside the body for at least a year in warm moist soil.

EPIDEMIOLOGY. *Toxoplasma* infection is a world-wide zoonosis. Natural infection occurs by ingestion of cysts or oocysts and by transplacental transmission. In nature the cycle of infection is probably maintained by cats and birds and small mammals. Primary human infection usually occurs by accidental ingestion of infected cat feces or by consumption of inadequately cooked meat. The relative importance of these primary routes probably depends on the amounts of rare meat consumed, hygienic practices, and the proximity of a feline population. When cats consume infected animals or inadequately cooked meat scraps they become infected and excrete oocysts. Children are particularly likely to come into contact with contaminated cat feces when playing in sand, or to inhale aerosolized dried feces under dusty conditions. Cockroaches and flies have also been shown to transfer oocysts to uncovered food.

In North America and Western Europe where many cats are confined to the home and eat only processed foods, and where food is usually covered and refrigerated, the consumption of rare meat is probably of greater epidemiologic importance than contact with cats or insects. Pork and lamb are more likely to contain cysts than is beef. If meat is not cooked to 60°C, or frozen to −20°C (a temperature not reliably reached by most commercial freezers), the cysts will be infective.

Toxoplasma has been transmitted rarely by needle stick accidents involving laboratory workers, by accidental inoculation during autopsy procedures, and by transplantation of an infected heart or kidney. Some immunodeficient patients (particularly those with chronic myelogenous leukemia) have parasitemia, and persistent parasitemia for a year has been described in an apparently healthy individual.

Secondary *Toxoplasma* infection can occur by transplacental transmission. Such transmission occurs only if the mother acquires *Toxoplasma* infection during the pregnancy or perhaps during the few months prior to conception. The frequency of congenital toxoplasmosis is thus dependent on the frequency with which women of childbearing age acquire *Toxoplasma* infection. In the United States and Europe 0.5 to 1 per cent of women show high or rising antitoxoplasma titers during pregnancy. The likelihood of transmission increases progressively during successive trimesters of pregnancy from 17 to 65 per cent.

The frequency of *Toxoplasma* infection in any population depends on a variety of sociologic, economic, and environmental factors. Among both men and women there is increasing prevalence of positive serologic results with increasing age. In the United States less than 1 per cent of infants have congenital *Toxoplasma* infection; there is an abrupt rise in incidence during teenage years; and from age 15 to 50 years there is an increase of approximately 1 per cent per year. Thus, about 20 to 70 per cent of adults in this country have positive serologic tests for *Toxoplasma* infection, the precise number depending on the specific population studied. Individuals in cold, arid, or mountainous regions tend to have a lower frequency than those in tropical areas. There are isolated communities that have little or no *Toxoplasma* infection. The regional variations cannot all be explained on the basis of meat-eating habits, the presence of felines, or climatic extremes.

PATHOGENESIS AND PATHOLOGY. *Toxoplasma* are liberated from cysts or oocysts in the gastrointestinal tract where they multiply in the mucosal cells. Trophozoites then disseminate via the bloodstream or lymphatics to infect any nucleated host cell. Multiplication of the trophozoites within host cell vacuoles does not appear to disturb host cell function until the dividing organisms cause the cell to rupture. As adjacent cells are infected and they are themselves ruptured, progressive tissue necrosis occurs and an inflammatory response is elicited. The inflammatory response typically consists of mononuclear cells, a few polymorphonuclear cells, and edema. How extensive the tissue necrosis and dissemination become depends on the effectiveness of both humoral and cellular immune mechanisms. Although any organ can be involved, small foci of infection are most often established in lymph nodes, skeletal muscle, myocardium, and brain. Even after effective immunologic response the organisms are not eradicated: A few cysts form in these organs as early as the first week of infection and remain dormant for the lifetime of the host unless host immunity is diminished, in which case active proliferation of the organisms can again cause substantial local disease and dissemination. In some patients primary infection can be associated with widely disseminated disease: Most of these patients have defects in cell-mediated immune mechanisms.

Histopathologically the changes in lymph nodes are so characteristic of toxoplasmosis that they are virtually diagnostic even in the absence of a visualized or cultivated organism. The lymph node shows reactive follicular hyperplasia with irregular clusters of epithelioid histiocytes. Trophozoites or cysts are rarely seen in lymph nodes, although promptly performed cultures will grow the organism in many cases.

When other organs are involved, the pathologic findings can vary from a few isolated cysts to a marked inflammatory response associated with extensive necrosis. In skeletal muscle or brain an isolated cyst can be found unassociated with any inflammatory response or with any clinical manifestations of organ dysfunction; this response is most often seen in someone with chronic latent infection but no active disease. In patients with disseminated disease, however, the heart, brain, liver, spleen, kidney, pancreas, or other organs can manifest an intense inflammatory response surrounding areas of necrosis that can vary greatly in size. The inflammatory response consists of lymphocytes, plasma cells, and monocytes in associated with edema. Perivascular mononuclear inflammatory changes are often seen contiguous to the necrotic areas. Intracellular and extracellular trophozoites are usually found in the periphery of the lesion rather than in the necrotic center; these trophozoites can be very difficult to distinguish from inflammatory debris.

In the central nervous system the necrotic lesions with margins of mononuclear cell infiltrate may be single or multiple. Periaqueductal and periventricular necrosis in congenital infection may lead to obstruction of the aqueduct of Sylvius or the foramen of Monro, resulting in obstructive hydrocephalus. The necrotic areas may ultimately calcify. In the eye, single or multiple necrotic lesions in the retina are the first manifestations of *Toxoplasma* infection. Mononuclear cell infiltrates are seen in association with cysts or trophozoites. Granulomatous inflammation occurs secondary to the necrotizing retinitis. The disease involves the posterior chamber almost exclusively and may be complicated by iridocyclitis, glaucoma, or cataracts.

In immunocompetent patients primary *Toxoplasma* infection is associated with both a humoral and cellular immune response. Antibodies against various *Toxoplasma* antigens can be detected in the blood. Subsequently, lymphocytes become responsive to *Toxoplasma* antigens and produce lymphokines. These lymphokines enable mononuclear phagocytes to inhibit *Toxoplasma* replication and to kill the intracellular organisms. Even immunocompetent individuals are not able to eliminate all *Toxoplasma* organisms from the body: Cysts characteristically form in brain and muscle and remain viable for the lifetime of the host. With the exception of the retina these cysts do not cause disease unless host immune function is altered.

CLINICAL MANIFESTATIONS. *Acquired Toxoplasmosis in the Immunocompetent Individual.* The vast majority of individuals who are infected with *T. gondii* after birth have no apparent clinical symptoms. In the small number of individuals with a symptomatic illness lymphoadenopathy (90 per cent), fever (40 per cent), and malaise (40 per cent) are the common manifestations. The lymphadenopathy classically occurs symmetrically in the posterior auricular, anterior cervical, or posterior cervical chains. Generalized lymphadenopathy or localized unilateral enlargement or enlargement of a solitary node can also be seen. The nodes are characteristically rubbery and nontender. Splenomegaly occurs in about 30 per cent of patients. The fever is usually low grade, but on occasion can be high, rapidly fluctuating, and prolonged. Fatigue can be a prominent feature. A minority of patients have a sore throat, maculopapular rash, myalgias, arthralgias, urticaria, or headache. The sore throat presents as hyperemia rather than as an exudative pharyngitis. For most patients with clinically apparent disease toxoplasmosis is self-limiting over a period of several weeks. Toxoplasmosis can, however, be a prolonged, severely debilitating disorder that may prevent the patient from working for many weeks or months. The lymph nodes may fluctuate in size during the recovery period.

In immunocompetent adults specific organ involvement can lead to clinically significant disease involving the lungs, myocardium, pericardium, liver, skin, and skeletal muscle. These manifestations may dominate the clinical picture. Glomerulonephritis has been reported. Death due to toxoplasmosis in immunocompetent individuals is extremely rare.

Laboratory evaluation reveals a normal leukocyte count with a slight lymphocytosis or monocytosis. When atypical lymphocytes are present they are found only in small numbers. The hemoglobin is usually normal, although a Coombs-negative hemolytic anemia has occasionally been reported. Serum transaminases are rarely elevated to more than twice normal. The chest radiograph is usually normal; hilar adenopathy is unusual. On the electrocardiogram ST and T wave abnormalities may be seen if myocarditis is present.

Ocular Involvement in the Immunocompetent Individual. *Toxoplasma* has been estimated to cause 20 to 35 per cent of cases of retinochoroiditis in children and adults. This ocular disease is almost always a consequence of congenital infection: there are very few well-documented cases of eye disease caused by infection acquired after birth.

Symptoms of retinochoroiditis are usually noted initially during the second or third decade of life. Symptoms and the degree of visual loss depend on the location and the extent of retinal involvement. Patients may complain of blurred vision, scotomas, pain, or epiphora. Strabismus may be an early sign in children. The lesions appear acutely as white or yellow cotton-like patches that have indistinct, elevated margins. Inflammatory exudate in the vitreous may obscure visualization of the fundus. As the lesions age they become atrophic with whitish-gray plaques, more distinct borders, and black spots of choroidal pigment. Lesions may be peripheral, but characteristically they occur near the posterior pole of the retina. They are usually multiple and vary in age, but single lesions do occur. Panuveitis and papillitis with optic atrophy can occur. Exclusively anterior uveitis has never been proven to be caused by *Toxoplasma*.

Patients with *Toxoplasma* retinochoroiditis have an unpredictable clinical course. Episodes of active disease may occur once or many times but usually stop after the age of 40. Recurrent episodes are often associated with progressive loss of vision.

Toxoplasmosis in the Immunodeficient Patient. Toxoplasmosis can occur as a disseminated disease in patients with immunodeficiencies. The disease occurs with particular frequency in patients with AIDS, but is also seen occasionally in patients with hematologic malignant conditions (particularly Hodgkin's disease) and organ transplants. The clinical manifestations are variable. Fever, hepatosplenomegaly, pneumonitis, maculopapular rash, myositis, myocarditis, meningoencephalitis, and central nervous system mass lesions may be seen. The lymphadenopathy characteristic of acquired disease in the immunocompetent patient is often absent. This syndrome is usually fulminant and rapidly fatal. It is very difficult to distinguish from numerous other infectious and noninfectious processes that can present in a similar fashion. The most common manifestation, particularly in patients with AIDS, is central nervous system involvement with fever, headache, confusion progressing to coma, focal neurologic signs, and seizures. The cerebrospinal fluid shows nonspecific changes that usually include pleocytosis and moderately increased protein and normal glucose content. Computed tomography usually shows one or more lesions that are contrast enhancing in a ring or nodular pattern.

Toxoplasmosis has been serologically associated with progressive polymyositis. It is unclear whether the association reflects the etiology of the muscular disorder or whether the disorder activates *Toxoplasma* infection. A few patients with polymyositis and high antitoxoplasma antibody titers have responded symptomatically to antitoxoplasma therapy.

Congenital Disease. Congenital toxoplasmosis is the result of acute infection acquired by the mother just before or during gestation. These *Toxoplasma* infections acquired by the mother are usually asymptomatic, as is *Toxoplasma* infection acquired by other immunocompetent hosts, and thus there is nothing to make the mother or her physician suspicious unless serologic testing is routinely performed. The likelihood that the fetus will become infected and the severity of the congenital infection are largely dependent on when during the gestation the infection is acquired. In cases in which the infection occurs late during gestation or involves very few organisms, the infant will probably have no immediate clinical manifestations, but will have positive humoral and cellular immune responses to *Toxoplasma*. Cysts of *Toxoplasma* will persist in the retina, brain, myocardium, and/or skeletal muscle for the infant's lifetime. If the infant remains immunocompetent during its lifetime, the subsequent clinical manifestations that might occur are retinochoroiditis, which usually flares during the second or third decade of life; seizures; and mild retardation. In infants who are infected early during gestation or with large inocula, the clinical sequelae can be severe. Spontaneous abortion, stillbirth, and prematurity may result. The infant may be born with microphthalmia, microcephaly, seizures, cerebral calcifications, bilateral retinochoroiditis, rash, lymphadenopathy, pneumonitis, fever, or hepatosplenomegaly, which can result in severe incapacity. If the cerebral inflammatory response involves the aqueduct of Sylvius, hydrocephalus may result. Clinical manifestations of these complications may be apparent at birth or may become obvious several months later when the infant fails to reach normal milestones.

DIAGNOSIS. The diagnosis of toxoplasmosis can be based on serologic tests, lymph node histology, the demonstration of trophozoites in body tissues or fluids, or isolation of *T. gondii* from certain sites. Which diagnostic test is most appropriate depends on the clinical situation.

Serology. Measurement of antitoxoplasma antibody titers is the most commonly employed mechanism for diagnosing toxoplasmosis. The *Sabin-Feldman dye test* is a highly sensitive and highly specific dye exclusion test that uses live *T. gondii*. This test is the reference procedure with which other tests must be compared. The Sabin-Feldman dye test and the indirect fluorescent antibody (IFA) test give comparable titers: Titers begin to rise one to two weeks after infection and reach a peak after two to eight weeks that is almost always ≥ 1:1000. Titers drift down slowly over several years and persist at low levels (1:16–1:64) for the patient's lifetime. The height of the initial peak does not correlate with severity of clinical disease. Sabin-Feldman dye test titers are positive at stable low levels in adults with reactivated ocular disease and in most immunoincompetent patients with disseminated toxoplasmosis. Titers in infants may be elevated because of passively transferred maternal antibodies. Sequential studies over four to six months must be performed to determine if the infant's titers are rising, suggesting that the infected infant is producing antibody, or if they are falling (usually by 50 per cent per month) and attributable to passively transferred maternal antibodies.

Tests for IgM antibody (IgM fluorescent antibody or double-sandwich ELISA techniques) are particularly useful for establishing recent *Toxoplasma* infection because titers appear early (as early as five days after infection) and disappear within several months. IgM tests have not been carefully standardized: The significance of specific titers needs to be evaluated by the laboratory performing the test. IgM titers are elevated in acute disease in immunocompetent individuals and in infants with congenital disease, but are not elevated in adults with reactivated ocular disease or in most immunoincompetent individuals with disseminated toxoplasmosis.

The complement fixation test using soluble *Toxoplasma* antigen becomes positive three to six weeks after infection, rises for the succeeding two to eight months, and falls to very low levels after one to two years. This test can be useful for documenting a titer rise in someone whose Sabin-Feldman dye test titer has already peaked and whose IgM-IFA or IgM-ELISA peak has already occurred, i.e., a patient whose infection occurred more than two to four months previously but less than six to eight months previously. Titers are often elevated in infants with congenital disease and in some immunologically abnormal patients with disseminated disease. Titers are not elevated in adults with reactivated ocular disease.

The indirect hemagglutination (IHA) test as performed in most laboratories measures antibodies that increase very late in the course of infection and persist for years. Titer rises occur so late that the test has very little clinical utility and is particularly poor for use as a screening device to identify pregnant women who have acquired *Toxoplasma* infection early during gestation and who might therefore elect abortion if still medically feasible. The IHA tests that are available in commercial kits are often poorly standardized and are therefore difficult to interpret.

False-positive results are not known to occur with the Sabin-Feldman dye test. The IFA and IgM-IFA tests may produce false-positive results if antinuclear antibody is present. Rheumatoid factor can also cause false-positive IgM-IFA titers.

In general, acute acquired toxoplasmosis is suggested serologically by Sabin-Feldman dye test or IFA titers ≥ 1:1000

and proven convincingly by the documentation of elevated IgM-IFA or IgM-ELISA titers, or the documentation of a two-tube (or greater) titer rise in the Sabin-Feldman dye test, IFA test, complement fixation test, and perhaps the indirect hemagglutination test. Congenital toxoplasmosis in infants is documented by demonstrating elevated complement fixation or IgM-IFA titers or by showing that Sabin-Feldman dye test or IFA titers are stable or rising over four to six months. Ocular toxoplasmosis or toxoplasmosis in the immunoincompetent host cannot be diagnosed with certainty by antibody testing. A negative Sabin-Feldman dye test result or IFA test titer excludes *Toxoplasma* as a cause of the ocular disease.

Isolation of the Organism. *T. gondii* can be isolated from leukocytes, body fluids, or tissue by direct inoculation of the specimens subcutaneously or intraperitoneally into mice. The mice are then examined periodically for the presence of antibody to *Toxoplasma*, for the presence of trophozoites in the peritoneum, or for the presence of cysts in the brain. The isolation of the *Toxoplasma* from leukocytes or body fluids is convincing evidence of acute infection, although parasitemia persisting for a year has been described. The isolation of *Toxoplasma* from tissue does not provide convincing evidence of acute infection because a tissue cyst may have been present for many years and may be irrelevant to the active disease process. *Toxoplasma* isolation requires several weeks to carry out.

Histologic Diagnosis. The histologic findings in the lymph nodes of patients with acute toxoplasmosis, described earlier, are so characteristic as to be diagnostic. The inflammatory reaction in other tissues is much less specific. In these other tissues free or intracellular trophozoites must be demonstrated for the diagnosis of toxoplasmosis to be established. The demonstration of *Toxoplasma* cysts proves that the patient was infected by *T. gondii* at some time in the past, but does not document that the current clinical disease is related. Histologic diagnosis is the preferred technique for patients with urgent clinical syndromes, especially immunoincompetent patients with cerebral mass lesions. Diagnosis of cerebral toxoplasmosis can be established by assessing empiric response to a two-week course of pyrimethamine (Daraprim) and sulfadiazine, but performing a guided needle biopsy (if such a procedure is technically feasible) is far preferable.

DIFFERENTIAL DIAGNOSIS. The differential diagnosis of a patient with lymphadenopathy includes lymphoma, Hodgkin's disease, AIDS, sarcoidosis, mycobacterial disease, cytomegalovirus disease, mononucleosis, brucellosis, tularemia, cat-scratch disease, and many other infectious processes. Toxoplasmosis can be distinguished from mononucleosis by the absence of atypical lymphocytosis, exudative pharyngitis, increased serum transaminases, and heterophile antibodies. Appropriate serologic tests, cultures, and lymph node biopsies are necessary to distinguish the other processes. Toxoplasmosis in immunosuppressed patients may mimic other disseminated infections: The central nervous system mass lesions need to be distinguished by biopsy from neoplastic or other infectious processes.

Toxoplasma retinochoroiditis needs to be distinguished on the basis of lesion morphology, serology, and appropriate cultures from cytomegalovirus, herpes, tuberculosis, histoplasmosis, syphilis, and sarcoidosis. Congenital toxoplasmosis must be distinguished from cytomegalovirus disease, syphilis, *Herpes simplex* infection, rubella, erythroblastosis fetalis, and bacterial sepsis.

THERAPY. The need and duration of therapy depend on the clinical setting. Most immunocompetent adults with lymphadenopathic disease do not need specific antitoxoplasma therapy. Patients with severe or prolonged constitutional symptoms, patients with specific organ dysfunction, immunoincompetent patients, and probably patients infected by direct inoculation (laboratory workers and transfusion recipients) merit treatment. Treatment for patients with retinochoroiditis or for pregnant patients is more controversial.

A combination of pyrimethamine and sulfadiazine is effective in inhibiting the replication of trophozoites. There are no drugs that will kill trophozoites or eradicate the cyst form. Pyrimethamine can only be given orally: In adults an initial dose of 75 mg is given, followed by 25 mg daily. Infants should be given 1 mg per kilogram for three days followed by 0.5 mg per kilogram per day. Sulfadiazine 1 gram orally every six hours is the adult dose. Infants should receive 100 mg per kilogram per day. Triple sulfonamides can be substituted for sulfadiazine, but sulfisoxazole (Gantrisin) is ineffective. Good urine flow should be maintained by adequate fluid intake to prevent crystalluria. Since sulfa drugs and pyrimethamine inhibit folate synthesis, folinic acid (leucovorin) 5 to 10 mg should be administered two to three times weekly to reduce bone marrow toxicity. Platelet counts and white blood cell counts should be monitored at least twice weekly during therapy. Pyrimethamine is a potential teratogen and should not be used in pregnant women.

Evaluation of the effectiveness of sulfadiazine and pyrimethamine therapy has been limited by the marked variability in clinical course and the frequency of spontaneous improvement. There is considerable anecdotal experience, however, that specific therapy can shorten the symptomatic period of fever and fatigue (although not the lymphadenopathy) in immunocompetent patients with acquired disease and is probably effective in hastening the resolution of serious organ dysfunction. Often a four- to six-week course of therapy is given and then the clinical situation re-evaluated. In *Toxoplasma* retinochoroiditis primary therapy should be directed at controlling the hypersensitivity response with anti-inflammatory drugs such as corticosteroids if the lesions are extensive or central. Pyrimethamine and sulfadiazine should be used to prevent local proliferation of the organisms and potential dissemination during periods when corticosteroids are given.

Sulfadiazine and pyrimethamine have been effective in a number of immunosuppressed patients in controlling systemic symptoms and specific organ dysfunction. Long-term therapy should be strongly considered for the duration of immunosuppression; for AIDS patients, therapy should probably be continued for life. Bone marrow toxicity and skin rash are major management problems in many of these patients, particularly those with AIDS or those treated with antineoplastic chemotherapy.

In pregnant women who plan to complete their pregnancy despite the acquisition of *Toxoplasma* infection during gestation, pyrimethamine is dangerous because of its teratogenic potential. There is some evidence that sulfadiazine alone may be effective therapy. In Europe spiramycin* has been used, but its efficacy has not been clearly established. Congenital toxoplasmosis should be treated aggressively whether or not the infant is symptomatic, because organism proliferation can continue after birth. Antitoxoplasma therapy will not reverse damage that has already occurred.

For patients who cannot tolerate sulfadiazine and pyrimethamine, there are no clearly effective alternatives. Pyrimethamine alone, clindamycin, or spiramycin has antitoxoplasma activity in preclinical studies, but evidence for their clinical efficacy in any form of human toxoplasmosis is not yet convincing.

PREVENTION. Toxoplasmosis is usually transmitted by the consumption of undercooked meat or exposure to oocyst-infected cat feces, so effective prevention should be directed against minimizing exposure to these two sources. Meat should be cooked as mentioned earlier. Pet cats should be kept in the house, and they should not be fed raw meat or have access to wild rodents or birds. Particularly susceptible individuals or pregnant women who are seronegative should avoid sandboxes or moist soil where outdoor cats may defecate.

Congenital toxoplasmosis can be largely avoided if pregnant women follow the aforementioned precautions carefully. Serologic testing at the time of the mother's first prenatal examination and again at 16 to 18 weeks of gestation permits recognition of mothers who have acquired toxoplasmosis early in pregnancy and allows consideration of therapeutic abortion.

Desmonts G, Couvreur J: Congenital toxoplasmosis. A prospective study of 378 pregnancies. N Engl J Med 290:110, 1974. *The risk of of congenital toxoplasmosis is documented in this prospective study.*

Dorfman RF, Remington JS: Value of lymph node biopsy in the diagnosis of acute acquired toxoplasmosis. N Engl J Med 289:878, 1973. *The specific histologic characteristics of toxoplasma lymphadenitis are documented.*

Navia BA, Petito CK, Gold JWM, et al.: Cerebral toxoplasmosis complicating the acquired immune deficiency syndrome. Clinical and neuropathological findings in 27 patients. Ann Neurol 19:224, 1986. *A comprehensive assessment of the presentation, clinical course, and outcome of AIDS patients with cerebral toxoplasmosis.*

Schlaegel TF Jr: Ocular Toxoplasmosis and Pars Planitis. New York, Grune & Stratton, 1978. *This detailed volume comprehensively covers ocular toxoplasmosis.*

Welsh PC, Masur H, Jones TC, et al.: Serologic diagnosis of acute lymphadenopathic toxoplasmosis. J Infect Dis 142:256, 1980. *The usefulness of different serologic techniques is assessed for diagnosing acute lymphadenopathic toxoplasmosis.*

Wilson CB, Remington JS, Stagno S, et al.: Development of adverse sequelae in children born with subclinical congenital *Toxoplasma* infection. Pediatrics 66:767, 1980. *An analysis of the sequelae that congenital* Toxoplasma *infection produced in 24 children.*

386 PNEUMOCYSTOSIS
Henry Masur

Pneumocystosis is a pulmonary disease characterized by dyspnea, tachypnea, and hypoxemia that occurs in immunodeficient patients and in malnourished or premature infants. It is caused by species of the genus *Pneumocystis*, organisms that are probably protozoa. *Pneumocystis* organisms probably cause asymptomatic infection in healthy mammalian hosts. They are seen extracellularly in the pulmonary alveoli.

ORGANISM. The life cycle of *Pneumocystis carinii* is not known with certainty. Morphologic data suggest that a thick-walled cyst and a thinner-walled trophozoite are the major stages in the life cycle of this extracellular organism. The cyst is 5 to 6 μ in diameter, and usually contains a cluster of six to eight round sporozoites (1 to 2 μ in diameter). When the sporozoites are released by the cyst, they develop into the trophozoites (1 to 5 μ in diameter). Under certain conditions, the trophozoites undergo a series of changes, including loss of internal structure, appearance of villous projections on the outer membrane, and development of an unusual trilaminar membrane, changes which transform the trophozoite into the cyst stage. A trophozoite-to-trophozoite cycle may also occur. The intra-alveolar exudate contains a mixture of cysts and trophozoites, as well as cellular and microbial debris and plasma proteins. The cyst is the stage of the organism usually identified in clinical specimens by means of the characteristic outer membrane staining with methenamine silver nitrate (Color plate 5G), Gram-Weigert, or toluidine blue O stains. With Giemsa stain, sporozoites can be identified within the cyst, as can the trophozoites, especially in touch preparations of fresh lung tissue or in bronchial secretions (including sputum).

EPIDEMIOLOGY. *Pneumocystis* species are widely distributed, infecting rodents, rabbits, dogs, goats, horses, sheep, and other mammals, including humans. There is no evidence

---

*Spiramycin is available from the National Center for Orphan Drugs and Rare Diseases (703–522–2590) in Virginia and (1–800–336–4797) in Washington, D.C.

that animals serve as a reservoir for infection of humans. Experimental animal models and epidemiologic investigations of human disease best support the theory that transmission is by a respiratory route via droplet spray. In a few cases, congenital transmission has appeared to be the most likely route of infection.

Epidemiologic data suggest that *Pneumocystis* is infectious, that healthy or diseased individuals can transmit the infection, and that infection is usually persistent and asymptomatic. Epidemics of human disease occur in institutionalized malnourished infants, hospitalized immunodeficient patients, and family clusters.

Pneumocystosis occurs most commonly in malnourished infants (especially in the second to fourth months of life when passively transferred maternal antibodies first reach low levels), patients with deficiency of immunoglobulins G or M, and patients with deficiencies in cell-mediated immune mechanisms. The vast majority of adult patients either have the acquired immune deficiency syndrome (AIDS) or have received chemotherapy for hematologic malignant disease or organ transplantation.

PATHOLOGY AND PATHOGENESIS. In the rat model, latent *Pneumocystis* infection can develop into active pulmonary disease after corticosteroid or cyclophosphamide therapy, but not after irradiation, splenectomy, or neonatal thymectomy. In humans, the relative importance of specific predisposing factors is less clear. When the *Pneumocystis* organisms are able to multiply, the inflammatory response includes transudation of fluid into the alveoli and a mononuclear cell infiltrate of interstitial spaces. The alveoli become filled with a foamy, proteinaceous material that contains clumps of both trophozoites and cysts. In malnourished or premature infants with pneumocystosis, the interstitial spaces contain predominantly plasma cells and alveolar epithelial cells—hence the pathologic description, interstitial plasma cell pneumonia. In immunodeficient children and adults, however, the inflammatory response consists of lymphocytes, macrophages, and occasionally eosinophils. Polymorphonuclear leukocytes are not seen, even in patients with normal white blood cell counts. The lung is usually involved diffusely, although localized disease has occasionally been described. The lung is usually firm and rubbery in consistency. Other pulmonary processes are occasionally found in association with pneumocystosis, including neoplastic, viral (particularly cytomegalovirus), bacterial, and fungal diseases. Rarely, *Pneumocystis* may occur outside the lungs, involving lymph nodes, spleen, bone marrow, skin, or external auditory canal.

CLINICAL MANIFESTATIONS. The major symptoms of pneumocystosis are dyspnea, tachypnea, chest tightness (which may be substernal and pleuritic), and a nonproductive cough. Fever and cyanosis are often present. The clinical syndrome can progress rapidly over several days or can appear insidiously over weeks or months. The rapidly progressive form is characteristic of patients with malignant neoplasms, especially during corticosteroid withdrawal. The insidious form is typically seen in children with congenital immunodeficiencies and in adults with AIDS.

On physical examination, the patient usually shows signs of respiratory distress (tachypnea, dyspnea, and cyanosis) associated with fever, but some patients, particularly those with AIDS, may have a paucity of signs. Auscultation of the lungs usually reveals no abnormalities, although scattered rales and rhonchi may be heard.

Routine laboratory tests are not generally helpful in distinguishing pneumocystosis from other pulmonary processes that are common in immunodeficient patients. Leukocytosis can be seen, but most often the white blood cell count reflects the underlying disease or the effects of chemotherapy. Eosinophilia has been reported, especially in children with humoral immune deficiencies. In AIDS patients the T4 lymphocyte count is characteristically below 200 per cubic millimeter. The

arterial blood gases will demonstrate decreased oxygen content and hyperventilation despite continuous oxygen therapy, consistent with alveolar capillary block. A mild respiratory acidosis may be seen. Early in the course of the disease the chest radiograph usually shows a perihilar interstitial or patchy reticulogranular infiltrate with peripheral sparing. At the time of presentation some patients, particularly those with AIDS, may have normal arterial blood gases and/or normal chest radiographs. As pneumocystosis progresses, diffuse alveolar infiltrates with air bronchograms usually involve the entire lung fields. Pleural reaction, pleural effusion, asymmetry of infiltrates, or nodular infiltrates are unusual manifestations of pneumocystosis alone, but can be seen in up to one half of cases, since more than one disease process is often present in the lungs.

COURSE. The course of untreated pneumocystosis is almost always one of progressive pulmonary consolidation, hypoxemia, and death. After institution of appropriate specific therapy, improvement usually occurs in five to ten days. The clinical and radiologic findings may become transiently worse after institution of therapy, but will then improve over one to three weeks in most patients who have a successful outcome. An association of pneumocystosis with interstitial fibrosis or emphysema has been reported, but the etiologic role of pneumocystosis has been difficult to document in view of the many factors that could lead to pulmonary changes in these patients.

DIAGNOSIS. Once the suspicion of pneumocystosis is raised by the clinical setting of immune deficiency and progressive pulmonary symptoms, pulmonary secretions (including sputum) or lung tissue should be examined by methenamine silver, Gram-Weigert, Giemsa, or toluidine blue O stains. When an AIDS patient with pneumocystis pneumonia is able to produce an adequate sputum specimen, organisms can be identified in more than 50 per cent of cases. Bronchoscopy is the preferred invasive technique for establishing the diagnosis if sputum examination is unrevealing. Bronchoalveolar lavage and transbronchial lung biopsy each have a diagnostic sensitivity over 90 per cent. When used together the two techniques enhance sensitivity further. Transbronchial biopsy has the added advantage of being able to recognize other processes such as cytomegalovirus infection or certain tumors that cannot be unequivocally diagnosed by lavage or brushings. Open lung biopsy provides the optimal chance for complete and accurate diagnosis, but should rarely be necessary to establish a diagnosis of pneumocystosis. Establishing a specific cause for pulmonary dysfunction permits institution of specific therapy, thus avoiding the complications of prolonged broad-spectrum antimicrobial therapy. If a diagnostic procedure cannot be performed because of technical or medical contraindications, a therapeutic trial that includes antipneumocystis therapy is warranted in appropriate clinical settings.

Reliable serologic techniques have not yet been developed for diagnostic purposes. Serology may, however, be useful in the epidemic infantile form of pneumocystosis and in epidemiologic investigations.

TREATMENT. If started early in the course of the disease, therapy for pneumocystosis is quite successful. Pentamidine isethionate was used to treat pneumocystosis in the United States for more than a decade; its use decreased mortality from nearly 100 per cent to less than 50 per cent, particularly if the patient survived long enough to receive the drug for nine or more days. Pentamidine has now been supplanted by co-trimoxazole, the fixed combination of trimethoprim and sulfamethoxazole, which appears to be as effective as pentamidine and less toxic. This drug combination interferes with the synthesis of folinic acid. Adults should be given at least a 14-day course of 20 mg per kilogram per day of trimethoprim and 100 mg per kilogram per day of sulfamethoxazole in three or four equal oral or intravenous doses. Serum concentrations should be monitored because critically ill patients may not absorb orally administered drugs optimally and because factors such as abnormal renal function or unusual volumes of distribution may make levels unpredictable even after intravenous administration. Peak levels of 5 to 10 μg per milliliter of trimethoprim and 100 to 150 μg per milliliter of sulfamethoxazole, in serum drawn 90 minutes after drug administration, have been documented in some successfully treated patients. Folinic acid can be administered orally or intravenously to prevent or to treat folate deficiency; a reasonable dosage is 10 mg two to three times weekly, although the efficacy of such therapy for preventing or treating adverse reactions is unclear. Hypersensitivity rashes and leukopenia occur with high frequency in AIDS patients, but are unusual in patients with malignant neoplasms.

If the patient is unable to tolerate co-trimoxazole, or if the patient has not responded after seven to ten days, then the use of pentamidine should be considered. The mechanism of action of pentamidine on *Pneumocystis* is unknown; with other protozoa, pentamidine binds to DNA, inhibits RNA polymerase, and alters synthesis of proteins, nucleic acids, and folic acid. Pentamidine is administered once daily intramuscularly or by slow intravenous infusion (over at least 60 minutes) for 10 to 21 days. The dose of pentamidine isethionate, the only form of the drug available in the United States, is 4 mg per kilogram per day. In more than 40 per cent of patients, pentamidine causes adverse effects, including renal insufficiency, abnormal liver function, and disturbances in bone marrow function or glucose metabolism (hypoglycemia or hyperglycemia). These adverse effects are usually reversible. Intramuscular administration often results in large and painful sterile abscesses. Intravenous administration has been associated with significant hypotension in the past, but increasing the infusion time and volume (100 to 150 ml of 5 per cent dextrose in water administered over 60 minutes) has substantially reduced the risk of this adverse effect. No therapeutic alternatives to co-trimoxazole and pentamidine have been approved by the Food and Drug Administration. Experimental trials have demonstrated potential roles for dapsone (with or without trimethoprim), trimetrexate, and alpha-difluoromethylornithine.

Repeat episodes of pneumocystosis have been documented after pentamidine and after co-trimoxazole therapy, particularly in patients with AIDS.

PREVENTION. Since the diseased patient may be able to transmit the infection to other immunosuppressed patients, it seems prudent to avoid respiratory contact between patients with pneumocystosis and other susceptible individuals, although such precautions are not recommended by the Centers for Disease Control. Such precautions may prevent hospital clusters of pneumocystosis. For certain highly susceptible patient populations such as children with acute lymphoblastic leukemia at institutions with high attack rates, and perhaps for patients with AIDS, continuous prophylactic treatment with co-trimoxazole is beneficial. The preventive dosage is trimethoprim, 5 mg per kilogram per day, and sulfamethoxazole, 25 mg per kilogram per day, in two equally divided doses.

Hughes WT, Kuhn S, Chaudhary S, et al.: Successful chemoprophylaxis for *Pneumocystis carinii* pneumonitis. N Engl J Med 297:1419, 1977. *This randomized, double-blind study demonstrates the efficacy of co-trimoxazole for the prevention of pneumocystosis in a high-risk pediatric population.*

Kovacs JA, Hiemenz JW, Macher AM, et al.: *Pneumocystis carinii* pneumonia: A comparison between patients with the acquired immunodeficiency syndrome and patients with other immunodeficiencies. Ann Intern Med 100:663, 1984. *The clinical presentation of pneumocystis pneumonia in AIDS is more subtle than in other disease states. Efficacy of therapy is similar in the two groups, but adverse reactions to trimethoprim-sulfamethoxazole are more common in AIDS patients.*

Ognibene FP, Shelhamer JH, Gill V, et al.: The diagnosis of *Pneumocystis carinii* pneumonia in patients with the acquired immunodeficiency syndrome using subsegmental bronchoalveolar lavage. Am Rev Respir Dis 129:929, 1984. *This study demonstrates the high sensitivity of bronchoalveolar lavage*

compared with transbronchial biopsy for establishing a diagnosis of pneumocystis pneumonia in AIDS patients.

Pearson RD, Hewlett EL: Pentamidine for the treatment of *Pneumocystis carinii* pneumonia and other protozoal diseases. Ann Intern Med 103:782, 1985. *This thorough review summarizes knowledge about pentamidine's pharmacology, mechanism of action, adverse effects, and theraputic indications.*

Walzer PD, Perl DP, Krogstad DJ, et al.: *Pneumocystis carinii* pneumonia in the United States. Epidemiologic, diagnostic, and clinical features. Ann Intern Med 80:83, 1974. *This article summarizes 194 confirmed cases of pneumocystosis in terms of information supplied to the Centers for Disease Control. Its data are useful and well organized.*

Wharton JM, Coleman DL, Wofsy CB, et al.: Trimethoprim-sulfamethoxazole or pentamidine for *pneumocystis carinii* pneumonia in the acquired immunodeficiency syndrome—a prospective randomized trial. Ann Intern Med 105:37, 1986. *A small but helpful assessment of the relative merits of two conventional regimens used to treat AIDS patients with pneumocystosis.*

387 CRYPTOSPORIDIOSIS
Rosemary Soave

Cryptosporidiosis is a gastrointestinal tract infection characterized by watery diarrhea, abdominal cramps, malabsorption, and weight loss. It is usually a severe, unrelenting illness in immunocompromised patients, particularly those with the acquired immunodeficiency syndrome (AIDS), and a self-limited disease in the immunologically normal host. It is caused by the coccidian protozoan, *Cryptosporidium*, long associated with disease in animals. In 1981–1982, identification of *Cryptosporidium* in 47 AIDS patients with severe enteritis brought the protozoan to the attention of the medical community. As more physicians have looked for this parasite, the number of reported cases of cryptosporidiosis has continued to rise, and it has come to be recognized as an important public health problem worldwide. There is currently no

THE PROTOZOAN. *Cryptosporidium* is assigned to the class Sporozoa in the order Eucoccidiorida and is thus taxonomically related to other coccidia that infect man, including *Toxoplasma gondii*, *Isospora belli*, and *Plasmodium spp*. However, morphologically and in its ability to parasitize the immunocompromised host, it most closely resembles the unclassified protozoan *Pneumocystis carinii*. The *Cryptosporidium* oocyst is 2 to 5 μ in diameter and is the stage identified in clinical specimens by means of its characteristic acid-fast positivity. When fully sporulated (mature) the oocyst contains four naked (without sporocysts) sporozoites that are elliptical (2 to 4 × 6 to 8 μ), flat, motile, and thought to be the infective form of the organism (Fig. 387–1). Sporozoites are released (excystation) and implant on intestinal epithelium where they develop into trophozoites, followed by asexual and sexual endogenous stages, finally resulting in the production of oocysts that are released in feces and are immediately infective. The ability of *Cryptosporidium* to develop completely within a single host (monoxenous life cycle) distinguishes the

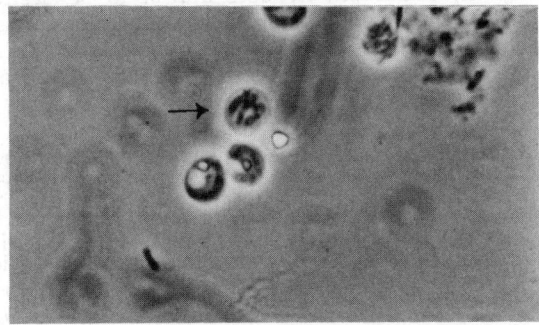

FIGURE 387–1. Wet mount of human stool showing three cryptosporidial oocysts, one of which is fully sporulated (*arrow*). (×630).

organism from other coccidia and imparts to it a tremendous potential for reinfection within the same host. This may help explain the persistent illness of AIDS patients infected with *Cryptosporidium*.

EPIDEMIOLOGY. The prevalence of human cryptosporidiosis is not yet known. Although initially recognized as a cause of gastroenteritis in immuosuppressed patients, *Cryptosporidium* should not be considered an opportunistic pathogen. Since 1983 there have been more than 25 published surveys of cryptosporidial infection, mostly emanating from the developing world. The studies have been primarily based on examination of stool specimens submitted to parasitology laboratories by persons with diarrhea and therefore do not reflect true prevalence. Nevertheless, the findings indicate that *Cryptosporidium* is a common cause of infection worldwide (Table 387–1). The data also suggest that cryptosporidiosis is more common in children than in adults and that breast feeding may be protective. The latter issue is debatable, since decreased susceptibility in breast-fed infants could also be explained by decreased exposure to potentially contaminated food or water.

Approximately 3 to 4 per cent of AIDS patients in the United States have been reported to have cryptosporidiosis. This is undoubtedly an underestimate, since not all AIDS patients are examined for *Cryptosporidium*. By contrast, more than 50 per cent of AIDS patients in Haiti have cryptosporidiosis, and another 15 per cent are infected with *Isospora belli*. Cryptosporidiosis does not appear to occur commonly in either organ transplant recipients or patients with neoplasms; however, this observation has not been confirmed with controlled investigations. Asymptomatic carriage of the parasite is rare.

Cryptosporidial infection has been documented in many species of animals, including mammals, birds, reptiles, and fish. Although 17 species of *Cryptosporidium* have been named, several cross-transmission studies have shown that the organism lacks host specificity, and indeed, there may be only one species able to parasitize many different hosts. Animal-to-human transmission has been well documented, placing animal handlers at high risk for infection. However, most humans do not acquire the parasite from infected animals. Nosocomial spread of cryptosporidiosis as well as common occurrence of the infection in day-care centers and in household or other close contacts of index cases indicate that person-to-person spread is important. Cryptosporidiosis has been reported in homosexual men without AIDS, but the role of sexual transmission in the spread of this disease is still uncertain. Infection with *Cryptosporidium* has also been described in travelers, particularly those returning from developing countries; in residents of San Antonio, Texas, who were exposed to a common water supply; and in children in Soledad, Mexico, where both animals and water were found to harbor the parasite. These findings suggest that *Cryptosporidium* may also be transmitted by indirect exposure to contaminated surfaces, food, or water. The cryptosporidial oocyst is quite hardy. It is resistant to a number of laboratory disinfectants, but infectivity does appear to be destroyed by ammonia, full-strength commercial bleach, formol-saline, and temperatures less than 0°C and greater than 65°C. For reasons that are not understood, cryptosporidiosis appears to occur more commonly in the tropics and in summer and autumn.

Animals and both immunocompetent and immunocompromised humans develop an antibody response to *Cryptosporidium*. There is a surprisingly high incidence of seropositivity in the immune normal healthy population. Seroepidemiologic studies are currently ongoing and should aid in determining the true incidence of human cryptosporidiosis.

PATHOLOGY AND PATHOGENESIS. *Cryptosporidium* has been found in the pharynx, esophagus, stomach, duodenum, jejunum, ileum, appendix, colon, rectum, gallblad-

TABLE 387–1. SURVEYS OF *CRYPTOSPORIDIUM* INFECTIONS IN 1985 IN PATIENTS WITH DIARRHEA

Location	No. of Persons	Per Cent Positive
USA (Massachusetts)	1290	2.6
Finland	4545	2.6
Spain	91	1.0
United Kingdom	213	3.2
France	190	2.1
Canada (British Columbia)	7300	0.6
Haiti	824	16.7
Brazil	117	7.7
Venezuela	120	9.2
Mexico	57	32.0
Bangladesh	578	4.3
India	687	11.1

der, and bile ducts of infected immunocompromised (primarily AIDS) patients. The parasite has also been found on bronchial epithelium and in sputum, but it may have reached there because of vomiting. Ultrastructural studies have revealed endogenous stages of the organism adherent to the enterocyte surface and enveloped by a membrane, believed by some to be derived from the host cell. Thus the position of the organism within a parasitophorous vacuole is considered to be intracellular, but extracytoplasmic and unique. Despite the presence of numerous organisms there is usually a remarkable absence of inflammatory changes. In fact, the lesions most resemble those described for giardiasis, i.e., villous atrophy, crypt elongation, and minimal subjacent inflammatory infiltrates of the lamina propria. Similar histopathologic findings have been described for only three immunocompetent patients with cryptosporidiosis.

Biliary cryptosporidiosis has been documented in at least five AIDS patients; it has not been reported in immunologically normal persons. The pathologic findings have included organisms in bile and adherent to gallbladder and biliary duct epithelium, with edema, lymphocytic infiltration, and destruction of the underlying mucosa. Two patients were concomitantly infected with cytomegalovirus (CMV).

The pathogenesis of cryptosporidial enteritis has not yet been delineated. A toxin-mediated mechanism is suggested by the secretory nature of the diarrhea and the absence of inflammation. Malabsorption has been documented in several cases of chronic cryptosporidiosis.

CLINICAL MANIFESTATIONS. Persons infected with *Cryptosporidium* have watery diarrhea, cramping upper abdominal pain (often exacerbated by food ingestion), weight loss, and flatulence. Nausea, vomiting, anorexia, myalgias, and malaise may also be present.

Physical examination is usually not remarkable except for dehydration. Fever and leukocytosis are not common. Examination of feces reveals many cryptosporidial oocysts and absence of leukocytes and blood. Reversible lactase deficiency and fat malabsorption have been documented in several cases.

The severity and course of cryptosporidiosis are determined by immunocompetence. In the immunologically normal host, infection is often explosive in onset and lasts an average of 10 to 14 days. Clearance of the parasite from stool lags behind clinical resolution by two to three weeks, thus creating problems for infection control. Although self-limited, symptoms are often severe enough to justify therapeutic intervention, were it available.

Infection in AIDS patients often begins insidiously and escalates in severity as the underlying immune defect becomes more profound. Frequent (6 to 25), voluminous (1 to 25 liters) daily bowel movements, weight loss, and stool oocyst shedding persist for months until the patient dies. Although in most cases, death is not directly attributable to cryptosporidial enteritis, the morbidity of this infection is devastating.

AIDS patients with documented biliary cryptosporidiosis have all had right upper-quadrant pain and persistent nausea and vomiting in addition to severe enteritis. Laboratory studies have revealed an elevated alkaline phosphatase level and minimally elevated serum transaminase values. Thickening of the gallbladder wall and dilation of bile ducts with distal duct strictures and luminal irregularities have been seen on radiologic examination.

Severe persistent cryptosporidiosis has also been described in patients with congenital hypogammaglobulinemia or severe combined immunodeficiency disease and in those receiving cytotoxic therapy. In the last group, illness resolves when the cytotoxic agents are discontinued.

DIAGNOSIS. Microscopic examination of a wet preparation of feces will usually reveal cryptosporidial oocysts, but they may be easily confused with yeasts, which are similar in size and shape. Since 1981, various staining techniques for detecting oocysts have been popularized, including several modifications of the acid-fast stain (Kinyoun, Ziehl-Neelsen), the fluorescent auramine-rhodamine stain, and the PAS and carbol fuchsin–negative stains. With the acid-fast stain, acid fast–positive (red) oocysts may be easily distinguished from acid fast–negative (green) yeast. Although the sensitivity and specificity of stool examination compared with intestinal biopsy have not been determined, stool examination appears to be more sensitive. Autolysis of tissue specimens during processing and the patchy distribution of cryptosporidial infection with absence of inflammatory changes to guide the endoscopist may result in false negative intestinal biopsies. Regardless of the staining method used, experienced observers have little difficulty in identifying oocysts. Since the pattern of fecal oocyst shedding in human cryptosporidiosis has not been determined in detail, the optimal number of negative stool specimens required to confirm the absence of cryptosporidial infection is unknown. Stool concentration techniques (e.g., Sheathers sucrose flotation method, the formalin-ether method of Ritchie) to optimize detection of fecal oocysts do not appear to be necessary for diagnosis during acute illness. Such techniques may have a role in detecting oocysts in follow-up specimens, asymptomatic contacts, or environmental samples. Special caution is advised, since these techniques expose laboratory workers to the risk of aerosolization or leakage of the specimen.

TREATMENT. There is currently no known effective therapy for human cryptosporidiosis. Identification of potentially active compounds has been severely hampered by the absence of an animal model of the chronic disease and inability to cultivate the organism in vitro.

Investigational therapy has not been given to the immunocompetent host with cryptosporidial enteritis, since illness in these patients is usually self-limited. Persons receiving corticosteroids or cytotoxic drugs may be successfully managed by discontinuation of the immunosuppressive agents.

Because of the severe nature of the illness in AIDS patients with cryptosporidiosis, a vast array of antidiarrheal, antimicrobial, and immunomodulating agents have been administered, but with no documented benefit. The macrolide antibiotic spiramycin is currently being used extensively in AIDS patients because of its possible value in palliating diarrheal symptoms and its lack of toxicity. Spiramycin* may be obtained from Rhône-Poulenc Pharmaceuticals, Monmouth Junction, NJ, and dispensed with FDA permission. It is given orally in a dose of 3 to 4 grams per day. Adverse effects, including hypersensitivity reactions and gastrointestinal irritation, are seen rarely. A multicenter, placebo-controlled clinical trial designed to test the efficacy of spiramycin in AIDS patients with chronic cryptosporidiosis is currently ongoing.

Alpha-difluoromethylornithine is an irreversible ornithine decarboxylase inhibitor with activity against a number of protozoa. It has demonstrated modest efficacy for crypto-

sporidiosis, but toxicity (bone marrow suppression and gastrointestinal irritation) has limited its use.

Other agents currently being evaluated include oral bovine transfer factor, hyperimmune bovine colostrum, and recombinant interleukin-2, and cow's milk globulin.

Fayer R, Ungar BLP: *Cryptosporidium* spp. and cryptosporidiosis. Microbiol Rev 50:458, 1986. *This thoroughly referenced review emphasizes the biological and veterinary aspects of* Cryptosporidium.
Jokipii L, Jokipii AM: Timing of symptoms and oocyst excretion in human cryptosporidiosis. N Engl J Med 315:1643, 1986. *A clinical and parasitologic study of 68 immunocompetent patients with cryptosporidiosis in Finland.*
Navin TR: Cryptosporidiosis in humans: Review of recent epidemiologic studies. Eur J Epidemiol 1:77, 1985. *This article discusses 14 recent studies of the occurrence of cryptosporidiosis throughout the world. The article provides documentation about probable routes of transmission.*
Soave R, Armstrong D: Cryptosporidium and cryptosporidiosis. Rev Inf Dis 8:1012–1023, 1986. *This thoroughly referenced review summarizes the literature to date.*

388 GIARDIASIS
David P. Stevens

DEFINITION. Giardiasis is an infection of the small intestine caused by the flagellated protozoan *Giardia lamblia*. When symptomatic, it results in diarrhea, malabsorption, and weight loss.

INCIDENCE AND PREVALENCE. Giardiasis is present in all climates. It is particularly prevalent in developing regions of the world where water supplies are not treated or where they overlap with sewage disposal systems such as local streams. Endemic giardiasis, however, is also found in industrialized countries. Examples of the latter include the municipal water supply of Leningrad and many of the pristine streams of the Rocky Mountains. The incidence of giardiasis in the United States has been estimated to be 7.4 per cent. *Giardia lamblia* is the most commonly identified cause of waterborne infectious diarrhea and the most frequently isolated stool parasite in the United States.

ETIOLOGY. The organism exists either as the motile, flagellated, pear-shaped trophozoite, 12 to 15 μm in length, or as the smaller, tough-walled oval cyst. Infection occurs in the small intestine of the host. Trophozoites either attach to the microvilli of the intestinal epithelium or move about in the unstirred layer of mucus just above the epithelial surface. The trophozoites, carried caudally by peristalsis, eventually encyst and are passed out into the environment. The cyst is resistant to many environmental stresses, including concentrations of chlorine normally found in treated municipal water supplies. It is ingested eventually by a subsequent host. Excystation occurs in the acid environment of the stomach, and infection is again established in the small intestine.

EPIDEMIOLOGY. *Giardia* spreads by two routes: waterborne infection, particularly in contaminated community water supplies, and direct person-to-person transmission. Dozens of epidemics have been described in the United States consequent to breakdown of community water filtration systems. Epidemics in daycare centers for children and among promiscuous male homosexuals indicate that direct person-to-person spread can occur.

A role for animal reservoirs of infection has been suggested by the demonstration of *Giardia*-infected beaver upstream from communities where outbreaks of human infection have occurred. It is likely that both beaver and dogs carry *Giardia* species infectious for humans.

Giardia is a frequent source of diarrhea in travelers returning from endemic areas. Twenty-three per cent of North American travelers returning from Leningrad have been shown to have giardiasis. Typically the infected traveler develops symptoms

---

*Investigational drug for this purpose.

several weeks after returning home, and on this basis the infection may be distinguished from that caused by toxigenic *Escherichia coli* and other forms of infectious traveler's diarrhea with shorter incubation periods.

PATHOGENICITY. Jejunal mucosal biopsies from infected persons range in appearance from normal to marked subtotal mucosal atrophy with submucosal inflammatory cell infiltration, reduced villous height, and elongated crypts. Electron microscopic observation of epithelial cells beneath overlying adherent trophozoites shows deformation and blunting of the individual microvilli. The mechanisms for these changes remain unknown. Possible hypotheses include mechanical interference by *Giardia* overlying the epithelium, elaboration by the parasite of an unidentifiable soluble toxin, competition between the parasite and host for nutrients, direct damage of the epithelium by adherent trophozoites, concurrent abnormal small-intestinal bacterial overgrowth, invasion of submucosa by *Giardia* trophozoites with consequent elicitation of cellular inflammation, and immunopathogenic mechanisms mediated by the host's immune system.

CLINICAL MANIFESTATIONS. The majority of infections with *Giardia* are asymptomatic. In those persons who are ill, disease ranges from mild diarrhea to severe debilitating malabsorption and weight loss. Reversible lactase deficiency as well as malabsorption of fat and vitamin B_{12} have been documented. The majority of symptoms result from malabsorption and include abdominal distention, cramps, nausea, flatulence, borborygmi, and frequent loose, bulky, foul, and urgent stools. Upper gastrointestinal symptoms such as nausea and epigastric pain may distinguish giardiasis from infectious disorders of the colon. Although some persons have a self-limited infection of several weeks' duration, many have a prolonged indolent illness with waxing and waning symptoms and progressive weight loss.

DIAGNOSIS. The diagnosis is established by demonstration of cysts or trophozoites in stools, or trophozoites in small-bowel contents. Because excretion of the organism in stool is episodic and its demonstration elusive, at least three stool specimens should be examined before a negative conclusion is drawn. If no organisms are seen the small-bowel contents may be sampled. This can be achieved by aspiration or passage of a string that will absorb sufficient jejunal fluid for examination. Microscopic examination of a wet preparation of jejunal contents will usually reveal motile organisms in the infected person. Small-bowel biopsy may be reserved for situations when these measures are unsuccessful. The small-bowel roentgenogram will usually show an edematous mucosa, but this finding is nonspecific. Hematologic studies are normal. Eosinophilia should not be expected, since this is a finding associated with infections by worms, not protozoa.

TREATMENT. All infected persons should be treated. There is occasional justification for a trial of therapy in the patient with typical signs and symptoms of giardiasis but in whom efforts to demonstrate the organism fail. Therapy is achieved with quinacrine hydrochloride, 100 mg three times daily for ten days. When this drug is contraindicated, metronidazole,* 250 mg three times daily for seven days, is an alternative. Treatment with either drug may be unsuccessful in 5 to 20 per cent of patients, requiring a second course of therapy. Resolution of symptoms is often slow, in spite of effective therapy.

---

*This use is not listed in the manufacturer's directive, but is recommended by the Centers for Disease Control.

Hoskins LC, Winawer SJ, Bortman SA, et al.: Clinical giardiasis and intestinal malabsorption. Gastroenterology 53:265, 1967. *Virtually every aspect of the clinical presentation of giardiasis is described in this series of case reports.*

Stevens DP: Selective primary health care: Strategies for control of disease in the developing world: XIX. Giardiasis. Rev Infect Dis 7:530, 1985. *A review of epidemiologic, clinical, and therapeutic aspects of giardiasis.*

Stevens DP: Giardiasis: Host-pathogen biology. Rev Infect Dis 4:851, 1982. *A detailed review of the sparse knowledge available on the pathogenesis of this infection.*

389 BABESIOSIS

Morton N. Swartz

DEFINITION. Babesiosis is a tick-borne malaria-like acute febrile illness caused by protozoa of the genus *Babesia* and usually occurring in sharply circumscribed endemic areas. Infection with *Babesia* was first recognized in animals, in which primary symptomatic illness (babesiosis) may be followed by persistent low-grade infection manifested only by the presence in blood of the parasites. Transmission of infection to humans is usually effected by ticks, rarely by transfusion of blood from an asymptomatic carrier.

PROTOZOAN AND VECTOR. *Babesia* is a protozoan that in mammalian hosts propagates only in erythrocytes: The majority of trophozoites differentiate into merozoites and undergo asexual reproduction. A small percentage of trophozoites undergo change to gametocytes identifiable on electron microscopy by a distinctive "arrowhead" organelle. Different species of *Babesia* have been described in specific vertebrate hosts, e.g., *B. canis* (dogs); *B. bovis* and *B. divergens* (cattle); *B. equi* (horses); *B. microti* (rodents). The latter has been the cause of most reported human cases, particularly those recently observed in the northeastern United States; rare cases in Europe have been due to *B. bovis* and *B. divergens*.

Ixodes dammini (northern deer tick), the same tick that is the vector of Lyme disease, is responsible for the spread of babesiosis from rodents to humans. In development through its three stages (larva, nymph, adult) the tick requires three animal hosts (of the same or different species), each as a source of a blood meal. Deer are the usual hosts for the adult tick, and the abundance of *I. dammini* in an area appears to depend on the presence locally of white-tailed deer. *I. dammini* appeared in adjoining areas of southeastern Massachusetts, Rhode Island, Connecticut, and New York in the 1930's to 1940's following reintroduction of deer into that area. By the 1980's the range of this tick had extended to include foci just north of Boston (particularly about the town of Ipswich); in Westchester County, New York; in southern New Jersey; in eastern Maryland; and in Wisconsin and Minnesota.

The initial step in the cycle of transmission occurs when larvae feed on infected rodents (white-footed mice in endemic areas of Massachusetts and New York) and acquire *B. microti* in the process. Infection in this rodent population can be extensive in endemic areas (60 per cent of white-footed mice on Nantucket Island harbor this protozoan). Infection in the larvae ultimately involves the salivary glands. Nymphs, the next stage, are the most abundant ticks on rodent reservoir hosts and usually feed from May through September. When an infected nymph takes its blood meal from rodents or man (requiring a period of at least 48 hours of feeding during which sporozoites replicate, mature, and become infectious), infection of these hosts ensues. Although transovarial transmission of other babesial species in other tick hosts occurs, there is no evidence that *B. microti* is transmitted in this way in *I. dammini*.

EPIDEMIOLOGY. Seven cases of babesiosis have been reported from Europe and about 120 additional human infections have been documented in the United States. The European cases have been caused by bovine *Babesia* (primarily *B. divergens*), have all occurred in splenectomized individuals, and have represented serious illness (71 per cent mortality). With the exception of two splenectomized patients in California who had infections thought to have been caused by equine *Babesia*, a patient in Georgia who harbored *Babesia* that were not defined as to species but were morphologically distinct from *B. microti*, and two patients with intraerythrocytic parasitosis due to a morphologically similar *Entopolypoides* species (family Babesiidae), the infections in the United States have all been caused by *B. microti*. The endemic area for human infection during the summer months includes circumscribed adjoining areas of Massachusetts (Nantucket Island, Martha's Vineyard, Cape Cod), Rhode Island, Connecticut, and New York (Shelter Island, Fire Island, eastern Long Island). Babesiosis has recently been reported in Wisconsin.

About 5 per cent of nymphal *I. dammini* on Nantucket are infected with *B. microti*. This finding, plus the fact that at least 48 hours of attachment and feeding are needed for transmission of infection, may account for the fact that infection is not more prevalent in endemic areas. However, the high frequency of parasitemia in white-footed mice in the offshore islands and the replacement of other rodent ticks by the newly dominant *I. dammini* may account for the increasing occurrence of human babesiosis in the endemic areas of the Northeast.

Subclinical infection occurs in humans: 4 to 7 per cent of asymptomatic individuals spending time outdoors in endemic areas during the summer months had significant IFA antibody titers to *B. microti*, and seroconversion had occurred in most. This appreciable rate assumes importance in view of the occurrence of transfusion-induced babesiosis in five patients. In several instances asymptomatic blood donors had been in endemic areas and had significant IFA titers against *B. microti*; *B. microti* was isolated on intraperitoneal inoculation of hamsters with blood from one such donor.

CLINICAL MANIFESTATIONS. The incubation period following a tick bite is one to six weeks. However, since the engorged nymph is only 2 mm in diameter, its presence may be easily overlooked. The incubation period for blood (or platelet) transfusion–induced babesiosis has been long (six to nine weeks) in five cases. Unlike the European cases, which were very severe and uniformly occurred in splenectomized patients, 70 per cent of clinical cases from the United States have occurred in patients with intact spleens. Most patients have been over 50 years of age and, with two exceptions, all recovered. The youngest patient was an infant of 10 weeks who developed transfusion-induced babesiosis and recovered with treatment.

The initial symptoms are nonspecific: malaise, fatigue, anorexia, headache, weakness. Fever (39 to 40° C), drenching sweats, chills, myalgias, and arthralgias then develop. Nausea and vomiting may occur; mental depression, mood lability, photophobia have been noted in some patients, but meningeal signs have been absent. The onset may occur acutely over a period of a few days or may be more protracted over several weeks. Lymphadenopathy is absent, but splenomegaly is detected in some patients. Rash is not observed. However, the simultaneous occurrence of Lyme disease and babesiosis has been observed in two patients; also, in endemic areas about one half of the patients with babesiosis, but without overt Lyme disease, have antibodies to *Borrelia burgdorferi*.

More severe disease occurs in splenectomized patients: Of 26 asplenic patients, six died (including five Europeans infected with bovine strains) with prominent hemolytic anemia, hemoglobinuria, jaundice, and renal insufficiency.

Occasional asymptomatic cases of human babesiosis have been described in the known endemic areas and elsewhere (Georgia, Mexico) in which the protozoan has been identified on blood smear or on animal inoculation of the individual's blood.

In addition to renal failure, occasional clinical complications of babesiosis have included pulmonary edema, adult respiratory distress syndrome, disseminated intravascular coagulopathy, and retinopathy ("cotton-wool" spots) in one patient. A nonsplenectomized pregnant woman who developed mild (4.3 per cent parasitized erythrocytes) symptomatic infection with *B. microti* during the fifth month of gestation recovered without specific treatment. Her infant daughter was delivered at term, had no detectable IgM antibody to *B. microti*, and exhibited neither clinical nor hematologic evidence of babesiosis.

Unlike certain malarial infections, relapses do not occur following recovery from babesiosis even though clearance of parasitemia may have been slow.

Hematologic changes consist of a hemolytic anemia with reticulocytosis, reduced serum haptoglobin level, normal or slightly reduced leukocyte count, and mild to moderate thrombocytopenia. Rarely, disseminated intravascular coagulation has developed in severe cases. In some patients with clinical babesiosis, tests for globulin on red blood cells give positive results as in patients with malaria. Usually, from 1 to 10 per cent of erythrocytes on peripheral blood smears contain the parasite. Parasitemias well below 1 per cent and as high as 85 per cent have been reported in patients with clinical illness. Mild elevations of serum bilirubin, SGOT, and alkaline phosphatase are common. Urinalysis shows proteinuria and hemoglobinuria.

Rarely babesiosis may present with a hematologic picture of pancytopenia and with bone marrow showing increased numbers of macrophages and marked hematophagocytosis, suggesting a diagnosis of malignant histiocytosis.

IMMUNITY. Babesiosis in humans caused by *B. microti* is a self-limited disease in most instances, presumably because of control exercised by the host immune defenses. IgM and IgG antibodies are detectable within a few days of the initial clinical manifestations, probably reflecting the relatively long prepatent period. However, parasitemia continues in the presence of such antibodies during the course of the clinical illness and after subsidence of symptoms. Considerable evidence indicates a role for the spleen in the host defense against *Babesia*: (1) increased severity of illness in asplenic humans, (2) increased level of parasitemia in experimental animals splenectomized before or during infection, and (3) recrudescent parasitemia following recovery from babesiosis in hamsters subsequently splenectomized.

The cellular immune response plays an important role in protection. Administration of antilymphocyte serum (ALS) to hamsters prior to infection with *B. microti* results in failure to induce specific antibody, exaggerated parasitemia, and death; in animals that have successfully handled infection, later administration of ALS results in recrudescent parasitemia and some mortality despite high serum antibody levels.

DIAGNOSIS. The diagnosis of babesiosis should be considered in a febrile patient from an endemic area in the tick season or in one who has received a blood transfusion (including platelet infusions or transfusions of frozen-thawed blood). The diagnosis is established by finding characteristic intraerythrocytic forms (pyriform, ring, tetrad) on thin or thick Giemsa-stained blood smears. Parasitized red blood cells are not larger than normal as they are in *Plasmodium vivax* infection. Ring forms of *Babesia* (often several in a single red cell) may be mistaken for *P. falciparum*, but can be distinguished by the presence of pigment deposits in erythrocytes parasitized by older forms of the latter. (However, small chromatin dots can be seen as part of the ring forms of *B. microti*.) Also, schizonts and gametocytes are not observed in *Babesia* infection but may be present in blood smears of patients with malaria. Tetrad (maltese cross) forms are uncommonly present in human blood smears, but are sufficiently distinctive when present to indicate babesiosis. With intense parasitemia, extraerythrocytic parasites (merozoites) in clusters may be seen occasionally in blood smears. Since parasitemia may vary, smears should be obtained over several days in suspected cases. Confirmation of diagnosis can be made by demonstration of IFA antibody (Centers for Disease Control) to *B. microti* in sera of patients; titers rise to 1:1024 or greater within the first few weeks of illness and then fall gradually over the next six months. Confirmation of the diagnosis can also be made by demonstration of parasitemia in blood smears of hamsters inoculated intraperitoneally with a patient's blood.

THERAPY. Patients with intact spleens, low-level parasitemia, and mild symptoms often recover without specific treatment. In adults with serious babesiosis, quinine (650 mg orally every six to eight hours) combined with clindamycin (300 to 600 mg intravenously every six hours) for seven to ten days is the current treatment of choice. This drug combination has been used successfully in treating at least five markedly symptomatic adults with prominent parasitemia and one heavily infected infant. In the hamster model of *B. microti* infection, clindamycin plus quinine also proved effective in rapidly clearing the infection. Other antimalarial drugs (pyrimethamine-sulfadoxine, primaquine) have no effect on parasitemia in animals.

The response to therapy is best followed by evaluating clinical parameters (fever, hemoglobinuria, etc.) and hematologic findings (anemia, reticulocytosis, serum haptoglobin levels, etc.) and by determining daily the percentage of red blood cells parasitized. Exchange transfusions have been very helpful in several ill patients with intense degrees (40 to 60 per cent) of parasitemia and hemolysis.

PREVENTION. Prevention consists of avoiding contact with nymphal *I. dammini* in endemic areas during May through September. If tick-infested areas are to be entered, use of repellents containing diethyltoluamide is advisable. Also, careful daily examination for ticks should be performed, and any found to be attached should be removed by fine forceps placed close to the site of attachment. Asplenic patients particularly should avoid endemic areas where they might come in contact with ticks.

In view of the cases of transfusion-induced babesiosis, current policy is not to accept as blood donors anyone with a history of babesiosis or any permanent residents of endemic areas (Shelter Island, Nantucket, etc.).

Auerbach M, Haubenstock A, Soloman G: Systemic babesiosis. Another cause of the hemophagocytic syndrome. Am J Med 80:301, 1986. *An interesting report of a patient with babesiosis with pancytopenia and prominent hemophagocytosis in bone mrrow suggesting the diagnosis of malignant histiocytosis.*

Marcus LC, Steere AC, Duray PH, et al.: Fatal pancarditis in a patient with coexistent Lyme disease and babesiosis. Ann Intern Med 103:374, 1985. *Report of a nonsplenectomized patient with dual infection with* Babesia microti *and* Borrelia burgdorferi *acquired on Nantucket Island.*

Rosner F, Zarrabi MH, Benach JL, et al.: Babesiosis in splenectomized adults. Am J Med 76:696, 1984. *Helpful summary of the 22 reported cases of human babesiosis that have occurred in splenectomized patients.*

Ruebush TK II, Cassaday PB, Marsh HJ, et al.: Human babesiosis on Nantucket Island. Ann Intern Med 86:6, 1977. *Good description of the clinical illness.*

Spielman A, Wilson ML, Levine JF, et al.: Ecology of Ixodes dammini–borne human babesiosis and Lyme disease. Ann Rev Entomol 30:439, 1985. *An excellent review of the epidemiology of babesiosis with particular emphasis on the association of* I. dammini *with its various hosts.*

Sun T, Tenenbaum MJ, Greenspan J, et al.: Morphologic and clinical observations in human infection with *Babesia microti*. J Infect Dis 148:239, 1983. *Detailed electron and light microscopic studies of Babesia infection in a patient with 85 per cent parasitemia.*

Wittner M, Rowin KS, Tanowitz HB, et al.: Successful chemotherapy of transfusion babesiosis. Ann Intern Med 96:601, 1982. *An important paper describing a case of transfusion-induced babesiosis successfully treated with the combination of quinine and clindamycin.*

390 AMEBIASIS

Donald J. Krogstad

DEFINITION. Amebiasis is defined as infection with the protozoan parasite *Entamoeba histolytica*.

ETIOLOGY. *E. histolytica* exists in both cyst and trophozoite forms. Motile trophozoites (12 to 50 μm) are found typically in the bloody and mucoid stools of patients with active disease. Cysts are smaller (10 to 20 μm) and nonmotile. They are the infectious form of the parasite and are found charac-

teristically in the formed stools of asymptomatic patients and those with minimal disease. Their double cyst membrane is an adaptation that protects them from desiccation and from gastric juice after ingestion. In contrast, trophozoites (which do not have this protective double membrane) disintegrate rapidly after excretion into the external environment. Trophozoites are not infectious on oral ingestion except in patients taking antacids or those with achlorhydria.

PREVALENCE. The data available suggest that less than 1 per cent of the United States population is infected with this organism (by stool examination) or has serologic evidence of previous infection (a positive antibody titer). The 5 to 10 per cent prevalence estimates of 50 to 70 years ago are no longer valid, although they are applicable in some developing countries.

EPIDEMIOLOGY. In most developed countries amebiasis is a mixture of indigenous and imported disease. Because the organism does not require a soil phase in its life cycle, it is not restricted to warmer climates. Thus, it may be transmitted by the fecal-oral route in areas far from the tropics. For example, there have been well-described outbreaks of amebiasis in the northern United States and Europe, including a relatively recent outbreak that was transmitted by the practice of colonic irrigation. Amebiasis may also be transmitted by sexual activity and is an important public health problem among homosexual populations.

Imported disease may result from the immigration of infected persons or from foreign travel by tourists. Although many refugees who come to the United States are screened for amebiasis, most returning tourists and their physicians are unaware of this risk. Thus, these patients may be mistakenly diagnosed as having ulcerative colitis and inappropriately treated with steroids.

In developing countries, the lack of sanitation and the high prevalence of infection combine to produce a greater risk of transmission than in developed countries. In both developing and developed countries, patients severely ill with amebiasis are less likely to transmit the infection than infected persons who are well or asymptomatic because ill patients excrete the more fragile trophozoite form in their stool. Thus, the epidemiology of amebiasis is complicated by the fact that the persons most important for transmission are minimally symptomatic or asymptomatic and are thus less likely to seek medical help.

PATHOGENESIS AND MECHANISMS OF DISEASE. *E. histolytica* directly invades the intestinal mucosa to cause amebic colitis and may also travel via the bloodstream to produce metastatic infections in the liver and at other sites. Although the mechanism(s) by which *E. histolytica* produces disease is incompletely defined, important factors include direct contact between the parasite and the mammalian target cell, calcium, phospholipase A, and an acid pH in the parasite's intracellular vesicles. Normal colonic mucin contains a glycoprotein that inhibits the adherence of *E. histolytica* to mammalian cells. This suggests that changes in colonic mucus may play an important role in the transition of *E. histolytica* from a commensal to a pathogenic organism.

PATHOLOGY. Amebic colitis is characterized by flask-shaped ulcers that contain pus and amebic trophozoites. On histologic examination with routine hematoxylin and eosin staining, trophozoites are usually identifiable at the periphery of these ulcers. Except for the presence of *E. histolytica* and the shape of the ulcers, these lesions may be mistaken for the colitis of inflammatory bowel disease. By contrast, amebic abscesses in the liver and elsewhere usually contain few identifiable amebae, typically found at the border between the abscess and normal tissue.

CLINICAL MANIFESTATIONS. The vast majority of persons infected with *E. histolytica* have few or no detectable symptoms from their infection. In a minority of patients, this commensal relationship breaks down for unknown reasons and the organism becomes a pathogen. The manifestations of amebic colitis may be subtle or severe and range from mild watery diarrhea to explosive, bloody dysentery with a fulminant course. In addition, it is not uncommon for the disease to wax and wane. The same patient may experience both exacerbations and remissions over a period of months to years without treatment.

Outside the gastrointestinal tract, amebic disease typically presents as a slowly expanding mass lesion. Abscesses are most frequently found in the liver, where right-sided lesions are much more common than left-sided ones (presumably owing to the vascular supply of the liver). For reasons that are not clear, amebic liver abscesses are much more common in males than females (6 to 7:1). Important clues to the presence of an amebic liver abscess include elevation of the right hemidiaphragm, right upper quadrant pain, and fever.

Although amebic abscesses are most common in the liver, the infection may also extend to the lung or pericardium and may metastasize to more distant sites, such as the central nervous system. Less frequently, lesions may present in the anogenital area. These lesions have been confused with squamous cell carcinoma of the rectum, penis, and cervix on the basis of their macroscopic appearance, although histologic examination typically reveals *E. histolytica* trophozoites.

DIAGNOSIS. *Stool Examination.* Stool examination for *E. histolytica* (Color plate 5H) is one of the most difficult tests to perform correctly in the clinical laboratory. False-negative results are common because morphology is insensitive. In addition, false-positive test results have been reported by inexperienced observers who have confused both white blood cells and other amebae with *E. histolytica. Entamoeba hartmanni* is a particular problem, because the only criterion by which it can be distinguished from *E. histolytica* is size. It tends to be smaller in diameter (cyst 5 to 8 μm, trophozoites 6 to 10 μm) than *E. histolytica*. This distinction is difficult even for experienced observers and is impossible without the use of an ocular micrometer to measure parasite size accurately.

In patients with severe intestinal disease, *E. histolytica* trophozoites tend to be large (25 to 50 μm in diameter) and actively motile. Another useful clue is the presence of ingested red blood cells, which are characteristic of *E. histolytica* but not of nonpathogenic protozoa. However, ingested red blood cells are not diagnostic of amebiasis. Macrophages may ingest red blood cells and have often been misdiagnosed as amebae on this basis in patients with shigellosis. Although material should be preserved in polyvinyl alcohol fixative for a permanent record, supravital stains such as methylene blue are often invaluable because they permit one to distinguish *E. histolytica* from white cells and other actively motile cells in the stool (by nuclear morphology) at the time of the initial stool examination.

The most important cause of false-negative stool examinations for *E. histolytica* is the presence of interfering substances. These include particulate material that obscures the parasite (barium sulfate, bismuth, and kaolin compounds), agents that lyse trophozoites (soap and tap water enemas), and antimicrobials that decrease the number of parasites excreted in the stool (tetracycline, sulfonamides, antiprotozoal agents). After excluding these substances (for 7 to 10 days prior to stool examination), there are several additional procedures worth considering in patients with negative stool examinations who are suspected of having amebiasis. Because long delays in transporting specimens to the laboratory may produce false-negative results, the next step should be to obtain fresh material from the patient and to examine it directly. If these examinations are negative, one may often increase the yield by examining pus or exudate taken at proctoscopy or sigmoidoscopy. This material should be taken with a glass rod or metal spatula, because parasites tend to adhere to cotton swabs. If the results are negative, biopsy of a rectal valve is frequently diagnostic. Even when all efforts to make a morphologic diagnosis are unsuccessful, serology is often positive.

Serology. Because most patients develop symptomatic amebiasis over months to years, the usual two- to four-week delay for the development of antibodies is not a significant problem. In the United States, where amebiasis is rare, a positive antibody titer is strong suggestive evidence for amebiasis. Most patients (≥ 80 per cent) with active intestinal disease have a positive indirect hemagglutination (IHA) test result. The sensitivity of this test is even greater in extraintestinal (metastatic) disease; 96 to 100 per cent of patients with amebic liver abscesses have positive titers (≥ 1:128). In areas where amebic infection is common, a positive titer is less useful because titers may remain elevated for years after resolution of the acute infection.

Many patients with active amebic disease have circulating immune complexes that contain amebic antigen. The titers of these immune complexes may decrease rapidly with treatment—in contrast to IHA titers, which tend to fall more slowly.

Radiology. Radiologic examination is often abnormal in amebic colitis. It may reveal mass lesions (ameboma), ulcerations, pseudomembranes, or toxic megacolon. However, these lesions are nonspecific and may also be produced by cancer or inflammatory bowel disease. Their lack of specificity emphasizes the need for a specific diagnosis based on morphology, i.e., microscopic identification of the parasite, or a positive serology.

A number of radiologic techniques have been used to demonstrate extraintestinal amebic disease. The most frequently used is technetium-99 scanning, which characteristically reveals an area of decreased uptake in amebic liver abscess. However, amebic liver abscesses have also been visualized by ultrasonography, gallium scanning, and computed tomography. In selecting a radiologic technique, observer experience is a more important variable with ultrasonography than with the other techniques. We recommend technetium scanning as the initial radiologic test for liver abscess and computed tomography or ultrasonography if the technetium scan is normal and for disease outside the liver.

TREATMENT. The treatment of amebiasis remains unsatisfactory. It is complicated because different forms of the infection require different treatment regimens (Table 390–1) and because several antiamebic drugs have significant toxicity.

TABLE 390–1. TREATMENT OF PATIENTS WITH AMEBIASIS*

Intestinal Infection

Cysts in stool (patients with few or no symptoms):

Diloxanide furoate (Furamide)†	500 mg three times a day for 10 days
Diiodohydroxyquin‡	650 mg three times a day for 20 days
Paromomycin	8–12 mg per kg three times a day for 7 days

Trophozoites in stool (patients with symptomatic disease):

Metronidazole (Flagyl)	750 mg three times a day for 10 days
Dehydroemetine†	1.0 to 1.5 mg per kilogram per day for 10 days intramuscularly or subcutaneously

Extraintestinal Infection

Metronidazole (Flagyl)	750 mg three times a day for 10 days
Chloroquine plus diiodohydroxyquin‡	500 mg a day for 10 weeks, plus 650 mg three times a day for 20 days
Dehydroemetine† plus chloroquine	As above, plus 500 mg a day for 2 to 3 weeks
Dehydroemetine†	As above

*Doses suggested are for adults: Unless otherwise noted, doses are for oral administration.

†Available from the Parasitic Disease Drug Service, Centers for Disease Control, Atlanta, Ga 30333 (404-329-3670; nights and weekends, 329-2888).

‡Now used less frequently because a close congener (iodochlorhydroxyquin-Entero-Vioform) has been associated with subacute myelo-optic neuropathy. Available from Panray Division of Orment Drug and Chemical, Englewood, NJ 07631, and Glenwood Laboratories, Tenafly, NJ 07670.

Adapted with permission from The New England Journal of Medicine (from Krogstad et al., 1978).

Emetine and dehydroemetine are cardiotoxic; metronidazole is mutagenic in bacteria and produces tumors in rodents.

Although susceptibility testing is not yet practical for individual patients, it is nevertheless important to individualize the treatment of patients with amebiasis. For instance, metronidazole penetrates the blood-brain barrier well and is an excellent choice for patients with suspected central nervous system involvement. Conversely, diloxanide furoate is the preferred agent for patients with minimal or no symptoms who are passing cysts in their stool.

PROGNOSIS. The prognosis of amebic infection is usually excellent if it is recognized before the patient is critically ill. However, steroids have been shown to enhance the pathogenicity of *E. histolytica* in animals and may interfere with the response to therapy in man. In addition, peritonitis may result from colonic perforation in amebic colitis or from rupture of an amebic liver abscess and clearly results in a worse prognosis.

Although high IHA antibody titers are associated with active disease, patients whose titers fall more slowly after therapy do not necessarily have persistent disease. Therefore, we recommend that patients be followed clinically and that those with persistently high titers not be re-treated on this basis alone.

PREVENTION. Amebiasis can be prevented by careful hygiene. Because amebic cysts are killed by cooking, only uncooked foods such as salads or those contaminated after cooking can transmit the infection. In endemic areas, it is best to avoid fresh, uncooked vegetables and fruits that cannot be peeled. The concentration of chlorine necessary to kill amebic cysts (≥ 10 ppm) is substantially greater than the levels used for water purification (1 to 2 ppm) and is unpalatable. Therefore, most water systems depend on sedimentation and filtration to remove amebic cysts.

Healy GR, Kraft SC: The indirect hemagglutination test for amebiasis in patients with inflammatory bowel disease. Am J Dig Dis 17:97, 1972. *Indirect hemagglutination antibody titers to E. histolytica are reliable in screening patients with inflammatory bowel disease for amebiasis.*

Istre GR, Kreiss K, Hopkins RS, et al.: Outbreak of amebiasis spread by colonic irrigation at a chiropractic clinic. N Engl J Med 307:399, 1982. *This outbreak demonstrates the potential danger of such practices (presumably including penile-rectal intercourse) that transfer colonic contents from one person to another.*

Krogstad DJ, Spencer HC Jr, Healy GR, et al.: Amebiasis: Epidemiologic studies in the United States, 1971–1974. Ann Intern Med 88:89, 1978. *This study demonstrates that lack of diagnostic skill in the United States produces both false-positive and false-negative laboratory results that lead to inappropriate therapy and increased morbidity and mortality. It also emphasizes the difficulty of distinguishing clinically between inflammatory bowel disease and amebic colitis.*

Mirelman D: *Entamoeba histolytica:* Effect of bacterial associates and culture conditions on isoenzyme patterns. Parasitol Today 3, 37, 1987. *This paper demonstrates that one can change the pathogenicity of E. histolytica by manipulating culture conditions in vitro.*

Pillai S, Mohimen A: A solid-phase sandwich radioimmunoassay for *Entamoeba histolytica* proteins and the detection of circulating antigens in amebiasis. Gastroenterology 83:1210, 1982. *This report suggests that the disappearance of circulating immune complexes from the serum may be a clinically useful indicator of successful treatment.*

Ravdin JI, Schlesinger PH, Murphy CF, et al.: Acid intracellular vesicles and the cytolysis of mammalian target cells by *Entamoeba histolytica* trophozoites. J Protozool 33:478, 1986. *An uninterrupted acid pH in the intracellular endocytic vesicles is necessary for amebic cytolysis of mammalian target cells.*

AMEBIC MENINGOENCEPHALITIS AND KERATITIS

Amebic meningoencephalitis is an infection of the brain and meninges caused by free-living amebae. It has been associated with *Naegleria, Acanthamoeba, Hartmanella,* and other free-living amebae. (*Acanthamoeba* may also cause a keratitis that is difficult to diagnose and treat. Amebic keratitis is associated with ocular trauma, including that caused by contact lenses, and may respond to topical and/or systemic treatment with the imidazoles.)

Amebic meningoencephalitis is a rare disease; only 100 to 200 cases have been reported. However, its prevalence has probably been underestimated because of difficulty in making the diagnosis. There are two different forms of primary amebic meningoencephalitis. One occurs primarily in young, healthy individuals who have been swimming in artifical fresh water lakes and is typically caused by one of the free-living *Naegleria* species. The other is more subacute and is associated with immunocompromised hosts. It is usually caused by *Acanthamoeba, Hartmannella,* or other free-living amebae, but not *Naegleria.*

In both of these infections, the morbidity and mortality are caused by meningitis and a hemorrhagic encephalitis. Inflammatory and hemorrhagic changes along the olfactory tract are often prominent in disease caused by *Naegleria.* This infection is thought to gain access to the central nervous system by crossing the cribriform plate from the nose during swimming exposure in fresh water. The pathogenesis of disease caused by *Acanthamoeba* and the other free-living amebae not associated with fresh water exposure is less clear. However, several investigators have described other amebic infections in these patients at distant sites such as the lung and have postulated hematogenous spread to the central nervous system.

Both types of amebic meningoencephalitis are characterized by fever, meningismus, and obtundation. The major distinctions between them are in the epidemiologic history and the tempo of the disease. Infections caused by *Naegleria* tend to be more fulminant, with a course of several days to a week and a half. In contrast, disease among immunosuppressed hosts tends to be more subacute.

The diagnosis of amebic meningoencephalitis is often missed because the amebae are mistaken for lymphocytes in the cerebrospinal fluid. In previously healthy young patients, the disease is also confused with viral meningitis. In compromised hosts, it may be confused with toxoplasmosis, cytomegalovirus infection, and other opportunistic pathogens. The diagnosis is best made by careful examination of spinal fluid wet mounts for motile trophozoites, 8 to 15 μm in size.

The outlook for patients with this infection is grim. There are only a few known survivors. The limited data available suggest that intravenous and intrathecal amphotericin B and miconazole, plus oral rifampin, may be effective. However, serologic studies in areas with known cases suggest that subclinical illness and spontaneous recoveries do occur with this infection. Although the only preventive measure is to avoid swimming in lakes epidemiologically associated with this infection, the risk is low (probably less than one in a million).

Cohen EJ, Buchanan HW, Laughrea PA, et al.: Diagnosis and management of *Acanthamoeba* keratitis. Am J Ophthalmol 100:389, 1985. *This paper stresses the difficulty of making an accurate diagnosis in these patients.*

Seidel JS, Harimatz P, Visvesvara VS, et al.: Successful treatment of primary amebic meningoencephalitis. N Engl J Med 306:346, 1982. *The in vitro susceptibility studies included in this report suggest that the combination of amphotericin B and miconazole may be synergistic against* Naegleria.

391 OTHER PROTOZOAN DISEASES

David P. Stevens

The human host provides an everchanging environment for protozoan infections. With the increasing prevalence of immune deficiency, caused by either immunosuppressant drugs or the acquired immunodeficiency syndrome (AIDS), protozoan infections that were previously considered rare or exotic are now observed more frequently. With this changing epidemiologic setting, additional protozoa will play the opportunist's role as pathogenic agents.

Protozoa that cause these infections should be distinguished, however, from the numerous nonpathogenic protozoa that may be found in the stool of apparently healthy persons. Notable among them are *Entamoeba coli, Endolimax nana, Iodamoeba butschlii, Dientamoeba fragilis, Trichomonas hominis,* and *Chilomastix mesnili.* The clinician must rely on a skilled laboratory technician to differentiate these agents from pathogenic species such as *Entamoeba histolytica* and the organisms discussed in the following chapters.

TRICHOMONIASIS

Trichomonas vaginalis is the only species of the trichomonads that is pathogenic for humans. *T. tenax* and *T. hominis* infect the human gastrointestinal tract, but as harmless commensals. *T. vaginalis* is a 10- to -20 μ motile flagellated organism that ordinarily inhabits the urethra, urinary bladder, vagina, and prostate. Nearly half of infections are asymptomatic. Recognized symptoms include a yellow creamy vaginal discharge associated with itching and burning. Dysuria may be prominent. Infection in the male is generally asymptomatic. Occasionally, however, it is associated with mild urethral burning of brief duration.

Diagnosis is made microscopically by identification of the organism in a wet preparation of the exudate. Long-term complications are unrecognized in otherwise healthy persons. Treatment of both partners is advised for this sexually transmitted disease. Treatment with a single 2-gram dose of metronidazole is as effective as metronidazole 250 mg three times daily for seven days. It is frequently associated with side effects of nausea, a metallic taste, or alcohol intolerance.

Lossick JG: Sexually transmitted vaginitis. Urol Clin North Am 11:141, 1984. *An authoritative clinical report for further detailed study.*

BALANTIDIASIS

Balantidium coli is a large, motile, oval ciliate, some five to ten times the size of an erythrocyte. The trophozoite form resides as a facultative anaerobe in the colon. The great majority of infections in humans are noninvasive, asymptomatic, and self limited. Infrequently a cause of disease, this protozoan can penetrate the colonic mucosa with formation of deep ulcers. Illness consists of dysentery, usually bloody, often with resulting dehydration and prostration. Complications include colonic perforation at the site of the ulcers. Infection may extend to mesenteric lymph nodes and, less commonly, the appendix and terminal ileum. Isolated reports of infection of vagina, liver, lung, and pleura have documented that extraintestinal migration of the organism is rare.

Balantidia infect numerous nonhuman reservoirs, particularly swine. It is said that 80 per cent of pigs in England carry this organism. The relevance of various other animal reservoirs, such as rats, to human infection is debated. The importance of porcine infections to human disease is borne out, however, by the documented high incidence of balantidiasis in communities where swine and humans live together closely, e.g., in New Guinea, Micronesia, Peru, and southern Russia. Poor nutrition and debilitating illness seem to predispose to symptomatic balantidiasis. Person-to-person spread probably occurs in settings where crowding and poor hygiene exist.

Ingestion of *Balantidium* cysts leads to infection in the susceptible host. Excystation occurs at an unknown location in the gastrointestinal tract, and multiplication occurs in the colon. An immune response develops in humans when tissue invasion occurs and is demonstrated by the presence of circulating immunofluorescent antibodies. Encystation occurs in the distal colon or after expulsion into the environment. The cyst, resistant to drying and other environmental stresses, becomes again the infectious form for the subsequent host.

The diagnosis is confirmed by microscopic demonstration of trophozoites in fresh wet preparations of liquid stool or scrapings of colonic ulcers. Cysts are less frequently observed in stool, and concentration techniques are usually required. Differentiation from amebiasis and idiopathic ulcerative colitis must always be considered.

Therapy is reserved for the patient with symptomatic infection and consists of tetracycline, 500 mg four times daily for ten days. Metronidazole, 250 mg four times daily for seven days, is probably effective and may serve as alternative therapy when tetracycline is not tolerated.

Knight R: Giardiasis, isosporiasis, and balantidiasis. Clin Gastroenterol 7:31, 1978. *There are few timely clinical reviews on balantidiasis; this is the best of the lot.*

SARCOSPORIDIOSIS

Infections with *Sarcocystis hominis* (previously designated *Isospora hominis*) may be associated with abdominal pain, diarrhea, and nausea. The human is the definitive host with sexual reproduction taking place in the small intestine; cattle are the intermediate host where the sarcocyst resides in the skeletal or cardiac muscle with little or no reaction. While infection in humans is relatively common in areas of the world where undercooked beef is ingested, the definition of the precise role of this agent in human disease remains clouded by its frequent coincidence with other pathogenic agents.

Beaver PC, Gadgil RK, Morera P: Sarcocysts in man: A review and report of five cases. Am J Trop Med Hyg 28:810, 1979. *This reference provides a good starting point into the available clinical literature.*

SECTION TWO / HELMINTHIC DISEASES
The Cestodes

Martin S. Wolfe

392 INTRODUCTION

More than 30 species of tapeworms, or cestodes, may infect man. They are dorsoventrally flattened and creamy white, and their habitat is the intestinal tract of vertebrates. With the exception of *Hymenolepis nana*, which can be passed directly from person to person, all the species that parasitize man require at least one intermediate host to complete their life cycle.

Adult cestodes range in size from the smallest, *Echinococcus* species of 2 to 9 mm long, to the largest, *Diphyllobothrium latum,* which ranges in size from 3 to 10 meters long. They all have characteristic morphologic and biologic features that differentiate them from other helminths and from each other. Most adult tapeworms consist of a head or scolex for attachment to the intestinal wall of the host, followed by an unsegmented narrow neck from which immature segments or proglottides develop progressively to fully developed mature proglottides. Most distal are the oldest and gravid segments, which are essentially a sac of eggs. The entire worm, from the scolex to and including the distal gravid proglottides, is called the strobila. Each mature proglottid has both sets of sex organs, nerve trunks, and an excretory canal. There is no alimentary canal in tapeworms, and food is absorbed directly from the cuticle, which has a microvillous surface similar to intestinal mucosa of vertebrates. Diagnosis of certain species can be made from the gravid segments, which may have particular branchings and shape of the uterus or position of the genital pore.

Eggs are passed from the bowel either in the segment or free in the stool and contain a form infective for an intermediate host. Eggs may be operculate, an adaptation for hatching in water, or nonoperculate, which usually develop in soil. Operculate eggs, exemplified by *D. latum,* are undeveloped when passed and develop into a free-swimming larva or coracidium that hatches in 9 to 12 days. This is ingested by a copepod, in which further development takes place to a procercoid larva; this in turn is ingested by an appropriate fish, in whose flesh the infective or plerocercoid larva is found. When man ingests fish with a plerocercoid larva, the larva adheres to the small intestinal wall, where it develops. When nonoperculate eggs of other species are ingested by an appropriate intermediate host, an embryo or oncosphere is released, which has the capability of penetrating the intestinal mucosa. Oncospheres of *Taenia* species penetrate the intestinal wall of the intermediate host and develop into small, fluid-filled structures called cysticerci, which are distributed in various tissues and cause the disease cysticercosis. *H. nana* oncospheres penetrate only into the villi of the small intestine and develop into cysticercoids, which eventualy break out into the lumen of the intestine and attach and develop into adults. With *Echinococcus granulosus* usually only one oncosphere develops into a cyst in the intermediate host, but this hydatid or echinococcal cyst is capable of producing daughter cysts, each containing many scolices, from an internal germinating membrane.

Pathogenesis and symptomatology are determined by the various forms of development. Humans are the definitive host of adult *D. latum* and *Taenia* worms, but the most serious effects occur when man becomes an accidental intermediate host of *Taenia solium* and cysticerci lead to many small lesions in the muscle and brain. The cysticercoids and adults of *H. nana* and adults of *Taenia* species may cause irritation of the small intestine. *Echinococcus* and *Multiceps* species produce large, space-occupying cysts with symptoms depending on their location.

In the following chapters, geographic distribution, essential biology, epidemiology, pathogenesis, symptomatology, diagnosis, and prevention will be described for each of the common and some less common cestode species that parasitize man. A final chapter will deal with the treatment of tapeworms.

Beaver PC, Jung RC, Cupp EW: Clinical Parasitology. 9th ed. Philadelphia, Lea & Febiger, 1984, Ch 29–31. *An encyclopedic review of both common and very rare tapeworms of man.*

Marcial-Rojas RA (ed.): Pathology of Protozoal and Helminthic Diseases with Clinical Correlations. Baltimore, Williams & Wilkins Company, 1971, pp 585–657. *A well-illustrated and very complete discussion of pathologic and clinical aspects of the major tapeworms.*

393 DIPHYLLOBOTHRIUM LATUM (The Fish Tapeworm)

This parasite is most prevalent in parts of the northern and southern temperate zones where freshwater fish are commonly eaten. The highest incidence of infection of humans is in the countries bordering the Baltic Sea, particularly Finland and Sweden. In North America, a high incidence of *D. latum* infection occurs in Alaska, Canada, and the smaller lake areas of northern Michigan and Minnesota. A related species carried by marine fishes, *D. pacificum,* has been described from coastal Peru.

D. latum adults are the largest tapeworms of man and may reach 10 meters in length with up to 4000 proglottides. The scolex has two deep sulci or bothria, one dorsal and one ventral, for attachment to the wall of the ileum. The last four fifths of the worm consists of maturing and gravid proglottides. The mature proglottid is broader than it is long, and in its middle is a dark, rosette-shaped, coiled uterus, which is of diagnostic value. The distalmost proglottides gradually disintegrate and release eggs in the bowel lumen, rather than separating from the parent worm like *Taenia* segments. Eggs are yellowish-brown, ovoid, and operculated and measure 56 to 76 μ long by 40 to 56 μ wide. They contain immature embryos when discharged into the feces, and under favorable conditions they mature and hatch into a ciliated coracidium in 9 to 12 days. This is ingested by the first intermediate host, a freshwater copepod of the genus *Cyclops* or *Diaptomus,* wherein it develops into a procercoid larva. The copepod is in turn ingested by the second intermediate host, certain freshwater fish species, including pike, perch, and salmon. The procercoid larva develops into a plerocercoid larva (sparganum) within the muscle and viscera of the fish in 7 to 30 days. Man becomes infected by eating raw or insufficiently cooked fish. The sparganum adheres to the wall of the small intestine and becomes a mature worm in three to six weeks, and eggs begin to appear in the feces. Inadequate sewage disposal allows pollution by human feces of fresh water containing suitable intermediate hosts. The fish of small lakes are more important sources of infection than those of the Great Lakes, since the cold deep waters of the latter inhibit the hatching of eggs. Women of particular ethnic groups, such as Jews, Russians, and Scandinavians, are more frequently infected, by eating raw or undercooked fish in the preparation of ethnic foods such as gefilte fish. Dishes made from raw fish (particularly salmon and herring) such as sushi, sashimi, and ceviche, can be a source of infection. *D. latum* may live for up to 20 years.

The great majority of infections are with a single worm in the ileum. Most infected persons are asymptomatic, but some may experience intestinal symptoms from mucosal irritation. A moderate eosinophilia may be present. The most harmful effect of the fish tapeworm is vitamin B_{12} malabsorption and, rarely, a megaloblastic anemia. The exact mechanism is not certain, but it is related to the absorption of vitamin B_{12} by the worm. This is reported primarily in Scandinavians.

Diagnosis can be made by recovering characteristic eggs in the feces, or from the typical proglottides, which are broader than long and have a characteristic rosette-shaped uterus. There is no satisfactory serologic method of diagnosis.

Prevention begins with adequate disposal of raw sewage. Fish from known or suspected infected waters must be thoroughly cooked at 56°C for at least five minutes or frozen at −10°C for 72 hours or brined to ensure destruction of the infective larvae.

SPARGANOSIS

Sparganosis is an uncommon infection of man with larval diphyllobothroid tapeworms closely related to *D. latum*. It is caused by the sparganum or plerocercoid larva of the genus *Spirometra*, which measures up to several centimeters in length. Most human infections have been encountered in the Orient and are caused by *S. mansonoides*. Very rarely, infection is with a budding larval tapeworm, *S. proliferum*. The life cycle is similar to that of *D. latum*. Adult worms are found in dogs and cats, and in man only the larval form occurs. Eggs hatch in water and develop into procercoid larvae in *Cyclops* species, which are swallowed by the secondary intermediate host—a frog, snake, bird, or mammal. A plerocercoid larva develops in the muscle and is ingested by the definitive host. Humans usually become infected by ingesting infected copepods containing the procercoid larvae. Infections in the Far East may occur from the ingestion of infected raw flesh of amphibians and reptiles or by the use of these animals' flesh for medicinal skin or eye poultices. After penetrating the intestinal wall, the larvae usually migrate through the tissues and localize in the subcutaneous or muscular tissues. When infected poultices are applied to the eye, localization and edema may occur around the eye. A slowly growing, pruritic nodule develops over a three- to ten-month period, eventually measuring up to 3 cm. Local indurations, periodic urticaria, edema, erythema, chills, fever, and marked peripheral eosinophilia may occur. The parasite should be considered in anyone with a localized subcutaneous swelling and a possible exposure history. Diagnosis is by finding the characteristic larvae in the removed nodules. Infection can be prevented by avoiding untreated drinking water in endemic areas and avoiding the ingestion of uncooked flesh of amphibians and reptiles or the use of this flesh for poultices in the Far East.

Pathogenesis of tapeworm anemia (editorial). Br Med J 2:1028, 1976. *A brief update on this most intriguing aspect of fish tapeworm infection.*

Ruttenber AJ, Weniger BG, Sorvillo F, et al.: Diphyllobothriasis associated with salmon consumption in Pacific Coast states. Am J Trop Med Hyg 33:455, 1984. *A hazard from eating raw salmon, an increasingly popular delicacy.*

Swartzwelder JC, Beaver PC, Hood MW: Sparganosis in southern United States. Am J Trop Med Hyg 13:43, 1964. *A number of interesting case reports.*

Von Bonsdorff B: Diphyllobothriasis in Man. London, Academic Press, 1977. *Written from a medical rather than parasitologic viewpoint. A useful reference book that covers developments in diphyllobothriasis since Birkeland's monograph of 1932.*

Weinstein P, Krawczyk HG, Peers JH: Sparganosis in Korea. Am J Trop Med Hyg 3:112, 1954. *Three case reports and discussion of snake eating among Koreans and its possible relationship to sparganosis.*

394   TAENIA SAGINATA (The Beef Tapeworm)

Cattle are the most important intermediate hosts. In Africa cattle are frequently and heavily infected, and human infection rates may exceed 10 per cent in some areas. The parasite occurs throughout Asia, there is a low level of endemicity in Latin America and Europe, and rare cases are indigenously acquired in the United States. *Taenia saginata* is one of the most frequently diagnosed tapeworms in the United States, usually being acquired abroad.

The adult worm ranges from 4 to 10 meters in length and consists of 1000 to 2000 proglottides. The scolex has four prominent muscular suckers for attachment to the small intestinal wall. Proglottides are usually detached singly and have muscular power that allows them to move through the anal sphincter, or they may be carried out with the feces. The eggs are liberated from the proglottid. They are yellow-brown and cannot be morphologically differentiated from those of *Taenia solium*. Eggs become mature in approximately two weeks and are then infective to the intermediate hosts, primarily cattle. After hatching in the intestine, the oncospheres penetrate the intestinal wall and eventually localize in the skeletal muscles of cattle, where they develop in 60 to 75 days into small cysticerci having an opaque invaginated neck and a scolex with four suckers. In about 12 months the cysticercus degenerates and calcifies. Humans are the only definitive host and become infected by ingesting raw or undercooked beef containing cysticerci. The scolex evaginates and attaches to the jejunal mucosa, where in 8 to 12 weeks it develops into an adult worm. *Taenia* worms may live up to 25 years in man. Human infection is favored by the ingestion of meat in the form of beef tartare, rare steak, and undercooked shashlik or kabobs.

Usually only one worm is present, but multiple infections can occur rarely. In most cases the adult worms are in the upper jejunum and cause no damage or symptoms. Irritation, however, may cause flatulence, cramps, or diarrhea. Eosinophilia occurs in almost half of those infected and is usually less than 10 per cent. Infection is usually recognized by the spontaneous passage of gravid proglottides out of the anus or in the feces.

Diagnosis is made by pressing the passed proglottid between two large glass slides and counting the number of lateral uterine segments. *T. saginata* usually has 15 to 30 of these uterine segments, whereas the only other similar-appearing segment, that of *T. solium*, usually has less than 13 and an average of 9 uterine segments. Identification of lateral uterine segments can be made only on mature proglottides. In doubtful cases, diagnosis may require fixation and staining of the segments. Typical *Taenia* ova may be found on stool examination, but differentiation between *T. saginata* and *T. solium* cannot be made on egg morphology alone. Eggs may also be recovered from the perianal region with use of a cellophane tape swab. Serologic tests have not proved useful in the diagnosis of *T. saginata*.

Infection can best be prevented by avoiding rare or raw beef in highly endemic areas such as Africa. Thorough cooking of beef at 56°C for five minutes or freezing at −10°C for ten days will kill cysticerci.

Pawlowski Z, Schultz MG: Taeniasis cysticercosis (*Taenia saginata*). Adv Parasitol 10:269, 1972. *Detailed coverage of all aspects of this parasite.*

Penfold HB: The signs and symptoms of *Taenia saginata* infection. Med J Aust 1:531, 1937. *Common and uncommon findings in 100 patients.*

395 TAENIA SOLIUM (The Pork Tapeworm; Human Cysticercosis)

Human infection with *Taenia solium* is especially prevalent where man commonly consumes raw or insufficiently cooked pork. Infections with both adult worms and tissue larvae are particularly common in India, Africa, Mexico, and Latin America, but are rare in the United States and western Europe where most recognized cases are imported.

The adult worm is smaller than *T. saginata*, measuring 2 to 7 meters long and contains 800 to 1000 segments. The scolex has four cup-shaped suckers and differs from *T. saginata* in having a double crown of between 25 and 30 hooks on a low, rounded rostellum. Mature proglottides are flabby, have less muscular action than those of *T. saginata*, and have 7 to 12 lateral branches. The ova are morphologically identical to *T. saginata* ova. Gravid proglottides or eggs are ingested by the usual intermediate host, the hog, and less frequently by other intermediate hosts, including wild boars, sheep, camels, and humans. Eggs must first be digested by gastric juice before they hatch and liberate oncospheres, which then penetrate the intestinal wall and are carried throughout the body. They typically are filtered out in the muscles but can also reach other organs. In 60 to 70 days cysticerci develop that contain an invaginated scolex with hooks and suckers. Cysticerci may remain viable in the hog for three to six years or, rarely, longer. Man is the only natural definitive host and becomes infected by eating raw or undercooked pork. The cysticerci are dissolved by gastric juices, and the larval worm attaches to the upper jejunum by its evaginated scolex. In 5 to 12 weeks it develops into an adult worm. Human infection with *Cysticercus cellulosae* occurs when people ingest eggs in contaminated food or water or eggs transferred from the anus to the mouth, or, rarely, by the regurgitation of ova into the stomach by reverse peristalsis associated with vomiting in the presence of an adult worm. Human infection is most common in populations with a preference for pork, thus being rare in Moslems and Jews. Infection is also related to general poor hygienic conditions in which hogs are allowed to have frequent contact with infected feces. As it often takes some years for cysticerci to develop, die, and lead to overt symptoms, most cases are recognized in adulthood.

Intestinal infection is usually with one adult worm, and this seldom causes anything more than local irritation and mild eosinophilia. Cysticerci may develop in any tissue or organ of the body. The cysticercus matures in man in a few months and forms a translucent cyst, which gradually becomes surrounded by a fibrous capsule. Eventually the larvae die and calcify. No serious effects result from cysticerci in their most frequent locations, the subcutaneous tissue and skeletal muscles, although palpable or visible subcutaneous nodules can be recognized in approximately half of those with established infections. These are more frequently felt in the pectoral and abdominal superficial tissues than in the limbs and may simulate neurofibromatosis. The invasive stage often causes no symptoms, but fever, eosinophilia, muscle aches, and fatigue have been described. In the brain, cysticerci may be present in the cortex, meninges, ventricles, or substance of the cerebrum. Cysts in the ventricle may cause hydrocephalus. When parasites die in the brain, they provoke a severe inflammatory reaction that can lead to increased pressure symptoms. Calcification occurs after the parasite has been dead for some years. Cerebrospinal changes occur more often in the presence of cysts in contact with the subarachnoid space rather than with parenchymatous cysts, and include pleocytosis, eosinophilia, increased protein, and decreased sugar. Patients with larvae in the brain may present with epilepsy, intracranial hypertension, and motor or sensory or personality changes many years after initial infection. *Cysticercus* is the most common larval tapeworm to invade the eye, which it reaches through the retinal artery. The unencapsulated larva is 6 to 14 mm in size and sausage shaped. It may lodge anywhere in the orbit, conjunctiva, or anterior chamber, but most commonly is subretinal in the vitreous. Reactions to live larvae are usually minimal, but dead parasites produce iridocyclitis, clouding of the vitreous, and severe retinal inflammation or detachment. Patients may present with intraorbital pain, light flashes, and absence of or blurred vision. Cysts may rarely localize in all layers of the heart tissue and may produce myocarditis or congestive heart failure.

Diagnosis of adult worms can be made by finding *Taenia* eggs or characteristic segments in the stool. Cysticercosis is suggested by a history of infection with an adult worm, the presence of multiple subcutaneous nodules, typical symptoms, earlier residence in a highly endemic area, and moderate eosinophilia. Definitive diagnosis is by removal of subcutaneous nodules or brain cysts. Ocular cysticercosis is confirmed from the characteristic movements and scolex of the worm. After calcification of larvae, roentgenologic diagnosis from typical lesions may be made, but this is usually not possible until after five years of muscle infection or until after ten years of brain infection. Brain scanning, EEG, CT, and MRI can confirm space-occupying lesions. With CT and MRI, the most useful diagnostic tests, different stages of development of the cysticerci may be seen in an individual patient. Cerebral cysticercosis must be differentiated from hydatid or coenurus cyst, brain tumors, and cerebral lues. An indirect hemagglutination test is presently the best available serologic test and is positive in a significant number of cases. However, a negative result cannot rule out cysticercosis. An ELISA or complement fixation test on CSF may be positive, particularly when inflammatory changes are present in the CSF.

Infection with adult worms can be prevented by heating pork from 49 to 53°C for at least a half-hour, or freezing at −5°C for three days, which kills larvae. Pickling and smoking are usually not sufficient to destroy cysticerci. Proper hygienic measures and disposal of human excrement can prevent human cysticercosis.

Bickerstaff ER: Cerebral cysticercosis. Common but unfamiliar manifestations. Br Med J 1:1055, 1955. *Illustrative case reports and good discussion.*

Byrd SE, Locke GE, Biggers S, et al.: The computed tomographic appearance of cerebral cysticercosis in adults and children. Radiology 144:819, 1982. *An excellent and more available method for diagnosis of brain cysts.*

Dixon HBF, Lipscomb FM: Cysticercosis: An Analysis and Followup of 450 Cases. London Privy Council, Med Res Special Rept Ser No 299, 1961. *A classic review of 450 cases in British troops returned from India.*

Nash TE, Neva FA: Recent advances in the diagnosis and treatment of cerebral cysticercosis. N Engl J Med 311:1492, 1984. *A recent, brief review emphasizing the diagnostic value of CT.*

Ramos OM, Stiebel-Chin G, Altman N, et al.: Diagnosis of neurocysticercosis by magnetic resonance imaging. Pediatr Infect Dis 5:470, 1986. *Cysticercus lesions are well demonstrated and need for intravenous contrast with CT is obviated.*

Reddy PS, Satyendran DM: Ocular cysticercosis. Am J Ophthalmol 57:665, 1964. *Ten cases and general review of subject.*

396 HYMENOLEPIS NANA (The Dwarf Tapeworm)

Hymenolepis nana has a worldwide distribution but is most prevalent in warm, dry climates. It is common in southern and eastern Europe, the Middle East, Africa, and Latin America. In the United States it is particularly common in the southeastern and southwestern states and in institutional populations.

This parasite takes its name of the dwarf tapeworm from the very small size of the adult worm, which measures 25 to 40 mm long by 1 mm wide. It has a minute scolex with four cup-shaped suckers and a short rostellum armed with 20 to 30 small hooks. Individual segments are not seen in the stool, and mature proglottides are approximately 0.85 mm long by 0.22 mm wide. Eggs are set free by gradual disintegration of the distalmost proglottides. Eggs are characteristic in having a clear area between the shell and an inner envelope, and four to eight threadlike filaments arising from each of two polar thickenings of the inner envelope. They measure 45 by 35 μ. Eggs are immediately infective when passed in the feces. No intermediate host is required, and upon ingestion of the eggs by the definitive host (man, mouse, or rat), oncospheres hatch in the small intestine and penetrate into the villi, where they develop into cysticercoid larvae. In about four days these break out into the intestinal lumen and attach to villi in the upper two thirds of the ileum, where they become adults in 10 to 12 days. Internal autoinfection may lead to continued heavy infection. The life duration of the worm is only a few months. Infection is transmitted directly from hand to mouth and also by contaminated food and water. Children are infected more often than adults, as resistance increases with age.

Infections with over 1000 worms can occur in man. In most light infections no injury is caused to the mucosa and there are no symptoms, but mucosal irritation from heavy worm loads may lead to anorexia, abdominal pain, and diarrhea. Mild eosinophilia is often present.

Diagnosis is by the recovery of characteristic double membrane eggs in the stool. Personal hygiene, particularly in families and institutions, is the most effective method of prevention.

Buscher HN, Haley AJ: Epidemiology of *Hymenolepis nana* infections of Punjabi villagers in West Pakistan. Am J Trop Med Hyg 21:42, 1972. *Epidemiology of this parasite in a typical semiarid endemic area.*

397 ECHINOCOCCOSIS (Hydatid Disease)

Three main species of *Echinococcus* infect man. *Echinococcus granulosus* is by far the most common with a worldwide distribution, especially in sheep-raising areas. Sheep are the main intermediate hosts, with dogs being the definitive host. Human infection rates are highest in southern Europe, the Mediterranean littoral, the Middle East, eastern Africa, Australia and New Zealand, and Latin America. The majority of cases in the United States are found in immigrants from endemic areas, but autochthonous cases are found in sheep-raising areas of western states. Another strain variant, *E. granulosus var. canadensis*, has a sylvatic cycle with wild animals as the main hosts and occurs in Alaska and Canada.

Alveolar hydatid disease, caused by *E. multilocularis*, is restricted to the Northern Hemisphere, occurring in Europe, north central United States, Canada, and Alaska, with foxes as definitive hosts and rodents as intermediate hosts. A related species, *E. vogeli*, with dogs as normal hosts and the paca as the main intermediate host, has been described in a few human cases in Panama and Colombia. The following discussion will refer primarily to *E. granulosus*.

Adult worms of the three species can be differentiated morphologically and are the smallest of the tapeworms, measuring from 2 to 9 mm long and consisting of a scolex, a neck, and usually three segments, the last of which is gravid. Adult worms inhabit the upper jejunum of the definitive host, principally dogs, wolves, coyotes, foxes, and cats. In dogs, their lifespan is three to six months. Ova, similar to those of *Taenia* species, are evacuated in the feces of the definitive host and are ingested by the intermediate host, primarily sheep and rodents, and less commonly by man. Eggs can live for some months in moist, shady soil. The shell is digested in the duodenum, and the freed embryo penetrates into the intestinal mucosa and is carried by the bloodstream until it is filtered out in a small capillary. This usually occurs in the liver, the first capillary filter; next most commonly in the lung; and less frequently in other tissues and organs of the body. The parasite then develops into a bladder-like cyst, which increases at a rate of approximately 1 cm per year. As the cyst grows, a fibrous connective tissue cyst wall is formed by reaction of the host. Inside this is a germinal layer from which budding secondary daughter cysts develop. Hydatid fluid fills the cyst, which in the case of *E. granulosus* is unilocular. With *E. multilocularis*, multilocular or alveolar cysts occur, owing to the very thin laminated membrane, which is not sharply separated from the surrounding tissue and allows for exogenous budding and malignant-like growth. Metastases may occur via the circulation. *E. vogeli* cysts also tend to be multilocular. When dogs or other definitive hosts eat the infected flesh or offal of intermediate hosts, embryonic tapeworms within developed cysts are freed in the duodenum and attach by their scolices to the intestinal wall, becoming adult worms.

Man is infected only by the larval or hydatid cyst stage through intimate contact with infected dogs or other definitive hosts. Infection of dogs and other reservoir hosts depends upon the dog-sheep (or rarely cattle) or wild animal-moose or rodent relationship, whereby reservoir hosts are infected by consuming infected carcasses or offal. Most *E. granulosus* infections occur in childhood by hand-to-mouth transmission of eggs picked up from the fur of dogs.

Pathology in man depends upon the location of the cyst. About 65 per cent of unilocular and 90 per cent of multilocular cysts occur in the liver, usually in the right lobe. *E. granulosus* cysts are multiple in about one quarter of patients. Lung cysts account for approximately 20 per cent of total *E. granulosus* infections, whereas the remaining 15 per cent may involve almost any other body organ or tissue. Physical signs and symptoms do not usually occur until cysts are at least 10 to 20 cm in diameter, about 10 to 20 years after initial infection. Rupture or leakage of viable cysts may lead to secondary multiple implantations of the peritoneum or other organs. Cysts may lead to compression or atrophy of surrounding tissue. Cysts may become inactive and calcify without ever causing symptoms, although there may still be some viability in a calcified cyst. There is less resistance to spherical growth in the lung than in the liver, and lung cysts may attain greater size more rapidly and rarely calcify. Brain cysts usually present at a younger age because of increased intracranial pressure, and they rarely calcify.

As many as 20 per cent of *E. granulosus* cysts may never cause symptoms. Symptoms related to liver cysts include right upper quadrant pain, hepatomegaly, and jaundice. Approximately one half of patients with pulmonary cysts are asymptomatic, but cysts may cause chest pain, cough, and hemoptysis. Brain cysts may give signs of increased intracranial pressure and convulsions. With slow leakage of a cyst, urticaria and other allergic symptoms may occur, whereas rupture or needle puncture of a cyst may lead to anaphylaxis, which is often fatal. When eosinophilia is present, it is usually related to some leakage of fluid.

Echinococcosis must be suspected in anyone with a history of a slow-growing cystic tumor, particularly in the liver or lung, who has lived in an endemic area. A characteristic physical sign over a hepatic cyst on ballottement is the hydatid thrill. Liver function tests are usually normal with hepatic cysts except for a frequent increase of alkaline phosphatase. Radiography may show older calcified lesions in the liver, spleen, or kidney. Echinococcal cyst is the leading cause of a round, reticulated calcified lesion in the liver, but the differential diagnosis includes calcified hemangiomas, metastases, and old amebic or bacterial abscesses. Radioactive scanning, CT, MRI, or sonography is useful in localizing noncalcified cysts. Invasive angiographic techniques are rarely required. Pulmonary cysts present as regular, well-defined, round shadows, which cannot be differentiated from a tumor. If a pulmonary cyst becomes detached from the adventitia, the so-called *water lily sign* is produced. Immunologic techniques are quite valuable and should always be employed preoperatively to alert the surgeon to the likely presence of a hydatid cyst. When the Casoni skin test, using an antigen with an appropriate nitrogen content, shows an immediate negative reaction, this is good but not absolute evidence of the absence of hydatid disease. False-positive test results may occur. Serologic procedures include indirect hemagglutination, bentonite flocculation, latex or complement fixation, and immunoelectrophoresis. Immunoelectrophoresis is the only one absolutely specific for hydatid disease, but it is presently not readily available. The diagnosis is confirmed by the finding at surgery of daughter cysts and scolices in the cyst fluid. Closed needle aspiration of a lesion with any possibility of its being a hydatid cyst should never be performed before radiologic and immunologic studies have been done.

In endemic areas, infected dogs should be treated with a taeniafuge such as arecoline or niclosamide, and stray dogs should be destroyed. Dogs should be kept from eating uncooked carcasses or offal.

D'Alessandro A, Rausch RL, Cuello C, et al.: *Echinococcus vogeli* in man, with a review of polycystic hydatid disease in Colombia and neighboring countries. Am J Trop Med Hyg 28:303, 1979. *A discussion of 14 cases and a general review of this form of multilocular hydatid infection.*
Gamble WG, Segal M, Schantz PM, et al.: Alveolar hydatid disease in Minnesota. First human case acquired in the contiguous United States. JAMA 241:904, 1979. *Case report and literature review with particular reference to the disease in North America.*
Langer JL, Rose DB, Keystone JS, et al.: Diagnosis and management of hydatid disease of the liver. A 15-year North American experience. Ann Surg 199:412, 1984. *A review of 40 cases from Toronto, mostly in patients of Greek and Italian origin.*
Wolcott MW, Harris SH, Briggs JN, et al.: Hydatid disease of the lung. J Thorac Cardiovasc Surg 62:465, 1971. *A series of 37 Tunisian cases treated by Hope Ship physicians. Emphasizes the need for surgery in diagnosis and treatment.*

398 OTHER, RARER TAPEWORMS

Hymenolepis diminuta, a common tapeworm of rats and mice, infrequently infects man. It has a cosmopolitan distribution worldwide, and the few cases reported in the United States have mostly been from the South. Various species of larval and adult insects are intermediate hosts and become infected by taking in eggs deposited in rodent stool. Man and dog are incidental hosts, becoming infected by ingesting one of the insects containing a cysticercoid larva, usually by eating stale

grains or cereals infested with insects. The majority of human infections are in young children. Adult worms are 20 to 60 cm long and reside in the small intestine. No pathologic changes are recognized, but bowel irritation may cause minor gastrointestinal symptoms. The eggs resemble those of *H. nana*, differing in having no filaments at the pointed poles of the inner membrane. Diagnosis is by finding typical eggs in the stool.

Dipylidium caninum is the most common tapeworm of dogs and cats worldwide. Adult worms measure 15 to 80 cm in length and reside in the small intestine. Eggs, passed onto the ground in packets or in proglottides by infected animals or man, are ingested by larval fleas in which they hatch and develop into cysticercoid larvae. Humans having close contact with dogs or cats are infected by ingesting an infected flea. Human infection is infrequent, and small children are usually infected. The majority of cases are asymptomatic, but diarrhea, abdominal pain, restlessness, and eosinophilia have been reported. Diagnosis is by finding characteristic cucumber seed-shaped proglottides or characteristic eggs singly or in packets in the stool. Proglottides are motile and may migrate from the anus and can be mistaken for pinworms by history.

Coenurosis is a well-recognized disease of the central nervous system of animals. Humans are rarely infected. The adult tapeworm of the genus *Multiceps* is a common parasite of dogs and wolves. *Taenia*-like eggs are passed in the host's feces and are ingested by an intermediate host, a sheep or other ruminant, and occasionally by humans. After hatching, larvae lodge primarily in the brain and central nervous system but may also involve the eye or subcutaneous tissue, where they metamorphose into a coenurus, a bladder worm with multiple scolices. Infections in temperate climates are probably due to *Multiceps multiceps*, usually involve the central nervous system, and may lead to increased intracranial pressure. The majority of subcutaneous cysts have been described from East Africa where the prevalent species is *Multiceps (Taenia) brauni* and are manifested by a solitary tender subcutaneous nodule on the trunk or rarely by an eye cyst within the vitreous chamber, attached to the retina or choroid. Diagnosis is possible only with surgery. Both clinically and microscopically it is often difficult to distinguish coenurosis of the central nervous system from hydatid cyst or cysticercosis.

Hermos JA, Healy GR, Schultz MG, et al.: Fatal human cerebral coenurosis. JAMA 213:1461, 1970. *The cerebral form of this disease seems to occur only in temperate climates and must be differentiated from hydatid cyst and cysticercosis.*
Templeton AC: Anatomical and geographical location of coenurus infection. Trop Geogr Med 23:105, 1971. *Review of 14 cases from Uganda involving subcutaneous nodules.*
Turner JA: Human dipylidiasis (dog tapeworm infection) in the United States. J Pediatr 61:763, 1962. *This tends to be primarily a disease of childhood but may not be as rare as earlier supposed.*
Turton JA, Williamson JR, Harris WG: Haematological and immunological responses to the tapeworm *Hymenolepis diminuta* in man. Tropenmed Parasitol 26:196, 1975. *A general review and detailed description of self-infection.*

399 TREATMENT OF TAPEWORM INFECTIONS

The present drug of choice for *Diphyllobothrium latum*, *Taenia* species, *Hymenolepis* species, and *Dipylidium caninum* is niclosamide (Niclocide). For *D. latum*, *Taenia saginata*, *T. solium*, and *D. caninum*, adults are given a single 2-gram dose. The tablets are chewed thoroughly in the morning and followed by water. No fasting or purging is necessary. The head and much of the worm disintegrate so that proof of cure depends on a negative stool examination for eggs at three months. For *Hymenolepis nana* and *H. diminuta* the adult dose is 2 grams daily for seven days. Side effects are rare. Another effective drug against *D. latum, Taenia* species, and *H. nana* is paromomycin (Humatin), a poorly absorbed antibiotic that is considered an investigational drug for tapeworms in the United States. For *H. nana,* the adult dose is 45 mg per kilogram once a day for five to seven days, while for the other worms 1 gram every 15 minutes for four doses is administered. Quinacrine hydrochloride had formerly been used for these parasites but is most effective when administered through a duodenal tube, and cure rates are lower than with niclosamide. The anthelmintic drug mebendazole (Vermox) is effective against *Taenia* species in a dose of 300 mg twice daily for three days but is not yet approved for this indication in the United States. Praziquantel, in a single dose, 10 to 20 mg per kilogram, is very effective against intestinal *Taenia, Hymenolepis,* and *Diphyllobothrium* infections in humans but is also not yet approved for cestode infections in the United States.

Praziquantel has also been shown to be effective against human cysticercosis of the brain and subcutaneous and muscle tissue. This has greatly improved the prognosis for this infection, formerly treated only surgically, with many cases being inoperable. The recommended dose is 50 mg per kilogram per day in three divided doses for 14 days. To prevent potential immunologic reactions in the brain tissue caused by death of parasites, steroids are administered concurrently. Calcified cysticerci do not respond to this treatment, and when they cause seizures, anticonvulsants must be used for control. Ocular cysticerci must be removed surgically; praziquantel is not recommended for treatment of ocular cysticercosis because of concern about ocular damage after parasite destruction in the eye. There are recent reports from Mexico of metrifonate being effective for ocular as well as cerebral and subcutaneous disease.

Surgery is recommended for accessible symptomatic *Echinococcus granulosus* cysts. Sterilization of cysts should be performed at surgery by scolecidal solutions, such as hypertonic saline or a 10 per cent formaldehyde solution. Cysts may also be marsupialized, or cryosurgery may be used. For multiple cysts, poor surgical risk patients, and inaccessible cysts,

mebendazole in large doses for several months has led to subjective improvement in cases of *E. granulosus* infection and evidence of regression of cysts in some; in other patients, cysts continued to grow or were proved viable even after lengthy treatment. Hepatic lobectomy is the only operation for *E. multilocularis,* but complete removal is usually difficult. In patients with inoperable *E. multilocularis* cysts, the progressive course of the disease can be arrested by mebendazole, but treatment apparently has not killed the parasite. Related benzimidazole drugs—flubendazole, fenbendazole, and albendazole—also appear to be promising in inoperable hydatid infections.

Symptomatic coenurosis must be managed surgically. Complete surgical excision is the treatment of choice for sparganosis; if it is inoperable, injections of alcohol into the lesion will kill the parasite.

Davis A, Pawlowski ZS, Dixon H: Multicentre clinical trials of benzimidazole-carbamates in human echinococcosis. Bull WHO 64:383, 1986.

Groll E: Praziquantel for cestode infections in man. Acta Trop 37:293, 1980. *Single-dose treatment of intestinal cestodes.*

Jones WE: Niclosamide as a treatment for *Hymenolepis diminuta* and *Dipylidium caninum* infection in man. Am J Trop Med Hyg 28:300, 1979. *Effective treatment of these uncommon cestodes.*

Peña Chavarria A, Villaraejos VM, Zeledon R: Mebendazole in the treatment of *Taenia solium* and *Taenia saginata.* Am J Trop Med Hyg 26:118, 1977. *An alternative treatment for the more common intestinal cestodes; not yet an approved indication in the United States.*

Perera DR, Western KA, Schultz MG: Niclosamide treatment of cestodiasis. Clinical trials in the United States. Am J Trop Med Hyg 19:610, 1970. *An early review of this drug, which has been further substantiated, showing it to be safe, simple, and effective.*

Sayek I, Yalin R, Savac Y: Surgical treatment of hydatid disease of the liver. Arch Surg 115:847, 1980. *A review of 100 surgically treated cases in Turkey.*

Schantz PM: Effective medical treatment for hydatid disease? JAMA 253:2095, 1985. *Summary and references on newer treatments with mebendazole and albendazole.*

Sotelo J, Escobedo F, Rodriguez-Carbajal J, et al.: Therapy of parenchymal brain cysticercosis with praziquantel. N Engl J Med 310:1001, 1984. *Promising new drug treatment of neurocysticercosis.*

Sotelo J, Torres B, Rubio-Donnadieu F, et al.: Praziquantel in the treatment of neurocysticercosis: Long-term follow-up. Neurology 35:752, 1985. *Benefits of treatment were sustained for at least one year.*

Wittner M, Tanowitz H: Paromomycin therapy of human cestodiasis with special reference to hymenolepiasis. Am J Trop Med Hyg 20:433, 1971. *Successful treatment of various common cestodes with an alternative to niclosamide.*

The Trematodes

400 SCHISTOSOMIASIS (Bilharziasis)

Adel A. F. Mahmoud

DEFINITION. Schistosomiasis, a chronic worm infection, affects more than 200 million people in the world; several hundred million more live in endemic areas and are at risk of exposure to the parasites. In view of its prevalence and the morbidity it causes, schistosomiasis ranks among the most important public health problems of tropical and subtropical areas. The schistosomes are blood flukes that parasitize the venous channels of the definitive human host; infection is transmitted via fresh-water snails. Man may be infected by one of five species: *Schistosoma haematobium, S. mansoni, S. japonicum, S. intercalatum,* or *S. mekongi.* Each species is endemic in specific geographic areas of the world and results in defined clinical syndromes which, if left undiagnosed and untreated, may cause major morbidity or mortality. Other species that occasionally infect man include *S. bovis, S. matthei,* and some avian schistosomes. In many parts of the world,

enhancing agricultural productivity by developing and expanding water conservation schemes is an economic necessity. Inadvertently, these projects created ideal breeding places for the snail intermediate host, thus increasing prevalence of schistosomiasis in the population and possibly causing its spread to new areas. Currently, schistosomiasis is endemic in various areas of Africa, Asia, South America, and the Caribbean islands. In the United States, there are approximately 400,000 cases; these usually occur in Puerto Rican immigrants or travelers who have been infected while in endemic areas. Because of the absence of susceptible snails, the life cycle of the schistosomes cannot be established in this country.

ETIOLOGY. The schistosomes are the most significant trematode parasites of man. They differ from other trematodes that infect humans in having separate sexes. The species of schistosomes that infect humans share some common features, although they are morphologically distinctive. Each worm has two suckers (anterior and ventral), and the bifurcate intestinal ceca unite posteriorly. The larger male (0.6 to 2.2 cm × 2 to 4 mm) has a ventral gynecophoric canal in which the female is held during copulation. The slender female worm (1.2 to 2.6 cm × 1 to 2 mm) has a rounded body with pointed ends.

Adult schistosome worms parasitize defined sites of the venous vasculature of humans. *Schistosoma haematobium* worms inhabit the venous plexus around the lower end of the ureters and the urinary bladder, whereas *S. mansoni, S. japonicum, S. intercalatum,* and *S. mekongi* are located in the mesenteric veins. Sexual maturity of female worms requires the presence of living mature males; when ready to deposit eggs, the worms move against the bloodstream toward the small venous radicles. The female schistosomes deposit ova singly or in bunches, depending on the species of the parasite, and retreat in the direction of blood flow. Egg deposition has been estimated at 300 per day for female *S. haematobium* and *S. mansoni* worms and 3000 per day for those of *S. japonicum.* The ova of each species have characteristic morphologic features, which are of diagnostic importance. Once deposited in the host, the eggs attempt to penetrate the venous capillaries and escape to the bladder or intestinal lumen; enzymatic secretions are thought to aid egg migration. The proportion of ova escaping from infected individuals varies in each species and also may depend on the extent of pathology and state of resistance in the host. Eggs that fail to reach the lumen of urinary tract or gut are trapped in these organs or may be carried by portal blood to the liver; these ova result in inflammatory and immunopathologic changes that are a major cause of disease in schistosomiasis.

The schistosome eggs, upon deposition by female worms, contain immature miracidia; they take approximately 10 to 12 days to develop while migrating through the host tissues. Once mature, miracidia have a mean lifespan of 11 to 12 days. Promiscuous urination and defecation by infected individuals result in dissemination of the parasite eggs in the environment. In fresh water the schistosome ova hatch within a few hours. Miracidia escape head first and swim, usually near the surface of water; they remain infective to the snail intermediate host for approximately eight hours. On encountering the specific snail, the miracidia penetrate its tissues and undergo tremendous asexual multiplication and transformation into hundreds of cercariae. Schistosome infection of snails causes varying degrees of pathology in their liver and sexual organs and reduces their lifespan. Development of schistosomes inside the snail takes approximately four to six weeks, but it varies with the species of the parasite and mollusc and with changes in environmental conditions. Cercariae, the infective forms to humans, emerge from the snails under specific conditions of light and temperature; they are elongate with a pear-shaped body and a long forked tail, and measure approximately 400 to 600 μm in length. They can survive in fresh water for almost 72 hours, but lose their infectivity considerably within the first 24 hours. Cercariae attach to skin of mammalian hosts by their oral or ventral suckers. Burrowing of the skin is helped by vertical vibratory movements of their bodies and secretions of the cephalic penetration glands; the process is usually completed within a few minutes. During penetration, the cercariae shake off their tails and change into the next stage of life cycle, the schistosomula, which lie in tunnels in the stratum corneum parallel to the skin surface. Schistosomula are anaerobic organisms with heptalaminar membrane (instead of the trilaminar cercarial membrane) and can no longer survive fresh water. They are thought to remain in the skin for one to three days before migrating to the lungs, finally reaching the liver in two to four weeks. In the intrahepatic portal system the worms complete the major digestive and sexual stages of their development. Adult worms start their migration to their final habitat in two weeks and mate; viable eggs can be seen in the excreta five to nine weeks after cercarial penetration.

The mean lifespan of adult schistosome worms inside the human host is not exactly known. Several individual case reports indicate that worms may live 20 to 30 years. This, however, represents extreme cases, as examination of infected individuals who migrated to nonendemic areas indicate that the mean lifespan of the worms is in the range of three to ten years.

EPIDEMIOLOGY. The endemicity of schistosomiasis in any specific area is dependent upon the unsanitary disposal of urine and feces, the presence of suitable snail hosts, and human exposure to cercaria-infected water bodies. Furthermore, the epidemiology of schistosomiasis is complex because of the existence of several stages of the life cycle of the parasite and the multitude of factors affecting each. Since adult schistosomes, like many parasitic worms, do not multiply in the human body, close correlation between worm load and fecal or urinary egg counts has been shown; estimates of intensity of infection can therefore be obtained by ova-enumerating procedures. Quantifying worm loads is important epidemiologically as well as for the individual patient, as it determines the potential of participation in transmission of schistosomiasis and predicts, to a large extent, the risk of morbidity and pathologic outcome.

In endemic areas, schistosomiasis incidence and intensity show characteristic association with age. Schistosomiasis is acquired early in childhood; incidence and intensity gradually increase to a peak in the second decade of life. In older individuals, a modest reduction of incidence may be seen along with a sharp fall in intensity of infection. The marked drop in intensity in adults may be due to a decrease in their water-related activities. Development of immunity may also explain age-related decrease in intensity, although there is not yet convincing evidence for acquisition of resistance against schistosomiasis in man. Intensity of infection in endemic communities shows another characteristic feature: most infected individuals harbor low worm loads, and only a small proportion acquire heavy infection. The underlying mechanism of this clustering of heavy infection in schistosomiasis is not known, but may be due to varying degrees of susceptibility and/or response of humans to the parasites.

Determination of the incidence and rate of acquisition of schistosomiasis in populations of endemic areas is important for risk assessment and planning control strategies. The incidence and intensity of infection peak in the age group 10 to 20 years in spite of the presumed multiple reexposures to the parasite. These observations suggest that the schistosomiasis transmission rate in endemic areas is slow. Several ecologic as well as host factors help maintain these features. For example, the incidence of schistosomal infection in the snail intermediate host is usually low, ranging between 0.6 and 2 per cent. Cercarial dispersion in water bodies is considerable; they appear in significant numbers only during certain hours of the day and lose their infectivity shortly thereafter. Once on their way to invade a certain host, no more than 40 per cent of cercariae mature into adult worms. In addition, attempts to measure incidence rates in endemic areas have confirmed the relatively slow rate of transmission, ranging from 2 to 4 per cent per year.

In some areas, the endemicity of schistosomiasis may be maintained by animal reservoirs; this is especially the case with *S. japonicum,* which infects dogs and cows. Although both *S. haematobium* and *S. mansoni* can infect primates and rodents, the role of these animals as reservoirs does not seem to be epidemiologically important.

PATHOGENESIS. Schistosomiasis is initiated by cercarial penetration of skin; inside the host three maturational forms of the parasite evolve: schistosomula, adults, and eggs. These stages are associated with morphologic, biochemical, and antigenic changes of the worm, which add to the complexity of host-parasite relationship. Disease caused by schistosomiasis occurs mainly in those with high eggs counts. This relationship, however, is not exact, as the roles of other factors such as genetic background and immunologic modulatory mechanisms are now being elucidated.

Three distinct disease syndromes caused by schistosomiasis have been described; each corresponds roughly to a stage in the parasite development in the host. Cercarial dermatitis, or swimmer's itch, may be seen in infections with human schistosomes but more commonly when avian or other nonhuman cercariae penetrate the skin. Swimmer's itch caused by nonhuman schistosomes is commonly seen in the north central United States where some lakes are infected. The condition has also been reported in subjects exposed to S. mansoni or S. haematobium but rarely after exposure to S. japonicum. Primary exposure to these larvae results in either no reaction or immediate pruritic macular rash. On repeated exposures, sensitization occurs, and a more pronounced papular eruption develops with erythema, edema, and pruritus. Histopathologically, edema, round cell infiltrate, and eosinophilia can be seen in the dermis and epidermis. Although the mechanism of this reaction is not known, it is probably due to host response to dying larvae and the subsequent development of humoral and cellular immunity.

Acute schistosomiasis, or Katayama fever, is a serum sickness–like syndrome that occurs three to nine weeks after infection. This period coincides with the onset of egg production and its associated increase in antigenic challenge to the host. Clinically significant acute schistosomiasis occurs more often with S. japonicum infections, but has also been reported with the other species. It is seen in previously unexposed individuals; the severity of symptoms and signs correlates with intensity of infection. There is very little known of the mechanism of this syndrome; it manifests itself as fever, abdominal pain, and headache with hepatosplenomegaly and eosinophilia. Elevations of serum IgG, IgM, IgE, and specific antischistosomal antibodies have also been observed, leading to the suggestion that the syndrome is a form of immune complex disease.

The basic pathologic lesion in chronic schistosomiasis is the egg granuloma. Although the schistosomes do not multiply in the definitive host, they continually produce eggs; some of these are trapped in the tissues. Enzymes and antigens are subsequently released from the eggs to facilitate their migration out of the body. These parasite products sensitize the host lymphocytes, which migrate to areas of egg deposition and recruit other cells through the secretion of lymphokines, and a compact cellular infiltrate "granuloma" is formed. Several cell types are prominent in the schistosome egg granuloma: lymphocytes, macrophages, eosinophils, and fibroblasts. Granuloma formation around the schistosome eggs leads to the development of lesions far bigger than the parasite ova. The extent of these granulomas along with fibrosis leads to most of the chronic fibro-obstructive lesions in schistosomiasis. In S. haematobium infection, granulomas at the lower end of the ureters impede urine flow and cause hydroureter and hydronephrosis. In infections with other schistosome species, granulomas in the intestinal wall are associated with the abdominal manifestations of the disease, and those in the liver result in presinusoidal obstruction of portal blood flow, portal hypertension, splenomegaly, and esophageal varices. Less commonly eggs may be carried to almost any organ or tissue in the body, eliciting granuloma formation and its pathologic sequelae. The size of the granulomatous response represents a delicate balance between sensitizing and modulating mechanisms. In chronic schistosomiasis, granulomas spontaneously modulate—i.e., their size decreases significantly—and may result in slowing the progression of disease manifestations. Modulation has been shown to be mediated by several arms of the host's immune system, including serum antibodies, anti-idiotypic antibodies, immune complexes, suppressor lymphocytes, and macrophages. Functionally, granulomas serve to destroy the parasite eggs. Among the cells constituting the granulomatous response, eosinophils play a key role in egg destruction.

The immune response of individuals with schistosomiasis includes humoral as well as cellular components. The degree and extent of these responses provide the balance that may result in either asymptomatic infection or disease manifestations. Furthermore, mechanisms that control the host immune response such as genetic background have been demonstrated to influence the extent of granuloma formation and consequently disease. The host immune response to schistosome antigens also is inversely related to intensity of infection; impaired responses are seen only in those with heavy worm loads. Whether the defect in immunity is a cause or consequence of infection is not yet clear. Another aspect of the host's immune response in schistosomiasis relates to the development of peripheral blood as well as tissue eosinophilia. Schistosomiasis, similar to other worm infections with tissue phases, results in significant increase of peripheral blood eosinophils, especially during the acute phase of infection. Later, in the chronic stage, the eosinophil count may not be significantly elevated. Eosinophils are seen in subcutaneous tissues around the entry points of cercariae, and they constitute approximately 50 per cent of the cells in egg granulomas. Eosinophils have been shown to play a central role in host defenses against the invading stage of the parasite (schistosomula) and the phase (ova) retained in the tissues.

The occurrence of immunity to schistosomiasis in humans has not convincingly been shown; Although the drop in intensity and incidence of infection in older individuals in endemic areas may reflect the development of resistance, these phenomena may be explained equally by the differences in patterns of contact with infected waters, or by changes in the rate of egg production by adult worms. Studies in vitro have demonstrated that several human cells—eosinophils, neutrophils, basophils, monocytes, and cytotoxic T lymphocytes—may alone or in combination with complement components or antischistosomal antibodies damage the larval stage of the parasite. The biologic relevance of these observations in humans is not yet clear.

MANAGEMENT. Diagnosis of schistosomiasis must be based on the clinical presentation, positive geographic history, and finding the parasite eggs in the excreta or biopsy material. Quantification of infection and assessing viability of the eggs are important procedures not only for planning therapy but also for prognostic evaluation. Serologic tests for schistosomiasis are not yet at the stage at which they can be used on a routine basis. Safe chemotherapeutic antischistosomal agents are now available and provide high cure rates (see Management of Schistosomiasis, below.). None of these drugs has any effect on cercarial penetration, on swimmer's itch, on the course of acute schistosomiasis, or as a prophylactic measure. Their major action is on the adult egg-producing worms. Appropriate management of patients with schistosomiasis must take into consideration the extent of disease and intensity of infection. Antischistosomal therapy, if given early enough during the course of disease, may lead to reversal of pathologic lesions. In late cases, chemotherapeutic measures may be useful only in preventing further damage resulting from the presence of the parasite.

CONTROL. The intimate relationship between humans and bodies of water in their environment leads to schistosomiasis endemicity. In addition, the lack of precise knowledge of the epidemiology of infection and disease in schistosomiasis has hampered efforts for its control. Several developments such as single oral-dose chemotherapeutic agents and better appreciation of transmission dynamics have led to clearer definition of strategies for control of schistosomiasis. Ideally, eradication of infection should be the target, but this is impossible to achieve with the currently available tools and the economic and social structure of the endemic areas. A more realistic approach is based on control of disease and reduction of transmission. The most cost-effective measure currently advocated is targeted mass chemotherapy, combined with focal mollusciciding if needed. Because of the specific features of infection dynamics, treated individuals remain with low egg counts for a few years. In addition, health education, attempts at raising socioeconomic standards, providing privies, and abandoning obsolete agricultural practices offer additional means for achieving progress in containing this infection.

Those traveling to endemic areas should be given proper advice. There are virtually no safe freshwater bodies in most of the areas endemic for schistosomiasis. Avoiding contact with these water sources is to be strongly recommended.

Butterworth AE, Taylor DW, Veith MC, et al.: Studies on the mechanisms of immunity in human schistosomiasis. Immunol Rev 61:5, 1982. *A detailed description of in vitro evidence and components of protective effector mechanisms against schistosomiasis.*

de Brito PA, Kazura JW, Mahmoud AAF: Host granulomatous response in schistosomiasis mansoni: Antibody and cell-mediated damage of parasite eggs in vitro. J Clin Invest 74:1715, 1984. *An examination of effector mechanisms that are responsible for elimination of schistosome eggs in vitro.*

Ellner JJ, Olds, GR, Osman GO, et al.: Dichotomies in the reactivity to worm antigen in human schistosomiasis mansoni. J Immunol 126:309, 1981. *Demonstration of an inverse relationship between intensity of infection and immune response to schistosome antigens.*

Iarotski LS, Davis A: The schistosomiasis problem in the world. Bull WHO 59:115, 1981. *An attempt to determine the global prevalence of schistosomiasis.*

Mahmoud AAF, Arap Siongok TK, Ouma J, et al.: Effect of targeted mass treatment on intensity of infection and morbidity in schistosomiasis mansoni. Lancet 1:849, 1983. *Evaluation of the clinical and parasitologic effects of targeting chemotherapy to those with hepatosplenomegaly and heavy infection.*

Mahmoud AAF, Warren KS, Peters PA: A role for the eosinophil in acquired resistance to *Schistosoma mansoni* infection as determined by anti-eosinophil serum. J Exp Med 142:805, 1975. *Demonstration of the in vivo protective function of eosinophils in animals with schistosomiasis.*

Warren KS: Regulation of the prevalence and intensity of schistosomiasis in man: Immunology or ecology? J Infect Dis 127:595, 1973. *A lucid discussion of the factors controlling transmission, and regulation of infection in schistosomiasis.*

World Health Organization: The Control of Schistosomiasis. Technical Report Series 728, pp 1–113, World Health Organization, Geneva, Switzerland, 1985. *An up-to-date examination of the epidemiology, morbidity, and methods of control of schistosomiasis. The report also includes a summary of control programs in endemic areas and an outline for a strategy of morbidity control.*

SCHISTOSOMIASIS HAEMATOBIA
(Urinary Bilharziasis)

Schistosomiasis haematobia is due to human infection with the trematode *S. haematobium*; adult worms reside in the venous plexus around the urinary bladder. *S. haematobium* infection is endemic in Africa and some parts of the Middle East; it is highly prevalent in the Nile valley and extends along the Mediterranean coast of the continent. In West Africa it is more widely disseminated than *S. mansoni*; its distribution in East and South Africa is patchy. The parasite is endemic also on the islands of the Malagasy Republic. In southwest Asia the endemic area includes most countries of the Middle East and Arabian peninsula. Clinically, infection with *S. haematobium* is the most significant of human schistosome infections. Symptoms and signs of disease occur in over half of the infected individuals, including those with light worm loads. Because of the anatomic location of the pathologic lesions, gross urinary tract disease can result from a few granulomas at the lower end of ureters. In endemic areas, extensive hydroureters and hydronephrosis can be demonstrated in a considerable proportion of infected children; the natural history of these lesions and the course of disease in adults have not been clearly defined.

Adult male *S. haematobium* worms are distinguished by their finely tuberculate surface and by the presence of four to five large testes. The ovaries are found in the posterior half of the female body and contain 20 to 30 eggs. Mature *S. haematobium* eggs measure approximately 143 × 50 µm and are spindle shaped with a rounded anterior end and a conical posterior end that tapers to a terminal delicate spine. Eggs are mainly found in urine of infected individuals, but may occasionally be seen in stools or rectal biopsies. The main intermediate hosts of *S. haematobium* in North Africa and the Middle East are freshwater snails of the genus *Bulinus*; in Africa south of the Sahara they belong to the subgenus *Physopsis*.

PATHOLOGY AND CLINICAL MANIFESTATIONS. Ova of *S. haematobium* pass from the venules of the vesical plexus into the bladder wall and the lower end of ureters, where most of the pathologic changes in infected individuals are seen. In the urinary bladder, the formation of egg granulomas leads to hyperemia, tubercles, ulcers, and polyps; as healing proceeds, sandy patches and scarring may be seen. Obstructive uropathy is the main functional disturbance caused by schistosomiasis haematobia. Other urinary tract lesions such as bacteriuria, calculi, and bladder cancer have been epidemiologically associated with *S. haematobium* infection, but no causal relationship has yet been confirmed. Ova of *S. haematobium* have occasionally been found in the lungs with subsequent focal pulmonary arteritis and diffuse hypertensive arteriolar changes; chronic cor pulmonale may occur in these patients.

Swimmer's itch and acute schistosomiasis have rarely been described in *S. haematobium* infection. By contrast, symptoms caused by egg deposition in the urinary tract occur in a large proportion of infected individuals. In endemic areas, 50 to 90 per cent of infected subjects complain of dysuria, hematuria, or frequency. Hematuria is characteristically terminal, but with extensive ulceration the whole stream of urine may be bloody along with passage of clots. In late cases, symptoms related to secondary infection of the urinary tract, severe obstructive uropathy, or neoplasia may appear. Urine examination reveals proteinuria and hematuria; both signs are closely related to intensity of infection. An association between *S. haematobium* infection and bacteremia, mainly caused by *Salmonella* organisms, has been reported. Renal function may be compromised in patients with obstructive uropathy; both minimum urine osmolality and the ability to excrete an ingested water load are reduced, but these are nonspecific changes. Cytoscopic examination shows some degree of pathology in almost all infected individuals, the most common being hyperemia near the ureteral openings and the bladder trigone. Sandy patches, tubercles, ulcers, and polyps are less frequently seen. Radiographically, bladder calcification is a characteristic feature of urinary schistosomiasis; it is found in approximately 50 to 80 per cent of infected individuals. Other pathologic lesions are also frequently seen in 40 to 60 per cent of patients, including obstructive uropathy, hydroureters, hydronephrosis, and filling defects in the bladder and ureters. The severity of most of these symptoms and signs of schistosomiasis haematobia correlates with intensity of infection; however, in individuals with light infection, considerable pathologic changes can still be demonstrated.

DIAGNOSIS. Urine examination for *S. haematobium* eggs can be performed by direct or concentration methods. Excretion of the parasite eggs is maximal around midday, when samples should optimally be obtained. Diagnosis and quantification of infection can be achieved by filtering 10 ml of urine through Nuclepore membrane. Examination of more than one urine sample may be necessary to establish the diagnosis; rectal biopsy may alternatively be obtained in suspected cases with negative urine results. Once *S. haematobium* infection is diagnosed, assessment of urinary tract pathology by ultrasonography is recommended. In addition, care must be taken in some endemic areas for early detection of bladder cancer by appropriate cytologic and histologic examinations.

TREATMENT. See Management of Schistosomiasis, below.

Lehman JS Jr, Farid Z, Smith JH, et al.: Urinary schistosomiasis in Egypt: Clinical, radiological, bacteriological and parasitological correlations. Trans R Soc Trop Med Hyg 67:384, 1973. *A complete clinical description of 200 individuals infected with* S. haematobium.

Mott KE, Dixon H, Osei-Tutu E, et al.: Relation between intensity of *Schistosoma haematobium* infection and clinical haematuria and proteinuria. Lancet 1:1005, 1983. *Correlation of proteinuria and hematuria to counts of* S. haematobium *eggs in urine.*

Peters PA, Mahmoud AAF, Warren KS, et al.:* Field studies of a rapid, accurate means of quantifying *Schistosoma haematobium* eggs in urine samples. Bull WHO 54:159, 1976. *Simple quantitative technique for urine examination.*

Smith JH, Kamel IA, Elwi A, et al.: A quantitative post mortem analysis of urinary schistosomiasis in Egypt. I. Pathology and pathogenesis. Am J

Trop Med Hyg 23:1054, 1974. *Description of the pathology of schistosomiasis haematobia as it relates to egg counts and parasite load.*
Warren KS, Mahmoud AAF, Muruka JF, et al.: Schistosomiasis haematobia in Coast Province, Kenya. Am J Trop Med Hyg 28:864, 1979. *Correlation of morbidity with egg counts in schistosomiasis haematobia; even in lightly infected children disease manifestations are significant.*

SCHISTOSOMIASIS MANSONI
(Intestinal or Hepatosplenic Bilharziasis)

Schistosomiasis mansoni is due to human infection with the blood fluke *S. mansoni*, which parasitizes the inferior mesenteric venous channels. Parasite eggs are detected in stools of infected individuals, and far less commonly in their urine. Infection with *S. mansoni* is endemic in Africa, the Middle East, South America, and some Caribbean islands. The distribution of schistosomiasis mansoni in Africa overlaps with that of schistosomiasis haematobia; it is prevalent in the Nile delta in Egypt, in the Sudan, in Ethiopia, and in a broad belt across central Africa. In southwest Asia, it occurs in Yemen and Saudi Arabia. *S. mansoni* is sporadically distributed all over the northern part of South America and is endemic in several Caribbean countries and islands and in many parts of Puerto Rico.

Adult male *S. mansoni* worms have a grossly tuberculate surface and usually contain seven small testes. In the female, the ovary occupies the anterior half of its body, with a short uterus containing one to four ova. Mature eggs measure 155 × 66 μm and are oval with a lateral, long spine. *Schistosoma mansoni* infects man and primates and is found also in rodents such as mice and hamsters, but none of these animals plays an important role as a reservoir for the infection. The intermediate snail hosts of *S. mansoni* are species of the genus *Biomphalaria* in Africa and *Australorbis tropicorbis* in the Americas.

PATHOLOGY AND CLINICAL MANIFESTATIONS. Cercarial dermatitis may occur following skin penetration by these larvae, but is uncommon. Acute schistosomiasis mansoni appears between three and seven weeks after exposure; the presenting symptoms, in their order of occurrence, are fever, anorexia, abdominal pain, and headache. Less often, diarrhea, nausea, and vomiting may occur. Hepatosplenomegaly, eosinophilia, and increased serum immunoglobulins are the main clinical signs. Most of these manifestations correlate significantly with intensity of infection as evaluated by stool egg counts.

Schistosoma mansoni eggs are primarily deposited in the small veins around the large intestine; some of the eggs may be trapped in the gut wall or break loose into the portal circulation to be carried to the small intrahepatic portal venules. On examination, the intestinal mucosa appears red and granular with pinpoint elevations surrounded by hyperemic zones. There may be minute hemorrhages and ulcerations. Sessile and pedunculated polyps, mainly in the rectosigmoid area, have been reported in Egyptians infected with *S. mansoni*, but not from other endemic areas. Pathologic examination of the liver in lightly infected individuals shows schistosome eggs with and without granulomas and mild portal inflammation. In advanced cases, the typical picture of Symmers' fibrosis is seen; the eggs are concentrated in and around large portal tracts with marked fibrosis and obstructive portal venous lesions. The lobular arrangement of liver parenchyma and its function are usually maintained. However, these structural changes lead to marked alteration of hepatic hemodynamics such as obstruction of portal blood flow through the liver and increase in number and size of intrahepatic arterial branches, thus shifting the blood flow through the liver from mainly portal to arterial sources. Portal hypertension leads to congestive splenomegaly and formation of portosystemic venous shunts at the lower end of the esophagus and other sites. In these patients, schistosome eggs may find their way to the pulmonary circulation, bypassing the obstructed portal blood flow. In the lungs, granulomas form around the trapped eggs, leading to arteriolar fibrosis and pulmonary hypertension.

Nervous system involvement in schistosomiasis mansoni is rare; the main clinical presentation, as in schistosomiasis haematobia, is transverse myelitis. The preferential involvement of the spinal cord may be due to the anatomic location of adult worms; both species rarely produce cerebral lesions. The underlying pathologic lesions are usually granulomas forming around eggs in the spinal cord.

Infection with *S. mansoni* does not have characteristic or specific symptomatology, in contrast to schistosomiasis haematobia. In several studies, infected individuals had a slightly higher incidence of crampy abdominal pain (21 to 48 per cent) and bloody diarrhea (4 to 28 per cent) than matched uninfected controls from the same endemic area. Examination of stools demonstrates an association between intensity of infection and the amount of blood detected. Other frequently mentioned nonspecific symptoms and signs, such as weakness, inability to work, or diarrhea, have not been convincingly demonstrated in any controlled studies. Significant enlargement of the liver is seen in 4 to 11 per cent of infected subjects, and splenomegaly occurs in 3 to 7 per cent. Patients with schistosomal hepatosplenomegaly present with a unique form of liver disease. The pathophysiologic changes are based on alteration of hemodynamics, fibrosis of large portal tracts, and very little derangement of liver function. Enlargement of the liver usually occurs in the left lobe, but later, in the course of infection and particularly in adults, uniform hepatomegaly may be seen. Simultaneously, gross enlargement of the spleen may occur; the organ is characteristically rubbery hard. Laboratory examination may show indications of anemia and a low degree of eosinophilia but no changes in liver function tests until late in the course of disease. Total serum proteins are usually normal, but gamma globulin increases are common. An association between schistosomal hepatosplenomegaly and hepatitis B antigen and antibody presence has been described, but its pathophysiologic significance is not clear. Although hepatosplenomegaly usually occurs in heavily infected individuals, other underlying mechanisms may be involved. An association between HLA haplotypes and schistosomal hepatosplenomegaly has been demonstrated. In patients with pure schistosomal fibrosis uncomplicated by cirrhosis or viral hepatitis, liver function is preserved for a long time. These individuals often present clinically with an episode of hematemesis caused by rupture of esophageal varices without prior complaints. Bleeding may recur several times while the liver parenchyma maintains its normal functions. Finally, however, symptoms and signs of liver cell failure ensue, along with the development of stigmata of chronic liver disease and ascites.

Several less-defined clinical syndromes have been associated with schistosomiasis mansoni. Formation of antigen-antibody complexes and their deposition in the kidney glomeruli have been demonstrated in infected laboratory animals as well as in individuals with chronic schistosomiasis mansoni. However, the prevalence of this syndrome and the rate at which it occurs in schistosomiasis are unknown, since proteinuria and nephrotic syndrome are not particularly prevalent in schistosomiasis-endemic areas. Schistosomiasis cor pulmonale is a better-defined disease entity, although its incidence is not known. It usually occurs in patients with advanced hepatosplenic schistosomiasis mansoni or japonica because of the development of collateral circulation. In *S. haematobium*–infected individuals, the anatomic location of adult worms may help eggs reach the systemic circulation directly and become trapped in the pulmonary arterioles. Patients with schistosomal pulmonary hypertension present clinically with symptoms and signs similar to those in cor pulmonale of other causes. Aneurysmal dilation of the pulmonary artery and its branches, along with right ventricular hypertrophy, may occur.

DIAGNOSIS. Stool examination for the characteristic *S. mansoni* eggs is the definitive diagnostic procedure. Since assessing intensity of infection is essential, quantitative techniques are recommended. The Kato thick smear method involves examination of sieved 50-mg stool samples placed on glass slides and spead under a cellophane cover slip presoaked in 50 per cent glycerol. The slides should be left at least 24 hours to allow for clearing of fecal material; the embryo within the ova also clears, but the characteristic shape of the egg shell is retained. Rectal biopsy may be used for diagnosis of stool-negative cases, particularly in lightly infected individuals.

TREATMENT. See Management of Schistosomiasis, below.

Abdel-Salam E, Abdel Khalik A, Abdel-Meguid A, et al.: Association of HLA class I antigens (A1, B5, B8, and CW2) with disease manifestations and infection in human schistosomiasis mansoni in Egypt. Tissue Antigens 27:142, 1986. *A large-scale, population-based study of association between certain HLA haplotypes and hepatosplenomegaly due to schistosomiasis mansoni.*

Cheever AW: A quantitative post mortem study of schistosomiasis mansoni in man. Am J Trop Med Hyg 17:38, 1968. *Correlation of worm loads with egg counts in tissues and feces, and detailed description of pathology of S. mansoni infection.*

Peters PA, El Alamy M, Warren KS, et al.: Quick Kato smear for field quantification of *Schistosoma mansoni* eggs. Am J Trop Med Hyg 29:217, 1980. *Detailed description of the Kato thick smear technique for quantification of S. mansoni eggs.*

Siongok TKA, Mahmoud AAF, Ouma JH, et al.: Morbidity in schistosomiasis mansoni in relation to intensity of infection: Study of a community in Machakos, Kenya, Am J Trop Med Hyg 25:273, 1976. *Correlation of symptoms and signs of S. mansoni with fecal egg counts.*

SCHISTOSOMIASIS JAPONICA

Schistosomiasis japonica, or Oriental schistosomiasis, is due to human infection with the fluke *S. japonicum*. This schistosome species characteristically infects humans and domestic animals such as cats, dogs, and cattle, thus providing reservoir hosts which may contribute to its endemicity in certain areas of the Far East. On the main Asian continent, schistosomiasis japonica is prevalent in some parts of China, Thailand, Laos, Cambodia, and Malaysia. It is also endemic in Taiwan, Japan, the Philippines, and Celebes.

Adult *S. japonicum* male worms have a nontuberculate surface and seven medium-sized testes. The ovary occupies the middle part of the body of female worms and contains 50 to 100 ova. *S. japonicum* eggs are found in stools of infected individuals; they measure 89×67 μm and are oval or rounded with a lateral short, sometimes curved spine. The intermediate hosts for *S. japonicum* are snails of the genus *Onchomelania*. They are amphibious and have separate sexes, and each infected snail sheds an average of two cercariae daily. These organisms emerge in the evening and lie very close to the surface film of water; they can penetrate mammalian skin within a minute.

PATHOLOGY AND CLINICAL MANIFESTATIONS. *S. japonicum* infection results in pathologic lesions in the human definitive host which generally follow the same time course as described for schistosomiasis mansoni. Cercarial dermatitis is not a prominent feature of schistosomiasis japonica. Katayama fever, or acute schistosomiasis, was named after the district in Japan endemic for *S. japonicum* infections. Symptoms usually begin five to seven weeks after infection and are similar to those associated with schistosomiasis mansoni. The clinical features usually subside in a few days but may last for several months, and fatalities have been reported. The chronic manifestations of schistosomiasis japonica are related to ova deposited in the intestines and liver; adult worms produce ten times more eggs than those of *S. mansoni*. These ova are laid in aggregates and remain so in the intestinal wall or when carried to the liver by the portal blood flow. In addition, *S. japonicum* eggs differ from *S. mansoni* in their tendency to calcify in tissues. Schistosomiasis japonica granulomas vary in size tremendously and tend to show signs of necrosis.

The major pathologic lesions in schistosomiasis japonica are seen in the intestines, liver, lungs, and occasionally brain. Morphologically these lesions are initiated by the presence of eggs and proceed to granuloma formation and fibrosis as in schistosomias mansoni. Individuals with chronic schistosomiasis japonica may present with no symptoms or several nonspecific complaints. Controlled surveys in endemic areas have shown no particular increase in complaints of weakness, abdominal pain, or diarrhea in infected individuals. Clinical signs of hepatosplenomegaly are more frequently seen in infected rather than uninfected individuals, but they were not uniformly correlated with intensity of infection. Severe hepatosplenic disease caused by schistosomiasis japonica may be seen in endemic areas, but its prevalence and relationship to intensity of infection and other complicating factors are unknown.

Cerebral schistosomiasis japonica is a unique syndrome reportedly occurring in 2 to 4 per cent of infected individuals in the endemic countries. *S. japonicum* infection of the central nervous system preferentially affects the brain. The lesions consist of large aggregates of eggs in the cerebral venous system, but adult worms have never been found in the brain. Cerebral schistosomiasis japonica presents clinically early in the course of the infection; the most frequent manifestation is focal jacksonian epilepsy; less commonly, generalized encephalitis may be the presenting feature.

DIAGNOSIS. Stool examination for *S. japonicum* eggs is the only reliable diagnostic procedure. The Kato thick smear technique provides both diagnosis and quantitative assessment of infection. Rectal biopsy may be used in individuals with light infections, particularly when a less common manifestation, such as cerebral schistosomiasis, is encountered.

TREATMENT. See Management of Schistosomiasis, below.

Domingo EO, Tiu E, Peters PA, et al.: Morbidity in schistosomiasis japonica in relation to intensity of infection: Study of a community in Leyte, Philippines. Am J Trop Med Hyg 29:858, 1980. *A controlled study of the correlation between symptoms and signs of schistosomiasis japonica and fecal egg counts.*

Warren KS, Su DL, Xu CY, et al.: Morbidity in schistosomiasis japonica in relation to intensity of infection; study of 2 royal brigades in Anhui Province, China. N Engl J Med, 309:1533, 1983.

OTHER HUMAN SCHISTOSOMES

Endemic foci for *S. intercalatum* are found in Central and West Africa. Adult worms inhabit the mesenteric blood vessels, and terminal spine eggs are seen in stools of infected individuals. No controlled studies have been performed to delineate the specific symptoms and signs in infected individuals. Symptoms usually ascribed to this species of human schistosomes include abdominal pain, diarrhea, and blood in stools. Diagnosis is based on positive geographic history and finding parasite ova upon fecal examination.

S. mekongi is the most recent of schistosome species that have been described to infect and cause disease in humans. The parasite is endemic in some parts of the mainland of Southeast Asia. Adult worm and eggs are similar to those of *S. japonicum*; ova of *S. mekongi* are, however, smaller. In symptomatic patients a syndrome not unlike that due to *S. japonicum* has been observed. It includes abdominal pain, diarrhea, and heptosplenomegaly. Diagnosis is established by fecal examination for parasite ova.

Hofstetter M, Nash TE, Cheever AW, et al.: Infection with *Schistosoma mekongi* in Southeast Asian refugees. J Infect Dis 144:420, 1981. *Description of clinical and parasitologic features of schistosomiasis mekongi.*

MANAGEMENT OF SCHISTOSOMIASIS

Chemotherapy is the major antischistosome strategy for eradication of parasites in infected individuals and for reducing incidence, intensity, and morbidity in populations of endemic areas. The current drug of choice is praziquantel, a pyrazinoisoquinoline derivative that is effective against all species of schistosomes that infect humans. Praziquantel has several advantages as the chemotherapeutic agent of choice, including oral administration, low incidence of toxicity and side effects, and marked antiparasitic activity. The recommended dose of praziquantel for treatment of infections with *S. haematobium*, *S. intercalatum*, or *S. mansoni* is 40 mg per kilogram of body weight once. For *S. japonicum* infection it is recommended to administer 30 mg per kilogram twice in one day, and for *S. mekongi* 20 mg per kilogram three times in one day. These dosages have been shown to result in parasitologic cure in approximately 80 per cent of treated individuals and a highly significant reduction of intensity of infection. Side effects of praziquantel are rare, usually mild, and self-limiting. These include abdominal pain, headache, dizziness, and skin rashes.

Metrifonate* and oxamniquine are two additional antischistosome chemotherapeutic agents that are orally administered and have therapeutic efficacy similar to those of praziquantel. Metrifonate is an organophosphorous compound that is effective against *S. haematobium* infection. It is given as a single oral dose of 10 mg per kilogram; the dose is repeated twice at two-week intervals. Oxamniquine is 2-aminomethyltetra-hydroquinoline derivative. It has been extensively used for treating individuals infected with *S. mansoni* in Brazil. Oxamniquine is administered orally, 20 mg per kilogram† as a single dose.

The effect of antischistosome chemotherapeutic agents on disease manifestations is variable. It is dependent on the duration of infection and extent of disease. Treatment is expected to result in reversal of pathology, e.g., hematuria, hepatosplenomegaly, in infected children. By contrast, adults with established fibro-obstructive disease in the liver and urinary tract may not show significant clinical improvement following chemotherapy. Other therapeutic or surgical methods may therefore be necessary to correct the anatomic lesions. Furthermore, medical management of the chronic sequelae of schistosomiasis, such as liver fibrosis, portal hypertension, and esophageal varices, should be conducted according to established practices and taking into consideration the unique pathophysiologic characteristics of disease due to schistosomiasis.

---

*Investigational drug. Available from the Centers for Disease Control, Atlanta, GA.
†Dosage exceeds manufacturer's recommendations.

Mahmoud AAF: Praziquantel for the treatment of helminthic infections. Adv Intern Med 32:193, 1987. *A summary of the known antihelminthic effects of praziquantel in experimental animals and humans.*

---

401 HERMAPHRODITIC FLUKES

S. K. K. Seah

The hermaphroditic flukes, unlike *Schistosoma* flukes, have male and female sex organs in the same worm, and self-fertilize. Those of medical importance are (1) flukes that parasitize the biliary tract, i.e., *Clonorchis sinensis*, *Opisthorchis* spp., *Fasciola hepatica*, *Dicrocoelium dendriticum*, and *Metorchis conjunctus*; (2) flukes that parasitize the intestinal lumen, i.e., *Fasciolopsis buski*, *Heterophyes heterophyes*, *Echinostoma ilocanum*, *Gastrodiscoides hominis*, and *Metagonimus yokogawai*; (3) flukes that parasitize the lung, i.e., *Paragonimus westermani* and other species; and (4) the mesocercarial stage of *Alaria americana*, which causes generalized systemic infection.

All of these flukes parasitize other mammals, and some of them, such as *Fasciola hepatica*, are of major importance in veterinary medicine. Most of these flukes have limited geographic distribution. However, with the migration of people around the world, human infections are often seen in nonendemic areas.

The hermaphroditic flukes are leaf-like, nonsegmented, and bilaterally symmetrical, ranging in size from a few millimeters to several centimeters. On one end is the anterior or oral sucker and just behind it the ventral sucker or acetabulum. The acetabulum acts as a holdfast to the epithelial tissue of the final host.

Eggs appear in bile and stool and, in the case of the lung fluke, in sputum and stool. The eggs are operculated. Some are fully embryonated when passed; others may require time for embryonation. The embryonated egg contains the first stage larva or miracidium. After hatching in fresh water the miracidium penetrates, or is ingested by, a suitable first intermediate host, a snail. In the snail the miracidium develops into thousands of cercariae, which are released into the water. The cercariae attach themselves to or penetrate into the second intermediate hosts, which, depending on the flukes, may be freshwater fish, crustaceans, frogs, or aquatic plants. The final definitive hosts (man or animals) acquire the infection by ingesting encysted metacercariae.

The treatment of digenetic trematodes is by the broad-spectrum anthelminthic praziquantel. Personal prevention of infection includes eating only well-cooked fish or crustaceans and avoiding raw watercress in endemic areas. Community prevention consists of cleaning up the environment and preventing infection of the intermediate hosts.

Seah SKK: Digenetic trematodes. Clin Gastroenterol 7:98, 1978. *A good review of all the hermaphroditic flukes up to date and well referenced.*

HEPATIC HERMAPHRODITIC FLUKES
Clonorchiasis (Clonorchis sinensis)

This infection is common in the Far East, especially southern China, Hong Kong, Taiwan, Japan, and Korea, where raw or undercooked fish have long been considered a delicacy. More than 40 species of freshwater fish, mainly the carp and salmon group, harbor metacercariae.

Clonorchis sinensis has a very long lifespan (probably up to 50 years), and this parasitic infection will likely be important in these areas for many years. Clonorchiasis occurs in all parts of the world where there are Asian immigrants from endemic areas. Over one-half million Southeast Asian refugees have come to North America in the past few years, and surveys show that a large percentage of these have asymptomatic liver fluke infection.

After ingestion of the contaminated fish, the metacercariae excyst in the duodenum. Most of the larval flukes ascend the biliary tree directly, but some may pass via the portal circulation to the liver. During maturation of the fluke there is marked desquamation of biliary epithelium. The fluke matures in two to three weeks and begins to lay eggs. Flukes prefer to reside in the second-order bile ducts, but in heavy infection they are found throughout the biliary system, including the gallbladder, and sometimes in the pancreatic duct. Adult flukes are grayish-brown, 15 × 3 mm. They feed on secretions from the bile duct mucosa. They cause low-grade inflammatory changes of the biliary tree, proliferation of the biliary epithelium, and progressive portal fibrosis. As a rule there is no parenchymal damage, and cirrhosis does not result from uncomplicated clonorchiasis.

CLINICAL MANIFESTATIONS. *Acute clonorchiasis* occurs one to three weeks after the ingestion of encysted metacercariae. There may be fever, chills, abdominal pain, diarrhea, tender hepatomegaly, and mild jaundice. The white blood cell count is raised with marked eosinophilia, and serum alkaline phosphatase, SGOT, SGPT, and bilirubin levels are elevated. The clinical presentation is often confused with acute viral hepatitis and seldom recognized. The ova of *C. sinensis* appear in the stool or bile three or four weeks after ingestion of the metacercariae. The history of eating raw fish in the endemic area and the eosinophilia should suggest the diagnosis.

The majority of people with ova of *C. sinensis* in their stools have no symptoms even when heavily infected. It is impossible to predict who will develop the complications of chronic clonorchiasis. *Acute suppurative cholangitis* is a severe febrile illness often associated with hypoglycemia and *Escherichia coli* bacteremia. The biliary system is blocked by numerous flukes and becomes secondarily infected. This condition carries a very high mortality rate. *Recurrent pyogenic cholangitis* is a recurrent febrile illness associated with clonorchiasis and intrahepatic bile duct calculi. During surgical operation or autopsy, *Clonorchis* flukes are not consistently found as in the case of acute suppurative cholangitis. With recurrent pyogenic cholangitis cirrhosis may eventually develop. The flukes occasionally block the pancreatic ducts and induce pancreatitis. Cholangiocarcinoma is a late complication of chronic clonorchiasis. Clonorchiasis has no causal relationship with hepatocellular cancer.

DIAGNOSIS. The diagnosis is made by finding the small operculated eggs in the stool or duodenal aspirate. The eggs average 29 × 16 μ; they are light brown and ovoid. Unfortunately the *C. sinensis* egg is almost identical to those of *Opisthorchis*, *Heterophyes*, and *Metagonimus*. To be absolutely certain of the diagnosis one must examine the adult fluke. However, geographic distribution may help in separating *Clonorchis* from *Opisthorchis*. Expulsion and eradication of the flukes by a course of bephenium hydroxynaphthoate will indicate whether the ova are *Heterophyes* or *Metagonimus*. In a patient with abdominal or other symptoms and *C. sinensis* eggs in the stool, it is often difficult to decide if the complaints are due to clonorchiasis. It is often necessary to eliminate other current illnesses before attributing the symptoms to clonorchiasis. As a rule in uncomplicated established clonorchiasis, there is no eosinophilia, elevation of sedimentation rate, anemia, or abnormal liver function test results, and radioisotope scan and ultrasound (B scan) of the liver are normal.

In acute clonorchiasis, leukocytosis, marked eosinophilia, and abnormal liver function test results are present. This condition must be distinguished from hepatic amebiasis and visceral larva migrans. In the former, eosinophilia is absent and serology for amebiasis is positive. In the latter, the serology for toxocariasis is positive. The presence of the flukes in the liver provokes irregular antibody response, and a large variety of serologic and skin tests is available in some centers. However, these are not sufficiently specific and sensitive for clinical use.

TREATMENT. Praziquantel has revolutionized the treatment of this condition. The recommended dosage is 75 mg per kilogram of body weight,* divided into three doses on the same day. Praziquantel is well tolerated, and no long-term toxicity has been shown. At the dose recommended there may be some gastrointestinal disturbance and transient headaches. Because this drug is safe, it is recommended that all cases of clonorchiasis whether symptomatic or not be treated. The cure rate of a single-day treatment is almost 100 per cent. Stool should be checked for ova of the fluke one month, six months, and one year after treatment. Re-treat if necessary. The cost of this drug may limit its use in mass chemotherapy in the endemic area.

The treatment of complications such as calculi, suppurative cholangitis, recurrent pyogenic cholangitis, and pancreatitis is both medical and surgical. Conservative treatment consists of broad-spectrum antibiotics and intravenous fluids. If this is not effective, a permanent and adequate drainage procedure, such as choledochoduodenostomy, is required. Suppuration usually kills many flukes, and medical treatment is not urgent. At surgery as many flukes as possible should be

removed from the biliary tree. A course of praziquantel should be given when the patient is able to swallow the tablets.

PREVENTION. In the endemic areas, freshwater fish must be well cooked before eating.

Opisthorchiasis (Opisthorchis viverrini and felineus)

Opisthorchis felineus is common in eastern Europe, the USSR, India, Japan, the Philippines, and Vietnam. *Opisthorchis viverrini* is common in northern Thailand and Laos. In northeastern Thailand 90 per cent of the people over the age of ten have *O. viverrini* infection. The life cycles of these flukes are similar to those of *C. sinensis*. Infection is acquired by eating undercooked freshwater fish. Many animals, especially the cat, are natural reservoirs.

The pathology, clinical manifestations, and complications of opisthorchiasis are similar to those of clonorchiasis. Cholangiocarcinoma can also result from chronic opisthorchiasis. The eggs of *Opisthorchis* are almost identical to those of *Clonorchis*. This emphasizes the importance of geographic history, for the only other way of distinguishing the parasites would be by examination of the adult flukes. The treatment is the same as for clonorchiasis.

Dicroceliasis

Dicrocoelium dendriticum is a lancet-shaped fluke, measuring 10 × 2 mm, that normally inhabits the biliary tract of sheep and cattle. Man is occasionally infected by ingesting ants that have eaten slime balls containing cercariae secreted by the snail. This occurs in Europe, in Asia, and around the Mediterranean basin. Infection is usually asymptomatic, and there is little information on the pathologic changes in man. It is important for the physician to recognize the small (40 × 25 μ), fully embryonated, thick-shelled operculated eggs for what they are. This infection requires no treatment.

Fascioliasis (Fasciola hepatica)

This is a common parasite in the bilary tract of sheep and cattle, but it may infect all types of mammals, including man. It has worldwide distribution in sheep, and is prevalent in low wet pastures where suitable species of snails are present. The cercariae, discharged from the snails, attach themselves to the water plants and encyst as metacercariae. Man is infected mainly as a result of eating watercress and other aquatic plants gathered in these pastures. In the duodenum the immature fluke penetrates the mucosa, enters the abdominal cavity, and through some unexplained hepatotropism penetrates Glisson's capsule. The immature flukes migrate throughout the liver for some weeks until they reach the biliary tract, where they mature in about two months. The fluke measures 3 × 1.3 cm, and the eggs are large, ovoid, and operculated, measuring 140 × 75 μ.

CLINICAL MANIFESTATIONS. *Acute Fascioliasis.* Invasion and maturation occur during the first three months after ingestion of the metacercariae. The immature flukes produce small necrotic foci along the migration paths. There may be no significant symptoms, or there may be abdominal pain, hepatomegaly, fever, vomiting, and jaundice. Leukocytosis and marked eosinophilia are present, but *F. hepatica* eggs are not found in the stool at this stage.

Established Infection. The mature flukes now produce metabolites that irritate the bilary passages, resulting in hyperplasia. Obstruction and dilation of the biliary passage and cholecystitis may occur. There may be abdominal pain, hepatomegaly, recurrent urticaria, jaundice, irregular fever, diarrhea, and weight loss. Anemia from blood loss can be severe. The obstruction and irritation may produce thickening of the biliary tree, atrophy of the hepatic cells, and biliary cirrhosis. Cholelithiasis is common. A relationship of fascioliasis and biliary cancers is not proved.

Extrabiliary Fascioliasis. Ingestion of raw sheep and goat

---

*Dosage exceeds manufacturer's recommendation.

liver containing young flukes causes the condition called halzoun (suffocation). This pharyngeal fascioliasis is due to lodgment of flukes in the upper respiratory and digestive tracts. Inflammation and edema may lead to dysphagia, dyspnea, and even asphyxiation. Cutaneous fascioliasis, usually in the upper abdomen, presents as migratory nodules that are pruritic, painful, and inflamed, and vary in size from 2 to 5 cm. Rarely the flukes may be found in the lung, peritoneum, muscles, eye, and brain.

DIAGNOSIS. In acute infection the diagnosis is made in an endemic area by a high index of suspicion and the clinical triad of fever, hepatomegaly, and marked eosinophilia. A history of ingestion of wild watercress supports the diagnosis. At this stage the stool does not contain eggs. Serologic tests, such as the complement fixation test, are helpful. In chronic infection the stool contains the characteristic large operculated eggs (140 × 75 μ). Duodenal and biliary aspirate will provide a higher yield than fecal examination. Liver function test results reflect the degree of hepatic cellular damage and biliary obstruction. Intravenous or percutaneous cholangiography may show abnormalities and filling defects. The diagnosis is often made during surgical operation for biliary disease. The diagnosis of halzoun in an endemic area is made by the history of ingestion of raw liver and the finding of a pharyngeal mass.

TREATMENT. In the past, bithionol,* emetine, dehydroemetine,* and chloroquine were used with some success in this condition. Praziquantel is now the drug of choice in fascioliasis. The recommended dosage is 75 mg per kilogram of body weight† divided into three doses per day for two days. Ectopic flukes are removed surgically. Prevention consists of not eating raw watercress and raw sheep and goat liver in the endemic areas.

Fasciola gigantica

This large fluke is a liver parasite of herbivorous animals and occasionally of man in Asia and Africa. The life cycle, mode of infection, clinical manifestations, and treatment are similar to those of *F. hepatica.*

---

*Available only from the Centers for Disease Control, Atlanta, GA.
†Dosage exceeds manufacturer's recommendation.

CLONORCHIASIS

Flavell, DJ: Liver fluke infection as an aetiological factor in bile duct carcinoma of man. Trans Roy Soc Trop Med Hyg 75:814, 1981. *Reviews the evidence of liver flukes as factors in causing bile duct cancer.*
Gibson JB, Sun T: Clonorchiasis. In Marcial-Rojas RA (ed.): Pathology of Protozoal and Helminthic Diseases. Baltimore, Williams & Wilkins Company, 1971, pp 546–566. *Profusely illustrated; very good on all aspects, especially on epidemiology and pathology as seen in Hong Kong.*
Hsu CCS, Kron MA: Clonorchiasis and praziquantel. Arch Intern Med 145:1002, 1985. *Summary of treatment of clonorchiasis.*
Schwartz DA: Cholangiocarcinoma associated with liver fluke infections: A preventable source of morbidity in Asian immigrants. Am J Gastroenterol 81:76, 1986. *Reviews and emphasizes the importance of early diagnosis and treatment of all liver fluke infections in the prevention of bile duct neoplasms in high-risk population.*
Sun T: Pathology and immunology of Clonorchis sinensis infection of the liver. Ann Clin Lab Sci 14:208, 1984. *A good review of the pathology of this fluke and its relationship with cholangiocarcinoma.*
Weniger BG, Schantz PM: Praziquantel and refugee health. JAMA 251:2391, 1984. *Reviews the use of praziquantel in the various helminthic infections.*

OPISTHORCHIASIS

Viranuvatti V: Liver fluke infection and infestation in Southeast Asia. Progr Liver Dis 4:537, 1972. *Concise review of liver flukes, especially Opisthorchis.*

FASCIOLIASIS

Condomines J, Rene-Espinet JM, Espinos-Perez JC, et al.: Percutaneous cholangiography in the diagnosis of hepatic fascioliasis. Am J Gastroenterol 80:384, 1985. *Emphasizes the importance of considering parasitic infections in the differential diagnosis of images obtained by direct visualization of the bile duct either by endoscopic retrograde cholangiography or percutaneous cholangiography.*
Jones EA, Kay JM, Milligan HP, et al.: Massive infection with Fasciola hepatica in man. Am J Med 63:836, 1977. *Report of an unusual case with a prolonged course of illness. Illustrates many of the complications of this disease.*
Marcial-Rojas RA: Fascioliasis. In Marcial-Rojas RA (ed.): Pathology of Protozoal and Helminthic Disease. Baltimore, Williams & Wilkins Company, 1971, pp 490–497. *Good on the epidemiology and pathology of this disease.*
Park CI, Ro JY, Kim H, et al.: Human ectopic fascioliasis in the cecum. Am J Surg Pathol 8:73, 1984. *Ectopic Fasciola in the cecum presenting as carcinoma of the colon.*

LUNG-HERMAPHRODITIC FLUKES (Paragonimiasis)

Paragonimiasis is due to infection with the adult *Paragonimus westermani* and other species. As a rule the infection is in the lung, where the flukes are encapsulated in the parenchyma. The disease is also called pulmonary distomiasis, endemic hemoptysis, and Oriental lung fluke disease. Human paragonimiasis occurs most commonly in the Far East, especially central China, Japan, Korea, Vietnam, Laos, Thailand, and the Philippines. It also occurs in the Indian subcontinent, Central and South America, and West Africa. In addition to *P. westermani,* over 30 species may affect man. Most of these flukes are parasites of mammals, especially of the cat family (cat, tiger, leopard), foxes, dogs, cattle, and pigs.

The adult flukes lives singly or in pairs encapsulated in the cystic spaces of the lung. They are ovoid, plump, and leaf-like, and measure about 1 × 0.5 × 0.4 cm. Oval yellowish-brown operculated ova (90 × 55 μ) are coughed up and expelled in the sputum or are swallowed and passed in the feces. The flukes have a lifespan of five to six years. In fresh water the miracidia escape from the ova and penetrate the first intermediate host, a suitable snail. After several weeks the cercariae emerge and penetrate the second intermediate host, the crayfish or crab. Man or animal acquires the infection by eating raw meat or viscera of the freshwater crustacean. In Korea and West Africa, fresh crab juice is used as a home remedy in the treatment of measles. In the duodenum the metacercariae excyst, enter the abdominal cavity, migrate through the diaphragm into the pleural space, and end up in the lung parenchyma, where they mature and begin to lay eggs about two months after ingestion of the crayfish. This circuitous route of migration explains the extrapulmonary cysts of *Paragonimus.*

PATHOLOGY. The migratory larval flukes tunnel into the lung at the periphery. This is accompanied by inflammatory reaction with many eosinophils. They finally encyst with a fibrous tissue wall. The cyst may communicate with a bronchus and may often be secondarily infected with abscess formation. The death of the fluke is followed by calcification. Flukes in the abdominal cavity may cause abscess and adhesion and intestinal ulceration, resulting in bloody diarrhea with mucus and ova. In the brain the temporal and occipital lobes are the favored sites of eosinophilic granulomas containing the flukes or ova. Lodgment of the flukes in the spinal cord causes transverse myelitis. Adult flukes have been found in other organs, including the genitalia and muscle. Some species are prone to cause ectopic paragonimiasis. Thus the characteristic feature of *P. skrjabini* is migratory subcutaneous nodules containing active flukes.

CLINICAL MANIFESTATIONS. In the rare case of acute paragonimiasis there may be fever, chills, and chest pain. The symptoms and physical findings are indistinguishable from those of bronchopneumonia. As a rule the onset is insidious and the symptoms are those of chronic bronchitis and bronchiectasis. Cough, especially in the morning, productive of thick, gelatinous, blood-tinged sputum, is the most prominent symptom. Exertional dyspnea and night sweats are common. Frank hemoptysis often occurs after a paroxysm of coughing. Chest pain and pleural effusion may be present, and clubbing of fingers may occur. The most characteristic physical finding is persistent moist, coarse rales over the area of involvement. Chest radiographs early in the disease show patchy, cloudy infiltrations, but later dense nodular opacities or ring shadows indicate the site of the cysts. Pleural thickening and calcification may be seen late in the disease.

Abdominal paragonimiasis occurs when the flukes localize in the abdomen. The symptoms are nonspecific dull ache, tenderness, and diarrhea, which may be bloody and accompanied by mucus. An abdominal mass with lung disease in a patient from an endemic area should raise this suspicion. On rare occasions the fluke localizes in the brain, resulting in a seizure disorder similar to cysticercosis. There may be pareses of varying degrees and optic atrophy with papilledema. The cerebrospinal fluid shows a raised protein concentration, and eosinophils are present. Children with cerebral paragonimiasis are usually mentally retarded. Subcutaneous localization of the fluke results in abscess formation.

DIAGNOSIS. This rests mainly on finding ova in the sputum. In more than half of the cases stools will also reveal the ova, especially after concentration. The main differential diagnoses in the chest radiographs are bronchopneumonia, bronchiectasis, tuberculosis, tumor, and the rarer fungal infections. In practice the most important differential diagnosis is tuberculosis. Active tuberculosis and paragonimiasis often are present in the same individual from the endemic area.

Abdominal paragonimiasis must be differentiated from intestinal parasitic and nonparasitic infections and other intra-abdominal disorders. The finding of the ova in the stool does not necessarily indicate abdominal paragonimiasis. The cerebral presentation must be differentiated from other causes of seizure disorder, space-occupying lesions, cysticercosis, hydatid disease, and meningoencephalitides.

Moderate eosinophilia is usual in the early cases, but in established cases there may be no abnormal hematologic findings. Serology, as a rule, is not useful in helminthic infections, and this is also true in paragonimiasis. The complement fixation test, using extract of the adult fluke as antigen, is positive when the fluke is alive, but the skin test may remain positive long after the fluke is dead.

TREATMENT. Praziquantel, because of its safety, ease of use, and high degree of efficacy, has replaced bithionol and niclofolan as the treatment of choice in pulmonary paragonimiasis. The recommended dosage of praziquantel in this infection is 75 mg per kilogram of body weight* divided into three doses daily for two days.

Paragonimiasis of the central nervous system requires surgery. Praziquantel should be given before the operation. Subcutaneous flukes should also be surgically removed.

PREVENTION. In theory prevention is simple. Freshwater crustaceans must be well cooked before eating, and hands and utensils should be thoroughly washed after contact with raw crabs and crayfish. However, in endemic areas it is difficult to persuade people to relinquish long-established cooking and eating habits and the use of raw crab juice for medicinal purposes.

Chung CH: Human paragonimiasis. In Marcial-Rojas RA (ed.): Pathology of Protozoal and Helminthic Diseases. Baltimore, Williams & Wilkins Company, 1971, pp 504–535. *Very detailed description of the pathologic changes of this disease. Well illustrated.*

Monson MH, Koenig JW, Sach R: Successful treatment with praziquantel of six patients infected with the African lung fluke Paragonimus uterobilateralis. Am J Trop Med Hyg 32:371, 1983. *Describes the usefulness of this drug in the common West African species of* Paragonimus.

Spitalny KC, Senft AW, Meglio FD, et al. Treatment of pulmonary paragonimiasis with a new broad-spectrum antihelminthic, praziquantel. J Pediatr 101:144, 1982. *Report of an Indochinese refugee to America with pulmonary paragonimiasis successfully treated with this drug.*

Yokogawa M: Paragonimus and paragonimiasis. Adv Parasitol 7:375, 1969. *Good review of the finer parasitologic points on this fluke.*

INTESTINAL HERMAPHRODITIC FLUKES
Fasciolopsiasis (Fasciolopsis buski)

Fasciolopsis buski is the largest intestinal fluke and is normally a parasite of pigs. Human infection is widespread in southern China, Southeast Asia, and the Indian subcontinent. The eggs are passed in the feces, and the miracidia are released to penetrate a snail. The cercariae encyst as metacercariae on edible water plants. Often the infected plants are peeled by using the teeth to remove the "skin," and the metacercariae are swallowed in the process. The larvae attach themselves to the upper small intestine, where they mature in about four weeks. The adult fluke has an average size of 3 × 1.2 cm.

CLINICAL MANIFESTATIONS. Many light infections are asymptomatic, but heavy loads of flukes produce symptoms, especially in children. The worm load may be up to several thousand. The flukes attach themselves to the duodenal and jejunal mucosa and produce symptoms by trauma, obstruction, and toxin production. There may be abdominal pain, gastrointestinal hemorrhage, diarrhea, and intestinal obstruction. In severe cases there may be edema of the face, trunk, and legs, as well as ascites.

DIAGNOSIS. This rests on finding the large ova (135 × 80 μ) or recovering of characteristic adult flukes in the stool. Difficulty may be encountered in distinguishing the ova of *F. hepatica* and *F. buski*. Eosinophilia is common and may exceed 50 per cent of the white cell count. Serologic tests, such as the indirect fluorescent antibody test, are available in some centers. The specificity of serologic tests is unproved, and definitive diagnosis cannot be based on serologic tests alone. This is also true of skin tests. Facial edema may require differentiation of fasciolopsiasis from trichinosis or the nephrotic syndrome.

TREATMENT. Praziquantel is the drug of choice in this condition. The dosage is 75 mg per kilogram of body weight* divided into three doses per day for one or two days. Personal prevention consists of cooking aquatic plants before eating. Community prevention entails eradication of the snails with molluscacides, public education, and prevention of fecal contamination of ponds.

Other Intestinal Hermaphroditic Flukes

Heterophyes heterophyes and *Metagonimus yokogawai* are small flukes that are acquired be eating raw or undercooked fish that contain the metacercariae. The former is found in Egypt, Tunisia, South China, India, and the Philippines, and the latter in the Far East and Indonesia. The adult flukes are 2 to 3 mm long and attach themselves to the intestinal mucosa. Usually the infection is light, and there are few symptoms. Very rarely the eggs gain access to the circulation and may be found in the organs. As a rule the eggs are passed in the stool; they closely resemble *Clonorchis* eggs. Both flukes can be treated with praziquantel. Differentiation of the two species requires examination of the adult flukes by experts. Many species of the genus *Echinostoma* infect man in the Far East, but they rarely produce symptoms. *Gastrocoides hominis* occurs in India and Malaysia, and may cause diarrhea. In western Canada the eggs of *Metorchis conjunctus*, which are somewhat similar to those of *Clonorchis*, are occasionally found in the stools of humans who eat raw fish. If treatment is called for, praziquantel (75 mg per kilogram of body weight* in three divided doses for one day) is the treatment of choice.

Alaria americana is an intestinal trematode of carnivores, such as the fox, wolf, lynx, or skunk. Two cases of human infection by the mesocercariae of this fluke have been reported in Ontario. Mesocercaria is a stage of development between the cercaria and the metacercaria. The cercariae emerging from the snail penetrate tadpoles. As the tadpole grows into a frog the mesocercariae tend to concentrate in the hind legs. When the frog is eaten by a carnivore, the mesocercariae develop into metacercariae and adult flukes in the lung and the gut, respectively. When man, who is not the normal host, eats the frog the mesocercariae migrate all over the body. In

*Dosage exceeds manufacturer's recommendation.

*Dosage exceeds manufacturer's recommendation.

the first reported case the mesocercaria was surgically removed from the retina of the eye. The second case was a fatal systemic infection manifested by severe respiratory distress, coma, a coagulation abnormality, and vasculitis. At autopsy mesocercariae were found in all organs. The diagnosis is by biopsy of affected organs. There is no known treatment, although praziquantel may be useful.

Faust EC, Beaver PC, Jung RC: Intestinal flukes. In Faust EC, Beaver PC, Jung RC: Animal Agents and Vectors of Human Disease. 4th ed. Philadelphia, Lea & Febiger, 1975, pp 134–141. *Emphasis is on the parasitology, life cycles, and morphology. A good reference for the less important parasites.*

Fernandes BJ, Cooper JD, Cullen JB, et al.: Systemic infection with *Alaria americana* (Trematoda). Can Med Assoc J 115:1111, 1976. *This is the first report of generalized infection with mesocercariae of this fluke. Good description of the clinical course and autopsy findings.*

The Nematodes

402 INTRODUCTION

Daniel S. Blumenthal

Nematodes are primitive, elongated, unsegmented worms, with a body cavity that is not lined with a peritoneum of mesodermal origin as is the body cavity of higher animals. The sexes are separate, but parthenogenesis occurs in some parasitic forms. The class includes half a million species; some are free-living, while others are parasitic for plants, invertebrates, and both wild and domestic vertebrates.

Eleven species are important parasites of humans. These may be classified as either intestinal or tissue parasites. The former include the hookworms *Ancylostoma duodenale* and *Necator americanus*, the large roundworm *Ascaris lumbricoides*, the whipworm *Trichuris trichiura*, the pinworm *Enterobius vermicularis*, and *Strongyloides stercoralis*. The adult *Trichinella spiralis* also inhabits the human intestine, but it is classified as a tissue nematode because its clinical manifestations are produced by larvae invading the tissues. The filariae are also tissue parasites; species commonly causing serious disease in humans include *Onchocerca volvulus*, the agent of river blindness; *Dracunculus medinensis*, the Guinea worm; *Loa loa*; and *Wuchereria bancrofti*. Several other nematodes are human parasites of lesser importance, and a variety of nematodes that ordinarily infect nonhuman species may occasionally infect people, sometimes causing serious disease.

The parasitic nematodes have evolved a great variety of mechanisms by which they are transmitted from one definitive host to another. Some (such as *Enterobius*) produce ova that may be passed from person to person, whereas the eggs of others (for instance, *Ascaris* and hookworm) must incubate in the soil before they become infective. Some, such as *Trichinella*, require an intermediate host that is eaten by the definitive host, whereas the intermediate hosts of some nematode parasites of animals release infective larvae. The filariae are transmitted by insect vectors.

Of the major nematode parasites of man, only *Strongyloides stercoralis* is capable of reproducing in the definitive host. Most other helminths are also incapable of reproducing in the definitive host; this distinguishes helminthiases from infections with viruses, bacteria, and protozoa. As a consequence, it is not usually necessary to seek total elimination of the parasite in a patient (or a community), since a light infection is not generally clinically significant. An exception is ascariasis, in which a single worm can cause serious morbidity or mortality.

It is hard to overestimate the amount of worldwide morbidity caused by parasitic nematodes. There are an estimated 1 billion cases each of infection with *Ascaris* and *Trichuris*. Approximately 600 million persons are infected with hookworm and 300 million with filariae. Nematode infections are still found in many communities in the United States and are particularly common in recent immigrants from tropical countries. There are perhaps 4 million persons infected with *Ascaris*

in this country; 2.2 million with *Trichuris*, 700,000 with hookworm, and 400,000 with *Strongyloides*.

In areas where soil and climatic conditions are suitable, nematode infections are a marker of rural poverty. Only when this poverty, with its accompanying inadequate levels of sanitation and education, has been alleviated, will the prevalence of these parasites be reduced to unimportant levels.

Major nematode infections; other nematode infections. In Intestinal Protozoan and Helminthic Infections. Report of a WHO Scientific Group. Technical Report Series 666. Geneva, World Health Organization, 1981. *A comprehensive public health approach.*

Markell EK: Intestinal nematode infections. Pediatr Clin North Am 32:971, 1985. *Reviews the major intestinal nematodes, with illustrations and case reports.*

Warren KS: The control of helminths: Nonreplicating infectious agents of man. Ann Rev Public Health 2:101, 1981. *A thoughtful commentary on efforts to control nematode and other helminth infections in developing countries.*

Intestinal Nematodes

Daniel S. Blumenthal

403 STRONGYLOIDIASIS

DEFINITION. Strongyloidiasis is infection with the parasitic phase of *Strongyloides stercoralis*. Clinical manifestations may be caused by adult worms in the small intestine or by migrating filariform larvae.

ETIOLOGY AND LIFE CYCLE. The adult female *Strongyloides* is about 2 mm long and lives in the mucosal epithelium of the duodenum and jejunum, extending above or below in the gastrointestinal tract in heavy infections. There is no parasitic male; reproduction in the parasitic phase is parthenogenic.

The life cycle of this parasite is complex and proceeds by several alternative pathways. Each worm produces fewer than 100 eggs daily. They hatch in the intestine of the host, and rhabditiform larvae are passed in the stool. These may metamorphose in the soil into infective filariform larvae or may mature into free-living adults that reproduce bisexually. They may then give rise to infective larvae in a later generation. The infective larvae invade the human host by penetrating the skin, travel through the venous circulation to the lungs, migrate through the alveolar capillary walls, ascend the respiratory tree to the epiglottis, and are swallowed to reach the small intestine where they mature.

Alternatively, *Strongyloides* larvae may develop to the infective stage in the intestine, penetrate the intestinal wall to reach the circulation, and enter the cycle of infection. This process of *internal autoinfection* is unique to this species among nematodes. Infective larvae may also penetrate the perianal skin after being passed with the stool to enter the host by *external autoinfection*. These processes may enable an infection to persist 30 to 40 years in the absence of re-exposure of the host.

In immunosuppressed or malnourished patients, internal autoinfection may assume massive proportions with ectopic migration of the larvae, resulting in the *hyperinfection syndrome*.

EPIDEMIOLOGY. *Strongyloides* is found in warm climates throughout the world, but, except in institutions for the retarded, high community prevalence rates have not been reported. In the United States, strongyloidiasis is most common in Southern Appalachia, but occasional autochthonous cases have been found in northern cities. Homosexual males may be at increased risk of harboring this parasite. There is at least one report of transmission from dog to man. *Strongyloides fulbornii*, a parasite of monkeys, has been reported to infect people in Africa.

PATHOLOGY. As the larvae migrate through the lungs, they sometimes cause a pneumonic process similar to Löffler's syndrome in ascariasis.

In the small intestine, microscopic abnormalities include stunted, swollen, or fused villi; eosinophilic infiltration of the lamina propria; and mononuclear infiltration of the mucosa.

In the hyperinfection syndrome and in other severe cases of strongyloidiasis, intestinal changes are more pronounced. Parasites may be found in all layers of the intestinal wall, which is thickened by edema and fibrosis. An inflammatory response is seen, but without eosinophilia, and there may be microscopic and macroscopic ulcerations. Pulmonary involvement in the hyperinfection syndrome is characterized by extensive larval migration and hemorrhagic pneumonia. Larvae may be found throughout the body, especially in the kidneys, brain, and heart.

CLINICAL MANIFESTATIONS. As the larvae penetrate the skin, particularly in cases of external autoinfection, they may cause a migratory pruritic eruption known as *larva currens*. Larvae migrating through the lung may cause pneumonia with cough, dyspnea, and hemoptysis, but this is not common. Infection may be accompanied by recurrent urticaria.

Mild intestinal infections are often asymptomatic. Moderate infections generally result in epigastric pain and intermittent diarrhea, whereas heavy infections may cause significant malabsorption with bulky, foul-smelling stools, abdominal distension, and hypoproteinemia with edema. In patients who are malnourished, malabsorption may persist even after the infection is adequately treated.

COMPLICATIONS. The hyperinfection syndrome occurs in hosts with altered immune status, in those with malignant disease or malnutrition, and rarely in those who are otherwise normal. The onset of symptoms in this complication is characteristically relatively abrupt, with fever and severe abdominal pain and distension, often accompanied by shock. Gram-negative sepsis frequently ensues; intestinal ulcerations caused by the parasite are thought to permit the entry of enteric pathogens into the circulation. When larval invasion of the lungs is severe, dyspnea and cough productive of blood-tinged sputum may be prominent.

DIAGNOSIS. *Strongyloides* ova do not appear in the stool; diagnosis is dependent on the identification of larvae. Multiple stool examinations, using concentration techniques, are generally necessary in light or moderate infections. Larvae may be identified in duodenal fluid when they cannot be found in stool specimens; the string test (Enterotest) is useful for obtaining samples of duodenal fluid for this purpose. In cases of hyperinfection, larvae may often be found in the sputum.

The ELISA test has a sensitivity of about 90 per cent. Eosinophilia is often present, but may be absent in cases of hyperinfection. Chest radiographs in patients with hyperinfection may show patchy infiltrates.

TREATMENT. The drug of choice, in both ordinary intestinal strongyloidiasis and hyperinfection, is thiabendazole, 25 mg per kilogram twice a day for two to five days. Nausea,

vomiting, drowsiness, and vertigo are common side effects. Other drugs that have been used include pyrvinium pamoate,* mebendazole, diethylcarbamazine,* and levamisole (not available in the United States). None of these drugs is recommended for pregnant women. A follow-up stool examination should be obtained two to six weeks following treatment, and stool examinations should also be obtained on other family members.

PREVENTION. This parasite, like the other soil-transmitted nematodes, is associated with rural poverty and its attendant conditions of poor sanitation and inadequate education. Alleviation of these conditions interrupts transmission. The wearing of shoes protects against infection.

Secondary prevention of the hyperinfection syndrome is important in persons from endemic areas who have altered immune status. Patients who exhibit suggestive gastrointestinal symptoms and/or eosinophilia should be studied for possible *Strongyloides* infection.

---

*Production of this drug has been discontinued in the United States.

Davidson RA, Fletcher RH, Chapman LE: Risk factors for strongyloidiasis—A case-control study. Arch Intern Med 144:321, 1984. *Identifies some interesting epidemiologic aspects of strongyloidiasis in the United States, including an increased relative risk among men, whites, and older patients.*
Igra-Siegman Y, Kapila R, Sen P, et al.: Syndrome of hyperinfection with *Strongyloides stercoralis*. Rev Infec Dis 3:397, 1981. *Reviews 103 cases of hyperinfection syndrome reported in the English language literature since 1964.*
Neva FA: Biology and immunology of human strongyloidiasis. J Infect Dis 153:397, 1986. *A lively review of the pathogenesis and immunologic features of this infection.*

404 HOOKWORM DISEASE

DEFINITION. Two species of hookworm infect man: *Ancylostoma duodenale*, the so-called Old World hookworm, and *Necator americanus*, the so-called New World hookworm. Both species attach themselves to the mucosa of the small intestine and ingest blood. When this results in anemia, hypoproteinemia, and clinical symptoms, the condition is termed hookworm disease. If these findings are lacking, the host is said merely to have hookworm infection.

ETIOLOGY AND LIFE CYCLE. Hookworms are about 1 cm long; the female is slightly larger than the male, and *Ancylostoma* is slightly larger than *Necator*. *Ancylostoma* bears two pairs of upper teeth in its mouth, whereas *Necator* has a pair of upper and a pair of lower cutting plates.

The female *Ancylostoma* produces about 25,000 eggs per day; *Necator*, about 7000. These eggs are passed in the stool of the host and hatch in the soil within 48 hours. The emerging rhabditiform larvae molt twice within five to ten days and become infective filariform larvae, which may survive for several months in the soil.

Upon coming in contact with the skin of man, the filariform larvae penetrate, enter the venous circulation, and are carried into the lungs. There they migrate across the alveolar capillary walls, ascend the respiratory tree, and are swallowed to reach the small intestine. Infection with *Ancylostoma* may also be acquired by ingesting the filariform larvae; *Necator* is not infective by this route. The life span of *Necator* in the human host is two to six years; that of *Ancylostoma* is probably less.

EPIDEMIOLOGY. *Necator americanus* was once endemic throughout the southeastern United States, where it caused considerable disability among the rural poor. Its prevalence was greatly reduced by the work of the Rockefeller Sanitary Commission from 1910 to 1920 and has continued to decline. *Necator* was originally imported to the New World from sub-Sahara Africa and has, in the past, been described as the predominant species in that part of the world, as well as in most of South and Central America. *Ancylostoma* was previously found exclusively in the Mediterranean basin, Asia, and parts of coastal South America. In more recent years, this distribution has become blurred.

In endemic areas, the highest prevalence is found in school-age children. During the time when hookworm was widespread in the southeastern United States, whites were more susceptible than blacks.

PATHOLOGY. A local inflammatory response occurs at the site of skin penetration by the filariform larvae, and as the larvae migrate through the lungs, an eosinophilic and mononuclear infiltration takes place along with local hemorrhages. A heavy passage of larvae through the lungs may cause a pneumonic process similar to Löffler's syndrome in ascariasis.

In the intestine, the adults attach themselves to the mucosa and actively suck blood. *Ancylostoma* ingests more blood (0.15 ml per worm per day) than *Necator* (0.03 ml per worm per day). The wall of the intestine becomes edematous, and a mononuclear and eosinophilic infiltrate surrounds each parasite.

CLINICAL MANIFESTATIONS AND COMPLICATIONS. Light infections, such as those generally found in the United States, are usually asymptomatic. In tropical countries, where worm burdens are often in the thousands, clinical manifestations of hookworm disease are frequent.

A pruritic vesicular or papular eruption, known as ground itch, may develop at the site of larval invasion. This is particularly pronounced after multiple exposures to the parasite. The passage of larvae through the lungs is sometimes associated with wheezing, dyspnea, and cough productive of blood-streaked sputum.

Abdominal pain and diarrhea may be caused by the adult worms in the intestine, particularly as the parasites attach themselves to the mucosa. The most important clinical manifestations, however, are those of anemia and hypoalbuminemia resulting from chronic blood loss. Weakness, fatigue, lassitude, and growth retardation are characteristic findings in patients with hookworm disease. Signs and symptoms of high-output congestive heart failure may be present, and peripheral edema may occur as a result of heart failure and hypoalbuminemia. The severity of anemia depends on the adequacy of dietary iron intake. Residents of communities endemic for hookworm often have inadequate diets and may be anemic independent of hookworm infection. On the other hand, an adequate diet may prevent anemia and hypoproteinemia despite significant infection.

DIAGNOSIS. The diagnosis of hookworm infection is made by finding characteristic ova in the stool. The ova of *Necator* and *Ancylostoma* are identical, but species differentiation is not necessary for appropriate treatment and follow-up.

Other laboratory findings include eosinophilia, Charcot-Leyden crystals in the stool, and, in heavy infections, hypoalbuminemia and anemia as low as 2 grams of hemoglobin per deciliter of blood.

TREATMENT. In holoendemic areas in the tropics, where resources are limited, it has generally been the practice to treat only moderate or heavy infections. In the United States, however, light infections should also be treated when discovered, and measures should be taken to prevent reinfection.

The drug of choice is pyrantel pamoate,* which is given in a single dose of 11 mg per kilogram of body weight (maximum, 1 gram). Mebendazole, 100 mg twice a day for three days, is equally effective. Neither drug should be used in pregnant women; mebendazole should be used with caution in children less than two years old. The anemia should be treated with oral iron supplementation; in cases of severe

anemia with hypoalbuminemia, transfusion may be necessary.

A follow-up stool examination should be performed two to six weeks after treatment; stool examination should also be performed on other family members.

PREVENTION. Hookworm, like the other soil-transmitted nematodes, is prevented by alleviating the conditions of rural poverty with which it is associated. The most important factors in this regard are the construction of sanitary facilities for the disposal of human wastes and community education regarding the etiology of the infection. The wearing of shoes is also important. Iron supplementation of the diet in endemic areas will prevent most cases of anemia.

Gilles HM: Selective primary health care: Strategies for control in the developing world: XVII. Hookworm infection and anemia. Rev Infect Dis 7:111, 1985. *A thorough review that focuses attention on appropriate approaches to this problem in developing countries.*
Gillman RH: Hookworm disease: Host-pathogen biology. Rev Infect Dis 4:824, 1982. *A concise review of the topic.*

405 CUTANEOUS LARVA MIGRANS

DEFINITION. Cutaneous larva migrans (creeping eruption) is infection with a larval nematode that wanders in the subcutaneous tissues. The most common agent is *Ancylostoma braziliense*, a hookworm of dogs and cats.

ETIOLOGY AND EPIDEMIOLOGY. In addition to *A. braziliense*, the larvae of several other nematodes can cause cutaneous larva migrans. These include *Ancylostoma caninum* (a dog hookworm) and several other species of hookworm and *Strongyloides* that ordinarily infect nonhuman hosts. The larvae of these species penetrate human skin if it is exposed to soil contaminated with the feces of infected animals. Rather than complete their life cycle, however, the larvae continue to migrate in the subcutaneous tissues.

The infection is most common in tropical and subtropical areas, particularly on beaches frequented by dogs. The coasts of the gulf of Mexico and Florida are common locales in the United States. Children, farmers, plumbers (working under beach houses), and sunbathers are most often affected.

The larvae of *A. braziliense* tunnel in the epidermis just above the basal layer, rarely penetrating into the dermis. The tunnel is surrounded by eosinophil and round cell infiltration.

CLINICAL MANIFESTATIONS. An erythematous pruritic papule or nonspecific dermatitis occurs at the site of skin contact. In two or three days (occasionally weeks or months), this becomes a slightly elevated, serpiginous track or burrow 2 to 3 mm wide. The patient experiences intense itching.

DIAGNOSIS AND TREATMENT. The diagnosis is clinical. There are no diagnostic tests and usually no eosinophilia.

Topical application, four times a day, of the commercially available 10 per cent suspension of thiabendazole* appears to work as well as giving the drug orally. If the oral route is elected, the dosage is 25 mg per kilogram in two divided doses for two to five days.

*This form is not listed in the manufacturer's directive.

Edelglass JW, Douglass CM, Stiefler R, et al.: Cutaneous larva migrans in northern climates. A souvenir of your dream vacation. J Am Acad Dermatol 7:353, 1982. *A good review with typical case presentations in United States tourists. The literature on topical and oral therapy is discussed.*

---

*Considered investigational for this use by the FDA.

406 ASCARIASIS

DEFINITION. Ascariasis is infection with the large round-worm *Ascaris lumbricoides*. Clinical manifestations may result from the migration of larvae through the lungs, from the presence of adult worms in the lumen of the small intestine, or from extraintestinal migration of the adults.

ETIOLOGY AND LIFE CYCLE. *Ascaris* is the largest of the intestinal nematodes. Adult females measure 20 to 45 cm in length; adult males are about three fourths as large. Worm loads in the intestine may range from only one or two to hundreds; the life span of the parasite averages about 18 months.

The female produces about 200,000 ova per day. These are passed by the host in the stool and become infective after an obligate period in the soil of about ten days. The eggs are killed by direct sunlight and temperatures above 45° C, but under proper soil and climatic conditions they may remain viable for years.

After ingestion by the host, the eggs hatch in the duodenum, and the larvae penetrate the intestinal wall, enter the venous circulation, and are carried to the lungs, where they migrate across alveolar capillary walls. They then travel up the respiratory tree to the epiglottis and are swallowed, returning to the small intestine, where they mature. The worms begin producing eggs in about two months.

EPIDEMIOLOGY. It is estimated that a quarter of the world's population is infected with *Ascaris*. The parasite occurs throughout the world but is most common in warm climates. In the United States, ascariasis is common in many rural parts of the southeast. The prevalence of the infection is greatest in children 1 to 13 years of age.

PATHOLOGY. As the larvae pass through the lungs, they may cause an eosinophilic pneumonitis known as *Löffler's syndrome*. The pathologic process appears to be a combination of physical damage to the alveoli caused by the migrating larvae and exudative interstitial pneumonia.

The adult worms in the small intestine do not invade the mucosa, but maintain their position by bridging across the lumen. Nonetheless, they may cause mucosal damage. Microscopically, this damage is seen as broadening and shortening of villi, elongation of crypts, and round-cell infiltration of the lamina propria. Mucosal disaccharidase deficiency has been described.

The adult worms may migrate to extraintestinal sites in response to drug administration, intercurrent illness in the host, or unknown causes, and in so doing may cause considerable damage.

CLINICAL MANIFESTATIONS AND COMPLICATIONS. The *Ascaris* pneumonia caused by the migration of the larvae through the lungs is characterized by cough, fever, and malaise and, in severe cases, by chest pain, dyspnea, and hemoptysis. Patchy pulmonary infiltrates are seen on chest x-ray examination.

Various nonspecific gastrointestinal symptoms have been described in association with worms in the intestine. These include abdominal pain, diarrhea, vomiting, irritability, and anorexia.

Malnutrition in children has been associated with ascariasis, but the amount of malnutrition caused by infection is controversial. Lowered serum vitamins A and C and protein values have been reported in infected children. Improvement in growth rates have also been reported following de-worming. The nutritional effects of ascariasis seem to stem more from malabsorption of fats, protein, and carbohydrate caused by mucosal damage than from ingestion of host nutrients by the parasite.

Serious and life-threatening complications of ascariasis include intestinal obstruction by a bolus of worms, intussusception, volvulus, appendicitis, intestinal perforation, hepatic abscess, aspiration of a worm, cholangitis secondary to bile duct obstruction, and pancreatitis secondary to pancreatic duct obstruction. Of these, intestinal obstruction is the most common; it occurs particularly in children under age six.

DIAGNOSIS. Infection is diagnosed by the finding of ova on microscopic examination of the stool. Often the patient will describe a typical worm passed in the stool; in endemic areas, this is sufficient evidence of ascariasis to warrant treatment. Eosinophilia is an inconstant feature of intestinal ascariasis.

Ascaris pneumonia is not associated with eggs in the stool unless adult worms are simultaneously present in the host intestine. A marked peripheral eosinophilia provides evidence for the etiology of the pneumonia, but may not be present until late in the course of the illness. Larvae may sometimes be identified in the sputum.

TREATMENT. Pyrantel pamoate is the drug of choice; it is administered in a single dose of 11 mg per kilogram (maximal dose, 1 gram). Mebendazole is equally effective and is particularly useful in mixed *Ascaris-Trichuris* infections; the dosage is 100 mg twice a day for three days. It should be used with caution in children less than two years old. Piperazine citrate, in a dosage of 75 mg per kilogram daily for two days (maximal daily dose, 3.5 grams), is another effective drug; it is contraindicated in persons with seizure disorders or impaired renal or hepatic function. Levamisole is also effective, but is not available in the United States.

Because the goal in treatment of ascariasis is complete elimination of the parasite, a follow-up stool examination should always be obtained two to six weeks after treatment. Stool examinations should also be performed on other members of the patient's household.

No specific treatment is available for *Ascaris* pneumonia. Oxygen and steroids may be indicated in severe cases.

Intestinal obstruction caused by ascariasis should be treated conservatively with nasogastric suction, intravenous fluids, and the instillation of an anthelmintic via the nasogastric tube. Surgery is indicated only in the event of failure of medical management.

PREVENTION. *Ascaris*, like the other soil-transmitted nematodes, is a marker of rural poverty in areas of suitable soil and climatic conditions. Primary prevention is largely dependent on the alleviation of poverty with its accompanying inadequate levels of education and sanitation.

Secondary prevention is possible through the periodic mass treatment of all children or all persons in an endemic community. Such a program may result in the near-eradication of the infection, but in the absence of improved hygiene and education, it is likely that the parasite will eventually become reestablished.

Arfaa F: Selective primary health care: Strategies for control of disease in the developing world: XII. Ascaris and trichuriasis. Rev Infect Dis 6:364, 1984. *Reviews the basics and discusses approaches to control in the Third World.*
Pawlowski ZS: Ascariasis: Host-pathogen biology. Rev Infect Dis 4:806, 1982.
Schultz MG: Ascariasis: Nutritional implications. Rev Infect Dis 4:815, 1982. *Two companion papers that together constitute a comprehensive review of the topic.*
Stephenson, LS: The contribution of *Ascaris lumbricoides* to malnutrition in children. Parasitology 81:221, 1980. *Argues that ascariasis negatively affects growth in children and that mass treatment of children should be undertaken in endemic areas.*

407 TOXOCARIASIS

DEFINITION. Toxocariasis is infection with larvae of the dog ascarid, *Toxocara canis*, or less often, the cat ascarid, *Toxocara cati*. The larvae do not complete their life cycle in humans, but migrate through the body, invading various organs, and producing a syndrome known as *visceral larva migrans*. When the eye is involved, other organs are usually spared; this is known as *ocular larva migrans*. The raccoon ascarid, *Baylisascaris procyonis*, has been reported to cause a particularly severe form of visceral larva migrans.

ETIOLOGY. Humans become infected by ingesting soil contaminated with the feces of infected dogs or cats. Swallowed ova hatch in the small intestine, and the larvae penetrate the intestinal wall to enter the circulation. When they reach a blood vessel with a diameter smaller than their own, they bore into the surrounding tissue. Larvae have been found in the liver, lungs, heart, and brain, as well as the eye.

EPIDEMIOLOGY. Toxocariasis is predominantly a childhood infection; fewer than 20 per cent of cases occur in adults. Visceral larva migrans tends to occur in younger children, whereas the ocular form of the infection tends to occur in older children. When both syndromes coexist, however, the patient is usually very young (under five years of age). Most cases are reported from the southern states. There is a strong association with the presence of a dog (especially a puppy) in the household. Serosurveys in the United States demonstrate a prevalence of antibodies to *Toxocara* of 15 to 25 per cent in black children age 1 to 11; white children have a prevalence of 4 to 5 per cent. This suggests that the vast majority of infections are asymptomatic.

PATHOLOGY. Migrating larvae leave tracks of hemorrhage, necrosis, and inflammatory cells. Eosinophilic granulomas or abscesses remain at the site of destruction of larvae; other larvae are walled off and may resume their migration up to years later.

CLINICAL MANIFESTATIONS. Common symptoms of visceral larva migrans are fever, coughing, wheezing, malaise, and weight loss. Physical findings commonly include wheezes, rales, and hepatosplenomegaly. Occasionally the central nervous system is involved, resulting in seizures or behavior disturbances. The white count may be greatly elevated (30,000 to 100,000) with 50 to 90 per cent eosinophils. Serum IgG, IgM, and IgE are usually elevated, as are isohemagglutinins.

In ocular larva migrans, the presentation may be one of visual loss, strabismus, or less often, eye pain. Funduscopic findings may range from a retinal granuloma to severe exudative endophthalmitis with retinal detachment. The condition often mimics retinoblastoma and must be distinguished by serologic testing to avoid needless enucleation.

DIAGNOSIS. Visceral larva migrans should be considered in any child with persistent eosinophilia, especially if there is a history of pica and/or a household dog. Diagnosis may be confirmed by enzyme-linked immunosorbent assay (ELISA).

TREATMENT AND PREVENTION. Most cases of visceral larva migrans are mild and self-limited, and no treatment is indicated. In severe cases, thiabendazole in a dose of 25 mg per kilogram twice a day for five days may be given, although its benefits remain controversial. Corticosteroids should also be given in severe cases to alleviate symptoms and to limit eye damage in ocular larva migrans.

Household dogs should be examined by a veterinarian for intestinal nematodes and treated as necessary. Leash laws and control of stray dogs may reduce fecal contamination of public parks and playgrounds.

Glockman LT, Schantz PM: Epidemiology and pathogenesis of zoonotic toxocariasis. Epidemiol Rev 3:230, 1981. *An extensive review with emphasis on the seroepidemiology of toxocariasis.*

408 TRICHURIASIS

DEFINITION. Trichuriasis is infection with the whipworm *Trichuris trichiura*. Clinical manifestations are caused by parasites in the cecum and large intestine; migration of larvae or adults elsewhere in the body has not been reported.

ETIOLOGY AND LIFE CYCLE. Both male and female adult *Trichuris* are about 30 to 50 mm long and have an elongated whiplike anterior portion that is embedded in the submucosa of the host's colon. The female produces 5000 to 10,000 eggs per day; these are passed in the stool and must incubate in the soil for at least three weeks. Embryonated eggs can survive in the soil for years.

Upon ingestion, the ova hatch in the small intestine, and the larvae proceed to the cecum and colon, where they mature. Egg production begins in two to three months. Adult worms survive for three to ten years in the host. Worm loads may number in the thousands.

EPIDEMIOLOGY. Trichuris is found in warm climates throughout the world. In the United States, it is estimated that 2.2 million persons are infected; over 40 per cent of children and adolescents in some rural communities in the southeastern United States harbor the parasite. Soil and climatic requirements for this parasite are similar to those for *Ascaris*, and infections with both worms often coexist in the same host.

PATHOLOGY. Pathologic findings are limited to the large intestine. Light infections cause little tissue reaction. Heavier infections cause edema and hyperemia of the mucosa; microscopically, there is a plasma cell, eosinophil, and polymorphonuclear infiltrate.

CLINICAL MANIFESTATIONS AND COMPLICATIONS. Light infections are often asymptomatic. Heavy infections are accompanied by abdominal pain and diarrhea, which may be severe and prolonged. Since the infection is limited to the large intestine, however, true malabsorption does not occur.

Rectal prolapse is a complication of heavy infection. Worms have also been reported to obstruct the appendix and cause acute appendicitis. The question whether trichuriasis causes intestinal bleeding is unresolved. Two studies using similar techniques have reached differing conclusions.

DIAGNOSIS. Characteristic eggs may be found on direct fecal smear. In light infections, stool concentration techniques are helpful in making the diagnosis.

Worms may be observed directly on proctosigmoidoscopy. An eosinophilia frequently accompanies infection.

TREATMENT. The drug of choice is mebendazole, 100 mg twice a day for three days regardless of body weight; even light asymptomatic infections may be treated. However, mebendazole should be used with caution in children under two years, and it should not be given to pregnant women. Oxantel is also effective; it is not available in the United States. A follow-up stool examination should be performed following treatment, and stool examinations should be obtained on other family members.

Reduction of rectal prolapse may be accomplished with a tissue paper–covered finger; the tissue paper, which facilitates withdrawal of the finger, remains in the rectum and is later expelled. The buttocks may be taped together for a day or two after the prolapse is reduced.

PREVENTION. As with the other soil-transmitted nematodes, this parasite is associated with rural poverty. The provision of sanitary means for the disposal of human feces, combined with community education regarding the transmission of worms, is essential in prevention.

Arfaa F: Selective primary health care: Strategies for control of disease in the developing world: XII. Ascaris and trichuriasis. Rev Infect Dis 6:364, 1984. *Discusses current thinking on approaches to the control of trichuriasis (and ascariasis) in developing countries.*

Chanco PP, Vidad JY: A review of trichuriasis, its incidence, pathogenicity and treatment. Drugs 15 (Suppl. 1):87, 1978. *A historical review.*

Greenberg ER, Cline BL: Is trichuriasis associated with iron-deficiency anemia? Am J Trop Med Hyg 284:770, 1979. *A slight reduction in hemoglobin levels was found in* Trichuris-*infected children compared to controls. Reviews the articles relevant to the controversy concerning trichuriasis and gastrointestinal blood loss.*

409 ENTEROBIASIS

DEFINITION. Enterobiasis is infection with the pinworm *Enterobius (Oxyuris) vermicularis*. This is a generally benign, although often symptomatic, parasitosis.

ETIOLOGY AND LIFE CYCLE. The adult female pinworm is about 1 cm long, the male, one fourth to one third as large. The parasites inhabit the cecum and colon. Gravid females emerge from the anus while the host sleeps, each female depositing several thousand eggs on the perianal skin. These are transmitted by person-to-person contact via the host's hands. Alternatively, they may be transmitted by bedclothes or become airborne. They remain viable in the environment only a few days. Swallowed eggs release larvae in the small intestine; these pass directly to the colon, where they mature.

EPIDEMIOLOGY. Pinworms are common throughout the world, in urban as well as rural populations and in the affluent as well as the poor. They are particularly common in group living situations, and their prevalence in institutions for the mentally retarded often exceeds 50 per cent. Adults are affected less often than children.

PATHOLOGY. The parasites in the intestine provoke little or no inflammatory response. Worms sometimes migrate into the appendix or fallopian tubes or escape into the peritoneum or elsewhere in the body, where they cause an inflammatory or granulomatous reaction.

CLINICAL MANIFESTATIONS. Many infections—perhaps the majority—are asymptomatic. The characteristic manifestation of symptomatic infections is pruritus ani caused by the deposited ova. This itch may result in restlessness or insomnia.

Nocturnal enuresis has been attributed to enterobiasis, and there are documented cases of bedwetting that resolved promptly upon treatment of concurrent pinworm infection. Most cases of enuresis are not associated with enterobiasis, however.

Numerous other symptoms in children have been attributed to this parasitosis, but no cause-and-effect relationship has been demonstrated. These include tooth-grinding, nose-picking, sleeping in the knee-chest position, anorexia, and abdominal pain.

COMPLICATIONS. Perianal scratching may result in excoriations or impetigo. Young girls may suffer bouts of cystitis or vaginitis caused by pinworms which enter the urethra or vagina during their nocturnal wanderings, carrying enteric bacteria. Thus, it is worthwhile to perform cellophane tape tests on girls with urinary tract infections. Pinworms have also been found in inflamed appendices. Rare manifestations of migrating pinworms include salpingitis, pelvic granulomas, and intestinal perforation. Syndromes resembling regional enteritis or carcinoma have been reported as resulting from enterobiasis.

DIAGNOSIS. Pinworm ova are usually not found in the stool but may be identified with a cellophane tape test. This test is performed by pressing the gummed side of a piece of cellophane tape to the perianal area, and then sticking the tape to a glass slide. The preparation is then examined microscopically for ova. At least three tests, performed on three different mornings before bathing, are necessary to attain a sensitivity of 90 per cent. On occasion, the worms may be seen if the suspected host's perianal area is inspected during sleep.

TREATMENT. A single-dose treatment with any of three drugs is effective in enterobiasis: pyrantel pamoate, 11 mg per kilogram (maximum, 1 gram); pyrvinium pamoate,* 5 mg per kilogram (maximum, 350 mg); or mebendazole, 100 mg regardless of body weight. Patients should be warned that pyrvinium stains stools red. Mebendazole should be used with caution in children less than two years of age; none of these drugs should be given to pregnant women.

Treatment should be repeated in two weeks. Since this parasite is readily transmitted from person to person, it is best to treat the entire household in which a single case is identified. Treatment should be accompanied by the washing of bedclothes, but further environmental measures, such as the scrubbing of floors and toilet seats, should be discouraged. Parents should be reassured about the relative harmlessness of this infection.

PREVENTION. Residents of institutions should be examined periodically for this and other intestinal parasitoses. However, no effective measures for preventing enterobiasis in the general population have been described.

---

*Production of this drug has been discontinued in the United States.

Sachdev YV, Howards SS: *Enterobius vermicularis* infestation and secondary enuresis. J Urol 113:143, 1975. *Describes several cases of nocturnal enuresis that resolved after treatment of pinworm infections.*

Kropp KA, Cichocki GA, Bansal NK: *Enterobius vermicularis* (pinworms), introital bacteriology and recurrent urinary tract infection in children. J Urol 120:480, 1978. Simon RD: Pinworm infestation and urinary tract infection in young girls. Am J Dis Child 128:21, 1974. *Two papers that provide evidence that pinworms play a role in causing urinary tract infections in girls.*

410 OTHER ANIMAL NEMATODIASES

Man may serve as a paratenic host for a number of nematodes that ordinarily parasitize the intestine of other species.

Several species of the genus *Trichostrongylus* infect both man and domestic ruminants. The infection is found widely in the Middle and Far East and Australia. The prevalence reported from Iran has been particularly high.

Ova are passed in the stool and hatch in the soil; larvae are ingested with leafy vegetables. The adult worms live in the intestines and suck small amounts of blood; heavy infections result in anemia. Diagnosis is made by identifying ova, which resemble those of hookworm, in the stool.

Treatment is with thiabendazole, 25 mg per kilogram twice a day for two days, or with pyrantel pamoate in a single dose of 11 mg per kilogram.

Anisakis sp. is an intestinal nematode of marine mammals. Several species of fish, including herring, serve as intermediate hosts, and human infection may be acquired when raw fish is eaten. The larvae of both *Anisakis* and *Phocanema decipiens* have been implicated. Most cases have occurred in Japan or western Europe, particularly Scandinavia and the Netherlands. Fewer than 35 cases have been reported from the Western Hemisphere.

The larvae invade the wall of the small intestine or stomach, causing pain and, rarely, intestinal obstruction or perforation. Gastric anisakiasis can be diagnosed endoscopically and treated by removal of the worms. Intestinal anisakiasis often resembles an acute abdomen leading to laparotomy. Thiabendazole, 25 mg per kilogram twice a day for three days, may be given if surgical intervention is not required. The disease may be prevented by cooking or freezing fish prior to eating.

Capillaria philippinensis infection has been reported from the Philippines and Thailand. At least 1500 cases have been reported, with a case-fatality rate of about 10 per cent. This nematode is thought to parasitize birds, with fish and crustaceans serving as intermediate hosts. Humans are infected by eating the raw intermediate hosts. The ingested larvae mature and live in the crypts of the small intestine, where they reproduce. (*Strongyloides* is the only other nematode that reproduces in man.) The result is often a heavy infection; up to 40,000 adult worms have been recovered at one autopsy. The clinical syndrome is one of severe malabsorption and protein-losing enteropathy. The diagnosis is made by finding eggs or larvae in the stool; an intradermal test is also available. The treatment of choice is mebendazole, 200 mg twice a day for 20 days; an alternative is thiabendazole, 25 mg per kilogram daily for 30 days. Fluid and electrolyte replacement and a high protein diet are also important.

Capillaria hepatica is a parasite of rats that occasionally infects the liver of man. The result is an acute or subacute hepatitis with eosinophilia. Diagnosis is made on liver biopsy; there is no known treatment.

Gnathostoma spinigerum is an intestinal nematode of dogs and cats for which fish serve as an intermediate host. Infective larvae are ingested by humans when raw or undercooked fish is consumed. The larvae do not complete their life cycle in humans but migrate through the body.

The infection is found throughout the Far East; the greatest number of cases has been reported from Thailand. Cases have also been reported from South America.

The larvae most often migrate to the subcutaneous tissues, where they are found in eosinophilic granulomas. In central nervous system gnathostomiasis, hemorrhagic tracks may be found in the brain. Fever, vomiting, and abdominal pain occur a few days after ingestion of the infective fish. A few weeks later, skin lesions appear; these consist of subcutaneous nodules or swellings that may be either pruritic or painful and are often migratory. Abscesses may form. In the CNS variety, there is paralysis of the extremities, encephalitis, and subarachnoid hemorrhage. Eye involvement with uveitis and orbital cellulitis represents a third variety. Gnathostome larvae have also been reported in many other parts of the body.

Peripheral eosinophilia is usual in cutaneous gnathostomiasis; the diagnosis is usually established by biopsy. In central nervous system infection, peripheral eosinophilia is an inconstant feature, but there are many eosinophils in the cerebrospinal fluid. This must be distinguished from the eosinophilic meningitis caused by *Angiostrongylus*, which is usually less severe. Diagnosis may be assisted by an enzyme-linked immunosorbent assay (ELISA). Treatment of subcutaneous lesions consists of surgical removal. For central nervous system infection, mebendazole* 200 mg every three hours for six days may be given. The infection may be prevented by cooking fish thoroughly before eating.

Several nematodes that ordinarily parasitize the intestine of monkeys occasionally infect man. *Oesophagostomum* sp. has been reported from Africa, Asia, and Brazil; it is responsible for the formation of granulomas in the intestinal wall. *Ternides deminutus* is sometimes found in the human colon in Africa and Asia; a heavy infection may cause anemia. *Physaloptera mordens*, also reported from Africa, may attach itself to the esophagus, stomach, or small intestine of humans.

The definitive host of *Lagochilascaris minor* is unknown. About 30 human cases have been reported from Central and South America, usually with worms invading the soft tissues of the neck and throat and sinuses.

Barrowclough H, Crome L: Oesophagostomiasis in man. Trop Geogr Med 31:183, 1979. *Presents a case, discusses the difficulties in diagnosis, and reviews the literature.*
Botero D, Little MD: Two cases of human *Lagochilascaris* infection in Colombia. Am J Trop Med Hyg 33:381, 1984. *Includes a review of the literature on this unusual parasite.*
Boogird P, Phuapradit P, Siridej N, et al.: Neurological manifestations of gnathostomiasis. J Neurol Sci 31:279, 1977. *A clinical and epidemiologic description of a series of 24 cases of CNS gnathostomiasis.*
Daengsvang S: Gnathostomiasis in Southeast Asia. Southeast Asian J Trop Med Public Health 12:319, 1981. *A review of the literature on both human and animal gnathostomiasis.*
Smith JW, Wootten R: Anisakis and anisakiasis. Adv Parasitol 16:93, 1978. *An exceptionally complete review.*

Tissue Nematodes

411 TRICHINELLOSIS (Trichinosis)

Donald W. Hoskins

DEFINITION AND ETIOLOGY. Trichinellosis is an intestinal and tissue nematode disease resulting from the ingestion of inadequately cooked meat containing larvae of *Trichinella spiralis*. The chief sources are pork, pork products, and bear or walrus meat. The enteral phase of the infection is largely unnoticed. Diffuse tissue invasion by *Trichinella* larvae, the result of the intestinal union of the adult worms, produces the trichinellotic syndrome of muscle pain and tenderness, fever, periorbital edema, and petechiae. The severity of an infection is directly related to the number and strain of *T. spiralis* larvae ingested, the duration of larval production, and poorly defined host factors.

The ingested larvae, resistant to acid-pepsin digestion, penetrate the villi of the small intestine, molt, and develop into mature adults within 48 hours. After fertilization, the gravid female burrows deep into the mucosa, discharging larvae (500 to 1500 per female) beginning 5 to 46 days after infection and continuing for 2 to 4 weeks or occasionally longer. Widely disseminated via lymphatics and the bloodstream, *Trichinella* larvae (0.1 mm) enter most organs, but persist only in individual skeletal muscle fibers. Increasing almost ten-fold in size (to 1.0 mm) over succeeding weeks, larvae gradually become surrounded by a cyst wall of muscle origin. Although the capsules calcify within six months to two years, the larvae within remain viable for months to years, rarely for decades.

The adult worms are usually expelled from the intestinal tract after the third or fourth week of infection, the result of immunologic mechanisms, including mast cell degranulation and B and T lymphocyte activity.

The definitive hosts of this infection include numerous carnivorous and omnivorous mammals, although the hog remains the single most important source of human infection.

EPIDEMIOLOGY. Approximately 28 million people worldwide are infected with this parasite, close to 75 per cent of whom reside in the United States. The disease is most prevalent in the temperate zones. Most infections are mild and go unrecognized or misdiagnosed. At present, approximately 100 cases are reported annually in the United States; this represents a significant decrease (except for occasional outbreaks—Louisiana, 44 cases 1979–80) from earlier decades. From 1940 to 1970, autopsy studies of human diaphragm

---

*This use and dosage are not listed in the manufacturer's directive.

revealed a drop in the incidence (16.1 to 4.2 per cent) and severity of infection. The current infection rate is 1.6 to 2.2 per cent. This decline is largely attributable to laws prohibiting the feeding of raw garbage to swine.

Pork and pork products, especially sausage, account for 75 per cent of all human *Trichinella* infection; nonpork products account for 13 per cent, and in 12 per cent the source is undetermined. Ground beef contaminated by pork (e.g., in the meatgrinder) is a common source of nonpork-induced disease. Bear and walrus meat account for less than 6 per cent of the reported cases of trichinellosis in this country.

PATHOLOGY AND PATHOGENESIS. Microscopic ulceration, mucosal hyperemia, localized edema, punctate hemorrhages, and intestinal inflammation may result from the penetration of the adult *Trichinella* into the mucosa of the small intestine.

The larvae produce basophilic granular alteration of muscle fibers within 48 hours of invasion. The fibers enlarge, and edema, nuclear proliferation, and interstitial inflammation ensue. Later, fatty metamorphosis is followed by atrophy and fibrosis. Larvae may produce a severe myocarditis with focal necrosis and eosinophilic infiltration, but encystment does not occur in cardiac muscle. Eosinophilic infiltration of the endocardium with fibrosis has been reported in fatal trichinellosis. Nonpurulent encephalomeningitis with larvae in the cerebrospinal fluid, choroid, and retina may also occur.

CLINICAL MANIFESTATIONS. The vast majority of persons infected with *T. spiralis* exhibit few or no symptoms. Less than 12 per cent have gastrointestinal symptoms. Heavy infection may produce acute enteritis (abdominal discomfort, diarrhea) one to two days following ingestion, with systemic symptoms beginning five to seven days later. The usual incubation period is 7 to 14 days, extending to 3 weeks or more in mild infections.

The onset of the trichinellotic syndrome is often acute with fever, muscle pain and tenderness, weakness, malaise, bilateral periorbital edema, and headache. Subungual, retinal, and subconjunctival petechiae and hemorrhage may be present, and a macular, petechial, or urticarial rash is not uncommon. Within the first two weeks of severe systemic disease, allergic phenomena such as edema, pneumonitis, and pleural transudate may occur.

Serious complications, including myocarditis, pneumonitis, and meningoencephalitis, occur most often in the third to ninth week of the disease. Mortality is less than 1.5 per cent and is almost always related to complications.

DIAGNOSIS AND DIFFERENTIAL DIAGNOSIS. Once considered, the diagnosis is not difficult. The trichinellotic syndrome coupled with marked peripheral blood eosinophilia (20 to 70 per cent), increase of muscle enzymes in serum (CPK, LDH, aldolase, and transaminases), and normal sedimentation rate should strongly suggest the diagnosis. Finding encysted larvae in any remaining suspected food source would be additional evidence.

Confirmation of the diagnosis is often accomplished by serologic testing, skin test, or muscle biopsy. Serologic testing is simple, highly sensitive, and specific. Antibodies are not detected, however, until three weeks or more after the onset of infection. Available tests include rapid screening counterimmunoelectrophoresis (CIE) and enzyme-linked immunosorbent assay (ELISA), passive hemagglutination (PHA), and indirect immunofluorescence (IF). The bentonite flocculation test is the most widely used; a titer of one to five or greater is considered positive, although a four-fold rise in the titer is more convincing. False positives do occur; 13.5 per cent of typhoid-paratyphoid sera may react positively. Two independent methods are often required to establish serodiagnosis of trichinellosis. Skin testing does not distinguish between past and present infection and therefore does not prove active disease.

Muscle biopsy may be positive as early as the second week of infection but is often not required. A small amount of muscle is excised under local anesthesia from a tender, painful, swollen muscle; a portion is sent for routine pathologic examination; and a small amount is crushed between glass slides and examined directly under a scanning or low power objective for motile larvae. Pepsin–hydrochloric acid digestion of 1.0 gram of muscle may also be performed and larvae sought microscopically.

The differential diagnosis in a disease with multisystem involvement is extensive. Common misdiagnoses include viral syndromes (influenza, gastroenteritis, various exanthems), connective tissue disease (periarteritis, dermatomyositis, sepsis (typhoid, pneumonitis, meningitis), allergic phenomena, and polymyositis.

TREATMENT. Rarely, infection with *T. spiralis* is suspected within hours or days of ingestion of infected meat. Treatment of the immature worms in the small intestine is usually successful and will abort or markedly inhibit systemic disease. Furthermore, given the relationship of the severity of infection to continued larval production by the adult female *T. spiralis* and the unknown duration of its fecundity, treatment of the intestinal phase in all cases up to six weeks after infection is advisable. Thiabendazole (Minetezol) 25 mg per kilogram twice daily (maximum 3.0 grams per day) for one week has been replaced by another benzimidazole, mebendazole (Vermox) 200 mg daily for four days, largely because of improved patient tolerance and increasing experimental evidence (in rodents) of a significant effect on migrating and encysted larvae. Alternatively, pyrantel pamoate (Antiminth) 10 mg per kilogram (maximum 1.0 gram per day) for four days has been used with similar results on the enteral phase. Should a hypersensitivity reaction (Jarisch-Herxheimer) occur on day three or four of benzimidazole treatment, corticosteroids may have to be given and/or the drug stopped. Although none of these drugs is advocated during pregnancy, mebendazole is specifically contraindicated.

Mild to moderate systemic infection is treated with rest and analgesics; recovery may take weeks and complications are rare. All patients must be carefully observed, especially in the first two weeks following onset of systemic symptoms, for progression to a more acute and severe form of trichinellosis.

Acute severe trichinellosis will require corticosteroids in high doses (prednisone, 60 mg daily) for two or more weeks, primarily for inhibition of host response. Since the enteral phase of *T. spiralis* may be prolonged (and larval production extended) with the use of corticosteroids, the concomitant administration of a benzimidazole (mebendazole, 5 mg per kilogram daily for five to ten days) is advisable. Adverse effects of the benzimidazoles include headache, nausea, vomiting, dizziness, rash, and agitation.

PREVENTION. Thorough cooking of infected meat kills larvae; a temperature of 58.3°C throughout the meat is adequate. Freezing meat at −32°C for 24 hours or at −15°C (home freezer) for three weeks is also effective. Government inspection of meat in the United States does not exclude *Trichinella* infection, nor does the smoking, salting, or drying of meat.

The application of an enzyme-linked immunosorbent assay (ELISA) for the detection of antibody to *T. spiralis* in pooled hog sera at slaughter may be practical in the detection of infected sources.

Campbell WC (ed.): *Trichinella* and Trichinosis. New York, Plenum Press, 1983. *An expensive but highly valuable update on all aspects of parasite and pathogen. The practicing physician will especially appreciate the chapters on chemotherapy, clinical aspects, and immunodiagnosis. Extensively referenced work.*

McCracken RO, Taylor DD: Mebendazole therapy of parenteral trichinellosis. Science 207:1220, 1980. *Experimental evidence in mice of the high degree of effectiveness of mebendazole on the enteral phase and the significant reduction in muscle larvae possible with treatment.*

Most H: Current concepts in parasitology. Trichinosis—preventable yet still with us. N Engl J Med 298:1178, 1978.

412 ANGIOSTRONGYLIASIS
Daniel S. Blumenthal

The larvae of two rodent parasites, *Angiostrongylus cantonensis* and *A. costaricensis*, may infect man. The pathology and clinical findings caused by the two species are quite different. The genus is also known as *Morerastrongylus*.

ANGIOSTRONGYLUS CANTONENSIS. Eosinophilic meningitis caused by larvae of the rat lungworm occurs in southeast Asia and many Pacific islands. The first cases in the Western Hemisphere were reported in 1981 from Cuba.

Humans are infected by ingesting, in an uncooked state, the snails, slugs, and crustaceans that serve as intermediate hosts. The infective larvae migrate to the capillaries of the meninges, where they cause an eosinophilic inflammatory response with granuloma formation. Sometimes the eye, brain, or spinal cord is invaded. Clinically there are signs of meningeal irritation, and there may be localizing neurologic findings, including paresthesias and cranial nerve palsies. There is peripheral and cerebrospinal fluid eosinophilia. The eosinophilic meningitis of angiostrongyliasis must be differentiated from that caused by gnathostomiasis, cysticercosis, and other parasitoses. Most cases resolve uneventfully, but some result in permanent sequelae or death. The diagnosis may be confirmed by ELISA. Brain lesions may be seen on CT. Thiabendazole has been given for this infection, but there is no convincing evidence that it is effective. Steroids may control symptoms.

ANGIOSTRONGYLUS COSTARICENSIS. Human larval infection with this species has been reported in children in Central America, Mexico, and Venezuela. Adult *A. costaricensis* live in the mesenteric arteries of rats and other rodents; a slug serves as intermediate host. Larvae are shed in the slime of the slug, and children may become infected by handling slugs and then putting their hands in their mouths. Vegetables on which slugs have crawled may also be infective. Once ingested, the larvae travel to the mesenteric arterioles, where they cause edema of the wall of the cecum, appendix, and ascending colon. Yellow granulations of the subserosa and eosinophilic infiltrates are common pathologic findings. There may be ulcerations, peritonitis, and fistula formation. The clinical picture is similar to that of acute appendicitis, with fever and right lower quadrant pain and tenderness. A tumor-like mass may often be palpated in the right lower quadrant. There is usually marked eosinophilia. Contrast studies of the gastrointestinal tract may show abnormalities of the cecum, ascending colon, and terminal ileum. The diagnosis is usually established at surgery. If surgery is not required, thiabendazole may be tried, but its efficacy is in doubt.

Prevention of both types of infection is dependent on education and rodent control.

Chin-Yun Y: Clinical observations on eosinophilic meningitis and meningoencephalitis caused by *Angiostrongylus cantonensis* on Taiwan. Am J Trop Med Hyg 25:233, 1976. *A series of 125 cases of this infection, including four deaths and three with permanent sequelae.*
Loria-Cortes R, Lobo-Sanahuja JE: Clinical abdominal angiostrongylosis. Am J Trop Med Hyg 29:538, 1980. *The largest series of A.* costaricensis *infection to date (116 children), with clinical and epidemiologic findings.*

413 FILARIASIS

413.1 Introduction
Eric A. Ottesen

Eight filarial parasites commonly infect humans (Table 413–1), but three are responsible for most of the pathology associated with these infections. These are the lymphatic dwelling filariae *Wuchereria bancrofti* and *Brugia malayi* and the subcutaneous filarid *Onchocerca volvulus*.

All eight species are transmitted by biting arthropods (Table 413–1) and go through complex life cycles that include a slow maturation phase of 3 to 18 months from the time infective larvae are introduced by the vector until the adult worms mature and reside in the lymph nodes, subcutaneous tissue, or body cavities. The offspring of these adults (microfilariae) are 200 to 300 μm long and 5 to 7 μm wide. They either circulate in the blood or migrate through the skin, awaiting ingestion by the appropriate arthropod in which they develop over one to two weeks to infective forms capable of initiating this life cycle again. Adult worms are long lived (probably up to 15 years), while microfilariae probably live about 6 months. Patent infection is generally not established unless exposure to infective larvae is intense and prolonged, and manifestations of disease usually develop slowly.

Diagnosis can be extremely difficult because it relies almost exclusively on parasitologic techniques to demonstrate microfilariae in the blood or tissue. At present, there are no completely satisfactory methods for making a definitive diagnosis in states of "amicrofilaremic filariasis" (before or after the microfilaremic state). When microfilariae circulate in the blood, they do so with or without a distinct periodicity (Table 413–1). Some are garbed in sheaths while others are sheathless. These two features, as well as other more subtle morphologic distinctions, are helpful diagnostically. Microfilariae can be identified either by direct observation of Giemsa-stained blood smears or, more sensitively, by concentration techniques using Knott's method (examination of centrifuged

TABLE 413–1. THE COMMON FILARIAL PARASITES OF MAN

Species	Distribution	Vector	Primary Pathology	Microfilariae Primary Location	Microfilariae Periodicity	Microfilariae Presence of Sheath
Wuchereria bancrofti	Tropics worldwide	Mosquitoes	Lymphatic, pulmonary	Blood, hydrocele fluid	Nocturnal, subperiodic	+
Brugia malayi	Southeast Asia	Mosquitoes	Lymphatic, pulmonary	Blood	Nocturnal, subperiodic	+
Brugia timori	Indonesia	Mosquitoes	Lymphatic	Blood	Nocturnal	+
Onchocerca volvulus	Africa; Central and South America	Black fly	Skin, eye, lymphatic	Skin, eye	None or minimal	−
Loa loa	Africa	Horse fly	Allergic	Blood	Diurnal	+
Mansonella perstans	Africa; South America	Midge	? Allergic	Blood	None	−
Mansonella streptocerca	Africa	Midge	Skin	Skin	None	−
Mansonella ozzardi	Central and South America	Midge	Vague	Blood	None	−

sediment after mixing 1 ml of blood with 9 ml of 2 per cent formalin) or membrane filtration of 1 ml or more of blood through a 3-μm or 5-μm pore Nuclepore membrane filter. Skin microfilariae are best sought by performing skin snips either as described in Ch. 413.4 or using a corneal-scleral biopsy punch. Antibody detection, although helpful in certain situations, is generally nondiagnostic because it cannot differentiate current from past infection or exposure and because of antigenic cross-reactivity between the filariae and other helminth parasites.

Diethylcarbamazine (DEC)* has been the single mainstay of treatment for all filarial infections since the late 1940's; however, it shows variable effectiveness for the different conditions. Suramin,† although extremely toxic, is also used for onchocerciasis. The new drug ivermectin,‡ because of greater efficacy and fewer side effects, likely will replace DEC as the drug of choice for onchocerciasis; it is currently under evaluation for use in lymphatic filariasis.

---

*Not commercially available in the United States, but may be obtained in special circumstances from Lederle Laboratories, Pearl River, NY.

†Available from the Centers for Disease Control, Parasitic Disease Drug Service, Atlanta, Ga.

‡Not commercially available, but may be obtained in special circumstances from Merck Sharp & Dohme Research Laboratories, West Point, PA.

Ciba Found Symp: Filariasis. 127:305, 1987. *A multiauthored compendium of the current forefronts of understanding in most aspects of the filarial diseases.*

Goodwin LC: Recent advances in research on filariasis—Chemotherapy. Trans R Soc Trop Med Hyg 78(Suppl):1, 1984. *A concise summary of what is old and what is new in the chemotherapy of filarial infections.*

Ottesen EA: Filariasis and tropical eosinophilia. In Warren KS, Mahmond AA (eds.): Tropical and Geographical Medicine. New York. McGraw-Hill Book Company, 1983, pp 390–412. *Detailed clinical, parasitologic and epidemiologic discussion of filarial disease.*

413.2 Lymphatic Filariasis

Eric A. Ottesen

ETIOLOGY. There are three lymphatic-dwelling filarial parasites of man, *Wuchereria bancrofti*, *Brugia malayi*, and *Brugia timori*. Adult worms are threadlike in form (2 to 10 cm long by less than 0.4 cm wide) and usually reside in the lymph nodes or afferent lymphatic channels. The female worms produce large numbers of microfilariae (200 to 300 μ long), which circulate in the peripheral blood awaiting ingestion by mosquito intermediate hosts, which are necessary to continue the parasite's life cycle. After about two weeks in these mosquitoes, the microfilariae develop into infective third stage larvae (L_3's). When infected mosquitoes feed, these L_3's leave the mosquito mouth parts and come to rest on the surface of the host's skin. Only if they manage to penetrate the skin through the puncture at the site of the bite can transmission be successful; after a further developmental period lasting as long as 4 to 12 months, adult worms can again be found in the lymphatic tissues, where they mate and produce another generation of microfilariae. The adult parasites may remain viable in the human host for decades.

EPIDEMIOLOGY. For *W. bancrofti* man is the only definitive host and thus the natural reservoir for infection. Indeed, considerable experimental effort to establish the parasite in a wide variety of mammalian hosts has met with minimal success. *W. bancrofti* is found throughout the tropics and subtropics, including areas of South America and the Caribbean, Africa, Asia, and the Pacific. Two forms of the parasite are distinguished by the periodicity of their circulating microfilariae. Nocturnally periodic forms have microfilariae detectable in peripheral blood primarily at night, whereas in the subperiodic forms the microfilariae are usually present in the blood at all hours but with maximal levels often in the late afternoon. Generally, subperiodic bancroftian filariasis is found only in the Pacific islands east of 160 degrees E longitude (including New Caledonia, Fiji, Samoa, Ellis and

Cook Islands, Society Islands, and the Marquesas); elsewhere *W. bancrofti* is nocturnally periodic. The natural vectors are *Culex fatigans* in urban settings and usually anopheline or aedean mosquitoes in rural areas.

The distribution of brugian filariasis is much more restricted, being limited primarily to parts of Malaysia, Indonesia, India, China, Korea, the Philippines, and Japan. Again, there are both nocturnally periodic and subperiodic forms of the parasite. The former is more common and is transmitted in coastal rice fields primarily by mansonian and anopheline mosquitoes; mansonian mosquitoes, found in swamp forests, are the major vectors of the subperiodic form. Unlike *W. bancrofti*, *B. malayi* can be a natural infection of cats and can be established in a number of laboratory animals. *B. timori* has been described from only two Indonesian islands.

PATHOLOGY. Most of the pathology of bancroftian and brugian filariasis is initiated in the lymphatics. Although details of the pathogenesis are lacking, the progression of pathologic changes is clear. Damaged lymphatics lead first to reversible lymphedema and then to chronic obstructive changes (elephantiasis) in the limbs, breasts, or genitalia, or to chyluria. The location of lymphatic damage determines the site and type of pathology expressed.

Adult worms, residing in the afferent approaches or cortical sinuses of the lymph nodes, induce local reactions by undefined mechanisms that result in dilatation of the lymphatics and hypertrophy of the vessel walls. Endothelial and connective tissue proliferation leads to polypoid growths that protrude into the lymphatic lumen; but so long as the worms remain alive, the vessel appears to stay patent. Patency, however, does not assure normal lymphatic function, as lymphangiographic studies have clearly documented the development of a characteristic tortuosity of the lymph vessels with loss of valvular function and backflow of lymph leading to lymph stasis and lymphedema even during this "preobliterative phase."

Death of adult worms is accompanied by local inflammatory and granulomatous reactions around the parasite with infiltration of plasma cells, eosinophils, and giant cells. Fibrosis occurs, and the fragmented parasites are either completely resorbed or partially calcified. Lymphatic obstruction develops, and associated endophlebitis may further complicate the lymphatic obstruction. Although there is subsequent formation of collateral lymphatics and some recanalization of obstructed vessels, lymphatic function remains compromised. Repeated infection with increasing host response to the parasite leads to the chronic changes of advanced elephantiasis.

CLINICAL MANIFESTATIONS. The three most common clinical presentations of the lymphatic filariases are asymptomatic microfilaremia, "filarial fever," and lymphatic obstruction. A fourth presentation, the tropical eosinophilia syndrome, is considered in Ch. 413.5.

Patients with asymptomatic microfilaremia rarely come to the physician's attention except through an incidental finding of microfilariae in the peripheral blood smear during mass surveys in endemic regions, or when blood eosinophilia leads to a diagnostic evaluation for filariasis. Such asymptomatic persons appear to be clinically unaffected by the parasites. It is likely that in some of these individuals the infections clear spontaneously, whereas the infections of others subsequently progress and become symptomatic, but what determines such clinical changes is unclear.

"Filarial fevers" are acute febrile episodes characterized by high temperature (often with shaking chills), lymphatic inflammation (i.e., lymphadenitis and lymphangitis), and transient local edema. They occur as often as six to ten times per year in affected persons and usually last three to seven days before subsiding spontaneously. The factors that initiate these episodes are unknown, but they are definitely parasite related. The lymphangitis characteristically develops in a retrograde fashion, extending peripherally *from* the draining node where the adult parasites reside. Regional nodes are enlarged and painful, and the entire lymphatic tract often becomes indurated and inflamed. Concomitant local thrombophlebitis is common. In brugian filariasis especially, a single local abscess may form along the inflamed lymphatic and subsequently rupture to the surface, leaving a characteristic scar whose presence has been used epidemiologically as an indication of the clinical "activity" of filarial infection in *Brugia* endemic regions. Neither the lymphatic inflammation nor the characteristic abscesses appear to be bacterially induced. Such lymphadenitis and lymphangitis occur in the upper and lower extremities with both bancroftian and brugian filariasis, but involvement of the genital lymphatics is almost exclusively a feature of *W. bancrofti* infection. Thus, acute *bancrofti* episodes may also involve funiculitis, epididymitis, scrotal pain, and tenderness. Patients with filarial fevers may be microfilaremic but more often are not.

As lymphatic damage progresses, the edema and anatomic distortion that were initially transient develop into the permanent changes of elephantiasis. Pitting edema yields to brawny edema, and there are both thickening of subcutaneous tissue and hyperkeratosis. Fissuring of the skin develops along with nodular and papillomatous hyperplastic changes. Superinfection (especially with the dermatophytes) becomes a problem. In addition, in bancroftian filariasis, obstructed genital lymphatics may lead to scrotal lymphedema or hydrocele, whereas obstruction of the retroperitoneal lymphatics can increase hydrostatic pressure in the renal lymphatics, causing their rupture into the renal pelvis or tubules and leading to chyluria. Characteristically chyluria is intermittent, sometimes lasting for days or weeks before abating spontaneously and then recurring; often it is most prominent in the morning after the patient first arises.

DIAGNOSIS. Definitive diagnosis of filariasis can be made only by the demonstration of parasites, either adult worms associated with the lymphatics (rarely observed) or microfilariae in the blood, hydrocele fluid, or chylous urine. These fluids can be examined directly (20 cu mm on a slide with or without red blood cell lysis), after concentration of the parasites by centrifugation in 2 per cent formalin (Knott's technique), or after filtration through a membrane (3- to 5-μm Nuclepore) filter. The time of blood collection should take into account the parasite's possible nocturnal periodicity.

Because many persons with filariasis (especially those with chronic pathology) are not microfilaremic, diagnosis must often be made clinically. The differential diagnosis is broad, but in the acute episodes primarily includes thrombophlebitis, infection, and trauma. The edema and other lymphatic obstructive changes associated with chronic filariasis must be distinguished from the manifestations of congestive heart failure, malignant disease, trauma, postsurgical scarring, and a number of less common congenital and idiopathic abnormalities of the lymphatic system. The many disorders associated with serum IgE and blood eosinophil elevations must be considered in evaluating asymptomatic filarial infections. Several specific points may help in this differential diagnosis: (1) Exposure to filariae must be prolonged or intense (for at least several months) before persons become infected; (2) the physical finding or history of *retrograde* lymphangitis can often aid in distinguishing filarial from bacterial lymphangitis; (3) although lymphadenopathy is characteristic of filariasis, alone it is never diagnostic; (4) lymphangiographic patterns of elephantiasis and chyluria are well defined so that even though not always diagnostic, lymphangiography is sometimes useful in distinguishing filarial from congenital or neoplastic lymphatic abnormalities; (5) although total serum IgE and blood eosinophil levels are elevated in all filarial infections, they cannot distinguish filarial from other helminth infections except in the case of the tropical eosinophilia syndrome (see Ch. 413.3); and (6) because most residents of endemic regions have been immunologically "sensitized" to

filarial antigens through years of bites by infected mosquitoes and because filarial antigens cross-react extensively with those of other nematode parasites, positive results in the numerous serologic and skin tests that have been developed are of little diagnostic value *except* in those who are not native to endemic areas.

TREATMENT. Available chemotherapy for lymphatic filariasis is both limited and inadequate. Diethylcarbamazine* (DEC, 5 mg per kilogram per day given in single or divided doses for two to three weeks) rapidly kills microfilariae in vivo, but its effect on adult parasites is less dramatic. Thus, following treatment with DEC, although the blood is temporarily free of microfilariae, the infection itself has often not been terminated, and several courses of DEC or long-term intermittent treatment with low doses of DEC are often required to kill the adult parasites. There are no other clinically useful drugs available for eradicating the infection, though early trials with ivermectin† look promising.

Side effects of DEC treatment, although not so frequent or severe as those seen in onchocerciasis, can be troublesome, especially in brugian filariasis. These include fever, chills, headache, dizziness, nausea, vomiting, and arthralgias, all usually occurring in the first 24 to 36 hours. Both the likelihood of developing such reactions and the degree of their severity are directly related to the number of circulating microfilariae. Thus, the side effects of DEC administration at these dosage levels are due not to direct drug toxicity but to allergic or immunologic responses of the host to dying parasites. To avoid these reactions in highly parasitemic persons, one can initiate treatment with very small doses of DEC or premedicate the patients with steroids, as suggested for onchocerciasis (see Ch. 413.4). A very few patients may also develop filarial fever episodes with lymphangitis and lymphadenitis in the first days after DEC treatment. All of these side effects occur early in treatment and generally subside even with continued administration of the drug.

Severe chronic lymphatic damage has recently been shown to have a surprising degree of reversibility. All such affected patients should receive long-term low-dose DEC (to eradicate persistent or new filarial infections) and diligent attention to local care of the lymphedematous extremity through limb elevation, use of special massage techniques and elastic stockings, and prevention of superficial bacterial and fungal infection. More severely affected patients may benefit remarkably from surgical decompression of the lymphatic system through "nodovenous shunt" surgery followed by excision of redundant tissue. Hydroceles can be repeatedly drained or managed surgically. Chyluria also can sometimes be corrected surgically, but, interestingly, many cases have been reported in which diagnostic lymphangiography itself appears to have terminated the leak of chyle into the urine, probably as a result of its sclerosing effects.

PREVENTION. Because DEC kills developing preadult forms of many filarial species, it is used in veterinary practice as a prophylactic agent to prevent filarial infection of dogs. Its potential for prophylaxis in man, however, has not been evaluated. In public health programs DEC has been used successfully as a protective measure to reduce infection rates in selected populations. Because of its microfilaricidal effects small doses administered intermittently to all residents of an endemic region‡ (e.g., 3 mg per kilogram monthly) reduce the number of blood-borne microfilariae in the community to levels so low that successful transmission of the infection by mosquitoes cannot occur. Other approaches to filariasis control designed to eradicate the mosquito vectors have also proved effective.

---

*Not commercially available in the United States, but may be obtained in special circumstances from Lederle Laboratories, Pearl River, NY.

†Not commercially available, but may be obtained in special circumstances from Merck Sharp & Dohme Research Laboratories, West Point, PA.

‡This use is not listed in the manufacturer's directive.

Ciba Found Sym: Filariasis. 127:305 1987. *A multiauthored compendium of the current forefronts of understanding in most aspects of the filarial diseases.*

Gooneratne BWN: Lymphangiography—Clinical and Experimental. London, Butterworths, 1974. *General description of lymphangiographic techniques, edited by a physician with great personal experience in the lymphangiography of filarial lymphatic obstruction. Three chapters are devoted exclusively to the lymphatic lesions seen in filariasis.*

Ottesen EA: Efficacy of diethylcarbamazine in eradicating infection with lymphatic-dwelling filariae in humans. Rev Infect Dis 7:341, 1985. *A thorough review of observations from the literature, finally concluding that the more DEC administered (preferably over an extended period), the greater the likelihood that lymphatic filarial infections will be eradicated.*

World Health Organization: Lymphatic pathology and immunopathology in filariasis: Report of the twelfth meeting of the scientific working group on filariasis. TDR/FIL-SWG(12)/85.3, 1986, p. 33. *A report available through WHO that summarizes the most recent advances in understanding the pathogenesis and optimal management of the consequences of filaria-induced lymphatic obstruction.*

413.3 Tropical Eosinophilia

Eric A. Ottesen

Tropical eosinophilia is a syndrome of acute and chronic lung disease first defined in the 1940's but not generally recognized as being of filarial etiology until the 1960's. Its main clinical features are a history of residence in a filaria-endemic region; paroxysmal cough and wheezing, which generally occur at night; scanty sputum production; occasional weight loss, low-grade fever, and adenopathy; and extreme blood eosinophilia (>3000 per microliter). It appears to be more common in Indians than in persons of other nationalities and more common in men than in women. Chest roentgenograms can be normal, but generally show increased bronchovascular markings, diffuse miliary lesions, or mottled opacities primarily involving the mid and lower lung fields. Tests of pulmonary function almost always indicate restrictive abnormalities and often show obstructive defects as well. The association of the syndrome with filarial infection was first recognized by finding very high levels of antifilarial antibody in these patients and by noting the favorable response to treatment with antifilarial drugs (now diethylcarbamazine* [DEC], 5 to 6 mg per kilogram per day for two to three weeks]). Later, several reports described microfilariae or their degenerating remnants in lung biopsy specimens. Most recently, extremely high levels of total serum IgE (usually 10,000 to 100,000 ng per milliliter) have been found in these patients, and an appreciable fraction of this IgE has been shown to be directed against filarial antigens.

Because of these and other findings, tropical eosinophilia is now considered to be a form of "occult filariasis" in which host immunologic hyper-responsiveness to the parasite results in such rapid clearance of microfilariae from the blood that this stage of the parasite is essentially never detectable. Generally this microfilarial clearance takes place in the lungs, and the clinical symptoms appear to result largely from the allergic and inflammatory reactions elicited by the cleared parasites. In some subjects, however, trapping of the microfilariae occurs predominantly in other organs of the reticuloendothelial system (liver, spleen, lymph nodes), and in these persons the major clinical manifestations are those resulting from hepatomegaly, splenomegaly, or lymphadenopathy. It has been postulated that infection with nonhuman filarial parasites is the major cause of tropical eosinophilia. More likely, however, the syndrome is caused not by an "abnormal parasite" but rather by an abnormal host response to those same parasites (*Wuchereria bancrofti* and *Brugia malayi*) that commonly cause lymphatic filariasis (see Ch. 413.2). In this respect, tropical eosinophilia may be similar to another pulmonary eosinophilic disorder, allergic bronchopulmonary aspergillosis, both in its clinical expression and in its pathogenesis (see Ch. 376).

Diagnosis depends primarily on distinguishing tropical eosinophilia from the other important eosinophilic syndromes with pulmonary involvement, namely, Löffler's syndrome, chronic eosinophilic pneumonia, allergic aspergillosis, certain vasculitic syndromes, the idiopathic hypereosinophilia syndrome, drug allergies, and some helminth infections. Although there is no one clinical or laboratory criterion that will distinguish tropical eosinophilia from these other conditions, a history of residence in the tropics along with high levels of specific filarial antibodies and response to DEC therapy are the most helpful differential points. Within three to seven days following administration of DEC, there is almost always marked improvement or disappearance of symptoms. Relapse may occur, however, months to years later and require retreatment. DEC will not, of course, reverse permanent pulmonary damage (primarily an interstitial fibrosis), which frequently develops prior to successful diagnosis and treatment of the disorder.

Pinkston P, Vijayan VK, Nutman TB, et al.: Tropical pulmonary eosinophilia: Characterization of the lower respiratory tract inflammation and its response to therapy. J Clin Invest 80:216, 1987. *Clinical and bronchoalveolar lavage studies probing the pathologic and immunopathologic mechanisms of the pulmonary pathology in this disorder.*

Udwadia FE: Pulmonary Eosinophilia. Progress in Respiration Research, Vol 7. Basel, S Karger, 1975. *Extensive review of tropical eosinophilia by a physician operating a chest clinic in Bombay, India, who has studied over 450 patients with this disease. Rich in clinical detail and perspective.*

413.4 Onchocerciasis (River Blindness)

Bruce M. Greene

Onchocerciasis is a disease, most commonly manifest by skin and ocular damage, resulting from chronic infection with the filarial parasite *Onchocerca volvulus*.

ETIOLOGY. Onchocerciasis is a vector-borne disease, transmitted from person to person by the bite of the blackfly, *Simulium* species. The female blackfly ingests microfilariae from the skin of an infected person while taking a blood meal. Within the vector, microfilariae develop into infective larvae over a period of six to eight days, and these larvae are transmitted to another person when the fly bites again. Over a period of several months, the larvae undergo a series of transformations leading to the development of adult worms that coil up into spherical bundles located in the subcutaneous tissues and deeper fascial planes. After a prepatent period of 9 to 18 months, the adult male and female worms reproduce sexually to yield millions of microfilariae that migrate through the skin and ocular tissues.

Microfilariae are highly motile, unsheathed, and measure 210 to 320 μm in length and 6 to 9 μm in width. Infective larvae measure approximately 600 μm in length, and in the human host undergo a molt to stage 4 larvae after a period of several days. Adult female worms are 23 to 70 cm in length, while the males are 3 to 6 cm long and weigh only 1 per cent as much as the female.

The lifespan of the adult worm in humans is known not to exceed 18 years, and the average survival is probably eight to ten years.

PREVALENCE AND EPIDEMIOLOGY. *Onchocerca volvulus* infects an estimated 20 to 40 million persons, principally in equatorial Africa in a broad belt extending from the Atlantic coast on the west to the Red Sea and Indian Ocean on the east. In the Western Hemisphere, the major focus is in Guatemala, on the Pacific slope of the Sierra Madre. Additional foci exist in Yemen, southwestern Saudi Arabia, southern Mexico, Venezuela, and northwestern Brazil, Colombia, and Ecuador.

Endemicity of *O. volvulus* in human populations is dependent upon habitation of fly-infested areas by sufficient, but not

---

*Not commercially available in the United States, but may be obtained in special circumstances from Lederle Laboratories, Pearl River, NY.

excessive, numbers of people who are exposed to man-biting flies during daily activities such as farming, fishing, bathing and washing, and water collection. Blackflies deposit eggs on vegetation, rocks, sticks, and debris in freely flowing streams and rivers, and these develop into larvae and pupae that attach to vegetation and continuously filter the water to obtain oxygen and nutrients. Because of the dependency of the fly on waterways for reproduction, flies concentrate around streams and rivers. As a result, infection in human populations and disease tends to be similarly distributed; hence the term *river blindness*. The vector usually flies only a few kilometers from waterways, but may fly as many as 20.

Approximately 1 to 4 per cent of infected persons become blind, and onchocerciasis ranks as the fourth leading cause of blindness in humans. In hyperendemic areas, over one half of adults become blind. A much higher percentage of persons develops skin disease and/or some ocular involvement. Because blindness or serious ocular involvement, or severe debility resulting from skin disease, typically occurs during the third and fourth decades of life, the impact of the disease on the community is particularly devastating, frequently incapacitating the heads of households.

PATHOLOGY AND PATHOGENESIS. The disease affects primarily the skin, lymph nodes, and ocular tissues. In the skin, histopathology reflects a low-grade chronic inflammatory process. The end stage shows loss of elastic fibers, atrophy, and fibrosis. The onchocercomata, which are fibrous subcutaneous nodules containing adult worms, show a rim of chronic inflammation with fibrosis and extensive capillary infiltration surrounding the worms themselves. Lymph nodes show chronic inflammatory changes and, in some cases, fibrosis and atrophy. In the eye, neovascularization and scarring of the cornea lead to loss of transparency and blindness. The remainder of the eye is frequently involved by a chronic nongranulomatous inflammatory process that leads to anterior uveitis and associated chronic complications, chorioretinitis with damage to the retinal pigment epithelium, and optic atrophy.

The basis for the pathologic changes of onchocerciasis is believed to be the host reaction to chronic infestation with microfilariae. A multiplicity of factors appears to contribute to the pathologic changes; these include toxic or tissue-altering products of host granulocytes and lymphoid cells, which are reacting to the parasite, and perhaps products of the microfilariae themselves.

CLINICAL MANIFESTATIONS. The earliest signs of infection include pruritus and intermittent papular rash with some thickening of the skin, which may be localized to one area of the body, and conjunctivitis. In nonresidents of endemic areas, who are usually lightly infected, these are frequently the only manifestations. Onchocercomata are firm 0.5- to 3-cm subcutaneous nodules that are nontender and freely movable if not attached to periosteum. These frequently occur in clusters that can be disfiguring. Common locations include the skin overlying bony prominences, including the superior iliac crests, the coccyx, the greater trochanter of the femur, the bony thorax, and the scalp and head region. With chronic infection, permanent skin changes occur, including loss of elasticity, a chronic, scaling hyperkeratotic maculopapular pruritic rash with mottled hypopigmentation or hyperpigmentation, and finally, atrophy, leading in some cases to areas of breakdown with the risk of superinfection. Chronic skin manifestations are unpredictably punctuated by transient episodes of localized rash, erythema, and edema. In Central America the dermal manifestations are most prominent around the head and neck, while in Africa they more commonly involve the trunk, buttocks, and lower extremities. Lymph node involvement is usually manifested by enlargement, particularly in the inguinal and femoral regions, and in some cases by secondary obstructive changes in the groin region or in an extremity. Early ocular manifestations include

punctate keratitis and anterior uveitis. Chronic changes include sclerosing keratitis, chorioretinitis (which leads to progressive constriction of visual fields), optic atrophy, and complications due to persistent anterior uveitis, including meiosis, pupillary distortion, and glaucoma. In general, the severity of disease correlates with intensity and duration of infection.

DIAGNOSIS. The diagnosis can be made clinically by the presence of onchocercomata, typical skin changes, or eye findings of onchocerciasis, including microfilariae in the cornea or anterior chamber in otherwise normal-appearing eyes. The diagnosis is confirmed by finding microfilariae of *O. volvulus* in the skin of the patient. This is done by biopsy, using a corneoscleral biopsy instrument or a razor blade, to yield approximately 1 to 2 mg of skin, including superficial dermis. The skin is weighed, incubated in tissue culture medium or saline, and the microfilariae that emerge are counted after a three-hour or overnight incubation. These must be distinguished from the smaller *Mansonella streptocerca* microfilariae. The skin-snipping technique has the inherent advantage of providing a measure of intensity of infection, with less than ten microfilariae per milligram of skin constituting a light infection, and greater than 100, heavy. For greatest reliability, four to six biopsies are done in different areas, including the hips, calves, and shoulders. Although elevated titers of antifilarial antibodies may support the diagnosis of onchocerciasis, a reliable and useful immunodiagnostic technique has not yet been developed.

TREATMENT. Diethylcarbamazine citrate* (DEC) is the standard drug used to treat onchocerciasis. Although well tolerated in uninfected persons, DEC frequently causes complications and side effects when given to individuals infected with *O. volvulus*; these complications appear to result in part from the massive killing of microfilariae that occurs over a few days following initiation of DEC therapy. This results in fever, intense pruritus, lymph node pain and swelling, prostration, hypotension, and arthralgias. In the eye a worsening of ocular inflammation occurs transiently, and permanent sight-threatening lesions may occur in the posterior segment of the eye. In an effort to minimize these complications, patients should be given corticosteroids (e.g., prednisone 40 to 60 mg per day) starting the day before initiation of DEC therapy and continuing for four to seven days as needed. DEC therapy should be started with a test dose of 25 to 50 mg, then increased to 4 mg per kilogram per day to complete a ten-day course. Re-treatment may be necessary after 6 to 12 months, since DEC does not substantially affect adult worm viability or reproductivity. To kill adult worms, suramin† must be used, but it is a toxic drug and should be employed only with a full understanding of the indications for use and the dangers involved. In general, it should be reserved for moderately or heavily infected persons who are leaving the endemic area. Ivermectin,‡ a newly developed microfilaricidal agent, shows considerable promise, and, because it is well tolerated and given as a single oral dose, it may soon replace DEC as the standard therapy.

Removal of nodules containing adult worms in the head region is indicated because of the increased risk of ocular involvement. Other palpable nodules should also be removed if feasible.

PROGNOSIS. With treatment, the early ocular and cutaneous changes are reversible, but for persons living in an endemic area, therapy must be given repeatedly, since neither DEC nor ivermectin is curative of the infection, and reinfection usually occurs continuously. The atrophic skin changes, scle-

---

*Available in the United States from Lederle Laboratories, Pearl River, NY.

†Available in the United States from the Centers for Disease Control, Atlanta, Ga.

‡Available in the United States from Merck Sharp & Dohme Research Laboratories, West Point, Pa.

rosing keratitis, and disease in the posterior segment of the eye are not helped by therapy.

PREVENTION. There is no proven chemoprophylaxis. Vector control is difficult and expensive, but has achieved remarkable success in some areas of Africa. Protective clothing, insect repellents, and avoidance of areas harboring the vector are useful measures for visitors to endemic areas.

Anderson J, Fuglsang H, Hamilton PJS, et al.: Studies on onchocerciasis in the United Cameroon Republic: II. Comparison of onchocerciasis in rain-forest and sudan-savanna. Trans R Soc Trop Med Hyg 68:209, 1974. *Detailed analysis of clinical manifestations with comparison of forest and savanna types of disease.*

Greene BM, Taylor HR, Cupp EW, et al.: Comparison of ivermectin and diethylcarbamazine in the treatment of onchocerciasis. N Engl J Med 313:133, 1985. *Shows that ivermectin is better tolerated, more effective, and safer than diethylcarbamazine.*

WHO Expert Committee on Onchocerciasis: Third Report. Technical Report Series No. 752. Geneva, World Health Organization, 1987. *Comprehensive summary of the disease and its distribution and impact.*

413.5 Loiasis
Eric A. Ottesen

Loa loa is indigenous only to the rain forest belt of western and central Africa. Mature female parasites, about twice the size of the males, are 50 to 70 mm long and 0.5 mm wide. They live wandering through the subcutaneous tissue in humans, usually attracting attention only when they cross the eye subconjunctivally. The sheathed microfilariae produced by these females circulate with a diurnal periodicity that peaks about noon.

Clinical loiasis presents in two primary forms, one more common among individuals native to endemic regions and the other more common in visitors to these areas who acquire infection. Among the natives, loiasis is often entirely asymptomatic until an adult worm appears moving across the eye or blood examination reveals microfilaremia. Such individuals may also have occasional episodes of Calabar swellings. These are characteristic localized areas of erythema and angioedema (up to 5 to 10 cm in diameter) that occur primarily on the extremities and last one to three days before regressing spontaneously. These swellings appear to be a hypersensitivity reaction to the adult worm, whose presence can also be detected in some patients by either a subcutaneous crawling sensation or the appearance of a fine vermiform hive in the skin. When the inflammation extends to nearby joints or peripheral nerves, corresponding symptoms may develop. Rarely, nephropathy (probably immune complex mediated) and encephalopathy have been reported.

The major difference between this presentation and that seen in outsiders who acquire infection is the greater predominance of allergic or hyper-reactive symptoms in the latter. Episodes of angioedema are likely to be more frequent and debilitating, and patients are much less likely to have microfilariae in the blood. In addition, they often present with extensive blood eosinophilia (30 to 60 per cent of an elevated total leukocyte count), much like patients with tropical eosinophilia (Ch. 413.3). Diagnosis in these patients often cannot be made parasitologically and must be based on the characteristic history, clinical presentation, blood eosinophilia, and elevated filarial antibody titers. If untreated, a small (but undefined) percentage of such patients develops severe cardiomyopathy, presumably secondary to the hypereosinophilia elicited by the infection.

Treatment is with diethylcarbamazine* (DEC, 6 to 10 mg per kilogram per day for two to three weeks). The drug is extremely effective against microfilariae, but less so against adult worms, so that multiple courses of treatment are often necessary before there is complete resolution of signs and symptoms. In cases of heavy microfilaremia (greater than several hundred microfilariae per milliliter of blood), allergic and other inflammatory side effects of treatment may be so severe that a regimen of 0.5 to 1.0 mg per kilogram DEC per dose (with or without simultaneous steroids) is safer for initiating treatment. Some evidence exists that DEC is effective in preventing loiasis when taken in doses of 5 mg per kilogram per day for three days each month, but large trials of this prophylactic regimen have yet to be carried out.

Duke BOL: Studies on the chemopophylaxis of loiasis. II. Observations on diethylcarbamazine citrate (Banocide) as a prophylactic in man. Ann Trop Med Parasitol 57:82, 1963. *The only published experience on the potential chemoprophylactic effects of diethylcarbamazine in human loiasis.*

Nutman TB, Miller KD, Mulligan M, et al.: *Loa loa* infection in temporary residents of endemic regions: Recognition of a hyperresponsive syndrome with characteristic clinical manifestations. J Infect Dis 154:10, 1986. *A thorough clinical description of a series of 20 patients with this syndrome and a review of previously published similar individual case reports.*

413.6 Dracunculiasis
Donald R. Hopkins

Dracunculiasis, or guinea worm disease, is caused by infection with the parasite *Dracunculus medinensis*. It occurs in the Indian subcontinent and Africa, where up to 10 million persons living in rural areas are thought to be affected annually and over 100 million persons are at risk of infection.

Diagnosis of patent infections is easy. The thin adult female worms, each up to 1 meter long, emerge directly through the skin, usually of the lower leg, ankle, or foot. The worms emerge 10 to 14 months after victims have drunk water containing infected *Cyclops*, a barely visible crustacean that serves as the parasite's intermediate host. When persons harboring such emerging worms enter a stagnant source of drinking water such as a step well or pond, larvae are released into the water where some are ingested by *Cyclops*. When humans drink water containing *Cyclops* with infective larvae, the larvae penetrate the intestinal or stomach wall, mature, and mate, after which the male worms die.

The adult worms emerge slowly, over a period of weeks or months. Emergence may be preceded by generalized allergic symptoms and is usually accompanied by a blister that ruptures to form an ulcer at the site of emergence. Some worms present first as a serpentine cord just beneath the skin or at the center of an abscess. No immunity develops, so persons in endemic areas are infected year after year.

The great social and economic significance of dracunculiasis, which rarely is fatal, derives from the fact that emergence of the worm is very painful and is often associated with swelling, local arthritis, and secondary infection. Thus, victims are often unable to farm or sometimes even walk for weeks or months. Over half of the adults in a village may be crippled at the same time, and the seasonal infection tends to occur precisely when villagers need to harvest or plant their crops. School attendance is also affected.

Treatment is difficult because anthelmintics such as thiabendazole or metronidazole only marginally reduce the duration of emergence and associated pain. Aspirin can help relieve the pain. Emerging worms are best rolled around a small stick as their predecessors have been for centuries, care being taken not to break the worm (which would exacerbate the inflammation). Some worms can be removed surgically. Victims should be immunized against tetanus, which is an all too frequent complication caused by secondary infection of the ulcer around the emerging worm. Persons at risk should be taught to boil their drinking water or filter it through a cloth and to avoid entering sources of drinking water when the infection is patent.

Since the most effective intervention against this infection is to provide safe drinking water, efforts are under way to

---

*Available in the United States from Lederle Laboratories, Pearl River, NY.

take advantage of the International Drinking Water Supply and Sanitation Decade (1981–1990) to provide safe water to dracunculiasis-endemic areas as a priority, and thereby eliminate the disease. By the end of 1986, India had reduced its reported dracunculiasis cases by 35 per cent, Ivory Coast had almost eliminated the disease altogether, and over one half of the remaining major endemic countries had begun programs to control the disease.

Hopkins DR: Dracunculiasis: An eradicable scourge. In Epidemiologic Reviews. Vol 5. Baltimore, The Johns Hopkins School of Hygiene and Public Health, 1983, pp 208–219. *A recent review of all aspects pertaining to control and eradication of dracunculiasis.*

Muller R: *Dracunculus* and dracunculiasis. In Dawes B (ed.): Advances in Parasitology. Vol 9. New York, Academic Press, 1971, pp 73–151. *A thorough consideration of the parasite's biology, life cycle, and the disease it produces.*

413.7 Other Filarial Infections

Eric A. Ottesen

PERSTANS FILARIASIS

Mansonella perstans (formerly *Dipetalonema perstans, Acanthocheilonema perstans*) is distributed in a broad belt across the center of Africa and in northeast South America. Adult worms, up to 70 to 80 mm long, reside in the body cavities (pleural, peritoneal, and pericardial) and in the mesentery, perirenal, and retroperitoneal tissues. Microfilariae are liberated *unsheathed* from the females and circulate in the blood without regular periodicity.

M. perstans infection was long thought to be asymptomatic, because up to 90 per cent of individuals with the parasite appeared to have no difficulty with it. Subsequent studies, however, indicate clearly that *M. perstans* is capable of inducing a variety of symptoms, including angioedematous swellings much like the Calabar swellings of loiasis; fever; headache; pain in bursae and/or joint synovia, in serous cavities, or over the liver; neurologic or psychologic symptoms; and extreme exhaustion. There is some evidence that symptoms are more prominent in outsiders coming to endemic regions, but in all series at least a quarter of the patients were asymptomatic despite persistent microfilaremia.

Treatment with diethylcarbamazine* (DEC, 5 to 6 mg per kilogram per day for two to three weeks) is often ineffective, with multiple courses usually necessary to achieve cure. When the parasites are eliminated, however, patients characteristically lose their symptoms (no matter how vague), lose their eosinophilia, and regain a sense of well-being.

Adolph PE, Kagan IG, McQuay RM: Diagnosis and treatment of *Acanthocheilonema perstans* filariasis. Am J Trop Med Hyg 11:76, 1962. *Results from a series of patients observed in the United States after returning from missionary work in Africa.*

Clarke V deV, Harwin RM, MacDonald DF, et al.: Filariasis: *Dipetalonema perstans* infections in Rhodesia. Cent Afr J Med 17:1, 1971. *Discussion of the clinical expression of* M. perstans *filariasis in Africans and Europeans living in east Africa.*

STREPTOCERCIASIS

Mansonella streptocerca is transmitted by midges, especially *Culicoides grahami*. It occurs in the tropical forest belt of Africa from Ghana to Zaire. The adult worms are subcutaneous, especially over the torso; and the microfilariae, which have shepherd's-crook tails, are found in the skin (see Ch. 413.4 for skin-snipping technique).

Infection is usually symptomless, but the adult worms may produce hypopigmented macules (to be distinguished from leprosy), and the microfilariae occasionally cause itching papular rashes similar to those of onchocerciasis. Both adult worms and microfilariae are killed by diethylcarbamazine citrate* (e.g., seven to ten days of treatment at 6 mg per kilogram per day).

Meyers WM, Connor DH, et al.: Human streptocerciasis: A clinicopathologic study of 40 Africans (Zairians) including identification of the adult filaria. Am J Trop Med Hyg 21:528, 1972. *Covers the clinical aspects and gives references to other aspects.*

MANSONELLA OZZARDI INFECTION

M. ozzardi is restricted in distribution to Central and South America and certain islands of the Caribbean. Adult worms have been recovered in humans only twice, both times from the peritoneal cavity. *Unsheathed* microfilariae circulate in the blood with little or no periodicity.

Many investigators consider these parasites to be nonpathogenic, but in one of the fullest clinical studies of an affected population it was asserted that the major clinical presentation is severe articular pain or dysfunction, especially in the arms and shoulders. Headache, fever, pulmonary symptoms, adenopathy, hepatomegaly, and pruritic skin eruptions also occurred in a small number of patients with a frequency greater than that in nonparasitized individuals in the same population. Diethylcarbamazine* has little or no effect on this infection.

Marinkelle CJ, German E: Mansonelliasis in the comisaria del Vaupes of Colombia. Trop Geogr Med 22:101, 1970. *A very complete and interesting account of clinical manifestations ascribed to* M. ozzardi *infections in South American Indians.*

Weller PF, Simon HB, Parkhurst BH, et al.: Tourism acquired *Mansonella ozzardi* microfilaremia in a regular blood donor. JAMA 240:858, 1978. *Evidence for the ineffectiveness of diethylcarbamazine in* M. ozzardi *infections.*

HUMAN DIROFILARIASIS

Dirofilaria species are filarial parasites mostly of dogs, cats, and raccoons that sometimes infect man but almost never fully develop to complete their life cycles in this abnormal host. The distribution of cases is worldwide and reflects the distribution of the parasites in animals.

Two general types of clinical presentation predominate. Pulmonary dirofilariasis, caused by the dog heartworm *D. immitis*, usually presents as an asymptomatic solitary pulmonary nodule but occasionally with chest pain, cough, or hemoptysis. Microscopically there is local eosinophilia and granuloma formation accompanied by infarction and thrombosis around an impacted, immature worm. The second common clinical presentation is that of a subcutaneous nodule found anywhere on the body (or within the eye) that results usually from infection with the subcutaneous dwelling filarids of dogs (*D. repens*) or raccoons (*D. tenuis*) but occasionally from infection with *D. immitis*. Local lesions again are granulomatous and eosinophilic and are sometimes accompanied by bacterial superinfection.

Definitive diagnosis and treatment most often result from the same surgical (excisional) procedure. Eosinophilia is not a regular finding in these patients nor are detectable antifilarial antibodies. Furthermore, since the worms are usually incompletely developed, microfilaremia occurs only in the rarest of circumstances. These "abnormal" parasite infections do not respond to diethylcarbamazine, and their treatment is primarily surgical.

Dissanaike AS: Zoonotic aspects of filarial infections in man. Bull WHO 57:349, 1979. *A scholarly, readable discussion of man's interaction with zoonotic filarial infections.*

Gershwin LJ, Gershwin E, Kritzman J: Human pulmonary dirofilariasis. Chest 66:92, 1974. *Description of the 35th of the more than 100 cases now reported, with a good discussion.*

*Not commercially available in the United States, but may be obtained in special circumstances from Lederle Laboratories, Pearl River, NY.

SECTION THREE
ARTHROPODS AND ANIMAL POISONS

414 ARTHROPODS AND LEECHES

William L. Krinsky

ARTHROPODS AS AGENTS OF DISEASE

Disease associated directly with arthropods results from toxic or allergic responses to the organisms or their products when humans are exposed by bites or stings, simple contact, or invasion through the skin or natural orifices. Arthropods most often involved in these types of exposure are listed in Table 414–1.

Physicians usually become aware of insects and their relatives (spiders, mites, ticks, scorpions, millipedes, and centipedes) when patients present with skin lesions caused by arthropods, when infestations of the creatures themselves are seen, when foreign bodies extracted from skin or sense organs are identified as arthropods, or when respiratory symptoms develop in response to arthropods or their products. Dermatoses associated with arthropods and human infestations with arthropods (e.g., lice, mites, fly larvae) are discussed in detail in this chapter. Arthropods as vectors are mentioned here; detailed discussions of arthropod-borne pathogens may be found elsewhere in this book.

Alexander JO: Arthropods and Human Skin. Berlin, Springer-Verlag, 1984. *This is the first comprehensive text devoted to dermatologic problems associated with arthropods.*

Harwood RF, James MT: Entomology in Human and Animal Health. 7th ed. New York, The Macmillan Company, 1979. *This is a comprehensive textbook that provides detailed references to the diverse arthropod-associated problems discussed here.*

Biting Arthropods

Louse Infestations (Pediculosis)

Pediculosis is infestation of the body with lice. Louse eggs (nits) seen cemented to hairs of the scalp or the observation of lice themselves confirm the diagnosis of head lice (*Pediculus capitis*). Nits (or lice) attached to the seams of clothing (often in undergarments) indicate the presence of body lice (*P. humanus*), and nits or lice attached to pubic hairs indicate a pubic (crab) louse (*Phthirus pubis*) infestation.

The eggs are pearly yellow-white and opaque, elongate-oval, about 0.8 mm long and 0.3 mm wide, and are attached singly to each hair or clothing fiber. After hatching, the nits appear translucent and opalescent. Although nits may be numerous, usually not more than 10 to 20 lice are associated with infested persons. The head louse egg is cemented on a hair about 1 mm above the scalp surface. Because hair grows 0.4 to 0.6 mm a day and most eggs hatch within five to ten days after deposition, nits attached over 7 mm from the surface are usually nonviable.

Head and body lice are very similar in appearance. Adult head lice are 2.5 to 3.5 mm long and adult body lice are 3 to 4.5 mm long. Immature and adult head and body lice each have three pairs of about equal-sized legs bearing claws for gripping hairs or fibers. Adult pubic lice, somewhat crablike in appearance, are 1 to 2 mm long, about as broad, grayish-white or yellowish-brown, and have forelegs narrower than the other pairs. All louse immatures (three stages in each species) resemble their respective adults except in size, and

all immatures and adults are obligate bloodsucking ectoparasites. The body louse is the only known natural vector of the pathogens of louse-borne typhus, trench fever, and louse-borne relapsing fever.

Head lice and their nits are found most frequently in the hair over the postauricular and occipital regions. Body lice are usually seen in clothing, with nits in the seams and creases in areas that contact the body. Crab lice and nits are found on hairs in the pubic and perianal regions, sometimes on hairs on the thighs and abdomen, less commonly on axillary hairs, beard, mustache, eyebrows, eyelashes, and rarely on the scalp. Pubic infestations are found only in postpubertal individuals.

The skin lesions produced by the bites of lice are erythematous papules that may be accompanied by urticaria or lymphadenopathy. Extensive erythema and pruritus result from hypersensitivity to louse saliva. Crab lice typically induce nonpruritic small gray-blue macules (0.3 to 1 cm diameter) with irregular borders (maculae ceruleae) that may persist for months. The lesions produced by any of the species may be covered with hair matted with eggs, dried serous secretions, and dark louse excrement. The latter, seen on the body or in underclothing, should trigger a search for lice. Excoriations from scratching disguise bite lesions and may lead to impetigo, furuncular, or eczematous lesions. The possibility of louse infestation should be considered when pyoderma is seen. The lichenification and pigmentation in chronically infested individuals is called vagabond's disease (morbus vagabondus). A nondescript macular or papular erythematous rash on the trunk may be the presenting sign for an undiscovered head louse infestation. Postauricular and posterior cervical lymphadenopathy in the absence of other node enlargement should suggest head lice. Body louse infestation may be differentiated from scabies by the absence of lesions on the hands and feet and the common occurrence of lesions in the intrascapular region. The differential diagnosis of louse-

TABLE 414–1. ARTHROPODS CAUSING HUMAN PATHOLOGY

Human Exposure	Arthropod	Antigens or Toxins
Bites	Insects (lice, bedbugs and other true bugs; fleas; flies including mosquitoes, black flies, biting midges, sandflies, horse and deer flies, stable flies, tsetse flies, keds; ants)	Salivary secretions, venoms
	Arachnids (chigger and other rodent and bird mites; ticks; spiders)	
	Centipedes	
Stings	Insects (some ants, wasps, and bees)	Venoms
	Arachnids (scorpions)	
Invasion	Insects (fly larvae, *Tunga* fleas)	Salivary secretions, excretions
	Arachnids (scabies mites)	
Simple contact	Insects (caterpillars, pupae or adults of moths and butterflies; blister and some rove beetles)	Setae, spines, secretions (venoms) and excretions
	Arachnids (stored product mites)	
	Millipedes	

induced dermatitis from various mite-induced lesions or non-arthropod-associated dermatoses is made by finding nits or lice.

Treatment for lice includes shampoos, creams, and lotions containing insecticides. The most often used preparations contain lindane (gamma benzene hexachloride) or pyrethrins with piperonyl butoxide. Malathion lotion has been approved for use in the United States. One effective treatment for head lice or pubic lice is a four-minute shampoo of the affected areas with about 25 ml of 1 per cent lindane shampoo. This may not be ovicidal; therefore, the treatment may be repeated seven to ten days later, if lice or new nits are seen. Patients infested with body lice may apply lindane (1 per cent) lotion or cream to affected areas. This should be thoroughly washed off six to eight hours later. Lindane should be used with caution on infants, children, and pregnant women. Infested clothing and linen should be washed in hot water (60°C) for 20 minutes or dry cleaned.

After being treated, lice and nits can be removed with a metal comb with teeth 0.1 mm apart. Moisture or oil rinses may make removal easier. Mechanical removal is recommended for facial pubic lice infestations. Lice and nits may be removed from eyelashes with a trachoma (roller) forceps. This may be followed by treatment with one of various pediculicide ointments, such as pyrethrin in Vaseline (1:8), or petrolatum, applied twice a day for seven to ten days. Blepharitis and other secondary infections associated with lice may require specific antibiotic therapy.

Prevention of recurrence involves treatment of infested human contacts and materials (fomites). Pillow cases, hats, scarves, and other items should be washed or cleaned. Infested combs and brushes should be cleaned and boiled or soaked for one hour in lindane shampoo or Lysol (2 per cent). Head and body lice will survive only about three days (ten days maximum) away from the body. Sexual partners of persons with pubic lice should be treated, and bedding, towels, and clothing should be washed or dry cleaned. Pubic lice will not survive longer than 24 hours away from a body; transmission via toilet seats is unlikely. Fumigation after any louse infestation is unnecessary, but vacuuming is helpful to remove stray lice and shed hairs with affixed nits.

Domonkos AN, Arnold HL, Odom RB: Andrews' Diseases of the Skin. 7th ed. Philadelphia, W. B. Saunders Company, 1982, pp 554–557. *This text has excellent photographs of nits, lice, and skin lesions seen in pediculosis.*

Raber IM: Pediculosis cilaris. In Parish LC, Nutting WB, Schwartzman RM (eds.): Cutaneous Infestations of Man and Animal. New York, Praeger, 1983, pp 138–143. *This is a lucid description of the clinical aspects and treatment of pubic louse infestation of the eyelashes.*

Witkowski JA, Parish LC: Pediculosis. In Parish LC, Nutting WB, Schwartzman RM (eds.): Cutaneous Infestations of Man and Animal. New York, Praeger, 1983, pp 125–137. *A concise, well-documented discussion of clinical louse infestations.*

Flea Bites

Most fleas, unlike lice, do not infest the body. The common flea species that suck blood from humans visit the body for a few minutes to hours, during which time feeding occurs. As in louse infestations, flea bites generally cause pruritus. Each bite lesion is an erythematous papule with a hemorrhagic punctum. Sensitization of an individual to flea saliva may result in papular urticaria (common in affected children), bullous eruptions, or erythema multiforme–type lesions. Bites are usually multiple and irregularly grouped. Bites in adults appear as widespread papules that become lichenified or as grouped papules overlying erythema or edema. Persons entering a previously infested room that has been vacant for weeks or months often suffer from multiple bites on the ankles and legs as hungry fleas emerge from pupal cocoons in floor crevices, debris, or carpeting. As with louse bites, excoriated lesions may become infected and furuncular.

Flea eggs are usually laid off the host, and larvae live off the host, feeding on organic debris. Adults reach their hosts by jumping. Flea species that most often bite humans are the cat flea (*Ctenocephalides felis*), the dog flea (*C. canis*), and somewhat less commonly the so-called human flea (*Pulex irritans*). Occasionally household infestations with fleas may arise from abandoned wild animal nests built near houses.

Treatment of flea bites is symptomatic and involves the use of antipruritic and anti-inflammatory creams or lotions, or oral antihistamines. Secondary infections may require antibiotic therapy. Infested pets should be treated with specific insecticides. Floors, carpets, upholstered furnishings, and pets' sleeping quarters should be sprayed or dusted with insecticides to kill larval, pupal, and adult fleas. Thorough cleaning, including vacuuming, of infested premises should eliminate the insects. Because fleas at all stages can live for weeks or months, a repeat insecticide application may be necessary.

Persons may protect themselves from fleas with repellents containing diethyl metatoluamide. Wild animal (especially rodent) fleas that feed on humans may transmit the bacilli of plague or tularemia, as well as the less virulent rickettsia of murine (flea-borne) typhus. Less common pathogens transmitted by accidental ingestion of fleas (mostly by children) are the dwarf tapeworm *Hymenolepis diminuta* and the dog tapeworm *Dipylidium caninum*.

Bagnall B, Rook A: Arthropods and the skin. In Rook A (ed.): Recent Advances in Dermatology. No. 4. Edinburgh, Churchill Livingstone, 1977. *This review includes information about the ecology of fleas and pathogenesis and clinical features of infestations.*

Smit FGAM: Siphonaptera (Fleas). In Smith KGV (ed.): Insects and Other Arthropods of Medical Importance. London, British Museum (Natural History), 1973. *This is a careful overview of the medical importance of fleas.*

Bedbugs and Kissing Bugs

Bedbugs (Cimicidae) are flat, mahogany-brown, wingless insects (5 to 7 mm long). Most species are blood sucking ectoparasites of birds and bats. Two species (*Cimex lectularius* and *C. hemipterus*) feed almost exclusively on humans; the former is cosmopolitan; the latter has a tropical distribution. Both species cause irritating, pruritic bite lesions in sensitized individuals. The bugs become engorged with blood in 3 to 15 minutes and feed only at night or in subdued light. They hide in crevices of bedding, beds, floors, and furnishings and in wood and paper trash accumulations during the day. The bites are often seen in short linear groups and vary from small urticarial lesions to large erythematous papules or bullae. The lesions are often excoriated, and eczematous reactions and pyoderma may be seen. Hypersensitivity reactions may include asthma, generalized urticaria, and arthralgia. While some affected persons complain of being awakened at night, most are troubled by the lesions on arising in the morning. Treatment is symptomatic. Prevention includes removal of debris that harbors the bugs, use of insecticides in crevices and cleaning of infested furnishings.

Triatomine kissing bugs (Reduviidae) that suck blood from a diversity of hosts are found in the New World subtropics and tropics and in Asia. Most of these cone-nosed bugs (8 to 38 mm long) are tan, brown, or black, with yellow or red spots around the dorsal edge of the abdomen. The bugs feed rapidly at night. Sensitive individuals may develop papular lesions, small vesicles or, in the extreme, large urticarial or hemorrhagic nodular to bullous lesions. Generalized anaphylactoid reactions, including shock and angioneurotic and laryngeal edema, have occurred. Kissing bugs may feed anywhere on the body. Domesticated species in the tropics are found most often in thatched houses or those with mud floors. In the southwestern United States, a species (*Triatoma protracta*) living in wood rat nests in desert areas occasionally invades homes. Treatment of bites or allergic reactions is symptomatic. In Central and South America these insects are vectors of Chagas' disease trypanosomes.

Crissey JT: Bedbugs—an old problem with a new dimension. Int J Dermaol 20:411, 1981. *This review article discusses bedbug biology and the possible role of these bugs in human disease.*

Ryckman RE: Host reactions to bug bites (Hemiptera, Homoptera): A literature review and annotated bibliography. Parts I, II. Calif Vector Views 26:Nos. 1–2, 1979. *This is an excellent source of specific references about all bugs that prey on humans.*

Mosquitoes and Other Bloodsucking Flies

Mosquitoes (Culicidae) are found worldwide, breeding wherever there is stagnant water. While biting, a female mosquito (3 to 6 mm long) induces a pruritic wheal that becomes an erythematous papule within 24 hours of the bite. In sensitive persons, bullous lesions, cellulitis, or hemorrhagic necrotic reactions may follow the bites. Systemic anaphylactic reactions are rare. The most serious medical problems associated with mosquitoes relate to their transmission of the agents of yellow fever, dengue, arboviral encephalitides, malaria, and filariasis.

Biting midges (Ceratopogonidae), also called punkies or no-see-ums because of their minute size (most are 0.6 to 2 mm long), give a painful bite. The resulting erythematous punctiform lesions may become papular and pruritic. Vesicles may develop that ooze fluid for days. These midges, especially *Culicoides* species, bite mostly on exposed parts of the body and may be pestiferous in sandy seashore or marshy areas where they breed. Biting occurs mostly at dawn or dusk.

Black flies (Simuliidae), also called buffalo gnats, are small (1 to 5 mm long), humpbacked, tan to black insects that breed only in running water. They are troublesome bloodsuckers in northern temperate regions. The bites may become hemorrhagic papules that ooze blood for hours. These lesions may be painful and cause recurrent pruritus. Lymphadenopathy is common in sensitive individuals, who may develop localized edema. Cephalalgia, fever, and nausea may occur following large numbers of bites. Black fly species found at high elevations in Central and South America and along rivers in Africa transmit *Onchocerca volvulus*, the etiologic agent of river blindness.

Phlebotomine sand flies (Psychodidae) are delicate, small (2 to 3 mm long), hairy flies found mainly in subtropical and tropical areas. Various species are abundant in rain forests in the New World and in arid areas in the Mediterranean region and Asia. Biting occurs at night or in subdued light. The bites may be painful, occur usually on the extremities, and cause pruritus and elevated pale urticarial lesions that become papular. Vesicular or bullous lesions may occur. Phlebotomine flies are vectors of sand fly (pappataci) fever, bartonellosis, and leishmaniasis.

Other flies that may attack man and cause painful bites are horse and deer flies (Tabanidae), stable flies, and tsetse flies. Tsetse flies, found only in Africa, transmit the trypanosomes of African sleeping sickness.

Treatment of any of these fly bites is symptomatic and includes the use of topical corticosteroids and oral antihistamines to reduce itching. Personal protection from biting flies involves the use of screen enclosures, headnets, and insect repellents. Protective clothing and open mesh jackets impregnated with repellents are effective.

Allen JR: Mosquitoes and other biting flies. In Parish LC, Nutting WB, Schwartzman RM (eds.): Cutaneous Infestations of Man and Animal. New York, Praeger, 1983, pp 344–355. *This is a concise, clearly presented review of pathogenesis and clinical aspects of fly bites.*

Chiggers and Other Biting Mites

Chiggers are the larvae (six-legged stage) of trombiculid (itch or harvest) mites. These larvae (0.15 to 0.40 mm long) are white to yellow or orange-red, and are found on many vertebrates. Human infestation occurs following contact with grassy or shrubby vegetation inhabited by the mites. First exposure may not produce dermatitis or may produce only slightly irritating, transient erythematous macules or papules (1 to 2 mm). The more commonly seen skin reactions to chigger feeding are extremely pruritic, papular, papulovesicular or papulourticarial lesions (4 to 20 mm) that persist with burning and itching for days to weeks. The lesions may fade and flatten or become hemorrhagic, purpuric, or vesicular. Diagnosis is dependent upon morphology and distribution of lesions, exposure history, and observation of the mites. Engorging chiggers may be apparent as minute reddish blebs embedded in hair follicles. The mites most often attach to skin covered by clothing, especially near belts, straps, or elastic bindings. Scrub itch mites of Asia and South Pacific Islands usually do not cause dermatitis, but they are vectors of scrub typhus rickettsiae.

Other mites that bite humans but that are rarely recovered from the lesions they cause are pyemotid (straw, hay, or grain itch) mites, cheyletiellid (cat or dog fur) mites, and dermanyssid (chicken, red, house mouse, tropical rat, fowl, and rodent) mites. All of these mites are extremely small (about 0.4 to 1 mm long), and depending on the species, the six-legged larvae or eight-legged nymphs and adults may attack humans. The resulting skin lesions may be extremely variable.

Differential diagnosis of mite-induced dermatitis depends on associating the patient with a source of mites. Sources include wild and domestic animals, agricultural commodities, infested furniture, and, in chigger-associated cases, particular outdoor habitats.

Treatment of dermatitis associated with biting mites is symptomatic. Antipruritic lotions and creams or oral antihistamines are useful. Secondary infections may require antibiotic therapy. Rare allergic reactions, including edema and asthma, require emergency treatment.

Prevention of recurrences is dependent on destruction or fumigation of the mite source. Personal repellents (containing sulfur or diethyl toluamide) are helpful in preventing chigger infestation, although avoidance of infested areas is the best prevention. *Rickettsia tsutsugamushi* is the only pathogen of major medical importance specifically associated with mite transmission. *R. akari*, the etiologic agent of rickettsialpox, is transmitted by the house mouse mite.

Krinsky WL: Dermatoses associated with the bites of mites and ticks (Arthropoda: Acari). Int J Dermatol 22:75, 1983. *This review includes a list of mites causing human dermatitis and discusses clinical findings.*

Parkhurst HJ: Trombidiosis (infestation with chiggers). Arch Dermatol Syphilol 35:1011, 1937. *This is an extensive review of the biology and clinical importance of chiggers.*

Tick Bites and Tick Paralysis

Ticks, like mites, are arachnids that have six-legged larvae and eight-legged nymphs and adults. Ticks, found worldwide, are grouped in two major families, soft ticks (Argasidae) and hard ticks (Ixodidae). The former, which have rugose integuments, are associated with restricted habitats, such as rodent burrows and bird nests, and rarely feed on humans. When they do, most attach for only a matter of minutes and produce maculate, erythematous lesions (6 to 30 mm in diameter). Some species in Africa cause extensive ecchymosis; pain, pruritus, edema, ulceration, and necrotic lesions have also been observed. The pajoroello (talaja) tick (*Ornithodoros coriaceus*), found in Mexico, California, and Oregon, is known to produce hemorrhagic, painful lesions. Soft ticks are of primary medical importance as vectors of the borreliae of relapsing fevers.

Hard ticks have smooth, hard, shiny integuments and are found on a diversity of animals and in tall grass and forests. Ticks carried on dogs, cats, or other animals sometimes drop off and attach to man. Hard ticks remain embedded in the skin for days while becoming engorged with blood and usually do not cause pain or discomfort. Engorging ticks, mistakenly identified as pedunculated moles or warts, are usually noticed only by chance observation. Typical tick bite lesions are small indurations with peripheral erythema. Unusual manifestations of hard tick bites include various forms of nonspecific dermatitis, acrodermatitis chronica atrophicans, necrotic ulcers, and alopecia. Most hard ticks attach, feed, drop off, and are never noticed. Nodular lesions that may persist for years at the sites of bites must be differentiated from malignant conditions, such as lymphomas. Hard ticks are vectors of the etiologic agents of various arboviral hemorrhagic fevers and encephalitides, several kinds of tick-borne typhus (including Rocky Mountain spotted fever), tularemia, babesiosis, and Lyme disease. An engorging tick itself may induce tick paralysis (discussed below).

Attached soft ticks may be easily removed by gentle traction with a forceps. Hard ticks require strong constant traction. Use of heat, flames, or caustic substances is ill-advised and may cause unnecessary damage to the patient. Hard ticks, embedded in sensitive sites, such as the ear canal or genitals, may be covered with petrolatum. The ticks then detach within about two hours and can be gently removed. Complete extraction of the mouthparts lessens the chance of secondary infection. Persistent nodules that cause discomfort should be surgically excised.

Tick paralysis is an unusual form of ascending flaccid paralysis that occurs while a tick is attached to the body. Mostly children (especially girls) are affected. Tick paralysis in humans has been associated with only a small number of hard tick species in North America, Europe, South Africa, and Australia. Most cases have been caused by female wood ticks, the Rocky Mountain wood tick (*Dermacentor andersoni*) in western North America and the common dog tick (*D. variabilis*) in eastern North America. Although nonspecific numbness or irritability may occur before the onset of paralysis, the initial consistent sign is *weakness in the legs*. Leg tendon reflexes are reduced or absent, and Romberg's sign is often present. Sensory changes are rarely noted. Blood counts and lumbar puncture usually give no indication of the disease. Complete paralysis of the extremities may occur within a few days after a tick attaches. If the cause is unrecognized, paralysis usually progresses, causing speech dysfunction, dysphagia, and ultimately death from aspiration or respiratory paralysis. If a tick is found, removal usually results in reversal of paralysis with a return to normal function in hours to weeks, depending on the severity of the neurologic deficit. The patient should be examined for other ticks, with special attention to concealed areas such as the scalp, ear canals, axillae, popliteal fossae, anus, and genitals. Even after all ticks are removed, death may occur in patients who exhibit bulbar or respiratory paralysis.

The clinical presentation of tick paralysis may suggest poliomyelitis, Guillain-Barré syndrome, diphtheritic polyneuropathy, transverse myelitis, botulism, or other acutely developing neuropathies. The specific etiologic agent of *Dermacentor* tick paralysis is unknown.

Prevention of tick bites and tick paralysis includes avoidance of tick-infested habitats. Individuals and their pets who enter such habitats should be thoroughly examined for ticks. Personal measures that may prevent ticks from reaching the skin include wearing long-sleeved shirts and long pants, tucking pants legs into socks, and using chemical repellents.

Gothe R, Kunze K, Hoogstraal H: The mechanisms of pathogenicity in the tick paralyses. J Med Entomol 16:357, 1979. *This review lists the tick species that have been associated with paralysis, general clinical aspects and experimental observations.*

Krinsky WL: Dermatoses associated with the bites of mites and ticks (Arthropoda: Acari). Int J Dermatol 22:75, 1983. *This is a review of skin lesions caused by acarines and epidemiologic and clinical factors helpful in diagnosis.*

Spider Bites

All spiders are eight-legged arachnids that use venom to immobilize their prey. Relatively few species have mouthparts (chelicerae) large and strong enough to inject venom into human skin. Among the better known spiders that cause

moderate to severe reactions in man are the widows (*Latrodectus* species) of the Old and New World, brown spiders (*Loxosceles* species) of the Americas, wandering spiders (*Phoneutria* species) and wolf spiders (*Lycosa* species) in South America, species of *Chiracanthium* in both hemispheres, funnel web spiders (*Atrax* species) in Australia, and *Harpactirella* species in South Africa.

The black widow (shoe button) spider (*Latrodectus mactans*) female may bite if it or its web is disturbed. Its abdomen is 6 mm wide and 9 to 13 mm long and is shiny black with a reddish hourglass marking or less well defined markings on the underside. The spider lives in sheltered, dark, dry places such as garages and in old stone walls and out-houses. The bite, which may not be felt, may become slightly swollen and appear as two erythematous puncture marks. Within a few hours, a bitten person develops intense muscle pains and commonly a tightening feeling in the chest. Abdominal (board-like) rigidity and waves of excruciating cramping pain are characteristic. Respiratory distress, nausea, vomiting, profuse perspiration, headache, vertigo, paresthesias of the extremities, and hyperactive reflexes are common. Speech difficulty and visual dysfunction may occur. In untreated adults, the pathologic effects of the venom usually disappear within two to three days. Death from cardiac or respiratory arrest occurs mostly in very young children and elderly or hypertensive persons.

Differential diagnosis requires consideration of various abdominal and vascular crises, such as perforated ulcer, acute appendicitis or pancreatitis, cholelithiasis, nephrolithiasis, splenic, renal, or mesenteric embolism, volvulus, porphyria, tetanus, and strychnine and lead poisoning. The generalized muscle pain, lack of abdominal tenderness, and the peripheral sensory changes help to differentiate the widow spider bite.

Treatment with muscle relaxants temporarily relieves muscle pains. A specific antivenin available from Merck Sharp and Dohme is effective against all *Latrodectus* venom and neutralizes the effects of the venom. Because the antivenin is derived from horses, horse serum sensitivity testing is required before the antivenin is administered.

The brown (violin or fiddleback) spiders, including *Loxosceles reclusa* (brown recluse) and *L. laeta* of the western hemisphere, are also secretive, living in secluded places in houses and nesting in clothing, and may bite when disturbed. They are 10 to 15 mm long and have a dark violin-shaped mark on the brown to gray cephalothorax. Their bites are most often recognized when a serious condition, *necrotic arachnidism*, is the result. The sometimes painful lesion that develops two to six hours after a bite is a bulla or pustule surrounded by concentric rings of ischemia and erythema. Within 24 to 48 hours the lesion becomes cyanotic, and a central necrotic area begins to form. This area may slowly expand (up to 20 cm) over days to weeks. The resulting ulcer may not heal for weeks or months. Systemic reactions to the bite include fever, chills, edema, nausea, vomiting, dizziness, myalgias, and arthralgias; morbilliform and petechial eruptions may occur within 48 hours of the bite. A fatal complication, most often seen in children, is *intravascular hemolysis*, followed by hemoglobinuria and acute renal failure.

Treatment of necrotizing lesions is mainly symptomatic and may include surgical debridement and antibiotic therapy for secondary infection. Systemic corticosteroid therapy has been successful in reducing symptoms and skin destruction. Skin grafts may be needed to promote healing of chronic lesions.

Maretic Z, Lebez D: Araneism with Special Reference to Europe. Belgrade, Yugoslavia, Nolit Publishing House, 1979. *This book has extensive clinical information about* Latrodectus *envenomation and biological and clinical discussions relevant to other spider bites.*

Millikan LE: Loxoscelism and other arachnid problems. In Parish LC, Nutting WB, Schwartzman RM (eds.): Cutaneous Infestations of Man and Animal. New York, Praeger, 1983, pp 284–295. *This chapter includes excellent photographs of the necrotic lesions caused by recluse spider bites and a discussion of pathophysiology and treatment.*

Southcott RV: Arachnidism and Allied Syndromes in the Australian Region. Rec Adelaide Child Hosp 1:99, 1976. *This detailed review treats basic biology and clinical aspects of arachnid bites and infestations and is relevant to much of the world's fauna.*

Centipede Bites

Centipedes are multilegged, elongated (up to 30 cm) arthropods with one pair of legs on each body segment. The first pair of legs is modified as poison claws that are used to inject venom into prey. Centipedes, which shun the light and are found under rocks and forest litter, rarely bite. The characteristic bite lesion has two punctate hemorrhages in the center of an erythematous swelling. Centipede bites may cause severe (fiery) local pain that may be followed by inflammation, edema, and superficial necrosis. Systemic reactions may include headache, dizziness, and vomiting. The transient effects of a bite may be accompanied by irregular pulse, muscle spasm, or lymphadenopathy. In general, centipede bites cause no long-term pathologic effects.

Southcott RV: Arachnidism and allied syndromes in the Australian region. Rec Adelaide Child Hosp 1:99, 1976. *This includes a careful review (pp 174–177) of clinical aspects of centipede bites and some case histories.*

Stinging Arthropods

Bee, Wasp, and Ant Stings

Bees, wasps, and ants (order Hymenoptera) are insects that include solitary and social species. Females have an egglaying tube (ovipositor) that has been modified as a sting that secretes venom from abdominal glands. Social bees include honeybees and bumblebees that all have two pairs of membranous wings, are stocky, hairy, and often yellow and black or brown. The honeybee (*Apis mellifera*) and its close relatives are found worldwide and often are responsible for human sting reactions. The honeybee has a barbed sting that becomes embedded in skin and, as the bee tries to escape, it leaves its venom apparatus and other abdominal organs and soon perishes. Vespid wasps (yellowjackets, hornets, paper wasps) are smooth insects, sleeker than bees and often yellow and black or with combinations of yellow, red, brown, or black. These wasps make the paper nests found in trees, under eaves of houses, or underground. Honeybees and bumblebees may sting when disturbed while seeking nectar or pollen at flowers. Vespid wasps may become pestiferous around food, being especially attracted to sweet or fermented liquids, fruit, and meats. Mutillid wasps (velvet ants, cow killers), which are hairy and wingless, sometimes sting persons in sandy, arid environments.

Human reactions to stings usually include intense local pain, followed by the appearance of a red punctum surrounded by a blanched area and erythema. A wheal forms and the swelling and erythema, accompanied by pruritus, may last for a few hours. Multiple stings, especially on the face, may cause extensive edema, severe skin lesions such as multiple vesicles or bullae, or purpura. Treatment includes gentle removal of the sting by scraping with a sharp blade (in cases of honeybee envenomation), application of ice, and topical hydrocortisone or oral antihistamines. Severe and sometimes fatal allergic reactions to stings of bees and wasps that occur in sensitized individuals are discussed in Ch. 423.

Ants (Formicidae) of some species can sting, causing severe pain. Two groups of New World stinging ants are the fire ants (*Solenopsis* species) and harvester ants (*Pogonomyrmex* species). These ants build ground nests that protrude as large mounds. An ant may grip the skin with its mandibles and then insert its sting. The ant may pivot and sting many times. This behavior, compounded by the common occurrence of mass attacks, leads to a clustering of lesions. The usual reaction to the sting is fiery, sharp pain, followed by a wheal and flare response. A clear vesicle appears that becomes pustular after about 24 hours. This sterile pustule may persist for three to ten days and dry as a crust that sloughs, leaving

a macule, scar, or fibrous nodule. Systemic reactions such as dizziness, nausea, vomiting, profuse perspiration, cyanosis, and asthma occur in allergic individuals, but may also be seen in cases of multiple stings. Symptomatic treatment of local reactions is similar to that for bee and wasp stings.

Harwood RF, James MT: Venoms, defense secretions, and allergens of arthropods. In Entomology in Human and Animal Health. 7th ed. New York, The Macmillan Company, 1979. *This is a review of the biology and clinical importance of stinging Hymenoptera.*
Paull BR: Imported fire ant allergy. Perspectives on diagnosis and treatment. Postgrad Med 76:155, 1984. *A well-illustrated review of the distribution and clinical aspects of fire ant stings.*

Scorpion Stings

Scorpions are mostly subtropical and tropical arachnids that have a pair of lobster-like claws (pedipalps) anteriorly and a curved spine posteriorly that is an outlet for the proteinaceous venom produced by a pair of venom glands. Scorpions are nocturnal predators that sting quickly and repeatedly when disturbed in their hiding places under rocks, lumber, vegetation or in shoes, bedding, or clothing left on the ground. In the United States, one scorpion species, *Centruroides sculpturatus*, of about 40 native species causes severe pathologic effects in humans. This small (about 6 cm long), straw-colored species is found only in Arizona. The arid regions that extend from North Africa to India are inhabited by the most abundant and dangerous scorpions.

The nature and severity of human reactions to scorpion stings are not consistent with the size, appearance, or aggressiveness of different species. Intense and immediate pain at the site of a sting is common to all cases. When a mildly toxic scorpion such as *C. vittatus*, a common southern United States species, is involved, the pain may be followed by local swelling and perhaps skin discoloration, regional lymphadenopathy, pruritus, or paresthesias, and less commonly by nausea and vomiting. These reactions are transient, lasting for minutes to as long as 24 hours. The more toxic species cause local pain but little or no skin response, and systemic effects are usually noted within a few minutes to 24 hours after the sting. Symptoms may include anxiety, drowsiness, syncope, increased salivation, lacrimation, perspiration, diminished vision, photophobia, numbness and sluggishness of the tongue, vomiting, diarrhea or involuntary defecation and micturition, priapism, muscular fibrillations or spasms, and convulsions. Clinical signs may include hypotension or hypertension, irregular pulse, tachycardia and arrhythmias, irregular respiration, rapid shifts in body temperature, oliguria or polyuria, and hemiplegia. Laboratory tests may reveal hyperglycemia, glycosuria, SGOT increase, hematuria, and melena. Pathologic changes that may lead to death include myocarditis, pulmonary edema, and shock. Respiratory paralysis is the usual immediate cause of death. In the most toxic cases, death may occur within minutes of the sting or not for over 40 hours later, but most deaths occur in 2 to 20 hours after the sting. The mortality is highest in children. Close monitoring of affected patients is important because sudden relapses, often involving acute respiratory distress, may occur after a patient's condition seems to have stabilized.

The most important treatment for moderate to very toxic stings is administration of an antivenin. Antivenin to *C. sculpturatus* is available in Arizona from the Antivenom Production Laboratory, Arizona State University, Tempe, Arizona 85281 (602-965-3116; outside of business hours 602-965-3456; ask for Dr. William Northey). Antivenins against other species are available from laboratories in Mexico, Brazil, Europe, Africa, and Asia.

Early treatment of stings may include cooling of the sting site for up to two hours and use of a local anesthetic. Oxygen administration or artificial respiration, sodium phenobarbital injection, and parenteral solutions, including blood plasma, may be needed to treat respiratory distress, convulsions, and shock, respectively. Calcium gluconate (10 ml of 10 per cent solution) given as a slow intravenous injection will reduce muscle spasms. In the United States, morphine and meperidine are contraindicated because they enhance the toxic effects of *C. sculpturatus* venom. Morphine and barbiturates are not recommended for treatment of any scorpion stings because these drugs inhibit the bulbar respiratory centers.

Personal protection includes wearing heavy gloves and boots when reaching into hidden areas in which scorpions may hide. Shaking out shoes and other materials left on the ground before using them is essential. Removal of litter from around houses, sealing cracks in foundations, and selective use of pesticides are helpful means of preventing scorpions from inhabiting houses and gardens.

Chippaux JP, Goyffon M: Producers of antivenomous sera. Toxicon 21:739, 1983. *Addresses of antivenom suppliers are listed in this article by type of venomous animal and continent.*
Keegan HL: Scorpions of Medical Importance. Jackson, University of Mississippi Press, 1980. *This book reviews scorpion morphology, taxonomy, biology, and geographic distribution, and clinical aspects and prevention of scorpion envenomation.*

Invasive Arthropods
Scabies

The scabies mite (*Sarcoptes scabiei*), unlike the other mites discussed, burrows into the skin and, because it reproduces on humans, can maintain a continuous infestation. Fertile female mites burrow into the skin and lay their eggs as they tunnel. Immature stages (larvae and nymphs) move out to the surface and enter hair follicles. Further development and mating take place near the skin surface. The mite burrows are slightly raised, curved, or tortuous gray lines, 5 to 15 mm long, and at the end of each is a female, a minute pearly bleb. The burrows are restricted to the horny layer of the skin and occur most often in the sides of the fingers, the interdigital webs, flexor surfaces of the wrists, elbows, skin around the nipples, and penis. Other lesions, including erythematous papules, lichenified patches, and pustules, which occur in sites other than the burrows, may be seen on the abdomen, thighs, and buttocks. In infants and young children, burrows may occur in the palms and soles, and papular lesions may be seen on the scalp, face, and neck.

Intense pruritus begins from two to six weeks after first exposure to the mite. Definitive diagnosis of the lesions is often difficult because of excoriations. In very clean individuals, few lesions may be present, and burrows may not be clearly visible. Generalized urticarial papules may result from previous treatment with fluorinated corticosteroids. Some patients have pruritic inflammatory nodules ($\le$ 12 mm in diameter) that occur on covered skin, especially the axillae, abdomen, scrotum, and penis. A severe form of scabies most often seen in immunologically compromised persons is called *crusted scabies* (originally called Norwegian scabies). As the name implies, warty plaques occur frequently on the hands and feet, and extensive scaling covers the scalp to the trunk or below. Horny debris collects under the fingernails, which are usually distorted and thickened. Pruritus, erythema, and lymphadenopathy may occur.

Diagnosis of any scabies infestation depends on observation of a mite in skin scrapings of a burrow or in situ, by gently raising the top of a burrow with a sterile needle and looking with a magnifier. In most scabies cases, only 10 to 15 mites are present on the body. In crusted scabies, large numbers of mites are present. To obtain a scraping of a burrow, an area suspected of infestation is scraped with a scalpel blade. The scaped material is examined at 50 to 100 times magnification. The movements of a living mite may be observed if the material is placed on a slide without any mounting media. Otherwise the scraping may be cleared in potassium hydroxide (20 per cent) or suspended in mineral oil under a coverslip on the slide. The adult female mite is about 300 to 400 μm long, oval, with the dorsum convex and venter flattened. It

has four pairs of legs, two pairs directed anteriorly and two posteriorly. Each anterior leg ends in an unjointed stalk with a distensible thin-walled sac at its tip; each posterior leg ends in a long, thick bristle. The size of the mite egg is about 100 × 150 μm.

Scabies lesions initially may be diagnosed as those of other skin conditions, e.g., neurodermatitis, dermatitis herpetiformis, lichen planus, and various other kinds of mite-associated dermatitis, such as that caused by *Cheyletiella* fur mites. The distribution of lesions and observation of the mite will rule out these other diagnoses. Secondary infections appearing as pyoderma are common, and nephrogenic strains of streptococci infecting the lesions may cause acute glomerulonephritis.

Treatment of uncomplicated scabies involves application of one of various acaricides. Lindane (1 per cent) cream or lotion is often used in a manner similar to that suggested for pediculosis; namely, an 8- to 12-hour treatment for adults, followed by thorough washing. The treatment should not be repeated more than once in seven days. Use of lindane on infants and pregnant women is discouraged. Pruritus and dermatitis may persist for days after adequate treatment. Antipruritic medications are often prescribed. Topical corticosteroids are contraindicated because of the urticarial reaction they sometimes cause.

Transmission occurs during contact with infested persons or with clothing recently worn by such persons. Transmission between bed partners is common and does not require bodily contact. All household and intimate contacts should be treated to prevent recurrence or continued transmission. The female mite will survive for only two to three days away from a host; therefore, as with louse infestations, fumigation of premises is unnecessary. Clothing, especially undergarments, bedding, and towels, should be laundered in hot water.

Scabies mites infesting domestic animals, including dogs and cats, occasionally cause dermatitis in humans, but the lesions are usually limited to the areas that contact the animals. These mites are usually not recovered from humans.

Burkhart CG: Scabies: An epidemiologic reassessment. Ann Intern Med 98:498, 1983. *This article reviews clinical and epidemiologic aspects of scabies.*
Mellanby K: Scabies. Middlesex, England, E. W. Classey (1943), 1972. *This classic work available in this reprinted form is a comprehensive review of the basic biology, clinical evolution, and treatment of scabies.*

Myiasis and Tungiasis

Myiasis is the infestation of living vertebrate tissue by fly larvae. Many flies (order Diptera) that normally deposit eggs or larvae on carrion, manure, or decaying organic matter sometimes deposit their immature stages in open wounds or infected human tissues. These include blow flies, also called greenbottle or bluebottle flies (Calliphoridae), flesh flies (Sarcophagidae), and house flies (Muscidae). The larvae of some of these flies are attracted to draining infections, or clothing stained with urine or feces.The larvae crawl into lesions or natural orifices when an infected person sleeps on the ground or is otherwise exposed to flies. Individuals immobilized because of physical illness or old age who have such open lesions or infections, and especially those who are living in poor sanitary conditions, are particularly susceptible. Urogenital myiasis may cause dysuria, hematuria, and pyuria.

Some fly larvae always invade intact skin of domestic animals or humans; species in this group include the human bot fly (*Dermatobia hominis*) found in Central and South America, the African tumbu fly *Cordylobia anthropophaga*, and some species of *Wohlfahrtia* that have a predilection for the tender skin of infants.

Fly larvae that live in food, e.g., vinegar flies (Drosophilidae) and cheese skippers (Piophilidae), are sometimes accidentally ingested and may cause gastrointestinal discomfort.

Wound or dermal myiasis often results in furuncular lesions, and an infested individual notices a swelling and feels pain or movement under the skin where the larvae are feeding on tissue fluids. Careful observation of the top of a lesion enables one to see two dark respiratory openings (spiracles) through which the larva breathes. Treatment consists of gentle compression of the swelling and removal of the larva with a forceps. A local anesthetic may be helpful because recurved spines may hold the larva tightly under the skin. Topical antibiotics are used to control or prevent secondary infections. Removal of larvae that crawl into sensory openings or urogenital and anal orifices may require irrigation or surgical intervention. Intestinal myiasis is usually self-limited, ceasing when the larvae are passed in the stool. Dermal myiasis of most kinds, if untreated, progresses until the mature larvae back out of the skin and drop to the ground to pupate. The physical and emotional distress caused by the presence of living larvae can be prevented if a physician considers the possibility of such an infestation and removes the larvae early in the infestation. Warble fly larvae, which normally migrate from the legs of cattle through the body to the back, in human infestations will also migrate dorsally and, unless they reach a cutaneous exit site, may cause extensive tissue damage that leads to chronic illness or death.

Prevention of myiasis requires frequent changing of dressings on wounds and use of screening.

Tungiasis is the infestation of vertebrate, including human, skin by the female flea *Tunga penetrans* (chigoe, jigger, or sand flea). This flea occurs in sandy soil in subtropical and tropical regions of the Americas, the West Indies, and Africa. It usually feeds between the toes, under a toenail, or in the sole of the foot, and becomes embedded as it gorges on blood. The flea, which remains embedded permanently, may cause irritation, pain, or pruritus, and the resulting swelling is often pustular. Secondary skin infections and tetanus are complications of infestations, and autoamputation of digits in Africans is apparently caused by inflammatory reactions to the flea.

Treatment of tungiasis includes removal of the flea with a sterile needle or blade, tetanus vaccination, and application of topical antibiotics. Personal protection against *T. penetrans* includes wearing footwear and using insect repellent. Sleeping above the ground surface usually prevents the flea from reaching the body.

Brothers W, Heckmann R: Tungiasis (*Tunga penetrans*) in Utah. J Parasitol 65:782, 1979. *This note succinctly describes the clinical problem and gives references to cases.*
Harwood RB, James MT: Myiasis. In Entomology in Human and Animal Health. New York, The Macmillan Company, 1979. *This is a thorough review of different clinical forms of myiasis.*

Arthropods and Contact Dermatitis

Various species of nonbiting mites found in stored products may cause dermatitis when they contact human skin. These microscopic foodstuff mites (Acaridae, Glycyphagidae) are found in commodities, including grains, cereals, seeds, bulbs, dried herbs, copra, dried vegetables, cured meats, mushrooms, humus, cheese, and animal and plant material used for stuffing furniture, pillows, and mattresses. Dried fruit mites (Carpoglyphidae) are found not only in dried fruits but also in jams, jellies, spoiled fruit, wine, caramel, flour, and dried milk products. The skin reactions to these mites vary, but pruritic diffuse erythema with urticarial wheals or erythematous papular eruptions are common. Laborers in granaries, food processing plants, and commercial kitchens and dockworkers are most susceptible.

Another form of pruritic dermatitis is caused by contact with various caterpillars, pupae, adults, and some egg masses of moths and butterflies (order Lepidoptera). Urticating setae and spines on these life stages may cause mechanical irritation of the skin or may have toxic effects. Contact with setae, spines, or hairs may cause intense stinging or fiery pain, followed by the formation of wheals, local edema, erythema,

and pruritus. Less common reactions include lymphadenopathy, cephalalgia, shocklike symptoms, or convulsions.

Treatment of dermatitis caused by foodstuff and dried fruit mites or lepidopteran spines or setae is symptomatic. Antipruritic substances, including antihistamines, corticosteroids, and anesthetics, have been used. Commodities containing mites must be fumigated or destroyed. Spines or setae of lepidopterans may be removed from the skin with fine forceps. Use of protective clothing and thorough washing of exposed materials will help prevent continuation of these forms of dermatitis.

A third form of contact dermatitis results from vesicants produced by blister beetles (Meloidae) and some rove beetles (Staphylinidae). Cantharidin, first isolated from the meloid called the Spanish fly, is found in all species of blister beetles. Contact with this substance causes mild to severe vesicular dermatitis.

Similar lesions, which usually follow a burning sensation and tanning of the skin, result from contact with millipedes. Some species of these herbivorous myriapods exude a fluid from pores along the length of the body. Secretions from the aforementioned beetles or millipedes will cause burning pain and conjunctivitis if they are rubbed into the eyes.

Treatment of toxic dermatitis associated with beetles or millipedes includes rapid washing of the skin or eyes, if affected, and use of local anesthetics. The dermal reactions caused by contact with mites, lepidopterans, beetles, and millipedes are usually transitory and do not have long-lasting effects.

Harwood RB, James MT: Vesicating Coleoptera. In Entomology in Human and Animal Health. New York, The Macmillan Company, 1979, pp 441–443. *This section discusses the nature of vesicant chemicals from beetles and reviews clinical cases.*
Radford AJ: Millipede burns in man. Trop Geogr Med 27:279, 1975. *Geographic distribution, toxicology, pathogenesis, clinical features, and treatment of millipede envenomation are carefully reviewed.*
Southcott RV: Lepidoptera and Skin Infestation. In Parish LC, Nutting WB, Schwartzman RM (eds.): Cutaneous Infestations of Man and Animal. New York, Praeger, 1983, pp 304–343. *This chapter gives a comprehensive review of worldwide lepidopterism, including pathogenesis and clinical presentations.*

PENTASTOMIASIS (Linguatuliasis)

Pentastomiasis is infestation with pentastomids, little-known invertebrates called tongue worms, which have been variously classified as arthropods or helminths. These blood-sucking endoparasites are found as adults in the lungs of reptiles and birds or in the nasal cavity of carnivores, especially cats and dogs. Herbivores are normal intermediate hosts, but humans and other mammals can be dead-end aberrant hosts for the larvae. Ingested eggs hatch and the larvae burrow through the intestine and migrate to diverse tissues where they molt several times and become encysted as third-stage larvae.

Human infestations have occurred in Europe, Africa, and North, Central, and South America. Two species account for most cases, *Armillifer armillatus*, found in pythons and other vipers in tropical Africa, and *Linguatula serrata*, found in canids in Europe and the Near and Middle East.

Infection occurs by accidental ingestion of tongue worm eggs contaminating food or drink, by ingestion of eggs picked up on fingers from handling infected snakes or lizards, or by ingestion of improperly cooked or raw reptiles. The third-stage larvae (20 to 25 mm long) encysted in fibrous capsules occur most often in the liver and are rarely noted except incidentally at autopsy or as calcified cysts (3 to 6 mm in diameter) on x-ray examination. Rarely, a mass of cysts in the intestinal wall may cause obstruction. Cysts compressing vital structures such as bile ducts or bronchi may lead to infections or obstructions.

Linguatuliasis, the direct infection of humans with third-stage larvae of *Linguatula* species, occurs most often in Lebanese people who eat raw or inadequately cooked liver or lymph nodes of goats and sheep. The ingested larvae migrate to the nasopharynx from the stomach. These larvae (5 to 10 mm long) cause Halzoun's syndrome, characterized by paroxysmal coughing, sneezing, nasal and lacrimal discharge, accompanied by pain and itching in the throat. Other symptoms may include hoarseness, dyspnea, dysphagia, and vomiting. Submaxillary and cervical lymph nodes may be enlarged. Recovery in most cases is spontaneous in seven to ten days; however, death from asphyxiation due to tonsillar edema has been reported. A similar syndrome seen in Sudan, Turkey, and Greece is called Marrara's syndrome.

Prevention of pentastomiasis includes proper cooking of exotic foods such as herbivore organs and reptiles, improved hygiene of persons handling reptiles, and ingestion only of clean water and thoroughly washed raw vegetables.

Herzog U, Marty P, Zak F: Pentastomiasis: Case report of an acute abdominal emergency. Acta Trop 42:261, 1985. *This report reviews clinical and epidemiologic information.*

Hopps HC, Keegan HL, Price DL, Self JT: Pentastomiasis. In Marcial-Rojas RA (ed.): Pathology of Protozoal and Helminthic Diseases. Baltimore, Williams & Wilkins Company, 1971, pp 970–989. *This is a comprehensive review that includes basic biologic and clinical information.*

LEECHES AS AGENTS OF DISEASE (Hirudiniasis)

Leeches of medical importance are bloodsucking annelid worms. Each has a ventral anterior or posterior sucker. The former encloses teeth that cut through the skin after the leech attaches. Feeding occurs within a half hour or more.

The leeches most often feeding on humans are aquatic (fresh water) species of *Hirudo,* the cosmopolitan medicinal leeches; *Limnatis,* the nasal leeches found from the Canary Islands east through Europe, Africa, and Asia; *Dinobdella,* found in Asia; and terrestrial species of *Haemadipsa,* found in Asia, Indonesia, Australia, Pacific Islands, and Central and South America. Humans are subject to attack by large leeches in tropical rain forests or infestation with aquatic species while wading or swimming.

Wounds produced by leeches often go unnoticed, except for the oozing blood or prolonged bleeding caused by an anticoagulant, hirudin. Pruritus is common at bite sites, and although leeches are not known to transmit any human pathogens, secondary infections may occur. Immature aquatic leeches may be ingested with water and infest the upper respiratory and digestive tracts or may invade the mouth, nose, eyes, vagina, urethra, or anus of swimmers.

Attachment of leeches to the nasal passages may cause epistaxis. Attachment to the larynx may cause hoarseness, dyspnea, and hemoptysis, and attachment to the pharynx or esophagus may cause dysphagia and hematemesis. Hemorrhaging from leech infestations may be so severe, especially in children, that anemia occurs that leads to death.

Techniques used for removing leeches from the respiratory and digestive tracts include a steady pull on the specimen with a forceps or hemostat, or narcotizing the leech with a spray of 5 per cent cocaine hydrochloride before removal. In genitourinary infestations, irrigation with a strong salt solution may cause the leeches to detach. A leech attached to skin or respiratory or digestive tract surfaces may be induced to release its grip by holding it in a hemostat and touching the exposed part of the worm with a small flame or other cauterant.

Prevention of attack by aquatic and land leeches includes use of protective clothing and of insect repellents. Repellents applied to boots, trouser legs, and exposed skin are quite effective, but, because they are water soluble, must be reapplied every few hours in wet tropical regions where leeches are commonly found.

Keegan HL, Radke MG, Murphy DA: Nasal leech infestation in man. Am J Trop Med Hyg 19:1029, 1970. *This paper discusses two cases and reviews other clinical reports and treatment.*

415 SNAKE BITES
Jay P. Sanford

EPIDEMIOLOGY. Of the nearly 3500 species of snakes, fewer than one tenth are venomous. The poisonous varieties belong to five families (Table 415–1). Throughout the world, snake bites are estimated to account for 30,000 to 40,000 deaths annually. The largest number occur in Burma and Brazil. In the United States the number of snake bites is estimated at 8000 per year. Some 20 to 30 per cent of the bites by venomous snakes in the United States do not result in envenomation (poisoning). Most bites occur in the states bordering on the Gulf of Mexico. Despite the large number of bites with envenomation, fewer than 15 deaths occur, and almost all of these are due to rattlesnake bites. This low case fatality ratio reflects the virtual absence of members of the species Elapidae and Hydrophidae in the United States.

Coral snakes, eastern and western varieties, are found in southern and western states (North Carolina, South Carolina, Georgia, Florida, Alabama, Mississippi, Louisiana, Arkansas, Texas, New Mexico, Arizona). Their fangs are short and permanently erect. They envenomate through chewing movements. Since they are nocturnal and shy, they rarely bite humans.

The pit vipers (Crotalidae) are identified by a small depression between the eyes and nostrils. Their fangs are long and hinged, folding back when the mouth is closed and erect when open. Upon contact, venom is expressed by muscular contraction. The pit vipers are generally aggressive. The eastern (*Crotalus adamanteus*) and western (*C. atrox*) diamondback rattlesnakes are the largest and most dangerous in the United States. Their distribution includes the aforementioned states plus California, Nevada, and Oklahoma. Cottonmouths (*Agkistrodon piscivorus*), or water moccasins, are found along streams in the southern and southeastern states. They may inflict facial bites when disturbed while resting on tree branches. Contrary to lore, they can bite under water. Copperheads (*A. contortrix*), or highland moccasins, have a geographic distribution similar to the cottonmouths. Their bite is painful but rarely fatal.

PATHOGENESIS. Snake venoms are probably the most complex of all poisons. Because of the heterogeneous composition and multiplicity of effects, snake venoms cannot be classified simply as neurotoxic, cardiotoxic, myotoxic, or hematotoxic on the basis of the snake family (Table 415–2).

Venoms from Elapidae and Hydrophidae contain basic polypeptides that produce presynaptic and/or postsynaptic neuromuscular block with resultant flaccid paralysis, including respiratory paralysis. Cobra cardiotoxin, an additional basic polypeptide, depolarizes cell membranes of skeletal, cardiac, and smooth muscles, thus contributing to paralysis.

TABLE 415–1. VENOMOUS SNAKES OF THE WORLD

Family	Common Varieties	Geographic Distribution
Crotalidae	Pit vipers (rattlesnakes, water moccasins, copperheads), fer-de-lance, bushmaster	Americas, Asia
Elapidae	Cobras, kraits, mambas, coral snakes, death adder	Worldwide except Europe
Colubridae	Boomslangs, bird snakes	Africa
Hydrophidae	Sea snakes	Indo-Pacific waters
Viperidae	True vipers, puff adder	Worldwide except Americas

TABLE 415–2. BIOCHEMISTRY OF SNAKE VENOMS

Toxins	Family	Mechanism of Injury-Death
Neurotoxin (basic polypeptide)	Elapidae, Hydrophidae, South American rattlesnake (Crotalus durissus terrificus), Palestine viper (Vipera palestinae)	Respiratory paralysis
Cardiotoxin	Elapidae	Cardiovascular depression
Enzymes Phospholipase A 5-Nucleotidase Phosphodiesterase Deoxyribonuclease II Ribonuclease Adenosine-triphosphatase Nucleotide pyrophosphatase Exopeptidase Hyaluronidase L-amino acid oxidase	Elapidae, Hydrophidae, Crotalidae, Viperidae (Absent in spitting cobra)	Hemolysis
Proteases	Crotalidae, Viperidae	Hypotension due to release
Acetylcholinesterase	Elapidae (absent in spitting cobra, mamba, coral)	
Alkaline phosphatase		
Acid phosphatase		

Venom of the South American rattlesnake contains an acidic protein with nondepolarizing curare-like neuromuscular blocking effects. Viperatoxin isolated from the Palestine viper causes a peripheral nerve conduction block. A variety of enzymes, mostly hydrolases and phospholipase A, are present in most venoms. Bradykinin is released from bradykininogen by most crotalid and viperid venoms but not by Elapidae except the king cobra (Ophiophagus hannah). The venom of a single snake seldom contains all of the toxins. The composition and potency of venom is highly variable and differs not only among species but even among individual snakes.

SYMPTOMS AND SIGNS. *Pit Viper Envenomation.* In the United States, most victims reach a physician within 15 minutes to 3 hours. At that time it is essential to determine whether or not envenomation has occurred and, if it has occurred, to determine the severity; this has important therapeutic implications. The clinical effects are summarized in Table 415–3. The most important early findings of envenomation are swelling at the bite, usually occurring within ten minutes, and pain, although pain may be absent. Mild envenomation is characterized by local edema (one to five inches in diameter) and pain without systemic symptoms or signs. With moderate envenomation, local findings are more extensive—edema of six to twelve inches in diameter. Systemic

findings occur: weakness, sweating, nausea, faintness, dizziness, ecchymoses, and tender regional lymph nodes. With severe envenomation systemic involvement includes tachycardia; tachypnea; hypothermia; hypotension; ecchymoses; paresthesias of the scalp, finger and toe tips; and muscle fasciculations. With very severe envenomation, gingival bleeding, hematemesis, hematuria, melena, oliguria, and coma occur.

Over the first 12 hours, the skin develops a tense discolored appearance and bullae, which may be either serous or hemorrhagic.

Coral Snake Envenomation. The bite wound usually resembles scratch marks and is somewhat painful, but there is little or no edema. The onset of systemic manifestations is usually delayed one to six hours. Paresthesias around the bite may occur within several hours. Systemic symptoms may include weakness, apprehension, giddiness, nausea, vomiting, excess salivation, and even a sense of euphoria. Bulbar and cranial nerve paralysis may develop with ptosis, diplopia, papillary dilation, excess salivation, dysphagia, dysphonia, and respiratory failure.

LABORATORY FINDINGS. Proteolytic enzymes in venoms produce not only tissue damage but have a marked effect on coagulation, thrombin-like activity being most prominent. Within the first few hours there is a drop in platelets due to local consumption (occasionally to less than 10,000 per milliliter), a decrease in fibrinogen, and an increase in fibrin degradation products. Striking increases in prothrombin time and partial thromboplastin time occur with severe envenomation. Erythrocytes show a peculiar ''burring'' indicating membrane damage, and drops in hematocrit and hemoglobin concentration occur.

With pit viper envenomation, baseline laboratory tests should include complete blood count, platelet count, prothrombin time, partial thromboplastin time, bleeding time, urinalysis, and serum electrolytes. Blood should be obtained for typing and cross matching. In patients with envenomation of moderate or greater severity arterial blood gas determinations and an electrocardiogram are indicated. Hematologic studies should be repeated every four to six hours for the first day or until the coagulopathy has stabilized. With coral snake envenomation, repetitive coagulation studies are not indicated.

TREATMENT. *First Aid.* The initial goal of first aid is to minimize systemic absorption of the toxin. This is accomplished by restraining the patient to minimize muscular activity, application of compressive dressings, and transport to the hospital with as little patient effort as circumstances permit. With neurotoxic venoms, absorption may result in respiratory arrest for which resuscitation is essential. The snake should be killed if this can be done quickly and safely and taken along with the patient to allow accurate identification; this may obviate unnecessary therapy. The dead snake must be handled with care since the head of an apparently dead snake can deliver a venomous bite for up to an hour after being severed. The potential value of incision and suction is less than the risks, which include delay in antivenom administration. The site of the bite should be wiped but not incised.

TABLE 415–3. PIT VIPER ENVENOMATION: SYMPTOMS AND SIGNS (PERCENTAGE)

Local		Generalized		Systemic Hematologic		Neuromuscular	
Fang marks	100	Weakness	70	Thrombocytopenia	42	Paresthesia scalp, fingertips	63
Edema	74	Tachycardia	60	Increased clotting time	37	Faintness, dizziness	57
Pain	65	Hypotension	54	Decreased hemoglobin	37	Paresthesias of affected part	57
Vesicles	40	Sweating	43	Burring of RBC	18	Fasciculations	41
Necrosis	27	Nausea/vomiting	42	Thrombocytosis	16		
		Hypothermia	42	Bleeding	15		
		Tachypnea	40				
		Regional adenopathy	40				

Adapted from Russell FE: Snake venom poisoning in the United States. Ann Rev Med 31:247, 1980.

Incisions can aggravate bleeding, damage nerves and tendons, introduce infection, especially with mouth suction, and delay healing. An absorption-delaying compressive bandage, preferably crepe (not a tourniquet) should immediately be applied firmly, as for a sprain, over the bite site and up the entire limb. The affected part should be immobilized (splinted) promptly. If available, an inflatable splint will provide both compression and immobilization. The patient should be promptly transported to the nearest medical treatment facility. The compressive bandage should not be released during transit. The affected area should not be placed on ice. Cryotherapy results in greater tissue damage with the potential for necessitating amputation.

Hospital Care. On admission it is important to determine, if possible, if the bite was inflicted by a pit viper or a coral snake and whether envenomation has occurred. The mainstay of therapy is antivenom (antivenin), which is a horse serum product; hence it has a high potential of causing serum sickness later. There are two antivenoms: one polyvalent for North American pit vipers and another for eastern coral snakes. For minor envenomation, antivenin is not indicated. For more serious envenomation, antivenin should be administered. For mild pit viper envenomation, three to five ampules of antivenin should be diluted (10 ml each), then added to 500 ml of intravenous fluid. Skin or conjunctival sensitivity tests are unreliable in predicting early reactions to antivenom. Treatment should not be delayed 20 to 30 minutes awaiting results. All patients given antivenom should be regarded as likely to have a reaction; incidence ranges from 3 to 54 per cent. Epinephrine should be available in a syringe before the infusion is started. At the first sign of anaphylactoid reaction, bronchospasm, hypotension, or angioedema, the infusion should be stopped and 0.5 ml of 1:1000 epinephrine injected intramuscularly. This is almost always effective, and the antivenom infusion can be. restarted. A history of allergy to horse serum contraindicates antivenom unless the risk of death from envenomation is high, and the patient is pretreated with epinephrine. The 500 ml should be given intravenously over 60 minutes. If the amount is adequate, the swelling will not progress and paresthesias will decrease. If progression occurs, the dose should be repeated. For moderate envenomation 5 to 10 vials, for severe envenomation 10 to 20 vials, and for very severe envenomation up to 40 vials (400 ml) may be required. In one series, the average dose required for adults with severe bites was 16 vials. Larger doses are required for bites in children and for those involving the fingers. Antivenin neutralizes both the local and systemic effects of the venom.

In coral snake bites, if any symptoms or signs develop within the first several hours, 3 to 5 vials of antivenin (*Micrurus fulvius*) should be given intravenously. Even in the absence of symptoms, patients should be observed in the hospital for approximately 48 hours because onset of symptoms may be delayed and insidious. If neurotoxic signs appear (Table 415–3) an edrophonium test should be done: atropine sulfate (0.6 mg) by slow intravenous infusion followed by edrophonium chloride (10 mg) intravenously over two minutes. If improvement occurs, neostigmine methylsulfate should be administered (beginning with 25 μg per kilogram of body weight per hour) by continuous infusion.

Antibiotics are usually recommended. Bacteriologic cultures of rattlesnake venom and fangs show growth from over 90 per cent. Aerobic gram-negative bacilli (*Enterobacter* sp., *Pseudomonas* sp., and *Citrobacter* sp.) and histotoxic clostridia (*Clostridum perfringens*) are the predominant isolates. On the basis of the microbiologic results, administration of one of the newer beta-lactam antibiotics, piperacillin or azlocillin, is most appropriate. A tetanus toxoid booster is recommended.

In the severely envenomated patient, concurrent supportive measures include the management of shock and respiratory and renal failure. Glucocorticoids have been recommended,

but a controlled trial of prednisone therapy helped neither local nor systemic effects of viperine poisoning. Despite the hypofibrinogenemia and increase in fibrin degradation products, heparin is not of benefit.

Decompressive fasciotomy is indicated only if edema within closed muscular compartments is inadequately controlled and arterial blood supply is compromised. From the end of the first to the third week the majority of patients will develop serum sickness, the prevalence approximating 1 per cent per milliliter of horse serum administered. Steroids are useful for treatment of serum sickness reactions.

PROGNOSIS. If adequate antivenom was administered intravenously, mortality is virtually nil. If cryotherapy was avoided, amputation or serious resultant deformities are uncommon.

Curry SC, Kraner JC, Kunkel DB, et al.: Noninvasive vascular studies in management of rattlesnake envenomations to extremities. Ann Emerg Med 14:1081, 1985. *Provides details for monitoring, using noninvasive arterial studies. All but one of 25 patients received antivenin, and none underwent early surgical decompression.*

Jimenez-Porras JM: Biochemistry of snake venoms. Clin Toxicol 3:389, 1970. *A detailed review of the enzymatic and toxic properties of smake venoms with an extensive bibliography.*

Malasit P, Warrell DA, Chanthavanich P, et al.: Prediction, prevention and mechanism of early (anaphylactic) antivenom reactions in victims of snake bites. Br Med J 292:17, 1986. *A study demonstrating the futility of intradermal and conjunctival tests for hypersensitivity.*

Reid HA, Theakston RDG: The management of snake bite. Bull WHO 61:885, 1983. *An excellent, concise summary of epidemiology, pathophysiology, and treatment of snake bite.*

Russell FE: Snake venom poisoning in the United States. Ann Rev Med 31:247, 1980. *An excellent general review by one of the foremost authorities on the subject in the United States. An excellent source of clinical features.*

Simon TL, Grace TG: Envenomation coagulopathy in wounds from pit vipers. N Engl J Med 305:443, 1981. *This study on experimental envenomation in rabbits enables a sequential assessment of the clotting abnormalities that occur.*

Warrell DA, Looareesuwan S, Theakston RGD, et al: Randomized comparative trial of three monospecific antivenoms for bites by the Malayan pit viper (Calloselasma rhodostoma) in southern Thailand: Clinical and laboratory correlations. Am J Trop Med Hyg 35:1235, 1986. *The authors' clinical observations are very helpful in understanding management and complications.*

416 VENOMOUS AND POISONOUS* MARINE ANIMALS

John Williamson

The world's seas contain a formidable array of venomous and poisonous marine creatures capable of harming or even killing the human intruder. The story of their relationship to humankind dates from antiquity but their scientific study remains relatively neglected. The animals are found in greatest variety and profusion in warmer tropical and subtropical waters—the very seas that attract human activities. Communities dependent on the seas as a food source or as a tourist attraction are typically foremost in studying the subject. Current research is being conducted in Australia, French Polynesia, Japan, Southeast Asia, Greece, India, and the United States (including Hawaii). Although the subject has now emerged from the realm of folklore, lack of objectivity still causes misconceptions. *Human injury by venomous marine creatures results from accidental or intentional human interference with the animal or its territory.*

TAXONOMIC CLASSIFICATION

Taxonomic classification has been customary, but is of limited practical value to those responsible for treatment and

---

*The currently held view is that the administration of venoms requires mechanical penetration, whereas the term *poison* implies oral ingestion. The term *toxins* (here marine zootoxins) refers to both venoms and poisons.

**TABLE 416–1. MARINE ANIMALS
CAUSING HUMAN FATALITIES**

I. **From Envenomation**
  A. Invertebrates
    1. Box jellyfish (*Chironex fleckeri, Chiropsolmus quadrigatus*)
    2. Blue-ringed octopuses (Family *Octopodidae*)
    3. Venomous cone shells (Family *Conidae*)
  B. Vertebrates
    1. Venomous sea snakes (Family *Hydrophidae*)
    2. Scorpionfishes, including stonefishes (Family *Scorpaenidae*)
    3. Catfish (Suborder *Siluroidei*)
    4. Stingrays (Order *Rajiformes*)
II. **From Poisoning**
  A. Ciguatoxic fishes
  B. Tetrodotoxic fishes
  C. Shellfish
  D. Sea turtles
  E. Viscera of whales, porpoises, polar bears, walruses, seals

prevention of marine envenomation. The animals listed in Table 416–1 have accounted for the majority of human deaths and a significant number of the poisonings and injuries that are documented to date.

ANIMALS CAUSING HUMAN FATALITIES

Table 416–1 lists invertebrates and vertebrates that have caused fatalities by envenomation and animals responsible for fatal poisonings in humans.

Box Jellyfish

The northern Australian box jellyfish (*Chironex fleckeri*) and the Phillipines' closely related *Chiropsolmus quadrigatus*, the world's only coelenterates known to be lethal to humans, have been responsible for 74 documented human deaths since 1884; many more fatalities remain unconfirmed. Found only in tropical West Indo-Pacific waters, they are true jellyfish, carrying up to 60 extendable tentacles. These tentacles bear a vast number of nematocysts (stinging capsules, including microbasic mastigophores) that discharge massively when a person blunders into them and becomes entangled. The animals are difficult to see under natural conditions. This massive envenomation produces rapid systemic absorption that is enhanced by struggling, and collapse occurs within minutes in serious cases. Seventy per cent of fatalities occur in women and children (small body mass and hairless skin). The venom of *Chironex fleckeri* at least is a high-molecular-weight protein mixture containing "lethal" and dermatonecrotic factors. Research into the toxic and immunologic properties of this venom is proceeding.

The densely adherent tentacles produce whip wheals with a diagnostic ladder pattern on the envenomated skin. Treatment is immediate resuscitation on the beach, vinegar dousing, compressive bandaging, and injection of the specific antivenom, intravenously if possible, in a dosage large enough to be effective. The antivenom is sheep antiserum; therefore, appropriate precautions are necessary.

Blue-Ringed Octopus

At least two species (*Hapalochlaena maculosa* and *H. lunulata*) have produced morbidity and mortality. The venom is located in the salivary glands and is injected by a bite that may be painless. The salivary toxin contains tetrodotoxin (M.W. 319), a unique biologic material also found in the flesh of puffer fish (see below). It inhibits action potentials (Fig. 416–1) by specific blockade of sodium ion transport and is thus in addition a valuable physiologic research tool. Clinically the danger is respiratory failure and hypoxia. Airway protection and expired air resuscitation will be lifesaving. There is no antivenom. First aid is as for snakebite (see Ch. 415), and must include compression-immobilization bandaging.

Venomous Cone Shells

There are 37 cases of cone shell envenomation in the literature, eight of them fatalities. Seven species of cone shells are considered dangerous. The injected venom produces postsynaptic neuromuscular blockade (Fig. 416–1) and thus death from hypoxia (respiratory failure). On-the-spot airway protection and expired air resuscitation will be lifesaving. No antivenom presently exists, but research is promising. First aid is identical to that for snakebite, and must include compression-immobilization bandaging.

Venomous Sea Snakes

Apart from the predominance of these snakes in warmer waters, the proven lethality of several species, and the availability of a specific antivenom (*Enhydrina schistosa* antivenom—Melbourne and Bombay), the subject of sea snakebite can be considered in the same manner as land snakebite. Early application of compression-immobilization bandages to the bite site is crucial first-aid treatment for sea (and most terrestrial) snakebite.

Scorpionfishes and Stonefishes

Deaths from zebrafish stings have been documented. No firm record of a fatality from stonefish (*Synanceja*) stings has been located from Australia, where these stings are not uncommon. In this group of animals dorsal spines inject the venom. The ensuing pain is a devastating experience, with intense local tissue swelling and discoloration. Immersion of the envenomated part in hot water offers partial pain relief. Medical management is concerned with pain relief (conduction anesthesia), prevention of wound infection, and in the case of stonefish stings specific antivenom injection, with appropriate precautions. Tourniquets or compressive bandages should not be used.

Catfish and Stingrays

Despite their ubiquity, these animals rarely cause human death. Pieces of the brittle stingray spines may break off in wounds, necessitating careful exploration under anesthesia.

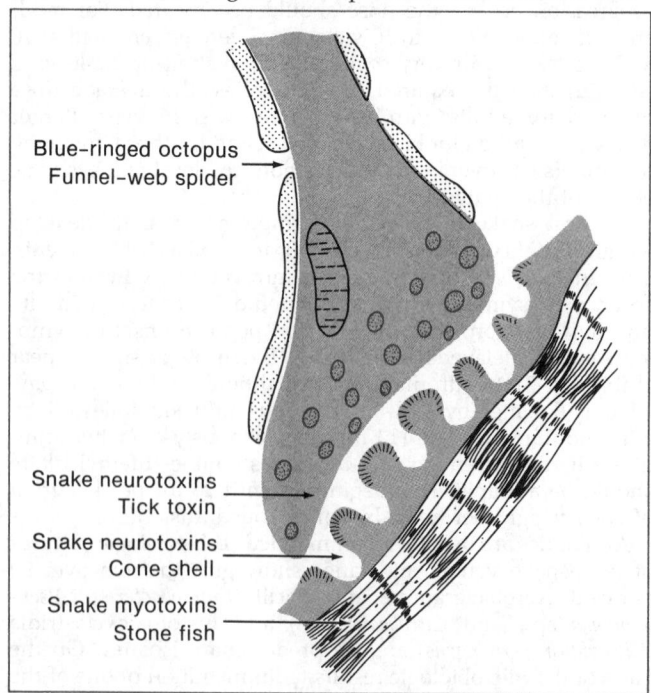

FIGURE 416–1. Scheme of a somatic neuromuscular junction, showing sites of action of a number of animal toxins. (Courtesy of Dr. V. Callanan, Townsville, North Queensland, Australia.)

Ciguatera (Poisoning by Fish in the Tropics)

This occurs in all tropical and subtropical seas and is a major public health and economic problem in the Pacific. About 1500 cases of ciguatera poisoning occur annually in the South Pacific alone. Deaths have been reported. The search for a simple chemical test of fish flesh to reveal the presence of ciguatoxin is proceeding. The most common symptoms are gastrointestinal (nausea, abdominal pain, vomiting, and diarrhea) and peripheral neurologic (paresthesias, especially circumoral and intraoral, dental discomfort, and a classic confusion of peripheral temperature sense; that is, hot and cold are confused). A generalized skin itch that is dramatically potentiated by alcohol consumption has been described.

Ciguatoxin is believed to be passed along in the food chain, and at least one source has been traced to a dinoflagellate, *Gambierdiscus toxicus.* There is no antidote, and treatment is symptomatic. Symptoms can persist for months. The precise chemical structure of ciguatoxin remains to be elucidated.

Tetrodotoxic Fishes

These include toad fish and puffer fish. Ingestion of the toxin in the fish flesh produces symptoms and signs characteristic of tetrodotoxin's action potential blockade (Fig. 416–1), viz: numbness, motor weakness, ataxia, and respiratory failure. Tetrodotoxin is one of the most toxic of known poisons and is the active component in blue-ringed octopus envenomation (see above). There is no specific antidote, so management of a patient is symptomatic.

Shellfish Poisoning

Paralytic shellfish poisoning is due to the ingestion of saxitoxin and is associated with a fatality rate of about 8.5 per cent. This condition should be distinguished from the gastrointestinal and the allergic types of shellfish poisoning. Like ciguatoxin (see above), saxitoxin is thought to originate in dinoflagellate organisms, at the beginning of the marine food chain. Treatment is symptomatic. No specific antidote is known.

Whales, Porpoises, Polar Bears, Walruses, and Seals

Poisoning results from the ingestion of the viscera of these animals, notably liver or kidneys. The intoxication from such organs of polar bears, walruses, and seals is believed to be due to hypervitaminosis A.

SOME NONFATAL ENVENOMATIONS (Table 416–1)

Nonfatal envenomations have occurred from true jellyfish (Class *Scyphozoa*), including *Carybdeid medusae* (notably *Carukia*

barnesi—"*Irukandji*"), and the "hydroids" '(Class *Hydrozoa*), including *Physalia* species (bluebottle, Portuguese man-of war), sea nettle (*Chrysaora quinquecirrha*), and mauve stinger (*Pelagia noctiluca*). Others have included corals and anemones (Class *Anthozoa*), and toxic sponges (Class *Demospongiae*).

A vast array of marine animals continues to be involved in less serious human envenomations, ranging from mild local itching to serious allergic manifestations. Certain treatment principles are becoming established.

1. Household vinegar inactivates undischarged nematocysts of several medically significant species of jellyfish (*Physalia, Irukandji, Carybdia tamoya,* and *Chironex*). Vinegar does nothing for the pain of these stings.
2. In general, ethyl alcohol should not be applied to serious marine stings.
3. Nematocyst inhibition appears to be a "species-specific" phenomenon.
4. Allergic phenomena can play a significant role in some marine envenomations, such as jellyfish stings and toxic sponge contacts.
5. Immediate pain relief continues as a major research goal; immunologic research holds promise here. Local cooling (ice) helps in some jellyfish stings.

Burnett JW, Calton GJ, Burnett HW: Jellyfish envenomation syndromes. J Am Acad Dermatol 14:100, 1986. *A state-of-the-art summary of the clinical applications of recent toxic and immunologic research in the field.*

Edmonds C: Dangerous Marine Animals of the Indo-Pacific Region. Newport, New South Wales, Wedneil Publications, 1975. *A readable and well-illustrated overview of the subject.*

Fenner PJ, Williamson JAH, Callanan V, et al.: Further understanding of, and a new treatment for, "Irukandji" (*Carukia barnesi*) stings. Med J Aust 145:569, 1986. *Confronts the reader with the complexities that presently face the clinician in the management of serious jellyfish envenomations. Contains a useful list of references.*

Gillespie HC, Lewis RJ, Pearn JH, et al.: Ciguatera in Australia: Occurrence, clinical features, pathophysiology and management. Med J Aust 145:584, 1986. *A useful summary of current research findings.*

Halstead BW: Paralytic shellfish poisoning guide. Geneva, WHO Publication, 1982. *A good review of the subject.*

Hartwick R, Callanan V, Williamson J: Disarming the box jellyfish. Nematocyst inhibition in *Chironex fleckeri*. Med J Aust 1:15, 1980. *Demonstrates the value of vinegar and the problems of alcohol application in the first aid treatment of box jellyfish stings.*

Sutherland SK: Australian Animal Toxins. Melbourne, Australia, Oxford University Press, 1983. *This detailed and profusely illustrated work is the most recent hallmark in the subject of animal envenomation and poisoning, both marine and terrestrial. Destined to become a classic work. The definitive work on snake and spider bite management.*

Torda TA: Tetrodotoxic fish—clinical management. In Sutherland SK (ed.): Australian Animal Toxins. Cambridge, Oxford University Press, 1983, pp 458–459. *A recent update on a potentially dangerous clinical situation.*

Williamson J: Some Australian Marine Stings, Envenomations and Poisonings. 3rd ed. Brisbane, Surf Life Saving Association of Australia, Queensland State Centre, 1984. *A concise illustrated account at the level of first aiders and paramedics.*

417 THE IMMUNE SYSTEM: INTRODUCTION

William E. Paul

The immune system consists of the recirculating pool of *lymphocytes* and *monocytes* and of cells in the bone marrow and in the organized lymphoid tissues, including the *lymph nodes*, *spleen*, *Peyer's patches*, and the *thymus*. The principal cells that comprise this system are the *B* and *T lymphocytes* and cells of the *monocyte-macrophage* lineage. These cells and their products, most notably *antibodies* and *lymphokines*, are responsible for the protective immunity that is so critical for survival of humans in the sea of potentially pathogenic microorganisms in which we live. The consequences of the failure to make an immune response or of major dysfunction in the immune system is graphically and tragically demonstrated by the fate of infants with severe combined immunodeficiency disease or of adults with acquired immunodeficiency syndrome.

The immune response is initiated by introduction of an immunogenic substance into an immunocompetent individual. Such immunization results in activation and proliferation of T and B lymphocytes that bear membrane receptors specific for antigenic determinants (epitopes) on the immunogen. This leads to the selective expansion of clones of specific lymphocytes that initially represented a very small fraction of the total lymphocyte population.

Stimulated B lymphocytes differentiate into antibody-secreting cells, of which plasma cells are a major morphologic type. Antibody-secreting cells produce *immunoglobulin* (Ig) molecules with antigen-combining sites that are identical to the antigen-combining sites of the membrane receptors expressed on their B lymphocyte progenitors. Ig's exist in a series of structurally distinct classes, including IgM, IgD, IgG, IgA, and IgE. Each of these types of Ig molecules has a distinctive function.

Stimulated T lymphocytes may differentiate into effector cells, such as specific cytotoxic lymphocytes. Other members of the T cell population play critical roles in regulation of the immune system. Among these regulatory cells are *helper* T lymphocytes, which interact with B lymphocytes and aid them to develop into antibody-secreting cells, and *suppressor* T cells, which inhibit immune responses, principally by diminishing the action of helper T cells.

The negative regulatory aspects of the immune system, as exemplified by suppressor cells, are necessary to prevent the uncontrolled growth of individual B or T cells that might result as a consequence of continued antigenic stimulation. An equally critical need of the immune system is to limit the production of antibodies specific for *self* antigenic determinants and the appearance of effector T lymphocytes with self-specificity. Lymphocytes potentially capable of such self-specific responses are eliminated or their activation inhibited by the establishment of immunologic tolerance. Disorders in immunoregulation or of tolerance induction are a major feature of autoimmune diseases, such as systemic lupus eythematosus.

This Introduction will serve to describe briefly the principal cell types that participate in the immune response, the means through which these cells are activated, how they communicate with one another, the nature of the antibodies and other soluble products that they secrete, and how these cells mediate their immunologic functions.

B LYMPHOCYTES

B lymphocytes are precursors of antibody-secreting cells. They are found in all of the peripheral lymphoid tissues and in the recirculating pool of lymphocytes. In lymph nodes, B cells are mainly located in primary follicles within the subcapsular cortex. B cells bear membrane receptors through which they recognize foreign antigens. These receptors are Ig molecules, mainly of the IgM and IgD classes, that are specialized for expression within membranes. All of the membrane receptors of any individual B cell have the same binding specificity. When these cells differentiate into antibody-secreting cells, they produce antibodies with specificity identical to that of the membrane Ig (mIg) of the B cells. Thus, the extremely large number of distinct antibodies that may be produced in the course of immune responses represents the existence of a correspondingly large number of antibody-secreting cells, each of which produces antibody of only a single specificity.

ONTOGENY, MOLECULAR GENETICS, AND DIVERSITY OF B LYMPHOCYTES. B lymphocytes are derived from hematopoietic stem cells. These cells are found in embryonic life within the blood islands of the yolk sac, later in gestation within the liver, and in postnatal life principally within the bone marrow. The earliest identifiable member of the B lymphocyte lineage is the *pre-B* cell. This cell lacks mIg, but expresses in its cytoplasm one of the two constituent polypeptide chains of IgM molecules, the μ heavy (H) chain. Early pre-B cells rapidly cycle, but more mature pre-B cells are small and quiescent.

Within pre-B cells a series of remarkable genetic translocations occur, involving the genes coding for both of the polypeptide chains of Ig's (H and light [L] chains). Both H and L chains consist of amino-terminal regions, which are highly variable and which form the walls of the antigen-combining sites of Ig's, and of carboxy-terminal regions, which, for a given H chain class or L chain type, are essentially constant, except for allotypic variation (Fig. 417–1). These regions are designated the variable (V) and constant (C) regions of the H and L chains respectively. The H chain V region is encoded by three distinct genes, the *V, D,* and *J* genes (Fig. 417–2). In the germline DNA and in DNA of nonlymphoid cells, the H chain *V, D,* and *J* genes, which are on chromosome 14, are widely separated from one another, but in the course of pre-B cell development, two separate

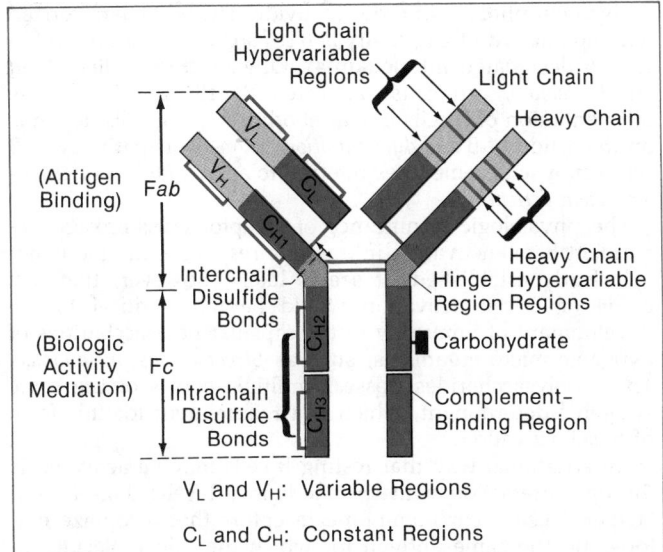

V_L and V_H: Variable Regions

C_L and C_H: Constant Regions

FIGURE 417–1. Structure of an Ig molecule. A schematic representation of an IgG molecule indicating the chain and domain structure of the molecule and the existence of hypervariable regions within variable regions of both H and L chains. Fab and Fc refer to fragments of the IgG molecule formed by papain cleavage. The former contains the V_H and C_{H1} H chain regions and an intact L chain; the latter consists of C_{H2} and C_{H3} region of two H chains, linked to one another by disulfide bonds. (From Wasserman RL, Capra JD: Immunoglobulins. In Horowitz MI, Pigman W (eds.): The Glycoconjugates. New York, Academic Press, 1977, pp 323–348.)

translocation events occur that bring these genes together to produce a single *VDJ* gene. This *VDJ* gene specifies an individual H chain V region. Germline DNA contains a large number (~300) of distinct V genes, a large but not yet determined number of D genes, and four functional J genes. It appears that these genes can be randomly combined, making possible the formation of a large number, probably more than 10,000, *VDJ* genes simply by combinatorial association. Furthermore, there are opportunities for somatic genetic changes, both in the translocation process and due to mutation and gene conversion events, so that the actual number of distinct *VDJ* genes that may be formed is much

greater. Within any individual cell, only one functional set of *VDJ* translocation events appears to occur. The *VDJ* gene is initially assembled near the gene encoding the μ constant region (*Igh-Cμ* gene). This leads to the expression within pre-B cells of μ H chains.

The L chain V region is also constructed by the translocation of distinct genes. L chain V regions are encoded by V and J genes, which are brought into apposition with one another; no D gene exists for L chains. L chains are of two different types, κ and λ. The V and J genes for κ (V_κ and J_κ) as well as the gene for the κ constant region (C_κ) are found on chromosome 2. The comparable λ genes (V_λ, J_λ, and C_λ) are on chromosome 22.

Translocation of H chain *V, D,* and *J* genes appears to precede translocation of L chain V and J genes; V_κ, J_κ translocation appears to precede translocation of V_λ, J_λ. In general, if V_κ and J_κ translocation events are successful and lead to an active κ gene, λ gene translocation events are not observed. Thus, an individual cell expresses only κ or λ chains but not both. Furthermore, a set of translocation events leading to the formation of active H or L chain genes generally occurs on only one of the two allelic chromosomes that specify H or L chains. Thus, Ig H and L chains produced by any individual cell are derived from only one of the allelic chromosomes, resulting in the phenomenon of *allelic exclusion*.

The completion of functional H and L chain genetic translocation within a pre-B cell is associated with the appearance of mIg on the surface of the cell and thus with the differentiation of the pre-B cell into a B cell. Immature B cells express mIg only of the IgM class. As these cells mature further, they also express mIgD. This expression of mIgD, in addition to mIgM, by developing B cells appears to be associated with acquisition of new immune functions, such as resistance to tolerance induction and responsiveness to polysaccharide antigens.

Mature B cells express a series of other markers that have potential functional significance. These include receptors for the Fc portions of Ig's (*Fc receptors*), receptors for complement components (i.e., for the C3b and C3d fragments of C3), and class II *major histocompatibility complex* (MHC) molecules. (A complete discussion of the MHC is found in Ch. 425.) Although the precise physiologic roles of Fc and C3 receptors are still uncertain, class II MHC molecules on B cells are involved in the process by which helper T cells recognize and

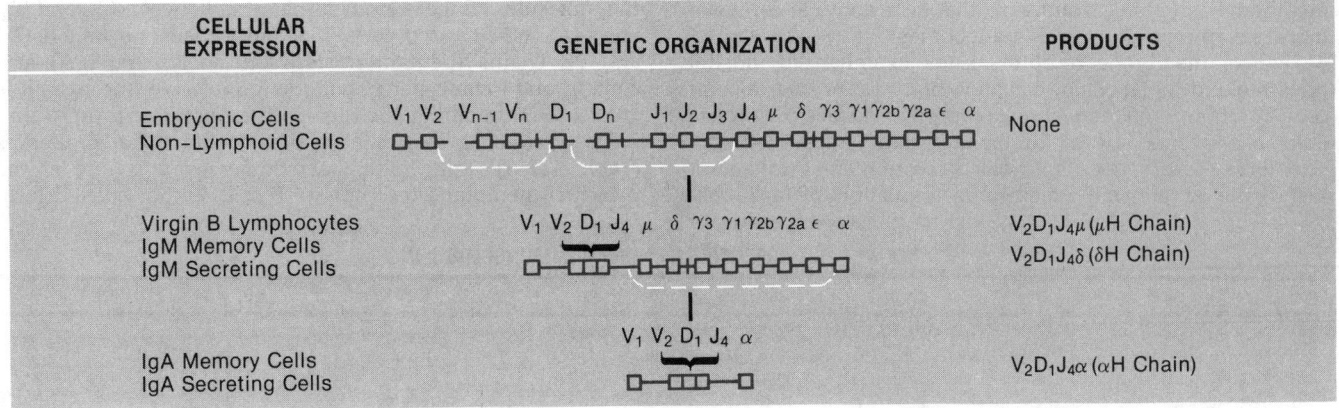

FIGURE 417–2. Organization and translocation of Ig genes. Immunoglobulin H chains are encoded by four distinct genetic elements: *Igh-V(V), Igh-D(D), Igh-J(J),* and *Igh-C* genes. The *V, D,* and *J* genes together specify the variable region of the H chain. The *Igh-C* gene specifies the C region. The same V region can be found in association with each of the C regions (e.g., in the mouse, μ, δ, γ3, γ1, γ2b, γ2a, ε, and α). A generally similar situation exists for human C region genes. In the germline genome, the *V, D,* and *J* genes are far apart, and there are multiple forms of each of these genes. In the course of lymphocyte development, a *VDJ* gene complex is found by translocation of individual *V* and *D* genes so that they lie next to one of the *J* genes, with the excision of intervening genes. This *VDJ* complex is initially expressed with μ and δ C genes, but may be subsequently translocated so that it lies near one of the other C genes (e.g., α) and in that case leads to the expression of a VDJα chain. (From Paul WE: The immune system: An introduction. In Paul WE (ed): Fundamental Immunology. New York, Raven Press, 1984, p 8.)

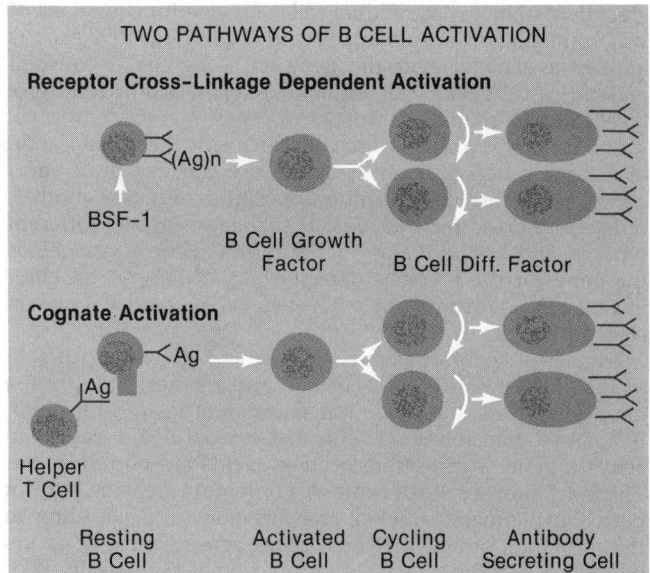

TWO PATHWAYS OF B CELL ACTIVATION

Receptor Cross-Linkage Dependent Activation

BSF-1

B Cell Growth Factor

B Cell Diff. Factor

Cognate Activation

Helper T Cell

| Resting B Cell | Activated B Cell | Cycling B Cell | Antibody Secreting Cell |

FIGURE 417–3. B cell stimulation. Resting B cells may be stimulated to proliferate and then to differentiate by two distinct mechanisms. One mechanism is designated receptor cross-linkage dependent activation. In this pathway, resting B cells are activated to an excited, or G_1, state by the action of agents that appropriately cross-link their respectors. Excited cells are acted upon by soluble factors, including B cell growth factor, and enter the S phase. Differentiation factors act upon these cells to cause them to synthesize and secrete Ig. The second major pathway involves the interaction of "histocompatibility-restricted" helper T cells with resting B cells. These T cells recognize antigen and class II molecules on the B cell surface and stimulate the cell to enter an excited state. This activation pathway is often designated cognate activation. The subsequent progress of the excited B cell may depend upon further interaction with helper T cells or soluble factors. Differentiation factors are probably necessary for differentiation of these into cells secreting Ig.

interact with B cells in the course of B cell responses to antigenic stimulation.

The events in pre-B cell and B cell development described thus far are antigen independent. Subsequent events in B cell development appear to require antigenic stimulation or stimulation by soluble factors made by antigen-activated T cells.

CONTROL OF B CELL RESPONSES. Resting, mature B cells can be activated as a result of cross-linkage of their membrane receptors by antigens that bear multiple copies of the same epitope or by anti-Ig antibodies (Fig. 417–3). Cross-linkage of membrane receptors leads to enhanced inositol phospholipid metabolism, elevation of cytosolic free calcium concentration, and activation of protein kinase C. These metabolic events appear to be important steps in B cell activation. Resting B cells activated through cross-linkage of membrane Ig generally require costimulation by a T cell-

derived lymphokine in order to divide. The best characterized lymphokine with this activity is *B cell stimulatory factor-1* (BSF-1, also designated interleukin-4). Other factors, called *B cell growth factors*, can cause activated B cells to divide. The differentiation of B cells into antibody-secreting cells depends on the action of B cell *differentiation factors*. This pathway of B cell response is sometimes referred to as *receptor cross-linkage–dependent activation*.

The physiologic significance of receptor cross-linkage–dependent B cell activation in immune responses in vivo is not yet clearly established. It seems likely, however, that this mode of B cell activation would be most critical to the development of immunity to the capsular polysaccharides of pyogenic micro-organisms, such as *Streptococcus pneumoniae*. These polysaccharides possess multiple copies of the same antigenic determinant, which is a requirement for this form of B cell activation.

An additional way that resting B cells may be activated is through interaction with specific helper T cells (Fig. 417–3). Helper T cells bear membrane receptors that recognize epitopes on the same antigen for which the mIg molecules of the B cells are specific. However, the T cell receptors recognize such antigenic determinants in association with polymorphic structures of class II MHC molecules. Interactions between T and B cells that depend upon the T cell's corecognition of antigen and class II molecules on the B cell membrane are referred to as *cognate* or *MHC restricted* T cell–B cell interactions. B cells activated as a result of cognate interaction with MHC–restricted T cells also appear to require the action of growth and differentiation factors to proliferate and to develop into antibody-secreting cells. Whether BSF-1 and the growth and differentiation factors important in factor-dependent responses also participate in cognate B cell responses has not been established. Cognate responses appear to be of principal importance in antibody responses to protein antigens.

IMMUNOGLOBULINS. Antibodies are Ig molecules. They exist in a series of classes that, as already noted, have distinct functions. Ig's are composed of one or more units, each of which consists of two identical H and two identical L chains. Both H chain and L chain polypeptides are divisible into a series of regions of 100 to 110 amino acids in length (Fig. 417–1). L chains consist of two such regions, an amino-terminal V region and a single carboxy-terminal C region. H chains consist of a V region and three or four C regions (C_{H1}, C_{H2}, . . .), depending on H chain class. Some classes of Ig's also have a hinge region, imparting segmental flexibility to the molecule. Hinge regions are located between C_{H1} and C_{H2} regions. The Ig's that consist of more than one unit of 2H and 2L chains (pentameric IgM and polymeric IgA) also contain one J chain per polymeric Ig molecule; the J chain is critical to maintaining such Ig's in their polymer form.

The various Ig classes have distinct functional properties (Table 417–1). IgM, in its membrane form, is one of the principal membrane receptors of B cells. In its secreted form

TABLE 417–1. PROPERTIES OF HUMAN IMMUNOGLOBULINS

	IgG	IgA	IgM	IgD	IgE
H chain class	γ	α	μ	δ	ε
H chain subclass	γ1,γ2,γ3,γ4	α1,α2	μ1,μ2		
L chain type	κ and λ	κ and λ	κ and λ	κ and λ	κ and λ
Molecular formula	$\gamma_2 L_2$	$\alpha_2 L_2$* or $(\alpha_2 L_2)_2 SC†J$‡	$(\mu_2 L_2)_5 J$‡	$\delta_2 L_2$	$\epsilon_2 L_2$
Molecular weight (approximate)	150,000	160,000 400,000§	900,000	180,000	190,000
Complement fixation (classic)	+	0	+ +	0	0
Serum concentration (approximate; mg/dl)	1,000	200	120	3	0.05
Serum half-life (days)	23	6	5	2–8	1–5
Placental transfer	+	0	0	0	0
Reaginic activity	?	0	0	0	+ +

*Monomeric serum IgA; † secretory component; ‡ J chain; § secretory IgA.

Adapted from Goodman JW: Immunoglobulins, I. In Stites DP, Stobo JD, Fudenberg HH, et al. (eds.): Basic and Clinical Immunology. Los Altos, Lange Medical Publications, 1982, p 34.

and when cross-linked by antigen, IgM activates complement and thus is important in lysis and opsonization of bacteria and other foreign particles. IgG exists in a series of subclasses (IgG$_1$, IgG$_2$, IgG$_3$, and IgG$_4$). IgG$_3$ and IgG$_1$ are efficient complement-fixing antibodies when cross linked and are the most efficient IgG subclasses in binding to Fc receptors. IgG molecules are capable of crossing the placenta and thus provide neonates with "preformed" antibodies during a period when their own immune systems are immature. IgA antibodies are the major Ig's found on mucosal surfaces and appear to play a major role in preventing initial access of microorganisms to portals of entry. Secreted IgA is locally synthesized and is transported through epithelial cells in association with a specialized 70,000-dalton polypeptide, secretory component. IgE molecules are principally responsible for immediate-type allergic reactions. They are secreted at a relatively low rate and are tightly bound to specialized Fc receptors (Fc$_\epsilon$ receptors) on mast cells and basophils. Antigens capable of binding to and cross-linking IgE bound to basophil and mast cell Fc$_\epsilon$ receptors cause the rapid release of vasoactive amines and other mediators from such cells; this mediator release is responsible for allergic and *anaphylactic* responses. IgD, as already mentioned, functions almost exclusively as a membrane receptor. Although it is secreted in small amounts, no specific function has been identified for IgD as a secretory Ig.

The initial Ig's expressed by any cell are mIgM and mIgD. The descendants of such cells may secrete antibody of any of the other Ig classes. Such Ig possesses the same V region as did the mIg of the progenitor B cell. The change in Ig class expression that occurs during B cell differentiation is known as "switching" and is dependent on a genetic translocation event, in which the chromosomal segment containing the assembled *VDJ* gene is moved from its location proximal to the C$_\mu$ gene into a new position proximal to the C gene for the Ig H chain constant region that will be expressed by the cell (i.e., C$_{\gamma 1}$, C$_{\gamma 2}$, C$_{\gamma 3}$, C$_{\gamma 4}$, C$_\alpha$, C$_\epsilon$) (Fig. 417–2).

T LYMPHOCYTES

T cells mediate both effector and regulatory functions. In general, these distinct functions are mediated by separate subpopulations of T cells. The principal T cell effector functions are the destruction of antigen-bearing target cells by specific "killer" T cells and the production of potent mediators. These mediators are responsible for induction of a variety of inflammatory phenomena, such as delayed-type hypersensitivity that is associated with activation of macrophages and with the chemotaxis of granulocytes and monocytes.

As regulatory cells, T cells function in a variety of distinct ways. They produce *interleukin-2* (IL-2), a T cell growth factor, which is critical to the development of cytotoxic T cell responses. They act as helper cells, collaborating with B cells and enabling them to produce antibodies to thymus-dependent antigens. Helper T cells play an important role in determining the class and idiotype of antibody produced in an immune response. A separate set of regulatory T cells, suppressor T cells, inhibit both antibody synthesis and cell-mediated immune responses, including delayed-type hypersensitivity.

T lymphocytes can be identified and quantitated because they bear specific membrane molecules that can be detected with *monoclonal antibodies*. (Monoclonal antibodies are homogeneous populations of antibody molecules, generally produced by somatic cell hybrids between activated normal B cells and a plasmacytoma cell line. Such hybrids are referred to as *hybridomas*.) All peripheral human T cells bear CD3, a determinant recognized by the monoclonal antibodies OKT3 and Leu 4. This determinant is borne on one component of a membrane complex (the T3 complex) that is closely associated with the T cell receptor and that plays an important role in

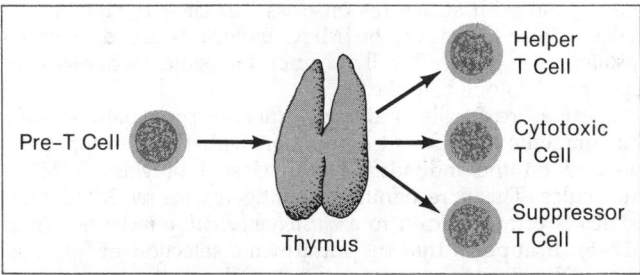

FIGURE 417–4. T cell differentiation. Precursors of T cells found in the hematopoietic tissue enter the thymus, where they undergo differentiation and emerge into the periphery as cells of distinct function, bearing markers that allow their characterization. Whether a single pre–T cell can develop into each of the three T cell lines illustrated here or whether there are distinct sets of pre–T cells has not yet been elucidated.

the process through which T cells are activated. Mature T cells may be subdivided into two major groups, distinguished by the membrane markers CD4 (T4) and CD8 (T8). CD4–positive cells generally include helper T cells, and CD8-positive cells include cytotoxic and suppressor T cells, although exceptions to this generalization exist. Measurement of the numbers of T cells in each of these subpopulations and their responsiveness to several mitogenic lectins, such as phytohemagglutinin (PHA), concanavalin A (con A), and pokeweed mitogen (PWM), provides a convenient *initial* means to assess certain aspects of T cell function. More specific and complex in vitro assays can be performed to measure helper and suppressor function. CD4 has been shown to be the membrane molecule that acts as the receptor for human immunodeficiency virus (HIV, the virus that causes AIDS). Only cells that express CD4 appear susceptible to infection with HIV.

T CELL DEVELOPMENT. T cells originate from hematopoietic stem cells. In contrast to B cells, T cell precursors undergo critical aspects of their differentiation in a specific central lymphoid organ, the thymus (Fig. 417–4). T cell precursors enter the thymus where an extensive series of proliferative events occurs and where these cells develop into mature, antigen-reactive T cells that are seeded into the peripheral lymphoid tissue. Much of the functional repertoire of possible T cell responses seems to be formed within the thymus. T cell receptors have a complex specificity pattern. Their receptors corecognize epitopes of foreign antigens in

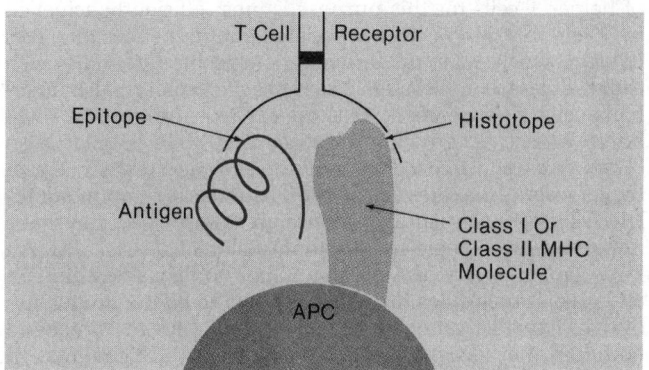

FIGURE 417–5. Corecognition of epitopes and histotopes by "MHC-restricted" T cell receptors. T cells that express histocompatibility-restriction in their interactions with B cells and macrophages have a complex antigen recognition system. These cells corecognize an antigenic determinant on a foreign molecule (an epitope) and a site on a self-MHC molecule (a histotope). Helper T cells generally corecognize epitopes with histotopes of class II MHC molecules. Cytotoxic T cells and their precursors generally corecognize epitopes with histotopes of class I MHC molecules. APC = Antigen presenting cell.

association with structures on class I or class II MHC molecules. These structures on MHC molecules are designated *histotopes*. A single T cell receptor molecule recognizes an epitope-histotope complex.

The mature T cells of an individual are principally specific for antigenic epitopes in association with the histotopes expressed on the individual's own class I or class II MHC molecules. This corecognition of antigen with *self*-MHC molecules is often referred to as *histocompatibility restriction* (Fig. 417–5). It appears that the intrathymic selection events that shape the T cell repertoire are based on the capacity of developing thymocytes to recognize histotopes of self-class I or -class II MHC molecules on thymic epithelial cells or thymic macrophages. Such events lead to the development of mature populations of T cells that have partial specificity for self-MHC molecules. It also appears that tolerance to many self-antigens may be established within the thymus.

Upon leaving the thymus, T cells are found in all the peripheral lymphoid tissues and in the blood and lymph. Within lymph nodes they tend to be principally found in the paracortex.

ANTIGEN RECOGNITION BY T CELLS. T cell receptors for antigen are disulfide-linked heterodimers of α and β chains, both of which contain amino-terminal variable regions and carboxy-terminal constant regions. Both chains are membrane glycoproteins, which possess membrane-spanning regions. The T cell receptor heterodimer is noncovalently linked to the T3 complex. Although the genes for α and β chains are distinct from Ig genes, T cell receptor genes and Ig genes have considerable sequence homology. Both sets of genes are members of the Ig supergene family.

The variable regions of T cell receptor genes are assembled from *V*, *D*, and *J* genes, just as IgV region genes are assembled. One important difference between T cell receptor genes and Ig genes is that the latter undergo somatic hypermutation in the course of immune reponses while the former do not.

A small subset of T cells possesses receptors composed of distinct chains, γ and δ. The functional properties of γ-expressing T cells have not yet been determined.

HELPER T CELLS. Helper T cells play a critical role in antibody responses to many antigens. They provide B cells with critical signals enabling them to respond to typical protein antigens. As discussed in Control of B Cell Responses, T cells may help B cell responses in several ways. Cognate T cell help depends upon the corecognition by T cells of antigen bound to the B cell as a result of interaction with its receptor, and of histotopes of class II MHC molecules. The activation of helper T cells for this purpose is most efficiently achieved by their interaction with specialized *antigen-presenting cells* (APC), which take up antigen nonspecifically and which express class II molecules. Macrophages, epidermal Langerhans cells, and dendritic cells appear to be important APC, but evidence is growing that activated B cells may also function as effective APC. Indeed, keratinocytes and endothelial cells can express class II MHC molecules upon stimulation by agents such as γ-interferon. These cells may have important physiologic and pathophysiologic roles as APC. An important property of APC, in addition to displaying antigen and class II molecules to T cells, appears to be the production of II-1. T cell activation of helper function appears to depend both on the recognition of complexes of antigen-class II molecules and on the presence of II-1 or a comparable factor.

Helper T cells may also function to help B cells respond to antigen by producing BSF-1, which is important in B cell proliferation, and by secreting a series of B cell differentiation factors. Stimulated T cells produce IL-2 and thus play a critical role in proliferation of cytotoxic T cells. Evidence is accumulating that there is a segregation of helper T cells with regard to the lymphokines that they produce and, thus, with regard to their functional properties.

T cells also play an important role in regulating the class of

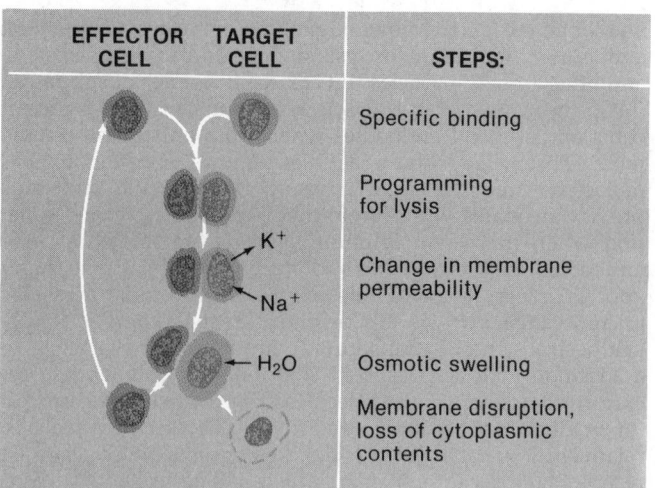

FIGURE 417–6. Stages in T cell–mediated lysis. (From Henry CS, Gillis S: Cell-mediated cytotoxicity. In Paul WE (ed.): Fundamental Immunology. New York, Raven Press, 1984, p 676.)

Ig synthesized and in the selective expansion of clones of B cells that express certain unique antigenic determinants (*idiotopes*) on their receptors and on the antibodies that their descendants secrete. Some of these T cells appear to function by recognizing Ig determinants on the B cell rather than by recognizing antigen. Our understanding of the physiology and relative importance of "receptor-specific" helper T cells is much less complete than is that of cognate and factor-producing helper cells (see Idiotypic Networks).

SUPPRESSOR T CELLS. Suppressor T cells play important roles in the immune system both by inhibiting immune responses against self-components and by regulating responses to conventional antigens. The suppressor system is highly complex, consisting of a series of cell types that act sequentially. Several distinct suppressor systems have been described by investigators working with different experimental models and a consensus suppressor pathway has not yet been agreed upon. The sequential action of the cells that are members of suppressor pathways appears to have an important amplification effect; the final cell in the pathway inhibits the function of helper T cells. The action of such *suppressor-effector* cells on antibody-secreting cells and on cytotoxic T cells or their precursors has been less intensively studied, but evidence exists to suggest that these cells are also important sites of suppressor action.

CYTOTOXIC T CELLS. Cytotoxic T cells recognize, interact with, and destroy cells bearing specific foreign antigens. Cytotoxic T cells play a major role in the destruction of virally infected cells, which bear viral antigens on their membranes. In addition, they may be very important in destroying tumor cells, which display unique tumor-associated antigens on their surfaces. Cytotoxic T cells generally corecognize foreign antigens together with histotopes on class I MHC molecules. Since essentially all cells express class I MHC molecules, cytotoxic T cells are capable of destroying cells of any type that express appropriate foreign antigens. The bulk of cytotoxic T cells are CD8 positive.

Cytotoxic T cells appear to lyse their target cells through a series of steps, including recognition and binding to the target cell and subsequent formation of "holes" in the membrane of the target cell. After this has been accomplished, the cytotoxic T cell may detach from its target and is free to attack other antigen-bearing cells. The cell in which membrane lesions have been induced will then undergo osmotic lysis (Fig. 417–6).

IDIOTYPIC NETWORKS

Since distinct antibodies have variable regions of different structure, it is hardly surprising that the antibodies themselves express unique antigenic determinants on their variable regions against which specific antibodies may be produced. These determinants are designated *idiotopes*, and the complement of idiotopes expressed by an individual Ig is its *idiotype*. The clonotypic antigenic determinants of T cells should be regarded as functionally equivalent to idiotopes of Ig. A provocative and influential theory holds that the immune system exists in a dynamic equilibrium in which members of each clone within the system are recognized by members of other clones (or by their products) through idiotope–anti-idiotope interactions. A key postulate of this theory is that there is considerable structural similarity between many of the epitopes on exogenous antigens and the idiotopes of Ig's or T cell receptors. Such idiotopes have sometimes been designated internal images of antigen. Thus, individual B cells and T cells may recognize internal images of antigen and may themselves be recognized by antibodies and T cells specific for the idiotopes they express. Such an interrelated system can allow an immune regulation based on recognition of receptors, without need for exogenous antigen, and can lead to dominance of a given immune response by cell types expressing particular idiotopes because of the action of idiotope-specific T cells or antibodies. Idiotopes that are dominantly expressed in immune responses because of such regulatory action have been designated *regulatory idiotopes*. The idiotope regulatory mechanism may offer opportunities for manipulation of the immune system to either enhance or suppress specific response. Furthermore, these idiotopes, as unique clonal markers, may also have value as specific markers of clonal malignant lymphoid disease.

MACROPHAGES

Cells of the monocyte-macrophage lineage play an important role in several aspects of the immune response. They have a critical function in (1) degrading complex structures, such as intact microorganisms, (2) processing the resulting antigens, and (3) presenting these antigens, in association with class II MHC molecules, to T cells that act as helper cells and that participate in cellular immune responses such as delayed hypersensitivity. This function depends upon the expression of class II MHC molecules on the macrophage. γ-Interferon, which is a product of activated T cells, can induce class II MHC molecules in macrophages. Thus, interactions between antigen-presenting macrophages and specific T lymphocytes are dynamic processes in which an initial activation step leads to the production of soluble factors capable of rendering many other macrophages competent to act as APC. A second important element in antigen presentation and T cell activation appears to be the production by macrophages if IL-1, a substance that has effects in many systems but that appears critical to activation of some resting T cells.

Macrophages also function as phagocytic cells. They recognize and ingest foreign particles that are coated by antibodies or complement components (Ch. 148). Macrophages possess membrane Fc receptors, which bind avidly to the aggregated Ig found in antigen-antibody complexes; they also bear receptors for fragments of the third component of complement. These complement fragments are generated in the course of the activation of the complement cascade and are found on opsonized microorganisms and in association with immune complexes.

Whether phagocytosed microorganisms and tumor cells are destroyed depends on both the nature of the ingested particle and the state of activation of the macrophage. Phagocytosis itself appears to be associated with a respiratory burst that enhances the bactericidal activity of the macrophage. Furthermore, T cell products, such as γ-interferon, increase the capacity of macrophages to destroy ingested microorganisms and cells.

NATURAL KILLER CELLS AND ANTIBODY-DEPENDENT CELLULAR CYTOTOXICITY

Natural killer (NK) cells are lymphoid cells from normal individuals that can lyse certain cell types, particularly members of certain long-term tumor cell lines. The NK cells in human peripheral blood are large lymphoid cells with prominent granules and are referred to as large granulocyte lymphocytes. However, their precise cellular lineage remains uncertain; they may be members of the T cell lineage, of the monocyte–macrophage lineage, or of an independent lymphoid lineage. Some patients with severe combined immunodeficiency have depressed NK activity while others display normal NK activity.

The cytotoxic mechanism employed by NK cells is probably very similar to that of specific cytotoxic T lymphocytes. It has been proposed that NK cells play an important role in surveillance mechanisms postulated to destroy emerging clones of malignant cells, but firm evidence for this view is still lacking.

Antibody-dependent cellular cytotoxicity (ADCC) is the destruction of antibody-coated cells by cytotoxic cells that possess Fc receptors. Evidence suggests that NK cells, or closely related cells, mediate ADCC. In general, the ADCC effector cells recognize the Fc region of IgG (Fc$_\gamma$) on the target cell, but Fcμ- and Fc$_\epsilon$-specific ADCC has been described.

ADCC almost certainly has immunopathologic significance. It appears to be important in autoimmune states in causing lysis of autoantibody-coated cells, in destruction of antibody-coated tumor cells, and in destruction of antibody-coated parasites.

CONCLUSIONS

The basic elements of the immune system, working together in a regulated manner, allow a rapid, specific, and highly protective response against foreign substances such as those associated with pathogenic microorganisms and against neoantigens expressed by tumor cells. Disorders, both qualitative and quantitative, in this system can have profound effects. It is clear that deficient immune responses may expose the individual to potentially devastating consequences. Furthermore, much of the tissue damage that occurs in a wide range of diseases is due to abnormal action of immune mechanisms. The subsequent chapters of this part, Diseases of the Immune System, outline in detail the pathophysiology of the immune system itself, describing disorders that directly relate to its function. Chapters in Part XXI, Musculoskeletal and Connective Tissue Diseases, describe many key examples in which disordered immune responses or, perhaps, normal responses to abnormal stimuli lead to profound disruption of normal function. Furthermore, immunologically mediated inflammation and tissue damage are key features of many diseases, affecting virtually every organ system. Progress in preventing and treating these disorders will require clear understanding of the nature of the immunologic abnormalities in each case. In turn, this will require a much deeper understanding of the normal physiology of the immune system than is now available to us.

Annual Review of Immunology, 1983–1987, Vol. 1–5. *A yearly series of reviews on topics in fundamental and clinical immunology aimed at providing a means of keeping up with this rapidly developing field.*

Paul WE (ed.): Fundamental Immunology. New York, Raven Press, 1984. *A general textbook of basic immunologic mechanisms.*

Stites DP, Stobo JD, Wells JV (eds.): Basic and Clinical Immunology. 6th ed. Los Altos, Lange Medical Publications, 1987. *A good introductory text.*

418 COMPLEMENT

Douglas T. Fearon

GENERAL CONSIDERATIONS. Complement functions as part of the immune system to protect the individual from microbial infection by mediating a variety of biologic reactions: opsonization, chemotaxis of leukocytes, increased vascular permeability, and cytolysis of target organisms. These activities of complement that promote an inflammatory reaction also carry the potential for damaging the host. Human disease related to complement may manifest itself either as defective resistance to infection secondary to impaired activation of the system or as hypersensitivity states caused by excessive complement activation. Paradoxically, impaired complement activation may also manifest as autoimmune disease.

The complement system consists of 18 proteins (Table 418–1) found in highest concentrations in plasma. These proteins are said to be in the *classic pathway* or *alternative pathway*, names that arose from common usage rather than considerations of relative importance or phylogenetic priorities. The proteins of the classic pathway are designated by letter C and a number: C1 (which comprises three distinct proteins, C1q, C1r, and C1s, that are held together by calcium), C4, C2, C3, and C5 to C9. Proteins of the alternative pathway are designated by capital letters: B, D, P, H, and I. Although C3 has been found to be an essential constituent of the alternative pathway, it has retained its classic pathway nomenclature. Cleavage fragments of components are denoted by lower case letters, as in C3a, C3b, Ba, and Bb, and inactive components are signified by the letter i, as in C3bi and Bbi. An overbar, as in C$\overline{1}$, indicates that a component has been converted to its enzymatically active form.

ACTIVATING AND EFFECTOR PATHWAYS OF COMPLEMENT. The cleavage of C3 by complement enzymes, termed *C3 convertases*, is the most critical reaction in the complement system for the elaboration of its biologic activities. There are two pathways, the classic and alternative, by which C3 convertase enzymes may be formed. The classic pathway is initiated by certain antigen-antibody complexes that confer immunologic specificity on this system. The phy-

logenetically older alternative pathway is activated by a variety of cell surfaces (including those of some bacteria, parasites, fungi, and mammalian cells) that possess certain biochemical characteristics. The alternative pathway is not necessarily dependent on antibody for recognition of the target. Both pathways may efficiently activate C3 and C5–C9 of the "effector" proteins from which are derived the biologically active peptides and complexes of complement.

Classic Pathway (Fig. 418–1). Only IgM and IgG can activate the classic pathway, as other antibody classes are not capable of binding C1 and converting it to its active form, C$\overline{1}$. Binding of the C1q subcomponent of C1 to the Fc regions of one IgM or of at least two adjacent IgG molecules within an antigen-antibody complex induces a conformational change in C1q that leads to autoactivation of a dimer of C1r, C1r$_2$. This subcomponent then proteolytically activates C1s$_2$ to C$\overline{1}$s$_2$. The C$\overline{1}$s$_2$ subcomponent of C$\overline{1}$ sequentially cleaves C4, whose major C4b fragment covalently binds to the immune complex, and C2 to generate C2a, which is taken up by C4b to form C4b,2a, the classic pathway C3 convertase. The site for proteolysis of C3 resides in C2a, which also acquires C5–cleaving activity after the major cleavage fragment of C3, C3b, covalently binds to adjacent sites on the target. The C4b,2a enzyme undergoes spontaneous decay of C3– and C5–cleaving activities by release of C2a, which immediately becomes inactive C2ai.

Three plasma proteins regulate activation of the classic pathway. The C$\overline{1}$ inhibitor (C$\overline{1}$INH) irreversibly binds to and blocks the enzymatic sites on C$\overline{1}$r and C$\overline{1}$s, which prevents activation of C1s by the former and cleavage of C4 and C2 by the latter. C$\overline{1}$INH also retards spontaneous activation of C1. The C4 binding protein (C4bp) binds to C4b to prevent uptake of C2 or to dissociate C2a that is already complexed to C4b. Binding of C4bp also makes C4b susceptible to proteolytic inactivation by C3b/C4b inactivator (I), which yields two degradation fragments, C4c and C4d.

Alternative Pathway (Figure 418–2). The alternative pathway is more complex than the classic pathway, since two C3 convertases are formed. The *"priming" C3 convertase*, C3,Bb, is assembled by the slow interaction in the fluid phase of C3 (in which the internal thiol ester has been hydrolyzed), B, D, and properdin regardless of the presence of activating substances, and it continuously provides small amounts of C3b that can initiate formation of the *"amplification" C3 convertase*, C3b,Bb. This amplification C3 convertase is responsible for effective C3 cleavage by the alternative pathway, and the adjective "amplification" is used because C3b is both a subunit and a product of this enzyme. C3b that has attached covalently to cell surfaces binds B, and the latter is cleaved by D to uncover the C3 cleaving site on the Bb fragment. C3b,Bb rapidly loses activity by spontaneous dissociation of the catalytic Bb subunit, which becomes inactive Bbi. Properdin serves to stabilize C3 convertase activity by binding to the C3b subunit and retarding dissociation of Bb. C3b,Bb acquires C5 convertase activity after cleavage of additional C3 and deposition of C3b at an adjacent site on the activating target. Regulation of the amplification C3 convertase is essential because of its positive feedback potential and is effected by two control proteins, H and I. The capacity of H to bind to C3b endows it with three inhibitory effects: blocking formation of C3b,Bb, dissociation of Bb that is already bound to C3b, and increasing the susceptibility of C3b to proteolysis by I, which yields C3bi, an inactive form of the protein.

The outcome of the competition between B and H for uptake by C3b on a cell membrane determines whether that cell activates the alternative pathway. C3b that is in the fluid phase or affixed to the surface of a nonactivator of the pathway binds H with almost 100-fold greater affinity than that with which it binds B, whereas C3b on the surface of an activator binds H less effectively, and uptake of the control protein is not favored relative to uptake of B. The latter circumstance

TABLE 418–1. PROTEINS OF THE COMPLEMENT SYSTEM

Name*	Former Designation	Molecular Weight	Serum Concentration (μg/per ml)
C1q	—	400,000	70
C1r	—	95,000	35
C1s	—	85,000	35
C4	—	209,000	400
C2	—	117,000	25
C3	—	185,000	1500
C5	—	200,000	85
C6	—	128,000	75
C7	—	121,000	55
C8	—	153,000	55
C9	—	80,000	200
B	C3 proactivator, glycine-rich β glycoprotein	95,000	250
D	C3 proactivator convertase	25,000	2
P	Properdin	160,000	25
C$\overline{1}$ inhibitor	—	105,000	180
C4-binding protein	—	$1.2 – 1.5 \times 10^6$	250
H	β1H	150,000	400
I	KAF, C3b inactivator	90,000	50

*This nomenclature for the alternative pathway proteins has been submitted by the Nomenclature Committee of the International Union of Immunology Societies to the World Health Organization for final approval and adoption.

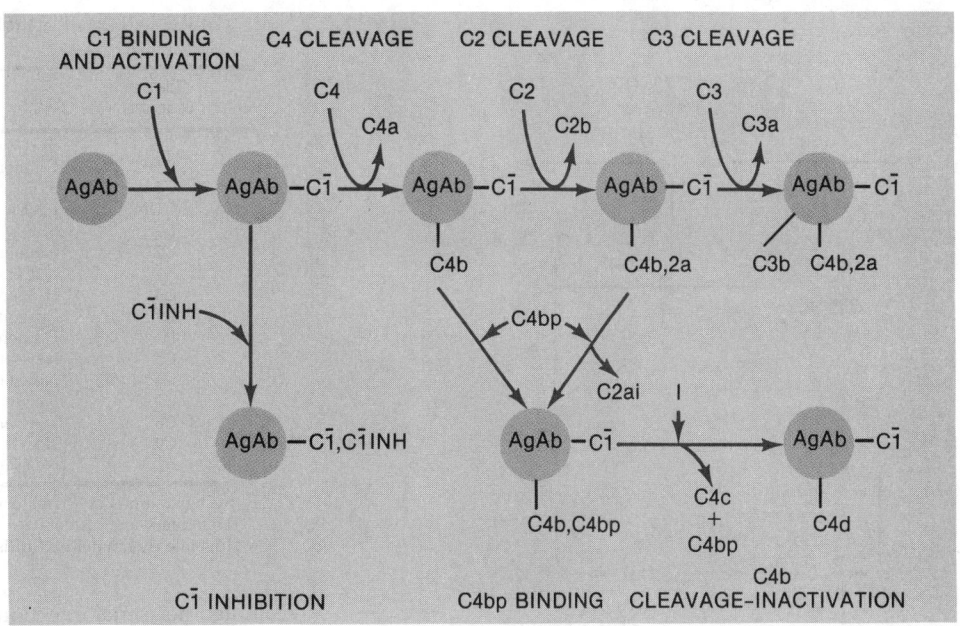

FIGURE 418–1. The classic pathway of complement activation. An antigen-antibody complex (AgAb) initiates the reaction by binding C1, which then self-activates. The C$\overline{1}$ cleaves C4 and C2, whose major fragments form a bimolecular complex, C4b,2a, the classic pathway C3 convertase. Formation of the C3 convertase is regulated by the control proteins C$\overline{1}$INH,C4bp, and I.

results in formation of C3b,Bb on the surface of the activating cell and amplifies the reaction by cleavage of additional C3.

A biochemical characteristic of cell membranes that influences the affinity of cell-bound C3b for H is the relative amount of sialic acid that is present in membrane-associated glycoproteins and glycolipids. This carbohydrate increases the affinity of C3b for H but not for B so that its presence on a cell membrane prevents alternative pathway activation. Conversely, the absence of cell surface sialic acid permits activation to occur on a membrane.

The capacity of the alternative pathway to respond to cells that are deficient in sialic acid residues may be relevant to its role in natural resistance to infection, since most bacteria, some parasites, and all plants lack this carbohydrate. Moreover, some of the bacterial species having capsular sialic acid, such as Type III Group B *Streptococcus*, Groups B and C *Neisseria meningitidis*, and K1 *Escherichia coli*, are pathogenic for man, suggesting that capsular sialic acid facilitates evasion of host defense. The capacity of antibody to enhance activation of the alternative pathway by bacteria and mammalian cells without involvement of classic activating components also

has been demonstrated and may be related to alteration of the distribution of membrane structures capable of regulating the uptake and function of cell-bound C3b.

Effector Sequence (Fig. 418–3). Assembly of C5 convertases by the two activating pathways provides the enzyme specificity that is necessary to continue the complement reaction through the effector sequence. Proteolytic cleavage of C5 liberates the C5a peptide that has anaphylatoxic and chemotactic activities and yields the major C5b fragment that initiates assembly of the membrane attack complex of C5b–9. C6 and C7 bind to C5b to form a trimolecular complex with exposed hydrophobic regions that inserts partially into the membrane of the target cell bearing the C5 convertase. The uptake by membrane-associated C5b–7 of C8 initiates the binding and polymerization of C9, and the latter forms a transmembrane "pore" through which water, salt, and even small proteins may pass. Cytolysis may ensue, caused either by osmotic changes or by metabolic alterations. Autologous cells are protected from these effects of complement activation by certain proteins that impair formation of the C3 convertase and binding of C9. Erythrocytes from patients with paroxys-

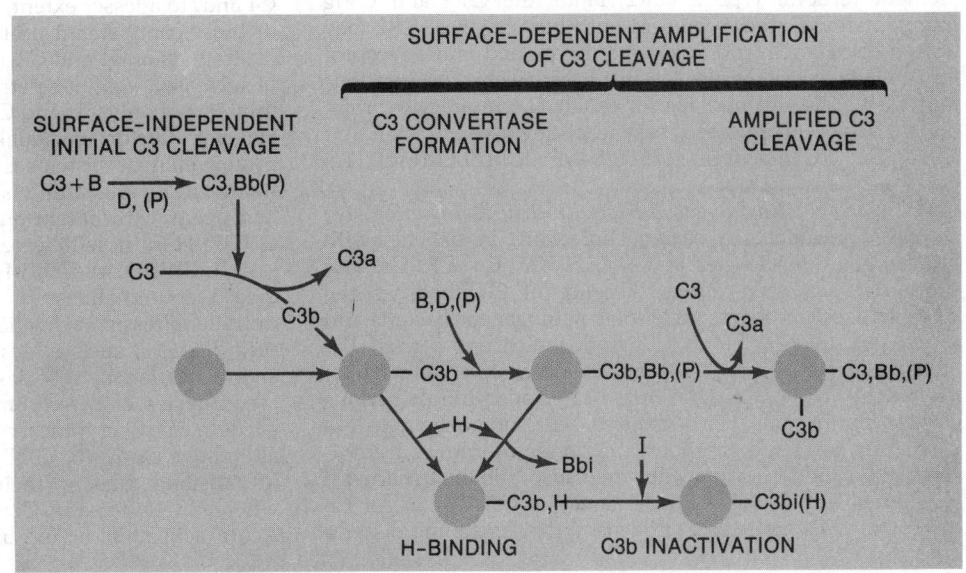

FIGURE 418–2. The alternative pathway of complement activation. C3b, which is slowly and continuously generated by a "priming" C3 convertase, C3,Bb(P), may attach to bystander cells. If the cell is an activator of the pathway, the amplification C3 convertase, C3b,Bb(P), is formed and catalyzes cleavage and deposition of additional molecules of C3b. In contrast, C3b bound to a nonactivator binds the regulatory protein, H, and is converted to inactive C3bi by I. P is shown in parentheses to indicate that it augments C3 convertase activity but is not required for alternative pathway activation.

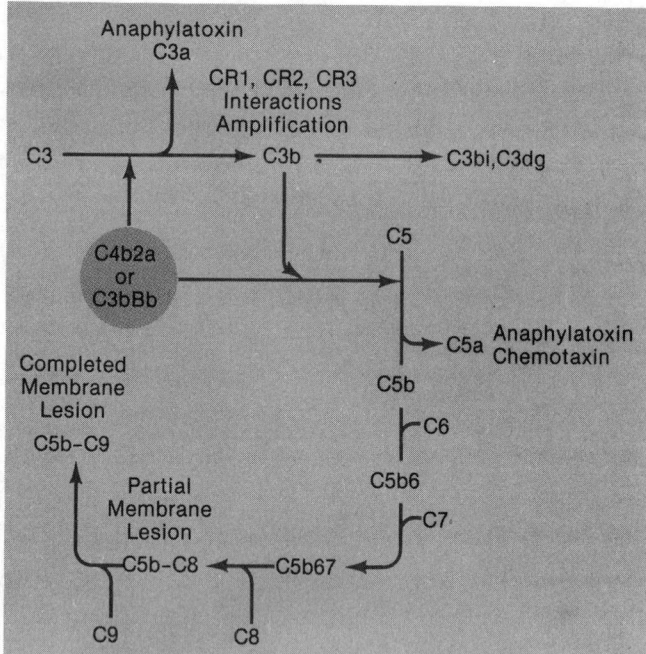

FIGURE 418–3. The effector sequence of complement, which is activated by the C3/C5 convertases of the classic and alternative pathways. Some of the prominent biologic activities associated with cleavage fragments and multimolecular complexes are shown.

TABLE 418–2. DISEASES ASSOCIATED WITH DEFICIENCIES OF COMPLEMENT

Deficient Component	Disease
C1q	SLE, vasculitis
C1r	Glomerulonephritis, SLE*
C1s	SLE
C1INH	HAE†, discoid LE, SLE
C4	SLE
C2	Glomerulonephritis, SLE, discoid LE, purpura, dermatomyositis, hemolytic anemia, JRA‡
C3	Pyogenic infections
I	Pyogenic infections
H	Pyogenic infections
C5	Neisserial infections, SLE
C6	Neisserial infections, Raynaud's phenomenon
C7	Neisserial infections, Raynaud's phenomenon
C8	Neisserial infections
C9	None
P	Neisserial infections

*Systemic lupus erythematosus
†Hereditary angioedema
‡Juvenile rheumatoid arthritis

mal nocturnal hemoglobinuria are deficient in the protein, decay-accelerating factor, that inhibits formation of C4b,2a and C3b,Bb (Ch. 145).

Other biologic effects of complement depend on the interaction of the activation fragments of individual components with specific cellular receptors. For example, the C5a peptide binds to receptors on neutrophils and monocytes to cause their adherence to endothelial cells, migration into the extravascular tissue and chemotaxis to the site of complement activation. The C3b and C3bi fragments of C3 that are covalently attached to targets of complement activation, such as bacteria and immune complexes, bind to complement receptor type 1 (CR1) and type 3 (CR3) on myelomonocytic cells to promote phagocytosis of the particles. CR1 is also present on erythrocytes, where it may mediate the uptake of immune complexes in the circulation and transport to reticuloendothelial cells. Partial deficiency of this receptor in patients with systemic lupus erythematosus may contribute to elevated concentrations of immune complexes in their plasma. Complement receptor type 2 (CR2) binds the C3bi and C3dg fragments of C3 and is present on B lymphocytes. CR2 may have a role in activation of this cell type and is the receptor for the Epstein-Barr virus, the agent responsible for infectious mononucleosis and perhaps for certain B lymphocyte–proliferative disorders and nasopharyngeal carcinoma.

INHERITED ABNORMALITIES OF COMPLEMENT (Table 418–2).

Association with Increased Susceptibility to Infection. An increased incidence of bacterial infections in patients with homozygous deficiencies of C3, I, H, C5, C6, C7, C8, and properdin has been noted. Absence of C3 abolishes the capacity of serum to opsonize some pathogenetic bacteria and prevents activation of C5–C9, from which are derived the chemotactic and cytolytic activities of complement. Thus, individuals with this deficiency have had multiple serious pyogenic infections. Two patients with homozygous deficiency of I or H and secondarily depressed serum concentrations of C3 and B also have increased susceptibility to bacterial infections. Individuals with deficiency of C5, C6, C7, or C8 appear to have a selective propensity for developing dissem-

inated neisserial infections without experiencing an increased incidence of infections with other pyogenic organisms, suggesting that cytolysis rather than phagocytosis is the primary host mechanism for defense against gonococci and meningococci.

Associations with Immunologic Disease. A variety of diseases with immunologic bases have been found in association with inherited deficiencies of C1q, C1r, C1s, C4, C2, and C3 components of the classic activating pathway. Possible consequences of these deficiencies that may predispose to diseases associated with elevated levels of circulating immune complexes include impaired solubilization of immune complexes, impaired clearance of immune complexes, and lack of generation of peptide fragments of C3 that have immunoregulatory functions. The relatively low frequency of infectious diseases in persons lacking C1, C4, or C2 has led to the proposal that the alternative pathway is primarily responsible for the host defense function of complement, while the classic pathway may be important for the processing of potentially noxious products of the immune response, such as immune complexes.

Hereditary Angioedema (see also Ch. 420). Episodic, occasionally trauma-induced attacks of subcutaneous and submucosal edema of the respiratory and gastrointestinal tracts occur in patients with heterozygous deficiency of C1INH. The diminished plasma concentration of this protein results in the continual presence of small amounts of C1, which consumes C4 and, to a lesser extent, C2, causing secondary depressions or these complement proteins. During acute attacks the concentrations of C4 and C2 are further depressed. The mediator of increased vascular permeability is not known. As C1INH inhibits not only C1r and C1s of complement but also activated Hageman factor and kallikrein, regulation of several plasma protein enzyme systems is impaired in those patients. Current treatment is the administration of low doses of impeded androgens with potent anabolic effects to increase synthesis of C1INH in these heterozygous individuals.

ACQUIRED ABNORMALITIES OF COMPLEMENT. Acquired abnormalities of serum complement levels usually indicate excessive activation of the system. In immune complex diseases, such as systemic lupus erythematosus, excessive activation of the classic pathway results in depressed serum levels of these components. In severe gram-negative bacteremia or cryptococcemia, organisms that activate the alternative pathway, C3, B, and properdin, may be consumed in plasma, causing their concentrations to be lowered, whereas C1, C4, and C2 may remain within normal limits. Acute activation of the alternative pathway occurs also in patients undergoing hemodialysis with cellulosic membranes. The C5a that is generated during this procedure causes aggregation of neutrophils and their sequestration within the pulmonary vasculature. Some studies suggest this effect of C5a may have a role in the adult respiratory distress syndrome.

An unusual mechanism for alternative pathway activation occurs in some patients with membranoproliferative glomerulonephritis and in most patients with partial lipodystrophy with or without glomerulonephritis. Their sera have low levels of C3, normal concentrations of C1, C4, and C2, and an IgG autoantibody, termed C3 nephritic factor, which is specific for antigenic determinants on the amplification C3 convertase. Binding of this autoantibody to C3b,Bb creates a stable trimolecular complex that is resistant to dissociation of its catalytic Bb subunit by H, causing deregulated consumption of C3 by the alternative pathway. An IgG autoantibody to the classic pathway C3 convertase with analogous stabilizing activity has been described in a few patients with systemic lupus erythematosus.

CLINICAL MEASUREMENTS OF COMPLEMENT. Activation of the complement system causes accelerated metabolism of the activated components and the generation of activation peptides such as C3a, C4a, and C5a. Thus, clinical assessment of complement activation involves assays that detect decreased levels of whole complement function or of individual components, or increased concentrations of activation peptides. The latter assay is most readily performed by radioimmunoassay for the C4a or C3a peptide in plasma or other fluids; the C5a peptide is usually too rapidly cleared by binding to specific high-affinity receptors on neutrophils for detection by this assay. The most frequently employed functional assay of complement activity is the determination of the amount of serum or other body fluid required to lyse 50 per cent of a sample of sheep erythrocytes that has been sensitized with rabbit antibody, and is reported as CH50 units. The test measures the overall activity of C1–C9; is not influenced by the alternative pathway proteins B, D, or properdin; and is relatively insensitive to a modest decrease in the activity of a single component. However, the CH50 is useful as an initial screen to detect marked consumption of complement proteins or homozygous deficiencies of individual components. Specific functional assays for all components of both pathways require specialized reagents that are not available in most clinical laboratories, and individual components are usually measured by immunoprecipitation. For the evaluation of patients with hypocomplementemia, determination of the C4 and C3 protein concentrations is most informative. Low concentrations of C4 indicate that classic pathway activation has occurred, since C4 is extremely sensitive to C̄1. Depressed levels of C3 suggest that rather intense activation of either pathway is occurring, and, if found to be associated with normal levels of C4, indicate that exclusive activation of the alternative pathways is occurring. Finally, the involvement of complement in a pathologic process is most directly assessed by immunofluorescent staining of individual complement proteins in the involved tissue.

Fearon DT, Wong WW: Complement ligand receptor interactions that mediate biological responses. Ann Rev Immunol 1:243, 1983. *Review of cellular receptors for complement proteins, an aspect of complement that is the basis for many of the biologic effects of this system.*

Joiner KA, Brown EJ, Frank MM: Complement and bacteria: chemistry and biology in host defense. Ann Rev Immunol 2:461, 1984. *A review of the biochemistry of complement, especially in relation to its bactericidal function.*

Ross SC, Densen P: Complement deficiency states and infection: Epidemiology, pathogenesis and consequences of neisserial and other infections in an immune deficiency. Medicine 63:243, 1984. *A review of the clinical consequences of inherited deficiencies of complement proteins that provides insight into the biologic functions of this system.*

Schifferli JA, Ng YC, Peters DK: The role of complement and its receptor in the elimination of immune complexes. N Engl J Med 315:488, 1986. *An analysis of the role of complement in preventing immune complex–mediated disease.*

419 PRIMARY IMMUNODEFICIENCY DISEASES

Rebecca H. Buckley

Since the first genetic defect in immunity was described in 1952, more than three dozen different primary immunodeficiency syndromes have been reported. Such diseases may involve all components of the immune system, including lymphocytes, phagocytic cells, and the complement proteins. This chapter will focus on abnormalities of lymphocytes. Deficiencies of the complement system (see Ch. 418) are mentioned briefly. A review of neutrophil dysfunction syndromes is presented in Ch. 149 and an overall review of the compromised host is given in Ch. 258. The acquired immunodeficiency syndrome (AIDS) is described in Ch. 346.

Despite the large body of knowledge gained regarding functional derangements and cellular abnormalities in the various primary disorders of lymphocytes, the fundamental biologic errors for most of them remain unknown. Exceptions include two defects accompanied by purine salvage pathway enzyme deficiencies—adenosine deaminase in some cases of autosomal-recessive severe combined immunodeficiency and purine nucleoside phosphorylase in some patients with Nezelof's syndrome. In addition, the absence of a 95 Kd beta chain common to three different leukocyte surface glycoproteins is the basis of a condition characterized by defective cytolytic lymphocyte and phagocytic cell functions. The genetic errors in many other immunodeficiencies are known to be on the X chromosome, and some progress has been made in localizing the abnormal regions in both X-linked agammaglobulinemia and chronic granulomatous disease. None of the primary defects studied has been found to have associated deficiencies of particular HLA antigens; thus they are unlikely to represent defects involving HLA-linked immune response genes on chromosome 6. However, immune deficiency can be associated with broad deficiencies of HLA class I and II antigens. Since trace amounts of immunoglobulins of all five isotypes can usually be found in the serum of most agammaglobulinemics, it is also unlikely that immunoglobulin deficiency states are due to deletions of genes encoding for immunoglobulin heavy chains. This does not, however, exclude the possibility of regulatory gene defects.

Various classifications of immunodeficiency disorders involving lymphocytes have attempted to postulate the cellular levels at which the defects occur. Cells with mature differentiation markers of both T and B lymphocytes, however, have been found in most of the known defects, despite profound deficiencies of T and/or B cell function. Thus, in most cases the suspect cell lineage is not missing but malfunctional. Table 419–1 lists the most prominent functional abnormalities and the presumed cellular level of the defect in 19 primary immunodeficiency syndromes.

In contrast to the acquired immunodeficiency syndrome (AIDS), which has a new case acquisition rate of more than 50 per week, primary immunodeficiency diseases are rare. The incidence of agammaglobulinemia is estimated at 1 in 50,000. Selective absence of serum and secretory IgA, the most common, has a reported prevalence of 1 in 333 to 1 in 700.

APPROACHES TO THE PATIENT WITH SUSPECTED IMMUNODEFICIENCY

The number of patients suspected of having primary immunodeficiency will far exceed the incidences of these dis-

TABLE 419–1. CLASSIFICATION OF PRIMARY IMMUNODEFICIENCY DISORDERS

Disorder	Functional Deficiencies	Presumed Cellular Level of Defect
X-linked agammaglobulinemia	Antibody	Pre-B cell
Common variable ("acquired") hypogammaglobulinemia	Antibody	B lymphocyte
Selective IgA deficiency	IgA antibody	IgA B lymphocyte
Secretory component deficiency	Secretory IgA	Mucosal epithelium
Selective IgM deficiency	IgM antibody	T helper cells
Immunodeficiency with elevated IgM	IgG and IgA antibodies	IgG, IgA B lymphocytes; switch T cell
Transient hypogammaglobulinemia of infancy	None; immunoglobulins low, but antibodies present	Unknown
Antibody deficiency with near-normal immunoglobulins	Antibody	Unknown; ?B cell
X-linked lymphoproliferative disease	Anti–EBV nuclear antigen antibody	B cell; ?also T cell
DiGeorge's syndrome	T cellular; some antibody	Dysmorphogenesis of 3rd & 4th branchial pouches
Nezelof's syndrome (including with PNP deficiency)	T cellular; some antibody	Unknown; ?thymus; ?T cell; metabolic defects
Severe combined immunodeficiency syndromes (autosomal recessive; ADA deficiency; X-linked recessive; defective expression of HLA antigens; reticular dysgenesis)	Antibody and T cellular; phagocytic in reticular dysgenesis	Unknown; metabolic defect(s); ?T cell; ?stem cell; ?thymus
Wiskott-Aldrich syndrome	Antibody; T cellular	Unknown
Ataxia-telangiectasia	Antibody; T cellular	B lymphocyte; helper T lymphocyte
Cartilage-hair hypoplasia	T cellular	G1 cycle of many cells
Immunodeficiency with thymoma	Antibody; some T cellular	B lymphocyte; excessive T suppressor cells
Hyperimmunoglobulinemia E syndrome	Specific immune responses; excessive IgE	Unknown
Chronic mucocutaneous candidiasis	Variable cellular	?Antigen overload
Lymphocyte function antigen 1 (LFA-1) deficiency	Cytotoxic lymphocytes; phagocytic cells	95 Kd beta chain of LFA-1, CR3, and p150, 95

eases. So it is important that the tests selected for immunologic assessment be broadly informative, reliable, and cost effective. Familiarity with certain clinical guidelines will aid in the initial selection. Patients with antibody-, phagocytic-cell–, or complement deficiencies have recurrent infections with high-grade encapsulated bacteria. Therefore, those with only repeated viral respiratory infections are not likely to have any of these disorders. By contrast, patients with deficiencies in T cell function usually manifest opportunistic infections. Most defects can be ruled out at little cost to the patient if the proper choice of screening tests is made (Table 419–2). Among the most informative are the complete and differential blood counts and the sedimentation rate. Examination of red cells for Howell-Jolly bodies will help exclude asplenia. A normal platelet count rules out Wiskott-Aldrich syndrome. If the sedimentation rate is normal chronic bacterial infection is unlikely. If the absolute neutrophil count is normal congenital and acquired neutropenia and severe chemotactic defects are eliminated. If the absolute lymphocyte count is normal a severe T cell defect is unlikely. Beyond this, it is well to keep in mind that tests of immune function are far more informative and cost effective than those measuring immunoglobulin concentrations or enumerating lymphocyte subpopulations.

In assessing B cell function, determination of antibody titers to type A and B red blood cells (usually IgM antibodies) can be carried out in most community blood banks. Further, the Schick test is still a very useful in-office test to detect the presence of IgG antibodies (to diphtheria toxin). As a rule,

TABLE 419–2. APPROACHES TO THE PATIENT WITH SUSPECTED IMMUNODEFICIENCY

Suspected Deficiency	Tests
All immunodeficiency	Complete and differential blood counts; platelet count; examination of red cells for Howell-Jolly bodies
Antibody deficiency	Isoagglutinin titers (anti-A, anti-B) by blood bank; Schick test; immunoglobulin quantification (particularly IgA) on antibody agar plates
T cell deficiency	Absolute lymphocyte count; intradermal skin test to *Candida albicans* 1:1000
Phagocytic cell deficiency	Absolute neutrophil count; nitroblue tetrazolium slide or tube assay
Complement deficiency	Freeze serum at −70° C immediately for CH50

patients with B cell defects for which there is an effective or indicated treatment do not have IgM or IgG antibodies. However, the finding of such antibodies does not exclude IgA deficiency, which would also be missed on a serum electrophoretic analysis. Immunoelectrophoresis is not quantitative and, for that reason, is not useful in evaluating immune competence. However, IgA can be quantified easily on antibody-agar plates in the office. If the IgA concentration is normal, this rules out not only IgA deficiency but all of the permanent types of agammaglobulinemia, since IgA is usually very low or absent in those conditions as well. A particularly uneconomical study is IgG–subclass measurement. It is far more helpful to know the results of pre- and postimmunization titers after administration of pneumococcal, *H. influenzae*, and diphtheria-tetanus vaccines.

The most cost-effective test for assessing T cell function is an intradermal skin test with 0.1 ml of a 1:1000 dilution of a known potent *Candida albicans* extract. If the test is positive, as defined by erythema and induration of 10 mm or more at 48 hours, virtually all primary T cell defects are excluded and the need for more expensive in vitro tests, such as lymphocyte enumeration on a cell sorter or assessments of responses to mitogens, is obviated. Killing defects of phagocytic cells, which should be suspected if the patient has problems with staphylococcal or gram-negative infections, can be screened for in the office by a nitroblue tetrazolium slide or tube assay. Complement defects can be most effectively screened for in a CH50 assay, which measures the intactness of the entire complement pathway. If these tests are abnormal, or even if they are normal and clinical features of the patient still strongly suggest a host defect, the patient should be evaluated at a center where more definitive immunologic studies can be done before any type of immunologic treatment is begun.

ANTIBODY DEFICIENCY DISORDERS

Antibody deficiency may occur either as an apparent congenital disorder or as an "acquired" abnormality. Most patients are recognized because they have recurrent infections, but some individuals with selective IgA deficiency or infants with transient hypogammaglobulinemia may have few or no infections. Table 419–3 lists some of the general features of these disorders.

X-LINKED AGAMMAGLOBULINEMIA. A majority of boys afflicted with this malady remain well during the first six to nine months of life, presumably by virtue of maternally

TABLE 419–3. CLINICAL CHARACTERISTICS
OF ANTIBODY DEFICIENCY DISORDERS

**TABLE 419–3. CLINICAL CHARACTERISTICS
OF ANTIBODY DEFICIENCY DISORDERS**

1. Recurrent infections with high-grade extracellular encapsulated pathogens
2. Few problems with fungal or viral (except enterovirus) infections
3. Chronic sinopulmonary disease
4. Growth retardation not striking
5. Antibody deficiency in serum and secretions
6. May or may not lack B lymphocytes with surface immunoglobulins or complement receptors
7. Absence of cortical follicles in lymph node and spleen in X-linked agammaglobulinemia
8. Paucity of palpable lymphoid and nasopharyngeal tissue in X-linked agammaglobulinemia
9. Compatible with survival to adulthood or for several years after onset except for those with persistent enterovirus infections, autoimmune disorders, or malignancy

transmitted immunoglobulin. Thereafter they repeatedly acquire infections with high-grade extracellular pyogenic organisms such as pneumococci, streptococci, and *Hemophilus* unless given prophylactic antibiotics or gammaglobulin therapy. The most common types of infections include sinusitis, pneumonia, otitis, furunculosis, meningitis, and septicemia. Chronic fungal infections are usually not present, and *Pneumocystis carinii* pneumonia rarely occurs unless there is an associated neutropenia. Viral infections and live virus vaccines are also usually handled normally, with the notable exceptions of hepatitis and enterovirus infections. Several examples of paralysis after polio vaccine administration have occurred, presumably because of mutation of persistent vaccine virus to a more neurotropic form. In addition, a dermatomyositis-like syndrome accompanied by chronic, eventually fatal central nervous system disease caused by various echoviruses has occurred in more than 40 patients. Approximately 20 per cent of patients have an arthritis resembling juvenile rheumatoid arthritis.

The diagnosis of X-linked agammaglobulinemia is suspected if serum concentrations of IgG, IgA, and IgM are below the 95-per-cent confidence limits for appropriate age and race-matched controls (usually there is <100 mg per deciliter total immunoglobulin). The demonstration of antibody deficiency in serum and in external secretions is of great importance in distinguishing this disorder from transient hypogammaglobulinemia of infancy. Tests for natural antibodies to blood group substances, for antibodies to antigens given during standard courses of immunization (e.g., diphtheria, tetanus, *H. influenzae*, or *Pneumococcus*) and for antibodies to and ability to clear bacteriophage $\phi \times 174$ are markedly abnormal. Polymorphonuclear functions are usually normal, but some patients with this condition have had transient, persistent, or cyclic neutropenia.

Lymphopenia is uncommon, and the percentages of T cells and T cell subsets have been found to be normal or elevated in most instances. In contrast, blood lymphocytes bearing surface immunoglobulin, "Ia-like" antigens or the EBV receptor, or reacting with a specific anti-B cell serum are absent or present in very low numbers. Hypoplasia of adenoids, tonsils, and peripheral lymph nodes is the rule; germinal centers are not present, and plasma cells are rarely found. Conversely, normal numbers of pre-B cells are found in the bone marrow. Mixed lymphocyte responsiveness and lymphocyte responses to antigens and mitogens are normal. Cell-mediated immune responses can be detected in vivo, and the capacity to reject allografts is intact. The thymus has appeared normal in all autopsied cases, and lymphoid cells are abundant in thymus-dependent areas of peripheral lymphoid tissues.

Except in those unfortunate patients who develop polio, persistent echovirus infection, or lymphoreticular malignancy (an incidence as high as 6 per cent has been reported), the overall prognosis is reasonably good if humoral replacement therapy is instituted early. Systemic infection can be prevented by administration of intravenous immune serum globulin (ISG, primarily IgG) at a dose of 400 mg per kilogram every three to four weeks. Such preparations are known to be free of hepatitis antigens and the AIDS virus. Many patients go on to develop crippling sinopulmonary disease despite this therapy, since no effective means exists for replacing secretory IgA at the mucosal surface. Intermittent or chronic antibiotic therapy is often necessary in addition for the management of such patients.

COMMON VARIABLE ("ACQUIRED") AGAMMA-GLOBULINEMIA (CVAγ). Patients with this condition may appear similar clinically in many respects to X-linked agammaglobulinemia. Although this disorder may occur in infants and young children, most patients present with a history of recurrent infection beginning several years after birth. CVAγ is distinguished from X-linked agammaglobulinemia by later age of onset, somewhat less severe susceptibility to infections, and almost equal sex distribution. In contrast to patients with the X-linked form, patients with CVAγ may have normal sized or enlarged tonsils and lymph nodes, and the latter may have cortical follicles. Additionally, such patients often have normal or near-normal numbers of circulating immunoglobulin-bearing B lymphocytes. Nevertheless, the serum immunoglobulin and antibody deficiencies are usually just as profound by measurement, and the bacterial etiologic agents are the same as in the X-linked disorder. Echovirus meningoencephalitis is rare in patients with CVAγ.

This condition has been variably associated with a spruelike syndrome, with or without nodular follicular lymphoid hyperplasia of the intestine; thymoma; alopecia areata; and autoantibody formation leading to hemolytic anemia, gastric atrophy, achlorhydria, and pernicious anemia. Frequent complications include giardiasis (seen far more often here than in X-linked agammaglobulinemia), bronchiectasis, gastric carcinoma, lymphoreticular malignancy, and cholelithiasis. Lymphoid interstitial pneumonia, pseudolymphoma, amyloidosis, and noncaseating granulomas of the lungs, spleen, skin, and liver have also been seen.

Despite normal numbers of circulating immunoglobulin-bearing B lymphocytes and the presence of lymphoid cortical follicles, the lymphocytes do not differentiate in vivo or in vitro into immunoglobulin-producing plasma cells, even in the presence of the polyclonal B cell activator, pokeweed mitogen. Although the primary biologic error responsible for this defect is unknown, in most patients it appears to be due to abnormal terminal differentiation of the B cell line. Because this disorder occurs in first-degree relatives of patients with selective IgA deficiency, and some patients with hyper–IgM have later become panhypogammaglobulinemic (or vice versa), it is possible that these diseases all belong to the same spectrum of B cell maturation arrests. The treatment of CVAγ is the same as that for the X-linked disorder.

SELECTIVE IgA DEFICIENCY. An isolated near-absence (i.e., <10 mg per deciliter) of serum and secretory IgA is the most common primary immunodeficiency disorder, a frequency of 1:333 being reported among some blood donors. Although IgA deficiency has been observed in apparently healthy individuals, it is commonly associated with ill health. The kinds of health problems experienced often reflect the type of clinic from which the patients are drawn. Among 75 from an allergy-immunology clinic, there were high frequencies of chronic or recurrent respiratory tract infection and atopic diseases. In contrast, 30 IgA–deficient patients drawn from a rheumatology clinic had a high frequency of autoimmune and/or collagen vascular disease.

IgA is the major immunoglobulin of external secretions. As would be expected, its deficiency is associated with infections occurring predominantly in the respiratory, gastrointestinal, and urogenital tracts. Bacterial agents responsible are essentially the same as in other types of antibody deficiency syndromes. A high incidence of viral hepatitis was noted in one group of IgA–deficient patients, but there is no clear evidence that patients with this disorder have an undue susceptibility to other viral agents. Children with IgA deficiency produce local IgM and IgG antipolio antibodies to killed vaccine given intranasally and IgM and IgG antirubella antibodies during convalescence from natural rubella. The compensating IgM seems to be locally synthesized and capable of combining with secretory piece for local secretion similar to IgA. Serum concentrations of other immunoglobulins are usually normal in patients with selective IgA deficiency, although an IgG_2 subclass deficiency has been reported in some, and IgM (usually increased) may be of the low-molecular-weight variety.

In addition to limiting the attachment of infectious agents to mucosal surfaces, secretory IgA antibodies probably act to prevent absorption of other foreign antigens, such as those in the diet. There is a high incidence of allergy and of IgG antibodies against cow's milk and ruminant serum proteins in patients with IgA deficiency. The antiruminant antibodies often falsely detect "IgA" in immunoassays which employ goat (but not rabbit) antisera. Intestinal nodular hyperplasia has been seen in a few such patients. A spruelike syndrome may occur in adults with selective IgA deficiency and sometimes responds to a gluten-free diet.

The basic defect leading to selective IgA deficiency is unknown. IgA-bearing blood B cells from most such patients also coexpress surface IgM and IgD, similar to cord blood B cells, suggesting maturation arrest. In addition, the B lymphocytes fail to secrete IgA in vitro. Studies of T cell function have been normal in most patients. The defect may not always be permanent. The occurrence of IgA deficiency in both males and females and in families suggests autosomal inheritance.

Serum antibodies to IgA are found in as many as 44 per cent of such patients. This observation is of possible etiologic and great clinical significance. At least seven IgA–deficient patients have had severe or fatal anaphylactic reactions after intravenous administration of blood products. For this reason, only multiply washed erythrocytes or blood products from other IgA–deficient individuals should be administered to these patients; ISG (which contains a small amount of IgA) is contraindicated.

Currently the only treatment for IgA deficiency is vigorous treatment of specific infections with appropriate antimicrobial agents. Even if serum IgA could be replaced (in the face of anti–IgA antibodies), it would not be transported into the external secretions, since the latter is an active process involving only locally produced IgA.

SECRETORY COMPONENT DEFICIENCY. A patient with chronic intestinal candidiasis and diarrhea was found to lack IgA in his external secretions, despite having a normal concentration of serum IgA. This was traced to a lack of secretory piece, which prevented the normal secretion of locally produced IgA.

SELECTIVE IgM DEFICIENCY. There are very few well-documented cases of this entity (IgM < 10 mg/ml). Fatal septicemia caused by meningococci and other gram-negative organisms, pneumococcal meningitis, tuberculosis, recurrent staphylococcal pyoderma, periorbital cellulitis, bronchiectasis, and recurrent otitis have all been reported. There is no specific therapy; early and vigorous treatment with antibiotics is recommended.

IMMUNODEFICIENCY WITH ELEVATED IgM. This disorder is characterized by very low serum IgG and IgA but markedly elevated polyclonal IgM. Some patients have low-molecular-weight IgM molecules. Like patients with X-linked agammaglobulinemia, those with this defect commonly become symptomatic during infancy with recurrent pyogenic infections, including otitis media, sinusitis, pneumonia, and tonsillitis. In contrast to patients with X-linked agammaglobulinemia, however, the frequent presence of lymphoid hyperplasia often leads away from a diagnosis of immunodeficiency. There is an increased frequency of autoimmune

disorders, such as hemolytic anemia and thrombocytopenia, and transient, persistent, or cyclic neutropenia is common. Thymic-dependent lymphoid tissues and T cell functions are usually normal, but several patients have had partial T cell deficiencies. A sex-linked mode of inheritance has been proposed, but several examples of the disorder in females now seem to make this less certain.

Normal or only slightly reduced numbers of Ig-bearing B lymphocytes have been found in the blood; however, cultured B cell lines from most such patients have shown the capacity to synthesize only IgM, suggesting a B cell maturation defect. Some patients with this condition have, however, been characterized as having normal B cells but a deficiency of "switch" T cells. Plasma cells in lymph nodes contain only IgM. Because these patients are unable to make IgG antibodies, the treatment is the same as for agammaglobulinemia.

TRANSIENT HYPOGAMMAGLOBULINEMIA OF INFANCY. Unlike patients with X-linked or common variable agammaglobulinemia, those with this condition can synthesize antibodies to human type A and B erythrocytes and to diphtheria and tetanus toxoids, usually by six to eleven months of age, well before immunoglobulin concentrations become normal. The finding of only eleven cases of transient hypogammaglobulinemia of infancy among over 10,000 sera tested by the author over a 12-year period suggests that this is not a common entity.

Gamma globulin replacement therapy is not indicated in this condition. In addition to the known risks of inducing anti-IgG allotype antibodies, passively administered antibodies could block endogenous primary antibody formation in the same manner that RhoGAM suppresses anti-D antibodies in Rh-negative mothers delivering Rh-positive infants.

ANTIBODY DEFICIENCY WITH NEAR-NORMAL IMMUNOGLOBULINS. The author and her associates have studied the antibody-forming capacities of twelve patients with deficient antibody responses despite apparently normal T cell function and normal or near-normal immunoglobulin concentrations. Blood group antibody titers were absent in all but two, diphtheria titers were low in all, and tetanus titers were low in ten. Geometric mean antibody titers to 13 pneumococcal serotypes were significantly lower than those of normal controls before and after immunization with tridecavalent pneumococcal polysaccharide vaccine. All patients cleared bacteriophage $\phi \times 174$ normally, but all primary immune responses were far below the normal range. Secondary responses to $\phi \times 174$ were also below the normal range in all but two, but, in both cases, most of the secondary response was IgM rather than IgG. This problem would not be detected unless functional tests of antibody-forming capacity are conducted. It may represent an early stage of "acquired" agammaglobulinemia. Patients with this disorder are candidates for immunoglobulin replacement therapy.

X-LINKED LYMPHOPROLIFERATIVE DISEASE. This disorder, also referred to as *Duncan's disease* (after the original kindred in which it was described), is characterized by an impaired immune response to Epstein-Barr virus (EBV). Affected persons are apparently healthy until they experience infectious mononucleosis. Two thirds of the more than 100 patients studied thus far died of overwhelming EBV–induced B cell proliferation during mononucleosis. A majority of the survivors developed hypogammaglobulinemia or B cell lymphomas or both. Such individuals have marked impairment in production of antibodies to the EBV nuclear antigen whereas titers of antibodies to the viral capsid antigen have ranged from zero to markedly elevated. Antibody-dependent cell-mediated cytotoxicity against EBV–infected cells and natural killer function are depressed, and there is a deficiency in long-lived T cell immunity to EBV. Despite normal numbers of B and T cells, there is an elevated percentage of lymphocytes of the suppressor (CD8) phenotype. In addition, lymphocyte immunoglobulin synthesis in response to polyclonal B cell mitogen stimulation in vitro is markedly depressed. Thus, both EBV–specific and nonspecific immunologic abnormalities occur in these patients.

CELLULAR IMMUNODEFICIENCY DISORDERS

Some important clinical characteristics of cellular immunodeficiency disorders are listed in Table 419–4. In general, patients with partial or absolute defects in T cell function have infections or other clinical problems for which there is no effective treatment or which are often of a more severe nature than in those with antibody deficiency disorders. It is therefore rare that such individuals survive beyond infancy or childhood.

THYMIC HYPOPLASIA (DIGEORGE'S SYNDROME). This condition results from dysmorphogenesis of the third and fourth pharyngeal pouches, leading to hypoplasia or aplasia of the thymus and parathyroid glands. Other structures forming at the same age are also frequently affected, resulting in anomalies of the great vessels (right-sided aortic arch), esophageal atresia, bifid uvula, congenital heart disease (atrial and ventricular septal defects), a short philtrum of the upper lip, hypertelorism, an antimongoloid slant to the eyes, mandibular hypoplasia, and low-set (often notched) ears. The diagnosis is usually first suggested by the presence of hypocalcemic seizures during the neonatal period. DiGeorge's syndrome has occurred in both males and females, and there is little evidence that it is heritable.

A variable degree of hypoplasia is more frequent than total aplasia of the thymus and parathyroid glands. Some children with the features of this syndrome have little trouble with infections and show evidence of some cell-mediated immunity. They are often referred to as having partial DiGeorge's syndrome. Those with marked thymic hypoplasia may resemble infants with severe combined immunodeficiency in their susceptibility to infection with low-grade or opportunistic pathogens (i.e., fungi, viruses, and *Pneumocystis carinii*) and to graft-versus-host (GVH) disease from nonirradiated blood transfusions.

Serum immunoglobulins are usually normal for age, but some fractions, particularly IgA, may be diminished and IgE may be elevated. T cell numbers are decreased, and there is an increased number of B cells. Responses of peripheral blood lymphocytes following mitogen stimulation, like the intradermal delayed hypersensitivity response, have been absent, reduced, or normal. Careful postmortem studies have sometimes revealed tiny nests of thymic tissue containing Hassall's corpuscles and a normal density of thymocytes. Lymphoid follicles usually appear normal, but lymph node paracortical areas and thymus-dependent regions of the spleen show variable degrees of depletion, depending upon the degree of thymic hypoplasia. Because of variability in the severity of the immunodeficiency, it is difficult to evaluate claimed benefits of fetal thymus transplantation.

CELLULAR IMMUNODEFICIENCY WITH IMMUNO-GLOBULINS (NEZELOF'S SYNDROME). This syndrome is characterized by lymphopenia, diminished lymphoid tissue, abnormal thymus architecture, and the presence of normal or increased immunoglobulins. Children with this condition may have recurrent or chronic pulmonary infections, failure to

TABLE 419–4. CLINICAL CHARACTERISTICS OF CELLULAR IMMUNODEFICIENCY DISORDERS

1. Recurrent infections with low-grade or opportunistic infectious agents such as fungi, viruses, or *Pneumocystis carinii*
2. Delayed cutaneous anergy
3. Accompanied by growth retardation, short life span, wasting, and diarrhea
4. Susceptible to graft-versus-host (GVH) disease if given fresh blood, plasma, or unmatched allogeneic bone marrow
5. Fatal reactions from live virus or BCG vaccination
6. High incidence of malignancy

thrive, oral or cutaneous candidiasis, chronic diarrhea, recurrent skin infections, gram-negative sepsis, urinary tract infections, severe varicella, or combinations of these. An autosomal-recessive pattern of inheritance has been suggested in some cases, but an X-linked mode seemed more likely in others. Other findings include neutropenia and eosinophilia.

Studies of cellular immune function have shown delayed cutaneous anergy to ubiquitous antigens and low to absent in vitro lymphocyte responses to mitogens and allogeneic cells. Such patients have profound deficiencies of total T cells and T cell subsets, with usually a normal helper (CD4+) to suppressor (CD8+) cell ratio, in contrast to patients with AIDS who characteristically have marked inversion of the CD4:CD8 ratio due to selective deficiency of CD4+ cells. Peripheral lymphoid tissues demonstrate paracortical lymphocyte depletion. The thymuses are very small and have a paucity of thymocytes and usually no Hassall's corpuscles; however, again in contrast to AIDS, thymic epithelium is present. These could all be useful in distinguishing Nezelof's syndrome from pediatric AIDS, since it is the primary immunodeficiency disorder most likely to be confused with it. Fatal or serious infections have included varicella, vaccinia, *Pneumocystis carinii*, cytomegalovirus, rubeola, *Pseudomonas*, and *Mycobacterium kansasii*. Antibody-forming capacity has been apparently normal in roughly one third of the reported cases. Plasma cells are usually abundant in the lamina propria and lymph nodes. Although very few patients have been reconstituted by bone marrow transplantation most other forms of therapy have also been unsuccessful.

With Purine Nucleoside Phosphorylase Deficiency. More than fourteen patients with Nezelof's syndrome have been found to have purine nucleoside phosphorylase (PNP) deficiency. In contrast to patients with adenosine deaminase (ADA) deficiency, serum and urinary uric acid are markedly deficient, and no characteristic physical or skeletal abnormalities have been noted. Three patients have suffered from a progressive neurologic disorder with spastic tetraplegia, two developed an autoimmune hemolytic anemia, and one, idiopathic thrombocytopenic purpura. Deaths have occurred from generalized vaccinia, varicella, lymphosarcoma, and GVH disease following blood transfusions. In contrast to a majority of patients with Nezelof's syndrome, the thymuses of PNP–deficient patients have had some Hassall's corpuscles, reminiscent of some patients with ADA deficiency. Analyses of lymphocyte subpopulations with monoclonal antibodies in two such patients revealed marked deficiencies of T cells and T cell subsets but increased numbers of cells with natural killer (NK) phenotype and function. Attempts to correct the immunologic and enzymatic deficiencies of PNP–deficient patients by enzyme replacement or deoxycytidine therapy have not been successful.

SEVERE COMBINED IMMUNODEFICIENCY (SCID) DISORDERS

The syndromes of SCID are characterized by their apparent congenital absence of all adaptive immune function and a great diversity of genetic, enzymatic, hematologic, and immunologic features. Unless immunologic reconstitution can be achieved through immunocompetent tissue transplants or enzyme replacement therapy or unless gnotobiotic isolation can be carried out, death usually occurs before the patient's first birthday. The major subcategories of this disorder are discussed below.

AUTOSOMAL-RECESSIVE SEVERE COMBINED IMMUNODEFICIENCY DISEASE. Within the first few months of life, infants affected with this first-described SCID syndrome have frequent episodes of otitis, pneumonia, sepsis, diarrhea, and cutaneous infections. Growth may appear normal initially, but extreme wasting soon develops. Infections with opportunistic organisms such as *Candida albicans*, *Pneu-*

mocystis carinii, varicella, measles, cytomegalovirus, and BCG frequently lead to death caused either by difficulties encountered in diagnosis or by a lack of effective treatment. These infants also lack the ability to reject foreign tissue and are therefore at risk for GVH disease. GVH reactions can result from maternal immunocompetent cells crossing the placenta or from the administration of blood products containing viable histoincompatible lymphocytes.

Immunologic evaluation reveals serum immunoglobulin concentrations to be diminished, and no antibody formation occurs following immunization. There is a lack of cellular immune function, with lymphopenia and absence of lymphocyte responses to mitogens or allogeneic cells, delayed cutaneous anergy, and inability to reject foreign tissues. Marked heterogeneity of lymphocyte subpopulations exists among SCID patients, even among those with similar inheritance patterns. Despite the uniformly profound lack of T or B cell function, some patients have had low numbers of both B and T lymphocytes, whereas others have had elevated numbers of B cells. Cytofluorographic studies with monoclonal antibodies to mature T cells and subsets have generally revealed very small numbers of cells reacting with such reagents; however, there is no increase in cells bearing the T6 antigen present on immature cortical thymocytes. Thus the lymphocytes present appear to have acquired surface markers characteristic of mature T cells. In contrast to similarly lymphopenic patients with AIDS, SCID patients rarely have an inverted ratio of helper (CD4 +) to suppressor (CD8 +) cells. A new phenotype of SCID was characterized in which virtually all of the lymphocytes of some infants with SCID are large granular lymphocytes with NK cell phenotype and function. NK function has been totally lacking in other SCID patients, again illustrating the striking heterogeneity at a cellular level. Typically, these patients have very small thymuses (less than 1 gram), which usually fail to descend from the neck, contain few thymic lymphocytes, lack corticomedullary distinction, and usually lack Hassall's corpuscles (see exception below). Despite the profound thymocyte depletion in SCID patients, thymic epithelium is present—in contrast to the situation in AIDS in which there is marked epithelial atrophy. Both the follicular and paracortical areas of the peripheral lymph nodes are depleted of lymphocytes. Tonsils, adenoids, and Peyer's patches are absent or extremely underdeveloped.

ISG fails to halt the progressively downhill course of SCID. Transplantation of bone marrow cells from HLA genotypically identical or D locus–compatible donors has resulted in apparent complete correction of the immunologic defect in a number of these patients, with some 50 known long-term survivors since 1968. More recently, techniques to deplete all post-thymic T cells from donor marrow have also allowed the use of haploidentical (half-matched) bone marrow cells for correction of SCID. These employ either a combination of soy lectin agglutination and sheep erythrocyte rosetting (the most successful method) or incubation with monoclonal antibodies to human T cells and complement. Both methods leave the stem cells intact. To date, over 75 infants with SCID who would have otherwise died because of lack of an HLA–identical donor have been treated successfully with T cell–depleted haploidentical bone marrow with few signs of GVH reaction.

With Adenosine Deaminase (ADA) Deficiency. Absence of the enzyme ADA has been observed in approximately 40 per cent of patients with the autosomal-recessive form of SCID. A marked accumulation of deoxyadenosine and its triphosphate may provide the biochemical mechanisms responsible for the immunodeficiency. Deoxyadenosine is an apparent suicide inactivator of the enzyme S-adenosylhomocysteine (SAH) hydrolase and could alter methylation in a manner which would lead to cell death. Although most such patients have had profound lymphopenia from the earliest age studied, a few have had early normal or fluctuating lymphocyte counts that declined by six weeks to two years of life. In marked contrast to "classic" SCID, some ADA–deficient patients have been found to have a few Hassall's corpuscles in their thymuses and changes suggestive of early differentiation. Other distinguishing features of ADA-deficient SCID patients have included the presence of rib cage abnormalities similar to a rachitic rosary and multiple skeletal abnormalities of chondro-osseous dysplasia on radiographic examination.

Both matched sibling and haploidentical post-thymic T cell–depleted bone marrow transplants have resulted in lymphocyte chimerism and partial or complete correction of the immunologic defect in ADA-deficient SCID. Enzyme replacement therapy with irradiated packed normal erythrocytes or polyethylene-glycol–modified bovine adenosine deaminase on a continuing basis has resulted in improvement in some patients. This condition is likely to be the first in which gene insertion therapy will be attempted, as the entire ADA gene has been cloned.

X-LINKED RECESSIVE SEVERE COMBINED IMMUNODEFICIENCY DISEASE. This is thought to be the most common form of SCID in the United States. Clinically, immunologically, and histopathologically, these patients appear similar to those with the autosomal-recessive form.

DEFECTIVE EXPRESSION OF MAJOR HISTOCOMPATIBILITY COMPLEX (MHC) ANTIGENS. There are two main forms: MHC class I antigen deficiency ("bare lymphocyte syndrome") and MHC class I antigen deficiency plus absence of MHC class II antigens. These autosomal-recessive conditions are thought to be due to regulatory gene defects, as cultured lymphocytes can be induced to express both class I and II antigens, and sera from affected individuals contain normal quantities of MHC class I antigens and beta 2 microglobulin. Patients (usually of North African descent) present with persistent diarrhea in early infancy and have oral candidiasis, bacterial pneumonia, pneumocystis, septicemia, and undue susceptibility to enteroviruses, herpes, and other viral agents. Those with both class I and II antigen deficiencies also have malabsorption. There is variable hypogammaglobulinemia with decreased serum IgM and IgA and poor to absent antibody production. B cell percentages are usually normal, but plasma cells are absent in tissues. Lymphopenia is only moderate; T cell functions in vivo and in vitro are decreased but not absent. The thymus and other lymphoid organs are severely hypoplastic. A majority of affected infants die in the first three years of life. The associated defects of both B and T cell immunity and HLA expression reinforce the important biologic role for HLA determinants in effective immune cell cooperation.

SEVERE COMBINED IMMUNODEFICIENCY WITH LEUKOPENIA (RETICULAR DYSGENESIS). In 1959, identical twin male infants were described who exhibited a total lack of both lymphocytes and granulocytes in their peripheral blood and bone marrow. Seven of eight infants reported died between three and 119 days of age from overwhelming infections; the eighth underwent complete immunologic reconstitution from a bone marrow transplant. Autosomal inheritance seems likely from reports of familial occurrences.

Serum immunoglobulins were very low, and no lymphocyte responses to mitogens occurred in the four patients in whom immunologic evaluations were conducted. The thymus glands all weighed less than 1 gram, and no Hassall's corpuscles and few thymocytes were seen.

PARTIAL COMBINED IMMUNODEFICIENCY DISORDERS

IMMUNODEFICIENCY WITH THROMBOCYTOPENIA AND ECZEMA (WISKOTT-ALDRICH SYNDROME). This X-linked recessive syndrome is characterized clinically by the triad of eczema, thrombocytopenic purpura, and undue susceptibility to infection. Often there is prolonged oozing from the circumcision site or bloody diarrhea during infancy. Atopic dermatitis and recurrent infections usually develop during the first year of life. Infections are caused by pneumococci and other bacteria with polysaccharide capsules, resulting in episodes of otitis media, pneumonia, meningitis, and sepsis. Later, infections with *Pneumocystis carinii* and the herpesviruses become more frequent. Survival beyond the teens is rare; major causes of death are infections or bleeding, but a 12-per-cent incidence of fatal malignancy also occurs in this condition. A papovavirus has been recovered from a reticulum cell sarcoma of the brain and from the urine of patients with this syndrome.

The earliest evidence of immunodeficiency is an impaired humoral immune response to polysaccharide antigens. Absent or markedly diminished isohemagglutinin titers are uniformly found, and poor or no responses are seen following immunization with polysaccharide antigens. Antibody titers to protein antigens also fall with time, and anamnestic responses are often poor or absent. Studies of immunoglobulin metabolism have shown an accelerated rate of synthesis—as well as hypercatabolism—of albumin, IgG, IgA, and IgM, resulting in highly variable immunoglobulin concentrations. The predominant dysgammaglobulinemia is a low IgM, elevated IgA, and IgE, and a normal or slightly low IgG concentration. Lymphocyte responses are moderately depressed, and cutaneous anergy is a frequent finding. Analyses of blood lymphocytes with monoclonal reagents have revealed low percentages of cells reacting with antibodies to all T cells and to the helper (CD4 +) and suppressor (CD8 +) subsets. However, as with the other primary cellular immunodeficiencies, there is usually no imbalance in the CD4:CD8 ratio.

The thrombocytopenia appears to be due to an intrinsic platelet abnormality, since antiplatelet antibodies are not usually demonstrated and survival times of homologous but not autologous ^{51}Cr-labeled platelets have been normal. Megakaryocytes are present in normal number in the bone marrow, but platelet size is small.

Treatment has been directed primarily toward control of bleeding with platelet transfusions, splenectomy, or both and of infections by intravenous administration of ISG. Several patients have had complete corrections of both the platelet and immunologic abnormalities by HLA–matched sibling bone marrow transplants after being conditioned with irradiation or busulfan and cyclophosphamide.

ATAXIA-TELANGIECTASIA. This is a complex syndrome with neurologic, immunologic, endocrinologic, hepatic, and cutaneous abnormalities. The most prominent clinical features are progressive cerebellar ataxia, oculocutaneous telangiectasias, chronic sinopulmonary disease, a high incidence of malignancy, and variable humoral and cellular immunodeficiency. Ataxia typically becomes evident soon after the child begins to walk. Telangiectasias usually develop by three to six years of age. Recurrent, usually bacterial, sinopulmonary infections occur in roughly 80 per cent of these patients; common viral exanthems have not usually resulted in untoward sequelae, but varicella was fatal in one of the author's patients.

The malignant tumors reported have usually been of the lymphoreticular type, but others have been seen. Cells from patients and heterozygous carriers have been reported to have increased sensitivity to ionizing radiation, defective DNA repair, and frequent chromosomal abnormalities. An autosomal recessive mode of inheritance seems operative.

The most frequent immunologic abnormality is selective absence of IgA, found in from 50 to 80 per cent of these patients. IgG$_2$ or total IgG may also be decreased. IgE concentrations are usually low, and the IgM may be of the low-molecular-weight variety. Specific antibody levels may be decreased or normal. In vivo, there is impaired but not absent cell-mediated immunity, as evidenced by delayed cutaneous anergy and prolonged allograft survival. Death from GVH

disease has not been reported. Enumeration of blood T cells and subsets reveals reduced percentages of total T cells and T cells of the helper (CD4) phenotype, with normal or increased percentages of cells of the suppressor (CD8) phenotype. In vitro studies of lymphocyte function have shown moderately depressed proliferative responses to mitogens, decreased T helper cell function, and an intrinsic defect in B cell IgA synthesis. The thymus is very hypoplastic and lacks Hassall's corpuscles. No satisfactory treatment has been found.

CARTILAGE HAIR HYPOPLASIA. An unusual form of short-limbed dwarfism with frequent and severe infections has been reported among the Amish. Features include short and pudgy hands; redundant skin; hyperextensible joints of hands and feet but an inability to completely extend the elbows; and fine, sparse light hair and eyebrows. Severe and often fatal varicella infections appear to be a particular hazard. Progressive vaccinia and vaccine-associated-poliomyelitis have also been observed.

The severity of the immunodeficiency varies; in one series, 11 of 77 patients died before age 20, but two were still alive at age 76. Three patterns of immune dysfunction have emerged: defective antibody-mediated immunity, defective cellular immunity, and severe combined immunodeficiency. The most striking abnormality appears to be one of defective cell proliferation due to an intrinsic defect related to the G1 phase, resulting in a longer cell cycle for individual cells. The trait appears to be autosomal recessive with variable penetrance.

IMMUNODEFICIENCY WITH THYMOMA. These patients are adults who almost simultaneously develop hypogammaglobulinemia, deficits in cell-mediated immunity, and benign thymoma (see Ch. 428). The thymomas are predominantly of the spindle cell variety. Eosinophilia or eosinopenia, aregenerative or hemolytic anemia, thrombocytopenia, or pancytopenia may also occur. Antibody formation is poor, although percentages of immunoglobulin-bearing B lymphocytes are normal, and progressive lymphopenia develops. Several patients with this disorder have been shown to have excessive suppressor T cell activity.

HYPERIMMUNOGLOBULINEMIA E SYNDROME. The hyper–IgE syndrome is a primary immunodeficiency characterized by recurrent staphylococcal abscesses and markedly elevated serum IgE concentrations. The disorder was first reported by the author and her coworkers in two young boys in 1972. These patients all have lifelong histories of severe recurrent staphylococcal abscesses involving the skin, lungs, joints, and other sites. Persistent pneumatoceles develop as a result of their recurrent pneumonias. The pruritic dermatitis that occurs is not typical atopic eczema and does not always persist; respiratory allergic symptoms are usually absent. An autosomal-dominant form of inheritance with incomplete penetrance seems possible. Laboratory features include exceptionally high serum IgE concentrations but usually normal IgG, IgA, and IgM concentrations; pronounced blood and sputum eosinophilia; abnormally low anamnestic antibody responses; and poor antibody and cell-mediated responses to neoantigens. In vitro studies have shown normal percentages of CD2–, CD3–, CD4–, and CD8–positive lymphocytes, and there is no increase in the percentage of IgE–bearing B lymphocytes. Lymphocyte responses to mitogens are normal, but responses to antigens or to related allogeneic cells have been absent or very low. Histologic sections of lymph nodes, spleen, and lung cysts show striking eosinophilia.

Phagocytic cell ingestion, metabolism, and killing mechanisms and total hemolytic complement have been normal in all patients. Defects of mononuclear and/or polymorphonuclear chemotaxis are present in some but not most patients and thus are not the basic problem in this syndrome.

The most effective therapy is long-term administration of a

penicillinase-resistant penicillin, with the addition of other antibiotic or antifungal agents as required for specific infections.

CHRONIC MUCOCUTANEOUS CANDIDIASIS. This clinical syndrome, probably of multiple causes, is associated with chronic candidal infection of the skin and mucous membranes but only rarely life-threatening systemic infections of the types seen in patients with severe T cell dysfunction. Some patients have endocrinopathies involving the parathyroid, thyroid, adrenal, and/or pancreatic glands (see Ch. 241); however, many have neither associated endocrinopathy nor any demonstrable immunologic abnormality. Ketoconazole (Nizoral) has been found to be the single most effective form of therapy.

LYMPHOCYTE-FUNCTION–ASSOCIATED ANTIGEN TYPE 1 (LFA-1) DEFICIENCY. This condition is due to an autosomal codominant or recessively inherited deficiency of a 95 Kd MW beta chain structure. The latter is linked noncovalently to each of three distinct alpha chain types to form different cell surface glycoproteins: LFA-1 on B, T, and natural killer (NK) lymphocytes; complement receptor type 3 (CR3) on neutrophils, monocytes, macrophages, eosinophils, and NK cells; and p150,95 (function unknown). Patients have histories of delayed separation of the umbilical cord, omphalitis, gingivitis, recurrent skin infections, repeated otitis media, pneumonia, peritonitis, perianal abscesses, and impaired wound healing. They do not have increased susceptibility to viral infections or malignancy. All cytotoxic lymphocyte functions are markedly impaired due to a lack of the adhesion protein LFA-1; deficiency of LFA-1 also interferes with immune cell interaction and immune recognition. CR3 binds fixed iC3b fragments of C3 and beta glucans; its absence causes abnormal phagocytic cell adherence and chemotaxis and a reduced respiratory burst with phagocytosis. Blood neutrophil counts are usually elevated. Deficiencies of these glycoproteins can be screened for by cytofluorography of blood leukocytes with appropriate monoclonal antibodies.

PRIMARY DEFICIENCIES OF THE COMPLEMENT SYSTEM

In addition to congenital or hereditary disorders of lymphoid cells, there are several well-defined primary immune defects involving the complement system. Genetically determined deficiencies have been described for all of the components of complement, and undue susceptibility to infection is a characteristic of deficiencies of C2, C3, C5, C6, and C7. The types of infections experienced in C2, C3, and in some with C5 deficiency are with gram-positive encapsulated organisms, whereas those in patients with deficiencies of the terminal components are usually meningococcal or gonococcal. A normal CH50 would exclude all heritable complement deficiencies. The complement system is discussed in detail in Chapter 418.

Buckley RH: Normal and abnormal development of the immune system. In Joklik WK, Willett HP, Amos DB (eds.): Zinsser Textbook of Microbiology and Immunology. 19th ed. New York, Appleton-Century-Crofts, 1988, in press. *A concise review of ontogeny of the normal human immune system as well as the primary immunodeficiency disorders.*

Buckley RH, Sampson HA: The hyperimmunoglobulinemia E syndrome. In Franklin EC (ed.): Clinical Immunology Update. New York, Elsevier North Holland, 1981, pp 147–167. *A review of the clinical and immunologic features of 21 well-studied patients with the hyper-IgE syndrome.*

Buckley RH, Schiff SE, Sampson HA, et al.: Development of immunity in human severe primary T cell deficiency following haploidentical bone marrow stem cell transplantation. J Immunol 136:2398, 1986. *A review of the time course and extent of immune reconstitution in 17 patients with severe T cell defects given haploidentical stem cell transplants.*

Childhood immunodeficiency disorders: Diagnosis, prevention, and management. Clin Immunol Immunopathol 40:1, 1986. *This multiauthored issue is the most current treatise on primary immunodeficiency and includes the latest World Health Organization Committee report on these diseases.*

Purtillo DT: Epstein-Barr virus–induced diseases in the X-linked lymphoproliferative syndrome and related disorders. Biomed Pharmacol Ther 39:52, 1985. *An update on EBV–induced immunodeficiency.*

Rosen FS, Cooper MD, Wedgewood RJP: The primary immunodeficiencies. N Engl J Med 311:235, 300, 1984. *An excellent Medical Progress article that presents an overview of the basic biology and the clinical manifestations of these disorders. 260 references.*

Ross GD: Clinical and laboratory features of patients with an inherited deficiency of neutrophil membrane complement receptor type 3 (CR3) and the related membrane antigens LFA-1 and p150,95. J Clin Immunol 6:107, 1986. *An excellent review of a new immunodeficiency syndrome for which the molecular basis is known.*

Ross SC, Densen P: Complement deficiency states and infection: Epidemiology, pathogenesis and consequences of neisserial and other infections in an immune deficiency. Medicine 63:243, 1984.

---

420 URTICARIA AND ANGIOEDEMA

Nicholas A. Soter

DEFINITION. Urticaria and angioedema are commonly encountered clinical entities that occur as evanescent areas of cutaneous edema. Urticaria appears as circumscribed elevated erythematous and usually pruritic areas of edema involving the superficial portions of the dermis. When the edema extends into the deep portions of the dermis or subcutaneous and submucosal tissues or both, it is designated angioedema and appears as large erythematous areas with diffuse borders. In addition to the skin, the respiratory and gastrointestinal tracts as well as the cardiovascular system may be involved singly or in any combination. The etiology of urticaria-angioedema is frequently unknown; however, its pathogenesis in many instances is believed to be related to activation of mast cells and/or basophils and release of their products. Similar symptoms and signs may occur with the participation of other inflammatory systems, such as the arachidonic acid metabolic pathways, the complement system (see Ch. 418), and the Hageman factor–dependent pathways of coagulation, fibrinolysis, and kinin generation, with or without the participation of mast cells.

INCIDENCE AND PREVALENCE. Urticaria-angioedema may develop at any age. The highest incidence is in young adults (approximately 15 to 20 per cent). In patients with urticaria-angioedema, about 50 per cent will have both; 40 per cent, urticaria alone; and 10 per cent, angioedema alone. Approximately 50 per cent of patients with urticaria alone are free of lesions within one year, but 20 per cent continue to experience lesions for more than 20 years. Of patients with both urticaria and angioedema, 75 per cent experience symptoms for more than one year; 50 per cent, for more than five years; and 20 per cent, for more than 20 years. Age, race, sex, occupation, geographic location, and season of the year are involved as factors only insofar as they may contribute to exposure to an eliciting cause.

PATHOGENESIS AND PATHOLOGY. Urticaria-angioedema is often attributed to an immediate-type immunologic reaction (Type I, anaphylactic, or IgE–mediated hypersensitivity) produced by the antigen-induced release of biologically active materials from mast cells sensitized with specific IgE. Antigen-dependent activation and secretion in mast cells is initiated by bridging of pairs of adjacent IgE molecules and is dependent upon several subsequent cell-membrane and intracellular events that are regulated by cyclic nucleotides (see Fig. 60–3). Urticaria-angioedema may also occur after mast cell degranulation induced by complement factors C3a and C5a, kinins, insect venoms, highly charged polyanions, or certain therapeutic and diagnostic agents. Physical stimuli such as trauma, pressure, cold, light, and heat may affect the mast cell via IgE or by unknown mechanisms.

The skin is rich in mast cells; the mean number is 7000 to

12,000 per cubic millimeter (see Fig. 427–1). The biologic effects of mast cells (described more fully in Ch. 427) are produced by the release of mediators, which alter venular permeability, contract smooth muscles, influence the motility of leukocytes, affect the generation and release of biologically active materials from other cell types, and enzymatically degrade complex substrates (see table in Ch. 427).

Urticaria-angioedema occurring after mast cell–mediated reactions traditionally has been attributed primarily to the release of *histamine*, although other mediators may play a role. Two tissue receptors, classified as H_1 and H_2, mediate the biologic activities of histamine. Inasmuch as the human skin vasculature contains both H_1 and H_2 receptors, vascular permeability may depend on the effect of histamine on both.

Skin biopsy specimens show edema involving the superficial portion of the dermis in the case of urticaria and the deeper dermis and subcutaneous tissue in the case of angioedema. Both urticaria and angioedema are associated with dilation of the venules, with or without tissue infiltration by various numbers of lymphocytes and/or eosinophils and neutrophils. In some instances, necrotizing vasculitis with fibrinoid necrosis of the venule is present. In individuals with hereditary angioedema, examination of biopsy specimens from skin, larynx, and jejunum has shown subcutaneous or submucosal edema without infiltrating inflammatory cells.

CLINICAL MANIFESTATIONS. Urticaria and angioedema may occur together or individually in any location; however, angioedema most commonly affects the face. Episodes of urticaria-angioedema appear suddenly, usually persist fewer than 24 hours, and may recur. Recurrent episodes of fewer than four to six weeks' duration are considered acute, whereas those persisting longer are chronic.

Urticaria-angioedema can be classified in five groups that include those types that are IgE dependent or complement dependent, those that are due to a direct action on mast cells, those that occur after presumed alterations of the arachidonic acid metabolic pathways, and those that are idiopathic (see Table 420–1).

Idiopathic Urticaria-Angioedema. In at least 70 per cent of individuals with chronic episodes of urticaria-angioedema the cause is unknown. Since this clinical condition is common, is easily recognized, and manifests a capricious course, it is often associated with concomitant events. Although viral, fungal, bacterial, and helminthic infections, foods, medications, diagnostic agents, metabolic and hormonal abnormalities, malignant conditions, and emotional factors are frequently claimed as causes, proof of their etiologic relation often is lacking. An idiopathic syndrome of episodic urticaria-angioedema with fever, weight gain, and peripheral blood and tissue eosinophilia has been described. Although idiopathic urticaria-angioedema is the most prevalent form, the diagnosis is one of exclusion and can be made only after the other types of urticaria-angioedema, discussed below, are eliminated. The laboratory studies to be considered in patients with urticaria-angioedema are noted under Laboratory Findings, below.

TABLE 420–1. CLASSIFICATION OF URTICARIA-ANGIOEDEMA

  I. **Idiopathic urticaria-angioedema**
 II. **IgE–dependent urticaria-angioedema**
    A. Atopic diathesis
    B. Specific antigen sensitivity
    C. Physical stimuli
    D. Contact urticaria
III. **Complement-mediated urticaria-angioedema**
    A. Hereditary angioedema
    B. Acquired C1 inhibitor abnormalities associated with angioedema
    C. Necrotizing venulitis
    D. Serum sickness
    E. Reactions to the administration of blood products
IV. **Urticaria-angioedema due to agents with a direct action on mast cells**
 V. **Urticaria-angioedema dependent on agents that alter the arachidonic acid metabolic pathways**

IgE–Dependent Urticaria-Angioedema. ATOPIC DIATHESIS. A history of acute episodes of urticaria-angioedema may be elicited in individuals with a personal or family history of asthma, rhinitis, or eczema. The prevalence of chronic urticaria, however, is not increased in atopic individuals.

SPECIFIC ANTIGENS. IgE–mediated urticaria-angioedema occurs after exposure to agents that include foods, diagnostic and therapeutic agents, aeroallergens, and Hymenoptera venoms.

PHYSICAL STIMULI. Physical urticaria-angioedema occurs after a variety of stimuli, some of which are IgE dependent as demonstrated by passive transfer of the cutaneous response with serum given to normal individuals (Prausnitz-Küstner reaction).

Dermographism. Dermographism occurs in 1.5 to 4.2 per cent of the normal population. It is usually recognized as a linear wheal appearing after the skin is briskly stroked with a firm object; however, its configuration depends on the eliciting stimulus. The transient pruritic wheal appears rapidly and fades within 30 minutes. Dermographism has been passively transferred to the skin of normal persons with both serum and its IgE fraction. Elevations in blood histamine levels have been detected after experimental scratching.

Pressure Urticaria-Angioedema. Pressure urticaria appears as erythematous, deep, often painful swelling that arises within minutes or up to six hours after sustained pressure, such as occurs under shoulder straps and belts, on the soles of the feet after running, and on the palms after manual labor. The delayed form may be associated with fever, chills, and arthralgia. Although pressure urticaria-angioedema often occurs in individuals with dermographism or chronic idiopathic urticaria, an IgE–dependent mechanism has not been documented.

Vibratory Angioedema. Angioedema occurring after a vibratory stimulus has been reported with an autosomal-dominant pattern of inheritance. It occurs also after several years of occupational exposure to vibration. In the heritable form, the swelling appears rapidly, is transient, and is accompanied by facial flushing. A transient rise in plasma histamine was noted during experimental induction of vibratory angioedema, both in the hereditary form and in those patients with acquired disease.

Cold-Induced Urticaria-Angioedema. There are both inherited and acquired forms of cold-induced urticaria-angioedema. The acquired form is more common. After exposure to changes in ambient temperature or direct contact with cold objects, patients experience a pruritic, urticarial eruption that may evolve into angioedema. Headaches, syncope, or wheezing may accompany an attack. If the entire body is cooled, as in swimming, hypotension and collapse, a potentially lethal event, may occur. Passive transfer with serum and its IgE fraction to the skin of a normal recipient has been documented, and the release into the serum of histamine and other mast cell–derived products has been detected after experimental challenge. Also, successful passive transfer with serum containing IgM antibody has been accomplished. In rare instances, acquired cold urticaria has been associated with underlying cryoglobulins, cryofibrinogens, cold hemolysins or cold agglutinins, especially in patients with viral illnesses, notably infectious mononucleosis. The mechanism by which cryoproteins induce cold urticaria may be activation of the complement system.

Dominantly inherited cold urticaria has been described in immediate and delayed forms. In the immediate or familial type, the eruption appears as erythematous macules or papules which manifest a burning sensation and which are accompanied by pyrexia, arthralgias, and a neutrophilic leukocytosis. In the delayed form, erythematous deep swellings develop 9 to 18 hours after cold challenge. This disorder is infrequently recognized, and its pathogenesis is unknown.

Light Urticaria. Idiopathic light- or solar urticaria is a rare condition manifested by pruritus and urticaria-angioedema developing within minutes after exposure to the sun or to artificial light sources. Light urticaria also occasionally occurs in patients with systemic lupus erythematosus and erythropoietic protoporphyria. Classification of the urticarial response into subtypes is based on the reaction to specific portions of the light spectrum; however, individuals may respond to more than one portion of the spectrum. Histamine and factors chemotactic for eosinophils and neutrophils have been detected in serum after experimental exposure to UVB (290–320 nm), UVA (320–400 nm), or visible (400–700 nm) light. In some individuals the response has been passively transferred; in other subjects a serum factor induced by irradiation has been implicated in the development of the lesions.

Cholinergic Urticaria. Cholinergic urticaria is a distinctive eruption that develops after stimuli that allegedly raise core body temperature, such as a hot shower, exercise, or episodes of pyrexia. After an initial sensation of warmth, pruritic wheals 1 to 2 mm in size appear, surrounded by extensive areas of erythema. Wheezing has been noted, and obstructive alterations in pulmonary function have been documented during experimental induction of the clinical syndrome by exercise. Elevations in serum histamine and the appearance of factors chemotactic for eosinophils and neutrophils have been noted. Although injection of cholinergic agents such as methacholine into the skin has been employed as a diagnostic test, in only one third of individuals with cholinergic urticaria does this maneuver reproduce the skin lesions. There is an exercise-related physical allergy with pruritus, urticaria-angioedema, and syncope that is distinct from cholinergic urticaria.

Heat Urticaria. Heat urticaria is a rare disorder in which urticaria-angioedema develops within minutes after exposure to locally applied heat. Elevations in plasma histamine levels have been noted after experimental challenge.

Aquagenic Urticaria and Aquagenic Pruritus. Contact of the skin with water of any temperature may result in pruritus alone or, more rarely, urticaria. The eruption consists of small wheals reminiscent of cholinergic urticaria. After experimental challenge, elevations of blood histamine have been noted in both aquagenic urticaria and aquagenic pruritus.

Contact Urticaria. Urticaria may occur after direct local contact with a variety of chemical substances. The eruption appears within minutes and is transient. Occasionally, systemic manifestations have been noted. Although passive transfer has been documented in some instances, agents such as stinging nettles, arthropod hairs, and chemicals may directly release histamine from mast cells.

Complement-Mediated Urticaria-Angioedema. HEREDITARY ANGIOEDEMA. Hereditary angioedema (HAE) occurs as episodes of edema of the skin and of the upper respiratory and gastrointestinal tracts. Episodes of swelling are self-limited, subside within 72 hours, and may occur over any area of the body, particularly on the face or an extremity. Urticaria is not a manifestation of HAE. Swelling of the face or buccal mucosa may progress to involve the larynx, with the danger of death by asphyxiation. The severity of the abdominal pain mimics surgical abdominal conditions.

HAE is transmitted as an autosomal dominant trait, and afflicted individuals are heterozygotes; however, the absence of a family history does not exclude the diagnosis. There are two forms of this inherited disease, each of which is characterized by the absence of function of the inhibitor (C$\overline{1}$INH) of the activated form of the first complement protein (C$\overline{1}$) of the classic activating pathway (see Ch. 418). Either the C$\overline{1}$INH protein and its function are lacking or normal levels of C$\overline{1}$INH protein without function are present. The absence of C$\overline{1}$INH provides a genetic marker for HAE. Levels of the fourth complement protein (C4) are also low, and levels of C4 and of the second complement protein (C2) diminish during clinical attacks. With the possible exception of post-traumatic attacks, the reasons for the episodic activation of C1 are

unknown. In the absence of the C$\overline{1}$INH, the activation of Hageman factor after tissue trauma may lead to the conversion of plasminogen to plasmin, which subsequently activates C1. Moreover, incubation of plasma spontaneously generates smooth-muscle contracting activity that may be involved in the production of angioedema. Urinary histamine levels are increased during attacks, presumably reflecting the degranulation of mast cells by C3a anaphylatoxin. Kallikrein has been found in the fluid of blisters induced over areas of edema, and increased bradykinin levels have been detected in plasma during attacks.

ACQUIRED C$\overline{1}$INH DEFICIENCY. The acquired depletion of the C$\overline{1}$INH sometimes associated with angioedema has been observed in patients with different types of lymphoproliferative disorders, in a patient with a rectal adenocarcinoma, and in some individuals with lupus erythematosus. In addition to low serum levels of C$\overline{1}$INH and C4, C1 and C1q levels are also reduced, thus permitting its differentiation from HAE. Abnormalities of complement in family members have not been reported.

NECROTIZING VENULITIS. Recurrent episodes of urticaria-angioedema may be manifestations of cutaneous necrotizing venulitis and may occur in individuals with systemic lupus erythematosus, Sjögren's syndrome, or hepatitis B–virus infection. An idiopathic clinical syndrome occurs primarily in women. The episodes of urticaria are chronic; individual lesions are transient, but last in many instances up to three to five days. Most patients experience transient arthralgias of the peripheral joints. In some instances, diffuse glomerulonephritis has been noted as well as pyrexia, lymphadenopathy, obstructive pulmonary disease, and benign intracranial hypertension. These cases have been described under the terms atypical erythema multiforme, lupus erythematosus-like syndrome, and hypocomplementemia-vasculitis-urticaria syndrome. Although some patients manifest serum hypocomplementemia with circulating C1q precipitins, many do not.

SERUM SICKNESS. Serum sickness is a self-limited clinical symptom complex occurring after the administration of serum or drugs. The clinical manifestations include pyrexia, urticaria, lymphadenopathy, myalgia, and arthralgia. Urticaria is seen in over 70 per cent of patients with serum sickness and often occurs at the site of injection.

REACTIONS TO BLOOD PRODUCTS. Urticaria-angioedema frequently occurs after the administration of blood products. Both the urticarial and the anaphylactic reactions noted after the transfusion of blood, serum, or IgG fractions are usually the result of immune complex formation with complement activation. Such immune complex reactions are especially prevalent in patients with IgA deficiency, in whom antibodies against IgA are present.

Urticaria-Angioedema Due to Agents with a Direct Action on Mast Cells. The administration of opiates, polymyxin B, curare and tubocurarine, or radiocontrast media may be associated with the idiosyncratic release of histamine from mast cells. Between 5 and 8 per cent of individuals receiving radiocontrast media experience urticarial reactions.

Agents Which Presumably Alter Arachidonic Acid Metabolism. Urticaria-angioedema in response to administration of aspirin or nonsteroidal anti-inflammatory agents occurs commonly. Aspirin intolerance in patients with chronic urticaria is reported to be as high as 20 to 50 per cent. Patients intolerant to nonsteroidal anti-inflammatory agents also react to azo dyes, notably tartrazine, as well as to benzoates used as preservatives. Such reactions are often unrecognized, may serve to aggravate preexisting urticaria, and may occur from 15 minutes to 20 hours after ingestion. In patients intolerant to aspirin, reactions do not occur after exposure to structurally related compounds such as sodium or choline salicylate, whereas structurally unrelated agents such as indomethacin may precipitate the response.

LABORATORY FINDINGS. Laboratory evaluation is usually not helpful in patients with acute episodes of urticaria-angioedema. Historical information and physical findings offer better diagnostic clues.

Evaluation of chronic episodes of urticaria-angioedema requires more extensive laboratory analysis. In those patients whose urticaria-angioedema suggests an IgE-mediated allergic process, prick skin testing or assessment in vitro by radioallergosorbent test (RAST) of specific IgE antibody may be indicated; however, the likelihood of obtaining diagnostically relevant information from unselected prick skin tests or RAST is minimal. Prick skin testing is unreliable in the presence of dermographism. Eosinophilia, when present, is a helpful feature in implicating a drug reaction or parasitic infestation as a cause of urticaria. Antinuclear antibody is helpful in detecting associated lupus erythematosus. Total serum concentrations of IgE in the absence of atopy are normal in patients with chronic urticaria-angioedema.

Assessment of the serum complement system is of value in detecting patients with hereditary and acquired forms of angioedema. In patients with HAE, immunochemical measurements of both C$\bar{1}$INH and C4 are low with normal levels of C1 and C3. If the C$\bar{1}$INH protein level is normal and the C4 low, functional assessment of C$\bar{1}$INH may be performed to confirm the diagnosis.

In patients with chronic idiopathic urticaria-angioedema the finding of an elevated erythrocyte sedimentation rate should prompt a biopsy of an urticarial lesion to search for underlying cutaneous necrotizing venulitis. In some patients with necrotizing venulitis hypocomplementemia may be detected. As not all patients with necrotizing venulitis manifest hypocomplementemia, the sedimentation rate has proved to be a more sensitive screening test than serum complement analysis.

DIAGNOSIS AND DIFFERENTIAL DIAGNOSIS. Urticaria and angioedema are easily recognizable. Urticarial eruptions are episodic and evanescent, with multiple lesions occurring in various stages of evolution and resolution. The differential diagnosis of urticaria includes papular urticaria, which consists of small wheals occurring after insect bites; the eruption of erythema multiforme that includes iris or target lesions; the early urticarial stages of the Henoch-Schönlein syndrome that evolve into palpable purpura; urticaria pigmentosa, which is a generalized, pigmented, papular, or even nodular mast cell infiltration in which the skin lesions become urticarial upon rubbing (see Fig. 427–2); and the syndrome of perceptive deafness, fever with urticaria, and renal insufficiency consequent to amyloidosis.

Disorders included in the differential diagnosis of angioedema are contact dermatitis appearing as recurrent episodes of eyelid and facial swelling; cellulitis and erysipelas, which may at times resemble angioedema; lymphedema occurring after cutaneous pyoderma or surgery; and congestive heart failure, renal insufficiency, obstruction of the superior vena cava, myxedema, thrombophlebitis, and stasis, which may produce recurrent swelling. The Melkersson-Rosenthal syndrome consists of swelling of the lips, facial paralysis, and a fissured tongue.

TREATMENT AND PREVENTION. When urticaria-angioedema is due to a known agent, avoidance is the therapeutic choice. Since patients may respond to the administration of placebos and the disease tends to remit spontaneously, evaluation of therapeutic intervention is difficult. Avoidance of aspirin or food additives has been claimed to help many patients. Recurrent episodes of idiopathic urticaria-angioedema are most effectively treated by the prophylactic administration of H$_1$ antihistaminic agents. A variety of H$_1$-type antihistamine preparations exist, which are used empirically. These agents are administered in divided doses; representative examples are chlorpheniramine maleate, 4 to 8 mg, or diphenhydramine hydrochloride, 25 to 50 mg, every four to six hours. The combination of H$_2$ antihistamines with H$_1$ agents is of value in a small number of individuals. The role of dietary manipulation is difficult to assess. Epinephrine is rarely required, and the chronic systemic administration of corticosteroid preparations creates risks out of proportion to the therapeutic benefits. The treatment of physical urticaria includes avoidance of the precipitating stimulus and the empiric administration of antihistamines.

The treatment of HAE can be divided into management of the acute episode, preoperative prophylaxis, and long-term prevention of spontaneous attacks. Specific therapeutic measures to interrupt spontaneous attacks are not available. The primary maneuver is to maintain the airway. Preoperative preparation of patients with antifibrinolytic agents suppresses attacks of angioedema. Nonandrogenic or impeded anabolic steroids, such as oxymetholone, danazol, and stanozolol, are effective in prevention of spontaneous attacks. Toxicity caused by attenuated androgens is dose related; however, the adverse effects that occur with daily therapy subside with alternate-day therapy. Impeded androgens have also been used to treat acquired C$\bar{1}$INH deficiency with recurrent angioedema. There is no proven effective treatment for the urticaria-angioedema that occurs as a manifestation of underlying necrotizing venulitis, although some patients benefit from the administration of antihistamines, nonsteroidal anti-inflammatory agents, colchicine, or prednisone.

Brickman CM, Hosea S: Hereditary angioedema. Int J Dermatol 22:141, 1983. *A useful review of hereditary angioedema with emphasis on its pathogenesis and treatment.*

Champion RH, Greaves MW, Kobza Black A, et al.: The Urticarias. Edinburgh, Churchill Livingstone, 1985. *The proceedings of a symposium on urticaria-angioedema.*

Jorizzo JL (ed.): Symposium on urticaria and the reactive inflammatory vascular dermatoses. Dermatol Clin, Vol 3, No 1, 1985. *A collection of papers on various aspects of urticaria.*

Kaplan AP: Exercise-induced hives. J Allerg Clin Immunol 73:704, 1984. *A review of the types of urticaria-angioedema induced by exercise.*

Neittaanmäki H: Cold urticaria: Clinical findings in 220 patients. J Am Acad Dermatol 13:636, 1985. *A thorough study of cold urticaria in a large number of patients annotating both clinical features and natural history.*

421 ALLERGIC RHINITIS

John E. Salvaggio

DEFINITION. Allergic rhinitis is an IgE–mediated, inflammatory disease of the nasal mucous membranes characterized by paroxysms of sneezing; itching of the nose, eyes, palate, pharynx, and conjunctivae; nasal stuffiness with partial or total obstruction of air flow; and mucous secretion often accompanied by postnasal drainage. The disease is often seasonal, depending on the pollination patterns of inhalant allergens that have direct impact on the respiratory mucosa. The condition may be perennial when due to nonseasonal allergens such as dust, animal danders, some plant products, and molds.

Patients with allergic rhinitis have an increased number of mast cells in nasal secretions. When appropriately sensitized with specific IgE molecules, mucosal mast cells can interact with allergenic airborne particles that initially affect the respiratory mucosa and release water-soluble allergens during inhalation. Mast cells and basophils concentrate IgE on their surfaces, which may have up to 500,000 IgE molecules per cell. The IgE fixes to a glycoprotein receptor site on the membrane by its Fc fragment, resulting in an arrangement that permits exposure of the antibody combining sites (or Fab) to the surrounding milieu. Cross-linking of two IgE antibody molecules by specific antigen aggregates the corresponding receptor sites and results in initiation of a series of cellular biochemical events that culminate in the expulsion of secretory granule contents. Among the important mast cell–derived mediators, either preformed within their granules or generated from precursor molecules, are histamine; bradykinin; thromboxanes; leukotrienes C, D, and E, which are derived from arachidonic acid released during the allergic reaction; eosinophil chemotactic factors of anaphylaxis (ECF-A), which are derived from the mast cell granule; heparin, which makes up 30 per cent of the dry weight of mast cell granules; superoxide dismutase (SOD), which is formed by the univalent reduction of oxygen; prostaglandins, which are C_{20} unsaturated fatty acid derivatives of arachidonic acid; platelet activating factor (PAF), a small phospholipid derivative of phosphoryl choline released from rabbit basophils; neutrophil chemotactic factor of anaphylaxis (NCF-A); inflammatory factors of anaphylaxis, which are constituents of the mast cell granules that induce a "late-phase" allergic inflammatory reaction; and a number of enzymes that are found in mast cell granules, such as chymotrypsin and trypsin. These enzymes may contribute to the tissue destruction accompanying various "late-phase" allergic reactions.

ETIOLOGY. The most apparent seasonal allergens acting as etiologic agents in allergic rhinitis are pollens such as ragweed and mold spores. Tree pollens are usually released during the spring, and in most parts of the country the peak of the grass pollen season is late spring to midsummer. Much of the nasal symptoms caused by airborne weed pollens occur in late summer and early fall. Ragweed pollen is by far the worst offender in the eastern, midwestern, and southern United States. Many individuals with allergic rhinitis have an IgE–mediated response to crude house-dust antigen, which is a mixture of lint, danders, insect parts, fibers, and other particulate matter. In many geographic areas and household situations, mites, including *Dermatophagoides farinae* and *D.*

petronyssimus, appear to be the primary sources of antigen in house dusts. Animal danders, particularly cat dander, may be especially potent in inducing sudden, violent nasal symptoms, even when there is contact only with the dander, saliva, or urine of the animal. In certain persons other inhalant allergens, including cotton seed and flax seed, which may be constituents of animal feeds, fertilizers, and inexpensive upholstery, may cause perennial or sporadic symptoms. Mold spores can be very important perennial allergens, since they are found in both outdoor and indoor environments.

INCIDENCE AND PREVALENCE. Approximately 9 per cent of all patients who seek care at a physician's office do so for one of the common allergic diseases. It is estimated that 40 million Americans have allergic diseases: an estimated 10 million suffer from asthma with or without allergic rhinitis, over 15 million have allergic rhinitis alone, and over 12 million have other allergic manifestations, such as urticaria, angioedema, eczema, or food-, drug-, or insect hypersensitivity. Stated another way, 17 per cent of all Americans have at least one common allergic disease, and 7 per cent have allergic rhinitis alone. These incidence figures are deceptively low, since they approximate only the number of patients who, at the time of the particular study, are actually afflicted with the condition and they do not include the large numbers of individuals who have had diseases such as allergic rhinitis in the past but have since "recovered."

PATHOGENESIS AND MECHANISMS. The pathogenesis of allergic rhinitis including IgE–allergen interaction, mast cell–mediator release, sensory nerve stimulation, and CNS–mediated reflex activity is illustrated in Figure 421–1. The nasal cavity is lined with airways epithelium of the ciliated

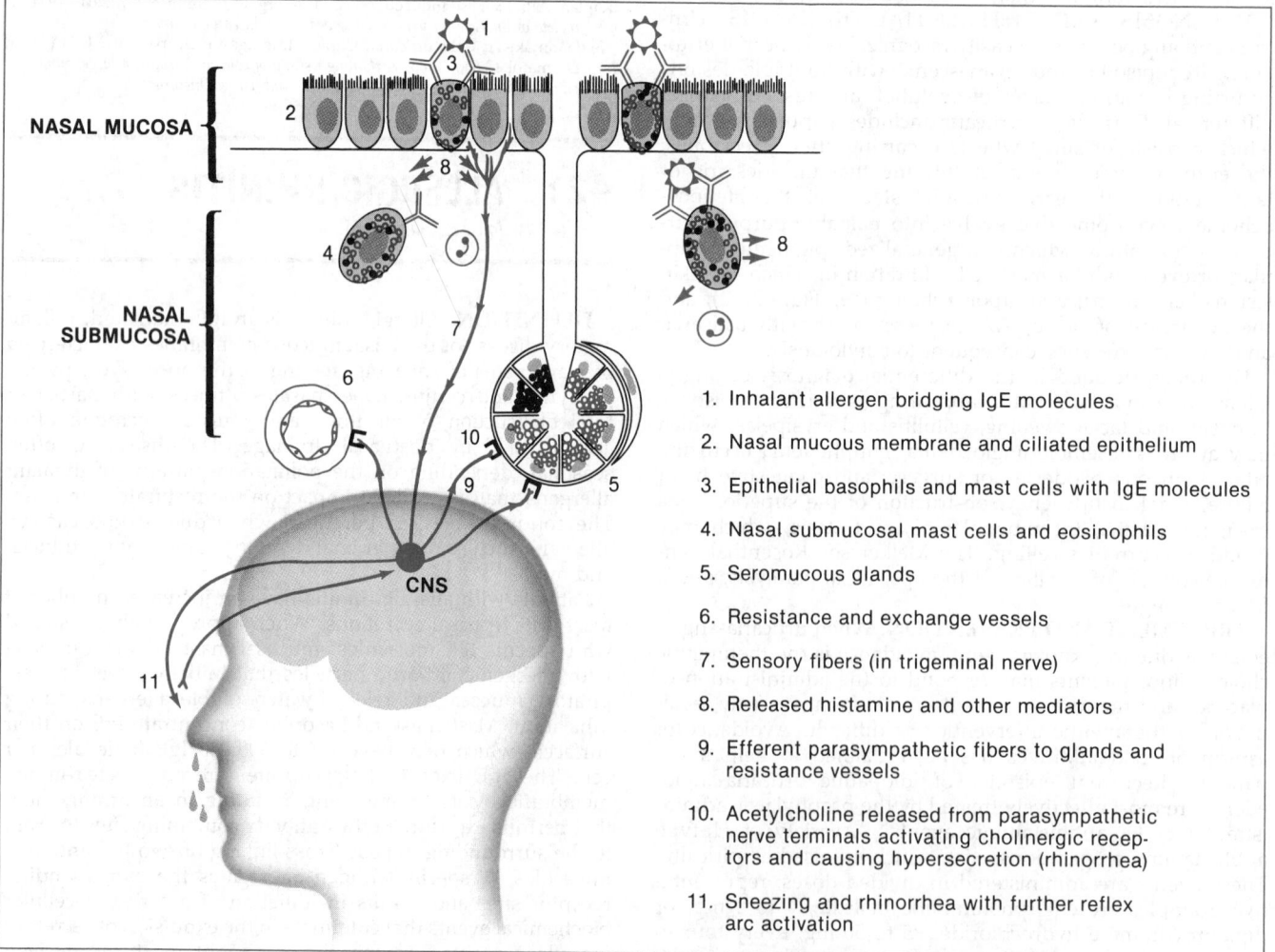

NASAL MUCOSA

NASAL SUBMUCOSA

CNS

1. Inhalant allergen bridging IgE molecules

2. Nasal mucous membrane and ciliated epithelium

3. Epithelial basophils and mast cells with IgE molecules

4. Nasal submucosal mast cells and eosinophils

5. Seromucous glands

6. Resistance and exchange vessels

7. Sensory fibers (in trigeminal nerve)

8. Released histamine and other mediators

9. Efferent parasympathetic fibers to glands and resistance vessels

10. Acetylcholine released from parasympathetic nerve terminals activating cholinergic receptors and causing hypersecretion (rhinorrhea)

11. Sneezing and rhinorrhea with further reflex arc activation

FIGURE 421–1. Pathogenesis of allergic rhinitis; antigen-antibody interaction and mediator release.

pseudostratified type. The lamina propria in the anterior part of the nose contains large numbers of seromucous and serous glands. Postganglionic sympathetic nerves emerge from the stellate ganglion in the neck and reach the nose along arteries. Most of the parasympathetic fibers to the nose travel via the vidian nerve. The parasympathetic fibers are part of a reflex arc with sensory fibers in the trigeminal nerve. The nasal sensory nerves are exposed to stimulation from unconditioned and polluted inhaled air, and there is constant reflex activity in the nerves.

There are immunologic as well as nonimmunologic triggers of this mast cell degranulation process. It is common for patients to note associations between symptoms and exposure to certain nonspecific irritants, such as strong odors, insecticides, and cigarette smoke. Histamine sprayed into the nose causes itching, sneezing, discharge, and blockage, and directly increases endothelial- and epithelial-cell permeability. This facilitates further allergen penetration into the submucosal areas. Histamine also has a direct effect on vascular H_1- and H_2 receptors, resulting in edema formation. In addition, when released from epithelial basophils, histamine indirectly stimulates sensory nerve H_1 receptors, resulting in a CNS–mediated parasympathetic reflex in the trigeminal and vidian nerves with subsequent itching, sneezing, and increased nasal discharge. Finally, repeated allergen exposure likely results in increased mucosal reactivity, and in association with production of "late-phase mediators" can result in chronic mucosal inflammation.

CLINICAL MANIFESTATIONS. Common symptoms include *nasal stuffiness*, paroxysms of *sneezing*, profuse *mucous secretion*, and frequent *itching* of the nose, eyes, posterior pharynx, or conjunctivae. Soreness or inflammation of the conjunctivae with excessive *tearing* and mucoid conjunctival discharge may be present in severe cases, and it is not uncommon for patients with recurrent symptoms to note a certain degree of fatigue, malaise, anorexia, and irritability. Many offending plants pollinate during the early morning hours. Thus, morning symptoms may be followed by improvement during the day, as exposure lessens. Repeated upward rubbing of the nose to relieve itching may cause a crease to develop across the nose, especially in children. Mouth breathing is common, as are typical dark, discolored infraorbital "shiners" (Fig. 421–2).

Examination of the nasal mucous membranes characteristically reveals bluish, edematous, boggy, pale nasal turbinates, often coated with clear secretion; but many persons with allergic rhinitis have an erythematous, boggy nasal mucosa that can easily be confused with that seen in infectious rhinitis. At times the nasal airways may be completely obstructed as a result of accumulation of mucous and turbinate swelling. Scleral and conjunctival injection and edema plus periorbital swelling and tearing may be noted. Nasal polyps are relatively uncommonly associated with uncomplicated rhinitis. They may, however, be associated with aspirin intolerance. Since asthmatics with aspirin intolerance often have severe disease, visualization of even small polyps in patients with rhinitis and asthma may provide important diagnostic leads.

In *seasonal rhinitis*, symptoms recur each year with regularity during the pollination season characteristic for a given area. IgE–mediated perennial rhinitis presents with continued low-grade symptoms which may improve only if the patient leaves the region of the inciting causes. *Perennial rhinitis* of unknown cause (also called *vasomotor rhinitis*) also produces persistent symptoms without correlation to any specific allergen exposure. This type of perennial rhinitis is often worsened by changes in temperature or humidity or with exposure to irritants or other types of air pollutants. It is also often associated with profuse nasal discharge after the patient eats chilled, highly spiced, or very hot foods, and such symptoms may be erroneously attributed to food allergy.

Serous otitis media may be superimposed upon the symptoms

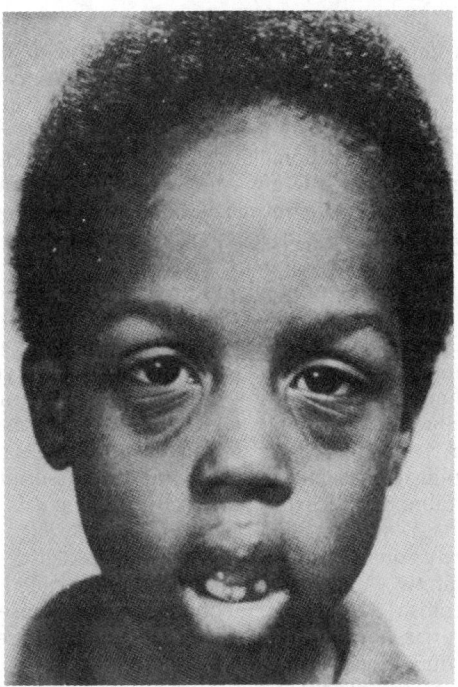

FIGURE 421–2. Typical appearance of highly allergic 6-year-old child. Note dark circles under eyes ("allergic shiners") and mouth breathing. Allergic nasal crease from constant "saluting" was also present. (Reprinted with permission from Mathews KP: Respiratory atopic disease. JAMA 248:2588, 1982.)

of seasonal or perennial allergic rhinitis. In many instances of serous otitis media, allergic factors cannot, however, be identified. Serous otitis, which can be an important complication in children, may result from nasal obstruction or obstructive dysfunction of the eustachian tube as a result of mucosal edema and secretions. It can also lead to hearing loss with adverse effects on cognition or speech development in the young child. The diagnosis of serous otitis media is suggested by a history of symptoms such as delayed speech development or decreased auditory perception. The tympanic membrane on physical examination is frequently amber colored and retracted, and shows decreased motion if there is negative middle-ear pressure, or no motion at all if there is a severe effusion.

Chronic sinusitis may be another complication, often manifested by the presence of chronic nasal discharge, nocturnal cough associated with postnasal discharge, pain, fever, headache, and recurrent otitis media. In adults, however, pain, headache, and low-grade fever are the most common signs. Chronic sinusitis as a complication of seasonal allergic rhinitis should be considered whenever symptoms of allergic rhinitis are more protracted than expected, when the patient has severe dull-to-intense throbbing pain over the involved sinus area, or when prolonged or persistent cough develops that is suggestive of bronchitis that has failed to respond to appropriate therapy.

DIAGNOSIS (WITH DIFFERENTIAL DIAGNOSIS). A good history is most important in correctly diagnosing rhinitis. In addition to the history of classic physical signs and symptoms, careful skin testing with common inhalant preparations together with positive and negative control substances is a mandatory procedure in diagnosing specific allergic factors associated with rhinitis. Direct skin tests of the scratch, prick, and intradermal variety are the least expensive and time consuming. The intradermal test should never be performed without prior performance of negative scratch or prick tests. In general, negative skin test responses with common inhalant allergens indicate that rhinitis is of nonallergic origin. Methods of detecting IgE antibodies in vitro have now been available for several years. In patients who are receiving medications that might prevent skin reactivity or in those with extensive eczema or dermatographia that negates the use of skin tests, these in vitro assays for serum IgE antibodies can be of diagnostic aid. Total serum IgE levels are elevated in only 30 to 40 per cent of patients with allergic rhinitis. They may also be elevated in many nonallergic conditions. Although frequently elevated in allergic rhinitis, the peripheral blood eosinophil count may be normal. A high peripheral eosinophil count may also be seen in nonallergic perennial rhinitis associated with nasal polyps, hyperplastic sinusitis, and idiopathic asthma. Of more significance is a smear of nasal secretions for eosinophils.

Clear-cut seasonal allergic rhinitis due to inhalant allergens seldom presents a differential diagnostic problem. Symptoms of the common cold may, however, be quite similar, although they usually last less than a week and are often associated with fever, pain, and the presence of considerable numbers of neutrophils in nasal secretions. Symptoms associated with structural abnormalities of the nasal area, such as polyps, deviated nasal septum, enlarged tonsils, or foreign bodies, are relatively constant rather than episodic in classic seasonal allergic rhinitis. A suspected diagnosis of so-called rhinitis medicamentosa due to the rebound effects of nose drops, sprays, ovarian hormonal agents (such as oral contraceptives), reserpine derivatives, or hydralazine can often be confirmed when symptoms gradually improve following avoidance of the suspected agent. Nasal symptoms may accompany metabolic disorders such as hyperthyroidism or emotional states, but the relationship is unclear. During pregnancy and the premenstrual period hormonally related rhinitis may occur. A condition known as nasal mastocytosis is associated with symptoms of perennial allergic rhinitis; the diagnosis can be made by nasal mucosal biopsy.

TREATMENT. Three basic principles are important in the treatment of allergic rhinitis: avoidance of offending allergens; use of symptomatic treatment, such as antihistamines, sympathomimetic drugs, and topical steroids; and allergenic extract immunotherapy.

Avoidance. When practical, avoidance of aeroallergens is the treatment of choice, since it removes the cause of difficulty and prevents symptoms. When a specific food, drug, occupational allergen, or animal dander is involved, it is the only measure that serves both to prevent and to treat disease. All physicians should be familiar, for example, with standard antidust regimens for use in home environments. Although avoidance of outdoor exposure to ubiquitous seasonal and perennial pollens is virtually impossible, common-sense measures to avoid heavy exposure often help to prevent severe exacerbations of symptoms. For example, mold-sensitive patients should avoid barns, working with hay, raking leaves, and mowing grass. Simply keeping doors and windows closed significantly decreases indoor pollen and mold spore concentrations, and air conditioning makes a closed environment more tolerable. Although electrostatic air-purifying devices do not provide cooling or dehumidification, they are quite efficient in removing pollen grains and other large mold spores. In certain cases a patient may choose to leave an area of exposure during a particularly symptomatic season. Such measures may be applicable when well-defined seasons, such as the late-summer–early-fall ragweed season, are involved. Only rarely should consideration be given to making a permanent move from an area of exposure to particularly aggravating allergens, since, with time, allergic individuals generally tend to acquire new sensitivities to allergens in their adopted environment.

Symptomatic Treatment. Although, in general, antihistamines are only partially effective and often produce drowsiness as a side effect, they are often used alone or in combination with oral sympathomimetic agents, anticholinergics, cromolyn sodium, and topical corticosteroids. The H_1 antihistaminics often control symptoms of profuse nasal itching and sneezing. They act as competitive inhibitors for histamine at its H_1 receptor site. Since receptor sites can be effectively blocked prior to histamine release, better results are often obtained when these drugs are administered on a regular basis rather than intermittently. Antihistamines have been classified into six groups on the basis of chemical structure. Some antihistamines representative of each group are listed in Table 421–1. These include the ethanolamines, such as diphenhydramine (Benadryl); the ethylenediamines, such as tripelennamine (Pyribenzamine); the alkylamines, such as brompheniramine (Dimetane) and chlorpheniramine (Chlortrimeton); the piperazines, such as hydroxyzine (Atarax, Vistaril); the phenothiazines, such as promethazine (Phenergan);

TABLE 421–1. H_1 ANTIHISTAMINE CLASSIFICATIONS

Class (Nonproprietary Name)	Trade Name	Dosage Adult	Dosage Child
Ethanolamines			
Diphenhydramine hydrochloride	Benadryl	25–50 mg, 3 or 4 times daily	5 mg/kg/day in 3 or 4 divided doses
Carbinoxamine maleate	Clistin	4 mg, 3 or 4 times daily	0.4 mg/kg/day in 3 or 4 divided doses
Ethylenediamine			
Tripelennamine	PBZ	25–50 mg, 3 or 4 times daily	5 mg/kg/day in 3 or 4 divided doses
Methapyriline hydrochloride	Histadyl	25–50 mg, 4 or 5 times daily	5 mg/kg/day in 3 or 4 divided doses
Alkylamines			
Chlorpheniramine maleate	Chlor-Trimeton, Teldrin, CTM (delayed action), Cosea, Histadur, Rhinihist	4 mg, 3 or 4 times daily 12 mg, 2 times daily	0.4 mg/kg/day in 3 or 4 divided doses
Brompheniramine maleate	Dimetane Dimetane (delayed action) Extentabs	4 mg, 3 or 4 times daily 12 mg, 2 times daily	0.4 mg/kg/day in 3 or 4 divided doses
Piperazines			
Hydroxyzine	Atarax, Vistaril	25–100 mg, 3 or 4 times daily	2 mg/kg/day in 4 divided doses
Phenothiazines			
Promethazine hydrochloride	Phenergan	12.5–25 mg, 2 or 3 times daily	1 mg/kg/day divided into half dose at bedtime and quarter dose every 6 hours in daytime
Trimeprazine tartrate	Temaril	2.5 mg, 4 times daily	2.5 mg in 3 divided doses (3-yr-olds only) 1.5 mg in 3 divided doses (6 mo to 3 yr)
Miscellaneous			
Terfenadine	Seldane	60 mg, 2 times daily	No recommendation
Cyproheptadine hydrochloride	Periactin	4 mg, 3 or 4 times daily	0.25 mg/kg/day in 3 or 4 divided doses
Azatadine maleate	Optimine	1–2 mg, 2 times daily	No recommendation
Clemastine fumarate	Tavist	2.68 mg, 2 times daily	No recommendation

and a miscellaneous group including cyproheptadine (Periactin), and azatadine (Optimine). In a typical case, one might start with one of the alkylamines such as chlorpheniramine maleate or brompheniramine maleate 4 mg three or four times a day in the adult (0.4 mg per kg per day in three or four divided doses in children). Both of these compounds are also available in long-acting preparations that can be given in 8- to 12-mg doses two times a day. A new generation of H_1 antihistamines is currently under development. They lack a direct chemical relation to histamine, but have as a common structure an aromatic nitrogen in the form of a piperidine, piperazine, or pyridine. They have limited access to the central nervous system, thereby reducing or eliminating drowsiness as a side effect. The first of these new drugs marketed in the United States have been terfenidine and astemizole.

The most commonly employed sympathomimetic nasal sprays and drops that contain alpha-adrenergic agonists are phenylephrine hydrochloride, a short-acting agent, and longer-acting preparations such as oxymetazoline hydrochloride. In most cases, use of these compounds for more than a few days will result in progressively severe nasal obstruction secondary to rebound swelling of the nasal mucosa that may be a self-perpetuating process (known as rhinitis medicamentosa). Thus these agents are not recommended for long-term use in allergic rhinitis. Sympathomimetic agents administered orally, such as pseudoepinephrine and phenylpropanolamine, may also reduce nasal congestion, although when used alone they may have significant CNS effects, often leading to insomnia and nervousness. A 4-per-cent solution of cromolyn sodium (Nasalcrom and Opticrom) applied topically can also be of benefit in the treatment and prevention of allergic rhinitis and conjunctivitis if administered frequently. The effect of treatment with Nasalcrom in typical dosage of one spray per nostril four times per day may not be noted until two to four weeks after initiation of treatment. Thus there may be an initial need for an antihistamine or decongestant before cromolyn's preventive effect becomes apparent.

Topical corticosteroids are widely used and highly successful in the symptomatic treatment and prevention of allergic rhinitis. These usually include the highly potent and rapidly metabolized corticosteroids such as beclomethasone dipropionate (Vancenase and Beconase) and flunisolide acetate (Nasilide). These agents act primarily topically, and have relatively few systemic effects, which is most advantageous. Although of substantial value in treating seasonal allergic rhinitis, these may not work well in acute, severe cases associated with considerable nasal mucosal edema and obstruction. They also do not relieve ocular symptoms. If used intermittently on a regular basis, they can help in perennial allergic rhinitis and vasomotor rhinitis. In addition, they may be of some help in weaning patients from excessive use of vasoconstrictor nasal sprays. The rule for use of corticosteroids is "as much as necessary but as little as possible."

Dose-response investigations in hay-fever patients have shown total control of nasal symptoms in about 30 per cent of patients treated with 200 or 300 μg of beclomethasone dipropionate per day. The rate increases to 60 per cent with 400 μg per day. Seasonal treatment on a daily basis with 400 μg per day is recommended and is considered to be quite harmless. (Each puff of beclomethasone dipropionate from a nasal inhaler is equal to approximately 42 μg of beclomethasone dipropionate, USP). Thus, one puff per nostril four times per day from the nasal inhaler would be a typical dosage. Some attention should be paid to the frequency of prescription; for example, when 400 μg is recommended, one aerosol container will last approximately four weeks. In all cases, clinical improvement is usually apparent within several days, but symptomatic relief may not occur in some patients for as long as two weeks. In adults and children, the inhalation of 400 μg daily is without risk of systemic steroid side effects. There is also substantial evidence that this is the case in adults

who use up to 800 μg daily (approximately 16 inhalations). In addition, cushingoid changes probably do not occur until the very large dose of approximately 1 mg* (20 inhalations or more) is reached. When the drug is used it should be remembered that, in regard to therapeutic potency, eight inhalations is roughly equivalent to 7.5 mg of oral prednisone. These drugs should be used with caution in the presence of viral and fungal nasal diseases such as ocular herpes or related diseases in which there appears to be an associated defect in cell-mediated immunity.

Inhalant Allergen Immunotherapy (Desensitization or Hyposensitization). With this form of therapy, one attempts to alter the immunologic reactivity of an allergic individual so that there is less response upon natural re-exposure to the offending allergen. The clinical decision to use immunotherapy in the patient with allergic rhinitis depends on several factors: (1) the existence of clinically important rhinitis should be confirmed; (2) maximal environmental control procedures should be utilized; and (3) the response to medication should be well defined. Immunotherapy is usually employed in patients who have substantial allergic components to their illness and who are attaining satisfactory clinical improvement with environmental control and symptomatic treatment. The technique involves injecting increasing amounts of allergen subcutaneously, usually at weekly intervals, starting with a very low dose and gradually increasing (usually a double dose) at each subsequent injection. One should always carefully monitor for the development of untoward reactions. After incremental increases in the amount of injected allergen, a maintenance dose is achieved, which is injected at intervals of two to six weeks, depending upon individual patient activity and requirements. In most cases a decrease in nasal symptoms following immunotherapy is obvious during the first six months to one year and is maximal by three years of therapy. There are no universally accepted guidelines for the duration of therapy, and many physicians attempt trials of discontinuation after approximately four years of a successful program.

Symptomatic improvement with immunotherapy has been clearly shown in hay fever due to ragweed, grass, mountain cedar pollen, or birch pollen and in asthma due to house dust mite, ragweed pollen, grass pollen, or cat dander. Beneficial results depend on a sufficiently high dose of antigen; relapse may occur once continuing maintenance injections are abandoned. Results are specific for particular antigens employed. A variety of immunologic changes have been demonstrated following immunotherapy, but it is not known which are responsible for clinical improvement. Among these changes are a rise in serum IgG-blocking antibodies against the allergens employed; suppression in the usual seasonal rise in IgE antibodies, which normally follows environmental seasonal exposure; increase of blocking IgA and IgG antibodies in secretions; reduced basophil reactivity and sensitivity to allergens; reduced in vitro lymphocyte responsiveness to allergens; and an increase in specific T suppressor cells following immunotherapy.

New experimental approaches to the therapy of allergic rhinitis include the use of altered antigens (such as allergoids and polymerized forms of antigen) that ultimately result in a heightened degree of immunization, with considerably less chance to trigger sensitized mast cells and produce local or systemic reactions. The use of other routes of antigen administration (e.g., intranasal) has also been attempted, as have efforts to depress specific IgE antibody synthesis, with or without effects on suppressor T cells, by linking allergens to certain agents such as polyethylene glycol, with subsequent production of tolerance. Still other efforts are directed toward such novel ideas as inhibition of IgE receptors on mast cells, basophils, and other IgE receptor–bearing cells.

---

*Exceeds dosage recommended by manufacturer.

Gershwin ME (ed.): Clinical Reviews in Allergy, Vol. 2, No. 3. New York, Elsevier Scientific Publishing Company, 1984. *A 250-page review of nasal physiology, acute and chronic rhinitis, clinical evaluation, rhinitis therapy, and diagnostic tests.*

Kaplan AP (ed.): Allergy. New York, Churchill Livingstone, 1985. *A comprehensive practical text stressing diagnosis and therapy of common allergic diseases. Diseases based on immediate hypersensitivity are stressed. Chapter on allergic and nonallergic rhinitis by KP Matthews is practical and well illustrated.*

Lichtenstein L, Fauci A: Current Therapy in Allergy, Immunology and Rheumatology. Toronto, B.C. Decker Inc., 1985. *A concise text devoted entirely to the therapy and diagnosis of a wide range of immunologically mediated diseases. Three excellent sections are devoted to allergic rhinitis.*

Middleton E Jr, Reed CE, Ellis EF: Allergy: Principles and Practice. 2nd ed. St. Louis, C.V. Mosby Company, 1983. *A multi-authored, two-volume reference work, stressing immunologic, pharmacologic, and clinical aspects of the common allergic diseases.*

Mygind N (ed.): Nasal Allergy. Oxford, Blackwell Scientific Publications, 1978. *A complete text devoted entirely to the structure, function, immunology, diagnosis, and therapy of rhinitis.*

Salvaggio J (ed.): Primer on allergic and immunologic diseases. JAMA 248:2579, 1982. *Compact article on the essentials of respiratory atopic diseases in a setting of other articles that stress the clinical implications of immunology for the medical student and resident.*

Stites D, Stobo J, Fudenberg H, et al. (eds.): Basic and Clinical Immunology. 5th ed. Los Altos, Lange Medical Publishers, 1986. *A text outlining relevant features of basic immunology, immunologic laboratory tests, and clinical immunology. Clinical chapters focus on primary immunology diseases and disorders with important immunopathologic characteristics.*

422 ANAPHYLAXIS*

Lawrence M. Lichtenstein†

Systemic anaphylaxis is the most dramatic example of an immediate hypersensitivity reaction. The first known report of this syndrome describes the sudden death of King Menes of Egypt from the sting of a wasp during the twenty-sixth century B.C. The experiments of Richet and Portier in the early 1900's, which gained them the Nobel Prize, showed that dogs who survived a large dose of sea anemone toxin died within a few minutes when given a minute dose some weeks later. They coined the term *anaphylaxis* to describe how this type of immunization led to a lack of protection rather than the expected immunity (i.e., prophylaxis).

Human anaphylactic reactions are uncommon but have always received considerable medical attention because of their unexpected nature and occasionally fatal outcome. They occur in previously sensitized individuals after re-exposure to foreign antigens or low-molecular-weight substances that act as haptens. These reactions are mediated by IgE antibody, begin a few minutes after antigen exposure, and result from the release of basophil and mast-cell mediators. Other "anaphylactoid" reactions probably involve the nonimmunologic release of the same chemical mediators. Systemic anaphylactic reactions involve the cutaneous, respiratory, circulatory, gastrointestinal, and hematologic systems. They range in severity from distressing but self-limited, generalized urticarial reactions to sudden death.

ETIOLOGY. During the early part of this century, anaphylaxis was most often seen as a reaction to the proteins of horse serum, which was used in the preparation of diphtheria and tetanus antitoxins. Table 422–1 lists the inciting agents that are now most common. Proteins likely to cause these reactions are hormones, enzymes, Hymenoptera venoms (in insect stings as described in Ch. 423), pollen extracts, and various foods (seafood, eggs, wheat products, nuts). Polysaccharides such as dextran are rarer causes of anaphylaxis. The most common etiologic agents are drugs, low-molecular-weight substances that are not antigenic in themselves but

*Supported by Grant AI 08270 from the National Institute of Allergy and Infectious Diseases, National Institutes of Health.

†I would like to thank my colleague, Eugene R. Bleecker, M.D., for his aid in the preparation and writing of this chapter.

TABLE 422–1. AGENTS CAUSING ANAPHYLAXIS

Type	Common	Rare
Proteins	Venoms (Hymenoptera)	Hormones (insulin, ACTH, vasopressin, parathormone)
	Pollens (ragweed, grass, etc.)	Enzymes (trypsin, penicillinase)
	Foods (eggs, seafood, nuts, grains, beans, cottonseed oil, chocolate)	Human proteins (serum proteins, seminal fluid)
	Horse and rabbit serum (antilymphocyte globulin)	
Haptens and other low-molecular-weight substances	Antibiotics (penicillins, cephalosporins, tetracyclines, amphotericin B, nitrofurantoin, aminoglycosides)	Vitamins (thiamin, folic acid)
	Local anesthetics (lidocaine, procaine, etc.)	
Polysaccharides		Dextrans, iron-dextran

act as haptens, combining with native proteins to form an antigen. Antibiotics (penicillin, cephalosporins, tetracycline, nitrofurantoin), local anesthetics, vitamins, and some diagnostic agents are thought to act by this mechanism. Some substances (Table 422–2) that are administered by intravenous injection (iodinated radiopaque dyes or hypertonic solutions [mannitol]) as well as some nonsteroidal anti-inflammatory agents (acetylsalicylic acid, aminopyrine, indomethacin) may induce mediator release by nonimmunologic mechanisms that are poorly understood, or vascular shock by direct systemic vasodilatation. Although the parenteral administration of these agents is the cause of most reactions, oral and topical exposure can also cause systemic anaphylactic reactions in highly sensitive individuals.

In the two best-studied situations, penicillin and insect-sting anaphylaxis, the incidence of sensitivity (e.g., a positive skin test) is not greater in patients with a familial or personal history of atopy. However, not all individuals with a positive skin test, indicating the presence of specific IgE antibody, are at risk of an anaphylactic reaction although their risk is very much higher than that of skin test–negative patients.

PATHOGENESIS. In a susceptible individual, exposure to an antigenic agent causes the production of IgE antibodies. With repeat exposure, the antigen combines with IgE antibodies on the surface of basophils and mast cells to initiate a sequence of biochemical reactions that result in the active secretion of mediators such as histamine, arachidonic acid metabolites, and factors that attract and activate platelets, eosinophils, and neutrophils (see Table 427–1). These mediators constrict bronchial smooth muscle, increase vascular permeability, affect systemic and pulmonary vascular muscle tone, induce platelet aggregation and degranulation, attract inflammatory cells to the reaction site, and, in general, are responsible for the manifestations of anaphylaxis. Elevated levels of histamine have been measured during human anaphylactic shock, and the intravenous injection of this mediator causes urticaria, bronchospasm, vasodilation, hypotension, and vomiting. It is certain, however, that other mediators are also involved. It is not yet possible to describe the mechanisms involved in anaphylaxis in detail. The alterations in coagulability which have been reported, for example, may be due to platelet activating factors or to an enzymatic mediator that activates Hageman factor.

CLINICAL FEATURES. The onset and clinical manifesta-

TABLE 422–2. AGENTS CAUSING ANAPHYLACTOID REACTIONS*

Curare
Hypertonic solutions (mannitol)
Nonsteroidal anti-inflammatory agents (acetylsalicylic acid, aminopyrine, indomethacin)
Radiopaque contrast material

*Reactions to these low-molecular-weight compounds may not be due to IgE-mediated immunologic mechanisms (see text).

tions of systemic anaphylaxis vary, depending on the route of administration of the antigen or hapten. The physiologic features are also determined by the type, quantities, and sites of release of pharmacologic mediators, by factors that control releasability, and by differing sensitivity of the organs to the released mediators.

There is no universal response pattern or "shock" organ that is always involved in man. Individuals do, however, have a characteristic pattern of response which tends to repeat. This pattern is often preceded by an aura that is also characteristic and well recognized by the patient. Attention to these subjective symptoms, which precede the physiologic events by one to two minutes, may be valuable. The most common manifestations of systemic reactions are *cutaneous:* erythema, pruritus, urticaria, and angioedema, often of the eyes, lips, or tongue. In adults, the cutaneous symptoms are usually accompanied by one or more other features. There are two patterns of respiratory failure. The first is *upper airway obstruction* owing to edema of the larynx and/or epiglottis, which can cause acute distress and death by suffocation. The second involves *diffuse lower airway bronchoconstriction* similar to the respiratory abnormalities observed in status asthmaticus. Such air flow limitation is not relieved by endotracheal intubation and may lead to abnormalities of pulmonary gas exchange with subsequent hypoxemia and hypercarbia.

Perhaps the most severe clinical manifestation of anaphylaxis is *hypotensive shock,* which can develop with or without other symptoms. The cause is thought to be either peripheral vascular pooling of blood resulting from vasodilation or increased capillary permeability with functional loss of intravascular blood volume into the interstitial spaces. Electrocardiographic abnormalities, including conduction disturbances, arrhythmias, and ischemic or infarction patterns, have been noted during anaphylactic shock. These changes may reflect myocardial ischemia and arrhythmias caused by decreased coronary perfusion and oxygenation.

Rarely, other symptoms are associated with systemic anaphylactic reactions. These include gastrointestinal (vomiting, nausea, and diarrhea) and central nervous system symptoms. Prolonged hypotension or anoxia can, of course, cause a variety of secondary, more permanent changes.

Metabolic abnormalities in severe human anaphylactic shock include increased blood histamine levels, which correlate with the duration and severity of shock. There is also depletion of clotting factors V, VII, and fibrinogen; activation of complement; and loss of high-molecular-weight kininogen. The utilization of these coagulation factors is consistent with acute intravascular coagulation and may account for clotting defects observed in clinical anaphylactic syndromes.

DIFFERENTIAL DIAGNOSIS. The diagnosis of systemic anaphylaxis is generally easy owing to the characteristic history of immediately antecedent exposure to foreign antigenic material and appropriate evidence of systemic involvement on physical examination. The presentation may, however, involve a patient unable to provide a history and suffering the secondary effects of shock (e.g., a myocardial infarction or an arrhythmia). Occasionally, this syndrome must be distinguished from other related clinical conditions (i.e., sudden acute bronchospasm in an asthmatic, vasovagal syncope, acute drug toxicity, hereditary angioedema, cold or idiopathic urticaria). Nonimmunologic "anaphylactoid" reactions to radiopaque dyes, hypertonic solutions, and nonsteroidal anti-inflammatory agents (indomethacin, aminopyrine, acetylsalicylic acid) have a similar clinical presentation and require an identical therapeutic approach, even though they may not be mediated by IgE antibody.

Because of the rapid onset of these reactions, initial laboratory testing is not helpful in making a diagnosis. The retrospective diagnosis of specific allergic sensitivity is by skin testing or the measurement of specific IgE antibody by the radioallergosorbent test.

PREVENTION AND TREATMENT. The sudden, usually unexpected onset of human anaphylaxis with a rapid clinical course that leads to either swift recovery or death has provided little opportunity for prospective, controlled, therapeutic studies. Even when anaphylaxis is treated in an intensive care unit by trained personnel with a well-planned therapeutic approach, severe systemic reactions often do not respond to medical treatment. Therefore, every attempt must be made to prevent these reactions. A careful medical history should include inquiry about any previous allergic drug reactions. Patients who have previously experienced anaphylactic episodes should wear a Medic-Alert bracelet and be instructed in the importance of relating details of their specific drug allergies before taking medications; their medical records should prominently state the patient's allergic history. The physician should be aware of which medications, proprietaries, and foods contain allergens or cross-reacting antigens. Sensitization may occur in the absence of clinical symptoms; previous tolerance of a substance provides no guarantee that an anaphylactic reaction will not occur.

If diagnostic tests are not available, as with most drugs, it is appropriate to substitute another therapeutic agent for the treatment of a patient with a history of sensitivity to a particular drug. Again, knowledge of cross-reactivity is necessary. If, for example, cephalosporins are substituted for penicillin, there is a significant risk of reaction, since these agents share a common β-lactam ring. Penicillin causes more anaphylactic reactions than any other drug, but at least 80 per cent of patients with a history of a previous reaction will have negative skin tests (to penicilloyl-polylysine and a mixture of haptens [MDM]) and can tolerate the drug with impunity. This is an important consideration, since penicillin is a relatively nontoxic drug and most antibiotics that would be substituted have a significant incidence of side effects. (See Ch. 426 for a further discussion of penicillin allergy.) When penicillin or other allergens must be used in a sensitive patient, an effort can be made to desensitize the patient by the use of sequential low doses, initially intradermally, then subcutaneously, and finally intramuscularly into the peripheral part of an extremity. Such a procedure should be carried out by experienced personnel, and potentially allergenic substances should be administered in a setting where anaphylactic reactions can be effectively treated.

Early recognition of anaphylaxis is critical, since death or irreversible anoxic organ damage can occur rapidly. When an anaphylactic reaction is initiated by an injection into the arm or leg, a tourniquet should be placed around that extremity to stop antigen absorption. The initial pharmacologic treatment is the subcutaneous administration of 0.2 to 0.5 ml of a 1:1000 solution of epinephrine, which may be repeated at 20 to 30-minute intervals for three doses as necessary. This is the agent of choice, antihistamines and corticosteroids play *no* role in the treatment of an acute reaction, although some physicians believe they limit late or recurrent cutaneous manifestations. Extrathoracic upper airway obstruction must be differentiated from diffuse bronchospasm, since severe laryngeal and epiglottic edema may require careful endotracheal intubation or an emergency tracheostomy to facilitate ventilation. Bronchospasm can be handled in a manner similar to the therapy for status asthmaticus, by the administration of inhaled B-2 sympathomimetics or by intravenous aminophylline at 6 mg per kilogram loading dose over 20 to 30 minutes, followed by 0.5 to 1 mg per kilogram per hour (see Ch. 60). Hypoxemia should be treated with supplemental oxygen. Hypovolemic shock requires rapid intravenous fluid administration (normal saline and colloid) to maintain blood pressure. Additionally, epinephrine at a dose of 5 ml of a 1:10,000 solution repeated every 5 to 10 minutes as needed can be given intravenously in severe shock. In addition, a vasopressor such as dopamine, 2 to 50 μg per kilogram per minute, is indicated to manage hypotension unresponsive to volume expansion. If severe vascular anaphylactic shock does not respond immediately to these measures, supportive treatment should be continued, preferably in an intensive care setting where vascular monitoring is available to guide additional therapy. Any patient who has had significant shock or airway obstruction should be hospitalized for at least 24 hours after the acute episode is handled, since these symptoms may recur many hours after an initial favorable response.

Parker CW: Systemic anaphylaxis. In Parker CW (ed.): Clinical Immunology. Philadelphia, W. B. Saunders Company, 1980, pp 1208–1218. *A textbook review of what is known about etiology, pathogenesis, and treatment.*

Peters SP: Systemic anaphylaxis. In Lichtenstein LM, Fauci AS (eds.): Current Therapy in Allergy, Immunology and Rheumatology, 1985–1986. Toronto, B.C. Decker Inc., 1985, pp 75–80. *A detailed description of how to treat this serious disorder.*

Smith PL, Sobotka AK, Bleecker ER, et al.: Physiologic manifestations of human anaphylaxis. J Clin Invest 66:1072, 1980. *Physiologic and biochemical changes monitored in human anaphylaxis occurring during a trial of therapy for insect allergy. Includes comments on therapy.*

423 INSECT STING ALLERGY*

Lawrence M. Lichtenstein†

The stings of insects of the order Hymenoptera have long been recognized as a potential cause of severe, often life-threatening reactions in susceptible individuals. These reactions are unrelated to the toxic chemicals in the venoms, being due to allergic sensitization. Insect sting allergy has recently become the most intensely studied mode of anaphylaxis in man, resulting in important advances that have had rapid clinical application.

EPIDEMIOLOGY. The incidence of immediate hypersensitivity to insect stings based on history is 4 per cent; more than 20 per cent of the population, however, has positive skin test reactions to insect venoms without having had a reaction. Other allergies do not seem to predispose to insect sting sensitivity. The frequency varies with exposure and is therefore greater in children and males as well as those inclined to outdoor activities or beekeeping. Insect stings cause few fatalities, but the morbidity, fear, and change in life style caused by these reactions is significant. A large number of people suffer prolonged and unusually large local inflammatory reactions to insect stings, which are allergic in nature. As with other allergies, there appears to be an inherited predisposition, since multiple family members are often affected.

ETIOLOGY. The only insects possessing true stingers are those of the order Hymenoptera. There are two families of importance, the bees (honeybees, bumblebees) and the vespids (yellow jackets, hornets, wasps). The bees have barbed stingers which remain in the skin after a sting. Yellow jackets are the most common culprits, but honeybees are more commonly implicated in the western United States. Wasps are more common in the south central United States (especially Texas). Sensitivity develops to antigens in the insect venom, most of which have enzymatic activity. A major allergen in both insect families is phospholipase A, but they do not cross-react with one another.

PATHOGENESIS. The injection of foreign proteins commonly causes the production of specific antibodies of the IgE and IgG classes. Individuals may develop venom-specific IgE antibodies after any sting, this response sometimes persisting

for less than three months and in other instances persisting for more than 25 years. Tissue mast cells and circulating basophils bind IgE antibody, thereby becoming sensitized so that a repeat encounter with the offending allergen will trigger release of the mediators of anaphylaxis (see Fig. 60–3). The initiation and persistence of this sensitization are related to inheritable and other unknown determinants. Sensitization may occur at any time in life, even after many uneventful stings. The sensitizing sting itself causes no unusual reaction, and is often so remote as to evade recollection.

Generalized mediator release from sensitized basophils and mast cells causes the many manifestations of anaphylaxis (see Table 427–1). Localization of symptoms to specific target tissues is not well understood. The pathology observed in fatal cases includes upper airway edema and obstruction, the visceral consequences of hypotension, or occasionally no discernible abnormality (see Ch. 422 for a discussion of anaphylaxis).

Large local reactions most often appear to be IgE dependent, but their prolonged time-course is not typical of immediate hypersensitivity. These reactions may involve a cascade of events beginning with mediator release from mast cells and culminating with local inflammation involving many cell types and numerous mechanisms. The potential roles of eosinophils, neutrophils, basophils, lymphocytes and lymphokines, complement, and mediators with prolonged release or activity have not been elucidated.

The venom-specific IgG antibody response to a sting is usually short lived, lasting only a few months. Repeated stings (as in beekeepers) are associated with high titers of IgG antibodies, which protect against allergic reactions. Beekeepers who do not have anaphylactic reactions have high IgG titers, as do affected individuals immunized with venoms. Passive transfer of these IgG antibodies protects sensitive patients from a sting. These protective antibodies are thought to block the allergic reaction by competing with IgE for the allergenic venom proteins and have therefore been termed "blocking" antibodies.

CLINICAL MANIFESTATIONS. Allergic reactions to insect stings are either generalized (systemic) or large local reactions. *Systemic sting reactions* present the classic manifestations of anaphylaxis described in Ch. 422. The observed frequency of the most common symptoms in adult patients is presented in Table 423–1. The risk of a fatal outcome increases, as might be expected, with age. Fatal anaphylaxis may occur without a history of sting allergy.

The onset of systemic symptoms is rapid, within two to three minutes, and rarely occurs more than 30 minutes after a sting. Symptoms presenting hours later (except large local reactions) are not usually associated with immediate hypersensitivity or IgE antibodies. Unusual reactions such as vasculitis, nephropathies, encephalitis, and other neurologic manifestations have been reported, but no causal relationship has been established. Allergic respiratory symptoms may occur in beekeepers and their families owing to sensitization to the dust in the hives that contain bee body proteins. This sensitivity is unrelated to sting reactions.

Large local reactions are slow in onset and occur with or without concomitant early systemic reaction. The area of induration increases in size progressively for the first 24 to 48 hours, and then resolves gradually over several days. These

*Supported by Grant AI 08270 from the National Institute of Allergy and Infectious Diseases.

†I would like to express my thanks to my colleague, David B. K. Golden, M.D., for his aid in the preparation and writing of this chapter.

TABLE 423–1. SYMPTOMS REPORTED BY 245 PATIENTS

Symptom	Per Cent
Cutaneous only	14
Urticaria-angioedema	78
Dizziness-hypotension	61
Dyspnea-wheezing	53
Throat tightness-hoarseness	40
Loss of consciousness	33

reactions may be so large as to immobilize an entire limb, and are a significant cause of morbidity in sensitive individuals. Red streaks resembling lymphangitis may be observed and are often treated with antibiotics despite a lack of evidence for true cellulitis. Some individuals develop large local sting reactions in the absence of allergic sensitivity. These are exaggerated reactions to the toxic and inflammatory venom components, and often occur in persons who report similar large swellings to mosquito or fly bites, or who have cutaneous sensitivity to many irritants.

NATURAL HISTORY. The natural history of insect sting allergy has been incompletely documented. The incidence of venom sensitization in the general population was noted above. It is estimated that about 20 per cent of those at risk by virtue of positive skin tests (with no history of a systemic reaction) will react on sting. There is considerable variability in the reaction to a sting among those who are clearly allergic as demonstrated by positive skin tests and a history of a previous reaction. In a small study 60 per cent of adults had a systemic reaction when stung by the appropriate insect. In children a repeat sting causes a reaction in only 8 per cent. The incidence in adolescents and young adults must lie between these extremes. This variability confounds the prediction of risk associated with sensitization.

Many patients and physicians believe that allergic sting reactions become progressively more severe with every sting. Although some patients progress from large local through mild systemic reactions to life-threatening anaphylaxis, most of those affected maintain a similar pattern of symptoms with every sting. Less than 10 per cent of those experiencing large local reactions will subsequently have systemic reactions. Factors favoring a systemic reaction include multiple stings, or stings in close temporal proximity (only weeks apart).

Sensitization may decrease or disappear in time, more commonly in children. However, resensitization has been observed upon resting.

DIAGNOSIS. The acute presentation of anaphylaxis is easily diagnosed by the presence of classic symptoms and signs. The insect sting may be inapparent. Differential diagnosis is more difficult in localized reactions such as acute chest pain and dyspnea or syncope without urticaria.

The diagnosis of insect sting allergy currently rests on a convincing history and positive skin tests. Demonstration in vitro of venom-specific IgE by the radioallergosorbent test (RAST) is less sensitive than skin tests, but may be useful in equivocal cases.

Skin tests are performed intradermally with venoms diluted to concentrations in the range of 1 to 1000 ng per milliliter. Five venoms are used: honeybee (HB), yellow jacket (YJ), yellow hornet (YH), white-faced hornet (WH), and *Polistes* wasp (POL). Positive intradermal skin tests develop, within 20 minutes, a wheal greater than 5 mm in diameter with at least 20 mm of erythema. The degree of skin test sensitivity does not correlate with clinical sensitivity. Within a few months after a systemic sting reaction, skin tests are almost uniformly positive. Stings more remote in time are more commonly associated with an apparent loss of sensitivity (similar to the situation in penicillin-related anaphylaxis).

Honeybee venom sensitivity occurs independent of other venom allergies, but about 10 per cent of patients are sensitive to both bee and vespid venoms. The vespid venoms are highly cross-reactive, so that almost all vespid-sensitive patients have positive YJ, YH, and WH skin tests even though most have been stung only by YJs. Half of these patients are also sensitive to POL venom. A few individuals are allergic to only one or two of the vespid venoms. In vitro RAST inhibition techniques are useful to distinguish cross-reactivity from specific sensitivity. This is clinically relevant in patients with a positive skin test to *Polistes*. This is usually due to cross-reactivity and the patient may be spared considerable

expense and unnecessary immunization by RAST inhibition analysis.

TREATMENT. The treatment of choice for anaphylactic reactions is subcutaneous epinephrine 1:1000, 0.5 ml initially and repeated twice at ten-minute intervals, if necessary, to reverse the progression of symptoms. Sublingual isoproterenol is probably ineffective. Antihistamines and glucocorticoids do not contribute to the management of life-threatening symptoms but may reduce the duration and severity of cutaneous manifestations. Their use should not be considered until the termination of the acute episode. Intravenous volume expansion or airway maintenance may be necessary. In a few individuals, the process is resistant to epinephrine; in such instances an alpha-adrenergic agent (i.e., norepinephrine) may be tried. Affected persons not yet protected by immunotherapy are advised to carry, and are instructed in the use of, a kit containing a syringe device preloaded with one or two recommended doses of epinephrine.

Venom immunotherapy is successful in virtually all patients. Less than 3 per cent of those immunized have any systemic symptoms after a challenge sting, and these are uniformly less severe than their previous reactions. The indications for venom immunotherapy are currently based on an incomplete understanding of the natural history of the disease. Those with a history of life-threatening reactions should be treated. The risk of progression from strictly cutaneous to life-threatening respiratory or vascular reactions is uncertain. Cutaneous reactors who are more likely to be stung in their daily activities or who for a variety of reasons (location, age, cardiovascular disease), can ill afford a more severe reaction should be treated. The cost and inconvenience of treatment may deter other cutaneous reactors from undergoing immunotherapy. Children, much more commonly than adults, have cutaneous symptoms only. These children may be left untreated. Venom immunotherapy is contraindicated in the absence of positive skin tests. Treatment is currently recommended using all venoms causing a positive skin test (for *Polistes*, see above). While other mechanisms may contribute, the induction of increased serum levels of venom-specific IgG antibodies is the most apparent mechanism of protection for venom immunotherapy; about 5 μg per milliliter is required.

Rapid immunization in six to eight weekly visits is recommended, since it is associated with a significantly greater and more rapid immune response and with fewer adverse reactions than a slower (more than 20 weeks) regimen. The maintenance dose of 100 μg of each venom is repeated monthly for at least six months, and is then continued at six- to eight-week intervals for five years or longer. After five years patients can usually stop therapy and suffer a sting without sequelae. If treatment is interrupted for more than three months, it is likely that protection will diminish to inadequate levels. Although unusual in adults, loss of sensitivity during maintenance immunotherapy may occur. Skin tests should, therefore, be repeated every two years.

Adverse reactions to venom immunotherapy may be early or late. Immediate reactions include all the manifestations of anaphylaxis. During the initial course of treatment, 10 to 15 per cent of patients report systemic complaints, only half of which require epinephrine. At maintenance doses, systemic reactions occur rarely. After a systemic reaction, the dose should be reduced by up to 50 per cent on the subsequent visit, and then increased gradually toward 100 μg again.

Large local reactions occur frequently. Fifty per cent of treated patients experience at least one such reaction. These occur after 10 out of every 100 injections in the induction phase, most commonly in the midrange of doses (10 to 50 μg) and much less often at maintenance doses. Large local reactions do not presage systemic reactions and require a reduction of dose only for the most severe reactions. Long-term side effects have not been observed with venom immunotherapy or in beekeepers stung frequently for over 30 years.

Golden DBK, Johnson K, Addison BI, et al.: Clinical and immunologic observations in patients who discontinue venom immunotherapy. J Allerg Clin Immunol 77:435, 1986. *Studies of when and how to discontinue venom immunotherapy.*

Golden DBK, Lichtenstein LM: Insect sting allergy. In Kaplan AP (ed.): Allergy. New York, Churchill Livingstone, 1985, pp 507–524. *A review of diagnostic and therapeutic problems in insect allergy.*

Hunt KJ, Valentine MD, Sobotka AK, et al.: A controlled trial of immunotherapy in insect hypersensitivity. N Engl J Med 299:157, 1978. *A comparison of venom immunotherapy with whole body extract and placebo. Demonstrates efficacy of venom therapy and the clinical consequences of challenge stings.*

Schuberth KC, Lichtenstein LM, Kagey-Sobotka A, et al.: Epidemiologic study of insect allergy in children. II. Effect of accidental stings in allergic children. J Pediatr 102:361, 1983. *A prospective epidemiology study of repeat stings in children. Has implications for young adults.*

424 IMMUNE COMPLEX DISEASES

Charles G. Cochrane

DEFINITION. Immune complex diseases are caused by the deposition or formation of antigen-antibody complexes in tissues. Inflammation results and leads to acute or chronic disease of the organ system in which the immune complexes have been deposited. The antigen-antibody complex localizes in a particular organ by two major mechanisms: (1) when antigens in that organ are exposed to antibodies entering from the circulation; and (2) when antigen-antibody complexes that form in the circulation are deposited in renal glomeruli, arteries, or venules, inducing inflammatory disease of each structure. Thus immune complexes are capable of causing severe inflammation in many organs of the body. For example, immune complexes may contribute to the pathogenesis of systemic lupus erythematosus (SLE), serum sickness, acute and chronic glomerulonephritis, rheumatoid arthritis, arteritis, vasculitis, and tissue injury associated with a wide spectrum of infectious agents (Table 424–1).

This chapter will examine the mechanisms by which the interaction of antigens and antibodies may form immune complexes and how this process may be injurious to the host.

PATHOGENESIS. The pathogenesis of immune complex diseases is best understood by examining several well-studied experimental models that closely mimic human diseases.

Immune Complex Disease with Tissue-Fixed Antigen. When the antigen is bound in an organ or is released locally from a tissue, the antibodies react with antigen at the locus to induce local inflammatory injury. As an example, antibodies in the circulation may react with antigens in the glomerular basement membrane of the kidney and result in inflammation of the glomerulus (glomerulitis) with acute or chronic injury. In human beings this takes the form of Goodpasture's disease. Similarly, when antigen-antibody complexes form in a joint space, synovitis results. This may play an important role in the pathogenesis of rheumatoid arthritis, in which antibodies have been found in the joint fluid complexed with many host proteins, especially IgG itself.

Immune Complex Disease Caused by the Deposition of Circulating Immune Complexes in Tissues. Acute immune complex disease, or serum sickness, can be produced in experimental animals by injection of serum protein antigens. The associated lesions are generally those of arteritis, glomerulonephritis, endocarditis, cutaneous rash, and synovitis. A mechanism for the production of immune complex disease is given in Figure 424–1. A chronic disease follows injections of the serum protein antigens for 30 days. In this form of the disease, chronic glomerulonephritis most characteristically

TABLE 424–1. DISEASES ASSOCIATED WITH IMMUNE COMPLEXES*

I. Autoimmune diseases
Rheumatoid arthritis, Felty's syndrome, SLE, cutaneous vasculitis, Sjögren's syndrome, MCTD, periarteritis nodosa, systemic sclerosis

II. Glomerulonephritis
Acute, subacute, chronic

III. Infectious diseases
Bacterial
Meningococcal, disseminated gonorrheal, streptococcal, leprous, and spirochetal infections; infectious endocarditis
Viral
Dengue hemorrhagic fever, cytomegalovirus infections, viral hepatitis, infectious mononucleosis, SSPE
Parasitic
Malaria, trypanosomiasis, schistosomiasis, filariasis, toxoplasmosis

IV. Neoplastic Diseases
Solid and lymphoid tumors

V. Other conditions
Dermatitis herpetiformis and celiac diseases; ulcerative colitis and Crohn's disease; myocardial infarcts; idiopathic interstitial pneumonia; cystic fibrosis; sarcoidosis; multiple sclerosis; amyotrophic lateral sclerosis; myasthenia gravis; uveitis; otitis media; atopic diseases; arthritis associated with intestinal bypass procedure for morbid obesity; sickle cell anemia; TTP; primary biliary cirrhosis; kidney and bone marrow transplantation; pregnancy, pre-eclamptic and eclamptic syndrome; Lyme arthritis; steroid-responsive nephrotic syndrome; xanthomatosis; vasectomy; oral ulceration and Behçet's syndrome; pemphigus and bullous pemphigoid; IgA deficiency; thyroid disorders; ankylosing spondylitis; iatrogenic diseases

*MCTD, mixed connective tissue disease; SLE, systemic lupus erythematosus; SSPE, subacute sclerosing panencephalitis; TTP, thrombotic thrombocytopenic purpura

(Adapted from Dixon FJ, Cochrane CG, Theophilopoulos A: Immune complex injury. In Samter M (ed.): Immunological Diseases. 4th ed. Boston, Little, Brown & Company, 1987.)

results, often without the other lesions of the acute disease. In cases in which a large antibody response occurs, pulmonary inflammation and fibrosis of the lung result. The glomerular lesions of chronic immune complex disease contain lumpy deposits rich in antigen, immunoglobulin, and complement along the outer edge of the basement membrane (Figs. 424–2 to 424–4). These morphologic characteristics have formed the diagnostic features of immune complex glomerulonephritis of human beings. However, in contrast to the lesions of chronic serum sickness of experimental animals, the amount of the inducing antigen (when known, as in poststreptococcal glomerulonephritis) is infinitesimal in concentration. By contrast, the IgG–anti-IgG complexes and cryoglobulins may dominate, suggesting that a nonspecific stimulation of the immune

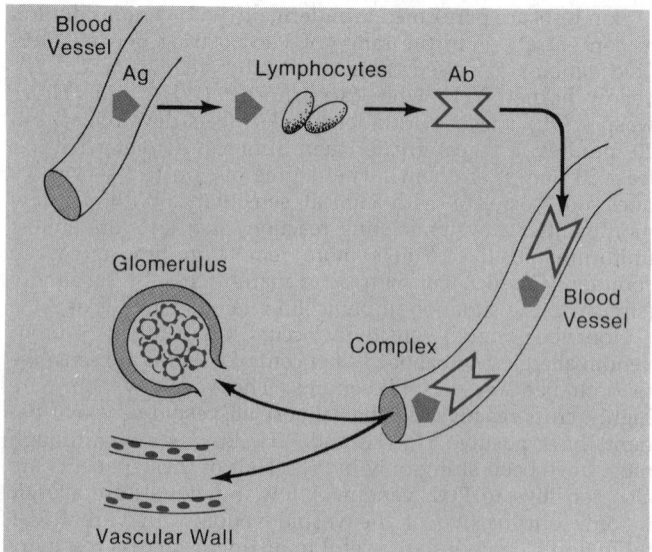

FIGURE 424–1. Schematic mechanism of the production of antibody by an antigen, the formation of antibody-antigen complexes in the circulation, and the localization of the complexes in tissues where inflammatory injury develops. Ag = antigen; Ab = antibody.

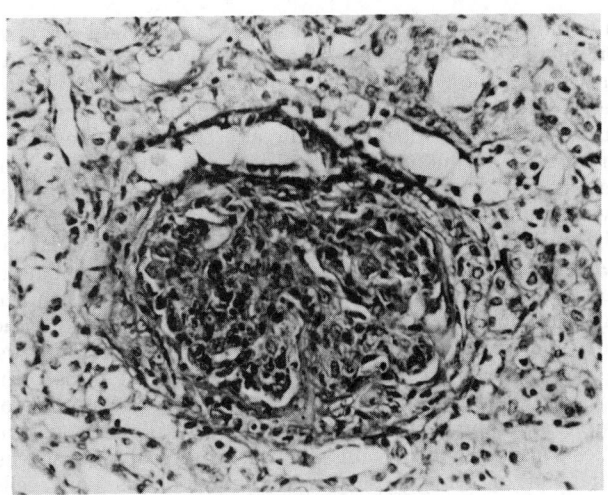

FIGURE 424–2. Glomerulus of a rabbit with subacute immune complex–induced glomerulonephritis. Inflammatory cells have accumulated, and injury of the glomerular basement membrane was evidenced by marked proteinuria. (× 150.)

system followed the initial exposure to antigen. Possibly a polyclonal stimulation of B lymphocytes and diminished activity of immune-suppressor systems are important pathogenic mechanisms in these human autoimmune diseases. Some antibodies to IgG proteins are anti-idiotypic; they form complexes with the immunoglobulin of the appropriate idiotype.

The Mechanism of Deposition of Circulating Immune Complexes. Several factors determine the ability of circulating complexes to localize in the vessel walls of a particular organ. Important among these factors are the quantity of complexes and the size of the complex. No definite minimal concentration of the complexes in the circulation has been established, but there seems to be a requirement for the complex to be of a particular size (19S or greater) for its deposition in blood vessel walls. The size of the three-dimensional lattice of antigen-antibody complexes depends largely upon the affinity of the antibody for the antigen. For example, in experimental animals complexes of intermediate size circulate and cause tissue injury, whereas larger complexes are insoluble and are rapidly cleared from circulation by the reticuloendothelial system. Another factor that may play a role in the deposition of immune complexes is electrical charge. By virtue of the overall anionic charge of the glomerular basement membrane,

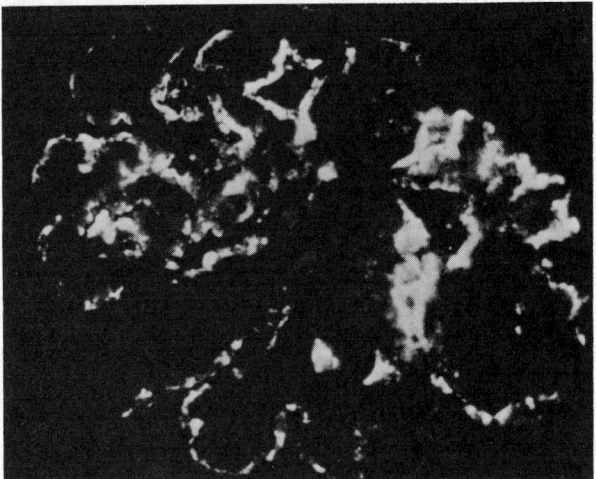

FIGURE 424–3. Fluorescent photomicrograph of a glomerulus similar to that in Figure 424–2, showing the presence of rabbit immunoglobulin along the glomerular basement membrane. The specific antigen and the third component of complement were localized in the same pattern.

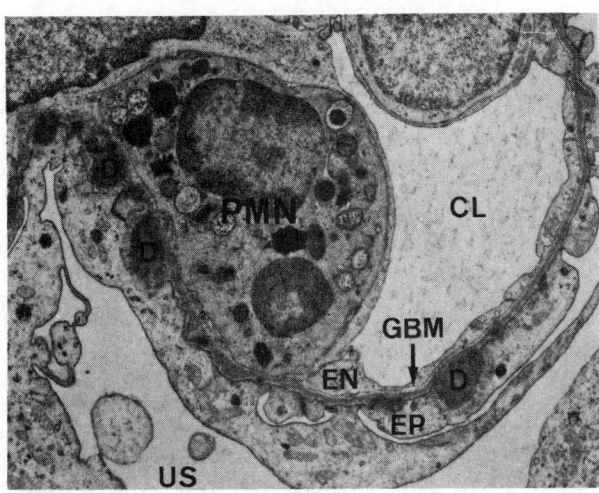

FIGURE 424–4. A polymorphonuclear leukocyte (PMN) is seen closely approximated along the glomerular basement membrane (GBM) in proximity to subepithelial (EP) electron dense deposits (D) in a rabbit with chronic serum sickness glomerulonephritis. The deposits are rich in antibody, complement, and, to a lesser extent, antigen by fluorescent antibody microscopy. Similar or identical deposits are observed in human immune complex glomerulonephritis. The endothelial cell (EN) has been displaced. Other abbreviations: CL = capillary lumen; US = urinary space.

cationic immune complexes or free antigens possess an affinity for glomeruli and are retained longer than neutral or anionic molecules.

An increase in vascular permeability is required for circulating immune complexes to be deposited in tissues and to initiate acute injury. The local release of vasoactive amines appears responsible for this increased permeability. Circulating antigen reacts with specific surface IgE on sensitized basophils to release an array of constituents, including histamine and a platelet activating factor (PAF). This latter factor causes clumping and degranulation of platelets and release of platelet histamine and serotonin. Thus an allergic reaction induces deposition of the circulating complexes in blood vessel walls. The anaphylatoxins C3a and C5a, generated by complement activation (see Ch. 418), also degranulate basophils and mast cells to liberate vasoactive amines and other substances. These may augment the increase in vascular permeability and facilitate the deposition of immune complexes along vascular basement membranes. In immune complex disease of man, the role of increased vascular permeability in the local deposition of circulating immune complexes has been documented in cutaneous vasculitis. In addition, in patients with active systemic lupus erythematosus, the circulating basophils undergo loss of granules and contain diminished levels of PAF. Basophils from patients with quiescent systemic lupus degranulate and release PAF upon exposure to DNA.

Host Factors Responsible for the Inflammation Caused by Immune Complexes. Immune complexes deposited in tissues activate mediator systems. These mediators are the cellular and humoral effectors of inflammatory injury—activated enzymes, biologically active peptides, oxidizing substances, polyamines, and prostaglandins—that are released in the tissues as a consequence of antigen-antibody complex deposition. The classic and (to a lesser extent) the alternative pathway of the complement system is activated by the complexed Ig molecule to initiate the complement cascade. This leads to the limited proteolytic cleavage of C3 and C5 to liberate small peptides, C3a and C5a and the fragment C3b, which rapidly bind to tissue structures such as vascular basement membrane. As noted, the peptides also degranulate basophils and mast cells releasing histamine, slow-reacting substance, and other substances that cause increased vascular permeability, smooth muscle contraction, and hypotension (see Table 427–1). C5a is also a potent chemoattractant for leukocytes. The remaining portion of the C3 molecule, C3b, binds white blood cells, thus facilitating phagocytosis and discharge of lysosomal granules. Short-lived oxidants (usually free radicals of oxygen) are generated in vivo in inflammatory foci and produce injury. Of particular interest, antioxidants have a profound therapeutic effect in experimental inflammatory disease.

White blood cells, platelets, and macrophages specifically bind the Fc portion of the antigen-antibody complex and in the process are stimulated to generate injurious oxidizing radicals (e.g., superoxide anion and H_2O_2) and to release their lysosomal granules containing proteolytic enzymes, peptides, and vasoactive amines into the surrounding fluid. The C5a peptide has a similar effect on leukocytes. The discharge of these effector molecules results in the inflammatory tissue injury characteristic of immune complex disease.

Acute immune complex-mediated injury depends, therefore, upon an interaction of the complement system and neutrophils at the local site. This has been clearly demonstrated in experimental studies of the Arthus reaction, pneumonitis, and arteritis in serum sickness; of immunologic synovitis; and of at least one form of experimental glomerulonephritis. In each reaction, an antigen-antibody complex is formed in the tissues, complement is rapidly activated, and neutrophils accumulate at the site. Inhibition of complement activation prevents the accumulation of neutrophils and prevents injury. Production of neutropenia also prevents the development of experimental immune complex injury. The release of mediators of inflammatory injury by neutrophils at the site of antigen-antibody complex deposition has been described above. Mononuclear leukocytes are also capable of generating oxidizing radicals and of releasing lysosomal constituents.

Experimental immune complex disease is capable of destroying several tissues through these mechanisms. In joints, glycosaminoglycans and cartilage are destroyed; in blood vessels and glomeruli, the basement membranes are hydrolyzed. Fragments of the injured glomerular basement membrane may be excreted in the urine. Elastic fibers of arteries are destroyed, and connective tissues, including collagen in the lung, are damaged by proteolytic cleavage. In man the histologic features of arteritis, acute streptococcal glomerulonephritis, acute homograft rejection, and some aspects of rheumatoid arthritis imply a similar mechanism of tissue destruction. Loss of elastin and collagen in the lungs is a hallmark of emphysema.

Chronic immune complex disease may call into play other mechanisms of injury. For example, the glomerulonephritis of experimental chronic serum sickness, which shows the typical lumpy appearance of antigen-antibody deposits of immunofluorescence, occurs independently of both complement and neutrophils. Macrophages, which may be attracted by chemotactic factors from neutrophils and by other substances, probably play an important role in this lesion. There is increasing evidence for an important role for the macrophage in both experimental models of chronic immunologic diseases and in immunologic lung disease in man. In a model of chronic membranous nephritis, marked by immune complex information along the epithelial side of the glomerular basement membrane, complement appears to play an essential role in the development of proteinuria independently of leukocytes. In this lesion, which closely resembles membranous nephritis of humans, the immune complexes and activated complement components lie on or adjacent to the delicate slit-pore diaphragm that bridges the space between epithelial food processes. This diaphragm may be an essential barrier to the passage of protein molecules, and its disruption may constitute a major cause of the glomerular dysfunction in chronic membranous nephritis.

DETECTION OF IMMUNE COMPLEXES. In tissues, conventional immunohistochemical assays at the light- or electron-microscopic level reveal the deposition of immunoglobulins, complement components, and, at times, antigen at the site of the lesion. This has been beneficial in determining pathogenetic mechanisms in acute and chronic glomerulonephritis, SLE (cutaneous and renal lesions), cutaneous vasculitis, arteritis, and other conditions. The immune complexes have been eluted from the tissues and further analyzed.

The detection of immune complexes in body fluids has been extensively developed (see References). These methods allow the detection of specific antigen in complex with immunoglobulins or simply of the immune complexes in the fluid. Since antigens are frequently unknown, the latter methods have been more useful. The detection of immune complexes in fluids are based on the physical properties of complexed immunoglobulin, the interactions of immune complexes with plasma proteins such as complement, and the interaction of the complexed immunoglobulins with cells having Fc or complement receptors on their surfaces.

The Significance of Circulating Immune Complexes in Human Disease. Circulating immune complexes have been detected in a wide variety of human diseases. Nevertheless, in diseases such as chronic glomerulonephritis, which is most probably caused by immune complexes, circulating complexes frequently cannot be detected. In other diseases in which immune complexes do not appear to play a role in pathogenesis, complexes may be readily measured in plasma. Thus the mere detection of circulating immune complexes does not necessarily imply that they play a role in the pathogenesis of the disease. Nevertheless, since the potential of immune complexes to deposit and establish inflammatory injury is established, their detection in the circulation should alert the physician to seek evidence of their pathogenicity in the individual patient.

Cochrane CG, Koffler D: Immune complex disease in experimental animals and man. In Dixon F, Kunkel H (eds.): Advances in Immunology Vol. 6. New York, Academic Press, 1973, pp 185–264. *This chapter reviews in detail many of the pathogenic mechanisms behind immune complex diseases, both experimental and human.*

Lambert PH, Dixon FJ, Zubler RH, et al.: A WHO collaborative study for the evaluation of eighteen methods for detecting immune complexes in serum. J Clin Lab Immunol 1:1, 1978. Theofilopoulos AN, Dixon FJ: The biology and detection of immune complexes. Adv Immunol 28:89, 1979. *These two references cover the mechanisms available for detecting immune complexes in the circulation of patients with a wide variety of disorders. The later reference offers, in addition, useful information on the effects of immune complexes on the host's response.*

Schraufstatter IU, Revak SD, Cochrane CG: Proteases and oxidants in experimental pulmonary inflammatory injury. J Clin Invest 73:1175, 1984. *This article provides evidence that oxidants are generated in situ in inflammation, and reviews the available data on oxidants and proteases in human pulmonary inflammatory disease.*

425 THE MAJOR HISTOCOMPATIBILITY COMPLEX AND DISEASE SUSCEPTIBILITY

Benjamin D. Schwartz

The existence of a human major histocompatibility complex (MHC) was first suggested in the mid 1950's when leukoagglutinating antibodies were discovered in the sera of multiparous women and multiply transfused leukopenic patients. Each serum would react with the cells of some but not all individuals; different sera reacted with the cells of different but overlapping populations of individuals. This pattern suggested that these antisera were detecting alloantigens (i.e.,

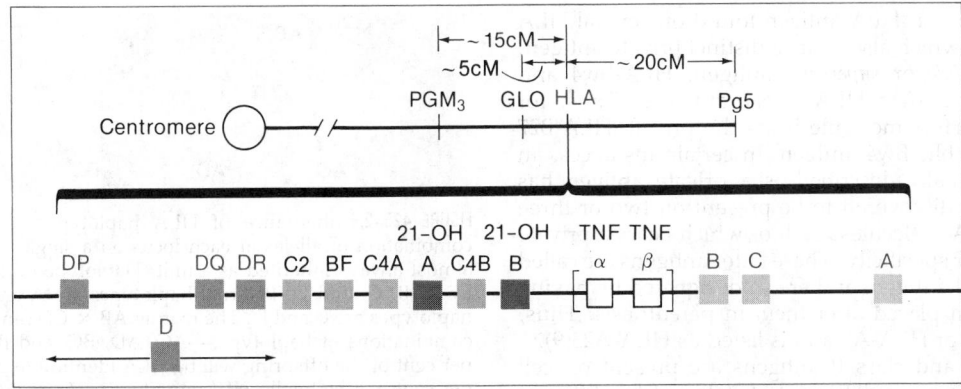

FIGURE 425–1. The current concept of the HLA complex. The upper part of the figure shows the position of the HLA complex in relation to other markers on the short arm of chromosome 6. PGM₃ = phosphoglucomutase 3; GLO = glyoxylase; Pg5 = urinary pepsinogen. Approximate distances are given in centimorgans (cM). The lower part of the figure shows the HLA complex itself. Class I loci are light red, class II loci are dark red, the complement class III loci are light gray, and the 21-hydroxylase loci are dark gray. Although the relative order of the class III loci is correct, the orientation of the entire class III region with respect to its centromeric and telomeric ends is not yet clear. Two additional loci for tumor necrosis factor (TNF-α) and lymphocytotoxin (TNF-β) may map close to HLA-B.

antigens that were present on the cells of some individuals of a given species) which were the products of a polymorphic genetic locus. These human leukocyte antigens (HLA) were found to have a major role in determining the success of organ transplants, and this finding spurred the initial study of these antigens. A second impetus for the study of the HLA complex derived from observations that certain HLA antigens are associated with specific diseases and that the HLA complex regulates several aspects of the human immune response. The reaction patterns of literally thousands of anti-HLA allo-antisera have now been codified by computer and have made possible the delineation of the HLA system. The application of molecular biologic technology to the study of the HLA complex over the past few years has allowed enumeration of the HLA genes and the determination of the amino acid sequence of many HLA molecules.

NOMENCLATURE AND GENETIC ORGANIZATION OF THE HLA COMPLEX

The genes for the HLA complex are located on the short arm of chromosome 6 (Fig. 425–1). Genes at the HLA-A, -B, and -C loci encode the class I or classic histocompatibility molecules; genes at the HLA-DR, -DQ, and -DP loci determine the class II or -Ia molecules; and genes at the C2, BF, C4A,

C4B, 21-OHA, and 21-OHB loci encode the class III molecules, including the second and fourth components of complement, properdin factor B, and 21-hydroxylase. Molecular biologic studies of the HLA complex will undoubtedly lead to recognition of other loci that map to this region. For example, the genes encoding human tumor necrosis factor (TNF-α) and lymphocytotoxin (TNF-β) will most likely map close to HLA-B.

At each locus, one of several alternative forms (alleles) of a gene may be found. Alleles at each locus are designated by the locus letter and a number; thus, for example, the number one allele at the HLA-A locus is designated HLA-A1. Alleles that have been assigned to a given locus but are not yet officially recognized are signified by a w (for *workshop*) placed before the number (e.g., HLA-DRw1). Official recognition results in the removal of the w (e.g., HLA-DR1).

The HLA system is highly polymorphic, having numerous different alleles at each locus (Table 425–1). For example, there are at least 23 distinct alleles at the HLA-A locus and at least 47 distinct alleles at the HLA-B locus. Each functional allele determines a glycoprotein product. The same designation is used for the HLA allele and its product, the HLA antigen. An HLA antigen found on a molecule determined by a single allele and no other is termed an HLA *private*

TABLE 425–1. CURRENT LISTING OF RECOGNIZED HLA ANTIGENS

HLA-A	HLA-B	HLA-C	HLA-D	HLA-DR	HLA-DQ	HLA-DP
A1	Bw4	Bw47	Cw1	Dw1	DR1	DQw1	DPw1
A2	B5	Bw48	Cw2	Dw2	DR2	DQw2	DPw2
A3	Bw6	B49(21)	Cw3	Dw3	DR3	DQw3	DPw3
A9	B7	Bw50(21)	Cw4	Dw4	DR4		DPw4
A10	B8	B51(5)	Cw5	Dw5	DR5		DPw5
A11	B12	Bw52(5)	Cw6	Dw6	DRw6		DPw6
Aw19	B13	Bw53	Cw7	Dw7	DR7		
A23(9)	B14	Bw54(w22)	Cw8	Dw8	DRw8		
A24(9)	B15	Bw55(w22)		Dw9	DRw9		
A25(10)	B16	Bw56(w22)		Dw10	DRw10		
A26(10)	B17	Bw57(17)		Dw11(w7)	DRw11(5)		
A28	B18	Bw58(17)		Dw12	DRw12(5)		
A29(w19)	B21	Bw59		Dw13	DRw13(w6)		
A30(w19)	Bw22	Bw60(40)		Dw14	DRw14(w6)		
A31(w19)	B27	Bw61(40)		Dw15			
A32(w19)	B35	Bw62(15)		Dw16			
Aw33(w19)	B37	Bw63(15)		Dw17(w7)	DRw52		
Aw34(10)	B38(16)	Bw64(14)		Dw18(w6)	DRw53		
Aw36	B39(16)	Bw65(14)		Dw19(w6)			
Aw43	B40	Bw67					
Aw66(10)	Bw41	Bw70					
Aw68(28)	Bw42	Bw71(w70)					
Aw69(28)	B44(12)	Bw72(w70)					
	B45(12)	Bw73					
	Bw46						

antigen. In contrast, an HLA antigen found on several HLA molecules, each of which also bears a distinct private antigen, is known as a *public* or *supertypic* antigen. HLA-Bw4 and -Bw6 are the best known HLA public antigens. Thus, for example, a single HLA molecule bears the private HLA-B27 antigen and the public Bw4 antigen. In certain instances, an HLA antigen originally described as a private antigen has been subsequently discovered to be present on two or three closely related HLA molecules, each of which bears a private antigen of narrower specificity. These latter antigens are called *splits* of the original antigen, and are so designated by having the original antigen placed after them in parenthesis. Thus, HLA-A23 is a split of HLA-A9 and is listed as HLA-A23(9).

All HLA class I and class II antigens are present on cell surface molecules but are defined and detected by different methods. The HLA-A, -B, -C, -DR, and -DQ class II antigens are defined and detected by serologic reactions. HLA-DP antigens, although originally defined and still typed by a cellular reaction known as the primed lymphocyte test (PLT), can now be detected serologically using monoclonal antibodies. In contrast, the HLA-D antigens are defined and detected solely by another cellular reaction known as the mixed leukocyte reaction (MLR). There is no known HLA-D molecule or HLA-D locus per se. Responder cells in the MLR appear to be detecting an array of antigenic determinants present on the HLA-DR, -DQ, and/or -DP molecules. In most cases, it is felt that antigenic determinants on HLA-DR molecules contribute most significantly to the MLR. As a result, HLA-D types tend to be most highly correlated with HLA-DR types.

Certain of the HLA-DR types have been organized into "supertypic" groups based on serologic reactions. Thus, for example, DR3, DR5, DRw6, and DRw8 have been grouped into the DRw52 supertypic group. It was initially thought that DRw52 was a public antigen on the molecules bearing the private antigens DR3, DR5, DRw6, and DRw8, but it is now known that DRw52 is on a separate DR molecule determined by a gene distinct from but tightly linked to the gene determining the molecule bearing the private DR antigen (see below). Similar comments apply to the DRw53 supertypic group composed of DR4, DR7, and DRw9. The DQ antigens have also been associated with particular sets of DR antigens. These associations are most likely secondary to the phenomenon of linkage disequilibrium (see below).

The products of the C2, C4, and BF loci are complement proteins that can be detected serologically and functionally and also display polymorphism (Chapter 418). The product of the 21-hydroxylase locus is an enzyme in the adrenal steroid synthetic pathway. The C4B-linked 21-hydroxylase gene is functional, while the C4A-linked 21-hydroxylase appears to be a pseudogene, that is, it is not expressed. A defective 21-hydroxylase B gene can therefore lead to congenital adrenal hyperplasia.

HAPLOTYPE

Because of their close linkage, the alleles at each locus on a single chromosome are usually inherited in combination, as a unit. This combination is referred to as the *haplotype*. Because each individual inherits one set of chromosomes from each parent, each individual has two HLA haplotypes. HLA genes are codominant; therefore, both alleles at a given HLA locus are expressed, and two complete sets of HLA antigens will be detected on cells. By simple mendelian genetics, there is a 25 per cent chance that two siblings will share both haplotypes and be fully HLA compatible, a 50 per cent chance that they will share one haplotype, and a 25 per cent chance that they will share no haplotype and thus will be completely HLA-incompatible (Fig. 425–2).

LINKAGE DISEQUILIBRIUM

Because of random matings, the frequency of finding a given allele at one HLA locus associated with a given allele

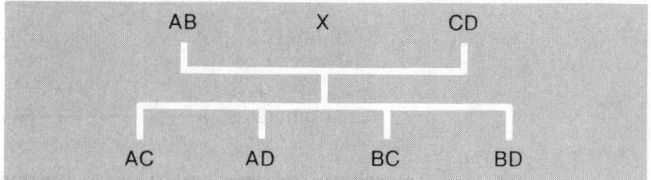

FIGURE 425–2. Inheritance of HLA haplotypes. A haplotype is the combination of alleles at each locus on a single chromosome and is almost always inherited as a unit. Haplotype designations are given by A, B, C, and D. Paternal haplotypes are A and B, and maternal haplotypes are C and D. The mating AB × CD can yield four possible combinations of haplotypes—AC, AD, BC, and BD. Statistically, 25 per cent of the offspring will be HLA identical (e.g., AC and AC), 25 per cent will be totally HLA nonidentical (e.g., AC and BD), and 50 per cent will be HLA-haploidentical (e.g., AC and AD).

at a second HLA locus should simply be the product of the frequencies of each allele in the population. However, certain combinations of alleles are found with a frequency greater than expected. This phenomenon is termed *linkage disequilibrium* and is quantitated as the difference (Δ) between the observed and expected frequencies. As an example, the HLA-DR3 allele and the HLA-DQw2 allele are found in the Caucasian population with frequencies of 0.118 and 0.179, respectively. Thus, the expected frequency with which the HLA-DR3, DQw2 haplotype should be found is 0.118×0.179, or 0.0221. However, this haplotype is found with a frequency of ~0.0585, almost three times the expected frequency, for $\Delta = 0.0585 - 0.0211 = 0.0374$. Table 425–2 lists some common examples of linkage disequilibrium. Several hypotheses have been put forth to explain linkage disequilibrium including a selective advantage of a given haplotype and recent admixture of two inbred populations.

HLA TYPING

Typing of the HLA-A, -B, -C, -DR, and -DQ antigens can be readily accomplished by a serologic assay known as microlymphocytotoxicity. Although some monoclonal antibodies are available for particular HLA antigens, the majority of serologic typing is still done with sera obtained from multiparous women. Typing for the HLA class I molecules is done on purified populations of lymphocytes. Typing of the HLA-DR and -DQ class II antigens is performed on purified populations of B lymphocytes. Alternatively, a two-color dye procedure is used which allows B cells to be distinguished from T cells. Although DP molecules can be detected by monoclonal antibodies, the HLA-DP antigens are typed by the primed lymphocyte test (PLT). The HLA-D antigens are typed by the mixed leukocyte reaction (MLR). HLA typing is used primarily for determination of HLA compatibility prior to transplantation and platelet transfusion, for paternity testing, and for establishing HLA disease associations.

Class I Molecules

TISSUE DISTRIBUTION AND FUNCTION. The class I antigens are found on virtually every human cell (Table 425–3). This tissue distribution is well suited to the physiologic

TABLE 425–2. EXAMPLES OF LINKAGE DISEQUILIBRIUM IN CAUCASIANS

Haplotypes	$\Delta(\times 10^{-3})$
HLA-A1, B8	53.2
HLA-A2, B44 (12)	14.8
HLA-A3, B7	32.4
HLA-B8, DR3	61.3
HLA-B7, DR2	36.8
HLA-DR2, DQw1	93.6
HLA-DR3, DQw2	37.4
HLA-DR7, DQw2	96.7
HLA-DR4, DQw3	87.5
HLA-A1, B8, DR3	28.0
HLA-A3, B7, DR2	11.5

TABLE 425–3. COMPARISON OF HLA CLASS I AND CLASS II MOLECULES

	Class I	Class II
Molecules included	HLA-A, B, C	HLA-DR, DQ, DP
Structure	44,000 MW heavy chain	~34,000 MW α Chain
	12,000 MW β$_2$-microglobulin	~29,000 MW β Chain
Tissue distribution	On virtually every cell	Normally limited to immunocompetent cells, particularly B cells, macrophages, activated T cells
Function	Restrict cytotoxic T cell killing of virus-infected cells	Restrict helper T cell recognition of foreign antigen

role of the class I antigens in which they function to present foreign antigens, for example, viral antigens to cytotoxic T lymphocytes (CTLs). Precursors of CTLs are specific for a particular viral antigen in the context of a particular class I molecule. When the precursors encounter this particular combination of the viral antigen and the class I molecule, they will proliferate and differentiate to mature CTLs. The mature CTLs are restricted in their killing to those target cells that bear both the same viral antigen and the same class I antigen as were present on the sensitizing cells. That particular CTL will not kill a target cell with the same class I molecule infected with a different virus, nor will it kill a target cell with a different class I molecule infected with the same virus. Thus, CTL killing is both antigen specific and class I restricted. In the nonphysiologic situation of a tissue or organ graft, the class I antigens are the principal antigens recognized by the host's CTLs during graft rejection.

STRUCTURE. The class I molecule consists of an HLA encoded polymorphic glycoprotein of 44,000 molecular weight known as the heavy chain, in noncovalent association with a 12,000 molecular weight nonpolymorphic protein known as β$_2$ microglobulin (Fig. 425–3). The β$_2$ microglobulin is encoded by a gene on chromosome 15 and not by the HLA complex. The entire molecule is anchored in the cell membrane only by the heavy chain. This chain contains ~338 amino acids and can be divided into three regions. Starting from the

amino-terminal end of the molecule, these regions are an extracellular hydrophilic region (amino acids 1–281), a transmembrane hydrophobic region (amino acids 282–306), and an intracytoplasmic hydrophilic region (amino acids 307–338). The extracellular hydrophilic region in turn can be divided into three domains, each of ~90 amino acids, designated from the amino terminal end α$_1$, α$_2$, and α$_3$. The α$_3$ domain and β$_2$ microglobulin have structural homology with the constant region of immunoglobulin, identifying the class I molecule as a member of the immunoglobulin supergene family. The HLA molecule somewhat resembles a mushroom, the α$_3$ domain and β$_2$ microglobulin forming the stalk and the α$_1$ and α$_2$ domains forming the cap. The majority of alloantigenic determinants recognized both by antibodies and by T cells are located in the α$_1$ and α$_2$ domains. The α$_1$ and α$_2$ domains interact with foreign antigen and together with the foreign antigen are recognized by antigen-specific class I restricted T cells.

The hydrophobic transmembrane region contains 24 amino acids, enabling it to span the cell membrane. The intracytoplasmic hydrophilic region can be phosphorylated, and it has been speculated that class I molecules may transduce external events across the cell membrane.

A schematic representation of a gene determining a class I molecule is shown in Figure 425–4. It consists of seven exons (transcribed regions of DNA) separated by introns (nontranscribed regions of DNA). Each exon encodes a particular portion of the HLA molecule.

Class II Molecules

TISSUE DISTRIBUTION AND FUNCTION. In contrast to the HLA class I molecules, the HLA class II molecules have a limited distribution (Table 425–3). They are found predominantly on immunocompetent cells including B cells, monocytes, dendritic cells, and activated T cells. Gamma-interferon can induce increased expression on macrophages and also induces expression of class II molecules on cells where they are not normally expressed (e.g., endothelial, thyroid, epidermal, and renal cells).

The physiologic role of the class II molecules parallels that of the class I molecules. Just as killer T cells recognize foreign antigen in the context of a class I molecule, helper T cells recognize foreign antigen in the context of a class II molecule. Indeed, the processed foreign antigen with class II molecules comprises the ligand recognized by the T cell receptor on helper T cells. In nonphysiologic states such as graft transplantation, the class II molecules present on donor cells can initiate an immune response in the host by stimulating the host's helper T cells.

STRUCTURE. The structure of a class II molecule is schematically depicted in Figure 425–5. Each class II molecule consists of two glycoprotein chains, an α-chain of 34,000 daltons and a β-chain of 29,000 daltons. The α-chain bears two N-linked oligosaccharides and has one disulfide-bridged domain, whereas the β-chain bears a single N-linked oligosaccharide and has two disulfide-bridged domains. Both of the chains span the membrane and therefore serve to anchor the molecule. Each chain can be divided into three regions. Beginning at the amino-terminal end, there is an extracellular hydrophilic region, a transmembrane hydrophobic region, and an intracytoplasmic hydrophilic tail. Each extracellular region has been further divided into two domains of ~90 amino acids each. For the α-chain, these are designated α$_1$ and α$_2$ and for the β-chain, β$_1$ and β$_2$. The α$_2$ and β$_2$ domains, like the α$_3$ domain of the class I molecule and β$_2$-microglobulin, show homology with the constant region domain of immunoglobulin, thus indicating the class II molecules are also members of the immunoglobulin supergene family. It is most likely that the α$_1$ and β$_1$ domains interact with foreign antigen.

The current concept of the HLA class II or HLA-D genetic

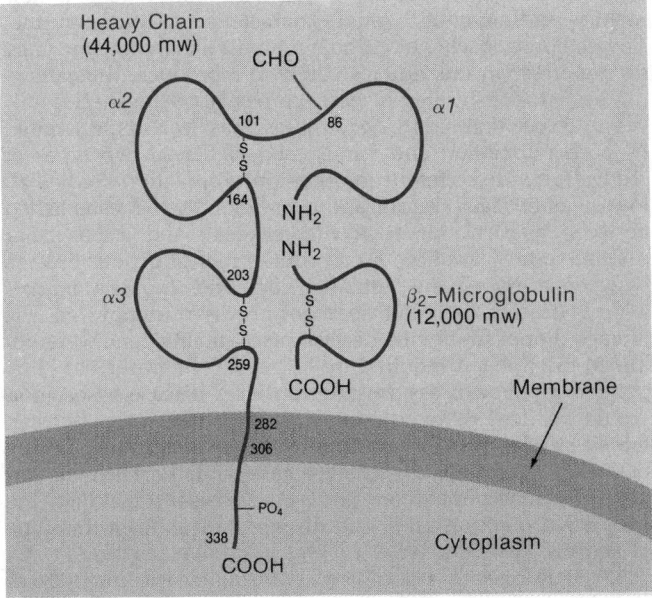

FIGURE 425–3. A schematic representation of an HLA class I molecule. The molecule consists of a heavy chain, which anchors the molecule in the membrane, noncovalently associated with β$_2$-microglobulin. Numbers indicate amino acid residues where certain features are found. NH$_2$ = Amino terminus; COOH = carboxy terminus; CHO = carbohydrate; PO$_4$ = phosphate. α$_1$, α$_2$, and α$_3$ are the three extracellular domains.

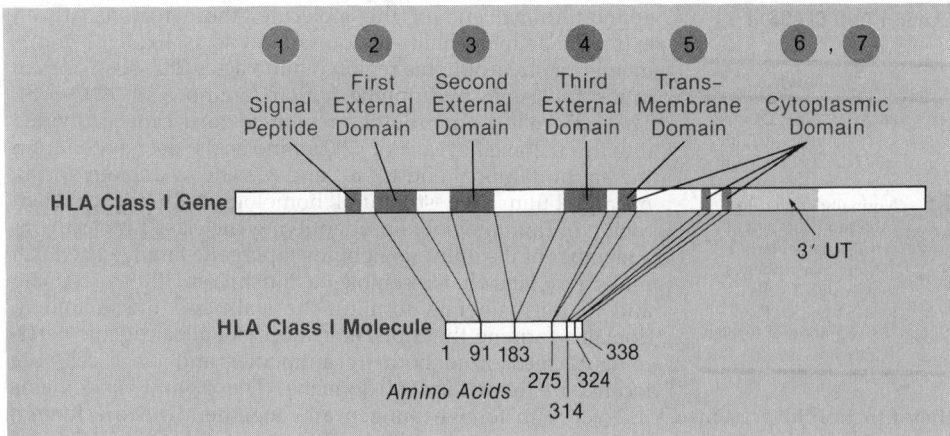

FIGURE 425–4. Schematic representation of an HLA class I gene, showing the organization of the exons and introns. The encircled numbers give the number of each exon (shaded), and the description below each exon gives the portion of the molecule each exon encodes. 3'-UT is the 3' = untranslated region.

region is shown in Figure 425–6. The region is divided into three subregions: DP, DQ, and DR. Each of these regions contains at least one functional α-chain and one functional β-chain gene. When these genes are expressed they lead to the formation of the class II αβ molecule. The HLA-DR region contains a single DRα chain gene and in most DR types, three β chain genes. In most DR types the DRβ$_{II}$ gene is a pseudogene; that is, it is not expressed. However, both the DRβ$_I$ and DRβ$_{III}$ genes are expressed. The DRα chain can combine with either the DRβ$_I$ chain or the DRβ$_{III}$ chain to produce the DRαβ$_I$ and DRαβ$_{III}$ molecules. The DRαβ$_I$ molecule is thought to bear the "private" DR antigen (e.g., DR3 or DR5), while the DRαβ$_{III}$ molecule is thought to bear the "supertypic" antigen (e.g., DRw52 or DRw53). The DQ subregion contains two pairs of αβ chain genes. One pair, designated DX, is a set of pseudogenes and not expressed. The other pair is expressed and results in the formation of the DQ αβ molecule. Likewise, the DP subregion contains two pairs of αβ chain genes. One pair, designated SX, contains pseudogenes. The other pair, designated DPα and DPβ, encode the DPα and β chains which form the DPαβ molecule. The polymorphism of the three sets of class II molecules (DR, DQ, and DP) varies somewhat for each set. For the DR molecules, the DRα chain is relatively nonpolymorphic between different DR types and the DRβ chain is highly polymorphic. For the DQ molecules, both the DQα and DQβ chains demonstrate a high degree of polymorphism. For the DP molecules, the DPα chains show

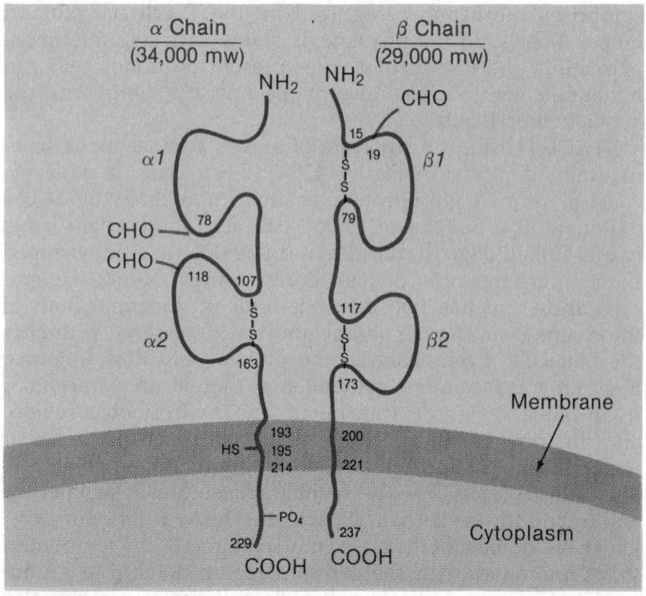

relatively limited polymorphism, while the DPβ chains are again highly polymorphic.

IMMUNE RESPONSE (IR) GENES IN MAN. The products of immune response (Ir) genes that were discovered in mice and guinea pigs are the class II molecules themselves. There is now a substantial body of evidence that suggests that human Ir genes do exist. Allergy to ragweed antigen Ra5 has been found to be highly associated with HLA-Dw2 and immune response to tetanus toxoid in the Japanese population has been found to be associated with a Japanese HLA-D allele. Additional evidence for the presence of human Ir genes derives from the observation that many HLA-associated diseases are associated with class II antigens.

HLA ASSOCIATION WITH DISEASE

The discovery in 1973 that ankylosing spondylitis was highly associated with HLA-B27 stimulated an intense search for other HLA disease associations. Well over 100 diseases from virtually all fields of medicine have now been associated with HLA. Despite this broad range of diseases, HLA-associated diseases for the most part share certain common characteristics. In general, these diseases have an hereditary tendency but weak penetrance and do not follow simple mendelian segregation. Their etiology and pathophysiology are unknown. They are associated with immunologic abnormalities and many of them are characterized as autoimmune. They follow subacute or chronic courses. Finally, they usually do not affect an individual's ability to reproduce, thus allowing the HLA-associated diseases to persist in the species.

The association of HLA and disease has been demonstrated by both population and family studies. These two types of studies provide different information. Population studies allow a statistically significant correlation to be established between a particular HLA marker gene and a particular disease state. They do not constitute proof of genetic linkage between a disease susceptibility gene and the HLA marker gene because correlation does not necessarily imply genetic linkage. For example, if a disease susceptibility gene were not linked to HLA but required the presence of a particular HLA antigen for its expression, then an HLA disease association would be demonstrated in population studies. In contrast, family studies provide an opportunity to determine linkage between a disease susceptibility gene and the HLA marker gene. Because population studies are easier to conduct, the majority of data on HLA and disease derives from this type of study.

No HLA-disease association is absolute. The majority of individuals with a given disease-associated HLA antigen do not contract the disease, and a given HLA associated disease can occur in individuals who lack the usual disease-associated HLA antigen. A combination of a particular HLA antigen, other genetic influences, and environmental agents seems to be necessary for the disease to be manifest.

The strength of the association of a particular disease with

FIGURE 425–5. Schematic representation of an HLA-DR molecule. The molecule consists of an α chain transmembrane glycoprotein noncovalently associated with a β chain transmembrane glycoprotein. For explanation of symbols, see Figure 425–3.

FIGURE 425–6. The current concept of the HLA-D region, showing the organization of the three subregions, DP, DQ, and DR. SXα, SXβ, DXα, DXβ, and DRβ$_{II}$ are pseudogenes and not expressed. Pairs of expressed genes (DPα and DPβ; DQα and DQβ; DRα and DRβ$_I$; and DRα and DRβ$_{III}$), which encode class II molecules, are indicated. DZα and DOβ are not currently known to be transcribed in vivo. Arrows under genes give the direction of transcription (5′ to 3′).

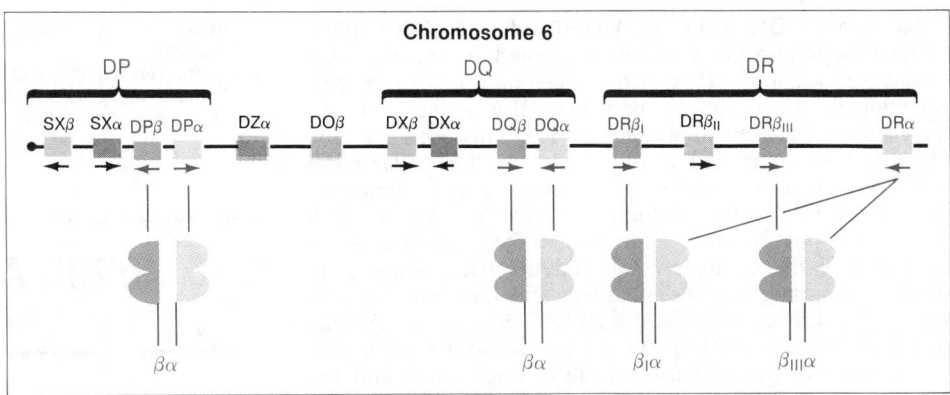

a particular HLA antigen is quantitated by calculating the relative risk. The relative risk (RR) is defined by the formula $RR = (P^+ \times C^-)/(P^- \times C^+)$, where P^+ is the number of patients possessing the disease-associated HLA antigen, C^- is the number of controls lacking that particular HLA antigen, P^- is the number of patients lacking that HLA antigen, and C^+ is the number of controls possessing that HLA antigen. The higher the relative risk above 1, the stronger the association between the HLA antigen and the disease. The relative risk can be stated as the chance of developing the HLA-associated disease for an individual with the disease-associated HLA antigen compared to an individual without the HLA antigen. Because there is usually a significant difference in the frequency of a given antigen among different racial groups, it is mandatory to compare a patient group with a control population of the same race. Thus, for example, HLA-B27 is found in 88 per cent of American Caucasian patients with ankylosing spondylitis and ~8 per cent of American Caucasian controls, yielding a relative risk of ~90. In contrast, HLA-B27 is found in 48 per cent of American black patients with ankylosing spondylitis but in only 2 per cent of American black controls, giving a relative risk of 37. Table 425–4 gives the relative risk for selected significant HLA disease associations.

Because of the phenomenon of linkage disequilibrium and the order in which the HLA class I and class II antigens were defined, a particular disease may have appeared to be asso-

ciated with a particular antigen at a given HLA locus when in actuality it is more highly associated with a particular antigen at a different HLA locus. Thus, for example, HLA-DQw2, HLA-DR3, and HLA-B8 are known to be in linkage disequilibrium. Before any of the HLA class II antigens were well defined, celiac disease was associated with HLA-B8. The definition of the DR antigens allowed a stronger association to be established between celiac disease and HLA-DR3. The subsequent definition of the HLA-DQ specificities suggested an even more significant association between celiac disease and HLA-DQw2. With the application of molecular biology techniques to the study of HLA and disease associations, restriction endonuclease fragments have been identified in the HLA-D region that may yield yet more significant associations. Thus, for example, 90 per cent of patients with celiac disease have a genomic DNA fragment that can be detected using a DQβ chain cDNA probe. Individuals with this fragment have a relative risk of 46 for contracting celiac disease.

In addition, because of linkage disequilibrium, a number of diseases have been associated with what has been termed extended haplotypes. Two such examples are the association of C2 deficiency with the haplotype Aw25, B18, C2*QO, BF*S, C4A*4, C4B*2, DR2, and systemic lupus erythematosus with the haplotype A1, B8, BF*S, C2*C, C4A*QO, C4B*1, DR3.

The majority of HLA-associated diseases have been associated with the class II antigens, consistent with the concept that class II molecules are the products of immune response genes and somehow predispose to disease. HLA-DR3, for instance, appears to be associated with hyperimmune responsiveness, even in normal individuals. An interesting finding in this regard is that several documented or presumed autoimmune diseases have been found associated with HLA-DR3 (Table 425–5).

For certain diseases it appears as if gene complementation between two different class II genes plays a role in disease predisposition. For example, the antibody response to Ro and La antigens in patients with Sjögren's syndrome is highest in patients who are DQw1/DQw2 heterozygotes. Insulin-dependent diabetes mellitus has been associated with both DR3 and with DR4 but is most highly associated with DR3/DR4 heterozygosity. Seropositive juvenile rheumatoid arthritis (JRA) has been associated with HLA-DR4 and with two particular subtypes of DR4, Dw4, and Dw14, but seropositive JRA is most highly associated with the Dw4/Dw14 heterozygous state. The molecular basis for this phenomenon has not yet been established.

TABLE 425–4. SELECTED HLA AND DISEASE ASSOCIATIONS IN CAUCASIAN PATIENTS

Disease	Antigen	Approximate Relative Risk
Ankylosing spondylitis	B27	81.8
Reiter's syndrome	B27	40.4
Acute anterior uveitis	B27	7.98
Reactive arthritis (*Yersinia*)	B27	17.6
Rheumatoid arthritis	DR4	6.4
Juvenile rheumatoid arthritis		
Seropositive	DR4	7.2
	Dw4	25.8
	Dw14	47
	Dw4/Dw14	116
Pauciarticular	DR5	2.9
Systemic lupus erythematosus	DR3	2.7
Behçet's disease	B5	3.3
Sjögren's syndrome	DR3	5.6
Graves' disease	DR3	3.8
Insulin-dependent diabetes mellitus	DR3	3.0
Celiac disease	DR3	13.3
Psoriasis vulgaris	B13	4.5
	B17	3.1
	Cw6	7.2
Pemphigus vulgaris	DR4	21.4
Dermatitis herpetiformis	DR3	18.2
Idiopathic hemochromatosis	A3	6.6
	B14	3.7
Goodpasture's syndrome	DR2	19.8
Multiple sclerosis	DR2	2.8
Myasthenia gravis (without thymoma)	B8	3.3
Narcolepsy	DR2	129

TABLE 425–5. DISEASES ASSOCIATED WITH HLA-DR3

Systemic lupus erythematosus
Sicca syndrome
Insulin-dependent diabetes mellitus
Graves' disease
Idiopathic Addison's disease
Celiac disease
Myasthenia gravis
Dermatitis herpetiformis

EXPLANATION FOR HLA-DISEASE ASSOCIATION. Several hypotheses have been suggested to explain HLA disease associations: (1) HLA molecules may act as receptors for etiologic agents. If only particular HLA antigens can act as receptors for agents that cause particular diseases, then the HLA-disease association would result. (2) "Molecular mimicry": the disease-associated HLA antigen may be immunologically similar to the etiologic agent for the disease, with one of two possible alternative results. First, because of the similarity of the etiologic agent and the HLA antigen, no immune response may be mounted, and therefore the etiologic agent can cause disease unabated. Second, a vigorous immune response may be mounted against the etiologic agent, but because of the similarity of the etiologic agent and the HLA antigen, the immune response is turned against the HLA antigen, and the resulting autoimmune response will produce disease. (3) The actual disease susceptibility genes may not be the HLA genes themselves but rather T cell receptor α- and β-chain genes. This hypothesis suggests that because a particular T cell receptor α- and β-chain combination that predisposes to disease recognizes only a particular HLA antigen (or a foreign antigen only in the context of that HLA antigen), an *apparent* association with the HLA antigen is seen. (4) For diseases associated with HLA class II antigens, the class II antigens may be merely markers for the immune response gene effects of the molecules on which they are borne.

Other mechanisms besides those noted above have also been suggested. Obviously, different mechanisms may be operating to predispose to different diseases, and more than one mechanism may be operating concurrently to produce disease.

CLINICAL IMPLICATIONS OF HLA-DISEASE ASSOCIATIONS. The association of HLA and disease has a number of theoretical clinical implications with respect to disease classification, diagnosis, prognosis, predictive risk of disease development, genetic counseling, and therapeutics. However, only a limited number of these have been realized to date. The finding that a number of diseases previously classified as rheumatoid arthritis variants were associated with HLA-B27 allowed these diseases to be reclassified as the B27-associated spondyloarthropathies. The high associations of HLA-B27 with ankylosing spondylitis and Reiter's syndrome can aid in the diagnosis of these two diseases. However, because of the lack of absolute association, the absence of HLA-B27 in a patient with suspected disease should not be interpreted to exclude the diagnosis, nor should the presence of B27 be used to make the diagnosis in a patient who lacks a strong clinical picture for the disease. In cases where HLA-associated diseases have been found in a family member and a particular disease susceptibility gene is known to map to the HLA complex, HLA typing of cells obtained during amniocentesis could be performed to determine whether the fetus will be at risk for the disease. Congenital adrenal hyperplasia attributed to 21-hydroxylase deficiency is an example of this potential application of HLA-disease associations. Further progress in elucidating the basis for HLA disease associations may allow additional theoretical implications to become reality.

Kaufman JA, Auffray C, Korman AJ, et al.: The class II molecules of the human and murine major histocompatibility complex. Cell 36:1, 1984. *A short review of the biochemistry and function of the class II molecules.*

McDevitt HO: The HLA system and its relation to disease. Hosp Pract 20:57, 1985. *A clearly written introduction for the neophyte.*

Moller G (ed.): HLA and disease susceptibility. Immunol Rev, Vol 70. Copenhagen, Munksgaard, 1983. *An overview of the data supporting the models for HLA-disease associations.*

Moller G (ed.): Molecular genetics of class I and II MHC antigens. Parts I and II. Immunol Rev, Vol 84 and 85. Copenhagen, Munksgaard, 1985. *A detailed discussion of the organization and basis for polymorphism of the HLA genes.*

Ploegh HL, Orr HT, Strominger JL: Major histocompatibility antigens: The human (HLA-A, -B, -C) and murine (H-2K, H-2D) class I molecules. Cell 24:287, 1981. *A brief review of the structure and biology of the HLA class I molecules.*

Tiwari JL, Terasaki PI (eds.): HLA and Disease Associations. New York, Springer-Verlag, 1985. *A comprehensive volume describing virtually all known HLA-disease associations. An excellent reference source.*

426 DRUG ALLERGY

Charles E. Reed

An allergic cause of a drug reaction is suspected when an inflammatory lesion characteristic of those provoked by immunologic mechanisms follows administration of the drug. The variety of drug allergies gives the initial impression that any drug can cause any reaction; in fact, distinct patterns are the rule. Any particular drug tends to cause a similar reaction in different subjects. Typical examples include urticaria after penicillin, lymphocytic pneumonitis after nitrofurantoin, or contact dermatitis from an ointment containing ethylenediamine. Allergic drug reactions need to be distinguished from expected side effects, idiosyncratic reactions of unknown cause, toxic reactions, psychophysiologic reactions, and also from immunologic manifestations of the underlying disease. A further distinction is made between allergic inflammation initiated by a ligand reacting with an antibody or a specifically reacting lymphocyte and similar inflammation initiated by a pharmacologic reaction. Unfortunately these distinctions are not always easily made at the bedside, and there are few reliable clinical or laboratory tests.

Many patients relate a history of allergy to one or more drugs, often without an objective basis. Usually this history can be accepted and serves as a deterrent to excessive drug therapy. Sometimes, however, it is important to evaluate the possibility of allergy to a potentially life-saving drug for which there is no substitute, since many patients with a history of a reaction will tolerate the drug, particularly if several years have passed. If the allergy is still present, taking the drug can be disastrous with fatality from anaphylaxis, Stevens-Johnson syndrome, exfoliative dermatitis, interstitial pneumonitis, or vasculitis. A decision for a particular course of action often rests on judicious weighing of the potential benefits and risks rather than on a definitive diagnosis.

INCIDENCE AND PREDISPOSING FACTORS. Allergic reactions constituted about 6 per cent of all adverse drug reactions in 1968. The frequency is thought to be less today, except for reactions to radiographic contrast agents, which now account for about 60 per cent of drug-induced anaphylaxis and about 20 per cent of all cases of anaphylaxis.

Several predisposing factors exist. Previous drug allergy to the same or a related drug is most important, and the frequency of allergy increases with multiple courses of treatment. Topical administration is the route most likely to sensitize; oral administration, least; and parenteral, intermediate. Parenteral administration provokes more severe reactions, especially anaphylaxis. Children are less likely than adults to react, and men less than women. Persons with history of atopic allergy may be at increased risk of anaphylaxis or urticaria but not of other kinds of allergic drug reactions. The antigenic determinant in drug allergy is often a metabolite rather than the drug itself; genetic differences in drug metabolism therefore influence allergic reactions. For example, persons with reduced acetyltransferase activity are more likely to develop drug-induced systemic lupus erythematosus from hydralazine.

MECHANISMS. Foreign macromolecules acting as complete antigens are the most likely to sensitize, eliciting an IgE or IgG antibody response that on a subsequent administration causes anaphylaxis, serum sickness, or vasculitis. Classic serum sickness after injections of large amounts of rabbit or horse serum requires large amounts of antigen and relatively high concentrations of circulating immune complexes. Most episodes of urticaria, fever, and arthralgia after relatively small doses involve a combination of IgE– and IgG–initiated events.

Low-molecular-weight drugs and diagnostic agents elicit an immune response only after reacting covalently with proteins. This hapten may be the drug itself, or a metabolite. The hapten-protein carrier then functions as the complete antigen, both initiating sensitization and eliciting the reaction. An allergic reaction requires a multivalent ligand to cross-link antibody molecules either in fluid phase or bound to cell surface receptors. Univalent haptens actually inhibit cross-linking by occupying the antigen-binding sites. Some chemicals may react with host proteins in such a way that the tertiary structure is altered and the new antigenic determinant is not the hapten itself but the altered structure of the host protein. Drug allergy may take any of the forms of allergic reaction described in Part XX. The mechanisms of immune defense and hypersensitivity, like many other biologic functions, exhibit redundancy such that a drug reaction may involve more than one allergic mechanism at the same time. The fact that the hapten often is a drug metabolite may explain the characteristic involvement of some particular organ where the metabolism occurs; alternatively, the hapten may react with a specific organ protein to account for the location of the reaction.

PREVENTION. Avoiding drugs with high sensitizing potential reduces frequency of drug allergy, so many drugs that formerly caused allergy are no longer used. Interrupted treatment is more likely to sensitize than is continuous treatment, especially with insulin. Beef insulin is more allergenic than pork or human insulin. Recurrence of drug allergy can be reduced by taking a careful history; by exercising a high index of suspicion when fever, rash, or organ damage occurs during treatment; by careful recording of manifestation of drug reactions and diagnosis in the chart when they do occur; and by proper instruction of the patient.

DIAGNOSIS. The history and physical examination provide the essential information for pattern recognition. A key point of the history is the time course of the reaction. Anaphylactic reactions follow within minutes; drug fever, within an hour or two; contact dermatitis, in a day or two; but cholestatic jaundice requires several days or a week. The character of the lesion is also important. Ampicillin characteristically causes a morbilliform rash that may be delayed for two days after the drug is stopped. All penicillins may cause urticaria within ten minutes, but the urticaria may not occur for several days. This distinction is important because the immediate reactions are more likely to be associated with anaphylaxis. A physician observing a drug reaction should record the physical findings for future use. For example, by history alone it is difficult to distinguish between laryngeal edema from anaphylaxis and the hyperventilation syndrome, but the presence of stridor and swelling of pharyngeal or laryngeal mucosa makes the distinction clear. Distinction between a drug reaction and an immunologic event from the underlying disease is important. For instance, many children with viral respiratory infections have transient urticaria that can be mistaken for a penicillin rash. Or, on the first or second day of penicillin treatment a patient with endocarditis may have a macular hemorrhagic rash and fever, reflecting a reaction to antigens released from the bacteria rather than drug allergy.

Some of the most important patterns of drug reactions are summarized in Table 426–1. For some of the drugs on this list there is no proof that the drug actually caused the reaction. The association is plausible but not certain.

Skin tests may be helpful in predicting anaphylaxis from macromolecules and are usually positive in patients with allergy to foreign sera, insulin, vaccines, and similar complex materials. With the important exception of penicillin, skin or in vitro allergy tests with low-molecular-weight drugs are not reliable for detecting anaphylactic (IgE-mediated) drug allergy, although positive skin tests have occasionally been reported after anaphylaxis from local anesthetics, cisplatin, and a few other drugs. Patch tests with single components are useful for identifying contact allergens. Ethylenediamine, one of the ingredients of many creams and ointments, is currently the most frequently encountered contactant. Attempts to adapt lymphocyte transformation tests for diagnosis of drug allergy have been unsuccessful. Eosinophilia, when otherwise unexplained, provides evidence of allergy. Deliberate trial of small doses of the drug strictly for diagnostic purposes is unwise and unnecessary. It may be indicated as a precaution in situations in which the diagnosis of drug allergy is uncertain and no chemically unrelated substitute is available for an urgently needed drug.

MANAGEMENT. In addition to stopping use of the offending drug, symptomatic or supportive treatment of the reaction may be indicated. As a rule it is unwise to attempt to continue using the offending drug under a protective shield of antihistamines or glucocorticoids, although occasional desperate situations may justify an exception. The emergency treatment of anaphylaxis is described in Ch. 422.

SPECIFIC DRUG ALLERGIES. *Penicillin.* Penicillin is one of the most common drugs causing allergy, and being the most fully understood it serves as a model for other drugs. Penicillin reactions include anaphylaxis, urticaria, vasculitis, dermatomyositis, maculopapular rashes, hemolytic anemia, drug fever, interstitial nephritis, pneumonitis, and contact dermatitis. Airborne penicillin can cause asthma in workers who produce or use it. The nature of the reaction is determined not only by the specific metabolite that becomes the hapten but also by the carrier molecule. For example, the penicilloyl determinant commonly evokes IgE antibody in cases of urticaria, but it also evokes IgG, and after complexing with red cell–membrane protein, it may be responsible for hemolytic anemia during intravenous penicillin treatment. Many patients who claim to be allergic to penicillin tolerate it without adverse effect. In such patients, treatment with more expensive or toxic antibiotics would be unnecessary. Reliable tests are available for predicting which patients with a history of penicillin allergy are at risk of immediate allergic reactions. Cautious skin testing with dilute solutions of the antibiotic itself and with commercially available benzylpenicilloyl-polylysine (Pre-Pen) will provide guidance. If skin test reactions are negative to these reagents and to the "minor" determinants (the plain drug, penicilloate, and penilloate), the probability of a mild allergic reaction is about 2 per cent, no higher than in subjects receiving penicillin for the first time. The minor determinants are as yet available only in research settings, but only about 7 per cent of patients react to this reagent alone. Therefore, for patients who give a history of a penicillin reaction and need a penicillin drug for a serious infection, tests with the available reagents interpreted in the light of the history will allow appropriate treatment to proceed. The skin test with penicilloyl-polylysine begins with a prick of the 6.0×10^{-5} M solution, and, if negative in 20 minutes, one proceeds to intradermal testing. Skin testing with the penicillin solution starts with a prick test with a solution containing 6000 units per milliliter of penicillin G or 4 mg per milliliter of other penicillins. Similar testing with cephalosporin is feasible. The frequency of reactions to cephalosporins in patients allergic to penicillin is controversial. About 50 per cent of subjects with positive skin test to penicillin reacted to cephalothin.

Desensitization can be undertaken when skin test reactions are positive or when there are other reasons for suspecting an appreciable risk of anaphylaxis but the patient has life-

TABLE 426–1. ALLERGIC DRUG REACTIONS

I. **Systemic**
  A. *Anaphylaxis*
    1. Macromolecules
      Allergenic extracts
      Dextrans (including
        iron dextran)
      Enzymes
        Asparaginase
        Chymopapain
        Chymotrypsin
        Trypsin
      Heparin
      Hormones (ACTH, in-
        sulin, etc.)
      Human gamma globu-
        lin
      Organ extracts
      Protamine
      Vaccines
      Xenogenic sera
    2. Diagnostic agents
      Fluorescein
      Iodinated contrast me-
        dia
    3. Antimicrobials
      Amphotericin B
      Cephalosporins
      Clindamycin
      Ethambutol
      Kanamycin
      Lincomycin
      p-Aminosalicylic acid
      Penicillins
      Streptomycin
      Sulfonamides
      Tetracyclines
      Vancomycin
    4. Other drugs and other
        nonsteroidal anti-in-
        flammatory drugs
      Aspirin
      Benzyl alcohol
      Bleomycin
      Cisplatin
      Colchicine
      Cromolyn
      Cytarabine
      Dantrolene
      Ethylenediamine
      Glucocorticoids
      Indomethacin
      Local anesthetics
      Mephyton
      Meprobamate
      Mercurials
      Niacin
      Opiates
      Pentamidine
      Probenecid
      Sulfite
      Tolmetin
      Triamterene
      Tubocurarine and other
        muscle-relaxing
        agents
      Vitamin B_{12}
  B. *Serum sickness*
    1. Macromolecules
      Dextrans
      Heparin
      Hormones (insulin,
        ACTH, etc.)
      Vaccines
      Xenogenic sera
    2. Antimicrobials
      Cephalosporins
      Griseofulvin
      Lincomycin
      Minocycline
      Penicillins
      Streptomycin
      Sulfonamides

    3. Other Drugs
      Barbiturates
      Cholecystographic dyes
      Hydantoins
      Hydralazine
      Mercurial diuretics
      Phenylbutazone
      Procarbazine
      Thiouracils
  C. *Drug fever*
    1. Antimicrobials
      Cephalosporins
      Chloramphenicol
      Erythromycin
      Isoniazid
      Kanamycin
      Nitrofurantoin
      p-Aminosalicylic acid
      Penicillins
      Pyrazinamide
      Quinine
      Streptomycin
      Sulfonamides
      Tetracyclines
    2. Other drugs
      Allopurinol
      Captopril
      Heparin
      Hydantoins
      Hydralazine
      Iodides
      Mercurial diuretics
      Methyldopa
      Penicillamine
      Phenobarbital
      Pneumococcal vaccine
      Procainamide
      Propylthiouracil
      Quinidine
  D. *Vasculitis*
      Allopurinol
      Busulfan
      Colchicine
      Diphenhydramine
      Ethionamide
      Furosemide
      Hydantoins
      Hydroxyurea
      Ibuprofen
      Indomethacin
      Iodides
      Isoniazid
      Meprobamate
      Methamphetamine
      Penicillins
      Phenothiazines
      Phenylbutazone
      Propranolol
      Propylthiouracil
      Sulfonamides
      Tetracyclines
      Thiazide diuretics
      Vaccines
  E. *Systemic lupus erythemato-
      sus syndrome*
      Chloroquine
      Chlorpromazine
      Ethosuximide
      Griseofulvin
      Hydralazine
      Isoniazid
      Methyldopa
      Nitrofurantoin
      p-Aminosalicylic acid
      Penicillins
      Penicillamine
      Phenytoin
      Procainamide
      Quinidine
      Tetracycline
      Thiouracils
      Trimethadione

II. **Skin**
  A. *Urticaria and angioedema*
    1. Antimicrobials
      Aminoglycosides
      Cephalosporins
      Ethambutol
      Isoniazid
      Metronidazole
      Miconazole
      Nalidixic acid
      p-Aminosalicylic acid
      Penicillins
      Quinine
      Rifampin
      Spectinomycin
      Sulfonamides
    2. Other drugs
      Asparaginase
      Aspirin and other non-
        steroidal anti-inflam-
        matory drugs
      Calcitonin
      Chloral hydrate
      Chlorambucil
      Cimetidine
      Cyclophosphamide
      Daunorubicin
      Doxorubicin
      Ergotamine
      Ethchlorvynol
      Ethosuximide
      Ethylenediamine
      Glucocorticoids
      Melphalan
      Methaqualone
      Penicillamine
      Phenothiazines
      Procainamide
      Procarbazine
      Quinidine
      Tartrazine and other
        dyes
      Thiazides
      Thiotepa
      Tragacanth
  B. *Morbilliform-maculopapular
      rash*
    1. Antimicrobials
      Erythromycin
      Gentamicin
      p-Aminosalicylic acid
      Penicillins
      Streptomycin
      Sulfonamides
    2. Other drugs
      Allopurinol
      Barbiturates
      Captopril
      Gold salts
      Hydantoins
      Thiazides
  C. *Erythroderma and exfolia-
      tive dermatitis*
      Allopurinol
      Amikacin
      Carbamazepine
      Chloral hydrate
      Chlorpromazine
      Ethambutol
      Ethylenediamine
      Glutethimide
      Gold salts
      Hydantoins
      Hydroxychloroquin
      Iodides
      Penicillin
      Phenobarbital
      Streptomycin
      Sulfonamides
      Trimethadione
  D. *Erythema multiforme*
      Acetaminophen

      Barbiturates
      Chloroquine
      Chlorpropamide
      Clindamycin
      Ethambutal
      Ethosuximide
      Gold salts
      Hydantoins
      Hydralazine
      Hydroxyurea
      Mechlorethamine
      Meclofenamate
      Mithramycin
      Penicillins
      Phenolphthalein
      Phenylbutazone
      Rifampin
      Streptomycin
      Sulfonamides
      Sulfonylureas
      Sulindac
      Vaccines
  E. *Photosensitive*
    1. Topical
      Fluorouracil
      Halogenated salicylani-
        lides
      Hexachlorophene
      Para-aminobenzoic acid
        esters
      Promethazine
      Sulfanilamide
    2. Systemic
      Carbamazepine
      Chlorpromazine
      Griseofulvin
      Imipramine
      Lincomycin
      Nalidixic acid
      Phenothiazines
      Quinethazone
      Sulfonamides
      Sulfonylureas
      Thiazide diuretics
  F. *Fixed drug eruptions*
      Acetaminophen
      Aspirin
      Barbiturates
      Chloroquin
      Dapsone
      Digitalis
      Diphenhydramine
      Gold salts
      Hydralazine
      Iodides
      Meprobamate
      Methanamine
      Mercurials
      Metronidazole
      p-Aminosalicylic acid
      Penicillins
      Phenacetin
      Phenolphthalein
      Phenothiazine
      Phenylbutazone
      Quinine
      Saccharin
      Streptomycin
      Sulfonamides
      Tetracyclines
  G. *Erythema nodosum*
      Bromides
      Iodides
      Oral contraceptives
      Penicillin
      Sulfonamides
  H. *Contact dermatitis*
      Antihistamines
      Bacitracin
      Benzalkonium chloride
      Benzocaine
      Benzyl alcohol

TABLE 426–1. ALLERGIC DRUG REACTIONS *Continued*

H. Contact dermatitis *Continued*
- Cetyl alcohol
- Chloramphenicol
- Chlorpromazine
- Ethylenediamine
- Fluorouracil
- Formaldehyde
- Glucocorticoids
- Glutaraldehyde
- Hexachlorophene
- Idoxuridine
- Iodochlorhydroxyquin
- Lanolin
- Local anesthetics
- Mechbrethamine
- Mercury salts
- Neomycin
- Nitrofurazone
- Opiates
- Para-aminobenzoic acid
- Parabens
- Penicillins
- Phenothiazines
- Propylene glycol
- Streptomycin
- Sulfonamides
- Thimerosal

III. Lung
A. Asthma
- Aspirin and other nonsteroidal anti-inflammatory drugs
- Cromolyn
- Pituitary snuff
- Sodium glutamate
- Sulfite
- Tartrazine and other dyes
- Occupational exposures to:
  - Cephalosporins
  - Glutaraldehyde
  - Pancreatic enzymes
  - Papain
  - Penicillins
  - Phenylmercurials
  - Psyllium

B. Eosinophilic pneumonitis
- Azathioprine
- Carbamazepine
- Chlorpropamide
- Cromolyn
- Gold salts
- Imipramine
- Mephenesin
- Nitrofurantoin
- p-Aminosalicylic acid
- Penicillins

- Phenytoin
- Sulfonamides

C. Fibrotic and pleural reactions
- Bleomycin
- Busulfan
- Cyclophosphamide
- Ganglionic-blocking drugs
- Gold salts
- Hydralazine
- Hydrochlorothiazide
- Melphalan
- Methotrexate
- Methysergide
- Mitomycin
- Nitrofurantoin
- Procarbazine

IV. Liver
A. Cholestatic
- Chlorzoxazone
- Erythromycin estolate
- Ethchlorvynol
- Imipramine
- Nalidixic acid
- Nitrofurantoin
- Phenothiazines
- Sulfamethoxazole
- Sulfonylureas
- Troleandomycin

B. Hepatocellular
- Amphotericin B
- Ethacrynic acid
- Furosemide
- Gold salts
- Griseofulvin
- Halothane
- Hydantoins
- Isoniazid
- Methyldopa
- Monoamine oxidase inhibitors
- Nitrofurantoin
- p-Aminosalicylic acid
- Propylbutazone
- Propylthiouracil
- Pyrazinamide
- Quinidine
- Rifampin
- Sulfonamides
- Trimethadione

C. Chronic active hepatitis
- Methyldopa
- Nitrofurantoin

V. Kidney
A. Glomerulitis
- Allopurinol

- Captopril
- Gold salts
- Mercurials
- Methoxyflurane
- Nonsteroidal anti-inflammatory agents
- Penicillamine
- Penicillins
- Phenytoin
- Probenecid
- Sulfonamides
- Thiazides

B. Interstitial nephritis
- Allopurinol
- Captopril
- Cephalosporins
- Chloramphenicol
- Cimetidine
- Colistin
- Furosemide
- Nonsteroidal anti-inflammatory drugs
- Penicillins, especially methicillin
- Phenytoin
- Polymyxin B
- Rifampin
- Sulfonamides
- Tetracycline
- Thiazides

VI. Bone Marrow and Blood Cells
A. Bone marrow aplasia
- Chloramphenicol
- Gold salts
- Mephenytoin
- Penicillamine
- Phenylbutazone
- Trimethadione

B. Anemia
- Acetaminophen
- Captopril
- Cephalosporins
- Chlorpromazine
- Cisplatin
- Hydantoins
- Ibuprofen
- Insulin
- Isoniazid
- Levodopa
- Mefenamic acid
- Melphalan
- Methyldopa
- Methysergide
- p-Aminosalicylic acid
- Penicillins
- Phenacetin

- Quinidine
- Quinine
- Rifampin
- Stibophen
- Sulfonamides
- Sulfonylureas

C. Thrombocytopenia
- Acetaminophen
- Acetazolamide
- Acetylsalicylic acid
- Carbamazepine
- Cephalothin
- Chloramphenicol
- Chlorpheniramine
- Digitoxin
- Ethchlorvynol
- Gold salts
- Heparin
- Hydantoins
- Isoniazid
- Levodopa
- Meprobamate
- Methyldopa
- p-Aminosalicylic acid
- Penicillamine
- Phenacetin
- Phenylbutazone
- Procainamide
- Quinidine
- Quinine
- Rauwolfia alkaloids
- Rifampin
- Stibophen
- Sulfonamides
- Sulfonylureas
- Thiazide diuretics

D. Granulocytopenia
- Captopril
- Cephalosporins
- Chloral hydrate
- Chlorpropamide
- Dipyrone
- Mercurial diuretics
- Methimazole
- Penicillins (semisynthetic)
- Phenothiazines
- Phenylbutazone
- Phenytoin
- Procainamide
- Propranolol
- Sulfamethoxypyridazine
- Sulfapyridine
- Tolbutamide

E. Lymphoid hyperplasia
- Phenytoin
- Mephenytoin

---

threatening infection with an organism for which no alternative antibiotic is available. Oral desensitization is preferred, except in comatose patients when the same principle can be followed parenterally (Table 426–2).

Radiographic Contrast Agents. Iodinated contrast agents injected for radiographic examination are now the most common cause of anaphylactic drug reactions. These reactions are not truly anaphylactic, for these materials do not combine with proteins to act as haptens but rather appear to act pharmacologically. As yet these reactions are not fully understood, but it is known that these drugs activate complement and release anaphylatoxin. Skin tests or small test doses do not predict reactivity. Persons who have had a previous reaction are at increased risk of a similar reaction from a subsequent injection. When a second examination is necessary, the patient should be given prednisone 50 mg every six hours for three doses, ending one hour before the procedure, and an antihistamine shortly before.

Local Anesthetics. Most adverse reactions to local anesthetics are either toxic or psychophysiologic, but allergic reactions can occur. The most frequent is contact dermatitis; anaphylaxis is more serious though quite rare. It has not yet been determined that skin testing with local anesthetics is useful in predicting anaphylaxis in patients with a history of reactions to local anesthetic. When local anesthesia is needed, an anesthetic as unrelated as possible to the one suspected of causing the reaction should be chosen, and a small test dose should be given first. Lidocaine seems to carry a low risk of allergy.

Aspirin and Other Nonsteroidal Anti-inflammatory Drugs. Shortly after its introduction in the late nineteenth century, aspirin was observed to provoke severe asthma in some asthmatic patients. Such patients react in the same way to other nonsteroidal anti-inflammatory agents. The typical reaction consists of acute bronchospasm, rhinorrhea, and occasionally urticaria. Most of the asthmatic patients who react to these agents also have nasal polyps and lack IgE-mediated allergy to common airborne allergens. In some patients with chronic urticaria but no respiratory disease, urticaria is the only manifestation of the reaction. The mechanism of this adverse response to aspirin is not allergic; extensive search for IgE antibodies has been unrewarding. Rather, it is presumably due to the inhibition of cyclo-oxygenase, but the precise mechanism is still undefined. Patients who have reacted to

TABLE 426–2. ORAL DESENSITIZATION PROTOCOL FOR PENICILLIN

Dose*	Units	Route†
1	100	P.O.
2	200	P.O.
3	400	P.O.
4	800	P.O.
5	1,600	P.O.
6	3,200	P.O.
7	6,400	P.O.
8	12,800	P.O.
9	25,000	P.O.
10	50,000	P.O.
11	100,000	P.O.
12	200,000	P.O.
13	400,000	P.O.
14	200,000	S.C.
15	400,000	S.C.
16	800,000	S.C.
17	1,000,000	I.M.

*Interval between doses, 15 min.
†P.O. = oral; S.C. = subcutaneous; I.M. = intramuscular.
From Sullivan TJ, Yecies LD, Shaty GS, et al.: Desensitization of patients allergic to penicillin using orally administered β lactam antibiotics. J Allergy Clin Immunol 69:276, 1982.

aspirin need not avoid other salicylates (except methylsalicylate), and salicylate-free diets are unnecessary. A few aspirin-reactive subjects react similarly to tartrazine (FD&C yellow no. 5) added to foods or drugs. Skin tests to aspirin and similar agents are not useful and may be dangerous. No biochemical tests are available for diagnosis.

American Academy of Pediatrics Committee on Drugs: "Inactive" ingredients in pharmaceutical products. Pediatrics 76:635, 1985. *A useful source of information about allergic reactions to drugs caused by ingredients other than the active drug itself.*
Van Arsdel PW: Adverse drug reactions. *In* Middleton EJ, Ellis FF, Reed CE (eds.): Allergy Principles and Practice. 2nd ed. St. Louis, C. V. Mosby Company, 1983. *A detailed review and extensive listing of agents and reactions.*

427 MASTOCYTOSIS

Robert A. Lewis

DEFINITION. Mastocytosis is a rare disease of mast cell proliferation, which occurs in both cutaneous and systemic forms. The mast cell is a connective tissue cell normally found in most organs. It is not surprising, therefore, that systemic mastocytosis has been reported to involve virtually all tissues except the central nervous system, most commonly the skin, bones, gastrointestinal tract, liver, spleen, and lymph nodes. Mast cell leukemia and malignant transformation of solid tumors have been described in a few cases.

Mast cells are generally identifiable by their metachromatic granules (Fig. 427–1), which contain histamine, heparin, tryptic and chymotryptic proteinases, and a number of acid hydrolases, the last of which defines the granules as modified lysosomes. Mast cells, activated by either immunologic or nonimmunologic stimuli, secrete their lysosomal contents into the microenvironment and additionally liberate arachidonic acid from their membrane phospholipid stores, metabolizing it selectively to prostaglandin D_2 (PGD_2), and the sulfidopeptide leukotriene, LTC_4. LTC_4 is then further metabolized to its peptide cleavage products, LTD_4 and LTE_4, extracellularly. (A discussion of arachidonic acid metabolism is presented in Ch. 420.) Several of the clinical manifestations of mastocytosis as well as the choice of some therapeutic agents are based on the pathophysiologic actions of these substances, termed *mediators of immediate hypersensitivity*, owing to their suspected roles in allergic diseases (Table 427–1).

INCIDENCE AND PREVALENCE. The reported cases of mastocytosis demonstrate an approximately equal occurrence in men and women. Familial incidence, although unusual, has been reported in nearly 50 families. As the hallmark of this disease is based on cutaneous manifestations, mastocytosis is said to involve the skin in over 95 per cent of patients. The actual frequency with which mastocytosis involves other organs with sparing of the skin may thus be underestimated because of the bias of ascertainment. Cutaneous lesions begin more frequently in early childhood than after maturity. Visceral disease is not commonly associated with single isolated skin lesions, especially those arising in infancy or early childhood. However, approximately one quarter of adults with cutaneous lesions have visceral involvement.

CLINICAL MANIFESTATIONS. The most common type of involvement of the skin in mastocytosis is termed *urticaria pigmentosa*. The lesions may be isolated mastocytomas or generalized and multiple (Fig. 427–2); they are usually reddish-brown and plaquelike or nodular. More rarely, telangiectatic or doughy-feeling erythrodermic forms of the skin lesions occur. When a cutaneous lesion is stroked firmly, it becomes pruritic and raised with surrounding erythema (Darier's sign). In many patients, stroking of seemingly uninvolved skin produces a wheal of dermographism, owing to microscopic dermal mastocytosis. Generalized pruritus and flushing may occur in the systemic disease, with or without cutaneous lesions.

Acute symptomatic episodes may occur, marked by systemic vasodilation with headache, dizziness, tachycardia, hypotension, syncope, and even frank shock. Rarely, such attacks may be fatal. These acute symptoms do not necessarily

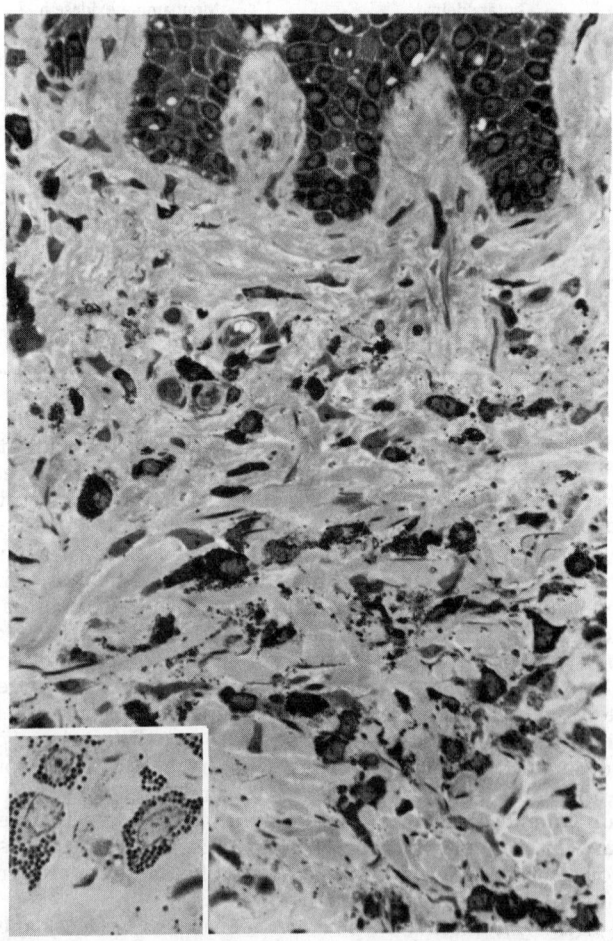

FIGURE 427–1. Mast cell proliferation in the dermis (Giemsa-stained lesional skin biopsy; × 520). Inset of dermal mast cells (× 1310). (Courtesy of J. Caulfield and A. Hein.)

TABLE 427–1. HUMAN MAST CELL–DERIVED PRODUCTS

Mediator	Function
Histamine	Increased vasopermeability; nonvascular smooth muscle contraction
Heparin	Anticoagulation; inhibition of complement activation
Prostaglandin D_2	Vasodilation; nonvascular smooth muscle contraction
Eosinophil and neutrophil chemotactic factors*	Eosinophil and neutrophil chemotaxis
Tryptase, chymotryptic proteinase, arylsulfatase, N-acetyl-β-D-glucosaminidase, β-glucuronidase	Enzymatic degradation of proteoglycans and glycoproteins
Sulfidopeptide leukotrienes	Vasoconstriction; increased vasopermeability; nonvascular smooth muscle contraction (LTC_4) Vasodilation; increased vasopermeability; nonvascular smooth muscle contraction (LTD_4 and LTE_4)

*Evidence for association with human mast cell granule is indirect.

indicate systemic mastocytosis, since extensive cutaneous lesions are capable of releasing large amounts of the potent mediators summarized in Table 427–1. Even the diagnostic test of stroking a cutaneous lesion to whealing may provoke systemic symptoms, especially flushing and colic in affected infants. Ingestion of alcohol may degranulate mast cells and provoke acute symptoms.

Gastrointestinal symptoms may dominate the clinical picture. Anorexia, nausea, vomiting, diarrhea, and a possible predilection for peptic ulceration, with or without hyperchlorhydria, may complicate mastocytosis whether or not mast cells have proliferated in the gastrointestinal tract. Some patients have developed the malabsorption syndrome (see Ch. 104), which may be due to the release of mediators from mast cells infiltrating the small bowel mucosa and lamina propria. Hepatomegaly or hepatosplenomegaly may result from mast cell infiltration. The liver in mastocytosis may also be fibrotic and sometimes exhibits piecemeal inflammation. Rarely there is associated portal hypertension and gastroesophageal varices.

Osseous lesions occur in approximately 10 per cent of all patients with mastocytosis, or two thirds of those with systemic disease. These lesions, most commonly found in the pelvis, ribs, vertebrae, skull, and proximal long bones, may

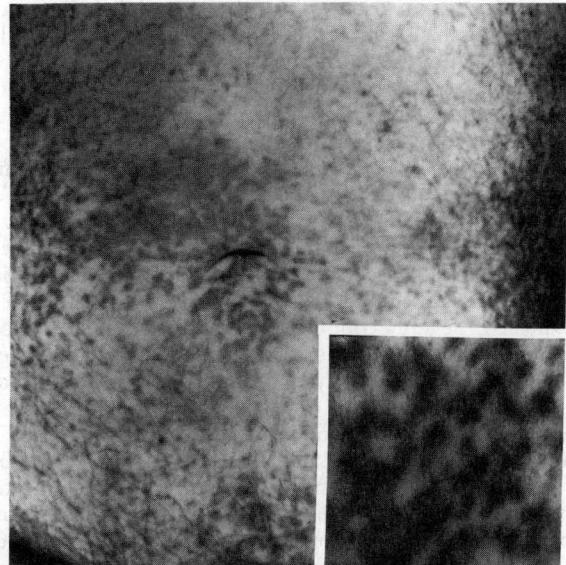

FIGURE 427–2. Skin lesions of mastocytosis (urticaria pigmentosa). Inset showing close-up view. (Courtesy of N. Soter.)

occasionally resemble Paget's disease radiologically. Bone pain may occur with or without pathologic fractures.

Occasionally rhinorrhea and rarely audible wheezing occur, reminiscent of the signs of allergic rhinitis and asthma, respectively. Ill-defined neuropsychiatric symptoms, ranging from malaise to decreased attention span and irritability, have been described. Anemia, leukopenia, thrombocytopenia, and even a rare incidence of mast cell leukemia have been reported in association with severe bone marrow infiltration by mast cells. Modest blood eosinophilia occurs occasionally, and the coagulation abnormalities of prolonged prothrombin and bleeding times related to heparin release, although uncommon, have also been reported.

DIAGNOSIS. The cutaneous lesions of urticaria pigmentosa in conjunction with Darier's sign are pathognomonic for mastocytosis. In their absence, additional criteria are necessary for the diagnosis. Osseous infiltration by mast cells may be suspected from radiologic lesions with adjacent areas of osteoporosis and mottled osteosclerosis. Bone marrow biopsy of involved areas demonstrates abnormally high numbers of mast cells, usually accompanied by eosinophils and lymphocytes, and rarefaction of the spongiosa or, alternatively, myelofibrosis and sclerosis. In the absence of radiologic abnormalities, ^{99}Tc bone scans may define areas of increased radionuclide uptake to guide the site of the biopsy. Increased urinary excretion of histamine and, more reliably, of its metabolites, N-methylhistamine and N-methylimidazoleacetic acid, is common among patients with extensive cutaneous and/or visceral disease and is quantitatively related to the total mast cell burden. Several PGD_2 metabolites, which are either undetectable or only minimally present in normal urine, have been described in urine specimens from patients with systemic mastocytosis. Where the assay is available, it can provide another sensitive diagnostic test.

For the patient with flushing, intermittent hypotension, diarrhea, tachycardia, and possibly hepatomegaly and peptic ulceration, the main differential diagnosis is with the carcinoid syndrome. The most direct criterion is a biopsy demonstrating mast cell proliferation as opposed to argentaffin cell infiltration in an involved organ. Failing this, the measurement of grossly elevated levels of histamine and its metabolites in the urine favors mastocytosis, whereas elevated urinary levels of 5-hydroxyindoleacetic acid (5-HIAA) are noted in the carcinoid syndrome. It must be recalled, however, that marked increases of urinary histamine may occur in gastric carcinoid (see Ch. 243), and elevated urinary excretion of serotonin metabolites may rarely occur in mastocytosis.

In addition to other clinical and laboratory manifestations, histopathology will differentiate the skin lesions of mastocytosis from those of histiocytosis X, myelomonocytic leukemia, cutaneous myelosarcoma, granular cell tumor, and dermatofibroma.

PATHOPHYSIOLOGY AND TREATMENT. When mast cells degranulate, they release their preformed granule-associated mediators and also generate newly formed PGD_2 and LTC_4. The mast cell in mastocytosis releases normal mediators in approximately normal amounts per cell. The most striking abnormalities seem to lie in the sensitivity of the degranulation response of the neoplastic cell to numerous physical stimuli, including not only gentle stroking (Darier's sign) but usually also moderate heat or cold. Once a skin lesion urticates, it requires up to three days to regenerate adequate granule histamine to form a second wheal.

In the past, the majority of the symptoms and signs of mastocytosis were ascribed to the effects of released histamine. Histamine is probably the major cause of local cutaneous whealing and pruritus. Vasodilation and gastrointestinal symptoms in this disease probably have a more complex pathogenesis. The combined use of antihistamines of both the H_1 antagonist group, such as chlorpheniramine maleate, and the H_2 antagonists, exemplified by cimetidine, may be effective in some patients with cutaneous disease, but fails to control either the gastrointestinal symptoms or the hypotension in some patients with systemic mastocytosis.

The identification of a vasodilating prostaglandin (PGD_2) formed by mast cells may therefore be relevant both to the pathophysiology of mastocytosis and to the development of effective therapy. Aspirin and other nonsteroidal anti-inflammatory compounds inhibit prostaglandin synthesis. It is therefore reasonable to try the use of such agents in mastocytosis. Aspirin therapy should be started in very small initial doses of 16 mg four times daily, with the dose doubled on each subsequent day for one week until either symptomatic relief is achieved or the side effects of salicylism supervene. The minimal therapeutic aspirin dose should then be maintained indefinitely. Aspirin should be given only after first initiating treatment with oral therapeutic doses of H_1 and H_2 antihistamines, such as 8 mg of chlorpheniramine maleate and 300 mg of cimetidine four times daily for an adult patient. The caution employed in initiating aspirin therapy follows from reports of a few patients with mastocytosis who have sustained precipitous hypotension after aspirin ingestion, suggesting the possibility that massive release of mediators may occur, including enhanced LTC_4 synthesis when nonsteroidal anti-inflammatory agents inhibit the cyclo-oxygenase pathway of arachidonate metabolism to prostaglandins.

The heparin released from islands of mast cells has been implicated in the prolonged local bleeding time at the sites of excised lesions, the occasionally reported purpura underlying cutaneous mastocytomas, and the rare incidence of significant gastrointestinal bleeding related to local mast cell infiltration. The development of osseous lesions that are both porotic and sclerotic may relate to the combined capacities of mast cell acid hydrolases and proteinases for proteoglycan degradation that precedes collagenolysis, followed by tissue repair. Heparin has also been reported to cause osteopenia. Hepatic fibrosis when documented may also be a product of altered tissue repair in the presence of these enzymes. Therefore, drugs known to cause mast cell degranulation, such as alcohol, morphine, and codeine, are to be prohibited.

Disodium cromoglycate (cromolyn),* given as 100 mg orally four times daily, has been used successfully, particularly for the gastrointestinal symptoms. Cromolyn is thought to reduce mast cell degranulation by interfering with cellular calcium uptake. As little of the drug is absorbed, its local action on the gastrointestinal mast cells probably occurs without directly preventing histamine release from other mast cell infiltrated organs. Histaminuria is not modified by successful therapy with cromolyn. Less easily explained are the therapeutic effects of this agent in decreasing cutaneous symptoms of pruritus, whealing, and flushing, as well as in relieving some of the neuropsychiatric complaints. Cromolyn may be given in combination with antihistamines and aspirin.

PROGNOSIS. Isolated cutaneous mastocytomas of infancy commonly involute spontaneously. If this does not occur, the single lesions may be excised surgically. None of the suggested medical therapies reduces the number of mast cells in either cutaneous or visceral lesions.

Malignant mastocytosis is a very rare disorder with high mortality within two years of diagnosis. It is most likely to occur in systemic disease of adult onset lacking cutaneous involvement and reportedly may appear by malignant transformation of a small minority of the clinically benign mastocytomas, especially of the systemic variety. Oligoclonal increases in IgG are suggestive of malignancy. Special histopathologic techniques may be necessary to detect the immature granules of malignant cells. Leukemia is associated with mastocytosis in fewer than 5 per cent of cases and may be monocytic, mastocytic, or myeloid, in approximately equal frequencies.

---

*Approved for investigational use only.

Parker CW, Cryer PE, Kissane JM: Clinicopathologic conference: Systemic mastocytosis. Am J Med 61:671, 1976. *An excellent review of the signs and symptoms of mastocytosis.*

Roberts LJ II, Sweetman BJ, Lewis RA, et al.: Increased production of prostaglandin D_2 in patients with systemic mastocytosis. N Engl J Med 303:1400, 1980. *Important for future diagnostic and therapeutic considerations.*

Stevens RL, Katz HR, Seldin DC, et al.: Biochemical characteristics distinguish subclasses of mammalian mast cells. In Befus AD, Bienenstock J, Denburg JA (eds.): Mast Cell Differentiation and Heterogeneity. New York, Raven Press, 1986, pp 183–203. *A detailed review of the biochemistry and biology of mast cell–derived mediators.*

Travis WD, Li C-Y, Hoagland HC, et al.: Mast cell leukemia: Report of a case and review of the literature. Mayo Clin Proc 61:957, 1986.

---

428 DISEASES OF THE THYMUS
Daniel P. Stites

DEVELOPMENT, STRUCTURE, AND FUNCTION. The thymus, a central lymphoid organ, functions in the development and maintenance of immunologic competence. Arising embryologically from the third and fourth branchial clefts, it migrates caudad, as a bilobed organ, to the anterior mediastinum. Ectopic thoracic and cervical thymic rests are present in 30 per cent of normal individuals. The thymus enlarges until late puberty and then involutes, the lymphocytes and epithelial cells being nearly completely replaced with fat by the fifth or sixth decade. The normal thymus varies greatly in size. It is uniquely susceptible to marked involution within hours owing to the stress of serious illness or to treatment with glucocorticoids. The thymus is composed primarily of lymphocytes encased in a lattice of epithelial cells. It also contains a few myoid cells, macrophages, and plasma cells. The thymus is arranged into discrete lobules containing a cortex and medulla. Hassall's corpuscles are specialized aggregates of epithelial cells whose function is unknown.

The thymus begins to function by about ten to twelve weeks of gestation when immunocompetent T cells can first be detected. Undifferentiated stem cells migrate to the thymus from fetal liver and bone marrow prenatally and from the bone marrow postnatally. Local influences, probably from epithelial cells, induce maturation of thymic lymphocytes, which then divide in the cortex, migrate to the medulla, and emigrate to the peripheral lymphoid tissue as mature T cells. The cortex is also the site of intense lymphopoiesis. The thymus secretes a variety of incompletely defined hormones which maintain T cell competence in peripheral lymphoid organs. The immunosuppressive effects of thymectomy vary with age, being most pronounced at younger ages (see below). The thymus also appears to play an important role in maintenance of tolerance to various antigens, in immune surveillance, and possibly in leukemogenesis (as judged by animal experiments).

THYMIC HYPOPLASIA. Hypoplastic thymus may be either congenital or acquired. In neonates and infants, *congenital thymic hypoplasia* is expressed as marked T cell and variable B cell immunodeficiency. Resulting diseases include reticular dysgenesis, severe combined immunodeficiency disease, DiGeorge's and Nezelof's syndromes, and ataxia-telangiectasia (see Ch. 419). Essentially all of these patients are diagnosed in childhood; the severity of the thymic lesion, if untreated, rarely allows survival beyond age ten or twelve years. Congenital thymic hypoplasia has been treated by thymic or bone marrow transplantation and by thymic hormone injections with variable success. *Acquired hypoplasia* or thymic involution occurs normally with age or results from stress (within hours or days), malnutrition, pregnancy, x-rays, glucocorticoids, or cytotoxic drugs. AIDS and graft-versus-host disease commonly produce severe thymic dysplasia.

THYMIC HYPERPLASIA. An enlarged thymus is very difficult to evaluate accurately because of its large normal variability in size. In the past, so-called status thymolymphaticus, a condition diagnosed with respiratory distress and large thymic shadow on chest roentgenogram, frequently led to unnecessary removal or radiation of normal thymuses. Individuals who received thymic irradiation for "enlarged thymus" have had significant increases in the incidence of thyroid cancer or adenoma. Extrathyroid tumors also increased slightly but there have been no increases in lymphoreticular malignancy, suggestive of immunodeficiency. The concept of status thymolymphaticus has been abandoned. The thymus may rarely enlarge in thyrotoxicosis, Addison's disease, anencephaly, acromegaly, castration or tumors (see below). Thymic cysts are usually asymptomatic and the occasional association with neoplasia warrants resection.

THYMUS AND MYASTHENIA GRAVIS. Myasthenia gravis is an autoimmune disease caused by the presence of antiacetylcholine receptor (AchR) antibodies (see Ch. 518). In myasthenia gravis there is a 10-per-cent incidence of thymoma. In fact detectable enlargement of the thymus in myasthenia gravis usually heralds the presence of a thymoma. In 65 per cent of cases the thymus is hyperplastic with increased numbers of germinal centers but not clinically enlarged. In the remaining 25 per cent of patients the thymus is normal. In large series of thymomas, 30 to 60 per cent of patients have myasthenia gravis. Rarely myasthenia gravis develops years after total thymectomy for thymoma, which militates against an absolute requirement for thymoma in the pathogenesis of this disorder. Neonatal myasthenia gravis occurs without any thymic abnormality, presumably owing to transplacental transfer of maternal antibody. There is little correlation with serum levels of anti-AchR antibody and clinical improvement in myasthenia following thymectomy. Damage to AchR antigen shared between muscles and thymic epithelial or myoid cells may explain the rather obscure relationship of the thymus to this autoantibody disorder.

EFFECTS OF THYMECTOMY. Total removal of the thymus during the neonatal period in rodents results in severe immunodeficiency, loss of T cells, and a wasting disease, a result of chronic unopposed infection. Thymectomy in adult animals, however, is associated with much subtler changes in T cell function. What is the effect of thymectomy in man? Because of the high incidence of extramediastinal thymic rests (30 per cent), thymectomy can rarely be considered total. Total thymectomy intentionally done during cardiothoracic surgery in children does not appear to result in compromised transplantation immunity. In patients with thymoma, a transient decrease in circulating lymphocytes and T cell functions is noted. Following thymectomy for myasthenia gravis, functional loss in some T cell populations occurs. However, the long-term effects of thymectomy, either in immunologically normal patients during cardiac surgery or in cancer patients with thymomas, is not known. These individuals should be carefully observed for development of autoimmune disease, infection, certain malignancies, or other signs of T cell deficiency.

THYMOMA. *Definition.* A thymoma is a neoplasm of thymic epithelial cells. This definition excludes other tumors that may affect the thymus such as lymphoma, germ cell tumors, and carcinoid. Thymomas are rare; fewer than 1000 cases have been reported. Nevertheless, it is the most common tumor of the anterior superior mediastinum (see Ch. 71).

Pathology. Thymomas contain various proportions of epithelial cells and lymphocytes. The latter are T cells and may constitute a large proportion of cellular content of the tumor; hence the term *lymphoepithelioma.* Although their significance is unknown, the activated appearance of these lymphocytes suggests a host reaction to neoplastic epithelial cells. These T cells all have the surface characteristics of thymocytes rather than peripheral blood T cells. Various histologic degrees of

malignancy from minimal cytologic atypia to undifferentiated carcinoma exist. However, correlation of microscopic appearance with clinical malignancy is notoriously poor. In fact, local invasion of pleura, pericardium, vessels, and nerves is the major criterion for determining clinical malignancy of the tumor.

Clinical Manifestations. Median age of patients with thymoma is about 50 years, and no sex predominance is noted. About 30 per cent of patients present with myasthenia gravis; another 30 per cent are asymptomatic, and the diagnosis is suggested by an anterior mediastinal mass on chest roentgenogram. The remaining 30 to 40 per cent of patients have a variety of symptoms and medical syndromes associated with the tumor (Table 428–1). Symptoms and signs include cough, chest pain, dysphagia, dyspnea, hoarseness, neck mass, and superior vena cava syndrome.

A few patients with spindle cell thymomas have marked *hypogammaglobulinemia.* Whether the relationship is causal is not established. The rare occurrence of red cell aplasia with or without immunodeficiency and thymoma raises the possibility of T cell–mediated suppression of erythropoiesis or immunoglobulin synthesis. Direct evidence to support these notions is only fragmentary.

Diagnosis. The presence of a round or oval anterior mediastinal mass visualized in posteroanterior and lateral chest roentgenograms in the presence of myasthenia gravis or of some other known systemic manifestations is suggestive of thymoma. Computed tomographic (CT) imaging is useful in defining the size and location of thymomas and is occasionally useful in differentiating various thymic lesions. Thymic biopsy has no place in evaluation of anterior mediastinal masses, and mediastinoscopy is of little or no value. Some centers claim success with fine needle aspiration and cytology. Thoracotomy with adequate exposure to determine whether capsular invasion has occurred is needed for diagnosis of any thymic tumor. Differential diagnosis includes other primary or secondary thymic tumors (see below), cysts, post-traumatic hemorrhage, aneurysm, or other abnormalities of the anterior mediastinal contents including metastatic tumors, giant lymph node hyperplasia, mesothelioma, thyroid and parathyroid tumors, and paragangliomas (see Ch. 71).

Treatment. Surgical removal of tumor followed by local irradiation if extracapsular extension has occurred is the treatment of choice. Distant metastases are rare; the tumor spreads mainly by local invasion of adjacent structures.

Prognosis. The prognosis is nearly entirely dependent on presence of local invasion and cannot be predicted by histologic appearance of the tumor. Noninvasive thymomas are usually cured by excision. Patients with invasive thymoma have about 50 per cent five-year survival.

OTHER TUMORS OF THE THYMUS. *Thymolipoma* probably represents a lipoma arising within normal thymus. This tumor is usually radiolucent and asymptomatic and has not been associated with myasthenia gravis. *Carcinoid tumor* of the thymus arises from neuroendocrine cells within the thymus (see Ch. 243). Fifty per cent produce ACTH-like mole-

---

TABLE 428–1. DISEASES ASSOCIATED WITH THYMIC TUMOR

I. **Thymoma**
    Myasthenia gravis
    Red cell aplasia
    Hemolytic anemia
    Neutrophil agranulocytosis
    Hypogammaglobulinemia (Good's syndrome)
    Systemic lupus erythematosus
    Polymyositis
    Pemphigus vulgaris
    Chronic mucocutaneous candidiasis
II. **Carcinoid**
    Cushing's syndrome
    Multiple endocrine neoplasia syndromes (see Ch. 241)

cules and cause Cushing's syndrome or hyperparathyroidism, or are associated with multiple endocrine adenomatosis; 30 per cent are malignant and metastasize. Surgery and radiotherapy are indicated. *Carcinomas*, particularly squamous cell types, may rarely occur. *Germ cell tumors* rarely occur: seminoma, teratoma, teratocarcinoma, choriocarcinoma, embryonal cell carcinoma, and yolk sac tumors. The thymus may be involved by *malignant lymphomas*. T cell lymphomas with acute lymphoblastic leukemia occur in the second decade. Cells from these tumors may have C receptors and are positive for terminal deoxynucleotidyl transferase. Hodgkin's disease usually is of nodular sclerosing type (see Ch. 158 and 160).

Day DL, Gedgudas E: The thymus. Radiol Clin North Am 22:519, 1984. *A thorough review of thymic anatomy and function. Special emphasis on use of imaging techniques such as CT scans, sonography, and NMR is presented.*

Namba T, Brunner NG, Grob D: Myasthenia gravis in patients with thymoma with particular reference to onset after thymectomy. Medicine 57:411, 1978. *Excellent review of literature on relationship of thymoma to myasthenia gravis with 72 locally studied cases.*

Salyer W, Eggleston JC: Thymoma. A clinical and pathological study of 65 cases. Cancer 37:229, 1976. *Clinicopathologic description of a large series of thymoma patients, annotating association with other medical syndromes.*

Shore RE, Woodard E, Hildreth N: Thyroid tumor following thymus irradiation. JNCI 74:1177, 1985. *Case control study of 2650 individuals who received thymic irradiation in infancy shows 30 cancers and 59 benign thyroid adenomas in an average of a 29-year follow-up period. No evidence for compromised imune function was detected based on absence of lymphoreticular malignancy.*

PART XXI

MUSCULOSKELETAL AND CONNECTIVE TISSUE DISEASES

429 APPROACH TO THE PATIENT WITH MUSCULOSKELETAL DISEASE

James F. Fries

The rheumatic diseases present a major challenge to clinical judgment. The chronicity, variability, tendency to exacerbate and remit, biochemical and immunologic complexity, unknown pathogenesis, variable response to specific treatment, and myriad effects upon the patient's lifestyle, family relationships, self-image, and employability combine to complicate the therapeutic equation. Difficult therapeutic decisions often must be made without adequate experimental justification and evaluated against a poorly understood natural history.

Balanced against these tremendous uncertainties, contemporary management is relatively straightforward but has recently changed substantially. The therapeutic strategy has shifted from dogma to flexibility. Good management now requires that therapeutic decisions be based upon individual circumstances rather than upon diagnosis per se. Further, decisions are never final but are modified in a continuing feedback between application of treatment and observation of response. Decisions change over time as appropriate to the trends, tempo, and previous response of the particular patient. Clinical judgment is essential to good outcome. The art of medicine is reborn in the approach to a patient with a chronic disease. The principles underlying contemporary management strategy are set forth in this chapter and are divided into six major facets. The medical history, the physical examination, and the laboratory data, which are discussed in following chapters, are integrated into decisions regarding these six areas.

DETERMINING THE PATHOPHYSIOLOGY

Modern management individualizes therapy within diagnostic categories, based upon subgroups of patients with differing prognoses and different therapeutic requirements. Patients with the same diagnosis often should be managed very differently. Rheumatic disease patients frequently have features of several diagnostic entities at the same time.

Diagnosis is *not* the most important factor in selecting management in rheumatic disease. Management in musculoskeletal disease is more closely linked to the underlying pathophysiologic process than to the disease entity. Reversal of the pathophysiologic process (or negation of its impact) requires a clear visualization of that process. Even such a basic pathophysiologic concept as "inflammation" has different therapeutic implications. The inflamed synovial membrane (synovitis) typical of rheumatoid arthritis responds to a different spectrum of anti-inflammatory agents than does the inflammation of ligamentous insertions (enthesitis) typical of ankylosing spondylitis or the inflammation within the joint space induced by microscopic crystals.

Eight specific types of musculoskeletal problems are readily distinguished by history and physical examination in most patients and provide a framework for pathophysiologic categorization. These categories are not mutually exclusive, but identification of the predominant pathophysiology in a given patient is usually straightforward. The eight categories are discussed in the following paragraphs and are listed in Table 429–1 together with the prototype disease of the category, examples of the most useful laboratory tests for that category, and the typical treatments required. Management implications for each category are surprisingly distinct and provide guidelines for laboratory investigation and initial treatment. Location of the process is shown in Figure 429–1.

SYNOVITIS. Inflammation of the synovial membrane, with gradual damage to surrounding joint structures, is most strikingly manifested in rheumatoid arthritis. The synovium is tender, thickened, and palpable and may demonstrate warmth and, less often, redness. Joint destruction is caused by the enzymatic products of inflammation and develops slowly over many years. Management is based upon reducing the *rate* of damage to joint structures. The sedimentation rate is consistently elevated with significant synovitis, and the latex fixation or other tests for rheumatoid arthritis are often useful for further categorization. A wide range of pharmacologic and other treatments may be required, and many patients require sequential trials with a variety of agents. Some useful drugs, such as gold, penicillamine, and hydroxychloroquine, are not proven therapeutically effective in any other category, and others, such as aspirin, find their greatest use here.

ENTHESOPATHY. Inflammation in certain diseases is most marked at the enthesis, that transition region where ligament attaches to bone. Such inflammation is the hallmark of a family of rheumatic diseases typified by ankylosing spondylitis and linked to the HLA-B27 antigen. The distribution of involvement in these diseases follows the location of regions of enthesis throughout the body. The marked predilection for the sacroiliac joints, heels, and spine identifies a process affecting areas characterized by ligament and tendon attachment. This newly recognized specific pathophysiology provides a unifying basis for the clinical features of the diseases and their typical response to specific therapy. Rheumatoid factor is predictably absent from the serum. Nonsteroidal anti-inflammatory agents, in particular indomethacin, phenylbutazone, and naproxen, are therapeutically effective and usually are well tolerated over the long term. The spectrum of effective anti-inflammatory drugs used for enthesopathy is different from that in synovitis. Prednisone, for example, is neither indicated nor effective in most patients.

TABLE 429–1. CATEGORIES OF RHEUMATIC DISEASE

Pathology	Prototype	Most Useful Tests	Typical Treatment
Synovitis	Rheumatoid arthritis	Latex, erythrocyte sedimentation rate	Acetylsalicylic acid, gold
Enthesopathy	Ankylosing spondylitis	Sacroiliac radiographs, HLA-B27	Indomethacin
Cartilage degeneration	Osteoarthritis	Radiographs of affected area	Analgesic
Crystal-induced synovitis	Gout	Joint fluid crystal examination	Colchicine
Joint infection	Staphylococcal	Joint fluid culture	Antibiotics
Myositis	Dermatomyositis	Muscle enzymes, muscle biopsy	Corticosteroids
Focal conditions	Tennis elbow	None, radiographs of affected area	Localized
Generalized conditions	Fibrositis	Erythrocyte sedimentation rate	Conservative

CARTILAGE DEGENERATION. Degenerative and other processes can cause fraying and destruction of the articular cartilage, with subsequent injury to the underlying subchondral bone. This occurrence is usually termed osteoarthritis (or osteoarthrosis), and a group of specific syndromes is recognized within this category. Narrowing of the apparent joint space and development of bony spurs make radiography the most useful investigative procedure; other ancillary tests are usually negative. Few patients have significant inflammation, and it is not surprising that anti-inflammatory treatment is not frequently useful. The analgesic effects of aspirin or nonsteroidal anti-inflammatory agents may be helpful; doses required for optimal effect are often considerably less than doses required for anti-inflammatory effects with the same compound. Medical treatment is symptomatic and is seldom dramatically effective.

CRYSTAL-INDUCED SYNOVITIS. Microcrystalline arthritis occurs when crystals forming in the synovial fluid (or injected therein) induce an acute inflammatory reaction in the joint fluid and the surrounding synovium. Gout is the prototype disease, with inflammation induced by crystals of monosodium urate. Similar syndromes may occur with crystals of several other types. The inflammatory response increases to very intense inflammation within a period of hours and spontaneously resolves without treatment over a period of a few days to a few weeks; this resolution is markedly accelerated with treatment. The physical factors underlying crystal formation determine that only one or, at most, a few joints are involved at a time. The crucial laboratory observation is inspection of the aspirated joint fluid for crystals under polarized light microscopy. Drugs inhibiting polymorphonuclear leukocytes are particularly effective, as exemplified by colchicine, a drug with little effect in any other rheumatic disease category.

JOINT INFECTION. The synovium encloses a body space that can be the site of direct infection by microorganisms. Critical to investigation of the patient with suspected joint infection is aspiration and culture of the joint fluid and, in many instances, culture of other body fluids as well. Treatment consists principally of prescribing an antibiotic specific for the microorganism involved. Drainage may be required.

MYOSITIS. Inflammation of muscle occurs in two closely related diseases, dermatomyositis and polymyositis, and in an unrelated condition, polymyalgia rheumatica. Determination of muscle enzyme levels and histologic examination of involved muscle may be the critical laboratory observations. In polymyalgia, the sedimentation rate is greatly elevated and is often the sole objective finding. Temporal artery biopsy may be useful when giant cell arteritis is demonstrated. Corticosteroids are almost always required in inflammatory muscle disease and, in contrast to every other rheumatic disease category, are usually required from the outset.

FOCAL CONDITIONS. A wide variety of conditions affecting the musculoskeletal system do not truly warrant the term "disease." Tendinitis, bursitis, low back strain, calcific tendinitis, and other entities can affect almost any area of the body and are the most common of all medical problems. Laboratory aids are few, although radiography occasionally may be useful in locating calcium deposits or spurs or in ruling out fracture. The therapeutic imperative in localized problems (unfortunately often neglected) is to emphasize localized rather than general treatment measures. Treatment of the entire organism for a problem in one local area is seldom rewarding. Splints, slings, heat, and local injection are usually the most reasonable initial approach.

GENERALIZED CONDITIONS. A variety of ambiguous entities fall into this poorly defined category. Terms such as "fibrositis" and the "chronic muscle contraction syndrome" are sometimes used to indicate the likelihood of organic disease. The terms "psychogenic rheumatism," "nonarticular rheumatism," and "depressive equivalent" are frequently used to suggest an emotional component to such complaints. These patients are rich in symptoms but poor in objective evidence of pathology. The conditions may be extremely troublesome for the individual but are not progressive and do not result in physical crippling. Laboratory tests, such as the sedimentation rate, give normal results and are employed only to rule out other categories of illness. Treatment is best termed "conservative." The therapeutic approaches listed for other categories are unlikely to be beneficial, and the physician who attempts pharmacologic intervention rather than reassurance, lifestyle counseling, and support often ends with a drug-dependent patient who gets no better.

These eight categories and the brief descriptions presented are supported by generalizations to which there are some exceptions. However, Table 429–1 suggests quite specific directions in which laboratory investigation and the therapeu-

SITES AND TYPES OF RHEUMATIC DISEASE
[SITE: PATHOPHYSIOLOGY (Typical disease)]

JOINT SPACE:
JOINT INFECTION

MUSCLE INFLAMMATION:
(Myositis)

SYNOVIAL MEMBRANE:
SYNOVITIS
(Rheumatoid arthritis)

TENDON

BURSA

MUSCLE

BONE   BONE

LOCALIZED SITE:
(Bursitis)

JOINT CAPSULE

ENTHESIS:
ENTHESOPATHY
(Ankylosing spondylitis)

CARTILAGE:
CARTILAGE DEGENERATION
(Osteoarthritis)

JOINT SPACE:
MICROCRYSTALLINE ARTHRITIS
(Gout)

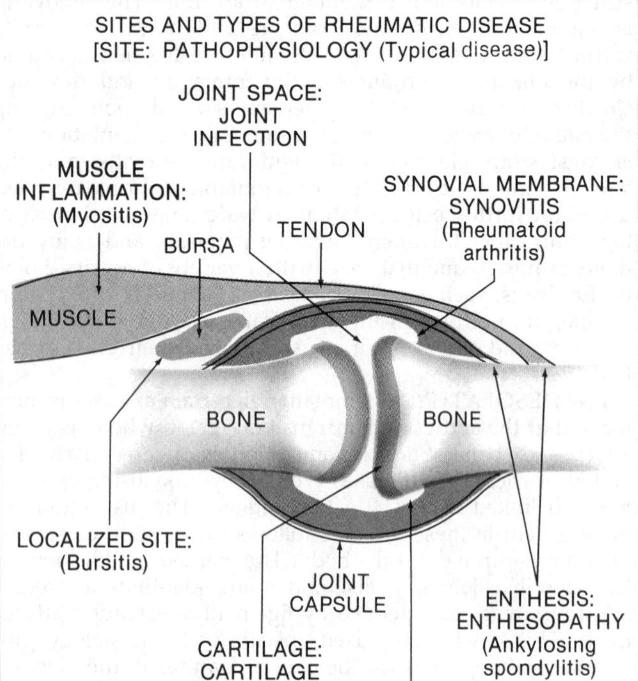

FIGURE 429–1. Location of musculoskeletal disease processes.

tic approach should begin. The experienced physician soon moves far beyond this table, but it provides a particularly useful framework upon which to place the more detailed clinical knowledge of following chapters.

USING THE LABORATORY SELECTIVELY

Laboratory tests in the rheumatic diseases usually provide confirmatory data rather than conclusive evidence. After the three exceptions of (1) the sacroiliac radiograph in ankylosing spondylitis, (2) the identification of specific crystals within the joint fluid, and (3) a positive bacteriologic culture from joint fluid, laboratory tests have varying degrees of lack of sensitivity and lack of specificity and, except in the unusual case, add relatively little to clinical assessment. As a result, the majority of patients presenting with musculoskeletal problems do not require any laboratory evaluation whatsoever. The key to appropriate use of the laboratory is selective use. Every test should have a specific indication, and blind "surveys" or "panels" should not be used.

One in six visits by a patient to a health professional is for a musculoskeletal complaint. The great majority of such physician visits occur for the common "focal conditions" of life. Low back pain, sprained ankles, tennis elbows, and other common musculoskeletal complaints account for most initial visits. The overwhelming majority of such problems are easily identified as self-limited. Optimal management includes ruling out more significant illness, advice about activity or rest, reassurance, occasionally symptomatic medication, and transmission of the expectation that the natural healing process will resolve the difficulty. The usual healing period for local musculoskeletal problems ranges from two to six weeks, depending upon the magnitude of the often inapparent injury, with the healing process beginning again from the start if there is reinjury during this period. Healing cannot be pharmacologically accelerated. Thus, optimal treatment usually requires "masterly inactivity," with confident reliance upon the natural healing process. Inappropriate rigor with test or treatment can lead to investigative mishaps, therapeutic side reactions, and an intensity of focus upon the problem entirely inappropriate to its magnitude. The careful rheumatic disease clinician uses time to establish the trends and tempo of the condition in the individual; time is used to demonstrate the self-limited condition while avoiding the hazards of inappropriate response.

The critical initial decision, therefore, is whether the problem requires immediate action or whether the decision to investigate or treat can be postponed until the course of the disease and the magnitude of the appropriate response may be better estimated. A six-week "rule of thumb" is appropriate. In the absence of specific indication or immediate threat, a waiting period of six weeks from onset of symptoms serves to minimize inappropriate use of laboratory tests or treatment. Four major exceptions to the six-week rule obtain. First, a condition that is severe and involves a single joint (or, at most, a few joints) is much more likely, paradoxically, to require immediate attention than is a widespread polyarthritis. Acute gouty arthritis and infections, the usual causes of the "single hot joint," require immediate attention. By contrast, in rheumatoid arthritis, a period of six weeks is required even before the criteria for diagnosis can be met, and management in the first days of disease is most appropriately conservative. Many "probable rheumatoid arthritis" patients actually have minor problems that disappear as the viral or minor hypersensitivity reaction subsides. They need not be given the emotional burden of a "serious" diagnosis.

Second, a patient who is febrile, systemically ill, and otherwise showing signs of major disease deserves immediate attention. Endocarditis, neoplasm, tuberculosis, and other illnesses are frequently identified through musculoskeletal clues, and a connective tissue disease with systemic manifestations deserves immediate attention.

Third, if the problem is associated with significant trauma, the possible need for immediate orthopedic management should be considered. Fourth, an associated neurologic problem such as carpal tunnel syndrome, sciatic nerve compression, or cervical nerve root compression may be benefited by immediate attention.

In practice, these four indications for action are relatively unusual. The large majority of patients with initial complaints of the musculoskeletal system are not found to have conditions requiring either intensive efforts at diagnosis or employment of hazardous therapy.

ESTABLISHING MANAGEMENT GOALS

Disease impact has too often been defined in terms of numerically expressed test results. The level of autoantibodies, titer of rheumatoid factor, number of radiographic erosions, and sedimentation rate often become the criteria for therapeutic success. The patient and family are more directly interested in a different list of disease endpoints: in survival, in normal mobility and function, in absence of pain and other symptoms, and in the ability to remain solvent through the duration of a chronic illness. These five "D's" (death, disability, discomfort, drug toxicity, and dollar cost) are the major dimensions of patient outcome in the patient's own terms.

In the rheumatic diseases the frequent "trade-offs" among several outcomes must be based upon the values perceived by the particular patient. For example, pain may be reduced by narcotics but disability increased; disability may be reduced by cyclophosphamide but a risk of death incurred; or short-term symptomatic relief by plasmapheresis may be obtained at very high cost.

Establishment of goals must precede development of the individual management strategy. In some instances, a limited goal, such as regaining the ability to walk, may be dramatically useful to the patient and far more valuable than a modest reduction in the general severity of the disease. Some worthy goals may not be achievable in a particular instance, and their pursuit may only increase therapeutic toxicity. The question of what is desirable is subordinate to the question of what is achievable.

PLANNING FOR OPTIMAL LONG-TERM OUTCOME

Hospital-based training tends to focus attention on improving the patient's status by the time of discharge. In chronic illness, such short-term benefits may be desirable but illusory. Corticosteroids, narcotic analgesics, and intra-articular injections often provide obvious short-term benefit. Unfortunately, the agent that provides the best initial response sometimes may lead to iatrogenic disaster over the longer term.

The basic therapeutic strategy holds that simple and nontoxic measures should be used first, and hazardous medications withheld unless the simpler approaches fail. But the individual patient frequently has special considerations requiring modification of such progressions. Thus, the tempo of disease may be such that joint destruction is developing over a short period of months; the therapeutic progression then requires acceleration. Or a major therapeutic attempt with gold, penicillamine, or an immunosuppressant agent may require months until the expected date of response. Meanwhile, the patient may have exhausted sick leave prior to forced retirement because of disability. Addition of a generally contraindicated agent, such as prednisone, might, under such circumstances, provide temporary support for the individual. In a patient of advanced age, concern about the eventual hazard of malignancy secondary to a drug might well be small. In a vigorous and active male patient, there may be less concern about corticosteroid osteopenia. For a young patient, the expectation for patient outcome should be integrated over perhaps 20 to 30 years. In the older patient, both the risks and the benefits of treatment might be reduced, but not by the same amount. Again, the necessity for the individual program is seen.

The inexperienced clinician is often trapped by taking the short view of a chronic illness. A chronic disease cannot be managed by short-term tactics; it requires a long-term strategy, shared and negotiated with the patient.

Such a strategy requires tactical modification at nearly every physician-patient encounter At each visit, new information is always present, even if it is only the information about what has transpired in response to the last set of decisions. A decision is thus followed by observation, then by further decision, then by another period of observation. The decision strategy is flexible and, in the final analysis, frequently empiric.

USING A COMPLETE CLINICAL REPERTOIRE

Treatment of musculoskeletal disease is frequently discussed in terms of pharmacologic agents. This myopic view neglects the dominant contributions often afforded by reconstructive surgical procedures, by the use of appliances and devices to allow handicapped individuals to function more normally, by exercise to strengthen bones and tissues, or by personal interaction to increase the motivation and self-image of the patient.

A drug-based strategy tends to find its greatest use in early, systemic, inflammatory disease processes. Orthopedic approaches tend to have the greatest utility if the number of joints or regions involved is small, if major problems are concentrated in a single anatomic region, or after an inflammatory process has "burned out." Improvement after occupational therapy is often seen in patients with moderate to major disability who require adaptive devices to render the environment more friendly. Confidence in the ability to live an independent life sometimes can be more important than any specific therapy, and patient confidence (personal efficacy) is a useful therapeutic adjunct. Medical therapy that interferes with mental or emotional adaptation frequently makes things worse.

The novice at managing rheumatic diseases employs only a limited therapeutic repertoire. Typically, the patient requires a diverse program individualized to specific needs and making use of a variety of different disciplines. Development of rational strategies requires intimate knowledge of the strengths and weaknesses of all therapeutic modalities. The physician cannot manage chronic musculoskeletal diseases effectively without knowledge of the techniques of complementary disciplines or a good working relationship with individuals who possess these skills.

ACHIEVING PATIENT UNDERSTANDING

The informed patient is the physician's greatest single asset in managing chronic illness. Consider even the recommendation that a patient should take aspirin. The lay media describe the hazards of aspirin, colloquialisms associate aspirin with physician neglect, and the over-the-counter availability suggests a minor remedy. Yet, for anti-inflammatory treatment with aspirin, the physician may aim for a narrow therapeutic range just below toxicity and far above the dose the patient expects. While establishing dosage, the patient is almost certain to encounter one or another side effect, even though the aspirin later may be well tolerated. The informed patient must know that anti-inflammatory and analgesic activities of aspirin are different, that a particular therapeutic range is important, that the drug is active against the inflammatory process itself, and that several weeks may be required to see the full effects of the drug. In the absence of such understanding, it is unusual for a patient to do well on aspirin; patient education is a prerequisite for therapeutic success.

Most clinicians believe that patients with positive expecta-

tions have better outcomes. While causality is not established from this observation, it is reasonable to assume that restoration of hope and a positive self-image are beneficial parts of the treatment program. The patient with arthritis is under intense psychologic pressures. Self-image is threatened by diseases that may cripple and prevent remunerative employment. The fear of dependence upon others is often present. Yet prognosis is generally better than that anticipated by the patient. The physician who is unaware that every patient with arthritis has significant fears may do great harm by inadvertently increasing those fears.

Additionally, the informed patient is more likely to comply with a particular therapeutic regimen. The patient's report of success or failure with previous recommendations is essential for the next clinical decision and must be as accurate as possible, again emphasizing the need for direct patient-physician communication. Unrealistic expectations followed by perceived therapeutic failures are a major cause of a burgeoning business in quack treatment. The patient must be educated to recognize the falsity of overstated claims and the losses in courage, independence, and money that may result. The obscenity of the quack who makes a living by defrauding patients focuses the attention upon the outrage. At the more important level, however, the patient susceptible to the claims of the quack does not have a confident and informed relationship with his or her personal physician.

The management of musculoskeletal disease is directed in large part at maintenance of the independence of the individual. Most persons with arthritis can be independent and healthy individuals despite their musculoskeletal condition. This independence is the final goal of the individualized management strategy.

Fries JF: Toward an understanding of patient outcome measurement. Arthritis Rheum 26:697, 1983. *Review of the concepts and practice of assessment of long-term outcome and the clinical implications thereof.*

Fries JF, Holman HR: Estimating prognosis in systemic lupus erythematosus. Am J Med 57:561, 1974. *Introduction to the concepts of subsets of disease and individualization of prognosis and treatment choice.*

Fries JF, Mitchell DM: Joint pain or arthritis. JAMA 235:199, 1976. *Flow charts and discussion of the approach to the patient with rheumatic disease.*

Kelley WN, Harris ED, Ruddy S, et al.: Textbook of Rheumatology. 2nd ed. Philadelphia, W.B. Saunders Company, 1985. *Definitive textbook of 2000 pages and many thousand references covering all aspects of rheumatology.*

Rodnan GP, Schumacher HR (eds.): Primer on the Rheumatic Diseases. Atlanta, Arthritis Foundation, 1983. *Classic, authoritative, current descriptions of all rheumatic diseases and indeed of all rheumatology, available as a public service at nominal cost.*

430 CONNECTIVE TISSUE STRUCTURE AND FUNCTION

Stephen M. Krane

Connective tissues are responsible for the form and shape of the animal body and, in addition, provide protection for vital organs and facilitate locomotion. The term connective tissue is also applied in a more restricted sense to structures such as dermis, tendons, fascia, bone, cartilage, and the capsules of the joint. All cells, however, make contacts with surrounding structures that involve connective tissues as components of the extracellular matrix. The matrix possesses chemical, physical, and mechanical properties uniquely suited to the function of tissues and organs of which the cells are a part. The extracellular matrix may be rigid (e.g., bone), elastic (e.g., blood vessel walls), compressible (e.g., cartilage), or liquid (e.g., synovial fluid). Most connective tissue matrices derive these properties by virtue of the content of fibrillar proteins, nonfibrillar macromolecules, and low molecular weight proteins and electrolytes. The properties of the matrix are therefore determined predominantly by the function of cells, specific for each tissue, which are responsible for syn-

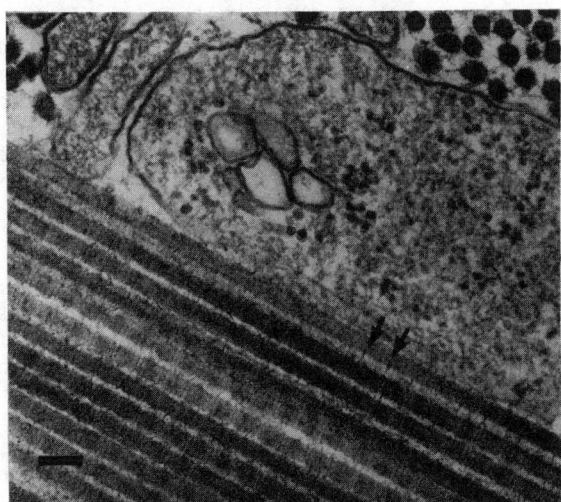

FIGURE 430–1. Electron micrograph of sections of 17-day-old chick Achilles tendon. Collagen fibrils are seen in longitudinal section in the lower left portion of the figure. These fibrils have a period of ~67 nm, as indicated by the distance between the two arrows. Fibrils seen in cross-section at the upper portion of the figure have an average diameter of ~50 nm. Collagen fibers, which are made up of many fibrils, have diameters that range from 0.1 to 15 μm. Bar = 100 nm. (Courtesy of Dr. Romaine Bruns.)

thesis of the matrix components. Many of the functions of the component cells, in turn, are influenced by the character of the extracellular matrix. The properties of connective tissues are also influenced by their relationships to the vascular system from which critical components are derived, such as water, electrolytes, and proteins. Indeed, the walls of blood vessels may themselves be considered as connective tissues. However, although some connective tissues are highly vascular (e.g., bone), others are essentially avascular (e.g., cartilage).

COMPOSITION OF EXTRACELLULAR MATRICES. The major components of the extracellular matrix are fibrillar proteins (collagens and elastin), globular proteins, complex carbohydrates, and, in the case of bone, the inorganic mineral phase. In most connective tissues the fibrillar proteins make up the bulk of the organic material. The *elastic fibers* consist of two distinct protein components. The most abundant is an amorphous protein (elastin) with no distinct periodicity by electron microscopy. The minor component associated with the elastin is a microfibrillar glycoprotein. Elastic fibers are most abundant in walls of large arteries and in some tendons and ligaments. In joints, however, collagens are the major fibrillar proteins. Collagens belong to a family of proteins that have similar chemical and structural properties. The term "collagen" is also used to refer to fibers or fiber bundles observed in tissue sections. The form of collagens in tissues is determined by the type of molecule that predominates and by interactions with other components of the matrix. Collagen fibers usually have diameters of 0.1 μm to 10 to 15 μm. The most abundant species, the interstitial collagens, such as those that predominate in tissues such as dermis, tendon, bone, and cartilage, have a characteristic banding pattern seen on electron microscopy with major periods of approximately 64 to 70 nm (Fig. 430–1). Some collagens, such as those comprising basement membranes or others that are deposited pericellularly, appear amorphous and do not have a banded structure detected by electron microscopy. The collagen molecules of most collagens consist of three polypeptides (α chains) that have a characteristic and unique helical structure determined by the amino acid sequence. The collagen molecules of the interstitial collagens can be solubilized from some tissues. In solution these molecules behave as long, rigid rods with dimensions of approximately 300 × 1.5 nm. Each of the

collagen polypeptide chains contains a glycine residue at every third position and is rich in amino acids such as alanine and proline. Collagens contain little phenylalanine and tyrosine and essentially no tryptophan, and, with the exception of type III collagen and the basement membrane collagens, usually lack cysteine in the body of the helical portion.

Collagen chains in the course of synthesis also undergo unique post-translational modifications of several component amino acids. The most important of these modifications involves the introduction of a hydroxyl group in the 4 position of specific prolyl residues. The 4-hydroxyproline residues are considered to be responsible for stabilization of the collagen helix. In addition, there is a small amount of 3-hydroxyproline in most collagens whose function is not known. Specific lysyl residues also are modified by hydroxylation in the 5 position to form hydroxylysine. The hydroxyproline and hydroxylysine of collagens liberated by proteolytic cleavage of the polypeptide chains in the course of physiologic remodeling or pathologic degradation are not reutilized for collagen biosynthesis. Quantitation of the urinary excretion of these amino acids therefore provides some index of collagen turnover. Certain ε-amino groups of lysines as well as hydroxylysines are oxidized to their respective aldehydes to form derivatives known as allysines and hydroxyallysines, respectively. Lysine, hyroxylysine, and their derivatives are involved in crosslinking between the chains that constitute the collagen molecules (intramolecular) as well as crosslinking one collagen molecule to another (intermolecular).

In the case of the interstitial collagens the characteristic banding pattern is accounted for by an ordered staggered arrangement of the collagen molecules within the collagen fibrils and the collagen fibers. The manner of molecular packing within the fibril in turn is determined by the amino acid sequence. The way the molecules are staggered in the fibril, however, gives rise to regions in which the molecules overlap and others in which there is no overlap (Fig. 430–2). It is probable that the mineral phase of bone is deposited predominantly within the voids or holes of the nonoverlap region. The macromolecular structure of type IV collagen, the major fibrillar component of basement membranes, is very different from that of the interstitial collagens. Type IV collagen structure consists of a network of individual 390 nm-long molecules that are aggregated and crosslinked via identical ends to form a distinctive lattice.

These proteins with structural homologies make up the collagen family. The different homologous species are referred to as types, with each type the product of a different (nonallelic) genetic locus. The 12 collagen types identified and characterized so far are listed in Table 430–1. Some tissues are characterized by a marked predominance of one type— e.g., types II, IX, X, and XI in cartilage and type I collagen in bone. It is likely that each of these collagen types is largely responsible for the functional and morphologic properties of each connective tissue, although it has not yet been possible to relate function to a particular chemical modification.

There is considerable information concerning the pathways of synthesis of various collagens. Even the genes from several animal species for the component polypeptide chains of

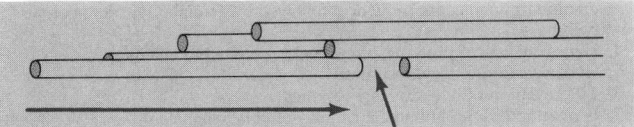

FIGURE 430–2. A model of the packing of the collagen molecules within the collagen fibril. The molecules, each consisting of three helical polypeptide chains, are depicted as long rigid rods and are represented here by the cylinders. The length of the molecules is indicated by the long arrow. The structure gives rise to regions where adjacent molecules are in contact and others in which there are holes, indicated by the short arrow. It is suggested that the inorganic crystals of bone are located predominantly in these holes.

TABLE 430–1. GENETICALLY DISTINCT MAJOR TYPES OF COLLAGEN

Type	Chains	Characteristics	Major Tissue Localization
I	α1(I), α2(I)	Most abundant	Bone, dermis, tendon, fascia, arteries, parenchyma
II	α1(II)	Most abundant	Cartilage, vitreous
III	α1(III)	Abundant	Dermis, blood vessels, parenchyma
IV	α1(IV), α2(IV)	Basement membrane	All basement membranes
V	α1(V), α2(V), α3(V)	Abundant small fibers	Most interstitial tissues
VI	α1(VI), α2(VI), α3(VI)	Microfibrils	Most interstitial tissues
VII	α1(VII)	Long chains—anchoring fibrils	Most interstitial tissues
VIII	α1(VIII)	Small tandem helices	Endothelial cells
IX	α1(IX), α2(IX), α3(IX)	Interrupted helix— interacts with type II collagen and proteoglycan	Cartilage
X	α1(X)	Short chain	Ossifying cartilage
XI	1α, 2α, 3α	Small fibers—type V homologue	Cartilage
XII	?	Type IX homologue	Tendon, bone

several collagen types have been partially characterized, illustrating the enormous progress that has been made in the study of these molecules. Although the chains of the interstitial collagen molecules contain approximately 1000 amino acids, and the procollagen precursor contains additional polypeptide sequences at either end which would require a messenger RNA of approximately 4500 bases, the genes coding for each of the proα1 and proα2 chains have lengths of approximately 18,000 and 38,000 bases, respectively. The enormous size of the genes is due to the presence of approximately 50 intervening DNA sequences (introns), which do not code for amino acid sequences of the mature collagen chains. A possible sequence of events in the course of synthesis of the collagen molecule is shown in Table 430–2. Further complexities are illustrated by the finding that, in the case of type I collagen, the genes coding for the constituent chains are not even on the same chromosome. In humans, the gene for the α1 chain is on chromosome 17 and that for the α2 chain on chromosome 7.

Despite the complexity of this synthetic process, there are several heritable disorders of connective tissue in which it is possible to demonstrate abnormalities in biosynthesis. Defects in synthesis of a particular type of collagen, type III collagen, have been demonstrated in a form of the Ehlers-Danlos syndrome (type IV), characterized by tissue friability and rupture of viscera and major blood vessels. Defects in hydroxylation of lysine have also been noted, which gives rise to another clinical form (type VI) of the Ehlers-Danlos syndrome. In addition, defects in processing of the procollagens

TABLE 430–2. SEQUENCE OF CELLULAR COLLAGEN BIOSYNTHESIS

1. Transcription of the gene for each collagen chain
2. Processing of collagen messenger RNA by removing ~ 50 noncoding sequences
3. Initiation of polypeptide α chain synthesis by formation of hydrophobic amino terminal leader sequence, followed by assembly of proregion and helix
4. Hydroxylation of prolyl residues begins on nascent chains
5. Hydroxylation of lysyl residues
6. Glycosylation of hydroxylysyl residues
7. Formation of –S–S– bonds at carboxyterminal extension
8. Formation of triple helix
9. Packaging for secretion
10. Amino terminal extension cleavage
11. Carboxy terminal extension cleavage
12. Formation of microfibril
13. Lysyl and hydroxylysyl oxidation
14. Formation of reducible crosslinks
15. Maturation and growth
16. Further crosslinking and interaction with other components

have been demonstrated (Ehlers-Danlos syndrome type VII) as well as problems with crosslinking accounted for by failure to oxidize critical lysine and hydroxylysine residues (certain forms of cutis laxa). Insufficient synthesis of type I collagen has also been found in certain forms of osteogenesis imperfecta, particularly the classic dominant variety of moderate severity, associated with deafness and blue sclerae. In other cases of osteogenesis imperfecta, which fall into a different clinical and genetic grouping, additions or deletions of portions of the coding region for the procollagen extensions or the helical portions have been described. In one extraordinary case, no α2 chains are present in skin and bone nor are such chains secreted by fibroblasts. The defect lies in a portion of the extension peptides that does not permit normal assembly of the procollagen trimer. Thus, absence of α2 chains is not lethal; trimers of α1 chains can be formed.

Other major components of connective tissues include the *high molecular weight carbohydrates* that make up the so-called ground substance of the interfibrillar matrix. These macromolecules, formerly known as mucopolysaccharides, are composed of a glycosaminoglycan portion (the complex carbohydrate itself) linked to a core protein. The core protein with the glycosaminoglycans attached is termed the proteoglycan subunit. In articular cartilage, proteoglycans constitute approximately half the dry weight of the tissue. Another abundant complex carbohydrate present in many tissues and the major polysaccharide of synovial fluid is hyaluronic acid. The complex carbohydrates of cartilage are composed of high molecular weight polymers of the proteoglycan subunits, with the polysaccharide side chains of chondroitin sulfate and keratan sulfate linked to serine residues of the core protein. The polymeric components consist of these proteoglycan subunits bound to high molecular weight hyaluronic acid chains through interactions with another glycoprotein, called link protein. These proteoglycan aggregates are envisioned as occupying the spaces in cartilage surrounded by the collagen fibers and other components of the matrix. Both the proteoglycans and the collagens are synthesized by the articular chondrocytes.

In general, the cells of the connective tissues interact with the complex carbohydrates and the collagen fibers through glycoproteins, which are probably specific for each type of connective tissue. For example, the cell membranes of epithelial cells interact with a glycoprotein known as laminin, which by interacting with type IV collagen, a unique heparan sulfate glycoprotein, and another protein, nidinogen, together make up the structure of the basement membrane. Many connective tissues and other cells interact with collagens through the protein fibronectin. Many cells have specific receptors for fibronectin which bind specifically to regions of this glycoprotein which contain the amino acid sequence Arg-Gly-Asp-Ser. Chondrocytes interact with their extracellular matrix through another glycoprotein called chondronectin.

STRUCTURE AND FUNCTION OF JOINTS. The structure and characteristics of the diarthrodial joints are determined by the function of specific cells, which produce unique extracellular matrices. A typical joint such as that depicted schematically in Figure 430–3 has its characteristic components. The joint is ideally suited for the demands of weight bearing and motion, which must be operational with a minimum of wear over the lifetime of the individual. The functional properties of the joint are dependent upon a compressible, deformable cartilaginous surface that is properly lubricated and supported by relatively rigid subchondral bone. The stability of the joint, in turn, is determined by the connective tissue structure of the joint capsule, tendons, and ligaments and is influenced by function of muscles concerned with movement or support of that joint. The joint cavity is lined by a synovial membrane, which normally consists of one or two layers of cells. Some tendency to piling up of the cells is observed at the margins of the joint where the synovium is reflected. The

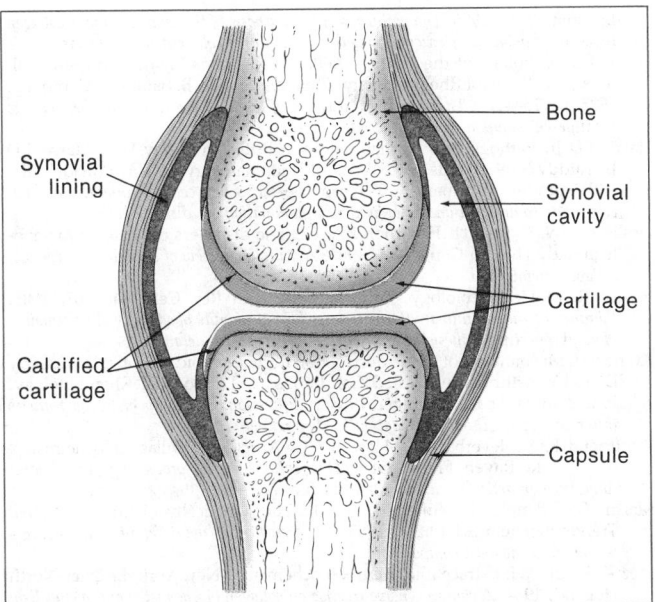

FIGURE 430–3. A schematic view of a diarthrodial joint.

synovial lining cells are derived from connective tissue (they are not epithelial) and do not rest on a continuous basement membrane. In the normal synovium, at least two types of cells have been recognized. The type A cell is a phagocytic cell possibly related to macrophages; the type B cell is fibroblast-like.

The joint cavity contains a characteristic synovial fluid. Its high viscosity is due to the presence of hyaluronic acid, which is probably synthesized by the synovial lining B cells. Water, electrolytes, and some low molecular weight serum proteins such as albumin are derived by filtration from the subsynovial capillaries. Glucose and electrolytes are present in normal synovial fluid at concentrations similar to those in plasma. In inflammation of the synovium, glucose entry is impaired and utilization increased to account for the lower synovial fluid glucose concentrations in some forms of arthritis, such as rheumatoid and septic arthritis. The concentration of proteins in normal synovial fluid is inversely proportional to their molecular weights. Albumin is therefore the most abundant protein. Plasma α_2-macroglobulin, IgM, and fibrinogen are essentially excluded from normal fluids, possibly owing to molecular sieving effects of the hyaluronic acid in the interstitial regions of the synovium and the synovial fluid. In joint inflammation, there is increased entry of the high molecular weight proteins into the synovial fluid. These pathologic fluids may thus form a *fibrin* clot, whereas normal fluids do not. This is to be distinguished from the so-called *mucin* clot, which is composed of a protein–hyaluronic acid complex that can be produced by the addition of dilute acetic acid to synovial fluid. A tight, ropy mucin clot is characteristic of normal or traumatic fluids, whereas inflammatory fluids tend to produce a fragmented clot or a dispersed sediment upon addition of acetic acid. The clinical diagnostic usefulness of the mucin clot test is not uniformly accepted, however.

The cartilage of the diarthrodial joint is avascular, and the chondrocytes must receive their nourishment from the synovial fluid; products of their metabolism are in turn disposed of through the synovial fluid. The function of the articular cartilage is critically dependent upon the interaction of the fibrillar collagenous matrix and the proteoglycans. By virtue of the highly negative charge on the proteoglycans, these molecules occupy a large domain. The extent to which articular cartilage is deformed on compression and the ability of the cartilage to regain its shape following release from compression is determined by interactions of the proteoglycan aggregates with the fibrillar matrix. It is envisioned that alternate compression and relaxation of the cartilage during motion and weight bearing are responsible for movement of fluid and electrolytes in and out of the cartilage interstitium and provide a mechanism for the nutrition of the chondrocytes. The properties of articular cartilage with its surface in contact with synovial fluid account for the extraordinarily low coefficient of friction upon movement of the joint. The viscous hyaluronic acid that serves a lubricating function for the synovial membrane is probably not responsible for lubrication of the articular cartilage itself. Other components such as lubricating glycoproteins interact with components on the surface of the articular cartilage, providing a so-called boundary type of lubrication. The very fact that the cartilage is capable of deforming under load and regaining its shape following release of the load also contributes to the low coefficient of friction of moving joints. This elastic, spongy nature of cartilage allows it to weep fluid when squeezed under high loads, which, in part, creates a film of lubrication at the head of the moving surfaces. It is also postulated that the highly ordered structure of the cancellous bone supporting the articular cartilage dissipates the shock of impact under loading and permits some of the mechanical forces to be dispersed away from the articular cartilage.

ALTERATION OF STRUCTURE AND FUNCTION OF JOINTS IN DISEASE. When joints are subjected to mechanical or chemical trauma, there are several predictable responses that occur in the articular cartilage and surrounding structures. Repeated mechanical trauma is associated with loss or decrease of the proteoglycan of the cartilage matrix, which can be appreciated histologically as a loss of the staining properties (e.g., metachromasia) attributed to this component. The mechanism for the proteoglycan loss probably involves the secretion of proteolytic enzymes, by the chondrocytes or by cells in the synovial fluid or the synovial lining, which, at neutral pH, cleave the core protein of the proteoglycans near the linkage region with the hyaluronic acid. Following cleavage of the core protein, the partially degraded proteoglycan is leached from the matrix. Alterations of this type have been observed following arthrotomy or bleeding into the joint. Since the articular chondrocytes have the capacity to resynthesize proteoglycans, if the mechanical injury is only temporary, some structure of the matrix can be restored. However, persistent deficiency of cartilage proteoglycan is accompanied by alteration in mechanical properties of the matrix manifested by an increased tendency of the cartilage to deform under load and a decreased ability to regain form following removal of the load. Only late in the course of injury is the collagenous component of the matrix affected. Although articular chondrocytes have retained the capacity to replicate and to increase, often in clusters, in response to chronic injury, these cells have a limited capacity to resynthesize type II collagen and reconstitute the normal fibrillar matrix. The proliferation of cartilage cells in response to trauma and mechanical stress may also be followed by vascularization and activation of the endochondral sequence, resulting in formation of osteophytes, usually at the margin of joints. Trauma may also produce reactions in the synovium, probably mediated by altered vascularization in addition to increased numbers and activity of the synovial lining cells. These synovial reactions may in turn result in the formation of increased synovial fluid, manifested clinically as effusions. The composition of these synovial fluids closely resembles that of normal synovial fluid with respect to viscosity (the concentration of hyaluronic acid) and the type and relative concentration of the protein components (predominance of albumin and absence of high molecular weight plasma proteins such as fibrinogen, IgM, and α_2-macroglobulin). Thus, a mild degree of "synovitis" may be a component of either acute or chronic injury. Under these circumstances, however, few cells (100 to 500 per cubic millimeter) are present in the synovial fluid; lymphocytes and monocytes predominate, whereas polymorphonuclear leukocytes are scarce.

In almost all types of joint inflammation, however, whether acute, as in urate gout or pseudogout (calcium pyrophosphate deposition disease), or chronic, as in typical rheumatoid arthritis, there is an exudation of cells, particularly polymorphonuclear leukocytes, into the synovial cavity. In these inflammatory joint diseases, the synovial fluid usually is characterized by a decreased viscosity, an inability to form a normal tight mucin clot, and an increased concentration relative to normal of macromolecules such as immunoglobulin, α_2-macroglobulin, and fibrinogen. Enzymes released from the inflammatory cells have the capacity to degrade the proteoglycan core protein and collagen of the articular cartilage and surrounding structures if their concentrations (activities) exceed those of inhibitors present in synovial fluid and synovial tissues.

The synovitis seen, for example, in rheumatoid arthritis may be particularly intense with chronic inflammatory cells present, especially at the margins of the joint where the synovial membrane is reflected. With persistent synovial inflammation, a mass of proliferating cells (pannus) may burrow beneath the articular cartilage and subchondral bone or appear to work its way over the surface of the articular cartilage, degrading matrix structures in its wake. These degradative processes are probably mediated by metalloproteinases, which can specifically degrade components of the extracellular matrix such as native collagen (collagenase), denatured collagen (gelatinase), and the core protein of the proteoglycans (stromelysin). Serine proteinases also play a role in this process. These degradative enzymes are produced not only by inflammatory cells but also by mesenchymal cells such as synovial fibroblasts and articular chondrocytes. The activity of the latter cells is markedly influenced by inflammatory cytokines such as interleukin 1 and tumor necrosis factor. Alterations also occur in the subchondral bone in joint disease. In the noninflammatory forms, the subchondral bone may increase in mass by new bone formation (sclerosis). In contrast, in inflammatory joint disease, subchondral bone is frequently resorbed, producing the typical radiologic appearance of juxta-articular osteoporosis. Diaphyseal cortical bone is usually not thinned until late in rheumatoid disease; in some subjects, it may even be increased in thickness owing to periosteal new bone formation. When the inflammation subsides, bony erosions may heal, and some restoration of the diffuse juxta-articular bone loss may also occur. Defects or clefts in articular cartilage, on the other hand, generally do not heal with restoration of the original form because of the limited capacity of chondrocytes to resynthesize the specific collagenous fibrillar component of extracellular matrix.

Each of the extracellular components of the matrix of the joint structures has its unique pattern of composition with respect to the collagen type, proteoglycan, and glycoprotein component. The composition of these matrices must in turn determine their function. Return of function with healing of disease therefore requires restoration of the original composition, which, in turn, is dependent upon the ability of the tissue to undergo remodeling. The limited capacity for remodeling of some tissues, such as articular cartilage, therefore accounts for disability in several of the rheumatic diseases. Thus, in instances in which structure is sufficiently distorted and return of function impossible, the only alternative may be to use the artificial surfaces of joint prostheses to permit or regain motion and weight-bearing capacity and to alleviate pain.

Brandt KD: Glycosaminoglycans. In Kelley WN, Harris ED Jr, Ruddy S, et al. (eds.): Textbook of Rheumatology. Philadelphia, W. B. Saunders Company, 1985, pp 237–253. *A review of the structure and biology of the complex carbohydrates, with particular reference to cartilage.*

Cheah KSE: Collagen genes and inherited connective tissue disease. Biochem J 229:287, 1985. *The structure and regulation of the collagen genes are reviewed, particularly with reference to disorders such as osteogenesis imperfecta and Ehlers-Danlos syndrome.*

Fessler JH, Doege KJ, Duncan KG, et al.: Biosynthesis of collagen. J Cell Biochem 28:31, 1985. *The pathways of biosynthesis of the more abundant collagen types are considered, particularly with respect to the role of disulfide bonds.*

Harris ED Jr: Biology of the joint. In Kelley WN, Harris ED Jr, Ruddy S, et al. (eds.): Textbook of Rheumatology. Philadelphia, W. B. Saunders Company, 1985, pp 254–271. *The anatomical features of the joint are related to chemistry of the different components and these to function.*

Harris ED Jr: Pathogenesis of rheumatoid arthritis. In Kelley WN, Harris ED Jr, Ruddy S, et al. (eds.): Textbook of Rheumatology. Vol. 1. Philadelphia, WB Saunders Company, 1985, pp 886–915. *The cellular interactions that contribute to destruction of the joint in inflammation are discussed.*

Hollister DW, Byers PH, Holbrook KA: Genetic disorders of collagen metabolism. Adv Human Genet 12:1, 1982. *A complete review of heritable disorders of collagen metabolism.*

Hynes R: Molecular biology of fibronectin. Ann Rev Cell Biol 1:67, 1985. *Fibronectin and laminin are the major members of a family of adhesive glycoproteins. How fibronectin synthesis is controlled is considered in detail.*

Krane SM: Mechanisms of tissue destruction in rheumatoid arthritis. In McCarty DJ (ed.): Arthritis and Allied Conditions. A Textbook of Rheumatology. Philadelphia, Lea and Febiger, 1985. *A discussion relating the histologic features to the connective tissue degradation in rheumatoid arthritis.*

Kuettner KE, Schleyerbach R, Hascall VC: Articular Cartilage Biochemistry. New York, Raven Press, 1986. *This volume is the proceedings of a recent conference on articular cartilage and its diseases.*

Martin GR, Timple R, Muller PK, et al.: The genetically distinct collagens. Trends Biochem Sci 10:285, 1985. *The structure of the different collagen types is related to chemical composition.*

Piez K, Reddi AH: Extracellular Matrix Biochemistry. New York, Elsevier-North Holland, 1984. *A comprehensive treatise on collagen biochemistry and metabolism as well as discussions of alterations in heritable and acquired diseases.*

Poole AR: Proteoglycans in health and disease: Structures and functions. Biochem J 236:1, 1986. *This review article supplements and updates the material discussed by Brandt.*

Prockop DJ, Kivirikko KI: Heritable diseases of collagen. N Engl J Med 311:376, 1984. *The authors update the material in their 1979 review on collagen structure and disease.*

Prockop DJ: Mutations in collagen genes. J Clin Invest 75:783, 1985. *Mutations in collagen genes are related to different clinical phenotypes of heritable disorders.*

Ruoslahti E, Pierschbacher MD: Arg-Gly-Asp: A versatile cell recognition signal. Cell 44:517, 1986. *An excellent review of how cells interact with the fibronectin of their extracellular matrix.*

Tsipouras P, Myers JC, Ramirez F, et al.: Restriction fragment length polymorphism associated with the proα2 (I) gene of human type I procollagen. J Clin Invest 72:1262, 1983. *An example of the kind of investigations that are currently being conducted in human beings using probes for the collagen genes.*

431 MECHANISMS OF INFLAMMATION AND TISSUE DESTRUCTION IN THE RHEUMATIC DISEASES

Ralph Snyderman

Immunologic processes mediate the localization and destruction of substances that, if disseminated, could disrupt the host's complex internal milieu. The immune system has several unique features that permit it to combat microbial invasion and provide resistance against the spread of cancer. Unlike other tissues, the immune system consists not only of fixed structures (i.e., thymus, spleen, and lymph nodes) but also of motile cells that wander throughout the body, performing surveillance. It is also the only tissue able to destroy other components of the host. Both the protective and destructive abilities of immunologic processes relate largely to their inflammatory potential. Understanding how inflammation is initiated is thus essential for understanding the mechanisms of immunologically mediated resistance and for comprehending how tissue destruction occurs in the rheumatic disorders.

To fulfill its function of host defense, the immune system must differentiate self from nonself and then rapidly destroy substances recognized as nonself. A progression of immunologic recognition, amplification of the immune reaction, accumulation of inflammatory cells, and finally destruction of the inciting agent is an ongoing subclinical process. Inflammatory reactions can be initiated by either specific or nonspe-

TABLE 431–1. COMPONENTS OF THE INFLAMMATORY RESPONSE

Function	Mediator
Recognition	
Specific	Immunoglobulins
	Lymphocyte receptors
Nonspecific	Macrophages*
	Polymorphonuclear leukocytes
	Alternative complement pathway
	Hageman factor
Amplification	Complement
	Cytokines—lymphokines, monokines, and
	interleukins
	Kinin-forming system
	Lipid mediators
	Mast cell products
Destruction of	Macrophages
antigen	Polymorphonuclear leukocytes
	Cytotoxic lymphocytes

*Macrophages are also involved in specific recognition, since they are required for antigen presentation to lymphocytes.

cific means (Table 431–1). Recognition of unique determinants (epitopes) on antigens by antibodies or by receptors on lymphocytes initiates immunologically mediated inflammation. Nonspecific recognition can be initiated by components of the immune system that bind to materials based on their charge, hydrophobicity, or lectin composition. Nonspecific recognition is mediated in part by phagocytic cells, such as polymorphonuclear leukocytes and macrophages, as well as by C3b, an initiator of the alternative pathway of the complement system (see Ch. 418), and by Hageman factor.

Following recognition of nonself, amplification systems are activated and lead to the production of mediators of inflammation. The type of amplifier involved depends upon the recognition component and the nature and location of the inciting material. Amplification components of the immune system such as complement cleavage products, cytokines, and other phlogistic factors magnify the initial response to nonself. Inflammatory reactions can also be initiated by non-

immunologic means. For example, inflammation following tissue necrosis results from the direct cleavage of complement components by lysosomal proteases released by injured cells. This phenomenon may play a role in extending cardiac tissue damage following myocardial infarction. In gout or pseudogout, inflammation follows the phagocytosis, by polymorphonuclear leukocytes, of monosodium urate or calcium pyrophosphate dihydrate crystals. Ingestion of these agents by leukocytes leads to the release of lysosomal hydrolases as well as the production of chemotactic factors, which attract other inflammatory cells into the joint.

Regardless of the type of inflammatory response, the accumulation of granulocytes and macrophages can result in phagocytosis and degradation of the material that initiated the inflammatory event. The factors that determine whether an inflammatory response will be protective or destructive depend in part upon the nature and location of the inciting agent, its quantity, digestibility, the genetic makeup, and the immunoregulatory competency of the host. In general, when the antigen or other inciting agent is rapidly disposed of, the inflammatory process is self-limited. When antigen persists or is excessive in amount, the inflammatory response can be locally destructive and become clinically apparent.

RHEUMATOID SYNOVITIS AS A MODEL OF INFLAMMATORY-MEDIATED TISSUE DESTRUCTION

A chronic, locally destructive inflammatory reaction in humans is exemplified by the synovitis present in some connective tissue disorders. The prototype disease is rheumatoid arthritis. The diarthrodial joint has several features that influence inflammatory processes that occur there. The synovial membrane is highly vascular and lines all intra-articular structures, except for cartilage. The synovial lining is devoid of a basement membrane and thus permits relatively free diffusion of soluble substances. Moreover, the synovium lines a closed

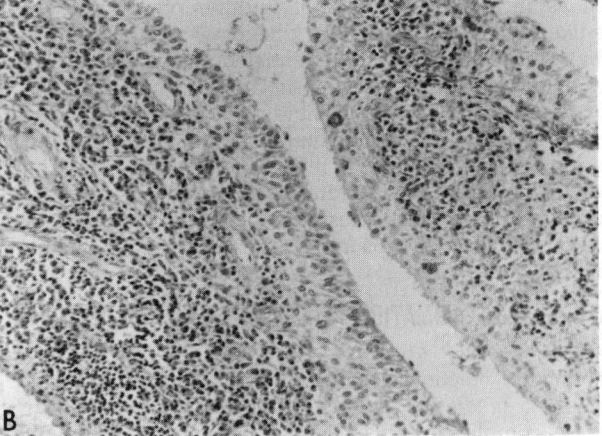

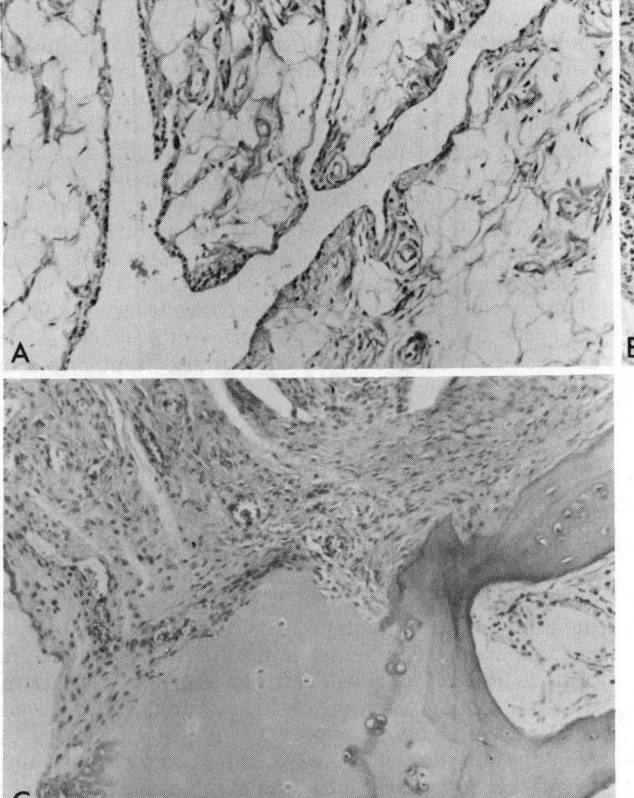

FIGURE 431–1. Normal synovium and synovitis of rheumatoid arthritis. *A,* A delicate network of connective tissue supports a thin layer of synoviocytes in the normal synovium. *B,* The thickened rheumatoid synovium with villous projections is composed of hyperplastic, hypertrophic synoviocytes and is infiltrated with lymphocytes, plasma cells, macrophages, and occasional multinucleated giant cells. *C,* Rheumatoid synovium invading articular cartilage and subchondral bone. (This figure is taken from the Clinical Slide Collection of the Arthritis Foundation with its kind permission.)

cavity, the joint space; therefore any reactive materials gaining entrance to the joint space are difficult to remove.

Normal synovium is a thin layer of tissue whose lining is composed of two principal cell types supported by a loose connective tissue stroma (Fig. 431–1A). The Type A cell is rich in surface pseudopodia, and its cytoplasm has many lysosomes and prominent Golgi complexes but little rough endoplasmic reticulum. Type A synoviocytes have many characteristics of macrophages and are phagocytic, and ultrastructural studies have implied a secretory role for these cells as well. The Type B synoviocyte exhibits prominent rough endoplasmic reticulum but few vacuoles, lysosomes, or cell processes. This cell is primarily a secretory cell, hyaluronic acid being an important product. Synoviocytes may, however, be multipotential, with their morphology reflecting the net result of stimuli present in the local milieu. Beneath the synovial membrane there are collagen fibrils, fatty tissue, and an extensive capillary network. Fibroblasts in this area produce Types I and III collagen. Lastly, the dense fibrous joint capsule provides support for the synovial lining membrane and separates the articular space from surrounding structures.

Rheumatoid synovitis exhibits three main components: inflammation, proliferation, and infiltration. In early stages, both Types A and B cells proliferate and increase in size. Fibrin deposits are frequently present on the inner synovial lining. Polymorphonuclear leukocytes predominate in the synovial fluid exudate, but cells are seen as infiltrates only in the superficial synovial layer. The supporting stroma beneath the lining cell layer becomes edematous and develops an increase in the number of small blood vessels. Concurrently, there are focal accumulations of inflammatory cells consisting of lymphocytes, plasma cells, macrophages, and occasionally mast cells. If the inflammatory synovitis persists, a proliferative lesion develops, characterized by synovial membrane thickening and projection of villous formations into the articular cavity (Fig. 431–1B). There is a concomitant increase in supporting connective tissue, small blood vessels, mononuclear cell infiltrates, and occasional multinucleated giant cells, as well as increased numbers of undifferentiated mesenchyme-like cells that have both phagocytic and synthetic potential. Clusters of poorly differentiated synovial cells may be found invading cartilage and subchondral bone. As the proliferative lesions progress, fibrous-mesenchymal tissue (pannus) begins to invade and replace cartilage and bone at the periphery of the synovial reflection (Fig. 431–1C). The invasion of cartilage, subchondral bone, and tendon by inflammatory synovial tissue results in collagen destruction, degradation of proteoglycans in the cartilage matrix, and bony resorption.

MEDIATORS OF INFLAMMATION THAT PARTICIPATE IN THE RHEUMATIC DISEASES

Inflammatory reactions result from the local production of a number of mediators derived from humoral or cellular sources. A complex interplay of activation and suppression mechanisms modulates the type and magnitude of the inflammatory response.

LIPID MEDIATORS. Phospholipids are major constituents of cell membranes, including those of leukocytes and platelets, and are subject to degradation by cellular phospholipases under certain conditions such as exposure of cells to inflammatory or noxious stimuli. Cleavage of phospholipids results in the release of arachidonic acid, which can be further metabolized into a number of biologically potent mediators and modulators of inflammation. Prostaglandins (PG) are synthesized from arachidonic acid following the action of the enzyme cyclo-oxygenase, which forms PGG_2, which is then reduced to PGH_2. Depending upon the isomerase enzymes present in the particular tissue, prostaglandins (PGE_2, $PGF_{2\alpha}$), thromboxanes, or prostacyclins will be formed. Leukocytes and explants of rheumatoid synovia produce predominantly

PGE_2, platelets produce thromboxane A_2, and endothelial cells produce prostacyclin. Thromboxanes are vasoconstrictors, whereas prostacyclins are vasodilators. PGE_2 appears to modulate a number of inflammatory events. It enhances vascular permeability, is pyrogenic, and increases sensitivity to pain. PGE_2 also stimulates formation of cAMP in many types of inflammatory cells and thereby suppresses a number of immunologic responses, including release of mediators from mast cells, lymphocyte blastogenesis, and lymphocyte-mediated cytotoxic reactions. An important source of PGE_2 in immunologic reactions is the macrophage. Supernatant fluids from explants of rheumatoid synovium stimulate bone resorption by enhancing osteoclast activity and release of bone calcium. This phenomenon is probably mediated in large part by PG, since it is inhibitable by indomethacin, which blocks their formation.

Arachidonic acid can also be metabolized into another class of biologically active derivatives by the enzyme lipoxygenase. The hydroxy-eicosatetraenoic acids (HETEs) and the derivatives of 5-hydroperoxy-eicosatetraenoic acid (termed leukotrienes) are examples of these arachidonic acid metabolites and are synthesized by granulocytes, macrophages, and basophils. 5,12-HETE, also termed leukotriene B_4 (LTB_4), is a potent chemotactic factor, whereas leukotrienes C and D stimulate bronchoconstriction. LTB_4 has been identified in the synovial effusions of patients with rheumatoid arthritis and ankylosing spondylitis. Large amounts of LTB_4 are produced when granulocytes phagocytize monosodium urate crystals, and production of LTB_4 is inhibited by colchicine. This chemoattractant may, therefore, be important in the pathogenesis of gouty inflammation. Platelet-activating factors (PAF) are a group of acetyl-alkylglycerol ether analogues of phosphatidylcholine. PAF causes platelet aggregation and is a potent leukocyte activator and chemoattractant. Leukocytes produce PAF following their stimulation by inflammatory mediators.

BIOLOGICALLY ACTIVE AMINES. *Histamine and Serotonin.* Histamine is derived from the decarboxylation of histidine by the enzyme L-histidine decarboxylase. The majority of histamine is stored in mast cells and basophils and is complexed with mucopolysaccharides such as heparin. Stimulation of mast cells and basophils by a number of mechanisms causes secretion of histamine. This agent has diverse biologic activities, including constricting smooth muscle, enhancing vascular permeability, depressing leukocyte chemotaxis, blocking T lymphocyte function, and depressing further histamine release from mast cells and basophils. Histamine thus may modulate both acute and chronic inflammatory responses. Serotonin (5-hydroxytryptamine) is produced by the decarboxylation of 5-hydroxytryptophan. More than 90 per cent of body stores of serotonin are found in the gastrointestinal tract and the central nervous system; the remainder is present in the dense granules of platelets. The biologic role of serotonin in inflammation is not well understood, but it enhances the chemotactic responses of leukocytes and increases fibroblast growth in vitro. It also stimulates collagen formation.

BIOLOGICALLY ACTIVE PEPTIDES. *Complement Cleavage Products.* The complement (C) system functions as an important amplifier of inflammatory events initiated by immunoglobulins IgG and IgM as well as inflammatory reactions initiated by release of hydrolytic enzymes from traumatized cells or by leukocytes. The biology and biochemistry of this complex series of proteins are described in Ch. 418. Two complement cleavage products, C3a and C5a, derived from the third and fifth C components, respectively, are mediators of inflammation in rheumatic disorders such as rheumatoid arthritis and will thus be described in greater detail here.

C3a: Enzymatic cleavage of the α chain of C3 by the earlier-acting C components or by other proteases releases C3a, a peptide consisting of 77 amino acids. C3a mediates a number of biologic responses, including smooth muscle contraction, vasodilatation, enhanced vascular permeability, the degranulation of mast cells and basophils, and the secretion of lysosomal enzymes by leukocytes. C3a also has immunoregulatory effects and suppresses humoral immune responses in vitro by affecting T lymphocytes. C3a is the most abundant of the C peptides released upon activation of C in serum. The COOH-terminal arginine of C3a is required for its biologic activity, and cleavage of this amino acid by a carboxypeptidase-B–like enzyme in serum renders the peptide inactive.

C5a: C5a has a number of structural and biologic similarities to C3a. C5a consists of 74 amino acids, the COOH-terminal constituent also being arginine. C5a is derived from cleavage of the α chain of C5. In addition to having all the biologic activities of C3a, C5a is also an extremely potent chemoattractant for polymorphonuclear leukocytes, monocytes, and macrophages. C5a is the major source of chemotactic activity generated in serum treated with immune complexes or endotoxin and is also an important source of chemotactic activity in rheumatoid synovial fluids. In contrast to C3a, C5a potentiates humoral immune responses in vitro. Cleavage of the terminal arginine of C5a by a serum carboxypeptidase-B markedly diminishes its biologic activity.

Crystal-Induced Chemotactic Factors. Leukocytes accumulate in the synovial fluid of individuals with gout or pseudogout following the ingestion by neutrophils of monosodium urate or calcium pyrophosphate dihydrate crystals, respectively. Incubation of neutrophils with these crystals in vitro results in the production by the cells of LTB$_4$ and a polypeptide chemoattractant (CCF) with a molecular weight of 8400. The production of these chemoattractants is blocked by colchicine. A mechanism by which colchicine abrogates acute gouty arthritis may be its ability to inhibit the synthesis of chemoattractants by neutrophils.

Kinin-Forming System. An intimate association exists between the activation and regulation of the intrinsic clotting, fibrinolytic, and kinin-forming systems. Hageman factor (HF) (Factor XII of the clotting system) is central to the activation of all three systems. HF is activated nonspecifically by a number of agents, including exposure to crude preparations of collagen, vascular basement membranes, monosodium urate crystals, calcium pyrophosphate crystals, and endotoxin. Negatively charged surfaces also activate HF. Upon activation, HF (an 80,000-dalton β globulin) is cleaved, and its active form HF$_A$ initiates the conversion of Factor XI of the clotting pathway to XIa, and the conversion of prekallikrein to kallikrein. Kallikrein activates plasminogen, an enzyme important in fibrinolysis. Kallikrein also cleaves serum kininogen to form bradykinin, a nonapeptide with potent biologic activities. C1 esterase inhibitor (C1INH), a protein that inhibits activated C1, is also an important inhibitor of HF$_A$ and kallikrein. Bradykinin and two other kinins produced by tissue kallikreins from kininogen induce smooth muscle contraction, increase vascular permeability, and induce pain. Cleavage of fibrinogen by plasmin results in production of a number of products, including fibrinopeptide B, which potentiates the action of bradykinin and has chemotactic activity.

Interleukins and Other Cytokines. Interleukins are immunoregulatory molecules synthesized by mononuclear leukocytes. Stimulation of macrophages by antigens as well as by factors from lymphocytes initiates the secretion of interleukin 1 (IL-1), a 15,000-dalton peptide with diverse biologic activities. Macrophages are required for many of the activities of lymphocytes, and certain of the "helper" functions of macrophages are mediated by IL-1. IL-1 may be identical to a factor termed mononuclear cell factor (MCF), which stimulates synovial cells to produce collagenase. IL-1 may also be identical to leukocytic pyrogen. Tumor necrosis factor-α (TNF-α) is a macrophage product with IL-1–like activities plus the ability to kill many types of tumor cells (see Ch. 257).

Interleukin 2 (IL-2), previously termed T-cell growth factor, is a 15,000-dalton polypeptide produced by T lymphocytes, which stimulates the continuous proliferation of activated T lymphocytes in culture. Transforming-growth factor-β (TGF-β) is a 25,000-dalton homodimeric protein found in platelets and produced by stimulated lymphocytes. TGF-β inhibits further lymphocyte division and regulates differentiation of many cell types including fibroblasts. Interferon-γ (IFN-γ) is a 50,000 dalton protein produced by stimulated lymphocytes. IFN-γ activates macrophages and synergizes with other immunomodulators.

LYSOSOMAL ENZYMES. Lysosomal enzymes are contained in subcellular organelles termed lysosomal granules. These enzymes degrade complex macromolecules. Lysosomal granules also contain antimicrobial constituents such as myeloperoxidase and lactoferrin. Leukocytes contain several types of lysosomal granules, two of which (primary and secondary) are differentiated by their staining characteristics. Lysosomal enzymes digest antigens following phagocytosis. However, since these enzymes may also be released during phagocytosis or upon cell death, they can cause tissue destruction. Lysosomal proteases found in leukocytes include collagenase, elastase, cathepsin D, cathepsin G, and gelatinase. These enzymes are capable of destroying extracellular structures and may participate in mediating tissue injury in the rheumatic diseases. Cathepsin D cleaves cartilage proteoglycan, whereas granulocyte collagenase is active in cleaving Type I and, to a lesser degree, Type III collagen of bone, cartilage, and tendon. Substrates of granulocyte elastase include collagen crosslinkages and proteoglycans, as well as elastin components of blood vessels, ligaments, and cartilage. Lysosomal hydrolyases also produce mediators of inflammation through their direct action on C components such as C5. Leukocytic hydrolyases can liberate kinin from kininogen. Plasminogen activator, an enzyme that converts plasminogen to plasmin (which stimulates fibrinolysis) is found in both granulocyte and macrophage lysosomes. Rheumatoid synovial collagenase is usually present as an inactive lysosomal proenzyme that requires plasminogen activator for conversion to its active form.

Regulation of tissue destructive potential of the lysosomal proteases is mediated by protease inhibitors such as α$_2$ macroglobulin and α$_1$ antiprotease. These antiproteases are present in serum and in synovial fluids and inhibit proteases by binding to them and covering their active sites.

PHYSIOLOGIC MECHANISMS OF INFLAMMATORY CELL ACCUMULATION

The accumulation of inflammatory cells at sites of antigen is central to the inflammatory process. Polymorphonuclear leukocytes and macrophages are motile cells that have many common physiologic characteristics. Both can perceive gradients of chemoattractant molecules and migrate directionally along such gradients. They also perform endocytosis (ingestion), secrete lysosomal enzymes, and generate superoxide anions (see Ch. 148). Polymorphonuclear leukocytes and macrophages have specific surface receptors that perceive C5a, CCF, and LTB$_4$ as well as synthetic polypeptide chemotactic factors. Binding of chemoattractants to the surface of phagocytes results in orientation of the cells toward the source of the chemotactic gradient. The cells lose their round configuration and become triangular, with the base of the triangle facing toward the chemoattractant gradient (Fig. 431–2). This change in cell shape requires rearrangement of intracellular cytoskeletal elements. Microtubules provide a front-to-back polarization, whereas actin filaments accumulate at the front and back of the cells and provide the contractile forces required for movement. Attachment of leukocytes to the vascular endothelium and other surfaces is a requirement for cellular motility. Chemoattractants stimulate the appearance of several adhesive proteins on the surface of phagocytes. These proteins include the iC3b receptor (mac 1, mo 1), LFA 1, and glycoprotein 150/90. These proteins are heterodimers

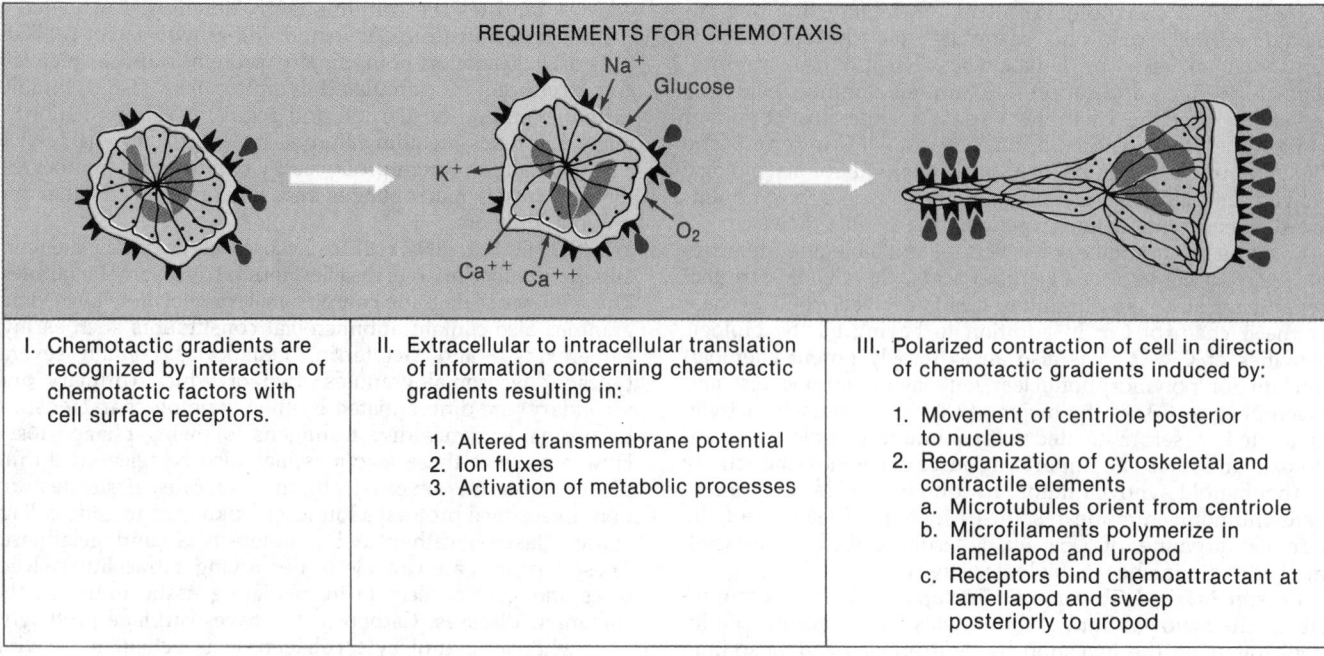

REQUIREMENTS FOR CHEMOTAXIS

| I. Chemotactic gradients are recognized by interaction of chemotactic factors with cell surface receptors. | II. Extracellular to intracellular translation of information concerning chemotactic gradients resulting in:

 1. Altered transmembrane potential
 2. Ion fluxes
 3. Activation of metabolic processes | III. Polarized contraction of cell in direction of chemotactic gradients induced by:

 1. Movement of centriole posterior to nucleus
 2. Reorganization of cytoskeletal and contractile elements
   a. Microtubules orient from centriole
   b. Microfilaments polymerize in lamellapod and uropod
   c. Receptors bind chemoattractant at lamellapod and sweep posteriorly to uropod |

FIGURE 431–2. The interaction of chemotactic factor receptors with chemotactic factors triggers the indicated cellular responses.

that serve a number of adhesive functions. They consist of individual α-chains and a common β-subunit. Their appearance on the surface of phagocytes enhances the cells' binding to endothelial cells, tumor cells, and other surfaces. Deficiency of these proteins is associated with a severe defect of leukocyte function and a marked increase in susceptibility to infection. Chemotactic factors can also initiate other cellular responses by leukocytes, such as superoxide anion production and lysosomal enzyme secretion. The concentration of chemotactic factors required to initiate these latter processes is approximately 10-fold greater than that required for the induction of chemotaxis. Thus, release of potentially toxic products from the cells may not occur until they arrive at the inflammatory site where the concentration of chemoattractants is high.

Chemoattractants activate leukocytes through their binding to cell surface receptors. Occupancy of chemoattractant receptors causes a guanine nucleotide regulatory (G) protein to become activated through the dissociation of GDP, followed by the binding of GTP. The activated G protein lowers the calcium concentration required to stimulate a membrane-associated phospholipase C, which in turn hydrolyzes a membrane phospholipid termed phosphatidylinositol 4,5-bisphosphate. This hydrolysis leads to the production of two second messengers, the calcium mobilizer inositol 1,4,5-trisphosphate (IP_3) and the protein kinase C activator, 1,2-diacylglycerol. When the dose of chemotactic factor is sufficient, protein kinase C becomes translocated from the cytosol to the plasma membrane of the phagocyte and activates the respiratory burst. Feedback inhibition of this activation pathway is mediated by transient cAMP elevation, which inhibits IP_3 production, as well as by protein kinase C, which uncouples the ability of the activated G protein to stimulate phospholipase C.

Lymphocytes are also motile cells, but they do not respond to the same chemotactic factors as polymorphonuclear leukocytes and macrophages. The migration of lymphocytes is stimulated by specific antigens, mitogens, and other undefined factors produced by lymphocytes.

Phagocytosis is initiated by binding of a particle to the surface of phagocytic cells. Particles carrying bound immunoglobulin or the complement fragments C3b or C3bi are more readily phagocytosed, since they bind to Fc and C3b receptors on both polymorphonuclear leukocytes and macro-phages. However, phagocytosis can occur in the absence of receptor involvement. Particle ingestion results from the envelopment and fusion of phagocytic cell membrane around the foreign material (Fig. 431–3). Intracellular lysosomes migrate to the phagocytic vesicle, fuse with it, and empty their contents, thus forming a phagolysosome. Within the phagolysosome, antigenic digestion and microbial killing generally occur. During phagocytosis, lysosomal hydrolases and toxic oxygen radicals may be released.

IMMUNOLOGICALLY MEDIATED TISSUE INJURY

Inflammatory responses can produce adverse reactions ranging from minor local tissue irritation to selective destruction of organs or even sudden death. The nature of immunologically mediated inflammatory responses depends upon the immunologic recognition component that identifies the antigen. Four general types of immunologically mediated inflammatory reactions have been defined (Table 431–2). In clinical and experimental situations it is not infrequent to have more than one, and even all types, of these immune reactions operative simultaneously.

TYPE I REACTIONS: INFLAMMATION INITIATED BY REAGINIC (IgE) ANTIBODIES. IgE antibodies bind to mast cells and basophils by means of their Fc portion, which allows the Fab portion to be available for binding to specific antigen. Shortly after the appropriate antigen binds, the cells degranulate and secrete their intracellular products, which include histamine, eosinophil chemotactic factors (ECF-A), and heparin. Release of mediators from basophils or mast cells causes an increase in local vascular permeability within seconds and produces vascular stasis and smooth muscle contraction. Type I reactions are responsible for such allergic phenomena as urticaria, seasonal rhinitis, asthma, and systemic anaphylaxis (see Ch. 420 to 423).

TYPE II REACTIONS: TISSUE DESTRUCTION MEDIATED BY CYTOTOXIC ANTIBODY. The development of antibody to antigens on the surface of a host's own cells can lead to tissue destruction. Injury results from the binding of C-fixing antibodies to host tissue cells. Activation of the C cascade leads to the release of inflammatory mediators and the accumulation of inflammatory cells. Release of lysosomal enzymes and toxic oxygen radicals by inflammatory cells and direct cytolysis of target cells through C action contribute to

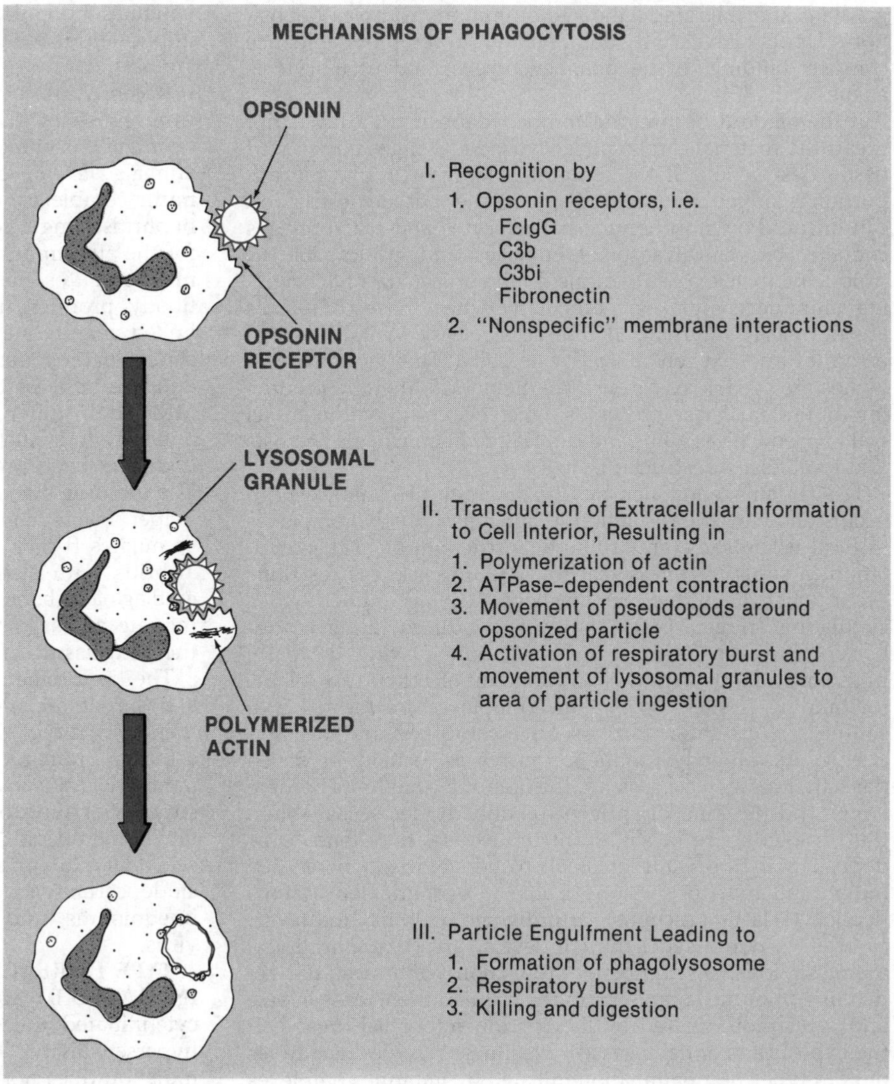

MECHANISMS OF PHAGOCYTOSIS

OPSONIN

OPSONIN RECEPTOR

LYSOSOMAL GRANULE

POLYMERIZED ACTIN

I. Recognition by
  1. Opsonin receptors, i.e.
    FcIgG
    C3b
    C3bi
    Fibronectin
  2. "Nonspecific" membrane interactions

II. Transduction of Extracellular Information to Cell Interior, Resulting in
  1. Polymerization of actin
  2. ATPase–dependent contraction
  3. Movement of pseudopods around opsonized particle
  4. Activation of respiratory burst and movement of lysosomal granules to area of particle ingestion

III. Particle Engulfment Leading to
  1. Formation of phagolysosome
  2. Respiratory burst
  3. Killing and digestion

FIGURE 431–3. Requirements for phagocytosis. Particulate antigen binding to the membrane of phagocytic cells initiates cellular responses that lead to envelopment of the antigen. The process is enhanced when the antigens have bound opsonins.

tissue destruction. A human disease resulting from antibody directed toward self tissues is Goodpasture's syndrome (see Ch. 63). The result of antibody deposition on pulmonary and glomerular basement membranes is the explosive onset of hemorrhagic pneumonitis and rapidly progressive glomerulonephritis. Spontaneous development of antibody to tissues characterizes certain rheumatologic disorders, particularly systemic lupus erythematosus (SLE). Autoimmune hemolytic anemia occurs following the deposition of C-fixing antibodies plus C3 cleavage products on circulating red blood cells. As a consequence, the cells are rapidly destroyed either by macrophages in the reticuloendothelial system (particularly in the spleen) or, less commonly, by intravascular hemolysis mediated by C. Also common in SLE is idiopathic thrombocytopenic purpura, in which antibody develops against platelet antigen and leads to thrombocytopenia.

TYPE III REACTIONS: INFLAMMATION INITIATED BY

IMMUNE COMPLEXES. The formation or deposition of certain types of immune complexes in local tissues produces an inflammatory response characterized by the accumulation of polymorphonuclear leukocytes within hours, followed by the influx of macrophages. Several mechanisms exist by which immune complexes initiate this reaction. The combination of IgM or IgG (subclasses 1, 2, or 3) antibodies with antigen leads to binding and activation of the first component of C. As a result, C4 and C2 are cleaved and activated, and then C3 is cleaved into two fragments. The larger fragment (C3b) binds to the immune complex; the smaller fragment (C3a) diffuses away. C3a enhances vascular permeability, contracts venular smooth muscle, and degranulates mast cells and basophils. Cleavage of C5 releases the potent inflammatory polypeptide C5a. Diffusion of C5a from the site of immunologic reactions establishes a gradient of this chemoattractant. Polymorphonuclear leukocytes and macrophages detect this

TABLE 431–2. TYPES OF IMMUNOLOGICALLY MEDIATED INFLAMMATION

Type of Inflammation	Recognition Component	Soluble Mediator	Inflammatory Response	Disease Example
I. Reaginic, allergic	IgE	Basophil and mast cell products (ECF)	Immediate flare and wheal, smooth muscle constriction	Atopy, anaphylaxis
II. Cytotoxic antibody	IgG, IgM	Complement	Lysis or phagocytosis of circulating antigens, acute inflammation in tissues	Autoimmune hemolytic anemia, thrombocytopenia associated with systemic lupus erythematosus
III. Immune complex	IgG, IgM	Complement, lipid mediators	Accumulation of polymorphonuclear leukocytes and macrophages	Rheumatoid arthritis, lupus erythematosus
IV. Delayed hypersensitivity	T lymphocytes	Cytokines	Mononuclear cell infiltrate	Tuberculosis, sarcoidosis, polymyositis, granulomatosis, vasculitis

gradient and migrate to the site of immune complex deposition. Upon arrival, Fc, C3b, and iC3b receptors enhance complex binding to the phagocytic cells, and phagocytosis ensues (Fig. 431–3).

If the amount of immune complex deposited locally is not great, the material can be phagocytized and digested without tissue destruction. If the amount is large or if a significant portion is lodged in vessel walls, permanent tissue destruction can ensue. Polymorphonuclear leukocytes and macrophages contain abundant lysosomal enzymes and are capable of producing toxic oxygen radicals. In the process of phagocytizing immune complexes, particularly when these complexes are not easily internalized, the cells release their lysosomal enzymes and oxygen radicals externally. The lysosomal enzymes are capable of cleaving additional C5, thereby producing more C5a. These processes, when occurring within vessel walls, produce vasculitis and can lead to hemorrhagic necrosis and local tissue destruction.

Tissue damage initiated by C-fixing immune complexes can occur following the formation of antigen-antibody complexes in local tissue sites (an Arthus-type reaction) or in the circulation (a serum sickness reaction). Serum sickness reactions occur when an individual develops C-fixing antibody to a circulating antigen. As antibody is produced, antigen-antibody complexes form in the circulation. During the early phase of antibody synthesis, the amount of antibody available for binding is small so that the complexes are formed in a setting of great antigen excess. Such complexes are not pathogenic. As antibody production increases, usually by seven days after antigenic exposure, the immune complexes become larger and the ratio of antigen to antibody decreases. When the complexes are in slight antigen excess, they tend to be deposited in the walls of small blood vessels, where they initiate inflammatory lesions. Palpable purpuric skin lesions (leukocytoclastic vasculitis), arthritis, glomerulitis, and fever, as well as depressed serum C levels, are common clinical manifestations. As antibody production continues, the remaining immune complexes in the circulation increase in size and are rapidly cleared by the reticuloendothelial organs. If the exposure to antigen ceases, the illness resolves. Examples of both types of inflammation initiated by immune complexes are common in rheumatic diseases such as rheumatoid arthritis and SLE.

Certain animals develop spontaneous immune complex diseases that bear striking similarities to human SLE. The F₁ hybrid cross between New Zealand Black (NZB) and New Zealand White (NZW) mice (NZB/W F₁) develops an immunologic disorder characterized by circulating antibody to nuclear proteins, glomerulonephritis, autoimmune hemolytic anemia, and vasculitis. In contrast to the NZB/W F₁ hybrids, NZB mice develop severe autoimmune hemolytic anemia but insignificant glomerulonephritis. NZW mice do not develop spontaneous autoimmune disease.

NZB/W disease illustrates the contribution of genetic, immunologic, and infectious factors to the production of a spontaneous immune complex disease. Genetically, multiple autosomal genes appear to be involved. Immunologically, the animals have heightened B-cell activity and abnormalities of regulatory T-cell function, including depressed suppressor function. A direct role of helper T cells in stimulating autoantibody responses has also been inferred, since therapy of mice with monoclonal antibodies to helper cells ameliorates disease. The disease itself appears to occur when the NZB/W mice produce unusually large amounts of antibody to Gross leukemia virus, an agent that infects many normal mouse strains but usually produces no disease. In the NZB/W mice, however, antigen-antibody complexes develop and deposit in a granular "lumpy-bumpy" immunofluorescent pattern in the renal glomerulus, leading to immune complex–induced glomerulonephritis. The circulating immune complexes cause a fall in the serum C titer, and a systemic vasculitis occurs.

Unique subpopulations of anti-DNA antibodies have also been implicated in renal immune complex deposition in these animals.

Recently, mice with genetic backgrounds quite different from those of NZB/W have also been shown to develop spontaneous immune complex disease. MRL-lpr/lpr and BXSB animals develop an illness characterized by circulating immune complexes, depressed serum C, and immune complex nephritis. Single gene abnormalities appear to be responsible for the autoimmune disease in mice of these strains. In MRL mice, an autosomal recessive gene termed *lpr* leads to autoantibody production, while in BXSB mice a Y-chromosome linked gene termed Yᵃᵃ, for autoimmune accelerator, plays a similar pathogenetic role. As in the NZB/W mice, one of the antigens appears to be an oncornavirus protein. Mice of the MRL strain differ from the NZB/W F₁ in that they produce antibody to a nuclear antigen termed Sm. This type of antibody has been previously found only in humans with SLE. The immune defect in MRL mice is associated with increased helper T cell activity and elaboration of a T cell factor that stimulates B cells. MRL-lpr/lpr mice also develop an erosive arthritis with similarities to rheumatoid arthritis. Prior to cartilage and bone destruction, dedifferentiated synovial cells migrate across cartilaginous surfaces and ultimately invade the hard tissues of the joint.

The requirement for a genetic predisposition along with exposure to the appropriate infectious agent or other environmental factor is also likely in human SLE and rheumatoid arthritis. Humans with SLE usually share similar histocompatibility antigens at the DR locus. Moreover, abnormal T cell suppressor function is seen not only in patients but also in family members. Other human illnesses that appear to occur secondary to circulating or localized immune complexes include certain adverse reactions to drugs, hypersensitivity pneumonitis, and reactions to viruses such as hepatitis B virus.

TYPE IV REACTIONS: INFLAMMATORY REACTIONS INITIATED BY MONONUCLEAR LEUKOCYTES. Lymphocyte-initiated inflammatory reactions are termed "delayed hypersensitivity" because maximal inflammatory cell accumulation does not appear for 48 to 72 hours after secondary antigenic exposure. For example, if an individual previously sensitized to the tubercle bacillus is injected locally with antigen from this organism, a delayed type of inflammatory response ensues. The foreign material is encountered first by macrophages and dendritic cells, which partially digest the antigen. This altered form of antigen is recognized by small lymphocytes that contain specific surface receptors for the antigen. Exposure to the antigen initiates synthesis and release of cytokines (Table 431–3), which diffuse to areas of the vessel wall closest to the immunologic event. Increased vascular permeability ensues; chemotactic gradients that attract macrophages and other lymphocytes result in inflammatory cell accumulation. Granulocytes precede the mononuclear cell influx, but their number is far less than in the inflammatory response mediated by immune complexes. Lymphokines also activate the macrophages, which become more metabolically active, develop higher levels of hydrolytic enzymes, and are better able to bind to and destroy tumor cells or many intracellular parasites.

Lymphocytes at the inflammatory site release lymphokines that recruit other nonsensitized lymphocytes, thus expanding the clones of cells capable of recognizing and responding to the specific antigen. If successful in complete destruction of the antigen, the inflammatory response resolves and produces no tissue necrosis. However, if the antigen is large in quantity or is difficult to digest, the inflammatory process continues. New cells arrive to replace the dying cells already present, resulting in the release of proteolytic enzymes and toxic oxygen radicals. Lesions typical of delayed hypersensitivity reactions are seen in mycobacterial and fungal diseases, sar-

TABLE 431–3. EFFECTOR MOLECULES RELEASED BY MONONUCLEAR LEUKOCYTES

Monocyte Products	Function
Colony-stimulating factors	Myeloid differentiation
Complement components	Inflammatory mediators
Interleukin-1 (IL-1)	Multiple activities including lymphocyte activation, pyrogenicity, stimulation of synovial dendritic cells
Leukotrienes	Inflammatory mediators
Lysosomal hydrolases	Proteolytic functions
Prostaglandins	Immunomodulation, bone resorption
Tumor necrosis factor-α (TNF-α)	Tumor cytolysis, IL-1–like activities
Lymphocyte Products	
Interleukin-2 (IL-2)	Lymphocyte proliferation
Interleukin-3 (IL-3)	Myeloid differentiation
Interleukin-4 (IL-4)	Lymphocyte proliferation
Interferon-γ	Immunoregulation, antiviral
Lymphocyte-derived chemotactic factor (LDCF)	Chemotaxis of mononuclear phagocytes
Osteoclast-activating factor (OAF)	Bone resorption
Transforming-growth factor-β (TGF-β)	Modulation of cellular growth and differentiation
Tumor necrosis factor-β (TNF-β)	Tumor cytolysis, IL-1–like activities

coidosis, and a number of rheumatologic disorders, including polymyositis and the granulomatous vasculitides.

MECHANISM OF TISSUE DESTRUCTION IN RHEUMATOID ARTHRITIS

The characteristic tissue reaction in rheumatoid arthritis is synovitis, in which the normally thin, loose connective tissue is replaced by a rich infiltrate of lymphocytes, macrophages, and plasma cells (see Fig. 431–1B). In the synovial fluid, the predominant inflammatory cells are the polymorphonuclear leukocytes. The cells are metabolically active: The plasma cells produce rheumatoid factors, and the mononuclear cells produce cytokines. Rheumatoid factors are immunoglobulins of the IgM, IgG, or, rarely, IgA class. These factors bind to the Fc portion of IgG antibodies, which either have combined with antigen or have been aggregated or denatured. Polymorphonuclear leukocytes taken from synovial fluids contain inclusions of immune complexes, many of which contain rheumatoid factors. Synovial fluid C levels are depressed in relation to serum levels. The turnover of C components, particularly of the classic pathway, is markedly enhanced in rheumatoid synovial fluid. Cleavage products such as C5a are present in rheumatoid synovial fluid, as are hydrolytic enzymes derived from inflammatory cells, kinins, LTB_4, and the inflammatory neuropeptide, substance P.

The sequence of events leading to synovitis and destruction of surrounding structures in rheumatoid arthritis can be envisioned as follows: Some as yet undefined antigen localizes in the synovium and is phagocytized by Type A synovial cells. The antigen is not completely destroyed and diffuses into the joint space, where it may adhere to cartilage. Binding of the processed antigen to B lymphocytes induces their differentiation to plasma cells, which then produce antibodies including rheumatoid factors upon chronic stimulation. Activation of T lymphocytes triggers lymphokine synthesis followed by blastogenesis. The role of viruses as stimulators of the immune response in rheumatoid arthritis must be considered. Rheumatoid synovial explant cells established in permanent lines exhibit many characteristics of virally transformed lymphocytes. Cell lines of the B lymphocyte variety frequently contain antigens of the Epstein-Barr virus (EBV). Sera from approximately 65 per cent of patients with rheumatoid arthritis contain antibody, called a rheumatoid arthritis precipitin (RAP), to nuclear antigens present in human lymphoblastoid cell lines infected with EBV. The antigens have been termed rheumatoid arthritis nuclear antigens (RANAs). RAPs are commonly present in sera of patients who are rheumatoid factor positive but are also found in the sera of

patients who are rheumatoid factor negative. The specificity of RAPs for rheumatoid arthritis has been questioned, as RAPs can be present in up to 20 per cent of normal individuals. In rheumatoid arthritis, there is no firm evidence to relate EBV causally to the disease, and serum antibody levels to EBV are not increased in the sera of rheumatoid arthritis patients. However, EBV does act as a polyclonal stimulator of antibody production and increases the mitogenic activity of lymphocytes. Another potential viral etiology may be related to parvovirus infection. This virus has been isolated from rheumatoid synovia, and acute parvovirus infection can cause at least a transient polyarthritis. Regardless of the initiating agent, combination of antibody with antigen, as well as combination of antigen-antibody complexes with rheumatoid factors, or self-association of rheumatoid factors, activates C as well as the kinin-forming system. This results in the production of inflammatory products such as C5a, arachidonic acid metabolites, kinins, and fibrinopeptides, which diffuse into the synovial fluid and to synovial blood vessels. These phlogistic agents enhance vascular permeability and attract polymorphonuclear leukocytes and macrophages. Polymorphonuclear leukocytes ingest the abundant immune complexes in the fluid, release lysosomal enzymes, and generate superoxide anions. This causes destruction of hyaluronate polymers in the joint fluid, as well as injury to cartilage. Cytokine and growth factor (i.e., interleukins, TNF, TGF-β, and platelet derived growth factor [PDGF]) production in the synovium leads to the further accumulation and activation of macrophages, fibroblasts, and lymphocytes.

The unique structure of the joint space is important, as enzymes present in synovial fluid or released and synthesized locally by the cells of the proliferative synovial lesion contribute to the pathology. The cartilage-degrading lysosomal enzymes collagenase and elastase are primarily derived from inflammatory cells. Proteinases released by dying cells may aid in superficial cartilage destruction by virtue of their role in uncrosslinking collagen fibrils, thus increasing their susceptibility to enzymatic degradation. Macrophages produce prostaglandins, hydrolytic enzymes, collagenase, plasminogen activator, IL-1, TNF-α, and TGF-β. The most abundant source of collagenase in the rheumatoid synovium is a synovial cell that has an unusual dendritic appearance, expresses Ia antigen, and is adherent to glass but is nonphagocytic. Collagenase synthesis by this cell is greatly enhanced by IL-1. With ongoing synovitis, early changes in cartilage involve the loss of proteoglycan content, often manifested microscopically as diminished metachromatic staining. In addition to collagenases, lysosomal proteinases can degrade aggregates of proteoglycans, and, once released from cartilage, these solubilized components are then sensitive to further enzymatic attack. The migration of the synovium (pannus) onto cartilage may be directed by the deposition of antigen there. In some synovial biopsies from patients with rheumatoid arthritis, tumor-like proliferations of dedifferentiated synovial cells can be found migrating across and into cartilage. The histopathology in these instances is similar to that seen in MRL mice.

The final stage of the destructive process, demineralization of bone, may result from combined elements present initially in the inflammatory and later in the proliferative responses. Demineralization must occur in bone before tissue is susceptible to collagenolytic enzymes. In rheumatoid synovitis, prostaglandins stimulate calcium release from bone matrix; other arachidonic acid metabolites are responsible for long-term leaching of mineral from bony matrix. In addition, bone demineralization is enhanced by heparin, which is released upon the degranulation of mast cells. Cellular mechanisms may also be operative in demineralization in that lymphocytes produce an osteoclast-activating factor (OAF). In addition, connective tissue activating peptides (CTAPs) and specific lymphokines such as lymphocyte-derived chemotactic factor

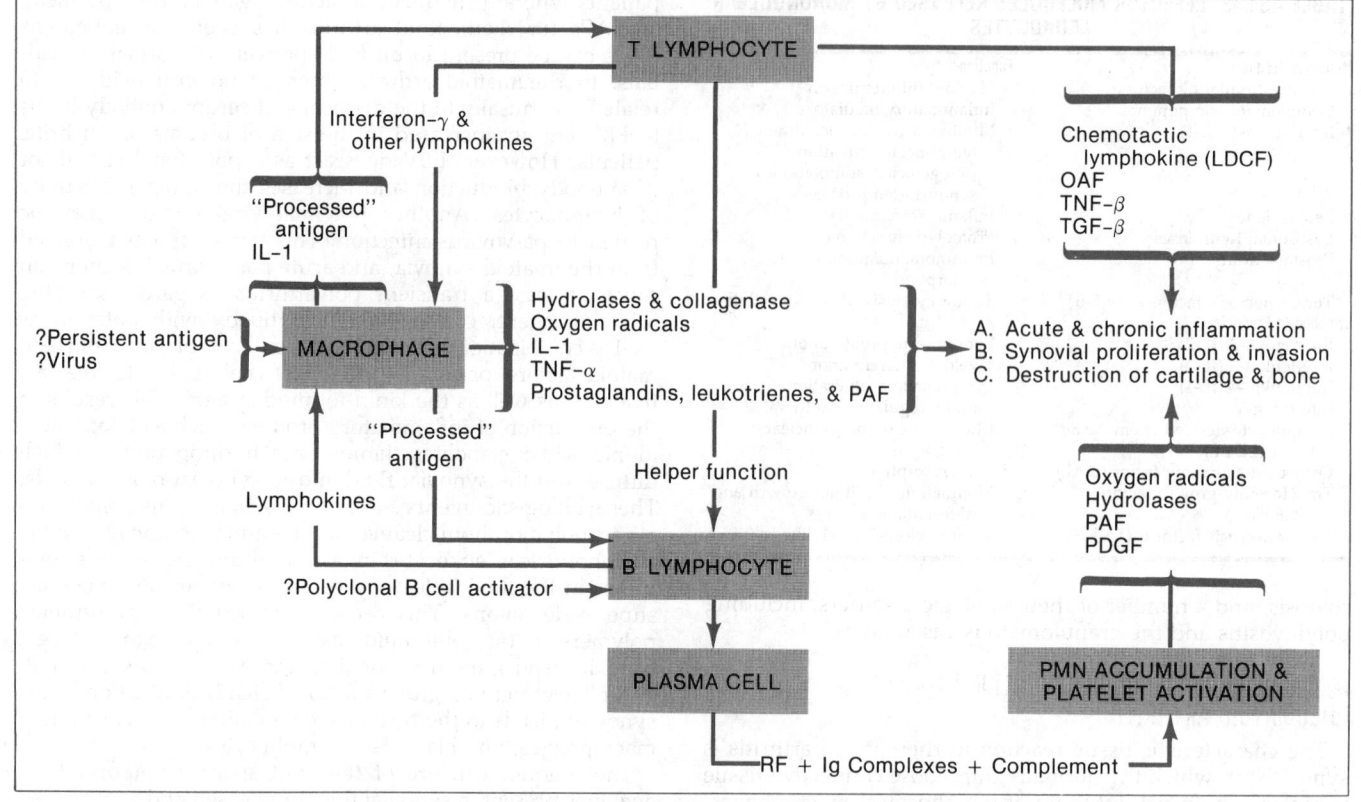

FIGURE 431–4. Model for inflammation and tissue destruction in rheumatoid arthritis. IL-1 = Interleukin 1; LDCF = lymphocyte-derived chemotactic factor; OAF = osteoclast-activing factor; PAF = platelet-activating factor; PDGF = platelet-derived growth factor; PMN = polymorphonuclear neutrophil; RF = rheumatoid factor; TGF = tumor growth factor; TNF = tumor necrosis factor.

for fibroblasts (LDCF-F) attract and stimulate fibroblasts to produce collagen and may contribute to the ultimate fibrosis in the destroyed ankylosed joint.

The net effect, resulting from either persistence of antigen or disordered regulation of T and B cell activation, is a chronic inflammatory response in the synovium (Fig. 431–4). Continued cellular proliferation and influx lead to synovial proliferation and its invasion into surrounding structures. Diffusion of collagenase, PGEs, hydrolytic enzymes, and lymphokines into cartilage and bone results in erosion of these tissues. Rheumatoid arthritis thus illustrates the devastating local tissue destruction that results from chronic inflammatory reactions produced by the immune complex and delayed hypersensitivity types of immune responses.

Alspaugh MA, Tan EM: Serum antibody in rheumatoid arthritis reactive with a cell associated antigen. Demonstration by precipitation and immunofluorescence. Arthritis Rheum 19:711, 1976. *The initial description of rheumatoid arthritis precipitins.*

Bomalaski JS, Williamson PK, Zurier RB: Prostaglandins and the inflammatory response. Clin Lab Med 3(4):695, 1983. *A detailed review of the role of prostaglandins in inflammation.*

Krane SM, Simon LS: Rheumatoid arthritis: Clinical features and pathogenetic mechanisms. *In* Snyderman R (ed.): Advances in Rheumatology. Med Clin North Am 70:263–284, 1986. *A concise review of potential pathogenetic mechanisms of rheumatoid arthritis as well as clinical features.*

McPhail LC, Snyderman R: Oxygen-dependent microbicidal activity of leukocytes. *In* Snyderman R (ed.): Contemporary Topics in Immunobiology, Vol. 14. "Regulation of Leukocyte Function." New York, Plenum Press, 1984, pp 247–281. *A comprehensive overview of oxygen metabolism in phagocytes.*

Pisetsky DS, Caster SA, Roths JB, et al.: lpr gene control of the anti-DNA antibody response. J Immunol 128:2322, 1982. *Evidence concerning the genetic regulation of anti–DNA-antibody production and an autoimmune disease is presented.*

Samuelsson B: The leukotrienes: An introduction. *In* Samuelsson B, Paoletti R (eds.): Leukotrienes and Other Lipoxygenase Products. New York, Raven

Press, 1982, pp 1–27. *An excellent review of the biochemistry of the leukotrienes and their potential biological roles.*

Smith HR, Steinberg AD: Autoimmunity—a perspective. *In* Paul WE, Fathman EG, Metzgar H (eds.): Annual Review of Immunology, Vol. 1. Palo Alto, Annual Reviews Inc., 1983, pp 175–210. *A very readable review of human and animal autoimmune disease mechanisms. Many references.*

Snyderman R, Smith CD, Verghese MW: A model for leukocyte regulation by chemoattractant receptors: Roles of a guanine nucleotide regulatory protein and polyphosphoinositide metabolism. J Leuk Biol 40:785, 1986. *A review of how chemoattractant receptors activate leukocytes. Details concerning guanine nucleotide regulatory proteins and phosphoinositide metabolism are given.*

Snyderman R, Pike MC: Transductional mechanisms of chemoattractant receptors on leukocytes. *In* Snyderman R (ed.): Contemporary Topics in Immunobiology, Vol. 14. "Regulation of Leukocyte Function." New York, Plenum Press, 1984, pp 1–28. *An up-to-date review of the biochemistry and biology of chemotactic factors and their receptors on leukocytes. Many references on inflammatory mechanisms.*

Theofilopoulos AN, Dixon FJ: Etiopathogenesis of murine SLE. Immunol Rev 55:179, 1981. *Interesting concepts and a good review of animal models of systemic lupus erythematosus.*

Theofilopoulos AN, Dixon FJ: Immune complexes in human diseases. Am J Pathol 100:531, 1980. *A comprehensive review of the role of immune complexes in human diseases.*

Wasserman SI: Mediators of immediate hypersensitivity. J Allergy Clin Immunol 72(2):101, 1983. *An exposition of the physiologic aspects of immediate types of hypersensitivity reactions.*

Weissmann G: Pathways of arachidonate oxidation to prostaglandins and leukotrienes. Sem Arth Rheu 13:123, 1983. *A recent review of arachidonate metabolism and its relevance to inflammation.*

Wofsy D, Seaman WE: Successful treatment of autoimmunity in NZB/NZW F₁ mice with monoclonal antibody to LTB₄. J Exp Med 161:378, 1985. *This provocative report, documenting the role of T cells in disease in NZB/NZW F₁ mice, suggests novel approaches to the therapy of autoimmunity.*

Wooley DE, Harris ED Jr, Mainardi CL, et al.: Collagenase immunolocalization in cultures of rheumatoid synovial cells. Science 200:773, 1978. *This article stresses the importance of the dendritic cell as a source of collagenase in rheumatoid synovium.*

Zvaifler NJ: Pathogenesis of the joint disease of rheumatoid arthritis. Am J Med 75:3, 1983. *A review of the role of various components of the immune response in rheumatoid arthritis.*

432 SPECIALIZED DIAGNOSTIC PROCEDURES IN THE RHEUMATIC DISEASES

Alan S. Cohen

An increasing number of specialized procedures are available for evaluation of patients with articular disease. Although many are useful, very few are diagnostic of a specific disorder. Laboratory data must be combined with clinical evaluation in order to arrive at a working diagnosis.

SYNOVIAL FLUID. In the patient with undiagnosed articular disease and an associated joint effusion, examination of the synovial fluid is mandatory. The preferred method of joint aspiration (most frequently the knee) is through the extensor surface, where major blood vessels and nerves are sparse and the synovial pouch is more superficial. If the synovial fluid sugar is to be measured, the patient should have fasted for six hours if possible. Careful sterile technique virtually precludes infection, the one very rare complication of arthrocentesis. The needle should be at least 19 gauge. After appropriate draping and intracutaneous instillation of 1 to 2 per cent procaine or Xylocaine, the needle is inserted through skin and subcutaneous tissue. It meets a small amount of resistance when it reaches the capsule and finally passes easily into the joint cavity. Although minimal amounts of fluid will suffice for basic studies, as a rule 6 to 10 ml will allow the necessary laboratory testing.

The synovial fluid is then ideally allocated as follows: (1) an aliquot (1 to 3 ml) in a sterile tube with heparin—for bacteriologic studies (cultures and Gram stain) or direct plating of an aliquot on appropriate culture medium; (2) an aliquot (1 ml) in a clean nonsterile tube with heparin—for routine cytology, white cell count, and differential (can also be used for mucin test and crystal examination); (3) an aliquot (2 to 3 ml) without anticoagulant in a clean nonsterile tube—for color, viscosity, clot turbidity, mucin clot test and crystals (as well as proteins, if indicated); and (4) an aliquot (2 ml) in a clean nonsterile tube with preservative—for glucose analysis with parallel determination of serum glucose.

Cultures must be obtained on all synovial fluids, since indolent bacterial infections can mimic or be superimposed on well-defined articular disease. Blood agar medium should be used; but if gonococcal infection is suspected, chocolate agar or its equivalent should be inoculated at the bedside. Appropriate cultures should be obtained if tuberculosis or fungal infection is suspected. A direct Gram stain should be performed on a concentrated specimen from the first tube, spun for 20 minutes in a clinical centrifuge.

Normal synovial fluid is a clear, pale yellow, viscous liquid that does not clot. It was appropriately named by Paracelsus because of its viscosity and physical resemblance to egg white. The few cells normally present (less than 200) are mononuclear. Although serous cavity fluids are plasma ultrafiltrates, synovial fluid is unique owing to the presence of hyaluronic acid (about 0.3 gram per deciliter) produced by the synovial lining cells. This large asymmetric molecule further influences the composition of synovial fluid, for because of its steric structure, some solute passage through the water surrounding the molecules may be hindered. Thus, according to the concept of excluded volume, the size and shape of the molecule play a large role; i.e., large molecules such as fibrinogen and macroglobulin would be excluded, and small molecules would more easily enter the compartment. The state of hyaluronate (as roughly determined by the mucin clot test) may be a primary determinant of the nature of the synovial fluid in various pathologic conditions.

When a synovial membrane is inflamed for any reason, the white cell count in the synovial fluid increases. In a rough fashion one can classify this fluid into four groups (Table 432–1). Noninflammatory effusions (Group I) occur when the white cell count is normal or minimally increased, as in traumatic arthritis or degenerative joint disease. Only rarely will such fluid have white cell counts of over 2000 cells per cubic millimeter. Noninfectious mildly inflammatory effusions (Group II) with white cell counts rarely over 5000 occur in systemic lupus erythematosus (SLE) and scleroderma. In noninfectious acute inflammatory effusions (Group III) characteristic of classic rheumatoid arthritis, gout, pseudogout, and rheumatic fever, the white cell count varies from 5,000 to 25,000 but may exceed 50,000 or even 100,000 cells per cubic millimeter. Finally, in inflammatory effusions caused by infection (Group IV) the white cell count commonly varies from 25,000 to over 100,000 cells per cubic millimeter and in some instances resembles frank pus. As the white cell count becomes elevated, the percentage of polymorphonuclear leukocytes generally increases, the hyaluronate becomes degraded, and the synovial fluid sugar falls.

Normal synovial fluid does not clot owing to the absence of several clotting factors, including fibrinogen. Pathologic fluids do contain clots, and their size is roughly proportional to the degree of inflammation. Hyaluronate degradation can be roughly assessed by diluting 1 ml of joint fluid with 4 ml of 2 per cent acetic acid solution. When the mucin is normal, a tight ropy mass forms in a clear solution. This is termed a "good" mucin. A softer mass with shreds is a "fair" mucin, whereas a "poor" mucin shows shreds and soft small masses in a turbid solution.

Under normal conditions, the total synovial fluid protein is about one quarter that of the blood. Multiple studies have been performed to assess whether specific fractions might be related to specific disease states, but findings in general are nonspecific. One may conclude that if the synovial fluid total protein is over 2.5 grams per deciliter, the fluid is not normal, and that if it is over 4.5 grams per deciliter, there is significant inflammation.

Rheumatoid factors (antigamma globulins) are also found in the synovial fluid, occasionally when they are absent from the serum. Their presence and presumed local manufacture in the synovial membrane may be of diagnostic value. Antinuclear antibodies have been found not only in the synovial fluids of patients with SLE but also in those of patients with rheumatoid arthritis and several other connective tissue diseases. Since DNA, especially in the native form, can be found free in synovial fluids from individuals with a variety of disorders, it is probable that its presence may reflect nonspecific tissue damage.

Complement levels in the synovial fluid depend upon rates of synthesis, catabolism, and local consumption and have little clinical value. The only tests widely available are immunoassays for C3 and C4 and functional assays for total complement (CH50). In rheumatoid arthritis the *serum* complement is not depressed, whereas in SLE it is low. Cryoproteins, predominantly of fibrinogen but including cryoglobulins with DNA and IgG, are also found in synovial fluids of patients with rheumatoid arthritis and other types of synovitis, and rheumatoid fluids may contain complexes with Igs, rheumatoid factors, complement, and DNA.

The intense inflammatory activity of various synovial diseases is associated with the presence of a variety of enzymes in the synovial fluid. Some, but not all, investigators have implicated lysosomal enzymes (e.g., myeloperoxidase, lactoferrin, lysozyme, chymotryptic cationic protein) in the process of joint destruction. Collagenase, collagen, and antibodies to collagen have also been extensively studied. Such investigations have advanced our concepts of the pathogenesis of synovitis (especially rheumatoid), but generally measurements of these substances have not reached the routine clinical

TABLE 432–1. SYNOVIAL FLUID ANALYSIS

Diagnosis	Appearance	Total White Cell Count per Cubic Millimeter*	Polymorphonuclear Cells	Mucin Clot Test	Synovial Fluid-Blood Glucose Difference (Mean Milligrams per Deciliter)	Miscellaneous (Crystals, Organisms)
Normal	Clear, pale yellow	0–200 (200)	<10%	Good	No significant difference†	—
Group I (noninflammatory effusions)						
Degenerative joint disease; traumatic arthritis	Clear to slightly turbid	50–4000 (600)	<30%	Good	No significant difference	—
Group II (noninfectious, mildly inflammatory effusions)						
Systemic lupus erythematosus; scleroderma	Clear to slightly turbid	0–9000 (3000)	<20%	Good (occasionally fair)	No significant difference	Occasional LE cell; decreased complement
Group III (noninfectious severe inflammatory effusions)						
Gout	Turbid	100–160,000 (21,000)	~70%	Poor	10	Monosodium urate crystals
Pseudogout	Turbid	50–75,000 (14,000)	~70%	Fair-poor	Not enough data	Calcium pyrophosphate dihydrate crystals
Rheumatoid arthritis	Turbid	250–80,000 (19,000)	~70%	Poor	30	Decreased complement
Group IV (infectious inflammatory effusions)						
Acute bacterial	Very turbid	150–250,000 (80,000)	~90%	Poor	90	Culture positive for gram-positive or gram-negative bacteria
Tuberculosis	Turbid	2500–100,000 (20,000)	~60%	Poor	70	Culture positive for *M. tuberculosis*

*Averages in parentheses.
†Less than 10 mg per deciliter difference.

domain. Other proteins and peptides (C-reactive protein, plasminogen, fibronectin, vasoactive peptides, and oxygen-derived free radicals) have also been measured in synovial fluid, but their precise role in diagnosis is not clear.

Synovial fluid normally contains little lipid, but it demonstrates increased lipid content in rheumatoid effusions. Prostaglandin E_2 appears to be elevated in the fluid of patients with inflammatory synovitis. The glucose content of synovial fluid, which normally approximates that of serum, is markedly diminished in the presence of infection and may show a modest decrease (10 to 30 mg per deciliter) in other inflammatory effusions. Several of these nonspecific parameters are collectively useful in evaluating the degree and type of inflammatory synovitis (Table 432–1).

Several types of crystals have been found in synovial fluids (Table 432–2). The two most important are monosodium urate, characteristic of gouty effusions, and calcium pyrophosphate

TABLE 432–2. SYNOVIAL FLUID CRYSTALS

Crystal	Polarization Microscopy	Other Identification
Monosodium urate	Strong negative birefringence, needle-shaped, long	Uricase digestion X-ray diffraction
Calcium pyrophosphate dihydrate (CPPD)	Weak positive birefringence, rhomboid or small rods, pleomorphic	X-ray diffraction
Calcium phosphate (hydroxyapatite)	Not easily visualized	Electron microscopy X-ray diffraction
Cholesterol	Rhombic or platelike, notched corners, multicolored, occasionally small and needle-like	Chemical determination
Corticosteroids	Pleomorphic; variable birefringence	Follows intra-articular steroid treatment

dihydrate (CPPD), characteristic of the effusions of pseudogout (crystal deposition disease). Crystals that cause inflammation are usually 0.5 to 20 μm in length, sparingly soluble in water, and capable of being phagocytized. At the peak of inflammation most are intracellular. Other crystals such as calcium hydroxyapatite, calcium oxalate, cholesterol, and corticosteroid esters may also be associated with inflammatory effusions.

Crystals are demonstrated in synovial fluid (collected without oxalate) by examining a drop of synovial fluid placed on a slide and covered with a thin glass coverslip for examination in the polarizing microscope. Birefringent materials demonstrate two refractive indices when plane polarized light passes through them. The birefringence is termed positive when the crystals (which then appear blue) are aligned parallel to the slow rays of the retardation plate (first-order red plate compensator) and negative when the crystals appear yellow when in parallel alignment (blue when perpendicular). On polarization microscopy the monosodium urate crystals demonstrate strong negative birefringence and are usually long (8 to 10 μm) and needle-like in appearance. They may occur extracellularly or within polymorphonuclear or mononuclear cells. They are almost invariably in effusions associated with acute gout and are virtually diagnostic. They may, however, be present in gouty fluids between attacks. The CPPD crystals are often broader than urate crystals, may show a faint "line" down their center, appear parallelopiped, and in the polarizing microscope exhibit a weak positive birefringence. They have a significant association with acute attacks of arthritis in patients with chondrocalcinosis (articular cartilage calcification).

Other crystals identified in synovial fluid include hydroxyapatite (calcium phosphate) crystals, which are minute and identified only with special techniques; plate-like cholesterol crystals seen in some rheumatoid effusions; and the rare corticosteroid crystals found after intra-articular steroid treatment. All are capable of inducing a synovitis.

Under certain circumstances joint fluids, when nontraumatically aspirated, may demonstrate gross blood. One must consider bleeding disorders such as hemophilia, overdosage with anticoagulants, rare lesions such as pigmented villonodular synovitis and joint tumor, as well as neuropathic and traumatic forms of arthritis.

Careful examination of synovial fluid may on occasion reveal malignant cells, LE cells, sickled RBCs, fat droplets suggestive of fracture, or amyloid fragments.

SYNOVIAL MEMBRANE HISTOPATHOLOGY. Synovial membrane is a non–basement membrane–lined, highly vascular structure consisting of several cell types (macrophages, fibroblasts, and possibly intermediate cells). It proliferates extensively during inflammation, such that synovial biopsy is often useful in establishing a diagnosis. The procedure is simple and may be an extension of the synovial fluid aspiration technique, using a wider bore Parker-Pearson needle. A specimen can also be obtained by arthroscopy or open surgical biopsy.

Although in the common rheumatic diseases (rheumatoid arthritis, degenerative joint disease, SLE) there are no common pathognomonic synovial membrane findings, the patterns of histologic involvement may be diagnostically useful. For example, severe synovial lining proliferation and especially the presence of lymphoid follicles are characteristic of rheumatoid arthritis, whereas the SLE membrane shows only minimal hyperplasia but may show dense surface fibrin and perivascular mononuclear infiltrates; rarely a pathognomonic hematoxylin body will be seen.

The procedure is very useful in the diagnosis of tuberculosis, atypical mycobacterial disease, or fungal disease; the demonstration of an organism in section (or in culture) or a caseating granuloma with giant cells virtually establishes the diagnosis. Other instances in which the synovial biopsy could be helpful include hemochromatosis (in which iron is seen in the synovial lining cell), pigmented villonodular synovitis (villous hypertrophy, hemosiderin deposits with numerous giant cells), tumors (malignant cells in synovium), and ochronosis (fragments of pigmented cartilage in synovium). Although in properly fixed tissue (use of absolute alcohol) one can observe the crystals associated with gout on histologic examination, the procedure is not necessary to establish this diagnosis, since examination of synovial fluid so commonly demonstrates the crystals.

ACUTE PHASE PHENOMENA. The ancient Greeks observed the sedimentation of blood following venesection and used it as a basic diagnostic tool. It was reintroduced by Fahraeus and refined by Westergren, whose method is in common use today. The sedimentation rate is only one, albeit the most popular, of the acute phase phenomena utilized by rheumatologists to follow inflammation in their patients. Acute phase reactions refer to the increases in certain plasma proteins that occur after an extraordinary variety of tissue damage, i.e., toxic, chemical, infectious, inflammatory, or malignant. The functions of most of these proteins are not known, although presumably the damage led to increased protein synthesis via macrophage-derived mediators. Only the sedimentation rate and C-reactive protein (CRP) will be briefly discussed here.

The basic measurement in the Westergren sedimentation rate is the rate of fall of erythrocytes in plasma; when rouleaux formation occurs owing primarily to increases in asymmetric proteins such as fibrinogen or macroglobulins (that alter the red cell zeta potential), the red cells sediment more rapidly. The original normal values are a 1 to 3 mm fall in one hour for men and a 4 to 7 mm fall in one hour for women. These levels may be elevated during menses or by certain drugs and appear to increase with aging. The cause of the last-named phenomenon is not clear despite several reports that seem to

document it well. Many now accept sedimentation rates of 0 to 10 mm per hour for men and 0 to 15 mm per hour for women and suggest that the values may be as much as 10 mm per hour higher after age 50. Whether these represent changes in serum proteins with aging or undetected disease in the normal person is not yet clear. In the rheumatic diseases, however, the value of this determination is that when elevated (and it is often in the 30 to 100 mm per hour range), it can be an index for following the severity of inflammation and, when falling, for following the response to therapy. In addition, disorders such as temporal arteritis are often associated with sedimentation rates of over 100 mm per hour.

One must be constantly aware, however, of the lack of specificity of this determination and that in selected series highly elevated sedimentation rates (over 100 mm per hour) are more commonly due to infections or malignancies. It is also documented that a small number of patients can have an active rheumatic disease (i.e., rheumatoid arthritis) with a normal sedimentation rate.

The CRP until recently has played little role in the evaluation of rheumatic diseases, although it has been the prototype acute phase reactant—virtually absent in normal conditions and appearing in large quantities in inflammation. It was named for its property of precipitating with pneumococcal cell wall polysaccharide. In recent years it has been isolated and characterized as a pentameric structure, and its molecular weight and primary structure have been determined. It has many homologies with a protein (AP) found uniquely in amyloid disease but is immunologically distinct.

Along with SAA (an acute phase reactant first identified in amyloidosis), CRP is an inducible acute phase protein, and both are quantitative and specific markers of inflammation. Their extremely short half-lives result in rapid evidence of response to treatment or detection of flares, whereas proteins such as fibrinogen and macroglobulins which bring about alterations in sedimentation rate have plasma half-lives approximately 50-fold greater than SAA and CRP. Unlike CRP, technical aspects of SAA measurement make it unavailable for routine clinical use.

RHEUMATOID FACTORS. Fifty years ago, when Cecil and coworkers found high titers of "streptococcal agglutinators" in the sera of some rheumatoid patients, they were actually alluding to rheumatoid factors. Such factors are now defined as antibodies (present largely in the IgM fraction, but in other Ig fractions as well) to determinants of the Fc fragment of numerous animal (especially human and rabbit) IgGs. As antibodies they possess the characteristics of such proteins. They were named when their frequency in the sera of patients with rheumatoid arthritis (about 70 per cent) was observed. They lack both sensitivity and specificity in the detection of rheumatoid syndromes.

Most clinical tests depend upon the detection of IgM antibodies. In such assays particles (red blood cells or latex or bentonite particles) are coated with immunoglobulin G, mixed with the test serum, and observed for appropriate agglutination or flocculation. Various standardization procedures exist as well as different tube dilutions that are interpreted as positive. Internal standardization as well as the use of cross-reference laboratories is important.

The IgM antibody reacts with IgG to form a soluble complex that sediments in the ultracentrifuge with a coefficient of 22. In addition, IgG-IgG complexes sedimenting at an intermediate range can also occur, as well as larger, insoluble IgM-IgG complexes. In some instances the IgM rheumatoid factor is firmly bound to autologous IgG such that it is not detected on routine agglutination tests. Gel filtration under mildly acid conditions dissociates these IgG and IgM fractions. When the rheumatoid factor activity is found in such instances, the term "hidden rheumatoid factor" is sometimes applied.

Rheumatoid factors are uncommon in children with chronic

arthritis. High titers have been correlated with severe progressive rheumatoid arthritis in patients with multiple rheumatoid nodules, vasculitis, skin ulcers, and other visceral manifestations. Rheumatoid factors are found in many diseases other than rheumatoid arthritis (other connective tissue diseases, leprosy, leishmaniasis, liver disease, tuberculosis). In some series of subacute bacterial endocarditis 50 per cent of the patients will transiently show rheumatoid factors in their sera. Family studies of seropositive rheumatoid propositi suggest that there is a higher incidence in its members.

Since rheumatoid factors have been induced experimentally with bacterial antigens and since they are so commonly associated with chronic infectious diseases, the concept that an as yet unknown infectious agent or agents may play a pathogenetic role in rheumatoid disease is still under active investigation. Data thus far suggest that rheumatoid factor is an epiphenomenon and not a direct cause of rheumatoid arthritis.

The absence of rheumatoid factors in well-defined groups of rheumatoid variants has led to the classification of seronegative spondyloarthritis for disorders such as psoriatic arthritis, ankylosing spondylitis, forms of juvenile chronic polyarthritis, and Reiter's syndrome.

ANTINUCLEAR ANTIBODIES AND THE LE CELL. The discovery of the LE cell by Hargraves in 1948 and subsequent studies demonstrating a lupus factor that reacted with nuclear material opened the door to a series of immunologic investigations that have led to new concepts of pathogenesis, diagnosis, and clinical course of SLE and related disorders. The LE factor was initially regarded as a 7S immunoglobulin, but it is now known that this is only one of many autoantibodies in lupus sera, and that these occur in all immunoglobulin classes, although most are IgGs.

The prototype LE cell is a phagocytic polymorphonuclear cell containing (on Wright's stain) a homogeneous purple nuclear inclusion surrounded by a rim of cytoplasm and a compressed nucleus. It is produced in vitro from blood samples but can be found on direct examination of synovial, pleural, peritoneal, and pericardial fluid. It represents phagocytized deoxyribonucleoprotein (DNA-histone complex) and has as its tissue equivalent the isolated hematoxylin body. The LE cell can be present in other connective tissue diseases. However, it is technically a time-consuming test and has been largely replaced by other immunologic procedures.

The fluorescence of isolated nuclear constituents or cells (especially the nuclei) on tissue slides after exposure to test sera was found to provide the most practical method for defining these antigen-antibody interactions (antinuclear antibodies) in a simple and reproducible fashion (Table 432–3). This approach led to the general concept of multiple antibodies to nuclear antigens (ANAs) and to the use of various cell substrates, i.e., rat liver cells, mouse kidney or liver cells, or human tissue culture cell lines. The test is usually performed in two steps: first the screening of the serum with rat liver tissue or more recently the human cell line (Hep-2) as the substrate, and the pattern identification and then the use of one or more specific procedures to define the nature of the

antigen. A homogeneous pattern of nuclear fluorescence indicates the presence of an antideoxyribonucleoprotein (LE cell factor), a peripheral (rim) pattern suggests the presence of anti-DNA antibody, and a speckled pattern reflects a variety of extractable nuclear antigens (ENA) that can be solubilized from the nucleus. By appropriate dilution of sera, titers of antibody can be determined. Unfortunately the use of a variety of kits and of various substrates (mouse liver cells, buccal cells, tissue culture cells) has made standardization difficult. Recently, however, reference sera have been made available from the Centers for Disease Control (Atlanta)—Arthritis Foundation.

Certain generalizations can be made, although the correlations are not absolute and exceptions occur. Indeed, there are patients with SLE in whose sera antinuclear antibodies cannot be identified. These patients are few (2 to 15 per cent), usually owing to the use of a less sensitive substrate, presence of autoantibodies against cytoplasmic rather than nuclear antigens, or inactive disease. It is truly rare for an SLE patient to have a negative immunofluorescence test when the Hep-2 cell substrate is used. In the identification of the specific antibody, methods such as double gel diffusion (Ouchterlony), counter immunoelectrophoresis, enzyme-linked immunoassays (ELISA), radioimmunoassays (RIA), and passive hemagglutination (PHA) may be of value.

From a pathogenetic point of view it is likely that multiple immunologic aberrations, seen particularly in SLE, do mediate certain aspects of the disease and may be responsible for renal and other tissue damage. Anti-DNA antibodies are heterogeneous and can have different specificities to distinct antigenic sites on the DNA molecule (Table 432–3). Of diagnostic, therapeutic, and prognostic importance is the presence of antibodies to double-strand DNA (dsDNA). They are closely associated with SLE and are related to active renal disease. Anti-dsDNA can be identified by an indirect immunofluorescence method using the kinetoplast of the hemoflagellate *Crithidia luciliae*, by PHA, or by RIA employing radiolabeled DNA. Antibodies that react only with single-stranded DNA are not highly specific and have been observed in patients with Sjögren's syndrome, rheumatoid arthritis, SLE, and a number of nonrheumatologic conditions associated with tissue damage.

Antibodies to deoxyribonucleoprotein are present in many patients with SLE, but they also occur in other connective tissue diseases and in unaffected relatives and may be present in moderate titers for years in asymptomatic SLE patients. They are the antibodies related to the LE cell phenomenon. Autoantibodies reactive with histones are detectable in more than 95 per cent of patients with drug-induced LE, in SLE, and in RA patients (Table 432–3). Anti-histone antibodies can have class specificity in certain diseases; for instance, in procainamide-induced LE, the antibodies are frequently directed to the complex H2A-H2B, and in the hydralazine-induced LE, the histone antibodies appear to be against the individual histones H2A and H3. Patients with SLE in general have a wider variety of antibodies and can react with all major classes of histones.

The study of the ENA, an acidic component, has led to the discovery that it contains several constituents. Antibodies against one, termed Sm antigen, are specifically associated with SLE but are found in only 20 to 30 per cent of such patients. Another, antiribonucleoprotein (anti-N1-RNP), has led to the identification of mixed connective tissue disease (MCTD). Anti-U1-RNP is also found in SLE, scleroderma, and polymyositis, as well as in MCTD (Table 432–4). Even more recently, antigens associated with Sjögren's syndrome—SS-B, an acidic nuclear antigen (cross-reactive with Ro antigen of cytoplasmic extracts), and SS-A antigen, a similar antigen (cross-reactive with La cytoplasmic antigen)—have been described. They occur in about 60 per cent of patients with Sjögren's syndrome and in smaller subsets of patients with

TABLE 432–3. AUTOANTIBODIES TO DNA AND HISTONES

Antibody Reactive with	Clinical Association
Double-strand DNA only	SLE. Rare cases reported.
Double/single-strand DNA with reaction of immunologic identity	SLE (60–70%). Rarely in other diseases where it is usually in low titer
Single-strand DNA only. Antigenic determinants related to exposed purines and pyrimidines	SLE, other rheumatic diseases, and certain nonrheumatic diseases
Histones (H1, H2A, H2B, H3, H4)	Drug-induced LE (95–100%), rheumatoid arthritis (15–20%), and SLE (30%)

Reprinted with permission from Tan EM: Autoantibodies to nuclear antigens (ANA): Their immunobiology and medicine. Adv Immunol 33:172, 1982.

TABLE 432–4. AUTOANTIBODIES TO NONHISTONE NUCLEAR PROTEINS AND RNA-PROTEIN COMPLEXES

Antibody Reactive with	Clinical Association
*Sm antigen	SLE (30–40%). Marker antibody
Nuclear ribonucleoprotein (nRNP) or U1-RNP	MCTD (95–100%), other ANAs absent; in SLE, usually other ANAs present
SS-A/Ro antigen	Sjögren's syndrome (60–70%), SLE (30–40%); neonatal lupus syndrome
SS-B/La antigen	Sjögren's syndrome (50–60%), SLE (10–15%)
*Scl-70	Scleroderma (15–20%). Marker antibody
*Centromere/kinetochore	CREST (70–90%). Marker antibody
RANA (rheumatoid arthritis associated nuclear antigen)	RA (90–95%)
Ma antigen	SLE (20%), severe course
PCNA (proliferating cell nuclear antigen)	SLE (5–10%)
PM-1	Polymyositis/scleroderma overlap (87%) Dermatomyositis (17%)
Mi-1	Dermatomyositis (11%)
*Jo-1	Polymyositis (31%). Marker antibody
Ku	Polymyositis/scleroderma overlap (55%)

Reprinted with permission from Tan EM: Autoantibodies to nuclear antigens (ANA): Their immunobiology and medicine. Adv Immunol 33:173, 1982, with modification

*Marker antibody.

SLE (SS-A in 30 to 40 per cent; SS-B in 10 to 15 per cent). SS-A (Ro) can cross the placental barrier and is regarded as a marker for neonatal lupus, often with complete heart block. Other significant associations and possibly marker antibodies exist. In scleroderma, the Scl-70 antibody (topoisomerase 1), while present in only 15 to 20 per cent of such patients, is relatively specific. Anti-kinetochore (centromere) antibody occurs in about 30 per cent of such patients but appears in over 90 per cent of those with CREST subset. Antibodies to Jo-1 are present in about 30 per cent of patients with polymyositis but may recognize a subset with interstitial pulmonary fibrosis. The accepted antigens and antibodies and an estimate of their prevalence in disease are listed in Tables 432–3 and 432–4.

In addition to these, another nuclear antigen, termed RANA, has been found to have a close association with the Epstein-Barr virus (EBV) and also a high association with rheumatoid arthritis. Whether this simply represents a marker for rheumatoid arthritis or implicates the EBV in the pathogenesis of the disease remains to be seen.

Tests for cell-mediated immunity and for circulating immune complexes (CIC) are of interest, but currently their significance in the rheumatic diseases is not well defined. CIC occur in infectious diseases, neoplastic states, and glomerulonephritis as well as rheumatic diseases. Methods of measurement are multiple and include the Raji cell assay, C1q binding assay, bovine conglutinin assay, and staphylococcal binding assay. Levels often correlate with disease activity but have no demonstrated value over other rheumatologic tests and should not be part of a routine evaluation.

RADIOGRAPHIC TECHNIQUES IN THE DIAGNOSIS OF ARTICULAR DISEASES. *Clinical Radiology of Joints.* Skeletal radiographs can contribute to the diagnosis of articular diseases because the bone and joint changes reflect the basic pathology. Proper integration depends upon an understanding of the pathophysiology of the various diseases and an appreciation of the typically affected areas. This discussion will highlight general patterns and differential diagnostic aspects of major diseases. The simplest classification is that used in assessing synovial fluid, i.e., inflammatory and noninflammatory articular disease.

General radiologic features of noninflammatory disease (such as degenerative disease) include uneven narrowing of the joint space, sclerosis of juxta-articular bone, and the presence of bone spurs and cysts. Target areas include the distal interphalangeal and first carpometacarpal and metatarsophalangeal joints, acromioclavicular joint, vertebral column, hip, and knee, with the appearance of genu varum.

Inflammatory joint disease (such as rheumatoid arthritis) is generally characterized by local bony demineralization, erosions, and uniform narrowing of the joint space. The pattern includes bilateral symmetry with involvement of the metacarpophalangeal joints, ulnar styloid area, and glenohumeral and atlantoaxial joints, as well as metatarsophalangeal joints. Involvement of the knees leads to genu valgum.

In addition there are patterns of change that assist in the differentiation of several types of inflammatory articular disease. For example, in tophaceous gouty arthritis the eroded joint may demonstrate an "overhanging ledge," as opposed to the erosion of rheumatoid arthritis. It may show asymmetric intra- and extra-articular erosions, as opposed to the marginal intra-articular erosions of rheumatoid arthritis. Gout does not lead to osteopenia, and joint space narrowing will be a late phenomenon rather than an early manifestation as it is in rheumatoid arthritis.

In the seronegative spondyloarthropathies (e.g., psoriatic arthritis) the articular involvement is less likely to be symmetrical, the interphalangeal joints of the feet may be more involved than the metatarsophalangeals, osteopenia is uncommon, and periosteal new bone formation may be seen as well as bony ankylosis. Finally, evidence of sacroiliitis with narrowing, erosions, sclerosis, and ultimate obliteration of the sacroiliac joint is common. Descriptions of specific changes, such as calcinosis in scleroderma and polymyositis and aseptic necrosis (osteonecrosis) associated with SLE, are detailed in the chapters devoted to the individual disease entities.

Several additional principles should be stressed in the radiographic examination of joints. First, films are of little value if they are not of good technical quality. Occasionally, for fine points, microradiography (high resolution magnification radiography) can clarify whether or not an erosion or lesion is present. Second, the use of radiography must be selective and usually can be limited both for safety and cost effectiveness. For example, in evaluating rheumatoid arthritis: (1) in the upper extremities, the key films are those of the hands (including the wrists) in posteroanterior and 15 degree oblique views; (2) in the neck, a lateral view in flexion alone will give sufficient data; and (3) in the feet, posteroanterior and lateral views without the oblique will often suffice. To assess degenerative joint disease of the knee, it is vital to include a standing anteroposterior view of both knees in one frame. For examination of the patient with seronegative spondyloarthropathy, limited views of the spine—i.e., a posteroanterior view of the pelvis to visualize the sacroiliac joints, anteroposterior and lateral views of the lumbosacral spine, and a lateral view of the neck in flexion—may suffice.

Joint Scintigraphy—Radioisotopes in the Evaluation of Articular Disease. The use of labeled isotopes in tracer amounts to measure their accumulation over normal and pathologic joints for the assessment of articular disease was introduced in the 1960's. The isotope evaluated first was technetium-99m (^{99m}Tc) pertechnetate, which largely binds to serum protein and is localized in areas of increased tissue vascularity. These scans correlate well with clinical assessment of joints and routine radiography, and on occasion allow the earlier detection of inflammation (increased blood flow). However, they are nonspecific, usually do not add significantly to routine radiography, and add (albeit a small amount) to the total body exposure.

The introduction of the bone seeking isotope ^{99m}Tc-diphosphonate added a new dimension to scintigraphy, since this allowed better evaluation of the axial skeleton. In many centers this has become the scan of choice. It can on occasion localize early sacroiliac inflammation prior to routine radiography, since new bone is laid down in the involved sacroiliac joint. However, it, too, gives nonspecific results (the lesions of degenerative joint disease are often not distinguishable from those of rheumatoid arthritis), and the other problems noted above pertain. A negative scintigram is believed to be predictive of the absence of serious articular disease. However, in assessments of normal individuals an occasional joint has appeared positive. Scintigraphy has an important role in the detection of osteomyelitis, bone tumors, and metabolic bone disease.

The routine history, physical examination, selected laboratory studies, and selected routine radiographs make the use of joint scintigraphy a procedure to be chosen by experts for a specific purpose rather than a routine part of the work-up of a patient with arthritis.

Arthrography (Synoviography). The injection of a contrast medium, often together with air or carbon dioxide, to visualize a joint space has become an accepted diagnostic procedure. Its value lies in the assessment of internal derangements of a joint space (usually a knee or shoulder) rather than in diagnosing inflammatory disease. The usual contraindications are infection or a bleeding diathesis. The radiopaque dye is introduced and the radiograph obtained promptly to determine its dispersion.

Orthopedists use the technique widely (as well as arthroscopy) in the diagnosis of cartilage tears in the knee and rotator cuff injuries of the shoulder. It is of great value medically in assessing masses in the popliteal area. When the differential diagnosis of deep venous thrombosis versus a ruptured popliteal cyst arises, venography is almost always indicated as a prior procedure.

Synovial cysts in rheumatoid disease, e.g., popliteal (Baker's) cysts, may rupture and lead to pain and discomfort about the knee and in the gastrocnemius area. Often the differential diagnosis is between acute thrombophlebitis and ruptured synovial cyst. When thrombophlebitis has been excluded, arthrography can often define the medical problem. On occasion, large synovial cysts can be instrumental in the development of thrombophlebitis caused by the pressure effect. Synovial cysts can occur about other joints but usually are asymptomatic.

Arthroscopy. Arthroscopy is an endoscopic procedure that has widespread orthopedic use. Its major application is in injuries about the knee joint, especially meniscal and cruciate tears. With advancing technology the procedure has also been utilized in other articular spaces.

It is occasionally used by the rheumatologist in undiagnosed monarticular knee disease as a method of obtaining a selective biopsy from a local area of the joint under direct observation. It is not, however, a routine procedure and should only be performed by those with appropriate expertise.

Miscellaneous. Other technologies have been applied to the diagnostic evaluation of articular disease. These include angiography (useful in defining synovial tumors), ultrasonic scanning (increasingly helpful in the assessment of intact popliteal cysts), and, most recently, computed tomography of the joint space. All these procedures have limited utility.

Bartfield H, Epstein WV: Rheumatoid factors and their biological significance. Ann NY Acad Sci 168:1, 1969. *A volume devoted to clinical and investigative aspects of the nature of rheumatoid factors and their relevance to disease.*

Cohen AS (ed.): Laboratory Diagnostic Procedures in the Rheumatic Diseases. 3rd ed. Orlando, FL, Grune & Stratton, Inc., 1985. *A definitive review of the methodology and interpretation of laboratory tests in rheumatology.*

Dixon AS, Rasker JJ: Synoviography. Clin Rheum Dis 2:129, 1976. *A fine exposition of synoviography (arthrography) of various joints and the information to be gleaned from these procedures.*

Egeland T, Munthe E: Rheumatoid factors. Clin Rheum Dis 9:135–160, 1983. *A thorough and up-to-date review of the history of RFs, their specificity, assay, biologic and pathologic effects, and clinical significance.*

Forrester DM, Brown JC (eds.): Radiologic investigation in rheumatology. Clin Rheum Dis 9:289–488, 1983. *Eleven papers covering scintigraphic imaging,* computed tomography, sonography, arthrography, and standard radiography in the rheumatic diseases. A British view.

Fritzler MJ: Antinuclear antibodies in the investigation of rheumatic diseases. Bull Rheum Dis 35:1–10, 1985. *Excellent review including an algorithm to indicate the diagnostic approach to the use of ANAs in clinical rheumatology.*

Goldenberg DL, Cohen AS: Synovial membrane histopathology in the differential diagnosis of rheumatoid arthritis, gout, pseudogout, systemic lupus erythematosus, infectious arthritis and degenerative joint disease. Medicine 57:239, 1978. *An analysis of synovial membrane histopathology in the common inflammatory articular diseases, pointing out patterns that are diagnostically useful even though individual pathognomonic findings are rare.*

Hadler NM, Spitznagel JK, Quinet RJ: Lysosomal enzymes in inflammatory synovial effusions. J Immunol 123:572, 1979. *A useful study of lysosomal enzymes of synovial fluid that discusses both sides of the question as to whether these enzymes are major causes of articular tissue destruction.*

Harris ED Jr, Krane SM: Collagenases. N Engl J Med 291:557, 605, 652, 1974. *A scholarly review of an increasingly important enzyme (collagenase) that might itself (or through its inhibitor) play a role in cartilage destruction.*

Jackson RW, Dandy DJ: Arthroscopy of the Knee. New York, Grune & Stratton, 1976. *A simple text that outlines the advantages and hazards of arthroscopy.*

Kushner I, Volanakis JE, Gewurtz H: C-reactive protein and the plasma protein response to tissue injury. Ann NY Acad Sci 389:1–482, 1982. *The latest update of the chemistry and significance of C-reactive protein.*

Nakamura RM, Peebles CL, Rubin RL, et al.: Autoantibodies to Nuclear Antigens. 2nd ed. Chicago, American Society for Clinical Pathology Press, 1985. *An authoritative review of antinuclear antibodies and their clinical significance by major contributors.*

Ng KC, Brown KA, Perry JD, et al.: Anti RANA antibody: A marker for seronegative and seropositive rheumatoid arthritis. Lancet 1:447, 1980. *An interesting test relating to rheumatoid arthritis that may have pathogenetic significance.*

Resnick D, Niwayam G: Diagnosis of Bone and Joint Disorders with Emphasis on Articular Abnormalities, Vols 1–3. Philadelphia, W. B. Saunders Company, 1981. *An extensive review of the radiologic findings in articular diseases.*

Ropes MW, Bauer W: Synovial Fluid Change in Joint Disease. Cambridge, MA, Harvard University Press, 1953. *The definitive work on synovial fluid analysis in various articular diseases. The data on synovial fluid white counts, differentials, mucin, clot, etc., of 35 years ago are still valid and represent the basis for most subsequent joint fluid analyses.*

Rosenspire KC, Kennedy AC, Russomanno L, et al.: Comparisons of four methods of analysis of ⁹⁹ᵐTc pyrophosphate uptake in RA joints. J Rheumatol 7:461, 1980. *One of the first critical comparisons of the value and limitations of various methods of joint scintigraphy.*

---

433 RHEUMATOID ARTHRITIS

J. Claude Bennett

Rheumatoid arthritis (RA) is a chronic systemic inflammatory process characterized by a pattern of morbidity in diarthrodial joints. Tendons, ligaments, fascia, muscle, and bone can be jeopardized by the inflammatory process. Mediators of inflammation can extend the involvement into many different organ structures.

For uniformity in investigative protocols and epidemiologic studies, the American Rheumatism Association (ARA) has established a set of diagnostic criteria (Table 433–1). These criteria are not based on theoretic knowledge of the etiology and pathogenesis of RA; current knowledge is insufficient for such a purpose. Accordingly, criteria developed to ensure the absence of bias from statistical summaries should not be taken as definitive in case-by-case clinical practice.

Also established in the same source are 20 criteria that exclude a diagnosis of RA. These criteria indicate other rheumatic diseases that mimic some of the early signs of RA. Advances in rheumatology since these criteria were revised (1958) would make it possible to extend the list considerably today.

RA occurs worldwide in all races and ethnic groups. By the usual diagnostic criteria the disease (or family of diseases?) is two or three times more prevalent among females than among males, but application of narrower criteria such as seropositivity (presence of rheumatoid factors [RF]; see below under Etiology) or roentgenographic indications of tissue erosion show less association with gender. The peak incidence of

TABLE 433–1. ARA DIAGNOSTIC CRITERIA FOR RA

Among these criteria only the finding of morning stiffness can be based on patient's report. The first five criteria must be found continuously for at least six weeks. Classic RA requires 7 of the 11. Definite RA requires 5 of the 11.

Morning stiffness
Pain on motion or tenderness in at least one joint
Swelling in at least one joint
Swelling in a second joint (any interval free of joint symptoms between the two joint involvements may not be more than three months)
Simultaneous involvement of the same joint on both sides of the body
Subcutaneous nodules on bony prominences or extensor surfaces or in juxta-articular regions
Roentgenographic findings typical of RA
Positive agglutination test result for rheumatoid factor
A poor mucin precipitate (with shreds and cloudy solution) obtained on adding synovial fluid to dilute acetic acid
Characteristic histologic changes in the synovium
Characteristic histologic changes in subcutaneous nodules

onset is between the fourth and sixth decades, but the prevalence continues to increase into the seventh decade. Determinations of overall prevalence in various studies of various populations have ranged from 0.3 to 1.5 per cent. We may take 1 per cent as a rough figure for the prevalence of RA in the general adult population.

ETIOLOGY. The etiology of RA is currently the subject of much research, as it has been for decades. Little of substance has been definitely established. Metabolic, endocrine, nutritional, genetic, geographic, occupational, and psychosocial factors have been considered, as has, of course, the possibility of an origin in infection. The areas in which research is most active today are abnormalities in the regulation of the immune system, and infection by one or more agents.

Rheumatoid factors (RF) are antibodies against an antigenic site located on the Fc portion of IgG molecules. They are produced by B cells in the blood and other tissues, including synovial tissue. They occur in the circulating blood in approximately four out of five patients. These cases are called seropositive. RF also occur in a variety of other diseases usually associated with hyperglobulinemic states such as cirrhosis, leprosy, schistosomiasis, and sarcoidosis, and in 1 to 5 per cent of normal subjects with an increasing incidence in older individuals.

High titers of RF are associated with more severe and active joint disease and with the presence of rheumatoid nodules. RF may react only with autologous IgGs or with isologous ones and sometimes even with the IgG of other species (heterologous) as well. IgM RF can react with five IgG molecules to produce very large complexes with sedimentation constants of 22S. Intermediate-size complexes (between 7S and 19S) containing only IgG molecules, some of which have rheumatoid activity against self and usually consist of three molecules, can be discerned. There is some evidence that these complexes occur to a greater extent in those individuals with widespread systemic disease and vasculitis.

Seropositive RA, at least, clearly can be classified as an autoimmune disorder, since RF are antibodies against autologous IgG. The cause of their production remains unknown. The antigenic epitope on the Fc portion of the IgG molecule appears to be absent or inaccessible in normal IgG. Alteration in the IgG could be caused by its binding to some specific antigen. Some evidence for this is provided by findings of RF in bacterial endocarditis and in other diseases involving chronic antigenic stimulation. Association has been found between RA and the Epstein-Barr virus, a polyclonal stimulator of B cells. It has been suggested that RF may be produced in certain individuals as a result of a special host response to this virus.

Despite the extremely strong association of RF with RA,

they clearly do not cause the disease, since they occur with other diseases and sometimes in healthy individuals, and furthermore because transfusion of RF into normal volunteers does not initiate inflammation. Nonetheless, the association indicates some fundamental process taking place within the synovial tissues. Multicentric immunoreactivity in various synovial tissues, with a dependence on the total available clonal repertoires, may be involved. The B lymphocytes of susceptible individuals may react in special ways against a variety of antigens and subsequently stimulate the production of RF.

There are numerous examples of polyarthritis in association with microorganisms, including the streptococci, clostridia, diphtheroids, and mycoplasmas. Associations of several viral diseases with inflammatory rheumatic syndromes suggest that RA itself could be caused by a virus. The striking synovitis sometimes seen following rubella infections and the arthritis that may precede the onset of jaundice in infectious hepatitis are interesting examples of such associations. The Ross River virus can produce an epidemic syndrome that clinically resembles systemic-onset juvenile chronic arthritis. Profound joint manifestations can be produced by the arboviruses, particularly of the togavirus family. Recently considerable interest has centered on the possibility that a parvovirus may be associated with an RA-like disease. Lyme arthritis, which is caused by a spirochete, can become a chronic rheumatoid disease, although clearly separable from RA. Many animal models of RA are caused by microorganisms or their products. Others involve immunologic reactivity against adjuvant or against bacterial cell wall peptidoglycans. All of these models involve erosive, destructive, fibrosing joint pathology.

The MRL-1 mouse provides an interesting animal model in which a syndrome closely resembling RA is evidently genetic in origin, without apparent dependence on any infectious agent. Further, a great deal of intensive research has failed to produce any direct evidence for an infectious origin of RA.

PATHOLOGY. The first apparent events in the rheumatoid synovium include microvascular injury and moderate proliferation of synovial lining cells. These are generally taken to be cause and effect, but opinions differ as to which is which. They are accompanied by edema or inflammation. Polymorphonuclear leukocytes (PMNs) appear in the synovial lining, and in its small blood vessels inflammatory cells and tiny thrombi can often be found. Phagocytosis involving large mononuclear cells accompanies the proliferation. Collagenase, elastase, cathepsins, and prostaglandins are released. Fibrin is formed at the synovial lining and incorporated into the synovium, which thus begins to encroach into the joint cavity. Some of the fibrin can break loose and form "rice grains" in the joint cavity. The interior surface of the synovium becomes villous, thus increasing its surface area more than proportionally to its increasing volume. The synovium proliferating in this manner is referred to as the pannus. Hyperplasia and hypertrophy occur among the lining cells, of which the number of layers is doubled or trebled. Soon the proliferating synovium is vascularized by arterioles, capillaries, and venules, sustaining the pathologic process. Segmental vascular changes occur, often accompanied by venous distention and infiltration of the arterial walls by PMNs and by areas of thrombosis and perivascular hemorrhage. The normally acellular subsynovial stroma becomes packed with inflammatory cells, largely mononuclear, which may collect into aggregates or follicles. In rare cases one can find true germinal centers. Follicles are usually dominated by lymphocytes surrounded by a layer of plasma cells. Immunofluorescence shows large numbers of Ig-secreting B cells, but the majority of lymphocytes in the RA synovium are T cells. Eventually some synovial cells differentiate to fibroblasts.

The formation of the pannus, with inflammatory destruction of soft tissues, causes laxity of ligaments and tendons and thus, with aggravation by mechanical pressure and regular use, typical deformities occur. Ultimately there is erosion of juxta-articular bone around the margins of the pannus and invasion by the pannus of subchondral tissue. Although cysts and loss of cartilage can generally be observed roentgenographically, the erosion of bone so characteristic of advanced RA is less commonly seen.

PATHOGENESIS. Two general ideas have dominated the discussion of pathogenesis. One is that extravascular immune complex formation incites the inflammatory response; the other attributes the inflammation to cellular hypersensitivity. According to the latter, an accumulation of activated T cells in the synovium produces soluble factors, specifically lymphokines, which stimulate the proliferation of the synovium and the general inflammation. The occurrence of an arthritic syndrome similar to RA in some agammaglobulinemic children suggests an important role for the cellular immune reaction in rheumatoid synovitis.

According to the concept of inflammation based on the formation of immune complexes, the immune response is triggered sufficiently, and perhaps specifically, against some foreign antigen. This must involve a host response determined by the genotype of the individual. Thus an association with histocompatibility markers may be expected, as has been noted between seropositive RA and the HLA-D4 and HLA-DR4 markers. Studies using DNA restriction fragment length polymorphisms appear to have revealed more specific molecular genetic markers associated with RA. The host response seems to involve a local reaction within a subset of the synovial joints. RA appears to be a multicentric immune response, with variables that differ from one joint to another determining the reaction of the synovial tissue at each joint. Therefore different B cell clonal reactivity might be found in different joints of one individual.

Antigen-antibody complexes formed within the joint cavity in this process can become trapped in hyaline cartilage and fibrocartilage, where they can cause changes in matrix macromolecules. Within the synovial fluid, the immune response activates the complement system, kinins, phagocytic cells, and lysosomal enzyme release. Mediators produced in this process stimulate synovial cells to proliferate and to produce proteinases and prostaglandins. These products cause dissolution of the connective tissue macromolecules within the associated connective tissue and the articular cartilage. Mediators also activate fibroblasts to produce a denser, richer connective tissue matrix and further synovial proliferation. Complexes in the synovial fluid can fix and activate complement and perpetuate the inflammatory process. In order for destruction of joint tissue to progress, the usual control mechanisms that inhibit both degradative enzymes and their activators must be overwhelmed by saturation of the synovial fluid and the tissue inhibitors of specific enzyme systems. This course leads to a chronic proliferation of cells, stimulation of enzyme systems, and destruction of normal tissue matrices.

Collagenase production seems to be markedly stimulated in synovial sites in the presence of interleukin 1, derived from mononuclear macrophages. This enzyme is generally inactive when released from synovial cells but may be activated by appropriate proteolytic enzymes. Plasmin may be the key activator. Synovial cells produce a plasminogen activator that converts plasminogen in the circulation to plasmin, which then activates latent collagenase bound to collagen fibrils. This promotes rapid destruction of collagenous tissue.

CLINICAL FEATURES. A diagnosis of RA is compatible with a wide range of clinical courses, ranging from a few months of discomfort to decades of severe disability. Perhaps two thirds of cases begin with symptoms arising gradually over a period of weeks or months. Malaise and fatigue characterize this period, often in conjunction with diffuse musculoskeletal pain. As the disease advances specific joints exhibit pain, tenderness, swelling, and redness. The pattern of joint involvement is typically symmetric, involving the hands, wrists, elbows, and shoulders, but usually sparing the distal interphalangeal (DIP) joints. Symmetry and the sparing of the DIP joints are helpful in differentiating RA from other arthritides.

A frequent complaint is that of stiffness following inactivity. It can occur in the morning upon arising or following prolonged sitting. It is described by some as a "gelling" process and seems to be associated with edema within the inflamed tissues. So characteristic is this symptom that the duration of morning stiffness has been taken as a guide to the severity of the inflammatory process. In most clinical studies of RA, it is a useful bit of quantitative data with which to follow the activity of the disease. As the process evolves, the patient may have increasing difficulty with pain and stiffness. This limits the ability to move about, climb stairs, open doors, open jars, or to do detailed small movements, such as sewing. The patient may develop an associated psychologic depression and weight loss, and sometimes a low-grade fever may occur in association with the systemic manifestations of the disease.

An acute onset of disease is seen in about 20 per cent of patients. "Acute" refers to the rapid build-up of symptoms over a period of a few days. Occasionally an individual retires in the evening with no symptoms and wakes up the next morning with acute generalized RA. Such rapid onset of pain involving joints and surrounding soft tissues, as well as muscles, can mimic, and must be differentiated from, acute myositis, viral syndromes, or if focal, even septic arthritis.

RA typically is intermittent in early stages but becomes more sustained as it progresses. However, as remarked above, the course varies greatly. Some patients show an unrelenting progression to severe disability and even, rarely, mortality, but repeated periods of some degree of remission are the general rule. An ARA committee has proposed criteria for clinical remission of rheumatoid arthritis. At least five of the following requirements must be fulfilled for at least two consecutive months: (1) duration of morning stiffness not exceeding 15 minutes; (2) no fatigue; (3) no joint pain (by history); (4) no joint tenderness or pain on motion; (5) no soft tissue swelling in joints or tendon sheaths; and (6) erythrocyte sedimentation rate by Westergren method less than 30 mm per hour for females or 20 mm per hour for males.

Uniform standards for the evaluation of functional capacity may be particularly useful in dealing with patients with RA. Although there have been a number of suggested systems, we may accept the following for a rough division:

Class I—No restriction of ability to perform normal activities.

Class II—Moderate restriction but adequate for normal activities.

Class III—Marked restriction, inability to perform most duties of the patient's usual occupation or self-care.

Class IV—Incapacitation or confinement to a bed or wheelchair.

DIFFERENTIAL DIAGNOSIS. The differential considerations in the diagnosis of RA are numerous. Although there is seldom confusion in classic RA, diagnosis can be more difficult in patients with early acute polyarthritis or those with involvement of only a few joints. One must consider osteoarthritis, gout, chondrocalcinosis, systemic lupus erythematosus, and progressive systemic sclerosis as the more common diseases that might be confused with RA. In addition, a variety of systemic diseases, including sarcoidosis, inflammatory bowel disease, Whipple's disease, amyloidosis, chronic infection, and malignancies, can all be manifested by arthritic syndromes mimicking RA. Therefore, a complete medical evaluation is indicated in all patients with joint manifestations. One must assess the patient for general systemic diseases and also for curable causes, such as bacterial infections. The careful

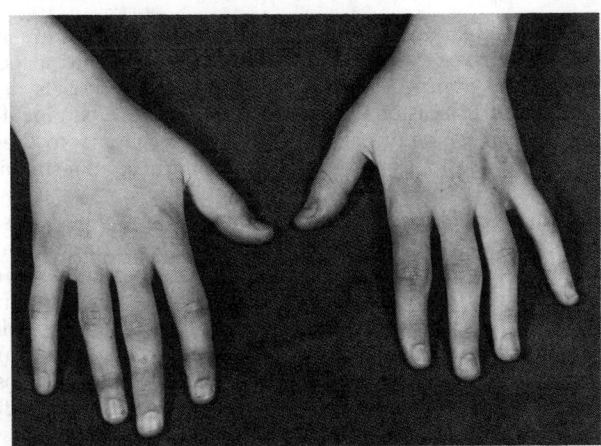

FIGURE 433–1. Early rheumatoid arthritis manifests as symmetrical swelling and slight flexion deformities of proximal interphalangeal joints of the hands. Roentgenograms were normal except for evidence of soft tissue swelling.

analysis of synovial fluid is critical in the differentiation of rheumatoid arthritis from chronic gout and chondrocalcinosis. Critical evaluation of inflammatory joint effusions is useful not only for diagnosis but also as a guide for therapeutic responses.

ARTICULAR MANIFESTATIONS. RA can affect any diarthrodial joint. Those most commonly involved are the small joints of the hands, wrists, knees, and feet. As the disease spreads it may involve elbows, shoulders, sternoclavicular joints, hips, and ankles. The temporomandibular and cricoarytenoid joints are less frequently involved. Spinal involvement in RA is generally limited to the upper cervical articulations, at least from the standpoint of clinically significant lesions.

Hands. One of the most common early signs of disease is swelling of the proximal interphalangeal (PIP) joints, giving the fingers a fusiform or spindle-shaped appearance. This is generally associated with bilateral and symmetric swelling of the metacarpophalangeal (MCP) joints (Fig. 433–1). Although the distal interphalangeal (DIP) joints can be involved, they generally are not, and this is useful in discriminating RA from osteoarthritis. Soft tissue laxity gives rise to ulnar deviation of the fingers (Fig. 433–2*A*), which is frequently accompanied by palmar subluxation of the proximal phalanges. Swan neck deformities develop through hyperextension of the PIP joints in conjunction with flexion of the DIP joints (Fig. 433–2*B*). Flexion deformity of the PIP joints and extension of the DIP joints give rise to the boutonnière deformity. These changes are associated with loss of strength in the hands and frequently loss of the ability to maintain a good pinch. Synovial erosions of tendons may lead to their rupture and thus to sudden loss of the ability to extend the fingers.

Wrists. The wrists are almost invariably involved in RA and frequently demonstrate easily palpable, boggy synovium. Such synovial proliferation on the volar aspect may compress the median nerve and produce the carpal tunnel syndrome. This consists of paresthesia and dysesthesia of the thumb and the second and third digits and the radial aspect of the fourth digit. It may also be accompanied by atrophy of the thenar eminence. Frequently, one of the first losses of motion in RA is the inability to dorsiflex the wrist fully. Normally the wrist should be able to move through nearly 180 degrees from palmar to dorsiflexion.

Knees. Synovial hypertrophy and effusion in these weight-bearing joints place them among the more frequently affected joints in RA. Effusions may be detected by balloting the patella or by observing a "bulge sign" along the patella when fluid is pushed into the suprapatellar pouch and then expressed back into the joint. One may expect to see quadriceps atrophy in association with chronic knee arthritis. Baker's cysts may form owing to enlargement of the semimembranous bursa into the popliteal space. Such synovial cysts may occasionally dissect and rupture and can give rise to symptoms mimicking acute thrombophlebitis. Sonograms and arthrograms may be useful for confirmation of the diagnosis. Destruction of soft tissue about the knee can also give rise to marked joint instability.

Feet and Ankles. Arthritis is common in the feet and may involve changes analogous to those described in the hands. Cock-up of the toes may produce subluxation of the metatarsal heads and finally a clawlike appearance.

Neck. Neck pain and stiffness are frequent in RA. As in other joints, the rheumatoid process can lead to the erosion of bone in the cervical vertebrae. Sustained erosion may produce atlantoaxial subluxation and thus cervical dislocation, spinal cord compression, and finally neurologic manifestations in rare cases. There is also a possibility of torsion and compression of the vertebral arteries, with vertebrobasilar insufficiency and syncope on downward gaze as symptoms. Occipital and occasionally more extensive headache is a frequent complaint. Localized tenderness, muscle spasm, and limitation of rotary motion may be found with neck involvement; limitations of flexion and extension of the cervical spine are less common. Uncontrollable head tilt may occur as a symptom of lateral mass collapse of the C1 and C2 vertebrae.

Elbows. Erosion around the margins of a pannus can easily eradicate the paraolecranon grooves. Often, even in early RA, the elbow does not relax into a fully extended position. Loss of joint space and deterioration of congruity occur as in other joints. Particularly in the elbow, this may facilitate dislocation of the joint.

Shoulders. Involvement of the glenohumeral, acromioclavicular, and thoracoscapular joints is a common feature of the advanced, but not the early, course of RA. Limitation of motion and tenderness just below and lateral to the coracoid

FIGURE 433–2. Hand deformities characteristic of chronic rheumatoid arthritis. *A*, Subluxation of metacarpophalangeal joints with ulnar deviation of digits. *B*, Hyperextension ("swan neck") deformities of proximal interphalangeal joints.

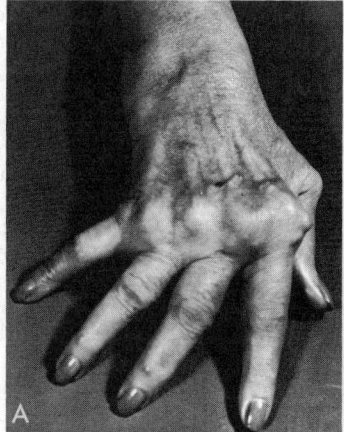

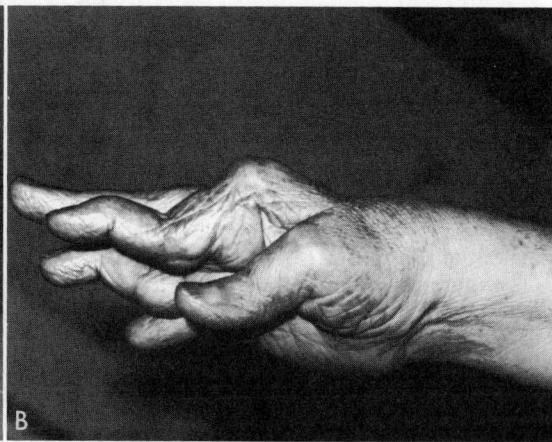

process are typical symptoms. Noticeable swelling is rare. Joint destruction typically involves rupture of the joint capsule and subluxation of the humerus.

Hips. The deep location of the joint may hide swelling and tenderness. Physician and patient should therefore be alert to limitation of joint motion, which may be manifested by a change of gait. Pain in the groin, or sometimes even the buttocks or lower back, may be symptomatic of hip involvement. Because the hip joint capsule has poor distensibility, great pain can result if a massive effusion occurs. Arthrocentesis should be done to rule out infection in such a case.

EXTRA-ARTICULAR MANIFESTATIONS. The occurrence of constitutional symptoms, occasionally a low-grade fever and minimal lymphadenopathy, are to be expected in RA. As the disease progresses, muscle atrophy, weakness, and sometimes the development of tremor can be seen. The latter is presumably caused by muscle fatigue and is usually associated with more severe disease and a poor prognosis.

Skin. Subcutaneous nodules may develop at some time in approximately 20 to 25 per cent of patients. They are nearly always associated with seropositive disease and are found most frequently in the rapidly progressive and destructive form of the disease. Periarticular structures and areas subject to pressure, such as the elbows, the occiput, or the sacrum, tend to be the primary sites for subcutaneous nodules. They may occasionally break down or become infected but generally are asymptomatic.

A vasculitic process in the skin often produces small brown spots or splinter-shaped lesions, frequently in the nail folds or in the digital pulp. Larger areas of ischemic involvement may occur in the lower extremities with infarction of a toe or the development of skin sloughs over the malleoli. Histologic examination of the involved area may show leukocytoclastic vasculitis, or only a mild venulitis with a relatively bland proliferation of affected digital vessels. It may also be a severe and widespread necrotizing vasculitis of the small and medium-sized arteries, indistinguishable from polyarteritis nodosa. Rheumatoid vasculitis is frequently associated with high fever and other manifestations of systemic disease, including a depression of serum complement.

Another common skin manifestation is a tendency to easy bruisability and production of ecchymotic lesions. This seems to be caused by the general fragility of the skin in RA and is possibly associated with the systemic manifestations of the inflammatory process.

Cardiac Manifestations. Although symptomatic cardiac disease is not common in RA, a relatively frequent symptomatic lesion is acute pericarditis. It is unrelated to the duration of the arthritis and seems to appear most often in seropositive disease. The pericardial fluid characteristics include a low glucose concentration, increased lactic dehydrogenase (LDH) level, elevated immunoglobulin levels, and low complement activity. Echocardiography is a sensitive diagnostic tool for pericarditis in RA. Pericardial disease may vary from a mild, fleeting process to a sizable effusion to cardiac tamponade and death. Some evidence of pericardial involvement with old fibrinous adhesions is found in about 40 per cent of RA patients at autopsy.

The rare pericardial tamponade is life-threatening. Typical symptoms are chest pain, dyspnea, and peripheral edema. A few cases have a pericardial friction rub. The pericardial fluid will generally have glucose levels below 15 mg per deciliter, protein levels above 4 grams per deciliter, and LDH levels greater than in serum.

The more common constrictive pericarditis is characterized by dyspnea, clinical right heart failure, peripheral edema, and increased jugular venous pressure. Fever, chest pain, pericardial friction rubs, Kussmaul's sign, and pulsus paradoxus can also occur. The definitive sign is the prominent y descent of the jugular venous pulse, demonstrated by right-side cardiac catheterization.

Lesions similar to rheumatoid nodules may be found involving the myocardium and the valves. Sometimes a focal interstitial myocarditis and arteritis of coronary vessels may be recognized. Occasionally valvular insufficiency, conduction abnormalities, and myocardial infarction secondary to these inflammatory lesions may be seen as clinical manifestations of rheumatoid heart disease.

Pulmonary Manifestations. Rheumatoid pleural disease, although frequently found at autopsy, is most commonly asymptomatic. Occasionally a pleural effusion may be of sufficient size to cause respiratory limitation. Neoplasm and infection should be ruled out based on a pleural tap. Typically the pleural fluid is exudative, and white cell counts vary greatly but generally are less than 5000 per microliter. Glucose levels tend to be low, and the LDH enzyme level is high. Total hemolytic complement, C3, and C4 levels are low. Immune complexes and RF are frequently found in the pleural fluid.

Intrapulmonary nodules may also be seen. Although they are usually asymptomatic, they may become infected and may cavitate or rupture into the pleural space with the production of a pneumothorax. Similar but distinct nodular infiltrates may also be seen in rheumatoid lungs in association with pneumoconiosis (Caplan's syndrome).

Finally one may see a diffuse interstitial fibrosis with pneumonitis. This may progress to a honeycomb appearance on the roentgenogram, bronchiectasis, chronic cough, and progressive dyspnea. Pulmonary function tests will show a diminished compliance and a restrictive ventilatory pattern. Large airways are not involved. An irreversible combination of respiratory insufficiency and resultant right-side cardiac failure is possible. Chronic inflammatory cell infiltration with neutrophils and eosinophils can forewarn of this possibility. Rarely small airway obstruction may develop into a necrotizing bronchiolitis. This has been associated with therapies with gold and D-penicillamine.

Neurologic Manifestations. Rheumatoid vasculitis is frequently associated with a mononeuritis multiplex syndrome in which there is patchy sensory loss in one or more of the extremities, frequently in association with foot drop or wrist drop. Biopsy of the sural nerve (when there is an abnormal conduction time) can confirm the diagnosis of vasculitis. As mentioned previously, neurologic complaints can also be produced in association with proliferating synovium causing compression of nerves. This can result in conditions such as a median neuropathy (carpal tunnel syndrome) or a tarsal tunnel syndrome with foot drop caused by an anterior tibial nerve palsy. Although the central nervous system is usually spared, rheumatoid vasculitis and rheumatoid nodule–like granulomas have been known to occur in the meninges.

Ophthalmologic Manifestations. Episcleritis is a self-limiting condition and may develop in association with mild pain and discomfort. Sjögren's syndrome can occur and cause corneal and conjunctival lesions associated with dryness of the eyes. Scleritis can be accompanied by severe pain and occasional visual impairment. Lesions may be found in the superior sclera as raised yellow nodules surrounded by a hyperemia of the deep scleral vessels. If this progresses over a period of time, allowing the dark blue color of the choroid beneath to show through, it is termed scleromalacia perforans. The histologic picture is similar to that of the rheumatoid nodule.

Felty's Syndrome. This syndrome is found in chronic RA associated with splenomegaly, lymphadenopathy, anemia, thrombocytopenia, and a selective leukopenia involving only the neutrophils. Most cases occur among seropositive patients with very active arthritis and systemic manifestations such as fever, fatigue, anorexia, and weight loss. Hyperpigmentation and leg ulcers can occur in association with Felty's syndrome. HLA-DR4 has been reported to characterize 95 per cent of patients. Although hypersplenism is proposed as one cause of the leukopenia, splenectomy fails to correct the abnormality in many patients. Gram-positive infections are common and frequently fail to respond to antibiotics. Interestingly, the incidence of infection may decline after splenectomy even when the neutropenia remains unaltered.

LABORATORY FINDINGS. A mild anemia, usually of the normocytic normochromic or hypochromic type, may be found. Sometimes there is a low serum iron level and normal or low iron binding capacity. The anemia, however, is generally resistant to iron therapy. The erythrocyte sedimentation rate tends to be elevated in most patients but only roughly parallels the disease activity. Although the white cell count and differential are usually normal, there may be a significant eosinophilia in association with systemic rheumatoid disease, especially vasculitis. The presence of RF by agglutination test is helpful in the clinical diagnosis of RA, and other serologic abnormalities, including antibodies against DNA and nuclear antigens in low titer, occur in a small percentage of patients. Although the finding of HLA-DR4 positivity by B cell typing is important for investigational purposes, it is not generally useful in the diagnosis of RA. Evidence now suggests that it is associated with a more aggressive disease, especially striking when found among seronegative patients.

Synovial fluid analysis generally shows white cell counts in the range of 5,000 to 20,000 per microliter, with approximately 50 to 70 per cent as polymorphonuclear leukocytes. Synovial fluid complement is usually low, rheumatoid factors are usually present, and there is evidence of hyaluronate degradation, as shown by a poor mucin clot test.

THERAPEUTIC MANAGEMENT. The prolonged and uncertain course of RA calls for special emphasis on the fact that most patients can continue their accustomed activities, with restrictions tailored to individual cases. Undue or excessive drug therapy, especially adrenocorticosteroids and immunosuppressive agents, can cause greater morbidity than the disease itself. Objectives of management include (1) relief of pain, (2) reduction of inflammation, (3) minimizing undesirable side effects, (4) preservation of muscle strength and joint function, and (5) return as rapidly as possible to a normal lifestyle. The basic initial program that achieves these objectives for the great majority of patients consists of (1) adequate rest, (2) adequate salicylate therapy, and (3) physical measures to maintain joint function.

Any confusion arising from the complementary requirements of rest and exercise should be promptly dispelled. As has been noted for many years, it is only a rare patient with RA who does not improve significantly upon being hospitalized. From this we have learned that bed rest tends to decrease the general systemic inflammatory response. Most patients will soon learn that their midafternoon fatigue is significantly reduced by a period of rest. This tends to give them a "second wind" for handling their functional requirements during the rest of the day. Thus a regularly disciplined midafternoon rest maintains the patient's overall sense of well-being. During acute attacks, longer rests and perhaps even remaining in bed for the duration of the attack may be required to treat the inflammation.

At the same time, full range of joint motion should be maintained. This can usually be accomplished by the patient through graded exercise programs. However, during acute attacks, passive range-of-motion exercises by a physical therapist or instructed layperson may be indicated. Physical overexertion will increase synovitis and inflammation in the RA joint, but this does not contradict the usefulness of appropriate exercise. Exercise, and heat treatments such as showers, baths, warm pools, paraffin baths, or hot packs, should be used to loosen the joints and relieve stiffness. Exercise following the heat treatment maintains motion of affected joints and prevents muscle atrophy. These goals can generally be achieved without aggressive overactivity and can

usually keep a patient fully mobile. Acutely inflamed joints may indicate total body rest or splinting.

Salicylate therapy is critical to the basic program. Salicylates are cheap, generally well tolerated, and demonstrably effective in controlling RA inflammation. The patient needs to understand that this requires a larger dose than would be used for analgesia alone. A constant blood level of 20 to 30 mg per deciliter is required. For most patients this will require between 3 and 6 grams of aspirin per day. All patients should be monitored for toxicity by blood tests and should be alerted to report deafness, ringing in the ears, or gastrointestinal intolerance. With the availability of buffered and coated aspirin, a suitable salicylate preparation can be found for almost any patient.

Nonsteroidal Anti-Inflammatory Drugs. Salicylate preparations often cause silent gastrointestinal bleeding. Fortunately, this is usually minimal and tolerable. Overt gastrointestinal tract hemorrhage caused by aspirin is rare, but if gastrointestinal bleeding is contributing to a constant anemia, the therapeutic regimen should be modified.

Many nonsteroidal anti-inflammatory drugs (NSAIDs) are available that are effective against pain, fever, and inflammation in RA. Indomethacin and phenylbutazone have been available for some time. Although they are more frequently used in osteoarthritis, they may also be effective in RA. Newer NSAIDs include derivatives of phenylacetic acid (ibuprofen, fenoprofen), naphthalene acetic acids (naproxen), pyrrolealkanoic acid (tolmetin), indoleacetic acid (sulindac), a halogenated anthranilic acid (meclofenamate sodium), piroxicam, zomepirac, and diflunisal. Most of these drugs are beneficial in RA. They are generally no more effective than aspirin but may be tolerated in the exceptional cases in which aspirin is not. Their major problem is high cost. Clinical experience suggests an occasional need to change from one to another of these drugs to minimize side effects and to give maximum benefit to the individual patient.

Other Therapies. If salicylates and NSAIDs fail to control the inflammation or are not tolerated, then one must consider the more slowly acting drugs, including antimalarials, gold, and penicillamine. Antimalarials are usually given as hydroxychloroquine 200 mg twice daily. This, or chloroquine, may cause retinal lesions and loss of vision; therefore the patient should be checked by an ophthalmologist at least twice a year.

Gold salts produce remission in many cases. Because of the potential toxicity to kidneys and bone marrow, frequent urinalysis and routine blood work (CBC) must be done, especially during early phases of treatment. The first gold treatment is usually a 10-mg test injection (Myochrysine or Solganal) for idiosyncrasy, then a 25-mg dose the second week, and a 50-mg injection weekly up to a total of about 1 gram. By this time usually a therapeutic response occurs, at which point the schedule of injections can be reduced to alternate weeks, and subsequently to every third or fourth week. Many patients have been on IM gold therapy for a number of years. A gold salt, auranofin, also is available for oral administration and is therapeutically effective. Side effects are common, causing as many as 30 per cent of patients to discontinue the therapy. The most common, and very annoying to the patient, are pruritic skin rashes. Mouth ulcers are even more painful. Severe manifestations include bone marrow suppression, usually leukopenia or thrombocytopenia, renal damage with proteinuria, and rarely a nephrotic syndrome.

Penicillamine may be used in the treatment of RA and is also quite effective in inducing improvements and sometimes even remissions. Like gold, however, it affects both the bone marrow and the kidneys, so that careful monitoring for toxicity is required.

Immunosuppressive agents such as azathioprine, cyclophosphamide, chlorambucil, and methotrexate have been used to treat especially severe unremitting RA. Currently the most effective form of immunosuppressive therapy for RA appears to be methotrexate.* Even once-a-week oral dosage of 7.5 mg seems efficacious.

For especially difficult-to-manage patients, experimental approaches include plasmapheresis, leukapheresis, and total lymph node irradiation. All of these procedures are experimental, and long-term effects are unknown.

Because of its side effects, long-term corticosteroid therapy is generally shunned by most rheumatologists. Patients with active rheumatoid disease do not tolerate alternate-day steroids well, and therefore one quickly gets into a pattern of daily therapy. Although they can be useful in patients with neuropathy, vasculitis, pleuritis, pericarditis, scleritis, and related conditions, for the usual patient with only joint disease it is wise to avoid them. Local steroid injections can sometimes be helpful for the relief of persistent effusions or to get patients more mobile in preparation for appropriate physical therapy.

Finally, reconstructive orthopedic surgery is of very great importance. Perhaps the greatest contribution of the last decade to the management of RA has been the development of superb techniques for joint replacement. The use of prosthetic devices for hip and knee joints has given excellent results, and the results for ankle, elbow, and shoulder replacement are improving rapidly.

JUVENILE CHRONIC ARTHRITIS

Rheumatic diseases are not rare in children, but they differ notably from RA. For this reason the term *juvenile chronic arthritis* (JCA) is used, rather than *juvenile rheumatoid arthritis*. The various subclasses have not yet been fully defined, but currently JCA is subdivided into systemic onset disease, polyarticular onset disease, and pauciarticular onset disease.

Systemic onset arthritis, or Still's disease, accounts for about 20 per cent of patients. It can begin at any age. RF and antinuclear antibody are generally not found. Clinical characteristics include a high intermittent fever, maculopapular rash, polyserositis, lymphadenopathy, hepatosplenomegaly, leukocytosis, and anemia. Although the disease is rarely life-threatening, it can be confused with leukemia or infection. A chronic polyarthritis usually develops in these patients within the first few months of the disease but sometimes not until years later.

Polyarticular onset disease without extra-articular manifestations occurs in approximately 40 per cent of patients. There is a female preponderance. The majority are seronegative. Seropositive patients are generally over eight years old at onset. Antinuclear antibodies are often found. These patients may have malaise, low-grade fever, adenopathy, anemia, and growth retardation. Cervical spine involvement is common, most typically at the C2–C3 apophyseal joints.

Pauciarticular onset disease accounts for the remaining 40 per cent of JCA patients. There are at least two subgroups within this group. One is characterized by early onset. It shows a female preponderance. The serum in this group is often positive for antinuclear antibodies but negative for RF. Some tend to develop inflammation of the anterior uveal tract (iridocyclitis). Occasionally this is the major manifestation; it can progress to blindness. Therefore evaluation of these children for progressive ophthalmologic manifestations is important. A second subgroup with pauciarticular onset has a strong male preponderance. Many of these patients are HLA-B27 positive and appear as young children with spondyloarthropathy.

Treatment is difficult, but fortunately most patients with JCA have a relatively benign course. Aspirin is a basic standby, and physical and psychosocial support are indicated.

---

*This use is not listed in the manufacturer's directive.

ADULT-ONSET STILL'S DISEASE

As already mentioned, Still's disease is one form of juvenile-onset chronic arthritis; adult-onset cases have also been found, with clinical features almost identical to those of juvenile-onset cases. Patients exhibit high fever, polyarthritis, tenosynovitis, and a salmon-colored maculopapular measles-like rash, particularly over the trunk and along pressure lines. Nodules sometimes occur. The fever and rash are most characteristic of the onset and point to the diagnosis of adult-onset Still's disease. Pericarditis and pleural effusions have been reported but are generally mild. Other systemic manifestations do occur. Acute symptoms generally respond to an adequate dose of salicylates, but occasionally NSAIDs or even prednisone may be necessary for short periods of time.

Alarcon GS, Koopman WJ, Acton RT, et al.: Seronegative rheumatoid arthritis: A distinct immunogenetic disease? Arth Rheum 25:502, 1982. *An interesting study of the association of histocompatibility markers and immunogenetic epidemiology in seronegative RA.*

Aptekar RG, Decker JL, Bujak JS, et al.: Adult onset juvenile rheumatoid arthritis. Arth Rheum 16:715, 1973. *An excellent clinical discussion of the adult-onset form of Still's disease.*

Fassbender HG: Normal and pathologic synovial tissue with emphasis on rheumatoid arthritis. In Cohen AS, Bennett JC (eds.): Rheumatology and Immunology. 2nd ed. Orlando, FL, Grune & Stratton, Inc., 1986. *Comprehensive discussion of the course of synovitis.*

Kay GN, Bennett JC: The heart in rheumatoid arthritis. In Hurst JW (ed.): Clinical Essays on the Heart. Vol. 3. New York, McGraw-Hill Book Company, 1986.

Krane SM: Aspects of the cell biology of the rheumatoid synovial lesion. Ann Rheum Dis 40:433, 1981. *Description of the biology of tissue destruction in the rheumatoid process dealing with both the enzymes involved and their regulation.*

Kremer JM, Lee JK: The safety and efficacy of the use of methotrexate in long-term therapy for rheumatoid arthritis. Arth Rheum 29:822, 1986.

O'Sullivan FX, Fassbender H-G, Gay S, et al.: Etiopathogenesis of the rheumatoid arthritis-like disease in MRL/1 mice: 1. The histomorphologic basis of joint destruction. Arth Rheum 28:529, 1985. *Discovery of an intriguing animal model of RA.*

Pinals RS, et al.: Preliminary criteria for clinical remission in rheumatoid arthritis. Arthritis Rheum 24:1308, 1981.

Southern P, Oldstone MBA: Medical consequences of persistent viral infection. N Engl J Med 314:359, 1986. *Considerations relating to possible infectious origin of RA.*

Strominger JL: Biology of the human histocompatibility leukocyte antigen (HLA) system and a hypothesis regarding the generation of autoimmune disease. J Clin Invest 77:1411, 1986. *Excellent review of concepts relating to autoimmune features of RA.*

Wees SJ, Sunwoo IN, Oh SJ: Sural nerve biopsy in systemic necrotizing vasculitis. Am J Med 71:525, 1981. *Description of a useful diagnostic procedure for vasculitis and peripheral neuropathy.*

Williams RC Jr, Sibbitt WL Jr, Husby G: Oncogenes, viruses, or rheumogenes? Am J Med 80:1011, 1986. *Extremely interesting reflections on etiology of RA.*

Ziff M: Systemic rheumatoid disease: Immunological aspects. Adv Inflam Res 3:123, 1982. *A comprehensive review of the immunologic mechanisms involving the pathogenesis of RA.*

---

434 THE SPONDYLARTHROPATHIES

Andrei Calin

The seronegative spondylarthritides are characterized by involvement of the sacroiliac joints, by peripheral inflammatory arthropathy, and by the absence of rheumatoid factor. Other features include (1) pathologic changes concentrated around the enthesis (i.e., the site of ligamentous insertion into bone) rather than the synovium. Nonenthesopathic changes may also develop in the eye, the aortic valve, the lung parenchyma, and the skin. (2) Clinical evidence of overlap among the various seronegative spondylarthritides. Thus, a patient with psoriatic arthropathy may well develop uveitis or sacroiliitis; a patient with inflammatory bowel disease may develop ankylosing spondylitis or mouth ulcers. (3) A tendency toward familial aggregation, with the suggestion that these entities "breed true" within families.

Types

The spondylarthropathies include ankylosing spondylitis, Reiter's syndrome (both the postvenereal, or endemic, and the postinfective, or epidemic, forms), the reactive arthritides (caused by infections with *Yersinia* and *Salmonella*), certain subsets of juvenile arthropathy (juvenile ankylosing spondylitis and the seronegative enthesopathic arthropathy syndrome), enteropathic sacroiliitis (ulcerative colitis and Crohn's disease), psoriatic arthropathy, and perhaps a group of rarer disorders (Behçet's syndrome, Whipple's disease, and pustulotic arthro-osteitis) (Fig. 434–1).

These disorders can be categorized according to the specific periarticular or articular involvement. The various spondylarthropathies can be distinguished from one another according to the particular peripheral joints involved, the associated clinical features (i.e., urethritis, conjunctivitis, skin involvement), and the manner in which the disease progresses (i.e., remission or relapse) (Table 434–1).

Hereditary Factors

Hereditary factors play an important role in the development of the spondylarthropathies. Some 10 to 20 per cent of HLA-B27–positive individuals develop ankylosing spondylitis following an unknown environmental event or develop Reiter's syndrome after exposure to *Shigella* or other environmental agents. The offspring of an individual with HLA-B27 have a 50 per cent chance of carrying the same antigen and, thus, an overall 10 per cent chance of developing ankylosing spondylitis or Reiter's syndrome if exposed to a specific arthritogenic trigger.

The explanation for the link between HLA-B27 and the spondylarthropathies remains unknown. Hypotheses include: (1) B27 acts as a receptor site for an infective agent; (2) B27 is a marker for an immune response gene that determines susceptibility to an environmental trigger; or (3) B27 may induce tolerance to foreign antigens with which it cross-reacts.

We now know that the risk of developing ankylosing spondylitis for a B27-positive relative of a B27-positive patient is 25 to 50 per cent compared with about 5 per cent for a B27-positive subject. This argues for genetic differences between the two B27 groups. Splitting of B27 by monoclonal antibodies and cytotoxic T cells has not provided an explanation for these differences, so there must be additional susceptibility

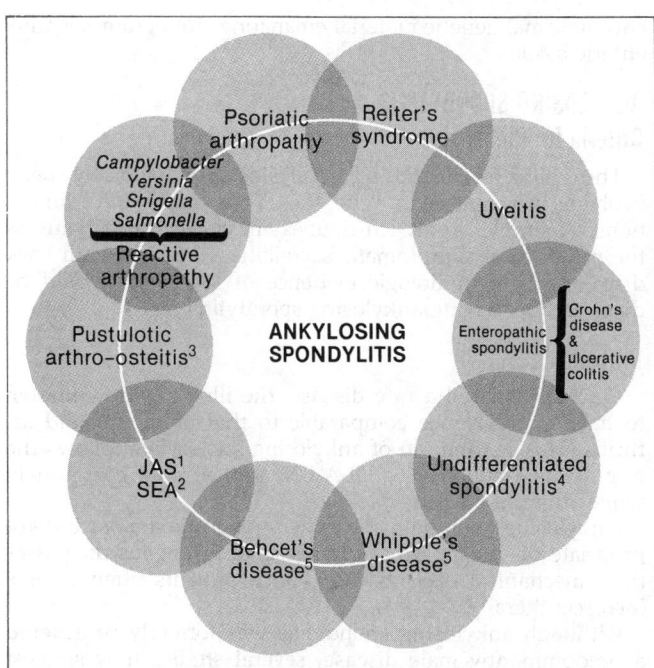

FIGURE 434–1. Individual conditions that overlap to form the spondyloarthritides. (1) Juvenile ankylosing spondylitis. (2) Seronegative enthesopathic arthropathy syndrome. (3) Considered by Japanese to be part of spondyloarthropathy spectrum (rare in United States and Europe). (4) Undifferentiated spondylitis (i.e., subset of patients who have spondyloarthropathic features but who fail to meet criteria for ankylosing spondylitis, Reiter's syndrome, or other condition, e.g., dactylitis, uveitis, plus unilateral sacroiliitis). (5) Not universally accepted as members of the spondyloarthropathy group.

(and perhaps severity) gene(s). Chromosomes 2, 14, and 19 may also be operative.

Etiologic Factors

Numerous infective triggers are recognized for the reactive arthropathies (*Shigella*, *Salmonella*, *Chlamydia*, etc.). By contrast, the arthritogenic environmental event in ankylosing spondylitis has not been adequately defined. However, much interest has focused on *Klebsiella* and plasmids or other extra-

TABLE 434–1. COMPARISON OF SERONEGATIVE SPONDYLOARTHROPATHIES

	Ankylosing Spondylitis	Reiter's Syndrome	Psoriatic Arthropathy	Enteropathic Spondylitis	Juvenile Arthropathy (JAS* subset)	Reactive Arthropathy
Sex	Male ≥ Female	Male ≥ Female	Female ≥ Male	Female = Male	Male > Female	Male = Female
Age at onset	20	Any age	Any age	Any age	<16	Any age
Uveitis	+ +	+ +	+	+	+	+
Conjunctivitis	–	+	–	–	–	+
Peripheral joints	Lower > Upper: often	Lower usually	Upper > Lower	Lower > Upper	Lower > Upper	Lower > Upper
Sex differences	Yes	No	No	No	No	No
Sacroiliitis	Always	Often	Often	Often	Often	Often
HLA-B27	95%	80%	20% (50% with sacroiliitis)	50%	90%	80%
Enthesopathy	+	+	+	+	+	+
Aortic regurgitation	+	+	? +	?	?	+
Familial aggregation	+	+	+	+	+	+
Risk for HLA-B27–positive individual	±20%	20%	?	?	?	20%
Onset	Gradual	Sudden	Variable	Gradual	Variable	Sudden
Urethritis	–	+	–	–	–	+/–
Skin involvement	–	+	+ +	–	–	–
Mucous membrane involvement	–	+	–	+	–	+
Symmetry (spinal)	+	–	–	+	+	–
Self-limiting	–	+/–	+/–	+/–	+/–	+/–
Remission, relapses	–	+/–	+/–	–	+/–	+/–

*JAS = Juvenile ankylosing spondylitis.

chromosomal genetic material emanating from gram-negative enteric bacilli.

ANKYLOSING SPONDYLITIS
Criteria for Diagnosis

The criteria for diagnosing ankylosing spondylitis have been evolving in recent years. The New York criteria have limitations. A simpler approach defines ankylosing spondylitis as the presence of symptomatic sacroiliitis. A patient with back discomfort and radiologic evidence of sacroiliitis would be diagnosed as having ankylosing spondylitis.

Prevalence

Once considered a rare disease, the illness is now known to have a prevalence comparable to that of rheumatoid arthritis. The distribution of ankylosing spondylitis follows the population frequency of HLA-B27 and is more common in whites than in blacks.

Ankylosing spondylitis has often gone undiagnosed; inappropriate diagnostic procedures lead to erroneous diagnoses (i.e., mechanical back disease). Such patients often receive incorrect therapy.

Although ankylosing spondylitis was formerly considered a predominantly male disease, several studies now suggest that there may be a more uniform sex distribution. Female patients are less frequently diagnosed, perhaps because physicians and radiologists may be reluctant to diagnose a disease that they consider to be rare in females. The disease may be milder in females and present with a greater number of peripheral joint manifestations. In the past, many women with ankylosing spondylitis were inappropriately diagnosed as having seronegative rheumatoid arthritis.

Clinical Presentation

A history of several of the following five features is suggestive of inflammatory spinal disease: insidious onset of discomfort, age less than 40 years, persistence for more than three months, association with morning stiffness, and improvement with exercise.

If this simple screening test is positive, radiologic evidence of sacroiliitis confirms ankylosing spondylitis. Many radiologists have been unfamiliar with rheumatologic joint disease and have diagnosed ankylosing spondylitis only when there was evidence of major ankylosis of the sacroiliac joints and spine. Ankylosing spondylitis can be diagnosed, however, in the presence of only minimal sacroiliitis. What determines whether a patient will have only mild pelvic disease, ascending spinal disease, extraspinal articular disease, or extra-articular symptoms remains unknown. Presumably, phenotypic expression depends on numerous interrelating genes.

Early change in the lumbar spine is manifested as squaring of the superior and inferior margins of the vertebral body. This phenomenon is caused by inflammatory disease at the site of insertion of the outer fibers of the anulus fibrosus (i.e., enthesopathy). Later changes result in the classic, though rare, bamboo spine. Comparable spinal changes are seen in primary ankylosing spondylitis and in the spondylitis associated with inflammatory bowel disease. In spondylitis associated with Reiter's syndrome and psoriatic arthropathy, however, the changes tend to be asymmetric and random.

Radionuclide scans, computed tomography, and other advanced radiologic techniques are usually unnecessary. A simple anteroposterior radiograph suffices.

Physical Examination

Examination of the spine may reveal muscle spasm and loss of the normal lordosis. The degree of restriction of forward flexion can be documented by measuring the distraction, on flexion, of two points—the lower point at the level of the lumbosacral junction and the upper point 10 cm above this level. In a normal individual, the distraction of this 10-cm line is 5 to 12 cm, compared with 0 to 7 cm in an untreated spondylitis patient. Lateral spinal flexion is measured by the distraction, on contralateral flexion, of a 20-cm line drawn in the midaxillary plane. In this case, normal distraction varies from 5 to 12 cm, compared with 0 to 7 cm in spondylitis patients.

Peripheral joint involvement, especially in the lower limb, occurs at some stage in approximately 20 to 30 per cent of cases; the frequency increases with the severity of the disease. Inflammatory disease of the hip and shoulder may produce progressive disability. Enthesopathic features include plantar fasciitis, costochondritis, and Achilles tendinitis.

Laboratory Findings

HLA-B27 testing should not be used as a routine screening procedure; it is expensive and usually unnecessary.

Other laboratory changes are less striking. Elevation of the erythrocyte sedimentation rate occurs in most patients but may be normal despite severe disease. Elevation of IgA levels and the presence of immune complexes suggest aberrant immunity. Serum creatine kinase and alkaline phosphatase activities may be elevated. Lymphocytes predominate in the synovial fluid, and synovial histologic findings are nonspecific.

Pathology

The synovial lesions of ankylosing spondylitis and rheumatoid arthritis share identical histopathologic characteristics: intimal cell hyperplasia; a diffuse lymphocyte and plasma cell infiltrate; formation of lymphoid follicles; and plasma containing IgG, IgA, and IgM. IgM is found less frequently in ankylosing spondylitis than in rheumatoid disease. Synovitis per se, however, does not explain the propensity toward ligamentous ossification and widespread new bone formation observed in ankylosing spondylitis. Inflammation at the enthesis accounts for the unique pathology, or enthesopathy, of ankylosing spondylitis; new bone formation appears to be a specific reparative process occurring at the enthesopathic site. Complications of severe spinal disease include fractures and spondylodiskitis after minimal trauma.

Extraskeletal Involvement

Extra-articular features include fatigue, weight loss, and low-grade fever. Cord compression resulting from spinal fractures or the cauda equina syndrome may cause neurologic symptoms. The negative effects of systemic involvement and of radiotherapy on the survival of patients with ankylosing spondylitis are well recognized.

EYE INVOLVEMENT. Uveitis develops in up to 25 per cent of patients during their illness. It occurs most often in HLA-B27–positive patients with peripheral joint disease but shows no correlation with the severity of the spondylitis. The visual episodes are usually self-limiting but may require local steroid therapy.

PULMONARY DISEASE. Patients with severe disease may exhibit chronic infiltrative and fibrotic changes in the upper lung fields that mimic tuberculosis. Pulmonary ventilation is usually well maintained by the diaphragm, despite the chest wall rigidity. The pulmonary fibrosis is occasionally clinically silent, but most affected patients present with cough, sputum, and dyspnea. Cyst formation and subsequent *Aspergillus* invasion may cause hemoptysis.

CARDIOVASCULAR DISEASE. Aortic incompetence, cardiomegaly, and persistent conduction defects occur in 3.5 to 10.0 per cent of patients with severe spondylitic disease. Cardiac involvement may be clinically silent or may dominate the clinical picture. Thickened aortic valve cusps and scar tissue in the root of the aorta represent the major histologic changes.

AMYLOIDOSIS. Amyloid deposition is an occasional complication of ankylosing spondylitis, particularly in Europe.

KIDNEY. In contrast to patients with rheumatoid arthritis who may show renal impairment as an expression of disease, renal glomerular function is apparently unimpaired in ankylosing spondylitis, despite recognized pathologic changes. An IgA nephropathy, however, has been described in patients with seronegative spondylarthropathy.

Treatment and Prognosis

Ankylosing spondylitis may be a mild or severe disease. We have recently shown that the younger the age at onset, the more severe the outcome. For example, in an analysis of 1500 cases, 15 per cent of those with onset between 15 and 16 years of age needed a total hip replacement within 15 years, compared to 10 per cent of those between 19 and 20 years and less than 1 per cent of patients with onset over 40 years of age (all cohorts followed for a similar period).

Ankylosing spondylitis is a gratifying condition to recognize and treat early: Much can be accomplished toward ameliorating symptoms and, perhaps, preventing spinal deformity. The primary objectives are to relieve pain, decrease inflammation, begin remedial strengthening exercises, and maintain good posture and function.

Anti-inflammatory agents relieve inflammation, pain, and spasm and permit patients to follow an adequate exercise program. There is some evidence that phenylbutazone decreases the rate of spinal fusion. Nevertheless, indomethacin is the drug of choice. Phenylbutazone, although more efficacious, may be more toxic. Indomethacin, started at a dosage of 25 mg three times a day, may be increased to a maximum of 150 mg daily. The dose should be titrated against response and side effects. Possible side effects include headache, vertigo, and depression, especially in older patients, and nausea, gastric discomfort, and diarrhea in all age groups. Phenylbutazone (100 mg t.i.d. or q.i.d.) is remarkably effective but must be used with caution. Dangerous side effects include agranulocytosis and aplastic anemia. Agranulocytosis is an idiosyncratic response, developing chiefly in young individuals within three to six weeks of the start of therapy. Aplastic anemia appears to be dose-related and occurs primarily in individuals more than 60 years of age.

Nonsteroidal anti-inflammatory drugs (NSAIDs) include ibuprofen, naproxen, fenoprofen, tolmetin, sulindac, meclofenamate sodium, and piroxicam. If indomethacin is efficacious but not tolerated, one of these NSAIDs may be given. In general, these agents play a minor role in the management of the spondylarthritides. Phenylbutazone should be tried when indomethacin is ineffective.

Gold and penicillamine have no role to play, but sulfasalazine may be effective. Radiotherapy, once the treatment of choice, is no longer practiced in view of the high risk of inducing leukemia.

The patient also needs remedial strengthening exercises and postural training. A firm mattress and small pillow are ideal when resting; attention to posture at work and at rest must be stressed. The best exercise regimen includes extension exercises and hydrotherapy; swimming is highly recommended.

In those few patients who, despite optimal management, develop an irreversible deformity, wedge osteotomy may be indicated. For those with destructive arthropathy of the hip, arthroplasty is useful.

REITER'S SYNDROME

The most common cause of an inflammatory oligoarthropathy in a young male is Reiter's syndrome. This classic triad of urethritis, conjunctivitis, and arthritis represents the one chronic rheumatic disorder related to both a specific genetic background (HLA-B27) and a specific infection. Reiter's syndrome is often not self-limiting. Progressive disease may result in major disability. The disease may be defined as "an episode of arthropathy within one month of urethritis or cervicitis."

Whether a dysenteric (epidemic) or a venereal (endemic) infection is the most common precipitating event is unclear. In young children, the former is the rule. In many cases, the distinction between urethritis as a precipitating factor and urethritis as an integral manifestation of the syndrome remains unclear. In postvenereal Reiter's syndrome both *Chlamydia* and *Mycoplasma* have been implicated. In a patient with a specific predisposing genetic background, a variety of different organisms may be responsible.

Prevalence

Reiter's syndrome develops in at least 1 per cent of patients with nonspecific urethritis. *Shigella* dysentery is followed by Reiter's syndrome in 1 to 2 per cent of cases (i.e., 20 per cent of B27-positive patients).

The sex distribution of Reiter's syndrome is difficult to define because the syndrome is diagnosed only with difficulty in females, in whom urethritis is often clinically inapparent. Formes frustes of the syndrome are now being recognized. A woman presenting with uveitis and an inflammatory arthropathy of the knee in association with the HLA-B27 antigen may have Reiter's syndrome. Similarly, the disorder is difficult to recognize in children; a diagnosis is usually made only if an epidemic of dysentery is present and Reiter's syndrome has been recognized in other family members. Postdysenteric Reiter's syndrome almost certainly has an equal sex distribution.

Clinical Picture

Reiter's syndrome should be considered a symptom complex rather than the association of three specific features. The syndrome may present as a tetrad (i.e., with the addition of buccal ulceration or balanitis to the classic triad); alternatively, only two of the three cardinal features may be present. Several of the classic features may appear insignificant and be overlooked. For example, the urethritis may be mild, perhaps forgotten; the discharge may be minimal and remembered by the patient only after direct questioning. Balanitis may not be evident unless the prepuce is retracted and the glans penis closely inspected. Buccal ulceration is usually painless and apparent only after close inspection. A red eye may be forgotten or considered irrelevant, and the various skin lesions typified by keratoderma blennorrhagicum may be misdiagnosed.

Rheumatologic features include arthralgias, tenosynovitic episodes, plantar fasciitis, and other enthesopathies, as well as frank arthritis. The typical sausage-shaped digit is a frequent occurrence related to the disorder's enthesopathic nature.

Some 20 per cent of patients with Reiter's syndrome develop sacroiliitis and ascending spinal disease. Other radiologic evidence of Reiter's syndrome includes plantar spurs and periosteal new bone formation. Cardiac complications similar to those in ankylosing spondylitis occur late in Reiter's syndrome.

The hyperkeratotic skin lesions seen in Reiter's syndrome cannot be distinguished from those in psoriasis.

Formerly considered a self-limited process, Reiter's syndrome is now known to be a more or less persistent disease in many patients. About 80 per cent of patients have evidence of disease activity when they are re-examined after a five-year period.

Laboratory Evaluation

It is unclear whether the presence of HLA-B27 correlates with increased severity of Reiter's syndrome. A patient with severe Reiter's syndrome may have an erythrocyte sedimentation rate in the normal range or one as high as 100 mm per hour or more. Synovial fluid analysis is rarely diagnostic, apart from the fact that it reveals a relatively high complement level (reflecting a nonspecific inflammatory reaction), rather than the low level seen in rheumatoid arthritis (reflecting immune complex disease).

Occasionally, the diagnoses of ankylosing spondylitis and Reiter's syndrome may prove difficult to disentangle. Some patients who are diagnosed as having ankylosing spondylitis may have presented originally with Reiter's syndrome, but the episodes of urethritis have subsequently been forgotten by the physician and patient. Similarly, patients diagnosed as having Reiter's syndrome may actually have ankylosing spondylitis with peripheral joint disease and a chance occurrence of urethritis.

Management

There is no cure for Reiter's syndrome. The patient's feelings of guilt and anxiety about sexual misconduct must be allayed. Although anecdotal evidence suggests that individuals with postvenereal Reiter's syndrome may develop a relapse following sexual activity, many individuals have spontaneous exacerbations. An explanation of allergic response may help the patient: Asthma may develop on exposure to a known or unknown allergen in sensitive individuals; in the same way, Reiter's syndrome may flare up following an unknown allergic event.

Symptomatic management includes the use of indomethacin, phenylbutazone, or other NSAIDs. Antibiotic therapy is too late and unnecessary. Patients with severe recurrent uveitis may require steroid eye drops or subconjunctival preparations. The syndrome may remit, recur, or continue unabated despite steroid or even cytotoxic therapy. For patients with progressive disease, azathioprine or methotrexate is effective.

THE REACTIVE ARTHROPATHIES

Reactive arthropathy refers to an inflammatory arthritis that follows an infection in which there is no microbial invasion of the synovial space. The B27-linked arthropathies following *Shigella, Salmonella, Yersinia,* and *Campylobacter jejuni* infections are in this group. Why some patients develop only an arthropathy whereas others have the full spectrum of Reiter's disease after exposure to one of these agents is unknown.

Yersinia Infection

Yersinia enterocolitica infection may produce the following: fever, mild gastrointestinal illness, and, after a latent period, polyarthropathy and erythema nodosum, especially in B27-positive individuals. The symptom complex may mimic acute rheumatic fever. The arthropathy may last for weeks or months, and in HLA-B27–positive individuals, sacroiliitis may occur.

Salmonellosis

An arthropathy associated with *Salmonella* infection mimics that caused by *Yersinia.*

Treatment of these disorders is the same as that of Reiter's syndrome.

JUVENILE CHRONIC ARTHROPATHY

Chronic arthritis in a child or teenager often persists into adulthood; therefore, an awareness of juvenile chronic arthropathy is relevant when attending adult patients. Until recently, the term juvenile rheumatoid arthritis was used, inappropriately, to describe all forms of childhood arthritis. As in adults, arthritis in children may be associated with psoriasis, inflammatory bowel disease, and other conditions.

The acute systemic form, Still's disease, presents with fever, rash, and toxicity in young children who are negative for B27 and rheumatoid factor (IgM-anti-IgG). Still's disease is also recognized in adults. Another subset (in the spondylarthropathy group) consists largely of adolescent males who predominantly exhibit oligoarthropathy affecting the large joints of the lower limbs: Such individuals are frequently positive for HLA-B27. This group may develop sacroiliitis or ankylosing spondylitis; the presence of B27 is associated with spinal disease involvement. Another group includes B27-negative individuals (usually females less than five years of age) presenting with an oligoarthropathy characterized by a positive fluorescent antinuclear antibody (FANA) test. These subjects are at risk for developing asymptomatic chronic iridocyclitis, in contrast with FANA-negative and B27-positive patients, who develop clinically obvious acute uveitis. A few older children (preponderantly females) develop a seropositive, nodular, and erosive disease that resembles adult rheumatoid arthritis. A B27-related syndrome known as seronegative enthesopathy and arthropathy (SEA syndrome) is now also recognized in children.

THE ENTEROPATHIC ARTHROPATHIES

Two major clinical patterns of arthopathy associated with inflammatory bowel disease (ulcerative colitis and Crohn's disease) are peripheral arthropathy and spondylarthropathy.

Peripheral Arthropathy

Approximately 20 per cent of individuals with severe Crohn's disease or ulcerative colitis develop an acute migratory inflammatory polyarthritis, often of abrupt onset and involving the larger joints of the lower extremities. The arthritis resolves in weeks or months. Arthritis flare-ups usually parallel exacerbations of the underlying disorder. The pathogenesis of the joint complication is unknown. B27 antigen is not present. Treatment is directed at the primary disorder and is more effective in ulcerative colitis than in Crohn's disease.

Spondylarthropathy

About one patient in five with inflammatory bowel disease develops sacroiliitis and, occasionally, severe ankylosing spondylitis. The spinal disease may precede the bowel disease or follow it. There is no correlation between the severity of the bowel disorder and the spondylitis, which mimics primary ankylosing spondylitis rather than the spondylitis associated with psoriasis or Reiter's syndrome. Therapy is the same as for classic ankylosing spondylitis. Despite the bowel disease, the NSAIDs are usually well tolerated.

About 50 per cent of individuals with both inflammatory bowel disease and ankylosing spondylitis are B27-positive, a percentage lower than that found in patients with primary ankylosing spondylitis.

A post–intestinal-bypass syndrome consisting of arthropathy and occasionally dermatitis is well recognized. Immune alterations have been described in these patients, and B27 is occasionally associated with this syndrome.

PSORIATIC ARTHROPATHY

Different subsets of psoriatic arthropathy are recognized, several forms of which appear to be enthesopathic rather than purely synovitic. Uveitis, sacroiliitis, and ascending spinal disease occur in up to 20 per cent of cases. Patients are seronegative for rheumatoid factor and exhibit sausage digits and characteristic radiologic changes. The disease may be markedly destructive.

Psoriasis itself is a genetically determined disease, associated with HLA-B13, HLA-Bw17, and HLA-Cw6. Moreover, HLA-B27 is present in approximately 20 per cent of individuals with psoriatic arthropathy even in the absence of sacroiliitis. HLA-Bw38, HLA-DR4, and HLA-DR7 appear to be genetic markers for patients with peripheral arthropathy. About 50 per cent of psoriatic spondylitis patients are B27-negative; thus, as with inflammatory bowel disease, other genetic or environmental factors are relevant.

Psoriatic arthropathy is a common disease, occurring in about 20 per cent of individuals with psoriasis, particularly in those patients with psoriatic nail disease. Women are affected only slightly more commonly than men, in contrast to the more marked sex distribution in rheumatoid disease. Several forms of psoriatic arthropathy, separated by indistinct boundaries, have been described.

1. Asymmetric oligoarthropathy. In general, there is little relationship between joint and skin activity. Patients with this common form of psoriatic arthropathy remain seronegative for rheumatoid factor. Asymmetric involvement of both large and small joints is seen; the sausage-shaped digit is common. A disparity is often observed between the clinical appearance and subjective symptoms. Any patient presenting with this form of arthropathy should be carefully examined for signs of psoriasis (scalp, umbilicus, gluteal region, and nails). In the past, many such individuals were considered to have seronegative rheumatoid arthritis.

2. Symmetric polyarthropathy resembling rheumatoid arthritis. Rarely, the pattern of arthritis may be indistinguishable from that seen in rheumatoid disease. This form may represent coincidental rheumatoid arthritis in a patient with psoriasis.

3. Arthritis mutilans. A resorptive arthropathy, arthritis mutilans is the severest form of destructive arthritis. The telescoping digits appear as the so-called opera-glass hand.

4. Psoriatic spondylitis. Approximately 20 per cent of subjects with psoriatic arthropathy have radiologic sacroiliitis (ankylosing spondylitis).

5. Psoriatic nail disease and distal interphalangeal joint involvement. Nail pitting, transverse depressions, and subungual hyperkeratosis often occur in association with distal interphalangeal joint disease. The relationship between the psoriasis and the arthritis remains unclear.

Laboratory Features

An elevated erythrocyte sedimentation rate, anemia, and rarely, hyperuricemia may occur. The frequency of positive tests for rheumatoid factor is the same as that found in the general population. The synovial tissue and fluid changes are nonspecific.

Radiologic Findings

Characteristic changes in this sometimes highly destructive disease include whittling of the distal ends of the phalanges, giving the joints a "pencil-and-cup" appearance; extensive bone resorption can result in an opera-glass hand. Erosions, ankylosis, periostitis, sacroiliitis, and ankylosing spondylitis are other typical radiologic findings.

Therapy

The skin and joints are treated separately. Improvement of the skin disease may be associated with amelioration of the joint inflammation. For mild arthropathy, indomethacin (25 to 50 mg t.i.d.) is the drug of choice. If this fails, phenylbutazone may be given. Gold and penicillamine may be useful, but few controlled studies have been done. Methotrexate is helpful in resistant cases.

Calin A (ed.): Spondylarthropathy. New York, Grune and Stratton, 1984, pp 1–427. *A multiauthored international text on spondylarthropathy including discussions on immunogenetics, the environment, and ethnic differences.*

Calin A, Marder A, Becks E, et al.: Genetic difference between B27 positive patients with ankylosing spondylitis and B27 positive healthy controls. Arthritis Rheum 26:1460–1464, 1983. *An up-to-date analysis of the genetics of B27-associated disorders.*

Fox R, Calin A, Gerber R, et al.: The chronicity of symptoms and disability in Reiter's syndrome: An analysis of 131 consecutive patients. Ann Intern Med 91:190–193, 1979. *A detailed evaluation of 131 consecutive patients with Reiter's syndrome.*

Wright V, Moll JMH: Seronegative Polyarthritis. Amsterdam, North Holland Publishing Company, 1976. *The best introduction to the concept of the spondylarthropathies.*

Ziff M, Cohen SB: The Spondyloarthropathies. Advances in Inflammation Research. New York, Raven Press. Vol 9, 1985. *An up-to-date series of research papers on epidemiology and pathogenesis.*

435 INFECTIOUS ARTHRITIS

Stephen E. Malawista

BACTERIAL ARTHRITIS

Bacterial arthritis usually results from bloodborne infection and much less commonly from direct penetration (e.g., needle aspiration) or contiguous osteomyelitis. Acute bacterial joint infections may be divided into two general groups, nongonococcal and gonococcal, based on their typically differing target populations, clinical characteristics, and ease of treatment. Differential features of these two classes of bacterial arthritis are presented in Table 435–1.

Nongonococcal Arthritis

Staphylococcus aureus heads the list of common infecting organisms in this group, followed by other gram-positive cocci (*Streptococcus pyogenes, pneumoniae, viridans*) and gram-negative bacilli (*Escherichia coli, Salmonella* sp., *Pseudomonas*, etc.); *Haemophilus influenzae* is unusual except in children under four years of age, before protective immunity develops. Patients are often very young, elderly, immunocompromised, or users of intravenous drugs. Risk factors for bacterial arthritis during septicemia include debilitating chronic disease, immunosuppressive therapy, previous joint damage (e.g., rheumatoid arthritis, neuropathic arthropathy, joint surgery), sickle cell anemia, hypogammaglobulinemia, and intra-articular corticosteroid injections. After prosthetic joint replacement, an increasing problem has been late infection by organisms of low virulence, such as *Staphylococcus epidermidis*.

CLINICAL MANIFESTATIONS. A patient may present typically with the abrupt onset of a single, severely tender, red-hot swollen joint, especially the knee or another weight-bearing joint; shaking chills and fever may occur. However, signs of inflammation may be masked in severely debilitated patients or in those receiving adrenocorticosteroids or immunosuppressive agents. Bacterial arthritis superimposed on a noninfectious inflammatory joint disease may also be easily overlooked. For example, infection in one or a few joints of a patient with rheumatoid arthritis may be mistaken for a flare in the chronic disease. An infected joint in a gouty individual may go unrecognized for too long, even when the patient

TABLE 435–1. DIFFERENTIAL FEATURES OF DISSEMINATED GONOCOCCAL INFECTION AND NONGONOCOCCAL BACTERIAL ARTHRITIS*

Disseminated Gonococcal Infection	Nongonococcal Bacterial Arthritis
Generally in young, healthy adults	Often in very young, elderly, or immunocompromised persons
Initial migratory polyarthralgias common	Polyarthralgias rare
Tenosynovitis in majority	Tenosynovitis rare
Dermatitis in majority	Dermatitis rare
>50% polyarthritis	>85% monoarthritis
Positive blood culture in <10%	Positive blood culture in 50%
Positive joint-fluid culture in 25%	Positive joint-fluid culture in 85–95%

*From Goldenberg DL, Reed JI: Bacterial arthritis. N Engl J Med 312:764–771, 1985.

does not respond to his usual regimen for acute gouty arthritis (a good clue that something else is going on). A high index of suspicion is essential in these circumstances, because delay can lead rapidly to destruction of cartilage and bone and eventual fibrous or bony ankylosis.

DIAGNOSIS. When bacterial arthritis is suspected, prompt joint aspiration and both Gram stain and culture of synovial fluid are imperative; most nongonococcal bacteria will be recovered. Cultures for both aerobic and anaerobic organisms should be made. Synovial fluid leukocyte counts are frequently greater than 50,000 per cubic millimeter, and the glucose level low and lactate level high compared with those of serum, but these findings are not specific for infection. Bacteriologic studies should of course be extended to blood and other material (sputum, urine, etc.) from which the infection may have disseminated. On x-ray, only soft-tissue swelling is likely to be seen during the first week, but evidence of loss of articular cartilage and erosion of bone may appear rather soon thereafter in untreated patients.

MANAGEMENT. Successful management of bacterial arthritis depends primarily on early institution of appropriate antimicrobial therapy and effective drainage of the joint space. The selection of antimicrobial agents and recommendations regarding dose and duration of therapy are discussed in other areas of the text (Part XVIII). Antibiotics are given parenterally, often in high doses, for two to four weeks or more, depending on the clinical situation and the patient's response. They generally attain adequate levels in joint fluid and need not be given intra-articularly; indeed, the latter procedure may induce a chemical synovitis. For drainage, daily (or even more frequent) closed joint aspiration through a large-bore needle is carried out until fluid no longer accumulates. Open surgical drainage usually can be avoided except when the hip or the shoulder is infected (difficult to evacuate completely by needle); when tissue debris or fibrin interferes with closed aspiration; or when loculations, gross joint destruction, or contiguous osteomyelitis is present. The affected joint should be at rest while inflamed, and mobilized to prevent atrophy when signs of acute inflammation have subsided.

Gonococcal Arthritis

Gonococcal infection is discussed in Ch. 306. The associated arthritis is by far the most common bacterial joint problem in generally healthy, sexually active teenagers and young adults, especially in urban populations. Gonorrhea is more likely to disseminate in women. The risk of dissemination is particularly high during menses and pregnancy, in the post-partum period, and in individuals with genetic deficiency in the terminal components of serum complement (C5, C6, C7, or C8). Additional features that help to distinguish gonococcal from other bacterial arthritides include a high frequency of associated tenosynovitis and rash and of multiple joint involvement, especially in the wrists and hands. Diagnosis is frequently presumptive because synovial fluid smear and culture—which requires special media—are often negative, and corroborating cultural evidence from urethra, cervix, throat, rectum, blood, or skin may be lacking. Highly suggestive diagnostically is a history of fever and migratory polyarthralgias that progress to frank oligoarticular arthritis and are associated with tenosynovitis and skin lesions. The latter are either vesiculopustular on an erythematous base, often with necrotic centers, or hemorrhagic. Similar lesions are seen with arthritis caused by the meningococcus. Response to (even oral) antibiotic therapy (Ch. 306) and drainage is usually dramatic. Resistance to penicillin of gonococci that disseminate is uncommon.

Tuberculous Arthritis

The general decline in the frequency of pulmonary tuberculosis in the western world is reflected in the relative rarity of tuberculous bone and joint disease. Infection usually reaches the joint from hematogenous dissemination to bone and direct extension from an osteomyelitic focus. Formerly, the classic presentation was chronic low back pain in a child because of involvement of lower thoracic or lumbar vertebrae, leading to collapse and sharp-angle kyphosis (Pott's disease). Currently, the typical target is a tuberculin-positive adult, often without evidence of pulmonary disease, who presents with chronic, insidious pain and swelling, usually in a single joint, especially the hip, knee, or wrist; this presentation is often mistaken for monoarticular rheumatoid arthritis. Tenosynovitis is common. Diagnosis depends upon culture of *Mycobacterium tuberculosis* from synovial fluid (positive in 80 per cent) or synovial biopsy (positive in 90 per cent). Sensitivities to chemotherapeutic agents must be determined; caseating granulomata and acid-fast bacilli are sometimes due to atypical mycobacteria resistant to the usual antituberculous drugs. Usual therapy for uncomplicated infections consists of long-term isoniazid and ethambutol or rifampin.

Goldenberg DL, Reed JI: Bacterial arthritis. N Engl J Med 312:764, 1985. *A compact, well-referenced review of the pathophysiology of bacterial arthritis, clinical and microbiologic characteristics of its common forms, and current approaches to diagnosis and therapy.*

VIRAL ARTHRITIS

Many specific viral infections are associated with polyarthritis, notably hepatitis B and rubella, but also mumps and vaccinia (and formerly, smallpox) and occasionally adenovirus type 7, Ebstein-Barr virus (EBV) (in infectious mononucleosis) and other herpes viruses, and certain enteroviruses. Polyarthritis may dominate the picture of various mosquito-transmitted arbovirus infections, especially epidemic polyarthritis of Australia (Ross River virus) and the dengue-like illnesses, chikungunya and o'nyongnyong.

In general, diagnosis is suggested by the exposure history (drug abuse for hepatitis B, immunization for rubella, epidemiologic considerations for arbo- or enteroviruses); recognition of the associated viral syndrome, which often includes fever, rash, and regional lymphadenopathy; brevity of the joint involvement (days to weeks); and changing antibody titers against specific antigens. Routine laboratory tests are nonspecific, and except for rubella, virus has rarely been recovered from synovial fluid. Little is known about pathogenesis, but studies of hepatitis B and rubella provide some clues.

Transient, often symmetric polyarthritis or arthralgias resembling acute rheumatoid arthritis may be associated with both hepatitis B and rubella infections. In the case of *hepatitis B*, 10 to 30 per cent of patients have arthritis, often accompanied by urticaria, fever, and lymphadenopathy, all occurring days to weeks before the onset of frank hepatitis. This prodromal syndrome typically occurs when hepatitis B surface antigen (HBsAg) is in excess over antibody, hypocomplementemia is present, and serum contains immune complexes composed of HBsAg and anti-HB, other immunoglobulins, and complement components. Similar material has been found in affected dermal blood vessels, and the antigen has been seen in synovial tissue. With the development of antibody excess, complexes disappear, the arthritis and rash resolve, and frank hepatitis may supervene. The process resembles experimental serum sickness and suggests an inflammatory pathogenetic mechanism driven by deposition of immune complexes. Joint symptoms may respond dramatically to salicylates.

Rubella arthritis is primarily a disease of adult women. It usually follows onset of the characteristic rash by a few days, but the rash may be absent and rheumatoid factor present, inviting diagnostic confusion. Arthritis is usually sudden in onset, symmetric and polyarticular in distribution (fingers, knees, wrists), brief in duration (less than a month), and without residua. Salicylates are useful for pain and stiffness.

Arthritis may also occur within a few weeks of vaccination by attenuated rubella virus. Again, attacks are brief but may recur periodically for a few years without permanent joint damage. Rubella virus has been recovered from synovial fluid in both the natural and vaccine-induced disease and more recently in a few patients with various chronic joint syndromes. It seems capable of replicating in synovium; whether its new association with chronic disease is critical or coincidental remains to be determined.

Steere AC: Viral arthritis. In McCarty DJ (ed.): Arthritis and Allied Conditions. 11th ed. Philadelphia, Lea & Febiger (in press). *Survey of common and uncommon arthrides associated with specific viral illnesses.*

Wands JR, Mann E, Alpert E, et al.: The pathogenesis of arthritis associated with acute hepatitis B surface antigen-positive hepatitis. Complement activation and characterization of circulating immune complexes. J Clin Invest 55:930, 1975. *Clinical description and characterization of immunologic aspects of the syndrome.*

OTHER FORMS OF INFECTIOUS ARTHRITIS

Lyme Disease (See Ch. 313.)

Syphilitic Arthritis

Syphilis is discussed in Ch. 310. Joint disease associated with congenital and acquired syphilitic infections is now rare. In infants with congenital disease, musculoskeletal complaints are related to periostitis and osteochondritis. About the time of puberty, painless knee effusions (Clutton's joints) may be confused with rheumatoid or pyogenic arthritis. With acquired infection, arthralgias, arthritis, or tenosynovitis may accompany classic signs of secondary syphilis: rash, mucous plaques, alopecia, or lymphadenopathy. In tertiary lues, gummatous arthritis or periostitis (tibia, clavicles) may occur. Neuropathic arthropathy (Charcot's joint) is reviewed in Ch. 482.

Fungal Arthritis

Any of the invasive mycoses can affect joints, usually by direct extension from bone. Frequent infectious agents include coccidioidomycosis and histoplasmosis—both of which may also be accompanied by erythema nodosum with joint involvement, sporotrichosis (often by direct penetration: rose thorns), blastomycosis, actinomycosis, and candidiasis. Clinically, the affected joint or joints resemble those in other forms of granulomatous arthritis (e.g., tuberculous). For diagnosis, the causative agent must be seen in appropriately stained synovial biopsy material or grown from synovial tissue or fluid.

436 SYSTEMIC LUPUS ERYTHEMATOSUS

Alfred D. Steinberg

Systemic lupus erythematosus (SLE) is a disease of unknown etiology characterized by inflammation in many different organ systems associated with the production of antibodies reactive with nuclear, cytoplasmic, and cell membrane antigens. Individual patients may have some, but not necessarily all, of the following: fatigue, anemia, fever, rashes, sun sensitivity, alopecia, arthritis, pericarditis, pleurisy, vasculitis, nephritis, and central nervous system disease. The course is often unpredictable with variable periods of exacerbations and remissions. There is no one clinical abnormality that definitely establishes the diagnosis, nor is there a single test for the disorder. As a result, criteria have been developed and modified in an attempt to include patients with SLE and to exclude patients with other disorders (Table 436–1). Although these criteria were developed for epidemiologic and research purposes, they are helpful in diagnosis as well. Nevertheless, it is possible to fulfill these criteria and not have SLE, and it is possible to fail to fulfill the criteria and still have SLE. Thus, a teen-age girl with a "butterfly" rash of the face, pleurisy, and large amounts of serum antibodies reactive with native DNA undoubtedly has SLE even if she does not yet manifest any other criteria. The disease derives its name (lupus =

TABLE 436–1. CRITERIA FOR CLASSIFICATION OF SYSTEMIC LUPUS ERYTHEMATOSUS*

Criterion		Definition
1. Malar rash		Fixed erythema, flat or raised, over the malar eminences, tending to spare the nasolabial folds
2. Discoid rash		Erythematous raised patches with adherent keratotic scaling and follicular plugging; atrophic scarring may occur in older lesions
3. Photosensitivity		Skin rash as a result of unusual reaction to sunlight, by patient history or physician observation
4. Oral ulcers		Oral or nasopharyngeal ulceration, usually painless, observed by a physician
5. Arthritis		Nonerosive arthritis involving two or more peripheral joints, characterized by tenderness, swelling, or effusion
6. Serositis	a)	Pleuritis—convincing history of pleuritic pain or rub heard by a physician or evidence of pleural effusion *OR*
	b)	Pericarditis—documented by ECG or rub or evidence of pericardial effusion
7. Renal disorder	a)	Persistent proteinuria greater than 0.5 gram per day or greater than 3+ if quantitation not performed *OR*
	b)	Cellular casts—may be red cell, hemoglobin, granular, tubular, or mixed
8. Neurologic disorder	a)	Seizures—in the absence of offending drugs or known metabolic derangements, e.g., uremia, ketoacidosis, or electrolyte imbalance *OR*
	b)	Psychosis—in the absence of offending drugs or known metabolic derangements, e.g., uremia, ketoacidosis, or electrolyte imbalance
9. Hematologic disorder	a)	Hemolytic anemia—with reticulocytosis *OR*
	b)	Leukopenia—less than 4000/mm^3 total on two or more occasions *OR*
	c)	Lymphopenia—less than 1500/mm^3 on two or more occasions *OR*
	d)	Thrombocytopenia—less than 100,000/mm^3 in the absence of offending drugs
10. Immunologic disorder	a)	Positive LE cell preparation *OR*
	b)	Anti-DNA: antibody to native DNA in abnormal titer *OR*
	c)	Anti-Sm: presence of antibody to Sm nuclear antigen *OR*
	d)	False-positive serologic test for syphilis known to be positive for at least 6 months and confirmed by *Treponema pallidum* immobilization or fluorescent treponemal antibody absorption test
11. Antinuclear antibody		An abnormal titer of antinuclear antibody by immunofluorescence or an equivalent assay at any point in time and in the absence of drugs known to be associated with "drug-induced lupus" syndrome

*The classification is based on 11 criteria. For the purpose of identifying patients in clinical studies, a person shall be said to have systemic lupus erythematosus if any 4 or more of the 11 criteria are present, serially or simultaneously, during any interval of observation.

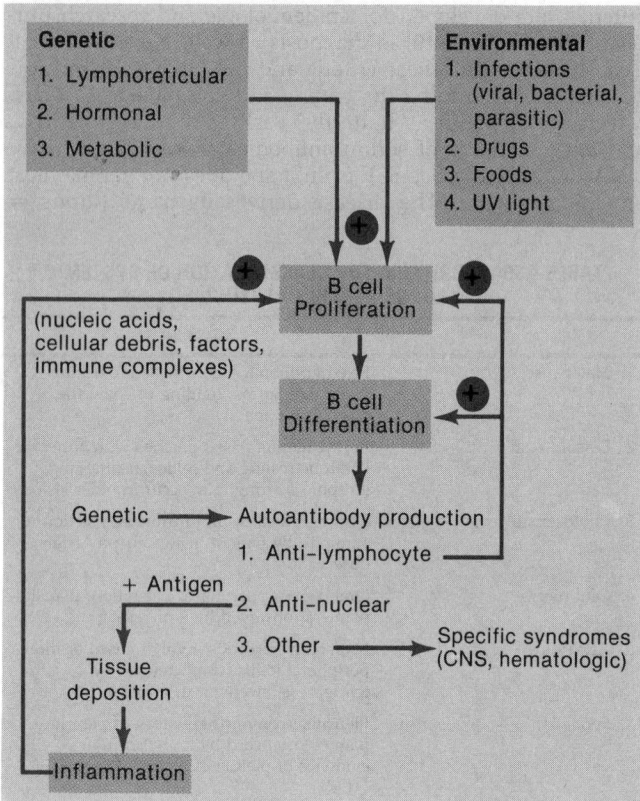

FIGURE 436–1. Initiation and perpetuation of systemic lupus erythematosus.

wolf) from the facial rash, which resembles the malar erythema of a wolf.

INCIDENCE. Although SLE can occur at any age (it has been diagnosed at birth and in individuals in the tenth decade of life), more than 60 per cent of patients experience the onset of disease between ages 13 and 40 years. Among children, SLE occurs three times more commonly in females than in males. In patients in their teens, twenties, and thirties, 90 to 95 per cent are female. Thereafter, the female predominance again falls to that observed before puberty.

The disorder is approximately three times more common among American blacks than American caucasians. Certain North American Indian tribes (Sioux, Crow, Arapahoe) have an even greater predisposition toward SLE. Orientals have been less well studied; however, the data suggest that they are affected to approximately the same extent as American blacks. The overall annual incidence of SLE is about 6 new cases per 100,000 population per year for relatively low-risk populations and approximately 35 per 100,000 for relatively high-risk populations. The chance of a black female developing SLE in her lifetime is approximately 1 in 250.

These data suggest that both genetic factors and sex hormones may affect the probability of developing SLE. If a family member has SLE, the likelihood of SLE increases (approximately 30 per cent for identical twins and 5 per cent for other first-degree relatives). Although males develop SLE less frequently than do females, their illness is not milder.

ETIOLOGY. The etiology of SLE is unknown. The signs and symptoms are thought to be caused by the autoantibodies that react with self constituents and initiate inflammatory responses. The initiation of this process may be multifactorial (Fig. 436–1) and may be different in different individuals. These factors are currently poorly understood. One or more genetic factors appear to be important in many individuals. These may be genes that allow augmented antibody responses following a variety of stimuli as well as genes that predispose to particular autoantibodies. In addition, hormonal, metabolic,

and environmental factors appear to act on the genetically conditioned immune substratum to predispose to or protect against disease expression. Males are protected against SLE by their androgens except in a subgroup of males who inherit a Y chromosome accelerating factor from their fathers. Estrogens probably predispose to SLE to a lesser extent than androgens protect against the expression of the illness. In general, factors that augment immunity favor disease expression, whereas those that retard immunity, especially antibody production, tend to protect. Any of a variety of bacterial, viral, or parasitic infections may stimulate the immune system, as may drugs or food additives.

Some patients may have a primary abnormality in the ability of their immune systems to perform normal self-regulatory functions. It is probably best to consider abnormal immune regulation as one of several factors that may contribute to illness. If any one is very abnormal, disease may occur. Under most circumstances, several defects probably combine to incite disease. However, once the process is initiated, impaired self-regulation would favor perpetuation of the disease-inducing abnormalities.

It has long been known that some individuals with SLE have disease exacerbations following exposure to ultraviolet light. Several different mechanisms are likely: UV light induces keratinocytes to secrete interleukin 1, which, in turn, stimulates B cells and induces T cells to produce growth factors (interleukin 2, B cell growth factors, B cell differentiation factors, interferon), which stimulate the immune system; UV light impairs processing of antigen and immune complexes, thereby increasing the load of pathogenic complexes on target organs; UV light induces cytosine and thymine dimer formation, which stimulates immune responses.

Certain drugs can cause an SLE-like illness in apparently healthy individuals. The drugs (Table 436–2) do not share common structural or chemical properties. The mechanisms of disease induction probably vary. Even chemicals in foods may induce SLE. For example, alfalfa sprouts contain L-canavanine, which can induce an SLE-like illness. The extent to which "idiopathic" SLE is triggered by such specific environmental factors is unknown.

A variety of complement deficiencies have been associated with SLE. The most common is C2 deficiency. It is not clear whether the association is one of genetic linkage or predisposition because of the deficiency itself. The latter might occur if the deficiency led to increased susceptibility to infections that trigger illness.

For many years it has been thought that there might be a "lupus virus," a particular virus that induces disease. Patients with SLE have, in the endothelial cells of their kidneys and in their lymphocytes, structures that resemble viral nucleocapsids. In addition, retroviruses have been implicated in the

TABLE 436–2. SOME DRUGS ABLE TO INDUCE FEATURES OF SLE

Related to Dose-Time Administration	More Idiosyncratic
Hydralazine	Aminosalicylic acid
Procainamide	D-Penicillamine
Alpha-methyldopa	Griseofulvin
Isoniazid	Penicillin
Chlorpromazine	Ampicillin
Chlorthalidone	Streptomycin
Phenytoin	Sulfonamides
Mephenytoin	Tetracycline
Trimethadione	Methylthiouracil
Primidone	Propythiouracil
Ethosuximide	Phenylbutazone
Carbamazepine	Oxyphenisatin
Phenylethylacetylurea	Practolol
	Tolazamide
	Methysergide
	Reserpine
	Quinidine
	Isoquinazepan
	Guanoxan

immune-complex renal disease of animals with SLE-like disorders. Nevertheless, even if such a virus is important, it is only one of many factors critical to the development of disease.

AUTOIMMUNITY AND DISEASE IN SLE. In past years it was believed that an anti-self response was harmful and that such responses did not occur normally. We now appreciate that normal immune responses involve self-self recognition. Moreover, many individuals produce nonpathogenic antibodies reactive with self antigens. As a result, disease occurs only when anti-self reactions are either excessive or productive of especially injurious immune responses. SLE is characterized by the production of large amounts of antibodies reactive with antigens having a great variety of specificities. Some antibody molecules cross-react with more than one antigen (DNA and cardiolipin or IgG and nucleoprotein). As a result, the true range of antibody molecules reactive with self-determinants may be less than the number of specificities as measured by the reactive antigens. Nevertheless, the range of determinants against which SLE antibodies may react is impressive (Table 436–3).

How could such self reactivity come about? It is believed that self-tolerance is a complex state brought about and maintained by several mechanisms. Very early in life, expo-

sure to antigens tends to produce tolerance rather than immunity. Subsequently, several immune mechanisms maintain self-tolerance. Although B lymphocytes and their progeny are responsible for antibody production, under most circumstances they require helper T lymphocytes for activation, proliferation, and differentiation into antibody-secreting cells. Moreover, specialized T cells (suppressor cells) appear capable of down-regulating immune responses. If the T cell population is self-tolerant, it may prevent B cells from proliferating and differentiating into autoantibody producing cells. A defect in self-tolerance mechanisms could occur at any of several steps in the immune pathway. In addition, strong immune stimulation can overwhelm normal regulatory mechanisms, rendering them incapable of regulating the immune stimuli. Strong immune stimuli such as graft-versus-host disease (as after allogeneic bone marrow transplantation) or stimulation by any of a variety of powerful polyclonal immune activators (endotoxin) or even viruses that stimulate B cells (Ebstein-Barr virus) may drive B cells to produce antibodies and autoantibodies without the usual requirements for or regulation by T cells. Individuals with B cells capable of producing pathogenic autoantibodies that had been previously held in check by T cells may, under such circumstances, be driven to produce large amounts of injurious antibodies. Since it is often the quantity of autoantibody that determines whether or not disease occurs, quantitative aspects of immune regulation and immune stimulation may be critical to the balance between disease and relative health with minor immune abnormalities.

PATHOGENESIS. Systemic lupus is often classified as an immune complex type disorder. This designation is, at best, an oversimplification. SLE is a disease primarily mediated by antibodies; however, the details of pathogenesis are not proven for many of the clinical and pathologic findings. It is clear that patients with SLE produce autoantibodies and that many of these are injurious. This has been well demonstrated for the renal disease associated with SLE. Antibody reacts with antigen either in the circulation or in the glomerulus, and complement is fixed, leading to release of chemotactic factors, attraction of leukocytes, and release of their injurious mediators of inflammation. The degree of pathology is determined, to a large extent, by the magnitude of the antibody deposition and the intensity of the inflammatory process initiated. Continued deposition of antibody and continued induction of inflammation ultimately leads to irreversible renal damage. Similar processes occur in other organs. However, antibody and complement may be deposited in the skin or in the choroid plexus with or without an attendant inflammatory response. The qualitative character of the antibody molecules (affinity, isotype, charge), the nature of the antigen or their combined properties (size, molecular configuration), or additional factors may be critical to pathogenesis.

It has long been taught that immunopathology of SLE results from the deposition of DNA–anti-DNA immune complexes. Although immune complexes may contribute to the immunopathology, it is likely that uncomplexed antibody may reach an organ where antigen is already present and there bind to antigen and initiate the inflammatory process. This idea is supported by demonstrations of DNA binding to basement membranes without antibody. Moreover, antibodies of other specificities appear to contribute to disease.

Antibody plays a role in SLE not only by depositing in vessels, but also by binding to the surfaces of cells. Patients with SLE produce antibodies to erythrocytes, granulocytes, lymphocytes, and macrophages. These antibodies can cause such cells to be removed from the circulation by the reticuloendothelial system or to be killed by complement-mediated cytotoxicity, or more likely, by the mechanism of antibody-dependent cellular cytotoxicity (ADCC). In this non-complement-mediated killing, leukocytes recognize antibody-coated target cells and kill them. ADCC may be responsible for some

TABLE 436–3. AUTOANTIBODIES FOUND IN PATIENTS WITH SLE

Specificity	Comments
Nuclear	Present in most but not all patients
Native DNA	Essentially restricted to SLE
Denatured (single-stranded) DNA	May also cross-react with double-stranded DNA. High titers in SLE; lower titers in other diseases
Histones H1, H3-H4	SLE
Histones H2A-H2B	More common in drug-induced SLE
Sm	In a minority of SLE patients, but not found in other diseases.
Nuclear ribonucleoprotein	Found in SLE, but highest titers in "mixed connective tissue disease." Multiple small proteins and combined RNA have been discovered.
Nucleolar antigens	Scleroderma, SLE, Sjögren's syndrome
SS-B (La, Ha)	Sjögren's syndrome, SLE
SS-A (Ro)	Sjögren's syndrome, SLE
Proliferating cell nuclear antigen	SLE
RANA	Especially in rheumatoid arthritis (Ebstein-Barr virus)
DNA-RNA hybrids, double-stranded RNA	SLE
Cytoplasmic	Less information available on these
Ribosomal ribonucleoprotein	SLE
Mitochondria	Primary biliary cirrhosis, SLE
Microsomal antigens	Chronic active hepatitis, malignancies
Lysosomes	SLE
Single-stranded RNA, tRNA	SLE
SS-B and SS-A	Sjögren's syndrome, SLE
Cell membrane determinants	Common in SLE
Red cells	May occur without important hemolysis
White cells	Granulocytes, T cells, B cells
Platelets	Common without thrombocytopenia
Lipomodulin	SLE, RA, others ?
Receptors	Insulin, IL-2, others
Ia	Interferes with immune functions
Others	
Mitotic spindle and intracellular supporting proteins	SLE and other rheumatic diseases
Immunoglobulins	JRA, RA, SLE, Sjögren's syndrome, others
Clotting factors	SLE and other diseases
Phospholipids (e.g., cardiolipin)	May cross-react with DNA
Thyroid antigens	Thyroid diseases, SLE, Sjögren's syndrome

of the pathology initiated in the kidneys and other organs by other antibody-mediated mechanisms. In addition, antibody directed against renal antigens, for example renal tubular or glomerular basement membrane, may be generated as a result of immunization by fragments released from the inflammatory process. Such antibody induces additional renal pathology and may account for much of the disease in some patients.

It appears that many of the inflammatory lesions that occur in SLE are initiated by antibody and that the injury occurs in small vessels. Thus, any organ so affected could be a site of inflammation with the possibility of scarring, dysfunction, or both. Many of the central nervous system problems of patients (seizures, psychoses) as well as hematologic (anemia, thrombocytopenia, leukopenia), cardiac (coronary artery disease), dermal (alopecia, sun sensitivity), and other clinical and laboratory abnormalities have additional pathogenetic mechanisms. The hematologic abnormalities could all be explained by antibodies specifically reactive with the formed elements of the blood; however, many relate to suppression at the level of the bone marrow. The central nervous system disorders are multiple, and each may have its own pathogenetic mechanism. Because central nervous system involvement in SLE is not a single entity, individual patients may require different approaches to understanding and therapy.

PATHOLOGY. The pathologic abnormalities of SLE follow directly from the pathogenetic mechanisms; moreover, the same degree of variability is encountered. In organs affected by small vessel vasculitis, the first lesions are usually characterized by granulocytic infiltration and periarteriolar edema. This is usually (except in some cases of leukocytoclastic involvement of the skin) followed by round cell infiltration and ultimately a relatively acellular eosinophilic material composed of fibrin, immunoglobulins, and complement (fibrinoid) containing scattered hematoxylin bodies. These basophilic-staining bodies are nuclear debris, often associated with antinuclear antibody, and represent a correlate of the LE cell in vivo. Immunofluorescence analysis demonstrates immunoglobulin and complement in the vessels in the affected areas. Arterioles, venules, and sometimes arteries and veins are involved.

Individual organs often have their peculiar abnormalities. The spleen has "onion skin lesions," concentric fibrosis of the walls and surrounding tissues of the central and penicilliary arteries. These lesions are thought to be diagnostic of SLE in patients with "idiopathic" thrombocytopenia. Nonbacterial verrucous endocarditis (Libman-Sacks) consists of vegetations on the heart valves or chordae tendineae; they can extend along the endocardium and become quite large.

The renal pathology varies from mild to severe glomerular inflammation and variable interstitial involvement. Most patients have relatively normal kidneys or a renal lesion consisting of minimal focal hypercellularity, thickening of the capillary basement membrane, and fibrinoid change. In clinically important glomerulonephritis, these lesions are more generalized and are usually a mixture of proliferative and membranous changes with increases in endothelial, mesangial, epithelial, and inflammatory cells, capsular inflammation leading to crescent formation, and focal thickening of the basement membrane and mesangial hypercellularity. Some kidneys have membranous glomerulonephritis with considerable thickening of the basement membrane. Basement membrane thickening, when associated with fibrinoid changes, results in the so-called wire loop lesions. There may also be hyaline thrombi in glomeruli, focal necrosis, hematoxylin bodies, and sclerosis in healed lesions. Tubular degenerative changes and mixed inflammatory interstitial inflammation are common. Some patients have primarily mesangial disease; this carries a better prognosis than does capillary loop involvement. Extensive crescent formation and substantial glomerular or interstitial scarring are unfavorable prognostic signs.

CLINICAL MANIFESTATIONS. SLE is a highly variable disease in onset and course. A young woman may present with a butterfly rash, a history of recent sun sensitivity, pleuropericarditis, arthritis, fever, extreme fatigue, seizures, and nephrotic syndrome. This "typical" presentation, which is easily recognized as SLE, occurs in only a minority of patients. More commonly, patients may have only one or two signs or symptoms of SLE, such as arthritis and fatigue. Only later do additional features of SLE occur. As a result, the initial presentation may not allow a definitive diagnosis nor insight into the organ systems that may become involved in the future. Many patients never develop major organ involvement. Some have kidney but not central nervous system involvement or vice versa. Thus, the clinical manifestations of one patient may be very different from those of another. Some associations between serologic findings and clinical features are valid on a statistical basis but may not hold for a given individual. Thus, patients with large amounts of anti-DNA, especially precipitating antibodies, are more likely to have renal disease. Those with antibodies to Ro (SS-A) and La (SS-B, Ha) are most likely to have sicca syndrome, muscle disease, lung disease, and inconsequential or no renal disease. In the paragraphs that follow, individual clinical features of patients with SLE are described (see also Table 436–4). Patients vary greatly in organ system involvement and also in the severity of disease when a given organ system is affected. Thus, most patients do not have many of the abnormalities described. In addition, SLE is characterized by periods of active disease followed by periods of less intense disease or even remission. In rare cases the patient has a rapidly progressive disease, but the majority can look forward to the time when the disease no longer interferes with their lives.

Constitutional Problems. The majority of patients have fatigue, fever, and weight loss at the time of diagnosis. However, before attributing these to SLE, a diligent search is necessary to rule out infection. Later in the illness, the recurrence of one or more of these findings often indicates an increase in disease activity. Fatigue, difficult as it may be to evaluate, often is the first sign that a flare is imminent.

Musculoskeletal Problems. Arthralgias are the single most common manifestation in SLE. They characteristically are much more transitory than in patients with rheumatoid arthritis (RA), lasting minutes to days in a given joint. With more long-standing or more severe disease, the pain may be constant and frank arthritis is observed. It is often symmetric, the proximal interphalangeal joints of the hands, metacarpophalangeal joints, wrists, and knees being most commonly affected. Morning stiffness is reported by many patients with SLE and joint disease. Although the bony erosions characteristic of RA do not occur, deformities similar to those in RA develop in 10 to 15 per cent of patients and are thought to result from tendon disease. Occasionally patients experience rupture of the Achilles or quadriceps tendons. Myalgias occur in approximately 30 per cent of patients; only a portion of these have muscle tenderness. Many patients with SLE and muscle disease do not have elevations of creatine kinase activity; some of these patients have an elevated aldolase value. Muscle samples from such patients may be normal or show perivascular infiltration or atrophy. Some patients have a vacuolar myopathy that is also observed in corticosteroid-treated individuals.

Skin and Mucous Membranes. The typical butterfly rash varies from a slight blush to a clear-cut and somewhat edematous nonpapular erythematous covering of both cheeks and the bridge of the nose. Patients with a butterfly rash often look as though they have applied too much rouge. This lesion may occur in the absence of sun exposure, but is often exacerbated by the sun. It often precedes other manifestations of disease. A maculopapular erythematous eruption is also common. Indistinguishable from a drug eruption, it is often induced or exacerbated by sunlight and sometimes by a drug (Gantrisin and ampicillin are common offenders). The palms

TABLE 436–4. COMMON CLINICAL ABNORMALITIES IN PATIENTS WITH SLE

Abnormality	Approximate Frequency (%)*
Constitutional	
Fatigue	90
Fever	80
Weight loss, anorexia	60
Musculoskeletal	
Arthritis, arthralgia	90
Myalgia, myositis	30
Skin and mucous membranes	
Butterfly rash	60
Alopecia	50
Photosensitivity	40
Raynaud's phenomenon	30
Mucosal ulcers	30
Discoid lupus	20
Urticaria	10
Edema or bullae	10
Eye (conjunctivitis/episcleritis/sicca syndrome	20
Gastrointestinal	30
Serosal (pleurisy, pericarditis, peritonitis)	50
Lymphoreticular	
Lymphadenopathy	50
Splenomegaly	30
Hepatomegaly	30
Hypertension	30
Bacterial infections	40
Pneumonitis (all)	30
"lupus"	10
Renal (all)	50
severe	20
Central nervous system	
Personality disorders	50
Seizures	20
Psychoses	20
Stroke or long tract signs	10
Migraine headaches	10
Cardiac	
Myocarditis	30
Murmurs and valvular disease	30
Coronary artery disease	20
Hematologic	
Anemia (all)	70
Hemolytic	10
Purpura (all)	50
Thrombocytopenia	10
Peripheral neuropathy	10

*Frequencies are compiled from a number of series and are rounded off to the nearest 10 per cent. There was some variation from series to series depending upon patient population, non-SLE therapy, and therapy for SLE. Some abnormalities are more common in younger patients than in older patients (e.g., splenomegaly and lymphadenopathy) and vice versa (e.g., muscle disease and sicca syndrome).

and soles are not always spared. Healing usually occurs without scarring. Urticaria and angioedema are more common than subepidermal bullae, which occur in only a few per cent of patients. Discoid lupus in SLE is indistinguishable from discoid lupus without systemic involvement; however, systemic disease may develop in patients with long-standing discoid lesions. In this rash, central atrophy, hyper- and hypopigmentation, telangiectasia, and follicular plugging accompany the usual stages of erythema followed by hyperkeratosis and then by atrophy. The hypopigmentation may be extensive and particularly disturbing to blacks.

Livedo reticularis occurs commonly in patients with SLE, but only rarely is it severe. Splinter hemorrhages, tender fingertip pulp lesions, and palmar erythema are sometimes remarkable. Purpura is more often secondary to vasculitis or capillary fragility (corticosteroid therapy is often responsible) than to thrombocytopenia.

Lupus profundus (relapsing nodular nonsuppurative panniculitis) occurs rarely in SLE patients. It may be limited to superficial panniculitis or may extend deeply into the thighs or buttocks. The overlying skin may ulcerate, and the deeper lesions often calcify.

One fifth of patients demonstrate vasculitic lesions of the skin. These can occur on the fingertips, forearms, lips, or lower leg (the latter may ulcerate). Although they are signs of disease activity, they do not usually imply impending disaster. The related mucosal ulcers are often painless and occur on the hard and soft palate, the nasal septum, other parts of the upper respiratory tract, and even the vagina. They are usually harmless, but occasional patients with involvement of the upper airway may require emergency tracheotomy.

Alopecia is usually diffuse; patients report increased hair on comb or brush or pillow. The hair will regrow in areas not scarred by discoid lesions.

Raynaud's phenomenon may be severe enough to cause digital gangrene and spontaneous amputation of the distal parts of the digits. More often it follows a more benign and variable course. Thrombophlebitis occurs in approximately 10 per cent of patients and may be accompanied by pulmonary emboli.

Eyes. Conjunctivitis or episcleritis or both are usually observed in younger patients at times of disease activity. Cytoid bodies (white exudates next to retinal vessels) are associated with active central nervous system involvement. Spasm of the retinal vessels may lead to transient or permanent blindness. Keratoconjunctivitis sicca occurs in 10 per cent of patients and is usually slowly progressive, but it often improves temporarily with therapy for other symptoms.

Gastrointestinal System. Anorexia, nausea, vomiting, and abdominal pain are observed in a minority of patients. Diffuse abdominal pain with or without rebound tenderness may be a manifestation of serositis or mesenteric arteritis. The latter can be complicated by intestinal infarct, which may lead to perforation and death. Corticosteroid therapy often improves symptoms in both situations; however, if perforation has already occurred, the symptoms may be blunted and therapy inappropriately delayed. Pancreatitis is occasionally due to SLE.

Dysphagia may be associated with reduced peristalsis, ulcerations of the esophagus caused by arteritis, or, more commonly, *Candida albicans* infection.

Liver. Liver enlargement is common but usually inconsequential. Fatty infiltration may rarely be associated with hepatic insufficiency. Liver enzyme elevations often occur early in the illness in the absence of therapy. Aspirin treatment may induce such enzyme elevations. Chronic hepatitis is only occasionally observed in patients with SLE.

Heart. Pericarditis is usually symptomatic but without consequence; however, an occasional patient may experience tamponade. The most common EKG abnormality is nonspecific T wave changes. A prolonged P-R interval or evidence of ischemia or infarction may be found. Myocarditis may be manifested by unexplained tachycardia or mild dyspnea on exertion. More severe involvement is associated with frank heart failure. Coronary artery disease, most often atherosclerotic but occasionally arteritic, can lead to myocardial infarction, even in women in their early twenties.

Lung. Pleuritic chest pain occurs more commonly than does x-ray evidence of effusion; however, massive effusions may occur. Pneumonitis in patients with SLE is often infectious; however a noninfectious syndrome occurs in SLE patients which varies from fleeting infiltrates (usually hemorrhagic) to marked consolidation and hypoxia. Diffuse interstitial pneumonitis also has been found in SLE.

Hematologic and Lymphoreticular Problems. Lymphadenopathy and splenomegaly may be sufficiently marked to suggest a lymphoproliferative disorder. Moreover, polyclonal immune hyperactivity in the lymph node may be mistaken for giant follicular or other lymphomas. Hematologic abnormalities are almost invariably present in patients with active disease. The most common is a normocytic anemia caused by impaired erythropoiesis. Hemolysis may occur in patients with or without a positive Coombs' test result, but significant hemolysis occurs in less than 10 per cent of patients. Iron deficiency often contributes to anemia. Many patients with lupus bruise easily; therapy and capillary fragility are more often the cause than a bleeding disorder. Mild thrombocytopenia occurs in a substantial proportion of patients; however, serious thrombocytopenia occurs in less than 10 per cent. Two types of "anticoagulants" occur. One is a laboratory finding caused by antibodies reactive with the phospholipids used in the partial thromboplastin time (PTT) test. This abnormality is not associated with prolonged bleeding and is not a cause of concern with regard to surgery or biopsies. Other antibodies may react with clotting factors (VIII, IX, XII, and others) and may be responsible for clinically important bleeding. It recently has become appreciated that patients with antibodies reactive with phospholipids often manifest a syndrome characterized by thromboses, repeated abortions, and lung disease. The thromboses may lead to severe central nervous system dysfunction.

Nervous System. Peripheral neuropathies have been observed in about 15 per cent of patients with SLE, sometimes in the absence of other nervous system involvement. In addition to a sensory neuropathy, a mononeuritis multiplex picture (e.g., footdrop) is notable. Central nervous system involvement is quite variable. Psychological problems include personality disorders of every variety and numerous forms of frank psychosis (depression, paranoia, mania, schizophrenia). Differentiating that caused by lupus and that caused by corticosteroids is often a challenge.

Seizures, often grand mal, are common, especially in younger patients. Migraine headaches and cytoid bodies may be indications of disease activity. An organic brain syndrome with impaired mentation can progress to coma. Recovery may be complete, or there may be residual impairment. Movement disorders are more common in younger patients: chorea, athetosis, and hemiballismus are observed. Cerebellar abnormalities may occur independently or with other defects.

Transverse myelitis occurs in patients with SLE. Paralysis may also occur following intracerebral hemorrhage or thrombosis. Sterile meningitis may be observed. Despite the large variety of lupus-related nervous system problems, bacterial and other non-lupus causes must be sought and treated.

Kidney Disease. The great majority of patients have some degree of renal involvement. In many, the degree of abnormality is mild enough to escape clinical detection. In others, it is clinically detectable but does not progress to functional impairment. Only a minority of patients has renal involvement that is threatening to the function of the organ. Hypertension and lupus renal involvement synergize in bringing about destructive changes. As a result, the presence of untreated hypertension poses a threat in patients with renal abnormalities.

The renal disease of SLE is of several types: rapidly progressive disease (a subacute glomerulonephritis picture), membranous involvement (usually with some mesangial hypertrophy) with nephrotic syndrome, a nephritic picture (mild to severe), and minimal abnormalities. Most patients have mesangial involvement. The progression to capillary loop pathology carries a worse prognosis. The biopsy picture can change from one form to another; as a result, the degree of active disease (e.g., necrosis) and scarring (glomerular hyalinization, interstitial) offers a much more useful measure than precise histologic classifications. The less scarring, the more there is to treat and preserve. If progression to renal failure occurs, chronic dialysis and renal transplantation are well tolerated. Most patients can be maintained with adequate renal function by modern therapy. Low-grade activity may be

associated with slow progression to renal failure. Complete remissions of renal disease occur.

Menses and Pregnancy. Disease activity in menstruating women tends to be greatest in the period between ovulation and menses. Flares generally occur or worsen in this period. Menses are frequently irregular during active disease. Bleeding may be increased in patients with antibodies to clotting factors or with thrombocytopenia. Repeated spontaneous abortions are common in some women. Others, especially when in remission, carry to term without difficulty. Patients in remission at the time of conception tend to have relatively normal pregnancies. Advanced cardiac, central nervous system, or renal disease is a contraindication to pregnancy. The risk of a disease flare after induced abortion is the same as after delivery. Patients with active renal disease often experience exacerbation during pregnancy and may develop preeclampsia. Patients without renal involvement tend to have calmer pregnancies, but the disease often flares following delivery or abortion. Increased dosage of corticosteroids during the time of delivery and for several weeks thereafter tends to reduce the likelihood of a disease flare. Babies of mothers with antibodies to SS-A may have congenital cardiac problems, including heart block.

LABORATORY FINDINGS. Specific tests for SLE are not available. The presence of large amounts of antibodies to native DNA is the single most useful diagnostic laboratory finding. A variety of abnormalities depend in large measure upon the organs involved. The lupus band test consists of a biopsy of nonlesional skin and staining for the presence of immunoglobulin and complement. This test is positive in about three fourths of patients with active SLE and one third of patients with inactive SLE; however, positive tests also occur in patients with rheumatoid arthritis, non-SLE renal disease, and certain dermatologic disorders. Many regard the test as not very helpful.

The LE cell consists of a nucleus that has been phagocytized. The phagocytosis requires antibodies reactive with DNA-histone and complement. In patients with extremely low complement, LE material that has not been phagocytized may be noted. About 80 per cent of patients with SLE are positive for LE cells. A small percentage of patients with related disorders are also positive: rheumatoid arthritis, especially with Felty's syndrome; Sjögren's syndrome; polymyositis-dermatomyositis. The fluorescent antinuclear antibody test (FANA or ANA) has been used as a screening test; however, many patients with related and unrelated diseases may also have positive tests. It is now possible to measure antibodies specifically reactive with various antigens (native DNA, Sm, various low molecular weight RNA species, SS-A, SS-B, etc.). These are much more informative than the FANA despite the improvement in usefulness of the FANA by virtue of analysis of patterns of staining.

Most patients with active SLE have impaired skin tests. Especially important is the common failure to respond to tuberculin in inactive patients as well.

Hematologic. Anemia usually is present in patients with active disease. Although leukopenia occurs in half of the patients, others may manifest leukocytosis. Corticosteroids may increase the white count. Infection in patients with SLE is to be suspected if there is an increase in percentages of granulocytes or immature granulocytes or both, even in the absence of leukocytosis. Thrombocytopenia may precede other features of SLE. Antibodies to coagulation factors may be measured in coagulation abnormalities. Antibodies to phospholipids, which prolong the PTT, do not cause bleeding. A false-positive serologic test for syphilis is also observed in 15 per cent of patients.

Immune. The erythrocyte sedimentation rate (ESR) is usually but not invariably elevated in patients with active disease. Serum albumin levels are usually near normal except in patients with renal disease. Hypergammaglobulinemia may be marked in an untreated patient. Cryoglobulins may be increased. Rheumatoid factor occurs in low titer in patients with SLE. Reduced hemolytic complement levels (CH_{50}) are common in active disease, especially with renal involvement. Some patients have specific congenital complement deficiencies. Immune complexes may be found in the serum or plasma. Antibodies reactive with leukocytes (granulocytes, B cells, T cells) are found in the majority of patients. Platelet-bound immunoglobulin often occurs in the absence of thrombocytopenia, as does a positive Coombs' test result in the absence of hemolysis. Antibodies are found that react with DNA, RNA, histones, nuclear ribonucleoprotein, and cytoplasmic antigenic determinants (see Table 436–3). Rarely, antibodies react with histamine (inducing acquired Type I hyperlipoproteinemia), insulin receptors (exacerbating difficulties in sugar regulation), and other functional molecules.

Renal. Proteinuria, granular or cellular casts, and cells (RBC, WBC) are found in the urine of patients with active kidney disease. Elevated serum creatinine levels may be reversible or fixed. Hypertension is common, even in the absence of renal failure. Renal biopsies are best used to determine therapy rather than to confirm the diagnosis.

Cardiac. Abnormal T waves are the most common EKG abnormality; evidence of coronary artery or hypertensive disease may be noted. Valvular abnormalities and pericardial fluid may be detected with echocardiograms.

Pulmonary. Pleural fluid may be seen on the x-ray film. It is usually an exudate; however, the protein content may not be very high in patients with hypoalbuminemia. The glucose level is usually much higher than that observed in rheumatoid effusions. LE cells may be seen in the fluid. Pleural biopsies can show varying degrees of fibrosis and infiltration. Lung biopsies may show alveolar hemorrhage only, alveolar damage with interstitial edema and hyaline membranes, hypertrophy with or without vasculitis, or acute alveolitis. There is mild to severe hypoxemia. Patients with interstitial fibrosis show decreased vital capacity; others have disproportionately impaired diffusing capacities.

Nervous System. The EEG most commonly shows diffuse slowing. Seizures often occur in the absence of the typical patterns observed in patients with foci. The cerebrospinal fluid may be normal or may have moderately elevated protein levels. The gamma globulin levels are not increased. Granulocytes are indicative of infection; some patients have small numbers of round cells. Aseptic meningitis with numerous lymphocytes in the CSF occurs occasionally. A loss of brain substance may be noted in patients with chronic disease. Isolated loss of cortical or cerebellar neurones occurs.

DIAGNOSIS. SLE should be suspected in any person with a multisystem disease including joint pain. For epidemiologic and study purposes, 4 of the 11 criteria listed in Table 436–1 are required; however, the diagnosis may be made for other purposes with fewer criteria. SLE should be suspected if any of the criteria shown in Table 436–1 are present and unexplained. The disorder should be considered if any of the following are present: unexplained fever, purpura, splenomegaly, adenopathy, pneumonitis, myocarditis, or aseptic meningitis. The presence of a single symptom, such as serositis, along with antibodies to native DNA in a young woman is highly suggestive of SLE.

Children are frequently misdiagnosed as having rheumatic fever or juvenile rheumatoid arthritis. Adults most commonly are misdiagnosed as having rheumatoid arthritis. Other diagnoses often applied to patients with SLE include Raynaud's disease, hemolytic anemia, idiopathic thrombocytopenia, thrombotic thrombocytopenic purpura, psychosis, vasculitis, progressive systemic sclerosis, lymphoma, autoimmune neutropenia, secondary syphilis, drug reaction, porphyria, multiple sclerosis, myasthenia gravis, polymyositis, glomerulonephritis, Henoch-Schönlein purpura, personality disorder, stroke, and seizure disorder.

In addition to those just listed, other diseases should be considered in patients suspected of having SLE: subacute bacterial endocarditis, bacterial peritonitis, gonococcal septicemia, meningococcal septicemia, tuberculosis, sarcoidosis, serum sickness, leukemia, leprosy, angioimmunoblastic lymphadenopathy, Wegener's granulomatosis, leptospirosis, Lyme arthritis, Rocky Mountain spotted fever, and acquired immune deficiency syndrome (AIDS).

Overlaps occur between SLE and other diseases such as progressive systemic sclerosis and Sjögren's syndrome. Some have defined these as "mixed connective tissue disease" or the "overlap syndrome"; others prefer less rigid categorizations.

THERAPY. The diagnosis of SLE often induces an emotional reaction. In addition, many patients with SLE have psychological problems that may be a result of the disease. Therefore it is necessary to provide effective emotional support. This includes an honest but optimistic assessment. Most patients with SLE can look forward to a normal lifespan, but with the requirement for periodic visits to the physician and treatment with various drugs. Many of the more serious problems do not affect most people. Renal failure can be handled by dialysis. Thus, although the patient must realize the presence of a serious and chronic disease, a dire prognosis should not be issued. Early involvement in educational programs and with physical therapists, dieticians, and occupational therapists may be helpful.

Patients with SLE usually need more than normal rest. Ten hours of sleep at night plus an afternoon nap would not be inappropriate. The more active the disease, the more rest needed. Ultraviolet light should be avoided: outdoor swimming should be limited to periods of reduced exposure (not at 1:00 PM ± 4 hours), and sunscreen should be used even for trips to the store. Drugs that augment the effects of UV light, such as tetracyclines and psoralens, should be avoided. The same is true of foods containing large amounts of psoralens (celery, parsnips, figs, and parsley). Exercise should be appropriate to the clinical situation, but exhaustion should be avoided. Stresses, including surgery, infections, childbirth, abortions, and psychological pressures, may exacerbate the process and dictate additional treatment.

Although certain drugs can induce a lupus-like syndrome, there is little evidence that those drugs are detrimental to patients with SLE. Therefore, such drugs as alpha-methyldopa and Dilantin may be used without undue concern. However, sulfonamides are often poorly tolerated; patients with active disease experience a rash up to one half of the time. Estrogens may worsen disease; therefore, birth control pills with minimum amounts of estrogens are preferred. Since hypertension is synergistic with immune-complex disease in bringing about pathology, the blood pressure should be kept in the middle of the normal range for age and sex.

Corticosteroids are frequently given. Short-acting drugs such as prednisone or methylprednisolone are preferred so that every-other-day therapy can be attempted (see Ch. 30) and the hypothalamic-pituitary-adrenal axis not disrupted. The side effects of every-other-day steroids are much less than those of daily therapy. Low doses are less than 30 mg per 1.7 square meters per day of prednisone, and every attempt should be made to maintain patients on less than 25 mg per 1.7 square meters every other day. Moderate doses are 30 to 50 mg per 1.7 square meters per day. Higher doses may be necessary. Patients with marked multisystem involvement may temporarily require corticosteroids in divided doses. Azathioprine has long been used to treat patients with SLE; its usefulness may be limited to a subset of patients with moderate kidney disease or those with intractable skin disease or arthritis. Heroic and experimental therapy includes boluses of very large doses of corticosteroids (1 gram or more of methylprednisolone) or of cyclophosphamide (0.85 to 2.0 grams per 1.7 square meters) and plasmapheresis.

A major problem in SLE is long-term management. The clinical picture (history plus physical examination) is usually a very good guide to therapy of nonrenal and nonhematologic problems. In the latter two situations, the laboratory measures are helpful. Anemia, fatigue, and hypergammaglobulinemia tend to weigh in favor of more therapy. The long-term toxicities of corticosteroids (cataracts, aseptic necrosis of bone, infections) must always be balanced against the benefits of continued vigorous therapy. In tapering corticosteroids, it is generally advisable to drop rapidly to 30 mg per 1.7 square meters per day and then to reduce dosage more slowly. The lower the dose, the slower the tapering process should be. Rapid tapering can cause a disease flare, which requires re-institution of high doses.

The variable severity and extent of involvement in SLE dictate individualized treatment. It is helpful to divide problems into those of major organs, which therefore are life threatening, and those that are unpleasant but not life threatening (Table 436–5). The major exception to this division is a syndrome of acute toxic lupus observed primarily in precorticosteroid times: a young woman with high fever, serositis, rash, and arthritis might succumb to SLE in the absence of major organ involvement. This syndrome is usually responsive to therapy with corticosteroids in modest doses.

Non–major-organ involvements are best handled with symptomatic therapy: the less medicine the better. Hydroxychloroquine (200 to 600 mg per day) is effective for skin involvement; it also may help treat arthritis and other manifestations. Nonsteroidal anti-inflammatory drugs (NSAIDs) such as aspirin and ibuprofen are useful for arthritis, serositis, and fever. Some patients tolerate one NSAID better than another—bizarre neurologic reactions may occur in SLE patients receiving ibuprofen; liver enzyme abnormalities may follow aspirin treatment; gastrointestinal tolerance varies. The combination of hydroxychloroquine and NSAID may be sufficient. The addition of low doses of corticosteroids may be necessary. Initial every-other-day therapy may not be possible; however, a subsequent switch to alternate-day treatment reduces steroid-induced side effects. In patients with continued disease activity, symptoms may be prominent every other day, necessitating return to daily steroids. Even in the face of corticosteroid therapy, NSAID and hydroxychloroquine may add substantial benefit and allow a lower steroid dosage. Fevers occurring in spite of daily corticosteroids may respond to NSAIDs. Indomethacin may be especially effective in pericarditis.

The management of major organ involvement is usually directed at preservation of function and prevention of organ failure and disability or death. Myocarditis usually responds to the symptomatic treatment of SLE, but occasional patients may require specific treatment; moderate doses of corticosteroids are usually adequate. Thrombocytopenia and hemolytic anemia are treated more or less as they are in the absence of SLE. Administration of plasma or plasma exchange may be helpful in patients with features of thrombotic thrombocytopenia (look for fragmented RBC on the peripheral smear). Patients with Factor VIII deficiency caused by specific antibodies should be treated with plasmapheresis and immunosuppression. Mild pneumonitis usually responds to moderate doses of corticosteroids; severe disease requires heroic measures. Central nervous system involvement may require moderate to high corticosteroid therapy; in patients with severe involvement, intravenous cyclophosphamide* (0.85 to 2.0 grams per 1.7 square meters) can be lifesaving. Seizures require treatment with both corticosteroids and anticonvulsants.

The most studied and controversial area is the treatment of SLE kidney disease. If there is active disease on biopsy and little scarring, high-dose corticosteroids or corticosteroids plus an oral immunosuppressive drug (e.g., azathioprine*) may be sufficient. If there is active disease and more scarring, vigorous therapy may be considered. The currently available data suggest that renal function can be preserved for long periods with cyclophosphamide therapy. Intermittent boluses are safer than daily oral therapy. Randomized trials to determine the relative efficacy of multiple doses of intravenous cyclophosphamide and intravenous methylprednisolone are in progress. Despite substantial loss of renal function, a patient with quiescent disease and moderate scarring will usually not benefit from aggressive and potentially toxic therapy.

---

*This use is not listed in the manufacturer's directive.

Am J Kidney Dis 11 (Suppl 1) (July, 1982). *Devoted to a symposium on SLE.*

Balow JE: Lupus nephritis. Ann Intern Med 106:79, 1987. *A symposium devoted to pathogenesis and therapy.*

Decker JL: Systemic lupus erythematosus: Evolving concepts. Ann Intern Med 91:587, 1979. *The experiences of a leading center for SLE research and patient care.*

DuBois EL: Lupus Erythematosus. Los Angeles, University of Southern California Press, 1978. *A lengthy monograph citing many case reports. Extensively referenced.*

Koffler D: Current perspectives on the immunology of systemic lupus erythematosus. Arthritis Rheum 25:721, 1982. *Devoted to a symposium on SLE.*

Ropes MW: Systemic Lupus Erythematosus. Cambridge, Harvard University Press, 1976. *Observations of a physician with over 40 years' experience with SLE patients.*

Smith HR, Steinberg AD: Autoimmunity—A perspective. Ann Rev Immunol 1:175–210, 1983. *Discussion of theoretical aspects of autoimmune diseases as well as their classification and pathogeneses.*

Steinberg AD: Therapy of lupus nephritis. Kidney Int 30:769, 1986. *A completely referenced discussion and thorough analysis of difficult problems.*

Winchester RJ: New directions for research in systemic lupus erythematosus. Arthritis Rheum (Supplement to June 1978 issue). *Proceedings of a multicenter conference on systemic lupus.*

TABLE 436–5. MAJOR VERSUS NON–MAJOR ORGAN INVOLVEMENT IN SLE

Non–Major Organ SLE*	Major Organ SLE†
Alopecia	Glomerulonephritis
Fever	Central nervous system disease
Fatigue	Myocarditis
Anorexia	Pneumonitis
Arthritis	Thrombocytopenic purpura
Myalgia	Hemolytic anemia (marked)
Pleurisy	Severe granulocytopenia (rare)
Pericarditis	Mesenteric vasculitis
Peritonitis	
Rash	
Skin vasculitis	
Raynaud's phenomenon	
Mucosal ulcers	
Splenomegaly	
Lymphadenopathy	
Peripheral neuropathy	
Episcleritis	
Hepatitis	

*Usually does not require high-dose corticosteroids or other vigorous treatment. In all cases, a careful search for infection is carried out.

†Usually requires high-dose corticosteroids or other vigorous treatment. Individual patients vary greatly and some do not require vigorous therapy.

---

437 SYSTEMIC SCLEROSIS (Scleroderma)

E. Carwile LeRoy

Scleroderma (hard skin) is an uncommon disease marked by increases in fibrotic connective tissue of skin and often of visceral organs as well. It varies widely in extent and severity from isolated hardened skin patches of largely cosmetic importance to a life-threatening, generalized condition that can restrict movement "by an ever-tightening case of steel" (Osler) and lead to insufficiency of the peripheral circulation, the lungs, the gut, the heart, and/or the kidneys. Fortunately,

TABLE 437–1. DIFFERENTIAL DIAGNOSIS OF SYSTEMIC SCLEROSIS

Vascular Changes
Peripheral vasospasm
  Idiopathic Raynaud's phenomenon (Raynaud's disease)
  Occupational Raynaud's phenomenon
    Vibration and physical trauma (e.g., jackhammer operator)
  Chemical exposure
    Vinyl chloride (plastics industry)
    Mining exposure (coal, silicates, gold, heavy metals)
    Organic solvents (trichloroethylene, others)
  Environmental and drug-associated Raynaud's phenomenon
    Toxic oil syndrome
    Arsenic
    Bleomycin
    Cisplatin
    Ergotamine
    Beta-blockers (high dose)
    5-Hydroxytryptophan and carbidopa
  Reflex sympathetic dystrophy (shoulder-hand, thoracic outlet)
  Other diffuse connective tissue diseases (systemic lupus erythematosus,
    polyarteritis nodosa, dermatomyositis/polymyositis)
  Intravascular causes (cryoglobulinemia, cold agglutinins, nondistensible
    RBCs, intravascular coagulation)
  Telangiectasia
    Hereditary telangiectasia (Osler-Weber-Rendu syndrome)
    Hepatic and hormonal spiders (cirrhosis, contraceptives)
Skin Changes
Localized scleroderma
  Morphea (circumscribed, guttate)
  Generalized morphea
  Linear (with hemiatrophy)
  Other localized hamartomas (collagenoma, tuberous sclerosis, keloids,
    hypertrophic scars)
  En coup de sabre (with or without facial hemiatrophy)
Scleroderma-like skin changes
  Inflammatory-immunologic
    Undifferentiated connective tissue syndromes (mixed)
    Eosinophilic fasciitis
    Overlap syndromes (SSc with SLE, RA, DM/PM, Sjögren's syndrome
      [sicca complex and its overlaps])
    Chronic graft vs. host disease (CGVHD)
  Occupational, environmental, and drug-associated (see Vascular Changes
    above)
  Metabolic-genetic (pseudosclerodermas)
    Porphyrias
    Phenylketonuria
    Carcinoid syndrome
    Scleredema with or without paraproteinemia
    Scleromyxedema with or without paraproteinemia
    Lichen sclerosus et atrophicus
    Insulin-dependent diabetes mellitus (digital sclerosis)
    Acromegaly
    Amyloidosis
    Heritable premature aging syndromes (Werner's, progeria,
      Rothmund's)
Visceral Disease
Esophageal hypomotility (diabetes mellitus, aging)
Idiopathic pulmonary fibrosis
Sarcoidosis
Amyloidosis
Infiltrative cardiomyopathies
Intestinal hypomotility syndromes
Malignant hypertension (hyper-reninemic, accelerated)
Occupational, environmental, and drug-associated interstitial pulmonary
  disease (see Vascular Changes above)

---

most persons with scleroderma are not at risk for the most severe of its consequences. Since the cause is unknown and no cure is available, the physician must distinguish as early as possible the attendant risks for each patient and manage these prospectively.

Distinctions between localized (skin only) and generalized scleroderma and the conditions that mimic each are shown in Table 437–1. Subsets of generalized scleroderma (systemic sclerosis, SSc) are outlined in Table 437–2. SSc is a multisystem, multistage disorder in which each target organ progresses through stages of inflammation, induration (fibrosis), and atrophy, although not always at the same pace.

DEFINITION. SSc is a generalized disorder of small arteries, microvessels, and the diffuse connective tissue characterized by scarring (fibrosis) and vascular obliteration of the skin, gastrointestinal tract, lungs, heart, and kidneys in which hidebound skin is the clinical hallmark and organ compromise the prognostic keystone.

PATHOGENESIS AND PATHOLOGY. The mechanism(s) of fibrosis in SSc is not understood. Mesenchymal cells (fibroblasts, smooth muscle cells, and endothelial cells) become activated by unknown stimuli, resulting in the deposition of increased amounts of the usual components of connective tissue (types I and III collagen, proteoglycan, fibronectin) in the interstitium and in the intima of small arteries. Endothelial cell changes, vasomotor and permeability changes, platelet activation, and perivascular mononuclear cell infiltrates are present in target tissues before fibrosis is prominent.

In SSc scar tissue, lesional fibroblasts can be shown to produce increased quantities of these connective tissue components on a per cell basis even after removal from the patient and propagation in vitro. These same cells show a growth regulatory abnormality characterized by insensitive responses to growth factors and a persistent state of competence, something of a partially transformed state. Gene expression in these cells is unusual and as yet incompletely characterized. Understanding the regulatory defect of fibroblast growth may be a key to understanding the unregulated fibrosis in SSc, and perhaps also in liver cirrhosis, atherosclerosis, and other examples of unregulated fibrosis.

Prominent vascular and microvascular lesions dominate the early stages of both limited cutaneous and diffuse forms of SSc (Table 437–2). The unusual cyclic vasoconstrictive-vasodilatory features of Raynaud's phenomenon are present in more than 90 per cent of all SSc patients (Table 437–3). Edema is prominent, often occurring episodically, especially in the diffusely involved patient. Circulating evidence of endothelial cell perturbation (elevated levels of Factor VIII—von Willebrand factor) and of platelet activation (elevated levels of beta-thromboglobulin, controlled with platelet factor IV levels to detect ex vivo platelet release) is present in many, but not all, patients. Histologically, vascular lesions are widespread. The small artery lesion in SSc, similar to the lesions seen in chronic homograft rejection, in hemolytic-uremic syndrome, and in chronic thrombocytopenic purpura, has three major characteristics: (1) intimal proliferation with smooth muscle cell migration centripetally and the deposition of a mixed mucoid and fibrous connective tissue matrix, (2) medial thinning, and (3) an adventitial cuff of primarily type I collagen, a virtually unique characteristic of the SSc lesion. Cellular proliferation and matrix deposition are prominent in the small arteries of all target organs; when renal involvement, hyper-reninemia, and hypertension characterize the clinical course, fibrinoid

TABLE 437–2. SUBSETS OF SYSTEMIC SCLEROSIS (SSc)

Diffuse Cutaneous SSc (dcSSc)
Onset of Raynaud's phenomenon within one year of onset of skin changes
  (puffy or hidebound)
Truncal and acral skin involvement
Presence of tendon friction rubs
Early and significant incidence of interstitial lung disease, oliguric renal
  failure, diffuse gastrointestinal disease, and myocardial involvement
Absence of anticentromere antibodies (ACA)
Limited Cutaneous SSc (lcSSc)*
Isolated Raynaud's phenomenon for years (occasionally decades)
Skin involvement limited to hands, face, feet (acral)
A significant late incidence of pulmonary hypertension, trigeminal
  neuralgia, skin calcifications, telangiectasia
A high incidence of anticentromere antibodies (ACA, 70–80%)
Dilated nailfold capillary loops without capillary dropout
Systemic Sclerosis *sine* Scleroderma (ssSSc)
Visceral disease without cutaneous involvement
Examples: (1) Esophageal hypomotility, duodenal dilatation with
  malabsorption, wide-mouthed colonic sacculations; (2) Raynaud's
  phenomenon, dilated nailfold capillary loops, esophageal hypomotility,
  oliguric renal failure; (3) Raynaud's phenomenon, dilated nailfold
  capillary loops, esophageal hypomotility, pulmonary hypertension and/or
  interstitial lung disease

*Also termed CREST syndrome, i.e., *C*alcinosis, *R*aynaud's phenomenon, *E*sophageal hypomotility, *S*clerodactyly, and *T*elangiectasia.

TABLE 437–3. RAYNAUD'S PHENOMENON IN MUSCULOSKELETAL DISEASE*

Systemic sclerosis	>90%
Overlap, mixed, undifferentiated	80%
Systemic lupus erythematosus	30%
Dermatomyositis, polymyositis	20%
Rheumatoid arthritis	10%

*From Black CM: Scleroderma, dermatomyositis, and polymyositis. *In* Dieppe PA, et al.: Atlas of Clinical Rheumatology. Philadelphia, Lea and Febiger, 1986, with permission.

necrosis is also present. In the nutrient microvascular beds, capillaries are sparse (up to 70 per cent absent), their endothelium is swollen and disrupted, and endothelial basement membranes may be frayed and separated from their cell attachment. Although the endothelial cells bear the brunt of the injury pattern, the basis of this all-out attack on vascular structures in SSc is not known.

Selected immune events, other than the autoimmune antinuclear antibodies, point also to the vascular structures. Three of the four defined antigens to which SSc patients show enhanced immune responsiveness are type I collagen, type IV collagen, and laminin (the fourth being topoisomerase I), all three components of blood vessels and the second and third being specific for basal lamina, of which the endothelial basement membrane is a prototype. Could a heightened immune response to basement membrane antigens select those persons destined to develop SSc and perpetuate the disease in these immunogenetically selected persons? As in the other rheumatic or diffuse connective tissue disorders that show manifestations of autoimmunity, antinuclear antibodies are prominent in SSc. With the recent introduction of rapidly proliferating, human cell substrates (particularly the human laryngeal carcinoma cell line, HEp-2), greater than 90 per cent of SSc patients have circulating antinuclear antibodies in significant titer. The most sensitive and specific of these is the anticentromere antibody (ACA) pattern, a B cell immune response to a major organizing structure of the chromosome called the centromere. ACA patterns are clinically useful in detecting the limited cutaneous type of SSc. Antibodies to a soluble nuclear isomerase, topoisomerase I, are currently emerging as the newest autoimmune serologic "find" in SSc; both clinical and biologic relevance remains to be determined.

THE PATIENT. *Diffuse SSc.* The usual age of onset is the fourth decade but may range from the first to the eighth. There is no sex, race, or geographic predilection. The onset may be abrupt and may present as swollen hands, face, and feet associated with Raynaud's phenomenon (episodic pallor of the digits, nose, or ears following cold exposure or stress associated with cyanosis and followed by erythema, suffusion, tingling, and pain). Fatigue is common; overt weakness may be present. The skin reveals a nonpitting fullness, an inability to pinch skin folds, and the loss of skin lines and creases in involved areas. These changes may evolve over 12 to 18 months to include the fingers, hands, forearms, arms, face, thorax, and abdomen, as well as the toes, feet, legs, and thighs. The fingers and toes may be dusky or overtly cyanotic and are usually cool to the touch. Blood pressure and pulse may be elevated, and evaluation of swallowing, breathing, urinary excretory, and cardiac functions may reveal abnormalities. Patients with diffuse SSc should be followed closely for visceral involvement (see Table 437–2 and Fig. 437–1).

Limited Cutaneous SSc. The typical patient with limited cutaneous SSc is a female (or a male who has worked with vibrating machines, plastics, or in mining), aged 30 to 50, who presents with a 10- to 15-year history of numbness and a "dead" or "wooden" sensation associated with color changes (often pallor only) of, at first, the second and third fingers of the dominant hand. Full-fledged Raynaud's phenomenon usually develops symmetrically in both hands, fingers 2 through 5, with increasing frequency, especially in winter; there may be a history of hard crusting lesions on the

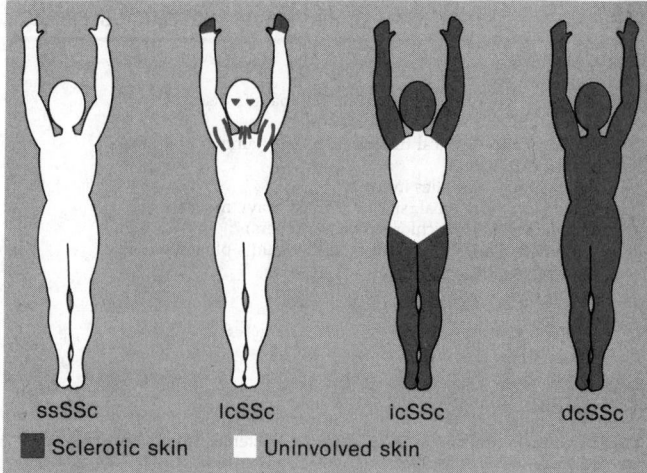

FIGURE 437–1. A pictorial representation of skin involvement in systemic sclerosis. Note that the limited cutaneous SSc patient (Table 437–2) may have subtle thickening of eyelid, neckfold, and armpit skin. Abbreviations: ssSSc = systemic sclerosis *sine* scleroderma; lcSSc = limited cutaneous systemic sclerosis; icSSc = intermediate cutaneous systemic sclerosis; dcSSc = diffuse cutaneous systemic sclerosis. (Reprinted with permission from Giordano M, et al.: J Rheumatol 13:911, 1986.)

fingertips, initially healing in warm weather. General stamina may be decreased, and there may be breathlessness with minimal exertion (see Table 437–2).

DIAGNOSIS. The annual incidence of Raynaud's phenomenon is substantially greater than the incidence of all diffuse connective tissue syndromes combined (Table 437–4). To select those Raynaud's patients destined to develop scleroderma and related disorders when a careful history and physical examination reveal no features of connective tissue disease, including no signs of peripheral ischemia, the single best test is widefield nailfold capillaroscopy—a noninvasive, reproducible, cost-effective, permanent identification of the connective tissue disease–prone patient. Coupled with autoimmune serology and possibly a test of vascular injury or platelet activation/release (such as plasma beta-thromboglobulin levels), capillary examination is an important procedure in the early detection of connective tissue disease.

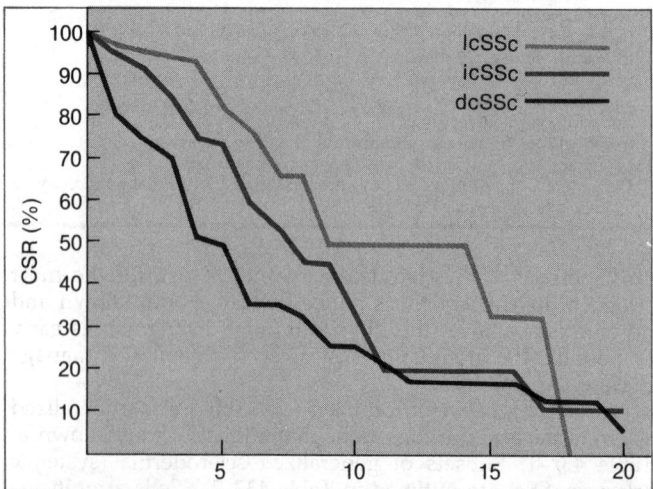

FIGURE 437–2. The cumulative survival rate (CSR, age-adjusted survival) in per cent plotted against time in years for diffuse cutaneous SSc and limited cutaneous SSc (crest syndrome) patients, showing the substantially reduced survival of diffuse cutaneous SSc patients (Table 437–2). An intermediate group with both intermediate survival and extent of skin involvement has been identified by Giordano et al. For abbreviations, see Figure 437–1. (Reprinted with permission from Giordano M, et al.: J Rheumatol 13:911, 1986.)

TABLE 437–4. POPULATION INCIDENCE OF MUSCULOSKELETAL DISEASE*

Raynaud's phenomenon	1000†
Rheumatoid arthritis	750
Systemic lupus erythematosus	75
Dermatomyositis, polymyositis	10
Systemic sclerosis	10

*From Kammer G: Raynaud's phenomenon. In Andreoli TE, et al.: Cecil Essentials of Medicine. Philadelphia, W. B. Saunders Company, 1986, with permission.

†New cases per million adults per year.

The diagnosis of diffuse SSc is straightforward. A previously well person is now sick with the triad of Raynaud's phenomenon, nonpitting edema, and hidebound skin that may eventually cover virtually the entire body, sparing only the back and buttocks. There are very few alternative diagnoses that must be seriously entertained. Other causes of Raynaud's phenomenon are not usually accompanied by edema, and other causes of edema are not usually associated with Raynaud's phenomenon. The key questions in such patients are (1) Are features of other connective tissue diseases present? and (2) What internal organs are affected?

If symmetric, erosive polyarthritis is present, an overlap between SSc and rheumatoid arthritis should be considered; if fever and a characteristic malar rash are present, overlap with systemic lupus erythematosus is likely. Most often these features are not present, and the second question represents the primary focus. Each visceral target organ (esophagus, lungs, kidneys, heart) of SSc deserves screening.

Abnormal skin texture provides the definitive diagnostic criterion of SSc in over 90 per cent of patients. When distal to the metacarpophalangeal (MCP) joints only, it is called sclerodactyly and is *not* diagnostic of SSc. Firm, taut, hidebound skin proximal to the MCP joints represents the major diagnostic criterion. Skin biopsy is usually *not* more sensitive diagnostically than the experienced touch. Skin changes also distinguish the three prognostically different subsets. If truncal skin changes are present, the patient has diffuse cutaneous SSc, and close surveillance of visceral function is indicated. If skin changes are limited to the hands, fingers, and face, limited cutaneous SSc is present, yearly evaluation is adequate, and management should focus on the Raynaud's phenomenon. If the skin is of normal texture, two possibilities are suggested: the patient formerly had abnormal skin changes—either diffuse or limited cutaneous—which have subsided (regressive systemic sclerosis); or the patient has visceral disease in the absence of skin changes which occurs in at least 5 per cent of SSc patients (Table 437–2, SSc *sine* scleroderma).

DIFFERENTIAL DIAGNOSIS. Connective tissue disorders are constellations of organ system involvements (skin, lungs, intestinal tract, serosal surfaces, joints, heart, central nervous system); each system involved can present immune-inflammatory, proliferative-erosive, or fibrotic-atrophic-insufficiency changes at different stages of the syndrome or disorder. Virtually none of the systems involved or the stages of involvement of those systems are entirely specific for the particular syndrome or disorder. It is not surprising, therefore, that the nomenclature is confusing. Terms such as mixed connective tissue disease (MCTD), undifferentiated connective tissue syndromes (UCTS), and overlap syndromes have emerged to describe the same patients.

MCTD was introduced to describe anew the already well-known overlap patients with features of myositis, lupus, and scleroderma. The early features of such patients were largely inflammatory and therefore briefly responsive to glucocorticoid therapy; proliferative and fibrotic features were not responsive to treatment. Neither the clinical syndromes, the laboratory tests proposed (antibodies to extractable nuclear antigen [ENA] or to ribonucleoprotein [RNP]), nor the response to therapy was specific. Therefore, the introduction of MCTD provided no new understanding beyond the time-honored overlap syndrome, which remains the preferred term for established, stable connective tissue disorders with features of more than one traditional disorder (such as rheumatoid arthritis–lupus overlap). In the early patient with inflammatory or edematous features that are insufficient for an established diagnosis, the term undifferentiated connective tissue syndrome (UCTS) is preferred. Some use UCTD here as a hybrid acronym.

Eosinophilic fasciitis is a syndrome that, when acute, is distinct from scleroderma and that blends into the scleroderma spectrum of disorders in its chronic form. Young, vigorous persons note, often after strenuous exertion, the onset of swelling and tautness of the skin of the trunk and proximal extremities with a brawny texture that may be tender. Raynaud's phenomenon is usually absent, and the hands and feet are usually spared. Initially, visceral disease is absent. Deep skin and subcutaneous biopsies show inflammatory changes including the deep fascia, the subcutis, and the dermis. Eosinophilia is present and eosinophils may or may not be present in the skin lesions. Symptoms subside with glucocorticoid therapy and also with no therapy over time. Eosinophilic fasciitis has been associated with aplastic anemia. In a substantial proportion of chronic patients, the visceral involvement of systemic sclerosis has been documented.

CLINICAL MANIFESTATIONS. *Peripheral Vascular System.* Pallor is the most definitive of the triphasic responses of Raynaud's phenomenon. In the presence of constant or episodic cyanosis alone, the diagnosis should be suspect. The circumstances that provoke pallor and the "dead" sensation of the fingers are usually reproducible in the individual patient (handling cold or frozen items, emotional disturbances). Persistent Raynaud's attacks may lead to a webbing phenomenon (like the frenulum of the tongue) binding the finger nail to the finger tip skin of involved fingers. This is evidence of structural vascular and persistent ischemic disease, as are the more obvious finger tip calluses, digital ulcerations (of finger tips or over dorsal proximal interphalangeal joints), overt ischemic tissue, or calcification; the toes, the nose, and the ears may be affected in Raynaud's attacks as well. The more widespread the areas involved, the more likely is systemic disease.

The Skin. The skin is the most distinctive diagnostic feature of SSc; the diagnosis can be made unequivocally by the texture and location of hidebound skin. In patients with diffuse SSc, skin tautness can limit movement at the wrists, elbows, shoulders, mouth, and thorax (less frequently the hips, knees, and ankles). When fully hidebound, the skin appears to become paper-thin over points of bony protrusion, such as the proximal interphalangeal joints, the ulnar styloid process, the olecranon process, the bridge of the nose, and the cheekbones. Gentle pressure over these areas removes all blood from the capillaries; the refilling time can be used as a rough approximation of the degree of ischemia and the propensity to ulcerate.

Gastrointestinal System. If sensitive diagnostic techniques are used, esophageal hypomotility, by far the most common manifestation of gastrointestinal SSc, can be documented in over 90 per cent of patients with both diffuse and limited cutaneous SSc. Many patients do not notice the subtle symptoms of esophageal SSc, which include a vertical substernal burning pain particularly at night, the occasional sense that a pill or large bit of meat "has not gone all the way down," or "heartburn" on lying down soon after a full meal. The single best screening test for esophageal hypomotility is the radionuclide esophageal transit time; it is noninvasive, safe, and can be relied upon when negative. Because severe esophageal complications, including stricture, can be prevented by early management and because intestinal involvement with SSc does not occur without esophageal involvement, the esophagus of all patients suspected of SSc should be examined for hypomotility. Patients with slow transit times should be further studied with both barium swallow (using light barium and the recumbent position) to detect structural abnormalities (hiatus hernia), and with esophageal motility studies, the definitive procedure for esophageal SSc. The earliest detectable abnormality is a reduction in resting lower esophageal sphincter (LES) pressure, which may be an isolated early finding or may be associated with reduced smooth muscle contraction (secondary and tertiary waves) of the distal two thirds of the esophagus. Upper third, striated muscle dysfunction suggests an overlap syndrome with dermatomyositis. If peptic esophagitis with mucosal ulceration is well-established, LES pressure may be increased and the diagnosis of achalasia could be incorrectly entertained. The presence of other features of SSc and reduced LES pressure after treatment are helpful.

Gastric hypomotility may be present but is not often of clinical significance. Small intestinal hypomotility, determined by upper GI series with small bowel follow-through, occurs in 10 to 20 per cent of patients, all of whom have esophageal hypomotility; these may occur in the absence of cutaneous scleroderma. It need not be searched for in the asymptomatic patient because it consistently declares its presence by postprandial bloating, abdominal distention with diffuse pain, intermittent diarrhea with or without steatorrhea, and weight loss from malabsorption. Abdominal attacks with adynamic ileus may mimic mechanical obstruction and lead to surgical intervention, from which some patients recover poorly and slowly, if at all.

Pulmonary System. Although renal failure was formerly the major threat to life in SSc, the combined impact of several pulmonary abnormalities now seems to be the number one cause of fatal involvement in this disease. Pleurisy and pleural effusions, pulmonary hypertension, interstitial lung disease with fibrosis, and ultimately obstructive pulmonary disease all may be a part of pulmonary SSc. Because the patient is often sedentary from skin or joint restrictions, shortness of breath or dyspnea on exertion are surprisingly late complaints; also, standard chest roentgenography is not a sensitive screening procedure. More than half of SSc patients selected for the absence of pulmonary symptoms and for a normal chest radiograph show reproducible abnormalities on pulmonary function tests. Patients who smoke show a much higher positive proportion. The single breath diffusion capacity, which measures the balance between ventilation and perfusion, is a sensitive pulmonary screening tool. Mild reductions in vital capacity are common as well. In smokers, there may be evidence of small airway obstruction.

Pleural effusions are usually silent and bland. They take on clinical significance primarily in the patient with established restrictive lung disease (decreased vital capacity) in whom the aspiration of an effusion may improve ventilation. They are present in two thirds of patients at postmortem examination. In the immunosuppressed patient, infection may present with "silent" empyema.

Pulmonary hypertension may be sudden in onset and constitutes a medical emergency. All patients with SSc should be followed closely for changes in the second heart sound over the pulmonic area and for the pulmonic valve closure component of that second sound, detected by the splitting of S2 on deep inspiration. The appearance of tricuspid regurgitation or right ventricular enlargement is evidence of established pulmonary hypertension. The chest x-ray may provide evidence of enlarged pulmonary arteries but often does not; the echocardiogram, while key in detecting cardiac SSc, has been disappointing in detecting pulmonary hypertension. Doppler techniques measuring tricuspid insufficiency (present in most patients with increased right ventricular pressures) are promising in the early detection of pulmonary hypertension. Aggressive attempts to lower pulmonary artery pressure should be instituted (see Ch. 48).

Renal System. At one time, the abrupt onset of accelerated hypertension and oliguria ("scleroderma renal crisis") accounted for the majority of deaths in SSc. Fortunately, with early identification and treatment with inhibitors of angiotensin-converting enzymes (captopril, enalapril), the incidence of renal involvement and its consequences have been greatly improved. All patients fulfilling the criteria for diffuse SSc should be suspect for renal involvement and should be followed with 24-hour urine collections for protein excretion and creatinine clearance three to four times a year. Excretion of greater than 750 mg of protein per 24 hours or clearances of less than 60 ml per minute, or distinct changes in either proteinuria or glomerular filtration rate (GFR), should initiate measurements of resting renin and, if elevated, treatment. Increases in blood pressure, pulse rate, accelerated increases in edematous skin tightening (rapidly increasing skin score), or the appearance of microangiopathic hemolytic anemia or disseminated intravascular coagulation (see Ch. 167) may also herald the onset of renal involvement.

The sudden appearance of renal SSc when other features of the disease appear more indolent is a characteristic of the kidney's unique ability to autoregulate its own blood flow. The typical small artery lesion of intimal proliferation develops slowly in the kidney of SSc patients with gradual reduction in renal blood flow, until both renal and glomerular flow drop abruptly and renal failure ensues. A rapid acceleration of these changes is associated with the onset of hyper-reninemia. It is during this accelerated phase that hypertension, funduscopic vascular changes (hemorrhages and exudates), and microangiopathic hemolytic anemia appear. The key to successful management of renal SSc is to identify the population at risk (those with diffuse SSc), to detect declining GFR early, and to treat expectantly.

One remarkable feature of renal SSc is the ability of some patients to regain renal function after months to years (up to four years) of end-stage renal disease and hemodialysis. Very little is known of the mechanisms of this slow reparative process. Whatever the reason, it stays the hand that would undertake nephrectomy.

Cardiac System. More than 90 per cent of patients with diffuse SSc (truncal skin involvement) have some form of cardiac involvement. Rarely, acute pericarditis with a friction rub is present; more frequently, a silent pericardial effusion appears slowly with ankle edema and shortness of breath as the presenting features. Echocardiography is the diagnostic procedure of choice. Pericardial effusions may predispose to renal failure by unknown mechanisms. By electrocardiographic monitoring and electrophysiologic studies, 80 per cent of diffuse SSc patients *without* cardiovascular symptoms have evidence of cardiac involvement; in more recent studies, 95 per cent show abnormalities of thallium reperfusion. Intermittent myocardial ischemia with the acute pathologic concomitant of contraction band necrosis seems to precede fibrosis, suggesting that spasm of the intramyocardial vessels plays a role in cardiac SSc. Most, but not all, of these patients have normal coronary arteries by coronary angiography.

Articular and Musculoskeletal. Approximately 10 per cent of SSc patients present with a symmetric small joint polyarticular synovitis indistinguishable from rheumatoid arthritis. Within a year, the pattern changes abruptly with subsidence of joint complaints and the appearance of Raynaud's phenomenon, edema, and diffuse cutaneous SSc. The presence of scleroderma-pattern nailfold capillary changes and a positive antinuclear antibody pattern can identify these patients during their polyarticular phase, prior to the development of cutaneous changes, as destined to develop SSc.

About one half of SSc patients develop stiffness and swelling of the fingers, wrists, knees, and ankles, concomitant with cutaneous changes. Morning stiffness may be present. Signs of inflammation are usually mild. Polymorphonuclear leukocytes are usually present in synovial fluid. On biopsy, the synovium is mildly inflamed, with a distinctive deposition of fibrin throughout the synovium. Obliterative microvascular disease and diffuse fibrotic changes occur at a later stage.

Indolent myopathy is common in SSc. It is difficult to distinguish from atrophy caused by taut skin. Most patients show diffuse atrophy of the extremities with slight elevations of muscle enzyme levels (CPK and aldolase); these features are refractory to glucocorticoids or to immunosuppressive therapy. Mild myositis of SSc is best left untreated. Less frequently, abrupt proximal muscle weakness develops and is associated with 10- to 50-fold increases in muscle enzymes, electromyographic features of acute myositis, and lymphoid cell infiltration with muscle fiber necrosis on biopsy. These patients generated the initial confusion regarding mixed, overlap, or undifferentiated connective tissue syndromes; they usually respond to glucocorticoid therapy.

Other. In the second and third decades following the onset of Raynaud's phenomenon, a small but significant proportion of patients with limited cutaneous SSc develop unilateral or bilateral trigeminal neuralgia, which can be disabling.

An increasing number of male SSc patients, especially those with diffuse disease, experience impotence after one or two years of the disease. Impotence is thought to have an organic neurovascular cause, because of diminished or absent nocturnal tumescence. It is refractory to treatment.

Dry eyes (keratoconjunctivitis sicca), dry mouth (xerostomia), or both occur in approximately one fourth of SSc patients. Salivary gland biopsies may show mononuclear cell infiltrates or replacement fibrosis. Supportive care with secretion substitution (artificial tears) and stimulation (lemon candy) provides some relief.

TREATMENT. No therapy has been shown to halt the progression of cutaneous or visceral SSc in a controlled, prospective study. A major source of confusion in assessing therapy is the dependence on softening skin as a key outcome measurement and the natural tendency for hidebound skin to soften after several years (dubbed regressive systemic sclerosis). Skin changes cannot be used as indications of the lessening of the vascular and microvascular disease.

The most distinctive change in the natural history of diffuse cutaneous SSc in the last decade has been the reduction in the proportion of patients who develop renal failure. This change has occurred with the advent of more powerful agents to control the accelerated hypertensive phase of renal failure, especially inhibitors of the angiotensin-converting enzyme, captopril and enalapril. Indications for immediate treatment are hypertension (an increase of 30 mm Hg systolic or 15 mm Hg diastolic blood pressure, no matter what the absolute level); a reduction in creatinine clearance of 30 ml per minute or to a clearance below 60 ml per minute; and microangiopathic anemia. If the serum creatinine value is less than 4.0 mg per deciliter, the crisis of renal scleroderma can often, but not always, be averted. Continued intensive treatment is indicated even if hemodialysis is instituted, since some patients can regain function sufficient to obviate dialysis after as long as four to five years.

D-Penicillamine* has been strongly advocated on the basis of retrospective studies that showed skin softening after two years. The proportion of patients who develop significant side effects is 30 to 40 per cent. It is a difficult drug to tolerate. Colchicine* has also been proposed as capable of influencing cutaneous changes in SSc. Brief cross-over studies were inconclusive, and longer open studies were promising but uncontrolled. Colchicine is better tolerated than D-penicillamine.

Glucocorticoids in moderate doses (30 to 40 mg per day in divided daily doses) effectively reduce the inflammatory and edematous changes in SSc but have no effect on the fibrotic features. When pulmonary SSc can be shown to have an active inflammatory component by bronchoalveolar lavage or gallium/indium scans, a brief trial of high-dose (60 to 80 mg in divided daily doses) glucocorticoids is indicated. Also, it may help to reduce pulmonary hypertension if used early in the course of its development, usually in conjunction with calcium channel blockers.

The management of Raynaud's phenomenon has improved in recent years (see Ch. 57); nonetheless, even the most successful management of the vasoactive features of SSc does not appear to slow or stop the continuing appearance of new fibrotic or visceral manifestations. Sometimes a change in life style is sufficient. Clothing should protect the trunk to encourage heat dissipation via peripheral vasodilatation. Extremes of cold, exhaustion, or stress should be avoided. Nitroglycerin ointment applied locally along the course of the digital arteries to those fingers showing severe ischemia is helpful. Selective sympathetic blockade, especially postganglionic alpha blockade with prazosin, usually reduces symptoms but may be difficult to tolerate due to palpitation and orthostatic hypotension. Inhibitors of the slow calcium channels of cell membranes have been a significant advance in the management of Raynaud's phenomenon. At present, nifedipine in gradually increasing doses is popular, but verapamil and diltiazem have their proponents as well. When tissue necrosis is present (gangrene), prompt hospital admission for stellate ganglion blockade or epidural blocks is indicated.

As an example of how therapeutic trials in SSc must be conducted to provide meaningful results in this indolent, variable disorder, the negative trial of chlorambucil by Furst and colleagues is cited. The agent was not better than placebo. Fifty-two patients, with a mean of 7.2 years of symptoms, were treated for three years each. Extensive inpatient evaluation of involvement was carried out at 6, 12, 24, and 36 months, evaluating skin, skeletal, pulmonary, cardiac (left and right heart), renal, upper and lower gastrointestinal, muscular, and global involvement. "Slope estimates" for each patient and each organ system were constructed and compared. It is a testimony to how much more we need to understand about SSc that a drug which has been as carefully evaluated as was chlorambucil by Furst et al., has been shown not to change the course of the disease.

Campbell PM, LeRoy EC: Pathogenesis of systemic sclerosis: A vascular hypothesis. Semin Arthritis Rheum 4:351, 1975. *A concise statement of the vascular pathogenesis of SSc.*

Campbell PM, LeRoy EC: Raynaud's phenomenon. Semin Arthritis Rheum 16:92, 1986. *A practical guide to the management of Raynaud's phenomenon in the office practice setting.*

Cohen S, Laufer I, Snape WJ, et al.: The gastrointestinal manifestations of scleroderma: Pathogenesis and management. Gastroenterology 79:155–166, 1980. *A thorough review of gastrointestinal SSc.*

Crystal RG, Bitterman PB, Rennard SI, et al.: Interstitial lung disease of unknown cause. Disorders characterized by chronic inflammation of the lower respiratory tract. N Engl J Med 310:154–165, 1984. *Pathogenetic considerations concerning inflammatory factors in pulmonary fibrosis.*

Follansbee WP: The cardiovascular manifestations of systemic sclerosis (scleroderma). In O'Rourke RA (ed.): Current Problems in Cardiology. Vol XI, No 5. Chicago, Year Book Medical Publishers, Inc., 1986. *An excellent review of the heart in scleroderma by an active investigator in the field. A scholarly work.*

LeRoy EC: Scleroderma (systemic sclerosis). In Kelly WN, Harris ED Jr, Ruddy S, et al. (eds.): Textbook of Rheumatology. 2nd ed. Philadelphia, W. B. Saunders Company, 1985, pp 1183–1205. *A more extensive and referenced treatment of the same topics covered briefly in the present chapter.*

Medsger TA Jr: Systemic sclerosis (scleroderma), eosinophilic fasciitis, and calcinosis. In McCarty DJ (ed.): Arthritis and Allied Conditions. 10th ed. Philadelphia, Lea and Febiger, 1985, pp 994–1036. *A thorough and fully referenced chapter emphasizing localized forms of scleroderma, calcifications, and therapy of SSc.*

Rocco VK, Hurd ER: Scleroderma and scleroderma-like disorders. Semin Arthritis Rheum 16:22, 1986. *An exhaustively referenced review of the history, clinical spectrum, and management of scleroderma.*

Tan EM: Systemic autoimmunity and antinuclear antibodies. Clin Aspects Autoimmun 1:2–8, 1986. *Detailed correlation of immunofluorescent patterns with morphologic/molecular epitopes in SSc in the context of autoimmunity in general.*

Traub YM, Shapiro AP, Rodnan GP, et al.: Hypertension and renal failure (scleroderma renal crisis) in progressive systemic sclerosis. Review of a 25-year experience with 68 cases. Medicine 62:335, 1983. *An extensive clinical experience with renal scleroderma.*

*This use is not listed in the manufacturer's directive.

Whitman HH, Case DB, Laragh JH, et al.: Variable response to oral angiotensin-converting enzyme blockage in hypertensive scleroderma patients. Arthritis Rheum 25:241, 1982. *Experience with 12 patients emphasizing the need for early, aggressive intervention in SSc renal crisis.*

438 SJÖGREN'S SYNDROME

Norman Talal

TABLE 438–1. CLINICAL PRESENTATION OF SJÖGREN'S SYNDROME

1. Sicca complex—dry eyes and dry mouth
2. Rheumatoid arthritis—or other connective tissue disease
3. Salivary gland enlargement
4. Purpura—nonthrombocytopenic; hyperglobulinemic; vasculitis
5. Renal tubular acidosis—or other tubular disorder
6. Polymyopathy; neuropathy—trigeminal
7. Central nervous system disease
8. Chronic liver disease
9. Chronic pulmonary disease
10. Lymphoma—local or generalized
11. Immunoglobulin disorder—cryoglobulinemia; macroglobulinemia

DEFINITION. Sjögren's syndrome is a chronic inflammatory and autoimmune disease in which the salivary and lacrimal glands undergo progressive destruction by lymphocytes and plasma cells, resulting in decreased production of saliva and tears. The term autoimmune exocrinopathy has been introduced. The spectrum of this illness includes a primary form (sicca complex), a secondary form accompanying rheumatoid arthritis (or occasionally another connective tissue disease), and a form characterized mainly by lymphoproliferation of either a benign infiltrative or a malignant nature. Females are involved 10 times more commonly than males.

PATHOGENESIS. The several factors involved in the etiology of autoimmune diseases such as Sjögren's syndrome include genetic, immunologic, hormonal, and probably infectious (? viral). The discovery of the immune response (IR) genes, which exist in linkage disequilibrium with other genes in the major histocompatibility complex, has helped distinguish primary from secondary Sjögren's syndrome. The former is associated with HLA B8 DR3, whereas the latter is associated with DR4 (when rheumatoid arthritis is the accompanying illness). Recently, gene interaction between DQ1 and DQ2 has been associated with marked hypergammaglobulinemic and high-titered autoantibody responses. The presence of Ia molecule and Ebstein-Barr virus (EBV) in salivary gland epithelium has also been noted. The predominant female incidence of Sjögren's syndrome may relate to the ability of sex hormones to modulate the immune response, with estrogen contributing to immune hyperactivity.

CLINICAL MANIFESTATIONS. The varied clinical presentations of Sjögren's syndrome are shown in Table 438–1.

Ophthalmologic (Keratoconjunctivitis Sicca). The patient may notice accumulation of thick ropy secretions along the inner canthus owing to a decreased tear film and an abnormal mucus component. Related complaints include a characteristic foreign body sensation ("sandy or gritty eyes"), photosensitivity, eye fatigue, decreased visual acuity, and the sensation of a "film" across the field of vision. Desiccation can cause small superficial erosions of the corneal epithelium. Slit lamp examination may reveal filamentary keratitis (filaments of corneal epithelium and debris) in severe cases.

Salivary. Complaints resulting from dryness of the mouth are varied. The "cracker sign" describes the difficulties encountered in trying to eat dry foods without sufficient lubrication. Many subjects require frequent ingestion of liquids. They may resort to carrying water bottles or candy in purse or pocket. Additional features include oral soreness, adherence of food to buccal surfaces, fissuring of the tongue, and dysphagia. Angular cheilitis resulting from superimposed candidiasis may occur. Patients may lose the ability to discriminate foods on the basis of taste and smell. Dental caries are accelerated. The parotid gland enlarges in many patients secondary to cellular infiltration and ductal obstruction. Usually asymptomatic and self-limited, the enlargement can be recurrent and associated with pain and erythema. Focal infiltrates of lymphocytes are also found in the minor salivary glands of the lower lip. When biopsied, these lesions provide histologic confirmation and quantification of the degree of infiltration.

Other Symptoms. Dryness may also involve the nasal mucosa, leading to recurrent epistaxis, and may extend throughout the upper respiratory tract, causing hoarseness, recurrent bronchitis, and pneumonitis. Eustachian tube blockage can result in conduction deafness and chronic otitis. Dysphagia may be ascribed to several causes: decreased saliva, infiltration of the glands of the esophageal mucosa, esophageal webbing, and abnormal motility. Other exocrine gland functions may be affected, leading to loss of pancreatic secretions, hypo- or achlorhydria, dermal dryness, and lack of vaginal secretions.

Extraglandular Involvement. Extraglandular involvement occurs more frequently in patients with primary than secondary Sjögren's syndrome. Dependent nonthrombocytopenic purpura is generally associated with hyperglobulinemia. Raynaud's phenomenon is present in 20 per cent of patients. A diffuse interstitial pneumonitis resulting from lymphocytic infiltration may cause dyspnea. Obstructive disease (in the absence of smoking) may result from lymphocytic infiltration surrounding small airways. The most common renal abnormalities involve the tubules, particularly overt or latent renal tubular acidosis and hyposthenuria. The presence of glomerulonephritis should suggest coexisting systemic lupus erythematosus (SLE), cryoglobulinemia, or immune complex deposition. Peripheral and cranial neuropathy have been associated with vasculitis involving the vasa nervorum. A variety of CNS manifestations has recently been described.

Lymphoproliferation and Lymphoma. The incidence of lymphoma is increased 44-fold in Sjögren's syndrome. Pseudomalignant or malignant lymphoproliferation may be present initially or may develop later in the illness. Most lymphomas belong to the B cell lineage, as demonstrated by immunophenotyping and immunogenotyping. Monoclonal immunoglobulin B cell proliferations in Sjögren's syndrome patients include Waldenström's macroglobulinemia, light chain myeloma, and non-IgM monoclonal gammopathies (IgG κ and IgA λ). A diminution of a previously elevated Ig class may signify malignant transformation. Pseudolymphoma is an intermediate stage in this transition from benign to malignant lymphoproliferation.

Other clinical indications of an increased risk of malignancy include persistent or greatly increased parotid swelling, generalized lymphadenopathy, and splenomegaly.

DIAGNOSIS. *Clinical.* The presence of dry eyes is suggested by a positive Schirmer test (less than 5 mm of wetting per five minutes, unanesthetized), but the frequency of both false-negative and false-positive results is high. The pattern and intensity of staining with rose bengal dye and slit lamp examination are more reliable in diagnosis. The presence of filamentary keratitis and corneal ulcerations indicates advanced keratoconjunctivitis sicca.

Diminution in stimulated parotid flow rate (PFR) (<5 ml per gland in 10 minutes) is a sensitive indicator of xerostomia. Salivary scintigraphy, which measures the uptake, concentration, and excretion of ^{99m}Tc-pertechnetate by the major salivary glands, is a sensitive index of glandular function. Scintigraphy is expensive, however, and offers no advantage in diagnostic sensitivity over minor salivary gland biopsy. Lip biopsy is a sensitive and specific diagnostic procedure, is well tolerated by the patient, and causes no disfigurement. In addition to confirming the diagnosis, biopsy allows quantification of the degree of lymphocytic infiltration and tissue damage. Aggregates of lymphocytes within the acinar tissue are scored, each aggregate of 50 or more cells representing a focus. The number of foci within 4 sq mm of glandular tissue is determined and constitutes the focus score. A focus score of more than 1 is characteristic of Sjögren's syndrome and is seen in less than 1 per cent of both normal and autopsy controls. The diagnosis of Sjögren's syndrome is based upon the presence of two of the following three criteria: (1) focus score of more than 1 in the labial salivary gland biopsy, (2) keratoconjunctivitis sicca, and (3) an associated connective tissue or lymphoproliferative disorder.

Clinically, a "sicca-like" syndrome may be caused by a number of other disease processes, including hyperlipoproteinemias IV and V, hemochromatosis, sarcoidosis, and amyloidosis. Use of anticholinergic drugs as well as a number of other medications may be the single most frequent cause of xerostomia. Thus, it is essential to establish the presence of focal lymphoid infiltrates and autoimmunity in a patient suspected of having Sjögren's syndrome.

Laboratory. Autoantibodies are common in Sjögren's syndrome. Rheumatoid factor may be found in 75 to 90 per cent; antinuclear antibodies may be positive in 50 to 80 per cent. Multiple organ-specific antibodies are noted, including antibodies directed against gastric parietal, thyroid microsomal, thyroglobulin, mitochondrial, smooth muscle, and salivary duct antigens.

An autoantibody to a nucleoprotein antigen called SS-B (also termed La) occurs in up to 90 per cent of patients with primary Sjögren's syndrome and to a lesser extent in Sjögren's syndrome accompanied by SLE. Antibodies to a related nucleoprotein SS-A (also termed Ro) are less specific for Sjögren's syndrome, also occur in SLE, and are associated with vasculitis. An antibody (RAP) to an EBV–related nuclear antigen (RANA) occurs in secondary Sjögren's syndrome with RA.

Persons with Sjögren's syndrome manifest B cell hyperactivity. Evidence for this includes the polyclonal hyperglobulinemia seen in over 50 per cent of patients and the presence of numerous autoantibodies and circulating immune complexes. The lymphoid infiltrates in the salivary glands synthesize immunoglobulins locally. Serum hyperviscosity may result from either macroglobulinemia or polymerizing IgG with rheumatoid factor activity which forms intermediate complexes. Cryoglobulinemia may be present, as well as vasculitis and glomerulonephritis. A high proportion of patients with Sjögren's syndrome have circulating immune complexes as measured by C1q binding and Raji cell assays. Serum levels of complement are only infrequently low.

Peripheral blood T lymphocytes are decreased in about one third of patients. Immunoglobulin-positive lymphocytes in peripheral blood may be increased slightly. Abnormalities in T cell function may be present, particularly in patients with lymphoproliferative or other systemic features. These patients tend to have alterations in T cell subsets and decreased autologous mixed lymphocyte responses. Natural killer (NK) cell activity is also diminished and may contribute to the emergence of lymphoid malignancy.

TREATMENT. Treatment of Sjögren's syndrome is aimed at symptomatic relief and limiting the damaging local effects of chronic xerophthalmia and xerostomia. Ocular dryness responds to the use of artificial tears, which can be applied every one to three hours. A slow-release tear is also available. Soft contact lenses may be used to protect the cornea but increase the risk of infection. Saran Wrap occlusion or diving goggles may be worn at night in an attempt to prevent tear evaporation. Topical steroid use should be avoided unless specifically indicated, because corneal thinning and subsequent perforation may occur. The use of diuretics, many antihypertensive drugs, and antidepressants may further diminish lacrimal and salivary gland function. Xerostomia is

difficult to treat but may be relieved with water, chewing gum, or sugar-free candies given as sialagogues. Scrupulous care of teeth is imperative; patients should avoid a high sucrose intake or the frequent use of sugar-containing candies to decrease oral dryness. Vigorous dental plaque control and topical application of fluoride should be used regularly. Oral candidiasis may be treated with Mycostatin tablets for a prolonged course, with separate treatment of dentures. Vaginal dryness can be treated with propionic acid gels.

Only those patients with severe functional disability or life-threatening complications warrant corticosteroid or immunosuppressive therapy. Prednisone may suppress parotid swelling and improve the restrictive component of pulmonary disease. Cyclophosphamide has decreased extraglandular lymphoid infiltrates and improved exocrine gland function in some individuals. Its use has been restricted to those patients with severe renal, skin, or pulmonary manifestations.

Talal N: Sjögren's syndrome. In Rose N, Mackay I (eds.): The Autoimmune Diseases. New York, Academic Press, 1985, pp 145–159. *An up-to-date concise review of this disease.*

Talal N: The biological significance of lymphoproliferation in Sjögren's syndrome. In Brooks PM, York JR (eds.): Rheumatology—85. The Netherlands, Elsevier Science Publishers, 1985, pp 365–369. *A review of this subject to date with a theoretic discussion of predisposing factors and an analogy to AIDS.*

Talal N: Sjögren's syndrome. In Fauci AS, Lichtenstein LM (eds.): Current Therapy in Allergy, Immunology and Rheumatology. Philadelphia, B. C. Decker Inc., 1985, pp 237–240. *A guide to systemic and local treatment of this disease.*

439 THE VASCULITIC SYNDROMES

Sheldon M. Wolff*

Vasculitis is a clinicopathologic process characterized by inflammation of the blood vessel itself. Associated with this inflammation may be compromise of the vessel lumen with resulting ischemic changes in the tissues supplied by the vessel. Any size, location, and type of blood vessel may be involved, including large muscular arteries, medium-sized and small arteries, arterioles, capillaries, postcapillary venules, and veins. This heterogeneous category of diseases comprises unique syndromes as well as diseases with overlapping clinical and pathologic features. The vasculitis may be the primary process, or it may be a component of another underlying disease. Furthermore, vasculitis varies considerably in its clinicopathologic manifestations. Certain of the vasculitic disorders are rarely life threatening (e.g., the hypersensitivity vasculitic syndromes in which cutaneous involvement usually predominates). Other vasculitic syndromes may be fulminant and, if untreated, rapidly fatal diseases (e.g., Wegener's granulomatosis and polyarteritis nodosa).

The vasculitic syndromes are generally thought to result from immunopathogenic mechanisms; however, the evidence for this varies among the different syndromes. Among these mechanisms, the deposition of circulating immune complexes with subsequent vessel damage has emerged as the major immunopathologic event associated with most of the vasculitic syndromes. The presence of circulating immune complexes does not prove that the associated vasculitis is caused by them, since many nonvasculitic diseases are also associated with circulating immune complexes, and complexes per se need not result in vasculitis, even in diseases in which vasculitis is present. In only a few diseases has the actual antigen involved in the immune complex been identified. The most noted of these is the hepatitis B surface antigen that has

---

*This chapter is an updated revision of one by A. S. Fauci that appeared in the 17th edition of this textbook.

been demonstrated in the circulating immune complexes, cryoprecipitable serum components, and involved tissues of certain patients with hepatitis B antigenemia–associated vasculitis.

The mechanism of tissue damage from immune complexes is thought to be similar to serum sickness. In this model, soluble immune complexes are formed in antigen excess and deposited in blood vessel walls in areas of increased vascular permeability. The increased permeability is attributed to release of vasoactive amines from platelets or mast cells under the influence of specific IgE. Following deposition of complexes, various components of complement are activated, particularly C5a, which is strongly chemotactic for neutrophils. The neutrophils infiltrate the vessel wall at the site of immune complex deposition and release intracytoplasmic enzymes such as collagenase and elastase that directly damage the vessel wall. Compromise of the lumen occurs with resulting ischemic changes.

Certain of the vasculitides are characterized by granulomatous inflammation in and around the blood vessels. Although granulomatous responses are generally of the delayed hypersensitivity type, immune complexes themselves can trigger granuloma formation and thereby produce granulomatous vasculitis.

Why certain persons develop vasculitis and others do not is an extraordinarily complex issue and likely involves a number of host factors such as genetic predisposition, immunoregulatory mechanisms, and the integrity of the reticuloendothelial system, which clears the complexes from the circulation. In addition, the reasons that certain complexes cause vasculitis and that certain types of vessels and not others are involved probably relate to the size and physicochemical properties of the immune complex and to other physical factors such as turbulence of blood flow, hydrostatic pressure within vessels, and previously damaged vessel endothelium.

CLASSIFICATION OF THE VASCULITIC SYNDROMES

The heterogeneity and the obvious overlap among the vasculitis syndromes have led to difficulties in classification of this group of diseases. The first report of a vasculitic syndrome was in 1866 by Kussmaul and Maier, who described the clinicopathologic features in a patient with what is now recognized as classic polyarteritis nodosa. It became evident that there were numerous vasculitic syndromes with diverse clinical and pathologic manifestations, but diagnostic criteria were controversial. More precise and accurate classification schemes now have emerged, based upon reexamination of clinical, pathologic, and immunologic features as well as responses to certain therapeutic regimens. Table 439–1 illustrates one such classification scheme.

The first group of vasculitides is the polyarteritis nodosa group. This syndrome is described in detail in Ch. 440. It is the prototype of the serious systemic necrotizing vasculitides and manifests certain features such as small and medium-sized muscular artery involvement, hypertension, visceral vessel involvement, and a noticeable lack of lung involvement. Eventually physicians recognized a systemic vasculitis that resembled classic polyarteritis nodosa except that lung involvement was a prominent feature and the patients generally manifested eosinophilia, granulomatous reactions, and a strong allergic diathesis, usually severe asthma. Most of these patients had what is now referred to as allergic angiitis and granulomatosis of the Churg-Strauss type. This disease is quite similar to classic polyarteritis nodosa except for the divergent features mentioned above. Many systemic necrotizing vasculitides manifest clinicopathologic characteristics that overlap these two syndromes as well as the hypersensitivity group of vasculitides (discussed below). This subgroup has been referred to as the "polyangiitis overlap syndrome" of systemic necrotizing vasculitis.

TABLE 439–1. THE CLINICAL SPECTRUM OF VASCULITIS

1. Polyarteritis nodosa group
    Classic polyarteritis nodosa
    Allergic angiitis and granulomatosis (Churg-Strauss disease)
    Overlap syndrome
2. Hypersensitivity vasculitis
    Henoch-Schönlein purpura
    Serum sickness and serum sickness–like reactions
    Vasculitis associated with infectious diseases
    Vasculitis associated with neoplasms
    Vasculitis associated with connective tissue diseases
    Vasculitis associated with other underlying diseases
    Congenital deficiencies of the complement system
    Erythema elevatum diutinum
3. Wegener's granulomatosis
4. Giant cell arteritides
    Cranial or temporal arteritis
    Takayasu's arteritis
5. Other vasculitic syndromes
    Lymphomatoid granulomatosis
    Mucocutaneous lymph node syndrome (Kawasaki's disease)
    Behçet's disease
    Vasculitis isolated to the central nervous system
    Thromboangiitis obliterans (Buerger's disease)
    Miscellaneous vasculitides

In addition to the polyarteritis nodosa group of systemic necrotizing vasculitides, certain other vasculitides are systemic and involve multiple organ systems. However, they are referred to by different names, since they possess characteristic clinical and/or pathologic features. This is true of diseases such as Wegener's granulomatosis (see Ch. 441) and the giant cell arteritides. In the latter group, the two major subcategories—cranial or temporal arteritis (see Ch. 442) and Takayasu's arteritis (see Ch. 56)—are systemic diseases involving large muscular arteries with mononuclear cell and often giant cell infiltration within the walls of the involved arteries. Despite the predisposition for certain vessels in these diseases (temporal artery in cranial arteritis and subclavian artery in Takayasu's arteritis), these are systemic diseases which involve multiple arteries. Lymphomatoid granulomatosis (see Ch. 441) is generally considered in the differential diagnosis of systemic necrotizing vasculitis with lung involvement such as Wegener's granulomatosis. However, it is not strictly speaking an inflammatory response in vessels but an infiltration of blood vessel walls with atypical and often neoplastic-looking lymphoid cells.

The hypersensitivity vasculitides include a broad and heterogeneous group of disorders which have often caused confusion in categorization. These are discussed in detail in this chapter.

Other vasculitic syndromes can be considered under the category of "miscellaneous" for want of a better term. These include Behçet's disease, the major pathologic feature of which is a true vasculitis (see Ch. 453), and thromboangiitis obliterans, which is an inflammatory and occlusive disease of arteries and veins, although its true vasculitic character has been questioned. In addition to the granulomatous vasculitis of the central nervous system, which is seen in association with certain lymphoproliferative malignancies, there is also a rare syndrome of isolated vasculitis of the central nervous system that occurs in the apparent absence of systemic vasculitis or other systemic disease.

HYPERSENSITIVITY VASCULITIS

Hypersensitivity vasculitis is a term applied to a heterogeneous group of disorders that are thought to represent a hypersensitivity reaction to an antigenic stimulus such as a drug or an infectious agent; hence the word "hypersensitivity." Although the antigenic stimuli associated with this group are heterogeneous, these disorders generally share the characteristic of involvement of small vessels. They can be subdivided into two basic groups. The vast majority of the patients manifest involvement of the postcapillary venules, and hence have a venulitis. A smaller group of patients falls into the second category, in which arterioles are predominantly involved (arteriolitis). Most importantly, there is a predominant and often exclusive involvement of the vessels of the skin. Confusion in the literature generally resulted from grouping this category of vasculitis with the more serious systemic varieties such as classic polyarteritis nodosa and related diseases. It is true that the hypersensitivity vasculitides may have variable degrees of organ system involvement other than of the skin. However, this is usually less severe than that of typical systemic vasculitis of polyarteritis nodosa and Wegener's granulomatosis. Most frequently, the skin is exclusively involved or, if other organ systems are involved, the cutaneous disease still dominates the clinical picture.

ETIOLOGY. As indicated by the terminology, the etiology is usually a recognizable antigenic stimulus such as a drug, microbe, toxin, or foreign or endogenous protein. From an etiologic standpoint the hypersensitivity vasculitides segregate into two distinct groups, depending on the source of the sensitizing antigen. In the classic original group, the antigen is foreign to the host. In the second group the antigen is endogenous. For example, certain connective tissue diseases may manifest a typical hypersensitivity small vessel vasculitis. These diseases are generally characterized by circulating immune complexes in which one of the components is an endogenous protein to which antibody is directed. This is true of patients with systemic lupus erythematosus who develop immune complexes composed of endogenous DNA and anti-DNA antibodies; in addition, patients with rheumatoid arthritis may develop immune complexes of rheumatoid factor with antibody activity against endogenous immunoglobulin. Thus, in most of the hypersensitivity vasculitides, the identity of the etiologic agent which triggers the formation of immune complexes is at least strongly suspected.

INCIDENCE AND PREVALENCE. It is difficult to determine an accurate incidence for the hypersensitivity group of vasculitides owing to the marked heterogeneity among these diverse syndromes. However, the hypersensitivity group of vasculitides is much more common than the polyarteritis group and other syndromes such as Wegener's granulomatosis and Takayasu's arteritis. The disease can be seen at any age and in both sexes; however, this varies considerably with the particular subgroup in question.

PATHOLOGY AND PATHOGENESIS. The histopathologic hallmark of the hypersensitivity vasculitides is a leukocytoclastic venulitis. The term leukocytoclasis refers to nuclear debris derived from the neutrophils that have infiltrated in and around the involved vessels. In skin biopsies, this type of involvement is most common in the postcapillary venules just beneath the epidermis. When biopsies are obtained in the acute phase of active disease, the typical pattern of neutrophil infiltration is readily observed. In the subacute or chronic stages, biopsies often reveal mononuclear cell infiltration. In the second and smaller category of hypersensitivity vasculitis, arterioles and capillaries are predominantly involved. In the typical case of hypersensitivity vasculitis with a predominance of cutaneous involvement, the lesions are usually found in the lower extremities or in the dependent areas such as the sacrum in supine patients. This is most likely due to the increase in hydrostatic pressure within the postcapillary venules in these areas.

Although immune complex deposition is widely considered to be the pathogenic mechanism of this group of vasculitis, not every case of hypersensitivity vasculitis has had immune complexes demonstrated, even when carefully sought, as mentioned above.

CLINICAL MANIFESTATIONS. Just as the broad group is etiologically heterogeneous, so too are the clinical manifestations. However, the hallmark of the group is the predominance of cutaneous involvement. The skin lesions may appear as the classic palpable purpura which results from the extrav-

asation of erythrocytes into the tissue surrounding the involved venules. In addition, one may see macules, papules, vesicles, bullae, subcutaneous nodules, ulcers, and even recurrent or chronic urticaria.

Even though skin lesions generally dominate, various organ system involvements can be seen. Certain constellations of clinicopathologic findings define relatively distinct syndromes. For example, in *Henoch-Schönlein purpura* the typical syndrome consists of palpable purpura (usually over the buttocks), arthralgias, gastrointestinal symptoms, and glomerulonephritis. Henoch-Schönlein purpura is usually seen in children; however, adults of any age may be affected. The disease usually remits spontaneously after one week. However, the disease is remarkable for its tendency to recur a number of times over weeks to months before remission is complete. The characteristic skin lesions are present in virtually all patients. The majority of patients also have arthralgias involving multiple joints, but frank arthritis is rare. The gastrointestinal involvement is usually manifested as colicky abdominal pain which may mimic an acute surgical abdomen. Patients may experience nausea, vomiting, diarrhea, constipation, and occasionally the passage of blood and mucus per rectum. In the more severe and rare case, bowel intussusception may occur. Renal disease is a glomerulitis (see Ch. 81), which is usually expressed as microscopic hematuria without significant renal functional impairment. However, in rare cases renal failure can occur. Most frequently, patients recovery spontaneously and completely.

Other groups within the hypersensitivity category include *serum sickness and serum sickness–like reactions*. The classic manifestations are fever, urticaria, arthralgias, and lymphadenopathy occurring seven to ten days after primary exposure to the antigen in question, which for serum sickness is usually a heterologous serum protein and for serum sickness–like reactions is usually a drug such as penicillin. Most of the manifestations of this disorder are not the result of vasculitis. However, in rare cases cutaneous vasculitis typical of the hypersensitivity group is documented. In addition, patients may rarely progress to a typical systemic necrotizing vasculitis involving multiple organ systems.

A number of disorders have vasculitis as a manifestation of an underlying primary disease. Included in these diseases are *systemic lupus erythematosus, rheumatoid arthritis, mixed cryoglobulinemia,* and *other connective tissue diseases.* In these disorders, the manifestations of the underlying disease usually predominate. When vasculitis is observed, it is generally of the small vessel cutaneous type, which is virtually indistinguishable from the vasculitis seen in the hypersensitivity group with recognized exogenous antigens. However, patients with these disorders, particularly systemic lupus erythematosus and rheumatoid arthritis, may also develop a systemic necrotizing vasculitis which closely resembles the polyarteritis nodosa group in manifestations and severity. Nevertheless, in the typical case, the cutaneous vasculitis usually dominates the clinical picture with respect to the vasculitic process.

Other diseases which may fall into this category of small vessel hypersensitivity vasculitis are the *vasculitis associated with congenital deficiencies of various complement components* such as Clr, Cls, and C2, *erythema elevatum diutinum; hypocomplementemic vasculitis;* the *vasculitis associated with certain neoplasms, particularly of the lymphoid type;* and the *vasculitis associated with other primary disorders such as ulcerative colitis, Crohn's disease, biliary cirrhosis,* and *retroperitoneal fibrosis.*

DIAGNOSIS. The diagnosis of hypersensitivity vasculitis rests on the demonstration of vasculitis on biopsy. Since the predominant organ involved is the skin, histopathologic material is usually readily available. Because cutaneous involvement is often present in severe systemic vasculitides, one should undertake a systematic workup of other organ systems in patients who present with apparently isolated cutaneous vasculitis.

TREATMENT AND PROGNOSIS. Therapy of the hypersensitivity group of vasculitides has in general been unsatisfactory. Since most cases resolve spontaneously, the lack of response to therapeutic regimens is of less importance. However, in those patients who go on to develop persistent cutaneous disease or serious organ system involvement, several regimens have been tried with variable results. In cases in which a recognized antigenic stimulus is present, the first order of therapy is to remove the antigen; e.g., to remove sensitizing drugs or responsible organisms by appropriate antibiotic therapy when possible. In situations in which disease appears to be self-limited, no specific therapy is indicated. However, when disease persists or results in organ system dysfunction, a glucocorticosteroid is the drug of choice. Prednisone is usually administered in doses of 1 mg per kilogram per day with rapid tapering when possible, in some instances directly to discontinuation or initially to an alternate-day regimen followed by ultimate discontinuation (see Ch. 30). In cases that prove refractory to corticosteroid therapy, cytotoxic agents such as cyclophosphamide have been used. The efficacy of these regimens has not yet been fully evaluated in hypersensitivity vasculitis. Thus, one should be reluctant to institute cytotoxic agents in persons with disease limited to the skin, particularly since the response of the cutaneous variety of hypersensitivity vasculitis to cytotoxic agents has not been as dramatic as the response of the systemic vasculitides such as Wegener's granulomatosis (see Ch. 441) and the polyarteritis nodosa group.

The prognosis of most of the diseases in this category is generally excellent, with spontaneous and complete remissions in most patients. However, certain patients may develop persistent and debilitating cutaneous disease, and others may evolve a typical systemic vasculitis with a serious prognosis.

Christian CL, Sergent JS: Vasculitic syndromes: Clinical and experimental models. Am J Med 61:385, 1976. *Excellent review of the vasculitic syndromes with emphasis on the pathophysiologic mechanisms in several of the human diseases as well as in animal models of vasculitis.*

Cupps TR, Fauci AS: The Vasculitides. Philadelphia, W. B. Saunders Company, 1981, pp 1–21. *Comprehensive treatise on the entire spectrum of the vasculitic syndromes. Pathogenesis, clinicopathologic manifestations, and updated therapeutic approaches are discussed in detail.*

Fauci AS, Katz P, Haynes BF, et al.: Cyclophosphamide therapy of severe systemic necrotizing vasculitis. N Engl J Med 301:235, 1979. *One of the first papers to show that aggressive therapy could lead to dramatic and long-term remissions in these diseases.*

Leavitt RY, Fauci AS: Pulmonary vasculitis. Am Rev Resp Dis 134:149, 1986. *An up-to-date review of the pathogenesis, classification, and treatment of the pulmonary vasculitides.*

Zeek PM: Periarteritis nodosa and other forms of necrotizing angiitis. N Engl J Med 18:764, 1953. *Classic article which represents the first well-organized approach to the rational classification of the vasculitic syndromes. It is still employed as the backbone of most classification schemes.*

440 POLYARTERITIS NODOSA GROUP

Sheldon M. Wolff*

DEFINITION. In 1866 Kussmaul and Maier described for the first time a patient with polyarteritis nodosa. They introduced the term *periarteritis nodosa* to describe segmental nodules of medium-sized muscular arteries. Because the swelling of the arterial walls often led to occlusion, many of the clinical manifestations were secondary to necrosis. Hence, polyarteritis nodosa is often classified as one of the systemic necrotizing vasculitides. Classic polyarteritis does not involve the lung as compared to allergic angiitis and granulomatosis of Churg-

Strauss, which some writers call *polyarteritis with pulmonary involvement.*

Polyarteritis associated with hepatitis B antigenemia and extending from the medium-sized muscular arteries to arterioles and venules was described in 1970 by Gocke and colleagues. The association of hepatitis B antigen-antibody complexes and polyarteritis provides strong support to the hypothesis that the vasculitides in general are secondary to the deposition of soluble immune complexes. On clinical grounds no criteria have been identified to distinguish between the hepatitis B positive and negative patients except that all positive hepatitis B antigenemia patients had abnormal liver chemistry test results.

In some patients there are manifestations of both classic polyarteritis nodosa and allergic angiitis and granulomatosis of Churg-Strauss. Such patients are classified as being in the group with the so-called overlap syndromes. Their diagnosis, work-up, and management are no different from those of other patients in the polyarteritis nodosa group.

The incidence, age distribution, and male-to-female ratio of polyarteritis nodosa are difficult to determine because a diagnostic serologic procedure is lacking, and the spotty distribution of lesions makes biopsy uncertain. Nonetheless, the condition occurs from infancy to old age, with a peak incidence in the fifth and sixth decades of life, and the male to female ratio has been estimated at from 2 to 3:1.

PATHOLOGY. The lesions of polyarteritis involve arteries of medium and small caliber, especially at bifurcations and branchings. The segmental process involves the media, with edema, fibrinous exudation, fibrinoid necrosis, and infiltration of polymorphonuclear neutrophils and extends to the adventitia and intima. Thrombosis and infarction or hemorrhage occur at this stage. Subsequently, the regions of fibrinoid necrosis are replaced by cellular granulation tissue, and the intima proliferates. Finally the involved segment is replaced by scar tissue with associated intimal thickening and periarterial fibrosis. These changes produce partial occlusion, thrombosis and infarction, and palpable or visible aneurysms with occasional rupture.

In allergic angiitis and granulomatosis the acute fibrinoid necrosis with cellular infiltration involves arterioles and venules as well as medium-sized muscular arteries, whereas in classic polyarteritis such vessels are spared except in areas contiguous to involved medium-sized muscular arteries. It is characteristic of the polyarteritis nodosa group for the vascular lesions to be in different stages of evolution, i.e., acute, subacute, and healed. In allergic angiitis and granulomatosis the pulmonary granulomatous lesions in vascular and extravascular sites are accompanied by an intense eosinophilic infiltration. The granulomas often include an eosinophilic core of altered collagen and necrotic eosinophils surrounded by radially arranged macrophages, lymphocytes, plasma cells, and varying numbers of polymorphonuclear leukocytes, both neutrophilic and eosinophilic.

In patients with polyarteritis associated with hepatitis B antigenemia, the specific antigen has been recognized in immune complexes present in the circulation and deposited in affected vessels along with complement proteins. It is presumed that this pathogenetic mechanism prevails in the entire polyarteritis nodosa group, but the basis for arterial deposition is unknown. The deposition of immune complexes in venules and glomeruli is attributed to changes in permeability and to physical trapping.

CLINICAL MANIFESTATIONS AND DIAGNOSIS. The widespread distribution of the arterial lesions produces diverse clinical manifestations, which reflect the particular organ systems in which the arterial supply has been impaired. Among the early symptoms and signs of polyarteritis nodosa are fever, weight loss, and pain in viscera and/or the musculoskeletal system so that the differential diagnosis is of fever of unknown origin. Striking and specific presenting signs may

---

*This chapter is an updated revision of one by K. F. Austen that appeared in the 17th edition of this textbook.

relate to abdominal pain, acute glomerulitis, polyneuritis, or myocardial infarction. Pulmonary manifestations, especially intractable bronchial asthma, would indicate allergic angiitis and granulomatosis rather than classic polyarteritis nodosa.

Renal. Renal involvement in two forms, renal polyarteritis and a glomerulitis, may occur separately or together. Approximately 70 per cent of patients with polyarteritis nodosa and renal disease have renal vasculitis, whereas the other 30 per cent have glomerulitis. Renal polyarteritis is the most common lesion seen at postmortem examination. Manifestations of the renal involvement include intermittent proteinuria and microscopic hematuria with occasional hyaline and granular casts. The glomerulitis is manifested by marked microscopic and even macroscopic hematuria, proteinuria, cellular casts, and progressive renal failure. Hypertension reflects healing renal polyarteritis, progressive glomerulitis, or both. Renal involvement is the cause of death in about two thirds of patients with classic polyarteritis nodosa and about one third of those with allergic angiitis and granulomatosis.

Gastrointestinal. Arterial lesions are commonly found in one or more abdominal viscera. The principal manifestation is pain, especially in the umbilical region or right upper quadrant; anorexia, nausea, and vomiting are less prominent. Impaired arterial supply to the bowel can produce mucosal ulcerations, perforation, or infarction with melena or bloody diarrhea. Involvement of appendix, gallbladder, or pancreas can simulate appendicitis, cholecystitis, or hemorrhagic pancreatitis. Liver involvement can range from hepatomegaly with or without jaundice to the signs of extensive hepatic necrosis. Splenomegaly is uncommon. There has been no consistent relationship between the development of necrotizing angiitis and the appearance of liver disease in patients with hepatitis B antigenemia. Some of the observed combinations include necrotizing angiitis as the initial clinical finding, superimposed upon chronic active hepatitis, or appearing simultaneously with an acute hepatitis.

Central and Peripheral Nervous System. Neurologic manifestations are generally late occurrences in the course of polyarteritis nodosa, and their particular presentation reflects the specific brain area compromised. Headache, seizures, and retinal hemorrhages and exudates occur with or without localizing signs referable to the cerebrum, cerebellum, or brain stem; meningeal irritation may occur as a result of subarachnoid hemorrhage. Multiple mononeuropathy, i.e., involvement of several or even many individual nerves at the same or different times, is a common finding and is attributed to arteritis of the vasa nervorum. The peripheral neuropathy is usually asymmetrical with both sensory and motor distribution. The former can be extremely painful, but the latter, with attendant muscular degeneration, has on occasion been so severe as to dominate the clinical presentation.

Articular and Muscular. Arthralgias and myalgias are frequent in polyarteritis nodosa. Arthralgias are migratory, generally without swelling, and apparently due to small localized arterial lesions. Muscle pain or weakness reflects either direct involvement of the arterial supply or a peripheral neuropathy.

Cardiac. Polyarteritis of the coronary arteries and their branches has a frequency approaching that of renal polyarteritis, and heart failure is responsible for or contributes to death in one sixth to one half of the cases. The clinical manifestations of cardiac involvement are those of partial or complete arterial occlusion as modified by the superimposition of renal hypertension and an appreciable incidence of acute pericarditis without effusion. Whereas the combination of infarction and hypertension commonly leads to left-sided failure, an occasional patient with allergic angiitis and granulomatosis will present with predominantly right-sided decompensation.

Genitourinary. Involvement of the ovaries, testes, and epididymis is frequent, though usually asymptomatic. Mucosal ulceration in the bladder can occasionally precipitate gross hematuria with dysuria.

Cutaneous. Cutaneous involvement of some form is believed to occur in over 25 per cent of those affected with polyarteritis nodosa. The acute cutaneous manifestations include polymorphic exanthemata—purpuric, urticarial, and multiform in character—and severe subcutaneous hemorrhage, resulting from necrotizing arteritis, with secondary gangrene. Ulcerations and a persistent livedo reticularis are associated with the more chronic stage of the disease. A most characteristic but uncommon finding is cutaneous and subcutaneous nodules; these occur at any time in the disease course. The nodules tend to group, appear in crops, are usually movable, may regress in days or persist for months, range in size from a pea to a walnut, and may cause the overlying skin to become reddened or to ulcerate.

Pulmonary. Although the bronchial arteries can be involved in classic polyarteritis, only allergic angiitis and granulomatosis which involves the pulmonary arteries and parenchyma with granulomatous lesions give rise to clinical manifestations. Asthma, when present, is intractable and associated with a marked peripheral eosinophilia. Pneumonic episodes are transient or progressive and may be accompanied by hemoptysis and/or pleuritic pain. Respiratory involvement accounts for about one half of the mortality, with the remainder being attributable to the polyarteritic process in other organs.

COURSE UNTREATED. The course of polyarteritis nodosa is progressive with destruction of vital organs. Intermittent acute episodes resulting from thrombosis of vital or nonvital structures are prominent. Death is most frequently attributed to renal involvement in cases of classic polyarteritis nodosa and to pulmonary lesions in those cases classified as allergic angiitis with granulomatosis. Cardiac failure caused by a combination of infarction and renal hypertension is an additional frequent cause of death in both groups, and acute vascular accidents in the gastrointestinal tract or central nervous system account for much of the remaining mortality. In the retrospective postmortem study of Rose and Spencer, the five-year survival rate was about 10 per cent in classic polyarteritis nodosa, and about 25 per cent in allergic angiitis and granulomatosis if onset was dated from the start of respiratory symptoms. The report of the British Medical Research Council in 1960 placed the 54 months' survival rate in polyarteritis nodosa at nearly 50 per cent. Rare patients with polyarteritis limited to nonvital sites have been reported to experience an unusually long course or even a lasting remission.

LABORATORY FINDINGS. Leukocytosis, predominantly polymorphonuclear, is apparent in over 75 per cent of the cases of polyarteritis nodosa or allergic angiitis and granulomatosis, eosinophilia often being marked in the latter group. Hypocomplementemia, which has not been observed in classic polyarteritis nodosa, has been present in patients with hepatitis B antigenemia. The erythrocyte sedimentation rate is customarily elevated. Abnormalities in the urine sediment, especially hematuria and proteinuria, reflect renal involvement. Abnormalities of the electrocardiogram and electroencephalogram are those expected on the basis of arterial occlusive disease or those secondary to the metabolic disturbances of uremia. Lesions apparent on chest roentgenograms are the rule in patients with allergic angiitis and granulomatosis. The findings range from transient or progressive infiltration to consolidation, cavitation, or scarring; upper and lower lobes are involved with equal frequency. As none of these findings is specific, antemortem diagnosis of polyarteritis depends upon biopsy. Since the arterial involvement is segmental and spotty in distribution, it is advisable to obtain tissue from a symptomatic site, and it is essential to section completely the entire specimen. A deep, open surgical biopsy, including subcutaneous tissue and underlying muscle, should be obtained whenever possible from a skeletal muscle exhibiting pain and tenderness. Involvement of the epididymis and testes is sufficiently common to make this a useful biopsy site if palpation reveals the typical nodularity of segmental vascular lesions. Needle and surgical biopsies of internal organs with clinical involvement, such as liver or kidney, are gaining in favor. As an alternative or additional procedure, angiography to detect aneurysms of medium-sized muscular arteries in renal, hepatic, or intestinal sites may be helpful.

DIFFERENTIAL DIAGNOSIS. The differential diagnosis of the polyarteritis group includes not only the constituent syndromes but also all those conditions associated with systemic necrotizing vasculitis. The key differences between classic polyarteritis nodosa and other causes of necrotizing vasculitis include the absence of extravascular granulomas, sparing of the pulmonary arteries, failure of venous involvement except by contiguous spread, and predilection for medium-sized arteries. For allergic angiitis and granulomatosis the striking granulomatous response excludes all but Wegener's granulomatosis. The prominence of bronchial asthma, peripheral eosinophilia, and the usual absence of necrotizing lesions in the upper respiratory tract permit a tentative clinical distinction between allergic angiitis and granulomatosis and Wegener's granulomatosis. Underlying connective tissue diseases are still recognized by their clinical characteristics even when necrotizing arteritis becomes prominent. For example, cases of rheumatoid arthritis with ulcerating cutaneous lesions and peripheral neuropathy often exhibit prominent rheumatoid nodules and a high titer of rheumatoid factor. The specificities of the immunoglobulins which accompany active systemic lupus erythematosus or mixed cryoglobulinemia are distinctive; in addition, in the presence of active renal disease both entities manifest a reduced serum complement level not generally observed in classic polyarteritis nodosa. The giant cell arteritides (i.e., temporal arteritis, Takayasu's arteritis) lack the glomerulitis, peripheral neuropathy, and cutanous manifestations notable in polyarteritis nodosa. The combination of progressive nephritis and pulmonary hemorrhage seen in Goodpasture's syndrome is unlike polyarteritis nodosa. The drug-induced hypersensitivity vasculitis group may be difficult to separate on purely clinical grounds, although the history of antecedent drug administration, infrequency of gastrointestinal manifestations, and absence of nodules along arteries are useful points. The clinical presentation in Henoch-Schönlein purpura is distinctive.

TREATMENT. The commonly employed nonsteroidal anti-inflammatory agents have little or no effect on the polyarteritis group; thus, corticosteroids have been employed most widely. Large doses, in the range of 40 to 60 mg of prednisone per day, afford symptomatic relief but probably have little effect on the one-year survival statistics. In our series of 17 patients falling within the polyarteritis group, including two with allergic angiitis and granulomatosis and six with hepatitis B-associated polyarteritis, 14 experienced dramatic remission with the introduction of cyclophosphamide at a dose of 2 mg per kilogram per day. It was subsequently possible to reduce the cyclophosphamide and to taper the steroids to every other day and yet maintain a remission and in some instances resolution of microaneurysms on repeat celiac axis angiography was noted.

Churg J, Strauss L: Allergic granulomatosis, allergic angiitis, and periarteritis nodosa. Am J Pathol 27:277, 1951. *This is the classic reference to the polyarteritis nodosa subgroup termed allergic angiitis and granulomatosis, and describes the cardinal clinical and pathologic manifestations.*

Collagen Diseases and Hypersensitivity Panel: Report to Medical Research Council. Br Med J 1:1399, 1960. *This is the classic reference on the natural history of the polyarteritis nodosa group, untreated and with steroid intervention.*

Cupps TR, Fauci AS: The Vasculitides. Philadelphia, W. B. Saunders Company, 1981. *An excellent and up-to-date general review of different diagnosis, classification, and treatment.*

Fauci AS, Katz P, Haynes BF, et al.: Cyclophosphamide therapy of severe systemic necrotizing vasculitis. N Engl J Med 301:235, 1979. *A most important contribution dealing with the effectiveness of cyclophosphamide therapy in the management of a series of patients falling within the polyarteritis group and including such subgroups as allergic angiitis and granulomatosis and hepatitis B-associated polyarteritis.*

Leavitt RY, Fauci AS: Polyangiitis overlap syndrome. Am J Med 81:79, 1986. *Patients are being seen with increasing frequency who do not fit into one of the*

well-defined vasculitic entities. This is a useful paper that describes 10 such patients.

Rose GA, Spencer H: Polyarteritis nodosa. Q J Med 26:43, 1957. *This classic article argued most effectively that allergic angiitis and granulomatosis was not a distinct entity from classic polyarteritis nodosa but could most easily be considered polyarteritis nodosa with pulmonary involvement.*

Sergent JS, Lockshin MD, Christian CL, et al.: Vasculitis with hepatitis B antigenemia. Long-term observations in nine patients. Medicine 55:1, 1976. *This represents the five-year experience of the group which originally described the association of hepatitis B antigenemia with necrotizing vasculitis and contains important information with regard to the natural history and clinical course of the disease.*

441 WEGENER'S GRANULOMATOSIS AND MIDLINE GRANULOMA

Barton F. Haynes

WEGENER'S GRANULOMATOSIS

DEFINITION. Wegener's granulomatosis is a distinct clinical form of systemic necrotizing vasculitis consisting of (a) necrotizing granulomatous vasculitis of the upper and lower respiratory tracts, (b) focal necrotizing glomerulonephritis, and (c) systemic small vessel vasculitis involving numerous organ systems.

ETIOLOGY. The cause of the disease is unknown. It is thought to be a hypersensitivity reaction to unknown inhaled antigen(s). No familial, geographic, or occupational exposure factors have been associated with the disease. The incidence of HLA B8 antigen may be increased in patients with the disease.

INCIDENCE AND PREVALENCE. Wegener's granulomatosis is an uncommon but not rare disease that can affect any age-group. The mean age at onset is 40 years, with a male:female ratio of 3:2.

PATHOLOGY AND PATHOGENESIS. The typical histopathologic lesion is necrotizing vasculitis of small arteries and veins, usually with granuloma formation in the surrounding cellular infiltrates.

Biopsy of paranasal sinus, nasopharyngeal, or tracheal lesions may show acute or chronic inflammation or frank vasculitis with or without granulomas. Pansinusitis, nasal crusting with drainage, and serous otitis may result, as well as nasal septal perforation and saddle nose deformity.

Pulmonary lesions are present in 95 per cent of patients, with granulomas and vasculitis the common findings in biopsy material. Lung infiltrates are typically multiple, nodular, bilateral lesions that frequently cavitate. Less frequently, obstructive endobronchial lesions that lead to airway obstruction and atelectasis, or pleural lesions leading to pleural effusions, are found. Renal involvement is due to focal segmental glomerulonephritis that can lead to glomerular necrosis, crescent formation, and rapidly progressive renal failure. Any other organ system, most commonly skin and eyes, can be involved, with small vessel vasculitis with or without granuloma formation.

Although the specific mechanisms that lead to granulomatous vasculitic lesions in Wegener's granulomatosis are poorly understood, there is considerable evidence suggesting that disordered immunity with both antibody and cell-mediated tissue damage occurs. Approximately 50 per cent of patients have elevated levels of circulating immune complexes, and positive rheumatoid factor and hypergammaglobulinemia with elevations of serum IgA and IgG are common. Deposition of IgG and complement components as well as fibrin can be found in some renal biopsies. Pulmonary infiltrates show predominantly T cells and macrophages in the granulomatous lesions as well as polymorphonuclear cells (PMN) in and around inflamed vessels. Some studies have suggested an abnormality of PMN's in this disease with chemotactic defects, antineutrophil antibodies, and intravascular lysis of leukocytes.

It is likely that there are more than one immunologic mechanism occurring, such that an abnormal or exaggerated antibody response to an inhaled antigen could lead to an immune-complex triggered macrophage–T cell granulomatous response centered in and around vessels.

CLINICAL MANIFESTATIONS. The most common presentation of Wegener's granulomatosis is with upper and lower airway disease (90 to 95 per cent). Multiple organ systems may be involved during the course of the disease, including kidneys, joints, ears, and eyes. Common signs and symptoms include purulent nasal discharge, fever, cough, hemoptysis, paranasal sinus pain, nasal mucosal ulceration, and saddle nose deformity. Lung involvement can be asymptomatic, with nodular infiltrates seen on routine radiograph.

Renal disease is seen in 85 per cent of patients and is a critical determinant of the clinical outcome. Renal manifestations include hematuria, azotemia, proteinuria, and pedal edema. Renal disease can be smoldering, but more often when untreated rapidly progresses to irreversible renal failure.

Nearly 70 per cent of patients have some form of joint involvement during the course of the disease. Of these, one third have a nondeforming arthritis, usually in ankles and knees. The remaining two thirds have symmetric polyarticular arthralgias. Eye involvement occurs in 60 per cent of patients and is manifested as proptosis, scleritis, conjunctivitis, uveitis, dacryocystitis, and retinal or optic nerve vasculitis. Corneoscleral ring ulcers may progress to scleral perforation. Proptosis is usually due to contiguous sinus involvement with extension of granulomatous inflammation into the orbit.

Nervous system disease occurs in 20 per cent of patients, with mononeuritis multiplex the most common manifestation. Central nervous system involvement can be in the form of cranial nerve dysfunction, diffuse cerebral vasculitis, or hypothalamic granulomas with diabetes insipidus.

Heart involvement is manifested by pericarditis or coronary vasculitis. Less common manifestations include thyroiditis, mastoiditis, parotid masses, nasolacrimal duct obstruction, ear pinna and tympanic membrane granulomas, ulcerating breast masses, and anosmia.

Characteristic laboratory abnormalities include elevated erythrocyte sedimentation rate, neutrophilic leukocytosis, anemia, and positive test for serum rheumatoid factor. Serum antineutrophil antibodies against a cytoplasmic antigen have been reported to be useful for diagnosis and monitoring disease activity.

DIAGNOSIS. The diagnosis should be strongly considered when findings of upper or lower respiratory tract disease, renal disease, and vasculitis involving other organ systems are present. The disease should also be considered when any of the typical disease manifestations occur as an isolated finding (such as proptosis due to granulomatous inflammation and vasculitis) in an otherwise well patient.

To establish a definitive diagnosis, a patient should have evidence of clinical disease in at least two of the following three areas: upper airways, lung, and kidney. Biopsy results should show disease in at least one and preferably two of these organ systems, with lung tissue providing the source of highest diagnostic yield. Open lung biopsy is the procedure of choice to obtain adequate tissue for diagnosis. Percutaneous renal biopsy is important for both diagnosis and documentation of extent of renal disease. Differential diagnosis should include other diseases that can cause pulmonary-renal syndromes such as Goodpasture's syndrome (see Ch. 62 and 81). Idiopathic midline granuloma (see below) destroys facial and palate bones and cartilage but is not a systemic vasculitis and does not involve lungs or kidneys. Lesions of Wegener's granulomatosis do not perforate the palate or erode through major bony structures of the face and upper airway, although they may destroy the medial wall of the orbit, called the lamina papyracea.

Another disease frequently confused with Wegener's granulomatosis is *lymphomatoid granulomatosis*. This disease is characterized by infiltration of various organs with a polymorphic cellular infiltrate consisting of atypical lymphoid and plasmacytoid cells together with granulomatous inflammation in an angiocentric pattern. The disease primarily involves lungs, skin, kidneys, and central nervous system, but not upper airways. Renal involvement is not a glomerulonephritis, but rather is due to interstitial infiltration with masses of atypical lymphoid cells. Lymphomatoid granulomatosis, unlike Wegener's granulomatosis, is not an inflammatory vasculitis, but more likely represents invasion of vessels with premalignant T cells. Up to one half of cases evolve into a frank T cell lymphoma that responds poorly even to combined chemotherapy regimens for non-Hodgkin's lymphoma.

TREATMENT AND PROGNOSIS. The treatment of choice for Wegener's granulomatosis is a combination of corticosteroids and a cytotoxic agent, of which the most efficacious is cyclophosphamide. Irreversible organ system dysfunction can occur if conservative therapy (such as with corticosteroids alone) is attempted. In patients with active but stable multisystem disease, oral cyclophosphamide should be given in a dose of 1 to 2 mg per kilogram per day, with the dose adjusted to maintain the total leukocyte count above 3000 per cu mm and the PMN count above 1000 to 1500 per cu mm. Weekly monitoring of the white blood cell count is essential to avoid severe leukopenia and infectious complications. In patients with fulminant disease, such as CNS vasculitis, severe pulmonary involvement with hypoxemia, rapidly progressive peripheral neuropathy, or rapidly progressive renal failure, cyclophosphamide may be given intravenously in a dose of 4 mg per kilogram per day for three days, with change to the lower oral dose regimen thereafter. Patients should be treated for one year after remission has been achieved, then cytotoxic drug therapy stopped and the patient re-evaluated periodically for disease relapse. Because of the risk of serious complications with cytotoxic therapy (see Ch. 176) and frequent symptomatic infection of damaged respiratory tracts with microorganisms such as *Staphylococcus aureus*, the presence of persistent vasculitis should be documented prior to continuation of long-term cytotoxic therapy (greater than one year) for presumed active disease.

Corticosteroids should be administered in an oral daily dose regimen (usually prednisone 1 mg per kilogram per day) or in divided doses (every six hours) for fulminant cases for an initial one to two weeks, followed by tapering to an alternate-day regimen (see Ch. 30). After three to six months, corticosteroids can usually be discontinued altogether. With this regimen remissions can be obtained in 90 per cent of patients with Wegener's granulomatosis. Those patients who have gone on to end-stage renal failure have had successful renal transplants while on this regimen. Patients who relapse while on little or no medication require diagnosis of the cause of relapse. In a previously treated patient with a new pulmonary infiltrate, it is critical to distinguish between a lung infection and a recurrence of pulmonary vasculitis.

Fauci AS, Haynes BF, Katz P: The spectrum of vasculitis. Clinical, pathologic, immunologic, and therapeutic considerations. Ann Intern Med 89:660, 1978. *Comprehensive review of all vasculitic syndromes with emphasis on the relationship of Wegener's granulomatosis to other diseases with vessel inflammation.*

Fauci AS, Haynes BF, Katz P, et al.: Wegener's granulomatosis: Prospective clinical and therapeutic experience with 85 patients for 21 years. Ann Intern Med 98:76, 1983. *Long-term follow-up is presented for a large group of patients, detailing presentation, clinical course, and treatment strategy.*

Fauci AS, Haynes BF, Costa J, et al.: Lymphomatoid granulomatosis. Prospective clinical and therapeutic experience over 10 years. N Engl J Med 306:68, 1982. *Report differentiating lymphomatoid granulomatosis from Wegener's granulomatosis and describing the treatment regimen and outcome for lymphomatoid granulomatosis.*

Haynes BF, Fishman ML, Fauci AS, et al.: The ocular manifestations of Wegener's granulomatosis. Fifteen years experience and review of the literature. Am J Med 63:131, 1977. *A detailed account of the clinical forms and therapy of a difficult-to-treat manifestation of Wegener's granulomatosis.*

Haynes BF, Allen NB, Fauci AS: Diagnostic and therapeutic approach to the patient with vasculitis. Med Clin North Am 70:355, 1986. *A concise review that summarizes in detailed tabular form for easy reference the diagnostic and therapeutic approach to patients suspected of having a vasculitic syndrome such as Wegener's granulomatosis.*

MIDLINE GRANULOMA

DEFINITION. Idiopathic midline granuloma, also known as idiopathic midline destructive disease, is a progressive, localized process that predominantly involves the nose, paranasal sinuses, and palate, with erosion through bone and soft tissues, frequently involving the face.

ETIOLOGY. The cause of idiopathic midline granuloma is unknown. No primary infectious or neoplastic cause has been found. An exaggerated hypersensitivity reaction to unknown inhaled antigens has been postulated.

PATHOLOGY. Biopsy demonstrates necrosis and acute and chronic inflammation. Mucosal surfaces of the nose and paranasal sinuses are frequently ulcerated, and inflammation invades and destroys adjacent cartilage and bone. The cellular infiltrate comprises polymorphonuclear leukocytes, lymphocytes, macrophages, plasma cells, and less frequently multinucleated giant cells with well-formed epithelial granulomas. Although perivascular infiltrations and vessel destruction due to widespread inflammation are common, a primary vasculitis is generally not seen. Foci of atypical lymphocytes or histiocytes suggest an underlying lymphoma or other midline neoplasm, rather than midline granuloma.

CLINICAL MANIFESTATIONS. Most patients with idiopathic midline granuloma have active sinusitis with superimposed bacterial infections. Symptoms begin with nasal stuffiness and crusting and progress to purulent nasal discharge and bleeding. Ulcerations may appear on the nasal septum, palate, or nose. Perforation and destruction of the nasal septum can occur, resulting in a saddle nose deformity. Destruction of the soft and hard palate permits reflux of food into the upper airway during eating. Paranasal inflammation with swelling frequently results in nasolacrimal duct obstruction and dacryocystitis. Relentless midline inflammation with necrosis can result in widespread, mutilating destruction of facial bones and tissues, with erosion into the central nervous system leading to meningitis, or into major blood vessels leading to life-threatening hemorrhage. Erosion can cause retro-orbital masses, orbit destruction, and blindness. Loss of smell is common, and recurrent sinus infection with *Staphylococcus aureus* is routine. Most patients are free of systemic signs and symptoms except when superimposed bacterial infections occur. There are no characteristic laboratory findings. Computerized tomograms and radiographs of the mid-line structures often show dramatic destruction of facial bones with evidence of widespread sinus inflammation.

DIAGNOSIS. The diagnosis is made from the characteristic clinical presentation of locally destructive lesions restricted to the upper respiratory tract and absence of histologic evidence of Wegener's granulomatosis or lymphoma. Although midline granuloma is a distinct disease, the diagnosis is made by excluding other diseases with similar findings.

While a large number of infectious, connective tissue, and inflammatory diseases can cause ulcerations of the nose and midline structures, the three entities that most often comprise the differential diagnosis are those listed in Table 441–1. Midline granuloma is a locally destructive disease that is relentlessly progressive over months to years. It is not a primary vasculitis and thus is clearly distinct from *Wegener's granulomatosis*, in which the lesions are not progressive, erode only cartilage and thin facial bones, and frequently heal spontaneously. *Malignant midline reticulosis* is a pleomorphic lymphoma, frequently of the T cell type, that presents with extensive mucosal ulceration, tissue necrosis, bone destruction, and fistula formation in facial midline tissues. The tempo of the disease is rapid, and, on repeat biopsy, atypical lymphoid cells or frank lymphoma is found. The diagnosis is a difficult one, however, since the clinical picture may suggest an inflammatory process rather than a tumor, and on biopsy the malignant nature of the process may be obscured by an intense inflammatory infiltrate, presumably in reaction to tumor antigens.

Rarely, other lymphomas, mycosis fungoides, and nonkeratinizing squamous cell carcinomas can produce midfacial destructive lesions. Other less destructive diseases in the differential diagnosis are *sarcoidosis* (Ch. 69), *relapsing polychondritis* (Ch. 445), and *necrotizing sialometaplasia*, a self-healing process of six to eight weeks' duration which presents with large ulcerations of the hard palate and a necrotizing process in minor salivary glands. Infectious diseases that should be ruled out include chronic bacterial infections, tuberculosis, syphilis, rhinoscleroma (due to *Klebsiella rhinoscleromatis*), actinomycosis, leprosy, phycomycosis, blastomycosis, candidiasis, histoplasmosis, coccidioidomycosis, and leishmaniasis.

TREATMENT AND PROGNOSIS. Radiation therapy, approximately 5000 rads, to the midfacial area is the treatment of choice. Prednisone and cytotoxic drug regimens have generally not been successful. Surgical procedures on involved tissues can accelerate the destructive process. However, following radiation therapy, surgical debridement and aggressive local care measures, such as routine upper airway irrigation and treatment of bacterial superinfections, can aid the healing process. Reconstructive plastic surgery and prosthesis placement for patients with extensive facial disfigurement are often of benefit. In long-term survivors, close mon-

TABLE 441–1. COMPARISON OF CLINICAL FEATURES OF IDIOPATHIC MIDLINE GRANULOMA WITH WEGENER'S GRANULOMATOSIS AND MALIGNANT MIDLINE RETICULOSIS

Feature	Idiopathic Midline Granuloma	Wegener's Granulomatosis	Malignant Midline Reticulosis
Types of upper airway disease	Destructive lesions of sinuses, palate, nose, and facial bones with soft tissue erosions—progresses over months to years	Inflammatory upper airway disease of sinuses and nasal mucosa. Palate ulcerations occur without perforation. Erosion of medial wall of orbit frequent; otherwise facial bone and soft tissue erosion does not occur.	Destructive lesions of sinuses, palate, nose, and facial bones with soft tissue erosion—progresses over weeks to months
Systemic involvement	Disease localized only to upper airway	Systemic involvement of multiple organs characteristic	Destructive lesion local; systemic disease related to disseminated lymphoma
Association with malignancy	None	None	Likely a midline T cell or histocytic lymphoma
Pathology	Acute and chronic inflammation, with or without granuloma	Necrotizing granulomatous vasculitis	Atypical and pleomorphic cells or frank lymphoma
Treatment	Radiation therapy	Cyclophosphamide and corticosteroids	Radiation therapy and/or combination chemotherapy

Adapted from Batsakis JG: Midfacial necrotizing diseases. Ann Otol Rhinol Laryngol 91:541, 1982, and Fauci AS, et al.: Radiation therapy of midline granuloma. Ann Intern Med 84:104, 1976.

itoring for radiation-induced upper airway neoplasia is essential.

Batsakis JG: Midfacial necrotizing diseases. Ann Otol Rhinol Laryngol 91:541, 1982. *A concise paper summarizing the distinguishing features of idiopathic midline granuloma compared to other syndromes.*

Fauci AS, Johnson RE, Wolff SM: Radiation therapy of midline granuloma. Ann Intern Med 84:104, 1976. *Classic paper describing the distinct clinical features of idiopathic midline granuloma and outlining successful treatment and management strategies.*

Fechner RE, Lamppier DW: Malignant midline reticulosis. A clinicopathologic entity. Arch Otolaryngol 95:467, 1972. *Detailed report characterizing this midfacial neoplasm and outlining diagnostic and histopathologic criteria.*

Fu YS, Perzin KH: Non-epithelial tumors of the nasal cavity, paranasal sinuses, and nasopharynx: A clinicopathologic study. X. Malignant lymphomas. Cancer 43:611, 1979. *An important study comparing the features of malignant midline reticulosis with other lymphomas of the head and neck.*

Tsokos M, Fauci AS, Costa J: Idiopathic midline destructive disease (IMDD) a subgroup of patients with the "midline granuloma syndrome." Am J Clin Pathol 77:162, 1982. *Paper in which clear diagnostic guidelines are emphasized and a more precise term for idiopathic midline granuloma proposed.*

442 POLYMYALGIA RHEUMATICA AND GIANT CELL ARTERITIS

Louis A. Healey

POLYMYALGIA RHEUMATICA

Polymyalgia rheumatica is a syndrome consisting of pain and stiffness in pelvic and shoulder girdles, very rapid erythrocyte sedimentation rate, and a prompt response to a small dose of corticosteroid. For reasons unknown, it is a disease of older patients. The diagnosis is made with reluctance in anyone less than 50 years old, and most patients are over age 60. It is seen more often in women than in men (2.5:1). Almost all patients affected are Caucasian.

Patients experience pain in the neck, back, shoulders, upper arms, and thighs. The onset may be gradual but at other times is so abrupt that patients go to bed well and awaken in the morning stiff and sore as though they had chopped wood or shoveled snow. Morning stiffness and jelling after prolonged sitting are essential features of the history. Patients graphically describe how a spouse has to pull them out of bed or, if they are alone, how it is necessary for them to wiggle like a snake and then push themselves up from a kneeling position. Although such a story may initially suggest weakness, the limitation is actually due to pain and stiffness rather than lack of strength. Some patients experience widespread symptoms and complain that they hurt all over. In others the pain and stiffness is in either shoulders or hips, but in all it is symmetric. Low grade fever, malaise, apathy, and weight loss are sometimes present. Carpal tunnel syndrome has been noted.

Despite the severity of complaints, the physical examination of these patients is surprisingly normal. Tenderness or limitation of shoulder and hip motion may be detected; effusions are present in the knees at times. Muscle strength is normal when tested. Radiographs are unremarkable. The clue to the diagnosis is the erythrocyte sedimentation rate, which is usually elevated, often very high, and may exceed 100 mm per hour (Westergren method). Slight anemia may be present. Rheumatoid factor and antinuclear antibodies are not present, and serum complement is normal. Serum levels of muscle enzymes, electromyograms, and muscle biopsies are normal. Arthroscopy and biopsy of the shoulder show that the symptoms of pain and stiffness are due to synovitis.

Although polymyalgia rheumatica appears to be a distinct clinical entity, it is obvious from this description that it is not a specific one, and as such it is often necessary to exclude other diseases in order to make the diagnosis. The sedimentation rate indicates that this is an inflammatory disease and serves to separate it from osteoarthritis or the functional musculoskeletal pain of fibrositis. Difficulty in getting out of bed or rising from a chair may suggest the weakness of polymyositis, but, as mentioned, muscles are normal. The common diagnostic problem is to differentiate polymyalgia rheumatica from the onset of rheumatoid arthritis. Patients with rheumatoid arthritis tend to have synovitis of the distal joints—wrists, metacarpophalangeal, and metatarsophalangeal. When present, the rheumatoid factor is helpful, but at times the diagnosis only becomes evident with follow-up visits.

The response of the pain and stiffness of polymyalgia rheumatica to 10 to 20 mg of prednisone may truly be described as dramatic. Many patients are well by the next day; improvement is so invariable that if it does not appear within one week, the original diagnosis should be questioned. After two to four weeks, the dose can be tapered and patients remain free of symptoms on 5 to 7.5 mg of prednisone daily, without risk of steroid side effects. The duration that therapy will be required is uncertain. Some patients can stop after one year, but others will have to continue. The duration can be determined only by attempting to withdraw the drug and observing for a recurrence of stiffness and pain. Aspirin and other nonsteroidal anti-inflammatory drugs provide partial relief but are not so effective as small doses of steroid.

GIANT CELL ARTERITIS

Since the recognition that any of the larger arteries may be involved, the term *giant cell arteritis* has been preferred to the original names *temporal* or *cranial arteritis*. In contrast to polyarteritis, smaller arterioles are not affected; thus pulmonary and renal complications are not seen, and stroke or myocardial infarction does not occur more frequently than would be expected in this age group.

Clinical manifestations may conveniently be divided into localized or systemic. Local manifestations depend on the artery involved. Inflammation of the temporal artery produces severe headache, most often in one temple. The artery may be tender and swollen. Sudden unilateral blindness is due to occlusion of the terminal branches of the ophthalmic artery. Since blindness is irreversible, this is the most dreaded complication of the disease. Pain in the masseter muscles with chewing is attributed to involvement of the facial artery. This "jaw claudication" is a pathognomonic symptom of giant cell arteritis. Transient diplopia from ischemia of extraocular muscles is important to recognize, since it may lead to early diagnosis, steroid treatment, and preservation of vision. Arteritic involvement of the aorta can cause aortic arch syndromes with claudication in the arms and unequal pulses or, rarely, aneurysm formation. Systemic manifestations include fever, anemia, weight loss, and malaise. Some or all of these may be present in varying degree. If headache and other cranial symptoms are either not present or minimal and if systemic symptoms predominate, the patients may present such diagnostic problems as fever of unknown origin, unexplained anemia, or possible occult carcinoma.

As with polymyalgia rheumatica, the only laboratory abnormality is the rapid erythrocyte sedimentation rate. Anemia is usually mild but can be more significant with hematocrit as low as 28 per cent. Red blood cell indices are normal, and there is a failure to utilize iron despite the presence of normal stores in the marrow. Tests of liver function, particularly the alkaline phosphatase, may show slight to moderate abnormalities, but biopsy of the liver shows normal tissue or slight fatty changes.

The diagnosis is established by biopsy of the temporal artery, which is safe and convenient to perform as an office procedure. The characteristic histologic picture shows zones of inflammatory infiltrate composed of histiocytes, lymphocytes, and giant cells surrounding markedly fragmented internal elastic lamina with intervening segments of normal artery. When headache, visual symptoms, or other signs of cranial artery involvement are present, the diagnosis may be suspected and the biopsy is usually positive. However, the characteristic arteritis has also been found in some patients with polymyalgia rheumatica, fever, or other systemic symptoms even when the temporal artery appears clinically normal.

Giant cell arteritis responds well to steroid treatment, but higher doses are needed to suppress the inflammation. When cranial arteritis is diagnosed or even suspected, treatment should be started immediately with at least 50 mg of prednisone in order to preserve vision. If the diagnosis is proved by biopsy, this dose should be continued for four weeks before gradual reduction is instituted with the aim of achieving the same maintenance dose and duration of therapy as described for polymyalgia rheumatica. Such a program carries a risk of steroid toxicity, particularly osteoporosis and vertebral collapse, which must be balanced against the risk of blindness. If the patient has been treated with high-dose steroid for one month, it is preferable to follow the clinical response as the dose is tapered. The risk of steroid toxicity from treating the sedimentation rate is greater than the risk of a complication of arteritis in a patient whose sedimentation rate increases somewhat as the steroid dose is lowered.

The nature of the relation between polymyalgia rheumatica and giant cell arteritis is uncertain. Both are diseases of older patients, the vast majority of whom are Caucasian. Both frequently are seen in the same patient. Sixty per cent of patients with giant cell arteritis experience polymyalgia rheumatica at some time during their illness. Conversely, of patients with polymyalgia rheumatica and normal-appearing temporal arteries, only 10 per cent show arteritis on biopsy. The majority of polymyalgia patients respond well to low-dose prednisone and never develop clinical evidence of arteritis.

Chuang T-Y, Hunder GG, Ilstrup DM, et al.: Polymyalgia rheumatica. A 10-year epidemiologic and clinical study. Ann Intern Med 97:672, 1982. *Based on an entire county population, this study gives the best information on incidence. The 10-year follow-up provides a look at the course of the disease, response to treatment, outcome, and complications.*

Healey LA, Wilske KR: Polymyalgia rheumatica and giant cell arteritis [medical progress]. West J Med 141:64–67, 1984.

Hunder GG, Michet CJ: Giant cell arteritis and polymyalgia rheumatica. Clin Rheum Dis 11:471–483, 1985. *These two articles review current concepts of the two syndromes, their manifestations, relation to one another, prognosis, and treatment. Recent references are included.*

443 POLYMYOSITIS

Ronald P. Messner

DEFINITION. Polymyositis is an inflammatory disease of skeletal muscle of unknown etiology, characterized by symmetric weakness of the limb girdles, neck, and pharynx. Patients with this illness can be divided into five clinical categories (Table 443–1).

In this chapter the term "polymyositis" is used to characterize the whole group of patients, while "adult polymyositis" is used to denote type I patients.

INCIDENCE. Polymyositis has an annual incidence of approximately five cases per million population. There is no relationship to birth order, family size, socioeconomic level, or geographic location. Familial cases are unusual. Age distribution is bimodal, with a small peak between ages 10 and 14 and a larger peak around age 50. Patients with myositis associated with malignancy are slightly older, with a mean age just over 60. In adult polymyositis and dermatomyositis,

TABLE 443–1. CLASSIFICATION OF POLYMYOSITIS

Type I	Adult polymyositis
Type II	Dermatomyositis
Type III	Myositis with malignancy
Type IV	Childhood myositis
Type V	Myositis associated with other connective tissue diseases (overlap syndromes)

females outnumber males by two to one. In cases associated with overlap syndromes the female dominance is even more pronounced. The sex ratio is equal in myositis associated with malignancy.

PATHOLOGY AND PATHOGENESIS. The characteristic features of polymyositis on muscle biopsy include (1) degeneration of individual fibers, sometimes with vacuolation; (2) regeneration indicated by sarcoplasmic basophilia, large vesicular nuclei, and prominent nucleoli; (3) necrosis of part or all of a muscle fiber (moth-eaten fibers) and phagocytosis of the debris by macrophages; (4) increased variation in fiber size without hypertrophy of individual fibers; (5) interstitial and/or perivascular mononuclear cell infiltrate; (6) perifascicular atrophy; and (7) interstitial fibrosis. These findings may vary from patient to patient and even on multiple biopsies of a single patient. Approximately 15 per cent of initial muscle biopsies are normal, and the full picture of typical changes can be expected in about 50 per cent. Biopsy should be performed on a muscle that is involved but not totally weakened. Electromyography may aid in localizing an involved area, but the biopsy should not include the exact site of the electromyograph needle puncture, for the needle may cause focal fiber destruction.

Biopsy of involved skin shows marked dermal edema, basal vacuolation, and colloid bodies. Similar changes occur in the skin in systemic lupus erythematosus, but in dermatomyositis the basement membrane is normal in thickness and does not stain for immunoglobulin or complement in indirect immunofluorescence studies.

The leading theory of the pathogenesis of polymyositis attributes muscle damage to cell-mediated autoimmunity. Several lines of evidence support this hypothesis. In adult polymyositis approximately one third of the cells invading the muscle are macrophages and two thirds are lymphocytes. The intensity of the inflammatory infiltrate increases from perivascular through the perimysial to the endomysial area. Lymphocytes directly in contact with viable muscle fibers are predominantly cytotoxic/suppressor (T8) in phenotype and often send finger-like projections into the muscle cells. Lymphocytes expressing the helper (T4) phenotype are found in the areas surrounding these invading cells. Studies of the ability of mononuclear cells from polymyositis to kill or damage muscle cells in vitro have yielded conflicting results, but sensitivity of these cells to muscle antigens has been demonstrated both by proliferation and lymphokine production. Soluble mediators released include a factor that inhibits calcium binding by normal sarcoplasmic reticulum. Class I major histocompatibility (MHC) antigens that are crucial to the interaction of T8 lymphocytes with target cells are poorly expressed in normal sarcolemma, but their expression is greatly enhanced in areas adjacent to infiltrating lymphocytes in polymyositis. The increase in Class I MHC antigens is apparently mediated by interferon produced by the infiltrating lymphocytes. Thus, many of the elements needed for cell-mediated injury have been identified at the site of pathology in polymyositis.

Further evidence for an autoimmune process in polymyositis comes from the multitude of autoantibodies present in the serum. Antimyosin antibodies occur in 90 per cent and antimyoglobin antibodies in 70 per cent of patients. While not specific for polymyositis, their prevalence is considerably higher than in other muscle diseases. Evidence for antibodies against structures on the surface of muscle cells is less plentiful, but IgG from polymyositis sera can accelerate degradation of acetylcholine receptors of cultured muscle cells. Antinuclear antibodies demonstrated by immunofluorescence on human tissue culture cells (HEp-2) or by precipitation with calf thymus nuclear extract occur in 90 per cent of patients. Specificities for a variety of discrete nuclear components have been identified. Two antibodies, anti-Jo-1 and PL-7, react with histidyl-tRNA synthetase and threonyl-tRNA synthetase, respectively. Anti-Jo-1 antibodies are found in 30 per cent of type I and less than 10 per cent of type II patients but in 50 to 100 per cent of patients with adult polymyositis and interstitial lung disease. It is postulated that these unusual antibodies may be the footprints of a preceding viral infection. Certain enteroviruses can mimic tRNA and interact with aminoacyl-tRNA synthetase enzymes. This interaction might render the enzyme immunogenic and account for the presence of the autoantibodies. Anti-PM-Scl antibodies react with a nucleolar antigen and anti-Ku with a novel non-histone DNA-binding protein. Both are found in patients with polymyositis and scleroderma overlap. Anti-Mi-1 and Mi-2 antibodies react with nuclear components and occur in 3 and 20 per cent of dermatomyositis patients, respectively. A small number of polymyositis patients also have antibodies to nRNP, and almost two thirds of the sera react with intermediate filaments of the cytoskeleton. Anti-Jo-1 is associated with HLA-DR3, suggesting a genetic basis for the expression of at least some of these autoantibodies.

Vascular damage is also implicated in the pathogenesis of polymyositis, particularly in children, and in dermatomyositis. In a subset of children with dermatomyositis, cutaneous ulceration, and intestinal infarction, the clinical picture suggests necrotizing vasculitis. Examination of tissue, however, reveals primarily noninflammatory endarteropathy and lymphocytic perivasculitis. The terminal membrane attack complex of the complement system is deposited, bound, and activated to completion in muscle microvasculature in most patients with childhood myositis and a smaller portion of adults with dermatomyositis. Correlation with immunoglobulin deposition is poor, suggesting an antibody-independent mechanism of complement activation. In addition, replication of capillary basement membrane and alterations in endothelial cells are frequently seen on electron microscopy. Loss of capillaries also occurs. It characteristically starts in the periphery of the fascicles and is more pronounced in children than in adults. These changes are probably not due to muscle atrophy, because the ratio of capillary lumina to muscle cell area does not change in Duchenne dystrophy and increases in denervation atrophy.

Infection caused by a virus or an organism such as *Toxoplasma gondii* has been postulated as a cause of polymyositis. The prevalence of IgM anti-*Toxoplasma* antibodies is increased in patients with polymyositis, and *Toxoplasma* organisms have been identified in a few cases of adult polymyositis, but treatment for toxoplasmosis has had little effect on the muscle disease. These cases may represent secondary infection with *Toxoplasma*. Coxsackievirus has been isolated from a few cases of polymyositis, and the prevalence of antibodies to Coxsackievirus B is increased in children with dermatomyositis. The recently described myositis that occurs in newborn mice after injection with Coxsackievirus B1 might provide a system to study the role of both infection and cell-mediated immunity in muscle damage.

CLINICAL MANIFESTATIONS. Weakness of the proximal muscles occurs in nearly all patients and is the presenting complaint in 93 per cent. The typical case begins with gradual onset of weakness in the hip girdle and proximal leg muscles. Muscle pain and tenderness are absent or mild. Weakness of the shoulders, proximal arm muscles, and neck flexors follows. Involvement of the pharyngeal muscles may occur with dysphagia, dysphonia, and dysarthria. Early symptoms include inability to rise from a low chair, to climb stairs without the use of a railing, or to raise the arms above the head to comb the hair. In advanced cases, the patient may be unable to lift the limbs against gravity. Muscular wasting is variable and frequently minimal until late in the disease. Contractures are almost exclusively associated with long-standing disease. The ocular muscles are almost never involved, and weakness of distal muscles occurs in less than 20 per cent of cases. Asymmetric weakness, weakness of isolated muscle groups, and acute onset with global weakness are unusual. Deep tendon reflexes are normal or slightly reduced. Muscle symptoms of childhood polymyositis are similar to those of the adult form, but fever, weight loss, rash, contractures, and subcutaneous calcification are more common.

Arthralgias occur in about one quarter of patients with adult polymyositis or dermatomyositis. True arthritis is usually mild; begins prior to or coincident with weakness; involves the hands, wrists, and knees; and responds quickly to steroid treatment. Synovial fluid has good viscosity and mononuclear cells. Synovial biopsy reveals fibrin deposition, focal loss of lining cells without proliferation, and mild inflammation. Patients with myositis and overlap syndromes may have joint involvement typical of rheumatoid arthritis or systemic lupus erythematosus. A peculiar arthritis of the hands with erosions, periosteal calcification, and instability of the interphalangeal joints of the thumb has also been described.

An erythematous skin rash occurs on the forehead, neck, shoulders, trunk, and arms of about one third of patients and distinguishes those with dermatomyositis. A lilac or heliotrope rash occurs on the upper eyelids and face in 15 per cent. The rash may be associated with edema. Reddened, elevated, scaly patches are characteristically seen over the extensor surfaces of the small joints of the hands (Gottron's sign), the elbows, the knees, and the medial malleoli. Nailfolds may show periungual telangiectasia, dilated and distorted nailfold capillary loops alternating with avascular areas, or thickening and roughening without redness. In some patients, the finger pads become shiny and atrophic with constant peeling. Patients with myositis and overlap syndromes may display the whole spectrum of dermatologic changes associated with connective tissue diseases. Raynaud's syndrome occurs in one half of the patients with overlap syndrome and one fifth of those with adult polymyositis and dermatomyositis. It is less common in children and in patients with malignancy.

Dysphagia in polymyositis is primarily due to weakness of the striated musculature of the posterior pharynx. Dysphagia may also result from cricopharyngeal obstruction secondary to inflammation or fibrosis of the cricopharyngeus muscles. In this case, surgical division of the involved muscles provides prompt relief of the symptoms. Dysfunction of the esophagus and stomach occurs but is usually overshadowed by pharyngeal dysfunction. Hypomobility and poor absorption in the small intestine have been seen in a few patients without symptoms of frank scleroderma. Vasculitis associated with the childhood form of the disease may lead to mesenteric thrombosis.

Asymptomatic electrocardiographic abnormalities are common in polymyositis, but cardiac involvement manifested by congestive heart failure or symptomatic heart block occurs in only 10 per cent of patients. Inflammatory cardiomyopathy, fibrosis, and small vessel disease have been found in some of these patients at autopsy. Interstitial pneumonitis occurs in 10 to 15 per cent of the patients. Cough and dyspnea precede muscle weakness in one half of the cases of interstitial pneumonitis. No relationship is apparent between the severity of the lung and muscle involvement. Vasculitis is not characteristic of this lesion, and pleurisy is uncommon. The presence of active inflammation on lung biopsy correlates well with steroid responsiveness. Renal involvement is rare. When renal failure occurs, it is usually attributable to myoglobulinuria.

About 13 per cent of patients with adult-onset polymyositis

2036 / XXI MUSCULOSKELETAL AND CONNECTIVE TISSUE DISEASES

have coexistent malignancy. Females are affected as frequently as males. Several recent studies have found an equal incidence of malignancy in adult polymyositis and dermatomyositis, but the combined data of large series in the past 10 years suggest that patients with dermatomyositis are at greater risk. Myositis precedes or occurs simultaneously with the diagnosis of malignancy in two thirds of patients, and in most instances the two diagnoses are made within the span of a year. Tumors of the breast and lung are the most common. Those of the ovary and stomach occur more frequently than in the general population, whereas tumors of the colon and rectum are less frequent. Polymyositis associated with malignancy has no clinical features that differentiate it from polymyositis alone. Extensive undirected radiographic screening of these patients for cancer has proved unrewarding. Clues to the coexistence of a malignancy are almost always present on history, physical examination, or routine laboratory tests.

CLINICAL COURSE AND PROGNOSIS. The five-year survival rate is approximately 80 per cent. The best survival rate occurs in children. Diagnosis at age 45 or above and the presence of cardiac involvement are associated with shorter survival. Death within the first year is often from pneumonia associated with dysphagia and aspiration. The leading causes of death are malignancy, infection, and cardiovascular disease. About half of the surviving patients will attain almost complete recovery of muscle strength.

LABORATORY DATA. Serum levels of muscle-derived enzymes, principally creatine kinase (CK), transaminases (SGOT, SGPT), lactate dehydrogenase (LDH), and aldolase, are elevated at some time during the course of the disease in 99 per cent of the patients and will be normal at any one time in about 10 per cent. CK and aldolase are the most sensitive, but it is wise to obtain all five enzymes on initial screening. The MB isoenzyme of CK is occasionally elevated in the absence of cardiac involvement owing to its increase in regenerating muscle. The levels of these enzymes correlate reasonably well with disease activity and can be used as guides to therapy. Approximately one half of patients have elevated serum levels of myoglobin or an abnormal erythrocyte sedimentation rate. Neither test can be relied upon as an index of disease activity. With few exceptions, complement studies are normal. Radionuclide scanning with ^{99m}Tc-polyphosphate may reveal increased uptake in areas of active myositis.

The electromyogram (EMG) is abnormal in almost all patients. The most common abnormalities, reduction in amplitude and duration of motor unit potentials, occur in 90 per cent of cases but are not specific for polymyositis. Evidence of membrane irritability, including fibrillation, positive sharp waves, and increased insertional activity, occurs in one half to three quarters of the EMG's. Spontaneous bizarre high-frequency discharges are also characteristic. Electromyographic patterns do not differ among the clinical types of disease. In some patients the characteristic pattern is present only in certain muscle groups. The paravertebral musculature is frequently involved and should be included in diagnostic electromyography.

DIAGNOSIS AND DIFFERENTIAL DIAGNOSIS. In order to standardize diagnosis of these patients a set of criteria has been proposed (Table 443–2). The reliability of the diagnosis depends upon the number of criteria met. Patients are classified as having definite disease with four, probable disease with three, and possible disease with two criteria. The presence of proximal muscle weakness is established both by

TABLE 443–2. PROPOSED CRITERIA FOR DIAGNOSIS OF POLYMYOSITIS

1. Symmetric proximal muscle weakness
2. Elevation of muscle enzyme activities in serum
3. Typical EMG abnormalities
4. Positive muscle biopsy
5. Typical rash of dermatomyositis

TABLE 443–3. CLINICAL GRADING OF MUSCLE STRENGTH

0	No evident contraction
1	Contraction but no movement
2	Movement with gravity eliminated
3	Movement against gravity
4	Movement against resistance
5	Normal

the history and by objective testing. One scheme for grading muscle strength utilizes a five-point scale (Table 443–3). This scheme works well with severe weakness but is relatively insensitive to clinically important changes in the range of grades 4 and 5. A test using 10 timed chair stands offers a reproducible quantitative method to assess lower extremity strength in this critical area.

Polymyositis is but one of a variety of diseases that may be present as muscle weakness with or without muscle pain. Neurologic disease is a primary concern in the evaluation of these patients. The history and physical examination will usually establish the neurologic origin, and EMG will show neuropathic changes. In muscular dystrophy a family history is often present and the symptoms progress over years rather than months. The CK may be elevated and may decrease on treatment with corticosteroids, but clinical improvement does not occur. The early involvement of the ocular and facial muscles helps differentiate myasthenia gravis.

Steroid myopathy begins insidiously in the proximal leg and hip muscles and spreads to involve the shoulders and arms. Other signs of glucocorticoid excess are usually present, but there is a poor correlation between the actual dose of corticosteroids and this syndrome. Raising the dose over a previously tolerated level may induce myopathy, and decreasing it to the previous level may relieve the symptoms. The combination of elevated urinary creatine and normal serum enzyme activities has been suggested as a useful differential point in favor of steroid myopathy. Other drugs that may cause myopathy include alcohol, clofibrate, penicillamine, azathioprine, phenytoin, polymyxin, chloroquine, and emetine.

Both hyper- and hypothyroidism may cause proximal muscle weakness. In hypothyroidism, serum creatine kinase may reach very high levels, and the electromyogram may mimic that in polymyositis. Hyperparathyroidism may also cause proximal muscle weakness, an abnormal electromyogram, and muscle atrophy without an inflammatory infiltrate.

Weakness and myalgia may occur after exercise in McArdle's syndrome, carnitine palmityl transferase deficiency, myoadenylate deaminase deficiency, or renal tubular acidosis. Acute exertional rhabdomyolysis is characterized by muscular pain, swelling, and weakness and is associated with heme pigment in the urine. It occurs after strenuous exercise in apparently healthy individuals.

Infectious causes of chronic myositis include trichinosis and tropical pyomyositis. In the latter, staphylococcal abscesses deep within muscles cause subacute pain and firm swelling, primarily in the gluteal, quadriceps, or trunk muscles. Serum muscle enzymes are normal, and blood cultures are usually negative. Inclusion body myositis is a rare disease that causes slowly progressive weakness of both proximal and distal muscles, usually most pronounced in the lower extremities. It affects primarily middle-aged men, and the response to steroids or immunosuppressive therapy is poor. Diagnosis is made on muscle biopsy, which reveals eosinophilic inclusions in both the nucleus and sarcoplasm of muscle cells. Other causes of muscle weakness and pain include the hypereosinophilic syndrome, diffuse fasciitis with eosinophilia, microemboli from atheromatous plaques or nonbacterial endocarditis, diabetic amyotrophy, and phosphate depletion secondary to the use of nonabsorbable antacids.

Polymyalgia rheumatica occurs in the elderly and is characterized by proximal muscle pain and stiffness (see Ch. 442).

The only laboratory abnormality is a striking elevation of the erythrocyte sedimentation rate. The absence of muscle weakness and prompt relief after treatment with a small dose of corticosteroid differentiate this disease from polymyositis. Other connective tissue diseases may have myositis as part of the symptom complex. These patients should be labeled as having polymyositis only if they meet the independent criteria for the diagnosis.

TREATMENT. Bed rest is necessary during the active stage of the disease. Active physical therapy should be reserved until the inflammation has subsided.

In spite of a lack of adequately controlled therapeutic trials, corticosteroids are generally accepted as the drug of choice. Prednisone, 50 to 100 mg, is given daily in divided doses and continued until definite improvement occurs. Serum enzymes typically decrease to half their pretreatment values one month after initiation of therapy and reach normal values in two to three months. Muscle strength usually shows definite improvement in two months. Attempts to decrease steroid dosage rapidly or discontinue treatment prematurely may lead to a recurrence of the disease. A single daily dose or alternate-day steroid therapy may be tried in order to decrease the side effects but should be attempted only when the disease is under good control. Maintenance therapy will be necessary for years in many cases. Failure to respond to steroids occurs in about 20 per cent of patients. Immunosuppressive drugs such as methotrexate and cyclophosphamide, or plasma exchange, may be beneficial in these instances, but controlled studies to substantiate their efficacy are not available. Combined therapy with azathioprine and prednisone has been shown to reduce steroid requirements and improve function in long-term treatment compared with steroid alone.

Arhata K, Engel AG: Monoclonal antibody analysis of mononuclear cells in myopathies III: Immunoelectron microscopy aspects of cell-mediated muscle fiber injury. Ann Neurol 19:112, 1986. *Detailed immunopathologic study of the muscle lesion in polymyositis.*
Bunch TW: Prednisone and azathioprine for polymyositis. Arthritis Rheum 24:45, 1981. *A three-year controlled study suggesting that the addition of azathioprine to conventional treatment with prednisone may have long-term benefits.*
Callen JP: Myositis and malignancy. Clin Rheum Dis 10:117, 1984. *Contains practical advice on the question of how extensively polymyositis patients should be investigated for malignancy.*
Csuka M, McCarty DJ: Simple method for measurement of lower extremity muscle strength. Am J Med 78:77, 1985. *Provides description and standardization of a simple quantitative clinical test of muscle strength.*
Fudman EJ, Schnitzer TJ: Clinical and biochemical characteristics of autoantibody systems in polymyositis and dermatomyositis. Sem Arthritis Rheum 15:255, 1986. *Concise review of autoantibodies in polymyositis.*
Hochberg MC, Feldman D, Stevens MB: Adult onset polymyositis/dermatomyositis: An analysis of clinical and laboratory features and survival in 76 patients with a review of the literature. Sem Arthritis Rheum 15:168, 1986. *An up-to-date clinical review with emphasis on factors influencing outcome.*

444 CALCIUM CRYSTAL DEPOSITION ARTHROPATHIES

H. Ralph Schumacher, Jr.

At least three different calcium-containing crystals are now known to deposit in joints and to be associated with a variety of patterns of arthritis in much the same way as urate crystals cause the various features of gouty arthritis. Calcium pyrophosphate and occasionally calcium oxalate produce linear or punctuate calcifications in menisci and articular cartilage that can be readily seen on roentgenograms. These calcifications are termed chondrocalcinosis. Both these crystals and calcium apatite can also deposit diffusely in synovium and periarticular tissues, giving a soft tissue pattern on roentgenograms. X-rays may not show obvious calcifications when crystals are

relatively few. Definitive diagnosis is made only by aspiration of synovial fluid for identification of the crystal type.

Dieppe PA, Calvert P: Crystals and Joint Disease. London, Chapman and Hall, 1983, p 282. *The most comprehensive recent review.*

CALCIUM PYROPHOSPHATE DIHYDRATE (CPPD) CRYSTAL DEPOSITION DISEASE (Pseudogout Syndrome)

This is defined by the identification of rod- or rhomboid-shaped 2- to 25-μ long, weakly positively birefringent crystals in synovial fluid or articular tissue. This is a common cause of arthritis; it is most frequent in the elderly. Up to 27 per cent of nursing home patients in their 80's have x-ray evidence of chondrocalcinosis on this basis. Familial cases have been described in populations of various ethnic origins. Both sexes are affected.

The cause of CPPD crystal deposition is not established, but local overproduction of pyrophosphate related to excessive activity of nucleoside triphosphate pyrophosphohydrolase, deficiency of phosphatases, and local connective tissue changes are probably important. CPPD crystals deposit only in joints and adjacent tendons or bursae, where they produce hematoxyphilic clumps replacing the normal tissue. Virtually any joint can be involved, but knees, wrists, and second and third metacarpophalangeal joints are most common so that chronic cases can be confused with rheumatoid arthritis. Acute bouts of crystal-induced arthritis at one or more joints can mimic gout and lead to "pseudogout." CPPD crystal deposition often complicates osteoarthritis; these crystals were seen in 42 per cent of osteoarthritic knee effusions in one series. Whether crystals contribute to cartilage degeneration in osteoarthritis is not yet clear. Occasional severe arthritis mimics the destruction seen in neuropathic joints. Radiographic evidence of calcification can be present in some cases for years without inducing any symptoms. Others may have crystals in joint fluid with osteoarthritis-like x-ray changes but no visible chondrocalcinosis.

Synovial effusions are generally inflammatory with leukocyte counts up to 100,000 per cu mm and with 80 to 90 per cent neutrophils during acute attacks. Between attacks crystals can be seen in clear, noninflammatory joint effusions.

CPPD crystal deposition can be an important clue to a number of associated diseases, many of which have specific treatments that can control systemic features if not the arthropathy. Associated diseases include hyperparathyroidism, hemochromatosis, myxedema, ochronosis, hypophosphatasia, hypomagnesemia, and perhaps acromegaly and Wilson's disease. CPPD crystal deposition may complicate other advanced arthritides such as gout and rheumatoid arthritis.

Treatment of inflammatory episodes with thorough aspiration and use of nonsteroidal anti-inflammatory agents is generally successful. Intra-articular steroid injections may provide relief in refractory involvement of individual joints. Intravenous colchicine may also be helpful. Recent studies show that chronic therapy with 0.6 to 1.2 mg colchicine per day can greatly decrease the frequency of acute attacks. Otherwise the prognosis is for slow progression. Joint replacement has been successful when needed.

Alvarellos A, Spilberg I: Colchicine prophylaxis in pseudogout. J Rheum 13:804–806, 1986. *Colchicine seems well worth trying to prevent acute exacerbations.*
Gibilisco PA, Schumacher HR, Hollander JL, et al.: Synovial fluid crystals in osteoarthritis. Arthritis Rheum 28:511–515, 1985. *The association of CPPD and apatite crystals with osteoarthritis.*
McCarty DJ (ed.): Proceedings of a conference on pseudogout and pyrophosphate metabolism. Arthritis Rheum (Suppl) 19: 1975. *Multiple authors discuss clinical picture, pathogenesis, and management.*
Rachow JW, Ryan LM: Partial characterization of synovial fluid nucleotide pyrophosphohydrolase. Arthritis Rheum 28:1377–1383, 1985. *Overproduction of pyrophosphate by this soluble extracellular enzyme is one possible factor in CPPD crystal deposition.*

APATITE CRYSTAL DEPOSITION DISEASE

Individual apatite crystals can be seen only by electron microscopy (EM), but clumps of these crystals appear as 2- to

15-μ shiny (but not generally birefringent) globules that can suggest the diagnosis. Apatite crystal deposition and crystal-induced inflammation are common findings in bursitis and periarthritis. Apatite also occurs in some otherwise unexplained acute arthritis and, like CPPD, is common in osteoarthritic joint effusions. Most joints or bursae can be involved, with more common sites including shoulders, hips, knees, and digits. Joint or periarticular inflammation can be acute or chronic. An extremely destructive arthritis has been noted especially at shoulders ("Milwaukee shoulder"), hips, and knees. X-rays can also show soft tissue calcifications with or without bony erosions. Definitive diagnosis of the crystal type is only by EM with electron probe elemental analysis, x-ray diffraction, or infrared spectroscopy. Other basic calcium phosphates such as octacalcium phosphate can be seen along with the apatite. Synovial or bursal effusions can have many or few leukocytes. Serum studies are generally normal except that phosphate levels are often elevated in renal dialysis patients who are at high risk of apatite deposition.

Apatite deposition can also be associated with scleroderma and the other connective tissue diseases and with high-dose vitamin D therapy. In most instances the cause of soft tissue apatite deposition is not known. Treatment for acute arthritis or periarthritis is with nonsteroidal anti-inflammatory agents or colchicine. Aspiration of crystals and local injection with depot corticosteroids can also be effective.

Doherty M, Holt M, MacMillan P, et al.: A reappraisal of "analgesic" hip. Ann Rheum Dis 45:272–276, 1986. *Destructive hip arthritis like the "Milwaukee shoulder" is felt to be related to apatite crystal deposition.*

Paul H, Reginato AJ, Schumacher HR: Alizarin red S staining as a screening test to detect calcium compounds in synovial fluid. Arthritis Rheum 26:191–200, 1983. *This describes a simple office screening test for apatite and other calcium-containing crystals.*

Pinals RS, Short CL: Calcific periarthritis involving multiple sites. Arthritis Rheum 9:566–574, 1966. *This recurrent calcific periarthritis is related to apatite crystals.*

Schumacher HR, Somlyo AP, Tse RL, et al.: Arthritis associated with apatite crystals. Ann Intern Med 87:411–416, 1977. *Clinical picture, diagnostic evaluation, and review.*

OXALATE CRYSTAL DEPOSITION DISEASE

Calcium oxalate deposition can occur in joints along with other tissues of renal failure patients on chronic hemodialysis, producing x-ray evidence of soft tissue calcification and chondrocalcinosis. Acute or chronic joint effusions with intracellular crystals can be seen. Diagnosis is made by identification of typical bipyramidal crystals. When less characteristic crystals are seen, other techniques as described under apatite deposition can be used. There is some recent suggestion that vitamin C may potentiate oxalate deposition so this might be avoided.

Hoffman EC, Schumacher HR, Paul H, et al.: Calcium oxalate microcrystalline-associated arthritis in end stage renal disease. Ann Intern Med 97:36–42, 1982. *Three cases with oxalosis and arthritis are described. Methods to identify oxalate crystals are included.*

Reginato AJ, Ferreiro Seoane JL, Alvarez CB, et al.: Arthropathy and cutaneous calcinosis in hemodialysis oxalosis. Arthritis Rheum 29:1387–1396, 1986. *Extensive oxalosis can involve skin, bursae, tendon sheaths, and joints.*

445 RELAPSING POLYCHONDRITIS

H. Ralph Schumacher, Jr.

This uncommon disease is characterized by recurrent inflammation and destruction of cartilaginous and other connective tissue structures. Frequently involved cartilages are the pinnae of the ears, nasal cartilages, and tracheal rings.

Polychondritis occurs nearly equally in both sexes and at any age, but with a peak of onset between the ages of 40 and 60.

The pathologic lesion seen by light microscopy consists of loss of matrix staining, predominantly superficial infiltration with polymorphonuclear neutrophils or lymphocytes, and eventual destruction of normal structures followed by fibrosis. Electron microscopy in addition shows alterations of superficial chondrocytes, matrix, and elastic fibers. The cause of polychondritis is unknown, but the location of lesions and frequency of associated systemic diseases suggest the importance of systemic factors. Antibodies to type II collagen and the presence of cell-mediated immunity to proteoglycan and type II collagen are evidences of immunologic aberrations.

Inflammation of the cartilaginous structures of the ears is the most common initial finding. There may be acute onset of pain and tenderness with erythema and swelling of one or both helices. The lobe is spared. Inner and middle ear involvement can occur, causing hearing loss or vertigo. Nasal cartilage involvement can produce a saddle nose. Laryngeal and tracheal disease can cause hoarseness or life-threatening upper respiratory obstruction. Ocular manifestations are common and include conjunctivitis, episcleritis, iridocyclitis, proptosis, and rarely other problems such as optic neuritis. Antigens in the eye that are cross-reactive with cartilage proteoglycans and their link protein have been identified.

Cardiac involvement, especially of the aortic root with aortic insufficiency, is seen in up to one fourth of cases. There may also be aortic aneurysms. Arthritis is reported in about three fourths of cases. This is generally nondestructive. Fever, rashes, oral or genital ulcers, and neurologic and renal disease can occur.

There are no diagnostic laboratory tests, although the erythrocyte sedimentation rate is often elevated. There may be anemia and leukocytosis. Roentgenograms can detect advanced tracheal narrowing. Cine CT scans and pulmonary function tests can detect more subtle airway obstruction.

Relapsing polychondritis is associated with other diseases in one third or more of cases. These include rheumatoid arthritis, systemic lupus erythematosus, Sjögren's syndrome, thyroid disease, ulcerative colitis, vasculitis of various types, cryoglobulinemia, diabetes mellitus, biliary cirrhosis, malignancies, sinusitis, and mastoiditis.

In mild cases nonsteroidal anti-inflammatory agents can be used for symptomatic treatment, although adrenocorticosteroids in the range of 30 to 60 mg prednisone per day are generally needed for acute inflammatory episodes and severe respiratory involvement. There is no evidence that steroids alter the long-term course of the disease. Immunosuppressives and recently cyclosporin A have been used with apparent benefit. Dapsone has been used with variable results in several series.

The course is unpredictable, with about 55 per cent of subjects surviving for 10 years. Infection and systemic vasculitis caused more deaths than did airway obstruction in a recent series. Remissions do occur. Aortic valve disease has required surgery.

Conn DL, Dickson ER, Carpenter HA: The association of Churg-Strauss vasculitis with temporal artery involvement, primary biliary cirrhosis and polychondritis in a single patient. J Rheum 9:744–748, 1982. *Vasculitis and other associated diseases are common.*

Ebringer B, Rook G, Swana T, et al.: Autoantibodies to cartilage and type II collagen in relapsing polychondritis and other rheumatic diseases. Ann Rheum Dis 40:473–479, 1981. *Immune mechanisms are described and discussed.*

Govet D, Marechaud R, Neu JPH, et al.: Relapsing polychondritis. A critical analysis of the therapeutic effectiveness of dapsone. Presse Med 13:723–726, 1984. *This interesting agent is not invariably effective.*

Michet CJ, McKenna CH, Luthra HS, et al.: Relapsing polychondritis. Survival and predictive role of early disease manifestations. Ann Intern Med 104:74–78, 1986. *Anemia, saddle nose deformity, and vasculitis appear to be poor prognostic signs.*

Ruhlen JL, Huston KA, Wood WG: Relapsing polychondritis with glomerulonephritis. Improvement with prednisone and cyclophosphamide. JAMA 245:847–848, 1981. *Renal involvement can occur. Drug therapy can include immunosuppressives.*

446 OSTEOARTHRITIS (Degenerative Joint Disease)

David S. Howell

Osteoarthritis (OA) is a complex response of joint tissues to aging and to genetic and environmental factors, characterized by degeneration of cartilage, bony remodelling, and overgrowth of bone. Idiopathic osteoarthritis refers to the common variety encountered during aging that is unrelated to known systemic or local diseases and includes certain hereditary and erosive subsets. *Secondary* osteoarthritis refers to the form indistinguishable from the idiopathic (primary) type on a pathologic basis but clearly provoked by antecedent events, such as an inflammatory, metabolic, endocrine, developmental, or heritable connective tissue disorder (Table 446–1). Effects of a macrotrauma, repeated microtrauma, or prolonged immobilization on normal joints may dispose the joints to secondary osteoarthritis.

When bony hypertrophy estimated by roentgenographic changes is used as a criterion, the majority of the population over 50 years of age is afflicted with osteoarthritis. By the eighth decade there is evidence of disease in 90 per cent of persons. It is the leading cause of joint pain and related disablements in middle-aged and elderly patients.

PATHOLOGY. Minor cartilage softening in non–weight-bearing sites and hypertrophic bony changes may persist a lifetime without producing symptoms. Osteoarthritis depends on development of progressively deepening clefts and erosions typically in weight-bearing sites. The disease advances over a period of years but rarely reaches the level of severity seen in rheumatoid arthritis; i.e., there is rarely joint fusion or pannus formation, and major subluxations are uncommon.

The earliest histologic changes may be documented in the surface, subsurface, and deep zones of articular cartilage. These changes include loss of staining reactions for proteoglycans, with areas of cell injury, or loss followed by proliferation. On electron microscopic views, lipid accumulations, reduced cartilage collagen fibril size, edema, and surface irregularities are found. Clefts, microcysts, and erosions arise at the site of these changes. Aggressive lesions consist usually of vertical clefts in cartilage, which progress to deep erosions and exposure of subchondral bone. Bony thickening, eburnation, cysts, and bone-on-bone contact across the joint surface typify end-stage disease.

ETIOLOGY. The most accepted premise is that primary changes in articular cartilage underlie development of osteoarthritis. Nevertheless, in a substantial subset of patients, biomechanical deficiencies arising from dysplasias of major or minor nature are causative. Similar biomechanical deficiencies may arise related to adolescent and adult remodelling of bones and abnormal distribution of weight-bearing forces (Table 446–1).

Repeated industrial or sports-invoked macro- and microtraumatic events may produce excessive wear and hypertrophic remodelling responses. Evidence has been obtained for reduced biomaterial properties of cartilage as a function of aging and for possible metabolic disturbances in cartilage metabolism, as in diabetes mellitus, acromegaly, and ochronosis.

The subchondral bone table is disturbed by tissue remodelling early in the disease or by such afflictions as Paget's disease or hyperparathyroidism with subchondral cysts. Hyperlaxity of ligaments per se or as part of certain overt (heritable) disorders of connective tissue can lead to osteoarthritis.

TABLE 446–1. ETIOLOGIC CLASSIFICATION OF OSTEOARTHRITIS*

Idiopathic (primary)
 Localized
  Hands: Heberden's nodes, erosive interphalangeal arthropathy
  Feet: hallux valgus, hammer toes; talonavicular osteoarthritis
  Knees: medial, lateral, patellofemoral compartments
  Hips: sites of cartilage loss—eccentric (superior), concentric (axial, medial), diffuse
  Spine: zygoapophyseal joints, osteophytes, intervertebral discs (spondylosis); ligaments, e.g., disseminated idiopathic skeletal hyperostosis
  Other single sites: shoulder, temporomandibular, carpometacarpal joints
 Generalized—Includes three or more areas listed above (described by Kellgren and Moore)
 Mineral deposition diseases
  Calcium pyrophosphate deposition disease
  Hydroxyapatite arthropathy
  Destructive disease (e.g., Milwaukee shoulder)

Secondary
 Post-traumatic
 Congenital or developmental
  Legg-Calvé-Perthes hip dislocation
  Epiphyseal dysplasias
 Disturbed local tissue structure by primary disease, e.g., ischemic necrosis, tophaceous gout, hyperparathyroid cysts, Paget's disease, rheumatoid arthritis, osteopetrosis, osteochondritis
 Miscellaneous additional diseases
  Endocrine: diabetes mellitus, acromegaly, hypothyroidism
  Metabolic: hemochromatosis, ochronosis, Gaucher's disease
  Neuropathic arthropathies
  Miscellaneous: frostbite, Kashin-Beck disease, caisson disease
  Mechanical: obesity, unequal lower extremity length; valgus/varus deformities, ligamentous laxity

*Compiled by Osteoarthritis Diagnostic Criteria Committee. American Rheumatism Association, 1983.

PATHOGENESIS. As a result of a multiplicity of etiologic factors, an apparent final common pathway of disease expression involves breakdown of cartilage both by direct physical injury and by enzymatic degradation resulting from injury to chondrocytes and indirectly by subchondral bone stiffening from remodelling. Most important in this context is injury of the collagen network or framework that holds together articular cartilage. This network retains in a semidehydrated conformed state the abundant, intensely hydrophilic, charged, proteoglycan macromolecules. The latter exert an osmotic pressure of several atmospheres against the network. Ungluing or cleavage of the collagen network by maldistributed or excessive weight-bearing forces, or degradation of the network by enzymes elaborated by injured cartilage cells may occur. This response to various precipitating events leads to loss of essential elastic properties.

In early osteoarthritis, repair responses by local chondrocytes are usually of a poor quality, leading to almost no replacement of lost tissue. From advanced erosions penetrating the marrow, tissue repair is more effective and consists of mixtures of fibro- and hyaline cartilage. Normal rugged biomaterial properties are never recovered by the repair cartilage. As degeneration proceeds, wear particles and matrix degradation products are released from both original and repair cartilages. These fragments are carried to the synovial lining membrane where a phagocytic response engenders low-grade inflammation and synovial effusion, proliferation of synovial cells, and thickening of the synovial membranes. Much evidence has accumulated that membrane-engendered inflammatory factors amplify cartilage breakdown.

Several biochemical abnormalities have been noted in osteoarthritic cartilage: increased water content, decreased aggregation and content of proteoglycans, decreased chain length and altered profiles of glycosaminoglycans, and increased proteolytic enzyme levels.

CLINICAL MANIFESTATIONS. The clinical presentation may be divided into early and late stages. Throughout these stages, there is deep, aching pain in the afflicted joints, morning stiffness of short duration, and variable joint thickening and effusion. Early stages are dominated by pain on motion with stiffness, night pain, and responsiveness to anti-inflammatory medication. The late stages are dominated by joint instability, predominance of pain at rest accentuated on weight-bearing, and failure of responsiveness to anti-inflammatory agents. The present description of clinical features is developed largely on an anatomic basis inasmuch as signs and symptoms reflect regional patterns of involvement. Roentgenographic and laboratory work-up and treatment are discussed later.

Hands. Heberden's nodes refer to the osteoarthritic disfigurements of distal interphalangeal joints, and Bouchard's nodes signify equivalent lesions of the proximal interphalangeal joints of the hands (Fig. 446–1). Early Heberden's nodes have a soft consistency and may be associated with prominent inflammatory signs. In the chronic stage, they are characterized by bony enlargement and angular deformities with variable symptoms. Heredity and sex, in addition to microtrauma, are prominently involved in the development of Heberden's nodes, which are more common in women at menopause or late middle age. The only other common hand lesion involves the first carpometacarpal joint. Such lesions are associated with pain in the radial side of the wrist, intensified by physical activities such as golf, tennis, and knitting.

Knees. The commonest source of major disability in osteoarthritis is from knee involvement. At any one time, heat, synovial thickening, or effusions have been documented in at least 50 per cent of cases. Elicitation of crepitus, which persists on repeated flexion and extension of the knee, bony marginal overgrowth, mediolateral instability (in the late stages), and synovial effusion are important diagnostic aids. Degenerative changes are usually more prominent in the medial compartment of the knee, leading to varus (bowleg) deformities. Developmental defects, i.e., knock-knee or bowleg deformity, predispose to OA.

Degenerative alteration of the patellofemoral joint is termed chondromalacia patellae. This syndrome of mild effusion and knee pain is usually associated with trauma and occurs predominantly in young adults. It is usually preceded by developmental biomechanical disturbances influencing knee flexion. There is often spontaneous remission of symptoms, but some cases progress to irreversible patellofemoral osteoarthritis.

Malum Coxae Senilis (Coxarthrosis). Clinical manifestations of primary hip joint disease appear usually in late middle or old age. Perhaps one third or more of cases arise from acetabular dysplasia, as well as growth or maturational disturbances in the femoral neck and head. Altered bone growth as well as developmental thickening at the zenith of the acetabulum may be causative in less than 5 per cent of cases. Beyond these factors, there is a background of adult bone remodelling and altered joint incongruity, which may further compromise normal weight-bearing patterns and chondrocyte nutrition. In addition, a variety of acquired disorders such as rheumatoid arthritis and ischemic necrosis of the femoral head are important etiologically.

Groin pain on weight-bearing or motion is a dominant symptom and is usually referred to the anterior aspect of the thigh above the knee. Over a period of months or a few years, invalidism from severely restricted mobility and pain is a common outcome of untreated disease.

Spinal Osteoarthritis (Including Herniated Disc Syndrome). Throughout the spine, weight-bearing compressive forces are largely supported by one set of articulations—the intervertebral discs. These are elastic organs similar to articular cartilage in respect to the fact that they depend on properties of the semi-dehydrated proteoglycan molecules. A high osmotic pressure at rest results from proteoglycan confinement by cartilage end-plates in two dimensions and the annulus fibro-

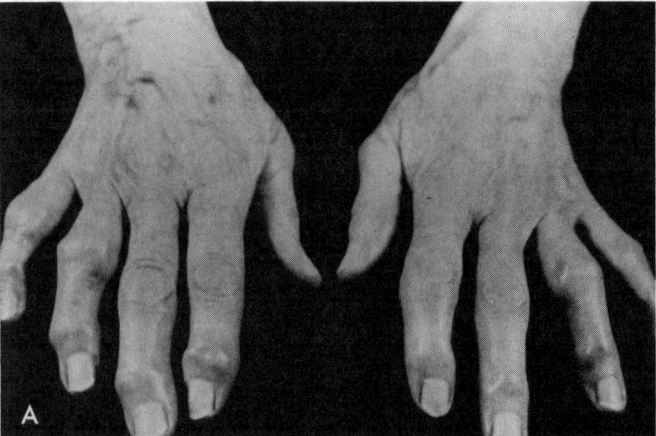
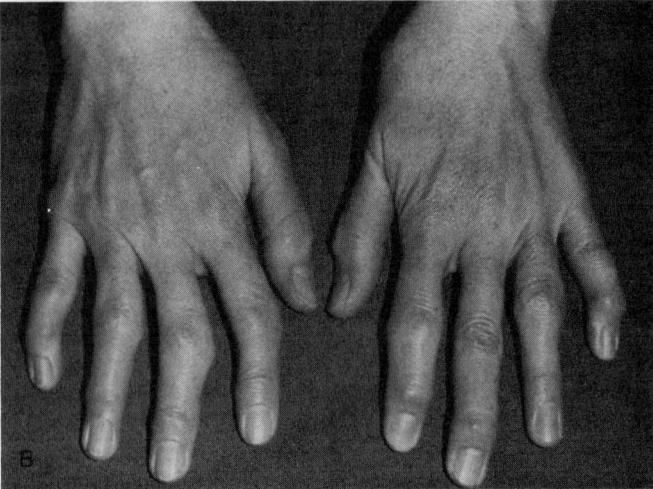

FIGURE 446–1. Typical hand deformities in osteoarthritis. *A*, Typical Heberden's and Bouchard's nodes comprise hypertrophic joint capsular and bony enlargement of the distal and proximal interphalangeal joints, respectively. *B*, Prominent Bouchard's nodes and minor subluxations may cause misdiagnosis of rheumatoid arthritis.

sus in the third. An additional important elastic component is provided by the annulus fibrosus. Rotary motions in the back and neck depend upon the zygoapophyseal joints. All of these joints undergo osteoarthritic changes almost identical in nature to those of the peripheral joints (see Ch. 448 for specific clinical features). Ordinarily, the former joints protect the latter against severe torsional trauma; under certain conditions, especially flexion of the lumbosacral spine, the rotary joints are of much less protectional value, and annular tears may occur under these (and several other) conditions. Resultant displacement of discal products into the spinal foramen adjacent to nerve rootlets and/or spinal canal occurs, depending on the conditions of damage. Injury of these structures both by mechanical trauma and by activated inflammatory pathways constitutes one of several causes of neural dysfunction leading to symptoms. The relationship of the posterior zygoapophyseal joints in the cervical, thoracic, and lumbar spines to their respective nerve roots as they traverse the intervertebral foramina, and the proximity of an additional set of *joints of Luschka* in the cervical spine (segments C2 to C7) have similar importance because of potential damage to nerves by inflammation secondary to mechanical irritation.

Notably, symptoms of osteoarthritis in the cervical spine depend upon the neural segment involved. Pain, aggravated by motion, often radiates into the supraclavicular and upper trapezius regions, as well as the occiput and distal upper extremities. Overgrowth of bone in either the cervical or lumbar spine can cause narrowing of the spinal canal and encroachment on the spinal cord rather than the nerve roots. In the neck, a myelopathy of a painless nature may result.

Constriction of the spinal cord by surrounding bone, disc, or ligamentous thickening leads to the syndrome of spinal stenosis most common in the lumbosacral spine. Neurogenic claudication pain (resembling vascular claudication) is an important symptom in this condition and must be differentiated from vascular insufficiency (see Ch. 448 for management of discogenic claudication).

Diffuse Idiopathic Skeletal Hyperostosis. This is characterized by a flowing ligamentous calcification along the anterolateral aspects of vertebral bodies. Symptomatology is variable and focused in the spine or multiple tendon osseous junctions (e.g., at the heel); ankylosis of apophyseal and sacroiliac joints is absent. The thoracic spine is most often affected without intervertebral disc narrowing.

LABORATORY FINDINGS. There are no specific abnormalities in osteoarthritis. The sedimentation rate is usually within normal limits, synovial fluid is clear and exhibits a normal range of viscosity, and there is a negative mucin clot test result. Leukocyte counts in synovial fluid generally vary from 150 to 1500 per cu mm; wear particles including whole fragments containing proteoglycans and collagen fibers as well as mineral particles are often identified in the fluid.

ROENTGENOGRAPHIC FEATURES. There is usually narrowing of the radiolucent interosseous joint space resulting from destruction of articular cartilage. Bony cysts varying in size may be seen in subchondral or denuded bone, which may be densely sclerotic. Osteophyte formation at the margins of affected joints is the basis for the most striking roentgenographic findings. Degeneration of lumbar and cervical intervertebral discs results in narrowing of the interspaces. A vacuum sign or marked translucency in the disc may be seen. Evidence for disc degeneration is usually documented in anteroposterior and lateral roentgenograms. For visualization of osteophytes blocking foramina, particularly in the cervical spine, oblique views are mandatory. Oblique views are also valuable for defining bony sclerosis and joint-space narrowing of the zygoapophyseal joints of the lumbar spine.

DIFFERENTIAL DIAGNOSIS. Osteoarthritis and rheumatoid arthritis are readily distinguished in terms of their usual clinical presentation. The latter is generally associated with prominent signs of joint inflammation, characteristically afflicting the hands and wrists symmetrically, especially the metacarpophalangeal joints. These joints almost never are affected in osteoarthritis.

Differentiation of these disorders is more complicated when seronegative rheumatoid arthritis involves only (or predominantly) the lower extremities. The presence of a normal erythrocyte sedimentation rate, negative serum rheumatoid factor test result, and minimal synovial fluid change supports the diagnosis of osteoarthritis. Despite severe deformities, occasionally seen with Heberden's and Bouchard's nodes, the lack of ulnar drift and metacarpophalangeal and diffuse wrist involvement help to rule out rheumatoid arthritis. Erosive osteoarthritis characteristically shows bony destruction and inflammatory changes in the proximal and distal interphalangeal joints but not in the metacarpophalangeal joints.

Secondary osteoarthritis must be considered in the presence of joint hypermobility, chondrocalcinosis, heritable disorders such as the Ehlers-Danlos syndrome, mechanical derangements of the joints, metabolic bone disorders, ochronosis, neuropathies, and hemochromatosis. Spinal involvement in osteoarthritis is distinctly different from that in ankylosing spondylitis; the latter predominantly afflicts young men and has characteristic and distinctive roentgenographic features involving sacroiliac sclerosis and fusion, calcification and ossification of the annulus fibrosus and adjacent paravertebral ligaments, and formation of bridging syndesmophytes (bamboo spine).

TREATMENT. Although treatment depends in large measure on the site and severity of joint involvement, the outlook with a multidisciplinary long-term management program is relatively optimistic for functional restoration and symptomatic improvement.

Early disease with signs of mild to moderate inflammation but without joint instability can usually be managed successfully with a combination of measures: (1) Relief of pain with mild analgesics (e.g., acetaminophen 500 mg three or four times a day) or nonsteroidal anti-inflammatory agents (e.g., aspirin 2400 to 3600 mg daily) or both. Indomethacin, ibuprofen, naproxen, fenoprofen, piroxicam, sulindac, and tolmetin are alternative agents, advantageous as substitutes for aspirin. Where possible, intermittent rather than continuous usage is encouraged to avoid gastrointestinal side effects, especially acid peptic disease. (2) Revision of daily schedule of activities, increased joint rest, and selected avoidance of activities unfavorable to the symptomatic joints. (3) Protection of joints with relevant devices, i.e., splints, crutches, walkers, canes, etc. (4) Use of weight-reducing diets. (5) Diazepam, 5 mg three to four times daily or another suitable agent may be used sparingly for acute episodes of muscle spasm. (6) Application of moist heat or cold packs may help. (7) Symptomatic response, in refractory cases, to intra-articular or para-articular injections of small amounts of corticosteroid at infrequent intervals is useful. (8) Once pain and muscle spasm have been relieved, a formalized program of physical therapy followed by a prolonged home exercise program is often recommended in the hope of retarding further joint deterioration.

In the case of cervical osteoarthritis, hyperextension and hyperflexion should be avoided. The patient should sleep flat on one pillow and employ intermittent traction devices available for home use. A cervical collar restricts motion and minimizes pain. (See Ch. 448 for treatment of osteoarthritis in the lumbar spine.)

The principal anatomic regions that are most benefited by orthopedic surgery are the knee, hip, and spine. Several surgical procedures are appropriate for patients with severe hip involvement, including osteotomy, mold arthroplasty, total joint replacement, and arthrodesis. For the knee, debridement, either through an arthroscope or via open surgery, osteotomy, and a variety of partial or complete arthroplasties are used for treatment. Tibial or femoral osteotomies may be of long-term benefit by realigning weight-bearing forces, but considerable follow-up rehabilitation is required. Otherwise, joint replacement is the treatment of choice for many cases of advanced osteoarthritis of the knees characterized by intractable pain, loss of function, instability, or all three. Some indications for spinal surgery are: (1) advancing intractable nerve deficits, (2) spinal instability, and (3) spinal stenosis affecting bladder or rectal function because of autonomic nerve involvement.

Brandt KD: Chapters 88–90: In Kelley WN, Harris ED Jr, Ruddy S, et al. (eds.): Philadelphia, WB Saunders Company, 1985, pp 1417–1456. *Especially clear concepts of pathophysiology woven into diagnosis and management readily understood and applicable from an internist's standpoint.*

McCarty DJ (ed.): Arthritis and Allied Disorders. Philadelphia, Lea and Febiger, 1985, pp 1377–1442. *A comprehensive coverage of multiple new topics of concern, especially well illustrated with radiograms and cogent clarifying tables.*

Moskowitz RW, Howell DS, Goldberg VM, et al. (eds.): Osteoarthritis: Diagnosis and Management. Philadelphia, WB Saunders Company, 1984. *Detailed reference emphasizing both medical and surgical approaches of regional and general importance, readily individualized to the patient.*

447 THE PAINFUL SHOULDER

David S. Howell

Shoulder pain is a common source of incapacitation and can result from numerous causes. Intrathoracic, diaphragmatic, and cervical pathologic lesions all can cause pain referred to the shoulder, a fact that deserves early consideration and strong emphasis. A characteristic of intrinsic painful disorders is that they often originate in periarticular soft structures—synovial membranes, tendons, and associated muscles. These structures have a unique role in joint stabilization. Loading forces are attenuated by the action of muscles across the coordinated bearings—glenohumeral, acromioclavicular, and sternoclavicular joints—as well as across the scapulothoracic surfaces. Multiple bursae and tendons near their attachment sites, particularly the rotator cuff tendons, are subject to microinjury and inflammation. Secondary recurrent pain and muscle spasm occur, followed by atrophic or reflex dystrophic responses or both. The most common disorders afflicting these structures are briefly reviewed in this chapter.

CALCIFIC TENDINITIS. A frequently encountered cause of painful shoulder is focal injury or degeneration of the rotator cuff tendons. Roentgenograms reveal calcium-containing minerals in the tendons of the rotator cuff in roughly 3 per cent of middle-aged persons, usually from prior insults. Mineral deposits in tendinous sites may engender bursal inflammation of variable intensity. Acute shoulder pain with radiation into the upper arm and neck is common. Associated muscle hypertonicity with limitation of shoulder motion and guarding, exquisite local tenderness over the inflamed site, and pain on motion or during prolonged rest are prominent. Most often roentgenograms show linear densities in the supraspinatus, infraspinatus, or subscapularis tendons. Occasionally, a diffuse calcific pattern in the subacromial bursa is seen. Evidence of acute inflammation usually subsides within one week, but subacute rotator cuff tendinitis may persist or recur for months to years.

Management is conditioned by the duration and intensity of attacks. Adequate early pain relief is of paramount importance and is usually attainable by use of moist heat or ice compresses; rest, including arm support; analgesics; and a nonsteroidal anti-inflammatory agent. Newer agents are discussed in Ch. 433. In most patients, pain and muscle spasm subside with variable reduction of mineral deposits. Injection of an adrenocorticosteroid derivative commonly hastens symptomatic recovery.

Follow-up evaluation is important to assess completeness of recovery. Residual loss of strength or joint motion or chronic pain deserves a conscientious program of active exercises, including both supervised therapy in a physical medicine facility and a home program of daily exercise. Long-term physical therapy or surgical excision of mineral deposits is seldom necessary.

BICIPITAL TENDINITIS. Inflammation of this tendon and synovial sheath is a frequent cause of shoulder pain. The tendon through attrition may subluxate from the bicipital groove or rupture. Localized tenderness on palpation with accentuation of pain by flexion or extension of the elbow against resistance or by internal rotation and abduction distinguishes the diagnosis clinically.

Treatment includes moist heat or ice compresses, rest, and nonsteroidal anti-inflammatory agents in the acute stages, and frequently the instillation of corticosteroids. Chronic recurrent disease is suggestive of the aforementioned mechanical derangements or an additional rotator cuff tear. Surgical transfer of the tendon may lead to satisfactory recovery.

ROTATOR CUFF TEARS. After heavy work, sports, or accidental injury, degenerative lesions in the rotator cuff often engender breakdown with moderate to major tendinous and ligamentous tears, predominantly in middle-aged persons. Complete rupture of the rotator cuff renders the arm incapable of abduction to 90 degrees. With mild tears, there is pain between 60 and 90 degrees abduction. Either preceding or following these tears, an impingement syndrome frequently occurs at the coracoacromial arch. Often this is associated radiographically with cysts or sclerosis of the greater tuberosity of the humerus, osteophytes at the anterior margin of the acromion, and narrowing of the distance between the humeral head and acromion. These changes are related to trauma from impingement of the aforementioned bones. Since the rotator cuff forms, in part, the roof of the glenohumeral joint and floor of the subacromial and subdeltoid bursae, tears in the cuff permit synovial joint fluid extrusion into these bursae—demonstrable by arthrogram.

Primary treatment of rotator cuff tears consists of heat and aspirin, 2.4 to 3.6 gm per day, or other nonsteroidal anti-inflammatory agents such as ibuprofen, 1200 to 2400 mg per day. Partial immobilization and exercise programs are indicated for incomplete tears. When these measures fail, surgical repair is often required.

ADHESIVE CAPSULITIS. This (frozen shoulder) disability of middle-aged persons develops more commonly in women than in men and is of unknown etiology. The diagnosis is suspected when persons with no primary shoulder disease develop active and passive restricted motion of the glenohumeral joint attended by increasing pain in the shoulder over a period of weeks to months, and it is more certain when an arthrogram shows a contracted joint capsule. Fibrosis is seen on pathologic study. Rotator cuff tears, hemarthroses, anterior shoulder capsule tear, psychophysiologic shoulder dysfunction, and shoulder-hand syndrome can all cause immobile painful shoulders and may be confused with adhesive capsulitis.

The key feature of management is prevention of severe pain through early use of heat, analgesics, range of motion exercises, and, if these are unsuccessful, the judicious use of intra-articular or systemic corticosteroids.

Manipulation mobilization under general anesthesia followed by a course of intensive physical therapy rarely is required for advanced disease.

SHOULDER-HAND SYNDROME. Shoulder pain and stiffness concurrent with pain, swelling, and vasomotor changes in the hands, wrists, and arms of various intensity and duration characterize this syndrome. Thickening of the skin and edema may follow, resembling Sudeck's atrophy. A small percentage of cases eventually develop adhesive capsulitis and sclerodactyly. This syndrome, which affects patients over age 50 years and follows acute severe illness such as cerebral vascular accident, myocardial infarction, and trauma to the distal upper extremity, is believed to be caused by reflex sympathetic stimulation. Associated changes of cervical osteoarthritis probably have a minor role if any. When the disease is bilateral, the differentiation from acute rheumatoid arthritis or polymyalgia rheumatica may be difficult. The most important feature of treatment is aggressive physical therapy assisted by analgesics and prednisone in a short, moderate-dosage trial of 20 to 30 mg per day for three weeks, tapered at the end of the course. Stellate ganglion blocks and local corticosteroid injections are sometimes employed.

AMYLOID ARTHROPATHY. In two thirds of patients, there is shoulder involvement usually secondary to myeloma. There is para-articular infiltration with amorphous amyloid fibers causing the "shoulder pad sign." Acute inflammatory signs are usually absent (see Ch. 210).

ISCHEMIC NECROSIS. This disease is half as common in the humeral head as in the hip. Diffuse shoulder pain precedes conventional radiologic changes, the most helpful of which is an irregular translucent band localized in subchondral bone.

POLYMYALGIA RHEUMATICA. This syndrome is often characterized by severely painful shoulders and upper arms in aged persons with anemia, high sedimentation rates, and negative rheumatoid factor test, and in a small percentage of cases temporal arteritis and retinal ischemia threatening to vision (see Ch. 527). Dramatic response of shoulder pain to low-dose corticosteroid administration (prednisone 10 mg per day) is characteristic.

MILWAUKEE SHOULDER. This syndrome consists of a painful, destructive, bilateral arthropathy in middle-aged and elderly patients with capsular calcification, joint effusions, and a high frequency of eroded rotator cuff tendons. Synovial fluids are virtually free of inflammatory cells despite a reported high collagenase activity.

Kozin F: Painful shoulder and the reflex sympathetic dystrophy syndrome. In McCarty DJ (ed.): Arthritis and Allied Conditions. Philadelphia, Lea and Febiger, 1985, pp 1322–1355. *An extremely concentrated and detailed coverage, especially useful as a reference for differential diagnosis.*

Post M: The painful shoulder. Clin Orthop 173:2, 1983. *A symposium by multiple authors on various clinically important syndromes and discussion of current management.*

448 THE PAINFUL BACK
David S. Howell

The back is a complex structure serving weight-bearing and locomotor functions. It provides for major support of body structures and transmission of loading forces through the sacroiliac joints to the lower limbs. The fundamental functioning unit is an articular triad composed of two zygoapophyseal joints posteriorly and the intervertebral disc anteriorly. The disc is composed of a nucleus pulposus encompassed by the annulus fibrosus. These structures are arranged in a series and stabilized throughout the spine by ligaments. The spinal bones also encase the spinal cord and the cauda equina, and through successive foramina rootlets connect the spinal cord with peripheral neural pathways. (See Ch. 446 for detailed discussion of the cervical spine, Ch. 434 for the spondyloarthropathies, and Ch. 499 for intervertebral disc disease.)

ETIOLOGY OF BACK PAIN. In Table 448–1, the numerous causes of back pain are displayed according to disease subgroups. Although all vertebral levels can be affected, pain in the low back is most prevalent. The majority of patients present with problems relating to functional or mechanical disturbances, and these must be distinguished from a wide variety of diseases either of focal origin or referred from multiple organ systems. Among degenerative diseases, low back pain is a leading cause of industrial absenteeism and chronic disablement.

MEDICAL HISTORY. *Sex.* Compression vertebral fractures from osteoporosis have their highest prevalence in postmenopausal women. Gynecologic pathology such as endometriosis is the basis for some referred patterns of back pain. Reiter's disease, ankylosing spondylitis, and back injuries are found more commonly in males.

Age. Young people with back pain most commonly suffer from muscle or ligament strains, congenital abnormalities, injury, spondyloarthropathies, and herniated disc syndromes. In middle and old age, osteoporosis, vertebral collapse, degenerative states, including spinal stenosis, and malignant lesions are common.

Family History. Familial patterns of segregation are often detected in respect to spondyloarthropathies and uncommonly in respect to spinal degenerative conditions.

Nature of Pain. Events or conditions that accelerate or retard symptoms should be explored. The chronic inflammatory diseases (spondyloarthropathies) are associated with increased pain and stiffness on inactivity. Patients with lumbar disc protrusion and radicular pain generally are relieved by lying flat with the knees flexed and are uncomfortable sitting.

Sudden or acute onset of symptoms is suggestive of a mechanical or infectious origin of symptoms respectively. Constitutional symptoms such as fever, weight loss, and fatigue are important clues to infectious, inflammatory, or neoplastic disorders.

In regard to localization, the dorsal segment suggests osteoarthritis, vertebral fracture, neoplasm, herpetic radiculitis, or referred pain from the viscera (see later paragraph). Localization of pain in the low back is usually of little help in regard to differential diagnosis.

Claudication-type pain, with onset after sustained walking, suggests either spinal stenosis or arterial insufficiency. The former condition often refers pain to the thigh and is poorly relieved by standing still. Usually neurogenic claudication is relieved by sitting, whereas vascular claudication is reduced by standing.

Referred Pain. A deep aching pain referred to various sites in the upper and midback may be engendered by lesions in the upper gastrointestinal tract. Pain of malignancy (whether local or referred) is typically severe and unrelieved by change of position or mild analgesics.

In respect to neuropathic symptoms, alteration of the structure of the vertebral foramina may lead to radicular dissemination of pain. In such instances, compression or traction of nerve rootlets or extension of inflammation to them can lead to sensory and motor nerve symptoms and signs, i.e., paresthesias, hypoesthesias, and muscle weakness.

Symptomatology. Discogenic pain is characteristically aggravated by cough or sneeze. Rarely, loss of bowel or urinary sphincter function can result from cord compression or bilateral involvement of sacral nerve roots from spinal stenosis, tumors, or infectious lesions.

PHYSICAL EXAMINATION. General examination of the

TABLE 448–1. ETIOLOGY OF BACK PAIN

Mechanical or Traumatic
  Paraspinal ligaments and musculature
    Myofascial syndrome, sacroiliac strain
  Spondylogenic
    Osteoarthritis-related lesions—zygoapophyseal joints
    Degenerative lesions—intervertebral discs
    Mechanical insufficiency, congenital and acquired, of ligaments and bones
    Spondylolisthesis
    Spinal stenosis
    Fractures
Metabolic
  Vertebral bodies, partial collapse and distortion—osteoporosis; osteomalacia—Paget's disease—often with secondary osteoarthritis
Tumors
  Neural tumors, osteosarcoma, metastatic tumors, e.g., from breast, thyroid, kidney
  Myeloma, lymphoma, leukemia
Systemic Inflammatory Disease
  Spondylitis (ankylosing)—Reiter's disease; psoriatic or enteropathic arthropathy
  Disseminated ankylosing skeletal hyperostosis
Infections
  Pyogenic, fungal, tuberculous disc infection, herpes zoster infection, paraspinal abscesses
Referred Pain
  Vascular—aneurysms, sclerosis of aorta and branches
  Tumors or inflammation of pleural, pulmonary, pericardial, cardiac, or neck origin
  Viscerogenic disease of gallbladder, pancreas, stomach, intestines, kidneys, ureters, bladder, prostate, uterus
  Pelvis or retroperitoneal tumors or inflammation
Nonorganic Components
  Hysterical conversion
  Learned painful behavior
  Psychosis
  Litigation neurosis, malingering
  Chronic pain syndrome
  Substance abuse

back is discussed in Ch. 429. Descriptions here are confined to vertebral compression fractures, degenerative disc disease, and lumbosacral strains and sprains.

Lumbosacral Strain. This and related myofascial syndromes are the most common ailment seen in office practice of rheumatology. A history of injury is often followed by prompt or delayed low-back pain. Transient disc prolapse, subluxation of facet joints, and injury to muscles or ligaments are diagnostic considerations. Physical signs are usually limited to paravertebral muscle spasm, tenderness, and restricted lower back motion without evidence of nerve root involvement.

Vertebral Compression Fractures. These are the most common complication of osteoporosis with the resultant traction or compression of rootlets adjacent to collapsed vertebrae. Severe pain may begin suddenly associated with the postural strain of lifting heavy objects or hyperflexing the trunk. Major physical findings consist of localized tenderness and muscle spasm related to the level of the nerve roots affected. Poorly localized back pain may be associated with osteoporosis in the absence of vertebral collapse. Metastatic tumor, myeloma,, and metabolic bone disease, especially osteopenia of aging, are common underlying conditions.

Discogenic Disease. The most common form of low back pain with radiculitis is associated with prolapse, protrusion, or extrusion of intervertebral disc substance (see Ch. 499). Usually the onset of acute symptoms is preceded by chronic intermittent low back pain, although a discrete injury may precipitate an attack. Ninety per cent of disc herniations are localized at L4–L5 or L5–S1 levels. Discs involving the L4 nerve root may cause pain referred along the course of the femoral nerve upon hip extension and knee flexion. Knee extension may be weak and the patellar reflex reduced or absent. Patients with L5 nerve root disturbance complain of classic sciatic distribution of pain, i.e., radiating to the posterior thigh and the anteromedial leg and foot, in association with weakness of the toe extensors. First sacral radiculopathy is associated with pain over the posterior thigh, calf, and heel, weakness of the ankle and toe flexors, and reduced or absent Achilles tendon reflex. Frequently, loss of neurologic function is subtle and requires repeated testing to document. A positive response to straight leg-raising is most frequently indicative of L4–L5 or L5–S1 disc protrusion. Usually there is pain on hip flexion with the knee extended and absence of pain on repetition of hip flexion with the knee flexed (Lasègue's sign). The cauda equina syndrome is a form of spinal stenosis and is an uncommon but important complication of massive disc prolapse. In the cauda equina syndrome, central midline disc displacement causes paralysis of the sacral root with bladder and bowel dysfunction. It is characterized by severe bilateral leg pain, urinary retention, weakness of the anal sphincter, and bilateral nerve root abnormalities. Once complete neurologic block has occurred, deceptively pain is often alleviated, and the patient will require a neurologic examination to verify the need for emergency surgery.

Spondylolisthesis. This condition, which refers to forward displacement of one vertebra on another, commonly involves the L4–L5 and L5–S1 levels. Bursts of segmental severe girdle pain are typical, often worse on activity and relieved by rest.

LABORATORY PROCEDURES. These are dictated by the results of medical history and physical examination. Simple x-rays of the back may suffice if a traumatic injury is causative. In instances of suspected metabolic disturbance, appropriate screening tests such as serum calcium, phosphorus, and alkaline phosphatase measurements should be obtained. Complete blood counts, sedimentation rate, urinalysis, and automated serum chemical profiles are sometimes justified to clarify the diagnosis. Anemia and an elevated sedimentation rate should prompt a more extensive search for infectious, inflammatory and neoplastic diseases.

X-RAY STUDIES. *Routine X-ray Studies.* These include frontal, lateral, and oblique films of the lumbosacral spine, which can demonstrate foraminal encroachment, compression fractures, degenerative changes, and subluxation of zygoapophyseal joints, as well as interspace narrowing (see Ch. 446). There may be severe degenerative changes by x-rays with few or no relevant symptoms, and severe back pain may occur in the absence of significant radiographic signs and be of discogenic origin.

Additional Imaging Procedures. When surgical intervention is planned or a diagnosis remains questionable and requires an imperative answer and high resolution, computed tomography (CT) and magnetic resonance (MR) imaging (noninvasive) are increasingly preferred to myelography. It is not usually necessary to perform a discogram (injection of radiopaque dye directly into the disc). When osteomyelitis or neoplastic involvement is likely, radionuclide bone scans are helpful. A percutaneous vertebral biopsy under fluoroscopic guidance may be performed to establish histopathologic diagnosis or bacteriologic diagnosis at highly suspicious sites obvious from scans or x-rays. Epidural venography scans have become an additional useful tool in precisely delineating sites of discogenic disease. Electromyography can confirm the presence of nerve root deficits.

MANAGEMENT. Conservative therapy for mechanical disorders of the spine and disc herniation focuses on bedrest, analgesics, muscle relaxants, and anti-inflammatory medication. Pelvic traction is also of benefit in some patients. Application of moist heat, e.g., hydrocollator packs wrapped with a wet towel, may relieve pain and muscle spasm. Cyclobenzaprine (10 mg) or diazepam (5 mg) three to four times daily serves as a useful muscle relaxant. The amount of bedrest is dependent on the severity of symptoms. After bedrest, gradual ambulation and a program of exercises together with back protection including a lumbosacral support are recommended. Most cases of disc herniation respond to conservative therapy; those unresponsive require further measures, including intrathecal and epidural steroids, nerve root or sleeve infiltrations with steroids, and injections of chymopapain into the disc space. Before surgery is indicated, a psychological assessment, a thorough program of muscle relaxants, and exercises emphasizing back stretching and abdominal strengthening should be attempted.

Progressive muscular weakness and progressive neurologic deficit despite bedrest and other aforementioned measures, as well as the cauda equina syndrome, are indications for surgery. Relative indications for laminectomy are severe pain, unrelieved by bedrest, and recurrent episodes of incapacitating pain. Ninety to 95 per cent improvement following surgery is anticipated, although 70 per cent of patients experience relief of pain whether or not the disc is removed.

Following either conservative therapy or surgery, a program of prophylactic management includes postural education, performance of daily exercise program to strengthen the lumbar and abdominal muscles, and avoidance of lower spine stress. Besides laminectomy, joint fusion for spondylolisthesis and discogenic disease or unroofing procedures for spinal stenosis are sometimes necessary. Myelography, CT scans, or MRI are indicated preoperatively to establish definitively the nature and extent of disease as well as the level of vertebral involvement.

Acute symptoms from compression fractures require appropriate rest and relief of pain with analgesics. Activities must be selected to avoid additional compression fractures. (See Ch. 250 for management of osteoporosis.)

Brown MD, Jackson C (eds.): Back Schools (Symposium). Clin Orthop Rel Res 179:2–85, 1983. *An overview of current noninvasive treatment of low back pain. Emphasis is on results of controlled trials with evaluation of exercise programs and other modalities.*

Lipson SJ: Low back pain. In Kelley WN, Harris ED Jr, Ruddy S (eds.): Textbook of Rheumatology. Philadelphia, WB Saunders Company, 1985, pp 448–468. *A useful reference; concisely written orthopedic diagnostic and therapeutic steps.*

Rothman RH, Simeone FA (eds.): The Spine. 2nd ed. Philadelphia, WB Saunders Company, 1982, Vol. 2, p 1131. *Excellent treatise on injuries, sepsis, metabolic bone disease, arthritis, tumors, spinal pain, psychiatric aspects, and rehabilitation; a detailed reference book.*

449 DISEASES WITH WHICH ARTHRITIS IS FREQUENTLY ASSOCIATED

Giles G. Bole

Arthritis can be a significant feature of each of the diseases discussed in this chapter. Description of the disorder is brief and limited to the rheumatic manifestations of the disease. More detailed discussion of each entity is found in other chapters devoted to these diseases.

SARCOIDOSIS

The most common rheumatic manifestation of sarcoidosis is an acute, symmetric polyarthritis associated with erythema nodosum and hilar adenopathy (Löfgren's syndrome). The ankles are most frequently involved, followed by the wrists, the proximal interphalangeal joints, and the elbows. Arthritis and the other acute manifestations usually resolve spontaneously within a few weeks without sequelae. Circulating immune complexes and an increased frequency of HLA-B8 are found in these patients. Treatment with salicylates or corticosteroids has been symptomatically beneficial in individual cases. Chronic granulomatous sarcoid synovitis is an uncommon form of oligoarthritis that can cause joint destruction. It is less responsive to drug treatment and follows a variable clinical course.

HEMOCHROMATOSIS

Joint involvement has been observed in approximately one half of patients with idiopathic hemochromatosis. Joint swelling with bony enlargement is particularly common in the small joints of the hands, but the wrists, hips, and knees may also be affected. The clinical and roentgenographic features resemble osteoarthritis more than inflammatory joint disease. There is roentgenographic evidence of narrowing of the joint space with subchondral erosions and sclerosis. Chondrocalcinosis is present in about 50 per cent of patients with arthropathy and may lead to acute episodes of crystal-induced synovitis (see Ch. 444). Management of this arthropathy includes the use of a nonsteroidal anti-inflammatory drug and prosthetic weight-bearing joint replacements in advanced disease.

SICKLE CELL DISEASE AND OTHER HEMOGLOBINOPATHIES

Severe polyarthralgia is a frequent manifestation of the crises of sickle cell disease. Occasionally the pain is accompanied by transient joint effusions. Skeletal abnormalities result from widening of bone marrow spaces and focal sickle cell thrombosis in bone. The most common bony lesion is avascular osteonecrosis of the femoral head; less commonly the humerus and vertebral bodies are involved. This complication is also associated with sickle cell trait, hemoglobin C disease, sickle cell disease, and sickle cell–thalassemia disease. In children, periostitis may result in transient diffuse swelling of the hands and feet (dactylitis). Sickle cell disease is associated with an increased incidence of bacterial arthritis and osteomyelitis, especially those caused by gram-negative organisms. Arthropathy in patients with the thalassemia syndromes is attributed to stress fractures of weakened subchondral bone.

HYPERLIPOPROTEINEMIA

In familial hypercholesterolemia (type II hyperlipoproteinemia) recurrent episodes of acute migratory polyarthritis occur in homozygous cases. In heterozygous patients Achilles tendinitis, monoarthritis, or polyarthritis of brief duration and variable severity can involve both large and small joints. Tendinous xanthomas appear in late stages of this disease. In some individuals with hypertriglyceridemia (type IV hyperlipoproteinemia) a mild asymmetric oligoarthritis of chronic or recurrent type has been observed. Several of these patients have had periarticular bone cysts identified in joint radiographs. Certain of the reported cases may have occurred in association with familial combined hyperlipidemia, which includes individuals with both of these plasma lipoprotein profiles. Several authors have reported gradual reduction in the severity and frequency of articular symptoms after correction of the plasma lipid abnormalities by appropriate dietary and drug therapy.

HYPOGAMMAGLOBULINEMIA

A polyarthritis, rarely deforming in character, has been observed in as many as one third of patients with congenital or acquired hypogammaglobulinemia. The pattern of joint involvement resembles that of rheumatoid arthritis; in addition, other connective tissue diseases such as systemic lupus erythematosus, systemic sclerosis, and dermatomyositis have been associated with immune deficiency states. A variety of autoimmune phenomena and connective tissue syndromes, including juvenile arthritis, have been observed in patients with selective IgA deficiency. Regression of arthritis has been observed following institution of gamma globulin therapy (see Ch. 419).

HYPERPARATHYROIDISM

Patients with hyperparathyroidism are subject to a variety of associated rheumatic disorders that may occur singly or in combination. These include hyperuricemia and gouty arthritis, chondrocalcinosis with episodes of calcium pyrophosphate dihydrate crystal-induced synovitis (CPPD disease), and osteoarthritis resulting from deformation of atrophic subchondral bone. Rheumatic symptoms, particularly those associated with CPPD disease, may be the first manifestations of hyperparathyroidism.

ACROMEGALY

The majority of patients with acromegaly develop an atypical form of osteoarthritis. Increased levels of growth hormone result in hypertrophy of articular cartilage, subchondral bone, and periarticular tissues. Hypermobility of joints, a common manifestation, may contribute to degenerative change. The fingers and knees are most frequently affected. Pathognomonic radiographic features include overgrowth of bone and cartilage. Median nerve entrapment (carpal tunnel syndrome) secondary to wrist synovitis can occur.

FAMILIAL MEDITERRANEAN FEVER

Joint involvement is second only to peritonitis as the most common manifestation in this disease. The arthritis is usually monoarticular and acute in onset and most commonly affects the large weight-bearing joints. The articular attacks remit in a few days, and only in a few cases do joint symptoms persist for weeks to months. Arthritis, like other manifestations of this syndrome, is recurrent, but permanent damage to joints other than the hip is rare. (For a more complete discussion, see Ch. 209.)

WHIPPLE'S DISEASE

This disease represents an unusual host response to a bacterial infection. It is characterized by diarrhea, malabsorption, fever, anemia, increased skin pigmentation, and migratory polyarthralgia or polyarthritis. Permanent joint damage is rare, and the disease is suppressed by chronic antibiotic therapy (see Ch. 104).

450 MISCELLANEOUS FORMS OF ARTHRITIS

Giles G. Bole

NEUROPATHIC JOINT DISEASE (Charcot Joints)

This chronic progressive degenerative arthropathy can be a complication of a variety of neurologic disorders. Impairment of proprioceptive and pain sensations deprives the affected joint of the normal protective reactions that ordinarily modulate the forces of weight bearing and motion. Diabetic neuropathy is now the most common and syphilitic tabes dorsalis the second most common cause of this joint disorder. Syringomyelia, myelomeningocele, and congenital indifference to pain are less frequent causes of neuropathic arthropathy. The basic neurologic lesion determines the distribution of the affected joints. In tabes dorsalis, the knees, hips, ankles, and vertebrae are frequently involved. In diabetic neuropathy, the changes are limited to the distal lower extremities, and in syringomyelia the shoulder and elbow joints are most commonly affected.

Although pain is generally present, discomfort tends to be mild relative to the degree of joint destruction. Clinical, pathologic, and roentgenographic features of chronic neuropathic joint disease reflect severe degrees of destruction and disorganization of the involved joints. Synovial fluid is usually noninflammatory, but it can be hemorrhagic and contain destructive debris (fragments of cartilage or bone). In the early stages, differentiation from other causes of joint derangement depends upon demonstration of a sensory neuropathy.

Management includes immobilization of affected joints and restriction of weight-bearing activities with crutches, splints, and braces. Surgical arthrodesis, although frequently unsuccessful, is indicated in selected individuals. Total joint replacement has been attempted, but success has been limited and most consider this approach contraindicated.

HEMARTHROSIS

Recurrent or chronic hemarthrosis is the most common complication of a group of heritable disorders of blood coagulation (see Ch. 167). Hemarthrosis can be a complication of anticoagulant therapy or severe trauma to a normal joint.

In hemophilia, joint bleeding usually begins before the age of five and tends to recur repeatedly during childhood in response to even minor injury. The most common sites are the knees, elbows, and ankles, but any joint can be involved.

Acute hemarthrosis usually results in marked local inflammation and joint symptoms that can last for days to weeks. Approximately one half of patients with hemophilia develop chronic deformities in one or more joints. Some of them develop a chronic progressive synovitis, restricted to one or a few joints, which clinically and roentgenographically resembles rheumatoid arthritis. In chronic cases there is marked synovial membrane hyperplasia, destruction of articular cartilage, and erosions of subchondral bone. This chronic progressive pattern probably results from a low level of continuous or intermittent bleeding into involved joints. Joint fluid, in chronic cases, usually contains blood and very high levels of leukocyte-derived proteases. Other musculoskeletal manifestations of hemophilia include bleeding into muscle and bone. The resolution of large hematomas can produce chronic cysts within these tissues.

The first principle in management is to prevent trauma, a goal not easily achieved in children. Acute hemarthrosis should be managed by immobilization, analgesic therapy, and the administration of appropriate plasma concentrates that contain the required coagulation factor. Aspirin and other nonsteroidal analgesics that alter platelet function should be avoided. If there is marked distention of a joint or bursa, aspiration can be accomplished after the defect in coagulation has been corrected. When pain and acute inflammation have subsided, an exercise program to restore range of joint motion should be initiated. For the patient with severe chronic deforming joint disease, the availability of potent plasma concentrates has made it possible to perform synovectomy and arthroplasty in selected instances.

HENOCH-SCHÖNLEIN PURPURA

Polyarthralgia and a nondeforming arthritis, most frequently affecting knees and ankles, are common manifestations of this disorder. Other features include nonthrombocytopenic purpura, abdominal pain, and glomerulonephritis. The syndrome is rare in adults. (For a more detailed discussion see Ch. 166.)

MULTICENTRIC RETICULOHISTIOCYTOSIS (Lipoid Dermatoarthritis)

This rare disorder usually begins in the middle decades of life and affects females three times more frequently than males. It is characterized by the development of multiple histiocytic nodules in the skin and severe polyarthritis that may simulate rheumatoid arthritis. The firm reddish-brown or yellow papular nodules are most commonly found on hands, forearms, head, neck, and chest. Mutilating joint destruction, especially in the interphalangeal joints, occurs in approximately one half of patients with this syndrome. Diagnosis is made by demonstration of histiocytes and multinucleated giant cells containing PAS-positive material in skin or synovium. Similar infiltrates have been observed in other organs. Reports of apparent benefit from adrenocorticosteroid or immunosuppressive therapy are difficult to interpret because of the tendency for spontaneous remission in this disorder.

HYPERTROPHIC OSTEOARTHROPATHY

This term refers to a syndrome that includes clubbing of fingers and toes, periostitis at the ends of long bones, arthritis, and in some cases signs of autonomic dysfunction such as flushing, blanching, and profuse sweating of the extremities. The syndrome occurs with a wide variety of underlying disease states. There is a rare hereditary and idiopathic form (pachydermoperiostosis) of this disorder. The fully expressed pattern is usually associated with intrathoracic disease: lung carcinoma, lung abscess, emphysema, bronchiectasis, chronic interstitial pneumonitis, or mesothelioma. Clubbing, usually without periostitis, can be seen with cyanotic heart disease, cystic fibrosis, bacterial endocarditis, biliary cirrhosis, ulcerative colitis, regional enteritis, or thyroid disease.

The distal joints (wrist, elbows, ankles) and long bones of the forearms and legs are most frequently affected. There are inflammatory changes in the periosteum, synovial membrane, and periarticular structures. The periosteum is "lifted" by the deposition of new bone matrix and subsequent mineralization. Clubbing results from edema, cellular infiltration, and connective tissue proliferation in the nailbeds.

Pain, tenderness, and enlargement of the distal portions of extremities may be accompanied by an acute polyarthritis that superficially resembles rheumatoid arthritis. Correct diagnosis of the acute polyarthritis syndrome is established by the recognition of digital clubbing and roentgenographic evidence of periostitis and intrathoracic disease.

The production of a humoral substance that mediates increased vascularity or connective tissue proliferation or both has long been suspected as the pathogenic factor in hypertrophic osteoarthropathy, but no such factor has been demonstrated. Evidence that neural factors are involved is derived from observations of striking resolution of signs and symptoms after denervation of the hilum or vagotomy on the same side as the thoracic lesion. Regression of osteoarthropathy has also been observed after resection of pulmonary neoplasms.

Aside from therapy directed at the associated disease, there is no effective treatment for hypertrophic osteoarthropathy. Symptomatic benefit may be obtained from salicylates, other analgesics, or adrenocorticosteroids.

PALINDROMIC RHEUMATISM AND INTERMITTENT HYDRARTHROSIS

These terms describe two different constellations of clinical findings in which no pathogenic mechanism or mechanisms have been defined and in which the symptoms are often the prodrome of another rheumatic disease. *Palindromic rheumatism* is a term applied to a recurrent pattern of polyarthritis that in individual cases is quite constant. The episodes are usually of brief duration. Many patients eventually develop typical features of rheumatoid arthritis. *Intermittent hydrarthrosis* is typified by recurrent joint effusions, usually occurring in young females at menstruation and involving the knee. Like palindromic rheumatism, there is a strong tendency for cases to evolve into rheumatoid arthritis. Diagnostic arthrocentesis is justified in each condition based upon the local joint findings during an acute attack. Since each of the disorders remits spontaneously for variable periods of time, there is no uniform opinion regarding treatment, which is strictly symptomatic.

451 NONARTICULAR RHEUMATISM

Giles G. Bole

This term designates a group of painful disorders resulting from involvement of tendons, bursae, and other periarticular structures. Conditions causing shoulder pain are considered separately in Ch. 447.

BURSITIS

Bursae are closed synovial spaces located at sites of friction between skin, ligaments, tendons, muscles, and bones. Trauma is the most common cause of acute bursitis, but almost any illness characterized by joint synovitis can be associated with inflammation in the lining of bursae. Bursae commonly involved include the following: subdeltoid, trochanteric, olecranon, and prepatellar. Septic or gouty bursitis can be documented by appropriate studies of aspirated fluid. Protection of an inflamed bursa from friction and trauma is the most important aspect of treatment, but moderate doses of salicylates or other nonsteroidal anti-inflammatory drugs can be helpful. Local injection with an adrenocorticosteroid preparation is indicated if symptoms are severe or refractory to other treatment.

TENOSYNOVITIS

Tendon sheaths, like bursae, have synovial linings and can be involved by any process capable of inducing joint synovitis. Transient tenosynovitis in the hand or foot is a frequent manifestation of gonococcemia. Calcific tendinitis, a common source of shoulder pain (see Ch. 447), can be associated with severe inflammation and can simulate acute gout. Focal thickening of a tendon sheath and adjacent tendon can result in "locking" or "trigger" phenomena. This problem, termed stenosing tenosynovitis, is most common in the flexor tendons of the fingers. Involvement of the abductor pollicis longus and extensor pollicis brevis tendons of the thumb (De Quervain's syndrome) produces pain and tenderness at the radial aspect of the wrist. There are few generalizations regarding management, since tenosynovitis can be a manifestation of various disease states, including rheumatoid arthritis and other connective tissue syndromes, infection, crystalline synovitis, or hyperlipidemia. The most common form of tenosynovitis, unassociated with systemic disease, often subsides with rest of the part. If symptoms are severe or recurrent, local injections of adrenocorticosteroid preparations are usually effective. Surgical excision of the affected tendon sheath is indicated for those patients with persistent disability.

TENNIS ELBOW (Epicondylitis)

This common disorder is characterized by pain over the lateral aspect of the elbow. Tenderness is localized at the site of origin of the extensor communis apparatus at the lateral epicondyle. The problem, most common in middle-aged males, is related to sports activities or occupations that involve repetitive wrist extension or pronation-supination. Pain is accentuated by resisted wrist extension. If symptoms fail to respond to rest, local injection of an adrenocorticosteroid preparation is usually successful. An exercise program designed to stretch and strengthen the forearm extensor muscles may also be required.

Medial epicondylitis, sometimes referred to as golfer's elbow, is associated with pain and tenderness over the medial aspect of the elbow, at the site or origin of the wrist flexors. Therapy is similar to that for tennis elbow.

CARPAL TUNNEL SYNDROME

This problem results from entrapment of the median nerve as it passes deep to the transverse carpal ligament at the wrist. Inflammation of the adjacent flexor tendons and their sheaths, the most common basis for median nerve entrapment, can be a feature of rheumatoid or other forms of arthritis, but in most patients the tenosynovitis is localized and unassociated with systemic disease. The syndrome can be seen in endocrine disorders, granulomatous infections, amyloidosis, and pregnancy. The most consistent symptoms are dysesthesia, paresthesia, and hypesthesia in the middle three digits of the hand. Referred pain to the more proximal upper extremity is common. Symptoms are usually intermittent, occurring most frequently during the night. Forced flexion of the wrist or nerve compression locally (Tinel's sign) can induce characteristic symptoms. In a minority of patients, there is progressive wasting of the muscles of the thenar eminence. Conservative management consists of fitting a removable wrist splint and the local injection of an adrenocorticosteroid preparation. Surgical release of the transverse carpal ligament is indicated for patients with persistent disability.

TIETZE'S SYNDROME

This anterior chest wall disorder is characterized by painful enlargement of the upper costal cartilages. It is usually unilateral and limited to a single costochondral juncture. Occasionally the manubriosternal and sternoclavicular joints are affected. The disease may be recurrent, but remission is the rule. If discomfort is severe or recurrent, analgesics, heat, or local infiltration (adrenocorticosteroid or local anesthetic agents) may be beneficial. The condition is distinct from costochondritis, which occurs at multiple sites lower in the anterior rib cage and is unattended by local palpable swelling of a costochondral junction.

FIBROSITIS

This term has been applied to a symptom complex that is characterized by pain and stiffness in varying areas, most commonly in the neck, shoulder girdle, and posterior aspect of the trunk. Physical signs except for questionable nodules or thickening of the deep fasciae are lacking, and results of laboratory and roentgenographic studies are normal. Localized areas of tenderness, commonly in the paravertebral areas medial to the scapula, have been termed tender or "trigger points." The syndrome usually begins in the middle years of life and is more common in females. Because the majority of patients appear tense and anxious and have no recognizable objective basis for their symptoms, the syndrome is often considered psychogenic. Patients with fibrositis frequently report difficulty with sleep, and electroencephalographic studies have demonstrated disturbances in slow wave non-REM sleep in some cases. Since pain and stiffness can be manifestations of a variety of musculoskeletal, neurologic, and systemic disorders, the diagnosis of fibrositis requires the exclusion of more specific disease entities. Patient and physician tend to share an unhappy experience in efforts to control symptoms. The results of strong reassurance that serious disease is lacking are variable, as are the results of therapy with salicylates, sedatives, tranquilizers, and muscle relaxants. Some authors favor the use of moderate doses of one of the tricyclic antidepressants to control the patient's reported sleep disturbance and other symptoms.

452 SYNOVIAL TUMORS

Giles G. Bole

Primary malignant tumors of joints are rare. Synovioma is a highly malignant fibroblastic sarcoma that usually originates in the knee or periarticular structures of the thigh. This neoplasm is most common in late childhood or early adult life. The recommended therapy is wide excision (frequently requiring amputation), irradiation, or systemic chemotherapy or all three. Synovial chondrosarcoma is a rare neoplasm that may simulate synovial chondromatosis. It most frequently involves the knee and is slow in producing distant metastases. Radical excision or amputation is the treatment of choice.

Benign tumors arising within joints include lipoma, chondroma, hemangioma, and xanthoma. These neoplasms are rather uncommon and are most frequently found in or around the knee.

Synovial chondromatosis is uncommon. It is characterized by multiple foci of cartilage metaplasia in the synovial tissues. The metaplastic growths form nodules and can detach and grow as loose bodies in the joint space. The lesions can also undergo ossification. The latter condition is referred to as synovial osteochondromatosis. The knee is the most common site of involvement; the disease is rarely polyarticular. Symptoms include crepitation, swelling, limitation of motion, and intermittent locking of the affected joint. Treatment is surgical synovectomy.

Pigmented villonodular synovitis is the most common term applied to a disorder characterized by villous or nodular growths that invade the synovial lining of joints, bursae, or tendons. It has a characteristic histopathologic picture, i.e.,

presence of inflammatory granulomas that contain hemosiderin, cholesterol crystals, and multinucleated giant cells. Authorities disagree whether the condition should be classified as a form of chronic synovitis or as a true neoplasm. The knee is most frequently involved, but it can occur in the hip, elbow, ankle, or foot. Synovial fluid is usually hemorrhagic or xanthochromic. The inflammatory granuloma frequently invades the cartilage, subchondral bone, and periarticular structures. Localized pigmented villonodular synovitis can affect extra-articular bursae or tendon sheaths or occur as a solitary nodule in a single joint. The treatment of choice for each of these conditions is synovectomy or local excision of the tumor masses. Recurrence is uncommon.

453 BEHÇET'S DISEASE

Ralph Snyderman

DEFINITION. Behçet's disease is an inflammatory disorder of unknown etiology characterized by recurrent oral and genital aphthous ulcers, ocular inflammation, and skin lesions of erythema nodosum and acneiform eruptions. Behçet's disease also frequently involves the joints, the central nervous system, and the gastrointestinal tract.

INCIDENCE AND PREVALENCE. Behçet's disease is common in northern Japan, Korea, China, and the Middle East. In Japan the current prevalence is 1 per 10,000. The frequency in the United States is far less. An annual incidence of 1 per 300,000 was determined for Olmstead County, Minnesota. The disease does not occur frequently in Japanese Americans, perhaps suggesting environmental factors in addition to genetic predisposition in the etiology of this illness.

ETIOLOGY AND PATHOGENESIS. No infectious agent has been consistently isolated, although a viral etiology is suspected. Sera frequently contain circulating immune complexes of the IgA and IgG variety, as well as elevated levels of chemotactic activity for leukocytes. Antibodies reactive against oral mucosal cells have been found, and factors produced by patient's lymphocytes are toxic for oral mucosal cells. However, these findings are also present in individuals with recurrent aphthous stomatitis alone. Serum complement levels in Behçet's disease are usually elevated, particularly levels of C9. Most patients with neurologic involvement have demyelinating antibodies in their sera. There is a strong association of HLA-B5 with Behçet's disease in Japan and in the Mediterranean area. Heavy metal exposure, certain foods (particularly English walnuts), and toxic factors such as organophosphates have initiated attacks in some individuals.

PATHOLOGY. Behçet's disease is primarily an inflammatory disorder involving small blood vessels, particularly venules. Areas of ulceration initially show an intense mononuclear cell infiltration around blood vessels. As the lesion evolves, polymorphonuclear leukocytes and plasma cells predominate. The early lesions resemble a delayed hypersensitivity reaction, the later lesions an immune complex–Arthustype reaction. The role of immune complexes in causing the venulitis is, however, questionable, since immunoglobulins are not routinely found in vessel walls.

CLINICAL MANIFESTATIONS. Behçet's disease can occur in many forms, but recurrent oral aphthous ulcers are present in 99 per cent of patients, and in almost 70 per cent of these they are the initial symptoms. Ocular symptoms occur in 90 per cent, skin lesions in 85 per cent, and genital ulcerations in nearly 70 per cent. Arthritis is present in approximately one half of the patients with Behçet's disease. The onset is usually in the third or fourth decade. Behçet's disease affects men and women approximately equally. Indi-

TABLE 453–1. DIAGNOSTIC CRITERIA OF BEHÇET'S DISEASE (SYNDROME)*

Major criteria
1. Recurrent oral aphthous ulcers
2. Eye lesions
   a. Recurrent hypopyon, iritis, or iridocyclitis
   b. Chorioretinitis
3. Genital ulcerations
4. Skin lesions
   a. Erythema nodosum–like eruptions
   b. Superficial thrombophlebitis
   c. Pustular skin lesions
   d. Hyperirritability of the skin (pathergy)

Minor criteria
5. Arthritis
6. Gastrointestinal lesions
7. Epididymitis
8. Vascular lesions (occlusion of blood vessels, aneurysms)
9. Central nervous system involvement
   a. Brainstem syndrome
   b. Meningoencephalomyelitic syndrome
   c. Organic confusional states

*Modified from the recommendations by the Behçet's Syndrome Research Committee of Japan (1972).

cations of poor prognosis include neurologic and posterior uveal tract involvement. In the absence of these, the disease tends to be unpredictable and remitting. In Japan, the mortality is approximately 4 per cent, with blindness occurring in as many as 65 per cent of untreated individuals. Young males have the worst prognosis.

The diagnosis of Behçet's disease is based upon the criteria listed in Table 453-1. Complete Behçet's syndrome is associated with all four major criteria. Persons with three major sites of involvement, or ocular lesions plus one other major site, have incomplete Behçet's disease. The diagnosis should be suspected when two major sites are affected. Since all manifestations need not appear, some investigators have grouped this illness into subtypes based upon the primary tissue involvement (i.e., neuro-Behçet's, oculo-Behçet's).

The oral aphthous ulcers are painful, unlike those of Reiter's syndrome, and occur singly or multiply on the lingual, gingival, buccal, or labial mucosal membranes. In Reiter's and Stevens-Johnson syndromes, the ulcers occur on the palate, pharynx, and tonsils, structures rarely involved in Behçet's disease. The aphthae of Behçet's disease usually last for approximately a week and may heal with or without scarring. Ulcers can also appear on the scrotum, vulva, penis, vaginal mucosa, or perianal areas. These lesions may be painless in women. Their gross appearance is similar to that of the oral aphthous ulcers. Vulvar lesions frequently occur premenstrually. Other types of cutaneous involvement are common. Painful, recurrent lesions of erythema nodosum may appear in crops over the tibia. Superficial thrombophlebitis can occur in the upper or lower extremities. Skin eruptions resembling acne vulgaris frequently appear on the upper thorax and face.

Approximately 40 per cent of patients with Behçet's disease exhibit a cutaneous phenomenon termed "pathergy" and develop sterile pustules at sites of trauma. Venipuncture or injection of sterile saline into the skin of these patients results in the formation of a pustule. This phenomenon is not pathognomonic for Behçet's disease.

Ocular lesions may consist of anterior or posterior uveitis. Anterior uveitis frequently produces hazy vision as an initial manifestation. The development of a hypopyon is not unusual. Recurrent posterior uveitis (retinal vasculitis) is an ominous expression of Behçet's disease which, if untreated, frequently leads to bilateral blindness. Choroidal exudates and bleeding may be seen.

Articular manifestations consist of arthralgias and arthritis. The involvement is usually asymmetric, affects one to several large joints such as the knees, ankles, elbows, and wrists, and resolves during remissions. Permanent joint damage is rare.

Gastrointestinal involvement during acute attacks, present in approximately 50 per cent of patients, is most commonly manifested by vomiting, abdominal pain, diarrhea, flatulence, or constipation. More specific for Behçet's disease are erosions or superficial ulcers in the terminal ileum or colon. Intestinal ulcers occasionally perforate. Differentiation of Behçet's disease from ulcerative colitis or regional enteritis may be difficult.

Nervous system involvement occurs in approximately 10 per cent of patients and can be extremely severe, explosive, and associated with a poor prognosis. Manifestations include hemiplegia, paraplegia, cerebellar dysfunction, and psychologic changes.

Superficial venous occlusions, perhaps related to abnormalities in the blood fibrinolytic system, occur in up to 40 per cent of patients. Inferior or superior vena caval obstructions can lead to death. Occlusive lesions have also occurred in the aorta and other large arteries. Epididymitis occurs in approximately 6 per cent of male patients.

TREATMENT. No therapy has been proved uniformly effective. Since the illness is unpredictable and frequently remitting, long-term continuous therapy with potentially dangerous drugs is not justified except in specific situations. Chlorambucil* (0.1 to 0.2 mg per kilogram per day) has been reported to prevent blindness in patients with posterior retinal involvement. Other immunosuppressive agents such as azathioprine,* cyclophosphamide,* and 6-mercaptopurine* have also been used. Cyclosporin* is reported to be effective in abrogating ocular as well as other disease manifestations. Since neuro-Behçet's syndrome is life-threatening, immunosuppressive agents are frequently used for this manifestation. Corticosteroids are strictly palliative for the inflammatory lesions (i.e., anterior uveitis) and should not be used except during acute flares of the disease. Avoidance of factors known to precipitate attacks (i.e., particular foods or toxic materials) should be encouraged. Colchicine* (0.6 mg orally twice a day) is sometimes effective in treating the mucocutaneous and cutaneous lesions. Transfer factor has not been effective in double-blind clinical trials. In patients with gastrointestinal manifestations, a trial of sulfasalazine* (2 to 4 gm per day) is warranted. Sulfasalazine may also be useful in patients without obvious gastrointestinal complaints. Fibrinolytic agents have been recommended for patients with occlusive vascular disease. Because the disease is remitting in nature, the efficacy of therapy is difficult to evaluate.

---

*This use is not listed in the manufacturer's directive

Chajek T, Fainaru M: Behçet's disease. Report of 41 cases and a review of the literature. Medicine 54:179, 1975. *Concise but thorough review of clinical features in a large number of patients with Behçet's disease.*

Jorizzo TL: Behçet's disease. Arch Dermatol 122:556, 1986. *A brief update of the 1985 International Conference on Behçet's Disease.*

Marquardt JL, Snyderman R, Oppenheim JJ: Depression of transformation and exacerbation of Behçet's syndrome by ingestion of English walnuts. Cell Immunol 9:263, 1973. *An immunologic study of Behçet's disease with a potential clue for pathogenesis.*

Michelson JB, Chisari FV: Behçet's disease. Surv Ophthalmol 26:190, 1982. *An up-to-date review of Behçet's disease, particularly good for ocular manifestations.*

Shimizu T, Ehrlich GE, Inaba G, et al.: Behçet's disease (Behçet syndrome). Semin Arthritis Rheum 8:223, 1979. *Comprehensive review of clinical features, pathology, and potential pathogenic mechanisms of Behçet's disease.*

454 PANNICULITIS AND DISORDERS OF THE SUBCUTANEOUS FAT

Gerald S. Lazarus

INTRODUCTION. The subcutaneous tissue is a fibrofatty layer spread between skin and muscles. It functions not only as a thermal and mechanical insulator but also as an active metabolic organ. The characteristic signet ring lipocytes are organized into lobules by fibrous septa, which are continuous with the dermis and contain the blood and lymph vessels and reticuloendothelial cells.

The diagnosis of panniculitis frequently requires deep skin biopsy. The most important histologic characteristic is the location of the inflammatory process. Inflammation primarily in the septa is designated *septal panniculitis*, whereas inflammatory cells primarily in the fat lobules designate *lobular panniculitis*. The presence or absence of vasculitis further differentiates panniculitis into the four major groups.

LOBULAR PANNICULITIS WITHOUT VASCULITIS. *Nodular Panniculitis—Weber-Christian Disease.* Nodular panniculitis describes a group of syndromes or diseases characterized by subcutaneous nodules and inflammatory cells in the fat lobules. The term Weber-Christian disease is applied when cutaneous lesions are associated with systemic complaints.

The etiology of this group of diseases is unknown. In the early stages the fat lobules are infiltrated with polymorphonuclear leukocytes. Later, macrophages appear and ingest fat, producing the characteristic lipophagic granuloma. The lesions heal with lobular fibrosis. Modest septal vasculitis may be observed.

Lobular panniculitis most commonly presents in females between the ages of 30 and 60, although cases have been reported in all age groups. The lesions begin as red, slightly tender nodules deep in the skin. They appear more or less in symmetric crops on thighs and lower legs, but lesions may also occur on arms, trunk, and face. The number of lesions may vary enormously. The lesions become firmer, less red, and less tender over a period of weeks. They heal, leaving a depressed hyperpigmented scar. *Liquefying panniculitis* is a variant in which the lesions become necrotic and drain an oily, yellow-brown fluid. *Rothmann-Makai syndrome* is a very rare variant of lobular panniculitis, affecting children with numerous large lesions; the lesions do not liquefy, and healing usually occurs within 12 months.

Systemic nodular panniculitis or *Weber-Christian disease* is a widespread process affecting cutaneous and visceral fat. Patients usually present with unequivocal cutaneous nodules and arthralgias, malaise, fatigue, weight loss, and abdominal pain. Involvement of the bone marrow may produce anemia, leukocytosis or leukopenia, and bone pain. Hepatomegaly, steatorrhea, and intestinal perforation have also been reported. Inflammation may occur in other internal organs such as lungs, pleura, pericardium, spleen, kidney, and adrenal glands. Visceral involvement may be confined to the retroperitoneal space, producing abdominal pain, nausea, and vomiting. Alpha$_1$-antitrypsin deficiency is associated with this syndrome not infrequently. Malignant histiocytosis (cytophagic histiocytic panniculitis) may present as Weber-Christian disease.

The prognosis of nodular panniculitis is good in patients with only cutaneous involvement. There are frequent remissions and exacerbations of the lesions. Some patients recover after a few months, and permanent remission is usual after several years. On rare occasions visceral involvement may be fatal.

There is no specific therapy for this disease. Saturated potassium iodide, increasing from 5 drops three times daily by 1 drop per day to 30 drops three times daily, has been suggested. Hydroxychloroquine,* 200 mg twice per day, has also been advocated as treatment. High dose prednisone, 40 to 60 mg for one to two weeks with gradual tapering over six to eight weeks, has also been reported to be of value in patients with severe disease; steroids should be used only for acute attacks and for limited periods of time.

Lobular Panniculitis Associated with Pancreatic Disease. The diagnosis is made by skin biopsy, which discloses acute fat necrosis with characteristic ghost cells. These patients often have associated arthritis, ascites, and eosinophilia. Acute pancreatitis, trauma to the pancreas, chronic pancreatitis, pancreatic cysts, and pancreatic carcinoma have been reported to be associated with this syndrome. Diagnosis depends upon the histologic findings at skin biopsy and documentation of a specific pancreatic abnormality. Therapy is directed at the underlying pancreatic disease.

Poststeroid Lobular Panniculitis. Children who receive large doses of steroid for a short period of time, followed by abrupt discontinuance, may develop lobular panniculitis. Lesions may occur in the viscera, and a fatal case has been reported.

Physical Lobular Panniculitis. Physical trauma of any kind and cold injury, especially in children, can produce lobular panniculitis. A unique traumatic panniculitis occurs in the obese breasts of women in their 50's. Injection of silicones or other foreign materials into female breasts or buttocks and into the male genitalia may induce a granulomatous foreign body nodular panniculitis. Similar inflammatory lesions may be seen following injections of Talwin.

Lobular Panniculitis Associated with Systemic Disease. Lupus erythematosus, sarcoidosis, granuloma annulare, Sweet's disease, acute sudden weight loss from gastrointestinal surgery, and infections including deep fungi and pyogens may present as lobular panniculitis. Lymphoma or leukemia may also present as panniculitis; histologically, these lesions demonstrate malignant cells in the fat lobules. Lupus erythematosus confined primarily to the fat is known as lupus profundus. The skin may be exclusively involved, or the panniculitis may be associated with systemic disease.

LOBULAR PANNICULITIS WITH VASCULITIS. This category of disease includes *nodular vasculitis* and *erythema induratum*. The eruption consists of recurring, tender, painful nodules on the calves, which often ulcerate and heal with scarring. It is much more common in females than in males. Increased erythrocyte sedimentation rate and hypertension have been associated with this syndrome. Bazin gave the name erythema induratum to this disease when histologic examination revealed caseation necrosis and the lesions were associated with tuberculosis.

There is no specific therapy. Most patients have remission of lesions with bed rest. Severe cases have been successfully treated with nonsteroidal anti-inflammatory drugs, dapsone, and prednisone. In the very rare case of nodular vasculitis associated with tuberculosis, appropriate antituberculous therapy is indicated.

SEPTAL PANNICULITIS WITHOUT VASCULITIS. This histology in a patient with nodular, painful, tender lesions, especially on the anterior leg, is diagnostic of *erythema nodosum*, which is discussed in Ch. 534. A chronic disease similar to erythema nodosum clinically and histologically except that the lesions spread peripherally over months, forming rings, is called *subacute migratory panniculitis*. This disease responds to therapy with increasing doses of saturated

---

*This use is not listed in the manufacturer's directive.

potassium iodide as described for nodular panniculitis. Septal panniculitis without vasculitis can also be seen in scleroderma, eosinophilic fasciitis, dermatomyositis, and necrobiosis lipoidica diabeticorum.

SEPTAL PANNICULITIS WITH VASCULITIS. *Thrombophlebitis* may present with subcutaneous nodules. Histology reveals inflammation of veins with adjacent panniculitis (see Ch. 57).

Cutaneous polyarteritis is a chronic, recurring, painful nodular eruption, primarily of the legs. There is often an associated mottled livedo vascular pattern. Cutaneous polyarteritis is associated with myalgias, arthralgias, and increased erythrocyte sedimentation rate. Histologic examination demonstrates leukocytoclastic vasculitis of medium-sized arterioles. This disease is usually not associated with systemic involvement. It has a benign course, but lesions may recur for years.

Therapy includes nonsteroidal anti-inflammatory agents and short courses of corticosteroids. Cutaneous polyarteritis associated with granulomatous bowel disease has responded to short courses of Cytoxan.

LIPOATROPHY. Loss of subcutaneous tissue can occur as a consequence of healing in almost any of the panniculitides described previously. The most common diagnosable cause of lipoatrophy is recurrent insulin injection. Insulin lipoatrophy is usually associated with repetitive injections of high doses of insulin in exactly the same location in females. Talwin injections may also produce panniculitis and severe lipoatrophy.

Total lipoatrophy associated with diabetes may occur in children and adults. The clinical picture is dramatic, and there is almost complete loss of subcutaneous fat. Partial lipoatrophy usually begins in children or young adults. It is five times more common in females than in males. Patients often lose the fat in the face and the upper half of the body. In some cases, there is hypertrophy of the fat on the lower half of the body. Patients with partial lipodystrophy often develop progressive mesangiocapillary glomerulonephritis and hypocomplementemia. Diabetes develops in one third of these patients. Retinitis pigmentosum has also been reported with this disease. The prognosis depends upon the severity of the renal disease.

Ackerman AB: Panniculitis. In Ackerman AB: Histologic Diagnosis of Inflammatory Skin Diseases. Philadelphia, Lea & Febiger, 1978, pp 779–826. *An outstanding review of the classification and histopathology of panniculitis.*

Barron DR, Davis BR, Pomeranz JR, et al.: Cytophagic histiocytic panniculitis. Cancer 55:2538–2542, 1985. *Excellent study of a serious disease.*

Bennett WM, Bardana EJ, Wuepper K, et al.: Partial lipodystrophy, C3 nephritic factor and clinically inapparent mesangiocapillary glomerulonephritis. Am J Med 62:757, 1976. *Description of the association of lipodystrophy with glomerulonephritis.*

Bleumink ET, Klokke HA: Protease inhibitor deficiency in a patient with Weber-Christian panniculitis. Arch Dermatol 120:936, 1984. *Growing evidence that serum proteinase inhibitor deficiency is associated with panniculitis.*

Bondi EE, Lazarus GS: Panniculitis. In Fitzpatrick TB, Eisen AZ, Wolff K, Freedberg IM, Austen KF (eds.): Dermatology in General Medicine. 3rd ed. New York, McGraw-Hill Book Company. In press. *A complete overview of panniculitis, emphasizing clinical description, mechanisms, and treatment.*

Panush RS, Yonker RA, Dlesk A, et al.: Weber-Christian disease. Medicine 64:181–191, 1985. *Excellent review of 15 patients and the world literature.*

455 MULTIFOCAL FIBROSCLEROSIS

H. Ralph Schumacher, Jr.

In rare instances the delicate fibrous areolar tissue in a certain anatomic region becomes the site of a chronic low-grade inflammatory process, leading to deposition of dense sclerotic plaques, which may obstruct or limit the movement of adjacent viscera. When the process is in the active phase, there are characteristic findings of chronic or granulomatous inflammation, featured by mononuclear cell infiltration and occasional giant cells. In the end stages the pathologic lesion is simply that of scar tissue, so that by the time this process causes clinical manifestations there may be little evidence of the initial inflammatory reaction. In at least some cases there is an accompanying vasculitis. As a general rule the process tends to originate in the midline, around the great vessels, and then to spread laterally. In most cases a clue to the inciting mechanism is lacking.

Syndromes that have been considered as manifestations of multifocal fibrosclerosis include retroperitoneal fibrosis, mediastinal fibrosis, sclerosing cholangitis (see Ch. 130), Riedel's thyroiditis (see Ch. 229), pseudotumor of the orbit, Peyronie's disease (a sclerotic induration of the corpora cavernosa of the penis), and sclerosing peritonitis. Other sites of a similar fibrosis such as the testes, vagina, and suprasellar area have also rarely been reported. Pulmonary and myocardial fibrosis syndromes have generally not been seen as related to multifocal fibrosclerosis.

Although most of these syndromes have been described as separate entities, several anatomic areas may become affected in one person. For example, retroperitoneal fibrosis and sclerosing mediastinitis may be present at the same time. Comings and his associates reported two brothers, offspring of a consanguineous marriage, who exhibited varying combinations of retroperitoneal fibrosis, mediastinal fibrosis, sclerosing cholangitis, Riedel's thyroiditis, and pseudotumor of the orbit. This suggests a possible genetic predisposition to disease of this character. This possibility is supported by an association between fibrosing syndromes and alpha$_1$-antitrypsin deficiency. Recent reports have also described familial mediastinal or retroperitoneal fibrosis associated with HLA-B27 and seronegative spondyloarthropathies.

Comings DE, Skubi KB, Van Eyes J, et al.: Familial multifocal sclerosis. Ann Intern Med 66:884, 1967. *Description of multiple sites of fibrosis in two brothers.*

Goldbach P, Mohsenifar Z, Salick AI: Familial mediastinal fibrosis associated with seronegative spondyloarthropathy. Arthritis Rheum 26:221–225, 1983. *Two siblings with both diseases but HLA-B27 negative.*

RETROPERITONEAL FIBROSIS

In retroperitoneal fibrosis the process usually begins over the promontory of the sacrum and extends laterally across the ureters and as high as the second or third lumbar vertebra. Less commonly, the lesion develops in other extraperitoneal areas, for example, contiguous with the kidneys, duodenum, descending colon, or urinary bladder. In some cases there has been an associated vasculitis in the skin and subcutaneous tissue, manifested by the formation of nodules, erythematous discolorations, and ulcerations. Similarly, inflammatory changes in small vessels at the sites of the sclerosis have been noted. Glomerulonephritis has been seen in a few patients.

The occurrence of retroperitoneal fibrosis in patients taking methysergide for migraine has been reported with greater frequency than could be due to chance. Occasional cases have been reported after use of other drugs such as ergotamine, various beta-adrenergic blocking agents, hydralazine, or methyldopa. Associated diseases in patients with retroperitoneal fibrosis have included systemic lupus erythematosus, vasculitis, scleroderma, rubella-associated arthritis, and carcinoid. Retroperitoneal tumors, trauma, or surgery may be a factor in some cases.

The disorder is about twice as common in males as in females, and the peak incidence is in the fifth and sixth decades. Cases have been reported in children. The manifestations are variable, depending on the anatomic location of the process. Pain is the most common symptom; it is vague, tends to be located in the low back, and may be accompanied by symptoms referable to the gastrointestinal tract. The patient is likely to lose weight and have low-grade fever. There may be some anemia and elevation of the erythrocyte sedimentation rate. Although the ureter is the structure most often affected, symptoms referable to the urinary tract are uncommon until obstructive uropathy has led to azotemia and other clinical manifestations of renal insufficiency. The fibrosing process may surround the inferior vena cava, but obstruction of that vessel is uncommon. Thromboembolism and hypertension can be complications. Arterial invasion has been described. Retroperitoneal fibrosis occasionally develops in association with abdominal aortic aneurysm or aortitis.

Diagnosis of retroperitoneal fibrosis is difficult because of the lack of localizing manifestations. It is most often suggested by the findings at intravenous pyelography: displacement of the ureters toward the midline and evidence of obstruction, usually at the level of the pelvic brim. One or both ureters may be affected. In rare instances a mass can be palpated in the pelvis or on the posterior abdominal wall. Ultrasonography, CT scanning, and magnetic resonance imaging (MRI) can also identify the fibrosing masses. Once a mass has been disclosed, the main problem in differential diagnosis lies in distinguishing retroperitoneal fibrosis from retroperitoneal tumor. For that reason it is advised that multiple deep biopsies should be made at the time of laparotomy.

Surgical treatment, if employed before there has been severe renal damage, is often highly successful. Inasmuch as the fibrosing process is seldom invasive, the constricted organ can usually be freed by blunt dissection so that normal movement or flow is restored. Relief of ureteral obstruction is usually achieved by bringing the ureter out on the anterior surface of the sclerotic mass. Occasionally, however, the obstruction recurs months or years after such treatment. Some surgeons wrap the ureters in omentum to try to decrease recurrent obstruction. Steroid therapy may be helpful in the rare case detected early or may be employed as an adjunct to surgical measures. Azathioprine has been used successfully in a few cases. Other drugs such as penicillamine, colchicine, and gamma interferon with theoretic ability to limit clinical fibrosis have not been studied in this disease.

Progesterone has been used with some apparent success in Latin America. When the inferior vena cava is obstructed, surgical relief is technically difficult and risky; here it may be preferable to temporize in the hope that development of collateral pathways may alleviate the circulatory block.

The long-term outlook is fairly good if the disease is recognized and if its obstructive consequences can be treated by surgical means. The disease often tends to run its course and subside. Most deaths have been caused by renal failure.

Cogan E, Fastrez R: Azathioprine. An alternative treatment for recurrent idiopathic retroperitoneal fibrosis. Arch Intern Med 145:753–755, 1985. *A case report describing successful therapy.*

Hricak H, Higgins CB, Williams RD: Nuclear magnetic resonance imaging in retroperitoneal fibrosis. Am J Radiol 141:35–38, 1983. *Documentation of the increasing value of CT scans and MRI in diagnosis.*

Littlejohn GO, Keystone E: The association of retroperitoneal fibrosis with systemic vasculitis and HLA-B27: A case report and review of the literature. J Rheum 8:665–669, 1981. *Vasculitis has been documented histologically in 37 of 500 cases reviewed and may be much more common. An association with HLA-B27 and sacroiliitis is seen in this case.*

MEDIASTINAL FIBROSIS

Taut bundles of collagenous tissue form in the superior and anterior mediastinum with impingement on the aorta, trachea, bronchi, esophagus, and pericardium, but the predominant manifestations are those caused by obstruction of the superior vena cava: puffy, suffused appearance of the face and conjunctivae; nonpitting edema of the face, neck, and upper extremities; and distended veins in the neck and upper extremities. Rarely the principal vessels affected are the pulmonary arteries, causing pulmonary hypertension. More frequently the pulmonary veins are involved, and here severe hemoptysis may be the most prominent manifestation. Pericardial fibrosis can lead to constrictive pericarditis. The main task in differential diagnosis is to distinguish this relatively benign condition from obstruction caused by tumor. Roentgenographic examination of the chest may reveal little or no abnormality, but angiographic studies will show obstruction of the affected vessels. Thoracotomy may be required for histologic diagnosis.

Histoplasmosis and possibly tuberculosis may cause some mediastinal fibrosis. Mediastinal hemorrhage can lead to fibrosis, and cases have been associated with methysergide use. Some patients with this syndrome have shown gradual improvement over months or years, presumably because of development of collateral circulation. Successful superior vena cava bypass surgery has been described. Steroid and other drug therapy as used with retroperitoneal fibrosis seems reasonable if infection is excluded, but such treatment has not been studied.

Dye TE, Saab SB, Almond MD, et al.: Sclerosing mediastinitis with occlusion of pulmonary veins. J Thorac Cardiovasc Surg 74:137, 1977. *An unusual but serious and treatable cause of hemoptysis.*

Goodwin RA, Nickell JA, Dez Prez RM: Mediastinal fibrosis complicating healed primary histoplasmosis and tuberculosis. Medicine 51:227, 1972. *Excellent review, certainly implicating histoplasmosis.*

SCLEROSING PERITONITIS

An unusual fibrotic syndrome has been observed primarily in patients treated with the β-adrenergic blocking drug practolol. Only a few cases have been reported with propranolol or other beta blockers. Sclerosing peritonitis with many similarities has also been seen in patients treated with chronic ambulatory peritoneal dialysis and in an idiopathic form. Practolol peritonitis seldom manifests itself in less than 12 months after beginning treatment. Some cases have developed a year or longer after cessation of therapy. Thus, although practolol has been withdrawn from use, occasional late-occurring cases may still be seen. The peritonitis consists of a thick fibrous encasement of the small intestine, and the symptoms include abdominal fullness, back pain, ascites, weight loss, and signs of subacute obstruction. It has usually been possible to relieve the symptoms by surgery, with blunt dissection to peel away the fibrous tissue. Some improvement occurs with time. A few patients treated with practolol have developed apparently related pericardial or lung disease, conjunctivitis, and dermatitis.

Pussteri R, Ross R, Marshall R, et al.: Sclerosing encapsulating peritonitis; report of a case with small bowel obstruction managed by long term hyperalimentation, and a review of the literature. Am J Kidney Dis 8:56–60, 1986. *This is a serious complication of peritoneal dialysis. Improvement in this patient occurred during parenteral nutrition.*

PART XXII

NEUROLOGIC AND BEHAVIORAL DISEASES

SECTION ONE / CLINICAL STUDY OF THE PATIENT WITH NEUROLOGIC SYMPTOMS

456 CLINICAL STUDY OF THE PATIENT

456.1 Approach to the Patient

GENERAL MANAGEMENT

Fred Plum

Patients with symptoms and signs referable to the nervous system place special requirements on the physician's clinical approach. The most immediate task is to consider whether the symptoms are merely the nonspecific signals of a systemic disorder or reflect intrinsic neurologic disease. Pain, headache, nausea, dizziness, fatigue, and weakness all lack specificity until taken in context with the rest of the history and physical findings; as often as not, such symptoms can reflect the emotional ravages of disturbed psychologic adjustment. To understand and treat human beings requires that the doctor know *who* is sick as much as or more often than *what* is sick. Put in Peabody's words, "The secret of the care of the patient is caring for the patient."

A second major consideration is to realize that although all patients are to some degree frightened of illness, concern over the possibility of paralysis, severe pain, or mental impairment instills an especial terror which requires the doctor's attention and reassurance. When examining such patients, if at all possible follow Osler's dictum: "Do the kind thing and do it first."

The third major consideration stems from the nervous system's vulnerability to damage and its inability to repair itself. In a broad sense, the purpose of the practice of medicine is to protect the brain. Man's brain makes him human. Damage it and life loses its meaning in direct proportion, no matter what other physiologic recoveries may parallel the process. The brain cannot be regenerated, repaired, or homotransplanted. It accumulates no metabolic debts, and, unless supplied continuously by an effective circulation carrying a large volume of oxygen and substrates, it digests itself promptly and irreparably. The doctor's mandate is clear: in seriously and acutely ill patients with neurologic abnormalities, life- or brain-threatening complications must be treated even while proceeding with diagnostic procedures that may take several more minutes, hours, or days to complete.

Wise and sensitive management of the neurologic patient requires attention to both disease and humane need. In general, the more specific and acute the illness, the less immediately important become the broad concerns of the patient. By contrast, patients whose diseases lack quick and specific remedies (e.g., most degenerative diseases, most residua of severe trauma) usually need far more from the doctor than the local pharmacy can supply. Three important maxims apply to all treatment situations: protect the brain first, no matter what successive steps must follow; relieve pain even while proceeding with diagnosis; and give reassurance, hope, and explanation at every step along the way. In order to plan long-term management effectively and economically, try to construct an accurate prognosis as early as possible. In acute, self-limited illnesses, such as meningococcal meningitis or most acute inflammatory polyneuritis, for example, one knows the probable outcome within a few days of onset. One even knows for most such patients the difference in convalescent time required before they will return to their former occupations. However, with diseases with intermediate outcomes such as multiple sclerosis, full recovery is less certain and the risk of relapse or chronic disability may require the physician to appraise all aspects of the patient's life in order to give proper guidance. At the third extreme are patients who become severely aphasic and hemiplegic from stroke or demented from Alzheimer's disease. They may never recover independence, and their proper early management requires that one guide whole families through major social and financial readjustments in planning for the future. How the doctor manages such complexities determines to a considerable degree his effectiveness as a physician.

Bennett AE: Communication Between Doctors and Patients. London, Oxford University Press, 1976. *A series of essays with a particularly good chapter by Maguire and Rutter on interviewing techniques for medical students.*

DeJong RN: The Neurological Examination. 4th ed. Hagerstown, MD, Harper & Row, 1979. *A comprehensive and detailed explanation of the technique and physiology of the examination.*

Emerson CP: Reminiscences of Sir William Osler. Int Assoc Med Museums Bull 1926, p 294. *A volume of gems on teaching, care, and scholarship by America's greatest clinician.*

Mayo Clinic and Foundation: Clinical Examinations in Neurology. Philadelphia, W.B. Saunders Company, 1981. *A useful compendium of clinical and electrophysiologic approaches to neurologic diagnosis.*

Peabody FW: The care of the patient. JAMA 88:877, 1927. *A thoughtful and compassionate statement about the doctor-patient relationship.*

PRINCIPLES OF DIAGNOSIS

Fred Plum

Two major, alternative strategies underlie the way that most physicians approach the process of diagnosis. One, *pattern recognition*, is the classic technique of putting together the symptoms and signs into a syndrome and determining that the result conforms to a condition that the doctor has read about, has previously observed, or can ferret from the medical literature. The method profits by experience and specialization and relies relatively less on an analytic consideration of basic mechanisms in disease. The other, *logic and probability*, consists of analyzing signs and symptoms as manifestations of disordered physiology and deducing their meaning in terms of the anatomic structures involved and the way diseases affect these structures. The reliability of the resulting diagnostic hypothesis is tested by estimating the probability that certain abnormalities in bodily mechanisms will accompany one another and by the knowledge of the frequency with which such involvements occur. History, physical examination, and laboratory tests serve as constant back-checks and extensions of the deductive process. Skillful physicians utilize both pattern recognition and logic-probability in varying measure. The pattern-recognizing qualities of astute clinicians can reach legendary quality, but even the most experienced doctors usually mentally test their diagnostic impressions against a physiologic benchmark to see if the implied pathophysiology "makes sense" (i.e., fulfills physiologic probabilities). For the young physician, especially as scientific knowledge grows in medicine, a logical approach based on deductions from pathophysiology is imperative, for it focuses attention on the patient's main problem and avoids the pitfall of treating minor symptoms or small laboratory perturbations that provide no threat to the patient's health. Particularly in neurologic diagnosis the strong communicative power of the nervous system and its reflections of the patient's inner self mean that information derived from the history and neurologic examination usually lends itself to logical analysis and probability testing (e.g., is it likely that *this* patient would have *this* disorder at *this* time with *this* combination of symptoms?). Armed with a provisional diagnostic formulation in anatomic and physiologic terms, the physician then should require only a limited number of laboratory tests to establish the precise mechanism of disease or to rule out the presence of some other, unsuspected condition or illness. One should recall, however, that the complexity of disease is such that even the most exhaustive efforts accurately diagnose only about 85 per cent of first time admissions to major medical centers. The number of relatively trivial uncertainties and errors probably rises higher in ambulatory patients with self-limited problems which inherently receive less attention or disappear without causing serious disability.

The first step in neurologic diagnosis is anatomic. To arrive at a regional diagnosis one asks: Does the patient have a structural disease (i.e., is the process organic, physiologic-functional, or psychiatric)? If a disease is present, is it monofocal or diffuse? Given the likelihood that a neurologic disorder is present, one asks in succession: Are the lesions peripheral (i.e., at the receptor, muscle effector, synapse, or nerve) or central (i.e., in the spinal cord or brain)? If central, does the disease affect structures above or below the foramen magnum, above or below the tentorium, on the right or the left side? Is the process static, worsening, or improving? Given the answer or answers to these questions, one can then formulate a pathologic-etiologic diagnosis according to whether the evidence suggests a disorder that is genetic, developmental, traumatic, environmental-toxic, infectious, immunologic, degenerative, neoplastic, metabolic, nutritional, physiologic (e.g., epilepsy, migraine), or psychophysiologic (e.g., tension backache, vasodepressor syncope). One then proceeds to nonspecific and specific laboratory tests in order to confirm the clinical diagnostic hypotheses.

THE NEUROLOGIC EXAMINATION

Fred Plum

Several texts can be consulted for the detailed techniques of bedside neurologic examinations. The necessary length of the complete examination and the potentially bewildering complexity of detailed neuroanatomy sometimes intimidate students and general physicians. This is unfortunate, because an understanding of a few fundamental principles about the nervous system plus the mastering of a relatively brief but systematically thorough approach to the examination can give a working knowledge that allows for the reliable and effective practice of medicine. The secret is to learn a relatively rapidly applied approach that covers the main elements of nervous system function and to be familiar with how to apply more exhaustive evaluations to selective functions if and when material in the history or the baseline examination suggests abnormalities in special parts.

An effective neurologic examination proceeds from general to specific in its principles and rostral to caudal in its anatomy. Such an examination checks on the integrity of major functions and yet avoids bogging down in details which do not relate to the complaints of most patients. In awake and talking patients, listen to them as they give their histories. Begin at that point to evaluate mental status and language (inconsistencies? vagueness on important points? word-blocking? circumlocutions? paraphasias? agrammaticisms?). Apply at least a brief mental examination on everyone, but be gentle and understanding: "How has your memory been? Can I just check a couple of points with you?" Check orientation. Examine memory for recent events, for public figures, and for three unrelated words at five minutes. Review the capacity to handle abstractions (boy—dwarf, small tree—bush, proverbs). Provide a problem in simple arithmetic (nickels in $1.35). Check serial sevens. Have the patient repeat five numbers backwards or the spelling of "world." But be patient and remember that anxiety can occlude the performance of even a normally good mind. Have the patient stand and walk; remember that the nervous system is the organ of communication and behavior, and that one learns most about man while watching him attempt natural tasks. To detect possible apraxia, watch the patient at least partially dress and undress; remark on alertness-dullness; hyperactivity-apathy; adventitious movement–akinesia; visible deformities, asymmetries, or weaknesses in functional tasks; hypertrophies-atrophies; cutaneous abnormalities (pox, birthmarks, café au lait spots, pigmented or hair spots over spinal defects); a straight, flat, or crooked spine. In other words, learn to observe constantly and closely, comparing always what you see with what you already have seen in thousands of people living everyday lives.

Examine cranial functions, screening certain structures and innervations in every patient. Palpate the skull and test the neck gently for suppleness and length. Then examine in everyone vision (rough fields and acuity), the optic fundi, pupillary activity, ocular movements, corneal reflexes, jaw movement, facial movement, bilateral hearing, swallowing, speaking, and breathing. One can omit or defer from most routine examinations such tests as those of smell, taste, facial sensation, labyrinthine-vestibular activity, sternocleidomastoid function, or the integrity of detailed tongue movements unless symptoms suggest the involvement of these bodily areas. Examine in everyone the extremities and trunk for symmetry (hypertrophy or atrophy), size, at least grossly for strength, muscle tonus, adventitious movements (e.g., tremors, fasciculations, tics), coordination (rhythmic movements and point-to-point tests), and reflexes. If the patient has no sensory symptoms, he is unlikely to have abnormal sensory signs. Nevertheless, make a brief check of the distal extremities for the threshold perception of vibration and pin prick before deciding that things are normal. Examine the plantar responses. Evaluate autonomic and sphincter functions as part of the general medical examination. Get in the habit of examining the neck over the carotid arteries for bruits that may herald partial stenoses. Above all, be systematic and consistent in the approach and *do not jump at diagnosis until all the evidence is in.* Doctors often make diagnoses quickly and surrender wrong ones reluctantly. By contrast, they view even partial unknowns as challenging problems. Try to choose the latter approach until matters become certain.

USE OF LABORATORY TESTS. Advances in laboratory methods during recent years have remarkably increased the accuracy of diagnosis and physiologic evaluations. At the same time, excessive technology raises the costs of medical care unnecessarily. More than anything else, the physician's ordering practices influence this aspect of health care costs. The doctor must recognize the precise advantages for both positive and negative knowledge that derive from each test, and order only those which add substantially to the patient's evaluation and treatment. To give an example: when managing an adult with recent onset of headache, the results of a computed tomographic scan, whether normal or abnormal, commonly help the doctor's management and provide the patient with great reassurance. However, to repeat the scan just to intensify reassurance for a querulous patient or an insecure physician wastes the time and resources of all concerned.

THE NEUROLOGIC HISTORY

Jerome B. Posner

In most respects, the neurologic history is similar to the general medical history. However, the neurologic history usually supplies a greater proportion of the diagnostically relevant information than does a medical history; many neurologic diseases (e.g., migraine and, often, epilepsy) are not accompanied by abnormal physical or laboratory findings, and in these instances the physician must depend solely on the history to reach an appropriate diagnosis. Even when the patient suffers from a neurologic disease marked by physical signs and/or laboratory abnormalities, the history usually supplies about 80 per cent of the total diagnostic information. Furthermore, because neurologic abnormalities affect such important functions as thinking, moving, and feeling, it is unusual to have significant abnormal signs which have not been reflected in symptoms. (Exceptions occur in demented patients and those with lesions of the nondominant parietal lobe, characterized by denial of disability. In these instances, abnormal behavior is recognized by family and friends.) Thus, findings on examination not recognized by the patient (or his family) are likely to be irrelevant or even misleading. By contrast, symptoms complained of by the patient, such as mild weakness or alterations of sensation, are probably significant even if too subtle to be detected by the most meticulous neurologic examination. Because patients so keenly appreciate neurologic symptoms, a meticulous history often allows a physician to localize the disease anatomically and to understand its pathophysiology even before he begins the physical examination.

Taking the neurologic history does (or should) occupy the majority of time spent with a patient suffering a neurologic disorder. At the completion of the history, the physician should be able either to make a definite diagnosis or to formulate three or four hypotheses which can be tested by the physical and laboratory examinations. Because there are an almost infinite number of potential questions which might be asked of a patient with a neurologic disorder, the physician must develop a strategy that allows him to achieve the maximal useful information in a reasonable period of time. Elements of that strategy are listed below.

BE INTERESTED AND SUPPORTIVE. The purpose of the neurologic history is not only to gain diagnostic information but also to learn enough about the patient's psychologic and social background to establish a satisfactory doctor-patient relationship. Diagnostic information is often lost when the patient does not volunteer symptoms that he believes would not interest the physician or that are too intimate or embarrassing to tell to an "unsympathetic stranger." Such information will be volunteered to the physician who demonstrates by his attitude his interest, reassurance, and support.

BE ALERT TO NONVERBAL CUES. What the patient does is often as important as what he says. The patient's overall appearance and demeanor, his tone of voice, or a sigh or a tear in discussing what appear to be relatively trivial symptoms may be important clues to an underlying depression or severe anxiety over those symptoms.

REQUIRE PRECISION. Interviewers should not accept jargon or names of diseases from the patient. Jargon terms such as "dizziness" or diagnostic appellations such as "sinus headache" require a thorough exploration of the exact nature of the symptom and its effect on the patient.

MAINTAIN A BALANCE BETWEEN LISTENING AND ASKING. Physicians should elicit the history in the patient's own words and, whenever possible, should allow the patient to tell the story without interruption. Excessive interruptions indicate to the patient that the physician is in a hurry or disinterested, and may lead the patient to exclude vital information. However, the physician must ask direct questions to encourage relevance, achieve precision, and place each symptom in its correct context. If not volunteered, the physician must ask about the intensity and frequency of the complained symptoms, their duration, events and factors that precipitate or relieve them, and any other symptoms associated in time with the patient's major complaint.

FORM HYPOTHESES. The physician cannot be a passive recipient of the patient's story. The patient supplies too much information, much of it not diagnostically relevant to recall at a later time, even with notes. Thus, while taking the history, one must sift and distill the information in order to retain what is relevant and discard the irrelevant. Concurrently, he must form hypotheses about the nature of the patient's symptoms as they are presented, and test those hypotheses by asking pertinent questions. Hypotheses are tested and refined during the course of taking the history, so that by the end the physician has three or four potential diagnoses to guide his physical and laboratory examinations. The best hypotheses are broad explanations of the patient's symptoms in anatomic and/or pathophysiologic terms, which are gradually refined into etiologic terms as the history develops. Hypotheses should give preference to those illnesses that are probable (i.e., common diseases are more likely than rare diseases), serious (e.g., brain tumors should be considered before tension headache), treatable (e.g., spinal cord meningioma and vitamin B_{12} deficiency should be ruled out before making a diagnosis of multiple sclerosis), and novel (some patients have rare diseases, and these should not be forgotten).

ALWAYS TAKE A COMPLETE HISTORY. Even if the diagnosis seems clear from the chief complaint and the present illness, other aspects of the patient's history must be elicited to ensure that other physical or psychologic disabilities are not playing a role in the patient's discomfort. In particular, inquiry must be made about the patient's mood (e.g., is he depressed or suicidal?), his usual daily activities (and whether the illness interferes with them), his sexual activities, the nature of psychologic and physical support at home, and his view of the illness and how it affects him.

END BY SUMMARIZING. At the end of the history it is useful to summarize the history as the physician understands it, asking the patient if the summary is correct and if anything has been missed.

OBTAIN FURTHER HISTORY FROM THE PATIENT'S FAMILY AND FRIENDS. If the history appears incomplete, and particularly if part of the illness involves changes in mental state or episodic unconsciousness, family, friends, and colleagues should be asked to supply missing elements, giving their views on how the signs and symptoms affect the patient's daily life.

GEAR THE NEUROLOGIC EXAMINATION TO THE HYPOTHESES. It is neither possible nor desirable to perform all elements of the neurologic examination on every patient. Thus, the hypotheses generated during the course of the history determine which of the nonroutine neurologic maneuvers the physician will carry out during the course of his examination. In similar fashion, hypotheses generated during the history direct the laboratory examination even in the presence of a normal neurologic examination. For example, if the history gives strong evidence of a left hemispheral mass lesion, failure to find a hemiparesis on examination does not rule out a brain tumor, and MR or CT scans should be performed. Even if the tests are initially uninformative, a strongly suggestive history requires that the doctor follow the patient closely.

456.2 Neurologic Diagnostic Procedures

Samuel Rapoport

LUMBAR PUNCTURE

With the advent of modern brain imaging devices, lumbar puncture now is performed far less often than in the past. Nevertheless, sampling the cerebrospinal fluid (CSF) remains an indispensable step in diagnosing several infectious diseases and is an emergency procedure in cases of suspected bacterial meningitis. Table 456–1 gives other indications and contraindications. Other considerations of when and when not to do lumbar puncture can be found in Chapter 462. Postlumbar puncture headache is discussed in Chapter 466.2.

ELECTRODIAGNOSTIC STUDIES

ELECTROENCEPHALOGRAPHY (EEG). The EEG is a record of the electronically amplified dendritic activity of the superficial layers of the cerebral cortex. The instrument is

TABLE 456–1. INDICATIONS AND CONTRAINDICATIONS FOR LUMBAR PUNCTURE

Diagnostic	Known or suspected meningitis-encephalitis
	Acute: bacterial, viral
	Subacute: tuberculous, syphilitic, fungal, neoplastic
	Chronic: syphilitic, granulomatous, neoplastic
	Intracranial-intraspinal hemorrhage (when no CT is available)
Useful	Multiple sclerosis
	Acute polyneuropathy
	Suspected benign intracranial hypertension (CT negative)
Contraindicated	Noninfectious states of undiagnosed increased intracranial pressure
	Thrombocytopenia or anticoagulated states
	Local skin or epidural infections
Therapeutic	Antimicrobial or anticancer therapy

indispensable for documenting the presence and type of epileptiform discharges, aiding the diagnosis of seizure disorders. In patients with altered states of consciousness, EEG helps differentiate seizures from metabolic encephalopathy and aids in distinguishing between organic and psychogenic causes of unresponsiveness. When seizures develop in comatose or therapeutically paralyzed patients, the EEG can delineate the response to the treatment, making it possible to titrate anticonvulsant dosage against cessation of epileptiform discharges. Absence of EEG activity supports the diagnosis of brain death.

SENSORY EVOKED POTENTIALS. Measurement of the EEG time-locked to a visual, auditory, or somatosensory stimulus generates modality-specific potentials that are highly reproducible and provide information on the integrity of the pathway carrying the signal.

Visual Evoked Potentials (VEP). VEPs usually are performed by having the subject fixate on a reversing black-white checkerboard pattern. Electrodes placed over the scalp record a positive potential (P_{100}), with mean latency of 100 msec from stimulus onset. The latency of the P_{100} is related to conduction in the optic nerve and central visual pathways. The method is highly sensitive for detecting demyelination of the optic nerve, whether produced by compression, toxic agents, metabolic abnormalities, or multiple sclerosis. P_{100} latency prolongation can occur when intracranial pressure is elevated and in the presence of degenerative neurologic disorders.

Brain-Stem Auditory Evoked Potentials (BAEP). Presentation of a white noise click stimulus to the ear generates a series of potentials from the brain-stem auditory relay pathway, which can be recorded over the scalp at the vertex. Five clinically relevant potentials occur within the first 10 msec following the stimulus. The first potential recorded is generated by the auditory nerve, and subsequent potentials are generated, respectively, in the auditory nuclei, superior olive, lateral lemniscus, and inferior colliculus. The results provide a measure of conduction between various points along the auditory pathway between the eighth nerve and colliculus. BAEPs detect abnormalities due to demyelinative, destructive, or compressive lesions affecting these pathways. In the appropriate clinical setting, absence of BAEP potentials rostral to the auditory nuclei (wave II) supports the diagnosis of brain death.

Somatosensory Evoked Potentials (SEP). Stimulation of a peripheral nerve by pulses of constant voltage or constant current gives rise to potentials that can be recorded over the spine and scalp. The median or peroneal nerves are most often stimulated. Stimulation of a lower-extremity nerve, such as the peroneal, gives rise to a volley whose transit can be recorded at all levels of the spine. If bipolar electrode arrays are placed over the spine, the latency of the recorded potential increases progressively from lumbar to cervical spine and brain. Measurement permits calculation of a conduction velocity that is thought to reflect conduction in the posterior columns of the spinal cord. The time interval between the potential recorded at the cauda equina and over the scalp measures total conduction time in the somatosensory pathway. Any lesion, whether demyelinative, nutritional, compressive, or destructive, that affects this ascending pathway in spinal cord or brain-stem can delay the total conduction time. The technique can also be used to measure conduction velocity in the most proximal segments of nerves and can supplement other studies (see below) in the diagnosis of radiculopathies, plexopathies, or proximal nerve entrapments such as occur in the thoracic outlet.

ELECTROMYOGRAPHY AND NERVE CONDUCTION STUDIES. Appropriate percutaneous electrical stimulation of a peripheral nerve excites the nerve to generate an action potential. When stimulating motor nerves, one places recording electrodes over a muscle and records the evoked muscle action potential on an oscilloscope. The nerve innervating

TABLE 456–2. PATTERN OF EMG AND NERVE CONDUCTION ABNORMALITIES IN MONONEUROPATHY, POLYNEUROPATHY, RADICULOPATHY, AXONOPATHY, AND MOTONEURON DISEASE

	EMG Abnormality	Nerve Conduction Abnormality
Mononeuropathy	Limited to muscles innervated by damaged nerve	Limited to damaged nerve
Polyneuropathy	Diffuse	Diffuse
Radiculopathy	Limited to muscles innervated by damaged root	Usually none
Axonopathy/motoneuron disease	Diffuse	None

that muscle is stimulated at various points along its length. The time from each site of stimulation to onset of the evoked muscle response is recorded and the conduction velocity is determined by dividing the time difference between different stimulation sites into the distance that separates them (meters per second). To record conduction velocity in sensory nerves, one stimulates cutaneous nerve branches distally and places recording electrodes over the nerve at various proximal sites; conversely, proximal nerve branches can be stimulated and potentials recorded over distal branches. Time interval divided into distance again provides the conduction velocity. The F-response gives an indication of conduction in motor nerves from the site of stimulation antidromically to the motoneuron and orthodromically back to the site of recording; when analyzed in conjunction with the conduction velocity of the more distal portions of the nerve, it provides a measure of conduction in the proximal portions of a motor nerve and ventral root. The H-reflex provides the electrical equivalent of the stretch reflex by stimulating sensory fibers of the posterior tibial nerve in the popliteal fossa at low intensities and recording the muscle evoked action potential from the soleus muscle.

Electromyography (EMG) is performed by inserting a needle electrode into the muscle to record the structure's electrical activity (Fig. 456–1). Under normal circumstances muscle at rest is silent, but in denervated or diseased muscle the membranes become spontaneously excitable, generating fibrillation potentials of small amplitude and injury currents, which are recorded as small-amplitude, sharp, positive potentials. When the nerve itself is diseased, entire motor units may become spontaneously active. The resulting fasciculations are often visible percutaneously and can be detected by the electrode. Furthermore, when damaged axons cease to innervate muscle fibers, remaining axons gradually sprout collaterals that reinnervate the denervated fibers; consequently the size of the few remaining motor units increases. As a result in partially denervated muscles one records during voluntary contraction a decrease in the number and an increase in the size of the electrical potentials generated by the activated motor units. By contrast, as muscle fibers degenerate in primary disease of muscle, the size of motor units decreases, since each nerve now innervates fewer fibers: during voluntary contraction the number of activated units is normal but their amplitude is smaller. The anatomic distribution of abnormalities helps differentiate a mononeuropathy from a generalized neuropathy and radiculopathy from a neuropathy. In primary myopathies, the distribution of abnormality helps in characterizing the myopathy itself. Tables 456–2 and 456–3 provide guides to the usefulness and pertinent changes in electrophysiologic tests in various neuromuscular disorders.

These peripheral nerve and muscle electrophysiologic studies assist in determining whether disease involves nerve, muscle, or both and in determining the distribution of abnormality. They facilitate the differentiation of demyelinating neuropathy from axonal neuropathy, neuropathy from radiculopathy, and primary muscle disease from disease of the motor unit. Demyelinating neuropathies affect mainly large fibers and slow the conduction velocity. When disease damages axons in addition to myelin, there is a decrease in the number of axons that can be electrically activated, resulting in a diminution in the site of the compound action potential.

NEUROMUSCULAR TRANSMISSION STUDIES

Diseases of the neuromuscular junction (Ch. 518) are characterized by normal nerve conduction velocity and usually a normal EMG. Repetitive electrical activation of the neuromuscular junction, however, will produce either an abnormal diminution or an abnormal facilitation of the evoked muscle action potential. In myasthenia gravis repetitive stimulation of a peripheral nerve most often causes a rapid progressive decrement of the amplitude of the muscle evoked action potential owing to rapid saturation of the small number of

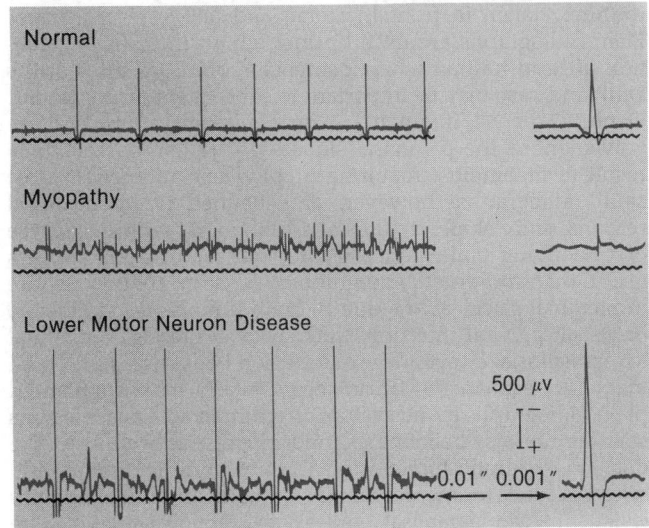

FIGURE 456–1. Diagram of muscle electrical activity showing motor action potentials during weak voluntary contraction of the biceps brachii. Note the normal amplitude and duration of the potentials on the top line compared to small, short duration potentials in muscular dystrophy and the enlarged amplitude and duration in amyotrophic lateral sclerosis. (From Aronson AE, Anger RG, et al.: Clinical Examinations in Neurology. 5th ed. Mayo Clinic and Mayo Foundation, 1981.)

TABLE 456–3. DIFFERENTIATION AMONG MYOPATHY, AXONOPATHY, MYELINOPATHY, AND RADICULOPATHY USING ELECTROPHYSIOLOGIC STUDIES

	Myopathy	Axonopathy	Myelinopathy	Radiculopathy
Nerve conduction velocity	Normal	Normal	Slow	Normal
F-response	Normal	Normal	Delayed/absent	Delayed/absent
H-reflex*	Normal	Normal	Delayed/absent	Delayed/absent
EMG				
Voluntary contraction	Predominance of small motor units	Predominance of large motor units	Normal	Normal/some large motor units
Spontaneous activity	Fibrillations	Fibrillations, fasciculations	Normal	Fibrillations, fasciculations

*Usually studied with posterior tibial nerve stimulation, recording the soleus contraction, thus providing an index of S1 root function only

postsynaptic receptors by the released acetylcholine. In botulism and Eaton-Lambert myasthenic syndrome, where the defect is on the presynaptic membrane, repetitive stimulation of the nerve overcomes the presynaptic blockade of acetylcholine release and usually elicits an increase in the size of the muscle evoked action potentials.

Single-fiber EMG (Jitter studies), using specially designed needle electrodes, positioned between two muscle fibers innervated by similar length branches of the same axon, permits detection of conduction failure at the neuromuscular junction.

Aminoff MJ (ed.): Electrodiagnosis in Clinical Neurology. 2nd ed. New York, Churchill Livingstone, 1986. *Twenty-two authoritative but introductory chapters cover most topics in the discipline including EEG, evoked responses, EMG, and others.*

Chiappa KH: Evoked Potentials in Clinical Medicine. New York, Raven Press, 1983. *A good summary of its topic.*

Kimura J: Electrodiagnosis in Diseases of Nerve and Muscle. Philadelphia, F. A. Davis, 1983. *This monograph provides the most thorough and clear description of the physiology and application of neuromuscular electrical studies.*

Spehlmann R: EEG Primer. New York, Elsevier, 1981. *An excellent general reference on electroencephalography.*

456.3 Radiologic Imaging Techniques in the Diagnosis and Care of the Neurologic Patient

Michael Deck

THE SKULL AND BRAIN

PLAIN RADIOGRAPHY. Plain radiographs of the skull are routinely taken in frontal, lateral, and half-axial projection. Plain radiographs are useful principally in the initial evaluation of head trauma where demonstration of fractures of the vault and base may be important to subsequent management. Depressed bone fragments may require elevation, and involvement of the paranasal sinuses or mastoid air cells may result in meningitis, requiring prophylactic antibiotics. Most skull radiographs, however, are obtained for medicolegal reasons, since skull fractures correlate poorly with the degree of underlying brain injury. Plain skull radiographs are less useful than computed tomographic (CT) scans to demonstrate intracranial calcifications due to brain tumors or to parasitic, bacterial, or viral infections such as cysticercosis, congenital toxoplasmosis, or cytomegalic inclusion body disease. CT and magnetic resonance (MR) images similarly have supplanted plain radiographs in the evaluation of intracranial mass lesions such as tumors, hematomas, and infarcts, as well as in the detection of optic foramen enlargement due to tumors and sclerosis due to meningiomas. Tumors and inflammatory lesions of the paranasal sinuses and abnormalities of the craniovertebral junction are also demonstrated better by CT or MRI.

COMPUTED TOMOGRAPHY. CT scanning has had a major influence in the evaluation of the patient with a neurologic disorder, supplanting radiographs of the skull and rendering pneumoencephalography obsolete. It has also reduced the need for cerebral angiography. CT images from current equipment demonstrate anatomical structures in the skull and brain with high spatial resolution. Fresh hemorrhages within the brain, subarachnoid, subdural, or epidural spaces are demonstrated because of the greater x-ray attenuation of clotted blood. The appearances of areas of calcification may be similar but are usually more irregular and have a higher attenuation value. Contrast enhancement with intravenous iodinated material is used in many CT examinations to demonstrate normal vascular structures as well as the abnormal endothelial permeability that accompanies certain types of tumors and inflammatory processes.

Although contrast material can add critical information in many CT examinations of the brain, it also carries a risk of adverse reactions due to anaphylaxis. The general population has about a 1:10,000 chance of serious anaphylactic reaction and a 1:40,000 chance of death. These dangers increase fourfold in patients with a previous allergic history to iodinated contrast material, iodine, or shellfish. The risks may be reduced by administering an antihistamine drug immediately before or 50 mg of prednisone orally 12 to 24 hours before the injection.

Special techniques can be used to improve resolution and generate physiologic data. These include:

- *Coronal projections* to image the floor of the skull, the sella turcica, and the petrous bones.
- *Image reformatting* for the generation of coronal or sagittal images from multiple axial images. The technique depends on absolute immobilization of the patient; it produces good resolution but results in greater amounts of radiation to the brain and, potentially, the eye.
- *Ultrathin sections* of 1.5 mm or less for examining areas requiring high detail, such as the sella turcica and petrous bones.
- *Bone targeting* employing a special reconstruction algorithm so as to demonstrate fine anatomy such as the ossicles and osseous labyrinth of the petrous bone.
- *Dynamic scanning* achieved by performing rapid sequence scans after rapidly injecting a bolus of contrast agent. The subsequent contrast enhancement and wash-out can help to differentiate an aneurysm or arteriovenous malformation from a vascular tumor.
- *CT cisternography and myelography* performed by injecting water-soluble nonionic contrast material (Iohexol or Iopamidol) into the subarachnoid space and running the contrast material to the area of suspected abnormality for scanning. This technique may help to delineate tumors of the sella region, the foramen magnum, and spinal canal.

MAGNETIC RESONANCE IMAGING (MRI, NUCLEAR MAGNETIC RESONANCE IMAGING). MRI is a rapidly developing technology that, in the near future, will probably replace CT as the examination of choice for most neurologic conditions (Table 456–4). Nuclear magnetic resonance occurs when hydrogen atoms or certain other elements with an odd number of nuclear particles, such as sodium or phosphorous, are placed in an intense magnetic field varying between 3,000 and 15,000 gauss (0.3–1.5 tesla). The nuclei behave like small magnets and align themselves in the field. When stimulated by a pulse of specific radio frequency energy, determined by the intensity of the main magnetic field, the nuclei flip off axis. While in this energized state, the nuclei spin in phase;

TABLE 456–4. IMAGING MODALITIES OF CHOICE IN DISEASES OF THE BRAIN

	Primary	Supplementary
Supratentorial tumor	MRI >* CT	Often arteriogram
Vascular lesions		
Infarcts	MRI = CT	Occasionally arteriogram
Hematoma	MRI > CT	
Aneurysm and AVM	MRI > CT	Usually arteriogram
Trauma		
Acute	Plain film	CT > MRI
Subacute	MRI >> CT	
Chronic	MRI = CT	
White matter disease	MRI >> CT	
Inflammatory disease		
Encephalitis	MRI > CT	
Abscess	MRI > CT	
Acute meningitis	MRI = CT	
Chronic meningitis	MRI = CT	
Congenital abnormalities	MRI > CT	
Sellar and parasellar tumor	MRI >> CT	Often arteriogram
Posterior fossa	MRI >> CT	Occasionally arteriogram
Base of skull	MRI > CT	

*> = better than

they then emit a small radio frequency signal, as they subsequently relax, into their original alignment with the main magnetic field. The MR image is produced from multiple MR phenomena, transformed by a computer using techniques similar to those employed in computerized tomography. The resulting images demonstrate a high contrast between various tissues due largely to differences at which magnetized nuclei reassume their original state. MR images may be obtained in axial, coronal, sagittal, or oblique planes simply by changing the switching of the instrument's several magnetizing coils. Paramagnetic contrast agents developed for use with MR imaging contain elements such as gadolinium that have a marked effect on the T_1, or spin-lattice relaxation time of protons. The agents, used in a manner similar to iodinated contrast media in CT, demonstrate in the tissue, areas of increased vascularity and/or permeability. Recently, MRI methods have been developed to quantify pulsatile and nonpulsatile flow of blood within the arteries and veins. The resulting images have a resolution similar to that obtainable with intravenous digital subtraction angiography techniques. In the future similar approaches may allow quantitation of the flow of cerebrospinal fluid through the aqueduct and posterior fossa in various disease entities such as aqueduct stenosis and transtentorial brain herniation.

CEREBRAL ANGIOGRAPHY. Most cerebral angiograms are performed with an intra-arterial catheter inserted over a guide wire into the femoral artery and passed upward to the aortic arch or into the carotid or vertebral arteries.

Although cerebral angiography is a relatively safe procedure in experienced hands, complications, including arterial damage, emboli to the brain, and contrast neurotoxicity, can occur in one to two per cent of patients. New less toxic nonionic contrast agents are now replacing traditional contrast materials.

Digital Subtraction Angiography (DSA). Arterial DSA uses computerized imaging enhancement to improve the contrast of the injected agent and lower the dose of the contrast agent.

Intravenous DSA is performed using similar equipment and rapid injections of contrast material into a peripheral vein or the right atrium. Intravenous DSA may be performed as an outpatient procedure for demonstrating the aortic arch and great vessels in the neck and the intracranial cerebral arteries and veins. It is not satisfactory for demonstrating small aneurysms of the circle of Willis or intracranial arterial abnormalities such as occlusions from emboli or vasculitis. Its rate of complications is about the same as that of arterial angiography.

THE SPINE

RADIOGRAPHY. *Conventional radiography* (plain films) *of the spine* demonstrates bony abnormalities such as degenerative disc disease, primary and metastatic tumors, and fractures of the vertebral bodies. Plain radiographs are the best method for demonstrating osteophytes in the neural foramina in the cervical, thoracic, and lumbar spine. Plain films should be obtained prior to myelography to identify skeletal anomalies at the thoracolumbar and lumbosacral junction.

CT. CT of the spine demonstrates abnormalities of the spinal cord, meninges, vertebral bodies and intervertebral articulations, and paravertebral and prevertebral soft tissues. CT supplemented with intravenous contrast enhancement may be used to demonstrate vascular tumors of the spinal cord and meninges and can be valuable in differentiating recurrent herniation of lumbar intervertebral discs from postsurgical scarring.

CT plus myelography gives improved delineation of subtle nerve root displacement due to herniated discs and osteophytes. It has been useful in demonstrating cysts and syringomyelia of the cord, where entry of water-soluble contrast

agent into the cavity may be detected by CT performed 12 to 24 hours after myelographic injection.

MRI. *MRI of the spine* is rapidly replacing CT because it gives better resolution of the spinal cord, subarachnoid space, and vertebral anatomy, particularly in sagittal and coronal planes. Surface coils can even image the internal structure of the spinal cord.

MYELOGRAPHY. Myelography is the most sensitive examination for demonstrating mass lesions of the spinal canal and for localizing them in the extradural, intradural, or intramedullary compartments. Contrast agents containing iodine, including water-soluble nonionic materials, are introduced by lumbar or cervical puncture. These agents are hyperbaric and flow under the influence of gravity. By tilting the patient on a radiographic table, the contrast may be manipulated under fluoroscopic control from the lumbosacral region to the base of the skull.

Complications of myelography include rare toxic reactions from the contrast material, injury to nerve roots by the lumbar puncture needle, bleeding into the spinal canal, infection, and aggravation of spinal cord compression by mass lesions, due to change in the pressure in the subarachnoid space. With new contrast agents, myelography is now sufficiently safe to perform as an outpatient procedure.

IMAGING TECHNIQUES IN SPECIFIC DISEASE CATEGORIES
(Table 456–4)

TUMORS OF THE CEREBRAL HEMISPHERES. MRI is often superior to computed tomography, being more sensitive in detecting small lesions and usually better able to demonstrate whether a tumor is intra- or extra-axial in location. The extent of cerebral edema is better discerned on MR than on CT images.

Coronal and sagittal MR images permit more accurate anatomic localization. The use of paramagnetic contrast agents increases the sensitivity of MR for detecting meningiomas and multiple metastatic foci.

VASCULAR BRAIN LESIONS. *Cerebral Infarcts.* In acute stroke, CT scanning is currently the imaging procedure of choice. It best determines whether a stroke consists of a frank hematoma or is due to a hemorrhagic or nonhemorrhagic infarct. These considerations may guide therapy using anticoagulants. After 48 hours MRI becomes more sensitive to blood than CT. In the future, novel image-aquisition techniques may improve the sensitivity of MRI during the early stages of hemorrhage or hemorrhagic infarct. MRI is superior to CT in demonstrating occlusions of the sagittal or other major venous sinuses. MRI is also superior to CT in demonstrating narrowing or occlusion of major arteries that may cause the infarct.

Arteriography is generally required if one wishes to confirm that infarction is due to an embolus or to primary intracranial arterial disease. Such considerations, however, are not of concern in managing most cases.

Hematomas and Hemorrhage. MRI is superior to CT in the demonstration of extra-axial subdural, extradural, and intraparenchymal hemorrhage because, after the first 48 hours, the presence of methemoglobin greatly increases the MR signal. The high contrast of the hemorrhagic collection remains for six to eight weeks on MRI, whereas the increase in density by CT images generally disappears by ten to 14 days. Late in the evolution of a hematoma, a low signal rim of hypointensity appears on MRI probably from a paramagnetic effect of hemosiderin deposits in macrophages.

MRI is very sensitive and fairly specific for demonstrating recurrent hemorrhage due to cryptic arteriovenous malformation or cavernous hemangiomas. Cerebral arteriography is necessary to diagnose or exclude an arteriovenous malformation or arterial aneurysm as the underlying cause of an intracranial hemorrhage.

Aneurysm and Arteriovenous Malformation. MRI is superior to CT for demonstrating aneurysms and arteriovenous malformations that have not bled. Before surgical intervention, however, cerebral angiography is essential for demonstrating the precise anatomy of the aneurysm and for detecting multiple feeding and draining vessels that often characterize an arteriovenous malformation.

HEAD TRAUMA. Conventional radiographs of the skull should be obtained to detect fractures of the skull and to identify associated fractures of the facial bones or cervical spine.

Computed tomography is the best method for demonstrating acute brain contusion or intracranial hemorrhage during the first 48 hours. Later, MRI is superior for showing small hemorrhagic collections, cerebral contusions, and axonal shearing injuries.

CT and MRI are probably equally effective in detecting late consequences of head trauma such as atrophy, hydrocephalus, and encephalomalacia.

WHITE MATTER DISEASE. (Multiple sclerosis, multiple infarctions, various leukoencephalopathies).

MRI is considerably more sensitive than CT in detecting abnormalities in the cerebral white matter. The MRI appearances are not specific, however, and their presence often correlates poorly with the clinical status of the patient. MRI can play a confirmatory role in the clinical diagnosis of multiple sclerosis. Other white matter diseases are diagnosed by morphologic configuration and appropriate associated clinical findings.

INFLAMMATORY BRAIN LESIONS. Both MRI and CT can demonstrate the changes of herpes simplex encephalitis, progressive multifocal leucoencephalopathy (PML) or cytomegalic inclusion body disease.

MRI is superior to contrast-enhanced CT in demonstrating intracranial abscess formation. Typically, an abscess is best shown on a T_2 image owing to the hyperintensity of the central purulent collection and surrounding edema, with a hypointense rim representing the abscess wall. MRI is substantially more sensitive than CT in detecting granulomas, particularly in immunosuppressed patients, and is the procedure of choice to study patients suspected of having toxoplasmosis.

In chronic or carcinomatous meningitis, both MRI and CT may demonstrate changes in the appearance of the meninges, but they play no role in the diagnosis of acute bacterial meningitis.

CONGENITAL ANOMALIES. Both MRI and CT can demonstrate agenesis of the corpus callosum, Dandy Walker cysts, and congenital hydrocephalus. MRI is superior in cases of aqueductal stenosis and Chiari I and II malformations because the technique can produce sagittal images.

SELLAR AND PARASELLAR TUMORS. MRI is superior to CT in delineating many tumors in or adjacent to the sella turcica because of its excellent resolution in the coronal and sagittal planes. There are good demonstrations of the carotid arteries and relatively specific appearances of hemorrhagic pituitary tumors and craniopharyngiomas. The capacity of

TABLE 456–5. IMAGING MODALITIES OF CHOICE FOR DISEASE OF THE SPINE

	Primary	Supplementary
Metastatic bone disease	Plain film and radionuclide scan	MRI and CT myelography
Degenerative disc disease	Plain film (MRI > CT)	Myelogram
Spinal cord tumor	Plain film and (MRI >> CT)	Myelogram
Spinal AVM	(MRI = CT) and myelogram	Arteriogram
Meningeal carcinomatosis	Myelogram	CSF cytology

MRI to detect pituitary microadenomas has not yet been fully determined.

POSTEROR FOSSA TUMORS. MRI is superior to CT in imaging both intra-axial and extra-axial tumors of the posterior fossa because of the absence of bone-induced artifacts, superior resolution in coronal and sagittal planes, and relatively high contrast between normal and abnormal tissues.

THE SPINE (Table 456–5). Conventional radiographs are essential to the detection of spinal deformity, bone destruction, degenerative changes at the intervertebral articulations and congenital anomalies.

With the increased resolution provided by surface coils, MRI is superior to CT in the evaluation of degenerative and neoplastic disorders of the spinal cord and canal as well as detecting intrinsic cord lesions such as cysts and syringomyelia.

Degenerated and herniated intervertebral discs are demonstrated accurately with MR images in the sagittal and axial planes. Cord compression due to metastatic disease is well shown by MRI, making myelography unnecessary in many cases. MRI is more sensitive in its detection of intraosseous metastases than is plain film, CT, or radionuclide scanning.

Myelography is superior to MRI and CT in the detection of small intradural masses such as neurofibromas and meningeal carcinomatosis, although in the latter condition even myelography may remain normal in more than half the cases.

Myelography is more sensitive than MRI or CT in detecting arteriovenous malformations of the spinal cord. In such cases, selective spinal arteriography is required as a preoperative measure in order to demonstrate the feeding arteries and draining veins.

Bradley WG, Waluch V, Yadley RA, et al.: Comparison of CT and MR in 400 patients with suspected disease of the brain and cervical spinal cord. Radiology 152:695, 1984.

Brant-Zawadski M, Normal D (eds.): Magnetic resonance imaging of the central nervous system. New York, Raven Press, 1987. *An up-to-date atlas of MRI demonstrating the classic appearances of a variety of brain lesions.*

Franken EA, Berbaum KS, Dunn V, et al.: Impact of MR imaging on clinical diagnosis and management: a prospective study. Radiology 161:377, 1986.

Newton TH, Potts, DG (eds.): Advanced Imaging Techniques. Modern Neuroradiology, vol. 2. San Anselmo, Clavedel Press, 1983. *Contains, among other useful information, an excellent description of the physics and techniques of various imaging modalities written for the nonphysicist.*

Masters SJ, McClean PM, Arcaresa JS: Skull x-ray examinations after head trauma. N Engl J Med 316:84, 1987. *A multidisciplinary, prospective study of 7035 patients with acute head trauma identified as (a) high-risk patients with severe head injuries and prominent accompanying clinical abnormalities and (b) low-risk patients who were asymptomatic or had mild symptoms. CT scanning was useful only in the high-risk group; skull radiographs could have been safely omitted in a prospectively identified low-risk group.*

SECTION TWO / DISORDERS OF CEREBRAL FUNCTION

457 DISTURBANCES OF CONSCIOUSNESS AND AROUSAL

Fred Plum and Jerome B. Posner

DEFINITIONS AND MECHANISMS OF ALTERED CONSCIOUSNESS

DEFINITIONS. Consciousness is a state expressed in two dimensions: wakefulness and the self-aware cognition of past events and future anticipations which accompanies the normal wakeful state. Disease or dysfunction that impairs this combination usually causes readily identifiable conditions as defined in Table 457–1. Occasionally, however, either certain forms of neurologic damage or the presence of a severe psychiatric disorder can mimic an unconscious state. Table 457–2 defines these potentially deceptive states of pseudocoma.

Impaired consciousness can be *sustained*, i.e., prolonged for periods lasting for hours or much longer, or *brief*, with the lapse enduring for no more than a few seconds to an hour or so. The longer the duration of an abnormal state of consciousness, the more likely it is to reflect structural damage to the brain rather than a transient alteration in its function. The following sections will discuss these states in greater detail.

The normal capacity to awaken and direct attention depends upon anatomic-vegetative arousal mechanisms lodged within or in close association with the ascending reticular activating system (ARAS). The ARAS consists of a loosely organized, fairly dense column of neurons which extends forward along the brain's central core from approximately the upper third of the pons to the deep reaches of the hypothalamus and the thalamus. Thus far it has not been possible to identify a single neurochemical anatomy for the system. The self-aware, cognitive aspects of consciousness depend largely on the interconnected neural networks of the cerebral hemispheres, especially their cortical mantles. Normal conscious behavior depends on the continuous, effective interaction of these cortical systems with the subcortical activating mechanisms.

TABLE 457–1. STATES OF ALTERED CONSCIOUSNESS OR UNRESPONSIVENESS

Coma: A state of unarousable unresponsiveness; even strong stimuli fail to elicit recognizable psychologic responses.
Stupor: Spontaneous unarousability interruptable only by vigorous, direct external stimulation.
Hypersomnia, pathologic drowsiness, obtundation: Terms applied to an increase above the patient's normal sleep/wake ratio, often accompanied by reduced attention and interest in the environment.
Delirium: An acute or subacute reduction in awareness, attention, and perception ("clouding of consciousness") usually fluctuating and accompanied by abnormal sleep/wake patterns and, often, psychomotor disturbances
Syncope: Brief loss of consciousness due to failure of global cerebrovascular perfusion.
Dementia: A sustained or permanent multidimensional or global decline in cognitive functions without a reduction in the level of arousal during wakefulness.
Vegetative state: A sustained, complete loss of self-aware cognition with wake/sleep cycles and other autonomic functions remaining relatively intact. The condition can either follow acute, severe bilateral cerebral damage or develop gradually as the end stage of a progressive dementia.

Impaired consciousness can be partial or complete, acute or occasionally chronic. By definition, there is at least some change of the normal wake-sleep cycle toward a reduction in alertness and attention. These reductions often are accompanied by diffuse impairments of normal cognitive activity, reflecting the close interaction between cortical and cognitive mechanisms and the ascending activating systems. Accordingly, acute lesions that affect either the ascending system or diffusely impair large amounts of the cortex will reduce the level of consciousness. Since its anatomic subcortical cross-sectional area is small, yet projects diffusely to the cortex, acute damage to or depression of the ARAS carries a high risk of blocking cortical arousal. By contrast, any given region of cortex feeds back to only a limited area of the activating system so that disease at the cerebral level usually must produce extensive and bilateral cortical dysfunction to cause stupor or coma. The tempo of the damage also is important. With disease that gradually affects either the cortex or the ascending activating mechanisms alone, arousal mechanisms tend to adapt rapidly. Slowly advancing, diffuse cerebral disease causes a multifaceted dementia rather than the clouded consciousness with fluctuating or reduced arousal that results from acute disturbances. In the subcortical reticular system, posterior hypothalamic damage is essentially the only locus where a chronic lesion will produce a permanent loss or severe reduction of the capacity to reawaken.

Loss of consciousness from medical causes can be brief, a matter of minutes to an hour or so, or it can be sustained for many hours, days, or sometimes even weeks. Between sustained and brief impairment of unconsciousness, the causes, management, and prognosis tend to differ importantly. Accordingly, the following sections discuss these conditions separately.

SUSTAINED IMPAIRMENTS OF CONSCIOUSNESS

ETIOLOGY. Three kinds of disorders produce sustained impairment of consciousness. All act either by (1) directly impairing ascending activating mechanisms, (2) affecting the cerebral cortex diffusely and bilaterally, or (3) causing simultaneous abnormalities in both processes. The three classes include (a) supratentorial mass or destructive lesions if they either secondarily compress or directly destroy deep midline thalamic-hypothalamic activating structures, (b) posterior fossa mass or destructive lesions that compress or destroy the brain stem's central reticular formation, or (c) metabolic diffuse abnormalities that acutely or subacutely interfere widely and bilaterally with the functions of the cerebral hemispheres. Metabolic abnormalities especially tend to affect both cerebral

TABLE 457–2. PSEUDOCOMA: STATES RESEMBLING ACUTE UNCONSCIOUSNESS BUT WITH SELF-AWARENESS PRESERVED

Locked-in state: Preservation of intellectual activity accompanied by severe or total incapacity to express voluntary responses due to damage to or dysfunction of descending motor pathways in the brain or peripheral motor nerves. Most but not all such patients can use vertical eye movements to signal by code.
Psychogenic unresponsiveness
1. *Catatonic States.* Uncommon conditions in either schizophrenic or severe depressive illness which resemble organic stupor. Mutism, bilateral motor resistance, hypokinesia, and even rigidity are common. Pathologic reflexes as well as abnormal brain images, EEGs, or laboratory chemical tests all are absent.
2. *Hysteria-malingering.* Unarousable unresponsiveness, usually of brief duration, unaccompanied by physiologic abnormalities and often associated with obviously factitious responses to stimulation.

TABLE 457–3. THE COMMON CAUSES OF STUPOR AND COMA

Supratentorial lesions (causing secondary upper brain stem dysfunction)
  Cerebral hemorrhage
  Large cerebral infarction
  Subdural hematoma
  Epidural hematoma
  Brain tumor
  Brain abscess (rare)
Subtentorial lesions (compressing or destroying the rostral reticular formation)
  Pontine or cerebellar hemorrhage
  Brain stem infarction
  Brain stem or cerebellar tumor
  Cerebellar abscess
Metabolic and diffuse lesions (see also Table 457–4)
  Anoxia or ischemia
  Hypoglycemia
  Nutritional deficiency
  Endogenous toxin due to organ failure or deficiency
  Exogenous poison
  Infections
    Meningitis
    Encephalitis
  Ionic and electrolyte disorders
  Concussion and postictal states
Psychogenic unresponsiveness

and ascending arousal mechanisms concurrently. Table 457–3 enumerates the common specific causes of stupor and coma according to these mechanisms.

PATHOPHYSIOLOGY OF MASS LESIONS. Intracranial mass and destructive lesions initiate a characteristic chain of events whose outcome and effects depend on (1) the anatomic locus of the abnormality, (2) its size and rate of enlargement, and (3) the degree of associated reactive changes they engender in adjacent cellular and intercellular spaces. The major factors include surrounding intra- and extracellular edema, local vasodilatation, and the inflammatory and glial reaction infiltrates that especially surround local areas of hemorrhage, necrosis, or infection. In many instances these secondary responses create the largest part of shift and compression of normal brain tissue that accompanies intracranial mass lesions.

As mass lesions form and enlarge within the cranial cavity, local intracranial compliance declines so that adjacent and, eventually, remote tissues become distorted and compressed, and the intracranial pressure rises. The pressure rise occurs, first in microportions of the region of local enlargement and then more generally. Gradually, the disease process interferes with the ventricular and subarachnoid fluid outflow. Eventually, the intracranial distortion and pressure increase sufficiently to impede the blood supply in areas of compressed tissue. When this occurs, arteriolar resistance intermittently fails, leading to temporary increases in intracranial blood volume which produce episodes of increased intracranial pressure (plateau waves) that last for seconds to minutes and may worsen neurologic function.

Functional neurologic abnormalities accompanying the above pathophysiologic changes occur earliest in tissue in and adjacent to the primary lesion but also gradually develop in more remote brain areas that are especially vulnerable to being compressed against unyielding edges of bone or dura. Particularly at risk are structures that become squeezed against the falx cerebri or the restricted apertures of the tentorial notch or the foramen magnum, into which impaction or actual herniation can occur.

With enlarging *supratentorial lesions* (i.e., those that affect the cerebral hemispheres or diencephalon), the process that most often causes stupor or coma consists of first lateral and then downward enlargement of the mass lesion so as to compress and displace the diencephalon. Sooner or later, and especially if the condition occurs rapidly (e.g., with acute, large cerebral hemorrhage) or remains untreated, either the diencephalon impacts across the tentorial opening against the midbrain or the medial temporal lobe shifts laterally into the

tentorial notch. When this occurs, the temporal lobe either compresses its hippocampus against the ipsilateral midbrain or squeezes the contralateral cerebral peduncle against the opposite tentorial edge. These potentially catastrophic herniations are late changes and generally are prevented by present-day intensive treatment.

The scenario with *subtentorial lesions* differs somewhat from the above. Subtentorial abnormalities, such as infarcts or hemorrhages, that directly damage or destroy the midbrain or upper pontine reticulum will produce coma from the start. Expanding lesions that lie outside this restricted brain stem area also can cause coma if they either directly compress the vital midbrain-pontine arousal mechanisms or push the midbrain upward toward the tentorial notch so that it impacts against the lower diencephalon. Acute downward herniation impacting the cerebellum and medulla into the foramen magnum is uncommon except when a deep cerebellar hemorrhage suddenly enlarges or bleeds into the fourth ventricle or when lumbar puncture is performed in the presence of an expanding posterior fossa lesion. The latter, by lowering spinal fluid pressures below the foramen, invites descent and impaction of the cerebellar tonsils.

Clinical Features of Supratentorial Mass Lesions Causing Stupor or Coma. The clinical picture of supratentorial mass lesions producing stupor or coma has several distinctive features. Localizing symptoms such as frontal headache, focal seizures, or other changes consistent with unilateral hemispheric disease almost always precede the development of unconsciousness. Physically, most patients demonstrate a combination of *focal* hemispheral signs, e.g., sensorimotor defect, aphasia, and visual field defect, reflecting the site of the original pathologic process, plus signs of *diffuse* supratentorial dysfunction, indicating that the lesion is exerting remote effects on the opposite hemisphere and the deep-lying diencephalon. Occasionally, however, supratentorial masses can begin and enlarge in neurologically silent areas such as the frontal lobes or the subdural space. In any event, CT scan or MR images will disclose a large, space-occupying lesion, characteristically associated with evidence of displacement of adjacent tissues caudally or across the midline. An important negative finding is that, unless the patient has already deteriorated into an advanced stage of illness, no evidence of direct subtentorial brain stem dysfunction can be found: pupillary and oculovestibular reflexes remain intact. As a supratentorial lesion progresses, however, the neurologic signs and symptoms evolve in a characteristic, rostral-caudal pattern.

Stupor or coma with supratentorial lesions is ominous because the changes imply that the deeply located diencephalon is already compressed or distorted and that the serious complication of midbrain compression or diencephalic herniation into the tentorial notch threatens to occur. Such impaction-herniation begins either with downward displacement of the diencephalon (central herniation) or with the uncus of the temporal lobe squeezing into the tentorial notch and against the midbrain (uncal herniation). Either way, if the hernia develops fully and is allowed to persist, it usually impacts itself upon the midbrain and nearly always results in permanent brain damage or death. A characteristic constellation of symptoms heralds each of these patterns of transtentorial herniation. As the central activating system becomes impaired with impending *central* herniation, stupor becomes gradually deeper, and the subjects sigh, yawn, or develop periodic respirations. The pupils shrink to 1 to 2 mm in diameter, reflecting hypothalamic dysfunction, but retain their light reflexes. Later, one or both pupils may ominously dilate. Loss of forebrain inhibition on the brain stem results in the development of brisk oculomotor reflexes (see Ch. 464). Oculovestibular reflex responses (cold caloric test) are marked by tonic deviation of the eyes toward the stimulated side. Because of bilateral dysfunction in corticospinal motor pathways, the extremities stiffen into bilateral rigidity or spasticity, combined with extensor plantar responses. With *uncal* herniation, signs are in many ways similar to the above except that as the uncus slides over the tentorial edge, it often compresses the third nerve ahead of it, even before the diencephalon is squeezed. As a result, the pupil on the side of the herniation begins to dilate more than its fellow. Eventually, the pupil dilates widely and becomes light-fixed, and the patient declines into stupor. Shortly afterward, somatic oculomotor functions of the third nerve are usually impaired, and the involved eye turns outward. If the herniating process continues, the opposite third nerve becomes involved, and then the brain stem. If at all possible, effective treatment of impending diencephalic-midbrain compression-herniation should be initiated before these late signs of deterioration appear. Emergency measures consist of reducing the bulk of the brain with hyperventilation to lower blood volume and giving osmotic agents such as mannitol intravenously to shrink the brain. Any possible specific therapeutic measures can then follow.

Clinical Features of Subtentorial Mass or Destructive Lesions Causing Coma. The characteristic clinical feature of subtentorial destruction or compression causing coma consists of evidence of focal, parenchymal, brain stem dysfunction, usually asymmetric, which frequently can be anatomically pinpointed by the clinical findings. The pupils are almost always abnormal, because either pontine or medullary sympathetic pathways or third nerve nuclei or fibers are destroyed. Dysconjugate eye movements are common, and bizarrely or independently moving eyes, ocular bobbing, or rotating ocular deviation often are present and indicate primary brain stem dysfunction. Unilateral facial anesthesia involving both the brow and lower face, absent caloric responses to one side, and conjugate eye deviation toward the paralyzed arm and leg all suggest a subtentorial lesion. The combination of flaccidity in the arms and flexor responses in the legs signifies pontine-midbrain damage. CT scans will reveal cerebellar or pontine hemorrhage as well as expanding cerebellar hematomas, neoplasms, or, sometimes, infarctions. MR imaging detects all these lesions and, in addition, can identify relatively small brain stem infarctions. In any event, the discrete, localizing signs of structural posterior fossa lesions differ from what occurs with metabolic lesions causing coma. There, the signs commonly indicate incomplete but bilateral dysfunction at several different levels of the brain. The focal signs of primary posterior fossa disease also are unlike the secondary brain stem dysfunction and coma that follow supratentorial herniation, in which *all* function at any given level tends to be lost as the pathological process advances from rostral to caudal along the neuraxis.

Purely compressive lesions of the posterior fossa rarely cause coma until late in their course when the patient is near death. The pathologic process involved is usually a hemorrhage, abscess, or tumor of the cerebellum or fourth ventricle. In such instances, occipital headache, nystagmus, diplopia, nausea, vomiting, cranial nerve signs, and ataxia usually precede unconsciousness. Neuro-ophthalmologic findings are of great help in distinguishing destructive and compressive posterior fossa lesions from metabolic depression of the brain stem. In metabolic depression, other than that caused by sedative drugs, oculovestibular responses are generally preserved until the advanced stages, and pupillary light reflexes are nearly always retained. By contrast, structural brain stem lesions causing coma always disrupt the oculovestibular responses, and those involving the midbrain also interrupt the pupillary reflexes.

Delirium and Exogenous Metabolic Brain Dysfunction

DEFINITIONS. *Metabolic encephalopathy* is a term applied to the altered consciousness and behavioral changes that result from diffuse or widespread multifocal failure of cerebral

metabolism. Such disorders usually begin acutely or subacutely and often subside with time or treatment, or both. The clinical picture is one in which confusion, thinking errors, behavioral abnormalities, disorders of consciousness, and abnormal motor activity predominate. In some instances (e.g., vitamin B_{12} deficiency or hypothyroidism) metabolic encephalopathy has an insidious, slow onset. The usual clinical findings then resemble dementia rather than delirium. However, the brain disorder remains reversible by appropriate treatment. Some causes of metabolic encephalopathy are listed in Table 457–4. The table also includes some primary disorders of the central nervous system such as encephalitis, meningitis, concussion, and seizure disorders, because these develop acutely, affect brain function diffusely, are reversible with appropriate treatment, and clinically resemble acute metabolic brain disease.

Metabolic brain disease is common and often underdiagnosed. When mild, it produces intellectual dullness, social indifference, and vague perplexity easily mistaken by observers for psychogenic depression or simply low intelligence. More severe encephalopathy elicits either a florid picture of tremulous agitation, rich and frightening hallucinations, and periods of seemingly complete loss of contact with the environment, or a more quiet, withdrawn, akinetic state that may fade into stupor or coma. The former, classically called *delirium* or *toxic psychosis*, may be confused with a functional psychosis, and the latter, often called *acute* or *subacute confusional state*, is likely to be mistaken for structural brain disease or psychologic depression. Although certain specific systemic disorders characteristically cause one or another of the aforementioned syndromes, each can occur with any of the metabolic brain diseases; thus the terms *delirium, toxic psychosis* and *confusional state* are used interchangeably in this chapter to describe the wakeful stage of metabolic encephalopathy.

Demented patients usually do not have the clouding of consciousness associated with delirium. However, an insidiously developing, quiet delirium may be clinically indistinguishable from the early stages of dementia.

CLINICAL FEATURES OF METABOLIC BRAIN DISEASE. Clinical evaluation of a patient with suspected metabolic brain disease has two goals: first, to determine if the observed changes in consciousness are due to metabolic brain disease (i.e., to rule out structural brain disease or psychiatric dysfunction); and second, to determine exactly the type of metabolic defect causing the delirium. In general, evaluation of the state of consciousness, motor activity, and autonomic activity, as detailed below, helps answer the first question, whereas the general physical examination, examination of ventilation, and laboratory examination (the latter two detailed below) help answer the second question. Despite the difficulties of examining a delirious patient, a thorough and systematic general physical, neurologic, and laboratory examination *must* be undertaken if a definitive diagnosis is to be established and specific treatment applied. Some principles of the examination are outlined in Table 457–5.

State of Consciousness and Mental Content. Disorders of attention are the earliest sign and the hallmark of metabolic brain disease. The patient may appear quietly perplexed or preoccupied and be unable to concentrate sufficiently to deal with significant stimuli in the environment. Conversely, he may appear hypervigilant and distractible, attending briefly to each new environmental stimulus no matter how trivial or irrelevant. Attentional defects may be subtle at onset and are easily mistaken for normal if slightly odd behavior. At about the same time, restlessness or lethargy, emotional lability, insomnia or drowsiness, and vivid nightmares may appear. Patients often appear fearful and anxious, or depressed. Some express the fear that they are "going crazy." They may be restless, irritable, and easily distracted. Conversely, they may lie quietly or sleep when left alone, and rarely read or attend to the world around them. With more severe metabolic

TABLE 457–4. SOME CAUSES OF METABOLIC BRAIN DYSFUNCTION

I. **Deprivation of oxygen, substrate, or metabolic cofactors**
  *A. Hypoxia (interference with oxygen supply to the entire brain—cerebral blood flow normal)
    1. Decreased oxygen tension (usually PaO_2 <35 mm Hg) and content of blood
      Pulmonary disease
      Alveolar hypoventilation
      Decreased atmospheric oxygen tension (e.g., high altitude)
    2. Decreased oxygen content of blood—normal tension
      Anemia (<40% normal)
      Carbon monoxide poisoning
      Methemoglobinemia
  *B. Ischemia (diffuse or widespread multifocal interference with blood supply to brain)
    1. Decreased cerebral blood flow resulting from decreased cardiac output
      Stokes-Adams syndrome, cardiac arrest, cardiac arrhythmias
      Myocardial infarction
      Aortic stenosis
      Pulmonary embolism
    2. Decreased cerebral blood flow resulting from decreased peripheral resistance in the systemic circulation
      Syncope: orthostatic, vasovagal
      Carotid sinus hypersensitivity
      Low blood volume
    3. Decreased cerebral blood flow due to generalized or multifocal increase in cerebrovascular resistance
      Hyperventilation syndrome
      Increased blood viscosity (polycythemia, cryo- and macroglobulinemia, sickle cell anemia)
      Bacterial meningitis and encephalitis
      Subarachnoid hemorrhage
    4. Decreased local cerebral blood flow due to widespread small vessel occlusion or tissue necrosis
      Disseminated intravascular coagulation
      Systemic lupus erythematosus
      Subacute bacterial endocarditis
      Cardiopulmonary bypass
      Small emboli (fat, fibrin, platelets)
      Acute viral encephalitis
    5. Alterations of blood flow due to failure of autoregulation
      Hypertensive encephalopathy
  *C. Hypoglycemia
      Resulting from exogenous insulin
      Spontaneous (endogenous insulin, liver disease, etc.)
  D. Cofactor deficiency
      Thiamine (Wernicke's encephalopathy)
      Niacin
      Pyridoxine
      Vitamin B_{12}
      Folate
II. **Diseases of organs other than brain**
  *A. Diseases of nonendocrine organs
      Liver (hepatic coma)
      Kidney (uremic coma)
      Lung (CO_2 narcosis)
      Pancreas (exocrine pancreatic encephalopathy)

II. **Diseases of organs other than brain** (*Continued*)
  *B. Hyper- and/or hypofunction of endocrine organs
      Pituitary
      Thyroid (myxedema-thyrotoxicosis)
      Parathyroid (hyper- and hypoparathyroidism)
      Adrenal (Addison's disease, Cushing's disease, pheochromocytoma)
      Pancreas (diabetes, hypoglycemia)
  C. Other systemic diseases
      Diabetes
      Cancer
      Porphyria
      Sepsis
III. **Exogenous poisons** (see also Ch. 32)
  *A. Sedative drugs or their withdrawal
  B. Acid poisons or poisons with acidic breakdown products
      Paraldehyde
      Methyl alcohol
      Ethylene glycol
  C. Psychotropic drugs
      Ethyl alcohol
      Tricyclic antidepressants and anticholinergic drugs
      Amphetamines
      Lithium
      Phenothiazines
      LSD-mescaline
      Monoamine oxidase inhibitors
  D. Others
      Penicillin
      Anticonvulsants
      Steroids
      Cardiac glycosides
      Cimetidine
      Heavy metals
      Organic phosphates
      Cyanide
      Salicylates
IV. **Abnormalities of fluid, ionic, or acid-base environment of CNS**
  A. Water and sodium (hyper- and hyponatremia) (hypo- and hyperosmolality)
  B. Acidosis (metabolic and respiratory)
  C. Alkalosis (metabolic and respiratory)
  D. Magnesium (hyper- and hypomagnesemia)
  E. Calcium (hyper- and hypocalcemia)
  F. Phosphorus (hyper- and hypophosphatemia)
  G. ? Trace metal deficiency or excess
V. **Disordered temperature regulation**
  A. Hypothermia
  B. Heat stroke, fever
VI. **Infections or inflammation of CNS**
  A. Leptomeningitis
  B. Encephalitis
  C. Acute "toxic" encephalopathy
  D. Parainfectious encephalomyelitis
  E. Cerebral vasculitis
  F. Subarachnoid hemorrhage
VII. **Miscellaneous diseases of unknown cause**
  A. Seizures and postictal states
  B. Concussion
  C. Acute delirious states
      Sedative drug withdrawal
      "Postoperative" delirium
      Intensive care unit delirium
      Chronic drug intoxications

*Alone or in combination, the most common causes of delirium seen on medical or surgical wards.

disturbances, patients become drowsy and finally stuporous or comatose. The particular affect that prevails in patients with metabolic encephalopathy depends partly on the nature of the illness and partly on the rapidity of its development; previous personality often has surprisingly little influence. Thus, barbiturate- or alcohol-withdrawal syndromes, acute liver necrosis, and porphyria often cause an agitated delirium, whereas uremia, pulmonary encephalopathy, and anoxia usually produce a more quiet illness. Rapidly developing metabolic abnormalities are more likely to produce agitated delirium than those that evolve more slowly.

Disturbances in cognition appear along with altered alertness and awareness and are characterized by difficulties with immediate recall and the ability to abstract. Normal subjects readily recall and repeat 6 or 7 digits forward and 5 or 6 backward and can identify the common denominator between such pairs as an apple and an orange or a fly and a tree, but delirious patients cannot. However, innate intelligence and education also determine cognitive abilities and, unless the physician has examined the patient previously, it is difficult to attribute mild disturbances to a metabolic defect. An early sign of delirium is impairment of memory and orientation. Loss of memory for recent events is a hallmark of organic brain disease. Orientation to place and time should be specifically tested by asking the date and year, the day of the week, and the present location. Orientation for time, particularly the year, is lost early in patients with delirium.

Perceptual errors, e.g., mistaking the physician for someone else, as well as illusions and hallucinations, are common accompaniments of delirium. They frighten and agitate some patients, but are tolerated quietly by others. A quiet, withdrawn patient must be specifically asked about hallucinations,

TABLE 457–5. PHYSICAL EXAMINATION OF PATIENTS WITH SUSPECTED METABOLIC BRAIN DISEASE

History (from relatives or friends)
  Previous medical illness (diabetes, uremia, heart disease)
  Previous psychiatric history
  Access to drugs (sedative, psychotropic drugs)
  Recent complaints (headache, depression)
General physical examination
  Evidence of trauma
  Evidence of chronic or acute systemic illness
Neurologic examination
  Mental status
    Affect (agitated, depressed, apathetic)
    Alertness (delirium, obtundation, stupor, coma)
    Memory (recent events, recall of objects)
    Orientation (time, place, person)
    Perceptual abnormalities (illusions, delusions, hallucinations)
    Psychomotor activity
  Motor examination
    Focal weakness
    Tremor
    Asterixis
    Myoclonus
    Seizures
  Autonomic examination
    Pupillary size and responses
    Temperature
    Heart rate and rhythm
    Diaphoresis
    Ventilation

because he often fails either to volunteer the information or to behave as if he were hallucinating. Hallucinations of metabolic origin may be visual, auditory, tactile, or a combination, contrasting with those of schizophrenia, which are usually auditory only.

Fluctuations of the mental status are common in metabolic encephalopathy. Patients may be totally out of contact one moment and lucid the next. Lucid intervals appear unpredictably and last for minutes or hours. Some of the fluctuation is environmentally related. Thus delirious patients characteristically become more disoriented at night, in unfamiliar surroundings, and in situations in which restraints, background noise, and unfamiliar activity replace familiar sensory stimuli. One study demonstrated a higher incidence of postoperative delirium in patients treated in a windowless intensive care unit than in those treated in a similar setting but with openings to the surrounding world.

Motor Activity. Tremor, asterixis, and multifocal myoclonus are characteristic of metabolic brain disease, and the specificity of the latter two makes them the most important physical signs that distinguish metabolic encephalopathy from psychiatric illness or from structural brain disease.

The *tremor* of delirious patients is coarse and irregular at a rate of about eight to ten per second. It is usually absent at complete rest. It is best seen in the fingers of the outstretched hands.

Asterixis is an abnormal, involuntary jerking movement, elicited in the hands by asking patients to dorsiflex the pronated wrist and spread the extended fingers. With fully developed asterixis there is sudden palmar flexion of the fingers at the metacarpophalangeal joints and of the wrist. The movements are asynchronous in the two hands and nonrhythmic. They occur every 2 to 30 seconds, recover quickly, and cannot be controlled even by the patient's effort. Bilateral asterixis almost universally accompanies metabolic encephalopathy at some stage of the illness. It is absent in patients with psychiatric disorders unless they are taking large amounts of drugs, and is encountered rarely, and then unilaterally, in patients with structural brain disease such as decompensating subdural hematomas or deep hemispheral infarcts, especially involving the basal ganglia.

Multifocal myoclonus consists of sudden nonrhythmic, nonpatterned gross contractions affecting a resting group of muscles. The movements are most common in the face and

shoulders but can occur anywhere in the body. Multifocal myoclonus can often be elicited, if not present at rest, by passive or active movements of the shoulder, upper arm, face, or tongue. Myoclonus occurs in a later and more severe stage of metabolic illness than does asterixis. Multifocal myoclonus makes its most frequent appearance in uremia, hypercarbic-anoxic encephalopathy, and penicillin overdose, but can occur in virtually all metabolic encephalopathies.

Psychomotor activity ranges from extreme hyperactivity to total immobility. Delirious patients may be unwilling or unable to stay in bed, pacing the halls, in constant movement, with outbursts of aggressiveness which may culminate in attacks on others. With more severe delirium, there may be groping movements, picking at the bedclothes, and constant tossing and turning. Affected patients may fall or attempt to climb out of bed and injure themselves. Increased psychomotor activity is typically observed in acute deliria such as delirium tremens and drug withdrawal states. More commonly, delirium is manifested by reduced activity, with the patient lethargic, drowsy, and generally bradykinetic. The same patient may run the gamut from psychomotor overactivity to quiet apathy during the course of the delirium. *Speech* is often abnormal. Patients with increased psychomotor behavior often speak rapidly, with a muttering or slurred speech that, because of its speed, is incomprehensible. Patients with reduced psychomotor activity may speak slowly, monotonously, and so softly as not to be clearly heard.

Seizures, hyperactive stretch reflexes, and *focal signs* frequently accompany severe metabolic brain disease. The seizures are usually generalized and the motor abnormalities usually symmetric. Nevertheless, focal paresis and focal seizures can occur, especially with anoxia, hypoglycemia, or hyperosmolar states. Signs of focal disturbance make it more difficult to distinguish between metabolic and structural brain disease. However, in metabolic brain disease the focal signs are usually mild and fleeting, and they are accompanied by more widely distributed neurologic dysfunction than occurs with gross structural disease.

Autonomic Activity. Pupillary light reactions are preserved in metabolic coma with rare exceptions, and their absence strongly suggests a structural lesion. The exceptions include the ingestion of drugs with an anticholinergic action which produce midposition or fixed, dilated pupils; and exposure to severe anoxia or asphyxia, which produces fixed dilated pupils that, if sustained, imply the presence of irreversible brain damage. The pupils, whatever their size and reaction to light, are usually symmetric in metabolic brain disease, but often asymmetric in patients comatose from structural brain disease.

Hypothermia is common in delirious patients with myxedema, hypoglycemia, and barbiturate intoxication. Hyperthermia with profuse perspiration and tachycardia accompanies most agitated deliria and is especially common with delirium tremens. Hyperthermia without perspiration sug-

TABLE 457–6. LABORATORY EVALUATION OF METABOLIC BRAIN DISEASE

Test	Reason for Test
Immediate	
Glucose	Hypoglycemia, hyperosmolar coma
Na$^+$	Osmolar abnormalities
Ca^{++}	Hyper- or hypocalcemia
BUN	Uremia
Arterial blood pH, P$_{CO_2}$, P$_{O_2}$	Acidosis, alkalosis, hypoxia
Lumbar puncture	Infection, hemorrhage, meningeal carcinomatosis
Later	
Liver function tests	Hepatic coma
Sedative drug levels	Overdose
Blood and CSF culture	Sepsis, encephalitis, meningitis
Full electrolytes, including Mg^{++}	Electrolyte imbalance
Coagulation profile	Intravascular coagulation
EEG	Seizure disorder

gests anticholinergic drug ingestion, infection or heat stroke. Hyperthermia also marks salicylate and occasionally phenothiazine overdosage.

LABORATORY TESTS. The causes of metabolic coma are legion, and a final diagnosis usually depends on extensive laboratory tests and history (e.g., of drug abuse, systemic disease, exposure to toxins, etc.). The tests that should be performed immediately to establish the presence of life-threatening metabolic defects are listed in Table 457–6, along with those whose results are not available immediately but should be done as soon as possible if the diagnosis is unclear. Brain imaging shows no immediately pertinent abnormalities in metabolic encephalopathy, although pre-existing abnormalities that predispose to the process may be detected.

PSYCHIATRIC DISORDERS

Psychiatric disorders, including acute schizophrenic or manic attacks, severe depression, catatonia, hysteria, and malingering can mimic physiologic alterations in consciousness. Patients with psychiatric disorders may complain of memory loss, confusion, and/or hallucinations. Patients with psychiatric amnesia, however, unlike those with metabolic or structural brain disease, often claim disorientation for self (i.e., they deny that they know who they are), even though they may be oriented for place and time. Furthermore, if the patient's cooperation can be elicited, recent memory and cognitive functions are usually preserved. Hallucinations are auditory rather than visual or tactile, and asterixis and multifocal myoclonus are never present. Patients with extreme anxiety may hyperventilate, producing respiratory alkalosis and a diffusely slow electroencephalogram. Except for that problem, however, the physical and laboratory evaluations are generally normal.

In patients with psychiatric unresponsiveness, the segmental neurologic examination is likewise normal. Breathing is eupneic or voluntarily hyperneic. Such patients are quietly unresponsive, with all their limbs either flaccid or resisting movement in unpredictable patterns. Eyes are usually closed and resist eyelid opening. In some patients, the eyes may deviate toward the bed when the patient is turned on his side. Furthermore, the eyelids are incapable of the slow closure of the passively opened eyelids which accompanies true coma. Pupils are briskly responsive or, if cycloplegics have been self-instilled, widely dilated. Oculocephalic responses are unpredictable, but if the diagnosis is doubtful, irrigating the tympanum with 50 ml of cold water produces physiologic nystagmus rather than the tonic eye deviation of the comatose patient with structural or metabolic disease. At times the diagnosis may be difficult because psychiatric pseudodelirium or unresponsiveness can be superimposed on underlying physical illness (e.g., a patient hospitalized with a severe medical or neurologic illness may be so anxious that he is unable to cope with his environment and thus withdraws psychologically to the point of unresponsiveness). In instances in which there is serious doubt about the diagnosis, slow infusions of small amounts of sodium amobarbital (Amytal interview) may allow the physician to establish contact and rapport with such psychiatrically withdrawn patients. The drug may be similarly used to awaken patients rendered unconscious by continuous focal seizures.

DIAGNOSTIC APPROACHES TO ALTERED CONSCIOUSNESS

HISTORY. Several questions must be asked and answered in attempting to diagnose and manage the patient with severe brain dysfunction of unknown cause. First one must determine if the disease is focal (i.e., structural) or multifocal-diffuse. If focal, is it (1) supra- or subtentorial in distribution? (2) arrested, improving, or worsening? (3) best treated medically or surgically? If apparently multifocal-diffuse, is the disorder due to (1) exogenous drugs, (2) endogenous meta-

TABLE 457–7. SYSTEMIC CLUES TO THE DIAGNOSIS OF STUPOR AND COMA

Fever—infection, inflammation, neoplasm (less often), anticholinergics

Hypothermia (30–36°C)—hypoglycemia, depressant drugs, myxedema, brain stem damage

Hypertension—cerebral hemorrhage, hypertensive encephalopathy

Hypotension—low blood volume (shock or nutritional), myocardial infarct, depressant drugs

Tachycardia— > 180/min
Bradycardia— < 44/min

Petechiae—thrombocytopenic purpura; meningococcemia, bacterial endocarditis, rickettsia

Bruises—trauma, nutritional deficiency, purpura, hypercorticism

Cherry red color—carbon monoxyhemoglobin

Cyanosis—hypoxemia, methemoglobinemia

Funduscopic abnormalities—increased pressure, hypertensive encephalopathy, subarachnoid hemorrhage, advanced diabetes, bacterial endocarditis, collagen vasculopathy

bolic error, (3) CNS infection or hemorrhage, or (4) psychogenic unresponsiveness? Given the answers to these questions, what is the specific etiologic diagnosis? However, even before pursuing this logical approach, the physician must ensure that the brain and other vital organs receive no further injury while he obtains whatever history, examination, or laboratory data are required. This means that in critical situations, lifesaving measures should be underway while methodical clinical and laboratory steps are undertaken to reach an accurate diagnosis and initiate definitive treatment. Nevertheless, one must be deliberate: the urge to act without delay is understandably strong but potentially dangerous.

Inquiry into both the past medical history and the circumstances under which the patient lost consciousness generally discloses more of diagnostic value than any other maneuver. Could head trauma have occurred recently? Is there chronic renal, hepatic, or myocardial disease? Could a seizure have preceded the present unconsciousness? Has the subject been taking insulin? Have there been recent changes in mood, behavior, or neurologic function to suggest an evolving intracranial process? Was the subject "blue," depressed, or moody, and did he have access to depressant drugs? Is he a "spree" drinker? These and other questions must be covered comprehensively with relatives, past physicians, friends, police, or ambulance personnel. Remember: *most cases of "coma of unknown cause," whether found at home or encountered in the emergency room of a busy hospital, are due to self-induced drug intoxication.*

PHYSICAL FINDINGS. To evaluate the possible presence of conditions listed in Table 457–3 and, especially, 457–4, one must perform both a meticulous neurologic examination and a thoughtful physical review of every body system. Disease in remote organs often causes or accentuates dysfunction in the brain. Some immediate clues to systemic mechanisms causing coma are given in Table 457–7. In addition, a number of the potential causes of acute encephalopathy are associated with abnormalities in ventilation and systemic acid-base balance, as indicated in Table 457–8.

During the neurologic examination, certain potentially informative steps are sometimes overlooked. The skull should always be palpated and inspected meticulously. Edema of the scalp commonly overlies fresh fracture lines, and basal skull fractures predispose to blood pigment stains behind the ear (Battle's sign) and about the orbit (raccoon eyes). Blood also may escape from basal fractures into the ear canals, the middle ears, or the nostrils. The skull should be percussed, because focal or unilateral skull tenderness, manifested by grimacing or withdrawal in a stuporous subject, often overlies an intracranial mass lesion. The neck should be tested carefully: stiff neck can reflect meningitis, cerebellar tonsillar herniation, or,

TABLE 457–8. ACUTE ACID-BASE DISORDERS ASSOCIATED WITH ENCEPHALOPATHY

Metabolic acidosis—diabetic ketoacidosis, uremia, lactacidosis, poisoning (methanol, paraldehyde, ethylene glycol, salicylates in children), severe convulsions

Metabolic alkalosis—corticosteroid excess (ingested or secreted), severe chloride or potassium depletion

Respiratory alkalosis—hepatic encephalopathy, pulmonary infiltration, congestive failure, sepsis, upper brain stem disease. If $PaO_2 < 60$: pulmonary infarction, miliary carcinoma of lung

Respiratory acidosis—hypercarbic-anoxic encephalopathy, pulmonary insufficiency, central or peripheral ventilatory paralysis

Mixed defect—sepsis, salicylism (adult), fulminant hepatic encephalopathy

---

occasionally, simply skeletal muscle spasm. The stiff neck of acute bacterial meningitis is rarely equivocal; that of impending herniation is commonly less severe and lacks accompanying signs of infection or a prominent Kernig sign. Subarachnoid blood usually requires several hours or a day or more to degenerate sufficiently to produce stiff neck.

Table 457–9 gives a profile of neurologic functions useful for clinically evaluating patients with acute brain dysfunction. As the table indicates, certain signs discriminate among normal, impaired, or absent cerebral hemispheric functions, whereas others point toward the presence of moderate or severe brain stem dysfunction. This fundamental examination is easily completed within a few minutes in most patients and can be employed both for making an immediate anatomic diagnosis and, subsequently, for indicating whether the patient is improving or worsening as time and treatment transpire.

Laboratory Tests. A *CT scan* or an *MR image* often resolves much of the issue of the diagnosis of impaired consciousness, particularly in potentially lethal but surgically treatable diseases. If the diagnosis is in doubt, an emergency scan should be obtained as soon as possible. An abnormal scan that identifies a supratentorial or subtentorial mass lesion indicates that urgent treatment must be applied. A negative scan reassures the physician that he can safely perform a lumbar puncture and informs him that no tissue-displacing mass lesion exists, greatly narrowing the choices and suggesting metabolic or diffuse brain disease.

When to do a lumbar puncture is always a serious question. All physicians are aware that in patients with increased intracranial pressure the procedure sometimes induces fatal herniation of the brain through the tentorium or foramen magnum. For this reason, lumbar puncture is best avoided if

---

TABLE 457–9. THE NEUROLOGIC EXAMINATION OF THE PATIENT WITH ACUTELY ALTERED OR CHANGING CONSCIOUSNESS*

Verbal function—oriented, syntactically normal; confused; aphasic; incomprehensible sounds only; mute
Spontaneous eye movements—conjugate pursuit; roving conjugate; dysconjugate; none
Eye opening†—spontaneous; in response to verbal stimuli; in response to noxious stimuli; none
Corneal response to stimulation—present; *absent*
Pupillary (note size) response to light stimulation—brisk; *unequal* (test directly and consensually); *sluggish; absent*
Oculocephalic-oculovestibular response—quick phase nystagmus present; tonic conjugate; *dysconjugate; absent*
Motor response to noxious stimulation—appropriate; stereotyped withdrawal; asymmetric; abnormal flexor ("decorticate"); abnormal extensor ("decerebrate"); *flaccid*
Breathing pattern—eupneic; rhythmic hyperpnea or hypopnea; regularly irregular (Cheyne-Stokes); *ataxic or bizarrely irregular; absent*

*Each function is subdivided in best-worse order and roughly indicates the rostral-caudal level of impairment. Signs of impaired or absent brain stem function are italicized. (For details consult Plum F, Posner JB: Diagnosis of Stupor and Coma. 3rd revised ed. Philadelphia, F. A. Davis Company, 1982.)
†Note that eye opening reflects only the state of arousal and not necessarily the presence of psychologic awareness or interaction.

---

the physician strongly suspects his patient of having an expanding intracranial mass, particularly in the posterior fossa. Such temporary forbearance is particularly advisable when an immediately available CT scan can give a definitive answer. Certain treatable diseases such as meningitis, however, can be diagnosed only by lumbar puncture, and in many others such as encephalitis or subarachnoid hemorrhage the procedure yields valuable preliminary diagnostic information. When the advice of neurologic specialists is unavailable, the doctor has no choice but to proceed with lumbar puncture if the diagnosis is in doubt and he believes the procedure has a reasonable chance of offering valuable information. Certain steps minimize the risk. One is to use a small (No. 20 or 22) needle. Another is to attach the manometer to the needle before releasing fluid, a technique that prevents sudden subarachnoid pressure shifts. Jugular manometrics should *never* be performed, for they offer little useful data and increase the risk of impacting potential intracranial herniations.

The *electroencephalogram* (EEG) has a limited use in evaluating patients with alterations in consciousness. In patients with metabolic brain disease, the EEG is usually slow but symmetric and bilateral synchronous paroxysmal bursts of 1 to 3 per second (Hz) activity are frequently superimposed upon the slow background. The degree of slowing roughly parallels the severity of the encephalopathy. Patients with agitated delirium are often exceptions, and particularly those suffering from drug withdrawal may have rapid rather than slow EEGs. Normal 8 to 13 Hz activity, however, is usually absent. In patients with supratentorial structural disease, the slow activity is usually more prominent on the side of the lesion. In some patients, alteration of consciousness is caused by a continuously discharging focal lesion (focal status epilepticus), and such abnormalities may be detected by the presence of focal spikes or sharp waves.

EMERGENCY MANAGEMENT OF COMA

The definitive treatment of altered states of consciousness requires removing, correcting, or halting the specific process responsible to whatever degree possible. Often, however, accurate diagnosis and specific therapy require time to complete. Meanwhile, one must move immediately to protect the brain against permanent damage.

Certain general measures apply to the care of all patients:

1. *Assure an adequate airway and oxygenation.* Immediately check and clean out the upper airway. If the patient is entirely unresponsive, arrange for the skillful insertion of an endotracheal airway, but first give 1 mg of atropine intravenously to guard against hypoxigenic vagal cardiac arrest. Be sure that no neck fracture exists before extending the head for intubation. Auscultate both lung bases after inserting the tube to assure that the lower airway is open. If a ventilator is used, choose a rate less than 16 per minute and adjust the volume and FIO_2 to give arterial blood gases of PaO_2 greater than 80 mm Hg and $PaCO_2$ 30 to 35 mm Hg. It is difficult to avoid leaving the patient supine while diagnosis is pursued; but once the diagnosis of metabolic encephalopathy is made, place the patient in mild Trendelenburg position and turn from side to side each hour.

2. *Maintain circulation.* Check the blood pressure and pulse frequently (insert a venous line immediately to replace volume loss), and infuse vasoactive agents to keep mean blood pressure at 80 to 90 mm Hg or more.

3. *Give glucose.* Draw blood for emergency blood gas and chemical determinations (see Table 472–4) and, if hypoglycemia is a possible diagnosis, immediately give 50 ml of 50 per cent glucose. (Blood is drawn first in order not to lose evidence for the diagnosis.) The glucose will not appreciably intensify hyperosmolality. Since, however, there is evidence that hyperglycemia may enhance the damage of anoxic encephalop-

athy, glucose should be withheld pending colorimetric estimation of finger blood when such a diagnosis appears likely.

4. *Give thiamine, 50 to 100 mg intravenously.* Many patients admitted to emergency rooms in stupor or coma are malnourished and therefore vulnerable to Wernicke's encephalopathy, especially if loaded with glucose.

5. *Stop generalized seizures.* Repetitive convulsions can result from either intracranial mass lesions or metabolic-diffuse encephalopathies. In either event, status epilepticus can cause coma and within a short period of time produces irreversible brain damage as well. Start treatment with intravenous diazepam. Give 5 to 10 mg or more, if necessary, at a rate of 1 to 2 mg per minute, keeping a ventilator available to treat depressed breathing. As soon as convulsions stop, give between 500 and 1000 mg of phenytoin intravenously at a rate of less than 50 mg per minute. If seizures continue, give more diazepam or resort to barbiturate general anesthesia. Repetitive focal seizures and myoclonus are potentially less damaging to brain, and their continuation does not require the use of general anesthesia.

6. *Restore blood acid-base and osmolar balance.* Extremes of either acidosis or alkalosis usually reflect profound metabolic problems, severe circulatory insufficiency, the postictal state (muscular lactic acidosis), or hyperadrenocorticism. Since severe metabolic acidosis can precipitate cardiovascular irregularity and alkalosis depresses breathing, they should be corrected. Extreme hypo- and hyperosmolality are equally dangerous to brain and should be corrected, the first by withholding fluids (except water by mouth) and stopping diuretics and the second by administering fluids (and insulin for hyperglycemia). Beware of too rapid reversal, however. Osmotic delays across the blood-brain barrier during treatment can lead to large fluid shifts in or out of brain. Also, too rapid correction of hyponatremia can produce central pontine myelinolysis (Ch. 467). A reasonable goal in treating osmolal shifts is to correct blood by about 12 to 15 mOsm in 24 hours.

7. *Treat infection.* Several kinds of infection can cause or intensify delirium and coma. Obtain nose, throat, blood, and wound cultures, and perform lumbar puncture if indicated. With any sign of infection, begin antimicrobial treatment after obtaining the cultures cited above, based on either the results of smears or the most probable clinically suggested organism.

8. *Treat extreme body temperatures.* Hyperthermia above 40° C or hypothermia below 34° C should be brought to within 3° C of normal.

9. *Consider specific antidotes.* Many, if not most, patients admitted to emergency rooms in coma will have taken an overdose of drugs, often in combination. For narcotic overdose, give 0.4 mg of naloxone intravenously every five minutes until the subject awakens. If the subject may be an addict, dilute the dose in 10 ml of saline and give slowly, trying to minimize withdrawal phenomena. Remember that naloxone's duration of action of two to three hours is shorter than that of several narcotics, and the dose may require repeating.

10. *Control agitation,* avoiding barbiturates but employing diazepam or haloperidol as necessary.

11. *Protect the corneas against abrasions,* using ophthalmic ointment and, if necessary, taping the lids shut.

Plum F, Posner JB: The Diagnosis of Stupor and Coma. 3rd rev. ed. Philadelphia, F.A. Davis Co, 1982. *Comprehensively outlines pathophysiology, diagnosis, and emergency management in acutely altered states of consciousness.*

Sterns RH, Riggs JE, Schochet SS: Osmotic demyelination syndrome following corrections of hyponatremia. N Engl J Med 314:1535, 1986. *Among 60 patients with serum sodium less than 116 mmol per liter, 8 developed central pontine myelinolysis. Both in the study group and in literature descriptions, the complication was always associated with correcting hyponatremia by more than 12 mmol per day.*

ACUTE CENTRAL NERVOUS SYSTEM POISONING

At one time sedative drugs, especially the barbiturates, were the chief causes of acute (and chronic) overdose but both patients and industry have become more imaginative in their choices, and the list of common agents has lengthened. To find descriptions of poisons not included in this section, especially chronic neurotoxic agents, the reader should consult the textbooks listed in the references.

Table 457–10 lists the most frequent acute neurotoxic poisonings in the United States, gives their principal signs of toxicity, and outlines their treatment. Almost all drugs in overdose amounts are likely to be mixed with intoxicating amounts of alcohol, thereby making their clinical signs more difficult to appraise. Nevertheless, clinical appraisal must be used to diagnose the specific agent causing several of these reaction patterns, since chemical tests are in many instances either unavailable or impractically slow. When any doubt exists, one should keep admission serum samples for possible later analysis. Blood levels and size of the dose are unreliable guides to the potential depth of coma or other complications with most of the drugs because tolerance develops to chronic ingestion and individuals may react differently to similar doses. The mixing of agents adds to the unreliability. Only the opiates and some of the sedatives create an immediate risk of death; concurrent alcohol ingestion enhances both these risks. Opiate poisoning is discussed in greater detail in Ch. 16.

PATHOGENESIS. All sedative drugs depress the central nervous system, although not equally on a gram-molecular weight basis, and not to the same degree so far as different central structures are concerned. The duration of action varies widely and depends largely on how the particular drug is detoxified or eliminated. The short-acting barbiturates, pentobarbital, secobarbital, and amobarbital, are detoxified by the liver, as is methaqualone. They exert their maximal effects promptly after being absorbed and, even in huge doses, seldom cause neurologic depression lasting longer than three to five days. Barbital and phenobarbital are partially detoxified by the liver and partially excreted in the urine. Severe poisoning with the latter agent can cause coma lasting 10 to 14 days. Glutethimide, nowadays seldom used, has a short duration of action comparable to that of secobarbital, but it is poorly absorbed from the gut and may degenerate into more longlasting neurotoxic metabolites. Meprobamate has an intermediate duration of effect lasting for days. Bromide rarely causes full coma, but, once it reaches high levels, it replaces chloride in the blood and tissues and persists for weeks to cause symptoms without further ingestion.

Although the sedatives have few important effects outside the nervous system, barbiturates, glutethimide, and meprobamate in toxic doses tend to produce hypotension. Glutethimide possesses anticholinergic properties and is the only sedative that predictably produces light-fixed pupils in relatively light anesthetic doses.

A withdrawal syndrome consisting of tremulousness, agitation, and sometimes delirium, and convulsions can develop after prompt withdrawal from chronic exposure to any of the hypnotic sedatives. Convulsions are a particular problem after withdrawal from meprobamate and methaqualone.

CLINICAL MANIFESTATIONS. Stupor or coma caused by depressant drug poisoning usually presents the characteristic picture of acute general anesthesia. The depression of the central nervous system tends to be bilateral and symmetric, and the drug affects simultaneously many levels, including the spinal cord. Respiratory and circulatory controlling mechanisms in the lower brain stem are affected only with very high doses or not at all, and, except with glutethimide or extremely large, doses of the barbiturates, the pupillary

TABLE 457–10. COMMON DRUG POISONINGS, SIGNS OF TOXICITY, AND TREATMENT

Drug	Signs and Symptoms Mild	Severe	Diagnostic Test	Treatment
Opiates Heroin Morphine Meperidine Methadone Hydromorphone Oxycodone Levorphanol	"Nodding" drowsiness, small pupils, urinary retention, slow and shallow breathing; skin scars and subcutaneous abscesses; duration 4–6 hours; with methadone, duration to 24 hours	Coma; pinpoint pupils, slow irregular respiration or apnea, hypotension, hypothermia, pulmonary edema	Response to naloxone Urine	Naloxone, 0.4 mg intravenously or intramuscularly; repeat at 15-minute intervals if responds and gradually increase intervals; repeat in 3 hours if necessary; if no response by second dose, suspect another cause; treat shock; find and detect infection
Depressants Alcohol Barbiturates Chloral hydrate Glutethimide (Doriden) Meprobamate (Equanil)	Confusion, rousable drowsiness, delirium, ataxia, nystagmus, dysarthria, analgesia to stimuli	Stupor to coma; pupils reactive, usually constricted; oculovestibular response absent; motor tonus initially briefly hyperactive, then flaccid; respiration and blood pressure depressed; hypothermia; with glutethimide, pupils moderately dilated, can be fixed; with meprobamate, withdrawal seizures common; with methaqualone, coma, occasional convulsions, tachycardia, cardiac failure, bleeding tendency	Blood, urine, breath Blood Blood Blood	Intubate, ventilate, lavage; drainage position; antimicrobials; keep mean blood pressure above 90 mm Hg and urine output > 300 ml per hour; avoid analeptics; hemodialyze severe phenobarbital poisoning
Methaqualone (Quaalude, Sopor, Mandrax)	Hallucinations, agitation, motor hyperactivity, myoclonus, tonic spasms		Blood	As above; diuresis of little help
Benzodiazepines (Librium, Valium, Tranxene, Ativan, Dalmane, etc.) Ethchlorvynol (Placidyl)	Usually taken with another sedative if poisoning is attempted		Blood	As above; diuresis of little help
Stimulants Amphetamines Methylphenidate	Hyperactive, aggressive, sometimes paranoid, repetitive behavior, dilated pupils, tremor, hyperactive reflexes; hyperthermia, tachycardia, arrhythmia Acute torsion dystonia	Agitated, assaultive and paranoid excitement; occasionally convulsions; hypothermia; circulatory collapse	Blood	Chlorpromazine
Cocaine	Similar but less prominent than above; less paranoid, often euphoric	Twitching; irregular breathing, tachycardia, arrhythmia, occasionally convulsions	Blood; urine	Diazepam plus specific symptomatic
Psychedelics (LSD), mescaline, psilocybin, phencyclidine (PCP, angel dust)	Confused, disoriented, perceptual distortions, distractable, withdrawn or eruptive, leading to accidents or violence; wide-eyed, dilated pupils; restless, hyperreflexic; less often, hypertension or tachycardia	Panic		Reassure; diazepam satisfactory; avoid phenothiazines
Scopolamine-atropine (knockout drops, Transderm delirium)	Agitated or confused, visual hallucinations, dilated pupils, flushed and dry skin	Florid toxic disoriented delirium, visual hallucinations; later, amnesia, fever, dilated fixed pupils, hot flushed dry skin, urinary retention		Reassure; sedate lightly, (1) avoid phenothiazines; (2) do not leave alone
Antidepressants Tricyclics (Tofranil, Elavil, Desipramine, etc.)	Restlessness, drowsiness, tachycardia, ataxia, sweating	Agitation, vomiting hyperpyrexia, sweating, muscle dystonia, convulsions, tachycardia or arrhythmia	Blood	Symptomatic; gastric lavage. Intensive care, anticonvulsants, and antiarrhythmics for severe cases
MAO inhibitors (Parnate, Nardil, Eutonyl, etc.)	Hypertensive crises, agitation, drowsiness, ataxia	Hypotension; headache; chest pain; agitation; coma, seizures and shock	Clinical	Symptomatic; gastric lavage

Table continued on following page

TABLE 457–10. COMMON DRUG POISONINGS, SIGNS OF TOXICITY, AND TREATMENT *Continued*

Drug	Signs and Symptoms		Diagnostic Test	Treatment
	Mild	*Severe*		
Antidepressants (*Continued*)				
Neuroleptics (phenothiazines, butyrophenones, etc.)	Acute dystonia, somnolence, hypotension	Coma; convulsions (rare); arrhythmias; hypotension	Blood	Anticholinergics; diphenhydramine; symptomatic; gastric lavage
Lithium	Mild lethargy	Sustention-intention tremor, lethargy; muteness with appearance of distraction; coma; multifocal seizures; slow or fluctuating course	Blood	Hydrate if mild; hemodialyze for delirium, coma, or convulsions
Acid-forming intoxicants				
Methanol (formic); ethylene glycol (oxalic and hippuric); other organic alcohols	Inebriation with hyperpnea	All produce progressive hyperventilation, drunkenness, stupor, eventually convulsions and death. Early blindness with methanol	Blood shows increasingly severe anion-gap acidosis	Inhibit hepatic alcohol dehydrogenase by giving alcohol until acidosis controlled; treat acidosis vigorously
Salicylate				
Aspirin	Tinnitus, dyspnea	Older persons: confusional state or toxic delirium leading to stupor, convulsions, coma	Blood salicylate > 60 mg/dl	Alkaline diuresis

light reflexes are preserved. Early in the course of acute poisoning, patients can demonstrate muscular hypertonus or even spasticity as the result of uneven depression of different neurologic levels. Within a short time, usually an hour or less, flaccidity supervenes, and the stretch reflexes tend to disappear. Even moderate degrees of drug depression can depress or block the oculovestibular reflexes.

As mentioned, blood levels are a poor index to the depth of coma. Generally speaking, however, blood levels of short-acting barbiturates of more than 2.5 mg per deciliter and phenobarbital blood levels of more than 12 mg per deciliter are associated with very deep coma to the level at which apnea and hypotension become management problems. Apnea rarely supervenes with the benzodiazepines.

DIAGNOSIS. The combination of acutely occurring unresponsiveness, with preserved or sluggish pupillary reactions, absent oculovestibular reactions, motor areflexia, hypothermia, and relative depression of respiration and circulation is clinically diagnostic of sedative-anesthetic drug poisoning. Only infarction or hemorrhage of the pons resembles this clinical state, and with lesions of the pons the pupils are usually small or pinpoint, the stretch reflexes are generally preserved or hyperactive, and the plantar responses are extensor. Specific chemical tests will detect barbiturates, glutethimide, meprobamate, methaqualone, and bromides in blood or urine, and can be done as emergency measures.

MANAGEMENT OF COMA. Treat the patient first, not the drug. Except for the antiopiate, naloxone, there are no specific antidotes, but certain precautions must be taken. First comes general physiologic support. Patients with drug overdose can sink rapidly and unexpectedly to deeper levels of anesthesia and should never be left alone with unskilled attendants.

Assure the Airway First and Throughout. Depressant drugs suppress the cough reflex and the ciliary action of the tracheal and bronchial mucosa. Give atropine, 1 mg intravenously and place a cuffed endotracheal tube before attempting gastric lavage. Subsequently, deflate the endotracheal cuff hourly, replace the tube at 48 to 72 hours, and consider tracheostomy at 10 to 14 days if no signs of awakening have occurred.

To empty the stomach in still arousable subjects, give apomorphine subcutaneously, 6 mg for adults and 1 to 2 mg for children. If apomorphine is not available, ipecac 20 ml may be given orally, followed with glasses of water to induce vomiting. Place vomiting subjects prone to avoid aspiration. For patients already in coma, once the endotracheal tube is in place, gavage the stomach until clear, using a large double-barreled tube and plain water or half-normal saline for the irrigating solution. To absorb remaining drug in the gut, instill

2 tablespoons of activated charcoal before withdrawing the tube. Repetitive dosing with charcoal may accelerate phenobarbital elimination if coma lasts longer than 12 hours.

Start moistened oxygen 25 per cent via a suitable nonobstructing airway connector. Treat any evidence of hypoventilation immediately with an automatic ventilator. Shallow breathing in a deeply comatose patient frequently reflects no more than the subject's depressed metabolism; if the rate falls below 12 per minute or the physician entertains serious doubts as to the adequacy of ventilation, artificial respiration is indicated. Measure arterial blood gases and initiate artificial respiration if the arterial P_{O_2} falls below 100 mm Hg on 25 per cent oxygen or if the P_{CO_2} climbs above 45 mm Hg. High concentrations (greater than 30 per cent) of oxygen therapy should be confined to patients receiving artificial respiration; such treatment increases the risk of CO_2 retention in nonventilated subjects.

Treat the Circulation. Maintain the blood pressure, but avoid overhydration. Shock is rare with depressant poisoning, but the action of the drugs on smooth muscle commonly produces moderate hypotension, which in turn impairs glomerular infiltration and renal clearance of drugs. Beware of patients with tricyclic antidepressant poisoning. These drugs cause bizarre and sometimes fatal arrhythmias whose treatment may require an experienced cardiologist. A widened QRS or QT interval may particularly predispose to ventricular tachycardia.

For all patients with depressant poisoning give fluids and pressor agents so as to maintain mean blood pressure at 80 to 90 mm Hg and a urine flow approaching 300 ml or more per hour. Dopamine will be sufficient to attain perfusion in many patients. Norepinephrine can be used cautiously if less vigorous agents fail to maintain ideal systemic pressures. Judge fluid intake by urine output, after first inserting a catheter for accurate collections. If hour-by-hour fluid excretion does not match intake by the third hour of treatment, try raising the blood pressure with a pressor agent before adding more fluids. Oliguric renal failure almost never occurs except in patients who have been in profound shock. Remember, however, that patients who have been in coma for several hours before reaching hospital may have shifted enough of their blood volume into extravascular compartments to be seriously hypovolemic. Check electrolytes at intervals of 12 hours; once diuresis is attained, replace sodium with half-normal saline and potassium at a rate of 80 to 120 mEq or more per day. Digitalis or other cardiac drugs are useful only for patients with heart disease.

Monitor blood pressure, pulse, and respiration every half hour. In the unventilated patient, the presence of a breathing rate above approximately 20 implies either pneumonitis or, less often, incipient pulmonary edema. Most patients with drug poisoning are hypothermic, and, except with the anticholinergics, body temperatures above 37.5°C generally imply infection. Hypothermia, as long as it remains above 33°C, requires no special treatment.

Prevent Complications. Keep unconscious patients semiprone in the drainage position and change their position from side to side, but never place them fully supine. Treat potential pulmonary infection with a broad-spectrum antibiotic. These patients will be unconscious for only a few days, and the risk of emergence of drug-resistant bacterial infections is of less concern than is pneumonia caused by already aspirated material.

Hemodialysis is not necessary to treat poisoning with the short-acting hypnotics. Hemodialysis may shorten the duration of coma for patients who have ingested large amounts of long-term barbiturates such as barbital or phenobarbital. Dialysis also is indicated for severe lithium or bromide poisoning.

Analeptics and pharmacologic stimulants are contraindicated for coma caused by depressant drug poisoning. Most carry the risk of overstimulating or producing convulsions in lightly poisoned patients.

RECOVERY AND PROGNOSIS. Patients recovering from coma require close medical supervision. Severe pneumonitis can develop as late as three to four days after recovery. If antimicrobial drugs were started during coma, they are best continued for at least 48 hours after it ends. Permanent physical sequelae are rare. Among 356 of our own such cases, residual brain injury was observed only once (in a patient who suffered an acute cardiac arrest). Peripheral nerve injuries from pressure developed in 6 subjects, and 14 subjects had pressure skin lesions leaving scars. There were no other physical residua.

Convalescent management varies according to the patient's underlying psychiatric disorder and attitudes. Suicide attempts are never accidents, and reports of near-fatal ingestion caused by misunderstanding the dose or forgetting previous doses carry little validity. The expert opinion of a psychiatrist should be sought before deciding whether to release or to institutionalize a patient. The immediate prognosis is good, but there is a high incidence of recurrent attempts over the years.

Dreisbach RH: Handbook of Poisoning. 10th ed. Los Altos, CA, Lange Medical Publishers, 1980. *Succinct and handy, an excellent quick source to consult in emergencies.*

Gilman AG, Goodman LS, Rall TW, et al. (eds.): Goodman and Gilman's The Pharmacological Basis of Therapeutics. 7th ed. New York, Macmillan, 1985. *The "bible" of pharmacology and associated toxicology addresses major drug poisonings in authoritative chapters.*

Goetz CG: Neurotoxins in Clinical Practice. New York, SP Medical and Scientific, 1985. *A useful guide, classified by agent and syndrome, to all forms of exogenous toxins affecting the nervous system.*

Spencer PS, Schaumberg HH: Experimental and Clinical Neurotoxicology. Baltimore, Williams and Wilkins, 1980. *A valuable compendium to nervous system poisons, mostly by the chronic variety.*

PROGNOSIS IN SEVERE BRAIN DAMAGE

An important part of the physician's responsibility includes forecasting the outcome of illness. Modern medical advances currently save many lives that only a few years ago would have been lost to severe disease or trauma. Unfortunately, however, when severe brain dysfunction accompanies acute illness, these advances create the risk that if the brain does not recover, vigorous treatment may be followed by an unwanted outcome. Many persons would prefer death over a life of overwhelming and permanent neurologic disability and often express this view in the form of a living will. These considerations have resulted in the development of several empirically based guidelines to help the physician predict between possibly good and almost certainly very poor neurologic outcomes following severe illnesses causing severe brain damage or coma.

Nontraumatic Coma

The outcome from severe medical coma depends (a) upon its cause, and, (b) with the exception of depressant drug poisoning, upon the initial severity and extent of neurologic damage as revealed by clinical neurologic signs obtainable at onset and within the first few days of illness.

Depressant drug poisoning, no matter how deep the coma, reflects a state of general anesthesia. Barring severe complications, almost all such patients who survive drug intoxication to reach medical attention can recover physically unscathed. This favorable prognosis applies even when coma is so profound that normal brain stem reflexes and the EEG temporarily disappear. Since most comas of unknown origin leading to emergency house calls or emergency room visits will be due to drug ingestion, such initially undiagnosed patients should receive maximal treatment unless direct evidence points to severe structural brain damage or systemic disease and the use of drugs by ingestion or for therapy has been ruled out.

Aside from drug poisoning, the acute or subacute development in the course of medical illness of loss of consciousness lasting more than a very few hours carries a poor prognosis, with only about 15 per cent of patients making a good recovery. The major problem in making early treatment decisions lies in attempting to discriminate between patients who have a chance of reaching a good outcome and those whose chances of a self-rewarding neurologic recovery are extremely small. In making such early decisions, clinical signs of abnormal forebrain and/or upper brain stem function have been found to be the most powerful available discriminating indicators. The nature of the underlying illness has a secondary influence on whether or not a good outcome occurs but does not modify the accuracy of predictions between the extremes of good and bad prognosis as indicated by early signs. No laboratory determinants have been found to predict outcome accurately, nor does age significantly influence the quality of survival of adults in medical coma.

The clinical tests most valuable for estimating the capacity for recovery after medical coma are identical to those used in making the initial diagnosis and in following the later course of the patient in coma. In most instances functional changes evolve so rapidly that one cannot reliably estimate the outcome of coma within the first minutes to hours, a time when improvement often occurs. After about six hours, however, so long as the patient has not received heavy doses of sedative drugs or alcohol, certain neurologic findings begin to correlate increasingly strongly with the potential for neurologic recovery and also confidently predict the outcome of about one third of patients who ultimately will do badly. By the end of the first day, clinical signs accurately predict about two thirds of the patients who actually will do well. With each successive day, the signs develop greater predictive power. When considered appropriate to the patient's expressed wishes, treatment can be adjusted accordingly.

Figure 457–1 provides a series of algorithms that describe the actual outcome of 500 patients in medical comas as related to their neurologic findings at six hours and on days one, three, and seven following onset. Reference to the charts discloses that signs of brain stem dysfunction (absent pupillary or corneal responses, imperfect or absent oculocephalic responses, or abnormal motor responses to stimulation) worsened the prognosis and, in combination, indicated a nearly hopeless outlook when they persisted beyond the third day.

Following an acute diffuse brain injury such as follows cardiac arrest, a few patients become immediately vegetative following the ictus and remain so as the days pass into weeks. Most who fail to speak until after the end of the second week are left with prominent intellectual defects, especially in recent

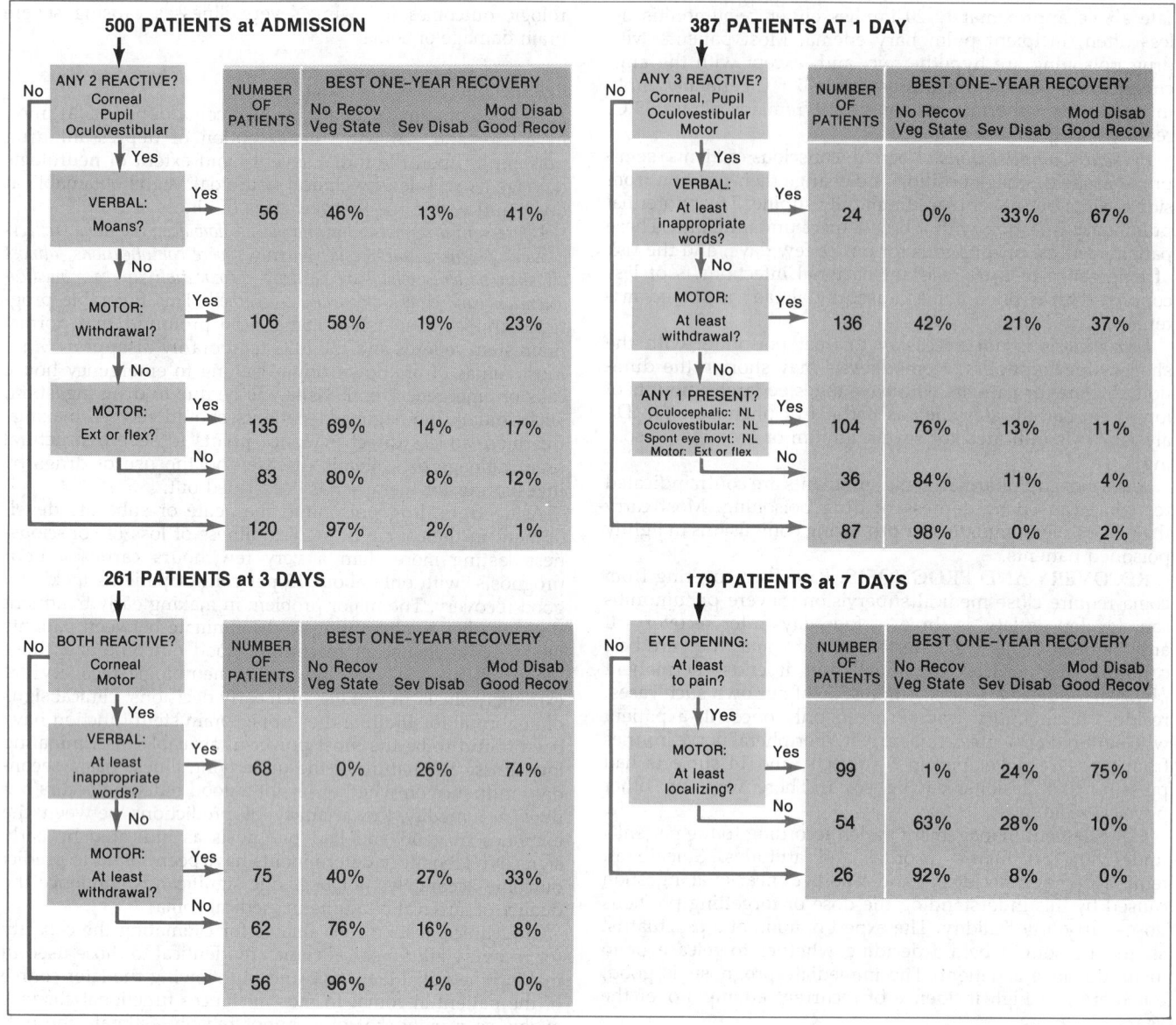

FIGURE 457–1. The best one-year outcome for 500 optimally treated patients in coma from nontraumatic causes. For each time period following onset, the diagram correlates the degree of recovery with clinical signs observed at that point. Although the diagrams describe actual events in a specific population, the numbers in most instances are sufficiently large to provide a basis for estimating prognosis among similarly affected patients in the future. (From Levy DE, Bates D, Caronna JJ, et al.: Prognosis in nontraumatic coma. Ann Intern Med 94:293, 1981, with permission.)

and anterograde memory, even if sensorimotor activities return to normal. Persistence of coma or the vegetative state in an adult for more than four weeks almost never is associated with later complete recovery and the longer the mindless state lasts, the greater the chance of permanent disability. Care must be taken in such instances, however, to rule out a locked-in state (see Table 457–1).

Traumatic Coma

Coma following head injury enjoys a somewhat more favorable outcome than that associated with medical illness. About 50 per cent of patients in coma from head injury die. Acute treatment may somewhat improve that figure. Recovery in traumatic cases is closely linked to age: the younger the better. As with medical coma, severely abnormal neuro-ophthalmologic signs reflecting brain stem dysfunction carry from the start a poor prognosis, with approximately 90 per cent of such patients either dying or remaining in near-vegetative states.

Brain Death

Modern resuscitative devices can maintain the functions of the heart, lungs, and visceral organs for hours or days after the life-maintaining brain stem tissue. The economic waste of this hopeless condition, as well as the increasing success of organ transplant programs, has led countries worldwide to adopt the principle that death of the person occurs when either the brain or the heart irreversibly fails in its functions. In the United States the time of brain death has been accepted as the time of the person's death in legal terms. Many states accept the brain death concept by statute, and in no state has the principle been successfully challenged legally. The Presidential Commission set as the criterion for brain death the "irreversible cessation of all functions of the entire brain, including the brain stem." Guidelines for the practical application of these principles are listed in Table 457–11. One of the supplementary criteria often is particularly desirable when making decisions at six hours to facilitate organ transplant.

Certain points in the diagnosis of brain death must be

TABLE 457–11. CRITERIA FOR DIAGNOSIS OF BRAIN DEATH

1. **Nature and duration of coma is known**
   a. Known structural disease or irreversible systemic metabolic cause
   b. No chance of drug intoxication or hypothermia; no paralyzing or potentially anesthetizing drugs recently given for treatment
   c. Six-hour observation of no brain function is sufficient in cases of known structural cause when no drug or alcohol is involved in causation or treatment; otherwise, 12 hours plus negative drug screen required
2. **Absence of cerebral and brain stem function**
   a. No behavioral or reflex response to noxious stimuli above foramen magnum level
   b. Fixed pupils
   c. No oculovestibular response to 50 ml ice water calorics
   d. Apneic during oxygenation for 10 minutes
   e. Systemic circulation may be intact
   f. Purely spinal reflexes may be retained
3. **Supplementary (optional) criteria**
   a. EEG isoelectric for 30 minutes at maximal gain
   b. Brain stem–evoked responses reflect absent function in vital brain stem structures
   c. No cerebral circulation present on angiographic examination

emphasized. *Recoverable drug depressant poisoning can in all ways resemble brain death and must be explicitly ruled out.* In any doubtful case, any evidence of EEG activity or of reflex activity of the brain stem means that the brain is not dead and contravenes immediate discontinuation of life support. However, purely spinal reflex activity can persist after brain death, including reflexes of the limbs and even some upper cervical–controlled trunk movements.

In these controversy-laden and litigious times, it is recommended that physicians faced with applying and acting upon the diagnosis of brain death familiarize themselves with the additional pertinent material listed in the references.

Abrams MB, et al.: Deciding to Forego Life-Sustaining Treatment. A Report on the Ethical, Medical, and Legal Issues in Treatment Decisions. President's Commission for the Study of Ethical Problems in Medicine and Biomedical and Behavioral Research. Washington, D.C., United States Government Printing Office, March, 1983. *A long and thoughtful report on the problems associated with the terminally ill and the neurologically hopelessly damaged patient.*

Barber J, et al.: Guidelines for the determination of death: Report of the medical consultants on the diagnosis of death to the President's Commission for the Study of Ethical Problems in Medicine and Biomedical and Behavioral Research.. Neurology 32:395, 1982. *The detailed report describing that cardiac death and brain death are equivalent and giving criteria for each.*

Levy DE, Bates D, Caronna JJ, et al.: Prognosis in nontraumatic coma. Ann Intern Med 94:293, 1981. *Provides detailed information correlating nature of illness and early clinical neurologic signs with best one-year outcome in 500 patients with loss of consciousness due to medical illness.*

Levy DE, Caronna JJ, Singer BH, et al.: Predicting outcome from hypoxic-ischemic coma. JAMA 253:1420, 1985. *Prospective correlations were obtained between early neurologic signs and eventual course in 210 patients, mostly with cardiac arrest. By 72 hours, signs accurately selected between good or poor eventual outcome in over 75 per cent of patients.*

BRIEF LOSS OF CONSCIOUSNESS

Brief loss of consciousness, defined as loss of self-awareness lasting from a few seconds or minutes to an hour or more, is a relatively common symptom. If one excludes readily diag-

TABLE 457–12. PRINCIPAL CAUSES AND APPROXIMATE FREQUENCIES OF BRIEF LOSS OF CONSCIOUSNESS OF UNKNOWN ORIGIN

Syncope	
Primarily neurogenic-vasodepressor	55%
Primarily cardiogenic	10%
Central Nervous System	<10%
First seizure	
Cerebral vascular insufficiency	
Subarachnoid hemorrhage	
Intracranial pressure waves	
Drugs-Metabolic	<10%
Alcohol-sedative blackouts	
Narcotic overdose	
Hypoglycemia-exogenous or endogenous	
Diagnosis Unknown	15–20%

nosed causes such as acute traumatic concussion, a recurrence of known minor seizures, a sleep attack in a known narcoleptic, or accidental hypoglycemia in a known insulin-receiver, possible diagnoses become restricted to a limited number of causes (Table 457–12). *Syncope* turns out to be far and away the most common mechanism, with drug and alcohol "blackouts" possibly ranking a distant second. With any of the listed causes, however, unless either serious, new cardiovascular or neurologic changes outlast the episode, diagnosis depends almost entirely on a careful history plus whatever the physician can glean from witnesses, subsequent clinical medical findings, and a limited number of laboratory tests. Few episodes of brief loss of consciousness can be medically witnessed, and even prolonged follow-up often offers little help. Even with exhaustive evaluations, as many as one third of patients will elude precise diagnosis.

Certain immediate guidelines aid in differential diagnosis and prove valuable in deciding to what extent further laboratory investigations may be fruitful. Among patients younger than age 40 years, brief loss of consciousness is almost always either vasodepressor syncope or undiagnosable unless the history of physical findings explicitly indicate the presence of severe heart disease, systemic illness, a seizure disorder or epileptiform movements during the attack, or alcohol-drug abuse. Among patients older than age 40 years, cardiac causes of syncope increase in frequency; but even among them, if the history, physical, and standard laboratory evaluation disclose no evidence of severe cardiac, systemic, or neurologic illness, the symptom most often has benign implications. To prove such benignity with elaborate, expensive laboratory procedures is unwarranted. Cryptic thrombophlebitis producing pulmonary infarction is a threat at any age; hypoglycemia or other metabolic perturbations are rare causes of brief loss of consciousness in the absence of strongly suggestive associated symptoms.

Neurologic causes of brief loss of consciousness other than syncope are comparatively few and are usually diagnosable by history; CT scans and EEG's almost never provide the diagnosis in patients unsuspected clinically of neurologic disease. Drugs contribute importantly to loss of consciousness, some producing hypotension and others predisposing to withdrawal seizures at any age over about 25 years. Head injury seldom represents a diagnostic problem unless neither witnesses nor evidence of surface trauma are present. Malingering-hysteria is a possible explanation for unexplained loss of consciousness, but the diagnosis should be considered only when social circumstances are appropriate, when history reveals evidence of previous similar difficulties, or when the examiner witnesses a factitious attack. Even then, underlying associated physical disease should be ruled out.

Syncope

MECHANISMS OF SYNCOPE. Pathophysiologic changes in four systems, acting alone or together, can cause a transient reduction in global cerebral blood flow by the two thirds or more required to cause syncope (Table 457–13).

Neurogenic mechanisms include dysfunction of autonomic reflexes that act on the parasympathetic-sympathetic control of the heart and blood vessels so as to slow the heart (vagal hyperactivity) and impair the normal constriction of venous capacitance vessels of the trunk and lower extremities (reduced sympathetic outflow). The abnormal efferent pathways travel from medullary autonomic centers via vagal and sympathetic nerves and can be triggered from higher limbic-autonomic centers responding to stimuli of fear, pain, disgust, hunger, heat, or unknown (idiopathic) origin. Similar medullary efferent discharges can be reflexly activated by painful dilatation of visceral structures, following micturition, and excess carotid sinus stimulation (due to receptor hypersensitivity). The result in each case reduces right heart filling and induces orthostatic hypotension; positional failure of cerebral

TABLE 457–13. PRINCIPAL MECHANISMS OF SYNCOPE

I. Mainly impaired right heart filling
  A. Reflex abnormalities
    1. Vasodepressor ("vasovagal"): capacitance veins dilated, cardiac rate normal or slow
      a. Psychophysiologic (limbic) stimuli, including hyperventilation
      b. Visceral reflex (micturition, pain, gastrointestinal dilatation, acute labyrinthine vertigo)
      c. Carotid baroreceptor sensitivity
    2. Primary or secondary autonomic insufficiency (Ch. 463)
  B. Hypovolemia: hemorrhage, acute salt-water loss, protein loss, enteropathy, burns
  C. Mechanically impaired right heart return: Valsalva maneuver, tussive excess, abrupt chest compression; term pregnancy; pulmonary embolism; pericardial tamponade
II. Globally impaired cardiac output
  A. Reflex abnormalities
    1. Vagal sinus arrest
      a. Psychophysiologic (rare)
      b. Visceral stimulation: glossopharyngeal neuralgia, swallow syncope, direct tracheal stimulation, dilatation of hollow viscus
      c. Carotid baroreceptor sensitivity
  B. Intrinsic cardiac disease (with or without reflex enhancement) Table 457–14
III. Primary cerebral ischemia (uncommon)
  A. Multivessel cervical arterial obstructive disease
  B. Transient acute increase in intracranial pressure (plateau waves)
  C. Basilar migraine (rare in adults)
  D. Vertebral-basilar TIA's

perfusion either occurs abruptly or evolves over a 15 to 30 second period. Vagal influences on the heart occasionally can be sufficiently strong to produce syncope associated with severe bradyarrhythmia with pulse rates below 30 per minute in apparently healthy persons; more rarely and usually in older persons, atrioventricular arrest has been observed with vagal stimulation, e.g., associated with glossopharyngeal neuralgia or neck cancers involving the reflex arc itself. The latter mechanism of reflex atrioventricular arrest also has been incriminated in some instances of sudden death in overtrained athletes or on a psychophysiologic basis. Additional neurogenic mechanisms potentially causing syncope include the relatively common deconditioning of autonomic tone that follows prolonged bedrest or that marks the aging process. Autonomic insufficiency due to direct damage to medullary centers, descending autonomic pathways, or peripheral nerves can occur in several neurologic disorders, in all of which chronic orthostatic hypotension or syncopal attacks are common (Ch. 463).

Cardiac causes of syncope represent no more than perhaps 10 per cent of the total incidence but take on particular importance because they bespeak a poor prognosis, some studies indicating a one-year mortality as high as 25 to 30 per cent. To cause syncope, cardiac output must fall by at least half, and few such episodes have been directly monitored in the everyday situations in which most syncope occurs. In the erect position, asystole of greater than five seconds, bradycardia with a rate less than 30 to 40 per minute (depending on age), or tachycardia with rates greater than 160 to 180 per minute can by themselves produce either clouded consciousness or full syncope. In cardiac patients, however, an already damaged conduction system or myocardial reserve may predispose to an abnormally severe response to modest reflex vasodepression or vagal action that would fail to perturb a healthy cardiovascular system. Table 457–14 lists cardiac abnormalities particularly associated with syncopal attacks as detected by clinical evaluation, standard EKG, prolonged EKG monitoring, or invasive studies. The ingestion of hypotensive drugs adds to the risk of syncopal symptoms in cardiac patients.

Blood volume reduction can cause syncope with acute hemorrhage. Chronic hypovolemia is common in the chronically ill, in cardiac patients, and especially in hypertensives, in whom it represents a goal of therapy. The condition adds to the risk of syncopal symptoms accompanying either cardiac irregularities or the taking of antihypertensive drugs. Transient failure of blood to reach the heart also occurs in association with vigorous application of the Valsalva maneuver. The effect produces syncope during coughing, straining at stool, weight lifting, and the "fainting lark" of children.

Vascular disease, as such, is not a common cause of syncope. Deep vein thrombosis can lead to *pulmonary embolism* with transient failure of cardiac filling or asystole; brief loss of consciousness occasionally is the first symptom. *Dissecting aortic aneurysm* can severely reduce cerebral blood flow if it produces either pericardial hemorrhage with cardiac tamponade or chokes off the orifices of the great vessels in the neck. *Cervical atherosclerosis*, producing severe stenosis or occlusion of two or more of the four brain-supplying internal carotid-vertebral arteries, occasionally causes recurrent confusion or syncope when severe narrowing or a source of emboli develops in the remaining, still patent vessels. The same cervical atherosclerotic process can cause recurrent orthostatic symptoms, including syncope, in the absence of any change in systemic blood pressure. Noninvasive carotid ultrasound studies help to diagnose such instances. Despite their frequency, vertebrobasilar transient ischemic attacks only rarely cause loss of consciousness.

SYNCOPE DUE PRIMARILY TO IMPAIRED RIGHT HEART FILLING (Mainly Reflex Syncope). Most examples of syncope resulting from a failure of right heart filling are associated with abnormalities in the neural feedback loop, described above, which reflexly controls the systemic circulation.

Syncope resulting from failure of right heart filling nearly always reflects pooling of blood in the venous, capacitance vessels of the lower extremities or the splanchnic abdominal circulation. Relaxation of arterial resistance vessels plays a lesser role. Since gravitational factors contribute importantly to the impaired venous return, fainting caused by impaired right heart filling always occurs in the erect or, occasionally, sitting positions.

Acute Vasodepressor (Vasovagal) Syncope. This is the most common cause of fainting and typically is marked by a diphasic course. During an initial brief period of apprehension and anxiety, heart rate, blood pressure, total systemic resistance, and cardiac output all may increase. *This initial sequence, however, often is lacking.* The vasodepressor phase follows, during which heart rate slows and blood pressure falls, cardiac output declines, and the CBF eventually drops. Both sympathetic and parasympathetic abnormalities are involved, since atropine prevents the bradycardia but not the depressor response. Symptoms of palpitation, salivation, and anxiety characteristically mark the first phase, whereas progressive sensations of lightheadedness, giddiness, abdominal sinking sensations, nausea, urinary urgency, and finally "gray-out" or faintness accompany the vasodepressor component. Occasionally the reflex suppression of sympathetic tone comes so rapidly that the affected subject topples like a log. Rarely, with a severe attack of vasodepressor syncope, as with other forms of profound reduction of cardiac output and cerebral ischemia, brief tonic convulsive movements result (convulsive syncope).

During vasodepressor syncope, subjects appear pale (but not dead-white), rather than cyanotic, and the accompanying parasympathetic hyperactivity characteristically induces pilo-

TABLE 457–14. CARDIOVASCULAR ABNORMALITIES FREQUENTLY ASSOCIATED WITH SYNCOPAL ATTACKS

Myocardial infarction	Ventricular tachycardia
Aortic stenosis	Sick sinus syndrome
Severe cardiomyopathy	Complete heart block
Severe hypertension	Asystole (> ± 3 sec erect, ± 8
Pulmonary embolism	sec supine)
Pulmonary hypertension	Bradycardia 30–44/min
Dissecting aortic aneurysm	Tachycardia > 160–180/min
Pacemaker malfunction	

erection and sweating. Awareness and normal cardiovascular reflexes usually return promptly once the subject becomes supine. Vomiting or explosive diarrhea may follow. Occasionally dysautonomic influences on the heart are so profound as to induce arrhythmia. Engel and others have speculated that this is one mechanism causing sudden death associated with sudden grief or fright.

Fainting is more likely in hungry subjects, in a warm moist environment, and after prolonged standing. A few individuals give a history of lifelong susceptibility to fainting attacks, and rarely one gets a history of multiple family members in several generations who have been susceptible to recurrent vasodepressor syncope.

Visceral reflex syncope acts via the same medullospinal pathways as the examples cited above. A sense of faintness or even complete syncope can follow immediately after any of the following: emptying a full bladder from the standing position (micturition syncope), acute visceral pain (as occurs with a suddenly distended gut or an abrupt joint or ligament injury), an attack of severe vertigo (as occurs with Ménière's disease), or a migraine attack.

Carotid sinus syncope type 2 describes a severe vasodepressor response to carotid sinus massage. The condition is seldom a practical consideration except with neoplasms of the neck that directly irritate afferent glossopharyngeal fibers.

The diagnosis of vasodepressor syncope is made largely by history; rarely are the events medically witnessed. Among young persons who lack histories of neurologic or cardiovascular disease and have normal physical examinations, laboratory examinations beyond routine blood work and an ECG are almost always uninformative and therefore unnecessary. Treatment is symptomatic. Impending sensations of faintness should be treated promptly by placing the subject supine. Placing the head far forward in a sitting position is customary but less effective, because it fails to empty the enlarged pool of blood located in the muscles and veins of the lower extremities. If the heart rhythm is regular, no further resuscitative measures are needed. Subjects who have fainted should be mobilized slowly, because the reflex abnormality occasionally can persist for as long as two hours. Prophylactic treatment has little value except when fainting occurs in response to a disease or injury that requires attention. Occasionally, overtrained athletes with chronically slow hearts and a history of syncope during exertion are helped by a regimen of reduced training combined with oral anticholinergic agents.

Orthostatic Hypotension. Acute orthostatic hypotension occasionally can occur in normal persons after acute blood loss or following prolonged standing; affected subjects undergo a sudden collapse of sympathetic reflex tone, as with soldiers at parade rest in a hot sun. Recurrent symptoms of syncope or faintness accompanying the erect position, however, usually can be traced to the presence of the chronic use of vasodepressor drugs or to neurologic disorders involving the peripheral or central nervous system. Increased age tends to intensify the effects of either cause. Many drugs accentuate tendencies to orthostatic hypotension, including almost all of the antihypertensive agents and a large proportion of the antidepressants, phenothiazines, and sedatives. Any tendency to impaired sympathetic reflex control is accentuated by a reduced blood volume such as is caused by Addison's disease, protein loss, or enteropathy. The combination of chronic diuretic use and vasodepressant medication outnumbers all other causes combined.

Orthostatic hypotension sufficient to cause cerebral symptoms can occur either rapidly upon standing or develop insidiously over seconds or minutes. Although symptoms of faintness and giddiness predominate, some patients lack such warnings, presumably because of the absence of strong efferent parasympathetic activity. When patients in this latter group sit for long periods or stand, they may become confused or tremulous without the usual sensations of faintness. Mental cloudiness, staggering, or falling is more common than complete unconsciousness. Diagnosis comes from observing an acute or progressive decline in the mean blood pressure of more than 10 to 15 mm Hg in the erect position. Autonomic insufficiency can be inferred by observing an unchanging pulse rate despite the hypotension, and confirmed by tilt-table tests or by identifying other autonomic impairment. The simplest way to evaluate sympathetic tone at the bedside is to take the pulse while the supine patient performs a vigorous Valsalva maneuver; the normal response consists of a palpable post-Valsalva slowing of pulse and a 10 to 30 mm Hg rise in mean blood pressure.

Treatment of orthostatic hypotension depends upon the cause. Symptomatic treatment requires eliminating drugs that cause hypotension, searching for and correcting causes of blood volume depletion, and applying elastic stockings to the lower extremities. When other measures fail, an increased salt intake and, subsequently, administering the salt-retaining steroid fludrocortisone, 0.3 to 0.8 mg per day in divided doses, can be cautiously initiated. The chronic use of vasopressor agents seldom helps. Just as vasomotor reflexes can be deconditioned by excess bed rest, they can be at least partially reconditioned by erect activity. Every effort should be made to keep affected patients up and walking.

SYNCOPE DUE PRIMARILY TO IMPAIRED LEFT HEART OUTPUT (Mainly Cardiac Syncope). *Vagovagal attacks* consist of reflexly induced changes in the cardiac rhythm, including nodal or sinus arrest, atrioventricular asystole, atrioventricular block, sinoatrial block, and ventricular arrhythmias. Usually these are accompanied by relatively minor vasodepressor changes in the peripheral vasculature, implying a lesser sympathetic component. Most but not all patients with vagovagal attacks belong to the older population and have associated heart disease. Most vagally induced cardiac arrhythmia or arrest represents an abnormally intense cardiac response to a relatively normal degree of increased parasympathetic stimulation or sympathetic inhibition. Vagal bradycardia or arrest occasionally is induced by sudden emotional stimuli, but more commonly follows acute noxious or abnormal visceral stimulation. Severe bradycardia or arrest especially accompanies glossopharyngeal neuralgia, swallowing in patients with mechanical esophageal lesions, sudden painful dilatations of a hollow viscus, prostatic manipulation, tracheal stimulation, or visceral wounds. *Carotid sinus syncope type 1* is a rare phenomenon in which massage or pressure of the sinus induces transient asystole.

Cardiac syncope almost always reflects serious heart disease. Analyses of large series of patients show that serious associated risk factors include those listed in Table 457–14. In the case of patients over 40 years of age or those showing risk factors in Table 457–14, prolonged (Holter) monitoring of cardiac activity is indicated. In the absence of specific predisposing abnormalities discovered by history, physical examination and such EKG monitoring, direct electrophysiologic studies of the heart, cardiac catheterization, coronary or cerebral angiography, brain CT scanning, and electroencephalography seldom add helpful information. Management of cardiac syncope depends upon the nature of the underlying heart disease, although affected persons should be considered for pacemaker insertion.

Other Causes of Brief Alterations of Consciousness

Hyperventilation is mechanistically closely related to syncope in that a globally reduced cerebral blood flow gives rise to sensations of giddiness, faintness, and other distress. Full unconsciousness rarely occurs without some additional abnormal maneuver. The abnormal state is most often part of an anxiety response and often is accompanied by sensations of suffocation, pressure on the chest, and a sense of being unable to obtain the satisfaction of a lung-filling deep breath.

Extreme or prolonged hyperventilation can produce feelings of unreality with anxiety bordering on panic.

In healthy subjects, only a modest increase in respiratory rate and depth is required to drop $Paco_2$ levels promptly to 25 mm Hg or less; once a new steady state develops, little more than the normal level of breathing is sufficient to match bodily CO_2 production and maintain hypocapnia. Casual inspection may show no more than a respiratory rate of 16 to 18 per minute, interrupted perhaps by occasional sighs. Hypocapnia induces cerebral vasoconstriction, which reduces the amount of oxygen delivered to the brain and is the presumed basis of the accompanying sensations.

Symptoms and signs include feelings of unreality, difficulty in concentrating, and several hard-to-explain sensory complaints, such as unilateral or bilateral chest pain or paresthesias involving the body and extremities. Symptoms of facial twitching, carpal spasm, and perioral paresthesias are more easily understood as part of alkalotic tetany.

Diagnosis is easy when otherwise structurally healthy patients complain of the aforementioned symptoms in settings of anxiety of dyspnea, but necessarily is conjectural when made in retrospect. Some patients can reproduce their symptoms by voluntarily overbreathing, and the maneuver can be helpful in guiding treatment. Most often the symptoms are observed as part of a larger pattern of anxiety and must be treated accordingly.

Hyperventilation occasionally precipitates syncope under special circumstances. Children sometimes voluntarily hyperventilate, then perform a vigorous Valsalva maneuver to induce syncope (fainting lark). Athletes may repeat a similar sequence in contests such as weight lifting or squat jumps. More dangerous is a pattern wherein underwater swimmers hyperventilate before diving, then exhaust their oxygen reserves before producing sufficient carbon dioxide to produce dyspnea. The ensuing cerebral hypoxia can induce fatal submersion syncope.

SEIZURE DISORDERS. Seizure disorders, discussed fully in Ch. 493, produce a diagnostic problem under four principal circumstances:

1. *Rapid, profound syncope* may induce a single brief tonic seizure or series of clonic twitches as a result of abrupt cerebral ischemia (convulsive syncope). The response is more likely when the subject has made maximal effort to stand or sit despite premonitory symptoms. Differential diagnosis rests on identifying the following as more consistent with syncope than epilepsy: the attendant psychologic circumstances and physical appearance, the associated medical conditions and body position, the brief quality of the seizure, rapid recovery, and the presence of a normal neurologic examination and interictal EEG.

2. *Akinetic seizures* consist of suddenly falling or pitching to the ground, starting in early childhood. Similar attacks occur in the supine position and are marked by unresponsiveness accompanied by generalized muscular hypotonia or brief body spasm. Diagnosis rests on the typical history, the age of onset, and the presence of an abnormal EEG. *Absence (petit mal) seizures* rarely provide a diagnostic problem, since the child, although out of contact during the attacks, neither falls nor turns pale and usually has no memory of the episode. The EEG is abnormal and frequently diagnostic.

3. *Partial complex (psychomotor) seizures* sometimes include brief behavioral automatisms in which the subject recalls only being out of contact and may retrospectively consider himself to have suffered a state of unconsciousness. Usually the presence of a characteristic, self-recognized aura or set of incipient symptoms indicates the diagnosis. Falling to the ground rarely occurs unless a generalized seizure develops. Witnessed attacks and the EEG usually are typical.

4. *Postictal unresponsiveness* from grand mal attacks produces unconsciousness lasting minutes, the duration usually depending on the severity of the preceding convulsion. Diag-

nosis is a problem only if the seizure was unwitnessed, in which case the state may look like concussion or profound fainting. However, the postictal state is marked initially by flushing (cyanosis), giving way to pallor, hyperpnea, and deep unresponsiveness, none of which occurs in syncope.

HYPOGLYCEMIA (see Ch. 232). Hypoglycemia, usually caused by excess exogenous insulin, less often by insulin secreted from endogenous tissues, can produce a variety of relatively brief episodes of neurologic dysfunction. These can consist, variably, of brief confusional episodes, seizures of a variety of types, narcolepsy-like syndromes, and focal or tetraparetic weakness with or without coma but not resembling syncope. Diagnosis depends on suspicion plus the detection of blood sugars of less than 30 to 40 mg per deciliter during an attack.

DRUG OR ALCOHOL BLACKOUTS. Drug or alcohol blackouts consist of episodes of such severe intoxication that they anesthetize memory for the event, leaving the subject with an episode of focal amnesia. Many are accompanied by "passing out," consisting of deep, barely arousable sleep.

CONCUSSION-POSTCONCUSSION AMNESIA. Variable periods of memory loss for immediate subsequent events can follow brief periods of concussive unconsciousness. The usual question is whether an intrinsic malady caused the fall or whether the fall represented the whole illness. Only diagnostic diligence can solve the issue.

ACUTE INTRACRANIAL HYPERTENSION. Plateau waves, associated with this condition, can produce brief episodes of loss of consciousness that resemble syncope, as described above. Occasionally, such brief unconsciousness may accompany the onset of acute subarachnoid hemorrhage. The unconscious episode, which is syncopal in its abruptness and often accompanied by either a tonic extensor spasm or brief clonic jerks, is most often due to an acute cardiac arrhythmia or asystole accompanying the onset of bleeding. Cerebral hemorrhage with intraventricular rupture can produce similar events.

Conditions Sometimes Resembling Loss of Consciousness

DROP SPELLS. As discussed in Chapter 465, these are poorly understood attacks affecting older persons. The legs suddenly and unexplainedly give way, and the women fall, often injuring themselves but experiencing no observed interruption of consciousness. The cause is unknown.

CONVERSION REACTIONS OR MALINGERING (Pseudosyncope). Hysterical or other forms of psychogenic unresponsiveness are almost impossible to diagnose in retrospect. If such a condition occurs during the physical examination, however, the diagnosis is based on the absence of physiologic abnormality and the presence of additional, often bizarre features. Most subjects awaken with gentle but firm confrontation. A few do so only when advised that psychiatric admission lies in store. Mutilating stimuli are unjustified and often unsuccessful as ways to prove the diagnosis.

Day SC, Cook ET, Funkenstein H, et al.: Evaluation and outcome of emergency room patients with transient loss of consciousness. Am J Med 73:15, 1982. *An analysis of 198 patients, giving differential diagnosis, identifying low- and high-risk groups, and indicating relative value of laboratory tests.*

Engel GL: Psychological stress, vasodepressor (vasovagal) syncope and sudden death. Ann Intern Med 89:403, 1978. *Must reading for the internist by one of the pioneers in understanding of both the physiology and emotion of cardiovascular responses.*

Evans DW, Lum LC: Hyperventilation: An important cause of pseudoangina. Lancet 1:155, 1977. *A clinical article, emphasizing the often misleading symptoms of the disorder.*

Kapoor WN, Karpf M, Maher Y, et al.: Syncope of unknown origin. The need for a more effective approach to its diagnostic evaluation. JAMA 247:2687, 1982. *Among 121 older patients with syncope, cardiac monitoring, cardiac electrophysiologic studies, and cardiac catheterization provided diagnostic evidence in only 13. Glucose tolerance tests, head CT, brain scans, lumbar puncture, and skull x-ray aided diagnosis in none.*

Kapoor WN, Karpf M, Wieand S, et al.: A prospective evaluation and follow-up of patients with syncope. N Engl J Med 309:197, 1983. *Among 204 mainly older patients with syncope, 40 per cent of whom were hospitalized from the start, diagnosis could be made in 53 per cent. Twenty-six per cent had a cardiovascular cause. At one year half the cardiovascular group had died, compared to 12 per cent with noncardiovascular causes and 6 per cent in the idiopathic group.*

Parsons M: Fits and other causes of loss of consciousness while driving. Q J Med 227:295, 1986. *Among 223 retrospectively reviewed examples, myocardial infarctions most often caused the condition but because of premonitions resulted in few accidents fatal to nondrivers. Falling asleep at the wheel accounted for 27 per cent of the series but 83 per cent of associated deaths. Alcohol levels were not reported.*

Savage DD, Corwin L, McGee DL, et al.: Epidemiologic features of isolated syncope: The Framingham study. Stroke 16:626, 1985. *In a population of 5209 men and women aged 30 to 62 years and then followed for a mean of 26 years, 3.3 per cent developed syncope without evidence for concurrent cardiovascular or neurologic disease. Such isolated syncope was not associated with any subsequent increased incidence of stroke, cardiovascular disease, or early mortality compared to the remainder of the cohort.*

458 SLEEP AND ITS DISORDERS

J. Allan Hobson

Sleep is a complex biologic function that normally varies among individuals, lasting between four and ten hours. Short sleepers tend to be hyperactive but productive and well-adjusted, whereas long sleepers tend to be low-key, under-achieving, and may be mildly depressed. Different species of animals also show marked differences in sleep length. Accordingly, sleep duration as such cannot be taken as an index of pathology, and the physician should beware of pushing patients against powerful biologic gradients.

Sleep varies according to age. The neonate sleeps two thirds of the time. At sexual maturity, this duration has fallen by half, but the capacity for deep, fulfilling sleep is still robust. By age 40 sleep normally becomes more shallow, and by age 60 sleep length may decrease further. The older the person the more the awakenings.

Sleep also varies within individuals from one sleep-wake cycle to the next. During highly productive periods, sleep need may decrease; sleep length may also undergo unwanted shortening during periods of anxiety and stress. Within limits—to be judged by the individual's adaptive responses—these variations should be regarded as signals to be understood and dealt with during the awake state rather than symptoms of disease needing to be extinguished via sedation.

Activity patterns also influence sleep variables. Animal experiments indicate that moderate exercise reduces sleep latency while also increasing sleep length and depth. Good sleep can be expected to follow poor. Despite highly publicized initial results, sleep deprivation studies have not revealed specific or long-lasting ill effects, so that conservative management is not likely to be dangerous even to the patient who may ultimately need pharmacologic treatment.

PHYSIOLOGY AND PHARMACOLOGY OF SLEEP. Normal circadian rhythms oscillate at slightly more than 24 hours in length and are reset each day by light and other time cues. The circadian oscillator appears to include the suprachiasmatic nucleus of the hypothalamus. The hypothalamus receives a direct input from the optic tract, which delivers the light pulses that reset the rhythm each day. Lesions of the posterior hypothalamus produce hypersomnia, whereas lesions of the anterior hypothalamus produce insomnia.

Each normal sleep period consists of a series of biphasic 90- to 100-minute cycles. A non–rapid eye movement (NREM) phase initiates sleep and each subsequent cycle. It is characterized by progressive EEG slowing and corresponding decreases in muscle tone, heart rate, respiratory rate, and blood pressure. When this deactivation process is maximal—at about mid-cycle—subjects are difficult to rouse and may be disoriented or may even confabulate when asked to report their mental activity. A typical night's sleep pattern is diagrammed in Figure 458-1.

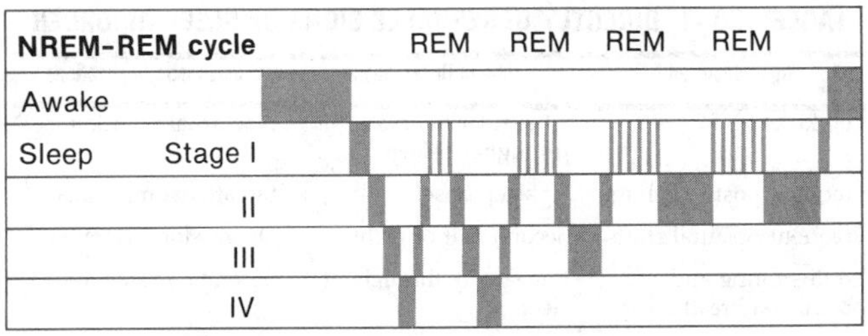

FIGURE 458–1. A typical night's sleep pattern.

The rapid eye movement (REM) phase follows NREM and ends each cycle. It is characterized by progressive reactivation of the EEG and autonomic functions. Muscle tone is actively inhibited in REM, paralyzing all but the ocular musculature. During REM, the eyes execute spectacular runs of nystagmiform movement behind still-closed lids. Heart and respiratory rates quicken and blood pressure rises. Subjects are easily aroused from REM sleep and often report detailed and vivid dreams.

The NREM-REM cycle repeats itself four or five times each night with postural shifts occurring at transitional points.

Lesion and ablation studies in animals indicate that the system controlling the EEG sleep cycle is located in the pontine brain stem. Single cell recordings suggest that two interconnected neuronal populations fluctuate periodically and oppositely owing to the reciprocal interaction of their excitatory and inhibitory neurotransmitters. During waking the resting activity level of aminergic inhibitory neurons is high. The nuclei containing these "waking" cells include the noradrenergic locus ceruleus and the serotonergic dorsal raphe nucleus. As a consequence of aminergic inhibition, the resting activity level of cholinergic neurons in many brain stem reticular nuclei is low in waking. During the NREM phase of the sleep cycle, aminergic inhibition gradually declines; simultaneously, cholinergic excitation increases and at mid-cycle the balance between aminergic inhibition and cholinergic excitation shifts. The REM period occurs when aminergic inhibition has fallen to its low point and cholinergic excitation becomes maximal.

THE EVALUATION OF SLEEP COMPLAINTS. Subjective disturbances in sleep can take a variety of forms—some distressing mainly to the sleeper, others bothering partners more than the sleeper. Table 458–1 lists the most frequent complaints offered by patients or their partners. Studies in sleep laboratories bring out two major features regarding patient complaints in relation to actual difficulties. One is that most who complain of insomnia far overestimate their actual time awake. The other is that patients with obstructive sleep apnea often are unaware of their many sleep-time obstructive arousals, some of which may lower arterial oxygen saturation to 50 per cent or less. In any event, in the presence of persistent complaints of difficulty sleeping, patients and, preferably, their partners as well should keep a reliable log of the disturbances so as to provide a quantitative estimate. Patients with protracted or recurrent sleep apnea may require the special expertise offered by a sleep laboratory.

CLASSIFICATION OF SLEEP DISORDERS. *The Insomnias* (Table 458–2). Current trends, spurred by the discovery of side effects of sedative medication, are toward a conservative, behaviorally oriented management approach of disorders of initiating and maintaining sleep. To be successful, this approach must first emphasize careful diagnostic study to determine specific underlying causes. In the most common, nonspecific cases, patients need education in the multifactorial determinants of sleep quality and duration, support in their behavioral and pharmacologic potentiation, and close follow-up monitoring of these interventions.

MEDICAL INSOMNIA. Many medical conditions exert specific and nonspecific effects on sleep. These include fever (which immediately suppresses REM sleep) and pain (which pro-

TABLE 458–1. DIRECTLY OBSERVABLE SIGNS OF SLEEP DISORDER

Signs Reported	Time of Observation	Diagnostic Implications
Leg kicks	At regular intervals throughout sleep	Nocturnal myoclonus
Frequent postural shifts	At sleep onset	Situational insomnia
Frequent postural shifts	Second half of night	Depression insomnia
Loud snoring and obstructed breathing	Repeatedly throughout sleep	Secondary sleep apnea
REM's with frightening dreams	At sleep onset	Narcolepsy
Arousal in fear (poor recall)	From NREM sleep, first half of night	Night terrors and nightmares
Arousal in fear (good recall)	From REM, second half of night	Frightening dreams
Coordinated mobility but unresponsive	From NREM sleep	Somnambulism (sleep walking)
Tooth grinding	From NREM sleep	Bruxism
Vocalization	From NREM sleep	Somniloquy (sleep talking)
Urination	From REM or NREM sleep	Enuresis
Uncoordinated mobility but unresponsive	From REM sleep	REM sleep without atonia
Quiet cessation of breathing	Deep sleep or initiating sleep	Primary sleep apnea

duces a general increase in arousal level). Sleep loss is common in hospital settings, where sleep-disruptive procedures can combine with anxiety to make night life miserable. Patients with coronary or pulmonary insufficiencies may decompensate during the autonomic storm of REM sleep. The patient with congestive heart failure or emphysema may be aware or unaware of the frequent interruptions of sleep which are caused by anoxic stimulation of the reticular formation and which may be lifesaving. Before prescribing sedatives, specific treatment of the underlying medical disease and manipulation of environmental variables must be vigorously pursued.

PSYCHIATRIC INSOMNIA. A variety of neurotic and psychotic disorders, all known to be associated with disturbances in balance of central sympathetic and cholinergic activity, are characterized by difficulty falling asleep and staying asleep.

The management of chronic anxiety, always notoriously difficult, is now further complicated by the discovery of three undesirable properties of the benzodiazepine class of hypnotic agents. One is a subtle but pernicious addiction syndrome, associated with the long-term use of diazepam. Another is rebound insomnia, a worsening of sleep following intermediate term use of nitrazepam,* flunitrazepam,* temazepam, and triazolam. The third is an interference with daytime functioning caused by the cumulative build-up of active metabolites of such "long-acting" agents as flurazepam, diazepam, and flunitrazepam, whose products have half-lives of

---

*Investigational drug in the United States.

TABLE 458–2. THE INSOMNIAS

Specific
    Circadian rhythm shift
    Nocturnal myoclonus
    Sleep apnea
Nonspecific
    Medical
        Fever
        Pain
        Cardiopulmonary disease
    Psychiatric
        Anxiety, stress
        Alcohol and drugs
        Depression
        Schizophrenia

---

36 to 48 hours. Short-acting agents, with half-lives of 10 to 12 hours, are less liable to suppress daytime effectiveness (lorazepam, triazolam, and temazepam).

GUIDELINES FOR PRESCRIBING SEDATIVES. A versatile and flexible approach to sedative prescription is needed. For example, when the desired relief of acute anxiety and insomnia has been obtained from a diazepine such as diazepam (Valium), 2 to 5 mg at bedtime, patient and physician can expect some temporary worsening of sleep when the drug is withdrawn. One should not attempt to suppress this time-limited effect of the treatment itself by increasing drug administration. The other agents (e.g., triazolam [Halcion], 0.125 to 0.250 mg at bedtime) tend not to produce rebound and are effective hypnotics. In cases of persistent or recurrent insomnia, intermittent and alternating drug use reduces the problems of habituation and withdrawal. Barbiturates are ill advised in view of their low margin of safety and addictive potential.

Chloral hydrate (0.5 to 1.0 gram at bedtime) deserves consideration. Amitriptyline (50 mg at bedtime) can enhance sleep even in patients who are not depressed. The tricyclic antidepressants also improve the sleep of severely depressed patients who may complain of sudden worsening of sleep when effective treatment is stopped. During such withdrawal, frightening hallucinations, occurring on awakening, may mislead both patient and doctor into thinking that psychosis is recurrent when, in reality, a time-limited and transitory pharmacodynamic intensification of REM sleep is the cause. This complaint demands reassurance, not reinstitution of medication.

Alcohol is a self-administered CNS depressant with profound short- and long-term effects on sleep. The REM phase of the cycle is suppressed during the first part of the night when sleep may be unusually sound. An associated suppression of normal postural shifts may explain the Saturday night paralysis that results from nerve compression occurring in alcoholic sleep. Later in the night, when metabolic breakdown products accumulate, sleep is fitful and more REM deprivation is incurred. Hangover includes a feeling of sleepiness and fatigue which alcohol may temporarily reverse only to perpetuate and intensify.

NOCTURNAL MYOCLONUS. In late middle-aged and elderly patients, rhythmic muscle twitches may cause sleep-disturbing involuntary movements of the extremities. Clonazepam (0.5 to 1.0 mg at bedtime) can be effective.

The Hypersomnias (Table 458–3). NARCOLEPSY. Narcolepsy is a syndrome in which patients complain of persistent drowsiness and one or more of a tetrad of specific signs: (1) *Sleep attacks*, which occur suddenly, are often REM sleep attacks. (2) *Cataplexy* is an equally sudden muscle weakness akin to atonia which normally occurs only in nocturnal REM. Cataplexy is often precipitated by surprise, mirth, or anger. (3) *Hypnagogic hallucinations* are vivid and frightening illusions associated with partial arousal from the sleep-onset REM period. (4) *Sleep paralysis* is an abnormal extension of REM sleep atonia into the waking state.

Narcolepsy is a relatively common disorder, affecting men more than women and displaying a strong hereditary pattern, suggesting the action of an autosomal dominant trait with variable expression. The disorder characteristically arises in the teens and may continue throughout life, although symptoms often become less incapacitating in late middle age.

TABLE 458–3. THE HYPERSOMNIAS

Primary
    Narcolepsy
    Kleine-Levin syndrome
    Sleep apnea
Secondary
    CNS lesion
    Pickwickian syndrome
    Depression

Sleep attacks tend to come on during periods of quiet semiattention such as when driving a car, listening to a lecture, or engaging in dull conversation. In any event, the attacks often are uncontrollable, and their unwarned appearance can lead to great social embarrassment and even injury.

Treatment of narcolepsy is only partially successful. Amphetamines or methylphenidate brings moderate relief from drowsiness, while the antidepressant amine oxidase inhibitors have been reported to ameliorate cataplectic attacks.

KLEINE-LEVIN SYNDROME. This is a rare disorder that occurs primarily in adolescent males and is characterized by episodic periods of excessive sleep and overeating, lasting up to several weeks. The cause is unknown. There is no specific treatment, although anecdotal reports describe relief with clonazepam.

DEPRESSION. Not only do asymptomatic long-sleepers tend to be depressed, some clinically depressed patients also tend to hypersomnolence (as well as to difficulty falling asleep). This depressive sleep disorder is best treated with amine reuptake blockers (which are also anticholinergic) and is aggravated by physostigmine.

PICKWICKIAN SYNDROME. Hypersomnia is integral to the obesity-hypoventilation syndrome and is a primary result of the anoxemia and hypercarbia consequent upon waking state hypoventilation. Waking arterial oxygen levels are often normal in the sleep apnea syndromes, and the hypersomnia seen in those conditions is, in part, secondary to the sleep disturbance.

The Parasomnias (Table 458–4). The parasomnias feature loss of control of some neural subsystem during sleep. All are age, sex, and sleep stage dependent.

ENURESIS. Bedwetting is a troublesome sleep disorder occurring predominantly in preadolescent males. Because the full bladder does not trigger an awakening, enuresis has been conceived of as a disorder of arousal. The beneficial effects of imipramine (25 to 50 mg given at bedtime) have been attributed mainly to peripheral anticholinergic effects on the bladder. Because of the risks of using drugs and even behavioral treatment in children, only the most persistent and severe cases should be treated.

NIGHT TERRORS, NIGHTMARES, SLEEP WALKING, SLEEP TALKING, AND BRUXISM. In night terrors, there is a partial arousal, in panic, from Stages III and IV of NREM sleep, associated with tachycardia and tachypnea. Although capable of coordinated motor behavior and responsive to sensory input, the affected child may hallucinate and thus terrify his parents as much as himself. Fortunately night terrors are benign and short lived, so that reassurance is both appropriate and adequate. Nightmares also occur in older subjects but tend to decline or disappear by middle age. They can be precipitated from NREM sleep when they are characterized by pure fear (without visual hallucinoid imagery) or from REM sleep (when vivid frightening dreams are reported). In both types, intense autonomic storm is measurable. Nightmares of the NREM type have been reported to respond to benzodiazepines such as diazepam, 2 to 5 mg. Age is also helpful, since Stage IV declines markedly in the fourth decade.

In sleep talking and sleep walking, automatic motor activity begins in Stages III and IV of NREM sleep without full arousal and without accompanying mental activity; bruxism occurs in Stage I of NREM sleep. Sleep talking is entirely benign and should not be treated; disturbed roommates may have to

TABLE 458–4. THE PARASOMNIAS

Motor
    Enuresis
    Sleep walking
    REM sleep without atonia
    Sleep talking
    Night terrors
    Bruxism
Respiratory
    Sleep apnea

make adjustments. A boxer's mouthpiece prevents enamel destruction in bruxism, and a child's stairway gate or other physical restraint may avoid embarrassment and injury in somnambulism. There is no evidence that these conditions are psychologically determined, and all are age related.

REM SLEEP WITHOUT ATONIA. Males over age 50 may injure themselves or their bed partners by performing dreamed motor acts of a vigorous or violent nature. These episodes occur in REM sleep (from which the patient does not arouse) owing to failure of the spinal inhibition which normally quells the movements commanded by the brain. Clonazepam 0.5 to 1.0 mg at bedtime can be effective.

THE SLEEP APNEA SYNDROMES. Sleep apnea occurs in two forms. Obstructive apnea occurs chiefly as a complication of obesity. Central apnea is a genetically determined failure of CNS drive in males. A combination of the two can be fatal. Primary sleep apnea also can occur as a complication of CNS disease affecting the lower brain stem and upper cervical spinal cord.

Middle-aged male patients who complain of either excessive daytime sleepiness or incapability of staying asleep at night should be considered as possibly suffering from the sleep apnea syndrome. If they are obese and snore, descriptions on tape recordings of their obstructive apneic spells—which occur on the order of 300 times per night—may be obtained from a bed partner. These peripherally mediated events are due to collapse of a fat-compromised airway by the negative intrathoracic pressure of inspiration; the situation is often made worse by the vigorous compensatory respiratory effects that ensue, accompanied by strained grunts. Observable cyanosis may develop and recovery occurs only with arousal. The frequent awakenings contribute to the excessive daytime sleepiness.

Even the peripheral obstructive type of apnea, which is often relieved by tracheostomy, an airway prosthesis, or a continuous positive-pressure nasally delivered airstream, may have a central component, since neither surgery nor weight loss always eliminates the sleep apnea episodes. Cases of pure central apnea are uncommon and difficult to diagnose—an important point, since sedative medication, prescribed as a well-intentioned response to the complaint of insomnia, may depress the respiratory centers. Patients suspected of having clinically significant sleep apnea are best referred for diagnosis and treatment to a sleep laboratory with pulmonary recording capability.

Cardiac abnormalities can complicate the pickwickian syndrome and the sleep apneas. Marked sinus arrhythmias may accompany the apneic spells, and extreme bradycardia, asystoles, second-degree atrioventricular block, premature ventricular contractions, atrial flutter, and ventricular tachycardia have all been reported. The abnormalities clear if night-time apnea and its associated hypoxemia are prevented.

At all ages males are more prone than females to intrinsic sleep abnormalities. The tendency to snore, to stop breathing, and to collapse and/or obstruct the airway in sleep has a genetic component and is greater in men of the same family. The times in life at which pathologic consequences are most likely to emerge are infancy (sudden infant death syndrome), puberty (chubby puffer syndrome), and late middle age (sleep apnea syndrome).

Cardiorespiratory arrest is a likely cause of *sudden "crib" death* in infancy. In those infants who are "near-miss" for sudden infant death, apneas occur with increasing frequency at four and one half months of age, predominantly during NREM sleep. The period of greatest risk for fatal accidents is between birth and six months of age, and respiratory infection is thought to be a contributing factor. Home-monitoring systems have been developed to detect apneas and alert parents to the need for resuscitative maneuvers.

In the *chubby puffer syndrome*, obese prepubescent males may resemble adult pickwickians whose symptoms are ascribed to primary alveolar hypoventilation, and this sign may persist after temporary relief has been provided by adenotonsillectomy. These facts imply a central respiratory abnormality whose neural basis is as yet obscure. Treatments designed to increase central respiratory drive with aminophylline and progesterone have not been generally effective. Recent reports claim that the antidepressant tricyclic agent protriptyline has been effective.

PHYSIOLOGY AND PHARMACOLOGY

Hobson JA, Steriade M: Neuronal basis of behavioral state control. In Mountcastle V (ed.): Handbook of Physiology. Section I. The Nervous System. Vol IV. Intrinsic Regulatory Systems of the Brain. Bethesda, MD, American Physiological Society, 1986, pp 701–823. *A comprehensive review of the basic science literature on sleep, which includes a systematic pathophysiologic approach to the sleep disorders.*

SLEEP DISORDERS

Hauri P: The Sleep Disorders. 2nd ed. Kalamazoo, MI, Upjohn, 1982. *A concise, complete, and sensible summary with excellent illustrations; for medical students, house officers, and practitioners.*
Hobson JA: The Neurobiology and Pathophysiology of Sleep and Dreaming. Discussions in Neurosciences, Vol 2, No 4, pp 1–50. Geneva, FESN, December 1985. *A clinically oriented discussion.*
Roffwarg H: Diagnostic classification of sleep and arousal disorders. Sleep 2:1, 1979. *A comprehensive diagnostic inventory that constitutes an invaluable reference for the sleep disorders specialist.*

459 REGIONAL DIAGNOSIS OF CEREBRAL DISORDERS

Antonio R. Damasio

The localization of the site of neurologic dysfunction based on clinical signs and symptoms is a crucial step in the assessment of neurologic diseases. Although advanced and noninvasive neuroimaging methods will localize many brain lesions, the abnormalities associated with some diseases continue to elude all but reseach-level imaging methods. For instance, in most degenerative diseases, the regional anatomical defect can be defined only on the basis of clinical signs. The regional diagnosis of most epileptogenic foci, a key element in the therapeutic management of epileptic patients, is another example. Also, an adequate regional diagnosis based on signs of higher nervous dysfunction is an important aspect of modern investigations on the neural basis of cognition.

The accuracy of regional clinical diagnosis depends on numerous factors. First, elementary motor and sensory disorders, which are related to dysfunction in motor and sensory pathways and in primary motor and sensory cortices, can be detected earlier than disorders of higher integrative processes such as language or thinking, which result from dysfunction in association cortices. The localization of the underlying lesions is generally more precise in the former than in the latter. This difference reflects the fine anatomical and functional modularity of the primary sensory and motor systems and the fact that integrative processes are distributed over a far larger number of neuron ensembles and networks of such ensembles. Furthermore, the neural substrate for integrative processes is prone to vary individually, different individuals having different endowments for specific abilities. For instance, language or visuospatial skills are linked to a variety of genetic and epigenetic factors and are influenced by age, educational background, and even gender. Second, the pathologic type of lesion and its rate of development influence the rate of appearance and the extent of symptoms. Most infarcts cause their damage rapidly and lead to a rapid onset of signs followed by at least some improvement. In contrast,

most intracranial tumors generate symptoms gradually and the brain adapts to their enlargement. Some slow-growing meningiomas can reach the size of a small orange before they cause detectable dysfunction, while small brain metastases from a carcinoma elsewhere in the body may rapidly cause major symptoms. Thirdly, the mass effect of some lesions (e.g., the edema that accompanies large infarcts or some tumors), may cause a topographic shift of brain structures and thereby compress remote and otherwise intact areas of the brain against the rigid frame of the skull and dural meninges. Compression can generate false localizing signs and lead to impairment in attention, motivation, and wakefulness which can, in turn, mask or aggravate other symptoms (see Ch. 457).

OCCIPITAL LOBES

The occipital cortices are solely dedicated to visual processing. Information from both lateral geniculate nuclei arrives in each primary visual cortex (Brodmann's area 17) which occupies the superior and inferior banks of the calcarine fissure (see also Ch. 464.2). This region contains a retinotopic projection of visual information. The inferior visual field maps onto the superior calcarine fissure and vice versa; the right visual field maps into the left calcarine region and conversely for the left visual field; the central part of the retina projects onto the caudal part of the calcarine region, at the occipital pole, while progressively more peripheral sectors of the retina project to more anterior sectors of the calcarine region. Beyond area 17, visual information is widely distributed by a large number of functionally distinct regions, located within the association cortices of Brodmann's areas 18 and 19. The main goal of these parallel processing units are: (1) to generate representations of the form, volumetric shape, texture, movement, color, and spatial location of stimuli in the external world, and (2) to serve as the distributed storage sites for the records of visual perception that become committed to memory and are later used in the processes of visual recall, recognition, imagetic thinking, and dreaming.

Damage to the calcarine cortices (Table 459–1) or to the optic radiations as they approach the calcarine region, causes varied field defects for form vision (hemianopias or quadrantanopias) depending on the region affected (e.g., damage to the left superior calcarine region causes a right inferior quadrantanopia; damage to an entire calcarine region leads to a hemianopia). When damage is confined to inferior occipital cortices but spares the calcarine regions, patients may develop achromatopsia, a disturbance of color perception without compromise of form vision (damage to the left side causes right hemiachromatopsia and vice versa). Damage to left occipital cortices and underlying periventricular white matter

TABLE 459–1. CHARACTERISTIC MANIFESTATIONS OF OCCIPITAL LOBE DAMAGE

Sign	Qualification	Lesion
Hemiachromatopsia	Right or left field (whole hemifield affected)	Left or right inferior mesial cortex and white matter
Pure alexia	Noted anywhere in intact field	Left inferior cortex and white matter (including outflow of callosum)
Color anomia	Seen only in left visual field (in combination with right hemianopia)	Left inferior and mesial
Visual agnosia	Noted anywhere in intact field	Bilateral inferior
Visual disorientation	Noted anywhere in intact field	Bilateral superior
Astereopsis	Noted anywhere in intact field	Bilateral superior
Impaired movement detection	Noted anywhere in intact field	Bilateral superior

combined with destruction of the interhemispheric visual pathways, often causes a disorder of reading without concomitant impairment of writing (alexia without agraphia). This is often accompanied by an impairment of color naming without impairment of color perception (color anomia). Bilateral damage to inferior visual association cortices causes agnosia, a selective impairment of visual recognition (see Ch. 460). Bilateral damage to superior visual association cortices leads to disturbances of visual attention (visual disorientation or simultanagnosia), stereo vision (astereopsis), and movement detection. Visual disorientation can also result from bilateral superior parietal lesions, as a component of Balint syndrome (see Parietal Lobe, below). Infarctions in the territory of one or both posterior cerebral arteries are by far the most common cause of pathology in the occipital lobes.

TEMPORAL LOBE

The temporal lobes contain structures necessary for visual and auditory perception, language, memory and affect. The most characteristic signs of temporal lobe damage are impairments of memory, which can be caused by lesions of either side, and impairments of language, generally related to dominant hemisphere lesions (see Ch. 460). The cortical structures related to vision are located in the inferior and lateral aspects of the lobe (part of area 37, areas 20 and 21). They are higher order association cortices that receive information from the occipital association cortices and further refine the processes of visual perception and memory. Those same cortices also process auditory information and should be seen as sensory integration units. Their damage leads to a combination of fine perceptual defects and memory impairments. A subcortical pathway (Meyer's loop) related to vision is the inferior component of the geniculocalcarine pathway, which courses in the depth of the temporal lobe (see Ch. 464).

The primary auditory cortices (areas 41 and 42) are located in the first temporal gyrus at the end of the most complex chain of subcortical processing stations of any sensory portal of the brain. Their purpose is the representation of acoustic frequencies and intensities for a large range of pitched and unpitched sounds (speech, music, environmental noises) so as to permit their recognition and spatial localization. The record of those representations is contained in the auditory association cortices which surround the primary cortices bilaterally, in the anterior, posterior, and lateral superior temporal gyrus (largely area 22). Although the auditory input from the contralateral ear prevails functionally over the ipsilateral input, each cortex receives information from both ears, so unilateral temporal lesions never cause deafness.

The medial and anterior temporal lobes contain cortical and subcortical structures of the limbic system (the entorhinal cortex, area 28, located in the anterior part of the parahippocampal gyrus; the hippocampal formation; and the amygdala). These highly interconnected structures are privy to information emanating from all sensory cortices as well as the diencephalon, and they project back to both. They integrate perceptual inputs, ongoing verbal and nonverbal thought operations, and the status of the internal milieu. This integration is indispensable for the processes of memory, affective

TABLE 459–3. ICTAL MANIFESTATIONS OF TEMPORAL LOBE EPILEPTIC FOCI

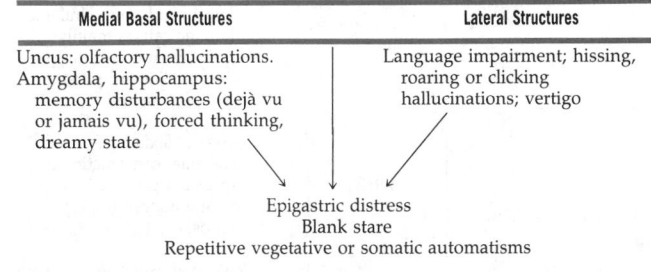

Medial Basal Structures	Lateral Structures
Uncus: olfactory hallucinations. Amygdala, hippocampus: memory disturbances (déjà vu or jamais vu), forced thinking, dreamy state	Language impairment; hissing, roaring or clicking hallucinations; vertigo

Epigastric distress
Blank stare
Repetitive vegetative or somatic automatisms

experience, and emotional expression. Lesions of this area severely compromise those functions.

The temporal lobes can be compromised by numerous pathologic processes. Epileptogenic scars and intracranial tumors are common; head injury often damages anterior temporal structures, and herpes simplex encephalitis has a predilection for the region; the highest and earliest concentration of cytoskeletal pathology in Alzheimer's disease is in entorhinal cortex and hippocampus; the hippocampus is selectively vulnerable to anoxia. Patients with temporal epileptogenic lesions experience a variety of affective, sensory, and visceral disturbances and exhibit emotional and motor disturbances that can appear before or during a seizure. In some patients, more subtle but longer lasting behavioral changes develop between seizures. Tables 459–3 and 459–4 list the major ictal and interictal symptoms. Although violent behavior is often blamed on temporal lobe dysfunction the evidence indicates that temporal lobe epilepsy should not be regarded as a medical explanation for criminal aggression. Bilateral removal of this region in animals causes the Kluver-Bucy syndrome, a multimodal disorder of memory characterized by indiscriminate sexual behavior, excessive orality, and placidity. The full syndrome rarely, if ever, develops in humans, but some components are often noted in patients with extensive bilateral temporal damage caused by herpes simplex encephalitis and dementias of degenerative or post-traumatic etiologies.

PARIETAL LOBE

The anterior aspect of the parietal lobe contains the postcentral gyrus where Brodmann's areas 3, 1, and 2 receive a convergence of somatosensory information obtained from nerve terminals in the contralateral half of the body (the projections are somatotopically organized with the largest share given to the phonatory apparatus and hand). These cortices are interlocked with the primary motor cortex in the precentral gyrus (area 4), and project to the superior parietal lobules (area 5 and 7), and inferior parietal lobules (areas 39 and 40, respectively, the angular and supramarginal gyri). A second source of somatic sensation is area S2, located in the upper bank of Sylvian fissure, which receives bilateral information and distributes it to ipsilateral parietal cortices. These cortices generate representations of the perceiver's body and of three-dimensional stimuli as apprehended by somatosensory processing and interweave such representations with pertinent visual and auditory information as well as appropriate motor programs.

Damage to the hand projection sector of the postcentral somatosensory cortex in either hemisphere impairs the ability to recognize form (astereognosia), scale, texture, and weight

TABLE 459–2. MANIFESTATIONS OF TEMPORAL LOBE DAMAGE

	Unilateral	Bilateral
Posterolateral	Aphasia* Pure-word deafness*	Auditory agnosia (includes aphasia and amusia)
Medial	Verbal* or nonverbal memory impairment Complex seizures	Amnesia
Anterolateral and inferior	Verbal* or nonverbal memory impairment Complex seizures	Amnesia

*Dominant hemisphere only

TABLE 459–4. INTERICTAL TRAITS OF PATIENTS WITH TEMPORAL LOBE EPILEPTIC FOCI

Lack of humor
Obsessiveness
Metaphysical preoccupation
Dependence
Sadness
Hyposexuality

TABLE 459–5. MANIFESTATIONS OF PARIETAL LOBE DAMAGE

Superior parietal lobule		Bilateral damage causes Balint syndrome. Unilateral damage causes mainly optic ataxia and transient abnormalities of pursuit eye movements.
Inferior parietal lobule	left	Aphasia; alexia; agraphia; acalculia; constructional apraxia; right/left disorientation; finger agnosia
	right	Neglect; anosognosia; inappropriate affect
Post-Rolandic cortices		Subjective alterations in somatic sensation. Astereognosia

of objects in the contralateral hand. (The thresholds for touch, pain, vibration, and temperature are generally not disturbed.) By contrast, damage to the dominant or nondominant inferior parietal lobule causes diverse manifestations. The dominant somatosensory cortex develops representations of the body and of its movements (especially those of the hand and phonatory apparatus), as well as shapes located within arm's reach, the so-called intrapersonal space. Dysfunction in the general area of the dominant angular gyrus disrupts reading and writing, planning and execution of representational hand movements in specific contexts (apraxia), arithmetic skills (acalculia), finger recognition (finger agnosia), right-left orientation and the ability to copy drawings, diagrams, and execute three dimensional constructions (constructional apraxia). Damage to the dominant supramarginal gyrus is mainly associated with aphasia (Table 459–5).

The nondominant parietal cortices hold a dynamic representation of extrapersonal space (the space beyond arm's reach) based on visual, auditory and somatosensory cues. *Both* hemispaces are represented in this region. The attentional survey of external sensory events and projected movements in both hemispaces also depend on this large nondominant region, damage to which leads to complex defects in spatial processing. The defects are especially pronounced in the hemispace opposite the lesion and cause the commonly encountered neglect syndrome. Not only is the left hemispace inappropriately attended to but the left side of the body itself may be neglected and left hemiplegia or hemisensory loss may be ignored or actively denied (anosognosia). The ability to negotiate a route without hitting obstacles placed to the left side of the body, the skill to follow a previously known and automated route (in a house or town), or the capicity to learn a new route, are all compromised by nondominant inferior parietal lesions. So is constructional ability, which is far more disturbed than with equivalent lesions on the dominant side. Unlike their counterparts with left-sided lesions, patients with such nondominant injuries show little concern for their condition and often offer an indifferent affect. An adequate rehabilitation program must take into account this reduced motivation. When these lesions are part of extensive cerebrovascular damage affecting the nondominant middle cerebral artery territory (involving the nearby auditory cortices), patients may become acutely confused.

Bilateral damage confined to superior parietal lobules causes ocular apraxia (the inability to direct gaze voluntarily toward new visual stimuli appearing in the periphery of the visual field), bilateral optic ataxia (the inability to generate precise contralateral hand movements toward an outbound target under visual guidance), and an impairment of visual attention, a breakdown in the ability to apprehend the visual panorama

in a cogent, seamless manner (visual disorientation or simultanognosia). The combination of ocular apraxia, optic ataxia, and visual disorientation, constitutes the Balint syndrome. Common causes are bilateral infarctions in the border zone between the posterior and middle cerebral artery territories, and bilateral metastases in this region. Unilateral damage to the superior parietal lobule causes optic ataxia and may cause defective pursuit eye movements.

FRONTAL LOBES

The human frontal cortices encompass almost half of the entire cortical mantle and integrate a large number of different anatomical fields. Their functions include movement control; higher problem solving; regulation of social behaviors, emotion, affect, and autonomic function; planning of goal-oriented behaviors and generation of willful responses; and higher regulation of language and thought processes. Understanding of the correspondence between structure and function is less advanced for frontal cortices than for any other cerebral region. Furthermore impairments of the functions outlined above are far easier to detect in real life than in clinical and laboratory settings.

The motor sector of the frontal lobe (the precentral and premotor cortices) is located mainly in the lateral frontal surface but spills into the mesial surface as well. The precentral cortex (area 4 or M1) contains a somatotopic representation of contralateral body movements in which the phonatory apparatus and hand are accorded the largest share. It is the principal target of re-entrant projections from cerebellum and motor thalamus. The premotor region (area 6) is part of a network for motor programming and it receives re-entrant projections from basal ganglia as well as projections from the posterior sensory cortices. It integrates incoming movement-related information for final transmission to the corticospinal tract. Part of the nearby area 8, known as the frontal eye field, controls voluntary eye movements (seizures originating in this area cause the eyes to deviate away from the lesion; damage by an infarction makes the eyes deviate toward the side of the lesion). The mesial aspect of area 6 is the supplementary motor area (SMA or M2). The SMA is anatomically contiguous with the rest of the premotor cortex but constitutes a functionally separate region. (It contains a whole body representation in its relatively small cortical surface.) Damage to area 4 causes varied degrees of focal paralysis in the contralateral side of the body or face (involvement of corticospinal projections in corona radiata or internal capsule cause progressively more widely distributed paralysis). Damage to the lateral aspect of area 6 causes impairments of motor

TABLE 459–6. MOTOR SYMPTOMS OF FRONTAL LOBE DISEASE*

	Structural Damage	Seizure
Precentral gyrus	Focal distal weakness, maximal in lower face, hand, less often foot; increased reflexes, mild spasticity, Babinski sign	Jacksonian: focal onset on face, thumb, foot. "March" toward proximal limb and trunk.
Corona radiata or internal capsule	Hemiplegia; increased spasticity	
Premotor (lateral)	Ocular ipsiversion; paratonic resistance to passive motion; grasping; hypokinesia; optic ataxia, aphasia	Adversive: ocular contraversion.
Premotor (mesial)	Mutism	Involuntary synergies (elevated arm and leg, body turning); speech arrest and/or vocalization

*All arise contralateral to the brain lesion.

learning and execution as well as transient forms of neglect, while involvement of the SMA leads to mutism and contralateral akinesia. Infarctions and parasagittal tumors in this region often compromise part of both SMA and the nearby cingulate gyrus (area 24) located immediately beneath the cingulate sulcus. The cingulate is a limbic cortex and its acute damage also causes akinesia, mutism, transient neglect, and an impairment of motivation (abulia). Tumors impinging in this region may cause speech arrest, seizures characterized by vocalization, and may trigger involuntary movement synergies involving contralateral limbs and trunk.

The frontal lobes contain limbic cortices in the posterior orbital surface. Selective involvement of this region is associated with disturbances of social behavior. These include inability to recognize the social value of real life situations, inability to plan future social actions appropriately, and inappropriate demeanor (facetiousness, sociopathic acts). During the acute phase of frontal limbic damage patients are generally akinetic, inattentive, and may exhibit inappropriate behavior regarding their sphincters. They may urinate or defecate in public although sphincter function per se is preserved.

Areas 44 and 45 lie between the premotor and the prefrontal cortices, in the lower lateral surface of the lobe. In the dominant side, this sector of the frontal operculum is known as Broca's area and its damage causes aphasia (see Ch. 460). Damage to the nondominant side of this area alters the prosodic qualities of speech. The most anterior regions of the frontal lobe accommodate the prefrontal cortices (areas 46, 9, 10, 11, 12), damage to which impairs the governance of higher behavior, resulting in a reduced ability to plan or implement goal-oriented behaviors, a reduced creativity or problem solving ability, or an impaired regulation of emotion and affect. With permanent damage, the magnitude of the deficit relates directly to the bilaterality or unilaterality of the lesion, the size of the lesion, and the previous intellectual caliber and occupation of the patient. Relatively small unilateral lesions may produce minor impairments that are difficult to detect and quantify. Large bilateral prefrontal lesions, however, although they leave motor, perceptual, and language functions intact, are incompatible with maintaining a high level, creative, self-conscious personality. The defects are most noticeable in patients who undergo bilateral prefrontal ablations for the treatment of large midline brain tumors. Even then, however, the impairments can be better sensed by appraising social and occupational behavior than by neuropsychologic tests, most of which may be passed flawlessly.

The frontal lobes are especially vulnerable to closed head injury which may, in turn, lead to the formation of cortical scar tissue and to the appearance of seizures. The lateral sector is frequently compromised by infarctions and meningiomas. The mesial sector is often struck by infarctions or hemorrhages mostly as a consequence of ruptured anterior communicating or anterior cerebral artery aneurysms. Meningiomas arising in the falx are another common cause of damage. The posterior orbital sector is often involved by herpes simplex encephalitis, by hemorrhages from ruptured anterior circulation aneurysms, and by meningiomas arising in the sphenoid and ethmoid regions. The brunt of the effects of normal pressure hydrocephalus reflect damage to the white matter of frontal lobe. Finally, all prefrontal cortices are involved in Pick's disease, and both prefrontal and frontal limbic cortices are involved in Alzheimer's disease. When involvement of frontal lobe structures is caused by large tumors, especially by malignant gliomas which often arise in the white matter of one hemisphere but traverse the corpus callosum to involve the other, patients exhibit not only florid disturbances of the functions outlined above but also impairments of attention and balance (see Ch. 465), along with primitive reflexes (grasp reflex, Gegenhalten or paratonia, echopraxia).

Bear DM, Fedio P: Quantitative analysis of interictal behavior in temporal lobe epilepsy. Arch Neurol 34:454, 1977. *An effort to quantify the personality traits of epileptics.*

Damasio AR: Disorders of complex visual processing. In Mesulam M-M (ed.): Principles of Behavioral Neurology. Philadelphia, F. A. Davis Company, 1985, p 259. *A review of the clinically relevant manifestations of dysfunction in the human visual system.*

Eslinger PJ, Damasio AR: Severe disturbance of higher cognition after bilateral frontal lobe ablation. Neurology 35:1731, 1985. *An example of the extreme dissociation of behavior caused by frontal lobe damage. The lesions prompted a variety of socially unacceptable behaviors but did not interfere with language or memory. The intelligence quotient remained superior.*

Gazzaniga M, Le Doux J: The Integrated Mind. New York, Plenum Press, 1978. *A brief and lucid survey of the integration of higher functions and of the role the cerebral commissures play in it.*

Heilman K, Valenstein E (eds.): Clinical Neuropsychology. Oxford, Oxford University Press, 1985. *A multiauthored collection of essays on major aspects of neuropsychology.*

Hier DB, Mondlock J, Caplan LR: Behavioral abnormalities after right hemisphere stroke. Neurology 33:337, 1983. *An analysis of a large series of patients with damage to the right parietal lobe.*

Mesulam M-M: A cortical network for directed attention and unilateral neglect. Ann Neurol 10:309, 1981. *A thoughtful discussion of the anatomic and physiologic underpinnings of attentional defects in man.*

Penfield W, Jasper W: Epilepsy and the Functional Anatomy of the Human Brain. Boston, Little, Brown, and Company, 1954. *The classic monograph on what epilepsy and the electrical stimulation of the cerebral cortex, tell us about the neural substrates of higher brain function.*

Roland PE: Astereognosis. Arch Neurol 33:543, 1976. *A confirmation that stereognosis depends on mechanisms related to the immediate postcentral cortex.*

Stevens JR, Hermann BP: Temporal lobe epilepsy, psychopathology, and violence: The state of evidence. Neurology 31:1127, 1981. *A vigorous defense against the view that psychopathology and temporal lobe epilepsy are directly linked.*

460 FOCAL DISTURBANCES OF HIGHER FUNCTIONS

Antonio R. Damasio

The designation *higher nervous function* stands for such complex cerebral abilities as the acquisition and categorization of knowledge (learning and memory), the translation of knowledge in a verbal code (language), the manipulation of nonverbal and verbal knowledge in thought processes, the learning and execution of representational movements (praxis), and the reflection upon ongoing cognitive activities as they relate to an autobiographical self (consciousness). These functions presume the normal operations of attention (the ability to concentrate willfully on a specific mental content to the exclusion of others), as well as motivation (the affective impetus to sustain a given mental activity or action). Because of their clinical importance, this section concentrates on disturbances of learning, memory, and language.

MEMORY AND ITS IMPAIRMENTS. Memory encompasses the ability to analyze (encode) and store perceptions of the external world, the perceiver's body, and the perceiver's own movements, to store concepts derived from the categorization of those perceptions, and to manipulate the memorized records internally for recall and recognition. The terms "learning" and "memory" are used almost interchangeably although learning should be used only to mean "memory acquisition."

The memory of a stimulus as perceived through a given sensory modality, for instance, the *sensory* record of the physical properties and structure of a human face, must be distinguished from the memory of a unique and specific episode that involves the face of a particular person. The latter is an *episodic* memory that binds the strictly visual record of one person's face with a variety of pertinently associated memories, visual or not. Each is different from the concept of human face, a *generic* memory that is applicable to any instance of human face whether or not its possessor is known to the perceiver. All these types of memory pertain to factual knowledge and are known as *declarative* memory. Another important type of memory, however, is based on procedures rather than facts, and consists of motor or perceptual skills rather than knowledge of the implements necessary to practice those skills. Dancing, the playing of instruments, typing or swimming, are examples of *procedural* memory. Procedural memory is spared in most amnesias.

Most sensory stimuli, polymodal or single modality, are retained only briefly, less than 60 seconds. Material held for that period, e.g., during digit span testing, is said to be in *immediate* memory, a term that has become largely synonymous with *short-term memory*. (Immediate memory is preserved in most amnesias.) If those sensory materials are to be consolidated into permanent or *long-term* memory, an active physiologic process must start promptly. The process of consolidation takes time, and recently acquired memories are more vulnerable than those that have been held long and internally rehearsed (most remote memories can be recalled better than recent ones; standard psychometric testing, because of its dependence on verbal and nonverbal knowledge acquired in youth, is a poor indicator of the extent of amnesia). Newer memories are known as *recent* or *intermediate* memories, and older memories as *remote*. In relation to the time of onset of memory impairment, the terms *anterograde* and *retrograde* are commonly used. Anterograde designates the time compartment since the amnesia began and denotes materials that have been improperly learned or not learned at all. Retrograde refers to the time compartment prior to the onset of amnesia and to materials previously acquired that may not be retrievable in recall or recognition. Retrograde amnesia can be as short as hours or days, as is often the case in post-traumatic situations, or extend back years or even decades as in Korsakoff's amnesia or that which follows herpes simplex encephalitis.

MEMORY MECHANISMS

The thesaurus of facts and rules acquired in a lifetime is stored in the association cortices of every lobe of both hemispheres. Memories are dynamically and flexibly distributed in overlapping neuron groups linked by patterned and highly specific corticocortical and commissural connections. Single modality memories appear to be distributed closer to the primary sensory cortex which conveyed the information in the first place (the impaired access or partial destruction of those stores causes an *agnosia*; see Agnosia below). Polymodal events are stored farther from sensory sources. Unique and elaborate polymodal episodes depend especially on the inferior and anterolateral temporal cortices (the impaired access or partial damage to such stores causes *amnesia*).

The ability to lock sensory events into neural structures to form a permanent record depends on the normal operation of the hippocampal system, the basal forebrain and diencephalon, and several brain-stem nuclei. The elucidation of the respective roles of these components is imperfect but it appears that the hippocampus, which is informed about relationships between components of an event via connections from the higher order association cortices, binds and stabilizes information according to its appropriate temporal and spatial links. Hippocampal action also is mediated by subcortical connections to diencephalon. Through the interconnected amygdala the hippocampus also influences basal forebrain and brain-stem nuclei. The basal forebrain and brain stem, in turn, provide the cerebral cortex with neurochemical inputs that act to stabilize memory at the cellular level (acetylcholine from the nucleus basalis of Meynert in the basal forebrain, noradrenaline from the locus ceruleus in the brain stem, and other, still ill-defined, mediators and modulators). The hippocampal interconnections with the diencephalon sample the status of the internal milieu at the time of a given sensory experience, informing on the value of a particular stimulus or event in the context of instinctual goals. Finally, the ascending brain stem reticular formation contributes importantly because most learning presumes attention and arousal. The neural structures and systems involving the acquisition of procedural memories are somewhat different. Most motor skills remain intact and new motor skills can be learned after major bilateral damage to hippocampus and basal forebrain. The motor and sensory cortices generate those memories and so do the cerebellum, the neostriatum, and the motor nuclei of the thalamus.

The understanding of the cellular physiology and molecular biology of learning is just beginning. Work in simple invertebrate systems indicates that classic conditioning is associated with presynaptic increases in neurotransmitter output. On the other hand, the phenomenon of long-term potentiation has been identified in the hippocampal formation and may relate to memory consolidation.

MEMORY DISORDERS

Some middle-aged and elderly persons have an increasing but isolated difficulty in recalling proper names and recent events of limited importance. This "benign forgetfulness" is not a predictor of the progressive dementias and is best treated with prompt and vigorous reassurance. As discussed in Chapter 461, the most frequent causes of incapacitating memory loss are the degenerative dementias, head injury, brain anoxia or ischemia, nutritional impairment, encephalitis, and surgical excisions of vital areas during the treatment of tumors or seizures. *Korsakoff's syndrome* is a severe amnesia that compromises both anterograde and retrograde memories and is accompanied by lack of insight and confabulation. It is caused by attacks of severe thiamine deficiency, generally in the setting of alcoholism, and often accompanies or follows acute Wernicke's encephalopathy (Ch. 467), or delirium tremens (Ch. 15), although it can occur whenever thiamine-free calories are the mainstay of nutrition. Thiamine deficiency results in bilateral damage to diencephalic structures, including the dorsal medial nucleus of the thalamus and the hypothalamic mamillary bodies. The consistent presence of these lesions in Korsakoff's amnesia established the diencephalon as a crucial component of the memory-related network.

The discovery of the critical contribution to memory of the hippocampal formation and its input and output stations came from patients who underwent *bilateral medial temporal lobe resection* to treat epilepsy. Several of them became severely amnesic and have remained unable to learn factual memories to this day. Their severe anterograde amnesia contrasts with a largely spared retrograde memory and with preserved generic memories and procedural learning. The amnesias caused by *postanoxic encephalopathies*, in which anterograde memory is also involved, are also caused by hippocampal damage in which the CA1 sector is selectively damaged. Together with the finding that specific areas of the entorhinal cortex and subiculum are damaged in amnesic patients with *Alzheimer's disease*, these findings underscore the importance of hippocampus in memory. *Herpes simplex encephalitis* commonly damages the hippocampal region bilaterally but it involves other, anterolateral and inferior regions, of the temporal cortices. Such patients suffer not only an anterograde memory defect but also a severe retrograde amnesia that can span virtually all of their life, especially when the right side is more heavily involved than the left. Bilateral damage to hippocampus can also be caused by infarctions in the territory of the posterior cerebral arteries. Infarctions in the area of the basal forebrain (septal nuclei, nucleus accumbens, nucleus basalis of Meynert) due to ruptured aneurysms in the anterior circulation are also associated with amnesia. Both anterograde and retrograde memory are involved, but unlike temporal lobe amnesia, the defect is mild, tends to improve, and appropriate cueing helps recall. *Head injury* is another cause of amnesia. Even modest head trauma results in transient dysfunction of hippocampus and diencephalon.

Transient global amnesia (TGA). TGA is a self-limited memory impairment during which the patient can identify himself but is unable to recall events preceding the episode and generally cannot recognize places. Patients with TGA remain attentive, have normal language and reasoning, and are generally distressed by their disorientation. They tend to ask repeatedly where they are, what they have been up to, and what is going on. Most TGA episodes last less than 12 hours, often about four or five, and the disorientation gradually clears. The attacks leave no residual impairment and are generally nonrecurrent. Status epilepticus with partial complex or petit mal seizures may mimic TGA but can be distinguished because patients with seizures are generally noninquisitive and inattentive. Most TGA attacks occur in middle-aged or older persons and presumably reflect transient vascular insufficiency affecting memory-related areas in temporal lobe or thalamus.

PSYCHOGENIC AMNESIA. Psychogenic amnesia generally has a recognizable pattern. Emotional upheaval often impairs attention and produces inconsistent performance in psychological testing. Depression may reduce communication to monosyllables. In organic amnesias emotionally reinforced material tends to be recalled better than neutral events, and disorientation is worst for time, less for place and persons, and never for self. By contrast, psychogenic amnesia is greatest for emotionally important events, may erase circumscribed epochs of the past while leaving intact epochs immediately preceding or following the alleged amnesia, affects remote as much as recent memories, and may include disorientation to self. Questions such as "Who am I?" or "What is my name?", unless uttered during delirium or a seizure, raise the strong suspicion of a psychogenic process.

TREATMENT. Patients with acute post-traumatic amnesia tend to recover spontaneously. The same is true of amnesia caused by overmedication or transient deliria. Memory loss caused by depression (pseudodementia) has a good prognosis when psychiatric treatment is effective. A less fortunate prognosis accompanies amnesia following prolonged post-traumatic coma. When coma lasts more than two or three weeks, most patients, particularly those over 25 years old, never fully recover from the memory loss. Patients with amnesia due to herpes encephalitis recover only when the lesions are mostly or solely unilateral and most retain some impairment. In most amnesias the recovery is inversely proportional to the initial severity, and is constrained by the extent and placement of lesions. Any important improvement usually takes place within the first year after onset, especially the first six months. Neuroactive peptides, neurotransmitter precursors, neurotransmitters, and special dietary agents have no proved usefulness in chronic organic amnesia.

AGNOSIA. Agnosia is the inability to recognize a previously familiar sensory stimulus despite the intactness of elementary perception of the stimulus and the absence of defects of intelligence, motivation, or attention. It is "a percept stripped of its meaning." The disorder is best considered as a form of monomodal amnesia, a disability that prevents a perceived stimulus from triggering pertinent, previously acquired information whose evocation would reveal its identity. Agnosia results from dysfunction of association cortices of the affected sensory modality, which contain records of purely modal processing. *Visual agnosia* is the most frequent example. It consists of the failure to recognize familiar faces (prosopagnosia) or objects (visual object agnosia), despite the ability to describe their physical structures, copy them, or recognize the stimulus by sound (prosopagnosics can recognize the possessor of a face by voice). The phenomenon is generally associated with bilateral occipitotemporal lesions, although visual object agnosia can be caused by *left* unilateral lesions

of the occipital lobe, and *right* unilateral lesions reduce the efficiency of face recognition.

LANGUAGE AND ITS DISORDERS

Verbal languages are arbitrary symbolic codes in which words stand for properties of external stimuli, actions, and relationships, as well as for the intellectual and emotional reactions that such stimuli evoke in the perceiver. The normal brain acquires and stores a dictionary of such words in at least one language, a lexicon, and develops a highly automated process of two-way translation between word representations and nonverbal representations of objects, actions, or concepts. The process of language comprehension is the translation of sentences (sequences of verbal representations) into sequences of more or less approximate nonverbal counterparts whose ongoing manipulation is known as thought. Nouns, verbs, or adjectives have fairly direct referential nonverbal equivalents. On the contrary, functor words (conjunctions, prepositions and adverbs, verb endings) refer to abstract relationships among stimuli or their representations. Functors, together with word order, are the key to the syntactic organization of sentences and their nonverbal counterparts in thought. The operation of language formulation into speech or writing is the rendering of a nonverbal thought process in a syntactical frame filled up with appropriate lexical elements. The lexical and syntactical operations of language depend on phonemic and graphemic devices, which can enact correspondences between sounds, their visual representations, and the articulatory patterns that permit their sensorimotor implementation in phonetic utterances or writing. Oral verbal expression also depends on word stress and the intonational contour of sentences, i.e., the fundamental frequency of the sounds in an utterance as well as the durational elements of speech. The term prosody subsumes the latter qualities of verbal expression.

NEURAL SUBSTRATES OF LANGUAGE. Verbal language is characteristically human and its experimental study is restricted to human beings. Considerable knowledge has been gathered about the neural substrates of language from the cognitive and neuroanatomical study of patients with acquired impairments caused by focal brain lesions (aphasias). Most such studies have relied largely on postmortem, CT, and MRI analysis, although more recent evaluations have been conducted using emission tomography devices. Electrical stimulation of different regions of the cerebrum during surgery for seizures or motor disorders, also has provided information on the neural representation of language. The preoperative precaution of pharmacologically inactivating part of the hemispheres with the intracarotid injection of a barbiturate (Amytal) has also contributed important clues. A salient finding, first noted more than a century ago and thoroughly confirmed since, is that the left hemisphere of more than 95 per cent of individuals is especially adroit at language processing. In left language-dominant persons all aspects of language depend largely on left-hemisphere processing, with the partial exception of some aspects of prosody. Handedness is an imperfect but clinically useful indicator of language dominance. In almost all right-handed persons the left hemisphere is dominant for language and its damage in key areas leads to severe aphasia. Most left-handed and ambidextrous persons (about 70 per cent) are also left language-dominant although they may have additional language representation in the right hemisphere. About one third of left-handers have either bilateral language representation or right-hemisphere language representation. Such persons are at a disadvantage in that lesions of either side can cause aphasia although the disability tends to be less severe and to improve. Even extreme right-handed individuals with full language dominance in the left hemisphere possess some language representation in the opposite hemisphere (especially for nouns and verbs; adjectives are poorly represented and functor words probably not at all). The right hemisphere of such a person has little access to speech output and little syntactical capability. It has been suggested that gender is an important variable in language representation, but the available data do not permit conclusive statements. Certainly both men and women can develop aphasia with similar signs and following similar lesions. Language representation is definitely different in children, however. Most children who suffer severe brain lesions up to age five or six can recover from aphasia and continue to develop language to nearly normal levels. Left-hemisphere lesions sustained later, especially after puberty, have the same consequences as for adults.

Some asymmetric abilities of the cerebral hemispheres have been related to neuroanatomic asymmetries. The left planum temporale, the area of association cortex located immediately behind the transverse gyrus (the primary auditory cortex), is far larger than the right in about 70 per cent of individuals. The sizable difference is visible on gross inspection and in the microscopic cytoarchitectonic structure of the area. In the same individuals, the left sylvian fissure is longer on the left than on the right so as to accompany the larger extent of the posterior temporal region, and more horizontally placed so as to accommodate a more voluminous left lower parietal lobule (supramarginal gyrus and angular gyrus). Fetuses show these anatomical symmetries as early as the sixteenth week of gestation, and the changes can be identified by MRI as well as in the vascular patterns of cerebral angiographies.

Language depends on a wide network of cortical and subcortical processing units, and its knowledge and operations are distributed *within* key cortical regions. The principal set of language areas is located around the left sylvian fissure (the perisylvian language region). In its posterior aspect lies Wernicke's area (the posterior auditory association cortex, or Brodmann's area 22; it includes the planum temporale and the posterior portion of the first temporal gyrus). Immediately below and behind, lies area 37, the lateral aspect of which, in the posterior sector of the second and third temporal gyri, is committed to language. Above and behind the sylvian fissure lie the supramarginal gyrus (area 40) and the angular gyrus (area 39). In the anterior aspect of the perisylvian region in the inferior and posterior aspect of the frontal operculum, lie areas 44 and 45, also known as Broca's area. Between sit the motor and sensory regions associated with sensory motor phonatory representations. Also part of the language network, are components of the basal ganglia (especially in the head of the caudate nucleus and parts of the putamen), some

thalamic nuclei, the supplementary motor areas (especially the one on the left), and the anterior cingulate gyri.

THE APHASIAS. Aphasia (or dysphasia) is a disturbance of one or more aspects of the comprehension or formulation of verbal messages caused by newly acquired brain disease. Although developments in cognitive science have led to a linguistic-based approach to aphasia, Geschwind's diagnosis of aphasic disorders in terms of the comprehension of language, the fluency of output, and the ability to repeat sentences, remains clinically useful because of the strong relationship between these traits and the anatomical sites of the underlying lesions. Table 460–1 summarizes the important clinical clues.

Damage to the posterior sector of the left superior temporal gyrus and its surround causes *Wernicke aphasia*. Patients speak fluently, with normal melodic contour, and even a normal syntactical frame. However, the words they select are the wrong words (semantic paraphasias), so the intelligibility of their otherwise well formed verbal messages may be low (jargonaphasia). Likewise, their comprehension of verbal message is poor because of their inability to translate words into nonverbal meanings. Wernicke aphasics with severe comprehension defects may develop paranoid reactions and become homicidal or suicidal. Wernicke's aphasia must be distinguished from *auditory agnosia*, the inability to recognize objects or actions by the characteristics sounds they make (due to bilateral lesions in auditory cortex), and *pure word deafness*, an agnosia restricted to words that allows patients to recognize nonspeech sounds and to produce normal speech (owing to dominant lesions undercutting the auditory cortex). It is also different from the logorrhea of manic states, the logical thought derailment of schizophrenia, or the rare verbal salads of chronic schizophrenics.

Posterior lesions outside the Wernicke area produce more restricted disturbances. Lesions of the supramarginal gyrus give rise to *conduction aphasia*, a disorder in which the patient speaks fluently, has relatively preserved comprehension, but makes sound substitution errors (phonemic paraphasias). The major impairment of repetition stands out among these comparatively milder defects. Other strategically placed lesions of the posterior dominant hemisphere selectively compromise reading or writing. *Alexia* (inability to comprehend written language while retaining relatively normal vision) without concomitant writing impairment, results when a lesion destroys the left visual cortex and, in addition, involves the outflow of the splenium of the corpus callosum. This placement cuts off projections that otherwise connect the unaf-

TABLE 460–1. DIAGNOSTIC POINTERS TO THE MOST FREQUENT APHASIA TYPES

	Speech	Comprehension	Repetition	Other Signs	Localization
Broca	Nonfluent; effortful	+	−	Right hemiparesis worse in arm; aware of defect; frustrated	Lower posterior frontal
Wernicke	Abundant; fluent; well articulated	−	−	Often none; may be euphoric and/or paranoid	Posterior and superior temporal
Conduction	Fluent with some articulatory defects	+	−	Often none; cortical sensory loss in right arm	Usually supramarginal gyrus; may extend to insula and primary auditory cortex
Global	Scant; nonfluent	−	−	Right hemiparesis worse in arm; may present *without* hemiparesis	With hemiparesis: massive perisylvian lesion; without hemiparesis: separate Broca and Wernicke area damage
Transcortical motor	Nonfluent; explosive	+	+		Anterior or superior to Broca area
Transcortical sensory	Scant; fluent	−	+		Surrounding Wernicke area, posteriorly or inferiorly
Atypical ("basal ganglia")	Fluent dysarthric	−	−/+	Right hemiparesis worse in arm	Head of caudate; anterior limb of capsule
Atypical ("thalamus")	Fluent	−	+	Attentional and memory defects in acute phase	Anterolateral thalamus

+ = Intact or largely preserved
− = Impaired

fected right visual cortex to language areas of the left. Despite their inability to comprehend the written word, patients with "pure" alexia can speak and write normally, in contrast to those with a combination of *alexia with agraphia* (impairment of writing despite normal motor function of the hand), in whom both reading and writing are compromised. In its pure form the abnormality is rare and follows lesions of the left angular gyrus. More frequently alexia and agraphia are accompaniments of Wernicke aphasia.

Broca aphasia is characterized by nonfluent, effortful, melodically flat speech, often shorn of functor words and marred by poor word order. The syntactical defect far outweighs the lexical impairment. Comprehension is well preserved in conversation. Broca aphasia must be distinguished from dysarthria, a disorder of speech articulation that does not impair the linguistic structure of communication. Many Broca aphasics are mute in the first hours or days after the onset of the disorder and only gradually develop characteristic signs. The intent to communicate, however poorly, is rarely in question. The lesion compromises Broca's area and adjacent cortical and subcortical territories. Because of patterns of vascular supply, many patients also have a contralateral hemiplegia. Apraxia is added, when the lesion involves the adjacent premotor cortex. Aphasia caused by lesions confined to Broca's area has an especially good prognosis.

Global aphasia consists of a severe loss of all aspects of language operation. Acutely, patients are often mute and have a right hemiplegia. The paucity of speech may become chronic, the patient being able neither to comprehend nor produce language (except in the form of expletives or brief phrases). Despite rehabilitation efforts, the prognosis is poor, and patients often become depressed and listless, more so than Wernicke aphasics. Two major localizations are associated with global aphasia (see Table 460–1).

With all the aphasias described above, patients are unable to repeat long sentences after the examiner. With some language defects, however, repetition is preserved. The dissociation between intact repetition and disturbed comprehension or speech output implies that Wernicke and Broca regions, as well as their interconnections, must be intact and that the causative lesions may lie near but outside those areas. There are two frequently encountered aphasias of this type: *transcortical motor* and *transcortical sensory* (Table 460–1).

Mutism accompanies a variety of conditions. It may describe the initial state of patients who evolve into Broca or global aphasia, but produce no speech at all acutely. It may describe patients with bilateral premotor lesions who often remain chronically mute. Mutism has been applied to the paroxysmal speech arrest caused by seizures arising out of the supplementary motor or Broca areas, generally as an irritative response to an overlying tumor, or to describe the absence of speech in acute psychoses. Prominent mutism affects patients with lesions of supplementary motor area and/or nearby cingulate, who not only do not speak but show no inclination to communicate through facial expression or gestures. Those patients also are generally motionless and when they recover do not exhibit aphasic symptoms. Mutism is not *anarthria*, a severe impairment of articulation, that prevents speech but allows both the vivid expression of the intent to communicate and the frustration of not being able to do so (anarthria is caused by bulbar or pseudobulbar defects and can be confirmed by the presence of other signs of nuclear and supranuclear paralysis). Nor is mutism the same as *aphonia*, in which the phonatory apparatus is locally inoperative for mechanical or psychogenic reasons.

Some aphasias can be caused by infarcts in the dominant basal ganglia, especially when they involve the head of the caudate and the anterior limb of the internal capsule, and by infarcts in anterolateral nuclei of the dominant thalamus. Their appearance indicates that subcortical structures contribute to language processing, probably by assisting cortical units. The basal ganglia aphasias most often show a combination of fluent, dysarthric speech accompanied by impaired auditory comprehension and a right hemiparesis. The thalamic aphasias resemble transcortical sensory aphasia.

Although seizures or transient vascular insufficiency can cause brief language disturbances, the development of a selective disturbance in language that lasts more than a few hours always reflects a structural and focal lesion. The most common causes are infarction and hemorrhage, in the distribution of a major cortical artery branch. Less frequent causes are head trauma and space-occupying lesions.

APRAXIA

Apraxia describes the inability to perform learned and representational movement acts under verbal or visual command, despite retention of intact motor function and the comprehension of the command. Apraxia cannot be explained by weakness, incoordination, akinesia, or impaired auditory visual or tactile perception. Apraxia bespeaks dominant hemisphere dysfunction and is mostly encountered together with aphasia. In stroke victims it accompanies the acute phase and diminishes within weeks of onset. In patients with degenerative dementia, however, apraxia is a persisting sign. Although the phenomenon of apraxia provides important clues regarding the learning and execution of different types of movement, its value for clinical localization is limited, and its meaning for rehabilitation is small. The interested reader may wish to consult Geschwind's article for details.

Damasio AR, Geschwind N: The neural basis of language. Annu Rev Neurosci 7:127, 1984. *A description of different aphasia types and their localization.*

Damasio AR: Prosopagnosia. Trends Neurosci 8:132, 1985. *A discussion of the cognitive and neuropsychologic aspects of this intriguing phenomenon with information applicable to the understanding of other agnosias and memory.*

Geschwind N: The apraxias. Neural disorders of learned movement. Am Sci 63:188, 1975. *The use of apraxia for the understanding of cerebral organization of movement.*

Geschwind N: Disconnection syndromes in animals and man. Brain 88:237; 585, 1965. *A seminal discussion on the anatomic basis of cognition.*

Kandel ER: Cellular mechanisms of learning and the biological basis of individuality. In Kandel ER (ed.): Principles of Neural Science. New York, Elsevier, 1985, p 816. *Learning and memory at cellular and molecular levels. A review of key developments.*

Scoville WB, Milner B: Loss of recent memory after bilateral hippocampal lesions. J Neurol Neurosurg Psychiatr 20:11, 1957. *Removal of the uncus and underlying amygdaloid complex resulted in little behavioral change. When the hippocampus was removed bilaterally memory loss ensued.*

Squire LR: Mechanisms of memory. Science 232:1612, 1986. *An update on cognitive research in memory.*

Victor M, Adams RD, Collins GH: The Wernicke-Korsakoff Syndrome. Philadelphia, F.A. Davis Company, 1971. *The classic monograph on the subject provides evidence for the role of diencephalon in memory.*

461 THE DEMENTIAS

Fred Plum

GENERAL CONSIDERATIONS

DEFINITION AND PREVALENCE. Dementia is a clinical term describing a sustained or permanent decline in several dimensions of intellectual function so as to interfere with the individual's normal social or economic activity. Loss of a single psychologic property, such as language function or an isolated amnesia, usually is not considered dementia as the term is commonly employed. Dementia must be differentiated from *amentia*, or mental retardation, in which normal intellectual function fails to develop, and *delirium*, a reversible state of diffuse mental impairment usually unaccompanied by permanent neuropathologic abnormalities.

The symptoms of a *static dementia* can follow any disease that permanently structurally damages large portions of the

TABLE 461–1. MAJOR CAUSES AND APPROXIMATE FREQUENCIES OF PROGRESSIVE DEMENTIAS

1. Senile dementia, Alzheimer type	50%
2. Multi-infarct (arteriosclerotic or other vascular cause)	20%
3. Combination of 1 and 2	
4. Communicating hydrocephalus	5%
5. Alcoholic–post-traumatic	5%
6. Huntington's	5%
7. Intracranial mass lesions	5%
8. Uncommon or mixed with above:	10%
Chronic drug use; Creutzfeldt-Jacob; metabolic (thyroid, liver, nutritional); degenerative (spinocerebellar, amyotrophic lateral sclerosis, parkinsonism, multiple sclerosis, Pick's, Wilson's, epilepsy); static dementia	

association areas of the cerebral hemispheres. Thus, for example, single episodes of severe head injury, global brain ischemia from cardiac arrest, large intracranial neoplasms or hemorrhages with their surgical removal, or infections such as severe encephalitis or meningitis each can injure the brain sufficiently to prevent intelligence from ever returning to a pre-illness level. Such conditions, however, represent only a fraction of the number of *progressive dementias* that affect increasing numbers as the average life span lengthens. In the United States alone estimates indicate that close to a million persons are incapacitated by a fixed or progressive dementia. Present population age trends indicate that this number will double or triple within 40 years unless scientific research slows or halts the epidemic. Table 461–1 indicates the most common causes and approximate frequencies of the progressive dementias.

EARLY CLINICAL MANIFESTATIONS. The component symptoms of dementia vary as broadly as do the underlying components of the damaged mind whose worsening they reflect. Acute, static dementia seldom provides a problem in diagnosis. Almost as soon as the acute illness passes, family, employers, and sometimes even the patient recognize that something is wrong, that things are different. Problems with social relationships, or employment soon follow, and when no improvement takes place within weeks or months, the diagnostic problem becomes not whether a mental decline has occurred but to what degree and how the patient can restructure his world to his new, possibly permanent limitation.

Early diagnosis in the progressive dementias is less certain and more difficult. Initial symptoms especially involve deterioration in mood, personality, recent memory, judgment, and the capacity to form abstractions, none of which is easily quantified, especially in the elderly. In general, families or work associates notice a change before the patient does, and persons who live by intellectual efforts show their limitations earlier than do those with routine or manual jobs. Danger signals in mood and behavior consist of a loss of vitality, of curiosity, and of mental energy—of "sparkle." Some patients become so apathetic as to seem depressed, while in others great anxiety or increased irritability disrupts a once pleasant personality. Affective responses lose their depth; some early dements become paranoid. Loss of recent memory and impaired judgment are universal features of the progressive dementias. One notes in affected patients an increasing tendency to make lists, then to forget where they left them. Appointments are missed, plans forgotten, stories of recent events become narrated repeatedly with no insight. Eventually orientation fails, first for days, then years, then months, and finally for place but never for self. Interest lags—first in papers, books, and new challenges, later in work, and eventually in friends and family. Debts may be accumulated silently, property unwisely sold, accounts lost, meals cooked twice over or served half-cold. In a curious, even startling way mental capacities may fluctuate suddenly and widely without apparent relationship to external events. In Alzheimer's disease and some of the other primary progressive dementias, social amenities tend to be retained until late in the course. Incontinence, soup on the shirt, and a disheveled appearance are more characteristic of frontal lobe disease and intracranial mass lesions than of the diffuse cortical and subcortical cellular diseases that produce progressive dementia.

DIAGNOSIS AND DIFFERENTIAL DIAGNOSIS. The three principal questions are (1) Does a true decline in intellect exist? (2) If so, what is its probable cause? (3) Can any aspect be treated effectively? Bedside testing answers the first, while the second and third require laboratory assistance.

The clinical examination of any patient with subacute or chronic central nervous system disease should include at least a brief evaluation of mental function. The test should be given gently and the results interpreted with due allowance for the patient's social background, schooling, innate capacities as judged by life attainments, and probable anxiety provoked by the interview and fear of failure. The standard examination measures orientation, language, and memory-retention by identifying recent major current events, the spelling of w-o-r-l-d backwards, and recalling three unrelated words at five minutes. Asking the subject to perform serial sevens backwards tests attention span, while proverbs and definitions (e.g., river from canal) give some idea of abstract capabilities. The Minimental Status examination (Table 461–2) provides valuable help in quantifying mental capacity. The evaluation usually requires considerably less than 10 minutes. Normals score 27 to 30, while clinically demented persons usually score less than 20. Psychologically depressed patients generally have intermediate scores.

When a quantitative baseline is desired against which to compare the effects of treatment or the rate of future deterioration, the Wechsler Adult Intelligence Scale (WAIS) provides useful information but requires the assistance of a trained psychologist. In mild to moderate dementia the verbal score of the WAIS provides an index of learning capacity, while the performance part reflects current mental abilities. A discrepancy of more than 15 points between the two provides a strong indication of structural brain damage. Special tests are required to evaluate selective memory failure.

The laboratory evaluation of dementia is guided by the combined results of the history, general physical and neurologic examinations, and preliminary laboratory results. In the absence of important leads from these sources (e.g., signs of chronic liver disease, uremia, severe vascular disease, bacterial endocarditis, a space-occupying intracranial lesion, etc.), the laboratory tests listed in Table 461–3 will detect nearly all of the treatable causes of dementia. The laboratory yield will be low in suspected degenerative cases, but the seriousness of the problem deserves the dignity of careful evaluation.

The term *pseudodementia* denotes reversible states in which reduced cognitive functions are caused by chronic drug intoxication (including prescribed agents) or depressive illness. The

TABLE 461–2. OUTLINE OF MINIMENTAL STATUS EXAMINATION*

Test	Score
What is the *year, season, date, day, month*	5
Where are you: *state, county, town, place, floor*	5
Name three objects: State slowly and have patient repeat (Repeat until patient learns all three)	3
Do reverse serial 7's (five steps) or spell "WORLD" backwards	5
Ask for the three unrelated objects above	3
Name from inspection a pencil, a watch	2
Have patient repeat "No ifs, ands, or buts"	1
Follow a three-stage command (1 pt each)	3
("Take a paper in your hand, fold it, and put it on the floor.")	
Read and obey, "Close your eyes"	1
Write a simple sentence	1
Copy intersecting pentagons	1

*From Folstein MF, Folstein SE, McHugh PR: Minimental state. A practical method for grading the cognitive state for the clinician. J. Psychiatr Res 12:189, 1975. The authors found that out of a possible total score of 30, mean score for dementia was 9.7, depression with cognitive impairment was 19.0, and uncomplicated affective depression was 27.6.

TABLE 461–3. LABORATORY TESTS MOST USEFUL IN EVALUATING DEMENTIA OF UNKNOWN ORIGIN

Blood: CBC and ESR, serologic test for syphilis (STS)
Metabolic screen (SMA 12–16)
Serum thyroxine, B_{12} level
Chest x-ray and brain CT or MRI
Lumbar puncture: cells (cytologic analysis if present), protein, STS

aging brain is especially susceptible to both conditions. Diagnosis in the first instance comes by taking a meticulous history of medications and reducing all potential offenders gradually so as to judge their effects on symptoms. Barbiturates, benzodiazepines, butyrophenones, tricyclic antidepressants, MAO inhibitors, anticholinergics, corticosteroids, and digitalis are most often responsible.

Psychologic depression (Ch. 462) is a common response to the physical and emotional deprivation of elderly life. The associated apathy, semi-mutism, akinesia, anxiety, and indifference often can resemble a dementia. Careful evaluation, however, quickly brings out differences. In contrast to demented patients, those with depression complain repeatedly of their poor memory. Patients with depression commonly eat little, often are severely constipated, sleep less than normal, and tend to behave best at night. They may answer questions slowly or reluctantly, but when they do, they respond to factual queries relatively well, revealing proper general orientation and understanding of commands. Errors occur because of indifference or obstinate refusal rather than poor comprehension. Depressed patients may stumble over tests requiring attention, but they rarely forget major recent events or political figures, and when they cooperate, they do not fail either simple tests or language or two- or even three-stage verbal commands. By contrast, patients with incapacitating dementia are disoriented, their nights are more agitated and confused than their days, they have difficulty following commands, both attention and recent memory are severely impaired, and many of them suffer difficulties in language and specific learned motor functions. Differences on mental status examinations usually are readily apparent. Laboratory tests add differentiating points. Brain imaging procedures show anatomic abnormalities in many of the dementias, and the EEG is slow in most of the dementias but not in depression.

Depression sometimes accompanies dementia, especially that associated with multiple strokes, head trauma, and Huntington's disease, all conditions in which insight tends to be relatively preserved. The diagnosis of an associated psychologic problem is suggested by the patient's mood and complaints and by behavior that is disproportionally withdrawn and mute for the degree of cognitive loss.

ALZHEIMER'S DISEASE

This most common of the progessive dementias affects both men and women, beginning in rare instances as early as the late teens or 20's and increasing in frequency progressively with age to affect approximately 5 per cent of persons over age 65 years and over 20 per cent of those who reach 80 or more. In past years, patients younger than age 65 were classified as having Alzheimer's presenile dementia, while older ones were believed to have a different illness, termed senile dementia. Clinical and biologic evidence, however, indicates that both terms describe the same disease, irrespective of age.

ETIOLOGY. The cause of Alzheimer's disease (AD) is unknown. The disease exists worldwide, and nothing suggests a relationship to nutritional factors, infection, toxins, or other environmental factors. A history of affected family members occurs in about a quarter of cases. This plus the fact that almost all patients with Down's syndrome develop Alzheimer's changes in the brain suggests a genetic susceptibility, perhaps transmitted as an autosomal dominant trait on chromosome 21. Other influences must be important, since identical twins show less than 50 per cent concordance for the illness, and when such cases have appeared, several years often separate the onset of clinical disease within the affected pair.

PATHOLOGY AND PATHOPHYSIOLOGY. AD produces a progressive neuronal degeneration of selective cells in the association and memory areas of the cerebral cortex, combined with similar abnormalities in certain subcortical nuclei. Some of the latter, in turn, cause a secondary degeneration of the ascending cholinergic and adrenergic pathways that diffusely connect the basal forebrain and locus ceruleus with the cerebral hemispheres.

By the time of death, the temporal lobe in AD is usually smaller than normal. Gross, more generalized atrophy sometimes is seen in younger, chronic victims of the disease. Histologic examination discloses characteristic abnormalities. Neuronal loss affects especially the large pyramidal cells of the hippocampus, the amygdala and the parietal and frontal association areas. The cholinergic basal forebrain nucleus of Meynert suffers severe degeneration. Silver-staining plaques containing degenerating neuronal products clustered around an amyloid core are scattered prominently in the cortex and subcortex. Many of the degenerating nerve cells contain tangles of twisted intracellular fibrils of a unique protein configuration related to altered neurofibrillary protein. Recent studies suggest that both the cerebral amyloid and the altered neurofibrillary protein are linked to the genetic error that predisposes to the disorder.

The pathologic changes of AD are more quantitatively than qualitatively different from those in other disorders, including uncomplicated aging. Neuronal loss, plaques, and tangles, usually in lesser degrees, can be found in the brains of many intellectually intact elderly persons. The functional importance of the reduced autonomic innervation remains unclear. Cell loss in the hippocampus and amygdala correlates with the prominent amnesia of the disease. The pyramidal cell dropout in areas of association cortex explains many of the early psychologic symptoms and correlates with recent research studies that show that brain metabolism is moderately reduced in early cases of AD, with the temporal-parietal-occipital association areas suffering the greatest decline.

SIGNS AND SYMPTOMS. Failure of recent memory for events, and, often, names is the earliest prominent symptom. Disturbances in emotional behavior often appear, consisting of either a reduction in affect or an increase in anxiety. Focal psychologic deficits are prominent, demonstrated by difficulty in managing spatial relationships or in initiating motor skills. The nominal amnesia may become so severe as to resemble a specific aphasia. Primary motor and sensory functions are spared. Similarly, social amenities are preserved until very late; even with moderately advanced, incapacitating dementia almost all AD patients continue to dress well, to maintain neat appearances, and to avoid incontinence. Seizures are rare and their occurrence prompts search for another etiology.

AD usually begins insidiously, although hints of abnormal behavior sometimes appear several years before sustained clinical changes allow a firm diagnosis. Among older victims a suddenly unexpected delirious or paranoid reaction associated with a minor febrile illness or an operation such as cataract extraction may be the first harbinger. The early progressive loss of recent memory can be difficult to distinguish from the "benign forgetfulness" for names and trivial events which affects many older persons in their seventh or eighth decades. When the defect extends to a failure to keep appointments, to initiate or keep track of business or domestic matters, or becomes coupled with a progressive loss of interest, early AD should be suspected. Less frequently, isolated psychologic deficits producing spatial disorientation, apraxia, syntactic aphasia, or acalculia may be prominent. The time course of evolution varies widely from patient to patient. In younger individuals a period of years sometimes separates the first suggestions of "peculiar" behavior from the advent of a readily diagnosed dementia.

Except for the signs of abnormal mental status, the physical and neurologic examinations remain normal in early or intermediate state AD. Laboratory tests are not helpful except in a negative sense. CT scans of the brain may or may not show moderate cortical atrophy but are otherwise unremarkable; blood and CSF studies are uninformative. The EEG usually is moderately but nonspecifically slow.

DIFFERENTIAL DIAGNOSIS. Diagnosis in AD is made by exclusion and largely on clinical grounds. No specific laboratory determinants exist, and brain biopsy is unjustified. The main problem occurs when laboratory tests, including brain imaging, show no abnormality. Psychologic depression, drug intoxication, some of the diffuse angiopathies, metabolic deficiency, chronic meningitis, Pick's disease, or early stages of diffuse primary or metastatic brain tumor sometimes may create diagnostic errors. Within a matter of weeks to a very few months most of these conditions clarify their nature, the exceptions being mainly neuropathologic rarities or another form of primary degenerative dementia such as the rare Pick's disease.

MANAGEMENT. There is no specific treatment, and neither diet nor drugs will slow the steady intellectual deterioration. The brunt of care usually falls on family or social agencies during the early and intermediate stages of illness. Institutionalization often is required in the late stages when patients may sink to a purely vegetative level. Occasionally depression is a prominent early symptom; it responds to small doses of the usual antidepressants. Sedatives or tranquilizers tend to make matters worse. With restless, agitated patients, tasteless liquid haloperidol can be given in doses of 0.5 to 1 mg two to three times daily as needed. The Alzheimer's Disease Foundation can provide the family with useful advice. Mace and Rabin's valuable guide is listed in the references.

OTHER PRINCIPAL DEMENTIAS

MULTI-INFARCT DEMENTIA (MD). This term describes diffuse mental impairment resulting from cerebral vascular disease. The condition is much less common than Alzheimer's disease and usually is readily distinguishable clinically. A general decline in intellectual function results from multifocal occlusion of cerebral arteries and arterioles either from remotely arising emboli or from intrinsic cerebral arteriolar occlusive disease. The condition appears most often in association with diabetic or hypertensive vascular disease, producing large and small infarcts that involve specific sensorimotor areas as well as areas of cortex dealing with specific and nonspecific cognitive functions. As a result, disturbances in gait, station, and skeletal motor function accompany abnormalities in language, praxis, gnosis, mood, abstract thinking, and attention. Lesions can affect any area of the brain but are most frequent in the distribution of the middle and anterior cerebral arteries. Pseudobulbar palsy is common, as is pathologic crying and laughing and abnormal motor reflexes. A high incidence of frontal lobe infarction is accompanied by a reduction in attention as well as emotional lability, often coupled with a disregard for neatness and social niceties. Insight often is retained and accompanied by depression of mood. Many patients develop urinary incontinence. MD characteristically progresses in steps, with each new bite out of the brain accompanied by an abrupt minor or major worsening, sometimes with modest improvement between. Occasionally, the individual infarcts of hypertensive arteriolar disease may be so small (lacunae) that the effect of their successive appearance gives the impression of an insidiously developing and gradually progressing process. Nevertheless, the presence of prominent motor changes and abnormal motor reflexes almost always differentiates the process from Alzheimer's disease; imaging studies usually disclose multiple brain infarcts and rule out a space-occupying lesion or communicating hydrocephalus. CSF analysis eliminates infection as the mechanism of the mental decline. Signs of systemic vascular disease are almost invariably present.

HYDROCEPHALIC DEMENTIA. Chronic communicating hydrocephalus, sometimes called normal pressure hydrocephalus (Ch. 495.3) occasionally produces an insidiously beginning and gradually progressive dementia, with forebrain functions becoming especially impaired by the abnormal hydrodynamic process. Affected persons may give a history of remote subarachnoid hemorrhage, recurrent head trauma, or meningeal infection, but the cause of hydrocephalus often lies in the remote past and remains unknown. The condition is most frequent in late middle-aged or elderly men. In hydrocephalic dementia, CT scans or other imaging studies show marked enlargement of the cerebral ventricular system, especially the lateral and third ventricles. Sometimes one finds narrowing of the aqueduct of Sylvius, but more frequently there is dilatation of all of the ventricles with reduced or absent sulcal markings over the surface of the hemispheres, especially at the vertex. The periventricular white matter often appears abnormally lucent owing to an increased water content. The cerebrospinal fluid pressure sometimes lies in the range of 180 to 220 mm H_2O, but lower levels often are found. CSF contents are normal and the presence of an elevation of cell count or protein immediately suggests a more active meningeal abnormality.

The typical signs and symptoms of hydrocephalic dementia comprise a triad of frontal-type dementia, broad-based ataxia, and urinary incontinence. Attention declines, abstract reasoning and the capacity to anticipate future events decay in parallel, and patients become careless in appearance and attire. Motor dysfunction is prominent and consists of a rigid-spastic increased resistance to passive movement of the extremities, especially the lower, coupled with a stiff, broad-based, hesitating, small-stepped gait, often accompanied by palmar and plantar grasp reflexes. Diagnosis depends principally on the clinical picture and characteristic brain imaging. Surgical CSF-shunting procedures are followed by intellectual and motor improvement in about half the cases. The operation is most often successful when the cause of the meningeal obstruction is evident or improvement follows a brief trial of spinal drainage by lumbar puncture.

HUNTINGTON'S DISEASE. Huntington's disease (HD), an inherited disorder transmitted as an autosomal dominant trait with close to complete penetrance, produces a combination of a choreiform movement disorder and dementia, as discussed in Ch. 470. The brain at autopsy shows prominent gross atrophy of the caudate, putamen, and, to a lesser degree, globus pallidus, with loss of the small neurons of the caudate and putamen being the most prominent cellular change. Studies of brain oxidative metabolism of asymptomatic family members at risk for HD have shown selective hypofunction in the region of the caudate possibly heralding onset of the disease. Early symptomatic patients show hypometabolism in both caudate and putamen but not at the cortical level. Postmortem pharmacologic studies of the striatum and its connections in HD have shown prominent decreases in the content of the synthesizing enzymes for GABA and acetylcholine, as well as decreases in the peptide neurotransmitters, substance P, enkephalin, and cholecystokinin. These changes relate more firmly to our understanding of the pathophysiology of the movement disorder than to the dementia, which currently lacks a satisfactory mechanistic explanation. The recent apparent identification of the locus of the Huntington gene suggests that preclinical diagnosis and genetic counseling may soon be a 100 per cent accurate opportunity for family members.

The earliest certain abnormalities in HD are usually those of the movement disorder. Early cognitive changes consist of a difficulty in anticipating and planning the future combined with a patchy memory loss, especially for serial tasks or memorization. Word memory and language functions are relatively well retained, as is spatial recognition. Later, the dementia takes on a more general quality. Prominent psychiatric symptoms mark the early stages in about two thirds of cases. Depression or schizophreniform behavior is common, and approximately 10 per cent of patients with HD commit suicide.

CREUTZFELDT-JAKOB DISEASE. Creutzfeldt-Jakob disease (CJD) is an infrequent disorder transmitted by a submicroscopic agent of unknown type ("slow virus") (Ch. 488.2). The cardinal clinical features are the early appearance and rapid progression over several months of signs of upper motor neuron dysfunction coupled with increasing dementia, focal motor or myoclonic convulsions, and prominent changes in the EEG. Brain images are normal. These features distinguish CJD from the other dementias described in this chapter.

PICK'S DISEASE. This is a rare cortical atrophy of unknown cause with an age incidence that overlaps that of AD. The illness usually develops insidiously and progresses slowly for a period of three to ten years or more. Severe atrophy affects the cerebral cortex, especially in the frontal and temporal regions. Microscopic examination shows neuronal loss, extensive gliosis, and characteristic swollen, pear-shaped "Pick cells." Plaques and tangles are unusual. The caudate, globus pallidus, and thalamus show less consistent cellular losses. Brain images reveal frontotemporal atrophy. In keeping with the pathologic findings, early clinical signs and symptoms include prominent disturbances in memory and in the anticipation and regulation of planned activities. Affected patients are apathetic, slovenly, and hypoactive and tend to forget the purpose of their acts, yet they retain spatial orientation and direction. Incontinence develops early and vocal productivity declines, often to the level of mutism. Signs of extrapyramidal and corticospinal motor dysfunction develop late, but the clinical findings are seldom diagnostically distinctive. There is no treatment.

Blackwood W, Corsellis JAN: Greenfield's Neuropathology. Chicago, Arnold-Yearbook, 1976. *The standard reference for the classic morphology of the dementias.*

Cummings JL, Benson DF: Dementia: A Clinical Approach. Boston, Butterworths, 1983. *The best current monograph on the subject, discussing all etiologies.*

Katzman R, Terry R: The Neurology of Aging. Philadelphia, FA Davis, 1983. *This recent monograph discusses many aspects of the needs of the aging patient, including conditions that must be differentiated from dementia.*

Katzman R: Alzheimer's disease. N Engl J Med 314:964, 1986. *The most recent comprehensive, clinically oriented review.*

Mace NL, Rabin PV: The 36-hour Day. A family guide to caring for persons with Alzheimer's disease, related dementing illnesses, and memory loss in later life. Baltimore, Johns Hopkins University Press, 1981. *An invaluable book for families and friends of the affected.*

Martin JB, Gusella JF: Huntington's disease: Pathogenesis and management. N Engl J Med 315:1267, 1986. *A recent review clearly summarizes new information on genetics, pathogenesis, and features of the disorder.*

462 PSYCHIATRIC DISORDERS IN MEDICAL PRACTICE

Gary J. Tucker

Perhaps of most concern to the nonpsychiatric physician is the process of psychiatric diagnosis. When does the wide range of human behavior become a pathologic process needing intervention and when is it a variation of normal response to life events? Lacking clear laboratory tests, precise anatomic dysfunctions, or specific pathologic findings, the diagnostic process in psychiatry has followed traditional medical practice for such conditions, i.e., to delineate syndromes and to categorize patterns of symptomatology. However, these syndromes and categories until recently have been broad, often

regional, and idiosyncratic. A massive revision of diagnostic practice in psychiatry occurred in 1980 with the publication by the American Psychiatric Association of the third edition of the *Diagnostic and Statistical Manual of Mental Disorders (DSM III).* The key components of this nomenclature represent diagnostic criteria that are descriptive and data based, and they require that the clinician view psychiatric disorders from a number of different aspects or axes. The specific symptoms not only include those that must be present but also identify explicit symptoms that must be excluded before a diagnosis can be made. For example, to make the diagnosis of "schizophrenia," one must exclude depressive illness. The clinician must also stipulate the role of biologic, characterologic, and sociologic factors that affect the illness in terms of five axes. Axis I is the specific syndrome, such as schizophrenia, affective disorder, etc. Axis II includes specific personality disorders such as antisocial, dependent, and specific developmental disorders, language disorders, reading disorders, etc. Axis III consists of contributing physical disorders and medical conditions. Axis IV consists of psychosocial stressors. Axis V designates the highest level of adaptive functioning the patient manifested in the past year. All of these axes add to the diagnostic description of the patient and are important in understanding and treating the specific condition. For example, a 50-year-old lawyer with a major depression may be described as follows: Axis I—major depression; Axis II—obsessive personality; Axis III—diabetes, hypertension; Axis IV—marital discord; Axis V—good social and work functioning.

At various times most people will experience anxiety, depression, sleep disturbance, and/or somatic preoccupation. In most cases such symptoms are transient, and the precipitants to such symptoms are often evident—an upcoming examination, a new job, marriage, divorce, work or family problems. In these instances the physician has no difficulty in reassuring the patient that the symptoms are transient and situational. However, when these symptoms persist and/or when they occur in situations that have no clear precipitants, they should become of concern to the physician. In order to classify someone as having a psychiatric illness, one must consider the following factors: (1) Do the signs and symptoms fit a psychiatric diagnosis? For example, when patients say they are sad or depressed, do they meet the diagnostic criteria for a diagnosis of depression or dysthymic disorder? (see Tables 462–7 and 462–9). (2) Is there a family history of similar symptoms? Many psychiatric illnesses tend to have a genetic incidence. (3) Is the longitudinal pattern of the symptoms consistent with the natural history of a psychiatric disorder? Emotional symptoms associated with specific situations are usually classified as reactions to the situation (see grief reactions); they do not usually become psychiatric disorders. (4) Are the symptoms incapacitating? All persons have enduring patterns of relating, perceiving, and reacting to others. These constitute various components of a person's personality and may take the form of such patterns as obsessive, passive, or antisocial personality traits. When such characteristics interfere with the individual's ability to function, however, the condition is regarded as a personality disorder, named for the predominant personality characteristic. (5) Do delusions and hallucinations exist? Delusions and hallucinations in the absence of other medical causes always indicate major psychiatric illness. While illusory phenomena can often occur at times of tiredness, intoxication, fever, etc., their occurrence in clear states of consciousness should alert one to the presence of major psychiatric illness.

The proper delineation of psychiatric disorders from normal emotional reactions rests on a careful history, a mental status evaluation, and a knowledge of psychiatric syndromes. If the findings of the history and mental status evaluation do not fit into any of the known psychiatric syndromes, the physician should reserve judgment and follow the patient. In many cases, the symptoms will neither persist nor return and all can be reassured. If the symptoms continue, one may recognize a clear psychiatric syndrome. With all persistent emotional and behavioral symptoms, however, the physician must first rule out systemic medical disorders.

DIFFERENTIATING PSYCHIATRIC DISORDERS FROM MEDICAL DISORDERS

While it has always been evident that the central nervous system mediates behavior, there has been a reluctance to look at major psychiatric illnesses as disorders of the central nervous system. However, as biologic studies of psychiatric patients progress and specific psychopharmacologic agents are found to affect behavior, it becomes increasingly evident that psychiatric disorders are disorders of central nervous system functioning. This awareness includes recognition that the central nervous system has a limited number of ways of responding to stress. For example, hallucinations can arise from psychologic causes, from toxins in the blood, from head trauma, from seizure disorders, and from fever. With such potentially diverse etiologies, it is imperative that the physician seek clues to differentiate the causes of the behavior change (Table 462–1).

Many clues in the history can suggest something other than an intrinsic psychiatric illness as a cause of abnormal behavior. Most patients with psychiatric illnesses have had psychiatric symptoms or reveal seeds of the current disturbance in their histories. When a patient presents with a good premorbid social history, a good work history, a warm and supportive family, and well-preserved sociality, one should seek nonpsychiatric factors to explain the behavior change. Many physicians tend erroneously to view behavior changes only in a psychologic framework. Abrupt changes in behavior, personality, mood, or ability to function should be evaluated for possible organic causes. As indicated, most decompensating patients with psychiatric illness describe similar, albeit less severe, symptoms in the past. To give an example: A 60-year-old man who has been stiff and proper his entire life but abruptly becomes bawdy and flirtatious is probably not experiencing the onset of a major psychiatric illness but rather is showing personality changes associated with an organic process, such as brain tumor, vascular disease, endocrine abnormality, or drug reaction. Rapid fluctuations in mental status also suggest an organic rather than a psychiatric disorder. Patients with psychiatric disease seldom are delusional and hallucinating in the morning but free of these symptoms the same evening (or vice versa). By contrast, the resolution of the delusions and hallucinations associated with schizophrenia typically requires days to weeks. Similarly, motor behavior does not change rapidly in psychiatric illness. Patients with organic encephalopathies, by contrast, often have a "motor driveness" with episodic desires to move about, to get up and walk. This restlessness is particularly prominent in delirious states. Lastly, and perhaps most subtly, when a patient does not respond to the usual interventions one should suspect the possibility of an incorrect diagnosis. For example, when a patient with hallucinations and delusions has been treated unsuccessfully with adequate doses of neuroleptic medications for an appropriate period of time with no change in the symptoms, one should consider the possibility of a disorder other than schizophrenia. These simple

TABLE 462–1. CLUES TO NONPSYCHIATRIC DISORDERS AFFECTING BEHAVIOR

1. The signs and symptoms do not fit into an established psychiatric diagnostic category.
2. There is no prior psychiatric history or symptoms.
3. The patient demonstrates an abrupt change in behavior or personality.
4. Signs and symptoms fluctuate rapidly.
5. The condition does not respond to treatment.

guidelines will often alert the clinician to multiple diagnostic possibilities.

Goodwin D, Guze S: Psychiatric Diagnosis. 3rd ed. New York, Oxford University Press, 1984. *An excellent overall text on descriptive psychiatry and the basis for diagnostic groupings.*

Jefferson J, Marshall J: Neuropsychiatric Features of Medical Disorders. New York, Plenum Press, 1981. *A comprehensive presentation of behavioral and psychiatric concomitants of medical illnesses.*

Lishsman W: Organic Psychiatry. Oxford, Blackwell, 1978. *A comprehensive description of neurologic and medical complications of behavioral disorders.*

Pincus J, Tucker G: Behavioral Neurology. 3rd ed. New York, Oxford University Press, 1985. *This monograph discusses differential diagnosis and behavioral aspects of neurologic disease as well as neurologic aspects of psychiatric disorders.*

Spitzer RL (ed.): Diagnostic and Statistical Manual of Mental Disorders. 3rd ed. Washington, D.C., American Psychiatric Association, 1980. *A useful, widely accepted outline of diagnostic features of the gamut of psychiatric disorders.*

SCHIZOPHRENIC DISORDERS

Schizophrenia and some forms of affective disorders comprise the major psychotic illnesses. (Psychosis is defined as the presence of hallucinations and/or delusions.) Kraepelin, a noted German psychiatrist, observed that among hospitalized psychotic patients there were two types of course. The first seemed to be characterized by exacerbations and remissions in mood and cognitive functioning which he labeled "manic depressive illness," and the second was characterized by a chronic psychotic course with its onset in youth and deteriorating social function, which he labeled "dementia praecox" (a dementing illness of young people). In 1911 Eugene Bleuler, a Swiss psychiatrist, changed the name of dementia praecox to "schizophrenia." He described the central features of schizophrenia as a psychotic process manifested by disturbed thinking, changes in the emotional responsiveness of the patient, and a preoccupation with their own inner life, or autism. By schizophrenia he did not mean a "split personality" but more a splitting of psychologic functions. While some functions, such as the ability to communicate, were often impaired, others, such as memory and mathematical abilities, were sustained. In essence, this early concept remains a good definition of the schizophrenic process.

Schizophrenia most often has its onset in late adolescence. The course of the illness is usually marked by a decline in psychosocial functioning, with a tendency for the patient to become downwardly mobile in social class. The introduction of neuroleptics in 1954 brought about some improvement in the treatment of these patients, but the observations of Kraepelin of an ultimate deteriorating course still hold true. Current treatment aims toward shorter hospitalizations for schizophrenics with more vigorous attempts to retain the patient in a community setting. Physicians encounter two principal groups of schizophrenic patients, one with an acute florid psychotic illness and the other suffering chronic illness with less florid symptoms. The care of these two groups differs in that the acute management is simple, whereas the care and rehabilitation of the chronic patient can be extremely difficult. The nationally pursued process of "deinstitutionalization" has thrust this latter patient population into our everyday world.

DIAGNOSTIC CRITERIA AND CLINICAL SIGNS AND SYMPTOMS. Table 462–2 lists the clinical symptoms of schizophrenia. Note the emphasis on hallucinations and delusions. The ones cited are typical of schizophrenia, although similar hallucinations and delusions can occur in affective disorders and organic conditions; however, the course of these later illnesses is different. A recent study by Cloninger et al. (1985) demonstrates the importance of the presence of delusions and hallucinations in the diagnosis of schizophrenia. They found that the greater the number of delusions and hallucinations present, particularly persecutory delusions, delusions of control, firmly fixed mood incongruent delusions, and auditory hallucinations, the more likely was the person to progress to a chronic psychotic condition. Other prominent

TABLE 462–2. SCHIZOPHRENIA*

A. Characterized by psychotic symptoms during the active phase of illness. One of the major symptom categories below must be present for at least one week (or less if symptoms respond to treatment):
  1. Two of the following:
     a. Delusions
     b. Prominent hallucinations (throughout the day for several days or several times a week for several weeks; each hallucinatory experience is not limited to a few brief moments)
     c. Incoherence of speech or marked loosening of verbal associations
     d. Catatonic behavior
     e. Flat or grossly inappropriate affect
  2. Bizarre delusions (i.e., involving a phenomenon that the individual's subculture would regard as totally implausible, e.g., thoughts being broadcast out loud, being controlled by a dead person)
  3. Prominent hallucinations of a voice keeping up a running commentary on the individual's behavior or thoughts, or two or more voices conversing with each other
B. During the course of the disturbance, a decrease in functioning in such areas as work, social relations, and self-care.
C. Major depressive or manic syndrome and medical conditions ruled out.
D. Continuous psychiatric symptoms for at least six months.

*Modified from American Psychiatric Association: Diagnostic and Statistical Manual of Mental Disorders, Third Edition. Washington, DC, APA, 1980. Used with permission.

symptoms of schizophrenia are the presence of incoherence and the inability of the patient to communicate with others in a logical and goal-directed fashion. As an example of the speech of a schizophrenic, the patient may respond as follows when asked why he was brought to the hospital: "You are a Nazi; God sent me to save the world; I have a lovely apartment; your eyes are blue."

The stipulation that these criteria must last for a six-month period (demonstrating a deterioration from a previous level of functioning) defines a more chronic population (Table 462–3). When the duration of symptoms is shorter than six months, it is inadvisable to use the diagnosis of schizophrenia. This allows the clinician to withhold judgment and encourages a search for other disorders. This is particularly important with the first episode of psychotic illness, in that it is difficult to differentiate an acute manic episode from an acute schizophrenic episode. Psychotic episodes due to toxic drug reactions, sleep deprivation, and medical causes invariably last less than six months (Table 462–4).

In the past many subtypes of schizophrenia have been described, but their predictive validity has been poor except for catatonia and paranoia. Catatonic symptoms include either markedly retarded motor behavior (often to the point of no voluntary movement, the patient retaining any posture into which he is passively placed) or markedly agitated motor behavior. The importance of a catatonic diagnosis, in either the retarded or the agitated form, has retained some validity in conferring a better prognosis, but there is also evidence that catatonia may be more related to affective disorders than to schizophrenia. The paranoid forms of schizophrenia also

TABLE 462–3. PRODROMAL OR RESIDUAL SYMPTOMS IN SCHIZOPHRENIA*

1. Marked social isolation or withdrawal
2. Marked impairment in role functioning as wage-earner, student, or homemaker
3. Markedly peculiar behavior (e.g., collecting garbage, talking to self in public, hoarding food)
4. Marked impairment in personal hygiene and grooming
5. Blunted, flat, or inappropriate affect
6. Digressive, vague, overelaborate, or circumstantial speech; poverty of speech; or poverty of content of speech
7. Odd beliefs or magical thinking, e.g., superstitiousness, belief in clairvoyance, telepathy, "sixth sense," "others can feel my feelings," overvalued ideas, ideas of reference
8. Unusual perceptual experiences, e.g., recurrent illusions, sensing the presence of a force or person not actually present
9. Marked lack of initiative, interests, or energy

*Modified from American Psychiatric Association: Diagnostic and Statistical Manual of Mental Disorders, Third Edition. Washington, DC, APA, 1980. Used with permission.

TABLE 462–4. USUAL SYMPTOMATIC PATTERNS OF PSYCHOTIC DISORDERS

	Acute Schizophrenia	Mania	Major Depression	Delirium
Delusions	++++	++++	+++	++
Hallucinations	++++	++	++	+++
Disorientation/confusion	0	0	0	++++
Incoherent speech	++++	+++	0	++++
Depressed mood	+	0	++++	+
Grandiosity	++	++++	0	0

show some unique features in that the paranoid delusions are often the only major symptoms and they tend to remain stable over time.

EPIDEMIOLOGY. The prevalence of schizophrenia in the general population is about 1 per cent for lifetime risk, or about an 0.5 in 1000 incidence of recorded or treated cases per year in the United States. The schizophrenic syndrome has a similar worldwide incidence, the only cultural difference being that prognosis for recovery seems better in rural environments than in urban settings. The prevalence rate is eight times higher in the lower than in the higher socioeconomic classes. Since the parents of schizophrenics have a social class distribution similar to that of the general population, the lower position of the patients appears to be a result of the illness rather than the cause of it.

Since the highest incidence of schizophrenia is in younger people, whose illness often becomes chronic, the number of cases is constantly increasing. Seventy per cent of schizophrenics become ill between ages 15 and 35, and the illness affects males slightly more than females. Peak onset in males lies between 15 and 24 years and in females between 25 and 34 years. There are slight ethnic differences with a higher incidence in Scandinavian countries and in nonwhites. The chronicity of the illness presents an enormous cost. A recent study notes that although schizophrenia affects only one-twelfth as many persons as does myocardial infarction, the cost is six times as great.

PATHOPHYSIOLOGY. The pathophysiology of schizophrenia is unknown, nor has an anatomic origin of the symptoms been determined. Nevertheless, a number of conditions (including trauma, seizure disorders, and Huntington's disease) can produce schizophrenia-like hallucinations and delusions. Many authors have reported a higher than normal incidence of nonlocalizing neurologic abnormalities in schizophrenia, changes that are not present in other psychiatric conditions. These include defects in stereognosis, graphesthesia, and various skilled motor activities. Minor vestibular system defects, usually consisting of a reduction in the nystagmus response unrelated to medication use, have been noted in schizophrenic patients. Deficits in smooth-pursuit eye movements during pendulum tracking have been reported in schizophrenia as well as in other psychoses. Other evidence of organic damage, including EEG abnormalities, is tantalizingly frequent.

Twenty-five per cent of hospitalized schizophrenic patients show abnormally slow EEG tracings using standard recording techniques; with more complex instrumentation the incidence rises as high as 80 per cent. Recently developed imaging techniques have confirmed an increase in cerebral ventricular size in subgroups of schizophrenic patients. Reduction of cerebral blood flow in the frontal lobes using xenon inhalation and PET scanning has been described inconsistently. Neuropsychologic testing shows a great deal of overlap between the findings in patients with clear-cut organic disease and those with schizophrenia to the point where the tests often fail to distinguish between the two conditions.

Most of the above described dysfunctions imply an abnormality in the functional integration of sensory and cognitive information in schizophrenia.

Strong evidence implicates a genetic factor in schizophrenia

TABLE 462–5. DRUGS COMMONLY USED FOR TREATMENT OF SCHIZOPHRENIA*

	Daily Dosage Range (mg)
Phenothiazines	
Chlorpromazine (Thorazine)	300–1500
Thioridazine (Mellaril)	150–800
Perphenazine (Trilafon)	8–64
Trifluoperazine (Stelazine)	4–60
Fluphenazine (Prolixin)†	
Butyrophenones	
Haloperidol (Haldol)	2–40
Thioxanthenes	
Thiothixene (Navane)	6–60

*Owing to untoward extrapyramidal reactions, one often needs to administer these drugs along with such drugs as benztropine mesylate (Cogentin), trihexyphenidyl HCl (Artane), diphenhydramine HCl (Benadryl).
†Comes in two injectable slow-release forms that can be given every 10 days to 3 weeks.

to a degree that 10 to 15 per cent of the offspring of a schizophrenic parent are at risk for the disease. Furthermore, the coincidence of schizophrenia in monozygotic twins is roughly 60 per cent. Additional evidence for a genetic factor comes from studies of children of schizophrenic parents, who are raised by either their natural or adoptive, nonschizophrenic parents: The chance of developing the disease is identical, regardless of the developmental environment. While genetic factors are evident in the transmission of schizophrenia, the family has been implicated in other ways in its development. Previous theories relate to the "schizophrenogenic mother," but little scientific documentation has been provided. A more likely hypothesis of family interaction was developed by Leff and others, who noted that certain family environments had a great deal of "expressed emotion." In these families with much highly charged emotional interaction, schizophrenic patients seemed to do very poorly. Those environments that were less stimulating emotionally allowed the schizophrenic to function better. Hogarty et al. discuss these familial factors more extensively.

Additional indirect evidence for biologic mechanisms in schizophrenia derives from pharmacologic studies: (1) Most of the neuroleptic drugs effective in controlling schizophrenic symptoms act as dopamine blockers in the central nervous system. (2) Many psychoactive drugs such as LSD, mescaline, and amphetamines are dopaminergic and also have the potential for creating psychotic reactions. Further suggestions of altered dopamine metabolism in schizophrenic patients come from the inconsistent findings of both elevated and reduced levels of homovanillic acid, its major metabolite in the CSF and urine. As yet, most of these biologic findings, as well as the results of parallel animal studies, are too inconsistent or incomplete to permit unifying hypotheses.

PROGNOSIS AND TREATMENT. Prognosis in schizophrenia is poor and specific therapy lacking. Over a 25- to 30-year period, approximately one third of cases show some recovery or remission, and the remainder either have major residual symptoms or are still hospitalized. The major treatment is neuroleptic medication.

Table 462–5 lists the drugs most commonly used in the treatment of schizophrenia. The goal of treatment is to decrease as many of the symptoms as possible. As long as hallucinations, delusions, and disorganized thinking persist, the accepted practice is to increase the dose of medication until reaching a maximum decrease in symptoms. The most frequent limiting factor is the appearance of extrapyramidal side effects, the most common of which are dystonia, akathisia (restlessness), and parkinsonism. These occur most commonly in the first two to four months of drug use.

There is little difference in efficacy in the neuroleptics (Table 462–5), and lack of efficacy usually reflects too low a dose. If, however, no response occurs to a phenothiazine-type drug (e.g., chlorpromazine), one usually changes to another class

of neuroleptics, such as a butyrophenone (haloperidol) or a thioxanthene. The physician should become familiar with one drug from each of these classes of neuroleptics for acute and maintenance use. The major long-term hazard in the use of these medications is tardive dyskinesia.

Tardive dyskinesia is a syndrome of choreoathetoid and/or involuntary movements that may affect the mouth, lips, tongue, extremities, or trunk. Although usually associated with use of neuroleptics for six months or more, tardive dyskinesia can occur with shorter administration. Patients on neuroleptics should be periodically evaluated for these abnormal movements. A frequent early sign consists of vermicular movements of the tongue. Anticholinergic drugs do not help this condition. The symptoms may decrease with an increase of the medication, but such improvement usually is only temporary and may lead to a vicious circle of worsening chorea and increased drug dosages. The cause of tardive dyskinesia is not known, but it is believed to represent the development of dopaminergic hypersensitivity. While no effective treatment has been found, in many instances gradually decreasing the dose of neuroleptics induces a slow remission of the symptoms (see also Ch. 470).

Despite the above conditions, the use of neuroleptics is effective, and the drugs should be used to help the patient function with as few symptoms as possible despite the potential side effects. Removing schizophrenic patients from medication greatly increases the chances of hospitalization within the following six months. This lag represents a major problem in that most patients immediately feel and do better without the medications. As a result, families and patients often fail to associate the cessation of medication with the subsequent relapse.

Most criteria for judging prognosis in schizophrenia are related to short-term outcome and can be summarized by saying that the more acute and florid the early symptoms or, as some have phrased it, the more the patient has "positive" symptoms (delusions, hallucinations, agitation, and depressive symptoms), the more likely he is to recover from the acute episode. The more insidious the onset and the more lacking in emotional display (negative symptoms), the worse the short- and long-term prognoses. The natural history of the illness (even in treated patients) seems to be of two major types: (1) an episodic, relapsing course with each episode resulting in a lower level of psychosocial functioning; and (2) a gradual, slow decline in functional ability. Both courses eventually result in a progressive loss of psychosocial capacities (see Table 462–3). Recent treatment efforts in schizophrenia have taken a rehabilitative, or psychoeducational, approach in which the family is educated about the problems of schizophrenia and issues of living are openly dealt with.

ACUTE USE OF NEUROLEPTIC MEDICATION. Neuroleptic drugs are also useful for patients who are markedly agitated with or without delusions and hallucinations (Table 462–6). They also help to control agitated states associated with organic delirium and dementia. In elderly patients and in those with delirium and/or dementia, the doses should be much lower until the patient's reaction is ascertained. Since acutely agitated psychotic patients will respond to lorazepam as well as to neuroleptics, the initial use of benzodiazepines is probably safer in cases in which the source of the agitation

TABLE 462–6. DRUGS USED IN ACUTELY AGITATED STATES

Drug	Dose*	24-hr Maximum
Haloperidol (Haldol)	5–10 mg every 1–2 hr I.M. or P.O.	50 mg
Thiothixene (Navane)	5–10 mg every 2–4 hr I.M. or P.O.	40 mg
Lorazepam (Ativan)	0.5–1.0 mg every 1–2 hr I.M. or P.O.	10 mg

*Doses should be 50 to 75 per cent reduced in the elderly or medically ill.

is not known and in manic states for which long-term neuroleptic medication is not planned.

Bellack A (ed.): Schizophrenia. Orlando, Grune & Stratton, 1984. *Gives general and specific aspects of the treatment of schizophrenia.*

Cloninger C, Martin R, Guze S, et al.: Diagnosis and prognosis in schizophrenia. Arch Gen Psychiatry 42:15–25, 1985. *An excellent study of the implications of symptoms for prognosis in schizophrenia.*

Henn F, Nasrallah H (eds.): Schizophrenia as a Brain Disease. New York, Oxford University Press, 1982. *An overview of organic factors in schizophrenia.*

Hogarty G, Anderson C, Reiss A, et al.: Family psychoeducation, social skills training, and maintained chemotherapy in the aftercare treatment of schizophrenia. Arch Gen Psychiatry 43:633–642, 1986. *A convincing review and study of the role of psychosocial factors in the treatment of schizophrenia.*

Kaplan H, Saddock B: Comprehensive Textbook of Psychiatry. 4th ed. Baltimore, Williams & Wilkins, 1983. *An excellent and detailed overview of all aspects of schizophrenia.*

Strauss J, Carpenter W: Schizophrenia. New York, Plenum Press, 1981. *A comprehensive presentation of major aspects of schizophrenic disorders.*

AFFECTIVE DISORDERS

A difficulty in clinical psychiatric diagnosis is that similar terms are used to describe feeling states that differ greatly in degree and sometimes in kind. Such is the case with the term *depression*. In common use the meaning may extend from a description of a brief pang of regret to profound feelings of futility and suicidal despair. At what point along this spectrum does one label the condition "illness"? When does normal grief become pathologic? This section discusses these questions.

Many have attempted to classify depressive illnesses based on *symptomatology*, e.g., psychotic vs. neurotic; *supposed etiology*, e.g., endogenous vs. reactive; or *age*, e.g., childhood, involutional. None of these distinctions has resisted careful investigation. The most recent characterization of depressive illness has been simplified into *bipolar disorders*, identifying wide swings of mood; *major depressive illness*, marked by severe depressive symptoms but without manic swings; and two milder forms, *cyclothymic disorder* (formerly called depressive neurosis) and *dysthymic disorder*. These latter two terms describe milder forms of bipolar disorders and depression that fall short of the specific diagnostic criteria for the more serious disorders.

Symptoms of depression also are classified by the company they keep. The psychiatric condition alone would be classified as a primary affective disorder, but when symptoms of affective disorders accompany medical conditions, they are termed secondary affective disorders. Marked depressive symptoms have been noted with various endocrine disorders, tumors, seizure disorders, vitamin deficiencies, and particular neurologic disorders such as multiple sclerosis, Parkinson's disease, and stroke. Depressive symptoms also can be associated with drugs used to treat medical conditions. In at least some instances, the consistency of the symptoms may reflect the fact that similar neurotransmitter systems are altered in both the primary and secondary affective disturbances.

Major Depression

The symptomatology and diagnostic criteria for major depression are listed in Table 462–7. While many patients have single episodes of major depressive illness, the condition also can be repetitive, and this recurrent condition is frequently called unipolar depressive illness. Fifty per cent of patients with a single episode of major depression will eventually have another depressive episode.

The key features of major depression are a markedly gloomy mood in which there is a loss of interest in life, a lack of pleasure in almost all activities, and a general feeling of hopelessness and worthlessness. The illness takes the form of a cognitive change in which the patient seemingly looks at the world with "black glasses," and everything thought about or accomplished is minimized or negated: The wealthy and successful career person will talk about his or her impending financial doom and general lack of accomplishment in life;

TABLE 462–7. MAJOR DEPRESSIVE EPISODE*

A. At least five of the following symptoms have been present during the same two-week period; at least one of the symptoms was either 1 or 2 below and not related to a physical condition. These symptoms can be subjective reports or reported by others and must occur nearly every day.
  1. Depressed mood most of the day (e.g., the patient feels "down" or "low")
  2. Loss of interest or pleasure in all or almost all activities
  3. Significant weight loss or weight gain when not dieting or binge-eating (e.g., more than 5 per cent of body weight in a month), or decrease or increase in appetite
  4. Insomnia or hypersomnia
  5. Psychomotor agitation or retardation
  6. Fatigue or loss of energy
  7. Feelings of worthlessness or excessive or inappropriate guilt (which may be delusional)
  8. Diminished ability to think or concentrate, or indecisiveness
  9. Thoughts that he or she would be better off dead, or suicidal ideation, nearly every day; a suicide attempt
B. 1. An organic etiology has been ruled out
   2. Not a normal reaction to the loss of a loved one
C. Not superimposed on schizophrenia

*Modified from American Psychiatric Association: Diagnostic and Statistical Manual of Mental Disorders, Third Edition. Washington, DC, APA, 1980. Used with permission.

the gifted artist dismisses his creations as trivial. When vegetative functions (sleep, appetite, psychomotor activity) are markedly impaired and a complete loss of pleasure accompanies almost all activities with no reactions to pleasurable stimuli, we often add the term *melancholia*.

Depressive symptoms range in severity from mild mood swings to severe delusions about self-worth, accomplishments, and the future. The "blackness" of the presentation in the depressed patient is most often accompanied by severe motor retardation with profound sleep and appetite disturbance and suicidal ideation. Nevertheless, some severe depressions can present in a highly anxious, agitated state. The history of previous episodes (either manic or depressive) aids in the diagnosis.

DIAGNOSIS. The diagnosis is made on clinical grounds as discussed above. Many tests to aid the diagnosis of depression have been introduced, including the dexamethasone suppression test (DST), the thyroid-stimulating hormone (TSH) response (see below), and many measures of disturbed sleep function such as rapid eye movement (REM) latency. Unfortunately, none has proved to be diagnostically reliable or specific for affective disorder. In diagnosing depression, the interview is central.

EPIDEMIOLOGY. The sex distribution of major depression is almost two-to-one female to male. The peak incidence for women is 35 to 45 years, whereas the age pattern is less clear for men. There may also be an increased incidence in women in their early 50's. The prevalence is about 3.2 per 100 males and about 4.5 to 9.3 per 100 females. Incidence is 82 to 201 new cases per 100,000 for men and 247 to 598 new cases per 100,000 for women. The mean duration of first attack of an untreated depressive illness is about 13 months. The episodes, if they recur, are likely to be similar in nature and respond to treatment in a similar fashion. As with bipolar illness, alcoholism is a frequent complication of depressive illness, particularly when it has a recurring course.

PATHOPHYSIOLOGY. Pathophysiologic theories of affective disorders have developed along three major lines: (1) endocrine studies; (2) neurotransmitters; and (3) electrophysiologic studies. Depressed patients frequently have elevated levels of cortical steroids in the blood and urine and at least half fail to suppress cortisol secretion after dexamethasone administration. Thyroid-stimulating hormone (TSH) response to thyrotropin-releasing hormone also has been found to be aberrant in many depressed patients, even though their blood T_3 and T_4 levels are normal. Growth hormone, prolactin, gonadal hormones, CRF, and melatonin have all been shown to have diminished responses in subgroups of affective disorders. While none of these findings is specific for any type of depressive illness or consistent in all depressive illnesses, they nevertheless suggest the presence of pituitary-hypothalamic dysfunction in affective disorders.

Studies of neurotransmitters in depression have been stimulated largely by the success of pharmacologic agents used to treat affective disorders. Many of the tricyclic compounds and the MAO inhibitors effective in the treatment of depression increase the availability of catecholamines and indolamines in the central nervous system. Drugs such as reserpine and phenothiazine reduce the amounts of these neurotransmitters, and their use is associated with an increase or onset of depressive symptomatology. L-Dopa, used to treat Parkinson's disease, is a major catecholamine (dopamine) precursor and may in itself induce mania. These and other observations have given rise to the catecholamine-indolamine hypothesis of depression. The theory postulates that a certain level of amines and/or receptor sensitivity to catecholamines functions to generate a normal mood. Receptor insensitivity, a depletion of amines, or a decrease in their synthesis or storage leads to depression. Conversely, if the amines are in excess or the receptors are hypersensitive, mania may develop. Recently, the acetylcholine system has also been implicated in affective disorders, a "balance" between adrenergic and cholinergic function being postulated as necessary for the stabilization of mood. Neither theory, however, is entirely satisfactory, since it has been found that the tricyclic drugs affect many receptor systems and that their main action may be one of changing or regulating the sensitivity of the receptor rather than acting directly as neurotransmitters. Furthermore, newer drugs that have antidepressant effects do not affect these transmitter systems. One study, for example, has found that the anticonvulsant carbamazepine favorably affects the course of certain patients with bipolar illness.

Electrophysiologic studies on affective illness have concentrated on changes in sleep functions, especially the presence of changes in the REM sleep pattern during episodes of active illness. A subgroup of patients with affective disorder shows a shortened REM latency. Furthermore, analyses of circadian rhythms provide increasing evidence for autumn and winter precipitation of some bipolar disorders, with depressive illnesses apparently related to diminished ambient light in winter climates. The change has been correlated with alterations of melatonin metabolism.

TREATMENT. In most cases the physician is presented with someone who seems mildly sad and self-deprecating, with perhaps slight sleep and appetite disturbances. In such patients an attempt at counseling about the events in their lives and helping delineate appropriate priorities and activities, along with prescriptions for adequate exercise, diet, rest, and general health measures, may suffice. When symptoms become more marked, particularly when they disturb sleep and appetite, and the person becomes unable to perform work, school, or household tasks, one should consider adding antidepressant medication to the above regimen (Table 462–8). If the mild symptoms have been present for a number of years, a trial of medication may be in order. With prominent depressive symptomatology hospitalization may be necessary, the major indication being to prevent suicide (15 per cent of patients with major affective disorders commit suicide). As discussed in a later section, it is a wise step in medicine to ask all patients with depression of mood, apathetic fatigue, or ill-defined somatic symptoms if they have ever considered the situation sufficiently unbearable that suicide becomes an option.

The approach and response to drug therapy in depression vary considerably among both physicians and patients. Perhaps the best prediction of a favorable response is if a blood relative has responded well to a similar agent. In patients who present primarily with insomnia and marked vegetative disturbances as well as some agitation, amitriptyline is somewhat more sedating, particularly if given at bedtime. Imipra-

TABLE 462–8. ANTIDEPRESSANT DRUGS

Dose	Daily Dosage Range (mg)*	Anticholinergic Effects
Tricyclics		
Imipramine (Tofranil)	50–150	+ +
Amitriptyline (Elavil)	50–150	+ + +
Nortriptyline (Aventyl)	50–150	+ +
Desipramine (Norpramin, Pertofrane)	50–150	+
Doxepin (Sinequan)	150	+ +
Tetracyclic		
Maprotiline (Ludiomil)	50–225	+
Other		
Trazodone (Desyrel)	150–600	0
MAOI's†		
Phenelzine (Nardil)	15–90	+ +
Tranylcypromine (Parnate)	20–30	+ +

*In most cases the dose should be reduced 30 to 50 per cent in the elderly and medically ill.
†Monoamine oxidase inhibitors.

mine is less sedating and often avoids the drowsiness that amitriptyline causes. After initial CBC, liver profiles, and in older patients an EKG, it is best to start these medications in single doses at bedtime. An initial starting dose of 50 mg may be rapidly increased every several days until a total dosage of 150 mg per night is reached. As stated earlier, with elderly patients all psychotropic drugs should be used cautiously, and doses of antidepressants should be decreased by 30 to 50 per cent from the above. For example, one would start an elderly patient on 10 or 25 mg of an antidepressant such as amitriptyline at bedtime or even every other night. For prolonged treatment the elderly may often respond to smaller doses (10 to 75 mg). However, if after six weeks the elderly patient has not responded to doses as high as 75 mg and there are no marked side effects, doses can be slowly increased. In the normal adult without medical illness, if there is no response to 150 mg per day within six weeks, then the dosage can often be increased to as much as 200 to 300 mg (this is beyond manufacturers' guidelines). It is wise, however, to obtain the counsel of a specialist prior to using these doses. If there is still no response one could switch to another tricyclic or immediately to an MAOI. Blood level measurements are available for most of the tricyclic antidepressants, although their main usefulness is to indicate that the person is taking and absorbing the drug. Only nortriptyline has had an effective therapeutic window (50 to 140 ng per milliliter) established.

It is useful to caution patients that the antidepressants do not produce an immediate response, although if given at bedtime they may improve sleeping immediately. Also, the prominent anticholinergic side effects and hypotension are often a bother, and patients should be forewarned. Some of the supposed side effects of the medication are also accompaniments of the depressive illness, and patients, if questioned, may reveal that they have had many of the symptoms prior to taking the medication. As with any class of drugs, the physician should have knowledge of several drugs of the same class. One must recognize that the tricyclics have a quinidine-like effect and have been used to treat some cardiac arrhythmias.

For patients who fail to respond to tricyclic antidepressants, psychiatric consultation is critical. However, some have found it useful to add 0.25 μg per day of triiodothyronine (T_3) to the tricyclic dosage, particularly in female patients. Also, the addition of lithium to tricyclic regimens has been found to have a marked augmenting effect on the response to antidepressant tricyclics (neither of the above is an FDA-approved use).

The monoamine oxidase inhibitors (MAOI's) have enjoyed a return to usage recently. They had been under-utilized in the United States owing to their tendency to cause hypertensive crises following the ingestion of foods containing tyramine. However, for patients not responding to tricyclic medications or those with atypical depressions marked predominantly by anxiety symptoms, they are quite effective. Patients can be started on MAOI drugs immediately following tricyclic cessation. The reverse, however, does not hold, and patients stopping an MAOI drug must wait 7 to 14 days before starting a tricyclic antidepressant. If dietary restrictions are followed and sympathetic amine medications are avoided, MAOI's are usually safe, their major side effects being hypotension and insomnia. They have milder anticholinergic effects and often are easier to tolerate than the tricyclic antidepressants.

In older patients, in those who fail to respond to pharmacotherapeutic interventions, and in those with complicated medical conditions which the drugs might adversely affect, electroconvulsive therapy (ECT) is probably the safest treatment. Whereas 60 per cent of most affective disturbances will respond to pharmacotherapy, close to 80 per cent improve after ECT. There are few contraindications: When ECT is administered in association with modern anesthetic techniques, the morbidity is reduced to that of the anesthesia alone. With careful monitoring, even patients with recent cerebral or myocardial insults can be treated with ECT.

PROGNOSIS. Antidepressant drugs should be continued for 6 to 20 weeks after patients become free of symptoms. More prolonged treatment is desirable for those who have had recurrent episodes. Many patients have been maintained for years on tricyclic antidepressants and MAOI's without major impairment. Nevertheless, in spite of the best treatment, between 15 and 20 per cent of depressives go on to a chronic course. Most patients with a single episode will continue to function well and, in fact, often tend to use the depressive episode as a chance to reorient and reorganize their lives and proceed to function better than they had previously.

Dysthymic Disorder (Depressive Neurosis)

DEFINITION. The symptoms consist of a depressed mood of long-standing duration with a severity less intense than in a major depressive disorder. These patients often seem to have situational reasons for their illness. Many present primarily with physical complaints to physicians. Substance and drug abuse, as well as personality profiles that involve dependency and obsessional symptomatology, are often part of the clinical picture. The diagnostic criteria are outlined in Table 462–9.

EPIDEMIOLOGY. As this condition is treated in many settings, the epidemiologic distribution is difficult to determine. One estimate of prevalence is 60 per 1000. Women predominate and familial patterns have not been established.

TABLE 462–9. DYSTHYMIA*

A. At least two years (one year for children and adolescents) during which there has been depressed mood most of the day, more days than not (either by subjective account, e.g., feels "down" or "low," or is observed by others to look sad or depressed) and at least two of the following:
  1. Poor appetite or overeating
  2. Insomnia or hypersomnia
  3. Low energy or fatigue
  4. Low self-esteem
  5. Poor concentration or difficulty making decisions
  6. Pessimism
B. During that two-year period the patient is never without the above symptoms for more than two months at a time.
C. No clear evidence of a major depressive episode during the first two years of the disturbance.
D. Has never had a manic episode.
E. No psychotic symptoms and symptoms not the residual phase of schizophrenia.
F. Not sustained by a specific organic factor or substance, e.g., prolonged administration of an antihypertensive medication.

*Modified from American Psychiatric Association: Diagnostic and Statistical Manual of Mental Disorders, Third Edition. Washington, DC, APA, 1980. Used with permission.

PATHOPHYSIOLOGY. There is evidence that various personality conflicts and situational precipitants are related to these conditions more than to the other affective disorders.

TREATMENT. Many types of short-term psychotherapy have been effective in treating these conditions. Patients who respond poorly to psychotherapy often benefit from antidepressant medication.

Grief Reactions

Physicians often find it emotionally difficult to deal with the relatives of patients who have died or been seriously injured, yet such contacts provide important preventive medicine. Grief should be looked upon as a biologic process with psychologic roots. Issues of loss and attachment are extremely prominent in bereavement. In normal bereavement 50 per cent of persons experience depressed mood, sleep disturbances, and crying lasting anywhere from two to six months. Furthermore, many grief reactions resolve only slowly over a number of years. This is particularly true in older persons who have lost spouses of many years' duration.

During bereaved states general health deteriorates, and there is often an increase in serious illness. A decrease in lymphocyte responses in husbands during mourning has been described. Some persons lose contact with reality and blame themselves, constantly asking "Why did this happen?" Others even have difficulty in accepting that the person is dead. Anger and withdrawal can prevail. Some survivors, particularly when the death was violent, experience stress responses similar to those of combat veterans, who in addition to the symptoms related above may have frequent and often violent intrusive mental images.

These normal reactions can blur into a more serious state with intense and prolonged symptoms lasting six months or more. Some survivors undergo a delayed response, functioning well immediately after the event but experiencing later symptoms of bereavement, often precipitated by the death of another person or the anniversary of the death of the loved one. Others can develop hypochondriacal symptoms resembling those of the deceased. Panic attacks and depressive illness may develop also in prolonged grief reactions.

The prevention and treatment of grief reactions can often be undertaken by the physician in his normal contact with the bereaved survivor. Lindeman has outlined several valid principles: (1) Allow the patient to share his feelings about the death of the relative. The physician can be extremely helpful in discussing the normal process of grief and the reactions that people experience. (2) Review the relationships of the deceased with the important people in their lives. (3) Help grieving persons to accept their feelings and fears about things such as their ability to cope, their fears about "going crazy," anger, etc. (4) Discuss with the bereaved how they are adapting to the stress and what modes they are using to cope. (5) Attempt to formulate the future relationships between the bereaved and others in their lives. (6) Find new persons with whom the bereaved can develop relationships.

While the above matters can only be touched on in the acute situation, they often can be dealt with over time. Even the gathering of information about these areas is often seen as useful by the patient. If the condition progresses to an abnormal degree, the use of medications for the appropriate conditions, e.g., affective disturbance or panic disorder, is indicated. The use of mild sedation and hypnotics at the acute stage is also useful. Support groups have been organized to deal with both the normal and excessive processes of grieving and appear to be useful.

Suicidal Behavior

About 75 per cent of patients who actually commit suicide will have seen a physician within the previous six months. Most practicing physicians encounter half a dozen potentially suicidal patients per year, among whom 10 to 12 will actually do away with themselves over the ensuing years. The figures illustrate how important it is for the physician to detect various clues. Suicide is higher in patients with psychiatric problems, with the highest incidence occurring in those with affective disorders or alcoholism or those who are in the early post-hospital phase of schizophrenic disorders.

The typical patient who makes a suicide attempt is a white female, 20 to 40 years of age, who ingests pills, usually after an interpersonal conflict. By contrast, the typical successful suicide victim is a white male, 45 years of age or older, often separated, widowed, or divorced, who lives alone and may be unemployed or retired. Patients who commit suicide suffer a high incidence of poor physical health, medical care within the past six months, and evidence of some psychiatric disturbance. Many have a previous history of suicide attempts or threats.

Doctors often feel more awkward than their patients in discussing suicidal thoughts or intent. It must be done gently and understandingly, but almost all adult patients who are ill should be asked gently if they have had thoughts about death or suicide. Comments patients make about feeling they would be "better off dead" or "people would be better off without me" should be taken seriously. Preoccupations with funerals, cemetery lots, and the buying of weapons should make one suspicious. Any patient who presents with vague complaints should be asked about his or her emotional state. If any indication of suicidal intent is forthcoming, one must immediately evaluate its seriousness, inquiring about the following: (1) Has the person considered actual suicide? If so, what plans have been made and how specifically? The more specific, the more worrisome. (2) What other psychopathology exists? Is the patient agitated, seriously depressed, etc.? (3) What precipitating stresses exist? (4) Are there people in the environment whom the person trusts and who could help? (5) Will the person agree to work with you and contact you if his suicidal feelings intensify? (6) If no reassurance comes from the patient or relatives that the situation can be managed at home, hospitalization may be necessary.

An even more difficult evaluation is how to treat those who have made a recent unsuccessful suicide attempt. After a suicide attempt there often is a brief period of days to weeks of lightening of the depressive mood, after which strong self-destructive feelings reappear. The more lethal the risk (i.e., the higher was the potential risk of death in the initial suicide attempt), the more determined should be the effort to provide psychiatric treatment, preferably in a hospital. If patients express an explicit intent to die, often stated with determination and conviction, there is no question about the necessity for hospitalization.

Most patients after suicide attempts should have a psychiatric consultation, but sometimes this may not be possible and the nonpsychiatric physician will have to assess the suicidal potential. Part of the evaluation of the patient can also serve as the initial formation of a doctor-patient relationship. If they have a supportive environment and will keep contact, some of these patients can be managed as outpatients. Physicians should be aware of writing potentially lethal prescriptions for patients who may have suicidal tendencies. For example, for a routine dosage schedule of tricyclic antidepressants (150 mg per day), even a week's supply provides a potentially lethal overdose.

Bipolar Disorders

Bipolar disorders (previously called manic-depressive disorders) are probably the most homogeneous diagnostic grouping in psychiatry, as they consist of a marked change in mood that varies from major depressive episodes (as discussed) (see Table 462–7) to significant manic episodes as defined below. There is usually a return to normal behavior between episodes. There is little difficulty in recognizing the illness if one looks at the longitudinal course. However, if patients are examined only briefly, at a particular moment in time, manic excitement can be confused with schizophrenic psychosis. The depressive phase of bipolar illness can also be misconstrued as a catatonic state.

DIAGNOSTIC CRITERIA AND CLINICAL SIGNS AND SYMPTOMS. The manic phase of the illness is characterized by an expansive euphoric mood in which grandiose plans and ideas predominate. It is important to be aware that despite this expansiveness and grandiosity, patients who are frustrated or disagreed with can often become quite irritable and at times aggressive. The major diagnostic criteria are listed in Table 462–10. The patient can be psychotic in the manic phase, with delusions and hallucinations that are consistent with the grandiosity; however, persecutory delusions, feelings of being controlled, etc., can also be present. At times it is difficult to distinguish an excited schizophrenic patient from a manic one. As already stated, one must examine the longitudinal course of the illness, either until the occurrence of a depressive episode or a deteriorating course after remission of the acute symptom, in order to diagnose a schizophrenic process. In all instances, it is crucial to rule out organic factors.

The average age of onset of bipolar disorder is about 30 years, but about 20 per cent of patients have an onset below the age of 20. In females, the onset of the condition seems to have a bimodal distribution, with one peak falling between 20 and 30 years and the other between 40 and 50 years. The peak age of onset of schizophrenia is much younger, but the age of onset of bipolar illness overlaps enough so that the differential diagnosis of a psychotic illness in a young person is difficult and may change as the clinical picture evolves over time. Almost half the patients with bipolar disorders will have at least two to three episodes of illness, and as many as one third will experience seven or more episodes of illness once the pattern has started. Each episode of illness, whether it is a manic or a depressive phase, can last from 4 to 13 months; some of these will go on to chronicity and some will be over much sooner. The course of the illness, however, has been modified significantly with the advent of lithium therapy, especially with respect to diminishing both the severity and the frequency of the episodes. The shorter durations are usually related to the effectiveness of the treatment. While some patients will rapidly alternate between extremes over two to four days, most episodes have a longer duration and, frequently, after a manic phase there can be a subsequent

---

TABLE 462–10. MANIC EPISODE*

A. A distinct period (lasting at least one week) when mood was abnormally and persistently elevated, expansive, or irritable.
B. During the period of mood disturbance, at least three of the following symptoms have been present to a significant degree:
  1. Inflated self-esteem (grandiosity, which may be delusional)
  2. Decreased need for sleep, e.g., feels rested after only three hours of sleep
  3. More talkative than usual or pressure to keep talking
  4. Flight of ideas or subjective experience that thoughts are racing
  5. Distractibility, i.e., attention too easily drawn to unimportant or irrelevant external stimuli
  6. Increase in activity (either socially, at work, or sexually) or physical restlessness
  7. Excessive involvement in activities that have a high potential for painful consequences which is not recognized, e.g., buying sprees, sexual indiscretions, foolish business investments, reckless driving
C. The episode of mood disturbance was sufficiently severe to cause marked impairment in occupational functioning, usual social activities, or relationships with others.
D. At no time during the disturbance have there been delusions or hallucinations for as long as two weeks in the absence of prominent mood symptoms (i.e., before the mood symptoms developed or after they have remitted), which would be more indicative of schizophrenia.

*Modified from American Psychiatric Association: Diagnostic and Statistical Manual of Mental Disorders, Third Edition. Washington, DC, APA, 1980. Used with permission.

depressive phase. Chronicity, again as opposed to schizophrenia, is not a major problem with manic-depressive illness, being cited as low as 1 per cent in some studies. Mortality with bipolar illness averages between two and two and one-half times the expected rate for that age; suicide occurs in about 8 to 10 per cent.

EPIDEMIOLOGY. The lifetime risk for developing bipolar illness ranges from 0.6 to 0.9 per cent of the population. The incidence per hundred thousand per year in men is from 9 to 15 new cases and for women from 7.4 to 32 new cases. The risk increases with a family history of bipolar illness. The exact mechanism of the genetic transmission in bipolar illness is uncertain but suggests autosomal dominance with incomplete penetration. There is a 72 per cent concordance in monozygotic twins and a 19 per cent concordance in same-sex dizygotic twins. Both the course of illness and the response to treatment are similar among blood relatives. In one well-studied Amish family, the abnormal gene has been identified on chromosome 11. Other families with equally strong genetic patterns, however, have not possessed this particular chromosomal alteration.

PATHOPHYSIOLOGY. Even though the phenomena of acute mania are so different from depression, most of what is known about the pathophysiology of bipolar illness is similar to what is known about the biology of the major depressive disorders.

DIAGNOSIS AND TREATMENT. The treatment of bipolar disorders has three distinct aspects: the manic episode, the major depressive episode, and long-term maintenance therapy. Prior to any specific therapy, an adequate medical workup is necessary in order to be certain that the patient suffers from a primary affective illness. The patient in an acute manic state is delusional, grandiose, and hyperactive and in this condition looks similar to any patient with psychosis. If this is the first episode, one cannot differentiate this state phenomenologically from the first episode of schizophrenia or a psychosis due to physical illness. The major differential diagnosis of the first episode rests on a careful history, family history, and physical and laboratory examination (see Table 462–3). The past history and the nature of onset of the illness are important, as noted previously. Furthermore, most psychiatric disorders have a familial pattern. A psychiatrist should be involved in the evaluation of patients who present with their first psychotic episode.

The treatment of the acute manic phase is usually undertaken in the hospital, as it is imperative to protect the patient from his own misdeeds, e.g., spending inordinate amounts of money, making embarrassing speeches, etc. If the family is supportive, however, and feels it can control the situation, treatment can be started outside of the hospital. Lithium is not useful for the acute management of mania and if the patient is severely agitated, sedation is necessary. Neuroleptics are not used in the long-term treatment of bipolar illness, but the use of benzodiazepines, particularly lorazepam, effectively controls most acute manic states (see Table 462–4). If the agitation is marked and not controlled with medication, one should obtain psychiatric consultation to consider using ECT to control the manic excitement. Manic excitement creates a medical emergency in which patients can die from exhaustion.

While most general physicians will treat acute mania rarely, the use of lithium is something they may encounter more often. Lithium effectively prevents relapses in over 60 per cent of bipolar illnesses. The drug is slightly more effective in preventing manic relapses than the depressive episodes, and its most specific use seems to be in preventing manic recurrences. Nevertheless, its use should be considered with any repetitive affective disturbance.

Prior to the beginning of lithium therapy, a CBC, urinalysis, electrolytes, creatinine, BUN, thyroid studies, and a baseline EKG and EEG should be obtained. Chronic medical illnesses, especially renal insufficiency, can contraindicate use of the agent. Lithium has a half-life of 24 to 36 hours, and it takes at least four days to achieve a steady state. The specific therapeutic effectiveness is not evident until at least four to ten days after institution of therapy. Consequently, lithium is not a good medication for the acutely agitated or manic patient but should be started early in anticipation of maintenance use. It is necessary to monitor the serum level of lithium, adequate levels for acute illness being in the range of 0.8 to 1.4 mEq per liter. For maintenance therapy, satisfactory responses accompany blood levels of 0.4 mEq per liter. Dose and blood level, however, should be titrated against clinical effectiveness for each patient. Once maintenance levels are reached patients usually can be maintained for long periods with minimal contact. Doses usually are given twice daily, as absorption from the gastrointestinal tract is rapid and the drug peaks in the serum within one to two hours. Serum lithium levels of more than 2 mEq per liter are highly dangerous and represent a medical emergency requiring immediate hospitalization and, sometimes, hemodialysis. Of most concern with regard to side effects in the long-term use of lithium is the development of mild leukocytosis, hypothyroidism, diabetes insipidus, and, occasionally, renal tubular damage. While these long-term side effects are not trivial, they are uncommon and must be weighed against the propensity of untreated patients to be chronically hospitalized. For patients who do not respond to lithium therapy or cannot tolerate it, increasingly encouraging reports describe the effective use of carbamazepine and other anticonvulsants in treating bipolar conditions.

The depressive phase of bipolar illness is treated the same as any major depressive disorder, as outlined previously.

Patients with bipolar disorders are often reluctant to continue with their medications, particularly lithium, as they feel it inhibits them, decreases their energy, or even affects their creativity. Consequently, a good deal of discussion about these issues is pertinent for the patient and especially for the family. The enlistment and assistance of the family of the patient with bipolar disorder are important. During either acute mania or severe depressive reactions, verbal interventions are often difficult, and it is useful simply to repeat some major reassuring statements—that they are a patient, that they are going to get better, and that this is not their normal state. While the role of precipitants is not clear in the onset of bipolar illness, it is important for patients to remain in treatment, and this can often be accomplished by helping them understand what situations seem to be stressful in their lives. Family and marital counseling often is useful.

PROGNOSIS. The more episodes a patient has had, the more likely he is to have another. Nevertheless, if one takes as indices of outcome successful marital and occupational adjustment, approximately two thirds of patients will do well. About 15 per cent will have some improvement, and the remainder will do poorly. While manic or depressive episodes may cause much acute social disruption, including job loss and marital strife, the wide spacing of episodes often spares long-term social decay. Patients with bipolar disease usually function normally between episodes. Accordingly, a major goal of treatment is to protect the patient during episodes so as to minimize social disruption. Nevertheless, while the prognosis is not as devastating as in schizophrenia, it is still fraught with a significant amount of periodic and, sometimes, long-term functional disability.

Conte H, Plutchik R, Wild K, et al.: Combined psychotherapy and pharmacotherapy for depression. Arch Gen Psychiatry 43:471–480, 1986. *A good review of treatment of unipolar depression.*

Egeland JA, Gerhard DS, Pauls DL, et al.: Bipolar affective disorders linked to DNA markers on chromosome 11. Nature 325:783, 1987. *Linkage analysis places the gene predisposing to autosomal dominant manic-depressive illness on chromosome 11 in a large, closely studied Amish family of 12,000 members, all of whom stem from 30 original progenitors.*

Hodgkinson S, Sherrington R, Gurling H, et al.: Molecular genetic evidence for heterogeneity in manic depression. Nature 325:805, 1987. *Study of three large Icelandic kindreds indicates that although a single autosomal dominant allele predisposes to bipolar illness, linkage analysis does not incriminate the abnormal gene locus on chromosome 11. Genetic heterogeneity appears to underlie the expression of the manic-depressive phenotype.*

Lindeman E: Symptomatology and management of acute grief. Am J Psychiatry 101:141–148, 1944. *A classic and still useful article on the diagnosis and treatment of grief reactions.*

Litman R, Farberow N: Emergency evaluation of self-destructive potentiality. *In* Farberow N, Schneidman E. (eds.): The Cry for Help. New York, McGraw-Hill, 1961, pp 48–59. *The most useful article on the evaluation of suicide.*

Michels R (ed.): Psychiatry. Philadelphia, J.B. Lippincott Company, 1985. *Excellent and detailed overview of affective disorders, especially with respect to treatment.*

Post RM, Ballenger J: Neurobiology of Mood Disorders. Baltimore, Williams & Wilkins, 1984. *A comprehensive overview of biologic and pharmacologic aspects of affective disorders.*

Schileifer S, Keller S, Camerino M, et al.: Suppression of lymphocyte stimulation following bereavement. JAMA 250:374–377, 1983. *A good introduction to immunologic factors in affective disorder.*

Shucter S, Zisook S.: Treatment of spousal bereavement. Psychiatr Ann 16:295–308, 1986. *An excellent discussion of treatment of bereavement.*

Simons A, Murphy G, Levine J, et al.: Cognitive therapy and pharmacotherapy for depression. Arch Gen Psychiatry 43:43–50, 1986. *A study of the use of cognitive therapy in depression.*

ANXIETY DISORDERS

Anxiety is the most ubiquitous psychiatric symptom. It occurs as part of most major psychiatric syndromes, particularly depressive ones, and represents several semidistinct entities. Anxiety also accompanies at least some aspects of most normal lives, and it can be an effective stimulus to improved performance. The performance curve follows an inverted U: A little anxiety can improve performance, performance then plateaus as the anxiety increases, and eventually too much anxiety causes a decrease in the ability to function. Currently, anxiety disorders are divided into two major categories: (1) panic disorders, which are episodic, "attack-like" symptoms; and (2) generalized anxiety disorder, which is a persistent state of anxiety.

Most patients with anxiety symptoms, including those with panic disorder, will consult a general physician first. Such patients, who are extremely high users of medical services, usually complain vaguely that "something is wrong." A retrospective study of 55 patients with panic disorder referred for psychiatric consultation from primary care physicians revealed that 89 per cent initially presented with one or two somatic complaints and, in most, somatic misdiagnoses continued for months or years. The most frequent symptom patterns were (1) cardiac (chest pains, tachycardia, irregular heartbeat); (2) gastrointestinal (epigastric distress); and (3) neurologic (headache, dizziness/vertigo, syncope, or paresthesias). In a random survey of 195 patients in a primary care practice screened with structured interviews, 13 per cent met DSM-III criteria for panic disorder.

DIAGNOSTIC CRITERIA AND CLINICAL SIGNS AND SYMPTOMS. A panic attack produces a distinct symptomatic event. There is a precipitous sensation of feelings of fear, impending doom, or imminent death, accompanied by a potential host of physical symptoms (Table 462–11). Affected patients often complain of the physical symptoms in an agitated state. These circumstances differ markedly from chronic anxiety states, in which symptoms are more gradual and do not create life-threatening fears. Generalized anxiety disorder is a pervasive feeling of anxiety or "nervousness" that lacks the attack-like characteristics of panic disorder. The symptoms of generalized anxiety disorders are mainly muscle tension, autonomic hyperactivity, and apprehensive hypervigilant behavior.

A strong association links agoraphobia and panic attacks. Agoraphobia is defined as a morbid fear and avoidance of being alone or being in public places, resulting in a marked

TABLE 462–11. PANIC DISORDER*

A. At some time during the disturbance, one or more panic attacks (discrete periods of intense discomfort or fear).
B. Either four attacks within a four-week period, or one or more attacks were followed by a period of persistent fear of having another attack.
C. At least four of the following symptoms during the attacks:
   1. Shortness of breath (dyspnea) or smothering sensations
   2. Choking sensation
   3. Palpitations or accelerated heart rate (tachycardia)
   4. Chest pain or discomfort
   5. Sweating
   6. Dizziness, unsteady feelings, or faintness
   7. Nausea or abdominal distress
   8. Depersonalization or derealization
   9. Numbness or tingling sensations (paresthesias)
  10. Flushes (hot flashes) or chills
  11. Trembling or shaking
  12. Fear of dying
  13. Fear of going crazy or of doing something uncontrolled
D. An organic etiology (e.g., amphetamine or caffeine intoxication, hyperthyroidism) has been ruled out.

*Modified from American Psychiatric Association: Diagnostic and Statistical Manual of Mental Disorders, Third Edition. Washington, DC, APA, 1980. Used with permission.

restriction of travel, often to the point of becoming housebound. In many cases the agoraphobia is secondary to panic attacks: The patient restricts activities for fear of having a panic attack and thereby develops an agoraphobic profile. Consequently, one looks for the presence of panic attacks or panic attack–like symptoms in patients with agoraphobia, as they will often respond to the same treatment given for panic attacks. Simple phobias, e.g., fear of flying, heights, snakes, respond better to behavioral management than to drug treatment and are usually associated with generalized anxiety rather than panic-like episodes.

EPIDEMIOLOGY. Recent epidemiologic studies of panic disorder have noted a prevalence rate of 0.4 to 1.2 per 100. The rates are highest in persons aged 25 to 44 years and in the separated and divorced. The rates are lowest in persons over the age of 64 and bear no relationship to race or education. For agoraphobia the prevalence rates are between 2.5 and 5.8 per 100. There is a marked prevalence for women (two to four times that of men), with an age range of 18 to 64 years. The rates for generalized anxiety disorder range from 2.5 to 6.4 per 100, again slightly more common in young women. Genetic studies have shown that monozygotic twins have higher concordance for anxiety disorders than do dizygotic twins when the proband has panic disorder but not when he has a generalized anxiety disorder.

PATHOPHYSIOLOGY. Panic attacks can be precipitated in susceptible patients by sodium lactate infusions, caffeine (P.O.), CO_2 inhalation, yohimbine (P.O.), isoproterenol (I.V.), and benzodiazepine receptor antagonists. All of these agents interact with the noradrenergic system and particularly the locus ceruleus system, which contains most of the brain's noradrenergic cell bodies. Recent studies of cerebral blood flow and metabolism in patients with panic disorder show asymmetric changes in the parahippocampal region.

TREATMENT. There are two major treatments available for panic attacks, one pharmacologic, the other psychologic. The key to treatment is the establishment of a supportive relationship with the patient. Affected patients are often frightened, concerned about "going crazy" and/or dying, and somewhat ashamed of the symptoms. It is useful for the physician immediately to reassure the patient by clarifying that what he experiences is part of a well-known illness that causes these feelings. It is often useful to educate patients with appropriate reading material.

Well-controlled studies have demonstrated the effective treatment of panic attacks with tricyclic antidepressants (particularly imipramine), MAOI's (particularly phenelzine), and the benzodiazepines (particularly alprazolam). The doses and treatment pattern of the tricyclics and the monoamine oxidase inhibitors are similar to those used for affective disorders, and the dose of alprazolam is usually between 4 and 6 mg per day.* At times the beta-blocking agents will offer relief, but they are not as dramatic and effective as the antidepressants and alprazolam. The doses of the antidepressants may need to be somewhat higher for these conditions than for affective disorders (tricyclics are usually used in the range of 150 to 300 mg; the MAOI's in the range of 60 mg or more per day—both higher than manufacturers' guidelines). Pharmacologic treatment should last for six months to one year after response, with the drugs then gradually tapered. Beta-blocking agents can be useful for treating the tachycardia and palpitations associated with panic attacks. Beta blockers can also be used to decrease the cardiac symptoms associated with tricyclic use, which is often reassuring to the patient.

The treatment of generalized anxiety disorders has less clear guidelines. Although benzodiazepines and psychologic interventions are commonly emphasized, their benefit is more difficult to evaluate. Furthermore, one must be concerned and cautious about the addicting potential of the benzodiazepines and to some extent the tricyclics. Consequently, the treatment of generalized anxiety disorders should rely heavily on counseling, relaxation techniques, behavioral modification, exercise, etc., rather than on prolonged pharmacologic interventions.

Certain medical conditions can simulate panic attacks and must be excluded. These include arrhythmias, angina, respiratory illnesses, asthma, obstructive pulmonary disease, various endocrine disturbances (hyperthyroidism, pheochromocytoma), seizure disorders, vertiginous conditions, and pharmacologic stimulants and caffeine. Withdrawal syndromes can simulate panic-like states, particularly withdrawal from central nervous system depressants (e.g., barbiturates and, occasionally, benzodiazepines). Medical conditions that are often noted in patients with severe panic attacks include episodic hypertensive episodes, peptic ulcer disorder, and mitral valve prolapse.

Owing to the sequelae of the Vietnam conflict, a great deal of interest has been focused on *post-traumatic stress disorders.* The basic differentiation of post-traumatic stress disorder from generalized anxiety disorder is the presence of a clear antecedent that is recognizable as potentially causing symptoms of distress in almost anyone. Another major characteristic of post-traumatic stress disorder is the feeling of re-experiencing the trauma, through either recurring or intrusive recollections, dreams, or sudden feelings that the event is about to recur. Patients often exhibit a lack of emotional responsiveness or involvement with the world after the trauma. Other symptoms may include hyperalertness, "startle responses," sleep disturbance, guilt, and memory and concentration difficulties. Affected persons may avoid activities that could evoke recollections of the traumatic event. While medications are sometimes useful for acute symptoms (especially if accompanied by panic attacks or depressive symptoms), the major treatment of post-traumatic stress is psychotherapeutic, particularly group sessions. At times narcosynthesis has been used successfully.

PROGNOSIS IN ANXIETY DISORDERS. The ubiquity of anxiety symptoms and the blurring of panic disorder into generalized anxiety or chronic anxiety and phobic states, as well as a strong association with depressive illness, make a prognosis difficult to establish. In general, panic disorder may run a limited course with episodic patterns; long periods of remission can intervene with no symptomatology at all. Only about one quarter of patients with panic disorder are treated, implying a high incidence of spontaneous remission in cases that do not come to medical attention. Nevertheless, many patients become housebound for a significant part of their lives. Follow-up studies of 5 to 20 years' duration show that

about 50 to 60 per cent of the patients recovered or were much improved. Drug abuse and alcoholism are potentially serious complications

Katon W: Panic disorder and somatization. Am J Med 77:101–106, 1984. *An excellent overview of the relation between anxiety and somatic symptoms.*
Klerman G (ed.): Update on anxiety and panic disorders. J Clinic Psychiatry, Supplement to Vol. 47, 1986. *This whole issue is an up-to-date review of all aspects of anxiety disorders, diagnosis, treatment, and research.*
Sonnenberg S, Blank A, Talbott J: The Trauma of War. Washington DC, American Psychiatric Press, 1985. *A good review of current knowledge on post-traumatic stress disorder.*
Zales M (ed.): Stress and Health in Disease. New York, Brunner/Mazel, 1985. *Good overview of stress and medical illness.*

SOMATIZATION DISORDERS

Somatization disorders consist of psychologically engendered symptoms suggesting organ dysfunction for which associated physical or laboratory dysfunction is either absent or trivial in relation to the degree of complaint. If physicians can find no clear biologic mechanism for a set of symptoms because they are too vague, diffuse, or disparate (or even anatomically impossible) and the symptoms could fulfill some purpose in the patient's life (e.g., would help to avoid some area of responsibility, deny failure, evoke increased attention by the family or others, etc.), they should have a high index of suspicion of a purely psychologic disorder. However, these patients should not be treated lightly. Many vague symptoms arise early in organic disease, and patients must be examined carefully, supported, and followed. For example, among one group of 85 patients diagnosed as hysterical, 42 were given a diagnosis 10 years later of an organic disease that could have explained their initial symptoms. In a similar manner patients with unfounded symptoms should also be evaluated for major depression and panic disorder, as those conditions can present primarily with somatic complaints. Patients who tend to present with somatization often have histories that are characterized by disturbed interpersonal relations and emotional disruptions (Table 462–12).

Diverse disorders can present with medically unfounded somatic symptoms, including such disparate conditions as somatization disorder (Briquet's syndrome), hypochondriasis, conversion disorder (hysteria), psychogenic pain disorders, factitious disorders, and malingering. What ties these conditions together are the following characteristics: (1) symptoms that suggest a physical disorder; (2) no demonstrable clinical signs or clear physiologic mechanism evident; (3) some evidence that the symptoms may be associated with psychologic factors; (4) symptoms that do not seem to be under voluntary control (except in malingering and factitious disorder).

Somatization disorder, or Briquet's syndrome, has been studied in most detail and is a condition manifested by frequent and recurrent multiple somatic complaints, usually beginning before the age of 30.

DIAGNOSTIC CRITERIA AND CLINICAL SIGNS AND SYMPTOMS. If one looks at the diagnostic criteria for somatization disorder, the number and variety of somatic symptoms are impressive (Table 462–13). It is also evident from the range of these symptoms that patients meeting these criteria

TABLE 462–12. COMMON FEATURES IN THE HISTORIES OF PATIENTS WITH SOMATIZATION SYMPTOMS

1. Developmental histories of gross neglect, child abuse, and/or sexual abuse
2. Unstable adult relationships characterized by multiple divorces and often physical violence
3. Past family histories of alcoholism
4. A past history of alcohol abuse prior to the start of somatization
5. Past history of substance abuse
6. A positive review of systems on medical history
7. A polysurgery history
8. A history of litigious relationships with authority figures
9. Past history of psychiatric illness
10. Modeling of pain behavior in their families as ways of solving problems and coping with intimate relationships

*Exceeds manufacturer's recommended dosage.

TABLE 462–13. SOMATIZATION DISORDER*

A. Many physical complaints or a belief that he or she has been sickly, for several years beginning before the age of 30.
B. At least 13 symptoms from the following list:
   1. *Gastrointestinal symptoms*, e.g., vomiting (other than during pregnancy), abdominal pain (other than when menstruating), nausea (other than motion sickness), bloating (gassy), diarrhea, intolerance of (gets sick on) several different foods
   2. *Pain symptoms* such as pain in extremities, back pain, joint pain, pain during urination, other pain (other than headaches)
   3. *Cardiopulmonary symptoms*, e.g., shortness of breath when not exerting oneself, palpitations, chest pain, dizziness
   4. *Conversion symptoms*, e.g., amnesia, difficulty swallowing, loss of voice, deafness, double vision, blurred vision, blindness, fainting or loss of consciousness, seizure or convulsion, trouble waking, paralysis or muscle weakness, urinary retention or difficulty urinating
   5. *Psychosexual symptoms*, e.g., burning sensation in sexual organs or rectum (other than during intercourse), sexual indifference, pain during intercourse, impotence
   6. *Female reproductive symptoms*, e.g., painful menstruation, irregular menstrual periods, excessive menstrual bleeding, vomiting throughout pregnancy

*Modified from American Psychiatric Association: Diagnostic and Statistical Manual of Mental Disorders, Third Edition. Washington, DC, APA, 1980. Used with permission.

have all types of somatic symptoms, from conversion reactions to pain syndromes; it is the number of symptoms over time and their persistence that are important diagnostically. While the minor symptoms may seem common to everyone, they are reported with such vigor and intensity that the physician almost feels obligated to investigate them. This constellation of symptoms was described in 1859 by Briquet and has been confirmed over and over again, most convincingly in a series of studies by Guze in the early 1960's.

EPIDEMIOLOGY. The syndrome occurs mostly in females. About 1 per cent of the population is estimated to suffer from somatization disorder. The condition runs in families, but in males it correlates significantly with the occurrence of sociopathy and alcoholism rather than somatic symptoms.

PATHOPHYSIOLOGY. The condition is marked by an empiric collection of symptoms, the exact etiology and pathophysiology of which are not understood. Most patients come from a low education level and lack sophistication; however, there are many exceptions to this characterization. Most explanations have been sociologic and psychologic and center on the somatization as a signal of personal distress. Consequently the behavior is often interpreted as a way to obtain help from caregivers or as a mechanism of obtaining social supports and, perhaps, manipulating relationships. It has also been postulated to represent a cognitive style whereby somatic symptoms are used in place of emotional expression.

TREATMENT. These patients are difficult to treat. Perhaps the most important factor should be the attempt to rule out depressive disorders, as there is a high correlation of depressive symptomatology with many of these conditions. Patients with somatization disorders can make the physician feel that there is an urgent need to intervene; however, this temptation should be resisted. Careful evaluation of the history is extremely important for, as is evident, most of them will not respond to treatment. It is not that these patients enjoy their pain but that they are seeking other things, e.g., attention, relief from other problems. Perhaps the most important thing the physician can convey to patients is that they will neither seriously worsen nor die, and although the physician may not know the cause of the complaint he is willing to see them through the illness episode. In fact, it is almost paradoxic that by scheduling these patients for frequent regular visits the physician often not only saves time but may decrease the patient's need to develop symptoms in order to be seen. After one becomes certain of the diagnosis and of the absence of a pathologic process, the diagnostic work-up should be kept to a minimum, as the more the physician investigates the more the patient becomes convinced that something is wrong. There is a tendency to dispense medications to these patients,

and one of the complications is not only addiction but such a confusion and plethora of drugs that they become a cause of untoward symptoms. The major goal of treatment should be to keep to a minimum the medical and surgical interventions. A general attempt should be made to substitute inquiry into the patient's life as opposed to procedures. A helpful attitude on the part of the physician is that he is more interested in maintaining the relationship than in curing the symptoms and that a successful outcome is the reduction in the number of physicians the patient sees and medications prescribed.

In summary, treatment of these difficult patients should include (1) recognizing the disorder; (2) listening to the patient to determine what has been helpful or harmful in the past; (3) defining a clear contract for continued supervision with no assurances for dramatic cure (or attempts at dramatic intervention beyond what the symptoms warrant). The scheduling of visits can be based on the frequency of visits over the past two- to three-month period; (4) empathizing with patients about their suffering, avoiding statements such as "It's all in your head" or "There is nothing wrong with you"; (5) openly discussing the risks of too much medical intervention and avoiding opiates and benzodiazepines owing to their potential for abuse. Tests should be ordered on the basis of objective symptoms, not just complaints; and (6) expecting a long-term relationship with slow improvement.

PROGNOSIS. Somatization disorders are more a way of life than a discrete episodic illness. The patient maintains a propensity for expression of emotional need or distress with somatic symptoms. While the episodes may wax and wane, it is clear that these patients are wedded to the medical establishment.

Other Conditions Associated with Somatic Symptoms

Somatization disorder has been extensively studied, but there are other conditions that are similar to somatization disorder that can be confusing to the physician. Although the term *hysteria* has been dropped from official use and such conditions are now termed *conversion reactions*, such patients present commonly to physicians and make up about 1 per cent of a neurologist's practice. The predominant disturbance in conversion disorder is a loss or alteration in physical functioning suggesting a physical disorder. Often the loss or distortion of neurologic function is not fully explained by any known disease process as determined by physical and laboratory examination. Much of what has been covered with regard to somatization disorder is true of hysterical conditions. These patients do not necessarily have histrionic personalities (overly dramatic, attention seeking, shallow manipulative relationships, etc.). They do have physical complaints, but when examined closely their symptoms conform more to a psychologic than a physiologic reaction.

Hypochondriasis is often simple to recognize in that the patient presents with a belief that a disease is present for which diagnosis and treatment are necessary. The complaints are more circumscribed, with often minute examination and description of bodily functions to the physician. As the physician talks to the patient he becomes increasingly aware that the patient is more concerned about the belief of illness than the discomfort from symptoms. In fact, the symptoms are not especially distressing or painful. This is in marked contrast to the patient with chronic pain whose pain is often out of proportion to the physical findings.

In patients with chronic pain, the continuation of the pain often allows the avoidance of activities in the patient's life or the obtaining of emotional or financial support from others. Affected patients frequently have histories of addiction, seeing many physicians, and undergoing multiple surgical procedures.

The genesis of many of the above conditions lies at an involuntary level in that the symptoms and the motivation for them are not in the control of the patient. Two conditions, factitious disorder and malingering, are voluntarily controlled by the patient. These patients, often described as having *Münchausen's syndrome*, induce illnesses in themselves, e.g., fevers (by injection), dermatitis, blood disease (anemia), or seizures. Affected patients are often associated with the health professions, and one can discern no clear goal or gain from their behavior. They frequently are peripatetic, traveling from hospital to hospital. When a factitious disorder is diagnosed, these patients should be confronted openly as to their behavior and what treatment (as some may be necessary) will be provided and not provided. In true malingering, the goal of the illness behavior is often evident (or evident after extensive inquiry), and the condition is usually less a chronic than a factitious disorder. In most cases we see partial malingering, in which an individual exaggerates symptoms of a real disease or attributes a voluntarily induced disability to an accident or injury. In both these conditions there is a tendency to be angry with the patient, but it is best to confront him about the situation in a nonjudgmental rather than an angry manner. Particularly when compensation issues surround the case, treatment is pointless until any legal questions or damage awards are settled.

Katon W, Egan K, Miller D: Chronic pain: Lifetime psychiatric diagnosis and family history. Am J Psychiatry 142:1156–1160, 1985. *An interesting study of the relationship between pain syndromes and psychiatric problems.*

Lipsitt P: Medical and psychologic characteristics of "crocks." Psychiatry Med 1:15–25, 1970. *Still one of the best discussions of the management of patients with many somatic complaints.*

Marsden CD: Hysteria—A neurologist's view. Psychol Med 16:277–288, 1986. *An excellent review of hysteria.*

Quill T: Somatization disorder. JAMA 254:3075–3079, 1985. *A good discussion of the physician's role in the treatment of patients with somatic disorder.*

Ries R, Balcon J, Katon W: The medical abuser: Differential diagnosis and management. J Fam Pract 3:257–265, 1981. *Good differential diagnosis of somatic complaints.*

Slater E, Glithero E: A followup of patients diagnosed as suffering from "hysteria." J Psychosomatic Res 9:9–13, 1965. *A classic article discussing the potential hazards in the diagnosis of hysteria.*

SECTION THREE / PATHOPHYSIOLOGY AND MANAGEMENT OF MAJOR NEUROLOGIC SYMPTOMS

463 AUTONOMIC DISORDERS AND THEIR MANAGEMENT

Fred Plum

THE NONENDOCRINE HYPOTHALAMUS

To survive in a constantly changing, often threatening environment, humans must continuously and automatically adjust the activity of both their internal organs and their outward behavior. The task of maintaining a stable internal environment falls largely on the endocrine and the autonomic nervous systems. The hypothalamus (HT) serves as an integrating command center for both. Chapters 222, 226, 228, and 243 discuss additional aspects of neuroendocrine regulation.

The tightly packed, interwoven contents of the hypothalamus make it difficult or impossible to assign specific signs and symptoms to any but a few local areas (Table 463–1). Ventromedial and posteriorly located lesions tend to produce greater functional abnormalities than those located elsewhere, because their position inevitably interrupts fibers leading to the endocrine and descending autonomic nervous systems, respectively. Except in unusual cases when they affect unilateral descending sympathetic projections, clinically detectable changes in autonomic function due to HT disorders always imply the presence of bilateral lesions. Table 463–2 lists the principal diseases that attack the structure.

COGNITIVE AND BEHAVIORAL ABNORMALITIES. Severe retrograde and anterograde memory loss and even a chronic delirium can accompany ventromedial hypothalamic destruction in man. Outbursts of fear and rage sometimes accompany lesions in this region, whereas lateral-posterior damage tends to be associated with apathetic hypoactivity.

Disorders of specific neurotransmitter systems have not, as yet, been linked successfully to these functional changes. Loss of libido in the male frequently accompanies structural HT disease but usually reflects associated gonadotropic or autonomic deficiency.

DISTURBANCES OF SLEEP AND AROUSAL. In animals, stimulation of the anterior HT produces behavioral sleep, whereas destruction of that area results in chronic insomnia. Limited evidence suggests that similar effects apply in humans. Selective anterior HT destruction in man is too uncommon to permit conclusions, but posterior hypothalamic destruction or inflammation frequently produces sleep disorders, including hypersomnolence or circadian reversals of sleep pattern. Chronic, sleeplike stupor or coma lasting longer than three to four weeks are pathognomonic for damage or dysfunction in the posterior hypothalamus.

HEAT REGULATION. The preoptic anterior HT contains separate receptors for warmth and cold as well as for pyrogens. Diurnal changes in central excitability and in the level of circulating ovarian hormones provide additional nonspecific stimuli. In turn, the HT activates varying combinations of behavioral, autonomic, and endocrine responses that conserve or dissipate body heat. Diseases in the region can be responsible for hypothermia or, rarely, hyperthermia.

Hypothermia. RELATIVE POIKILOTHERMIA. Poikilothermia, defined as a fluctuation in body temperature of greater than 2° C with changes in ambient temperature, is the most common central abnormality of heat regulation in man. Most such cases are detected by a lowered body temperature. Severe poikilothermia results from damage to the posterior HT and rostral mesencephalon. Damage to this area impairs not only autonomic heat-regulating pathways but those that control the sense of thermal discomfort and the behavioral regulation of body temperature as well. As a result, many patients with poikilothermia are unaware of their condition and do little to avoid it. At ordinary ambient temperatures of 20 to 25° C, the

TABLE 463–1. REGIONAL SYNDROMES OF THE HYPOTHALAMUS*

	Preoptic Anterior Hypothalamus	Tuberal and Ventromedian Hypothalamus	Posterior Hypothalamus
Integrates	Endocrine, thermal, parasympathetic autonomic	Cognition; endocrine; sympathetic autonomic caloric balance; fluid balance	Consciousness; cognition; complex endocrine; autonomic; thermal
Contains	Sleep-inducing mechanism; forebrain parasympathetic paths; thermal sensing areas	Final common endocrine paths	Reticular activating system; regulatory and outflow autonomic effectors
Acute lesions	Insomnia; hyperthermia; diabetes insipidus; inappropriate ADH	Hyperthermia; diabetes insipidus; hypothalamic-endocrine disorders	Hypersomnia; poikilothermia; autonomic storm
Chronic lesions	Insomnia; complex endocrine changes (e.g., precocious puberty); endocrinotropic abnormalities; hypothermia; hypodipsia	Medial: memory loss; emotional disorders; hyperphagia and obesity; endocrinotropic abnormalities Lateral: emotional disorders; emaciation	Memory loss; apathy; hypersomnia; poikilothermia; autonomic incoordination; complex endocrine disorders (e.g., precocious puberty)

*As indicated in the text, functional localization is more precise for some activities than for others.

degree of hypothermia tends to be proportional to the degree of functional hypothalamic impairment. Relative poikilothermia resulting from impaired hypothalamic-autonomic function frequently affects elderly persons (*senile hypothermia*), making them dangerously susceptible to lowered environmental temperatures. Chronic poikilothermia also accompanies several degenerative disorders that affect the HT in children and adults. Poikilothermia regularly follows extensive damage to the posterior HT or midbrain by stroke, trauma, neoplasm, encephalitis, or thiamine deficiency. Such central hypothermia must be differentiated from that caused by metabolic disorders such as acute or chronic sedative drug ingestion, hypoglycemia, and myxedema.

PAROXYSMAL HYPOTHERMIA. Sustained hypothermia (as opposed to relative poikilothermia) is rare in humans. Less uncommon is paroxysmal hypothermia consisting of attacks of lowered body temperature that vary widely in frequency from daily to more than a decade apart. Such attacks usually begin abruptly, last from minutes to days, and are characterized by sweating, flushing of the skin, and a fall in body temperature, usually to 32° C or lower. Fatigue, decreased mental responsiveness, hypoventilation, hypotension, cardiac arrhythmias, ataxia, lacrimation, and asterixis may accompany the temperature drop. The attacks subside either slowly (hours to days) or rapidly with shivering and peripheral vasoconstriction. During hypothermia, mechanisms for both heat production and heat dissipation respond normally, but around a lower temperature set-point. Most affected patients have had direct evidence for hypothalamic disease; several have suffered from congenital agenesis of the corpus callosum. In some instances anticonvulsant therapy stops the attacks.

Hyperthermia. Chronic fever never results from HT disease, and even acute neurogenic fever is rare. The most frequent causes of acute neurogenic hyperthermia include gross head injury, surgical trauma or spontaneous bleeding into the region of the anterior hypothalamus, and hemorrhage in the adjacent meninges or the third ventricle. With neurogenic hyperthermia, the body temperature can rise to potentially fatal levels of 42° C or higher as a result of active heat production unbalanced by heat dissipation. The cardiovascular changes that normally accompany fever are disproportionately lacking. If standard cooling measures fail, small (2 mg) doses of morphine can ameliorate dangerously high neurogenic fevers.

TABLE 463–2. PRINCIPAL CAUSES OF INTRINSIC HYPOTHALAMIC DISEASES IN ADOLESCENTS AND ADULTS

Congenital midline brain defects (e.g., agenesis of corpus callosum)
Stroke: basilar artery occlusion, subarachnoid hemorrhage
Tumors: craniopharyngioma, glioma, hamartoma, dysgerminoma, dermoid, lipoma, lymphoma or leukemia, meningioma
Trauma
Encephalitis
Granulomas: sarcoid, tuberculosis, histiocytosis X
Wernicke's polioencephalopathy (thiamine deficiency)
Progressive idiopathic degeneration (rare, childhood)

DISORDERS OF FEEDING BEHAVIOR AND CALORIC BALANCE. Psychologic influences of complex origins provide the major influences on feeding behavior in man; primary hypothalamic error accounts for no more than a tiny fraction of human obesity or emaciation, making it all the more important to recognize when it occurs.

In experimental animals, stimulation of the ventromedian region of the HT inhibits feeding, whereas lesions destroying this region produce hyperphagia and a weight gain that later stabilizes at a new elevated set-point. Evidence suggests that the changes are mediated by autonomic influences on the digestive tract and on insulin secretion to enhance appetite. Conversely, stimulation of the lateral hypothalamus induces feeding in excess of caloric requirement, whereas damage to this region results in a temporarily severe aphagia that slowly recovers to maintain a chronically lowered body weight. Both hyperphagia and hypophagia due to HT dysfunction occasionally can be observed in man.

Hypothalamic Obesity. Most patients with hypothalamic obesity have diffuse or large lesions of the structure. A few, however, have suffered from precisely placed abnormalities damaging the ventromedian HT. Examples include leukemic infiltration as well as discrete tumors in this area. Affected patients have experienced remarkable combinations of food-seeking behavior, including ravenous hyperphagia, decreased motor activity, and sometimes enormous obesity.

The hypothalamus integrates a set-point that roughly regulates the individual's body weight. Whether or not hyperphagia continues or disappears in patients who develop hypothalamic obesity depends upon whether (a) the neurologic abnormality is fixed and (b) the new disease-related set-point for weight has been reached. Patients with obesity following surgical procedures or severe closed head trauma that affects the hypothalamus illustrate this principle. Characteristically, such persons eat ravenously and gain weight quickly following the injury until they reach their new set-point, at which point they become normophagic and stabilize at a new, higher weight.

Emaciation sometimes accompanies hypothalamic disease in man, but the associated lesions usually have been large and their specificity uncertain. Efforts to link hypothalamic disease and anorexia nervosa have been unsuccessful.

WATER BALANCE. The HT controls body water content and osmolality via coordinated mechanisms regulating affective thirst, drinking behavior, and the release of vasopressin (ADH) via the paraventricular (PV) and supraoptic (SO) nuclei. Hypothalamic or limbic system disease can produce four principal disorders of water balance, including ADH deficiency (diabetes insipidus), inappropriate ADH secretion, neurogenic (essential) hypernatremia, and episodic hyperdipsia. Chapters 77 and 227 discuss much of the pathophysiology of these disorders. Important from the neural standpoint is to understand that the brain's osmoreceptors and volume receptors appear to reside in different areas of the HT. Osmoreceptors and central thirst receptors have been identified within the preoptic region. These respond to afferent stimulation from peripheral thirst receptors as well as to local sodium concentrations and circulating levels of the peptide angiotensin. Volume receptors appear to lie more laterally in the HT and project to the PV and SO nuclei by pathways different from those that carry osmoreceptor signals. Peripherally, thirst is stimulated or quenched by signals arising from receptors lying within the mouth and interstitial fluids, while different receptors arising from heart, large capacitance systemic veins, and carotid baroreceptors signal volume control needs. Differential peripheral stimulation of the two systems or selective damage to the central osmoreceptor-thirst area explains some examples of inappropriate ADH secretion and most if not all cases of neurogenic (essential) hypernatremia.

Neurogenic (Essential) Hypernatremia. This disorder is marked by four features: (1) elevated serum sodium unaccompanied by circulating volume deficiency, (2) a preserved renal tubular responsiveness to ADH, (3) in most but not all instances, an inadequate secretion of ADH in response to osmotic stimuli, and (4) the absence or deficiency of appropriate thirst (hypodipsia) despite otherwise relatively normal conscious behavior. True essential hypernatremia is rare; most cases of serum hyperosmolarity accompanying intracranial disease result from a nonspecific combination of dehydration and impaired drinking behavior due to stupor or organic hypodipsia.

Essential hypernatremia in its milder and more chronic forms often elevates the serum sodium only modestly, and such patients characteristically lack symptoms except for a remarkable lack of thirst. Close attention often discloses considerable fluctuation in daily serum sodium values above the 150 mmol per liter mark. When sodium levels climb to the 160 to 170 mmol per liter range, affected patients develop weakness and sometimes fever as well as muscle tenderness and cramping that may progress to fatigue, ataxia, and even myoglobinuria. Mental symptoms include lethargy, anorexia, depression, and irritability. With elevations of serum sodium above 180 mmol per liter, most patients become confused or stuporous, and some will die. Patients with essential hypernatremia fail to experience thirst, but many retain persistent habitual drinking, although at a volume insufficient to maintain a normal serum osmolality. They commonly lack clinical evidence of dehydration; only mild hypovolemia or even normovolemia can accompany serum sodium levels of 200 mmol per liter or more. An associated hypokalemia usually contributes to the muscular symptoms. Urine volumes may be low or normal but are always more dilute than appropriate for the serum hyperosmolality. The administration of arginine vasopressin induces a more concentrated urine. Either an acute water load or a hypertonic saline load, however, can produce an increase in free water clearance, reflecting the failure of central osmoreceptors to respond to the latter stimulus.

The hypothalamic defect that produces essential hypernatremia is inexactly localized. Almost all affected patients have had associated neurologic or endocrine abnormalities, but many have lacked radiographic evidence of central nervous system abnormalities. Some give a history of diffuse head trauma, while in others space-occupying lesions destroy the entire hypothalamic region by the time of death. In a few patients, restricted tumors have involved the preoptic and tuberal region. The mechanisms of essential hypernatremia remain unsettled. The absence of thirst is critical. Direct measurements showing that in many cases serum vasopressin levels fail to increase when sodium levels rise but fall when blood volume increases, indicates either that osmoreceptor function is selectively uncoupled from the behavioral and hormonal control of water balance or that mechanisms that regulate natriuresis are distinct from ADH control.

Treatment consists of lowering the serum sodium and raising the potassium by manipulating the diet and conditioning the patient automatically to drink several liters of water each day regardless of thirst. Spironolactone, chlorpropamide, and the thiazide diuretics may help to achieve fluid balance. Treatment of hypernatremic crises must be initiated slowly: symptoms of water intoxication can develop if serum sodium is reduced by more than 20 mmol per liter per day.

Hyperdipsia and Self-induced Water Intoxication. Excessive water drinking in the absence of either hypovolemia or serum hyperosmolality is termed primary hyperdipsia and must be differentiated from the compensatory hyperdipsias of conditions such as diabetes insipidus, diabetes mellitus, or polyuric renal failure. In the absence of inappropriate ADH secretion, symptoms of severe hyperdipsia, i.e., hypervolemia, hyponatremia, and clinical water intoxication accompanied by stupor, delirium, and convulsions, are infrequent. The problem never arises, to our knowledge, as the result of primary central nervous system disease. Most severe hyperdipsia occurs in persons with acute psychiatric disorders who drink excessively to overcome delusional fears. Occasionally, acute water intoxication occurs in alcoholics with gastritis or in youngsters drinking huge amounts of fluids on a dare, e.g., during ritual hazing or tea-party games.

DISORDERS OF PERIPHERAL AND CENTRAL AUTONOMIC FUNCTION

Centripetal parasympathetic influences emanate largely from the anterior HT, whereas sympathetic descending pathways take their origin mainly in the posterolateral reticulum of the structure. Work of recent years has shown that peripheral as well as central autonomic pathways cosecrete neuropeptides as well as classic neurotransmitters at their synapses. The functional and dysfunctional role of these newly discovered agents remains to be clarified. Autonomic control extends to almost every organ of the body and symptoms resulting from perturbations in these regulatory systems probably take more American patients to doctors than all other conditions combined. The large number of autonomic drugs annually prescribed for functional cardiovascular, gastrointestinal, pulmonary, and genitourinary disorders affirms this premise.

Most *psychosomatic disorders* produce their symptoms at least partly and often predominantly through the limbic-autonomic system. As John Hunter said of his angina pectoris, "My life is in the hands of any rascal who chooses to annoy and tease me." (He subsequently died during an argument at a hospital board meeting.) Autonomic influences act in subtle ways, and abnormal responses to life stress are often highly individual matters, not easy to separate from the nervous system's routine adjustments to living. Clinical sensitivity to the possibility that the brain rather than the target organ sometimes

TABLE 463–3. PRINCIPAL DISORDERS OF THE AUTONOMIC NERVOUS SYSTEM

Central Nervous System
Primary, selective autonomic failure (e.g., Shy-Drager)
Associated with other disorders (e.g., multisystem atrophy, parkinsonism, olivopontocerebellar atrophy, etc.)
Thiamine deficiency (e.g., Wernicke's encephalopathy)
Syringomyelia-syringobulbia

Peripheral Nervous System
Primary or predominantly autonomic failure
    Selective autonomic neuropathy (rare)
    Familial dysautonomia (Riley-Day)
    Familial amyloid disease
Disorders with prominent, generalized autonomic components
    Acute inflammatory neuropathy
    Diabetic neuropathy
    Syphilis (tabes)
    Alcoholic-nutritional neuropathy
    Lambert-Eaton myasthenic syndrome
Focal disorders with autonomic components
    Causalgia
    Shoulder-hand syndrome
    Sudeck's atrophy
    Primary hyperhidrosis

causes the symptoms represents perhaps the most important first step in detecting pathologic autonomic adjustments to life stress.

Diffuse, moderate sympathetic-parasympathetic dysfunction can accompany occasional cases of otherwise typical parkinsonism and is seen as a component to several of the late-life cerebellar or olivopontocerebellar degenerative disorders. Similarly, many elderly patients gradually lose the briskness of their autonomic reflexes and suffer an insidious decline in orthostatic circulatory control, sexual function, heat regulation, urinary and rectal sphincter continence, and bowel motility, all of which must be treated symptomatically. More severe diffuse autonomic dysfunction occurs in two major forms: one accompanying chronic or acute disease of the peripheral nerves; the other consisting of a progressive, central autonomic degeneration, arising either alone or accompanied by degeneration of corticospinal, extrapyramidal, or cerebellar pathways. Table 463–3 lists the principal causes of autonomic disorders.

Peripheral Autonomic Insufficiency

Involvement of autonomic fibers is prominent in several axonal diseases and peripheral neuropathies, including, especially, acute poliomyelitis, acute inflammatory neuropathy, diabetic neuropathy, tabes dorsalis, and poisoning with the toxic chemical acrylamide. Autonomic impairment with predominantly sympathetic dysfunction accompanies the peripheral neuropathy of inherited amyloid disease.

A small number of patients have been recorded as suffering from a variably complete degree of acutely or subacutely developing failure of peripheral sympathetic and parasympathetic function without accompanying somatomotor or sensory changes (*acute pandysautonomia*). Most but not all cases have been in children. Recovery has been the rule, and the disorder generally is regarded as a selective variant of idiopathic inflammatory neuropathy, a condition in which more restricted autonomic signs and symptoms in the form of tachycardia, hypertension, sweating impairment, and gastrointestinal atony commonly accompany the more prominent motor and sensory changes. Similarly restricted adrenergic abnormalities also accompany the motor polyneuropathy of acute intermittent porphyria. The treatment in all instances is symptomatic.

FAMILIAL DYSAUTONOMIA. This disorder, also called Riley-Day syndrome, is a rare autosomal recessive disorder that predominantly affects Ashkenazi Jewish children and is characterized by several developmental defects, prominently including abnormalities in peripheral and, probably, central adrenergic and cholinergic neurotransmission.

Idiopathic Autonomic Insufficiency (Idiopathic Orthostatic Hypotension, Shy-Drager Syndrome)

This is a rare degenerative disorder of unknown etiology that strikes during middle age, causing progressive autonomic dysfunction; severe debility or death may occur within 5 to 15 years of onset. Associated cerebellar or, especially, extrapyramidal abnormalities sometimes play a prominent role.

Pathogenesis and Pathology. Histologic examination at autopsy has disclosed various changes, ranging from the severe to the barely detectable. Degenerative morphologic and neurochemical abnormalities may affect autonomic ganglia in the periphery, the preganglionic intermediolateral cell column in the spinal cord or autonomic centers in the hypothalamus, nigrostriatal system, pontine nuclei, and globus pallidus. The pathogenesis of the disease is unknown. The degree of clinical overlap is consistent with the existence of a broad continuum rather than distinct entities. Even at postmortem, the extent of neurologic abnormalities varies widely from selected degeneration of autonomic systems alone to varying degrees of extrapyramidal and cerebellar system damage.

Clinical Manifestations. The disorder begins mainly between the ages of 40 and 60 years, more often in men. Symptoms of autonomic dysfunction predominate early in the course. Characteristically, initial difficulties consist of sexual impotence; urinary hesitancy, urgency, or incontinence; and/or anhidrosis. These early symptoms are frequently unrecognized and their cause misdiagnosed. Within months to years, the hallmark of the disorder, postural hypotension, appears. This may be manifested as dizziness, giddiness, or frank syncope upon standing. Less frequently, patients complain of generalized weakness, cervico-occipital discomfort, or leg weakness upon standing. Attendant autonomic symptoms include intermittent diplopia, dysphagia, and diarrhea, fecal incontinence, or constipation. A parkinsonian disorder, consisting of bradykinesia, coarse tremor, and rigidity, is common, and tends to progress inexorably. Myoclonus, gait disturbance, and signs of olivopontocerebellar dysfunction may also occur.

Physical signs of autonomic dysfunction parallel the aforementioned symptoms. Orthostatic hypotension, a greater than 30/20 mm Hg fall in blood pressure upon assumption of the erect position, constitutes the fundamental sign. Other signs include absence of sinus arrhythmia and absence of the normal overshoot in diastolic pressure during phase IV of the Valsalva maneuver. There may be Horner's syndrome, in parasympathetic pupillary changes, or as anhidrosis even with elevated ambient temperature. Muscle wasting, fasciculation, and extensor plantar responses occasionally have been observed.

A variety of clinical laboratory tests can be employed to evaluate autonomic function, and only the simplest will be delineated here. *Miosis* in response to ocular administration of dilute solutions of methacholine, or *mydriasis* after instillation of dilute epinephrine, suggest, respectively, parasympathetic or sympathetic denervation supersensitivity. On the other hand, absence of mydriasis after ocular instillation of cocaine or hydroxyamphetamine suggests that endogenous norepinephrine stores are defective. Absence of sweating with elevation of the ambient temperature and absence of the axon reflex after intradermal histamine suggest peripheral autonomic denervation. An abnormally accentuated blood pressure response to the intravenous infusion of norepinephrine is consistent with widespread denervation supersensitivity.

Differential Diagnosis. Orthostatic hypotension itself may accompany intravascular hypovolemia (as with massive hemorrhage or adrenal insufficiency), vasodepressor syncope, acute cardiac failure from a variety of causes, familial hyperbradykininism, and intracranial posterior fossa mass or vascular lesions. In these conditions other signs of autonomic dysfunction are absent. Autonomic insufficiency, including orthostatic hypotension, also may occur with any disease that alters peripheral or central autonomic pathways. Many disorders conform to this description. A variety of peripheral neuropathies may be accompanied by dysautonomia, including the acute Guillain-Barré syndrome; the chronic neuropathies of diabetes mellitus, amyloidosis. Wernicke's disease, and porphyria; and the congenital Riley-Day syndrome. Ganglion dysfunction may result from ingestion of ganglioplegic drugs. Tabes dorsalis is commonly accompanied by autonomic signs. Autonomic dysfunction may result from interruption of descending pathways in the spinal cord, as observed with syringomyelia, trauma, or spinal tumor. Pontine hemorrhage can interrupt descending sympathetic pathways in the brain stem, thereby causing sympathetic dysfunction. Differentiation from these diseases is readily accomplished by suitable history, examination, and laboratory tests.

Course and Treatment. Although treatment does not alter the underlying pathologic process, it may allow an otherwise symptomatic semi-invalid to lead a considerably improved life. Orthostatic hypotension may be treated with a variety of measures, dictated by the severity of the problem. The head of the bed should be raised during recumbency, including sleep. Antigravity Jobst stockings minimize pooling of blood in the lower extremities upon standing. In moderately severe cases, intravascular volume expansion may be achieved by using the mineralocorticoid desoxycorticosterone acetate or 9-α-fluorocortisone plus sodium chloride, with potassium supplementation. In severe cases, oral sympathomimetic agents, including ephedrine or hydroxyamphetamine sometimes help. Indomethacin may be effective in selected patients for the treatment of orthostatic hypotension. Inadvertent ingestion of microgram quantities of vasoactive amines in the diet may result in alarming elevation of blood pressure in patients being treated with monoamine oxidase inhibitors for widespread sympathetic denervation. Although the diet may be rigorously regulated in the hospital setting, this is rarely possible on an outpatient basis. For example, such foods as cheese, broad beans, Chianti wine, raisins, bananas, and aged or smoked meat contain significant quantities of vasoactive amines.

Parkinsonian signs and symptoms may be successfully treated with L-dopa and the customary anticholinergic agents.

ABNORMALITIES OF SWEATING. *Primary anhidrosis*, a relatively uncommon complaint, occurs as part of a rare, probably autosomal recessive disorder in which it is associated with congenital insensitivity to pain. Anhidrosis due to congenital absence of the sweat glands is similarly rare. *Secondary anhidrosis* also follows pre- or postganglionic sympathetic denervation produced by disease or surgical procedures and can occur in the appropriate territorial distribution of any diseased or damaged peripheral nerve.

Hyperhidrosis, defined as sweating in excess of apparent thermal requirements, is a common response to anxiety, especially among persons less than 30 years old. Longstanding severe hyperhidrosis causing constantly dripping hands and feet is an uncommon but socially troublesome disorder of unknown cause. Emotional factors seem to contribute little. Severe cases can be relieved by sympathectomy directed at the upper extremities. The procedure is best limited to either the upper or lower extremities, since compensatory accentuation of pre-existing sweating tends to affect nondenervated parts. Total sympathectomy produces too many undesirable side effects to be recommended. Focal hyperhidrosis localized to a particular body part occasionally occurs in association with irritation of the related preganglionic fibers or ganglia by an infection or neoplasm and deserves careful attention from that standpoint.

Urinary Bladder Control

Abnormalities in micturition arise from four principal causes: local disease in the bladder and urethra, neurologic disorders, drug effects, and psychologic perturbation. Table 463–4 outlines a differential diagnosis of these conditions based on the predominant symptoms, while the following paragraphs briefly discuss neurogenic mechanisms.

The bladder is a hollow pelvic structure composed of the interlacing smooth muscle fibers of the detrusor covered by its internal mucous membrane and outer serosa. The bladder is smooth muscle and its resistance to stretch is determined predominantly by the viscoelastic properties of its wall rather than by direct neurogenic mechanisms. With progressive filling, the normal intravesical pressure rises slowly, remaining below about 15 cm of water until average capacities are reached, between 250 and 450 ml, at which point the intravesical pressure rises either abruptly, owing to the onset of the micturition reflex, or more gradually, owing to reaching the elastic limits of the wall itself. Normal adult micturition volumes average between 200 and 400 ml, but with acute urinary retention the structure can stretch abnormally to accommodate one or more liters, while chronic infection and hypertrophy may contract it to a capacity of no more than 60 to 100 ml.

Urine enters the bladder from the paired ureters and normally leaves via the membranous urethra. In both sexes the lower detrusor musculature joins with elastic tissue to form an involuntary internal

TABLE 463–4. SYMPTOMS OF URINARY DIFFICULTY

Painful Urination
  Cystourethral inflammation (Ch. 86)
  Urethral stricture
  Psychogenic

Increased Frequency-Urgency
  Increased fluid intake of any cause (e.g., diabetes, alcoholism)
  Cystourethral inflammation
  Psychogenic
  Partial outlet obstruction (e.g., prostatic hypertrophy)
  Neurogenic
    Damage to prefrontal or spinal inhibitory pathways
    Spinal reflex facilitation

Incontinence
  Stress: Small volumes, event-related, women more than men
    Normal in 50 per cent of giggling girls
    Multiparas with cystocele, other outflow damage
    Increases with normal aging
  Retention-overflow: Dribbling or small volumes, pain in pelvis or flanks, palpable bladder
    Causes as listed with retention, below
  Confusional: Small or large volumes, usually shameless
  "Spastic": Variate volumes, sporadic occurrence, prominent urgency, emptying complete
    Prefrontal lesions
    Extramedullary advanced spinal compression
    Occasionally partial outlet obstruction
    Severe cystitis (small bladder volume)
    Circumstance: bedridden or crippled elderly with facilities remote
  Intraspinal Lesions: Moderate volumes, brief urgency, frequent occurrence, high residual urine
    Intramedullary cervical-thoracic-lumbar lesions (multiple sclerosis, neoplasms, etc.)
    Occasionally with partial peripheral denervation

Retention
  Acute or chronic outflow obstruction
  Acute neurologic disease
    Peripheral: Autonomic polyneuropathy, pelvic trauma, cauda equina compression, conus lesions
    Central: Poliomyelitis, spinal transection
  Drugs (usually plus local structural problems)
    Anticholinergics, antidepressants, opiates
  Psychogenic
  Postanesthetic

sphincter that normally can resist passively induced intra-abdominal–intravesical pressures as high as 150 mm Hg. The more distal urethra is encircled by voluntarily controlled striated muscle innervated by the somatomotor pudendal nerve. More competent in men than in women, this external sphincter can withstand briefly the intraurethral detrusor-induced pressure of normal micturition but is unnecessary to normal urinary continence.

The act of voiding represents a stretch-induced parasympathetic reflex of smooth muscle facilitated by brainstem and spinal mechanisms. The latter normally are inhibited or released by forebrain regulatory influences. The actual neuromuscular sequence consists of an initial voluntary relaxation of the skeletal muscle of the pelvic floor followed by the disinhibited autonomic reflex discharge, which contracts the detrusor, assimilates and relaxes the musculoelastic tissue of the internal sphincter, and empties the organ by a fusion of successive detrusor contractions.

The complete reflex mechanism for micturition exists within the spinal cord. The afferent route of the arc depends upon fibers that originate in stretch receptors in the bladder wall and travel centrally via sacral roots 2 to 4. Efferent preganglionic fibers arise in the lateral columns of the sacral segments of the conus medullaris, whence they travel in the cauda equina to and through the lower sacral foramina to synapse with their final ganglia over the outer surface of the bladder and the region of the proximal urethra. Centrally, afferent proprioceptive signals travel rostrally via the lemniscal system while descending inhibitory influences originate in the paramedian prefrontal cerebral cortex. These latter pathways are joined in the brain stem and upper spinal cord by reflex-facilitating fibers that enhance complete reflex bladder emptying. The pathway descends in the spinal cord within the lateral funiculus to synapse upon the sacral preganglionic neurons.

CEREBRAL DISTURBANCES IN MICTURITION. Damage to the bilateral prefrontal area lowers the micturition reflex threshold, resulting in a proportionately smaller bladder capacity. The chief symptoms are sudden, sometimes uncontrollable urgency with moderately large volumes, usually of less than 250 ml, but complete bladder emptying. The cystometrogram shows a normal bladder pressure-volume filling curve but a reduced micturition reflex threshold, with a comparably reduced threshold to filling sensation. Clinical evaluation or CT scanning of the head readily discloses evidence of structural frontal lobe disease.

Dementia leads to an incontinence of indifference (a loss of bladder training) in which visceral physiology remains intact but social restraints depart. Patients with severe physical disabilities such as hemiplegia, advanced arthritis, etc., may develop *pseudoincontinence* due to difficulty in reaching the toilet or, occasionally, as a depressed, angry, and frustrated response to the limitations of their condition.

SPINAL DISTURBANCES OF MICTURITION. Gradual *extramedullary* spinal cord compression produces few changes in bladder function until late in the course when the reflex is facilitated along with somatic motor reflex pathways. Urgency with moderately reduced voiding volumes results. Incontinence occurs only with advanced or sudden cord compression. *Intramedullary* spinal lesions can directly affect the descending parasympathetic pathways, releasing the reflex from higher inhibition and impairing pathways originating in the brain stem that facilitate complete detrusor emptying. The reflex threshold drops, and urgency-frequency with moderate volumes results, often leaving a high postvoiding residual volume. Sporadic reflex incontinence is common.

Acute spinal transection produces reflex inhibition in the distal segment ("spinal shock"), with loss of voiding reflexes as well as of somatomotor ones. Acute retention develops, stretching the smooth muscle wall and producing a flat pressure-volume curve with no reflex. Overflow dribbling incontinence ensues. Reflex recovery is marked by increasingly large, randomly spaced, reflex partial bladder emptyings that in many instances can be trained by skill and patience into complete self-stimulated reflex voidings.

PERIPHERAL (PREGANGLIONIC OR SOMATIC AFFERENT) DEFECTS IN VOIDING. These can result from disease of either efferent or afferent peripheral nerves (e.g., occasional inflammatory neuropathy, diabetic neuropathy, tabes dorsalis, pelvic carcinoma), of the cauda equina, or of the conus medullaris. Depending upon the rate of neuritic progression, the bladder gradually dilates, with sensations of fullness disappearing commensurately with the degree of mechanical stretching. Normal sensations of urgency disappear, and the reflex progressively loses its effectiveness. Residual urine volumes increase. Ultimately, moderate to severe retention occurs, with or without spontaneous dribbling or occasionally spurting, small-volume overflow incontinence. In the absence of cystitis, the cystometrogram shows a flat filling curve on which, in time, autonomous ganglion-induced local detrusor contractions increasingly become superimposed. Spontaneous parasympathetic activity eventually leads to nearly continuous autonomous local detrusor activity, producing a hypertrophied bladder wall with a decreased bladder capacity and a steep pressure-volume curve.

TREATMENT OF NEUROGENIC BLADDER DIFFICULTIES. This varies according to the anatomic distribution of the cause. Urinary tract infections intensify all neurogenic functional abnormalities and should be treated promptly and effectively. Urgency or urgency-incontinence due to cerebral lesions or spinal extramedullary compression sometimes is aided by antispasticity drugs such as baclofen or parasympathetic blocking agents such as oxybutynin chloride 5 mg bid or tid. Often such symptoms are relatively minor and can be treated by addressing the neurologic abnormality and forcing fluids in an attempt to stretch the bladder wall so as to raise the threshold for the voiding reflex. Urgency-retention-incontinence due to intramedullary spinal lesions can be difficult to manage, especially when a high residual urine volume leads to recurrent urinary tract infection. Many women and

some men can be taught clean self-catheterization to assure complete bladder emptying every four to six hours, thereby minimizing infection. Effective control is more difficult to attain in persons who suffer damage to the conus or peripheral micturition pathways; they usually require the assistance of an experienced urologist to develop effective bladder care.

Male Sexual Function

Organic disturbances of male sexual function are limited almost entirely to loss of libido, failure to attain an erection of sufficient strength to carry out sexual intercourse (impotence), and failure to attain normal ejaculation-emission. Kolodny et al. define impotence somewhat generously as greater than a 25 per cent failure during attempted intercourse. Failure to reach orgasm or the presence of premature or delayed ejaculation with normal libido and erectile capacity almost always reflects a psychogenic rather than an organic problem.

Neural control over male sexual activities arises within forebrain limbic areas, generating sexual drives that, in turn, are chronically stimulated by the effects of circulating androgens. Descending pathways travel with the parasympathetic outflow. Parasympathetic sacral efferents control penile tumescence by inducing vascular engorgement and also stimulate a large proportion of the severally originating pelvic contractions that initiate ejaculation and lead to the sensation of orgasm. Sympathetic stimulation contracts the seminal vesicles and closes the bladder neck to prevent retrograde emission, thereby guaranteeing anterograde ejaculation. Genital sensory fibers reach the spinal cord via the S2 to S4 dorsal roots and thenceforth ascend in the lemniscal system. Considerable evidence gained from the study of sexual function in paraplegics with high spinal lesions indicates that the distal thoracic and lumbosacral spinal cord contains all the necessary reflexes to complete sensory-induced erection and ejaculation.

Male impotence is common and increases with age to affect at some time almost half the population over 55 years; at that age psychogenic causes appear to be primary in only about 25 per cent. Therapeutic drugs and alcohol excess represent the most frequent causes of male impotence. Aging itself, however, eventually becomes a cause, and about 25 per cent of males of 70 years or more have erection failure attributable to aging alone.

Impotence has several possible causes, as indicated in Table 463–5, and more than one can affect a given patient. In perhaps 10 per cent of cases no satisfactory explanation can be found. Psychologic factors are always important. They

TABLE 463–5. PRINCIPAL ORGANIC CAUSES OF MALE SEXUAL FAILURE

Drugs (Table 463–6)

Endocrine
Secondary: pituitary adenoma; idiopathic or acquired hypogonadotropic hypogonadism; hyperprolactinemia
Primary gonadal failure
Advanced diabetes mellitus
Hypothyroidism, hyperthyroidism (rare)

Chronic Systemic Illnesses
Cirrhosis
Chronic renal failure
Disseminated malignancy, etc.

Neurogenic
Temporal lobe disorders: trauma, epilepsy, neoplasm, stroke
Intramedullary spinal lesions: paraplegia; demyelinating disorders; neoplasms; syrinx; Shy-Drager dysautonomia
Peripheral nerves. Somatic or autonomic neuropathies; pelvic neoplasms, granulomas, trauma; structural lesions of cauda equina or conus medullaris

Urologic
Complete prostatectomy; priapism; local trauma or neoplasms; Peyronie's disease; rectosigmoid "cleanouts"

Vascular
Severe aortic atherosclerosis; lower aortic bypass

account for most of the younger cases and influence many of the older ones as well. They must be inquired into carefully even when adequate organic reasons for sexual failure appear to exist.

Differential diagnosis begins with a careful history. Does the patient's complaint reflect a recent change in libido and performance or a longstanding pattern that has finally proved more troublesome to a sexual partner than to self? Longstanding absence or low level of libido can reflect either psychologic factors, chronic temporal lobe disease, or primary or secondary androgenic failure. If the disease is recent in origin, does it relate entirely to a specific partner? Such instances are usually psychogenic and best managed by a sex therapist if a careful history, physical examination, and tumescence studies provide no suggestion of the organic disorders listed in Table 463–5. If recent in onset, did libido remain high as potency declined? The latter pattern is more common among drug-induced or neurologic disorders than among endocrine ones.

Specific drugs most often causing impotence are listed in Table 463–6. Among the endocrine disorders, most that are severe enough to cause impotence are readily recognized. Pituitary tumors and hypothalamic lesions impairing gonadotropic release usually give prominent additional symptoms (Ch. 226). Hypo- or hyperthyroidism similarly generates other systemic symptoms. In doubtful cases, measurement of serum prolactin, testosterone, thyroxin, and triiodothyronine should settle the question. Borderline changes of a single serum hormone value, however, seldom provide evidence for a disorder of potency that will be reversed by giving hormone therapy.

Neurologic disturbances cause only about 10 per cent of all cases of impotence, although the symptom affects patients with a number of neurologic diseases and deserves compassionate inquiry. Temporal lobe disease affecting limbic systems is associated with reduction in male libido, while structural lesions involving descending parasympathetic systems commonly interfere with the capacity to gain and maintain an erection. Peripheral neurologic disorders, as Table 463–5 indicates, are the commonest neurologic offenders and should be approached as indicated in Section 16.

Aside from a record of sexual inadequacy limited to a specific partner, little in the history alone guarantees psychogenic causes. Since patients with physical illness may suffer psychogenic impotence (e.g., postmyocardial infarction or poststroke sexual failure) while others with prominent psychiatric disorders may have unsuspected physical illness (e.g., depressives with diabetic neuropathy), objective testing measures are valuable in differential diagnosis. Useful in this regard is the measurement of nocturnal penile tumescence (NPT), which, taken during sleep monitoring, records the frequency and intensity of the erections that normally accompany rapid eye movement sleep. When matched suitably for age with normal controls, the results correlate highly although not completely with psychogenic (no appreciable decline in NPT) versus organic (moderate to marked decline in NPT) impotence. The intracorporeal injection of vasodilators such as papaverine to induce erection can be both diagnostically and therapeutically useful.

TABLE 463–6. DRUGS OFTEN REPORTED TO INTERFERE WITH MALE POTENCY

Alcohol	Clonidine
Anticancer chemotherapy	Guanethidine
Anticholinergics	Immunosuppressives
Antiparkinson agents	Lithium
Barbiturates and congeners	Opiates
Benzodiazepines	Phenothiazine
Beta blockers	Several antihypertensive ganglionic blockers
Bethanidine	Several diuretics
Cannabis	Tricyclic and MAO-inhibitor antidepressants
Cimetidine	

Treatment of male impotence depends upon the cause. Drug avoidance or readjustment can benefit many cases, as can substitution therapy when endocrine failure is demonstrated. Local genital abnormalities should be approached surgically. A variety of surgically implantable prostheses to assist erection have become available in recent years to aid the patient affected with impotence caused by neurogenic or locally severe vascular disease. Thus far, attempts at revascularizing the penis have met with only limited success. Testosterone therapy given in the absence of a demonstrated androgen deficiency almost never provides more than placebo benefit and creates a carcinogenic risk as well.

HYPOTHALAMUS AND ITS DISORDERS

Greenberg HS, Rocher LL, Clavin DB, et al.: Episodic hyperhidrosis, hypothermia, and agenesis of the corpus callosum. Neurology 33:1122, 1983. *The most recent comprehensive review of this uncommon condition, with the addition of new material.*

Martin JB, Reichlin S: Clinical Neuroendocrinology. 2nd ed. Philadelphia, F. A. Davis Company, 1987.

Plum F, Van Uitert R: Non-endocrine diseases and disorders of the hypothalamus. Res Publ Assoc Res Nerv Ment Dis 56:415, 1977. *A comprehensive review of the clinically important autonomic functions of the hypothalamus written at the dawn of the peptide era. Extensively referenced.*

PERIPHERAL AND CENTRAL AUTONOMIC FUNCTIONS

Appenzeller O: The Autonomic Nervous System. 3rd ed. Amsterdam, Elsevier North Holland, 1982. *The only available comprehensive monograph of recent origin.*

Bannister R: Autonomic Failure: A Textbook of Clinical Disorders of the Autonomic Nervous System. New York, Oxford University Press, 1983. *A multiauthored monograph providing excellent summaries of particular disorders.*

Bradshaw MJ, Edwards RTM: Postural hypotension—pathophysiology and management. Q J Med 231:643, 1986. *A careful review of the most common of the autonomic insufficiencies. Well referenced.*

Hines S, Houston M, Robertson D: The clinical spectrum of autonomic dysfunction. Am J Med 70:1091, 1981. *An analysis of 297 patients with various forms of autonomic insufficiency of both secondary and primary causes.*

URINARY BLADDER CONTROL

Andersson K-E, Sjögren C: Aspects on the physiology and pharmacology of the bladder and urethra. Prog Neurobiol 19:71, 1982. *Describes bladder-urethral innervation and comprehensively lists drugs that have been used to treat bladder dysfunction.*

Boyarsky S, Labay P, Hanick P, et al.: Care of the Patient with Neurogenic Bladder. Boston, Little, Brown and Company. 1979. *A well-balanced monograph describing all aspects of this difficult subject.*

Williams ME, Pannill FC: Urinary incontinence in the elderly. Physiology, pathophysiology, diagnosis and treatment. Ann Intern Med 97:895, 1982. *A thorough, highly practical guide with an extensive bibliography.*

MALE SEXUAL FUNCTION

Bennett AH (ed.): Management of Male Impotence. Baltimore, Williams and Wilkins, 1982. *A useful multiauthored monograph that covers the organic causes of the problem.*

Kaplan HS: Disorders of Sexual Desire. New York, Brunner/Mazel, 1979. *A detailed review of the most frequent psychogenic sexual dysfunctions.*

Kolodny RC, Masters WH, Johnson VE: Textbook of Sexual Medicine. Boston, Little, Brown and Company, 1979. *A good textbook of sexual medicine designed for students and general physicians.*

Slag MF, Morley JE, Elson MK, et al.: Impotence in medical clinic outpatients. JAMA 249:1736, 1983. *Among 1181 men attendees at a VA Hospital, 34 per cent with a mean age of just over 60 years had erectile dysfunction.*

464 THE SPECIAL SENSES

Robert W. Baloh

Smell and Taste

Approximately two million American adults suffer from disorders of taste and smell, yet there is relatively little information available on how to evaluate or treat these patients. These disorders have been neglected because they are seldom fatal and, unlike abnormalites of vision and hearing, are not considered serious handicaps. Chemosensory disorders, however, often reduce the enjoyment and quality of life and are important to patients who suffer from them. Disorders of taste interfere with digestion because taste stimulants alter salivary and pancreatic flow, gastric contractions, and intestinal motility. Smell also contributes to the anticipation and ingestion of food since much of what we taste derives from olfactory stimulation during ingestion and chewing. The inability to detect noxious tastes and odors can result in food- or gas poisoning, particularly in elderly subjects. In the extreme, chemosensory disorders can lead to overwhelming stress, anorexia, and depression.

DEFINITIONS. Disorders of taste and smell are defined as follows: *Ageusia*, absence of taste; *hypogeusia*, diminished sensitivity of taste; *dysgeusia*, distortion of normal taste; *anosmia*, absence of smell; *hyposmia*, diminished sensitivity of smell; and *dysosmia*, distortion of normal smell. *Hypergeusia* and *hyperosmia* (increased sensitivity of taste and smell) also occur, but little is known about their cause or significance.

ANATOMY. The sensory receptor for taste, the taste bud, is made up of approximately 50 cells arranged to form a pear-shaped organ. The life span of these cells is about ten days, and they are constantly being renewed from dividing epithelial cells surrounding the bud. Taste buds are located on the tongue, soft palate, pharynx, larynx, epiglottis, uvula, and the upper one third of the esophagus. The taste buds located on the anterior two thirds of the tongue and on the palate are innervated by the seventh cranial nerve. The ninth cranial nerve innervates the posterior one third of the tongue and the folds or clefts on the lateral border of the tongue. The ninth and tenth nerves innervate taste buds in the pharynx. Afferent signals from the taste buds project to the nucleus of the solitary tract in the medulla and then via a series of relays to the thalamus and postcentral somatosensory cerebral cortex. Free nerve endings of the fifth cranial nerve are found on the tongue and in the oral cavity, and lesions involving these pathways also can alter taste perception.

Olfactory receptors lie in a roughly dime-sized area of specialized pigmented epithelium that arches along the superior aspect of each side of the nasal mucosa. Specialized bipolar sensory cells in this region thrust short receptor hairs into the overlying mucosa to detect aromatic molecules as they dissolve. As with taste buds, the specialized receptor portion of the bipolar neuron undergoes continuous renewal, turning over approximately every 30 days. Thin axons of the bipolar neurons course through small holes in the cribriform plate of the ethmoid bone to form connections in the overlying olfactory bulb on the ventral surface of the frontal lobe. From here second- and third order neurons project directly and indirectly to the prepiriform cortex and parts of the amygdaloid complex of both sides of the brain, representing the primary olfactory cortex.

PATHOPHYSIOLOGY OF CHEMOSENSORY DISORDERS. Disorders of taste and smell can be divided into local, systemic, and neurologic (Table 464–1). The taste buds and the specialized receptor portion of the bipolar olfactory cells are constantly being renewed, and the process of renewal can be affected by nutritional, metabolic, and hormonal states, therapeutic radiation, drugs, and age. For example, with interruption of mitosis by antiproliferative agents, a return of

normal taste function takes a minimum of 10 days, while a return to normal olfactory function takes more than 30 days. Numerous local conditions such as colds and allergies, chronic sinusitis, and nasal polyposis can influence the sense of smell by restricting airway patency. Accidental blows to the head can shear the fine axons of the bipolar olfactory neurons resulting in loss of smell. Lesions of the fifth, seventh (*chorda tympani),* and ninth nerves can lead to disordered taste sensation. Olfactory and gustatory disturbances can serve as important diagnostic signs for focal neurologic lesions (e.g., frontal lobe tumors). Hallucinations of smell and taste occur with epileptogenic lesions affecting the mesial temporal lobe and insular region, respectively. Finally, olfactory disturbances and hallucinations occur with a number of psychiatric illnesses (particularly depressive illness and schizophrenia).

EXAMINATION OF TASTE AND SMELL. Olfaction can be tested grossly at the bedside with a few easily recognized odors such as coffee, chocolate, and the roselike aroma of the compound phenylethyl alcohol. (Avoid nasal irritants.) Each nostril is tested separately to determine whether the problem is unilateral or bilateral. More detailed testing can be obtained in specialized clinics in which a variety of qualitatively distinct substances that span a number of established odor classes are presented with a forced-choice paradigm. Gustatory sensation is typically tested with weak solutions of sugar, salt, and acetic acid, or vinegar. The patient must keep his tongue protruded and respond to questions either by nodding the head or pointing to names of the tastes written on cards. The protruding tongue is dried and a drop of test solution is applied to the lateral border of each side. The anterior two thirds and posterior one third of the tongue should be tested separately.

COMMON CAUSES OF LOSS OF SMELL AND TASTE. The most frequently encountered causes of loss of smell are: local obstructive disease, viral infections, head injuries that sever the neurons crossing through the cribriform plate, and normal aging. Patients can lose their sense of smell not only from chronic allergies and sinusitis but also from the nasal sprays and drops that they use to treat these conditions. The most common cause of loss of the sense of taste is drug ingestion, particularly antirheumatic and antiproliferative drugs and drugs containing sulfhydryl groups in their molecular structure, such as penicillamine and captopril. Patients with poor dental hygiene commonly complain of distortions of taste. Many of the systemic disorders listed in Table 464–1 probably have their effect by decreasing the rate of turnover of sensory receptors on the tongue and olfactory epithelia. Disturbances of smell and taste in malnourished patients have been attributed to specific deficiencies in vitamins and minerals, such as zinc. However, it is possible that the loss of protein and calorie intake impairs the functioning of taste buds and olfactory cells in the same manner that it impairs the regeneration of intestinal epithelia. Viral illnesses such as influenza and viral hepatitis produce disorders of both taste and smell. The loss of olfactory sensation after viral illnesses may be due to scarring of the subepithelial tissue and the replacement of olfactory epithelium with respiratory epithelium. Multifocal neurologic disorders such as multiple sclerosis can affect the central olfactory and gustatory pathways at multiple levels, and therefore abnormalities of taste and smell are common in such patients. Treatment, other than avoiding drugs known to affect taste or smell, is unsatisfactory.

TABLE 464–1. COMMON CAUSES OF LOSS OF TASTE AND SMELL

	Taste	Smell
Local	Radiation therapy	Allergic rhinitis, sinusitis, nasal polyposis, bronchial asthma
Systemic	Cancer, renal failure, hepatic failure, nutritional deficiency (B_3, zinc), Cushing syndrome, hypothyroidism, diabetes mellitus, infection (influenza), drugs (antirheumatic and antiproliferative)	Renal failure, hepatic failure, nutritional deficiency (B_{12}), Cushing syndrome, hypothyroidism, diabetes mellitus, infection (viral hepatitis, influenza), drugs (nasal sprays, antibiotics)
Neurologic	Bell's palsy, familial dysautonomia, multiple sclerosis	Head trauma, multiple sclerosis, Parkinson's disease, frontal tumor

Henkin RI, et al.: The role of zinc in taste and smell. In Prusad AS (ed.): The Clinical Biochemical and Nutritional Aspects of Trace Elements. New York, Alan R. Liss, 1982. *Reports that some zinc-deficient patients with decreased olfactory ability can be helped with zinc administration. A controversial issue.*

Schellinger D, Henkin RI, Smirnolopoulous JG: CT of the brain in taste and smell dysfunction. AJNR 4:752, 1983. *Report of structural abnormalities identified in patients with smell and taste disorders.*

Schiffman SS: Taste and smell in disease. N Engl J Med 308:1275; 1337, 1983. *A well-referenced two-part review.*

Neuro-ophthalmology

The mechanistic understanding of vision impairment along with disturbances of pupillary and oculomotor control lies close to the heart of diagnosing neurologic disorders. Diseases of the eye itself are further considered in Part XXIII.

VISION

One of the most difficult diagnostic problems is vision loss that cannot be explained by obvious abnormalities of the eye. In order to properly evaluate such a patient the examining physician must be familiar with the anatomy and physiology of the afferent visual system. The afferent visual pathways cross at right angles to the major ascending sensory and descending motor systems of the cerebral hemispheres and in their anterior portion are intimately related to the vascular and bony structures at the base of the brain. Not surprisingly, localization of lesions within the afferent visual pathways has great localizing value in neurologic diagnosis.

DEFINITIONS. *Amblyopia* refers to dimness or partial loss of vision, *amaurosis* to blindness. *Scotomas* are areas of relative or complete vision loss isolated within a comparatively better total field of vision for the particular eye. Involvement of the macular area or its projections produces *central scotomas*. Scotomas that lie near the macular visual area are sometimes called *paracentral*, whereas those that extend into macular vision from the more peripheral field may be termed *cecocentral*.

Visual field defects impairing half or nearly half of a field are termed *hemianopic*. Those affecting less than this extent are called *partial field defects*, often with the additional designation of *quadrantic* or *altitudinal* (superior or inferior), depending on the abnormality. A vision defect that affects similar points of the right or left half-field in both eyes is called *homonymous*; identical areas of involvement from the two eyes are termed *congruent*.

ANATOMY OF THE VISUAL PATHWAYS. Light entering the eye falls on the retinal rods and cones, which transduce the stimulus into neural impulses to be transmitted to the brain. The distribution of visual function across the retina takes a pattern of concentric zones increasing in sensitivity toward the center, the fovea. The fovea consists of a "rod-free" central grouping of approximately 100,000 slender cones. The ganglion cells subserving these cones send their axons directly to the temporal aspect of the optic disk, forming the papillomacular bundle. Axons originating from ganglion cells in the temporal retina must curve above and below the papillomacular bundle, forming dense arcuate bands.

The arteries supplying the optic nerve and retina both derive from branches of the ophthalmic artery. The central retinal artery approaches the eye along each optic nerve and pierces the inferior aspect of the dural sheath about 1 cm behind the globe to enter the center of the nerve. The artery emerges in the fundus at the center of the nerve head, from which it nourishes most of the retina by superior, medial, inferior, and lateral branches. Anastomotic branches derived from the choroidal and posterior ciliary arteries supply the nerve head itself and the macular region. Venous drainage from the retina and nerve head flows primarily via the central retinal vein, whose course of exit from the eye parallels that of the entry of the artery. The venous anatomy explains why inflammatory lesions of or adjacent to the optic nerve head cause venous distention and ipsilateral papilledema (optic neuritis), whereas inflammation lying posterior to the point where the vein leaves the nerve produces only visual loss without swelling of the nerve head (retrobulbar neuritis).

What each eye "sees" is termed its visual field (Fig. 464–1). The nasal side of the left eye and the temporal side of the right eye see the left side of the world, and the upper half of each retina sees the lower half of the world. Behind the eye, the optic nerve passes through the optic foramen and sphenoid bone to reach the optic chiasm. In the chiasm, nerves from the nasal half of each retina decussate and join the fibers from the temporal half of the contralateral retina. From the chiasm, the optic tracts pass around the cerebral peduncles to reach the lateral geniculate ganglia of either side. At the

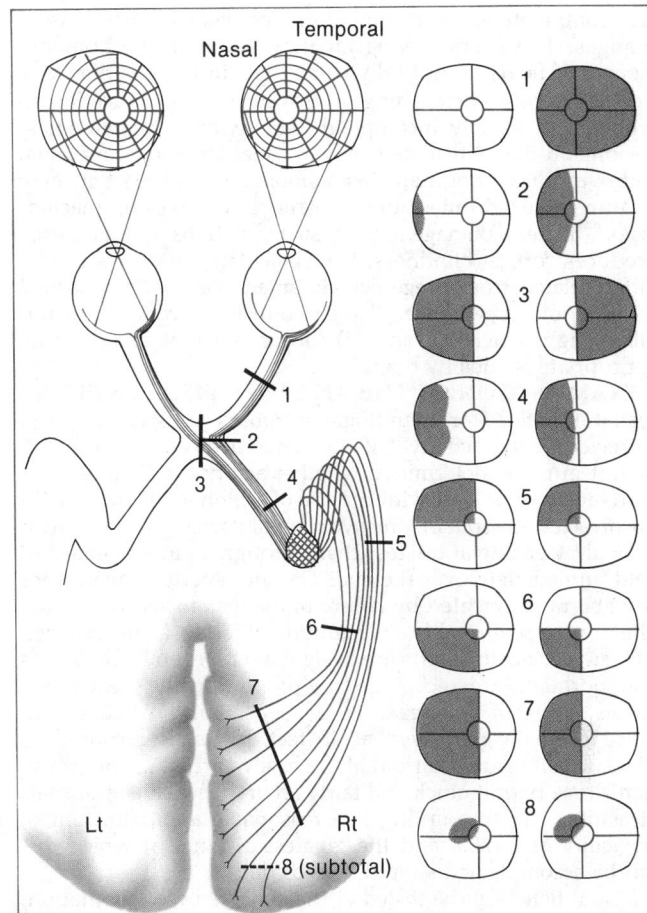

FIGURE 464–1. Visual fields that accompany damage to the visual pathways. 1. Optic nerve: Unilateral amaurosis. 2. Lateral optic chiasm: Grossly incongruous, incomplete (contralateral) homonymous hemianopia. 3. Central optic chiasm: Bitemporal hemianopia. 4. Optic tract: Incongruous, incomplete homonymous hemianopia. 5. Temporal (Meyer's) loop of optic radiation: Congruous partial or complete (contralateral) homonymous superior quadrantanopia. 6. Parietal (superior) projection of the optic radiation: Congruous partial or complete homonymous inferior quadrantanopia. 7. Complete parieto-occipital interruption of optic radiation. Complete congruous homonymous hemianopia with psychophysical shift of foveal point often sparing central vision, giving "macular sparing." 8. Incomplete damage to visual cortex: Congruous homonymous scotomas, usually encroaching at least acutely on central vision.

level of the geniculus, fibers serving corresponding points in each retinal half visual field lie adjacent to each other, and this proximity is maintained in the subsequent relay to the calcarine cortex. The geniculocalcarine radiation initially fans out into superolateral and inferolateral projections, the latter passing around the lateral ventricle and for a short distance into the temporal lobe (Meyer's loop) before turning posteriorly to head for the striate cortex of the occipital lobe. At the occipital pole, the striate cortex (Area 17) lies along the superior and inferior bands of the calcarine fissure, with macular fibers projecting most posteriorly to the occipital pole and more peripheral retinal projections lying more anteriorly. Each occipital pole "sees" the opposite half of the world. Fibers serving the superior retinal quadrants project to the superior bank of the calcarine fissure, and those from the inferior quadrants project to the inferior bank. The macular field is represented strictly unilaterally.

LOCALIZATION OF LESIONS WITHIN THE VISUAL PATHWAYS. Monocular vision loss is due to a lesion of one eye or its retina or optic nerve. Binocular visual loss, on the other hand, can result from disease located anywhere in the visual pathways from the retinae to the occipital poles. Lesions involving or compressing the optic chiasm produce nonhomonymous visual abnormalities that affect the unilateral visual fields incongruously (e.g., the bitemporal hemianopia illustrated by Lesion 3 in Fig. 464–1). Optic tract abnormalities are comparatively rare but produce characteristic visual changes. The fibers serving identical points in the homonymous half fields do not fully commingle in the anterior optic tract, so lesions encroaching on this structure produce incongruous and usually incomplete homonymous hemianopias. Lesions on the geniculate ganglia, visual radiations, or visual cortex produce congruent hemianopic field defects that may go unrecognized unless the hemianopia intrudes on macular vision. Bilateral damage to the visual radiations or optic cortex produces cortical blindness. Postgeniculate amaurosis can be differentiated from pregeniculate amaurosis by (1) a normal funduscopic appearance (2) intact direct and consensual pupillary light reactions, and (3) the presence of anatomically appropriate lesions by brain imaging.

EXAMINATION OF THE AFFERENT VISUAL SYSTEM. Visual function for neurologic purposes consists of "best corrected visual activity." If the visual acuity is not normal, then it must be determined whether acuity can be improved with lenses or at least with the use of a pinhole. Patients with uncorrected myopia or presbyopia will correct vision to near normal by gazing at the test chart through a pinhole in a card held immediately over the eye. The tiny aperture overcomes any aberration created by failure of the lens to accommodate. The normal reference is a recognition of letters at an idealized 20 feet, and acuity charts are designed with even larger letters that normally are recognized at proportionally greater distances. Thus, if one reads at 20 feet letters no better than those normally perceived at 40 feet, vision is recorded as 20/40. Small visual charts that are easily carried in the physician's case permit quick and fairly accurate bedside appraisals of acuity. Finger counting is a reasonable approximation of an acuity of 20/200, and the greatest distance at which this can be accomplished should be recorded.

Visual fields can be tested at the bedside by confrontation, and rough estimates of their integrity can be made even in patients with reduced alertness. The fields should be tested individually for each eye, since the pattern of visual field defects can provide important localizing information. A quick screen of the visual fields can be made by having the patient fixate on the examiner's nose and identify the number of fingers flashed in each of the four visual field quadrants. With practice and a cooperative subject, accurate confrontation fields can be obtained that outline even scotomas. The examiner should place the test object (e.g., a red match head) midway between his eye and the patient's eye and test the patient's unilateral visual field against his own. Ophthalmoscopic examination permits direct visualization of the cornea, lens, vitreous, retina, and optic disk. Ophthalmologists routinely dilate the pupil to examine the optic fundus, but this step should be avoided in acutely ill patients or those suspected of neurologic diseases until one is certain that an intrinsic pupillary abnormality will not be important in reaching a diagnosis or in following the patient's course. Corneal, lenticular, or vitreous opacities large enough to produce visual symptoms almost always can be detected with the ophthalmoscope.

COMMON CAUSES OF VISUAL LOSS. Eye. The cause of monocular vision loss due to ocular and retinal lesions often can be detected with ophthalmoscopic examination or with measurement of intraocular pressure. *Glaucoma* caused by impaired absorption of the aqueous humor results in a high intraocular pressure that usually produces gradual visual loss with reduced nighttime vision, "halos" seen around illuminated lamps, and, often, pain and redness in the affected eye. Infrequently, rapid vision loss can occur with few premonitory symptoms. Diagnosis comes from the tonometric measurement of a high intraocular pressure and may be suspected by palpating an abnormally firm globe and observing a deep, pale optic cup and attenuated blood vessels. *Retinal tears and detachments* give rise to unilateral distortions of the visual image seen as sudden angulations or curves of

objects containing straight lines (metamorphopsia). *Hemorrhages* into the vitreous humor or unilateral *infections* or *inflammatory lesions* of the retina can produce scotomas that in all ways resemble those resulting from primary disease of the central visual pathway.

Binocular vision loss due to retinal disease in younger subjects is usually due to *heredodegenerative conditions*. Vascular diseases, diabetes, idiopathic (senile) macular degeneration, and bilateral retinal detachments are causes in older age groups. In the *pigmentary retinal degenerations* visual loss begins peripherally and proceeds centrally, and often very slowly, before acuity (central vision) is impaired. By contrast, *macular degenerations* impair central vision early in their course. Most of the retinal degenerations produce characteristic and recognizable ophthalmoscopic appearances. With pigmentary degenerations the visual fields shrink progressively in size. With macular degenerations, on the other hand, the fields show noncongruent central scotomas.

Optic Nerve. Acute or subacute monocular vision loss due to optic nerve disease is most commonly produced by demyelinating disorders, vascular obstruction, or neoplasm. Demyelinating disease of the nerve head (*optic neuritis* or *papillitis*) produces papilledema along with loss of central vision in the affected eye only; subjectively unrecognized scotomas sometimes may be found in the other eye. Demyelination in the optic nerve behind where the retinal vein emerges (*retrobulbar neuritis*) initially leaves a normal-looking disk but a central or paracentral scotoma. With chronic demyelinating disorders the optic disk becomes pale and atrophic. More than 50 per cent of patients who initially present with optic neuritis or retrobulbar neuritis go on to develop typical symptoms and signs of multiple sclerosis. Vascular lesions produce either total amaurosis or a sector field defect consistent with an intraocular arterial occlusion (*ischemic optic neuropathy*). The common causes of transient monocular vision loss and their differential features are listed in Table 464–2. *Tumors* invading the optic nerve or space-occupying lesions compressing it anywhere between the orbit and the chiasm cause gradually decreasing central vision (intrinsic or far advanced lesions) or a sector defect of the peripheral visual field. With such chronic lesions the affected optic nerve becomes visibly atrophic.

Acute binocular vision loss due to bilateral optic nerve disease is most often caused by demyelinating disease and less frequently by optic nerve or retinal vascular disease or by toxic or nutritional optic neuropathies. In younger persons and those lacking a clear history of toxic exposures demyelinating lesions overwhelmingly predominate (optic neuritis). Symptoms are of abrupt or subacute onset with visual blurring or loss of acuity, which may progress rapidly to blindness

TABLE 464–2. COMMON CAUSES OF TRANSIENT MONOCULAR VISION LOSS

Category/ (Typical Duration)	Causes	Differential Features
Thromboembolism (1–5 min)	Atherosclerosis	Other atherosclerotic vascular disease, associated crossed hemiparesis, angiography (carotid atheromata)
	Cardiac	Valvular disease, mural thrombi, atrial fibrillation, recent MI
	Blood dyscrasia	Blood tests + for sickle cell anemia, macroglobulinemia, multiple myeloma, polycythemia, etc.
Vasospasm (5–30 min)	Migraine	Ipsilateral headache, other classical aura, and family history
Vascular compression (few sec)	Papilledema	Precipitated by position change, Valsalva maneuver, or pressure waves
	Tumor	Associated slowly progressive monocular visual loss
Vasculitis (1–5 min)	Temporal arteritis	Associated headache, polymyalgia rheumatica, palpable temporal artery, elevated sed rate

TABLE 464–3. DIFFERENTIATION OF OPTIC NEURITIS FROM PAPILLEDEMA

	Optic Neuritis	Papilledema
Central-cecocentral vision loss	Present	Absent
Distribution	Usually unilateral	Usually bilateral
Ocular pain on movement	Present	Absent
Direct light reflex	± Reduced	Intact
CT scan of head	Normal	Often abnormal
Visual evoked responses	Abnormal	Normal
Lumbar puncture pressure	Normal	Elevated

within hours or days. There may be pain about the eyes, particularly on eye movement.

Papilledema resulting from increased intracranial pressure occasionally causes vision loss under one of three circumstances: (1) Acute transient episodes of amaurosis lasting a few seconds and attributable to acute increases in intracranial pressure (plateau waves) that interfere with retinal venous drainage into the cavernous sinus or with vascular irrigation of the occipital lobe; (2) acute bilateral sustained amaurosis following abrupt surgical relief of longstanding, severely increased, intracranial pressure (a rare cause); (3) progressive loss of peripheral vision with longstanding, severe papilledema, presumably owing to pressure atrophy of the most peripherally lying fibers in the tightly sheathed optic nerve. Table 464–3 gives the main differential points between papilledema and optic neuritis. Subacute or chronic binocular vision loss due to optic nerve disease results mainly from *toxic nutritional* causes and the *inherited optic atrophies*. The latter sometimes accompany spinocerebellar degeneration or selectively affect the optic nerves in both juveniles and adults (Leber's forms). With either cause visual loss is moderate or severe and primarily or initially affects central vision; ophthalmoscopy shows mild to moderate primary optic atrophy.

Chiasm and Optic Tract. Patients with lesions of the optic chiasm and optic tract are often unaware of visual impairment until the deficit encroaches on central vision in one or both eyes. Intrinsic or extrinsic neoplasms and parachiasmal arterial aneurysms are the most common lesions in this location. *Gliomas* that arise in the chiasm are rare in adulthood but, when they occur, impair central vision early. Extrinsic space-occupying lesions compressing the chiasm can arise from the superior, lateral, or inferior aspect and include *dysgerminomas, craniopharyngiomas, pituitary adenomas, meningiomas* arising from the sphenoid bones, and large *aneurysms* of the carotid artery. The diagnosis rests on finding the characteristic visual field abnormalities (bitemporal hemianopsia for chiasm and incongruous homonymous hemianopsia for optic tract lesions) and identifying the specific lesion with computed tomography (CT) or magnetic resonance imaging (MRI). Pituitary apoplexy (due to acute hemorrhage into the gland, occurring most frequently in patients with unrecognized pituitary adenomas) can result in sudden vision loss. Prompt neurosurgical intervention under steroid coverage is required for most patients.

Visual Radiations and Occipital Cortex. Lesions involving the postgeniculate visual pathways most often result from *vascular damage, traumatic injuries, neoplasms* or, rarely, *inflammatory* or *degenerative disorders* involving the cerebral white matter. Their localization can be deduced by the resulting visual field defects (see Fig. 464–1). Vascular disease of the occipital lobes is the most common cause of homonymous visual field defects in the middle-aged and elderly population. Typically, the onset of such field defects is associated with other signs and symptoms of transient ischemic episodes in the vertebrobasilar distribution. Bilateral damage to the visual radiations or occipital cortex produces *cortical blindness*. Most often, there are other signs of vascular disease including focal neurologic findings. *Anton's syndrome* refers to cortical blindness with denial of visual defect. Affected patients not only deny the fact that they are blind but confabulate details of their visual environment from memory. Autopsy studies

reveal lesions of the medial, temporal, and parietal lobes as well as the calcarine cortex. *Tumors* are rarely confined to the limits of the occipital lobes, therefore neurologic deficits with occipital tumors are rarely only visual.

PUPILLARY CONTROL

The neuromechanisms that control pupil size and reactivity are complex, yet they can be evaluated by simple clinical procedures. The diameter of the pupil is determined by the antagonistic actions of the iris sphincter and dilator muscles with the latter playing a minor role. If the sphincter muscle is severed or ruptured it does not retract toward one quadrant but rather continues to function except in the altered segment. Therefore, the pupillary response can be evaluated even in the presence of significant damage to the iris.

DEFINITIONS. A difference in the size of the pupils is called *anisocoria*. *Mydriasis* refers to a dilated pupil while *miosis* refers to a constricted pupil. *Hippus* refers to a pupil that is constantly changing in size (a physiological phenomenon that has no pathological significance). *Light-near dissociation* refers to a pupil that responds to accommodation but not to light. An *afferent pupil* is a pupil that responds poorly, or not at all, to direct light but has a normal consensual response when a light is shined in the opposite eye.

ANATOMY AND LOCALIZATION OF LESIONS WITHIN PUPILLARY PATHWAYS. The size of the pupil is governed by tonic balance between sympathetic and parasympathetic innervation of the muscles of the iris. Sympathetic stimulation dilates the pupil, and parasympathetic stimulation constricts it. In the normal resting state, light entering the eye provides the major stimulus governing the size of the pupil. Light activates the retinal rods and cones with maximal sensitivity in the macular area. The optic nerve fibers follow the crossed and uncrossed visual pathways to the pregeniculate portion of the optic tracts, where the receptor fibers for light diverge to the pretectal nucleus located at the midbrain diencephalic junction. Interneurons project from this nucleus to the Edinger-Westphal nuclei atop the midbrain third nerve complex of either side. From that point paired parasympathetic efferents leave the midbrain with the third nerves to travel in the interpeduncular space across the petroclinoid ligament and edge of the tentorium, where, after traversing the cavernous sinus, they enter the superior orbital fissure. In the orbit the parasympathetic efferents synapse in the ciliary ganglion from which short ciliary nerves enter the eye to reach the pupillary muscles.

Lesions of the retina or optic nerve results in an ipsilateral afferent pupillary defect. Midbrain lesions in the region of the third nerve nuclei destroy the preganglionic parasympathetic neurons but also interrupt descending sympathetic pathways, resulting in irregular, often unequal and fixed, midposition pupils of 3 to 5 mm diameter. Damage to a third nerve or its parasympathetic postganglionic fibers results in a dilated pupil that does not respond to direct or consensual stimulation.

The principal sympathetic control of the pupil originates in the ventral lateral hypothalamus (first-order neuron) from which fibers descend ipsilaterally to the lower brain stem tegmentum and thence to the cervical cord, where they lie superficially and synapse with the preganglionic neurons in the intermedial lateral column of the upper three thoracic segments. Preganglionic fibers (second-order neurons) emerge with the ventral roots of C8, T1, and T2 and ascend in the neck to synapse in the superior cervical ganglion adjacent to the base of the skull. Postganglionic (third-order neurons) pupillary fibers accompany the internal carotid artery through the skull leaving it to follow the ophthalmic branch of the trigeminal nerve to reach the pupillodilator muscle of the eye.

Sympathetic paralysis of the eye with ptosis and miosis (Horner's syndrome) can result from lesions anywhere along the course of the pathway described above. Topical diagnosis is made best by identifying associated signs in the brain stem or neck or along the carotid artery.

EXAMINATION OF THE PUPIL. The pupillary response to light should be examined in a dimly lighted room, in which case the pupils will be in a semidilated state. First, the size and symmetry of the pupils are assessed by shining a dim light onto the face from below so that both pupils are seen simultaneously in the indirect illumination. To test light reactivity gaze is directed at a distant object and first one and then the other pupil is illuminated with a very bright light source. If a pupil reacts poorly to direct light, it is observed as the opposite eye is illuminated (consensual response). Pupils that react poorly to light should be tested for activity to the near reflex. This is done by first having the patient gaze at a distant object and then quickly fixate on his fingertip just in front of his nose.

COMMON CAUSES OF PUPILLARY ABNORMALITIES. The differential features for distinguishing between several common causes of a dilated pupil are illustrated in the logic tree shown in Figure 464–2. With so-called benign pupillary dilatation or *physiological anisocoria* there is a lifelong difference in the size of the two pupils with normal reflex reactions; the disparity remains constant during constriction and dilatation. Lesions compressing or damaging the tectal region interrupt the afferent light reflex bilaterally to produce dilated (>5 mm) and light-fixed pupils. Pupillary constriction on accommodation is preserved until late stages. Tumors of the pineal gland (e.g., dysgerminomas) and *localized infarctions* are the most common lesions in this location. *Adie's tonic pupil* is a medium-to-large (3 to 6 mm) pupil that constricts little or not at all to light and slowly to accommodation but constricts with the instillation of dilute pilocarpine (0.0125 per cent). The abnormal pupil is associated with diminished or absent deep tendon reflexes in the extremities. The condition usually affects one eye (occasionally both), is more common in women 25 to 45 years of age, and carries no serious implications. Its cause is unknown. Unexplained unilateral or bilateral dilated pupil as an isolated finding can result from the *accidental or intentional instillation of mydriatics*. The recent widespread use of transdermal scopolamine has increased the problem. Failure of the pupil to constrict promptly with pilocarpine (1 per cent) gives the diagnosis if the history is unclear. Interruption of the emerging third nerve in the ventral midbrain or along the proximal part of its course produces a mid-dilated pupil 6 to 7 mm in diameter. Important causes of compression of the third nerve in this region are: *aneurysms, neoplasia,* and *brain herniation* due to increased intracranial pressure. In nearly all cases the pupillary involvement is associated with other signs of third nerve involvement (see p. 2115). Rarely, compressive

lesions such as a posterior communicating artery aneurysm can present with an isolated dilated pupil.

As noted above, the causes of *Horner syndrome* are numerous because of the long course of sympathetic innervation to the eye. It is unlikely that a patient with a central nervous system lesion will present with an isolated Horner syndrome. The most common lesions producing Horner syndrome involve the ascending second order neuron in the neck or the extra-cranial postganglionic neuron; *malignant tumors in the apex of the lung* are by far most common. *Argyll-Robertson pupils* are small (1 to 2 mm), unequal, irregular, and fixed to light; they constrict to accommodation. Their principal cause is tertiary neurosyphilis, although partial Argyll-Robertson changes occur with diabetes and certain of the autonomic neuropathies.

OCULOMOTOR CONTROL

Abnormal eye movements can result from disturbances at several levels. Disconjugate eye movements result from lesions of the individual ocular muscles, the myoneural junctions, the oculomotor nerves and their three paired nuclei in the brain stem and the internuclear medial longitudinal fasciculus (MLF) that yokes the eyes in parallel movements. Supranuclear lesions typically produce disorders of conjugate gaze (gaze palsies).

DEFINITIONS. The term *strabismus* describes an involuntary deviation of the eye from its normal physiological position. *Nonparalytic strabismus* is due to an intrinsic imbalance of ocular muscle tone and is usually congenital. *Paralytic strabismus* results from defects in ocular muscle innervation. Strabismus is called *comitant* when the relationship between the two ocular axes remains constant in all directions of gaze, *noncomitant* when they change, and *latent* when the imbalance is brought out only by covering one eye to prevent fixation. Latent strabismus can become *manifest* during great fatigue or in association with high fever in systemic illness. Congenital comitant strabismus present at birth or soon thereafter carries with it the strong risk that if uncorrected the subject will suppress vision in the nondominant eye during the developmental period when it usually forms its connections with the visual cortex. The result is unilateral, permanent reduction of vision in the nondominant eye (*amblyopia ex anopia*). Strabis-

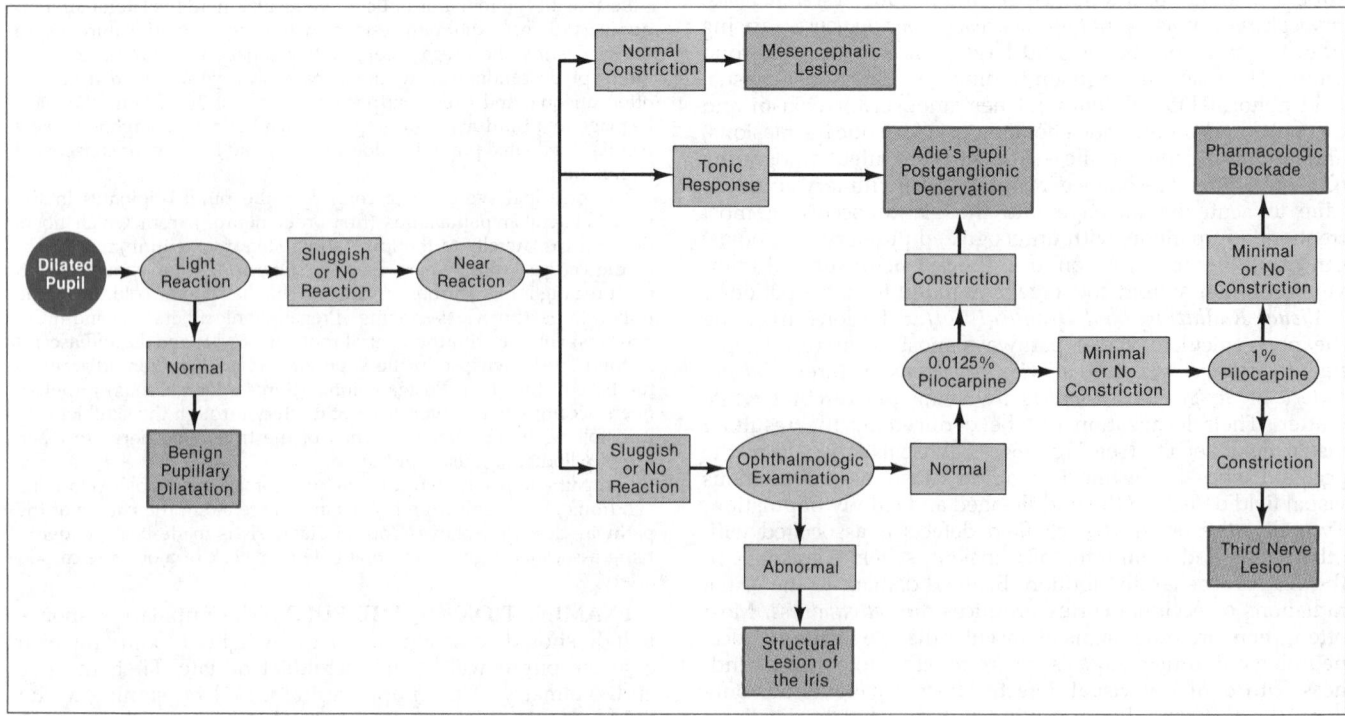

FIGURE 464–2. Evaluation of a dilated pupil.

mus beginning after binocular fusion has developed does not lead to permanent visual loss. *Nystagmus* is an involuntary rhythmic oscillation of the eyes that usually has clearly defined fast and slow components. By convention, the direction of the fast component defines the direction of nystagmus. Physiologic nystagmus refers to nystagmus that occurs in normal subjects, while pathologic nystagmus implies an underlying abnormality. *Physiologic nystagmus* may be vestibular induced (rotatory or caloric), visual induced (optokinetic), or end point (occurring on extreme lateral gaze). *Pathologic nystagmus* may be spontaneous (present in the primary position with the patient seated), positional (induced by change in head position), or gaze evoked (induced by change in eye position).

ANATOMY AND LOCALIZATION OF LESIONS WITHIN THE OCULOMOTOR PATHWAYS. *Nuclear and Internuclear Pathways.*

The abducens nerve supplies the lateral rectus muscle. Selective involvement of the abducens nerve anywhere along its pathway leads to isolated weakness of abduction of the affected eye. Destruction of the abducens nucleus in the brain stem leads to a conjugate gaze paralysis (ipsilateral) because, in addition to oculomotor neurons, the nucleus contains interneurons destined for the contralateral medial rectus nucleus. The trochlear nucleus supplies the contralateral superior oblique muscle which intorts the eye and moves it down. Patients with superior oblique weakness note an increase in diplopia with head tilt toward the side of weakness and often tilt the head in the opposite direction. At rest there is slight upward deviation of the involved eye and downward movement is impaired when the affected eye is turned in. The third cranial nerve supplies the remaining ocular muscles. Involvement of the third nerve nucleus in the midbrain always produces at least some bilateral oculomotor weakness; the superior rectus division of the nucleus supplies the contralateral superior rectus muscle (all other divisions supply ipsilateral muscles). Peripheral third-nerve paralysis can result from lesions damaging the structure anywhere from its origin from the ventral midbrain to where it enters the orbit via the superior orbital fissure. Depending on its completeness, a third nerve palsy produces a widely dilated pupil, severe ptosis, and an externally deviated eye held in position by the unopposed contraction of the lateral rectus muscle. In such conditions, the continued trochlear action reveals itself by intorsion of the eye when the subject attempts to look down and in.

The MLF interconnects the abducens nucleus in the pons with the contralateral oculomotor nuclear complex in the midbrain. It terminates cephalad in the interstitial nucleus in the rostral midbrain and can be traced as far caudad as the thoracocervical region of the spinal cord (co-ordinating nuchal-ocular control). Lesions involving the MLF characteristically produce an internuclear ophthalmoplegia (INO) with which the eyes are conjugate in the primary position but disconjugate on lateral gaze. With a fully developed INO on lateral gaze away from the side of the lesion the contralateral eye abducts and shows nystagmus whereas the ipsilateral adducting eye partially or completely fails to move nasally because of failure of ascending impulses to reach the third nerve nucleus. Adduction for convergence is usually relatively maintained. Upbeat gaze-evoked nystagmus typically occurs with INO.

Supranuclear Pathways. The pathway descending from the frontal eye fields in the frontal lobe regulates rapid voluntary eye movements (*saccades*). A signal from the frontal eye field activates a burst of firing in the contralateral horizontal gaze center in the paramedian pontine reticular formation. This high frequency burst (or pulse) of neuronal firing is transmitted directly to the nearby sixth nerve nucleus and via MLF to the contralateral third nerve nucleus. For voluntary vertical gaze both frontal eye fields send signals to the vertical gaze center in the pretectum (probably the interstitial nucleus of the MLF). Acute lesions involving a frontal eye field (e.g., hemorrhage or infarction) result in transient (24 to 72 hours) inability to direct the eyes contralaterally. Vertical eye movements are not affected by unilateral frontal lobe lesions. Bilateral damage to the frontal eye fields or their descending pathways may produce the inability to move the eyes voluntarily (horizontal or vertical) despite preserved reflex eye movements, a condition called *oculomotor apraxia*. Lesions involving the horizontal-gaze center in the pons produce an ipsilateral paralysis of conjugate gaze and tonic deviation of the eyes to the contralateral hemiorbit. Lesions of the pretectum selectively impair vertical gaze with the vertical up-gaze center being slightly rostral and dorsal to the vertical down-gaze center.

Pathways descending from the parieto-occipital region of the two hemispheres subserve slow visual tracking or *smooth pursuit move-*

ments. The exact location of these descending pursuit pathways is not completely known, but there are strong projections to the ipsilateral superior colliculus and ipsilateral pons. The cerebellar flocculus is also a critical relay station for smooth pursuit pathways. Lesions of the parieto-occipital region, pons, and cerebellum impair smooth pursuit and optokinetic slow phases when the target moves ipsilateral to the lesion. The *convergence* center is located in the rostral-dorsal midbrain near the vertical gaze center. Lesions in this region typically impair convergence and voluntary vertical gaze (particularly up-gaze). Pathways for cortical control of vergence have not been identified. The fourth supranuclear oculomotor control system, the *vestibulo-ocular reflex*, and its examination are discussed in Section 464.3.

EXAMINATION OF EYE MOVEMENTS. Fixation and gaze holding are tested by having the patient, look center, right, left, up, and down. Each position should be held steady and unwavering with the observer documenting carefully abnormal movements or ocular disconjugacies. Each supranuclear oculomotor control system is examined separately. *Saccades* are tested by having the patient fixate alternately on two targets such as the examiner's finger and nose; the speed and accuracy are noted. *Smooth pursuit* is tested by slowly moving a target back and forth and up and down and observing the patient's ability to produce smooth tracking movements. It the target velocity is low (less than 30 degrees per second) normal subjects should be able to pursue without requiring catch-up saccades. *Convergence* is tested by having the patient follow a target moving from far to near. The degree of normal convergence varies considerably and depends on the cooperation of the patient. A clear sign that the patient is attempting to converge is simultaneous pupillary constriction.

COMMON CAUSES OF ABNORMAL OCULOMOTOR CONTROL. *Strabismus.* The flow chart in Figure 464–3 outlines the logic for determining the common causes of strabismus. A comitant strabismus present since childhood is usually a benign *congenital disorder.* As noted earlier, latent congenital strabismus can become manifest in adulthood in association with a systemic illness. An acquired skew deviation (vertical displacement of the ocular axes) can result from any number of lesions involving the brain stem and has little localizing value. Noncomitant strabismus can result from restrictive disease of the orbit or from abnormal muscle or oculomotor nerve function. The presence of mechanical restriction is confirmed by the use of forced duction testing. (After a topical anesthetic is applied to the eye the ophthalmologist grasps the muscle insertion with a large blunt-toothed forceps and identifies mechanical restriction.) Common causes of *orbital restrictive disease* include dysthyroid ophthalmopathy, orbital pseudotumor, trauma, and orbital mass lesions. Variable strabismus that increases with fatigue suggests the likelihood of *myasthenia gravis.* A Tensilon test can usually confirm the diagnosis (see Ch. 518 for description of Tensilon test). If both restrictive disease and myasthenia gravis have been excluded most patients with noncomitant strabismus will have processes affecting the oculomotor nuclei, their fascicles, or the cranial nerves themselves. Common causes of an *isolated third nerve palsy* in an adult include aneurysm, vascular occlusive disease (including diabetes mellitus), trauma, and neoplasm. Typically, but not always, third nerve lesions due to vascular disease spare the pupil. Vascular disease and trauma are by far the most common causes of *isolated trochlear nerve palsies.* The abducens nerve is particularly vulnerable to isolated traumatic involvement because of its long pathway outside the brain stem. Lesions at distant sites that produce increased intracranial pressure can lead to abducens nerve dysfunction producing a "false localizing sign." Other common causes of *isolated sixth nerve palsies* are vascular disease, trauma, and neoplasm. About one fourth of cases with cranial nerve palsies (third, fourth or sixth nerves) remain undiagnosed.

Internuclear Ophthalmoplegia (INO). INO may be unilateral or bilateral, partial or complete, depending on the location of the lesion and the degree of damage to the MLF. *Demyelinating*

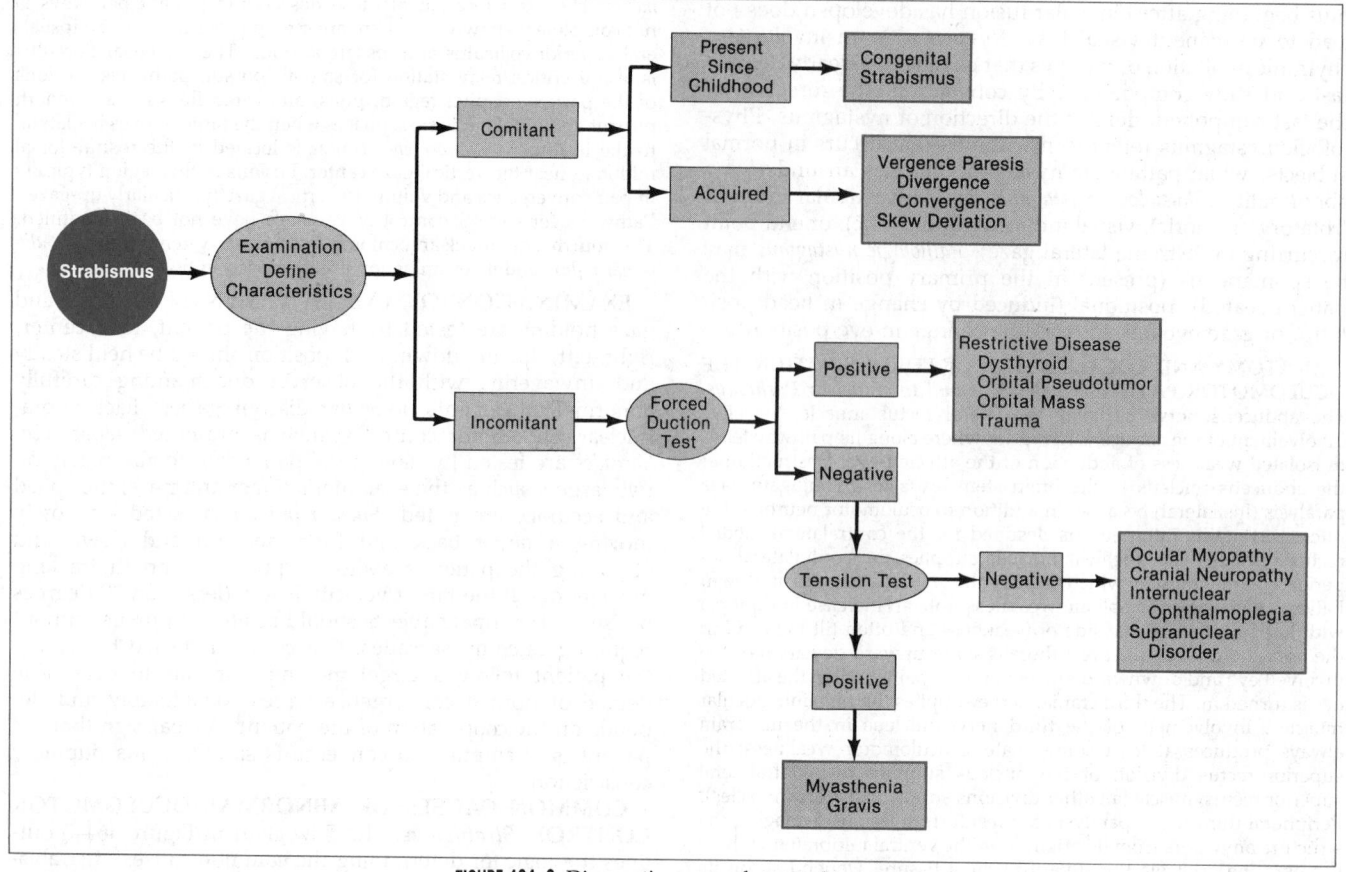

FIGURE 464–3. Diagnostic approach to strabismus.

and small *vascular lesions* are the most common cause of unilateral INO unaccompanied by other ocular palsies or brain-stem signs. Larger brain-stem lesions that damage one or more oculomotor nuclei plus the MLF often produce bizarre combinations of disconjugate eye movements coupled with nuclear oculomotor palsies. Myasthenia gravis can produce an ophthalmoparesis resembling INO owing to the greater involvement of the medial rectus compared to the lateral rectus. Demyelinating diseases are by far the most common causes of bilateral INO involvement.

Disorders of Conjugate Gaze. As noted earlier, infarction of the frontal cortex results in transient contralateral gaze paresis. Tumors and infarction of the paramedian pontine reticular formation produce ipsilateral horizontal gaze paralysis. With the so-called locked-in syndrome (secondary to basilar artery thrombosis) voluntary horizontal eye movements are absent; the patient's only remaining motor functions are vertical eye and lid movements. Lesions of the pretectum typically affect only vertical eye movements, although the descending pathways from the frontal eye fields to the horizontal gaze centers in the pons can also be affected. With the *dorsal midbrain syndrome* (Parinaud syndrome) patients present with a conjugate up-gaze paresis. When they attempt to make upward saccades they develop convergence retraction nystagmus. As noted earlier, impaired convergence and light-near dissociation of the pupillary reflexes are also part of the syndrome. The most common causes of the dorsal midbrain syndrome include tumors of the pineal gland (dysgerminomas), aqueductal stenosis, and localized infarction.

Nystagmus. *Spontaneous nystagmus* can be congenital or acquired. *Congenital nystagmus* typically has a high frequency and variable wave form (occasionally pendular) and is highly fixation-dependent. It is usually not associated with a structural brain lesion. The lifelong history confirms the diagnosis. Spontaneous nystagmus due to a *peripheral vestibular* lesion (i.e., in the labyrinth or vestibular nerve) usually has com-

bined horizontal and torsional components and is strongly inhibited with fixation (Table 464–4). Acquired persistent spontaneous nystagmus that is not inhibited by fixation indicates a lesion in the brain stem and/or cerebellum (*central vestibular*). The latter is often purely vertical or horizontal, since the vertical and horizontal vestibulo-ocular pathways separate beginning at the vestibular nuclei. Spontaneous *downbeat nystagmus* is commonly seen with lesions of the medulla or cervicomedullary junction (e.g., Arnold-Chiari malformation).

Gaze-evoked nystagmus is always in the direction of gaze and is usually present with and without fixation. It is most commonly produced by ingestion of *drugs* such as phenobarbital, phenytoin, alcohol and diazepam. It can also occur in patients with such varied conditions as myasthenia gravis, multiple sclerosis, and cerebellar atrophy. Asymmetrical horizontal gaze-evoked nystagmus indicates a structural brain-stem or cerebellar lesion (particularly at the cerebellopontine angle) with the lesion usually being on the side of the larger amplitude nystagmus. *Rebound nystagmus* is a type of gaze-

TABLE 464–4. KEY DISTINGUISHING FEATURES OF PERIPHERAL AND CENTRAL TYPES OF SPONTANEOUS AND POSITIONAL NYSTAGMUS

Type of Nystagmus	Peripheral (End Organ and Nerve)	Central (Brain Stem and Cerebellum)
Spontaneous	Unidirectional, fast phase away from lesion, combined horizontal torsional, inhibited with fixation	Bidirectional or unidirectional; often pure horizontal, vertical, or torsional; *not* inhibited with fixation
Static positional	Direction-fixed or direction-changing, inhibited with fixation	Direction fixed or direction-changing, *not* inhibited with fixation
Paroxysmal positional	Vertical-torsional occasionally horizontal-torsional, vertigo prominent, fatigability, latency	Often pure vertical, vertigo less prominent, no latency, nonfatigable

evoked nystagmus that either disappears or reverses direction as the eccentric gaze position is held. When the eyes are returned to the primary position nystagmus occurs in the direction of the return saccade. Rebound nystagmus occurs in patients with cerebellar atrophy and focal structural lesions of the cerebellum; it is the only variety of nystagmus thought to be specific for cerebellar involvement. *Disconjugate gaze-evoked nystagmus* most commonly results from lesions of the MLF (see above), but it can also occur with other lesions of the brain stem involving the oculomotor nuclei. Positional nystagmus is discussed on page 2121.

Other Ocular Oscillations. Ocular bobbing consists of a fast conjugate downward eye movement followed by a slow return to the primary position. The phenomenon accompanies severe displacement or destruction of the pons or, much less often, metabolic CNS depression. *Ocular myoclonus* consists of continuous rhythmic pendular oscillations, most often vertical, with a rate of 2 to 5 beats per second. Often it accompanies palatal myoclonus and has a similar pathogenesis. *Square wave jerks* and *ocular flutter* consist of brief, intermittent, horizontal oscillations (saccades) arising from the primary gaze position. These types of ocular oscillation are most commonly seen with cerebellar disease but can also accompany more diffuse central nervous system disorders. *Opsoclonus* consists of rapid, chaotic, conjugate, repetitive, saccadic eye movements (dancing eyes). One type of opsoclonus accompanies cerebellar dysfunction, but the most chaotic varieties are associated with brain-stem encephalitis or the remote effects of systemic neoplasm, especially neuroblastoma in children. *Ocular dysmetria* refers to over- and undershooting of saccadic eye movements often followed by multiple attempts at refixation. It reflects cerebellar dysfunction.

Burde RM, Savino PJ, Trobe JD: Clinical Decisions in Neuro-ophthalmology. St. Louis, The C. V. Mosby Company, 1985. *Liberal use of flow charts to help the clinician answer the question, "Given the symptom and signs, what is the disease?"*

Glaser JS: Neuro-ophthalmology. Hagerstown, MD, Harper & Row, 1977. *An excellent one-volume didactic introductory text.*

Zee DS, Leigh RJ: Disorders of Ocular Movement. Philadelphia, F. A. Davis Company, 1983. *An up-to-date monograph that gives the clinical and physiological details of modern investigations on ocular control.*

Hearing and Equilibrium

The neural pathways subserving hearing and those most important for equilibrium and spatial orientation are anatomically proximate in much of their course from their end organs in the inner ear to their termination in the superior portion of the temporal lobe. Because of the close anatomic linkage, disorders that affect hearing often affect equilibrium, and vice versa. For this reason they are considered together here. Despite their anatomical propinquity, however, substantial pathophysiologic differences make clinical examination of the two systems quite different. The auditory system is physiologically relatively isolated, so that its function and dysfunction can be tested independently of other neural systems. The vestibular system, in contrast, has many close physiologic links with the motor system (particularly the cerebellum, oculomotor system, and autonomic nervous system) and can be tested only indirectly by noting secondary effects on oculomotor and cerebellar functions. Abnormalities of the auditory system lead to only a few well-defined and unique symptoms (i.e., hearing loss or tinnitus). Abnormalities of the vestibular system can cause symptoms that mimic disorders of the other neural structures. Such symptoms include dizziness, ocular abnormalities (nystagmus), motor abnormalities (including ataxia or sudden falls), and autonomic abnormalities (including nausea, vomiting, and even syncope).

HEARING

DEFINITIONS. *Hearing loss* is usually expressed in terms of the ability to hear *pure tones*, which are defined by their frequency and intensity. In order to quantify the magnitude of hearing loss, normal hearing levels are defined by an international standard. These levels approximate the intensity of the faintest sound that can be heard by normal ears. A patient's hearing level is the difference in decibels (dB) between the faintest pure tone that he can hear and the normal reference level given by the standard. *Tinnitus* refers to noises that arise spontaneously in one or both ears. With *diplacusis* the tonal quality of a pure tone is distorted so that it may sound like a complex mixture of tones.

ANATOMY AND PHYSIOLOGY OF HEARING. In normal hearing, sound waves are transmitted from the tympanic membrane via the three ossicles of the air-filled middle ear (air conduction) to the oval window and the basilar membrane of the fluid-sealed cochlea. The ossicles serve to increase the gain from the tympanum to oval window about 18-fold, compensating for the loss that sound waves moving from air to fluid would otherwise suffer. In the absence of this system, sound may reach the cochlea by vibration of the temporal bone (bone conduction) but with much less efficiency (approximately 60 dB loss). Hair cells lying along the cochlear basilar membrane detect the vibratory movement of that membrane and transduce vibration into nerve impulses. The nerve impulses are relayed via nerve cells that synapse at the base of hair cells and have their bodies in the spiral ganglion to the cochlear nucleus of the ipsilateral pontine tegmentum. The spiral cochlea mechanically analyzes the frequency content of sound. For high frequency tones only sensory cells in the basilar region are activated, whereas for low frequency tones all or nearly all sensory cells are activated. Therefore, with lesions of the cochlea and its afferent nerve the hearing levels for different frequencies are usually unequal, typically resulting in better hearing sensitivity for low frequency than for high frequency tones. Within the brain stem, auditory signals ascend from the ventral and dorsal cochlear nuclei to reach the superior olivary nuclei of both sides. Thus nervous system lesions central to the cochlear nucleus do not cause monaural hearing loss, and, conversely, unilateral central lesions do not cause deafness. From these structures the pathway projects by way of the lateral lemnisci to the inferior colliculi. Each inferior colliculus transmits to the other and to its ipsilateral medial geniculate body, which in turn sends the final projection to the transverse auditory gyrus lying in the superior portion of the ipsilateral temporal lobe.

The normal ear can detect sound frequencies ranging between 20 to 20,000 Hertz (Hz); the upper range drops off fairly rapidly with advancing age. The ear is most sensitive between 500 and 4,000 Hz, which roughly corresponds to the frequency range most important for understanding speech. The hearing level in this range has several practical implications in terms of the degree of handicap and the potential for useful correction with amplification. A 30 to 40 dB hearing level in the speech range would impair normal conversation, whereas an 80 dB hearing level would make everyday auditory communication almost impossible (the social definition of deafness).

LOCALIZATION OF LESIONS WITHIN THE AUDITORY PATHWAYS. *Conductive hearing loss* results from lesions involving the external or middle ear. It is typically characterized by an approximately equal loss of hearing at all frequencies and by well preserved speech discrimination once the threshold for hearing is exceeded. Patients with conductive hearing loss can hear speech in a noisy background better than in a quiet background because they can understand loud speech as well as anyone.

Sensorineural hearing loss results from lesions of the cochlea and/or auditory division of the eighth cranial nerve. With sensorineural hearing loss the hearing levels for different frequencies are usually unequal, typically resulting in better hearing for low- than for high-frequency tones. Patients with sensorineural hearing loss often have difficulty hearing speech that is mixed with background noise and may be annoyed by loud speech. Three important manifestations of sensorineural lesions are diplacusis, recruitment, and tone decay. Diplacusis and recruitment are common with cochlear lesions; tone decay usually accompanies eighth nerve involvement.

Central hearing disorders result from lesions of the central auditory pathways. As a rule patients with central lesions do not have impaired hearing for pure tones, and they can understand speech as long as it is clearly spoken in a quiet environment. If the listener's task is made more difficult with the introduction of background noise or competing messages, performance deteriorates more markedly in patients with central lesions than in normal subjects.

EXAMINATION OF HEARING. *Bedside Test.* A quick test for hearing loss in the speech range is to observe the response to spoken commands at different intensities (whisper, conversation, shouting). Tuning fork tests permit a rough assessment of the hearing level for pure tones of known frequency. The clinician can use his own hearing level as a reference standard. In the Rinne test nerve conduction is compared to bone conduction by holding a tuning fork (preferably 512 Hz) against the mastoid process until the sound can no longer be heard. It is then placed 1 inch from the ear and in normal subjects can be heard about twice as long by air as by bone. If bone conduction is better than air conduction, the hearing loss is conductive, but care must be taken to assure that the bone conduction is not heard in the normal ear. In the Weber test, the tuning fork is placed on the patient's forehead or upper teeth. Normally this sound is referred to the center of the head. If it is referred to the side of unilateral hearing loss, the hearing loss is conductive; if it is referred away from the side of unilateral hearing loss, the loss is sensorineural. The Weber test is often unreliable in conductive hearing loss because the patient cannot accept the fact that he hears better in what he knows to be the diseased ear.

Audiometry. *Pure tone testing* is the nucleus of most auditory examinations. Pure tones at selected frequencies are presented via either earphones (air conduction) or a vibrator pressed against the mastoid portion of the temporal bone (bone conduction), and the minimal level that the subject can hear is determined for each frequency. Two speech tests are routinely used. The *speech reception threshold* (SRT) is the intensity at which the patient can correctly repeat 50 per cent of the words presented. The SRT is a test of hearing sensitivity for speech and should reflect the hearing level for pure tones in the speech range. The *speech discrimination test* is a measure of the patient's ability to understand speech when it is presented at a level that is easily heard. In patients with eighth nerve lesions speech discriminations can be severely reduced, even when pure tone thresholds are normal or nearly normal, whereas in patients with cochlear lesions discrimi-

nation tends to be proportional to the magnitude of hearing loss.

Recruitment is usually measured by the alternating binaural loudness balance (ABLB) test (if the hearing loss is unilateral). This test compares the loudness for tones of varied intensities as perceived by the pathologic ear and the normal ear. Recruitment is present if smaller increases in stimulus intensity are required in the poorer ear than in the better ear to maintain equal loudness. Otologists employ a variety of special tests to evaluate hearing loss, including the fistula test, tone decay, distorted speech testing and dichotic stimulation, acoustic impedance, tympanometry, and stapedius muscle contraction. The text by DeWeese and Saunders gives details.

Brain stem auditory evoked responses (BAER) can be recorded from scalp electrodes at 0 to 10 msec (early), 10 to 50 msec (middle), and 50 to 500 msec (late) following a click stimulus. The early potentials reflect electrical activity at the cochlea, eighth cranial nerve, and brain stem; the later potentials reflect cortical activity. Computer averaging of the responses to 1,000 to 2,000 clicks separates the evoked potential from background noise. Early evoked responses may be used to estimate the magnitude of hearing loss and to differentiate among cochlea, eighth nerve, and brain-stem lesions.

CAUSES OF HEARING LOSS. *Conductive Hearing Loss.* The logic for identifying common causes of hearing loss is shown in Figure 464-4. The history, examination, and audiometry usually provide the key differential features. The most common cause of conductive hearing loss is *impacted cerumen* in the external canal. This benign condition is usually first noticed after bathing or swimming when a droplet of water closes the remaining tiny passageway. The most common serious cause of conductive hearing loss is inflammation of the middle ear, *otitis media*, either infected (suppurative) or noninfective (serous). Fluid accumulates in the middle ear impairing the conduction of airborne sound. Since the air cavity of the middle ear is in direct connection with the mastoid air cells, infection can spread through the mastoid bone and, occasionally, into the intracranial cavity. Chronic otitis media with perforation of the tympanic membrane can result in an invasion of the middle ear and other pneumatized areas of the temporal bone by keratonizing squamous epithelium (*cholesteatoma*). Cholesteatomas can produce erosion of the ossicles and bony labyrinth resulting in a mixed conductive sensorineural hearing loss. *Otosclerosis* commonly produces progressive conductive hearing loss by immobilizing

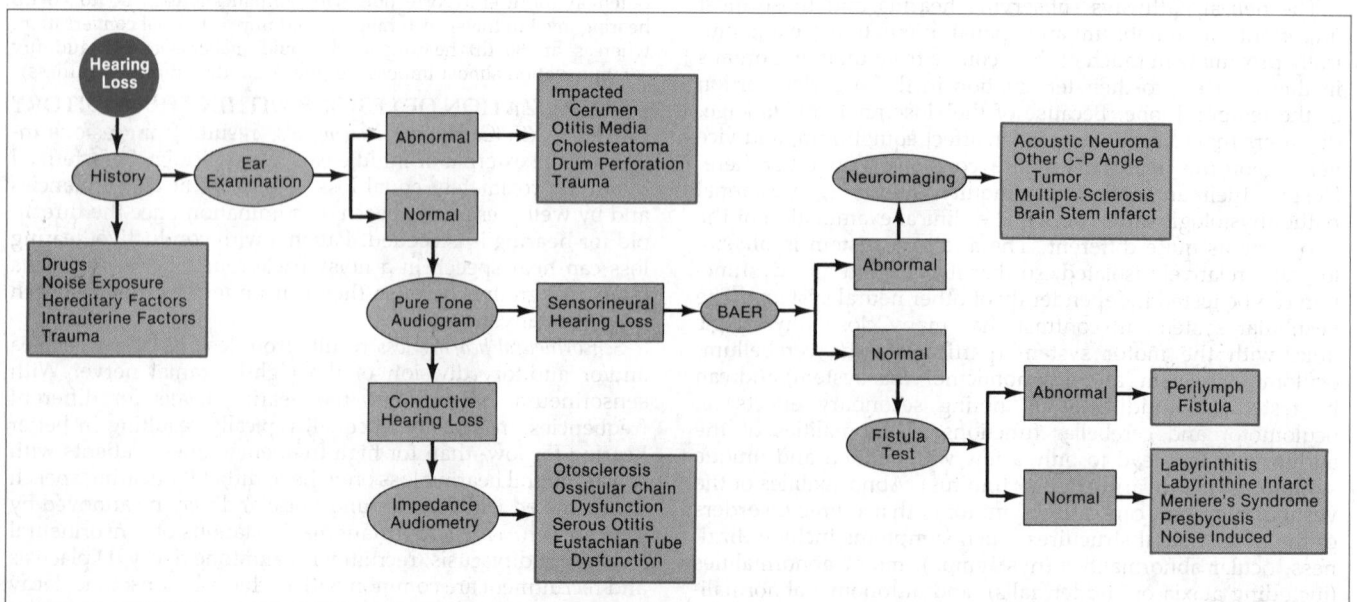

FIGURE 464-4. Evaluation of deafness.

the stapes with new bone growth in front of and below the oval window. The hearing loss is typically conductive, although in some persons the cochlea may be invaded by foci of otosclerotic bone producing an additional sensorineural hearing loss. Otosclerosis usually stabilizes when the hearing level reaches 50 to 60 dB and rarely progresses to deafness. Other common causes of conductive hearing loss include trauma, congenital malformations of the external and middle ear, and glomus body tumors.

Sensorineural Hearing Loss. Genetically determined deafness, usually from hair cell aplasia or deterioration, may be present at birth or may develop in adulthood. The diagnosis of *hereditary deafness* rests on the finding of a positive family history. In many instances the inheritance is through a recessive gene or a dominant gene with low penetrance, making it difficult to determine the genetic nature of the disorder. *Intrauterine factors* resulting in congenital hearing loss include infection (especially rubella); toxic, metabolic, and endocrine disorders; and anoxia associated with Rh incompatibility and difficult deliveries.

Acute unilateral deafness usually has a cochlear basis. *Bacterial or viral infections* of the labyrinth, *head trauma* with fracture or hemorrhage into the cochlea, or *vascular occlusion* of a terminal branch of the anterior inferior cerebellar artery all can damage extensively the cochlea and its hair cells. An acute idiopathic, often reversible, unilateral hearing loss strikes young adults and is presumed to reflect an isolated viral infection of the cochlea and auditory nerve terminals. Sudden unilateral hearing loss often associated with vertigo and tinnitus can result from a *perilymphatic fistula.* Such fistulae may be congenital or may follow stapes surgery or head trauma. *Drugs* cause acute and subacute bilateral hearing impairment. Salicylates, furosemide, and ethacrynic acid have the potential to produce transient deafness when taken in high doses. More toxic to the cochlea are aminoglycoside antibiotics (gentamicin, tobramycin, amikacin, kanamycin, streptomycin and neomycin). These agents can destroy cochlear hair cells in direct relation to their serum concentrations. Some antineoplastic chemotherapeutic agents, particularly cisplatin, cause severe ototoxicity.

Subacute relapsing cochlear deafness occurs with *Meniere syndrome,* a condition associated with fluctuating hearing loss and tinnitus, recurrent episodes of abrupt and often severe vertigo, and a sensation of fullness or pressure in the ear. Recurrent endolymphatic hypertension (hydrops) is believed to cause the episodes. Pathologically, the endolymphatic sac is dilated, and the hair cells become atrophic. The resulting deafness is subtle and reversible in the early stages but subsequently becomes permanent and is characterized by diplacusis and loudness recruitment. The disorder is usually unilateral, but in about 20 to 40 per cent of patients bilateral involvement will occur.

The gradual, progressive, bilateral, hearing loss commonly associated with advancing age is called *presbycusis.* Presbycusis is not a distinct disease entity but rather represents multiple effects of aging on the auditory system. It may include conductive and central dysfunction, although the most consistent effect of aging is on the sensory cells and neurons of the cochlea. The typical audiogram of presbycusis is a symmetrical high-frequency hearing loss gradually sloping downward with increasing frequency. The most consistent pathology associated with presbycusis is degeneration of sensory cells and nerve fibers at the base of the cochlea. The recurrent trauma of *noise-induced hearing loss* affects approximately the same cochlear region and is almost as common, particularly among those with exposure to loud explosive or industrial noises. Loud, blaring, modern music has become a recent offender. The loss almost always begins at 4,000 Hz and does not affect speech discrimination until late in the disease process. With only brief exposure to loud noise (hours to days) there may be only a temporary threshold shift, but with

continued exposure permanent injury begins. The duration and intensity of exposure determine the degree of permanent injury.

Hearing loss from direct damage to the acoustic nerve in the petrous canal occasionally results from infection within or trauma to the surrounding bone; severe deafness of abrupt onset marks the event and is usually associated with acute vertigo due to concurrent vestibular nerve injury. Progressive unilateral hearing loss that arises insidiously and worsens by almost imperceptible degrees is characteristic of benign neoplasms of the cerebellopontine angle, such as *acoustic neuromas.* In about 10 per cent of cases the hearing loss can be acute, apparently owing to either hemorrhage into the tumor or compression of the labyrinthine vasculature.

Central Hearing Loss. Central hearing loss is unilateral only if it results from damage to the pontine cochlear nuclei on one side of the brain stem. Such can occur with *ischemic infarction* of the lateral brain stem (e.g., occlusion of the anterior inferior cerebellar artery), a plaque of *multiple sclerosis,* or, rarely, invasion or compression of the lateral pons by a *neoplasm* or *hematoma.* Bilateral *degeneration* of the cochlear nuclei accompanies some of the rare recessive inherited disorders of childhood. As noted, clinically important unilateral hearing loss never results from neurologic disease arising rostrad to the cochlear nucleus. Although bilateral hearing loss could, in theory, result from bilateral destruction of central hearing pathways, in practice this is rare since involvement of neighboring structures in brain stem or hemisphere would usually produce overwhelming neurologic disability.

TREATMENT OF HEARING LOSS. If an underlying disorder has not yet destroyed the auditory system and can be ameliorated medically or surgically, hearing may be improved or preserved. Most patients with otosclerosis respond to stapedectomy. Closure of a perilymph fistula may improve hearing. Antibiotic and decongestive treatment of otitis media should prevent permanent hearing loss. A low-salt diet and diuretics are effective in selective cases of Meniere syndrome, particularly if episodes are precipitated by premenstrual water retention. The surgical treatment of Meniere syndrome is still controversial. Hearing aids amplify sound, usually with the goal of making speech intelligible. Patients with conductive hearing loss require simple amplification, but those with sensorineural hearing loss often need frequency selective amplification in order to make hearing aids useful. Recent advances in acoustic technology have markedly improved the outlook for the latter. Monitoring audiograms in patients with noise- or ototoxic drug exposure are critical for prevention of permanent hearing loss.

TINNITUS. The flow chart in Figure 464–5 outlines the logic for determining the common causes of tinnitus. A careful history should be taken to identify common offending drugs (Table 464–5). With *objective tinnitus* the patient hears a sound arising external to the auditory system, a sound that can usually be heard by the examiner with a stethoscope. Objective tinnitus usually has benign causes such as noise from temporomandibular joints, opening of eustachian tubes, or repetitive muscle contractions. Sometimes, in a quiet room, the patient can hear the pulsatile flow in the carotid artery or a continuous hum of normal venous outflow through the jugular vein. The latter can be obliterated by compression of the jugular vein or extreme lateral rotation of the neck. Pathological objective tinnitus occurs when patients hear turbulent flow in vascular anomalies or tumors (e.g., glomus jugulare tumor). Objective tinnitus may also be an early sign of increased intracranial pressure. Such tinnitus, which is usually overshadowed by other neurologic abnormalities, can be obliterated by pressure over the jugular vein. It probably arises from turbulent flow through compressed venous structures at the base of the brain.

Subjective tinnitus can arise from sites anywhere in the auditory system. The sounds most frequently complained of

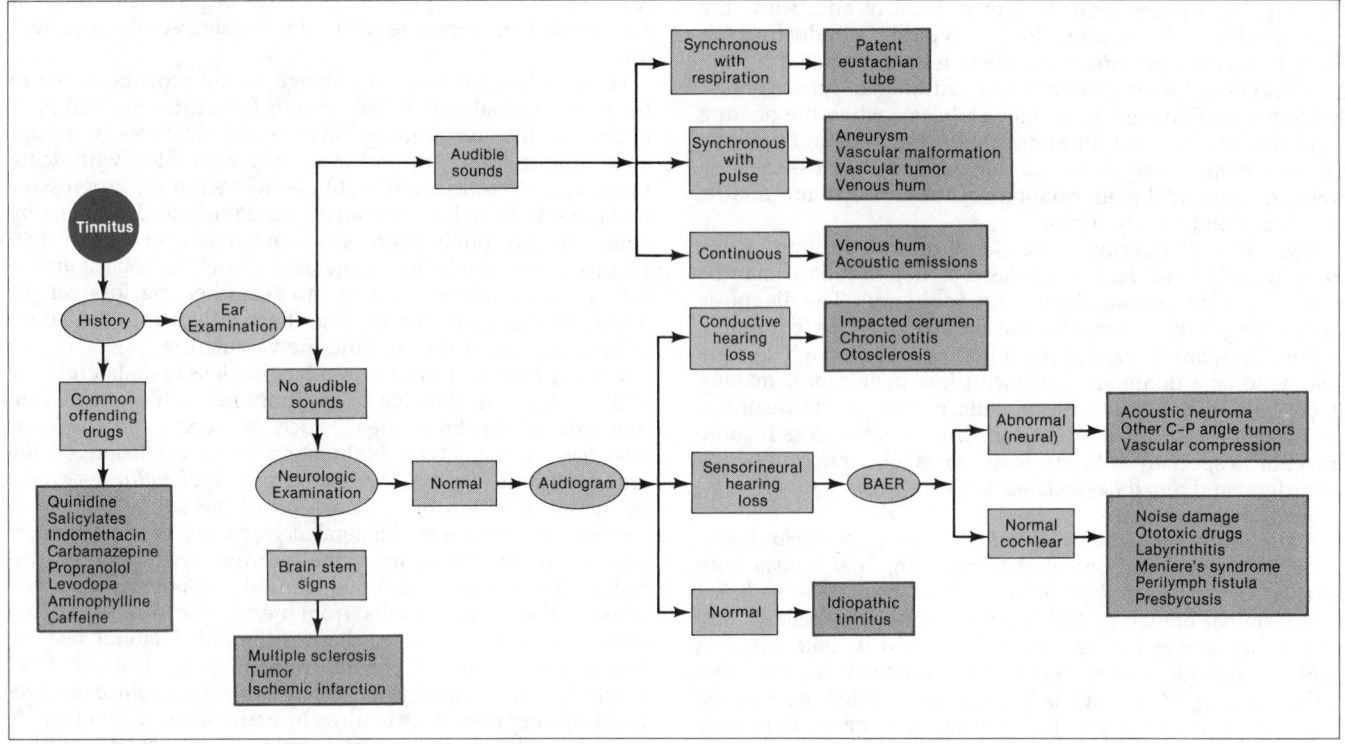

FIGURE 464–5. Evaluation of tinnitus.

are metallic ringing, buzzing, blowing, roaring, or, less often, bizarre clanging, popping, or nonrhythmic beating. Tinnitus heard as a faint, moderately high-pitched, metallic ring can be observed by almost anyone who concentrates attention on auditory events in a quiet room. Sustained louder tinnitus accompanied by audiometric evidence of deafness occurs in association with both conductive and sensorineural hearing loss. Tinnitus observed with otosclerosis tends to have a roaring or hissing quality, while that associated with Meniere syndrome often produces sounds that vary widely in intensity with time and quality, sometimes including roaring or clanging. Tinnitus with other cochlear or auditory nerve lesions tends to be higher pitched and ringing in quality. Audiometric and brain-stem evoked response testing can help distinguish betwen lesions involving the conducting apparatus, the cochlea, and the auditory nerve.

Tinnitus without observable deafness appears sporadically and for variable lengths of time in many persons without other evidence of an ongoing pathological process. In many instances one suspects that the auditory experience is no more than an anxious preoccupation with normal auditory physiology.

TREATMENT OF TINNITUS. Most patients with tinnitus can be helped by detailed interview together with the relevant examination and laboratory investigations followed by reassurance where this can be given. Often exacerbating factors such as chronic anxiety and depression can be identified. In patients with hearing loss and tinnitus a hearing aid may improve communication in two ways, as amplification of ambient sound may effectively mask the tinnitus. This mechanism probably explains the frequent observation that removal of cerumen from the external auditory canal to improve ambient hearing also improves tinnitus. Also, when cerumen is attached to the tympanic membrane, tinnitus may result from local mechanical effects on the conductive system. For

patients who find their tinnitus most obtrusive when trying to sleep, a bedside FM clock radio tuned between stations can provide an effective masking sound that will switch itself off after the patient falls asleep. A careful drug history should be taken, and a drug-free trial period should be considered when possible. Some patients who notice that caffeine, alcohol, or nicotine exacerbates their tinnitus, experience significant relief when these drugs are discontinued.

Surgical treatment of tinnitus has been disappointing. Even when a lesion can be localized to the inner ear or cochlear nerve, removing these structures often has little effect on the tinnitus. A single exception to the generally dismal record of surgical treatment of tinnitus is complete cure of objective tinnitus after surgical correction of a vascular malformation or tumor in the mastoid.

EQUILIBRIUM—VESTIBULAR SYSTEM

DEFINITIONS. *Vertigo* is a subtype of dizziness in which there is an illusion of movement, most commonly rotation. *Physiologic vertigo* occurs in normal subjects when there is a mismatch among the vestibular, visual, and somatosensory systems induced by some external stimulus. The most common example is coming to a sudden stop after several whirling turns. The vestibular signals arising from the semicircular canals are in conflict with the visual signals that indicate a stable surround. *Pathological vertigo* occurs when there is an imbalance in the vestibular system caused by a lesion within the vestibular pathways anywhere from the inner ear to the cerebral cortex. *Oscillopsia* refers to an illusion of oscillation of the environment.

ANATOMY AND PHYSIOLOGY OF THE VESTIBULAR SYSTEM. The paired vestibular end organs lie within the temporal bones next to the cochlea. Each organ consists of three semicircular canals that detect angular acceleration and two otolith structures, the utricle and saccule, that detect linear acceleration (including gravitational). Like the cochlea, these organs possess hair cells that act as force transducers converting the forces associated with head acceleration into afferent nerve impulses. The hair cells of the three semicircular canals, each of which is oriented at right angles to the others, are concentrated in the crista, where they are embedded in a gelatinous mass called the cupula. Movement of the head causes the endolymph to flow either toward or away from the cupula, bending the hair cells

TABLE 464–5. DRUGS COMMONLY ASSOCIATED WITH TINNITUS

Quinidine	Propranolol
Salicylates	Levodopa
Indomethacin	Aminophylline
Carbamazepine	Caffeine

and, depending on the direction of endolymphatic movements, either exciting or inhibiting the afferent nerve firing. Since the afferent nerves arising from the semicircular canals are tonically active, the baseline activity can be increased or decreased depending on the direction of hair cell bending. Furthermore, the two sets of semicircular canals are approximately mirror images of each other, so that rotational movement of the head that excites one canal will inhibit the analogous canal on the opposite side. The hair cells of the utricle and saccule are concentrated in an area called the macule. The macule of the utricle lies approximately in the plane of the horizontal canal and the macule of the saccule is approximately in the plane of the anterior canal. The hair cells are imbedded in a membrane that contains calcium carbonate crystals or otoliths; the density of otoliths is considerably greater than that of the endolymph. Linear accelerations of the head combine with the linear acceleration of gravity to distort the otolith membrane thereby bending the underlying hair cells and modulating the activity of the afferent nerve terminals at the base of the hair cells.

The afferent vestibular nerves have their cell bodies in Scarpa's ganglion. The nerve fibers travel in the vestibular portion of the eighth cranial nerve contiguous to the acoustic portion. Fibers from different receptor organs terminate in different vestibular nuclei at the pontomedullary junction. There are also direct connections with many portions of the cerebellum, the greatest respresentation being in the flocculonocular lobe, the so-called vestibular cerebellum. Efferent fibers from the brain stem travel through the vestibular nucleus to reach hair cells of the semicircular canals and macules. Efferent fibers are inhibitory in nature and, like the efferent fibers of the cochlea, may function to enhance inputs to which the brain will attend. From the vestibular nuclei second order neurons make important connections to the vestibular nuclei of the other side, to the cerebellum, to motor neurons of the spinal cord, to autonomic nuclei in the brain stem, and, most importantly for the examining clinician, to the nuclei of the oculomotor system. Fibers from the vestibular nuclei also ascend through the brain stem and thalamus to reach the cerebral cortex bilaterally. The exact site of cortical representation is unclear. Clinical evidence points to both superior temporal and inferior parietal lobes as likely sites.

LOCALIZATION OF LESIONS WITHIN THE VESTIBULAR PATHWAYS. Vertigo can be caused by either the peripheral or central vestibular apparatus. In general, peripheral vertigo is more severe, is more likely to be associated with hearing loss and tinnitus, and often leads to nausea and vomiting. Nystagmus associated with peripheral vertigo is usually inhibited by visual fixation. Central vertigo is generally less severe than peripheral vertigo and is often associated with other signs of central nervous system disease. The nystagmus of central vertigo is not inhibited by visual fixation and frequently is prominent when vertigo is mild or absent.

EXAMINATION OF THE VESTIBULAR SYSTEM. Most vestibular problems presenting to the physician are episodic, and often there are neither symptoms nor signs when the physician examines the patient. The history, therefore, can become paramount for identifying vestibular dysfunction. The history should attempt to distinguish vertigo (the illusion of movement in space) from light-headedness (presyncope), ataxia (disequilibrium of the body without true movement in space), and psychogenic symptoms (the feeling of dissociation or, sometimes, dysequilibrium). If the history is not clear, bedside provocative tests to mimic the symptom may assist in making a pathophysiological diagnosis. Hyperventilation, which lowers the $PaCO_2$ and decreases cerebral blood flow, causes a light-headed sensation associated with syncope. Ask the patient to hyperventilate maximally for 1 to 3 minutes to cause light-headedness. If the episode mimics the patient's symptoms it suggests that anxiety and hyperventilation may be playing an important role. In addition, during the course of hyperventilation the patient may suffer dry mouth, chest tightness, and paresthesias, which he may recognize as part of his spontaneous attacks, thus helping in diagnosis.

Bedside tests of vestibulospinal function are often insensitive because most patients can use vision and proprioceptive signals to compensate for any vestibular loss. Patients with acute unilateral peripheral vestibular lesions may past point

or fall toward the side of the lesion, but within a few days balance returns to normal. Patients with bilateral peripheral vestibular loss have more difficulty compensating and usually will show some imbalance on the Romberg and tandem walking tests, particularly with eyes closed.

The vestibulo-ocular reflex can be tested at the bedside by inducing physiological nystagmus and searching for pathological nystagmus. In an alert human, rotating the head back and forth in the horizontal plane induces compensatory horizontal eye movements that are dependent on both the smooth pursuit and vestibular systems. Because of the combined visual and vestibular input, a patient with complete loss of vestibular function and normal pursuit may still have normal compensatory eye movements on this test. The doll's-eye test is a useful bedside test of vestibular function in a comatose patient, however, since such patients cannot generate pursuit or corrective fast components. In this setting slow conjugate compensatory eye movements indicate normally functioning vestibulo-ocular pathways. Since the vestibulo-ocular reflex has a much higher frequency range than the smooth pursuit system, a qualitative bedside test of vestibular function can be made by having the patient shake his head back and forth at frequencies above 1 Hz while reading a standard visual acuity chart. A decrease in visual acuity of more than one line compared to testing with the head still indicates an abnormal vestibulo-ocular reflex.

The caloric test uses a nonphysiologic stimulus to induce endolymphatic flow in the horizontal semicircular canal and horizontal nystagmus by creating a temperature gradient from one side of the canal to the other. With a cold caloric stimulus the column of endolymph nearest the middle ear falls because of its increased density. This causes the cupula to deviate away from the utricle (ampullofugal flow) and produces horizontal nystagmus with the fast phase directed away from the stimulated ear. A warm stimulus produces the opposite effect causing ampullopedal endolymph flow and nystagmus directed toward the stimulated ear (mnemonic: COWS—cold opposite, warm same). Because of its ready availability ice water (approximately 0° C) is usually used for bedside caloric testing. To bring the horizontal canal into the vertical plane the patient lies in the supine position with head tilted 30 degrees forward. Infusion of 10 ml of ice water induces a burst of nystagmus usually lasting from 1 to 3 minutes. A comatose patient shows only a slow tonic deviation toward the side of stimulation. Greater than a 20 per cent asymmetry in nystagmus duration suggests a lesion on the side of the decreased response. This should always be confirmed, however, with standard bithermal caloric testing and electronystagmography (see below).

Examination for pathological vestibular nystagmus should include a search for spontaneous and positional nystagmus (see Table 464-4). Since vestibular nystagmus secondary to peripheral vestibular lesions is inhibited with fixation, the yield is increased by impairing fixation (such as with +30 lenses, Frenzel glasses). Two general types of positional nystagmus can be identified on the basis of nystagmus regularity: static and paroxysmal. One induces static positional nystagmus by slowly placing the patient into the supine, then right lateral, and then left lateral position. This type of positional nystagmus persists as long as the position is held. Since direction-changing and direction-fixed static positional nystagmus occur with both peripheral and central vestibular lesions, their presence indicates only a dysfunction somewhere in the vestibular system. As with spontaneous nystagmus, however, lack of suppression with fixation and signs of associated brain-stem dysfunction suggest a central lesion.

Paroxysmal positional nystagmus is induced, after a brief delay, by a rapid change from erect sitting to supine headhanging left, center, or right position (the so-called Hallpike maneuver). It is initially high in frequency but dissipates rapidly (within 30 seconds to 1 minute). The most common variety of paroxysmal positional nystagmus, benign positional nystagmus, usually has a 3 to 10 second latency before onset and rarely lasts longer than 30 seconds. The nystagmus is always torsional with fast phase directed upward (i.e., toward the forehead). It is usually prominent in only one head-hanging position, and a burst of nystagmus in the reverse direction occurs when the patient reassumes the sitting position. Another key feature is the severe vertigo and nystagmus that the patient experiences with the initial positioning which, with repeated positioning, rapidly disappear (fatigability). Benign positional nystagmus is a sign of vestibular end-organ disease (probably damage to the posterior semicircular canal, see p. 2123).

Electronystagmography (ENG) is a technique for recording eye movements that allows precise quantification of both physiologic and pathologic nystagmus. A standard ENG test battery includes: (1) Tests of visual ocular control (saccades, smooth pursuit, and optokinetic nystagmus); (2) a careful search for pathologic nystagmus with fixation and with eyes open in darkness, and (3) measurement of induced physiological nystagmus (caloric and rotational). ENG can be helpful in identifying a vestibular lesion and localizing it within the peripheral and central pathways.

EVALUATING THE "DIZZY" PATIENT. Figure 464–6 summarizes the evaluation for several common types of dizziness. The history is key, since it determines the type of dizziness (vertigo, light-headed, feeling of dissociation, disequilibrium), associated symptoms (neurologic, audiologic, cardiac, psychiatric), precipitating factors (position change, trauma, stress, drug ingestion), and predisposing illness (systemic viral infection, cardiac disease, cerebrovascular disease). The examination should include complete neurologic, head and neck, and cardiac assessments. When focal neurologic signs are found, neuroimaging usually leads to specific diagnosis. When vertigo is present without focal neurologic symptoms or signs, audiometry and electronystagmography aid in localizing the lesion to the labyrinth or eighth nerve. Patients with hyperventilation syndrome and/or acute anxiety should be identified after the history and examination so that needless tests are not obtained. A detailed cardiac evaluation (including Holter monitoring) often identifies the cause of episodic presyncopal light-headedness. Patients complaining of disequilibrium without focal neurologic signs require ENG assessment to rule out bilateral vestibular loss.

COMMON CAUSES OF VERTIGO. *Physiologic Vertigo.* Physiologic vertigo includes common disorders such as *motion sickness*, *space sickness*, and *height vertigo*. In these conditions vertigo (defined as an illusion of movement) is minimal or absent while autonomic symptoms predominate. With height vertigo, patients often experience acute anxiety and panic reaction. Subjects with motion sickness and space sickness typically develop perspiration, nausea, vomiting, increased salivation, yawning, and generalized malaise. Gastric motility is reduced and digestion, impaired. Even the sight or smell of food is distressing. Hyperventilation is a common sign, and the resulting hypocapnia leads to changes in blood volume with pooling in the lower parts of the body predisposing to postural hypotension and syncope. An unusual variant of motion sickness continues when the subject returns to stationary conditions after prolonged exposure to motion. Typically, affected patients report that they feel the persistent rocking sensation of a boat long after returning to solid ground. Rarely, the syndrome can last for months to years after exposure to motion and can even be incapacitating. The cause is unknown.

Physiologic vertigo can often be suppressed by supplying

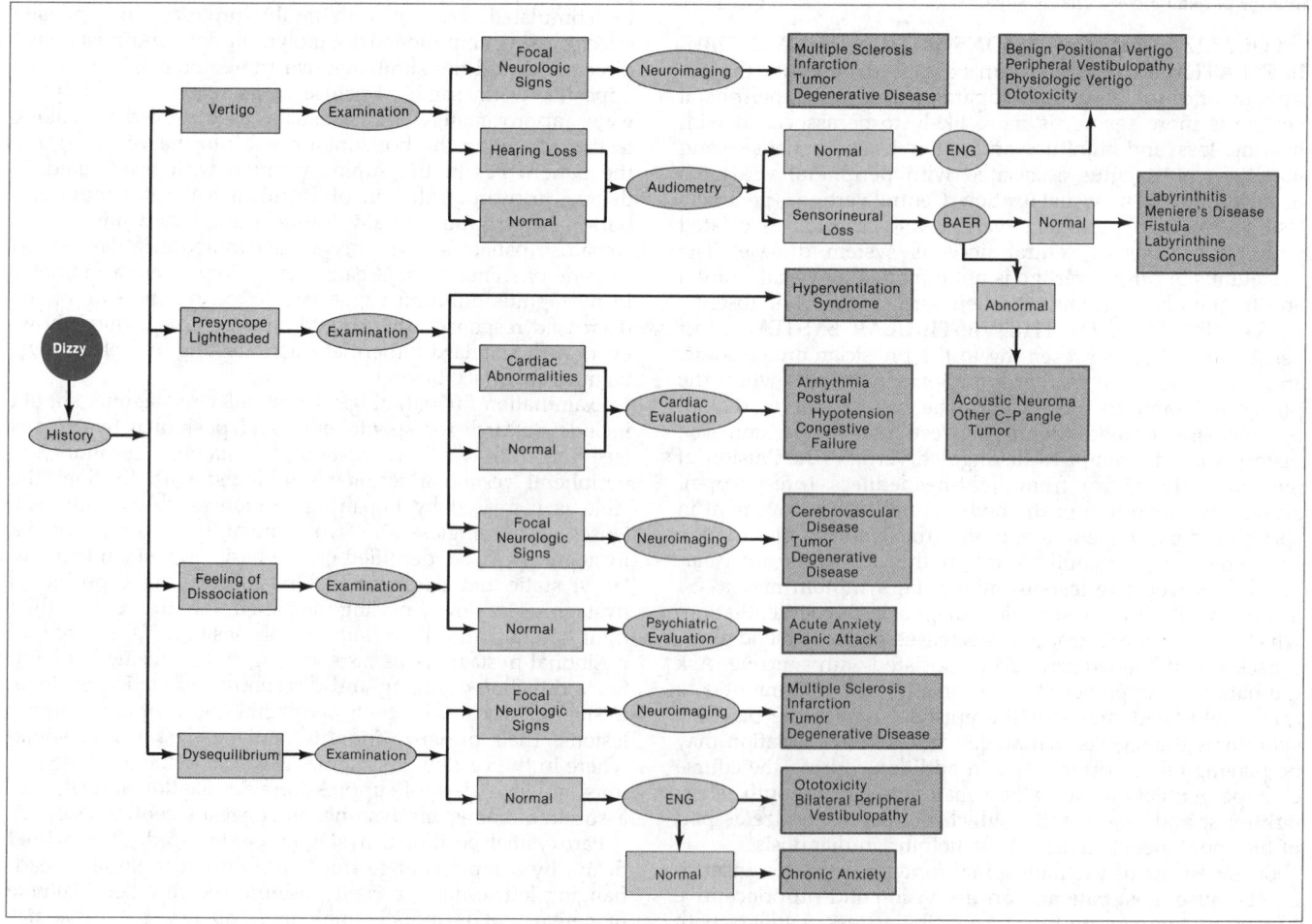

FIGURE 464–6. Evaluation of dizziness.

sensory cues that help to match the signals originating from different sensory systems. Thus, motion sickness, which is exacerbated by sitting in a closed space or reading (giving the visual system the miscue that the environment is stationary), may be improved by looking out at the environment and watching it move. Height vertigo, caused by a mismatch between sensation of normal body sway and lack of its visual detection, can often be relieved either by sitting or by visually fixating a nearby stationary object.

Benign Positional Vertigo (BPV). BPV is by far the most common cause of pathologic vertigo. Patients with this condition develop brief episodes of vertigo (less than 1 min) with position change, typically when turning over in bed, getting in and out of bed, bending over and straightening up, or extending the neck to look up. BPV can result from *head injury, viral labyrinthitis,* and *vascular occlusion,* or it may occur as an isolated symptom of unknown cause (in about 50 per cent of cases). The latter is particularly common in the elderly. This syndrome is important to recognize, since, in the vast majority of patients, the symptoms spontaneously remit within 6 months of onset. It does commonly recur, however. The diagnosis rests on finding characteristic fatigable paroxysmal positional nystagmus after a rapid change from the sitting to head-hanging position (described on p. 2121). The pathophysiology of BPV is not established, but some investigators have postulated that debris from the utricular macule may become attached to the cupula of the posterior semicircular canal and artificially stimulate that canal when it is in the dependent position. Consistent with this theory, the burst of paroxysmal positional nystagmus is in the plane of the posterior canal of the "down ear," and the positional nystagmus disappears after the ampullary nerve has been surgically resected from the posterior canal on the diseased side. If the history and physical findings are typical, no further evaluation is necessary. If the history or findings are atypical, the condition must be distinguished from other causes of positional vertigo that may occur with tumors or infarcts of the posterior fossa. Typical BPV is rarely associated with such conditions. The treatment for most patients is simple reassurance. Since the vertigo can be extinguished by fatigue many patients find that exercises involving repetitive position changes that initially produced the vertigo will provide prolonged relief.

Acute Peripheral Vestibulopathy ("Acute Labyrinthitis"). One of the most common clinical neurologic syndromes at any age is the acute onset of vertigo, nausea, and vomiting lasting for several days and not associated with auditory or neurologic symptoms. Most affected patients gradually improve over one to two weeks, but some develop recurrent episodes. A large percentage report an upper respiratory tract illness one to two weeks prior to the onset of vertigo. This syndrome occasionally occurs in epidemics (epidemic vertigo), may affect several members of the same family, and more often erupts in the spring and early summer. All of these factors suggest a viral origin, but attempts to isolate an agent have been unsuccessful, except for occasional findings of a herpes zoster infection. Pathologic studies showing atrophy of one or more vestibular nerve trunks, with or without atrophy of their associated sense organs, are evidence of a vestibular nerve site and, probably, viral etiology for many patients with this syndrome (*viral neurolabyrinthitis*). In some patients attacks of acute vestibulopathy (usually less severe) recur over many months or years. There is no way of predicting whether a person who suffers a first attack will have repetitive attacks.

Meniere Syndrome. The typical clinical features of Meniere syndrome are described on page 2119. This disorder accounts for about 10 per cent of all patients with vertigo. The diagnosis is based on documenting episodic severe attacks accompanied by more or less continuous tinnitus and fluctuating hearing levels on audiometric testing.

Post-traumatic Vertigo. Vertigo, hearing loss, and tinnitus often follow a blow to the head that does not result in temporal bone fracture, the so-called *labyrinthine concussion.* Although they are protected by a bony capsule the delicate labyrinthine membranes are susceptible to blunt trauma. Blows to the occipital or mastoid region are particularly likely to produce labyrinthine damage. *Transverse fractures* of the temporal bone typically pass through the vestibule of the inner ear, tearing the membranous labyrinth and lacerating the vestibular and cochlear nerves. Complete loss of vestibular and cochlear function is the usual sequela, and the facial nerve is interrupted in approximately 50 per cent of cases. Examination of the ear often reveals hemotympanum, but bleeding from the ear seldom occurs, since the tympanic membrane usually remains intact. As noted above, *benign positional vertigo* is also a common sequela of head trauma. *Fistulae* of the oval and round windows can result from impact noise, deep-water diving, severe physical exertion, or blunt head injury without skull fracture. The mechanism of the rupture is a sudden negative or positive pressure change in the middle ear or a sudden increase in cerebrospinal fluid pressure transmitted to the inner ear via the cochlear aqueduct and internal auditory canal. Clinically, the rupture leads to the sudden onset of vertigo or hearing loss, or both. Surgical exploration of the middle ear is warranted when there is a clear relationship between the onset of vertigo or hearing loss, or both, and the onset of severe exertion, barometric change, head injury or impact noise.

Postconcussion Syndrome. The so-called postconcussion syndrome refers to a vague dizziness (rarely vertigo) associated with anxiety, difficulty in concentrating, headache, and photophobia induced by a head injury resulting in concussion. Occasionally, similar, less pronounced symptoms are associated with mild head injury judged to be trivial at the time. The cause is unknown, but animal studies indicate that small multifocal brain lesions (petechiae) commonly occur after concussive brain injury.

Other Peripheral Causes of Vertigo. Vertigo can be associated with *chronic bacterial otomastoiditis,* either from direct invasion of the inner ear by the bacteria or by erosion of the labyrinth by a cholesteatoma. Radiographic studies of the temporal bone readily identify these disorders. Just as *otosclerosis* can result in sensorineural hearing loss it can also produce vertigo by involving the bony labyrinth. The typical audiometric findings of a combined conductive and sensorineural hearing loss should suggest this diagnosis. Several *drugs* that damage the auditory system (see p. 2119), such as the aminoglycosides, may also damage the vestibular labyrinth. The patient may suffer acute vertigo, either along with or independent of hearing loss and tinnitus, if the toxic effect is asymmetrical. More often there is a progressive symmetrical loss of vestibular function leading to imbalance but not vertigo. Unfortunately, many patients being treated with ototoxic drugs are initially bedridden and unaware of the vestibular impairment until they recover from their acute illness and try to walk. Then they discover that they are unsteady on their feet and that the environment tends to jiggle in front of their eyes (*oscillopsia*). Younger patients adapt after weeks to the labyrinthine failure; older ones may be left permanently disabled. Usually there is no nystagmus (because of the symmetrical involvement), but the patient is ataxic. Caloric and rotational tests during electronystagmography can document impairment or absence of vestibular function. The best treatment is prevention. If the drug is discontinued early during the course of symptoms the disorder may stabilize or improve.

Vascular Insufficiency. Vertebrobasilar insufficiency is a common cause of vertigo in the elderly (see also Ch. 479). Whether the vertigo originates from ischemia of the labyrinth, brain stem, or both structures is not always clear since the blood supply to the labyrinth, eighth cranial nerve, and vestibular nuclei originate from the same source, the basilar vertebral circulation. Vertigo with *vertebrobasilar insufficiency* is abrupt in onset, usually lasting several minutes, and is frequently associated with nausea and vomiting. Associated symptoms resulting from ischemia in the remaining territory supplied by the posterior circulation include visual illusions and hallucinations, drop attack and weakness, visceral sensations, visual field defects, diplopia, and headache. These symptoms occur in episodes either in combination with the vertigo or alone. Vertigo may be an isolated initial symptom of vertebrobasilar ischemia, but repeated episodes of vertigo without other symptoms should suggest another diagnosis. Vertebrobasilar insufficiency usually is caused by atherosclerosis of the subclavian, vertebral, and basilar arteries. Occasionally, episodes of vertebrobasilar insufficiency are precipitated by postural hypotension, Stokes-Adams attacks, or mechanical compression from cervical spondylosis. Diagnostic studies including CT scans are usually normal, since the vascular insufficiency is transient and function returns to normal between episodes. Angiography can be helpful in confirming the diagnosis but carries a risk and rarely leads to definitive therapy.

Vertigo is a common symptom associated with *infarction of the lateral brain stem or cerebellum*, or both. The diagnosis usually is clear, based on the characteristic acute history and pattern of associated symptoms and neurologic findings. Occasionally cerebellar infarction or hemorrhage presents with severe vertigo, vomiting, and ataxia without associated brain-stem symptoms and signs that might suggest the erroneous diagnosis of a acute peripheral vestibular disorder. The key differential point is the finding of clear cerebellar signs (extremity- and gait ataxia) and gaze-evoked nystagmus. Such patients must be watched carefully for several days since they may develop progressive brain-stem dysfunction owing to compression by a swollen cerebellum.

Cerebellopontine-Angle Tumors. Most tumors growing in the cerebellopontine angle (e.g., *acoustic neuroma, meningioma, epidermal cyst*) grow slowly, allowing the vestibular system to accommodate so that they produce a vague sensation of disequilibrium rather than acute vertigo. Occasionally, however, episodic vertigo or positional vertigo heralds the presence of a cerebellopontine-angle tumor. In virtually all patients, retrocochlear hearing loss is present, best identified by an abnormal brain-stem auditory evoked response. Magnetic resonance imaging (MRI) of the cerebellopontine angles is the most sensitive diagnostic study for identifying a cerebellopontine-angle tumor.

Other Central Causes of Vertigo. Acute vertigo may be the first symptom of *multiple sclerosis*, although only a small percentage of young patients with acute vertigo eventually develop multiple sclerosis. Vertigo in multiple sclerosis is usually transient and often associated with other neurologic signs of brain stem disease, in particular, internuclear ophthalmoplegia or cerebellar dysfunction. Vertigo may also be a symptom of *parainfectious encephalomyelitis* or, rarely, *parainfectious cranial polyneuritis*. In this instance the accompanying neurologic signs establish the diagnosis. The *Ramsay-Hunt syndrome* (geniculate ganglion herpes) is characterized by vertigo and hearing loss associated with facial paralysis and, sometimes, pain in the ear. The typical lesions of herpes zoster, which may follow the appearance of neurologic signs, are found in the external auditory canal and, sometimes, over the palate. Rarely is herpes zoster responsible for vertigo in the absence of the full-blown syndrome. *Granulomatous meningitis* or *leptomeningeal metastasis* and cerebral or systemic *vasculitis* may involve the eighth nerve, producing vertigo as an early symptom. In these disorders cerebrospinal fluid analysis usually suggests the diagnosis. Patients suffering from *temporal lobe epilepsy* occasionally experience vertigo as the aura. Vertigo in the absence of other neurologic signs or

symptoms is never caused by epilepsy or other diseases of the cerebral hemispheres.

TREATMENT OF VERTIGO. Treatment of vertigo can be divided into two general categories; specific and symptomatic. Specific therapies include antibiotics for bacterial or syphilitic labyrinthitis, anticoagulants for vertebrobasilar insufficiency, and surgery for acoustic neuroma. When possible, treatment should be directed at the underlying disorder. In most cases, however, symptomatic treatment is either combined with specific therapy or is the only one available (e.g., with acute peripheral vestibulopathy). Many different classes of drugs have been found to have antivertiginous properties, and in most instances the exact mechanism of action is uncertain. All of these agents produce potentially unpleasant side effects, and the decision on which drug or combination to use is based on their known complications and on the severity and duration of the vertigo. An episode of prolonged, severe vertigo is one of the most distressing symptoms that one can experience. Affected patients prefer to lie still with eyes closed in a quiet, dark room. Antivertiginous drugs with sedation such as phenergan (25 mg four times daily [q.i.d.]) or diazepam (5 mg q.i.d.) may be helpful. Prochlorperazine suppositories (25 mg) may stop vomiting. In more chronic vertiginous disorders, when the patient is trying to carry on normal activity less sedating antivertiginous medications such as meclizine (25 mg q.i.d.) or transdermal scopolamine (0.5 mg every 3 days) may provide relief. Transdermal scopolamine has also been shown to prevent motion sickness. To be most effective, the patch must be in place several hours before exposure to motion. Scopolamine should be used cautiously in elderly subjects because it tends to produce confusion, memory loss, and even hallucinations.

Baloh RW: Dizziness, Hearing Loss and Tinnitus: The Essentials of Neurotology. Philadelphia, F. A. Davis Company, 1984. *More details in a similar format.*

Baloh RW, Honrubia V: Clinical Neurophysiology of the Vestibular System. Philadelphia, F. A. Davis Company, 1979. *Monograph reviewing basic and clinical aspects of vestibular function.*

DeWeese DD, Saunders WH: Textbook of Otolaryngology. 6th ed. St. Louis, The C. V. Mosby Company, 1982. *A good text with chapters on hearing loss, tinnitus, dizziness, and vertigo.*

Tinnitus. Ciba Foundation Symposium. London, Pitman Books, 1981. *A nice collection of articles on the diagnosis and treatment of tinnitus.*

465 DISORDERS OF MOTOR FUNCTION

465.1 Asthenia, Fatigue, and Weakness

Fred Plum

The closely related symptoms of asthenia, fatigue, and weakness relate to motor activity in different ways. *Asthenia* describes an anticipatory experience, sensed in advance of the act. It consists of an inner sense of usually subacute or chronic lassitude in which persons feel weak before they start or expect that greater than normal effort will be required to perform tasks. Affected persons hesitate to undertake motor activity, fearing that strength or endurance may be insufficient to the requirement. Small reductions in motor power or impaired endurance can be difficult to measure, so that asthenia sometimes reflects the presence of clinically undetectable motor weakness as in mild myasthenia gravis or in the early course of acute polyneuropathy. Similarly, asthenia can be an early, prominent symptom of thyrotoxicosis. The symptom can accompany acute lateral cerebellar dysfunction, presumably due to impairment of neocortical long loop feedback control, and emerges with the complex difficulty in initiating movement that accompanies parkinsonism. Most asthenia, however, is non-neurogenic and accompanies several psychologic and systemic disorders.

Most organically based asthenia has a relatively recent onset and arises in association with other symptoms, signs, or laboratory findings of physical illness. Subacute or chronic asthenia (neurasthenia, formerly called "effort syndrome") is one of the major symptoms of anxiety or depression. Its physiology is little understood. The symptom may be accompanied by signs of autonomic imbalance, including tachycardia, recurrent sighing, multifocal blushing, and inappropriate sweating. Neurasthenia is difficult to treat; affected patients often tenaciously regard their symptom and its accompaniments as expressions of some still-undiscovered organic disease rather than as a reflection of psychologic maladjustment.

Fatigue refers to an abnormal rate or degree of exhaustion during or following motor activity. Abnormal fatigue can be local or generalized; acute, subacute, or chronic. Many systemic illnesses produce at least briefly a sense of generalized lassitude, purposelessness, and easy exhaustion, including bacterial and influenzal infections, hepatitis, infectious mononucleosis, myocardial infarction, endocrine disorders (e.g., Addison's disease, panhypopituitarism, and hypo- or hyperthyroidism), severe anemia, malnutrition, disseminated malignancy, and anticancer chemotherapy. Fatigue is a prominent symptom of certain chronic neurologic disorders such as parkinsonism and multiple sclerosis. A distressing sense of purposelessness, easy tiring, and lack of initiative characterize the postconcussion syndrome and states of chronic sedative drug ingestion. The management of such complex mixtures of psychic and somatic reactions provides a major challenge for the physician. It is best to approach the matter directly, as the symptoms are common and easily self-reinforced if not managed effectively in their early stages. *Local* fatigability with a rapid decline in strength after repeated movement of a particular group of muscles is characteristic of myasthenia gravis. Less easily measurable feelings of muscle tiredness also accompany local peripheral motor neuropathy or radiculopathy. Chronic fatigue that remains unexplained by a careful search for systemic or neuromuscular causes often has a psychogenic basis.

Most acute fatigue states have a metabolic or musculoskeletal origin and can be related to a recent illness or to episodes of unusual exercise or muscular hyperactivity. Almost all kinds of muscular or neuromuscular weakness lower the threshold for the exercised part to tire, but persistent somatic fatigue rarely can be attributed to mere chronic overwork. Organically engendered fatigue states are worse in the evening than in the morning. They are accentuated by further activity and typically relieved by sleep. Psychogenic fatigue follows the opposite pattern, being maximal in the morning and declining in the evening as the social pace increases.

Weakness refers to a specific loss of strength in voluntary muscle movement, usually complained of as an inability to complete a specific and familiar act. The symptom can be subtle. Patients sometimes ignore even prominent degrees of weakness until noticed by friends or family ("your foot drags" or "why are you limping?") or brought out by the examiner's tests. The presence of weakness can reflect disease or dysfunction at any level of the nervous system: muscle, neuromuscular junction, peripheral nerve or root, anterior horn cell, descending motor systems, basal ganglia or cerebellum, as well as hysteria or malingering. Muscular weakness can develop from generalized metabolic dysfunction as with hyponatremia, hyper- or hypothyroidism, certain drug intoxications, and in the setting of starvation or cancer. Painful areas of bone and joint inflammation can induce local, non-neurogenic weakness as a protective response against the further discomfort of movement.

465.2 Ataxia and Related Gait Disorders
Fred Plum

Any neurologic illness that affects sensorimotor functions in the lower extremities can interfere with the coordinated act of walking. Accordingly, an introductory analysis of the differential features of certain gait abnormalities may prove helpful in diagnosis. Other chapters provide descriptions of the specific abnormalities that characterize parkinsonism, chorea, athetosis, spastic paraparesis, and various forms of poly- and mononeuritic motor weakness.

ATAXIA. Ataxia is a failure of muscular coordination expressed as irregularity or awkwardness of movement. Common usage has applied the term most often to an unsteadiness of walking, but the same principles apply to disturbances in coordinated movements affecting the upper extremities, the speech mechanisms, or even the eye movements. In the literal sense, ataxia can result from any abnormality in motor function, whether induced by faulty peripheral sensory mechanisms or by disturbances of descending corticospinal, basal ganglion, or cerebellar control. Most often the analysis of ataxia as a diagnostic problem lies in distinguishing disturbances in proprioceptive control from those caused by weakness, cerebellovestibular abnormalities, or the influence of toxic drugs.

PROPRIOCEPTIVE (SENSORY) ATAXIA. Proprioceptive ataxia can result from diseases of the large afferent fibers of the peripheral nerve, dorsal root, or the dorsal spinal funiculus, and less often from lesions of the brain-stem lemniscal system or the sensory projection from the thalamus to the parietal lobe cortex. The functional defect results from a variable loss of knowledge of the location of the body part combined with relatively preserved strength in the member. Afferent peripheral nerve, dorsal root, and spinal lesions most often result from inflammatory-demyelinating neuropathy, diabetic neuropathy, syphilitic tabes dorsalis, or meningomyelopathy, and any of several inherited forms of spinocerebellar degeneration. Cyanocobalamin (B_{12}) deficiency involves both the peripheral nerve and the dorsal column of the cord, whereas multiple sclerosis and allied demyelinating diseases affect the cord alone.

Nerve or root lesions cause a bilateral defect that characteristically (1) affects the lower more than the upper extremities; (2) involves position as much as or more than vibratory sensation but may sometimes be difficult to verify; (3) shows absent or greatly reduced deep tendon reflexes; and (4) produces a broad-based, weaving gait that with severe sensory loss becomes lurching, sometimes leg flinging, or pounding, and is worse in the dark (rombergism). Spinal dorsal column lesions produce similar symptoms except that position loss may be more profound, the signs may be less equally symmetrical, the tendon reflexes can be preserved, and pathologic reflexes may be present if the abnormality also involves the descending corticospinal tract. Brain-stem lemniscal involvement resembles spinal impairment but is seldom bilateral. Position sense loss may outstrip vibratory impairment. Patients with peripheral or spinal sensory ataxia are subjectively well aware of their deficits. They are also aware that their lack of coordination is not due to "dizziness," which distinguishes them from patients with vestibular disorders. Parietal or thalamoparietal proprioceptive impairment produces an ataxia that is usually unilateral and (1) affects the contralateral upper extremity as severely as the lower, (2) impairs position sense disproportionately more than vibration, and (3) may go partially unrecognized or be denied by the patient (anosognosia).

CEREBELLAR ATAXIA. The motor abnormality associated

with cerebellar lesions depends on the localization of the abnormality in the cerebellum and on whether or not adjacent or related neural structures are involved. Thus midline, lateral-hemispheric, and cerebellar outflow lesions each tend to produce somewhat distinct syndromes. These differences become less typical and more individualized when cerebellar tumors compress the adjacent brain stem to produce additional dysfunction or when diseases such as disseminated sclerosis or spinocerebellar degeneration affect neurologic structures that lie remote from the cerebellum.

Spinocerebellar disorders produce a predominantly sensory ataxia superimposed on which is a variable degree of cerebellar dyssynergia, depending on the extent to which specific cerebellar inflow and outflow pathways are affected in the particular disease in question.

Midline cerebellar dysfunction results principally from degenerative (nutritional-alcoholic, remote effects of carcinoma) or neoplastic disease (e.g., medulloblastoma, hemangioblastoma, metastasis). The gait is characteristic with legs thrust widely apart and extended, the arms extended in compensatory balance, and walking accomplished by short steps. Affected patients usually look at the ground for additional sensory stabilization and turn en bloc. With extension into the anterior midline cerebellum, stretch reflexes become hyperactive. In the early stages of the illness, the upper extremities and cranial nerves can be affected little or not at all, even in the presence of substantial lower extremity ataxia. As the disorder advances, truncal titubation appears, as can difficulty in rhythmic movements of the upper extremities and, eventually, even nystagmus. Posterior midline space-occupying lesions may add retropulsion (see below) to this symptom complex.

Lateral cerebellar hemispheric abnormalities produce ipsilateral hypotonia and incoordination marked by an irregular swaying gait and a tendency to drift toward the side of the lesion. The feet are spread apart, although not so broadly as with midline lesions, and patients characteristically cannot manage close-footed tandem walking. Rombergism is absent, but, as with all ataxias, distorted vision or closing the eyes moderately accentuates the patient's unsteadiness. Rhythmic movements and point-to-point tests are impaired in both the upper and lower extremities. If classic intention tremor appears, it implies that the abnormality includes the outflow from the dentate nucleus or its projection through the superior cerebellar peduncle to the red nucleus of the midbrain.

DRUNKENNESS. Drunkenness, whether due to alcohol or depressant drug intoxication, results mainly from bilateral labyrinthine-vestibular dysfunction and is accompanied by sensations of both vertigo and dizziness. Few patients with cerebellar disease walk the streets with as much incapacity as the reeling, lurching, twisting, and falling inebriate. Lesser degrees of intoxication produce unsteadiness, a tottering, cautious gait with the feet placed moderately widely apart, clumsiness, dysarthria, and nystagmus in all directions.

VESTIBULAR ATAXIA. Chronic unilateral impairment of the vestibulosensory system can occur with lesions anywhere along the peripheral pathway from labyrinth to brain stem. Patients with such abnormalities tend to drift toward the side of impairment and then quickly correct the deviation in the opposite direction. Turning accentuates their unsteadiness and induces missteps. Bilateral damage or degeneration of the vestibular nuclei in the brain stem results in a narrow-based ataxia with poor compensating movements in the limbs, drifting or falling to either side, and a tendency to retropulsion and falling backward. Patients with vestibular dysfunction depend heavily on visual proprioception, so closing the eyes accentuates the gait disorder.

SPASTIC ATAXIA. Combined abnormalities of the spinal dorsal columns and cortical spinal tracts produce a characteristic broad-based tottering and sometimes pounding gait with the knees held high but the legs moving stiffly. The condition occurs with demyelinating diseases and other intrinsic spinal disorders such as vascular malformations, cyanocobalamin deficiency, arachnoiditis, and, occasionally, neoplasms.

FRONTAL LOBE GAIT DISORDERS. Patients with frontal lobe disease can suffer any of several gait disorders, depending upon the anatomic distribution of the lesions. Unilateral injury to the foot-leg area of the somatosensory cortex produces a focal monoparesis, whereas bilateral motor-premotor damage results in a relatively narrow-based, stiff-legged impairment, sometimes with scissoring of the legs. More anteriorly placed premotor and prefrontal abnormalities arise in association with deep bilateral tumors, multiple cerebral infarctions, or communicating, "low pressure" hydrocephalus. The ensuing ataxia sometimes (and probably erroneously) is called "gait apraxia." It consists of a severe difficulty in walking or otherwise using the lower extremities so long as the patient is in the erect position. The feet appear glued to the floor (magnet reaction), and attempts to walk often consist of short shuffles or even hops, before the legs get moving. Walking, once (or if) it begins, proceeds as a halting and broad-based movement made easier by guidance or support. Advanced cases may be unable to get under way and, unless supported, increasingly tend to retropulse or fall backward, even from a sitting position. A degree of clinically obvious dementia accompanies the gait disorder.

Patients with frontal ataxia of this type show a greater ability to move their legs on command when lying supine than when standing. Examination of the lower extremities discloses an increased paratonic resistance to passive movements coupled with bilateral plantar grasp responses, extensor thrust responses, and usually accentuated tendon reflexes. These reflex abnormalities and physiologic dysfunctions best explain the difficulty in movement.

HEMIPARESIS. Both pyramidal-corticospinal and extrapyramidal motor disorders sometimes have a hemiparetic pattern and in their early stages can be confused with one another clinically. Severe spastic hemiplegia from damage to the corticospinal tract or the full-blown stooped, festinating, semishuffling gait of parkinsonism is so well known and readily recognized as to require no discussion. More subtle hemiparesis, however, can easily be overlooked, especially when it reflects the akinesia of early parkinsonism. In their initial stages, both pyramidal and extrapyramidal disorders produce mild or inconstant weakness, a susceptibility to easy fatigue in the affected member, and a sense of stiffness. Both corticospinal and parkinsonian hemiparesis incipiently produce a gait disorder marked by a slack arm and a reduction of other automatic accessory movements on the affected side, a tendency to scuff the toe, and a measure of bodily akinesia. Both may result in an increase in muscular resistance to passive stretch on the involved side; in the early stages it may be difficult clinically to distinguish between pyramidal spasticity and extrapyramidal rigidity. The following points help in differential diagnosis. Patients with early pyramidal tract dysfunction tend to have unilaterally increased reflexes on the affected side. When walking, they flex the wrist and fingers, circumduct the lower extremity, and hold the foot in an equinovarus position. Patients with early hemiparetic parkinsonism, on the other hand, tend to have greater facial and bodily hypokinesia, to stoop, and to show at least some cogwheel resistance on rotary movements of the elbow or wrist. They extend the affected wrist and step the weak foot forward rather than circumducting it. The foot itself is held in simple varus position. The deep tendon reflexes may or may not be slightly asymmetrical.

GAIT DISTURBANCES IN THE ELDERLY. Any of several specific visual, somatosensory, or motor diseases may impair walking in elderly persons. Less easily classified but fairly typical walking difficulties include a tendency to walk with slow, short, mincing, and unsteady steps (marche à petits pas). Fairly common is a stooped position coupled with a moderately broad-based, unsteady gait, sometimes associated with computed tomographic evidence of a chronic communicating hydrocephalus (see Ch. 495.3).

RETROPULSION. A tendency to step backward from the standing position or to fall backward while sitting can be a symptom of several serious, acquired midline abnormalities of the brain. The physiology is poorly understood. It accompanies midline tumors of the posterior cerebellum as well as degenerative disorders affecting the central vestibular mechanisms bilaterally, and has been reported in association with bilateral lesions affecting the sides of the third ventricle, the basal ganglia, and the frontal lobes. Occasionally the abnormality is associated with large, unilateral frontal lobe neoplasms that produce an increase in intracranial pressure and intracranial shift. Retropulsion of posterior fossa origin is especially dangerous, as it often comes on suddenly and is accompanied by a loss of the normal postural protective mechanisms that guard against injury during falling.

HYSTERICAL GAIT. Hysteria can mimic a variety of hemiparetic, steppage, or ataxic gait disorders. With a hemiparetic type, the pattern usually gives itself away by an atypical dragging behind of the affected leg during a series of hops or supported steps. The most obviously factitious hysterical disorder is a lurching, irregularly based, sometimes bent-forward walk in which the patient grasps any object in reach for support and reels from side to side inconsistently. Such patients may sink to the floor, but almost never endure an unsupported, self-injuring fall. Signs of altered muscular tonus or abnormal reflexes are absent, and the bizarre movements not only differ from the expected pattern of sensory or cerebellar dysfunction but often change from examination to examination.

Garcin R: Coordination of voluntary movement and the ataxias. In Vinken PJ, Bruyn GW, Garcin R (eds.): Handbook of Clinical Neurology, Vol 1, Disturbances of Nervous Function. Amsterdam, North Holland, 1969, pp 293, 309. *A detailed and thoughtful exposition of clinical and physiologic principles.*

Kremer M: Sitting, standing and walking. Br Med J 2:63, 1958. *A succinct and readable analysis, still pertinent.*

Plum F, Posner JB: Motor system. In Smith LH, Thier SO (eds.): Pathophysiology. The Biological Principles of Disease. 2nd ed. pp 1036–1072. Philadelphia, W B Saunders Company, 1985. *Discusses the pathophysiology of human motor dysfunction in its various forms.*

465.3 Episodic Loss of Motor Function

Jerome B. Posner

Sometimes patients report episodic loss of motor function affecting one or more extremities which, although severe, is brief in duration and is quickly followed by a return to normal. Such episodic loss of motor function can be caused by a variety of pathophysiologic abnormalities. Because the symptoms are episodic, the patient is usually normal when he presents to the physician; therefore, preliminary diagnosis depends on obtaining an accurate description of the event. The paragraphs below describe the potential causes of episodic loss of motor function.

Drop Attacks

PATHOPHYSIOLOGY. The most perplexing diagnostic problem associated with episodic loss of motor function is the so-called drop attack (Table 465–1). A patient, usually in the later decades of life, who is standing or walking suddenly

TABLE 465–1. CAUSES OF DROP ATTACKS IN ADULTS

Consciousness lost: syncope, seizures (rare)

Consciousness retained: idiopathic (aging reflexes?); basilar ischemic attacks; acute labyrinthine vertigo; cataplexy; cerebral plateau waves

falls to the ground. In a classic drop attack, the patient does not lose consciousness, has not tripped or otherwise lost his balance, and is able to resume normal activity immediately or shortly following the fall. Affected persons suffer no accompanying neurologic signs but often fall with sufficient suddenness and force to cause injury.

Pathophysiologically, most drop attacks without loss of consciousness are poorly understood. Abnormal tonic, long-loop, posture-controlling reflexes to extensor muscles have been postulated, but the mechanism lacks proof. *Transient ischemia* produces bilateral leg weakness when motor pathways are involved bilaterally but only rarely causes sudden collapse. Bilateral weakness is likely only when the ischemia occurs in the distribution of either the anterior spinal or the vertebrobasilar arterial system. Episodic spinal cord ischemia is usually accompanied by sensory as well as motor symptoms, and with vertebrobasilar ischemia, most patients suffer other signs of brain stem ischemia as well (Ch. 479).

As the above implies, most drop attacks do not have the implication of severe spinal or brain stem ischemia. *Cryptogenic drop attacks* occur in many middle-aged and elderly individuals whose evaluation reveals no evidence of either cardiac or central nervous system vascular disease. The attacks are more common in women and can occur episodically for months or years without the development of other nervous system disease. Nothing is known of their pathophysiology.

Cataplexy, the sudden loss of motor tone without paralysis or change in consciousness, is an occasional cause of drop attacks. The fall to the ground is usually slower than with the classic drop attack, and the patient rarely hurts himself (Ch. 458). Occasionally cataplexy occurs as an isolated symptom of the sudden rises of intracranial pressure (*plateau waves*) that sometimes accompany brain tumors or hydrocephalus (Ch. 495). Because there are important connections between the vestibular system and pathways controlling muscle tone, sudden *vestibular failure* can cause drop attacks. Such episodes are almost always accompanied by vertigo and usually by nausea and vomiting as well. *Akinetic* or *myoclonic seizures* causing drop attacks are common in childhood but rare in adults. However, drop attacks occasionally have been reported in adults that appear to be epileptic in origin and respond to anticonvulsant drugs.

DIAGNOSIS. The first task is to determine whether the patient was truly unconscious at any time during the episode. If so, the first diagnosis should be syncope, and the diagnostic evaluation is directed toward that disorder (Ch. 457.4). If it is clear that the patient is conscious throughout the episodes and that the disorder cannot be attributed to tripping or loss of balance, the physician should probe carefully for accompanying symptoms or signs that may help to localize the cause. Back pain, lower extremity paresthesias or sensory loss, or sudden changes in bladder or bowel function accompanying the drop attacks suggest spinal cord dysfunction. Headache, diplopia, and dysarthria accompanying the attack suggest brain stem dysfunction, probably caused by vertebrobasilar arterial insufficiency. Tinnitus or vertigo suggests a vestibular disorder. Severe headache, particularly if accompanied by nausea and vomiting, suggests plateau waves from increased intracranial pressure.

Computed tomography (CT) or magnetic resonance imaging (MRI) will rule out brain tumor or hydrocephalus leading to plateau waves. In the absence of demonstrated syncope or a cause of increased intracranial pressure, the most serious potential diagnosis is vertebrobasilar transient ischemic attacks. Patients in whom no other diagnosis can be made should be treated for cerebral vascular disease until proved otherwise. Most often, however, no diagnosis can be made and no definitive treatment prescribed. Elderly patients with drop attacks not due to cerebral vascular disease sometimes benefit by carrying a cane, which may prevent or lessen the force of the fall.

TABLE 465–2. CAUSES OF TRANSIENT FOCAL MOTOR PARALYSIS

Transient carotid or basilar ischemia
Nonconvulsive seizures
Complicated migraine
Plateau waves (rare)

Other Transient Paralyses

Episodic loss of motor function in one or more extremities can be a perplexing problem (Table 465–2). Affected patients may complain of sudden or rapid loss of motor function involving an arm or a leg or both, with or without associated sensory symptoms, but without abnormal motor movements of either the arm or the leg. The most common cause is transient cerebral ischemia in the distribution of the internal carotid artery. All patients suffering episodic loss of motor function on one side of the body should be considered to be suffering from transient ischemic attacks until proved otherwise. In transient ischemic attacks and the much less frequent plateau waves of increased intracranial pressure, there is usually sudden loss of motor function lasting 5 to 15 minutes and, in the instance of plateau waves, often an accompanying headache and sometimes some clouding of consciousness. With atonic seizures and migraine, the onset of motor dysfunction is usually but not always slower, but it too persists for 5 to 20 minutes. The motor weakness in late-life migraine may or may not be accompanied by a contralateral headache that appears as the paralysis disappears.

In differential diagnosis, CT or MRI will identify intracranial abnormalities while noninvasive ultrasound or angiography can detect carotid vascular lesions. Electroencephalography may assist in the diagnosis of a seizure disorder, but the EEG is often normal between episodes. A past or family history of migraine assists in the diagnosis of late-life migraine. Therapeutic trials directed successively at treatment of the several causes of these episodic attacks sometimes help in reaching a definitive diagnosis.

Fisher CM: Late-life migraine accompaniments as a cause of unexplained transient ischemic attacks. Can J Neurol Sci 7:9, 1980.

Meissner I, Wiebers DO, Swanson JW, et al.: The natural history of drop attacks. Neurology 36:1029, 1986.

466 DISORDERS OF SENSATION

Jerome B. Posner

Major Sensory Symptoms

An organism perceives its environment through its sensory systems. When a sensory system is disordered, sensation may be diminished, increased, or distorted. Table 466–1 lists definitions for major sensory abnormalities.

Anatomy and Physiology of Sensory Pathways

Two major sensory pathways subserve exteroception and conscious proprioception. The first pathway subserves the sensations of pain, temperature, and crude touch. It begins as free nerve endings of small myelinated and unmyelinated fibers.

The receptors are connected to small (5μ), thinly myelinated, "A delta" fibers, which conduct at about 35 meters per second, and to unmyelinated "C" fibers (1 to 2 μ), which conduct at about 0.5 meter per second. This dual set of fibers explains the phenomenon of "double pain." A noxious stimulus elicits first a sharp, pricking, well-localized pain mediated by the more rapidly conducting fibers, and the C fibers mediate a burning, poorly localized, exceedingly unpleasant "second pain."

After synapsing in the dorsal horn, the ascending pain pathways in the spinal cord divide into two groups: the neospinothalamic tract, which is believed to subserve the perception of intensity and localization of pain, temperature, and crude touch, and the phylogenetically older paleospinothalamic tract, which is believed to subserve the arousal and emotional components of pain. The axons of the neospinothalamic tract arise from the dorsal horn, cross the anterior commissure, and ascend in the anterolateral quadrant of the spinal cord. The axons terminate in the ventral basal complex of the thalamus, principally within the ventral posterolateral nucleus (VPL) ipsilateral to the side of their ascent. The thalamic terminations of these fibers coincide to a large extent with those of the dorsal column. Third-order neurons from the thalamus project to somatosensory area 1 (sensorimotor cortex), with the same somatotopic localization as other sensory modalities. Lesions at the brain-stem or thalamic level often lead to chronic so-called "thalamic pain." The paleospinothalamic tract, whose cells of origin in the dorsal horn receive C-fiber input, also crosses in the anterior commissure and ascends in the spinal cord closely applied to but more ventral than the neospinothalamic tract. Many of the fibers of the paleospinothalamic tract send collaterals to the reticular formation of the brain stem.

The second system consists predominantly of larger myelinated fibers and subserves the functions of light touch, position sense, and tactile localization. The central nervous system begins where these large fibers enter the spinal cord via the dorsal root ganglion, lying in a position medial to the smaller fibers that subserve pain and temperature. Most of the large fibers ascend without synapsing in the posterior and to a lesser extent lateral columns of the spinal cord to reach the gracile and cuneate nuclei in the low brain stem. Second-order neuron fibers then decussate and ascend in the medial lemniscus to reach the contralateral ventral posterolateral thalamus. Third-order neurons projected from the thalamus terminate in the cerebral cortex, predominantly in the sensorimotor strip surrounding the Rolandic fissure. Lesions of this system lead to loss of sense of position of the limbs and body in space, inability to localize tactile stimuli or to distinguish between one and two closely placed stimuli (two-point discrimination), and inability to describe accurately the size, shape, and texture of objects (stereoanesthesia). Subcortical lesions of the system also cause loss of the ability to recognize vibratory sensation (pallesthesia).

The two major exteroceptive systems are anatomically separated through much of their course, particularly in the spinal cord, and they differ physiologically as a result of fiber size. Thus, lesions at different sites in the nervous system and lesions of different physiologic natures cause unique sensory syndromes that assist in localizing the site and nature of the disorder. A discussion of the principles of pain management can be found in Chapter 27.

Localization of Sensory Disorders

PERIPHERAL NERVES. Sensory perception begins when a physical or chemical stimulus alters the activity of a *sensory*

TABLE 466–1. MAJOR SENSORY SYMPTOMS DEFINED

Hyperesthesia, anesthesia: reduction, loss of exteroceptive sensation
Hyperesthesia: lowered exteroceptive sensory threshold
Hypalgesia, analgesia: reduction, loss of pain sensation
Paresthesias: spontaneously arising exteroceptive sensation (e.g., pins and needles sensations, burning sensations)
Dysesthesias: unpleasant distortion of afferent stimuli
Hyperpathia: elevated threshold to noxious stimuli with accentuated discomfort above the threshold
Causalgia: a continued spontaneous sense of burning pain

receptor in such a way that the stimulus is transduced into an electrical potential (receptor potential). Many diseases of peripheral nerves affect both large and small fibers, leading to a diminution of all sensory modalities to approximately equal degree. In some disorders of peripheral nerves, however, small or large fibers can be involved preferentially, leading to a "dissociated sensory loss." When small fibers are predominantly affected, one finds pin and temperature sensation involved out of proportion to light touch, vibration, and position sense. Because autonomic fibers are also small, trophic changes in skin and joints may accompany such a small-fiber peripheral neuropathy, but because motor fibers and the afferent portion of the stretch reflex are subserved by large fibers, these functions are relatively preserved despite sometimes profound loss of pain and temperature sensation. Such selective small fiber damage is sometimes encountered in diabetes and is common in some of the hereditary neuropathies as well as in toxic-nutritional neuropathies (Ch. 508 and 509). Large fiber loss is more common in demyelinating neuropathies and may lead to profound loss of localizing touch and proprioception, with relative preservation of crude touch, pin, and temperature sensation. Such disorders are commonly accompanied by paresthesias and sometimes spontaneous pain. The deep tendon reflexes are lost because of damage to large afferent fibers from muscle, and there is usually weakness as well. The diagnosis of a peripheral neuropathy involving sensory fibers is established by the distribution of the sensory loss, which may be in the distribution of a single nerve, multiple individual nerves, or a symmetrical distal stocking-and-glove distribution. Polyneuropathies are distributed distally because longer axons are more vulnerable to disease than shorter ones. In general, mononeuropathies are caused by local disease (e.g., compression entrapment), mononeuritis multiplex by vascular disorders (e.g., polyarteritis), and polyneuropathies by immunologic or metabolic disorders (e.g., demyelination-inflammatory neuropathy, diabetes, uremia, nutritional neuropathy).

SPINAL CORD. True dissociation of sensory loss is more common in spinal cord disorders than in those originating in peripheral nerves or roots. Lesions of the posterolateral columns produce profound loss of position and vibration sense with normal crude touch, pin, and temperature sensation. Usually corticospinal tracts are involved as well as sensory pathways, and thus many such patients often have hyperactive reflexes and extensor plantar responses. Lesions of the spinothalamic tract or of crossing fibers from the posterior horn to the spinothalamic tract cause loss of pain and temperature sense with preservation of vibration, position, and localizing touch. Such dissociated sensory loss is common in syringomyelia and may occur with infarction of the anterior portion of the spinal cord from occlusion of the anterior spinal artery. In both of these disorders, motor function may be relatively well preserved. When only one side of the spinal cord is involved, one finds loss of proprioceptive sensation on the ipsilateral side and loss of pin and temperature sensation on the contralateral side, both below the level of the lesion. There is usually a small band of decreased sensation to all modalities resulting from damage to the posterior horn at the level of the lesion. This so-called Brown-Séquard syndrome is sometimes seen with tumors either compressing or invading the spinal cord and is a common presenting syndrome in radiation myelopathy. Lesions of the spinal cord are rarely confused with those of peripheral nerves, even when the latter show dissociated sensory loss, because the sensory loss in spinal cord lesions is usually proximal as well as distal and restricted to those segments below the spinal cord level damaged. Thus, by the time a polyneuropathy causes substantial sensory loss above the knees, nerve fibers supplying the fingertip are usually involved as well, whereas with a thoracic spinal cord lesion the arms are always spared.

Furthermore, motor signs of upper motor neuron disease, particularly extensor plantar responses, usually correctly identify the central nature of a spinal cord disorder rather than pointing to a peripheral disturbance.

BRAIN STEM. In the lower brain stem, spinothalamic and proprioceptive pathways remain separated, lateral lesions of the medulla causing loss of pin and temperature sensation on the ipsilateral side of the face (a result of damage to the descending root of the trigeminal nerve) and the contralateral side of the body. This sensory abnormality is usually accompanied by other signs of lateral medullary damage (Wallenberg's syndrome) and spares proprioceptive pathways. Higher in the brain stem, as the two pathways converge in their route toward the thalamus, damage causes contralateral sensory loss to all modalities, usually accompanied by cranial nerve palsies, ataxia (from the cerebellar outflow), and motor weakness.

CEREBRUM. In the thalamus, damage to the ventral posterolateral nucleus causes decreased sensation of all modalities on the contralateral side of the body and face. Sensory loss is often accompanied by dysesthesias. A *thalamic syndrome* often appears 4 to 6 weeks after acute thalamic damage and has been attributed to denervation hypersensitivity of sensory neurons in the midbrain reticular formation. The patient develops spontaneous pain in the distribution of the sensory loss, usually associated with a dysesthetic response to touch and a hyperresponsiveness to pinprick once threshold is exceeded. The thalamic syndrome is rare but causes a particularly unpleasant pain intractable to most therapeutic endeavors. Conversely, surgical lesions of the intralaminar nuclei, which receive fibers from the paleospinothalamic tract, often decrease pain without affecting sensory thresholds.

Kandel ER, Schwartz JH: Principles of Neural Science. New York, Elsevier, 1985. *Excellent chapters on the anatomy and physiology of sensory systems.*

Headache and Other Head Pain

Headache ranks ninth among the causes of visits to physicians and is a major source both of time lost from work and of medical diagnostic procedures. The frequency of disabling headache is explained in part by the rich nerve supply to the head (including afferent nerve fibers from trigeminal, glossopharyngeal, vagus, and upper three cervical nerves) and in part by the psychologic significance of head pain, causing anxiety about even modest discomfort, whereas a pain of equal severity elsewhere in the body might be ignored. Head pain can result from distortion, stretching, inflammation, or destruction of pain-sensitive nerve endings as a result of intra- or extracranial disease in the distribution of any of the aforementioned nerves. However, most head pain arises from extracerebral structures and carries a benign prognosis. The physician's twofold task is first to distinguish the commoner, benign head pain from more serious causes and then to administer appropriate treatment. The diagnosis can usually be established by history and physical findings alone; skull radiographs, computed tomographic (CT) and magnetic resonance (MR) images, and other diagnostic tests are seldom required. Table 466–2 is a simplified classification of the pathogenesis of head pain; the overwhelming majority of headaches are either muscle-contraction or common migraine headaches, with both abnormalities frequently playing a role in a given individual. The other forms of headache are much less common.

Migraine and Other Vascular Headaches

The term *vascular headache* applies to a group of clinical syndromes of unknown etiology in which the final step in

TABLE 466–2. PATHOPHYSIOLOGIC CLASSIFICATION OF HEADACHE

Vascular Headache
  Migraine Headache
    Classic migraine
    Common migraine
    Complicated migraine
    Variant migraine
  Cluster Headache
    Episodic cluster
    "Chronic" cluster
    Chronic paroxysmal hemicrania
  Miscellaneous Vascular Headaches
    Carotidynia
    Hypertension
    Orgasmic, exertional, and cough headache
    Hangover
    Toxins and drugs
    Occlusive vascular disease

Muscle Contraction (Tension) Headache
  Common tension headache
  Depressive equivalent
  Conversion reaction
  Temporomandibular joint dysfunction
  Atypical facial pain

Traction-Inflammation Headache
  Cranial arteritis
  Increased or decreased intracranial pressure
  Extracranial structural lesions
  Pituitary tumors

Extracranial Structural Lesions
  Paranasal sinusitis and tumors
  Dental infections
  Otitis
  Ocular lesions
  Pituitary tumors
  Cervical osteoarthritis

Cranial Neuralgias

pathogenesis of the pain appears to be dilatation of one or more branches of the carotid artery, leading to stimulation of nerve endings supplying that artery. There may be a release of noxious substances by either the arterial wall or nerve endings, causing a substantially lowered pain threshold. Such substances as serotonin, substance P, bradykinin, histamine, and prostaglandins alone or in combination have all been implicated in the pathogenesis of vascular headache. Most vascular headaches are unilateral in distribution and often but not always throbbing in quality, and they recur over months or years. Individual headaches are frequently precipitated by identifiable environmental or psychologic factors. During the course of a vascular headache, the involved arteries may be tender to the touch, and pain may be relieved temporarily by compression of the carotid artery, only to return with increased severity when compression is released. Most vascular headaches can be relieved by prompt administration of vasoconstrictive agents, and many recurrent headaches can be prevented by one of several vasoactive drugs. So-called common migraine may affect as many as 25 per cent of the population. Other vascular headache syndromes are less common, but each has distinctive clinical findings.

Classic Migraine

Classic migraine is distinguished by well-defined symptoms of neurologic dysfunction that precede or, less often, accompany the headache. Neurologic symptoms are usually visual, consisting of bright flashing lights (scintillation or fortification scotomata) beginning in the center of a homonymous visual half-field and radiating over 10 to 30 minutes outward toward the periphery. Less commonly, the visual abnormalities are monocular (retinal) or consist of hemianoptic loss of vision in place of or following the scintillating scotomata. Other neurologic disturbances that can occur in classic migraine include unilateral paresthesias, usually involving the hand and perioral area, aphasia, hemiparesis, and hemisensory defects. An uncommon variant named *basilar artery migraine* occurs pre-

dominantly in children and adolescents and is characterized by vertigo, ataxia, and diplopia, along with hemiparesis or hemisensory changes. Rarely, confusion, stupor, or even coma may develop. Neurologic symptoms of classic migraine usually last no longer than 30 minutes and generally clear before the headache phase begins. However, in some instances neurologic signs may persist for hours or, rarely, for days, throughout and even beyond the headache phase of the illness.

The pathogenesis of the neurologic dysfunction is not fully understood. Measurements of regional cerebral blood flow during episodes of classic migraine have shown a wave of focal hyperemia followed by abnormally low flow spreading from posterior to anterior over the cerebral cortex. The flow reduction is not sufficient in and of itself to produce the neurologic symptoms, nor is it always accompanied by neurologic symptoms. One explanation is that there may be a wave of physiologic depression that spreads across the cortex, accounting for both the neurologic symptoms and the changes in blood flow. Changes in brain blood flow do not accompany common migraine, even though the headache phase of the illness is similar. Thus, it is likely that if "spreading depression" is the cause of the neurologic symptoms of migraine, it is only one of several precipitating factors that may produce the headache.

The syndrome of classic migraine has four parts: (1) The *prodromal phase* occurs in a minority of patients and consists of an alteration of mood, often occurring for 24 or more hours before the headache. Patients may complain of increased hunger or thirst, drowsiness, euphoria, or depression. In some patients, known precipitants such as red wine commonly induce an attack. (2) The second phase consists of the *neurologic symptoms* described above. The neurologic symptoms may occur without subsequent headache (termed migraine equivalent), particularly in older people. (3) The third phase usually begins as the neurologic symptoms clear and characteristically consists of a unilateral throbbing frontotemporal *headache* on the side opposite the neurologic symptoms. The headache is frequently accompanied by nausea, photophobia, vomiting, diarrhea, phonophobia (noise intolerance), and a general feeling of being unwell. The headache commonly lasts 4 to 6 hours but may persist for 1 or more days. If the headache is prolonged, it may change into a dull, aching, bilateral pain extending back into the neck and shoulders. The headache phase is often terminated either by vomiting or by a period of sleep. (4) The *postheadache* phase is characterized by a feeling of exhaustion, tenderness of the scalp at the site of the headache, and recurrence of headache on sudden head movement.

The diagnosis of classic migraine is made by history; physical findings are absent, and laboratory evaluation is not helpful. When the attacks are atypical, particularly when neurologic disability is severe or prolonged, CT or MR imaging may be required to rule out structural lesions of the brain. However, such instances are rare. The treatment of classic migraine is similar to that of common migraine (see below), except that classic migraine attacks usually occur no more than four or five times a year and rarely more than once a month.

Common Migraine

Common migraine is similar to classic migraine except that neurologic symptoms are absent. Many patients with classic migraine also have episodes of common migraine. Common migraine is characterized by recurrent headaches, often severe, frequently beginning unilaterally, and usually associated with malaise, nausea and/or vomiting, and photophobia. The disorder often begins in childhood, affects women more often than men, and runs in families (70 per cent of patients give a family history). Characteristically, the headache affects individuals with perfectionistic and "driven" personalities. Identifiable factors that often precipitate individual headaches are holidays and weekends, menstrual periods, foods (especially red wine, chocolate, nuts, and aged cheese), environmental stimuli (such as bright sunlight, too much sleep, and undue emotional stress or resentment). Medical conditions and their treatment may also precipitate attacks. Vasodilators such as nitroglycerin and antihypertensives and serotonin releasers such as reserpine, as well as estrogens and oral contraceptives, have been reported to cause migraine attacks in susceptible individuals. The diagnosis of common migraine is usually made by the history. Important historical points that help distinguish migraine from the equally common tension headaches (see below) include their unilaterality, their association with nausea or vomiting, the tendency of migraine to awaken one from sleep, a positive family history, and a positive response to ergot preparations. When the diagnosis is in doubt, treatment of the patient for common migraine often clarifies the issue.

TREATMENT. The best treatment for migraine is prevention. Whenever possible, the patient should avoid precipitating factors. Medications known to cause migraine should be withdrawn if others can be substituted. Foods commonly implicated may also be withdrawn and, if withdrawal is effective, replaced one at a time to determine the specific precipitant. The patient should attempt to avoid undue stress or fatigue and not to sleep excessively on weekends. If these methods fail and severe headaches occur frequently (once a week or more), pharmacologic prophylaxis is indicated. Several agents have been reported effective in the prophylaxis of migraine, but not every patient responds to each agent. Perhaps the safest and most effective class of drugs are the beta-adrenergic blockers, particularly propranolol. The drug is begun at a dose of 80 mg a day in divided doses, and increased as tolerated until headaches are controlled. Recent reports suggest that calcium channel blockers such as verapamil* (80 mg three to four times daily) sometimes are effective. Methysergide, a serotonin antagonist, is effective at a dose of 2 mg three to four times daily. Methysergide must be employed cautiously because it can cause serious side effects, including vascular insufficiency, retroperitoneal or pleural fibrosis, and fibrotic thickening of heart valves. The side effects can be minimized by gradually withdrawing the drug for 1 month after every 4 to 6 months of treatment. Amitriptyline* in gradually increasing doses from 25 to 125 mg daily may be useful if the above drugs fail.

Acute attacks, if mild, often respond to analgesic agents and bedrest. More severe attacks are best treated by ergot preparations such as ergotamine tartrate. The drug, given parenterally, is sufficiently effective (85 to 90 per cent) to be useful as a diagnostic test. Oral ergot 1 to 2 mg given at the onset of a headache is effective in about 50 per cent of patients. However, during the headache, absorption of the oral form of the drug is often poor, and better results can be achieved with sublingual or rectal preparations. The best nonparenteral results are generally achieved by the insertion of half of a 2-mg ergotamine rectal suppository. The side effects of *ergotism* (muscle pain, vasoconstriction, mottled skin, peripheral gangrene, multifocal encephalopathy) make it unwise to treat frequent migraine headaches in this way, and one should switch to prophylaxis if the headaches occur more than once a week.

Migraine Variants

Several migraine syndromes differ sufficiently from classic and common migraine to earn separate names. *Ophthalmoplegic migraine* is the name given when an ocular motor palsy develops during the course of a severe migraine attack. Ophthalmoplegic migraine usually begins in childhood and is characterized by unilateral pupillary dilatation, ptosis, and paralysis of ocular muscles occurring 12 to 24 hours *after* the beginning of an attack of severe migraine. The ophthalmoplegia usually clears within hours to days but frequently recurs. Angiography (usually DIVA) may be required to rule out a carotid aneurysm. *Hemiplegic migraine* is a familial syndrome in which aphasia, confusion, and hemiparesis or hemiplegia precede or more often accompany the migraine attack. Repetitive episodes alternating from side to side may occur over many years. *Complicated migraine* is a term applied to attacks of migraine prodromes in which the focal neurologic defects may last for the entire headache attack and may even leave permanent residua. The few available anatomic studies of such patients have shown ischemic brain infarction involving the functionally impaired region.

Cluster Headache

Cluster headaches are short-lived attacks of severe, acute, and intense unilateral head pain that occur in clusters lasting several weeks, only to disappear for months or years on end. The disorder affects men much more than women and usually first begins between the third and sixth decades. Clusters characteristically occur in the spring and fall and last 3 to 8 weeks. The individual headaches occur one to several times a day, particularly at night, awakening the victim from sleep. They frequently have a clock-setting predictability. Each attack, which lasts 30 minutes to 2 hours, is characterized by rapid onset of a knife-like pain in the nostril or behind the eye which spreads to involve the forehead. During the attack, the ipsilateral nostril may water and the eye tear. In about 20 per cent of instances, a homolateral Horner syndrome develops. During the course of the headache, the patient is usually unable to lie still (the opposite of the situation with migraine) and restlessly paces the floor. The pain may be so severe that the patient bangs his head against the wall or threatens suicide. The headache disappears as abruptly as it arises, usually leaving no residua. Unlike the patient with migraine, the patient with cluster headaches does not feel systemically ill, and there is no nausea, vomiting, or sense of exhaustion when the headache ceases. During the time when clusters are occurring (but not between) alcohol will invariably induce an attack. When the headaches occur frequently, the Horner syndrome may outlast the head pain.

The pathogenesis of cluster headache is unknown, although it is believed to be a vascular headache related to migraine. The diagnosis is established by the characteristic history. Treatment of an acute attack is usually not worthwhile, since by the time the patient absorbs the analgesic agents the attack is over. In some patients the headache rapidly responds to oxygen inhalation. Several drugs prevent attacks of cluster headache. Ergotamine tartrate given prophylactically in a dose of 1 mg four times a day, or 2 mg at bedtime if the attacks are all nocturnal, is often effective. The drug should be withdrawn every seventh day to prevent the symptoms of ergotism and to see if the cluster has ceased. Methysergide 2 mg three to four times daily is also often effective; since the cluster rarely lasts more than 8 weeks, the drug can be discontinued and therefore is safe. Prednisone 40 mg daily in divided doses may also work and can be added to methysergide if the former is only partially effective. Lithium carbonate in daily doses of 0.9 to 1.5 grams sometimes works.

Cluster Variants

Several variants of cluster headache should be recognized by the physician, since their treatment may be different. The most striking is *chronic paroxysmal hemicrania*, a rare disorder consisting of painful episodes similar to cluster headaches that appear many times a day and recur unremittingly for years. There may be as many as 10 to 20 headaches daily, each lasting 10 to 30 minutes. Indomethacin* orally in doses

---

*This use is not listed in the manufacturer's directive.

*This use is not listed in the manufacturer's directive.

of 75 to 150 mg daily has relieved all subjects. A cluster variant characterized by daily cluster headache without remission, multiple brief jabs of pain in the head, and a background of continuous unilateral headache of variable severity exacerbated by exertion has recently been described and is said to respond to indomethacin in most instances. Patients who did not respond to indomethacin did so to tricyclic antidepressants.

Other Vascular Headaches

Several vascular headache variants deserve mention so that the physician may recognize them as benign and treat them appropriately. Included are *orgasmic headaches,* several short-lived bilateral throbbing headaches occurring in either sex and appearing abruptly at orgasm. The attack can be differentiated from subarachnoid hemorrhage because the headache usually disappears within minutes to an hour or more and may recur repetitively. Usually the illness is self-limited, but if not it may respond to 1 mg of ergot given an hour before sexual activity. *Exertional headache* occurs, as the name implies, during active exercise. Like orgasmic headaches, these are usually bilateral and throbbing, and may last several hours. They respond well to indomethacin. Vascular headaches have been reported to follow minor *trauma* to the carotid artery in the neck and to *carotid endarterectomy.* These headaches are unilateral, recurrent, and severe and usually respond to prophylaxis with propranolol. *Carotidynia* is the name given to spontaneous vascular headaches associated with unilateral anterior neck pain and/or carotid tenderness. They usually respond to the same treatment as vascular headaches. When attacks of carotid pain and/or headache recur, the diagnosis is not difficult, but the first attack must be distinguished from a spontaneous dissection of the carotid artery and may require intravenous angiography for diagnosis.

Hangover headache is part of a larger syndrome, usually including premature awakening from an evening of overindulging and often accompanied by a fine tremor of the extremities and mild gastric distress or nausea, mental dulling, and mild incoordination. The pathogenesis is related to alcohol withdrawal, dehydration, and the toxic effect of various congeners found with different intoxicants. *Nitrites* can induce pulsating headache and, occasionally, facial flushing, most often after the ingestion of processed foods ("hot dog" headache). *Monosodium glutamate* has been blamed for the "Chinese restaurant syndrome," characterized by postprandial headache, tight sensations about the face and head, and, less often, giddiness and diarrhea.

Cough headache is, as the name implies, sudden and often severe headache related to cough. The headache may last only seconds or may persist minutes to hours after a single cough or a coughing paroxysm. In some patients, cough headache is a symptom of an intracranial mass lesion. Most patients, however, do not have underlying structural disease; in these patients the disorder is probably similar to exertional and orgasmic headaches and has a vascular origin.

Hypertensive headaches occur only in patients with very severe or episodic hypertension. They are characterized by early-morning, usually throbbing, occipital headache that responds to the treatment of the hypertension.

Muscle Contraction (Tension) Headache

Muscle contraction or tension headaches are characterized by a steady, nonpulsatile, unilateral, or bilateral aching pain, usually beginning in the occipital regions but also often involving frontal or temporal regions as well. The headaches are so named because they are frequently accompanied by tight and tender muscles at the site of the most severe pain. They are probably the commonest cause of headache in the adult. Tension headaches are recurrent, often present every day, and usually begin in early afternoon or evening, with a dull occipital or frontal pain that may spread to grip the entire head "in a vise." Unique among headaches, the pain may be constantly present for days, weeks, or months and is often associated with tenderness in the posterior cervical, temporalis, or masseter muscles. The pain may be quite severe, but patients rarely complain of nausea, vomiting, or malaise, although modest dizziness, blurring of vision, and sometimes tinnitus may occur. These headaches are more frequent in women, in individuals who are tense and anxious, and in those whose work or posture requires sustained contraction of posterior cervical, frontal, or temporal muscles. The symptoms of common migraine and tension headaches overlap, and many patients suffer from both. The distinguishing features favoring tension headaches include pressure or tightness, which is worst at the back of the neck, increased severity of pain as the day progresses, and pain that is preceded by or associated with anxiety-producing situations. Tension headaches are less commonly unilateral than migraine and less commonly associated with nausea and vomiting. They seldom awaken the patient from sleep and do not respond to ergot preparations.

The pathogenesis of tension headaches is unclear. They are commonly accompanied by skeletal muscle contraction about the neck, face, and jaw, and palpation of those muscles may reveal sharply localized painful areas or nodules, injection of which with local anesthetics transiently relieves the headache. Sometimes massage has a similar effect. Patients are frequently aware that sustained contraction of muscles leads to headache. The contracting muscles or the nerves supplying them may release vasoactive substances such as lactate, serotonin, bradykinin, and prostaglandins, which lower pain threshold. Thus, some of the same substances implicated in migraine may also play a role in tension headache and explain the frequent overlap between the two syndromes. Muscle contraction headache may also be a result of sustained contraction of the head as a consequence of structural disease of the eye, ear, nose, paranasal sinuses, teeth, scalp, or intracranial contents.

TREATMENT. The first step in treatment is to identify causal factors. If these include abnormalities of posture leading to sustained muscle contraction, they should be corrected. Many patients with tension headache, particularly chronic ones, are depressed and respond to treatment with antidepressant agents such as amitriptyline. Others are tense and anxious and respond to anti-anxiety agents such as diazepam. This drug, in a dose of 15 to 20 mg a day for 2 to 3 weeks, is often effective as a diagnostic test. The relief of chronic headache establishes the diagnosis for the physician and helps to convince the patient that tension and anxiety are playing a major role in the headache. In addition, these drugs frequently break up a cycle of anxiety–muscle tension–anxiety, so that a short course may give prolonged relief. Addiction, however, is a potential complication of chronic use.

An individual headache may be treated with aspirin. This drug is probably more useful for tension headaches than acetaminophen because of its anti-prostaglandin properties. Vasoactive agents used for the treatment of migraine have no role in this disorder unless vascular headaches are concomitantly present. Some clinics report that biofeedback treatments effectively relieve muscle contraction and thus the headache.

Tension Headache Variant

Several rather characteristic headache syndromes of unknown cause may have muscle contraction and psychologic tension as part of their pathogenesis. The syndrome most clearly related to muscle contraction headache is the so-called "temporomandibular joint syndrome." Patients complain of unilateral or bilateral head pain, usually in the temporal region and in the jaw, often radiating into the ear. The pain is often associated with tenderness of the masseter and temporalis muscles and may be exacerbated by chewing. Accompanying symptoms often include limitation of full movement at the temporomandibular joint when opening the jaw, bruxism, and malocclusion. The disorder sometimes responds to dental manipulation, particularly use of a mouth guard during sleep that prevents bruxism. However, for most patients analgesics and anxiolytic agents effectively treat muscle-contraction head pain. *Post-traumatic headaches* are dull, generalized, aching head pains that follow head injury. The injury is often mild. The patient suffering the "post-traumatic syndrome" complains of headache often coupled with unsteadiness, giddiness, difficulty concentrating, insomnia, and fatigue. Contrary to popular belief, the syndrome is not more common in patients seeking compensation for the injury. It often persists for months or years. Treatment, like that of muscle contraction headaches, consists of psychologic support and reassurance and the use of mild analgesics and sometimes anxiolytic agents. Patients should be encouraged to return to work as soon as possible and to try to live a normal life despite the symptoms. The disorder can blend into *depressive headache*, a chronic generalized headache, usually vaguely described, sometimes associated with giddiness and unsteadiness, that occurs as a frequent and sometimes predominant manifestation of depression. The headache may have muscle contraction and tension as its pathogenesis or may be a *somatic delusion* in a severely depressed patient. In either event, the treatment of choice is an antidepressant drug.

Atypical Facial Pain

Atypical facial pain or atypical facial neuralgia is a term used to describe a syndrome characterized by steady aching facial pain, usually unilateral, localized to the lower part of the orbit, maxillary area, and sometimes the jaw. The pain begins without a known precipitating episode and may last for hours to days. It may spread to involve the head or neck, and muscles of the jaw and neck are often tender. Sometimes autonomic symptoms including sweating, flushing, rhinorrhea, and pallor are present. The disorder usually affects women, often in early middle age. Patients affected with the disorder are tense, anxious, and often chronically depressed. The pathogenesis of the illness is unknown. The autonomic changes have led some to suggest that the syndrome is a migraine variant, and the muscle tenderness and depression have led others to suggest that it be classified with musculoskeletal tension pain. Patients suffering from atypical facial pain should be examined carefully for local pathology of the eyes, nose, teeth, sinuses, and pharynx, but such is rarely found. Careful psychologic evaluation will often reveal a masked depression. Treatment is usually unsatisfactory. Analgesic agents are usually not helpful, and patients respond poorly to psychotherapy. In some patients, ergot preparations or propranolol are effective, suggesting a vascular pathogenesis for the face pain. Others respond to physical methods such as massage and biofeedback. Antidepressants sometimes help. It is important to recognize that the syndrome is not caused by structural disease and that patients require no invasive diagnostic or therapeutic procedures. Dental extraction does more harm than good. This disorder should not be confused with trigeminal neuralgia, discussed below; carbamazepine is ineffective.

Traction/Inflammation

Cranial Arteritis

This condition receives detailed consideration in Ch. 442 but deserves mention here as an important cause of headache in the elderly. The illness almost always appears after age 60 and usually later. It usually begins with unilateral or bilateral temporal, occipital, or fronto-occipital head pain of variable intensity, often coupled with tenderness of the painful areas.

Many patients have pain in the jaw muscles, making chewing uncomfortable. Nodules occasionally are palpable on affected vessels. The great risk is occlusion of retinal arteries secondary to untreated inflammation. Diagnosis depends on suspicion and usually on the presence of an elevated erythrocyte sedimentation rate. Diagnosis should be confirmed by arterial biopsy because definitive steroid treatment, once started, often must be maintained for many months. Since migraine-vascular headaches and depressive headaches also can have their onset in the elderly, a confirmed diagnosis is essential.

Meningitis and Subarachnoid Hemorrhage

Acute and subacute meningitis cause headache by inflammation of the pain-sensitive meninges surrounding the brain. The headache is usually generalized, throbbing, and very severe. It may be rapid or gradual in onset, and by the time it is fully developed is associated with nuchal rigidity. The diagnosis is established by lumbar puncture. In patients suspected of harboring an intracranial mass lesion, CT scan of the brain should be performed first and lumbar puncture deferred, unless the physician suspects that the patient is suffering from acute bacterial meningitis, in which case lumbar puncture must be done immediately. In *subarachnoid hemorrhage*, the initial sudden headache is caused by alteration of intracranial pressure. This headache is succeeded by a chronic persistent headache, often accompanied by nuchal rigidity that results from inflammation of the meninges caused by the blood. In a patient suspected of having suffered a subarachnoid hemorrhage, a CT scan should be performed first. The presence of extravascular blood establishes the diagnosis and obviates the need for lumbar puncture, which may exacerbate the bleeding by altering intracranial dynamics. The absence of identifiable hemorrhage on CT scan, however, does not rule out a small subarachnoid hemorrhage, and lumbar puncture then must be performed to establish or rule out the diagnosis definitively.

Alterations of Intracranial Pressure

Headache from altered intracranial pressure is caused by compression or traction of pain-sensitive vascular and neural structures over the apex and base of the brain. In the instance of *intracranial hypotension*, the loss of spinal fluid decreases the buoyancy of the brain so that the organ descends when the upright position is assumed, exerting traction on structures at its apex and compression on structures at its base. (In rare instances, the small bridging veins that enter the sagittal sinus may rupture and cause subdural hematomas.) In *intracranial hypertension*, the source of pain is probably compression of vascular and neural structures at the base of the brain by tumor or edematous brain.

INTRACRANIAL HYPERTENSION. Increased intracranial pressure per se does not lead to headache unless pain-sensitive structures are distorted. Many patients with high intracranial pressure from brain tumors, jugular venous obstruction, hydrocephalus, or pseudotumor cerebri do not suffer headache. If headache is present, it may be mild or severe, throbbing or steady, localized or generalized. When localized, it usually overlies the site of the lesion, but posterior fossa lesions may cause bifrontal headache. The headache is characteristically at its worst early in the morning, although, unlike cluster headache, it usually does not awaken the patient from sleep. It is exacerbated by stooping, coughing, moving the head suddenly, or straining at stool. Many patients prefer to sleep in the sitting position. The headache is rarely continuously intense. Transient rises of intracranial pressure called plateau waves (see Ch. 457) sometimes cause 5 to 20 minutes of severe headache accompanied by nausea, vomiting, or other neurologic signs. These episodes are commonly precipitated by assuming the upright posture but can also be precipitated by coughing, sneezing, or straining.

The treatment of headache related to increased intracranial pressure is the treatment of the underlying disease. Mild analgesics produce temporary relief; narcotic analgesics should not be used because of their tendency to produce respiratory depression and further raise the pressure in neurologically compromised individuals.

INTRACRANIAL HYPOTENSION (see Ch. 495.4) AND LUMBAR PUNCTURE HEADACHE. Intracranial hypotension usually follows a lumbar puncture and is due to continued leakage of cerebrospinal fluid through a rent in the dural sheath. The syndrome develops 12 hours to several days after the lumbar puncture and is characterized by headache that occurs on assuming the upright position. There is no evidence that a period of recumbency after a lumbar puncture prevents subsequent development of the headache. The headache usually begins as a dull ache in the posterior cervical area, radiating laterally toward the shoulders and cephalad toward the frontal area. It persists, often growing more severe, as long as the patient remains upright, and when most severe it may be associated with perspiration, nausea, and vomiting. Persistent headache of intracranial hypotension can lead to diplopia, probably a result of traction on the abducens nerves. The diagnosis of post–lumbar puncture headache is made by history; spontaneous intracranial hypotension is suspected by the history of positional headache and confirmed by low (<30 mm H₂O) or even negative CSF pressure on attempted lumbar puncture. The fluid is usually normal, but there may be an elevated protein concentration if the needle has entered a subdural or epidural fluid collection. Analgesics relieve the mildest headaches; the most severe ones can be controlled only by assuming the recumbent position. The headaches usually clear within a few days to a few weeks; in rare instances, surgical repair of the torn dura is necessary.

Extracranial Structural Lesions

Nasal and Sinus Headache

Although acute or chronic inflammation and neoplasms of the paranasal sinuses can cause headache, most patients who have been physician- or self-diagnosed as having sinus headaches are in fact suffering from either vascular or muscle contraction headache. Most true paranasal sinus headaches result from acute inflammation of the paranasal sinuses, which produces pain localized over the involved sinus and is associated with the stigmata of acute infection, including fever, swelling, and tenderness over the sinus and engorgement of the turbinates, ostia, nasofrontal ducts, and superior nasal spaces. Most of the discomfort comes from the ostia, which are many times more sensitive than the poorly innervated walls of the sinuses. Typically, "sinus" headache commences in the morning (frontal) or early afternoon (maxillary) and subsides in the early or late evening. The pain is dull and aching, is made worse by changing head position, and is seldom associated with nausea and vomiting. Sinus headache is best treated with decongestants and analgesics. Persistent purulent discharges should be cultured and appropriate antimicrobial drugs employed. Chronic suppurative disease in the frontal, ethmoid, and sphenoid sinuses, or in the mastoid air cells, may result in osteomyelitis and inflammation of adjacent cranial tissues. Headache persisting after surgical drainage of the diseased sinus is evidence for extradural and possibly subdural infection. More chronic inflammation and neoplasms, particularly when they occur in the sphenoid sinus, may not be accompanied by the usual physical signs of sinusitis. In such instances, sinus radiographs or CT scan may be required to establish the diagnosis.

Dental Pain

Noxious stimuli in a tooth usually evoke local toothache, but severe dental pain can be extremely difficult to localize. Afferent fibers for sensation in the teeth are contained in the second and third divisions of the trigeminal nerve. Headache in the areas supplied by the latter is, in rare instances, associated with prolonged, intense toothache or follows a tooth extraction. More commonly, in association with toothache, tooth extraction, or a tender, diseased tooth, distant tissues exhibit surface hyperalgesia, tenderness, and vasomotor reactions, such as tender eyeballs, reddening of the conjunctivae, and tenderness of the auricular and temporal tissues. Because of secondary muscle contraction, other sites of tenderness and pain may be noted behind the ears, behind the lower border of the mastoid process, and in the muscles of the occiput, neck, and shoulders. The upper teeth frequently hurt in association with disease of the nasal and paranasal structures. Occasionally, in coronary insufficiency, pain is experienced in the lower jaw. One should beware of ascribing bizarre pains in and around the jaws to a dental origin unless unequivocal acute inflammatory dental lesions are present. Dental extraction rarely ameliorates neuralgias or atypical facial pain. However, hysterical or delusional face pain is often attributed by the patient to prior dental work. Headache may not be attributed to a diseased tooth unless the injection of procaine into the tissues about the suspected tooth greatly reduces the intensity of, or eliminates, such headache.

Aural Pain

Severe pain in the vicinity of the ear can be caused by disease of the teeth, acute tonsillitis, inflammatory and neoplastic disease of the larynx and nasopharynx, temporomandibular joint disorders, tumors, inflammation in the posterior fossa, and disease of the cervical spine and its soft tissues. Pain in the ear is also associated with vascular headaches, atypical facial pain, and herpes zoster of the fifth and seventh cranial nerves and, rarely, the glossopharyngeal nerve. True glossopharyngeal neuralgia causes severe pain radiating from the tonsil into the ear. It has the usual timing feature of "tic" (see Cranial Neuralgias, below).

Primary ear disease is an infrequent but important source of headache, because it almost always indicates inflammation or destructive disease. Acute otitis media (purulent or nonpurulent), furunculosis of the ear canal, traumatic rupture of the tympanum, and fracture of the anterior wall of the bony canal all cause pain in the ear associated with sustained tender contraction of adjacent skeletal muscles. Osteomyelitis of the mastoid bone may be associated with inflammation of the nearby periosteum as well as of dura and adjacent tissues (epidural abscess)—both sources of pain in or behind the ear. Pain in this region also accompanies tumors of the acoustic nerve and inflammation and thrombosis of the lateral sinus.

Eye Pain and Headache

Errors of refraction (hypermetropia, astigmatism, anomalies of accommodation), disturbances of ocular muscle equilibrium, and glaucoma are universally described as causing headache, but most such headaches are probably tension headaches rather than truly related to "eye strain." Refractive errors are also said to give origin to such other symptoms as aching of the eyes, "sandy" feeling in the eyes, pulling sensations in and about the orbit, and conjunctival congestion. Headache is mild in degree and usually starts around and over the eyes and subsequently radiates to the occiput and back of the head.

The pain of glaucoma at first remains localized in the eyeball, then extends along the rim of the orbit and, finally, throughout most of the area supplied by the ophthalmic division of the trigeminal nerve. Nausea and vomiting sometimes accompany such headaches, which can become prostratingly severe if not treated promptly.

Simple myopia does not evoke headache because the myope, in attempting to improve his vision by the contraction of his eye muscles, actually makes his vision worse and soon abandons the attempt.

With inflammation of the iris and ciliary body, light may cause intense pain in the eye and adjacent areas because of movement of the inflamed iris. When the iris is immobilized, pain is allayed.

Pituitary Pain

Headache caused by pituitary tumors is the result of compression and distortion of pain-sensitive structures at the base of the skull, particularly the diaphragma sella. Pain is generally referred to the frontal or temporal regions bilaterally and may on occasion be referred to the vertex or occipital regions. Because the pain is not related to intracranial pressure, it does not have the same temporal characteristics of most brain tumor headaches and instead can occur at any time and is frequently chronic and unremitting. The diagnosis can be established by endocrine examination and by CT scan of the pituitary fossa. Acute headache occurring with known pituitary lesions (*pituitary apoplexy*) usually results from infarction or hemorrhage into the tumor. Sudden expansion of the tumor may compromise the overlying optic chiasm, leading to visual loss, or invade the laterally lying cavernous sinus, producing ocular palsies. Pituitary apoplexy should be treated surgically by emergency drainage of the hemorrhagic or infarcted material.

Neck Pain

Osteoarthritis of the zygapophyseal joints of the upper cervical spine is an occasional cause of perplexing headache. The pain is generally constant, aching, and perceived in the upper cervical and occipital areas. It may radiate to the vertex of the head or even the orbit. At times, vertex or orbital pain is more severe than occipital and neck pain, leading to confusion in diagnosis. The pain probably results from entrapment of the C3 root by overgrowth of the C2 zygapophyseal joint. A syndrome of unilateral upper nuchal and occipital pain accompanied by ipsilateral numbness of the tongue occurring on sudden turning of the head, is probably explained by compression of the second cervical root in the atlanto-occipital space. Such acute pain can be prevented by restricting neck movement with a cervical collar. Upper cervical nerve blocks relieve more chronic pain and are useful diagnostically as well as therapeutically. A few reports suggest that severe headache and neck pain affecting young male weight lifters (weight-lifter's headache) may result from pull or tear of cervical ligaments during the strain of exertion.

Cranial Neuralgias

The term cranial neuralgias refers to several distinctive head pains that appear to result from sudden and excessive discharge from the involved nerve. The best-known cranial neuralgia is trigeminal neuralgia. The concept of cranial neuralgias has been expanded to include the chronic burning pain that frequently follows herpes zoster infection of the nerve. Some also include atypical facial pain and temporomandibular joint syndrome under the cranial neuralgias, but these probably have muscle contraction or vascular disturbances as their pathogenesis and in this chapter are included under those headings.

TRIGEMINAL NEURALGIA. Trigeminal neuralgia (tic douloureux) is characterized by sudden, lightning-like paroxysms of pain in the distribution of one or more divisions of the trigeminal nerve. Most trigeminal neuralgia is caused by compression of the trigeminal nerve by arteries or veins of the posterior fossa. In some patients there is no identifiable structural disease. Occasionally trigeminal neuralgia may be a symptom of a gasserian ganglion tumor, multiple sclerosis, or a brain-stem infarct involving the descending root of the trigeminal nerve.

The history is diagnostic. The pain occurs as brief, lightning-like stabs, frequently precipitated by touching a trigger zone around the lips or the buccal cavity. At times, talking, eating, or brushing the teeth serves as a trigger. The pains rarely last longer than seconds, and each burst is followed by a refractory period of several seconds to a minute in which no further pain can be precipitated. The pains, however, often occur in clusters so that the patient may report somewhat erroneously that each pain lasts for hours. The pain is limited to one or more divisions of the trigeminal nerve, usually the second, or third, or both. Spontaneous remissions and exacerbations are common, the exacerbations tending to occur in spring and fall. Between paroxysms of pain, the patient is asymptomatic. Tic pain rarely occurs at night. In idiopathic trigeminal neuralgia, the neurologic examination is entirely normal. In symptomatic trigeminal neuralgia, there may be sensory changes in the distribution of the trigeminal nerve, and such a finding should prompt a careful search for structural disease of the nervous system.

Carbamazepine is the drug of choice for the treatment of trigeminal neuralgia. The anticonvulsant drug is given in doses varying from 400 to 800 mg a day, but because of its sedative properties the initial dose is 100 mg twice daily, gradually increased to the required maintenance dose. No more than 1200 mg should be taken daily. The drug is not an analgesic and is only effective for specific kinds of pain such as trigeminal neuralgia, glossopharyngeal neuralgia, and the lightning pains of tabes dorsalis. Side effects include dizziness, sedation and, rarely, aplastic anemia. Phenytoin* in doses of 400 mg a day is also effective in trigeminal neuralgia but less so than carbamazepine. Occasionally the two drugs appear to be synergistic. Baclofen* 60 to 80 mg daily has also been found to be a useful agent. If medical treatment fails, surgical intervention is necessary.

The most popular operations consist of lesioning of the gasserian ganglion (either by radiofrequency or glycerol injections) and posterior fossa craniotomy to relieve the compression of the trigeminal nerve by vascular structures. Gasserian ganglion lesions can be made under local anesthesia, are generally effective initially, but have a high relapse rate. Posterior fossa craniotomy is as effective as gasserian ganglion lesions and appears to have a lower relapse rate. The purpose of both operations is to relieve pain with little or no loss of sensation, thus preventing the dreaded complications of anesthesia dolorosa. Either of these operations is preferable to section of the nerve root proximal to the ganglion. However, that operation affords permanent relief. If surgery on the ganglion is contemplated, a prior test of local anesthesia of the ganglion or the peripheral branches of the nerve is desirable because some patients find the sensory loss less tolerable than the pain itself.

GLOSSOPHARYNGEAL NEURALGIA. Glossopharyngeal neuralgia is characterized by pain similar to that of trigeminal neuralgia but in the distribution of the glossopharyngeal and vagus nerves. The trigger zone is usually in the tonsil or posterior pharynx, and the pain spreads toward the angle of the jaw and the ear. Occasional patients suffer cardiac slowing or arrest during these attacks as a result of the intense afferent discharge over the glossopharyngeal nerve. Carbamazepine is often effective, but if it fails, glossopharyngeal nerve roots are sectioned in the posterior fossa. Symptomatic glossopharyngeal neuralgia is occasionally the presenting complaint of a tonsillar tumor, and careful examination of the pharynx and tonsillar fossa must be carried out.

OTHER NEURALGIAS. Similar but much rarer disorders than trigeminal or glossopharyngeal neuralgia have been reported to involve the greater occipital nerve and the nervus intermedius portion of the facial nerve. The clinical features

---

*This use is not listed in the manufacturer's directive.

and treatment of these rare disorders are similar to those for trigeminal neuralgia.

Diagnostic Evaluation

Headache is an extremely common disorder, and the excessive application of expensive and highly technical laboratory procedures to the diagnosis and management of benign head pain has been a substantial cause of unnecessary medical costs. Set against this truism is the fact that in some instances a timely CT scan, MRI, or lumbar puncture can give life-saving information about an otherwise undiagnosable problem. Given these antitheses, the following principles may help in the management of the individual patient:

1. Patients with chronic classic or common migraine or with chronic tension headache rarely require more than a careful history and examination. Even when the unilateral prodromes and headache of longstanding, classic migraine consistently affect the same side, the incidence of associated intracranial lesions remains so low that scans are unnecessary and arteriography unjustified.

2. Headaches that are of recent origin or progression deserve investigation. This principle especially applies to headaches that have a consistently focal distribution, follow trauma, or begin after the age of 30 years. MRI, if available, is probably more sensitive than CT scan, but the additional expense may not be justified.

3. The EEG is almost never useful in the diagnosis of diseases causing headache and can be omitted. Skull radiographs are useful in diagnosing headache only (a) when searching for abnormalities involving the base of the brain such as sellar and suprasellar lesions or (b) immediately following head trauma. CT scans have discriminating capacities superior to those of plain films and, when available, make radiographs unnecessary.

4. Diagnostic lumbar puncture should be performed with any acute headache that (a) is accompanied by fever or (b) is explosive or the most severe headache ever suffered (a history typical of acute subarachnoid hemorrhage). Lumbar puncture should, if possible, be deferred until after CT scanning with other forms of acute headache, especially if stiff neck but no fever is present. (This combination may indicate partial herniation of cerebellar tonsils into the foramen magnum secondary to an intracranial mass lesion.)

5. Now that CT and MRI are widely available, radioisotopic brain scanning almost never adds useful information and is expensively superfluous.

Diamond S, Dalessio DJ: The Practicing Physician's Approach to Headache. 3rd ed. Baltimore, Williams & Wilkins, 1982. *This short, up-to-date monograph describes the practical approach to the management of headache. The book is beautifully illustrated.*

Headache and *Cephalgia* *Two journals which publish original articles concerning new developments in the diagnosis and management of headaches and other types of head pain.*

Packard RC: Symposium on Headache. Neurol Clin Vol 1, No 2, May, 1983. Philadelphia, W. B. Saunders, 1983. *A comprehensive and up-to-date review of headache and its management.*

Some Specific Pain Syndromes

Some disorders causing pain produce a specific constellation of signs and symptoms. Many of these pain syndromes often respond completely to treatment with nonanalgesic medications. Thus, it behooves the physician to recognize these disorders and to prescribe appropriate treatment.

LIGHTNING PAINS OF TABES. Tabes dorsalis can produce acute, short-lived, intense pains in the trunk or lower extremities due to structural lesions of the dorsal roots. Lightning pains are analogous to trigeminal and glossophar-yngeal neuralgia. Like those two disorders, the pain usually responds to carbamazepine. There is no surgical therapy.

"REFLEX SYMPATHETIC DYSTROPHIES." This is a term that applies to pain, hyperalgesia, hyperesthesia, and autonomic changes, usually after injury to an extremity. If the injury has involved a peripheral nerve, particularly the sciatic or median nerve, the syndrome is called *causalgia* (hot pain). If the injury has not involved a peripheral nerve, such terms as post-traumatic painful osteoporosis, Sudeck's atrophy, post-traumatic spreading neuralgia, minor causalgia, shoulder-hand syndrome, and reflex dystrophy have been applied, the particular term depending on the outstanding symptom. Whatever the term, the pathophysiology of all these disorders appears to be the same, as do their clinical manifestations and response to therapy.

The disorder may follow either a major or a minor injury to an extremity, after which severe pain, usually of a burning quality, develops in the extremity. The pain is continuous but exacerbated by emotional stress and is associated with severe hyperpathia, so that moving or touching the limb is often intolerable. At first the pain is localized to the site of the injury or the distribution of the nerve injured, but with time it spreads, often to involve the entire extremity. Along with the pain there are vasomotor changes, first of vasodilatation (warm and dry skin) but later a change to vasoconstriction (edema, cyanosis, cool skin). Other autonomic disturbances include either hyper- or hypohidrosis; trophic changes in the skin, subcutaneous tissue, and muscles; and osteoporosis. The entire symptom complex is rarely present in any one patient, and one sign or symptom usually predominates. Untreated, severe reflex sympathetic dystrophy leads to muscle atrophy, fixation of joints, osteoporosis, and a useless extremity. The mechanism of the pain and sympathetic changes is not understood.

The earlier the treatment, the more effective it will be. Treatment begins with local anesthetic infiltration of the painful site, using 2 to 5 ml of 0.5 per cent lidocaine, repeated frequently enough to maintain relief of pain. When local measures fail, most patients are relieved by sympathetic ganglionic block with lidocaine. This procedure often gives permanent relief, but if repeated local anesthetics produce only transient benefit, surgical sympathectomy should be considered. A short course of corticosteroids has been reported to be effective if used early.

POSTHERPETIC NEURALGIA. Postherpetic neuralgia refers to severe and prolonged burning pain with occasional lightning-like stabs in the involved dermatome after an attack of herpes zoster. Severe postherpetic neuralgia is usually a disease of elderly patients and, like most chronic pain, is exacerbated by emotional upset and relieved to some degree by distraction. Touching the involved area usually exacerbates the pain. Treatment of postherpetic neuralgia is not entirely satisfactory, but the initial treatment should be directed toward stimulating the painful area. Brisk rubbing applied repeatedly with a terrycloth towel or stimulation of the dermatome with a cutaneous electrical stimulator often brings relief which long outlasts the stimulus. Initially, when therapy is undertaken, the hyperpathia may be so severe that the patient is unwilling to have the area stimulated. One can then spray the area with a local anesthetic (e.g., ethyl chloride) before stimulation is undertaken. During the first 48 to 72 hours, stimulation should be done as often as possible when the patient is awake and then decreased gradually. Care must be taken to keep the rubbing light so as not to excoriate friable skin. Relief of pain may take several weeks. Analgesic drugs are sometimes beneficial, and psychotropic drugs (amitriptyline, up to 75 mg daily, and fluphenazine, 1 to 3 mg daily) have been reported to be useful. Recent evidence suggests that nerve blocks using agents injected paraspinally or epidurally may relieve postherpetic neuralgia if given early in its course. There is also some evidence that adrenocorticosteroids and interferon used for the treatment of acute herpes zoster may diminish the incidence of postherpetic neuralgia. In many patients the disease runs its course, and after a year or two the pain disappears spontaneously. Ablative and other surgical procedures are ineffective.

PHANTOM LIMB PAIN. Phantom limb pain is a chronic and severe pain appearing to be localized in an amputated or totally denervated limb. All patients suffer phantom sensations after amputation, but in only about 10 per cent is it painful, usually when there has been severe preamputation pain. The pain is frequently similar to that suffered before amputation, or at times it may resemble muscle pain with the phantom seeming to be in a cramped or uncomfortable position. In most instances, the pain lessens and disappears with time, but occasionally it is a chronic and severe problem. Therapy is difficult. A search should be made for painful neuromas, but these are an uncommon cause, and even if small neuromas are found and removed, the pain is not usually relieved. Surgical procedures directed at the central nervous system are often not helpful. The pain may be triggered by touching the amputation stump, and eventually even touching healthy areas may trigger pain. Phantom pain is sometimes permanently abolished by cutaneous stimulation, either rubbing or electrical stimulation, or by repeated anesthetic blocks of peripheral nerves proximal to the stump. Narcotic analgesics may be helpful; other analgesic agents are usually not helpful. Sympathetic blocks have been reported to relieve pain in some patients for prolonged periods, but sympathectomy rarely produces relief.

MYOFASCIAL PAIN SYNDROMES. Pain arising from skeletal muscle is common. Unaccustomed exercise causes soreness and tenderness in the involved muscles but is rarely a source of patient complaint. Prolonged tonic contraction of skeletal muscles, however, has an underlying pathogenesis of psychologic tension, resentment, and anxiety, and may produce pain whose cause is not immediately apparent to the patient. Examples are tension headache arising from chronic contraction of paraspinous muscles at the base of the skull, anterior chest pain from contraction of pectoralis major, posterior thoracic or lumbar pain from paraspinous muscle contraction, and abdominal pain from rectus muscle retraction. The pain is initially localized over the area of muscle contraction but may spread widely into a distribution characteristic for the muscles involved. The muscles are usually tender to palpation, and there is often a particular tender area somewhere in the muscle, called a trigger area, which, when palpated, reproduces the entire distribution of the spontaneous pain. When the pain is acute, it may be treated with rest, local heat, and mild analgesic drugs, along with muscle relaxant drugs such as diazepam or meprobamate. When the pain is chronic or severe, particularly when a trigger area is found, local anesthesia with ethyl chloride spray or local injection of 0.2 per cent lidocaine or physiologic saline sometimes affords relief. At times, a single injection breaks the pain–muscle tension–pain cycle and permanent relief is achieved. At other times, repetitive injections with the addition of analgesic agents and muscle relaxants are required.

Payne R: Neuropathic pain syndromes, with special reference to causalgia and reflex sympathetic dystrophy. Clin Pain 2:59, 1986. *A thorough review of the pathogenesis and management of a very perplexing pain problem.*

Travell JG, Simons DG: Myofascial Pain and Dysfunction. The Trigger Point Manual. Baltimore, Williams & Wilkins, 1983. *An analysis of myofascial pain syndromes of the upper half of the body. The volume on the lower half of the body was to be published April 1987.*

Wall PD, Melzack R: Textbook of Pain. London, Churchill Livingstone, 1984. *A comprehensive monograph describing basic clinical and therapeutic aspects of all varieties of pain.*

SECTION FOUR / ALCOHOL AND NUTRITIONAL COMPLICATIONS

467 NUTRITIONAL DISORDERS OF THE NERVOUS SYSTEM
Ivan Diamond

The neurologic effects of either general or specific nutritional deprivations are common worldwide (Table 467–1). In the developed countries of Western Europe and North America, many of these disorders are observed most frequently in association with chronic alcohol abuse. Other major causes include food faddism; chronic starvation such as can occur with cancer, infantile malnutrition, or psychiatric illness; intestinal malabsorption or the complicated postoperative state. The conditions are relatively common, especially in large public hospitals that serve the underprivileged. More importantly, they often go undiagnosed. One recent study, for example, determined that only 20 per cent of patients found at autopsy to have Wernicke's encephalopathy were correctly diagnosed and treated during life.

Although conditions such as Wernicke's encephalopathy can develop in as little as a few weeks after an acute illness such as hyperemesis gravidarum, most nutritional syndromes among alcoholics develop only following prolonged severe abuse with years of proportional semistarvation. Binge drinkers who eat well between bouts of intoxication seldom suffer neurologic complications. Genetic predisposition also may contribute to neurologic vulnerability. Chapters 214 and 217 more extensively discuss nutritional requirements and the systemic effects of their deprivation.

THE WERNICKE-KORSAKOFF SYNDROME
Wernicke's Encephalopathy

This acute disorder occurs most commonly in chronic alcoholics but also can accompany other conditions listed in Table 467–2. This is the only alcohol-related neurologic disorder that can be corrected by a specific vitamin—thiamin.

CLINICAL MANIFESTATIONS. A clinical triad of ophthalmoplegia, ataxia, and global confusion is characteristic, although the condition should be suspected and treated in any chronically malnourished subject suffering from a confusional state of recent onset. Affected patients may complain of double vision or difficulty with balance. There is almost always horizontal nystagmus on lateral gaze. Vertical nystagmus, usually on upward gaze, occurs in about 50 per cent of cases. Bilateral, often asymmetric, lateral rectus palsies are characteristic and may develop rapidly. Defects in conjugate

TABLE 467–1. MAJOR ACQUIRED NUTRITIONAL SYNDROMES AFFECTING THE NERVOUS SYSTEM

Vitamin A (carotene)	Night blindness, possibly pseudotumor in children
Vitamin B	
B₁ (thiamin)	Peripheral neuropathy, Wernicke-Korsakoff syndrome
	Possibly amblyopia, cerebellar degeneration, cerebral atrophy
B₂ group	
Pantothenic acid	Possibly burning feet syndrome
Nicotinic acid	Pellagra, polyneuropathy, spastic ataxia, amblyopia, psychosis-dementia
Riboflavin	Possibly burning feet syndrome, amblyopia
B₆ (pyridoxine)	Convulsions in B₆-deprived babies and older children, possibly peripheral neuropathy
B₁₂ (cyanocobalamin)	Combined systems disease, peripheral neuropathy, dementia
Folic acid	Impaired peripheral nerve function, possibly neuropathy and encephalopathy
Vitamin C (ascorbic acid)	Retinal and occasionally cerebral hemorrhages
Vitamin E (α-tocopherol)	Peripheral neuropathy and cerebellar degeneration
Starvation	Possibly developmental neurologic defects in infants

gaze are common. Bilateral ptosis and total external or an apparent internuclear ophthalmoplegia occurs rarely. Light-fixed pupils should suggest an alternate or additional diagnosis.

Virtually all patients have an ataxic gait due to cerebellar involvement. This can vary widely in severity. Peripheral neuropathy and vestibular dysfunction frequently complicate Wernicke's encephalopathy. Intention tremor is less common, and speech disturbances are rare.

Most patients have an acute confusional state characterized by inattention, disorientation, and sleepiness. Stupor or coma occurs but is rare. Sometimes patients may be hyperactive and agitated (alcohol withdrawal, see Ch. 15) but most are apathetic, indifferent, and amnesic.

Associated physical abnormalities related to chronic alcoholism or poor nutrition are often present (Ch. 122). Tachycardia and orthostatic hypotension are common. Hypothermia occurs less frequently; any fever should prompt a search for concomitant infection. Patients with Wernicke's encephalopathy do not develop beriberi heart disease (see Ch. 217).

PATHOLOGY. The major lesions occur in the periventricular regions of the diencephalon, mid-brain, and brain stem, and in the superior vermis of the cerebellum; they may consist of areas of demyelination and glial proliferation. Microglia are prominent in acute lesions and fibrous astrocytes in older ones. Acute lesions show capillary dilation with occasional petechial hemorrhages. In experimental animals, defects in serotonergic transmission can be demonstrated in affected areas.

TABLE 467–2. CONDITIONS PREDISPOSING TO WERNICKE'S ENCEPHALOPATHY

Chronic alcoholism
Starvation
Persistent vomiting
  Hyperemesis gravidarum
  Gastric malignancy
  Gastritis
  Intestinal obstruction
  Digitalis intoxication
Systemic diseases
  Malignancy
  Hepatic failure
  Disseminated tuberculosis
  Uremia
Iatrogenic
  Inadequate parenteral nutrition
  Chronic hemodialysis

TREATMENT. Thiamin is specific. Because intestinal absorption is impaired in malnourished alcoholics, thiamin (50 to 100 mg) is given parenterally before starting infusions. Glucose given prior to giving thiamin can precipitate or worsen the encephalopathy. Recovery begins promptly. Ophthalmoplegia and gaze palsies often begin to resolve during the first day. Nystagmus, gait ataxia, and confusion may improve within days to weeks although many patients are left with residual nystagmus or gait ataxia. Nearly all patients with Wernicke's encephalopathy recover from the global confusional state, but many are left with a residual disorder of memory—Korsakoff's amnestic syndrome.

Korsakoff's Syndrome

CLINICAL MANIFESTATIONS (see also Ch. 463). There is a characteristic defect in forming new memories (anterograde amnesia) and in summoning previously established memories (retrograde amnesia). Patients are usually disoriented for place and time. Immediate recall is intact, but patients are unable to remember the same items several minutes later. Unhesitating confabulation often occurs early in the course. Other aspects of cognitive function, including arousal, language, praxis, and judgment, are spared.

PATHOLOGY. The findings are of active or remote Wernicke's encephalopathy. Damage to the dorsal medial nucleus of the thalamus probably accounts for the memory deficits.

TREATMENT. Patients with Korsakoff's syndrome should be given thiamin to treat coexistent Wernicke's encephalopathy and to prevent progression of the amnesia. About 20 per cent of patients recover completely, but more than half show little or no change. Improvement may take one to three months to be recognizable.

METABOLIC CONSIDERATIONS. Thiamin (vitamin B₁) in human tissues is derived entirely from dietary sources, is absorbed in the small intestine (Ch. 217), and transported into the brain by a saturable, energy-dependent transport system. A series of reactions produces phosphorylated thiamin derivatives, and thiamin pyrophosphate (TPP) is a required co-factor for certain enzymes in carbohydrate and amino acid metabolism. In addition to its role as a co-factor, thiamin and thiamin triphosphate (TTP) may also be important in the electrical function of neural membranes. Defects in some of these thiamin-dependent activities may underlie the acute symptoms of Wernicke's encephalopathy or Korsakoff's syndrome.

The confusional state and oculomotor disturbances seen in Wernicke's encephalopathy respond to thiamin treatment, and it is said that recovery may proceed during thiamin therapy whether or not alcohol consumption continues. However, calorie-containing ethanol appears to be an important contributing factor to the neurologic deficits. Calorie-deprived prisoners of war who developed Wernicke's encephalopathy rarely exhibited the irreversible amnestic syndrome. Moreover, nystagmus, ataxia, and the memory deficits often fail to improve after thiamin therapy, indicating that some areas of the brain have become irreversibly damaged. The molecular metabolic defect that precedes tissue damage in Wernicke's encephalopathy and Korsakoff's amnestic syndrome is not known.

ALCOHOLIC CEREBRAL ATROPHY

Many chronic alcoholics develop cerebral atrophy that increases with age and that can be visualized on CT scans of the brain. There is usually symmetrical enlargement of the lateral ventricles and an increase in the size of cerebral sulci and the width of interhemispheric and sylvian fissures. The abnormalities may lessen if drinking is discontinued. Many chronic alcoholics also show deficiencies on psychometric examination. The CT scan abnormalities, however, correlate poorly with such specific cognitive defects. The specific mechanisms of these cerebral abnormalities are not known.

ALCOHOLIC-NUTRITIONAL NEUROPATHY

CLINICAL MANIFESTATIONS. Polyneuropathy is common among alcoholic patients. The most typical complaints are weakness, pain, and paresthesias in the hands and especially the feet. Symptoms usually begin insidiously in the legs and progress proximally and symmetrically. Abnormal motor and sensory signs develop concomitantly. Patients may complain of burning pain and heat sensations on the plantar surfaces of the feet and aching pain in the calves. Dysesthesias can become so severe that light touch and deep pressure are intensely unpleasant. Burning pain made worse by contact can interfere with walking despite adequate strength.

On examination muscle weakness and wasting are usually more prominent distally, affecting legs more than arms and never the latter exclusively. The muscles may feel tender to pressure. Weakness can be so severe that contractures develop at the ankles and knees. Sensory abnormalities usually involve all modalities, but especially the pain and temperature modalities early in the course, and are more prominent distally. The deep tendon reflexes are usually absent to diminished in a distal to proximal distribution. Even asymptomatic patients often show mild sensory loss in the feet and absent Achilles tendon reflexes.

Involvement of the vagus nerve and thoracoabdominal sympathetic chain occurs rarely and can produce hoarseness, dysphagia, vocal cord paralysis, and hypotension. Cerebrospinal fluid protein levels are usually normal.

PATHOPHYSIOLOGY AND TREATMENT. The classic pathologic findings in alcoholic neuropathy are axonal degeneration and demyelination. Alcoholic-nutritional neuropathy, since it first affects smaller sensory fibers, is characterized by axonal degeneration with electromyographic signs of denervation and normal nerve conduction velocities often present at an early stage. Later, additional nutritional change may result in slow nerve-conduction velocities.

A specific vitamin deficiency has not been identified in alcoholic neuropathy. Treatment consists of a balanced diet with supplemental B vitamins. Recovery is slow and often incomplete. Several weeks may be needed for motor improvement to begin, and it may take a year before patients with marked weakness begin to walk.

ACUTE AND CHRONIC ALCOHOLIC MYOPATHY

ACUTE MYOPATHY. This is a dramatic and life-threatening condition that develops in chronic alcoholics during prolonged heavy drinking. Symptoms begin abruptly with pain, cramps, tenderness, weakness, and swelling of the legs. Muscle involvement may be generalized or confined to one limb. Creatine phosphokinase activity in blood is elevated, and muscle biopsy shows acute rhabdomyolysis. Myoglobinuria often occurs and may lead to acute renal failure, hyperkalemia, and death. Electromyography usually shows evidence of a primary myopathy (Ch. 456.2). Recovery usually follows days to weeks of abstinence, occasionally leaving residual proximal muscle weakness in its wake.

CHRONIC MYOPATHY. This is a chronic, painless disorder of proximal muscle weakness and atrophy that occurs rarely in alcoholics. It can be mild or severe. Muscles of the pelvic girdle and thighs are involved most frequently; weakness of shoulder girdle muscles is less common. Improvement usually occurs within two to three months after ethanol withdrawal. A coexistent peripheral neuropathy may contribute to the weakness.

ALCOHOLIC CEREBELLAR DEGENERATION

Cerebellar cortical degeneration occurs frequently in chronic alcoholics and in several presumably nutritional disorders in underdeveloped countries. About half the patients have an associated peripheral neuropathy. Men are affected more often than women. Most patients give a history of episodic binge drinking superimposed on heavy consumption extending over many years. Some complain of progressive unsteadiness and difficulty in walking, but these more insidiously developing symptoms often reflect a superimposed peripheral neuropathy that may clear with treatment. Abnormalities of gait and station are the most common findings. Initially, unsteadiness occurs during rapid turns, and tandem walking is difficult or impossible. Gradually, the feet become more widely based, walking becomes hesitant, and truncal ataxia is added. Ataxia of the legs may be demonstrable on heel to shin tests, but nystagmus, dysarthria, and tremor are rare. Often the syndrome develops abruptly or rapidly over several weeks and then remains stable. Sometimes the disorder evolves more slowly, with exacerbation following a binge or during an intercurrent illness. The most prominent pathologic abnormality is degeneration of the neurons of the anterior and superior cerebellar vermis with loss of Purkinje cells. CT or MR images confirm cerebellar vermis atrophy. Abstinence, dietary treatment, and supplemental B vitamins may produce moderate improvement in the gait ataxia as peripheral neuropathy recovers.

NUTRITIONAL AMBLYOPIA

The condition involves retrobulbar neuritis affecting maculopapillary fibers, caused by a nutritional deficiency and encountered primarily in alcoholics. Patients complain of dim or blurred vision that evolves gradually over weeks to months. Decreased visual acuity occurs in one or both eyes, accompanied by bilateral symmetrical central or centrocecal scotomas. Peripheral visual fields are usually unaffected, and funduscopic examination is normal. Treatment consists of abstinence, diet, and supplemental B vitamins. The extent of recovery varies inversely with the severity of impairment before therapy.

CENTRAL PONTINE MYELINOLYSIS

Central pontine myelinolysis (CPM) is a rare disorder that affects alcoholics primarily but also occurs in children and adults with severe electrolyte disorders, liver disease, malnutrition, anorexia, burns, cancer, Addison's disease, sepsis, and Wilson's disease.

PATHOPHYSIOLOGY, SIGNS, AND SYMPTOMS. The signs and symptoms relate closely to the pathologic change, which consists of a varying extent of symmetrical focal myelin destruction involving the basal central pons, with similar lesions occasionally affecting extrapontine areas (Fig. 467–1).

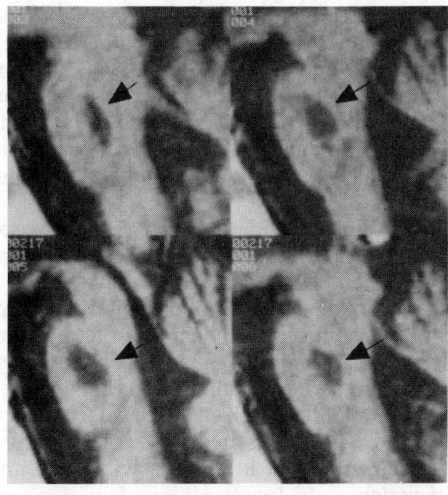

FIGURE 467–1. Central pontine myelinolysis. Magnetic resonance images were obtained in the sagittal plane using a "T₁-weighted" pulse sequence. An area of decreased signal is seen in the pons (*arrows*). (Photographs courtesy of Drs. Michael E. Charness and Robert L. DeLaPaz.)

There is no associated inflammation or nerve cell destruction, and the lesions appear to be reversible with time and proper nutritional and fluid balance.

Typically CPM evolves within days or weeks in severely ill patients. Almost always the condition follows by one to three days a period of profound hyponatremia followed by rapid osmolal correction of greater than 20 mEq per liter. Mental symptoms often are prominent and consist of clouded consciousness or exacerbation of pre-existing delirium. Reflecting interruption of corticospinal pathways in the pons, a flaccid or spastic quadriparesis ensues, accompanied in many instances by bulbar difficulties of speaking and swallowing. Some patients develop a supranuclear ophthalmoplegia and the mortality is high. Reflecting the sparing of the pontine tegmentum, sensory abnormalities usually fail to develop. The characteristic story has recently led to many cases being diagnosed during life, confirmed by abnormalities on CT or MRI scan. Some patients recover; others remain tetraplegic. Treatment consists of meticulous maintenance of electrolytes, especially sodium balance and adequate nutrition.

MARCHIAFAVA-BIGNAMI DISEASE

This is a rare disorder consisting of symmetrical demyelination of the corpus callosum and adjacent white matter. The lesions can be imaged by CT scan. The disorder affects mainly middle-aged men, severely addicted to various kinds of alcoholic beverages. Patients may have a progressive dementia accompanied by agitation or apathy, hallucinations, and emotional disorders until seizures, stupor, and coma supervene. Clinical findings such as rooting and sucking responses, grasp reflexes, paratonic rigidity, incontinence, and a slow hesitant gait suggest bilateral frontal lobe involvement. Recovery is rare, and the specific etiology unknown.

VITAMIN E DEFICIENCY

Vitamin E deficiency is a complication of intestinal malabsorption in patients with chronic steatorrhea often due to cholestatic liver disease or cystic fibrosis (Ch. 66). Patients with vitamin E deficiency develop a slowly progressive, distinctive neurologic syndrome with areflexia, cerebellar ataxia, ophthalmoplegia, pigmentary retinopathy, loss of vibratory sensation, and muscle weakness. Neurologic signs usually begin in childhood or adolescence with a loss of deep tendon reflexes followed by mild reduction in vibratory sensation; position sense is less affected, and pain and temperature sensation may be normal. Babinski signs are variable. A progressive external ophthalmoplegia is commonly associated with limitation of upward gaze. There may be impaired visual acuity and night vision because of pigmentary retinopathy. Muscle weakness and atrophy is often a late complication, affecting muscles diffusely, distally, or in a proximal myopathic distribution. Untreated patients can become severely disabled. Vitamin E deficiency probably is responsible for the similar neurologic syndrome which develops in abetalipoproteinemia (Ch. 473).

Vitamin E is an antioxidant which appears to protect unsaturated fatty acids of membrane phospholipids from oxidative degradation. The major pathologic findings in vitamin E deficiency are axonal degeneration of peripheral nerves and dorsal columns, reduced numbers of large myelinated fibers in peripheral nerves, and breakdown of the outer rod segments of the retina. Deposition of lipopigment, perhaps due to polymerization of peroxidized fatty acids, occurs in selected neurons and non-neural tissue. Similar neurologic abnormalities have been produced in animals with experimental vitamin E deficiency.

Serum vitamin E levels are low, particularly when related to serum lipids or cholesterol. Neurophysiologic studies usually show evidence of an axonal neuropathy with abnormal sensory nerve conduction velocities or amplitudes, and abnormal H-reflexes. Motor nerve conduction is altered less often or less severely, but evidence of denervation may be found in the tongue and somatic muscles. Central somatosensory conduction is often delayed, consistent with posterior column axonal degeneration. Electroretinograms and visual evoked potentials are abnormal according to the severity of the neurologic findings.

Treatment with vitamin E often improves the neurologic condition but high oral doses or parenteral administration may be necessary. Early treatment of unaffected children with cholestasis probably prevents the neurologic complications of vitamin E deficiency (Ch. 217).

VITAMIN B₁₂ DEFICIENCY

Vitamin B_{12} deficiency causes subacute degeneration of white matter in the dorsal and lateral columns of the spinal cord, peripheral nerves, optic discs, and cerebral hemispheres. The neurologic findings usually accompany a macrocytic (pernicious) anemia, but anemia need not be present. Hematologic and pathophysiologic considerations of vitamin B_{12} deficiency and details of treatment are discussed in Ch. 217.

CLINICAL MANIFESTATIONS. Neurologic symptoms develop in most patients with long untreated pernicious anemia, especially those in whom anemia has been masked by folate ingestion. Occasional examples can occur with B_{12} deficiency due to intestinal malabsorption, gastrectomy, or inadequate diet. Patients first complain of paresthesias in the hands or legs, such as tingling, numbness, and "pins and needles" sensations. Stiffness and weakness of the legs with unsteadiness in walking may be bothersome, particularly in the dark. Neurologic symptoms progress relentlessly if untreated; ataxia and stiffness eventually are followed by paraplegia and dysfunction of bowel and bladder. Psychologic symptoms are frequent and include apathy and depression, irritability and paranoid tendencies, nocturnal confusion, and dementia. Intellectual deterioration does not usually develop in the absence of other neurologic signs. Failing vision with central scotomas occurs rarely.

Initially one may find few objective changes despite complaints of paresthesias. Later, symmetrical distal impairment of vibratory sensation occurs, usually first in the legs but eventually reaching the trunk and arms. Position sense is affected less prominently, although Romberg's test may be positive. The earliest changes are those of a peripheral neuropathy. The patellar and Achilles tendon reflexes are diminished or absent, and there may be decreased perception of touch, pain, and temperature in the feet and ankles. In the intermediate advanced case, one finds symmetrical weakness in the legs associated with spasticity, clonus at the knees and ankles, increased or decreased deep tendon reflexes, and extensor plantar responses. Tingling distal paresthesias may follow flexion of the neck (Lhermitte's sign).

PATHOLOGY. The most prominent findings are in the peripheral nerves and dorsal and lateral columns of the spinal cord. Fragmentation and spongy degeneration of myelin usually begin in the lower cervical and upper thoracic regions; in untreated patients the disease progresses up and down the spinal cord and reaches into the ventral columns. Myelin sheaths and axons are destroyed, and Wallerian degeneration is found in the spinal cord funiculi. Cerebral white matter is affected late. Peripheral nerves may show distal degeneration.

DIAGNOSIS AND PATHOPHYSIOLOGY. Serum vitamin B_{12} levels are low and appear to correlate with the severity of the neurologic findings. The CSF protein concentration may be increased slightly. Neurologic disorders that can be confused with vitamin B_{12} deficiency include multiple sclerosis, cervical spondylosis, spinal cord tumors, and syphilitic meningomyelitis. A virtually identical syndrome has been reported after chronic abuse of nitrous oxide.

PATHOGENESIS. The molecular pathogenesis of the neurologic lesion in vitamin B_{12} deficiency is unknown. Vitamin B_{12} exists in different forms, some of which are required for at least two enzymes: N5-methyltetrahydrofolate homocysteine methyltransferase, which catalyzes the synthesis of methionine and regeneration of tetrahydrofolate, and methylmalonyl-CoA mutase, which generates succinyl-CoA. Prolonged exposure to nitrous oxide, which produces a neurologic disorder resembling combined system disease, also inhibits methionine synthesis.

TREATMENT. Intramuscular administration of vitamin B_{12} is the only treatment for vitamin B_{12} deficiency due to pernicious anemia or other malabsorptive states. Therapy should be started immediately and continued throughout the patient's lifetime. Early neurologic changes can be rapidly and completely reversed if treatment with vitamin B_{12} is begun promptly within the first few weeks or months of symptoms. If the neurologic manifestations have reached the stage of spinal cord dysfunction, therapy will halt progression, but improvement cannot be guaranteed.

Charness ME, Diamond I: Alcohol and the nervous system. Current Neurology 5:383, 1984. *A discussion of recent advances in many alcohol-related neurologic disorders.*

Dreyfus PM, Geel SE: Vitamin and nutritional deficiencies. In Albers RW, Siegel GJ, Katzman R, Agranoff BW (eds.): Basic Neurochemistry. 3rd ed. Boston, Little, Brown and Company, 1981. *A clear discussion of the basic neurochemistry of the vitamins.*

Greenberg DA, Diamond I: Wernicke-Korsakoff syndrome. In Tartar RE, Van Thiel DH (eds.): Alcohol and the Brain: Chronic Effects. New York, Plenum Publishing Corp., 1984. *A discussion of recent advances.*

Harper CG, Giles M, Finlay-Jones R: Clinical signs in the Wernicke-Korsakoff complex: A retrospective analysis of 131 cases diagnosed at necropsy. J Neurol Neurosurg Psychiat 49:341, 1986. *In this large series from Australia, correct antemortem diagnosis was reached in only 20 per cent of cases; most of the missed cases lacked ophthalmoplegia.*

Satya-Murti S, Howard L, Krohel G, et al.: The spectrum of neurologic disorders from vitamin E deficiency. Neurology 36:917, 1986. *A recent study of nine patients with more variable features. A helpful bibliography.*

Sterns RH, Riggs JE, Schochet SS: Osmotic demyelination syndrome following correction of hyponatremia. N Engl J Med 314:1535, 1986. *A recent report of eight patients and a review of the literature suggests that to avoid myelinolysis serum sodium should be raised by less than 12 mmol per liter per day.*

Vinken PJ, Bruyn GW: Handbook of Clinical Neurology. Vol. 28, Metabolic and Deficiency Diseases of the Nervous System. Amsterdam, North Holland Publishing Co., 1976, Ch. 1–14. *A comprehensive review of nutritional diseases of the nervous system.*

SECTION FIVE / THE EXTRAPYRAMIDAL DISORDERS

Stanley Fahn

Extrapyramidal disorders are associated with abnormalities of the basal ganglia and are characteristically manifested by a combination of alterations in muscle tone, disturbances in postural stability, and abnormal involuntary movements or a paucity of movement. Included are the syndromes of parkinsonism, tremor, chorea, athetosis, dystonia, and hemiballism, collectively referred to as *movement disorders*, a heading which also encompasses the syndromes of myoclonus and tics, maladies that probably arise from sites outside the basal ganglia. Usually, diagnosis of the particular abnormal involuntary movement depends more on careful clinical observation than on laboratory study. The age and mode of onset, genetic traits, exposure to drugs and toxins, progression of symptoms, and development of other neurologic features (e.g., dementia) provide the most important clues to etiology.

ANATOMIC, PHYSIOLOGIC, AND BIOCHEMICAL CORRELATES. The basal ganglia comprise five paired nuclei: caudate nucleus, putamen, globus pallidus (or pallidum), subthalamic nucleus, and substantia nigra (Fig. 1). The first three lie deep within the cerebral hemispheres and collectively are referred to as the corpus striatum. The subthalamic nucleus is in the diencephalon, and the substantia nigra is located in the midbrain.

Although separated by the internal capsule, the caudate and putamen are similar microscopically, chemically, and physiologically and are considered collectively as the neostriatum or striatum. The striatum serves as the main site of neural input into the basal ganglia, receiving afferents from all parts of the cerebral cortex and from the nucleus centrum medianum of the thalamus. The major output of the neostriatum is to the pallidum and the zona reticulata portion of the substantia nigra. The pallidum and zona reticulata are also separated by the internal capsule, and are similar microscopically, chemically, and physiologically. These two regions serve as the major site of neural output from the basal ganglia,

with the principal neural efferent pathway going to the ventral anterior (VA) nucleus of the thalamus and thence to the premotor cortex. The premotor cortex is one source of the corticospinal tract (pyramidal tract), the major descending cortical efferent pathway controlling motor function.

The subthalamic nucleus receives afferents from the pallidum and sends its efferents back to the pallidum. Thus, it can be considered to function as a modulator of the globus pallidus and probably regulates the basal ganglia output to the VA nucleus of the thalamus. In an analogous fashion, the substantia nigra can be considered to modulate the neostriatum. The dorsal part of the substantia nigra (zona compacta) sends efferents to the neostriatum (the dopaminergic nigrostriatal pathway), and the ventral part of the substantia nigra (zona reticulata) receives fibers from the neostriatum.

Considerable progress has been made in identifying and understanding the neurotransmitters of some of the neuronal pathways in the basal ganglia. The nigrostriatal pathway contains dopamine and may inhibit the striatum. The other inputs to the striatum (the thalamostriatal pathway and the glutamate-containing corticostriatal pathway) are excitatory. The GABA-containing efferents from the neostriatum to the pallidum and substantia nigra are inhibitory. Lesions of the substantia nigra with resulting loss of dopamine in the striatum result in the bradykinetic syndrome of parkinsonism. Drugs that deplete dopamine (e.g., reserpine) and drugs that block striatal dopamine receptors (e.g., phenothiazines) can also cause parkinsonism. By contrast, excessive dopamine activity (e.g., levodopa overdosage) produces the hyperkinetic state of chorea. A lesion of the subthalamic nucleus produces contralateral hemiballism. It is generally believed that such a lesion removes an inhibitory influence on the pallidum (disinhibition). Lesions in the corpus striatum produce inconsistent patterns of dyskinesias, depending on particular sites and mode of involvement. Athetosis and dystonia can follow

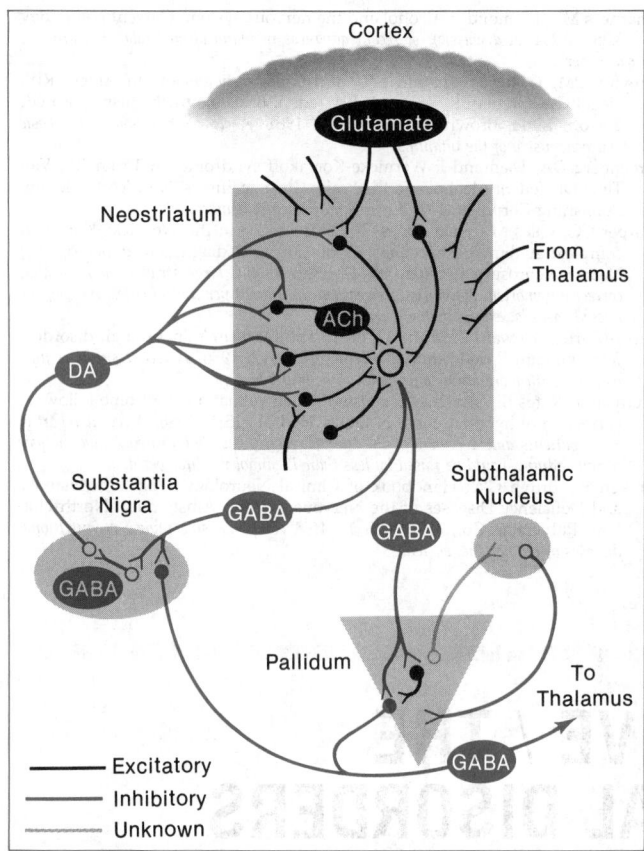

FIGURE 1. A simplified scheme of the neuronal pathways in the basal ganglia, depicting their function and suspected neurotransmitters. DA = dopamine; ACh = acetylcholine; GABA = gamma-aminobutyric acid.

trauma and vascular lesions of the striatum, whereas chorea accompanies degenerative loss of neurons in this structure (e.g., Huntington's chorea).

The basal ganglia serve as a major input to the pyramidal tract motor system. In fact, a lesion of the pyramidal tract sufficient to cause paralysis will eliminate existing dyskinesias, such as tremor and chorea. The term extrapyramidal system was originally coined to denote a motor system operating in parallel with and independent from the pyramidal tract. This is incorrect, but the long use of the term "extrapyramidal" in clinical medicine has embedded it as synonymous with the basal ganglia system. The extrapyramidal system is believed to be involved in automatic movements (e.g., walking, swinging arms when walking, feeding), control of muscle tone, and maintenance of posture. Much of our knowledge of the function of the basal ganglia has been derived from clinicoanatomic correlations in humans.

ABNORMAL INVOLUNTARY MOVEMENTS. Movement disorders can be divided into *bradykinesia* (or *akinesia*), a paucity of automatic and spontaneous movement, and *hyperkinesia* (or *dyskinesia*), which is excessive or abnormal involuntary movements. Bradykinesia is a feature of parkinsonism and is virtually specific for that syndrome, whereas the dyskinesias are subdivided into specific types, depending on their rhythmicity, speed, duration, repetitiveness, and other characteristics. As a general rule, dyskinesias are absent during sleep, reduced with relaxation, and increased with stress.

Tremor refers to relatively rhythmic oscillatory movements. These can result from alternating contractions of opposing muscle groups (e.g., parkinsonian tremor) or from simultaneous contractions of agonist and antagonist muscles, with one group more forceful than the other (e.g., essential tremor). Clinical examination of tremor can aid in the etiologic

diagnosis (Table 1). One should seek for (1) tremor at rest (hands in lap when patient is sitting or at side when patient is lying supine), (2) postural tremor (arms outstretched in front of body), (3) action tremor (when patient is moving arms or using hands to write or lift a cup of water to the mouth), and (4) intention tremor (finger-to-nose maneuver).

The classic parkinson tremor is present at rest. In the limbs, it is almost always distal, being present in the hands (pill-rolling) and feet. Tremor can also involve the tongue, lips, and chin, but rarely the head or neck. The rate of parkinsonian tremor is from 3 to 7 Hz. Characteristically, the tremor at rest transiently disappears when the patient initiates movement of the involved part. Some patients with parkinsonism may have an action tremor in addition to or instead of tremor at rest.

Postural and action tremors are more rapid than tremor at rest (rate between 7 and 11 Hz) and are also more severe distally than proximally. Drugs, metabolic illnesses, and essential tremor are common causes. These tremors can usually be suppressed by beta-adrenergic blockers such as propranolol. Intention tremor (rate: 1.5 to 3 Hz) is a manifestation of cerebellar pathology, especially in the major outflow pathway, the superior cerebellar peduncle. The most common cause is multiple sclerosis; unfortunately, no effective drug is available for this problem. Thalamotomy may bring relief of all types of tremor.

Chorea refers to brief, irregular, nonrhythmic contractions that can involve any or all parts of the body. In disorders such as Huntington's disease and Sydenham's chorea, the choreic movements are not repetitive; instead, they flow from one muscle to another. This can be an important distinction from tardive dyskinesia, in which the brief movements are rhythmic and repetitive (stereotypic). In chorea, patients frequently try to mask the abnormal jerks by carrying out voluntary movements, so-called semipurposeful movements. Patients with chorea cannot maintain a sustained, even contraction, as manifested by "milkmaid" grips, inability to keep the tongue protruded, stuttering gait, and clumsiness with dropping of objects.

Ballism is a form of chorea in which the brisk, involuntary, large-amplitude contractions affect proximal muscles, causing wild, flinging movements of the limbs. The movements usually occur unilaterally (hemiballism).

Athetosis refers to continual slow, writhing movements that can involve limbs (distal and proximal), trunk, head, face, and tongue. When the movements are brief, the term choreoathetosis is commonly applied; when sustained contractions occur at the end of an athetotic movement, the term athetotic dystonia can be used. It is common to see an increase of athetotic movements when the patient carries out voluntary movements (overflow phenomenon).

Dystonia refers to involuntary movements with sustained contractions at the end of the movement. The positions can be prolonged (dystonic postures) but usually last only a second or less (dystonic movements). Dystonic movements are usually of a twisting nature; hence the term torsion dystonia. They may be brisk from the beginning to peak of

TABLE 1. A CLASSIFICATION OF COMMON ABNORMAL TREMORS

   I. Tremor at rest
      A. Parkinsonism
  II. Postural and action tremor
      A. Essential tremor
      B. Accentuated physiologic tremor
         1. Epinephrine, amphetamines
         2. Thyrotoxicosis
         3. Anxiety, fatigue
         4. Lithium, tricyclics
         5. Alcohol withdrawal
 III. Intention tremor
      A. Multiple sclerosis
      B. Wilson's disease
      C. Phenytoin toxicity

the contraction, and a misdiagnosis of chorea is not uncommon. However, if a twisting aspect is present, a diagnosis of dystonia is appropriate even if sustained contractions are not obvious. Action dystonia refers to dystonic movements that occur only when the affected part of the body is in voluntary motion. For example, twisting movements of a leg or foot may appear only when the patient attempts to walk. As the dystonia becomes more severe, the involuntary contractions appear at rest as well. Another peculiar but characteristic feature of dystonia is the lessening of abnormal contractions by tactile or proprioceptive input. For example, patients with torticollis will frequently place a hand on the mandible to provide some relief from the involuntary muscular contractions. Dystonic movements may be generalized or limited to only one part of the body. The focal dystonias include spasmodic torticollis, writer's cramp, blepharospasm, and spastic dysphonia.

Myoclonus refers to shock-like or lightning-like movements due to muscular contractions or inhibitions (the latter is referred to as negative myoclonus). Myoclonic jerks can involve a single muscle or a group of muscles, with the amplitude ranging from a small muscular flicker to a large body-moving synchronous jerk. The myoclonus that accompanies the initial stage of normal sleep is an example of the latter. Asterixis, which resembles a tremor, is an example of negative myoclonus. It occurs in metabolic encephalopathies and is due to brief periods of electrical silence in muscles.

Tics are complex coordinated movements that appear suddenly and transiently. Head shaking, eye blinking, shoulder shrugging, and complex facial contortions are examples. In addition to motor tics, vocal tics are common, and when present indicate a diagnosis of Tourette's syndrome (Ch. 471).

ALTERATIONS IN MUSCLE TONE. Increased muscle tone (rigidity) and decreased muscle tone (hypotonia) are common components of extrapyramidal disorders. Tone is determined by the examiner who manipulates the passive limb, neck, and trunk of the patient. Rigidity is most commonly encountered in parkinsonism, and must be differentiated from spasticity. The latter accompanies corticospinal tract lesions and is manifested by increased tone in either flexion or extension of a limb, with sudden relaxation as the muscle continues to be stretched (clasp knife phenomenon). Spasticity is also associated with weakness, increased tendon reflexes, and a Babinski sign. In contrast, rigidity is present in both flexion and extension and continues throughout the length of muscle stretch. Most often it is jerky (cogwheeling) owing to an underlying tremor rhythm, but it can be smooth (lead-pipe rigidity). Electromyographic recordings reveal that the agonist and antagonist muscles contract simultaneously, even when the patient attempts to relax. Hypotonia occurs characteristically in chorea and may also be present in patients with torsion dystonia at a time when the muscle is not involuntarily contracting.

DISTURBANCES OF POSTURAL REFLEXES. Normally, an individual can recover balance quickly if thrown off his center of gravity. Such postural reflexes tend to be lost in parkinsonism, Huntington's disease, and Wilson's disease. The effect leads to falling when the patient attempts to walk or stand. Such reflexes can be tested by pulling the standing patient backward or forward toward the examiner with a quick tug on the shoulders. One must prepare to catch the patient should he not be able to recover owing to loss of postural reflexes.

Postural changes, such as stooping and kyphosis, are encountered in parkinsonism. Torsion dystonia can lead to deformities such as scoliosis, tortipelvis, and lordosis. Eventually, fixed postures develop as a result of contractures.

DeLong MR, Georgopoulos AP: Motor functions of the basal ganglia. In Handbook of Physiology. The Nervous System II. 2nd ed. Bethesda, MD, American Physiological Society, 1982, pp 1017–1061. *A review of basal ganglia physiology in terms of motor behavior.*

Findley LJ, Capildeo R (eds.): Movement Disorders: Tremor. London, The Macmillan Company, 1984. *The most complete, but discursive, treatise on tremors of all types.*

Jankovic J, Fahn S: Physiologic and pathologic tremors: Diagnosis, mechanism, and management. Ann Intern Med 93:460, 1980. *An etiologic classification of tremors and their mechanisms and treatment.*

Martin JP: The Basal Ganglia and Posture. Philadelphia, J. B. Lippincott Company, 1967. *An outstanding discussion of the role of the basal ganglia in postural mechanisms in normal and disease states.*

Penney JB Jr, Young AB: Striatal inhomogeneities and basal ganglia function. Movement Disorders 1:3, 1986. *The latest review of neurotransmitter pathways within the basal ganglia and their role in motor function.*

468 PARKINSONISM

Parkinsonism is a clinical syndrome consisting of four cardinal signs: tremor at rest, rigidity, bradykinesia, and loss of postural reflexes. Not all patients have all four cardinal signs. Bradykinesia refers to a paucity of automatic and spontaneous movements and difficulty in initiating voluntary movement. Bradykinesia is almost always present in parkinsonism and is virtually synonymous with this diagnosis. Bradykinesia accounts for the majority of parkinsonian symptoms and signs: a general slowing down of movement, masked face (hypomimia), decreased frequency of blinking with a staring expression, decreased swallowing resulting in drooling of saliva, soft voice (hypophonia), loss of speech modulation, impaired handwriting with micrographia, decreasing amplitude in performing rapid repetitive movements (such as opening and closing the hand or tapping the foot), difficulty in arising from a chair and turning in bed, loss of armswing on walking with a tendency to take short steps or shuffle, and loss of spontaneous gesturing when speaking.

Parkinsonism is the most common extrapyramidal disorder. Its prevalence has been placed at close to 1 million individuals in the United States, with the addition of 50,000 new cases each year. It is a prominent cause of disability.

Parkinsonism can be categorized into three etiologic groups (Table 468–1): (1) the primary or idiopathic disorder referred to as Parkinson's disease, (2) secondary or acquired parkinsonism, and (3) "parkinsonism-plus" syndromes, in which additional neurologic findings are present. A history of encephalitis, exposure to drugs or toxins, surgical removal of the parathyroid glands, or previous strokes suggests one of the secondary forms of parkinsonism. The presence of impaired ocular movements, orthostatic hypotension, cerebellar ataxia, or dementia suggests one of the "parkinsonism-plus" syndromes.

In parkinsonism, dopamine activity in the striatum is deficient. In Parkinson's disease, there is a loss of pigmented neurons in the substantia nigra and locus ceruleus with

TABLE 468–1. A CLASSIFICATION OF COMMON FORMS OF PARKINSONISM

I. **Primary**
   Idiopathic parkinsonism (Parkinson's disease)
II. **Secondary**
   A. Infectious: postencephalitic parkinsonism
   B. Toxins: manganese, carbon monoxide, MPTP
   C. Drugs: antipsychotics, reserpine
   D. Hypoparathyroidism
   E. Vascular
III. **Parkinsonism-plus**
   A. Striatonigral degeneration
   B. Progressive supranuclear palsy
   C. Shy-Drager syndrome
   D. Normal pressure hydrocephalus
   E. Alzheimer's disease
   F. Wilson's disease
   G. Huntington's disease

subsequent loss of their dopamine and norepinephrine neurotransmitters. In postencephalitic parkinsonism, the midbrain is particularly affected, with loss of substantia nigra neurons. In these two conditions degeneration of the dopaminergic nigrostriatal pathway leads to striatal dopamine deficiency. Reserpine depletes striatal dopamine, and antipsychotic drugs (e.g., phenothiazines and butyrophenones) block dopamine receptors. In other conditions (e.g., lacunar infarcts, hypoparathyroidism, striatonigral degeneration, and progressive supranuclear palsy), it is suspected that striatal dopamine receptors are directly affected. Reduction or blocking of dopamine receptors renders treatment with levodopa or dopamine agonists ineffective.

PRIMARY PARKINSONISM (Parkinson's Disease)

The incidence of Parkinson's disease increases with age, reaching a maximum at about 75 and declining after that. Idiopathic parkinsonism can occur in younger adults and, rarely, in children. (Juvenile parkinsonism is often a feature of Wilson's disease, Huntington's disease, or rarer forms of pallidal degeneration.) Both sexes are affected, males more than females by a ratio of 3:2. Familial parkinsonism sometimes occurs, but the lack of concordance in twins indicates the absence of a strong genetic factor.

Parkinson's disease begins insidiously, most commonly with tremor or bradykinesia in one limb. The symptoms then involve the other limb on the same side and tend to remain unilateral for several years before spreading to the opposite side. Rigidity, masked face, and soft voice appear early, and the patient reports a slowness in carrying out the day's activities. The gait becomes short stepped and shuffling. Loss of postural reflexes with unsteadiness on turning and festination (the need to walk faster and faster to avoid falling forward) appears as the disease progresses. Postural deformities appear: the head is flexed forward, the trunk is stooped and may be tilted to one side, the hands develop ulnar deviation with flexion at the metacarpophalangeal joints and extension at the interphalangeal joints, and the arms are adducted at the sides with elbows flexed. This characteristic posture plus masked face often allows first inspection to make the diagnosis even if tremor is not present.

As the disease progresses, patients develop gait hesitation ("freezing") on initiating gait (start-hesitation), when approaching a target (terminal-hesitation), and when trying to walk in a crowded area, as if the feet are glued to the ground. With progressive bradykinesia and loss of postural reflexes, the patient eventually becomes wheelchair bound. Swallowing difficulty with choking becomes a problem. Parkinson's disease is not lethal, but increased mortality occurs because of debility, aspiration pneumonia, urinary tract infections, and decubitus ulcers. The rate of progression varies. Disability seldom ensues until 10 to 15 years after onset.

Other symptoms include personality changes: patients become less assertive and more passive, dependent, fearful, and indecisive, disabling qualities for those in an executive position. Depression is common, and dementia may ensue as the disease progresses. Some patients complain of pain, tingling, numbness, and burning sensations, usually on the side of initial symptoms. These are frequently misdiagnosed as arthritis or bursitis. Primitive reflexes, such as Myerson's sign (repetitive blinking on repetitive tapping of the glabella), snout reflex, and palmomental reflex, are commonly found.

Pathologically, depigmentation of the normally pigmented brainstem nuclei is characteristic, and cytoplasmic eosinophilic inclusions (Lewy bodies) are seen microscopically in substantia nigra and locus ceruleus neurons. The initiating cause is unknown.

SECONDARY PARKINSONISM

This category comprises numerous disorders in which parkinsonism provides the predominant symptoms or in which

it plays a smaller role in the clinical picture. The list includes poisonings with manganese, carbon monoxide and a synthetic opiate by-product (MPTP), brain tumors affecting basal ganglia function, cerebral trauma, intoxication with neuroleptic drugs, encephalitis, hypoparathyroidism and basal ganglia calcification, chronic hepatocerebral degeneration, and cerebrovascular disease. Most frequent are drug-induced parkinsonism, postencephalitic parkinsonism, and vascular parkinsonism.

DRUG-INDUCED PARKINSONISM. Drug-induced parkinsonism rivals idiopathic parkinsonism as the most common form of this syndrome. High dosages of both reserpine and the antipsychotic drugs (e.g., phenothiazines and butyrophenones) cause parkinsonism. Reserpine is now usually used only in low dosage to treat hypertension, making the antipsychotic agents the predominant offending agents. Reserpine depletes the storage of dopamine in the dopaminergic nerve terminals in the striatum; the antipsychotic agents and the gastrointestinal-active drug, metoclopramide, block postsynaptic dopamine receptors in the striatum to produce several extrapyramidal syndromes: (1) Acute *akathisia* (motor restlessness) can occur as the dosage is increased; sometimes anticholinergics relieve this symptom. (2) Acute *dystonic reactions* can appear with the initial doses, especially in children and young adults. These dystonic postures can be relieved with parenteral administration of anticholinergics (benztropine, 2 mg intramuscularly), antihistamines (diphenhydramine, 50 mg intravenously), or diazepam (5 to 7.5 mg intravenously). (3) *Oculogyric crisis*, in which the eyes are deviated in a fixed posture for minutes to hours, is a form of dystonia, but occurs in adults as well as children. It can be relieved by the drugs described above. (4) *Parkinsonism* can appear as a toxic reaction and resembles idiopathic parkinsonism in all the cardinal signs of the syndrome. Levodopa will not reverse this complication, probably because the dopamine receptors are blocked and occupied by the antipsychotic agent. Oral anticholinergic drugs are effective (e.g., trihexyphenidyl, 2 mg three times a day). If the antipsychotic drug is withdrawn, the symptoms clear over several weeks to months. (5) *Tardive dyskinesia*, a chorealike disorder presenting predominantly as an oral dyskinesia, can appear after long-term use of antipsychotic drugs. The condition may be irreversible and can worsen when the drugs are withdrawn. (6) *Tardive dystonia*, a persistent dystonic disorder, predominantly affecting the upper part of the body, often with retrocollis and opisthotonus. In contrast to choreic tardive dyskinesia, this complication occurs in children as well as adults. (7) *Tardive akathisia*, a persistent motor restlessness often accompanying tardive dyskinesia and tardive dystonia.

POSTENCEPHALITIC PARKINSONISM. The pandemics of encephalitis lethargica (von Economo's encephalitis) that occurred between 1919 and 1926 caused a variety of extrapyramidal disorders. Parkinsonism sometimes began years after the encephalitis. A viral etiology was suspected but never established.

Clinically, postencephalitic parkinsonism progressed more slowly than Parkinson's disease. Affected patients could have oculogyric crises and a variety of neurologic deficits, such as hemiplegia, ocular palsies, dystonia, chorea, tics, or behavioral disorders. Postencephalitic parkinsonism is more sensitive to levodopa therapy than is Parkinson's disease. The condition has been reported in association with coxsackieviruses, Japanese B encephalitis, and western equine encephalitis. In most cases, the parkinsonian syndrome either improves or remains stable.

VASCULAR PARKINSONISM. Most parkinsonism among persons over age 70 is of the idiopathic variety. However, vascular or arteriosclerotic parkinsonism does occur in middle life as well as in old age. Occasionally it follows a stroke, but more often it appears as a complication of multiple small infarctions involving the striatum and is diagnosed by CT and

MR imaging. Gait disturbance is the most frequent complaint, with short steps, "freezing," and unsteadiness on turning common. Increased muscle tone and loss of postural reflexes are present, but tremor is rare, as are masked facies and classic bradykinesia. Dementia may be present, as well as hyperactive tendon reflexes and Babinski signs. Antiparkinson drugs have little benefit.

MPTP-PARKINSONISM. Drug addicts and chemists exposed to the synthetic opiate MPTP have developed parkinsonism. In glial cells, MPTP is metabolized to MPP+, which is taken up into dopamine neurons and damages them irreversibly. Patients respond to levodopa. This entity raises the possibility that exogenous toxins may contribute to the cause of Parkinson's disease.

PARKINSONISM-PLUS (Multisystem Degenerations)

The clinical signs of parkinsonism can accompany other neurologic deficits in several multisystem degenerative diseases including striatonigral degeneration, olivopontocerebellar degeneration (with cerebellar ataxia), progressive supranuclear palsy (with ophthalmoplegia), and Shy-Drager syndrome (with orthostatic hypotension). Parkinsonism with profound dementia can occur in patients in whom cerebral pathology reveals features of both Alzheimer's disease and Parkinson's disease. The parkinsonism-dementia complex is also seen in some patients with normal pressure hydrocephalus, which typically presents as a triad of gait disturbance, dementia, and urinary incontinence. Rarely, parkinsonian features, with or without associated dementia, accompany otherwise typical amyotrophic lateral sclerosis.

STRIATONIGRAL DEGENERATION. This rare disorder presents clinically as Parkinson's disease. As the disease progresses, however, signs of cerebellar ataxia and laryngeal stridor may appear. Loss of neurons occurs predominantly in the substantia nigra and putamen, with additional degeneration in other basal ganglia and the cerebellum. This disorder may be one of the many types of the olivopontocerebellar degenerations (see Ch. 475). The diagnosis can be suspected clinically by its failure to respond to levodopa, explained by the loss of dopamine receptors with the neuronal loss in the striatum.

PROGRESSIVE SUPRANUCLEAR PALSY. Progressive supranuclear palsy can resemble Parkinson's disease, but tremor is rare. Additional distinguishing features are external ophthalmoplegia, nuchal dystonia (especially neck hyperextension), and a dystonic facial smile with deep nasolabial folds (rather than the flattened folds seen in Parkinson's disease). The presence of ophthalmoplegia is required for the diagnosis, but may not appear until late in the course. Initially vertical eye movements are lost. Whereas upward gaze alone is limited in Parkinson's disease, downward gaze is also impaired in progressive supranuclear palsy. Eventually, horizontal eye movements become limited. A full range of reflex eye movements can be detected by the doll's-eyes test. Pathologically, basal ganglia, brain stem, and cerebellum contain neuronal loss and neurofibrillary tangles. There is no effective treatment.

MANAGEMENT OF PARKINSONISM

GENERAL PRINCIPLES. The overall goals of therapy should be directed toward keeping the patient functioning independently as long as possible. Although symptoms can often be suppressed, at least for a short period of time, the consequences of chronic drug administration must be considered, since long-term levodopa use may be accompanied by disabling effects. It is best to individualize therapy in treating parkinsonism; one must constantly adjust drug dosage and timing to achieve the optimal balance between amelioration of symptoms and avoidance of unacceptable adverse reactions.

Parkinsonism is frequently accompanied by fearfulness, passivity, dependence, and depression, and affected patients need repeated encouragement and reassurance in meeting the stresses of everyday life and their all-too-realistic fears of the future.

PHYSICAL THERAPY. Patients must be encouraged to be as active as possible; the family must participate in this as well. Maintaining employment as long as feasible, taking long walks, gardening, and becoming active in hobbies are among the possibilities. As the disease advances, more formal home exercise programs with a physiotherapist can be arranged. Appropriately placed hand bars enable patients to arise unassisted from toilet seats or beds. Patients should be encouraged to carry out daily activities as independently as possible. For gait difficulty and unsteadiness, a cane is not useful but may serve as a warning that the patient is handicapped, thereby avoiding unnecessary jostling and preventing falls and fractures. Pain from rigid cervical muscles may be relieved by heat and massage.

DRUG THERAPY. When the disease is mild and symptoms not troublesome, drugs are not necessary. The physician can explain that the symptoms may progress very slowly in the first few years, that drugs can be utilized at the appropriate time, and that regular evaluations will be carried out. As symptoms become annoying or restrict activities, drug therapy becomes necessary.

Direct-acting dopamine receptor agonists have less antiparkinsonian effect than levodopa (see below). Bromocriptine (Parlodel) is commercially available; other agonists are limited currently to investigational studies. Bromocriptine is used alone in the initiation of drug therapy or later in combination with levodopa, preferably in low doses (up to 40 mg per day). Using the drug before adding levodopa appears to minimize the fluctuations associated with the latter. Higher doses of bromocriptine often produce adverse reactions, including hallucinations, delusions, and confusion. These tend to be more severe and longer lasting than those induced by levodopa. Other adverse effects seen with levodopa also occur with bromocriptine, including anorexia, nausea, vomiting, postural hypotension, and abnormal involuntary movements. In addition, erythromelalgia can occur in the extremities, probably related to an ergot effect of bromocriptine, which is an ergot derivative. Erythromelalgia disappears when the drug is discontinued. Bromocriptine unfortunately tends to lose its effect with long-term use, and levodopa will need to be added.

The antiviral agent amantadine HCl (Symmetrel) has an antiparkinsonian effect in approximately two thirds of patients. The usual dosage is 100 mg twice a day, and any benefit becomes evident within two to three days. Effectiveness may persist in mild disease, but in more advanced stages it decreases unless levodopa has been given concomitantly. Amantadine is believed to act by enhancing the release of dopamine stored in presynaptic terminals. The most common adverse effect is livedo reticularis, a medically unimportant reddish mottling of the skin around the knees. If pronounced erythematous edema of the ankles occurs, amantadine should be discontinued. Amantadine also can cause nonfrightening visual hallucinations, usually of people and animals. Lowering the dosage usually provides relief. If amantadine is not effective within three days, it should be discontinued.

Anticholinergics are useful as adjuncts to levodopa, especially to suppress tremor. They are also the agents of choice in drug-induced parkinsonism. Commonly employed anticholinergics are trihexyphenidyl (Artane), available in 2- and 5-mg tablets; benztropine mesylate (Cogentin), as 1- and 2-mg tablets; ethopropazine (Parsidol), as 50- and 100-mg tablets; cycrimine (Pagitane), as 1.25- and 2.5-mg tablets; procyclidine (Kemadrin), as 2- and 5-mg tablets; and biperiden (Akineton), as 2-mg tablets. Treatment should be initiated with small doses (e.g., trihexyphenidyl, 2 mg three times daily), and gradually increased until further increases yield no additional benefit or side effects occur. Peripheral anticholinergic adverse effects include blurred vision, dry mouth, anhidrosis, hyperthermia, constipation, and urinary urgency or sometimes retention. The central side effects are forgetfulness, confusion, delusions, hallucinations, somnolence, and rarely coma. The last of these can be treated with physostigmine, 0.5 to 2 mg intramuscularly. Anticholinergics tend to produce mental disturbances in the elderly and should be avoided in patients older than 70.

When parkinsonian symptoms cannot be adequately suppressed by bromocriptine, amantadine or anticholinergics (alone or in combination), levodopa is employed. Peripheral adverse effects (anorexia, nausea, vomiting) can be largely avoided if levodopa is taken concomitantly with a peripheral dopa decarboxylase inhibitor. In the United States this combination is marketed as Sinemet, which contains carbidopa and levodopa. The combinations available are 10/100-mg, 25/100-mg, and 25/250-mg (carbidopa/levodopa) tablets. The more decarboxylase inhibitor used, the less likely are peripheral adverse effects. However, the potency of levodopa is enhanced, increasing the possibility of central adverse effects such as abnormal involuntary movements (chorea and dystonia), confusion, hallucinations, delusions, somnolence, and postural hypotension. One method is to begin treatment with carbidopa/levodopa, 10/100 mg three times daily. If peripheral adverse reactions appear, change to 25/100-mg tablets. There is usually a latency period before maximal benefit at a given dose is encountered. The dosage can be increased gradually, utilizing half-tablets in the incremental build-up, in order to "fine tune" the response. Low dosage may prevent complications seen with chronic use. Therefore, the patient who is retired from his occupation can be brought to a level approximately 80 to 85 per cent free of symptoms, rather than totally free, which may require higher dosages. Concomitant administration of bromocriptine, amantadine, and anticholinergics may allow for smaller doses of levodopa and may be especially valuable to control symptoms such as tremor. Levodopa can control tremor but is especially effective in eliminating rigidity and reducing bradykinesia. Loss of postural reflexes may be ameliorated in the early but not advanced stages of the disease. With long-term treatment central adverse effects are usually more troublesome than peripheral ones. In such situations, it may be necessary to change from carbidopa/levodopa to levodopa alone. Levodopa is available in capsules and scored tablets in strengths of 100, 250, and 500 mg. Since the potency of levodopa is increased about fourfold if given as carbidopa/levodopa, levodopa alone allows for finer adjustments of the central effects of the drug.

Levodopa is contraindicated in patients with a history of malignant melanoma and in those with psychosis or profound dementia. In the presence of cardiac arrhythmias, as much as 200 mg per day of carbidopa (available as Lodosyn from Merck) should be given to block peripheral formation of dopamine; antiarrhythmic agents or digoxin should be used as indicated. Levodopa can be administered safely in hepatic, renal, and hematopoietic disorders. With a history of peptic ulcer, carbidopa/levodopa is preferred over levodopa alone.

In more advanced stages of parkinsonism or with chronic administration of levodopa, central adverse effects may appear with doses that are insufficient to control the symptoms of the disease. Since both levodopa and other commonly used drugs must be reduced in this situation, drugs with mild anticholinergic properties can be employed. These include diphenhydramine (Benadryl), orphenadrine (Disipal), and chlorphenoxamine (Phenoxene). Dosages of 50 mg three times daily may prove helpful. In contrast to the more powerful anticholinergic agents, these three drugs tend not to produce mental disturbances.

Tricyclic antidepressants may help to relieve the depressive symptoms that often accompany parkinsonism. Amitriptyline, 50 to 75 mg at bedtime, and imipramine, 25 mg three times daily, are commonly used. For tremor incompletely relieved by antiparkinson drugs and aggravated by stress or anxiety, anxiolytic agents such as diazepam and beta-adrenergic antagonists such as propranolol may provide some relief.

Clinical fluctuations from levodopa therapy usually begin after taking the drug for two years or longer and appear in at least 40 per cent of patients on long-term therapy. These troublesome fluctuations may prevent employment and are resistant to control. There are two predominant forms: the "on-off" phenomenon and the "wearing-off" or "end-of-dose" effect. The on-off phenomenon consists of sudden loss of the antiparkinson effect of levodopa. Symptoms of severe parkinsonism may produce immobility from severe bradykinesia and rigidity. They appear irregularly, may last up to several hours, can recur several times daily, and disappear ("on" effect) as suddenly as they appear, even without more levodopa. Higher doses of levodopa or bromocriptine can prevent the episodes, but usually induce continuous and distressing dyskinesias.

The wearing-off phenomenon comes on gradually, as plasma levels of levodopa fall. The phenomenon is a pharmacokinetic effect due to reduced bioavailability of levodopa as a result of its short half-life in plasma (30 to 45 minutes). Spacing the doses more closely is a partial remedy, and some patients take levodopa every three hours, every two hours, or even more frequently to prevent the "off" periods. Unfortunately, the price may be a state of continual dyskinesia. Longer-acting dopamine agonists reduce this problem. Some patients with severe wearing-off phenomena are unable to miss a single dose of levodopa without being in an "off" state, and if awakened in the middle of the night are immobile. These "dopa addicts" require levodopa before retiring and perhaps during the night. Patients who are free of clinical fluctuations do not usually require bedtime medication and can be maintained on three doses a day. Suddenly discontinuing levodopa carries considerable risk and should be avoided except for severe toxicity, and then confined to the hospital to protect against immobility and aspiration.

Treatment of postencephalitic parkinsonism usually requires smaller dosages of levodopa than does idiopathic parkinsonism. Drug-induced parkinsonism responds well to anticholinergics. Striatonigral degeneration may respond to levodopa in the early stages of the disease, but then becomes resistant to therapy, as does progressive supranuclear palsy. Anticholinergics, the drugs of choice in these conditions, offer only modest relief.

SURGICAL MEASURES. Stereotactic lesions of the ventrolateral thalamus can alleviate tremor, rigidity, and dyskinesias of the contralateral limbs. This approach is not useful for bradykinesia and loss of postural reflexes, which are the predominant causes of disability, nor does it halt progression of the disease. Bilateral surgery to relieve tremor on both sides usually results in impaired speech. With the introduction of levodopa therapy, surgical therapy has almost entirely been discontinued.

COURSE OF THE PARKINSONIAN SYNDROME. Although levodopa and other drugs do not alter the progression of the disease, they do increase survival time because of improved functional capacity. The mortality rate has been reduced by half since the introduction of levodopa. The symptom that becomes least responsive is loss of postural reflexes, and falling with resultant hip fracture is a potential consequence. Although chronic levodopa therapy may bring troublesome adverse effects of clinical fluctuations, dyskinesias, mental disturbances, and loss of efficacy, many patients continue to have a substantial response to the drug for a decade or more.

Ballard PA, Tetrud JW, Langston JW: Permanent human parkinsonism due to 1-methyl-4-phenyl-1,2,3,6-tetrahydropyridine (MPTP): Seven cases. Neurology 35:949, 1985. *Describes the clinical features of MPTP-parkinsonism.*

Burke RE, Fahn S, Jankovic J, et al.: Tardive dystonia: late-onset and persistent dystonia caused by antipsychotic drugs. Neurology 32:1335, 1982. *Describes the clinical and pharmacologic features of a persistent complication of dopamine-receptor-blocking drugs.*

Maher ER, Lees AJ: The clinical features and natural history of the Steele-Richardson-Olszewski syndrome (progressive supranuclear palsy). Neurology 36:1005, 1986. *The clinical findings and the progression of this disorder are characterized.*

Marsden CD, Fahn S (eds.): Movement Disorders. 2nd ed. London, Butterworth Scientific, 1987. *A multi-authored, well-edited monograph that discusses most aspects of these conditions with a welcome clinical slant.*

Rinne UK: Combined bromocriptine-levodopa therapy early in Parkinson's disease. Neurology 35:1196, 1985. *Reports that if parkinsonism patients are first treated with bromocriptine, and later with levodopa when the first drug is no longer effective, the clinical fluctuations commonly encountered with levodopa alone are largely prevented.*

Ward DC, Duvoisin RC, Ince SE, et al.: Parkinson's disease in 65 pairs of twins and in a set of quadruplets. Neurology 33:815, 1983. *They report that Parkinson's disease is discordant in twins, indicating the lack of a strong genetic factor in its etiology.*

469 ESSENTIAL TREMOR (Familial or Senile Tremor)

Essential tremor is a monosymptomatic disorder, expressed as tremor of the hands, head, and, least frequently, voice. The hand tremor is usually more rapid than that of parkinsonism and occurs with volitional movement instead of at rest. It is aggravated by handwriting and suppressed by the use of alcohol. The age of onset varies, often beginning mildly before the age of 25 and persisting throughout life with some increase in intensity and spread to other body parts. Physical and social disability may result. There is a strong familial incidence distributed as an autosomal dominant trait. With late-life onset, the tremor is commonly called *senile tremor*. No specific neuropathologic lesion has been reported. An occasional patient may develop Parkinson's disease on top of a long history of essential tremor. Beta-adrenergic blocking agents are useful in some patients, but dramatic relief of tremor is not achieved. Propranolol in a dosage of 120 to 240 mg per day in three or four divided doses has been most commonly used. The selective beta-1 adrenergic blocker metoprolol, 50 mg three times daily, can be used in patients with bronchospasm or asthma. Beta-adrenergic blockers should be avoided in patients with congestive heart failure or heart block. The anticonvulsant primidone can sometimes be very effective. Because many patients are sensitive to this drug, it should be started at a dose of 25 mg h.s. The dosage may need to be increased gradually up to 250 mg three times daily. It can be given concomitantly with propranolol. It is probably safer to avoid the use of drugs in the elderly population. Light wine with meals offers sufficient relief to aid dining. The major differential diagnosis is parkinsonism, but the lack of bradykinesia, rigidity, and postural abnormalities, as well as the presence of tremor with action instead of at rest, rule out that disorder.

Findley LJ, Calzetti S, Cleeves L: Primidone in essential tremor. In Findley LJ, Capildeo R (eds.): Movement Disorders: Tremor. London, The Macmillan Company, 1984. *A double-blind study shows the effectiveness of primidone.*

Wilson JF, Marshall RW, Richens A: Essential tremor: Treatment with beta-adrenoceptor blocking drugs. In Findley LJ, Capildeo R (eds.): Movement Disorders: Tremor. London, The Macmillan Company, 1984. *Reviews the mechanism of action of these drugs and the properties required for beneficial effect.*

470 THE CHOREAS

Many disorders can cause choreic movements (Table 470–1), having in common brief, involuntary contractions. It is important to determine whether the movements are fluid (flowing from one location to another), as in classic chorea, or rhythmically repetitive in the same site (stereotypy), as in tardive dyskinesia. The presence of other neurologic deficits (gait disturbance, dementia) assists in the diagnosis of Huntington's disease, and a detailed family history and drug history are essential for reliable diagnosis. A difficult diagnostic problem can arise when a patient with Huntington's disease has been treated with antipsychotic drugs causing tardive dyskinesia.

HEREDITARY CHOREA (Chronic Progressive Chorea, Huntington's Disease)

Huntington's disease, the most common of the hereditary choreas, is a progressive degenerative disorder predominantly affecting the basal ganglia and the cerebral cortex. Clinically, it is manifested by a triad consisting of choreic movements, intellectual decline leading to dementia, and emotional disturbances. The disease is transmitted as an autosomal dominant trait with complete penetrance. Both sexes are equally affected, and each offspring has a 50 per cent chance of becoming affected. In the United States the prevalence ranges from 4 to 8 per 100,000 population. The disease usually begins in adulthood after childbearing, with a peak age at onset of 40 years; it can begin at any age, however, and approximately 10 per cent of cases start before age 20. Often, juvenile cases exhibit bradykinesia and rigidity, rather than chorea and hypotonia. The presence of a movement disorder is essential to the disease; emotional and cognitive disorders are common problems in the general population and hence insufficient for the diagnosis. Motor symptoms begin with clumsiness and the dropping of objects followed by typical chorea, consisting

TABLE 470–1. A CLASSIFICATION OF COMMON CAUSES OF CHOREA

  I. **Hereditary**
    A. Huntington's disease
    B. Wilson's disease
    C. Ataxia-telangiectasia
    D. Lesch-Nyhan syndrome
    E. Chorea-acanthocytosis
    F. Benign hereditary chorea
 II. **Secondary**
    A. Infections
      1. Sydenham's chorea
      2. Encephalitis
    B. Drugs
      1. Levodopa
      2. Estrogen (oral contraceptives)
      3. Phenytoin
      4. Antipsychotic drugs
    C. Metabolic and endocrine
      1. Chorea gravidarum
      2. Thyrotoxicosis
    D. Vascular
      1. Lupus erythematosus
      2. Polycythemia vera
      3. Hemichorea-hemiballism
III. **Unknown**
    A. Senile chorea

first of brief, low-amplitude movements of the fingers, but spreading to involve arms, legs, trunk, neck, and face. The limb movements can be proximal as well as distal and flow from one site to another. In the face they are more common in the forehead than around the mouth (the latter being more common in tardive dyskinesia). Sustained postures are difficult: often, the tongue cannot be protruded steadily nor can a steady grip be maintained. An abnormal gait is characterized by hesitation and stuttering steps and postural instability can lead to frequent falls. Choking is common and sometimes fatal.

Emotional disorders are common and may precede choreic movements. Personality changes, mania, hallucinations, delusions, paranoia, schizophreniform thinking, impulsiveness, hostility, and agitation can develop. Most common are apathy and withdrawn behavior with a decrease in conversation and inattention to personal hygiene. Depression is frequent as is an increased incidence of suicide. Cognitive changes tend to appear later with impairment of recent memory and judgment, loss of capacity to plan and organize, and intellectual decline. Dementia leads to urinary and fecal incontinence and an inability to handle activities of daily living.

Pathologically, there is loss of neurons with reactive gliosis predominantly in the striatum and cerebral cortex. The most consistent neurotransmitter change is a marked reduction of GABA and its synthesizing enzyme, glutamic acid decarboxylase, in the basal ganglia. Acetylcholine, substance P, cholecystokinin and Met-enkephalin also decline, as do dopamine, acetylcholine, and serotonin receptors. Somatostatin, thyrotropin-releasing hormone, and neurotensin show a relative increase. Treatment with GABA agonists or cholinergic agonists has not led to clinical improvement.

The triad of chorea, progressive dementia, and emotional disturbances strongly suggests Huntington's disease. The diagnosis is confirmed by a positive family history, but such may be lacking if a parent is unavailable, has disappeared, or died before symptoms appeared. The lack of a positive family history in the presence of longevity and good health of the parents raises questions of paternity, spontaneous mutation (rare), or misdiagnosis. Computed tomography of the head eventually will reveal atrophy of the caudate nuclei; this may assist in the diagnosis. Positron emission scanning with fluoro-2-deoxyglucose reveals hypometabolism in the basal ganglia. Accurate diagnosis of affected persons and carriers may soon be possible by identifying a marker on the short arm of Chromosome 4 linked to the Huntington gene.

Treatment of Huntington's disease should extend to the family as well as the patient, since this is a hereditary disorder and since the mental symptoms create enormous family stress. Explanation and nondirective genetic discussion are important and will enable family members at risk or who are known carriers to reach a decision about having children. Therapy is available for many of the symptoms. Presynaptic dopamine-depleting agents (reserpine* and tetrabenazine) can reduce chorea. Reserpine therapy should begin with a small dose (0.25 mg per day); the daily dosage is then increased weekly by 0.25 mg until chorea declines. As much as 8 to 10 mg per day may be required. A slow buildup in dosage will usually avoid nasal stuffiness and depression. Postural hypotension and increased apathy may necessitate a reduction in dosage. Dementia is not treatable, but emotional disturbances can be ameliorated. Tricyclic antidepressants are useful for depression, and antipsychotic agents can treat psychosis.

Chorea-acanthocytosis (also called neuroacanthocytosis) is rare in the United States but more common in Japan. It is manifested by mild chorea and tics, self-mutilation (usually of lips and tongue), loss of tendon reflexes, elevated serum creatine phosphokinase, presence of acanthocytes in the blood, and atrophy of the caudate nuclei. *Benign hereditary chorea* is an autosomal dominant disorder in which choreic movements begin in childhood and do not progress; there is no dementia or disability. Wilson's disease is described in Ch. 205, ataxia telangiectasia in Ch. 477, and Lesch-Nyhan syndrome in Ch. 196.

Gusella JF, Wexler NS, Conneally PM, et al.: A polymorphic DNA marker genetically linked to Huntington's disease. Nature 306:234, 1983. *Reports the localization of the gene for Huntington's disease to chromosome 4.*

Kuhl DE, Phelps ME, Markham CH, et al.: Cerebral metabolism and atrophy in Huntington's disease determined by 18-FDG and computed tomographic scan. Ann Neurol 12:425, 1982. *Position emission tomography reveals hypometabolism of striatum in patients with Huntington's disease and in some at-risk individuals.*

Martin JB: Huntington's disease: New approaches to an old problem. Neurology 34:1059, 1984. *A concise review of the clinical, pathologic, genetic, and chemical abnormalities.*

Sakai T, Mawatari S, Iwashita H, et al.: Chorea-acanthocytosis: Clues to clinical diagnosis. Arch Neurol 38:335, 1981. *Descriptions of the clinical features of chorea-acanthocytosis.*

Shoulson I: Care of patients and families with Huntington's disease. In Marsden CD, Fahn S (eds.): Movement Disorders. London, Butterworth Scientific, 1982, pp 277–290. *Describes a practical approach to the diagnosis genetic counseling, and management of families.*

SECONDARY CHOREA

The several causes (see Table 470–1) of acquired chorea, except for tardive dyskinesia, cause similar abnormal movements.

SYDENHAM'S CHOREA (St. Vitus' Dance). This is an acute chorea encountered primarily during childhood, with the greatest incidence between the ages of five and fifteen. Later occurrence can be associated with pregnancy (chorea gravidarum). There is a female preponderance after the age of ten. A close relationship exists with rheumatic fever, and the condition has declined substantially during the antibiotic era.

The choreic movements in this disorder are usually generalized, and only 20 per cent of patients have hemichorea. The brief, involuntary movements flow from site to site, and the patient has difficulty sitting quietly. Fidgety behavior, clumsiness, dropping of objects, dysarthria, and an awkward gait are common. Other neurologic symptoms are infrequent.

Sydenham's chorea is not fatal, and recovery occurs in 2 to 6 months. The few pathologic studies have disclosed scattered vasculitis in the cortex, basal ganglia, cerebellum, and brainstem. There are no specific laboratory abnormalities. Differential diagnosis depends on eliminating other causes of chorea by history and laboratory studies.

Recurrence, with as many as two or three attacks over a period of years, occurs in almost one third of the patients. Since the disease is self-limited, specific drugs may not be necessary. If the chorea is disabling and interferes with school work, short-term treatment with perphenazine (12 to 16 mg per day in divided doses) or haloperidol (3 to 6 mg per day in divided doses) can be effective. Some patients with Sydenham's chorea may have residual deficits of valvular heart disease, behavioral problems, mild motor abnormalities, and a poor performance in psychometric testing.

HEMIBALLISM. Hemiballism is a forceful, violent form of hemichorea manifested by flinging movements of the limbs on one side of the body. The most common cause is a hemorrhage or infarct involving the contralateral subthalamic nucleus. Tumors rarely are involved. Most hemiballism or hemichorea develops on recovery from a hemiparesis and hemisensory deficit secondary to stroke. Occasionally the sensorimotor deficits are minor, and ballism occurs as the initial event. Like other abnormal involuntary movements, ballism disappears during sleep. In most instances, the intensity of hemiballism decreases gradually to hemichorea and then fades away after several weeks, but in some patients the movements persist. Severe movements can be exhausting but can be controlled with drugs such as reserpine or antipsychotic agents. Because of the self-limiting nature of hemiball-

---

*This use is not listed in the manufacturer's directive.

ism, it is reasonable to use antipsychotics for their rapid onset of action and then slowly withdraw the drug to avoid producing tardive dyskinesia.

SENILE CHOREA. Occasional patients older than 60 years present with generalized chorea resembling Huntington's disease, but with no associated dementia, emotional disturbance, available family history, or evidence of other etiologies. Postmortem studies reveal striatal pathology identical to Huntington's disease. It has been speculated that senile chorea is a late-onset form of Huntington's disease in which cognitive symptoms have not developed because of the advanced age of onset. No definitive genetic studies are available.

Aron A, Freeman J, Carter S: The natural history of Sydenham's chorea. Am J Med 38:83, 1965. *One third of patients evaluated an average of 29 years after the initial episode of chorea were found to have valvular heart disease.*

Bird MT, Palkes H, Prensky AL: A follow-up study of Sydenham's chorea. Neurology 26:601, 1976. *An average of an eight-year follow-up evaluation revealed that some individuals have behavioral disorders, abnormal electroencephalograms, and poorer performance on psychometric testing.*

Johnson WG, Fahn S: Treatment of vascular hemiballism and hemichorea. Neurology 27:634, 1977. *Reports on the effectiveness of the antipsychotic drug perphenazine in eight cases of hemiballism.*

Klawans HI, Moses H, Nausieda PA, et al.: Treatment and prognosis of hemiballism. N Engl J Med 295:1348, 1976. *Report on the effectiveness of haloperidol and chlorpromazine in 11 cases.*

Nausieda PA, Grossman BJ, Koller WC, et al.: Syndenham's chorea: An update. Neurology 30:331, 1980. *This survey points out the marked decrease in the incidence of the disorder in recent years.*

TARDIVE DYSKINESIA

This most feared complication of antipsychotic drug therapy can persist indefinitely. The disorder is associated with chronic administration of these drugs (hence the name "tardive"), but there are reports of its occurring after exposure of only several weeks. Tardive dyskinesia is more common in women and the elderly, and more likely to occur with exposure to high dosages and prolonged treatment. The drugs themselves mask the symptoms so that onset is not clearly recognized. Withdrawal of the drug exposes rhythmically repetitive, rapid movements that can occur in most parts of the body. The lower part of the face is involved most often; this oral-lingual-buccal dyskinesia resembles continual chewing movements, with the tongue intermittently darting out of the mouth ("fly-catcher" tongue). In the trunk the movements usually assume a repetitive flexion and extension pattern ("body-rocking"). The distal limbs may flex and extend incessantly ("piano-playing"), whereas the proximal muscles are usually spared. Standing may induce repetitive movements of the legs ("marching in place"). The arms tend to swing to a larger degree than normal and the stride may elongate. The patient may be unaware of the movements unless there is an associated akathisia (a subjective feeling of restlessness), characterized by the need to move about and walk back and forth. Sometimes patients describe feeling as if they were going to jump out of their skin. This most distressing symptom resembles the acute akathisia that sometimes accompanies an initial administration of antipsychotic drugs, but disappears when the drug is withdrawn. In contrast, akathisia in tardive dyskinesia lasts chronically and is made more severe by drug withdrawal; hence it is analogous to the dyskinesia. Both tardive akathisia and tardive dyskinesia can be largely suppressed by antidopaminergic drugs.

The major differential diagnoses are Huntington's disease (Table 470–2) and a focal form of facial and mandibular dystonia referred to as Meige's syndrome (see Ch. 471). Patients with known Huntington's disease also may develop tardive dyskinesia if antipsychotic drugs are used in its treatment. A drug-free history eliminates tardive dyskinesia by definition.

In addition to the classic form of tardive dyskinesia described above, there are two clinical variations. One is the self-limiting "withdrawal emergent" syndrome more common in children, in which choreic movements resembling those

TABLE 470–2. DIFFERENTIAL DIAGNOSIS OF TARDIVE DYSKINESIA AND HUNTINGTON'S DISEASE*

Clinical Features	Tardive Dyskinesia	Huntington's Disease
Akathisia	Present	Absent
Body-rocking	Present	Absent
Marching-in-place	Present	Absent
Oral-lingual-buccal dyskinesia	Present	Sometimes present
Darting tongue	Present	Rarely present
Repetitive movements	Present	Absent
Flowing movements	Absent	Present
Forehead chorea	Absent	Present
Saccadic eye movements	Normal	Abnormal
Protrusion of tongue	Maintained (normal)	Not maintained
Milkmaid grip	Absent	Present
Postural stability	Normal	Impaired
Walking	Reduces chorea	Increases chorea
Gait	Normal	Stuttering, ataxic

*Although the tabulated clinical features may be found in any individual patient, they are not always present in every patient.

seen in Sydenham's chorea or Huntington's disease appear when an antipsychotic drug is suddenly discontinued. There are flowing, rather than repetitive, choreic movements. Reintroducing the antipsychotic drug and tapering it slowly may eliminate the symptoms. The other variant is the presence of sustained dystonic rather than choreic movements. This variant (tardive dystonia) can affect any age.

Tardive dyskinesia is believed to be caused by the development of supersensitive dopamine receptors as a result of chronic blockade by antipsychotic drugs. In some patients who remain drug free for several months or years the syndrome resolves, and withdrawal of the offending agents is the treatment of choice. But many patients, particularly those with psychosis or severe tardive akathisia, must continue to take antidopaminergic drugs. If the patient does not have psychosis, then dopamine-depleting drugs (reserpine and alpha-methylparatyrosine) that act presynaptically are the preferred agents and can relieve both the dyskinesia and akathisia. The dosages are increased slowly, as in the treatment of Huntington's chorea. Anticholinergics sometimes help tardive dyskinesia.

The incidence of tardive dyskinesia appears to be increasing owing to widespread administration of antipsychotic drugs. It is important to consider this complication before prescribing these agents. Such drugs should be used only in clinical situations in which no satisfactory alternatives exist.

Baldessarini RJ, Tarsy D: Tardive dyskinesia. In Lipton J, DiMascio A, Killam KF (eds.): Psychopharmacology. A Generation of Progress. New York, Raven Press, 1978, pp 993–1004. *A concise review of the clinical features and the pharmacology of tardive dyskinesia.*

Fahn S: The tardive dyskinesias. In Matthews WB, Glaser GH (eds.): Recent Adv Clin Neurol 4:229, 1984. *A thorough review of the clinical spectrum of these disorders, along with their epidemiology and pharmacology.*

Fahn S: A therapeutic approach to tardive dyskinesia. J Clin Psychiat 46:19, 1985. *Describes the results of treating patients with reserpine and alpha-methylparatyrosine, including the chance for remission.*

471 THE DYSTONIAS

TORSION DYSTONIA (Dystonia Musculorum Deformans, Torsion Spasms)

The torsion dystonias comprise a group of disorders in which sustained contractions, usually of a twisting nature (torsion spasms) are characteristic. Slow, continual torsion spasms are called athetotic dystonia or athetosis, but torsion spasms can also be rapid. Contractions sustained for minutes to hours are called dystonic postures. Ultimately joint contractures can occur, leading to permanent deformity, especially in the growing child. Both agonist and antagonist muscles contract simultaneously in dystonia. Dystonia can be present at rest or during attempted movement (action dystonia). In carrying out a voluntary movement, inappropriate muscles contract when they should be quiescent. Dystonic movements are sometimes broken up into a tremor pattern (dystonic tremor), which may reflect an attempt to resist the abnormal pulling and maintain a more normal posture. Dystonia varies with change of posture, worsens with stress, decreases with relaxation or hypnosis, disappears with sleep, and is modified by tactile or proprioceptive input.

The torsion dystonias can be etiologically divided into primary and secondary types (Table 471–1). The first is more common and includes hereditary forms and those that are sporadic or idiopathic. The disorder has a higher prevalence in Ashkenazi Jews, but both Jews and non-Jews appear to be susceptible to an autosomal-dominant trait that has a low rate of penetrance and produces a similar clinical illness. Often, formes frustes appear in other members of the family: club foot, scoliosis, torticollis, writer's cramp, and essential tremor. The disease commonly begins between the ages of five and fifteen. The legs are typically affected first, starting with action dystonia. At rest the patient may seem normal, but when he stands or walks, one or both feet assume an equinovarus posture, and the leg executes a bizarre stepping twisting movement. As the disease progresses, the other leg and other parts of the body become involved. Lordosis, scoliosis, torti-pelvis, and torticollis can appear. Because of modification by proprioceptive input, walking backward or running may be less abnormal than walking forward. Action dystonia of the arms interferes with handwriting and other manipulations. Dystonic movements appear at rest, and eventually dystonic postures may develop. When movements are absent, muscle tone is normal or hypotonic; hypertonia accompanies movements. Mentation, sensation, strength, and tendon reflexes remain normal. Many patients tend to plateau after a period of progression.

As a general rule, childhood onset of dystonia is likely to begin in the feet and legs and become progressive and generalized: juvenile onset tends to begin in the hands and arms and plateaus after involving several segments; adult onset tends to remain focal, the neck being the most common site (spasmodic torticollis). Other common varieties of focal dystonia are blepharospasm, facial and mandibular dystonia (Meige's syndrome), spastic dysphonia, and writer's cramp. Primary dystonia with childhood onset is also referred to as dystonia musculorum deformans.

No clear-cut pathologic lesions have been discerned in the brain in primary torsion dystonia. It is assumed that the lesion is of a chemical and physiologic nature, affecting the basal ganglia, since this is the area of pathology in secondary or acquired forms of dystonia. Moreover, lesions in, and drugs that affect, the basal ganglia (i.e., levodopa, antipsychotic agents) can induce dystonic movements and postures.

TABLE 471–1. A CLASSIFICATION OF COMMON DYSTONIC STATES

I. **Primary**
  A. Hereditary
  B. Idiopathic
II. **Secondary**
  A. Associated with other neurologic syndromes
    1. Wilson's disease
    2. Huntington's disease
    3. Hallervorden-Spatz disease
    4. Leigh's disease
  B. Environmental causes
    1. Perinatal cerebral injury
    2. Encephalitis
    3. Head trauma
    4. Focal cerebrovascular injury
    5. Toxins: manganese, carbon monoxide
    6. Drugs: phenothiazines, levodopa

A variety of drugs have been proposed to treat torsion dystonia, but none has been consistently effective. High-dose anticholinergics are often effective and are well tolerated in children if the daily dose is increased gradually. A recommended schedule is to begin with trihexyphenidyl (Artane), 2.5 mg twice daily, and increase the daily dose at a rate of 2.5 mg weekly. The dosage should be increased until there is satisfactory improvement or intolerable adverse effects. As much as 50 mg per day in four divided doses may be necessary. Unfortunately, most adults cannot tolerate high dosages of anticholinergics. Common adverse effects are dry mouth, blurred vision, forgetfulness, and confusion. Other compounds that may provide some benefit are baclofen (Lioresal, up to 60 mg per day), carbamazepine (Tegretol, 400 to 800 mg per day), and diazepam (Valium, 30 to 60 mg per day). Stereotactic thalamotomies can be effective for limb dystonia, but several repeat procedures may be necessary, and bilateral surgery entails a high risk of producing a major speech deficit. Patients should not undergo such surgery unless they are well aware of the risks, have had an adequate trial of pharmacologic agents, and have intractable, disabling symptoms.

SPASMODIC TORTICOLLIS

Spasmodic torticollis is the most common focal torsion dystonia. It usually begins in adulthood and remains limited to this region of the body. Occasionally there is spread to involve the vocal cords (spastic dysphonia) and one or both arms (segmental dystonia). The patient notices a pulling sensation in the neck musculature turning the chin toward one shoulder. Usually that shoulder is elevated as well. When the symptom is mild, the patient can easily straighten the neck; when severe, the head may be held in prolonged twisted postures. In some patients the head may be flexed (antecollis), extended (retrocollis), tilted, or shifted instead of rotated or twisted. These are all examples of spasmodic torticollis. A concomitant head tremor is frequent. In many patients the tremor is most pronounced when the patient attempts to keep the head straight (i.e., a dystonic tremor); in others tremor persists irrespective of the position of the head, and therefore represents essential tremor that may also be present in the hands. Placing a hand on the jaw tends to provide some relief of the torticollis.

In spasmodic torticollis, multiple and bilateral neck muscles, including the sternocleidomastoids, trapezius, and scalenus muscle, are involved in the involuntary contractions. In most patients, spasmodic torticollis persists and can be painful. In addition to pharmacologic therapy (discussed above under Torsion Dystonia) sensory biofeedback therapy has had some success in patients with spasmodic torticollis. Surgical section of the spinal accessory nerve and selective cervical nerves can be effective. Initial therapy should utilize anticholinergics along with other drugs, if necessary, such as baclofen, diazepam, and carbamazepine. Many patients improve moderately with drug therapy.

CRANIAL DYSTONIA

Cranial dystonia (blepharospasm, Meige's syndrome) is the second most common form of adult-onset focal dystonia. It usually begins with increased blinking and then worsens, and forced contractions of the orbicularis oculi eventually develop. Frequently, other muscles innervated by the facial nerve are also involved, including those around the lips. The contractions sometimes spread to involve mandibular muscles and even the tongue and neck. When the dystonia spreads to involve the jaw muscles, the "blepharospasm-plus" has been called Meige's syndrome. Bright light usually aggravates the blepharospasm. When severe, blepharospasm can result in functional blindness, preventing many activities, such as reading, driving, watching movies, and shopping. Pharmacotherapy is frequently unsuccessful. Surgical therapy, such as sectioning the branches of the facial nerve, can be helpful; regrowth of the branches frequently leads to eventual return of symptoms. Injections of small doses of botulinum toxin into the eyelid muscles provides relief in about 70 per cent of patients for up to 3 months and can be repeated. This approach is also useful for hemifacial spasm.

Eldridge R, Fahn S (eds.): Dystonia. Adv Neurol Vol 14, 1976. *Summarizes the state of the art up to the date of publication.*

Fahn S: High dosage anticholinergic therapy in dystonia. Neurology 33:1255, 1983. *Reports the successful use of very high dosage of anticholinergic agents in children with dystonia.*

Jankovic J, Ford J: Blepharospasm and orofacial-cervical dystonia: Clinical and pharmacological findings in 100 patients. Ann Neurol 13:402, 1983. *A thorough review of the clinical features of blepharospasm and associated dystonic movements.*

Lal S, Hoyte K, Kiely ME, et al.: Neuropharmacologic investigation and treatment of spasmodic torticollis. Adv Neurol 24:335, 1979. *Study revealed that anticholinergic drugs can be effective in reducing torticollis.*

Marsden CD: Dystonia: The spectrum of the disease. In Yahr MD (ed.): The Basal Ganglia. New York, Raven Press, 1976, pp 351–367. *Discusses the different forms of dystonia.*

Mauriello JA Jr: Blepharospasm, Meige syndrome, and hemifacial spasm: Treatment with botulinum toxin. Neurology 35:1499, 1985. *Injecting small doses of botulinum toxin subcutaneously over contracting facial muscles can relieve symptoms of blepharospasm and hemifacial spasm for several months.*

472 OTHER EXTRAPYRAMIDAL DISORDERS

MYOCLONUS

Myoclonic jerks are sudden, shocklike muscular contractions or inhibitions (the latter are called negative myoclonus). They can be singular or repetitive, rhythmic or arrhythmic, symmetrical or asymmetrical, synchronous or asynchronous, and generalized, segmental, or focal. Typically, myoclonic jerks occur unpredictably and irregularly. However, regular and rhythmic myoclonus exists, associated with lesions in the brain stem or spinal cord. The most common is *palatal myoclonus*, which results from infarction or degeneration involving the anatomic triangle that links the dentate nucleus, red nucleus, and inferior olivary nucleus. This form is categorized as myoclonus (rather than tremor) because of its synchronous (instead of alternating) contractions. Lesions in many parts of the nervous system, including spinal cord, brain stem, cerebellum, and cerebral cortex, can give rise to myoclonus. Myoclonus is most often a symptom of an irritable nervous system. It is present in many diseases (Table 472–1) but can also occur as an isolated phenomenon (essential myoclonus).

TABLE 472–1. A CLASSIFICATION OF COMMON FORMS OF MYOCLONUS

I. **Benign myoclonic jerks**
   A. Physiologic: sleep jerks, anxiety
   B. Essential myoclonus: familial or sporadic
   C. Periodic movements of sleep
   D. Associated with petit mal or grand mal seizures

II. **Symptomatic myoclonus**
   A. Myoclonus epilepsy
   B. Dementias: Creutzfeldt-Jakob, Alzheimer's
   C. Infectious: subacute sclerosing panencephalitis
   D. Lipidoses
   E. Cerebellar degenerations
   F. Hypoxia
   G. Toxins: methyl bromide, strychnine
   H. Drugs: levodopa, tricyclics
   I. Systemic illnesses: uremia, hepatic, dialysis encephalopathy
   J. Metabolic: biotin-responsive

III. **Rhythmic myoclonus**
   A. Palatal myoclonus
   B. Ocular myoclonus
   C. Spinal myoclonus

When associated with objective neurologic findings, it is usually progressive. In contrast, essential myoclonus (familiar or sporadic) tends to be stable and nonprogressive. Nocturnal myoclonus, now called "periodic movements of sleep" because of its regularity, may awaken patients from sleep; it is often associated with "restless legs syndrome," dysesthesias, and mild dyskinesias while awake.

One form of progressive encephalopathy characterized by myoclonus, seizures, deafness, and ataxia has been found to be responsive to biotin. Most cases occur in infants or young children and are associated with biotinidase deficiency or carboxylase deficiency, but it has also been reported in an adult.

Clonazepam is the drug of first choice to treat myoclonic syndromes, especially posthypoxic action myoclonus. Drowsiness and ataxia are common adverse effects, and the dosage should be increased gradually until improvement or adverse effects are encountered. A dosage as high as 8 mg per day (in four divided doses) may be necessary. Valproate is also useful alone or in combination with clonazepam; the dosage should be increased gradually until it is effective or toxic. As much as 3000 mg per day may be necessary. The combination of clonazepam and valproate can be particularly effective. Carbamazepine, diazepam, and the serotonin precursor 5-hydroxytryptophan also have been tried. The last-named drug is not available commercially in the United States.

Fahn S, Marsden CD, Van Woert MH (eds.): Myoclonus. Adv Neurol, Vol 43, 1986. *A detailed monograph devoted to the topic.*

TICS (Habit Spasms, Gilles de la Tourette's Syndrome)

A tic is a sudden rapid series of involuntary movements that are usually complex and coordinated. For example, an irregular sequence of movements can contain such diverse movements as eye blinking, head shaking, shoulder shrugging, and limb and facial gestures. Patients usually describe a compelling need to make these movements. Tics can be voluntarily controlled for brief intervals, but such efforts are usually followed by more intense and frequent contractions. Stress and anxiety aggravate tics, and psychotherapeutic management may diminish them.

In some individuals tics reflect recurrent nervous mannerisms appropriately called habit spasms. Other tics are caused by neurologic disorders. They may be present in the acute phase of encephalitis or as a sequela of encephalitis. Most tics are of unknown etiology and are sometimes familial occurring in an autosomal-dominant pattern and associated with compulsions. Males are more often affected. Tics can be considered in a spectrum, from transient tics of childhood, through persistent tics, to the most severe type in which vocal tics are also present. This last form is known as Gilles de la Tourette's syndrome. Vocalizations occur as various involuntary and compulsive sounds (barking, sniffing, throat clearing, yelping). Obscene words or gestures are often part of the clinical picture. The age of onset is usually between 2 and 15 years. Often, there are remissions and exacerbations, and the tics move from one part of the body to another. The tics tend to become less severe and more controllable with age. Patients are hesitant to be seen in public, and avoid areas where silence is required (cinema, theater, library). They are frequently misunderstood, teased, or insulted by schoolmates, teachers, and strangers. No anatomic abnormalities have been observed in the brain, but the consistency of the clinical syndrome implies that Tourette's syndrome is an organic disorder.

Haloperidol appears to be the most effective drug for treating tics and is given in divided doses up to 20 mg or more a day. Treatment is begun with a low dosage and increased slowly until control is achieved or adverse affects are obtained. Unfortunately, haloperidol affects personality ("zombie" effect) and school performance. Furthermore, there is a danger of inducing tardive dyskinesia or its variants.

Other drugs should be tried initially, such as clonazepam (3 to 6 mg a day) and clonidine (up to 0.6 mg daily) in divided doses.

Friedhoff AJ, Chase TN (eds.): Gilles de la Tourette syndrome. Adv Neurol, Vol 36, 1982. *The proceedings of the first international symposium on this subject. It provides reports of many studies on tic disorders.*

Kurlan R, Behr J, Medved L, et al.: Familial Tourette's syndrome: Report of a large pedigree and potential for linkage analysis. Neurology 36:772, 1986. *The largest reported kindred links motor tics, vocal tics, compulsions, and attention deficits in an autosomal-dominant pattern.*

Shapiro AK, Shapiro ES, Bruun RD, et al.: Gilles de la Tourette Syndrome. New York, Raven Press, 1978. *Thorough review of the literature and an analysis of the large number of cases personally observed by the authors.*

ATHETOSIS (Mobile Spasms)

Athetosis falls between the rapid movements of chorea and the sustained movements of dystonia. The term is applied to constant writhing and twisting movements without fixed postures. Yet as the spectrum of torsion dystonia becomes better appreciated, athetosis increasingly seems to be part of the dystonic syndromes; athetotic dystonia may therefore be a more appropriate name. Athetosis is most frequently en-countered in patients who suffered perinatal brain injury, usually from hypoxic damage (athetotic cerebral palsy). Athetosis has also been reported in kernicterus, in rare childhood degenerative diseases of the basal ganglia, in glutaric aciduria, and after hemiplegia secondary to strokes in childhood. Athetosis thus appears to be the expression of basal ganglia damage at an age when the nervous system is still developing. In athetotic cerebral palsy pathologic studies reveal either status marmoratus of the striatum or status dysmyelinatus of the globus pallidus.

Athetosis involves the limbs (distal and proximal), trunk, neck, face, and tongue. The movements are enhanced when the patient attempts to speak ("overflow"). Speech is impaired with poor articulation, in part because of continual tongue movements and facial movements. Stress and attempted voluntary movements also bring out an overflow of writhing movements throughout the body. There is no satisfactory treatment.

Spiegel EA, Baird HW: Athetotic syndromes. In Vinken PJ, Bruyn GW (eds.): Handbook of Clinical Neurology, Vol 6. Amsterdam, North-Holland, 1968, pp 440–475. *The best and most thorough clinical review of athetosis in a relatively sparse literature on this subject.*

SECTION SIX / DEGENERATIVE DISEASES OF THE NERVOUS SYSTEM

Robert B. Layzer

The term degenerative diseases refers to a varied assortment of central nervous system disorders characterized by gradual and progressive loss of neural tissue. This section deals with several degenerative diseases of unknown cause: the hereditary ataxias, paraplegias, and amyotrophies; the phakomatoses; syringomyelia; and amyotrophic lateral sclerosis. Several important diseases are discussed in other chapters concerned with dementia, extrapyramidal diseases, and autonomic disorders. Some degenerative diseases are difficult to classify because they involve multiple anatomical locations; these *multisystem atrophies* have arbitrarily been assigned to the chapters that deal with their principal symptom (see Table 473–1).

473 HEREDITARY CEREBELLAR ATAXIAS AND RELATED DISORDERS

The symptoms of hereditary ataxia may be intermittent or progressive. *Intermittent or periodic ataxia* occurs in children with a variety of recessively inherited biochemical disorders such as aminoacidurias and disorders of pyruvate metabolism. A rare, autosomal-dominant disease known as hereditary periodic ataxia is characterized by attacks of vertigo, nystagmus, ataxia, and dysarthria, lasting several hours; it responds to prophylactic treatment with acetazolamide.

Progressive ataxia occurs in children with known biochemical disorders such as abetalipoproteinemia and some of the lipidoses, but most diseases in this category are of unknown etiology. Those that begin before age 20, including Friedreich's ataxia and ataxia-telangiectasia, are usually inherited in an autosomal-recessive fashion, while most adult-onset types are autosomal dominant.

FRIEDREICH'S ATAXIA

This autosomal recessive disease, with a carrier frequency of nearly 1 in 100 and a prevalence of 2 in 100,000, is probably the most common type of hereditary ataxia. The biochemical mechanism is unknown; reports describing reduced activity of pyruvate dehydrogenase or of mitochondrial malic enzyme have not been confirmed independently.

PATHOLOGY. At autopsy the spinal cord is atrophic. There is loss of nerve cells in the dorsal root ganglia and Clarke's columns, and 'dying-back' degeneration of nerve fibers in the dorsal columns, pyramidal tracts, spinocerebellar tracts, and peripheral nerves. Minor changes are present in the brain stem and cerebellum. The heart shows chronic interstitial fibrosis and ventricular hypertrophy.

CLINICAL MANIFESTATIONS. Progressive ataxia of gait usually begins in childhood or adolescence and within a few years is accompanied by loss of deep reflexes, limb ataxia, Babinski signs, and cerebellar dysarthria. The ability to walk is lost about 15 years after onset. Most patients eventually exhibit scoliosis, pronounced impairment of vibration and position sense in the lower extremities, and pes cavus. Some develop wasting of distal limb muscles, a stocking-glove deficit of superficial sensation, nystagmus, deafness, or optic atrophy. Intellect remains normal. A hypertrophic cardiomyopathy is present in most patients and often leads to supraventricular arrhythmias; heart failure is probably the major cause of death. Insulin-dependent diabetes mellitus develops in 10 to 20 per cent of patients. The mean age at death is 37 years.

TABLE 473–1. THE MULTISYSTEM ATROPHIES

Disease	Heredity	Principal Feature	Associated Features	Chapter
Shy-Drager syndrome	Sporadic	Autonomic insufficiency	Parkinsonism, cerebellar ataxia, dysphagia, laryngeal stridor, amyotrophy	463
Progressive supranuclear palsy	Sporadic	Ophthalmoplegia, especially vertical	Gait ataxia, axial dystonia, parkinsonism, pseudobulbar palsy, dementia	471
Kearns-Sayre syndrome	Sporadic	Ptosis and ophthalmoplegia	Short stature, cerebellar ataxia, retinal degeneration, heart block, deafness, mitochondrial myopathy, mental deficiency, Babinski signs	513
Hereditary ataxias, adult type	Autosomal dominant	Cerebellar ataxia	Ophthalmoplegia, dementia, parkinsonism, dystonia, optic atrophy, retinal degeneration, dysphagia, amyotrophy	473

DIAGNOSIS. Sensory nerve action potentials are small or absent. Electromyography may show signs of denervation in distal limb muscles, but motor nerve conduction velocities are normal. The cerebrospinal fluid is normal except for mild elevation of the protein content in a few cases. Computed tomographic brain scans may show mild cerebellar atrophy late in the disease. Electrocardiography often shows inverted T-waves, right or left axis deviation, and right or left ventricular hypertrophy; conduction disturbances are uncommon. There is no treatment.

DIFFERENTIAL DIAGNOSIS. The constellation of progressive ataxia, areflexia, Babinski signs, and onset before age 25 is usually diagnostic. However, a similar picture can occur in vitamin B_{12} deficiency and in vitamin E deficiency (including abetalipoproteinemia). True Friedreich's ataxia is sometimes confused with a less common autosomal recessive type of early-onset progressive ataxia, in which the tendon reflexes are preserved; in the latter syndrome, optic atrophy, scoliosis, and electrocardiographic abnormalities are rare.

ATAXIA-TELANGIECTASIA

Ataxia-telangiectasia is an autosomal-recessive, multisystem disease affecting the skin, nervous system, and immune system. Its prevalence has been estimated at 1 to 2 per 100,000. Although the precise genetic defect is not known, it appears to involve defective DNA repair, with an increased frequency of chromosomal breakage and translocations. The main neuropathological abnormality is a severe loss of neurons in the cerebellar cortex, dentate nuclei, and inferior olives. The level of alpha-fetoprotein in the blood is elevated in nearly all cases.

Beginning at a few years of age, affected children show progressive cerebellar ataxia and incoordination, choreoathetosis, and a peculiar incoordination of head and eye movements known as oculomotor apraxia. Some develop opsoclonus. Later, fine venous telangiectases appear on the conjunctivae, ears, face, and skin creases. The thymus gland and lymph nodes are underdeveloped, and serum IgA levels are usually low; the resulting impairment of immunity leads to repeated bacterial infections in the respiratory tract. An axonal polyneuropathy appears late in the disease. Lymphoreticular malignancies and other forms of cancer develop in 10 to 20 per cent of patients. Most patients die from infection or neoplasm in the second or third decade of life.

ADULT-ONSET CEREBELLAR ATAXIA

Hereditary ataxia starting in adult life is nearly always an autosomal-dominant disorder with multiple neurologic manifestations, among which cerebellar signs are prominent. The classification of these diseases is difficult because the clinical features vary greatly even within the same family, and there is no agreement as to how many genetically distinct diseases exist in this category. In southern England cases of this type

are about one tenth as numerous as cases of Friedreich's ataxia. There are several reports of reduced activity of glutamate dehydrogenase in leukocytes and other tissues in some patients.

PATHOLOGY. Many cases have the pathologic features of olivopontocerebellar atrophy, with loss of neurons in the inferior olives and pontine nuclei (which provide major afferent pathways to the cerebellum), as well as degeneration of the spinocerebellar tracts, corticospinal tracts, and posterior columns. Neuronal degeneration is sometimes found in the cerebellar cortex, dentate nucleus, basal ganglia, midbrain, cerebral cortex, and spinal cord, including the anterior horns. The pathology, however, is as variable as the clinical findings, even within a given family. In cases of Azorean origin (Machado-Joseph disease) the cerebellar cortex and olives are spared.

CLINICAL MANIFESTATIONS. The age of onset, though quite variable, is usually between 20 and 50. Cerebellar ataxia of gait, dysarthria, and incoordination of the limbs usually dominate the clinical picture, so that the ability to walk is lost within 15 years. The other manifestations are extremely variable. Babinski signs and increased reflexes are commonly present, and some patients have spastic weakness in the legs. Vibration and position sense are sometimes lost as the disease advances, and the reflexes may disappear as the primary sensory neurons degenerate. Extrapyramidal findings may include impassive facies, cogwheel rigidity, chorea, athetosis, dystonia, and facial dyskinesia. Many patients have supranuclear oculomotor disorders such as lid retraction, ptosis, nystagmus, slow eye movements, and gaze paresis, especially upgaze. Optic atrophy, with pale discs, is common. Personality change or dementia, muscle wasting, and fasciculation in the tongue and distal extremities, and bulbar symptoms of dysphagia or hoarseness, are other common manifestations. Death occurs approximately 20 years after onset, at an average age of 57.

Pigmentary degeneration of the retina, beginning in the macula, is an early and constant feature in some families, suggesting that these cases may be genetically distinct. A few families seem to have a "pure" cerebellar syndrome beginning in the seventh decade of life. There is much controversy about the status of Machado-Joseph disease, which affects mainly people of Portuguese and Azorean descent. Although the range of clinical manifestations in these patients is similar to that of patients who have typical olivopontocerebellar atrophy, the pathologic features are said to be distinct because the inferior olives are spared. However, only a few cases have come to autopsy.

DIAGNOSIS. CT or MR images may show atrophy of the cerebellar folia and pons, with enlargement of the fourth ventricle and pontine cisterns. The cerebrospinal fluid is usually normal. Sensory nerve action potentials are small or absent in patients with absent reflexes; in patients with preserved reflexes, somatosensory evoked potentials may be abnormal.

DIFFERENTIAL DIAGNOSIS. Nonhereditary cases of late-onset cerebellar degeneration are at least as common as the hereditary kind. Some are associated with alcoholism or a visceral malignancy, but in many, no apparent cause can be established. These patients' cerebellar symptoms tend to begin between the ages of 40 and 60 and may be accompanied by dementia, extrapyramidal signs, or Babinski signs. Some cases of this kind have the pathological features of olivopontocerebellar atrophy, but whether there is any genetic link to the autosomal-dominant ataxias is unclear. It should be noted that patients presenting with ataxia may later develop the typical signs of progressive supranuclear palsy or one of the other multisystem atrophies listed in Table 473–1.

Harding AE: The Hereditary Ataxias and Related Disorders. Edinburgh, Churchill Livingstone, 1984. *A detailed review of the hereditary cerebellar ataxias and spastic paraplegias, including the author's own study of several hundred patients and family members. A modern classic.*

474 HEREDITARY SPASTIC PARAPLEGIAS

This is a diverse group of uncommon diseases whose main symptom is an insidiously beginning, progressive spasticity of the lower extremities. Families with "pure" hereditary spastic paraplegia (Strümpell's disease) are the most numerous, but many rare variants have been reported in which spasticity is associated with other neurologic, ocular, or cutaneous manifestations, overlapping with the spinocerebellar degenerations. The prevalence of these diseases is not well established. Harding found 29 families with hereditary spastic paraplegia in southern England, compared with 11 families of autosomal-dominant late-onset cerebellar ataxia. Rare examples of *primary lateral sclerosis*, although sporadic in incidence, may belong to this class.

PATHOLOGY. In the pure form, the spinal cord shows degeneration of the lateral corticospinal tracts and posterior columns, most severe in the thoracic region. Less often there is minor degeneration of the spinocerebellar tracts, anterior corticospinal tracts, anterior horn cells, and cortical Betz cells. The dorsal root ganglia, posterior roots, and peripheral nerves are normal, suggesting that the dorsal column degeneration is caused by "dying-back" of the central processes of the sensory neurons.

CLINICAL MANIFESTATIONS. Most patients with pure hereditary spastic paraplegia continue to walk for many years and have a normal life span. Many cases begin in infancy with delayed walking, but the onset can be as late as the seventh decade. Spasticity of the legs and a stiff, slow gait are the main symptoms. Affected persons walk on their toes, trip easily, and are unable to run. About one fourth have pes cavus. The legs are spastic with hyperactive reflexes, clonus, and Babinski signs, while the arms are usually normal. Later the legs may become weak, the arms may show increased reflexes, and distal muscle wasting may develop, especially in the hands. Vibration and position sense may become impaired in the legs, and many patients develop urinary frequency, urgency, and precipitancy, although sexual function remains normal. Most patients become unable to walk sometime in the sixth or seventh decade.

DIAGNOSIS. The cerebrospinal fluid is normal. Electromyography may show denervation in the distal limb muscles, but the sensory nerve action potentials are preserved, even

in patients showing decreased vibration and position sense. Somatosensory evoked potentials, however, are consistently small or unobtainable, reflecting a degeneration of dorsal column fibers.

DIFFERENTIAL DIAGNOSIS. Hereditary spastic paraplegia must be distinguished from nonhereditary causes of slowly progressive myelopathy such as cervical spondylosis, intraspinal tumor, arteriovenous malformation of the spinal cord, multiple sclerosis, and amyotrophic lateral sclerosis. MR imaging has simplified the diagnosis of many of these conditions.

Harding AE: The Hereditary Ataxias and Related Disorders. Edinburgh, Churchill Livingstone, 1984. *A detailed review of the hereditary cerebellar ataxias and spastic paraplegias, including the author's own study of several hundred patients and family members. A modern classic.*

475 HEREDITARY AND ACQUIRED INTRINSIC MOTOR NEURON DISEASES

Degenerative diseases of several presumed causes can attack the large motor neurons on the spinal cord or the brain to produce selective impairment of motor strength and/or skill. Those of childhood are largely hereditary with clinically evident genetic expression, while the major adult disorder, amyotrophic lateral sclerosis, appears overwhelmingly in a sporadic pattern with few clues illuminating either its etiology or molecular pathogenesis. Table 475–1 lists the major disorders in this category and the references provide greater detail on the many subtypes.

HEREDITARY AMYOTROPHIES

Hereditary spinal muscular atrophy is a syndrome of progressive muscular weakness and atrophy resulting from selective degeneration of the motor neurons of the spinal cord. A comparable disorder of the lower brain stem nuclei produces progressive bulbar palsy. Many different clinical syndromes have been delineated based on the age of onset, the pattern of muscular weakness, the rate of progression, and the mode of inheritance. Using this approach, at least 15 separate genetic disorders can be recognized. Pearn (1980) has estimated that 1 in 40 Caucasians carries a gene for spinal muscular atrophy. No consistent biochemical defect is known, although hexosaminidase deficiency has been identified in a few cases.

PATHOLOGY. At the time of post mortem examination in the spinal cases, the anterior horns show gliosis and loss of large neurons, and many of the remaining motor neurons are

TABLE 475–1. THE MAJOR INTRINSIC MOTOR NEURON DISEASES

Hereditary
Spinal muscular atrophy
   Type I. Acute, infantile (Werdnig-Hoffman disease)
   Type II. Late infantile and childhood type
   Type III. Juvenile and adult types
Familial amyotrophic lateral sclerosis
Acquired
Acute: anterior poliomyelitis
Chronic:
   ALS alone
   Anterior horn cell degeneration associated with: spinocerebellar
     degeneration, Shy-Drager syndrome, parkinsonism, Creutzfeld-Jacob
     disease
   Remote neoplasms, other
Primary lateral sclerosis (rare)

undergoing degeneration. The ventral roots are atrophic owing to loss of myelinated nerve fibers. Similar changes are observed in the motor nuclei of the brain stem in bulbar cases.

In the well developed infantile and childhood types, microscopic examination of the skeletal muscles using histochemical techniques shows large groups of round, atrophic muscle fibers and large groups of hypertrophied fibers staining uniformly as either type 1 or type 2. These features reflect the continuing process of denervation and reinnervation. However, at an early stage of infantile spinal muscular atrophy the only finding may be uniform atrophy of all muscle fibers, with preservation of the normal "checkerboard" fiber-type pattern. In slowly progressive cases of juvenile or adult onset, atrophic muscle fibers are found mainly in small groups; most muscle fibers are of normal size but are arranged in groups of uniform fiber type. After many years some muscle fibers show secondary myopathic changes such as internal nuclei, splitting, or degeneration.

ACUTE INFANTILE SPINAL MUSCULAR ATROPHY

Werdnig-Hoffman disease is a fatal, early infantile form of spinal and bulbar muscular atrophy that appears to be a single genetic entity. Inherited as an autosomal recessive trait, it is one of the most common fatal hereditary diseases of childhood, with an annual incidence of 1 in 20,000 live births and a carrier frequency in the general population of about 1 in 80.

In at least one third of the cases there is a prenatal onset, with reduced fetal movements, weakness at birth, or congenital joint deformities. The remaining infantile examples become apparent in the first two or three months of life. There is progressive, flaccid weakness of the trunk and limbs with severe hypotonia, poor head control, and diminished movements of the limbs, more severe in the proximal muscles. Weakness of the intercostal muscles causes retraction of the chest during inspiration; the cry is weak, and coughing is ineffective. Bulbar weakness causes difficulty sucking and swallowing. The tendon reflexes are usually absent. Death occurs before three years of age; half of the patients die in the first 7 months of life, 95 per cent in the first 18 months.

The serum creatine kinase activity and the cerebrospinal fluid are normal. Electromyography shows reduced activation of motor unit potentials, many of which are of increased size, duration, and complexity. Fibrillations may be present, and in the majority of cases there is a spontaneous, regular discharge of motor unit potentials at a frequency of 5 to 15 Hz. It is important to distinguish this disease from treatable disorders such as infant botulism and chronic inflammatory polyneuropathy. The former is identified by repetitive nerve stimulation tests showing abnormal neuromuscular transmission and the latter, by abnormalities of nerve conduction and increased protein levels in the cerebrospinal fluid.

PROGRESSIVE MUSCULAR ATROPHY IN CHILDREN

Proximal Type. Clinically this is a rather diverse disorder, but most cases are now thought to be caused by a single autosomal-recessive gene. The incidence of this syndrome is 1 in 24,000 live births, and the carrier rate is approximately 1 in 90. A milder, autosomal-dominant form is also known.

Weakness starts any time from birth to eight years of age, usually before one year of age. The weakness affects the trunk and limbs and initially is more severe in proximal muscles. The limb muscles become atrophic, the tendon reflexes are lost, and joint contractures may develop. Fasciculations are not prominent but may be apparent in the fingers, producing a fine, irregular tremor. The face and jaws may be weak, and the tongue may be atrophic and show fasciculation.

Children with early onset may never be able to walk and often develop severe scoliosis, limb deformities, and respiratory insufficiency. Many eventually die of pulmonary infec-

tion, but some very weak patients survive into adult life, the progress of the disease apparently having arrested early in childhood. Children with a later onset of weakness tend to have a milder course, with slowly progressive proximal weakness, increased lumbar lordosis, and a waddling gait. Those with autosomal-recessive inheritance rarely walk after age 20, while those with the rare autosomal dominant form may still be walking in middle age.

Serum creatine kinase activity may be mildly or moderately increased in patients with slowly progressive weakness, apparently because of secondary myopathic changes in muscle. The cerebrospinal fluid is normal. Electromyography shows the typical changes of chronic denervation and reinnervation as well as fibrillations and fasciculations, serving to distinguish these patients from similar patients with muscular dystrophy. Spontaneous, regular discharges of single motor unit potentials, like those found in infants with Werdnig-Hoffman disease, are seen in children whose weakness began before age two, but not in those with onset later in childhood.

Many of these children benefit from active and passive physical therapy and the judicious use of light-weight braces. Special attention should be given to spinal support to counteract scoliosis. Later in childhood, surgical immobilization of the spine may be indicated.

Distal Type. This category includes both dominant and recessive disorders and accounts for about 10 per cent of all cases of spinal muscular atrophy. Distal limb weakness and muscle wasting, more severe in the lower extremities, usually begins in early childhood and tends to be mild and slowly progressive. Three quarters of the patients have pes cavus, and, except for the absence of sensory deficits, the disorder is often clinically indistinguishable from Charcot-Marie-Tooth disease. However, patients with spinal muscular atrophy have normal conduction in motor and sensory nerves. A rare scapuloperoneal type, with autosomal-recessive inheritance, is characterized by distal leg weakness and scapular winging, starting in infancy; there may also be bulbar symptoms such as laryngeal stridor.

Bulbar Type. The Fazio-Londe syndrome is a rare, fatal disorder of young children characterized by degeneration of the motor neurons of the brain stem resulting in progressive paralysis of the face, throat, larynx, and tongue and sometimes the ocular and jaw muscles. The cases have occurred sporadically or among siblings, suggesting autosomal-recessive inheritance.

SPINAL MUSCULAR ATROPHY OF ADOLESCENT OR ADULT ONSET

Patients with late-onset spinal muscular atrophy have slowly progressive muscular weakness and usually continue to walk for two or three decades or more. Although much less common than the infantile and childhood types, the adult types include at least four clinical and eight genetic categories.

Proximal Type. These patients resemble patients with muscular dystrophy, and clinical examination may offer few clues to the neurogenic character of the proximal weakness. Fasciculations and muscle cramps are usually not prominent, and the serum creatine kinase activity may be substantially increased. To add to the confusion, males with onset of symptoms in their teens may have large calves. Some patients eventually develop mild bulbar symptoms such as dysphagia. Electromyography serves to establish the neurogenic nature of the disorder, and muscle biopsy is rarely needed. Families with autosomal dominant, autosomal recessive, and X-linked recessive inheritance have been described.

Scapuloperoneal and Facioscapulohumeral Types. Both myopathic and neurogenic scapuloperoneal syndromes are known, and several varieties begin in the second or third decade of life. Autosomal-dominant, autosomal-recessive, and X-linked recessive forms have been described. The common feature of these disorders is progressive atrophy and weakness of the shoulder girdle and lower leg muscles, though weakness eventually may spread to the other limb muscles. Electromyography and muscle biopsy can distinguish the anterior horn cell diseases from the muscular dystrophies, but the prognosis is similar in both groups. A few families have an autosomal-dominant form of spinal muscular atrophy resembling facioscapulohumeral muscular dystrophy.

Distal Type. This is usually a childhood disorder, but there are a few families with distal amyotrophy beginning in the third or fourth decade of life, inherited as an autosomal dominant trait. Some familial as well as adult cases exhibit onset in middle age and such a slow progression as never to be incapacitating, even in old age.

AMYOTROPHIC LATERAL SCLEROSIS

Amyotrophic lateral sclerosis (ALS) is a fatal degenerative disease of the central nervous system characterized by slowly progressive paralysis of the voluntary muscles. The French neurologist Charcot gave a detailed clinical and pathologic description in 1865. Little substantive knowledge about the cause and treatment of the disorder has been added since.

INCIDENCE. The annual incidence is about 1 case per 100,000 population, the prevalence being 4 to 6 cases per 100,000. Geographical pockets of much higher incidence in Guam, the Kii peninsula of Japan, and western New Guinea suggest possible, still unknown, exogenous causes. Ninety-five per cent of cases in the United States are sporadic, but a few families have several members with the typical clinical picture of sporadic ALS arising in an autosomal-dominant pattern. Males are affected slightly more often than females. Although the disease can appear as early as the third decade of life, most cases begin after the age of 40, and the incidence increases with age into the eighth decade.

PATHOLOGY. Degeneration of the motor neurons of the spinal cord and lower brain stem is marked by extensive cell loss and astrocytic gliosis. Swellings containing neurofilaments are often found on axons close to their cell bodies. As the Betz cells and large pyramidal neurons of the motor cortex disappear the corticospinal tracts degenerate, leaving gliosis of the lateral columns of the spinal cord. The ventral spinal roots are depleted of large myelinated nerve fibers, but surviving axons develop distal sprouts that reinnervate some muscle fibers, so that skeletal muscle histopathology shows both muscle fiber atrophy and fiber-type grouping.

ETIOLOGY. Few clues exist to the cause of ALS. Some authors regard the disease as a manifestation of premature aging or a deficiency of a neurotrophic factor. Other speculations include toxic exposure to minerals such as lead or aluminum, deficiency of calcium or magnesium, infection by an unidentified virus, and autoimmunity. Benign paraproteinemia has been encountered in a small proportion of patients, but the significance of the association is unclear.

CLINICAL MANIFESTATIONS. The major symptom consists of slowly progressive muscle weakness involving the limbs, trunk, breathing muscles, throat, and tongue. Most patients have a mixture of lower and upper motor neuron symptoms, although either may predominate. The former include muscle weakness, wasting, fasciculations, and cramps; the latter include stiffness and slowness of movement, slow and clumsy speech, and explosive release of laughter and crying (pseudobulbar palsy). The ocular muscles are not affected except in patients who survive long times after bulbar paralysis has begun. No impairment affects bladder, bowel, or sexual function. The stretch reflexes are diminished in severely denervated muscles, but more often signs of lower motor neuron weakness are combined with brisk reflexes, a finding nearly specific to ALS. Babinski signs are often present. Sensation is normal except for an expected diminution of vibration sense in the feet in older patients, and mental function is nearly always normal.

The onset is insidious, and initial symptoms may be confined to a single limb (especially the distal muscles), a side, or to lower cranial nerves. Gradually, however, the patchy and asymmetrical weakness becomes widespread, and the patient becomes unable to walk, dress, or feed himself. There is loss of weight because of muscle atrophy and impaired swallowing; the speech becomes unintelligible; choking interferes with eating and sleeping; and breathing becomes difficult even at rest. Pulmonary infection and insufficiency is the usual cause of death. The average survival is three years after onset of symptoms, but a few patients live for ten years or longer in a severely debilitated state.

DIAGNOSIS. Because there are no specific laboratory tests, the diagnosis is based principally on clinical criteria. The disease to be diagnosed as ALS should have a relentlessly progressive, gradual course; lower motor neuron signs should exist at widely separate levels of the nervous system, or upper motor neuron signs should be found well above the level of the lower motor neuron signs; and no conflicting findings such as sensory loss, incontinence, or ocular weakness should be present. The cerebrospinal fluid is normal except for a mild elevation of protein concentration in some cases. CT and MR imaging of the brain and spinal cord are unrevealing. Electromyography shows active and chronic denervation in multiple muscles of the brain stem, upper and lower extremities and trunk; motor nerve conduction velocity is normal or slightly reduced, and sensory nerve conduction is normal. Serum creatine kinase activity is normal or moderately increased.

DIFFERENTIAL DIAGNOSIS. Although ALS is nearly always fatal, a few patients stop deteriorating or even recover normal strength, but such cases are extremely rare. Other motor neuron disorders, treatable myelopathies, and even thyrotoxic myopathy must be distinguished from ALS (see Table 475–2).

TREATMENT. With a disease as grim as ALS, the physician must be careful to avoid premature misdiagnosis. Once the diagnosis is certain, however, some explanation must be given to the patient and his family. This requires considerable tact and gentleness; often it is best to convey the information gradually on successive visits, allowing the relentless progression of weakness to speak for itself.

No medication has been shown to be beneficial, and physical therapy does not delay the neuromuscular deterioration. Quack remedies surface periodically; for their own protection, patients who wish to try experimental forms of treatment should be referred to a reputable academic center.

Patients with impaired gait may benefit from using a cane or a walker, and patients who suffer from severe dysphagia without other disabling symptoms can be offered nasogastric

TABLE 475–2. DIFFERENTIAL DIAGNOSIS OF AMYOTROPHIC LATERAL SCLEROSIS

Disease	Distinguishing Features
Benign fasciculations	No weakness, atrophy, or EMG abnormality
Motor neuron diseases	
*Lead or mercury toxicity	Increased lead or mercury levels
Benign focal amyotrophy	Onset in youth, strictly focal, no upper motor neuron signs
Postpolio progressive muscular atrophy	Slow course, no upper motor neuron signs
Subacute motor neuronopathy in lymphoma	Plateau in few months, later improvement
*ALS in lung cancer or B-cell dyscrasia	Improves on treatment of tumor
Hereditary spinal muscular atrophy	Symmetric, slow course, no upper motor neuron signs
*Thyrotoxic myopathy with fasciculations	Myopathic EMG
*Compressive myelopathy due to cervical spondylosis or extramedullary tumor	Sensory symptoms. No lower motor neuron signs in legs. Cord compression on MRI or myelography

*Treatable conditions

tube feeding or a gastrostomy. The most difficult medical question, however, involves the therapeutic role of artificial ventilation. Most patients, understanding the hopeless prognosis, prefer not to be kept alive artificially in a state of total paralysis, unable to communicate except with eye movements. Nevertheless, some patients have survived for several years in this fashion, living at home with the help of a devoted and intelligent family. It is important to discuss these issues when patients are in the early stages of respiratory involvement, so that they can make decisions in advance about whether or not to accept emergency resuscitation during a respiratory crisis.

Dubowitz V: Muscle Disorders in Childhood. London, WB Saunders Company, 1978, pp 146–90. *A rich compendium of clinical observations on the spinal muscular atrophies, by a leading neuromuscular expert. Superb illustrations.*

Pearn J: Classification of spinal muscular atrophies. Lancet 1:919, 1980. *This brief article, based on the author's own study of 240 consecutive patients, is a valuable source of references on the clinical and genetic features of spinal muscular atrophies.*

Rowland LP (ed.): Human Motor Neuron Diseases. New York, Raven Press, 1982. *Results of an international symposium summarizing research into the cause of ALS. Little has changed since then.*

Tandan R, Bradley WG: Amyotrophic lateral sclerosis: Part 1. Clinical features, pathology, and ethical issues in management; Part 2. Etiopathogenesis. Ann Neurol 18:271; 419, 1985. *A recent review of research and treatment, with an important discussion of the ethical issues involved in the use of respirators.*

476 SYRINGOMYELIA

Syringomyelia is a spinal-cord, and, often, lower brainstem, disorder characterized by slowly progressive enlargement of a fluid-filled cyst (syrinx) within the cord or medulla. Most cases are congenital in origin, related to maldevelopment of the cervicomedullary junction; others are caused by arachnoiditis, intraspinal tumor, or trauma. A prevalence of 8.4 cases per 100,000 has been suggested.

PATHOLOGY. The most common type is "communicating" syringomyelia, or hydromyelia, where the fourth ventricle communicates with the spinal cord cavity, which is thought to represent an enormously dilated remnant of the fetal central canal. The cyst is lined by glial tissue, and in places by remnants of ependyma, and contains clear fluid identical to cerebrospinal fluid. Extending from the high cervical level or medulla to the thoracic or lumbar cord, the cyst varies in shape and size at different levels, and is variably associated with damage to the anterior horns, crossing spinothalamic fibers, and lateral columns. Most patients have a Chiari type of congenital cerebellar malformation, in which the flattened ectopic tonsils descend caudally and press against the dorsal aspect of the upper cervical cord so as to obstruct both the exit foramina of the fourth ventricle and the subarachnoid space at the foramen magnum. About 15 per cent of patients show a basal arachnoiditis without cerebellar ectopia but with similar obstruction of the cerebrospinal fluid pathways.

Noncommunicating syringomyelia develops in a segment of the cord rendered abnormal by an intramedullary tumor, spinal arachnoiditis, or severe traumatic injury. In nontumor cases the cavity is lined only by glia, whereas in tumor cases the cyst wall may contain both tumor and glial cells. The cyst fluid may have an increased protein concentration in post-traumatic and tumor cases.

PATHOGENESIS. The mechanism of cyst formation and expansion is poorly understood. In communicating syringomyelia the cavity probably originates before birth as a dilatation of the primitive central canal, which remains in communication with the fourth ventricle. Fluid pressure from the ventricular system is probably transmitted to the spinal cyst

as a result of obstruction of the exit foramina of the fourth ventricle. When cerebellar ectopia is present it may intermittently obstruct the subarachnoid space at the cervicomedullary junction, causing a pressure gradient between the cyst and the subarachnoid space, especially during straining, coughing, or sneezing. In arachnoiditis cases the cyst may originate in an area of ischemic myelomalacia, and in cases associated with tumor or severe injury there is cystic degeneration of the spinal cord before the syrinx starts to expand. Why the cyst continues to enlarge in these noncommunicating cases is hard to understand, since there is no apparent pressure gradient between the cyst and the subarachnoid space.

CLINICAL MANIFESTATIONS. The classic clinical picture of communicating syringomyelia is of a slowly progressive, asymmetric, destructive process in the central portion of the cervical and thoracic spinal cord, damaging the anterior horn cells, the crossing spinothalamic tract fibers, and the lateral corticospinal tracts. This causes muscle weakness and wasting in the hands and arms; scoliosis owing to denervation of paraspinal muscles; loss of arm reflexes; spastic weakness of the lower extremities; and a *dissociated sensory loss* with impaired perception of pain and temperature in the neck, arms, and upper trunk and preserved light touch perception and proprioception. Some patients experience a deep, aching pain in the neck or arms. Symptoms usually begin between 25 and 40 years of age and advance relentlessly for decades, although one third of the patients have long periods of stability. The deficits may worsen suddenly after a fall or after coughing or sneezing. Ten per cent of patients develop a painless arthropathy (Charcot joint) of the shoulder, elbow, or hand. Extension into the medulla may cause nystagmus, dysphagia, or wasting of the tongue, and some patients have hydrocephalus or cerebellar signs related to an associated Chiari malformation.

The manifestations of noncommunicating syringomyelia depend on the segment of the spinal cord affected. Congenital syringes produce predominantly cervical-thoracic symptoms, as noted. Post-traumatic syringomyelia, developing in paraplegic or quadriplegic patients months or years after the injury, is revealed by weakness and sensory impairment rising craniad from the transected level. The cases associated with

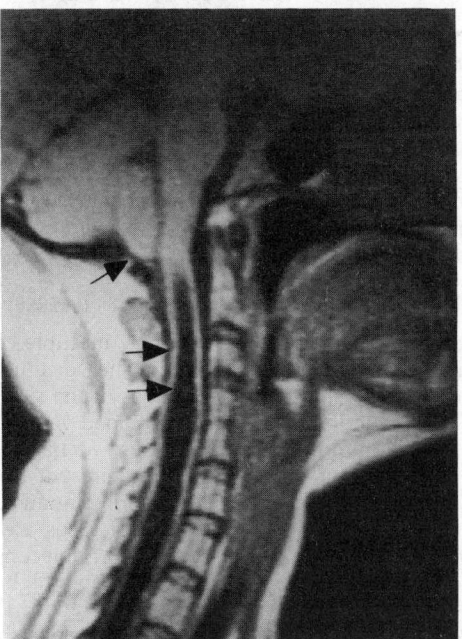

FIGURE 476–1. Magnetic resonance image of upper spine and foramen magnum in a patient with syringomyelia and a small Chiari I malformation (*single arrow*). The syrinx appears as a dark central area in the cervical and thoracic spinal cord (*double arrows*).

arachnoiditis following previous purulent meningitis, subarachnoid hemorrhage, surgery, trauma, or spinal anesthesia tend to involve the thoracic and lower cervical segments. Syringes associated with intramedullary spinal cord tumor extend for variable distances rostrad or caudad to the tumor.

DIAGNOSIS. Myelograms, once widely employed, have been rendered largely obsolete by MR imaging, which is both safer and more informative. Such images outline the size and extent of the cavity as well as the presence of cerebellar ectopia, arachnoiditis, or an intraspinal tumor (Fig. 476–1). Electromyography reveals active and chronic denervation in wasted upper extremity muscles, but sensory nerve conduction is normal in the analgesic hand, since the lesion is located proximal to the dorsal root ganglia. The cerebrospinal fluid is normal except for a raised protein content in some cases associated with tumor or arachnoiditis.

TREATMENT. Various surgical procedures have been devised in the hope of arresting the neurologic deterioration, but none has been reliably successful. For communicating syringomyelia, Gardner performed a posterior decompression of the foramen magnum and plugged the opening into the fourth ventricle that communicated with the syrinx. In recent years this operation has been generally abandoned in favor of a syringopleural or syringoperitoneal shunt, applicable to either communicating or noncommunicating cases. It has not been satisfactorily established that the outcome of any of these procedures is superior to the natural history of the disease. Several neurosurgical reports, however, suggest that such shunting reduces or halts chronic pain in the disease. Similarly, decompression of a foramen magnum obstructed by ectopic cerebellar tonsils sometimes may arrest progression of neurologic symptoms.

Barnett HJM, Foster JB, Hudgson P (eds.): Syringomyelia. London, WB Saunders Company, 1973. *Although written before CT and MRI, this book is still the best account of the clinical and pathological basis of congenital and acquired syringomyelia.*

Suzuki M, Davis C, Symon L, et al.: Syringoperitoneal shunt for treatment of cord cavitation. J Neurol Neurosurg Psychiat 48:620, 1985.

477 THE PHAKOMATOSES

The phakomatoses, or neurocutaneous syndromes, are congenital disorders characterized by disordered growth of ectodermal tissues, producing distinctive skin lesions and malformations or tumors of the nervous system. More than 20 syndromes have been described, the most important of which are neurofibromatosis, tuberous sclerosis, and Sturge-Weber disease.

NEUROFIBROMATOSIS (von Recklinghausen's Disease)

Neurofibromatosis is characterized by multiple café-au-lait spots on the skin, multiple peripheral nerve tumors, and a variety of other dysplastic abnormalities of the skin, nervous system, bones, endocrine organs, and blood vessels. It is one of the most common genetic diseases, occurring approximately once in every 3,000 births and present in about 30 persons per 10,000 population. It is inherited as an autosomal-dominant trait, but 40 to 60 per cent of cases are clinically sporadic. Even allowing for the difficulty of detecting the trait in mild cases, there seems to be a remarkably high mutation rate, on the order of 10^{-4} per locus per generation. The nature of the genetic defect is unknown; reports of elevated levels of nerve growth factor in the serum have not been independently substantiated. The syndrome of bilateral acoustic neuromas, with few café-au-lait spots, appears to be a separate autosomal dominant disorder with a prevalence of only 0.1 per 100,000.

PATHOLOGY. The peripheral nerve tumors are of two types, schwannomas and neurofibromas, the latter derived from both Schwann cells and perineural fibroblasts. Neurofibromas of sensory nerve twigs produce the distinctive subcutaneous nodules; in peripheral nerve trunks the tumor appears as a fusiform enlargement or plexiform neuroma. Schwannomas arise in cranial and spinal nerve roots and also in peripheral nerve trunks. Both types of tumor occasionally become malignant. The brain may show disordered architecture, hamartomas, gliomas, and meningiomas.

CLINICAL MANIFESTATIONS. Some manifestations are congenital, but most appear gradually during childhood and adult life. Café-au-lait spots become larger and more numerous with age; the majority of patients eventually have more than six spots greater than 1.5 cm in diameter. Other skin lesions include freckles (axillary freckles being specific to this disease); soft, pedunculated, cutaneous neurofibromas; and firm, subcutaneous neurofibromas.

Plexiform neurofibromas may grow to lemon or even melon size, leading to grotesque overgrowth of soft tissues and bone in a limb or around the orbit. Enlarging nerve trunk tumors may cause pain and impairment of motor and sensory function; intraspinal nerve root tumors do the same, and also compress the spinal cord. Gliomas of the optic nerve and chiasm are the most frequent intracranial tumor; they usually behave in an indolent fashion as hamartomas do. A hamartoma of the hypothalamus may cause precocious puberty.

About 10 per cent of children are mentally deficient and about 10 per cent develop seizures, half in association with an intracranial tumor. Kyphoscoliosis, dysplasia of the skull, bowed legs, and other bony abnormalities are common. Pheochromocytoma occurs in about 5 per cent of patients, usually in adult life, and hypertension may result from renal artery dysplasia.

DIAGNOSIS. The diagnosis of neurofibromatosis is usually evident on clinical grounds, but biopsy of a neurofibroma can be diagnostic in otherwise cryptic cases. Spinal nerve root tumors often have a dumb-bell shape, with intraspinal and extraspinal components; these are most readily identified by MR imaging. For diagnosis of intracranial tumors and hamartomas either CT or MR images are suitable.

TREATMENT. Most patients live a normal life with few or no symptoms. Small cutaneous or subcutaneous neurofibromas can be removed if they are painful or frequently irritated, but large plexiform neurofibromas should usually be left alone. A few become malignant with continued invasion and fatal outcome. Asymptomatic peripheral nerve trunk schwannomas can sometimes be removed safely by an experienced surgeon. Intraspinal and intracranial schwannomas are approached in the usual surgical fashion. Optic nerve gliomas are generally treated with radiation, but it is not clear whether this improves the outcome.

TUBEROUS SCLEROSIS

The typical clinical triad of tuberous sclerosis consists of mental deficiency, epilepsy, and a characteristic facial eruption known as adenoma sebaceum. The disease is inherited as an autosomal-dominant trait, but about 80 per cent of the cases are sporadic, due to new mutations. The incidence is about 3 cases per 100,000 births, the prevalence is about 10 per 100,000 population, and the mutation rate is 10.5×10^{-6} per gene per generation.

PATHOLOGY. The facial papules of adenomas sebaceum are angiofibromas. The cerebral hemispheres contain multiple hamartomas or tubers, which give the disease its name; these are characterized by disordered architecture, proliferating and abnormal astrocytes, and deposits of calcium. Occasionally a subependymal nodule forms a giant-cell astrocytoma, obstructing the foramen of Monro. The common retinal hamartomas are also probably of glial origin. Visceral lesions include multiple rhabdomyomas of the heart, multiple angiomyo-lipomas of the kidneys, and cystic transformation of the lungs by proliferating fibrous, muscular, and vascular tissue.

CLINICAL MANIFESTATIONS. Mental deficiency may be mild or severe, but one third of affected individuals have normal or even superior intelligence. Seizures occur in 80 per cent of cases, usually starting before the age of 5, and are often difficult to control with medication. In infants the seizures often take the form of infantile spasms; these children tend to be more severely impaired mentally. Occasionally, diagnosis escapes attention until late adolescence or adult life, when investigation of a new onset seizure disorder turns up subtle skin lesions or multiple retinal or intracranial hamartomas.

Nearly all patients have distinctive skin lesions. Hypopigmented spots are present from the time of birth in nearly 100 per cent of patients; they are more numerous on the trunk and are easier to see with a Wood's lamp. The next most common is adenoma sebaceum, a papular, salmon-colored eruption on the center of the face, especially in the nasolabial folds. It usually appears around 4 years of age and becomes more prominent after puberty. Leathery "shagreen" patches over the lower back, and fibromas of the nailbeds, affect perhaps 40 per cent of patients.

Retinal hamartomas are present in about half the patients. About 30 per cent of patients have cardiac rhabdomyomas, which sometimes cause arrhythmia or congestive heart failure. Rental tumors occur in two thirds of patients and are usually asymptomatic, though pain and bleeding can occur. Cystic disease of the lungs, an uncommon complication, mainly affects women over the age of 20; the symptoms include pneumothorax, dyspnea, cyanosis, and cor pulmonale.

DIAGNOSIS. Calcified cerebral lesions and subependymal nodules are well seen on brain CT, but uncalcified cortical tubers may show up better with MRI. Adenoma sebaceum, ungual fibromas, and hypopigmented spots are diagnostically specific, but retinal hamartomas also occur in neurofibromatosis. In 85 per cent of patients the EEG is abnormal, most often showing epileptiform activity.

Treatment is confined to symptomatic control of the epilepsy and to surgical therapy of the occasional hamartoma that undergoes gliomatous changes and enlarges to produce symptoms.

STURGE-WEBER SYNDROME

The Sturge-Weber syndrome is a nonhereditary, congenital disorder of facial and cerebral blood vessels characterized by a facial angioma (port-wine stain), seizures, and mental deficiency. The condition involves a defect of embryonic development, with persistence of a vascular plexus in the cephalic portion of the neural tube. The incidence is about 5 in 100,000 births.

The facial angioma is usually unilateral but may extend to the other side and conforms largely but not strictly to trigeminal nerve subdivisions. There may be cavernous angiomas of the tongue, gums, or mouth, and choroidal angiomas may cause congenital glaucoma. An angioma of the occipital and parietal leptomeninges accompanies the facial nevus on the same side, and the underlying cerebral hemisphere is atrophic, with degenerative changes and deposits of iron and calcium in the superficial layers of the cerebral cortex. The cortical calcifications and atrophy are easily seen on brain CT. Neurologic symptoms develop in infancy or early childhood, consisting of focal or generalized seizures. Half of the children become mentally impaired, and one third develop a hemiparesis. When seizures are difficult to control with medication, early surgical removal of the affected part of the brain may improve control and prevent intellectual deterioration.

Carey JC, Lamb JM, Hall BD: Penetrance and variability in neurofibromatosis: a genetic study of 60 families. Birth Defects: Original Article Series XV (5B): 271, 1979. *The most accurate information available on the incidence of various clinical manifestations of neurofibromatosis.*
Gomez MR (ed.): Tuberous Sclerosis. New York, Raven Press, 1979. *A compilation of the Mayo Clinic experience, with excellent illustrations of the skin and retinal lesions.*

SECTION SEVEN / CEREBROVASCULAR DISEASES

478 INTRODUCTION

H. J. M. Barnett and I. Meissner

Vascular stroke represents the most common devastating disease affecting the central nervous system. In developed countries it is the third leading cause of death, ranking behind heart disease and cancer. Among white populations in the U.S. and Canada the annual incidence rate is between 1 and 2 per 1000, the death rate is between 0.5 and 1 per 1000, and the prevalence is between 4 and 6 per 1000. Blacks have a higher incidence. Encouragingly, in both North America and Western Europe the incidence of stroke is declining at a rate approaching 5 per cent per year, a change attributed mainly to the improved control of hypertension and rheumatic fever.

Vascular stroke occurs as a result of two major causes: *ischemia* and *hemorrhage*.

ANATOMY AND SUPPLY OF THE MAJOR CEREBRAL ARTERIES

Interference with the blood supply to the brain by occlusion and stenosis, and to some degree as a consequence of arterial rupture, produces neurologic syndromes related to arterial territories rather than to specific neuroanatomic and physiologic systems. The interpretation of vascular syndromes is based on a working knowledge of these arterial territories.

Four large arteries supply the brain, the two common carotid and the two vertebral arteries (see Fig. 478-1). The left common carotid artery arises from the aortic arch and the right from the innominate artery in the upper thorax. The two vertebral arteries originate from the left and right subclavian arteries respectively. Each common carotid artery bifurcates into the internal and external carotid arteries at the level of the upper border of the thyroid cartilage. No branches arise from the extracranial internal carotid artery. Each internal carotid artery enters the skull through the ipsilateral foramen lacerum, passes through the cavernous sinus, and gives off

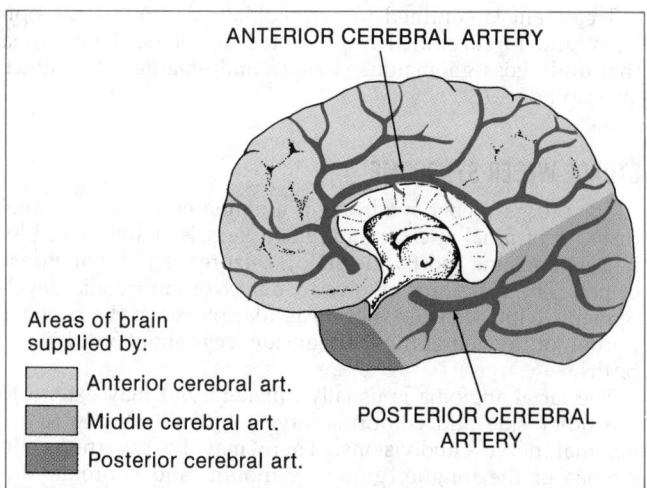

FIGURE 478–1. The medial surface of the cerebral hemisphere, showing the course of the anterior and posterior cerebral arteries and the medial area of brain supplied by them and the small area of medial supply of the middle cerebral artery.

the ophthalmic, posterior communicating, and anterior choroidal arteries and terminally bifurcates into the anterior and middle cerebral arteries.

ANTERIOR CEREBRAL ARTERY. As Figures 478–1 and 478–2 show, the anterior cerebral artery supplies the medial and superior surfaces of the cerebral hemisphere and the entire most anterior portion of the frontal lobes. This area contains the motor and sensory cortex for the foot and leg and the supplementary motor cortex. The anterior cerebral artery, through medial lenticulostriate and Heubner's arteries, also supplies several deep structures of importance, including the anterior nucleus of the thalamus with contributions to the corona radiata, the anterior limb of the internal capsule, the head of the caudate nucleus, and the putamen. The first part of either of the paired anterior cerebral arteries is vestigial or absent in 3 to 4 per cent of normal individuals, its cortical portion being supplied from the opposite normal side by the anterior communicating artery. The anterior cerebral artery's strategic location between the two cerebral hemispheres makes it an important angiographic midline marker, and moderately sensitive to compression by midline and frontal cerebral mass lesions.

MIDDLE CEREBRAL ARTERY. With the exception of the occipital and frontal poles, the middle cerebral artery (Figs. 478–2 and 478–3) supplies most of the lateral surface of the

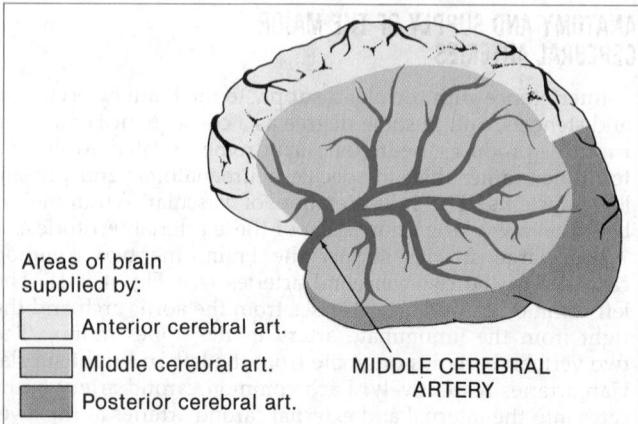

FIGURE 478–2. The lateral surface of the cerebral hemisphere and the course of the middle cerebral artery. The middle cerebral artery has been elevated from the Sylvian fissure to better illustrate its course. (For clarity the shadings differ from those in Figure 478–1.)

cerebral hemisphere, the primary motor and sensory areas for the face, throat, hand, and arm; the optic radiations; and, in the dominant hemisphere, the cortical areas for speech. The perforating (lenticulostriate) branches of the middle cerebral artery reach the depths of the cerebral hemisphere supplying the posterior limb of the internal capsule, basal ganglia, and corona radiata. Branches of the middle cerebral artery form the angiographic Sylvian triangle, the displacement of which provides important information regarding lesion localization.

VERTEBRAL AND BASILAR ARTERIES. The vertebral arteries arise from the subclavian arteries and after a short, free course ascend through the transverse foramina of C6 to C1 (atlas), entering the skull through the foramen magnum. In the majority, the left vertebral artery is dominant. Individual variations are common, including in 10 per cent of cases, a vestigial vertebral artery with basilar blood supply provided by a single vertebral artery. Upon entering the skull, each vertebral artery gives off a medial branch, which unites with its opposite counterpart to form the anterior spinal artery. The posterior inferior cerebellar arteries arise rostrad to this point.

At all levels of the brain stem the ventral medial portion is supplied by short paramedian vessels; the ventrolateral portion, by short circumferential branches from the vertebral or basilar arteries; and the dorsolateral portion and cerebellum, by long circumferential branches: the posterior inferior, the anterior inferior, and the superior cerebellar arteries.

The vertebral artery lies on the lateral surface of the medulla oblongata ventrally, and from it and the anterior spinal artery short paramedian branches supply the pyramids, the inferior olives and medial lemnisci, the medial longitudinal fasciculi, and the emerging fibers of the hypoglossal nerve (Fig. 478–4).

The dorsolateral medulla contains the spinothalamic tract, the vestibular nuclei, the sensory nucleus of the fifth cranial nerve, descending fibers of the sympathetic nervous system, the restiform body, and the emerging fibers of the vagus and glossopharyngeal nerves; these structures are supplied by longer branches from the vertebral artery and posterior inferior cerebellar artery branches. The most cephalad and dorsal segment of the medulla includes the vestibular and cochlear nuclei, which, along with the posterior portion of the cerebellum, are supplied by the posterior inferior cerebellar artery.

The basilar artery, formed at the ventral lower pontine border by the midline union of the two vertebral arteries, supplies perforating branches as it spans the ventral midline pons and midbrain. These short perpendicular branches supply paramedian structures, including the corticospinal tracts, the pontine nuclei, the medial lemnisci, the medial longitudinal fasciculi, and the pontine reticular nuclei (Fig. 478–5). The anterior inferior cerebellar artery, the long circumferential branch at this level, supplies the lateral pons, including the emerging seventh and eighth cranial nerves, the trigeminal nerve root, the vestibular and cochlear nuclei, and the spinothalamic tracts. It also branches to the most dorsal and lateral of these structures on its dorsal course to supply the cerebellum.

At the midbrain level the basilar artery lies in the midline in the peduncular fossa (Fig. 478–6). Short branches pass laterally and dorsally to both sides to supply the cerebral peduncles, the emerging fibers of the third nerve, medial portions of the red nuclei, the medial longitudinal fasciculus, the oculomotor nuclei, and the midbrain reticulum. Branches of the posterior cerebral artery supply the lateral portions of the peduncles, the red nuclei, and the medial lemnisci. The superior cerebellar arteries contribute to the dorsal midbrain supply, including that of the colliculi and of the superior portion of the cerebellum on each side.

POSTERIOR CEREBRAL ARTERY. Cortical branches supply the posterior pole and the posterior medial and inferior hemispheric surfaces, including the calcarine cortex (the pri-

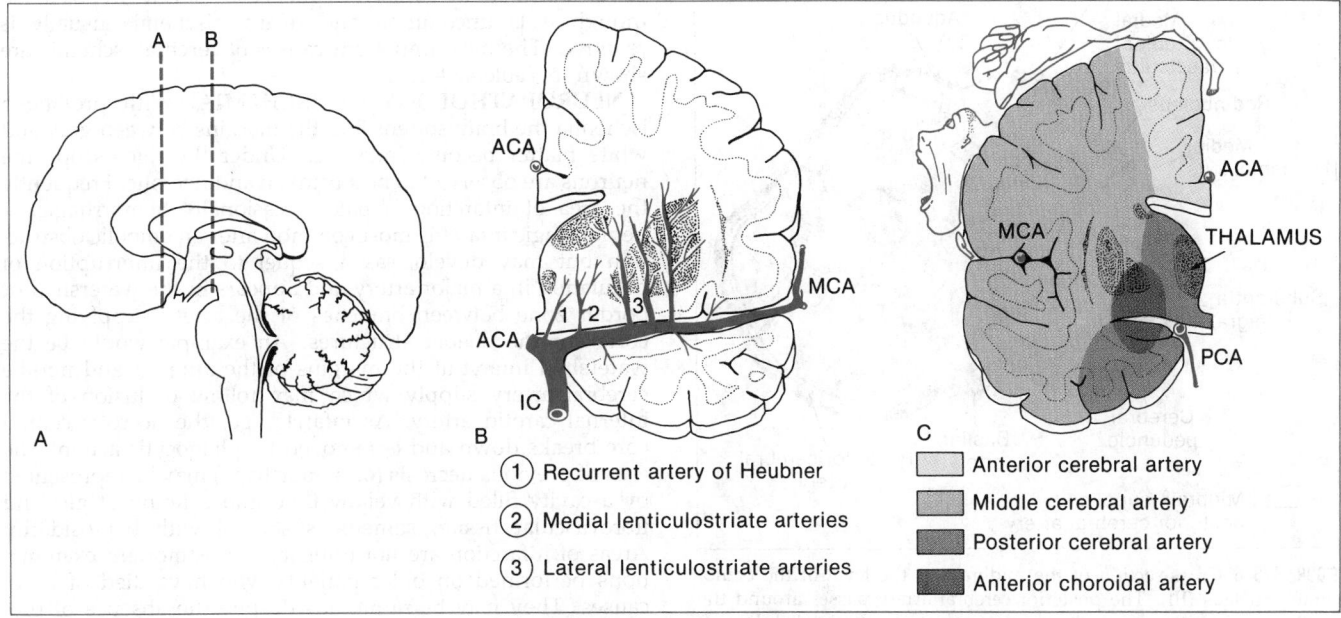

FIGURE 478–3. *A*, The lateral surface of the cerebral hemisphere showing the planes through which *B* and *C* were taken. *B*, Coronal section through the left hemisphere demonstrating the thalamostrate arteries and the recurrent artery of Heubner. *C*, Coronal section through the right hemisphere showing the area of the brain supplied by the anterior (ACA), middle (MCA), and posterior (PCA) cerebral arteries and the anterior choroidal artery. The "homunculus" overlies the cortex, illustrating the area of representation of movements and the proportional cortical allocations to the motor functions. (Adapted from Penfield and Rasmussen, 1950.)

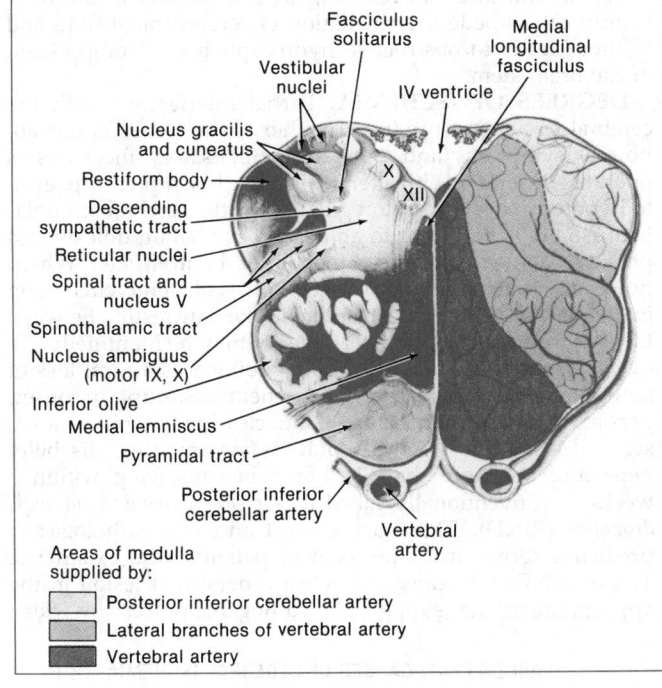

FIGURE 478–5. Cross-section of mid-pons. The medial portion receives blood supply from short perforating basilar artery branches. More laterally, the blood supply comes from lateral basilar artery branches.

FIGURE 478–4. Cross-section of the medulla oblongata at the level of the hypoglossal nuclei (XII). Short branches of the vertebral and anterior spinal arteries supply the medial medulla. Longer circumferential branches, including the posterior inferior cerebellar artery, supply the lateral portions of the medulla.

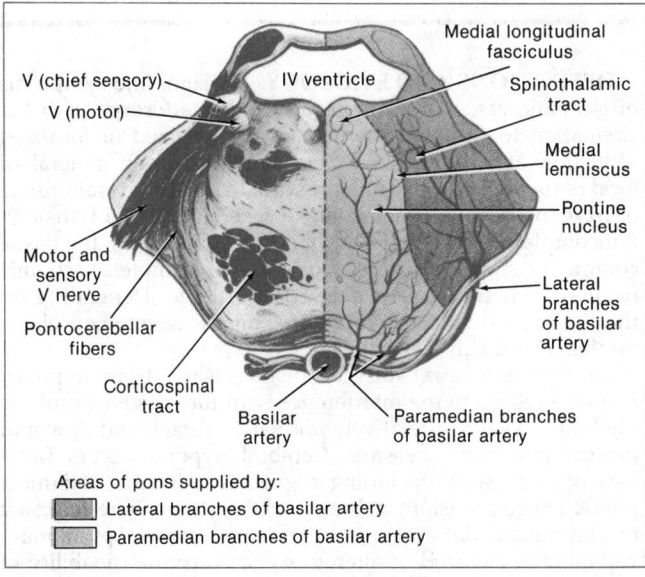

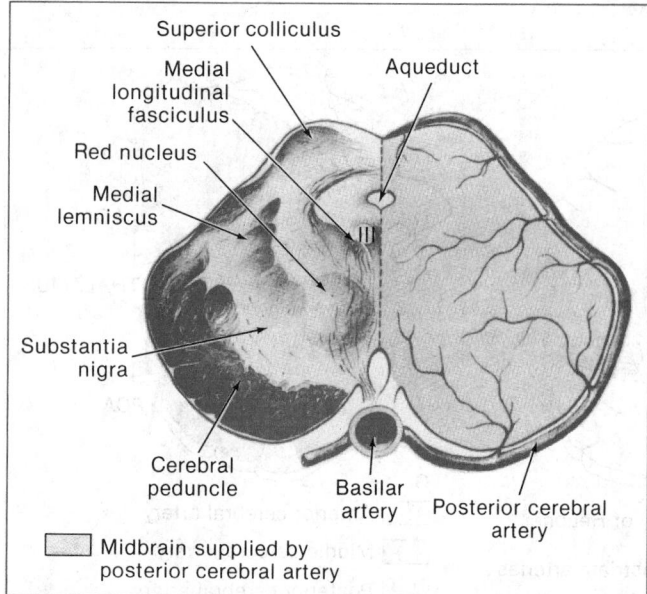

FIGURE 478–6. Cross-section of the midbrain at the level of the oculomotor nucleus (III). The posterior cerebral artery passes around the midbrain and gives off short branches supplying the medial, lateral, and dorsal regions.

mary visual receptive area) and the hippocampus (see Figs. 478–1 and 478–2). Short perforators supply the midbrain, including the cerebral peduncle and red nucleus, subthalamic area, thalamus, posterior internal capsule, and contribute to the optic pathways and hypothalamus.

Anatomic variation in the origin of the posterior cerebral artery is common. In approximately 70 per cent of cases both posterior cerebral arteries originate from the basilar artery apex with small posterior communicating arteries which connect to the carotid arteries. In 5 to 10 per cent of cases, dominant posterior communicating arteries provide the major blood supply to the posterior cerebral arteries. In the remaining, one posterior cerebral artery originates from the basilar artery and the other, from the posterior communicating artery.

479 CEREBRAL ISCHEMIA AND INFARCTION

H. J. M. Barnett

DEFINITIONS AND ETIOLOGY. The signs and symptoms of ischemic vascular stroke result from interference with the circulation to the brain owing to a generalized or localized reduction of blood flow. Ischemia follows upon general or local reductions in perfusion pressure that deprive brain tissue of oxygen and other metabolites. Ischemia may be transient; if incomplete and lasting less than 10 to 15 minutes, the tissue commonly survives. More prolonged or complete ischemia results in infarction, i.e., death of the tissue. Depending on the site and extent of the infarction, mild to severe neurologic disability or death will follow.

Cerebral ischemia must be distinguished from hypoxia. Hypoxia relates to the interference with the oxygen supply to the brain, despite a relatively normal cerebral blood flow and normal perfusion pressure. Cerebral hypoxia occurs for a variety of reasons, including a general reduction of atmospheric oxygen tension, pollution of the atmosphere (e.g., by carbon monoxide), chronic pulmonary disease, pulmonary emboli, and reduced or altered oxygen-carrying capability of

the blood (e.g., anemia, methemoglobinemia). Ischemic infarction will occur as a consequence of severe hypoxia, although it is uncommon and relative ischemia usually is required. The most important causes of cerebral ischemia are shown in Table 479–1.

NEUROPATHOLOGY OF ISCHEMIA. With prolonged ischemia the brain softens and the margins between gray and white matter become indistinct. Under the microscope the neurons are observed to be shrunken and necrotic. Frequently the area of infarction is pale, occasionally hemorrhagic. A hemorrhagic infarct is most common after an embolic obstruction but may develop as a sequel to the interruption of circulation in a major artery and appears in the watershed or border zone between branches of the artery supplying the cortex or the deeper structures. An example would be the watershed infarct at the margins of the anterior and middle cerebral artery supply which may follow occlusion of the internal carotid artery. As infarcts age, the necrotic central core breaks down and is removed by phagocytic action. The area of previous necrosis (or hemorrhage) may be represented by a cavity filled with yellow fluid and a lining of glia and fibrovascular tissue, sometimes stained with hemosiderin. Areas of infarction are not unusual in postmortem examinations performed on older patients who have died of other causes. They may be numerous despite the absence of previous clinical symptoms.

Cerebral edema, variable in amount and dependent on the extent of the infarction, accompanies cerebral infarction. If edema is extensive, it produces distortion of the hemisphere or cerebellum with a shift medially beneath the falx, downward or upward through the tentorium cerebelli, or downward through the foramen magnum. The effects of such compression shifts (Ch. 456) are visible on CT.

Edema and swelling resulting from infarction in the cerebellum can impede the circulation of cerebrospinal fluid and at times leads to obstructive hydrocephalus or compression of the brain stem.

DEGREES OF ISCHEMIA. Partial interference with the cerebral circulation produces neither tissue ischemia nor abnormal symptoms and signs if compensatory mechanisms operate efficiently. With altered systemic blood pressure, even to hypotensive levels, autoregulation by the cerebral arteriolar bed usually is sufficient to adjust the circulation quickly and preserve the vitality and function of brain tissue. When, however, ischemia is prolonged and collateral circulation inadequate, a major catastrophic stroke can result. Between these extremes, gradations of severity may be identified:

A transient ischemic attack (TIA) is defined as a focal loss of neurologic function caused by ischemia, abrupt in onset, persisting for less than 24 hours, and clearing without residual signs. Most such TIAs last only a few minutes; disability persisting for more than 24 hours but resolving within 3 weeks is conventionally called a *reversible ischemic neurologic disability* (RIND). These are clinical and not pathologically predictive terms; in 15 per cent of patients who experience TIA or RIND, CT scans will detect a persistent lesion in the appropriate arterial supply. The pathogenic process by which

TABLE 479–1. CAUSES OF CEREBRAL ISCHEMIA

1. Arterial disease: (a) Atherothrombosis in the intra- and extracranial arteries; (b) emboli from the extracranial and larger intracranial arteries
2. Emboli of cardiac origin
3. Pulmonary embolism: paradoxic emboli
4. Cardiac disease causing reduced cerebral blood flow
5. Lacunar infarction
6. Generalized cerebral hypoxia
7. Cerebral artery thrombosis due to nonarteriosclerotic vasculopathies
8. Cerebral artery thrombosis due to coagulation abnormalities (polycythemia, thrombocytosis)
9. Cerebral arterial spasm following subarachnoid hemorrhage
10. Cerebral arterial vasoconstriction associated with migraine
11. Cerebral vein and sinus thrombosis

TIA or RIND occurs is the same as that which produces clinical signs of persistent stroke; only the size and location of the lesion make the difference.

An ischemic event leaving persistent disability but short of a calamitous stroke, is defined as a *partial nonprogressing stroke* (PNS). More severe ischemia producing major permanent neurologic disability is termed a *completed stroke*. These levels of disability have varying temporal profiles, most often reaching maximum in a few minutes, but in approximately 15 per cent of patients there will be worsening gradually or stepwise over hours to weeks as a *progressing stroke* or a *stroke-in-evolution*.

ATHEROTHROMBOTIC STROKE. *Sites of Occlusion.* Arteriosclerosis of the major extracranial cerebral arteries to the brain accounts for most strokes. The most common site for obstructive disease (bifurcation) of the carotid artery is the region of its bifurcation followed by the intracavernous sinus portion. In Caucasians, the carotid artery is responsible for atherothrombotic stroke six to seven times more frequently than is the main trunk of the middle cerebral artery. In Asians the ratio of carotid to middle cerebral disease is reversed.

The extracranial vertebral artery is commonly diseased at its origin and at the C1–C2 level. Intracranially, the most common site for vertebral artery disease and occlusion is within 1 to 2 cm of the termination of the artery, just beyond the origin of the posterior inferior cerebellar artery. Basilar artery disease usually occurs at the middle level (Fig. 479–1).

Anastomotic Circulation. The manifestations of stroke are commonly described in terms of the arterial territories supplied by the internal carotid and vertebral basilar arterial branches. It is now recognized that obstruction in the more proximal, commonly extracranial, arterial brain supply often presents a picture indistinguishable from that of more distal obstructions. For example, internal carotid artery occlusion compensated by intracranial anastomoses can be asymptomatic. Without protection by collaterals, carotid occlusion commonly results in focal middle cerebral artery territory ischemia.

Collateral supply for the internal carotid artery can come from: the ipsilateral basilar circulation via the posterior communicating artery; ipsilateral leptomeningeal communications between the cortical branches of the posterior cerebral artery and those of the middle and anterior cerebral arteries; the ipsilateral external carotid artery by retrograde flow through the ophthalmic artery and, of less importance, through the middle meningeal and ascending pharyngeal arteries; and via the contralateral communicating artery.

The vertebral artery forms anastomoses with branches of the occipital artery and of ascending and deep cervical arteries arising from the thyrocervical and costocervical trunks. Vertebral artery occlusion near its origin is commonly asymptomatic because of the development of an extensive cervical anastomotic network. More significant deficits result from more distal vertebral artery occlusion. At any level, obstruction to one or even both vertebral arteries may be asymptomatic. Commonly, a modified ischemic syndrome appears owing to the protective effect of collaterals.

Although basilar artery occlusion usually produces serious consequences, collateral supply may modify the extent of ischemia or, rarely, allow asymptomatic occlusion. Midbasilar artery occlusion or severe stenosis may cause flow reversal from the anterior circulation via the posterior communicating artery. Potential collaterals exist between the large vertebral and basilar arterial branches, particularly the superior, anterior inferior, and posterior inferior cerebellar arteries.

Watershed Infarction. Following internal carotid artery occlusion, circulation may be least effective in the arterial border zone or watershed between the anterior and middle cerebral arteries. Severe impairment of cerebral perfusion, such as occurs with cardiac arrest, tamponade, and exsanguination, predisposes these border zones to infarction. Watershed infarcts tend to be hemorrhagic since, with flow restoration, blood passes into the surrounding tissues through hypoxic, damaged capillaries.

STROKE DUE TO EMBOLI OF CARDIAC ORIGIN. The incidence of embolic cerebral infarction is generally greatly underestimated in most populations. The use of improved technical diagnostic skills to identify potential embolic sources has raised the estimated 3 to 5 per cent cardioembolic stroke incidence of 20 years ago to a more probable 20 per cent. Endocardial mural thrombus related to myocardial infarction is an important source, accounting for 8 to 10 per cent of strokes. At least 5 per cent of patients with a myocardial infarction have clinical evidence of cerebral embolization. Postmortem studies of patients who succumbed to myocardial infarction identify systemic emboli in 45 to 60 per cent, half of which are cerebral. Emboli after myocardial infarction are most common in the second week. In one large series 84 per cent occurred in the first 4 weeks; 6 per cent in the second month, and 8 per cent in the third month. Embolism strikes the left hemisphere slightly more often than the right, the carotid circulation more often than the vertebrobasilar, and the middle cerebral artery more than other intracranial arteries. Postischemic akinetic segments of the left ventricle and ventricular aneurysms are other, uncommon, sources of thromboembolism. Occasionally postischemic rhythm disorders, particularly atrial fibrillation, will precipitate embolic strokes.

Since the decline in incidence of rheumatic fever, mitral stenosis has become a less common cause of thromboembolic stroke. Of the systemic embolic events developing in 20 per cent of patients within 5 years of the diagnosis of mitral stenosis, approximately half are cerebral; recurrent emboli occur in half of these patients, most commonly within the first year after the initial event. The association of atrial fibrillation increases the risk of stroke. The Framingham Study disclosed a 17-fold increase in stroke risk in rheumatic heart disease-related atrial fibrillation and a six fold increase for atrial fibrillation alone.

Careful cardiac history and physical examination, supplemented when indicated by ECG monitoring, two-dimensional echocardiography, wall-motion studies, and, in certain selected cases, ventricular angiocardiography, identify the less

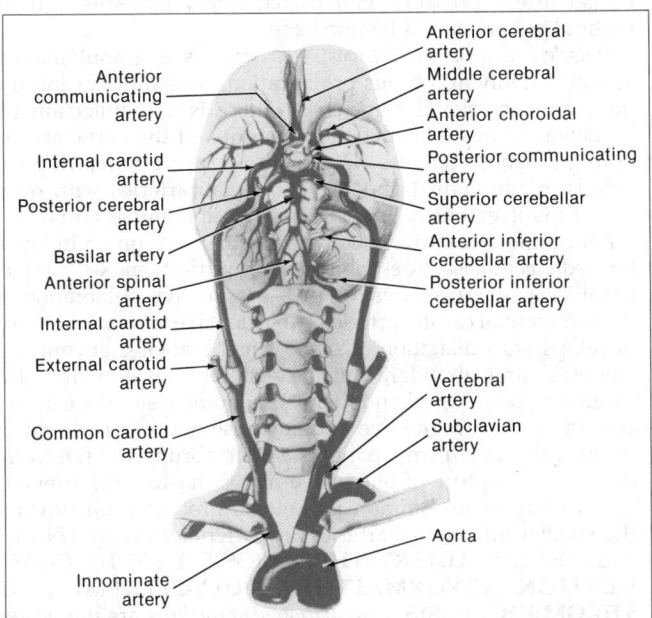

FIGURE 479–1. The light bands around the arteries indicate the sites of predilection for atheroma. The two most common sites to cause symptoms are the region of the carotid sinus and the intracranial portion of the carotid artery.

Labels from figure:
Anterior communicating artery
Internal carotid artery
Posterior cerebral artery
Basilar artery
Anterior spinal artery
Internal carotid artery
External carotid artery
Common carotid artery
Innominate artery

Anterior cerebral artery
Middle cerebral artery
Anterior choroidal artery
Posterior communicating artery
Superior cerebellar artery
Anterior inferior cerebellar artery
Posterior inferior cerebellar artery
Vertebral artery
Subclavian artery
Aorta

TABLE 479–2. CARDIAC LESIONS PRODUCING CEREBRAL THROMBOEMBOLIC EVENTS

1. Myocardial infarction—mural thrombosis
2. Postinfarction aneurysms and akinetic segments—stasis thrombi
3. Postinfarction atrial fibrillation—atrial thrombi
4. Mitral stenosis with or without atrial fibrillation—atrial and auricular thrombi
5. Atrial fibrillation of any cause—persistent or paroxysmal thrombi
6. Mitral regurgitation with atrial mural "jet lesions"—small mural thrombi
7. Bacterial endocarditis—valvular mycotic thrombi
8. Nonbacterial thrombotic endocarditis—valvular thrombi
9. Prolapsing mitral valve—valvular thrombi
10. Mitral annulus calcification—? degenerate valve fragments
11. Calcific aortic stenosis—? degenerate valve fragments
12. Atrial myxoma–neoplastic tissue—? attached thrombi
13. Prosthetic heart valve—attached thrombi

common cardiac conditions associated with cerebral thromboembolism listed in Table 479–2.

Certain valvular and mural lesions cannot be identified with certainty by physical examination, ECG, and routine radiography. These include atrial myxoma, mitral annulus calcification (a degenerative process in older subjects), and the myxomatous degeneration of the mitral valve, the most common cause of "ballooning" or "prolapse" of the mitral valve (PMV). Such lesions, identified by echocardiography, are being increasingly recognized as causes of ischemic events, in younger patients in the case of PMV, and in older subjects with mitral annulus calcification. Since PMV exists asymptomatically in 6 to 8 per cent of normal persons, its implication in cerebral ischemic disease provides a diagnostic challenge. Several epidemiologic studies indicate a 20 to 30 per cent incidence of PMV in patients under the age of 45 who present with focal ischemic symptoms, as compared with a 6 to 8 per cent incidence in age- and sex-matched asymptomatic controls. Familial PMV is well recognized, with documented strokes in several young family members. In juveniles with Marfan's syndrome, PMV is more common. Its causative relation to stroke in this setting is probable in the absence of other recognizable etiologic factors.

CARDIAC DISEASE CAUSING REDUCED CEREBRAL BLOOD FLOW. Disorders of cardiac output and serious hypotension result in diffuse disturbances of brain function. The most common manifestation is the syncopal Stokes-Adams attack caused by heart block, but similar clinical pictures can accompany sinoatrial node disorders, intermittent ventricular arrhythmias, or a variety of conditions producing severe orthostatic hypotension. Clinical signs reflecting a diffuse reduction of cerebral perfusion include syncope, convulsions, visual blurring, nonspecific dizziness, and occasionally vertigo. Discrete focal hemispheric events, characteristic of thromboembolic ischemia, are uncommon with these hemodynamic events.

LACUNAR INFARCTION. Lacunar infarction is a condition most commonly associated with longstanding hypertension in which multiple small infarcts occur in the region of the corona radiata, internal capsule, striatum, thalamus, basis pontis, and cerebellum. The distribution of the infarcts favors the territory of the penetrating branches of the middle and posterior cerebral arteries and the median branches of the basilar artery. The infarcts soften, are absorbed by phagocytosis, and leave small (1 to 3 mm diameter) residual cavities (lacunae). Similar lesions occasionally result from emboli passing distally from atheromatous lesions in the large arteries, but in most instances the pathologic cause is fibrosing hyaline degeneration ("lipohyalinosis"), followed by thrombotic occlusion in distal arteries 50 to 150 μm in diameter. The lesions are in the same small arteries which rupture in primary spontaneous intracerebral hemorrhage. It is not known why these vessels develop thrombosis in some hypertensive individuals and become necrotic and rupture in others.

The incidence of lacunar infarction is uncertain. The Harvard Stroke Registry, a prospective study of stroke in the Boston region, estimated that 19 per cent of strokes were of lacunar origin. A decline of such cases is now evident as part of the reduction in deaths resulting from hypertension.

NONARTERIOSCLEROTIC VASCULOPATHIES. *Fibromuscular hyperplasia* is the most common nonarteriosclerotic disorder affecting the large arteries, predominantly in their extracranial course. It is of unknown etiology, first described in the renal arteries with a predilection for middle-aged females. Although it is most commonly asymptomatic, minor or major thromboembolic events occur; the long-term prognosis is good, and late recurrence of ischemic events is uncommon. An increased incidence of berry aneurysm is reported with the condition.

Dissecting aortic aneurysm consequent upon the medial necrosis related to hypertension and occurring in middle life rarely may cause obstruction to the innominate, common carotid, and subclavian arteries. Stroke developing in association with crushing pain in the chest radiating to the back and possibly into the abdomen, with obliteration of some upper or lower limb pulses, suggests this diagnosis. Affected patients who are normotensive and under middle age should be examined for features of Marfan's syndrome.

Traumatic and spontaneous dissection of carotid and vertebral-basilar arteries is a disorder distinct from aortic dissection. Dissections have been described as a sequel to trauma, including direct blows to the neck, fracture dislocations that injure the vertebral artery in its bony canal, and indirect damage such as follows neck manipulations or other violent twisting or severe cervical hyperextension movements. Most dissections develop spontaneously without recognizable disease in the arterial wall. In a minority there is detectable medial degeneration, fibromuscular dysplasia, or advanced atheroma. The condition occurs in both sexes from childhood to middle life. Internal carotid artery dissection is most common and is characterized by neck, ear, face, or head pain. Focal cerebral ischemic symptoms, Horner's syndrome, bruits, or lightheadedness also commonly occur. Bilateral carotid and associated vertebral dissection may occur. Common angiographic manifestations include elongated tapered luminal narrowing, abrupt luminal reconstitution, aneurysms, intimal flaps and distal branch occlusions. Resolution of angiographic abnormalities and clinical recovery is to be expected in over 85 per cent of cases. A similar rare condition involving the basilar artery presents with basilar artery ischemia with or without subarachnoid hemorrhage.

Pulseless disease or *Takayasu's arteritis* is a granulomatous angiitis, involving fibrous proliferation, mononuclear infiltration, and occasional giant cells. There is a predilection for involvement of the media and adventitia of the aortic arch in young Japanese females. Occlusion or severe narrowing develops in the cranial and the subclavian arteries with occasional involvement of branches of the abdominal aorta. Another proliferative arteriopathy, particularly common in Japan termed *moyamoya* (describing its "puff-of-smoke" angiographic appearance), results in a progressive obliteration of the intracranial carotid arteries. An extensive vascular network develops with dilatation of many small branches beyond the stenoses, and abundant small collaterals develop from the ascending pharyngeal and meningeal branches of the external carotid artery. Progressive and stepwise neurologic disability is the rule, and many patients suffer abrupt worsening or death from rupture of one of the many anastomotic arteries.

A variety of uncommon pathologic processes can involve the smaller intracranial arteries and arterioles (Table 479–3).

CEREBRAL ARTERY THROMBOSIS DUE TO COAGULATION ABNORMALITIES, POLYCYTHEMIA, OR THROMBOCYTOSIS. *Coagulation abnormalities* are implicated in a variety of conditions which produce cerebral hemorrhage; they are less often associated with thrombotic events in the cerebral circulation. Some of these, such as consumption coagulopathies and thrombotic thrombocytopenic purpura

TABLE 479-3. NONARTERIOSCLEROTIC ANGIOPATHIES CAPABLE OF CAUSING TIA AND STROKE

Large Arteries
1. Fibromuscular hyperplasia
2. Dissecting aortic aneurysm
3. Traumatic and spontaneous carotid and vertebrobasilar artery dissection
4. Takayasu's arteritis (pulseless disease)
5. Moyamoya

Smaller Arteries and Arterioles
6. Collagen vascular disease
7. Giant cell ("temporal") arteritis
8. Meningovascular syphilis
9. Allergic vasculitis
10. Congophilic angiopathy
11. Vasculitis with homocystinuria
12. Vasculopathy resulting from drug abuse
13. Vasculitis with Behçet's disease
14. Granulomatous angiitis

(TTP), can produce combinations of hemorrhage and thrombosis in the same individual. The phenomena are confined to patients with serious systemic illness.

There are a variety of less devastating clinical states in which abnormalities of the coagulation process may be accompanied by cerebral ischemic events and stroke (Table 479–4). Venous thrombosis is more common than arterial in some of these conditions. Nevertheless the gamut of ischemic phenomena, varying from TIA to devastating stroke with massive infarction, may complicate any of these conditions.

The angiographic study of patients with these conditions tends to indicate branch arterial occlusions rather than large extracranial artery lesions. However, the initiating thrombus that eventually produces the thromboembolic intracranial occlusion may begin in the large aortic branches or in the pulmonary veins and pass cephalad from these sites.

Thrombocytosis, whether alone or with other features of polycythemia, is a rare but recognized platelet abnormality sometimes accompanied by transient and major persistent cerebral and retinal ischemia.

INTRACRANIAL VENOUS AND SINUS THROMBOSIS. Septic venous and sinus thrombosis complicating middle ear, sinus, and facial infection and aseptic venous and sinus thrombosis are discussed in Chapter 481.

SYNDROMES AND SYMPTOMS OF CEREBRAL ARTERIAL ATHEROTHROMBOSIS AND THROMBOEMBOLISM. Distinction between thrombotic and embolic arterial disease on clinical grounds alone can be difficult. Furthermore, variability of collateral circulation often precludes clinical differentiation of main-artery from branch occlusions. With these caveats, this section discusses features of stroke in individual arterial territories.

Internal Carotid Artery. The most common site for atheroma leading to stroke or threatening stroke is at the common carotid artery bifurcation. Minor lesions, smooth or ulcerative stenosis, and sometimes complete occlusions can be present without symptoms.

TABLE 479-4. CONDITIONS IN WHICH ALTERED BLOOD COAGULATION MAY PRODUCE CEREBRAL ISCHEMIA

Nonspecific:
The postpartum period
Pregnancy
Ingestion of oral contraceptives
Manifest and occult cancer
Postoperative and post-traumatic states
Paroxysmal nocturnal hemoglobinuria
Hyperviscosity syndromes
Polycythemia rubra vera
Sickle cell disease
Macroglobulinemia
Homocysteinuria

Specific:
Antithrombotic III deficiency
Protein C deficiency
Protein S deficiency
Lupus anticoagulant

Internal carotid artery stenosis is frequently accompanied by transient events, the most characteristic being ipsilateral monocular vision loss. Common symptoms are episodic weakness and/or sensory disturbance of the contralateral arm, leg, or face, at times causing a transient hemiplegia and hemisensory defect that returns to normal within minutes, hours (TIA), or days (RIND). Slurring of speech (dysarthria) or dysphasia, with dominant hemisphere involvement, may be present. Consciousness is preserved during carotid territory ischemia unless an uncommon convulsive episode is precipitated. Vertigo, diplopia, and simultaneous bilateral vision loss are not symptoms of carotid artery disease.

Carotid artery occlusion may occur asymptomatically, or it may be heralded by a series of transient or minor persisting events followed by a major hemisphere stroke. Fifty per cent of major strokes from carotid artery occlusion occur with no warning episodes. The motor and sensory cortex may be involved with impaired motor and sensory function of the face, arm, and leg. Speech impairment reflects dominant hemisphere dysfunction. Large infarcts can cause severe brain edema producing secondary herniation syndromes.

Approximately one third of patients complain of mild to severe ipsilateral or, occasionally, contralateral frontal and orbital pain coincident with the onset of the occlusion. The mechanism is probably related to distention of pain sensitive collateral arterial channels. Approximately 15 per cent of patients with internal carotid artery occlusion develop an ipsilateral Horner's syndrome. Some of these cases occur without significant evidence of cerebral ischemia and may reflect involvement of the vasa nervorum to the periarterial sympathetic fibers or possibly, ischemia of the hypothalamic cells of origin of the sympathetic pathway.

Firm palpation of the carotid artery in the neck is undesirable as it may dislodge an intra-arterial clot with subsequent ischemic deficit; it can be diagnostically misleading because of potential external carotid artery contribution to the carotid pulse. Gentle palpation is useful in the identification of complete loss of pulsation in common carotid occlusion, complemented by the observation of an absent facial or superficial temporal artery pulse.

Bruits are common over an internal carotid stenosis and are heard loudest at the bifurcation (i.e., at the level of the upper border of thyroid cartilage). *To identify a bruit as being of carotid origin, one must trace its disappearance down the artery, thereby separating it from transmitted heart sounds.* Although the carotid bruit is a well recognized marker for generalized atherosclerosis, its presence or absence often does not reflect the degree or nature of the underlying pathology. Substantial stenosis, ulcerative disease, or complete occlusion may be present without an audible bruit. External carotid artery stenosis can produce a local bruit despite internal carotid occlusion. An orbital bruit may represent severe intracavernous carotid stenosis or compensatory arterial collateralization accompanying severe ipsi- or contralateral internal carotid system occlusive disease.

Stenosis of an internal carotid artery is more likely to be associated with recurrent ischemic events than is an occluded artery. Nevertheless, with occlusion, recurrent ischemic events may continue from thromboembolism from the distal soft "tail" of the thrombus in the cavernous sinus portion of the carotid artery; from ulcerative atheroma in the ipsilateral, common, or external carotid arteries; or from a residual "stump" of the occluded internal carotid artery. If such a "stump" remains open, it provides a site for turbulent flow, predisposing to the accumulation of platelet-fibrin thrombus material. From these neck sources the intracranial circulation is embolized through retrograde flow in the ophthalmic artery or through meningeal and ascending pharyngeal anastomoses.

Middle Cerebral Artery. The middle cerebral territory is the most common site for cerebral infarction. The main trunk of the middle cerebral artery is occasionally the site of severe atheroma out of proportion to that of the other intra- or extracranial arteries, at times in excess of that affecting the internal carotid artery. Most often, however, occlusion of the main stem of the middle cerebral artery and of its major branches reflects embolic disease. Experimental emboli placed in the carotid artery or the aorta have a predilection to lodge in the middle cerebral as opposed to other intracranial arteries. In a young person with a middle cerebral artery occlusion or occlusion of one or more of its branches, a cardiac source should be sought. In older patients, either a cardiac or an internal carotid source for thromboembolism is more probable than intrinsic disease of the middle cerebral artery. When recurrent ischemia, persistent or transient, involves the middle cerebral artery distribution in both hemispheres or in one hemisphere and the posterior circulation in quick succession, cardioembolic events should be suspected.

The cortical distribution of the middle cerebral artery supplies the areas representing movements and higher sensory functions for the upper limb and face, sparing the leg. Dominant hemisphere involvement produces aphasia. Posterior parietal lesions may result in a lower quadrantanopia. The capsular and ganglionic branches, including particularly the lenticulostriate branches, supply a major amount of the posterior limb of the internal capsule, and infarcts in this territory produce hemiplegia with variable sensory components and with a possible accompanying homonymous hemianopia—all contralateral to the lesion.

Anterior Cerebral Artery. The clinical presentation of occlusion of the anterior cerebral artery depends on the involved segment of the artery and on the availability of collateral circulation. Proximal occlusions may produce no symptoms because of adequate flow through the anterior communicating artery. At the opposite extreme, occlusion of an artery responsible for the complete supply to both anterior cerebral arteries because of a vestigial proximal portion of the opposite anterior cerebral artery may result in drop attacks, or the rare syndrome of bilateral leg paralysis, urinary incontinence, and serious personality change. Intermediate between these extremes is the usual picture of an occlusion producing partial contralateral leg weakness and sensory loss, minimal arm involvement, and a sparing of face and speech function. Voluntary control of urination is commonly disturbed; mental confusion and behavioral disorders may be encountered. Since the ganglionic branches contribute to the supply of the subcortical white matter beneath the motor speech area, dysphasic symptoms may result from occlusion of the proximal part of the anterior cerebral artery.

Vertebral-Basilar (Posterior) Circulatory System. Occlusion of one or both vertebral arteries in the face of good collateral circulation may occur without causing clinical or pathological damage. A more common clinical syndrome following unilateral vertebral artery occlusion is the lateral medullary syndrome (Wallenberg's syndrome), caused by ischemia in the posterior inferior cerebellar artery territory. The ipsilateral findings include limb ataxia; Horner's syndrome; loss of appreciation of facial pain and temperature (trigeminal nerve); paralysis of larynx, pharynx, and palate (ninth and tenth nerve); and nystagmus. Intense vertigo and vomiting are common at the outset. Contralateral findings consist of impaired pain and temperature sensations, sparing only the face (see Fig. 478–4).

If one vertebral artery is vestigial, the remaining one becomes the main supply of the medulla. Depending on the condition of the posterior communicating artery, it may be the origin of much of the basilar artery flow. Under these anatomic circumstances, more serious brain-stem infarction can result from a single vertebral artery occlusion.

Occlusion of the subclavian artery at its common site proximal to the origin of the vertebral artery can cause reversal of ipsilateral vertebral artery flow into the subclavian artery distal to the occlusion, as demonstrated angiographically. In most patients this diversion is not clinically significant but on rare occasions it may produce symptoms of brain-stem ischemia aggravated by arm exercise, a phenomenon called the "subclavian steal."

Basilar Artery. Basilar artery occlusion results in variable degrees of infarction of pons, midbrain, cerebellum, and occipital and medial temporal lobes determined, as elsewhere in the brain, by the availability and adequacy of collateral circulation. The usual and frequently fatal presentation of basilar artery occlusion includes the sudden development of sustained coma from ischemia of the midbrain reticular activating system, accompanied by bilateral third nerve palsies proceeding to fixed and dilated pupils and paralysis of the face, bulbar muscles, tongue, and all extremities. Incomplete presentations include bilateral, usually asymmetric corticospinal tract limb involvement; limb ataxia; variable sensory loss; and a variety of cranial nerve lesions frequently contralateral to the hemiparesis ("crossed" syndromes).

On occasion, the basilar collateral circulation confines the infarction to unilateral ventral structures with a resultant hemiparesis difficult or impossible to distinguish from that of a more rostrad capsular or cortical lesion. Although such partial brain-stem lesions may result from total occlusion of the main basilar artery trunk, they are more often due to atherothrombotic, lacunar or embolic occlusion of the median and short circumferential basilar artery branches.

Posterior Cerebral Artery. The site of occlusion, anatomic variations, and the availability or lack of collateral supply determine the clinical syndromes arising from posterior cerebral artery atherothrombosis or embolism. Infarctions from proximal branch obstruction include the "thalamic syndrome" and complex midbrain syndromes, including several of the eponymic "crossed syndromes." Hemiballismus or hemichoreoathetosis, intention tremor, and ataxia may be encountered. Conjugate gaze palsies including vertical gaze paresis, skew deviation, and retraction nystagmus, may be seen.

Cortical branch arterial lesions result most often in homonymous hemianopia, but an upper quadrantanopia may result from interference with the lower optic radiation fibers in the temporal lobe. Dyslexia and a variety of visual hallucinations and distortions follow ischemia of visual association cortex.

Bilateral cortical lesions produce cortical blindness and in confused subjects are commonly accompanied by denial of the blindness. Preservation of central vision occurs if anterior and middle cerebral leptomeningeal collaterals supply the occipital pole.

Amnestic syndromes result from bilateral interruptions of the posterior cerebral arteries, producing ischemia in the hippocampal formations of the temporal lobes, or from thalamoperforating branches of the posterior cerebral arteries causing bilateral paramedian thalamic infarctions.

Lacunar Strokes. Several acute stroke syndromes have been delineated in association with small vessel disease producing areas of infarction and subsequent cavitation (lacunae). The lacunar lesions are less than 3 mm in diameter but may be multiple and occasionally coalesce to form larger areas visible by CT. Identical CT lesions and clinical syndromes are produced by embolic occlusion of the appropriate small arteries. The most important of the clinical syndromes related to these lacunar infarcts are outlined in Table 479–5.

PATHOGENESIS OF THREATENED STROKE. Stroke prevention has become a realistic goal; thus an appreciation of the way in which stroke presents is important. A "threatened stroke" may be regarded as any ischemic cerebral or retinal event that causes a TIA, RIND, PNS, or progressing stroke, each condition having the potential to evolve into a devastating stroke. Since it is common for patients with early TIA to go on to develop RIND or PNS prior to a complete stroke, we will discuss together the pathogenesis of all the

TABLE 479–5. CLINICAL SYNDROMES RELATED TO LACUNAR INFARCTION

Lacunar Syndrome	Location of Pathology
Pure motor hemiplegia	Internal capsule, basis pontis
Pure sensory stroke	Thalamus
Ataxic hemiparesis	Basis pontis corticospinal and cerebellar peduncle tracts
	Internal capsule, posterior limb
Dysarthria—clumsy hand	Anterior limb of internal capsule (rarely basis pontis)
Lacunar state	Diffuse deep white matter

earlier warning conditions. Such warning ischemic events result from a variety of conditions, listed in relative order of importance, in Table 479–6.

Artery-to-Artery Emboli. The retina, in which the arterioles are visible at the bedside, provides a microcosm reflecting the circulatory dynamics and pathology of the cerebral arterioles and arteries. Patients under study for recurrent unilateral visual loss *(amaurosis fugax)*, a particular variety of TIA, have been observed with three kinds of material located in the retinal arterioles coincident with the development of this symptom. First, grayish-white material composed of platelets and fibrin has been noted passing in the arterioles from the central disc region out to the periphery over a 5- to 45-minute period. Second, fragments of atheromatous debris in the form of bright yellowish amorphous material have been noted. These "bright plaques" may pass through reasonably quickly or lodge and be visible for days or weeks before disappearing (Fig. 479–2). They may persist and become surrounded by white fibrous scar. Finally, pure crystals of cholesterol may be visualized, caught at the bifurcation of a retinal arteriole.

Platelet-fibrin emboli originate in the heart valves and chambers or attached to its walls, or in the arteries which lead from it to the brain and retina. Emboli of atheromatous debris and pure cholesterol crystals come from the arteries but not from the heart. Surgeons at operation have observed both types of emboli lodging in the operative field of the exposed cortex in patients known to have irregular and ulcerative atheroma of the internal carotid or middle cerebral arteries. At postmortem examination, pathologists have identified atheromatous debris lodged in thrombi obstructing cortical and deep arteries and arterioles.

The onset of symptoms from major arterial disease may reflect the fact that the narrowing has become great enough to lead to platelet deposition in the area of turbulence beyond the stenosis. An alternative triggering mechanism is the occurrence of hemorrhage into an atheromatous plaque with a rupture into the lumen triggering thrombosis and embolism or resulting in the formation of a roughened surface upon which platelets and fibrin are deposited. Close scrutiny of patients affected with symptoms of threatened stroke reveals that many have atheromatous lesions in the arteries leading to the territory of the threatening symptoms. Whether the significance of such emboli to TIA in the carotid artery is greater than in the vertebral-basilar territory remains an open question. One of the difficulties in proposing a difference in pathogenesis in the two major arterial systems lies in the fact that vertebrobasilar symptoms are sometimes initiated by

TABLE 479–6. PATHOGENETIC MECHANISMS OF THREATENED STROKE

Arterial emboli
Cardiac emboli
Lacunar infarction
Arteriolar sclerosis
Hemodynamic factors
Nonarteriosclerotic vasculopathies
Mechanical interference with arteries
Coagulation abnormalities
Thrombocytosis
Cerebral venous and sinus thrombosis

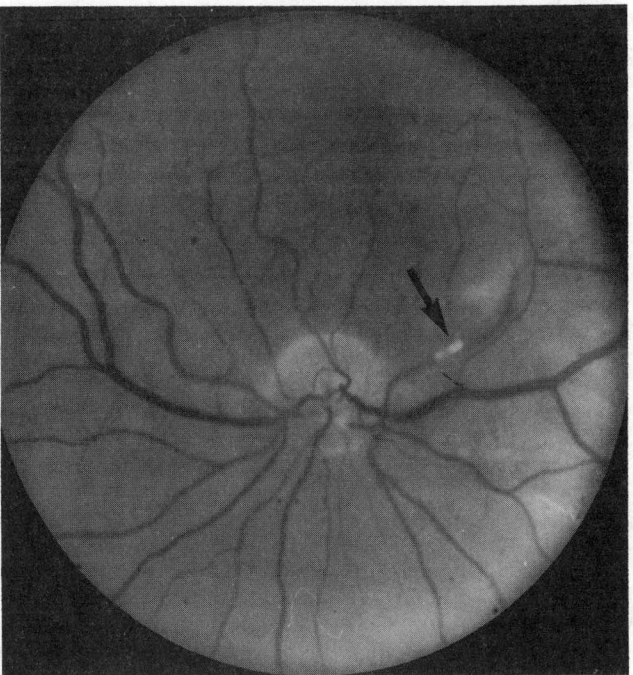

FIGURE 479–2. Atheromatous debris ("bright plaque") lodged in retinal arteriole in patient with history of attacks of amaurosis fugax. (From Barnett HJM: Med Clin North Am 63:649, 1979.)

cardiac and other systemic circulatory phenomena, and by a number of nonvascular conditions. Despite these limitations, in one study 78 per cent of cases with threatening stroke in the carotid artery territory and 82 per cent of vertebrobasilar cases had arteriographically detectable lesions appropriate to the symptoms.

Emboli of Cardiac Origin. In all age groups one must consider the heart as a source for symptoms and signs of threatening stroke. These have been discussed earlier (see Table 479–2).

Lacunar Infarction. Lacunar infarcts (lacunae) are preceded by transitory symptoms in about one quarter of the cases. Concurrent large-vessel occlusive disease in hypertensive patients can make clinical diagnosis of lacunar events difficult.

Hemodynamic Factors. Transient hemodynamic events such as cardiac arrhythmias tend to produce diffuse cerebral ischemic symptoms rather than focal ones. The evidence to support this statement comes from a variety of sources. In one study a series of 37 patients who had experienced focal TIA were exposed to a drop in blood pressure by pharmacologic and postural changes sufficient to induce syncope. Only one patient experienced focal symptoms. In a series of patients dying several days following global ischemia caused by cardiac arrest, the associated areas of cerebral infarction did not correspond to the sites of major atheromatous lesions. By contrast, old infarcts from previous cerebral events corresponded to arteriosclerosis in the appropriate arteries. A study of 290 patients who required a pacemaker because of heart block indicated that although 231 patients had suffered neurologic symptoms, only two had experienced focal ischemic events. Despite this, one sometimes encounters patients in whom a sudden impairment of cardiac output or an episode of severe hypotension (idiopathic cases, autonomic system dysfunction and disease, iatrogenic orthostatic hypotension, pulmonary emboli, carotid sinus hypersensitivity) has been accompanied by a focal ischemic event or a major stroke. Occasionally in the presence of a previously occluded major artery (internal carotid or basilar), a postural drop in blood pressure will result in symptoms that revert to normal when the patient reclines. When this happens, one usually finds that other major arteries are severely stenosed or occluded as well.

Arteriolar Sclerosis. Progressive fibrosis of the walls of small (<150 μm diameter) arterioles with luminal narrowing is accelerated in hypertension and diabetes. It is represented in most cases by small focal infarcts. "Binswanger's disease" (subcortical arteriosclerotic encephalopathy) is a term describing patchy or diffuse white matter degeneration associated with multifocal infarcts. The clinical picture is one of subacute progressive dementia without discrete neurologic symptoms. A lack of neuropathologic correlation and pathognomonic radiologic features makes this a controversial diagnosis. Only a handful of proven examples of the disorder are on record and the diagnosis should be entertained with great caution.

Nonarteriosclerotic Vasculopathies. Nonarteriosclerotic vasculopathies (Table 479–3) are rare but so diverse as to make a generic description of little value. Minor events in all of these disorders may precede major hemisphere or brain-stem ischemic infarction. Repetitive and multiple hemispheric events should always suggest a widespread vasculopathy or cardiac source.

Mechanical Interference with the Course of the Cerebral Arteries. The location of the common and internal carotid arteries renders them liable to direct trauma with rupture and hemorrhage and even more to injury and subsequent thrombosis. Occasionally violent hyperextension neck injuries can stretch the carotid arteries abruptly in their extracranial course, producing intimal damage, medial dissection, and thrombosis. Similar injury can damage the vertebral artery before its entry at the C6 level into its protective bony canal in the transverse processes of the cervical vertebral bodies. At the C1-C2 level, the artery is more mobile and may be levered into hyperextension and rotation by athletic injury, motor vehicle accident, or violent chiropractic manipulations. The trauma can lead to early thrombotic occlusion and the clinical picture of a vertebral artery ischemia, or may be followed by recurrent transient ischemic events reflecting a damaged endothelium with an irregular surface attracting thrombi and subsequent thromboembolic events.

Within the canal of the vertebral artery, there may be encroachment on the lumen of the vessel by osteophytes forming at the uncovertebral fissures, or "neurocentral joints" of the spine developing because of cervical spondylosis. Such conditions rarely cause symptoms, even when the artery must deviate around a large osteophyte. There is little movement at this site, and what there is requires lateral flexion to produce further narrowing of the affected artery. The popular concept of cervical spondylosis being a common cause of symptoms such as dizziness and vertigo is erroneous. At most this is a rare cause of ischemic events, and as a rule it occurs only after a severe neck injury.

The internal carotid artery below and adjacent to the cavernous sinus rarely may be distorted and encroached upon by tumors such as "en plaque" meningioma or extensions of nasopharyngeal cancer. Occasionally an odontoid dislocation, of traumatic origin or secondary to rheumatoid disease, will produce brainstem ischemic symptoms related to neck movement by compressing the lumen of the vertebral artery. Similarly, on very rare occasions benign tumors extending into the foramen magnum produce intermittent symptoms of vertebral artery insufficiency.

With routine activities involving neck hyperextension, elderly subjects may complain of episodes of blurred or lost vision, syncope, vertigo, or ataxia. Although some of these effects may reflect vertebral artery compromise, the mechanism is not clear.

TRANSIENT CAROTID AND VERTEBROBASILAR ISCHEMIA. *Symptoms and Signs.* TIA, RIND, and PNS warn of the possibility of a more significant stroke. It is essential for the physician to recognize the various expressions of TIA symptomatology, as the management of carotid and vertebro-

TABLE 479–7. SYMPTOMS OF CAROTID ARTERY DISEASE*

Symptoms	TIA AND RIND (208 Cases) (%)	PNS (103 Cases) (%)
Monocular visual	34	21
Paresis (mono-, hemi-)	59	88
Paresthesia (mono-, hemi-)	57	62
Facial paresis	22	43
Facial paresthesia	30	26
Dysphasia	21	30
Dysarthria	14	18
Headache	11	11
Binocular visual (hemianopsia)	7	10
"Dizziness"—nonspecific	6	2
Mental change	1	—
Convulsions		
Focal	—	—
Grand mal	1.5	2
Loss of consciousness	—	1
Visual hallucination	1	—

*From Barnett HJM: Clin Neurosurg 23:543, 1976.

basilar disease may differ, and both may mimic other nonvascular conditions. The initial symptoms experienced by 311 patients with associated internal carotid disease are given in Table 479–7.

Amaurosis fugax is highly suggestive of carotid disease. A possible hemianopic disturbance must not be mistaken for monocular visual loss. Having the patient cover one and then the other eye during subsequent attacks may permit this distinction. Frequently, the description is of a descending window blind obliterating vision. Positive phenomena such as flashing or shimmering sensations only seldom reflect retinal ischemia. The description of ocular and contralateral limb symptoms on separate occasions is highly suggestive of carotid artery symptom origin. It is rare for visual and limb symptoms to occur simultaneously.

Vertebrobasilar symptoms are more varied. Binocular visual loss is exceeded as a symptom only by vertigo and diplopia. The symptoms described in a series of 124 vertebrobasilar cases are outlined in Table 479–8.

The binocular visual symptoms frequently involve the entire vision, and descriptions vary from a complete blackness to a haziness of vision. At times a description is obtained of a veil over the vision with a random preservation of normal islands. Flashing and shimmering may occur as in migraine aura. Loss of consciousness is uncommon and did not appear in our patients. Syncope, however, is a common expression of cardiac arrhythmia producing diffuse reduction in cerebral perfusion.

Motor or sensory symptoms simultaneously involving both sides of the body are highly suggestive of vertebrobasilar ischemia; so, also, is unilateral weakness or sensory loss along

TABLE 479–8. SYMPTOMS OF VERTEBROBASILAR ARTERY DISEASE*

Symptoms	TIA or RIND (78 cases) (%)	PNS (46 Cases) (%)
Binocular visual	50	30
Vertigo	51	35
Diplopia	44	48
"Dizzy"	22	13
Ataxia	41	46
Paresthesia	44	54
Paresis	33	59
Dysarthria	21	37
Headache	18	33
Nausea and vomiting	14	17
Hearing loss	3	7
Mental change	8	8
Dysphagia	4	4
Dysphasia	3	4
Visual hallucinations	5	2
"Drop attacks"	4	4
Convulsions	—	2
Drowsiness	1	2

*From Barnett HJM: Clin Neurosurg 23:543, 1976.

TABLE 479–9. CORRELATION OF VERTEBROBASILAR ISCHEMIC SYMPTOMS WITH ANATOMIC STRUCTURES

Symptom	Anatomic Structure
Common symptoms:	
Bilateral visual blurring	Visual cortex—occipital lobe
Diplopia	Oculomotor nuclei—midbrain and pons
Vertigo	Vestibular nuclei—medulla and pons
Bilateral, alternating, or "crossed" motor and sensory symptoms	Long motor and sensory tracts, cranial nerve nuclei
Ataxia	Cerebellum or cerebellar connections
Less common symptoms:	
Episodic unconsciousness, drowsy state	Reticular activating structures of midbrain and rostral connections
Tinnitus and deafness	Cochlear nuclei
Dysphagia	Tenth nerve nuclei
Nausea and vomiting	Vagus nerve area
Confused episodes	Bilateral temporal lobe, upper brainstem
Amnestic episodes, transient global amnesia	Bilateral temporal lobe
Visual hallucinations	Parietal-occipital region
Symptoms less readily localized:	
Isolated monoplegia or hemiplegia and similar sensory phenomena	{ ? Possibly carotid { ? Possibly vertebrobasilar
Dysarthria	{ ? Possibly in brainstem { ? Possibly nondominant hemisphere
Drop attacks	{ ? Pontine reticular structures { ? Ventral corticospinal tract

with evidence of cranial nerve symptomatology, especially vertigo or oculomotor dysfunction producing diplopia. The variety of symptoms experienced by patients with vertebrobasilar disease reflects the anatomic substrate subserved by the vertebral and basilar arteries and their branches. A guide to the origin of common and uncommon symptoms is given in Table 479–9.

Certain symptoms cannot be accurately localized if they occur in isolation. For example, a transient monoplegia or even a hemiplegia may arise from dysfunction of the hemisphere, either cortical or capsular, but might originate from the corticospinal tract in the ventral brain stem. Corresponding sensory phenomena may be equally difficult to localize. The occurrence or recurrence of dysarthria may be due to the involvement of corticobulbar fibers coming from the nondominant hemisphere and proceeding from this area of carotid supply down to their location in the brain stem with its vertebrobasilar supply. In general, such isolated dysarthria is more likely to result from carotid than vertebrobasilar insufficiency.

Five to 10 per cent of patients with TIA experience symptoms that reflect abnormalities in both the carotid and vertebral-basilar arterial territories. Careful analysis of characteristic carotid symptoms such as amaurosis fugax or dysphasia, or of vertebrobasilar symptoms such as simultaneous bilateral long track involvement and dysfunction of cranial nerve nuclei, helps clarify the coincidence of anterior and posterior symptomatology.

Drop attacks are unheralded falling spells without change in sensorium and immediate righting. Their features and pathogenesis are discussed in Ch. 465.

Transient global amnesia (see Ch. 460) occurs fairly frequently in older persons. Episodes in conjunction with typical vertebrobasilar ischemic phenomena may be ischemic in origin; amnestic events during hemodynamic compromise may be related to bilateral medial temporal lobe ischemia.

Headache is common in cerebrovascular disease. It may accompany TIA and also stroke. It is most common on the side of the ischemia, frontotemporally, but may lie on the opposite side or in the occiput. As a rule such headaches are mild and nonthrobbing, lasting from a few minutes to a few hours. Violent headache sometimes occurs in association with an asymptomatic occlusion of the carotid artery and may be due to dilatation of anastomotic arteries.

A number of symptoms that sometimes accompany syndromes of cerebral vascular insufficiency bear much less specific connotations if they occur or recur in isolation. More common and prosaic conditions may be the cause. The list of such isolated symptoms of doubtful origin even in the face of known arterial disease, neck and orbital bruits, includes headache, episodic loss of consciousness, amnestic episodes, drop attacks, attacks of vertigo, deafness, diplopia, and dysarthria. Frequent but stereotyped recurrence of a single symptom weighs against ischemia and requires a search for alternative mechanisms.

DIFFERENTIAL DIAGNOSIS OF TIA. Transient episodes of hemispheric, brain-stem or retinal dysfunction cannot be automatically attributed to ischemia. Whereas other conditions may mimic ischemic disorders by the equally abrupt onset of symptoms, the temporal evolution may be a useful distinguishing feature. Ischemic events often evolve over seconds to minutes, seizures over 2 to 3 minutes, and migraine, over 15 to 20 minutes.

Every patient presenting with the symptom of thromboembolic amaurosis fugax requires close scrutiny for alternative primary ocular conditions such as muscae volitantes ("floaters"), vitreous hemorrhage, glaucoma, and retinal detachment. Cranial ("temporal") arteritis causing ischemic optic neuropathy also can cause transient visual obscurations, as can the plateau waves associated with increased intracranial pressure. Migrainous auras tend to be scintillating and hemianopic, although patients often mistakenly assume these symptoms are monocular.

Localized sensory ischemic events may be difficult to distinguish from focal sensory seizures. Both may occur in the same subject, if an area of focal ischemia becomes epileptogenic. The lack of a "march" in the ischemic episode is helpful in distinguishing it from sensory epilepsy.

Brain tumors, arteriovenous malformations, subdural hematomas, and on rare occasions multiple sclerosis may produce short-lived fluctuating symptoms, mimicking ischemia. A postictal paralysis (Todd's paralysis) must not be mistaken for a transient paresis of ischemic origin. Embolization from aneurysmal thrombi may produce carotid or vertebrobasilar symptoms indistinguishable from those of arteriosclerotic lesions.

Benign positional vertigo, Menière's disease, and other peripheral vestibular causes of vertigo can be mistaken for hindbrain ischemia, since there may be accompanying ataxia. Such patients often describe visual blurring in association with severe vertigo, and they may be syncopal, increasing the resemblance of their symptoms to those of a central lesion. The occurrence and aggravation of tinnitus and deafness with vertigo are useful in alerting the physician to a peripheral vestibular origin.

Vertigo, diplopia, slurred speech, and loss of consciousness may be manifestations of "basilar artery migraine." In such patients, motor and sensory phenomena may be due to hemisphere involvement ("hemiplegic migraine"). The diagnosis of these uncommon varieties of florid migraine must be made cautiously, particularly in the absence of an accompanying family history. Usually, with migraine other family members manifest an equally striking aura, with accompanying hemicrania, usually developing in late adolescence or early adult life. An important distinction is that migraine of this dramatic type rarely has its onset during the late adult years. Structural lesions are to be suspected and "hemiplegic migraine" becomes a diagnosis by exclusion in middle-aged or older subjects.

Of special importance in the differential diagnosis of vertebral basilar insufficiency are cardiac and circulatory hemodynamic crises producing diffuse disturbances of cerebral perfusion. Most patients who develop complete heart block, as well as some afflicted with a sick sinus syndrome and a variety of tachyrhythmias, experience neurologic symptoms. Sudden loss of consciousness, convulsions, vertigo, and nonspecific dizziness and, less commonly, confusion, amnesia, and diplopia may be described. Focal events mimicking TIA are uncommon.

COURSE AND PROGNOSIS. *The Prognosis of Threatened Stroke.* Prognosis for threatened stroke patients is multifactorial but especially dependent upon the presumptive mechanism of the threatening symptoms. Mortality following TIA is primarily due to cardiac disease with similar survival rates for patients with either carotid or vertebrobasilar TIA. A Rochester, Minnesota, population-based study identified a stroke probability of 8 per cent in the first year, 5 per cent for the next three years, and about 3 per cent per year thereafter for such patients. A comparable stroke rate of 5 per cent per year over 2.5 years was shown in patients with TIA, RIND, and minor stroke who received placebo in the aspirin-sulfinpyrazone clinical trial.

The Prognosis of Completed Stroke. About one fourth to one fifth of patients with thrombotic or embolic cerebral infarction die with their first attack. This figure varies somewhat with the cause of the infarction and especially with other factors such as age, cardiac status, and the degree of neurologic disability. The mortality rises sharply with increasing age: for patients over the age of 70 and those with marked neurologic defects, coma, or extensive systemic vascular disease, the initial mortality approaches 50 per cent. Infarction of the ventral portions of the brain stem after basilar artery occlusion, especially with quadriplegia, carries a poor outlook, although solicitous medical and nursing care may preserve a vegetative or severely disabled existence for long periods.

The prognosis for cerebral infarction is better in younger patients; in those with the least evidence of vascular disease at other sites, especially cardiovascular disease; and in those who do not have hypertension, diabetes, or severe neurologic defects.

About one fifth of patients who survive a cerebral infarction from atherosclerotic vascular disease suffer another stroke within the next 12 to 24 months. However, the most significant limiting factor on survival is not recurrent stroke but cardiovascular disease. About half of the patients who survive an initial cerebral infarction die at a later date from myocardial infarction or cardiac failure.

Recurrence of cerebral infarction is common with cerebral emboli of any cause. Estimates made over varying time periods indicate the rate of recurrent strokes caused by cerebral emboli from rheumatic heart disease to be between 30 and 70 per cent. Including extracerebral sites, nearly all patients have more than one embolus. In rheumatic heart disease, 40 per cent of the recurrences take place within the first month after the original episode and 50 to 60 per cent, within the first year. Each cerebral recurrence carries a strong chance of causing death or further neurologic disability.

Course of Completed Stroke. During the first 72 hours gradual worsening of neurologic deficits and incipient or increasing impairment of consciousness are frequent. Potential causes of deficit progression are listed in Table 479–10.

Patients whose course is not complicated by severe cerebral edema usually show an early improvement in neurologic function suggesting an excellent outcome. Slow return of function predicts less complete recovery. Persistent flaccid

TABLE 479–10. CAUSES OF POST-ONSET DETERIORATION

Necrotic cerebral edema
Progressive thrombosis
Recurrent emboli from a proximal arterial or cardiac source
Peri-infarct edema
Hemorrhage into the infarction
Concurrent febrile illness
Seizure disorder
Drug (sedative, tranquillizer, narcotic) effect
Circulatory or respiratory failure
Metabolic or electrolyte

paralysis without return of voluntary movement after 30 to 60 days suggests a poor functional prognosis. Substantial sensory loss impairs the chances of recovery of motor function and interferes with rehabilitation. The course of lateral medullary brain-stem infarction is usually one of gradual improvement. Symptoms of nausea, vertigo, diplopia, swallowing difficulty, hoarseness of voice, and ataxia lessen and may disappear.

MANAGEMENT OF CEREBRAL ISCHEMIA. *Investigation of Acute Stroke, PNS, RIND, and TIA.* The first step is to be sure that the description and findings of the acute illness fulfill the clinical and laboratory criteria for acute cerebral ischemia. That being established, the next is to determine whether the patient has suffered a completed stroke, is still progressing, or is already improving. Improvement indicates that the attack was an RIND or TIA. In patients who have suffered a complete major stroke, most of the neurologic damage will already be done. They necessarily will be subjected to less intense immediate attention and investigation than those whose disease is unstable, still progressing, or threatening to recur.

The non-neurologic history specifically should inquire for symptoms or previous diagnoses of heart disease, hypertension, diabetes, toxic drug exposure, alcoholism, or potentially precipitating metabolic problems. Thorough examination of the heart and peripheral vasculature is essential, as already mentioned. When any doubt exists about the pathogenesis of transient or partial cerebral attacks, 24-hour ECG monitoring, echocardiography, and cardiac wall motion studies should be obtained. In younger persons with stroke or in any with unusual features, laboratory evaluations should include an appraisal of coagulation factors and at least consideration of the thrombosis-predisposing conditions listed in Table 479–4.

In the neurologic evaluation, lumbar puncture is unnecessary unless syphilis or some granulomatous condition is suspected. Similarly, the EEG is not useful unless a question of seizures arises. A CT scan or MRI is desirable in all first-time acute strokes or stroke suspects to distinguish between ischemia and hemorrhage and to exclude other primary cerebral disorders. Isotope brain scanning is not useful diagnostically. Noninvasive Doppler sonography or ultrasound of the carotid arteries often provides information about the degree of atherosclerosis and, specifically, the presence or absence of carotid stenosis but offers no direct information about the intracranial vasculature. Direct carotid arteriography, preferably performed with digital enhancement, is reserved for the evaluation of unusual diagnostic problems or for the specific identification of major carotid bifurcation lesions that might be candidates for surgical endarterectomy.

Treatment of Threatened Stroke (TIA, RIND, PNS). Once an accurate individualized decision regarding the pathogenesis of the ischemia has been made, the possibilities for preventive treatment include risk factor management, vasoactive drugs, antithrombotic drugs, and surgical therapy.

Risk factors are not always amenable to successful manipulation. Heredity cannot be altered. It is not certain that the reduction of high blood lipids alters the outlook once symptoms develop. Although no data demonstrate a reduction of stroke with the elimination of hyperglycemia by rigid diabetic regulation in patients with cerebrovascular ischemia, control of both hyperlipidemia and diabetes mellitus is desirable. Cigarette smoking should be eliminated. Hypertension demands therapy, and in all age groups and both sexes the systolic and diastolic pressures must be kept at or below 160 and 90 mm Hg. Control of the diastolic value is especially important. An increase in hematocrit above 50 with an accompanying increase in blood viscosity has been identified as an added risk factor and probably should be controlled with the judicious use of phlebotomy. Cardiac abnormalities, whenever amenable to therapy, require careful attention. Although the carotid bruit is a marker for generalized atherosclerosis, evidence to date fails to prove that investigation and surgical treatment are justified.

Vasoactive drugs such as calcium channel blockers and free radical scavengers have shown variable promise in vitro in the treatment of focal ischemia; however, there is no current evidence for their usefulness in the clinical setting. Other "vasodilators" have never been shown to be of value.

Antithrombotic drugs, first introduced as heparin and Coumadin derivatives, remain controversial in stroke prevention. In cases of threatened stroke from emboli arising in mural thrombi following myocardial infarction, and in mitral stenosis with and without atrial fibrillation, their use has received fairly wide acceptance. In the former instance they need not be utilized after eight weeks. In the latter condition prolonged use is customary, since most cases of rheumatic heart disease with emboli have a high incidence of recurrent events over a long period of time, particularly within the year after the initial embolus.

Many authorities advise the use of anticoagulants for recently developed TIAs in carotid and vertebrobasilar territory, recommending them for two to three months or longer if a flurry of TIAs recurs and they are not relieved by platelet antiaggregant therapy. The data upon which this treatment is based are equivocal and the therapy is empirical. In progressing stroke, many workers advise the use of heparin followed by a few weeks of Coumadin treatment. Controlled studies with convincing data are lacking to establish this as a scientifically proven approach, and its use remains empirical. Anticoagulants alone or combined with platelet antiaggregant agents are usually recommended for the prevention of embolization following the insertion of a prosthetic heart valve. Anticoagulants are not of value in patients with a completed stroke. The administration of anticoagulants carries a risk of fatal intracerebral or systemic hemorrhage, and their administration always must be rigidly controlled.

Several clinical trials have evaluated platelet antiaggregants in TIA, RIND, and PNS. The weight of evidence indicates that aspirin is effective in preventing stroke and death in a significant number of patients at risk for atherothrombotic stroke. The benefit to females is uncertain: one large trial detected a male benefit only, while another appeared to indicate no particular difference in responsiveness by gender. No benefit has yet been demonstrated for the other known platelet antiaggregants, sulfinpyrazone and dipyridamole. Theoretical evidence, however, supports the hypothesis that the combination of aspirin with dipyridamole may be superior to either drug alone. Trials are under way to establish or disprove this possibility. The optimal dosage of aspirin is unsettled. Clinical studies in stroke prevention have employed 1 to 1.5 grams daily. The balance between the dose of aspirin that suppresses platelet production of the aggregating thromboxane A_2 via cyclo-oxygenase inhibition, and the dose that suppresses the production of antiaggregating prostacyclin by the vascular endothelial cells, through similar cyclo-oxygenase inhibition, is under active study. Theoretical evidence indicates that lower doses of aspirin may affect the platelet aggregation and spare the inhibition of the more beneficial prostacyclin production. In time the problem of optimal dosage will be settled by clinical trial. Present evidence from clinical trials favors the use of 1300 mg of aspirin daily. Little information exists on the use of platelet antiaggregants in cardioembolic threatened stroke.

Anticoagulant therapy in cerebral vein and sinus thrombosis is covered in Chapter 481.

Role of Surgery in Cerebral Atherothrombotic Disease. The realization that many patients with cerebral ischemia are afflicted with disease of the extracranial arteries, combined with the development of acceptably safe cerebral angiographic procedures and the development of surgical capability to operate on arterial lesions, culminated in the first carotid endarterectomy being carried out in 1952. The role of surgery in the management of lesions of the cerebral arteries continues to be under active study. The answers are not easily obtained, and it is well to weigh the decision carefully in all cases with the following guidelines:

1. Carotid endarterectomy has become common practice for patients with specific neurologic symptoms appropriate to a stenosed and/or ulcerated atheromatous lesion in the lower cervical portion of the internal carotid artery.

2. A single major randomized study carried out to determine the benefit of carotid endarterectomy found no advantage for surgery over standard medical therapy. However, the study was completed before the improved skills in angiography and surgery of the past decade were available. The results of such a study might be improved if the controlled trial were repeated.

3. Cerebral angiography and carotid endarterectomy carry a small but definite risk even in the most expert hands. If the combination of morbidity and mortality from these two procedures in a given institution exceeds 3 per cent, it is likely that the patient will fare as well by medical management alone. The risk-benefit ratio is too low to place either of these procedures in inexperienced hands.

4. In the presence of intracranial occlusive disease equal to or exceeding that in more proximal cervical lesions, the efficacy of carotid endarterectomy is dubious.

5. Patients with vertebral artery symptoms are not considered candidates for surgery at present. Proximal lesions in the vertebral artery may be accessible, but there is little evidence that such patients benefit by endarterectomy. Patients with vertebrobasilar symptoms do not benefit from surgery on simultaneously stenosed but asymptomatic carotid lesions.

6. Whether or not surgery is performed in suitable candidates, risk factor management and the utilization of appropriate antithrombotic treatment must not be overlooked. No controlled study to determine the benefit of endarterectomy has been pursued since the benefits of risk factor management and antihypertensive treatment have been established.

7. Carotid endarterectomy in the presence of a completed stroke or in the presence of a complete arterial occlusion appropriate to the symptoms has no demonstrated value.

Final conclusions about the role of carotid endarterectomy in extracranial symptomatic vascular disease await careful future evaluation. In the interim patients should be subjected to this procedure only after careful analysis of the appropriateness and significance of the symptoms and a full awareness of the angiographic and surgical risks in the particular institution concerned. It should be emphasized, however, that there is no evidence that endarterectomy benefits patients unless they show approximately 80 per cent or more stenosis of the internal carotid artery and have had neurologic symptoms ipsilateral to the lesion.

A recent multicenter randomized trial comparing surgical revascularization (superficial temporal to middle cerebral artery anastomosis) with medical therapy following TIA or minor stroke found no surgical benefit in these patients, reflected by poorer overall survival and higher stroke rates compared with medically treated patients. For any patients with arteriosclerotic disease causing middle cerebral artery or internal carotid occlusion or stenosis, no evidence has been advanced to indicate benefit for revascularization for stroke prevention.

The Asymptomatic Carotid Lesion. A bruit detected on routine physical examination, or stenosis revealed by carotid angiography in an artery from which no symptoms have arisen, presents controversial management questions. Long-term surveillance of several large series of patients with neck bruits has determined that although such bruits are associated with an increased stroke risk, the resultant stroke often develops in a vascular territory remote from that related to the bruit or from a cardiac source. The incidence of bruits increases with age and with the existence of hypertension. Evidence indicates that prophylactic endarterectomy has no value when performed on asymptomatic carotid lesions as a prelude to open-heart and aortic surgery. Until carefully conducted studies reveal convincing evidence to the contrary, conservative, nonsurgical management of asymptomatic carotid lesions and bruits is recommended.

Treatment of Completed Stroke. Treatment of cerebral infarction is designed to preserve life, limit the extent of the infarction, reduce disability, and prevent recurrences.

Stroke victims present with the same life-threatening circumstances as do patients with other serious neurologic illness. The principles of therapy are similar: the maintenance of a proper airway; adequate fluid, electrolyte, and caloric intake; and adequate urinary output. Constant vigilance is required to prevent aspiration pneumonitis and avoid necrotic skin lesions at pressure points.

The development of cerebral edema should be considered in a deteriorating patient who has suffered a recent cerebral infarct. Despite the lack of convincing benefit, hyperosmolar agents are often used in such patients. The use of corticosteroids has been largely discredited.

Although experimental evidence in animals suggested that deep barbiturate coma given immediately after stroke onset might reduce the ultimate cerebral damage, clinical trials have shown no advantage for the procedure, which cannot be recommended.

Efforts to increase cerebral blood flow to limit the amount of ischemic infarction have been attempted. Vasopressor as well as vasodilator regimens have been attempted by hyperoxygenation or by producing hypercarbia, neither with evidence of benefit.

Treatment in the later and convalescent stages of stroke should be directed toward lessening the deformity and disability with daily passive exercise of paretic limbs, and early ambulation with appropriate assistance.

Rehabilitation. Recovery from stroke depends mainly on spontaneous neurologic recovery. It may be assisted by learning to improve function and utilize alternatives, and this requires an active rehabilitation program. Programs of retraining should begin as soon as there is no longer evidence of increasing infarction. Stabilization of the neurologic findings for 12 to 24 hours is usually sufficient evidence to permit the start of rehabilitation. All programs have as their goal the exploitation of remaining functions for maximal effectiveness. Although a few patients require and benefit from special hospital facilities, most rehabilitation programs can be carried out on medical services without the aid of extensive equipment. An internist or general physician who is interested in rehabilitation can direct programs of activity and exercise, and can achieve results in rehabilitating hemiplegic patients which often are as effective as those of specialized centers.

The first requirement is to increase the patient's tolerance to sitting and standing, both of which are impaired by weakness and by changes in the sense of balance. Patients are allowed to sit up and then stand for increasingly long periods, beginning with five to ten minutes several times a day. During this period daily active and passive exercises of the weakened extremities are carried out. When patients begin to stand they need firm support and often splinting or bracing of the knee on the weakened side; marked quadriceps weakness may occasionally demand a long leg brace. Ambulation is one of the main goals of rehabilitation. Gait training should begin as soon as the patient can comfortably stand for 15 to 20 minutes without fatigue. The support of parallel bars or a walker should be depended upon at first. After ambulation begins, it may be necessary to brace the foot to avoid the foot drop and inversion that commonly occur after hemiplegia. At the same time that the patient is relearning to walk, he should be trained to develop new skills with his unaffected arm and

to improve the strength and function in the paretic arm. This is done by an active program of exercise and by retraining the patient in the activities of daily living such as eating, dressing and undressing, and personal hygiene. Usually the maximal effect of rehabilitation and recovery is gained in three to four months, but some patients continue to show improvement over periods lasting as long as two years. Passive exercise must be continued indefinitely for severely paralyzed patients if contractures are to be avoided.

A painful shoulder resulting from periarthritic changes is common after hemiplegia and may develop despite early passive motion of the member. Continued passive movements combined with heat and, if persistent, with subacromial steroid injection or a short course of systemic steroids will avoid additional pain and permanent fixation of the shoulder in adduction.

For patients with mild to moderate dysphasia, speech therapy may be helpful, encouraging patients and their families to be aggressive about the need to practice talking; speech therapy does not benefit severe dysphasia.

HYPERTENSIVE ENCEPHALOPATHY. Hypertensive encephalopathy is an uncommon acute neurologic disorder characterized by attacks of headache, nausea, vomiting, visual impairment, focal or generalized seizures, and drowsiness, which may proceed to stupor and coma. Transient focal deficits can include hemiparesis, dysphasia, and hemianopia. The blurred vision reflects cortical or local retinal ischemic changes, but it is not necessarily associated with retinal hemorrhage or papilledema. Although the latter retinal findings are present in many of the patients, others show no more than narrowing, often segmental, of the arterioles. The blood pressure as a rule is severely elevated. Some patients have had longstanding raised blood pressure with recent further elevation, whereas in others a markedly elevated pressure is a new development.

Hypertensive encephalopathy can complicate acute nephritis, chronic renal disease, eclampsia, and pheochromocytoma. Hypertensive crises and encephalopathy can follow the ingestion of a combination of monamine oxidase inhibiting drugs with food high in tyramine content. The crises can result from the abrupt withdrawal of antihypertensive therapy, particularly clonidine. In patients with acute and chronic spinal cord injuries, excessive autonomic stimulation by bladder or gastrointestinal distention can precipitate potentially fatal hypertensive encephalopathy.

At postmortem examination, the brain in hypertensive encephalopathy may appear grossly normal or swollen, with evidence of tentorial and cerebellar herniation. Edema is not a universal finding even with a history of increased intracranial pressure and papilledema. Cut section reveals small petechial hemorrhages and sometimes larger hypertensive hemorrhages. Microscopically, one finds scattered small areas of infarction accompanied, in patients with longstanding hypertension, by hyaline necrosis of the arteriolar walls.

The pathogenesis of hypertensive encephalopathy is thought to be a breakdown in the normal process of cerebral autoregulation, whereby the arterioles maintain a stable cerebral blood flow despite fluctuations in the mean systemic arterial pressure. The intensity and speed of blood pressure elevation exceeds the tolerance of the regulatory mechanisms, and a combination of segmentally narrowed and dilated arterioles results. Disruption of the blood-brain barrier results in cerebral edema. Necrotic arterioles may lead to the creation of petechial and larger hemorrhages.

Uremia closely resembles hypertensive encephalopathy in its symptoms. Once that condition is ruled out by determining a BUN below 100 mg per deciliter, the differential diagnosis includes the more usual complications of severe hypertension, including intracerebral hemorrhage, ischemic infarction related to atherothrombosis in large arteries, and lacunar infarction. These conditions are more likely to exhibit focal clinical signs that are florid and persistent. By contrast, the focal neurologic deficits in hypertensive encephalopathy tend to be transient, mild, and multifocal. Sudden increases in intracranial pressure from obstructive hydrocephalus, brain tumor, and subdural hematoma may precipitate severe hypertension, as may acute lead encephalopathy in children. All these conditions also cause papilledema and convulsions. A careful history and attention to the condition of the retinal arterioles, heart size, and the associated conditions in which hypertensive encephalopathy develops will be valuable in differential diagnosis.

Hypertensive encephalopathy is a medical emergency. Its treatment consists of the prompt lowering of the blood pressure over 30 to 60 minutes, taking great care to avoid hypotensive levels. The drug of choice is parenteral sodium nitroprusside. Hypercapnia can aggravate or precipitate hypertensive encephalopathy and is to be avoided. Both the (commonly) elevated intracranial pressure and seizures respond favorably to the lowering of systemic pressure. Convulsions may be additionally treated with intravenous diazepam, 10 to 20 mg, repeated every 30 minutes if need be until the seizures stop, taking care not to suppress respirations. The maximal dosage should be kept between 100 and 150 mg in 24 hours. An alternative is to give phenytoin (Dilantin) through a duodenal tube or intravenously in a dose of 0.5 to 1 gram per day, although that drug is less useful for immediately terminating seizures. Oral phenytoin, 300 mg daily, can be given prophylactically for a few weeks after the acute stage has passed.

The long-term prognosis of the patient with hypertensive encephalopathy is good provided that the blood pressure is manageable, that other organs are not in end-stage failure, and that the cause of the hypertension is remediable. Strict, continuing supervision and regulation of the blood pressure are mandatory. Hydrochlorothiazide, beta-blockers, and alpha-methyldopa, alone or in combination, are usually the most effective drugs.

Barnett HJM: Heart in ischemic stroke—a changing emphasis. Neurol Clin 1:291, 1983. *A description of the traditional and the more recently recognized cardiac sources for cerebral ischemia.*

Barnett HJM, and the EC/IC Bypass Study Group: Failure of extracranial-intracranial arterial bypass to reduce the risk of ischemic stroke. N Engl J Med 313:1191, 1985. *An already classic study evaluating a form of surgical reconstructive therapy in 1377 patients meticulously followed and showing no advantage of the treatment.*

Bousser MG, Eschwege E, Haguenau M, et al.: "AICLA" controlled trial of aspirin and dipyridamole in the secondary prevention of athero-thrombotic cerebral ischemia. Stroke 14:5, 1983. *The second large controlled trial of aspirin in stroke prevention, demonstrating a 50 per cent risk-reduction in stroke for both sexes.*

Brice JG, Dowsett DJ, Lowe RD: Haemodynamic effects of carotid artery stenosis. Br Med J 2:1363, 1964. *A landmark study which indicates that a residual lumen of the carotid artery greater than 2 mm does not compromise blood flow or produce a pressure gradient.*

Canadian Cooperative Study Group: A randomized trial of aspirin and sulfinpyrazone in threatened stroke. N Engl J Med 299:35, 1978. *The controlled trial which indicated the efficacy of aspirin in stroke prevention in males.*

Cerebral Embolism Task Force: Cardiogenic brain embolism. Arch Neurol 43:71, 1986. *A review of natural history, diagnosis, prevention and treatment of cardioembolic stroke.*

Chester EM, Dimitris P, Agamanolis DP, et al.: Hypertensive encephalopathy: A clinicopathologic study of 20 cases. Neurology 28:928, 1978. *A detailed study of the cerebral and systemic vascular changes found in patients dying with longstanding hypertension culminating in renal failure.*

Corrin LS, Sandok BA, Houser OW: Cerebral ischemic events in patients with carotid artery fibromuscular dysplasia. Arch Neurol 38:616, 1981. *A natural history study of patients with fibromuscular dysplasia indicative of a reasonably benign prognosis.*

Hypertension Detection and Follow-Up Program Cooperative Group: Five-year findings of the hypertension detection and follow-up program. 1. Reduction in mortality of persons with high blood pressure including mild hypertension. JAMA 242:2562, 1979. *The importance of mild to severe untreated hypertension carefully assessed in the best study to date.*

Mohr JP, Caplan LR, Melski JW, et al.: The Harvard cooperative stroke registry: A prospective registry. Neurology 28:754, 1978. *The report of a prospective registry to determine the incidence of the varieties of stroke in the Boston Hospitals.*

Mokri B, Sundt TM, Houser ON, et al.: Spontaneous dissection of the cervical internal carotid artery. Ann Neurol 19:126, 1986. *Describes clinical and angiographic manifestations of this disorder, often associated with good prognosis.*

Ross Russell RW: How does blood pressure cause stroke? Lancet 2:1283, 1975. *A thoughtful commentary on the modern concepts of the pathogenesis of the arteriolar reaction in the cerebral complications of hypertension.*

Sherman DG, Hart RG, Easton JD: Abrupt change in head position and cerebral infarction. Stroke 12:2, 1981. *An updated report on the risk of vertebral artery lesions producing stroke from neck manipulation.*

Soltero I, Liu K, Cooper R, et al.: Trends in mortality from cerebrovascular diseases in the United States, 1960 to 1975. Stroke 9:549, 1978. *A discussion of the declining incidence of stroke and the probable factors responsible for the phenomenon.*

Whisnant JP, Wiebers DD: Clinical epidemiology of transient cerebral ischemic attacks (TIA) in the anterior and posterior cerebral circulation. *In* Sundt TM (ed.): Occlusive Cerebrovascular Disease: Diagnosis and Surgical Management. Philadelphia, PA, WB Saunders Company, 1987.

480 SPONTANEOUS INTRACRANIAL HEMORRHAGE

H. J. M. Barnett

Spontaneous intracranial hemorrhage constitutes approximately 15 per cent of acute cerebrovascular disorders, usually with drastic consequences, due to an abrupt increase in the volume of the intracranial contents. Perhaps a majority of patients lose consciousness at least briefly, and many die without recovering awareness. The anatomic locations of the bleeding importantly influence the clinical picture, and these fall into the following general categories: (1) *Subarachnoid hemorrhage* for the most part results from bleeding of surface arteries, mostly at the base of the brain, and is limited to the space between the pial and the arachnoid membranes which contains the cerebrospinal fluid. (2) *Intracerebral hemorrhage* results from rupture of vessels within the brain substance. (3) Surface bleeding may extend into the brain, producing a combined *subarachnoid and intracerebral hemorrhage*. (4) *Intraventricular hemorrhage* results from the extension of intracerebral hemorrhage or subarachnoid blood into the ventricles. Traumatic epidural, subdural and intraparenchymal hemorrhage are discussed in Chapter 496.

ETIOLOGY. Bleeding from aneurysms of arteries composing the circle of Willis and bleeding from arterioles damaged by hypertension or arteriosclerosis are the two most common causes of intracranial hemorrhage. Table 480–1 lists the usual causes of spontaneous intracranial hemorrhage.

Arterial Aneurysms. "BERRY" ANEURYSMS. These round or saccular dilatations, characteristically found at arterial bifurcations on the circle of Willis and its major branches or connections, account for 80 to 90 per cent of all intracranial aneurysms. The pathogenesis of the berry aneurysm is controversial. The observation that the frequency of medial defects increases with age suggests that berry aneurysms are acquired rather than congenital. Muscle and elastic tissue defects in the media are subjected to the physical effects of pulsatile arterial pressure aggravated by turbulence in the circulation through the aneurysm. The result is a gradual

TABLE 480–1. CAUSES OF SPONTANEOUS INTRACRANIAL HEMORRHAGE

1. Arterial aneurysms
   a. "Berry" aneurysm
   b. Fusiform aneurysm
   c. Mycotic aneurysm
   d. Aneurysm with vasculitis
2. Cerebrovascular malformations
3. Hypertensive-atherosclerotic hemorrhage
4. Hemorrhage into brain tumor
5. Systemic bleeding diatheses
6. Hemorrhage with vasculopathies
7. Hemorrhage with intracranial venous infarction

distention and thinning of the weakened segment until the wall is no longer able to contain the blood under arterial pressure. In a natural history study of unruptured intracranial aneurysms a diameter greater than or equal to 1 cm was the single variable predictive of subsequent rupture. Some aneurysms reach a size of 2 to 3 cm or more ("giant aneurysm") before rupturing, or, with calcific hardening of the wall never rupture at all, acting rather as mass lesions compressing adjacent structures. Atheromatous plaques form in some aneurysms and may contribute to weakening of the wall. Larger aneurysms develop thrombi which may calcify. This process thickens the wall and may account for the growth of some to giant size without rupture.

Although hypertension is not a significant risk factor for aneurysmal subarachnoid hemorrhage, aneurysms have been known to rupture under conditions associated with sudden rise in blood pressure, including severe emotional excitement and physical exertion (e.g., athletic competitions or coitus). Associated medical conditions include coarctation of the aorta, polycystic renal disease, connective tissue disorders (Marfan's, Ehlers-Danlos), arteriovenous malformation, and fibromuscular dysplasia.

Intracranial aneurysms occur in all age groups but most commonly rupture in the fifth, sixth, and seventh decades. They are more common in women than in men (3:2). Approximately 85 per cent of berry aneurysms develop in the anterior part of the circle of Willis derived from the internal carotid artery and its major branches (Fig. 480–1). The most common site is at the origin of the posterior communicating artery from the internal carotid artery, followed in frequency by the middle cerebral and the anterior communicating arteries. Fifteen per cent of aneurysms arise from the vertebral or basilar arteries and their branches. Aneurysms are multiple in 15 to 20 per cent of patients.

FUSIFORM ANEURYSMS. These are spindle-shaped dilatations of arteriosclerotic origin arising along the course of the large arteries. They occur most commonly on the basilar artery and less frequently on the carotid artery. Small fusiform aneurysms are asymptomatic, but they can enlarge sufficiently to interfere with the function of surrounding structures, including the cranial nerves at the base of the brain; some compress the brain stem, others mimic cerebellopontine angle tumors, and still others simulate pituitary and suprasellar neoplasms. The underlying arteriosclerotic disease may be associated with ischemic attacks or infarction in the territory supplied by the

artery and its branches. Occasionally embolism may result from thrombi forming within a large fusiform aneurysm. Fusiform aneurysm rupture, although less frequent than that of saccular aneurysms, is more often fatal since it is not amenable to direct surgical management. Extreme basilar-artery arteriosclerotic elongation (ectasia) may be the precursor to a fusiform aneurysm. Rarely, ectasia or fusiform basilar aneurysm has been described in association with communicating hydrocephalus in which the dilated tip of the elongated basilar artery interferes with the normal cerebrospinal fluid outflow from the third ventricle and along the subarachnoid space.

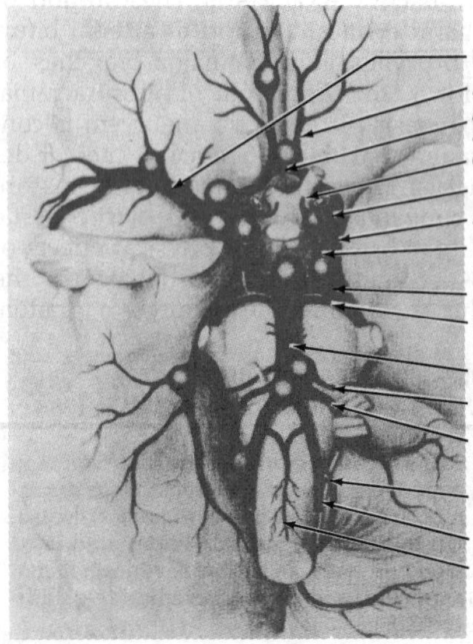

MYCOTIC ANEURYSMS. Septic emboli from acute and subacute bacterial endocarditis result in arterial necrosis, which may lead to thrombosis or aneurysm formation at the site of lodgment. Such aneurysms characteristically arise along the distal middle and anterior cerebral arterial branches, rather than at the base, and are frequently multiple.

ANEURYSMS WITH VASCULITIS. A rare form of aneurysm is associated with collagen vascular disease, usually polyarteritis nodosa. Recently a vasculitis has been described in intravenous-drug users, particularly with amphetamine abusers. The resultant arteriopathy produces irregularly dilated segments, some of which may rupture producing subarachnoid and intracerebral hemorrhage.

Cerebrovascular Malformations. Vascular malformations within and on the surface of the brain parenchyma constitute about 7 per cent of cases with subarachnoid hemorrhage. Four varieties are recognized: capillary telangiectasia, cavernous angioma, venous angioma, and arteriovenous malformation (AVM). Brain-stem capillary telangiectasiae, which occasionally bleed, are most commonly incidental postmortem findings. Venous angiomas are often associated with the Sturge-Weber syndrome. They occur twice as often in females as in males, and present most commonly with seizures, less often, with hemorrhage . Cavernous angiomas are the cause of many examples of cryptic intracerebral hemorrhage—*cryptic* since the vessels are not outlined by angiography. These lesions may be discovered at postmortem examination in the subcortical white matter or during the evacuation of a hematoma.

AVMs more often produce symptoms than the other types of cerebral vascular malformations. They consist of tangled, interconnected networks of vessels in which arterial blood passes directly to the draining veins without intervening capillaries. They range in size from barely detectable lesions to networks large enough to occupy an entire lobe or hemisphere. They occasionally involve the cerebellum and brain stem. AVMs tend to be supplied by more than one parent artery, and the draining veins may be as large as 1 cm in diameter. The frequency of AVM rupture is uncertain, but small bleeds occur in over 50 per cent of cases. Others declare themselves by producing recurrent unilateral migraine headaches, epileptic seizures, or a progressive neurologic defect. Once detected, most AVM's do not increase much in size. Enlargement is associated with small hemorrhage or with thrombosis of draining veins. Owing possibly to blood shunting into the malformation, progressive neurologic disability may occur either on a compressive basis or away from the underlying brain ("intracranial steal").

Hypertensive-Arteriosclerotic Hemorrhage. At least two thirds of parenchymatous cerebral hemorrhages in adults are accompanied by clinical or pathologic evidence of systemic hypertensive vascular disease. Most of the remainder occur in subjects showing atherosclerotic vascular changes, suggesting a common initiating arterial pathology in atherothrombotic and hypertensive vasculopathies. The ready availability of CT scanning has facilitated the diagnosis of small intracerebral hemorrhages that were previously misdiagnosed as ischemic lesions, or overlooked entirely.

Hemorrhage into Brain Tumor. Hemorrhage of apoplectic

Middle cerebral artery
Anterior cerebral artery
Anterior communicating artery
Ophthalmic artery
Internal carotid artery
Anterior choroidal artery
Posterior communicating artery
Posterior cerebral artery
Superior cerebellar artery
Basilar artery
Internal auditory artery
Anterior inferior cerebellar artery
Posterior inferior cerebellar artery
Vertebral artery
Anterior spinal artery

FIGURE 480–1. The common sites for berry aneurysms to develop at the bifurcation of arteries on the undersurface of the brain.

onset is most common in rapidly growing malignant gliomas and very vascular secondary tumors (e.g., melanotic, renal, thyroid, chorionic, and bronchogenic carcinoma). Bleeding complicates the clinical course in some benign brain tumors, including meningioma and pituitary adenoma, as well as some slowly growing gliomas, including oligodendroglioma.

Systemic Bleeding Diatheses. Intracerebral hemorrhage can complicate leukemia, aplastic anemia, thrombocytopenic purpura, hemophilia, and a variety of less common bleeding diseases. Usually there is systemic evidence of bleeding. The intracerebral hemorrhage involves more locations than is usual in hypertensive hemorrhage, including superficial cortical areas. Multiple hemorrhages may occur, particularly in thrombotic thrombocytopenic purpura and with the consumption coagulopathies. Thrombotic infarction may accompany the hemorrhagic tendency in some instances. The primary process may lie in the vessel wall rather than in the circulating blood.

Anticoagulant therapy can be complicated by intracerebral-traumatic as well as extradural, subdural, and subarachnoid hemorrhage. When the intracerebral hematomas are in the usual locations for hypertensive hemorrhages, the relation to the anticoagulation will be uncertain, possibly incidental. By contrast, subcortical location of a hematoma is uncommon in spontaneous hypertensive hemorrhage. Extension through the pia into the subarachnoid space is common in hematoma complicating anticoagulation therapy and uncommon with spontaneous hypertension.

Hemorrhage with Vasculopathies. Polyarteritis nodosa is the most significant nonarteriosclerotic degenerative disease of arteries producing intracerebral hemorrhage. The mechanisms include aneurysmal dilatation and necrotic arterial disruption. Cerebral hemorrhage with systemic lupus erythematosus is usually secondary to accompanying hypertension. Congophilic (amyloid) angiopathy, a special senile and presenile vasculopathy, is usually independent of systemic amyloidosis but is almost always coexistent with senile plaques in the brain. The usual presentation is a sudden apoplexy with signs of cerebral hemorrhage in a patient with a recent history of progressing dementia. Such hemorrhages are often multiple and occupy posterior white matter, sites not common in hypertensive intracerebral hemorrhage. "Lobar" (white matter) hematomas in older patients are more often associated with this vascular lesion than with any other pathologic entity. In patients over 60 years of age, the development of more than one lobar hematoma within days or weeks of the initial hemorrhage strongly suggests the diagnosis of congophilic angiopathy. This amyloid degeneration of the cerebral arterioles is six times more common in women than men and an infrequent but important cause of "multi-infarct dementia." Drug abuse, particularly the use of amphetamines, is associated with intracerebral hemorrhage. These hemorrhages are frontal, occasionally into the basal ganglia, may extend into the subarachnoid space or the ventricles, and are associated with drug-related vasculitis.

Hemorrhage with Intracranial Venous Infarction. This presents most commonly in association with the complex findings described for septic or nonseptic lateral, sagittal, and cavernous sinus thrombosis (see Ch. 481). The finding of blood in cerebrospinal fluid coupled with seizures at the onset sometimes makes it difficult to distinguish between this condition and an aneurysm rupture on clinical examination alone.

PATHOLOGIC CONSEQUENCES OF ANEURYSM RUPTURE. Aneurysms lie within the subarachnoid space, and their rupture introduces blood into this space under arterial pressure. The aneurysmal bleeding may be minimal and emerge through a very small tear in the sac or alternatively, can bleed sufficiently to fill the basal cisterns, or to produce a hematoma that distorts the subarachnoid space and the overlying brain. Such hemorrhages can be under sufficient pressure to cause reflux into the fourth ventricle through the

foramina of Magendie and Luschka and to fill and distend the ventricles with blood. Also, aneurysms usually send their jet of blood directly into the brain parenchyma. Anterior communicating artery aneurysms lying adjacent to the medial surface of the frontal lobes, and middle cerebral artery aneurysms within the sylvian fissure adjacent to the frontal and temporal lobes, are particularly prone to rupture into the brain. Anterior communicating aneurysms may rupture into both frontal lobes. Basilar artery aneurysms may rupture into the diencephalon or midbrain. Such intracerebral hemorrhages commonly extend through the brain substance, with secondary intraventricular rupture.

Aneurysm rupture may include hemorrhage into the adjacent cranial nerves. The most commonly involved is the third, owing to rupture or compression of an aneurysm at the point of origin of the posterior communicating artery from the internal carotid artery. Less often, third nerve palsy is due to a basilar artery aneurysm. The optic nerve commonly is involved with ophthalmic artery aneurysms, and carotid aneurysms in the cavernous sinus involve the three cranial nerves acting on the muscles of the eye (III, IV, VI) and the first division of the trigeminal nerve. The distortions resulting from increased intracranial pressure commonly result in unilateral or bilateral sixth nerve palsies. Most cranial nerve palsies that develop in patients with aneurysm result from bleeding in the nerve and not from compression of the nerve by the aneurysm. Large aneurysms, being as space-occupying lesions, may damage cranial nerves progressively by compression.

Adherence of the dome of the aneurysm to the arachnoid may result in rupture into the subdural space; a substantial quantity of subdural blood is present at postmortem examination in approximately 10 per cent of patients who die of ruptured aneurysm. Rarely, such a subdural hematoma occurs with little or no subarachnoid bleeding.

Rupture of an aneurysm produces a sudden increase in the intracranial pressure by several mechanisms. First, an expanding hematoma, whether intracerebral, intraventricular, subdural, or subarachnoid, represents an abruptly enlarging space-occupying lesion. Also, blood in the basal cistern interrupts the natural flow of cerebrospinal fluid. Finally, if the pacchionian granulations become distended with blood, spinal fluid reabsorption is impeded. Papilledema and subhyaloid hemorrhage in the retina follow, with coma, deterioration of brain-stem function, and secondary midbrain hemorrhages.

As a late sequel to subarachnoid hemorrhage, hydrocephalus may develop or persist. The cerebrospinal fluid pressure measurements, although moderately elevated, tend to approach normal—an example of so-called "normal-pressure" hydrocephalus. Some examples of this complication are known to be sequelae to a fibrosing reaction in the basal cisterns, in particular the cisterna ambiens, producing, in effect, an extraventricular obstructive phenomenon. Others may be associated with ventricular ependymal damage and a change in the hydrodynamics of cerebrospinal fluid circulation, with accumulation of interstitial fluid in the subependymal tissue. Both causes create a form of communicating hydrocephalus.

Ischemic infarction of the brain is common in patients with subarachnoid hemorrhage. Cerebral vasospasm, a segmental, often extensive, reactive narrowing of intracranial arteries, develops in more than one third of patients suffering aneurysmal subarachnoid hemorrhage. It has been angiographically demonstrated after 4 to 10 days, causing focal and neurologic deterioration in 20 per cent of individuals. Vasospasm is most marked in the arterial territory adjacent to the bleeding point, correlating also with the presence of blood in the basal cisterns. Vasoactive substances, including prostaglandins, serotonin, catecholamines, and methemoglobin, released by the blood in the subarachnoid space, are believed to precipitate this vasospastic response. Desquamation of the endothelial cells, followed by platelet-fibrin thrombogenesis in the affected arteries, has been described. Edema, necrosis of the media, and intimal proliferation have been reported as sequelae to the initial chemically induced vasospasm.

CLINICAL FEATURES OF SUBARACHNOID HEMORRHAGE. The location of the bleeding is the main determinant in the clinical presentation: aneurysms that rupture entirely into the subarachnoid space present with features of meningeal irritation or transiently increased intracranial pressure; with the formation of an intracerebral hematoma or with intraventricular rupture more devastating signs develop. Direct involvement of adjacent cranial nerves produces specific focal features (e.g., a third nerve palsy with posterior communicating and basilar aneurysms). Vasospasm and obstruction of the cerebrospinal fluid pathways impose new clinical signs. The most common symptom of subarachnoid hemorrhage is the sudden development of a violent headache. At the onset many patients localize the headache frontally or temporally. Soon it becomes occipital, spreads to involve the entire head and neck, and at times radiates down the spine and the backs of the legs. Arterial distortion and injury produce the initial head pain with spreading discomfort owing to increased intracranial pressure and meningeal irritation.

The initial hemorrhage may be minor, a "warning leak" characterized by the sudden development of a headache usually severe but sometimes only moderately intense, with or without associated neck stiffness. This type of headache in an adult not prone to headache may disappear in 2 to 3 days, but its presence demands that subarachnoid hemorrhage be considered. If hemorrhage is suspected, a diagnostic lumbar puncture must be done, since subsequent rupture is often devastating and potentially fatal. The initial hemorrhage often is preceded by no other warning symptoms, but some patients complain of minor neurologic symptoms in the days or weeks prior to the major event. Although emotional excitement and physical exertion are known to precipitate the hemorrhage in some patients, they can occur during sleep.

Brief loss of consciousness or seizures are common at the onset, preceded by an awareness of dizziness or vertigo and by vomiting. Persistent coma usually reflects massive intracerebral or intraventricular bleeding. Recovery of consciousness within minutes is the rule if the bleeding is confined to the subarachnoid space or is localized as a small intracerebral hematoma. The development of brain-stem signs commonly indicates transtentorial compression, but occasionally indicates a posterior fossa aneurysm with rupture into the brainstem.

Neck rigidity is the most common physical sign but it may not appear until 12 to 24 hours after onset; if severe bleeding has occurred, it produces retraction of the neck into hyperextension. Small, round hemorrhages observable by funduscopic examination over or near the optic nerve head have a "subhyaloid" or preretinal location and may be associated with the early development of papilledema. These changes reflect the fact that the optic nerve sheath is surrounded by an extension of the subarachnoid space and an abrupt rise in the cerebrospinal fluid pressure interferes with venous return from the retina.

When lateralizing signs, including hemiplegia, develop at the beginning or within a few hours, an intracerebral hematoma, a large subdural hematoma, or occasionally a subarachnoid hematoma is the usual cause. If such signs develop after several days without a fresh and violent headache, one suspects the presence of vasospasm producing ischemia and infarction. Delirium is a common and nonspecific symptom with subarachnoid hemorrhage; gradual deterioration of consciousness after 3 or 4 days, with or without an accompanying worsening of pre-existing neurologic deficits, suggests the development of hydrocephalus with increasing intracranial pressure.

Systemic signs include low-grade fever, glycosuria, albuminuria, and a peripheral white blood cell count up to 15,000. A massive outpouring of systemic catecholamines may cause multifocal myocardial micronecrosis producing ECG abnormalities that simulate the changes of myocardial infarction. An occasional patient with subarachnoid hemorrhage develops acute pulmonary edema. Others develop the syndrome of inappropriate antidiuretic hormone secretion (SIADH), nephrogenic salt wasting, or both.

Little other than the history clinically distinguishes the symptoms of subarachnoid hemorrhage resulting from the rupture of an AVM from those that emanate from a ruptured aneurysm. Intracerebral bleeding is more common with AVMs, however, since most of them lie within the brain. Accordingly, focal neurologic signs and evidence of the sudden development of a mass lesion are frequent accompaniments of a rupture. The presence of an AVM as the cause of subarachnoid hemorrhage is suggested by a history of previous focal seizures, by indolently or slowly stepwise progressing focal neurologic signs, and occasionally by recurrent unilateral throbbing headache suggesting migraine. In addition to meningeal irritation and focal neurologic signs reflecting bleeding, one finds a bruit over the orbit or skull in approximately 40 per cent of patients. Apart from occasional giant aneurysms, bruits are not audible with berry aneurysms.

LABORATORY INVESTIGATION OF SUBARACHNOID HEMORRHAGE. Computed tomographic diagnosis of a subarachnoid and/or parenchymal/ventricular bleed obviates the need for a potentially hazardous lumbar puncture (LP), except in select cases where a high index of clinical suspicion exists despite a negative CT scan. LP should be done if CT scan is unavailable, barring evidence for mass effect. CT evidence of bleeding disappears rapidly after the first week, at which times the examination should be supplemented with a lumbar puncture, seeking discolored fluid, increased cells, or protein.

The distinction between a traumatic LP and a spontaneous subarachnoid bleed is outlined in Table 480–2. Immediately after a subarachnoid hemorrhage, the proportion of white blood cells to red in the cerebrospinal fluid is the same as in the peripheral blood. After 12 hours or more, the white blood count rises owing to the meningeal irritation; in a few days, when the red cells have become crenated, there may be as many as 500 polymorphs and lymphocytes per mm^3, followed a few days later by lymphocytes alone. The protein content slowly increases to as high as 80 to 100 mg per dl; the glucose content declines slightly at most. During the first 2 weeks or so, the cerebrospinal fluid pressure commonly rises to levels of 200 to 300 mm, and at times readings as high as 500 mm will be recorded owing to an associated communicating hydrocephalus.

COMPUTED TOMOGRAPHY. The CT scan is invaluable in the detection of intracerebral, intraventricular, subdural, and (occasionally) subarachnoid hematomas, and has become an essential part of the evaluation of patients with subarachnoid hemorrhage. Immediate CT examination demonstrates blood in the subarachnoid space in about 95 per cent of cases of ruptured aneurysm or AVM. The technique will not demonstrate the high density of blood in cases in which the scan is delayed. Less than 30 per cent of cases of ruptured aneurysms show blood in the subarachnoid space four days after the hemorrhage. The finding of a subarachnoid clot in the CT

TABLE 480–2. "TRAUMATIC TAP" OR SUBARACHNOID HEMORRHAGE?

	"Traumatic Tap"	Spontaneous Subarachnoid Bleed
Xanthochromia	Absent	Onset: 4–6 hours Duration: approx. 6 wks.
Red-cell count (serial tubes)	Decreasing	Constant
Blood clot formation	Rapid	Slower

scan in the first 24 hours following a subarachnoid hemorrhage greatly increases the likelihood that vasospasm will complicate the patient's course. Aneurysms larger than 5 mm in diameter often are directly visualized by this technique, particularly after contrast enhancement. Serial CT studies help determine whether new symptoms are related to rebleeding, ischemia secondary to vasospasm, the development of edema surrounding previous intracerebral bleeding, or hydrocephalus.

ARTERIOGRAPHY. The cerebral angiogram remains the definitive procedure to identify aneurysms and AVMs. The procedure is performed in all cases of subarachnoid hemorrhage that are considered reasonable operative risks or when diagnostic doubt exists. Four-vessel angiography is mandatory for several reasons: 15 per cent of aneurysms occur in the posterior circulation, multiple aneurysms occur in another 15 per cent of patients, and bleeding is due to an AVM in a small but important number of patients. When aneurysms are multiple, the largest and most irregular is usually the source of the hemorrhage. Postoperative angiograms are imperative, again, for several reasons: (1) to ensure the entire base of the aneurysm was clipped, (2) to rule out inadvertent occlusion of perforator branches, particularly in giant aneurysm surgery, (3) to ensure a secure clip in the face of a giant-pulsatile or calcific-walled aneurysm, (4) to identify, at three to seven days, areas of local or diffuse vasospasm.

PROGNOSIS IN SUBARACHNOID HEMORRHAGE. Subarachnoid hemorrhage from ruptured aneurysm carries a grave prognosis. It has been estimated that 28,000 individuals per year in the United States experience a subarachnoid hemorrhage caused by a ruptured aneurysm and that 10,000 die or are disabled from the initial event without referral for treatment, 9,000 die or are disabled despite treatment, and 9,000 survive without major disability. In a 30-year survey of morbidity following aneurysmal subarachnoid hemorrhage conducted at Rochester, Minnesota, only 42 per cent of patients survived for as long as 30 days. Only 39 per cent of patients survived for six months, and of these, 25 per cent were disabled. Primary factors affecting survival following subarachnoid hemorrhage are the clinical grade of the patient and the duration of time from bleed onset to patient presentation for medical attention. Recurrence is most likely in the first two weeks after the initial bleed. Long-term studies of prognosis indicate that in patients who survive six months after the subarachnoid hemorrhage, rebleeding occurs at a rate of 3.5 to 4 per cent per year, with a mortality approaching 65 per cent.

The prognosis for bleeding from AVMs is better than that for aneurysm. Initial mortality is 10 per cent, with rebleeding in approximately 20 per cent at a rate for fatal recurrence of 1 per cent per year in one major series followed for 35 years. There is a slight increase in mortality for recurrent compared with initial bleeding. Neurologic disability in the patients who have bled is higher than in surviving aneurysm patients because of the usual intracerebral location of the malformations.

TREATMENT OF BERRY ANEURYSM. The goal of aneurysm treatment is to prevent further rupture of the aneurysm while maintaining normal cerebral perfusion. The logical approach to ruptured aneurysm is to exclude the thin-walled sac from the arterial circulation while maintaining the normal patency of the parent and adjacent branch vessels. This is best accomplished by surgically placing a small metal clip or ligature across the neck of the sac. Unfortunately, it has proved to be hazardous to proceed to immediate or emergency surgery following subarachnoid hemorrhage. At this point in time the brain is bruised and swollen, the normal arterial autoregulation is impaired, and surgical manipulation may hasten and aggravate the evolution of vasospasm. Accordingly, many surgeons delay eight to ten days before performing craniotomy, meanwhile reducing the patient's risk of

rebleeding by the judicious control of blood pressure and, sometimes, the giving of antifibrinolytic agents. Collaborative investigation is under way in an effort to identify patients for whom early operation may be a better approach. If the aneurysm cannot be directly obliterated, surgical ligation of a proximal vessel may be effective in reducing the risk of recurrent hemorrhage by reducing the pressure and turbulence within the sac. In the anterior circulation aneurysm, where the common or the internal carotid artery or one of the major intracranial branches must be ligated, some surgeons employ a preliminary superficial temporal to middle cerebral artery anastomosis to protect against the ischemic infarction that might otherwise develop.

Recent advances in technique, including the development of the operating microscope, improved angiography, the CT scan, improved anesthesia, controlled hypotension, and the modern management of vasospasm, have reduced the morbidity and mortality of patients considered appropriate for surgery. Nevertheless, many patients die first or never become suitable candidates for surgery so that aneurysmal subarachnoid hemorrhage retains a distressingly high morbidity and mortality. The risk of dying in the first eight weeks after rupture remains at 40 per cent. The following points are important in deciding on the management of these patients:

1. The best results from direct clipping of the neck of an aneurysm are obtained in patients who have no focal neurologic signs, have had no evidence of focal bleeding for seven to ten days, and have no evidence of vasospasm in an arteriogram performed immediately prior to surgery. Unfortunately by this time about 20 per cent of hospitalized patients have died or become disabled by rebleeding, infarction, or other complications.

2. A patient deteriorating from a hematoma or hydrocephalus may require urgent surgery to remove the mass and reduce the raised intracranial pressure. Usually the aneurysm will be dealt with at the same time. However, patients already in stupor or coma, or with major neurologic deficits, rarely do well with surgical treatment.

3. The presence of vasospasm requires delay of surgery until the spasm disappears or it is apparent that it is causing no further neurologic worsening. Blood volume expanders such as albumin or dextran with crystalloid are recommended to treat patients with evidence of spasm so as to improve intracranial blood flow.

4. During the period of delay prior to surgery careful pharmacologic control of the blood pressure and complete rest in a quiet environment must be sought. The use of epsilon-aminocaproic acid,* an inhibitor of fibrinolysis, administered in a dosage of 30 to 40 grams per day intravenously is controversial but believed by some to reduce the chance of rebleeding.

5. Occasional patients develop SIADH. Fluid and electrolyte intake should be monitored appropriately. The commonest electrolyte imbalance is the result not of excess antidiuretic hormone output but of excessive administration of 5 per cent dextrose solutions, causing iatrogenic hyponatremia.

6. Patients with subarachnoid hemorrhage are best treated in centers possessing experienced, collaborating teams of neurologists, neurosurgeons, and radiologists rather than by inexperienced and occasional operators. In the hands of skilled surgeons most aneurysms can be dealt with successfully, provided that the complications of vasospasm, intracerebral hemorrhage, hydrocephalus, or continuing comatose states can be prevented.

7. Giant aneurysms rebleed in 30 per cent of cases. Removal is more hazardous than with berry aneurysms even in the hands of skilled and experienced surgeons. However, no other treatment can assuredly prevent progressive and disabling neurologic signs or fatal hemorrhage.

---

*This use is not listed in the manufacturer's directive.

TREATMENT OF ARTERIOVENOUS MALFORMATION. Large unrupted AVMs, especially those in an area where a surgical approach might damage vital neurologic function, should not be removed. Some malformations can be dissected out and removed. Those located in the frontal or occipital poles can sometimes be safely excised by lobectomy. Ligation of the feeding vessels coupled with balloon catheter embolization and the injection of plastic polymers into anomalous vessels is being carried out in a few centers. Serious complications can occur, and its indications are regarded as uncertain and its value as unproved.

PATHOLOGY OF SPONTANEOUS HYPERTENSIVE-ARTERIOSCLEROTIC INTRACEREBRAL HEMORRHAGE. Arteriolar hypertensive disease is associated with five main regions of intracerebral hemorrhage in order of decreasing frequency: external capsule-putamen, internal capsule-thalamus, central pons, cerebellum, and subcortical white matter–centrum ovale. When older patients without hypertension exhibit hemorrhage in the centrum ovale, the possibility must be considered that the hematoma is the result of amyloid angiopathy.

Hypertension in many patients produces its most devastating effects on the arterioles. Those of the capsular and ganglionic (lenticulostriate) branches of the middle and posterior cerebral arteries, those supplying the central pontine structures (penetrating branches of the basilar artery), and those lying in the central cerebellum are the sites of predilection for the characteristic arteriolar changes. These distinct changes affect the small intracerebral arteries 50 to 150 μm in diameter. Microaneurysms (Charcot-Bouchard aneurysms) form with loss of lining endothelium, media, and elastic tissue, and all are replaced by fibrous tissue. Fibrin and fat constitute the hyaline tissue within the walls. The penetrating arteries subject to these changes are peculiar in that they do not divide into smaller branches, and the suggestion has been made that they are more vulnerable to the direct transmission of marked fluctuations of blood pressure. These same penetrating small arteries develop necrotic degeneration leading to rupture in some hypertensive patients, thrombosis and lacunar infarction in others.

Hypertensive-arteriosclerotic intracerebral hemorrhages tend to be catastrophic despite their origin from small arterioles. It is postulated that one arteriole ruptures, producing a small hemorrhage, and that this in turn compresses surrounding tissues leading to necrotic degeneration of adjacent arterioles. Hemorrhages in the cerebral hemisphere tend to dissect along fiber pathways and rupture into the ventricles. Relatively few extend directly into the subarachnoid space, although secondary drainage into the subarachnoid space from the ventricles is common. Pontine and cerebellar hemorrhages extend into the subarachnoid space either by direct extension or indirectly through the fourth ventricle. Massive intracerebral hemorrhage often shifts the brain tissue under the falx or downward through the tentorium, leading to secondary brainstem hemorrhage. Many small hemorrhages remain circumscribed but may be associated with extensive surrounding edema.

CLINICAL MANIFESTATIONS OF SPONTANEOUS INTRACEREBRAL HEMORRHAGE (Fig. 480–2). Intracranial bleeding develops abruptly and evolves over a period of minutes to hours. The ictus usually occurs while the patient is awake and active as compared to thrombotic obstructions, which more commonly occur during sleep. With a typical onset the patient cries out with the intensity of head pain or complains of distressing dizziness. Most will have a history of hypertension, and with the onset of bleeding the blood

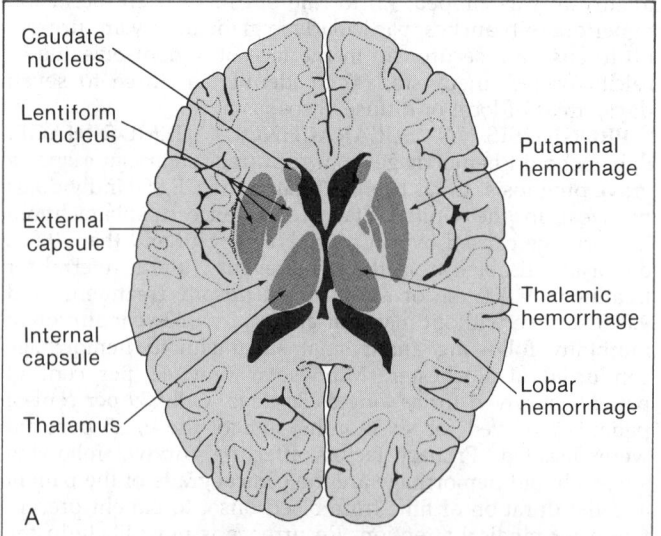

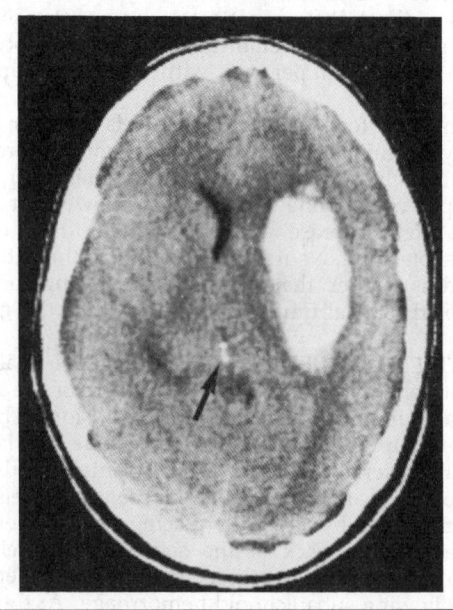

FIGURE 480–3. *A,* A horizontal section through the cerebral hemispheres illustrating thalamic, putaminal, and lobar hemorrhages. *B,* CT scan showing a putaminal hemorrhage. The ipsilateral lateral ventricle is obliterated by the mass effect and some blood is visible in the third ventricle (*arrow*).

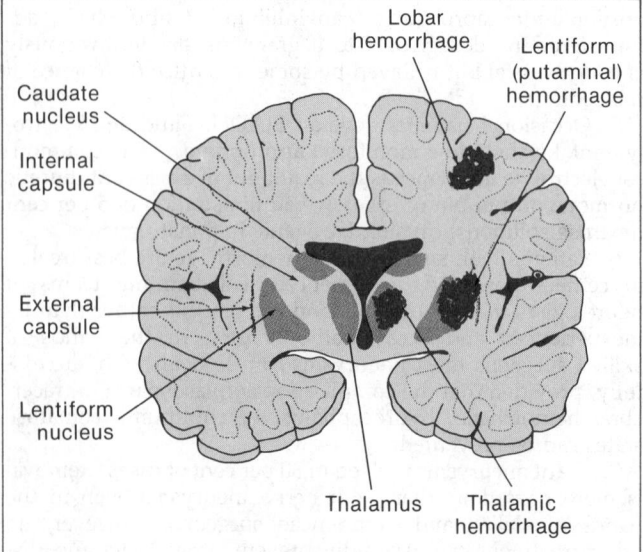

FIGURE 480–2. A coronal section through the cerebral hemispheres illustrating thalamic, putaminal, and lobar subcortical hemorrhages.

pressure can rise to excessively high levels. Cardiomegaly is common, and retinal arteriolar changes, although not always impressive, can be observed within minutes to hours; 75 per cent of patients with a large hemorrhage (greater than 2 to 3 cm diameter by CT scan) will lose consciousness (Fig. 480–3). The associated physical findings depend on the size and site of the bleeding.

External Capsular–Putaminal Hemorrhage. Affected patients are likely to lose consciousness within minutes to hours and quickly develop evidence of hemiplegia. Smaller lesions may produce drowsiness without loss of awareness and the rapid evolution of a hemiplegic stroke. Conjugate deviation of the eyes to the side opposite the paretic limbs is common; deviation toward the paralysis occasionally reflects the irritative effects of the blood. Larger lesions compress the upper brain stem so that coma deepens, with dilated and fixed pupils, bilateral motor hypertonus, Babinski signs, and intermittent or irregular respirations.

Internal Capsular–Thalamic Hemorrhage. The onset is often not distinguishable from the more laterally located hemorrhage described above. Some patients will be aware of sensory disturbances. A homonymous hemianopia may be detected because of the involvement of the optic radiation in the posterior limb of the internal capsule. The medial location of this hemorrhage and its compression of the tectal-midbrain area can produce a variety of conjugate gaze palsies, including defective vertical and lateral gaze, fixed downward deviation of the eyes, unequal pupils briefly nonreactive to light, skew deviation, and retraction nystagmus.

Pontine Hemorrhage (Fig. 480–4*A*). Coma, accompanied by quadriplegia, decerebrate rigidity, and breathing irregularities, often occurs at onset. The usual oculomotor sign is the finding of tiny pupils that are reactive to light; oculovestibular responses rapidly disappear. Most patients die after a few hours or days, although CT scanning has shown a larger number of nonfatal lesions than were previously recognized. Most who survive are quadriparetic and severely disabled.

Cerebellar Hemorrhage (Fig. 480–4*B*). The clinical picture begins with sudden occipital headache, diplopia, and incoordination. Early difficulty is experienced with stance and gait without prominent lateralizing ataxic signs. Vertigo is uncommon. The development is not as rapid as in pontine hemorrhage and usually evolves over several hours. Sixth nerve or conjugate lateral gaze palsies are common eye signs, but ocular bobbing and skew deviation can ensue, as can facial weakness, dysarthria, and dysphagia.

Progressive worsening can occur either from enlargement of the hematoma and edema in surrounding tissue, producing pressure on the brain stem, or from obstruction by the mass of the fourth ventricle, leading to a subacute hydrocephalus with equally serious implications. Recognition of the condition is crucial, since surgical treatment can be life-saving, as noted below.

Hemorrhage in Subcortical White Matter. A small number of intracerebral hemorrhages in hypertensive individuals occur in less vital areas of the brain, generally in the centrum ovale. Some of these small hematomas can be almost asymptomatic, others can produce the picture of progressing stroke. Many patients remain alert and do not develop evidence of subarachnoid bleeding. Spontaneous recovery with little or no disability is common. CT scans establish the diagnosis.

DIFFERENTIAL DIAGNOSIS OF HYPERTENSIVE HEMORRHAGE. In establishing a clinical suspicion of hypertensive intracerebral hemorrhage, the sudden onset and the evolution over a few minutes to hours are important. Such abrupt onsets also occur, however, with thrombosis and embolism. Headache is the predominant feature at the onset in at least one half of hemorrhages and in less than one fourth of cases of thromboembolism. Vomiting is prominent as an early symptom. Funduscopic examination will indicate reduced arteriolar caliber and, often, periarteriolar hemor-

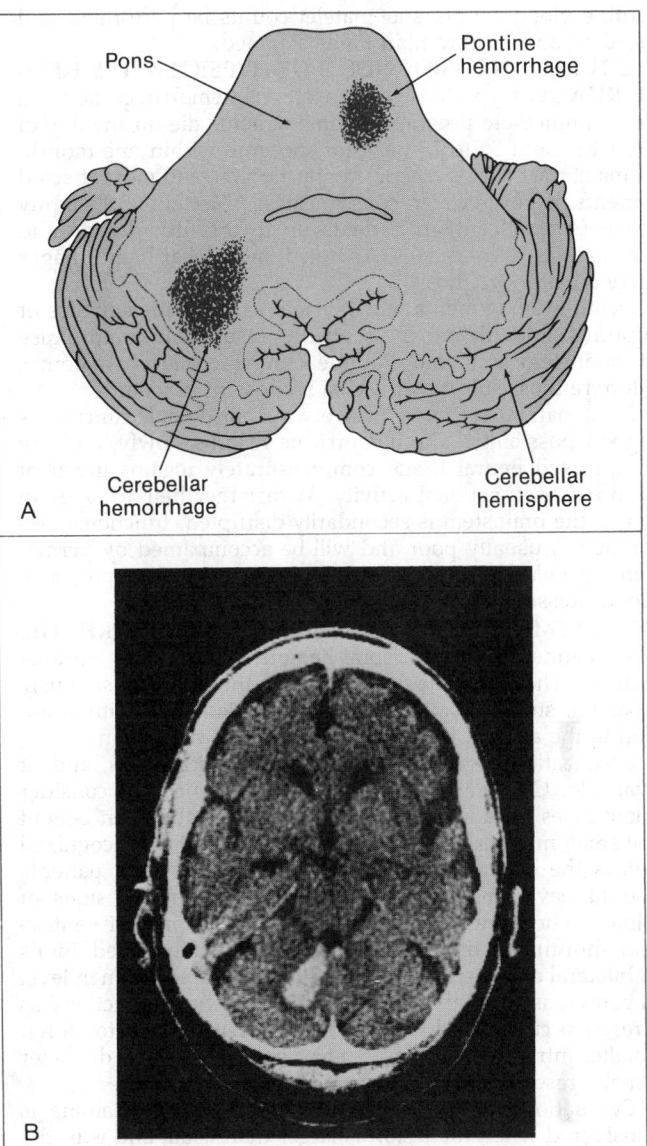

FIGURE 480–4. *A,* A horizontal section through the pons and cerebellum illustrating pontine and cerebellar hemorrhages. *B,* CT scan illustrating a hemorrhage in the right cerebellar hemisphere approaching the midline.

rhages. Nuchal rigidity is common with primary intracerebral as well as subarachnoid hemorrhage. It disappears as the depth of coma increases. Restlessness and vomiting are more common with hemorrhage than with infarction. Convulsions are common with intracerebral hemorrhage, are less frequent with subarachnoid hemorrhage, and are uncommon (<10 per cent) with cerebral infarction. The most important clues to the diagnosis of hypertensive hemorrhage are the explosive onset, an early decline of the level of consciousness, and the detection of meningeal irritation and blood in the cerebrospinal fluid (by CT scanning preferably) with the evidence of a focal lesion in the areas described.

INVESTIGATION OF INTRACEREBRAL HEMORRHAGE. CT will identify the size and exact location of the hemorrhage, as well as the degree of surrounding edema and the amount and location of any distortion of the brain. Lumbar puncture is potentially hazardous and should be avoided. Angiography should be performed only when a surgical lesion such as aneurysm, AVM, or a brain tumor might exist, and in the rare cases in which surgical drainage might be considered. The possibility of a bleeding disorder requires that routine blood counts and platelet counts be performed and bleeding and prothrombin times obtained.

COURSE AND PROGNOSIS OF HYPERTENSIVE HEMORRHAGE. Hypertensive intracerebral hemorrhage carries a grave immediate prognosis. Some patients die on the day of the ictus, and 50 to 75 per cent succumb within one month. Coma at the onset is a poor prognostic sign, and most affected patients never recover consciousness. Mortality is slightly lower (40 per cent) in patients up to the fifth decade and increases in later decades. As noted, most lobar hemorrhages carry a better prognosis.

Death occurs when a hemorrhage reaches sufficient size or ruptures suddenly into the ventricles, resulting in compromise of brainstem function. Pontine and cerebellar hematomas interfere most quickly with vital brain-stem functions.

If the patient survives, recovery of considerable function is a good possibility. The hemorrhage resorbs slowly, and the compressed neural tissue commensurately regains much of its previous functional activity. With larger hemorrhages in which the brainstem is secondarily disrupted, functional restoration is usually poor and will be accompanied by permanent sequelae. Subsequent bleeding is rare with appropriate blood pressure control.

TREATMENT OF INTRACEREBRAL HEMORRHAGE. The treatment of intracerebral hemorrhage is mostly unsatisfactory. The principles involved in the care of seriously disabled, stuporous, or comatose patients apply, with attention to the airway, fluids, electrolytes, and circulation.

Localization of the clot by history, physical signs, and, if available, CT scanning will determine the need to consider some cases for a surgical evacuation. Evacuation can benefit the small number of cases with *cerebellar hematoma* recognized before the onset of coma. If CT is available, such patients should have daily or more frequent CT scans. If signs of clinical worsening progress after admission, prompt ventricular shunting or direct removal of the clot is indicated. Signs of bilateral corticospinal tract dysfunction or reduction in level of consciousness imply that severe brainstem dysfunction has already occurred and that action has been delayed too long. Smaller intracerebellar hematomas less than 3 cm in diameter usually resolve without surgical evacuation.

Evacuation of the occasional supratentorial hematoma is considered when the lesion is larger than usual and is in the subcortical white matter, and the patient is not afflicted with calamitous hemiplegia and aphasia but is showing signs of progression with evidence of incipient deterioration of the level of consciousness. Evacuation of most examples of hypertensive intracerebral hematoma is a futile pursuit and may worsen prognosis since it inevitably removes some potentially recoverable tissue. The most satisfactory recoveries occur in patients who have not been submitted to operation.

Overzealous reduction of blood pressure while attempting to reduce the amount of bleeding may be dangerous. In the hypertensive patient the uninvolved brain requires a higher than normal perfusion pressure because of the intraluminal resistance of the widespread arteriolar disease. A dramatic reduction of blood pressure puts the patient at risk for the development of additional neurologic disability from ischemia. If the patient survives the ictus, gradual restoration of normal blood pressure and its maintenance at normal levels are mandatory.

Drake CG: Giant intracranial aneurysms: Experience with surgical treatment in 174 patients. Clin Neurosurg 26:12, 1979. *A comprehensive statement is provided on the surgical approach to an uncommon but distressing clinical condition.*

Drake CG: The treatment of aneurysms of the posterior circulation. Clin Neurosurg 26:96, 1979. *A review of a very large experience in this area.*

Drake CG: Cerebral arteriovenous malformations: Considerations for and experience with surgical treatment in 166 cases. Clin Neurosurg 26:145, 1979. *A comprehensive review of the clinical features and treatment possibilities.*

Gilbert JJ, Vinters HV: Cerebral amyloid angiopathy: Incidence and complications in the aging brain. I. Cerebral Hemorrhage. Stroke 14:915, 1983. *An update on these subcortical hemorrhages that occur in the aging brain*

Kassell NF, Drake CG: Review of the management of saccular aneurysms. Neurol Clin 1:73, 1983. *A contemporary discussion on the diagnosis of saccular aneurysm, the prevention of rebleeding, the problem of vasospasm, and early versus later surgical intervention.*

Ojemann RG, Heros RC: Spontaneous brain hemorrhage. Stroke 14:468, 1983. *A recent article on spontaneous brain hemorrhage and its management.*

Ott KH, Kase CS, Ojemann RG, et al.: Cerebellar hemorrhage: Diagnosis and treatment. A review of 56 cases. Arch Neurol 31:160, 1974. *A comprehensive review of a condition which must be recognized early for optimal management.*

Ropper AH, Davis KR: Lobar cerebral hemorrhages: Acute clinical syndromes in 26 cases. Ann Neurol 8:141, 1980. *A description of a series of patients with intracerebral hemorrhage located outside the usual locations common to the hypertensive patient. This paper reflects part of the new understanding of brain hemorrhage in normotensive and hypertensive patients diagnosed by CT scanning.*

Shenkin HA, Zavala M: Cerebellar strokes: Mortality, surgical indication and result of ventricular damage. Lancet 2:429, 1982. *A recent summary of the condition.*

Sundt TM Jr, Whisnant JP: Subarachnoid hemorrhage from intracranial aneurysms. Surgical management and natural history of disease. N Engl J Med 299:116, 1978. *A report of the progress being made to improve by surgery on the natural history of subarachnoid hemorrhage. The disease remains serious.*

Wiebers DO, Whisnant JP, O'Fallon WM: The natural history of unruptured intracranial aneurysms. N Engl J Med 304:696, 1981.

SECTION EIGHT / INFECTIOUS AND INFLAMMATORY DISORDERS OF THE NERVOUS SYSTEM

Bacterial Diseases

481 PARAMENINGEAL INFECTIONS

Donald H. Harter

Central nervous system infections caused by pyogenic bacteria other than acute meningitis include brain abscess, collections of pus enclosed within membranes covering the brain and spinal cord (subdural empyema, cerebral epidural abscess, spinal epidural abscess, spinal subdural empyema), and dural sinus infection and thrombosis. Most of these paracranial diseases are secondary to adjacent infections of the ear, sinuses, or bones of the skull or migrate from an infection elsewhere in the body.

The development of CT and magnetic resonance (MR) imaging has greatly improved the early diagnosis and treatment of localized central nervous system infections. The new imaging techniques also permit monitoring of the progress of the infection during treatment, a capability that should further reduce the mortality and morbidity.

BRAIN ABSCESS

DEFINITION. Brain abscess describes encapsulated or free pus in the substance of the brain. Abscesses may vary in size from a microscopic focus of inflammatory cells to a major encapsulated area of necrosis occupying a major part of a cerebral hemisphere. They may be single or multiple and caused by local extension or hematogenous spread.

INCIDENCE. Brain abscess is about one sixth as frequent as bacterial meningitis and consitiutes approximately 0.7 per cent of all neurosurgical operations. The condition occurs two to three times more frequently in males than in females.

PREDISPOSING FACTORS. The causes of brain abscess can be classified into those in which a primary focus of infection can be identified and those in which no extracranial focus can be found. In most cases a primary focus can be found at the time of initial presentation or at necropsy. The site of primary infection can be classified into otolaryngologic causes, metastatic infections, or trauma.

Otogenic Abscess. About 0.5 per cent of patients with acute otitis media and 0.3 per cent of patients with chronic otitis media will develop brain abscess. Middle ear infection, even in the antibiotic era, remains the most common single causative disease. Otogenic brain abscesses are usually located in the temporal lobe or cerebellum.

Infection spreads along the path of bony erosion; final intracranial spread is precipitated by an acute exacerbation of a chronic process. Spread to the posterior fossa may be through the lateral sinus or through the internal ear with erosion of the bony labyrinth and necrosis of the horizontal semicircular canal, oval window, or promontory. Involvement of the posterior fossa occurs quickly once labyrinthine fluid is infected. Alternatively, a cholesteatoma in the mastoid antrum and attic may erode through the antral roof, leading to infection. In cerebellar abscess there is often evidence of retrograde thrombosis from the lateral, petrosal, or superior petrosal venous sinuses. The duration of otorrhea preceding brain abscess caused by middle ear disease may vary from one month to as long as 20 years.

Infection of Paranasal Sinuses. Paranasal sinus infection accounts for about 5 to 10 per cent of all brain abscesses, usually extending directly from the frontal sinus into the anterior part of the frontal lobe. Rarely, infection of the ethmoid sinus can cause a deep temporal lobe abscess in the region of the uncus. Infection may erode the sinus wall and invade the brain directly or may spread by veins communicating with the cavernous sinus or brain.

Trauma to the Face and Skull. Brain abscess secondary to trauma is usually due to an unrepaired dural laceration in association with a compound depressed skull fracture. The abscess is always directly related to the site of injury. Penetrating gunshot wounds are often responsible for brain abscesses. In post-traumatic brain abscess a bone fragment or other foreign body may be found in the devitalized tissue. Sometimes the injury may be seemingly trivial and unsuspected. For example, penetration of the orbital roof and temporal bone by pencil tips has given rise to brain abscess. Brain abscess may also follow otolaryngologic or neurosurgical operations.

Metastatic Brain Abscess and Hematogenous Spread. Hematogenous brain abscesses usually originate from the heart, lungs, or pleura. Less frequently, septic foci in the skin, teeth, abdomen, or surgical wounds may be the origin. The incidence of metastatic abscess is less than that of otogenic or rhinogenic abscess.

The single most important cause of metastatic brain abscess is chronic infection of the pleura or lungs, including bronchiectasis, empyema, and lung abscess. Brain abscesses metastatic from the lung often lie in frontal, parietal, or deep cortical regions but are seldom in the cerebellum. They follow a more chronic course than abscesses of cardiac origin. Metastatic abscess is believed to originate from a transient bacteremia with release of infected material into the pulmonary venous and systemic circulations. A number of these patients have had thoracic surgery.

About 10 per cent of brain abscesses are associated with congenital heart disease. Affected patients often present with the sudden onset of a focal neurologic deficit in a strokelike manner. Paradoxical infected embolism, bacterial endocarditis, and primary thrombosis with secondary bacteremic infection have all been held responsible for the development of brain abscess. The mortality of brain abscess in association with pulmonary or cardiac disease is higher than that of abscess from other causes.

Metastatic brain abscess of pure dental origin is rare. There is often intervening cellulitis, sinusitis, and osteomyelitis of the mandible and base of the skull, permitting direct rather than hematogenous spread. Intrauterine contraceptive devices have been incriminated as an occasional source of metastatic brain abscess.

ETIOLOGY. Comprehensive statements about the bacteriology of brain abscesses are difficult to make because of diversity in the isolation methods used. Many bacteria, notably anaerobic species, have peculiar or particular growth requirements, making them difficult to cultivate. A lack of attention to detail can lead to a failure to isolate the responsible bacteria or microorganisms in as high as 60 per cent of cases. In many instances more than a single bacterial species is isolated from a brain abscess.

For best results a Gram-stained smear should be studied at the time of surgery. Aerobic and anaerobic bacterial and fungal cultures should be planted. Ideally, the bacteriologist should be on hand when the abscess is tapped in the operating room. If this is not possible, the neurosurgical team should know precisely how to inoculate suitable media as soon as the aspirate is available. Aspirated purulent material should be rapidly transported to the bacteriologic laboratory. Blood cultures should also be taken at the time of operation.

The most common microorganisms isolated from brain abscesses are aerobic or anaerobic streptococci. Nontraumatic brain abscess has become largely a disease of streptococci, more particularly of anaerobic or microaerophilic strains. *Bacteroides* and enteric bacteria are still recovered in a number of cases. *S. pneumoniae* is now a rare cause unless the abscess is the sequel to occult cerebrospinal fluid rhinorrhea or occurs in an elderly person in association with pneumococcal pneumonia. Staphylococcal abscesses are usually due to penetrating head trauma or bacteremia. Clostridial infections are posttraumatic. Gram-negative bacilli very rarely occur alone.

Rarely *Actinomyces* and *Nocardia* species may be recovered from an abscess cavity. Actinomycotic brain abscess may be secondary to infection elsewhere, particularly the chest and oropharynx. *Nocardia asteroides* is a rare cause of cerebral abscesses which are often multiple, multilocular, and thick walled. They almost invariably are associated with pulmonary infection. Aspergillosis of the central nervous system, occurring in association with leukemia, lymphoma, aplastic anemia, and other conditions, may produce microabscesses and focal neurologic findings. Cerebral infection with *Candida albicans* can also lead to abscess formation.

PATHOLOGY. Localized inflammatory changes with necrosis and edema, thromboses of vessels, and collections of degenerating leukocytes represent the early response to bacterial invasion. The histologic appearance of brain abscess includes an inner layer of pus surrounding a zone of inflammatory granulation tissue. In the early acute stage, granulation tissue may be absent and the limits of the abscess defined by a zone of infiltration by polymorphonuclear leukocytes and plasma cells. There is often surrounding edema of the white matter.

The acute area of local suppuration is followed in several weeks by encapsulation of the liquefied brain and accumulated pus. As encapsulation proceeds, a layer of granulation tissue merges with surrounding collagenous tissue. Active fibroblasts appear to infiltrate the surrounding brain, and a zone of avascular necrosis forms. The macroscopic appearance of a dormant smooth capsule at the time of excision is not confirmed histologically, because there is active vascular hyperplasia and perivascular cuffing about the capsule. Meninges adjacent to the abscess are often infiltrated by inflammatory cells.

Multiple satellite abscesses may develop and communicate with the principal cavity. Because abscess cavities may spread through the central white matter, they often extend through the ventricular wall, producing meningitis, and may rupture into the cerebral ventricles.

CLINICAL MANIFESTATIONS. Brain abscess may happen at any time of life, but the highest incidence of the disease occurs between the second and fifth decades.

General Features. The symptoms of brain abscess are generally those of a space-occupying intracranial lesion, the specific neurologic changes depending on the anatomic locus of the abscess in the brain. Systemically, the illness may be acute with fever, headache, nausea or vomiting, increasing obtundation, seizures, and localizing neurologic findings. As noted, occasional cases produce a strokelike onset. One should suspect brain abscess in the presence of chronic middle ear disease, congenital heart disease, sinusitis, or bronchiectasis. The diagnosis should also be considered in the presence of other forms of sepsis such as osteomyelitis, surgical wound infections, dental and periodontal disease, and pneumonia. Absence of a focus of infection, however, never excludes the possibility of brain abscess.

Symptoms of acute infection are often lacking unless the focus giving rise to the abscess is still active. Chills and fever at the onset of nervous system invasion may accompany an embolic lesion in the brain secondary to acute endocarditis. The body temperature may be elevated, normal, or subnormal. Approximately one third of patients remain afebrile during their illness.

Increased intracranial pressure usually develops rapidly. Headache, nausea, and vomiting are common early symptoms. Seizures, more often generalized than focal, are present in one quarter to one third of patients. The diagnosis of brain abscess can often be inferred because of past or present evidence of otitis media or sinusitis. Unexplained headache in a child with cyanotic congenital heart disease should be regarded as being due to brain abscess until proved otherwise. Headache may be localized to the side of the abscess, but it is often generalized and increases in severity as the abscess expands. Signs attributable to meningeal irritation may be present.

Increased intracranial pressure may lead to bradycardia, confusion, drowsiness, and stupor. Papilledema may be a relatively late event, but develops eventually in about half of cases. Signs of damage to the third or sixth cranial nerves may reflect an increased intracranial pressure and may not have localizing value. The course of untreated brain abscess is usually fulminating, ending fatally in five to fifteen days. In certain patients, however, the course may be prolonged and incorrectly regarded as a brain tumor until complications arise or a modern imaging device corrects the diagnosis.

LABORATORY DIAGNOSIS. Elevation of the white blood cell count is of limited value, being above 20,000 per cubic millimeter in only about 10 per cent of brain abscess patients. Lumbar puncture is unjustified when brain abscess is suspected, especially if CT scanning is available. If a lumbar puncture is inadvertently performed, cerebrospinal fluid pleocytosis greater than 5 cells per cubic millimeter is found in about two thirds of patients, a protein content greater than 100 mg per deciliter in two fifths, and a cerebrospinal fluid glucose level less than 40 mg per deciliter in about one fifth. Pressure usually is moderately elevated, and the fluid usually is sterile.

Radiographic studies of the skull, including mastoids and sinuses, may disclose evidence of otitic or paranasal sepsis.

CT or MR images give nearly definitive diagnosis, and their application has had a remarkable effect in changing the management and reducing the mortality of brain abscess. The most frequently observed CT appearance is a lucent area surrounded by a faint dense rim with a second lucent zone outside the rim. After intravenous administration of contrast material, dense ring enhancement is seen around an area of low attenuation with a lucent area of edema peripheral to the enhanced ring. Varying degrees of compression or shift of the ventricular system indicate mass effect (Fig. 481–1). The CT scan of patients with suspected brain abscess should be performed with and without contrast enhancement. Occasionally, one observes a patchy, nonuniform enhancement pattern. Ring enhancement is by no means diagnostic of

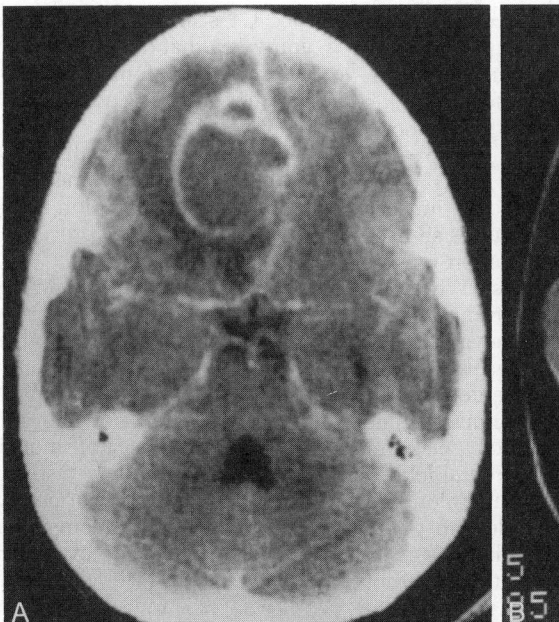 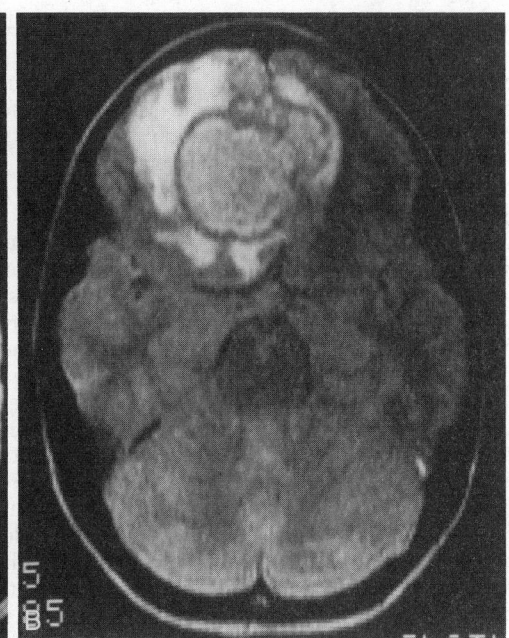

FIGURE 481–1. Frontal lobe brain abscess in a 13-year-old boy with headache and seizures but no systemic symptoms or abnormal signs. *A,* CT shows a contrast-enhanced ring lesion with a daughter ring, the larger ring being characteristically less dense medially. *B,* MRI of the same lesion. Note the characteristic hypointense ring, identical in contour to the contrast-enhanced CT ring. Edema-produced hypodensity by CT appears hyperintense on this T₂-weighted phase of MRI. Following limited surgical drainage and antimicrobial therapy, the boy recovered.

abscess: the differential diagnosis includes septic infarcts, tumors with cyst formation, and metastatic tumors.

Ring formation represents an area of hypercellularity and hypervascularity with varying amounts of fibrous tissue. Ring enhancement is neither synonymous with a well formed capsule nor related to the patient's clinical condition. Ring formation in abscesses may be seen in the stage prior to capsule formation and may persist after complete surgical excision and in clinically stable patients.

Brain abscess may also be identified by magnetic resonance imaging. Although the experience with MR imaging has been limited, there do not appear to be any specific features indicative of the infectious nature of the imaged lesion. Arteriography adds little to the diagnosis. The EEG in brain abscess is almost always abnormal, usually indicating only the presence of a space-occupying lesion.

TREATMENT. Early diagnosis and prompt initiation of antimicrobial therapy are crucial. Once antimicrobial agents are started, some authorities advocate giving parenteral corticosteroids, although in any but late cases their benefit is problematic. During the stage of acute focal suppuration or cerebritis, surgical intervention is contraindicated.

Recent evidence indicates that many brain abscesses can be treated by nonsurgical means if carefully monitored by CT or MRI. Treatment with antibiotics and other supportive medical measures alone is indicated before capsule formation has occurred or when an encapsulated abscess is small and produces no shift or compression of intracranial structures. Multiple brain abscesses may require medical treatment because of the anatomical location of the pus collections. Patients who improve on medical treatment alone all show a decrease in enhancement of ring formation on CT scan and, gradually, shrinking and disappearance of the lesion.

In all likelihood an increasing number of brain abscess patients will be nonsurgically managed in years to come. Because penicillin-susceptible organisms predominate in brain abscesses, the optimal antimicrobial regimen consists of giving 10 to 20 million units of penicillin intravenously daily in divided doses. If there is reason to suspect the presence of another organism not susceptible to penicillin, chloramphenicol or another drug can be given concurrently. If evidence suggests staphylococcal infection, adequate amounts of a penicillinase-resistant penicillin or a cephalosporin drug should be given. Antimicrobial drug therapy can be modified after the antibiotic sensitivity of the microorganism identified in abscess pus has been determined. Treatment should be continued for six weeks.

If, despite medical treatment, the patient's clinical status changes for the worse and/or the CT scan shows an increase in the size of the abscess and an increase in the intensity of ring enhancement, surgical treatment is commonly undertaken. However, heightened ring enhancement may occur after steroids have been discontinued; if the patient shows continued clinical improvement on antibiotic therapy, close, nonsurgical observation can continue.

Available surgical procedures include initial aspiration of the abscess cavity, followed in some cases by excision at a second operation, or primary total excision of the abscess. If the abscess is superficial and encapsulated, primary excision is the operation of choice. The abscess may be aspirated and drained by CT-guided percutaneous puncture if facilities are available. Persistence of a ring sign on CT scan after primary abscess excision does not imply that a residual abscess has formed. If the abscess is deep or affects a neurologically critical area, aspiration and injection of antimicrobial agents is the only operative possibility. Gas within an intracranial abscess as shown by CT scanning calls for total excision of the cavity and closure of a persistent extracranial communication.

PROGNOSIS AND OUTCOME. Mortality from all brain abscesses remained at 30 to 40 per cent after the use of antibiotics had become common practice. The use of the CT scan to assist diagnosis and to monitor the increasingly common use of predominantly or exclusively medical treatment has greatly reduced mortality. Although results are still incomplete, some place current mortality as low as 5 per cent. Mortality is greatest in patients with reduced consciousness at the time of admission.

Residual neurologic damage is frequent in survivors of brain abscess. Convulsive seizures are frequent and require continuous anticonvulsant medication.

SUBDURAL EMPYEMA

DEFINITION AND CAUSE. Subdural empyema refers to an intracranial collection of pus located between the inner surface of the dura and the outer surface of the arachnoid. The most common causes are infections of the paranasal sinuses or middle ear. Other causes include rupture of an intracerebral abscess, cranial osteomyelitis, infection of a subdural hematoma, penetrating wounds of the skull, leptomeningitis, and septicemia. An acute exacerbation of sinusitis just prior to the development of subdural empyema is common.

PATHOLOGY. Infection may enter the subdural space by direct extension following erosion of osteitic areas or by indirect extension through progressively infected mucosal veins and subsequent spread to dural veins, venous sinuses, and cerebral veins. The first route is more common in otitic infections, the second in paranasal infections. When the infection enters the subdural space, it elicits a prompt inflammatory response with rapid pus formation. Extension of pus depends on the primary site of infection. Dorsolateral and interhemispheric collections are common; those beneath the cerebral hemispheres are uncommon. After paranasal infection, subdural pus usually forms at the frontal poles and extends posteriorly over the convexity of the frontal lobe. It may reach into the parietal and occipital areas and along the falx and sylvian fissure. When a subdural collection occurs after ear infection, it passes posteriorly and medially over the falx to the tentorium. Pus may then climb above the tentorium and extend over the occipital poles.

Thrombosis or thrombophlebitis of superficial cortical veins is a common complication and produces hemorrhagic infarction of the area drained by the diseased vessels. The cerebral hemisphere under the pus collection is depressed and indented. Superficial layers of the cerebral cortex undergo ischemic necrosis. Microscopic studies disclose various degrees of organization of the exudate on the inner surface of the dura and infiltration of the underlying pia with inflammatory cells.

ETIOLOGY. The most common organism isolated from subdural pus is the streptococcus, often an anaerobe. Other frequent pathogens include staphylococci and gram-negative enteric organisms.

CLINICAL MANIFESTIONS. Symptoms and signs of antecedent sinusitis, otitis, or osteomyelitis often blend into those of subdural empyema. The usual clinical onset is with high fever, headache, and vomiting, followed by impaired consciousness and signs of meningeal irritation. The patient gradually or rapidly becomes irritable and drowsy. Stiff neck and Kernig's sign are present, and the area of the abscess is characteristically tender to percussion. Progression of the infection leads to confusion, stupor, or coma. Focal neurologic signs appear, including convulsions, hemiparesis, and aphasia, and may be the result of compression of the cerebral cortex underneath the pus collection or cortical thrombophlebitis and cerebral infarction. In the later stages, the intracranial pressure may rise. The entire clinical picture may evolve in as little as a few hours or may take as long as ten days or more. Without treatment, death usually occurs within a few days after the onset of focal neurologic findings.

LABORATORY DIAGNOSIS. A marked peripheral leukocytosis is usually present. X-rays of the skull may show infection of the mastoid, nasal sinuses or other bones. The cerebrospinal fluid is under increased pressure and usually contains a few hundred to 1000 or more cells per cu mm, an increased protein content, and a normal or near normal glucose level.

Spinal fluid is typically free of bacteria. There is potential danger in the performance of a lumbar puncture in patients with subdural empyema who have evidence of increased intracranial pressure, and the procedure should be avoided if the diagnosis can be reached or is strongly suggested by other procedures.

CT scan of the head characteristically depicts a crescent-shaped area of increased density at the periphery of the brain and mass displacement of the cerebral ventricles and midline structures. Contrast enhancement demonstrates a rimlike crescent adjacent to the cortex or a collection of pus near the

falx. CT scan may be more reliable in showing the subdural empyema that develops in patients after drainage of a chronic subdural hematoma than in showing the subdural empyema of other causes. Subdural collections may also be visualized by MR imaging.

In the absence of a diagnostic image, cerebral arteriography is the most reliable method for detecting a subdural mass lesion. The combination of CT scanning and cerebral angiography is the current procedure of choice for demonstration of subdural empyema.

Radionuclide scan is rarely helpful in diagnosing subdural empyema.

TREATMENT. Subdural empyema requires prompt surgical drainage of pus by burr holes or craniotomy. Vigorous systemic therapy with penicillin (10 to 20 million units daily) and other antimicrobials should begin before surgery and continue until the infection is brought under control. Antibiotics are commonly instilled into the subdural space at the time of operation. Surgical treatment of the accompanying sinusitis, frontal osteomyelitis, or mastoiditis, is usually postponed until the intracranial infection has subsided.

OUTCOME. Mortality from subdural empyema remains at between 25 and 40 per cent, usually because of delayed diagnosis. The main causes of death are thrombophlebitis associated with dural venous sinus thrombosis and massive cerebral infarction, fulminant meningitis, and multiple intracerebral abscesses. Progressive and uncontrollable cerebral edema can contribute to a lethal outcome.

CEREBRAL EPIDURAL ABSCESS

Cerebral epidural (or extradural) abscess is a collection of purulent material localized to the outer layer of the dura. It occurs in relationship to adjacent osteomyelitis, mastoiditis, or paranasal sinusitis. Epidural abscess may lead to sinus thrombophlebitis, subdural empyema, leptomeningitis, or brain abscess.

Signs and symptoms are nondistinctive and apt to be masked by primary disease of the ear, nasal sinuses, or skull, or by secondary complications. There may be ipsilateral headache, fever, localized pain, tenderness on local percussion, and swelling with pitting edema. Evidence of increased intracranial pressure is rarely present. Focal neurologic signs are uncommon. In most cases the cerebrospinal fluid is sterile, contains a few lymphocytic cells, and has a mild elevation of protein content. Many cerebral epidural abscesses are diagnosed at the time of operation for a subdural empyema or a brain abscess. Treatment is with surgical drainage plus appropriate systemic antibiotic therapy.

MAJOR DURAL SINUS THROMBOSIS

The large dural sinuses may become thrombosed spontaneously, when they are infected, or when there is infection in the adjacent epidural or subdural spaces. Although any dural sinus may be involved in intracranial infection, the paired sinuses (lateral, cavernous, and petrosal) are affected most often. Spontaneous or primary sinus thrombosis tends to favor unpaired sinuses, and occurs in association with pregnancy and the puerperium, malignancy, use of oral contraceptive agents, hematologic disorders, and collagen vascular diseases. Venous sinuses may become infected by contiguous spread from otorhinogenic foci of infection, by periphlebitis leading to the direct spread of infection through the sinus wall, by an infected draining vein, or by septic venous embolization. Inflammation may also spread from infected dural sinuses to the extradural and subdural spaces by direct extension or venous radicles, to the leptomeninges and adjacent brain, to the bloodstream, and to distant sites by embolism.

Thrombosis of major dural sinuses may result in increased intracranial pressure, multifocal regions of brain ischemia, or cerebral infarction, all because of obstruction to venous drainage from the brain.

LATERAL SINUS THROMBOSIS. Lateral sinus thrombosis is almost always a complication of acute or chronic otitis media, mastoiditis, or cholesteatoma formation. Infants and children are most commonly affected. The thrombosis may coincide with the acute attack of middle ear disease or may be delayed until the chronic stage of ear infection.

The classic symptoms of lateral sinus thrombosis are fever, headache, nausea, and vomiting. An increase of pain in the ear or cessation of aural discharge may point to sinus thrombophlebitis. Local venous distention and swelling, pain, redness, and tenderness indicate involvement of the mastoid emissary vein and may extend into the neck over the jugular vein. Pain in the neck with restriction of movement accompanies jugular vein involvement.

The intracranial pressure is typically increased and more apt to be high when the right lateral sinus is occluded, since it normally is the larger of the two. Papilledema is usually bilateral, but may be unilateral because of extension of the process to the ipsilateral cavernous sinus. Drowsiness and coma are common. Convulsive seizures occur, but focal neurologic findings are unusual.

Spread to the inferior petrosal sinus may lead to abducens nerve paralysis and trigeminal nerve involvement (Gradenigo's syndrome). Involvement of the ninth, tenth, and eleventh nerves may occur because of damage to the jugular bulb and related structures. The symptoms produced include pain on swallowing, dysphagia, dysarthria, hoarseness, weakness or spasms of the sternocleidomastoid and trapezius muscles, and changes in pulse and respiration. The incidence and mortality of lateral sinus thrombosis have been greatly reduced since the introduction and use of antibiotics for middle ear and mastoid infections. The differential diagnosis of lateral sinus thrombosis includes a flare-up of mastoiditis; a perisinus, subdural, or brain abscess; and leptomeningitis.

CAVERNOUS SINUS THROMBOSIS. Cavernous sinus thrombosis is usually due to a suppurative process in the orbit, nasal sinuses, or upper half of the face. Infection may reach the cavernous sinus by the anterior route (ophthalmic veins from orbit, frontal sinus, nasal cavity, and upper face); by the middle route (sphenoid sinus by direct spread or the pharyngeal and pterygoid plexuses from pharynx, upper jaw, and teeth); or by the posterior route (petrosal sinuses and occasionally ear and lateral sinuses). Spread by the anterior route follows the most acute course, and that by the posterior route the most protracted course. The initial infection is usually a furuncle, acute sinusitis, or ear infection. Most infections are due to *Staphylococcus aureus* and many spread by the anterior route to the contralateral cavernous sinus.

Cavernous sinus thrombosis usually produces an illness of desperate severity with high fever, headaches, malaise, prostration, nausea, vomiting, convulsions, tachycardia, and leukocytosis. Characteristically, the sensorium remains clear until late in the infection. Local changes include chemosis, edema, and cyanosis of the upper face, particularly of the eyelids and base of the nose. These are due to obstruction of the ophthalmic vein as it enters the cavernous sinus. Superficial veins over the forehead may be distended. Swelling of the lids, haziness of the cornea, local pain, and photophobia may make examination of the eyes difficult. Ophthalmoplegia, often first affecting the sixth nerve, is common. The pupil may be dilated from parasympathetic paralysis or may be small and immobile if both parasympathetic and sympathetic fibers are involved. Involvement of the first division of the trigeminal nerve may lead to eye pain and hyperesthesia of the forehead. Retinal hemorrhages and papilledema are late events. Visual acuity may be normal or moderately impaired. When the infection originates in the throat, sphenoids, or ear, the evolution of the disease is less acute, and the orbit becomes less engorged.

The differential diagnosis of cavernous sinus thrombosis includes orbital tumors, meningiomas and other tumors in the region of the sphenoid, trichinosis, malignant exophthalmos, and arteriovenous aneurysms.

SUPERIOR SAGITTAL SINUS THROMBOSIS. The superior sagittal sinus is less commonly involved than the lateral or cavernous sinuses in septic thrombosis. Infections may reach the superior sagittal sinus by extension from the nasal cavities, by secondary spread from the lateral or cavernous sinuses, or by extension from osteomyelitis or an epidural or subdural infection. The site of initial thrombosis depends on the source and route of infection.

General signs of superior sagittal sinus thrombosis are prostration, fever, headache, and papilledema. Local signs include edema of the forehead and anterior part of the scalp. At times, there is engorgement of the scalp veins. The neurologic symptoms include convulsive seizures and motor paralysis. Focal seizures which alternatively involve one and then the other side of the body are characteristic. One or both legs may be weak or paralyzed, but the motor loss may be hemiplegic in distribution with the leg and proximal arm involved. Some patients develop homonymous hemianopsia or quadrantanopsia, paralysis of conjugate ocular movements, visual disorientation, alexia, apraxia, or aphasia.

DIAGNOSTIC TESTS. X-rays of the skull may provide evidence of middle ear disease, sinusitis, osteomyelitis, fracture, or other conditions associated with dural sinus thrombosis. Radionuclide dynamic and static scans sometimes show termination of radionuclide activity in the mid-portion of the sinus. CT brain scan most frequently discloses hemorrhage, hyperdensity along the straight sinus, and linear hyperdensities consistent with thrombosed veins on the precontrast scan and a filling defect in the sinus after contrast enhancement (the "delta" sign).

Cerebral angiography is the most specific diagnostic test for the demonstration of venous sinus thrombosis. Particular attention must be paid to the late filling of the venous sinuses and veins. Sagittal sinus thrombosis has been demonstrated by digital subtraction angiography.

TREATMENT. Appropriate antimicrobial drugs in high dosage and surgical drainage with the removal of infected bone and extradural or intrasinus abscess constitute the proper treatment of the major sinus thrombosis secondary to infection. Ligation of the jugular vein in lateral sinus thrombosis to prevent the spread of septic emboli is usually unnecessary. Because of the frequent isolation of penicillinase-producing staphylococci, semisynthetic penicillins should be used until culture results are reported. Although the point is controversial, anticoagulants appear to be contraindicated because venous thromboses tend to produce hemorrhagic brain tissue. Prognosis for survival is fairly good when optimal treatment is given expeditiously, but residual neurologic deficits are frequent.

MALIGNANT EXTERNAL OTITIS

Malignant external otitis begins as an infection of the external auditory canal due to *Pseudomonas aeruginosa*. It affects mainly elderly patients with diabetes mellitus. The infection spreads from the outer ear to the soft tissues below the temporal bone and invades the parotid gland, temporomandibular joint, masseter muscle, and temporal bone. Necrotizing osteitis of the temporal bone develops. The high mortality rate originally reported for the condition (about 40 per cent) led to the use of the adjective "malignant" for this form of temporal bone infection.

The symptoms and signs include rapidly evolving pain in the ear, with or without purulent discharge, swelling of the parotid gland, trismus, and paralysis of the sixth to twelfth nerves. Death is usually caused by the development of meningitis.

Technetium-99m bone scanning is useful in the early detection of the disease. Gallium-67 citrate scanning is preferred for assessing resolution of infection. CT scanning is of use in following the progression of bone- and soft-tissue disease.

Patients with malignant external otitis should be treated with intravenous carbenicillin and gentamicin. Minor surgical debridement is helpful. Antimicrobial treatment should be continued for about a week after apparent cure in order to avoid recurrent disease.

CEREBRAL MANIFESTATIONS OF BACTERIAL ENDOCARDITIS

Neurologic symptoms and signs occur in 25 to 30 per cent of patients with subacute bacterial endocarditis (Ch. 270). Strokes are the most common complication, occurring in about half of the instances. Cerebral infarction, hemorrhage, or transient focal ischemic attacks are all seen and behave like similar lesions from other kinds of emboli. Another presentation consists of a subacute toxic encephalopathy, producing confusion, delirium, hallucinations, confabulation, disorientation, paranoid ideation, and other mental disturbances. Milder manifestations include drowsiness, insomnia, apathy, irritability, and personality changes. Autopsy studies suggest that these mental changes reflect the effects of multiple thromboemboli.

Mycotic aneurysms represent about 5 per cent of the neurologic complications, characteristically involving distal branches of the middle cerebral artery. They typically present with subarachnoid or intracerebral hemorrhage. Occasional mycotic aneurysms have been observed to disappear after antimicrobial therapy, but late rupture of a mycotic aneurysm after bacteriologic cure may occur. Infected embolic material carried to the nervous system may erode blood vessel walls and cause brain abscess or meningitis. There is a higher incidence of meningitis in acute bacterial endocarditis than in the subacute form. Brain abscess and embolic infarction of cerebral tissue may also complicate acute bacterial endocarditis.

SPINAL EPIDURAL ABSCESS

DEFINITION. Spinal epidural abscess describes a collection of purulent material located outside the dura mater within the spinal canal.

INCIDENCE. Epidural abscesses account for approximately one of every 20,000 admissions to United States hospitals. They make up two thirds of surgically treatable infections of the spinal cord and canal. Epidural abscesses occur at all ages, most affecting adults between 20 and 50 years of age.

PREDISPOSING FACTORS. Infections may reach the spinal epidural space by direct extension from an inflammatory process in adjacent tissues, by metastasis through the bloodstream from infections elsewhere in the body, or by perforating wounds. Bacteremia and resultant hematogenous dissemination appear to account for about one third of acute cases. Furuncles, urinary tract infections, dental infections, chronic pulmonary disease, and decubitus ulcers all have been implicated. Contamination of the epidural space by direct spread accounts for another third of acute cases and approximately one half of chronic cases in adults. The usual focus is an adjacent vertebral osteomyelitis with direct extension into the anterior epidural space. Surgical wounds, retroperitoneal abscesses, and lumbar punctures represent other potential causes. In children the usual sources of bacteremia are perineal skin infections, urinary tract infections, pharyngitis, and endocarditis.

Chronic debilitating diseases, diabetes mellitus alcoholism, immunosuppressive therapy, and heroin abuse are common contributing factors. About one quarter of patients give a history of recent back trauma.

ETIOLOGY. *Staphylococcus aureus* is the most common cause and accounts for 50 to 60 per cent of epidural abscesses. Other bacteria responsible for the infection include *E. coli* and other gram-negative organisms. Hemolytic and anaerobic streptococci have also been recovered.

PATHOLOGY. Infection in the epidural space may be acute or chronic. In acute cases, purulent necrosis of the epidural fat can extend over several segments, or the entire length of the cord. The pus is almost always posterior to the spinal cord, but may extend to the anterior surface as well. The epidural fat is hyperemic and infiltrated with numerous polymorphonuclear leukocytes. If the infection is of low virulence, the abscess may be circumscribed and have a granulomatous appearance. Necrosis in the periphery of the cord may result from pressure of the abscess; myelomalacia of one or several cord segments may occur when spinal veins or arteries are thrombosed. Ascending and descending degeneration of the spinal cord can extend above and below the level of the necrotic lesion. In chronic infections, the dura is thickened and gray. The epidural fat is missing and replaced by granulation tissue. In the absence of pus, the granulation tissue may be mistakenly identified as a neoplasm.

CLINICAL MANIFESTATIONS. The clinical course of spinal epidural abscess proceeds in four phases: back pain, radicular pain, muscular weakness, and paralysis. Back pain characteristically identifies the level of the major pathologic process. It is usually severe and localized to a small region of the spine. Movement of the spine in the anteroposterior direction is limited, and the spinous projections overlying the disease process are tender to percussion. Fever and malaise are the rule.

Two to four days later, irritation of nerve roots leads to radicular pains in the trunk or extremities. An erroneous diagnosis of neuritis may be made at this time. Meningeal signs evolve, and headache becomes a common symptom.

The illness then progresses to cause neurologic impairment at and below the level of the lesion. If the abscess compromises the spinal cord, paraparesis and sensory loss occur, accompanied by urinary and fecal incontinence. Abscesses in the lumbosacral spine compress the cauda equina and produce painful sensations in nerve root distribution, eventually resulting in weakness, depressed stretch reflexes, and sensory impairments. There is often erythema and swelling in the area of back pain and tenderness. If appropriate treatment is delayed, paralysis occurs within hours or at most a few days. Immediate surgery is indicated when any degree of weakness is detected, since most patients who become completely paralyzed will remain so permanently.

Evolution of a chronic epidural abscess is much slower. Fever and malaise are unusual. Weakness and paralysis may not develop for weeks or months.

LABORATORY DIAGNOSIS. The white blood cell count and erythrocyte sedimentation rate characteristically are elevated. X-rays of the spinal column may show osteomyelitis or a contiguous abscess, but are usually normal. If available, high-resolution CT scanning of the spine, supplemented by intravenous contrast agent is the diagnostic step of choice.

If CT or MRI is not available or gives equivocal results, one proceeds with lumbar puncture and, possibly, myelography. Lumbar puncture should be performed with caution when acute epidural abscess is suspected. The needle should be introduced slowly and suction applied with a syringe as the epidural space is approached. If the infection has extended to the level of the puncture, pus may be encountered; the needle should be withdrawn immediately at that point in order not to enter and possibly infect the subarachnoid space. Spinal fluid obtained from below the level of the abscess is xanthochromic or cloudy in appearance, with a cell count varying from a few to several hundred cells per cubic millimeter. The protein content is often between 100 and 1500 mg per deciliter. The spinal fluid sugar content is normal, and cultures of the fluid are usually sterile unless meningitis has developed. Chronic epidural abscess usually produces a complete or almost complete spinal block with an inconstant pleocytosis and an elevation of the protein content.

Myelography is abnormal in all cases. Complete extradural block is found in 80 per cent and the remainder have a partial block. Myelography should be performed by cervical subarachnoid puncture in patients in whom complete block or a lumbar abscess is suspected. Every effort should be made to define the entire extent of the abscess.

Enhancement around epidural abscess collections and in the epidural space is diagnostic. The MR image of vertebral osteomyelitis is also characteristic.

Acute spinal epidural abscess must be differentiated from acute or subacute meningitis, acute poliomyelitis, acute transverse myelitis, acute poliomyelitis, acute transverse myelitis or multiple sclerosis. The clinical and spinal fluid findings usually permit differentiation of these conditions. Chronic adhesive arachnoiditis and tumors within the epidural space may be confused with chronic epidural abscess; the myelogram should clarify the diagnosis.

TREATMENT. The usual treatment of spinal epidural abscess is immediate surgical decompression preceded and followed by appropriate antibiotic therapy. Aerobic and anaerobic cultures should be obtained at operation. The area of acute suppuration should be irrigated with an antibiotic solution. Large doses of penicillin are begun prior to surgery and continued postoperatively unless bacterial cultures and sensitivities indicate otherwise. A limited number of patients have been successfully treated by parenteral antibiotics alone after early recognition of the abscess by CT scanning, but the safety and comparative merits of this approach remain to be established.

PROGNOSIS AND OUTCOME. Mortality from epidural abscess is near 30 per cent. The most important determinant for recovery is the patient's neurologic status at the time of operation. Total recovery occurs in patients who have no total paralysis or whose weakness has lasted less than 36 hours. One half of patients paralyzed for 48 hours or more progress to permanent paralysis or death.

SPINAL SUBDURAL EMPYEMA

Infection beneath the dura, but outside the spinal cord, is called spinal subdural empyema. The condition is very rare and has a predilection for the cervical and thoracic spinal cord. The symptoms and signs are indistinguishable from spinal epidural abscess. Coexisting meningitis is common. There is often a greater degree of spinal tenderness than in spinal epidural abscess. Sudden transverse myelitis can occur, attributable to spinal cord infarction from vascular compromise caused by the pus collection. The lesion is best demonstrated by myelography. *Staphylococcus aureus* is the most commonly isolated microorganism. Prompt antimicrobial and surgical treatment is mandatory.

BRAIN ABSCESS

Boom WH, Tuazon CU: Successful treatment of multiple brain abscesses with antibiotics alone. Rev Infect Dis 7:189, 1985. *Describes the medical management of multiple brain abscesses in seven adults.*

Coin CG, Hucks-Folliss AG, Mehegan CC: Computed, tomographically guided percutaneous transmastoid drainage of a cerebellar abscess. Surg Neurol 20:387, 1983. *A technique that is being used more frequently in the management of brain abscess.*

Davidson HD, Steiner RE: Magnetic resonance imaging in infections of the central nervous system. AJNR 6:499, 1985. *Reports on the MR appearance of brain abscess and subdural empyema.*

deLouvis J: Bacteriological examination of pus from abscesses of the central nervous system. J Clin Pathol 33:66, 1980. *Discussion of the often elusive bacteriology of purulent CNS collections.*

Gruszkiewicz J, Doron Y, Peyser E, et al.: Brain abscess and its surgical management. Surg Neurol 18:7, 1982.

Nielsen H, Glydensted C, Harmsen A: Cerebral abscess: Aetiology and pathogenesis, symptoms, diagnosis and treatment: A review of 200 cases from 1935–1976. Acta Neurol Scand 65:609, 1982. *This and the above article*

emphasize the sharp reduction in mortality since CT scanning has allowed better diagnosis and monitoring.

Rosenblum ML, Hoff JT, Norman D, et al.: Nonoperative treatment of brain abscess in selected high-risk patients. J Neurosurg 52:217, 1980. *Reports successful treatment by antimicrobial agents alone in eight high-risk patients followed closely by serial CT scans.*

Young RF, Frazee J: Gas within intracranial abscess cavities: An indication for surgical excision. Ann Neurol 16:35, 1984. *A report of five patients with gas-containing brain abscesses.*

SUBDURAL EMPYEMA

Kaufman DM, Miller MH, Steigbigel NH: Subdural empyema: Analysis of 17 recent cases and review of the literature. Medicine 54:485, 1975. *A thorough consideration of the problem.*

Kaufman DM, Litman N, Miller MH: Sinusitis: Induced subdural empyema. Neurology (New York) 33:123, 1983. *Reviews experience in 17 patients, only 5 of whom had a history of sinusitis.*

Weisberg L: Subdural empyema: Clinical and computed tomographic correlations. Arch Neurol 43:497, 1986. *Reviews the clinical and CT findings in 15 patients with the condition.*

CEREBRAL EPIDURAL ABSCESS

Sharif HS, Ibrahim A: Intracranial epidural abscess. Br J Radiol 55:81, 1982. *Points up the potential value of CT imaging in detecting this uncommon disorder before serious neurologic damage occurs.*

MAJOR DURAL SINUS THROMBOSIS

Goldberg AL, Rosenbaum AE, Wang H, et al.: Computed tomography of dural sinus thrombosis. J Comput Assist Tomogr 10:16, 1986. *Describes the CT appearance of the brain in this condition.*

Kalbag RM, Woolf AL: Cerebral Venous Thrombosis. London, Oxford University Press, 1967. *The classic monograph on the subject.*

MALIGNANT EXTERNAL OTITIS

Mendelson DS, Som PM, Mendelson MH, et al.: Malignant external otitis: The role of computed tomography and radionuclides in evaluation. Radiology 149:745, 1983. *Outlines the use of CT and radioisotope scanning in the condition.*

Strauss M, Aber RC, Connor GH, et al.: Malignant external otitis: Long-term (months) antimicrobial therapy. Laryngoscope 92:397, 1982. *Six patients with this often fatal syndrome were treated successfully with long-term antimicrobials plus (in two) surgical debridement.*

CEREBRAL MANIFESTATIONS OF BACTERIAL ENDOCARDITIS

Churchill MA Jr, Geraci JE, Hunder GG: Musculoskeletal manifestations of bacterial endocarditis. Ann Intern Med 87:754, 1977. *Outlines the muscular, arthritic, and myalgic manifestations of the disorder. In 27 per cent of patients, musculoskeletal complaints were among the first symptoms.*

Pruitt AA, Rubin RH, Karchmer AW, et al: Neurologic complications of bacterial endocarditis. Medicine 57:329, 1978. *A comprehensive review of the subject.*

SPINAL EPIDURAL ABSCESS

Leys D, Lesion F, Viaud C, et al.: Decreased morbidity from acute bacterial spinal epidural abscesses using computed tomography and nonsurgical treatment in selected patients. Ann Neurol 17:350, 1985. *Medical management of four patients with spinal epidural abscess.*

Verner EF, Musher DM: Spinal epidural abscess. Med Clin North Am 69:375, 1985. *A recent review of the clinical condition and its microbiology.*

Whalen MA, Schonfeld S, Post JD, et al.: Computed tomography of nontuberculous spinal infection. J Comput Assist Tomogr 9:280, 1985. *Describes the CT findings in 16 patients with this illness.*

SPINAL SUBDURAL EMPYEMA

Fraser RAR, Ratzan K, Wolpert SM, et al.: Spinal subdural empyema. Arch Neurol 28:235, 1973. *A case report and review of 10 examples from the literature of this uncommon disorder.*

482 SYPHILITIC INFECTIONS OF THE CENTRAL NERVOUS SYSTEM

Kenneth P. Johnson

A general exposition of *T. pallidum* infection is presented in Ch. 310. The following presentation is restricted to a discussion of neurosyphilis.

Neurosyphilis is the invasion and persistent infection of the leptomeninges and, in some cases, brain parenchyma with the spirochete *Treponema pallidum*. Such persistent infection may be asymptomatic or may cause a wide spectrum of neurologic abnormalities.

PATHOLOGY. A meningitis of varying severity and extent is present in every case of active neurosyphilis. The cerebrospinal fluid (CSF) usually reflects this involvement even in cases of asymptomatic neurosyphilis.

Study of *acute syphilitic meningitis* has shown a meningeal inflammatory reaction in which lymphocytes and plasma cells predominate primarily about blood vessels, often with evidence of early arteritis. Reactive arachnoiditis, especially about the base of the brain, is also seen. This accounts for the cranial nerve palsies and for an impairment of CSF circulation that can sometimes result in increased intracranial pressure. A granular ependymitis is commonly present which rarely may obstruct CSF flow through the aqueduct.

In *meningovascular syphilis*, typically a more chronic disorder occurring months or a few years after the primary lesion, the inflammatory response is usually prominent. An associated arteritis predisposes to arterial occlusion and consequent infarction. When larger arteries become occluded, infarction of brain or spinal cord may be extensive.

In *general paresis* the spirochete directly invades the brain as well as the meninges. One finds meningeal thickening, atrophy of cerebral tissue (especially of frontal and temporal lobes), enlargement of ventricles, and a granularity of the ependymal surface. Microscopically, diffuse destruction and loss of neurons, especially in the cortex, are found. Special stains may demonstrate the presence of *Treponema pallidum*. Inflammation of the meninges is prominent.

In *tabes dorsalis* and primary optic atrophy, the pathogenesis of the neurologic lesion is unclear. Direct invasion by the spirochete and an immunologic reaction affecting the meninges may both occur. Grossly, atrophy affects the dorsal roots and the dorsal aspect of the spinal cord. Secondary demyelination of dorsal columns is readily demonstrated. Involvement of anterior roots with resultant amyotrophy occurs rarely.

Focal granulomatous accumulations (*gummata*) are rare, but may reach the size of clinical brain tumors. More diffuse granulomas of the dura (hypertrophic pachymeningitis) sometimes compress neural structures, especially the spinal cord.

CLINICAL SYNDROMES IN NEUROSYPHILIS. *Asymptomatic Neurosyphilis.* This is the most common form of neurosyphilis; it generally follows the acute infection within one to three years. As the term suggests, affected patients lack symptoms or signs of neurologic disease. The diagnosis rests on the finding in the CSF of a low-grade meningitis plus the immunologic abnormalities of syphilis. Adequate treatment prevents the development of neurologic symptoms.

Atypical Neurosyphilis. Primary syphilis occurs in as many as 70,000 persons per year in the United States and secondary syphilis in perhaps 13,000. The spirochete often invades the central nervous system (CNS) during early phases of infection, even though detectable neurosyphilis is rare. Large numbers of persons frequently receive antibiotics to which *T. pallidum* is sensitive for other conditions, but in doses inadequate to cure neurosyphilis. Such partial treatment can modify CSF and serologic reactivity, impairing diagnostic efficiency. Therefore, unusual or bizarre neurologic syndromes accompanied by some CSF abnormalities should at least raise the possibility of neurosyphilis. This is especially important in high risk groups such as homosexual males, in whom syphilis appears with increased frequency.

Symptomatic Neurosyphilis. MENINGITIS. An acute meningitis develops only rarely, although it seems likely that some patients with mild or even moderate symptoms go unnoticed. Symptomatic syphilitic meningitis usually occurs during the early weeks or months after infection, often during the period of the secondary rash or concurrently with a mucocutaneous relapse in a patient previously but inadequately treated. The full-blown illness usually lasts less than one month, but symptoms may persist for longer periods. Headache, vomiting, malaise, and irritability are prominent even though patients are afebrile. Kernig's and Brudzinski's signs develop. Occasionally, confusion, delirium, seizures, and cranial nerve palsies (seventh and eighth nerves most common) occur. Argyll Robertson pupils do not occur in acute syphilitic meningitis. Acute syphilitis hydrocephalus with increased intracranial pressure, including papilledema, may mimic other inflammatory and neoplastic conditions. The CSF always contains an increased number of white blood cells (average about 500 per cubic millimeter—usually mononuclear, rarely polymorphonuclear), an elevated total protein (average, about 100 mg per deciliter), and normal sugar concentrations (reduced rarely). An elevated gamma globulin concentration develops in 70 per cent of cases. The serum serologic tests for syphilis (VDRL and FTS-ABS) are usually but not always positive.

The response to therapy is generally prompt, although an occasional patient will subsequently develop some other form of neurosyphilis.

MENINGOVASCULAR SYPHILIS. Three to 10 per cent of patients with neurosyphilis develop this form of disease. Men are affected more often than women (3:1). Meningovascular syphilis occurs most commonly from two to ten years after the primary lesion. Symptoms and signs of meningitis are lacking, although headache is a frequent complaint. The neurologic deficits often are preceded by a nonspecific prodrome of vertigo, malaise, or mild psychiatric symptoms. Major symptoms can develop slowly or abruptly, and patients may develop hemiplegia, hemisensory defect, dysphasia, or homonymous hemianopia. Focal cerebral seizures develop occasionally. A transverse myelopathy may produce varying degrees of paraparesis, sensory loss, and impaired function of bladder and bowel. Infarction of the anterior two thirds of the cord, with resultant paraplegia and loss of pain sensation below the lesion, can follow occlusion of the anterior spinal artery. Sensory functions subserved by the posterior columns are usually preserved. Hydrocephalus and various cranial nerve palsies have been described.

A CSF lymphocytic pleocytosis (up to 100 cells per cubic mm) and an elevated protein concentration are characteristic. The CSF gamma globulin content is usually elevated. Angiographic studies may show focal arterial narrowing, and CT scans often indicate areas of infarction.

The progress of meningovascular syphilis can usually be halted by specific antibiotic treatment, but the degree of functional recovery depends upon the extent and location of the infarcts.

GENERAL PARESIS (DEMENTIA PARALYTICA, GENERAL PARALYSIS OF THE INSANE). General paresis can develop at any time from 2 to 30 (usually 10 to 25) years after the primary lesion. It appears more often in men than in women (4:1). About 60 per cent of paretics present with a progressive simple dementia; less than 20 per cent display manic symptoms and megalomania. Often faulty judgment, impaired memory (recent memory affected first), disturbed affect (depression or euphoria), or paranoia develops and progresses. The patient may complain of "nervousness," but characteristically lacks insight into the nature of his difficulty. Fine or coarse tremors, often affecting facial muscles and tongue, are present in about two thirds of the patients with fully developed general paresis. Abnormal pupillary response, including Argyll Robertson pupil (see Tabes Dorsalis, below), impassive facies, slurred or dysarthric speech, exaggerated stretch reflexes, and extensor plantar responses are additional abnormal neurologic signs. Convulsions occur in 10 per cent of patients, and strokes may develop secondary to vasculitis.

The CSF is always abnormal, containing a modest (15 to 100) increase in mononuclear cells and an elevated total protein concentration (greater than 50 mg per deciliter in 75 per cent, and 100 mg per deciliter or higher in about 20 per cent of cases). An elevated CSF gamma globulin level is routinely found in general paresis as well as the presence of oligoclonal IgG bands. Most patients have a positive VDRL and RPR (see below) test for syphilis in the CSF, and more than 90 per cent have a positive blood serologic test. Incomplete, prior treatment may modify the CSF abnormalities.

General paresis, once established, evolves rapidly. If untreated, the disease is universally fatal, usually within three years. If paresis is recognized early and treated vigorously, about 80 per cent of patients will improve, but only about one half completely recover neurologic function.

TABES DORSALIS (LOCOMOTOR ATAXIA). Tabes dorsalis develops in less than 5 per cent of patients with untreated syphilis, with symptoms beginning 10 to 30 years after the primary infection. Men are more often affected (7:1).

Dysfunction of affected posterior roots develops insidiously, usually first in the lower limbs. Impaired joint position sense results in stumbling and progressive sensory ataxia, especially in the dark when visual compensation is imperfect. Hypotonia, secondary to a lack of modulation of muscle tension by afferent fibers, accentuates the slapping gait. Paresthesias usually appear early.

Lightning pains, brief, sharp, burning, or aching jabs, sometimes flitting from one body region to another without predictable pattern are characteristic of tabes dorsalis but are nonspecific, occurring also in other diseases affecting dorsal roots (e.g., diabetic neuropathy). They are most common in the lower extremities. Involvement of thoracoabdominal nerve roots can produce visceral pains (gastric or visceral crises), which may simulate intrinsic visceral disease and lead to misdiagnosis of abdominal surgical disease.

As tabes advances, pain sensation is progressively lost and recurrent peripheral trauma goes unnoticed. Indolent ulcers of the skin develop; the toes and balls of the feet are especially vulnerable. Weight-bearing joints and adjacent bone, deprived of pain sensation, are destroyed by the constant trauma of use in 5 to 10 per cent of tabetic patients (Charcot joints).

Unless general paresis coexists, as it does in a small percentage of cases (taboparesis), tabetic patients are mentally normal. Optic atrophy complicates tabes dorsalis in about 10 per cent of cases or occurs as an isolated disorder. Argyll Robertson pupils that are small, irregular, and unequal, and respond poorly to light but constrict with accommodation, are present in most cases. Tonic pupils, large with slow constriction and redilation, also can occur. Occasionally, other oculomotor functions are involved as well. Hypotonia, ataxia, and a slapping broad-based gait are common. The deep tendon reflexes, especially the Achilles, are diminished or absent. The plantar responses are usually normal. Loss or diminution of position and vibratory sensation is found in every case. Increased swaying when the eyes are closed and the patient is standing with feet together (Romberg's sign) results from the impaired position sense. Variable degrees of hypoesthesia and hypalgesia occur in nerve root distribution. Isolated areas of hypalgesia sometimes affect the trunk or shoulders. Delayed perception (from one to several seconds) of pain stimuli delivered to a distal extremity provides a classic sign. Involvement of afferent autonomic fibers leads to impotence in males, and in both sexes constipation, urinary retention or incontinence, and orthostatic hypotension.

The course of tabes dorsalis is unpredictable, and the response to antisyphilitic therapy varies. Patients who have had symptoms for a few months or at the most a few years, with prominent CSF abnormalities and no prior therapy, often improve with treatment. In the absence of cells or increased protein in the CSF, treatment usually brings little benefit. Patients with severe degeneration of dorsal roots and who suffer from painful complications usually retain many of their troubles but progress relatively little after antisyphilitic therapy. Anticonvulsant doses of phenytoin or carbamazepine bring at least partial relief of lightning pains in most instances. Urologic complications, penetrating skin ulcers, and Charcot joints may require surgical treatment.

OPTIC ATROPHY. Visual impairment in syphilis may result from iritis, choreoretinitis, increased intracranial pressure, or primary optic atrophy. Optic atrophy occurs in 1 per cent of patients with untreated syphilis and is five times more common in males than in females.

Because the outer portions of the optic nerve are first affected, the initial visual impairment tends to be peripheral. Ultimately, however, the papillomacular bundle becomes involved, and impaired visual acuity with central and paracentral scotomas develops. It has been estimated that, without treatment, 50 to 90 per cent of patients will go blind. One eye is typically affected before the other. Optic pallor is usually present by the time symptoms appear, but in the early stages it is recognizable only by the reduced vascularity. The optic atrophy of syphilis is indistinguishable from that caused by other diseases. The CSF is abnormal in most patients with active disease of the optic nerve. Intensive antisyphilitic therapy may arrest the process, but return of vision cannot be anticipated.

GUMMA. This rare complication of syphilis usually presents as an intracranial or intraspinal mass lesion and behaves as a slowly growing neoplasm. The correct diagnosis may be suspected from a positive serum serologic test for syphilis or from CSF abnormalities. Removal of the tumor mass, supplemented by antimicrobial therapy, alleviates symptoms and prevents spread of the disease.

CONGENITAL NEUROSYPHILIS. Syphilis acquired in utero after the first trimester of pregnancy tends to be a fulminant disease. Miscarriages and stillbirths are common, and a wide spectrum of clinical manifestations may be recognized in the infant or child who survives. *Neurosyphilis* develops in an estimated 10 to 20 per cent of infants and children with congenital syphilis. *Asymptomatic neurosyphilis* may be diagnosed in the early months or years of life by routine CSF examinations on children of syphilitic mothers. But, as with the acquired disease, symptoms and signs of active neurosyphilis develop only after a latent period, which in the case of *juvenile paresis* may be as long as 20 years. More often, symptoms first appear late in the first decade or during adolescence. Clinical syndromes and CSF findings mirror those found with the acquired disease, except that *tabes dorsalis* is rare and *chorioretinitis* more common. Hydrocephalus, cranial nerve palsies (eighth cranial nerve especially), and seizures may complicate congenital syphilitic meningitis. Syphilis should be considered as a potential cause of stroke in children. More than a third of all children with juvenile paresis are mentally retarded.

Non-neurologic stigmata of congenital syphilis include dental deformities (Hutchinson's teeth), saddle nose, frontal bossing of the skull, saber shins, and interstitial keratitis (usually developing during the second decade). These signs are not seen in acquired syphilis. Fortunately, the current practice of obtaining routine serologic tests on all pregnant women and on infants of syphilitic mothers has almost eliminated congenital neurosyphilis in many areas of the world. It should be remembered, however, that the mother can acquire syphilis at any time during pregnancy and the negative serologic studies obtained early do not exclude the possibility of active syphilis later in pregnancy. Some institutions routinely test blood from the umbilical cord for the reagin of syphilis.

Early and intensive treatment of neonates with congenital syphilis materially reduces the morbidity (see Treatment) from neurologic complications. Results from even optimal treatment of patients with juvenile paresis remain poor.

LABORATORY DIAGNOSIS OF NEUROSYPHILIS. Laboratory studies can be of considerable aid in the diagnosis of neurosyphilis and in the evaluation of therapy. Nevertheless, both false-positive and false-negative results may occur with all assays currently available, so that the final diagnosis requires a consideration of clinical as well as laboratory data.

Cerebrospinal Fluid Changes. Neurosyphilis always includes meningeal inflammation and its accompanying abnormalities in the CSF. A modest increase in cells, predominantly lymphocytes, numbering from six to 100 per cubic millimeter, is noted. The cytologic identification of plasma cells may be useful. The total CSF protein is usually elevated moderately to between 40 and 100 mg per deciliter. The CSF glucose is almost always normal.

The presence of treponemes within the CNS stimulates a local immunologic response, including the production of immunoglobulins which leak into the CSF. This is expressed as an increase in the CSF immunoglobulin G (IgG) level, which can be measured either as the IgG percentage of total protein (usually above 12 per cent) or, more specifically, by an IgG index. The index formula

$$\frac{CSF\ IgG}{Serum\ IgG} : \frac{CSF\ albumin}{Serum\ albumin},$$

which requires assessment of albumin and IgG in both serum and CSF, can be used to determine a specific increase in CSF IgG, considered by most workers to be a measure of IgG synthesis within the CNS compartment. In most laboratories an IgG index above 0.7 is considered abnormal. Oligoclonal bands usually appear in the CSF with active neurosyphilis. Newly described methods also allow the determination of synthesis of both IgG and IgM antibodies to *T. pallidum* within the CNS. Such tests can be of considerable value in both the diagnosis of neurosyphilis and in judging the response to therapy. Spirochetes have been demonstrated directly in CSF of patients with secondary syphilis by immunofluorescent methods.

Serologic Tests. The serologic tests for syphilis are divided into two groups: those which are nontreponemal, and those which measure specific serologic reactivity to treponemal antigens. The nontreponemal tests use purified cardiolipin, which reacts with an antibody (formerly called reagin) in the serum or CSF to produce a serologic reaction. Presently, two flocculation tests, the Venereal Disease Research Laboratory (VDRL) and the rapid plasma reagin (RPR) tests, are routinely available and both can be accurately quantitated. Both are inexpensive and readily adapted to screening large numbers of serum specimens. Neither of these tests is as sensitive as the specific treponemal tests, and both may react in several nonsyphilitic disease states, especially the autoimmune disorders such as systemic lupus erythematosus. The specific treponemal serologic tests include the treponemal immobilization test (TPI), which is expensive, difficult to assay, and not routinely available, and the readily available indirect immunofluorescence assay, the fluorescent treponemal antibody-absorbed (FTA-ABS) test. The FTA-ABS test uses inactivated treponemes reacted with the patient's serum, which has been previously absorbed with an extract of nonpathogenic Reiter treponemes to remove nonspecific reactants. The other increasingly useful specific test is the treponemal hemagglutination test (TPHA), which employs sheep or turkey erythrocytes coated with antigens of *T. pallidum*.

In practice, the nontreponemal tests are used for screening purposes and the specific treponemal tests for confirmation of diagnosis. It should be noted that the nontreponemal assays may be incorrectly reported in 5 to as many as 25 per cent of cases; therefore, if a negative result is obtained in a suspected case of neurosyphilis or a positive result is unexpectedly found, the test should first be repeated. Following confirmation of the nontreponemal assays, a specific treponemal test can be used to confirm the diagnosis.

Both the nonspecific and the specific treponemal antibody assays are positive in serum by the secondary stage of syphilis when acute meningitis and meningovascular syphilis appear. In the majority of late asymptomatic cases as well as in tabes dorsalis and general paresis, the tests are also often positive, although late CNS involvement sometimes has been reported with negative serology. The serum FTA-ABS is usually reactive even if the VDRL is negative in these late cases.

The serologic assay of CSF in neurosyphilis is still controversial. Many authorities advocate the use of the CSF VDRL test, both as an aid in the diagnosis of neurosyphilis and as a rough evaluation of therapy. The CSF VDRL is rarely falsely positive during nonsyphilitic disease states. If the test is positive, it is assumed that the patient does have invasion of the CNS by *T. pallidum*, especially if there is confirmatory clinical or CSF evidence of neurosyphilis. Usually the CSF VDRL titer falls with adequate treatment, although it may remain positive for prolonged periods. Accordingly, therapy must also be monitored by the clinical response and by a decrease in the number of CSF cells, total protein, or IgG level. The specific serologic tests often remain reactive for long periods after an apparent cure.

The specific treponemal tests, especially the CSF FTA, have yielded conflicting results in the diagnosis of neurosyphilis. Contamination of CSF with a minute amount of blood has been shown to convert a negative CSF sample to a positive one, so that CSF containing any red blood cells cannot be reliably used. Estimation of specific IgG and IgM *T. pallidum* antibodies in CSF may provide better evidence of local invasion of the CNS by the organism.

The need for evaluation of CSF during late (over one year after contact) asymptomatic syphilis remains unclear. Most authorities advocate CSF examination in all cases of a positive serum FTA-ABS test with an unclear treatment history. Recent studies showed a very small yield of positive CSF findings in such patients. Therefore patients without neurologic signs or symptoms can probably be safely treated with three weekly intramuscular injections of 2.4 million units of penicillin G benzathine and followed for later evidence of neurologic disease. Of course, evaluation of any patient with a positive serum FTA-ABS and any neurologic abnormality, even if not typical of the classic neurosyphilis syndromes, requires CSF assay to rule out atypical neurosyphilis.

TREATMENT OF NEUROSYPHILIS. Penicillin is the antibiotic of choice for all forms of syphilis, and no resistant strains of *T. pallidum* are known. Because the organism divides slowly and penicillin is effective during the dividing stage, prolonged therapeutic blood and CSF levels are necessary to accomplish a cure. Table 482–1 defines a simplified schedule for treating all cases of suspected neurosyphilis. An alternative for proven neurosyphilis is aqueous procaine penicillin G,

TABLE 482–1. THERAPY OF LATE LATENT AND NEUROSYPHILIS

Stage	Definition	CSF	Treatment
Late latent	Serum serology positive, asymptomatic	Not done	Three weekly injections of 2.4 million units of penicillin G benzathine, maintain follow-up
Suspected neurosyphilis	Serum serology positive, neurologic abnormalities	Negative	Three weekly injections of 2.4 million units of penicillin G benzathine, maintain follow-up
		Positive	2–4 million units of crystallized penicillin G, IV, every 4 hrs. for 10 days
Neurosyphilis: penicillin allergy	Serum serology positive, neurologic abnormalities	Positive	Oral tetracycline or erythromycin, 500 mg q.i.d. for 30 days, maintain follow-up

9 million units total given intramuscularly in 15 daily 600,000-unit doses.

As mentioned above, therapy is monitored clinically and by repeating the CSF evaluation two to six months later. CSF leukocytes should decline, as should total protein and IgG levels and, usually, the CSF VDRL titer. If CSF cell, protein, or IgG abnormalities persist unchanged, retreatment should be considered.

Burke JM, Schaberg DR: Neurosyphilis in the antibiotic era. Neurology 35:1368, 1985. *A recent description of various forms of neurosyphilis and of CSF changes following therapy.*

Muller F, Moskophidis M, Prange HW: Demonstration of locally synthesized immunoglobulin M antibodies to *Treponema pallidum* in the central nervous system of patients with untreated neurosyphilis. J Neuroimmunol 7:43, 1984. *A new CSF method to determine which patients truly have neurosyphilis by measuring focal production of treponemal antibodies within the CNS.*

Prange HW, Moskophidis M, Schipper HI, et al.: Relationship between neurological features and intrathecal sythesis of IgG antibodies to *Treponema pallidum* in untreated and treated human neurosyphilis. J Neurol 230:241, 1983. *Improved CSF analysis to prove presence of neurosyphilis.*

Simon, RP: Neurosyphilis. Arch Neurol 42:606, 1985. *A major review of all facets of neurosyphilis.*

Traviesa DC, Prystowsky SD, Nelson BJ, et al.: Cerobrospinal fluid findings in asymptomatic patients with reactive serum fluorescent treponemal antibody absorption tests. Ann Neurol 4:524, 1978. *A study of the variations in the laboratory diagnosis of syphilis between different laboratories testing the same specimen. Test includes a helpful discussion of the use of lumbar puncture to detect neurosyphilis in asymptomatic patients.*

Venereal Disease Control Advisory Committee, Center for Disease Control, Atlanta, Georgia: Syphilis: Recommended treatment schedules, 1976. Ann Intern Med 85:94, 1976. *Current official recommendations for treatment of all forms of syphilis.*

Wiesel J, Rose DN, Silver AL, et al.: Lumbar puncture in asymptomatic late syphilis. Arch Intern Med 145:465, 1985. *Arguments for not doing lumbar punctures in seropositive asymptomatic patients.*

SECTION NINE / VIRAL INFECTIONS OF THE NERVOUS SYSTEM

483 INTRODUCTION

Richard W. Price

Agents belonging to nearly all the major groups of viruses can infect the central nervous system. The spectrum ranges from the large complex DNA herpesviruses to small, relatively simple viruses with DNA or RNA genomes such as the papovaviruses and retroviruses. Also included are agents not yet fully characterized which cause the spongiform encephalopathies in which the nature of "genetic material" remains uncertain. As a result, neurologic manifestations of viral infections can be almost equally diverse, extending from the typical acute febrile encephalitides to chronic progressive disorders which clinically resemble degenerative neurologic diseases.

In most cases, particularly in those infections presenting as acute encephalitis, nervous system involvement is an uncommon complication of a relatively common systemic infection. In adaptive terms, extension of infection to the central nervous system is "accidental" and may preclude survival of the virus and its transmission to a new host. For example, the polioviruses are enteric infections in which replication in the gut and fecal-oral transmission determine the essential survival and transmission of the organism; extension of infection to anterior horn cells of the spinal cord devastates the host but does not contribute to the "life-cycle" of the virus. By contrast, the neurotropic herpesviruses, including herpes simplex virus Type 1, are exquisitely adapted to cause latent and reactivated infection within the peripheral nervous system; in this case, the sensory neuron is the reservoir for latent virus and reactivated virus exploits axoplasmic transport to reinfect the epithelium and consequently induce local shedding of virus. However, even in the case of the herpesviruses, central nervous complications, such as acute herpes encephalitis, are "accidental" and not essential in the organism's adaptive strategy. Rabies illustrates an illness in which central nervous system infection plays a central role in the life cycle of the virus: involvement of the brain produces "rabid," biting behavior that actually contributes to virus transmission.

Viruses can enter the nervous system along a number of avenues. Transport up peripheral nerves can allow direct passage from epithelium or viscera to the central nervous system, and, once virus enters the brain, similar intraneural passage by axoplasmic transport can facilitate further spread. It has been demonstrated that a number of viruses are transported along nerve processes by both orthograde and retrograde axoplasmic transport systems. This allows rapid passage over long distances and also provides an avenue that is protected from immunologic interference. Many, if not most, viruses, however, enter the brain via hematogenous dissemination with passage across the vascular endothelium. As a general rule, agents that travel over neural routes tend to produce initially focal symptoms, while those that disseminate hematogenously cause more diffuse clinical changes. Exceptions exist, however. One lies in the selective vulnerability of particular nervous system structures or cells to infection with particular agents. Focal or multifocal disease can also follow general hematogenous dissemination in a random seeding of brain regions. Many viruses preferably infect the meninges rather than the brain, gaining access via the choroid plexus.

Thus, while within the nervous system a number of viruses appear not to discriminate among neurons, glial, or endothelial cells, others choose selective targets. Such selectivity is probably determined to a great extent by cell-surface molecules, principally glycoproteins, that serve as receptors for viruses and determine the character of attachment and subsequent entry into cells. Different cell types may also vary in their capacity to support virus-directed metabolism and replication.

The character of virus-cell interactions can assume a number of courses: *abortive infection* results in little or no change in the cell and no virus replication; *acute productive/lytic infection* is characterized by a full replication cycle with production of progeny and subsequent cell death; *chronic productive infection* may allow prolonged release of progeny virus without cell death; in *latent infection*, the viral genome resides in the cell, either integrated into the host genome or as a separate genomic fragment with little or no gene transcription or translation but retention of the capacity to subsequently reactivate; *transforming infection* results in increased and characteristically abnormal cell proliferation, usually in the absence of virus replication; *defective infection* may result in nonproductive infection or production of incomplete particles, yet cause varying degrees of cell alteration and viral antigen expression.

Diagnostic approaches to viral diseases depend on the clinical setting and specific agents involved. Available methods of diagnosis include: serologic assessment of host-antibody responses in serum or cerebrospinal fluid, direct identification of virus in brain or cerebrospinal fluid using viral isolation techniques or methods that identify viral antigens or nucleic acid, and histological examination of infected tissue for pathognomonic reactions (e.g., formation of inclusion bodies or other specific cell changes).

In the past, limitations of specific treatment made specific virologic diagnosis either largely an academic exercise or important principally for epidemiologic purposes. Efforts to combat viral disease consisted exclusively of prevention through active, or at times passive, immunization. These time-honored methods still predominate, and the prevention of poliomyelitis remains a landmark of biomedical research. In the last decade, however, antiviral chemotherapy has finally become a practical reality. Effective therapy is now available for neurotropic herpesviruses, and the promise exists not only for more effective treatments for this group of viruses, but also for the development of chemotherapeutic agents that will act selectively against several other important viruses causing neurologic diseases.

Johnson RT: Viral Infections of the Nervous System. New York, Raven Press, 1982. *An excellent introduction to all aspects of viral infection of the nervous system.*

484 ACUTE VIRAL MENINGITIS AND ENCEPHALITIS

Richard W. Price

DEFINITIONS. The terms *viral meningitis* and *viral encephalitis* refer to infections of the leptomeninges and brain parenchyma, respectively. When the spinal cord is involved along with brain, the term *encephalomyelitis* may be used. When both meninges and brain parenchyma appear to be involved, *viral meningoencephalitis* sometimes is employed, although viral encephalitis is almost always accompanied by meningeal inflammation. The nonspecific term *aseptic meningitis* refers to an inflammatory process of the meninges accompanied by a predominantly mononuclear cell pleocytosis and not caused by pyogenic bacterial infection. Although viral infections are the commonest cause of aseptic meningitis, infections by other types of organisms as well as chemical irritation of the meninges can cause a similar clinical picture and cerebrospinal fluid profile. Most viral meningitides are benign, self-limiting processes with a low acute morbidity and only rare long-term sequelae. Viral encephalitis, by contrast, often carries a high morbidity and mortality, with the long-term outcome of survivors ranging from full recovery to permanent disability.

Central nervous system infections caused by a variety of viruses are appropriately considered together because their clinical aspects can be largely indistinguishable. Viral infections causing more distinct neurologic symptoms and signs are considered separately in subsequent sections.

ETIOLOGIES. Many viruses can cause acute encephalitis or meningitis (Table 484–1). Table 484–2 indicates the most common viruses and the syndromes they produce.

Enteroviruses are small, nonenveloped RNA viruses of the picornavirus family. Over 50 serotypes have been associated with meningitis and encephalitis, the most frequent being

TABLE 484–1. VIRUSES ASSOCIATED WITH ACUTE CENTRAL NERVOUS SYSTEM INFECTIONS IN THE UNITED STATES

RNA viruses
  Picornaviruses (enteroviruses)
    Polioviruses
    Coxsackieviruses, Groups A and B
    Echoviruses
  Togaviruses
    Eastern encephalitis*
    Western encephalitis*
    Venezuelan equine encephalitis*
    St. Louis*
    Powassan*
    Rubella
  Reovirus
    Colorado tick fever*
  Bunyavirus
    California encephalitis*
  Arenavirus
    Lymphocytic choriomengitis
  Rhabdovirus
    Rabies
  Myxoviruses and paramyxoviruses
    Influenza
    Parainfluenza
    Mumps
    Measles
  Retroviruses
    Human immunodeficiency virus
DNA viruses
  Herpesviruses
    Herpes simplex, types 1 and 2
    Varicella-zoster
    Epstein-Barr
    Cytomegalovirus
  Adenoviruses

*Arthropod-borne viruses (arboviruses)

echoviruses 3, 4, 6, 9, 11, 18, and 30, coxsackievirus A9, and coxsackieviruses B1 through B5. Echovirus 9 has been associated with the largest epidemics.

The arboviruses include agents of several families that are transmitted by mosquitoes or ticks. More than 15 different arboviruses have been associated with encephalitis in varied geographic areas of the world; seven of these cause meningitis or encephalitis in the United States.

Adenoviruses are respiratory viruses that only rarely cause meningitis or severe childhood encephalitis. Aseptic meningitis has now been recognized as a complication of acute infection by the retrovirus causing the acquired immunodeficiency syndrome (AIDS, Ch. 488.1).

The acute neurologic disease associated with measles, vaccinia, rubella, and primary varicella (chickenpox) infections in most cases represents postinfectious encephalomyelitis (Ch. 489). This may also be true of the encephalitis that has occasionally been reported with influenza and parainfluenza virus infections.

EPIDEMIOLOGY. Viral meningitis and encephalitis are relatively common disorders. In Rochester, Minnesota, for example, the incidence rate of aseptic meningitis was nearly 11 per 100,000 person-years, while that of viral encephalitis was over 7 per 100,000 person-years. This compares with a rate of 8.6 episodes of bacterial meningitis per 100,000 person-

TABLE 484–2. RELATIVE FREQUENCY OF MENINGITIS AND ENCEPHALITIS OF KNOWN VIRAL ETIOLOGY

Viral Agent	Viral Meningitis (%)	Viral Encephalitis (%)
Enteroviruses	83	23
Arboviruses	2	30
Mumps	7	2
Herpes simplex	4	27
Varicella	1	8
Measles	1	<1

From Jubelt B.: Enterovirus and mumps virus infections of the nervous system. Neurologic Clinics, Symposium on Neurovirology 2:187, 1984.

years. No deaths followed meningitis, while the mortality from viral encephalitis was 3.8 per cent. The relatively low mortality may reflect the inclusion of milder cases in case finding. Also, the more severe arbovirus infections were not seen in this particular population. An etiologic diagnosis was identified in only 11 per cent of cases of meningitis and 14 per cent of encephalitis in the United States.

The incidence of viral meningitis and encephalitis peaks in the late summer, reflecting the relative seasonal frequency of enterovirus and arbovirus infections. Enterovirus epidemics in temperate climates characteristically occur in the late summer, with transmission occurring by the fecal-hand-oral route, often involving young children with rapid spread in family or social groups. The geographic and seasonal incidence of arbovirus infection relates to the life cycle of arthropod vectors and animal reservoirs (Ch. 359) and their contact with man. Eastern equine encephalitis virus is limited largely to the Atlantic and Gulf coasts, while Western equine encephalitis virus is confined to the western two thirds of the country. The latter virus causes many more human infections than does Eastern, but only 1 in 100 of those infected develops encephalitis. St. Louis encephalitis virus causes both rural and urban disease over a large area in the United States. In the rural areas the virus has the same pattern as Western encephalitis virus, but in urban areas more explosive outbreaks can occur. In recent years California encephalitis virus has been related to encephalitis every year over a wide geographic area of the eastern half of the United States with disease confined largely to children. Venezuelan encephalitis has spread into Florida and the southwestern states and in most of those infected produces an influenza-like illness, but about 3 per cent develop acute meningitis or encephalitis. Powassan virus is a rare cause of encephalitis in man in Canada and along the northern border of the United States. Colorado tick fever occurs in the Rocky Mountain area; about 18 per cent of infected patients develop meningitis, but encephalitis is rare.

Lymphocytic choriomeningitis virus is the major zoonotic virus causing meningitis and encephalitis. Man acquires the infection by contact with dust or food contaminated by excreta of the common house mouse. Human disease is more common in winter, when this natural host tends to move indoors. Lymphocytic choriomeningitis virus has also been found in hamsters, and human infections have been traced to laboratory and pet hamsters.

Mumps virus spreads by the respiratory route, occurring throughout the year but increasing in incidence during the spring. Although mumps virus equally infects the two sexes, males develop meningitis three times more frequently than females.

PATHOGENESIS. Events leading up to the development of the acute viral encephalitides and meningitides can be divided into three stages. The first involves exposure of an external body surface to the virus, usually with local replication of the "inoculum." The infecting virus may be contained in body fluids or excreta from infected patients and transferred by direct contact or within contaminated environmental materials, or it may be introduced by an arthropod bite. The next stage involves systemic viremia and amplification of virus in visceral organs; a secondary viremia may then lead to invasion of and replication within the nervous system or meninges. With the exceptions of rabies virus, the neurotropic herpesviruses and perhaps the polioviruses, agents that cause acute viral encephalitis or meningitis reach the nervous system hematogenously. This accounts for the widespread distribution of cerebral dysfunction associated with most of the encephalitides.

In viral encephalitis, infection of neurons as well as various glial cells and even vascular endothelium leads to cell dysfunction and, sometimes, cell death. Inflammatory responses follow, and lymphocytes and macrophages first line the blood vessels and then migrate into the parenchyma. Clinical symptoms and signs depend on the distribution of infection and on both the direct effect of the virus and the secondary reaction in the tissue. The relative contribution of direct viral infection or secondary host reactions to the genesis of brain dysfunction varies, depending on the particular infecting virus. The remarkable degree of recovery in many patients suggests that secondary immune responses play an important role in producing symptoms.

CLINICAL MANIFESTATIONS. The general features of most acute viral encephalitides and meningitides are similar. Often they are preceded or accompanied by systemic symptoms, including fever, malaise or myalgia, gastrointestinal disturbance, respiratory symptoms, or rash. These are followed in viral meningitis by the development of headache, photophobia, stiff neck, and other signs of meningeal irritation, usually but not always with an intensity milder than that of bacterial meningitis.

When encephalitis coexists, evidence of diffuse or, less commonly, focal brain dysfunction adds to the signs of meningeal irritation. Patients characteristically exhibit altered attention and consciousness, ranging from confusion to lethargy or coma. Movement may also be abnormal, with weakness, abnormalities in motor tone or incoordination, reflecting affliction of the cortex, basal ganglia, or cerebellum in varying degree. In severe cases, generalized or focal seizures may be difficult to control. Some patients exhibit myoclonus or tremor. Hypothalamic involvement may lead to hyper- or hypothermia, autonomic dysfunction with vasomotor instability, or diabetes insipidus. Abnormalities of ocular motility, swallowing, or other cranial nerve functions are uncommon. Likewise, spinal cord infection can result in flaccid weakness, with acute loss of reflexes in the most severe cases. Focal symptoms other than seizures are usually minor and overshadowed by generalized brain dysfunction, but in some patients hemiparesis, visual disturbance, or sensory loss may be prominent. Such focal abnormalities are particularly characteristic of herpes encephalitis (Ch. 485).

The time course of viral meningitis and encephalitis is variable. The onset may occur within a matter of hours or evolve more slowly over a few days. Usually maximum deficit appears within one to four days.

LABORATORY FINDINGS. Examination of the cerebrospinal fluid is essential. Characteristic is the presence of 10 to 1000 mononuclear cells per cubic mm. On occasion, early examination may show acellular fluid or polymorphonuclear leukocytes may predominate, but the typical mononuclear pleocytosis soon evolves. The pressure may be elevated, while the glucose is characteristically normal or modestly reduced. The protein is usually elevated (50 to 100 mg per deciliter) and may exhibit increased immunoglobulin concentration and the presence of oligoclonal bands. An increased protein content and number of cells may persist for weeks and perhaps months after convalescence, and the oligoclonal bands can be detected for an even longer period.

Systemic laboratory findings may vary depending on the etiologic agent. Generally the blood white-cell count is not elevated, but either elevations or depressions can be seen, usually with a lymphocytic predominance. Involvement of salivary glands or pancreas in mumps may elevate the serum amylase.

Neurodiagnostic tests usually yield nonspecific abnormalities, with notable exception in the case of herpes simplex encephalitis (Ch. 485). The electroencephalogram characteristically exhibits generalized slowing, but focal sharp-wave or spike activity can occur in association with seizures. Computerized tomography is usually normal early in the course of the nonherpetic viral encephalitides, but focal edema and contrast enhancement may appear in the more severe cases.

The greatest value of CT scanning lies in excluding alternative diagnoses. Experience with magnetic resonance (MR) imaging is too limited to judge its relative advantages. Cerebral angiography and radioisotope scans are of no specific value.

DIAGNOSIS. With a few exceptions, the neurologic and laboratory findings accompanying the acute viral meningoencephalitides are insufficiently distinct to allow an etiologic diagnosis, and it may even be difficult to distinguish these disorders from a number of nonviral diseases. More helpful in diagnosis are the epidemiologic setting (e.g., time of year, exposure to insects, the local community) and any accompanying systemic manifestations. Thus, involvement of the nervous system by mumps virus is usually suspected from associated clinical parotitis or pancreatitis, although the neurologic disease can be the sole or presenting clinical manifestation; conversely, a certain history of mumps eliminates this diagnostic possibility. Several enterovirus infections produce a rash which usually accompanies the onset of fever and persists for four to ten days. In infections by coxsackievirus A5, 9, and 16 and echovirus 4, 6, 9, 16, and 30 the rash is typically maculopapular and nonpruritic, and may be confined to the face and trunk or may involve extremities, including the palms and soles. Echovirus 9 infections can cause a petechial rash resembling meningococcemia. Herpangina, characterized by grayish vesicular lesions on the tonsillar fossae, soft palate, and uvula, can accompany Group A coxsackie infection. In coxsackievirus A16 and, rarely, other Group A serotype infections, a vesicular rash may involve hands, feet, and oropharynx. As discussed below, the encephalitis related to Epstein-Barr virus occurs in the setting of acute mononucleosis and the principally postinfectious encephalitides related to measles and varicella follow overt systemic diseases with characteristic rashes.

Because no specific treatment exists for viral encephalitis (except herpes), and their signs and symptoms are often nonspecific, exclusion of other diagnoses becomes important. Potentially confusing are partially treated bacterial meningitis, rickettsial infections, Lyme disease, meningitis caused by a variety of nonpyogenic organisms including *Mycobacterium tuberculosis* and *Cryptococcus neoformans* and other fungi, meningeal or parameningeal bacterial infections, brain abscess, or subacute bacterial endocarditis. Lacking cerebrospinal fluid examination, the differential diagnosis becomes even broader, encompassing additional toxic and vascular diseases. Most alternative diagnoses can be suspected or eliminated by the cerebrospinal fluid profile or by appropriate brain imaging.

Specific virologic diagnosis most often is established serologically, but direct detection of the organism either in the cerebrospinal fluid or systemically may also be achieved in some cases. Selection of tests and their interpretation depends upon the particular organism. Almost all acute viral syndromes occur in the setting of a first encounter with the agent which then results in lasting immunity. In these cases, seroconversion documented by a fourfold or greater rise in serum antibody titers between acute and convalescent sera is a principal means of diagnosis. A notable exception is herpes simplex encephalitis in which antibody titers must be more cautiously interpreted (Ch. 485). Attempts at direct viral isolation are of limited value in clinical management and must be tailored to the suspected agent. Arboviruses and enteroviruses can be isolated from the blood but are seldom recoverable at the time of clinical meningitis or encephalitis. During the acute disease, coxsackie- and echoviruses are most readily isolated from stool or cerebrospinal fluid and, in some cases, throat washings. Lymphocytic choriomeningitis virus can be isolated from blood or cerebrospinal fluid. Mumps virus may be isolated from saliva, throat washings, or cerebrospinal fluid. Type 2 herpes simplex virus and human immunodeficiency virus may also be cultured from the cerebrospinal fluid.

TREATMENT. Treatment of acute viral encephalitis and meningitis (except herpes) is directed at symptom relief, supportive care, and preventing and managing complications. Strict isolation is not essential, as most of the offending viruses are common in our environment. If an enteroviral infection is suspected, precautions in handling of stools and careful hand washing should be instituted. Measles, chickenpox, rubella, or mumps virus infections should receive the usual isolation from susceptibles.

The headache and fever of meningitis can usually be managed with judicious doses of acetaminophen. Severe hyperthermia (> 40°C) may require vigorous therapy, but modest temperature elevations may serve as a natural defense mechanism and are best left untreated.

Patients with severe encephalitis often become comatose. Since, however, they may well recover, vigorous support and avoidance of complications are essential. Intubation, tracheostomy, and even mechanical respiration to maintain the airway may be required. Although intravenous fluids may suffice for brief periods, more prolonged coma necessitates either total parenteral nutrition or cautious tube feeding. Blood glucose and electrolytes should be monitored to avoid osmotic fluid shifts. Comatose patients often develop infections in the respiratory tract, urinary tract, intravenous site, or skin. Prophylaxis or prompt treatment is paramount.

Although seizures sometimes complicate encephalitis, prophylactic anticonvulsants are not routinely recommended. If seizures develop, they can usually be managed with phenytoin and phenobarbital. If status epilepticus ensues, appropriate vigorous therapy should be instituted to prevent secondary brain injury and attendant hypoxia (Ch. 493).

Modest increases in intracranial pressure can be treated with mannitol or glycerol, but this is usually only of short-term benefit. Steroids should probably be avoided in the treatment of encephalitis because of their inhibitory effects on host-immune responses.

PROGNOSIS. Full recovery from viral meningitis usually occurs within 1 to 2 weeks of onset, although some patients describe persistent fatigue, lightheadedness, and asthenia that may persist for months.

The prognosis of encephalitis is dependent on the etiologic agent. Arbovirus encephalitides have variable mortality rates; that with Eastern encephalitis is approximately 50 per cent; with St. Louis, 10 per cent; with Western, 10 per cent; with Venezuelan equine, 1 per cent; and with California, less than 0.5 per cent. The mortality rates for Western encephalitis are greater in children under one year of age, and for St. Louis encephalitis they are greater in the elderly. Nonfatal encephalitis caused by Eastern, Western, and St. Louis viruses leaves a relatively high rate of neurologic sequelae. Encephalitis associated with mumps or lymphocytic choriomeningitis viruses is very rarely associated with death, and sequelae are infrequent. Hydrocephalus has been reported as a late sequela of mumps meningitis and encephalitis in children.

Johnson RT: Viral Infections of the Nervous System. New York, Raven Press, 1982. *A monograph reviewing the pathogenesis, epidemiology, and clinical features of acute central nervous system infections.*

Jubelt B: Enterovirus and mumps virus infections of the nervous system. Neurologic Clinics, Symposium on Neurovirology 2:187, 1984. *A well-done review of the pathogenetic and clinical aspects of enterovirus and mumps virus infections.*

Nicolosi A, Hauser WA, Beghi E, et al.: Epidemiology of central nervous system infections in Olmstead County, Minnesota, 1950–1981. J Infect Dis 154:399, 1986. *Provides incidence figures for viral meningitis and encephalitis.*

Rennels MB: Arthropod-borne virus infections of the central nervous system. Neurologic Clinics, Symposium on Neurovirology 2:241, 1984. *A review of the major epidemic arbovirus infections in the United States.*

485 HERPESVIRUS INFECTIONS OF THE NERVOUS SYSTEM

Richard W. Price

Three of the five human herpesviruses (see also Ch. 340–344) share an essential "neurotropism" in their adaptation for survival and transmission. Herpes simplex virus types 1 and 2 (HSV-1 and 2) and varicella zoster virus, all establish in sensory ganglion neurons a latent infection which can subsequently reactivate to release progeny virus into the territory of the ganglion's epithelial innervation. The major complications of these infections in adults include adult-type herpes simplex encephalitis caused by HSV-1, aseptic meningitis, radiculitis and autonomic insufficiency caused by HSV-2, and encephalitis, myelitis, radiculopathy, and vasculitis complicating herpes zoster. Prompt diagnosis of infections by these viruses is important since they are now amenable to selective antiviral drug therapy. The two remaining human herpesviruses, Epstein-Barr virus and cytomegalovirus, are largely lymphotropic but in the setting of systemic illness can also cause neurologic disease.

HERPES SIMPLEX ENCEPHALITIS (HSE)

Adult-type HSE is a sporadic disease with a severe morbidity and high mortality. Both HSV-1 and 2 are capable of causing encephalitis, but type 1 by far predominates. In contrast, type 2 herpes simplex virus accounts for the great majority of neonatal herpetic encephalitis, which is not considered here.

EPIDEMIOLOGY AND PATHOGENESIS. Although the commonest identified cause of severe sporadic viral encephalitis in the United States, HSE is nonetheless uncommon. The disease afflicts persons of all postneonatal ages, with peaks of incidence in late childhood and middle age. It occurs with approximately equal frequency throughout the year, and case-to-case transmission does not occur. Immunosuppression plays no apparent role.

HSV-1 is a ubiquitous organism; over 90 per cent of adults exhibit serologic evidence of exposure, and most harbor latent ganglionic infection. Recurrent cold sores resulting from viral reactivation occur in perhaps one fourth of adults. Although HSE may occur as a primary infection, evidence indicates that it more often results from reactivated virus.

The characteristic gross and microscopic pathology of herpetic infection distinguishes HSE from other encephalitides. Although often asymmetrical, the disease is usually bilateral and afflicts the medial temporal and inferior frontal lobes and related "limbic" structures, including the hippocampus, amygdaloid nuclei, olfactory cortex, insula, and cingulate gyrus. Necrosis with petechial hemorrhage is so intense that the disease was once called *acute necrotizing encephalitis*. Microscopically, hemorrhagic necrosis with mononuclear inflammation characterizes involved areas, with neurons and glia often containing Cowdry Type A intranuclear inclusions during the acute phase of infection. The gray matter is affected predominantly, but infection extends into the white matter as well.

CLINICAL MANIFESTATIONS. HSE most commonly presents as an abruptly beginning subacute illness causing local and diffuse cerebral dysfunction. Typically patients are febrile, although in as many as 10 per cent fever may be absent, and thus herpes encephalitis warrants consideration even in afebrile patients who present with an acutely altered mental status. Severe headache, focal or generalized convulsions, and alterations in consciousness and behavior comprise the most prominent symptoms. Common symptoms including disorientation, delusions, agitation, or personality changes sometimes lead erroneously to psychiatric referral. Motor paralyses are present in less than half.

DIAGNOSIS. Evaluation of suspected HSE proceeds in three stages: (1) considering the possible diagnosis on clinical grounds, (2) obtaining supportive evidence from neurodiagnostic procedures, and (3) establishing the diagnosis by viral isolation or by retrospective serologic testing in concert with a therapeutic antiviral drug trial.

Standard neurodiagnostic procedures are important to identify findings consistent with herpetic infection and, importantly, in ruling out alternative disorders. Most helpful in this regard are cerebrospinal fluid (CSF) analysis, electroencephalogram, and computed tomography (CT). The CSF is usually but not always abnormal. Protein levels are most often less than 100 mg per deciliter with cell counts usually greater than 50 leucocytes per 100 cu mm.

CT scans are at least initially normal in perhaps two fifths of patients. When present, CT abnormalities include evidence of localized edema, low-density areas, mass effect, contrast enhancement, and hemorrhages (most often in the temporal or, less commonly, the frontal lobes). The potential diagnostic value of magnetic resonance (MR) imaging awaits additional study; presently its technical requirements preclude its use in many acutely ill encephalitic patients. Cerebral arteriography may be helpful in suspected herpes encephalitis, principally in searching for alternative vascular diagnoses. In more than three fourths of patients, the electroencephalogram contains focal abnormalities, most often showing a spike and slow-wave pattern over the involved brain region.

Attempts at isolating HSV-1 from CSF rarely succeed. Isolation of the virus from the oropharynx is useless since no relationship exists between symptomatic or asymptomatic viral shedding at such peripheral sites and brain infection. HSV-1 is often reactivated by other neurologic diseases eliciting fever, creating a source of false-positive serologic responses in patients suffering nonherpetic encephalitis or meningitis.

Unlike the epidemic encephalitides in which documentation of seroconversion provides a major method of diagnosis, in HSE serologic testing is often inconclusive. This is particularly true at the onset, when prompt diagnostic decisions are critical. Even during convalescence analyses of blood and CSF antibody titers can give false-negative or false-positive results.

The imprecision of serodiagnosis, particularly at the onset of illness, has led some to advocate brain biopsy for diagnosis; the pros and cons of this approach continue to be debated. The principal argument favoring biopsy is that it remains the only available method to establish a certain diagnosis early in the course of the disease. Cultures of biopsied material characteristically produce virus within two to three days. Counterarguments center on the occurrence of false-negative biopsy results, the potential morbidity of biopsy, and the benignity of empiric antiviral therapy.

TREATMENT. The introduction of antiviral therapy has greatly improved the outcome of HSE. This was first demonstrated with vidarabine, and even greater benefit has been shown with acyclovir, which has become the treatment of choice. HSE is treated by an intravenous infusion of 10 mg per kilogram given over a one-hour period every eight hours for ten days. Because acyclovir is excreted principally by the kidney, caution must be exercised in patients with renal impairment. Side effects of acyclovir are generally few, although neurotoxicity rarely occurs, manifested as altered consciousness, tremors, hallucinations, and seizures. Other aspects of care also require meticulous attention. Optimally, patients with HSE should be managed in the intensive care setting of a tertiary referral center.

PROGNOSIS. Both age and initial neurologic status importantly influence prognosis in HSE; even with antiviral therapy patients who are comatose when first treated often fare poorly. Extensive infection and brain damage are present in most of these patients as a result of a more fulminant illness and, sometimes, delay in beginning therapy. Many patients, however, particularly those less than 30 years old who are neurologically intact when treatment begins recover normal or near normal function. Even patients with minor neurologic deficits may survive without severe long-term sequelae and return to normal function if diagnosis and specific treatment are instituted early in the course. In a few patients, and despite antiviral treatment, HSE can relapse within a few weeks after the acute disease, resulting in severe sequelae. The pathogenesis of such relapses is unknown.

HERPES ZOSTER (HZ)

HZ (shingles, zona) is a dermatomal cutaneous infection caused by reactivation of the varicella-zoster virus that normally lies latent in sensory ganglia following an early attack of varicella. In addition to its cutaneous manifestations, zoster is accompanied by neuritic symptoms and may be complicated by an array of neurologic sequelae. The varicella-zoster virus is distantly related to herpes simplex virus, sharing only minor antigen cross-reactivity.

INCIDENCE AND EPIDEMIOLOGY. HZ is a common disorder, with an annual incidence estimated at 3.4 cases per 1000 persons. Unlike varicella, HZ occurs throughout the year with neither significant clustering of cases nor seasonal or yearly preponderance. Case exposure in HZ is rarely identified. Two factors, age and immunosuppression, importantly influence its incidence. The disease is uncommon in childhood, relatively constant between 20 and 50 years of age (approximately 2.5 cases per 1000 annually), and thereafter doubles its incidence between the ages of 50 and 60 and redoubles it between age 80 and 90. Immunosuppression due to systemic disease (in particular Hodgkin's disease and other lymphoreticular malignancies), cytotoxic drugs, corticosteroids, radiation therapy, or acquired immunodeficiency syndrome (AIDS) predisposes. Zoster afflicts about 10 per cent of patients with Hodgkin's disease annually, the highest incidence being in those who have received recent radiation or chemotherapy. In some cases, a history of neoplasm, radiation, or physical injury in the proximity of the dorsal root ganglion or nerve is elicited.

Age is an important factor also in the development of postherpetic neuralgia, which develops almost exclusively in persons older than 50 years of age. Figures of incidence of postherpetic pain vary, ranging between 15 and 75 per cent depending on clinical definition of the syndrome and patient selection. Immunosuppression predisposes to spread of virus beyond the ganglion-nerve-dermatome unit into the central nervous system or systemically.

PATHOGENESIS AND PATHOLOGY. Once the reactivation of latent varicella-zoster virus occurs, it characteristically spreads within the sensory ganglion, and travels centrifugally over the peripheral nerve processes of this ganglion, eventually seeding the skin with the resultant dermatomal vesicular rash.

Cell-mediated defenses rather than humoral immunity are critically involved in protecting the host during herpes zoster. Pathologically, acutely infected dorsal root ganglia and nerve show the presence of a mononuclear inflammatory response, neuronal degeneration with intranuclear Cowdry type A inclusion bodies, and similar infection of surrounding satellite cells. The peripheral nerve may contain parallel changes. In more severe cases, dorsal root ganglia above and below the primarily affected ganglion also show active herpetic infection.

CLINICAL MANIFESTATIONS. Prodromal sensory symptoms include dermatomal pain, itching, or paresthesias, which often antecede by several days the eruption of the segmental rash. The early pain of zoster may be confused with other types of neuropathic or visceral pain. The most frequently involved dermatomes are those extending from the third

thoracic to the second lumbar segments and the first (ophthalmic) division of the trigeminal nerve. The rash itself initially consists of erythematous macules that vesiculate over 12 to 24 hours. Normally the vesicular fluid pustulates within 72 hours; in a week the pustules begin to dry, and crusting takes place by 10 to 12 days. The crusts, in turn, fall off in two to three weeks. In the immunocompromised host, this time course may be protracted. In uncomplicated cases, the rash heals with a variable degree of superficial scarring, at times leaving areas of hyperpigmentation or depigmentation which may be anesthetic. More severe cases may leave denervation of a large segment of the dermatome.

Zoster can affect any of several of the cranial nerves. The ophthalmic division of the trigeminal nerve is the most common and may be complicated by spread to orbital structures, resulting in acute and long-term ocular sequelae. Spread of cutaneous rash along the bridge of the nose to its tip should be taken as a signal of impending ocular infection, prompting early ophthalmologic consultation. Facial palsy, with or without accompanying loss of taste on the anterior two thirds of the tongue, may accompany either otic zoster (Ramsay-Hunt syndrome) with rash confined to a segment of the auricle, or the second and third cervical (cervical collar) zoster. Occasionally infection of the ninth and tenth or fifth cranial nerve may antecede facial weakness. As with other motor syndromes (see below), weakness is often delayed for a variable period after the rash. Eighth nerve dysfunction with sensorineural hearing loss or vertigo occurs in the same setting as facial palsy but with less frequency. HZ may rarely cause facial palsy in the absence of rash (*zoster sine herpete*). Zoster of the ninth and tenth cranial nerves is unusual and may be overlooked without a careful search for the pharyngeal rash or ipsilateral laryngeal or pharyngeal palsy.

Herpes zoster of the extremities or trunk can also be complicated by segmental motor weakness, the motor loss usually corresponding to the involved cutaneous dermatome. Weakness characteristically develops from a few days to two weeks after the onset of the rash, and longer delays are rare. Its onset is characteristically abrupt, occurring over hours or one or two days, with little or no subsequent deterioration. Weakness improves or recovers in about 85 per cent of cases.

Myelitis of variable extent is a less common complication of HZ and results from direct viral invasion of the spinal cord, perhaps augmented by local inflammatory responses. It occurs most commonly in the immunosuppressed and, like motor paresis, is characteristically delayed after the onset of the rash. The most common manifestation is bladder dysfunction. Other signs include mild or transient asymmetric reflexes, lower extremity weakness, or sensory disturbance. Severe myelopathy can produce a partial Brown-Sequard syndrome or total cord transection. Characteristically, involvement lies at the same spinal cord segment as the rash but may ascend to a higher level. Myelography may be needed to rule out coexisting epidural tumor.

At least three types of brain involvement may complicate zoster: diffuse encephalitis, focal parenchymal infection, and vasculitis. Headache, stiff neck, and mild diffuse encephalitis often accompany acute HZ but are difficult to distinguish from the effects of fever, sepsis, narcotic analgesics, and other underlying medical problems. Most such patients recover. In more severe diffuse encephalitis, chances for recovery may also be good if other complications of the disease do not intervene. The clinical picture is that of an acute or subacute delirium accompanied by cerebrospinal fluid pleocytosis with few focal features.

Focal varicella-zoster virus encephalitis is a rare complication in immunosuppressed patients that can resemble progressive multifocal leukoencephalopathy. The onset may be temporally remote from the cutaneous rash. The cerebral lesions involve principally the white matter; the varicella-zoster etiology can be identified by the presence of Cowdry type A intranuclear inclusions on microscopic examination, by specific viral antigens and by visualizing herpesvirus nucleocapsids by electron microscopy. Brain biopsy may be required for accurate diagnosis.

Cerebral vasculitis is probably the most common serious postzoster central nervous system complication. Affected patients develop delayed contralateral hemiplegic strokes following ophthalmic-division zoster owing to inflammation or occlusion of the internal carotid artery and its major branches ipsilateral to the rash. The delay between the rash and onset of cerebral dysfunction varies from none to as much as six months, with a mean interval of seven weeks. A more general cerebral vasculitis following zoster has also been reported. The pathogenesis is still incompletely understood, but the characteristic involvement of local vessels innervated by the infected ganglion in conjunction with reports suggesting the presence of viral nucleocapsids and viral antigens within vessels suggests that the arteries are directly infected. Additional contributions may be made by secondary local inflammatory responses and thrombosis, leading to vascular occlusion or distal embolization. Arteriographic evidence of vasculitis or occlusions in the involved vessels and the clinical setting usually allow diagnosis.

DIAGNOSIS. The clinical diagnosis of HZ is seldom difficult. The dermatomal distribution and the evolution of the vesicular rash is characteristic, and only rarely does herpes simplex infection assume a similar pattern and confuse diagnosis. Difficulty, however, may occur early in the disease, when pain or other sensory symptoms precede the rash. The rare case of zoster sine herpete may require additional methods of diagnosis, and, in cases with an occult rash, a careful search is necessary. When there is question of the diagnosis, the Tsanck test examining lesion scrapings, a direct culture, or immunohistochemical identification of infected cells, can provide specific identification of varicella-zoster virus. Serology may also be helpful, although the commonly used complement fixation test can cross-react between HSV and varicella-zoster virus.

THERAPY. The goals are to relieve the acute segmental infection, to curtail spread of infection either systemically or to other areas of the nervous system, and to prevent postherpetic neuralgia. The means available consist of using antiviral drugs to interrupt viral replication and perhaps corticosteroids to modify local inflammatory responses. Treatment of individual patients must take into account their background risk for particular complications.

Since involvement of the ophthalmic division of the trigeminal nerve risks spreading to orbital structures, such infections should receive early antiviral treatment. Systemic antiviral therapy should also be used for immunosuppressed patients, who are more susceptible to severe disseminated infection. In young patients with normal immune function, there is usually no requirement for specific therapy because zoster is usually mild with swift recovery and no residua. Older nonimmunosuppressed persons are susceptible to postherpetic neuralgia; two controlled studies of such individuals have suggested that a brief course of corticosteroids may reduce the subsequent incidence of pain without untoward complications. A reasonable course begins with a daily dose of 60 mg of prednisone (or the equivalent glucocorticoid) in four individual doses with rapid tapering so that patients are off medication within seven to ten days. Whether the addition of acyclovir to the corticosteroids is helpful has not been evaluated.

The antiviral treatment of choice for herpes zoster is acyclovir. The nucleoside can abort the rash and prevent systemic spread when administered promptly by the intravenous route. The recommended intravenous doses vary from 5 to 10* mg per kilogram infused every eight hours for five days. More

recently, the use of oral acyclovir has been suggested at a dose of 800 mg* every four hours with omission of the nighttime dose, particularly in individuals who are not at marked risk of developing viral complications.

Intravenous acyclovir is indicated for patients in whom VZV infection progresses to cause myelitis or encephalitis, although delay in institution reduces its overall effect. No satisfactory data indicate whether either acyclovir or steroids improves the outcome of HZ-associated motor weakness. Likewise, there is no proven effective treatment for zoster-associated cerebral vasculitis. Postherpetic neuralgia is discused in Ch. 466.3.

NEUROLOGIC COMPLICATIONS OF GENITAL HERPES

Genital herpes, most often caused by HSV-2, may be complicated by local or radicular pain, aseptic meningitis, autonomic (bowel, bladder, and sexual) dysfunction, and rarely myelitis. These complications are more common in association with primary genital herpes but may occur with recurrent disease as well. Prodromal neuritic symptoms commonly precede recurrences and may involve the buttock, groin, or, less commonly, the lower extremities.

Aseptic meningitis and autonomic dysfunction may occur either independently or together. Meningitic symptoms are associated with primary genital herpes in about one fourth of patients, but only a minority require hospitalization. Its course is benign, usually clearing in four to ten days without residua. The cerebrospinal fluid profile is typical of an aseptic meningitis with a mononuclear pleocytosis, mild protein elevation, and normal, or ocasionally reduced, glucose. When the history clearly implicates an epidemiologic and temporal relationship with genital herpes and the cerebrospinal fluid findings are those of a typical mononuclear profile, a clinical diagnosis can usually be made. Specific diagnosis can often be established by isolation of herpes type 2 at lumbar puncture.

Urinary retention, constipation, or sexual impotence in association with genital herpes are less common than meningitis. Symptoms and signs of a sacral sensory radiculopathy sometimes accompany the autonomic changes. The pathophysiology of this disorder is uncertain, but direct herpetic infection of nervous system structures is likely. Fortunately, autonomic dysfunction is reversible, and patients can be assured that their symptoms will probably clear. Although unusual, these autonomic symptoms can recur. It is important to consider and pursue the diagnosis of HSV-2 infection in patients who present with isolated bladder, bowel, or sexual dysfunction. It is critical not to make an inappropriate diagnosis of spinal neoplasm or, especially, early multiple sclerosis. When there is a clear history of genital herpes, the cause of autonomic dysfunction is usually readily established clinically. Inspection and viral culture of genital lesions plus accompanying antibody titers, which may appear and rise slowly only in primary HSV-2 infection, provide additional help.

In adults, HSV-2 only rarely produces adult-type herpes encephalitis indistinguishable from that caused by HSV-1. Transverse myelopathy due to HSV-2 is very rare.

Epithelial herpes simplex virus type 2 primary infections and recurrences can be treated with acyclovir, but the effect on the neurologic complications of genital herpes is uncertain. In the absence of adequate data, it appears appropriate to give acyclovir for neurological complications of primary genital herpes.

In patients with frequent recurrent attacks of genital herpes, early, self-initiated treatment of recurrent lesions with oral acyclovir has been advocated, beginning therapy at the onset of prodromal symptoms. This approach is probably appropriate for the rare patient with recurrent herpetic meningitis.

---

*Exceeds manufacturer's recommended dosage.

*Exceeds manufacturer's recommended dosage.

CYTOMEGALOVIRUS AND EPSTEIN-BARR VIRUS INFECTIONS

Both human cytomegalovirus and Epstein-Barr virus infections can cause neurologic disease. While in children cytomegalovirus is an important and relatively common cause of congenital neurologic deficit, central nervous system infection in adults occurs almost exclusively in the setting of immunosuppression. Central nervous system complications of Epstein-Barr virus occur in the setting of acute mononucleosis. Both viruses have been implicated in the Guillain-Barré syndrome.

Cytomegalovirus encephalitis and, less commonly, meningoencephalitis or myelitis have been reported as opportunistic infections in adults suffering from impaired cell-mediated immunity. Earlier these complications were reported most commonly in patients undergoing organ transplantation, but more recently their occurrence has been noted principally in association with AIDS. The clinical features of cytomegalovirus brain infection have been imprecisely characterized, but the major symptoms and signs appear to reflect diffuse brain dysfunction with concomitantly impaired levels of attention and cognition, paralleling the symptomatology of a metabolic encephalopathy. At times, focal deficits (e.g., hemiparesis) or seizures are superimposed. Pathologically, infection of the brain by this virus is marked by scattered microglial nodules, some of which contain typical cytomegalovirus intranuclear inclusions. As many as one fourth of autopsied AIDS patients have neuropathologic evidence of central nervous system cytomegalovirus infection, although in most the infection appears to be mild, and indeed its contribution to symptoms is uncertain. Scattered reports have described a variety of other neurologic complications of cytomegalovirus infection, including ventricular ependymitis, ascending polyradiculitis, myelitis, and aseptic meningitis.

Diagnosis of cytomegalovirus encephalitis is difficult. Most AIDS patients, particularly homosexual men, have circulating antibody to the virus, and in many it can be isolated from urine or blood, yet they do not suffer nervous system infection. For this reason, serologic evaluation or systemic virus isolation are not particularly helpful in diagnosis; rather one must rely on clinical suspicion and perhaps viral isolation from the cerebrospinal fluid. Recently, the antiviral nucleoside 9-(1,3-dihydroxy-2-propoxymethyl) guanine has been found effective in treating certain manifestations of cytomegalovirus infection, including particularly the retinopathy which sometimes complicates AIDS. Unfortunately, when the drug is discontinued, the retinopathy characteristically recurs. No information is yet available regarding the drug's efficacy in central nervous system infections caused by human cytomegalovirus.

The neurologic complications of Epstein-Barr virus infection range from symptoms of headache, photophobia, weakness, and fatigue which occur relatively frequently in infectious mononucleosis, to more serious, but uncommon, complications which have been described principally in the context of individual case reports. These include encephalitis, meningoencephalitis, Guillain-Barré syndrome, Bell's palsy, acute cerebellar ataxia, and transverse myelitis. It is likely that most of these neurologic complications result from immune-mediated injury rather than direct viral infection.

Bale JF Jr: Human cytomegalovirus infection and disorders of the nervous system. Arch Neurol 41:310, 1984. *A general review of the nervous system complications of human cytomegalovirus, including both congenital and adult infections.*

Collaborative DHPG Treatment Study Group: Treatment of serious cytomegalovirus infections with 9-(1,2-dihydroxy-2-propoxymethyl) guanine in patients with AIDS and other immunodeficiencies. N Engl J Med 314:801, 1986. *Describes the experience with a new antiviral drug in treating visceral and retinal cytomegalovirus infections.*

Corey L, Spear PG: Infections with herpes simplex viruses. N Engl J Med 314:749, 1986. *A review of the clinical spectrum and treatment of herpes simplex virus infections.*

Hilt DC, Buchholz D, Krumholz A, et al.: Herpes zoster ophthalmicus and delayed contralateral hemiparesis caused by cerebral angiitis: Diagnosis and management approaches. Ann Neurol 14:543, 1983. *A report of four cases and review of the literature related to herpes zoster–associated cerebral angiitis.*

Horten B, Price RW, Jimenez D: Multifocal varicella-zoster virus leukoencephalitis temporally remote from herpes zoster. Ann Neurol 9:251, 1981. *A report of two immunosuppressed patients with multifocal varicella-zoster virus encephalitis.*

Jemsek J, Greenberg SB, Taber L, et al.: Herpes zoster–associated encephalitis: Clinicopathologic report of 12 cases and review of the literature. Medicine 62:81, 1983. *A review of encephalitis complicating herpes zoster.*

Price RW: Neurobiology of human herpesvirus infections. CRC Crit Rev Clin Neurobiol 2:61, 1986. *A general review of the pathophysiology of neurotropic herpesvirus infections and their neurologic complications.*

Whitley RJ, Soong S-J, Dolin R, et al.: Adenine arabinoside therapy of biopsy-proved herpes simplex encephalitis. N Engl J Med 297:289, 1977.

Whitley RJ, Soong S-J, Hirsch MS, et al.: Herpes simplex encephalitis—vidarabine therapy and diagnostic problems. N Engl J Med 304:313, 1981.

Whitley RJ, Alford CA, Hirsch MS, et al.: Vidarabine versus acyclovir therapy in herpes simplex encephalitis. N Engl J Med 314:144, 1986. *This series of papers traces the progress made by a large collaborative study in establishing the efficacy of antiviral therapy for herpes simplex encephalitis.*

---

486 POLIOMYELITIS

Richard W. Price

DEFINITIONS. Poliomyelitis (acute anterior poliomyelitis, infantile paralysis) is an acute illness caused by the three strains of poliovirus. The disease selectively destroys the motor neurons of the spinal cord and brain stem to cause flaccid asymmetric weakness. Until recently one of the most feared of all human infectious diseases, poliomyelitis is now almost entirely preventable by vaccination.

ETIOLOGY. The three strains of poliovirus (types 1, 2 and 3) are classified in the genus *Enterovirus* within the family Picornaviridae. These are small (approximately 270 nm), roughly spherical particles with icosahedral symmetry. They contain a single-stranded RNA core and are surrounded by a protein capsid without an envelope. The molecular weight of a single-stranded RNA is approximately 2.5×10^6 Daltons, corresponding to about 7500 nucleotide sequences. This nucleic acid codes for a single protein precursor which is subsequently cleaved into at least four distinct viral proteins. Lacking a lipid envelope, the virus is resistant to lipid solvents and is stable at low pH. The three poliovirus strains can be antigenically distinguished.

INCIDENCE, PREVALENCE, AND EPIDEMIOLOGY. In the United States, the number of cases of paralytic poliomyelitis, which averaged 21,000 per year over the five years before the introduction of vaccines, has now fallen to just a few cases yearly. In less advanced regions of the world, polioviruses remain endemic and paralytic polio continues to occur with a seasonal incidence of infection in temperate zones, but a more even distribution throughout the year in tropical areas. Poliovirus is acquired by the oral route and subsequently replicates in the oropharynx and lower gastrointestinal tract. It may be secreted for a week or two in saliva and for more prolonged periods in feces, which provides the major avenue of host-to-host transmission. Spread of polioviruses is greatly influenced by standards of hygiene and greatest dissemination occurs within families or other crowded circumstances.

Paralysis is an unusual complication of poliovirus infection. During an epidemic, 95 per cent of infections are asymptomatic and only 1 to 2 per cent result in neurologic symptoms and signs; the remaining 4 to 8 per cent of affected individuals suffer nonspecific (minor) illness. Where poliovirus is endemic and among children during epidemics, the incidence of neurologic manifestations is even lower. A number of factors increase the incidence of paralytic disease, including advancing age, recent hard exercise, tonsillectomy, and pregnancy. Immunity to each of the three types of poliovirus is lifelong, but infection with one strain does not necessarily protect against subsequent infection by another.

PATHOGENESIS AND PATHOLOGY. Poliovirus is a prototype of a selective agent inducing highly stereotyped pathology, and in this manner contrasts with most of the viruses causing acute encephalitis or meningitis.

The poliovirus invades the nervous system only after prior systemic replication. An initial alimentary phase with local replication in the intestinal mucosa and spread to the local lymphatics is followed by a viremic phase which results in seeding of the nervous system. Once poliovirus gains access to the brain, it may disseminate along neural pathways, attacking highly specific neuronal populations. Infected motor neurons undergo characteristic sequential degenerative changes followed by cell loss and phagocytosis. The disease attacks principally and randomly the motor neurons of the spinal cord and lower brain stem, the brain stem reticular formation and, to a lesser extent, the precentral gyrus. Convalescent poliomyelitis is characterized by loss of motor neurons, and denervation atrophy of their associated skeletal muscles.

CLINICAL MANIFESTATIONS. Human poliovirus infection varies widely in its severity. In most persons, poliovirus either produces only minor nonspecific systemic illness or is asymptomatic; only a small percentage develop neurologic complications. The incubation period from exposure to the neurologic phase characteristically lasts between four and ten days but may be prolonged to four to five weeks. The major illness usually begins with fever and malaise, and is followed within hours by generalized headache, vomiting, and within another day by the development of neck and back stiffness. Patients at this time often are drowsy, but on arousal are irritable and apprehensive. Progression may stop at this point, making the illness indistinguishable from other enterovirus meningitides. When paralysis develops, it usually begins on the second to fifth day after the onset of headache. Weakness, however, may be among the initial symptoms, or rarely, especially in children, may be delayed for seven to ten days. Children generally exhibit less intense systemic symptoms than adults, who characteristically appear acutely ill and are tremulous, flushed, and agitated. Their muscles are often sensitive and stiff.

Poliomyelitis preferentially damages the larger somatic motor neurons. In all but the most severe cases, the involvement tends to include the lumbar segments to a greater degree than the cervical, and the spinal cord more than the brain stem. The damage and consequent paralyses are usually asymmetric, weakness characteristically being more proximal than distal, and in mild cases affecting parts of muscles rather than the entire muscle or the distribution of a single motor root. The asymmetry may be such that one member is rendered useless yet the contralateral one is spared entirely. About fifty per cent develop acute urinary retention. The trunk musculature is least commonly affected. The affected muscles are flaccid, and the deep tendon reflexes may be absent. Atrophy develops rapidly, usually beginning within a week in paralyzed muscles and progressing over the ensuing weeks. Once it starts, progression of the motor deficit for more than three to five days is rare.

About 10 to 15 per cent of cases affect the lower brain-stem motor nuclei. Involvement of the ninth and tenth cranial nerve nuclei leads to paralysis of pharyngeal and laryngeal musculature, with resultant difficulty in phonation and swallowing. Parts of the facial muscles can be involved, either unilaterally or bilaterally. Less often, the tongue and muscles of mastication will be partially paralyzed. External oculomotor weakness occurs only rarely and never permanently. The pupils are spared. Direct involvement of the brain-stem reticular formation can disrupt breathing and swallowing and can

produce serious disturbances in cardiovascular control. Poliomyelitis seldom causes permanent functional paralysis of the bulbar muscles, probably because of the relatively small size of the motor units served by brain-stem nuclei and because overwhelming disease in these critical segments usually kills the patient.

DIAGNOSIS AND DIFFERENTIAL DIAGNOSIS. Because of its rarity in the United States, poliomyelitis may present diagnostic difficulties. In its early phases, it may be difficult to differentiate from other acute meningitides, and when paralysis ensues, a major differential diagnosis is with the Guillain-Barré syndrome and other predominantly motor polyneuropathies. However, for practical purposes, no other acute disease produces headaches, stiff neck, fever, and asymmetrical flaccid paralysis without sensory loss coupled with an increase in white blood cells in the CSF. Diagnosis may be more difficult if these major findings are equivocal or lacking. The CSF rarely shows a persistence of significant pleocytosis in polyneuritis, and CSF protein levels above 100 mg per mililiter are frequent. Acute intermittent porphyria may cause an illness similar to that of postinfectious polyneuropathy. At times, acute transverse myelitis may be confused with poliomyelitis, but in the former a sensory and motor level at the appropriate spinal cord segment usually serves to separate an inflammatory cord transection from diffuse anterior horn cell involvement. Hysterical paralysis may mimic poliomyelitis during epidemics, but such patients do not usually appear acutely ill. Both epidemic neuromyasthenia (Iceland disease) and pleurodynia (Bornholm's disease) may be confused with mild attacks of poliomyelitis. The epidemiologic setting, the lack of CSF abnormalities, and the absence of clear motor paralysis serve to distinguish these entities. In rare cases, infection with other viruses can produce a paralytic illness resembling mild paralytic poliomyelitis. Both coxsackie- and echoviruses have been reported to cause encephalitides with prominent (but not extensive) motor neuron symptoms and signs. Diagnosis can be established by isolation of virus from blood or cerebrospinal fluid, or serologic evidence of acute poliomyelitis infection. In cases related to vaccine strains, viral isolates can be characterized epidemiologically.

TREATMENT. There is no specific treatment, but supportive care can be important in reducing suffering during the acute attack, in maintaining vital functions to assure survival, and perhaps in modifying the overall outcome and disability. Important measures include preventing contractures, maintaining airway and cardiovascular stability, and preventing excessive calcium mobilization and bed sores.

PROGNOSIS. Death in poliomyelitis is usually the result of bulbar involvement and attributable to respiratory and cardiovascular impairments. Death rates are higher in adolescents and adults than in children. Mortality also varies with individual epidemics and has been considerably reduced with modern management of respiratory insufficiency. Patients who survive an episode of acute paralytic poliomyelitis usually recover considerable motor function. Generally, motor improvement begins within the first weeks after onset, and 60 per cent of eventual recovery is achieved by three months and 80 per cent by six months. Minimal further improvement may continue over the next two years. The degree of permanent paralysis cannot be assessed accurately until two to three months have passed.

The Postpolio Syndrome. This is an important disorder characterized by progressive weakness beginning years after a severe attack of poliomyelitis. Clinicians in the United States are presently more likely to see this late complication of poliomyelitis than the initial paralytic disease. There is some controversy as to the course, prognosis, and pathogenesis of this disorder. Most commonly it presents many years after the acute disease as a late-life progression of weakness in already affected muscles, or, less often, in muscles previously thought to be normal. This weakness is often accompanied by fasciculations, and there may be additional atrophy. Muscle biopsy shows type grouping consistent with denervation-reinnervation. Overall, the prognosis is generally good, with only slow progression of further weakness, which may plateau and rarely leads to a major increase in disability or death. This development must be distinguished from motor neuron disease of a more malignant variety (Ch. 475), which has also been described many years after acute poliomyelitis but appears to be much less common than the above more gradual and benign syndrome.

PREVENTION. Poliomyelitis can be prevented by either live-attenuated or killed polio vaccines. These are now given routinely in Western cultures, although the practice of immunization has relaxed as the threat of developing paralytic poliomyelitis has become less conspicuous. If this trend is not reversed, a resurgence of the disease can be expected. An important consequence of accurate diagnosis of poliomyelitis is the prompt institution of local vaccination programs for communities at risk, including subcultures in which vaccination is avoided for religious or other reasons.

Dalakas MC, Elder G, Hallett M: A long-term follow-up of patients with post-poliomyelitis neuromuscular symptoms. N Engl J Med 314:959, 1986. *The authors conclude that new weaknesses develop late after the disease in slightly affected muscles, owing to eventual failure of earlier neural compensating mechanisms.*

Mulder DW, Rosenbaum RA, Layton DD: Late progression of poliomyelitis or forme fruste amyotrophic lateral sclerosis? Mayo Clin Proc 47:756, 1972. *Description of the progressive postpoliomyelitis syndrome that resembled motor neuron disease.*

Price RW, Plum F: Poliomyelitis. In Vinken PJ, Bruyn GW (eds.): Handbook of Clinical Neurology, Vol. 32, Part I. Amsterdam, Elsevier North-Holland, 1978. *A lengthy review of clinical and biologic aspects of poliomyelitis.*

487 RABIES

Daniel B. Fishbein and George M. Baer

DEFINITION. Rabies is a viral infection of humans and other warm-blooded animals most often caused by the bite of a rabid animal and manifested as an acute encephalomyelitis. In humans, the encephalitis often has distinct clinical features and progresses to coma or death within 14 days of onset of symptoms.

ETIOLOGY. Rabies viruses are classified as Lyssaviruses (Greek *lyssa:* frenzy) in the family Rhabdoviridae. The agent contains a cylindrical central ribonucleoprotein capsid composed of a helical, single-stranded RNA genome closely associated with nucleoprotein, nonstructural protein, and the RNA transcriptase. The nucleoprotein represents the group-specific antigen of the genus. The membrane protein and glycoprotein form a lipoprotein envelope through which knobbed spikes of glycoprotein project. These spikes attach to cell surfaces and contain the only antigenic sites that elicit the protective neutralizing antibody. Rabies glycoprotein cDNA, incorporated into the genetic material of vaccinia virus, protects a variety of animals against challenge with street strains of rabies virus.

Rabies virus is relatively fragile; it is usually inactivated by drying or heating to 60° C for 35 seconds, 54° C for 30 minutes, or to 40° C for 4 hours. The virus may survive for hours in saliva, depending on temperature and humidity. Rabies virus is also inactivated by many chemical agents, especially soap and other surface-active agents, organic solvents, oxidizing agents, acids (pH ≤3), and alkali (pH ≥11). It is stable for many years when frozen at −70° C or lyophilized and held at 0 to 4° C.

PATHOLOGY AND PATHOGENESIS. Almost all human rabies is caused by the bite of a rabid animal, although rare cases have resulted from non-bite contamination of mucous membranes or open wounds by the saliva of rabid animals, aerosols (produced in research laboratories or in bat caves), or by corneas transplanted from patients dying of undiagnosed disease. After its introduction, the virus becomes sequestered, probably in striated muscle cells at the site of the bite, and the infection may be aborted by immunization or host factors. Replication of virus in myocytes may amplify virus for invasion of the peripheral nervous system but fails to stimulate humoral or cell-mediated immune responses. After attaching to muscle spindles or motor end plates the virus genome ascends passively at about 3 mm per hour along axons to reach the central nervous system and is probably no longer susceptible to immunologic intervention. The initial central dissemination infects the limbic system generating the unusual behavior associated with the disease. The virus then spreads centrifugally via the efferent nerves to the mucous cells in the salivary glands and the outer nerve endings of most organs. The disease can sometimes be diagnosed at this stage by fluorescent antibody staining of the network of nerve endings around the hair follicles (e.g., in the nape of the neck). Neutralizing antibody and inflammatory infiltration appear only after the onset of encephalitic signs, and antibody may actually hasten the demise of the patient. Terminally, the virus reaches the neocortex, 'furious' rabies abates, and paralysis and coma set in.

Nonspecific pathologic findings in the central nervous system include congestion, perivascular cuffing, and lymphocytic and plasma-cell infiltrates, mostly in the grey matter of the brain stem and spinal cord. A specific finding in about 70 per cent of cases is the Negri body, a sharply defined neuronal eosinophilic intracytoplasmic inclusion composed mainly of viral ribonucleoprotein. There is a surprisingly mild degree of neuronal degeneration, in light of the severity of encephalitis. Virions can be detected in brain tissue by electron microscopy, but the immunofluorescent antibody technique is the preferred method of diagnosis.

EPIDEMIOLOGY. Rabies is primarily a disease of animals, humans being dead-end hosts. In North America rabies is primarily a disease of wildlife, especially red foxes (*Vulpes fulva*) in sub-Arctic Canada and the northeastern United States, striped skunks (*Mephitis mephitis*) in the midwestern part of the United States, and raccoons (*Procyon lotor*) in the South and Mid-Atlantic states. In Europe, the red fox is the predominant rabid animal. Bat rabies has been reported from almost all countries where surveillance has been conducted, and is present in a number of countries that do not report terrestrial rabies. In most developed countries the human disease has been almost completely eliminated by pet vaccination and elimination of stray dogs. Rabies in domestic animals in the United States is acquired from wild animals. In Africa and in much of Asia and Latin America, however, rabies is still endemic in dogs, which continue to be the most important source of human rabies.

The different possible sources of infection are reflected in the epidemiology. Of the 49 cases of human rabies in the United States reported between 1960 and 1986, 16 were acquired from foreign dog or cat bites; 13 resulted from exposures to bats, skunks, foxes, and bobcat; 10 had no known exposure; and only 7 acquired rabies from American domestic animals. The remaining 3 acquired rabies by exposure to a laboratory aerosol (two cases) or corneal transplant (one case). With the exception of rabies following corneal transplant, there have been no well-documented human-to-human transmissions of the disease.

Although a number of places in the world, including Hawaii and other insular areas, are classified as "rabies free," a case of human rabies attributed to a bat bite recently occurred in one of these countries, Finland. The experience emphasizes the need to maintain constant surveillance for the disease in animals.

DIAGNOSIS. *Clinical Manifestations.* During the *incuba-*

tion period, the time between exposure and the first neurologic symptoms, the virus probably remains confined to the muscle cells at the bite site, and the patient remains well except for symptoms from the bite. Although the extremes of incubation range from four days to 23 months about two thirds lie between one and three months, and about 99 per cent within a year. Short incubation periods are more common in children, in cases where large quantities of virus have been involved, or when the exposure site is close to the brain (e.g., with aerosol exposure or bites on the face, head, and neck).

The *prodromal symptoms* reflect viral invasion of the central nervous system. A specific symptom—pain, paresthesia, or pruritus at the exposure site—occurs in about half of the cases. However, common infections are initially suspected because of the rarity of rabies, the nonspecific nature of early complaints and findings (i.e., fever, chills, malaise, myalgia, headache, mood changes), or symptoms of upper respiratory or gastrointestinal dysfunction. By the time the patient deteriorates enough to warrant hospitalization, severe central nervous system disease is usually evident.

The *acute neurologic period* follows two to ten days of prodromal symptoms. Findings commonly include difficulty in swallowing, excitement, agitation, paralysis or weakness, and occasional disorientation, hallucinations, seizures, bizarre behavior, and meningismus. The disease often presents as one of two clinical syndromes, furious or paralytic (dumb). Characteristic of furious rabies are terrifying and sometimes painful spasms of the pharynx and larynx during which the patient chokes, gags, and may violently avoid liquids. Such episodes may be precipitated by drinking, or even seeing or hearing water (hydrophobia), feeling air blown on the face (aerophobia), or a variety of other cutaneous or sensory stimuli. Hydrophobia and aerophobia have been noted in only about one third of rabid patients in the United States since 1960. Associated with hydrophobic attacks are 1- to 5-minute periods of agitation and aggressive behaviors alternating with lucidity and calm. In paralytic rabies, a symmetrical or ascending paralysis dominates the clinical picture. In both forms, lability of blood pressure, respirations, and heart rate are common, often leading to sudden death. If the patient survives the early neurologic phase, paralysis replaces agitation. Four to 14 days after the first symptoms, *coma* develops with irregular breathing and flaccid paralysis, creating a picture virtually indistinguishable from other encephalitides. Potentially fatal complications include increased intracranial pressure, autonomic dysfunction, pulmonary congestion, arrhythmias, gastrointestinal hemorrhage, and renal failure. Intensive care can lengthen the average survival from 2 to 5 days to as many as 24. Recovery followed such treatment in three known cases, but partial vaccine-induced immunity may explain these exceptional events which have not been repeated.

Differential Diagnosis. Rabies should be considered in any patient with acute encephalitis of unknown etiology, especially when a patient has been bitten by an animal capable of transmitting rabies. Since, however, no history of exposure has been reported in 21 per cent of Americans with rabies since 1960, the diagnosis should always be considered when patients have suggestive symptoms or signs or die of encephalitis of undetermined origin. As noted, rabies routinely progresses to coma or death in four days to two weeks, and a failure of this progression excludes the diagnosis. Infectious diseases resembling clinical rabies include tetanus, cerebral malaria, typhoid, and many encephalitides. Potentially confusing noninfectious diseases include hysteria (a rabies phobia engendering the symptoms), intoxication with poisons or drugs, and withdrawal from alcohol. The differential diagnosis of paralytic rabies should include postvaccinal neuroparalytic reactions, poliomyelitis, acute inflammatory polyneuropathy (Guillain-Barré syndrome), and simian herpes virus (B) encephalitis.

Laboratory Diagnosis. Antemortem diagnosis depends on the isolation of rabies virus from the saliva or brain, detection of viral antigens in the brain or in nerves surrounding a hair follicle, or measurement of rabies neutralizing antibody in the serum or CSF. Routine laboratory tests offer no specific assistance in diagnosis. No technique will detect rabies virus before it reaches the central nervous system and causes clinical illness. Even when there is central nervous system involvement, the diagnosis is often complicated by the absence of antibody, viral antigen, or virus. Because the regions of the central nervous system available for biopsy are relatively unaffected, such examination often reveals only nonspecific changes. The most valuable specimens include serum and spinal fluid, saliva, and a 5- to 10-mm-thick skin biopsy from the nape of the neck just above the hairline. If all results are negative, another set of specimens may need to be examined five to seven days later, especially if the initial specimens are obtained in the first week of disease or the patient is immunosuppressed.

The only sensitive test during the first few days of illness is viral isolation from the saliva. The demonstration of rabies virus antigen by direct fluorescence of skin biopsy specimens may be useful in making the diagnosis late in the first and early in the second week of illness. Serum neutralizing antibody is found by the eighth day of illness in about half the cases and by the fifteenth in all who have not received immunosuppressive drugs. Cerebrospinal fluid neutralizing antibody becomes detectable a few days later and is a less useful diagnostic test, except in patients who have been vaccinated. (Vaccine-induced antibody does not enter the CSF.) Interferon or corticosteroid therapy may suppress the appearance of neutralizing antibody.

Postmortem diagnosis of rabies in humans and animals is readily accomplished by the immunofluorescent staining of fresh tissue from the hippocampus, brain stem, and cerebellum. The techniques are less sensitive on formalin-fixed material. An experienced laboratory should confirm the findings.

TREATMENT AND PROGNOSIS. Therapy with rabies immune globulin, vaccine, or human interferon does not alter the outcome, but may complicate the diagnosis and hasten death. Effective therapy awaits the development of antiviral or immunomodulating drugs capable of arresting the virus in the central nervous system. As noted, intensive care alone is probably insufficient.

PREVENTION. The cornerstone of prevention of human rabies is the vaccination of pets and elimination of strays. Even with the wildlife epizootics in North America and Europe, the spread of rabies to humans has been prevented by public education campaigns that stress the importance of vaccinating domestic animals and avoiding contact with wild animals. Rabies prevention through immunization represents one of the great achievements of the 19th century, and the rabies biologics currently used in developed countries are among the safest and most effective immunizing agents known for humans. Unfortunately, they are among the most costly. Because of the cost, deciding whether or not to vaccinate can be difficult when the risk of rabies is very low.

The decision to administer *postexposure prophylaxis* is based on the risk of the specific incident (Fig. 487–1). The initial step should be to determine if infectious material has contaminated an open wound or mucous membrane. Next, the epidemiologic status and clinical condition of the animal responsible for the exposure are considered. In the United States, treatment is usually begun as soon as possible following a bite by a skunk or raccoon, but is usually delayed pending a 10-day evaluation of healthy-looking dogs and cats (except strays). This is the maximum presymptomatic period during which virus can be found in the saliva. Ill or unwanted animals are usually killed and their brains examined for rabies. In wild animals the diagnosis must be based on tests of the animal's brain; if postexposure prophylaxis has been started

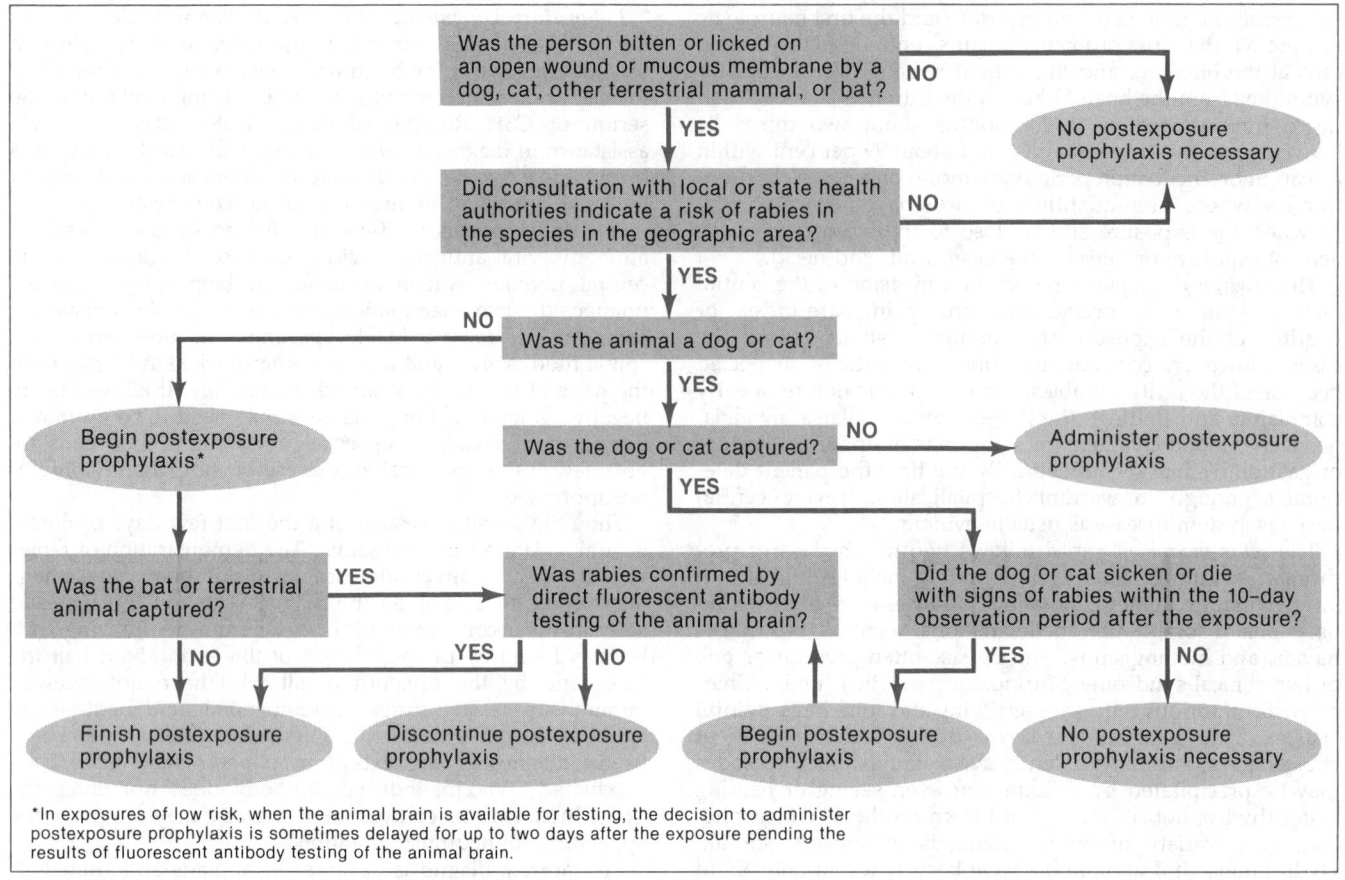

FIGURE 487–1. An algorithm for rabies postexposure prophylaxis administration in most developed countries.

empirically it can be stopped if the fluorescent antibody examination is negative. Exposures to rodents (except woodchucks) and lagomorphs almost never call for postexposure prophylaxis. Local public health officials should be consulted about the epidemiology of rabies and the need for therapy after exposures to animals that are not available for testing.

The best protection against rabies is local treatment of the wound followed by a combination of passive and active immunization. Two passive immunizing agents, rabies immune globulin of human origin (RIG) and antirabies serum of equine origin (ARS), are available in the United States, but the latter is associated with an unacceptably high incidence of serum sickness and is not recommended. Local wound care should be begun immediately. This consists of thorough washing of all wounds with soap and water (perhaps the most effective single measure in preventing rabies), tetanus immunization, and measures to control bacterial infection. RIG is administered once in a dose of 20 IU per kilogram of body weight. Up to half of the volume is infiltrated around the bite site; the rest is administered in the gluteal area, in divided doses if necessary.

The only rabies vaccine currently licensed in the United States is human diploid cell rabies vaccine (HDCV). Five 1-ml doses of HDCV are administered IM in the deltoid area on days 0, 3, 7, 14, and 28. HDCV and RIG should never be given in the same site. Persons who are exposed after having been previously immunized with a tissue culture rabies vaccine (or any other rabies vaccine if a response was documented by an acceptable neutralizing antibody titer) should receive two 1-ml IM doses of HDCV, one on day 0 and one on day 3. The importance of proper postexposure prophylaxis is underscored by the deaths of two persons who had received preexposure prophylaxis but failed to seek the necessary boosters, and another person who received all postexposure doses of HDCV in the gluteal area instead of the deltoid.

In most developing countries the main treatment is nerve tissue vaccine made from the brains of young sheep (Semple vaccine) or suckling mice. Such vaccination is associated with a 0.004 to 0.5 per cent incidence of neurologic reactions, about 15 to 30 per cent of which are fatal. Outside the United States, considerable savings have been achieved by using postexposure regimens that involve reduced dosages of HDCV administered intradermally (ID) or purified vaccines produced on an industrial scale from substrates that provide much higher virus yields such as VERO cells and chick embryo cells.

Preexposure prophylaxis is offered to persons at risk of inapparent or unrecognized exposure such as veterinarians, animal handlers, zoologists, workers in rabies research and diagnostic laboratories, and some international travelers. The recommended pre-exposure prophylaxis regimen consists of three 1-ml IM or 0.1-ml ID doses of HDCV administered over 28 days (day 0, 7, and 21 or 28). Depending on the nature of the continuing risk, booster doses are administered every 6 to 24 months, or not at all. Serum antibody titers to document seroconversion are recommended only for persons who are immunosuppressed by diseases or medication.

Pain, swelling, and itching are reported in up to 90 per cent of those vaccinated with HDCV, and mild systemic reactions of fever, malaise, headache, and nausea, by up to 50 per cent. Allergic reactions include a usually mild anaphylaxis in less than 0.1 per cent of vaccinations, and a serum-sickness–like illness that follows about 5 per cent of booster vaccinations. The only serious neurologic reactions that have been reported are two cases of Guillain-Barré syndrome that may or may not have been directly related.

Anderson LJ, Nicholson KG, Tauxe RV, et al.: Human rabies in the United States 1960–1979. Epidemiology, diagnosis, and prevention. Ann Intern Med 100:728, 1984. *Describes recent experience.*
Kaplan C, Turner GS, Warrell DA: Rabies: The facts. Oxford, Oxford University Press, 1986. *A brief text, very readable, with interesting anecdotes.*

Koprowski H, Plotkin S (eds.): World's debt to Pasteur. New York, Alan R Liss, Inc., 1985. *Proceedings of a symposium commemorating the first rabies vaccination. Contains a number of up-to-date chapters on selected aspects of rabies.*

Recommendations of the Immunization Practices Advisory Committee (ACIP). Rabies Prevention—United States, 1984. MMWR 33:393, 1984. *The United States Public Health Service's complete guidelines on prevention by vaccination.*

World Health Organization. WHO expert committee on rabies. Seventh Report. Geneva:World Health Organization, 1984. (Technical report Series 709). *A global view of rabies and its prevention.*

Kieny MP, Desmettre P, Soulebot J-P, et al.: Rabies vaccine: Traditional and novel approaches. Prog Vet Microbiol Immunol, 1987 (in press). *A current and thorough discussion of rabies immunology and vaccinology.*

488 SLOW VIRUS INFECTIONS OF THE NERVOUS SYSTEM

488.1 Introduction
Richard W. Price

The term *slow infections* was first applied by Bjorn Sigurdsson to a group of transmissible diseases of sheep characterized by an incubation period and course measured in months or years rather than hours or days as in typical acute viral or bacterial infections. Subsequently, several human diseases sharing these characteristics have been described. Although often considered together because of their chronic nature, these disorders are in fact heterogeneous with respect to their clinical manifestations, neuropathology, etiology, and pathogenesis. Although in some instances the infections are accompanied by inflammatory pathology, in several symptoms and signs typical of the acute encephalitides are absent, and both clinically and pathologically they resemble degenerative or hereditary diseases of the nervous system. Two of the sheep diseases upon which Sigurdsson based his concept of slow infections, *visna* and *scrapie*, have subsequently proved to have human counterparts. Visna is caused by a retrovirus and somewhat resembles the nervous system infection caused by the human immunodeficiency virus responsible for AIDS, while scrapie closely parallels human Creutzfeldt-Jakob disease and kuru.

The agents causing the slow infections are taxonomically diverse as are the mechanisms by which they maintain chronic progressive infection and cause clinical symptomatology (Table 488–1). Thus, the human immunodeficiency virus is an RNA-containing retrovirus which codes for a DNA intermediary that can integrate into the host genome and persist for the life of the cell, progressive multifocal leukoencephalopathy is caused by a small nonenveloped DNA-containing papovavirus, subacute sclerosing panencephalitis is due to the enveloped RNA measles virus, while Creutzfeldt-Jakob disease is caused by an agent which has not yet been characterized and, indeed, appears to fall outside of the classic definitions of a virus. Contributions of host immune responses to the development and symptomatology of these diseases are similarly varied. In the case of progressive multifocal leukoencephalopathy, a conventional virus that circulates commonly in the human community and is ordinarily associated with little if any disease, causes devastating central nervous system infection in the presence of depressed host cell-mediated immunity. Human immunodeficiency virus causes profound systemic disease by virtue of its predilection for infecting the helper-inducer (T4) subset of lymphocytes, with the resultant systemic immunosuppression perhaps playing a role in the subsequent development of progressive brain infection by this same virus. Subacute sclerosing panencephalitis appears to result from defective replication in the brain of a once-common conventional virus and is accompanied by an exuberant but ineffective antibody response. In the case of Creutzfeldt-Jakob disease, immunosuppression plays no role in the development or progression of the disease, and indeed there is little evidence that the host recognizes the infectious agent as foreign.

The diversity of the agents causing these slow infections, along with their variable cell and tissue tropism, host susceptibility, and pathologic reactions has led to speculation that viruses may play a role in many of the common neurodegenerative disorders, including multiple sclerosis, amyotrophic lateral sclerosis, parkinsonism, and Alzheimer's disease. To date, however, no direct evidence for such an infectious cause of any of these disorders has been identified.

Johnson RT: Viral Infections of the Nervous System. New York, Raven Press, 1982. *Contains sections dealing with the general background as well as the specific slow virus infections of the nervous system.*

488.2 AIDS Dementia and Human Immunodeficiency Virus Brain Infection
Richard W. Price

DEFINITION. The acquired immunodeficiency syndrome (AIDS) is caused by a human retrovirus recently renamed human immunodeficiency virus (HIV). As noted in Ch. 346, AIDS is transmitted by venereal or parenteral routes and is most common in homosexual men, intravenous drug abusers, and recipients of blood transfusions or blood products (including particularly hemophiliacs). Neurologic complications are frequent in AIDS and include opportunistic infections and neoplasms (Table 488–2). Far more common is a primary neurologic disorder that has been variously referred to as subacute encephalitis or encephalopathy, AIDS encephalopathy, and, more recently, the *AIDS dementia complex*.

ETIOLOGY AND EPIDEMIOLOGY. The first cases of AIDS appeared in the United States in the late 1970's, and by 1981 the disease was described. The AIDS virus was first identified in 1984, and by 1985 serologic tests for antibody to the virus were licensed and widely available. By 1986, over 21,000 cases of AIDS had been reported, and it has been

TABLE 488–1. HUMAN SLOW VIRUS INFECTIONS OF THE CENTRAL NERVOUS SYSTEM

Disease	Etiologic Agent		Pathogenetic Factors
	Name	*Classification*	
AIDS dementia complex	Human immunodeficiency virus	Retrovirus (RNA) (lentivirus)	Virus infects brain, ? prepares way by causing immunosuppression
Progressive multifocal leukoencephalopathy	JC virus	Papovavirus (DNA)	Opportunistic infection, depressed cell-mediated immunity
Subacute sclerosing panencephalitis	Measles virus	Myxovirus (RNA)	Defective viral gene expression
Progressive rubella panencephalitis	Rubella virus	Myxovirus (RNA)	
Creutzfeldt-Jakob disease		Spongiform encephalopathic agents (coding material unknown)	Nature of agent uncertain, immune response unimportant

TABLE 488–2. NERVOUS SYSTEM COMPLICATIONS OF AIDS

Brain
  AIDS dementia complex
  Cerebral toxoplasmosis
  Cytomegalovirus encephalitis
  Primary CNS lymphoma
  Progressive multifocal leukoencephalopathy
  Varicella-zoster virus encephalitis and vasculitis
  Fungal abscess: candida and cryptococcus
  Tuberculosis (*M. tuberculosis*)

Leptomeninges
  Cryptococcal meningitis
  Aseptic meningitis
  Lymphomatous meningitis

Spinal Cord
  Vacuolar myelopathy
  Viral myelitis: VZV, HSV, and CMV

Peripheral Nerve and Root
  Distal, predominantly sensory polyneuropathy
  Inflammatory demyelinating neuropathies
  Mononeuritis multiplex
  Herpes zoster

estimated that for every case of AIDS, perhaps 50 to 100 individuals have been infected by the virus. It has been estimated that perhaps 15 to 30 per cent of individuals with newly diagnosed AIDS exhibit neurologic symptoms on careful examination, and that ultimately as many as 90 per cent of AIDS patients may have neurologic involvement. Two thirds of these exhibit major symptoms and the remainder, mild cognitive or motor dysfunction. Although most infected individuals develop the neurologic symptoms after AIDS is diagnosed, some show neurologic manifestations before they develop the life-threatening opportunistic infections or neoplasms that define full-blown AIDS. Occasionally, neurologic dysfunction can precede even the less severe symptoms of HIV infection, such as chronic lymphadenopathy.

PATHOGENESIS AND PATHOLOGY. Neuropathologically, the AIDS dementia complex involves principally the subcortical white matter and deep gray nuclei of the brain, with relative sparing of the cortex. In the spinal cord, approximately one third of AIDS patients develop a vacuolar myelopathy in the white matter of the lateral and posterior columns.

Both direct and indirect evidence indicates that the AIDS virus infects the brain. Not entirely certain at present is which cell types are infected within the brain. A major component of the infection involves macrophages and multinucleated cells, but emerging evidence suggests additional participation in some cases of endothelial cells and perhaps glia and neurons as well. It is also uncertain when in the course of systemic HIV infection the virus usually enters the brain. Clear evidence, however, suggests that the virus may seed the brain relatively early after exposure.

CLINICAL MANIFESTATIONS. A self-limiting aseptic meningitis during which HIV can be recovered from the cerebrospinal fluid occurs in some patients early after viral exposure, even before seroconversion. This syndrome is indistinguishable from other, clinically benign, viral meningitides.

The AIDS dementia complex develops later and is characterized by a variable combination of cognitive, motor, and behavioral dysfunction. The disorder begins insidiously and usually pursues a steadily progressive course. Some patients, however, deteriorate only slowly in their neurologic condition extending over many months or even two or more years. In others, impairment may appear abruptly within a period of a few days, or the course may be punctuated by rapid deterioration over a similarly short period. Usually, rapid changes in symptoms occur within the setting of systemic illness with hypoxia or sepsis and may reverse when the metabolic disorder clears. More often no improvement occurs, and patients remain in a more advanced plateau of the disease.

The early mental impairment of AIDS may be mistaken for depression or systemic illness. Careful inquiry, however, usually discloses "organic" brain dysfunction. Most often, patients complain of poor concentration and memory. They begin to keep lists in order to keep track of appointments or perform daily responsibilities. Routine tasks require enervating concentration and effort. Patients lose track of conversations, and their thought processes slow down. Motor symptoms include gait unsteadiness and leg weakness. Coordination and handwriting suffer. Patients become apathetic and socially withdrawn, but most deny a dysphoric mood. Sometimes agitation, confusion, paranoia, or hallucinations ensue.

Early during AIDS dementia, mental status examinations may be within the normal range, but, even at this point, psychomotor slowing is usually evident. Of the routine tests, patients perform poorest on serial sevens and other tasks requiring concentration and complex sequencing. On neurologic examination, impaired rapid alternating movements of the fingers or feet and impaired ocular motility are common. Mild gait ataxia is accentuated during quick turns or when performing tandem walking.

As the disease advances, patients become distractible, circumlocutory, and may appear to be unaware of their illness. Ataxia gives way in many to overt leg weakness. Urinary and fecal incontinence commonly complicate management. Tremor is frequent, sometimes with myoclonus. About 10 per cent of patients develop an agitated psychosis. Eventually, psychomotor slowing evolves to near or complete mutism. Only the most rudimentary of social interactions remain. Despite this severe impairment, consciousness is usually spared until superimposed metabolic or systemic disease complicates the course, and lethargy, stupor, or coma ensues.

Other Neurologic Problems. Peripheral neuropathies of several types may complicate AIDS. A self-limited, demyelinating polyneuropathy indistinguishable from the Guillain-Barré syndrome or its more chronic variant may occur early. Occasionally mononeuritis multiplex appears and progresses, probably related to an immune-mediated vasculitis. The most common neuropathy is a chronic distal sensorimotor neuropathy which usually develops late in the course and produces painful dysesthesias accompanied by relatively mild sensory loss and motor weakness.

DIAGNOSIS. Individuals infected by HIV are susceptible both to the AIDS dementia complex and to a variety of opportunistic conditions involving the brain, leptomeninges, spinal cord, and peripheral nerve. Diagnosis of the AIDS dementia complex relies on the characteristic symptoms and signs, the epidemiologic setting, laboratory evidence of HIV infection, and neurodiagnostic studies. Diagnosis may be difficult in patients who develop neurologic disease but exhibit only mild (or no) systemic symptoms and signs related to immunodeficiency. A history of possible exposure to the virus through sexual or blood contact must be explored. Serologic testing may help by showing antiviral antibody: it is nearly always positive in infected individuals.

Among neurodiagnostic studies, imaging by CT or MRI is helpful in ruling out other central nervous system complications of AIDS and supporting the diagnosis of AIDS dementia. Almost all demented patients exhibit cerebral atrophy as an early finding. A small minority display white matter abnormalities on CT scan, while MRI detects patchy white matter abnormalities in a larger number. Routine cerebrospinal fluid analysis shows an elevated protein in the majority and a mild mononuclear pleocytosis in about one third.

In persons with AIDS, diagnosis revolves on distinguishing the primary dementia from the opportunistic infectious or neoplastic disorders to which these patients are susceptible. The opportunistic neurologic conditions complicating AIDS can be considered in two broad groups, those producing *predominantly focal* manifestations and those causing *predomi-*

nantly diffuse dysfunction. Among the focal disorders, the most common and important to recognize is cerebral toxoplasmosis, for which rapid diagnosis and therapy can allow an excellent symptomatic response. The diagnosis of toxoplasmosis and the other important focal disorders complicating AIDS, including primary central nervous system lymphoma, progressive multifocal leukoencephalopathy, and tuberculosis, can usually be suspected clinically by the presence of focal cerebral hemispheric symptoms and signs (e.g., hemiparesis, aphasia, hemisensory deficit) and corroborated by finding abnormalities on CT or MRI. Definitive diagnosis of toxoplasmosis is most often made by therapeutic trial, while the other disorders usually require brain biopsy to identify. The predominantly nonfocal opportunistic conditions include cryptococcal, lymphomatous, and tuberculous meningitis, in which cerebrospinal fluid analysis is critical for diagnosis. These processes may often be suspected when headache, nuchal rigidity, or cranial nerve palsies are present, but often such symptoms and signs are mild or absent. Since cryptococcal meningitis in AIDS patients can produce remarkably bland symptoms and spinal fluid findings, all patients suffering neurologic impairment should undergo spinal fluid analysis for cryptococcal antigen.

In patients not known to have AIDS, differential diagnosis can encompass a number of chronic neurologic disorders ranging from dementia of the Alzheimer type to multiple sclerosis or even schizophrenia, depending on the relative prominence of cognitive, motor, and behavioral manifestations. In most patients, however, the AIDS dementia complex can be readily distinguished by clinical and virologic analyses.

The aseptic meningitis of retrovirus infection is diagnosed principally by the epidemiologic setting and identifying infection by the virus. Because blood serology can be negative, direct isolation of the virus from the cerebrospinal fluid should be attempted. The peripheral neuropathies in patients infected by the AIDS virus may be difficult to distinguish from those associated with other conditions and must be identified by the clinical setting or other evidence of HIV infection.

TREATMENT AND PROGNOSIS. At present, management of the AIDS dementia complex is focused principally on symptom control and supportive therapy. Alprazolam sometimes reduces anxiety associated with early dementia, while butyrophenones, phenothiazines, or lithium may be required in psychotic patients. Tricyclics are of limited benefit.

Uncontrolled observations suggest that the demyelinating motor neuropathy complicating early HIV infection may respond to plasmapheresis or corticosteroids.

Cornblath DR, McArthur JC, Kennedy PGE, et al.: Inflammatory demyelinating peripheral neuropathies associated with HTLV-III infection. Ann Neurol 21:32, 1987. *A well-documented series describing demyelinating peripheral neuropathy in patients seropositive for human immunodeficiency virus and including experience with plasmapheresis.*

Navia BA, Jordan BD, Price RW: The AIDS dementia complex: I. Clinical features; II. Neuropathology. Ann Neurol 19:517, 525, 1986. *Companion articles describing the clinical and neuropathologic features of the AIDS dementia complex in an autopsy-based clinical series.*

Navia BA, Price RW: Central and peripheral nervous system complications of AIDS. Clin Immunol Allergy 6:543, 1987. *A general review of the neurologic complications of AIDS.*

Snider WD, Simpson DM, Nielsen S, et al.: Neurological complications of acquired immune deficiency syndrome: Analysis of 50 patients. Ann Neurol 14:403, 1983. *An early series outlining the spectrum of neurologic complications of AIDS.*

488.3 Creutzfeldt-Jakob Disease

Paul E. Bendheim

DEFINITION. Creutzfeldt-Jakob disease (CJD) is a central nervous system disorder characterized by a progressive dementia, myoclonus, and distinctive electroencephalographic and neuropathologic findings. Although uncommon, it is the most prevalent of the human subacute spongiform encephalopathies, fatal diseases caused by transmissible pathogens of uncertain type.

ETIOLOGY. CJD is closely related to kuru and scrapie. Scrapie is a spongiform encephalopathy of sheep experimentally transmissible to other animal species. The scrapie agent is not known to cause disease in humans. Kuru is a disease previously endemic among the Fore people inhabiting an area in the eastern highlands of Papua New Guinea. Cerebellar dysfunction, dementia, and progression to death within two years were typical. Women and children were affected much more frequently than men. Circumstantial evidence indicates that the kuru agent was transmitted to them through the ritual handling of affected tissues, especially brain, from deceased relatives. This cultural practice was discontinued and the incidence of kuru has decreased dramatically since 1959. Brain tissues from patients dying of kuru were inoculated into the brains of chimpanzees which, after a prolonged incubation period, developed a similar disease. Subsequently, the neuropathology of kuru and CJD were noted to be similar and experimental transmission studies using CJD-affected brain were undertaken. These experiments also were positive and CJD now has been transmitted to a wide range of laboratory animals.

The CJD, kuru, and animal spongiform encephalopathy agents are unlike any known virus or other well characterized transmissible pathogen. Their biochemical structures are incompletely known. This has resulted in the terms *slow spongiform encephalopathy virus*, *virino*, and *prion* being used interchangeably with *agent* to refer to them. The agents provoke no inflammatory response or specific antibody production. They are resistant to chemical and physical treatments that inactivate most viruses, including heat, formaldehyde, nuclease digestion, and ultraviolet and ionizing radiation. The agents can be inactivated by procedures that denature proteins. Unique fibrillar structures are observed in electron micrographs of samples prepared from CJD brain tissue. They resemble the abnormal fibrils that accumulate in scrapie-affected animals and may represent an aggregated form of the CJD agent.

INCIDENCE AND EPIDEMIOLOGY. On a worldwide basis the incidence of CJD is one case per million population. This incidence peaks in the fifth through seventh decades, although cases have been documented as early as the second decade. The sexes are equally affected. Approximately 250 deaths occur in the United States each year. Higher rates have been noted in Israel among Libyan-born Jews and in circumscribed areas of Czechoslovakia and Chile.

CJD usually occurs sporadically in middle-aged adults without known exposure. A family history is evident in 8 per cent of patients and suggests common exposure or a genetic susceptibility. Several reports document iatrogenic human-to-human transmission. CJD developed 18 months after surgery in the recipient of a corneal transplant whose donor had the disease. Two cases resulted from the use of stereotaxic electroencephalographic electrodes that had been used earlier to evaluate a patient with CJD. Additional clusters of cases have been reported suggesting neurosurgical transmission. Recently, CJD developed in four young adults who had received human pituitary gland growth hormone replacement therapy. It seems apparent that certain lots of the cadaveric hormone preparation were contaminated with the CJD agent. Incubation periods were between four and 21 years, emphasizing the astonishingly long incubation times of the spongiform encephalopathies. Additional cases may yet appear, since approximately 10,000 patients in the United States received this form of human growth hormone prior to its discontinuation in 1985.

PATHOLOGY. The pathologic findings in CJD are limited to the central nervous system, although the transmissible agent can be detected in many organs. Cortical neuronal depletion, marked reactive astrocytosis, intracellular vacuolar or spongiform change, and the absence of inflammation are the major features. Amyloid plaques occur in some cases.

CLINICAL MANIFESTATIONS. Vague psychiatric or behavioral symptoms suggesting a personality change often herald the onset of CJD, but within a few weeks or months a relentlessly progressive dementia becomes evident. Myoclonus is usually present at some time during the course. Deterioration is usually rapid, and 90 per cent of victims die within one year. CJD patients are afebrile and have normal blood and cerebrospinal fluid profiles. In the late stages, the electroencephalogram in at least 75 per cent of cases shows a diffusely slow background with superimposed complexes which may or may not be associated with myoclonus.

The dementia can be accompanied by signs of involvement of any part of the central nervous system. Signs of cerebellar and pyramidal tract dysfunction are found in most patients as the disease advances. Visual disturbances, extrapyramidal signs, and various dysphasias often occur. The terminal stage is marked by decorticate and decerebrate postures, stupor, and coma. Myoclonus may persist and massive myoclonic responses to auditory or other sensory stimuli may create the false impression that the patient is alert and responsive.

Subtypes of CJD based on distinctive clinical presentations have been delineated. The optic type features visual disturbances, usually cortical blindness. The dyskinetic form has prominent extrapyramidal signs, while the ataxic form resembles kuru with its marked cerebellar involvement. The Gerstmann-Sträussler syndrome is a familial form of CJD with slower progression and signs of spinocerebellar ataxia.

DIAGNOSIS. The diagnosis of CJD should be considered when a relatively rapid dementia and myoclonus develop in an adult patient with normal spinal fluid. The characteristic EEG recording is strongly supportive but often not present in early stages. Histopathologic examination of brain tissue is required for confirmation. Clinically, CJD can be mistaken for other dementing disorders, especially Alzheimer's disease (Chap. 461) which, however, usually has a more protracted course without either the myoclonus or the typical EEG. The recent development of scrapie antibodies that cross-react with CJD-specific proteins allows rapid immunologic confirmation of the diagnosis by brain biopsy or postmortem examination of specimens. Preliminary reports also indicate that a highly specific protein marker for CJD may exist in the cerebrospinal fluid of affected patients.

TREATMENT AND PROGNOSIS. No effective treatment is available and the disease appears to be uniformly fatal.

PREVENTION. Although CJD can be transmitted, the risk to health care workers and others having contact with patients is no higher than to the general population. Isolation of patients is not indicated, but certain guidelines should be followed. Hospital workers should wear gloves when handling tissues, blood, and spinal fluid. Accidental skin contact with possibly contaminated fluids or materials should be followed by washing with 1N sodium hydroxide or a 1:10 dilution of 5 per cent household chlorine bleach. All laboratory samples should be clearly marked and needles disposed of properly. The agent can be inactivated on contaminated surfaces using a 1:10 dilution of bleach for one hour. Surgical and pathologic instruments should be steam autoclaved for one hour at 132°C. No organs, tissues, or tissue products from patients with CJD or with any ill-defined neurologic disease should be used for transplantation or replacement therapy.

Bendheim PE, Bockman JM, McKinley MP, et al.: Scrapie and Creutzfeldt-Jakob disease prion proteins share physical properties and antigenic determinants. Proc Natl Acad Sci USA 82:997, 1985. *Experimental studies demonstrate that the scrapie and CJD agents contain antigenically similar proteins and aggregate into fibrillary structures visible by electron microscopy.*

Brown P, Cathala F, Castaigne P, et al.: Creutzfeldt-Jakob disease: Clinical analysis of a consecutive series of 230 neuropathologically verified cases. Ann Neurol 20:597, 1986. *Clinical features are detailed in this large series of documented cases.*

Brown P, Gajdusek DC, Gibbs CJ Jr, et al.: Potential epidemic of Creutzfeldt-Jakob disease from human growth hormone therapy. N Engl J Med 313:728, 1985. *This paper focuses on epidemiologic aspects of iatrogenic transmission.*

Carp RI, Merz PA, Kascsak RJ, et al.: Nature of the scrapie agent: current status of facts and hypotheses. J Gen Virol 66:1357, 1985. *A review that discusses the virus, virino, and prion models for the spongiform encephalopathies. Extensive references.*

Harrington MG, Merrill CR, Asher DM, et al.: Abnormal proteins in the cerebrospinal fluid of patients with Creutzfeldt-Jakob disease. N Engl J Med 315:279, 1986. *First report of a possible CSF diagnostic marker for CJD, which also cross-reacts with herpes simplex encephalitis fluid.*

Rosenberg RN, White CL III, Brown P, et al.: Precautions in handling tissues, fluids, and other contaminated materials from patients with documented or suspected Creutzfeldt-Jakob disease. Ann Neurol 19:75, 1986. *Safety guidelines for health care workers and specific decontamination protocols for surgical and pathologic instruments.*

488.4 Subacute Sclerosing Panencephalitis

Jerry S. Wolinsky

Subacute sclerosing panencephalitis is an uncommon disorder which primarily affects children but can have its clinical onset in early adult life. The archetypical patient with subacute sclerosing panencephalitis is a rural male with a known history of otherwise uncomplicated measles within the first two years of life. During the second decade, subtle behavioral abnormalities and neuropsychiatric disturbances emerge to imprecisely mark the onset of clinical disease. These progress in severity and are eventually replaced by a relentless neurologic syndrome characterized by dementia, motor impairment, and, often, visual disturbances. Myoclonus is a characteristic feature, usually accompanied by a distinctive electroencephalogram showing suppression of the normal background rhythm interrupted by synchronous bursts of high-voltage slow and sharp waves. Further clinical deterioration leads to a loss of useful motor function and produces a bedridden and preterminal vegetative state. Exceptions exist to this stereotyped pattern, and the tempo of progression can vary considerably. Most often, this disease follows a subacute course with a survival half-life of 12 months from first symptoms. However, five percent or more of all cases follow a protracted course lasting six or more years. Despite occasional extended remissions the disease is eventually fatal.

Diagnosis is straightforward once entertained. Computed tomographic scans or MRI can be normal early but show progressive cortical atrophy, ventricular enlargement, and multifocal low-density white matter lesions as the disease evolves. Most patients show remarkably elevated levels of immunoglobulins in their cerebrospinal fluid, reflecting the intrathecal synthesis of antibodies to measles virus. Diagnosis can be established with confidence based on the clinical course, the exclusion of mass lesions, an elevated cerebrospinal fluid gammaglobulin content, and a markedly increased cerebrospinal-fluid-to-serum ratio of measles virus antibody titers. Cerebral biopsy for confirmation of the diagnosis or virus isolation techniques are seldom justified as a routine approach.

Pathologic findings are limited to brain and consist of widespread perivascular infiltrates of mononuclear and plasma cells with gliosis in both grey and white matter. Demyelination is prominent. Glial cells and neurons contain intranuclear and intracytoplasmic (Dawson's) inclusions composed of viral nucleocapsids. Variable transcription and defective translation of measles viral mRNAs which code for membrane-associated viral gene products have been demonstrated in brain, but why this occurs in affected persons is unknown.

Progressive rubella panencephalitis is a rare slow virus disease which is similar to subacute sclerosing panencephalitis. Most patients show stigmata of the congenital rubella syndrome.

Neurologic symptoms and signs begin during the second decade and are similar to those of subacute sclerosing panencephalitis, except that disturbances of gait are prominent and myoclonus seldom is. The cerebrospinal fluid features resemble those of subacute sclerosing panencephalitis, but the elevated immunoglobulins are specific for rubella virus.

There is no generally accepted therapy for either subacute sclerosing panencephalitis or progressive rubella panencephalitis. Uncontrolled clinical trials have suggested that inosiplex or interferon may beneficially modify the course of subacute sclerosing panencephalitis. Myoclonus can often be managed with clonazepam.

Baczko K, Liebert UG, Billeter M, et al.: Expression of defective measles virus genes in brains of patients with subacute sclerosing panencephalitis. J Virol 59:472, 1986. *Detailed molecular analysis of restricted measles replication in the human disease.*

Waxham MN, Wolinsky JS: Rubella virus and its effects on the central nervous system. Neurol Clin 2:367, 1984. *Includes a recent review of progressive rubella panencephalitis.*

488.5 Progressive Multifocal Leukoencephalopathy

Richard W. Price

Progressive multifocal leukoencephalopathy is an uncommon demyelinating disorder resulting from opportunistic brain infection by a papovavirus which causes benign infection in the normal host. Early studies reported isolation of a simian papovarvirus, SV-40, from brains of patients with progressive multifocal leukoencephalopathy, but subsequent isolations have uniformly identified a previously unrecognized human papovavirus, JC virus (named after the patient from whom the first isolate was derived), as the major, if not the only, etiologic agent. Infection by JC virus is common worldwide; by the later teens more than 80 per cent of individuals in the United States exhibit serologic evidence of prior infection. Primary infection apparently results in little or no disease, and it is likely that the virus establishes a prolonged but innocent latent infection. Only rarely does depression of cell-mediated defenses related to some other condition result in viral reactivation with spread and consequent progressive central nervous system disease.

Until recently, the highest incidence of progressive multifocal leukoencephalopathy was in patients with Hodgkin's disease and chronic leukemias. The disease also was reported in patients with a variety of underlying conditions associated with depressed cell-mediated immunity as well as rarely in individuals without defined underlying disease. With the advent of the AIDS epidemic the incidence of this disorder has increased, although it still remains uncommon, having an autopsy incidence of less than 5 per cent of AIDS patients.

Progressive multifocal leukoencephalopathy usually has an insidious onset and steady progression. Symptoms and signs of cerebral dysfunction represent the commonest presentation and include gradually increasing hemiparesis, aphasia, cortical sensory impairment, or visual disturbance; posterior fossa involvement with cerebellar or brain-stem dysfunction occurs much less often. The disease typically begins with focal symptoms but proceeds to multifocal, bihemispheric abnormalities in most patients at the time of diagnostic evaluation. Steady progression characteristically leads to death within weeks to months after onset, although in non-AIDS patients spontaneous arrest of the disease has been reported.

Suspicion of diagnosis is based upon the presence of an underlying disorder with altered cell-mediated immunity and the characteristic clinical and laboratory findings. In the early stage, the CT scan typically shows one or more lucent areas in the subcortical white matter without contrast enhancement or mass effect. Initial experience with MRI indicates a greater sensitivity in detecting the characteristic white matter lesions. The cerebrospinal fluid is typically normal, except for occasional mild elevations of protein. Serum antibody titers against JC virus are not helpful in diagnosis because of the high seroprevalence in the community. Cerebrospinal fluid antibody against JC virus is almost invariably absent. Definitive diagnosis requires pathologic examination of a brain biopsy. Light microscopy of brain is usually adequate to establish the disease's unique histopathologic features, but immunohistochemical staining for viral antigen may be helpful for virologic confirmation.

At autopsy the gross appearance of the cut brain reveals multifocal lesions with a predilection for white matter. Microscopically the earliest lesions are most often observed in the subcortical white matter where small foci expand and coalesce, eventually giving rise to large confluent areas of demyelination. Little or no inflammation is present in the majority of cases.

There is no established treatment for this disorder. Several case reports have suggested that cytosine arabinoside may have a benefit, although no controlled trial has been undertaken. Where possible, the best therapeutic approach is to reverse the underlying immunosuppression.

Krupp LB, Lipton RB, Swerdlow ML, et al.: Progressive multifocal leukoencephalopathy: Clinical and radiographic features. Ann Neurol 17:344, 1985. *A description of seven cases of progressive multifocal leukoencephalopathy emphasizing the computer tomographic findings.*

Walker DL: Progressive multifocal leukoencephalopathy: An opportunistic viral infection of the nervous system. In Vinken PJ, Bruyn GW, Klawans HL (eds.): Handbook of Clinical Neurology. Vol. 34, Infections of the Nervous System, Part II. Amsterdam, Elsevier North-Holland, 1978. *A review that includes discussion of the virologic aspects of progressive multifocal leukoencephalopathy.*

489 CENTRAL NERVOUS SYSTEM COMPLICATIONS OF VIRAL INFECTIONS AND VACCINES

Central nervous system (CNS) symptoms and signs arising in the course of systemic infections usually reflect direct CNS invasion by the inciting organism. Less frequently, systemic infections, especially viral infections, or the administration of certain vaccines give rise to CNS abnormalities that do not appear to depend on direct invasion of the brain but rather to reflect dysfunction as the result of presumed autoimmune or toxic mechanisms selectively. Several reasonably distinct patterns of involvement have been delineated. Two of these, *acute disseminated encephalomyelitis* and *acute hemorrhagic encephalomyelitis*, appear to be mediated by immune mechanisms and have as peripheral nervous system counterpart, *acute inflammatory polyneuropathy* or the *Guillain-Barré syndrome*. The remainder, *Reye syndrome*, *acute toxic encephalopathy*, and *acute cerebellar ataxia of childhood*, are likely to be toxic in origin.

ACUTE DISSEMINATED ENCEPHALOMYELITIS (ADE)

DEFINITION. Acute disseminated encephalomyelitis (*parainfectious* or *postinfectious encephalomyelitis, acute demyelinating encephalitis, immune-mediated encephalomyelitis*) is an acute disease of the CNS that most commonly occurs in association with viral infections or as a complication of vaccination. Involvement of brain and spinal cord is usually widespread but may be limited to discrete areas such as the optic nerves, as in optic neuritis or papillitis, or to a single spinal cord level, as in acute transverse myelitis.

ETIOLOGY AND PATHOGENESIS. Table 489–1 lists principal predisposing factors to ADE.

The neurologic complications usually occur six to ten days after the appearance of the exanthem or onset of other specific symptoms. However, ADE can occur prior to or concomitantly with systemic symptoms of infection. Characteristically, ADE begins ten days to three weeks after initiation of the vaccination regimen. Perhaps the most easily understood form of ADE is that which followed vaccination against rabies with

TABLE 489–1. PRINCIPAL CONDITIONS PREDISPOSING TO ACUTE DISSEMINATED ENCEPHALOMYELITIS

Infections	
Measles	*Mycoplasma pneumoniae*
Varicella-zoster	Respiratory agents
Influenza	E-B virus
Rubella	

Vaccines: smallpox, measles, rabies (Semple vaccine)

(now obsolete) inactivated inoculum of fixed rabies virus propagated in animal brain. These early vaccines were contaminated with CNS proteins, including the antigens associated with myelin. Both complement-fixing antibody and specific lymphocyte blast transformation responses to crude and purified CNS antigens have been measured in blood of patients receiving rabies vaccine, and the responses were highest in those whose vaccination was complicated by ADE; the incidence of neuroparalytic accidents was reported to be as high as 1:600 to 1:6000 persons. Current rabies vaccines derived from virus grown in human diploid cells appear to be essentially free of neural complications (Ch. 487).

A compelling analogy links rabies vaccine-related ADE to the animal experimental disorder, *experimental allergic encephalomyelitis (EAE)*. In EAE, brain homogenates, highly purified myelin components, or peptides containing the encephalogenic sequences of myelin basic protein (MBP) can induce an acute CNS perivascular inflammatory and demyelinative reaction that is histologically identical to ADE. In affected animals, clinical disease begins 10 to 14 days after sensitization and is associated with both humoral and cellular immune responses directed against the inciting CNS antigen(s). Furthermore, EAE can be adoptively transferred to naive animals by T lymphocytes, suggesting that this cell type is of primary importance in the pathogenesis.

The occurrence of ADE following viral infections is more difficult to understand. Encephalitis is relatively frequent following measles (1:1000 cases), but there is little evidence to implicate invasion of the CNS by measles virus as an obligate prerequisite· and no compelling data support cross-reactivity between the antigens of measles virus and CNS proteins such as MBP. Nonetheless, very early in the course of measles ADE, specific blast transformation responses to MBP are apparent in the lymphocytes of children and measurable quantities of MBP are released into the cerebrospinal fluid (CSF). These findings support the hypothesis that acute measles transiently alters the immune system, which in some persons results in a breakdown of tolerance to CNS antigens. Despite the usual absence of CNS symptoms, this process appears to occur frequently, as reflected by a high incidence of abnormal appearing electroencephalograms (EEGs). Both EEG abnormalities and clinical ADE can occur after vaccination with live attenuated measles virus but at a markedly lower frequency, with ADE arising in about 1:1,000,000 vaccinated persons.

INCIDENCE. Valid incidence figures for ADE are difficult to derive. Encephalitis complicates about 1:1000 cases of measles. ADE following vaccination for smallpox is only of historical interest but occurred in the United States with a reported incidence of 2.9 per million primary vaccinations. ADE following other childhood viral illnesses or vaccinations is uncommon. Most adult cases of ADE have no identifiable antecedents.

PATHOLOGY. Neuropathologic changes consists of perivenular infiltration by lymphocytic and mononuclear cells and variable amounts of primary demyelination extending in centripetal manner from involved vessels of the white matter. The axons are relatively spared. This primary lesion can occur throughout the neuraxis but tends to be most prominent in the centrum semiovale of the cerebrum and in the pontine white matter. The brain may appear somewhat swollen or grossly normal. Repair occurs through remyelination. In certain cases, large confluent demyelination can take on a superficial resemblance to the plaques of multiple sclerosis, differing primarily in that all lesions reflect a similar age of onset.

CLINICAL MANIFESTATIONS. The clinical disorder can resemble almost any of the acute encephalitides. In adults neurologic symptoms often first suggest the illness. With the childhood exanthemata, CNS symptoms usually begin about five days after the onset of the rash (range 0 to 24 days, with rare examples of ADE preceding the rash). The course of the preceding illness is in no way atypical for patients who subsequently develop ADE. Fever or recrudescence of fever is nearly universal. Headache, with or without meningismus, and lethargy occur in from 20 to 80 per cent of cases. In about half of the cases there is one or more generalized seizure. Usually the onset of altered consciousness is abrupt, occurring within a few hours, but CNS symptoms sometimes evolve over several days. Stupor, delirium, or coma develops in severe cases. Multifocal motor and sensory deficits of varied severity are common and often asymmetrical.

The EEG is abnormal in appearance, with widespread slowing of background rhythms. The CSF in children almost invariably shows a modest mononuclear pleocytosis of 20 to 200 cells per cubic millimeter and occasionally higher. Adult CSF is sometimes acellular. The fluid contains a slight elevation of protein content, a normal glucose level, and a raised myelin basic protein level. After several days, CT or MRI may show scattered white matter lesions, at least some of which enhance with contrast during the acute phases of the disease.

The duration of active CNS disease varies from days to weeks, often with a protracted convalescence. The overall mortality is about 20 per cent. About 90 per cent of survivors recover completely or nearly completely, although severe residual deficits can occur.

DIAGNOSIS. Diagnosis in ADE is by exclusion. First encephalitis, meningitis, or meningoencephalitis must be excluded as a direct effect of a virus or other infectious agent. In the setting of a recent exanthematous illness or vaccination, ADE is more readily implied. However, in pathologic series of clinically diagnosed ADE occurring in the course of mass vaccination programs, postmortem examination proved the majority of patients to have had other illnesses, including potentially treatable CNS infections. Differentiation of an initial severe episode of multiple sclerosis can be challenging, but subsequent recurrences eventually make the proper diagnosis clear.

TREATMENT. Treatment consists of supportive care, including the use of anticonvulsants and, when necessary, intensive care monitoring. Neither corticosteroids nor other immunosuppressive drugs have proved benefit.

ACUTE HEMORRHAGIC LEUKOENCEPHALITIS

Acute hemorrhagic leukoencephalitis is a fulminant and fatal syndrome believed to have an immunopathogenesis similar to that of ADE. Typically, the illness arises either spontaneously or following an uneventful upper respiratory illness. Sudden headache precedes the neurologic symptoms, which include seizures and rapid progression from lethargy to coma in a matter of a few hours to several days. Major focal neurologic abnormalities are common and may suggest lateralized cerebral involvement. Systemic signs and symptoms include fever and marked peripheral leukocytosis. The accompanying CSF pleocytosis usually shows a preponderance of polymorphonuclear cells and sometimes evidence of minor degrees of hemorrhage into the subarachnoid space. More than 80 per cent of all recognized cases of acute hemorrhagic leukoencephalitis are fatal, although these findings may be biased by selective reports of postmortem studies. The brain is usually swollen, and examination shows bilateral but asymmetric abnormalities with petechial hemorrhages scattered throughout the white matter. Microscopic lesions consist of features reminiscent of hyperimmune forms of EAE. The clinical differential diagnosis includes ADE and acute viral encephalitis, especially herpes simplex encephalitis (see Ch. 485.1). Computed tomography may be diagnostically helpful in selected cases. Therapy is supportive.

Dunn V, Bale JF Jr, Zimmerman RA, et al.: MRI in children with postinfectious disseminated encephalomyelitis. Mag Res Imag 4:25, 1986. *Early examples of the potential contribution of magnetic resonance imaging to the diagnosis of ADE.*

Hemachudha T, Phanuphak P, Johnson RT, et al.: Neurologic complications of Semple-type rabies vaccine: Clinical and immunologic studies. Neurology 37:550, 1987. *A new look at a classic problem.*

Johnson RT, Griffin DE, Hirsch RL, et al.: Measles encephalomyelitis—Clinical and immunological studies. N Engl J Med 310:137, 1984. *A multifaceted study of ADE complicating natural measles which emphasizes possible mechanisms of disease pathogenesis.*

490 REYE SYNDROME

DEFINITION. Reye syndrome is a well delineated biphasic disease in which one of several common viral illnesses is followed by an acute and sometimes fatal encephalopathy associated with fatty infiltration and dysfunction of the liver.

ETIOLOGY AND PATHOGENESIS. Reye syndrome most commonly occurs following influenza A, influenza B, and herpes varicella-zoster virus infections. Many other common viral illnesses have been implicated, each at a much lower frequency. Little evidence links the precipitating viral infection directly to either the central nervous system or hepatic involvement. A toxic origin is proposed for both types of involvement. The hepatic dysfunction appears to be the primary error and the direct result of a mitochondrial disturbance that causes secondary metabolic derangements including hyperammonemia, lactic acidemia, and elevated levels of serum-free fatty acids. The latter derangements have been implicated in the pathogenesis of the brain swelling and increased intracranial pressure that dominate the clinical course of severe cases. What causes the mitochondrial impairment remains to be clarified. Available epidemiologic evidence suggests that aspirin plays a potentiating role in the pathogenesis of this syndrome.

INCIDENCE. Reye syndrome occurs most commonly among children between 1 and 15 years of age but has been reported in adolescents and rarely in adults. Inner-city black infants may be especially at risk for the disease. Prospectively derived incidence figures for susceptible age groups are as high as 6.2 per 100,000 children.

PATHOLOGY. The liver shows a noninflammatory, panlobular, hepatocellular accumulation of lipid droplets and both histochemical and ultrastructural evidence of inflammation. At postmortem examination, swelling of astrocytic foot processes and ultrastructural changes in mitochondria similar to those seen in hepatic mitochondria may be found in the greatly swollen brain.

CLINICAL MANIFESTATIONS AND COURSE. Reye syndrome is a biphasic disorder. As symptoms of the initial viral illness begin to wane or clear, the dramatic features begin, usually with intractable vomiting associated with lethargy or delirium. Early diagnosis is confirmed by the findings of nonicteric hepatic dysfunction, an elevated arterial blood ammonia level, and serum transaminase levels that exceed three times normal levels. Hepatic enlargement is present in about one half of the cases. Children under one year of age often show hypoglycemia. Signs of central nervous system deterioration include the development of generalized seizures, deepening obtundation, and transtentorial herniation. The cerebrospinal fluid is under increased pressure but is acellular, with otherwise normal constituents.

DIAGNOSIS. Diagnosis rests on the clinical findings and appropriate biochemical abnormalities. Liver biopsy usually is not necessary. Central nervous system infection or the presence of known toxins, particularly salicylate, must be actively excluded. A childhood syndrome, distinguishable from Reye syndrome only by the absence of hepatic involvement and a high incidence of acute convulsions, can follow both banal viral infections and vaccination.

TREATMENT. Affected patients require intensive care monitoring until the course of the disease is well established. Hypoglycemia and electrolyte abnormalities must be corrected. Many authorities suggest hydration with solutions of high glucose content. Appropriate measures should be taken to continuously monitor intracranial pressure in the more severely affected cases, as judicious control of intracranial hypertension contributes to a favorable outcome. Mortality is about 10 per cent.

Barrett MJ, Hurwitz ES, Schonberger LB, et al.: Changing epidemiology of Reye syndrome in the United States. Pediatrics 77:598, 1986.
DeVivo DC: Reye syndrome. Neurol Clin 3:95, 1985. *A comprehensive review including detailed recommendations for the medical management of affected children.*

491 NEUROLOGIC COMPLICATIONS IN THE IMMUNOLOGICALLY COMPROMISED HOST

Modern treatment of several previously fatal conditions in many instances leads to an immunocompromised state that is associated with opportunistic infections of the central nervous system (CNS). Such treatments include transplantation for organ failure; chemotherapy and radiotherapy of malignancies; and immunosuppressive treatment of autoimmune diseases. The epidemic emergence of the acquired immune deficiency syndrome (AIDS) also has been associated with a marked increase in the number of unusual CNS infections likely to be encountered in routine practice.

CENTRAL NERVOUS SYSTEM INFECTIONS IN TRANSPLANT RECIPIENTS. Renal transplantation is now commonplace, and bone marrow, cardiac, and other organ transplantations are performed with increasing effectiveness. Hospital-acquired bacterial species predominate in early infections in transplant recipients. Immunosuppression, especially lethal irradiation used in preparation for marrow transplantation from nonidentical donors, almost predictably gives rise to reactivation of herpes viruses: first herpes simplex viruses types 1 and 2 (HSV), then herpes varicella-zoster virus (HVZ), and finally cytomegalovirus (CMV). The systemic manifestations of each can be overwhelming, but symptomatic CNS dissemination has so far been remarkably infrequent. However, encephalitis or meningitis can complicate either HSV or HVZ infections. Also, while EEG, CT, or MRI findings evolve as anticipated in the intact host, the CSF pleocytosis is often absent, especially in patients with severe leukopenia.

CNS involvement by CMV has been pathologically documented in transplant patients but has not been associated with a recognizable clinical syndrome and presently appears to be asymptomatic. The availability of effective antiviral chemotherapy now makes it imperative to attempt early diagnosis in cases of suspected HSV or HVZ meningoencephalitis (see Ch. 483).

Transplant patients are at greatest risk of infection by opportunistic agents after the second month of the transplant. They remain at risk while they are on most immunosuppressive regimens, if they are azotemic, and when there are ongoing graft-versus-host or chronic rejection reactions. *Listeria monocytogenes, Cryptococcus neoformans,* and *Aspergillus fumigatus* account for the overwhelming majority of infections. *Toxoplasma gondii, Candida* species, *Nocardia asteroides,* the rhinocerebral phycomycoses, and *Coccidioides immitis* are less frequently encountered.

The acute or subacute development of fever in the transplant patient should suggest *Listeria* meningitis even in the absence of meningeal signs. The CSF has the characteristics of a purulent meningitis, although occasionally patients with *Listeria* infection have misleading mononuclear pleocytosis (see Ch. 272). Otherwise unexplained headache of acute to chronic duration, even in the absence of a febrile response or confusion, should suggest the possibilty of cryptococcal meningitis. A mononuclear pleocytosis with or without a low glucose content are the characteristic CSF findings (see Ch. 373). India ink preparations can provide immediate confirmation of diagnosis and tests for cryptococcus antigen can be more helpful than direct culture of the organism from the CSF. Since both listerial and cryptococcal meningitis represent some of the most frequently encountered and more manageable infections that affect the immunocompromised host, careful attention must be given to symptoms that suggest infection of the CNS.

Aspergillis fumigatus infections of the CNS usually are manifested as acute fulminant disease with seizures, obtundation, and, frequently, apoplectic onset of focal neurologic deficits. The propensity of *Aspergillis* to invade and destroy blood vessels underlies the frequent strokelike appearance of infected patients. Low density lesions with ill-defined, poorly contrast-enhancing borders may be seen on computed tomography, but diagnosis depends on brain biopsy in the absence of systemic disease. Current diagnostic and therapeutic approaches to this CNS infection are inadequate (see Ch. 376).

CENTRAL NERVOUS SYSTEM INFECTION IN PATIENTS WITH LYMPHOMA, LEUKEMIA, OR CHRONIC IMMUNOSUPPRESSIVE THERAPY. Splenectomy, often used in the staging of Hodgkin's disease, places patients at increased risk for conventional bacterial infections that may be complicated by meningitis. In community-acquired infections, *Hemophilus influenzae* and *Streptococcus pneumoniae* species predominate. Metastatic spread from various systemic sites by a wide spectrum of bacterial organisms is a continual threat for all immunosuppressed patients. The usual signs and symptoms of CNS infection can be obscured by the anti-inflammatory effect of therapy. The use of chronic immunosuppressive therapy for leukemia, lymphoma, or presumed autoimmune disorders can be complicated by *Listeria monocytogenesis* in a manner similar to that described for transplant patients. The emergence of listerial meningitis often follows an increase in the intensity of the immunosuppressive regimen.

Cryptococcal meningitis and *Aspergillus* meningoencephalitis are significant sources of morbidity for this group of patients. Their clinical appearances parallel those seen in organ-transplant patients. Segmental zoster, occasionally with dissemination, is a well recognized problem among these patients, and CNS toxoplasmosis is occasionally encountered. Of special interest is *progressive multifocal leukoencephalopathy (PML)* (Ch. 488.4), which may account for up to 10 per cent of all CNS infections in this patient group. Progressive deterioration in mental status and the evolution of focal neurologic deficits in the absence of meningismus or CSF abnormalities characterize the clinical symptomatology of PML. Serial computed tomographic scans are usually diagnostic, but the recent observation that some patients with CNS infections by HVZ can have a clinical course similar to that of PML must be considered because HVZ is potentially responsive to antiviral chemotherapy.

Hooper DS, Pruitt AA, Rubin RH: Central nervous system infection in the chronically immunosuppressed. Medicine 61:166, 1982. *Analysis of 10 years' experience with opportunistic CNS infections at a major hospital and comprehensive literature review.*

SECTION ELEVEN / THE DEMYELINATING DISEASES

492 THE DEMYELINATING DISEASES

Donald H. Silberberg

The demyelinating diseases affect myelin to a greater extent than other nervous system components. This section discusses disorders that primarily affect central nervous system (CNS) myelin; the demyelinating peripheral neuropathies are discussed in Ch. 506. A few disorders, such as the neurologic complications of vitamin B_{12} deficiency and some of the leukodystrophies, affect both central and peripheral myelin.

Since central myelin is an extension of the oligodendrocyte, which manufactures the myelin sheath, most demyelinating diseases include alterations in or disappearance of this glial cell. An oligodendrocyte process wraps around a segment of an axon in a concentric fashion to form myelin. One oligodendrocyte sends processes to as many as 20 or 30 axons within a surrounding area of several millimeters, myelinating axon segments of 1 mm or less on each fiber. The most active synthesis of myelin starts in utero and continues for the first two years of life; subsequently, slower synthesis continues until the adult CNS is achieved.

TABLE 492–1. DISORDERS SELECTIVELY AFFECTING MYELIN

I. Demyelinating diseases (acquired destruction of preformed myelin)
  A. Multiple sclerosis
    1. Uniphasic events presumably related to multiple sclerosis
      a. Optic neuritis
      b. Acute transverse myelopathy
  B. Parainfectious disorders
    1. Acute disseminated encephalomyelitis
    2. Acute hemorrhagic leukoencephalopathy
  C. Viral infections
    1. Progressive multifocal leukoencephalopathy
    2. Subacute sclerosing panencephalitis
  D. Nutritional disorders
    1. Combined systems disease (B_{12} deficiency)
    2. Demyelination of the corpus callosum (Marchiafava-Bignami)
    3. Central pontine myelinolysis
  E. Anoxic-ischemic sequelae
    1. Delayed postanoxic cerebral demyelination
    2. Progressive subcortical ischemic encephalopathy
II. Dysmyelinating diseases (developmental failure to form or maintain myelin)
  A. The leukodystrophies
    1. Metachromatic leukodystrophy
    2. Sudanophilic (Pelizaeus-Merzbacher disease)
    3. Globoid cell (Krabbe's disease)
    4. Adrenoleukodystrophy (Schilder's disease)
    5. Others (e.g., Alexander's, Canavan's, Seitelberger's disease)
  B. Aminoacidurias (e.g., phenylketonuria)
  C. Neonatal hypothyroidism

Each tightly compacted layer of mature myelin is a bimolecular lipid leaflet between parallel layers of hydrated protein, which is in close apposition to the polar groups of the lipid molecules. The lipids, which constitute about 75 per cent of the dry weight of myelin, include cerebroside, phospholipids, and cholesterol. Proteins include the distinctive molecule, myelin basic protein (the antigen capable of eliciting experimental allergic encephalomyelitis in experimental animals), proteolipid proteins, and many others detectable by electrophoretic separation but not yet well characterized. Turnover of the components of mature myelin continues at a slower rate than the rate during development. Both developing and mature myelin are readily susceptible to injury by many diseases.

CLASSIFICATION. Definitive classification awaits an understanding of the causes of these disorders. Failing that, a mixed temporal-etiologic-descriptive classification must serve as the scaffold. A useful distinction is to separate what seem to be acquired disorders from those which are errors in development (Table 492–1). Multiple sclerosis will be discussed first, since it is by far the most common of these problems.

MULTIPLE SCLEROSIS

DEFINITION. Multiple sclerosis (MS) is a disorder of unknown etiology, defined by its clinical characteristics and by typical scattered areas of brain, optic nerve, and spinal cord demyelination. Clinical diagnosis requires evidence on neurologic examination of two or more CNS white matter lesions, preferably with at least a month's interval between symptoms, in a patient of the appropriate age, in whom evidence is lacking of any other explanation for the signs and symptoms. MS usually produces its first clinical symptoms between ages 15 and 50 years. Occasional cases occur beyond these extremes, but the average age of onset is 33. Most patients recover clinically to some extent from individual bouts of demyelination, producing the classic remitting and exacerbating course of the early disease. Except for autopsy findings, presently available laboratory data may support the clinical diagnosis but cannot be used to define MS.

ETIOLOGY. The cause of MS remains unknown. The tissue response has features of an immunopathologic process, with perivenular mononuclear cell infiltration and absence of any overt histopathologic evidence of an infection. Two other lines of evidence point to either an immunologic cause or immunologic participation in the MS process; (1) the frequent elevation of cerebrospinal fluid (CSF) gamma globulin, and the common oligoclonal pattern in the gamma globulin region on CSF electrophoresis, apparently synthesized by plasma cells in areas of demyelination, and (2) changes in the proportion of lymphocyte subclasses in the peripheral blood,

CSF and brain lesions. These changes are, however, nonspecific and may be the consequence of demyelination induced by some other disease mechanism, rather than the cause of the demyelination.

Epidemiologic studies suggest an infectious etiology. Perhaps the best evidence for this is the outbreak of MS which occurred in the Faroe Islands during the 20 years following the start of World War II. The Faroes were occupied by British troops during the war. No cases of MS had occurred prior to the occupation. The sudden appearance of MS starting several years after the arrival of the troops strongly suggests the presence of an infectious agent. The geographic areas where MS is prevalent are more common farther from the equator, suggesting the presence of an environmental factor, presumably an infectious agent. Efforts continue without confirmed success to recover a virus from MS tissues. MS is among the diseases with a strong linkage to certain HLA haplotypes. The particular haplotype varies from one population group to another. In North America, haplotypes Dw2 and DR2, D locus markers, are found in about 65 per cent of MS patients, as compared with 15 per cent of control subjects. Additional evidence for an immunogenetic component in the etiology of MS is the increase in frequency of MS among close relatives and the fact that MS is rare among Orientals, even after emigration to the United States. A possible synthesis is that MS is an unusual consequence of infection by a common virus, or any of several viruses, with subsequent immunologic alterations in genetically susceptible individuals.

INCIDENCE AND PREVALENCE. The prevalence of MS in the northern United States and Canada and in northern Europe is about 60 per 100,000 population. In Denmark the chance of an individual developing MS in a lifetime is 1 in 500. The risk is somewhat higher for women. MS is almost unknown among Orientals and among African blacks. There is no evidence for changing incidence or prevalence, except where population patterns are undergoing changes as the result of immigration.

EPIDEMIOLOGY. MS is more common farther from the equator in North America, Europe, and in Australia and New Zealand. Regional population figures are punctuated by many reports of clusters of cases in a small area, such as particular cantons in Switzerland.

Many of the population studies were done before the availability of HLA typings, so that some of the observed regional differences may prove to have a genetic basis. Multiple sclerosis occurs in both members of about 50 per cent of monozygous twin pairs when the disease has been identified in one. This supports the concept that genetic susceptibility may increase the chances of developing MS but is not sufficient to cause it and may not be required for its development.

PATHOLOGY. The lesions of MS consist of scattered areas of dissolution of CNS myelin, within which the axons remain intact. The border between histologically normal myelin and myelin dissolution is often sharp, or may shade from normal to thinning before bare axons occur. Some areas show only partial myelin destruction. Lesions range in size from 1 mm to several centimeters in diameter, and occur throughout the brain, optic nerves (which are central tracts of white matter), and spinal cord. Although plaques may occur anywhere within CNS myelin, predilections involve the optic nerves, periventricular regions within the cerebrum, and cervical spinal cord. Most plaques occur near blood vessels.

Oligodendrocytes disappear from within plaques. Astrocytes proliferate forming the scar that lent the term "sclerosis" to multiple sclerosis. One always finds many more plaques at autopsy than could have been suspected on the basis of the clinical history and examination. Similarly, the sensitivity and resolution provided by magnetic resonance imaging (MRI) often reveal clinically unsuspected plaques. Occasionally, typical plaques of MS are found in previously asymptomatic individuals at autopsy. The acute lesion of MS may produce considerable edema, visible as cord swelling on myelography or optic nerve enlargement on imaging studies. Electron microscope examination of plaques shows evidence of attempts at remyelination. However, this is not nearly so complete as to explain the remissions of neurologic dysfunction that characterize MS and which remain unexplained.

Plasma cells appear to synthesize much of the excess of gamma globulin which is found in and around plaques and in CSF. Plasma cells occur throughout affected tissue, and persist in large numbers throughout a patient's lifetime, correlating with the observation that once CSF gamma globulin elevation appears, it persists. It is not known whether plasma cells and other mononuclear cells precede, accompany, or follow myelin and oligodendrocyte destruction.

LABORATORY ABNORMALITIES. *Cerebrospinal Fluid.* CSF gamma globulin elevation occurs in about 75 per cent of MS patients, more commonly after the first year following the appearance of symptoms. Normal CSF gamma globulin is less than 13 per cent of total CSF protein by most testing methods. The gamma globulin is mostly IgG, but often contains IgA and IgM as well. Separate discrete "oligoclonal" bands are seen in the gamma region on agarose or polyacrylamide gel electrophoresis in about 90 per cent of patients, including some with normal total IgG levels. These abnormalities are helpful when other causes of the phenomenon are excluded; these include CNS syphilis, subacute sclerosing panencephalitis, chronic meningitis, and any disease associated with a peripheral blood paraproteinemia. Other CSF abnormalities in MS can include elevation in total protein, usually to no more than 100 mg per deciliter, and an increase in the number of mononuclear white cells, usually to 5 to 15 per cu mm, rarely to more than 50 per cu mm. Myelin destruction releases myelin basic protein (MBP) into the CSF, which can be detected by radioimmunoassay. The amount present correlates wtih disease activity and lesion size and location; none is detectable normally, or during quiescent periods in MS patients. MBP levels rise in association with acute attacks or rapid progression. This serves as a valuable index of disease activity, but is not specific to MS. Myelin destruction from any other cause, such as acute infarction, causes a similar elevation of MBP.

Alterations in the ratio of subclasses of peripheral blood and of CSF lymphocytes occur at the time of acute exacerbations. These changes, which may indicate abnormalities of immunoregulation, are presently of investigative interest only.

Neurophysiologic Function Studies. The presence of myelin enhances the propagation of the nerve impulse along the axon. Loss of myelin, from any cause, slows conduction velocity. This alteration in conduction velocity can be measured by timing the appearance of an evoked potential (visual, auditory, or somatosensory) after an appropriate stimulus. Measurement of the latency of the visual evoked response (VER) is used most widely (Ch. 456.2). The normal latency from stimulus to evoked response in most laboratories is less than 102 to 105 milliseconds. A prolonged latency indicates an abnormality in the visual system, most commonly within the optic nerve in patients with MS. An abnormality of the visual, auditory, or somatosensory evoked response is used to detect dysfunction (prolonged conduction velocity) either as an objective measurement of what has already been detected clinically or for detection of a presumed subclinical abnormality.

CT and MR Scans. Hypodense areas seen with the CT scan reflect the presence of lesions in various stages, ranging from inflammation with edema to various degrees of demyelination. Edema, which may resemble a mass lesion, often occurs acutely. During this stage, leakage of intravenously injected iodinated contrast material into the lesion area reflects abnormal leakage of the blood-brain barrier. Atrophy is seen in those instances of severe demyelination.

TABLE 492–2. FIRST SYMPTOMS OF MULTIPLE SCLEROSIS IN 937 PATIENTS*

Symptom	Per Cent†
Weakness	48
Paresthesias	31
Visual loss	25
Incoordination	15
Vertigo	6
Sphincter impairment	6

*Combined series of Carter et al., Res Publ Assoc Nerv Ment Dis 28:471, 1950; Poser CM: Recent advances in multiple sclerosis. Med Clin North Am 56:1343, 1972; and McAlpine et al., Multiple Sclerosis: A Reappraisal. 2nd ed. Edinburgh, Churchill Livingstone, 1972.

†Many patients experience more than one symptom at onset.

MR imaging provides a much more sensitive method for detecting hypodense areas of demyelination, and often reveals many more areas of abnormality than were suspected clinically. The use of intravenously injected paramagnetic agents such as gadolinium permits detection of alterations in the blood-brain barrier with MRI. The abnormalities detected by CSF examination, neurophysiologic testing, and by imaging are not specific for MS (see Role of Laboratory Aids, p. 2214).

CLINICAL MANIFESTATIONS. *Onset.* The random distribution of MS lesions leads to a variety of initial symptoms and signs, alone or in combination. Further, it must be kept in mind that lesions occur in clinically silent areas of CNS white matter so that the first lesion that announces itself clinically may not be the first that has occurred in an individual. Common initial problems include weakness of one or more extremities, unilateral visual loss (optic neuritis), incoordination, and paresthesias (Table 492–2). Urinary frequency, incontinence, hesitancy, or retention; vertigo; hearing loss; facial, extremity, or truncal pain; dysarthria; and changes in intellectual function occur less commonly. Weakness most often affects the lower extremities and may produce a range of dysfunction from slight fatigability to paraparesis. The arm and hand may be involved alone or with the legs. Patients who develop paraparesis often develop urinary urgency and constipation. Incoordination as the result of cerebellar lesions, or loss of position sense, may occur independently of weakness and often leads to gait impairment or to tremor-like, clumsy movements of the arms and hands. Paresthesias range from the spontaneous perception of vague pins-and-needles discomfort, or girdle-like pressures, to the pain of classic trigeminal neuralgia. Loss of perception of vibration and position at the ankle and toes is common; loss of pain and touch perception is less frequent. Impairment of two-point discrimination over the palmar surface of the fingertips often accompanies cervical cord lesions.

Visual loss can vary in degree from slight blurring with a small central scotoma, slight decrease in acuity, and a slight impairment of color perception, to no light perception. The patient often reports pain on eye movement acutely. Other visual symptoms include blurring secondary to nystagmus on primary gaze, or explicit perception of nystagmus as spontaneous movement of objects (oscillopsia). Diplopia often occurs as the result of involvement of the pontine white matter. Horizontal nystagmus of the abducting eye on lateral gaze with paresis of the adducting eye, termed *internuclear ophthalmoplegia*, is common. It is often unilateral at first, and is due to lesions involving the median longitudinal fasciculus in the pons. In rare instances, extensive midline lesions lead to alterations of consciousness.

The speed of onset of symptoms varies from minutes to days, and in patients with a chronic progressive course symptoms may appear to increase gradually over many months. Recovery (remission) varies enormously, but usually occurs over the course of two to eight weeks following an acute bout.

Clinical Course. At least 70 per cent of patients improve in the days to months following their initial bout, the degree ranging from slight to virtual disappearance of the neurologic dysfunction. Whether or not a particular patient will improve, and to what extent, is as unpredictable as whether or not more lesions will occur and when. Overall, about three fourths of patients experience exacerbations and remissions early in their course. In many, however, as time goes by, the recovery from individual bouts decreases, disability results from accumulated failures to improve, and the course becomes chronically progressive.

About 30 per cent of patients develop successive disabilities without remission, often with long periods of clinical stability between periods of deterioration. This course occurs more commonly in patients experiencing their first neurologic manifestations after age 45. Older onset patients seem to compress the course of events, and often develop the same degree of dysfunction within a few years that takes decades to occur in a younger onset patient.

Most patients experience additional difficulties at some time after their initial symptoms; subsequent acute bouts or chronic progression may produce signs and symptoms in any combination. Several generalizations are of interest, but help little when counseling the individual. Ten years after onset about 50 per cent of patients are still able to carry out their household and/or employment responsibilities. Twenty years after onset about 25 per cent have these capacities. However, a fortunate few patients never develop significant disabilities, whereas others are bedridden within months after onset. One of the major psychologic burdens borne by patients with MS is the uncertainty about their future. Most neurologists find it useful to emphasize the hopeful possibilities, allowing the patient's course to reveal its own manner of progression.

The average interval from clinical onset to death is 35 years. Premature death is usually due to bacterial infection resulting from urinary retention, decubiti, or inability to handle pulmonary secretions. Rarely, primary respiratory failure from lower medullary lesions spells the terminal event.

FACTORS POSSIBLY AFFECTING THE CLINICAL COURSE. Elevation of body temperature by as little as 0.5°C noticeably reduces neurologic function in some patients, particularly those with recent disease activity. Reduction in visual acuity, incoordination or weakness, and sensory or bladder dysfunction can be affected. This is the result of slowed axonal conduction induced by heating, and the alterations disappear within hours of regaining normal body temperature. For this reason, many patients' conditions worsen with the fevers of an intercurrent infection. Patients should be instructed to rest and respond to respiratory infections with more care than they might otherwise exercise and to use aspirin to reduce fever.

Pregnancy makes neither exacerbations nor progression of MS more likely. Decisions regarding child bearing should be made on the basis of the patient's overall situation, rather than on the basis of this concern alone.

DIAGNOSIS. Despite the availability of increasingly complex laboratory aids, multiple sclerosis remains fundamentally a clinical diagnosis (Table 492–3). Physical signs on examination providing solid evidence for two or more lesions of central white matter occurring at least a month apart in a patient between age 10 and the early 50's, in the absence of any other possible etiology, are required. If the evidence for a second lesion is history or a laboratory abnormality alone, the diagnosis should be considered possible or probable,

TABLE 492–3. DIAGNOSTIC CRITERIA FOR MULTIPLE SCLEROSIS

Clinically Definite Multiple Sclerosis
Two attacks + clinical evidence of two lesions
Other conditions ruled out

Clinically Probable Multiple Sclerosis
Two attacks + clinical evidence of one lesion
or
One attack + clinical evidence of two or more lesions

rather than clinically definite MS. The differential diagnosis includes cervical cord compression resulting from tumor or cervical spondylosis; cerebral, cerebellar, brain-stem, and pituitary tumors; familial spinocerebellar degenerations; acute systemic lupus erythematosus (SLE); sarcoidosis; brain-stem atherosclerotic cerebrovascular disease; vitamin B$_{12}$ deficiency; chronic barbiturate or other intoxications; and psychogenic disturbances.

If all of the patient's signs can be attributed to a lesion in a single area of the nervous system, the working assumption must be that one is not dealing with MS. In patients with a persistent headache, seizures, persistent and progressive unifocal signs, or papilledema (without a central scotoma), CT scan or MRI is the most sensitive screening procedure. High-resolution CT or MRI examination of the spinal canal may obviate the need for myelography to exclude cervical mass lesions.

Spinocerebellar degenerative diseases differ from MS by having associated abnormalities (such as the areflexia commonly seen with Friedreich's ataxia), by progressing slowly within a given neuroanatomic system, such as the cerebellum and its connections, and by having an abnormal family history. However, MS occurs more commonly in first-degree relatives of patients with MS, so that family history alone is not sufficient to make the distinction. Neurologic presentation of SLE in young women can be distinguished by appropriate immunologic testing. The neurologic manifestations of B$_{12}$ deficiency may precede the peripheral red blood cell abnormalities by several years; the deficiency is detected by the serum B$_{12}$ level or Schilling test. The correct diagnosis of brain-stem arterial disease in patients in their fifties can sometimes be difficult; absence of CSF abnormalities associated with MS helps, as does the fact that all the abnormalities can be localized to a small anatomic area. The clinician's suspicion of chronic drug intoxication, often accompanied by nystagmus and ataxia, may be substantiated by appropriate blood levels or other evidence of disturbed behavior.

The total absence of objective neurologic signs at any time, together with symptom patterns or apparent weakness or sensory loss that fail to conform to known neuroanatomic systems, raise the suspicion of psychogenic illness. However, one must be wary, for many patients with urinary retention, urgency, or incontinence; ataxia; or vague sensory symptoms occurring in the early stages of MS have been misdiagnosed as psychoneurotic. Evoked response or CSF abnormalities will help exclude purely psychogenic disturbances, but must not be overinterpreted.

Role of Laboratory Aids. The rational use of laboratory abnormalities requires an awareness of their limitations. Elevation of the total CSF gamma globulin, or the appearance of an oligoclonal pattern within the gamma region on electrophoresis, is not specific for MS, although the non-MS causes can usually be readily excluded. However, these abnormalities fail to appear in 10 to 20 per cent of patients with clinically definite multiple sclerosis. Further, many patients who experience a single episode of neurologic abnormality, such as optic neuritis or transverse myelopathy, may exhibit CSF gamma globulin abnormalities, but do not develop a second clinically visible lesion after long follow-up. Thus it is not appropriate to make the diagnosis of MS with a first neurologic attack, even when one encounters CSF gamma globulin abnormalities.

Similarly, although evoked potential abnormalities serve to suggest the possibility of a lesion in that part of the CNS tested, the nonspecific nature of the electrophysiologic alterations makes it unwise to base a diagnosis on such data. A patient with paraparesis and prolonged latency of the VER may have MS, but could possibly have two tumors, pernicious anemia, systemic vasculitis, or a spinal cord tumor plus an uncorrected refractive error. Also, multiple lesions detected on CT or MRI may reflect another disease process. Despite these cautions, the discovery of CSF abnormalities commonly associated with MS, evoked potential evidence of a second lesion, or multiple lesions on CT or MRI help greatly to focus on MS as a possible or probable diagnosis.

TREATMENT. Management of MS requires a combination of an understanding of the personal problems posed by an unpredictable disorder of unknown etiology, an awareness of the measures available to alleviate spasticity, urinary incontinence, and other dysfunctions, and a skeptical approach to "definitive" treatments which are proposed to alter the course of the illness. The fact that over 70 per cent of patients experience spontaneous improvement following an acute bout makes evaluation of proposed treatment difficult, time consuming, and expensive. Nevertheless, carefully conducted controlled trials are the only means for deciding whether or not an agent helps patients with MS. Testimonial-style reports should not be accepted as evidence until a controlled study has confirmed the findings. At present, no method for prevention of MS is known.

Dealing with patients affected by a chronic, sometimes disabling disease for which there is no specific treatment is frustrating to many physicians. Patients with MS often report that they must help alleviate their physician's depression by denying problems. Most patients respond well to an explanation of the disease, a discussion of those things which can be done, and assurance that vigorous research is underway to develop better treatment.

Acute bouts of neurologic dysfunction may be treated with short-term administration of corticosteroids. There is evidence that administration of ACTH for 10 to 14 days somewhat shortens exacerbations, although the ACTH (or other corticosteroid) does not alter the long-term course of MS. From 40 to 80 units of ACTH per day may be used; prednisone, 40 to 60 mg per day, or equivalent doses of other oral corticosteroids are often employed as alternatives. The period of treatment should not exceed three or four weeks, with appropriate precautions to avoid steroid complications. It must be emphasized that there is no evidence that corticosteroids (or any other agent) modify the MS pathogenic process. Beneficial effects are most probably due to anti-edema and anti-inflammatory effects. Many responsible clinicians choose not to treat patients in this manner, believing that minimal evidence favors steroid use.

Therapeutic trials to evaluate various immunosuppressants, immunoenhancing agents, plasmapheresis, and other treatments are under way; none can be recommended at present.

Physical therapy plays an important role in several aspects of patient management, including developing alternative muscle strengths, preventing contractures, improving daily living, and providing supportive psychotherapy. A cool bath or swimming pool improves neurologic function transiently by lowering body temperature and improving axonal conduction. Occupational therapy is often a key to the patient's adjustment to MS.

Spasticity and flexor spasms can be alleviated with baclofen, or with diazepam, which inhibits central synaptic transmission. Individual responses vary sufficiently that one must start with very low doses and increase slowly if needed. Many patients depend on spasticity for support while walking, so that removal of this aid or induction of weakness or drowsiness as temporary side effects limits treatment. Occasionally, leg contractures occur despite physical therapy, and require orthopedic surgical relief for ease of handling the patient.

Bladder dysfunction is usually the result of incomplete emptying, accumulation of residual urine, and overflow frequency or incontinence and infection. Rational treatment requires careful urologic evaluation, often including urodynamic studies, in order to plan appropriate pharmacologic therapy. Uninhibited bladder contraction leading to urinary frequency or incontinence may be alleviated by controlling infection and restricting fluid intake prior to trips or several

hours before sleep. Imipramine, oxybutynin chloride, or pro-
pantheline may help patients who cannot initiate urination or
cannot fully empty their bladder. Attempts to void at fixed
intervals and the Credé maneuver often help. If catheterization becomes necessary, many individuals can learn self-
catheterization in order to avoid the complications of an
indwelling catheter. Long-term urinary bacterial suppressant
therapy is helpful in minimizing infection in patients carrying
residual urine. The possibility of an ascending urinary tract
infection must be sought and treated appropriately in any
patient with recurrent cystitis.

Constipation usually responds to stool softeners and laxatives. Many patients must be reassured that no harm arises
from the lack of a daily bowel movement.

Painful paresthesias and dysesthesias may occur, and fortunately are usually transient. Carbamazepine, diazepam, or
phenytoin will usually provide relief. Prevention of decubiti
in the paraplegic or desensitized patient requires constant
vigilance.

Specific psychiatric support is often needed to aid patients
and their families. The incidence of marital breakup, changes
in roles within the family, and financial problems is exceeded
only by the frequency of frustration over the unpredictability
of MS. The physician often must call on a range of associates,
including social workers, community agency workers, and
psychiatrists, in order to help these patients cope.

Brown FR, Beebe GW, Kurtzke JF, et al.: The design of clinical studies to assess
    therapeutic efficacy in multiple sclerosis. Neurology 29:1, 1979. *A thorough
    review of the many factors which must be taken into consideration in designing a
    study to determine whether or not a proposed treatment benefits patients with
    multiple sclerosis.*
Cohen SR, Herndon RM, McKhann GM: Radioimmunoassay of myelin basic
    protein in spinal fluid: An index of active demyelination. N Engl J Med
    295:1455, 1976. *This paper presents the first large series of patients in whom
    measurement of myelin basic protein in CSF was correlated with disease activity.*
Gonzalez-Scarano F, Grossman RI, Galetta S, et al.: Multiple sclerosis disease
    activity correlates with Gadolinium-enhanced MRI. Ann Neurol 21:300–
    306, 1987.
Kurtzke JF, Hyllested K: Multiple sclerosis in the Faroe Islands: I. Clinical and
    epidemiological features. Ann Neurol 5:6, 1979. *A lucid description of the
    remarkable, seemingly limited epidemic of multiple sclerosis in the Faroe Islands.*
McDonald WI, Silberberg DH (eds.): Multiple Sclerosis. London, Butterworths,
    1986.
Poser C, Presthus J, Horstal O: Clinical characteristics of autopsy-proved
    multiple sclerosis. Neurology 16:791, 1966. *A valuable analysis of the presen-
    tation and signs and symptoms which developed among a large series of patients
    in whom MS was proved by autopsy.*
Poser S, Raun E, Wikstrom J, et al.: Pregnancy, oral contraceptives, and
    multiple sclerosis. Acta Neurol Scand 59:108, 1979. *The largest study of the
    possible effect of pregnancy or oral contraceptives on the course of MS; this study
    shows no relationship.*
Williams A, Edrige R, McFarland H, et al.: Multiple sclerosis in twins. Neurol-
    ogy 30:1139, 1980.

MULTIPLE SCLEROSIS VARIANTS
Neuromyelitis Optica (Devic's Disease)

Neuromyelitis optica describes a syndrome characterized
by the occurrence of partial or complete transverse myelopathy and optic neuritis. Loss of vision and paraplegia may
occur in either disorder, and days or weeks may elapse
between the onsets of the two symptom complexes. It is best
considered a syndrome, in that it may occur as the result of
multiple sclerosis, acute disseminated encephalomyelitis, systemic lupus erythematosus, or sarcoidosis. When this symptom complex occurs in the course of multiple sclerosis, its
clinical and pathologic features are indistinguishable from
those of MS.

Diffuse Sclerosis, Transitional Sclerosis

These terms describe a group of progressive neurologic
disorders occurring primarily in young patients who manifest
severe neurologic deficits of various types with progressive
visual and mental deterioration. These are pathologists' terms,
which were first used in the late nineteenth century. Schilder
described three cases of what came to be known as Schilder's

cerebral sclerosis, or Schilder's disease. It is likely that three
separate conditions have been included as Schilder's disease
and that this eponymic designation should be discarded.
Some cases represent the result of severe confluent extensions
of large lesions of multiple sclerosis. Some represent white
matter disease of known viral origin, such as subacute
sclerosing panencephalitis and progressive multifocal
leukoencephalitis (see Ch. 488). A third group includes the
leukodystrophies (see later discussion). It is probable that
adrenoleukodystrophy was the disorder identified by Schilder
in one of his early cases.

Possibly Related Monophasic Disorders

ACUTE DISSEMINATED ENCEPHALOMYELITIS. This
disorder is discussed in Ch. 491. It can be noted here that an
episode of acute disseminated encephalomyelitis can closely
resemble an attack of multiple sclerosis. Distinction may be
impossible until sufficient time has elapsed to determine
whether or not a second bout occurs. The distinction between
ADEM and MS is blurred by the occurrence of typical exacerbations in the course of MS, concomitant with intercurrent
viral infection.

OPTIC NEURITIS. Optic neuritis denotes partial or complete loss of vision in one or both eyes, attributable to one or
more optic nerve lesions of unknown etiology. If a cause is
known, it is more precise to describe, for example, syphilitic
optic neuropathy, or optic neuritis or neuropathy secondary
to multiple sclerosis. Retrobulbar neuritis describes a lesion
in the posterior two thirds of the optic nerve. The term
papillitis indicates a lesion in the anterior portion of the optic
nerve, leading to an ophthalmoscopic appearance indistinguishable from that of acute papilledema but differing from
the papilledema of increased intracranial pressure by being
associated with reduction of visual acuity early in its course.
The visual loss usually, but not always, affects macular vision
with appearance of a central scotoma and a reduction in color
perception. Pain on eye movement is frequent during the first
few days of the event. Unless the patient has papillitis,
ophthalmoscopic examination is normal for the first two to
three weeks, after which disc pallor with loss of small vessels
on the disc or more severe atrophy may develop.

Visual loss occurs over the course of hours to several days,
and almost always recovers to some degree within several
weeks. Blindness as the result of the optic nerve demyelination of MS rarely occurs. Optic neuritis can occur as the
presenting sign of MS (see Table 492–2) or at any time during
the course of the disease. Practically all MS patients exhibit
optic nerve demyelination at autopsy, which underlies the
usefulness of the visual evoked response. Approximately one
third of patients who develop idiopathic optic neuritis will go
on to develop the clinical manifestations of MS. The presence
of the CSF abnormalities associated with MS makes this course
somewhat more likely, but does not have firm predictive
value; certainly MS may develop in the absence of CSF gamma
globulin abnormalities.

The illnesses which can mimic idiopathic optic neuritis
include optic nerve compression on any basis, neurosyphilis,
ischemic optic neuropathy (in older patients), pernicious anemia, Leber's optic atrophy (which is hereditary), tobacco-
alcohol amblyopia, and chronic papilledema with optic atrophy and visual loss, associated with prolonged increased
intracranial pressure.

LEUKODYSTROPHIES

These are diseases of dysmyelination, rather than demyelination, in that the normal formation of myelin is interfered
with by a genetically determined biochemical defect. The
classification of leukodystrophies is based on their histopathology. A biochemical defect is known for several, but they
remain relatively rare, incurable disorders, affecting individuals from the first months of life to the twenties.

Metachromatic Leukodystrophy

This, the most common of the leukodystrophies, describes diffuse dysmyelination, usually starting in the first ten years of life. It produces personality changes leading to dementia, convulsions, cranial nerve abnormalities, and finally severe spasticity or rigidity. Death usually occurs in from two to four years, although longer survival is reported. Juvenile and adult-onset cases have been reported.

The appearance of metachromatic material (staining red with toluidine blue) in the urinary sediment and in peripheral nerves usually allows diagnosis during life. The metachromatic material also collects in the liver, gallbladder, kidneys, and spleen. The CSF protein is usually elevated above 100 mg per deciliter.

Metachromatic leukodystrophy is usually inherited as an autosomal recessive trait. The pathogenesis of the widespread loss of normal myelin is accumulation of sulfatides in glial cells, in Schwann cells, within myelin lamellae, and in the cytoplasm of some nerve cells. The underlying biochemical defect is abnormally low activity of arylsulfatase A, an enzyme in the system which normally reduces the concentration of cerebroside sulfate.

Sudanophilic Leukodystrophy

This subset includes a heterogeneous group of diseases which have in common only the fact that extensive CSF myelin destruction occurs, associated with products of myelin breakdown, cholesterol esters which stain bright red with the usual fat stains. This staining quality distinguishes these diseases from the metachromatic leukodystrophies. These pathologic characteristics are found in aminoacidurias, adrenoleukodystrophy, and Pelizaeus-Merzbacher disease.

ADRENOLEUKODYSTROPHY. This disorder combines diffuse dysmyelination and myelin breakdown associated with idiopathic adrenocortical insufficiency. It occurs exclusively in males, inherited as a sex-linked recessive trait. The onset occurs most often in childhood, but has been reported in adults, with a progression of symptoms similar to those of metachromatic leukodystrophy. CSF protein is elevated in most patients. Endocrine testing reveals primary adrenal failure. Instances of adrenal failure alone have been reported in relatives of patients with adrenoleukodystrophy.

Pathologic examination reveals widespread changes in CNS myelin, and also peripheral nerve demyelination, with numerous lipid lamellar inclusions throughout the tissue. The underlying biochemical defect is not known.

PELIZAEUS-MERZBACHER DISEASE. This rare leukodystrophy affects males primarily, is inherited as a sex-linked recessive trait, and starts in early infancy. It progresses slowly, producing extensive, diffuse, symmetrical disturbances of myelin staining associated with gliosis within the cerebrum and cerebellum. The peripheral nervous system is not affected. The underlying biochemical defect is unknown. No treatment is available.

Globoid Cell Leukodystrophy (Krabbe's Disease)

This affects infants in the first two to three months of life, initially producing irritability and unexplained episodes of crying, sensitivity to light and noise, and failure to achieve developmental milestones. During the second year these children become opisthotonic, developing myoclonic jerks, atypical seizures, and optic atrophy. Rare instances occur in late infancy, or in adulthood.

Neuropathologic examination reveals marked loss of myelin throughout the brain with the presence of round or oval mononuclear cells the size of large glia or as large irregular multinucleated cells. These globoid cells contain galactocerebroside (galactosyl ceramide) which accumulates in abnormal quantities. The disorder probably is transmitted as an autosomal-recessive trait. No treatment is known.

Spongy Degeneration of White Matter

Many disorders can produce the pathologic changes leading to this label, including aminoacidurias and other metabolic disturbances. Instances affecting infants in whom no underlying metabolic defect is apparent are called Canavan's disease, with spastic paraplegia, severe mental retardation, optic atrophy, enlargement of the head and death occurring by 18 months. Spongiform degeneration is also produced by exposure to large amounts of hexachlorophine in infancy and by Creutzfeldt-Jakob disease in adults (see Ch. 488).

Austin J: Metachromatic form of diffuse cerebral sclerosis: II. Diagnosis during life by isolation of metachromatic lipids from urine. Neurology 7:716, 1957. *Description, clearly written, of methods for identifying metachromatic urinary sediment in children with this disorder.*

Moser HW, Moser AB, Singh I, et al.: Adrenoleucodystrophy: Survey of 303 cases, biochemistry, diagnosis and therapy. Ann Neurol 16:628, 1984.

Seitelberger F: Pelizaeus-Merzbacher's disease. In Vinken P, Bruyn G (eds.): Handbook of Clinical Neurology, Vol 10. Amsterdam, North-Holland, 1970, p 150. *An excellent review of this and related degenerative diseases of myelin.*

Suzuki K, Suzuki Y: Globoid cell leukodystrophy: Deficiency of galactocerebroside-galactosidase. Proc Natl Acad Sci USA 66:302, 1970. *This report describes the detection of the enzyme deficiency underlying this rare form of leukodystrophy.*

THE SYNDROME OF ACUTE TRANSVERSE MYELITIS

CLINICAL DESCRIPTION. Acute transverse myelopathy describes the rapid onset of paraparesis or paraplegia as the result of spinal cord dysfunction. The term transverse myelitis has a slightly more specific meaning, referring to acute transverse myelopathy of unknown etiology. The onset of weakness is often preceded by abrupt or rapidly developing, localized back pain or radicular pain, often in the thoracic region. This is followed by paresthesias of the toes and feet and rapidly ascending sensory loss and weakness. Urinary and fecal incontinence are common. The speed of progression varies from minutes, as with an infarction, to steady or stepwise progression over several days, as often occurs with compression due to a tumor or as a result of multiple sclerosis. It is often difficult to separate the patient who has developed an idiopathic transverse myelopathy from the one who has a detectable and often treatable underlying cause. Presentation of the syndrome of acute spinal cord dysfunction demands immediate and careful consideration of the differential diagnosis so as to undertake appropriate treatment if warranted.

DIFFERENTIAL DIAGNOSIS. Table 492–4 list disorders that produce an acute or subacute transverse myelopathy with varying degrees of frequency.

Bacterial infections of the spinal cord and its surrounding spaces are considered in Ch. 481.

Viral infection of the spinal cord occurs with direct extension by the varicella (herpes) zoster or other viruses. Alternately, spinal cord inflammation and demyelination may follow a viral infection, such as measles or other common viruses, either as an isolated phenomenon or as part of the more widespread acute disseminated encephalomyelitis.

TABLE 492–4. ACUTE OR SUBACUTE TRANSVERSE MYELOPATHY

Associated with infections
  Bacterial
  Spinal epidural abscess
  Intramedullary abscess
  Viral, e.g., herpes zoster
  Postviral, e.g., rubella with disseminated encephalomyelitis

Compression
  Tumor, especially metastatic
  Trauma
  Herniated intervertebral disc

Vascular
  Acute extradural, subdural, or parenchymal hemorrhage
  Dissecting aortic aneurysm
  Arteritis
  Lupus erythematosus

Idiopathic

Spinal cord compression from metastatic tumor may present acutely, even though the tumor has been present for a longer time. Centrally *herniating intervertebral discs* may lead to acute cord compression with or without local pain. In each instance, myelography is usually required for diagnosis, although CT scans or MRI may be sufficient. Trauma often leads to an acute transverse myelopathy in what is usually an obvious setting.

Rapidly progressing myelopathy in a previously healthy person should always raise the question of *spontaneous epidural, subdural, or intraparenchymal bleeding*, as may occur from an arteriovenous malformation, or as a complication of anticoagulation or blood dyscrasia. CT or MR imaging will visualize the blood. Surgical decompression is often appropriate. Other vascular causes of transverse myelopathy include interruption of spinal cord blood supply by dissecting aortic aneurysm or traumatic aortic rupture. Inflammatory disorders affecting blood vessels such as disseminated lupus erythematosus or giant cell arteritis may produce an acute myelopathy.

Subacute myelopathy is a common manifestation of multiple sclerosis, either as a first clinical manifestation or in a patient with previous clinical evidence of the disorder. Motor dysfunction is usually much more prominent than sensory loss, and complete cord transection syndrome only rarely occurs. When a patient with isolated transverse myelopathy has CSF oligoclonal bands, abnormal visual or brain-stem auditory evoked response values or MRI evidence of multiple lesions, one must suspect multiple sclerosis. However, the probability has not yet been established, and it is not appropriate to consider that combination as a single event as having established the diagnosis of multiple sclerosis (see Table 492–3).

In many instances no identifiable cause of acute transverse myelopathy is found even at autopsy, although some will prove to have an occult arteriovenous malformation or unsuspected multiple sclerosis. The degree of acute neurologic impairment among patients with the idiopathic syndrome ranges from partial to complete; the speed of onset ranges from hours to days. Patients who progress acutely to total paralysis are less likely to improve than those whose impairments develop over several days or longer. Idiopathic acute transverse myelopathy may leave a patient paraplegic regardless of treatment or may lead to complete or nearly complete recovery, probably depending on the degree of necrosis which occurs initially.

LABORATORY AIDS. An imaging procedure is essential in the evaluation of acute transverse myelopathy. Increasingly sensitive CT and MRI techniques are beginning to replace myelography. CSF exam is usually obtained as part of or following the appropriate imaging procedure and is essential in doubtful cases.

PATHOLOGY. Idiopathic acute transverse myelopathy is associated with destruction of neurons, glia, and tracts at the level involved. A range of inflammatory cells have been seen acutely. Invasion by macrophages with subsequent cord atrophy and hypertrophy, and adhesion of the meninges to the spinal cord occur and sometimes lead to spinal block. The pathology of instances secondary to known causes depends on the disorder in question.

TREATMENT. Time is of the essence. Treatment may halt progression but may not restore function already lost. Diagnostic studies must be undertaken on an emergency basis and, when cord compression is present, surgical decompression, treatment with antibiotics or with corticosteroids is needed quickly. In idiopathic transverse myelopathy, multiple sclerosis, or cord compression, corticosteroids may reduce edema and lead to earlier restitution of function, although the effect on long-term outcome is problematic. Treatment of specific recognized etiologies is covered elsewhere. Urinary retention must be treated symptomatically with intermittent catheterization. Fecal impaction must be prevented. Patients with cervical lesions may require ventilatory assistance.

Berman M, Feldman S, Alter M, et al.: Acute transverse myelitis: Incidence and etiological considerations. Neurology 31:966, 1981. *A retrospective study of a well-defined population.*

Ropper AH, Poskanzer DC: The prognosis of acute and subacute transverse myelopathy based on early signs and symptoms. Ann Neurol 4:51, 1978. *Reviews the experience of a large general hospital with an excellent description of the clinical findings and follow-up*

SECTION TWELVE / THE EPILEPSIES

493 THE EPILEPSIES

Jerome Engel, Jr.

DEFINITION AND PREVALENCE. Epilepsy is the term applied to a group of disorders, sometimes called *the epilepsies*, that are characterized by recurrent, spontaneous, transient paroxysms of hyperactive brain function resulting in epileptic seizures. The epileptic attack or seizure, the common denominator of all of these conditions, may appear as impaired consciousness, involuntary movement, autonomic disturbance, or psychic or sensory experiences. Epileptic disorders can be considered either primary (conditions of intrinsic, nonprogressive, and presumably hereditary cerebral hyperexcitability, with seizures as the only manifestation of disordered brain function) or secondary (epileptic attacks symptomatic of some known pathologic process affecting the brain).

Epileptic disorders most commonly begin in early childhood but can appear at any time. Epidemiologic surveys indicate that 0.5 per cent of the United States population have active seizures, 3 per cent have had a recurrent seizure disorder at some time in their life, and 9 per cent have experienced at least one epileptic seizure. Prevalence is greater in areas of the world that have a higher incidence of brain injury owing to high rates of infection, poor perinatal care, and frequent head trauma.

PATHOGENESIS. Most investigators believe that the fundamental abnormality in all epileptic conditions lies in the cerebral cortex, including the limbic cortex (hippocampus). In chronic epilepsy, the recurrent neuronal paroxysms that underlie ictal (seizure) events are transient expressions of a more permanently physiologically disordered cortex. Even though seizures themselves are intermittent, the physiological abnormality persists throughout the interictal (between seizures) period.

An epileptogenic cortex in the interictal state is characterized by the appearance of brief high-amplitude electrical discharges that usually can be recorded from the scalp by *electroencephalography (EEG)*. The typical interictal EEG discharge consists of a sharp negative transient followed by a slower wave, referred to as a *spike-and-wave complex*. Studies of well localized cortical epileptogenic lesions (epileptic foci) in animals indicate that the EEG spike-and-wave complex reflects the summation of highly synchronized abnormal neuronal membrane potentials. These abnormal events consist of large paroxysmal depolarization shifts followed by prolonged after-hyperpolarizations. The depolarization shift results in enhanced neuronal excitation, while the after-hyperpolarization represents inhibition that may prevent ictal development. Neurons in cortical areas adjacent to the epileptic focus may demonstrate paroxysmal hyperpolarization only, forming an *inhibitory surround* that appears to prevent epileptic spread during the interictal state. These abnormal membrane events reflect inherent pathologic properties of individual epileptic neurons as well as disturbances in interconnections of neuronal aggregates.

Many neuronal defects have been identified in experimental models of epilepsy that can destabilize the membrane or interfere with the balance of excitatory and inhibitory synaptic activity. However, the fundamental mechanisms that underlie spontaneous recurrent seizures in the various forms of chronic human epilepsy remain unknown. Whatever the precise mechanism, ictal symptoms in human seizures reflect the functions of the cortex from which they arise, and the symptoms may gradually progress as the local discharge spreads to adjacent areas. Propagation to distant brain areas can proceed along fiber tracts to produce additional symptoms. With widespread or bilateral involvement, consciousness becomes impaired and generalized tonic-clonic convulsions can occur.

Partial seizures are seizures initiated in only part of the cerebral cortex. They can, but do not always, spread to involve larger areas of the brain. *Generalized seizures* are seizures that begin bilaterally from the start, presumably as a result of normal synchronizing afferent influences from brain stem and diencephalon acting on diffusely epileptogenic cortex or on widespread, multiple cortical epileptogenic foci. This condition has been referred to as *corticoreticular epilepsy*.

The neuronal basis of seizure termination is also poorly understood. Seizures stop not merely as a result of neuronal exhaustion, but due to self-activating inhibitory mechanisms. These events can depress neuronal function after a seizure, producing prominent postictal symptoms. Generalized convulsions and partial seizures with impaired consciousness are followed by diffuse EEG suppression and periods of confusion and fatigue that can last minutes to hours. Partial seizures may also be followed by transient localized EEG suppression and focal neurological deficits, known as *Todd's paralysis*, that reflect postictal dysfunction of cortical structures involved in the ictal event.

ETIOLOGY. The causes of epilepsy are many (Table 493–1), and several factors may coexist in the same patient. Commonly, the combination of a cerebral insult and a genetic predisposition determines the appearance of epileptic seizures. Systemic illness or trauma may uncover a latent epileptic condition.

Genetic Factors. Genetic factors may contribute to the development of epilepsy in three ways: (1) an individual may inherit a low threshold for seizures; (2) genetic traits underlie certain specific primary epileptic conditions; and (3) many inherited diseases of the brain are associated with structural disturbances that produce seizures.

A number of poorly understood genetic factors determine the susceptibility of individual brains to the development of generalized convulsions. Under certain circumstances a single isolated generalized convulsion can occur as a natural reaction to physiologic stress or transient systemic injury such as sleep deprivation, alcohol or sedative drug withdrawal, use of

convulsant drugs, fever, and acute head trauma. Recurrent generalized convulsions may also be induced by reversible infectious, toxic, or metabolic processes and are limited to the period of systemic illness. Occurrence of such *reactive seizures* generally indicates an inherited lowered threshold for seizures and not a chronic epileptic condition. The most commonly encountered reactive seizures are the *benign febrile convulsions* of infancy and early childhood. Persons with lowered convulsive thresholds are also more likely to develop chronic recurrent seizures of all types if irreversible brain injury occurs for other reasons.

Inherited epileptic disturbances unassociated with other neurologic dysfunctions are referred to as *primary epilepsies*, and account for 30 per cent of chronic epileptic disorders. Autosomal dominant genetic traits have been identified as the basis of characteristic EEG patterns that underlie the generalized *petit mal epilepsy* and partial *sylvian epilepsy*, but not all individuals with these EEG traits have seizures. Most primary epilepsies are relatively benign and many remit spontaneously in adolescence or early adulthood.

Epileptic disorders that occur due to structural lesions of the brain are referred to as *secondary epilepsies*. Secondary epilepsies are most often due to acquired factors; however, inherited neurologic diseases can also produce brain lesions that give rise to chronic recurrent epileptic seizures. These include inborn errors of metabolism such as phenylketonuria and the lipidoses; other degenerative diseases, not only those that affect gray matter, such as the progressive myoclonus epilepsies, but also the leukodystrophies; and syndromes such as tuberous sclerosis and neurofibromatosis that are associated with the development of cerebral ectopic or alien tissue.

Acquired Factors. Congenital lesions due to pre- and perinatal injuries are commonly encountered in epileptic patients. Minor focal lesions that can give rise to partial seizures include microgyria, porencephalic cysts, areas of calcification, and atrophy. More severe trauma, anoxia, and infections such as toxoplasmosis, cytomegalic inclusion disease, rubella, herpes, and syphilis also can produce diffuse neocortical and hippocampal damage and secondary generalized seizure disorders.

Head trauma with cicatrix formation is an important cause of epileptic seizures. Chronic recurrent seizures occur in 30 per cent of patients with acute hematomas, 15 per cent of those with depressed skull fractures, and 5 per cent of those hospitalized for severe closed head trauma. Epilepsy is rare, however, after head trauma without loss of consciousness. Seizures occurring at the time of injury (contact seizures) or within the first week thereafter do not necessarily herald development of a recurrent epileptic disorder. Chronic posttraumatic seizures usually have a delayed onset, most often beginning 6 to 12 months following injury and occasionally starting even many years later.

Infectious processes involving the brain and its coverings can produce acute and chronic seizures. As with trauma, generalized seizures that occur during active meningitis and encephalitis may not indicate a recurrent epileptic condition. Acute and chronic recurrent generalized and partial seizures are seen with slow virus infections and are common late sequelae when adhesions or scars result from purulent meningitis, fungal infections, or destructive viral processes such as herpes simplex encephalitis. Partial seizures may be the first sign of focal bacterial encephalitis or abscess formation, lesions especially likely to produce chronic epilepsy. Other focal inflammatory processes such as tuberculomas and parasitic infestations, particularly cysticercosis and schistosomiasis, are common causes of partial seizures in many countries and because of increased international travel are sometimes found outside their endemic areas.

About half of all *brain tumors* located in the anterior and middle cranial fossae produce epileptic symptoms. Gliomas are most often implicated, but any neoplasm that impinges on the cortex can produce seizures. Partial seizures are com-

TABLE 493–1. CAUSES OF EPILEPSY

Type of Disorder	Genetic Factors	Acquired Factors
Reactive seizures (transient reaction to stress or insult, not epilepsy)	Lowered threshold	Physiologic stress Sleep deprivation Alcohol or sedative drug withdrawal Convulsant drugs Fever Acute head trauma Toxic, metabolic, and infectious processes
Primary epilepsy (without structural lesions, usually benign)	Genetic trait	Little or none
Secondary epilepsy (with structural lesions and associated neurologic disturbances)	Lowered threshold Inherited diseases associated with epilepsy: 　Inborn errors of metabolism 　Degenerative diseases 　Ectopic or alien tissue	Congenital lesion Head trauma Infections Brain tumors Systemic toxic and metabolic disorder Hippocampal sclerosis Miscellaneous disorders

mon with *Sturge-Weber syndrome* and often result from small cryptogenic hamartomas, ectopias, and angiomas.

Cerebral vascular diseases produce seizures in many ways. Partial seizures are rare during acute strokes and usually reflect embolic events with bleeding into the cortex rather than thrombosis. Completed strokes, however, often produce scar tissue that can become epileptogenic months or years later. Such a process is presumed to be the most common cause of unexplained recurrent partial seizures in the elderly. Partial and generalized seizures are early symptoms of cerebral venous thrombosis, cerebral arteritis, and hypertensive encephalopathy (now rare). Partial seizures often occur with arteriovenous malformations (AVMs), and small cortical hemorrhages of any cause can produce refractory partial seizures or focal myoclonic jerks.

Systemic toxic and metabolic disturbances caused by exogenous and endogenous substances that lower seizure thresholds or produce neuronal membrane instability as well as ionic imbalance, such as hyponatremia, can give rise to reactive generalized convulsions, but these are not considered epileptic conditions. Nevertheless, such metabolic causes occasionally can lead to status epilepticus with subsequent brain damage or death. It is important to recognize the rare reversible metabolic causes of seizures in infancy, such as hypocalcemia and pyridoxine deficiency, that can be treated easily by replacement therapy. Toxic or metabolic disturbances may occasionally cause partial seizures when superimposed on unsuspected focal cerebral lesions from old head injuries. These occur most commonly in alcohol and drug abusers who are undergoing withdrawal. Hyperosmolar conditions such as nonketotic hyperglycemia and uremia may also give rise to partial seizures, presumably because of brain shrinkage that tears bridging vessels and produces small areas of hemorrhage into the cortex.

Miscellaneous disorders that can cause seizures include systemic diseases that can give rise to cerebral pathology, such as the collagen vascular diseases and blood dyscrasias, and cerebral gray matter degenerative diseases, such as allergic encephalopathies, and, very rarely, the presenile and senile dementias. Demyelinating diseases occasionally produce lesions adjacent to cortex that cause epileptic attacks: seizures occur in 3 per cent of patients with multiple sclerosis.

Mesial temporal sclerosis, consisting of largely unilateral neuronal loss often accompanied by astrocytic proliferation in the hippocampus and adjacent limbic structures, is found in over half the patients who have undergone temporal lobe resection for complex partial seizures. This may be the most common pathologic finding in epilepsy, but it remains uncertain whether the lesion is the cause or the result of seizures. Prolonged convulsive seizures are known to produce cell loss in the hippocampus, the neocortex, and the cerebellum. Some authorities believe that prolonged convulsions (lasting more than 30 minutes), such as those that occasionally accompany fever in infancy or childhood exanthems, can produce mesial temporal sclerosis and that this lesion becomes epileptogenic later in life. In any event, this form of epileptic brain damage suggests that in some situations epilepsy itself becomes a cause of progressive symptoms. Even if mesial temporal sclerosis does not actually cause seizures, it may alter their manifestations and account for some interictal behavioral disturbances. For this reason convulsive seizures should be controlled as promptly as possible.

CLINICAL MANIFESTATIONS AND CLASSIFICATION. Epileptic seizures are classified by their clinical manifestations (Table 493–2), since precise anatomic and pathophysiologic correlates of specific ictal behaviors are still largely unknown. The classification plays an essential role in the diagnosis and management of epileptic disorders for four major reasons:

1. The diagnosis of epilepsy is often difficult because of the similarity between certain epileptic attacks and intermittent symptoms of nonepileptic disorders. Recognition that a patient's complaints are consistent with a known epileptic seizure pattern helps to determine whether the true nature of the condition is identified or even suspected. The classification of epileptic seizures by specific symptoms is particularly useful for this purpose.

2. Differentiation between partial and generalized seizures is of great clinical value. Partial seizures indicate the presence of a focal brain disturbance that may be a curable cause of epilepsy, such as a surgically resectable scar, or a focal progressive process that requires specific attention, such as

TABLE 493–2. CLASSIFICATION OF EPILEPTIC SEIZURES*

Partial seizures (focal, local)
　Simple partial seizures
　　With motor signs
　　With somatosensory or special sensory symptoms
　　With autonomic symptoms or signs
　　With psychic symptoms
　Complex partial seizures
　　Simple partial onset followed by impairment of consciousness
　　With impairment of consciousness at onset
　Partial seizures evolving to generalized tonic-clonic convulsions (secondarily generalized)

Generalized seizures (convulsive or nonconvulsive)
　Nonconvulsive seizures
　　Absence seizures
　　Atypical absence seizures
　　Myoclonic seizures
　　Atonic seizures
　Convulsive seizures
　　Tonic-clonic seizures
　　Tonic seizures
　　Clonic seizures

Unclassified epileptic seizures

*Modified from Commission on Classification and Terminology of the International League Against Epilepsy: Epilepsia 22:489, 1981.

TABLE 493–3. THERAPEUTIC CLASSIFICATION OF EPILEPTIC SEIZURES

Seizure Type	Preferred Drugs
Partial seizures and generalized convulsions	Carbamazepine
	Phenytoin
	Phenobarbital
	Primidone
	Valproic acid
Absences	Ethosuximide
	Valproic acid
	Clonazepam
Myoclonus	Clonazepam
	Valproic acid

an infection or neoplasm. Because the exact expression of a partial seizure is determined by the site of ictal onset and spread and not by the causative agent, additional clinical information is usually needed to identify the nature of the underlying lesion.

3. The choice of antiepileptic drugs is determined by the seizure type rather than by the specific cause or anatomic substrate. For example, the differential diagnosis between absence attacks and complex partial seizures and between myoclonus and convulsions is essential for determining appropriate drug therapy.

4. A number of epileptic syndromes have been defined on the basis of seizure manifestations and other clinical features. Although pathophysiologic mechanisms or underlying disease processes have yet to be identified for most, diagnosis of a specific syndrome usually has important therapeutic and prognostic implications. In particular, recognition of the benign inherited primary epileptic conditions such as petit mal, juvenile epileptic myoclonus, and sylvian epilepsy facilitates prompt control with the proper medication, spares the patient unnecessary tests, and relieves anxiety by assuring an excellent outcome. A diagnosis of medically intractable temporal lobe epilepsy suggests that surgical resection might be considered. Epileptic syndromes can be classified as reactive, primary and secondary, and also according to whether the underlying disturbance is partial or generalized (Table 493–3). Some of the more important syndromes are also described in this section (Table 493–4).

Partial Seizures. Although the expression of partial seizures depends on the areas of cerebral cortex that are involved, the precise anatomic origin of specific seizures cannot always be accurately inferred from ictal symptoms, since functional localization within the brain remains inexact. Moreover, epileptic manifestations may reflect dysfunction produced by propagation away from the primary focus as much or more than from the area where the lesion lies.

Partial seizures are classified as simple when consciousness is preserved. *Simple partial seizures* reflect an ictal discharge that is localized within one hemisphere. The ictal symptoms can take many forms.

Motor symptoms begin with clonic or tonic movements of a discrete body part. Areas of the body with large representation

TABLE 493–4. SOME DISTINCTIVE EPILEPTIC SYNDROMES

Type of Disorder	Partial	Generalized
Reactive seizures		Febrile convulsions
Primary epilepsy	Sylvian epilepsy	Petit mal epilepsies
		Juvenile myoclonic epilepsy
Secondary epilepsy	Temporal lobe epilepsy	Lennox-Gastaut syndrome
	Epilepsia partialis continua	Progressive myoclonus epilepsies
		West's syndrome

in the motor cortex, such as the face and hand, are involved most frequently. When spread occurs in an orderly fashion along the precentral gyrus, clonic motor symptoms can progress (e.g., from thumb or face) which is termed a *Jacksonian march*. More commonly, however, ictal discharges in frontal cortex activate multiple muscle groups to produce complex versive movements such as turning of the head, eyes, or body to one side and posturing with one or more extremities. Involvement of the supplementary motor cortex classically results in adversive seizures with turning of the head and eyes away from the epileptic focus and elevation of the contralateral arm. The arm position can vary, however, and the direction in which the head turns is not a good localizing or lateralizing sign. Other simple motor manifestations include speech arrest or vocalizations when language areas are involved; eye or lid twitching, which is most often initiated from frontal or occipital foci; and inappropriate laughter unassociated with humor (*gelastic epilepsy*). Simple partial clonic or tonic motor seizures can be followed by a transient *Todd's paralysis* of involved muscles, which rarely persists longer than 48 hours.

Sensory symptoms occur with lesions in or connected to primary sensory cortex. Thus, localized paresthesias or numbness arise with seizures emanating from the parietal lobe, unformed luminous visions occur with lesions of the occipital lobe, and unpleasant olfactory and gustatory sensations, vertigo, and sounds can result from lesions of appropriate areas of the temporal cortex. Postictal phenomena such as blindness, deafness, and anesthesia may occasionally follow simple partial seizures with sensory symptoms.

Autonomic symptoms often are due to ictal involvement of limbic structures in the mesial temporal and frontal lobes that project to the hypothalamus and brain stem and include feelings of epigastric rising or distress, nausea, or vague lightheadedness. Brief paroxysmal epigastric symptoms, including vomiting, can be the sole manifestation of an epileptic disorder (*abdominal epilepsy*). This condition has most often been identified in children, but it is rare and greatly overdiagnosed. In other autonomic seizures, ictal signs and symptoms such as pallor, flushing, sweating, piloerection, pupillary dilatation, cardiac arrhythmia, and incontinence may be apparent.

Psychic symptoms can accompany ictal discharges in limbic and association cortex and mimic features of psychiatric disorders. These include dysmnesic symptoms such as feelings of familiarity (deja vu) and unfamiliarity (jamais vu) and forced thinking; cognitive disturbances such as dreamy states, depersonalization, and time distortion; affective symptoms such as fear and rage, which often are associated with appropriate autonomic changes, depression, and on rare occasions elation; illusions such as multiple images (polyopia) or distortions of size (micropsia and macropsia); and hallucinations consisting of stereotyped mixed sensory experiences such as visions of well-formed recognizable faces or specific scenes accompanied by voices that can be understood, familiar smells, and emotional responses. Persistent psychic symptoms in epileptic patients may also be postictal.

Simple partial seizures are usually brief and do not interfere with daily living unless they occur frequently or evolve into other types of attacks. Simple partial seizures that consist only of experiential phenomena may be referred to as *auras* when the patient perceives them as a warning of impending more noticeable epileptic symptoms. Patients who complain only of simple partial seizures may report having many seizures a week or many a day, with each lasting a few seconds.

Partial seizures are classified as complex when they impair consciousness. Approximately 40 per cent of patients with epilepsy experience *complex partial seizures* with impaired consciousness ranging from amnesia for the ictal event to behavioral unresponsiveness. Complex partial seizures usually reflect bilateral ictal involvement of limbic structures, particularly the hippocampus, amygdala, and their connections. The seizure may begin with impaired consciousness from the start, or the spread of ictal discharge may result in evolution from a simple into a complex partial event. The evolution occurs most often when the simple partial seizure is caused by a lesion involving the mesial temporal lobe or a region of cerebral cortex directly connected to mesial temporal limbic areas. Autonomic auras most commonly precede complex partial seizures and include sensations of epigastric rising or distress and psychic experiences. Complex partial seizures preceded by olfactory auras are called *uncinate fits*. Such attacks may be more consistently associated with brain tumors than are other types of seizures.

The term complex partial seizure is not synonymous with *temporal lobe, psychomotor,* and *limbic seizures*. These latter designations have more specific anatomic implications and may involve ictal symptoms resulting from unilateral activation of mesial temporal limbic structures without impaired consciousness. Some complex partial seizures, on the other hand, may not reflect primary activation of the limbic system. The complex partial seizure that typifies the temporal lobe or psychomotor attack begins with a motionless stare at the time consciousness is impaired and purposeless movements called *automatisms*. Oroalimentary automatisms, such as chewing, swallowing, sucking, and lip smacking, are most common and presumably reflect amygdala involvement. Other examples of automatisms include verbal utterances of sounds or words; gestural movements such as fumbling, posturing, and picking at clothing; expressions of emotion; and ambulation. Ongoing activities such as washing dishes or even driving a car may continue automatically. Patients may undress, run, respond to commands, and demonstrate a variety of complicated automatisms that indicate a residual ability to relate to the environment despite the ictal state. In some types of complex partial seizures patients can display irregular thrashing movements of the extremities, scream, fall, or exhibit bizarre behavior that can be difficult to differentiate from hysteria.

Complex partial seizures usually last from a few seconds to a few minutes and are followed by confusion as well as amnesia for the ictal event, although most patients remember an aura. Postictal anterograde amnesia and automatisms are common, and aphasia often occurs when seizures begin in the dominant hemisphere. Other cognitive deficits and headache may occur during the postictal period. In cases of unusually prolonged or recurrent complex partial seizures, postictal anterograde memory disturbance may persist for hours or days.

Complex partial seizures and postictal symptoms can severely disrupt daily life. While it is not uncommon for patients to have many complex partial seizures a week and several auras a day, even one or two seizures a year may prevent them from driving a car or destroy a chosen career.

Both simple and complex partial seizures can evolve into *secondarily generalized tonic-clonic convulsions*. Most patients with partial seizures experience at least some secondarily generalized seizures, but generalization usually occurs infrequently and is more easily controlled by drugs than are partial ictal symptoms. Some patients, particularly those with lesions in the frontal lobes, have partial seizures that always generalize secondarily. When such secondarily generalized partial seizures begin in a silent area of the brain, their focal origin may be overlooked by both the patient and observers. When neither ictal symptoms nor signs provide a clue that a seizure is secondarily generalized, postictal focal or lateralizing signs and symptoms such as reflex asymmetry, focal weakness, or aphasia may indicate a partial seizure disorder. Differentiation from true generalized convulsions in these cases helps to identify potentially progressive or treatable focal lesions.

Partial Syndromes. Sylvian or *rolandic epilepsy* (benign partial epilepsy of childhood with centrotemporal spikes) is a familial disorder that may be the cause of as many as 20 per cent of childhood seizures. It is characterized by nocturnal generalized convulsions and simple partial seizures that occur during the day. Typically, the partial seizures begin with perioral or lingual paresthesias, although other sensory or motor symptoms may occur, especially involving the face. The EEG demonstrates centrotemporal interictal spikes that may be unilateral or bilaterally independent. Associated neurologic deficits are lacking, and the seizures respond well to medication. The disorder almost always disappears during adolescence.

Temporal lobe (psychomotor, limbic) epilepsy is the most common chronic epileptic syndrome and may account for 40 per cent of adult epilepsies. It is characterized by auras and complex partial seizures involving temporal lobe limbic structures either initially or occasionally by spread from other areas. Typically there are unilateral or bilateral independent anterior temporal EEG spikes. Patients may also have memory deficits and psychiatric symptomatology. Complex partial seizures, as described earlier, are often difficult to control medically but can be abolished by surgical resection. Patients with complex partial seizures that do not respond to appropriate medical therapy should be referred to a surgical facility for evaluation.

Epilepsia partialis continua also is often unresponsive to medication. This disorder occurs in adults after severe cerebral injury, such as anoxia or stroke—occasionally with brain tumors. It also can be seen in young children, particularly in those with a rare unilateral chronic cerebral inflammatory disorder of unknown cause. The continuous focal motor seizures reflect widespread or multiple rather than single lesions that usually are not amenable to localized surgical resection. Seizures can be abolished by large resections such as in hemispherectomy, and this may be indicated in some children who already have hemiatrophy and hemiparesis.

Epileptic acquired aphasia syndrome is a rare partial seizure disorder of unknown cause that appears as language deterioration in young children and is associated with bilateral temporal epileptiform EEG spikes. The disorder resolves spontaneously.

Generalized Seizures. Absences are brief losses of consciousness that can be of two types. Both begin almost exclusively in childhood and take the form of a blank stare, which can also be associated with mild clonic movements of eyelids and face, more generalized jerks, alterations in motor tone, and simple automatisms. *Petit mal absences* affect about 10 per cent of epileptic children, last less than 10 seconds, and begin and end abruptly without pre- or postictal EEG or clinical disturbances. *Atypical absences* also occur in about 10 per cent of epileptic children, can last longer than 10 seconds, and produce some degree of postictal confusion. Petit mal and atypical absences must not be confused with each other or with complex partial seizures consisting only of brief lapses of consciousness, since cause, prognosis, and treatment differ for the three seizure types.

Absences can occur spontaneously hundreds of times a day. Petit mal absences respond well to appropriate medications, tend to disappear during adolescence, and are rarely disabling. Atypical absences may be refractory to therapy and can disrupt normal function. Children with atypical absences, however, are usually hampered more by other seizures and by neurologic and mental deficits.

Myoclonic seizures are single, rapidly recurrent, bilaterally synchronous shock-like jerks of the face, trunk, and extremities that are not associated with loss of consciousness. A single myoclonic jerk that occurs while a person is falling asleep is a normal physiologic event. More frequent myoclonus implies a more serious problem. In most patients with myoclonic seizures, these events cluster shortly after waking or when falling asleep. A prolonged attack can terminate in a generalized tonic-clonic convulsion. Myoclonic seizures occur in certain rare benign genetic epileptic disorders of the primary generalized type such as *juvenile myoclonic epilepsy (impulsive petit mal)* and respond well to drug therapy.

In contrast to myoclonic seizures, there are many other types of myoclonic jerks that are not generalized and should not be considered epileptic. These include the asymmetric or sporadic jerks (involving first one area of the body and then another) that are spontaneous or induced by movement or sensory stimulation and that result from anoxic, toxic, and metabolic disturbances. Similar jerkings accompany the *progressive myoclonus epilepsies* associated with lesions of the diencephalon, brain stem, and cerebellar nuclei. Other myoclonic phenomena that are not epileptic seizures include regular rhythmic *palatal myoclonus* and *segmental myoclonus* that are caused, respectively, by medullary and spinal cord lesions and *benign familial (essential) myoclonus* of unknown origin.

Tonic-clonic (grand mal) convulsions occur at least once in 80 per cent of epileptic patients. Occasionally, such seizures can be epileptic responses of a normal brain to nonspecific physiologic stress or systemic disturbances. More often they represent the final form taken by partial seizures that secondarily generalize or are a manifestation of a generalized epileptic disorder. Convulsions that are not secondarily generalized from partial seizures never have auras, although patients may occasionally recognize nonspecific affective changes or experience a flurry of bilaterally synchronous myoclonic jerks some hours before a seizure occurs. The typical generalized convulsion begins with a sudden cry accompanied by loss of consciousness, falling, and bilateral tonic extensor rigidity of the trunk and extremities. After several seconds of rigidity, recurrent synchronous clonic muscular contractions ensue for one or two minutes, until the seizure ends, leaving the patient flaccid and unconscious. Cyanosis results from breath-holding during the tonic phase, and autonomic hyperactivity is prominent. The blood pressure increases abruptly, the body temperature rises, and patients salivate and may have urinary and fecal incontinence. Often they bite their tongue and the inside of their mouth. Occasionally generalized convulsive attacks consist of either tonic or clonic activity alone.

Postictal depression can last many minutes, occasionally hours, and rarely a day or more. During this period patients gradually regain consciousness but feel exhausted, frequently complain of headache, and wish to sleep. A few remain partially confused. Focal or lateralized postictal symptoms do not occur following true generalized tonic-clonic convulsions.

Grand mal convulsions rarely occur more than a few times a year in primary generalized epileptic disorders but can occur daily in severe secondary generalized disorders. In both situations, however, the attacks tend to respond well to antiepileptic drugs.

Atonic seizures (drop attacks), considered to be minor motor epileptic events, begin almost exclusively in childhood and are usually in association with diffuse lesions of the brain. The ictal episode consists of a sudden extremely brief loss of tone. In its simplest form, the child's head drops for a second or less. More severe forms cause tone to disappear in the entire body leading to collapse, sometimes with serious injuries such as concussion, broken bones, and lost teeth. This characteristic drop should be distinguished from the more gradual slump that can accompany partial seizures, the more rigid loss of balance that occurs during tonic or tonic-clonic convulsions, and the sudden impulsive falls that result from myoclonic jerks. Atonic seizures occur many times a day, are refractory to therapy, and can be the most debilitating ictal manifestation of the Lennox-Gastaut syndrome. Brief *tonic seizures* also occur as minor motor symptoms of secondary generalized epileptic disorders.

Generalized Syndromes. One or more *febrile convulsions* occur in 3 to 4 per cent of otherwise healthy children between the ages of six months and five years and consist of brief tonic-clonic generalized seizures. Although febrile convulsions can be recurrent, the syndrome is so benign that it is usually not considered an epileptic disorder, and treatment is usually not necessary. A genetic basis is certain but poorly defined. Affected children outgrow their vulnerability between three and five years of age, although 5 per cent develop seizures without fever later. Against the diagnosis of benign febrile convulsions are the following: seizures lasting longer than 10 minutes, focal abnormalities during or after the seizure, or an abnormal neurologic or mental status examination result. In such instances an underlying neurologic disorder is likely and treatment is required.

The *petit mal epilepsies* account for 10 per cent of childhood epilepsies. Several varieties are recognized depending on the age of onset, frequency of EEG spike-and-wave discharges, and occurrence of myoclonic seizures. Infrequent grand mal seizures can occur in all forms, or they may occur alone. They are characterized by frequent petit mal absences in an otherwise neurologically normal child. Response to appropriate medication is usually excellent, especially when onset is in early childhood. These disorders often remit in adolescence; juvenile onset or myoclonic seizures tend to worsen the prognosis.

The *Lennox-Gastaut syndrome* describes a nonspecific epileptic condition of children suffering from diffuse or multiple lesions of the brain. Although patients with the Lennox-Gastaut syndrome can have absences identical to the primary generalized type, usually they also have or develop additional neurologic impairment, mental subnormality, and multiple seizure types including drop attacks. Seizures associated with the Lennox-Gastaut syndrome and other secondary generalized epileptic disorders are difficult to control. The patients often become severely handicapped by the frequent attacks as well as other static or progressive interictal neurologic deficits.

Juvenile myoclonic epilepsy begins in mid- to late childhood with bilaterally synchronous myoclonic seizures. The paroxysms can be completely controlled with appropriate medication, and there are no other associated disturbances. The condition should not be confused with the myoclonic disorders characterized by sporadic, often stimulus-sensitive, myoclonic jerks, such as postanoxic myoclonus and the progressive myoclonus epilepsies. These last-mentioned sporadic myoclonic events are not epileptic, are extremely difficult to treat, and are usually associated with other evidence of diffuse cerebral injury.

The *progressive myoclonus epilepsies* comprise a group of familial cerebral degenerative disorders that affect both cortical and subcortical gray matter, leading to progressive neurologic deficits, dementia, sporadic multifocal myoclonic jerks, occasional epileptic myoclonus, and tonic-clonic convulsions. Whereas the epileptic myoclonus and convulsions respond well to medication, patients are severely disabled by the nonepileptic sporadic myoclonus and other handicaps. The course may be rapid with severe neurologic and mental impairment (*Lafora type*), intermediate (*Unverricht-Lundborg type*), or relatively slow with little mental impairment or EEG disturbance (*Ramsay Hunt syndrome,* which is associated with cerebellar disturbances and may be considered a separate entity). A benign familial myoclonic syndrome (*essential myoclonus*) also exists and is important to recognize because it has an excellent prognosis and responds readily to treatment with valproate.

Unclassified Seizures. *Infantile spasms* begin in the first year of life as brief intermittent ictal events that take a variety of forms, ranging from subtle twitches of the mouth or nose to violent jackknife or "salaam" movements. They result from severe diffuse disturbances of brain function from a variety of causes, are often associated with a severely abnormal interictal EEG pattern called *hypsarrhythmia*, and have a poor prognosis. Because infantile spasms may reflect subcortical disturbances similar to myoclonus or movement disorders, they have been removed from the current classification of epileptic seizures. However, children with this EEG and clinical symptom complex (*West's syndrome*) usually develop recurrent epileptic seizures as they get older, and their illness often evolves into the Lennox-Gastaut syndrome.

Because of an immature brain, *neonatal seizures* almost never generalize. Rather, they manifest themselves subtly as jitteriness, focal or multifocal twitches, clonic movements, and posturing. Benign as well as severely disabling forms of neonatal seizures can occur.

Patterns of Seizure Occurrence. Appreciation for precipitating factors and temporal patterns of certain epileptic seizures can influence approaches to management. In some of the primary generalized epileptic disorders, seizures may be induced by specific sensory stimuli, most commonly flashing light (*photosensitive epilepsy*). Reading, video games, music, and other specific complex stimuli may activate seizures in patients with rarer forms of *reflex epilepsy*. The seizures themselves range from brief absences through synchronous myoclonic jerking to occasional generalized convulsions. Partial seizures can occasionally be induced by specific sensory stimuli and are commonly provoked by emotional stress and drowsiness. *Hyperventilation* is a potent activator of petit mal absence seizures and sometimes will precipitate other types of ictal events as well. Possibly the associated respiratory alkalosis may explain why some patients report an increased incidence of seizures during exercise. Sleep deprivation and withdrawal from alcohol and sedative drugs are well-established precipitants of partial and generalized convulsive seizures in patients with chronic epilepsy. Some patients have seizures that occur only at night or only during the day. Others exhibit regular cycles of seizures over days or months or patterns of seizure clusters followed by prolonged seizure-free periods. The term *catamenial epilepsy* is used when seizures regularly recur in women around the menstrual period. Women with all forms of epileptic disorders commonly experience more frequent seizures at this time of the month, and seizures may worsen or disappear during pregnancy.

Status Epilepticus. Rapidly recurring or continuous ictal events are referred to as status epilepticus. *Epilepsia partialis continua* is a state of simple partial seizures that can last hours, days, weeks or, rarely, months. The focal clonic motor form resembles myoclonic jerks, while the rarer sensory and psychic forms may be difficult to differentiate from psychiatric disorders. Ictal EEG changes may be difficult to identify.

Complex partial status epilepticus is a rare condition of rapidly recurring seizures characterized by a fluctuating level of consciousness, automatic behavior, and ictal EEG discharges recorded over the temporal lobe. The condition may be confused clinically with a psychosis or metabolic disturbance and must be included in the differential diagnosis of altered states of consciousness; failure to treat it promptly can be followed by prolonged memory deficits.

Absence status or *spike wave stupor* consists of a continuous state of dulled mentation, which often has a subtle appearance. Eye blinking and other associated movements can occur, and there is a characteristic EEG pattern of diffuse spike-and-wave discharges. The condition occurs fairly often in patients with atypical absences and is also seen with a juvenile form of primary generalized petit mal epilepsy. A rare type of absence status of unknown cause also affects older adults with no previous history of epilepsy. Absence status is not a medical emergency, since no secondary brain damage occurs. The benign and adult forms respond well to antiepileptic

drugs, but atypical absence status associated with diffuse lesions of the brain may be extremely difficult to control.

Major motor status epilepticus exists when generalized tonic-clonic convulsions recur so frequently that consciousness is not regained between them. This can occur with the generalized disorders but is more commonly a result of partial seizures that secondarily generalize. In the latter instance, the partial onset often is not recognized because of the severity of the attacks. Toxic and metabolic disturbances, including drug and alcohol withdrawal, can precipitate major motor status epilepticus in epileptic patients as well as in nonepileptic individuals with genetically low seizure thresholds. Major motor status epilepticus can also be a presenting symptom of acute intracranial hemorrhage and infections, as well as brain tumors and other focal processes, especially in the frontal lobes. Major motor status epilepticus is a life-threatening situation demanding immediate treatment.

DIAGNOSIS. Diagnosis in epilepsy involves searching for treatable causes when possible and recognizing epileptic conditions that indicate a specific prognosis and therapy. When a treatable cause of epilepsy is not revealed, management of the seizures is determined by correct diagnosis of the type of epileptic disorder.

History. The history is overwhelmingly important. The patient's description of any auras should be recorded as well as the ictal behavioral changes observed by others. The occurrence of an aura or any focal signs at onset, during progression, or in the postictal period indicates a partial rather than a generalized seizure disorder. If more than one type of seizure occurs, each should be described separately. Often patients will report several seizure types, which after careful questioning are revealed to be variations of the same ictal phenomenon and not evidence for multiple lesions. For instance, when auras are not followed by further symptoms they may be recognized as one event, while the same aura that spreads to become a complex partial seizure may be reported as another phenomenon. If on occasion there is evolution to a secondarily generalized seizure without postictal recall of the aura, a careful description of the initial ictal events by an observer often will verify that the generalized convulsion is a manifestation of the same epileptogenic lesion. When patients report only seizures that are generalized from the start, an attempt should be made to determine whether convulsive and nonconvulsive ictal manifestations resemble those of benign genetic disorders, generalized disorders caused by diffuse or multiple brain lesions, or secondarily generalized partial seizures caused by a focal lesion. Clues to differential diagnosis derive from the circumstances and age of the patient at onset of seizures and how they may have changed with time or treatment. If the patient has been treated previously, it is important to know what drugs have been used and the specifics of their therapeutic and toxic effects.

The history can provide crucial etiologic information. In children, patterns of early development may delineate the difference between a progressive degenerative disorder and a static lesion. There may be evidence of specific predisposing factors such as perinatal injury, intracranial infections, or reactions to immunizations. A history of a prolonged childhood convulsion preceding the onset of complex partial seizures raises the possibility of mesial temporal sclerosis causing the subsequent chronic epileptic disorder. In older patients there may be hints of cerebral vascular disease or metastatic cancer. A history of head trauma at any age can be relevant but must be evaluated carefully because parents and patients often recall trivial injuries of no importance occurring days or weeks prior to the first seizure. In addition, a specific injurious event such as a fall may be mistakenly interpreted as having generated traumatic epilepsy when it actually represented the first seizure.

The family history can reveal important genetic factors. The existence of relatives with similar seizures or other neurologic symptoms suggests a specific primary epileptic disorder. A family history of individuals with isolated seizures or varied epileptic conditions may indicate the inheritance of a lowered threshold for seizures. Absence of left-handedness in the family of a left-handed patient may hint at early injury of the left cerebral hemisphere.

The psychosocial history can give important clues to diagnosis and indicate needs for more specific evaluations. Patients with benign inherited epileptic disorders usually have normal school and work histories and no evidence of mental disturbance. A history of specific cognitive deficits suggests a focal lesion, while more generalized mental impairment suggests a diffuse abnormality. When the latter is progressive, more detailed laboratory, EEG, and psychometric examinations can determine whether the patient has an underlying degenerative disease, increasing dysfunction because of recurrent seizures, or toxic symptoms of overmedication.

Physical Examination. A careful general medical examination should be done to seek for evidence of systemic diseases responsible for seizures as well as for stigmata of tuberous sclerosis, neurofibromatosis, hemangiomas, and other predisposing congenital disorders. Asymmetry (hemiatrophy) in the size of hands, feet, and face may indicate a long-standing abnormality in the contralateral cerebral hemisphere.

The neurologic examination can provide evidence for a specific diagnosis or reveal focal disturbances that differentiate partial from generalized seizure disorders. Findings of minimal brain dysfunction, such as clumsiness, posturing, and hyperreflexia, or more marked diffuse impairment indicate a secondary rather than a primary generalized seizure disorder.

The mental status examination can distinguish specific cognitive deficits caused by focal lesions from more general mental retardation or dementia. Poor attention span in patients on drug therapy may indicate side effects of medication rather than structural lesions. Increasing degrees of fixed neurologic and mental impairment confer a poor prognosis for both seizure control and psychosocial adaptation.

Many patients can be observed during a seizure. Status epilepticus usually lasts until hospitalization, absences can be provoked by hyperventilation, reflex seizures are easily induced (it is unwise to attempt to induce tonic-clonic convulsions), and spontaneous seizures may occur in the examining room. The initial manifestations and early development should be noted. Consciousness should be assessed by repeating a phrase to determine whether the patient can recall it after the seizure is over. Even if the seizure appears to be generalized at the start, postictal examination of neurologic and mental status may reveal focal deficits that indicate a partial seizure disorder. When circumstances make direct examination impossible, try to find a reliable witness who can describe the attack.

Laboratory Studies. Epilepsy provides no diagnostic hematologic or chemical laboratory tracers, but such tests can help to diagnose underlying disease processes that give rise to seizures. One or more generalized epileptic attacks can mildly increase protein content and white cell count in the cerebrospinal fluid for 24 to 48 hours. Although up to 100 white cells per cubic millimeter have been reported after major motor status epilepticus, a lumbar puncture revealing more than 10 white cells per cubic millimeter should initiate a search for an intracranial inflammatory process. In infants and young children with seizures, it is wise to test blood and urine for metabolic disorders. In older patients with refractory focal motor seizures, hyperosmolar syndromes such as hyperglycemia and uremia should be considered. Complete blood count, liver function tests; blood urea nitrogen, and urinalysis are necessary in all patients about to begin antiepileptic drug therapy to establish a baseline for evaluating possible subsequent toxic side effects.

Radiologic Studies. A computed tomographic (CT) scan is necessary for adolescents and adults with the recent onset of seizures but may be avoided in younger children when history and other examinations indicate a primary generalized disorder or a nonprogressive lesion. Cerebral angiography should be confined to cases in which surgery is considered or a primary vascular disorder is suspected.

Psychometric Studies. Psychometric testing, including standard tests of attention, performance and verbal IQ, memory, language, and personality can help verify the existence of a focal or diffuse brain disturbance. When there is evidence that mental function is deteriorating, serial testing can quantify the change and evaluate subsequent trends of disease or therapy. An astute psychometrician should also be able to offer advice for improving psychosocial adaptation.

Electroencephalography. The EEG is the most useful diagnostic laboratory test for epilepsy. However, overinterpretation of the EEG often generates an unwarranted diagnosis of epilepsy. A number of spike-like EEG events can be normal, and 2 per cent of the nonepileptic population may have true epileptiform spike-and-wave complexes on their EEGs but never develop seizures. Conversely, 20 per cent of patients with epilepsy do not demonstrate epileptic abnormalities on a routine interictal EEG. Whereas an EEG can help verify a clinical diagnosis of epilepsy, interictal epileptiform EEG abnormalities alone should be considered neither necessary nor sufficient information for arriving at this diagnosis. If a seizure occurs in the EEG laboratory, the association of an ictal EEG pattern with observed clinical behavior makes possible a definitive diagnosis.

The pattern of interictal EEG abnormalities may help determine the type of epileptic disorder. Focal spike-and-wave discharges or slow waves indicate a partial epileptic disorder. A diagnosis of benign sylvian epilepsy may be confirmed by characteristic centrotemporal spikes that are easily differentiated from the anterior temporal EEG transients of temporal lobe epilepsy. While bilaterally synchronous EEG discharges may also reflect a focal lesion (*secondary bilateral synchrony*), especially in the frontal lobes, such activity more often indicates a generalized epileptic disorder. Baseline nonepileptiform EEG abnormalities suggest a secondary epileptic disorder, although antiepileptic drugs can produce mild diffuse EEG slowing.

Typical petit mal absences are associated with symmetric, synchronous, and regular *three-per-second* (or faster) *spike-and-wave* discharges that begin and end abruptly without postictal EEG changes. This EEG pattern is usually easily distinguished from the *slow and irregular spike-and-wave* (2.5 per second or less) seen in the Lennox-Gastaut syndrome.

Activation procedures used in the EEG laboratory include hyperventilation for absences, photic stimulation for photosensitive epilepsy, and sleep. But there are major pitfalls: hyperventilation in children and some normal adults can induce high amplitude slowing resembling spike-and-wave discharges; photomyogenic responses of facial muscles to photic stimulation can occur in normal individuals and during drug and alcohol withdrawal and should not be considered evidence of epilepsy; a number of normal sharp transients that occur during sleep and on arousal often are misinterpreted as epileptic spikes.

Nonstandard techniques, available in some laboratories, may offer additional diagnostic advantages. Nasopharyngeal and sphenoidal electrodes can clarify interictal EEG spike patterns originating in mesial temporal structures, but the same information usually can be obtained more easily from ear lobe electrodes. Special epilepsy centers throughout the country offer prolonged EEG telemetry and television monitoring to provide a more precise description of specific ictal events when diagnosis is in doubt. Ambulatory EEG monitoring is being developed for outpatient evaluations.

A repeat EEG may be indicated to determine whether behavioral deterioration is due to an increase in subclinical seizure activity, an increase in drug side effects, or a progressive underlying lesion. If necessary, EEG telemetry combined with frequent antiepileptic drug level determinations or ambulatory monitoring can improve medical management by allowing dose schedules to be tailored to individual patients' needs.

The EEG is also essential for monitoring the progress of therapy for status epilepticus when clinical behavior is not a reliable guide. This is often true in stupor related to spike-and-wave discharge patterns and in complex partial status epilepticus and is always the case when anesthesia or paralysis is used to control major motor status epilepticus.

DIFFERENTIAL DIAGNOSIS. The diagnosis of epilepsy should be made only on firm clinical evidence. Such a diagnosis can have irreversible psychosocial effects resulting in the loss of a driver's license, a job, independence, and self-esteem. Consequently, a physician often does more harm by making an unjustified diagnosis than by reserving judgment until the nature of the disorder has declared itself adequately. When doubt exists injury can be minimized by warning the patient to avoid the conditions that might have precipitated the event and to be aware of potentially dangerous situations should another event occur.

Systemic Disturbances. *Syncope* is the most common systemic disturbance confused with epilepsy. Syncope can be associated with motor twitches and in rare instances may produce a tonic-clonic convulsion in susceptible individuals, *"convulsive syncope."* This condition must be treated as syncope, not as epilepsy. Because cardiogenic syncope can cause a convulsion while seizures may be associated with cardiac arrhythmias, diagnostic monitoring of blackout spells should ideally include both ECG and EEG recordings. Other intermittent systemic disorders that can be mistaken for epilepsy include breath-holding spells in early childhood, hyperventilation syndrome, alcoholic blackouts, intermittent porphyria, hypoglycemia, pheochromocytoma, tetanus, and toxic-metabolic abnormalities.

Neurologic Disturbances. Nonepileptic episodic neurologic disturbances are most often of vascular origin. Transient ischemic attacks must be considered when intermittent neurologic symptoms occur in older patients. Drop attacks beginning in adulthood usually are caused by posterior fossa vascular disturbances or cataplexy and are almost never epileptic. Transient global amnesia also is more likely to have a vascular than an epileptic cause. Prodromal migraine symptoms can resemble epileptic seizures, and the subsequent headache can be mistaken for a postictal headache. The distinction between migraine and epilepsy is not always completely clear.

Sleep disorders are also commonly mistaken for epilepsy. Narcolepsy is easily diagnosed when all four of the classic symptoms are present; however, if sleep attacks, cataplexy, sleep paralysis, or hypnogogic hallucinations occur alone, they can be confused with epileptic seizures. Careful questioning usually will elicit evidence for some of the other symptoms as well. Hypersomnia, as seen in Kleine-Levin and sleep apnea syndromes, as well as dyssomnias such as somnambulism, night terrors, and enuresis must be differentiated. On rare occasions epileptic seizures can be manifested as nocturnal ambulation, fear, and urinary incontinence; all-night sleep EEG recordings may be necessary to make the correct diagnosis in such instances.

Other neurologic symptoms that can masquerade as epilepsy include intermittent vertigo from a variety of causes and the episodic uncontrolled movements that occur with *Gilles de la Tourette's syndrome*, hemiballismus, chorea, athetosis, and other extrapyramidal disorders. Although the involuntary movements of paroxysmal choreoathetosis are not

epileptic, they can often be successfully treated with antiepileptic medication. The myoclonic disorders discussed earlier also should not be confused with epilepsy.

Behavioral Disturbances. It is both important and, sometimes, difficult to differentiate between true epileptic seizures and conversion reactions. Hysterical seizures (*pseudo seizures*) may be manifested in ways that have psychologic significance such as with pelvic thrusting, may involve motor symptoms that do not fit with known anatomic spread patterns, and only rarely result in injury to the patient despite risk. Nevertheless, it is impossible to make this diagnosis definitively from a description or even from observation of a seizure. Virtually any paroxysmal behavior, no matter how bizarre, could be a true epileptic seizure. The diagnosis of hysterical seizures may be made with some confidence, however, when ictal events are suggestive for the reasons just stated, EEG recordings are normal, antiepileptic medication is ineffective, and evidence of secondary gain is obtained during psychiatric interview. EEG telemetry and television monitoring of ictal events may help in this differential diagnosis: clear EEG changes or an elevated postictal serum prolactin can confirm the occurrence of an epileptic convulsion, but their absence does not necessarily rule out this possibility.

There are several considerations, however, which limit conclusions drawn from telemetry. Simple partial ictal events may have no EEG correlates that can be recorded from the scalp, EEG changes that accompany motor seizures may be obscured by muscle artifact (but postictal EEG suppression is evidence that a true epileptic seizure has occurred), and repeated bilaterally synchronous myoclonic jerks unassociated with loss of consciousness may be mistaken for psychogenic events. Even if a definite diagnosis of hysterical seizure disorder can be made, many such patients have epileptic seizures as well. When hysterical seizures and real seizures coexist, EEG and television monitoring may help to differentiate the two types and provide a basis for independently assessing the results of psychiatric and medical treatment.

Some true epileptic symptoms can be confused with behavioral disturbances. Frequently occurring absences in children can be mistaken for attentional deficits, learning disabilities, and disciplinary problems, but the EEG should provide the correct diagnosis. Certain simple partial seizures with sensory or psychic symptoms may be interpreted as psychotic hallucinations. Although these epileptic experiences can have an emotional content, they usually are more stereotyped and more likely to have visual components than are psychotic hallucinations. Rarely, *fugue states* may represent continuous epileptic seizures (*poriomania*) or prolonged periods of postical confusion.

Episodic dyscontrol is a poorly defined entity consisting of intermittent periods of inappropriately violent, occasionally destructive behavior. Confusion with epilepsy is compounded by the fact that some patients with this syndrome have epileptic seizures as well. If the episodic behavior lasts only several minutes, is uncharacteristic of the patient's interictal personality, and there is amnesia for the event with appropriate remorse afterward, this may possibly reflect an epileptic disturbance. Although ictal EEG recordings have not supported this contention, an occasional patient with episodic dyscontrol may be helped by antiepileptic medication. Organized and directed violence is not seen during the epileptic seizures described earlier, and epilepsy is never the cause of premeditated criminal acts.

Reactive Seizures. Single isolated generalized convulsions resulting from documented precipitating events such as sleep deprivation, alcohol or sedative drug withdrawal, use of convulsant drugs, fever, and acute head trauma, as well as recurrent convulsions induced by reversible infectious, toxic, or metabolic processes and limited to the period of systemic illness should not be considered evidence of an epileptic

TABLE 493–5. COMMONLY USED ANTIEPILEPTIC DRUGS

Drug	Seizure Type	Adult Dose (mg/kg)	Therapeutic Range (μg/ml)	Half-life (hours)	Peak Time (hours)	Daily Doses
Carbamazepine (Tegretol)	P, GC	15–25	8–12	12	2–6	4
Phenytoin (Dilantin)	P, GC	3–8	10–30	24	4–8	2
Primidone (Mysoline)†	P, GC	10–20	5–15	12	2–4	4
Phenobarbital	P, GC	2–4	15–40	96	6–18	1
Clorazepate (Tranxene)	P, GC	0.7–1.0	1–2*	30*	1*	2
Mephobarbital (Mebaral)	P, GC	4–10	10–30*	96*	6–18*	1
Mephenytoin (Mesantoin)	P, GC	2–10	10–40	100*	27*	1
Ethosuximide (Zarontin)	A	10–30	40–100	30‡	2–3	2
Trimethadione (Tridione)	A	20–40	500–1200*	240*	120–240*	1
Clonazepam (Clonopin)	A, M	0.03–0.3	0.01–0.05	30	1–2	2
Methsuximide (Celontin)	P, A	10–25	20–40*	40*	<3	2
Valproic acid (Depakene)	All	15–60	50–100	8	1–4	4

Modified in part from Leal KW, Troupin AS: Clin Chem 23, 1964, 1977.
*For derived metabolite.
†Substantial antiepileptic effect is obtained from derived phenobarbital.
‡For children (60 hours for adults).
Key: P = partial; GC = generalized convulsive; A = absence; M = myoclonus.

disorder. However, a chronic epileptic condition probably exists if there is an indication of focal ictal or postictal features; if there is evidence of an intracerebral lesion; or if seizures recur in the absence of the presumed cause.

TREATMENT. Treatable causes of epileptic seizures include intracerebral mass lesions that can be surgically removed and toxic, metabolic, infectious, and vascular diseases that require medical management. A treatable cause cannot be found in most patients with chronic recurrent seizures, however, and the objective of therapy is then to maximize useful function, ideally by complete eradication of seizures without introduction of unwanted side effects. Adequate control is usually possible with appropriate pharmacologic, surgical, and psychosocial management. Only about half of patients treated for chronic epilepsy can expect to become seizure free indefinitely.

Pharmacologic Therapy. Although many antiepileptic drugs are available, it is prudent to become familiar with and use the few that are most effective for each of the various seizure types (Table 493–5). Pharmacologic therapy is based on obtaining an accurate diagnosis of seizure type or epileptic syndrome, selecting the single most appropriate drug for that diagnosis (monotherapy), and correlating measurements of drug levels in the serum with patient reports in order to adjust dosages and dose schedules for the best control and fewest side effects. The best control does not necessarily mean the greatest reduction in seizure frequency. In certain patients, the disability caused by some continued seizures may be less than limitations induced by therapy. For example, a few absences a day for a child is preferable to an alternative of no seizures on a dose of medication that produces continuous sedation and impairs school performance. Similarly, aggressive therapy is not justified for a patient with refractory epilepsy when high drug levels exacerbate existing physical and mental handicaps without producing a worthwhile improvement in the seizure pattern.

PHARMACOKINETIC PRINCIPLES. Dose planning for individual antiepileptic drugs depends on pharmacokinetic factors that determine the amount of available drug in the blood. The therapeutic ranges for individual antiepileptic drugs refer to the ranges of steady state levels of each drug that by trial and error have been most effective in controlling seizures with minimal or no side effects. Average or approximate pharmacokinetic variables for the commonly used antiepileptic drugs appear in Table 493–5.

The proper dose schedule for a newly introduced drug depends on balancing the need for rapid control of seizures against the avoidance of side effects. If a patient has been warned about the possible occurrence of another seizure and takes appropriate precautions, it usually is not necessary to build a drug level rapidly at the risk of producing severe toxicity. It is more important that the patient accept the drug of first choice. Patients can be encouraged to remain on medication by beginning a drug regimen slowly, taking the medication with meals when nausea is anticipated, using higher doses at bedtime when sedation is anticipated, and reducing doses transiently when untoward side effects occur. Most unpleasant dose-related side effects are temporary, and an appropriate regimen eventually can be instituted. A loading dose can be given practically for some drugs (phenytoin and phenobarbital) when the risk of repeated seizures requires therapeutic levels to be achieved rapidly despite side effects. A loading dose of 1.5 (rather than 2) times the calculated total daily dose may be an adequate compromise between obtaining rapid seizure control and producing minimal side effects if the planned maintenance schedule is begun less than one half-life after the loading dose.

Although a maintenance steady-state level of a drug can be achieved with an interdose interval of approximately one half-life time, in this situation drug levels will fall below the protective range if a single dose is missed. However, a dose schedule that requires a drug to be taken too frequently may be inconvenient and reduce compliance. An interdose interval of 0.5 half-lives, which amounts to one to four times a day for the commonly used medications, is usually recommended. Therapeutic failure using recommended dose schedules most commonly reflects noncompliance by the patient, but also may result from aberrant absorption and metabolism, and dose schedules must then be determined individually from measurements of serum drug levels.

The recommended therapeutic range for a given drug is based on average measures. One should use these values as a guide rather than a goal; therapeutic drug levels in individual patients may be well above or below the average. Once an effective maintenance schedule has been achieved, determination of serum drug levels, always drawn at the same time after a given dose, provide a reliable long-term record in steady-state conditions. Such measurements are useful when recurrent seizures or side effects result from decreases or increases in available drug (Table 493–6).

Enzyme Induction and Inhibition. Failure of compliance and enzyme induction by the liver are the two most common reasons for the late appearance of subtherapeutic blood levels after an effective maintenance schedule has been achieved. If seizures recur following a period of control, owing to enzyme induction, the dose of the initial anticonvulsant should be increased gradually to the desired blood level or to toxicity rather than immediately adding a new drug. The latter may merely enchance enzyme induction and further decrease blood levels. Addition of a second drug can also inhibit liver

TABLE 493–6. INDICATIONS FOR SERUM ANTIEPILEPTIC DRUG LEVELS

To establish individual therapeutic range
    Initiation of treatment while seizures remain uncontrolled

To identify altered pharmacokinetics
    Loss of seizure control or appearance of toxic symptoms
    Addition of second antiepileptic drug or change in drug regimen
    Questionable change in drug efficacy during:
        Intercurrent illness
        Multiple drug therapy
        Altered physiologic state such as pregnancy or puberty
    Unexplained behavioral or neurologic symptoms that might be evidence of
        toxicity

To document compliance

enzymes and cause toxic effects owing to increased levels of the first drug. If it is necessary to add a second anticonvulsant, serum levels of both agents require checking so as to assure that adequate but not toxic levels of both have been attained. In general, if the first drug recommended for treatment has no effect on seizure control despite adequate serum levels or achieves control only at the expense of severe toxicity, it is best to replace it with a second drug. Gradual withdrawal of the first drug may induce a temporary exacerbation of seizure frequency, which does not necessarily indicate that the second drug is ineffective. Occasionally the use of more than one drug becomes unavoidable, particularly when patients have more than one type of seizure.

Selection of Antiepileptic Drugs. PREFERRED AGENTS. While specific types of seizures respond to specific drugs (Table 493–3), many factors determine the choice of the best single drug for an individual patient. The trend today is to treat generalized convulsive and partial seizures first with either carbamazepine or phenytoin. The idiosyncratic hematologic side effects of carbamazepine, which were generally feared when this drug was initially introduced, have proved to be rare, and carbamazepine often is preferred over phenytoin by epileptologists. While both drugs offer the same protection, phenytoin use is associated with a high incidence of disturbing cosmetic side effects.

The barbiturates primidone and phenobarbital are also used for convulsive and partial seizures. They are less effective than carbamazepine and phenytoin, but phenobarbital is the least expensive of the available antiepileptic drugs and has the fewest dangerous side effects. Sedation is common but may not be a problem at lower doses and may subside over time even at higher doses. Furthermore, both carbamazepine and phenytoin can dull mentation at high doses. Barbiturates are a problem in children, since these drugs commonly engender hyperkinetic activity and other undesirable behavioral disturbances. Most epileptologists now generally prefer carbamazepine for this age group because it does not seriously alter behavior. Phenobarbital should not be given to patients with depressive tendencies. It can exacerbate psychologic depression and is the most common instrument of suicide in the epileptic population.

Ethosuximide is still the drug of choice for absence seizures, since it is safer than valproic acid. Valproic acid can produce serious idiosyncratic hepatic side effects that laboratory tests may not predict. Fortunately, mortality from this complication is rare (1 per 35,000), and valproic acid is effective against a variety of seizure types. Valproic acid is the drug of choice for mixed seizure disorders because of its broad spectrum of action and for juvenile epileptic myoclonus. Valproic acid may be more effctive than ethosuximide for atypical absences and also is used widely as a second choice drug for other types of seizures. Enzyme inhibition occurs with valproic acid, which greatly increases serum levels of other antiepileptic drugs. This is a particular problem with the barbiturates and sometimes results in inadvertent sedation or even coma.

The drugs of choice for nonepileptic forms of myoclonus

are the benzodiazepine clonazepam, and valproic acid. Benzodiazepines tend to lose their effectiveness with time as tolerence develops. In progressive myoclonus epilepsy, where myoclonic jerks and seizures are both present, valproic acid may be the best hope for control with monotherapy. If this is unsuccessful, clonazepam plus carbamazepine or phenytoin may be required. Clonazepam and valproic acid given together may interact to make seizures worse and produce unpleasant side effects.

SECOND-LINE ANTIEPILEPTIC DRUGS. Clorazepate is a benzodiazepine currently used as an adjunctive medication for convulsive and partial seizures, although it may also be an effective primary antiepileptic. Other drugs that may be of value if first-line drugs fail include mephenytoin and mephobarbital for convulsive and partial seizures, and clonazepam and trimethadione for absences. Methsuximide is effective against absence and atonic and partial seizures and can be used alone or as an adjunctive medication. Acetazolamide may be a useful adjunctive medication, particularly for 10 days premenstrually through the end of menses for women with catamenial accentuation of epilepsy. Adrenocorticotropic hormone (ACTH) and adrenocorticosteroids have been found useful in the treatment of infantile spasms but not in other epileptic conditions.

SIDE EFFECTS. Almost all antiepileptic drugs potentially produce undesirable side effects, and physicians should consult the *Physicians' Desk Reference* or a current textbook before first use. Common dose-related side effects of carbamazepine and the hydantoins include nausea, dizziness, diplopia, and ataxia. Sedation, impaired mentation, and hyperactivity occur most often with the barbiturates and benzodiazepines. These symptoms may abate with time. Drug-induced folic acid deficiencies may reach symptomatic levels in some patients and require vitamin supplements. Idiosyncratic side effects that usually affect skin, blood, liver, and kidneys are potentially more serious. When a new drug is introduced, complete blood counts and appropriate blood chemistry analyses should be obtained every four weeks for several months, and then monitored every 3 to 12 months as long as therapy continues. Leukopenia as low as 3000 per cu mm can occur with carbamazepine and does not necessarily indicate impending agranulocytosis. Moreover, an elevated serum alkaline phosphatase level alone does not indicate a hepatotoxic reaction. Mild pruritus may be treated medically. Evidence of blood dyscrasias, liver or kidney damage, or more serious skin rash requires prompt discontinuation of medication and referral to the proper specialist. Cosmetic side effects commonly associated with phenytoin include hirsutism, gingival hyperplasia, and coarsening of features; weight gain and alopecia are occasionally seen with valproic acid therapy. Carbamazepine can cause water retention and is not used for patients with congestive heart failure. A paradoxic increase in seizure frequency may result from elevated drug levels, particularly with phenytoin, and can cause seizures to recur after a period of control.

Pregnancy presents certain problems for women with epilepsy. Seizures may become more frequent, and antiepileptic drug clearance may increase, requiring higher doses of medication. Hemorrhagic disease of the newborn occurs with phenobarbital and phenytoin and can be treated with vitamin K. A two- to three-fold drug-related increase in the incidence of birth defects has been documented for phenytoin, but the nature of all antiepileptic drugs is such that they may have teratogenic effects. Phenytoin is not recommended for women of childbearing age; however, there is little to be gained from discontinuing effective medication once pregnancy has been determined, especially after the first trimester has been completed. The risk to mother and fetus from seizures may be greater than the risk of teratogenicity. Maternal drug levels can cause sedation and withdrawal in the newborn but only rarely do they present a problem for breast-fed infants.

Surgical Therapy. Resective surgery has proved safe and beneficial and can cure a chronic epileptic condition when all else fails. At present it is a greatly underutilized therapeutic modality. Most surgical facilities will consider epileptic patients potential candidates for resective surgical therapy if (1) a partial seizure disorder has been documented, (2) seizures continue at a frequency that seriously interferes with daily living despite adequate levels of appropriate antiepileptic medication, and (3) there is not substantial interictal mental retardation or psychosis. Patients with complex partial seizures of temporal lobe origin are ideal candidates for surgery. Worthwhile improvement occurs in 85 per cent of such patients, and as many as two thirds may become seizure free after anterior temporal lobectomy. Local resection of an extratemporal focal epileptogenic lesion is also possible if the area of cortex can be identified precisely and removed safely. A history of generalized convulsions, a focus in the dominant hemisphere, or the presence of bilateral independent temporal spike foci on EEG do not contraindicate surgery.

Section of the corpus callosum has been particularly effective in controlling otherwise intractable drop attacks, and patients with other secondary generalized and partial seizure patterns have experienced improvement from this operation. While *hemispherectomy* is the most effective surgical procedure for epilepsy, it is justified only for children who have severely incapacitating unilateral seizures and hemiparesis. Destructive lesions and cerebellar stimulation are no longer routinely recommended.

Other Therapeutic Considerations. Patients with some types of seizures may benefit from special management. Reflex seizures induced by specific stimuli can be treated by avoiding the stimuli. For example, epileptic photosensitivity can be abolished by patching one eye or wearing colored glasses, and desensitization is possible for many forms of reflex seizures. Spread of some simple partial seizures may be aborted by strong or painful sensory stimulation administered at onset. Operant conditioning (biofeedback) can reduce seizures in some patients, but the approach is generally impractical. When seizures occur only at specific times of the day, medications can be adjusted to insure maximum levels at those times, and daily schedules can be altered so that the patient is home or in a safe environment when at risk. A *ketogenic diet* appears to have helped some children.

Patients with all types of seizures should remain active and maintain daily habits that insure regular meals, adequate sleep, and a reduction in unnecessary stress. Alcohol or sedative drugs can be taken sparingly, but excessive use can provoke seizures during withdrawal. Patients who have seizures associated with an alteration in consciousness, particularly those that occur without warning, should be counseled to avoid hazardous situations: they should not swim alone, should shower rather than bathe, should not climb to unprotected heights, and should not operate potentially dangerous power-driven machines, including automobiles.

Emergency Treatment. First aid for a generalized tonic-clonic convulsion consists of protecting the patient from self-injury. Clothing should be loosened, sharp objects removed from the area, and the patient's head cushioned from impact. Hard objects or fingers must not be inserted into the patient's mouth: patients do not choke on their own tongues. When the seizure is over, turn the patient's head to drain oral secretions. Have someone stay with the patient during the postictal period until full consciousness has returned. It is not necessary to call an ambulance unless the patient has never had a seizure before, the seizure lasts longer than ten minutes, another attack occurs before consciousness is regained, or there is evidence of injury, respiratory distress, or pregnancy. Patients should not be forcibly restrained during complex partial seizures but protected from surrounding hazards until ictal and postical symptoms cease and they can care for themselves.

Major motor status epilepticus is a medical emergency requiring immediate intervention to prevent permanent brain damage or death. A recommended approach appears in Table 493–7. As soon as the airway is secured, a quick neurologic examination should be performed to appraise critical forebrain and brainstem functions. There may be evidence of an acute intracerebral lesion with herniation or other life-threatening conditions. Because the effects of diazepam are shortlived, it should be administered simultaneously with a longer-acting antiepileptic drug. Phenytoin usually is preferred, since it produces no sedative effects. This allows the patient to regain consciousness when seizures are terminated and facilitates neurologic evaluation. If seizures have not stopped 60 minutes after the institution of therapy, high intravenous doses of phenobarbital or general anesthesia are recommended; some physicians prefer to use a 4 per cent intravenous solution of paraldehyde in normal saline solution, which can be titrated to maintain the desired therapeutic effect. If these latter approaches are necessary, intubation and ventilation should be used and the progress of treatment followed with EEG recordings.

Once status has been controlled, maintenance drug therapy is instituted. The most common cause of major motor status epilepticus is a sudden reduction or discontinuation of antiepileptic drugs in patients with known seizure disorders.

Psychosocial Considerations. To some extent, psychosocial disturbances among epileptics are situational. Because most seizures occur spontaneously and unpredictably, many patients spend their lives anticipating inappropriate behavior, embarrassment, or serious injury. Epileptics are frequently unable to find work if they admit to a seizure disorder, so that their opportunities for rewarding social relationships are reduced. In most states, patients with seizures that impair consciousness are not allowed to drive. These factors contribute to a higher incidence of depression and suicide among epileptics than in the general population.

Although the evidence is controversial, aberrant personality traits, affective disorders, and psychoses, including late paranoid schizophrenia, have been reported to be more common among patients with epilepsy, particularly those with complex partial seizures of limbic origin. It is unclear to what extent these disturbances result from the underlying pathologic lesions or specific seizure activity, how much can be attributed to the effect of long-term antiepileptic drug therapy, and how much relates to limitations imposed on daily living and the stigma of being epileptic.

Only about one in four patients with uncontrolled epilepsy is handicapped by seizures alone. The others have physical, intellectual, and/or psychiatric disabilities that disrupt their

TABLE 493–7. MANAGEMENT OF CONVULSIVE STATUS EPILEPTICUS

Treatment Goal	Cumulative Time Since Arrival in Emergency Room (minutes)
Restore homeostasis	
Check for airway obstruction; check blood pressure, nasal O_2; intubate as needed	0–15
Draw blood sample for glucose, blood urea nitrogen, electrolytes, complete blood count, drug level determination	0–15
Start administering isotonic saline solution, 1000 ml, IV	
Administer glucose 50%, 50 ml, IV; thiamine, 100 mg, IM	0–15
Stop convulsive seizures	
Give diazepam, 10 mg., IV; repeat administration of 10 mg with every seizure, up to 50 mg*	15–60
Give phenytoin, 20 mg/kg, IV (<50 mg/minute)	15–60
If seizures do not stop by 1 hour, give high doses of phenobarbital IV or general anesthesia	60–120

*Exceeds manufacturer's recommended dosage.
Modified from Wasterlain CG. In Engl J Jr, et al: Ann Intern Med *97*:584, 1982.

daily lives. Epileptic seizures, perhaps more than any other neurologic symptom, are modified by internal and external influences that are under the control of the patient and other persons. For these reasons, treatment of the epileptic patient requires more than manipulation of anticonvulsant drugs, and outcome depends upon more than just seizure control. The physician must come to know the patient and the patient's family, their psychologic interactions, and their social situation. Furthermore, improving psychosocial adaptation itself often leads to a reduction in seizure frequency. To provide the comprehensive care required by patients with seizure disorders, the physician must attend to the patient as well as to the neurological disorder. The doctor must be friend as well as therapist.

Commission on Classification and Terminology of the International League Against Epilepsy: Clinical and electroencephalographic classification of epileptic seizures. Epilepsia 22:489, 1981. *The currently accepted classification of epileptic seizures and definition of relevant terms.*

Engel J Jr (ed.): Surgical Treatment of the Epilepsies. New York, Raven Press, 1987. *A comprehensive presentation of modern surgical therapy for epilepsy.*
Epilepsy Abstracts 1947–present. *Published now by Excerpta Medica, this monthly journal contains abstracts of all epilepsy-related papers and is an easy introduction to the literature on any subject.*
Gumnit RJ: The Epilepsy Handbook, The Practical Management of Seizures. New York, Raven Press, 1983. *An excellent practical guide for the diagnosis and treatment of patients with epilepsy. Does not include references.*
Penfield W, Jasper H: Epilepsy and the Functional Anatomy of the Brain. Boston, Little, Brown and Company, 1954. *A classic by pioneers of modern epileptology; describes epileptic phenomena and applications of clinical data to the understanding of normal brain functions.*
Porter RJ: Epilepsy, 100 Elementary Principles. Philadelphia, W. B. Saunders Company, 1984. *A small volume of clinical pearls.*
Roger J, Dravet C, Bureau M, et al.: Epileptic Syndromes in Infancy, Childhood and Adolescence. London, John Libbey Eurotext, Ltd., 1985. *Detailed descriptions of the currently recognized epileptic syndromes.*
Spehlmann R: EEG Primer. Amsterdam, Elsevier/North Holland, 1981. *A simple straightforward introduction to clinical EEG.*
Woodbury DM, Penry JK, Pippenger CE (eds.): Antiepileptic Drugs. New York, Raven Press, 1982. *A multiauthored compendium of recent concepts of pharmacologic therapy of epilepsy.*

SECTION THIRTEEN /
INTRACRANIAL TUMORS AND STATES OF ALTERED INTRACRANIAL PRESSURE

---

494 INTRACRANIAL TUMORS
William R. Shapiro

Intracranial tumors include neoplasms, both benign and malignant, and space-taking lesions of chronic inflammatory origin (granulomas) that develop in brain, meninges, or skull. The present chapter concerns neoplasms; granulomas are covered elsewhere. Primary tumors of the central nervous system are the second most common cancer in children, and in adults they are more common than Hodgkin's disease. In 1986 there were approximately 12,000 new cases of primary central nervous system cancer in the United States. About 15 per cent of deaths from systemic cancer are directly associated with metastases to the nervous system, mostly from primaries in lung or breast, malignant melanoma, lymphomas, and leukemias.

PATHOGENESIS. *Intracranial Neoplasms as a Form of Cancer.* The cause of brain tumors is unknown, although genetic factors appear to be important in tumors such as hemangioblastoma, neurofibroma, and some gliomas. *Benign intracranial tumors* are slow growing, with few mitoses, no necrosis, and no vascular proliferation. They may arise in the meninges or as neuroectodermal tumors. *Malignant tumors* are characterized by more rapid growth, invasiveness, frequent mitotic figures, necrosis, vascular proliferation, and endothelial hyperplasia. However, "benign" brain tumors that cannot be entirely excised are lethal, and "malignant" brain tumors rarely metastasize out of the central nervous system. Thus, the distinction between benign and malignant is less important for intracranial tumors than for systemic cancer.

Intracranial tumors differ from systemic cancers in several other ways. Primary neuroectodermal tumors infiltrate the brain, whereas secondary metastatic brain tumors are partly encapsulated. The microenvironment of tumors in the brain—the blood-brain barrier—influences both diagnosis and therapy. The blood-brain barrier retards entry of many compounds, including radiologic contrast agents and chemotherapeutic drugs. The barrier appears to be intact in most benign neuroectodermal tumors, but it becomes progressively disrupted in malignant brain tumors. The breakdown of the barrier allows the entry of contrast agents and radioisotopes that permit the tumor to be imaged separately from the brain in scanning techniques. Both experimental and clinical studies suggest that the disruption of the barrier in malignant tumors also permits the entry of chemotherapeutic agents. Because the brain has no lymphatic system, fluid that accumulates from leaking capillaries within the brain tumor cannot be removed except via slow diffusion toward the cerebrospinal fluid (CSF) pathways. This fluid, or "cerebral edema," itself produces symptoms by adding to the mass effect of tumors. Central nervous system tumors rarely metastasize to the rest of the body, but infiltrate within the brain, and some tumors spread along CSF pathways, producing obstruction and hydrocephalus. Perhaps the most important difference between central nervous system neoplasms and systemic cancer is that large block "cancer operations" are not possible in the brain. Attempting to remove normal tissue margins in brain tumor can produce irreparable neurologic dysfunction. The neurosurgeon attempting to remove a primary neuroectodermal tumor must stay within the confines of the tumor in order to spare brain tissue. Often, tumor-infiltrated brain tissue must be spared because its removal would produce unacceptable neurologic dysfunction. Such considerations weigh heavily in the management of patients with intracranial neoplasms.

CLASSIFICATIONS AND PATHOLOGY. Table 494–1 depicts a classification of intracranial tumors by both pathology

TABLE 494–1. THE MAJOR INTRACRANIAL TUMORS

	Pathological Characteristics	Clinical Characteristics
Neuroectodermal		
Astrocytoma	Diffuse infiltration cerebrum and brain stem; microcystic, especially in cerebellum; occasionally calcifies; no mitoses; may become malignant	Slow growing, survival of 4 to 7 or more years possible
Oligodendroglioma	Circumscribed, globular mass, often cystic and often calcifies; cellular perinuclear halos; rarely becomes malignant	Slow growing, seizures common, calcification on CT, survival of 4 to 7 or more years possible
Anaplastic astrocytoma	Astrocytomas with increased cellularity, nuclear pleomorphism, increased mitoses, vascular hyperplasia, no necrosis; malignant	Moderately rapid growing, younger patients, survival of 1.5–2.5 years
Glioblastoma multiforme	Variegated, infiltrative; occasionally cystic, necrotic or hemorrhagic, mitoses present, highly malignant	Rapidly growing, older patients, survival usually under 1 year
Ependymoma	Most often fourth ventricle, demarcated; rarely malignant	Primarily children, good prognosis
Medulloblastoma	Usually arises in vermis of cerebellum; highly cellular, hyperchromatic nuclei; seeds the meninges via CSF	Primarily children, prognosis with RT to whole neuraxis = 60% 5-year survival
Mesodermal meningioma	Arises from dura on dorsal surface, along base of brain, from falx, sphenoid ridge; benign, variable pattern; rarely converts to malignant tumor	Adults, more common in women, curable by resection if not too large
Cranial nerves		
Acoustic schwannoma (acoustic neurilemoma), trigeminal neurilemoma	Nodular mass on cranial nerve; benign, Schwann cell proliferation	Usually curable by resection, especially if small
Neurofibroma	Nodular mass on cranial nerve; Schwann cell and fibroblast proliferation	More common in von Recklinghausen's disease
Pituitary tumors		
Adenomas	Sellar and suprasellar masses of various sizes; chromophobic, acidophilic, and basophilic; all may be secretory or nonsecretory	Common cause of amenorrhea/galactorrhea syndrome, usually curable
Craniopharyngioma	Sellar or suprasellar, often calcified and cystic; derived from Rathke's pouch	More common in children, often curable on resection
Pineal tumors	Germinomas, may produce endocrinopathy; may seed via CSF	Most common in children, good initial response to radiation, many cured, others recur
Metastatic tumors	Parenchymal, skull, meningeal, may seed via CSF (meningeal carcinomatosis)	Common with many cancers, respond to initial treatment
Primary lymphoma	Diffuse histiocytic, B cell; malignant; higher incidence after renal transplant and in AIDS	Good initial response to treatment, usually recur
Vascular tumors	Arteriovenous malformation; non-neoplastic. Hemangioblastoma (von Hippel-Lindau syndrome); neoplastic	Hemorrhage common
Congenital tumors	Craniopharyngioma, chordoma, dermoid, teratoma	Often curable by resection
Granuloma and parasitic cysts	Tuberculoma, toruloma (cryptococcosis), sarcoidosis, cysticercosis, toxoplasmosis (especially in AIDS)	

and general clinical characteristics. Neuroectodermal tumors, the most common primary parenchymal tumor, occur at any age. About half are relatively benign, infiltrating astrocytomas that may be cystic. Neuroectodermal tumors can arise in the cerebrum in the form of astrocytomas, oligodendrogliomas, and the more malignant glioblastoma multiforme. Childhood astrocytomas usually arise in the cerebellum and are frequently cured by surgical extirpation. Juvenile astrocytomas occur around the third ventricle, and most brain-stem gliomas are infiltrating astrocytomas. Adult astrocytomas may be calcified, and some undergo malignant degeneration. The oligodendroglioma is often calcified but only rarely becomes malignant. The classic malignant parenchymal brain tumor is the glioblastoma multiforme. This tumor may arise de novo or by progressive malignant degeneration of an astrocytoma. About half of all intracranial gliomas are glioblastomas; 20 per cent are astrocytomas. In children, astrocytomas represent half of the cerebellar tumors; medulloblastomas and ependymomas make up the rest of the intracranial tumors.

Astrocytomas are characterized histologically by increased numbers of uniform cells resembling fibrillary, gemistocytic, or, less commonly, protoplasmic astrocytes; mitoses are absent. Patients harboring this tumor commonly survive four to seven years or longer. *Anaplastic astrocytomas* contain astrocytic elements with considerable nuclear pleomorphism, markedly increased cellular density, increased mitotic figures, and endothelial hyperplasia, but no necrosis. These tumors are associated with survival of 1.5 to 2.5 years. *Glioblastoma multiforme* is characterized by heterogeneous cell populations with bizarre pleomorphic nuclei that make it difficult to identify their astrocytic origin. There is prominent endothelial hyperplasia

and areas of focal necrosis that often resemble palisades. Survival with this tumor exceeds a year in only a minority of patients.

Intracranial ependymomas occur primarily in children as fourth ventricle masses that obstruct the CSF pathways. *Medulloblastomas* arise from a primitive neuroectodermal cell, usually the cerebellum, and may seed throughout the CSF. They are highly malignant, although sensitive to radiation therapy and chemotherapy.

Mesodermal tumors are represented most commonly by the benign *meningioma*. Meningiomas arise in certain favored sites: along the dorsal surface of the brain, the base of the skull, the falx cerebri, the sphenoid ridge, or within the lateral ventricles. Although benign, these tumors often reach large size before discovery, making removal difficult. The most common cranial nerve tumor is the *acoustic schwannoma* (neorilemoma, neuroma). In recent years early diagnosis through refined auditory tests and computed tomographic (CT) scans have enabled removal via a translabyrinthine approach. *Pituitary adenomas* may appear as intrasellar masses extending into an extrasellar location. CT and magnetic resonance (MR) imaging have made it easier to diagnose microadenomas of the pituitary. *Craniopharyngiomas* are intrasellar or suprasellar developmental tumors derived from Rathke's pouch; they are frequently calcified and often cystic. *Pineal region tumors* occur primarily in children and rarely truly originate from the pineal gland; usually they are germinomas and may produce endocrinopathies. *Metastatic* tumors may invade the brain parenchyma, the skull, or the meninges; their pathology depends on the primary tumor. The benign *colloid cyst* usually grows in the anterior third ventricle. Vascular tumors include arte-

TABLE 494–2. GENERAL CLINICAL MANIFESTATIONS OF BRAIN TUMOR

Headache
Common; new or altered, worse in morning and in association with plateau waves
Mental changes
Common; psychomotor retardation, depression, social indifference, forgetfulness, sleepiness, confusion
Generalized convulsions
One third of patients; more common with slower growing tumors, focal seizures may generalize
Papilledema
Occurs in only 25% of brain tumor patients
Vomiting
Especially with subtentorial tumors
Vasomotor and autonomic changes
Late in course; bradycardia, hypothalamic symptoms
False localizing signs
Sixth-nerve palsy, ipsilateral hemiplegia

riovenous malformations, which are not truly neoplastic, and the *hemangioblastomas*, which are. The latter tumors, when located in the brain stem or cerebellum, may be part of the *von Hippel-Lindau* syndrome that includes hemangioblastomas elsewhere in the body. Congenital tumors include the craniopharyngiomas, *chordomas* (that arise from the primitive notochord), *dermoids*, and *teratomas*. Granulomas and parasitic cysts come from tuberculomas, cryptococcosis (toruloma), sarcoidosis, and cysticercosis.

PATHOPHYSIOLOGY. Brain tumors produce *generalized symptoms* because of their expanding size (Table 494–2) and *focal symptoms* by direct compression on or infiltration into specific areas of the brain (Table 494–3). As tumors grow, they raise the intracranial pressure because the volume of the intracranial cavity is fixed. The total mass effect is a sum of both the tumor size and the cerebral edema the tumor produces. Large tumor masses obstruct the CSF pathways, producing enlargement of and a pressure rise in the upstream ventricular system. As the primary or secondary mass produced by the tumor enlarges, brain tissue may be displaced through the fixed intracranial openings, producing various herniation syndromes as discussed in Chapter 457.

Focally, the mass of the tumor compresses and infiltrates the surrounding brain tissue. Edema, produced within a parenchymal brain tumor, increases the total size of the mass. Cerebral edema may also be produced from compression by an extra-axial tumor, in which case the edema comes from the brain itself. Focal symptoms occur as the tumor compresses surrounding brain, producing distortion and ischemia; such symptoms may be reversible if the pressure is relieved before tissue necrosis occurs. In addition, tumor tissue may infiltrate along nerve fiber tracts, interfering with neurologic function. Cyst formation within tumors provides another mechanism that compresses adjacent normal brain.

CLINICAL MANIFESTATIONS. The symptoms and signs of intracranial tumor depend on the size of the tumor and on its rate of growth. Characteristically, the clinical course is progressive, varying from an acute apoplectic onset such as follows hemorrhage or a seizure, to a slowly progressive mental deterioration associated with slower growing neoplasms. General clinical manifestations of brain tumors are outlined in Table 494–2; focal manifestations are outlined in Table 494–3.

Headache is common, especially with rapidly growing tumors. Of special importance are headaches that have begun recently or changed character, are worse in the morning, awaken the patient at night, or are recurrent.

Mental changes are frequent, but may not attract the attention of coworkers or family members until the patient's behavior changes substantially. Symptoms include impersistence in routine tasks, increased irritability, emotional lability, inertia, faulty insight and forgetfulness, reduction in the range of mental activity, indifference to social practices, reduced initiative and spontaneity, and blunted affect. The patient may complain of fatigue, dizziness, and lethargy. If the tumor continues to grow, such symptoms progress to confusion, dementia, and eventually stupor. Such personality changes are often initially diagnosed as anxiety or depression.

Seizures in brain tumor patients often follow alcohol use or withdrawal of barbiturates or other sedative drugs. They may be precipitated by intravenous contrast material given for CT scans. The onset of generalized convulsions in the adult or

TABLE 494–3. FOCAL CLINICAL MANIFESTATIONS OF BRAIN TUMORS

	Common Characteristics	Special Characteristics
Cerebrum		
Frontal lobe	Generalized or focal seizures, contralateral hemiparesis	Dominant hemisphere: language disorder Corpus callosum: mental changes, ataxia
Parietal lobe	Generalized or focal seizures, contralateral hemisensory defect, especially for "cortical" modalities (stereognosis and position sense, two-point discrimination)	Dominant hemisphere: language disorder, agraphia, agnosia Nondominant hemisphere: contralateral homonymous hemianopia, apraxia, and denial of illness Thalamus: contralateral cutaneous sensory impairment
Temporal lobe	Seizures most common, often no symptoms	Deep: contralateral hemianopia, psychomotor seizures with olfactory or complex visual aura Superficial dominant: expressive and receptive aphasias
Occipital lobe	Contralateral quadrantanopia or hemianopia	Seizures: unformed, flashing lights
Pituitary Adenoma	Neurologic: headache, bitemporal hemianopia; hypothalamic syndromes Endocrine: pituitary insufficiency, specific endocrinopathies	Secretory syndromes: Prolactin: amenorrhea, galactorrhea Growth hormone: gigantism before puberty, acromegaly after puberty ACTH: Cushing's syndrome
Pineal Tumors	Neurologic: hydrocephalus, paralysis of upward gaze	Germinomas, precocious puberty in boys
Posterior Fossa		
Brain stem glioma	Cranial nerve palsies, weakness, sensory disturbances, ataxia, nystagmus	Destroy cranial nuclei and nerves, motor and sensory pathways, and cerebellar connections
Fourth ventricle	Ependymoma, medulloblastoma: hydrocephalus, vomiting, brain stem/cerebellar signs	Interferes early with CSF circulation, producing increased intracranial pressure and hydrocephalus
Cerebellum	Astrocytoma, metastatic: cerebellar, brain stem signs	
Cerebellopontine angle	Acoustic schwannoma: tinnitus, hearing loss, nystagmus, vertigo; brain stem signs	Loss of vestibular response to caloric stimulation, high CSF protein
Optic nerve glioma	Childhood; monocular blindness, proptosis; may be associated with neurofibromatosis	Slow-growing astrocytoma; may invade chiasm and hypothalamus
Meningeal carcinomatosis	Carcinoma, sarcoma, lymphoma and leukemia, glioma	Symptoms and signs of cerebral dysfunction plus cranial nerve and spinal cord nerve root involvement
Skull	Malignant tumors of base: pain and cranial neuropathies	Glomus jugulare: deafness and red blush behind tympanum

focal seizures at any age should alert the physician to the possibility of a structural lesion. Intracranial tumors produce generalized major motor seizures and various forms of focal seizures. Minor temporal lobe seizures that occasionally resemble petit mal attacks may accompany temporal lobe tumors. Other lesions of the temporal lobe may give rise to psychomotor seizures that may be associated with olfactory hallucinations (uncinate fits), disorders of visual or auditory perception, episodes of "déjà vu" phenomena, or automatic behavior. Jacksonian seizures usually imply a lesion of the motor or sensory cortex.

Papilledema occurs in only about one fourth of patients with intracranial neoplasms, and its absence does not exclude increased intracranial pressure. It is more likely to accompany tumors that obstruct CSF flow and may be accompanied by visual phenomena, especially acute visual obscurations and "graying out."

Nausea and vomiting result from direct or reflex stimulation of the emetic center of the medulla. This most often accompanies increased intracranial pressure, particularly with brainstem displacement secondary to herniation or bleeding into the CSF. Vomiting may occur without preceding nausea.

Vasomotor and autonomic changes that accompany expanding intracranial tumors include bradycardia and hypertension, as well as respiratory abnormalities associated with brain-stem compression. Rarely, patients with brain tumor may have gastric ulceration (Cushing's ulcer) that may produce hemorrhage. Fortunately, the adrenal corticosteroids used for treating the edema of brain tumors rarely contribute to such hemorrhages. Other autonomic changes associated with hypothalamic compression include fever, hypothermia, hyperthermia, disturbances in eating and drinking, and occasionally more specific abnormalities such as diabetes insipidus, inappropriate antidiuretic hormone secretion, hypopituitarism, and precocious puberty.

False localizing signs may accompany prolonged elevation of intracranial pressure and reflect compression of remote neurologic structures due to intracranial tissue shift.

Focal clinical manifestations of intracranial tumors depend on localized impairment of nervous tissue function, and therefore vary with the location of the process. Of special interest are focal seizures, which imply specific localized cortical irritation from either a benign or a malignant condition. Other focal symptoms and signs are listed in Table 494–3. In general terms, all these changes tell is *where* a lesion lies, not its histology. In most brain tumors such changes evolve gradually, although the onset can be stroke-like in as many as 5 per cent. Ultimate diagnosis depends on brain imaging or other studies.

Clinical syndromes of tumors in specific sites are outlined in Table 494–3. A further discussion of the localized clinical manifestations of neurological disease states may be found in Chapters 459 and 460. Tumors of the cerebral hemispheres are characterized by progressive, focal neurologic deficits and commonly by generalized or focal convulsive seizures. In addition to those symptoms listed in Table 494–3, tumors of the frontal lobe, being in a "silent area," often first cause seizures or impairment of judgment and intellectual function. A tumor of the medial surface of the frontal lobe may cause urinary urgency or, occasionally, precipitate incontinence. Similarly, temporal lobe tumors, particularly in the nondominant hemisphere, are often relatively "silent" except when they cause convulsive seizures.

Cranial, extradural, or subdural metastatic tumors, by compression or invasion of the underlying brain tissue, produce the same localizing signs as those caused by primary tumors.

The most common endocrine abnormality associated with pituitary adenomas is hypersecretion of prolactin, producing amenorrhea and galactorrhea in women and, less frequently, impotence and gynecomastia in men. Many secretory tumors are microadenomas found only after an endocrine abnormality is discovered. Enlarging pituitary adenomas cause headache; as the tumor grows out of the sella, it compresses the optic chiasm, nerve, or tracts, and the hypothalamus. The most common visual field defect is bitemporal hemianopia, but unilateral optic atrophy, contralateral hemianopia, or any combination may occur. Hypothalamic compression usually causes diabetes insipidus from injury to the supraoptic-pituitary tract. The tumor may destroy functioning glandular tissue and cause pituitary deficiency. Skull x-rays show a characteristic balloon-shaped appearance of the sella, but microadenomas may produce no more than laterally placed focal bulging of the sellar floor, visible only on x-ray tomograms. A rare complication of pituitary adenoma, called *pituitary apoplexy*, is acute hemorrhagic necrosis of the tumor, producing sudden headache, vomiting, visual loss, ophthalmoplegia, and altered pituitary function.

Other tumors in the region of the sella turcica (e.g., meningiomas, craniopharyngiomas, metastases, dermoid cysts) or aneurysms may compress the optic chiasm, invade the sella, and produce symptoms similar to those of chromophobe adenoma.

In addition to the symptoms for pineal tumors listed in Table 494–3, germ-cell tumors in this region may secrete the beta subunit of human chorionic gonadotropin or alpha-fetoprotein into the CSF.

Diffuse meningeal neoplasm (meningeal carcinomatosis): Carcinomas, gliomas, sarcomas, melanomas, and lymphomas sometimes diffusely infiltrate the leptomeninges and subarachnoid space to produce a syndrome of chronic meningitis, which may simulate chronic meningitis caused by fungi, tuberculosis, sarcoidosis, and meningovascular syphilis. As noted in Table 494–3, there is involvement of more than one central nervous system region, i.e., brain, cranial nerves, spinal cord, and nerves. The CSF findings generally establish the diagnosis. The pressure may be normal or elevated, sugar content is often below 45 mg per deciliter, protein content is usually elevated, and cell counts may reveal an increased number of mononuclear cells or cytologic evidence of malignant cells. Cultures are negative. Biochemical tumor markers are present in many cases as discussed in Malkin and Posner's reference.

Other lesions that give x-ray evidence of bone destruction and that must be differentiated from skull tumors include Paget's disease, Hand-Schüller-Christian disease, eosinophilic granuloma, and cholesteatoma (epidermoids). As noted, metastases are common to the skull and will occasionally invade through the dura to produce subdural effusions indistinguishable in their manifestations from subdural hematoma.

DIAGNOSIS. Computed tomography and magnetic resonance (MR) imaging permit the diagnosis of most intracranial tumors at a high level of safety. MRI is especially useful in visualizing tumors in the posterior fossa. It is limited by poor distinction of tumor from surrounding edema. Such tumors produce abnormalities in the normal structures and may be visualized directly or after the intravenous infusion of iodide-containing contrast materal (Figs. 494–1 and 494–2). Skull tumors are seen as eroded regions of bone. Parenchymal lesions may distort the normal ventricular structures and produce cerebral edema visible as low-density (CT) regions in the brain's parenchyma. After intravenous contrast enhancement, the tumor may be visualized as a hyperdense region, frequently ringlike, around a central radiolucent area. The more malignant the tumor, the more contrast agent will enhance its image owing to breakdown of the blood-brain barrier. An exception is strong contrast enhancement in most meningiomas and schwannomas. Low-density lesions may imply cysts, necrotic tumor, or cerebral edema. Contrast-enhanced arteriography may be necessary as an aid to surgical treatment.

Lumbar puncture and examination of CSF rarely contribute

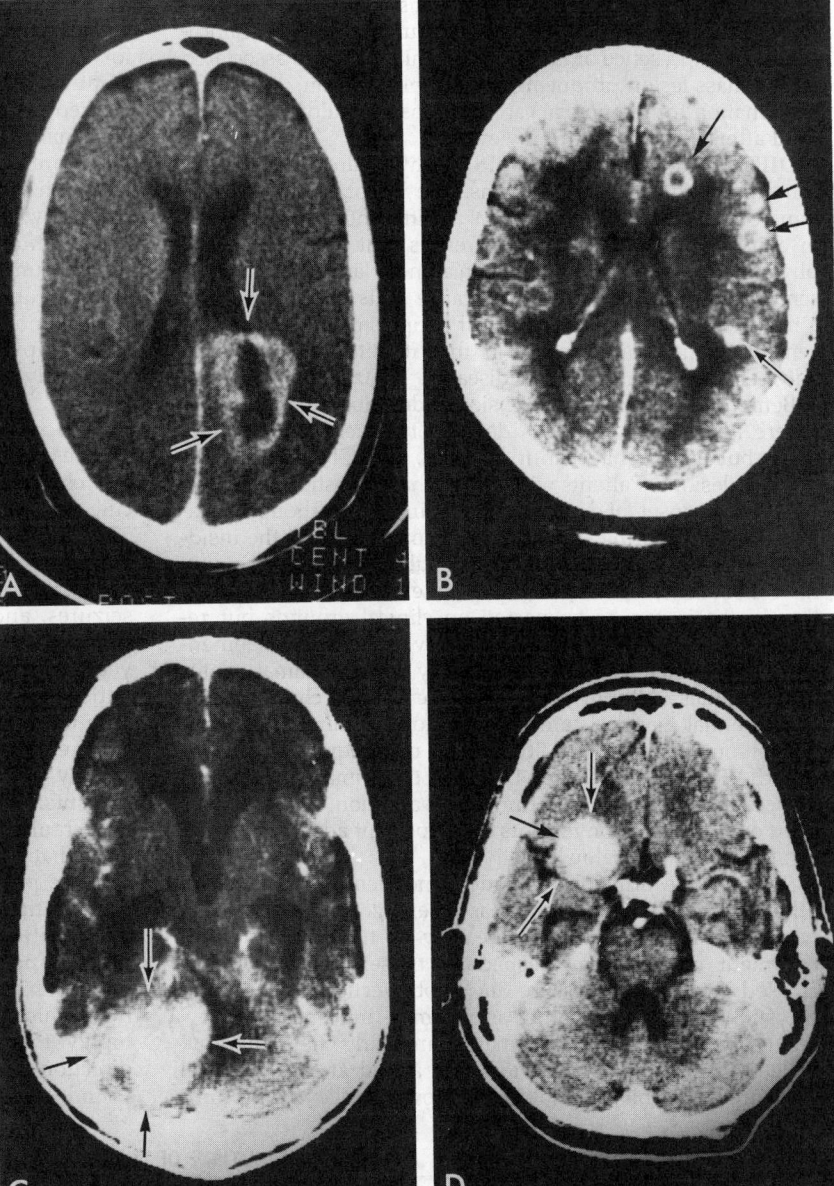

FIGURE 494–1. Computed tomographic scans of patients with intracranial tumors. *A,* Glioblastoma multiforme of the medial parieto-occipital lobes. Note the ring enhancement with central region of hypodensity (*arrows*). *B,* Multiple metastatic brain tumors from carcinoma of the lung. Each enhanced mass represents a brain tumor (*arrows*). *C,* Medulloblastoma of the right and mid-cerebellum. Note the displacement and encroachment of the fourth ventricle and hydrocephalus (*arrows*). *D,* Sphenoid wing meningioma. The lesion is diffusely contrast enhanced (*arrows*).

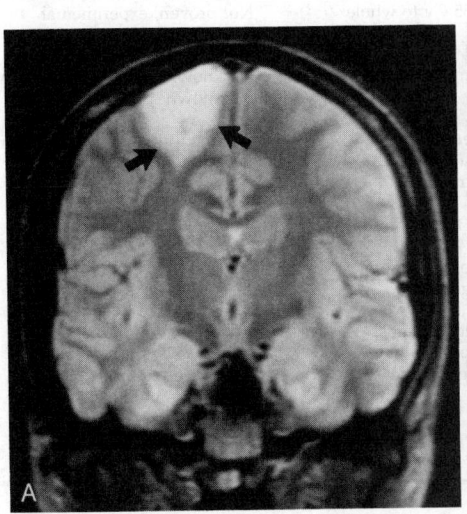

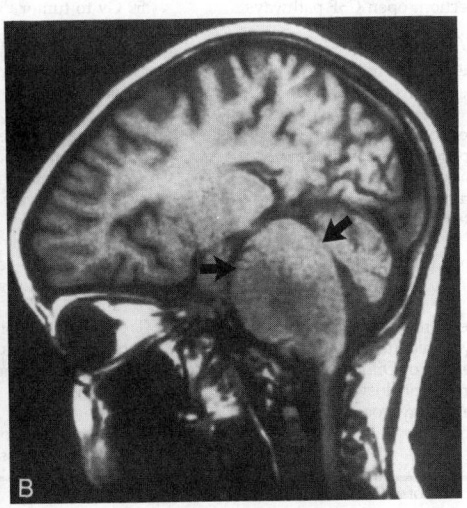

FIGURE 494–2. Magnetic resonance imaging scans of patients with intracranial tumors. *A,* Coronal T$_2$ weighted scan demonstrating low-grade astrocytoma of the posterior frontal lobe (*arrows*). The CT scan was normal. Note the increased signal representing increased water content in the tumor and surrounding edema. It is not possible to distinguish the tumor from the edema. *B,* Sagittal T$_1$ weighted scan demonstrating a large brain stem (pontine) glioma in a five-year-old child (*arrows*). The brain stem is diffusely swollen and is readily distinguished from the surrounding structures. Note the absence of bone artifacts in comparison to most posterior fossa CT scans (see Fig. 494–1*D*).

to the diagnosis of intracranial neoplasm except for diffuse meningeal carcinomatosis. Lumbar puncture is contraindicated in the presence of raised intracranial pressure associated with a mass lesion producing incipient herniation, and a CSF examination for meningeal carcinomatosis should be deferred until after CT findings are reviewed.

DIFFERENTIAL DIAGNOSIS. Many neurologic diseases can mimic intracranial neoplasms. The importance of considering other neurologic syndromes in differential diagnosis lies in emphasizing the clinical differences that should lead the physician to search for intracranial neoplasm. MRI is the screening procedure of choice; because of its great sensitivity, a negative image usually rules out neoplasm. CT scan is less sensitive, but more specific in that it better distinguishes between neoplasia and other diseases.

Benign intracranial hypertension is described in detail elsewhere (Ch. 495.1). Patients develop headache and papilledema but usually have no focal signs, and CT demonstrates no mass lesions. Patients with stroke characteristically present with acute onset of neurologic dysfunction, although occasionally a "stuttering" onset may be confused with the insidious history of tumor. Patients with subdural hematoma may have headache, drowsiness, papilledema, and hemiparesis; the diagnosis can be suspected on clinical grounds but requires CT or arteriography for certainty. Patients with dementia from Alzheimer's disease usually have minimal motor abnormalities. Although CT scans are usually characteristic, a differential diagnosis among granuloma, brain abscess and tumor sometimes can be difficult and may require biopsy.

TREATMENT. Table 494–4 outlines the primary therapeutic choices for the major CNS tumors. In addition, corticosteroid hormones and anticonvulsants are important adjunctive medical therapies (see below).

Surgery. The principles include tumor removal if possible, otherwise, palliation. Surgery has several goals: (1) diagnosis, which can be established in life only by tissue removal; (2) treatment of symptoms, especially those arising from increased intracranial pressure due to obstruction of CSF pathways; (3) debulking of tumor as a form of anticancer therapy; and (4) permitting time for radiation and early chemotherapy. Surgery for meningiomas should be aimed at total removal and cure if possible, and subtotal removal to relieve symptoms

in other cases. For subtentorial parenchymal tumors, surgery is necessary for diagnosis and to open CSF pathways. Surgery for benign cerebellar or acoustic schwannomas is potentially curative. Surgery for metastatic brain tumors should be considered in selective circumstances of single metastases if systemic disease is minimal or well controlled. Pituitary tumors are usually removed by trans-sphenoidal resection, although, if they are large, a transfrontal craniotomy may be necessary.

Radiation Therapy. Radiation is utilized primarily for malignant tumors. Radiation is often given for low-grade astrocytomas and oligodendrogliomas, although efficacy has not been demonstrated by prospective trials. Radiation therapy is the therapy of choice for most metastatic brain tumors and is frequently recommended for large pituitary tumors after surgery.

Medical Therapy. Corticosteroid hormone therapy usually relieves cerebral edema. Steroids almost always improve general clinical manifestations but are less effective against specific clinical manifestations. Dexamethasone in doses of 16 to 32 mg per day is recommended, although attempts should be made to reduce the doses slowly to a level of relatively stable symptoms. Anticonvulsants are given to patients who have seizures, and any patient who develops generalized or focal seizures should be placed on anticonvulsants for three to five years or permanently, if attacks continue postoperatively. Patients who do not have seizures usually do not require long-term anticonvulsant therapy. Since the likelihood of a seizure following clean neurosurgical intervention is low, it is usually not necessary to maintain such patients on anticonvulsants. Seizures occurring late after primary therapy for intracranial neoplasms imply recurrence of tumor and should immediately lead to re-evaluation of the patient's status. Because phenytoin reduces the bioavailability of dexamethasone, patients receiving both drugs may require higher doses of the latter. Several chemotherapeutic agents are useful in the adjunctive treatment of malignant astrocytomas. Two examples are bis-chloroethyl-nitrosourea (BCNU) and cyclohexyl-chloroethyl-nitrosourea (CCNU). These agents are highly toxic and should be administered only under the direction of physicians trained in their use.

Endocrine replacement is often necessary after treatment of

TABLE 494–4. OUTLINE OF THERAPY OF CNS TUMORS

	Surgery	Radiation Therapy*	Chemotherapy
Malignant glioma (glioblastoma and anaplastic astrocytoma)	Debulking, resection if possible	60 Gy to the tumor, 45 Gy to the rest of the brain	Nitrosourea: BCNU or CCNU every 6–8 weeks for 18 months
Astrocytoma, oligodendroglioma	Biopsy; resection if possible	50–55 Gy to the tumor only	No known role, but experimental chemotherapy may be offered on recurrence
Ependymoma	Resection, open CSF pathways	50 Gy to tumor, neuraxis RT if malignant or if subtentorial	No known role, but experimental chemotherapy may be offered
Medulloblastoma	Resection, open CSF pathways	50 Gy to tumor, 35 Gy to whole neuraxis	Not proven; experimental chemotherapy under investigation
Meningioma	Resection often curative	Utilized on recurrence	No known role
Cranial nerve tumors (e.g., acoustic schwannoma)	Resection usually curative	No known role	No known role
Pituitary adenoma	Resection via trans-sphenoidal approach for small tumors; larger tumors may require craniotomy	50 Gy may be used instead of resection or in addition if residual tumor remains postoperatively	Bromocriptine may be used for microadenomas
Craniopharyngioma	Resection usually curative	Used for residual tumor postoperatively	No known role
Pineal tumors	Biopsy if possible	Whole neuraxis for germinomas, focal for other germ cell tumors	Experimental use only
Metastatic parenchymal tumors	Resection of single metastases if systemic tumor under control	Treatment of choice for most tumors; 30 Gy over 10 days	Experimental use only
Meningeal carcinomatosis	Insertion of Ommaya reservoirs or ventriculosystemic shunts to relieve hydrocephalus	Irradiation of symptomatic regions	Intrathecal methotrexate or cytosine arabinoside
Primary lymphoma	Biopsy	55–60 Gy to tumor; whole brain RT often necessary	Experimental

*Radiation therapy generally administered at rate of 1000 cGy per week unless otherwise indicated pituitary adenomas and includes anterior pituitary hormones and vasopressin for diabetes insipidus as required.

OUTCOME OF THERAPY AND PROGNOSIS. For *malignant neuroectodermal tumors,* e.g., glioblastoma multiforme, therapy is palliative, almost never curative. Patients are often able to resume employment for a year or two, unless they have major residual neurologic deficits from the original tumor or from the surgery. Late radiation damage to the brain can occur and may be responsible for the return of symptoms, although tumor recurrence accounts for most patient worsening. Chemotherapy suppresses the immune system and the bone marrow, and may lead to systemic infection and bleeding. For malignant astrocytomas, most recent studies give a median survival time of 52 weeks following combined treatment with surgery, radiation, and BCNU chemotherapy; 25 to 30 per cent of patients survive 18 months. Factors favoring longer survival include age younger than 50, histopathology of anaplastic astrocytoma rather than glioblastoma multiforme, and minimal postoperative neurologic deficit. The prognosis for more benign intracerebral neuroectodermal tumors is better than for the malignant tumors. Radiation therapy is often helpful and patients frequently return to employment for several years. Seizures are likely, but control is usually possible. Patients may survive for three to seven years with relatively preserved neurologic deficit until tumor recurrence or progression occurs. With the advent of whole neuraxis radiation therapy of childhood medulloblastoma, five-year survival rates of 60 per cent are reported.

With a combination of steroids and either radiation therapy alone or a combination of surgery and radiation therapy, two thirds to three fourths of patients with *metastatic brain tumors* show substantive amelioration of presenting symptoms. Many are able to return to work for short periods of time. The median survival, however, is approximately six months, with survival at a year limited to 10 to 15 per cent. *Meningeal carcinomatosis* treated with combination radiation therapy and intrathecal chemotherapy often responds when the primary tumor is lymphoma or carcinoma of the breast. Both neurologic deficits and the CSF may improve for periods of up to a year or more. Affected patients usually die of their systemic disease.

Meningiomas are often curable. There may be residual neurologic deficits, including seizures, but overall the prognosis for survival is excellent, and that for neurologic recovery is good to very good. The prognosis of patients with *acoustic schwannomas* depends on the size of the tumor. For small acoustic schwannomas, especially those removed by translabyrinthine approach, the results are excellent, with a low mortality and a high percentage of cures. Eighth nerve deficits, including hearing loss and vestibular difficulty, may hinder overall functional capacity. Facial paresis is common, and occasionally functionally disturbing. In contrast, there is a 10 to 20 per cent mortality with surgical resection for large tumors and considerable morbidity. Many patients have residual neurologic deficits.

Pituitary tumors and *craniopharyngiomas* carry a fairly good prognosis. Fifty to 60 per cent of macroscopically obvious pituitary adenomas come to attention because of visual failure, whereas in 20 per cent headaches are the initial symptom. Less commonly, an endocrine abnormality is noted, although microadenomas, occurring primarily in women, are usually diagnosed because of infertility, galactorrhea, or amenorrhea. Adult craniopharyngiomas similarly have a good prognosis, although recurrence is somewhat more common than in children following therapy of such tumors. Pituitary tumors may be removed by trans-sphenoidal microsurgery or craniotomy. They may also be treated by irradiation alone or irradiation after surgery. Surgery is indicated if vision is threatened, but the method of treatment of microadenomas is controversial. Hyperprolactinemia from pituitary adenomas

may be treated effectively with bromocriptine, but resection or irradiation is necessary to treat the tumor itself.

Other intracranial tumors generally have a good prognosis, depending on their location. *Cholesteatomas* and *colloid cysts* are usually easily removed with little neurologic deficit, although some tumors may not be resectable because of danger to surrounding normal brain.

Bloom HJG: Medulloblastoma in children: Increasing survival rates and further prospects. Int J Radiat Oncol Biol Phys 8:2023, 1982. *A concise review of the problem of therapy in this disease by a recognized authority. Well referenced.*

Cairncross JG, Kim J-H, Posner JB: Radiation therapy for brain metastases. Ann Neurol 7:529, 1980. *One of the largest series of such cases yet reported.*

Kornblith PL, Walker MD, Cassady JR: Neoplasms of the central nervous system. In DeVita VT, Hellman S, Rosenberg SA (eds): Cancer, Principles and Practice of Oncology, 2nd ed. Philadelphia, J. B. Lippincott Company, 1985, pp 1437–1510. *A good review of the clinical presentation of central nervous system tumors.*

Malkin MG, Posner JB: Cerebrospinal fluid tumor markers for the diagnosis and management of leptomeningeal metastases. Eur J Cancer Clin Oncol 23:1–4, 1987.

Russell DS, Rubinstein LJ: Pathology of Tumours of the Nervous System. 4th ed. Baltimore, Williams & Wilkins Company, 1977. *An excellent, well illustrated textbook of tumors of the nervous system.*

Shapiro WR, et al.: Brain tumors. Semin Oncol 13:1, 1986. *The entire issue is devoted to a discussion of brain tumors, including chapters on biology, pathology, surgery, radiation, chemotherapy, immunobiology, PET studies, and childhood tumors. Both clinical and experimental studies are reviewed.*

Wasserstrom WR, Glass JP, Posner JB: Diagnosis and treatment of leptomeningeal metastases from solid tumors: Experience with 90 patients. Cancer 49:759, 1982. *A definitive review of wide-ranging experience with this disease, including its diagnosis and treatment.*

495 DISORDERS OF INTRACRANIAL PRESSURE

David A. Rottenberg

INTRACRANIAL HYPERTENSION

Cerebrospinal fluid (CSF) pressure in excess of 250 mm CSF is usually a manifestation of serious underlying neurologic disease. Intracranial hypertension is most often associated with rapidly expanding mass lesions, CSF outflow obstruction, or cerebral venous congestion; however, a variety of systemic and central nervous system disorders may be accompanied by an increase in intracranial pressure (ICP; Table 495–1). It should be emphasized that lumbar CSF pressure may not accurately reflect ICP. In patients with intracranial mass lesions and brain hernias, lumbar CSF pressure may be normal or low despite grossly elevated supratentorial CSF pressure. Kinking of the aqueduct of Sylvius or impaction of either the temporal lobes into the tentorial incisura or the cerebellar tonsils into the foramen magnum can impede the transmission of ICP into the lumbar subarachnoid space. Most of the signs and symptoms traditionally associated with intracranial hypertension are related to traction on cerebral blood vessels, distortion of pain-sensitive dura mater, impending herniation with intermittent vascular compression, midline shifts, or axial distortion of the brain stem and are not caused by increased ICP per se. Papilledema, when present, is the most reliable sign of intracranial hypertension; however, many patients with raised ICP fail to develop papilledema, and in some patients with pseudotumor cerebri (see later discussion), papilledema develops and then subsides spontaneously although CSF pressure remains elevated. Moreover, papilledema is not synonymous with raised ICP. Ocular hypotony, bilateral optic neuritis, orbital venous stasis, retrobulbar tumors, and granulomatous inflammation or cystic lesions of the optic nerve sheath may produce papilledema in the absence of intracranial hypertension. Retinal venous pulsations, when present, imply that CSF pressure is normal or

TABLE 495–1. PATHOGENESIS OF INCREASED INTRACRANIAL PRESSURE

Perturbation	Proximate Cause	Clinical Example
Increased dural sinus venous pressure	Sinus compression or occlusion	Sagittal sinus thrombosis Otitic hydrocephalus Brain tumors
	Increased sinus blood flow	CO₂ retention Arteriovenous malformation
	Increased peripheral venous pressure	Internal jugular vein occlusion Superior vena cava syndrome Congestive heart failure
Increased CSF outflow resistance	Ventricular outflow obstruction Obliteration of the cisternal and/or convexity subarachnoid space Plugging of the arachnoid villi	Brain tumors Aqueductal stenosis Meningitis Extra- or subdural masses Cerebral masses or edema Subarachnoid hemorrhage Infectious polyneuritis Spinal cord tumors
Increased rate of CSF formation	Increased choroidal CSF formation Increased extrachoroidal CSF formation	Choroid plexus papilloma Hypo-osmolality Cerebral edema
Unknown	Increased cerebral volume Increased sagittal sinus pressure Increased CSF outflow resistance	Pseudotumor cerebri

not significantly elevated, but the absence of spontaneous venous pulsations is not helpful diagnostically. In conditions associated with intracranial hypertension, various nonepileptic paroxysmal phenomena (e.g., crescendo headache, photopsia, visual obscurations) may accompany spontaneous elevations of ICP, referred to as *plateau waves*. The occurrence of plateau waves during sleep may explain why night-time deterioration and early morning headache are frequently reported by patients with raised ICP.

The initial treatment of any patient with increased ICP whose neurologic status is deteriorating is aimed at reducing the volume of the intracranial contents in an attempt to prevent irreversible brain damage (Table 495–2). Once the patient's condition has stabilized, additional treatment modalities are employed in an effort to consolidate the gains of emergency therapy and to allow the physician ample opportunity to deal with the underlying pathologic process. Almost always, ICP is not the actual cause of the patient's distress but a reflection of a pre-existing pathologic process; the definitive treatment of intracranial hypertension is ultimately determined by the nature of the underlying pathologic process.

TABLE 495–2. EMERGENCY TREATMENT OF IMPENDING HERNIATION IN ACUTELY DECOMPENSATING PATIENTS

Therapy	Dosage or Procedure	Onset (Duration) of Action
Hyperventilation	Lower PaCO₂ to 25 to 30 mm Hg	Seconds (minutes)
Osmotherapy	Mannitol, 0.5 to 2.0 gm/kg intravenously over 15 minutes followed by 25 gm as needed	Minutes (hours)
Corticosteroids*	Dexamethasone, 100-mg intravenous push followed by 100 mg daily in divided doses	Hours (days)

*Corticosteroids have no demonstrated benefit for the treatment of cerebral hemorrhage, ischemic edema, or head trauma. They may even accentuate the ischemic process.

James HE, Langfitt TW, Kumar VS, et al.: Treatment of intracranial hypertension. Acta Neurochirurg 36:189, 1978. *Based on an analysis of 105 consecutive recordings of intracranial pressure in 95 patients, the authors provide a touchstone for future therapeutic trials.*

Rottenberg DA, Posner JB: Intracranial pressure control. In Cottrell JE, Turndorf H (eds.): Anesthesia and Neurosurgery. St. Louis, C. V. Mosby Company, 1980, pp 89–118. *This well-referenced chapter provides a quantitative description of the CSF system. Some familiarity with the subject is helpful.*

PSEUDOTUMOR CEREBRI

DEFINITION. Pseudotumor cerebri is a syndrome of increased intracranial pressure unaccompanied by localizing neurologic signs, intracranial mass lesion, or CSF outflow obstruction in an alert, otherwise healthy-looking patient. Pseudotumor (also called *benign intracranial hypertension, serous meningitis,* or *otitic hydrocephalus*) can be associated with a variety of systemic and iatrogenic disorders (Table 495–3). Chronically increased ICP may give rise to the "primary empty sella syndrome," which refers to a radiographically globular enlargement of the sella turcica and an incompetent diaphragma sellae.

CLINICAL MANIFESTATIONS. Although pseudotumor cerebri may present as asymptomatic papilledema, most patients complain of headache. Other common early symptoms include nausea and vomiting, visual disturbances (blurring, obscurations of vision, scotomata), retro-ocular pain, diplopia, tinnitus, and vertigo. Bilateral papilledema, the cardinal feature, is almost invariably present and may be associated with peripapillary retinal hemorrhages, exudates or both. Visual loss, the only serious complication of pseudotumor, may occur either early or late in the course of the disease. Hypertension may be a risk factor for visual loss, but obscurations of vision do not predict subsequent visual failure. Characteristically, visual field testing reveals enlarged blind spots. Generalized constriction of the peripheral isopters and inferior nasal quadrantopsia are less frequently observed, as are central and paracentral scotomata. Diplopia, caused by unilateral or bilateral abducens palsy, may develop as a false localizing sign. The remainder of the neurologic examination is normal. Regarding the diagnosis of papilledema, it is important to distinguish *pseudopapilledema*—defined as an anomalous elevation of the optic disc—from true papilledema, which is prima facie evidence of increased intracranial pressure. Anomalous elevation of the optic papilla, which may be associated with identifiable hyaline bodies (*drusen*), should suggest the diagnosis of *retinitis pigmentosa*. Pseudotumor cerebri is generally believed to be a self-limited disease in which CSF pressure returns to normal as clinical symptoms remit; the illness is usually brief, lasting weeks to several months.

TABLE 495–3. SYSTEMIC AND IATROGENIC DISORDERS ASSOCIATED WITH PSEUDOTUMOR CEREBRI

Commonly Prescribed Drugs
Nalidixic acid
Nitrofurantoin
Phenytoin
Sulfonamides
Tetracycline
Vitamin A
Endocrine and Metabolic Disorders
Addison's disease
Cushing's syndrome
Hypoparathyroidism
Levothyroxine therapy
Menarche, pregnancy, oral contraceptives
Obesity and irregular menses
Steroid therapy/withdrawal
Hematologic Disorders
Cryoglobulinemia
Iron-deficiency anemia
Miscellaneous Disorders
Dural venous sinus obstruction/thrombosis
Head trauma
Internal jugular vein ligation
Lupus erythematosus
Middle ear disease

However, clinical improvement is not always accompanied by a reduction in CSF pressure, and there is a subgroup of pseudotumor patients whose pressure remains persistently elevated after neurologic signs and symptoms have resolved. The course of such cases implies that clinical symptoms may be independent of the absolute magnitude of CSF pressure and that chronically raised intracranial pressure may be totally asymptomatic. Also, despite persistently elevated CSF pressure, most patients with chronic pseudotumor do not become hydrocephalic. This observation suggests that whatever mechanism "resets" CSF pressure above normal does not necessarily predispose to the development of communicating hydrocephalus.

PATHOPHYSIOLOGY. In most cases, the causal mechanism is unknown. Chronically increased ICP necessarily implies an increase in dural sinus venous pressure, an increase in CSF outflow resistance, an increase in the rate of CSF formation, or some combination of these factors. One or more of these mechanisms must elevate CSF pressure in pseudotumor patients. Pathogenetic hypotheses that postulate an increase in brain bulk consequent to an increase in cerebral blood volume or in brain water content (interstitial brain edema) do not provide an adequate explanation for the intracranial hypertension of pseudotumor.

ASSOCIATED DISORDERS. The typical patient with pseudotumor is 20 to 40 years old, female, and obese. The frequency of menstrual irregularities in obese female pseudotumor patients may simply reflect the increased incidence of menstrual irregularities in obese females of child-bearing age. In addition to obesity, a wide variety of systemic and iatrogenic disorders has been associated with pseudotumor cerebri (Table 495–1).

DIAGNOSIS. The diagnosis of idiopathic pseudotumor cerebri is one of exclusion. Intracranial masses (tumors, hematomata, infections) and CSF outflow obstruction must be ruled out by appropriate neuroradiologic studies, including transmission computed tomography (CT) or magnetic resonance (MR) imaging, or both. Cerebral angiography is occasionally necessary in order to rule out dural venous sinus or cortical venous thrombosis. Lumbar puncture, which is usually deferred until CT or MR has revealed a normal or small ventricular system, is required to confirm the diagnosis of increased ICP. Lumbar spinal fluid pressure is elevated, frequently above 300 mm CSF, but the composition of the fluid is normal; the protein content is usually in the low normal range, below 20 mg per dl. Laboratory evidence of mild hypothalamic-hypophyseal insufficiency may be present, but the diagnostic significance of subclinical endocrinopathy in obese patients with increased intracranial pressure remains to be established. Pseudopapilledema can be distinguished from true disc edema by means of stereoscopic color fundus photography and fluorescein angiography.

TREATMENT. Although papilledema may persist for many years without visual impairment, visual failure occasionally may occur, sometimes without warning, often early in the course of the disease. Unfortunately, there is no convincing evidence that any of the frequently recommended treatment modalities are efficacious, and the high rate of spontaneous remission complicates the evaluation of various therapies. At present, four general approaches to symptomatic treatment are used: (1) repeated lumbar puncture, (2) ventriculosystemic or lumboperitoneal shunting, (3) medical treatment (with corticosteroids, glycerol, diuretics, acetazolamide), and (4) incision of the optic nerve sheath.

Although repeated (weekly) lumbar puncture may provide transient relief of symptoms and document the occurrence of remission, there is no convincing evidence that this therapeutic approach is beneficial. CSF shunting procedures are not without risk, and their long-term efficacy remains to be established. Corticosteroids (especially prednisone) have been the mainstay of medical treatment in many clinics, although

there is evidence to suggest that systemic corticosteroid administration, by raising intraocular pressure, may increase the risk of visual loss. Incision of the optic nerve sheath for the relief of papilledema is of unproved value and is performed infrequently because of the risk of postoperative blindness.

In conclusion, repeated lumbar puncture and the administration of diuretics (such as furosemide) are relatively safe and may provide temporary symptomatic relief. The use of corticosteroids, which can provoke pseudotumor cerebri in susceptible individuals and may raise intraocular pressure, seems to be contraindicated. The normal or small ventricles of patients with pseudotumor provide difficult targets for shunt catheters; thus, lumboperitoneal shunting is preferable to ventriculosystemic shunting and should be considered the treatment of last resort in patients with disabling symptoms or failing vision.

Ahlskog JE, O'Neill BP: Pseudotumor cerebri. Ann Intern Med 97:249, 1982. *A critical review of the clinical syndrome of pseudotumor cerebri. The section on patient management is particularly noteworthy.*

Bulens C, de Vries WAEJ, Van Crevel H: Benign intracranial hypertension. J Neurol Sci 40:147, 1979. *A careful clinical evaluation of 36 pseudotumor patients with long-term follow-up.*

Corbett JJ, Savino PJ, Thompson HS, et al.: Visual loss in pseudotumor cerebri. Arch Neurol 39:461, 1982. *This paper provides a detailed and definitive discussion of the only serious complication of pseudotumor cerebri, visual loss.*

HYDROCEPHALUS

Hydrocephalus refers to the net accumulation of CSF within the cerebral ventricles and their consequent enlargement. Although acute obstructive hydrocephalus usually produces a sudden increase in intraventricular pressure, CSF pressure is frequently normal (or low) in patients with chronic hydrocephalus. It is useful to distinguish between "noncommunicating" and "communicating" hydrocephalus; the former is produced by lesions that obstruct the intracerebral CSF circulation at or proximal to the foramina of Luschka and Magendie, the latter by obstruction of the basal cisterns or convexity subarachnoid space such that the ventricular system communicates with the spinal subarachnoid space, but CSF cannot drain through the arachnoid villi into the superior sagittal sinus. Ventricular dilatation associated with severe cerebral atrophy, sometimes called "hydrocephalus ex vacuo," must be distinguished from congenital or acquired obstruction of the CSF system.

DIAGNOSIS. Ventriculomegaly is readily diagnosed by means of CT or MR imaging. The diagnosis of hydrocephalus, however, must take into account the increase in ventricular volume that accompanies normal aging and the presence or absence of cerebral atrophy. Enlargement of the temporal horns and an inability to visualize the sylvian and interhemispheric fissures or cerebral sulci, plus the presence of periventricular lucencies (CT) or periventricular hyperintensity (MR), favor the diagnosis of hydrocephalus. A normal or small fourth ventricle in the presence of enlarged lateral and third ventricles suggests aqueductal stenosis.

ACUTE VERSUS CHRONIC HYDROCEPHALUS. Sudden complete ventricular outflow obstruction leads to acute hydrocephalus, coma and, if untreated, death; partial obstruction is more common and only moderately less dangerous (Table 495–4). Chronic hydrocephalus in the adult is most often caused by aqueductal stenosis or the complications of subarachnoid hemorrhage. Other reported causes and associations are listed in Table 495–4. In many instances, the cause of symptomatic chronic hydrocephalus ("normal-pressure hydrocephalus") cannot be determined. Unequivocally asymptomatic hydrocephalus may be found in approximately 4 per cent of patients over the age of 60 who consult a neurologist for assorted neurologic complaints and undergo CT scanning.

CLINICAL MANIFESTATIONS. The patient with acute obstructive hydrocephalus has severe headache, lethargy, signs of increased intracranial pressure (papilledema and/or

TABLE 495–4. POTENTIAL CAUSES OF HYDROCEPHALUS

Acute Hydrocephalus
Cerebellar hemorrhage/infarction
Colloid cyst of the third ventricle
Exudative meningitis
Head trauma
Intracranial tumor/hematoma
Spontaneous subarachnoid hemorrhage
Viral encephalitis
Chronic Hydrocephalus
Aqueductal stenosis
Ectasia and elongation of the basilar artery (rare)
Granulomatous meningitis
Head trauma
Hindbrain malformations
Meningeal carcinomatosis
Spinal cord tumors
Spontaneous subarachnoid hemorrhage
Syringomyelia

TABLE 495–5. CAUSES OF ABNORMALLY LOW (0–50 mm) CSF PRESSURE

Dehydration-hypovolemia
Cranial-intraspinal CSF block
Post–CNS surgery
CSF fistula
Post–LP drainage
Spontaneous-idiopathic; dural nerve sheath tear

abducens palsy), and signs of the causative lesion. Hyperactive reflexes and bilateral extensor plantar responses are almost invariably present. Ventricular CSF pressure is markedly increased, but if CSF pathways are blocked this increase may not be transmitted to the lumbar subarachnoid space. Patients with chronic communicating hydrocephalus, including normal-pressure hydrocephalus, have a progressive dementia, characterized by forgetfulness and psychomotor retardation, an unsteady gait, and urinary incontinence. Apathy, hypophonia, and bilateral pyramidal and extrapyramidal signs may be present. The lumbar CSF pressure is usually normal or near normal in range, although overnight recording of ventricular CSF pressure may reveal intermittent waves of elevated pressure.

TREATMENT. Acute hydrocephalus responds dramatically to ventricular drainage and CSF diversion. Treatment of the primary lesion is the treatment of choice, although temporary ventricular decompression or ventriculosystemic shunt may be necessary in some cases. Medical treatment for long-term symptomatic hydrocephalus is not efficacious. Ventricular shunting also has been employed for patients with chronic communicating hydrocephalus. Unfortunately not all respond, and response may be delayed for weeks or months; moreover, there are no reliable clinical or neuroradiologic predictors of shunt response. Absence of cerebral atrophy and temporary psychomotor improvement after lumbar puncture seem to correlate with, but do not guarantee, benefit from a shunt operation.

Adams, RD, Fisher CM, Hakim S, et al.: Symptomatic occult hydrocephalus with "normal" cerebrospinal-fluid pressure. N Engl J Med 273:117, 1965. *This classic account of normal pressure hydrocephalus is still worth reading.*
Petersen RC, Bahram M, Laws ER Jr: Surgical treatment of idiopathic hydrocephalus in elderly patients. Neurology 35:307, 1985. *A clinically oriented review of the indications for, risks of, and benefits to be expected from the surgical treatment of normal-pressure hydrocephalus.*
van Gijn J, Hijdra A, Wijdicks EFM, et al.: Acute hydrocephalus after aneurysmal subarachnoid hemorrhage. J Neurosurg 63:355, 1985. *A prospective study of 174 patients describing the association between acute hydrocephalus after aneurysmal subarachnoid hemorrhage and subsequent death from cerebral infarction.*

INTRACRANIAL HYPOTENSION

CSF pressure measured at lumbar puncture in the lateral decubitus position normally ranges from 70 to 200 mm CSF (5 to 15 mm Hg). Low or zero lumbar CSF pressure can be recorded under several circumstances as indicated in Table 495–5. Symptoms of the first two or three on that list are likely to be dominated by the underlying illnesses. The remainder tend to cause a consistent syndrome characterized by severe throbbing frontal and occipital headache, which usually appears within 30 seconds or so after the patient assumes an erect posture and which subsides completely when he lies down. Associated complaints may include dizziness, nausea, stiff neck, photophobia, and, rarely, diplopia due to an associated abducens palsy. The disorder often arises 3 to 21 days after lumbar puncture. Rarely, auditory symptoms such as buzzing, popping, humming, roaring, or frank hearing loss may supervene. Pathogenesis is as with lumbar puncture headache (Ch. 466.2).

The term *aliguorrhea* has been used to describe rare cases of CSF hypotension that occur spontaneously, producing symptoms similar to those already described in previously healthy persons. The onset can be acute or subacute and is occasionally precipitated by mild trauma such as a fall on the buttocks or a casual bump to the head. The cause usually remains unknown, although spontaneous rupture of a dural nerve sheath has been postulated. Erect headache can be prostrating. Diagnosis can be difficult, since spontaneous pressure in the lumbar subarachnoid space can be zero or even negative, giving the initial false impression of missing the thecal sac. Treatment is symptomatic; spontaneous recovery usually requires days to a few weeks. When post-lumbar-puncture symptoms are persistent, disabling, or both, an *epidural "blood patch"* may be indicated. This procedure involves the injection of 10 ml of the patient's own blood into the epidural space to seal a presumed dural leak. Rarely, in very long-lasting cases, surgical exploration has exposed the dural leak and closed it.

Bell WE, Joynt RJ, Sahs AL: Low spinal fluid pressure syndromes. Neurology 10:512, 1960. *A detailed clinical account of the neurologic manifestations of intracranial hypotension.*
Vandam LD, Dripps RD: Long-term follow-up of patients who received 10,098 spinal anesthetics. JAMA 161:586, 1956. *This prospective study of over 10,000 spinal anesthetizations documents the incidence of headache associated with lumbar puncture and describes the syndrome of decreased intracranial pressure.*

SECTION FOURTEEN / INJURY TO THE HEAD AND SPINE

Donald P. Becker

496 HEAD INJURIES

GENERAL CONSIDERATIONS

In Western nations trauma is the leading cause of death in persons aged 1 to 40 years, and head injury contributes to half that number. At least 50,000 Americans die each year as a direct consequence of traumatic brain injury, and another 50,000 to 60,000 who survive suffer from varying degrees of disability.

Brain injury represents the most serious sequela to head trauma, producing various degrees of pathologic damage, ranging from temporary cellular and subcellular injury to shearing and tearing of brain cells and even disruption of brain tissue by contusion, hemorrhage, or laceration. The lesions vary in location and degree from patient to patient. Following the initial insult, the brain may be further damaged by secondary hypoxemia from respiratory embarrassment, cerebral ischemia due to elevated intracranial pressure, or brain shift caused by accumulation of intracranial hematoma or brain swelling. In each patient management depends on the location, extent, and nature of the brain damage.

MECHANISMS OF TRAUMATIC PRIMARY AND SECONDARY BRAIN INJURY

PRIMARY BRAIN INJURY. This immediately follows impact. The most common mechanism is brain movement and deformation within the skull—the "acceleration-deceleration" injury. In *deceleration*, the rapidly moving skull is suddenly stopped, as in an auto-tree collision, but the gelatinous and viscoelastic brain continues to move during a 20-msec time period. In *concussion*, there is brief unconsciousness, but no clinical or radiographic evidence of residual structural damage can be found. The immediate loss of consciousness results from the deformation affecting the brain stem and its reticular activating system. Brief vegetative paralysis may occur at the moment of impact. Neither the loss of consciousness nor rapid recovery is well understood mechanistically; sudden, diffuse neurotransmitter release has been postulated.

Impact injury deforms different loci of the brain substance to different degrees, and internal shearing and stress can traumatize and even disrupt deep-lying cells and their processes. Diffuse axon and neuron cell body injury (reversible or permanent) may be scattered throughout. If blood vessels are not disrupted, there may be no intracerebral hemorrhage, even with severe injury leading to early death. The brain can move in the sagittal plane or rotate in the skull around the axis of the brain stem. Actual tissue disruption can affect almost any region, but contusions most commonly affect the inferior frontal lobe gyri and anterior temporal lobes. Contusions and hematomas of the brain stem accompany the most severe injuries and produce major neurologic deficits. Blood clots can accumulate in brain parenchma from vascular injury, in the subdural space from laceration of a bridging vein, or in the epidural space from disruption of a dural vessel (e.g., middle meningeal artery).

In *acceleration* injury, the head suddenly accelerates (e.g., during the boxer's upper cut when the head jolts back and inertial forces cause the still unmoving brain to strike the accelerating skull with varying degrees of possible injury resembling those above).

The remaining major mechanism of primary brain damage consists of direct tissue injury under the site of impact. Extensive local brain injury can occur even among patients who remain alert. For example, a crushing injury to the *fixed* head can drive a large plate of skull inward, destroying large areas of the underlying brain, such as the posterior parietal and occipital lobes, yet the patient need not lose consciousness despite suffering a homonymous hemianopsia and neurologic signs of injury to the sensory association cortex. Because only the directly traumatized cerebrum is damaged and the brain stem is not deformed, there is no loss of consciousness.

Gunshot wounds cause brain damage along the tract of the missile that extends radially outward from the path in proportion to the size and velocity of the missile. The shock wave can produce loss of consciousness if it reaches the brain stem with sufficient force.

SECONDARY BRAIN INJURY Traumatized brain is more sensitive and vulnerable to a supplemental injury than is normal, undamaged brain. Following brain trauma many recoverable cells remain in a metabolically dysfunctional state. In such areas, glucose may be metabolized incompletely so that lactate accumulates in brain tissue and the cerebrospinal fluid. Additional physiologic insults such as arterial hypoxemia ($Pao_2 < 60$ mm Hg), impaired cerebral blood flow from arterial hypotension, or severely elevated intracranial pressure can convert a reversible brain injury into an irreversible one so as to increase the patient's ultimate neurologic handicap or likelihood of death. Such complications are common and often preventable (Table 496–1).

Accumulating evidence indicates that toxic products resulting from trauma can secondarily damage tissue. These include breakdown products of blood as well as abnormal metabolites released from damaged brain cell membranes (Fig. 496–1). Examples of the latter include arachidonic acid, metabolism of which may release oxygen free radicals in the production of prostaglandins.

Elevations of intracranial pressure (ICP) provide an additional potential complication of severe head trauma. Cerebrovascular engorgement, brain edema, or an expanding intracranial hematoma or contusion can, alone or in combination,

TABLE 496–1. SYSTEMIC INSULTS OBSERVED ON ADMISSION IN SEVERE HEAD INJURY*

Systemic Insults	Patients (%)	Poor Outcome (%)
Arterial hypoxemia (Po₂ 60 mm Hg)	37	59
Arterial hypotension (systolic pressure <90 mm Hg)	16	65
Anemia (hematocrit 30%)	10	62
Arterial Hypercarbia (Pco₂ >45 mm Hg)	8	78
None	52	35

*Correlation between systemic insults observed on admission and outcome in the author's series of severe head injuries. Other unlisted examples of systemic complications causing delayed brain insults include septic shock, sudden gastrointestinal hemorrhage, severe hyponatremia, and myocardial infarction.

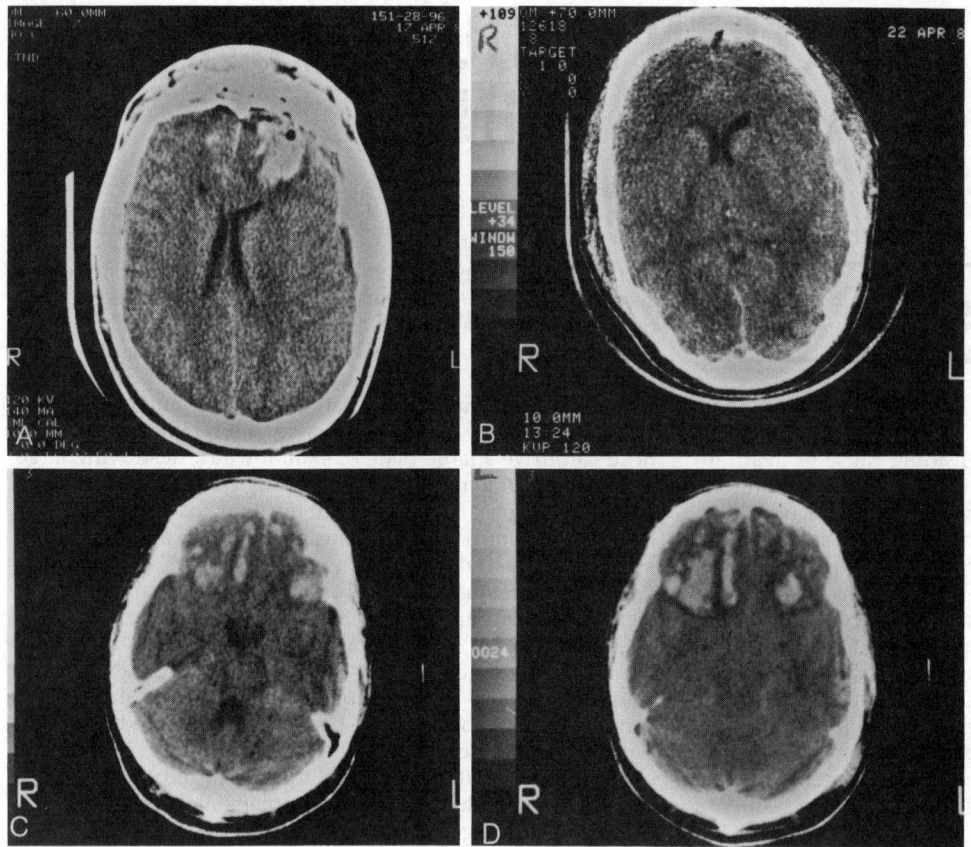

FIGURE 496–1. Brain contusions (disrupted brain and blood) contain metabolites toxic to surrounding brain. *A* and *B* are CT scans of a 19-year-old college student who fell one story, landing on his face, and entered the hospital in a coma. *A* is the initial scan. The subdural clot and intracerebral contusion were promptly removed. *B* is the scan at five days. He made an excellent recovery. *C* and *D* are scans of a 23-year-old man who fell backwards off a golf cart and entered the hospital slightly lethargic but oriented. *C*, Twenty-four hours later he was comatose, and *D* showed massive extension of contusion and edema. He remained severely disabled.

raise ICP well above the normal of up to 10 mm Hg, and sometimes to levels that impair blood flow. Several pathophysiologic factors contribute to this process. Thus, in patients with severe head injury, cerebrovascular blood flow autoregulation is usually impaired. In this situation, brain capillary flow may fall to critical levels below 20 ml per 100 grams of brain tissue per minute when the ICP reaches no more than 20 to 30 mm Hg. At this point, brain ischemia with neurologic worsening follows, producing gradual or abrupt deterioration of neurologic signs. Brain ischemia stemming from elevated ICP is an important problem in severe head injury. Most patients who have a large intracranial mass have elevated ICP during their postoperative course.

CLINICAL APPEARANCE OF THE PATIENT

MILD BRAIN INJURY. The mildest form is experienced by visual disturbance ("seeing stars") and a sensation of being dazed or stunned that lasts seconds to several minutes. The next degree is immediate unconsciousness. Boxers present a classic example of the phenomenon. A clean knockout blow produces acute generalized flaccidity, accompanied by apnea and bradycardia, with widely dilated pupils that are unresponsive to light. Rarely, a generalized seizure follows the blow. Oculovestibular reflexes may be lost transiently. The signs usually resolve over 30 to 60 seconds, and the individual gradually becomes oriented.

Within minutes after injury, patients with mild brain trauma are characteristically alert and oriented, can describe what they were doing up to the moments before the injury, and demonstrate little or no retrograde amnesia. They rarely remember the blow itself, however, and often cannot remember events that occurred for up to 10 minutes after the accident. This period of memory loss following the injury is called the time of antegrade or post-traumatic amnesia.

MODERATE BRAIN INJURY. Patients with moderate brain injury characteristically remain lethargic or stuporous after emerging from periods of unconsciousness lasting 5 to 10 minutes or more. During early recovery, they are often intermittently restless and sometimes combative but return to sleep if undisturbed. They may speak in short sentences or phrases and are able to follow at least a simple single-stage command. A mild focal neurologic deficit such as a hemiparesis or visual field deficit may exist. Over the following several days orientation and alertness gradually return. Mild focal neurologic deficits usually disappear. During the acute stages, however, these patients are potentially vulnerable to secondary brain insults from respiratory insufficiency and hypoxemia, the development of an intracranial blood clot, or the presence of brain edema.

SEVERE BRAIN INJURY. Such patients do not regain consciousness for at least 20 minutes and often much longer after injury. Acutely, they neither speak understandable words nor follow commands. This state remains after cardiopulmonary care. Other serious neurologic signs are common, and prognosis is related largely to what evidence exists of brain stem injury. Motor posturing (decorticate and decerebrate responses) indicating extensive deep cerebral injury occurs in 30 per cent; decerebrate (extensor) posturing implies a poorer prognosis. Impaired eye movements to the doll's-head maneuver (oculocephalic test) or ice water irrigation of the tympanum (oculovestibular test) affect about 40 per cent of patients in this group, and represents brain-stem damage or, less often, injury to the inner ear or to the third, fourth, sixth, or eighth cranial nerve. Bilateral pupillary unresponsiveness to light also signifies brain-stem damage. Bilateral decerebrate posturing with impaired or absent oculocephalic responses implies a very extensive brain injury involving both the hemispheres and brain stem. Four fifths of such patients die, and most survivors remain severely disabled or vegetative, even in the absence of an intracranial hematoma or elevated intracranial pressure.

Patients with decerebrate motor posturing who show normal eye movements sometimes make a good recovery because of the more limited extent of the brain damage. If they remain free of systemic complications such as septic shock or pulmonary edema, patients with severe head injury who have normal withdrawal or normal flexor response of their limbs to noxious stimuli can be expected to make a good recovery. Prognosis worsens, however, if they harbor an intracranial mass lesion that causes a major brain shift or produces a sustained elevation of intracranial pressure to over 40 mm Hg. The presence of flaccidity or paralysis of all four limbs to noxious stimuli may be caused by a concomitant spinal cord injury; if related to the brain injury, flaccidity is an ominous sign.

About 40 per cent of patients with severe brain injury harbor an intracranial hematoma causing brain compression and displacement as well as a high intracranial pressure. Such patients almost always require prompt surgery to evacuate the mass lesion. If the physician waits for signs of neurologic deterioration, further permanent brain damage usually occurs. Rarely, even patients who show bilateral decerebrate posturing, impaired eye movements, and pupils fixed to light can recover if they have a subdural or epidural hematoma and the clot is quickly evacuated.

POST-TRAUMATIC NEUROLOGIC DETERIORATION. Patients with mild, moderate, or severe brain injury may progressively worsen. If the vital signs and blood oxygen levels are satisfactory, such early deterioration usually reflects the effects of an expanding intracranial hematoma, usually in the subdural or epidural space, but sometimes from an intracerebral contusion or hematoma. Less frequent causes are progressive brain swelling or focal metabolic abnormalities. Unless checked by prompt treatment, expanding masses threaten to produce potentially fatal uncal or central transtentorial herniation with signs and symptoms as outlined in Ch. 457. The signs of impending transtentorial herniation ought to be recognized because even at this stage rapid appropriate treatment with osmotic diuretics and surgical evacuation of a mass can save life and, perhaps more important, brain function.

SKULL FRACTURES

The presence or absence of fractures often bears little relationship to the severity of underlying brain injury. Autopsy demonstrates an intact skull in 30 per cent of patients who die from severe head injury. Linear nondisplaced skull fractures may gain clinical importance if the crack extends across the groove of the middle meningeal artery in the temporal bone. Bleeding from this vessel is a common cause of extradural hematoma, a clot that characteristically causes brain compression within a few hours of injury. Most patients with a linear fracture of the temporal bone do not develop an epidural hematoma, however, and some patients who accumulate epidural blood clots do not have radiographically visible fractures of the temporal bone. CT scanning has largely replaced plain skull films in the evaluation of head injuries.

Fractures across the skull base create a potential cause of complications. The dura over the base is thin, firmly adherent to the bone, and easily lacerated. A fracture that traverses an air sinus or the middle or external ear canal risks producing intracranial infection, particularly meningitis. Clinical signs of communication include cerebrospinal fluid (CSF) rhinorrhea or otorrhea or the presence of intracranial air visible on radiography. With fractures of the floor of the anterior fossa, blood usually seeps into the loose periorbital tissue, producing the appearance of raccoon eyes. With fractures of the floor of the middle fossa, subcutaneous blood may accumulate over the mastoid bone just behind the ear (Battle's sign). Antibiotics used prophylactically do not reduce the incidence of meningitis. If traumatic CSF rhinorrhea or otorrhea occurs, it usually stops spontaneously or after treatment with repeated lumbar punctures. CSF leaks that persist for longer than seven to nine days should be surgically repaired.

The cranial nerves exit via the skull base and may be traumatized by a basal skull fracture. Post-traumatic nerve palsies involving the second, third, fourth, seventh, or eighth cranial nerves almost invariably reflect the presence of a fracture. A fracture may damage the olfactory or abducens nerve, but these structures have a long intracranial course and can be injured by brain movement and deformation.

In depressed skull fracture the outer table of one or more of the broken fragments is displaced below the level of the inner table of the surrounding intact skull. Open depressed fractures require cleansing and debridement of the wound to prevent infection. Post-traumatic epilepsy occurs in 15 to 60 per cent of cases, the higher number resulting when such fractures are complicated by a lacerated dura mater, when seizures develop in the first week after injury, or when a period of post-traumatic antegrade amnesia lasts more than 24 hours.

MANAGEMENT

Mild to moderately severe head injuries require close monitoring to prevent medical complications and to guard against the potential delayed effects of intracranial hemorrhage or cerebral edema. With severe mechanical brain injury, carefully and rapidly executed treatment can reduce mortality and improve recovery. For example, patients with subdural hematoma who arrive at their final hospital destination in less than two hours fare twice as well as those who are admitted four or more hours after the accident (Fig. 496–2).

AT THE SCENE OF THE ACCIDENT. Avoid flexing the spine by placing patients promptly in the supine, horizontal, neutral position. This allows examination and a direct approach to the airway. The mouth should be cleared.

Assisted ventilation is indicated for apnea or hypoventilation, using mouth-to-mouth assistance or positive-pressure ventilation via an oral airway and Ambu bag. Rescue teams

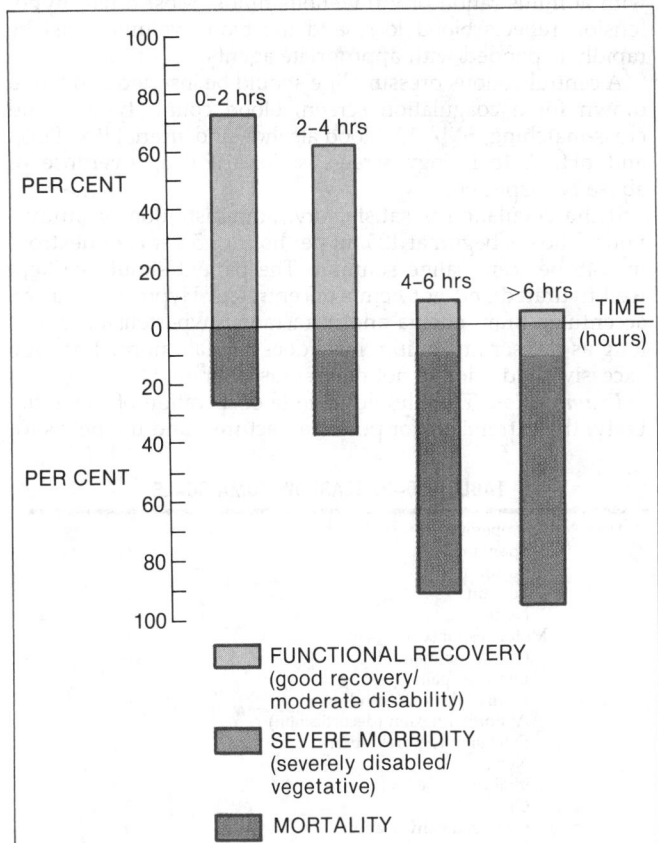

FIGURE 496–2. Influence of time delay from injury to surgical intervention on outcome in patients with acute subdural hematoma.

can apply face-mask positive pressure, an esophageal occlusive airway, or endotracheal intubation, depending on local expertise. One hundred per cent oxygen should be administered. Scalp bleeding can usually be controlled with firm pressure. The Glasgow Coma Scale (Table 496–2) plus examination of pupil size and reactivity to light provides an adequate emergency measure of brain function.

TRANSPORT. Given a skilled emergency crew, the patient should be transferred without delay to an optimal care hospital where CT scanning and neurosurgical care are available. Distance is not the primary consideration; only profound shock justifies initial transport to a local receiving hospital.

During transport of comatose patients, the following steps should be followed: insert an intravenous catheter, 16 gauge, for the possible administration of agents to maintain circulation. Initially, use a saline solution of Ringer's lactate, 100 ml per hour. Administer 100 per cent oxygen nasally or via intubation. Place a nasogastric tube and empty the stomach by suction. Place a cervical collar or sandbags to protect the neck. Make repeated assessment of pupils, eye opening, motor and verbal response, pulse, blood pressure, and breathing. Osmotic agents such as mannitol should be given for progressive neurologic deterioration consistent with a growing mass and tentorial herniation.

EMERGENCY ROOM CARE. *Ventilation.* Patients not talking or following commands should be intubated. When positive pressure ventilation is initiated early, progressive respiratory failure only rarely occurs, although ventilation often must be maintained for several days. Controlled hyperventilation producing mild hypocarbia often must be maintained for several days to keep brain CO_2 levels low and to counteract tissue acidosis.

Circulation. Hypotensive arterial blood pressures should be brought into the normal range (mean pressure, 90 to 100 mm Hg). Acute hypotension may result from the primary brain insult, but this should be transient or should reverse promptly with administration of intravenous fluids. Most often, hypotension reflects blood loss, and the blood volume must be rapidly expanded with appropriate agents.

A central venous pressure line should be inserted and blood drawn for a coagulation screen, blood count, typing, and cross-matching, SMA 12, blood alcohol, and arterial Po_2, Pco_2, and pH. A toxicology screen is done if drug overdose or abuse is suspected.

If the circulation is satisfactory, administration of intravenous fluids is begun at 125 ml per hour of 5 per cent dextrose in 0.45 per cent saline solution. The patient should be kept well hydrated and not hemoconcentrated. Hyponatremia can accentuate brain edema and intracranial hypertension but as long as the serum sodium level does not fall, normal or even excessive hydration is not dangerous to brain.

Examination. This should include observation of the entire body, the extremities for possible fractures, and the pelvis for

TABLE 496–2. GLASGOW COMA SCALE

Eye opening	
Spontaneous	4
To sound	3
To pain	2
None	1
Motor response	
Obeys commands	6
Localizes pain	5
Normal flexion (withdrawal)	4
Abnormal flexion (decortication)	3
Extension (decerebration)	2
None	1
Verbal response	
Oriented	5
Confused conversation	4
Inappropriate words	3
Incomprehensible sounds	2
None	1

stability, as well as an evaluation of the abdomen, chest, and cardiovascular system.

Neurologic examination includes estimating the Glasgow coma scale, plus appropriate evaluation of brain stem function. The pupils are evaluated for size, reactivity, shape, and position. If the cervical spine is in proper alignment, the oculocephalic reflexes are tested; otherwise, oculovestibular reflexes (cold calorics) are obtained. The motor system is evaluated for weakness and muscle tone, reflexes are tested for symmetry and response, a sensory examination is attempted, and the superficial reflexes are tested. (See Ch. 457 for evaluation of the comatose patient.)

TRIAGE ACCORDING TO SEVERITY OF INJURY. *Mild Injury (Grade I).* The concern is that Grade I patients may develop delayed damage from extradural or subdural hematoma. Most such patients, however, can be observed at home if results of their initial examination are normal, with warnings to the family to awaken the patient during the first night to check responsiveness. If there is severe headache, vomiting, or lethargy, a 24-hour period of hospital observation is advisable. CT scan is the procedure of choice.

Moderate and Severe Injury (Grades II and III). A CT head scan is indicated in all, and promptly in those with Grade III status. Assignment to the operating room or intensive care unit can then be made on the basis of the findings. Additional radiographs should include cervical spine: lateral (cross-table); and chest: anteroposterior (semi-upright if possible). Other x-rays will be guided by the physical examination. A diagnostic peritoneal lavage to detect cryptic abdominal hemorrhage is recommended if the patient has been hypotensive, has a hemoglobin level below 10 grams per deciliter, or has had violent body trauma.

Up to 40 per cent of patients in coma from head trauma will show an intracranial mass by CT scan. These should be operated on if they cause a midline shift of 5 mm or more, especially if the patient is deteriorating. Small mass lesions without midline shift and no counterforcing hematoma on the opposite side can be managed without surgery. Frequent neurologic examinations must evaluate the possible need for surgical therapy, however. Therapeutic decisions often benefit from ICP monitoring and repeated CT scanning.

INTENSIVE CARE AND MEDICAL MANAGEMENT. *Neurologic Monitoring and General Graphic Display.* A 24-hour clinical chart describing the neuro-ophthalmologic findings and the status of motor responses and voluntary motor strength usefully graphs the patient's course. The same side of the neurologic examination sheet can contain graphs or spaces for recording hourly pulse rate, arterial blood pressure, ICP (when appropriate), body temperature, respiratory state and rate, and central venous pressure.

Other important variables include hemoglobin and hematocrit levels, white blood counts, arterial blood gases, serum electrolytes, and other pertinent metabolic measurements. A radial arterial indwelling catheter can be used to monitor arterial blood pressure and to obtain blood samples. Specimens of urine, CSF (when available), and tracheal aspirate should be cultured at regular intervals.

Fluid and Electrolyte Management. Central venous pressure should be maintained at 8 to 12 cm H_2O. Urinary output should be about 30 ml per hour. Higher or lower output implies either improper fluid administration or a specific medical abnormality. Customary fluid therapy includes dextrose, 5 per cent in 0.45 per cent saline solution, plus 20 mEq of KC1 per 1000 milliliters. About 3000 ml per day is usually given to adults, but gastric, third-space, and diarrheal losses must be replaced. Serum and urine electrolyte levels should be checked at least daily.

Transient hyponatremia caused by inappropriate secretion of antidiuretic hormone (ADH) often develops as early as the second day after injury. Ideal treatment consists of fluid restriction and slow administration of 5 per cent dextrose and isotonic saline solution. Occasionally, severe hyponatremia may require hypertonic intravenous saline. If the central venous pressure is low and the patient is volume depleted, the hypertonic saline solution should not be accompanied by fluid restriction.

Feeding via nasogastric tube can usually begin after five days. Earlier efforts risk producing aspiration or vomiting. Total parenteral nutrition (TPN) can begin after five days if the patient cannot eat. Some evidence indicates that TPN, given to match metabolic needs, can reduce nitrogen loss and muscle wasting, can stimulate recovery of the immune system, and may reduce mortality. Since hyperglycemia may accentuate cerebral anoxic-ischemic lactic acidosis, blood sugar concentration should be maintained below 180 mg per deciliter.

Ventilation. Controlled ventilation should be used for all comatose head injury patients, employing a volume respirator initially set for adults at a rate of 12 per minute, with a tidal volume varying between 750 and 900 ml (13 ml per kilogram body weight). The slow rate permits adequate venous blood return to the heart, and the large volume helps re-expand collapsed alveoli. Minute volume is adjusted to bring the Pa_{O_2} above 70 mm Hg. Ventilatory control is continued until the patient follows commands or becomes neurologically stable. Most patients require this regimen for three or four days, but it can be used effectively for as long as two to three weeks.

Medications and General Care. Although early seizures are infrequent, convulsions can intensify the brain insult by increasing ICP, causing respiratory distress, or increasing cerebral metabolism. Accordingly, phenytoin sodium is usually begun on admission. Corticosteroids have no proven benefit and are contraindicated because of their complications. Cimetidine, 300 mg every six hours to inhibit gastric acid secretion, plus antacids may reduce serious gastric bleeding.

Elevation of the head 10 to 20 degrees, turning and changing position every hour, frequent pulmonary toilet, pulmonary physical therapy, long-leg antithrombus stockings, standard catheter care, decompressing the stomach by nasogastric tube, instilling artificial tears every four hours, oral hygiene, and range-of-motion exercises to the extremities are standard.

The role of ICP management is discussed in the appropriate references. Although barbiturate anesthesia reduces elevated intracranial pressure, no studies have demonstrated a benefit from anesthetic treatment.

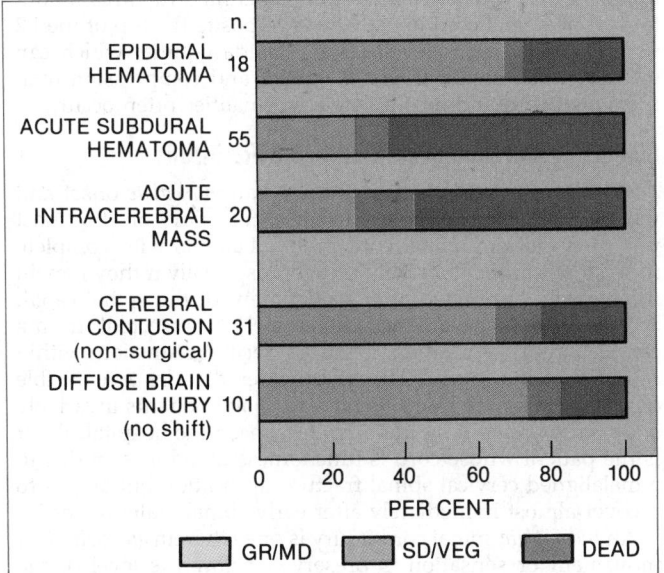

FIGURE 496–3. Distribution of outcomes in diagnostic groups of severe cerebral trauma.

RECOVERY AND SEQUELAE OF BRAIN TRAUMA

All injuries severe enough to interrupt consciousness probably cause at least some loss of brain cells. Although most patients with severe trauma rapidly regain independent function, some recover only slowly and others, never (Fig. 496–3). The punch-drunk boxer reflects the cumulative effect of recurrent brain damage to which is added the effects of a progressive communicating hydrocephalus.

Most patients with moderate brain injury make a reasonably satisfactory recovery, even when they have suffered subarachnoid hemorrhage, cerebral contusions, or a small intracerebral hematoma. Some, however, never overcome impairment of mental performance, and many have annoying subjective symptoms that last one to two years or longer.

Few patients with severe brain injury fully recover their neurologic and psychologic faculties. Most recovery from traumatic brain injury occurs in the first six months, although some neurologic improvement can continue for 12 to 18 months. Improvement thereafter is usually due to retraining or learning of special skills. Furthermore, the quality of ultimate outcome depends on the location and extent of the initial and secondary brain injuries. Somatic neurologic deficits such as hemiparesis or hemaniopsia are relatively uncommon. Most frequent are deficits and alterations in intellectual function, memory, and behavior, reflecting damage to frontal and temporal lobes and limbic structures.

Rehabilitation efforts after head injury should include neuropsychologic appraisal and therapy tailored to specific handicaps in the motor, emotional, behavioral, and mental spheres. Psychological depression is common, and drug treatment with antidepressants is often effective. Family counseling is critical.

POSTCONCUSSIVE SYNDROME. Many patients experience annoying symptoms following head trauma that may last for months or (rarely) years. Those with mild or moderate injury who expect an early complete recovery often complain the most. Characteristically, no obvious abnormal neurologic signs accompany the symptoms, which usually include headache, irritability, and a feeling of lightheadedness or dizziness but not true vertigo. Other complaints include difficulty with concentration, worry and apprehension, a preoccupation with self, a lack of interest in other's affairs, mild difficulty with memory, intolerance to loud noises and alcohol, insomnia, and loss of sexual interest. Quick movements or turning the head up or sideways may induce lightheadedness or a dazed weak feeling. Perhaps as many as half of these patients show subtle clinical abnormalities such as those revealed by electronystagmography. Otherwise, the mechanism of the postconcussive syndrome is not known. Associated neck injuries (whiplash) are often a part of the complex. The syndrome is so frequent, however, and the complaints so consistent that they imply a biologic substrate, but whether this is structural, neuropharmacologic, or psychologic remains unknown. The symptoms are not merely a reflection of compensation claims or pending litigation, although such concerns undoubtedly influence the length and degree of the complaints. The most important aspect of treatment consists of firm and immediate reassurance that the symptoms are not unusual, have no serious implications, and will eventually disappear. Advice that there is no reason for the complaints only intensifies self-preoccupation. Diazepam, 5 mg three or four times a day, helps some patients. Recovery within weeks or months is the rule, but some patients require as long as several years.

CHRONIC SUBDURAL HEMATOMA

Chronic subdural hematoma presents a problem apart from acute traumatic brain injury; the clinical syndrome develops weeks to many months after the original trauma. The clinical effects relate primarily to brain shift, although focal cortical compression, elevated ICP, and secondary cerebral vascular insufficiency occasionally contribute to the pathogenesis. Subdural hematoma follows mild more often than severe head trauma and occurs more frequently among alcoholics, the elderly, and those receiving anticoagulants. The minor head injury may not be remembered by the patient or the family. Headache is common and may be present almost from the time of injury. Subsequently, subtle mental changes may occur, and the patient may become somewhat lethargic with a loss of initiative. Following this stage, at six weeks or more after injury, fluctuating obtundation, somnolence, confusion, and memory loss often ensue, sometimes accompanied by hemiparesis or other mild focal changes. If untreated, patients may progress to signs and symptoms of tentorial herniation (see Ch. 457). Clinical diagnosis can be difficult, and CT or MRI is required.

Chronic subdural hematoma must be considered in the differential diagnosis of any new mental disturbance or gradually developing focal neurologic deficit in patients aged 40 years or older and in all patients with chronic alcoholism. Smaller hematomas may resolve spontaneously, but for larger lesions surgical drainage is the treatment of choice. Steroid therapy often improves symptoms and signs initially, but whether they reduce the need for surgical treatment is uncertain.

Becker DP, Miller JD, Gade G: Diagnosis and treatment of head injury in adults. In Youmans JR (ed.): Neurological Surgery. 3rd ed. Philadelphia, W.B. Saunders Company, 1988. *This chapter presents a comprehensive, detailed, and practical description of head injury management.*

Cooper P (ed.): Head Injury. 2nd ed. Baltimore, Williams & Wilkins, 1987. *This represents the most up-to-date and complete multiauthored text on the subject of human brain trauma.*

Jennett B, Teasdale GM: The Management of Head Injuries. Philadelphia, F.A. Davis Company, 1981. *A comprehensive monograph giving detailed statistics on the relation of outcome to early signs and to varied treatments.*

Kontos HA, Wei EP: Superoxide production in experimental brain injury. J Neurosurg 64:803, 1986. *Metabolites potentially damaging to healthy brain are released following brain trauma. This area represents a frontier in brain injury research.*

Rutherford W, Merrett JD, McDonald JR: Sequelae of concussion caused by minor head injuries. Lancet 1:1, 1977. *This brief paper places the postconcussive syndrome into perspective. The authors discuss the interplay between symptoms from organic brain damage and post-traumatic neurosis.*

Seelig JM, Becker DP, Miller JD, et al.: Traumatic acute subdural hematoma. N Engl J Med 304:1511, 1981. *This article clarifies the importance of prompt management and treatment of elevated intracranial pressure.*

497 INJURIES TO THE SPINE

GENERAL CONSIDERATIONS

The spinal column surrounds and encases the spinal cord, nerve roots, and cauda equina, providing the major support for the body as well as flexibility for the neck and back. Injury to the spine can cause severe pain, impair spinal support and flexibility, and create deformity. The greatest hazard, however, involves potential or actual damage to the enclosed spinal cord or nerve roots.

Spinal cord injury has a low incidence but a high residual morbidity. Each year in the United States, approximately 8000 new cases are admitted to hospital. There are about 200,000 survivors of severe traumatic spinal cord injury living in America today, half quadriplegic and half paraplegic. Slightly more are rendered quadriplegic at the time of injury, but a higher early death rate renders the ratio equal. Half of the initially quadriplegic and 60 per cent of the paraplegic patients remain completely paralyzed below the level of their spinal lesions. Only 17 per cent recover enough function to walk. Eighty per cent are under age 40, and half of all spinal injuries occur in persons 15 to 25 years of age.

MECHANISMS OF INJURY TO SPINE AND SPINAL CORD

Physical forces generally deform the spinal column in one of four ways: flexion injuries can fracture the vertebral body and cause acute disc rupture; extension deformation often fractures posterior bony elements (laminae and spinous processes) and disrupts the strong and stabilizing longitudinal ligaments that run along the anterior and posterior surfaces of the vertebral bodies; compression injuries cause explosion fractures of the vertebral body and tear surrounding ligaments; and rotational injuries can disrupt ligamentous structures. Flexion or extension injuries usually have a major rotational element that combines to produce extensive ligamentous and bony injury.

Deformation and dislocation of the spinal column at the time of injury can immediately injure the spinal cord. If the spinal column remains dislocated, additional continuing pressure on the cord and nerve roots may compound the problem. The maximal vertebral displacement that actually occurs at the moment of impact is greater than that seen on the initial x-ray, since the bone rebounds toward normal position.

The cervical spine is the least protected and most flexible portion of the vertebral column. It is relatively fixed to the thoracic spine below and its top end supports the head. As a result, only moderate trauma can cause a fracture or fracture dislocation. The cervical spinal canal normally is at least 30 per cent larger in diameter than the spinal cord. Individuals who have normal or large canals often can tolerate a considerable vertebral dislocation and show no spinal cord deficit. In contrast, patients with narrow canals or older individuals with osteoarthritic ridging that narrows the canal can develop major spinal cord deficits from flexion or extension injury with minimal or no spinal column malalignment. Since relatively low-energy forces can displace the cervical spinal column, more partial or reversible cord injuries occur in this region. In contrast, most thoracic cord injuries are complete and irreversible. The thoracic spine has additional fixation from the ribs and is the least flexible area of the spine. Tremendous force is required to malalign the thoracic spine; if dislocation occurs, the the spinal cord is subjected to a major impact. Additionally, the thoracic canal is normally small in relation to the spinal cord diameter, and malalignment that does not relocate is likely to cause continued compression of the cord.

The lumbar column is heavily constructed and gains additional support from the bulky paraspinal muscles. Here, also, massive energy forces are required to dislocate the spine. The lumbar canal widens relative to the neural structures it contains. The spinal cord usually ends opposite the top of the L2 vertebra. Below this level lies the cauda equina, which can tolerate much higher levels of trauma and compression than the spinal cord and incomplete abnormalities often occur.

COMPLETE AND INCOMPLETE SPINAL CORD INJURY

Whether the neurologic deficit had an *immediate* onset and whether it is *complete* below the level of injury are the most notable factors in spinal cord injury. Patients with complete functional transection rarely recover, especially if they remain functionally transected after realignment of the spinal canal. A patient may be rendered immediately "transected" from a cervical injury and then begin to recover function within minutes of the injury. This is considered to be a reversible *concussive* injury to the cervical cord. Such patients invariably show improvement by the time they reach the hospital. Rarer is the patient whose cord is functionless on admission due to a malaligned cervical spinal fracture-dislocation but begins to recover almost immediately after early spinal realignment.

An *incomplete* spinal cord injury is one wherein *any voluntary* movement or sensation is preserved below the level of the lesion. This may include no more than touch or pin sensation in the perianal region (termed sacral sparing; the sacral sensory fibers run in the most peripheral aspect of the ventral spinal cord). The distinction is important because some patients with incomplete lesions eventually improve remarkably. With trauma, all the compact bundles of ascending and descending long fiber tracts in the spinal cord tend to be damaged to the same degree. If one bundle or part of a fiber tract retains function across the injury site, there is a good chance that the remaining tracts have only been severely concussed and not disrupted. Occasional reports of spectacular recoveries following "complete" injuries with no distal normal neurologic function even after 6 to 24 hours probably represent failure of the examiners to test sensory function sufficiently. Retained function of distal motor reflexes, however, does *not* define an incomplete injury. Bulbocavernous reflex, full penile erection in males, anal wink, cremasteric reflex, reflex leg withdrawal, or downgoing toe movement to noxious stimuli can all represent reflex activity in an isolated cord. Spinal shock, defined as loss of reflex activity below the lesion, is usually present for three to six weeks after complete lesions, but in civilian spinal cord trauma, it may not develop at all. This is especially true with cervical cord damage.

The center gray matter is the part of the cord most sensitive and vulnerable to physical blows. As the force of the blow increases, increasing damage extends radially outward into the more lateral ascending and descending long white matter fiber tracts that carry information from brain to body and vice versa.

SYNDROMES OF SPINAL CORD INJURY

The *central cord syndrome* reflects cord damage from injury at or adjacent to the traumatic force. With increasing trauma, the lesion extends from central gray matter to the medial portion of the cord white matter, where voluntary myelinated motor fibers to the arms are located (Fig. 497–1; note that motor fibers to the legs lie more peripherally). The characteristic clinical syndrome is identified by lower motor neuron changes in the arms combined with spasticity in the legs, with the arms being weaker than the legs. Sensory modalities are variably involved, depending upon the extent to which injury involves the posterior and anterolateral columns; pain and temperature sensation are characteristically reduced in the hands. As in many or most intramedullary acute cord lesions, urinary retention-incontinence is often present. Striking neurologic recovery may be seen over time, although some permanent handicap often remains in arm and hand function.

In the *anterior cord syndrome*, voluntary motor function and pain and temperature sensation are lost, but distal position sense, light touch, and vibratory sensation remain. The anterior and lateral columns of the cord are dysfunctional, but the posterior columns are intact. Either anterior cord compression or a lesion involving the anterior spinal artery can be responsible. Prognosis in these cases is less hopeful than in the *posterior cord syndrome*, in which the opposite clinical picture is present.

Recovery with *Brown-Séquard syndrome* lies between the aforementioned extremes. Affected patients have dysfunction of half of the cord (the meridian defined in the sagittal plane), with distal motor weakness ipsilateral to the lesion and distal pain and temperature loss contralateral to the lesion. Also, ipsilateral loss of position and vibratory sense occurs if the injury represents a true "hemisection" of the cord. Improvement is the rule, usually accompanied by some permanent deficit.

Most patients with incomplete lesions show progressive improvement, but on occasion neurologic function worsens. Early after injury progressive loss of function is almost always due to continued or increased compression of the spinal cord by a protruded disc, bone spicules, or distortion of the spinal canal.

The level of the injury is critical. Complete lesions involving the cervical spine cause quadriplegia. When the lesion lies above the C4 cord level, many patients die of respiratory muscle paralysis. Patients with complete lesions in the C6 cord region may retain some biceps function but lack important arm extension, wrist extension, and finger flexion. If the injury is at C7–T1 spine level (C8 cord level), intrinsic hand function is impaired, but since the patient usually retains wrist extension, linkage splints applied to the wrist and fingers will give finger pincer function. Spinal cord injuries that last more than 24 hours will not improve distally, but neurologic function related to the level of injury may improve. Thus, a patient with a complete injury at C7 cord level might initially lack wrist extension and finger movement and have weak triceps function, yet over time may regain improved triceps function and recovery of wrist extension.

PATIENT MANAGEMENT

EMERGENCY AND EARLY MANAGEMENT. Most trained rescue teams can place patients carefully in a neutral supine position at the accident site and maintain that position during transport. During transport, the head should be kept in unchanging alignment with the spine. Nasal oxygen should be administered and artificial ventilation and cardiovascular support provided as needed.

In the emergency room cardiorespiratory resuscitation is often required. If intubation is necessary, nasotracheal or

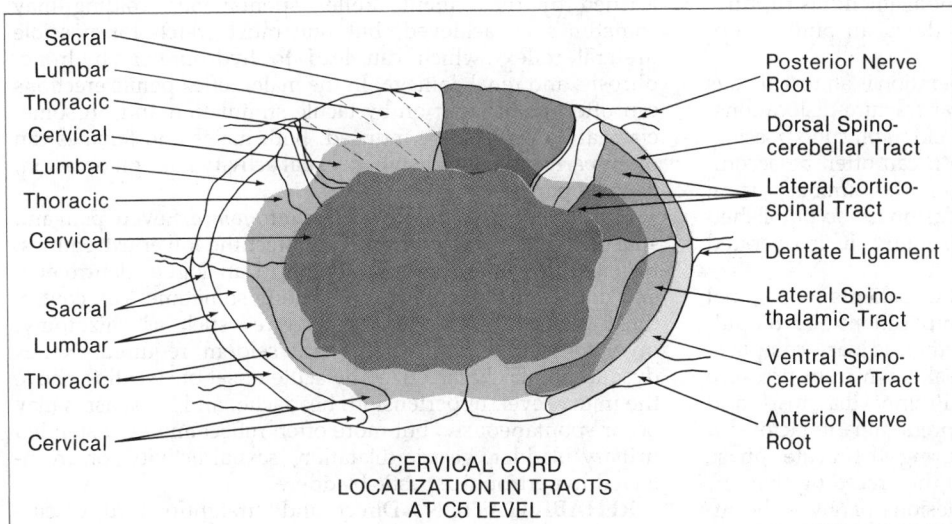

Sacral
Lumbar
Thoracic
Cervical
Lumbar
Thoracic
Cervical
Sacral
Lumbar
Thoracic
Cervical

Posterior Nerve Root
Dorsal Spinocerebellar Tract
Lateral Corticospinal Tract
Dentate Ligament
Lateral Spinothalamic Tract
Ventral Spinocerebellar Tract
Anterior Nerve Root

CERVICAL CORD
LOCALIZATION IN TRACTS
AT C5 LEVEL

FIGURE 497–1. Diagrammatic description of the spinal pathways at the lower cervical level showing the usual distribution of the contusion-hemorrhage that causes a central cord syndrome.

endotracheal intubation should be performed rather than tracheostomy. Following a major cervical or upper thoracic cord injury, signs of peripheral sympathetic nervous system denervation are common. Characteristically, patients have bradycardia, hypotension, and perhaps hypothermia. Immediately following the impact, there occurs a brief and temporary three- to four-minute episode of marked arterial hypertension secondary to cord sympathetic massive discharge. The subsequent hypotension can be reversed with alpha-adrenergic agonists such as metaraminol, and also responds to intravenous fluid administration. Hypoxemia is common after cervical and upper-thoracic cord trauma. The thoracic intercostal muscles are paralyzed, and diaphragmatic breathing initially may be inadequate to support adequate ventilation. Associated lung, chest, and abdominal injuries are frequent. After resuscitation a baseline neurologic examination can be completed and appropriate spine films obtained. The goals of treatment are to realign the spinal column, restore spinal canal diameter, stabilize the spine, and prevent a secondary or delayed cord injury.

Cervical Spine Injuries. Fracture-dislocations should be reduced promptly. These injuries often are unstable and threaten to produce worse cord damage. Skull tongs that can be placed without the necessity of a scalp incision or skull drill holes are now available in most emergency services. Initially, traction weights to pull the tongs rostrally are applied at 5 pounds per interspace (a C3–C4 dislocation would have 15 to 20 pound weights). Weights are increased progressively under radiographic control (a radiograph and neurologic examination are checked after each 5- to 10-pound addition of weight). With careful and judicious use of diazepam (Valium) or, in unusual cases when ventilation is controlled, neuromuscular junction blockade, most dislocations can be reduced with less than 60 pounds. Following reduction, further management concerning the need for restoration of canal diameter is controversial. Patients whose neurologic deficits remain complete do not ordinarily improve with surgical decompression of the spinal cord, and those whose injuries are incomplete generally improve without surgery. All agree, however, that the patient who demonstrates neurologic worsening should have the canal diameter defined and restored. The modern view that many specialists espouse is that the canal diameter should be defined radiologically in *all* cases and any pressure on the cord removed surgically so as to give the spinal cord maximal chance for recovery. Clinical evidence to support this aggressive approach is not available.

Myelography with or without CT and magnetic resonance (MR) imaging will define diameter and cord position. If extrinsic cord compression is present and surgery is to be performed, the operation must be tailored to the location of the intraspinal pressure and the type of ligamentous rupture. Anterior compression is best removed via an anterior approach to the spine.

Thoracolumbar Injuries. An open operation is almost always required to reduce thoracic and lumbar fracture-dislocations. This should usually be preceded by myelography and possibly CT. Surgical reduction and stabilization can often be accomplished with intraoperative traction on the laminae, using Harrington metal rods. Permanent fusion is accomplished with intraoperative bone grafting at the injury site in operated cases.

MEDICAL CARE. Over 40 per cent of patients with spinal cord injury have serious medical complications. Cardiopulmonary complications are the most lethal, urinary complications the most common, and skin breakdown from pressure the most intractable to treatment. Prompt diagnosis and treatment of complications are the predominant factors in early management. Medical care during the acute phase should follow the principles defined in the preceding chapter.

Cardiorespiratory. Because higher lesions paralyze the in-

tercostal muscles, vital capacity is impaired, and breathing is diaphragmatic-abdominal. Pressure on the abdomen must be avoided in prone patients. Patients often hyperventilate and reduce their $PaCO_2$. Ventilatory reserve is reduced, and a small pulmonary insult can cause hypoxemia.

The cardiovascular system may be very unstable. The combination of reduced arterial and venous tone from the traumatic sympathectomy results in profound peripheral muscle paralysis, pooling in the vascular compartment. Severe bradycardia can be life threatening. Anticholinergics such as atropine will help reverse this, but occasionally a cardiac pacemaker is temporarily needed. Although the hypotension will temporarily respond to alpha agonists such as norepinephrine, volume expansion with colloids and saline is imperative. Monitoring of the central venous pressure or wedge pressure and heart rate helps one gauge requirements. Venous stasis is responsible for a high incidence of venous thrombosis and pulmonary embolism, which may be countered by antiembolic stockings, continuous passive leg improvement, and subclinical heparinization.

Gastrointestinal. Paralytic ileus is common, and nasogastric suction is advisable for a minimum of 48 hours. Hyponatremia is common secondary to high sodium loss via nasogastric suction, diarrhea, and urinary loss, or loss into the gut in association with the adynamic ileus. Total parenteral nutrition, begun early, may minimize the complications of inanition. With extensive paralysis, metabolic and caloric requirements may be reduced below normal. Once eating begins, daily stool softeners and laxative suppositories given every other day will encourage spontaneous reflex defecation.

Skin. After two hours of pressure, anesthetic skin begins to develop ischemic changes that can lead to ulcer formation. Skin over the sacrum, ischial tuberosities, trochanters, and heels is prone to pressure sores. A prophylactic program should begin as soon as possible after admission.

Spinal Cord Injury Beds. Rotating bed frames that incorporate traction devices are commonly used to change patient position. Recently, a bed that places the patient in perpetual motion has been introduced. It is expensive and has not yet been widely applied, but the reported reduction of pulmonary complications, decubitus ulcers, and venous thromboembolism attests to the need for frequent turning, pulmonary toilet, passive range-of-motion exercises to extremities, and early mobilization. Halo traction for external cervical spine stabilization has permitted earlier mobilization for many patients.

Genitourinary Tract. A Foley catheter should remain in the urinary bladder for ten days, during which time chemoprophylaxis is recommended. After the tenth day, it is a good policy to discontinue straight drainage and begin an every-four-hour intermittent catheterization program, preferably learned by the patient. Reflex spontaneous voiding may sometimes be achieved, but one must watch for possible ureteral reflex, which can lead to hydroureter, hydronephrosis, and renal damage. In the male, reflex penile erections can often be brought on by tactile stimulation and, in some, ejaculation can also be induced. Both males and females can often participate in satisfying sexual activity and, on occasion, become parents.

Pain, Spasticity, and Reflex Dysautonomia. Severe pain and spasticity with flexor spasms can affect the lower extremities. Baclofen, a gamma-aminobutyric acid analogue, dantrolene, and diazepam alone or in combination sometimes can control these symptoms. Surgical procedures such as rhizotomy, myelotomy, and neurectomy are seldom required. Reflex dysautonomia characterized by acute onset of sweating above the injury level, hypertension, headache, and leg spasms may occur spontaneously, but more often reflect an overdistended urinary bladder, gastric dilatation, sexual activity, or an infected hypertrophic spastic bladder.

REHABILITATION. Direct and straightforward discussions with patient and family should begin immediately regarding the diagnosis and prognosis. Early, honest communication usually creates an optimal attitude for expeditious institution of a rehabilitative program. The common psychologic response to spinal cord injury is initial denial, followed by anger and then depression. The patient must be encouraged to cope and move quickly to retraining. Physical, occupational, and respiratory therapy should begin early. Furthermore, the restoration process should include psychologic, social, sexual, and vocational rehabilitation. Most patients can be brought back into competitive society. Life expectancy following spinal cord transection for those who survive the initial hospitalization period is only about 10 per cent less than for the population at large, but lifelong follow-up care is a necessary medical program. The major impediments to success are renal failure, decubitus ulcers, and psychosocial problems.

Bracken MB, Shepard MJ, Hellenbrand KG, et al: Methylprednisolone and neurological function 1 year after spinal cord injury. J Neurosurg 63:704, 1985. *A study of the outcome in 256 patients with partial and complete spinal cord injury shows no beneficial effect from steroid therapy.*

Cooper PR, Maravilla KR, Sklar FH, et al.: Halo immobilization of cervical spine fractures. Indications and results. J Neurosurg 50:603, 1979. *Halo immobilization is now in common use. Indications, complications, and contraindications are clearly outlined.*

Guttman L: Spinal Cord Injuries, Comprehensive Management and Research. 2nd ed. Oxford, Blackwell Scientific Publications, 1976. *This is the most comprehensive publication on spinal cord injury written by the man who pioneered the development of spinal cord injury centers.*

Yashon D: Spinal Injury. 2nd ed. New York, Appleton-Century-Crofts, 1986. *Modern diagnosis and management as practiced in the United States are clearly outlined in a practical manner. Common complications are discussed lucidly, and each chapter is well referenced.*

Young HF, Becker DP: Complications of spine surgery and trauma. In Greenfield LJ (ed.): Complications in Surgery and Trauma. Philadelphia, J. B. Lippincott Company, 1984. *Complications of spinal trauma and their management are covered in a comprehensive yet concise fashion.*

SECTION FIFTEEN / MECHANICAL LESIONS OF THE SPINE AND RELATED STRUCTURES

Jerome B. Posner

The vertebral column, its contents (spinal cord, exiting nerve roots) and surrounding structure (spinal ligaments, paraspinous muscles) are responsible for some of the most common afflictions of man. Neck and/or back pain originating from these structures affects almost every individual at some time of life. Each year 4 per cent of Americans suffer an episode of low back pain. The disorder ranks next to alcoholism as the leading cause of time lost from work. More than 200,000 spinal operations are performed in the United States annually. Most back and neck pain is transient and neither life-threatening nor associated with obvious pathologic abnormalities. However, in the small minority of patients suffering from serious structural disease of the spine or spinal cord, severe neurologic abnormalities may develop which, unless correctly diagnosed and treated, may lead to paralysis, sensory loss, and incontinence. Because the pathophysiology of most neck and back pain is poorly understood, the physician often encounters patients in whom he can neither make a certain diagnosis nor prescribe rational therapy. From this vast group he must cull the small number of patients suffering potentially remediable structural disease of the spine so that appropriate treatment can be instituted before permanent neurologic damage occurs.

498 ANATOMY, PHYSIOLOGY, AND DIFFERENTIAL DIAGNOSIS

ANATOMY AND PHYSIOLOGY OF THE SPINE

The spine is composed of two functional segments. The *anterior segment* contains two adjacent vertebral bodies separated by an intervertebral disc. The anterior segment bears weight and cushions the spine during such activities as walking and running. The posterior segment is composed of the vertebral arches, the transverse processes, the posterior spinous processes, and the paired articulations known as *facets* with the facet joint between them. The *posterior segment* is non-weight bearing but protects the contained spinal cord and nerve roots and allows the spine to move in extension and rotation. The midcervical and lower lumbar levels are particularly mobile and therefore susceptible to damage from mechanical lesions such as herniated discs (see Ch. 499). Several ligaments offer the spine passive support and paravertebral muscles support the spine actively by voluntary and automatic contractions.

Only parts of the spine are pain-sensitive (Fig. 498–1). The *periosteum* of the vertebral body is pain-sensitive. (Therefore, compression fractures are, at least initially, painful.) The *intervertebral disc* is not in itself pain-sensitive. However, if the disc bulges and compresses the posterior longitudinal ligament, pain may result even if the nerve root itself is not involved. Posteriorly, the synovium-lined *facet joints* are pain-sensitive and probably an important source of neck and back pain, although the intraspinal ligaments holding the posterior elements are not. Most of the pain-sensitive structures are innervated by the recurrent meningeal or sinuvertebral nerves, a branch of each spinal nerve that arises just distal to the dorsal root ganglion and reenters the spinal canal through the intervertebral foramen. The sinuvertebral nerves also receive fibers from neighboring grey rami or directly from thoracic sympathetic ganglia. *Sympathetic nerves* contain sensory fibers and probably play a role in the transmission of pain. The *paravertebral muscles* surrounding and supporting the spine are also pain-sensitive, particularly when overstretched or in spasm. These muscles are probably the commonest source of both acute and chronic neck and back pain (myofascial pain syndromes). The pain-sensitive nerve root usually occupies only a small portion of the intervertebral foramen through which it exits the spinal canal. When the spine is extended (i.e., hyperlordotic posture), the intervertebral foramen becomes smaller, potentially impinging on the nerve root and leading to overlap of the facet joints, giving potential irritation of pain-sensitive synovial membranes. Thus, pain in patients with intervertebral disc or facet joint disease may be exacerbated by extension and relieved somewhat by flexion of the spine. Additionally, hyperlordosis, a common postural abnormality, sometimes leads to chronic low back pain; most back exercises aim at developing a flat or slightly flexed, but not hyperlordotic, lumbar spine.

The spinal cord and its attached motor, sensory, and autonomic nerve roots are the primary occupants of the spinal cord. The spinal cord itself extends in the adult from the first cervical to the first lumbar vertebral body, and the spinal roots continue in the subarachnoid space to the second sacral vertebra. The caudal portion of the spinal cord is called the *conus medullaris*, and the bunched lumbar and sacral roots that exit below the cord are the *cauda equina*.

Within the canal several processes can compress or deform

the spinal cord and its roots. The resulting signs and symptoms depend on the location of the abnormality, its speed of development, and whether it affects the nerve roots or the spinal cord alone. In the cervical spine, the spinal cord and vertebral segments lie at approximately the same level; thus, the C5 vertebral body marks the C5 spinal segment and emerging nerve roots are virtually horizontal.

The more caudad spinal cord segments and vertebral segments move out of alignment so that thoracic spinal cord segments gradually become two to three levels higher than the corresponding vertebral segments (e.g., T8 vertebral body marks the T11 thoracic segment). Most of the lumbar and sacral cord is found between T10 and L1 lumbar segments. As a result, the nerve roots travel a descending pathway in the subarachnoid space before exiting via the vertebral foramen. In addition, because there is a C8 spinal segment and no C8 vertebral body, cervical spine nerve roots exit above the vertebral body with the same number (e.g., the C4 root exits between C3 and C4). Thus, a herniated C4–C5 disc may compress the C5 or C6 root but not the C4 root.

In the thoracic and lumbar spine, nerve roots leave the intervertebral foramen above the disc (e.g., the L4 root exits between L4 and L5 and the S1 root between L5 and S1) so that a herniated disc between L4–L5 vertebral bodies usually compresses the L5 nerve root; a herniated disc between L5 and S1 usually compresses the S1 root (Fig. 498–2). If the disc protrudes medially (less common than laterally protruding discs), an L4–L5 disc may compress sacral roots rather than the L5 lumbar root. Only if the disc completely extrudes into the vertebral canal will an L4–L5 disc compress the L4 root.

The size of the vertebral canal relative to the spinal cord varies from level to level and among persons. There is generally more space in the lumbar and cervical areas than in the thoracic area. Thus, herniated thoracic discs (uncommon) are more likely to cause myelopathy than cervical or lumbar herniations. In some individuals the spinal canal is congenitally small (spinal stenosis). Disc herniation or osteoarthritis is more likely to cause myelopathy in these individuals than in those with capacious canals.

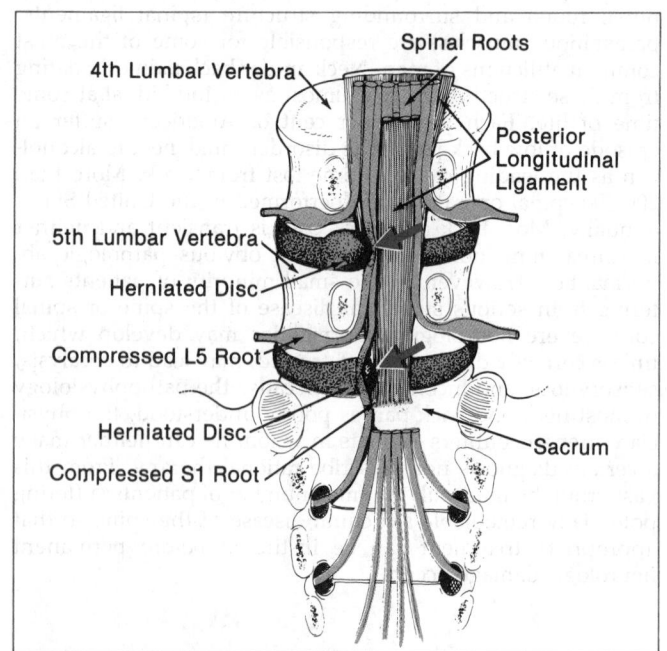

FIGURE 498–2. Nerve root compression by herniated disc. The figure illustrates that the posterior longitudinal ligament tapers as it reaches the lower lumbar area, leaving a weakened area laterally allowing disc herniation. An L4-L5 disc is shown lateral to the L5 root displacing it medially; a herniated disc between L5 and S1 displaces the root laterally. (From Posner JB: Back pain and epidural spinal cord compression. Med Clin North Am 71:185–205, 1987.)

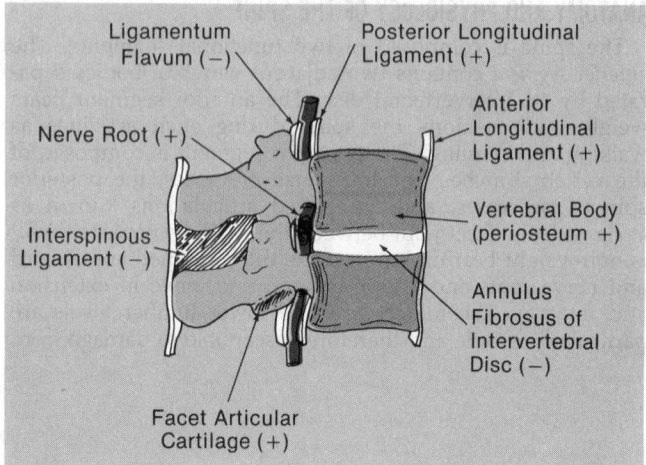

FIGURE 498–1. Pain-sensitive structures of the spine. This lateral view indicates the pain-sensitive structures with a plus sign (+) and those structures not pain sensitive with a minus sign (−). (From Posner JB: Back pain and epidural spinal cord compression. Med Clin North Am 71:185–205, 1987.)

TYPES OF PAIN

The cardinal symptom of lesions of the spine or its contents is pain. Pain from structures other than the spinal cord or nerve roots is of three types: local, referred, and muscular.

LOCAL PAIN. Local pain results from the irritation of nerve endings at the site of the pathologic process. Metastatic tumors and osteoporotic collapse of a vertebral body cause pain at the site of the lesion by irritation of nerve endings in the periosteum surrounding the vertebral body. Metastatic tumors involving the vertebral body that do not distort the periosteum are usually painless. Intervertebral discs cause local pain when they compress nerve endings in the anulus fibrosus or posterior longitudinal ligament. Local pain is usually steady and aching but may be intermittent, occurring particularly when the involved structure is moved. Local pain is usually associated with tenderness to palpation or percussion. The site of local pain is diagnostically helpful. Most spine pain from mechanical causes (e.g., herniated disc) occurs either in the neck or low back, since these structures are most mobile and more subject to injury. However, tumors often strike the thoracic area, and osteoporotic vertebral collapse also tends to affect the structurally weak thoracic vertebral bodies.

The *character* of the local pain is helpful diagnostically. Pain caused by lumbar muscle or ligamentous strain or by herniated disc usually disappears when the patient lies recumbent. Herniated lumbar disc pain is often exacerbated by sitting and relieved by standing or walking. The pain of spinal stenosis, on the contrary, is often absent when lying or sitting and occurs only when the patient walks. Vertebral metastases with or without epidural spinal cord compression cause pain that is often more prominent when lying and sometimes is relieved by sitting up; many patients with spinal cord compression elect to sleep in a sitting position. Even if pain is absent in the lying position, movement such as turning over in bed or arising may be particularly painful.

REFERRED PAIN. Referred pain is felt at a distance from the site of the local lesion but not in the dermatomal distribution of a nerve root (radicular pain, see below). Referred pain, like local pain, has a deep aching quality and is often associated with tenderness of subcutaneous tissues and muscles at the site of referral. Maneuvers that affect local pain usually have the same effect on referred pain. Pain referred from pathologic abnormalities of the cervical spine often is either just medial to the scapula or over the lateral aspect of the arm; pain referred from the low back is usually appreciated in the buttocks and posterior thighs, although rarely below the knees. Pain from the upper lumbar spine is often referred to the flank, groin, and anterior thigh. Pain also can be referred to the spine from lesions of thoracic or abdominal viscera, a prominent example being the back pain from pancreatic carcinoma.

MUSCLE PAIN. Muscle pain occurs when an injury to or structural abnormality of the spine induces paravertebral muscle spasm. Sustained contraction of paravertebral muscles gives rise to chronic aching pain, usually felt lateral to the midline of the neck or back. Palpation of painful muscles may reveal evidence of spasm and tenderness. At times, when areas of extreme sensitivity (trigger points) are palpated, the pain may be felt not only locally in the muscle but also may be referred to distant structures. These trigger points are thought to underlie many myofascial pain syndromes, common causes of neck and back pain without structural abnormalities of the spine.

RADICULAR PAIN. Injured spinal roots or spinal cord produce, respectively, radicular or funicular pain. Radicular pain is the prominent symptom of nerve root compression. Nerve roots are not usually pain-sensitive. However, chronic compression leads to edema and, perhaps, inflammation and demyelination; the root then becomes sensitive to stretching or compression. When compressed, the pain may be experienced only in the cutaneous distribution (dermatome) of the involved root or may be felt locally and deep in muscles that it supplies. Root pain is usually least severe in positions that minimize compression and most severe in positions that compress or stretch the root. Root pain is usually exacerbated by increasing intraspinal pressure by coughing, sneezing, and straining.

FUNICULAR PAIN. Funicular pain is caused by compression of the long tracts of the spinal cord. Funicular pain is less sharp than radicular pain and is often described as a cold, unpleasant sensation in the extremity. Its distribution is more diffuse than that of radicular pain but like root pain is usually exacerbated by movements that stretch the cord (neck flexion, straight leg raising) or that increase intraspinal pressure.

SIGNS OF NERVE ROOT AND SPINAL CORD DYSFUNCTION

In addition to pain, chronic compression of nerve roots can produce paresthesias, sensory loss, weakness, atrophy, and hyporeflexia in root-supplied tissues, thus localizing the lesion. Knowing the myotomal and dermatomal distribution of spinal roots (Table 498–1) often allows one not only to localize the lesion but also to suggest its etiologic diagnosis: involvement of a single root is more likely to occur with intervertebral disc herniation (Ch. 499), whereas multiple root dysfunction is likely to be caused by tumor or chronic inflammation. However, myotomal and dermatomal localization must be utilized cautiously. In the first place, not every body obeys the standard maps. Also, contiguous dermatomes and contiguous myotomes can develop, and the apparent size of a dermatome can vary between examinations, depending on central nervous system excitability. Mostly, however, the localizing diagnosis of root lesions is accurate.

Clinical signs of spinal cord compression depend on the speed with which the compression develops, the transverse and longitudinal site of the lesion, and the vulnerability of the individual spinal fibers. The spinal cord accommodates considerably to gradually developing compression (e.g., from meningiomas), and such disorders can cause the gradual onset of painless paraparesis or paraplegia. Because of this accommodation, subsequent decompression, even when patients are severely paraparetic, often leads to complete resolution of neurologic symptoms. On the other hand, rapidly developing lesions such as epidural hematomas, acute midline herniated discs, or epidural spinal cord compression from metastatic tumor cause rapidly developing neurologic signs that respond poorly to therapy once severe paraparesis has developed.

The site of compression in the transverse plane may determine clinical signs, particularly when the compression develops slowly. For example, laterally located lesions compressing one side of the spinal cord may cause the Brown-Séquard syndrome (ipsilateral hemiparesis, vibration and position sense loss, with contralateral pain and temperature loss); compression of the posterior portion of the cord may cause bilateral position and vibratory loss, with preservation of pain and temperature sensation and of motor power. However, most lesions twist the cord as they compress it and also interfere with the vascular supply to sites beyond the compression. Accordingly, one can depend only in a general way on the neurologic signs to evaluate the exact transverse site of compression. The longitudinal location of the lesion is more important. Cervical lesions cause quadriplegia, thoracic lesions, paraplegia; and upper lumbar lesions, normal motor function with bowel and bladder dysfunction and extensor plantar responses (conus medullaris syndrome). Lesions below the first lumbar vertebral body compress the cauda equina, causing loss of bowel and bladder function with lower motor neuron leg weakness and normal plantar reflexes.

Certain spinal tracts appear to be more vulnerable to

TABLE 498–1. DIAGNOSIS OF NERVE ROOT LESIONS

	C2–C3	C5	C6	C7	C8	Nerve T1
Pain	Back of head, lateral face, behind ear (occasionally vertex or orbit)	Medial scapula, lateral border of arm	Lateral forearm, thumb and index finger	Posterior arm, lateral hand, mid-forearm, and medial scapula	Medial forearm and hand	Deep aching in shoulder and axilla to olecranon
Sensory loss	Posterior scalp, pinna, lateral face	Lateral border of upper arm	Lateral forearm, including thumb	Mid-forearm and middle finger	Medial forearm and little finger	Axilla down to olecranon
Reflex loss	None	Biceps	Supinator	Triceps	Finger stretch	None
Motor deficit	None	Deltoid, supraspinatus, infraspinatus, rhomboids	Biceps, brachioradialis, brachialis (pronators and supinators of forearm)	Latissimus dorsi, pectoralis major, triceps, wrist extensors, wrist flexors	Finger flexors, finger extensors, flexor carpi ulnaris (thenar muscles in some patients)	*All* small hand muscles (in some thenar muscles via C8)
Some causative lesions	Tumor, injury	Brachial neuritis, cervical disc or spondylosis, upper plexus injury	Cervical disc or spondylosis	Cervical disc or spondylosis	Pancoast tumor, rare in disc lesions or spondylosis, metastatic tumor, thoracic outlet syndrome	Pancoast tumor, cervical rib, outlet syndromes, metastatic carcinoma in deep cervical nodes
Autonomic changes	Gustatory sweating					Horner's syndrome

compression than others. The corticospinal tracts and posterior columns are particularly vulnerable, the spinothalamic tracts and descending autonomic fibers less so. As a result, weakness, spasticity, and reflex hyperactivity tend to be the earliest signs of spinal cord compression, with paresthesias, and vibratory and position sense loss occurring soon thereafter. Loss of pain and temperature sensation and of bladder and bowel function usually occur late in the course of spinal cord compression. The spinocerebellar pathways are also sensitive to compression, and at times ataxia mimicking cerebellar disease may be the only sign of spinal cord compression.

APPROACH TO THE PATIENT

Most mechanical lesions of the spine and its contents begin with pain and only later produce other signs of neurologic dysfunction. There are many potential causes of neck or back pain. One survey listed over 100 cases (Table 498–2). The task for the physician is to separate those patients with potentially serious disease from those with more common, if unknown, causes of back pain who need only reassurance, sometimes coupled with bedrest, analgesics, and physical therapy.

HISTORY. The diagnostic evaluation begins with the history. Get a complete description of the pain. Most spine pain begins acutely or subacutely and often follows, by minutes to hours, some unaccustomed physical activity, particularly lifting or bending. Patients may awaken stiff and sore the morning after unusual exercise or may develop acute back pain on arising in the morning, without any obvious precipitating event. Most neck pain begins as a stiff neck, often on awakening, without a history of unusual activity. In many patients, neck or low back pain recurs episodically over many years. Most neck or back pain is dull and aching in quality, exacerbated by movement and relieved by rest. Pain that is present when the patient is immobile and cannot be relieved by positional manipulation should lead the physician to consider a more serious disorder (e.g., tumor or extruded disc). *Radicular pain*, particularly if accompanied by paresthesias or loss of sensation, indicates mechanical compression of the

nerve root supplying that dermatome and implies identifiable structural disease (e.g., herniated disc). *Referred pain*, however, does not imply compression of a root.

A history of serious systemic illness may suggest disease of vertebral bodies. Carcinoma of the breast or thyroid may cause back pain from bony metastases years after the primary tumor has been successfully treated. Previous systemic infection may lead to delayed onset of vertebral osteomyelitis or epidural abscess. A family history may also give clues to the etiology of back pain. Neurofibromas causing neck or back pain by compression of nerve root or the spinal cord may be associated with neurofibromatosis. Rheumatoid arthritis and ankylosing spondylitis are causes of familial back pain.

EXAMINATION. A careful general physical examination may reveal evidence of systemic disease such as cancer or infection. Urinary tract infections, pelvic disease, abdominal aneurysms, and other intra-abdominal or intrathoracic processes sometimes cause back pain by impinging on vertebral bodies or paravertebral structures. Special attention should be paid to mobility of the spine and paravertebral structures. Most patients who complain of a stiff neck have some limitation of movement of the cervical spine, but if gradual movement of the cervical spine causes intense pain, if pain on neck flexion is referred to the thoracic or lumbar area, or if neck flexion causes paresthesias radiating into the arms, legs, or back (Lhermitte's sign), spinal cord compression should be suspected. Most low back pain not caused by a herniated disc is exacerbated by flexion and relieved by lying down. The paravertebral muscles are often in spasm, straightening the normally lordotic lumbar spine, and tender to palpation. Almost any severe low back pain, particularly if it radiates into a lower extremity, can increase when the extended leg is raised from the bed (straight leg raising sign). However, pain referred to the contralateral back or leg when the non-painful leg is raised (crossed straight leg raising) implies root compression. Forced extension of the hip (reverse straight leg raising) can elicit pain from upper lumbar root disease (L4 and above). Point tenderness over a spinous process raises the suspicion of involvement of the vertebra by either tumor or infection.

TABLE 498–1. DIAGNOSIS OF NERVE ROOT LESIONS *Continued*

Roots T4	T10	L2	L3	L4	L5	S1	S2–S4
Anterior chest and/or upper back	Midback and/or anterior abdomen	Across thigh	Across thigh	Down to medial malleolus	Back of thigh, lateral calf, dorsum of foot	Back of thigh, back of calf, lateral foot	Buttocks, genitalia, back of thigh
Usually none (upper back and chest at nipple level)	Usually none (midback and abdomen at umbilicus level)	Often none	Often none	Medial leg	Dorsum of foot	Behind lateral malleolus	Buttocks, genitalia
None	Decreased abdominal reflex	None	Adductor reflex	Knee jerk	None	Ankle jerk	Bulbocavernosus
Not discernible	None	Hip flexion, adduction of thigh	Knee extension, adduction of thigh	Inversion of foot	Dorsiflexion of toes and foot (latter L4 also)	Plantar flexion and eversion of foot	Bladder and bowel
Intravertebral or paravertebral tumor, herpes zoster	Intravertebral and paravertebral tumor, herpes zoster	Neurofibroma, meningioma, neoplastic disease; disc lesions very rare except at L4 < 5 per cent			Disc lesions, metastatic malignancy, neurofibromas, meningioma		Tumor, midline disc
Chest wall, piloerection, hyperhidrosis, unilateral gynecomastia, galactorrhea	Chest wall, piloerection, hyperhidrosis, retrograde ejaculation	Alterations in temperature and color of all or parts of the leg or thigh					Incontinence, impotence, urinary retention

The neurologic examination is important. Sensory loss, reflex diminution, and weakness all suggest neurologic disease that requires further evaluation. The distribution of abnormalities localizes the lesion. Remember, however, that patients in severe pain may be reluctant to move the painful part, making normal neuromuscular structures appear to be weak. Likewise, guarding can affect deep tendon reflexes, either increasing or decreasing them with respect to the normal side. Repeating the neurologic examination after pain has been relieved by analgesics usually clarifies whether or not there is neurologic dysfunction. Clear and reproducible neurologic signs, particularly sensory loss in a dermatomal distribution or a diminished stretch reflex, imply root compression.

Careful examination can often reveal inconsistencies (leg pain on straight leg raising when the patient is recumbent disappears in the sitting position) that suggest a psychologic rather than a physiologic basis.

LABORATORY AIDS TO INVESTIGATION. In most patients with back pain, laboratory tests are not required.

DIAGNOSTIC IMAGING. *Radiography.* In patients suspected of harboring structural disease, *radiographs* of the spine should be the first test. For suspected cervical lesions, frontal, lateral, oblique, and open-mouth odontoid views are required. If the patient has a short neck, the lower cervical area on lateral view may be obscured by the shoulders and require tomography. Flexion and extension views of the neck often help to determine if subluxation is present. If the patient is allowed to control the degree of flexion and extension, these tests are not harmful. For the thoracic and lumbosacral spine, frontal and lateral views are usually sufficient. Flexion and extension views assess subluxation. Review the radiographs with a radiologist to assure that all potential lesions at the site in question have been assessed. Pay particular attention to the sagittal diameter of the cervical and lumbar canal, to the pedicles, and to the presence of osteophytes and loss of height in disc spaces. Congenital spinal anomalies should also be sought, but most are common and do not cause pain

or neurologic dysfunction. Similarly, most patients of middle age or older have evidence of cervical or lumbar osteoarthritis. Such abnormalities do not prove that the radiologic defect is responsible for the symptoms. However, changes such as significant spondylolisthesis, marked multiple disc narrowing, stenosis of the lumbar canal, or vertebral destruction from tumor or infection are likely to be responsible for pain, and often for neurologic disability. If back pain is referred to the lower extremities, radiographs of the pelvis and femora may reveal unsuspected abnormalities.

Computed Tomography (CT). CT can detect erosion of vertebral bodies not identified on a bone scan, can identify paravertebral masses, dumb-bell tumors growing through the intervertebral foramen, and herniated discs. With high-resolution CT scanners, tumors and syringes within the cord can sometimes be identified. Thus, CT is now the best easily available radiologic test for the diagnosis of spine, nerve root, and spinal cord disease.

Magnetic Resonance (MR) Imaging. MR using appropriate surface coils can identify most lesions seen on plain radiography or CT and can identify intramedullary lesions such as tumors and syringes not currently detected by other techniques. Although MR images delineate bone poorly, lesions involving the bone marrow (e.g., metastases) or compromising the spinal cord or intervertebral foramen are easily seen. MRI will probably replace invasive diagnostic tests such as myelography.

Radionuclide Bone Scans. Bone scans are often used for screening patients with known or suspected cancer. The test can identify lesions not recognized by radiographs, but is nonspecific and does not distinguish tumors from inflammatory or degenerative diseases.

Myelograms. Myelography, using either lipid- or water-soluble radiopaque material, reliably outlines lesions in the spinal canal and determines whether they are extradural, intradural, or intramedullary. If complete obstruction to the passage of the contrast material is encountered after lumbar injection, a cisternal or upper cervical injection of contrast

TABLE 498–2. SOME CAUSES OF BACK PAIN

Transitory Back Pain
Tumors
  Benign bone and neural tumors (e.g., neurinoma, ependymoma,
    meningioma, osteoid osteoma, hemangioma, osteoblastoma)
  Malignant bone and neural tumors
    Primary (e.g., multiple myeloma, osteosarcoma)
    Secondary tumors (metastases)
Congenital Disorders
  Facet tropism (asymmetry)
  Transitional vertebra
  Spondylolysis and spondylolisthesis
Trauma
  Lumbar strain* (acute or chronic)
  Compression fracture (vertebral body or transverse process)
*Degenerative Disorders**
  Osteoarthritis
  Herniated disc
  Spinal stenosis
  Nerve root entrapment
Metabolic Disorders
  (e.g., osteoporosis, gout, diabetic neuropathy, Paget's disease)
Inflammatory Diseases
  (e.g., ankylosing spondylitis, arachnoiditis, rheumatoid arthritis)
Infections
  (e.g., disc space infection, tuberculosis, epidural and subdural abscess,
    herpes zoster, meningitis, sacroiliac joint infection)
Mechanical Causes
  (e.g., poor muscle tone, chronic postural strain)
Postoperative
  (e.g., sequelae of scar formation, arachnoiditis)
*Psychosomatic**
  (e.g., myofascial pain syndromes, conversion reaction)
Scoliosis
  (e.g., idiopathic, postparalytic, aging)
Visceral Disease
  (e.g., visceral inflammation, female pelvic pathology, retroperitoneal
    pathology, aortic aneurysm, prostatic disease)

Persistent Back Pain
Psychophysiologic
  (e.g., myofascial pain syndromes, conversion reaction)
Degenerative Disorders
  (e.g., osteoarthritis, herniated disc, spinal stenosis, nerve root entrapment)
Trauma
  (e.g., acute lumbar strain, compression fracture—vertebral body or
    transverse process)
Mechanical
  (e.g., chronic lumbar strain, poor posture, scoliosis, congenital anomalies)
Tumors
  Benign bone and neural tumors (e.g., neurinoma, ependymoma,
    meningioma, osteoid osteoma, hemangioma, osteoblastoma)
  Malignant bone and neural tumors
    Primary (e.g., multiple myeloma, osteosarcoma)
    Secondary tumors (metastases)
Visceral
  (e.g., pelvic or retroperitoneal lesions, aortic aneurysm, prostatic disease)
Infections
  (e.g., disc space infection, tuberculosis, epidural and subdural abscess,
    herpes zoster meningitis, sacroiliac joint infection)
Inflammatory
  (e.g., ankylosing spondylitis, arachnoiditis, rheumatoid arthritis)

*Common cause

material will determine the upper extent of the lesion. Lumbar puncture detects the presence of malignant cells or infecting organisms in the cerebrospinal fluid. When a spinal mass lesion is suspected, a lumbar puncture should be performed only in conjunction with myelography.

Angiography. Spinal angiography is a specialized technique, sometimes essential for the detailed investigation of tumors and vascular malformations in the spinal cord. The technique is particularly useful to the surgeon who requires preoperative knowledge of the vascular supply.

Discography. Discography is a controversial technique for identifying clinically important herniated discs. Its advantage over modern imaging methods is unproved.

Electromyography. Electromyography can help identify the presence and site of anterior horn cell or central root damage. Somatosensory evoked potentials can be recorded along the spinal cord or in the brain after a peripheral nerve is stimulated. Abnormalities sometimes identify the approximate site of a spinal cord lesion (Ch. 456.2).

MANAGEMENT OF THE PATIENT WITH NECK AND BACK PAIN. If no clinical findings suggest serious structural disease of the spine, nerve roots, or spinal cord, patients should be treated as if they suffered from an acute neck or back strain, without further diagnostic evaluation. Because most patients recover within a few weeks without specific therapy, it is difficult to assess various therapeutic regimens. For severe pain, the best treatment probably consists of bed rest on a firmly supported mattress in the position most comfortable. The best positioning for low back pain is usually semi-Fowler's position (head slightly elevated with pillows under the knees). Bed rest may be combined with analgesic agents (usually aspirin or acetaminophen) and with local heat. Patients should be encouraged to stay recumbent except to go to the toilet until pain diminishes. Control studies indicate that two days of bed rest are generally as beneficial as seven or more. As pain subsides, patients should gradually ambulate and start strengthening exercises for the paravertebral muscles of the neck and back, to prevent recurrence of pain. Other treatment modalities, including physical therapy, traction, procaine or saline injection into trigger points, and spinal manipulation, have not been shown to be more efficacious than the regimen described above. Manipulation of the neck is potentially dangerous because it can occlude the vertebral arteries as they enter the skull. Using standard therapy, 70 to 80 per cent of patients will become free of pain and able to return to full activity within a four-week period. During the period of bed rest, repeated physical and neurologic examinations are unwise, since vigorous movement of the neck, back, and extremities can exacerbate pain and delay improvement. A small minority of patients continue to have chronic pain, and they, along with those whose initial examination has suggested more serious disease, need further evaluation.

For neck pain, a soft cervical collar is sometimes as effective in immobilizing the neck as is bed rest; transcutaneous nerve stimulation has been reported to be effective as well. The management of specific causes of nerve root and spinal cord compression, such as a herniated disc, is detailed in the chapters that follow.

499 INTERVERTEBRAL DISC DISEASE

HERNIATED DISC. Herniated intervertebral discs are the most common cause of neck or low back pain associated with a clearly defined structural abnormality. Lumbar and cervical strain and myofascial pain syndromes (see Ch. 498) are more common but not marked by clear pathological abnormalities. Between each two vertebral bodies is a fibrocartilaginous intervertebral disc. The disc consists of a soft inner nucleus pulposus (a remnant of the notochord) surrounded by thicker fibrous tissue (the anulus fibrosus). The nucleus pulposus is gelatinous in structure and acts as a shock absorber between adjacent vertebral bodies. With advancing age, the nucleus loses fluid, volume, and resiliency, and the entire disc structure becomes more susceptible to trauma and compression. Tears develop in the anulus fibrosus as a result of repeated minor trauma, and eventually, if the tears become large enough, a portion of the soft nucleus pulposus herniates through the anulus. Asymptomatic herniation may occur into the center of the vertebral bodies bordering the disc (Schmorl's nodules). However, if the disc material herniates into the vertebral canal, it compresses nerve endings and nerve roots, causing pain and other symptoms. Generally, the disc herniates lateral to the posterior longitudinal ligament, thus compressing spinal roots as they enter the intervertebral foramen. Occasionally the disc herniates more centrally, compressing either the spinal cord in the cervical or thoracic area or the cauda equina in the lumbar area. The term herniated disc refers to a disc that maintains continuity with the nucleus pulposus; extruded disc refers to a fragment within the spinal canal that has lost continuity with the disc itself. The signs and symptoms of herniated discs are caused by compression of either nerve roots or the spinal cord. The specific signs and symptoms depend in part on whether the predominant compression is spinal cord or nerve root, and in part on the level at which the neural structures are compressed (see Ch. 498). The most common sites of disc herniation are in the lumbar area, between L4 and L5 and between L5 and S1, compressing the L5 and S1 roots, respectively. L3–L4 herniations are less common. In the cervical area, the common herniations occur between C5 and C6 (C6 root) and, especially, C6 and C7 (C7 root). Less commonly, herniations appear between C3 and C4, C4 and C5, and C7 and T1. Thoracic discs are rare, but when they occur they usually compress the spinal cord as well as the emerging root because most of the thoracic vertebral canal is occupied by spinal cord. Although clinical localization in diagnosis of disc disease is usually quite accurate, at times an extruded disc fragment may be large enough to affect several roots, or may migrate from the disc space in which it herniated, to cause signs at a distance.

The most common symptom of a herniated disc is pain. Local pain is felt as a dull aching in the neck or back, with an associated stiffness of those structures, frequently occurring episodically in response to minor trauma (or no discernible trauma at all) months or years prior to the development of radicular pain. The exact pathogenesis of the local pain in disc disease is not known, but some believe that it results from compression of the sinuvertebral nerve, a recurrent branch of the nerve root that supplies the dura mater. Radicular pain may occasionally be the first sign of disc disease, but is far more likely to follow repeated bouts of local pain. Radicular pain is generally sudden in onset, often following minor trauma such as a twist, turn, or unusual bend. Radicular pain is perceived as sharp and well localized, and may radiate from the back along the entire distribution of the involved root or affect only a portion of the root. Both local and radicular pain have the characteristics of being exacerbated by activity and relieved by rest.

With cervical disc herniation, most patients hold their necks stiffly and resist passive movement. Lateral bending either to or away from the side of the herniated disc frequently exacerbates both the local and radicular pain. The patient may be more comfortable with his neck slightly flexed but is usually comfortable only in the recumbent position. Patients with lumbar disc disease are most comfortable lying, most uncomfortable sitting, and a little less uncomfortable standing. The back is held stiffly, so that the normal lumbar lordotic curve is no longer apparent, and pain is usually exacerbated by extension of the back. Slow forward bending sometimes relieves the pain. Muscle spasm is prominent with both cervical and lumbar disc disease. Raising the intraspinal pressure, as by coughing, sneezing, or straining, increases the pain sharply. Stretching the compressed root also aggravates the pain. In the upper extremities, extending the arm and laterally flexing the neck away from the extended arm often reproduces radicular pain. In the lower extremities, raising the extended leg with the patient in the recumbent position frequently reproduces the pain of an L5 or S1 radiculopathy and, if the pain is felt on the opposite side as well (crossed straight leg raising), the sign is very suggestive of herniated disc disease. Symptoms of L4 radiculopathy can often be reproduced by extending the hip (stretching the femoral nerve) when the patient is lying in the prone position. Often tenderness is present along the entire distribution of the nerve(s) supplied by the compressed root as well as in the

muscles supplied by the root. In patients with cervical disc disease, palpation or light percussion of the brachial plexus and the supraclavicular fossa or axilla often causes pain. In patients with lumbar disc disease, palpation over the femoral nerve (L4) in the groin or over the sciatic nerve (L5–S1) in the calf, thigh, or buttocks often causes severe pain. Occasionally tenderness in the calf (the posterior tibial nerve) is so striking as to suggest that the patient is suffering from thrombophlebitis rather than disc herniation. Other neurologic signs that commonly accompany disc disease include paresthesias and sensory loss in the distribution of the involved root and motor weakness in the myotome supplied by that root. The most important single sign is a diminished or absent reflex, giving objectively verifiable evidence of neurologic disease.

If an intervertebral disc herniates medially rather than laterally, it may spare the root and involve the spinal cord directly. When this occurs, there may be little or no pain or pain in a bilateral radicular distribution. Sometimes the pain is felt at a site far distant from the disc herniation as a result of compression of long sensory tracts in the spinal cord (funicular pain). The signs and symptoms of cord involvement are the same as those of compression of the spinal cord by other mass lesions. In contradistinction to diseases that arise within the spinal cord themselves, compressive lesions tend to spare bladder and bowel function until late. (The exception is when the compression occurs either at the conus medullaris or in the cauda equina.)

The diagnosis of herniated disc is deduced from the characteristic clinical symptoms and findings. In many patients with radiculopathy, findings are minimal and the history must establish the diagnosis. When the patient complains of back pain, with or without a radicular component, but has no motor, sensory, or reflex changes to suggest the site of a radiculopathy, the differential diagnosis includes pain arising from pain-sensitive nerve endings in the muscles, ligaments, and joints of the vertebral bodies and the paravertebral structures. These structures must be examined carefully to determine which of them is responsible. A high-resolution CT scan often establishes the diagnosis. MRI is also helpful.

There is controversy about the management of herniated discs. Most physicians believe that the first step is bed rest. Some investigators have reported that adrenocorticosteroids, either taken orally or injected into the epidural space, may hasten resolution of pain and other symptoms. No controlled studies support this recommendation. Steroids injected into the epidural or subarachnoid space are contraindicated and may produce severe inflammatory reactions. Surgery is indicated when (1) bed rest fails, and the patient is incapacitated by severe, intractable pain; (2) a centrally placed lumbar disc compresses the cauda equina, producing urinary dysfunction; (3) motor weakness (e.g., foot drop) is severe and gets worse on bed rest; or (4) acute cervical or thoracic discs cause substantial myelopathy. Myelography may be performed before surgical extirpation to localize the site of disc herniation and to determine whether other disc lesions or tumors are present as well, but in many cases the CT scan or MRI suffices. The best operation removes the involved disc, leaving as much bone as possible intact. Fusion of the lumbar spine is rarely necessary. Lumbar disc operations are done posteriorly via a laminotomy. Cervical disc operations may be done either posteriorly to decompress the cord or anteriorly across the neck to remove the disc without disturbing posterior bony elements. The surgical approach for myelopathy should probably be anterior if the disc is in the cervical area and lateral if the disc is in the thoracic area.

Disc dissolution by the injection of the enzyme chymopapain directly into a lumbar disc space has received enthusiastic support from some centers and, in the best hands, appears as effective as surgery. Occasional, serious anaphylactic reactions can occur and the procedure's role remains uncertain.

SPONDYLOSIS. Spondylosis is a term applied to chronic

degenerative disease of intervertebral discs associated with reactive changes in the adjacent vertebral bodies. Spondylotic changes in the neck and low back increase with age and are almost invariably present in the elderly. Spondylosis is usually asymptomatic except when the reactive tissue compresses a nerve root or the spinal cord. When this occurs, the signs and symptoms are similar to those of herniated disc disease, but the onset is less abrupt and the treatment often more difficult. In both the cervical and lumbar areas, spondylosis is more likely to produce spinal cord or cauda equina symptoms if the sagittal diameter of the spinal canal is congenitally narrow.

Cervical Spondylosis. Most patients suffer either radiculopathy or myelopathy, but not both. Pain is common but usually less acute and severe than with herniated discs. Even muscle spasm may be absent. However, the vertebral degenerative changes in the neck lead to limitation of movement in all directions. The classic picture of cervical spondylotic myelopathy is one of little or no pain but slowly developing weakness, atrophy, and fasciculations in the upper extremities, particularly the small muscles of the hand, accompanied by spastic paraparesis with decreased proprioception in the legs. At first the findings may suggest a diagnosis of amyotrophic lateral sclerosis. However, in cervical spondylosis there are sensory changes, particularly vibration loss in the lower extremities, and in amyotrophic lateral sclerosis fasciculations extend to innervated areas beyond the cervical level. The differential diagnosis also includes other compressive lesions of root and spinal cord as well as chronic multiple sclerosis.

Plain films of the cervical spine confirm the presence of cervical spondylosis, but many patients without symptoms have similar x-ray findings. Evidence that spondylosis is symptomatic is found by measuring the sagittal diameter of the cervical canal. When the diameter is less than 10 mm, cord compression is almost a certainty. If the diameter is over 13 mm, it is unlikely that cord compression is occurring, but a soft disc or tumor not seen on the x-ray may be impinging on the cord. CT or MR will delineate accurately the size of the cervical canal, and myelography determines the site of the lesion and the degree of obstruction.

The natural history of cervical myelopathy and radiculopathy is not well established. Many patients experience long periods of pain relief and remission or stabilization of neurologic symptoms, making it difficult to evaluate the effect of a particular treatment. Many physicians prefer, once having established the diagnosis, to begin with conservative treatment with a brief (7 to 10 days) period of bed rest accompanied by cervical traction and stabilization of the neck with a soft collar. If these latter approaches are successful, they should be continued. However, if the patient develops progressive neurologic signs in the face of conservative treatment, surgical therapy is indicated. Most neurosurgeons believe that if the spinal cord compression occurs at one or two segments, anterior removal of the disc material with spinal fusion is the preferred course. If more than a few segments are involved, laminectomy with foraminotomy is preferred.

In some patients with cervical spondylosis (or with congenital narrowing of the cervical spinal canal, or both), neurologic symptoms are exacerbated by exercise, with pain, numbness, and weakness appearing when a particular extremity is exercised. The pathogenesis is thought to be compression of the spinal cord so severe that the blood supply to the area cannot increase during its activity, leading to ischemia of cord and root structures (pseudoclaudication).

LUMBAR SPONDYLOSIS. Most of the considerations described above apply. The symptoms of lumbar spondylosis are similar to those of herniated disc, often occurring at multiple levels. One outstanding difference is the frequent presence of *pseudoclaudication* from cauda equina compression in patients with spinal stenosis due to either spondylosis or

congenital narrowing. Typically, symptoms and signs are evoked or accentuated by walking, and include pain, paresthesias, and weakness in the lower extremities. All of the symptoms may disappear when the patient ceases walking, even though he remains in the standing position. At times, however, the symptoms may be exacerbated by prolonged standing and relieved only by sitting or lying down. Pseudoclaudication of the cauda equina may be distinguished from intermittent vascular claudication in several ways: in vascular disease, the pulses in the lower extremities are usually absent or become absent as exercise begins. Also, the symptoms are usually reproducible and stereotypic, i.e., the patient can predict the exact distance he can walk at a given speed before symptoms develop. Symptoms of cauda equina pseudoclaudication are less stereotypic, so that on some days patients can walk much longer distances than on others. The reason for this variability is not known. In patients with pseudoclaudication, the lumbar canal is narrowed on either lateral radiographs or CT scan, and there is a substantial block to the passage of myelographic dye. With severe lumbar stenosis, conservative treatment usually fails, and decompressive laminectomy is the treatment of choice.

500 NEOPLASMS OF THE SPINAL CANAL

Neoplastic growths that cause nerve root or spinal cord compression can be paravertebral, extradural, intradural, or intramedullary (Fig. 500–1). Most of those causing spinal cord compression are extradural and metastatic. Most extradural neoplasms originate in the vertebral body surrounding the spinal cord and compress spinal roots or cord without invading them. Most intradural neoplasms also cause symptoms by compressing spinal roots or cord without invading, but unlike extradural neoplasms the majority are benign and slow growing. Intramedullary neoplasms cause symptoms both by invading and by compressing spinal structures; the tumors may be either benign or malignant.

PARAVERTEBRAL TUMORS. Neoplastic lesions that begin in or metastasize to the paravertebral space often cause serious and perplexing neurologic problems. The tumor may extend longitudinally within the paravertebral space, progressively compressing or invading nerve roots. At times, such tumors grow through an intervertebral foramen and compress not only the nerve root but also the spinal cord. Rarely, spinal cord symptoms may be caused by paravertebral tumors compromising radicular arteries that supply the spinal cord. If the tumor is more lateral than the immediate paravertebral space, the brachial, lumbar, or sacral plexus may be compressed, causing symptoms similar to root compression but with a different pattern of sensory and motor loss. The symptoms of extravertebral tumor begin insidiously with severe, unremitting pain, often with a burning quality and usually localized just lateral to the spine, radiating in a band-like pattern in the distribution of the involved dermatome(s). If the lesion involves abdominal or thoracic roots, motor and sensory changes are usually not appreciated by either the patient or the examiner. Autonomic changes may be a prominent or the only neurologic sign. Hyperhidrosis occurring in a band coinciding with the site of the pain strongly suggests the diagnosis. When the tumor involves cervical or lumbar roots, the pain may be soon followed by numbness in fingertips or toes, with accompanying weakness and reflex diminution, depending on the roots involved. Autonomic changes, including anhidrosis or hyperhidrosis, may affect the arm or leg. Horner's syndrome and/or diaphragmatic paralysis often

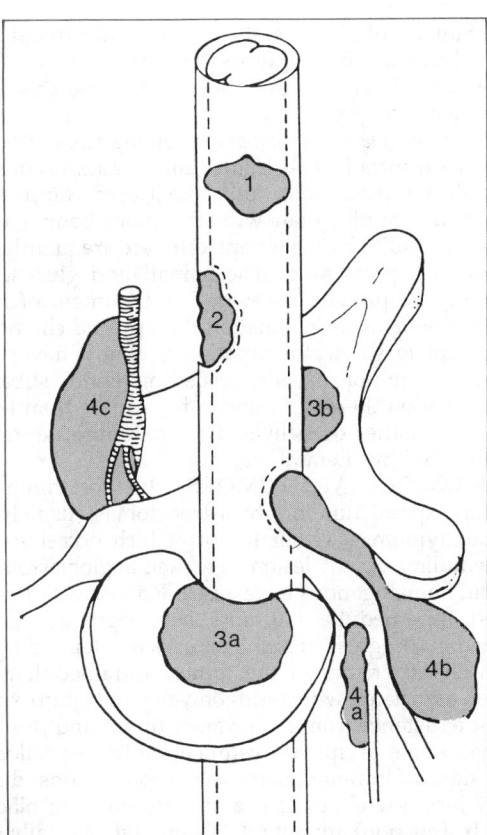

FIGURE 500–1. Pathophysiology of myelopathy caused by neoplasms. 1, The tumor may arise in or metastasize hematogenously to the substance of the spinal cord (intramedullary). 2, The tumor may be extraparenchymal but intradural. 3, The tumor may be extradural, extending either from the vertebral body (3a) or from a spinous process (3b), and cause symptoms by compressing the spinal cord. 4, The tumor may originate in or spread to the paravertebral space and produce its symptoms either by (4a) invading nerve roots, (4b) invading the epidural or subdural space through the intravertebral foramen, or (4c) compressing radicular arteries to cause spinal cord ischemia. (From Andreoli TE, Carpenter CCJ, Plum F, Smith LH Jr (eds.): Cecil Essentials of Medicine. Philadelphia, W. B. Saunders Company, 1986.)

accompany cervical or upper thoracic paravertebral tumors. The diagnosis is best established by CT or MR scan at the level suggested by the clinical findings. The scans can also determine whether the lesion has grown through the intervertebral foramen or has eroded vertebral bodies.

The differential diagnosis of paravertebral tumor includes disorders that cause paravertebral pain with or without compression of nerve roots. *Myofascial pain syndromes* cause low back or neck paravertebral pain with referred pain into arms or legs. On examination there is often marked tenderness of muscles and, sometimes, trigger points identified by either their hardness to palpation or their ability to reproduce symptoms when compressed. Relief of pain in these instances can be produced by injecting the trigger point with saline solution or a local anesthetic. Temporary relief of pain after such injection does not imply that structural disease is absent; the trigger points may be a reaction to spinal or nerve root disease. In myofascial syndromes, autonomic, sensory, or motor changes are never present. Disease of kidneys and other viscera lying in the retroperitoneal space may cause pain similar to that of paravertebral tumors, but the pain usually does not radiate and is not associated with autonomic, motor, or sensory changes. Percussion of the involved viscera reproduces the pain that is described as a dull ache rather than a neurogenic burning pain. Spontaneous or induced *entrapment neuropathies* not caused by tumor occasionally

mimic the symptoms of paravertebral tumor. Chronic pain after a thoracotomy (*post-thoracotomy pain*) probably results from entrapment of nerve roots at the time of surgery, perhaps with neuroma formation. The pain characteristically appears shortly after surgery and may be unremitting for many years. Motor, sensory, or autonomic changes are rare. The pain can sometimes be relieved by paravertebral anesthetic blocks.

The management of paravertebral masses depends on the diagnosis. In patients known to have cancer, particularly lymphomas or carcinomas of the breast or lung, the tumor can be assumed to be metastatic and should be treated with radiation therapy and, if available, chemotherapy. If the patient has no history of cancer, a biopsy is required and, depending on the site of the lesion, resection may be attempted both to establish a diagnosis and to decompress the nerve roots. Once the diagnosis is established by biopsy, further therapy such as radiation or chemotherapy may be indicated.

EXTRADURAL TUMORS. Extradural neoplasms compress spinal roots and cord in one of three ways. Either they arise in vertebrae surrounding the spinal cord and grow into the epidural space or they arise in the paravertebral space and grow through the intervertebral foramen to compress the cord laterally. Rarely, tumors may arise in the epidural space itself, without involving either vertebral or paravertebral structures. Most extradural neoplasms are metastatic (e.g., carcinomas of the breast, lung, prostate, or kidney). Some extradural neoplasms arise de novo in the vertebral bodies (e.g., chordoma, osteogenic sarcoma, myeloma, chondrosarcoma). A minority of extradural neoplasms are benign (e.g., osteoma, osteoid osteoma, angioma). Because extradural neoplasms usually destroy bone before producing spinal cord compression, local pain is the first symptom and may precede either radicular pain or other symptoms of spinal cord compression by weeks or months, depending on the rate of growth of the tumor. Rarely, extradural neoplasms may be painless and the first symptoms may be spinal cord dysfunction. As with other causes of spinal cord compression, extradural neoplasms cause symptoms first distally and later proximally. Thus, even thoracic and cervical neoplasms generally cause weakness and numbness in the legs before trunk and upper extremity muscles are involved. The diagnosis of extradural spinal cord compression must be suspected by the history of pain followed by signs and symptoms of spinal cord dysfunction and confirmed by radiographic study. In about 85 per cent of patients suffering from extradural spinal cord compression, there are bone lesions at the site of compression on plain radiographs. In a few patients with negative plain radiographs, radionuclide bone scan, CT or MR scan may demonstrate a bone lesion. The diagnosis of extradural spinal cord compression and its localization require myelography. A myelogram not only establishes the site of cord compression but also determines that the compression is extradural rather than intradural or intramedullary. The differential diagnosis of extradural neoplasms includes inflammatory disease of bone and epidural abscess (e.g., vertebral tuberculosis, bacterial osteomyelitis), acute or subacute epidural hematomas, herniated intervertebral discs, spondylosis, and, very rarely, extramedullary hematopoiesis (in patients with severe and chronic anemias) or epidural lipomatosis (in patients on chronic steroid therapy). Often definitive diagnosis can be made only by biopsy of the lesion either via decompressive laminectomy or by percutaneous needle biopsy.

The treatment of extradural neoplasms depends on the cause. Most neoplasms that cause extradural spinal cord compression are malignant and progress rapidly. Once spinal cord symptoms begin, paraplegia may develop in a matter of hours to days. Complete paraplegia is usually irreversible, whereas patients with mild to moderate spinal cord signs often can maintain or regain neurologic function. Thus, the early diagnosis and vigorous emergency treatment of extradural spinal cord compression is mandatory. The treatment of patients known to be suffering from cancer who develop signs and symptoms of spinal cord compression from extradural metastases is radiation therapy. Therapy should begin with corticosteroids (dexamethasone, 16 to 100 mg daily) to decrease spinal cord edema, followed immediately by radiation therapy. If effective chemotherapeutic agents are available, they should be used in conjunction with steroids and radiation therapy for the treatment of metastatic or primary malignant tumors of the extradural space. In patients not known to be suffering from a primary cancer, metastatic disease is the most common cause of extradural spinal cord compression, but in these instances a definitive diagnosis must be made by biopsy. Such patients should begin corticosteroid therapy followed by surgery with removal of as much tumor as possible for both diagnostic and therapeutic purposes. If a malignant neoplasm is encountered at operation, radiation therapy should be begun as soon after the surgery as is practical. In a few patients in whom radiation therapy and chemotherapy are ineffective, resection of the vertebral body involved by tumor may delay the development of paraplegia. In some patients with extradural tumors and destruction of the vertebral body, subluxation may compress the cord and may be relieved by surgery. Benign extradural tumors require surgery.

INTRADURAL EXTRAMEDULLARY TUMORS. Most intradural tumors are benign. Meningiomas and neurofibromas are the two most common types. Teratomas, arachnoid cysts, and lipomas are less common. *Meningioma* occurs in middle-aged and elderly women, predominantly in the thoracic region of the spinal cord. Another common site is at the foramen magnum. Meningiomas are benign, slow growing, and usually located on the posterior aspect of the spinal cord. Pain is the first symptom in the majority of patients, but in about 25 per cent the meningioma is painless, the first symptoms being those of spinal cord compression. Because they are often located on the posterior aspect of the cord, paresthesias and sensory changes beginning distally in the lower extremities are a frequent early symptom and are often mistaken for peripheral neuropathy. As the disease progresses, however, corticospinal tract signs betray the spinal origin. Even when spinal cord signs and symptoms are obvious, the lack of pain may lead one to suspect a degenerative or demyelinating disease such as multiple sclerosis rather than a neoplasm. In patients with meningiomas, the lumbar puncture reveals a spinal fluid protein content higher than that in degenerative or demyelinating disease. Myelography usually establishes the diagnosis of a tumor. Tumors located posteriorly, if small or near the foramen magnum, may be difficult to identify on the usual prone myelogram. A CT scan performed shortly after the myelogram, while the water-soluble contrast material is still visible, often delineates the lesions. The treatment of spinal cord compression from meningiomas is surgical removal. Because the tumor grows so slowly and the cord has an opportunity to adapt to compression, even patients with severe neurologic disability often make a full recovery after the lesion is removed.

The second common cause of intradural spinal cord compression is *neurofibroma*. Because these tumors usually arise from the dorsal root, radicular pain is often the first symptom, preceding signs of spinal cord compression by months or years. When spinal cord compression develops, it progresses slowly. Some patients with spinal neurofibroma suffer from neurofibromatosis. That diagnosis may be suspected either by a positive family history or by the cutaneous stigmata of the disease. A neurofibroma may extend on either side of the intervertebral foramen, involving the root both in the paravertebral space and within the spinal canal. As neurofibromas grow through the intervertebral foramen, they enlarge it, a finding appreciated by an appropriately posi-

tioned radiograph. The cerebrospinal fluid protein is almost always elevated. The diagnosis is established by CT, MRI or myelography. Surgical extirpation of the lesion usually leads to complete recovery.

Occasionally *metastatic tumors* involving the leptomeninges present with intradural extramedullary mass lesions. Pain is almost always prominent, and spinal cord compression develops more rapidly than with the more benign intradural tumors. In addition, malignant cells are frequently encountered in the spinal fluid. The spinal fluid glucose may be decreased, the protein elevated. The treatment of intradural malignant neoplasms is radiation therapy and chemotherapy, since complete surgical extirpation is almost never possible. Because the tumor usually seeds the entire subarachnoid space, radiation therapy, if it is to have more than temporary effect, must either be delivered to the entire neuraxis or be supplemented by chemotherapy.

INTRAMEDULLARY TUMORS. The most common intramedullary spinal tumors are astrocytomas (usually benign) and ependymomas. Other tumors which occasionally cause intramedullary spinal lesions are hemangioblastomas, lipomas, and hematogenous metastases. Pain is an early symptom of most intramedullary tumors, and signs of spinal cord dysfunction progress rapidly or slowly, depending on the growth characteristics of the tumor. Intramedullary tumors are often associated with syringomyelia, the syrinx sometimes being at a distance from the primary tumor and producing its own symptoms of spinal dysfunction. The so-called characteristic signs of intramedullary spinal cord lesions (dissociated sensory loss, sacral sparing, and early onset of bladder and bowel dysfunction) are not reliable enough clinically to distinguish intramedullary from extramedullary lesions; that diagnosis is established by CT, MR, or myelography. In some patients with longstanding benign intramedullary lesions, plain radiographs of the spine may show widening of the spinal canal and erosion of the pedicles. Myelography reveals an enlarged spinal cord, sometimes with complete block to the passage of myelographic contrast material. If a syrinx is suspected, a CT scan performed six hours after myelography with water-soluble contrast material usually reveals contrast material in the syrinx. MR scans often identify both tumor and syrinx, obviating the need for other studies. The differential diagnosis of intramedullary tumors includes intramedullary abscesses and syringomyelia without tumor. A definitive diagnosis is established by biopsy. Successful surgical removal of intramedullary tumors is possible, particularly with ependymomas and hemangioblastomas but sometimes with gliomas as well. Highly skilled and experienced surgeons are necessary for tumors to be removed without increasing neurologic symptoms. If the tumor cannot be totally excised, postoperative radiation therapy often delays recurrence.

Ependymomas have a predilection to involve the lower end of the spinal cord and the filum terminale. An unusual symptom sometimes produced by such tumors is hydrocephalus with headache, papilledema, and enlarged cerebral ventricles. The pathogenesis of the hydrocephalus is believed to be the plugging of pacchionian granulations by protein exuded from the tumor into the spinal fluid. CT or MRI of the head are negative; myelography establishes the diagnosis.

501 INFLAMMATORY DISEASES OF THE SPINAL CANAL

Inflammatory diseases that compress nerve roots and spinal cord can be extradural, intradural, or intramedullary. Extradural inflammatory lesions include vertebral tuberculosis or bacterial osteomyelitis with extradural extension and primary extradural bacterial abscesses. These entities are discussed in Ch. 481. Intradural but extramedullary inflammatory diseases include bacterial, fungal, and parasitic meningitis, inflammatory disease of the leptomeninges of unknown cause such as sarcoidosis or Behçet's syndrome, and reactions to foreign substances such as myelographic contrast material, spinal anesthetics, or steroids. Occasionally, leptomeningeal infiltration with tumor or subarachnoid hemorrhage causes an inflammatory response of the leptomeninges that mimics subacute or chronic infection. All of these inflammatory intradural lesions can lead to spinal arachnoiditis. *Spinal arachnoiditis* is characterized by neck and back pain and by radicular pain in the distribution of the roots involved in the inflammatory process. Dysfunction of multiple roots, particularly in the lumbosacral area, is common; occasional patients go on to develop signs of spinal cord dysfunction, which may progress to paraplegia. The diagnosis of spinal arachnoiditis is established by myelography. A myelogram reveals spotty and irregular collections of contrast material with impairment of the flow through the subarachnoid space. Sometimes there is a complete block to the passage of the myelographic contrast material. The spinal fluid may contain an increased cellular response and a decreased glucose concentration. The protein concentration is usually elevated. Sometimes a specific infectious organism can be identified either by microscopic examination or by culture. There is no therapy for spinal arachnoiditis unless a specific treatment-sensitive infective agent is identified.

Intramedullary infectious processes include bacterial and parasitic abscesses and acute transverse myelitis. These entities are discussed under the appropriate chapter headings.

502 VASCULAR DISORDERS OF THE SPINAL CANAL

Extradural, intradural, and intramedullary vascular disorders all can cause spinal cord compression. The most common and serious extradural vascular disease is *spinal epidural hematoma.* Hemorrhage into the spinal epidural space may occur spontaneously or be associated with trauma, a bleeding diathesis, or a vascular malformation. It is particularly common in patients being treated with anticoagulants. It may occasionally follow lumbar puncture, particularly in patients with bleeding abnormalities. Hemorrhage usually arises from the epidural venous plexus and tends to collect over the dorsum of the spinal cord covering several segments. The clinical picture is characterized by the sudden onset of severe localized back pain and the rapid development of spinal cord dysfunction, often leading to complete paraplegia in several hours. If the patient has a known bleeding disorder, the clinical diagnosis is easily established. In patients without known bleeding or clotting disorders, the differential diagnosis includes acute epidural abscess and acute transverse myelopathy. Although occasional patients recover from paraparesis related to epidural spinal cord compression spontaneously, the majority require emergency surgical evacuation if neurologic function is to be preserved. The more rapidly the paralysis develops and the longer the delay in decompression, the less likely is the patient to recover.

Intradural but extramedullary vascular lesions are usually caused by hemorrhage from *vascular malformations* on the surface of the spinal cord. Spinal subarachnoid hemorrhage is characterized by the sudden onset of back pain, often with a radicular component with or without the development of signs of spinal cord compression. Lumbar puncture reveals evidence of subarachnoid hemorrhage with red cells, xanthochromic spinal fluid, and usually an elevated protein concentration. In the absence of spinal cord signs, the differential diagnosis includes spontaneous intracerebral subarachnoid hemorrhage. Arteriovenous anomalies of the subarachnoid space and spinal cord can often be identified on supine myelography by the characteristic wormlike appearance of the surface of the spinal cord.

Vascular malformations also may lie within the substance of the spinal cord where they can give rise to intramedullary hemorrhage (hematomyelia) as well as subarachnoid hemorrhage. The sudden development of partial or complete transverse myelopathy is the most common onset. If blood leaks into the subarachnoid space, pain in the neck and back and other signs of meningeal irritation occur.

Arteriovenous malformations may also compress the spinal cord or give rise to hemodynamic changes that result in spinal ischemia. In such cases, distortion and compression of the cord by enlarged, abnormal vessels occur only gradually, producing slowly progressive symptoms of spinal cord dysfunction. Exacerbation of symptoms may accompany menstrual periods or pregnancy.

Complete or partial recovery of function can follow episodes of spinal cord ischemia or even small hemorrhages. The unchanging localization of the attacks and the prominence of pain help differentiate arteriovenous malformations from other recurrent neurologic disorders such as multiple sclerosis. Rarely, a bruit may be heard by auscultation over the site of the malformation, or injection of intravenous contrast agent for CT can induce spinal flexor spasms (presumably by accentuating vascular engorgement).

Angiography with regional catheterization of radicular vessels is necessary to establish the diagnosis of spinal vascular malformations and as a preliminary step to surgical treatment. Advances in microsurgery have increased the chances for satisfactory removal of these lesions. Embolization of the malformation or ligation of feeding arteries has been performed when the abnormality cannot be removed surgically.

503 CONGENITAL ANOMALIES OF THE CRANIOVERTEBRAL JUNCTION, SPINE, AND SPINAL CORD

Congenital anomalies of the spine are common and are often encountered on radiographs of patients suffering from neck or low back pain. Some congenital anomalies such as *spina bifida occulta* can be considered variants of normal and are probably never responsible in and of themselves for low back pain. Others such as the *Klippel-Feil syndrome* (congenital fusion of two or more cervical vertebrae) are not responsible for neck pain or other neurologic symptoms except when associated with coexisting congenital anomalies of the central nervous system. Congenital abnormalities of the spine that are common and usually asymptomatic but that must be considered potential causes of neck or back pain include *facet tropism* (misalignment of the facets on the two sides of the corresponding vertebral body; several authorities believe that this increases rotational stress on the facet joints and may cause back pain); *transitional vertebrae,* such as in sacralization to a lumbar vertebra or lumbarization of a sacral vertebra (these alter spinal mechanics and result in instability and stress, sometimes producing back pain); and *spondylolisthesis* (forward slipping of one vertebral body onto another caused by a defect between the articular facets). A third group of congenital anomalies of the spine consists of those that are likely to cause not only neck or back pain but also neurologic disability. These include *basilar impression*, which is often associated with *Arnold-Chiari malformation* (see later discussion). Severe spinal *scoliosis* or *kyphosis*, congenital *stenosis* of the lumbar or cervical spinal canal, anterior and lateral spinal *meningoceles*, and *diastematomyelia* are other causes of back pain and neurologic disability. Diastematomyelia is a bony abnormality that divides the spinal canal, leading to duplication of the spinal cord. It is usually associated with evidence of spina bifida on plain radiographs, and sometimes the bony septum can be identified as well. Patients who become symptomatic in adulthood almost always have some cutaneous abnormality, especially hypertrichosis over the sacral area. The disorder may be associated with other congenital abnormalities of the central nervous system as well.

ARNOLD-CHIARI MALFORMATION

INFANTILE FORM. The Arnold-Chiari malformation is characterized by downward displacement of the cerebellum through the foramen magnum of the skull and by similar caudal elongation of the medulla. The infantile form is commonly associated with other midline defects such as spina bifida and meningocele, hydrocephalus caused by aqueductal or fourth ventricular obstruction, and other congenital malformations of the brain and cord. The infantile form of the Arnold-Chiari malformation usually occurs because of hydrocephalus in the early months of life, with evidence of spina bifida or frank paraparesis resulting from meningomyelocele. Therapy is directed toward surgical relief of the hydrocephalus with a ventricular shunting procedure and repair of the meningomyelocele. Prognosis is poor for patients with extensive defects.

ADULT FORM. The malformation may be asymptomatic until adult life, when the patient gradually develops symptoms and signs of dysfunction of the cerebellum, lower cranial nerves, pyramidal tracts, and posterior columns. Posterior cranial displacement may occur with coughing or straining. Downbeat nystagmus is characteristic. At times the initial signs may be those of hydrocephalus secondary to obstruction of the cerebrospinal fluid pathways or to coexisting syringomyelia of the cervical spinal cord and medulla (Ch. 476). Commonly there is x-ray evidence of fusion of the cervical vertebrae, platybasia, or basilar impression, but MR scan establishes the diagnosis even when there are no coexisting bony abnormalities. The Arnold-Chiari malformation in adults may simulate syndromes produced by tumors near the fora-

men magnum or by multiple sclerosis. Surgical enlargement of the foramen magnum and decompression of the cervico-medullary junction benefit selected cases.

BASILAR IMPRESSION AND PLATYBASIA

Basilar impression refers to abnormal invagination of the cervical spine into the base of the posterior fossa of the skull. The diagnosis is made from lateral roentgenograms of the skull when there is excessive protrusion of the tip of the odontoid process of the axis above Chamberlain's line, i.e., a line drawn from the back of the hard palate to the posterior margin of the foramen magnum. Other radiologic criteria are also useful. *Platybasia* refers to flattening of the base of the skull, wherein lateral roentgenograms of the skull reveal flattening of the angle between the orbital plates of the anterior fossa and the clivus, the sloping anterior floor of the posterior fossa. The abnormality by itself has no clinical significance.

These malformations are usually developmental in origin, and there may be hereditary transmission. Occasionally, basilar impression may result from metabolic bone diseases such as rickets, osteitis deformans, osteomalacia, osteogenesis imperfecta, or fibrous dysplasia. Minor degrees of deformity of the base of the skull give rise to no symptoms. The neck appears shortened, and its movements may be limited. With more severe invagination, there may be signs of impaired function of the cerebellum, lower cranial nerves, pyramidal tracts, and posterior columns. Syringomyelia and syringobulbia may be present. Increased intracranial pressure may develop owing to obstruction of the foramina of the fourth ventricle and the basal cisterns. The clinical manifestations must be differentiated from those caused by neoplasms in the region of the foramen magnum and multiple sclerosis. When neurologic signs are progressive, surgical decompression of the posterior fossa and upper cervical cord may be indicated.

Aminoff MJ: Spinal Angiomas. Oxford, Blackwell Scientific Publications, 1976. *A comprehensive text on spinal vascular anomalies.*

Austin GM (eds.): The Spinal Cord. 3rd ed. New York, Igaku-Shoin, 1983. *The third edition of a comprehensive, multi-authored monograph describing the clinical findings and management of many disorders of the spinal cord, including lumbar and cervical disc disease.*

Vinken PJ, Bruyn GW: Tumours of the spine and spinal cord, I & II. Handbook of Clinical Neurology, Vol. 19, 20. New York, American Elsevier Publishing Company, 1975, 1976. *Comprehensive descriptions of benign and malignant tumors and herniated discs.*

Vinken PJ, Bruyn GW: Congenital malformations of the spine and spinal cord. Handbook of Clinical Neurology, Vol. 32. New York, American Elsevier Publishing Company, 1978. *Comprehensive essays on congenital anomalies of the spine and spinal cord, including chapters on stenosis of the lumbar and cervical spinal canal and spondylodysplasia.*

SECTION SIXTEEN / DISEASES OF THE PERIPHERAL NERVOUS SYSTEM

Herbert H. Schaumburg

504 INTRODUCTION AND BASIC TERMINOLOGY

The structure and function of the peripheral nervous system (PNS) appear deceptively simple when compared with the central nervous system (CNS). Actually, however, PNS dis-

eases represent a potentially confusing jumble of conditions whose only common thread appears to be PNS dysfunction. Thus, while the anatomic diagnosis of peripheral neuropathy is readily established in nearly 100 per cent of cases by symptoms and signs, the correct cause is determined in less than one half of cases except in a few special centers. Recent clinical and experimental studies suggest a simple, anatomic classification of most PNS disorders suggesting that a working knowledge of the common peripheral neuropathies can be easily mastered. However, since common diseases (diabetes or malignancy) produce more than one type of anatomic reaction in the PNS and most physicians are "etiology oriented," this chapter is organized according to individual diseases, stressing their common anatomic and pathophysiologic features whenever possible.

Certain terms associated with peripheral nerve disease have, by common usage, acquired set connotations. These include:

Neuropathy (peripheral neuropathy). This is the usual term for any disorder of peripheral nerves and replaces the term *peripheral neuritis.*

Polyneuropathy (symmetrical polyneuropathy). This designates a generalized process resulting in widespread and symmetrical effects on the peripheral nervous system.

Focal or multifocal neuropathy (mononeuropathy, mononeuropathy multiplex). These terms indicate local involvement of one or more individual peripheral nerves.

Dysesthesia. This term, like paresthesia, is poorly defined; it is commonly used to describe an unpleasant sensation produced by an ordinarily painless stimulus.

Paresthesia. This term indicates a spontaneous aberrant sensation such as pins and needles or tingling.

Hypoesthesia. This term refers to diminished sensation.

Hyperesthesia. This condition is an excessive response to sensory stimulus, even when the sensory threshold is elevated.

Asbury AK, Johnson PC: Pathology of Peripheral Nerve. Philadelphia, W. B. Saunders Company, 1970. *A concise, clearly written book covering the salient aspects of peripheral neuropathy.*
Dyck PJ, Thomas PK, Asbury AK, et al.: Diabetic Neuropathy. Philadelphia, W. B. Saunders Company, 1986. *A new book covering all aspects of diabetic neuropathy.*
Dyck PJ, Thomas PK, Lambert EH, et al. (eds.): Peripheral Neuropathy. 2nd ed. Philadelphia, W. B. Saunders Company, 1984. *A multiauthored and authoritative reference on peripheral nerve disease.*
Kelley, JJ: Peripheral neuropathies associated with monoclonal proteins. A clinical review. Muscle Nerve 8:138, 1985. *A clear overview of this heterogeneous group of disorders.*
Moore PM, Cupps T: Neurological complications of vasculitis. Ann Neurol 14:155, 1983. *A comprehensive review of the protean neurologic complications of these disorders, especially the neuropathies.*
National Institutes of Health, Consensus Development Panel: The utility of therapeutic plasmapheresis for neurologic disorders. JAMA 256:1333, 1986. *A recent consensus report that thoughtfully analyzes the role of plasmapheresis in neuropathies and other neurologic conditions.*
Schaumburg HH, Spencer PS, Thomas PK: Disorders of Peripheral Nerves. Philadelphia, F. A. Davis Company, 1983. *A short lucidly written monograph providing a good introduction to this complex subject.*
Spencer PS, Schaumburg HH: Experimental and Clinical Neurotoxicology. Baltimore, Williams and Wilkins, 1980. *A multiauthored comprehensive text with special emphasis on the peripheral nervous system.*
Sunderland S: Nerve and Nerve Injuries. New York, Churchill Livingstone, Inc., 1978. *A monumental monograph on nerve injury: The standard reference.*

---

505 ANATOMIC CLASSIFICATION OF NEUROPATHY

SYMMETRICAL GENERALIZED NEUROPATHY (Polyneuropathy)

DISTAL AXONOPATHY (DYING-BACK NEUROPATHY). This is the most common morphologic reaction of the peripheral nervous system (PNS) to toxins and probably underlies many metabolic and hereditary neuropathies.

The pathologic features include initial degeneration of the distal ends of large and long axons; the myelin sheath breaks down concomitantly with axonal disintegration. Axonal degeneration appears to advance slowly proximally toward the nerve cell body. Schwann cells and their connective tissue tubes remain in distal nerves, facilitating appropriate peripheral regeneration (Fig. 505–1).

Many prominent clinical phenomena closely correlate with the morphologic profile. Gradual onset reflects chronic metabolic disease or prolonged intoxication, stocking-glove sensorimotor loss reflects distal axonal degeneration in long nerves (sciatic, ulnar), normal cerebrospinal fluid (CSP) protein reflects the sparing of proximal sited nerve roots, and slow recovery corresponds to the indolent rate of axonal repair.

MYELINOPATHY. The term myelinopathy, when applied to the PNS, refers to conditions in which the lesion primarily affects myelin or the myelinating (Schwann) cell. The Guillain-Barré syndrome is the only frequently encountered disease that primarily affects PNS myelin. It is likely that the demyelination of spinal roots and nerves in this disorder results from an immune-system-mediated attack on PNS myelin.

The cardinal pathologic features, depicted in Figure 505–2, include primary destruction of the myelin sheath with the axon usually left intact. Demyelination initially affects multiple

FIGURE 505–1. The cardinal features of a toxic distal axonopathy. The jagged lines (lightning bolts) indicate that the toxin is acting at multiple sites along motor and sensory axons in the PNS and CNS. Axon degeneration has moved proximally (dying-back) by the late stage. (From Schaumburg et al., with permission.)

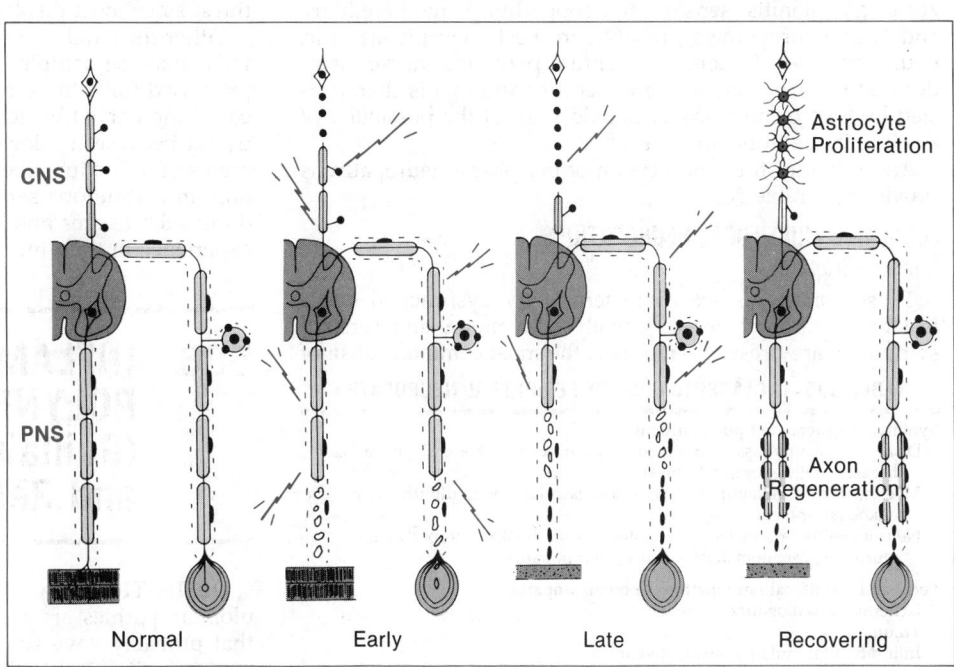

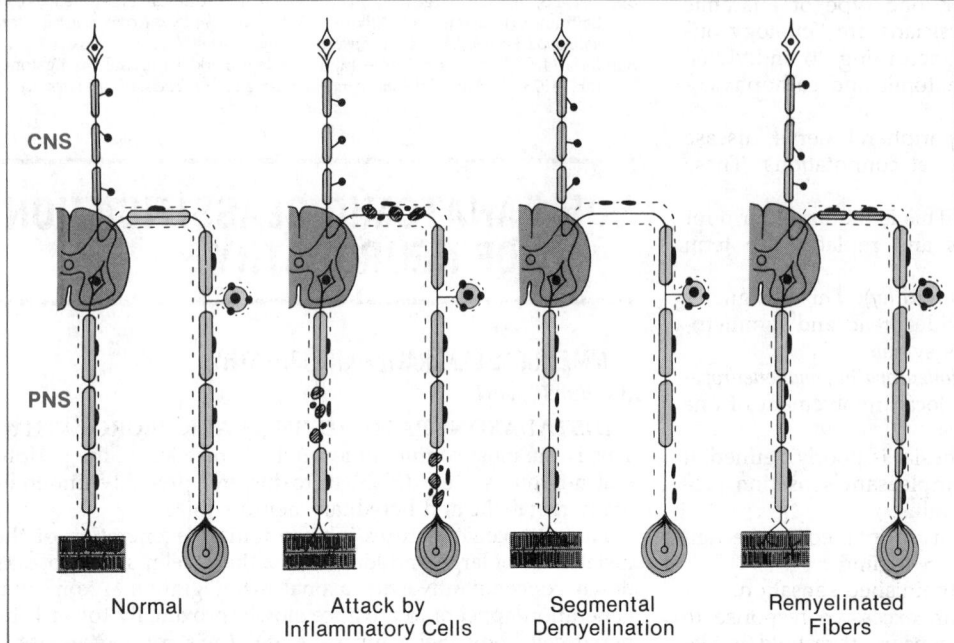

Normal | Attack by Inflammatory Cells | Segmental Demyelination | Remyelinated Fibers

CNS

PNS

FIGURE 505–2. The cardinal pathologic features of an inflammatory myelinopathy. Axons are spared as is CNS myelin. After the attack, the remaining Schwann cells divide and remyelinate the denuded segments of axons. (From Schaumburg et al., with permission.)

sites in nerves. The Schwann cell subsequently divides and rapidly remyelinates the axon to restore function.

Many prominent clinical findings correlate with the morphologic profile. Onset and recovery are rapid, reflecting the speed of demyelination and remyelination. Initial changes may be distal or proximal or may affect cranial nerves. Generalized weakness and reflex loss are dominant features, reflecting the vulnerability of long myelinated fibers, and the CSF protein is usually elevated because inflammation in spinal roots results in leakage of protein into the surrounding subarachnoid space.

NEURONOPATHY. This term describes conditions in which the initial morphologic or biochemical changes occur in the neuron cell body. If the changes are intense, the affected neuron dies and permanent total motor or sensory dysfunction in the affected segment follows. The neuronopathies are a heterogeneous, poorly understood group of conditions and include many disorders of motor, sensory, and autonomic neurons. Infectious neuronopathies include familiar conditions such as poliomyelitis (motor neuronopathy) and herpes zoster ganglionitis (sensory neuronopathy). Some hereditary and toxic neuropathies probably are best conceptualized as neuronopathies. In general, a diffuse peripheral nerve disorder that is exclusively motor or sensory and that is characterized by little or no recovery should suggest the possibility of a primarily neuronal disorder.

An outline of the classification of peripheral neuropathy is provided in Table 505–1.

FOCAL AND MULTIFOCAL NEUROPATHIES (Mononeuropathy)

These conditions are characterized by dysfunction of an isolated peripheral nerve. Usually both motor and sensory symptoms are present. Trauma is the most common cause of

TABLE 505–1. CLASSIFICATION OF PERIPHERAL NEUROPATHY

Symmetric generalized polyneuropathy
  Distal axonopathy (associated with drugs, industrial chemicals, metabolic
    diseases, deficiency syndromes)
  Myelinopathy (Guillain-Barré syndrome, associated with diphtheria, genetic
    leukodystrophies)
  Neuronopathy (associated with motor neuron diseases, herpes zoster
    neuronitis, carcinomatous sensory neuronopathy)

Focal and multifocal neuropathies (mononeuropathy)
  Ischemia (vasculopathy)
  Trauma
  Infiltration (granulomatous, malignancy)

monofocal neuropathy. Instances of nontraumatic focal neuropathies may pose formidable diagnostic problems and usually require extensive evaluation for the underlying cause (ischemia, infiltration by tumor, amyloid, leprosy, among others).

DIAGNOSIS. Nerve conduction studies performed by an expert in neuromuscular disease are the initial diagnostic procedures (Ch. 456). They are critical in determining the presence of neuropathy, whether suggested by clinical features or subclinical. Nerve conduction studies also establish the location of focal peripheral nerve lesions such as carpal tunnel or other entrapments. Also, they usually indicate whether a symmetrical polyneuropathy is axonal or demyelinating, a crucial first step in diagnosis.

Nerve biopsy is most useful in identifying the cause of multiple mononeuropathy syndromes (amyloidosis, sarcoidosis, leprosy, and vasculitis) and demyelinating neuropathies. Conditions readily diagnosed on clinical grounds, such as diabetic neuropathy and Guillain-Barré syndrome, do not require biopsy. Biopsy is seldom helpful in distal axonopathies, since most display similar nonspecific findings.

Either the sural nerve at the ankle or the radial nerve at the wrist may be sampled under anesthesia. Tissue should be processed for routine histopathologic study, electron microscopy, and nerve fiber teasing. The latter technique is especially useful because it allows the rapid examination of long segments of individual fibers. Nerve biopsy should be performed only in institutions served by a surgeon accustomed to handling such tissues and whose pathologists have considerable experience in their interpretation.

506 INFLAMMATORY POLYNEUROPATHY (Guillain-Barré Syndrome and Related Disorders)

DEFINITION. The inflammatory demyelinating polyradiculoneuropathies are a group of acute and chronic disorders that probably have similar pathologic bases but can differ in anatomic sites and temporal profile. The most common is the

Guillain-Barré syndrome (acute postinfectious polyneuropathy), a rapidly evolving paralytic illness of unknown origin. Its salient morphologic feature is widespread inflammatory peripheral nervous system (PNS) demyelination, presumably secondary to a hypersensitivity reaction. Other less common forms of inflammatory neuropathy include chronic inflammatory polyneuropathy (CIP), acute sensory neuropathy, and acute pandysautonomia. The Guillain-Barré syndrome is the most common acute paralytic illness in young adults and almost the only form of inflammatory polyneuropathy encountered in general medical practice.

PATHOLOGY, PATHOGENESIS, AND PREDISPOSING FACTORS. Inflammatory cell infiltration (lymphocytes and plasma cells) followed by segmental demyelination are the hallmarks of the Guillain-Barré syndrome. Axons are relatively spared and blood vessels are normal. These reactions are most pronounced in spinal roots, limb girdle plexuses, and proximal nerve trunks, but less intense changes are also present in distal nerves and autonomic ganglia. There is virtually no inflammatory change in the central nervous system (CNS). Within two to three weeks of the onset of acute demyelination Schwann cell proliferation occurs as a prelude to remyelination and recovery.

It is generally held that Guillain-Barré syndrome is an autoimmune disorder; however, its pathogenesis is unclear. There is evidence for both lymphocyte-mediated delayed hypersensitivity and for a humoral mechanism involving antibodies to peripheral nerve myelin.

Many predisposing events have been implicated in the Guillain-Barré syndrome, but a common antigen has not been identified, and HLA studies have not disclosed any predisposing pattern. Sixty per cent of cases have an antecedent upper respiratory infection or gastrointestinal illness within one month of onset; a host of common viral infections including infectious mononucleosis, hepatitis, and Epstein-Barr virus have been implicated. Other putative predisposing factors include vaccination against rabies and swine flu, surgery, pregnancy, and malignancy (especially lymphoma).

CLINICAL FEATURES. This is a worldwide illness and occurs throughout the year. It has a bimodal age distribution, with most cases in young adults and a lesser peak in incidence in the 45 to 64 age group.

The Guillain-Barré syndrome is a rapidly progressive, largely reversible, predominantly motor neuropathy. The cardinal clinical features are progressive and usually symmetrical weakness, combined with hyporeflexia. Weakness usually begins in the distal lower limbs and spreads upward (ascending paralysis); this pattern is not inevitable and patients may have weakness of the proximal upper limbs, face or even extraocular muscles. Most weakened individuals do not appear systemically ill, and constitutional signs such as fever, chills, and weight loss are unusual.

The degree of paralysis varies ranging from encompassing a mild footdrop to extreme weakness of all extremities and of the face. Severe involvement may lead to flaccid quadriplegia with inability to breathe, swallow, speak, or close the eyes. Limb weakness is generally symmetrical and early muscle atrophy mild. Tendon reflexes usually disappear.

The presence of facial weakness helps to distinguish the Guillain-Barré syndrome from most other neuropathies, apart from those related to sarcoidosis. Rarely, limb ataxia, paralysis of eye movements, and diffuse hyporeflexia may be the sole manifestations. Central nervous system involvement is not part of this illness. Increased intracranial pressure and papilledema rarely occur late.

Sensory symptoms, usually distal paresthesias, are present in most cases and rarely persist or progress (in contrast to the weakness). Mild impairment of distal position and vibration sensation and slight loss of pinprick sensation over the toes are common.

Autonomic dysfunction accompanies most cases. Relative tachycardia is universal. Orthostatic hypotension and hypertension are frequent, difficult to treat, and can complicate the management of patients with respiratory compromise. Death can occur suddenly following unexplained fluctuation in blood pressure or cardiac dysrhythmias.

Cerebrospinal fluid (CSF) and electrodiagnostic studies are helpful. The CSF protein concentration is usually normal during the first three days of illness; it then steadily rises and may exceed 500 mg per deciliter. The CSF protein level may remain elevated even after recovery is under way. Mononuclear cells, usually less than 10 per cubic millimeter, are present in up to one half of the cases.

Early in the illness, distal motor nerve conduction may be normal. Presumably, in such cases the disease process is confined to spinal roots and proximal nerves. If the demyelination affects distal nerves as well, slowing of motor conduction, characteristic of segmental demyelination, occurs. Analysis of the F response, a measurement of proximal motor conduction, can be useful in diagnosing patients who display normal distal motor conduction.

Differential diagnosis is not difficult, especially since the decline of poliomyelitis and diphtheria in North America. Hypokalemia, tick paralysis, botulism, acute myelitis, and cervical spine fracture should be ruled out rapidly.

COURSE AND PROGNOSIS. Rapid progression of weakness is characteristic of the Guillain-Barré syndrome. Paralysis is maximal by one week in more than half, by three weeks in 80 per cent, and by one month in 90 per cent. In the other patients, weakness may progress for variable intervals up to eight weeks.

Recovery usually begins two to four weeks after progression ceases. The pattern is variable, normally proceeding at a steady pace. Within six months 85 per cent of patients are ambulatory. Occasionally, individuals experience more rapid recovery and are able to return to work within two months following quadriparesis. Rare cases show little or no improvement.

Although most patients eventually recover, the illness is not benign. Five per cent will die and more than half suffer residual damage to the peripheral nervous system with one sixth remaining handicapped by weakness. Few initial features help in predicting the eventual outcome. In general, individuals who experience only mild distal extremity weakness and subsequently improve within weeks of the first signs do best.

TREATMENT. Early and accurate diagnosis is crucial since controlled trials indicate that plasmapheresis administered within the first two weeks significantly shortens the clinical course and reduces morbidity. A conservative regimen of 200 to 250 cc per kilogram is given in three exchanges within one week. Patients suspected of having the Guillain-Barré syndrome must be admitted to the hospital even if the involvement is minimal, since the neuropathy may evolve rapidly and unpredictably. In general, they should be admitted to a unit where respiratory care is available, to remain until their condition stabilizes or improves. The tidal volume, oxygen saturation, vital capacity, blood pressure, and ability to cough and swallow should be closely monitored, since they can change without warning.

If a need for mechanical ventilation is anticipated (as determined by the degree of respiratory effort, the vital capacity, and the blood gases), it should be instituted early without waiting for decompensation.

Autonomic dysfunction may produce pupillary disturbances, neuroendocrine disturbance, peripheral pooling of blood, poor venous return, cardiac arrhythmias, and low cardiac output. Beat to beat (R-R) variation of the heart rate during normal and deep breathing is a reliable index. Pharmacologic manipulation of blood pressure in Guillain-Barré syndrome patients is perilous and should be avoided unless absolutely necessary.

Some patients will be unable to swallow or to gag. Feeding should be done through a small nasogastric tube. The patient should be sitting when food is given and for 30 to 60 minutes thereafter to minimize the risk of aspiration.

If patients with the Guillain-Barré syndrome can be carried through the acute stage of progressive paralysis (usually two to three weeks), strength will gradually return. Since most patients achieve good recovery after months of weakness, the importance of fastidious supportive care in the acute stage cannot be overstressed. Glucocorticoids are contraindicated.

ACUTE INFLAMMATORY SENSORY POLYNEUROPATHY (Postinfectious Sensory Neuropathy or Neuronopathy)

This disorder is probably the counterpart of the motor polyradiculoneuropathy of Guillain-Barré. There are no histopathologic studies; it is suggested that inflammatory demyelination of the dorsal roots has also involved adjacent dorsal root ganglion cells. Thus this disease may be conceptualized as a combined myelinopathy-neuronopathy disorder to explain the rapid onset and poor recovery of many cases. An infection may antedate the neurologic syndrome by several weeks. Typically the onset is acute or subacute and marked by combinations of sensory dysfunction and pain. The sensory dysfunction is most commonly described as unsteadiness in gait or clumsiness in the use of the hands. Even more incapacitating are painful dysesthesias that develop in some patients. Varying combinations of lancinating pain, prickling hyperesthesia, constricting bandlike sensations, and burning or coldness of skin may be described. Any region of the body may be affected, and the disorder involves proximal as well as distal dermatomes. Lower limbs tend to be affected more than upper, and the various modalities of sensation may be affected to different degrees. Patients often exhibit sensory ataxia, and because of the severe impairment of joint position the limbs may be held in distorted positions. Tendon reflexes are characteristically diminished or absent.

Concurrent minor involvement of motor and autonomic function may occur. Cerebrospinal fluid changes are similar to those in the motor variety of the illness. Motor nerve conduction velocity may be within normal limits; by contrast, nerve action potentials cannot be elicited from stimulation of sensory nerve fibers, either because the afferent fibers have degenerated or because the action potential is so dispersed.

Prognosis for recovery is poor. Symptoms of cutaneous hyperpathia often persist or recur for many years. Sensory ataxia usually improves but may not recover completely. The neurologic deficit probably reflects irreversible damage of spinal ganglion neurons.

ACUTE INFLAMMATORY AUTONOMIC NEUROPATHY (Postinfectious Pandysautonomia)

Acute inflammatory autonomic neuropathy is a poorly understood, rare condition that may be the autonomic counterpart of the motor and sensory varieties already described. Pathologic studies are unavailable. The onset and time course are similar to those in the motor and sensory neuropathies. Principal symptoms include postural hypotension, cramping abdominal pain, and varying amounts of diarrhea and constipation. Hypotension may be so severe that the patient cannot sit up without losing consciousness. Affected subjects reportedly improve with time, but few long-term follow-up studies are available. (See also Ch. 463.)

CHRONIC INFLAMMATORY DEMYELINATING POLYNEUROPATHY

DEFINITION, PATHOLOGY, AND PATHOGENESIS. Affected individuals initially have an illness similar to the Guillain-Barré syndrome (although usually with a more gradual onset) but subsequently undergo either a chronic relapsing or progressive course. The salient histologic features of both chronic forms are similar to those of the Guillain-Barré syndrome. Segmental demyelination, onion bulb formation and lymphocytic infiltration are prominent findings.

CLINICAL FEATURES. Both the relapsing and progressive forms are uncommon, and there is rarely a temporal relationship to antecedent infections. The cardinal symptoms and signs reflect predominant motor involvement: weakness of the extremities, intercostal muscles, and lower cranial nerves. Sensory complaints are almost as common as weakness, and objective signs of sensory loss are more frequent in the chronic disorders than in the Guillain-Barré syndrome. Hyporeflexia or areflexia occur in almost all cases.

The development and course of illness are the salient features that distinguish between the relapsing and progressive variants. Each has a protracted onset and an indolent progression.

The course of the relapsing form may vary considerably in interval between episodes and rate and degree of recovery. Subsequent attacks usually resemble the initial one, and disability varies considerably. With treatment, improvement is generally good between episodes. Life-threatening episodes with respiratory insufficiency are more common early in the illness. The degree of disability following repeated attacks is variable, and the attacks often cease after a few years.

The course of the progressive form is usually stepwise but may be gradual. If untreated, this condition may become disabling or fatal; the prognosis is uncertain.

The CSF protein level is elevated at some stage of the illness in almost every case. Slowed nerve conduction, sometimes profound, in both motor and sensory nerves is characteristic, although this is not always present. Nerve biopsy may be extremely helpful in diagnosis if a diseased area can be located. The histologic picture is characteristic for these disorders. The differential diagnosis of the relapsing form is seldom a problem after several episodes have occurred. The differential diagnosis of the progressive disorder is sometimes extremely difficult. Unless a nerve biopsy displays characteristic changes, it may be indistinguishable from some hereditary disorders (see Ch. 508).

TREATMENT. Glucocorticoids are sometimes efficacious in treating chronic polyneuropathy, in contrast to the acute forms. Plasma exchange may produce dramatic improvement in the relapsing form and also is effective in the progressive disorder. Its value is less well established in chronic, end-stage polyneuropathy. It does offer a useful alternative for individuals who cannot tolerate long-term corticosteroids or other immunosuppressive therapy.

507 NEUROPATHY ASSOCIATED WITH ENDOCRINE DISEASES

THE DIABETIC NEUROPATHIES

A variety of peripheral nerve disorders may occur in diabetes mellitus. Diabetic neuropathies may be classified as either mononeuropathies or symmetric polyneuropathies, but neuropathy is frequent and mixed syndromes often occur. For instance, an individual with symmetric sensory polyneuropathy may develop acute third nerve palsy (a mononeuropathy). See Table 507–1.

Symmetric Polyneuropathy

PATHOLOGY. The experimental animal model of diabetic neuropathy exhibits only nerve conduction abnormalities

TABLE 507–1. CLASSIFICATION OF DIABETIC NEUROPATHIES

Symmetric polyneuropathies
 Distal primary sensory neuropathy
 Autonomic neuropathy
 Rapidly reversible neuropathy

Mononeuropathy and multiple mononeuropathies
 Cranial neuropathies
 Focal nerve lesions (other than cranial)
 Proximal painful lower limb neuropathy (diabetic amyotrophy)

without degeneration of nerve fibers, therefore, the early fundamental, pathologic diabetic changes in peripheral nerve are unclear. Previous human histopathologic studies were described in individuals with chronic neuropathy; nerves from biopsy or autopsy displayed a mixture of axonal loss and segmental demyelination. These observations suggested that axonal loss was primary and reflected an underlying metabolic disorder and that segmental demyelination was secondary to focal axonal change. Clearly fiber loss is the predominant change in chronic cases, restricting potential recovery. Recent postmortem histopathologic studies of long segments of nerves of diabetics indicate a multifocal pattern of fiber loss along nerves, suggesting that ischemia has a role in the symmetric neuropathies. Microangiopathic changes in the vasa nervorum are prominent in such nerve tissue but appear to occur with equal frequency in diabetics without neuropathy.

PATHOGENESIS. The clinical features of symmetric polyneuropathy, which often selectively involve particular fiber types, favor a metabolic basis. Elevated levels of neurotoxic ketones have been sought but not found. Distal axonopathy may be one of the mechanisms operating in individuals with the common progressive distal symmetric sensory neuropathy. No valid animal models are currently available to test this hypothesis.

Confounding a metabolic explanation is the inconsistent relationship of severity of neuropathy to control of blood glucose. There are many instances of "well-controlled" patients who develop severe sensorimotor neuropathy and others with "poor control" who have no evidence of neuropathy. The balance of recent evidence favors the notion that hyperglycemia is an important determinant of diabetic neuropathy and improved glycemic control is beneficial for nerve function. Current large-scale clinical trials that emphasize rigid glycemic control should determine whether prevention or amelioration of neuropathy is possible.

Glycemic control does help two types of symmetric diabetic neuropathy. One affects the newly diagnosed, insulin-dependent diabetic whose nerve conduction velocity and distal sensation loss improve following institution of therapy. The other occurs in individuals with acute painful neuropathy associated with rapid weight loss (diabetic neuropathic cachexia) in whom institution of glycemic control is followed by weight gain and recovery from neuropathy.

Among the proposed biochemical mechanisms underlying diabetic neuropathy, accumulation of nerve sorbitol and depletion of nerve myoinositol have received most attention. Sorbitol accumulates in the lens of the eye, alters the state of hydration, and may, by this mechanism, lead to cataract formation. Sorbitol also accumulates in nerve, but not in sufficient quantities to lead to osmotic damage unless it is confined to a particular cell compartment. Controlled clinical trials of aldose reductase inhibitors (the enzyme responsible for sorbitol accumulation) have been inconclusive at best.

Myoinositol is a cyclic hexitol normally present in nerve and is a precursor of membrane polyphosphoinositides that may regulate the patencies of ion channels. Nerve myoinositol concentration is reduced in both human and experimental diabetes. Although the addition of small quantities of myoinositol to the diet of animals with experimental diabetes may prevent reduction in nerve conduction velocity, the adminis-

tration of dietary inositol to humans with diabetic neuropathy has little beneficial effect.

CLINICAL FEATURES AND TREATMENT. *Distal Primary Sensory Neuropathy.* This is the commonest type of diabetic peripheral nerve disorder, estimated to be present in about 40 per cent of individuals with diabetes of 25 years' duration. It is present in less than 10 per cent of patients at the time of diagnosis (which it may antedate) and is uncommon in children.

Neuropathy may be asymptomatic, with abnormal signs first detectable on routine examination, or there may be a variety of symptoms. There appear to be three consistent patterns:

1. A "large-fiber" pattern with paresthesias in legs, absent ankle jerks, and impaired senses of light touch, vibration, and position in the lower limbs. Slight distal weakness is common and the hands may become involved.

2. A "small-fiber" pattern with dull aching pain and impaired cutaneous pain, touch, and temperature sensations. Position and vibration sense, deep tendon reflexes, and strength are usually spared. Autonomic nervous system dysfunction may accompany this variant.

3. A rare "pseudotabetic" pattern associated with long-term diabetes. Severe reduction of cutaneous and deep senses permits ulceration of the feet and distal joint deformity. Romberg's sign is present, tendon reflexes are absent in the legs, and hypotension and Argyll Robertson pupils may be observed.

The course is variable in sensory neuropathy. Most often it fluctuates and then plateaus. The pseudotabetic variety of the illness has an especially bad prognosis. Electrodiagnostic tests usually reveal changes in sensory conduction and variable alteration in motor conduction. The cerebrospinal fluid protein is usually elevated, sometimes to a very high level.

There is no specific treatment. Simple analgesics rarely help the severe pain that accompanies sensory neuropathy. Trial treatment with phenytoin, carbamazepine, phenothiazine, and tricyclic antidepressants is advocated. Persons with pain and temperature insensitivity of hands and feet are vulnerable to injuries that potentially can cascade into ulceration, cellulitis, lymphangitis, osteomyelitis, and osteolysis. Similar abnormalities are seen in syphilitic tabes, leprosy, inherited amyloidosis, and other inherited and acquired neuopathies, with the aforementioned sensory loss. The goal in treatment is to prevent the onset of tissue damage or, when it has occurred, to promote healing and prevent further damage. Persons with loss of pain and temperature sensation should not engage in most forms of manual labor or perform potentially bruising tasks with the hands and feet. Repeated inspection of hands and feet is necessary. If any bruise or ulcer appears, weight bearing or rough use should be stopped until healing occurs. Shoes should be wide and well constructed, with the insides inspected to remove retained objects or nails. Patients should soak the feet in lukewarm water for 15 minutes twice daily and cover them lightly with petrolatum lotion to retain moisture in the softened skin.

Autonomic Neuropathy. Diabetic autonomic neuropathy generally is associated with symmetrical sensory neuropathy and occasionally predominates. Autonomic involvement can be asymptomatic or cause incapacitating disability. Three types of dysfunction are prominent: gastrointestinal, cardiovascular, and genitourinary. The common gastrointestinal disturbances are gastroparesis, episodic nocturnal diarrhea, and colonic dilatation. Gastroparesis is often asymptomatic; it is best identified by radiographic or nuclear scans that demonstrate delayed emptying. Cardiovascular manifestations include impaired vasomotor reflexes (postural hypotension), elevated heart rate, and loss of respiratory sinus arrhythmia. Genitourinary disturbances are especially distressing and include disordered micturition with large residual volume, retrograde ejaculation, and impotence. Impotence is sometimes the initial manifestation of autonomic neuropathy. It usually steadily worsens and rarely, if ever, is reversed by control of hyperglycemia, the use of testosterone, or penile implants.

Treatment of autonomic disturbances is difficult. Gastroparesis secondary to vagal denervation can be treated with either neostigmine or metoclopramide. Diabetic diarrhea may be helped by codeine phosphate or diphenoxylate, but not all cases respond favorably. A single 250-mg dose of tetracycline, if given at the outset, sometimes aborts the attack. Simple cases of postural hypotension may be helped by support stockings. More severe cases may require supplemental sodium in the diet plus sodium-retaining steroids.

Rapidly Reversible Neuropathy. Newly diagnosed untreated diabetics may display asymptomatic slowing of nerve conduction velocity. This slowing is rapidly reversed by lowering blood sugar concentration to normal levels. It seems unlikely that this phenomenon is associated with structural breakdown in peripheral nerve fibers; it is not known whether such individuals are at greater risk of developing persistent symptomatic neuropathy.

MONONEUROPATHY AND MULTIPLE MONONEUROPATHY

PATHOLOGY AND PATHOGENESIS. It is believed that isolated peripheral nerve lesions in diabetics have a vascular basis. Several clinical facts support this notion: they have an abrupt onset, often recover spontaneously, and are most common in the elderly. Three careful autopsy studies, two of oculomotor palsy and one of femoral neuropathy, have demonstrated focal vascular lesions within the area of nerve damage.

CLINICAL FEATURES AND TREATMENT. *Cranial Nerve Lesions.* Isolated or multiple palsies of extraocular muscle nerves or lower cranial nerves may be the first indication of diabetes in asymptomatic older adults. The third nerve is most frequently affected. Onset is usually abrupt and is associated with an intense, retro-orbital aching sensation. Sparing of the pupillomotor fibers in diabetic third-nerve palsy helps distinguish this condition from lesions that compress the nerve, such as aneurysm. Satisfactory recovery of nerve function usually occurs within several weeks.

Isolated Peripheral Nerve Lesions (Other Than Cranial). Almost every isolated peripheral nerve can be affected by diabetic mononeuropathy. Lesions of the ulnar, radial, sciatic, peroneal, tibial, and lateral cutaneous nerves of the thigh are especially common. Diabetic nerves are especially vulnerable to compresson, and lesions frequently appear at such sites. Onset is abrupt and usually painful. Recovery is usually good in distally sited lesions and less satisfactory if the lesions are proximal. Treatment includes physical therapy and use of appropriate orthotic devices.

Proximal Lower Extremity Motor Neuropathy (Diabetic Amyotrophy). This syndrome usually appears after middle age, in the setting of substantial recent weight loss. Cardinal findings include progressive, painful, asymmetrical weakness of thigh muscles, loss of knee jerks, and few sensory abnormalities. The spinal fluid protein level is usually elevated, and the motor changes are usually bilateral, differentiating the condition from acute nerve root disease. Recovery is gradual. There is considerable variation in the clinical features, and many patients display distal weakness as well. As a result, the term diabetic amyotrophy has come to encompass a spectrum of illnesses that range from ischemic femoral or lumbar plexus neuropathy to symmetrical proximal metabolic neuropathy. Treatment includes major analgesics for relief of the self-limited pain and physical therapy directed at the weakness.

Hypothyroidism is associated with both mononeuropathy and symmetrical polyneuropathy. Clumsiness and limb ataxia of uncertain origin are common, probably due to cerebellar disease. Thyroid replacement therapy ameliorates the carpal and tarsal tunnel syndromes as well as the diffuse symmetrical neuropathy.

Acromegaly produces entrapment neuropathies at wrist and elbow and a distal symmetrical polyneuropathy. Proximal muscle weakness occurs independently of the peripheral neuropathies and may make the clinical profile confusing. The carpal tunnel syndrome presumably results from compression by acral soft-tissue hyperplasia and osteoarthritis. Improvement follows removal of the pituitary tumor; surgery of the carpal ligament is seldom necessary. Symmetrical polyneuropathy usually occurs late in the illness; it bears no relationship to plasma levels of growth hormone. No studies have been made on the effect of removal of the pituitary adenoma on neuropathy.

---

508 HEREDITARY NEUROPATHIES

Hereditary neuropathies represent a group of slowly progressive disorders characterized by the type of inheritance, their natural history, and the population of neurons involved. Predominant involvement of lower motor neurons (progressive muscular atrophy) is called *inherited motor neuropathy*; involvement of sensory neurons is *hereditary sensory neuropathy* (*HSN*); and involvement of both motor and sensory neurons is *hereditary motor and sensory neuropathy* (*HMSN*); and involvement of autonomic neurons is *dysautonomia*.

Expression of clinical symptoms varies widely from patient to patient and functional disability is frequently less than might be expected from the neurologic signs. Certain of these disorders (HMSN types I and II) are common and account for many cases of cryptogenic neuropathy. The number of correct diagnoses increases considerably when the patient's asymptomatic relatives are examined clinically and by nerve conduction studies.

HEREDITARY MOTOR AND SENSORY NEUROPATHY

These disorders, previously described by various eponyms (Charcot-Marie-Tooth disease, Roussy-Lévy syndrome, Dejerine-Sottas disease) are now numerically subdivided into types I, II, and III. Table 508–1 outlines their salient features.

DISORDERS OF PERIPHERAL SENSORY NEURONS

Patients with disorders of peripheral sensory neurons characteristically suffer from pain, cutaneous injury from lack of sensation, unsteady movement from kinesthetic sensory loss, or combinations of these conditions. Frequently they also have autonomic dysfunction. The nature of these symptoms and the associated sensory loss correspond reasonably well with the populations of fibers affected. Thus patients with loss of pain and temperature sensation and with autonomic impairment have degeneration mostly of unmyelinated and small myelinated fibers, whereas patients with loss of touch-pressure sensation have degeneration of large myelinated fibers of cutaneous nerves. In advanced disease this selectivity of involvement by fiber size tends to be lost.

HEREDITARY SENSORY NEUROPATHY, TYPE I. Hereditary sensory neuropathy, type I, is a dominantly inherited sensory radicular neuropathy. It has been variously termed as perforating ulcers of the feet, mutilating acropathy, acrodystrophic neuropathy, and hereditary sensory radicular neuropathy. The severity varies widely. Sensory loss is usually more severe over the feet and legs than in the hands and

TABLE 508–1. THE HEREDITARY MOTOR AND SENSORY NEUROPATHIES (HMSN)

Nomenclature	Heredity	Clinical Features	Pathology and Pathogenesis
HMSN type I (peroneal muscle atrophy; hypertrophic form of Charcot-Marie-Tooth disease)	Autosomal dominant	Common; many mild cases; childhood onset; slow progression; predominantly motor; deformed feet (pes cavus); extreme distal lower limb atrophy; very slow motor nerve conduction	Possibly a distal axonopathy but much segmental demyelination and remyelination ("onion bulbs"); nerves may be enlarged
HMSN type II (neuronal form of Charcot-Marie-Tooth disease or peroneal muscle atrophy)	Autosomal dominant	Less common than type I; onset in second decade; nerve conduction almost normal; otherwise, identical to type I	Possibly a motor and sensory neuronopathy syndrome; loss of fibers; little remyelination (no "onion bulbs")
HMSN type III (Dejerine-Sottas disease)	Autosomal recessive	Rare; infantile onset; short stature, scoliosis, pes cavus; steady progression to severe disability; very slow nerve conduction	Few studies; enlarged nerves; many "onion bulbs"; pathogenesis unclear

TABLE 509–1. PHARMACEUTICAL AGENTS ASSOCIATED WITH GENERALIZED NEUROPATHY

Chloramphenicol	Metronidazole-misonidazole
Dapsone*	Nitrofurantoin*
Disulfiram	Nitrous oxide
Dichloracetate	Phenytoin
Ethionamide	Platinum (cis-platinum)†
Gold	Pyridoxine†
Glutethimide	Sodium cyanate
Hydralazine	Taxol
Isoniazid†	Thalidomide†
Lithium	Vincristine

*Predominantly motor.
†Predominantly sensory.

forearms, and some patients have lancinating pains. Pain and temperature sensation are affected more than touch-pressure sensation. Nerve conduction of motor fibers is usually normal, as is life expectancy in most cases. Late in the disorder, perforating ulcers of the foot may develop, especially in patients with poor foot care.

HEREDITARY SENSORY NEUROPATHY, TYPE II. This is a recessively inherited disorder, also called congenital sensory neuropathy, that usually manifests itself in infancy or childhood with a mutilating acropathy characterized by paronychia, whitlows, ulcers of the fingers and plantar surfaces of the feet, and, frequently, unrecognized fractures of the extremities. Sensory loss affects all types of cutaneous and sometimes kinesthetic sensation and is most marked distally in all four limbs. Tendon reflexes are usually absent.

HEREDITARY SENSORY NEUROPATHY, TYPE III (Dysautonomia of Riley-Day). Familial dysautonomia is a recessively inherited disorder of Jewish infants and children. It affects peripheral autonomic neurons, peripheral sensory neurons, peripheral motor neurons, and probably other central nervous system neurons. Characteristics are onset in infancy, poor feeding, repeated episodes of vomiting and pulmonary infections, autonomic disturbances, and premature death. Autonomic abnormalities include defective lacrimation, defective temperature control, skin blotching, excessive perspiration, hypertension, and postural hypotension. There is insensitivity to pain, areflexia, corneal insensitivity, and absence of the fungiform papillae of the tongue. An abnormality of nerve growth factor is postulated.

509 TOXIC NEUROPATHIES

UREMIA

DEFINITION AND ETIOLOGY. Uremic polyneuropathy can be associated with chronic renal insufficiency of any type. The cause is unknown. It is believed that uremic neuropathy is related to dialyzable toxins or metabolites normally excreted by the kidneys. The responsible agent has a molecular weight exceeding that of urea or creatinine.

PATHOLOGY. Axonal degeneration is characteristic of this disorder, and the distribution suggests that it is a distal axonopathy. The nature of the axonal change is nonspecific.

CLINICAL FEATURES. Initially, sensory symptoms predominate, with especially frequent tingling paresthesias of the leg. Occasionally a "burning foot" or "restless leg" syndrome accompanies uremic polyneuropathy. Muscle cramps in the distal extremities are common. Diminished sensation in distal limbs is the most consistent feature, usually in combination with hyporeflexia and moderate weakness.

Uremic neuropathy has an insidious onset, and subclinical cases are common. Most cases progress over several months to reach a plateau despite worsening of the renal state. The prognosis of untreated uremic neuropathy is poor.

TREATMENT. Successful renal transplantation both prevents and reverses uremic polyneuropathy. Patients with mild cases display prompt relief of paresthesias and a steady return of strength. Recovery is more prolonged in advanced cases and is not always complete. Chronic hemodialysis is less helpful and often ineffective in reversing the neuropathy.

PHARMACEUTICAL AGENTS

GENERAL. New pharmaceutical agents are constantly being implicated on clinical-epidemiologic grounds as causes of peripheral neuropathy. Except for isoniazid, pyridoxine, and vincristine, few careful experimental studies of these substances have been conducted. Since following prolonged use most of the offending agents produce an insidious-onset distal axonopathy, little in the clinical diagnostic profile helps to identify the specific offending agent. The most important diagnostic factor in these disorders is a meticulous history of drug use. Table 509–1 lists pharmaceutical agents that are associated with generalized neuropathy. Treatment consists of withdrawing the drug if symptoms are prominent or progressive.

OCCUPATIONAL, BIOLOGICAL, AND ENVIRONMENTAL AGENTS

GENERAL. Many potential toxic chemicals are deployed in the work place and general environment, and several have

TABLE 509–2. AGENTS CAUSING SYMPTOMS ASSOCIATED WITH TOXIC NEUROPATHY

Acrylamide (truncal ataxis)
Arsenic (sensory, brown skin, Mees' lines)
Buckthorn toxin
Carbon disulfide
Cyanide
Dimethylaminopropionitrile (urinary complaints)
Biologic toxin in diphtheritic neuropathy (pharyngeal neuropathy)
Ethylene oxide
n-Hexane
Lead (wrist drop, abdominal colic)
Lucel-7 (cataracts)
Mercury
Methyl bromide
Organophosphates (cholinergic symptoms, delayed onset of neuropathy)
Thallium (pain, alopecia, Mees' lines)
Trichloroethylene (facial numbness)

been implicated as causes of peripheral neuropathy, usually of the distal axonopathy type. Since the various agents result in similar clinical syndromes, a careful occupational and environmental history is often the most important clue for diagnosis. The various agents are listed in Table 509–2, with prominent clinical features included in parentheses. *Buckthorn* and *diphtheritic neuropathies*, which are demyelinating conditions, are the sole examples of diseases in which biologic toxins are consistently associated with neuropathy. Diphtheria is further discussed in Ch. 277.

510 MISCELLANEOUS DISEASE-SPECIFIC NEUROPATHIES

NEUROPATHY ASSOCIATED WITH MALIGNANCY AND DYSPROTEINEMIA

Direct compression of nerves by metastatic tumors occurs within the spinal canal or invertebral foramina and behind tight fascial sheaths. Bronchogenic, renal, prostatic, and breast carcinomas are especially prone to such metastases. The direct and nonmetastatic neurologic effects of cancer are described in Ch. 174.

Polyneuropathy is more common in multiple myeloma than in most other malignancies; furthermore, subclinical neuropathy appears to be frequent. Recent evidence has demonstrated that the benign gammopathies are also associated with polyneuropathy, some examples of which can resemble motor neuron disease.

AMYLOID NEUROPATHY

Extracellular deposition of the fibrous protein amyloid is associated with peripheral neuropathy in both hereditary (nonimmunoglobulin-derived) amyloidosis and nonhereditary (immunoglobulin-derived) amyloidosis.

Hereditary amyloidosis is frequent only in endemic regions such as Portugal and Japan. Rare variants have also been described in Iowa and Indiana. In the Portuguese variety, which is inherited as an autosomal-dominant trait, the disorder usually begins in the third, fourth, or fifth decade and affects predominantly small sensory and autonomic fibers. Lumbosacral dermatomes show a syringomyelia-like loss of pain and thermal discrimination with preservation of touch-pressure sensation. Loss of potency in the male, postural hypotension, and bladder and bowel incontinence are common in advanced stages. The disorder tends to progress over a decade or so. Biopsied sural nerves show an endoneurial reduction in unmyelinated and small myelinated fibers with nodular deposits of amyloid among the nerve trunks.

Nonhereditary amyloidosis may be divided into primary and secondary varieties. The peripheral neuropathy of primary amyloidosis also affects the distal aspects of the lower extremities more than the upper and includes small fibers as much as or more than larger ones. When typical symptoms of neuropathy are associated with enlargement of the heart, nephropathy, and enlargement of the tongue, the diagnosis of primary amyloidosis should be strongly suspected and can be confirmed by histologic examination of rectal mucosa, kidney, carpal ligament, muscle, gingivae, nerve, or bone marrow. No effective treatment for the neuropathy is available.

Patients with multiple myeloma who develop a symmetrical carpal tunnel syndrome should be investigated for systemic amyloidosis.

NEUROPATHY ASSOCIATED WITH NECROTIZING ANGIITIS AND RHEUMATOID ARTHRITIS

No fewer than nine disorders are associated with vasculitis and ischemic neuropathy. These include: polyarteritis nodosa, rheumatoid arthritis, systemic lupus erythematosus (SLE), hypersensitivity angiitis, allergic granulomatosis (Churg-Strauss syndrome), Sjögren's syndrome, Wegener's granulomatosis, and cranial arteritis (temporal arteritis).

Only polyarteritis nodosa, rheumatoid arthritis, and lupus erythematosus are encountered with any frequency in clinical practice. Although the fundamental expression of these conditions varies considerably, they all produce similar clinical and pathologic syndromes of ischemic mononeuritis multiplex. The pathogenesis of nerve fiber destruction in each condition presumably relates to focal ischemia from arteriolar occlusion. The clinical features are similar to those depicted for the mononeuropathies associated with diabetes (Ch. 507.1).

Rheumatoid arthritis, in addition to producing a vascular mononeuropathy, may also cause entrapment neuropathy (reflecting prolonged immobilized postures and nerve compression by articular deformity) and a chronic symmetrical sensory neuropathy. This latter disorder develops with long-term rheumatoid arthritis and is characterized by mild, distal, symmetrical sensory loss. Although frequently painful, the condition is generally benign and improves spontaneously. Corticosteroid treatment is not indicated.

INFECTIOUS AND GRANULOMATOUS NEUROPATHY (Herpes Zoster, Leprosy, and Sarcoidosis)

HERPES ZOSTER. This viral disorder affects sensory ganglia of cranial or spinal nerves to produce characteristic disorders, which are discussed in Ch. 485.3.

LEPROSY. This remains one of the most common neuropathies on a worldwide scale. It is discussed in Ch. 304.

SARCOIDOSIS. Peripheral neuropathy of uncertain pathogenesis develops in 5 per cent of cases. Both multiple mononeuropathy and symmetrical polyneuropathy occur. A mixture of localized granulomatous infiltration and vascular compromise is probably the cause.

Mononeuropathy can affect either the spinal or the cranial nerves. Most cranial neuropathy with sarcoid involvement occurs as an acute facial (Bell's) palsy that is indistinguishable from the idiopathic variety, unless it causes an isolated bilateral facial paralysis that is almost pathognomonic. Simultaneous bilateral involvement is rare. Lower cranial nerves are less commonly involved. Severe paralysis is common and incomplete recovery the rule, even with corticosteroid therapy.

Distal symmetric polyneuropathy is a rare complication of sarcoidosis. Little is known about the specific cause, prognosis, or natural history of this neuropathy. Paradoxically, this form of neuropathy is usually not accompanied by prominent evidence of systemic disease.

NEUROPATHY ASSOCIATED WITH ALCOHOLISM, NUTRITIONAL DEFICIENCY, AND MALABSORPTION

See Ch. 467.

NEUROPATHY ASSOCIATED WITH ACQUIRED IMMUNE DEFICIENCY SYNDROME

See Ch. 346.

BELL'S PALSY (Idiopathic Facial Paralysis)

PATHOLOGY AND PATHOGENESIS. Neither the pathology nor the pathogenesis of this common illness are known. It is likely that mild cases with rapid recovery represent segmental demyelination and that axonal degeneration occurs in instances with prolonged dysfunction.

CLINICAL FEATURES. Idiopathic unilateral facial paralysis may develop rapidly within a few hours or evolve over one or two days and is often accompanied by pain behind the ipsilateral ear and excess tearing. Numbness of the face is a common complaint but inevitably refers to a proprioceptive sensation that accompanies weakness. Global facial muscle weakness is the hallmark of this condition. Hyperacusis, diminished lacrimation, and abnormal taste sensation are present to variable degrees. Untreated, 80 to 85 per cent of all patients with Bell's palsy recover completely or almost so. In a smaller number, persistent facial weakness ensues. Rarely, motor recovery fails completely. Aberrant regeneration is frequent. There may be embarrassing synkinetic movements (chewing producing eye winking) or excessive lacrimation.

Patients who are going to recover completely usually begin to show improvement during the first two weeks, while those destined to have permanent residual disability show no changes in status for three or more months. Except when paralysis is incomplete, there is little in the acute clinical profile to indicate prognosis. In patients who have complete paralysis from the onset, reliance must be placed on careful observation and electrodiagnostic tests of nerve excitability (performed at about one week after the onset).

Most authorities recommend treatment with prednisone, 1 mg per kilogram daily in two divided doses for four days, with dosage tapered to a total of 5 mg per day within ten days. It is claimed that prednisone therapy should be instituted as soon as possible if it is to have an effect in decreasing residual paralysis and synkinetic movements. In any event, pain usually subsides promptly. The unusual residual of a severe facial paralysis has a distressing cosmetic effect. Hypoglossal-facial nerve anastomosis will restore facial tone and is the operation of choice.

ACUTE BRACHIAL NEURITIS (Idiopathic Brachial Plexus Neuropathy)

PATHOLOGY AND PATHOGENESIS. There have been no thorough pathologic examinations of this condition, and the pathogenesis is unknown. Biopsy of cutaneous nerves has revealed nonspecific axonal degeneration. In most cases there is no common antecedent illness, immunization, or toxic exposure; some cases follow surgical procedures. The clinical profile is identical to that in certain serum vaccine paralyses, and a common immunologic basis has been suggested.

CLINICAL FEATURES. The condition arises as an acute, painful, and usually monophasic illness characterized by brachial plexus dysfunction. It is especially common in males aged 18 to 40. A cardinal feature is sudden severe shoulder girdle-scapular pain, occasionally extending into the arm or hand. The pain persists for a few days to a week and then subsides concomitantly with or shortly after the appearance of weakness, although it sometimes persists for several weeks. The serratus anterior is the single most commonly affected muscle. Distal weakness occurs less frequently. Rarely, the entire arm and ipsilateral diaphragm are affected. Uncommonly, weakness may appear in the other arm. Tendon reflexes are diminished in the involved extremity, but sensory loss is slight or negligible, being most commonly found at the apex of the shoulder. Involvement is usually restricted to muscles innervated by the brachial plexus. Weakness and atrophy of involved muscles lasts for months in many cases, but total recovery occurs in 90 per cent within two or three years. Treatment consists of physical therapy and orthotic devices to prevent joint damage. Corticosteroid therapy has no demonstrated value. There are occasional recurrences.

TRIGEMINAL NEUROPATHY

Rare cases are encountered of a slowly progressive bilateral sensory loss confined to the territory of the trigeminal nerve. This may lead to tissue destruction, particularly around the nostrils, as a result of repeated picking and scratching. Drug toxicity with trichloroethylene or stilbamidine may cause this syndrome. Sjögren's syndrome, systemic sclerosis, and trigeminal neurilemomas should be excluded. Some cases have been found at autopsy to have infiltration of the trigeminal ganglion with amyloid. The explanation for other cases is obscure.

---

511 ACUTE PHYSICAL INJURY AND CHRONIC COMPRESSION-ENTRAPMENT NEUROPATHIES

ACUTE PHYSICAL INJURY. The results of recent experimental studies suggest a simple classification for acute nerve injury in which the clinical features, including prognosis, closely approximate the nature of the acute injury. Basically there are three different types (classes 1 through 3). In mild injury (class 1) axonal integrity is maintained but myelin may be damaged. In more severe injury (class 2) axonal continuity is lost but the connective tissue framework of the nerve is maintained. In the most severe injuries (class 3), nerve fibers and connective tissue are damaged to varying degrees. Table 511–1 depicts the types of nerve injury and their corresponding anatomic and clinical features.

COMPRESSION-ENTRAPMENT NEUROPATHY. The pathophysiologic features of chronic compressions and entrapment are still debated. It is widely believed that demyelination initially occurs and, if the condition persists, axonal destruction may follow. Several clinical forms are common, including carpal tunnel syndrome, ulnar palsy, meralgia paresthetica, and cervical rib.

CARPAL TUNNEL SYNDROME. The median nerve becomes compressed at the wrist as it passes deep within the tissue to the flexor retinaculum. The usual symptoms include numbness, tingling, and burning sensations in the hand and fingers. The pain sometimes radiates up the forearm as far as the elbow or even as high as the shoulder or root of the neck. These sensations are occasionally restricted to the radial fingers but may affect all the digits. Pain and paresthesias are most prominent at night and often wake the patient from sleep. They may be relieved by shaking the hand. The hand tends to feel numb and useless on waking in the morning, but these sensations subside after brief use. The symptoms may recur following use or when the patient is sitting with the hands immobile. Such symptoms may persist for many years without objective signs of median nerve damage. In other patients, weakness of the thumb muscles develops in association with atrophy of the lateral aspect of the thenar eminence. Sensory loss may appear over the tips of the fingers. Occasionally, patients have motor symptoms of median nerve deficit in the hand without paresthesias, or motor and sensory signs may be discovered incidentally in the absence of symptoms, particularly in older individuals.

Most cases of carpal tunnel compression occur in middle aged and often obese females. In younger women it is

TABLE 511–1. TYPES OF NERVE INJURY

Type	Anatomic Lesion	Clinical Features	Course and Prognosis
Class 1	Either (A) transient conduction block due to ischemia or (B) demyelination	(A) Mild sensory loss and weakness (ischemic type) from transient abnormal posture (legs crossed) (B) Prolonged compression (Saturday night palsy) with paralysis and moderate sensory loss below site of lesion	(A) Rapid complete recovery (B) Gradual (lasting weeks) complete recovery
Class 2	Axonal interruption; connective tissue intact	Closed crush and percussion injury; loss of motor, sensory, and autonomic function below site of lesion; surgical exploration not indicated	Very slow recovery; prognosis best with distal lesions
Class 3	Transection of axons and connective tissue sheaths	Severe stretch injuries (heavy blows, motorcycle accidents) or penetrating wounds; total loss of all motor, sensory, and autonomic function; surgical intervention indicated for penetrating wounds	Little recovery even with surgical repair; poor prognosis

commonly associated with excessive use of the hands, and it may develop in males after unaccustomed use of the hands, such as in house-painting. The disorder may be caused by tenosynovitis at the wrist, by involvement of the wrist joint in rheumatoid arthritis, or as a consequence of osteoarthritis of the carpus, perhaps in relation to an old fracture. Other predisposing causes are pregnancy, myxedema, acromegaly, infiltration of the transverse carpal ligament in primary amyloidosis, and chronic hemodialysis treatments. Diagnosis is based on clinical symptoms, the finding of Tinel's sign over the median nerve in the tunnel, and demonstration of conduction block at the wrist by motor nerve velocity studies. Individuals with muscle weakness and wasting or prominent sensory loss should undergo decompression of the nerve by section of the transverse carpal ligament. In patients with paresthesias alone or when the cause is probably tenosynovitis at the wrist, a reduction in hand activity may be sufficient to allow the symptoms to subside. Injection into the carpal tunnel of a long-acting corticosteroid preparation sometimes gives temporary relief, as does splinting of the wrist to reduce movement. When troublesome symptoms persist, decompression is advisable.

For most patients with paresthesias, symptoms are relieved by decompression. Sensory impairment and cutaneous hyperesthesia, however, may persist postoperatively, and there may not be recovery after prolonged denervation of the thenar muscles.

ULNAR PALSY. The ulnar nerve may be injured at the elbow, especially in persons with a shallow ulnar groove, those who rest their weight on their elbows excessively, and those who are cachectic and lie in bed. Injury may occur years following a previously malunited supracondylar fracture of the humerus with bony overgrowth (*tardive ulnar palsy*). Contrary to the findings in the carpal tunnel syndrome, muscle weakness and atrophy characteristically predominate over sensory symptoms and signs. Patients notice atrophy of the first dorsal interosseous muscle or difficulty in performing fine manipulation. There may be numbness of the small finger, the contiguous half of the proximal and middle phalanges of the ring finger, and the ulnar border of the hand. Treatment in mild cases consists of prevention of further injury. A doughnut cushion for the elbow may be helpful. Mobilizing and transplanting the nerve to a position in front of the medial epicondyle sometimes prevents further progression.

LATERAL CUTANEOUS NERVE OF THE THIGH. *Meralgia paresthetica* is an entrapment neuropathy resulting from compression of this nerve as it passes under the inguinal ligament. Although the case often remains unexplained, obese persons wearing tight girdles, individuals with gun belts, and those with pendulous abdomens are especially prone to develop numbness or burning sensations over the lateral thigh. Sometimes prolonged standing or walking provokes the symptoms. Weight reduction may help, and in many cases the condition subsides spontaneously. Surgical decompression is rarely necessary.

CERVICAL RIB AND THORACIC OUTLET SYNDROME. Angulation of the brachial plexus over an abnormal rib or fibrous band can damage its lower fibers and lead to weakness and wasting of the small hand muscles. Numbness and pain may occur along the inner border of the forearm and hand. Surgical removal of the rib or fibrous band sometimes abolishes the pain and paresthesias, but the small muscles of the hand often fail to recover strength. Cervical rib compression is uncommon, and most patients with paresthesias of the fingers prove to have either root compression from a cervical disc or a carpal tunnel syndrome.

SECTION SEVENTEEN / DISEASES OF MUSCLE (MYOPATHIES) AND NEUROMUSCULAR JUNCTION

Andrew G. Engel

512 GENERAL APPROACH TO MUSCLE DISEASES

Muscle diseases are caused by derangements in the structure or function of the muscle fiber or in the innervation, blood supply, or connective tissue elements of muscle. A myopathy is a muscle disease not related to a demonstrable alteration in the innervation of muscle. Disorders that affect the innervation of muscle are considered in Ch. 504 through 511. Ch. 513 through 517 consider the myopathies. Ch. 518 deals with diseases of the neuromuscular junction. To facilitate the understanding of muscle diseases, this chapter begins with a brief overview of the structure and function of muscle.

BASIC STRUCTURE AND FUNCTION OF MUSCLE

Each voluntary muscle contains myriad muscle fibers. A small proportion of the fibers is confined to muscle spindles and innervated by gamma or beta motor neurons and by sensory neurons. These intrafusal fibers function as mechanoreceptors and participate in regulating the motor tone. Most muscle fibers are extrafusal and are innervated by alpha motor neurons. A *motor unit* consists of one alpha motor neuron and all muscle fibers innervated by that neuron. The peripheral axon of the motor neuron extends into muscle, where it divides into terminal branches that reach the neuromuscular junction on individual fibers. The number of motor units per muscle and the number of muscle fibers per motor unit vary from muscle to muscle. In general, motor units are smaller in small muscles subserving delicate movements (e.g., the external ocular, facial, and intrinsic hand muscles) than in large muscles maintaining posture or exerting strong force (e.g., biceps or quadriceps). The territory of a motor unit is a cylinder of the same length as the fibers and with a diameter that extends over a few millimeters. Muscle fibers belonging to different motor units intermingle with each other, so that the territories of individual motor units overlap. Many physiologic, biochemical, histochemical, and morphologic features of the muscle fibers are regulated by their innervation. Consequently, all muscle fibers in a motor unit share similar properties or are of the same type. Three major muscle-fiber (and motor-unit) types can be recognized: Type I, slow-twitch, fatigue-resistant fibers, high in oxidative enzymes but low in glycolytic enzymes; Type IIB, fast-twitch fatigable fibers, high in glycolytic enzymes and low in oxidative enzymes; and Type IIA, intermediate-twitch, fatigue-resistant fibers, high in glycolytic enzymes and with an intermediate content of oxidative enzymes. The myofibrillar ATPase, also different in the three fiber types, provides a convenient histochemical marker. In most human muscles the three fiber types occur in about equal proportions. Because the motor unit territories overlap, the fiber types intermingle randomly.

The muscle fibers of an adult are about 50 μm in diameter. Each fiber contains multiple subsarcolemmal nuclei. The myofibrils, which account for most of the fiber volume, are associated with mitochondria, glycogen granules, transverse (T) tubules and sarcoplasmic reticulum (SR). The myofibrils, 0.5 to 1.0 μm wide, consist of repeating units, or sarcomeres, limited by Z disks. The latter anchor 1-μm-long thin filaments that extend from each Z disk toward the center of the sarcomere. The thin filaments interdigitate with 1.6 μm–long thick filaments in the central region (A-band) of the sarcomere. That part of the sarcomere which contains only thin filaments is referred to as the I band. It is the sarcomeres of adjacent myofibrils lying in register that give the striated appearance to the muscle fiber. The thin filaments are composed of actin, troponin, and tropomyosin. The thick filaments are made up nearly entirely of regularly arrayed myosin molecules. The head of each myosin molecule projects laterally from the thick filament and can serve as a cross bridge between myosin and actin. The T-tubules are inward extensions of the muscle fiber surface membrane and propagate the action potential into the depth of the fiber. The SR abuts on the T-tubules and partially envelops individual myofibrils. In the resting state the SR sequesters calcium into its lumen by means of an ATPase and thereby maintains a very low calcium concentration (about 10^{-7} M) around the myofilaments.

Depolarization of the T-tubules by an action potential induces the release of calcium from the SR into the myofilament space. The released calcium binds to troponin on the thin filaments which then acts on tropomyosin to allow repeated binding of the myosin cross bridges to actin. Each binding is associated with a conformational change in the cross bridge that exerts a force on the thin filament toward the center of the sarcomere. The cross bridge cycle requires adenosine triphosphate (ATP), which is split by an ATPase on the cross bridge. If ATP is depleted, the cross bridges remain attached to the thin filaments and the muscle becomes stiff, as in rigor mortis. When ATP is available, the unloaded fiber shortens, the thin filaments are propelled into the A-band, and the Z disks are pulled closer together in every sarcomere. The active state subsides with calcium reuptake by the SR; interaction between actin and the cross bridges ceases and relaxation sets in.

THE DIAGNOSIS OF MUSCLE DISEASES

The diagnosis of a muscle disease rests on a tripod: the clinical data, the electromyogram (EMG), and the muscle biopsy. None of the three approaches is entirely adequate by itself, but their combined use yields the correct diagnosis in a very high proportion of cases. Examples of disorders that are similar by clinical criteria but require muscle biopsy and EMG for accurate diagnosis are polymyositis, limb-girdle dystrophy, and adult acid maltase deficiency; distal muscular dystrophies, progressive muscular atrophy, and the slow-channel myasthenic syndrome; benign congenital myopathies, mitochondrial myopathies, and childhood or juvenile spinal muscular atrophies.

CLINICAL DATA. *The Genetic History.* This is relevant to diagnosis as well as counseling in the muscular dystrophies, congenital myopathies, and inherited metabolic myopathies. A negative family history, however, does not exclude autosomal recessive inheritance, an incompletely penetrant autosomal-dominant gene in one parent, or a new mutation. In autosomal dominant disorders (e.g., myotonic and facioscapulohumeral dystrophy or the familial periodic paralyses) a negative family history needs to be validated by examination of both parents. The clinical examination or biochemical tests may help in detecting heterozygotes in autosomal-recessive or X-linked-recessive diseases.

The History of the Illness. AGE AT ONSET, DURATION, AND RATE OF PROGRESSION OF SYMPTOMS. Most benign congenital myopathies, congenital muscular dystrophy, congenital myasthenic syndromes, a number of inherited metabolic myopathies, and the acute form of spinal muscular atrophy present in infancy. Duchenne dystrophy usually presents in early childhood. Many inherited myopathies, inherited anterior horn cell diseases, and most hereditary peripheral neuropathies present in childhood or early adult life. Limb-girdle, Becker, and facioscapulohumeral dystrophy usually present in adolescence; myotonic, oculopharyngeal, limb-girdle, and distal dystrophies can present in adult life. Dermatomyositis and scleroderma can begin in childhood or adult life; pure polymyositis is unusual before adolescence; and inclusion-body myositis seldom presents before the fifth decade.

Muscle weakness evolving over a few hours suggests an exogenous intoxication (e.g., organophosphorus or barium poisoning), periodic paralysis, or rhabdomyolysis. An abrupt onset of symptoms also can occur in myasthenia gravis or with other defects of neuromuscular transmission. Acute muscle weakness appearing during or after recovery from a Reye syndrome–like metabolic crisis suggests an enzyme defect in organic acid metabolism associated with secondary carnitine deficiency. Weakness evolving over a few days to a few weeks can occur in acute postinfectious polyneuropathy (Guillain-Barré syndrome), toxic neuropathies, and in acute dermatomyositis. A subacute evolution, over a period of weeks to months, is seen in motor neuron disease; some metabolic myopathies, such as corticosteroid-induced or thyrotoxic myopathy; late-onset nemaline myopathy; and most cases of dermatomyositis and idiopathic polymyositis. A slow evolution over a number of years is typical of most dystrophies but can also occur in the inflammatory myopathies, such as inclusion body myositis, and in motor neuron disease.

EFFECTS OF EXERCISE, REST AFTER EXERCISE, DIET, AND TEMPERATURE. Weakness appearing or increasing during exercise suggests a defect of neuromuscular transmission or in muscle energy metabolism. Weakness that decreases with exercise but increases during rest after exercise is typical of the periodic paralyses. Depending on the type of periodic paralysis, alterations in sodium, potassium, and carbohydrate intake can improve or exacerbate the symptoms. Fasting or a high-fat diet may provoke or worsen symptoms in patients with defects of fatty acid oxidation. Exposure to cold worsens myotonia and can provoke weakness in periodic paralysis and paramyotonia congenita. Exposure to heat can increase neuromuscular transmission defects.

Symptoms in Muscle Diseases. Relatively few symptoms are associated with diverse muscle diseases: weakness, decrease of muscle bulk, increased fatigability, muscle pain, cramps, stiffness, and discoloration of the urine caused by myoglobinuria. The cardinal symptom is muscle weakness, but patients often describe its consequences instead of speaking of weakness. Patients complaining of cramps sometimes suffer from contractures or tetany. The term stiffness is used to describe a variety of conditions, such as the stiff-man syndrome, neuromyotonia, and myotonia.

MUSCLE WEAKNESS. Vague complaints, such as constant fatigue and exhaustion, or weakness of all muscles of uncertain duration in a patient who can carry out the tasks of everyday living suggest functional weakness. Patients with organic and evolving muscle weakness can always specify the tasks that they cannot do presently, but could a year, a month, or a few weeks before the examination.

Weakness of the cranial, cervical, torso, and limb muscles presents stereotypically. Weakness of muscles supplied by cranial nerves causes drooping of the eyelids (ptosis, third cranial nerve); double vision (diplopia, third, fourth, and sixth cranial nerves); failure of the eyelids to close at night, altered facial expression, difficulty in whistling or sucking from a straw (seventh cranial nerve); inability to close the jaw, difficulty in chewing hard food (fifth cranial nerve); difficulty in pronouncing words (dysarthria), hypernasal voice, nasal regurgitation of liquids, and difficulty in swallowing (dysphagia) (tenth and twelfth cranial nerves). Weakness of the cervical muscles is shown by difficulty in lifting the head from a pillow or holding the head erect, and weakness of the truncal muscles by difficulty in rolling over in bed or sitting up from the supine position. Weakness of the arm muscles is related as difficulty in holding the arms overhead, lifting heavy objects, or using the hands for motor tasks. Weakness of the pelvic girdle and of the proximal lower extremity muscles is reflected by difficulty in rising from sitting or squatting, climbing stairs, stepping in or out of the bathtub. Weakness of the distal lower extremity may cause flopping of the feet or difficulty in rising on the toes.

OTHER SYMPTOMS. In evaluating *abnormal fatigability*, it is important to define the duration and intensity of exercise that provokes it. Even mild exercise can induce fatigue in patients with defects of neuromuscular transmission or with mitochondrial myopathies that involve an electron transport complex. Brief periods of intense, anaerobic exercise precipitate fatigue in patients with glycolytic enzyme defects, but sustained exercise is required to induce fatigue in carnitine palmityltransferase deficiency.

Muscle pain (myalgia) at rest can occur in some of the inflammatory myopathies (especially dermatomyositis), during acute viral infections, in polymyalgia rheumatica, myxedema, myotonic disorders, necrotizing vasculitis, during attacks of myoglobinuria, and in neuropathies associated with vitamin-B_1 deficiency, arsenic intoxication, and alcoholism. *Muscle pain during and after exercise* is experienced when the energy supply to muscle is restricted, as with defects in glycolysis or fatty acid oxidation, AMP deaminase deficiency, ischemia (as in intermittent claudication, scleroderma, and amyloidosis involving muscle), or in normal subjects after unusually strenuous exercise.

Muscle cramps last from seconds to minutes, are associated with high-frequency (up to 150 Hz) discharges of the motor units, can be initiated by strong contractions and stopped by stretching the muscle. They occur with dehydration, azotemia, hyponatremia, in partially denervated muscles, and sometimes in normal individuals without known cause.

Muscle contractures are electrically silent, last from a few to more than 30 minutes, occur only in patients with glycolytic enzyme defects, are provoked only by exercise, and involve only those muscles that had been exercised.

The facial and carpopedal spasms of *tetany* occur with hypocalcemia or hypomagnesemia and are associated with high-frequency (up to 300 Hz) axonal discharges. High-frequency electrical discharges also occur in muscle in the *stiff-man syndrome, neuromyotonia,* and *myotonia,* arising in the spinal cord, the peripheral nerves, and in the muscle fiber surface membrane, respectively.

In *myotonic disorders* mechanical or electrical stimuli applied to any region of the muscle fiber surface membrane elicit repetitive spike discharges that wax and wane in amplitude and frequency. Mechanical deformation of the membrane during contraction acts as positive feedback, again depolarizing the membrane. This electrical activity, which is independent of the anatomic arrangement of the fibers in the motor unit, causes tetanic contraction of the individual fibers. The symptoms are stiffness, difficulty in relaxing muscles after a strong contraction, being muscle-bound at the beginning of exercise, and improvement with continued exercise.

Myoglobinuria follows the excessive release of myoglobin from muscle during a period of rapid muscle fiber destruction (rhabdomyolysis). Weakness, muscle pain, and malaise are associated features.

The Clinical Examination. INSPECTION. This can reveal muscle atrophy, hypertrophy, contractures, winging of the scapulas, fasciculations (twitching of portions of muscles at rest caused by single contractions of motor units), myokymia (fine undulating movements of muscles associated with sustained abnormal motor-unit activity). The examiner also notes the patient's stance and gait, ability to walk on toes and heels, hop on one foot, and rise from sitting, squatting, or lying supine.

Inspection provides information on the distribution of weakness, which is then confirmed by detailed manual muscle testing. For example, weakness of the pelvic girdle muscles causes a waddling gait; if there is also weakness of the back extensor muscles, the gait is also lordotic with hyperextension of the upper torso. Muscle atrophy consistently predicts muscle weakness, but not all weak muscles are atrophic, and muscle atrophy can be masked by obesity. Muscle hypertrophy not from voluntary exercise is common in myotonia congenita; it also occurs in the course of Duchenne and Becker and—less commonly—of limb-girdle dystrophy. Hypertrophy may appear with chronic partial denervation, acid maltase deficiency, the permanent myopathy of periodic paralysis, myxedema, sarcoidosis, amyloidosis, and cysticercosis. The nonspecific term *pseudohypertrophy* refers to enlargement of a weak muscle.

MANUAL MUSCLE TESTING. This part of the examination requires knowledge of the origin, insertion, action, and innervation of the muscles tested, a consistent technique, and a generally accepted rating scale. A commonly used scale is that adopted by the British Medical Research Council: 5, normal power; 4, active movement against gravity and resistance; 3, active movement against gravity; 2, active movement with gravity eliminated; 1, trace contraction; 0, no contraction. Experienced examiners further differentiate among slight, mild, and moderate weakness within Grade 4. The results are recorded and used for following the patient's clinical course.

The distribution of the weakness can help in formulating the clinical diagnosis, as shown by the following examples. Weakness greater in proximal than distal muscles suggests a myopathy rather than a neuropathy. Predominantly distal muscle weakness suggests a neuropathy but can also occur in myotonic and other distal dystrophies and inclusion body myositis. Selective involvement of some muscles with sparing of others is more likely to occur in dystrophy than in inflammatory muscle disease, but it can also occur in such diverse entities as adult acid maltase deficiency, focal myositis, or the slow-channel myasthenic syndrome. The external-ocular and other cranial muscles can be affected by the Guillain-Barré syndrome, neuromuscular transmission defects, some mitochondrial myopathies, oculopharyngeal dystrophy, and myotubular myopathy. Diffuse, symmetrical weakness of multiple cranial muscles with ptosis but with sparing of the ocular movements suggests myotonic dystrophy. Motor neuron disease can affect the bulbar muscles but spares the external ocular muscles except rarely in terminal stages. Selective weakness of the triceps, wrist extensor, finger extensor, iliopsoas, hamstring, anterior tibial, and peroneal muscles, with relative sparing of other muscles, suggests upper motor neuron involvement.

OTHER FINDINGS. *Action myotonia* is observed as an inability to open the fist or the eyes promptly after closing them tightly for a few seconds. *Percussion myotonia* appears as a local postpercussion contraction followed by abnormally slow relaxation. It can best be observed in the tongue, deltoid, thenar, and extensor digitorum communis muscles. A local swelling appearing for a few seconds at the site of percussion is not myotonia but *myoedema*, seen in myxedema and emaciation.

The *deep tendon reflexes* are diminished in proportion to the weakness in most myopathies; an early loss of tendon reflexes is observed in neurogenic diseases of muscle, inclusion body myositis, the Lambert-Eaton myasthenic syndrome, and in a number of benign congenital myopathies. Slow relaxation of the reflexes is typical of myxedema.

A complete *examination of the nervous system* is also relevant to the evaluation of muscle weakness. Table 512–1 lists clinical guidelines that differentiate nerve from muscle disease. Peripheral neuropathy, ataxia, neurosensory hearing loss, myoclonus, fluctuating neurologic deficits, and mental deterioration can be associated with mitochondrial myopathies.

Recognition of the *signs or symptoms of an associated illness* can point to the cause of the myopathy. Examples are collagen-vascular diseases, sarcoidosis, amyloidosis, the endocrine myopathies, and the mitochondrial myopathies with multisystem involvement. *Involvement of organs or tissues other than muscle* provides further diagnostic clues. For example, cardiomyopathy can be associated with myotonic dystrophy, Emery-Dreifuss dystrophy, certain types of periodic paralysis, thymomatous myasthenia gravis, familial limb-girdle myasthenia, and late-onset nemaline myopathy. Cardiomyopathy and/or hepatic enlargement can occur in sarcoidosis and in the myopathies associated with deficiencies of acid maltase, debranching enzyme, carnitine, acyl-CoA dehydrogenase, and of a mitochondrial electron transport complex.

SERUM ENZYMES OF MUSCLE ORIGIN. The serum creatine kinase (CK) level is elevated in many muscle diseases. The enzyme is released into serum from injured skeletal or cardiac muscle. CK is a dimer of muscle-specific (M) and brain-specific (B) monomers, and the different CK isoenzymes can be distinguished by electrophoretic analysis. Mature muscle contains predominantly the MM isoenzyme, whereas in mature cardiac muscle the MB form predominates. Accordingly, abnormal CK release from muscle increases mostly the MM isoenzyme, whereas CK release from heart increases the MB form in serum. Injured muscle releases other enzymes, such as aldolase, lactate dehydrogenase, and aspartate aminotransferase, but the increases are less marked and can derive from other tissues, such as the liver and erythrocytes. The serum CK level is a sensitive index of muscle fiber injury in a myopathy; it also can increase slightly or modestly in motor neuron disease, chronic peripheral neuropathies, after severe voluntary exertion, or following a convulsion.

ELECTROMYOGRAPHY (EMG). This test consists of the analysis of spontaneous, evoked, and voluntarily generated potentials from nerve and muscle. The procedure is useful in distinguishing between broad categories of disease, such as myopathy versus neuropathy, or demyelinating versus axonal neuropathy. In some instances the types of electrical potentials and the pattern of abnormality suggest a disease category, such as an inflammatory myopathy, a myotonic disorder, or a storage myopathy. A progressive decrease of the amplitude of the compound muscle action potential evoked by low-frequency repetitive nerve stimulation (decremental response) is observed with defects of neuromuscular transmission. Se-

TABLE 512–1. CLINICAL CLUES DIFFERENTIATING MUSCLE FROM NERVE DISEASE

	Myopathy	Neuropathy-Neuronopathy
Distribution	Mainly proximal and symmetric	Distal if symmetric; nerve or root distribution if mono- or multi-focal
Atrophy	Late and mild	Early and prominent
Onset	Usually gradual	Often rapid
Fasciculations	Absent	Sometimes present
Reflexes	Lost late	Lost early
Tenderness	Diffuse in myositis	Focal in nerve or root disease
Cramps	Rare	Common
Sensory loss	Absent	Often present
Muscle enzymes	Usually elevated	Usually not or slightly elevated

quential assessment of an EMG abnormality can provide useful information of the distribution, degree of activity, and progression of a disease. For example, persistent fibrillation potentials in polymyositis reflect continuing disease activity; the decremental response can be used to monitor the course of myasthenia gravis; and alterations in nerve conduction velocities are a guide to the progression of peripheral neuropathies. Further details of the usefulness of EMG are given in Ch. 456.2, 505, and 518.

THE MUSCLE BIOPSY. Biopsy specimens are used for light microscopic, ultrastructural, and biochemical studies. In most instances, light microscopic observations with enzyme histochemical studies are sufficient for diagnosis.

Muscles showing mild to moderate weakness are biopsied. Strong muscles may not show diagnostic pathologic change, and in more severely affected muscles excessive amounts of connective tissue may obscure the basic pathologic process. Muscles that have been injected (as is often the case for the deltoid) or recently examined by EMG are unsuitable for diagnosis.

Light Microscopy. The following pathologic alterations can be recognized in conventional paraffin sections of muscle: excessive variation in muscle fiber diameter; isolated or grouped atrophic fibers; target formations; increase in the number of internally located nuclei; focal loss of cross striations; loss of myofibrillar markings; cytoplasmic inclusions; vacuolar change; fiber necrosis and phagocytosis; inflammatory exudates; invasion of non-necrotic fibers by mononuclear cells; regenerating fibers; ring fibers (caused by aberrant myofibrils); and proliferation of connective tissue elements. Histochemical studies of fresh-frozen sections reveal the dimensions of the muscle fibers in the native state; the distribution and abundance of mitochondria, lipid, and glycogen in the muscle fibers; myofibrillar integrity; increased lysosomal activity; the presence or absence of certain enzymes (phosphorylase, phosphofructokinase, cytochrome c oxidase, AMP deaminase); the histochemical profiles of the muscle fibers; and the distribution of the histochemical fiber types.

Neurogenic alterations in muscle consist of the appearance of atrophic fibers, singly or in groups of varying size; target formations; and grouping of histochemical fiber types caused by reinnervation of previously denervated fibers by collateral nerve sprouts. Central nuclei, loss of cross striations, and hypertrophy and degeneration of nondenervated fibers also can occur in partially denervated muscle. Further details of muscle biopsy changes can be found in Dubowitz's monograph on the subject.

Electron Microscopy. This is primarily a research tool used in studying previously unrecognized syndromes, diseases of neuromuscular transmission, or in analyzing mechanisms of muscle fiber injury. However, in some instances electron microscopy does have a role in diagnosis (e.g., in identifying the filamentous inclusions in inclusion body myositis or in revealing capillary microtubular inclusions and necrosis in dermatomyositis when inflammation and perifascicular atrophy are absent).

Biochemical Studies. These are essential for defining the biochemical basis of those metabolic myopathies in which the clinical or histologic data suggest a defect in carbohydrate, lipid, or mitochondrial metabolism. The direct measurement of the glycogen and carnitine content of muscle, assays of enzymes associated with glycolysis or fatty acid oxidation, determination of various aspects of mitochondrial respiration, and analysis of cytochrome spectra are examples of biochemical procedures currently used in the diagnosis of metabolic myopathies.

Dubowitz V: Muscle Biopsy: A Practical Approach. Philadelphia, Baillière Tindall, 1985. *A well-illustrated guide to the processing and interpretation of the muscle biopsy specimen.*

Engel AG, Banker BQ (eds.): Myology. New York, McGraw-Hill Book Company, 1986. *A multiauthored book on the anatomy, physiology, and biochemistry of skeletal muscle, the approach to muscle diseases, and the clinical aspects of muscle diseases.*
Walton J (ed.): Disorders of Voluntary Muscle. 4th ed. New York, Churchill-Livingstone, 1981. *A popular, multiauthored book with excellent chapters on the basic science and clinical aspects of muscle diseases.*

513 MUSCULAR DYSTROPHIES

DEFINITION AND BASIC CONCEPTS. Muscular dystrophies are inherited myopathies of unknown etiology associated with progressive muscle weakness, destruction and regeneration of the muscle fibers, and eventual replacement of the muscle fibers by fibrous and fatty connective tissue. There is no accumulation of metabolic storage material in the muscle fibers. The possibility of an abnormal neural or vascular influence on the muscle fibers is still debated. Ultrastructural studies in Duchenne dystrophy indicate that breakdown of the muscle fiber plasma membrane is an early and possibly an initial abnormality in the course of muscle fiber destruction. This results in the influx of calcium-rich extracellular fluid and complement components into the fiber, activation of intracellular proteases and complement, and, eventually, removal of the necrotic fiber by macrophages. It is not yet known whether similar membrane lesions initiate muscle fiber destruction in the other dystrophies. Recognition of the molecular basis of the dystrophies awaits the identification of the primary product of the dystrophic genes.

The current classification of the muscular dystrophies is based on the mode of inheritance, age of onset and rate of progression, distribution of the involved muscles, and associated findings in muscle or other organs. This is not entirely satisfactory because some cases cannot be fitted into currently recognized groups, and some dystrophies, such as the limb-girdle, distal, and facioscapulohumeral types, are heterogeneous by clinical, pathologic, or genetic criteria. A classification of the muscular dystrophies based on the categories used by Gardner-Medwin (1980) is shown in Table 513–1. A more precise classification awaits the chromosomal assignment and mapping of the loci of dystrophic genes (thus far accomplished only in Duchenne, Becker, and myotonic dystrophy) and the availability of probes that can identify the presence of a given dystrophic gene in a given patient.

DUCHENNE DYSTROPHY. This is a lethal, X-linked recessive disorder of childhood. The abnormal gene is positioned on band Xp21 of the X chromosome. The incidence is close to 1 in 3300 male births; the mutation rate is about 1 in 10,000. The disease is present at birth, becomes symptomatic during early childhood, leads to failure of ambulation near the end of the first decade, and terminates fatally near the end of the second decade. Early symptoms are developmental delays, difficulty in running or climbing stairs, frequent falls, and enlargement of the calves. Initially the weakness is more proximal than distal. Except for the sternocleidomastoids, the cranial muscles and the external anal sphincter are spared. The proximal deep tendon reflexes disappear in about half the cases by the age of ten. Joint contractures, caused by uneven weakness of agonist and antagonist muscles, appear in the majority of patients between six and ten years of age. After ambulation is lost, all muscles decrease in size and paraspinal muscle weakness causes progressive kyphoscoliosis. Weakness of the respiratory muscles can be detected after the age of ten, but the diaphragm is relatively spared. Carbon dioxide retention and anoxemia occur terminally with respiratory infections. Pure respiratory failure without infec-

TABLE 513–1. CLASSIFICATION OF THE MUSCULAR DYSTROPHIES

X-linked Recessive Dystrophies
  Duchenne dystrophy
  Becker dystrophy
  Emery-Dreifuss dystrophy with joint contractures and atrial paralysis
    ? Scapuloperoneal syndrome variant
    ? Rigid-spine syndrome variant
Autosomal-recessive Dystrophies
  Autosomal-recessive childhood (limb-girdle) muscular dystrophy
  Scapulohumeral (limb-girdle) muscular dystrophy
  Autosomal-recessive distal muscular dystrophy
    With necrotizing features
    With rimmed vacuoles
  Congenital muscular dystrophy
    Without cerebral abnormalities*
    Fukuyama type with cerebral abnormalities
  ? Autosomal-recessive rigid-spine syndrome
Autosomal-dominant Dystrophies
  Facioscapulohumeral dystrophy
    With inflammatory changes in muscle
    With cochlear hearing loss and retinal telangiectasis
  Autosomal-dominant scapuloperoneal dystrophy (? related to
    facioscapulohumeral dystrophy)
  Dominantly inherited adult-onset limb-girdle dystrophy*†
  Oculopharyngeal dystrophy
  Myotonic dystrophy
  Autosomal-dominant distal dystrophy
    With onset in upper limbs (Welander type)
    With onset in lower limbs

*Variable clinical phenotypes suggest genetic heterogeneity.
†X-linked dominant form may also exist.

tion can also occur and is an irreversible terminal event. The heart is affected with scarring of the posterobasal portion of the left ventricle, producing tall right precordial R waves and deep left precordial Q waves in the electrocardiogram in 90 per cent of the patients. Clinically significant cardiomyopathy is uncommon and in only 10 per cent of cases is death related to cardiac dysfunction. Central nervous system involvement is indicated by lower than average intelligence and mild cerebral atrophy.

Infrequently, Duchenne dystrophy manifests in females who have Turner's (XO) or Turner's mosaic (X/XX or X/XX/XXX) syndrome, a structurally abnormal X chromosome, or an X-autosomal translocation. In a few female heterozygotes, the disease manifests because of incomplete inactivation of the maternal X chromosome.

BECKER DYSTROPHY. This is also an X-linked recessive disorder with an incidence of about 1 per 20,000 male births. The Becker and Duchenne genes have similar positions and may be alleles for the same locus, on the X chromosome. The manifestations of the two diseases are also similar, but Becker dystrophy begins later and evolves more slowly. In Becker dystrophy the mean ages for onset of symptoms, becoming chair-bound, and death are 12, 30, and 42 years, respectively. All patients show marked enlargement of the calves until the terminal stage. The serum creatine kinase (CK) level is markedly elevated in preclinical and clinical stages of the disease but begins to decline after the age of 20. Contractures develop at the wheelchair stage. Only some patients show electrocardiographic abnormalities, and only a minority are mentally retarded. The disease usually can be distinguished from Duchenne dystrophy by its more benign course, but it cannot be reliably distinguished from a limb-girdle dystrophy without evidence of X-linked inheritance.

X-LINKED MUSCULAR DYSTROPHY WITH EARLY JOINT CONTRACTURES AND CARDIOMYOPATHY (EMERY-DREIFUSS DYSTROPHY). The disease presents in childhood, progresses slowly, and involves distal or proximal muscles in the lower extremities and proximal muscles in the upper extremities. There is no muscle hypertrophy. The serum CK is moderately elevated. Contractures of the knees, elbows, and cervical and dorsolumbar spine appear early in the disease. Atrial conduction defects and paralysis, requiring treatment by pacemaker, appear later. The disorder has been

referred to as Emery-Dreifuss dystrophy and as X-linked scapuloperoneal myopathy, the distinction depending only on whether the proximal or distal muscles are affected in the lower limbs. The lack of muscle hypertrophy, early contractures, slow progression, relatively low serum CK, and overt cardiac involvement distinguish this disease from Duchenne dystrophy; all these features but the slow progression differentiate it from Becker dystrophy. When cardiomyopathy cannot be detected or the pedigree of X-linked inheritance is not established, the disease can be difficult to distinguish from the rigid-spine syndrome or other heterogeneous scapuloperoneal syndromes.

LIMB-GIRDLE SYNDROMES. The term *limb-girdle dystrophy* was applied by Walton and Nattrass in 1954 to a group of 18 patients (11 males and 7 females). The shoulder girdle was first affected in 13 cases (Erb type) and the pelvic girdle in 5 (Leyden-Möbius type). The face was spared. The onset was in the second decade in 7 patients and later in the others. Severe disability appeared over the next 20 years. An autosomal-recessive inheritance was postulated, though in one family the inheritance appeared to be autosomal dominant. Subsequently, a number of incompletely defined disorders were called limb-girdle dystrophy. The following diseases now appear to be reasonably distinct entities.

Childhood Muscular Dystrophy of Autosomal-Recessive Inheritance. This disease presents in the first or second decade, progresses slowly, and involves pelvic and pectoral girdle muscles without muscle hypertrophy. The serum CK level is moderately elevated (up to tenfold). Ambulation is lost near the end of the second decade. Cardiac abnormalities are absent. More severe variants, with muscle hypertrophy and death before the age of 20, have been described in inbred Amish and Tunisian kinships.

Scapulohumeral Muscular Dystrophy of Autosomal-Recessive Inheritance. Phenotypically this entity resembles that described by Erb in 1884. The onset is usually in the second decade. The shoulder girdle is initially affected; weakness then slowly extends to the pelvic girdle and to distal limb muscles. Facial muscles are spared. There is no muscle hypertrophy. The serum CK is moderately elevated at the onset but decreases with progression of the disease.

Adult-Onset Limb-Girdle Dystrophy of Dominant Inheritance. This is a rare condition with onset from the second through the sixth decade of life. It begins proximally and remains restricted to limb-girdle muscles. The serum CK level is normal or elevated. In some families there are rimmed vacuoles in the muscle fibers. In some kindreds the expression of the disease is restricted to either males or to females. Thus, this disease is also heterogeneous.

The Differential Diagnosis of Limb-Girdle Syndromes. All patients with limb-girdle syndromes need to be further investigated by EMG and muscle biopsy. Only a minority have a pedigree consistent with autosomal-recessive or -dominant inheritance and can be fitted into one of the above clinically distinct syndromes. The differential diagnosis in these patients includes inherited metabolic myopathies (e.g., acid maltase deficiency or a lipid storage myopathy); morphologically distinct congenital myopathies or their late-onset variants (e.g., nemaline, central core, and myotubular myopathies); or progressive muscular atrophy. In sporadic cases of a limb-girdle syndrome the differential diagnosis includes the same diseases, and also inflammatory myopathies (polymyositis, inclusion body myositis, or sarcoidosis confined to muscle), endocrine myopathies, sporadic Duchenne dystrophy, Duchenne dystrophy manifesting in female carriers, sporadic Becker dystrophy, and sporadic Emery-Dreifuss dystrophy before the appearance of joint contractures or cardiomyopathy.

FACIOSCAPULOHUMERAL DYSTROPHY. The inheritance is autosomal dominant with high penetrance and variable expression. The disease presents in childhood or adult life. It involves the facial muscles early and then descends to the scapular fixators, the muscles of the upper arm, and the anterior leg muscles. Characteristic early physical signs include failure to bury the eyelashes, an expressionless face, pouting lips, winging (upward and forward displacement) of the scapulas when the arms are raised, and an inward-sloping anterior axillary fold. The rate of progression and the extent to which pelvic girdle, forearm, and lower torso muscles are eventually affected vary considerably from family to family and sometimes even within a family. There is no muscle hypertrophy; joint contractures are uncommon; and the serum CK level is normal or shows mild elevation. A number of variants have been described. In some families a conspicuous inflammatory reaction appears in affected muscles, but the course of the illness is unaltered by corticosteroid therapy. In other families an associated sensorineural hearing loss occurs, with or without retinal telangiectasis and progressive painless blindness (Coats syndrome). The differential diagnosis includes progressive muscular atrophy, congenital myopathies (e.g., nemaline, central core, and myotubular myopathy), mitochondrial myopathies, sporadic cases of Emery-Dreifuss dystrophy before the appearance of joint contractures or cardiomyopathy, the scapuloperoneal syndrome, the slow-channel myasthenic syndrome, and polymyositis.

MYOTONIC DYSTROPHY. Transmission is by dominant inheritance with high penetrance and variable expressivity. The gene resides on chromosome 19 and shows linkage to the gene encoding complement C3. The incidence is about 1 in 7500 births. A typical distribution of the weakness, myotonia, and multisystem abnormalities characterizes the disease.

Myotonic dystrophy presents in childhood or adult life; the mean age at onset is 19 years. Myotonic symptoms either precede or accompany the muscle weakness. As the disease evolves, the myotonia diminishes in those muscles severely affected by the dystrophic process. Distal limb, levator palpebrae, masticatory, facial, cervical, pharyngeal, laryngeal, and upper esophagus muscles are commonly affected. External ophthalmoplegia is rare. Weakness can also appear in the proximal limb and respiratory muscles. The latter, when severe, results in alveolar hypoventilation, hypercapnia, arterial oxygen unsaturation, and increasing somnolence. Action myotonia is commonly observed in facial, lid elevator, and hand muscles; percussion myotonia is usually found in tongue, thenar, finger extensor, and selected proximal limb muscles.

A congenital form of myotonic dystrophy can occur in infants born to affected mothers. The onset is at birth with hypotonia, respiratory distress, and cranial muscle weakness. Myotonic phenomena, absent at birth, appear later in childhood. Motor development is delayed and mental retardation common.

Myotonic dystrophy produces systemic abnormalities including frontal baldness, subcapsular cataracts, testicular atrophy and ovarian dysfunction in adult life, extrathyroidal hypometabolism, end-organ unresponsiveness to insulin, mental changes, and hypercatabolism of IgG. Cardiac conduction defects are common and can cause sudden death. Gastrointestinal smooth muscle involvement results in reduced lower esophageal and gastric motility and dilatation of segments of the colon. Some patients have bouts of diarrhea alternating with constipation and colicky abdominal pain. Less frequent manifestations are pigmentary retinal degeneration and cranial anomalies (hyperostosis cranii, small sella turcica, large paranasal sinuses, and prognathism).

The pathologic alterations in the affected muscles are relatively distinct. These consist of very large muscle fibers with numerous central nuclei, sarcoplasmic masses, ring fibers, and variable type 1 fiber atrophy. Necrotic fibers are uncommon, which may explain why the serum CK level is normal or only slightly elevated.

DISTAL DYSTROPHIES. A number of genetically distinct entities has been recognized. An *autosomal dominant type*, initially described in a large Scandinavian kinship by Welander, presents between the fourth and sixth decades with selective weakness and atrophy of the forearm extensor and intrinsic hand muscles and then involves the anterior leg and small foot muscles. In patients homozygous for the dominant gene, the onset is earlier and proximal muscles are also affected. In other non-Scandinavian kinships with late onset and dominant inheritance, the disease first involves the lower extremities. The serum CK level is normal or slightly increased. Two varieties of *autosomal recessive distal muscular dystrophies* have been described. In both there is a juvenile onset and the lower limbs are affected before the upper. In one type there is frequent fiber necrosis and regeneration and the serum CK level is markedly increased. In the other type the muscle fibers harbor rimmed vacuoles and the serum CK level is only slightly increased.

The differential diagnosis of the distal muscular dystrophies includes myotonic dystrophy, inclusion body myositis, debranching enzyme deficiency, distal mitochondrial myopathy, distal chronic spinal muscular atrophy, and the neuronal form of peroneal muscular atrophy.

OCULOPHARYNGEAL MUSCULAR DYSTROPHY. The disease, inherited as an autosomal dominant, presents in the fifth or sixth decade with progressive ptosis and dysphagia. Later, all external ocular and other voluntary muscles may become affected. Death usually results from starvation or aspiration pneumonia. The serum CK level is normal or slightly increased. Muscle biopsy discloses intranuclear tubular filaments and rimmed vacuoles in the muscle fibers. This syndrome needs to be distinguished from mitochondrial myopathies that involve the external ocular muscles with or without affecting facial and limb muscles, and with or without multisystem features. In the mitochondrial myopathies, as discussed below, the age of onset and mode of inheritance are variable, and the muscle biopsy displays ragged red fibers.

SCAPULOPERONEAL SYNDROMES. These are heterogeneous disorders identified by the distribution of the affected muscles. An X-linked recessive form of scapuloperoneal myopathy with early joint contractures which also involves the spine and produces late cardiac atrial paralysis is essentially identical with Emery-Dreifuss dystrophy. An autosomal-dominant scapuloperoneal myopathy resembles facioscapulohumeral dystrophy except that the face is spared. Other autosomal-dominant forms of the scapuloperoneal syndrome are associated with chronic anterior horn cell disease (Stark-Kaeser syndrome) or with a hypertrophic sensorimotor neuropathy (Davidenkow syndrome).

THE RIGID-SPINE SYNDROME. This is also a heterogeneous disorder in which muscle contractures involve the spine as well as other joints. The X-linked recessive form with cardiomyopathy and scapuloperoneal weakness appears to be identical with Emery-Dreifuss dystrophy. An autosomal dominant form presenting with proximal muscle weakness in the first decade is also recognized. In most cases the disease is sporadic, begins in the first decade, and results in widespread muscle weakness and atrophy during the second decade.

CONGENITAL DYSTROPHIES. These present at birth with weakness and hypotonia, with or without multiple joint contractures. Most cases are sporadic; in some families several siblings are affected, suggesting autosomal-recessive inheritance. The weakness involves limb, torso, cervical, and sometimes the facial muscles. The serum CK level is normal or elevated. The subsequent course is one of slow or rapid progression, or the weakness increases only slightly during early childhood and then remains unchanged. The differential diagnosis includes Duchenne or autosomal-recessive limb-girdle dystrophy presenting at birth, morphologically distinct congenital myopathies, and acute infantile spinal muscular atrophy. The Fukuyama form of congenital dystrophy is associated with mental retardation, seizures, developmental abnormalities in the central nervous system, a progressive course, and death by the age of 10. The inheritance is autosomal recessive.

TREATMENT OF THE MUSCULAR DYSTROPHIES. There is no specific treatment of any of the muscular dystrophies. Physical therapy to prevent contractures, orthoses, and corrective orthopedic surgery can be used to improve the quality of life in some stages. The cardiac conduction defects in Emery-Dreifuss dystrophy and myotonic dystrophy may require treatment by pacemaker. The myotonia in myotonic dystrophy is rarely a clinical problem but can be treated with phenytoin (0.3 to 0.6 gram daily) or by quinine (0.3 to 1.5 grams daily).

Preventive treatment consists of prenatal diagnosis in families with known pedigrees, carrier detection, and genetic counseling. Cloned DNA sequences are now available for linkage analysis with the Duchenne locus and provide a powerful tool for carrier detection and prenatal diagnosis in families in which identified carriers are available for study. More importantly, a segment of the Duchenne gene has now been cloned, and cloning of the entire gene is in sight. When accomplished, this will provide reliable probes for identification of carriers, fetuses at risk, and sporadic male or female cases.

Chutkow JG, Heffner RR, Kramer AA, et al.: Adult-onset autosomal dominant limb-girdle muscular dystrophy. Ann Neurol 20:240, 1986. *A careful study of a dominant variety of limb-girdle dystrophy.*

Engel AG, Banker BQ (eds.): Myology. New York, McGraw-Hill Book Company, 1986. *An excellent, comprehensive description of the muscular dystrophies authored by multiple experts.*

Gardner-Medwin D: Clinical features and classification of the muscular dystrophies. Br Med Bull 36:109, 1980. *A revision of the classification proposed by Walton and Nattrass. Also contains concise and accurate summaries of the major clinical features of the different muscular dystrophies.*

Harper PS: Myotonic Dystrophy. Philadelphia, W.B. Saunders Company, 1979. *A modern classic—thorough in coverage, thoughtful in analysis, and written in a lively style.*

Miyoshi K, Kawai H, Iwasa M, et al.: Autosomal-recessive distal muscular dystrophy as a new type of progressive muscular dystrophy. Brain 109:31, 1986. *A well-documented study and a good review of the different types of distal muscular dystrophies.*

Monaco AP, Neve RL, Coletti-Feener C, et al.: Isolation of candidate cDNAs for portions of the Duchenne muscular dystrophy gene. Nature 323:646, 1986. *Provides the first glimpse of the Duchenne gene. An important step on the road to preventing the disease and identifying its molecular basis.*

Walton JN, Nattrass FJ: On the classification, natural history and treatment of the myopathies. Brain 77:169, 1954. *Presents a classification of muscular dystrophies based on a clinical survey of 105 personal cases. With minor modifications, the classification is still generally accepted.*

514 MORPHOLOGICALLY DISTINCT CONGENITAL MYOPATHIES

DEFINITIONS AND BASIC CONCEPTS. The diseases in this group are characterized by the following features:

• The course is nonprogressive or relatively nonprogressive. The prognosis is generally benign except in reducing body myopathy and in the X-linked form of myotubular myopathy.

• A distinct pattern of inheritance is observed in some diseases (e.g., central core disease, nemaline myopathy); others are genetically heterogeneous (e.g., myotubular myopathy).

• Muscle weakness is present at birth or appears in early childhood. It is proximal or diffuse and may or may not involve the cranial muscles.

• The muscle bulk is normal or reduced. There is no muscle hypertrophy.

• The deep tendon reflexes are reduced or absent in most cases.

• Skeletal abnormalities related to the weakness, such as a high-arched palate, kyphoscoliosis, dislocated hips, and pes cavus, are common.

• The serum CK level is normal, except in some older patients with myotubular or sarcotubular myopathy.

• The EMG is normal or suggests a myopathy. Spontaneous electrical activity is absent in all cases, except for fibrillation potentials and myotonic discharges in some cases of myotubular myopathy.

• Each disease has one or more distinguishing, but not specific, morphologic features. Type I fiber preponderance and small type I fibers occur in most disorders.

Central Core Disease. The disease is transmitted by autosomal-dominant inheritance. The cranial muscles are usually not affected. The core formations can be central or peripheral, extend through the length of the fiber, are devoid of mitochondria, and may show focal myofibrillar degeneration. T-tubules, SR profiles, and glycogen are decreased in the cores.

Nemaline (Rod) Myopathy. An autosomal-dominant inheritance with variable expressivity has been demonstrated in some families. Facial, masticatory, oropharyngeal, neck flexor, respiratory, and proximal and distal limb muscles are typically affected. An oval face, micrognathia, and malocclusion are common. The disease is most severe in the first few years of life because of feeding difficulty and respiratory infections. Subsequently, some increase in strength takes place, and the clinical course remains stable. The nemaline bodies represent a replicative anomaly of the Z disk.

Myotubular (Centronuclear) Myopathy. X-linked recessive, autosomal-recessive, and autosomal-dominant forms of the disease have been described. The X-linked type is associated with severe respiratory muscle weakness and leads to death in early infancy. The autosomal-dominant form is relatively mild and may not present until adult life. External ocular, facial, oropharyngeal, and neck muscles are often affected. In each disorder the muscle fibers contain rows of central nuclei surrounded by cytoplasmic material, reminiscent of maturing myotubes. Type I fiber atrophy and type II fiber hypertrophy are common associated features.

Multicore Disease. The onset occurs in the first few months of life. Weakness is greater in proximal than distal muscles and in the upper than lower extremities. Ptosis as well as weakness of external ocular, facial, and neck muscles can occur. The inheritance is autosomal recessive with rare families manifesting heterozygotes or autosomal dominant with marked variation in penetrance. Individual muscle fibers contain myriad small core formations devoid of mitochondria.

Congenital Fiber Type Disproportion. The disease may occur in successive generations, suggesting an autosomal-dominant inheritance. Weakness is usually present at birth and tends to improve after the age of two years. Muscle contractures, skeletal deformities, and short stature are common. There is type I fiber atrophy and type II fiber hypertrophy with or without type I fiber predominance.

Other Morphologically Distinct Congenital Diseases. These less frequently encountered entities are identified by their morphologic abnormalities in muscle: fingerprint body myopathy, sarcotubular myopathy, reducing body myopathy, trilaminar myopathy, myopathy with focal lysis of the myofibrils in type I fibers, and spheroid body myopathy.

Late-Onset Variants. Adult-onset cases of central core disease, nemaline myopathy, myotubular myopathy, and multicore disease also exist. In some of these cases mild disease probably has been present since birth but is recognized only after additional progression in adult life or when discovery of an affected younger relative prompts investigation of other family members.

Two other forms of late-onset nemaline myopathy are noteworthy. One is sporadic, evolves subacutely or chronically, affects the proximal limb and torso but not the cranial muscles, and may cause death from respiratory failure. The CK level is normal. In some cases there is an associated monoclonal gammopathy. The EMG shows myopathic changes and fibrillation potentials. Histologically, there is progressive accumulation of nemaline rods and progressive atrophy of rod-containing fibers. Another late-onset form occurs in a familial setting, is associated with cardiomyopathy, and can result in sudden death.

Banker, BQ: The congenital myopathies. In Engel AG, Banker BQ (eds.): Myology. New York, McGraw-Hill Book Company, 1986, pp 1527–1581. *A comprehensive, well-illustrated review. It raises numerous unanswered questions about etiology and nosology.*

515 INFLAMMATORY MYOPATHIES

DEFINITION AND CLASSIFICATION. Inflammatory myopathies represent a heterogeneous group of disorders. Most inflammatory myopathies are diffuse in distribution, but some are focal, affecting circumscribed regions in single or multiple muscles. Some are caused by bacterial, parasitic, or viral infections. In most other inflammatory myopathies the etiology is undetermined, but an autoimmune etiology is suspected, and in inclusion body myositis both an autoimmune and a viral etiology have been postulated. A classification of the inflammatory myopathies is shown in Table 515–1. This section focuses on selected aspects of the idiopathic inflammatory myopathies not covered in other chapters.

Autoimmunity in Idiopathic Inflammatory Myopathies. An autoimmune etiology in inflammatory myopathies has been inferred from one or more of the following observations: (1) The myopathy is associated with another identifiable autoimmune disease (e.g., systemic lupus erythematosus or rheumatoid arthritis). (2) Laboratory tests suggest an altered immune state (e.g., increased serum gamma globulins,

TABLE 515–1. CLASSIFICATION OF INFLAMMATORY MYOPATHIES*

Infections
Parasitic: toxoplasmosis, sarcosporidiosis, African trypanosomiasis, American trypanosomiasis, cysticercosis (*Taenia solium*), trichinellosis
Bacterial: pyomyositis, septic myositis, gas gangrene (*Clostridium welchii*), leprous myositis
Viral: acute myositis following influenza or other viral infections

Idiopathic, Autoimmune Origin Suspected
Pure polymyositis
Dermatomyositis
Inclusion body myositis
Scleroderma involving muscle
Inflammatory myopathy associated with another autoimmune disease (systemic lupus erythematosus; rheumatoid arthritis; Sjögren's syndrome; rheumatic fever; overlap syndromes; chronic graft-versus-host disease; polyarteritis nodosa)
Sarcoidosis involving muscle
Inflammatory myopathies with eosinophilia
  Eosinophilic polymyositis
  Localized eosinophilic myositis
  Eosinophilic perimyositis
  Diffuse fasciitis with eosinophilia
Focal myositis
  Focal proliferative myositis
  Localized nodular myositis
    Pseudothrombophlebitis of a calf muscle
  Orbital myositis
Polymyalgia rheumatica†

Other Inflammatory Myopathies
Localized myositis ossificans
Generalized myositis ossificans

*Adapted from Walton J (ed.): Disorders of Voluntary Muscle. Edinburgh, Churchill Livingstone, 1981.

†There are no inflammatory changes in muscle.

decreased total hemolytic complement in serum, and positive tests for antibodies against native DNA, other nuclear factors, or rheumatoid factor). (3) There is a predominantly mononuclear inflammatory exudate in muscle. (4) There is evidence of focal invasion and destruction of muscle fibers by antigen-specific cytotoxic T cells. (5) The diseases are responsive to corticosteroids or other immunosuppressants. The first criterion, if fulfilled, represents strong, but indirect, evidence for an autoimmune origin of the myopathy. Without a recognizable associated autoimmune disease, only the other criteria can be applied, and these may not suffice. Laboratory tests suggesting an altered immune state are usually negative in dermatomyositis and in polymyositis not associated with another autoimmune disease (i.e., "pure polymyositis"). A mononuclear inflammatory exudate also can occur in some genetically determined muscle diseases (e.g., Duchenne or facioscapulohumeral dystrophy). Inclusion body myositis, in which an inflammatory exudate is often prominent, is usually refractory to immunosuppressants; most cases of scleroderma and some cases of pure polymyositis and dermatomyositis also do not respond to immunosuppressants. Further, neither the factors that initiate self-sensitization nor the sensitizing antigen have been defined in any of the major inflammatory myopathies (idiopathic polymyositis, inclusion body myositis, dermatomyositis, and scleroderma). None has been transferred to an experimental animal.

Inclusion Body Myositis. This entity differs from the other idiopathic inflammatory myopathies in several respects. Clinically, it is not usually associated with another autoimmune disease, and it fails to respond to corticosteroids or other immunosuppressants. Most patients are older than 50, and there is male predominance. The disease evolves slowly, affecting the lower limbs first, involving both proximal and distal muscles, and resulting in selectively severe weakness and atrophy of the quadriceps. Facial, cervical, and pharyngeal muscles are spared. There is an early loss of deep tendon reflexes from the affected limbs. The serum CK level is mildly elevated or normal. The EMG indicates myopathic changes and abnormal electrical irritability, as in dermatomyositis or polymyositis, but there may be additional neurogenic features, such as an increase in the amplitude of motor unit potentials or mild slowing of nerve conduction velocities. Affected muscles show a typical pattern of histologic change: rimmed vacuoles in a significant proportion of the fibers; eosinophilic intranuclear and cytoplasmic inclusions in a few fibers; small groups of atrophic fibers without type grouping; and an endomysial and a lesser perivascular inflammatory exudate. The exudate is enriched in cytotoxic T cells that focally surround, invade, and destroy non-necrotic fibers. Necrotic fibers also occur but are less common than in polymyositis. Ultrastructural studies show that the rimmed vacuoles contain myeloid structures and other cytoplasmic degradation products and that the inclusions consist of microtubular filaments resembling paramyxovirus nucleocapsids. According to recent observations by Chou, the inclusions immunoreact with mumps virus antigens. The differential diagnosis of inclusion body myositis includes motor neuron disease, distal and other muscular dystrophies, peripheral neuropathies, and pure polymyositis. The diagnosis is usually clarified by a careful study of the muscle biopsy.

Differences Between Dermatomyositis and Pure Polymyositis. Dermatomyositis and pure polymyositis resemble each other in the predominantly proximal distribution of the muscle weakness, a mononuclear inflammatory exudate in muscle, myopathic changes and spontaneous electrical activity in the EMG, and responsiveness to corticosteroid therapy. Consequently, they are often treated as a single entity in evaluating their etiology, natural history, and therapy. However, several aspects of dermatomyositis differentiate it from pure polymyositis: (1) The characteristic rash of dermatomyositis is lacking in pure polymyositis. (2) Capillary injury and necrosis are constant findings in dermatomyositis. Many of the injured capillaries react for the membrane attack complex of complement whereas other vessels are found to be occluded by platelet thrombi or to harbor microtubular inclusions. (3) Muscle fibers at the periphery of the fascicles undergo selective degeneration and atrophy. (4) The inflammatory exudate is concentrated at perimysial and perivascular sites and is enriched in B cells and helper T cells. (5) There is no evidence for T-cell mediated cytotoxicity directed against the muscle fibers. These findings suggest that a humoral response against vascular elements plays an important role in the pathogenesis of dermatomyositis.

By contrast, in pure polymyositis there is no capillary necrosis or loss. The inflammatory exudate contains fewer B cells and helper T cells than in dermatomyositis, and B cells are virtually absent from the endomysium. There are focal invasion and destruction of non-necrotic muscle fibers by antigen-specific cytotoxic T cells accompanied by macrophages indicating cell-mediated cytotoxicity directed against the muscle fiber. Necrosis of isolated fibers also occurs. These findings suggest that a component of the muscle fiber surface membrane is a target of the immune effector response.

Differences Between Scleroderma and the Other Major Inflammatory Myopathies. In scleroderma, the serum CK level is either normal or only slightly elevated, spontaneous electrical activity is often absent from the EMG, and necrotic fibers are uncommon. The pathologic changes are those of fibrosis and inflammation involving the perimysium and the perimysial blood vessels. The inflammatory cells at these sites are predominantly T cells and macrophages. The findings suggest a cell-mediated immune response against a perimysial and/or vascular component in muscle.

Myositis Ossificans. The *localized form* appears as a tender swelling after trauma to a muscle. After a few months this becomes hard and ossified. Therapy consists of excision. The *generalized form* represents an autosomal-dominant disease with variable expressivity that begins in childhood, involves many muscles, and causes progressive rigidity of body parts. The initial lesions appear in fascia and dermis and are associated with inflammation, local hemorrhage, and connective tissue proliferation. Cartilage and bone formation occur at a later stage. Other congenital malformations (microdactyly of the great toe, exostoses, absence of upper incisors or of ear lobules, and hypogenitalism) are found in most patients. There is no effective therapy.

Banker BQ: Other inflammatory myopathies. In Engel AG, Banker BQ (eds.): Myology. New York, McGraw-Hill Book Company, 1986, pp 1501–1524. *A well-illustrated review of the myopathies associated with eosinophilia, focal myositis, orbital myositis, and myositis ossificans.*

Banker BQ, Engel AG: The polymyositis and dermatomyositis syndromes. In Engel AG, Banker BQ (eds.): Myology. New York, McGraw-Hill Book Company, 1986, pp 1385–1422. *A well-illustrated review. Presents arguments for viewing the two syndromes as distinct entities.*

Chou SM: Inclusion body myositis. A chronic persistent mumps myositis? Hum Pathol 17:765, 1986. *An excellent review of the clinical and pathologic aspects of the disease. The author shows immunolocalization of the mumps virus antigen in the inclusions.*

Engel AG, Arahata K: Mononuclear cells in myopathies: Quantitation of functionally distinct subsets, recognition of antigen-specific cell mediated cytotoxicity in some diseases, and implications for the pathogenesis of the different inflammatory myopathies. Hum Pathol 17:704, 1986. *Describes antigen-specific T-cell–mediated cytotoxicity against the muscle fiber in polymyositis and inclusion body myositis, but not in dermatomyositis or scleroderma.*

Mastaglia FL, Ojeda VJ: Inflammatory myopathies. Parts I and II. Ann Neurol 17:215; 317, 1985. *A comprehensive survey of the inflammatory myopathies. More than 200 references are cited.*

516 METABOLIC MYOPATHIES

GLYCOGEN STORAGE DISEASES. These are described in detail in Ch. 179. When muscle is involved, glycogen-filled vacuoles appear in the fibers; the glycogen excess can vary from slight to marked, and definitive diagnosis requires demonstration of a specific enzyme deficiency. Of the several glycogenoses, only glucose-6-phosphate dehydrogenase and liver phosphorylase deficiencies fail to affect muscle. All glycogenoses that affect muscle are transmitted as autosomal-recessive traits except phosphoglycerate kinase deficiency, which is X-linked recessive.

Acid Alpha-1,4-Glucosidase (Lysosomal Acid Maltase) Deficiency. The gene encoding the enzyme is mapped to chromosome 17. Various mutations affecting the synthesis, phosphorylation, and maturation of the enzyme have now been identified. Three major clinical variants exist. The *infantile type* presents in early infancy with generalized and rapidly progressive weakness and heart, tongue, and liver enlargement. There is widespread and marked glycogen excess in tissues, including lower motor neurons. Death occurs from cardiorespiratory failure before the age of two years. The *childhood type* presents in infancy or early childhood as a myopathy. Weakness is more proximal than distal, and there may be calf enlargement simulating muscular dystrophy. Glycogen excess is less marked and confined to muscle. Death occurs before age 20 of respiratory failure. The *adult type* presents between the second and seventh decade of life, either with slowly progressive limb muscle weakness that mimics limb-girdle dystrophy or polymyositis or with insidiously developing ventilatory insufficiency leading to respiratory failure. Whatever the early stage, the latter dysfunction is the usual cause of death. In all three types the serum CK level is increased, but to less than ten times normal. The EMG in affected muscles shows myopathic changes and excessive abnormal electrical irritability, including myotonic discharges (but there is no clinical myotonia). The muscle biopsy demonstrates a vacuolar myopathy with high glycogen content and acid-phosphatase reactivity in the vacuoles, an appearance that otherwise occurs only in chloroquine myopathy and a rare cardioskeletal lysosomal storage disorder without acid maltase deficiency.

Debranching Enzyme Deficiency. A clinically impairing myopathy affecting both proximal and distal muscles can appear in childhood or (more commonly) in adult life. Often there is a history of a protuberant abdomen and hypoglycemic episodes in childhood, along with muscle fatigue on exertion. Persistent hepatomegaly and biventricular cardiac hypertrophy are found in most cases. There is a diminished glycemic response to epinephrine and glucagon and an impaired rise of lactic acid after ischemic exercise. The EMG shows myopathic changes and abnormal electrical irritability in affected muscles.

Branching Enzyme Deficiency. The disease presents in infancy with progressive hepatosplenomegaly and failure to thrive. The abnormal starchlike glycogen, which resists diastase digestion, induces nodular cirrhosis and liver failure. Death occurs in early infancy from liver or heart failure. Muscle weakness is variable; if present, the tongue is severely affected.

Phosphorylase Kinase Deficiency. This is a recently recognized syndrome presenting in early childhood with muscle weakness with or without hepatomegaly. Muscle contractures and myoglobinuria have not been observed.

Glycolytic Enzyme Defects: Myophosphorylase, Phosphofructokinase (PFK), Phosphoglycerate Kinase (PGK), Phosphoglycerate Mutase (PGM), and Lactate Dehydrogenase (LDH) Deficiencies. The common features are muscle cramps and periodic myoglobinuria on strenuous exertion since childhood; easy fatigability; a venous lactate level that fails to rise after ischemic exercise in myophosphorylase and PFK deficiencies, and fails to rise or rises by less than 100 per cent in PGK, PGM, and LDH deficiencies. Muscle cramps are prominent. They are caused by electrically silent contractures and are not associated with ATP depletion; their mechanism is not understood. The muscle glycogen excess is slight to modest. Permanent muscle weakness and atrophy are also slight, but they may increase with age. Fatal infantile variants have been identified in myophosphorylase and PFK deficiency. In PFK deficiency hyperuricemia and gout occur in some cases, and there is mild hemolytic disease caused by a partial erythrocyte enzyme defect. PGK mutations result in severe hemolytic anemia and neurologic deficits but no myopathy, or produce a myopathy with only the features described above.

DISORDERS OF FATTY ACID METABOLISM.
Long-chain fatty acids taken up by muscle are utilized for energy metabolism or incorporated into triglycerides and stored as lipid droplets. Long-chain fatty acids entering the catabolic pathway are esterified with coenzyme A (CoA) to form acyl-CoAs. These react with carnitine to form acylcarnitines in a reaction catalyzed by carnitine palmityltransferase I, an enzyme positioned on the inner surface of the inner mitochondrial membrane. The acylcarnitines are transported through the inner mitochondrial membrane by a carnitine-acylcarnitine translocase and are then reconverted to acyl-CoAs by carnitine palmityltransferase II on the inner surface of the inner mitochondrial membrane. The acyl-CoAs undergo repeated cycles of beta-oxidation, generating acetyl-CoAs that enter the citric acid cycle or form ketone bodies. The inner mitochondrial membrane is impermeable to long-chain fatty acids, CoA, and acyl-CoAs. Consequently, carnitine, carnitine-acyltransferases, and carnitine-acylcarnitine translocase jointly regulate the oxidation of fatty acids and modulate the intramitochondrial CoA/acyl-CoA ratio. Excessive intramitochondrial accumulation of an acyl-CoA compound leads to its conversion to a corresponding acylcarnitine. The acylcarnitine so formed leaves the mitochondrion via the translocase, diffuses out from the cell, and is preferentially excreted by the kidney. If this process continues, the muscle and body carnitine stores become depleted.

Derangements in fatty acid oxidation produce a variety of syndromes that affect muscle and other organs. The possible consequences include one or more of the following: intermittent energy shortage in muscle causing *rhabdomyolysis* and *myoglobinuria*; intramitochondrial acyl-CoA excess and CoA deficiency, secondary carnitine depletion, and inhibition of multiple mitochondrial enzyme systems (these events trigger a *Reye syndrome–like metabolic crisis* associated with hypoglycemia, acute fatty infiltration of the liver, hyperammonemia, marked release of enzymes from muscle and liver into serum, and encephalopathy); and triglyceride accumulation in muscle producing a *lipid-storage myopathy*. Lipid storage myopathy is one expression of carnitine deficiency, and carnitine deficiency syndromes are the most common cause of lipid storage myopathy. Most carnitine-deficiency syndromes, however, are secondary to another metabolic defect in, respectively, fatty acid oxidation, branched-chain amino acid metabolism, or the respiratory chain (Table 516–1).

Carnitine Palmityltransferase Deficiency. The normal enzyme is a long-chain carnitine acyltransferase. The inheritance

TABLE 516–1. CAUSES OF SECONDARY CARNITINE DEFICIENCY

Organic Acidurias with Acyl-CoA Dehydrogenase Deficiencies
Long-chain acyl-CoA dehydrogenase deficiency
Medium-chain acyl-CoA dehydrogenase deficiency
Short-chain acyl-CoA dehydrogenase deficiency
Multiple acyl-CoA dehydrogenase deficiency

Organic Acidurias with Defects in Branched-chain Amino Acid Metabolism
Isovaleryl-CoA dehydrogenase deficiency*
Propionyl-CoA carboxylase deficiency
Methylmalonyl-CoA mutase deficiency
β-hydroxy-β-methylglutaric-CoA lyase deficiency

Defects in Mitochondrial Respiratory Chain or Energy Utilization†
Block at NADH-coenzyme Q reductase (Complex I deficiency)
Mitochondrial ATPase deficiency (Complex V deficiency)

Other Metabolic Disorders†
Methylenetetrahydrofolate reductase deficiency
Kearns-Sayre syndrome

Miscellaneous Disorders†
Idiopathic Reye syndrome
Valproate therapy
Renal Fanconi syndrome
Cirrhosis with cachexia

---

*This enzyme is also an acyl-CoA dehydrogenase.
†Only some patients develop carnitine depletion.

is autosomal recessive with reduced penetrance in women. The symptoms consist of muscle aching, fatigability, and periodic myoglobinuria on sustained exertion, especially if combined with fasting and exposure to cold. There are no symptoms between attacks, and the muscle lipid content is normal or only slightly increased. The mutant enzyme is not diminished in amount but is abnormally sensitive to inhibition by its own product and substrate, which explains why symptoms appear only when fatty acid metabolism is stressed and why little or no lipid accumulates in muscle.

Acyl-CoA Dehydrogenase Deficiencies. Deficiencies of the long-chain, medium-chain, and short-chain specific enzymes, and in the factors that transfer electrons from multiple acyl-CoA dehydrogenases to coenzyme Q (multiple acyl-CoA dehydrogenase deficiency), have been identified. Each syndrome causes secondary carnitine depletion, a lipid storage myopathy, and organic aciduria. The urinary organic acid and acylcarnitine profiles reflect the site of the metabolic block. *Short-chain acyl-CoA dehydrogenase deficiency* is associated with adult-onset lipid storage myopathy. Ketogenesis is not impaired and there are no metabolic crises. The other acyl-CoA dehydrogenase deficiencies produce intermittent metabolic crises resembling Reye syndrome. *Long-chain acyl-CoA dehydrogenase deficiency* usually has a neonatal onset and is associated with hepatomegaly and cardiomyopathy. *Medium-chain acyl-CoA dehydrogenase deficiency* presents in the first or second year of life with a metabolic crisis. Between attacks the patients are well or have mild weakness, easy fatigability, and mild hepatomegaly. *Multiple acyl-CoA dehydrogenase deficiencies* are genetically and biochemically heterogeneous. Severe neonatal forms with cardiomyopathy and milder late-onset cases have been described. Some cases respond to riboflavin therapy. The acyl-CoA dehydrogenase deficiencies are treated with a low-fat, high-carbohydrate diet and L-carnitine supplements (2 to 4 grams daily in adults and 100 mg per kilogram daily in infants and children). Crises can be prevented by avoiding fasting and maintaining alimentation at all times, especially during febrile illnesses. The crises are treated by intravenous therapy to correct the hypoglycemia and electrolyte abnormalities, and by L-carnitine, initially 100 mg per kilogram and then 25 mg per kilogram every four hours.

Primary Carnitine Deficiency Syndromes. Because many metabolic errors can cause secondary carnitine deficiency (Table 516–1), primary carnitine deficiency should not be diagnosed unless all currently recognized causes of secondary carnitine deficiency have been adequately excluded. A primary myopathic form, with lipid storage myopathy and muscle carnitine deficiency, and a systemic form, with lipid storage myopathy and intermittent metabolic crises, have been described. Cardiomyopathy may occur with either form. Some cases of muscle carnitine deficiency respond to prednisone; L-carnitine; a low-fat, high-carbohydrate diet; or a combination of these measures. It is probable that additional metabolic errors producing carnitine depletion will be identified in most or all patients who are now thought to have primary carnitine deficiency.

Other Lipid Storage Myopathies. Autosomal-recessive and -dominant lipid storage myopathies associated with lifelong weakness, myalgias, and electrical myotonia, but without carnitine deficiency, have been described. *Chanarin's disease* is a rare autosomal recessive condition with congenital ichthyosis, steatorrhea, and lipid storage in muscle fibers, hepatocytes, gastrointestinal epithelial cells, epidermal cells, monocytes, myelocytes, and fibroblasts.

MITOCHONDRIAL MYOPATHIES. These disorders are defined by a specific biochemical and/or a nonspecific morphologic abnormality in muscle mitochondria. The morphologic abnormality consists of too many and too large mitochondria in a substantial proportion of the muscle fibers ("ragged red fibers"); some of the mitochondria have abnormal cristae and harbor various inclusions. Because the morphologic abnormalities are not specific and are not found in all mitochondrial myopathies, a purely biochemical definition would be preferable, but the biochemical defect in many mitochondrial myopathies is still unknown. A current classification of mitochondrial myopathies is shown in Table 516–2.

From a clinical standpoint, in many mitochondrial myopathies there is slowly progressive weakness of limb and/or external ocular and other cranial muscles, abnormal fatigability on sustained exertion, and lactacidemia on exertion or even at rest. Some mitochondrial disorders affect multiple organs or systems, and the myopathy is but one facet of a multisystem disease.

Myopathies with Defective Energy Conservation. Luft syndrome is a hypermetabolic myopathy. Thyroid function studies exclude hyperthyroidism, but the basal metabolic rate is markedly elevated. The few patients observed to date had heat intolerance, hyperphagia, diaphoresis, polydipsia without polyuria, and progressive weakness since childhood. Oxidative phosphorylation was uncoupled, possibly because of abnormal recycling of calcium between the mitochondria and the cytosol.

Mitochondrial ATPase deficiency is a multisystem disease that presents in childhood. It produces muscle weakness associ-

TABLE 516–2. CLASSIFICATION OF MITOCHONDRIAL MYOPATHIES

Biochemically Distinct Disorders
  Defective energy conservation
    Hypermetabolic myopathy (Luft syndrome)
    Mitochondrial ATPase deficiency
  Impaired substrate utilization or transport
    Acyl-CoA dehydrogenase deficiencies
    Carnitine palmityltransferase deficiency
    Carnitine deficiency syndromes of undetermined cause
    Defects in the pyruvate dehydrogenase complex
  Defects in the mitochondrial respiratory chain
    Complex I (NADH-coenzyme Q oxidoreductase) deficiency
    Complex III (coenzyme Q-cytochrome c oxidoreductase) deficiency
    Complex IV (cytochrome c oxidase) deficiency
      Fatal infantile type
      Benign infantile type
      Benign with external ophthalmoplegia
      Necrotizing encephalomyelopathy (Leigh's syndrome)
      Trichopoliodystrophy (Menkes' disease)

Clinically Distinct but Biochemically Undefined Disorders
  Kearns-Sayre syndrome (retinitis pigmentosa, heart block, external ophthalmoplegia, plus other features)
  Myoclonus, generalized seizures, cerebellar syndrome, lactacidemia, plus other features
  Encephalopathy with strokelike episodes and lactacidemia, plus other features

Recognizable only by Morphologic Criteria

ated with a myopathy and peripheral neuropathy, high-tone hearing loss, frequent vomiting, increased spinal fluid protein, basal ganglia calcifications, retinopathy, ataxia, and dementia. Secondary carnitine deficiency and lipid storage in muscle can also occur.

Impaired Substrate Utilization Caused by Transport or Enzyme Defects. These disorders include the primary carnitine deficiencies, acyl-CoA dehydrogenase deficiencies, carnitine palmityltransferase deficiency (all dealt with above) and *defects in the pyruvate dehydrogenase complex.* The latter are associated with various neurologic syndromes that include movement disorders, ataxia, neuropathy, subacute necrotizing encephalomyelopathy (Leigh's syndrome), and fatal infantile lactic acidosis. The muscle biopsy shows ragged red fibers, lipid excess, or denervation atrophy.

Defects in the Mitochondrial Respiratory Chain. The mitochondrial respiratory chain includes four distinct enzyme complexes and also coenzyme Q and cytochrome c. The components are attached to the inner mitochondrial membrane and carry reducing equivalents from reduced nicotinamide adenine dinucleotide (NADH) or flavin adenine dinucleotide ($FADH_2$) to molecular oxygen. A fifth complex, an ATPase, uses released energy to phosphorylate ADP to ATP in a tightly coupled process. Mitochondrial ATPase deficiency was discussed above. Defects in the electron transport complexes are associated with marked clinical, biochemical, and genetic heterogeneity. The reasons for this are that each complex is composed of multiple subunits, different subunits of a given complex are encoded by different genes, some subunits of a given complex are encoded by mitochondrial rather than nuclear DNA, some subunits are tissue specific, and some subunits are developmentally regulated.

COMPLEX I (NADH-COENZYME Q OXIDOREDUCTASE) DEFICIENCY. Most of these begin in childhood and allow survival to adult life. Either muscular or central nervous system manifestations dominate the clinical picture. In the former group the findings include muscle weakness, exercise intolerance, exertional lactacidemia, and ragged red fibers in muscle. Headaches, progressive visual loss, hemiparesis, dysphasia, dementia, dystonia, and cerebral atrophy affect the latter group. A fatal infantile form also exists.

COMPLEX III (COENZYME Q-CYTOCHROME C OXIDOREDUCTASE) DEFICIENCY. These also begin in childhood or adult life. Muscle weakness, exercise intolerance, exertional lactacidemia, and ragged red fibers are constant findings. Some patients also have external ophthalmoplegia and/or dementia, myoclonus, ataxia, pyramidal signs, and loss of proprioception. The muscle symptoms in one patient were improved by treatment with menadione and vitamin C, agents that can function as electron transfer mediators instead of complex III.

COMPLEX IV (CYTOCHROME C OXIDASE) DEFICIENCY. Several syndromes are associated with this defect. A *fatal infantile mitochondrial myopathy* presents at birth or shortly thereafter with weakness, hypotonia, and lactacidemia. Renal Fanconi syndrome *or* cardiomyopathy *or* liver enlargement can be associated with the fatal infantile syndrome. Muscle contains large accumulations of mitochondria, lipid, and glycogen. The phenotypic variability is attributed to the existence of tissue-specific subunits of complex IV. A *benign infantile myopathy* with reversible complex IV deficiency presents neonatally with profound weakness of all but the ocular muscles, hepatomegaly, macroglossia, and severe lactacidemia. Spontaneous improvement begins after six months, and only mild weakness persists into later life. Complex IV deficiency in muscle, liver, and brain also has been described in some cases of *necrotizing encephalomyelopathy* (Leigh's syndrome) and *trichopoliodystrophy* (Menkes' disease).

Clinically Distinct but Biochemically Undefined Syndromes. KEARNS-SAYRE SYNDROME. The disease presents in childhood. Nearly all cases are sporadic, suggesting an exogenous influence or polygenic inheritance. The rate of progression, severity, and system involvement vary from case to case. The original description in 1958 was that of retinitis pigmentosa, heart block, and external ophthalmoplegia. Subsequently ataxia, hearing loss, short stature, and increased spinal fluid protein were noted in more than half of the cases. Muscle weakness, mental changes, pyramidal signs, hypogonadism, and diabetes occur in less than half of the cases. Serum and spinal fluid lactate and pyruvate levels are increased, and the muscle fibers contain morphologically abnormal mitochondria. The presence of heart block requires treatment by pacemaker.

MYOCLONUS, GENERALIZED SEIZURES, CEREBELLAR SYNDROME, MITOCHONDRIAL MYOPATHY, AND LACTACIDEMIA. The syndrome presents in childhood or adult life. The family history is often positive, and some kinships show evidence for maternal mitochondrial inheritance. Short stature, dementia, hearing loss, and optic atrophy are frequent; spasticity, central hypoventilation, endocrinopathies, and peripheral neuropathy occur less often.

MITOCHONDRIAL MYOPATHY, ENCEPHALOPATHY, LACTACIDEMIA, AND STROKELIKE EPISODES (MELAS). The main distinction between this syndrome and the preceding one is the occurrence in adolescence or young adulthood of strokelike episodes associated with intermittent vomiting. Brain imaging during the acute episodes discloses areas of encephalomalacia not in the territories of the main blood vessels. Other associated features include short stature, seizures, hearing loss, progressive dementia, macular degeneration, and calcification of the basal ganglia. Early development is normal, and the family history is often positive.

ENDOCRINE MYOPATHIES. Muscle weakness can be a symptom of any endocrine disorder. The term endocrine myopathy is therefore restricted to cases in which weakness is more prominent than usual, or selective in distribution, with or without muscle atrophy. The serum CK level is normal, except in myxedema and in uremic hyperparathyroidism. The EMG is normal or myopathic without spontaneous electrical activity. The histologic alterations in muscle are often nonspecific, such as type II fiber atrophy, focal increases and decreases in mitochondria, and focal myofibrillar degeneration. Fiber necrosis and regeneration and connective tissue proliferation are uncommon.

Glucocorticoid-Induced Myopathy. Muscle weakness commonly occurs in Cushing's syndrome and in patients receiving relatively high doses of glucocorticoids. Fluorinated drugs (dexamethasone, triamcinolone) are more pathogenic than nonfluorinated ones (prednisone). Considerable variation exists in the minimal dosage that induces myopathy. However, daily treatment for three months with 60 mg prednisone in divided doses induces some weakness in nearly all patients. Women are more susceptible than men, and divided daily doses are more pathogenic than single or alternate daily doses. The onset is usually insidious but occasionally sudden with diffuse myalgias. The weakness is more proximal than distal and affects the lower more than the upper limbs. Hip and ankle flexors are selectively severely affected. The cranial muscles are spared. The serum CK level remains normal. The biochemical basis of the disease is poorly understood. Reduced protein synthesis, accelerated protein degradation, and enhanced lysosomal protease activity all may contribute. Therapy consists of reducing the steroid dosage to the lowest possible level. Muscle strength returns to normal within one to four months after therapy is stopped.

Adrenal Insufficiency. Weakness is a typical feature, closely related to derangements in fluid and electrolyte balance and possibly to the associated hypotension. Joint contractures, especially of the knees and not related to muscle weakness, may also occur. Hyperkalemia in chronic adrenal insufficiency can be a cause of secondary periodic paralysis (discussed below).

Thyrotoxic Myopathy. Both acute and chronic forms have been described. The acute form, seldom seen, appears during a thyroid storm and is associated with bulbar weakness. Some patients have responded to anticholinesterases and may have had acute myasthenia gravis beginning during thyrotoxicosis. The chronic form appears in 80 per cent of untreated cases of hyperthyroidism. The hyperthyroid state can be mild and of long duration or present for only a few weeks before the onset of the weakness. Weakness is predominantly proximal, less often both proximal and distal. Although often out of proportion to the atrophy, severe muscle wasting can occur. The deep tendon reflexes are hyperactive or normal. The serum CK level remains normal. The EMG shows myopathic motor unit potentials but never fibrillation potentials. Indeed, an increased serum CK level or fibrillation potentials in a hyperthyroid patient with muscle weakness indicate an additional associated muscle disease such as polymyositis.

Graves' ophthalmopathy is described in Ch. 229. Thyrotoxic periodic paralysis is considered below.

Hypothyroid Myopathy. Muscle aching, cramps, slow relaxation of the reflexes, ridging of the muscles on percussion (myoedema), and an increase of the serum CK level are common findings in myxedema. Muscle enlargement and limb-girdle weakness occur only occasionally. The Debré-Semelaigne syndrome consists of muscle hypertrophy, weakness, and slow movements in the cretinous child. The same features and painful spasms in hypothyroid adults constitute Hoffmann's syndrome.

Muscle Symptoms in Hyperparathyroidism and Osteomalacia. Parathormone and biologically active forms of vitamin D are important regulators of calcium metabolism and the serum calcium level. Vitamin D also affects calcium metabolism, protein synthesis, ATP stores, and force generation in muscle. Furthermore, conditions that lead to osteomalacia (vitamin D deficiency, renal tubular acidosis, or chronic renal failure) are associated with secondary hyperparathyroidism. Proximal muscle weakness, fatigability, and muscle pain and tenderness, usually with bone pain and tenderness, can occur in primary and secondary hyperparathyroidism and in osteomalacia. The serum alkaline phosphatase activity is increased; the serum calcium level is increased in primary hyperparathyroidism but is low or normal in osteomalacia; phosphate levels tend to be low except in the presence of chronic renal failure.

A more malignant syndrome can appear in uremic hyperparathyroidism. Here, metastatic calcification of the media and proliferation of the intima of small blood vessels produce skin and visceral infarcts and a necrotizing myopathy with marked elevation of serum enzymes and myoglobinuria.

Muscle Symptoms in Hypoparathyroidism. The typical neuromuscular symptom is tetany. This is considered in Ch. 247.

Acromegaly and Hypopituitarism. Acromegaly initially causes muscle hypertrophy, particularly if the disorder begins before growth ceases. Later generalized weakness and atrophy develop. Muscle biopsies can show segmental muscle fiber degeneration, type I or type II fiber atrophy, or no pathologic change. The serum CK level remains normal. A hypertrophic distal neuropathy and nerve entrapment are common in acromegaly.

Hypopituitarism in children causes dwarfism and poor muscle development. Pituitary failure in adults results in weakness and fatigability with little muscle atrophy. The weakness itself may reflect the combined influence of thyroid, adrenal, and growth hormone deficiencies.

THE PERIODIC PARALYSES (PP). These disorders occur as either inherited (primary) or acquired (secondary) illnesses and can be further classified according to measurable alterations in the serum potassium level during attacks (Table 516–3). The primary types are transmitted by autosomal-dominant inheritance, but nearly a third of the cases arise sporadically. It is important to realize that in the primary

TABLE 516–3. CLASSIFICATION OF THE PERIODIC PARALYSES

Primary	Secondary
Hypokalemic	Hypokalemic
Normokalemic	Thyrotoxic
Hyperkalemic	Urinary potassium wastage
Without myotonia	Gastrointestinal potassium
With myotonia	wastage
With cardiac arrhythmia (hyper-,	Barium intoxication
hypo- or normokalemic)	Hyperkalemic
	Renal insufficiency
	Adrenal insufficiency

forms the serum potassium decreases or increases but may still remain within the normal range during attacks and is normal or low-normal between attacks. By contrast, in secondary PP caused by potassium wastage or retention the serum potassium is always markedly reduced or elevated during and even between attacks.

In each type of PP the propagation of the muscle fiber action potential fails during an attack. Recent studies indicate the presence of distinct abnormalities in the sodium channel of the muscle fiber plasma membrane in the primary periodic paralyses that tend to reduce the resting membrane potential. The action potential mechanism fails during the attack either because the resting membrane potential is so low that the sodium channel becomes inactivated or because the channel itself is abnormally sensitive to inactivation by even a minor membrane depolarization.

The different types of periodic paralysis share several common features: (1) The paralytic attacks last from less than an hour to as long as several days. (2) The weakness can be localized or generalized. (3) The deep tendon reflexes diminish and then disappear during attacks. (4) The muscle fibers become inexcitable to direct or indirect electrical stimulation during the attacks. (5) The generalized attacks begin proximally and spread distally. Respiratory and cranial muscles tend to be spared except in the most severe attacks. (6) Rest after exercise provokes weakness in the muscles that had been exercised. Continued mild exercise aborts attacks. (7) Exercise followed by rest of a single muscle can induce weakness of that muscle without any detectable change in the potassium level in the systemic circulation. (8) Exposure to cold can provoke weakness in the primary forms of the disease. (9) Complete recovery occurs after initial attacks. (10) In the primary disorders permanent weakness and a persistent vacuolar myopathy can develop after repeated attacks. Despite these similarities, the different forms of PP differ in their response to sodium, potassium, or carbohydrate loading, as well as their pattern of urinary electrolyte excretions during attacks, and in some of their clinical features.

Primary Hypokalemic Periodic Paralysis. The attacks begin in the first or second decade, increase in frequency during early adult life, and become less frequent or cease during the fourth or fifth decade. When attacks recur daily, the patient is weakest in the morning and becomes stronger as the day passes. High dietary sodium or carbohydrate intake as well as excitement provokes or exacerbates the episodes. Major attacks are associated with urinary retention of sodium, potassium, chloride, and water. The diagnosis is supported by a positive family history and a decrease in serum potassium during an attack. An abnormally low serum potassium level between attacks suggests secondary rather than primary PP. In diagnosing sporadic cases one must employ appropriate tests to exclude potassium wastage and thyrotoxicosis. The oral or intravenous administration of glucose, 2 grams per kilogram of body weight, combined with 10 to 20 units of insulin given subcutaneously, may provoke an attack within two to three hours. Depression of the serum potassium during the attack and a favorable response to 2.5 to 7.5 grams of potassium chloride (KCl) given orally must be demonstrated. Provocative tests must never be done in patients already

hypokalemic, and potassium chloride must not be given to patients unless they have adequate renal or adrenal reserve.

Thyrotoxic Periodic Paralysis. This disease resembles primary hypokalemic PP in the changes in serum and urinary electrolytes that accompany the attacks and in the response to glucose, insulin, potassium, and rest after exercise. However, 95 per cent of the cases are sporadic, the male to female ratio is six to one, most cases occur among Orientals, the onset is usually in adult life, and correction of the hyperthyroidism prevents further attacks.

Barium-Induced Periodic Paralysis. The accidental ingestion of absorbable barium salts such as barium carbonate induces hemorrhagic gastroenteritis, hypertension, cardiac arrhythmias, convulsions, hypokalemia, and muscle paralysis. Barium blocks potassium channels and thereby reduces potassium efflux from muscle; potassium uptake by muscle, mediated by the sodium-potassium pump, continues, and hypokalemia results.

Periodic Paralysis Secondary to Urinary or Gastrointestinal Potassium Loss. The differential diagnosis of hypokalemia resulting from urinary or gastrointestinal potassium depletion is discussed in Ch. 76. Paralytic attacks do not occur unless the serum potassium falls below 3 mEq per liter, and during the attacks the serum potassium decreases even further. Other neuromuscular complications of severe potassium depletion include a necrotizing myopathy, myoglobinuria, and latent or manifest tetany.

Primary Hyperkalemic Periodic Paralysis. The attacks begin in the first or second decade. They are often brief but can last up to several days. Between attacks the serum potassium is normal or slightly lower than normal. During major attacks the serum potassium increases but may not exceed the normal range, and the urinary potassium excretion increases. Myotonic and nonmyotonic forms of hyperkalemic PP can be distinguished. In *myotonic hyperkalemic PP* myotonia can be detected in facial, tongue, finger extensor, and thenar muscles between attacks; exposure to cold causes widespread and severe myotonia, and exercise in the cold is followed by prolonged weakness not reversed by rewarming. These features resemble those of *paramyotonia congenita*, which may be the same disease as hyperkalemic PP. In both disorders attacks are provoked by orally administered KCl, 50 to 100 mg per kilogram, given in an unsweetened solution in the fasting state. The test is contraindicated in subjects already hyperkalemic or those without adequate renal or adrenal reserve.

Secondary Hyperkalemic Periodic Paralysis. This can occur when the serum potassium level exceeds 7 mEq per liter. The usual cause is renal or adrenal insufficiency, but hyperkalemia from exposure to spironolactone and during attacks of malaria also have caused paralytic attacks. The diagnosis is suggested by the presence of a very high serum potassium level during attacks, persistent hyperkalemia between attacks, and the associated primary disorder.

Primary Normokalemic Periodic Paralysis. There are no consistent changes in the serum potassium during the attacks. The existence of the disease has been questioned because some patients are sensitive to potassium salts. However, in some kinships potassium loading does not provoke attacks. The observations suggest that normokalemic PP is a heterogeneous entity.

Primary Periodic Paralysis with Cardiac Arrhythmia. Affected patients suffer from PP and tachyarrhythmias that can cause sudden death. The cardiac symptoms are provoked or worsened by hypokalemia and digitalis; are refractory to disopyramide phosphate, propranolol, or phenytoin; but may respond to imipramine. Dysmorphic features, such as short stature, clinodactyly, and microcephaly can also occur. The PP has been clearly related to hyperkalemia in some patients, but hypokalemic and normokalemic PP were diagnosed in others.

Therapy of the Periodic Paralyses. In all forms of primary PP acetazolamide, from 250 mg to 2 grams daily, can prevent attacks or decrease their frequency. The metabolic acidosis induced by the drug may prevent sodium channel inactivation by small depolarizations. Prolonged exposure to the drug promotes the formation of renal calculi.

The treatment of attacks of *primary hypokalemic PP* consists of giving 2 to 10 grams of oral KCl. Preventive therapy includes acetazolamide, a low-carbohydrate and relatively low-sodium (2.3 grams per day) diet, and 2.5 grams of KCl taken orally three times daily. *Thyrotoxic PP* is treated by antithyroid therapy, KCl supplements, and a low-carbohydrate, low-sodium diet. Acetazolamide is ineffective.

In *primary hyperkalemic PP* one treats the acute attacks with 2 grams per kilogram of glucose by mouth and 15 to 20 units of crystalline insulin subcutaneously. The inhalation of 1.3 mg metaproterenol every 15 minutes for three doses, or of 0.18 mg albuterol repeated once after 10 minutes, has aborted acute attacks. Preventive treatment consists of acetazolamide or thiazide diuretics and frequent high-carbohydrate meals. Tocainide, 300 to 400 mg three to four times daily, prevents cold-induced stiffness and weakness in myotonic hyperkalemic PP. The drug acts by blocking sodium channels in muscle.

The periodic paralyses caused by excessive wastage or retention of potassium are treated by correcting existing electrolyte abnormalities and, if possible, removing the existing cause. In acute barium poisoning, 10 ml of a 10 per cent solution of sodium sulfate is administered intravenously every 30 minutes until symptoms subside.

NUTRITIONAL AND TOXIC MYOPATHIES. Although malnutrition is common in many parts of the world, its effects on skeletal muscle have not been well investigated. Diffuse muscle atrophy and weakness associated with type II fiber atrophy are commonly observed in malnourished or cachectic patients. The muscle weakness in nutritional osteomalacia has been attributed partly to disuse and partly to malnutrition.

Vitamin E Deficiency. This has now been implicated in progressive gait and limb ataxia, sensorimotor neuropathy, extraocular muscle paresis, and a myopathy in which giant abnormal lysosomes accumulate in muscle. The cause is a malabsorption syndrome, as detailed in Ch. 104 and 467. High doses of vitamin E may be of benefit.

Myopathy in Alcoholism. An acute necrotizing myopathy associated with myoglobinuria occurs in chronic alcoholics after a bout of drinking. Hypokalemia caused by sweating, vomiting, diarrhea, and renal wastage may act as a precipitating factor. The hypokalemia may be followed by hyperkalemia as myoglobinuria and renal failure develop. A subacute alcoholic myopathy with proximal muscle weakness and elevation of the serum CK level may also exist. If so, it is usually associated with a chronic neuropathy.

Chloroquine Myopathy. The side effects of the drug include macular and corneal degeneration, peripheral neuropathy, and myopathy. Muscle weakness appears when the daily dosage is 500 mg for a year or longer. Lower daily dosages are now used in clinical practice, making chloroquine myopathy uncommon. Pathologically, the condition produces a vacuolar myopathy and constitutes a prototype for myopathies due to an excited autophagic mechanism.

Emetine Myopathy. Emetine, an ipecac alkaloid, is used to treat amebiasis. Side effects include cardiotoxicity and muscle weakness. A reversible myopathy involving proximal limb muscles has been observed in patients with feeding disorders who abuse ipecac to induce vomiting and in alcoholics receiving emetine for aversion therapy. The pathologic findings include focal destruction of mitochondria and focal myofibrillar degeneration.

MALIGNANT HYPERTHERMIA. Susceptibility to the disorder is transmitted by autosomal-dominant inheritance with variable penetrance. In addition, the syndrome also can occur in myotonic disorders, Duchenne dystrophy, branchial hypertrophic myopathy, central core disease, and a congenital myopathy with dysmorphic features. It is not yet known what proportion of patients with these disorders is at risk.

The reaction is triggered by major inhalation anesthetics (e.g., halothane, ether, methoxyflurane, enflurane) or succinylcholine. Warning signs include tachypnea, tachycardia, increased carbon dioxide production, cyanosis, rising temperature, rigidity, sweating, and unstable blood pressure. Failure to obtain muscle relaxation with adequate doses of succinylcholine represents an early warning sign. Subsequently, body temperature rises rapidly (up to 1° C every five minutes), followed by a rapidly evolving lactic acidosis, respiratory acidosis from carbon dioxide overproduction, muscle rigidity, hyperkalemia, variable alterations in the serum calcium, and muscle fiber breakdown reflected by very high serum CK levels, myoglobinemia, and myoglobinuria. The postulated mechanism for these changes is failure of calcium homeostasis in the muscle fiber; a high intracellular calcium level activates phosphorylase kinase, saturates troponin, and overloads mitochondria with calcium. These events cause accelerated glycogen breakdown, ATP splitting, uncontrolled muscle contraction, uncoupling of oxidative phosphorylation, and excessive production of heat, lactate, and carbon dioxide.

Therapy of the acute syndrome consists of body cooling, hydration, sodium bicarbonate infusion, mechanical hyperventilation, and diuretics to maintain urine flow. More specific treatment consists of dantrolene, a medication that blocks excitation-contraction coupling between the T-tubules and the SR. The drug is given intravenously, 1 to 2 mg per kilogram, which may be repeated every five minutes to a total of 10 mg per kilogram. The mortality remains high. Screening of relatives of patients for the metabolic defect is important. Seventy per cent of those at risk have increased serum CK activity. If well standardized, an in vitro halothane contracture test on fresh muscle can also predict susceptibility. Preventive treatment of individuals at risk consists of dantrolene, 4 to 8 mg per kilogram per day in four divided doses for one to two days prior to surgery; and, if possible, alternative methods of anesthesia.

Other Hyperthermic States. Two other syndromes are associated with hyperthermia, autonomic instability, abnormal muscle rigidity, and myoglobinuria. The *malignant neuroleptic syndrome* occurs in less than 1 per cent of all patients exposed to neuroleptics, and especially in young men. It evolves over one to three days and lasts five to ten days after drug withdrawal. The mortality is about 25 per cent. A nearly identical *hyperthermic syndrome in Parkinson's disease* is precipitated by abrupt withdrawal of antiparkinson medications. The same treatment as in malignant hyperthermia, including the use of dantrolene up to 10 mg per kilogram per day, is beneficial in both disorders. Bromocriptine, 2.5 to 20 mg three times daily, may also help, but it acts more slowly than dantrolene.

MYOGLOBINURIA. The clinical syndrome of myoglobinuria is associated with brown discoloration of urine by myoglobin and metmyoglobin. Myoglobin, a 17,000-molecular-weight protein with a prosthetic heme group, is present in muscle at a concentration of 1 gram per kilogram. It has a lower renal excretory threshold than hemoglobin. Small amounts of myoglobin not sufficient to discolor urine are excreted in various necrotizing myopathies. The visible discoloration of urine by myoglobin indicates both massive and acute muscle destruction (rhabdomyolysis) and warns of impending renal damage. The pigment has to be distinguished from hemoglobin and porphyrins. If there is no hemoglobinemia or hematuria, a positive benzidine test strongly suggests myoglobinuria. However, myoglobinuria itself can induce microhematuria, and certain identification of myoglobin must be made specifically. The immunoprecipitation assay has the virtue of being simple and quantitative but is so sensitive that it detects the pigment in the absence of overt myoglobinuria.

Muscle pain, swelling, and weakness precede overt myoglobinuria by a few hours. In addition to myoglobin, phosphate, potassium, creatine, and muscle enzymes are released into the circulation. The heme pigment in the glomerular filtrate and casts in the tubules cause proteinuria, hematuria, and tubular necrosis. Renal failure is more likely if there are also hypotension, acidosis, and hypovolemia. With increasing renal insufficiency, hyperphosphatemia, hypocalcemia, tetany, and life-threatening hyperkalemia appear. Death results from renal or respiratory failure. Otherwise, the myoglobinuria and proteinuria disappear in three to five days. The marked hyperenzymemia decreases gradually, and muscle strength returns relatively slowly after major attacks. EMG abnormalities, and especially fibrillation potentials, can persist for several months.

Myoglobinuria can have many causes: metabolic, infectious, toxic, ischemic and/or traumatic, secondary to another myopathy, and idiopathic. It is likely that many of the so-called idiopathic cases have a metabolic or infectious etiology.

Myoglobinuria Caused by a Metabolic Disturbance. The common denominator is impaired substrate utilization for energy metabolism, or a critical substrate deficiency in the face of excessive demands for energy. Most diseases in this group were considered earlier in this chapter. Deficiencies of myophosphorylase, phosphofructokinase, phosphoglycerate mutase, phosphoglycerate kinase, and lactate dehydrogenase block anaerobic glycolysis, and carnitine palmityltransferase deficiency impairs fatty acid oxidation when it is most needed. Substrate deficiency in the face of excessive demands and derangements of muscle metabolism account for the myoglobinuria associated with malignant hyperthermia, the malignant neuroleptic syndrome, and the abrupt withdrawal of antiparkinson drugs. Substrate deficiency may also account for the myoglobinuria that occurs after severe exercise in untrained individuals, as in military recruits.

Almost any severe metabolic insult can cause myoglobinuria. These include carbon dioxide poisoning, extreme hypoglycemia, severe hypokalemia, hypernatremia, or water intoxication.

Postinfectious Myoglobinuria. This can occur after influenza A, herpes simplex, Epstein-Barr and Coxsackie virus infections. The precise mechanism of the rhabdomyolysis is not understood. Myoglobinuria also occurs with bacterial infections accompanied by high fever and sepsis, and with muscle gangrene caused by clostridial infection.

Toxic Myoglobinuria. The myoglobinuria associated with alcoholism was considered above. Barbiturate, narcotic, and amphetamine intoxication, especially if associated with coma, can produce myoglobinuria. In Haff disease, an unidentified toxin induced an epidemic of myoglobinuria along the Baltic coast. The toxin of the Malayan sea snake, *Enhydrina schistosa,* induces myalgias, trismus, flaccid paralysis, and myoglobinuria.

Ischemic and Traumatic Myoglobinuria. Massive ischemia of muscle from any cause (e.g., major vessel occlusions, angiopathy in uremic hyperparathyroidism), crush injuries, or prolonged pressure on dependent muscles in the immobile comatose patient can induce myoglobinuria. Localized ischemic necrosis of muscle and sometimes myoglobinuria occur in severe forms of the anterior tibial syndrome.

Myoglobinuria Secondary to Other Myopathies. Myoglobinuria has been observed infrequently in acute dermatomyositis (where the cause is probably ischemia), systemic lupus erythematosus, and muscular dystrophies.

Treatment. The acute episode is treated by rest, maintenance of adequate urine flow by hydration and diuretics, and alkalinization of the urine with sodium bicarbonate. Other measures consist of treatment of the renal insufficiency as required and removal of the offending cause if possible.

DiMauro S, Bonilla E, Zeviani M, et al.: Mitochondrial myopathies. Ann Neurol 17:521, 1985. *A complete and lucid review of the biochemical and clinical aspects of the mitochondrial myopathies.*

Eleff S, Kennaway NG, Buist NRM, et al.: ^{31}P NMR study of improvement of oxidative phosphorylation by vitamins K_3 and C in a patient with a defect in electron transport at complex III in skeletal muscle. Proc Natl Acad Sci USA 81:3529, 1984. *A remarkable example of how understanding the biochemical basis of a myopathy can provide a rational basis for its treatment.*

Engel AG, Banker BQ: Myology. New York, McGraw-Hill Book Company, 1986. *Chapters by DiMauro and Bresolin, DiMauro and Papadimitron, Engel, Gronert, Morgan-Hughes, Penn, Ruff, and Victor provide detailed reviews of several of the metabolic myopathies.*

Friedman JH, Feinberg SS, Feldman RG: A neuroleptic malignant-like syndrome due to levodopa therapy withdrawal. JAMA 254:2792, 1985. *Directs attention to a serious potential complication of the "drug holiday" in Parkinson's disease.*

Guzé BH, Baxter LR: Neuroleptic malignant syndrome. N Engl J Med 313: 163, 1985. *Clear description of the clinical aspects and treatment of this uncommon but highly lethal complication of neuroleptics.*

Ricker K, Rohkamm R, Böhlen R: Adynamia episodica and paralysis periodica myotonica. Neurology 36:682, 1986. *Highlights the clinical differences between nonmyotonic and myotonic hyperkalemic periodic paralysis and describes a useful diagnostic test.*

Rosing HS, Hokins LC, Wallace DC, et al.: Maternally inherited mitochondrial myopathy and myoclonic epilepsy. Ann Neurol 17:228, 1985. *A thorough clinical study of a biochemically undefined disorder.*

Rüdel R, Ricker K: The primary periodic paralyses. Trends Neurosci 8:467, 1985. *A concise review of the evidence that different abnormalities of the sodium channel condition membrane inexcitability in different types of primary periodic paralysis.*

517 MISCELLANEOUS MYOPATHIES

INFILTRATIVE MYOPATHIES. *Systemic Amyloid Myopathy.* The most common neurologic complication in various types of amyloidosis is a predominantly sensory-autonomic neuropathy. Amyloid deposition in muscle is frequent, but the muscle involvement is usually subclinical. Occasionally amyloidosis presents or is associated with an overt myopathy characterized by muscle enlargement, macroglossia, stiffness, exertional muscle pain, and proximal or diffuse weakness. Electromyography shows myopathic features in proximal muscles with or without changes of neuropathy distally. The amyloid deposits, identified by their metachromasia and affinity for Congo red stain, appear between and around the mural elements of the small vessels and extend into the interstitial spaces where they tightly surround individual muscle fibers.

Hypertrophic Branchial Myopathy. This sporadic illness presents between the second and fourth decades of life and is restricted to muscles that derive from the embryonic brachial cleft. The disease evolves with slowly progressive, asymmetric, bilateral enlargement of temporalis, masseter, and pterygoid muscles. Weakness is minimal or absent. The swelling itself is painless but may lead to pain with jaw opening. The EMG and muscle biopsy show nonspecific myopathic alterations in the affected muscles. There is no satisfactory treatment. When chewing is impaired, partial excision of the enlarged muscles has proved beneficial.

SYNDROMES ASSOCIATED WITH ABNORMAL MUSCLE ACTIVITY. These can be caused by (1) abnormal neural activity in the central nervous system (e.g., dystonia, tetanus, stiff-man syndrome); (2) abnormal excitability of the peripheral nervous system (neuromyotonia, tetany, cramps); (3) abnormal excitability of the muscle fiber surface membrane (myotonic disorders); (4) a defect within the muscle fiber resulting in abnormal mechanical activity (e.g., malignant hyperthermia, contractures without electrical activity, and slow relaxation of electrically silent muscle fibers). Dystonia, tetanus, and tetany are considered in Ch. 247, 281, and 472. The remaining entities were discussed earlier in this section or will be discussed below.

Stiff-Man Syndrome. This is a disease of adult life affecting men more frequently than women. Initially intermittent spasms of axial and limb muscles are followed by continuous stiffness that immobilizes the patient. Agonist and antagonist muscles are simultaneously affected, preventing voluntary movement. The EMG shows constant firing of normal motor unit potentials in the stiff muscles. There are no signs of cerebral or spinal cord disease. Spinal anesthesia relieves the spasms. The continuous alpha motor neuron activity has been attributed to abnormal gamma motor neuron activity caused by a suprasegmental drive. Relatively high doses of diazepam, which depresses facilitation of the gamma motor neurons by the reticular system, or baclofen, which inhibits spinal reflexes, may improve or relieve the symptoms.

Neuromyotonia. This can be generalized or focal. *Generalized neuromyotonia* is sporadic or familial. Some of the familial cases are associated with a peripheral neuropathy; some of the sporadic cases have an intrathoracic malignancy. Abnormal impulses arising in peripheral motor axons produce continuous muscle fiber activity that persists even during sleep. Depending on the site of origin in the axon, the abnormal activity is abolished by proximal nerve block or block of neuromuscular transmission. The EMG shows very high frequency (150 to 300 Hz) recurring bursts of motor unit potentials. The involuntary activation of multiple motor units causes stiffness and delayed relaxation of the affected muscles and continuous, small, undulating movements of the overlying skin (*myokymia*). Phenytoin or carbamazepine may inhibit the abnormal discharges and relieve the symptoms.

Similar high-frequency and rhythmically recurring bursts of motor unit potentials occur in *facial myokymia* seen with demyelinating or other lesions of the brain stem.

Focal neuromyotonia can occur following peripheral nerve lesions, but here the firing rate is slower (30 to 60 Hz). The delayed relaxation of an affected muscle after a willed contraction mimics action myotonia.

A benign syndrome of *muscle cramps, fasciculations, and myokymia* associated with low-frequency bursts of motor unit potentials also occurs and may incorrectly suggest the diagnosis of early motor neuron disease.

Schwartz-Jampel Syndrome. This is an autosomal-recessive disease that begins in early childhood. It is characterized by chondrodystrophy, bone and joint deformities, short stature, a doleful facial expression with blepharospasm, hypertrichosis, muscle stiffness, and muscle hypertrophy or atrophy. There is delayed muscle relaxation suggesting myotonia. The EMG, however, shows high-frequency repetitive discharges, not myotonic discharges. Muscle biopsy reveals neurogenic and myogenic features.

Myotonia Congenita. Autosomal-dominant (Thomsen's disease) and autosomal-recessive forms are recognized. Both are benign and associated with diffuse muscle hypertrophy and diffuse action, percussion, and electrical myotonia. Cold increases the myotonia, and sustained exercise improves it. The membrane defect consists of a markedly reduced chloride conductance. Quinine, 0.3 to 1.5 grams daily, or phenytoin, 0.3 to 0.6 gram daily, relieves the myotonia.

Paramyotonia Congenita. This autosomal-dominant disease resembles myotonic hyperkalemic periodic paralysis. However, there are cases in which potassium loading does not induce weakness. The myotonia is worsened rather than improved by exercise. Exercise in the cold causes prolonged electrically silent stiffness and weakness not relieved by rewarming. Although the membrane shows an abnormal increase in sodium conductance on cooling, this fails to explain the prolonged stiffness induced by cooling. Tocainide, 300 to 400 mg three to four times daily, prevents the cold-induced symptoms.

Slow Relaxation of Electrically Silent Muscle Fibers. This is a rare disease in which there is impaired muscle relaxation that is rapidly worsened by exercise. The slowly relaxing fibers are electrically silent. The defect lies within the calcium-pump ATPase of the sarcoplasmic reticulum.

Rippling Muscles. This is a benign and dominantly inherited disorder presenting in late childhood or adult life. Sporadic cases also occur. Local compression of a muscle evokes myoedema. This is replaced by a longitudinal depression parallel to the long axis of the muscle which then moves to the periphery of the muscle in 10 to 20 seconds in a wave that resembles the plucking of a chromatic scale on a harp. The response to percussion superficially resembles myotonia, but the rippling muscles are electrically silent. Mild muscle pain, stiffness at the beginning of exercise, and mild elevation of the serum CK level are associated features.

Alberca R, Rafee E, Castella JM, et al.: Increased mechanical muscle irritability syndrome. Acta Neurol Scand 62:250, 1980. *A clear description of an unusual disease with rippling muscles and a review of the relevant literature.*

Auger RG, Daube JR, Gomez MR, et al.: Hereditary form of sustained muscle activity of peripheral nerve origin causing myokymia and muscle stiffness. Ann Neurol 15:13, 1984. *An excellent discussion of the differential diagnosis of neuromyotonias and related syndromes.*

Ii K, Hizawa K, Nunomura S, et al.: Systemic amyloid myopathy. Acta Neuropathol (Berl) 64:114, 1984. *A clear clinical and pathologic description and review of the relevant literature.*

Karpati G, Charuk J, Carpenter S, et al.: Myopathy caused by a deficiency of Ca²⁺-ATPase in sarcoplasmic reticulum (Brody's disease). Ann Neurol 20:38, 1986. *Provides an explanation for the slow relaxation of electrically silent muscle fibers.*

Mancall EL, Patel AN, Hirschhorn AM: Hypertrophic branchial myopathy. Neurology 24:1166, 1974. *A classic account of a neglected myopathy.*

Miller F, Korsvik H: Baclofen in the treatment of the stiff-man syndrome. Ann Neurol 9:511, 1981. *A useful guide to treatment.*

Rüdel R, Lehmann-Horn F: Membrane changes in cells from myotonia patients. Physiol Rev 65:310, 1985. *An up-to-date account of the clinical features and membrane abnormalities in the myotonic syndromes.*

518 DISORDERS OF NEUROMUSCULAR TRANSMISSION

DEFINITION AND BASIC CONCEPTS. Disorders of neuromuscular transmission can be acquired or inherited and are associated with abnormal weakness and fatigability on exertion. In each disorder the safety margin of neuromuscular transmission is compromised by one or more specific mechanisms. The following paragraphs provide a brief review of the anatomic and physiologic aspects of neuromuscular transmission.

The motor end-plate consists of a nerve terminal separated from the postsynaptic region by the synaptic space. Acetylcholine (ACh) is stored in quantal packets (6,000 to 10,000 molecules per packet) in synaptic vesicles in the nerve terminal. The vesicles release ACh into the synaptic space by exocytosis. The postsynaptic region has junctional folds containing on their terminal expansions acetylcholine receptor (AChR) molecules packed at a density of about 10^4 sites per square micrometer. The binding of two ACh molecules to an AChR molecule opens the AChR ion channel, which subsequently closes again when ACh dissociates from AChR. Acetylcholinesterase (AChE) is distributed throughout the basal lamina of the synaptic space at a density of about 2,500 sites per square micrometer.

In the resting state single ACh quanta are randomly released into the synaptic space. The high local ACh concentration saturates all nearby AChE sites so that most ACh molecules can reach postsynaptic AChR's. The AChR packing density is so high that ACh needs to diffuse only 0.3 μm along the top and 0.3 μm down along the junctional folds before it meets all the AChR it can saturate. The resultant resting depolarizations of the muscle fiber are known as miniature end-plate potentials (MEPP's). The MEPP amplitude depends on the number of ACh molecules in the quantum, the number of available AChR's, the geometry of the synaptic space, and the average depolarization generated by the opening of an AChR ion channel. When ACh dissociates from AChR it is hydrolyzed by AChE to choline and acetate. Choline is taken up by the nerve terminal and is reutilized for ACh synthesis.

Depolarization of the nerve terminal by nerve impulse opens voltage-sensitive calcium channels in the presynaptic membrane. The calcium influx increases the probability of synaptic vesicle exocytosis. The exocytosis occurs adjacent to active zones in the presynaptic membrane. The voltage-sensitive calcium channels are thought to be associated with regularly arrayed large membrane particles in the active zones.

The quanta released by a nerve impulse generate an end-plate potential (EPP) the amplitude of which depends on the MEPP amplitude and the number of quanta (m) released by a nerve impulse. The value of m depends on the probability of release (p) and the number of quanta readily available for release (n) according to the relationship $m = np$. *The safety margin of neuromuscular transmission is defined as the difference between the actual EPP amplitude and the EPP amplitude required to trigger the muscle fiber action potential.*

Repetitive stimulation results in a frequency-dependent depression of the EPP amplitude and of the safety margin to a certain plateau. The decrease is mainly due to a decrease in n. Repetitive stimulation also can facilitate transmitter release by increasing p, or n, or both. The temporal profiles of the opposing processes are such that (1) a defect of neuromuscular transmission is most readily detected by a train of five to ten stimuli delivered at a low (2 to 3 Hz) frequency; (2) tetanic stimulation results in transient improvement and then a worsening of the defect.

Table 518–1 shows a classification of currently recognized defects of neuromuscular transmission. Botulism is described in Ch. 280, the others in this chapter.

MYASTHENIA GRAVIS (MG). This is an acquired autoimmune disorder associated with AChR deficiency at the motor end-plate. The safety margin of neuromuscular transmission is compromised by the small amplitude of the MEPP and consequently of the EPP. Circulating AChR antibodies are present in 80 to 90 per cent of the cases, and immune complexes (IgG and complement components) are deposited on the postsynaptic membrane. AChR deficiency results from complement-mediated lysis of the junctional folds, accelerated internalization and destruction of AChR cross-linked by antibody (modulation), and, to a lesser extent, by antibodies blocking the binding of ACh to AChR.

Clinical Features. The incidence is two to five per year per million and the prevalence 13 to 64 per million. The female to male ratio is six to four. The disease may present at any age, but the incidence in females peaks in the third decade and in males in the sixth or seventh decade.

The disease can involve either the external ocular muscles

TABLE 518–1. CLASSIFICATION OF DISORDERS OF NEUROMUSCULAR TRANSMISSION

Autoimmune
Myasthenia gravis
Lambert-Eaton myasthenic syndrome

Congenital
Familial infantile myasthenia*
End-plate acetylcholinesterase deficiency†
Slow-channel syndrome‡
End-plate acetylcholine receptor deficiency*

Toxic
Botulism
Drug-induced
Pesticide poisoning

*Autosomal-recessive inheritance
†Autosomal- or X-linked recessive inheritance
‡Autosomal-dominant inheritance

selectively or the general voluntary muscle system. The symptoms may fluctuate from hour to hour, day to day, or over longer periods. They are provoked or worsened by exertion, exposure to extremes of temperature, viral or other infections, menses, and excitement. Ocular muscle involvement is usually bilateral, asymmetric, and typically is associated with ptosis and diplopia. Weakness of other muscles innervated by cranial nerves results in loss of facial expression, everted lips, a smile that resembles a snarl, jaw drop, nasal regurgitation of liquids, choking on foods and secretions, and a slurred, hypernasal speech of a reduced volume. Abnormal fatigability of the limb muscles causes difficulty in combing the hair, lifting objects repeatedly, climbing stairs, walking, and running. Depending on the severity of the disease, dyspnea appears on moderate or mild exertion or is present even at rest. The abnormal fatigability can be demonstrated by asking the patient to look up without closing the eyes for a minute, to count loudly from one to one hundred, to hold the arms abducted to the horizontal position for a minute, or to perform repeated deep knee-bends. The deep tendon reflexes are normally active even in weak muscles. Atrophy of masseter, temporal, facial, or tongue muscles, and less often of other muscles, occurs in about 15 per cent of patients.

Initially, the symptoms are purely ocular in 40 per cent, generalized in 40 per cent, and involve only the extremities in 10 per cent, and only the bulbar or bulbar and eye muscles in another 10 per cent. Subsequently, the weakness can spread from ocular to facial to lower bulbar muscles and then to torso and limb muscles, but the sequence may vary. Proximal limb muscles are affected more than distal ones. In the most advanced cases the weakness is universal. By the end of the first year, the ocular muscles are affected in nearly all patients. The symptoms remain ocular in only 16 per cent. In nearly 90 per cent of those in whom the disease becomes generalized, this occurs within the first year after the onset. Progression is most rapid within the first three years, and more than half of the deaths caused by MG occur in that period. Spontaneous remissions lasting from weeks to years can occur. Long remissions are uncommon, and most remissions occur during the first three years.

Two thirds of patients with MG have thymic hyperplasia and 10 to 15 per cent have thymoma. A few with thymoma also develop myocarditis or giant cell myositis. In about 10 per cent the MG is associated with another autoimmune disease, such as hyperthyroidism, polymyositis, systemic lupus erythematosus, Sjögren's syndrome, rheumatoid arthritis, ulcerative colitis, pemphigus, sarcoidosis, pernicious anemia, and Lambert-Eaton myasthenic syndrome.

A clinical classification of MG, originally proposed by Osserman, is based on the distribution and severity of symptoms: group 1, ocular; group 2A, mild generalized; group 2B, moderately severe generalized; group 3, acute fulminating; group 4, late severe. Another classification, proposed by Vincent and Newsom-Davis, is according to the age of onset and the presence or absence of thymoma: Type 1, MG with thymoma: The disease is usually severe and the AChR antibody level is high; there is no association either with sex or HLA antigen. Type 2, no thymoma, onset before age 40: The AChR antibody level is intermediate; there is female preponderance and an increased association with HLA-A1, HLA-B8, and HLA-DRw3 antigens (HLA-B12 in Japan). Type 3, no thymoma, onset after age 40: The AChR antibody level tends to be low; there is male preponderance and increased association with HLA-A3, HLA-B7 or HLA-DRw2 antigens (HLA-A10 in Japan). Striated muscle antibodies are found in 90 per cent, 5 per cent, and 45 per cent, respectively, in the three types. The association with other autoimmune diseases is highest in Type 3 and lowest in Type 1. Both classifications are discussed further in the Engel chapters cited in the references.

TRANSIENT NEONATAL MG. Circulating AChR antibodies can

be detected in most infants born to myasthenic mothers, but only 12 per cent of such children develop MG, usually during the first few hours of life. The findings are feeble cry, feeding and respiratory difficulty, general or facial weakness, and ptosis. The mean duration is 18 days. There is no relation between the severity of MG in mother and infant. The disease is caused by the transfer of AChR antibodies or immunocytes from mother to infant, or perhaps fetal AChR damaged by maternal antibodies triggers a transient immune response in the infant.

Diagnosis. This is based on the characteristic history, physical examination, anticholinesterase tests, and laboratory studies. The latter include EMG studies, tests for AChR antibodies, and in selected cases, microelectrode studies in vitro of neuromuscular transmission and ultrastructural and cytochemical studies of the end-plate.

ANTICHOLINESTERASE TESTS. Edrophonium given intravenously acts within a few seconds, and its effects last for a few minutes. One to 2 mg of the drug is injected intravenously over 15 seconds. If there is no response in 30 seconds, an additional 8 to 9 mg is injected. The evaluation of the response requires objective assessment of one or more signs, such as degree of ptosis, range of ocular movements, and the force of the hand grip. Possible cholinergic side effects of the drug include fasciculations, flushing, lacrimation, abdominal cramps, nausea, vomiting, and diarrhea. The drug must be given cautiously to patients with cardiac disease, for it may cause sinus bradycardia, A-V block, and, rarely, cardiac arrest. Atropine is used to reverse toxicity. Intramuscular neostigmine, 0.5 to 1.0 mg, acts maximally in about 30 minutes, and its effects last up to two hours, allowing a more leisurely evaluation of changes in clinical status.

ELECTROMYOGRAPHY. Supramaximal stimulation of a motor nerve at 2 to 3 Hz results in a 10 per cent or greater decrement of the amplitude of the evoked compound muscle action potential from the first to the fifth response. The test is positive in nearly all patients provided that two or more distal and two or more proximal muscles are examined. The decrement is caused by a normally occurring decrease in the number of quanta released from the nerve terminal, and hence in the amplitude of the EPP, at the beginning of low-frequency stimulation. In MG the EPP amplitude is already reduced by the AChR deficiency, and the additional decrease during stimulation results in blocking of transmission at an increasing number of end-plates. Single-fiber EMG compares the timing of action potentials between pairs of closely adjacent muscle fibers in the same motor unit during a willed contraction. In MG the low amplitude and relatively long rise time of the EPP cause abnormally long interpotential intervals and intermittent blocking of action potential generation at some fibers.

SEROLOGIC TESTS. The usual AChR antibody test measures the binding of antibody to AChR labeled with radioactive alpha-bungarotoxin. The toxin itself is attached irreversibly to the ACh binding site of AChR. The antibody binding test is positive in nearly all patients with moderately severe or acute severe MG, in 80 per cent with mild generalized MG, in 50 per cent with ocular MG, but in only 25 per cent of those in remission. In a few patients only antibodies that block the binding of ACh to AChR can be detected. The antibody titer correlates only loosely with disease severity but in individual patients a greater than 50 per cent decrease in titer for more than 12 months is nearly always associated with sustained clinical improvement. Striated muscle antibodies also occur in MG patients. Their role remains unknown but they often are associated with thymoma.

OTHER DIAGNOSTIC STUDIES. Immune complexes can be localized at the MG end-plate in cryostat sections even when circulating AChR antibodies cannot be detected. C3 localization is technically the easiest and most convenient way to confirm the suspected diagnosis. Electrophysiologic studies

of neuromuscular transmission in vitro can distinguish between atypical cases of MG, the Lambert-Eaton myasthenic syndrome, and some of the congenital myasthenic syndromes.

Differential Diagnosis. This includes neurasthenia, oculopharyngeal dystrophy, mitochondrial myopathies involving the external ocular and/or other cranial and limb muscles, intracranial mass lesions compressing cranial nerves, drug-induced myasthenic syndromes, and other disorders of neuromuscular transmission listed in the table. Neurasthenia is recognized by giving way on muscle testing and the lack of objective clinical and laboratory findings. In myopathies involving the ocular muscles, the weakness does not fluctuate, diplopia is seldom a symptom, the muscle biopsy may show distinct morphologic abnormalities, and pharmacologic and laboratory tests for MG are negative. Drug-induced and other myasthenic syndromes are considered below.

Therapy. Anticholinesterases, alternate-day prednisone treatment, azathioprine, thymectomy, and plasmapheresis are currently used to treat MG. Anticholinesterases are useful in all clinical forms of the disease. Pyridostigmine bromide (Mestinon) (60-mg tablets) acts for three to four hours, and neostigmine bromide (15-mg tablets) for two to three hours. The former drug has fewer muscarinic side effects and is therefore more widely used. One half to four tablets of pyridostigmine bromide are given every four hours in the daytime. This medication is also available in 180-mg "timespan" tablets for use at bedtime and as a syrup for children and patients requiring nasogastric feeding. If troublesome muscarinic side effects occur, these can be treated with 0.4 to 0.6 mg atropine given orally two or three times daily. Postoperatively or in critically ill patients intramuscularly injectable pyridostigmine bromide (the dose is one thirtieth of the oral dose) and neostigmine methylsulfate (the dose is one fifteenth of the oral dose) can be used.

Progressive weakness despite increasing amounts of anticholinesterases signals the onset of a myasthenic or cholinergic crisis. Cholinergic crises are associated with muscarinic effects, such as abdominal cramps, nausea, vomiting, diarrhea, miosis, lacrimation, increased bronchial secretions, diaphoresis, and bradycardia. In a myasthenic crisis the muscarinic effects are not conspicuous, and 2 mg edrophonium given intravenously improves rather than worsens the weakness. In practice, however, the two types of crises often are difficult to distinguish, and overmedication of a myasthenic crisis can convert it into a cholinergic crisis. Therefore, patients who have increasing difficulty with respiration, feeding, or handling secretions and who are not responding to relatively high doses of anticholinesterases are best treated by drug withdrawal, tracheal intubation or tracheostomy, support with respirator, and intravenous feeding. Refractoriness to drug therapy usually disappears after a few days.

In patients with generalized disease not responding adequately to modest doses of anticholinesterases, other forms of therapy must be employed. Thymectomy increases the remission rate and improves the clinical course of MG. Although controlled clinical studies of thymectomy according to age, sex, and severity of disease have never been carried out, there is general agreement that the best response occurs in young women with hyperplastic thymus glands and high antibody titer. Thymoma represents an absolute indication for thymectomy because the tumor is often locally invasive. Chest radiographs combined with linear tomography detect most thymomas. Computed tomography of the mediastinum is a sensitive screening test, but it can give false-positive results.

Alternate-day prednisone treatment induces remission or significantly improves the disease in more than half the patients. The treatment is relatively safe provided that one institutes the usual precautions for patients taking corticosteroid therapy. With an average dose of 70 mg on alternate days, the average time for significant improvement is five months. After the improvement reaches a plateau the dose must be lowered gradually over several months to establish the minimum maintenance dose.

Azathioprine in doses of 150 to 200 mg per day also induces remissions or measurable improvement in more than half the treated patients. The minimum time for improvement is three months. Surveillance to detect side effects (pancytopenia, leukopenia, serious infection, and hepatocellular injury) must be maintained during therapy.

Plasmapheresis is indicated in severe generalized or fulminating MG refractory to other forms of treatment. Daily exchanges of two liters of plasma result in objective improvement and lower the AChR antibody titer in a few days. Plasmapheresis, however, is expensive and does not confer greater long-term protection than immunosuppressants alone.

LAMBERT-EATON MYASTHENIC SYNDROME. This is an acquired autoimmune disease associated with a reduced probability of quantal release from the nerve terminal by nerve impulse. Among patients over 40 years 70 per cent of males and 30 per cent of females will have an associated carcinoma, usually a small-cell carcinoma of the lung. The syndrome may predate tumor detection by up to three years. In one third of patients the syndrome is non-neoplastic and occurs at any age.

Patients have weakness and fatigability of proximal limb and torso muscles with relative sparing of extraocular and bulbar muscles. The lower limbs are more severely involved than the upper ones. On maximal voluntary contraction the force produced by a weak muscle increases for a few seconds and then again decreases. The tendon reflexes are hypoactive or absent in most patients. Autonomic manifestations (dry mouth, impotence, decreased sweating, orthostatic hypotension, or altered pupillary reflexes) occur in one half of the patients.

On EMG, the amplitude of the compound muscle action potential evoked by a single nerve stimulus from rested muscle is abnormally small. Repetitive stimulation at 2 Hz induces a further decrement, but stimulation at frequencies higher than 10 Hz or voluntary exercise for a brief period markedly facilitates the response so that the evoked potential attains normal amplitude.

Evidence for the autoimmune origin of the syndrome rests on its responsiveness to immunosuppressants and plasmapheresis, association of non-neoplastic cases with other autoimmune disorders and organ-specific autoantibodies, and the passive transfer with IgG of the electrophysiologic and morphologic features of the disease from human to mouse. Freeze-fracture electron microscopy reveals a paucity of presynaptic membrane-active zones and active zone particles. This suggests that the reduced quantal release by nerve impulse is related to reduced ingress of calcium into the nerve terminal and that the active zone particles are direct or indirect targets of the pathogenic autoantibodies.

Anticholinesterases are only slightly effective. Guanidine hydrochloride (10 mg per kilogram per day) or 3,4-diaminopyridine (1 mg per kilogram per day) increases quantal release from the nerve terminal and relieves the symptoms. However, the former drug has severe toxic side effects, and the latter is not yet available in clinical practice. Optimal treatment of non-neoplastic cases consists of modest doses of alternate-day prednisone and 2 mg per kilogram per day of azathioprine.

CONGENITAL MYASTHENIC SYNDROMES. *Familial Infantile Myasthenia.* This is an autosomal-recessive disorder characterized by fluctuating ophthalmoparesis since birth, feeding difficulty during early infancy, weakness after exercise, and attacks of apnea precipitated by crying, vomiting, or fever. The symptoms tend to improve with age. A decremental EMG response is present in muscles weak when examined. Weakness can be induced in some, but not all, muscles by exercise or repetitive stimulation at 10 Hz for a few minutes. Unlike in autoimmune MG, the postsynaptic region is intact and there is no AChR deficiency. The MEPP amplitude is normal in rested muscle but decreases to abnormally low values after 10-Hz stimulation for a few minutes. This suggests a presynaptic defect in ACh resynthesis or in ACh packaging into synaptic vesicles. Weakness, when present, responds to small or modest doses of anticholinesterases. Parenteral anticholinesterase therapy is indicated in crises. Parents of young patients must be taught to use a hand-assisted ventilatory device and to inject appropriate doses of neostigmine intramuscularly during crises.

Congenital End-Plate Acetylcholinesterase Deficiency. Sporadic cases in males have been observed to date. Severe weakness refractory to anticholinesterases and a decremental EMG response are present in all voluntary muscles from birth. There is total absence of AChE from all end-plates. ACh-AChR interaction and the duration of the EPP are prolonged, so that a single stimulus applied to a motor nerve evokes two or more compound muscle action potentials. The motor nerve terminals are small and contain a reduced number of releasable ACh quanta. AChR is preserved or reduced at the end-plate. The AChR loss, if present, is caused by degenerative changes in the junctional folds which can be accounted for by the ACh excess, but this in itself is mild because ACh release is also reduced. The safety margin of neuromuscular transmission is compromised by lack of releasable ACh quanta and by AChR deficiency.

Slow-Channel Syndrome. This is an autosomal-dominant disorder with high penetrance and variable expressivity. It presents in infancy or later life with selective weakness, fatigability, and atrophy of cervical, shoulder girdle, and forearm muscles. There is variable involvement of extraocular, other cranial, truncal, or limb muscles. The tendon reflexes are normal or hypoactive. Anticholinesterases are usually ineffective. A decremental EMG response appears in clinically affected muscles. The basic abnormality is slow closure of the AChR ion channel. This prolongs the duration of the EPP, causes a stimulus-linked repetitive compound action potential in all muscles, and allows abnormal accumulation of calcium in the postsynaptic region. The calcium excess results in destruction of the junctional folds, loss of AChR, and myopathic changes near the end-plates. The safety margin of neuromuscular transmission is compromised by the AChR deficiency and the altered end-plate geometry.

Congenital End-Plate AChR Deficiency. This is an autosomal recessive disorder that presents during infancy. The symptoms and electrophysiologic abnormalities resemble those in autoimmune MG and respond to anticholinesterases. Circulating AChR antibodies are absent, and no immune complexes are found at the end-plate. The cause has not been established. It could stem from decreased synthesis, impaired membrane insertion or accelerated degradation of AChR, or abnormal ACh-AChR interaction.

DRUG-INDUCED MYASTHENIC SYNDROMES. These are uncommon in clinical practice. Tetracycline, polymyxin and aminoglycoside antibiotics, antiarrhythmic agents (procainamide, quinidine), β-adrenergic blockers (propranolol, timolol), phenothiazines, lithium, trimethaphan, methoxyflurane, and magnesium given parenterally or in cathartics, reduce the safety margin of neuromuscular transmission. However, overt myasthenic symptoms do not usually appear unless an overdose of the drug is administered or the renal or hepatic elimination of the drug is impaired. The same drugs also can potentiate neuromuscular blocking agents used during surgical procedures and both may worsen or unmask pre-existing disorders of neuromuscular transmission. Calcium channel blocking drugs can worsen the transmission defect in the Lambert-Eaton myasthenic syndrome.

Succinylcholine, a depolarizing blocking drug, is used to induce muscle relaxation during anesthesia. A single dose of the drug sufficient to cause transient apnea is eliminated by plasma pseudocholinesterase in 2 to 10 minutes. In approximately 1 of 2500 patients receiving the drug, prolonged apnea occurs and persists up to several hours. Most of these patients have an autosomal-recessive abnormality of the plasma pseudocholinesterase. In some genetic variants the plasma pseudocholinesterase activity is abnormally low; in others the enzyme shows increased sensitivity to inhibition by dibucaine.

PESTICIDE POISONING. Poisoning with pesticides containing long-acting anticholinesterases causes ACh accumulation at central, muscarinic, and nicotinic cholinergic synapses. The intoxication is associated with alterations in sensorium, severe muscarinic effects, and muscle weakness from desensitization of AChR at the neuromuscular junction. Therapy consists of respiratory support, large doses of atropine (2 to 4 mg intramuscularly and repeated as necessary) and pralidoxime (1 gram intravenously, repeated in 20 minutes if necessary).

Engel AG, Banker BQ (eds.): Myology. New York, McGraw-Hill Book Company, 1986. *Chapters by Engel and Magelby ably discuss the detailed anatomy, physiology, and clinical dimensions of neuromuscular transmission.*

Grob D, Brunner NG, Namba T: The natural course of myasthenia gravis and effect of therapeutic measures. Ann NY Acad Sci 377:652, 1981. *A model clinical study.*

Lang B, Newsom-Davis J, Prior C, et al.: Antibodies to motor nerve terminals: An electrophysiologic study of a human myasthenic syndrome transferred to mouse. J Physiol (Lond) 344:335, 1983. *This work convincingly establishes the autoimmune basis of the Lambert-Eaton myasthenic syndrome.*

Nelson TC, Burritt MF: Pesticide poisoning, succinylcholine-induced apnea and pseudocholinesterase. Mayo Clin Proc 61:750, 1986. *A good description of pesticide poisoning and the different pseudocholinesterase deficiencies.*

Swift TR: Disorders of neuromuscular transmission other than myasthenia gravis. Muscle Nerve 4:334, 1981. *A thorough review of drug-induced myasthenic syndromes.*

PART XXIII
EYE DISEASES

John W. Gittinger, Jr.

Because many systemic diseases affect the eyes, ophthalmoscopy is a necessary skill for the physician. The pupil of the eye is a window opening onto the arterioles and venules of the retina, the optic disc, and the pigmented tissues of the fundus. Ch. 464 describes the autonomic and somatic motor disorders of ocular control and reviews the clinically important anatomy of the visual pathways.

The discussion that follows highlights the interrelationship between ocular and systemic disease, beginning with a discussion of transient visual loss, then a brief review of the two common ophthalmic disorders—cataract and glaucoma, before turning to ocular entities and ocular manifestations of medical disorders likely to present to nonophthalmic physicians.

519 TRANSIENT VISUAL LOSS

Transient monocular blindness is often referred to as *amaurosis fugax*, which literally means "fleeting blindness." Momentary loss of vision may be described as a transient obscuration. Many disorders can produce this symptom (Table 519–1), but the major clinical importance of transient monocular blindness in persons older than 40 years is as an indicator of embolic carotid or cardiac disease.

TABLE 519–1. CAUSES OF TRANSIENT MONOCULAR BLINDNESS

Common Causes
Carotid vascular disease
  Atherosclerosis, fibromuscular dysplasia
Embolic cardiac disease
  Rheumatic valvular disease, mitral valve prolapse, subacute bacterial
    endocarditis, atrial myxoma, mural thrombi
Local vascular phenomena
  Increased intracranial pressure—papilledema (usually bilateral visual loss)
  Migraine (usually bilateral loss)
Prodromes to prolonged or permanent visual loss
  Ischemic optic neuropathy
  Arterial or venous occlusion
  Optic neuritis
Unexplained or idiopathic

Uncommon Causes
Ocular anomalies
  Peripapillary staphylomas
  Optic disc drusen
  Recurrent hyphema
  Angle-closure glaucoma (transient)
Systemic vascular phenomena
  Hypotension and hypertension (usually bilateral visual loss)
  Hematologic abnormalities
    Polycythemia
    Thrombocytosis
    Anemia (usually bilateral loss)
    Macroglobulinemia
    Sickle cell trait
Orbital disease
  Optic nerve meningiomas
  Cavernous hemangiomas

In younger persons without risk factors, transient monocular blindness is often attributed to migraine, but probably should simply be considered idiopathic. The significance of mitral valve prolapse in this population is debated.

Monocular visual loss should be distinguished from the aura of classic migraine, which is another type of transient, usually homonymous, visual loss. The migranous aura consists of an expanding hemianopic scotoma with scintillating borders and characteristically lasts approximately 20 minutes. In classic migraine, the aura is followed by a headache, but many auras occur without headache. This type of *migraine equivalent* or *acephalgic migraine* may develop in middle aged or elderly persons who had classic migraine as youths or may present spontaneously at any age in isolation.

Migraine-like scotomata also are occasionally manifestations of systemic lupus erythematosus or can accompany arteriovenous malformations of the brain. Most, however, are independent phenomena of unknown cause; acephalgic migraine as an isolated symptom is an unlikely indicator of a hemispheric transient ischemic attack.

Adams HP Jr, Putman SF, Corbett JJ, et al.: Amaurosis fugax: The results of arteriography in 59 patients. Stroke 14:742, 1983. *Twenty of these patients had normal arteriograms, and only 15 had carotid stenosis. The remainder had a heterogenous group of disorders or no cause was found.*
Kunkel RS: Acephalgic migraine. Headache 26:198, 1986. *A brief review of purported migraine equivalents.*

520 CATARACT

A cataract is an opacity of the lens that produces painless, gradual loss of vision. Cataracts are described according to their location—nuclear (deep in the lens), cortical (more superficial), and subcapsular (immediately beneath the capsule). Cataracts are classified as immature, mature, or hypermature. An immature cataract has some clear cortex; a mature cataract is totally opaque—the pupil appears white (leukokoria). A hypermature cataract has liquefied cortex that leaks through the capsule and may excite destructive inflammation. Immature cataracts are usually removed for visual reasons. A mature or hypermature cataract in an eye with potentially useful vision should be removed to prevent irreversible damage.

ETIOLOGY. Congenital cataracts are a feature of rubella embryopathy and often are associated with other congenital malformations. Acquired cataracts may result from trauma, radiation, or metabolic disorder. Several examples of colorful cataracts have diagnostic, but little visual, significance. In Wilson's disease, orange copper deposits may appear on the anterior capsule—the sunflower cataract. Chlorpromazine administration may result in a brown or white dusting on the anterior lens surface. Red, green, and blue opacities in the lenticular cortex characterize myotonic dystrophy, but are occasionally encountered in its absence.

Hypocalcemia may be cataractogenic. Cataracts occur in disorders of carbohydrate metabolism: hypoglycemia, galactosemia, and diabetes mellitus. Diabetics do not necessarily have an increased incidence of cataracts, but theirs progress rapidly, perhaps because of variations in lens hydration.

Systemic corticosteroids promote formation of posterior subcapsular cataracts. Because of the path light takes through the lens, posterior subcapsular cataracts reduce vision more than similar, eccentric opacities. Central posterior opacities get in the way of light, especially when the pupil is small, as in bright light or with close work. Difficulties with driving and reading are often the first complaints.

Most cataracts have no known etiology. The common nuclear sclerotic cataract, or senile cataract, is often familial, but no specific factors have been proven to accelerate or retard its development.

TREATMENT. The treatment for cataract is surgical removal. With the exception of mature and hypermature cataracts and of immature cataracts that have swollen sufficiently to threaten to precipitate angle-closure glaucoma, most cataracts are removed for visual reasons. Considerations in planning cataract extraction are the patient's visual needs, the potential for improvement, and the risks of surgery. A person who drives will require surgery when the better eye is worse than 20/40, the legal minimum for a driver's license in most states. By contrast, an elderly patient with 20/200 vision and limited visual needs may be happy without intervention. Care must be taken to identify intercurrent ocular disease; removal of the lens of an eye with advanced glaucoma or macular degeneration does not improve vision.

The risk of cataract surgery itself is small. Despite the possibility of intraocular hemorrhage, postoperative infection, corneal decompensation, or problems with wound healing, the chances for a good visual outcome are excellent. Even successful cataract surgery, however, increases the likelihood of subsequent retinal detachment, and a small percentage of eyes postoperatively develop prolonged cystoid macular edema with reduced acuity.

General anesthesia constitutes a major portion of the risk. Cataract surgery, however, can usually be performed under local anesthesia, and this should be considered the method of choice in medically fragile patients.

Jaffe NS: Cataract Surgery and its Complications. 4th ed. St. Louis, The C. V. Mosby Company, 1984. *This profusely illustrated monograph addresses most of the issues of modern cataract surgery and includes extensive references.*

521 GLAUCOMA

Glaucoma comprises a group of disorders in which elevated intraocular pressure damages the optic nerve. The major types of glaucoma are open-angle, angle-closure, congenital, and secondary.

The dynamics of aqueous humor control intraocular pressure. The aqueous humor is derived from blood by a process of secretion and ultrafiltration in the ciliary body. Aqueous humor then passes from the posterior chamber through the pupil to fill the anterior chamber, the space between the back of the cornea and the plane of the iris and pupil. The aqueous humor is reabsorbed through the trabecular meshwork, located in the angle between the cornea and the iris, to enter Schlemm's canal, which connects with the venous system (Fig. 521–1).

OPEN-ANGLE GLAUCOMA

In chronic open-angle glaucoma, the most common type, a block in aqueous humor reabsorption exists at the level of the trabecular meshwork. Intraocular pressure rises above its normal maximum of 21 mm Hg and gradually destroys axons and supporting tissue on the optic disc.

The prevalence of open-angle glaucoma varies with the population studied and the diagnostic criteria employed. A conservative estimate of unequivocal glaucoma in American and European adults is 0.5 per cent. A larger number sustain increased intraocular pressure without signs of optic nerve damage—*ocular hypertension.* The patient with ocular hypertension is considered suspect for glaucoma.

Open-angle glaucoma is ordinarily asymptomatic until well advanced. Only rarely does the elevated intraocular pressure cause corneal edema, with the attendant perception of halos around lights. Pain is not characteristic of open-angle glaucoma. Initially only the peripheral visual field is lost; visual acuity remains normal until late in the course of the disease. Diagnosis is made by measurement of intraocular pressure, examination of the optic disc, and testing of the visual fields. Gonioscopy, the visualization of the angle structures under high magnifications with special contact lenses, can distinguish an angle-closure from an open-angle mechanism.

The treatment of open-angle glaucoma is primarily medical. Topical administration of parasympathomimetics (pilocarpine and carbachol), beta-adrenergic blockers (timolol, betaxolol, and levobunolol), and sympathomimetics (epinephrine and dipivefrin) decreases intraocular pressure. When these medications—individually and in combination—are ineffective in arresting progressive disc damage and visual field loss, indirect parasympathomimetics (echothiophate) and carbonic anhydrase inhibitors (acetazolamide and methazolamide) may be prescribed.

If maximum tolerated medical therapy fails to halt progression, surgery is indicated. *Laser trabeculoplasty* opens aqueous outflow channels by burning the surface of the trabecular meshwork. If all else fails, a surgical fistula can be created between the anterior chamber and the subconjunctival space, allowing direct absorption of aqueous humor by subconjunctival and episcleral vessels.

The management of open-angle glaucoma depends upon early recognition, careful follow-up, and patient compliance with therapeutic regimens. Routine measurement of intraocular pressures (*tonometry*) at general physical examinations is often advocated, but careful ophthalmoscopy with referral of patients whose central excavation ("cup") exceeds one third of the disc's area may be an equally effective screen.

ANGLE-CLOSURE GLAUCOMA

Angle-closure glaucoma develops when the normal path of aqueous flow is interrupted in an eye with a shallow anterior chamber, the consequence of a structurally anomalous anterior segment. Intraocular pressure is normal until resistance to aqueous flow through the pupil—pupillary block—bows the iris forward to obstruct the resorptive surfaces in the angle. The pressure then rises precipitously, often to above 50 mm Hg (Fig. 521–2).

Acute angle-closure glaucoma is generally monocular. The eye is red and painful and the pupil is about 6 mm and fixed. Vision is decreased. The patient is diaphoretic, nauseated, and often vomits.

Typical angle-closure glaucoma is easy to recognize. Occasionally, chronic or subacute angle-closure mimics open-angle glaucoma. Gonioscopy then distinguishes between the two mechanisms. The elderly often do not develop the full set of clinical signs and symptoms. Always consider angle-closure glaucoma in patients with a fixed, mid-dilated pupil and decreased vision.

Angle-closure can be precipitated in predisposed eyes by dilating the pupils. The risk of pharmacologic dilation is assessed by noting the depth of the anterior chamber. Eyes

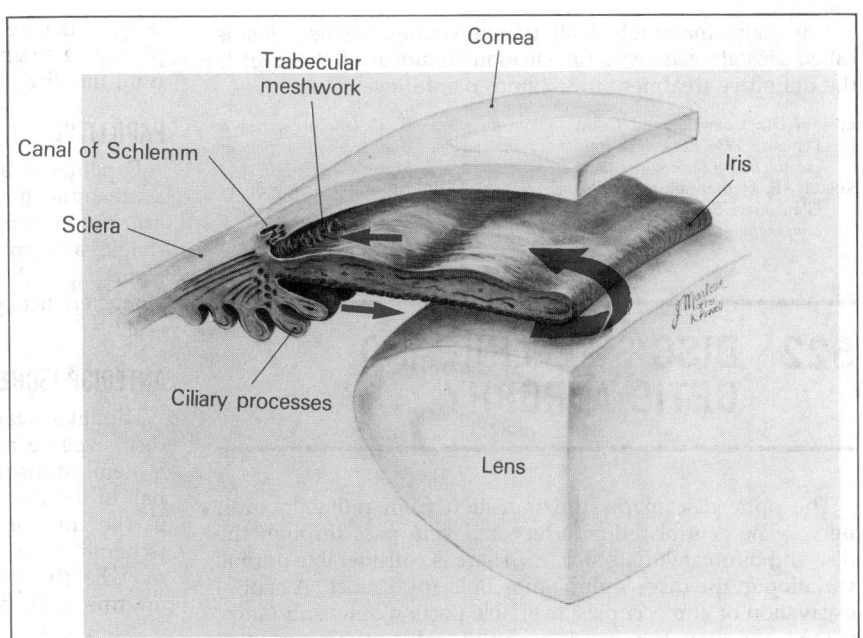

FIGURE 521–1. Circulation of aqueous humor in the normal eye. Aqueous is produced in the ciliary body and its processes, fills the posterior chamber (which also contains the lens), passes through the pupil (*large arrow*), and is reabsorbed through the trabecular meshwork into the canal of Schlemm.

with shallow anterior chambers are at risk for angle-closure. This distinction is not always easy to observe, and even an experienced ophthalmologist sometimes cannot determine whether an angle will close with dilation. The risk of dilation increases with age, and everyone over the age of 50 whose anterior chamber is less than full depth should be considered to have the potential for angle-closure. This does not mean that most patients should not be dilated, but rather that dilation should be performed with a short-acting mydriatic agent such as tropicamide or hydroxyamphetamine, and the patient observed until the mydriatic begins to wear off.

A nonophthalmologist should probably not routinely dilate adult outpatients. Children and in-patients may be dilated if there is no other contraindication such as recent head trauma, an iris-fixated intraocular lens, or impending general anesthesia. With these exceptions, the diagnostic benefits of dilation outweigh the risk of precipitating angle-closure. Should angle-closure glaucoma develop, it can be recognized and promptly treated.

An acute angle-closure attack is a medical emergency. Initial management consists of administration of parenteral acetazolamide, oral glycerol or intravenous mannitol, and topical

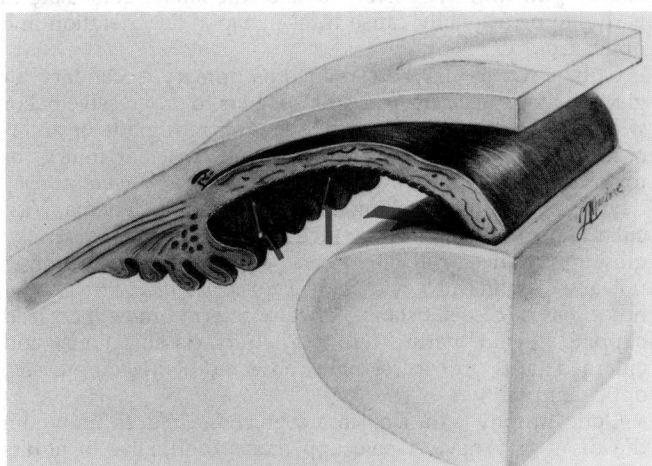

FIGURE 521–2. Angle-closure glaucoma. Owing to an anatomical anomaly in the anterior segment of the eye, the aqueous becomes trapped behind the pupil, bowing the iris forward (iris bombé) to cover the trabecular meshwork, which lies in the angle between the iris and the cornea.

pilocarpine and perhaps timolol. Once the attack has been broken, the anatomic predisposition can be circumvented by connecting the posterior and anterior chamber through the peripheral iris, either with a laser—*laser iridotomy*—or by surgical iridectomy. The anterior segment abnormality that underlies angle-closure glaucoma is bilateral, and prophylactic surgery on the other eye is usually indicated.

CONGENITAL GLAUCOMA

Congenital glaucoma is an open-angle glaucoma that results from dysgenesis of the angle structures. Increased intraocular pressure enlarges the immature eye (*buphthalmos*); a corneal diameter greater than 12 mm suggests congenital glaucoma. Progressive corneal enlargement disrupts the deeper layers of the cornea, with resulting corneal edema and loss of transparency. The cornea of a child with advanced congenital glaucoma is enlarged, with a ground-glass translucency.

Treatment of congenital glaucoma is both surgical and medical. The condition is fortunately rare and the prognosis for preservation of vision is only fair.

SECONDARY GLAUCOMA

Secondary glaucoma develops as the consequence of another ocular disease. Examples of secondary glaucomas are angle-closure glaucoma precipitated by intumescence of the lens, glaucoma developing as a result of formation of new vessels in the angle, and glaucoma in a chronically inflamed eye. Severe blunt trauma to the eye damages angle structures, predisposing to the subsequent development of open-angle glaucoma.

The treatment of secondary, lens-induced angle-closure glaucoma is surgical removal of the lens. Most other secondary glaucomas are managed in much the same way as primary open-angle glaucoma. Neovascular glaucoma is difficult to treat, and most eyes ultimately lose all useful vision. If the stimulus to neovascularization is ischemia, ablation of ischemic tissues by photocoagulation may halt progression. If neovascularization continues, medical control becomes ineffective. Filtering procedures generally fail because exuberant tissue growth closes the surgical fistula, a problem that may be avoided by connecting the anterior chamber and the subconjunctival space with a plastic valve. Destruction of the ciliary body by an externally applied liquid nitrogen probe—*cyclocryotherapy*—controls intraocular pressure but seldom preserves useful vision.

Any glaucoma in which all light perception has been lost is called *absolute glaucoma*. Enucleation (removal of the eye) is the definitive treatment for a blind, painful eye.

Epstein DL: Chandler and Grant's Glaucoma, 3rd ed. Philadelphia, Lea & Febiger, 1986. *Epstein's revision of this text adds an excellent section on examination of the eye in glaucoma.*
Kolker AE, Hetherington J Jr: Becker-Shaffer's Diagnosis and Therapy of the Glaucomas. St. Louis, The C. V. Mosby Company, 1983. *The best one-volume compendium on this subject. The illustrations are numerous and clear.*

522 DISC SWELLING AND OPTIC ATROPHY

The optic disc marks the transition from retina to optic nerve. The central retinal artery and vein pass through the disc and bifurcate on its surface. There is considerable normal variation in the disc's ophthalmoscopic appearance. A central excavation or cup occupies a variable portion of its substance; vessels are often seen curving over the edge of this cup.

Over one million axons originate in the ganglion cells of the retina and pass through each optic disc. Although these axons are nearly transparent, a bright ophthalmoscope will visualize fine reflective striations on the disc's surface and the immediately surrounding retina. Disc swelling can be a consequence of ischemia, infarction, infiltration, or local changes in tissue pressures (Table 522–1).

PAPILLEDEMA (Color plate 7B)

Disc swelling from increased intracranial pressure is termed papilledema. The swelling reflects a combination of increased back pressure to the central retinal vein and accumulation of axoplasm in and around the disc. The swelling appears ophthalmoscopically as a protrusion of the disc, most obvious just adjacent to the normal borders. When the increase in intracranial pressure is rapid, the veins become engorged, and hemorrhages appear on the disc or adjacent retina.

Papilledema is usually bilateral but may be asymmetrical. Visual acuity remains normal in acute papilledema. Only in long-standing papilledema does secondary optic atrophy, with decreased vision, ensue (see below).

PSEUDOPAPILLEDEMA

Because the common causes of papilledema include intracranial tumor and hemorrhage, its recognition and differential diagnosis are important. Various other disc appearances may be confused with papilledema. Hyperopic (farsighted) eyes are small, with axonal crowding at the disc. Drusen of the optic disc, depositions of hyaline material in the prelaminar optic nerve, appear as swollen discs in young persons. In time, the buried drusen become exposed and are visible ophthalmoscopically as refractile bodies that resemble rock crystals. Such anomalous discs are often discovered inciden-

TABLE 522–1. CAUSES OF DISC SWELLING

Increased intracranial pressure (papilledema)	Compressive optic neuropathy
	Graves' disease
Inflammatory optic neuropathy (papillitis)	Sphenoid wing meningioma
	Vasculopathies
Infiltrative optic neuropathy	Anterior ischemic optic neuropathy
Sarcoidosis	Central retinal vein occlusion
Leukemia and other malignancies	Malignant hypertension
Optic nerve tumors	Toxic-metabolic optic neuropathy
Angioma	Idiopathic
Optic nerve meningioma	Pseudopapilledema
Childhood optic nerve glioma	Optic disc drusen
Malignant optic nerve glioma	Hyperopia
Metastatic carcinoma	Other anomalies

tally. One clue to their nature is the frequent absence of the physiologic cup, for in true papilledema the cup is preserved until the disc swelling is far advanced.

PAPILLITIS

Papillitis is an anterior optic neuritis. In the majority of acute optic neuritides the disc appears normal—*retrobulbar neuritis*. In papillitis, the disc is swollen and may be hemorrhagic, an appearance ophthalmoscopically indistinguishable from papilledema. Unlike papilledema, however, acuity is characteristically reduced, and the condition is usually unilateral.

ANTERIOR ISCHEMIC OPTIC NEUROPATHY

Papillitis is largely a disease of the young. In older persons, disc swelling and loss of vision suggest infarction—anterior ischemic optic neuropathy. Often only the superior or inferior half of the disc is involved, with consequent loss of function in the inferior or superior visual field. Most instances of ischemic optic neuropathy are idiopathic, but the disorder may be the initial manifestation of giant cell or temporal arteritis, a disease of the elderly described in Ch. 442.

OTHER CAUSES OF DISC SWELLING

Papilledema often accompanies severe, untreated hypertension. The relative roles of local vascular changes and of increased intracranial pressure in the pathogenesis are uncertain. Decreased intraocular pressure, encountered after ocular surgery or injury, also produces disc swelling, and the disc may swell acutely during an attack of angle-closure glaucoma. Disc swelling is also a feature of some toxic and hereditary optic neuropathies.

Compression causes disc swelling only when the nerve is constricted. This occurs in some patients with the orbitopathy of Graves' disease (Ch. 525), pseudotumor of the orbit (Ch. 525), and sphenoid wing meningioma. Intrinsic tumors of the optic nerve, the most common being glioma and meningioma, may present as disc swelling and visual loss. Infiltration of the optic nerve heads is also encountered in leukemia, metastatic carcinoma, and sarcoid.

OPTIC ATROPHY (Color plate 7C and D)

Optic atrophy results from death of the axons in the retina and optic nerve. Disc pallor and optic atrophy are not synonymous; some temporal pallor is a feature of normal discs. A lesion anywhere from the retina through the optic tract will cause optic atrophy. Lesions behind the lateral geniculate in early life occasionally cause trans-synaptic degeneration and optic atrophy.

Optic atrophy may be classified as primary, secondary, or glaucomatous. *Primary optic atrophy* refers to progressive pallor without loss of disc substance, a sign of retrograde or anterograde degeneration from compression, vascular injury, or toxic metabolic injury to the axons. *Secondary optic atrophy* develops after disc swelling, as in chronic papilledema. Vascular and glial changes may give the disc an irregular, milky gray appearance with ill-defined borders. The distinction is not always clinically evident. *Glaucomatous optic atrophy* denotes loss of disc substance, already referred to as increased cupping. Again, nature rejects arbitrary classifications, and enlarged cups are occasionally observed with compressive optic neuropathy.

Optic atrophy is difficult to recognize in children, in whom the discs may have a pale appearance normally. In adults with nuclear sclerotic cataracts, pallor is masked by the lens acting as a yellow filter. The diagnosis of optic atrophy should not be made unless there is evidence of alteration in visual function: decreased acuity or field—or, in infants, nystagmus.

Ultimately, optic atrophy is not a clinical finding but a pathologic entity. In retinitis pigmentosa there is a primary dystrophy of the rods and cones. The ganglion cells remain intact, but there are secondary vascular and gliotic changes with a waxy pallor of the disc, but not a true optic atrophy since the axons are preserved. Disc pallor is a finding to be evaluated in the context of the entire ophthalmologic and neurologic examination.

Miller NR: Walsh and Hoyt's Clinical Neuro-Ophthalmology. 4th ed. Baltimore, Williams & Wilkins Company, 1982, Vol 1, pp 175–271, 329–342. *The most recent revision of a classic monograph. The pages cited contain a comprehensive review of the entities discussed here.*

523 UVEITIS

Uveitis denotes inflammation of the uveal tract—the iris, ciliary body, and choroid. There are two major clinical types, anterior and posterior (Table 523–1). Anterior uveitis, also known as *iritis* or *iridocyclitis,* has as its hallmark cells in the anterior chamber. Curiously, it is the rare case of iritis that displays any recognizable iris abnormality. Posterior uveitis may take the form of *chorioretinitis.* The choroid and retina are so intimately connected that it is difficult to have inflammation of one without the other.

Acute anterior uveitis presents with congestion of the eye, often in a perilimbal distribution described as ciliary flush. Frequently, the eye is painful, vision reduced, and the pupil small and poorly reactive. The diagnosis is confirmed on slit lamp examination by the presence of free cells in the aqueous humor, visible as bright points as the slit beam passes through the anterior chamber. In more severe inflammation, *keratitic precipitates,* cellular aggregates on the back of the cornea, appear.

Most cases of anterior uveitis are idiopathic. Rarely, anterior uveitis is a manifestation of a systemic inflammatory disease such as sarcoid, or an infection such as syphilis or tuberculosis. In such cases the inflammation may be marked, with large, oily keratitic precipitates classically described as resembling mutton fat. This variant of anterior uveitis is *granulomatous iritis.*

UVEITIS AND ARTHRITIS

Juvenile rheumatoid arthritis (see Ch. 433) and ankylosing spondylitis (see Ch. 434) are especially apt to be associated with uveitis. Young men with this disorder may have recurrent episodes that respond to standard treatments (see below). A majority are HLA-B27 positive. By contrast, the uveitis accompanying juvenile rheumatoid arthritis is chronic and may initially be subclinical. Young women with the pauciarticular form of juvenile rheumatoid arthritis who develop uveitis often have white and quiet eyes. With time, however,

TABLE 523–1. DISEASES ASSOCIATED WITH UVEITIS

	Infections	Other
Anterior (iridocyclitis)	Herpes zoster Herpesvirus hominis Hansen's disease	Ankylosing spondylitis Rheumatoid arthritis Reiter's syndrome
Posterior (chorioretinitis)	Toxoplasmosis Toxocariasis Histoplasmosis Measles	
Both anterior and posterior	Syphilis Coccidioidomycosis Onchocerciasis Brucellosis	Sarcoid Behçet's syndrome Vogt-Koyanagi-Harada syndrome Inflammatory bowel disease

adhesions, called posterior synechiae, form between the iris and lens, potentially causing secondary pupillary block glaucoma or occlusion of the pupil. The inflammation may lead to cataract formation and ectopic calcification in the corneal epithelium—band keratopathy. Physicians treating seronegative pauciarticular arthritis should schedule slit lamp and dilation examinations several times a year. Posterior synechiae are visible with a hand light after instillation of mydriatics as the pupil does not fully dilate and has an irregular, scalloped border.

REITER'S SYNDROME

The triad of arthritis, urethritis, and conjunctivitis suggests Reiter's syndrome (see Ch. 434). This develops most often in men between the ages of 20 and 40 as a nonbacterial urethritis followed by polyarthritis and ocular inflammation. The initial ocular manifestation is usually a mucopurulent conjunctivitis, followed in many cases by an anterior uveitis. Keratitis and episcleritis also occur. As in ankylosing spondylitis, with which it shares similarities, HLA-B27 is often positive.

BEHÇET'S SYNDROME

Uveitis (or retinitis) is a cardinal feture of Behçet's syndrome (see Ch. 453). In some cases a characteristic layer of white cells forms in the lower portion of the anterior chamber (*hypopyon*). In other patients the primary ocular manifestation is a retinal vasculitis and vitritis. Rarer neuro-ophthalmic manifestations such as cranial nerve palsies or homonymous hemianopias are part of a wider central nervous system involvement.

UVEOMENINGITIS—THE VOGT-KOYANAGI-HARADA SYNDROME

Another systemic disease with characteristic ocular inflammation is uveomeningitis (the Vogt-Koyanagi-Harada syndrome). This disease affects the uvea, retina, meninges, and skin and is more common in Orientals. Manifestations include meningeal signs, alopecia, poliosis, vitiligo, tinnitus, and dysacousis. There may be an anterior or a posterior uveitis with exudative retinal detachment.

MALIGNANCY MASQUERADING AS UVEITIS

A steroid-responsive exudative process simulating uveitis can occur in adults over the age of 40 as part of a lymphoreticular neoplasia (variously called reticulum cell sarcoma, histiocytic sarcoma, or—when the brain is involved—primary CNS lymphoma). Diagnosis may be made from the cytology of a vitreous aspirate. Radiation treatment has palliative value.

An apparent iritis developing during a course of treatment for leukemia may represent infiltration of the anterior segment. Diagnosis and therapy are similar to reticulum cell sarcoma.

TREATMENT

The treatment of uveitis consists largely of topical or, when the inflammation is prolonged or severe, systemic immunosuppression. Prednisolone or dexamethasone topically, or prednisone orally, is the preferred drug. Cytotoxic immunosuppressive agents are sometimes used in chronic, intractable uveitis. Mydriatic-cycloplegics in anterior uveitis reduce discomfort and retard posterior synechiae formation.

James DG, Spiteri MA: Behçet's disease. Ophthalmology 89:1279, 1982. *A review of Behçet's disease's multiple manifestations with excellent color illustrations.*

Kanski JJ, Shun-Shin GA: Systemic uveitis syndromes in childhood: An analysis of 340 cases. Ophthalmology 91:1247, 1984. *Uveitis under the age of 16 most often represents juvenile rheumatoid arthritis.*

Kraus-Mackiw E, O'Connor GR (eds.): Uveitis: Pathophysiology and Therapy. New York, Thieme-Stratton, 1983. *This and Smith's monograph discuss various aspects of evaluation and treatment.*

Rosenthal AR: Ocular manifestations of leukemia: A review. Ophthalmology

90:899, 1983. *This paper covers the retinal, orbital, optic nerve, and uveal manifestations of leukemia.*

Smith RE, Nozik RM: Uveitis: A Clinical Approach to Diagnosis and Management. Baltimore, Williams & Wilkins Company, 1983.

Snyder DA, Tessler HH: Vogt-Koyanagi-Harada syndrome. Am J Ophthalmol 90:69, 1980. *Clinical findings in 20 cases treated in the American midwest.*

524 OCULAR INFECTIONS

Ocular infections (or inflammations) are most sensibly grouped according to their locations. The most common and most superficial infection is a *blepharoconjunctivitis* or, more simply, *conjunctivitis*. Infection of the lacrimal gland is a *dacryoadenitis*; infection of the lacrimal drainage system, a *dacryocystitis*. When the cornea is involved, the infection is called *keratitis*. *Uveitis*, *scleritis*, and *episcleritis*, which are seldom infectious, are discussed elsewhere (see Ch. 523, 527). Infection or inflammation inside the eye is an *endophthalmitis*. An infectious *vitritis* is usually called an endophthalmitis. Some *chorioretinitis* is infectious.

CONJUNCTIVITIS

The etiologies for the conjunctivitides include allergic, viral, bacterial, chlamydial, and chemical. Mild acute viral conjunctivitis, with a watery discharge and lids that are sealed closed upon awakening, usually requires only symptomatic treatment—warm or cool compresses and a topical vasoconstrictor to whiten the eye. Antibiotics have no clear efficacy. Any severe or chronic conjunctivitis should be managed by an ophthalmologist.

GONOCOCCAL CONJUNCTIVITIS. Purulent conjunctivitis is usually bacterial and amenable to antibiotics. An important variety is gonococcal conjunctivitis, a disease of the newborn (*gonococcal ophthalmia neonatorum*) and of sexually active adults. The eye is markedly inflamed with a copious discharge and swollen lids, a picture described as hyperpurulent conjunctivitis.

The discharge should be Gram stained and cultured on Thayer-Martin medium. Treatment consists of parenteral penicillin, or an equivalent antibiotic, and saline lavage of ocular secretions. There is debate as to the necessity and efficacy of topical antibiotics. Untreated gonococcal infection can penetrate the intact eye and destroy it; treatment should be immediately initiated if there is a reasonable suspicion of the diagnosis.

CHLAMYDIAL CONJUNCTIVITIS. In some parts of the world, chronic chlamydial conjunctivitis leads to conjunctival scarring and corneal vascularization, a disease known as *trachoma*. The resulting blindness is an important international public health problem. In developed countries, chlamydial infection manifests as a subacute conjunctivitis, frequently with associated urethritis. Although a keratitis may be present, severe corneal damage does not ensue. Chlamydial conjunctivitis, also called *inclusion blennorrhea* because of the cytoplasmic inclusions found in Giemsa-stained conjunctival scrapings, is difficult to eradicate in adults unless treated with systemic tetracycline or erythromycin.

HERPESVIRUS HOMINIS KERATITIS

Viral keratitis is a common and potentially serious consequence of infection with *Herpesvirus hominis*. The corneal involvement may be recognized by the characteristic *dendrite*, a branching epithelial ulcer (Color plate 7*A*). Topical antivirals promote healing, but recurrence is frequent, with increasing risk of corneal stromal involvement and scarring. Topical steroids activate epithelial herpes infections and should not be used without ophthalmological consultation.

CORNEAL ULCERS

Bacterial and fungal infections of the cornea are a serious threat to vision. Corneal ulcers tend to develop in the context of ocular trauma or contact lens wear, after surgery, or with pre-existing corneal disease. Corneal ulceration appears as an area of white, gray, or yellow infiltrate that stains with fluorescein. Such patients should be referred promptly to an ophthalmologist for evaluation and treatment with topical antibiotics and other measures.

ENDOPHTHALMITIS

Infection inside the eye most often follows accidental or surgical perforation of the eye. Epidemics have occurred following use of contaminated solutions in intraocular surgery. Only rarely do infections elsewhere metastasize to the eye.

Bacterial endophthalmitis must be treated aggressively if there is to be any chance of preserving vision. When the infection is recognized, cultures and smears are taken from the anterior chamber and vitreous cavity by aspiration, and a course of systemic, topical, and periocular antibiotics is begun. The choice of antibiotics depends upon what organisms, if any, are found on the Gram stain.

***CANDIDA* ENDOPHTHALMITIS.** *Candida albicans* is the most prevalent organism causing metastatic (endogenous) endophthalmitis. Fungemia after prolonged use of intravenous catheters or parenteral drug abuse results in colonization of the eye, with multiple white, fluffy chorioretinal infiltrates. These often involve the macula, reducing central vision. Careful direct ophthalmoscopy through a dilated pupil is indicated in patients at risk. Most *Candida* endophthalmitis requires systemic administration of antifungal agents, although spontaneous resolution has been observed.

INFECTIOUS CHORIORETINITIS

CONGENITAL TOXOPLASMOSIS. A common type of infectious chorioretinitis is *toxoplasmosis*, acquired in utero. This protozoan parasite can remain dormant in large, pigmented chorioretinal scars for many years and then become active, with white infiltration at the border of the scar and an overlying vitritis. If a previously uninvolved macula is threatened, treatment with pyrimethamine and sulfa or with clindamycin may be indicated.

CYTOMEGALOVIRUS CHORIORETINITIS (Color plate 7*G*). Cytomegalovirus chorioretinitis appears in immunosuppressed hosts as a discrete area of white or yellow retinal opacification with associated hemorrhage and vascular sheathing. The ophthalmoscopic picture resembles that of a branch retinal vein occlusion (see Ch. 528), but in this instance, one eye often has multiple foci, and there is a tendency for bilaterality.

Diagnosis can be made clinically and by culture of throat and urine. Dosages of immunosuppressive drugs should be reduced, if possible. The efficacy of treatment with antiviral agents is being actively evaluated.

OTHER INFECTIOUS CHORIORETINITIDES. Syphilis and tuberculosis are now rarely encountered as chorioretinitis. *Herpesvirus* retinitis resembles that of cytomegalovirus. Cryptococcal meningitis may have an associated chorioretinitis. Focal chorioretinitis can accompany subacute sclerosing panencephalitis (Ch. 488).

Darrell RD (ed.): Viral Diseases of the Eye. Philadelphia, Lea & Febiger, 1985. *Individual chapters on herpesvirus, cytomegalovirus, and measles, among others.*

Ficker L, Peacock J: Infectious endophthalmitis. Trans Ophthalmol Soc UK 105:319, 1986. *Describes 28 cases and provides references to other series.*

Parke DW II, Jones DB, Gentry LO: Endogenous endophthalmitis among patients with candidemia. Ophthalmology 89:789, 1982. *A prospective study of 38 patients with fungemia. Over one third of patients with Candida had ocular lesions.*

Tabbara KF, Hyndiuk RA: Infections of the Eye. Boston, Little, Brown and Company, 1986. *Forty-three chapters cover most known infectious entities.*

Wilhelmus KR: Bacterial corneal ulcers. Int Ophthalmol Clin 24:1, 1984. *This practical clinical review can serve as a manual of diagnosis and management.*

525 ORBITAL DISEASE AND TUMORS

GRAVES' ORBITOPATHY

The orbitopathy of Graves' disease consists of inflammation and infiltration of orbital tissues, with characteristic enlargement and scarring of the extraocular muscles. The varied clinical manifestations include lid retraction, exophthalmos, and limitation of eye movement.

Graves' orbitopathy frequently develops in persons previously treated for hyperthyroidism. When the orbitopathy first appears, the patient may be hyperthyroid, euthyroid, or hypothyroid. A classic Graves' orbitopathy in the absence of a demonstrable thyroid abnormality, even to sophisticated testing, is referred to as *ophthalmic Graves' disease.* Computed tomography demonstrating enlarged ocular muscles is probably the most sensitive diagnostic maneuver.

Graves' orbitopathy is the most frequent cause of both unilateral and bilateral exophthalmos. Retraction of the upper lid to expose sclera above the cornea exaggerates the appearance of exophthalmos and predisposes to a major complication, corneal exposure. Tethering of the eye by fibrotic muscles produces a mechanical ophthalmoplegia. Movement up and out is often restricted; pure loss of abduction mimicking sixth nerve palsy occurs. Ophthalmoplegia is not necessarily accompanied by exophthalmos.

Enlargement of the ocular muscles at the apex of the orbit may lead to another major complication of Graves' orbitopathy—compressive optic neuropathy. Severe exposure or major visual loss from compressive optic neuropathy is an indication for treatment. Systemic steroids will reduce exophthalmos and relieve optic nerve compression temporarily. Surgical decompression of the orbit by one of several routes is one definitive therapy; orbital irradiation is also used. Direct surgery on the ocular muscles relieves diplopia and permanent lid retraction.

INFLAMMATORY PSEUDOTUMOR OF THE ORBIT

Orbital pseudotumor is an idiopathic inflammation that falls within the spectrum of lymphoproliferative disorders. Its clinical manifestations are pain, exophthalmos, and limitation of eye movement. There may also be erythema and swelling of the lids. Orbital pseudotumors can mimic orbital infection, true tumors, or the orbitopathy of Graves' disease. The major site of inflammation is muscle (myositis), nerve (perineuritis), sclera (scleritis), or lacrimal gland (dacryoadenitis).

If the inflammation is posterior to the orbital apex in the walls of the cavernous sinus, the painful ophthalmoplegia that results is called the *Tolosa-Hunt syndrome.* Orbital pseudotumor merges pathologically and clinically with orbital lymphoma, which in turn merges with systemic lymphoma.

Initial evaluation of a patient with clinical signs and symptoms of orbital pseudotumor includes orbital ultrasonography and computed tomography. A trial of high-dose systemic corticosteroids is usually indicated prior to biopsy. Orbital biopsy is not a trivial undertaking and should be reserved for steroid-unresponsive or recurrent processes. Some histologically benign infiltrations do not respond to corticosteroids. Biopsy in such cases reveals fibrous tissue—*sclerosing pseudotumor.* Occasionally, a patient with a histologically benign pseudotumor subsequently develops a systemic lymphoma.

A necrotizing vasculitis, Wegener's granulomatosis, must also be included in the differential diagnosis of orbital pseudotumor, especially when the inflammation is bilateral. Most cases of Wegener's granulomatosis involve contiguous sinus structures, but local ocular forms of the disease have been reported. The combination of progressive proptosis and sinus disease also suggests orbital aspergillosis, especially in residents of warmer climates.

RHABDOMYOSARCOMA

Rhabdomysarcoma is the most common malignant tumor of the orbit during the first decade of life and occurs during the second and third decades. The initial presentation is usually ptosis with lid infiltration and proptosis. Progression may be extremely rapid, the clinical picture mimicking trauma or cellulitis. Biopsy and prompt treatment with irradiation and chemotherapy results in a high percentage of survival, although vision in the eye on the side of the tumor is seldom preserved.

OTHER ORBITAL TUMORS

The variety of primary, secondary, and metastatic tumors in the orbit is large. Most present with exophthalmos, visual loss, and limitation of eye movement. High degrees of malignancy are rare with meningiomas, gliomas, hemangiomas/lymphangiomas, and dermoids. Carcinomas of the lacrimal or meibomian glands represent a serious threat to life, and some cases require the most distressing of all ophthalmologic surgery—*exenteration,* removal of the orbital contents. Carcinoma from contiguous sinuses invades the orbit, and breast carcinoma is especially likely to metastasize to the orbit.

Char DH: Thyroid Eye Disease. Baltimore, Williams & Wilkins, 1985. *Char reviews his subject comprehensively and recommends treatment emphasizing short-term steroids and high-voltage radiotherapy.*

Kennerdell JS, Dresner SC: The nonspecific orbital inflammatory syndromes. Surv Ophthalmol 29:93, 1984.

Mauriello JA Jr, Flanagan JC: Management of orbital inflammatory disease. A protocol. Surv Ophthalmol 29:104, 1984. *Consecutive papers that provide an overview of pseudotumor of the orbit. The authors of the first review discard the term pseudotumor, preferring nonspecific orbital inflammation.*

526 INTRAOCULAR TUMORS

RETINOBLASTOMA

Retinoblastoma, a malignancy of the retina, is the most common intraocular tumor of childhood (and one of the more common tumors at any site). One third are bilateral. About 6 per cent of retinoblastomas are inherited as an autosomal dominant disease; half of these are bilateral. Ninety per cent of retinoblastomas are discovered before the age of three.

MALIGNANT MELANOMA

Primary melanomas develop in the conjunctiva, iris, ciliary body, or choroid; skin melanomas have a predilection for metastasis to the eye and orbit. Malignant melanomas of the choroid are the most common primary intraocular tumor of adulthood. Most occur in middle-aged Caucasians.

The prognosis of malignant melanoma of the choroid depends upon size, cytology, and the presence or absence of extrascleral extension. Choroidal malignant melanomas often metastasize to the liver.

The differential diagnosis of a pigmented intraocular mass includes benign choroidal nevus, senile disciform macular degeneration (also known as central exudative hemorrhagic retinopathy), peripheral exudative hemorrhagic chorioretinopathy, choroidal hemangioma, and hypertrophy or hyperplasia of the retinal pigment epithelium. Many eyes have been removed because of the suspicion of malignant melanoma when the pathology revealed a benign condition.

Enucleation is the traditional treatment for malignant melanoma of the choroid. Other treatment modalities are photocoagulation, radiotherapy, and local resection. Many pigmented choroidal tumors are now followed without intervention, especially when they are found incidentally in the seeing eyes of elderly patients. The effect of enucleation on life expectancy is debated.

METASTATIC CARCINOMA TO THE EYE

Once considered rare, metastatic cancer has become the most common ocular malignancy of adulthood, its incidence exceeding that of choroidal melanoma. Most are carcinomas invading the choroid, the commonest coming from the breast. Next in frequency are carcinomas of the lung, followed by kidney, gastrointestinal tract, testis, and prostate. With lung or renal carcinoma, the primary site may be inapparent at the time the metastasis is detected.

If tumor is identified elsewhere, removal of the eye is seldom indicated. Enucleation should be performed only if the eye is completely blind and painful, as palliative radiotherapy or chemotherapy may preserve vision.

Mewis L, Young SE: Breast carcinoma metastatic to the choroid: Analysis of 67 patients. Ophthalmology 89:147, 1982. *The status of detection and treatment.*
Shields JA: Current management of posterior uveal melanomas. In Mizuno K (ed.): Ophthalmology. Amsterdam, Excerpta Medica, 1985, pp 154–161. *A brief review of current approaches by an authority.*
Yanoff M, Fine BS: Ocular Pathology: A Text and Atlas. 2nd ed. Philadelphia, Harper Medical, 1982. *A comprehensive textbook with clinicopathologic correlations.*

527 EPISCLERITIS, SCLERITIS, AND THE DRY EYE

To a neurologist, the eye is an anterior extension of the brain; to a rheumatologist, the eye is a joint. Medicine and ophthalmology come together in the diagnosis and management of rheumatoid and connective tissue disorders. Uveal manifestations are discussed in Ch. 523; the toxicity of drugs used in treatment in Ch. 529; and the retinal changes in Ch. 528.

EPISCLERITIS AND SCLERITIS

Inflammation of the collagenous shell of the eye is either superficial (*episcleritis*) or deep (*scleritis*). The transparent, avascular cornea is continuous with the opaque, vascular sclera and may be secondarily involved.

Episcleritis resembles a localized conjunctivitis. The inflammation is deeper, however, and the dilated vessels do not always blanch with topically applied phenylephrine 2.5 per cent, as in a pure conjunctivitis. Episcleritis usually is self-limited (although it may be recurrent) and does not permanently damage the eye. Most episcleritis is idiopathic, but it may be encountered in rheumatoid arthritis, polyarteritis nodosa, Wegener's granulomatosis, systemic lupus erythematosus, dermatomyositis, progressive systemic sclerosis, and relapsing polychondritis.

Scleritis is more likely than episcleritis to accompany a systemic disease, although the list of associations is about the same for the two disorders. Any portion of the sclera may be affected. The diagnosis is especially difficult with posterior scleritis, which may present as ocular pain or as an exudative retinal detachment. Anterior scleritis often consists of a prolonged, indolent inflammation with eventual permanent structural alteration of tissues. Pain may be prominent and severe.

Initially in scleritis the inflammation is localized and may be nodular or diffuse. With prolonged inflammation, scleral thinning results in a localized bluish discoloration as the underlying choroid becomes visible. Scleral necrosis with perforation is possible; this is especially frequent in rheumatoid arthritis. The adjacent cornea may melt away.

Management of scleritis is difficult. Local steroid injections may predispose to perforation. Systemic corticosteroids and other antirheumatic drugs are useful in some patients. The ocular process often closely parallels the activity of the underlying disease, and the best approach is systemic therapy.

KERATOCONJUNCTIVITIS SICCA

Corneal inflammation as the result of drying is referred to as *keratoconjunctivitis sicca*. Keratoconjunctivitis sicca, a dry mouth (xerostomia), and a connective tissue disorder constitute *Sjögren's syndrome*. The underlying pathophysiology appears to be an autoimmune reaction affecting the lacrimal and salivary glands. Sjögren's syndrome is common in patients with rheumatoid arthritis, especially middle-aged women. Complaints of burning, irritation, or excessive secretions suggest a dry eye but are notoriously nonspecific.

Diagnosis depends upon demonstration of tear hyposecretion (usually by decreased wetting of a strip of litmus or filter paper placed between the lower lid and the eye in the inferior cul-de-sac) accompanied by corneal and conjunctival epithelial damage. Once epithelial cells start to slough, the corneal surface will take up fluorescein instilled into the conjunctival sac. Devitalized cells that have not yet been sloughed stain with rose bengal, making this dye an even more sensitive test for keratitis sicca.

Treatment consists of tear replacement and reduction of tear turnover. Various preparations of artificial tears are available. Other therapeutic maneuvers include occlusion of the lacrimal puncta to reduce tear outflow and placement of contact lenses, moisture chambers, or goggles over the eyes to decrease evaporation. Such measures are reserved for severe keratitis.

Baum J: Clinical manifestations of dry eye states. Trans Ophthalmol Soc UK 104:415, 1985. *Outlines the clinical and laboratory signs and associations. Other papers in the same issue are relevant.*
Watson PG: The nature and treatment of scleral inflammation. Trans Ophthalmol Soc UK 102:257, 1982. *A review by an acknowledged expert.*

528 OCULAR VASCULAR DISEASE

SYSTEMIC HYPERTENSION AND ARTERIOSCLEROSIS

Although the retinal vascular abnormalities in hypertension are nonspecific and variable, they can be important diagnostically and therapeutically. The effects of blood pressure on the retinal vessels depend upon both its absolute level and duration. Although essential hypertension is a disease of arterioles, the retinal vascular bed lacks sympathetic innervation, and the fundus changes must be considered secondary.

Arteriolar narrowing is the commonest hypertensive change and the most difficult to differentiate as abnormal. The normal ratio of the diameters of the arteriolar and venous blood columns is 2:3 or 3:4. A decrease in this ratio can best be appreciated in the smaller branches away from the disc.

Other findings include microaneurysms, hemorrhages, lipid deposits, and edema. Retinal and disc edema usually follows a rapid increase in systemic blood pressure. Disc edema defines the entity *malignant hypertension*. By contrast, opacification (or sclerosis) of the vessel walls—described ophthalmoscopically as copper or silver wiring—accompanies longstanding hypertension.

Thickening of the arteriolar wall explains arteriovenous nicking and venous dilation distal to the crossing. Cotton-wool spots are signs of local ischemia; hemorrhages and hard exudates reflect vascular leakage. Microaneurysms indicate irreversible structural alterations in the capillary beds. Retinal vascular occlusions (see below) and ischemic optic neuropathy are potential consequences of hypertensive vascular changes.

The only pure arteriosclerotic funduscopic change is atheroma of the retinal arterioles. These are seen as yellow-white plaques in the central retinal artery or its first branches, where the arteries still have an internal elastic lamina. The plaques must be differentiated from calcific or lipid emboli, which are usually smaller or more peripheral. Hypertension accelerates atherosclerosis, but atherosclerosis does not require hypertension.

DIABETIC RETINOPATHY (Color plates 1 and 7E)

Diabetic retinopathy, the most common of the vascular retinopathies, shares many features with hypertensive retinopathy. The pathophysiologic defect in diabetic retinopathy appears to lie at the level of the retinal capillaries. Progressive degeneration of the capillary walls results in leakage (hemorrhages and exudates), diffuse and focal expansion (microaneurysms), and closure of small vessels. The ischemic retina in the focal areas of nonperfusion elaborates factors stimulating new vessel and fibrous ingrowth. (A similar retinopathy can follow radiotherapy given as part of the treatment for head and neck cancers, which damages the capillary wall cells.)

Diabetic retinopathy is classified as *background* or *proliferative*. Background retinopathy is further subdivided into *simple background*—with microaneurysms, dot/blot hemorrhages, and hard exudates—and a *preproliferative* form. In preproliferative background retinopathy there is beading of veins, cotton-wool spots, and many hemorrhages. Also characteristic is intraretinal new vessel pathology, so-called *intraretinal microvascular anomalies*.

In proliferative retinopathy, neovascularization appears on the disc and elsewhere, especially along the major vascular arcades. There may be fibrovascular proliferation and vitreous hemorrhages. Proliferative diabetic retinopathy confers a poor visual prognosis.

Background retinopathy alone reduces visual acuity when there is edema or exudation in the macula. More new cases of blindness result from background retinopathy with macular edema than from proliferative retinopathy, because the former is much more prevalent. Background retinopathy with macular edema is common in type 2 diabetics over age 50.

TREATMENT. Good diabetic control appears to retard the progression of retinopathy. Ablation of ischemic retina by panretinal photocoagulation helps preserve central vision in patients with early proliferative retinopathy, making this the current treatment of choice. Advanced proliferative retinopathy may require major intraocular surgery—*vitrectomy*. In such cases the visual prognosis is guarded but an estimated 50 to 75 per cent of operated patients experience some visual improvement.

OTHER VASCULAR RETINOPATHIES

SYSTEMIC LUPUS ERYTHEMATOSUS. The retinopathy is common but nonspecific: The most frequent findings are retinal hemorrhages and cotton-wool spots. Cotton-wool spots are not exudations but, rather, localized areas of axoplasmic stasis caused by ischemia, which may indicate active vasculitis. Patients with lupus often also have hypertensive retinopathy. Central nervous system involvement may be associated with optic and chiasmal neuropathy, papilledema, ocular motor cranial nerve palsies, hemianopias, and a migraine-like syndrome.

HEMATOLOGIC DISEASE. Anemia and thrombocytopenia predispose to retinal and subconjunctival hemorrhages. When these are the result of leukemia, the hemorrhages often have a white center—the classic, but nonspecific *Roth spot*. Roth spots also are encountered in subacute bacterial endocarditis and other conditions.

Leukemia can cause hyperviscosity retinopathy, characterized by venous tortuosity and dilation, retinal hemorrhages, and vascular occlusions. A chronically elevated leukocyte count also predisposes to capillary drop out and microaneurysm formation, but proliferative retinopathy is rare. Other causes of hyperviscosity retinopathy are Waldenström's macroglobulinemia, multiple myeloma, polycythemia, and sickle cell anemia. In extreme cases sludging of blood in the veins is visible ophthalmoscopically.

PERIPHERAL RETINAL NEOVASCULARIZATION. Diabetic retinopathy affects largely the posterior pole of the eye. The retinopathy of prematurity (retrolental fibroplasia) and sickle cell disease have their major impact on the peripheral retina.

The ocular and systemic manifestations of sickling hemoglobinopathies correlate poorly. In patients with sickle cell anemia, proliferative retinopathy is rare. Peripheral neovascularization is more common in sickle cell hemoglobin C disease (SC) and sickle cell thalassemia (S-thal). Patients with sickle cell trait usually have no ocular symptoms, although hypoxia encountered at high altitudes may precipiatate hemorrhages and vascular occlusions.

The ocular findings in sickle hemoglobinopathies include small, dark red, comma-shaped conjunctival vascular segments, best seen on the inferior bulbar conjunctiva after instillation of a topical vasoconstrictor. Ischemic infarction of iris segments is also observed. In addition to the "sea fan" peripheral neovascularization, other characteristic retinal findings include hemorrhages that have a salmon pink coloration from hemoglobin breakdown products and black chorioretinal scars with irregular borders in the equatorial periphery.

About one fifth of proliferative sickle retinopathy regresses spontaneously. The rest, if untreated, will progress to retinal detachment and vitreous hemorrhage. Treatment consists of photocoagulation or trans-scleral cryotherapy or diathermy.

RETINAL VASCULAR OCCLUSIONS

CENTRAL RETINAL ARTERY OCCLUSION (CRAO). The central retinal artery is a branch of the ophthalmic artery, in turn a branch of the internal carotid artery. Occlusion of the central retinal artery causes sudden, usually nearly complete, visual loss in one eye. Ophthalmoscopy reveals arteriolar narrowing and vascular stasis (most obvious as segmentation of the venous blood column—"boxcar" pattern).

Within hours the infarcted superficial layers of the retina lose their normal transparency to assume a milky white translucency. Because the thin retina over the fovea receives its oxygen from the underlying choroid, this region retains its normal reddish pink color. This contrasts with surrounding tissue, producing an appearance described as a cherry red macula. (A similar appearance is encountered in certain lipid storage diseases, in which abnormal metabolic products partially opacify the ganglion cell layer.)

Eventually arterial flow is restored, the edema resolves, and the fundus appearance returns to near normal. The disc, which is initially normal because it derives its blood supply from the surrounding choroid, gradually becomes pale and atrophic. After several weeks it is difficult to distinguish a central retinal artery occlusion from other causes of primary optic atrophy.

Acute central retinal artery occulsion is an emergency. Rarely, prompt action may dislodge an embolus and restore circulation in time to prevent retinal death and thus preserve vision. For a nonophthalmologist this action consists of firm, intermittent pressure on the globe with the heel of the hand to alternately raise and lower intraocular pressure. Ophthalmologists use other measures: retrobulbar injection of anesthetic and anterior chamber paracentesis to lower the pressure in the ocular vascular bed. Seldom does treatment save vision.

In some persons, portions of the retina are supplied by vessels arising from the choroidal circulation, and such areas may be spared if the central retinal artery alone is occluded. Most eyes with CRAO are deprived of useful vision.

CRAO's are the result of emboli (atheromatous, myxomatous, and material from diseased or artificial heart valves), of local small vessel disease, or of carotid occlusion. A CRAO is sometimes the initial sign of giant cell arteritis or polyarteritis nodosa. CRAO has been reported in patients with sickle cell trait after trauma or other stress.

BRANCH RETINAL ARTERY OCCLUSION (BRAO). Branch arterial occlusions present as sudden loss of vision in a sector of the field affected. Ophthalmoscopically one observes a wedge-shaped area of infarcted retina spreading outward from an arteriolar bifurcation. Branch retinal artery occlusions are almost always embolic in origin. By far the commonest source of emboli in older adults is the ipsilateral carotid artery. In children and young adults, migraine, coagulation abnormalities, increased intraocular pressure, and oral contraceptives may predispose to vascular occlusions.

CENTRAL RETINAL VEIN OCCLUSION (CRVO) (Color plate 7H). The dramatic ophthalmoscopic findings of dilated, tortuous veins, extensive retinal hemorrhages, and disc swelling in one eye have classically been called a central retinal vein occlusion. Actually there is evidence that such *hemorrhagic retinopathy* is the consequence of both arterial ischemia and venous disease.

A CRVO presents as sudden unilateral visual loss in older adults, but unlike a CRAO, a CRVO is not an emergency, as there is no accepted immediate therapy. There are also no specific accompanying diseases, although hypertension and diabetes are loosely associated, and hypercoagulable states must be considered.

Visual prognosis varies. In the fully developed form usually encountered in older persons, vision is poor and generally remains so. Panretinal photocoagulation may decrease the risk of subsequent neovascular glaucoma. A less severe ophthalmoscopic picture is encountered in younger patients. Acuity in such *partial central retinal vein occlusion* or *venous stasis retinopathy* is only slightly reduced, and the visual prognosis is good. Ischemic oculopathy after carotid occlusion produces a similar retinopathy; retinal arterial pressures measured by ophthalmodynamometry or oculopneumoplethysmography are low in such cases.

BRANCH RETINAL VEIN OCCLUSIONS. Patients with branch vein occlusions complain of blurred vision. In the fundus, hemorrhages and cotton-wool spots spread out in a wedge from an arteriovenous crossing. As in CRVO, there are few specific systemic associations. Neovascular glaucoma is rare, but vision may be persistently reduced by macular edema. Branch retinal vein occlusion must be distinguished from viral retinitis (see Ch. 524).

Asdourian GK: Peripheral retinal neovascularization—differential diagnosis. In Peyman GA, Sanders DR, Goldberg MF (eds.): Principles and Practice of Ophthalmology. Philadelphia, W. B. Saunders Company, 1980, pp 1277–1298. *A clear reveiw of clinical manifestations and pathogenesis.*

Brown GC, Magargal LE, Shields JA, et al.: Retinal arterial obstruction in children and young adults. Ophthalmology 88:18, 1981. *A report of 27 cases of BRAO or CRAO in patients under 30 years of age.*

Hall S, Buettner H, Luthra HS: Occlusive retinal vascular disease in systemic lupus erythematosus. J Rheumatol 11:846, 1984. *Two cases with large retinal vessel occlusion.*

Kearns TP: Differential diagnosis of central retinal vein obstruction. Ophthalmology 90:475, 1983. *This paper is one of four in the same issue that describes the work-up, differential diagnosis, and management of CRVO.*

Little HL, Jack RL, Patz A, et al.: Diabetic Retinopathy. New York, Thieme-Stratton Inc., 1983. *A collection of 31 position papers on various aspects of diabetic retinopathy.*

529 THE EYE AND MEDICATIONS

DRUGS WITH OCULAR SIDE EFFECTS

ANTICHOLINERGICS. A variety of systemic drugs have ocular side effects. Any medication with anticholinergic properties can dilate the pupil and diminish accommodation (the ability to focus at close range). The possibility of angle-closure is the basis for the caution that such medications are contraindicated in glaucoma. Patients on therapy for open-angle glaucoma are at little risk, as mydriasis will not usually affect intraocular pressure. If the patient has known angle-closure, previous iris surgery all but eliminates the danger of dilation. Only when there is a potential for angle-closure are such drugs contraindicated, and this is usually unrecognized. Of the systemic anticholinergic drugs, only transdermal scopolamine can dilate and fix pupils and paralyze accommodation, even in young persons.

CORTICOSTEROIDS. Prolonged administration of systemic dosages of corticosteroids often leads to the formation of posterior subcapsular cataracts. Topical corticosteroids increase intraocular pressure in genetically predisposed persons. Topical steroids also activate *Herpesvirus* keratitis and should be administered only under the supervision of an ophthalmologist.

QUININE AND CHLOROQUINE. Quinine may cause acute blindness, with narrowing of the retinal arterioles. An overdose increases the probability of toxic effects, but rare persons are sensitive even to therapeutic doses. Other symptoms of quinine toxicity include dizziness, tinnitus, and hearing loss. Central vision may improve, with persistent constriction of peripheral field and evolution of optic atrophy.

The synthetic antimalarials chloroquine and hydroxychloroquine have a specific retinal toxicity. This usually appears only after prolonged administration in doses exceeding 250 mg per day for chloroquine and 400 mg per day for hydroxychloroquine. Reduced visual acuity is the usual initial symptom, the parafoveal retina being most affected. Chloroquine binds to pigmented tissues, exerting a toxic effect on the retinal epithelium with loss of pigmentation in a target-like or bull's-eye pattern around the fovea. Discontinuation of the drug may result in improvement, but if the process is moderately advanced, visual loss may be progressive.

Chloroquine, hydroxychloroquine, and a variety of other drugs including the antiarrhythmic amiodarone cause whorl-like corneal epithelial deposits that are usually asymptomatic. Such deposits disappear after discontinuation of the drug.

THIORIDAZINE. Phenothiazines are potentially toxic to retina and retinal pigment epithelium, producing a coarse pigmentary degeneration. Of those now in common use, only thioridazine has clinically significant toxicity, and then only with dosages exceeding 1 gram per day for prolonged periods.

ETHAMBUTOL. Various drugs have been implicated in optic neuropathies. Only with ethambutol is the incidence of such side effects high enough that monitoring is considered mandatory. The physician administering ethambutol should perform monthly checks of acuity and color vision, especially when dosages exceed 15 mg per kilogram.

OCULOCUTANEOUS DISORDERS

A variety of related disorders (including erythema multiforme, Stevens-Johnson syndrome, and toxic epidermal necrolysis, or Lyell's syndrome) arise as idiosyncratic responses to drugs or infections. Their ocular manifestations are a bullous conjunctival eruption followed by a cicatricial conjunctivitis. Adhesions may obliterate the conjunctival sacs and prevent the normal production and distribution of tears. A severe dry eye may be the most disabling sequela.

Early treatment with topical steroids (and perhaps antibiotics to prevent secondary infection) sometimes limits damage. Sweeping the conjunctival fornices several times a day with a sterile glass rod inhibits adhesions.

SYSTEMIC SIDE EFFECTS OF TOPICAL OCULAR MEDICATIONS

Medications in solution are easily absorbed from the nasal mucosa, and systemic side effects are more likely with drops than ointments. Dilation of the pupil with 10 per cent phenylephrine solution has been known to precipitate severe hypertension, especially in infants and the elderly. Topical epinephrine increases ventricular extrasystoles in some patients. Timolol maleate causes bronchospasm in asthmatics.

Topical anticholinergics such as atropine, scopolamine, and cyclopentolate may contribute to confusional states in the elderly. Cyclopentolate is occasionally a cause of acute hallucinations and even psychosis in the young. Pilocarpine, used in large doses in the treatment of acute angle-closure glaucoma, has resulted in cholinergic overdose—nausea, vomiting, salivation, and gastrointestinal cramps. As these are also symptoms of the angle-closure attack itself, such toxicity may not be immediately recognized, leading to continued administration and cardiovascular collapse.

Echothiophate iodide, an organophosphate used in the treatment of some forms of childhood strabismus and of open-angle glaucoma, predisposes to cholinergic crisis, mimicking an acute surgical abdomen. Also, patients receiving echothiophate have impaired metabolism of succinylcholine. Use of succinylcholine during the induction of general anesthesia in a patient receiving echothiophate has caused death.

CARBONIC ANHYDRASE INHIBITORS

Acetazolamide and methazolamide inhibit aqueous production and are used systemically to reduce intraocular pressure when topical medications are inadequate. Most patients experience paresthesias; their absence is thought by some to indicate noncompliance. Carbonic anhydrase inhibitors also induce a systemic acidosis, with a syndrome of malaise and anorexia, depression, and weight loss that responds to concurrent administration of sodium bicarbonate, and may rarely cause blood dyscrasias. Acetazolamide increases the incidence of urolithiasis. The combination of a carbonic anhydrase inhibitor and a thiazide diuretic depletes body potassium. Carbonic anhydrase inhibitors should not be given to people with known allergy to sulfonamides.

Adler AG, McElwain GE, Merli GJ, et al.: Systemic effects of eye drops. Arch Intern Med 142:2293, 1982. *A brief review that serves as a cautionary tale.*
Fraunfelder FT, Meyer SM: Drug-Induced Side Effects and Drug Interactions. 2nd ed. Philadelphia, Lea & Febiger, 1982. *A compendium based on a collection of reports of side effects.*
Grant WM: Toxicology of the Eye. 3rd ed. Springfield, Charles C Thomas, 1986. *An enormous review with component parts that are coherent and readable.*

PART XXIV

SKIN DISEASES

Frank Parker

530 INTRODUCTION

An understanding of how the skin functions in health and disease is relevant to every physician for several reasons: First, the skin is the interface with our environment and serves many functions crucial to survival, such as protection against the elements and thermoregulation. Second, the psychologic role the skin and its appendages, the hair and nails, play in our appearance cannot be overestimated. Third, skin problems are exceedingly common, as some 30 per cent of Americans have dermatologic conditions requiring a physician's care. Ten common skin problems constitute 76 per cent of the burden of skin disease as established by population survey (Table 530–1). Fourth, the skin can be readily examined and biopsied and frequently provides evidence of internal disease. The trained examiner recognizes certain apparently insignificant skin findings as subtle signs of life-threatening disease.

Chapter 531 reviews the functions subserved by the skin and the local variations in skin structures which help to explain the localization of certain disease processes to specific areas. Chapter 532 discusses the examination of the skin and presents an approach to diagnosing skin diseases based upon clinical morphology. Nine major disease groupings are described, and the common dermatologic conditions and their etiologies are discussed (Ch. 534). Chapter 533 contains a guide to general principles of therapy. Chapter 534 describes skin diseases of general medical importance as well as specific therapy for each disease.

TABLE 530–1. PREVALENCE OF COMMON DERMATOLOGIC DISEASE IN THE UNITED STATES*

	Rate per 1000	Numbers (in 1000's)
Fungus infections	81.1	15,733
Tinea pedis	38.7	7509
Tinea unguium	21.8	4232
Tinea versicolor	8.4	1623
Tinea cruris	6.7	1301
Acne vulgaris	68.1	13,217
Cystic acne	1.9	375
Acne scars	1.7	321
Seborrheic dermatitis	28.2	5476
Verruca vulgaris	8.5	1684
Folliculitis	8.0	1553
Atopic dermatitis	6.9	1332
Lichen simplex chronicus	4.5	882
Hand eczema	1.6	311
Dyshidrotic eczema	2.1	405
Psoriasis	5.5	1070
Vitiligo	4.9	957
Herpes simplex	4.2	824

*Persons 1 to 74 years of age—noninstitutionalized.
Reprinted from the chapter by Dr. Marie-Louise Johnson in the 17th edition of the Cecil Textbook of Medicine, with her permission.

Callen JP: Cutaneous Aspects of Internal Disease. Chicago, Year Book Medical Publisher, 1981. *Discussions of skin disorders that confront the clinician which have underlying systemic disorders. Discussion of the pathogenesis of these disorders is provided by a number of contributing authorities.*

Fitzpatrick TB, Eisen AZ, Wolff K, et al.: Dermatology in General Medicine. New York, McGraw-Hill Book Company, 1987. *A detailed and well-illustrated textbook covering all aspects of dermatology. Two volumes.*

Hurwitz SH: Clinical Pediatric Dermatology. Philadelphia, W. B. Saunders Company, 1981. *A well-written and well-illustrated book of dermatology of children and adolescents.*

Lookingbill DP, Marks JG: Principles of Dermatology. Philadelphia, W. B. Saunders Company, 1985. *A concise, well-illustrated textbook covering major topics in general dermatology.*

Moschella SL, Pillsbury DM, Hurley HJ: Dermatology. Philadelphia, W. B. Saunders Company, 1975. *A useful textbook of dermatology in two volumes.*

Rook A, Wilkinson DS, Ebling FJG, et al.: Textbook of Dermatology. Oxford, Blackwell Scientific Publication, 1986. *This three-volume multi-authored text covers every aspect of dermatology in great detail. It is well written and referenced.*

531 THE STRUCTURE AND FUNCTION OF SKIN

The skin serves a variety of functions crucial to survival and health. In general, the functions may be correlated with specific properties of epidermal or dermal regions. The epidermis differentiates to form anucleate cornified cells that act as a relatively impermeable protective barrier to the outward loss of body fluids and the inward penetration of various substances and microorganisms. These lamellae of cornified surface cells together with the brown pigment melanin also play an important role in protecting against the carcinogenic effects of ultraviolet radiation. Two components of the dermis, the unique circulatory system and the specialized cutaneous appendages, the sweat glands, play a vital role in the body's thermoregulation. Finally, the skin is important immunologically. Both the epidermis (Langerhans' cells) and dermis (epidermodermal junction structures) are sites at which a number of immunologic reactions occur that can give rise to unique inflammatory skin diseases.

ANATOMIC CONSIDERATIONS

The skin is composed of two mutually dependent layers: the outer *epidermis* and inner *dermis*, both cushioned on the fat-containing subcutaneous tissue, the *panniculus adiposus* (Figs. 531–1 and 531–2).

EPIDERMIS. The stratified cellular epidermis contains two main zones of cells (keratinocytes), an inner region of viable cells, the *stratum germinativum*, and an outer layer of anucleate cells known as the *stratum corneum*, or horny layer. Three strata of cells are recognized in the germinativum: the *basal*, *spinous*, and *granular* layers, each representing progressive stages of differentiation and keratinization of the epidermal cells as they evolve into the dead, tightly packed stratum corneum cells on the skin surface.

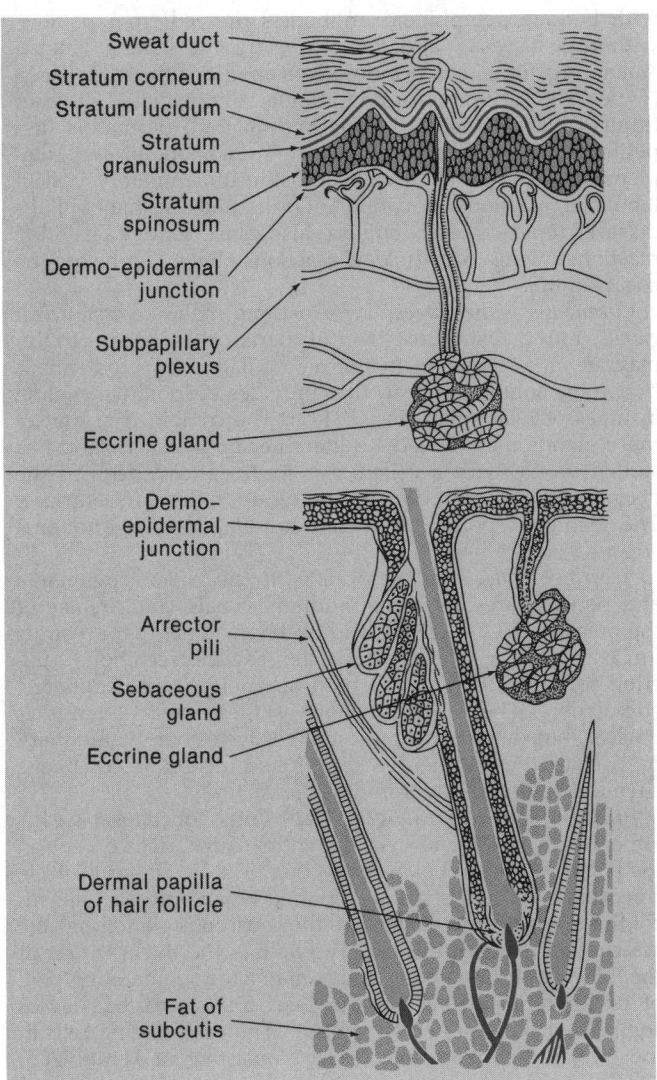

FIGURE 531–1. Structure of the skin. (Adapted from the 17th edition of the Cecil Textbook of Medicine with the permission of Dr. Marie-Louise Johnson.)

The epidermis is derived from the mitotic division of the columnar basal cells resting on the basement membrane (*basal lamina*), with the daughter cells moving outward to the surface, where they become polyhedral as they synthesize increasing quantities of intracellular insoluble protein, keratin. These *stratum spinosum cells* attach to one another mechanically by desmosomes, complex modifications of the cellular membranes that impart a spinous or quill-like appearance to the cells. Desmosomes play a crucial role in maintaining the adherence of the epidermal cells to one another. With further outward displacement the differentiating cells of the spinous layer become flattened, and refractile keratohyalin granules appear in the cytoplasm, accounting for the designation of *granular layer* that rests just below the stratum corneum.

The transformation from viable granular cells to anucleate, nonviable cornified cells is abrupt. The cornified layer consists of up to 25 layers of tightly packed, highly flattened horny cells.

The differentiation of the epidermal cells involves the formation of fibrous proteins known as *keratin*. The process of maturation of the epidermis (cornificiation) is complete in the stratum corneum, yielding cells with mature keratin, namely, a system of filaments embedded in a continuous matrix (which is probably derived from the keratohyalin granules) within a thickened cell membrane. The stratum corneum limits the

rate of passage of ions and molecules into and out of the skin.

The basal layer of epidermis has a permanent population of germinal cells whose progeny undergo the specific pattern of differentiation just described. The new keratinocytes require about 14 days to evolve into stratum granulosum cells and another 14 days to reach the surface of the stratum corneum and be shed. Proper control of proliferation of basal cells and their subsequent orderly differentiation into keratinized stratum corneum cells produces the smooth, pliable surface of the skin. Alterations in the homeostatic state of cell division, defects in differentiation, or changes in exfoliation from the surface can lead to irregularities in the skin surface, characterized as roughening, scaling, and hyperkeratosis (accumulation of excessive layers of stratum corneum).

Two other cell types are found in the epidermis, the *melanocyte* and the *Langerhans' cell*. Both are dendritic cells with cytoplasmic arms that stretch out to contact the keratinocytes in their vicinity. The melanocytes are pigment (melanin)-producing cells that are arrayed in the basal epidermal layer and hair follicles, whereas the Langerhans' cells are usually found in the suprabasal layers of the epidermis, and at times in the dermis. Each dendritic cell has a different origin and function.

Melanocytes evolve in the neural crest of the embryo and migrate to the skin in early embryonic life. These cells synthesize brown, red, and yellow melanin pigments that give

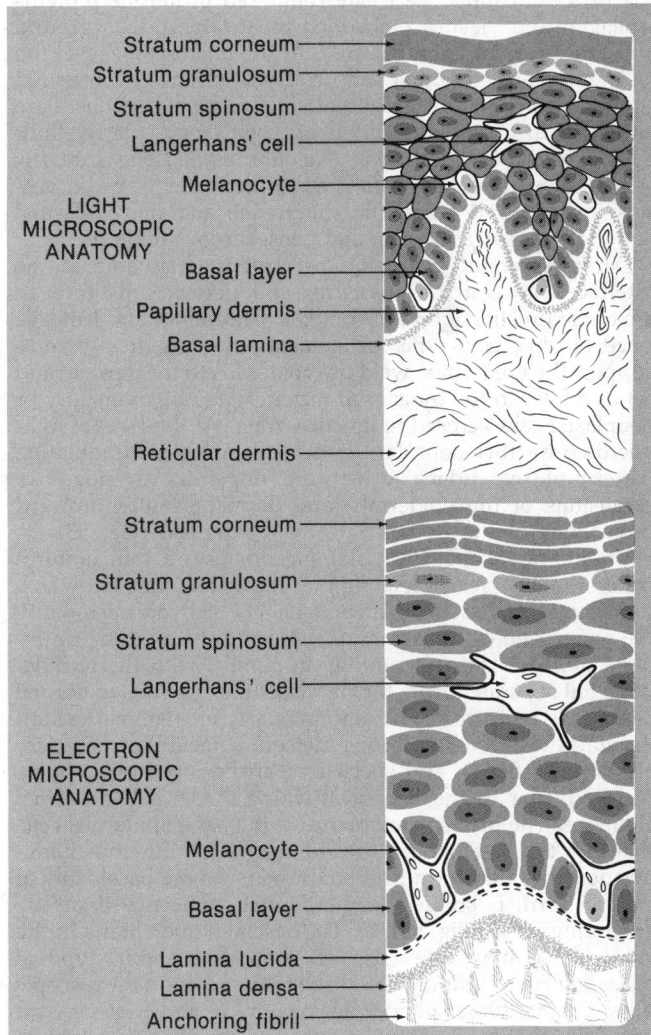

FIGURE 531–2. Diagrammatic representation of the light microscopic and electron microscopic anatomy of the skin.

us our distinctive skin coloration. Melanocytes contain distinctive submicroscopic organelles (melanosomes) within which melanin is synthesized. A specific enzyme, tyrosinase, found within the melanosome, oxidizes tyrosine to dihydroxyphenylalanine (DOPA) and then to DOPA quinone. Additional nonenzymatic oxidation and polymerization occur to form the final product, melanin. Two kinds of melanin are recognized: eumelanin (brown-black biochrome) and phaeomelanin (yellow-red biochrome that contains large quantities of cysteine). The genetic make-up of the individual determines which melanin is produced, thus providing the various colors and hues of our skin and hair. Once the melanosomes are fully melanized, the resulting melanin granules are transported out the dendritic processes of the melanocyte and transferred into the adjacent epidermal cells (or into hair in the case of hair follicles).

Langerhans' cells, derived from bone marrow, contain a unique submicroscopic racket-shaped organelle (Birbeck granule) and are now recognized as playing a major immunologic role in the skin (Fig. 531–2). They contain surface receptors for immunoglobulins, complement, and Ia-antigens and are able to capture external antigenic materials that contact the skin and to circulate to draining lymph nodes and there induce specific sensitization of immunocompetent T cells. Langerhans' cells thus play a central role in delayed hypersensitivity reactions of the skin (allergic contact dermatitis).

DERMIS. Beneath the epidermis is the principal mass of the skin, the dermis, which is a tough, resilient tissue with viscoelastic properties. It consists of a three-dimensional matrix of loose connective tissue composed of fibrous proteins (collagen and elastin) embedded in an amorphous ground substance (glycosaminoglycans). At the microscopic level the collagen fibers resemble an irregular meshwork oriented somewhat parallel to the epidermis. Coarse elastic fibers are entwined in the collagenous fibers, being particularly abundant over the face and neck. This fibrous and elastic matrix serves as a scaffolding within which networks of blood vessels, nerves, and lymphatics intertwine and the epidermal appendages, sweat glands, and pilosebaceous units rest.

Dermoepidermal Junction. The structures situated at the interface between the epidermis and dermis constitute an anatomic functional unit of complex membranes and lamellae laced by divergent types of filaments that together serve to support the epidermis, weld the epidermis to the dermis, and act as a filter to the transfer of materials and inflammatory or neoplastic cells across the junction zone. At the level of light microscopy, this boundary zone is seen as an undulating pattern of rete ridges (downward finger-like or ridge-like extensions of the epidermis) and dermal papillae (upward projections of the dermis into the epidermis) (Fig. 531–2). Periodic acid–Schiff (PAS) staining discloses a thin uniform zone of intense reaction along this undulating junction which represents the basement membrane. By electron microscopy the membrane (or basal lamina) is seen to be a dense continuous fibrillar structure running in parallel with the undulations but separated from the dermal surfaces of the epidermal basal cells by a thin clear amorphous space (lamina lucida). Several substructural fibrous elements, including collagen, elastic microfibrils, and specialized anchoring fibrils, course perpendicular to the lamina attaching epidermal to dermal elements. The plasma membranes of the basal epidermal cells that face the basal lamina are studded with numerous hemidesmosomes that form firm attachments to the basal lamina; this, in turn, is bonded to the dermal connective tissue by anchoring fibrils (Fig. 531–2). The basement membrane in the skin, like that in other tissues, contains a special type of collagen (Type IV) and is localized to the electron microscopic basal lamina. Other noncollagenous glyco- and proteoglycan proteins of the basement membrane zone include *laminin* (found in the lamina lucida), *bullous pemphigoid antigen* (identified in the lamina lucida of normal skin by their reactivity

with bullous pemphigoid antibodies derived from patients with this disease), and *fibronectins* (in the lamina lucida). Anchoring fibrils are composed of another type of collagen (Type VII). A number of immunologically mediated diseases (lupus erythematosus, bullous pemphigoid, dermatitis herpetiformis) involve deposition of immunoglobulin and complement in the junction zone, causing inflammatory vesiculobullous reactions; a variety of inherited mechanobullous diseases (epidermolysis bullosa) also cause serious blistering reactions owing to pathologic reactions above and below the basal lamina.

Cutaneous Appendages. Two to three million *eccrine sweat glands*, found distributed over all parts of the body surface, play an important part in thermoregulation by producing a hypotonic solution (sweat) that provides evaporative cooling in times of heat stress (Fig. 531–1). The combined output of these glands may exceed 1.5 liters per hour. Each gland is a simple tubule with a coiled secretory segment deep in the dermis and a straight duct extending up to the skin's surface. The glands respond to thermal stimulation and emotional stress.

Apocrine sweat glands are localized to the axillae, circumanal and perineal areas, external auditory canals, and areolae of the breasts. They secrete viscid, milky material that accounts for axillary odor when bacteria degrade the secretion. Apocrine secretion occurs with both adrenergic and cholinergic stimulation. The exact function of these sweat glands is unclear, but they may represent a vestige of our evolutionary past, since the odoriferous secretions function as cutaneous chemical communicators in other primates.

Pilosebaceous Appendages. Hair units, or pilosebaceous appendages, are found over the entire skin surface except on the palms, soles, and glans penis (Fig. 531–1). The hair follicle consists of the hair shaft surrounded by an epithelial sheath continuous with the epidermis, the sebaceous gland, and the arrector pili smooth muscle. The bulb is the thickest part of the follicle at its lower end and contains the proliferating pool of undifferentiated cells which gives rise to various layers comprising the hair and the follicle. The proliferating cells in the bulb differentiate into a hair consisting of keratinized, hard, imbricated, flattened cortex cells surrounding a central medullary space. The sebaceous glands are multilobular holocrine glands that connect into the pilosebaceous canal (hair canal) through the sebaceous duct. Germinative undifferentiated sebaceous cells at the periphery of each lobule of the gland give rise to daughter cells that move to the central areas of each acinus as they differentiate and form sebum (a complex oily substance composed of tri- and diglycerides, fatty acids, wax esters, squalene, and sterols). The sebaceous glands are usually associated with a hair follicle, although some glands open directly on the skin surface. Sebaceous glands are also found normally in the buccal mucosa (Fordyce's spots), around the female areola (Montgomery's tubercles), on the prepuce (Tyson's glands), and in the eyelids (meibomian glands). The sebaceous glands and certain hair follicles are androgen-dependent target organs. These appendages can reduce testosterone to dihydrotestosterone, convert testosterone to estradiol, and metabolize dehydroepiandrosterone to androstenedione and testosterone. The action of androgen on the pilosebaceous units is the sum total of effects of these various weak and strong androgens. Sebaceous gland growth and synthesis of sebum, as well as the growth of various hair follicles, are under the control of androgens. Various androgens produced by the testes, ovaries, and adrenal glands are converted to dihydrotestosterone (DHT) in these appendages by action of an enzyme, 5-alpha reductase. DHT combines with a specific cytosol receptor protein found in androgen-dependent tissues and is transported to chromosomal DNA where it initiates transcription of enzymes that stimulate sebaceous gland and follicular hair growth. Follicles particularly responsive to androgen stimulation are found over the frontal and vertex areas of scalp, beard, chest, axillae, and upper and lower pubic triangles.

The rate at which hair grows and the size of the hair shaft are modulated in some hair follicles by androgens. Hair follicles are formed in early embryonic life, and no more develop after birth. Males and females have approximately the same number of hair follicles distributed over the body, but the degree of hairiness depends on two distinct features of hair growth—the *hair cycle* and the *hair pattern*. Hair growth consists of recurring cycles of growth (anagen phase), regression (catagen phase), and resting (telogen phase). Throughout telogen the resting hair lies high in the follicle, where it forms a stubby hair bulb that is easily shed. When anagen begins there is a burst of mitotic activity and the follicle grows downward to reconstitute a new hair bulb. The hair bulb cells divide rapidly and keratinize to form a new hair shaft that dislodges the old resting club telogen hair. With a hand lens a fallen or plucked hair can be identified by inspection as having been resting (telogen, root of the hair is a rounded fine bulb) or actively growing (anagen, elongated root with fine white sheath). Catagen is the brief respite when mitosis ceases and the hair follicle pulls upward in the dermis as the hair shaft evolves into a telogen club hair. In the adult scalp 85 per cent of the hairs are in anagen at any given time, 14 per cent in telogen, and 1 per cent in catagen. Considerable variation in timing of the cycle occurs from one region of the body to another, and the length of anagen determines the length of hairs. Thus, short hairs are found on the arms and eyebrows with relatively short anagen periods (few months), while long anagen periods are seen in the scalp (up to six years).

Hair cycles also vary with the second important feature of hair growth, namely, hair pattern or the type of hair growing in each follicle. Two types of hairs are seen: vellus hair (fine, soft, short, nonpigmented, and common on "nonhairy" areas of the body) and terminal hair (coarse, long, pigmented, and found on hairy areas of the body).

The dramatic changes in both hair cycle and hair pattern which occur at puberty are selectively mediated by either testosterone or dihydrotestosterone. The characteristic increase in hairiness at puberty is not the result of formation of new follicles. Rather, the increased hairiness results from the conversion of vellus hair follicles to large terminal follicles. In the axillae and lower pubic triangle this conversion is mediated by testosterone and androstenedione. In other regions such as the beard, chest, upper pubic triangle, nostrils, and external ears, this conversion is mediated by dihydrotestosterone. Paradoxically, DHT also mediates the reverse process, namely, the miniaturization of large terminal follicles into vellus hairs. Such physiologic miniaturization occurs with the reshaping of the frontal hairline from a straight line to an M-shaped configuration at puberty. This occurs in all men and in the majority of women.

Maternal androgens ensure full development and function of sebaceous glands at birth. The vernix caseosa covering the neonate is mostly sebum. Normally sebaceous glands atrophy after birth, until puberty, when androgens again stimulate their activity. Acne is often one of the earliest signs of puberty. Disorders of androgen excess in adult women (e.g., polycystic ovary syndrome) are also associated with increased sebaceous activity and acne. Estrogens in large amounts decrease gland size and secretion.

FUNCTIONS OF THE SKIN

PROTECTION. Several structures in the skin, including the stratum corneum, melanin, cutaneous nerves, and the dermal connective tissue, provide protective functions of importance to our survival. The skin protects against the loss of essential fluids, the entrance of toxic agents and microorganisms, and damage from ultraviolet radiation, mechanical shearing forces, and extreme environmental temperatures.

The *stratum corneum* serves as a low-permeability barrier that not only retards water loss from the inner epidermal hydrated layers, but also shields against damage from the environment. The barrier properties of the horny layer are of practical importance from several points of view: First, excessive drying or inflammatory reactions in the skin (e.g., eczema) will lead to roughness and scaling as the normally compact layers of horny cells are disrupted. This leads to increased transepidermal water loss and, if extensive areas of the horny layer are disrupted (as in generalized exfoliative dermatitis, erythroderma, or burns), the total water loss can contribute to fluid and electrolyte imbalance. Second, with breaks in the horny layer, external substances more readily gain entrance to the underlying epidermis. Thus, various chemical substances, including medications placed on injured skin, have a greater opportunity for systemic absorption or a greater propensity to act as haptens or antigens, increasing the possibility of allergic contact dermatitis. Third, the disruption of the barrier increases the chance of colonization of pathologic bacteria in the skin, especially in the presence of tissue fluid exudates, which serve as excellent culture media. Fourth, percutaneous absorption of various topical medications used in treating skin conditions, such as topical steroids, can be enhanced by hydrating the stratum corneum with the use of occlusive plastic wraps.

The stratum corneum not only serves as a barrier to the invasion of various bacteria, it also harbors a number of aerobic and anaerobic resident organisms (i.e., *Staphylococcus epidermidis*, diphtheroids, *Proprionibacterium acnes*, and *Pityrosporon*). Breaks in the stratum corneum, poor hygiene, and excessive humidity with maceration (especially in intertriginous areas) all contribute to cutaneous infections such as impetigo, erysipelas, folliculitis, furunculosis, and ecthyma.

A second structural component that provides protection is the *melanocyte*, which produces melanin pigment. Melanin is a large polymer that has the unique capability of absorbing light over the broad range of 200 to 2400 nm wave lengths. It serves as an excellent screen against the untoward effects of solar ultraviolet radiation, such as aging and wrinkling of the skin and the development of cutaneous neoplasms. The importance of melanin is dramatically illustrated by the high incidence of skin cancers in sun-exposed areas of the body, particularly in light-skinned, blue-eyed, easily sunburned individuals and in albinos. Ultraviolet light exposure also causes aging and wrinkling of the skin. Neither sex nor race affects the number of melanocytes in the epidermis. Negroid skin contains the same number of melanocytes as Caucasian skin, but the pigmentation is more intense as a result of the synthesis of more melanin that is dispersed throughout the melanocytes and adjacent keratinocytes. Accordingly, black skin is much less likely to form skin cancers, and it ages more slowly than white skin.

A third structural component in the skin which plays a part in protection is the dermal *nerves*. Nerve endings are extensively distributed in the skin in two general morphologic types: free nerve endings and specialized endings (Pacini's and Meissner's corpuscles), which mediate many sensations including pain, pressure, and itch. Pain is important to our survival, since we pull away from the source of pain and avert further injury. Loss of sensation (e.g., diabetic neuropathy) may result in deep traumatic ulcers (trophic ulcers) without the patient's awareness of them. Damage to the dermatomal nerves (e.g., herpes zoster) may result in prolonged burning pain and hypesthesias.

Itch is another important sensation mediated by cutaneous nerves. It is the most common symptom in dermatology and may occur in conjunction with a number of dermatologic diseases or without clinically evident skin disease (pruritus) (Tables 531–1 and 531–2). Itch and pain are carried on unmyelinated C fibers found in the upper portion of the dermis of the skin, mucous membranes, and cornea. The afferent C

TABLE 531–1. SKIN DISEASES ASSOCIATED WITH ITCHING

Xerosis (dry skin)
Insect infestations (scabies, pediculosis, insect bites)
Dermatitis (atopic, contact, nummular)
Drugs (opiates, aspirin, quinidine)
Lichen planus
Urticaria
Dermatitis herpetiformis (burning itch)
Sunburn
Fiberglas dermatitis

fibers enter the dorsal horn of the spinal cord, synapse, cross the midline, and ascend the spinothalamic tracts to the thalamus. Then the impulse proceeds to the sensory area of the postcentral gyrus of the cortex. Cutting the spinothalamic tract, as in an anterolateral hemichordotomy, abolishes pain and itch. A variety of peripheral mediators stimulate the C fibers and induce itching. These include histamine, trypsin, proteases, peptides (bradykinin, vasoactive intestine peptide, substance P—all potent histamine releasers), and bile salts. Prostaglandins are modulators of pruritus rather than primary mediators, lowering the threshold to itching evoked by both histamine and pain. Central modulators of pruritus, such as systemic morphine, cause itch while relieving pain by acting on central opiate receptors.

Generalized itching in the absence of primary skin disease (pruritus) may be an important sign of internal disease (Table 531–2). Such diverse conditions as uremia, cholestatic biliary disease, lymphoma and myeloproliferative diseases, thyrotoxicosis, diabetes, carcinoma, iron deficiency anemia, and psychiatric disorders may cause severe pruritus. An important cause of pruritus is psychic stress. Some patients with psychogenic pruritus believe the itching is caused by invisible parasites in the skin. Such patients scratch until excoriations and prurigo papules (thickened papular areas of skin due to constant rubbing) evolve in areas that the patient can readily reach (extremities, scalp, upper back). Dry skin (xerosis) is a common cause of itching in older individuals. Certain drugs (aspirin, opiates) can cause itching without a visible rash. Patients with polycythemia vera display a unique type of

TABLE 531–2. PRURITUS ASSOCIATED WITH SYSTEMIC DISEASE

Systemic Disease	Postulated Etiology
Uremia	Secondary hyperparathyroidism, high skin calcium concentration, proliferation of mast cells, xerosis

Obstructive biliary disease
  Primary biliary cirrhosis
  Cholestatic hepatitis secondary to drugs (chloropropamide)
  Intrahepatic cholestasis of pregnancy
  Extrahepatic biliary obstruction
	High concentrations of bile salts in skin

Hematologic and myeloproliferative disorders Lymphoma Mycosis fungoides Polycythemia vera Iron deficiency anemia	Unknown

Endocrine disorders
  Thyrotoxicosis
  Hypothyroidism
  Diabetes
	Unknown

Carcinoid	Serotonin
Visceral malignancies Breast, stomach, lung	Unknown

Psychiatric disorders
  Stress
  Delusions of parasitosis
	Unknown

Neurologic disorders
  Multiple sclerosis (paroxysmal itching)
  Notalgia paresthetica—local itch of back, medial left scapula (local neuropathy)
  Brain abscess
  CNS infarct
	Unknown

pruritus, namely, itching triggered by sudden changes in temperature, especially as the patient emerges from a warm bath. The itch is prickly in nature and lasts minutes to hours.

The tough, viscoelastic properties imparted to the skin by the fibrous proteins (collagen and elastin) and amorphous ground substance that make up the dermis provide protection from shearing forces applied to the skin. The viscous and elastic properties of the ground substance allow it to resist compression and accept molding, thus serving to reduce point pressure on more sensitive skin structures.

THERMOREGULATION. Thermoregulation is subserved concomitantly by the cutaneous vasculature and the sweat glands. A massive network of interconnecting musculocutaneous arteries and venules, as well as capillaries, arteriovenous shunts, and small venules, plays a crucial role in the maintenance of body temperature (Fig. 531–1). The major fraction of the blood volume of the skin is contained in the large venous plexus, in which the blood moves with low velocity close to the surface, enabling maximal dissipation of heat. Equally important in thermoregulation is the formation of eccrine sweat, which provides cooling by evaporation from the skin's surface. For every gram of water that is evaporated from the skin, 580 calories of heat are lost.

Blood flow through the skin is 10 to 20 times that required to supply needed metabolites and oxygen. Under basal conditions 8.5 per cent, or 450 ml per minute of the total blood flow, passes through the skin, the control of flow being primarily by the sympathetic nervous system (via epinephrine and norepinephrine). Blood flow can increase up to 3.5 liters per minute with exercise in a warm environment. Because the heat conductivity and specific heat of blood are high, large amounts of heat can be dissipated through the skin. Both central (hypothalamic heating) and peripheral thermoreceptors stimulate sweating via the sympathetic nervous system, but in the case of sweat glands, acetylcholine is the postganglionic transmitter. Increase in body core temperature is the strongest stimulus for inducing sweating, whereas peripheral (cutaneous) thermoreceptors are only one tenth as effective in eliciting perspiration.

Response to cold begins when blood cooler than normal passes to the hypothalamus, which then elicits both heat conservation and heat production mechanisms. The sympathetics are excited, constricting cutaneous blood vessels and thereby reducing the transfer of heat to the body surface. Impulses from the hypothalamus also activate the motor center for shivering, which increases heat production by as much as 50 per cent. Conversely, when blood warmer than normal passes to the hypothalamus, the central heat production mechanism becomes inoperative, and cutaneous blood vessels dilate, allowing blood to accumulate near the skin surface and heat to be lost by conduction and convection. Vasodilatation also occurs reflexly through direct warming of the skin surface (in warm environments). In addition, stimulation of the hypothalamus produces sweating and increases evaporative heat loss. With periodic exposure to heat or to heat and work stresses (i.e. daily one- or two-hour exposures for 10 to 14 days), the secretory capacity of the eccrine sweat glands is enhanced (i.e., acclimatization).

One example of the crucial role of cutaneous vasculature in thermoregulation and in cardiovascular homeostasis is widespread inflammatory conditions of the skin causing *erythroderma*. In such diseases as generalized dermatitis, psoriasis, drug reactions, and underlying lymphomas, the inflammatory response in the skin can cause generalized cutaneous vasodilatation with diversion of 10 to 20 per cent of cardiac output through the skin. Central blood volume may be decreased. To maintain blood pressure, cardiac output must increase and in older individuals with impaired cardiac reserve high-output failure may occur in association with tremendous loss of body heat with wide swings in temperature and shivering.

THE SKIN AS AN ENDOCRINE ORGAN. Many metabolic

activities of the skin are under hormonal regulation to the extent that the skin is recognized as an important hormone end organ. Indeed, not only do sebaceous glands and certain hair follicles respond readily to androgens, but they are capable of many diverse steroid transformations, as described above.

Dihydrotestosterone causes sebaceous glands to enlarge at puberty, the growth of certain hair (male sexual hair of the beard, chest, upper pubic triangle, nose, and ears), and the growth and development of the external genitalia. Antiandrogens, drugs that block the conversion of testosterone to DHT, do this by competitively inhibiting either 5 alpha-reductase or the cytosol receptor protein for DHT. Drugs such as cimetidine and spironolactone have antiandrogenic activity and have been used to treat acne and hirsutism. In addition, thyroid hormones can regulate hair growth and alter the texture of the skin (fine, sparse hair and smooth, soft skin in hyperthyroidism; coarse hair and cool, rough, thick skin in hypothyroidism). Further, hormones affect melanin pigment formation, melanocyte stimulating hormone, and estrogen stimulating skin pigmentation.

THE SKIN AS AN IMMUNOLOGIC ORGAN. The epidermis and the dermoepidermal junctional area serve as active participants in immunologic reactions. The skin is composed of immunologically important cells including keratinocytes, Langerhans' cells, and melanocytes as well as immunologic structures such as the lamina lucida and basal lamina that are involved in a variety of bullous reactions of the skin.

Epidermal Immunologically Important Cells. Perhaps the most important immunologic cell in the epidermis is the Langerhans' cell, comprising 2 to 5 per cent of the total epidermal cell population. Langerhans' cells play a role in a number of immunologic reactions, including macrophage–T cell interaction, T and B lymphocyte interactions, graft versus host (GVH) reactions, and skin graft rejection. The Langerhans' cell synthesizes and expresses Ia antigens (Class II antigens, immune response gene–associated antigens) that are crucial in processing and presenting allergens to sensitized T lymphocytes critical in the elicitation of delayed hypersensitivity contact dermatitis. Lymphokines, made by the Langerhans' cells during these immunologic reactions, augment and enhance these processes and also contribute to the accompanying inflammatory response.

Keratinocytes also play a role in immunologic responses by expressing Ia antigens on their surfaces in such conditions as GVH reaction, mycosis fungoides, allergic contact dermatitis, lichen planus, and tuberculoid leprosy. In these conditions the keratinocytes make lymphokines, particularly interleukin 1 (ETAF, epidermal cell thymocyte factor), which provides a second signal supplementing macrophages (Langerhans' cells) in mitogen- and antigen-induced T cell activation. In addition, epidermal cells make other cytokines such as prostaglandin-E2 and leukotrienes that participate in inflammatory reactions in the skin. Keratinocytes are the immunologic target in the pemphigus group of diseases where circulating autoantibodies against intercellular antigen of the epidermis and mucous membrane epithelium initiate intraepidermal acantholytic bullae.

The Dermoepidermal Junction as an Immunologic Structure. A variety of inflammatory diseases often characterized by bullous reactions seem to be mediated by immunoreactants, including IgG, IgA, and IgM, and complement deposition along the dermoepidermal junctional area. The anatomic site of blister formation correlates with the position of deposition of these immunoreactants. The antigens in several diseases have been isolated and partially characterized. The use of immunofluorescent techniques at the light microscopic and especially the ultrastructural level has been very helpful in more precisely diagnosing these bullous conditions. These are summarized in Table 531–3, along with immunofluorescent skin findings in connective tissue diseases.

INFLAMMATORY REACTIONS IN THE SKIN AND WOUND HEALING. Cutaneous inflammation reflects the sum of the effects of biologic products of cells (mast cells,

TABLE 531–3. IMMUNOFLUORESCENT CUTANEOUS FINDINGS IN IMMUNOLOGICALLY MEDIATED SKIN DISEASE

Diseases	Biopsy Findings of Direct Immunofluorescence Immunoreactants (DII)	Ultrastructural Localization of Immunoreactants	Site of Blister Formation on Routine Light Microscopic Pathology	Serum Findings: Indirect Immunofluorescence (IIF)
Bullous Diseases				
Pemphigus (all forms)	Deposits of IgG intercellular areas between keratinocytes	Between keratinocytes	Suprabasilar in pemphigus vulgaris; substratum corneum in pemphigus foliaceus	IgG antibodies to intercellular areas of keratinocytes in 90% of patients
Bullous pemphigoid	IgG and/or complement (C) in basement membrane zone (BMZ)	Lamina lucida and hemidesmosomes—upper part lucida and sub-basal cells	Subepidermal	IgG Ab to BMZ in 70%
Cicatricial pemphigoid	IgG and/or C in BMZ	Lamina lucida	Subepidermal	IgG antibodies BMZ in 10%
Herpes gestationis	Complement in BMZ—occasionally IgG	Lamina lucida—close to lamina densa	Subepidermal—sub-basal cell—above lamina densa	IgG antibodies BMZ in 20% (HG factor in 25%)
Dermatitis herpetiformis	IgA and C in dermal papillae (granular deposits)	Granular IgA associated with microfibril bundles in dermal papilla	Subepidermal in dermal papillae—papillar dermal microabscesses	No circulating antibodies
Epidermolysis bullosa acquisita	IgG in BMZ	Sublamina densa amorphous granular deposits	Subepidermal	No circulating antibodies
Linear IgA bullous dermatosis in childhood	IgA and complement in linear deposition in BMZ	—	Subepidermal	No circulating antibodies
Connective Tissue Diseases				
Bullous SLE	IgG, IgM, and complement in BMZ in involved and normal skin—linear homogeneous	Just beneath lamina densa (basal lamina)	Subepidermal	No circulating antibodies to BMZ; ANA found in 90%
Discoid LE	IgG, other Ig, and C in lesional skin at BMZ	—	—	No circulating antibodies to BMZ, ANA titers normal
Systemic LE	IgG band at BMZ in normal skin (over 90% in sun-exposed areas)	—	—	Elevated ANA titers
Systemic sclerosis	Nucleolar IgG	—	Epidermal thinning and increased dermal collagen	ANA, speckled, 85%; centromere + in CREST syndrome
MCTD	IgG/IgM in BMZ in some patients; nuclear IgG in epidermis	—	—	Speckled ANA and ENA (extractable nuclear antigens)
Dermatomyositis	Negative	—	—	ANA often normal range

infiltrating neutrophils, monocytes/macrophages, lymphocytes) as well as the effects of the products of the complement system, membrane-derived arachidonic acid metabolic pathways (prostaglandins and leukotrienes) and the Hageman factor–dependent pathways of coagulation, fibrinolysis, and kinin generation. Early phases of wound healing also encompass many of these reactions.

Cutaneous Inflammation. A variety of pathophysiologic reactions initiate inflammation, including infectious, immunologic, and toxic processes that affect the epidermis or dermis, or both. Mast cells in the skin not only function as the sentinel cells in immediate-type hypersensitivity reactions but also as major effector cells in inflammatory reactions releasing (1) histamine, prostaglandin D2, and leukotrienes, which cause vascular dilatation and increased permeability, redness, swelling, pain, and itch; (2) chemotactic factors for eosinophils and neutrophils; (3) proteases that interact with the complement, kinin, and fibrinolytic pathways; and (4) heparin, which may play a role in local angiogenesis. Degranulation of mast cells occurs in response to various antigens that cross-link IgE on the mast cell surface (immediate hypersensitivity reactions), to by-products of complement activation C3a and C5a (as occurs in leukocytoclastic vasculitides), as well as to radiocontrast media, aspirin, insect venom, and various physical stimuli. Circulating peripheral blood cells infiltrate local tissue sites in response to chemotactic factors released by mast cells and other infiltrating cells. Basophils release histamine and chemotactic substances, such as those involved in allergic contact reactions, bullous pemphigoid, erythema multiforme, and inflammatory responses. Neutrophils release myeloperoxidase, acid hydrolases, and neutral proteases that are active against microbes and cause tissue destruction (dermatitis herpetiformis, psoriasis, leukocytoclastic vasculitis, and bacterial infections of the skin). Eosinophils release major basic protein and peroxidase (allergic drug reactions in the skin, bullous pemphigoid). Lymphocytes release lymphokines that modulate immunologic and inflammatory responses (lichen planus, lupus erythematosus, allergic contact dermatitis, tuberculoid leprosy). Monocytes and macrophages engulf foreign proteins and microorganisms (granulomatous reactions in the skin such as sarcoidosis, deep fungus and acid–fast bacilli infections, and cutaneous foreign body responses). In addition, both classic and alternate complement pathways release products that induce mast cell degranulation and induce inflammation. (The activation of the system seems to play a role in inflammatory reactions in hereditary complement deficiencies causing lupus erythematosus–like syndromes or pyodermas, as well as necrotizing vasculitis.)

Wound Healing in the Skin. Healing proceeds temporally in three phases: substrate, proliferative, and remodeling. The initial substrate phase, encompassing the first three to four days after wounding, is so named because the cellular and other interactions lead to preparation for subsequent events. During this phase vascular and inflammatory components prevail (vascular clotting in the severed vessels; leukocyte and macrophage chemotaxis into the area to ingest bacteria, debride the wound, and degrade collagen). The proliferative phase (10 to 14 days after wounding) results in regeneration of epidermis, neoangiogenesis, and proliferation of fibroblasts with increased collagen synthesis and closure of the skin defect. The final remodeling phase takes place over 6 to 12 months, during which time a more stable form of collagen is laid down to form a scar of progressively increasing tensile strength. In some instances so much collagen is deposited in the healing wound that an elevated *hypertrophic scar* (red, raised scar within the boundaries of the original wound) or keloid (scar tissue extending beyond the boundaries of original injury into surrounding normal tissue) is produced. Keloids, which occur most commonly over the anterior chest, upper back, and deltoid regions, rarely regress, and they recur after excision. Fibroblasts from keloid areas synthesize collagen at significantly greater rates than normal skin, even in tissue culture.

THE COSMETIC IMPORTANCE OF SKIN. With age virtually all the structures and functions of the skin change. Environmental insults, especially chronic sun exposure, cause far greater destruction of the skin than time itself. Sun exposure over a lifetime, especially in fair-skinned, easily sunburned individuals, accelerates the aging process, resulting in thin, wrinkled, skin in exposed areas. The major age changes in gross appearance of skin include roughness, wrinkling, laxity, uneven pigmentation, and a variety of benign and malignant proliferative lesions.

Changes with aging at the structural, physiologic, and biochemical level are as follows: (1) A decrease in epidermal turnover rate of approximately 50 per cent occurs between the third and seventh decades. Concurrent loss of dermal elastic and collagen fibers accounts for the paper-thin, transparent quality of aged skin and the easy rupture of dermal vessels. Further, with age there is increasing cross-linkage of collagen and elastin, making the dermis more rigid and therefore less able to withstand shearing forces. Aged skin, when "tented up," only slowly returns to its original form, whereas young skin readily snaps back. (2) Sun-damaged aged skin shows microscopic collagen damage. Dermal collagen is replaced by amorphous basophilic staining material. This condition, termed *elastosis*, results in deep wrinkling and furrowing, especially over the face and back of the neck, and yellow papules and nodules in a reticular pattern on the face. (3) Decreases in the number of functioning sebaceous and sweat glands contribute to the dryness of aged skin and to impaired thermoregulation in aged persons. (4) Reduction in the vascular network in the skin surrounding hair bulbs and eccrine and sebaceous glands may be responsible for the atrophy of these appendages with age. (5) A 50 per cent reduction in the number of Langerhans' cells may account in part for the age-associated decrease in immune responsiveness and allergic contact dermatitis reactions in the elderly. (6) Loss of enzymatically active melanocytes (10 to 20 per cent per decade) causes irregular pigmentation of the skin and graying of the hair. (7) Gradual reduction occurs in the number of body hairs, especially in the scalp, axillary, and pubic regions (related in part to decreased androgen production). (8) Linear growth of nails also decreases by 30 to 50 per cent between early and late adulthood. Often nails become brittle and thickened. (9) A number of proliferative growths are associated with aging skin, including skin tags (acrochordon), cherry angiomata, seborrheic keratosis, lentigenes, and sebaceous hyperplasia.

532 EXAMINATION OF THE SKIN AND AN APPROACH TO DIAGNOSING SKIN DISEASES

General considerations in history taking and physical examination:

THE DERMATOLOGIC HISTORY

A proper history includes the following: where the patient's skin condition first appeared; what it looked like and what symptoms, if any, were associated with it initially; how the skin disease progressed and changed and what has been done to treat the condition (by the patient or by other physicians).

A careful review of the systemic medications (both proprietary and prescribed) that the patient is taking, is in order. The relationship of the onset of the skin rash to the use of systemic internal medications is particularly crucial in evaluating the possibility of a drug reaction.

A history of atopic diseases or skin cancer and a careful family history of skin problems help to alert the physician to genetic and familial aspects of dermatosis.

If contact dermatitis is suspected, a detailed work and hobby history can identify exposure to allergens or irritants, for instance by noting the waxing of the skin condition in relation to time on the job and waning during time away from work, such as weekends and vacations. Environmental exposure to the elements such as sun, cold, and heat may be important in provoking skin reactions. Also, when dealing with possible infectious and parasitic processes of the skin, it is useful to determine whether family members or sexual partners are similarly affected.

Psychologic stress, although seldom a sole cause of cutaneous conditions, can exacerbate many dermatoses (e.g., acne, psoriasis, seborrhea, atopic eczema).

THE PHYSICAL EXAMINATION

Dermatology is a visual specialty, and because the identification of skin lesions is a crucial aspect of dermatologic diagnosis the examiner's eye and a magnifying lens are the most important tools. Good lighting is essential, either daylight or fluorescent light simulating daylight. At times side lighting in a darkened room is also useful for detecting minimally raised or depressed lesions.

The skin should be examined from head to toe in a systematic manner, so that all regions of the integument, including the nails and the mucous membranes, are evaluated. It is not unusual for the informed and observant physician to find some significant skin lesion, such as a basal cell carcinoma or even a melanoma, of which the patient is unaware. The general assessment of the entire skin, then, allows the examiner to determine the pattern of the skin problem before focusing on specific lesions. Distribution of the skin problem may follow neural (as in a dermatome) or vascular patterns (as in livedo reticularis). In addition, factors related to the patient's general medical condition can also be discerned in the skin by noting signs of aging, pigmentation, trauma, nutrition, and hygiene. Color changes related to underlying systemic conditions (e.g., jaundice with hepatobiliary conditions, cyanosis with various cardiopulmonary diseases, diffuse hyperpigmentation with Addison's disease, paleness with anemia) are important to the assessment.

In each region of the body the physical examination includes three maneuvers: (1) *Observation* for color or surface changes. (2) *Touch or light stroking* to perceive texture changes, warmth, and moisture. Smoothness or roughness of the skin depends on such things as normal keratinization, proper hydration of the stratum corneum, normal cutaneous blood flow. (3) *Palpation* to determine the consistency and pliability of the skin by stretching the integument between the fingers. Plasticity depends on the normal structure and function of dermal connective tissue and ground substance.

Because there are many hundreds of dermatoses, a logical process of elimination is required to narrow the possibilities, first to specific groups of diseases and finally to one condition. Such a diagnostic approach is based on specific morphologic descriptions of the skin lesions that the physician sees and feels, together with an appropriate history and laboratory tests. Three steps are involved in this systematic approach. First, the entire skin is examined for primary and secondary skin lesions that allow the examiner to place the patient in one of nine diagnostic groups (the second step) (Table 532–1). Many skin conditions are found in each group, but all of the conditions in a given group manifest the same primary and secondary lesions. The third step involves differentiating the one disease the patient has from the others in the group.

This is done by looking for several specific features, such as the distribution of skin lesions, any unusual shapes of the lesions or arrangement of several lesions (annular, serpiginous, dermatomal), color of the lesion including dominant hue and the color pattern, and the surface characteristics (particularly the appearance of scales or verrucous or vegetative changes).

STEP 1: DESCRIPTION OF PRIMARY AND SECONDARY SKIN LESIONS. Primary skin lesions are uncomplicated lesions that represent the initial pathologic change, uninfluenced by secondary alterations such as infection, trauma, or therapy. Secondary skin lesions are changes that occur as consequences of progression of the disease or scratching or infection of the primary lesions (Fig. 532–1). Most of the primary changes can also, at times, occur as secondary manifestations; for example, pustules may appear as primary lesions of folliculitis or as secondary lesions when scaling, itching lesions are scratched and infected. The trick is to recognize any single primary skin lesion as the initial change characteristic of the disease.

The terminology used to describe primary and secondary skin changes is the basic language of dermatology, the means by which one can accurately describe skin diseases to a colleague. If this terminology is not used correctly it will be difficult to arrive at the precise diagnosis of skin diseases. Each descriptive word is not only a short account of what is seen on the surface of the skin but also relays specific information about processes within the skin. A diagrammatic representation and description of primary and secondary skin lesions are presented in Figure 532–2.

STEP 2: ASSIGNMENT OF THE LESION TO A MAJOR GROUP OF DISEASES. Each disease within a given group shares the same primary and secondary skin lesions. Some diseases have overlapping traits so they may be assigned to more than one group. An arbitrary grouping that has proved to be of practical value is listed below and is used later in this chapter to discuss specific diseases within each group (Table 532–1).

STEP 3: NARROWING THE POSSIBILITIES TO THE EXACT DIAGNOSIS. Of great importance is the distribution of the skin disease, for many conditions have typical patterns or affect specific regions. For example, psoriasis commonly affects extensor surfaces and atopic eczema flexor areas of the extremities (Fig. 532–2). Photoreactions are confined to parts of the body exposed to sunlight. Involvement of the palms and soles is seen in erythema multiforme, secondary syphilis, psoriasis, and eczema. Contact dermatitis to exogenous allergens or irritants often presents with unusual patterns and distributions corresponding to the areas where the offending material came in contact with the skin. The best way to examine for distribution is to step away from the patient and view from a few feet away.

Another important clue in differentiating diseases in a given group is to consider the shape of the individual lesions and the arrangement of several lesions in relation to each other. A *linear* arrangement of lesions may indicate a contact reaction to an exogenous substance brushing across the skin, a pathologic process involving a vascular or lymphatic vessel, or a cutaneous nevus (Fig. 532–2). *Zosteriform* refers to lesions arranged along the cutaneous distribution of a spinal nerve. It is thus bank-like and unilateral and denotes herpes zoster and, occasionally, metastatic carcinoma of the breast or the dermatomal hemangiomatous growths of Sturge-Weber syndrome. *Annular* lesions are circular with normal skin in the center. Annular macules are observed in drug eruptions, secondary syphilis, and lupus erythematosus. Resolving hives may leave annular configurations. Annular lesions with scale suggest dermatophytosis or pityriasis rosea. *Iris* lesions are a special type of annular lesion in which an erythematous annular macule or papule develops a second red ring or a purplish papule or vesicle in the center (target or bull's-eye

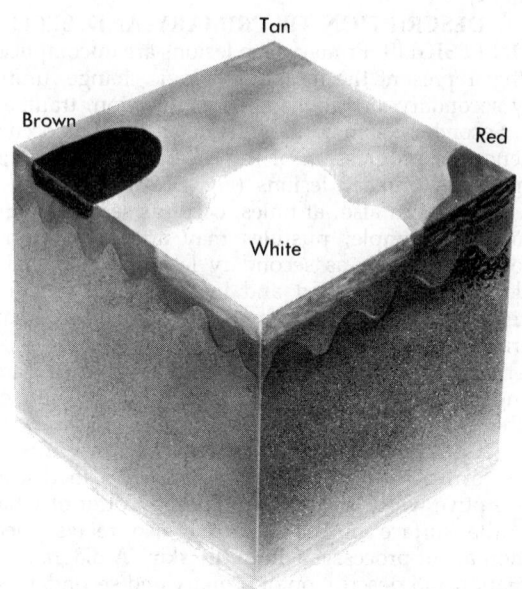

MACULE
A circumscribed color change

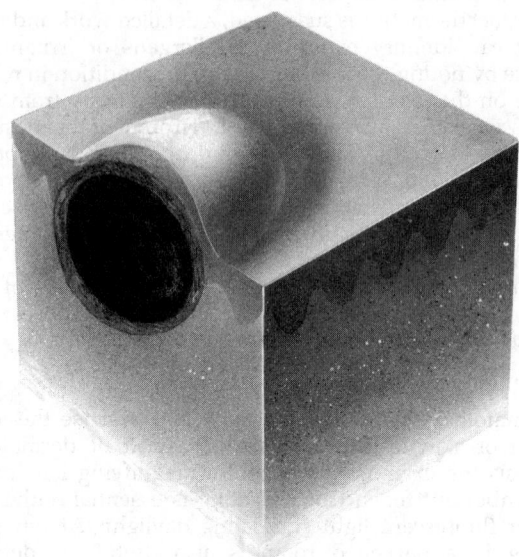

CYST
Semi-solid sac
Resilient

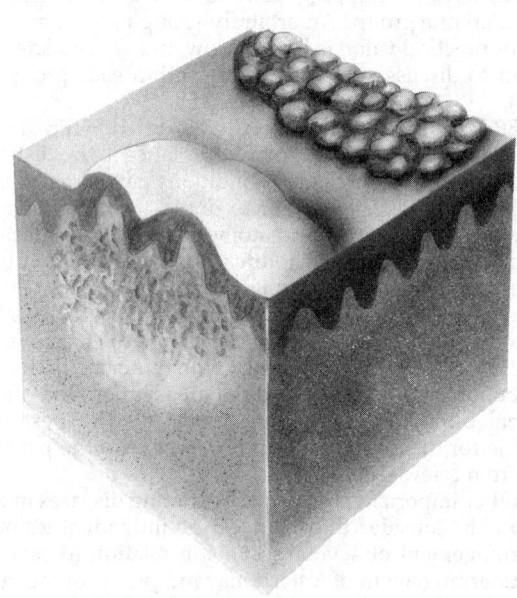

PAPULE
A solid elevation 1 cm or less
skin colored or not

PLAQUE
Raised, circumscribed,
extensive

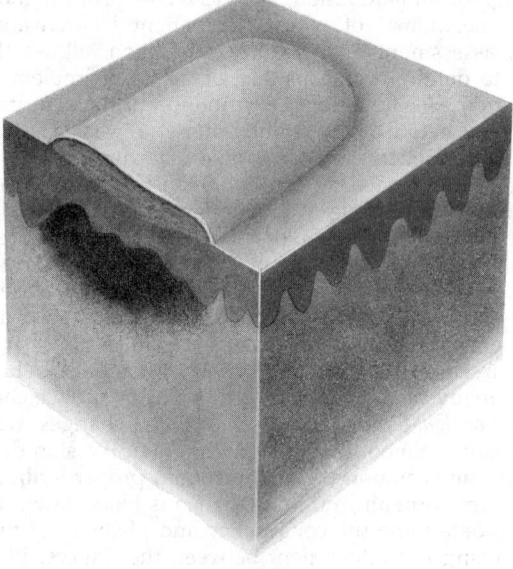

WHEAL
Evanescent
Edematous
Erythematous

FIGURE 532–1. Lesions of the skin. (From the 17th edition of the Cecil Textbook of Medicine, with the permission of Dr. Marie-Louise Johnson.)

Illustration continued on opposite page

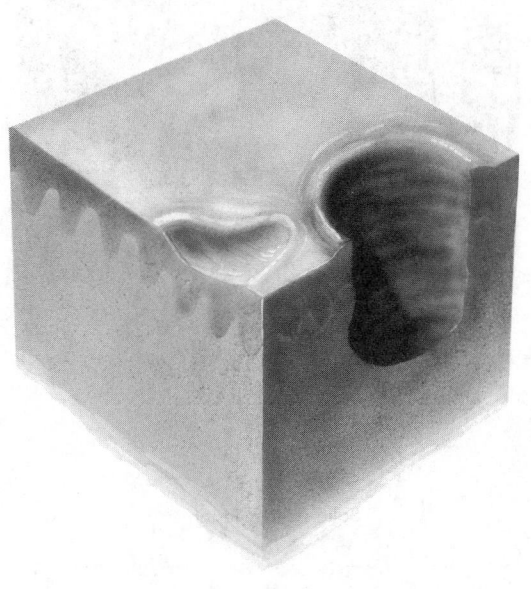

EROSION   ULCER
Superficial denudation Defect penetrates dermis

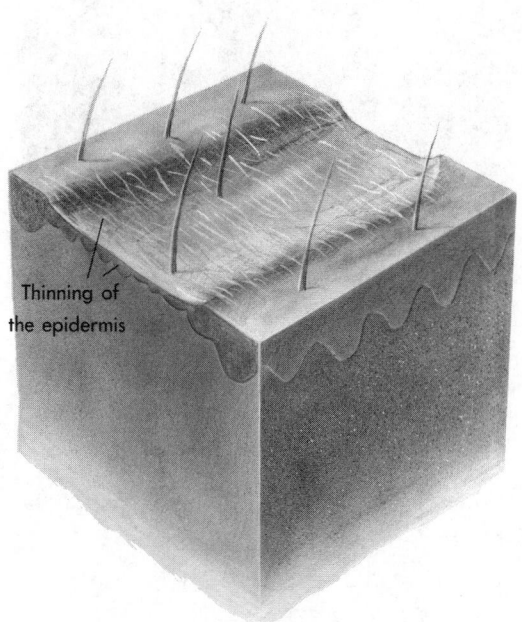

Thinning of
the epidermis

ATROPHY

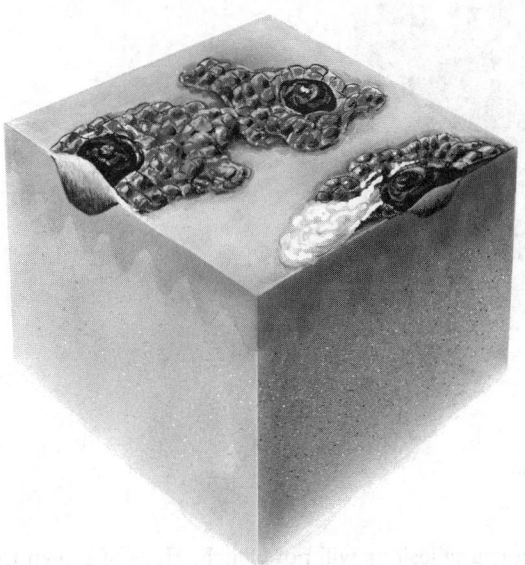

CRUST
Coagulated blood elements

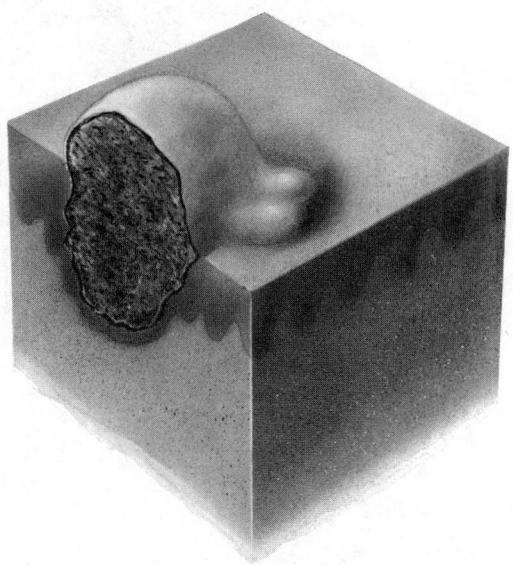

PUSTULE
Fluid-filled sac with
neutrophils

FIGURE 532–1. *Continued.*

Illustration continued on following page

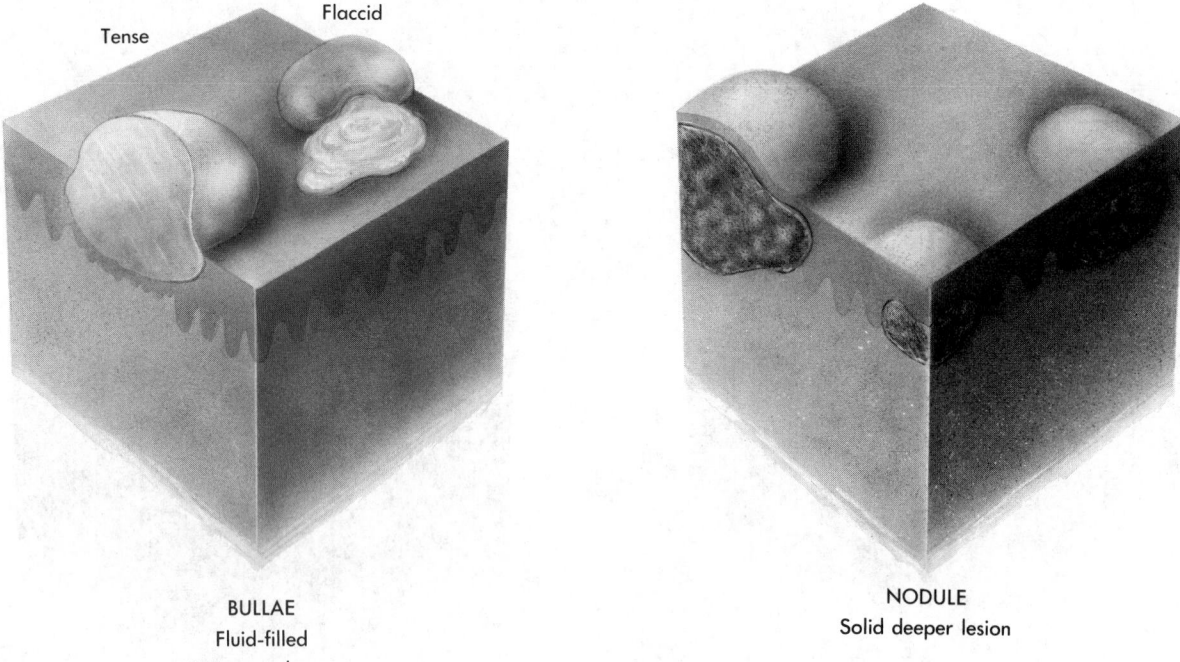

BULLAE
Fluid-filled
0.5 cm or larger

NODULE
Solid deeper lesion

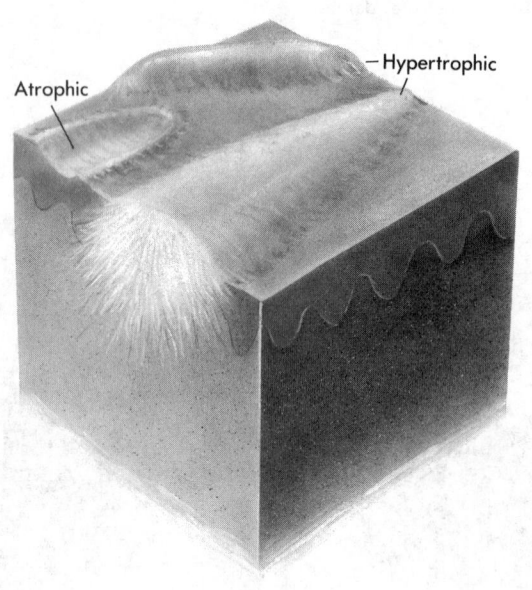

SCAR

FIGURE 532–1. *Continued.*

lesion). Iris lesions are seen in erythema multiforme. *Arciform* lesions form partial circles or arcs and may be seen in dermatophyte infections. *Polycyclic* patterns evolve when numerous annular lesions enlarge and run together. *Serpiginous* (snakelike, undulating, linear) patterns are seen in creeping eruptions and in psoriasis. *Herpetiform* refers to a grouping of lesions such as occurs in herpes simplex or dermatitis herpetiformis.

Other physical features are important in diagnosing skin diseases: Dry, lichenified lesions suggest a chronic state of a disease, whereas wet, weeping, macerated lesions suggest acute reactions. Abscesses are soft and fluctuant, whereas nodules are usually firm. Redness caused by dilatation of superficial blood vessels will blanch with pressure, whereas erythema caused by extravasated blood as occurs in petechiae

and purpuric lesions will not blanch. Hues of brown to black usually indicate melanin, although some drugs (e.g., tetracycline) cause brown-black pigmentation in the skin. The variation in color from melanin is related to the depth of the pigment in the skin—the deeper the pigment the more blue-black the color.

DIAGNOSTIC TESTS AND AIDS IN EXAMINATION OF THE SKIN

Certain technical, clinical, and laboratory aids and procedures, when combined with the history and physical examination, are indispensable in arriving at the correct diagnosis.

VISUAL AIDS. *Magnification.* Certain diagnostic findings are revealed by magnification of the skin lesions, for example,

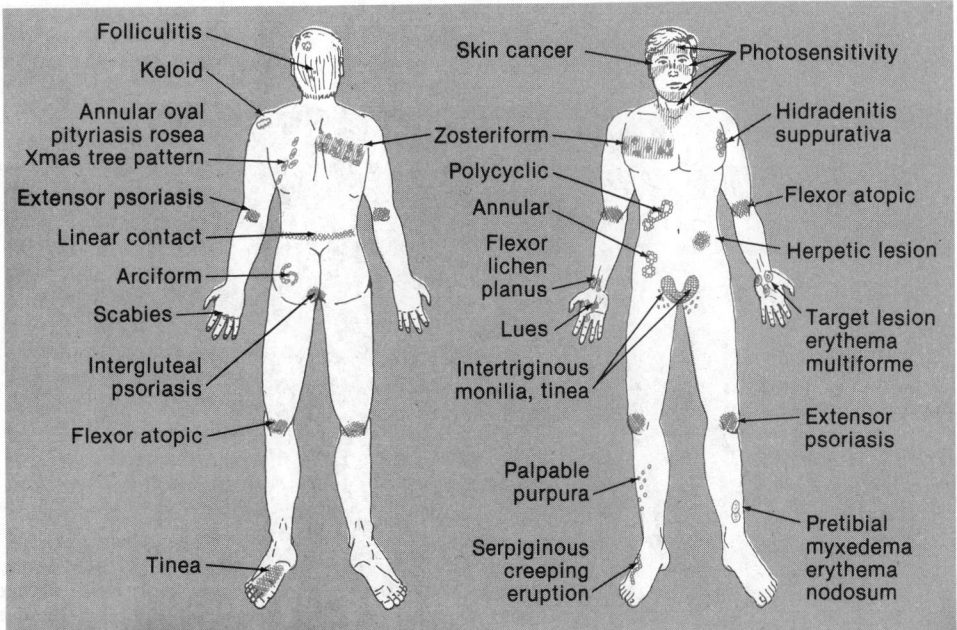

FIGURE 532–2. Configurational and regional diagnostic aids for the diagnosis of primary and secondary skin lesions.

TABLE 532–1. MAJOR GROUPS OF DERMATOLOGIC DISEASES BASED ON THE CLINICAL MORPHOLOGY OF THE SKIN CONDITION

Group	Clinical Morphology	Examples of Diseases in the Group
Eczema or dermatitis	Macules (erythema), papules, vesicles, lichenification, fine scaling, excoriations, crusting	Contact dermatitis, atopic dermatitis, stasis dermatitis, photodermatitis, scabies, dermatophytoses, exfoliative dermatitis, candidiasis
Maculopapular eruptions	Macules, erythema, papules	Viral exanthems, drug reactions, verruca vulgaris, Kawasaki's disease, vasculitic and purpuric eruptions
Papulosquamous dermatoses	Papules, plaques, erythema with unique scales	Psoriasis, Reiter's syndrome, pityriasis rosea, lichen planus, seborrheic dermatitis, ichthyosis, secondary syphilis, mycosis fungoides
Vesiculobullous diseases	Vesicles, bullae, erythema	Herpes simplex and zoster, hand-foot-and-mouth disease, insect bites, bullous impetigo, scalded skin syndrome, pemphigus, pemphigoid, dermatitis herpetiformis, porphyria cutanea tarda, erythema multiforme
Pustular diseases	Pustules, cysts, erythema	Acne vulgaris and rosacea, pustular psoriasis, folliculitis, gonococcemia
Urticaria, persistent figurate erythemas, cellulitis	Wheals and figurate, raised erythema, scaling	Urticaria, erythema annulare centrifugum, erysipelas, necrotizing fasciitis
Nodular lesions	Nodules and tumors, some associated with erosions and ulceration	Benign and malignant tumors—basal cell cancer, squamous cell cancer, rheumatoid nodules, xanthomas
Telangiectasias, atrophic, scarring, ulcerative diseases	Atrophic, sclerotic telangiectasias and ulcerative changes	Connective tissue diseases, radiation dermatitis, lichen sclerosus et atrophicus, vascular insufficiency (arterial and venous), pyoderma gangrenosum
Hyper- and hypomelanosis	Increased and decreased melanin deposition in skin	Acanthosis nigricans, café au lait spots, vitiligo, tuberous sclerosis, xeroderma pigmentosum, chloasma, freckles

the follicular plugging seen in discoid lupus erythematosus, or fine telangiectasias in the pearly, opalescent borders of basal cell cancers.

Transillumination. Oblique lighting in a darkened room can be useful in detecting slight degrees of elevation or depression of lesions as well as fine wrinkling or atrophy of the epidermis. In addition, the application of a penlight directly to nodular lesions in a dark room may give clues as to the density and make-up of such lesions. Cystic lesions allow transmission of some light, whereas nodules composed of cellular infiltrates do not.

Diascopy. Firm pressure with a microscope slide against skin lesions differentiates erythema of capillary dilatation from that of extravasated blood. Sarcoidosis, tuberculosis, and other granulomatous inflammatory reactions in the skin are suggested if diascopy of the lesions shows a characteristic "apple-jelly" or glassy, fawn-colored appearance.

Long-wave Ultraviolet or Wood's Light Examination. Long-wave ultraviolet light (UVA) (360 nm) is useful in evaluating several conditions of the skin. Wood's light is of great help in estimating subtle variations in pigmentation. It exaggerates the differences in the degree of pigmentation when the skin is examined with the lamp in a dark room. Melanin is a universal absorber of UV light, so decreased melanin shows more reflection (light color) and increased melanin less reflection (darker color). Pigment in the epidermis is exaggerated with UVA light, but that in the dermis is not, so a reasonable guess as to the site of melanin in the skin can be made. Wood's light may be the only means of recognizing the hypomelanotic ash leaf–shaped macules in tuberous sclerosis. The extent of vitiligo and melanotic nevi (which appear darker than surrounding normal skin) can also be determined. Some superficial fungal infections of the scalp fluoresce blue-green; erythrasma, a superficial intertriginous bacterial infection that produces a porphyrin, fluoresces a brilliant coral red; *Pseudomonas* infections may give off yellow-green color under a Wood's light.

CLINICAL TESTS. *Patch Tests.* Patch testing is used to validate a diagnosis of allergic contact sensitization and to identify the causative allergen. Since the entire skin of sensitized humans is allergic, the test reproduces the dermatitis in one small area where the allergen is applied, usually on the back. The suspected allergen is applied to the skin, occluded, and left in place 48 hours. A positive test reproduces an eczematous response at the test site from 48 hours up to a week after the test. The latter is a delayed hypersensitivity

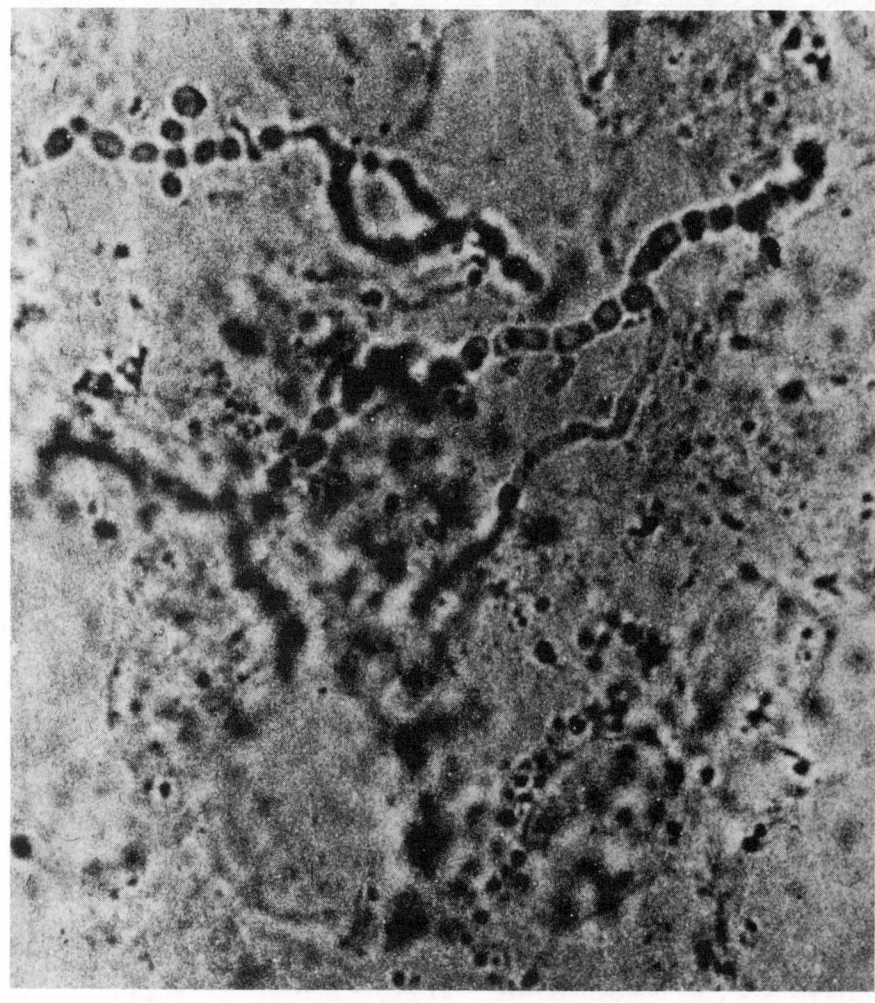

FIGURE 532–3. KOH preparation, high power. (From the 17th edition of the Cecil Textbook of Medicine, with the permission of Dr. Marie-Louise Johnson.)

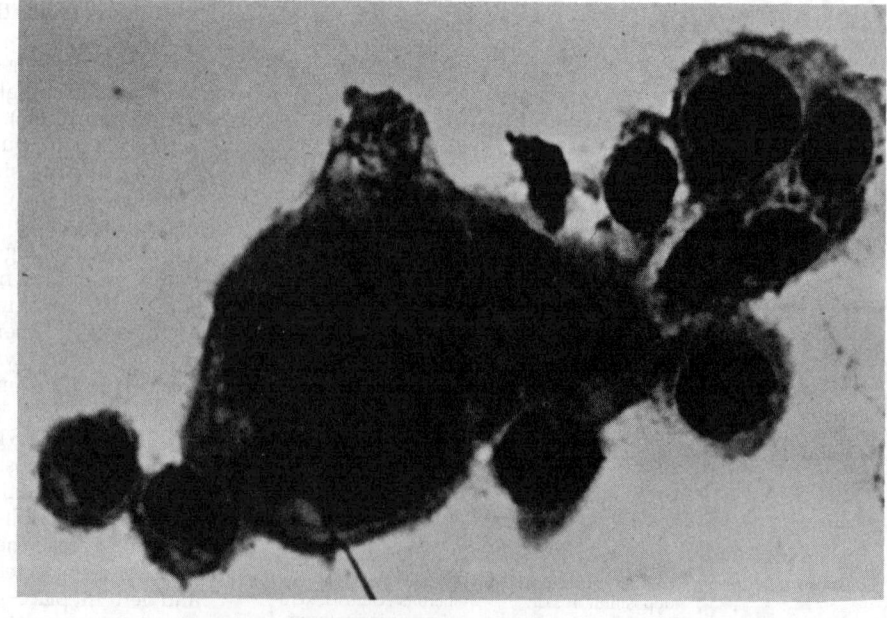

FIGURE 532–4. Positive Tzanck smear, herpes simplex. (From the 17th edition of the Cecil Textbook of Medicine, with the permission of Dr. Marie-Louise Johnson.)

reaction. Considerable experience is required to accurately perform and interpret patch tests. *Photopatch testing* is performed to detect photocontact allergy. Suspected photoallergens are placed on the skin in two sets. One set of allergens is irradiated with appropriate wavelengths of light after the patches are in place on the skin 24 hours; the second set of the same photoallergens is kept covered to serve as controls. Photoallergens cause an erythematous reaction that will be evident 24 hours after exposure to light.

Physical Contact Testing. Darier's sign is the development of an urticarial and flare reaction after vigorously rubbing cutaneous mast cell (urticaria pigmentosa) lesions of the skin. The rubbing degranulates the mast cells, releasing histamine.

Nikolsky's sign demonstrates disadherence of the epidermal cells to one another. Pushing, rubbing, or rotating normal skin near bullous lesions causes the epidermis to be dislodged, leaving a moist, glistening defect. This sign is present in various forms of pemphigus and in toxic epidermal necrolysis.

The *Koebner phenomenon* occurs in certain skin diseases that tend to evolve new skin lesions after traumatic injury in areas of apparently normal skin. Thus, psoriasis may evolve within surgical scars and after sunburn or in the wake of a drug reaction involving the skin. Lichen planus may also exhibit this phenomenon.

Pathergy, the development of pustular and ulcerative lesions at the site of needle puncture, is suggestive of Behçet's syndrome and pyoderma gangrenosum.

Hair-pull examination is done to assess hair loss in the scalp. It is often useful to pull vigorously on scalp hairs to (1) determine whether there is an increased number of falling hairs (normally only one or two can be removed with a tug of a group of hairs between the thumb and forefinger); (2) ascertain the ratio of anagen to telogen hairs; and (3) examine the hairs under a microscope for various congenital malformations of the shaft. Normally 10 to 15 per cent of scalp hairs are in telogen, whereas in telogen effluvium the percentage is greatly increased.

Paring Hyperkeratotic Lesions to Differentiate Warts from Calluses. After the hyperkeratosis is pared away, the wart displaces and obliterates epidermal ridges and small bleeding points, and black and red dots are seen in the wart. In calluses the epidermal ridges are not interrupted, and no vessels are seen within the callus.

LABORATORY PROCEDURES. *Gram's Stain and Cultures.* Gram's stain for bacteria and bacteriologic cultures are extremely important when the primary lesion is a pustule or furuncle or appears to be impetigo. When an unusual cutaneous infection is considered in an immunosuppressed patient, a skin biopsy specimen can be minced or ground in a sterile mortar and cultured for aerobic and anaerobic bacteria, including typical and atypical mycobacteria, deep fungi, and *Candida.* A more rapid method of screening for infectious agents in a skin infection in immunosuppressed patients (often the first sign of septicemia in such patients is pustules, nodules, or ulcerative lesions) is to perform frozen sections on a skin biopsy specimen taken from the lesion and to obtain Gram's stains, acid-fast bacterial stains, and PAS stains (to identify fungal and yeast elements). This may provide a diagnosis within a few hours.

Examination and Culture for Fungi and **Candida.** The presence of mycelia may be ascertained by applying 10 per cent potassium hydroxide to scale or exudative material scraped from suspected lesions and briefly heating the slide to dissolve the keratin. Hyphal elements can be observed by direct microscopic examination (Fig. 532–3). Dermatophyte hyphae appear as long, branching, refractile, walled structures; *Candida* appears as shorter, linear hyphae in association with budding yeast forms (see Fig. 534–2); tinea versicolor is seen as round yeast forms with short, club-shaped hyphae (so-called spaghetti and meatballs pattern) (see Fig. 534–4).

Tzanck Smear. The microscopic examination of cells from

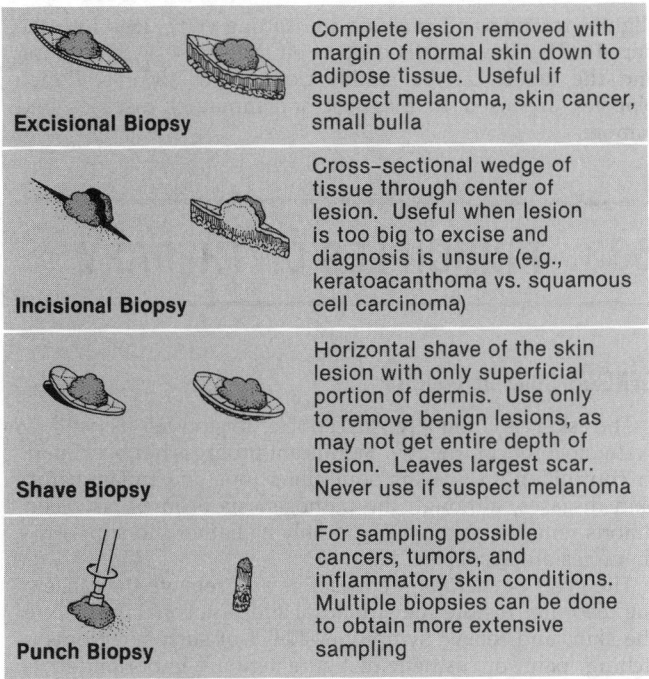

FIGURE 532–5. Methods of skin biopsy.

Excisional Biopsy	Complete lesion removed with margin of normal skin down to adipose tissue. Useful if suspect melanoma, skin cancer, small bulla
Incisional Biopsy	Cross-sectional wedge of tissue through center of lesion. Useful when lesion is too big to excise and diagnosis is unsure (e.g., keratoacanthoma vs. squamous cell carcinoma)
Shave Biopsy	Horizontal shave of the skin lesion with only superficial portion of dermis. Use only to remove benign lesions, as may not get entire depth of lesion. Leaves largest scar. Never use if suspect melanoma
Punch Biopsy	For sampling possible cancers, tumors, and inflammatory skin conditions. Multiple biopsies can be done to obtain more extensive sampling

the base of vesicles reveals the presence of giant epithelial cells and multinucleated giant cells in herpes simplex, herpes zoster, and varicella. Material is obtained from the base of a vesicle by gentle scraping with a scalpel and is spread on a glass slide and stained with Giemsa's or Wright's stain for the examination (Fig. 532–4).

Skin Biopsy. Lesions characteristic of the eruption (primary lesions) should be biopsied. Lesions altered by scratching, infection, crusting, or lichenification are not likely to provide useful information.

Clinical indications for biopsy include lesions thought to be malignant; lesions that fail to heal, increase in size, bleed easily, or ulcerate spontaneously; tumors or growths of uncertain nature; and many inflammatory conditions, especially those for which the diagnosis is uncertain.

Four types of biopsies can be performed. The choice of technique will determine the size and shape of the specimen obtained (Fig. 532–5). The procedure selected should secure the tissue most likely to contain the pathologic alterations and leave the smallest cosmetic defect. For the most complete histopathologic assessment an *elliptical, full-thickness excision* is best because, in one procedure, the entire lesion is removed and secured for diagnosis and the remaining defect is easily sutured. The excisional biopsy technique is indicated when malignant melanoma is suspected or when a lesion is deep in skin or subcutaneous tissue and its orientation in surrounding tissue is relevant for diagnosis. A second procedure is the *paramedian incisional biopsy*, in which a thin but deep elliptical section is taken through the center of the lesion including normal skin at each end. This is especially useful in diagnosing large keratoacanthomas. A third biopsy method is the *shave*, or *parallel incision*, in which Xylocaine is injected locally under the lesion to lift it above the skin surface, and a scalpel (the knife horizontal to the skin surface) is used to "shave" off the protruding part of the skin and lesion. This technique is useful for diagnosing malignant and benign tumors when subsequent treatment by curettage and electrodesiccation is anticipated. It should never be used when melanoma is suspected, because the specimen obtained is too superficial for adequate histologic grading. Shave biopsy is convenient for removing superficial benign tumors such as seborrheic keratoses or skin tags. The fourth technique, *punch biopsy*, utilizes a tubular blade to cut out a circular plug of skin by slightly rotating and pushing the cutting edge deep into the dermis. The specimen is clipped off at its base with scissors, and the defect can be readily closed with sutures. Punch biopsies are used to diagnose inflammatory diseases and tumors.

533 PRINCIPLES OF THERAPY

GENERAL CONSIDERATIONS

The skin is uniquely susceptible to topical as well as systemic forms of therapy. Significant progress has been made in controlling and curing some infectious and inflammatory skin diseases, although the pathogenesis of many skin conditions remains unknown, and only palliative and supportive therapies are available.

The goals of therapy are to define and remove the cause of the disorder, restore the structural and functional integrity of the skin, and relieve symptoms. Relief of such symptoms as itching, pain, or cosmetic disfigurement are important goals. Damaged skin needs protection, as its barrier function is impaired. This can be assured with dressings and by minimizing scratching and avoiding abrasive clothing and soaps or chemicals. Removal of debris, such as excessive scale, hyperkeratoses, crusts, and infection, is also a crucial goal of therapy if the skin is to heal. Topical and systemic medications, dressings, and other treatments can alter skin temperature and blood flow and thus favorably affect the metabolism of the skin.

Some topical and systemic forms of therapy that have proven beneficial are discussed in this chapter.

TOPICAL MODES OF THERAPY

SOAKS AND WET DRESSINGS. The use of water, with or without various additives, can provide many benefits to the skin, including soothing comfort, antipruritic effects, and increased rate of epidermal healing with hydration and debridement of crusts, dead skin, and bacteria.

Baths. When the area of involvement is too large to apply compresses, a bath is useful. Baths with whirlpool action are particularly useful for debridement of large or deep ulcers. Medicated baths can evenly distribute soothing antipruritic and anti-inflammatory agents to widespread lesions. Starch and oatmeal complexes are commercially available in forms suitable for tub baths. Tar bath preparations are available for use in conjunction with ultraviolet light treatments. Bath oil prevents drying by leaving a thin film of emollient on the skin. The tub should be one-half full, and the soak should last no longer than 20 to 30 minutes, to avoid maceration. Warm baths cause vasodilation and may increase itching; cool baths constrict vessels and usually sooth pruritus. The best time to apply lubricants is immediately after the bath so that they may hold water in the hydrated stratum corneum.

Wet Dressings. Water and medication can be applied to the skin with dressings (finely woven cotton, linen, or gauze) soaked in solution. As water evaporates, the skin is cooled and pruritus is soothed. For maximal benefit from evaporation, the dressing should be no more than a few layers thick and should be dipped in the solution and reapplied to the area of treated skin every few minutes for 15 to 30 minutes several times a day. Wet compresses, especially with frequent changes, provide gentle debridement, the cleansing resulting from transfer of crusts, scales, and cutaneous debris to the compress. If the compresses are permitted to dry (wet to dry compresses) and to become adherent, the debriding effect is greater and can even damage the skin. The dressing may need to be remoistened in place to facilitate removal. Wet compresses also leach water-binding proteins from the stratum corneum and epidermis, causing drying, a desirable effect for moist, oozing and weeping lesions. Wet compresses are therefore useful in treating acute vesicular, bullous, oozing or weeping conditions as well as crusty, swollen, and infected skin. There are two types of wet dressings, open or unoccluded and closed or occluded.

The *open wet dressing* is applied directly to the skin, leaving the dressing exposed to the air. The fluid is allowed to evaporate, providing a cooling, antipruritic effect. Frequent reapplication of the compresses debrides exudate, crust, and bacterial contamination and dries out the skin, rapidly decreasing oozing and weeping.

Closed wet dressings, in which the moist fabric dressings are applied to the skin and covered with an impervious material such as plastic, oil cloth, or Saran wrap, may be useful when some degree of maceration and heat retention is required. For example, if there is excessive keratin of the palms or soles or when an early abscess needs heat to help localize the infection, this form of dressing may be appropriate. Closed dressings are less frequently used than open dressings.

Dry dressings protect the skin, hold medications against the skin, keep clothing and sheets from rubbing, and keep dirt and air away. Such dressings also prevent patients from scratching and rubbing. In the case of neurodermatitis or stasis dermatitis, they are often left in place for several days. Soft casts or castlike boots (e.g., Unna boot) serve the same purposes.

The medication most commonly added to baths and dressings is aluminum acetate, which serves to coagulate bacterial and serum protein. As a 5 per cent preparation it is known as Burow's solution, and it must be further diluted for use. Burow's solution can be readily made by dissolving tablets or powder packets in appropriate amounts of water. (One tablet or packet in 500 ml = 1:20 concentration.) Potassium permanganate and silver nitrate are occasionally added to soak solutions for their antimicrobial properties, but they stain the skin, may be absorbed if used over large raw areas of skin, and may burn the skin if used in high concentrations. The question is often raised about the use of antimicrobial agents in wet dressings, but the quantities needed for adequate concentration in the dressing would make their use exceedingly inefficient and wasteful.

TOPICAL MEDICATIONS. Topical medications are the mainstay of dermatologic therapy. In general, topical medications consist of two major agents, the active ingredient or specific medication and the vehicle or base in which the active material is dissolved. Both are important in treating skin conditions.

Bases or Vehicles. Bases come in a variety of forms. *Powders* promote dryness by absorbing evaporative moisture. They are used to reduce moisture, maceration, and friction in intertriginous areas. Powders may be inert chemicals (corn starch, talcum), or they may contain medications. *Lotions* are suspensions of insoluble powders in water. As water on the skin surface evaporates, it cools, creating a feeling of dryness and leaving a uniform film of powder on the surface. The addition of alcohol increases the cooling effect. *Creams* are emulsions of oil in water (more water than oil). They vanish into the skin because water evaporates and the residual oil is spread thinly and imperceptibly over the skin. *Ointments* consist of oils with variable smaller amounts of water added in suspension. They have a pleasant lubricating effect on dry or diseased skin, but they may also give a greasy feeling to the skin and clothing. Oils in bases give a softening effect to the skin by forming an occlusive layer that traps water and retards evaporation through the stratum corneum. Thus, ointments with large amouts of oil in them give a more sustained, softening effect to the skin than creams or lotions. In fact, ointments with large percentages of inert oil in them may be occlusive and thereby retain heat, increase pruritus, and increase percutaneous absorption of added active ingredients. The more occlusive ointments should not be used on oozing or infected areas, as the resulting occlusion and warmth may increase bacterial growth. *Pastes* are mixtures of powder and ointment (e.g., zinc oxide paste). *Sprays*, another form of base, are freon-propelled aerosols.

Bases thus represent a spectrum of varying amounts of water and oil in emulsion. At one end of the spectrum are lotions with less than 5 or 10 per cent oil in water; creams are composed of relatively more oil dispersed in water, but water is still the continuous phase. As the oil-water ratio reverses and oil becomes the continuous phase, the preparation, considered an ointment, is more lubricating, leaving a noticeable greasy film on the skin. At the far end of the spectrum is inert mineral oil or petrolatum.

Selection of a base or emollient depends on the condition being treated and the needs of the patient. A powder in water, such as calamine lotion, permits evaporation and cooling with some drying. Lotions are useful for pruritic, oozing reactions. Petrolatum, by contrast, retains heat and promotes hydration and even maceration of the stratum corneum. Ointments are used most often on dry, scaling conditions in which endogenous hydration of the stratum corneum is defective. Between these two extremes there is a spectrum of possibilities that permit some cooling but add lubrication. Choice will depend on the needs of and cosmetic acceptance by the patient.

Active Agents—Specific Agents. Having made a judgment about the base or vehicle required, the physician makes a separate selection of active ingredients to be added.

Topical steroids have revolutionized the practice of dermatology, providing effective local anti-inflammatory and antipruritic effects. Topical steroids have two basic anti-inflammatory actions. First, they cause immediate and profound constriction of cutaneous blood vessels. This is believed to prevent mobilization of polymorphonuclear leukocytes and monocytes into the reaction site. Second, they directly interfere with the inflammatory activities of cells that are already present (e.g., mast cells). Corticosteroids used in topical preparations are intrinsically active without need for further metabolism; this accounts for their rapid effect on cutaneous blood vessels as manifested by blanching of the skin. Therapeutic action is also rapid. Topical steroids slow the mitotic rate of fibroblasts, decreasing collagen synthesis, and possibly enhance collagen catabolism. They further interfere with phagocytosis and the skin's ability to fight off bacterial, viral, and fungal infections. Topical corticosteroids that are effective in treating skin diseases all have the basic hydrocortisone structure. A 1 per cent concentration of hydrocortisone ointment or cream continues to serve as a norm for comparing potency of subsequently modified topical steroids. By fluorinating hydrocortisone or adding acetonide, the potency of the steroid is greatly enhanced. Occlusion increases the efficacy of most topical steroids. Topical corticosteroid preparations may be classified in a general way as of low, intermediate, or high potency (Table 533–1). The potency corresponds closely to the degree of anti-inflammatory effectiveness as well as to the incidence and severity of associated side effects. Although some corticosteroids (particularly fluorinated compounds) are more topically active than others, the potency of a preparation is also related to the concentration of active drug in the vehicle and to the nature of the vehicle in which the steroid is mixed. Since corticosteroids are poorly soluble in most vehicles, many preparations deliver only a fraction of the drug to target cells. Of the various types of vehicles used in steroid preparations, ointments are the most efficient by virtue of the excellent solubility of steroids in ointments and because the occlusive nature of ointments increases stratum corneum permeability. Second in order of efficiency is acetone-alcohol gel, whereas creams and lotions are less useful. Some examples of topical

TABLE 533–1. POTENCY RANKING OF SOME COMMONLY USED TOPICAL STEROIDS

Potency	Generic Name	Clinical Applications
High	Fluocinonide 0.05%; betamethasone dipropionate 0.05%; halcinonide 0.1%	Recalcitrant psoriasis; discoid lupus erythematosus; recalcitrant lichen planus
Intermediate	Triamcinolone acetonide 0.1%; betamethasone valerate (cream) 0.1%; fluocinolone acetonide 0.01%	Dermatitis—allergic contact, atopic; psoriasis; neurodermatitis
Low	Desonide 0.05%; hydrocortisone 1.0% or 2.5%	Intertrigo; pruritus ani; seborrheic dermatitis

steroids and their grouping according to potency are listed in Table 533–1.

The adverse effects of topical steroids relate almost exclusively to the intermediate and high-potency compounds. Epidermal and dermal atrophy can be a pronounced effect; decreased collagen synthesis and reduced stromal support for dermal blood vessels lead to telangiectasia, purpura, and striae. These are especially likely to occur in intertriginous "occluded" areas of the skin and on the face. Fluorinated steroids can cause a perioral scaling, papular and pustular dermatitis (perioral dermatitis), or facial redness, telangiectasia, and acne rosacea–like eruption. Potent topical steroids applied for prolonged periods around the eyes can occasionally cause glaucoma and even cataracts. Topical steroids can predispose to or worsen skin infections such as folliculitis, tinea, and candidiasis. Systemic absorption of potent topical steroids may lower plasma cortisol levels when they are used with occlusion over as little as 20 per cent of the body, but this is unusual.

The combined characteristics of drug potency and vehicle type should be used to advantage in treatment. Intermediate-potency steroids are useful in most dermatologic conditions. Ointments are useful for thickened skin or for dry, exposed areas where creams or gel preparations rapidly evaporate. Low-potency steroids are used to treat the face and the thin and occluded skin of the groin and genital area. Lotions and gels are best for hairy areas. High-potency steroid preparations should not be used to treat most dermatologic conditions. Their use is primarily reserved for areas of skin that have been substantially thickened by disease, such as dense plaques of psoriasis or chronic dermatitis. There is a substantial risk of local side effects with these high-potency steroids, and the onset of these effects is more rapid than with less potent drugs. Table 533–2 gives some guidelines for selecting the steroid potency and vehicle most useful in various areas of the body.

TABLE 533–2. GUIDELINES FOR SELECTING TOPICAL STEROIDS

Location or Type of Lesion	Suggested Potency of Steroid	Suggested Vehicle
Areas of Body		
Trunk, arms, legs	Intermediate or low	Ointment or cream
Palms, soles	Intermediate or high	Ointment
Scalp	Intermediate or low	Lotion, gel, aerosol
Intertriginous areas	Low	Cream, lotion
Face	Low	Cream, lotion
Area around eyes	Low	Cream or ophthalmic preparation
Ears	Intermediate or low	Cream, gel or lotion
Types of Lesion		
Dry, scaling, fissuring, lichenified lesion	Intermediate	Ointment
Thickened, hyperkeratotic skin patches	High	Ointment
Oozing, weeping lesions	Intermediate	Lotion, cream
Ulcerative lesions. Do not use topical steroids		

Topical steroids are usually applied once or twice a day. The stratum corneum acts as a reservoir and continues to release topical steroid into the skin after the initial application. Chronic dermatoses become less responsive after prolonged use of topical steroids. This phenomenon is referred to as *tachyphylaxis*. Changing to another topical steroid often overcomes this phenomenon.

Intralesional corticosteroids are used to shrink inflammatory acne cysts and hypertrophic scars and keloids. They are occasionally injected into unresponsive, localized dermatoses such as alopecia areata, granuloma annulare, discoid lupus erythematosus, psoriasis, and lichen simplex chronicus. Several types of steroids are used for this purpose, varying in their duration of action. Triamcinolone acetonide is the most widely used, and its maximal duration of action is four to six weeks. Triamcinolone hexacetonide is longer acting (six to eight weeks); injectables of shorter duration (two to four weeks) include Celestone and Decadron. The steroids should be diluted to less than 5 mg per milliliter to avoid the risk of causing significant skin atrophy. Since intralesional steroid preparations are crystalline and dissolve in the tissues very slowly over weeks to months, great care is necessary in using low concentrations and in shaking the diluted material just prior to injecting into the dermis to avoid the often disfiguring side effects of atrophy that can occur if precipitates settle in the solution.

Topical Antibiotics. These are used to help suppress bacteria in erosions or superficial infections and occasionally in chronic leg ulcers. Silver sulfadiazine preparations are particularly useful as an adjunct to currently accepted principles of burn wound care. The commonly used topical antibiotics are bacitracin, neomycin, clindamycin phosphate, erythromycin, and tetracycline hydrochloride. The latter three are used to treat acne vulgaris. All topical antibiotics have the potential to sensitize, but neomycin is particularly prone to do so, especially after long-term use on chronic stasis dermatitis and leg ulcers.

Topical Antifungal Agents. Antifungals are used to treat localized infections by superficial dermatophytes, *Candida*, and tinea versicolor. Topical broad-spectrum antifungal preparations effective against all of these organisms include clotrimazole, econazole, and miconazole creams and lotions used two times a day. Topical agents useful against dermatophytes but not *Candida* include haloprogin and Tinactin. Over-the-counter preparations, perhaps less effective against dermatophytes, are undecylenic acid and Verdefam. No topical preparations are useful against nail infections with these fungal organisms. Nystatin creams, oral suspensions, and vaginal tablets are effective against *Candida* infections in various areas of the body. Ketoconazole is a broad-spectrum imidazole antifungal agent highly effective against dermatophytes, *Candida*, and tinea versicolor. It is available in cream and oral forms.

Tars and Anthralin. Crude coal tar is often applied directly to the skin to treat psoriasis. Tars increase the effectiveness of ultraviolet light and reduce the accelerated mitotic rate of keratinocytes in psoriasis. Tars are often incorporated into shampoos for control of seborrheic dermatitis and in bath oils for use in psoriasis.

Anthralin is a synthetic coal tar derivative that is used in the treatment of psoriasis. Both tar and anthralin cause staining of clothing and skin. They can also be irritating. Anthralin must be started at the lowest concentrations (0.1 per cent) and initially left on the skin for short periods of time (one-half hour) to avoid irritation.

Antiparasitic Topical Medications. Antiparasitics are employed for the treatment of pediculosis capitis, pediculosis pubis, and scabies. The lice of pediculosis corporis live in the seams of clothes and bedding. These must be disinfected by washing or dry cleaning. One per cent gamma benzene hexachloride (lindane), cromatiton, and pyrethrin compounds (RID) all are useful in treating pediculosis and scabies. Lindane is not suggested for children less than six years of age or for pregnant or lactating women.

Sunscreens. Sunscreens help protect the skin from the acute and chronic effects of UV radiation. They are rated by their sun protective factor (SPF). The SPF, which ranges from 3 to 23, is the factor by which the product extends the period of exposure to reach the sunburn reaction that would have taken place without the sunscreen. The action of topical photoprotectives is to reduce penetration of photoactive nonionizing radiation. Such protection can be achieved by either absorbing or reflecting the radiation. No sunscreen enhances tanning. Rather, if partial block is achieved, it permits melanin production relative to the radiation transmitted and the inherent capacity of the partially protected skin to respond. Most sunscreens are less effective in blocking UVA (320 to 400 nm) than UVB (290 to 320 nm). Para-aminobenzoic acid and its esters protect the skin from UVB and allow UVA to pass. Other non-PABA chemical sunscreens such as benzophenones and cinnamates are also useful against UVB and, to some extent, UVA. If protection against UVA is required, a sunscreen containing benzophenones or anthranilate compounds should be sought. For complete protection or total blockade of UVB and UVA, physical sunscreens containing titanium dioxide, zinc oxide, or iron oxide are available as heavy creams or pastes that reflect ultraviolet light.

SYSTEMIC MODES OF THERAPY FOR DERMATOLOGIC CONDITIONS

ANTIHISTAMINES. By occupying histamine-receptor sites on various cell membranes, antihistamines interfere with one or more of the actions of histamine. Their most specific use is in the control of allergic disorders mediated by histamine, such as urticaria, angioedema, and allergic rhinitis. Non–histamine-induced itching is also suppressed by antihistamines by virtue of their sedative, soporific side effects. Antihistamines are of two major classes, the classic H1 blockers and the newer H2 blockers, which also decrease gastric acid secretion. H1 blockers have three problems: (1) They don't block all the effects of histamine. (2) They provide only limited protection against anaphylaxis because mediators other than histamine are involved in this reaction. (3) They are not selective in their effects (i.e., they also have anticholinergic and sedative effects). Antihistamines (H1 blockers) can be arranged into several groups depending on their molecular configurations (Table 533–3).

An effective agent for a given patient may be selected from one group or from a combination of groups, but its effects are unlikely to be enhanced by combining antihistamines

TABLE 533–3. ANTIHISTAMINES ARRANGED ACCORDING TO THEIR MOLECULAR CONFIGURATIONS

Antihistamine Group	Generic Name (Proprietary Name)
H1 receptor antagonists	
Ethanolamines	Diphenhydramine (Benadryl)
	Bromodiphenhydramine (Ambenyl)
	Clemastine (Tavist)
Piperidines	Cyproheptadine (Periactin)
	Azatadine (Optimine)
Phenothiazines	Promethazine (Phenergan)
	Trimeprazine (Temaril)
Alkylamines	Chlorpheniramine (Chlortrimeton)
	Dexchlorpheniramine (Polaramine)
	Parabromidylamine (Dimetane)
Ethylenediamines	Tripelennamine (Pyribenzamine, PBZ)
	Pyrilamine (Neoantergan)
Piperazines	Hydroxyzine (Atarax)
	Meclizine (Bonamine)
Miscellaneous H1 receptor antagonists	
Tricyclic compounds	Doxepin (Sinequan)
H2 receptor antagonists	Cimetidine (Tagamet)
	Ranitidine (Zantac)

within a given group. If response to one antihistamine is minimal, another from a different group should be added or substituted. Evidence that blood vessels in human skin have H2 as well as H1 receptors has led to the evaluation of H2-receptor antagonists such as cimetidine in combination with an H1 antagonist, and the combination has proved to be effective in the treatment of some cases of chronic urticaria otherwise unresponsive to H1 antagonists.

Antihistamines should be started in moderate doses until sufficient improvement occurs or until troublesome side effects develop. Generally, they are administered three or four times a day. Low doses should be given to elderly patients, as they are unusually sensitive to central nervous system side effects such as confusion, dizziness, and syncope, as well as to urinary retention, dry mouth, and blurred vision. In children, paradoxically, antihistamines may induce hyperactivity.

SYSTEMIC STEROIDS. Systemic steroids are used for a number of dermatologic conditions, but they have several drawbacks: (1) Prolonged administration leads to adrenal suppression and susceptibility to infection. (2) Many diseases such as psoriasis and atopic dermatitis may worsen after steroid withdrawal. (3) Safer and simpler therapy is available for most common dermatoses. Systemic corticosteroids are used in three types of situations. First, patients severely ill with life-threatening diseases known to be responsive to corticosteroids (anaphylactic reactions, extensive erythema multiforme, acute exfoliative dermatitis, pemphigus vulgaris) are initially given high doses—80 to 100 mg daily. Second, patients with conditions that are acute and severe but self-limited are treated with steroids to control or suppress the condition during a predicted period of activity. Examples include wide-spread poison ivy dermatitis, extensive sunburn, and acute generalized urticaria of known cause. Intermediate doses of 60 to 80 mg of prednisone daily are used initially and then tapered over one to two weeks. Third, steroids are used for patients with chronic dermatologic conditions that, because of periodic exacerbations, intermittently require low doses (15 to 20 mg) of prednisone together with supportive topical therapy. Examples include flares of chronic atopic dermatitis, pemphigoid, and some connective tissue diseases.

SYSTEMIC ANTIFUNGAL AGENTS. Two systemic agents are available for superficial fungal infections: griseofulvin and ketoconazole. *Griseofulvin* is active against dermatophytes but not against tinea versicolor or *Candida*. It is fungistatic, entering the horny layer of the skin via the sweat and the nails by incorporation into the keratinizing cells at the nail matrix. The entire nail must grow out with the griseofulvin incorporated into it before tinea at the distal end of the nail is affected. It is for this reason that griseofulvin must be given for many months before dermatophytic infections of the toenails are cleared. Less time is required for infections of fingernails and glabrous skin. Griseofulvin is the treatment of choice for tinea capitis, onychomycosis, and tinea corporis too extensive for topical therapy and for superficial fungal infections in immunosuppressed patients (Table 533–4).

Ketoconazole, a broad-spectrum imidazole antifungal agent, is effective against dermatophytes and, unlike griseofulvin, also against tinea versicolor and *Candida*. Several instances of anaphylactic reactions to ketoconazole have been recorded, as well as fatal hepatocellular toxicity, so ketoconazole should be used only for extensive cutaneous or systemic *Candida* infections and extensive dermatophyte infections unresponsive to griseofulvin. Liver enzyme levels should be determined before starting treatment and monitored at monthly intervals during treatment.

RETINOIDS. Retinoids are derivatives of natural vitamin A compounds. Two retinoids, isotretinoin and etretinate, are available for use in the treatment of dermatologic conditions. Retinoids decrease epidermal cell proliferation and keratinization and inhibit sebaceous gland activity. Etretinate has been found to be useful in severe psoriasis, especially the erythrodermic and pustular forms, as well as in several forms of ichthyosis. Isotretinoin has proved to be especially useful in severe cystic acne, often inducing prolonged remissions for several years after the drug is given for the usual three- to four-month course. The retinoids have many side effects, including cheilitis, conjunctivitis, dryness and fragility of skin, congenital malformations (heart defects, hydrocephalus, microtia), osteophytic growths on the vertebrae, epiphyseal closure in growing youngsters, corneal opacities, night blindness, and elevations of very low density and low density lipoproteins.

SYSTEMIC GOLD SALTS. Chrysotherapy has been useful in the treatment of autoimmune bullous disease, particularly pemphigus vulgaris. Intramuscular compounds have been used in the same manner as in rheumatoid arthritis. Remissions with a mean duration of 21 months or longer have been obtained in some patients with these bullous diseases. Generally a total dose of 400 to 600 mg of gold must be given before bullae respond.

SYSTEMIC ANTIBIOTICS. These are frequently used to treat cutaneous bacterial infections and conditions aggravated by bacterial overgrowth such as acne vulgaris, acne rosacea, and acute dermatitis. Because most bacterial infections of the skin involve *Staphylococcus aureus* or *Streptococcus pyogenes* (erysipelas, cellulitis, folliculitis, furunculosis, carbunculosis), the penicillins, cephalosporins, and erythromycins are commonly used in treating these conditions. In addition, erythromycin and tetracyclines are effective in controlling acne vulgaris and acne rosacea. Trimethoprim-sulfamethoxazole is used for pyodermas in patients allergic to penicillin, for pyodermas caused by methicillin-resistant *S. aureus*, as an alternative therapy for gonorrhea, and occasionally for the treatment of acne vulgaris. The sulfone antibiotic dapsone is occasionally used successfully in treating noninfectious diseases such as dermatitis herpetiformis, pyoderma gangrenosum, and leukocytoclastic cutaneous vasculitis. How dapsone brings about improvement in these conditions is not known.

ANTIMALARIALS. Chloroquine, hydroxychloroquine, and quinicrine are beneficial for cutaneous lupus erythematosus, polymorphic light eruption, solar urticaria, and porphyria cutanea tarda. Antimalarials bind DNA, inhibit the LE cell phenomenon and antinuclear antibody reactions, block chemotaxis, and antagonize histaminic responses, all of which may be related to the therapeutic effects on the diseases mentioned above. Cutaneous and mucous membrane pigmentation, nausea, diarrhea, and cycloplegia are common toxic effects, but retinopathy is the adverse reaction of greatest concern. Quinacrine does not cause retinopathy.

SYSTEMIC ANTIVIRAL AGENTS. Acyclovir and vidarabine are used for treating herpes simplex and zoster skin and systemic infections. These drugs can be given intravenously, and acyclovir is also administered orally. Intravenous acyclovir is utilized in severe primary genital herpes simplex, in neonatal herpes simplex, and in cutaneous herpes simplex and zoster infections in immunosuppressed patients. Oral acyclovir is also effective in primary and recurrent genital herpes simplex and eczema herpeticum. The usual oral dose

TABLE 533–4. SUGGESTED DOSAGE AND LENGTH OF TREATMENT WITH GRISEOFULVIN FOR DERMATOPHYTE INFECTIONS

Region of Dermatophyte Infection	Dose of Griseofulvin Ultrafine	Length of Treatment
Extensive or resistant tinea corporis	500 mg b.i.d.	30 days
Tinea pedis	500 mg b.i.d.	2–4 months
Onychomycosis		4–6 months
fingernails		12–18 months, but
toenails	500 mg b.i.d.	frequently cannot clear
	500 mg b.i.d.	toenail involvement
Tinea capitis	500 mg b.i.d.	4–6 weeks

is 200 mg five times a day for five to ten days; IV acyclovir is usually given at a dose of 15 mg per kilogram per day. Acyclovir is activated to acyclovir monophosphate by herpes simplex virus–coded thymidine kinase; the monophosphate is further phosphorylated to acyclovir triphosphate, which inhibits viral DNA synthesis. This antiviral agent is thus selectively activated only by virus-infected cells with little disruption of host cellular metabolism. This accounts for the low incidence of side effects. Acyclovir ointment is also available for mild primary genital and labial infections and for localized, chronic cutaneous lesions in immunosuppressed patients.

SYSTEMIC CYTOSTATIC DRUGS. Cytotoxic drugs such as methotrexate, cyclophosphamide, azathioprine, and hydroxyurea are used in a number of skin conditions when they cannot be controlled by more conventional means. Thus, psoriasis, when it is generalized, severe, and life-ruining, may be treated with modest doses of methotrexate, azathioprine, or hydroxyurea; life-threatening bullous diseases such a pemphigus vulgaris are occasionally treated with these agents as an alternative to high doses of corticosteroids.

ULTRAVIOLET LIGHT AS A THERAPEUTIC AGENT. UV phototherapy is used primarily in patients with psoriasis and vitiligo, but it may also help patients with nummular and atopic eczema, pityriasis rosea, the pruritus of uremia, and mycosis fungoides. UV light units are available in two wavelength ranges, UVB (the sunburn range of 280 to 320 nm) and UVA (long wavelength spectrum of 320 to 400 nm). The use of topical tar preparations, which "photosensitize" the skin to UVB wavelengths, adds to the effectiveness of treatment (the so-called Goekerman regimen).

UVA light units are employed by dermatologists (and also commercial suntan centers) to cause tanning rather than burning. The ability of UVA to evoke a sunburn is 1000 times less than that of UVB. The primary use of UVA is in the treatment of severe, extensive psoriasis and vitiligo, for which it is used in combination with topical or oral psoralen, a drug that binds to DNA in the skin and sensitizes it to the effects of UVA. The combination of psoralen with UVA light is called PUVA. The long-term side effects of PUVA therapy are unknown, although it seems to induce squamous and basal cell cutaneous carcinomas. The unprotected cornea and retina can be damaged by UV light, especially PUVA. Stringent guidelines for protecting the eyes, such as wearing special protective eye glasses for 24 to 48 hours after taking the psoralens as well as regular eye examinations, must be observed.

534 SKIN DISEASES OF GENERAL IMPORTANCE

In Chapter 532, an approach to diagnosing skin diseases was discussed in which the specific morphologic descriptions of primary and secondary skin lesions are used to place the condition into one of nine large diagnostic groups. These nine groups, encompassing the majority of skin diseases, are listed in Table 532–1. In this chapter, some of the diseases in each of these groups will be discussed, providing the clinician with a differential diagnosis of conditions within each group. As stressed in Ch. 532, the differential diagnosis within each major group depends on such things as variations in distribution; specific location and symmetry of lesions; and shape, arrangement, color, and texture of lesions.

THE ECZEMAS (DERMATITIS)

The term *eczema* is derived from the Greek word that means "to boil out," a reference to the fact that eczematous reactions

may be vesicular and oozing. Eczematous dermatitis is an inflammatory response of the skin to multiple exogenous and endogenous agents, although often the etiology is not clear. Eczemas are defined by their clinical appearance and are subdivided either by their pattern of distribution or by etiologic factors (when known). Many eczematous processes are related to immunologic reactions (Table 534–1).

The term *eczema* or *eczematous dermatitis* is applied to eruptions characterized histologically by epidermal intercellular edema, termed *spongiosis*. Eczemas can be acute, with marked spongiosis causing red papules and vesicles and oozing, weeping, and crusting, or they may be chronic, with redness, scaling, fissuring, and especially lichenification. Indeed, both acute and chronic forms of eczema may be seen in the same patient, with the acute reaction progressing to oozing and crusting; with continued pruritus, the patient's rubbing and scratching will convert the eczema to the chronic, dry, lichenified form. The hallmarks, then, of all types of eczematous dermatitis are (1) marked pruritus and (2) varying degrees of erythema along with papules, vesicles, fine scaling, or lichenification.

A number of the eczematous processes are listed in Table 534–1, along with some useful diagnostic findings that help to differentiate one from another. Histology of various types of eczemas is the same; skin biopsies will identify a lesion as an eczematous reaction, but it will not differentiate among the various types of eczema.

CONTACT DERMATITIS. Contact dermatitis is the best understood cause of eczematous reactions and potentially the most correctable. For any eczematous rash, the clinician should first determine whether it could be a contact reaction. If the cause can be identified, avoidance of the offending substance will be curative. There are two types of contact dermatitis, *irritant* and *allergic*. Irritant contact dermatitis is produced by substances that simply irritate or have a direct toxic effect on the skin, such as acids, alkalis, solvents, and detergents; no immunologic process is involved. Allergic contact dermatitis, on the other hand, is a delayed-type hypersensitivity reaction that occurs in response to a wide variety of allergens commonly found in the environment. The allergens consist of small molecular weight substances that act as haptens and bind to proteinaceous components of the skin to form the sensitizing antigen. The antigen is processed by the Langerhans' cells in the epidermis (see Ch. 530), which then present the antigen to T lymphocytes to elicit sensitization. Sensitization to the allergen requires 10 to 14 days to develop after the first encounter; subsequent exposure to the allergen elicits the eczematous response in one to three days (delayed hypersensitivity).

The onset of irritant reactions after exposure to the topical substance is variable. Skin damage is evident within hours after contact with a strong irritant. Weaker irritants may require multiple applications and days or weeks before the development of the eczema (e.g., housewife's eczema of the hands due to chronic exposure to water and detergents). Contact dermatitis accounts for more than 50 per cent of all occupational illnesses (excluding injury). In the industrial setting, approximately 70 per cent is irritant and 30 per cent allergic contact dermatitis.

Both irritant and allergic contact eczema are initially confined to sites of contact, and therefore unique patterns of distribution and configuration suggest contact dermatitis as well as provide clues to the contactant. Thus, allergic reactions to plants, such as poison oak or ivy, appear as linear, red, papular and vesicular streaks where the plant brushes across the skin. Allergies to metals (especially nickel) cause eczematous reactions under rings or watchbands or on the lobes of ears (earrings). Dermatitis under a ring may also stem from trapped water and irritating soap residues.

The most common allergens causing allergic contact dermatitis are pentadecylcatecol (allergen in poison oak, ivy, and

TABLE 534–1. ECZEMATOUS DERMATITIS SKIN ERUPTIONS

Clinical Type	Etiology or Suspected Cause	Distinctive Diagnostic Findings
Eczemas with Known Causes		
Contact dermatitis		
Irritant contact	Chemical agents that have direct toxic effects on skin	Contact precedes rash by hours to days
Allergic contact	Chemical agents that elicit type IV delayed hypersensitivity reaction on skin	Contact precedes rash by two or more days; in both instances site and configuration of eczéma reaction conform to site of contact with exogenous substances (plants, medicaments, cosmetics, metals); patch tests
Photodermatitis	Ultraviolet light exposure plus topical or systemic substances induce type IV delayed hypersensitivity	Eczematous reaction in sun-exposed areas of skin with sharp "cut off" borders, i.e., face, ears, V of neck, dorsum of hands, extensor surfaces of arms
Eczematous drug-induced reaction	Drugs such as penicillin taken internally	Generalized eczema reaction evolves after taking medications (usually 10 or more days after first beginning drug; sooner if previously exposed) and clears with stopping drug
Dermatophyte and *Candida* eczematous reactions	Dermatophytes and *Candida* induce eczematous inflammatory reaction	Dermatophyte or yeast found in scales or exudate
Infectious eczematoid dermatitis	Products from draining infected skin areas induce eczema reaction—linear infections, leg ulcers	Occurs near site of infection or other draining lesion; clears with treatment of infection
Dermatophytid	Hypersensitivity reaction occurring on distant areas of skin in response to products from fungal infection of other areas of skin	Often vesicular eruption of palms or fingers with dermatophyte infection of feet
Autosensitization	Hypersensitivity reaction to cutaneous or bacterial antigens released from area acute dermatitis	Generalized dermatitis following localized acute dermatitis
Xerotic eczema or eczema craquelé	Dry skin or xerosis	Can lead to redness and fissuring of skin that appear as cracks in dried mud
Eczemas with Unknown or Unclear Etiologies		
Atopic eczema	Hereditary disposition in association with familial tendency for asthma and allergic rhinitis	Eczematous reaction often localized to face, neck, antecubital, and popliteal areas
Stasis dermatitis	Chronic venous insufficiency	Associated with varicosities, leg edema, hyperpigmentation, and ulcers
Lichen simplex chronicus (neurodermatitis)	Repeated scratching leads to eczema	Lichenified patches in areas within reach of fingers (nape of neck, lower legs)
Nummular eczema	Dry skin, underlying infections; sometimes seen in atopic dermatitis	Coin-shaped patches on extensor areas of extremities and trunk
Seborrheic dermatitis	Occurs in areas of high concentrations of sebaceous glands; may be related to intrinsic yeast in skin (*Pityrosporon ovale*)	Inflammatory, yellow, greasy, scaling patches on scalp, retroauricular, eyebrows, nasolabial fold, and presternal areas
Dyshidrotic eczema	Emotional stress—unrelated to disturbances in sweating	Pruritic vesicles on palms, soles
Nonspecific eczematous dermatitis	No obvious cause—diagnosis of exclusion after above eczemas ruled out	Acute and chronic eczema patches anywhere on body; severe itching

sumac as well as in cashews, mangos, and ginko trees), paraphenylenediamine (a substance in hair dyes which cross-reacts with benzocaine and hydrochlorothiazide), nickel, mercaptobenzothiazol and thiuram (components in rubber), and ethylenediamine (a preservative in many medications and also found in industrial dyes and insecticides). Other common sources of contactants include topical medications (neomycin, anesthetics such as benzocaine, topical antihistamines), preservatives (ethylenediamine, merthiolate, parabens), vehicles (propylene glycol), and cosmetics (fragrances, preservatives, paraphenylenediamines). It is obvious that a detailed history of the patient's occupation, hobbies, habits, clothing, cosmetics, and medications applied to the skin is necessary to find the contactant. Careful detective work on the part of the physician and the patient will often bring to light the etiologic factor. One must not overlook the possibility that a topical medicine is perpetuating or exacerbating a pre-existing dermatitis.

There is no standard testing method available for diagnosing irritant contact dermatitis. For allergic contact eczema, the causative agent can be identified by patch tests, but these must be properly performed and interpreted by trained dermatologists.

Therapy of contact dermatitis is avoidance of the irritant or allergen if possible. This may require a change in lifestyle or occupation. Sometimes protective clothing is curative. Barrier creams are of little benefit. Acute, severe generalized contact dermatitis is treated with a short (10- to 14-day) course of systemic steroids and wet dressings or baths. Milder eczematous reactions respond to topical steroids and systemic antihistamines.

PHOTODERMATITIS. A variety of skin reactions, termed photosensitivity reactions, may occur in response to exposure to ultraviolet light. Some appear as eczematous reactions, so-called photoallergic dermatitis, which may occur in response to topical as well as systemic substances in the presence of UV light. The distribution of the eczematous eruption in light-exposed areas is an important feature in the differential diagnosis, with the cheeks, nose, forehead, and tips of ears as sites of predilection. The backs of hands and forearms are also frequently involved and, of course, the history of exposure to UV light prior to the onset of the reaction is important in identifying light sensitivity (see Fig. 532–2).

Photoallergic dermatitis is immunologic. Absorption of a specific wavelength of ultraviolet light by a topical substance or a systemic drug (which is deposited in the skin from the cutaneous circulation) causes chemical conversion of the substance or drug to a hapten that binds cutaneous proteins to become a complete antigen capable of eliciting a type IV delayed hypersensitivity reaction similar to an allergic contact dermatitis reaction. Photoallergic reactions appear only where the UV light hits the skin, even though the systemic drug or topical photoallergen is present in the skin all over the body; i.e., the reaction depends on UV light hitting the skin with the allergen in it. Long wavelength UVA light is usually responsible for these reactions. UVA light penetrates window glass (UVB light is blocked by glass), so the reaction often occurs even though the patient remains indoors. Such drugs as thiazides and phenothiazines can cause photoeczematous reactions; a number of topically applied substances, such as methylcoumarin, musk ambrette, halogenated salicylanilids, and topical sunscreening agents, can cause a similar reaction. Photopatch testing can identify substances in materials causing these reactions. Avoidance of the offending material is often curative. Oral or topical steroids will relieve the inflammatory reaction.

ATOPIC DERMATITIS. This chronic, eczematous condition of the skin is often associated with a personal or family history of atopic disease (asthma, allergic rhinitis, and atopic eczema). Pruritus is a prominent symptom, and the consequent scratching and rubbing lead to lichenification, most typically in the antecubital and popliteal flexural areas. The eczema usually manifests itself after the first few months of life, appearing on the face and extensor areas of the extremities as acute and subacute, red, vesicular and oozing dermatitis. Many cases resolve spontaneously by puberty only to recur in adolescence and adulthood as a chronic dermatitis with scaling, dryness, and lichenification over the face, neck, upper chest, and characteristically the antecubital and popliteal fossae (flexural dermatitis). Atopics have a readily identifiable facies with diffuse erythema, perioral pallor, and a redundant crease or fold below the lower eyelids (Dennie-Morgan fold). The palms often have an increased number of skin markings, noticeable as fine cross-hatched lines. Stroking the skin in atopic dermatitis causes a white line, or dermatographism, probably due to dermal edema and vasoconstriction.

The exact cause of atopic dermatitis is not known, but a number of immunologic and pharmacologic abnormalities are seen in association with the skin condition. For example, IgE reagenic antibodies are increased in 80 per cent of atopic patients, especially those with extensive skin disease (and such patients respond to many antigens applied by skin prick testing), but these antibodies seem to play no definitive role in *causing* atopic eczema. Avoiding antigens to which these patients react by scratch test does not improve the eczema. Patients with atopic eczema also have depressed cell-mediated immunity, with deficient T suppressor cells. This may account for the overproduction of IgE, resulting in unusual susceptibility to cutaneous herpes simplex, vaccina, molluscum contagiosum, and wart infections. Neutrophil and monocyte chemotaxis is reduced during exacerbations of eczema, explaining the frequent staphylococcal skin infections in these patients. Treatment with oral antibiotics to reduce staphylococcal flora (or overt staphylococcal infections such as folliculitis, furuncles, or cellulitis) often results in marked improvement in the eczema.

Atopic individuals are often tense, resentful, aggressive, and restless, but it is not clear whether this is a basic characteristic of the diathesis or the result of living with chronic, unremitting itching and skin inflammation. Whether these personality traits are primary or secondary, the physician must help the patient meet the stresses of life.

Keratoconjunctivitis and stellate anterior subcapsular cataracts are associated with atopic eczema, particularly in patients with extensive skin changes. The conjunctivitis and keratitis usually start in childhood. The cataracts may also begin at a young age and form rapidly, often by age 20. Keratoconus is seen in 25 per cent of atopics.

The treatment of atopic dermatitis is the same as for other eczematous eruptions and includes topical steroids, emollients, and systemic antihistamines. In some children (less than two years of age) food allergy can cause atopic dermatitis, but dietary factors remain controversial. Skin tests or RAST tests help identify which foods may be responsible. Positive results must be confirmed with controlled food challenges and elimination diets. Allergic immediate skin testing and desensitization have been of little value in atopic dermatitis.

Skin irritation must be avoided by wearing soft cotton clothing. Counseling, psychotherapy, and stress reduction may sometimes be helpful. Patients often worsen during the autumn and winter seasons when decreased humidity in homes associated with the use of central heating causes increased skin dryness and itching. The frequent use of emollients is the best treatment for skin dryness, especially immediately after bathing when the skin is hydrated. Topical corticosteroids are the most important means of controlling the inflammatory response, and the least potent forms should be utilized, usually in an ointment base. Systemic steroids should be used only in short courses to overcome exacerbations not controlled by topical steroids.

STASIS DERMATITIS. This is an eczematous eruption of the lower legs secondary to peripheral venous insufficiency. Venous incompetence causes increased hydrostatic pressure and capillary damage with extravasation of red blood cells and serum. These conditions seem to trigger an inflammatory, brawny, edematous, red, and hyperpigmented petechial scaling or weeping reaction, usually around the medial malleolus or distal one third of the lower leg. Secondary allergic contact dermatitis frequently complicates this problem when neomycin in used chronically to treat accompanying stasis ulcers. The cornerstone of managing stasis dermatitis is prevention of venous stasis and edema with the use of supportive hose while the patient is ambulatory. Weight reduction is helpful in obese patients. The eczema is treated with topical steroids and wet compresses when oozing and crusting are present. Occasionally chronic stasis dermatitis, when secondarily infected, can undergo exacerbation with spread of the acute inflammation to distant areas of the body, a condition known as *autosensitization dermatitis*. These secondary eczematous patches evolve on the face, neck, and extensor areas of the extremities. Control is achieved with topical steroids (occasionally oral steroids if the reaction is severe) and antibiotics to control the cutaneous infection.

NUMMULAR ECZEMATOUS DERMATITIS. This condition is defined by coin-shaped patches predominantly on the extensor surfaces of the arms and legs, but the trunk is often involved as well. Lesions appear as patches of minute vesicles and papules that spread to become scaling and thickened, occasionally clearing in the center so that they may resemble superficial fungal infections. Mild to severe pruritus accompanies the eczematous patches. Although the cause is unknown, many factors acting alone or in combination may play a role. Dry skin is a frequent accompaniment, and the disease reaches a peak in the winter months. Irritating substances such as wool and soap and frequent bathing may also contribute to the condition. The combination of topical steroids (usually of intermediate potency), 3 per cent crude coal tar, and ultraviolet light treatments is helpful in controlling this form of eczema. The condition tends to persist with remissions and recurrences.

LICHEN SIMPLEX CHRONICUS. Also known as neurodermatitis, this is a chronic, pruritic, lichenified eczematous eruption that results from constant scratching. Pruritus often precedes the scratching, and rubbing induces lichenification, initiating a vicious circle of itch-scratch-itch. In most patients it is a nervous habit. Patches of neurodermatitis commonly are found on the nape of the neck, lower legs, groin, or other regions of the body within easy reach of the hands. Occasionally constant scratching results in scaling, thickened, excoriated papules and nodules (prurigo nodularis). Treatment consists of explaining to the patient the cause and the need to stop rubbing. Topical steroids and antihistamines may also be helpful. Occasionally steroids injected into the lesion will break the itching cycle more successfully than topically applied steroids.

SEBORRHEIC DERMATITIS. Seborrheic dermatitis is characterized by erythematous, eczematous patches with yellow, greasy scales localized to hairy areas and regions of the skin with high concentrations of sebaceous glands, especially the middle of the face, nasolabial folds, eyebrows, ear canals, retroauricular folds, and presternal areas. Dandruff is scaling of the scalp without inflammation. In severe cases the axillae and groin regions can also be involved. Seborrheic dermatitis may appear in infants until about six months of age ("cradle cap"); after that it does not appear until after puberty. Patients with neurologic disorders, such as Parkinson's disease or stroke, may have a dramatic flare of their seborrhea. Although the precise cause of seborrhea is unknown, the exacerbations associated with emotional stress and neurologic disease suggest a role of the central nervous system. It is sometimes difficult to differentiate seborrhea from psoriasis when the latter is localized to the scalp, ears, and face.

Antiseborrheic shampoos containing tar, sulfur, salicylic acid, selenium sulfide, or zinc pyrithione are the most useful form of treatment. The shampoo should be used daily, rubbed into the scalp and left on for five minutes before rinsing. Inflammatory seborrhea that does not respond to shampoos alone will benefit from a topical steroid lotion or gel in hairy areas and hydrocortisone cream for facial glabrous skin. Continual use of shampoo and topical steroids is required to control this chronic dermatitis.

XEROTIC ECZEMA AND ECZEMA CRAQUELE. These conditions are characterized by chapping and symptomatic dryness that may lead to visible fissuring through the stratum corneum, giving criss-crossing cracks that resemble dried mud. Such changes occur most commonly in winter, and they respond to the frequent use of emollients and/or hydrocortisone ointments.

HAND ECZEMA. Hand eczema is most common in housewives, cooks, food handlers, and medical personnel. The most common etiologic factors are constant exposure to mild primary irritants (soap, water), frequent hand washing, atopy, and nummular dermatitis. Allergic contact dermatitis may be another cause. *Dyshidrotic eczema* (pompholyx), a relatively noninflammatory, recurrent, pruritic, vesicular eruption of the palms and soles of unknown etiology, differs from other hand eczemas in that the primary involvement is on the palm instead of the dorsum of the hands. The term *dyshidrotic eczema* suggests malfunction of the sweat ducts, but this is a misnomer. Pompholyx, from the Greek meaning bubble, is a more apt term. Emotional stress tends to be a trigger. Vesicles on the palms can also represent *dermatophytid*, an allergic reaction to a dermatophyte infection on the feet. If KOH examination of the feet is positive, treatment of the fungus will clear up the palmar reaction as well.

Treatment of hand dermatitis involves avoidance of primary irritants such as soap, solvents, detergents, and frequent exposure to water. The use of cotton gloves with rubber gloves over them is useful in protecting the hands in water. Topical steroids and emollients are also beneficial, and potent topical steroids are often required.

EXFOLIATIVE DERMATITIS (ERYTHRODERMA). Total body cutaneous erythema, edema, scaling, and fissuring may occur as an idiopathic entity without preceding dermatologic or systemic disease, or it may be the result of a variety of cutaneous diseases (atopic or contact dermatitis, psoriasis, seborrheic dermatitis, autosensitization, pityriasis rubra pilaris) or systemic disorders (mycosis fungoides, lymphomas, leukemias) as well as a reaction to a number of drugs (antibiotics, barbiturates, antiepileptic agents, gold) (Fig. 534–1). Other organ systems are affected by the general erythroderma and changes in the stratum corneum barrier function. For example, the diffuse redness and warmth of the skin reflect vasodilation and increased blood flow through the immense cutaneous vasculature. Blood flow may be increased 100-fold in erythroderma, and 5 to 8 per cent of the total cardiac output may be directed to the dilated, inflamed, cutaneous vasculature. This has two consequences. First, a compensatory increase in cardiac output occurs. In older individuals with underlying cardiac disease, heart failure may ensue. The second consequence is defective thermoregulation. Increased heat loss leads to decreased core temperature, shivering, and swings in temperature. When high-output failure occurs and/or thermoregulation is impaired, oral steroids will decrease the cutaneous inflammation and correct the abnormalities. In less acute situations total body applications of topical steroids with plastic sauna suit occlusion will reverse the erythroderma.

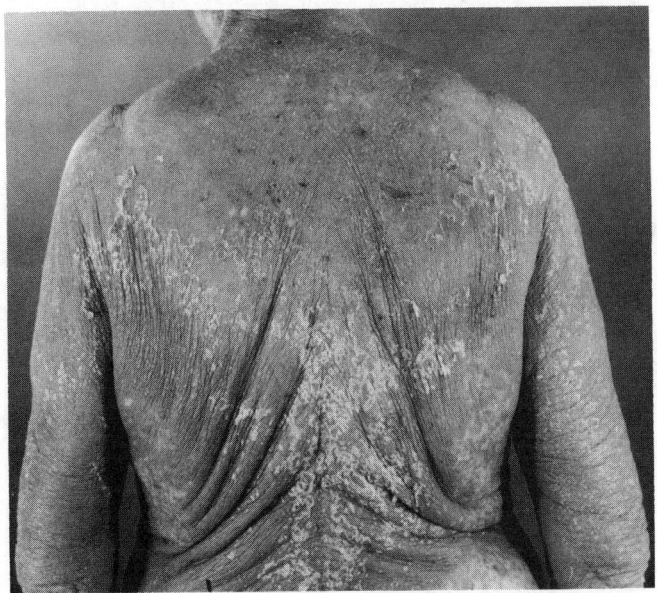

FIGURE 534–1. Exfoliative erythroderma. (From the 17th edition of the Cecil Textbook of Medicine, with permission of Dr. Marie-Louise Johnson.)

FUNGAL INFECTIONS OF THE SKIN. Fungal infections may be confused with eczematous conditions. These infections include dermatophytosis, candidiasis, and tinea versicolor. *Dermatophytes* are a homogeneous group of fungi that live on the keratin of the stratum corneum, nails, and hair and frequently provoke an inflammatory reaction in the skin with pruritus, redness, scaling, and vesiculation. Three genera of dermatophytes cause these infections: *Trichophyton, Microsporum,* and *Epidermophyton.* Dermatophytosis of the trunk (tinea corporis) can be caused by several species (*T. rubrum* and *T. mentagrophytes* are most common), resulting in annular inflamed patches with elevated scaling and, at times, vesicular borders with a tendency for central clearing. The eruption may be widespread and may mimic nummular eczema. Very extensive, red, scaling lesions with elevated serpiginous borders may occur in diabetic and immunosuppressed patients. The usual ringworm of the scalp appears as scaling areas of hair loss with black dots indicating breakage of hair shafts. Most infections are now due to *T. tonsurans* or *M. canis.* The latter agent may fluoresce under Wood's light, but this should not be used for diagnosis. Rather, examination with potassium hydroxide (KOH) preparations and cultures for fungi should be performed. Tinea cruris infection in the groin appears as red patches with elevated serpiginous and scaling borders. The scrotum is seldom involved. Erythrasma is still another type of intertriginous erythema caused by a *Corynebacterium* infection. It appears as velvety red patches with fine scale which, under Wood's light examination, fluoresce a diagnostic coral pink color. Erythromycin clears this infection. Tinea of the feet (pedis) and hands (manum) often present together. Infections of the feet appear in three forms: (1) interdigital maceration, scaling, and fissuring (*T. rubrum* and *T. mentagrophytes*); (2) diffuse, dry, scaling and mild erythema of the plantar surface, often extending onto the sides of the feet in a "moccasin" distribution, occasionally associated with dry scaling of one palm ("two foot–one hand syndrome"); (3) vesiculopustular lesions on the insteps of the feet. Involvement of the nails—onychomycosis—often accompanies hand and foot dermatophytosis.

Candidiasis, particularly involving *C. albicans* (Fig. 534–2), causes inflammatory skin reactions. Intertriginous moniliasis occurs in the groin, perineum, gluteal folds, inframammary areas, axillae, and digital webs. Typically, the folds become macerated and erythematous with small satellite papules and

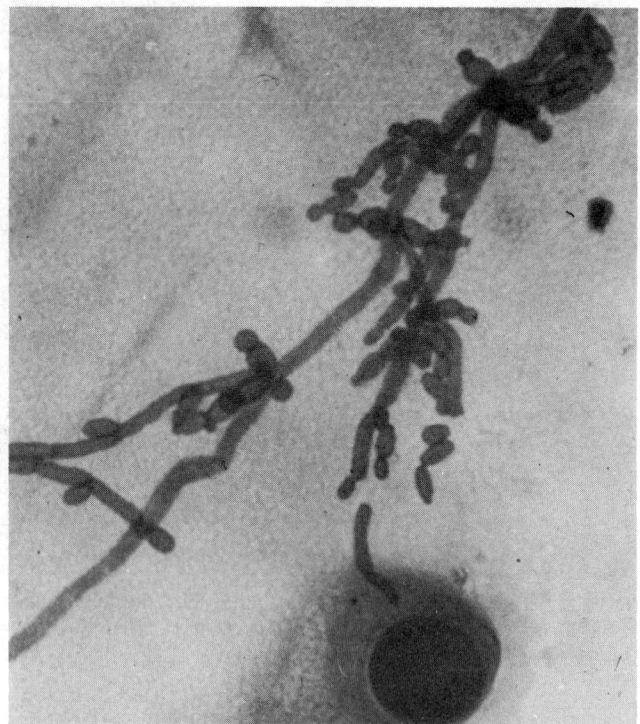

FIGURE 534–2. *Candida albicans.* (From the 17th edition of the Cecil Textbook of Medicine, with the permission of Dr. Marie-Louise Johnson.)

erosions around the periphery of the main lesion. Obesity, diabetes, and use of antibiotics may play a role in *Candida* infection. Chronic mucocutaneous candidiasis is a rare condition characterized by superficial *Candida* infection of the skin, nails, and oral and genital mucosal surfaces complicating a variety of systemic immunodeficiencies (see Ch. 375). *Tinea versicolor*, a common superficial fungus infection caused by *Pityrosporon orbiculare*, is identified by scaling, red to brown or white, oval patches over the neck, trunk, and upper arms. As the name versicolor implies, the lesions vary in color (Fig. 534–3). During the summer months when the skin is exposed to ultraviolet light, the lesions appear hypopigmented, as the infection prevents the involved skin from forming pigment. Examination of the lesion with KOH reveals budding yeast forms and club-shaped hyphae (Fig. 534–4).

Treatment of fungal infections of the skin can be accomplished with topical or systemic agents. If the dermatophytic or candidal glabrous skin infection is localized, econazole, miconazole, clotrimazole, and ciclopirox creams, ointments, and lotions are effective when applied two to three times a day for three to four weeks. Tinea versicolor also responds to these agents, but selenium sulfide antidandruff shampoo is less expensive and also effective. Application of the shampoo to the involved areas of skin for 10 minutes each night for three to four weeks will clear the disease, although the hypopigmentation will not resolve until the patient is exposed to the sun. Regular shampooing with selenium sulfide reduces reinfection rates. Widespread fungal lesions, or those resistant to topical therapy, may require systemic agents. Griseofulvin is an effective, safe agent and the treatment of choice for dermatophyte infections, but it is not effective for *Candida* infections. The drug must be given for varying periods of time, depending on the site of infection. The micronized form (Ultrafine, U/F) seems to be most consistently effective. Approximately 10 mg per kilogram per day is used in children and 1 gram per day in adults (see Table 533–4).

Ketoconazole is a second oral medication useful for dermatophytes, but it is also effective in *Candida* infections. Because ketoconazole occasionally causes severe liver damage,

it should not be used initially for dermatophyte infections. It is useful in mucocutaneous candidiasis at a dose of 200 to 400 mg per day in adults. Because of its toxicity, liver function tests should be performed every two to four weeks.

MACULOPAPULAR SKIN DISEASES

The rashes included in this group represent diverse cutaneous and systemic conditions characterized by widespread erythematous macules and papules. Some of the conditions also have associated petechiae or purpura (Table 534–2).

VIRAL EXANTHEMS. Because many *viral exanthems* are maculopapular, this group of skin diseases is often termed morbilliform, or measles-like. The clinical appearance of virus-induced erythema is not specific for a given etiologic agent; other signs and symptoms help to suggest a particular viral agent. Most viral exanthems are preceded by a prodrome of fever and constitutional symptoms. A history of previous exposure to infected individuals may be obtained. Incubation times vary from days to weeks depending on the virus. Drug history may also be important, especially with infectious mononucleosis, in which only 3 per cent of patients have a maculopapular or petechial eruption, but with the administration of ampicillin the frequency approaches 100 per cent. In measles (rubeola) and rubella, the erythematous macules and papules begin on the face and spread to the trunk and extremities, fading with desquamation in six days in rubeola and on the third day in rubella. The rashes associated with enterovirus infection are most commonly rubella-like but occasionally are purpuric. Exanthem subitum (roseola infantum) displays fleeting, discrete, red papules surrounded by a whitish halo that begins on the trunk and then evolves on the neck. Erythema infectiosum (fifth disease) is an alarming appearing red, "slapped cheek" rash over the face with reticulate maculopapular lesions on the extremities that clear in three to six days. Mucous membranes are sometimes involved. In rubella, red spots occur on the soft palate. In

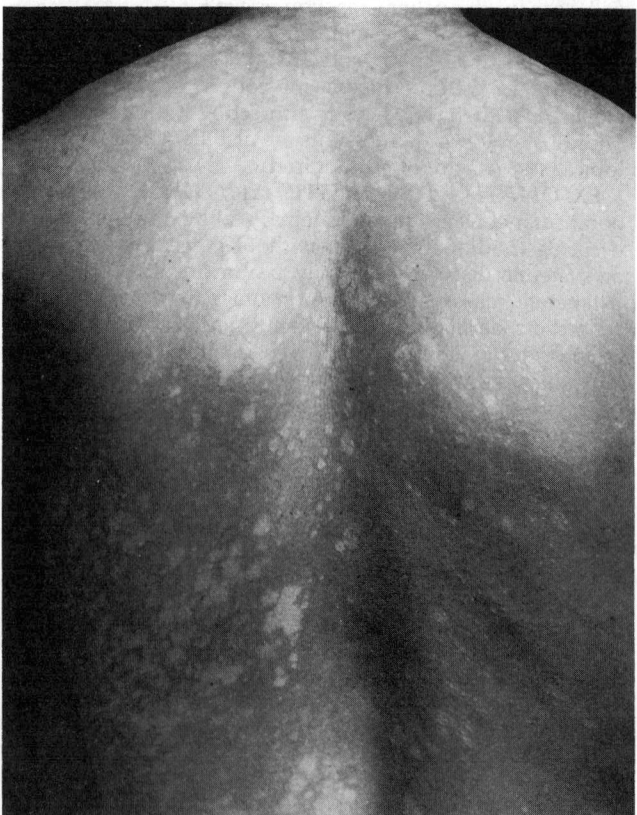

FIGURE 534–3. Tinea versicolor. (From the 17th edition of the Cecil Textbook of Medicine, with the permission of Dr. Marie-Louise Johnson.)

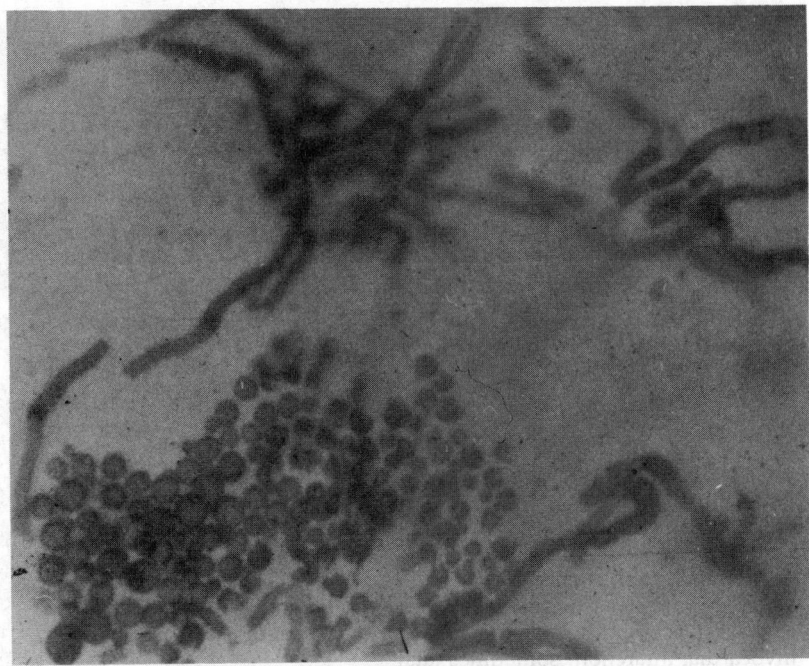

FIGURE 534–4. *Pityrosporon orbiculare.* (From the 17th edition of the Cecil Textbook of Medicine, with the permission of Dr. Marie-Louise Johnson.)

measles, Koplik's spots, tiny gray-white papules on an erythematous base, are found on the buccal mucosa opposite the molars. An erythematous, maculopapular rash that begins peripherally on the palms and soles and spreads to the trunk, often with a petechial component, is seen in *atypical measles.* This is a hypersensitivity reaction to wild measles virus in a partially immune host (one who has been vaccinated with killed measles virus).

TABLE 534–2. SOME MACULAR AND PAPULAR SKIN CONDITIONS

Clinical Condition	Etiology	Distinctive Diagnostic Features
Nonpetechial or Nonpurpuric		
Viral exanthem	Hematologic dissemination of virus to skin where vascular response is elicited	Rubella, rubeola—begin on face; mucous membranes often involved—Koplik spots; palate petechiae rash preceded by fever and prodromata
Scarlet fever	*Streptococcus* erythrogenic toxin	Sore throat preceding rash; bright erythema that feels like sand paper; desquamates; strawberry tongue
Kawasaki's disease	Unknown	Morbilliform or scarletiniform rash; red palms and soles; desquamation of hands and feet 10 to 18 days after fever
Toxic shock syndrome	*Staphylococcus aureus* toxin	Diffuse, maculopapular rash sparing areas where clothing presses on skin; associated with strawberry tongue, fever, vomiting, and renal insufficiency
Drug eruptions	Drugs	Often rash begins proximally and proceeds distally— legs involved last; no prodromata
Verruca vulgaris	Papillomavirus	Corrugated, hyperkeratotic papule
Molluscum contagiosum	Poxvirus	Smooth, dome-shaped, translucent papules with central umbilication
Petechial or Purpuric Component		
Nonpalpable Purpura		
Thrombocytopenic and blood clotting abnormalities	Thrombocytopenia	Petechiae and ecchymoses in dependent areas
Actinic (senile) purpura	Aging and chronic actinic damage to dermal collagen	Flat ecchymoses, usually on arms
Steroids	Thin dermis by decreasing dermal collagen	Flat ecchymoses on arms, legs
Amyloidosis of skin	Infiltrate of dermal vessels by amyloid makes them more fragile	Petechiae and purpura with or without waxy papules around eyes; can be precipitated by trauma, including pinching ("pinch" purpura)
Ehlers-Danlos syndrome	Several variants, all with defects in collagen formation leading to decreased support and increased fragility of cutaneous blood vessels	Easy bruising of skin and joint hyperelasticity
Shamberg's disease	Capillaritis of dermal vessels—usually unknown cause, occasionally due to drugs	Hyperpigmentation with petechiae superimposed, usually on legs
Hypergammaglobulinemic purpura	Hypergammaglobulinemia of variety of causes associated with immune complex damage to blood vessels	Purpura and petechiae on lower legs
Disseminated intravascular coagulation	Intravascular clotting causes thrombosis in blood vessels with subsequent purpura and skin necrosis; induced by infections, malignancies	Hemorrhagic and purpuric star-shaped ecchymoses with skin necrosis and deep hemorrhagic crusts
Infections Causing Purpura		
Meningococcemia, disseminated gonococcemia, Rocky Mountain spotted fever, subacute bacterial endocarditis	Direct invasions of blood vessels by infective organisms or hypersensitivity vascular damage to vessels— Shwartzman reaction or immune complex reactions	Varying forms of petechiae and purpura in skin and mucous membranes
Palpable Purpura		
Vasculitis	Immune complex disease	Palpable purpuric lesions, ulcers on legs can be seen with drugs, infections, collagen vascular disease and underlying malignancies

SCARLETINIFORM ERUPTIONS. Scarlet fever, *Kawasaki's syndrome*, and *toxic shock syndrome* also present with erythematous macular and papular eruptions. Group A streptococcal pharyngitis or tonsillitis with a strain producing erythrogenic toxin initiates a confluent, papular eruption with sandpaper texture that begins on the neck and upper chest and evolves over the abdomen and extremities. The face is flushed, and circumoral pallor is prominent. Extensive desquamation occurs in four to five days. Punctate redness of the palate is seen in scarlet fever along with strawberry tongue.

Kawasaki's syndrome, a condition of unknown cause, displays a morbilliform or scarletiniform eruption more prominent on the trunk than on the face. Most distinctive are magenta red discolorations of the palms and soles associated with indurative edema of the hands and feet. The skin and extremity changes occur within three to four days of the onset of fever, along with mucous membrane inflammatory changes consisting of conjunctivitis and strawberry tongue. Palm, sole, and finger tip desquamation occurs 10 to 18 days after the onset of fever. Asymmetric lymphadenopathy, especially in the cervical area, is seen in 75 per cent of patients—hence the name *mucocutaneous lymph node syndrome*. This is a disease of young children and occasionally young adults, and 1 to 2 per cent of these individuals develop coronary aneurysms or myocardial infarction, sometimes fatal.

Toxic shock syndrome is a serious condition arising from toxins elaborated by *Staphylococcus aureus* infections, often in menstruating women using tampons but also in patients with postsurgical infections. The rash is an erythematous, macular, diffuse eruption that blanches readily with pressure followed by desquamation of the affected skin, in association with fever, strawberry tongue, hypotension, vomiting, and renal insufficiency. The rash often spares the skin where clothing fits tightly with pressure on the skin, e.g., waistline where underwear elastic and belt press tightly.

DRUG REACTIONS. The most common forms taken by drug eruptions are hives and morbilliform rashes (Figs. 534–2 and 534–17). The erythematous macules and papules that often become confluent usually begin within a week of initiating the drug. Unfortunately, there are no laboratory tests to identify a responsible drug, so heavy reliance must be placed on the history. Often patients are taking several drugs. In trying to select the offending medication from the list, two variables to consider are (1) the temporal relationship between the initiation of the drug and the rash and (2) the odds that a given drug is likely to cause an eruption. Drugs most likely to cause maculopapular eruptions include trimethoprim-sulfamethoxazole, penicillin G, semisynthetic penicillins, ampicillin, quinidine, gentamicin sulfate, and blood products. Itching is common with drug reactions, and fever may occur. It is difficult to differentiate the maculopapular drug rash from viral exanthems except that viral prodromata and viral mucous membrane lesions are lacking in drug rashes (see section on drug reactions at the end of this chapter).

Verruca vulgaris and *molluscum contagiosum* are two examples of viral infections confined to the skin which elicit unique papular lesions. Wart papilloma virus induces various forms of warts: *common warts*, dome-shaped papules with corrugated, hyperkeratotic surfaces; *flat warts*, slightly raised, smooth, flat-topped papules often on the hands and face; *plantar warts*, painful papules on the soles of the feet covered by a thick callus with black puncta within the lesion; *condylomata acuminata*, or veneral warts, soft, moist, sessile, pedunculated and verrucous papules involving the perianal and genital areas. *Molluscum contagiosum* is caused by a DNA poxvirus that infects epidermal cells to induce smooth, dome-shaped, translucent papules with a central umbilication from which a cheesy core can be expressed. These lesions occur most commonly on the trunk, face, and genitals. The treatment of warts relies on a variety of nonspecific destructive techniques, including liquid nitrogen cryotherapy, salicylic

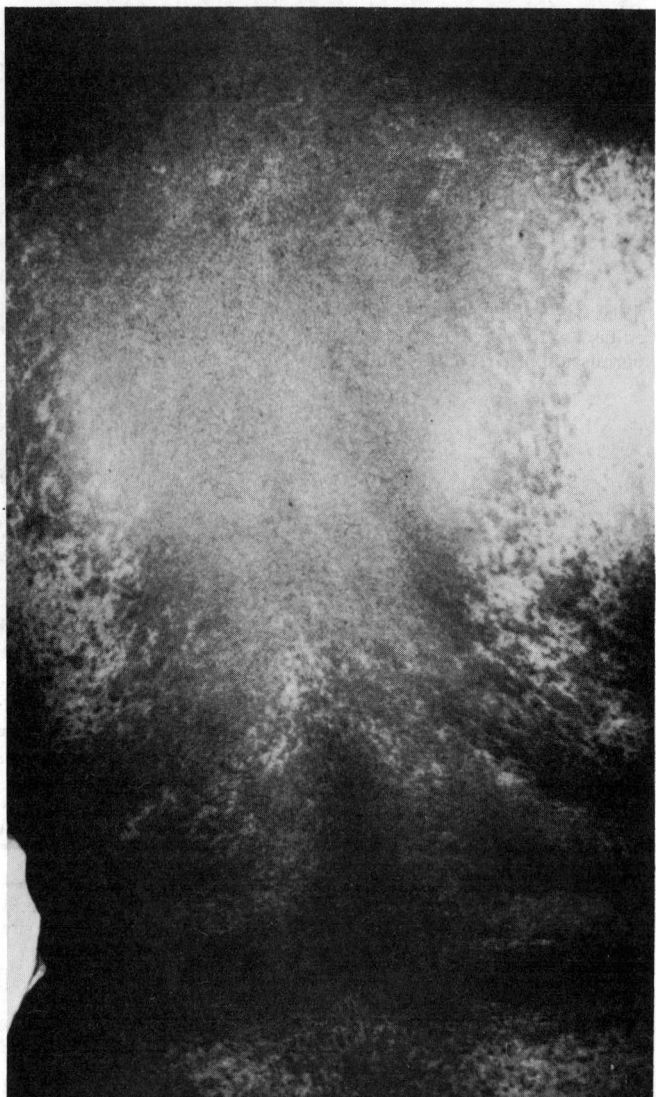

FIGURE 534–5. Drug eruption. (From the 17th edition of the Cecil Textbook of Medicine, with the permission of Dr. Marie-Louise Johnson.)

and lactic acid combinations, cantharidin, and podophyllin. Molluscum contagiosum lesions are removed by curettage of the central core, liquid nitrogen freezing, or cantharidin application for short periods of time (30 to 60 minutes).

Purpuric maculopapular skin lesions should cause the physician to consider a different group of conditions (Table 534–2). Purpura, because it represents extravasation of red blood cells outside the cutaneous vessels, cannot be blanched as erythema can. Purpura can be classified as nonpalpable (macular) and palpable (papular). Nonpalpable purpura results from bleeding into the skin without associated inflammation of the vessels and indicates either a bleeding diathesis or blood vessel fragility. Nonpalpable purpura can be *petechial* (macules less than 3 mm) or *ecchymotic* (macules larger than 3 mm). Thrombocytopenia causes petechiae, whereas abnormalities in the blood-clotting cascade commonly cause ecchymoses. Necrotic ecchymoses are found when thrombi form in dermal vessels, leading to infarction and hemorrhage as in disseminated intravascular coagulation (DIC). Palpable purpura results from inflammatory damage to cutaneous blood vessels, the inflammation causing elevated lesions as in vasculitis.

NONPALPABLE PURPURAS. Nonpalpable purpuras include thrombocytopenic conditions, senile or actinic purpura, blood clotting abnormalities, Schamberg's disease, hypergammaglobulinemic conditions, and disseminated intravascular coagulation. *Actinic (senile) purpura* is a common problem in older individuals, the result of increased vessel fragility reflecting dermal connective tissue damage from chronic sun exposure and aging. Minor trauma induces ecchymoses, usually on the dorsum of the hands and forearms. The skin in these areas is thin and fragile. Topically or systemically administered steroids can induce similar purpura. Other causes of vascular fragility of the skin include *amyloidosis* and the *Ehlers-Danlos* syndrome. *Schamberg's disease*, or *pigmented purpuric dermatitis*, is an idiopathic capillaritis that causes petechial lesions of the lower legs (occasionally the arms and trunk) in association with hyperpigmentation. The lesions have the appearance of cayenne pepper. Occasionally Schamberg's disease is secondary to a drug reaction. Petechiae and purpura also occur in *hypergammaglobulinemic purpura*, a syndrome characterized by episodes of fever and arthralgias which appear to be the result of immune complex–mediated damage to small blood vessels. *Disseminated intravascular coagulation* (DIC) refers to uncontrolled clotting within blood vessels with the formation of diffuse thrombosis. The skin is frequently involved with hemorrhage, ecchymosis, and infarction. DIC occurs in association with bacterial sepsis (particularly meningococcemia), as a postviral or poststreptococcal infection phenomenon (*purpura fulminans*), or in conjunction with malignancies such as prostatic carcinoma and acute myelocytic leukemia. The most distinctive hemorrhagic skin lesions are stellate (star-shaped) purpuric ecchymoses with necrotic centers. The center of the lesion is dark gray, indicative of necrosis and impending slough. Petechiae are seen, and hemorrhagic bullae, acral cyanosis, mucosal bleeding, and prolonged bleeding from wound sites can occur. Patients may be systemically ill with fever, shock, and renal failure.

A variety of infectious diseases cause cutaneous petechiae, purpura, or ecchymoses. Already mentioned is *meningococcemia*, in which the organisms produce acute vasculitis or local Shwartzman-like reactions with erythematous macules, petechiae, purpura, and ecchymosis on the trunk and legs. These may become confluent, often with central necrosis. Patients with acute meningococcemia are ill with fever, malaise, headache, meningeal signs, and hypotension. The skin lesions of *disseminated gonococcemia* begin as tiny red papules and petechiae and then evolve into painful purpuric pustules and vesicles scattered on the distal extremities. Fever, polyarthritis, or monoarticular arthritis may be present. The rash of *Rocky Mountain spotted fever* appears between the second and sixth day of the illness, initially as small, erythematous macules that blanch on pressure but then evolving into petechiae, purpura, and ecchymoses. The rash first occurs on the acral areas and then spreads to the extremities and trunk. Small areas of necrosis may occur on the fingers, toes, and ear lobes. Fever, severe headache, toxicity, confusion, and myalgias commonly occur. *Infective endocarditis* is associated with petechial and purpuric skin lesions. Petechiae appear in crops in the conjunctivae, buccal mucosa, upper chest, and extrem-

ities. Splinter hemorrhages (linear, red to brown streaks under the fingernails or toenails); Osler nodes (2- to 15-mm, tender, red nodules on the pads of the fingers and toes); and Janeway lesions (small, painless plaques and palpable, purpuric nodules on the palms or soles) may be seen. The skin lesions are related to immune complex vasculitis or septic emboli.

PALPABLE PURPURAS. *Vasculitis* and *necrotizing angiitis* are terms used in disorders in which there is segmental inflammation in the blood vessel wall with accumulation of neutrophils and fibrinoid necrosis. The vascular reaction is mediated by immune complexes. Papules with purpura result from extravasation of blood from the damaged vessels. Although all sizes of blood vessels may be affected, the vasculitis in the skin involves venules. If the process is extensive or if large vessels are involved, skin necrosis and ulceration may occur. Depending upon the size of the blood vessels affected, at least five types of vasculitis may involve the skin. The size and type of vessels in the skin, in turn, determine the kind of morphologic lesion (Table 534–3).

In general, as the vasculitis involves progressively larger and more deeply situated vessels, the skin lesions become more nodular, with larger ulcerative or gangrenous processes. The term *granulomatous vasculitis* refers to angiitis associated with a histiocytic proliferation that also involves necrotizing granulomas in the connective tissue of multiple organs, causing rhinorrhea, sinusitis, cough, arthralgias, and ocular and neurologic symptoms (Churg-Strauss vasculitis).

Necrotizing leukocytoclastic vasculitis can occur in a variety of settings including (1) sepsis, (2) connective tissue disease—especially systemic lupus erythematosus and rheumatoid arthritis, (3) cryoglobulinemia, (4) drug reactions, and, occasionally, (5) underlying carcinomas, lymphomas, or leukemias. In many instances no apparent cause is found.

Circulating immune complexes have been demonstrated in patients with necrotizing angiitis. Immunoglobulins and complement are found in the affected vessel wall by direct immunofluorescence. The immune complexes lodge in the small vessel walls and activate the complement system, forming the anaphylatoxins C3a and C5a, which recruit neutrophils that induce inflammatory and necrotic damage to the vessel with accompanying fragmented nuclei of the neutrophils (so-called nuclear dust).

Several syndromes are associated with leukocytoclastic vasculitis, depending on the organ systems affected. *Henoch-Schönlein syndrome* occurs most often in children, frequently preceded by an upper respiratory infection and accompanied by arthralgias, abdominal pain, and renal vasculitis. IgA is usually found along with complement in the involved vessels on direct immunofluorescence. *Hypocomplementemic vasculitis* is characterized by urticaria-like lesions, arthritis, and low serum complement. IgG and C3 are present in vessels taken from early skin lesions. Facial and laryngeal edema may also occur. A third form consists of purpura, arthralgia, weakness, and *mixed cryoglobulinemia* (mixed cryoglobulins contain IgG

TABLE 534–3. TYPES OF VASCULITIS AND ASSOCIATED SKIN LESIONS

Type of Vasculitis	Blood Vessels Involved	Type of Skin Lesion
Leukocytoclastic or hypersensitivity angiitis: Henoch-Schönlein purpura, cryoglobulinemia, hypocomplementemic vasculitis	Dermal capillaries, venules, and occasional small muscular arteries in internal organs	Purpuric papules, hemorrhagic bullae, cutaneous infarcts
Rheumatic vasculitis: systemic lupus erythematosus; rheumatoid vasculitis	Dermal capillaries, venules, and small muscular arteries in internal organs	Purpuric papules; ulcerative nodules; splinter hemorrhages; periungual telangiectasia and infarcts
Granulomatous vasculitis		
Churg and Strauss allergic granulomatous angiitis	Dermal small and larger muscular arteries and medium muscular arteries in subcutaneous tissue and other organs	Erythematous, purpuric, and ulcerated nodules, plaques, and purpura
Wegener's granulomatosis	Small venules, arterioles of dermis, and small muscular arteries	Ulcerative nodules; peripheral gangrene
Periarteritis: classic type limited to skin and muscle	Small and medium muscular arteries in deep dermis, subcutaneous tissue, and muscle	Deep subcutaneous nodules with ulceration; livedo reticularis; ecchymoses
Giant cell arteritis: temporal arteritis, polymyalgia rheumatica, Takayasu's disease	Medium muscular arteries and larger arteries	Skin necrosis over scalp

and IgM with anti-IgG or rheumatoid factor activity), which may be idiopathic or occasionally associated with systemic lupus erythematosus, infectious mononucleosis, lymphomas, or primary biliary cirrhosis.

If the vasculitis is idiopathic and cutaneous, the skin responds to prednisone (60 to 80 mg per day) or dapsone (100 to 150 mg per day). Systemic vasculitides may require prednisone and cyclophosphamide (2 mg per kilogram per day).

Necrotizing cutaneous vasculitis may occur in association with *hepatitis B* and in patients with *intestinal bypass surgery* for morbid obesity or in patients with jejunal diverticula or other gastrointestinal conditions characterized by bacterial overgrowth. An *arthritis-dermatitis syndrome* with intestinal bypass surgery may occur with polyarthritis and palpable purpura or purpuric nodules and pustules on the trunk, legs, feet, and arms. Antigenic components of the intestinal bacterial overgrowth lead to the formation of cryoprotein immune complexes that deposit in the skin and joints, causing a hypersensitivity vasculitis and nondeforming arthritis. Antibiotics such as chloramphenicol, sulfamethoxazole-trimethoprim, tetracycline, and metronidazole have been reported to improve the condition.

PAPULOSQUAMOUS SKIN DISEASES

Unique scales are the common characteristic of diseases in this group. *Squamous* refers to scaling that represents thickened stratum corneum and thus implies an abnormal keratinization process. The lesions, in addition to being scaly, are characterized by sharply demarcated, red to violaceous papules and plaques that result from thickening of the epidermis and/or underlying dermal inflammation.

The papulosquamous disorders have diverse etiologies and include psoriasis, Reiter's syndrome, pityriasis rosea, lichen planus, pityriasis rubra pilaris, secondary syphilis, mycosis fungoides, and ichthyosiform eruptions (Table 534–4).

PSORIASIS. Psoriasis is a genetically determined, chronic epidermal proliferative disease of unpredictable course. Onset is most frequent in early adult life, but it may begin at any age. Once the disease becomes manifest, it may remain localized to a few areas or may cause intermittent or continuous generalized disease.

The lesions appear as erythematous papules and plaques surmounted by silvery, thick scales that resemble mica (micaceous) and that are easily removed and may accumulate in the patient's clothing or bed (Fig. 534–6). In intertriginous areas maceration prevents scales from accumulating, but the lesions remain red and sharply defined. Classically, lesions are distributed symmetrically over areas of bony prominence such as elbows and knees. They also commonly occur on the trunk and scalp and in the intergluteal cleft. These latter two areas are frequently overlooked. Palms and soles may be involved, with diffuse redness, scaling, and, at times, pustular lesions. Nail involvement occurs in up to 50 per cent of patients. The nails may be pitted with small ice pick–like depressions on the surface of the nail plate. Onycholysis can also occur, in which a plaque of psoriasis in the distal nail bed causes a red-brown discoloration that is reminiscent of an oil stain under the nail. Another helpful diagnostic feature is the Koebner phenomenon, in which intense trauma to the skin induces new skin lesions. Thus, scratches or surgical incisions elicit linear papulosquamous lesions that should alert the physician to the diagnosis. This may also explain the high incidence of psoriasis on the elbows and knees. Other aggravating factors include streptococcal infections, emotional

TABLE 534–4. PAPULOSQUAMOUS SKIN DISEASES

Disease	Appearance of Lesion	Distribution	Mucous Membrane Involvement	Other Features
Psoriasis	Erythematous plaques with silvery, mica-like scales, usually nonpruritic	Anywhere: scalp, knees, elbows, intergluteal cleft favored; symmetric	None	Koebner phenomenon, nail involvement, arthritis
Reiter's syndrome	Erythematous, silvery scaled plaques; hyperkeratotic papules of palms and soles (keratoderma blenorrhagica)	Similar to psoriasis	Frequent: mouth, genitals; balanitis circinata	Nail involvement, arthritis, urethritis, conjunctivitis, iritis
Pityriasis rosea	Tannish pink, oval papules and plaques with delicate collarette scale; may or may not be pruritic	Rash preceded by herald patch, Christmas tree pattern on trunk; spares face, extremities	None	May be associated with upper respiratory infection; drugs may cause similar rash
Secondary syphilis	Ham red or copper colored scaling papules and plaques, sometimes annular	Generalized: palms and soles often involved	Mucous patches, often white or red; condyloma warts of anal area	Condylomata in genital area; serologic test for syphilis positive
Lichen planus	Violaceous polygonal, flat-topped papules with white scale or Wickham's striae. May be hyperkeratotic, annular, or bullous lesions; pruritic	Often on wrists and ankles, but can be generalized; Koebner reaction	Frequent reticulated white patches or erosive lesions in mouth or genital areas	Occasionally involves nails; drugs can cause similar reaction
Pityriasis rubra pilaris	Red, scaling plaques and patches with follicular horny excretions, especially on dorsum of hands and fingers; diffuse, yellow hyperkeratoses of palms and soles	Often diffuse, rough scaling erythema involving entire body with islands of normal skin within scaling scalp	Occasionally lacy white plaques in mouth	Remits spontaneously in 2-4 years; nail changes as in psoriasis
Pityriasis lichenoides et varioliformis acuta (Mucha-Habermann disease)	Red, discrete, palpable papules that vesiculate and then become hemorrhagic, crust, scale, and leave a scar	Scattered lesions over trunk and extremities	May resemble leukocytoclastic vasculitis	May resolve in a few months or persist for years
Pityriasis lichenoides et varioliformis chronica (chronic parapsoriasis)	Guttate to larger, red slightly scaling papules and plaques; nonpruritic	Usually on trunk	Some forms may represent early stages of mycosis fungoides	Responds to UVB light treatments
Mycosis fungoides	Persistent, pruritic, red, thickened plaques with fine scales as seen in eczema, or thick mica-like scales suggestive of psoriasis; may ulcerate	Scattered asymmetrically over trunk, extremities; girdle area often first area involved	Neoplastic T-cell lymphoma	May show islands of normal skin within red areas
Ichthyosis	A variety of syndromes with variation in scaling skin; fine light scales to large, thick, coarse, verrucous scales that resemble fish skin; hyperkeratosis of palms and soles	Variable distribution but can involve flexural or extensor surfaces of extremities or trunk	Autosomal dominant, recessive, and X-linked recessive conditions	See Table 534–5

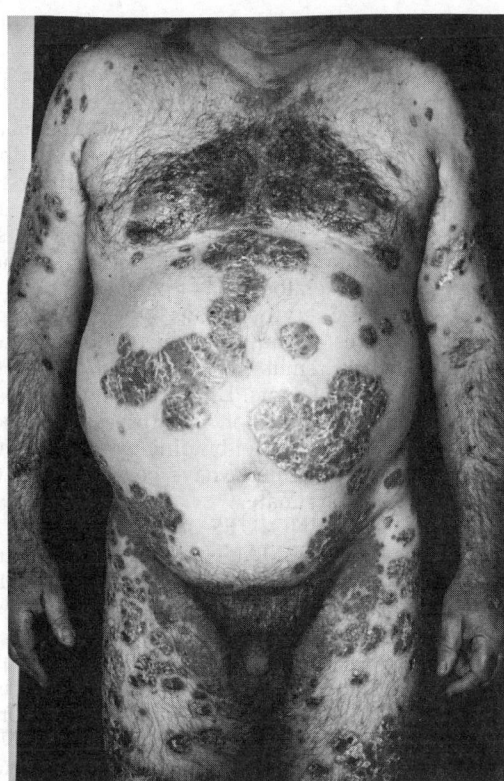

FIGURE 534–6. Psoriasis. (From the 17th edition of the Cecil Textbook of Medicine, with the permission of Dr. Marie-Louise Johnson.)

stress, overuse of alcohol, and drugs, including lithium and beta blockers. Several common variants of psoriasis may also be seen: (1) *guttate psoriasis,* in which numerous, small papular lesions with silvery scales evolve suddenly over the body, often one to three weeks following streptococcal pharyngitis; (2) *inverse psoriasis,* in which plaques evolve in intertriginous areas and thus lack the typical silver scale because of maceration and moisture; (3) *pustular psoriasis,* a form of the disease in which superficial pustules occur in one of three presentations—pustules studding typical plaques; pustules confined to the palms and soles; and a rare generalized eruption in which pustules evolve abruptly on large areas of erythematous skin accompanied by fever and leukocytosis; (4) *erythroderma*—occasionally the psoriasis can become generalized to involve erythema and scaling of the entire integument. This may occur secondary to a general Koebner phenomenon with overvigorous therapy, a drug reaction, or withdrawal of oral steroids; (5) *psoriatic arthritis*—arthritis may accompany psoriasis in 10 to 15 per cent of cases.

At times Reiter's syndrome may be confused with psoriasis. The skin lesions of the two disorders are indistinguishable clinically and histologically. In Reiter's syndrome pustular and hyperkeratotic papules and plaques commonly occur on the palms and soles (keratoderma blenorrhagica) and scaling, red patches evolve encircling the glans penis and within the groin (balanitis circinata). The presence of asymptomatic erosions on the tongue and buccal mucosa, urethritis, iritis or conjunctivitis, arthritis, and occasionally diarrhea should suggest the diagnosis.

The pathogenesis of psoriasis is unknown, but it appears to be a multifactorial disease in patients who are genetically predisposed. There is an increased prevalence of psoriasis in individuals with HLA antigens BW17, B13, and BW37. Thirty per cent of patients have a family history of disease. The basic alteration represents an accelerated cell cycle in an increased number of dividing cells, culminating in rapid epidermal cell proliferation. Cellular turnover is increased seven-fold, and the transit time from the basal layer to the top of the stratum corneum is three or four days rather than the usual 28 days. This rapid turnover of keratinocytes alters keratinization, resulting in thickened epidermis (seen as papules and plaques) and parakeratotic stratum corneum (silvery scales). The basic mechanism underlying this benign proliferative reaction is unknown.

The goal of therapy is to decrease epidermal proliferation and underlying dermal inflammation. There is no curative agent for psoriasis, and treatment suppresses the condition only as long as it is administered. Three types of topical therapies are employed: (1) topical steroids, usually with intermediate and strong potency agents administered once or twice a day; (2) topical tars and anthralin preparations, often used once a day in combination with topical steroids; (3) ultraviolet light, either UVB with tar or UVA with oral psoralens (see Ch. 533).

Two systemic types of therapy are available, but because of their side effects these should be reserved for severe widespread disease that is unresponsive to topical measures: (1) antimetabolites or antimitotic agents, including methotrexate, azathioprine, and hydroxyurea. The most commonly used is methotrexate in low doses, usually given on a weekly basis. Because these agents affect bone marrow and liver (in the case of methotrexate), complete blood counts and liver function tests should be performed regularly, together with intermittent liver biopsies. (2) Etretinate, a retinoid, is particularly useful in pustular and erythrodermic forms of psoriasis. Careful monitoring of blood counts, plasma triglycerides, and liver function is required, and avoidance of pregnancy during the use of this drug is mandatory.

PITYRIASIS ROSEA. Oval or round, tannish pink or salmon colored, scaling papules and plaques appear rapidly over the trunk, neck, upper arms, and legs (Fig. 534–7). Several features of this self-limited papulosquamous condition are unique. First, the generalized eruption is preceded by a single lesion, termed the "herald patch," that is commonly misdiagnosed as "ringworm." The herald patch can occur anywhere but often appears on the neck or lower trunk area and precedes the general rash by several days to a week. Second, the oval patches have an unusual fine, white scale located near the border of the plaques, forming a collarette. Third, the lesions follow skin cleavage lines, in a pattern likened to a Christmas tree. Last, the condition spontaneously involutes in one to two months. Recurrences are rare. Itching occasionally is a prominent symptom.

Pityriasis rosea occasionally is preceded by a mild upper respiratory infection, and its greatest incidence is in the winter months, suggesting a viral etiology. However, the disease does not occur endemically and is not transmitted person to person.

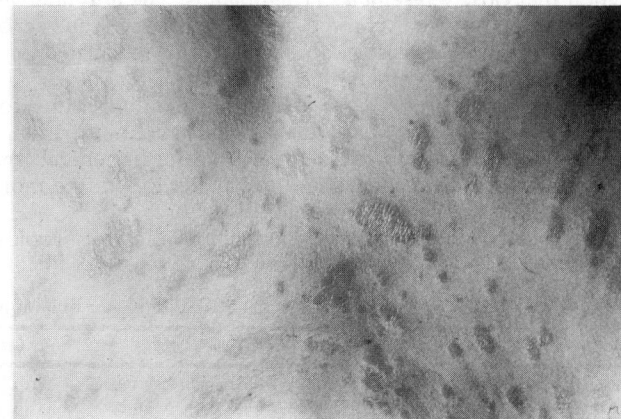

FIGURE 534–7. Pityriasis rosea. (From the 17th edition of the Cecil Textbook of Medicine, with the permission of Dr. Marie-Louise Johnson.)

Such conditions as tinea corporis and guttate psoriasis may be considered in the differential diagnosis, but two possibilities should always be entertained: drug eruption and secondary syphilis. If the rash persists longer than two or three months or generalizes to involve the trunk, extremities, and especially the face, a drug reaction should be considered. Such medications as gold compounds, barbiturates, captopril, clonidine, and tripelennamide can cause such a rash. Secondary syphilis should be suspected and a serologic test obtained if the rash involves palms and soles and if fever, coryza, or mucous membrane erosions (so-called mucous patches) are present.

Treatment of pityriasis rosea is usually not necessary, although topical corticosteroids and antihistamines may relieve itching and decrease erythema. Ultraviolet light (UVB), given as three to five treatments eliciting a mild erythema reaction, will often clear the rash.

LICHEN PLANUS. This idiopathic, pruritic, inflammatory condition of the skin is included in the papulosquamous group of diseases because the primary lesion is a unique papule. The papules are flat topped (planus) and polygonal in configuration (i.e., the sides conform to normal fine skin folds) and have a lilac or purple hue. They may have visible scales on their surface, but more characteristic are subtle, fine white dots or white reticulated lines (Wickham's striae) surmounting the shiny, flat tops (resembling the appearance of a lichen). Wickham's striae are more visible under a hand lens after the application of a drop of mineral oil to the surface of the papule. The Koebner phenomenon occurs in lichen planus, so linear streaks of papules at the sites of skin trauma may be noted.

Although lichen planus can occur anywhere on the body, typical locations are the ankles, wrists, mouth, and genitalia. There may be only a few papules or innumerable ones in a generalized distribution. Mucous membranes are commonly involved, the lesions appearing most frequently as asymptomatic white streaks in a reticulated pattern on the buccal mucosa, tongue, gums, or lips. At times blisters and erosions are superimposed (erosive lichen planus), causing severe discomfort. Lichen planus involving the male genitalia may appear as violaceous annular lesions. Rarely, lichen planus may appear as violaceous annular and polycyclic lesions on the legs and arms, or as hyperkeratotic, follicular, scarring alopecia. All lichen planus lesions leave residual hyperpigmented macules in their wake.

The etiology of lichen planus is not known, but two conditions may mimic lichen planus skin lesions and thus offer clues to an immune etiology. Certain drugs such as thiazides, phenothiazines, gold, quinidine, and antimalarials can cause lichen planus–like, generalized eruptions. Second, some patients with graft-versus-host disease also develop a skin reaction that closely resembles lichen planus. The eruption can evolve into the usual chronic graft-versus-host sequelae of diffuse dermal sclerosis, cicatricial alopecia, reticulated pigmentation, and ulceration.

Lichen planus tends to be a chronic condition lasting for months to years. Perhaps two thirds of patients experience spontaneous resolution in one to two years. In general, the more acute, intense, and widespread the eruption, the more likely it is that an early remission may occur.

Treatment is nonspecific and often unsuccessful. Topical steroids help suppress the inflammatory reaction and itching. Severe oral lichen planus may respond to etretinate.

PITYRIASIS RUBRA PILARIS. This idiopathic papulosquamous and keratotic disease has an uncertain and often chronic course. The condition can appear in a familial form (autosomal dominant) with onset in infancy or childhood or as an acquired disease evolving during the fourth to sixth decades. In either form the following features help in diagnosis: (1) diffuse salmon color of involved skin with sharply bordered residual areas of normal skin (so-called island sparing), (2) waxy, yellow keratoderma of palms and soles similar to carnauba wax, and (3) erythematous hyperkeratotic papules on the dorsal surfaces of the proximal portions of the phalanges. The condition remits spontaneously in two to four years in 80 per cent of patients. Differentiation from psoriasis may be difficult. The cause of this disease is unknown, although low levels of retinol-binding protein have been found. High doses of vitamin A have been reported to help the condition, as has etretinate.

PITYRIASIS LICHENOIDES ET VARIOLIFORMIS ACUTA (MUCHA-HABERMANN DISEASE). This unusual condition of unknown cause usually begins as widely scattered, red papules that may be purpuric and/or vesicular. Although not initially papulosquamous, the lesions evolve into scaling, eroded, and crusted papules that leave depressed scars in their wake. Lesions develop in crops, often in association with malaise and fever, and persist for months or years. Acute lesions show a lymphocytic vasculitis. No therapy is effective, although tetracycline, systemic corticosteroids, and cytotoxic agents may give short-lived remissions.

ICHTHYOSIS. A variety of inherited and acquired conditions cause rough, dry skin with retained scale simulating fish skin. On close inspection there may be fine scale with keratin-plugged follicles or large, polyhedral, loosely adherent scales.

A number of inherited ichthyosis conditions are recognized (Table 534–5), the most common being *ichthyosis vulgaris*, a dominant trait in which the cells of the stratum corneum are retained, forming fish-like or reptilian scales on the extensor surfaces of the extremities (Fig. 534–8). Other forms of ichthyosis such as *lamellar* and *epidermolytic hyperkeratoses* may be associated with considerable erythema and blistering of the skin. Lamellar ichthyosis may be present at birth (collodion baby). A deficiency of steroid sulfatase has been found in association with *X-linked ichthyosis*. Mothers of such babies often have a prolonged labor, as steroid sulfatase appears to play an important role in the parturition process.

Emollients and keratolytic agents (propylene glycol, salicylic acid, lactic acid) are often useful in softening the skin. In severe ichthyosis oral retinoids, especially etretinate, have been beneficial.

VESICULOBULLOUS DISEASES

Vesicles and bullae, when intact, are readily recognized primary skin lesions. Crusts or superficial erosions are secondary lesions that lead one to suspect a preceding fluid-filled primary lesion. The etiology of blistering disease includes bacterial and viral infections, contact dermatitis, and autoimmune and metabolic diseases. The pathogenesis of the blister formation is often helpful in understanding its anatomic location: Blisters occur either within the epidermis (intraepi-

TABLE 534–5. COMMON ICHTHYOSIFORM DERMATOSES

	Inheritance	Onset	Distribution	Clinical Associations	Kinetics
Lamellar ichthyosis	Autosomal recessive	Birth	Body, palms, soles	Ectropion	Increased
Epidermolytic hyperkeratosis	Autosomal dominant	Birth	Predominant flexural involvement	Blisters	Increased
X-linked ichthyosis (steroid sulfatase deficiency)	X-linked	Birth	Trunk	Corneal opacities	Normal
Ichthyosis vulgaris	Autosomal dominant	Childhood	Spares flexural areas	Atopy	Normal

Reprinted from the chapter by Dr. Marie-Louise Johnson in the 17th edition of the Cecil Textbook of Medicine, with her permission.

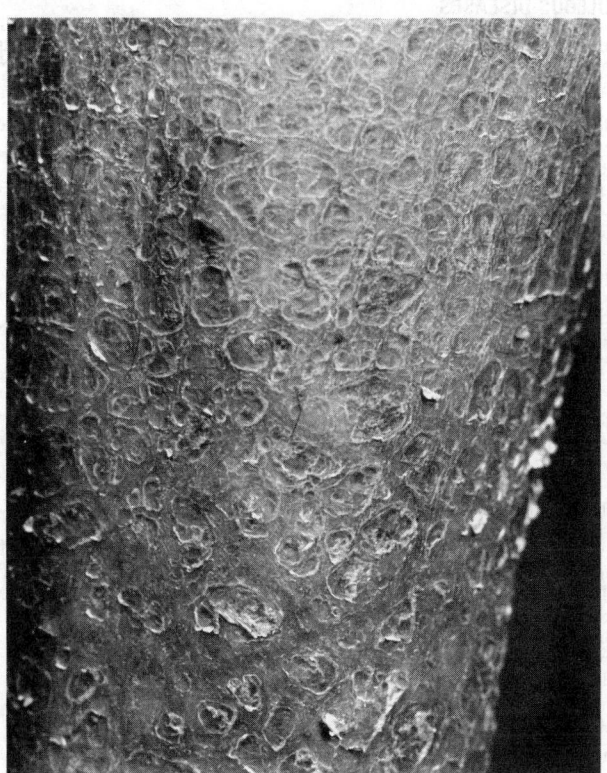

FIGURE 534–8. Ichthyosis. (From the 17th edition of the Cecil Textbook of Medicine, with the permission of Dr. Marie-Louise Johnson.)

dermal) or at the dermoepidermal junction (subepidermal) (Table 534–6).

Intraepidermal vesicles or bullae usually contain clear fluid (but may become filled with purulent material secondarily) and have very thin roofs, so they are flaccid in appearance and are easily broken. At times the blisters are difficult to recognize, and only erosions, crusts, or the thin shreds of the epidermal blister roofs remain. Subepidermal blisters have an epidermal roof and are tense and remain intact. Hemorrhagic fluid is common in subepidermal blisters because of their location close to dermal capillaries.

Biopsy of early vesicles or blisters is imperative in diagnosis. Immunofluorescence studies on biopsy material may differentiate certain immunologically mediated diseases. Pathologic studies are most informative when performed early, before therapy has been initiated.

INTRAEPIDERMAL VESICULOBULLOUS DISEASES. Pathologic processes involved in epidermal blister formation include spongiosis, primary cell damage, and acantholysis. Spongiosis, a common form of blister formation in eczematous processes, represents edema between cells of the prickle layer and liquefaction of cells which gradually increases the size of the fluid spaces. Primary epidermal cell damage with fluid accumulation is seen in viral infections and friction damage. Blisters may also occur when cellular desmosomal attachments and intercellular cementing substances are immunologically or chemically altered, causing dyshesion referred to as acantholysis (pemphigus).

Bullous impetigo, a subcorneal infection of the skin with staphylococcal and/or streptococcal organisms, causes large, fragile, clear or cloudy bullae that form thin, honey-yellow crusts and a delicate collarette-like remnant of blister roof after the blisters rupture. Autoinoculation results in satellite lesions. The superficial epidermal blistering is caused by the toxic effects of an epidermal toxin elaborated by certain strains of these bacterial organisms.

A more serious variant of bullous impetigo is *staphylococcal scalded skin syndrome,* usually affecting infants and characterized by the formation of rapidly progressive, painful, ery-

thematous patches in which large flaccid bullae evolve and shed as large sheets of skin, leaving a denuded, scalded-appearing surface. With only slight trauma the skin readily slides off, much like wet wallpaper slides off a wall (Nikolsky's sign—see Ch. 532). In contrast to localized bullous impetigo in which the *Staphylococcus aureus* may be recovered in the skin lesions, the bullae of scalded skin syndrome are sterile, although a staphylococcal infection may be found in the conjunctiva, nose, or pharynx. The widespread intraepidermal blistering results from an epidermal toxin elaborated by specific strains of *Staphylococcus* and hematogenously carried to the skin. These are penicillinase-resistant strains of *Staphylococcus* and therefore require methicillin-type antibiotics.

A somewhat similar condition, *toxic epidermal necrolysis* (TEN), occurs in adults, often secondary to drugs (e.g., ampicillin, allopurinol) and occasionally to *Staphylococcus* infections in an immunosuppressed patient. TEN is a reaction to a variety of antigenic materials that cause a suprabasilar split in the epidermis with necrosis of much of the overlying epidermis. Because of the more extensive destruction of epidermis and barrier stratum corneum layer (as opposed to staphylococcal scalded skin syndrome, in which the split is subcorneal), TEN is often fatal and, when extensive, should be treated as a widespread burn would be cared for. TEN also often involves the mucous membranes and therefore may be confused with Stevens-Johnson syndrome (see below).

Viral infections of the skin may cause vesicles and bullae by virtue of direct infection of the keratinocytes and the destructive effect on the cells. Vesicles caused by viruses often display two important characteristics: (1) they tend to occur in groups on an indurated erythematous base, and (2) they often take on an umbilicated appearance.

Herpes simplex is caused by two strains of DNA *Herpesvirus* (type 1, which commonly causes infections above the waist, and type 2, which most frequently is responsible for those in the genital region). Primary infections, gingivostomatitis, and vulvovaginitis, are extensive vesicular eruptions that quickly become necrotic, leaving painful, purulent erosions. The herpesvirus is highly contagious, spread by direct contact with infected individuals. The virus penetrates the epidermal cells, undergoes replicative cycles, and eventually lyses the host cell membrane. The virus is neuropathic, traveling up cutaneous nerves to dorsal nerve root sensory or autonomic ganglia, where it resides in a nonreplicative state. Reactivation of the replicative cycle triggers recurrence, and the virus spreads back down the nerve to induce grouped, umbilicated vesicles on an indurated, red base in areas of the skin innervated by the infected ganglia. Periods of latency vary, and recurrences have a shorter course than primary infections (one to two weeks versus three weeks). A number of factors seem to induce recurrences, including fever, ultraviolet light, physical trauma, menstruation, and emotional stress. Recurrences are most common on the lips and face (herpes labialis), genital regions (herpes genitalis), and fingers (herpetic whitlow). *Eczema herpeticum* is a generalized herpes simplex skin infection in areas of atopic dermatitis. Recurrent herpes infections are contagious from the time the vesicular lesions develop to the time the vesicles re-epithelialize. Between attacks there is little chance of causing infection, although perhaps 1 or 2 per cent of individuals may be chronically shedding the virus in the saliva or genital excretions (women may also have active herpes simplex infections of the cervix and be unaware of them).

A complication of herpes simplex infection, *erythema multiforme,* is a hypersensitivity skin and mucous membrane reaction that evolves one to two weeks following herpetic recurrences as a result of an immune complex reaction to the herpes antigen.

Diagnosis of herpes infections (including zoster and varicella) is made with a Tzanck preparation of material taken from the roof of vesicles. The contents are smeared onto a

TABLE 534–6. VESICULOBULLOUS DISEASES

Location of Blister in Skin	Etiology if Known	Important Physical Findings	Other Facts of Note in History or Laboratory Results
Intraepidermal Blisters			
Bacterial infectious processes			
Bullous impetigo (subcorneal)	Staph toxin	Large, fragile, clear or cloudy bullae that break to leave honey-yellow crusts on face, neck, extremities; erythematous areas that slough as superficial blisters	An initial site may be followed by multiple pruritic autoinoculated sites
Staph scalded skin syndrome—upper epidermal blisters	Staph toxin		
Viral infections			
Herpes simplex, eczema vaccination, herpes zoster varicella (ballooning degeneration)	Direct cell damage	Grouped umbilicated vesicles on erythematous base anywhere on body; diffuse umbilicated vesicles in sites of atopic eczema; unilateral grouped umbilicated, clear or hemorrhagic vesicles in dermatomal distribution	Frequently recurrent; respond to acyclovir
Insect bites	Insect toxins or proteases, delayed hypersensitivity	Papules, bullae—pruritic	Associated with radicular pain and hypesthesia of involved dermatome; respond to acyclovir
Eczema—acute contact (spongiosis)	Type IV hypersensitivity or irritant	Vesiculobullous lesions on red base; often form unusual patterns of contact with substances	
Autoimmune diseases			
a) Pemphigus vulgaris and vegetans (suprabasilar split)	a) Autoimmune interepidermal cell IgG and C3	a) Superficial, flaccid bullae that readily rupture, leaving nonhealing erosions over the body that can cause death; Nikolsky's sign prominent	a) 100% of patients develop mucous membrane blisters, erosions
b) Pemphigus foliaceus and erythematosus (subcorneal split)	b) Autoimmune IgG and/or C3 between cells in upper epidermis	b) Superficial blisters crusting, oozing over scalp and face in seborrhea distribution or butterfly-like rash	b) Seldom see mucous membrane involvement
c) Hailey-Hailey disease (suprabasilar split)	c) Genetically inherited—dominant	c) Superficial erosive blisters, vesicles, pustules in flexural areas of body	c) No mouth lesions
Subepidermal Blisters			
Autoimmune or immunologic			
Bullous pemphigoid	C3 in lamina lucida	Tense bullae on normal or erythematous skin	
Herpes gestationis	C3 in basement membrane zone	Erythematous plaques, tense vesicles, and pruritic bullae that evolve first on abdomen and then on extremities; often polycyclic	Develops during 2nd or 3rd trimester of pregnancy—clears with delivery; increased fetal wastage
Erythema multiforme	Hypersensitivity reaction in blood vessels of dermis to number of antigens—immune complexes seen	Multiforme lesions of red urticaria, papules and target lesions on extremities, palms	Can involve mouth, eyes (Stevens-Johnson syndrome)
Cicatricial pemphigoid	Subepidermal IgG linear in basement membrane zone	Scarring blisters in the mucous membrane; 25% have blisters on skin	Causes blindness; stenosis of urethra, anal areas
Dermatitis herpetiformis (vesicles in dermal papillae)	Immunologic deposition of IgA in dermal papillae	Grouped, symmetrically distributed vesicles and urticarial papules on scalp, scapulae, buttocks, elbows, knees	Intense burning, itch; high incidence of asymptomatic celiac sprue
Metabolic			
Porphyria cutanea tarda	Metabolic defect in porphyrin metabolism	Tense bullae that leave scars in sun-exposed areas; bullae induced by sun, trauma	May also see facial hirsutism and hyperpigmentation
Bullous disease of renal disease	Unknown	Bullae usually on extremities	
Bullous disease in diabetics	Unknown	Large bulla on acral areas	
Mechanicobullous diseases			
Epidermolysis bullosa (split above, below, and within dermal-epidermal zone)	Variety of inherited conditions	Tense blisters that erode and scar, especially in recessively inherited forms; can lead to severe scars covering digits	Severe forms may involve mouth, esophagus
Epidermolysis bullosa acquisita (blister below lamina densa)	Linear IgG and C3 deposits below lamina densa	Tense blisters that lead to scars and milia in pressure and trauma sites on hands, feet; scarring mucous membrane lesions also occur	Circulating antibody to sublamina densa antigen found

slide and stained with Wright or Giemsa stain to reveal multinucleated giant cells (see Ch. 532).

Acyclovir administered orally and intravenously is the most frequently used form of therapy for primary and recurrent forms of herpes (see Ch. 340 and Fig. 532–4).

Varicella infection, when initially encountered, causes chickenpox, a generalized pruritic eruption with widespread, delicate vesicles on an erythematous base which have been likened to a dew drop on a rose petal. They often become umbilicated, hemorrhagic, and pustular and may leave scars. Chickenpox lesions occur predominantly on the trunk but also involve the head, extremities, and mucous membranes of the mouth and conjunctiva. Successive crops of lesions evolve for a week. *Herpes zoster* is a recrudescence of latent varicella virus in persons who previously had varicella. It appears as grouped, umbilicated, and, at times, hemorrhagic vesicles and pustules on an erythematous base situated unilaterally along the distribution of cranial or spinal nerves. Frequently several immediately adjacent dermatomes are involved. Bilateral involvement is rare. Zoster is frequently

associated with a prodrome of severe radicular pain in the involved areas. A common useful sign in making the diagnosis is hypesthesia of the dermatomal areas—the patient often bitterly complains that the rubbing of clothing on the area is intolerable. Most patients with herpes zoster are over 50 years of age, and cancer patients (especially those with lymphomas such as Hodgkin's disease) are particularly prone to this infection. In such patients or in immunocompromised individuals, cutaneous dissemination from the original dermatome may occur, as well as visceral involvement of liver, lung, and central nervous system. Postherpetic neuralgia is common in individuals over 50. Treatment of herpes zoster is usually symptomatic with Burow's compresses, analgesics, and acyclovir, especially in immunocompromised patients.

Insect bites including flea and fire ant bites may also induce vesicles or bullae, a response to injected toxins or foreign chemicals or proteins in the bite or an allergic reaction to them.

Several unusual conditions, the *pemphigus diseases*, cause blistering in the epidermis by virtue of the process of acantholysis. Nikolsky's sign is commonly present in these conditions. *Pemphigus vulgaris* and a variant, *pemphigus vegetans*, which heals with hypertrophic, "vegetative" surfaces, are acquired autoimmune diseases of the skin and mucous membrane. The superficial bullae, evolving just above the basal layer, readily rupture, leaving denuded, bleeding, weeping and crusted erosions over the body which do not heal. The oral mucosa is almost always involved and is frequently the presenting site. The painful erosions characteristically spill over the vermilion border of the lips and onto the skin. Lesions of the skin occur anywhere but often in pressure and friction areas. The blisters arise on normal-appearing skin. The usual course of untreated pemphigus vulgaris is slow progression with extensive denudation, leading to fluid and electrolyte imbalance, sepsis, and death. Pain from mouth lesions prevents adequate food intake. Skin biopsy of early vesicles should be obtained for routine histologic examination. The edge of a bulla, including adjacent normal skin, should be examined by direct immunofluorescence to make the diagnosis. Immunofluorescence shows deposits of immunoglobulins (usually IgG) and/or C3 in the intercellular spaces around keratinocytes (see Table 531–3). Antibodies to the intercellular areas of the epidermis are found in the serum of patients with pemphigus vulgaris. High doses of systemic steroids (100 to 200 mg of prednisone per day) over prolonged periods usually control the disease. Methotrexate and other cytotoxic agents are useful as steroid-sparing agents. Treatment with intramuscular gold is often successful, occasionally inducing long-term remissions (Ch. 533).

Pemphigus foliaceus is a less severe disease in which the acantholytic separation within the epidermis is in the upper portion of the prickle layer. *Pemphigus erythematosus* may be a localized variant of pemphigus foliaceus presenting with superficial blisters, erosions, and crusting and oozing over the scalp and face in a seborrheic dermatitis–like rash or often simulating the butterfly rash of systemic lupus erythematosus. Mucous membrane involvement in pemphigus foliaceus and pemphigus erythematosus is unusual, and lower doses of systemic steroids generally control these conditions. Immunofluorescent studies on skin from the edge of lesions reveal immunoglobulin and/or C3 in the intercellular areas of the upper portions of the epidermis.

Familial benign pemphigus, or Hailey-Hailey disease, is a dominantly inherited disorder with suprabasal cell acantholysis, the groups of bullae arising on erythematous skin in the flexural areas (neck, axillae, groin). Spreading erosions display vesicles and pustules at the borders with a moist, granular center. Warm weather and superficial bacterial infections seem to cause flares with spontaneous exacerbations and remissions continuing for years. Familial benign pemphigus differs from other forms of pemphigus in its genetic pattern, absence of mouth lesions, benign course, and absence of intercellular antibodies. Antibiotics, both topical and systemic, may improve acute flares of the disease.

DERMAL-EPIDERMAL VESICULOBULLOUS DISEASES. Separation of the epidermis from the dermis occurs in a variety of bullous diseases resulting from autoimmune and immunologic reactions, metabolic disturbances, and a number of inherited mechanicobullous conditions (Table 534–6).

Bullous pemphigoid, a disease of the elderly, is an autoimmune disorder in which tense, large blisters occur on normal or erythematous skin, often in the groin, axillae, and flexural areas. Nikolsky's sign is not present, and only one third of patients have oral blisters. Healing usually occurs in some blisters without scarring while new lesions evolve. Itching may be severe or absent. Skin biopsy specimens display a subepidermal blister through the lamina lucida (at the electron microscopic level), and direct immunofluorescence reveals deposition of the IgG immunoglobulin and complement. Circulating antibodies to the lamina lucida zone are found in

70 per cent of patients (see Table 531–3). The prognosis is good, and the disease usually subsides after months or years. Widespread bullae require therapy with 40 to 60 mg of oral prednisone per day and occasionally with immunosuppressive agents.

Another subepidermal blistering disease, *herpes gestationis*, is a rare autoimmune condition that occurs during pregnancy and the postpartum period. The name of the disease is misleading, for it is not associated with *Herpes virus* infection. The blisters develop at any time throughout the course of pregnancy, although they most often begin during the second and third trimesters and subside a few weeks post partum. Some patients may experience transient flares or recurrences with each menstrual period or following the use of oral contraceptives. There are recurrences with subsequent pregnancies. Herpes gestationis is a pruritic condition with numerous tense vesicles arising on both normal-appearing and erythematous areas of skin. Arcuate and polycyclic red plaques with peripheral blistering are seen. The lesions first appear on the abdomen and then spread to involve the entire integument. Skin biopsy findings are indistinguishable from those of bullous pemphigoid by light microscopy, and examination of perilesional skin by direct immunofluorescence reveals C3 and less often an IgG linear band just below the epidermis. There is associated fetal mortality as high as 30 per cent, and there is also an increased rate of premature live births. Transient vesiculobullous lesions may infrequently occur in some otherwise healthy infants of affected mothers. Occasionally the patients' intractable pruritus and extensive bullae respond to high-potency topical steroid ointments and diphenhydramine, but most patients require oral prednisone (20 to 60 mg daily) throughout pregnancy with intermittent tapering.

Cicatricial pemphigoid (benign mucosal pemphigoid), another subepidermal blistering disease, has a predilection for mucous membranes, especially the conjunctiva where it causes scarring that leads to synblepharon and blindness. Subepidermal blisters also occur on the skin in one quarter of patients. Subepidermal IgG staining is seen on direct immunofluorescence, but circulating immunoglobulin antibodies are infrequently found. Therapy is unsatisfactory, although dapsone and gold may slow this chronic and progressive condition. Ophthalmologic care should be sought for the eye involvement.

Dermatitis herpetiformis is a chronic, intensely pruritic, vesicular disease that is identified by the bilaterally symmetric (herpetiform) grouping of papules, urticarial plaques, and vesicles over the elbows, knees, buttocks, low back, scapular areas, and scalp. The itching often has a burning quality. The blisters occur just below the epidermis, where collections of neutrophils are found in the dermal papillae. Direct immunofluorescence testing of perilesional normal-appearing skin reveals granular deposits of IgA at the tips of the dermal papillae. Approximately 75 per cent of patients have an associated gluten-sensitive enteropathy that is usually asymptomatic. A gluten-free diet strictly followed for at least 12 months causes remissions or significantly reduces the required dose of dapsone or sulfapyridine, either of which promptly clears the disease. The rash recurs when therapy is stopped.

Erythema multiforme is an immunologic reaction in the skin and mucous membranes often mediated by circulating immune complexes that evolve in response to a number of antigenic stimulae (infections, drugs, connective tissue disease). As the name implies, the skin reaction is characterized by a variety of lesions, namely, erythematous plaques, blisters, and target or bull's-eye lesions. The mucous membranes of the mouth and eye may also be involved, and this is referred to as *Stevens-Johnson syndrome*. Typically the cutaneous lesions favor the extremities (often the palms) and are symmetric. Target lesions are diagnostic and are recognized by a central, dark purple area or a blister surrounded by a pale, edematous, round zone, surrounded in turn by a peripheral rim of erythema. In Stevens-Johnson syndrome the skin disease is more widespread, with blisters and painful erosions in the mouth and eyes. The patients look and feel ill with fever, prostration, and difficulty in eating. Histologically, subepidermal separation is found in the blistering center of the target lesion, and when early lesions are biopsied, immunofluorescence reveals immunoglobulin and complement in the walls of the small dermal blood vessels; the inflammation and bulla form in response to vascular damage and leaking. In one half of cases no etiology is found for the reaction, but a cause should be sought in all cases, especially drugs (penicillins, barbiturates, phenytoin [Dilantin], and sulfonamides) and infections (herpes simplex, *Streptococcus*, *Mycoplasma pneumoniae*). Recurrent herpes simplex infection is the most common cause of recurrent erythema multiforme. It is not clear whether medical therapy favorably alters the course of idiopathic erythema multiforme, although treatment of a precipitating infection seems appropriate and acyclovir may prevent recurrences of herpes-associated erythema multiforme. Stopping suspected drugs is also imperative. The value of systemic steroids in erythema multiforme and Stevens-Johnson syndrome is controversial. In addition, IV fluids may be required in patients with severe oral involvement, and topical anesthetics (viscous Xylocaine) may help to decrease mouth discomfort.

An example of a bullous disease caused by a metabolic disorder is *porphyria*. Porphyria is a group of disorders characterized by abnormalities in the heme biosynthetic pathway, resulting in the excessive accumulation of various porphyrins (see Ch. 203). In several types of porphyria light reacts with photosensitizing porphyrins in the circulation and skin to cause both acute and chronic alterations in the integument. The onset of photosensitivity in childhood and severe scarring, hair loss, and discolored red teeth are recognized findings in the very rare *congenital erythropoietic porphyria*. Adult porphyrias causing skin changes are, at times, more subtle. Photodistributed skin fragility, with bullae and erosions that leave scars over the dorsum of the hands, forearms, and face, is a frequently missed sign of *porphyria cutanea tarda* (a familial or acquired deficiency in the enzyme uroporphyrinogen decarboxylase). Urinary uroporphyrins and coproporphyrins are markedly elevated, causing the urine to appear dark brown and fluoresce an orange-red color under Wood's light. Both sun exposure and mild trauma to the skin induce subepidermal bullae that leave scars (Fig. 534–9). Facial hair, predominantly on the temples and lateral cheeks, mottled facial pigmentation, and, at times, diffuse scleroderma–like changes on the face and neck also occur. Porphyria cutanea tarda is worsened by alcohol and birth control pills. There seems to be an associated iron overload syndrome with elevated liver stores and serum iron. The treatment of choice is phlebotomy to reduce hepatic iron. When used carefully, antimalarials are also effective.

Other metabolic bullous diseases are those seen with chronic renal disease and diabetes mellitus. Subepidermal bullae occasionally occur in association with hemodialysis in chronic renal failure. The bullae are found on light-exposed areas, primarily the dorsa of hands, and may be worsened by sunlight. A few such patients have elevated uro- and coproporphyrins, suggesting that porphyria cutanea tarda is unmasked by dialysis, but most patients have had no alterations in porphyrin metabolism. These latter patients with *bullous dermatosis of hemodialysis* have scarring, tense, asymptomatic bullae without surrounding erythema. High doses of furosemide have also been reported to produce a bullous eruption on light-exposed skin of patients on hemodialysis. *Bullosis diabeticorum* appears as tense, bullous lesions on a noninflammatory base, usually localized to the lower extremities. These are related to trauma in diabetic patients with small vessel disease.

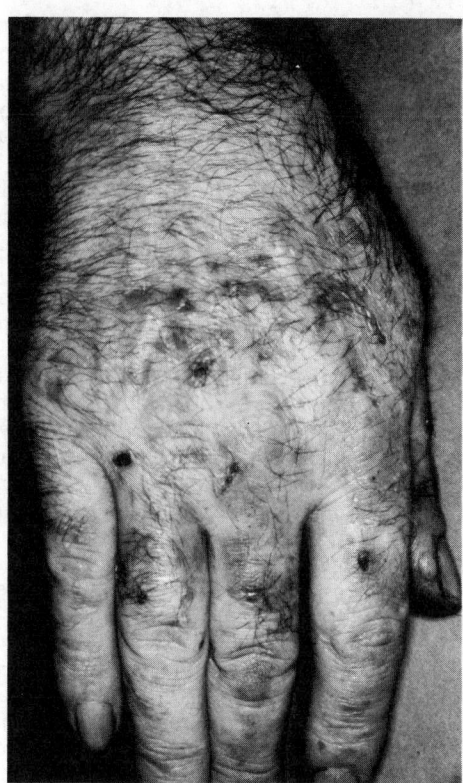

FIGURE 534–9. Porphyria cutanea tarda. (From the 17th edition of the Cecil Textbook of Medicine, with the permission of Dr. Marie-Louise Johnson.)

The last group of subepidermal bullous diseases is the *mechanobullous conditions*, a variety of inherited defects in various structures found within and above the dermal-epidermal junction *(epidermolysis bullosa)*. Blisters, erosions, ulcers, and varying degrees of scarring result from minor trauma to the skin. The forms vary by inheritance pattern, level of blister formation, and degree of scarring. Scars and milia at sites of repeated trauma are more common in the recessive dystrophic variants (anchoring fibrils are missing in these epidermolysis bullosa dystrophica patients). In severe forms the mouth and esophagus are involved, adhesions cover the digits, and growth is retarded. The more serious forms appear at birth, whereas milder types occur later in life. No therapy is available except in the severe dystrophic form in which two thirds of patients may be helped by phenytoin (Dilantin), which decreases the excess production of collagenase found in this condition.

An acquired type of epidermolysis bullosa (EB), *EB acquisita*, has recently been recognized. EBA occurs in adult life and is easily confused with EB dystrophica and/or bullous pemphigoid. It presents with bullous lesions and skin fragility to minor trauma over pressure points and on the hands and feet which heal with wrinkled scars and milia (yellow-white inclusion cysts). Oral lesions as well as extensive esophageal, laryngeal, and ocular scarring, features of cicatricial pemphigoid, may also be seen. The blisters occur below the lamina densa zone, where linear deposits of IgG and complement react with an EBA autoantigen. Circulating antibodies to this sublamina densa antigen are found in many patients. No satisfactory therapy is available.

PUSTULAR DISEASES OF THE SKIN

Pustules usually bring to mind infection, but not all pustular dermatoses are caused by pathogenic microorganisms. Pustular conditions often occur in association with erythematous papules, cysts, and nodules and may open to form crusts (Table 534–7).

NONINFECTIOUS PUSTULAR SKIN DISEASES. *Acne* is the most common pustular condition of the skin. It is an

TABLE 534–7. PUSTULAR DISEASES OF THE SKIN

Name of Skin Condition	Etiology	Important Physical Findings	Other Facts of Note in History or Laboratory Results
Noninfectious Pustular Diseases of the Skin			
Acne	Androgens; follicular orifice keratinization problem; *Propionibacterium acnes*	Open and closed comedones; red papules, pustules, cysts; scarring of face and upper trunk	Rule out acneiform eruptions such as caused by drugs, greasy cosmetics, endocrinologic abnormalities
Rosacea	Unknown	Red papules, pustules on background of erythema, telangiectasia; central face flushing is a common problem; rhinophyma; eye involvement	Seen in patients usually older than those with acne
Perioral dermatitis	May be caused by potent topical steroids; variant acne	Perioral and periorbital red scaling patches, papules, and pustules	
Pustular psoriasis	Variant of psoriasis	Sterile pustules localized to palms and soles or generalized over body	Patient is toxic with fever, leukocytosis; can die of generalized form
Miliaria pustulosa	Occlusion of sweat glands in hot environment	Discrete red papules or pustules with red base over trunk, especially back	
Infectious Pustular Diseases of the Skin			
Localized to the skin			
Folliculitis, carbuncles, furuncles	*Staphylococcus aureus* invasion of hair follicles	Discrete pustules with red base with centrally placed hairs on buttocks, thighs, beard, scalp	Gram's stain, culture
Candidiasis	*Candida* organisms	Satellite pustules around beefy red patches in moist intertriginous areas	KOH preparation; culture
Hot tub folliculitis	*Pseudomonas aeruginosa*	Widely scattered, pruritic pustules with red base over trunk and extremities	Gram's stain, culture; folliculitis resolves spontaneously in 10-14 days; *Pseudomonas* contaminates hot tubs, whirlpools, and swimming pools
Dematophytes-Kerion	Dermatophyte	Boggy patch with pustules in scalp	KOH, culture
Tinea barbae	Dermatophyte	Pustular inflammatory reaction in beard area	
Systemic infections (septicemias)			
Bacterial septicemia (gonococcal, streptococcal, fungal—*Candida*)	Gonococcus	Purpuric pustules—acral lesions in *Gonococcus*; *Staphylococcus aureus*; *Candida*	Associated with arthritis in *Gonococcus*; patients usually ill

inflammatory disorder affecting pilosebaceous units and hence is usually found over the face and upper trunk where the greatest concentration of these skin appendages is found. Several factors play a pathogenic role in acne as individuals enter puberty: (1) androgenic stimulation of the sebaceous glands and increased sebum production (see Ch. 531); (2) abnormal keratinization and impaction in the pilosebaceous canal (comedones) causing obstruction to sebum flow; (3) proliferation of anaerobic bacteria, *Propionibacterium acnes*, which predispose to rupture of the pilosebaceous unit with extravasation into the surrounding dermis, resulting in sterile, inflammatory papules, pustules, and cysts. The inflammatory lesions lead to disfiguring scarring. Therapy of acne is usually successful in controlling the disease until the patient "grows out" of this condition. Treatment is directed at correcting the three major factors that seem to cause acne. Thus, topical agents that remove comedones such as benzoyl peroxide and topical vitamin A preparations are particularly effective because their action allows sebum to flow freely onto the surface of the skin. Topical and oral antibiotics (tetracycline and erythromycin) are indicated in patients with inflammatory papules and pustules. Last, decreasing sebum production has beneficial effects, and oral 13-*cis*-retinoic acid decreases sebaceous gland size and sebum production. This drug should be used primarily for severe cystic acne. The clinician should recognize that other factors may play a role in exacerbating acne, including oil-based cosmetics and drugs (androgenic hormones, antiepileptics [phenytoin], high-progestin birth control pills, systemic corticosteroids, when taken in high doses, and iodide- and bromide-containing agents). Occasionally endocrinologic conditions characterized by excess androgen secretion may cause acne, i.e., polycystic ovarian disease, adrenal or ovarian tumors.

Rosacea is a chronic inflammatory disorder affecting the blood vessels and pilosebaceous units of the face in middle-aged individuals. Patients with rosacea have papules and pustules superimposed on diffuse erythema and telangiectasia over the central portion of the face. An important component of the patients' history is easy flushing and blushing of the face, and this is often accentuated when alcohol, caffeine-containing, or hot spicy foods are ingested. Hyperplasia of the sebaceous glands, connective tissue, and vascular bed of the nose sometimes causes *rhinophyma* or a large, red, bulbous nose (Fig. 534–10). Ocular complications occur in a small but significant number of rosacea patients; these include blepharitis, chalazion, conjunctivitis, and keratitis. Progressive keratitis can lead to scarring and blindness. Rosacea and the eye complications are usually dramatically responsive to tetracycline, but the antibiotic must be continued for life (at the lowest dose that suppresses the condition) because rosacea recurs when therapy is interrupted. High-potency topical corticosteroid preparations may induce or aggravate preexisting rosacea and should not be used for long periods of time on the face.

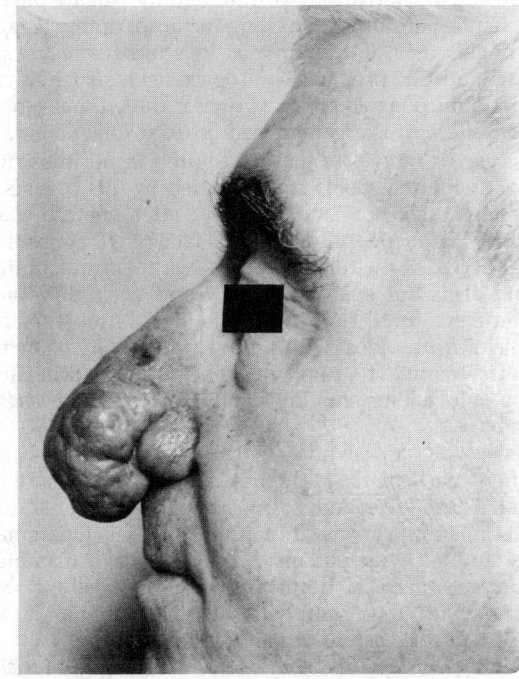

FIGURE 534–10. Rhinophyma. (From the 17th edition of the Cecil Textbook of Medicine, with the permission of Dr. Marie-Louise Johnson.)

Perioral dermatitis, as the name suggests, is a conspicuous affliction consisting of red papules, pustules, and fine scaling erythema in a concentric oval about the mouth, sparing the skin immediately adjacent to the lips. Perioral dermatitis is probably a variant of rosacea or acne, and is most often seen in women between 18 and 40 years of age. Tetracycline is the mainstay of therapy, usually requiring 250 mg twice a day for six to eight weeks.

Hidradenitis suppurativa is a chronic suppurative and scarring problem of the apocrine glands appearing as tense, draining lesions with retracted scars in the axillae and anogenital regions (Fig. 534–11).

Psoriasis can occasionally present in a pustular form, either localized to the palms and soles or as a generalized, total body reaction associated with fever and leukocytosis.

Miliaria, or heat rash, represents an inflammatory reaction caused by occlusion of sweat ducts with extravasation of their contents into the surrounding tissue. Occlusion of the duct at the level of the epidermal granular layer results in *miliaria rubra* (discrete, small, red papules), especially on the trunk and back. The presence of discrete lesions not associated with hair follicles suggests the diagnosis. In more deeply situated occlusion of the duct, *miliaria pustulosa*, or pustules with surrounding erythema, is seen. In the ambulatory patient miliaria results from exposure to hot, humid environment, while in bed-ridden patients fever, sweating, and occlusion of the skin on bed sheets are predisposing factors. The problem usually remits with cooling and ventilation of the patient's skin.

INFECTIOUS CAUSES OF SKIN PUSTULES. *Folliculitis*, a *Staphylococcus aureus* infection of the hair follicle, appears as pustules with a red rim with hair emanating from the center of the pustule. Folliculitis typically occurs in hairy regions where clothing rubs (buttocks, thighs) or on the face. The key to diagnosis is finding a central hair in the pustule. Occasionally the follicular infection can extend more deeply to form a larger, red, fluctuant nodule that "points" to drain pus from one (furuncle) or more follicles (carbuncle). Systemic antibiotics such as erythromycin or dicloxacillin usually clear extensive infections; topical antiseptic cleansers such as providone-iodine or chlorhexidine can resolve mild folliculitis and may be useful in preventing recurrences.

Candidiasis appears as beefy red patches in intertriginous, moist areas characteristically surrounded by satellite pustules. Paronychia, a painful red swelling in the periungual regions of the finger, may also drain pus in which *Candida* can be found with a KOH preparation. Topical agents such as clotrimazole and miconazole are used two or three times a day.

Hot tub folliculitis is a generalized, pruritic folliculitis caused by *Pseudomonas aeruginosa* that is acquired in hot tubs, whirlpools, or swimming pools contaminated by this organism. It usually begins six hours to five days after hot tub soaking and affects many people using the facility. It appears as a vesicular and then pustular eruption over the trunk, buttocks, legs, and arms but spares the head and neck. *Pseudomonas* can often be cultured from fresh pustules. In most instances the folliculitis resolves within seven to ten days without specific treatment. The tubs and pools implicated in causing this type of folliculitis should be cultured for *Pseudomonas* and disinfected.

Dermatophytes can, at times, infect hair follicles and result in pustules, particularly in the beard (tinea barbae) and scalp (kerions). These are readily confused with a bacterial folliculitis. Kerions appear as indurated, boggy, inflammatory plaques studded with pustules. These intense inflammatory reactions to superficial dermatophytes (especially *T. verrucosum*) respond to griseofulvin therapy, although a short course of oral corticosteroids is also useful.

Deep fungal infections such as *blastomycosis, sporotrichosis*, and *coccidioidomycosis* may cause pustules, as well as verrucous, ulcerative papules and nodules. Sporotrichosis charac-

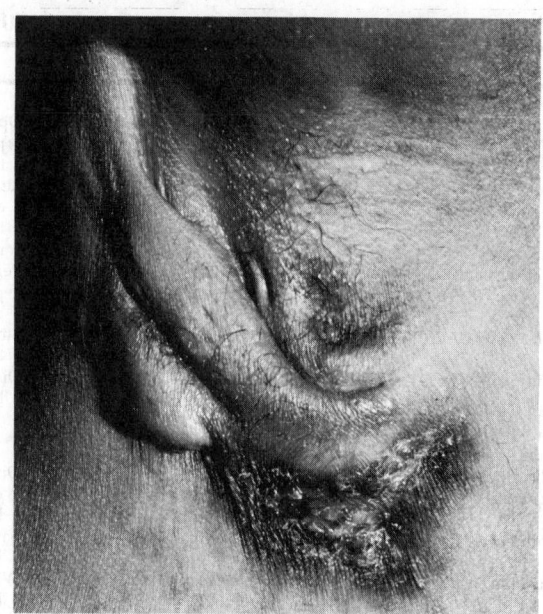

FIGURE 534–11. Hidradenitis suppurativa, axilla. (From the 17th edition of the Cecil Textbook of Medicine, with the permission of Dr. Marie-Louise Johnson.)

teristically spreads up cutaneous lymphatics and appears as nodular, pustular lesions in a linear distribution.

SYSTEMIC INFECTIONS CAUSING PUSTULES ON THE SKIN. A variety of septicemias including gonococcemia, staphylococcal septicemia, and *Candida* septicemia (in immunosuppressed patients) cause pustular lesions associated with purpura.

URTICARIA, PERSISTENT FIGURATE ERYTHEMAS, CELLULITIS

This group of skin lesions is of disparate appearance and etiology. The common feature is a raised edematous, red plaque with a sharply demarcated border (Table 534–8).

URTICARIAL REACTIONS. Urticaria, the most common condition in this group, appears as wheals, transient erythematous and edematous swellings of the dermis caused by local increase in permeability of capillaries and small venules. This increased permeability results from histamine and other chemical substances released from cutaneous mast cells by Type I IgE hypersensitivity reactions, as well as by nonimmunologic mechanisms (see Ch. 420). Certain agents such as aspirin, opiates, and some foods degranulate mast cells directly without an allergic mechanism. Other urticarial reactions are immunologically mediated by such allergens as infections (viral, i.e., hepatitis, sinus and tooth infections), infestations (systemic parasites), drugs, pollens, and injections (blood products, vaccinations). Other hives are caused by physical modalities: light (solar urticaria), cold (cold urticaria), heat or exercise (cholinergic urticaria), or pressure or rubbing of the skin (dermatographism). Hives are transient, any given lesion lasting less than 24 hours, although new hives may continuously evolve. Acute urticaria (i.e., lasting less than six weeks) often results from drugs and the cause is frequently identified. The etiology of chronic urticaria (lasting longer than six to eight weeks) is more difficult to identify. Hives covering large areas and producing deep tissue swelling are termed *angioedema*. This condition can involve the tongue and throat and threaten to close off the airway. In such patients a careful history about medications (including over-the-counter drugs, especially cold tablets or medications containing aspirin) should be elicited. Infections such as "silent" sinusitis or apical abscess of teeth must be looked for. In addition, physical types of urticaria should be considered: *cholinergic* urticaria is characterized by evanescent multiple,

TABLE 534–8. URTICARIA, PERSISTENT FIGURATE ERYTHEMAS, CELLULITIS

Skin Condition	Etiology	Important Physical Findings	Other Facts of Note
Urticaria-like Reactions			
Urticaria	Drugs, foods, infections, physical modalities (heat, cold, light)	Transient, red wheals that usually stay in one area of skin less than 6-8 hours	Occasionally chronic sinus infection or apical tooth abscess can be silent cause
Erythema marginatum	Associated with rheumatic fever	Transient annular lesions	Associated with carditis
Urticaria pigmentosa	Abnormal accumulation of mast cells	Pigmented papules of skin; Darier's sign present	In adult, mast cells may infiltrate lymph nodes, liver, spleen, GI tract
Figurate Erythemas			
Erythema annulare centrifugum	Occasionally an "id" reaction to tinea infection elsewhere on the body	Annular lesions with red border and trailing scale; persist for many days or months	May mimic ringworm
Erythema chronicum migrans	Part of Lyme disease caused by bite of tick and spirochete infection	One or more slowly expanding annular lesions	Arthritis, cardiac problems, Bell's palsy often part of Lyme disease
Cellulitis			
Erysipelas	Streptococcal infection of dermis	Erythematous, warm, painful area with sharply demarcated border	Responds readily to penicillin
Necrotizing fasciitis	Mixed, aerobic, and anaerobic infection in fascial plane	Deep red, painful cellulitis that causes purpura and then tissue necrosis; moves rapidly	Seen in immunosuppressed patients and diabetics

small wheals surrounded by a wide pink flare induced by heat and exercise; *solar* urticaria by large plaques in sun-exposed areas; *cold* urticaria by wheals that evolve with exposure to cold. Urticaria accompanied by fever and arthralgias occurs in serum sickness reactions and in the prodromata of viral hepatitis. Occasionally urticaria occurs in conjunction with internal conditions such as malignancies or connective tissue diseases. Hereditary angioedema, an autosomal dominant disorder, causes recurrent urticaria, angioedema, intestinal colic, and life-threatening laryngeal edema.

If the cause for the urticaria cannot be found or avoided, symptomatic control is achieved with antihistamines or oral steroids. Acute angioedema or laryngeal edema requires rapid systemic treatment with epinephrine and diphenhydramine (see Ch. 420).

Other urticaria-like skin lesions include *erythema multiforme* (see above); *juvenile rheumatoid arthritis skin lesions*—small, 2- to 3-mm, salmon-colored hives that last only a few hours appearing with fever spikes; *erythema marginatum*—lesions found in 10 per cent of patients with acute rheumatic fever (Ch. 269). *Urticaria pigmentosa* (mastocytosis), a disease caused by increased accumulations of mast cells in the skin and at times in lymph nodes, liver, spleen, bones, and gastrointestinal tract (see Ch. 427), presents with multiple tan to brown, papular spots that urticate when rubbed (Darier's sign) owing to the release of histamine from the mast cells. A skin biopsy specimen stained with Giemsa stain will readily identify increased numbers of mast cells in the dermis. When the lesions in the skin develop in early childhood, the condition is usually limited to skin and the lesions resolve by puberty, leaving only hyperpigmented macules. If the skin lesions evolve in adulthood there is a greater chance for mast cell infiltration of the organ systems noted above, and the skin lesions persist. Symptoms and findings in mastocytosis depend on the organ systems involved and the release of various vasoactive substances contained in the increased masses of mast cells. Hepatosplenomegaly, lymphadenopathy, and bone pain may occur secondary to infiltrates. Patients may experience flushing, palpitations, headache, syncope, hypotension, abdominal pain, and diarrhea, all related to histamine and prostaglandin release from the mast cells.

FIGURATE ERYTHEMAS. This is a group of uncommon conditions characterized by annular, polycyclic, and geographic erythematous skin lesions. These conditions, in contrast to the urticarial reactions, persist for many days or even years, moving slowly or rapidly over the skin surface (hence, the term sometimes used for these reactions—persistent figurate erythema).

The most common of these diseases, *erythema annulare centrifugum*, appears as one or more annular lesions with an elevated erythematous border and a fine scale on the inner aspect of the border (trailing scale).

Erythema chronicum migrans is the unique annular skin lesion found in Lyme disease caused by a spirochete inoculated by infected tick bites (see Ch. 313 and Color plate 4).

CELLULITIS. Although superficially resembling urticaria, these inflammatory infections of the dermis are readily distinguished from hives by their persistent, slowly enlarging nature as well as their pain and warmth. Group A streptococci and *Staphylococcus aureus* are the organisms most commonly responsible. *Erysipelas* is sometimes identified separately from cellulitis. It displays a sharply demarcated painful border and an "orange-peel" epidermal surface. Group A *Streptococcus* is the usual cause. Patients usually feel ill and are febrile. Cellulitis on the lower legs in adults may develop from fissures between the toes from tinea pedis. Systemic antibiotics, erythromycin, dicloxacillin, or the cephalosporins are the drugs most commonly used.

Necrotizing fasciitis is a special form of cellulitis involving the deep fascial structures underlying the skin. Rapidly evolving in enclosed fascial spaces, usually in diabetics or immunosuppressed patients, these infections are caused by a mixture of aerobic and anaerobic gram-negative organisms and must be diagnosed early by deep fascial biopsy and treated immediately with a broad spectrum of antibiotics and surgical debridement.

NODULES AND TUMORS OF THE SKIN

Nodular and tumorous lesions of the skin may evolve within the epidermis or the dermis and subcutaneous tissue, arising in various skin appendages and structures, including melanocytes. Such nodular lesions may represent benign or malignant growths, infiltrative or inflammatory reactions. In many instances the structures giving rise to the nodule will reflect the colors of these structures; i.e., vascular lesions appear red to purple, whereas lesions involving melanocytes will appear pigmented.

In general, epidermal nodules are recognized by localized thickening of the epidermis or corneum with hyperkeratosis or scale. Dermal or subcutaneous nodules appear as lumps, often with no alteration in the overlying epidermis.

Of primary concern in every patient with a nodule is whether it is benign or malignant. This is not always easy to discern, and therefore skin nodules and tumors often must be biopsied. Some clinical generalizations can be made in distinguishing benign from malignant tumors (Table 534–9).

Common nodular lesions of the skin are listed in Table 534–10.

NONPIGMENTED NODULES—BENIGN. *Warts* are be-

TABLE 534–9. CLINICAL FEATURES HELPFUL IN DISTINGUISHING BENIGN FROM MALIGNANT TUMORS

Clinical Feature	Benign	Malignant
Configuration	Symmetric, sharp borders	Asymmetric, irregular borders
Rate of growth	Slow	Slow or rapid
Friability	No friability	Often friable
Bleeding or ulceration	Seldom bleed or ulcerate	Often bleed and ulcerate
Consistency	Firm or soft	Usually firm to hard
Color	Uniform color and pigmentation	Irregularity of color and pigmentation

nign epidermal growths caused by papilloma viruses (see above, under Maculopapular lesions).

Sebaceous hyperplasia occurs as papular and occasionally nodular lesions on the faces of individuals past 50 years of age. This proliferation of sebaceous glands surrounding a hair follicle appears as groups of yellow papules evolving in an annular configuration with a central pore. Sebaceous hyperplasia is sometimes clinically difficult to differentiate from basal cell cancers, although the yellow discoloration and central pore may help. At times skin biopsy may be necessary. No treatment is generally required.

Keratoacanthomas, or self-healing epitheliomas, are rapidly

TABLE 534–10. NODULAR LESIONS OF THE SKIN

Lesion	Appearance	Distribution	Etiology	Other Factors
Nonpigmented Nodules—Benign				
Warts	Skin-colored, corrugated hyperkeratotic surface	Anywhere on body	Papillomavirus	Appearance may vary, depending on location of wart; i.e., plantar warts are flat with callus on surface; condylomata acuminata are soft, moist, cauliflower-like nodules
Sebaceous hyperplasia	Yellow, papular nodules, lesions	Face	Benign hyperplasia of sebaceous glands	
Keratoacanthoma	Rapidly growing nodule with keratin-filled central crater	Sun-exposed areas	Benign hyperplasia of keratinocytes	Resolves spontaneously leaving scars
Epidermal inclusion cyst	Flesh-colored, firm nodules with rubbery consistency and enlarged pore on surface	Often scalp, face, trunk	Epidermally lined cysts	Occasionally becomes secondarily infected
Lipoma	Multilobulated, firm nodule with normal overlying epidermis	Extremities, trunk	Benign localized hypertrophy of adipose tissue	
Neurofibroma	Soft, flesh-colored, protruding nodules that can be invaginated deeper into skin—buttonhole sign	Extremities, trunk	Hyperplasia of neural tissue in dermis	Can be associated with von Recklinghausen's disease and café au lait spots and axillary freckling
Nonpigmented Nodules—Malignant				
Basal cell carcinoma	Opalescent, waxy nodule often with ulceration	Sun-exposed areas, 97% face, neck, arms	Ultraviolet light and genetics play a role	Locally invasive—seldom metastasizes
Squamous cell cancer	Hard, smooth or verrucous nodules that often show hyperkeratinization	Sun-exposed areas	Ultraviolet light and genetics play a role	May be metastatic, especially those on lower lip
Pigmented Nodules—Benign				
Seborrheic keratosis	Light brown to black verrucous lesions with stuck-on appearance	Face, trunk	Seen in older people	Individual lesions of uniform color
Dermatofibroma	Firm dermal papules and nodules with overlying brown hyperpigmentation; dimple sign—dimpling of epidermis with pinching of skin	Usually legs	Trauma, insect bites induce dermal fibrosis	Can be flesh-colored or red
Nevi	Uniformly pigmented, flat to nodular symmetrically shaped lesions	Anywhere on body	Accumulation of benign pigmented nevus cells	Itching nevi or changes in color, size, or configuration are danger signs of melanoma
Pigmented Nodules—Malignant				
Melanoma	Flat to nodular, pigmented lesions with asymmetry of growth, irregular borders, variegation of pigmented, and diameter greater than 6 mm	Anywhere on body	Probably ultraviolet light exposure; genetic predisposition	Itching may be early sign of melanoma; melanoma can arise from pre-existing nevi
Vascular Tumors of Skin				
Hemangiomas	Flat to nodular, red, blue, purple, soft lesions	Anywhere on body	Proliferation of blood vessels of dermis	Strawberry hemangiomas usually regress; port-wine stains persist
Pyogenic granuloma	Bright red nodules that readily bleed	Extremities, hands, fingers	Proliferation of blood vessels following trauma	
Kaposi's sarcoma	Red, purple, brown papules and plaques	Legs, neck, trunk	Cytomegalovirus, AIDS	See most often with AIDS or immunosuppression
Inflammatory Nodules of Skin				
Erythema nodosum	Multiple, red, painful nodules; do not ulcerate; involute leaving bruises	Pretibial areas	Hypersensitivity reaction in subcutaneous fat	Number of antigenetic stimuli: drugs, infections, intestinal inflammatory disease
Subcutaneous fat necrosis	Red nodules, tender	Lower legs, thighs	Fat necrosis secondary to release of pancreatic lipase	Pancreatitis, pancreatic cancer
Rheumatoid nodules	Nonpainful, firm nodules	Elbows, knees, fingers	Unknown	Rheumatoid arthritic changes with high rheumatoid factor titer
Nodules Associated with Metabolic Conditions				
Xanthomas	Nontender, firm, yellow to red papules and nodules	Elbows, knees, Achilles tendons	Hyperlipoproteinemias	Xanthomas related to genetic disorders of lipoprotein metabolism (primary) or secondary to underlying diseases

growing neoplasms of epidermal keratinocytes that are biologically benign. These lesions resolve spontaneously, leaving a scar. Keratoacanthomas are usually found on sun-exposed areas and begin as flesh-colored papules that rapidly grow over a period of six weeks, evolving a central keratin-filled crater. The lesions remain for six to eight weeks and then subside. Such lesions are best excised because they leave unsightly scars and are difficult to differentiate from squamous cell cancer, even histologically.

Epidermal inclusion cysts appear as flesh-colored, firm nodules in the skin, particularly over the scalp and trunk. A helpful diagnostic sign is a central enlarged pore where the epidermis has invaginated to form the cyst. If the central pore is patent, slight squeezing will express white, cheesy, foul-smelling keratin and sebum. If the cyst is bothersome it can be excised.

Lipomas are more deeply situated than epidermal inclusion cysts; although they can feel firm and even rubbery, like a cyst, they usually are multilobulated and softer in consistency. If the diagnosis is in doubt and especially if the lesion is firm, a biopsy is indicated. Lipomas may be multiple, and familial multiple epidermal cysts and lipomas, fibromas, and osteomas associated with intestinal polyps are recognized as Gardner's syndrome.

Neurofibromas, focal proliferations of neural tissue within the dermis, may present in two forms: (1) soft, flesh-colored, protruding nodules that, on compression, can be invaginated into what feels like a defect in the skin (buttonhole sign), and (2) deep, firm, dermal or subcutaneous nodules. Neurofibromas may be solitary, but when they are multiple *von Recklinghausen's disease* should be considered, especially when café au lait spots (light brown macules) and axillary freckling are seen.

NONPIGMENTED NODULES—MALIGNANT. Malignant tumors of the epidermis—*basal cell* and *squamous cell carcinomas*—are related to the amount and intensity of electromagnetic radiation, including ultraviolet light and x-radiation, the skin has received over a lifetime. Such cancers are therefore found most commonly on sun-exposed areas, especially the face, neck, arms, and hands. The cancers are more common in patients living in southern latitudes of the northern hemisphere and in Australia in those with light complexions who sunburn easily, and especially in patients whose occupations keep them outdoors. In addition, these epidermal cancers are more common in immunosuppressed patients, attesting to the importance of the immune surveillance system in cancer etiology. A personal or family history of skin cancer should always make the physician more alert to the possibility of cancer.

Basal cell carcinoma is a malignancy arising from the basal cells of the epidermis. These tumors rarely metastasize, but they have considerable potential for extensive, local destruction. Four clinical forms should be recognized: (1) the *nodular* type, the most common, appears as a pearly or opalescent, irregularly shaped papule or nodule with a central depression or crater; telangiectasias and a rolled, waxy border are often in evidence. When ulceration and crusting occur, it is referred to as a rodent ulcer (Fig. 534–12). Many times the raised, waxy border is subtle and is observed more readily by stretching the skin. (2) *Superficial* basal cell carcinoma is recognized as a red, slightly scaling, eczematous plaque that may be slightly eroded and crusted. Careful examination reveals a threadlike, pearly, rolled edge. This is an easily overlooked neoplasm, frequently confused with psoriasis or eczematous patches, so that a high index of suspicion, along with skin biopsy, is needed to make the diagnosis. (3) *Pigmented* basal cell carcinoma appears as a blue-black nodule or plaque with a pearly, opalescent sheen as seen in other basal cell cancers. Melanocytes are not histologically involved in these cancers, merely stimulated to make more pigment, and the prognosis of these pigmented forms is the same as for other basal cell

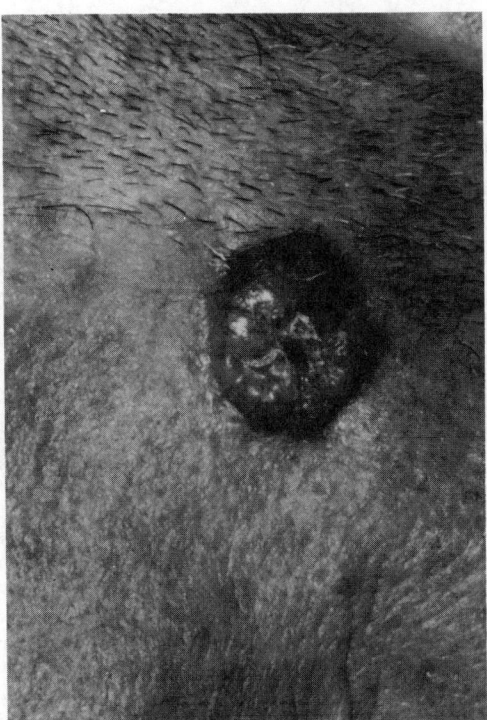

FIGURE 534–12. Basal cell epithelioma. (From the 17th edition of the Cecil Textbook of Medicine, with the permission of Dr. Marie-Louise Johnson.)

cancers. (4) *Scarring* or *sclerosing* basal cell cancers present as atrophic, white, sometimes slightly eroded or crusted plaques with telangiectasia. This is the most difficult form to cure because of its indistinct borders. The diagnosis of basal cell carcinoma should be confirmed by biopsy. Treatment will depend on the location of the lesion, the morphologic type, the size of the tumor, and whether it is primary or recurrent. Treatment modalities include curettage and electrodesiccation, scalpel excision, radiotherapy, and cryotherapy. When these are selected properly each modality has a cure rate of greater than 90 per cent. A specialized form of excision using careful histologic orientation and detailed mapping of the extent of the tumor is the Mohs surgical technique. This tedious form of surgery is used for recurrent basal cell cancers, sclerosing basal cell cancers, and large primary basal cell cancers in regions in which recurrences are likely (particularly in the nasolabial folds and the periorbital and immediate preauricular areas).

Squamous cell carcinoma, a malignant neoplasm of the keratinocytes, is a less common but more aggressive type of cancer than basal cell cancer. Squamous cell carcinoma is locally invasive and has the potential to metastasize. It occurs primarily on the head and neck, upper extremities, and trunk, presenting as firm, red, smooth or verrucous nodules. Hyperkeratoses may be prominent, and indeed "cutaneous horns" are often squamous cell carcinomas. The cancers also display increased friability, ulceration, and crusting (Fig. 534–13). *Bowen's disease* is a squamous cell cancer in situ, appearing as red, scaling, crusted, sharply demarcated plaques. Squamous cell cancer in situ on the penis in uncircumcised males evolves as velvety red patches on the glans and foreskin (erythroplasia of Queyrat). Bowen's disease and erythroplasia are banal, easily overlooked conditions that can metastasize if not diagnosed early. *Actinic keratoses*, precancerous lesions of atypical keratinocytes, appear as red, ill-marginated macules and papules with yellow-brown, adherent scales in sun-damaged skin. They may evolve into squamous cell cancers. Any lesion suspected of being a squamous cell cancer should be biopsied. Excision is the treatment of choice in squamous cell cancers. Actinic keratoses are treated with liquid nitrogen

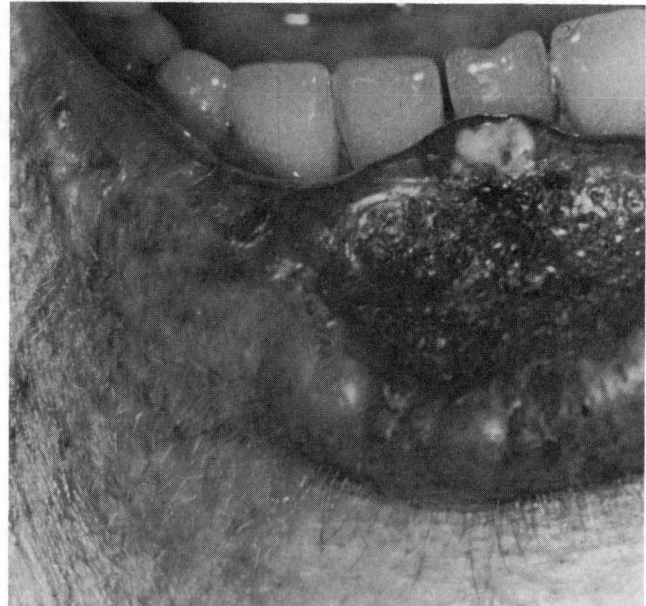

FIGURE 534–13. Squamous cell carcinoma. (From the 17th edition of the Cecil Textbook of Medicine, with the permission of Dr. Marie-Louise Johnson.)

freezing or, if numerous, with topical 5-fluorouracil applied as 1 or 5 per cent cream or solution.

PIGMENTED NODULES—BENIGN. *Seborrheic keratoses* are neoplasms of the epidermal cells that appear on the face and trunk in middle age. These 2-mm to 5-cm, elevated, tan to brown or occasionally black, round to oval lesions have a verrucous or crumbly, greasy surface and a stuck-on appearance. No therapy is necessary unless they are of cosmetic concern, and then liquid nitrogen cryotherapy or curettage is an effective means of removal.

Dermatofibromas are areas of focal dermal fibrosis accompanied by overlying epidermal thickening and hyperpigmen-

tation, appearing clinically as brown papules or nodules. A useful diagnostic test is the "dimple sign," in which pinching the lesion results in central dimpling of the overlying epidermis. Some dermatofibromas are dark brown in color and occasionally raise the concern of melanoma, but the fibromas are symmetric and uniform in color. The lesions occur frequently on the lower extremities and less often on the arms, and they may be multiple. Although therapy is usually not required, simple excision can be done.

Nevi, or *moles,* are benign accumulations of pigment-forming nevus cells. They may be congenital or acquired, and most nevi evolve before age 35, appearing sometime after the first year of life. There are three forms, representing various stages of biologic evolution and growth: *Junctional nevi* are light to brown macular lesions (Fig. 534–14). *Compound nevi* have flat, junctional portions along with brown papules with a smooth or rough surface; these evolve from junctional nevi in older children and young adults. Later, *intradermal nevi* evolve from the compound nevi as flesh-colored to brown papules or sessile growths (Fig. 534–15). Although nevi vary in appearance and color, individually they are uniform in color, symmetric in their growth and configuration, and usually less than 6 mm in diameter. Occasionally nevi darken in color or may itch, and new nevi may develop during pregnancy, but symptomatic nevi that change should be regarded suspiciously.

PIGMENTED NODULES—MALIGNANT. Malignant melanoma is the cutaneous neoplasm of melanocytes and nevus cells. Four important clinical features are useful in recognizing malignant melanoma, the so-called A-B-C-D's of diagnosis:

A = Asymmetry of the lesion is due to irregular, random growth of the malignant cells associated with irregular surface topography and papules and nodules.

B = Borders of the tumors are irregular with notching and pigment "spilling" out beyond the edges.

C = Color variegation consists of browns, blacks, blues, and even shades of red and white. The variations in color represent different depths of invasion of pigment cells along with inflammatory reaction and immunologic response to the malignant cells.

D = Diameter or size of melanomas tends to be greater than 6 mm before they are recognized.

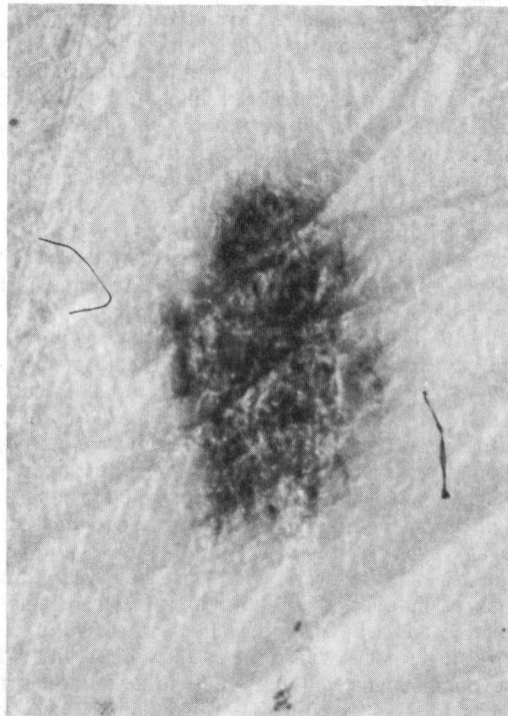

FIGURE 534–14. Junctional nevus. (From the 17th edition of the Cecil Textbook of Medicine, with the permission of Dr. Marie-Louise Johnson.)

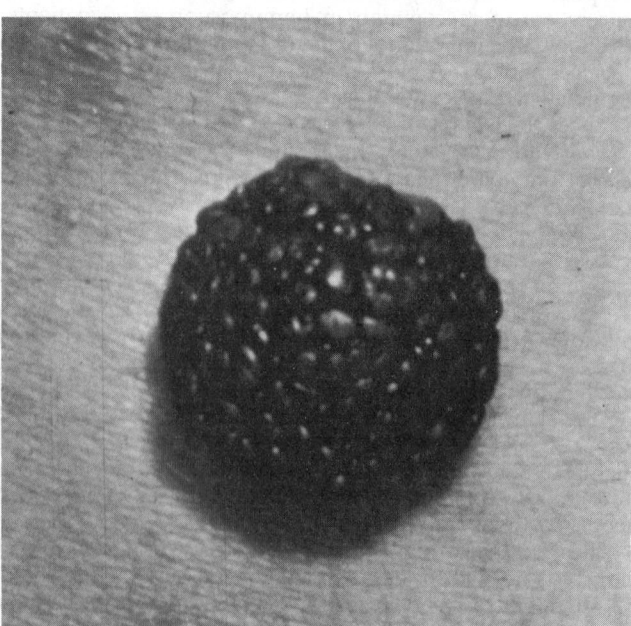

FIGURE 534–15. Intradermal nevus. (From the 17th edition of the Cecil Textbook of Medicine, with the permission of Dr. Marie-Louise Johnson.)

Several clinical forms or presentations of melanoma can be identified, each of these forms demonstrating the above characteristics. *Lentigo maligna melanoma* is a slowly evolving, multicolored lesion on the head and neck. It is preceded by lentigo maligna (in situ melanoma), which extends peripherally and is an unevenly pigmented, dark brown to black macule that can grow to a size of 5 to 7 cm over a period of many years before nodules develop, signifying dermal invasion (Fig. 534–16). *Superficial spreading melanoma* may occur on any area of the body, appearing as irregularly pigmented lesions with papules, nodules, and notched borders (Fig. 534–17). Invasion into the dermis occurs more rapidly than in lentigo maligna melanoma. *Nodular melanoma* appears as a rapidly growing, blue-black, smooth or eroded nodule (Fig. 534–18). It invades dermis early in its evolution, so it is less likely to be diagnosed in a premetastatic stage. *Acral lentiginous melanoma* occurs on the palms, soles, and digits. It evolves as an irregular, enlarging, variegate-colored, brown to black growth similar to lentigo maligna melanoma but more aggressive in its propensity for dermal invasion early in its course. Only minor degrees of papular elevation may be associated with deep invasion.

One third of melanomas may arise from existing nevi, so that a change in size, shape, and color or itching of a pigmented lesion (a common symptom in melanomas) should be carefully investigated. Early diagnosis is the key to survival of patients with melanoma. The deeper the malignant cells invade the dermis, the more likely is metastasis. The depth of dermal invasion can be microscopically measured from the granular cell layer in the epidermis to the deepest penetration of melanoma cells into the dermis. If the melanoma is thin (< 0.76 mm), there is a virtually 100 per cent cure rate. If the depth is greater than 1.6 mm, only a 20 to 30 per cent five-year survival is seen.

Any suspicious pigmented lesion must be biopsied, preferably by excision. Definitive, wide surgical excision should be undertaken only after confirmation of melanoma is established histologically. In large lesions such as lentigo maligna, it is acceptable to do incisional biopsy prior to definitive therapy. Suspicious pigmented lesions should never be shave-biopsied or shave-excised, nor should they be electrocauterized. Full-thickness tissue through the lesion is required for diagnostic and prognostic evaluation.

The precise cause of melanoma is unknown, but sunlight and heredity have been suggested as risk factors. The occurrence of melanoma has been increasing during the past few

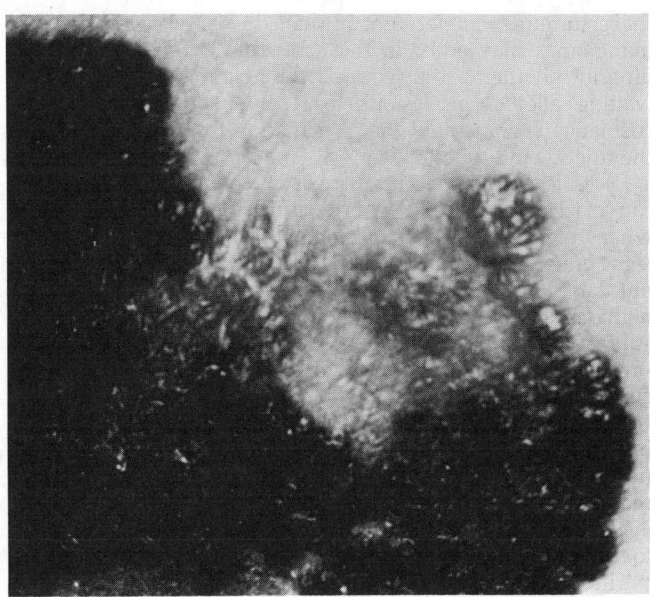

FIGURE 534–17. Superficial spreading melanoma. (From the 17th edition of the Cecil Textbook of Medicine, with the permission of Dr. Marie-Louise Johnson.)

decades. Familial occurrence of malignant melanoma is seen in families with the *dysplastic nevus syndrome*. Numerous atypical, haphazardly colored, red-brown nevi with irregular borders are found over the trunk, extremities, and scalp. Biopsy of these atypical nevi reveals disordered melanocytic proliferation. The nevi have an increased risk of developing melanoma, although the melanomas can also arise from normal skin in these individuals. Close clinical follow-up and excision of suspicious nevi are important.

VASCULAR TUMORS OF THE SKIN. *Hemangiomas*, benign proliferations of dermal vessels, appear as red, blue, or purple, flat to papular and nodular lesions present at or soon after birth. Their appearance depends upon the number, size, and depth of the proliferating vessels. Thus, capillary angiomas are composed of small, superficial vessels causing *nevus flammeus* and *strawberry hemangiomas*. *Cavernous hemangiomas* are made up of larger and deeper vessels. Cavernous and strawberry angiomas often enlarge at an alarming rate over the first year or two and then usually involute by age nine or ten. Cavernous hemangiomas are less likely to resolve and at times may be deeply situated, large lesions that, when located in strategic locations (around the eye and mouth), may require systemic steroids that, in some instances, shrink

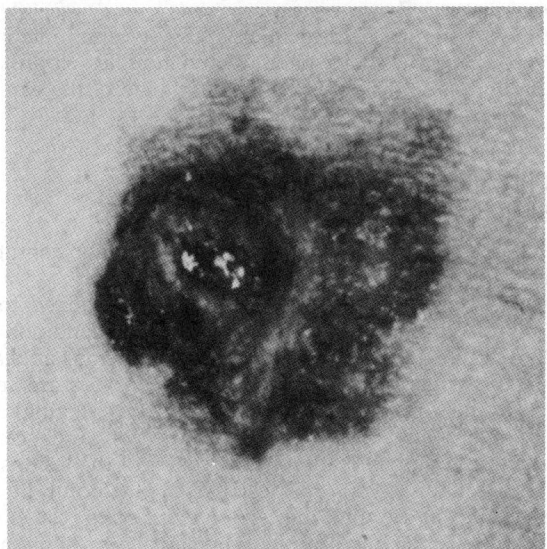

FIGURE 534–16. Lentigo maligna. (From the 17th edition of the Cecil Textbook of Medicine, with the permission of Dr. Marie-Louise Johnson.)

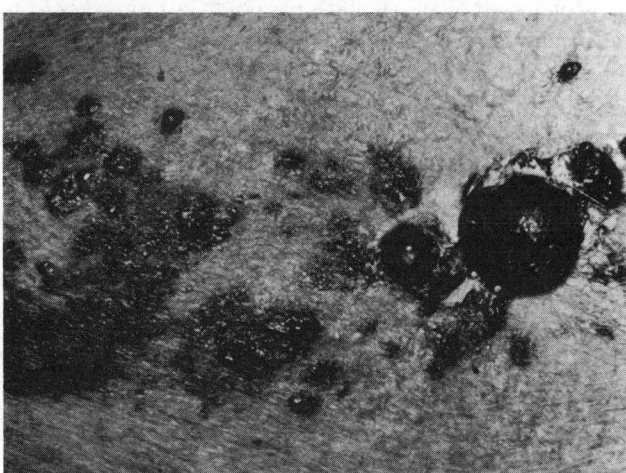

FIGURE 534–18. Nodular melanoma. (From the 17th edition of the Cecil Textbook of Medicine, with the permission of Dr. Marie-Louise Johnson.)

these tumors. Platelet consumption by large cavernous hemangiomas may occur in the *Kasabach-Merritt syndrome*. Ordinarily no therapy is required for hemangiomas; watchful waiting allows the lesions to resolve spontaneously, the cosmetic result usually being superior to that obtained by therapeutic intervention.

Pyogenic granuloma, a bright red, raspberry-like growth that can reach a centimeter in size, is friable and bleeds easily when traumatized. These lesions occur most often on arms, legs, fingers, and hands. They enlarge rapidly within weeks but have no malignant potential; they represent capillary hemangiomatous proliferation and occur following injury or surgery. The term *pyogenic* is a misnomer, as no infectious process is involved. These lesions are treated with excision, curettage and electrocauterization, or cryotherapy.

Kaposi's sarcoma is a rare neoplasm of multifocal origin which presents as red-purple to blue-brown macules, plaques, and nodules of the skin and other organs. The cutaneous lesions may be firm or compressible, solitary or numerous, and may even appear initially as a dusky stain, especially about the toes.

These round-cell and spindle-cell sarcomas are also found in viscera and until their association with AIDS was recognized, seemed to occur predominantly in older men, leading to their demise. In Europe and North America, where Kaposi's sarcoma is more frequently seen among Jews and those of Mediterranean descent, the lesions commonly affect the lower extremities, are indolent, and often are associated with chronic lymphedema, indicating tumor infiltration of the lymphatics. Men are affected 10 to 15 times more often than women, are usually in their seventh decade, and have an average survival time of approximately 10 years. The incidence of such Kaposi's sarcoma reported for the United States is less than 0.1 per 100,000 population and fewer than 0.02 per cent of all malignancies.

In tropical Africa, however, there is an endemic belt at an altitude of 1200 to 1500 meters where the disease accounts for 3 to 9 per cent of all malignancies, afflicting the black population while sparing white people and Indians. It has a peak incidence in the first decade, with most patients less than 20 years of age, and with survival of less than three years. Visceral rather than cutaneous involvement and marked lymphadenopathy are the predominant clinical signs in these African children, who exhibit a unique form of Kaposi's sarcoma found in no other population.

The selective geographic distribution of the lymphadenopathic type of Kaposi's sarcoma is remarkably similar to that of Burkitt's lymphoma. With electron microscopic studies that affirm an association between cytomegalovirus and Kaposi's sarcoma, another parallel is made with Burkitt's lymphoma, the malignancy so closely linked to the Epstein-Barr virus. In the acquiring of Kaposi's sarcoma, therefore, it would seem that infectious agents and immune status are of significance, as well as genetic and environmental factors. Kaposi's sarcoma has been observed to complicate systemic lupus erythematosus being treated with immunosuppression and to appear along with tumors of lymphoreticular origin in the immunosuppressed recipients of renal transplants. It is known to coexist with other primary malignancies. However, its appearance as an aggressive lethal tumor in the young male homosexual is the stunning observation of grave concern. Those affected have a mean age in the fourth decade. Their skin lesions are generalized in distribution and are smaller, softer, and lighter in color than the classic firm, indurated lesions of the legs. Mucous membrane tumors or symptomatic visceral or lung lesions may appear before the hemorrhagic sarcomas of the skin. Average survival time from onset of the disease is less than two years.

Such fulminant Kaposi's sarcoma appears alone or with *Pneumocystis carinii* pneumonia and other opportunistic infections in increasing numbers in male homosexuals and drug abusers. A small painless red nodule of the skin, easily overlooked, can signal a profoundly compromised immune state and grave prognosis (see Ch. 346 and Color plate 6D, E, and F).

INFLAMMATORY NODULES OF THE SKIN. *Erythema nodosum* is an inflammatory reaction in subcutaneous fat which represents a hypersensitivity response to a number of antigenic stimulae. These well-localized, multiple, tender, red, deep nodules, 1 to 5 cm in size, usually develop bilaterally over the pretibial areas. They eventually involute, leaving yellow-purple bruises. Ulceration does not occur. Immunoglobulin and complement deposition has been found in deep blood vessels in early lesions, and in some patients circulating immune complexes have been detected. The localization of the painful nodules to the lower legs may be related to hemodynamic factors. Although no cause can be found in many patients, the following etiologic factors have been identified: drugs, pregnancy, inflammatory bowel disease, sarcoidosis, streptococcal infection, *Yersinia* enterocolitis, deep fungus infections, and tuberculosis. If the etiology cannot be identified and eliminated, symptomatic therapy with aspirin, nonsteroidal anti-inflammatory medications, or occasionally short courses of systemic steroids may be useful.

Subcutaneous fat necrosis is a condition in which tender, red nodules occur on the lower legs and thighs in patients with pancreatitis or pancreatic carcinoma. The skin lesions may occur in the absence of signs associated with the internal carcinoma. Serum amylase and lipase values are elevated, and skin biopsy will provide diagnostic findings.

Rheumatoid nodules are subcutaneous inflammatory lesions usually found over elbows, knees, and fingers in patients with severe rheumatoid arthritis and high rheumatoid factor titer (see Ch. 433).

NODULES ASSOCIATED WITH METABOLIC DISEASES AND MISCELLANEOUS CONDITIONS. *Xanthomas* are focal collections of lipid-containing histiocytes in the dermis and tendon sheaths which appear as yellowish papules (eruptive xanthomas), plaques (xanthelasma), nodules (xanthoma tuberosum), and xanthomas in tendon and tendon sheaths (xanthoma tendinosum). Xanthomas often arise in association with inherited hyperlipoproteinemias (see Ch. 183) or in a variety of underlying metabolic diseases that alter lipoprotein metabolism, such as diabetes, hypothyroidism, cholestatic liver disease, pancreatitis, and renal disease, and in reaction to some drugs (e.g., 13-*cis*-retinoic acid). Xanthelasma usually develops in the absence of hyperlipidemia, although hypercholesterolemia (and increased low density lipoproteins) may be present.

Patients with gout occasionally deposit sodium urate in the skin, forming firm, hard papules and nodules (tophi) that may discharge whitish crystals in the pinnae of the ears and periarticular areas.

ATROPHIC SKIN CONDITIONS WITH SCARRING, INDURATION, ULCERATION, AND TELANGIECTASIAS

Connective tissue diseases are the most common conditions that lead to this spectrum of cutaneous changes.

SCARRING. *Lupus erythematosus* may be localized to the skin (discoid lupus) or present as a systemic condition (see Ch. 436) (Table 534–11). Discoid lupus skin lesions appear as red plaques with white, cohesive scales that often are accentuated in the follicular openings (follicular plugging). The plaques eventually atrophy, with depression and scarring along with hypopigmentation in the center of the lesions and a hyperpigmented rim. The lesions usually occur in sun-exposed areas and, when they involve the scalp, cause scarring alopecia. Systemic lupus erythematosus presents as an erythematous rash with a violaceous hue, accentuated in sun-exposed areas, especially the malar area, producing a butterfly configuration. Telangiectasias may also be prominent, and, at

TABLE 534–11. ATROPHIC SKIN CONDITIONS WITH SCARRING, INDURATION, ULCERATION, AND TELANGIECTASIAS

Condition	Etiology	Important Physical Findings	Other Facts of Note
Connective Tissue Diseases	Autoimmune conditions		
Discoid lupus		Plaques with atrophic centers, erythematous and telangiectatic borders; follicular plugging prominent	May rarely be associated with systemic LE
Systemic lupus	Unknown	Erythematous, scaling, telangiectatic rash in sun-exposed areas; butterfly configuration on face; periungual telangiectasias	Antinuclear antibodies plus arthritis and serositis
Dermatomyositis	Unknown	Heliotrope of eyelids; Gottron papules on knuckles, poikilodermatous changes on face, V of neck, elbows	Proximal muscle weakness; occasionally associated with underlying cancer
Morphea	Unknown	Localized patches of induration with erythematous borders	Seldom related to systemic sclerosis
Progressive systemic sclerosis	Unknown	Hidebound, indurated, tight skin over acral areas and face; periungual and matlike telangiectasias; ulcerations of fingertips	Raynaud's phenomenon common; lungs, heart, GI tract may also be involved
Lichen sclerosus et atrophicus	Unknown	Porcelain white, indurated plaques commonly on genitalia but may occur on trunk; follicular plugging may be seen	
Cutaneous Ulcers of Extremities			
Venous and arterial insufficiency	Impairment of vascular flow	Arterial insufficiency causes ulcers; gangrene acrally with associated claudication; venous ulcers usually around malleoli in association with stasis dermatitis	Lower leg and foot edema common in venous insufficiency
Hemoglobinopathies	Poor oxygenation of tissue	Sickle cell anemia and other hemoglobinopathies can cause ulcerations on lower third of leg	
Pyoderma gangrenosum	Hypersensitivity reaction	Deep, necrotic ulcer with undermined violaceous borders, usually on the legs	Associated with ulcerative colitis, rheumatoid arthritis, dysproteinemia
Ecthyma gangrenosum	*Pseudomonas* septicemia	Ulcers with erythematous borders, usually in body folds	Often early sign of *Pseudomonas* septicemia
Genital Ulcers			
Venereal diseases			
Herpes	*Herpes virus hominis*	Grouped vesicles that leave superficial erosions	
Syphilis	*Treponema pallidum*	Superficial, indurated, painless ulcer	VDRL may or may not be positive
Chancroid	*Haemophilus ducreyi*	Multiple, soft, painful ulcers with undermined edges	
Lymphogranuloma venereum	*Chlamydia trachomatis*	Transient, painless skin ulcer—inguinal bubo	
Granuloma inguinale	*Donovania granulomatis*	Nodules that erode with granulation tissue ulcer	
Behçet's disease	Autoimmune disease	Multiple shallow genital ulcers in association with oral aphthae and iritis	Erythema nodosum, arthritis, and CNS symptoms also seen

times, fine scaling is seen. Occasionally bullae, erosions, and ulcers also occur. Periungual telangiectasia is a prominent finding in systemic lupus as well as in other connective tissue diseases. Subacute lupus is a form in which psoriasiform skin patches are found on the face and trunk.

Dermatomyositis (see Ch. 443) findings include violaceous edema of eyelids (heliotrope), flat-topped papules over the knuckles (Gottron's papules), and reticulated patches of hyper- and hypopigmentation, erythema, and telangiectasia (poikiloderma) found on the V of the neck, face, elbows, and knees.

X-radiation can cause chronic skin changes of atrophy, telangiectasias, irregular pigmentation, and eventually ulceration. Within these areas malignant changes may later appear.

DERMAL INDURATIONS (SCLEROSIS). *Scleroderma* is a condition in which excessive collagen is found in the dermis (see Ch. 437). *Morphea* is localized scleroderma confined to the skin, whereas *systemic scleroderma,* or *progressive systemic sclerosis,* is a more extensive form in which fibrosis diffusely involves the skin as well as internal organs (see Ch. 437). Morphea lesions are asymptomatic, oval to irregular, whitish, firm, thickened patches with an erythematous border. The plaques are most often found on the trunk. The thickened skin in progressive systemic sclerosis is not sharply demarcated, but rather causes indurated, "hide-bound" tight skin over the fingers, toes, and extremities (acrosclerosis). Thickening of the facial skin causes smoothness and loss of wrinkles except for furrowing around the mouth. Ulcerations followed by pitted scars occur on the finger tips. Telangiectasia may be prominent, appearing as periungual telangiectasias and multiple, small punctate macules on the face and hands (matlike telangiectasia). A variant of systemic scleroderma, the *CREST syndrome,* displays extensive telangiectasias over face and hands. Patients with *hereditary hemorrhagic telangiectasia* also display telangiectasia, particularly around the mouth and nose and on the fingers as well as vascular malformations

in the gastrointestinal tract and, at times, the lung. No cutaneous induration is found in this condition.

Lichen sclerosus et atrophicus may be confused with morphea, presenting as porcelain white, atrophic, indurated plaques most commonly on the vulva or on the male genitalia (balanitis xerotica obliterans). At times it occurs as scattered patches on the trunk.

Myxedema may cause a doughy thickening of the skin from deposition of glycosaminoglycans in the dermis. This may be localized to the pretibial areas (pretibial myxedema) as firm, nonpitting plaques and nodules with accentuation of the follicular orifices giving a peau d'orange appearance.

CUTANEOUS ULCERS. Primary skin ulcers are caused by a wide variety of etiologies and conditions. The location of the ulcers, the symptoms associated with them, and the rapidity of their appearance are important clues in diagnosing their various etiologies.

Ulcers of the extremities are frequently associated with vascular disease. Sudden pain associated with numbness of an extremity and ulceration suggest arterial occlusion. Ulceration of digits associated with a purplish red color with dependency and pallor when the extremity is elevated suggests arteriosclerotic peripheral vascular disease. Brawny edema, brown discoloration, and dermatitis over the lower legs in association with ulcers around the malleoli are seen with venous insufficiency. Sickle cell anemia causes ulcerations in the lower third of the leg. Areas of pressure and trauma, particularly on the foot, in patients with peripheral neuropathy, are susceptible to neurotrophic ulcers (mal perforant), as in diabetes and leprosy. The skin around the ulcer is anesthetic and callused. Pressure sores or decubitus ulcers occur in immobilized debilitated patients. Shearing forces, friction, moisture, and pressure contribute to the development of these sores. The sacral and coccygeal areas, ischial tuberosities, and greater trochanters are favored sites. The best treatment of pressure sores is prevention by frequently moving immobilized patients, keeping the skin clean, and using air mattresses.

An unusual and dramatic ulcerative condition, *pyoderma gangrenosum*, often begins as an inflammatory nodule or pustule resembling a furuncle which breaks down, ulcerates, and gradually enlarges peripherally. Fully developed, the lesions are moderately deep, red, necrotic ulcers with undermined, violaceous, edematous borders. These lesions, which typically evolve on the lower legs, are postulated to represent a Shwartzman-like hypersensitivity reaction to a number of underlying internal conditions, including chronic ulcerative colitis, regional ileitis, rheumatoid arthritis, dysproteinemias, and occasionally leukemia or lymphoma. In over one half of the cases no etiology is identified.

Ecthyma gangrenosum is characterized by ulcerative lesions, often in the body folds (anogenital and axillary areas), in immunosuppressed patients with *Pseudomonas* septicemia. The painless lesions begin as hemorrhagic bullous patches that become necrotic and ulcerate and are surrounded by considerable erythema with a central gray to black eschar. *Pseudomonas* can be cultured from these skin lesions.

Ulcerations on the genitalia are suggestive of venereal disease, including herpes simplex (multiple grouped vesicles and erosions), syphilis (indurated, painless, round ulcer with a clean base), chancroid (single or multiple, soft, painful, purulent ulcers with undermined erythematous edges), lymphogranuloma venereum (transient, painless skin ulcer with associated inguinal bubo-adenopathy), and granuloma inguinale (small nodules on genitalia which erode and become filled with velvety red granulation).

Multiple genital ulcers also occur in *Behçet's syndrome* in association with oral ulcers and ocular disease (iridocyclitis). Erythema nodosum, arthritis, and neurologic and intestinal involvement may also occur. The oral and genital ulcers are small, painful aphthae. Occasionally sterile pustules and ulcers at the site of minor trauma such as blood sampling can occur (pathergy) (see Ch. 453).

Geometric, bizarre-shaped, angular ulcers are characteristic of a self-inflicted, factitial cause.

HYPER- AND HYPOPIGMENTATION OF THE SKIN

Disorders of melanin pigmentation can be classified as hypomelanoses (decreased or absent epidermal melanin) or hypermelanoses (increased epidermal or dermal melanin). Hyper- and hypomelanosis can be further subdivided into localized or generalized (total body) alterations of pigmentation (Table 534–12).

Hyperpigmentary Conditions

LOCALIZED PIGMENTARY CONDITIONS. *Freckles* (ephelides) are light brown-red macules found in sun-exposed areas which are caused by increased melanin production in normal numbers of melanocytes. These occur in fair-complexioned individuals with red or sandy hair. Ultraviolet radiation increases melanin production in these lesions.

Lentigines are also hyperpigmented macules, but they occur because of increased numbers of melanocytes in the basal layer of the epidermis. Two types are recognized: (1) *lentigo simplex*, which occurs in early life and is congenital, and (2) *actinic lentigines*, which are acquired in middle age and are related to sun damage over the face, arms, and dorsum of the hands. Actinic lentigines are sometimes difficult to distinguish from early lentigo maligna on the face, but actinic lentigines have no malignant potential. The *multiple lentigines syndrome* is a rare, dominantly inherited condition character-

TABLE 534–12. HYPER- AND HYPOPIGMENTATION OF THE SKIN

	Etiology	Important Physical Findings	Other Facts of Note
Hyperpigmentation			
Localized			
Freckles	Increased melanin synthesis in skin	Light brown macules on sun-exposed areas	UV light accentuates
Lentigines	May be congenital or related to chronic sun exposure	Flat, light brown, uniformly pigmented lesions	No malignant potential
Melasma	Hormonal changes (pregnancy, birth control pills) plus sunlight	Irregular, flat, light brown areas on malar areas, cheeks, forehead	May fade after delivery or coming off birth control pills
Café au lait spots	Dominantly inherited pigmented lesion	Single to multiple coffee-with-cream–colored macules; may be associated with neurofibromatosis	Six or more such lesions suggest neurofibromatosis
Generalized			
Addison's disease	Increased MSH, ACTH	Diffuse hyperpigmentation with accentuation in body folds, palmar creases	Similar pigmentation with lung cancer; Cushing's disease with pituitary tumor
Hemochromatosis	Deposition of iron in skin and increased melanin in skin	Metallic gray-brown hyperpigmentation	
Chronic arsenic exposure	Stimulation of melanin synthesis in skin	Generalized hyperpigmentation studded with small depigmented macules	Keratosis on palms and soles
Hypopigmentation			
Localized			
Vitiligo	Immunologically mediated loss of melanocytes	Symmetrically distributed depigmented macules around body orifices and over bony prominences	In small percentage of cases associated with pernicious anemia, diabetes, thyroiditis
Piebaldism	Failure of melanocytes to migrate to skin in embryologic development	White forelock and depigmented patch—midline forehead, thorax	
Pityriasis alba	Dry skin	Pink, oval hypopigmented patches that often scale on face, trunk	Often accompanies atopic eczema, dry skin
Tuberous sclerosis	Dominantly inherited condition	Ash leaf–shaped, white macules on trunk, extremities; often present at birth	Associated with adenoma sebaceum, tuberous sclerosis
Generalized			
Oculocutaneous albinism	Autosomal recessive traits with variable degrees of tyrosinase insufficiency	White skin, hair; no pigment in fundi oculi; translucent irides	Nystagmus and eye problems common
Phenylketonuria	Deficiency of enzyme converting phenylalanine to tyrosine, so decreased precursor for melanin synthesis	Generalized depigmentation of hair, skin, eye color	Severe mental developmental defects if not diagnosed early and treated with special diet

ized by hundreds of lentigines on the trunk, head, extremities, palms, and soles, and it is associated with *E*lectrocardiographic abnormalities, *O*cular hypertelorism, *P*ulmonary stenosis, *A*bnormal genitalia, *R*etarded growth, and *D*eafness (thus the acronym LEOPARD syndrome). Another dominantly inherited condition is *Peutz-Jeghers syndrome,* distinctive for its numerous lentigines occurring around the mouth, eyes, hands, and feet in association with gastrointestinal polyps, gastrointestinal hemorrhage, and occasionally malignant degeneration of the polyps.

Melasma (chloasma) of the face usually affects women, and in this instance the melanocytes produce more melanin than normal in response to hormonal factors (occurs during pregnancy or while on birth control pills) in association with ultraviolet radiation. This type of pigmentation occurs symmetrically over the malar eminences, forehead, and upper lip (Fig. 534–19). The lesions may fade with delivery but often persist and are accentuated when birth control pills are used. Hydroquinone, a bleaching agent (2 to 4 per cent creams), may help reduce the pigmentation. Sunscreens are also useful.

Postinflammatory hyperpigmentation is the term given to macular pigmentation following inflammatory skin diseases (lichen planus typically causes brown to blue pigmentation).

Café au lait spots are light brown (coffee-with-cream hue) macules that occur on the trunk and extremities in neurofibromatosis (Fig. 534–20). Six or more such lesions, each greater than 1.5 cm in diameter, are diagnostic for this dominantly inherited disease. Axillary freckling, discrete neurofibromas (Fig. 534–21), and large plexiform neurofibromas along with bony abnormalities combine to make this a disfiguring condition. Ten per cent of the normal population have isolated café au lait spots. In *Albright's disease* (polyostotic fibrous dysplasia) three or four large, irregularly shaped, hyperpigmented macules are usually found unilaterally distributed on the buttocks or cervical area.

Xeroderma pigmentosum is a rare, heterogeneous group of diseases with hereditary deficiencies of enzyme systems in the skin that repair ultraviolet-induced damage to keratinocyte

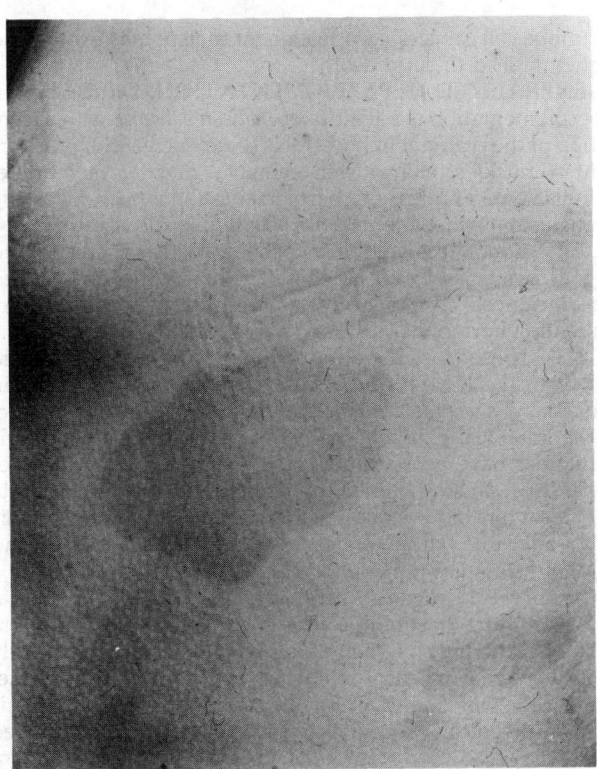

FIGURE 534–20. Café au lait spot. (From the 17th edition of the Cecil Textbook of Medicine, with the permission of Dr. Marie-Louise Johnson.)

and melanocyte DNA. This inability to maintain the integrity of DNA leads to extreme sun sensitivity and multiple freckles over the face, lips, conjunctivae, and extremities which evolve into variably sized pigmented patches interspersed with hypopigmented areas. Keratoses, keratoacanthomas, basal and

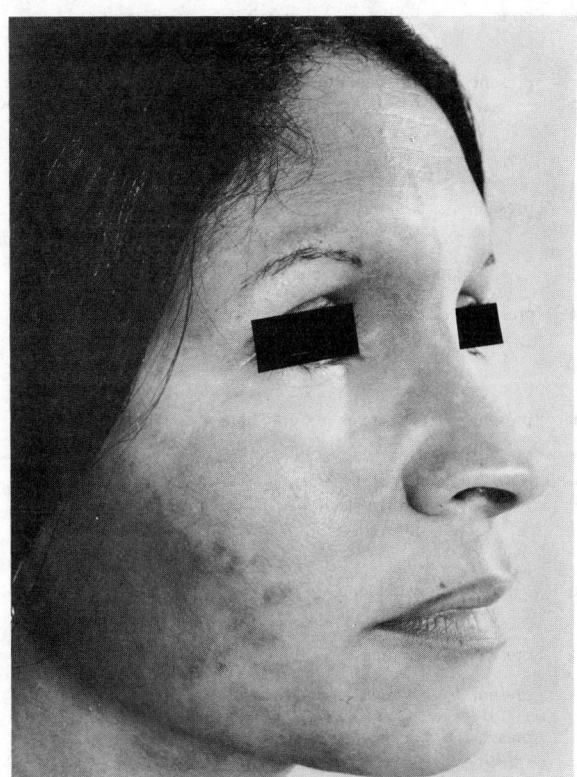

FIGURE 534–19. Melasma. (From the 17th edition of the Cecil Textbook of Medicine, with the permission of Dr. Marie-Louise Johnson.)

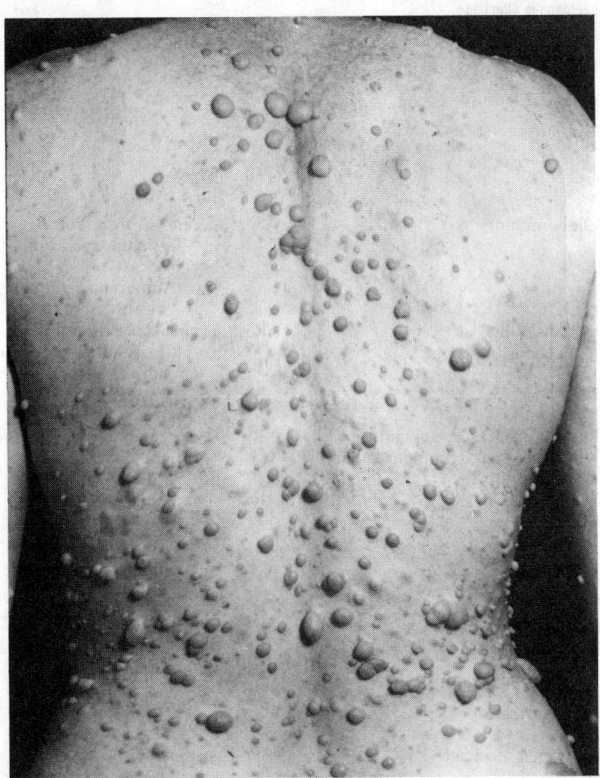

FIGURE 534–21. Neurofibromatosis—von Recklinghausen's disease. (From the 17th edition of the Cecil Textbook of Medicine, with the permission of Dr. Marie-Louise Johnson.)

squamous cell cancers, and malignant melanomas evolve and frequently lead to early death.

GENERALIZED HYPERPIGMENTATION. Diffuse brown hyperpigmentation is a feature of *Addison's disease* with accentuation of the pigment in body folds (palmar creases), pressure points (knuckles, elbows), and gingival mucous membrane. A similar type of diffuse hyperpigmentation is seen following adrenalectomy in patients with Cushing's disease due to a pituitary tumor, as well as in patients with pancreatic and lung carcinomas. In all of these instances the generalized hypermelanosis results from overproduction of melanocyte-stimulating hormone (MSH) and adrenocorticotropic hormone (ACTH). These trophic hormones share common amino acid sequences. Both MSH and ACTH secretions are increased in Addison's disease as a result of diminished output of cortisol by the adrenals. Oat cell cancers of the lung and pancreatic carcinomas have been found to excrete increased amounts of MSH, thus causing similar hyperpigmentation. Melanocyte MSH receptors bind MSH, which stimulates intracellular cyclic AMP, and this, in turn, increases tyrosinase activity and pigment formation in melanocytes.

A number of drugs can cause Addisonian-like hypermelanosis including busulfan, cyclophosphamide, and nitrogen mustard. Blue-gray pigmentation may occur either diffusely or in localized patches following use of chlorpromazine, minocycline, and antimalarial drugs. In addition, inorganic trivalent arsenicals (found in insecticides and contaminated water) may also produce a generalized brown pigmentation, but in this instance the hypermelanosis is studded with small, scattered, depigmented macules (likened to rain drops on a dusty road) and punctate keratoses on the palms and soles.

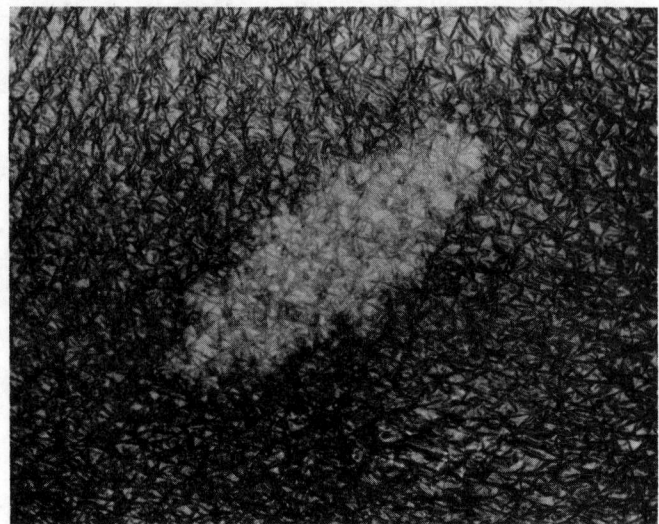

FIGURE 534–22. Tuberous sclerosis ash leaf. (From the 17th edition of the Cecil Textbook of Medicine, with the permission of Dr. Marie-Louise Johnson.)

Hemochromatosis causes a metallic gray-brown, generalized hyperpigmentation resulting from the combination of increased pigment formation in the skin and iron deposition.

Hypopigmentary Conditions

LOCALIZED PIGMENTARY CHANGES. *Vitiligo*, a circumscribed hypomelanosis of progressively enlarging amela-

TABLE 534–13. ALBINISM

	Inheritance	Frequency	Skin Color	Pigmented Nevi Freckles	Hair	Eyes Color	Red Reflex
Oculocutaneous Albinism							
Tyrosinase-negative	AR*	1 in 34,000	pink/wte	none	white	gray-blue	present
Tyrosinase-positive	AR	blk: 1 in 15,000 wte: 1 in 40,000	wte-cream	present	wte-yellow red-darkens	blue-yellow brown	present but may be absent in dark races
Yellow-mutant	AR	rare—Amish, Polish, German-American; blacks (American, Ceylonese, African)	wte at birth, slgt tan pos	present	wte-birth red/yellow 6 mos	blue at birth: darkens	present
Hermansky-Pudlak syndrome	AR	rare—cases from Puerto Rico; Southern Holland; Madras	cream-lgt normal	present	wte-red dk brown	blue-gray to brown	wte—present blk—absent
Cross-McKusick-Breen syndrome (oculocerebral hypopigmentation syndrome)	AR	extremely rare—3 in Amish family	pink/wte	present	wte-lt yel	gray-blue	?, cataracts
Chédiak-Higashi syndrome	AR	rare in most countries; none in blacks	pink/wte	present	blond-dk brown-steel gray	blue to brown	present but diminishes with time
Oculocutaneous Albinoidism	AD†		pink/wte	?	wte blond	blue	present
Ocular Albinism							
Vogt	X-linked	uncommon	normal	present	normal	blue	
Forsius-Eriksson	X-linked	less common	normal	present	normal	blue	
Autosomal recessive	AR	10 families	normal	present	normal	blue	present

*AR = Autosomal recessive.
†AD = Autosomal dominant.
Reprinted from the chapter by Dr. Marie-Louise Johnson in the 17th edition of the Cecil Textbook of Medicine, with her permission.

notic macules in a symmetric distribution around body orifices and over bony prominences (knees, elbows, hands), is familial in 36 per cent of cases. In one third of cases some spontaneous repigmentation occurs, particularly in sun-exposed areas. White hairs are common in the vitiliginous areas. Although most patients with vitiligo are healthy, there is an increased association with certain autoimmune conditions such as thyroiditis, hyperthyroidism, Addison's disease, pernicious anemia, and diabetes mellitus. Melanocytes are absent from the vitiliginous macules. Circulating complement-binding antimelanocyte antibodies have been found in some vitiligo patients. The use of PUVA may give some repigmentation, but it may require 200 or more such treatments.

Piebaldism is a local hypopigmentary condition representing an autosomal dominant hypomelanosis on the extremities, anterior surface of the thorax, and especially over the midline of the forehead and central scalp. A white forelock is typical. The hypomelanosis stems from the lack of normal migration of the melanocytes to these regions during embryologic development.

Waardenburg's syndrome, another autosomal dominant condition, may be confused with piebaldism, as a white forelock is seen, but other abnormalities are also found at birth, including perceptive deafness, heterochromia, and hypertelorism.

A common localized form of hypopigmentation, *pityriasis alba*, appears as slightly pink and hypopigmented, oval to round patches with mild, fine scaling. These occur on the cheeks of children, but they may also be found on the trunk, mimicking the hypopigmented, scaling patches seen in tinea versicolor (a KOH examination of the scales may be necessary to differentiate these two conditions). Pityriasis alba is most frequently seen in atopic dermatitis patients.

Tuberous sclerosis, an autosomal dominant condition, displays white macules in 98 per cent of cases. These depigmented macules characteristically are found on the trunk or buttocks in an oval or mountain ash–leaf configuration (Fig. 534–22). The presence of three or more of these macules is strongly suggestive of tuberous sclerosis, and because the hypomelanotic patches are present at birth, they represent one of the earliest signs of the condition. Examination with Wood's light is often useful in visualizing the lesions, which histologically contain melanocytes with decreased numbers of melanosomes. Newborns with unexplained seizures or mental retardation should be screened with a Wood's light for the presence of the white spots. CT brain scans are also useful in defining the tumorous dysplasia. Patients with tuberous sclerosis (epiloia) suffer from seizures, mental retardation (due to hamartomatous gliomas), phakomas (yellow-appearing gliomatous tumors of the retina), bilateral hamartomas of the kidneys, and a number of hamartomatous tumors of the skin. These cutaneous lesions include *adenoma sebaceum* (smooth, red to yellow papules over the butterfly area and nasolabial folds which appear by age four), shagreen patches (flesh-colored, lumpy plaques over the lumbosacral area), and ungual fibromas (firm, pink papules in the periungual areas of fingernails and toenails).

Certain chemicals, particularly phenol derivatives, when applied to the skin, may cause permanent depigmentation. Hypomelanosis has been observed on the hands of black-skinned individuals wearing rubber gloves in which hydroquinone is used as an antioxidant.

TABLE 534–13. ALBINISM *Continued*

Nystagmus	Photophobia	Eyes Visual Acuity	Pigment in Fundus	Other	Hair Bulb Incubation (Tyrosine)	Defect	Melanosome Maturation by Stage	Complications or Associated Problems
marked	severe	legally blind	none	–	negative	no tyrosinase	I-unmelanized II	skin malignancy basal cell ca squamous cell ca
present but less	present but variable	severe defect in children; may improve with age	none; some with age	pigment cartwheel pupil, limbus	positive	no access of enzyme to tyrosine	I, II, some III, rare IV	skin malignancy basal cell ca squamous cell ca
present but variable	present but variable	marked defect; may improve with age	none; some with age	pigment cartwheel effect	neg to pos ?	unknown ? pheomelanogenesis	I, II, III	unknown
present but variable	present, may be severe	normal or slight decrease	none; some with age	may have pigment cartwheel	positive	pleiotropic effect— single gene mutation	I, II, III	storage-pool defect platelets; ceroid-like material in RE system, oral mucosa, urine
marked	—	blind	?, cataracts	?, cataracts	weakly positive	decreased melanocytes	I, II, III, IV	oligophrenia, athetosis, severe mental retardation
absent or slight	absent or slight	normal or slight decrease	some; increase with age	normal or cartwheel effect	positive	giant melanosomes, lethal defect in leukocytes	I, II, III, IV	infections; hematologic and neurologic abnormalities; lymphoreticular malignancy
no	no	normal or slight decrease	punctate		positive	unknown	unknown	none
present	severe	marked decrease	reduced		positive			
latent	absent or slight	color blind			positive			
present	severe	marked decrease			positive			

GENERALIZED HYPOPIGMENTATION. *Oculocutaneous albinism,* a group of autosomal recessive traits, is recognized by generalized hypomelanosis of the skin, hair, and eyes (Table 534–13). The classic constellation of findings includes marked hypomelanosis or amelanosis of the skin, white or faintly yellow-blond hair, photophobia, nystagmus, and translucent irides. Albinism can be classified according to the presence or absence of tyrosinase, the enzyme crucial in the synthesis of eumelanin and pheomelanin. Normal plucked hair bulbs darken when incubated in vitro with tyrosine; tyrosinase-positive albinos display some minimal darkening (but not normal) of the hair bulb when incubated with tyrosinase, whereas tyrosinase-negative patients show no darkening of the hair bulb. These two types of albinism have separate gene loci. Although melanogenesis is deficient in both forms, persons with the tyrosinase-positive form develop some pigmentated nevi and less eye damage than tyrosinase-negative albinos. Persons with *phenylketonuria* have diffuse hypopigmentation, with light hair and blue eyes. This is an autosomal recessive disorder in which the enzyme that converts phenylalanine to tyrosine is deficient. Consequently, melanin synthesis is decreased (see Ch. 188).

REGIONAL DIAGNOSIS OF SKIN DISEASES—COMMONLY ENCOUNTERED PROBLEMS BY ANATOMIC REGION

Many skin diseases have a predilection for certain areas or regions of the body, often related to variations in the structure and function of the integument (Table 534–14).

Disorders of the Nails

The nail is a plate of hard keratin synthesized from an invagination of the epidermis. The proximal nail fold houses the matrix of the nail where basal cells rapidly proliferate and differentiate into the nail plate, which grows over the nail bed. Nails grow continuously throughout life. The average fingernail grows 0.5 to 1.2 mm per week, whereas toenails grow at one half to one third this rate. It takes a fingernail about five and one-half months and the toenails 12 to 18 months to regrow from the matrix, although rate of growth slows as the individual gets older. Defects in nail formation go by various terms useful in describing nail disorders:

1. *Brittleness*—easy breaking of nail tips
2. *Leukonychia*—white discoloration of nails
3. *Striations*—longitudinal ridges running parallel or perpendicular to the length of the nail
4. *Onycholysis*—separation of the nail plate from the bed
5. *Onychogryphosis*—hypertrophy and thickening of the nail
6. *Pitting*—discrete pitlike depressions in the nail surface
7. *Koilonychia*—spoon-shaped deformity of the nails (concave nail with everted edges)
8. *Pterygium formation*—growth of cuticle onto the nail plate.

SKIN DISEASES INVOLVING NAILS. Nail changes in *psoriasis* have been described above. Fingernails are more frequently involved than toenails. Fungal infection must be ruled out. Therapy of psoriatic nail changes is not satisfactory, although topical tar and steroid preparations may be of some help.

In 10 per cent of *lichen planus* patients, accentuated longitudinal nail ridging occurs as well as pterygium formation resulting from destructive focal scarring of the matrix. Early treatment with oral steroids is indicated to arrest the cicatricial course.

Nail pitting frequently occurs in *alopecia areata* along with onycholysis. The nail is susceptible to deformities when *eczematous* processes involve the periungual regions and matrix. *Atopic eczema* and other eczematous entities may cause pitting, transverse striations, and onycholysis.

Onychomycosis, or fungal infections of the nail, may be

TABLE 534–14. REGIONAL DERMATOLOGY

Region of Skin	Type of Skin Group	Disease Process
Scalp	Papulosquamous and eczematous	Psoriasis, seborrheic dermatitis, tinea capitis, eczema (atopic, contact)
	Pustular	Folliculitis, kerion
	Nodular	Nevi, seborrheic keratosis, pilar cysts, verruca
	Atrophic and telangiectatic	Connective tissue disease, scleroderma, discoid LE
Face	Pustular	Acne, rosacea, folliculitis, tinea
	Papulosquamous and eczematous	Psoriasis, seborrheic dermatitis, contact dermatitis (cosmetics), atopic dermatitis, impetigo, lupus erythematosus, photodermatitis
	Vesicular	Herpes zoster and herpes simplex, insect bites
	Nodular	Basal cell cancers, squamous cell cancers, melanomas, keratoacanthomas, nevis, actinic keratosis, tuberous xanthomas
Trunk	Papulosquamous and eczematous	Psoriasis, atopic and contact eczema, tinea versicolor, pityriasis rosea, scabies
	Vesiculobullous	Pemphigus, bullous pemphigoid
	Maculopapular	Secondary syphilis, drug reaction, viral exanthems
	Nodular	Nevi, seborrheic keratosis, lipoma, basal cell cancer, keloid, neurofibroma, angiomas, melanoma
	Pustular	Acne
	Urticarial	Hives
Arms and forearms	Eczematous and papulosquamous	Contact dermatitis—plants; atopic dermatitis, lichen planus
	Nodular	Nevi, warts, seborrheic keratosis, actinic keratosis
	Atrophic telangiectasia	Scleroderma, dermatomyositis
Legs	Eczematous and papulosquamous	Contact dermatitis, stasis dermatitis, atopic dermatitis, psoriasis, lichen planus
	Nodular	Erythema nodosum, dermatofibromas, nevi, melanoma, Kaposi's sarcoma, lipoma
	Maculopapular	Vasculitis, Schamberg's disease, actinic purpura, pretibial myxedema
	Atrophic, telangiectic, and ulcerative	Scleroderma, dermatostasis ulcers, arterial insufficiency
Genitalia and groin	Eczematous and papulosquamous	Contact dermatitis, seborrheic dermatitis, scabies, pediculosis pubis, psoriasis, Reiter's syndrome, erythrasma, tinea, candidiasis, lichen planus, intertrigo, lichen simplex chronicus
	Vesiculobullous	Herpes simplex, Stevens-Johnson syndrome
	Ulcerative and atrophic	Syphilis, chancroid, lymphopathia venereum, Behçet's syndrome
	Nodular	Verrucae vulgaris, erythroplasia of Queyrat, squamous cell cancer, sebaceous cyst, molluscum contagiosum
	Pustular	Hidradenitis suppurativa
Hands	Eczematous and papulosquamous	Allergic contact and irritant contact dermatitis, dyshidrosis, pyoderma, tinea, dermatophytids, scabies, atopic dermatitis, secondary syphilis
	Vesiculobullous, pustular	Erythema multiforme, hand-foot-and-mouth disease, porphyria cutanea tarda, psoriasis
	Nodular	Warts, squamous cell cancer, actinic keratosis, keratoacanthoma, pyogenic granuloma, granuloma annulare, synovial cysts
	Hypopigmented	Vitiligo
	Atrophic-telangiectatic	Scleroderma, dermatomyositis
Feet	Eczematous and papulosquamous	Contact dermatitis, atopic dermatitis, tinea, psoriasis, lichen planus
	Vesiculobullous	Tinea, epidermolysis bullosa, erythema multiforme
	Nodules	Verruca, corn, nevus
	Atrophic-telangiectatic	Scleroderma

caused by dermatophyte (tinea unguium) or candidal infections. Infection of toenails is more frequent than fingernails, but all nails may be involved. The nail plate is discolored (cloudy, yellowish or brown), thickened, crumbly, and onycholytic with accumulation of debris under the nail. White superficial onychomycosis appears as white patches in the toenail plate due to organisms growing on the surface barely penetrating the nail. Scrapings reveal hyphae upon KOH examination. An unusual condition, *chronic mucocutaneous candidiasis*, is caused by widespread *Candida albicans* infection leading to diffuse white thickening of all nails.

Topical antifungal therapy is ineffective, so oral griseofulvin is given for dermatophyte infection until the nails appear clear. Ketoconazole (200 mg daily) is an alternative should griseofulvin fail or when *Candida* is the causative agent. Oral therapy requires 4 to 6 months for fingernails and 12 to 16 months for toenails. In older individuals toenail problems may never be irradicated because the nails grow so slowly. Residual fungal spores in patient's shoes and environment are no doubt responsible for the high frequency of recurrence, and for this reason topical antifungal powders may be helpful in long-term prophylaxis.

Paronychia, or painful, red swelling of the nail fold, is usually caused by *Candida albicans*. At times a small abscess or purulent discharge is seen. This infection usually occurs in hands constantly exposed to a wet environment (bartenders, janitors). Therapy consists of avoidance of water and the use of antifungal solutions two or three times a day for a month or two.

EXOGENOUS FACTORS CAUSING NAIL CHANGES. Cosmetics, trauma, and occupational influences can all cause nail deformities. Nail hardeners, enamel removers, and stick-on nails all may cause reactions including onycholysis, subungual hyperkeratoses, paronychia, and contact dermatitis around the nails. Nail manipulation, biting, and tight-fitting shoes may induce nail injury. A variety of systemic drugs may induce color changes or other alterations in the nails (e.g., chronic arsenic ingestion causes transverse white lines—Mee's lines; antimalarials, blue-brown coloration; minocycline, variable brown discoloration).

NAIL DISTURBANCES IN SYSTEMIC DISEASES. *Splinter hemorrhages* result from the extravasation of blood from longitudinally oriented vessels of the nail bed. Although often thought to be associated with bacterial endocarditis, they are much more commonly associated with trauma to the nails. *Beau's lines* are commonly associated with systemic disease, but they are nonspecific, appearing as transverse depressions across the nail plates of all nails following any severe disability that temporarily interferes with nail growth, including systemic infections, myocardial infarction, and use of chemotherapeutic agents. *Longitudinal pigmented bands* occur most often in response to trauma or a nevus located in the matrix, but in white individuals a melanoma must be ruled out. *Yellow nail syndrome* exhibits yellow thickening of all the nails with absence of the lunula and variable degrees of onycholysis in association with a number of pulmonary conditions such as bronchiectasis, pleural effusion, and chronic obstructive pulmonary disease. Lymphedema of the extremities may be a third component of the syndrome. *Clubbing* of the nails (increased bilateral curvature of the nails with enlargement of the soft connective tissue of the distal phalanges resulting in the flattening of the obtuse angle formed by the proximal end of the nail and the digit) occurs most often with respiratory ailments, including bronchiectasis, lung abscess, and pulmonary neoplasms. Cardiovascular disease and chronic gastrointestinal diseases (ulcerative colitis, sprue) are also associated with clubbing. When clubbing is found with bone pain and proliferative periostitis, it is termed *hypertrophic osteoarthropathy*, and the condition is most often associated with bronchogenic squamous cell carcinoma. *Nail-patella syndrome* is a dominantly inherited condition affecting both mesodermal and ectodermal structures which causes defective growth of nails (often the nails are missing) in association with hypoplasia or absence of the patellae and enlarged, palpable iliac horns. *Hereditary ectodermal dysplasia* appears in two forms, hidrotic and anhidrotic. The teeth and hair are involved similarly in both (anodontia, hypodontia, and peg-shaped teeth in association with soft, downy, scant hair in the scalp and eyebrows), but in the hidrotic form sweat gland function is normal and the nails are small, thickened, and longitudinally striated.

TUMORS OF THE NAIL. A variety of benign tumors occur around the nail unit. These include *periungual fibromas*, *myxoid cysts*, and *subungual exostoses*. Surgical removal of the benign tumors is the only certain means of cure.

The main malignant tumor involving the nails is *melanoma*, which appears as a pigmented area at the base of the nail or as a longitudinal pigmented streak in the nail. Nevi can give the same appearance, and biopsy of the lesion in the matrix is the only absolutely certain way of making a diagnosis.

Disorders of the Mucous Membranes

Any abnormality of color, texture, or appearance of the mucous membranes should be investigated. Malignant changes should be suspected in infiltrated or ulcerated lesions and a biopsy performed.

ULCERATIVE AND BULLOUS LESIONS. *Acute ulcerative* lesions may be caused by trauma (from jagged teeth or ill-fitting dentures); bacterial infections such as acute necrotizing ulcerative gingostomatitis (Vincent's angina; infection with *Borrelia vincentii* and fusiform bacilli which cause punched-out ulcers in the interdental papillae and gingival inflammation; infections with *Staphylococcus* and gram-negative organisms in patients receiving chemotherapy; viral infections such as primary herpetic gingivostomatitis with small vesicles that rupture leaving shallow, discrete ulcers anywhere in the mouth; infectious mononucleosis, which frequently causes exudative tonsillitis and aphthous ulcers of the buccal and labial mucosae; a coxsackievirus infection termed herpangina which results in vesicles that rupture, leaving 1- to 2-mm ulcers with a grayish base over the pharynx; *Candida* infections causing white pseudomembranous lesions; drug reactions that can elicit oral ulcerations (salicylates, barbiturates, antiepileptic drugs, and particularly drugs used for chemotherapy such as methotrexate, actinomycin-D, and daunorubicin, which are extremely toxic to mucosal epithelium).

Chronic oral ulcerations are most frequently caused by bullous diseases (pemphigus, cicatricial pemphigoid, bullous pemphigoid—see above). Both discoid and systemic lupus erythematosus may have associated mouth lesions with central depressed erosions and elevated keratotic borders. Reiter's syndrome may include superficial erythematous erosions anywhere in the oral cavity. Any chronic, localized, erosive lesion in the mouth should be viewed with concern as a possible carcinoma.

Recurrent ulcerative conditions of the mouth are most commonly aphthous stomatitis or herpes simplex stomatitis. *Aphthous stomatitis* is manifested by multiple punched-out ulcers on the buccal and labial mucosae that may be grouped, simulating herpes. A severe form of aphthous stomatitis (periadenitis mucosa necrotica recurrens) with large, deep, recurrent painful ulcers may involve any area of the mouth. An immunologic reaction to intrinsic mouth bacteria may play a role in aphthous ulcers, as tetracycline suspension mouthwashes may reduce the duration, size, and pain of the oral ulcers.

Recurrent *herpes simplex* of the oral mucosa is unusual but should be differentiated from aphthous stomatitis by Tzanck preparation and herpes cultures. Another recurrent condition is Behçet's syndrome (see above). Erythema multiforme may present as an acute, recurrent, erosive stomatitis in association with target lesions of the skin.

WHITE PATCHES. Thrush (*Candida albicans* infection of the oral epithelium) appears as curdy white membranes that can be scraped away, leaving an inflamed base. It is most common in newborns and in immunosuppressed adults and is a common presenting symptom in AIDS, especially in Africa. KOH examination of material scraped from the white patch is diagnostic. Clortrimazole troches dissolved in the mouth twice a day are very successful in clearing such infections. The white oral lesions of lichen planus have been mentioned above. Leukoplakia is discussed in Ch. 97.

GLOSSITIS AND DISEASES AFFECTING THE TONGUE. Two common clinical varieties of glossitis (see Ch. 97) are geographic tongue and black hairy tongue. *Geographic tongue* is a recurrent condition characterized by loss of filiform papillae on the dorsum of the tongue. Typically, a white margin of desquamating epithelium surrounds a central, red, atrophic area. Lesions often migrate across the surface of the tongue, giving a maplike appearance. The lesions may be uncomfortable but are often asymptomatic. The cause is unknown, and no treatment is available. *Black hairy tongue* is a condition recognized by elongated black or brown filiform papillae that grow on the posterior tongue and extend toward the tip. The condition is seen in patients using systemic antibiotics and in those who smoke or chew tobacco and have poor oral hygiene, allowing an overgrowth of pigment-producing bacteria. Gentle brushing of the involved area with a soft tooth brush and hydrogen peroxide several times a day may be of some value.

Strawberry tongue is the name applied to the white exudative glossitis with prominent red papillae poking through the exudate. After several days the tongue becomes beefy red. Typically a strawberry tongue is found in scarlet fever, Kawasaki's disease, and toxic shock syndrome.

Atrophy of the filiform papillae occurs as a response to iron-deficiency anemia and vitamin B$_{12}$ and folate deficiency.

Glossodynia, or burning tongue syndrome, occurs in elderly women and is usually a psychological condition without mucosal abnormalities. Occasionally glossitis or stomatitis occurs as a result of irritant reactions to chewing gum, mouthwashes, and dentifrices.

CARCINOMA OF THE MUCOUS MEMBRANES. Squamous cell carcinoma is the most common oral malignancy, and its incidence increases with age (see Ch. 97). The sites of origin in order of decreasing frequency are the tongue, lower lip, oropharynx, floor of the mouth, gingiva, buccal mucosa, and hard palate. Predisposing factors include use of all forms of tobacco (especially smokeless) and alcohol. AIDS patients may develop Kaposi's sarcoma on the palate, and such patients have an increased number of squamous cell cancers, especially on the tongue. Premalignant and malignant mucous membrane cancers are usually painless and appear most commonly as red, erythroplastic lesions in two distinct forms. The first is a granular, red, velvety lesion with either stippled or patchy areas of (white) keratin within or peripheral to the lesion. The second appears as a smooth, nongranular lesion, primarily red, with minimal or no keratosis. Leukoplakia or white lesions may also be precancerous, but only 4 per cent of leukoplakias develop into cancer. Less than 5 per cent of patients have attendant bleeding, ulceration, or induration with early cancers. It is incumbent upon the practitioner finding such red or white lesions to remove irritants that might cause keratoses; if the lesions do not resolve over a two- to four-week period, they should be biopsied.

DISEASES OF THE LIPS. Irritant or allergic contact cheilitis with redness, scaling, and fissuring can result from topical medications (lip salves), cosmetics (lipsticks), mouthwashes and dentifrices, and various dental materials. A careful history may establish the probable cause, which must be confirmed by patch testing.

Angular cheilitis, or *perleche*, is an acute or chronic inflammation of the skin and contiguous labial mucous membrane at the angles of the mouth. Causative factors include poorly fitting dentures that permit saliva to accumulate at the angles of the mouth, riboflavin and iron deficiencies, and *Candida* infections.

Actinic cheilitis is a dry, scaling premalignant reaction, often with white, leukoplakic plaques most pronounced on the lower lip, in individuals chronically exposed to ultraviolet light.

Alterations of Hair Growth

The evaluation of patients with alopecia or hirsutism requires a detailed history, physical examination, and, at times, laboratory and biopsy examination. Important points in the history include age of onset, medications taken, recent emotional or physical stress, diet, grooming techniques, and family history of baldness or hair disorders.

Hair Loss (Alopecia)

In the growth phase, scalp hair grows about 10 to 15 mm every month. Physical, chemical, and emotional events cause fluctuations in hair growth and if severe enough may stop growth entirely. The physical examination is important in noting the pattern of hair loss and whether or not scarring is present. Nonscarring alopecia may be a temporary phenomenon, whereas scarring is indicative of permanent hair loss.

NONSCARRING ALOPECIA. *Localized Alopecia.* *Alopecia areata* is characterized by well-circumscribed, round or oval patches of nonscarring hair loss, usually over the scalp or in the beard, eyebrows, or eyelashes. Erythema may be present early in the course of the patches. Characteristically the periphery of patches of hair loss is studded with "exclamation point hairs," so named because these hairs are fractured, with tapered shafts resembling punctuation marks. Histologic features of this disease include small dystrophic hair follicles and a lymphocytic infiltrate around the hair bulbs. Occasionally all the scalp hair is lost (alopecia totalis), and all the body hair may fall out (alopecia universalis). Alopecia areata has a variable, unpredictable course. Most patients regrow hair within a few months, but one fourth of individuals experience recurrences. The more extensive the alopecia, the poorer the prognosis. Alopecia involving the occipital region or eyebrows, lashes, and nasal hairs portends a poor prognosis. Alopecia areata may be an autoimmune disease and is occasionally associated with Hashimoto's thyroiditis and pernicious anemia. Topical, intralesional, and systemic steroids give variable benefits. Recent modes of therapy include induction of allergic or irritant contact dermatitis (1 per cent anthralin, or topical dinitrochlorobenzene), photochemotherapy with PUVA, and topical minoxidil.

Tinea capitis is most likely to be confused with alopecia areata. However, tinea infection appears as one or more patches of hair loss with mild scaling and erythema and broken hair shafts leaving residual black stumps (black dot ringworm). Although Wood's light examination will cause hairs to fluoresce bright green with *Microsporum audouini* and *M. canis* infections, these are now rare causes of tinea capitis; rather, nonfluorescing *Trichophyton tonsurans* is the usual etiology. Griseofulvin is the drug of choice in treating these infections.

Trichotillomania refers to traumatic, self-induced alopecia and results from compulsive twisting and rubbing, which causes breaking and epilation of the hair shafts. The scalp is usually affected, less often the eyebrows and lashes. If the patient can be given insight into the nature of the condition it is self-limited, but when more severe emotional problems underlie the trichotillomania, referral for psychiatric evaluation should be considered.

Women who develop hair thinning at the margins of the scalp may be using excessive traction or other traumatic hair styling techniques (*traction alopecia*). Traction from overtight hair curling such as corn rowing and the use of hot combs to straighten hair leads to progressive hair thinning and even scarring.

Hair loss is sometimes seen in the scalp of patients with *secondary syphilis*. The hair loss is spotty, often "moth-eaten" in appearance.

Androgenic alopecia, or male pattern baldness, involves the frontal, vertex, and upper occipital regions of the scalp while sparing the posterior and lateral margins. The process may begin at any age after puberty, with temporal recession of hair usually noted first. There is no actual loss of hair but rather the conversion of thick terminal hairs to fine, unpigmented, poorly seen vellus hairs. Common baldness is genetically predetermined and androgen dependent. Males who are castrated prepubertally or men born with low testosterone production, as in Klinefelter's syndrome, do not become bald, regardless of their genetic predisposition to balding. Women may also show balding, but it is milder with only diffuse thinning. However, women with elevated androgen levels, as occur in masculinizing disorders, have baldness in a pattern similar to that in men. Topical minoxidil may slow androgenic hair loss. Surgical techniques such as hair transplants (plugs of hair-bearing areas from the sides of the scalp placed in the thinned frontal and crown areas) or scalp reduction may be useful in some patients.

Diffuse or Generalized Alopecia. *Stress alopecia,* or *telogen effluvium,* is a transient, reversible, diffuse hair loss of scalp hair that results from alterations in the normal hair cycle. Normally 80 to 85 per cent of scalp hair follicles are in the growing anagen stage, while 15 to 20 per cent are in the resting (telogen) stage of growth (Ch. 531). Severe emotional and physiologic stress (high fever, systemic illness, major surgery with general anesthesia, crash diet) and certain drugs (heparin, coumarin, allopurinol, amphetamines, beta-blocking agents, lithium, probenecid, thiouracil) may cause growing anagen hairs to convert prematurely to resting telogen hairs, which are subsequently shed. Pregnancy and oral contraceptives cause hairs to grow continually, rather than cycling at programmed times to telogen. After childbirth or discontinuation of oral contraceptives, anagen follicles "catch up" by simultaneously entering telogen, and shedding follows two to four months later. If the stress resolves, the hair regrows in four to six months. Diffuse hair loss may not be noticeable until there is greater than 50 per cent scalp hair loss. Therefore, the patient may only become aware of increased hair shedding (greater than 125 to 150 hairs per day) without thinning. Gentle pulling of the hair verifies the degree of shedding; if more than five hairs come out when a dozen are grasped, excessive shedding is present. All the hair bulbs that come out are telogen (i.e., a white bulb at the end of the shaft instead of an elongate white sheath as seen in anagen hairs).

Toxic alopecia, or *anagen effluvium,* occurs if hair growth is disrupted during anagen. The newly synthesized hair shaft is weakened and the hair breaks readily. Thinning may be extreme, occurring within a few weeks of an insult, involving all 80 per cent of follicles in anagen on the scalp. Chemotherapeutic agents, especially Adriamycin and related agents, exert their effect on rapidly growing cells in the hair bulb and commonly cause anagen hair damage in cancer patients receiving chemotherapy. Radiotherapy to the scalp area does the same thing. *Retinoids* and *hypervitaminosis A* cause hair loss owing to their interference with keratinization.

Diffuse hair loss over the scalp occurs in *hypothyroidism,* associated with hair that is dry and brittle. Nutritional deficiency (essential fatty acid, biotin, zinc, iron deficiency anemia) also cause diffuse alopecia.

Seborrheic dermatitis, with erythema and yellow, greasy scales throughout the scalp, may also be associated with mild, diffuse hair loss. Treatment of the seborrhea with tar shampoos and topical steroids to control the inflammatory response will reverse the hair loss.

Diffuse scalp hair loss also occurs because of *hair shaft weakness,* either acquired (due to braiding, permanent wave solutions, or excessive heat when drying or straightening hair) or resulting from congenital hair shaft weakness. Patients with congenital hair weakness have sparse fine or wiry hair from early childhood. A few of the more common conditions that can be identified with the naked eye, hand lens, or microscope include short beaded hair—monilethrix; twisted hair—pili torti; banded hair—low sulfur hair syndrome; and trichorrhexis nodosa—multiple hair shaft fractures.

SCARRING ALOPECIA. Scarring alopecias display atrophy of the scalp and absence of hair follicles. These cicatricial areas of hair loss can be the result of a variety of pathologic processes that permanently destroy the hair follicles.

Localized Scarring Alopecia. *Systemic lupus erythematosus* causes diffuse, nonscarring alopecia of the scalp in 20 per cent of patients, along with short, broken (lupus) hairs in the frontal margin, whereas *discoid lupus erythematosus* causes oval scarring areas of alopecia. Typical plaques have an active erythematous margin, white atrophic center, and telangiectasias and keratin-filled follicles.

Morphea, when it involves the scalp, causes firm, hairless, ivory colored, indurated lesions. At times morphea takes on linear patterns that simulate saber wound (en coup de sabre).

Aplasia cutis is a developmental, rectilinear defect in skin formation anywhere on the scalp but usually on the vertex in the newborn.

A number of *physical injuries* such as mechanical trauma, burns, and radiodermatitis may also cause local scarring alopecias.

Nonlocalized Scarring Alopecia. *Lichen planus* may cause diffuse, patchy scarring alopecia (*lichen planopilaris*). Typical lichen planus lesions are often found in other areas of the body. Biopsy of the affected areas may help in the diagnosis.

Poorly understood conditions of the scalp, *pseudopelade* and *folliculitis decalvans* cause oval, scarred, bald areas that are often multiple and may coalesce to form large, irregular, noninflammatory plaques, most often on the vertex. Pseudopelade may be the result of a variety of entities, including lupus erythematosus, lichen planus, or scleroderma. Folliculitis decalvans is characterized by follicular inflammation that leads to destruction of follicles and permanent alopecia. Small follicular pustules are usually seen.

Hirsutism (Excessive Hair Growth)

Excessive hair growth, usually a complaint of females, may be due to either endocrinologic or nonendocrinologic conditions. When women are affected in those areas of the body which normally develop hair as a secondary sex characteristic in males, their hirsutism generally reflects treatable endocrinopathy, as it is these follicles that are responsive to high concentrations of testosterone and are capable of converting various androgens to dihydrotestosterone (Ch. 531).

NONENDOCRINE HIRSUTISM. *Ethnic* or *racial hirsutism* is characterized by excessive hair growth on the upper lip, beard area, chest, nipples, or lower abdomen in women without menstrual abnormalities or masculization. Type of hair, rate of hair growth, and distribution of hair over the body differ among the races, relating to variations in the sensitivity of follicles to circulating androgens. A male pattern of hirsutism is more common in females whose ancestors came from the southern parts of Europe. Orientals and American Indians have less body hair. If endocrinologic abnormalities are not found (serum testosterone, dehydroepiandrosterone, and androstenedione are normal), bleaching or shaving may be sufficient to make the hair less noticeable. Electrolysis permanently destroys hair follicles but is time consuming and costly. Spironolactone,* which has antiandrogenic properties (200 mg per day), used for a period of 12 months is also useful in decreasing hair growth.

---

*This use is not listed in the manufacturer's directive.

Certain *drugs* may also increase hair growth. Androgenic or steroidal medications, such as anabolic steroids, corticosteroids, and contraceptives may cause increased hair growth in the beard, chest, and groin areas. Drugs such as phenytoin, phenothiazines, cyclosporin, and minoxidil cause excess hair in both men and women anywhere on the body.

Porphyria cutanea tarda causes increased hairiness of the face, especially on the temples and pinnae of the ears. Treatment of the condition results in decrease of hair growth.

ENDOCRINE HIRSUTISM. A distinction must be made between hirsutism caused by increased androgen production with and without virilization. In general, virilization is a sign of markedly elevated androgens derived from the adrenal glands or ovaries, especially adrenogenital syndrome, congenital adrenal hyperplasia, Cushing's disease or syndrome, Stein-Leventhal syndrome (polycystic ovarian syndrome), and occasionally malignant adrenal or ovarian tumors. Any woman with hirsutism and accompanying virilization should be tested for excess cortisol and androgen production.

Simple or *idiopathic hirsutism* is the designation given to those hirsute women in whom a specific etiologic diagnosis cannot be made and in whom normal or slightly elevated adrenal or ovarian androgens are found. The cause may be slightly increased production and metabolism of androgens or increased sensitivity of hair follicles to normal levels of androgens. Such patients have been successfully treated with cyclically administered birth control pills or with spironolactone.

PHOTOSENSITIVITY AND OTHER REACTIONS TO LIGHT

Certain wavelengths of light are capable of inducing a number of undesirable cutaneous reactions, including sunburn, skin aging, carcinogenesis, and a variety of photosensitivity reactions.

Clinically, photorelated conditions occur in a typical distribution of light-exposed areas which should make the diagnosis of light-related reactions apparent (see Fig. 532–2). Thus, maximal changes occur over the forehead, malar eminences, bridge of the nose, and pinnae of the ears, with sparing of the upper lip (shaded by the nose), periorbital areas, and submental region. The V of the neck, dorsum of the hands, and forearms are often involved, with a sharp demarcation where clothing and watch bands cover the skin. In addition, light must be suspected from historical evidence. Seasonal recurrences are seen, especially in the spring or early summer. The evoked reaction may be to light alone, to light in association with exogenous substances (taken internally, such as drugs or externally applied materials), or to abnormal metabolites as in porphyria.

The incidence of photoreactions depends on a number of factors such as the amount of light reaching the earth's surface, season of the year, latitude and weather conditions, and thickness of the ozone layer, as well as topographic features of the environment. There are some useful climatologic and environmental factors to keep in mind which have bearing on the amount of sunlight hitting the skin. For example, 50 per cent of the daily ultraviolet light is emitted between 11 A.M. and 2 P.M., so avoiding exposure to sunlight during this time may be useful in minimizing photoreactions. Sitting in the shade does not protect against UV exposure, because 50 per cent of the ambient ultraviolet light is received; 90 per cent of ultraviolet light penetrates clouds, so one can get sunburns even in the shade and on cloudy days.

Electromagnetic radiation (EMG) from the sun has been arbitrarily classified into spectral regions measured in nanometers, ranging from short cosmic rays to long radiowaves. The solar spectrum that commonly affects human skin is in the ultraviolet light range (290 to 400 nm), which is subdivided into three bands designated as UVC (shorter than 290 nm), UVB (290 to 320 nm), and UVA, or long-wave ultraviolet light

(320 to 400 nm). UVC does not reach the earth, being absorbed by ozone; UVB, or the sunburn spectrum, causes burning, tanning, aging, and carcinogenic changes in the skin. UVA is melanogenic and erythrogenic, but the amount of energy required to produce these effects is 1000 times greater than UVB. UVA causes skin reactions through window glass, and these wavelengths are often responsible for photoreactions in which chemical photosensitizers and UV radiation interact to cause inflammatory skin reactions.

The amount of UV light reaching various levels of the skin depends on wavelength. The longer wavelengths penetrate deeper into the dermis. Thus, depending on the wavelength of light and depth of penetration, the reactions may involve absorption by cellular DNA, RNA, and cutaneous proteins (keratin, collagen, etc.).

Direct Photo Effects on the Skin

ACUTE EFFECTS. Sunburning and tanning are common acute reactions to sun exposure and are attributed primarily to UVB light, although prolonged exposure to UVA can produce mild burn and marked hyperpigmentation. The sunburn reaction is a complex inflammatory process causing dyskeratotic cells, spongiosis, vacuolation of keratinocytes, and edema from capillary leakage, 12 to 24 hours after exposure to light. Occasionally, in addition to redness and pain, blisters may evolve. Prostaglandins may play a role in the burn reaction, as they are found in increased quantities in UV sunburned skin, and aspirin or indomethacin, prostaglandin synthesis inhibitors, can reduce the burn.

Three to four days after a sunburn, new melanin pigment is formed. Several cellular and molecular changes occur in the skin after each sunburn reaction which, if repeated, may lead to the chronic effects of UV light. A few days after UV light burning, epidermal mitosis and hyperplasia occur and DNA, RNA, and proteins in the skin are damaged.

CHRONIC EFFECTS. Degenerative changes of the skin consisting of wrinkling, telangiectasias, and keratoses are the long-term effects of chronic exposure to UV light. A furrowed and leathery condition of the skin may develop along with yellow papules and plaques due to solar degeneration of the dermal collagen, especially in fair-skinned individuals. These changes are caused by both UVB and UVA radiation. Such changes can be minimized by daily topical applications of effective sunscreens (see Ch. 533).

A number of malignant and premalignant skin lesions are associated with chronic sun exposure, including actinic keratoses, keratoacanthomas, basal cell and squamous cell carcinomas, and probably melanomas (see above).

Indirect Photo Effects on the Skin

Photoreactions that occur when systemic or topical chemicals induce photosensitivity or when there is an underlying immunologic, biochemical, or genetic abnormality that predisposes to sun sensitivity are considered indirect reactions; i.e., the sun alone does not cause photoreactions.

EXOGENOUS FACTORS CAUSING PHOTOSENSITIVITY. Chemical agents either taken systemically or placed topically on the skin can cause one of two general types of photoreactions: phototoxic and photoallergic. In these photosensitivity reactions, the absorption spectrum of a given drug, substance, or chemical is maximal at a certain wavelength of light that induces molecular changes in the exogenous material, which, in turn, initiates the cutaneous reaction. In most of the drug or chemical photosensitivity reactions, the wavelengths that evoke abnormal reactions are in the 320 to 400 nm (UVA) region. The reactions include acute, abnormal sunburn responses and eczematous and urticarial reactions.

Phototoxic reactions are those nonimmunologic cutaneous responses that occur in most individuals when enough light energy of a specific wavelength is absorbed by an appropriate concentration of drug or chemical in the skin. Free radicals are generated in the photosensitizer which damage cell membranes and lysosomes, inducing an exaggerated sunburn reaction, with intense redness, swelling, pain, and occasionally blistering. Most phototoxic agents absorb UVB light.

Photoallergic reactions to topical chemicals or internal drugs represent an acquired, altered response to light which involves immunologic mechanisms. Absorption of specific wavelengths of light by chemicals or drugs causes changes in their chemical configuration so that these substances become haptens that bind to proteins in the skin to become a complete antigen capable of eliciting a type IV delayed hypersensitivity immunologic response. The clinical manifestations of such photoallergic reactions are usually eczematous in nature (occasionally urticarial), evolving 24 hours after exposure to the sun in sun-exposed areas of the skin. The action spectrum is generally long-range UVA light, and less energy is required to elicit the reaction than for the production of phototoxic reactions.

Table 534–15 summarizes the differences between phototoxic and photoallergic reactions.

SYSTEMIC PHOTOSENSITIZERS. Drugs may cause either phototoxic or photoallergic reactions. Table 534–16 lists some of the drugs and chemicals that may induce photosensitivities and the type of reaction and action spectrum thought to induce them.

TOPICAL AGENTS CAUSING PHOTOSENSITIVITY. Most topical photosensitizing agents respond to the UVA action spectrum. Drugs and chemicals that induce *phototoxic contact reactions* include coal tar derivatives, topical drugs (phenothiazines, sulfonamides), dyes (eosins, methylene blue), and plant derivatives (furocoumarins). The photosensitive properties of coal tar derivatives and furocoumarins (psoralens) are utilized in treating certain skin diseases with ultraviolet light.

When plants, vegetables, or fruits containing a phototoxic chemical cause phototoxicity, the reaction is referred to as a *phytophotodermatitis*. Photocontact dermatitis develops with contact with plants in the Umbelliferae family, such as figs, cow parsnip, fennel, parsley, parsnip, and gas plant. Phyto-

TABLE 534–16. SYSTEMIC PHOTOSENSITIZERS

Name	Type of Photoreaction	Action Spectrum (nm)
Sulfonamides	Phototoxic and photoallergic	290–320
Sulfonylureas (tolbutamide, chlorpropamide)	Phototoxic	290–360
Chlorothiazides	Phototoxic and photoallergic	290–320 320–400
Phenothiazines	Phototoxic, urticaria eruption, gray-blue hyperpigmentation	290–400
Antibiotics (tetracyclines, griseofulvin, nalidixic acid)	Phototoxic and photoallergic bullae	320–400
Furocoumarins (psoralens)	Phototoxic	
Nonsteroidal anti-inflammatory agents	Phototoxic and photoallergic	Unknown
Anticancer drugs (DTIC, fluorouracil, methotrexate, vinblastin)	Phototoxic	Unknown
Estrogens, progestins, and other drugs	Phototoxic, melasma	?290–320
Chlordiazepoxide (Librium)	Photoallergic	290–360
Cyclamates	Phototoxic and photoallergic	290–360
Quinidine, quinine	Photoallergic	320–400

photodermatitis also occurs in individuals exposed to Persian limes and celery. Such reactions are caused by furocoumarin compounds found in the plant which readily penetrate the epidermis. Two things are needed for initiation of phytophotodermatitis: (1) contact with a sensitizing furocoumarin and (2) subsequent exposure to UV radiation greater than 320 nm. Phytophotodermatitis may take on unique clinical forms: (1) berloque dermatitis presents as streaky erythema followed by hyperpigmentation in areas where perfumes containing oil of Bergamot (a psoralen) are applied to the skin (e.g., on the neck); (2) criss-cross linear streaks of erythema, vesicles, and bullae that heal with hyperpigmentation where meadow grass or other related plants rub on the skin; (3) oil of the rind of a Persian lime causes erythema and pigmentation on the hands of bartenders.

Photoallergic contact dermatitis, a form of delayed allergic hypersensitivity, evolves in some individuals after exposure to such chemicals as fragrances (methylcoumarin and musk ambrette), halogenated salicylanilides, sunscreens, and blankophores, or optical whitening agents, used in laundry soaps and bleaches. These photoallergic responses appear as eczematous reactions. A number of perfumes (after-shave lotions, colognes, etc.) contain musk ambrette, a synthetic fragrance fixative that causes a photoeczematous reaction over the face and hands. Paradoxically, sunscreening agents containing PABA esters and cinnamates that readily absorb UV light may cause eczematous photoallergic reactions. A small number of individuals will have persistent chronic eczematous dermatitis after all exposure to the photosensitizing agent has ceased—so-called persistent light reactivity. Such patients may be so photosensitive that they react to artificial fluorescent light.

Identifying the cause of contact photoallergic reactions can be done with photopatch testing (Ch. 532). Treatment of photocontact sensitivity obviously begins by eliminating the photosensitizing agent and minimizing sunlight exposure (avoiding sun and use of sunscreens). Topical and, at times, oral steroids may be needed to decrease the cutaneous inflammatory response.

ENDOGENOUS CONDITIONS ASSOCIATED WITH PHOTOSENSITIVITY. Certain immunologic, biochemical, and genetic diseases display photoreactions as a prominent feature.

TABLE 534–15. CHARACTERISTICS OF PHOTOTOXIC AND PHOTOALLERGIC REACTIONS OF THE SKIN

Reaction	Phototoxic	Photoallergic
Clinical changes	Prolonged sunburn	Eczema or urticaria
Relative incidence	All people receiving chemical and exposed to appropriate wavelength of light	Few individuals exposed to chemical and appropriate wavelength of light
Concentration of drug necessary for reactions	High	Low
Reaction possible on first exposure	Yes	No
Incubation period necessary after first exposure	No	Yes
"Flares" at distant, previously involved sites possible	No	Yes
Cross-reaction to structurally related agents	No	Frequent
Immunologic mechanism involved	No	Yes—type IV delayed hypersensitivity
Cross-reactions to structurally related agents	Infrequent	Frequent
Concentration of drug or chemical necessary for reaction	High	Low

Immunologic diseases with photosensitivity include connective tissue conditions such as lupus erythematosus, both discoid and systemic, and solar urticaria. Solar urticaria, hives with itching and burning, evolves within minutes of sunlight exposure and lasts an hour or more. The inciting wavelength of light differs among patients.

Biochemical conditions associated with photosensitivity include two forms of porphyria: porphyria cutanea tarda and erythropoietic protoporphyria. These are discussed above (see Vesiculobullous Diseases).

Pellagra, once a common disease, especially in the southeastern United States, is caused by an inadequate diet and a deficiency of nicotinic acid. It is still seen occasionally with alcoholism, poor dietary intake in the elderly, and malabsorption. The carcinoid syndrome may also be associated with pellagra because tryptophan, the precursor of nicotinic acid, is diverted to serotonin production by the tumor. A scaly dermatitis on sun-exposed parts of the skin, especially on the face, the neck, and the back of the hands, is seen in association with diarrhea and dementia (the three D's). Low serum vitamin levels will establish the diagnosis of this condition, and dietary replacement will clear the skin and other signs of the disease.

Other Photosensitivity Conditions

A condition known as *polymorphous light eruption* (PML) presents with a variety of skin lesions, including eczematous patches, red to violaceous papules or plaques, and urticarial lesions over the face, the nape and V of the neck, and the back of the hands. The rash characteristically arises hours to days after sun exposure. The onset is frequently in early summer with some degree of resistance being acquired with continued sun exposure. Recurrences each spring and summer are common, and the eruption remits during the winter. The disease may begin at any age, but it is most frequent during the first half of life. The etiology is unknown, and its diagnosis is one of excluding other photosensitivity conditions.

PML may respond to the use of sunscreens with an SPF of 15 and, if elicited by UVA light, sunscreens with benzophenone or anthranilate to improve protection against the UVA spectrum. If sunscreens fail, the induction of tolerance by tanning with PUVA or UVB light or a short course of antimalarial agents or oral steroids may occasionally be needed.

Actinic reticuloid is another form of persistent photodermatitis of unknown etiology which occurs in middle-aged males and causes a most distressing photoreaction of red papules and pruritic eczematous patches. Both UVB and UVA appear to play a role. PUVA chemotherapy may help control the condition.

DERMATOLOGIC MANIFESTATIONS IN THE IMMUNOCOMPROMISED HOST

Immunosuppression causes an increase in benign and malignant skin growths as well as a variety of infections in the skin (see Ch. 258). Cutaneous neoplasms such as squamous cell and basal cell carcinomas occur with a much higher frequency than would be expected. Transplant patients have an estimated risk of skin cancer that is 7.1 times greater than normal. Most patients have multiple skin cancers.

Any skin lesion, no matter how innocuous, should be carefully evaluated in the immunosuppressed host. The gross morphology of infections is so frequently modified by the altered inflammatory response in the immunocompromised patient that early skin biopsies are essential for diagnosis. The array of potential pathogens is imposing in these patients, and even common infectious processes are greatly modified or obscured by immunocompromising illness. Skin infections are common, accounting for 22 to 33 per cent of infections in immunosuppressed patients.

Microbial involvement of the skin and subcutaneous tissue can be grouped into two major categories in immunocompromised patients: (1) *primary skin infections* that are typical of those occurring in nonimmunocompromised hosts, widespread involvement with infectious agents that commonly cause localized skin infection, and primary skin infections from opportunistic agents that rarely cause skin infection in normal patients; and (2) *disseminated systemic infections* metastatic to the skin from a noncutaneous portal of entry.

PRIMARY SKIN INFECTIONS. Typical primary infections, including group A streptococcal and *Staphylococcus aureus* cellulitis, are frequent, although more unusual causes of cellulitis in granulocytopenic patients must also be considered (*Pseudomonas*, anaerobic bacteria). Skin biopsy of the cellulitic areas for Gram's stain and culture is often helpful.

Unusually widespread, primary cutaneous infections by viruses and skin dermatophytes are also common. Warts caused by papillomavirus may be numerous, disfiguring, and difficult to remove. Malignant transformation has been documented in such warts in immunosuppressed individuals. Herpes simplex infections may present as chronic, large, ulcerated lesions persisting for weeks to months (herpes phagedena, especially in the genital areas), and there may be internal dissemination from cutaneous sites. Reactivation of herpes zoster infections is common in immunocompromised hosts, with systemic dissemination. Widespread dermatophyte infections of the skin appear as scaling, red patches that provide a portal of entry for bacterial infection.

Unusual opportunistic primary skin infections with atypical *Mycobacterium*, *Aspergillus*, *Rhizopus*, and *Candida* organisms cause cellulitis-like reactions that form a central pustule and eschar. Skin biopsy of such lesions with a portion of the biopsy processed by frozen section and specially stained for AFB and fungi may identify the pathologic organisms rapidly.

DISSEMINATED INFECTION METASTATIC TO THE SKIN. Hematogenous dissemination of infection to the skin from distant primary sites frequently occurs in patients with impaired host defenses. Three groups of organisms are responsible for this: (1) *Pseudomonas* and other gram-negative bacilli; (2) endemic systemic mycoses (*Histoplasma*, *Coccidioides*); and (3) opportunistic fungi (*Aspergillus*, *Candida*, Mucoraceae). The range of cutaneous clinical presentations of these infections is varied and mimicked by all of these infections, namely (a) *vesicles and bullae* that become hemorrhagic, (b) *gangrenous cellulitis* with necrotic ulcerations, and (c) widespread, red, warm, fluctuant *nodules* with pustules and purpura. Prompt biopsy of these lesions with frozen sections stained for bacterial and hyphal elements may provide rapid diagnosis.

CUTANEOUS DRUG REACTIONS

Rashes are among the most common adverse reactions to drugs and occur in 2 to 3 per cent of hospitalized patients. Any drug can potentially produce a rash, and over-the-counter preparations should be considered when defining drug reactions.

The causes of adverse drug reactions are multiple, including *toxic* (too much drug is given or degradation of the drug is slow owing to an underlying disease or action of another drug), *idiosyncratic* (unanticipated side effects), and *allergic* reactions. Because tests for drug allergy are not available, it is often difficult to be sure one is dealing with an allergic reaction. However, a hypersensitivity reaction can be suspected when (1) rechallenge or re-exposure to small amounts of the drug elicits the same response, (2) the reaction appears following several days to weeks of administration of the drug, (3) the reaction occurs when the patient is exposed to a structurally similar drug, and (4) the clinical response does not resemble the general pharmacologic effects of the drug.

TABLE 534–17. CUTANEOUS DRUG REACTIONS

Type of Skin Reaction	Drugs Likely to Cause Skin Reaction
Eczematous (allergic contact reaction)	Antihistamines, neomycin, formaldehyde, sulfonamides
Photodermatitis	
Phototoxic	Chlorpromazine, psoralens, demeclocycline, doxycycline
Photoallergic	Promethazine, griseofulvin, Diuril, hypoglycemic drugs
Exfoliative dermatitis	Carbamazepine, hydantoins, nitrofurantoin, isoniazid, gold, allopurinol, phenothiazines
Maculopapular eruption (exanthematous)	Penicillin, sulfonamides, hypoglycemic drugs, phenothiazines, allopurinol, phenytoin, quinine, gold salts, captopril, meprobamate
Papulosquamous reactions Psoriasiform, lichen planus, pityriasis rosea–like	Beta blockers, lithium (psoriasiform), thiazides, gold, phenothiazines, quinidine, antimalarials (lichen planus–like); gold (PR-like); others—practolol, dapsone, ethambutol, furosemide
Vesiculobullous reactions	Azapropazone, captopril, clonidine, furosemide, gold, psoralens, barbiturates, phenytoin, Hydrodiuril, penicillamine
Toxic epidermal necrolysis	Acetazolamide, allopurinol, barbiturates, carbamazepines, gold, hydantoin, nitrofurantoin, pentazocine, tetracycline, quinidine
Pustular—acneiform reactions	Androgen hormones, corticosteroids, iodides, bromides, hydantoin, lithium
Urticaria and erythemas	
Urticaria	May occur with anaphylaxis; penicillin, xenogenic sera, cephalosporins, sulfonamides, barbiturates, hydralazine, phenylbutazone, hydantoin, quinidine, x-ray contrast media
Erythema multiforme	Sulfonamides, hydantoin, barbiturates, penicillin, carbamazepines, allopurinol, amikacin, phenothiazides
Nodular lesions	
Erythema nodosum	Birth control pills, sulfonamides, diuretics, gold, clonidine, propranolol, furosemide, opiates, penicillin
Vasculitis reaction	Allopurinol, barbiturates, carbamazepine, chlorothiazide, cimetidine, gold, indomethacin, hydantoin, piperazine, sulfonamides
Telangiectatic and LE reactions	Procainamide, hydralazine, phenytoin, penicillamine, trimethadione, methyldopa, carbamazepine, griseofulvin, nalidixic acid, oral contraceptives, propranolol
Pigmentary reaction	Anticonvulsants, antimalarials, antitumor agents (Adriamycin, bleomycin, busulfan, cyclophosphamide, doxorubicin, melphalan), oral contraceptives, corticotropin, tetracyclines, phenothiazines, amiodarone
Other cutaneous reactions	
Fixed drug reactions	Phenolphthalein, barbiturates, gold, sulfonamides, meprobamate, penicillin, tetracyclines, analgesics
Alopecia	Alkylating agents, antimetabolites, heparin, coumarin, hydantoin, accutane, gold, nitrofurantoin, propranolol, colchicine, allopurinol
Hypertrichosis	Anabolic agents, diazoxide, minoxidil, phenytoin

Some of the most common drugs causing skin reactions in hospitalized patients are amoxicillin, trimethoprim-sulfamethoxazole, ampicillin, penicillin G, allopurinol, dipyrone, gentamicin sulfate, mefruside, nitrazepam, and barbiturates. Drugs least likely to cause allergic skin reactions include digoxin, antacids, promethazine, acetaminophen, nitroglycerin, aminophylline, propranolol, antihistamines, cromolyn, and emollient laxatives.

Table 534–17 lists the various morphologic types of drug reactions and some of the drugs capable of inducing each reaction.

Fixed drug eruptions are unique reactions that appear in the same area of the skin each time the responsible drug is administered. These appear as macular, eczematous, or even bullous, pink to dark red patches occurring as few or many lesions. When the drug is stopped the lesions fade, leaving postinflammatory hyperpigmentation. The lesions return in the same place within a few hours of taking the drug again.

Nonsteroidal anti-inflammatory drugs are being used with increasing frequency and may cause cutaneous reactions including vesiculobullous photosensitivity reactions, serum sickness, erythroderma, fixed drug reactions, and toxic epidermal necrolysis.

The treatment of drug reactions is discontinuation of the suspected agent. Often the patient is taking many drugs, and generally once a drug reaction is suspected all nonessential drugs should be stopped and appropriate substitutes used for the necessary medications. An asymptomatic eruption may require no therapy, or a mild reaction with pruritus may be controlled with topical steroid applications and antihistamines. In severe conditions such as exfoliative dermatitis, oral steroids are often indicated. Most drug eruptions resolve in one to two weeks after withdrawal of the drug, but some reactions take months to clear. While an occasional reaction may be fatal (e.g., toxic epidermal necrolysis), patients with drug eruptions usually have an excellent prognosis.

PART XXV

OCCUPATIONAL AND ENVIRONMENTAL MEDICINE

535 PRINCIPLES OF OCCUPATIONAL MEDICINE

Charles E. Becker

Occupational medicine is concerned with the physical and emotional safety and health of workers. It encompasses issues of public concern, particularly the quality of air and water, the degree of environmental pollution, and the complex mosaic of legal, economic, social, and ethical questions that are raised whenever human action produces human disorders.

Among the 100 million workers in the United States today, approximately 100,000 deaths per year are attributed to the workplace. Yet there are only 8000 physicians whose self-determined primary specialty is occupational medicine, and only 800 of these have subspecialty board certification. Primary-care internists, family physicians, and emergency physicians constitute the "front line" for identification of work-related disorders. Therefore, they must learn to target the medical history and to recognize classic signs and symptoms of occupational and environmental disorders.

Occupational medicine deals almost exclusively with diagnosis and prevention, not treatment. The diagnosis of an occupational disease may be difficult, since occupational diseases (1) may simulate many other disorders, (2) often lack unique pathology, and (3) may be marked by a long latency period between exposure and the manifestation of the disease.

Problems from chemical contamination do not always remain exclusively in the workplace; they may extend into the community: polychlorinated biphenyls (PCBs) in Japan; dioxin in Seveso, Italy; radiation exposure at Three Mile Island; mercury contamination in Minamata Bay; lead pollution in cities and around smelting plants; and nervous system, liver, and reproductive toxicity from chlordecone (Kepone) in Virginia. These events give rise to important political, social, and economic considerations that emphasize the need for specialized training in occupational medicine.

Competency in occupational medicine is best acquired from a base of general training in internal medicine, with extended knowledge and experience in epidemiology, industrial hygiene, biostatistics, and toxicology. The relationship between workplace-environmental exposure and disease centers on four basic concepts: recognition, prevention, exacerbation, latent manifestation. Workplace-associated diseases are presumed to be preventable when recognized and fully understood. Since the signs and symptoms of occupational diseases may be identical to those of many other diseases, a high level of suspicion is required for the recognition that allows prevention. Rather than causing an illness, occupational environ-

mental conditions may, in fact, exacerbate or compound a pre-existing condition. For example, a patient with toxicity from aminoglycoside antibiotics may have additional otologic injury from loud noises occurring at work. Although some environmental and occupational diseases become manifest acutely, many have a long latency period and may extend from the workplace into the family or society and thus pose important considerations in diagnostic and preventive strategies.

In occupational medicine there are four basic categories of hazard: physical, biologic, psychologic, and chemical. Physical hazards may include vibration, heat, noise, radiation, and trauma. Occupational injuries account for approximately 14,000 deaths, 245 million lost work days, and $25 billion in direct and indirect costs annually in the United States. Biologic hazards include the well-known occupational risks of hepatitis or tuberculosis, for example. Psychologic hazards of stress and work-shift changes are complex and will be discussed subsequently. Chemical hazards involve exposure to solvents, dusts, vapors, and gases. It is important here to distinguish between toxicity and hazard. *Toxicity* is the inherent capability of a material to cause injury to a living cell. *Hazard* is the chance of a resultant injury from use of such a material in a given setting. Asbestos, for example, is a useful fire retardant construction material with known basic toxicity that may become hazardous during repair or demolition work or fire, which may cause its release into the air.

In occupational medicine one is also concerned with the difference between exposure and dose. Exposure is determined by surveillance of the environment with the knowledge that a toxic agent(s) has had the potential of being delivered into the body. For example, environmental measurements of lead can provide an index of exposure. Dose, however, can be assessed only by biologic monitoring of blood, urine, and hair, and indices of enzyme systems that may be affected. In the case of lead, the total dose delivered is dependent on the amount that is respirable and the amount absorbed from the gastrointestinal tract. Figure 535–1 depicts the complex interactions in the field of occupational medicine.

This chapter outlines some of the basic concepts and a few selected disorders encompassed in occupational medicine. Other chapters in this section describe at length occupational diseases of the lung (Ch. 536) and of the skin (Ch. 538) and a variety of chemical and physical sources of injury. Some chapters in other parts of the book contain useful information related to the discipline: toxic nephropathies (Ch. 82), epidemiology of cancer (Ch. 170), painful back and painful shoulders (Ch. 447 and 448), and neuropathies associated with the workplace (Ch. 542).

THE OCCUPATIONAL-ENVIRONMENTAL HISTORY

Key elements of an occupational and environmental history should be added to the data base collected on all patients. In

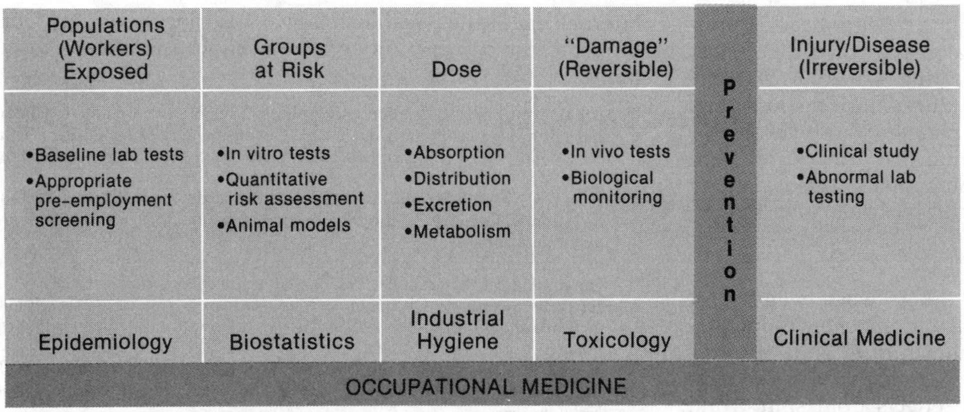

Populations (Workers) Exposed	Groups at Risk	Dose	"Damage" (Reversible)	P r e v e n t i o n	Injury/Disease (Irreversible)
•Baseline lab tests •Appropriate pre-employment screening	•In vitro tests •Quantitative risk assessment •Animal models	•Absorption •Distribution •Excretion •Metabolism	•In vivo tests •Biological monitoring		•Clinical study •Abnormal lab testing
Epidemiology	Biostatistics	Industrial Hygiene	Toxicology		Clinical Medicine
OCCUPATIONAL MEDICINE					

FIGURE 535-1. Multidisciplinary approach to occupational (environmental) medicine.

every problem-oriented assessment of a current illness, individual problem lists should include such questions concerning the occupational health history: Are symptoms associated with work, or do they improve during vacations and weekends? Are other workers similarly affected? Is there or has there been direct exposure to dust, fumes, and chemicals? Have there been work-related injuries? Is periodic testing and medical surveillance or routine industrial hygiene sampling of the workplace performed? A careful work history should include a chronologic list of all previous jobs with a reasonably detailed description of the work site, the scope of a typical work day, and such pertinent factors as protective equipment, ventilation, and pre-employment examinations.

A specific listing of the total number of days missed on each job and the reasons for the absences may be useful. Has a worker-compensation claim been filed in the past? Does the worker perform additional jobs, i.e., is he or she moonlighting? A patient may not relate work to health, and so the physician should obtain initially, on each examination, specific answers to common occupational problems, for example, Have you ever been exposed to loud noises, excessive vibration, or heat? Do you work with asbestos? Have you been exposed to radioactive chemicals? Have you had previous chemical exposure? During the military, what were your duties?

The environmental health history should include information about industries located in the neighborhood, exposure to hazardous waste or toxic spills, jobs of the spouse, degree of air pollution, and types of hobbies and recreational activities that also may contribute to health-related problems, such as painting, sculpturing, welding, or woodworking.

In addition, it may be important to elicit a description of home insulation or heating as well as exposure to cleaning agents and insecticides. Special questions should be directed toward unique workplace problems such as working hours and job schedule (Do these affect your sleep pattern? Are you bored on the job?). The reproductive history is essential: the number of miscarriages, children, stillbirths, previous pregnancies; difficulty in conceiving; and changes in libido and menses.

SIGNS AND SYMPTOMS OF OCCUPATIONAL AND ENVIRONMENTAL DISORDERS. Because occupational and environmental diseases have a long latency and may be synergistic with other causes for disease, the clinician should always consider that the signs and symptoms may be caused by occupational or environmental conditions. Sometimes it may be useful to identify all the signs and symptoms that could be associated with disease of the environment or the workplace. A useful handbook by Daugaard provides such a guide to signs and symptoms of both acute and chronic occupational diseases compiled from standard works on toxicology and occupational medicine. For instance, knowledge of exposure to certain substances may implicate or suggest the cause: chlorinated hydrocarbons and acne; arsenic and thallium and alopecia; solvent exposure and anosmia; chlori-nated hydrocarbons and arrhythmias; and aniline dyes and bladder or other cancers.

Reproductive hazards, noise-induced hearing abnormalities, work-shift changes, and ergonomics will be discussed as important occupational entities not covered specifically by other chapters in this section.

REPRODUCTIVE HAZARDS

Seven per cent of all newborns in the United States have birth defects, approximately 70 per cent of which are of unknown cause. The relationship between exposure to environmental and occupational agents and consequent development of male and female reproductive abnormalities is an area of intense study and interest. Animal studies have demonstrated the transmission to subsequent generations of chemically induced abnormalities of sperm and at a rate determined by mendelian principles. These observations have sparked interest in predicting and thereby preventing reproductive hazards from environmental agents. Short-term bioassays for mutagenesis, such as the Ames test, have been used to screen for teratogenic agents to predict reproductive outcome. These relatively inexpensive and rapid initial screening tests of chemicals can be performed in animals or bacteria. Agents encountered in the environment or the workplace can clearly cause reproductive hazards, i.e., testicular toxicity of dibromochloropropane (DBCP) recognized in California chemical workers in 1977. Male workers with sterility suffered no systemic illness and were working in an environment that was alleged to be safe. Previous laboratory tests in animals had suggested reproductive hazards from this chemical. The controversy surrounding this event sparked great interest in this subject. To date, the following environmental and occupational agents have been shown to cause adverse reproductive effects in men: anesthetic gases, carbon disulfide, diethylstilbestrol, toluene diamine, ethylene dibromide, chlordecone, and ionizing radiation. A much stronger data base is required to assess environmental effects on pregnancy outcome, spontaneous abortion, and stillbirth.

NOISE-INDUCED HEARING LOSS

More than five million people in the United States have noise-induced hearing loss. This most common form of hearing loss is associated with damage to, and loss of, hair cells in the organ of Corti. Early or moderately advanced, noise-induced hearing loss is associated with normal hearing in the low frequencies but gradually increasing loss of hearing at higher frequencies (with a maximum of 3, 4, or 6 kHz). There may be some return toward normal function at 8 kHz. The audiometric shape of this curve is not pathognomonic because other otologic disorders (e.g., that caused by aminoglycoside antibiotic therapy) can result in an identical audiogram. Some of the hearing loss attributed to aging (presbycusis) may be due to the nearly ubiquitous noise pollution in modern society. Epidemiologic studies suggest that aging individuals in a nonindustrialized society have much better hearing preservation than older Americans. Major individual differences in susceptibility to noise-induced hearing loss occur. Men are much more susceptible to noise-induced hearing loss than women. Smoking and lack of skin pigmentation may also be risk factors for noise-induced hearing loss. Hearing impairment from occupational and environmental factors is a major and entirely preventable public health problem.

WORK-SHIFT CHANGES

Twenty per cent of American workers work evenings or nights. In some industries, such as automobile production, petrol chemicals, and textile manufacturing, shift workers number nearly 50 per cent. There is growing evidence to suggest clinically significant health effects from shift work. Twenty per cent of workers are unable to tolerate shift work, tolerance for which also diminishes with increasing age. Daily physiologic variations known as circadian rhythms are distorted by shift work, which in turn alters the quality of sleep and causes important disturbances of the gastrointestinal tract and other organs. Diabetes mellitus and epilepsy may be aggravated by shift work, and the risk of accidents may be increased. Shift workers tend to have an increased number of subjective health complaints in general and may have enhanced risk factors complicating management of other medical disorders.

ERGONOMICS

Ergonomics is the interface of a worker with his or her work station, machine, or work environment. This interface may create physical and psychologic stresses that present as common diseases to internists. Physical factors may include repetitive motion disorders, back injuries, and musculoskeletal problems. Psychologic factors involve attention span, memory, vigilance, and behavior. They may play an important role in safety in the workplace and are often called *human error.* Ergonometric problems may progress from chronic discomfort of aches and pains to temporary disabling conditions, such as sprains, strains, tendinitis, and fibromyositis syndromes. These syndromes ultimately lead to long-term disabilities—nerve entrapment, chronic back pain, and musculoskeletal disorders. Careful history taking will suggest an ergonometric problem that frequently involves highly repetitive, monotonous work or fast-paced production jobs. Sometimes extremely sedentary work, such as word processing or microscopic inspection, may also cause a disability. It may be essential to make a plant visit to observe the work station in order to assist the patient in resolving an ergonometric problem. Reducing physical and psychologic stresses may have beneficial effects that seem out of proportion with the magnitude of the changes in the work practice.

CONCLUSIONS

Strictly speaking, all diseases that are not genetic in origin are "environmental." Even genetic disorders are not totally endogenous, since they most frequently alter the ability of the host to accommodate to the environment. Broadly conceived, even the infectious diseases and nutritional disorders are environmental in origin. In practice, however, the term *environmental medicine* is used in a much more restrictive sense to reflect the chemical and physical hazards to which an individual is exposed and the injuries that may result from that exposure. Occupational medicine is that subset of environmental medicine directly concerned with the hazards of the workplace. The following chapters will describe in greater detail some of the specific hazards and injuries incident to modern occupations. The topics selected cannot be inclusive, since the boundaries of occupational and environmental medicine are indistinct, merging into the traditional domains of internal medicine, epidemiology, toxicology, surgery, orthopedics, and many other clinical and basic science disciplines.

Department of Health, Education and Welfare, NIOSH Pocket Guide to Chemical Hazards. Washington, DC, U.S. Government Printing Office, Publication No. 78-210, September 1985. *Gives the chemical names, synonyms, exposure limits, and appropriate protections for many chemicals.*
Finkel AJ (ed.): Hamilton and Hardy's Industrial Toxicology 4th ed. Littleton, MA, John Wright PSG Inc., 1983. *This is an excellent, practical guide to industrial toxicology.*
Ladou J: Current Occupational Medicine: Diagnosis and Treatment. Los Altos, Lange Medical Publications, 1987. *A full review of key occupational topics.*
Morgan WK, Seaton A: Occupational Lung Diseases. 2nd ed. Philadelphia, W.B. Saunders Company, 1984. *Useful, conservative approach with easy readings for occupational lung disease.*
Rosenstock A, Cullen M: Clinical Occupational Medicine. Philadelphia, W.B. Saunders Company, 1986. *Useful, inexpensive guide to common occupational health problems.*
Selikoff I: The role of the internist in occupational medicine. Am J Indust Med 8:95, 1985. *An elder statesman of occupational medicine puts everything in perspective.*

536 OCCUPATIONAL PULMONARY DISORDERS

Dean Sheppard

The lung is the major interface between man and his external environment. As such, the lungs and airways have evolved an elaborate system to filter out the myriad of potentially toxic particles and gases present in inspired air in order to protect the delicate gas exchanging apparatus of the alveolar surface. This system is remarkably durable. The irritant gases and approximately 2 mg of dust inhaled daily by urban dwellers generally have no effect on lung function. Even the high concentrations of dust, irritants, and carcinogens present in cigarette smoke, inhaled daily for periods of 50 years or more, fail to cause disease in most smokers. Given the continuing contact between the lungs and the environment, however, it is not surprising that the lungs are the most common site of serious environmentally induced disease. Environmental pollutants are generally present in highest concentration at sites of industrial use or production. Thus, environmentally induced lung disease usually results from occupational exposure.

The major determinants of whether or not disease will occur in a given individual are the toxicity of the material inhaled, the dose and duration of exposure (including the duration of lung retention, which may be several years for some inhaled particles), and the individual's host defenses. One would like to be able to identify host factors that predispose to the development of occupational disease in order to advise individuals at risk to avoid particular occupations, but unfortunately this is rarely possible. A few notable exceptions are the increased susceptibility of cigarette smokers to asbestos-induced carcinoma of the lung and the increased susceptibility of atopic individuals to some types of occupational asthma. In general, a more fruitful approach to the prevention of occupational lung disease is protection of all workers from exposures that can be anticipated to cause disease in any. This approach is most likely to be effective if it includes a significant margin of safety, limiting exposures to levels considerably less than the exposure anticipated to cause disease. These principles underlie the workplace exposure standards promulgated by the American Council of Government Industrial Hygienists and more recently by the U.S. Occupational Safety and Health Administration. However, the standard setting process is a slow one and in the absence of adequate data, the assessments of disease probability on which they are based are necessarily subjective. Furthermore, as new data emerge, standards need to be continually revised, but this process too can take many years. Keeping these shortcomings in mind, physicians cannot assume that a given occupational exposure is not responsible for causing a disease, even if the exposure level was below the current standard.

Even if workplace standards could be set instantaneously with the emergence of new scientific data, individual practicing physicians would still play a critical role in the identification and ultimate prevention of occupational lung disease. Onset of occupational disease is often delayed long after exposure (e.g., up to 60 years for mesothelioma caused by asbestos exposure). Furthermore, the first cases of an occupational disease are rarely recognized as being caused by work exposure, especially when the disease is a common one, such as asthma or carcinoma of the lung. Thousands of new chemicals are introduced into the workplace each year without systematic screening for their ability to cause disease. Therefore, new causes of occupational lung disease will undoubtedly continue to emerge. Identification of these new causes of lung disease and prevention of additional cases will continue to be the responsibility of practicing physicians.

Even when adequate workplace standards exist, they are hard to enforce especially for workers who are self-employed or who work in small shops. Under these circumstances the identification of an individual worker with an occupationally induced lung disease can be the first indication of unsafe working conditions. Thus, a diagnosis of occupational lung disease necessitates a report to the appropriate public health agency and a thorough investigation of the workplace to identify additional cases and prevent future ones.

The lung responds to injury in a limited number of ways. Virtually any type of lung disorder can be caused by an occupational exposure. The specific type of disorder is determined by the site of deposition of the responsible agent, the dose and duration of exposure, the susceptibility of specific lung cells to the agent's toxic effects, and the nature of the interaction between the agent and local host defense mechanisms.

Gases are deposited in the respiratory system based on their water solubility. Water-soluble gases, such as ammonia and sulfur dioxide, are nearly entirely removed from inspired air by the aqueous layer lining the nose, oropharynx, and upper airways. These gases thus are most likely to cause disease in the airways. Relatively water-insoluble gases, such as nitrogen dioxide and phosgene, bypass the upper airways and injure the distal airways and alveoli. In contrast, particles are deposited based on size or, more accurately, on "aerodynamic diameter," which means that a particle is deposited out of a moving air stream in the same fashion as would be a perfect sphere of that diameter. During quiet breathing through the nose, essentially all particles with aerodynamic diameters in excess of 10 microns are deposited on the nasal mucosa. During strenuous exercise, however, because of increased air flow and mouth breathing, up to 20 per cent of particles between 10 and 20 microns in diameter are deposited within the airways. Particles between 3 and 10 microns in diameter can be deposited throughout the tracheobronchial tree. More central deposition is favored by high inspiratory flow rates, by airway obstruction, and by the presence of increased quantities of mucus. Particles between 0.1 and 3 microns in diameter can also be deposited in the airways, but are preferentially deposited within the alveoli. Smaller particles are mainly exhaled. A fiber (a particle whose length exceeds its width by at least three times) is also deposited on the basis of aerodynamic diameter and not length. This explains why fibers up to 25 microns long are often deposited in alveoli.

GENERAL APPROACH TO A PATIENT WITH SUSPECTED OCCUPATIONAL LUNG DISEASE

HISTORY. A thorough occupational history is the most important step in diagnosing any occupationally induced disease. The history must go beyond the patient's present job to a complete list of each job done throughout the patient's lifetime. Job titles often are not helpful. Rather, a detailed description of what the patient actually did and what materials he or she worked with should be elicited. The relationship of the patient's work site to other associated jobs is important, as is the use and adequacy of exhaust ventilation and personal protective devices. For instance, one electrician could develop asbestosis from working near insulators in the holds of ships while another electrician working outdoors on new-building construction might have no significant asbestos exposure. The presence or absence of special work clothes, lockers, and showers should be noted, since hazardous materials (e.g., asbestos) brought home by workers who have worked in their street clothes can cause disease in family members. Hobbies should also be described in detail; hazardous exposures in home workshops can cause disease (e.g., asthma from exposure to isocyanate varnishes). Each job and hobby should be recorded in chronological order to insure that all working years are accounted for. The temporal relationship between symptoms and exposure can also be important. This is especially true for disease with acute symptomatic exacerbations, such as occupational asthma and hypersensitivity pneumonitis. In all cases, it is important to determine that symptoms did not precede exposure. Because of the high prevalence of cigarette smoking, the important toxic effects of cigarette smoke itself on the lungs, and the possible interactions between smoking and occupational exposures, a careful quantitative smoking history is also important. Finally, it is important to seek out historical information that would suggest a nonoccupational cause for the patient's lung disease. For instance, a history of uveitis and parotid enlargement might suggest that sarcoidosis rather than asbestos exposure was responsible for a given patient's interstitial lung disease.

ROENTGENOGRAPHIC TECHNIQUES. Chest roentgenographs are important in the evaluation of patients suspected of having parenchymal lung disease and in detecting pleural abnormalities in workers exposed to asbestos. They can also be useful in surveillance of workers in hazardous occupations to detect subclinical abnormalities. For standardization of epidemiologic surveys, roentgenographic abnormalities should be characterized by trained and certified readers using the International Labor Office (ILO) classification system. In this system small parenchymal opacities are described by shape (irregular or rounded) and size. Profusion (the concentration of opacities) is scored on a 12-point scale (0/−, 0/0, 0/1, up to 3/3, 3/+). Large parenchymal opacities and the extent and width of pleural thickening are also quantified. This scoring system allows the clinician to make a reasonable assessment of prognosis in individual patients. Computed axial tomography is more sensitive and specific than standard chest radiographs in detecting pleural abnormalities. Nonetheless, this technique is seldom necessary in symptomatic individuals, and its expense does not justify its use in screening. Roentgenographs are not useful in evaluating patients with suspected occupational airway diseases.

PULMONARY FUNCTION TESTS. Tests of static lung function are important in evaluating patients suspected of having occupationally induced interstitial lung diseases or those with dyspnea of undetermined etiology. When these tests are abnormal, they provide information about the pattern and extent of lung dysfunction. Tests of static lung function do not provide information about the *cause* of lung dysfunction (occupational or not) or about dynamic abnormalities (e.g., bronchospasm or decreased pulmonary vascular reserve). Thus, for instance, many, if not most, patients with occupational asthma will have normal screening pulmonary function tests between symptomatic episodes. Special studies such as bronchial provocation tests (see below) may be required before a diagnosis of occupational lung disease can be excluded. An additional problem of tests of static lung function is the wide range of normal values seen among healthy individuals. For example, if an individual worker starts with a vital capacity near the upper limit of normal (120 per cent of predicted) his or her vital capacity would need to fall by one third (to 80 per cent of predicted) before it would be considered abnormal. If, as is often the case, a single measurement is made after many years of employment and a vital capacity of 90 per cent of predicted is recorded, a significant occupationally induced loss of lung function could easily be overlooked. To avoid this problem, serial measurements of lung function should be performed on the same equipment for surveillance of workers in occupations suspected of causing occupational lung disease. Accelerated rates of decline of lung function can thus be detected before the test results deviate from the predicted normal range.

In addition to tests of static lung function, pulmonary exercise testing can provide important information for the evaluation of any patient with unexplained dyspnea. This test can distinguish between cardiovascular and pulmonary limitations to exercise and can identify pulmonary vascular dysfunction (as occurs with interstitial fibrosis) in some patients with normal static lung function. In addition, exercise limitation can be measured and compared to the patient's actual job requirements.

EVALUATION OF THE JOB SITE. In the clinical evaluation of a worker suspected of having any occupationally induced disorder it is important to inspect and monitor his or her workplace. It is essential to do so if a diagnosis of an occupationally induced disorder has been established. Inspections usually require the assistance of a trained industrial hygienist who may be employed by the worker's company, the worker's compensation insurance company, a state or federal agency (e.g, the Occupational Safety and Health Administration) or a specialized occupational health clinic. In addition to a visual walk-through inspection and direct observation of each of the worker's job tasks (and adjacent workers' tasks) an inspection should include air sampling for agents suspected of being released by the work processes involved. Even if for some reason air sampling cannot be obtained, direct site inspection can provide important clues to the occupational etiology of a worker's disease. For example, a maintenance worker with asthma may be found to be working in a warehouse in which toluene di-isocyanate is used in manufacturing.

Morgan WKC, Seaton A: Occupational Lung Disease. 2nd ed. Philadelphia, W. B. Saunders Company, 1984. *A reasonably priced, up-to-date textbook.*

Parkes WR: Occupational Lung Disorders. 2nd ed. London, Butterworths, 1982. *A detailed and very well-referenced textbook by a single author.*

Rom WN (ed.): Environmental and Occupational Medicine. Boston, Little, Brown & Company, 1983. *A comprehensive review of occupational medicine with excellent introductory chapters covering issues of assessment and control of workplace hazards and broad coverage of individual exposures and diseases.*

Wiell H, Ziskind MM: Occupational pulmonary disorders. In Fishman AP (ed.): Pulmonary Diseases and Disorders. New York, McGraw-Hill Book Company, 1980, pp 754–792. *A comprehensive but concise review.*

AIRWAY DISORDERS
Occupational Asthma

Occupational asthma is defined as asthma that occurs in a previously healthy individual as a result of occupational exposure. This is usually distinguished from an exacerbation of pre-existing asthma on the basis of pre-employment history. Work-induced exacerbations of pre-existing asthma are also an important cause of morbidity and may qualify the affected worker for worker's compensation. Asthma is a

common disease (affecting 3 to 6 per cent of the United States population), but most patients with mild disease can function perfectly normally under most circumstances (Ch. 60). Thus, virtually every occupation includes a significant number of workers with asthma. Patients with asthma are extremely sensitive to bronchoconstrictor stimuli and may develop symptomatic attacks from exposure to occupational irritants (e.g., low concentrations of sulfur dioxide gas) that have no effect on their nonasthmatic coworkers. In this circumstance, although the worker's asthma may have antedated occupational exposure, management would be the same as for patients with true occupational asthma, including application for compensation and job retraining if these are required to avoid further exposure.

CAUSATIVE AGENTS. Well over 100 causative agents are now recognized, and the list continues to grow (Table 536–1). This list, necessarily incomplete, can be roughly divided into highly reactive low-molecular-weight chemicals (such as toluene di-isocyanate and trimellitic anhydride) that share the ability to cause acute airway injury, and complex organic materials such as animal dander and grain dust. Since asthma is common and usually of unknown cause, the occupational etiology of asthma is often missed. In addition, thousands of new chemicals are introduced into the workplace each year, but it takes many years for any association between exposure to a chemical and induction of asthma to be recognized. Finally, many workers are simultaneously exposed to dozens or even hundreds of different chemicals, so determining the single one responsible for causing asthma is often difficult. For all these reasons, a diagnosis of occupational asthma must often be considered on the basis of clinical characteristics even if a worker is not exposed to any agent already known to cause asthma. On the other hand, if it can be determined that a worker with asthma of recent onset *is* exposed to an agent known to commonly cause asthma (for instance, toluene di-isocyanate, grain dust, and western red cedar dust cause asthma in approximately 5 per cent of exposed workers), this information should increase the suspicion that the worker's asthma is occupationally induced.

PATHOPHYSIOLOGY. Organic materials such as animal excreta, green coffee beans, and shellfish extracts probably serve as antigens and cause asthma primarily as a result of repeated immediate hypersensitivity responses in the airways. Some of these agents (e.g., animal excreta) are most likely to affect individuals with a previously demonstrated predisposition to atopy. Most of the low-molecular-weight chemicals that cause asthma are too small to serve as antigens by themselves. These chemicals could trigger immediate hypersensitivity responses by combining with tissue proteins or by altering tissue proteins to create new antigenic determinants. Some of these agents (e.g., toluene di-isocyanate) can cause acute airway injury and inflammation in the absence of

TABLE 536–1. COMMON CAUSES OF OCCUPATIONAL ASTHMA

Agents	Occupational Exposure
Low-Molecular-Weight Chemicals	
Isocyanates	Plastics, varnishing, spray painting, foundries
Anhydrides: phthalic, trimellitic, tetrachlorophthalic	Plastics, epoxy resins
Soldering fluxes	Electronics, aluminum plants
Metal salts: platinum, chromium, nickel	Metal plating, refining, tanning
Wood dusts: red cedar, redwood, zebrawood	Sawmills, carpentry
Complex Organic Materials	
Plant dusts: grain, coffee bean, castor bean	Grain handlers, bakers, agricultural workers
Laboratory animals	Lab workers, animal handlers
Shellfish: crab, prawn, oyster	Shellfish processors
Biologic enzymes	Detergents, pharmaceuticals, chemical industry

immune sensitization. Asthma appears to be more common in workers exposed to repeated accidental spills, suggesting that this acute airway injury may contribute to the development of asthma.

CLINICAL MANIFESTATIONS. *Cough* is the most common initial manifestation of occupational asthma. This is often preceded by symptoms of *rhinitis*, which is associated with asthma in up to 70 per cent of affected workers. Intermittent *chest tightness, dyspnea,* and *wheezing* may be present initially or develop weeks to months after the onset of cough and rhinitis. Initially, these symptoms occur with a distinctive temporal relationship to work exposure. The three most common temporal patterns are: an immediate response characterized by short-lived symptoms occurring at the time of work exposure, a late response characterized by symptoms that begin 4 to 12 hours after exposure, and a dual response that combines elements of the first two (Fig. 536–1). Unfortunately, the immediate response—the pattern most commonly recognized as due to work exposure—is the least common. Furthermore, workers who experience dual responses are much more likely to notice the late response than the immediate one, because the late response is usually longer in duration and more difficult to treat. Thus, a typical history of occupational asthma would include symptoms that are most prominent in the evening or at night. Initially, improvement in these symptoms during weekends and vacations is the most important clue to their occupational origin. Eventually, however, as the worker's asthma becomes more severe, any temporal relationship with work may disappear and an affected worker may complain of persistent asthma indistinguishable from asthma of any other etiology.

Symptoms of occupational asthma can develop at any time after the onset of employment but usually appear after months to years of exposure to the responsible agent. When the diagnosis is suspected soon after the onset of symptoms and further exposure to the responsible agent is prevented, most affected workers gradually improve. Workers who are diagnosed after several years of symptomatic asthma, however, or who continue to be exposed after the diagnosis has been established can develop asthma that may persist for years (and perhaps indefinitely) even if further exposure ceases.

DIAGNOSIS. As noted above, a history of new onset rhinitis, cough, chest tightness, dyspnea, and/or wheezing in a previously healthy worker is essential. Screening pulmonary function tests are usually normal between symptomatic episodes but may reveal reversible (or fixed) airway obstruction. Measurement of spirometry (FEV_1 and FVC) before and after a work shift may reveal a more than 10 per cent decrease, but this test is insensitive because of inconsistent exposures over a single work shift and varied temporal patterns of response. If the worker is still actively employed, repeated measurements of peak expiratory flow can be performed and symptoms recorded at two-hour intervals over a two-week period that should ideally include at least two weekends. This method is sensitive to intermittent airway obstruction and provides information on the temporal relationship between obstruction and exposure. A 20 per cent difference between the best and worst value of peak flow during any 24-hour period is abnormal. If symptoms are recorded but peak flow does not vary, an explanation for the symptoms other than asthma should be sought.

A single measurement of nonspecific airway responsiveness (e.g., by methacholine or histamine challenge) can confirm a diagnosis of asthma but does not provide information about the occupational etiology. Furthermore, nonspecific airway responsiveness can be normal in workers with occupational asthma, especially during periods of minimal exposure to the responsible agent. Demonstration of a dramatic *increase* in airway responsiveness in association with work exposure does provide strong supportive evidence of an occupational etiology.

Skin testing and/or measurement of specific IgE antibody can be useful for selected causes of occupational asthma. These include animal exposures, green coffee beans, platinum salts, and trimellitic anhydride. For most causes of occupational asthma, however, the responsible antigens have not been sufficiently well characterized to allow definitive interpretation of these immunologic tests. Specific inhalation challenge testing is much more likely to be definitive, but such testing is time-consuming and expensive, requiring at least two days of hospitalization to evaluate sham and actual exposures, and should only be performed in specialized centers with experience in generating and monitoring stimulated exposures. For these reasons, specific inhalation challenge should be reserved for cases in which a specific agent rather than a work process must be identified and for research evaluation of previously unrecognized causative agents.

TREATMENT. Prevention of further exposure is the only effective treatment. Although this can occasionally be achieved by the use of improved workplace ventilation and/or personal respiratory protective equipment when exposure is intermittent, often affected workers are unable to continue to work anywhere in the vicinity of the responsible agent. This is especially true for vapors such as toluene di-isocyanate, where exposure to concentrations below the lower limit of detection (<1 ppb) can trigger severe asthma attacks in affected individuals. Asthmatic symptoms can often be suppressed with standard treatment for asthma (e.g., inhaled beta-adrenergic agonists and theophylline) or with inhaled cromolyn. Such an approach cannot be recommended, since continued exposure appears to increase the likelihood of persistent asthma.

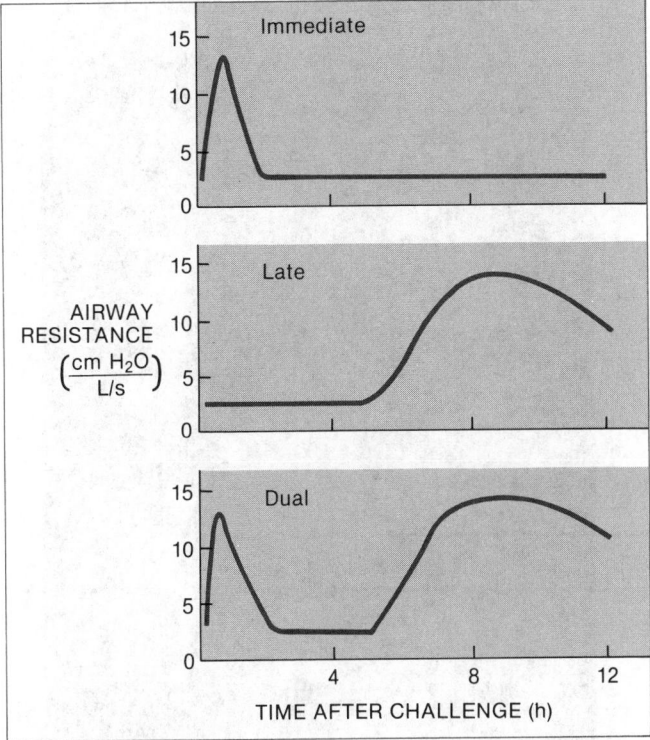

FIGURE 536–1. Temporal patterns of bronchoconstriction (as indicated by increases in airway resistance) after exposure to agents responsible for causing occupational asthma. Delayed responses that can begin from 4 to 12 hours after exposure tend to be more prolonged than immediate responses and thus often cause more prominent symptoms. (Reprinted by permission of the *Western Journal of Medicine*, from Sheppard D: Occupational asthma. West J Med 137:480, 1982.)

Chan-Yeung M, Lam S: Occupational asthma: State of the art. Am Rev Respir Dis 133:686, 1986. *A comprehensive and up-to-date review.*

Byssinosis

Byssinosis is an occupational airway disorder that occurs in workers exposed to dust generated during the handling of crude cotton, hemp, or flax. This disorder differs from other forms of occupational asthma in that symptoms of chest tightness and dyspnea are most prominent during the initial work shift following a weekend or vacation and tend to diminish over the course of each work week. Although the dust component responsible for these symptoms has not been definitively identified, contaminants such as bacterial endotoxins may play a prominent role. Steam cleaning crude cotton before it is carded and engineering controls to reduce airborne dust concentrations can both markedly reduce the incidence of acute symptoms. Long-term chronic exposure to cotton dust also appears to cause productive cough and accelerated loss of lung function in some workers.

Mundie TG, Ainsworth SK: Etiopathogenic mechanisms of bronchoconstriction in byssinosis: A review. Am Rev Respir Dis 133:1181, 1986.

Industrial Bronchitis

Workers in a number of dusty industries have an increased prevalence of chronic daily productive cough. This effect of occupational dust exposure has been most clearly demonstrated in workers exposed to coal, grain, and cotton dusts. A similar increased prevalence of productive cough has been reported in workers chronically exposed to high concentrations of sulfur dioxide gas in smelters and paper pulp mills and in welders who are chronically exposed to a variety of irritant gases. The high prevalence of cigarette smoking among industrial workers and the potent effect of smoking in causing bronchitis often make establishing an occupational cause of bronchitis difficult. Each of the exposures noted above has been reported to cause bronchitis even in nonsmokers. In the absence of smoking, lung function is usually normal in workers with industrial bronchitis. Nonetheless, the prospective demonstration of accelerated loss of lung function in grain workers and data demonstrating a high prevalence of airway obstruction in cotton workers suggest that these exposures can cause chronic air flow limitation.

PARENCHYMAL LUNG DISORDERS
Disorders Caused by Inorganic Dusts
Silicosis

DEFINITION. Silicosis is the parenchymal lung disease caused by inhalation of particles of crystalline silicon dioxide (SiO_2). Free silicon dioxide is usually encountered in nature as quartz. Other crystalline forms, cristobalite and tridymite, are most often encountered in industry as by-products produced when amorphous silicates are heated to high temperature. More complex silicates such as asbestos, talc, and kaolin cause clinically distinct pulmonary responses and will be discussed separately.

OCCUPATIONAL EXPOSURE. Silicon dioxide is widely deposited through the rock that makes up the earth's surface. Industrial activities that involve cutting, polishing, or shearing rock are thus all potential sources of respirable silica. These include mining, tunnelling, quarrying, and stone cutting. Industrial uses of sand, which is largely composed of quartz, can lead to exposure to high concentrations of respirable silica, especially the use of sand for abrasive blasting. Sand is also widely used in foundry work, glass blowing, and pottery making.

PATHOLOGY AND PATHOGENESIS. Three different forms of silicosis are roughly related to the intensity of exposure to respirable silica. *Chronic silicosis* is defined as radiographic abnormalities that are first noted 15 years or more after the onset of exposure. *Accelerated silicosis* resembles the chronic disease but occurs 5 to 15 years after the onset of exposure to high concentrations of silica. *Acute silicosis* occurs within 5 years of the onset of exposure, is virtually always caused by massive exposure, and is clinically and pathologically quite different from the other two forms.

Chronic silicosis is characterized by small nodules that may be diffusely distributed or present primarily in the upper lobes (Fig. 536–2). Nodules are also present in hilar lymph nodes. The nodules have an acellular core composed of concentric swirls of hyalinized collagen and are surrounded by a cellular capsule containing macrophages, plasma cells, and fibroblasts (Fig. 536–3). Silica crystals are often present in these nodules. In a minority of patients small nodules coalesce to form large masses that can compress and obliterate normal lung structures (so-called progressive massive fibrosis). These nodules occasionally cavitate in the absence of infection, but most often cavities result from infection with *Mycobacterium tuberculosis* and other mycobacteria. The appearance of accelerated silicosis is similar, but conglomerate nodules occur more commonly and giant cells may be seen. Acute silicosis is characterized by an eosinophilic exudate that fills alveolar spaces and resembles alveolar proteinosis.

Tissue injury from silica is probably initiated by the interaction between silica crystals and alveolar macrophages and appears to involve disruption of phagolysosomes and release of lysosomal contents into the extracellular space. Macrophages stimulated by silica also secrete factors that are chemotactic for other macrophages and neutrophils and that stimulate fibroblasts to proliferate and lay down collagen.

CLINICAL MANIFESTATIONS. Chronic silicosis most commonly causes radiographic abnormalities without symptoms. When symptoms do develop, dyspnea is the most common but it is usually severe only in patients with progressive massive fibrosis. Cough is commonly seen but is often attributable to chronic bronchitis in cigarette smokers or

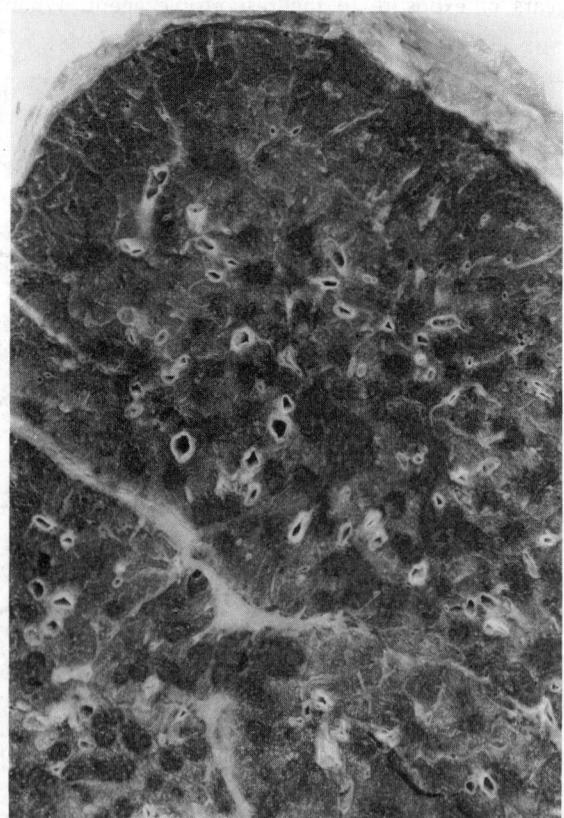

FIGURE 536–2. Close-up of the upper lobe of a slice of lung with marked simple silicosis. The rounded, sharply circumscribed black spots are silicotic nodules. The surrounding parenchyma is normal. (From Warnock ML, Kuwahara TJ, Wolery G: The relation of asbestos burden to asbestosis and lung cancer. Pathol Annu 18:109, 1983 (Part 2), reprinted with permission of Appleton-Century Crofts, Norwalk, CT.)

tests are useful in evaluating and quantifying pulmonary impairment in symptomatic workers. In patients with simple silicosis, severe air flow obstruction is usually due to another coexisting disorder (e.g., bronchitis and/or emphysema) not caused by silica. In accelerated or chronic silicosis, other causes of interstitial fibrosis should be considered in differential diagnosis. In patients with progressive loss of lung function in whom the diagnosis is uncertain, lung biopsy should be performed to look for other treatable causes. Silica crystals can be seen as birefringent by plane polarizing microscopy, but this feature is not specific for free silica. In patients with mixed dust exposure, energy dispersive x-ray analysis can identify silicon dioxide and other elements associated with silicates (e.g., calcium, magnesium, iron). Acute silicosis resembles other forms of alveolar proteinosis, but the history of massive silica exposure is usually obvious.

Antinuclear antibodies may be present in up to 40 per cent of patients with silicosis. This test is of no diagnostic value, however, since antibodies are also seen in a high percentage of exposed workers without silicosis. Rapid progression of conglomerate lesions, especially if this is unilateral, suggests coexisting mycobacterial infection or neoplasm and justifies aggressive efforts at diagnosis, as does the appearance of a new cavity. Some epidemiologic studies suggest that silica exposure increases the risk for pulmonary neoplasms, but most of these studies have involved workers exposed to other potential carcinogens, so the role of silica itself in pulmonary carcinogenesis remains controversial.

TREATMENT. There is no proven effective treatment for any form of silicosis. Patients with acute silicosis should probably be treated with sequential whole lung lavage as are other patients with alveolar proteinosis. Mycobacterial infections should be treated with standard chemotherapy (Ch. 302). Patients with silicosis and a positive PPD should all receive a year of prophylactic therapy with isoniazid (300 mg daily).

The major hope for reducing the prevalence of silicosis lies with prevention. Industrial processes that generate respirable free silica should be enclosed or modified; dust containing silica should never be swept dry, and workers should always use personal respiratory protective devices for unavoidable short-term exposures. In many countries (not including the United States) sand is no longer allowed for use in abrasive blasting because of the large quantities of respirable silica produced. Such a ban should be instituted worldwide, since a number of acceptable replacements are available (e.g., steel grit and coal ash).

Dauber JH: Silicosis. In Fishman AP (ed.): Pulmonary Diseases and Disorders. New York, McGraw-Hill Book Company, 1982, pp 149–166. *Excellent summary of pathogenesis.*
Goldsmith DF, Winn DM, Shy CM (eds.): Silica, Silicosis and Cancer. New York, Praeger, 1986. *Proceedings of an international conference. Includes several chapters summarizing present understanding of prevalence and pathogenesis of silicosis.*
Ziskind M, Jones RN, Weill H: Silicosis. Am Rev Respir Dis 113:643, 1976. *A classic comprehensive review.*

Coal Workers' Pneumoconiosis

DEFINITION. Coal workers' pneumoconiosis is the parenchymal lung disorder caused by inhalation of coal dust. A similar disorder occurs in workers exposed to graphite or carbon black. Coal dust inhalation also causes chronic bronchitis. These disorders occur primarily in coal miners but can occur in coal trimmers, graphite miners and millers, and workers involved in manufacturing carbon electrodes.

PATHOLOGY. The principal pathologic lesion in coal workers' pneumoconiosis is the coal macule, a small, heavily pigmented lesion that consists of a collection of macrophages filled with dust. These cells are distributed around terminal airways and often fill alveolar spaces, but there is remarkably little initial tissue reaction. Larger macules called coal nodules can also contain collagen. These lesions are usually more

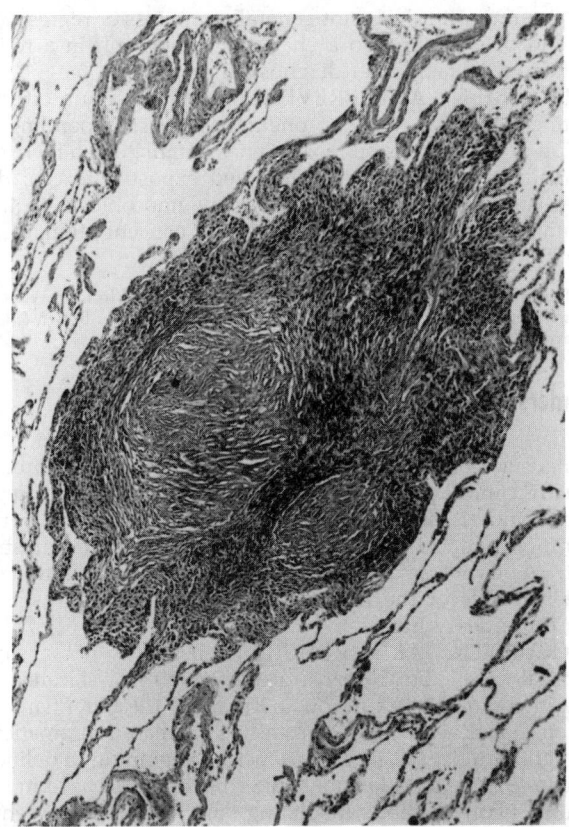

FIGURE 536–3. Light microscopic view of a typical silicotic nodule (original magnification, ×70). Note the whirled fibrous core. The surrounding alveoli are normal. (From Warnock ML, Kuwahara TJ, Wolery G: The relation of asbestos burden to asbestosis and lung cancer. Pathol Annu 18:109, 1983 (Part 2), reprinted with permission of Appleton-Century Crofts, Norwalk, CT.)

to superimposed infection. Patients with silicosis have an increased susceptibility to both tuberculous and nontuberculous mycobacterial infections; these should be suspected in affected workers who develop fever, weight loss, asymmetric upper lobe infiltrates, or cavitary lesions. Susceptibility to fungal infections is also increased. Chest pain and clubbing are not features of silicosis.

Chest radiographs usually show multiple small nodules that may be diffusely distributed but are often primarily in the upper lobes and are occasionally calcified. This pattern is called *simple silicosis*. Enlarged hilar lymph nodes may contain outer rims of calcium called *egg-shell calcification*. In patients with progressive massive fibrosis, large masses are usually seen in the upper lobes, often symmetrically distributed around the hilar regions in a so-called angel's wing distribution. In these patients compensatory emphysema is also common. Severe abnormalities in lung function are generally seen only in patients with conglomerate shadows who are said to have *complicated silicosis*. Because the airways and the pulmonary vascular bed are often distorted by these conglomerate masses, pulmonary function tests often reveal airway obstruction and a decrease in pulmonary diffusing capacity as well as the decrease in lung volumes commonly seen in patients with interstitial fibrosis.

Patients with rheumatoid arthritis who develop silicosis can present with multiple large pulmonary nodules that pathologically resemble extrapulmonary rheumatoid nodules. This presentation, called *Caplan's syndrome*, can also occur in workers with asbestosis or in coal workers' pneumoconiosis.

DIAGNOSIS. The diagnosis of silicosis is based on a history of significant occupational exposure to free silica and appropriate radiographic abnormalities. Pulmonary function tests are usually normal in patients with simple silicosis; they are not helpful in establishing the diagnosis. Pulmonary function numerous in the upper lobes but can be found throughout the lungs. As in silicosis a small minority of affected workers (~1%) develop progressive massive fibrosis. This complication appears to be related at least in part to heavy dust loads. Pathologically, large rubbery masses are seen, usually in the superior segments of the lower lobes and the posterior segments of the upper lobes. Microscopically, these masses resemble large coal nodules but contain considerably more collagen and are frequently associated with compensatory emphysema.

The pathogenesis of coal workers' pneumoconiosis remains controversial. The coal macules are probably produced by phagocytosis of overwhelming quantities of dust by air space macrophages. The interaction between coal dust and macrophages may not by itself be sufficient to explain the fibrosis and parenchymal destruction seen in patients with progressive massive fibrosis. Tissue injury may require concomitant exposure to silica, mycobacterial infection, or an immunologic abnormality such as rheumatoid arthritis. As noted above for silica, coal miners with rheumatoid arthritis can develop Caplan's syndrome, a distinctive pattern of multiple lung masses that resemble rheumatoid nodules. The mechanisms by which coal dust causes mucus hypersecretion (chronic bronchitis) and chronic air flow limitation require further investigation.

CLINICAL MANIFESTATIONS. Simple coal workers' pneumoconiosis most often consists of x-ray abnormalities without symptoms. Patients with complicated pneumoconiosis (progressive massive fibrosis) can develop progressive dyspnea, pulmonary hypertension, and respiratory failure. The risk of mycobacterial infection may be increased in patients with coal workers' pneumoconiosis, but not to the same extent as in patients with silicosis. Chest radiographs usually show small irregular opacities, especially in the upper lung zones. For epidemiologic studies these can be quantified by the ILO classification described above. In simple coal workers' pneumoconiosis the degree of profusion is well correlated with the dust burden, an observation that is not surprising since x-ray abnormalities are primarily due to retained dust. In complicated pneumoconiosis, radiographs show large conglomerate shadows and compensatory emphysema.

Chronic sputum production and chronic air flow limitation are also complications of coal mining related to the quantity of dust exposure but not to radiographic abnormalities. These effects are not entirely due to cigarette smoking and can be seen in nonsmoking miners, but abnormalities in air flow tend to be mild in nonsmoking miners in the absence of complicated pneumoconiosis. In an individual coal miner who smokes it is not possible to determine the relative contributions of coal dust and cigarette smoking to the development of chronic bronchitis and airway obstruction.

Pulmonary function tests in patients with simple coal workers' pneumoconiosis are usually normal. In patients with complicated pneumoconiosis both airway obstruction (characterized by decreases in the FEV_1 and other tests of maximal flow) and lung restriction (characterized by a decrease in total lung capacity) can occur. In addition, the diffusing capacity for carbon monoxide is often reduced as a result of obstruction or destruction of the pulmonary vascular bed. Some epidemiologic studies in coal miners have shown an increase in residual volume and a decrease in flow measured at low lung volumes in comparison to matched nonexposed control populations. These findings are consistent with mild airway obstruction caused by coal dust exposure.

DIAGNOSIS. The diagnosis of coal workers' pneumoconiosis is made on the basis of a history of exposure and appropriate radiographic abnormalities. In patients with large conglomerate shadows, mycobacterial infection needs to be excluded. Affected patients do not have an increased risk of lung cancer, but in smokers with unilateral enlarging masses, neoplasm must be excluded. The lesions of simple coal work-

ers' pneumoconiosis do not generally progress or regress after the end of exposure, so a changing radiograph in a retired worker suggests another diagnosis.

TREATMENT AND PREVENTION. There is no effective treatment for coal workers' pneumoconiosis. Impending depletion of the world's oil reserves has stimulated an increased demand for coal, insuring continued exposure to coal dust for years to come. Prevention of pneumoconiosis requires minimizing the airborne respirable dust concentration at each step in the extraction and processing of coal.

Merchant JA, Reger RB: Coal workers' respiratory disease. In Rom WN (ed.): Environmental and occupational medicine. Boston, Little, Brown & Company, 1983, pp 183–196.

Disorders Caused by Asbestos

Inhaled asbestos is a more potent stimulus to tissue injury than is silica or coal. Furthermore, asbestos causes a broader range of clinical disorders besides pulmonary fibrosis: pleural fibrosis and effusion; mesothelioma of the pleura and peritoneum; and cancer of the lung, larynx, and gastrointestinal tract. The term *asbestosis* is usually reserved for the nonmalignant response of the lung parenchyma to inhaled asbestos fiber (pulmonary fibrosis).

OCCUPATIONAL EXPOSURE. Asbestos is not a single chemical entity, but rather a group of mineral silicates that have in common their fibrous nature and the potential to be woven. Worldwide use of asbestos increased dramatically throughout most of this century before beginning to deline in the late 1970's. Asbestos fibers have been widely used in ship building, construction, insulating, and automotive vehicle clutch and brake manufacturing because they are highly resistant to heat, acid, and chemical degradation. For the same reasons, asbestos has also been used in the manufacture of textiles and building supplies. In the past, the heaviest occupational exposures have occurred in miners, millers, shipyard workers, and insulation workers; but because of the diverse uses of asbestos, cases of asbestos-induced disease are seen among a wide variety of other occupations. As the use of asbestos in new construction has been nearly eliminated in the U.S., continued exposure is likely to be due to demolition and renovation of buildings and ships containing asbestos. In developing countries application of new asbestos continues to be widespread. Since most asbestos-induced diseases have a long latency, the prevalence of asbestos-induced diseases is not likely to fall for many years despite a marked decrease in exposure. Nonoccupational exposure can also cause disease. For instance, cases of mesothelioma and an increased prevalence of pleural thickening have been reported among household contacts of asbestos workers (presumably due to exposure to fibers brought home on work clothes).

PATHOLOGY AND PATHOGENESIS. *Pleural Disease.* Asbestos can cause localized or diffuse areas of acellular pleural fibrosis that are usually bilateral and primarily on the parietal pleura. Asbestos fibers are often found in the adjacent visceral pleura, suggesting that injury from asbestos fibers that migrate out to the visceral pleural surface may injure the adjacent parietal pleura. Asbestos exposure can also cause benign exudative pleural effusions that usually contain a mixed population of inflammatory cells. The exudative lesion is nonspecific.

Pulmonary Fibrosis. Macroscopically, in advanced cases the lungs are small and stiff, and fibrous streaks are most prominent in the lower lobes and in subpleural locations. Honeycombing is occasionally seen (Fig. 536–4). Microscopically, asbestosis is indistinguishable from other causes of pulmonary fibrosis, except for the presence of asbestos fibers. A small percentage of asbestos fibers become coated with hemosiderin and form asbestos bodies that are visible under the light microscope. Identification of the more numerous uncoated

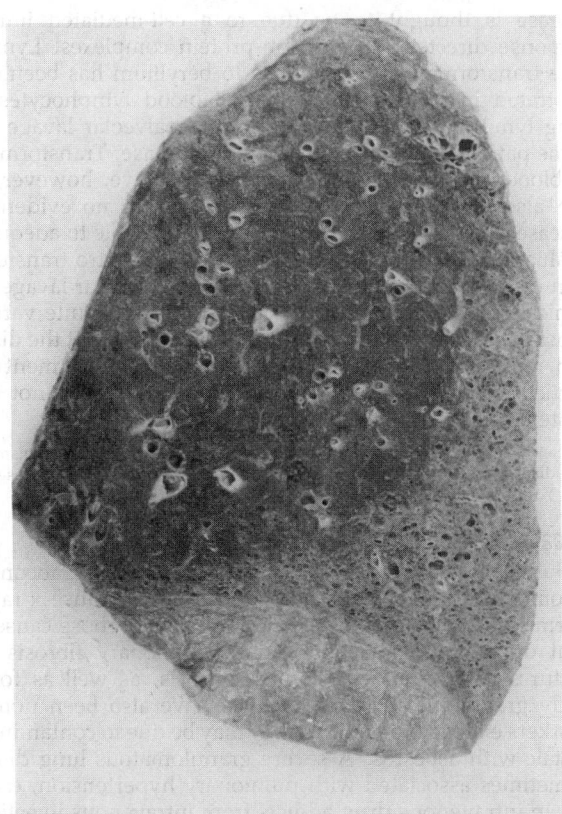

FIGURE 536–4. Slice of lower lobe from a patient with asbestosis. Note the thick pleural opacity at the base and the marked subpleural fibrosis with honeycombing. (From Warnock ML, Kuwahara TJ, Wolery G: The relation of asbestos burden to asbestosis and lung cancer. Pathol Annu 18:109, 1983 (Part 2), reprinted with permission of Appleton-Century Crofts, Norwalk, CT.)

fibers requires electron microscopy. The number of asbestos bodies recovered from dried lung correlates well with the total number of fibers (though there are several orders of magnitude more uncoated fibers). However, because asbestos bodies are not uniformly distributed throughout the lungs, examination of standard lung sections by light microscopy may not reveal asbestos bodies even from patients with a heavy asbestos burden and asbestosis. On the other hand, occasional asbestos bodies can be seen in urban dwellers without occupational exposure and are of little significance in the absence of associated pulmonary fibrosis.

In experimental animals exposed to asbestos, the earliest pathologic abnormality is an accumulation of inflammatory cells (especially macrophages) around asbestos fibers in the terminal airways. Similar lesions are also common in asbestos-exposed workers and may explain why exposure to asbestos reduces air flow at low lung volumes.

Malignant pleural mesotheliomas are bulky, slow-growing tumors that spread by local extension to encase the lung and mediastinum. They vary histologically and can be difficult to distinguish from metastatic adenocarcinoma even in large specimens obtained by open pleural biopsy. Lung cancer can be of any cell type. Asbestos exposure and cigarette smoking act synergistically in causing lung cancer, so that heavily exposed smoking workers have a risk of lung cancer 30 to 90 times higher than unexposed nonsmokers (Ch. 70).

Asbestos fibers appear to cause tissue injury by stimulating alveolar macrophages to secrete cytotoxic materials, inflammatory cell chemoattractants, and at least one factor that stimulates fibroblast proliferation. Because of their durability, individual fibers can repeatedly stimulate macrophages for many years without being degraded. This helps to explain the continued progression of asbestos-induced disease after exposure ceases and points out why the effective intensity of

exposure depends on *time* from first exposure as well as total lung fiber burden. Nonetheless, the enormous variability in disease severity seen among individuals with equivalent exposure histories and lung fiber burdens suggests an important role for as yet uncharacterized host factors.

CLINICAL MANIFESTATIONS. Pleural plaques are the most common manifestation of asbestos exposure. Patients with only pleural involvement are usually asymptomatic and have normal pulmonary function. Occasionally, patients with extensive pleural thickening develop extrapulmonary lung restriction that can cause dyspnea. The major significance of pleural plaques is that their appearance on a chest radiograph confirms a history of exposure. Diaphragmatic plaques are especially likely to calcify, and bilateral diaphragmatic calcification is almost always caused by asbestos exposure. Diffuse unilateral pleural thickening and/or pleuritic chest pain suggests the possibility of mesothelioma.

Asbestosis presents as do other forms of pulmonary fibrosis, with dyspnea that is initially most prominent with exertion and is often associated with cough. Bibasilar rales are a common finding, and clubbing can occur. The chest radiograph reveals linear and irregular opacities that are most prominent in the lower lung fields. Pleural thickening is often present but may not be radiographically apparent. As with other forms of pulmonary fibrosis, up to 10 per cent of patients with asbestos-induced fibrosis severe enough to cause lung restriction have normal chest radiographs. Progressive massive fibrosis is not seen. In patients with pulmonary fibrosis severe enough to cause dyspnea, pulmonary function tests usually show lung restriction (a symmetric reduction in all lung volumes) and a reduction in diffusing capacity. Flow-volume curves show reduced flow at low lung volumes, but marked airway obstruction as manifested by a marked reduction in FEV_1 per cent, usually has other causes, such as cigarette smoking. In an asbestos-exposed smoker, a decrease in total lung capacity cannot be caused by smoking, but decreases in diffusing capacity and flow at low lung volume could be due to cigarettes, asbestos, or the combined effects of both.

DIAGNOSIS. The diagnosis of asbestos-induced pleural plaques is made on the basis of the typical bilateral appearance and a history of exposure. In approximately 80 per cent of patients with bilateral pleural plaques, asbestos exposure is responsible. Oblique radiographs increase the likelihood of detecting plaques, and computed axial tomography is more sensitive than standard radiography and allows distinction between true plaques and subpleural fat. Since plaques themselves are rarely clinically significant, the considerable cost of these studies and the additional radiation exposure is difficult to justify, except for research purposes. The diagnosis of asbestos-induced pleural effusion depends on a history of exposure and exclusion of other causes of a pleural exudate.

Asbestosis is usually diagnosed on the basis of significant exposure, radiographic abnormalities, and pulmonary function studies showing lung restriction. Occasionally, in patients with early disease, radiographs or lung function studies may be normal, but exercise testing will reveal abnormalities in pulmonary gas exchange. Lung biopsy should be performed only in patients with progressive disease to exclude causes of pulmonary fibrosis that might respond to treatment. If sufficient lung tissue is available (from open lung biopsy or autopsy) asbestos burden should be estimated by counting asbestos bodies from ashed tissue or asbestos fibers by electron probe analysis. In patients with stable lung function, lung biopsy should not be performed merely to establish asbestos exposure as the cause of lung fibrosis, since such a diagnosis will not lead to any specific therapy whereas all biopsy procedures are associated with some risk.

Asbestosis usually does not develop before 15 years after the first exposure to asbestos and usually requires several years of exposure. However, workers have been reported to develop the disease 15 to 30 years after periods of very heavy exposure as short as 6 months.

A diagnosis of asbestos-induced lung cancer is based on a history of heavy exposure that should ideally be confirmed by quantification of asbestos fiber burden from resected lung or autopsy specimens. Like pulmonary fibrosis, lung cancer does not develop within 15 years of first exposure and has its peak incidence within 25 to 40 years. The distribution of tumor cell types is the same as that seen in the general population. Epidemiologic evidence suggests that an increased incidence of lung cancer requires a similar intensity of asbestos exposure to that required to increase the incidence of pulmonary fibrosis. These data do not imply that both abnormalities would occur in the same individuals. Thus, lung cancer of any cell type in an individual with a well-documented history of heavy exposure can be reasonably considered to be due, at least in part, to asbestos exposure irrespective of coexistent pulmonary fibrosis.

TREATMENT AND PREVENTION. There is no proven effective treatment for asbestosis. The major strategy for prevention is worldwide elimination of new asbestos use and replacement with synthetic substitutes that appear to be considerably less toxic. Continuing exposure to asbestos presently in use needs to be minimized by use of engineering controls, personal protection, and public education. For prevention of lung cancer, individuals with past exposure should be strongly encouraged to stop smoking, since the risk of lung cancer falls dramatically (but is not eliminated) within a few years of smoking cessation.

Becklake MR: Asbestos-related diseases of the lungs and pleura: Current clinical issues. Am Rev Respir Dis 126:187, 1982. *An update of a comprehensive 1976 review by the same author.*

Craighead JE, Abraham JL, Churg A, et al.: The pathology of asbestos-associated diseases of the lungs and pleural cavities: Diagnostic criteria and proposed grading system. Arch Path Lab Med 106:544, 1982. *A comprehensive report of a consensus committee.*

Murphy RL, Becklake MR, Brooks SM, et al.: The diagnosis of nonmalignant disease related to asbestos. Am Rev Respir Dis 134:363, 1986. *An authoritative consensus statement on evaluation of patients exposed to asbestos.*

Beryllium Disease

Beryllium is a rare metal that can cause both acute and chronic disease. Acute beryllium disease results from intense exposure and resembles acute lung injury from other massive toxic exposures. Clinical manifestations include upper airway injury, bronchiolitis, and pulmonary edema. Mortality has been reported to be as high as 10 per cent. Chronic beryllium disease can follow acute disease but more often occurs without antecedent symptoms from months to years after first exposure. Because beryllium salts are absorbed through the respiratory tract and distributed throughout the body, exposure causes a systemic disease. Pathologically, chronic beryllium disease is characterized by noncaseating granulomas in lung, lymph nodes, liver, spleen, adrenal glands, and kidneys. Granulomas in the skin are thought to be due to direct exposure.

Before 1949, most cases of beryllium disease were due to the use of beryllium in fluorescent lights. Since that time, when such use was discontinued, most cases have occurred in the manufacturing of metal alloys and x-ray tubes and in the mining and milling of beryllium. The number of new cases has progressively fallen as industrial hygiene measures have been improved in these industries, but occasional cases continue to occur.

The diagnosis of chronic beryllium disease is made on the basis of a history of exposure and demonstration of granulomas on tissue biopsy. The lung pathology is nonspecific and indistinguishable from sarcoid and hypersensitivity pneumonitis (Ch. 69). Involvement of the uvea, salivary glands, or central nervous system and the presence of erythema nodosum favor sarcoid. Demonstration of beryllium in urine confirms exposure but does not correlate with disease. The

disease is thought to be due to a cell-mediated immune response directed at beryllium-protein complexes. Lymphocyte transformation in response to beryllium has been demonstrated in vitro from peripheral blood lymphocytes and lung lymphocytes obtained by bronchoalveolar lavage from some patients with chronic beryllium disease. Transformation of blood lymphocytes is relatively insensitive, however, and can also be seen in exposed workers with no evidence of disease. Insufficient data are presently available to adequately evaluate the sensitivity and specificity of in vitro transformation of lymphocytes obtained by bronchoalveolar lavage. The clinical course of chronic beryllium disease is quite variable. Most patients remain stable if exposure ceases, but the disease can remit or progress in some individuals. Treatment with corticosteroids has been recommended but has not been systematically studied.

Daniele RP: Beryllium-induced lung disease: Immunologic mechanisms and diagnostic approaches. In Gee JBL (ed.): Occupational Lung Disease. New York, Churchill Livingstone, 1984, pp 183–192.

Diseases Caused by Other Inorganic Dusts

Silicates other than asbestos can also cause pneumoconiosis. Kaolin, mica, and vermiculite, for example, cause x-ray abnormalities and pathologic lesions similar to those caused by coal dust. Talc inhalation causes pulmonary fibrosis with features of both asbestosis and silicosis, as well as foreign body granulomas. Pleural plaques have also been noted in workers exposed to talc, but they may be due to contamination of talc with asbestos. A severe granulomatous lung disease, sometimes associated with pulmonary hypertension, can occur in intravenous drug addicts from intravenous injection of talc. Synthetic vitreous fibers such as fiberglass and glass wool are physically similar to asbestos, but evidence to date suggests that they are considerably less toxic. Because of the long latency of fiber-induced disorders, continued close surveillance of the effects of use of these fibers is essential. As new technologies evolve, it is likely that new reactions to inorganic dusts will be recognized. For example, exposure to the dust of a variety of metals (including tungsten carbide, cobalt, titanium, and tantalum) may cause acute and/or chronic injury to the airways and lung parenchyma.

Hypersensitivity Pneumonitis

Hypersensitivity pneumonitis is a parenchymal lung disorder that usually results from occupational exposure to organic dusts. The disease is characterized clinically by recurrent episodes of cough, dyspnea, and signs of systemic illness (fever, leukocytosis, and myalgias). After long-term exposure to the responsible dust, affected workers can develop pulmonary fibrosis often with noncaseating granulomas in lung tissue. This disorder is discussed in detail in Chapter 62.

Occupational Lung Cancer

As the site of entry of most airborne carcinogens, the lung is the organ most often affected by occupational carcinogenesis. Definitive identification of an occupational agent as a lung carcinogen is made difficult by the long latency period for most carcinogens (20 to 40 years), the high background incidence of lung cancer, and the potent confounding effect of cigarette smoke. Thus, of the more than 100 agents suspected of causing respiratory cancer in animals, only a few have been shown to cause cancer in humans, for example, arsenic, asbestos, cadmium, chloromethyl ether, chromates, coal tars, coke-oven emissions, mustard gas, nickel, and uranium and other sources of ionizing radiation. Chloromethyl ether appears to be especially likely to cause oat-cell carcinoma, but most occupational carcinogens increase the risk for lung cancer of all common cell types. Prevention of occupational lung cancer requires minimizing exposure to suspected carcinogens *before* they are definitively shown to cause cancer in exposed workers.

537 PHYSICAL, CHEMICAL, AND ASPIRATION INJURIES OF THE LUNG

James D. Crapo

The lung has an extremely large and delicate surface exposed to the environment. Extensive defense mechanisms protect the lung from inhaled pathogens and toxic substances. Under normal conditions, air is fully humidified and warmed to body temperature, and all large particulate substances are cleared by the upper airways. These defenses are not adequate to handle many physical and chemical substances that cause lung injury. This chapter deals with a variety of lung injuries that are initiated by external factors rather than being due to an intrinsic defect or failure of the respiratory system and its defenses.

PHYSICAL DISORDERS

Thermal Injuries

About 25 per cent of patients with major burns have pulmonary complications; these complications account for the majority of burn-related deaths. Thermal injury to the lung is associated with three groups of complications: (1) *Immediate reaction*—direct thermal injury to upper airways, leading to upper airway obstruction, carbon monoxide poisoning, and smoke inhalation (potent bronchoconstrictors and edemagenic substances). (2) *Adult respiratory distress syndrome* (ARDS) developing 24 to 48 hours after the thermal injury. (3) *Late-onset pulmonary complications*, which include pneumonia, atelectasis, thromboembolism, and chest-wall restriction caused by circumferential thoracic burns.

Few burns actually cause thermal injury to the lung parenchyma; the large capacity of the upper airways to humidify and modify the temperatures of inhaled air protects the alveolar tissue. Exceptions are steam burns and explosions in an enclosed space.

The initial symptoms are tachypnea, cough, dyspnea, wheezing, cyanosis, hoarseness, and stridor (an ominous sign). During the next 12 to 48 hours the patient may become increasingly hypoxic; lung compliance may decrease, and pulmonary edema may develop in the presence of normal pulmonary capillary wedge pressure. Roentgenograms of the chest may show no significant changes or a pattern of diffuse, patchy infiltrates. The major complication is infection, usually caused by *Pseudomonas aeruginosa* or *Staphylococcus aureus*. The lung defenses against infection are compromised by thermal injury to the airway epithelium and often by an endotracheal or tracheostomy tube. The pathway of infection may be either by inhalation of airborne organisms or by hematogenous spread from the burn.

The constituents of smoke are potent mucosal irritants and bronchoconstrictors and contribute to the upper and lower lung lesions. Typical constituents of smoke include oxides of nitrogen, sulfur and lead, ammonia, hydrochlorides, chlorine, and aldehydes. Acrolein, found in wood smoke, is a potent mucosal irritant which contributes to upper airway obstruction and to pulmonary edema. Carbon monoxide poisoning from inhaled smoke is discussed in Chemical Injury to the Lung.

The adult respiratory distress syndrome commonly develops 24 to 48 hours after the initial symptoms subside. The causes of adult respiratory distress syndrome in the burn patient are controversial, but possibilities include a chemical pneumonitis caused by constituents in smoke, a circulating burn toxin, disseminated intravascular coagulation, microembolism, or central neurogenic pulmonary edema. The extent of surface thermal injury does not correlate with the degree of respiratory distress that subsequently develops.

Late-onset pulmonary burn complications—atelectasis, thromboembolism, and pneumonia—are discussed in Ch. 62, 67, and 262 to 267, respectively.

THERAPY. Carbon monoxide poisoning and upper airway obstruction are the most immediate life-threatening complications in the patient presenting with major burns or with the history of smoke or steam inhalation. The patient should be closely observed for evidence of these complications and given high levels of inspired oxygen. Fiberoptic bronchoscopy may help detect laryngeal and tracheobronchial inflammation and evidence of smoke contamination in the lower airways. Arterial blood gases should be monitored and prompt intubation or tracheostomy performed if evidence of significant airway obstruction develops. Corticosteroids may be helpful to treat edema of the upper airways but must be used with caution since one of the major complications of both skin and lung thermal injury is infection. Prophylactic antibiotics are of no value in preventing pneumonia and may predispose to infection with resistant organisms. Careful pulmonary toilet, humidification, and sterile suctioning should be used to reduce the risk of pneumonia. Repeated bronchoscopy is often necessary to remove mucous plugs and thereby prevent segmental atelectasis and infection.

Crapo RO: Smoke-inhalation injuries. JAMA 246:1694, 1981. *A review of the clinical presentation and treatment of smoke inhalation injuries.*
Demling RH: Burns. N Engl J Med 313:1389, 1985. *A general review of the approach to the burn patient; 119 references.*
Trunkey DD: Inhalation injury. Surg Clin North Am 58:1133, 1978. *A detailed review of pulmonary damage caused by smoke inhalation; 16 references.*

Radiation Injury (See also Ch. 539)

The predominant factors determining the incidence of radiation pneumonitis are the total radiation dose, the number of fractions, and the duration of time over which the total dose is given. Some chemotherapeutic drugs may potentiate damage from radiation. A total lung dose of less than 2000 rads generally is not associated with severe radiation pneumonitis, whereas a total dose in excess of 4000 rads, even if distributed over as many as 30 fractions, has virtually a 100 per cent risk of radiation pneumonitis.

HISTOPATHOLOGIC CHANGES. The reaction of the lung to radiation injury can be divided into three phases: (1) The acute phase, occurring one to two months after radiation, is characterized by vascular damage, congestion, edema, and mononuclear cell infiltration. Alveolar Type II cells and alveolar macrophages are increased in number. (2) The subacute phase occurs two to nine months later. The alveolar walls become infiltrated with mononuclear inflammatory cells and fibroblasts. (3) The chronic or fibrotic phase generally occurs more than nine months after irradiation. Capillary sclerosis and alveolar fibrosis are its predominant histologic features.

CLINICAL PRESENTATION. Signs of bronchial irritation may appear immediately after radiation therapy and/or evidence of esophagitis shortly thereafter, but patients may have no symptoms for 6 to 12 weeks, at which time mild cough appears. If large volumes of lung have been irradiated, or if high radiation doses over short periods have been given, dyspnea, tachypnea, and fever, sometimes high and spiking, can develop. These symptoms can be extremely severe and will either progress to severe dyspnea and death or gradually subside, leaving varying degrees of respiratory impairment resulting from chronic lung fibrosis. The permanent changes of fibrosis take 6 to 24 months to evolve, and then usually remain stable after two years if no further exposure occurs. Auscultation of the chest is usually normal, although rales, signs of consolidation, and rubs may be found. Clubbing does not develop after radiation injury. Laboratory findings include a mild leukocytosis and an increased erythrocyte sedimentation rate. If the irradiated area is extensive, arterial hypoxemia may be found. Radiographic changes generally appear one to three months following treatment. After therapeutic thoracic irradiation the affected areas are generally demarcated by a sharp edge limited to the margins of the portal of irradiation and have a "ground-glass appearance"—a hazy increase in density with indistinct pulmonary markings. In the later phases of the radiation injury, fibrosis and contraction of the irradiated region are the predominant radiographic findings.

Pulmonary function testing shows no change until clinical symptoms appear, at which time a restrictive ventilatory defect is present. Capillary sclerosis is associated with a decrease in blood flow to the affected region and a decrease in carbon monoxide transfer capacity. Severe radiation injury is associated with a decrease in lung compliance and hypoxemia.

Complications of radiation pneumonitis include small pleural effusions and occasionally spontaneous pneumothorax. The cough may be severe enough to cause rib fractures.

The differential diagnosis of acute radiation pneumonitis is usually complicated by the immunocompromised state of many of the patients, by the presence of bacterial, fungal, and protozoan pneumonias, particularly *Pneumocystis carinii*, or by the signs and symptoms of the neoplasm being treated. Radiation pneumonitis has not been documented in parts of the lung outside the radiation portal.

TREATMENT. The best management of radiation pneumonitis is to avoid it when possible. The patient who develops radiation pneumonitis requires supportive care, including medication for cough suppression and often oxygen delivered by nasal catheter or mask for hypoxemia. Corticosteroids (prednisone, 1 mg per kilogram of body weight) are effective at the start of pneumonitis. On occasion the response may be dramatic, with complete resolution of symptoms within 24 hours. Corticosteroids should be tapered as rapidly as possible. There is no evidence that corticosteroids given at the time of irradiation have any protective effect. They are also ineffective in the late fibrotic phases of the disease.

Antibiotics have been tried both prophylactically and when pneumonitis develops. There is no evidence that this treatment modifies the clinical course; therefore antibiotic therapy should be reserved for patients in whom the findings suggest significant infection to be present. Since the lesion involves occlusion and thrombosis of many small blood vessels, anticoagulation has been suggested but without experimental evidence of its effectiveness.

Gross NJ: The pathogenesis of radiation-induced lung damage. Lung 139:115, 1981. *A review of the biochemistry and cell biology of irradiated lung and how these factors relate to the clinical syndrome.*

Disorders of the Lung Caused by Barometric Pressure

Altitude

The major physiologic effects of reduced atmospheric pressure are due to the resulting low partial pressure of oxygen. At 10,000 feet (3048 meters) the alveolar Po_2 is approximately 60 mm Hg, and some individuals will manifest impairment of recent memory, judgment, and the ability to perform complex calculations, and will demonstrate an increased heart rate and increased pulmonary ventilation. The time required for these symptoms to begin is partially related to age, physical fitness, and acclimatization. At 12,000 feet (3658 meters) the alveolar Po_2 is 52, and dyspnea, headache, nausea, and decreased visual acuity may occur. At 18,000 feet (5486 meters) the alveolar Po_2 is 40, and unacclimatized individuals will lose consciousness after several hours of exposure. At 22,000 feet (6706 meters) the alveolar Po_2 is 30, and almost all acutely exposed individuals become unconscious after sufficient time. The rapid change in physiologic functions that begins to occur at about 10,000 feet is due to the shape of the oxygen-hemoglobin dissociation curve, which has a steep

downslope below a Po_2 of approximately 60 mm Hg. A small drop in Po_2 below this level results in a relatively large decrease in arterial saturation.

In general, commercial aircraft cabins are maintained at a pressure greater than or equal to that encountered at 8000 feet so that no supplemental oxygen is required. Some patients with reduced cardiac reserve or with chronic obstructive lung disease may have difficulty tolerating even a small drop in arterial oxygen saturation and may require supplemental oxygen during flights. Aircraft regulations require that the flight crew receive supplemental oxygen when the cabin pressure drops below that at 10,000 feet, and that passengers receive supplemental oxygen should the cabin pressure drop below that at 15,000 feet.

ACUTE MOUNTAIN SICKNESS. This syndrome occurs in unacclimated persons who rapidly ascend to a high altitude. Symptoms can occur at altitudes as low as 7000 to 8000 feet in particularly susceptible individuals, usually those in poor physical condition, and during a rapid ascent requiring significant physical exertion. The symptoms are headache, exertional dyspnea, malaise, anorexia, nausea, vomiting, diarrhea, and abdominal pain. Judgment may be impaired. Inability to sleep is a common problem. Cyanosis, Cheyne-Stokes breathing, and tachycardia are commonly present. In untreated individuals, these signs and symptoms subside gradually over a period of several days. The treatment is oxygen therapy or descent to a lower altitude. The disorder is thought to be related to an increase in ventilation stimulated by hypoxia and resulting in hypocapnia and respiratory alkalosis. Acetazolamide, 250 mg every eight hours prior to and during the ascent to altitude, can prevent symptoms, presumably by increasing renal excretion of bicarbonate and reducing the extent of the respiratory alkalosis. Furosemide, 80 mg every 12 hours, has also produced relief of symptoms.

CHRONIC MOUNTAIN SICKNESS (MONGE'S DISEASE). Chronic mountain sickness occurs in people living at high altitudes, usually at over 14,000 feet, for many years. These "highlanders" have a blunted respiratory drive in response to hypoxia and have a lower minute ventilation at high altitudes than do those who normally reside at lower altitudes. Chronic mountain sickness is characterized by what appears to be an exaggerated adaptive response to altitude. This includes erythrocytosis with hemoglobin levels as high as 25 grams per deciliter, a decreased minute ventilation with an elevated Pco_2, low arterial oxygen saturation, and an impaired sensitivity of the respiratory center to hypoxia. Clinical manifestations are similar to those of polycythemia rubra vera and include cyanosis, dyspnea, cough, palpitations, headache, giddiness, muscular weakness, pain in the extremities, sensory and motor changes, and episodic stupor. The only therapy is to move the patient to a lower altitude. Subacute forms of this illness also occur in which the marked cyanosis and alveolar hypoventilation are absent. A similar syndrome, brisket disease, has been described in cattle.

HIGH-ALTITUDE PULMONARY EDEMA. Acute pulmonary edema is a potentially fatal complication of rapid ascent to altitudes of greater than 9000 feet. The mechanism is unknown, but clearly hypoxia is the provoking cause. Symptoms begin after 6 to 36 hours at high altitude and may follow an episode of acute mountain sickness. Rales, cyanosis, orthopnea, and hemoptysis commonly develop unless oxygen is administered or the patient is rapidly moved to a lower altitude.

At autopsy the lungs are typically heavy, congested, and edematous and have hyaline membranes in the small airways and alveoli. The cause of hyaline membrane formation is not known; this is not a characteristic finding in death caused by other forms of hypoxia. During a large military airlift in India, approximately 6 of each 1000 persons flown to an altitude of 11,500 feet developed this syndrome.

Hemodynamic studies have shown elevations of the pulmonary artery pressure with a normal pulmonary venous pressure. The pulmonary edema may be due to an increase in pulmonary capillary pressure in small regions of the pulmonary capillary bed, or to increased permeability in lung capillaries.

Increased Barometric Pressure

Pressure increases approximately one atmosphere for each 33 feet of descent in water. Direct body contact with increased barometric pressure under water is most commonly encountered during breathhold diving, when continuous consumption of oxygen and production of CO_2 lead to hypoxia and hypercapnia. The increasing serum carbon dioxide concentration causes an almost irresistible drive to breathe. Since hypoxia is a mild stimulation for ventilation, it is relatively easy to continue holding one's breath in the presence of profound hypoxia. A common hazardous error made by swimmers is to hyperventilate prior to a dive in an effort to increase the time of breath holding. This depletes the body of carbon dioxide stores, but does not significantly increase oxygen stores. In these circumstances hypoxia can cause unconsciousness before accumulation of carbon dioxide forces the termination of the dive. This is thought to account for many deaths in swimming pools. Decompression during ascent from a breathhold dive can cause a marked fall in alveolar Po_2, leading to the diver's losing consciousness just as the surface is reached.

DECOMPRESSION SICKNESS. Decompression sickness was first described in caisson workers in tunnel construction, where compressed air was used to exclude water and mud. The increase in military, commercial, and sport diving has made decompression sickness a relatively common clinical problem. When ordinary air is breathed under increased ambient pressure, inert gas, commonly nitrogen, dissolves in tissue and blood, reaching saturation equilibrium at the greater partial pressures. Upon rapid decompression to sea level, the inert gas may come out of solution to form intravascular bubbles. The onset of symptoms tends to be gradual, beginning minutes to hours after the termination of a dive. Manifestations include "bends" (deep pain in joints, aggravated by exercise), pruritus, cyanosis, substernal chest pain, dyspnea, nonproductive cough, evidence of spinal cord injury, confusion, blurred vision, visual field defects, paralysis, dysphasia, headache, vertigo, and seizures. In severe cases the symptoms may rapidly progress to shock and death. Symptoms of mild or early decompression sickness resemble and are often confused with acute alcohol intoxication.

The treatment of decompression sickness is recompression with a gradual return to sea level pressures over a period of days to weeks. Recompression decreases bubble size and permits their gradual resorption during the "ascent" to surface pressures.

Air embolism can occur in scuba divers who ascend without exhaling. Intrapulmonary gas expands and the high pressure may rupture a portion of the lung and introduce gas into the systemic circulation, mediastinum, pleura, or subcutaneous tissues. Gas bubbles may form arterial emboli to the brain and result in sudden unconsciousness, focal or generalized seizures, visual field loss or blindness, weakness, paralysis, hypoesthesia, or confusion. The therapy is rapid recompression similar to that employed to treat decompression sickness. Gas embolism has been reported during ascents of as little as 2.2 meters and is thought to be one of the most common causes of accidental death in divers.

THERAPEUTIC HYPERBARIC OXYGEN. Hyperbaric oxygen has been clearly proven to be beneficial in treating only a limited number of illnesses: acute carbon monoxide poisoning, acute cyanide poisoning, clostridial myonecrosis, decompression sickness, air embolism, and osteoradionecrosis. The hazards of oxygen toxicity limit the dose of oxygen that can be delivered by hyperbaric techniques. Central nervous

system toxicity, usually in the form of convulsions, occurs at oxygen pressures greater than 2.5 atmospheres if the exposure is maintained for a sufficient length of time. Thus, hyperbaric oxygen therapy is limited to a maximum of two to three atmospheres of oxygen and durations of no more than one to three hours.

Schoene RB: Pulmonary edema at high altitude, review, pathophysiology and update. Clin Chest Med 6:491, 1985. *A historical perspective and pathophysiologic review of high-altitude pulmonary edema including a review of evidence showing this is due to a permeability type of leak.*
Strauss RH: Diving medicine. Am Rev Respir Dis 119:1001, 1979. *A comprehensive state-of-the-art review on all aspects of diving medicine.*

CHEMICAL INJURY TO THE LUNG
Toxic Inhaled Gases

A large number of gases and chemicals, to which exposures most frequently occur in an industrial setting, can cause an acute and sometimes a chronic injury to the respiratory system.

A few agents cause an *"asthma-like"* reaction with cough, chest pain, and wheezing. Toluene di-isocyanate and other isocyanates (liberated as gas during the reaction of isocyanates with polyol in the manufacture of polyurethane foams), aluminum soldering flux, and platinum salts are typical examples. Reaginic and precipitating antibodies against platinum salts and soldering flux have been found in symptomatic individuals, suggesting an immunologic basis for the reaction. An allergic basis for the reaction to toluene di-isocyanate has not been demonstrated. The symptoms usually subside after removal from exposure; however, chronic lung injury may occur if the exposure is prolonged.

A number of highly irritating gases cause an *acute chemical pneumonitis*. Such gases include chlorine (used in the chemical and plastic industries and to disinfect water), ammonia (used in refrigeration), sulfur dioxide (used in paper manufacture and smelting of sulfide containing ores), ozone (generated in welding and in photochemical smog), nitrogen dioxide (released from decomposed corn silage), and phosgene (used in production of aniline dyes).

The prototype for injury of this type is *silo-filler's disease* (nitrogen dioxide). During the initial exposure there may be no symptoms, there may be tracheobronchitis with cough and shortness of breath, or there may be the immediate onset of acute pulmonary edema. Signs of ocular and oropharyngeal mucous membrane irritation may be present. The symptoms may rapidly progress, but commonly the initial symptoms resolve and are followed by a period of minimal symptoms (cough) lasting up to 48 hours. Fever, myalgias, dyspnea, and progressive hypoxemia then occur and the radiographic picture is that of pulmonary edema. These severe symptoms may resolve only to recur two to five weeks later and may lead to progressive pulmonary insufficiency with a picture of bronchiolitis obliterans. Treatment with corticosteroids (prednisone, 1 mg per kilogram per day) may dramatically improve the acute illness. Bronchodilators, mechanical ventilation, and supplemental oxygen may be necessary. Since there may be a period of temporary improvement following the initial exposure, observation for a period of 48 hours is advisable.

The clinical response caused by each irritant gas varies, but appears to be closely related to the degree of acute irritation it causes and to its water solubility. The less irritating gases, such as ozone and the oxides of nitrogen, phosgene, mercury, and nickel carbonyl, can be inhaled for prolonged periods of time and thereby cause injury throughout the respiratory system. Highly irritating and soluble gases, such as ammonia and hydrochloric acid, are less likely to be inhaled deeply and tend to result in immediate injury to the upper airways and have potential for obstruction secondary to mucosal edema. Less soluble substances, such as chlorine, cadmium, zinc chloride, osmium tetraoxide, and vanadium, can cause injury to the entire tracheobronchial tree and do not commonly present with upper airway obstruction. Bronchiolitis and pulmonary edema are common, ultimately leading to bronchiolitis obliterans. The long-term consequences vary with the gas. Cadmium, for example, can cause diffuse emphysema and severe airway obstruction but only minimal fibrosis.

Different mechanisms are involved in the injury caused by these gases. Most of them cause injury by acting as a strong acid, a strong base, or an oxidant. Gases of chemicals that are strong acids or bases in water solution, such as hydrogen chloride, sulfuric acid, sulfur dioxide, and ammonia, tend to react more in the upper airways where they change tissue pH and thereby cause cell damage.

Evans MJ: Oxidant gases. Environ Health Perspect 55:85, 1984. *A review of the effects of ozone, nitrogen dioxide, and oxygen on lung structure and the factors that can modulate the degree of damage.*

Summer W, Haponik E: Inhalation of irritant gases. Clin Chest Med 2:273, 1981. *A comprehensive review of gases that are toxic to the lung; 74 references.*

Pulmonary Oxygen Toxicity

Oxygen is used in extremely high concentrations in large numbers of patients in intensive care units, often with endotracheal intubation and mechanical ventilation. The toxic effects of hyperoxic atmospheres may not infrequently outweigh the potential therapeutic benefits. Superoxide, an unstable free radical produced by the single electron reduction of oxygen, is produced as a normal by-product of oxidative metabolism in almost every plant and animal tissue that uses oxygen as an electron sink. Superoxide dismutase is a protective enzyme that catalyzes the dismutation and therefore the detoxification of the superoxide free radical. If not scavenged by superoxide dismutase, this free radical can react with hydrogen peroxide to form the hydroxyl free radical (OH•) and free radical chain reactions can be initiated, resulting in the destruction of cell lipids and proteins. This "free radical injury" is the presumed chemical basis for oxygen toxicity (Fig. 537–1).

In the adult the major target tissue of oxygen injury is the pulmonary capillary endothelium. Other body organs are protected by the consumption of oxygen and the characteristics of the binding of oxygen to hemoglobin. The mixed venous P_{O_2} is maintained at about 40 to 50 torr even when the patient is breathing 100 per cent oxygen.

At autopsy the lungs are atelectatic, congested, and edematous and have hyaline membranes. The most serious injury appears to be destruction of the capillary bed with resultant interstitial and alveolar edema, hypoxemia, and sometimes death. Alveolar epithelium is also injured, causing hyperplasia of Type II cells. An acute tracheobronchitis also occurs, and histologic changes have been found in the ciliated epithelium and Clara cells in the small airways.

The typical presentation in the adult is that of an acutely ill patient who is receiving oxygen in high concentrations and mechanical ventilation for a lung injury that makes the onset of pulmonary oxygen toxicity difficult to detect. Lung compliance progressively falls; the patient develops tachypnea, substernal pain, and increased cough. The alveolar-arterial oxygen gradient gradually widens with progressive hypoxemia. Increasing concentrations of oxygen are needed to maintain adequate oxygenation of arterial blood, and the cycle progresses to pulmonary edema, respiratory failure, and death.

The earliest symptoms of oxygen toxicity are due to acute tracheobronchitis. A dry, hacking cough and substernal pain may occur within six to twelve hours while breathing pure oxygen. Nausea, vomiting, and paresthesias follow. Vital capacity decreases, and there is an increase in the respiratory rate.

The flow of tracheal mucus decreases after short exposures to excess oxygen, probably reflecting functional injury of airway epithelium. These patients are therefore more susceptible to mucus impaction and to infection caused by failure to clear inhaled pathogens adequately.

The only proven therapy is prevention of the insult by using high oxygen concentrations judiciously. Corticosteroids have no proven benefit and may actually enhance the lung injury caused by hyperoxia. It is usually impossible clinically to distinguish early oxygen toxicity because of the severity of the original lung insult. The physician often faces a dilemma in which increasing concentrations of oxygen are essential for immediate survival but its administration contributes to deterioration of the patient a short time later. Alternative methods to improve tissue oxygen delivery without using high inspired partial pressures of oxygen should be used whenever possible. These include transfusion of packed red cells to raise the serum hemotocrit to even supranormal levels, measures to improve cardiac output, and measures to decrease the tissue oxygen demand by reducing fever or intense agitation.

The safe maximal concentration of oxygen is not known.

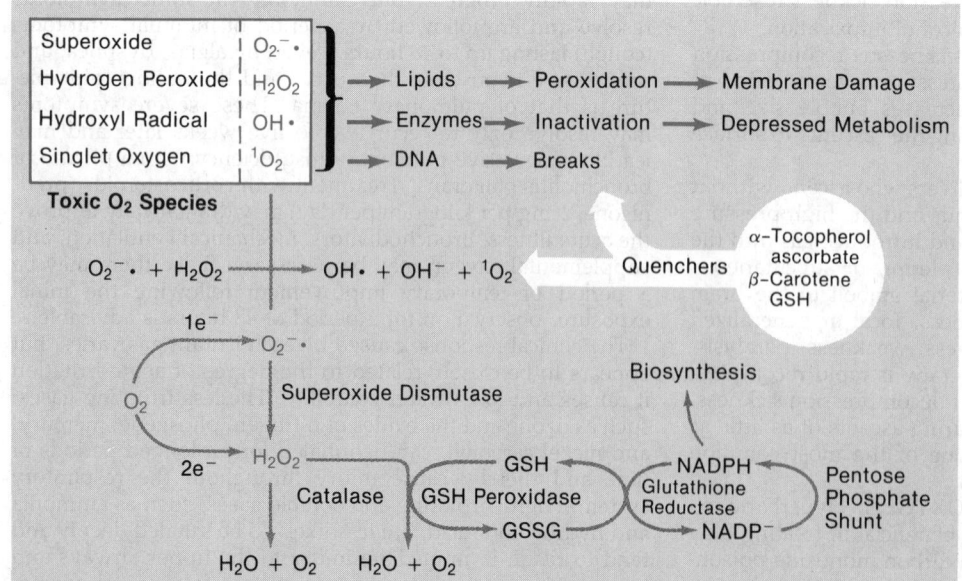

FIGURE 537–1. Toxic oxygen species and antioxidant defense systems. The incomplete reduction of oxygen produces superoxide and/or hydrogen peroxide. These species can react together in the presence of metal salts to form the hydroxyl radical and singlet oxygen. Free radical chain reactions can be initiated in lipid membranes, with enzymes and DNA also attacked by these reactive O_2 species. Quenchers interact with the oxygen species or with oxidized tissue components to block further tissue oxidation and to terminate free radical chain reactions. The antioxidant defense systems—superoxide dismutase, catalase, and glutathione peroxidase—function to detoxify superoxide and hydrogen peroxide, thus preventing the formation of other toxic O_2 species and the subsequent reactions with tissue. Glucose-6-phosphate dehydrogenase is the rate-limiting enzyme in the pentose phosphate shunt and thereby controls the availability of NADPH. This cofactor is essential both for the reduction of glutathione and for the biosynthetic pathways critical for repair processes. Net tissue injury represents the balance between the rate of production of partially reduced oxygen species, the rate at which these species are scavenged, and the rate of repair of any injury that occurs.

Many recommend the range of 40 to 50 per cent oxygen as safe because little injury has been demonstrated in normal animals or human volunteers breathing 40 to 50 per cent oxygen for prolonged periods. The diseased lung may be more susceptible to oxygen injury, however. Rather than identify an arbitrary oxygen concentration that should not be exceeded, rational therapy is to use only enough oxygen to provide adequate arterial blood saturation—an arterial Po_2 of 60 torr. Patients should not continuously be given 40 to 50 per cent oxygen under the assumption that this concentration is harmless. If the patient survives oxygen toxicity, some residual damage to the lung parenchyma may remain, with septal fibrosis replacing areas where the pulmonary capillary bed was destroyed by the hyperoxia.

Crapo JD: Morphologic changes in pulmonary oxygen toxicity. Annu Rev Physiol 48:721, 1986. *A detailed review of the time course and patterns of injury to the lung during exposure to hyperoxia.*

Deneke SM, Fanburg BL: Normobaric oxygen toxicity of the lung. N Engl J Med 303:76, 1980. *A comprehensive and well-written review.*

Jamieson D, Chance B, Cadenas E, et al.: The relation of free radical production to hyperoxia. Annu Rev Physiol 48:703, 1986. *A review of the pathogenesis of hyperoxic mediated cell injury.*

Carbon Monoxide Poisoning

Carbon monoxide is commonly produced by internal combustion engines, by poorly vented heating devices, and by gas refrigerators. Lower levels can exist in automobile repair shops, in areas of high automobile traffic density, and in arc welding. Natural gas is free of carbon monoxide, but its incomplete combustion by a faulty heating apparatus can produce carbon monoxide. The most common source of human exposure to carbon monoxide is smoking; cigarette smokers commonly have carboxyhemoglobin concentrations of 3 to 8 per cent. Endogenous carbon monoxide is normally produced from cleavage of the α-methylene bridge in the catabolism of heme, which results in a normal blood carboxyhemoglobin concentration of 0.5 to 0.8 per cent.

Carbon monoxide injures by causing tissue hypoxia. Carbon monoxide has an affinity for hemoglobin which is 218 times greater than that of oxygen. Thus, even small amounts of inspired carbon monoxide will have profound effects on the oxygen-carrying capacity of blood. An alveolar carbon monoxide tension of 0.5 torr and an arterial oxygen tension of 100 torr will produce blood concentrations of 50 per cent carboxyhemoglobin and 50 per cent oxyhemoglobin. In addition, carbon monoxide shifts the oxyhemoglobin saturation curve to the left and changes its shape, resulting in a further decrease in oxygen unloading in tissues.

The clinical picture of carbon monoxide poisoning is dependent upon the blood concentration of carboxyhemoglobin. Levels of less than 10 per cent carboxyhemoglobin produce few clinical symptoms. At 10 to 30 per cent carboxyhemoglobin, headaches and nausea occur and there may be mild dysfunction of the central nervous system with decreased visual acuity and impaired cognitive functions. Thirty to 40 per cent carboxyhemoglobin is associated with severe headaches, dyspnea on exertion, dizziness, nausea, vomiting, dimness of vision, ataxia, and possible collapse. Levels greater than 50 per cent carboxyhemoglobin cause tachypnea, convulsions, coma, and death from profound shock and respiratory and cardiovascular failure.

The diagnosis is confirmed by the determination of blood carboxyhemoglobin concentration. Carboxyhemoglobin has a characteristic cherry red color which can produce the classic bright red skin color in patients poisoned by carbon monoxide. This is in fact rare during life and is seen most often after death.

TREATMENT. The patient must be immediately removed from the contaminated environment. The specific therapy is administration of oxygen. Breathing normal air will result in a 50 per cent clearance of blood carbon monoxide in approx-

imately five hours. Administration of 100 per cent oxygen at sea level will achieve a 50 per cent reduction of carboxyhemoglobin in 80 minutes, whereas oxygen at three atmospheres of pressure will achieve the same clearance in approximately 25 minutes. The use of 95 per cent oxygen–5 per cent carbon dioxide will hasten oxygenation, largely by lowering the pH (Bohr effect). In the acutely ill patient the presence of metabolic acidosis is a contraindication to further reductions in pH by administration of carbon dioxide. The level of carboxyhemoglobin is not the sole determinant of the need for therapy. Patients with neurologic abnormalities should be considered for treatment with hyperbaric oxygen even if carboxyhemoglobin levels are low.

Patients who do not become comatose usually recover without permanent sequelae. Among those who survive more severe intoxication, some have residual neurologic symptoms such as seizures, dysphasia, parkinsonism, or mental impairment. Some resolution of neurologic symptoms will occur over a period of weeks, and maximal recovery should be expected within two years of the acute episode.

Dinman BD: The management of acute carbon monoxide intoxication. J Occup Med 16:662, 1974. *A good clinical review.*

Jackson DL: Accidental carbon monoxide poisoning. JAMA 243:772, 1980. *A brief review of the effects and treatment of carbon monoxide poisoning.*

ASPIRATION-RELATED INJURIES

Injury to the respiratory system by aspiration can be categorized by the nature of the aspirate: (1) *Infectious material.* Contamination of the lungs by aspiration of oropharyngeal bacterial flora is discussed in Ch. 64. (2) *Toxic or inflammatory substances.* Aspiration of gastric acid is the most commonly occurring example in an adult population; hydrocarbon aspiration occurs predominantly in children but is encountered in adults. Both these injuries can cause fulminant illness. By contrast, lipids (mineral oil, vegetable and animal fats) most often provoke a chronic inflammatory reaction. (3) *Inert matter.* The injury of drowning is predominantly secondary to asphyxia. Food particles can cause a fibrotic, granulomatous lesion or, if large enough to occlude the larynx or trachea, sudden death by asphyxiation ("café coronary").

Aspiration Pneumonitis

Aspiration pneumonitis refers to the caustic injury to the respiratory system caused by gastric acid. This is in contrast to "aspiration pneumonia," an infectious process caused by the contamination of the tracheobronchial tree by oropharyngeal flora. Aspiration of gastric acid can occur during vomiting or during regurgitation, and in the latter instance the event may go unnoted—i.e., "silent aspiration." The normal protective mechanisms of the upper airway include epiglottic closure during deglutition, glottic closure on contact with solids or fluids, the cough reflex, and the esophageal sphincters. Altered states of consciousness, anesthesia and surgery, neuromuscular disease, gastrointestinal disease, and medical devices (nasogastric tubes or uncuffed tracheostomy tubes) impair these defenses. The use of low pressure, high volume cuffs on endotracheal tubes serves to reduce the high incidence of aspiration of gastric contents in patients with predisposing disorders.

The main factors determining the extent of illness caused by gastric acid aspiration are as follows: (1) *pH of the aspirate.* The acidity of the material is the most important cause of lung injury, with a critical pH ≤ 2.5 inducing severe pneumonitis from acid aspiration. (2) *The presence of food particles.* Aspiration of gastric foodstuff has been shown to cause a severe pneumonitis and peribronchial inflammatory reaction in the absence of a low pH. (3) *Volume of the aspirate.* Aspiration of more than 0.4 ml per kilogram of body weight of gastric acid is sufficient to cause pneumonitis. (4) *Distribution of the aspirate.* Many patients who aspirate immediately begin to cough, which may expel the aspirate and thereby partially protect the lung from injury or may enhance dispersion of the acid over a greater area and turn a potentially localized lesion into a diffuse one. (5) *Contamination of the gastric contents with fecal matter,* as in intestinal obstruction. Such a soiling of the tracheobronchial tree is associated with a marked increase in mortality, but death presumably ensues from infection, not from acid injury.

PATHOPHYSIOLOGY. After intratracheal instillation, acid is rapidly distributed in the lungs, and can reach the pleura in 12 to 18 seconds. It is rapidly neutralized by bronchial secretions; in less than 30 minutes the pH at the bronchial surface will have returned to normal. The acid causes a chemical burn of the bronchi, bronchioles, and alveolar walls, with subsequent exudation of fluid into the lungs. Plasma volume may decrease by as much as 35 per cent in severe injury without fluid replacement, and cardiac output and systemic arterial blood pressure may fall. Pulmonary capillary wedge pressure is normal or low, indicating a nonhydrostatic cause of the pulmonary edema. The characteristics of phospholipids in the alveolar surface lining layer (surfactant) are altered, causing increased surface forces and promoting early airway and alveolar closure. Lung compliance decreases secondary to the increase in interstitial fluids and the alteration of surface forces. These disturbances of airways, alveoli, and vascular elements cause profound imbalance of the normal ventilation-perfusion relationships. Hypoxemia is invariably present and usually severe. Increased right-to-left shunting is commonly present.

CLINICAL MANIFESTATIONS. Some patients aspirate a large volume of gastric acid and almost immediately become apneic and hypotensive and die. More commonly a patient aspirates stomach contents and, with various amounts of coughing, survives the initial crisis, but later develops a fulminant illness marked by dyspnea, cough, and pink, frothy sputum. Alternatively aspiration may be secondary to regurgitation and not accompanied by immediate coughing and agitation. With this so-called silent aspiration the patient presents with acute respiratory failure but with no obvious reason for the precipitous deterioration in function. Within one to five hours after aspiration of gastric acid, tachypnea, rales, and rhonchi occur, and wheezing, cyanosis, cough, and hypotension may be present. Fever of 38 to 39° C in the first 36 hours occurs in about 50 per cent of patients.

Laboratory tests are nonspecific. A moderate leukocytosis with left shift develops early. Arterial blood gases, the best variable to follow, show hypoxemia, and the arterial oxygen tension does not reach predicted levels after the patient has been breathing 100 per cent oxygen for several minutes, indicating increased right-to-left shunting of blood. The arterial P_{CO_2} may be slightly elevated, normal, or mildly reduced, and pH will vary reciprocally. Abnormalities on chest roentgenograms are extremely variable, and there is no characteristic pattern. Extent of radiographic abnormalities does not correlate with clinical outcome. About 50 per cent of patients have roentgenographic changes consistent with pneumonitis, while about 30 per cent develop an abscess and 20 per cent show a necrotizing pneumonia. Although the distribution of the acid in some cases is preferentially to areas dependent at the time of aspiration, frequently the abnormalities are diffuse, presumably from enhanced dispersion of the acid during coughing. On radiographs taken early in the course, the majority of patients have perihilar or basilar infiltrates, usually bilateral or multicentric, with bilaterally symmetrical infiltrates in only about 40 per cent of cases. Pleural effusions and cavitation of infiltrates are not seen in uncomplicated cases. Bronchoscopic findings are diagnostic if food particles or gastric debris is seen in the trachea or bronchi. Subsegmental mucosal erythema in a suspected case is a supportive but not diagnostic finding.

The key to the accurate diagnosis of aspiration pneumonitis is a high index of suspicion for this entity in any patient with an abrupt respiratory deterioration, especially a patient with a condition that places him or her at increased risk of gastric acid aspiration. The differential diagnosis includes cardiogenic pulmonary edema, pulmonary embolus, bacterial pneumonia, and many of the causes of the adult respiratory distress syndrome such as sepsis, hypotension, amniotic fluid embolism, and increased intracranial pressure.

TREATMENT. Treatment of the individual whose aspiration was witnessed begins with the prompt establishment of an adequate airway. The airway should be suctioned to remove any particulate matter. A single lavage of 10 ml of saline may be used; larger volumes have been shown to increase the extent of injury in rabbits. Intratracheal instillation of sodium bicarbonate or of steroids is of no value.

General supportive measures include fluid replacement with crystalloid or colloid solution. Supplemental oxygen is given to maintain $Pa_{O_2} > 60$ torr. Bronchodilators (intravenous aminophylline) may help. Associated pulmonary edema is not cardiogenic in origin and is usually associated with intravascular volume depletion. Therefore, there is no place for the routine use of digitalis or diuretics.

The use of antibiotics is controversial. In general, antibiotics should not be used prophylactically for acid aspiration since they do not reduce morbidity or mortality and they increase the risk of subsequent infection with a resistant organism. The acid-damaged respiratory tract has an increased susceptibility to bacterial infection. In a patient who has been improving after aspiration, new deterioration, especially after the first three days, with increasing fever, leukocytosis, worsening hypoxemia, new infiltrates on chest x-ray, and the production of purulent sputum is suggestive of a secondary bacterial pneumonia. Management of the patient who has aspirated gastric contents that had been contaminated with fecal matter would include the early use of antibiotics providing activity against anaerobes and gram-negative organisms.

The role of systemic corticosteroids in aspiration pneumonitis is controversial. There have been no controlled human trials. Early anecdotal reports supported their use, but more recent retrospective and prospective but uncontrolled series totaling approximately 250 patients have failed to show any improvement in morbidity or mortality.

Positive-pressure ventilation is helpful, particularly when it is initiated early after the aspiration. Arterial oxygen tensions improve and mortality rates decrease with its use. Positive end-expiratory pressure (PEEP) to improve oxygenation has been beneficial in other forms of adult respiratory distress syndrome and is commonly used in the management of gastric acid aspiration. Caution should be used in applying PEEP, since in the acid-injured lung a marked increase in lung extravascular water content can occur, especially if PEEP >15 cm water is applied.

Aspiration pneumonitis carries a high mortality rate despite treatment, and because it largely occurs in a defined population at increased risk, efforts should be made at prevention. Elevation of the head of the bed will retard regurgitation. In intubated patients placement of a nasogastric tube to keep the stomach decompressed should be considered. Aspiration may occur even in the presence of a cuffed endotracheal tube. Elective general anesthesia should be given with the stomach empty, after at least a 12-hour fast. If anesthesia must be undertaken with a full stomach, consideration should be given to rapid induction and intubation while employing cricoid pressure. In recognition of the critical role of the degree of acidity of the aspirate, the pH of gastric contents can be raised by a single dose of cimetidine (300 to 400 mg orally two to four hours before surgery, given with minimal water) or by a single 10-ml dose orally of antacid, best given after premedication.

OUTCOME. Mortality from aspiration pneumonitis is high, reaching 28 to 62 per cent of cases. Factors associated with highest risk of death are age greater than 50 years, the early development of shock or apnea, severe and prolonged hypoxemia, pH of gastric contents ≤1.75 at the time of aspiration, and the development of secondary bacterial pneumonia. Most but not all survive the early moments. After the initial deterioration (24 to 36 hours), some then show steady improvement, with radiographic resolution within a week. Some have a second episode of deterioration, an event which should suggest a new problem such as bacterial infection, pulmonary embolism, heart failure, or another aspiration. Still others pursue a relentlessly worsening course to death. Few data exist regarding long-term clinical follow-up, but it is thought that pulmonary fibrosis of varying degrees ensues in some of these patients.

Bynum LJ, Pierce AK: Pulmonary aspiration of gastric contents. Am Rev Respir Dis 114:1129, 1976. *A retrospective analysis of the clinical features and outcome in 50 patients observed to aspirate gastric contents.*

Newman GE, Effman EL, Putman CE: Pulmonary aspiration complexes in adults. Curr Prob Diagn Radiol 11(4):1, 1982. *A thorough review of the mechanisms, diagnosis, and treatment of aspiration; 65 references.*

Drowning

Drowning accounts for about 7000 deaths annually in the United States, mostly in children and young adults. It is one of the three leading causes of accidental death. Pathophysiologically, drowning can be of four types: (1) *"Wet" drowning*—initial laryngospasm but early relaxation and subsequent aspiration of copious amounts of fluid. The majority of drownings are of this sort. (2) *"Secondary" drowning*—death occurs 15 minutes to 72 hours after extraction from the water, and is due to a form of adult respiratory distress syndrome. (3) *"Dry" drowning*—asphyxiation secondary to intense glottic spasm which persists beyond the point of apnea, so that when the muscles relax, no water is aspirated. This accounts for 10 to 20 per cent of drownings. (4) *Immersion syndrome*—cardiac arrest secondary to the intense parasympathetic discharge of the diving reflex.

The most important consequences of near-drowning are severe hypoxemia and metabolic acidosis. The difference between fresh water and salt water near-drowning appears to be of little significance. Life-threatening electrolyte disturbances caused by water aspiration in humans are rare, and the salt content of the aspirate is relatively unimportant. Hypoxemia is caused by occlusion of airways with fluid and particulate debris in the water, by changes in surfactant activity, by direct injury to the alveolar septa, and by bronchospasm. There is a marked increase in right-to-left shunting and an increase in physiologic dead space. Severe metabolic acidosis develops in most cases, presumably secondary to anaerobic metabolism in the asphyxiating victim, especially with the violent struggling that normally occurs. Cardiac arrhythmias, conduction disturbances, and central nervous system injury can occur in this setting. Cerebral edema is far more common than actual brain infarction.

Autopsies of drowned persons demonstrate wet, heavy lungs with varying amounts of hemorrhage and edema and some disruption of alveolar walls. In about 70 per cent, vomitus, sand, mud, and aquatic vegetation have been aspirated. Specimens from victims dying from "secondary drowning" show desquamation of alveolar epithelial cells, hemorrhage, hyaline membrane formation, acute inflammatory infiltrates, and foreign body reactions to particulate matter. Cerebral necrosis and edema are seen; changes of acute tubular necrosis are found sometimes in the kidneys.

CLINICAL MANIFESTATIONS, TREATMENT, AND OUTCOME OF NEAR-DROWNING. The initial appearance of the patient can vary widely, from coma to agitated alertness. Cyanosis, coughing, and the production of frothy pink sputum are common. Tachypnea, tachycardia, and a low grade fever in the first few hours are seen if the patient did not become hypothermic during submersion. Rales, rhonchi, and, less often, wheezes are heard. Neurologic signs vary between patients and can fluctuate in any given patient but usually derive from bihemispheric cerebral dysfunction. Signs of associated trauma should be sought.

Laboratory studies reveal mild hypokalemia, hypernatremia, and hyperchloremia, none of life-threatening magnitude. There may be a moderate leukocytosis. Hematocrit (Hct) and hemoglobin usually are normal on first measurement; in fresh water aspiration the Hct sometimes falls slightly in the first 24 hours. An increase in serum free hemoglobin is seen more often, without significant changes in Hct. Rarely the picture of disseminated intravascular coagulation has been reported in near-drowning. Arterial blood gases, usually obtained after preliminary resuscitation, show severe hypoxemia and metabolic acidosis. The most common electrocardiographic changes are sinus tachycardia and nonspecific S-T segment and T wave changes, which revert to normal within hours; however, other, more ominous abnormalities may occur—ventricular arrhythmias, complete heart block, or myocardial infarction. The chest x-ray may be normal initially in spite of severe respiratory disturbances. It often shows patchy infiltrates, and sometimes a classic pulmonary edema pattern is seen.

Treatment of the near-drowning victim begins with the establishment of an adequate airway and, if necessary, emergency cardiopulmonary resuscitation. Oxygen in high concentrations is necessary, since hypoxemia is present in essentially all victims. Even the patient who quickly becomes apparently normal should be hospitalized for 24 hours to watch for a subsequent picture of adult respiratory distress syndrome. During transportation to a hospital, supplemental oxygen should be continued, and precautions taken for potential cervical spine injury and other critical trauma.

In the hospital, subsequent therapy is dictated largely by the arterial blood gases and the degree of respiratory failure. Continuous positive airway pressure or PEEP is particularly helpful. Prophylactic antibiotics have not been shown to be beneficial. The use of corticosteroids for the pulmonary lesions of near-drowning remains controversial, and there have been no controlled prospective human studies of that therapy; animal models and retrospective studies in humans have failed to demonstrate any benefit.

If there is evidence of cerebral edema, intracranial pressure (ICP) monitoring can be used to guide therapy. In the event of increased ICP, PEEP should be minimized, since it increases ICP. Hyperventilation to maintain a Pa_{CO_2} of 25 to 30 torr will decrease cerebral blood flow and ICP. Mannitol or glycerol should be used. Corticosteroids (e.g., dexamethasone, 16 mg intravenously initially, then 4 mg intravenously every four hours) are beneficial for the central nervous system injury. Seizures, shivering, or random nonpurposeful movements can increase ICP and should be aborted with pancuronium bromide. If these maneuvers fail to lower ICP, then barbiturates (e.g., pentobarbital, 3 mg per kilogram) every hour intravenously to obtain a serum level of 2.5 to 4 mg per deciliter can be tried.

Outcome in near-drowning is best judged by the neurologic status. The shorter the interval between extraction from the water to first spontaneous gasp, the better the prognosis for recovery without chronic neurologic sequelae, which include mental subnormality, minimal brain dysfunction, spastic quadriplegia, extrapyramidal syndromes, optic and cerebral atrophy, and peripheral neuromuscular damage. Between 5 and 20 per cent of children who survive near-drowning have such residual deficits. Survival without neurologic damage is better in children who are hypothermic when recovered, and occurs even after 40 minutes of submersion. Similar information regarding adults is lacking.

Conn AW, Edmonds JF, Barber GA: Near-drowning in cold fresh water: Current treatment regimen. Can Anaesth Soc J 25:259, 1978. *This paper describes a treatment protocol designed to minimize brain edema, including deliberate hypothermia, hyperventilation, muscle paralysis, barbiturates, and corticosteroids.*

Hoff BH: Multisystem failure: A review with special reference to drowning. Crit Care Med 7:310, 1979. *An excellent, thoroughly complete review of the evaluation and care of the nearly drowned patient with attention to all critical organ systems.*

Redding JS: Drowning and near drowning. Can the victim be saved? Postgrad Med 74:85, 1983. *A review of current therapy.*

Hydrocarbon Pneumonitis

Hydrocarbon pneumonitis results from the direct toxic effects of volatile hydrocarbons on the respiratory epithelium and vasculature. It occurs in individuals who have ingested the hydrocarbons, but results almost exclusively from aspiration into the respiratory tract rather than from absorption from the gastrointestinal tract and systemic distribution. It does not occur from "sniffing" the compounds. The problem occurs most often in children, particularly those below the age of five years, in whom it is usually accidental. It is an uncommon problem in adults, occurring most often in industrial accidents, in patients attempting suicide, in siphoning of gasoline, and in uninformed alcoholics seeking an ethanol substitute.

Different hydrocarbons cause respiratory injury of varying extent, the critical parameters being the viscosity and volume of the aspirate. The lower the viscosity or the larger the volume, the worse the lesion. Being lipid solvents, all these compounds are directly toxic to respiratory tissues. The lungs of children dying from hydrocarbon pneumonitis demonstrate hemorrhage, pulmonary edema, atelectasis, hyaline membrane formation, and necrosis of airway epithelium and alveolar septa. In animal models the acute inflammation begins to resolve by the third day, and is followed by a proliferative response of alveolar lining cells, an increase in intra-alveolar macrophages, and a mononuclear cell infiltration in perivascular and peribronchiolar tissues. By six weeks there is partial clearing of these changes, although the alveolar walls remain thickened. These compounds have systemic toxicity, and in fatal cases degenerative changes in the liver and kidneys have been seen.

CLINICAL MANIFESTATIONS. Aspiration usually occurs at the time of hydrocarbon ingestion. There may be choking and coughing, with a burning sensation in the mouth and throat. A history of vomiting after hydrocarbon ingestion is obtained in less than half the patients. Dyspnea, tachypnea, tachycardia, and high fever quickly ensue. Sputum may be bloody. Lethargy is common, but more severe disturbances of consciousness such as confusion, coma, and seizures also occur. Auscultation is frequently normal, but rales and rhonchi may be present.

The chest radiograph is particularly helpful, since even before auscultation becomes abnormal, infiltrates frequently occur, developing as quickly as 20 to 30 minutes after aspiration of some types of hydrocarbons but later in others. The distribution of the multiple, fluffy, ill-defined infiltrates is preferentially in the dependent areas of the lungs, predominantly on the right side, but occurs bilaterally in about one fourth of cases. Some patients present a picture of bilateral perihilar infiltrates, a "pulmonary edema" pattern. Pleural effusions, pneumothorax, and pneumomediastinum occur but are uncommon. Pneumatoceles can form later, especially in children.

Laboratory tests give nonspecific results. A moderate leukocytosis with left shift is common. Arterial hypoxemia of various degrees develops owing to shunting and to ventilation-perfusion mismatching.

The differential diagnosis is that of respiratory distress of abrupt onset, frequently in a patient with an impaired sensorium at the time of presentation. In the adult this is often an alcoholic. Gastric acid aspiration, an intracranial catastrophe, cardiogenic pulmonary edema, pulmonary embolism, and acute bacterial pneumonia can all present similarly. The correct diagnosis requires the history of hydrocarbon ingestion or aspiration. The diagnosis is also suggested by the odor of the patient's breath and by extensive radiographic abnormalities in a patient with a clear chest by auscultation.

TREATMENT. Emesis to remove residual hydrocarbons is contraindicated. Gastric lavage by nasogastric tube may induce vomiting and should be performed only in the patient who has ingested a large volume of hydrocarbons and then only after placement of a cuffed endotracheal tube. Supplemental oxygen should be given to maintain Pa_{O_2} >60 torr. Mechanical ventilation and PEEP may be necessary. There are no data to show that the routine use of antibiotics modifies the course. The use of systemic corticosteroids is supported by anecdotal reports of improvement after their use in children and adults. Prednisone, 1 mg per kilogram per day, or its equivalent should be used during the acute illness, with termination as the patient improves.

OUTCOME. Hydrocarbon pneumonitis in adults is rare, so that morbidity and mortality estimates are not available. In children death occurs in as many as 10 per cent of cases, but most children have a prompt clinical recovery. Bronchiectasis, recurrent bronchitis, and/or pulmonary fibrosis ensues in an unknown portion of cases. After recovery from the initial illness, children frequently are asymptomatic and have normal chest examinations and radiographs. However, pulmonary function abnormalities suggestive of small airway (<2 mm diameter) disease have been found in asymptomatic patients as late as 8 to 14 years after the hydrocarbon pneumonitis.

Klein BL, Simon JE: Hydrocarbon poisonings. Pediatr Clin North Am 33:411, 1986. *A review showing that most ingestions can be managed by careful observation and respiratory support.*

Lipoid Pneumonia

Lipoid pneumonia is a chronic inflammatory reaction of the lungs that results from the aspiration of vegetable, animal, or (most commonly) mineral oils. This material differs greatly from the excessive accumulation of endogenous lipids in the lungs occurring in fat embolism, cholesterol pneumonitis, pulmonary alveolar proteinosis, and the lipid storage diseases.

The most frequently implicated agent is a mineral oil, which is used as a laxative and to reduce dysphagia, either in clear liquid form or as petroleum jelly. Mineral oil is bland and when introduced into the pharynx can enter the bronchial tree without eliciting the cough reflex. It also mechanically impedes the ciliary action of the airway epithelium. Risk of mineral oil aspiration is increased in the debilitated or senile patient, in those having neurologic disease that interferes with deglutition, and in patients with esophageal disease. Mineral oil taken as nose drops to relieve nasal dryness has caused lipoid pneumonia, and in earlier years was a frequent cause of the illness. Inhalation of mineral oil mists by airplane and automobile mechanics has been implicated as a cause of the problem. Aspiration of vegetable (e.g., castor, olive) or animal (e.g., cod liver oil, milk, butter, egg yolk) fats has been an infrequent cause.

Mineral oils, which are relatively inert, cannot be hydrolyzed in the body and provoke a chronic inflammatory reaction which may not become clinically overt until years later. The fat is emulsified in the alveolar spaces, where macrophages accumulate and phagocytize it. Some macrophages disintegrate, releasing their lysosomal enzymes and fat. The alveolar septa become thickened and edematous, containing lymphocytes and lipid-laden macrophages. Oil droplets are seen in the pulmonary lymphatics and hilar nodes. Later, fibrosis develops and the normal lung architecture is effaced. It is usual in a single specimen to find both the early inflammatory and the later fibrotic picture, in keeping with repetitive aspirations over many months or years. If nodular, the lesion may grossly resemble tumor and is called a paraffinoma.

CLINICAL MANIFESTATIONS, DIAGNOSIS, AND TREATMENT. Most patients are asymptomatic, coming to a physician's attention because of an abnormal chest radiograph, or the lesion is found unexpectedly at autopsy. When patients are symptomatic, the complaints are nonspecific, with cough and exertional dyspnea being the most frequent. Chest pain (sometimes pleuritic), hemoptysis, fever (usually low-grade), chills, night sweats, and weight loss may occur. The physical examination may be completely normal, or fever, tachypnea, dullness on percussion of the chest, bronchial or bronchovesicular breath sounds, rales, and rhonchi may be found. Clubbing is rare. Cor pulmonale uncommonly develops.

The erythrocyte sedimentation rate may be prolonged. In mild lipoid pneumonia arterial blood gases may be normal at rest but show hypoxemia after exercise. In more severe disease, resting hypoxemia, hypocapnia, and mild respiratory alkalosis develop. Pulmonary function testing reveals a restrictive ventilatory defect; static compliance of the lungs is decreased. The only specific laboratory finding is the presence in sputum of macrophages with clusters of vacuoles 5 to 50 μ in diameter that stain deep orange with Sudan IV, and extracellular droplets that similarly stain.

Radiographically, the earliest abnormalities are air space infiltrates, unilateral or bilateral, localized or diffuse, but most often in the dependent portions of the right lung. Air bronchograms may be seen. Hilar adenopathy and pleural reaction are rare. As fibrosis develops, there is volume loss and the appearance of linear and nodular infiltrates. A solid lesion may develop which closely resembles bronchogenic carcinoma.

The differential diagnosis is extensive, particularly in the late phase when multiple other causes of pulmonary fibrosis must be considered. Sarcoidosis, mycobacterial and fungal infection, chronic hypersensitivity pneumonitis, primary lung carcinoma, bronchiectasis, pneumoconiosis, pulmonary alveolar proteinosis, and pulmonary hemosiderosis are some of the major diseases that are a part of the differential diagnosis. The key to the correct diagnosis before biopsy is the history of chronic use of an oil or a lipid-based product, orally or intranasally, or an occupational exposure to oil mists. The presence of lipid-laden macrophages in the sputum confirms the diagnostic impression.

Once the diagnosis has been made and the aspiration stopped, the subsequent course is variable. Some patients will have no change in symptoms. Others will have improvement in some or all parameters, whereas a few patients continue to deteriorate with worsening pulmonary function and cor pulmonale.

Discontinuation of the use of the offending lipid is essential. Since the only way the body can dispose of mineral oil is by expectoration, the patient should be instructed in coughing exercises to be performed many times each day for months. Expectorants have not been shown to help. Systemic corticosteroids are recommended by some: prednisone, 40 mg orally each day at the beginning and then decreased to 10 mg daily until stabilization of clinical and radiographic signs (which might involve months of therapy). The use of steroids has been based on improvements seen in a very few patients in uncontrolled, anecdotal trials. The rationale has been that the cellular reaction, rather than the oil itself, is the destructive factor. Because of the well-recognized side effects from prolonged use of systemic corticosteroids, their use for lipoid pneumonia should be limited to those patients who have significant symptoms, and then for as brief a period as possible, to "buy time" while decreasing the lipid burden by expectoration.

Blöndal T, Hartvig P, Bengtsson A, et al.: An unnecessary case of paraffin oil pneumonia. Acta Med Scand 213:227, 1983. *The problems in diagnosis of mineral oil pneumonia are illustrated in a current case report.*

Heckers H, Melchar FW, Dittmar K, et al.: Long-term course of mineral oil pneumonia. Lung 155:101, 1978. *This case report documents persistence of oil in expectorated sputum for months after stopping the oil use and the sequential improvement in physiologic parameters.*

538 OCCUPATIONAL DISEASES OF THE SKIN

Edward A. Emmett

Occupational skin diseases are a group of heterogeneous conditions that share a common occupational etiology. They account for about one half of reported occupational disease in the United States. Occupational contact dermatitis, the prototypical disorder, makes up about 95 per cent of all occupational skin diseases; infections, about 2.5 per cent; and a large number of different, infrequent diseases, the remainder. The relative frequency of each of these diseases in any location depends largely on the pattern of industrialization.

Almost all occupational skin disease is due to external contact with chemical, physical, and biologic agents. The cause is often multifactorial. In relatively few instances are agents absorbed systemically (rather than locally) responsible.

OCCUPATIONAL CONTACT DERMATITIS

DEFINITION. Occupational contact dermatitis is an erythematous or eczematous response of the skin as a result of local contact with one or more irritating, allergenic, or photosensitizing chemical agents.

ETIOLOGY. Many chemicals from a wide variety of classes—alkalies, acids, volatile organic solvents, metallic salts, organic prepolymers, and many others—are capable of inducing contact dermatitis. The cause is often multifactorial; in addition to one or more chemicals, friction, abrasion, changes in temperature and humidity, and ultraviolet (UV) radiation may play a role. Superinfection may occur. Severe and persistent occupational contact dermatitis, particularly from irritants, is more frequent in those with an atopic diathesis.

INCIDENCE AND PREVALENCE. Bureau of Labor Statistics reports put the incidence in the United States at about 0.9 per 1000 full-time workers per year; because of substantial under-reporting, the true incidence is estimated to be from 10 to 50 times higher.

EPIDEMIOLOGY. The incidence of occupational contact dermatitis is generally highest in agriculture/forestry/fishing, followed by the manufacturing industries. The highest risks occur in poultry dressing plants, meat packing plants, fabrication of rubber products, leather tanning and finishing, manufacture of ophthalmic goods, plating and polishing, production of frozen fruits and vegetables, internal combustion engine manufacture, machining operations, and canning and curing of seafoods. Virtually no industry is immune.

PATHOGENESIS. Contact dermatitis may result from direct local irritation, cell-mediated immune reactions, or photosensitivity.

Direct local irritation may be immediate, as in irritation from strong acids or alkalies, or may be delayed and occur only after repeated or prolonged local application as cumulative insult dermatitis. The latter can occur from one or more relatively mildly irritating substances that are termed marginal irritants.

Allergic contact dermatitis occurs as a result of sensitization to specific haptens through a process of cell-mediated immunity. The hapten combines with protein in the skin to form a complete antigen that is processed and presented to T lymphocytes by epidermal Langerhans cells, specialized macrophages that form an intraepidermal network. Among the most frequent allergens are poison ivy/oak; rubber additives, particularly accelerators and antioxidants; monomers of plastics and resins, such as epoxies, acrylates, and di-isocyanates; nickel; chromium salts; paraphenylenediamine and derivatives; and formaldehyde. There are many more possible allergens. The number of substances reported to cause allergic contact dermatitis is very large.

Chemical photosensitivity results from the photochemical excitation of a UV-absorbing molecule with resultant tissue damage. In a photoirritant reaction there is direct damage to cellular components, for example, when psoralens irradiated with long UV bind covalently to DNA. Coal tar pitch, certain aromatic dyes, and UV absorbers used in printing processes also cause photoirritation. In the rarer photoallergic reaction, photochemical alteration of the inciting chemical either forms a hapten or leads to a hapten-protein combination in the skin, the subsequent steps are identical with those for allergic contact dermatitis.

A major factor in man's resistance to environmental chemicals is the barrier provided by the outer stratum corneum layer of the epidermis. Damage to this barrier by trauma, inflammation, or skin disease or by altering barrier conditions, for example by occlusion, may play an important role in the development of contact dermatitis.

CLINICAL MANIFESTATIONS. The clinical presentation is dominated by dermatitis that is confined, at least initially, to the region of contact. The morphology varies according to the concentration and duration of the exposure, the pathogenesis, and individual constitutional differences. Acute irritant dermatitis is characterized by erythema, perhaps edema, papules and vesicles, or in the more extreme instance one or more large bullae filled with purulent fluid. Postinflammation hyperpigmentation and hypopigmentation may occur; necrosis may leave scars. The cause of acute irritant dermatitis is usually obvious because of the rapidity with which the reaction develops.

Cumulative insult dermatitis may develop only after a long period of contact. On the hands it tends to start under rings or watchbands and to be somewhat patchy in distribution. Individual susceptibility varies widely. Initially, drying and fissuring may be seen with subsequent development of an eczematous response with papules and vesicles. Excoriations and lichenification are frequent if the process persists. Relapse may occur on relatively brief exposure to mild irritants, even when the dermatitis is clinically healed, especially if the epidermal barrier has not yet been fully reestablished.

Allergic contact dermatitis most often presents as an acute or chronic eczematous reaction with erythema, papules, vesicles, scaling, and pruritus. Characteristically there is a latent period of at least seven to ten days before the development of dermatitis following first exposure to the allergen. Recurrence usually occurs 24 to 72 hours after an eliciting exposure. Certain allergens, for example, epoxy resin monomers, have a tendency to produce severe acute reactions with significant edema.

Localization is important for diagnosis. Over 90 per cent of occupational contact dermatitis involves the hands, sometimes in conjunction with other sites. Where the eruption is due to contact with objects or contaminated surfaces, the pattern of contact will determine localization. Reaction to immersion of the hands in liquids generally involves the dorsum of the hands and palmar aspects of the wrists. Photosensitivity reactions on exposed sites may be distinguished from airborne contact dermatitis by the relative sparing of shaded areas such as the eyelids or behind the ears.

DIAGNOSIS. A good occupational history is the cornerstone of diagnosis. It is most useful to get a description of the worker's daily activities, including nonoccupational activities, with particular attention to contact of the skin with chemicals. The localization of the eruption at its onset, initial appearance of lesions, nature of progression, and circumstances of remissions and recurrences help determine occupational etiology. A personal or family history or both will confirm the presence of atopy, in which there is increased susceptibility to irritants, changes in heat and humidity, and other

factors. A complete examination of the skin will help rule out dermatoses other than contact dermatitis, including id reactions of the hands secondary to dermatophytosis of the feet. Allergic contact dermatitis is confirmed by diagnostic patch testing; photoallergy, by photopatch testing. Patch testing is relatively easy to perform, but the interpretation requires skill. There is no clinically useful confirmatory test for irritant contact dermatitis.

Other information may be necessary to make a precise diagnosis and formulate appropriate management. Toxicity information on industrial compounds can be obtained from Material Safety Data Sheets, which reveal the composition and properties of industrial materials. In the United States these are available to most employees and their physicians. A visit by the physician to the workplace allows the physician to view the work firsthand. If such a visit is made, opportunity for skin contact with hazardous agents should be explored as well as the use of protective measures.

Epidemiologic surveys to establish the prevalence of dermatitis in workers at similar jobs and industrial hygiene surveys to characterize the nature and amount of chemical exposure may occasionally be helpful. Public health authorities, university centers for occupational and environmental health, and sometimes concerned employers may be able to assist in such investigations.

TREATMENT. Symptomatic treatment is similar to that for dermatitis of other types. Acute contact dermatitis is treated with cold wet dressings of Burow's solution. Systemic steroids in rapidly tapering doses are indicated in severe acute widespread disabling eruptions; topical steroids and emollients, for dry and chronic eczema. Superinfection requires appropriate systemic antibiotics. Antihistamines may be given for sedation and are mildly antipruritic. The patient should be given careful instruction to avoid casual exposures, and should be alerted to the fact that even when the skin has apparently healed the barrier may not have returned to normal. A temporary or permanent change of job tasks may be necessary. If a permanent job change is necessary, vocational rehabilitation should be considered. Some states require reporting of occupational diseases.

PROGNOSIS. The prognosis of occupational contact dermatitis is surprisingly poor, especially if effective treatment is not given early and if the dermatitis is prolonged. The reasons for this are not entirely clear; however, surveys have shown that a high percentage of individuals still have dermatitis several years later, in many cases despite a change of employment. Those with atopy appear to have the worst prognosis. In allergic contact dermatitis the prognosis is dependent on the ease with which the allergen can be avoided.

PREVENTION. Preventive measures serve both to prevent recurrences and to halt the development of novel disease. These include elimination or substitution for strong irritants and sensitizers; education of workers as to skin care; avoidance of overly harsh skin cleansers; prompt reporting and treatment of dermatitis; engineering controls to minimize skin contact with potential hazards; appropriate impervious protective clothing; good personal hygiene with rapid effective removal of contaminants; and counseling of individuals with predisposing conditions, such as atopy, regarding career selection.

OTHER OCCUPATIONAL DERMATOSES

A relatively large number of other dermatoses can result from occupational exposure. In large part, management is dependent upon diagnostic recognition and on discontinuing further exposures, using measures outlined above.

Chemical burns result from corrosive agents that produce necrosis, ulceration, and subsequent scarring. Prompt removal of these agents (such as strong acids, alkalies, phenol, alkyl metal compounds, and metal chlorides) from skin, eyes, and mucous membranes is essential. Water is generally best for removal. Quicklime, tin tetrachloride, and titanium tetrachloride should be removed with mineral oil. Specific antidotes are few; these include topical or injected calcium gluconate for hydrofluoric acid burns.

Urticaria may occur from local contact with or systemic absorption of agents that elicit an immediate hypersensitivity reaction or directly release histamine and other vasoactive substances.

Fiberglass dermatitis causes intense pruritus; there may be no visible changes or it may be accompanied by excoriations, pinpoint petechial papules, or both. Microscopy of a cellophane tape stripping from the skin, which had been treated with 10 per cent potassium hydroxide, reveals the fibers.

Relatively deep indolent *ulcers* of skin and mucous membranes result from contact with arsenic, chromates, and lime.

Chemical acne and folliculitis may result from contact with greases and oils, coal tar pitch, creosote, and a number of cosmetics (acne cosmetica) and from ingestion of bromides, iodides, and isoniazid. These forms of acne typically commence with comedones or inflammatory papules.

Chloracne is due to halogenated aromatic compounds with specific molecular shape, including dioxin and related chlorinated aromatic hydrocarbons. The illness is characterized by small straw-colored cysts and comedones that first involve the malar crescent and behind the ear and may not spread beyond these areas. Inflammatory pustules, abscesses, and large cysts may be seen in severe cases. Chloracne is the first and most constant finding in chronic dioxin poisoning. More variable findings may include porphyrinuria, hyperpigmentation, hypertrichosis, central and peripheral nervous system effects, alteration of lipid metabolism, and mild hepatotoxicity. Experimentally observed effects include teratogenicity, immunosuppression, and tumor induction.

Cutaneous granulomas occur as slightly erythematous grouped flesh-colored papules, with or without inflammatory changes, from foreign body reactions at the site of contact with talc and silica or as an immunologic response to beryllium and zirconium.

Chemical leukoderma, which may mimic vitiligo but which is confined to the areas of skin contact, may result from a number of phenols and catechols, including hydroquinone, monobenzyl, and monomethyl ethers of hydroquinone (used as rubber additives) and *p*-tertiary butyl and related phenols (in disinfectants).

Basal and squamous cell carcinomas and keratoacanthomas result from prolonged exposures to ultraviolet radiation, ionizing radiation, polycyclic aromatic hydrocarbons (including coal tar pitches and related products), and arsenic. Exposures to arsenic may be associated with various internal malignant neoplasms.

Cutaneous T cell lymphoma (mycosis fungoides) may be more frequent in those who have worked in heavy industry or who have industrial chemical exposure, but the particular causal agents are uncertain.

INFECTIONS AND INFESTATIONS

The development of infections and infestations frequently depends on occupational factors, individual susceptibility, and the geographic distribution of the causal organism. Occupational associations include the following:

Viral. Herpes simplex (dentists, medical personnel), milkers' nodules and papular stomatitis (veterinarians, milk handlers), orf (farmers, shepherds, abattoir workers), viral warts (butchers), Rift Valley fever (shepherds).

Bacterial. Staphylococcal infections of hands (abattoir workers and butchers), erysipeloid (fish, fowl, rabbit, and pig handlers), anthrax (wool, hair, and hide handlers), tularemia (farmers), nontuberculous mycobacterial infections (aquarium workers and pet shop attendants). Bacterial and yeast infec-

tions and tinea versicolor are prominent where there are heat, humidity, and lack of hygiene.

Fungal. Dermatophyte infections are more frequent in farm workers, surveyors, zoo attendants, animal care technicians, and certain others. Particular examples include tinea verrucosum (farmers); infection due to *Trichophyton rubrum* (miners), *Microsporum canis* (pet shop workers), *Trichophyton violaceum* (wrestlers), and *Candida albicans* (those in wet work, particularly those in contact with sugar and fruit); sporotrichosis (mine workers); chromomycosis (agricultural workers); and actinomycosis (agricultural workers).

Protozoal. South American leishmaniasis (foresters).

Helminths. Creeping eruption (plumbers, gardeners, farm workers in the tropics), ankylostomiasis (miners), schistosomiasis and cercarial dermatitis (rice planters and canal workers).

In addition, bites and stings of arthropods and other creatures are common in those who work out of doors and in certain other occupations.

Adams RM: Occupational Skin Disease. New York, Grune & Stratton, 1983. *A comprehensive review of contact dermatitis and related conditions with descriptions of skin diseases caused by a variety of agents with detailed lists of agents encountered in various occupations.*

Maibach HI (ed.): Occupational and Industrial Dermatology. Chicago, Year Book Medical Publishers, 1987. *A multiauthor text that broadly covers occupational dermatoses and dermatotoxicology and describes the skin diseases caused by a number of specific agents.*

539 RADIATION INJURY

Theodore L. Phillips

DEFINITION. Radiation injury may be defined as any somatic or genetic disruption of function or form caused by electromagnetic waves or accelerated particles. Common sources of such injury include ultraviolet radiation from the sun and man-made sources, microwave radiation from radar, ovens, and other appliances, high-intensity ultrasound, and ionizing radiation from natural and man-made sources.

Ultraviolet radiation, produced by the sun, is largely absorbed by the atmosphere of the earth. It penetrates poorly in tissue and, so, is a threat only to exposed body surfaces. Injury occurs through direct chemical effects in molecules with high ultraviolet absorbance. Ultrasound and microwaves exert their effects by generating heat during absorption.

Radiation with wave lengths shorter than that of visible light has an additional property: the ability to displace electrons from their normal orbits. As these electrons traverse tissue, they generate ions and free radicals which then react with biologically important molecules leading to cell death. The ability of high-energy rays to penetrate and cause severe biologic damage after deposition of small amounts of energy is of concern.

Ionizing radiation, both natural and man-made, is of two types—photons (or waves) and accelerated particles. Photons, called *gamma rays*, are given off in many types of nuclear decay. Man-made ionizing rays, called x-rays, occur when an electron is stopped in a dense material. Accelerated particles include protons from solar radiation, heavy nuclei in cosmic rays, and beta and alpha particles given up in nuclear decay. These particles are charged, and they cause direct ionization. Neutrons are given off in nuclear decay and cause damage through secondary reactions in tissue in which protons are produced.

Radiation dose is defined in terms of energy deposition. The basic unit is the *Gray (Gy)* equal to 1 joule per kilogram. Radioactivity is defined in terms of the rate of decay; one disintegration per second is a *Becquerel (Bq)* (Table 539–1).

TABLE 539–1. RADIATION DOSE SPECIFICATION

Type	Dose Unit	Definition
Radioactivity	Becquerel (Bq)	One disintegration/second
Absorbed Dose	Gray (Gy)	Energy deposited in tissue (1 joule/kg)
Dose Equivalent	Sievert (Sv)	Absorbed dose weighted for the quality (damaging effect) of the radiation
Effective Dose Equivalent	Sievert	Dose equivalent weighted for the sensitivity of the organs
Collective Effective Dose Equivalent	Man Sievert	Effective dose equivalent applied to a population

Because radiations differ in the density of the ionization they cause, their biologic effects vary; densely ionizing radiations have more profound biologic effects. Thus, a unit called the Sievert (Sv) is used to express risk estimates in which a *quality factor* is applied to the absorbed dose. Additional weight may be applied depending on the specific organ(s) irradiated.

Absorption of charged particles and their range in tissue are determined by their charge and mass. Particles with high charge and mass give up their energy rapidly and penetrate only short distances, unless they are of extremely high energy. Photons are absorbed exponentially by electron or nuclear interactions. Because photons diverge as they leave the source, the dose decreases as the square of the distance from the source.

Injury from radiation may be either thermal or ionizing. Ionizing radiation injury expressed within a few hours or days is called *acute*; when expressed after months or years it is called *delayed*.

ETIOLOGY. *Biology of Ultraviolet Radiation.* Ultraviolet light photons are capable of generating chemical changes in DNA and other molecules, the most important of which is the production of pyrimidine dimers. Although these dimers may be excised and repaired, if unrepaired these lesions lead to reproductive cell death and desquamation after skin irradiation. Ultraviolet exposure also causes immediate effects such as vasodilatation and erythema. The limited penetration and the absorption by melanin limit human injury to the superficial layers of the skin and the eye. Solar carcinogenesis in the skin and eye is a major problem.

Biology of Ionizing Radiations. When electrons traverse a cell they cause the formation of ion pairs both in cell water and in the DNA. During such events reactive radicals are formed containing unpaired outer electrons. These radicals react with DNA or occur in the DNA itself. A radical may be repaired by reduction by SH groups or fixed by oxidation or electron transfer. If a free radical persists, it leads to a break in the DNA strand. Single-strand breaks are generally repaired, but if two occur side by side a double-strand break occurs. Unrepaired double-strand breaks lead to chromosome aberrations which are generally lethal.

Chromosome injury is expressed at the time of cell division, which causes most mammalian cells to die a mitotic death. Deletions and dicentric chromosomes lead to loss of genetic information at each cell division. Some cells may survive a few divisions but will be incapable of sustained reproduction. Intermitotic death occurs in some lymphocytes and gonadal cells, even after low radiation doses, but most cells will survive 10 to 30 Gy with no obvious damage until mitosis occurs.

Dose-Response Relationships. The percentage of cells that survive after exposure to ionizing radiation decreases logarithmically with dose. There are two components to the injury, reparable and irreparable, so that most dose-survival plots show a shallow slope at small doses and become steeper with increasing dose. Low-level effects are thus generally less than one would expect based on observations at high doses. Cells can repair radiation damage very effectively. Repair is primarily of single- and double-strand DNA breaks and requires only a few hours.

The radiation dose required to reduce survival in mammalian cells to 10 per cent is quite uniform. The most sensitive cells require 1 Gy to reduce survival to 10 per cent and the most resistant about 5 Gy. Changes in sensitivity by a factor of three occur under hypoxia and as cells traverse the mitotic cycle.

INCIDENCE AND PREVALENCE. *Background Radiation.* Both ionizing and ultraviolet radiations are ubiquitous in the universe because of the fusion processes in stars. Gamma rays, x-rays, and highly energetic particles are emitted by stars and by nuclear decay of isotopes produced by stellar processes. On the earth radiation comes from isotopes in the earth and construction materials and from the sun and other sources in space. The dose of radiation that one receives from this natural radiation depends on the altitude and the geologic nature of the region. The average annual exposure is 2.5 milli-Sievert (mSv), about 80 per cent of which is natural radiation, half of which is due to radon and 20 per cent of which is man-made.

Medical Exposure. Shortly after the discovery of x-rays by Roentgen in 1895 and the subsequent discovery of radioactivity, the first medical injuries occurred. The early workers were unaware of the injurious properties of the rays until damage to hands, eyes, and bone marrow were evident. After World War II the full hazards of radiation exposure were recognized and exposures were strictly limited. Currently injury of the acute and chronic types is rare after medical exposure but is a side effect of radiation therapy.

Radiation is used in the treatment of 50 to 60 per cent of patients with malignancy; 300,000 to 400,000 patients are exposed annually. Although every precaution is taken to avoid clinically important delayed effects, acute reactions to radiation therapy are common. Since most tumors require doses for cure close to organ tolerance the risk of injury is always present.

Rarely injuries occur to medical workers or patients during machine malfunction or repair operations. Workers and patients, as well as the general public, are also exposed to low-level radiation either while obtaining diagnostic studies or while working in medical radiation environments. Permissible exposures have been reduced to 50 mSv for workers and 5 mSv for the public; less than half that exposure is highly recommended. These rules keep the additional medical exposure of the population as a whole to less than half that of the background level.

Industrial and Military Exposure. High-level radiation to the largest populations occurred at the Hiroshima and Nagasaki fission weapon explosions in World War II. Although most casualties were due to blast and burns, 40 to 50 per cent of the survivors had radiation injury. Late effects have included several hundred cases of leukemia and other malignancies. Atomic weapons testing has led to the inadvertent exposure of 300 or more persons, about 25 per cent of whom show clinically detectable effects. The fallout from nuclear tests has also added about 0.02 mSv to the annual background radiation exposure. The Chernobyl reactor accident has also added to background exposure. Industrial and laboratory exposures occur both in the nuclear industry and through the use of industrial radiography, neutron activation, and x-ray spectroscopy devices.

Ingestion or inhalation of long-lived isotopes is also potentially injurious. About 5000 persons have been exposed to ingested radium, and at least 400 malignancies have occurred with increased incidence in the sinuses and in bone. Inhalation of plutonium and other alpha emitters is a problem in the nuclear industry.

EPIDEMIOLOGY. Radiation injury is not caused by a vector, and the source and nature of the exposure should be obvious. Persons may be exposed without awareness, and clinical symptoms must be identified in order to suspect an exposure. In other cases, psychologically deranged persons may have access to radioactive materials and ingest them or expose themselves but deny the exposure.

It is extremely important to determine the nature of the exposure and to reconstruct the dose distribution in order to predict the level of injury and the required treatment.

PATHOGENESIS. *Cell Kinetics and Radiation Effects.* Cells not subject to intermitotic death live out their normal life span after irradiation and their injury becomes apparent only because the dying cells cannot be replaced due to mitotic death. Organs are made up of several populations of cells, some of which do not normally divide and persist for many years after a radiation exposure. Other cells, such as the cells in the renal tubules and the liver, are replaced slowly, and eventually depopulation occurs. The endothelial cells of the capillary system are slowly replaced. Radiation causes gradual loss of capillary patency, and the number of capillaries decreases.

Specific Tissue Radiobiology. The tissues of the body can be divided into those critical to life and those whose injury by radiation may cause morbidity but is not fatal. The critical tissues for survival are discussed below. The doses quoted are single exposures to high-energy photons. Because of repair, doses two to four times higher are required for the same effect after fractionated exposures.

BONE MARROW. Because of the short life span and rapid renewal of most peripheral blood and marrow cells, this organ shows the most dramatic and acute clinical syndrome. Small lymphocytes die an intermitotic death and depletion is seen in a few hours. The half-life of platelets and granulocytes is one week, and depletion is maximal at three weeks. The half-life of red cells is about 100 days. There is a dynamic balance between the declining numbers of mature cells and regeneration. The marrow regenerates after single whole body exposures up to 6 Gy and can be repopulated by transplantation after doses up to 10 Gy.

INTESTINES. The mature surface and villus cells of the intestinal mucosa are replaced by the division of cells in the crypts which migrate up the villus. In contrast to this rapid renewal system, the muscular wall contains a slowly renewing capillary network. Doses as low as 1 Gy can reduce crypt cell survival to 50 per cent, but histopathologically detectable injury requires 10 Gy or more. After 15 Gy the cell kill in the crypt is sufficient to cause complete loss of the villus and in some cases denudation, followed by repopulation. Higher local doses cause these acute changes but also lead to late fibrotic changes in the muscular layer and serosa due to capillary injury.

CENTRAL NERVOUS SYSTEM. There are no rapid cell renewal systems in the CNS but the glial cells and the endothelial cells cycle slowly and can show injury. The neurons are not injured except secondarily at doses below 60 Gy. Large exposures of 50 to 500 Gy can produce acute functional changes and, at the highest doses, immediate death. After 15 Gy changes begin in four to five months and persist in development over one to two years. There are focal necrosis and calcification, demyelinization, and gliosis seen, particularly in the white matter (see Ch. 174).

SKIN. After exposure to between 3 and 9 Gy the skin can show transient vasodilatation, cessation of mitosis in the basal layer, and thinning of the prickle cell layer. At doses above 20 Gy denudation and ulceration occur before repopulation begins from either surviving basal cells or cells at the periphery of the exposed area. The cells of the hair follicles and sweat glands are often depleted and will not regenerate after 20 Gy. Late vascular damage can cause a second wave of ulceration.

LUNG (Ch. 537). In the lung, both the type II pneumocytes and the capillary cells, as well as the mucosal cells of the bronchial tree, regenerate slowly. About 90 days after a dose of 10 Gy, acute pneumonitis occurs, capillaries occlude, and endothelial cells are lost. This is preceded by depletion of surfactant and type II cells. Secondary influx of alveolar macrophages is seen. The acute phase is followed over the ensuing nine months by replacement of the capillaries and alveoli by collagen. Acute pneumonitis is reversible only at the lowest doses, 8 to 11 Gy in a single exposure.

HEART. The cardiac muscle cells do not proliferate, so almost all radiation changes occur primarily in the endothelium of the capillaries. Four to six months after exposure of up to 15 Gy or more the capillaries become occluded and show a dose-related reduction in number. This can lead to a secondary loss of muscle cells. The pericardium is also injured with resulting effusion and fibrotic thickening.

LIVER. The hepatocytes are normally replaced very slowly, but injury to the liver can induce a wave of cell division. There is also continuous replacement of the sinusoidal endothelium in the lobules. Six weeks after 10 Gy, central lobular occlusion occurs, and there is secondary hepatocyte loss and portal hypertension.

KIDNEY. After 10 Gy the tubule cells are reduced in number and exhibit flattening in the tubule lining. Whole nephrons are lost over the period of four to 18 months after exposure. At the same time many capillaries are occluded. At one year and beyond damage in the glomerulus with loss of foot processes and thickening of the basement membrane can be seen. Secondary hypertension is common.

GONADS. In contrast to most other tissues during fractionated exposure the gonads are quite sensitive to complete depopulation of the reproductive cells. Sterilization can occur after as little as 5 to 10 Gy and prolonged hypospermia, after even fewer Gy. The hormone secreting cells of the gonads are much more resistant, but, of course, ovarian hormone secretion is dependent on ovulation and is obliterated by sterilization.

CLINICAL MANIFESTATIONS. *Acute Whole-Body Exposures.* The classic acute whole-body radiation syndrome is usually seen after reactor accidents, after malfunction of large treatment or research accelerators or industrial irradiation facilities, and after nuclear explosions. It is also seen after total-body irradiation for bone marrow transplantation and treatment of malignancy. In the subsequent discussion, doses quoted are for single exposures. For fractionated exposures, two to four times higher doses are needed for the same effect because of repair.

The initial symptoms are directly related to the radiation dose. After 2 Gy about half of the patients exhibit nausea and vomiting two to six hours after exposure. After 3 Gy the incidence is 100 per cent. With doses above 3 Gy, three syndromes occur:

(1) *The hematologic syndrome* occurs in patients who receive up to 10 or 12 Gy. At these doses, although the small intestine is affected, there is usually little or no diarrhea, and the bowel is not denuded. The chief effects are in the bone marrow, although patients who survive the acute phase can develop lung or kidney injury months to years later. In the hematologic syndrome, the patient experiences the prodromal symptoms of nausea and vomiting, and in the most serious cases this is often associated with malaise and weakness. These symptoms subside over the first 24 hours and may be followed by salivary gland swelling in some patients. If the dose has been less than 5 Gy, there will then be a quiescent period of two to three weeks. At that point depopulation of the marrow and the resultant fall in granulocyte and platelet levels lead to infection and hemorrhage. Purpura, petechiae, and fever are common. Skin erythema and desquamation can occur, particularly if there are local areas of higher dose. Temporary epilation occurs if the patient survives. If the dose is 3 Gy or below, recovery is the rule, and patients who have received doses up to 5 or 6 Gy can recover if they have support.

(2) *The gastrointestinal syndrome* occurs at doses of 13 to 30 Gy. When the dose exceeds that needed to denude the small bowel, the gastrointestinal syndrome occurs before the he-

matologic syndrome, and, since it is usually fatal, is the dominant manifestation. After similar initial symptoms to the hematologic syndrome, a brief asymptomatic period will ensue although malaise and diarrhea may be persistent. Five to seven days after exposure, severe diarrhea and fluid loss occur, followed by infection with enteric bacteria. It is not possible to survive this syndrome after whole-body exposure, even with modern bone marrow transplantation techniques.

(3) *The cardiovascular–central nervous system syndrome* occurs following very large doses and is uniformly fatal. After 20 to 50 Gy, the patient will experience immediate nausea, vomiting, and diarrhea. This is followed rapidly by ataxia, sweating, prostration, and shock. Huge doses, such as 300 to 500 Gy, can cause immediate death due to generalized CNS dysfunction.

Local or Regional Radiation Injury. The clinical syndromes following whole-body irradiation are all associated with acute effects that subside within two months of exposure. Local or regional exposures to very high doses may not be immediately fatal, and delayed effects can be seen. Local irradiation of the bone marrow does not usually produce a detectable clinical syndrome. The peripheral white and red cell counts will be depressed, but more than half the marrow must be exposed to doses over 4 Gy before any clinical symptoms similar to the acute whole-body syndrome appear. Doses over 10 Gy in a single exposure or 25 Gy in a fractionated exposure produce prolonged aplasia of the marrow in the irradiated area. When the percentage of marrow irradiated is large, clinical symptoms of marrow hypoplasia will occur if additional radiation exposure, infection, or cytotoxic chemotherapy occur.

Abdominal irradiation can lead to signs and symptoms from the liver, kidney, and small bowel. The stomach and colon can be injured by doses of fractionated radiotherapy over 50 Gy. Radiation hepatopathy results in ascites with other signs of portal hypertension six to eight weeks after the exposure. Renal injury leads to edema and proteinuria six to eight months later. Hypertension, occasionally severe, can be seen one to ten years after exposure, as can renal failure. The acute small bowel or gastrointestinal syndrome can occur after abdominal exposure, but it is usually not fatal after local exposures. Delayed injury to the small bowel results in signs of intestinal obstruction, malabsorption, or diarrhea. Gastric irradiation produces signs of hypochlorhydria and at 15 Gy can lead to large greater curvature ulcers.

Local irradiation of the CNS produces late signs. Whole-brain irradiation with 10 Gy in a single exposure causes edema with transient nausea and vomiting. Doses of 15 to 20 Gy can be fatal in six to 18 months with generalized dementia. More focal irradiation can produce a mass lesion with focal signs, headache, and vomiting.

Injury to the skin results from local or regional exposures. This leads to transient erythema the first day. After three weeks, erythema, dry desquamation, or moist desquamation can occur. Epidermolysis and chronic ulceration occur with single exposures over 25 Gy.

Thoracic irradiation can lead to symptoms due to either cardiac or pulmonary damage. Pulmonary damage is first seen three to four months after a single exposure or six weeks to two months after a fractionated exposure. The patient experiences fever, dyspnea, and cyanosis. If the acute phase is survived there will be chronic signs of pulmonary constriction and fibrosis. Somewhat higher doses cause acute pericarditis with symptoms similar to a viral pericarditis with fever, malaise, and some dyspnea seven to 24 months after irradiation. Paradoxical pulse and cardiac tamponade can be seen with large pericardial effusions. Myocardial infarction and chronic myocarditis are sometimes seen.

Gonadal irradiation in the male rarely leads to symptoms. The patient becomes oligospermic after low doses and aspermic after higher doses about six weeks later. In the female, ovarian effects usually occur by the next menstrual cycle and result in amenorrhea which is rarely reversible after doses of 5 Gy in single exposures or 20 Gy in fractionated exposures.

Systemic Exposure to Radionuclides. Systemic isotopes cause whole-body exposure and specific organ exposure, depending on the concentration of the isotope by the organ and the nature and energy of the radioactivity. Ingestion of ^{131}I leads to a whole-body exposure and high doses in normal thyroid. There can be symptoms of nausea and vomiting, and the hematologic syndrome followed by hypothyroidism and pharyngitis. Plutonium concentrates in the pulmonary macrophages causing local fibrosis and malignancy. For each isotope it is necessary to know the distribution to predict the symptoms.

Delayed Effects of Low-Level Exposure. These effects are purely genetic and carcinogenic. If an exposure does not lead to sterilization, genetic damage can persist in the spermatogonia and oocytes. Experiments have shown point mutations in mice, but they have been difficult to prove in humans because of the background of about 10 per cent spontaneous abortions. The risk is estimated as being about one congenital abnormality per million live births per mSv exposure. The risk of carcinogenesis varies by organ and ranges from 70 to 1000 cases per Gy per million people exposed per year of follow-up.

DIAGNOSIS. It is essential that any facility likely to treat radiation injuries have a trained team on call. The physician should obtain as clear a history as possible about the exposure, including the nature of the radiation, the distance from the source, and any documentation such as monitors, badges, and witnesses. A preliminary estimate of the dose should be made from the history as well as from the symptoms. Malaise, nausea, and vomiting suggest an exposure over 1 Gy and occur in all patients who have been exposed to 3 Gy or more (Table 539–2). The physical examination should pay particular attention to the skin, conjunctivae, mucous membranes, and salivary glands. After high local doses there may be acute erythema; two to three weeks after exposure there may be signs of infection or hemorrhage.

TABLE 539–2. SYMPTOMS, THERAPY, AND PROGNOSIS AFTER RADIATION INJURY IN MAN

Dose range	0–1 Gy	1–2 Gy	2–6 Gy	6–10 Gy	10–20 Gy
Therapeutic needs	None	Obsevation	Specific treatment	Possible treatment	Palliative
Vomiting	None	5–50%	3 Gy = 100%	100%	100%
Time delay, nausea, and vomiting	—	3 hr	2 hr	1 hr	30 min
Main organ damaged	None	Lymphocytes	Bone marrow	Bone marrow	Small bowel
Symptoms and signs	—	Mod. leukopenia	Leukopenia, purpura, hemorrhage, epilation	Leukopenia, purpura, hemorrhage, epilation	Diarrhea, fever, electrolyte imbalance
Critical period	—	—	4–6 wk	4–6 wk	5–14 days
Therapy	Psychotherapy	Observation	Transfusion granulocytes, platelets; antibiotics	Transfusion; antibiotics; bone marrow transplant	Fluids and salts; possible marrow transplant
Prognosis	Excellent	Excellent	Guarded	Guarded	Poor
Lethality	None	None	0–80%	80–100%	100%
Time of death	—	—	2 months	1–2 months	2 wk
Cause of death	—	—	Infection, hemorrhage	Hemorrhage, infection	Enteritis, infection

Laboratory tests should include a complete blood count with differential. The total lymphocyte count directly reflects the whole-body dose within 24 hours. Elevation of the granulocyte count can occur transiently at 24 to 48 hours. If possible, a lymphocyte culture should be done by a cytogeneticist to determine the number of chromosome aberrations, which allows calculation of the dose received. Pulmonary function tests are useful after thoracic irradiation, as are lung scans and chest computed tomographs. Blood counts are essential one to three weeks after exposure to follow the pancytopenia and to direct therapy. In the gastrointestinal syndrome there may be findings of dehydration and electrolyte imbalances.

WHOLE-BODY EXPOSURE. The granulocyte count may rise transiently to 10,000 or more 24 to 48 hours after exposure, while the lymphocyte count falls close to zero with doses of 3 Gy or more. The granulocyte count hits a nadir at four weeks and then returns toward normal at eight weeks. The lymphocyte count may remain low for many years.

LOCAL OR REGIONAL EXPOSURE. Clinical findings after such exposure vary widely and reflect injury to the specific organ involved. CNS damage will be reflected in an abnormal neurologic examination, with signs of edema and enhancing areas on the CT scan months to years after irradiation.

Radiation injury to the thorax is usually detected on the chest x-ray, although CT yields more accurate information on the volume of lung affected. Initially areas of patchy or confluent pneumonitis conform to the shape of the exposed area. This progresses to stranded fibrosis and retraction. Cardiac injury may lead to transient ECG abnormalities, pericarditis with effusion detectable on ultrasound scans, and signs of myocardial ischemia.

Abdominal exposure leads to abnormal kidney and liver function tests. High doses to the pancreas can lead to diabetes and decreased pancreatic enzymes. Chronic diarrhea can occur due to malabsorption and bile salt irritation.

SYSTEMIC EXPOSURE TO RADIOISOTOPES. Large doses of gamma ray–emitting isotopes can cause symptoms and signs similar to those seen in the acute whole-body syndrome or local skin or mucosal injury. The most important diagnostic tests that must be obtained are radioactivity counts and spectroscopy in order to identify the isotope(s), predict the dose, and localize the injury. Urine and blood samples should be obtained (and, if possible, a whole body count in a suitable counter).

TREATMENT. *Acute Whole-Body Exposure.* The initial symptoms of whole-body exposure can be treated with antiemetics. The profound weakness seen at doses above 3 Gy can be reduced by a short course of intravenous corticosteroids. Further therapy is not needed for patients who have received 2 Gy or less. Above that, and up to 10 Gy, survival is possible with active medical management. Support similar to that used for the pancytopenic leukemia patient is required

including reverse isolation or life island–type support. Trauma and burns complicate the situation and may dominate in terms of survival. Antibiotics should be used if the granulocyte count is below 1000 per microliter or if there is infection, in which case granulocyte transfusions should be used as well. Platelet transfusions should be given if the platelet count is below 10,000 per microliter. The diarrhea seen at doses below 10 Gy is usually mild but may require intravenous fluid and electrolyte replacement.

Bone marrow transplantation may be a useful adjunct at doses of 5 Gy or more. Bone marrow samples and peripheral blood for tissue typing should be obtained early, before depletion occurs. Techniques should be similar to those used for leukemia (Ch. 165). Exposures above 12 Gy (which will lead to the gastrointestinal or CNS syndrome) are uniformly fatal. Palliative support is indicated with fluids, as is the treatment of infection or hemorrhage.

Local or Regional Exposure. Skin reactions are the most common injury requiring treatment. Dry or moist desquamation occurs and can be ameliorated with cleansing, using an antibacterial soap. Crusts should be soaked off and the open areas dressed with petroleum jelly or bacitracin ointment. Large areas can benefit from temporary lanolin closed dressings which should be changed daily, washing before each redressing (Table 539–3).

The electrolyte imbalances seen with nausea and vomiting must be corrected. Radiation pneumonitis can be reversed at borderline doses with prednisone 60 mg per day tapered over the ensuing month. The acute symptoms of pericarditis can be relieved by aspirin or other anti-inflammatory agents. Cardiac tamponade should be treated by pericardiocentesis or a pericardial window. Delayed effects of doses of 20 Gy or more may require skin grafts, resection of necrotic bone, and other surgical procedures, including resection of necrotic brain tissue.

Systemic Exposure to Radionuclides. After the victim has been given urgent first aid and has been decontaminated, the dose and nature of the exposure should be determined, making use of a whole-body counter if possible. Large body burdens should be treated by specific methods designed to remove the isotope or to block uptake. After iodine exposure, stable iodine should be given as 5 drops of potassium iodide. One gram of soluble phosphate should be given to patients ingesting ^{32}P. Radium ingestion can be treated with magnesium sulfate or epsom salts, 10 grams in 100 ml of water. Strontium exposure is treated with 100 ml of aluminum phosphate gel.

Pulmonary exposures to aerosols or dust can be treated by bronchial lavage, expectorants, or diethylenetriaminepentaacetic acid (DTPA) aerosol mist. DTPA products are available from the U.S. Department of Energy.

Gastrointestinal absorption can be reduced with mild laxatives. Sodium alginate and aluminum hydroxide gel may

TABLE 539–3. ORGAN DAMAGE, DYSFUNCTION, TREATMENT, AND PROGNOSIS AFTER LOCAL IRRADIATION

Organ	Acute Lesion	Delayed Lesion	Clinical Signs	Treatment	Prognosis
Bone marrow	Pancytopenia	Vascular occlusion Myelofibrosis	Infection Hemorrhage	Antibiotics Transfusion	Good if % of total marrow irradiation small
Intestine	Flattened villi	Fibrosis, obstruction	Diarrhea	Fluid, electrolyte acute Resection for obstruction	Good for acute Obstruction can be fatal
CNS	Edema	Necrosis	Headache Focal neurologic	Resection	Poor Fair
Skin	Desquamation	Ulcer, necrosis	Pain, oozing	Cleansing, ointments, graft	Good
Lung	Pneumonitis	Fibrosis	Cough, fever, cyanosis Dyspnea	Corticosteroids	Good at low dose Good if small volume
Heart	Pericarditis	Carditis	Fever, dyspnea	Anti-inflammatory, pericardiocentesis	Fair
Liver	Central venous thrombosis	Fibrosis	Ascites	Diuretics	Fair
Kidney	Tubular degeneration	Fibrosis	Proteinuria Hypertension, renal failure	Dialysis Transplant	Fair

reduce strontium uptake. Certain heavier isotopes including plutonium, americium, yttrium, lanthanum, cerium, scandium, zinc, and other fission products can be partially removed from the body by DTPA. A dose of 0.5 to 1 gram should be given intravenously in 250 ml of normal saline.

PROGNOSIS. *Acute Radiation Syndromes.* Survival with little or no treatment other than good hygiene and treatment of infections can be expected after exposures to 3 Gy or less. Between 3 and 6 Gy, therapy with antibiotics, platelets, and granulocytes allows for a high survival rate. Leukemic patients show 80 per cent survival after 10 Gy whole-body exposure at a dose rate of 4 Gy per hour when bone marrow transplantation is used. The use of all available methods will allow high survival after 5 Gy and some survival after acute exposures to 10 Gy.

Local Radiation Effects. Acute skin reactions usually heal completely. If the exposure has been over 20 Gy, late ulceration can be expected. Most delayed radiation injury is irreversible and slowly progressive as depopulation of stromal and capillary cells occurs.

Systemic Exposure. The prognosis will depend on the whole-body radiation dose and the isotope. Large whole-body doses result in a prognosis similar to that for whole-body external exposure. Thyroid ablation occurs after 50 to 100 millicuries of ^{125}I and bone marrow ablation after smaller doses of ^{32}P.

PREVENTION. Because radiation injury always has an irreversible component not subject to repair, prevention is essential. The largest population exposure is from natural background and can be limited by careful selection of building materials and good ventilation of the home.

The largest additional exposure is medical. This can be limited by careful selection of diagnostic tests. Optimal techniques and shielding of the gonads must be employed. Substitution of CT at some sites is helpful. The design of facilities must limit the exposure of public and monitored personnel to less than recommended levels. Proper training of workers using radiation is essential. Radiation treatment must be carried out by highly skilled specialists who limit the dose as much as possible to tumor areas.

The Effects on Populations of Exposures to Low Levels of Ionizing Radiations. Washington, National Academy of Sciences–National Research Council, 1980. *A detailed presentation and analysis of radiation exposure information and the incidence of malignancy induction with projections for large populations.*

Hall EJ: Radiation and Life. Elmsford, NY, Pergamon Press, 1976.*An introductory overview of radiation in the environment for the student and lay person.*

Hall EJ: Radiobiology for the Radiologist, 2nd ed. Hagerstown, MD, Harper & Row, 1978. *The best introductory text on the biologic effects of radiation for the medical worker.*

Johns HE, Cunningham JR: The Physics of Radiology. 4th ed. Springfield, IL, Charles C Thomas, 1983. *The most comprehensive text in the field of medical radiation physics.*

Principles and general procedures for handling emergency and accidental exposures of workers. Annals ICRP 2:1, 1978. *Detailed instructions and useful references for physicians who may be required to deal with victims of accidental exposure.*

Protection against ionizing radiation from external sources used in medicine. Annals ICRP 9:1, 1982. *The basic international manual which sets dose limits, protection standards, and monitoring standards. Essential for anyone employing radiation equipment.*

Radiation: Doses, Effects, Risks. United Nations Environment Programme. United Nations Publications, 1985. *An excellent yet simple manual with good illustrations of the effects of radiation and of environmental exposure levels.*

Shapiro J: Radiation Protection–A Guide for Scientists and Physicians. 2nd ed. Cambridge, MA, Harvard University Press, 1981. *The standard text for those using ionizing radiations in medicine with particular emphasis on radionuclides. Covers biologic, physics, and protection aspects.*

Thames HD, Withers HR, Peters LJ, et al.: Changes in early and late radiation responses with altered dose fractionation: Implications for dose-survival relationships. Int J Rad Oncol Biol Phys 8:219, 1982. *A detailed review of the factors influencing acute and late radiation injury. Some background in radiobiology needed.*

540 ELECTRIC INJURY
Basil A. Pruitt, Jr.

INCIDENCE AND PREVALENCE. Electricity produces a spectrum of injury ranging from sudden death caused by cardiopulmonary arrest to immediate tissue injury and necrosis caused by transformation of electric energy into heat. Delayed organ damage may also occur; its pathogenesis is incompletely defined. The number of electric injuries occurring annually in the United States and other industrialized countries has paralleled the use of electricity. It is estimated that in the United States approximately 1500 deaths occur from high voltage electricity and up to 300 from lightning injury each year. The incidence of electric injury is unknown, but the percentage of patients with high voltage electric injury admitted to burn centers in this country ranges from 0.04 to 6.7 per cent.

PATHOGENESIS. The effects of electricity on tissue depend upon current, voltage, type of current, i.e., direct or alternating and the frequency of the latter, pathway of the current, duration of contact, and environmental conditions. High tension is arbitrarily defined as voltage above 1000, apparently because the likelihood of sudden death and remote tissue injury is much less with lower voltage. However, any voltage above 40 should be considered potentially dangerous. In general, alternating current is considered more dangerous than direct current, in part because of the tetanic effect of the former, which may "lock" the patient to the source of electricity, and its likelihood of producing cardiac and/or pulmonary arrest. Injurious tissue effects decrease as the frequency of alternating current increases above 60 cycles per second, which is extremely dangerous to the heart and respiratory center. The points of contact and the current pathway through the body are important in determining tissue damage; passage of current through the heart or respiratory center is particularly dangerous. Current flow from a hand to the feet of only 100 ma is capable of producing ventricular fibrillation. The longer the duration of passage of the electric current, the greater will be the tissue damage, emphasizing the need for rapid separation of the victim from the source of electricity. Environmental conditions influence the resistance at the point of contact; dry thickened palmar skin is more resistant to the passage of current than is similar thickness skin when moistened by perspiration or other liquid.

In high voltage electric injury, heat is the principal mediator of tissue damage, and such damage is related to both voltage and duration of application. Because all body tissues and fluids are conductive, the body should be considered as a volume conductor. Heat is produced in this conductor as a function of voltage drop and current flow per unit cross-sectional area, i.e., current density. This characteristic accounts for the rarity of major injury to the trunk and frequency of severe injury to the digits and extremities in high tension electric injury. The skin is severely injured and chars at the points of contact, where current density is highest (Fig. 540–1). Charring of the skin may also occur from arcing across flexor surfaces of joints, and arcing can also ignite the patient's clothing and thereby produce associated flame burns. Below 1000 volts, when arcing and contact point

The opinions or assertions contained herein are the private views of the author and are not to be construed as official or as reflecting the views of the Department of the Army or the Department of Defense.

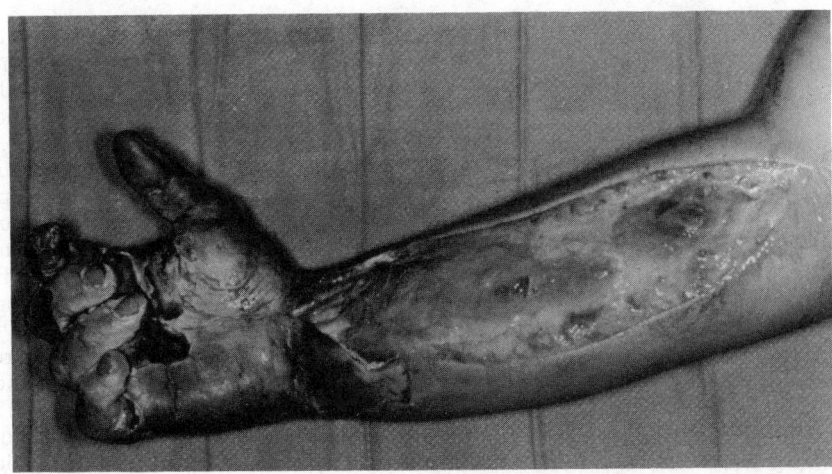

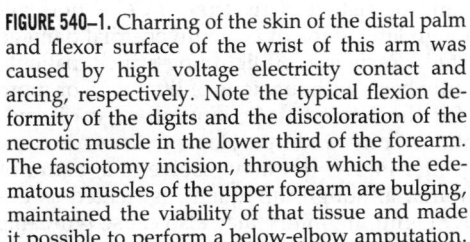

FIGURE 540–1. Charring of the skin of the distal palm and flexor surface of the wrist of this arm was caused by high voltage electricity contact and arcing, respectively. Note the typical flexion deformity of the digits and the discoloration of the necrotic muscle in the lower third of the forearm. The fasciotomy incision, through which the edematous muscles of the upper forearm are bulging, maintained the viability of that tissue and made it possible to perform a below-elbow amputation.

charring occur, resistance rises rapidly and limits subsequent current passage and tissue heating; in this sense, such electric injury is self-limiting. Above 1000 volts, arcing is intense, and relatively constant levels of current are maintained with an associated marked increase in tissue destruction. The heated tissue cools unevenly, the superficial portions cooling more rapidly than the deeper portions. Since tissue injury caused by thermal energy depends upon both temperature and duration of exposure, the deeper tissues are more liable to severe injury. These characteristics of tissue as a volume conductor and a volume radiator influence surgical treatment in patients with high voltage electric injury.

Low voltage direct current may also produce tissue damage, and focal injury has occurred at the contact sites of ground plates used with electrosurgical devices. Prolonged application of direct current of as little as 3 volts to such grounding plates can cause tissue injury either directly or as a result of electrolysis of the conductive materials used to ensure contact of the grounding plates and the skin surface.

CLINICAL MANIFESTATIONS. Cardiopulmonary arrest is relatively common in patients who have sustained high voltage electric injuries. Cardiac arrhythmias may occur after resuscitation and persist for a variable period thereafter or develop as late as 24 to 48 hours post-injury. The risk of renal failure is also great in patients with electric injury for two reasons. First, the extent of deep tissue injury may not be appreciated, which leads to underestimation of fluid needs, inadequate resuscitation, and oliguria. Second, the deep tissue injury may liberate myoglobin, which may precipitate in the renal tubules unless a brisk urinary output is maintained. Hyperkalemia may also occur as a result of extensive tissue destruction and reach sufficient levels to interfere with cardiac function.

The effects of electric injury on the deep tissues of a limb may produce sufficient edema beneath the investing fascia of an involved muscle compartment to impair nutrient blood flow and to reduce flow to distal unburned tissue, requiring fasciotomy to relieve pressure and restore circulation.

BURNS OF THE ORAL COMMISSURE IN CHILDREN. Burns of the oral commissure are frequently sustained by children, usually less than three years of age, as a consequence of sucking on the end of a live extension cord or biting the cord of a light or small appliance. Although these burns often have the pearly white appearance of an avascular full thickness burn and initially appear to be significantly deforming, most heal with minimal cosmetic defects when treated conservatively with periodic debridement of only nonviable tissue. Following spontaneous healing, residual functional or cosmetic defects can be repaired electively.

REMOTE ORGAN INJURY. Instances of intestinal perforation, focal pancreatic necrosis, focal gallbladder necrosis, and direct liver injury have been reported, but are uncommon.

Deficits of cerebral, cerebellar, spinal cord, and peripheral nerve function may be evident immediately following electric injury or may be delayed in onset. In all patients with high voltage electric injury, a thorough neurologic examination must be performed on admission and at scheduled intervals thereafter, and any nerve deficits must be fully documented. Return of function following direct nerve damage is uncommon. In general, immediate and early deficits involving nerves not directly injured (motor nerves appear to be more sensitive to current injury than sensory nerves) show spontaneous resolution. Late appearing peripheral nerve deficits may be part of a polyneuritic syndrome involving nerves far removed from the points of electric contact. The immediate symptoms of spinal cord injury are considered to result from direct neuronal insult and are more often transient than are those of later onset, which are more apt to be permanent. Spinal cord deficits of delayed onset may take the form of quadriplegia, hemiplegia, or localized nerve deficits with signs of ascending paralysis, transverse myelitis, or an amyotrophic-lateral-sclerosis–like syndrome.

Delayed hemorrhage from moderate- to large-sized blood vessels has occurred in many patients with high voltage electric injury and is ascribed by some to "arteritis" caused by electric injury per se. It has been our experience that such hemorrhage has occurred only when debridement has been inadequate or when the vessel wall underwent desiccation and necrosis secondary to exposure following debridement.

Fractures of long bones may result from falls following the electric shock, and compression fractures of vertebral bodies may result from tetanic contractions of the paraspinous muscles. Both types of fractures should be ruled out by indicated roentgenograms.

DELAYED ORGAN DAMAGE. In one group of 45 patients recurrent gastrointestinal dysfunction in three fourths and cholelithiasis in six were noted within two years following injury, but such has not been the general experience. Cataracts are common sequelae of high voltage electric injury and are most frequent in patients in whom the contact point has been on the head or neck. The formation of such cataracts may be quite rapid or may occur three or more years following high voltage electric injury.

TREATMENT. Cardiopulmonary resuscitation must be begun immediately in any patient with cardiopulmonary arrest following electric injury. All patients who have sustained high voltage electric injury should undergo continuous electrocardiographic (ECG) monitoring for at least 48 hours beyond the last ECG evidence of dysrhythmia, if such occurs. In those patients with high urinary hemochromogen concentrations, an hourly urinary output of 75 to 100 ml should be maintained. If the patient remains oliguric despite the administration of more than the estimated fluid resuscitation needs or the hemochromogens do not clear promptly, 12.5 grams of mannitol should be added to each liter of intravenous fluid given until the pigment has cleared from the urine. Hyperkalemia should be treated as in any other patient (Ch. 77).

The clinical indications for fasciotomy and surgical exploration of a limb include stony hardness of a muscle compartment to palpation, cyanosis of distal unburned skin, impaired capillary refilling of distal unburned skin or nails, and absent or diminished pulsatile flow in distal arteries on ultrasonic flowmeter examination. If large vessel pulses are intact but significant deep tissue injury is otherwise indicated by clinical signs, arteriography is helpful in determining the need for operation. Arteriographic evidence of large vessel thrombosis merely confirms clinical findings, but luminal irregularity, "beading," or narrowing may be identified in severely injured vessels that will subsequently be occluded by thrombosis, when the arteriogram is performed early following injury. Moreover, "pruning" (a decrease in the density of muscular nutrient arteries in a limb) helps define the level of amputation needed to remove muscle that has sustained inapparent but irreversible damage. [133]Xenon wash-out studies have also been used to assess the need for amputation. Muscle flow of less than 1 ml per minute per 100 grams of tissue has been proposed as the level below which amputation is required. An intramuscular compartment pressure of greater than 30 mm Hg, as measured by a wick-type catheter, has also been used as an indication for the need of immediate post-injury wound decompression. Technetium-99m pyrophosphate scintigraphy performed within 24 hours following injury has been suggested as a means to determine the extent of muscle damage, i.e., frankly necrotic tissue showed no perfusion and uninjured tissue showed normal perfusion, while areas of increased uptake of the radioactive material showed variable degrees of partial necrosis requiring operative exposure and debridement of a variable amount of tissue. Since repeated debridement was often required in patients in whom the scintigraphic findings of partial necrosis were present, the clinical reliability, accuracy, and usefulness of that diagnostic method remain uncertain.

Tissue damaged by high voltage electric injury should be explored as soon as the patient is hemodynamically stable. The viability of vital structures and deep muscle is assessed, with necrotic tissue debrided to reduce the risk of infection and eliminate a source of hyperkalemia. Extensive muscle necrosis and destruction of vital structures, such as nerves, tendons, and vessels, speak for amputation at a level proximal to the area of tissue death. Operative wounds following debridement or amputation are left open, and the patient is rescheduled for exploration of the wounds 24 to 72 hours later, at which time further debridement of any residual necrotic tissue is carried out. If no, or only minimal, debridement is required, the amputation wound can be closed by a sausage type of delayed primary closure.

Local flaps and vascularized free muscle flaps may be used for immediate coverage of deep electric injuries in which the tissues exposed following debridement, e.g., bone or tendon, do not have sufficient blood supply to support a skin graft. Early autogenous vessel grafts and delayed nerve grafts have been used to bridge focal areas of vessel or nerve destruction, respectively, but the functional success of such procedures is unconfirmed.

In those patients in whom electric injury is confined to the skin and subcutaneous tissue, bacterial control is best achieved by the use of Sulfamylon burn cream, the active ingredient of which (mafenide acetate) can diffuse into the nonviable tissue to exert its antimicrobial action.

LIGHTNING INJURY. A lightning bolt may have a voltage in the neighborhood of 1 billion volts and induce currents ranging from 12,000 to 200,000 amperes. Its duration is characteristically brief, ranging from one hundredth to one thousandth of a second. The temperature in a lightning bolt may be as high as 30,000° K, but dissipates in a few microseconds.

Cardiopulmonary arrest is common in patients struck by lightning and may be secondary to either asystole or fibrillation. Immediate cardiopulmonary resuscitation is life-saving in such patients, and persistent or recurrent ECG abnormalities are rare, although later signs of acute myocardial damage have been reported. Recovery of lightning-struck patients who have apparently been without signs of life for 15 or more minutes speaks for the immediate institution of cardiopulmonary resuscitation. Coma and neurologic deficits are common immediately after injury, but may resolve in a matter of hours. Myoglobinuria, although infrequent, is treated as described previously. Lightning injury may also cause tympanic membrane rupture and hearing loss. The cutaneous burns are characteristically superficial and present a "splashed-on" appearance of arborescent and spidery character. Signs of vasoconstriction and mottling of the skin, previously considered characteristic of lightning injury, typically relent with adequate resuscitation. Prompt treatment of the sequelae of lightning injury, including immediate cardiopulmonary resuscitation, has significantly decreased the mortality associated with this injury, and two thirds of lightning-injured patients now survive.

Amy BW, McManus WF, Goodwin CW Jr, et al.: Lightning injury with survival in five patients. JAMA 253:243, 1985. *The characteristics of lightning injury and its complications are presented and current treatment detailed.*

Holliman CJ, Saffle JR, Kravits M, et al.: Early surgical decompression in the management of electrical injuries. Am J Surg 144:733, 1982. *The management of electric burns of the extremities is detailed, and the use of radionuclide scanning in assessing extent of muscle injury is described.*

Hunt JL, Mason AD Jr, Masterson TS, et al.: The pathophysiology of acute electric injuries. J Trauma 16:355, 1976. *The experimental studies reported confirm that an electric injury is simply a thermal burn. The fact that tissue acts as a volume conductor is identified, as is the self-limiting nature of electric injury.*

Pruitt BA Jr: The burn patient: I. Initial care. In Ravitch MM (ed.): Current Problems in Surgery. Chicago, Year Book Medical Publishers, 1979, pp 43–52. *A thorough description of techniques of diagnosis and treatment of high voltage electric injury.*

Sances A Jr, Myklebust JB, Larson SJ, et al.: Experimental electrical injury studies. J Trauma 21:589, 1981. *Experimental studies of electric injury relate tissue damage to voltage, current flow, and tissue characteristics, including cross-sectional area.*

541 DISORDERS DUE TO HEAT AND COLD

James P. Knochel

To maintain a normal body temperature requires that heat gain equal heat loss. Heat is produced by metabolism or gained from the environment. Thermoregulation is heavily dependent upon blood flow to cutaneous vessels. Cutaneous flow is regulated by hypothalamic centers. Vasoconstriction reduces and vasodilatation increases delivery of heated blood to the skin. Heat is exchanged between the skin and the environment by radiation, conduction, or convection. If heat loss is inadequate by these means, active sweating begins, and cooling occurs by vaporization of sweat. If heat gain is necessary, metabolic heat production rises by a voluntary increase of physical activity or involuntarily by shivering. Body heat thus produced is retained by cutaneous vasoconstriction. *Acclimatization*, a term defining critical cardiovascular, endocrine, exocrine, and other physiologic adaptations to heat stress, requires one to two weeks to develop. Such adaptations permit one to work comfortably and safely under conditions of heat stress that were previously intolerable.

DISORDERS DUE TO HEAT

HEAT CRAMPS. Workers who sweat profusely and replace sweat losses with water but inadequate salt may experience excruciating muscle cramps. They are more common in acclimatized and physically fit men whose bodies are able to produce voluminous quantities of sweat. The cramps tend to occur in muscles used while working and often do not appear until the person relaxes after work. Cooling the muscles during a cold shower is likely to bring on an attack. Cramps in the abdominal wall may suggest a perforated viscus. Mild hyponatremia is a consistent finding. Severe cramps may cause rhabdomyolysis and modest serum elevations of muscle enzymes (creatine phosphokinase). Salted liquids taken orally or saline given intravenously leads to rapid improvement. Heat cramps are preventable by replacement of sweat with a solution containing about 2.5 grams (one half teaspoon) sodium chloride per liter of water, or merely by increasing dietary salt intake.

HEAT EXHAUSTION. Heat exhaustion is a common disorder that occurs after sustained heat stress of three or more days. Its cause is water or salt depletion or both.

Primary water loss heat exhaustion is particularly dangerous since it increases the risk of heat stroke. This form is seen most often in the elderly, infirm, obtunded, or very young who are unable to communicate their thirst. It is also seen in active persons who take salt supplements without adequate water. Deliberate efforts should be made to insure water intake by patients in nursing homes where summertime room temperatures are often too high. Hypernatremia of several days' duration may itself reduce secretion of antidiuretic hormone and recognition of thirst. Symptoms of heat exhaustion resulting from predominant water loss include intense thirst, fatigue, weakness, anxiety, and impaired judgment. Signs may include dehydration, hyperventilation, paresthesias, tetany, agitation, hysteria, muscular incoordination, and psychotic behavior. Body temperature may rise to 38.9°C. Delirium, rising temperature, coma, and frank heatstroke may follow. Laboratory findings include hemoconcentration, hypernatremia, mild azotemia, and oliguria.

Salt depletion heat exhaustion occurs mainly in unacclimatized persons in whom losses of thermal sweat are replaced with water but not adequate salt. Dehydration, weight loss, and thirst are absent in the pure form. Sweating and urinary output remain normal. Prominent symptoms include profound weakness, fatigue, severe headache, giddiness, and muscle cramps. In some patients, anorexia, myalgia, nausea, vomiting, and diarrhea may masquerade as a viral illness. Such patients appear haggard, with pale, clammy skin. Hypotension and tachycardia are common. Fever is notably absent.

Treatment of heat exhaustion should be individualized, depending upon symptoms and findings. Since kidney function is usually normal, most patients can be treated with lightly salted fluids, rest, and elimination of heat stress. Hypernatremic dehydration should be treated with isotonic dextrose at a rate sufficient to reduce serum sodium about 2 mEq per liter per hour. It is seldom necessary to administer hypertonic salt solutions to patients with hyponatremic heat exhaustion.

HEATSTROKE. Heatstroke is a catastrophic illness requiring immediate treatment for survival. It is convenient to subclassify heatstroke into two forms, classic and exertional (Table 541–1).

Classic heatstroke occurs especially in the poor, the elderly, the chronically ill, alcoholics, patients with advanced heart disease, and the obese. Hot, humid weather of three or more days' duration usually precedes epidemics of this disorder. Deaths due to myocardial infarction and congestive heart failure increase sharply during heat waves because of increased demands placed upon the heart by heat stress. Certain medications also increase the propensity to develop heatstroke. These include drugs that depress sweating (anticholinergics, phenothiazines, beta blockers, antihistamines), diuretics, drugs that may increase heat production (amphet-

amines, neuroleptics), and butyrophenone, which may depress thirst. Rarely, patients with classic heatstroke may recall a prodrome resembling heat exhaustion or cessation of sweating. Once sweating stops, body temperature mounts and collapse soon follows. Typical findings include profound central nervous system dysfunction, especially coma or bizarre behavior; hot, dry, flushed skin; and hyperpyrexia. Rectal temperature exceeds 40.6°C and may reach 44°C or more. Hypotension is common. It is probably due to redistribution of blood from the central to the peripheral circulation since it often responds to cooling alone. Convulsive seizures, fasciculations, and muscle rigidity are absent until active cooling is under way.

Exertional heatstroke is more likely to develop in laborers, farmers, military recruits, football players, long distance runners, and those who work in boiler rooms or foundries. They display physical findings in the acute phase similar to those of patients with classic heatstroke, with one common exception: About half of these patients continue to sweat. If this occurs, the skin may be deceptively cool despite a high core temperature.

Other major differences between classic and exertional heatstroke become apparent from laboratory measurements. In the classic form, respiratory alkalosis is usual, and circulatory collapse may cause modest increases of lactate, a particularly ominous sign. In contrast, *lactic acidosis* is the rule in exertional heatstroke, may exceed 20 mmol per liter, and is not a foreboding finding in this condition. Although serum creatine phosphokinase activities may be slightly increased in classic heatstroke (usually not greater than 1000 to 2000 IU per liter), clinically important rhabdomyolysis is exceptionally rare unless heatstroke occurs in an individual who has a preexisting myopathy, such as a chronic alcoholic. Major *rhabdomyolysis* and its associated complications such as hyperkalemia, hyperphosphatemia, hypocalcemia out of proportion to hypoalbuminemia, hyperuricemia, and myoglobinuria are almost invariable findings in exertional heatstroke. Both forms of heatstroke may be complicated by *hemorrhage* (resulting from *disseminated intravascular coagulation*, fibrinolysis, clotting factor deficiency due to hepatic injury, or *thrombocytopenia* due to bone marrow injury); *jaundice; acute renal failure; pancreatitis; brain damage; peripheral neuropathy; myocardial necrosis and arrhythmias*; and pulmonary capillary damage with *adult respiratory distress syndrome*. Hypokalemia in heatstroke usually results from respiratory alkalosis, but it may represent potassium deficiency in those who have performed hard work in the heat for one or two weeks. Hypoglycemia may also occur.

Treatment of heatstroke depends upon anticipation, prompt recognition, and rapid cooling. The importance of educating paramedical personnel, nurses, athletes, coaches, and trainers to prevent, accurately recognize, and initiate immediate cooling cannot be overestimated. Common mistakes include administration of fluids to comatose patients or delay of cooling.

Proper emergency management includes removal from direct sunlight, removal of clothing, wetting the body surface, and fanning to move air and thereby promote vaporization. When such simple measures are undertaken on the spot,

TABLE 541–1. MAJOR DIFFERENCES BETWEEN CLASSIC AND EXERTIONAL HEATSTROKE

	Classic	Exertional
Persons at risk	Infants, chronically ill, elderly	Laborers, soldiers, farmers, athletes
Skin	Usually hot, dry	Sweating may be present
Acid-base status	Repiratory alkalosis	Metabolic (lactic) acidosis
Rhabdomyolysis	Unusual	Major
Acute renal failure	Less than 5%	30% or more
Disseminated intravascular coagulation	Mild to moderate	Severe

some victims awaken. Most require aggressive cooling in the hospital. A thermistor probe temperature device should be inserted high in the rectum to ensure recording of core temperature.

Conventional cooling techniques include immersion in ice water while the skin is rubbed briskly or placing the patient on a stretcher, rubbing the skin with ice bags while keeping the skin wet, and moving air over the skin to promote vaporization of the water. Rapid cooling by ice water immersion may cause cutaneous vasoconstriction, shivering, and convulsions. Immersion in cool water (11°C) may facilitate cooling with equal speed by avoiding cutaneous vasoconstriction.

Hypotension often responds to cooling alone, but if it persists, 0.5 liter of normal saline should be infused. If additional quantities are necessary, one must guard against circulatory congestion. Hypotension not responding to such quantities of saline suggests myocardial injury or serious rhabdomyolysis, and vasopressor support may be necessary. The stomach should be emptied, since vomiting and aspiration often occur during cooling. Cooling should be stopped when core temperature reaches 39°C to avoid progressive hypothermia.

Steroids are unnecessary. Hypokalemia and hypophosphatemia are very common in the acute phase but usually resolve quickly without treatment. Glucose may be necessary for hypoglycemia. Although lactic acidosis usually responds to volume expansion, if it persists in the absence of hypotension, 44 to 88 mEq of sodium bicarbonate may be helpful. Other complications described earlier should be anticipated, and appropriate measures taken as necessary.

MALIGNANT HYPERTHERMIA. This rare but serious disorder, representing an idiosyncratic reaction to general anesthesia, is discussed in Ch. 516.

MINOR DISORDERS RELATED TO HEAT STRESS. *Heat edema* is a transient, benign disorder that occurs during initial exposure to hot weather. It appears to result from aldosterone-mediated salt and water retention (a physiologic adaptation) and usually disappears spontaneously with continued heat exposure. It seldom, if ever, requires treatment. Diuretics should not be administered. *Miliaria* (heat rash) is caused by sweat gland occlusion. Its medical importance is enhanced, since it may impair sweat formation and evaporative heat loss.

Heat syncope occurs when a healthy person squats for a minute and then suddenly stands, upon which a sensation of transient dizziness or visual blurring may occur. Such symptoms are exaggerated by salt and water losses induced by sweating and by heat-induced vasodilatation of the superficial blood vessels and may cause syncope in an individual unacclimatized to heat. When acclimatization occurs, the associated retention of salt and water corrects the problem. Besides syncope, findings usually include slight tachycardia and moist skin. Fever is absent. Recovery occurs rapidly if the patient is allowed to remain supine. Removal from the heat and administration of lightly salted liquids are helpful.

Hart GR, Anderson RJ, Crumpler CP, et al.: Epidemic classical heat stroke: Clinical characteristics and course of 28 patients. Medicine 61:189, 1982. *A detailed presentation of classic heatstroke, emphasizing the important roles of medications that impair heat loss and pre-existent disease in its pathogenesis. It also presents a detailed analysis of laboratory abnormalities commonly observed in this illness.*

Jones TS, Liang AP, Kilbourne EM, et al.: Morbidity and mortality associated with the July 1980 heat wave in St. Louis and Kansas City, Mo. JAMA 247:3327, 1982. *A report illustrating increased death rates during heat waves.*

Knochel JP: Environmental heat illness. Arch Intern Med 133:841, 1974. *A general review of heat stress injuries and description of exertional heatstroke.*

Knochel JP, Reed G: Disorders of heat regulation. In Maxwell MH, Kleeman CR, Narins RG (eds.): Clinical Disorders of Fluid and Electrolyte Metabolism. 4th ed. New York, McGraw-Hill Book Company, 1986, pp 1197–1232. *A review of environmental heat illness, pharmacologic and endocrine hyperthermia, malignant hyperthermia, and hypothermic disorders.*

HYPOTHERMIA

Hypothermia, defined as a core temperature of less than 35°C, is a medical emergency that occurs in both temperate and cold environments. Its prompt recognition is critical to avoid serious morbidity or death. When body temperature declines, heat production increases by shivering, and heat loss is reduced by decreasing cutaneous blood flow. Reduction of core temperature decreases the rate of chemical reactions so that cooling proceeds until a new equilibrium is established between the body and its environment.

As hypothermia develops, cerebral blood flow declines. The resulting fall in nutrient availability is offset by a reduction in brain metabolism. This fall in metabolic demand permits successful cerebral resuscitation of hypothermic patients even after prolonged periods of anoxia and circulatory arrest.

PATHOGENESIS. The causes of hypothermia seen in clinical practice are summarized in Table 541–2. Advanced age, disorders causing hypometabolism, central nervous system disease, malnutrition, a variety of drugs, and exposure commonly cause hypothermia. In elderly persons, hypothermia, hyperventilation, hypotension, and thrombocytopenia are common signs of bacteremia and sepsis.

CLINICAL MANIFESTATIONS. A decline in mental status, ataxia, tremulous speech, and hyperreflexia appear as temperature falls to about 32°C. At lower temperatures, hyporeflexia, stupor, dysarthria, and sluggish pupillary responses appear. Shivering usually stops below 32°C. Muscle rigidity becomes prominent. Established hypothermia reduces heart rate, blood pressure, peripheral vascular resistance, cardiac output, and central venous pressure. Creatine phosphokinase (MB isoenzyme) may increase with severe hypothermia without evidence of myocardial infarction, suggesting myocardial cellular damage. Cardiac arrhythmias are very common. Atrial arrhythmias are usually benign. Ventricular ectopic beats may herald ventricular fibrillation, an imminent danger if core temperature becomes less than 28°C. Stimulation, such as urethral catheterization, movement, endotracheal intubation, and vascular catheterization, also predisposes to the development of this arrhythmia. Osborn waves, characterized by a widening of the base of the QRS complex and J point deflection, are the most characteristic ECG findings. They can be seen with hypothermia from any cause and do not herald the onset of ventricular fibrillation. Early tachypnea and respiratory alkalosis are replaced by progressive hypoventilation. Advancing hypothermia leads to carbon dioxide retention and respiratory acidosis. Shivering increases lactic acid production and hypoxia in muscles and may cause severe lactic acidosis.

In early hypothermia, hypokalemia may be caused by respiratory alkalosis. Additional cooling corrects hypokalemia by reducing sodium-potassium transport. During therapeutic rewarming, sodium-potassium exchange accelerates, such

TABLE 541–2. CAUSES OF HYPOTHERMIA

Exposure plus:	
I. Central nervous system disease	III. Interference with muscle
Brain tumor, injury, seizure	movement
Cord transection	Paralysis, paresis
Hypoglycemia	Extremes of age
Thiamin deficiency	Drugs
Uremia	Alcohol
Hepatic failure	Phenothiazines
II. Interference with vasoconstriction	Hypothyroidism
Drugs	IV. Mixed causes
Alcohol	Starvation
Phenothiazines	Adrenal insufficiency
Sepsis	Hypothyroidism
Erythroderma	Hypopituitarism

From Fitzgerald FT, Jessop C: Accidental hypothermia: A report of 22 cases and review of the literature. Adv Intern Med 27:127, 1982. Reprinted with permission.

that hypokalemia may become important and contribute to arrhythmias. Hypophosphatemia may also occur during the recovery phase of hypothermia.

TREATMENT. Significant hypothermia is a medical emergency. When it is suspected, an estimate of core temperature should be obtained, by inserting a thermistor probe high into the rectum. Esophageal temperature probes are difficult to place properly and may precipitate ventricular arrhythmias or fibrillation.

Airway patency must be insured in comatose patients and steps taken to prevent aspiration of gastric contents. A large intravenous catheter should be inserted, and thiamine and glucose given immediately in appropriate situations. Stimulation of the patient should be minimized to avoid precipitating ventricular fibrillation. Blood pressure, pulse, temperature, electrocardiogram, neurologic status, and urine output should be monitored frequently during rewarming.

A warming rate of about 0.5°C per hour is generally accepted as optimal. Most shivering patients will spontaneously rewarm at a rate equal to or greater than this. *Passive* rewarming with blankets is ideal for hemodynamically stable, moderately hypothermic patients. This method will allow a rise of 0.5 to 1°C per hour if the initial core temperature is greater than about 27°C. It is especially effective in patients with acute hypothermia without underlying disease. *Active* rewarming becomes necessary in patients with severe hypothermia or cardiopulmonary arrest or both. This is especially important in patients with ventricular fibrillation or asystole because the hypothermic myocardium is resistant to mechanical or pharmacologic intervention until temperatures are above 28°C to 30°C.

"Rewarming shock" and accentuated lactic acidosis have been most commonly encountered with active external rewarming techniques, i.e., heat applied to the surface of the body with hot water bottles or immersion in warm water. To avoid these problems, rapid rewarming of core blood has been attempted by several means in patients with severe hypothermia or cardiac arrest. Most patients with hypothermia will tolerate warm intravenous fluids and heated oxygen. If rapid rewarming is required, peritoneal lavage with solutions warmed to about 40°C is effective.

Supportive measures may be very important. Because of the wide diversity of electrolyte derangements in hypothermic patients, no general recommendations can be made regarding fluid management other than warming the fluid to 37 to 40°C before administration. Plasma volume expanders may be given if the central venous pressure is low. Oxygen and bicarbonate should be given if serious metabolic acidosis exists. Subsequent metabolic alkalosis and its adverse effects on oxyhemoglobin dissociation, calcium, and ventricular irritability must be avoided. As patients are rewarmed, metabolic acidosis may worsen as lactate is washed out of previously hypoxic tissues. Recognition and treatment of this phenomenon are important to reduce the risk of ventricular fibrillation and cardiovascular collapse. Severe respiratory impairment with significant carbon dioxide retention should be treated with assisted ventilation. Ventilatory adjustments should be made with respect to reduced carbon dioxide production. Hypoglycemia should be suspected in any patient with hypothermia. Hyperglycemia should be treated only if severe and potentially life threatening. Vasopressors should be avoided if possible because of their ability to induce ventricular arrhythmias. Drugs with significant myocardial depressing effects such as quinidine and propranolol should be avoided. Thyroxine should be given only if significant hypothyroidism is suspected.

Fitzgerald FR, Jessop C: Accidental hypothermia: A report of 22 cases and review of the literature. Adv Intern Med 27:127, 1982. Reuler JB: Hypothermia: Pathophysiology, clinical settings, and management. Ann Intern Med 89:519, 1978. *These two articles are excellent clinical reviews of hypothermia*

as seen in medical practice, with discussions of differential diagnosis, clinical manifestations, and treatment.
Matz R: Hypothermia: Mechanisms and countermeasures. Hosp Pract 21:45, 1986. *This is a comprehensive presentation of the pathophysiology of hypothermia and its management.*

542 TRACE METAL POISONING
Donald B. Louria

Many trace elements, both metals and nonmetals, are capable of causing human disease. In some cases poisoning is a consequence of workplace exposure. In others the disease results from use of prescription or nonprescription medicines or as an adverse effect of medical procedures such as hemodialysis or insertion of prosthetic devices. Occasionally trace element poisoning results from attempts at suicide or homicide.

Over the past few decades, increased awareness of the health consequences of industrial substances, more stringent federal and state regulations, and fear of lawsuits have resulted in a healthier workplace. However, the majority of the potentially exposed work force is employed by small industries that may not have plant physicians or insist on proper worker protection.

We know a great deal about overwhelming exposure that results in acute illness, but our knowledge of the subtle consequences of chronic, low level trace element exposure is still grossly inadequate. This is well illustrated by lead exposure. Acute lead poisoning in children or adults is readily diagnosed, but we are only beginning to understand the consequences of increased body lead burdens in the absence of the anemia, colic, or clinically apparent encephalopathy.

The interrelationships between and among trace elements are also poorly understood. For example, copper smelter workers are exposed not only to copper but also to lead, zinc, arsenic, gold, silver, cadmium, and mercury; in these workers pneumonitis or other acute illnesses may result from two or more metals acting in concert. In other instances excesses or deficits of a trace element may act indirectly by inducing deficiency or toxicity of another trace element.

LEAD

ETIOLOGY. In the past lead poisoning was ascribed to pica (abnormal ingestion) among children living in dilapidated houses with peeling layers of lead-based paints. In the last two decades lead intoxication has occurred with increasing frequency in less socioeconomically deprived areas of the cities, as well as in more affluent suburbs. This may in part be related to environmental contamination from leaded gasoline; several studies relate environmental lead contamination to traffic density patterns. Contaminated soil is also a well-described source of lead.

In the United States, hundreds of occupations entail potentially significant exposure. Lead and other metal smelter workers or miners, welders, storage battery workers, and pottery makers are particularly heavily exposed. Workers in auto manufacturing, ship building, paint manufacture, and printing industries are also at substantial risk, as are house painters and those who repair old houses.

Lead-soldered kettles and cans and lead-glazed pottery can release lead when acidic fluids are stored or cooked in them. Demolition workers and those employed in firing ranges have become poisoned from intensive aerosol exposure. In the southern United States, moonshine whiskey is an important cause of poisoning. The stills are connected with lead solder, and old radiators containing lead are used as condensers; 20 to 90 per cent of moonshine samples contain lead in the potentially toxic range.

In past centuries lead was added to wine to sweeten it, a deception that was eventually made punishable by death. Recently, addition of lead to aphrodisiacs and various herbal and folk medicines has resulted in poisoning. Retained bullets can result in lead poisoning, especially if host metabolic changes favor lead mobilization or if a joint or bone is involved, since synovial fluid appears to be a good solvent for lead. The interval between lodging of the bullet and clinical evidence of lead poisoning has ranged from two days to 40 years.

Gasoline sniffing for hedonistic purposes can produce lead poisoning; the organic tetraethyl lead appears to have a proclivity for the nervous system.

In a sense we are all lead poisoned; prior to the Industrial Revolution the total body burden of lead was about 2 mg, whereas currently in industrialized societies the whole body content is about 200 mg. One hundred fifty to 250 μg per day is ingested, 5 to 10 per cent of which is absorbed. In children the percentage is higher and absorption is facilitated by iron, calcium, magnesium, and perhaps zinc deficiency. Aerosol exposure is especially likely to result in poisoning, since approximately 40 per cent of inhaled lead is absorbed.

CLINICAL MANIFESTATIONS. The major toxic effects of lead are referable to the abdomen, the blood, and the nervous system.

Gastrointestinal Tract. The exact pathogenesis of lead colic remains uncertain; in part it appears to be due to a direct effect of lead on smooth muscle. The crampy, diffuse, often intractable abdominal pain may be accompanied by nausea, vomiting, anorexia, constipation, or occasionally diarrhea. The pain may be confined to the epigastric, periumbilical, or other areas of the abdomen and may simulate a variety of surgical and nonsurgical diseases. Lead-induced megacolon has been reported.

Blood. Lead interferes with a variety of red cell enzyme systems, including delta-aminolevulinic acid dehydratase and ferrochelatase. The former is needed for the conjugation of levulinic acid to form porphobilinogen; the latter facilitates the incorporation of iron into protoporphyrin IX (see Fig. 135–2). The red cell abnormalities include punctate basophilic stippling and clover leaf morphology. Anemia is frequent and may be normocytic normochromic or microcytic hypochromic. An inherited deficiency in delta-aminolevulinic acid dehydratase can sensitize the individual to lead intoxication and result in the appearance of symptoms of acute lead poisoning at modest blood lead levels.

Nervous System. Either the brain or peripheral nerves may be involved. The CNS symptoms at first are vague and are often mistakenly disregarded. These manifestations include irritability, incoordination, memory lapses, labile affect, sleep disturbances, restlessness, listlessness, paranoia, headache, lethargy, and dizziness. In more serious cases manifestations include syncope-like attacks, disorientation, flaccidity, more intense headache, severe mental impairment, ataxia, vomiting, cranial nerve palsies, localized neurologic signs, psychosis, somnolence, seizures, blindness, and coma. Severe lead encephalopathy is not restricted to children. Occasionally the brain manifestations mimic a space-occupying lesion. The cerebrospinal fluid may be under increased pressure and may show an increased protein content, a modest pleocytosis (predominantly lymphocytic), and rarely diminished glucose levels. Papilledema has been reported, as have grayish deposits surrounding the optic disc and optic atrophy. Frank encephalopathy is an ominous prognostic sign in regard to both mortality and persistent brain damage. Most children who experience two or more bouts of clinically evident encephalopathy have neurologic residua.

The peripheral nerve involvement, seen more often in

adults than in children, is almost always exclusively motor and involves muscle groups used extensively. Wrist drop and foot drop are seen most often; the former, depending on type of occupation, may be asymmetrical and there may be paresthesias.

The spinal cord may also be involved, manifestations having some similarity to those of amyotrophic lateral sclerosis.

Tetraethyl lead poisoning causes euphoria, nervousness, insomnia, hallucinations, convulsions, and sometimes frank psychosis.

There is increasing evidence of subtle brain damage in the absence of clinical evidence of encephalopathy. Inordinate body burdens of lead may result in mentation difficulties, emotional lability, deficits in intelligence and memory, impaired psychomotor and visual motor function, slowed nerve conduction, and behavioral aberrations in both children and adults, even in the absence of overt evidence of poisoning. These changes often occur at blood levels of 25 to 60 μg per deciliter (or even less in very young children), and may improve substantially after reduction in exposure.

Other Clinical Manifestations. In adults the kidneys are often involved (see Ch. 82), the characteristic lesion being interstitial nephritis; as the disease progresses, glomerular filtration rate falls. In children, Fanconi's syndrome, characterized by glycosuria, aminoaciduria, and phosphaturia, may occur transiently; and occasionally, asymptomatic renal failure supervenes. Lead poisoning appears to be responsible for some cases of renal failure associated with either gout or hypertension and there is increasing suspicion based on epidemiologic studies that the level of systolic or diastolic blood pressure may be related to blood lead concentrations.

Polyarthralgias, mild hepatic dysfunction, and dysuria may occur. Occasionally arrhythmias and cardiomegaly have been reported as have abnormalities of liver function. A gingival blue, blue-black, or gray line is found in up to 20 per cent of adult patients but is infrequent in children.

Lead readily crosses the placenta and is thought to be responsible for an increased incidence of spontaneous abortion and miscarriage. Some studies suggest lead poisoning may result in hypospermia and other sperm abnormalities. Teratogenic effects occur in lead-treated animals, but congenital abnormalities have not been convincingly documented in humans. Lead exposure may also result in transient chromosomal breakage.

DIAGNOSIS. The interference with delta-aminolevulinic acid dehydratase results in marked increase in delta-aminolevulinic acid in the urine. Urinary coproporphyrin levels are also increased. Lead interferes with incorporation of iron into heme and zinc then replaces the iron to form zinc protoporphyrin (ZPP). The latter or its hydrolysis product erythrocyte protoporphyrin (EP) can be measured rapidly fluorometrically; both EP and ZPP are reliable indicators of lead poisoning. EP and ZPP elevations also occur in patients suffering from iron deficiency anemia or erythropoietic protoporphyria. Table 542–1 lists some indications of undue lead absorption.

Blood aminolevulinic acid dehydratase activity can also be measured directly. Blood lead levels are readily determined by atomic absorption spectrophotometry or anodic stripping voltometry. Specimens can be obtained by either venipuncture or finger stick; the latter technique is often difficult to interpret because of skin contamination. Urine lead concentrations can also be measured; if concentrations are normal, increased

TABLE 542–1. POSITIVE SCREENING TESTS INDICATING UNDUE LEAD ABSORPTION

Whole blood lead	Children	> 25 μg/dl
	Adults	> 40 μg/dl
Whole blood erythrocyte protoporphyrin or zinc protoporphyrin	Children	> 35 μg/dl*
	Adults	> 50 μg/dl

*This value is unsettled.

TABLE 542–2. CaNa₂ EDTA LEAD MOBILIZATION TEST

	Children	Adults
Normal premobilization test	< 100 μg/day	< 150 μg/day
	Normal	
Post-CaNa₂ EDTA 50 mg/kg IM or IV or 500–1000 mg/m² (children); or 1 gm IM* × 2, 12 hours apart, or 1–2 gm IV (adults)	< 0.60 μg Pb/mg CaNa₂ EDTA† administered over 8- to 24-hour collection period	< 650 μg/day
	Increased Body Burden	
	> 0.60 μg Pb/mg CaNa₂ EDTA administered	> 650 μg/day

*Procaine must be used with intramuscular injections.
†EDTA = edetate.

body burdens can still be detected by measuring urinary lead excretion after administration of calcium disodium edetate (Table 542–2). This test is particularly useful in assessing lead storage in bones. In children a blood level of 60 μg per deciliter or greater is considered evidence of definite lead poisoning; and concentrations of 25 μg per deciliter or greater, evidence of excessive absorption. For adults, who show less enzyme inhibition at a given blood lead concentration, the permissible industrial concentration is currently up to 50 μg per deciliter.

Additional industrial exposure should not be permitted if blood levels exceed 40 μg per deciliter or if there is any increase in EP or ZPP.

TREATMENT. Three agents are used that form tight complexes with lead and thus promote its elimination from tissues (Table 542–3). Dimercaprol (British antilewisite, BAL) is given in oil intramuscularly; calcium disodium edetate (calcium versenate) can be given either intramuscularly or intravenously; and D-penicillamine is administered by mouth. Chelation should be undertaken only after careful consideration in those with milder evidences of poisoning, because each of the agents may be associated with significant adverse effects. Occasionally chelation may be complicated by acute renal failure. Because most of the body lead is stored in the bones, clinical improvement and reduction in blood lead levels (or reduction in EP or ZPP) may be followed by increases in blood lead concentrations and clinical evidence of repoisoning owing to mobilization of lead from bone. In such cases chelating agents should again be administered.

Treatment is ordinarily successful in extra-CNS disease, but is not predictably effective in patients with encephalopathy. Various degrees of mentation deficits may remain in both children and adults. Among adults the frequency of residual brain deficits is not clearly established.

TABLE 542–3. CHELATION REGIMENS

	Children*	Adults*	Duration
CaNa₂ EDTA	50 mg/kg/day IM† or IV, or 1500 mg/m²/24 hours (severe disease); 1000 mg/m²/day (mild-moderate intoxication)	1.0 gram IV in 5% dextrose twice daily, or 2.0 grams/day IM in divided doses; longer-term, 1 gram IM 3 × per week† until lead burden reduced to satisfactory levels	Three to five days
BAL	3 mg/kg/dose IM, or 300–450 mg/m²/24 hours IM	2.5 mg/kg/dose IM	Three to five days
	(Given in divided doses every four hours)		
Penicillamine	30 mg/kg/day PO	1.0–1.5 grams/day PO	Until blood lead and FEP‡ levels approach normal§

*CaNa₂ EDTA and BAL are ordinarily used together for symptomatic illness.
†Procaine must be used for IM injections of CaNa₂ EDTA.
‡FEP, free erythrocyte protoporphyrin.
§Must be monitored carefully, since toxicity occurs in up to 20% of cases.

Baker EL, White RF, Pothier LJ, et al.: Occupational lead neurotoxicity: Improvement in behavioral effects after reduction of exposure. Br J Indust Med 42:507, 1985. *This is one of a growing number of articles that together offer a reasonably persuasive argument that significant defects in brain function occur in lead-exposed persons who do not exhibit evidence of obvious poisoning and whose blood lead levels in the past would have been considered in the acceptable range. Thirty-one references.*

Batuman V, Landy E, Maesaka JK, et al.: Contribution of lead to hypertension with renal impairment. N Engl J Med 309:17, 1983. Batuman V, Maesaka JK, Haddad B, et al.: The role of lead in gout nephropathy. N Engl J Med 304:520, 1981. *These two articles present reasonably compelling evidence that renal dysfunction associated with either hypertension or gout may be related to lead intoxication in a small but important percentage of such cases.*

Bellinger D, Leviton A, Waternaux C, et al.: Longitudinal analyses of prenatal and postnatal lead exposure and early cognitive development. N Engl J Med 316:1037, 1987. *A prospective study of 249 newborns followed for mental development for two years. Those with higher (though normal) cord blood lead levels scored lower on the developmental tests. A provocative study requiring at least several other investigations with convergent data.*

Needleman HL, Gunnoc C, Leviton A, et al.: Deficits in psychologic and classroom performance of children with elevated dentine lead levels. N Engl J Med 300:689, 1979. *This important, although controversial, article gives substantial support for the notion that subtle lead poisoning can result in significant psychosocial defects. Based on comparison of 58 children with high dentine levels and 100 with low levels.*

Piomelli S, Rosen JF, Chisholm JJ Jr, et al.: Management of childhood lead poisoning. J Pediatr 105:523, 1984. *This is an excellent, up-to-date summary of the treatment of lead poisoning. Thirty-five references.*

Whitfield CL, Ch'ien LT, Whitehead JD: Lead encephalopathy in adults. Am J Med 52:289, 1972. *Twenty-three adults exposed to moonshine developed encephalopathy, manifestations ranging from confusion to coma, seizures, and death. This article emphasizes that encephalopathy can be a major problem in adults. Chelation therapy appeared to be effective.*

MERCURY

ETIOLOGY. Mercury has been used for at least 2000 years. At present more than 60 occupations involve mercury exposure. These include chloralkali work; manufacture of pesticides, insecticides, and fungicides; manufacture of mercury-containing instruments, lamps, neon lights, batteries, paper, paint, dye, electrical equipment, and jewelry; and dentistry.

In addition to occupational or industrial exposure, poisoning has resulted from inadvertent contamination of grains by mercury-containing pesticides; and accidental or intentional ingestion or injection of elemental mercury or mercury-containing compounds. In the past mercury was administered medicinally as a component of cathartics, teething powders, and anthelmintics. Mercury compounds are now rarely used as diuretics.

CLINICAL MANIFESTATIONS AND TREATMENT. The biologic effects, tissue distribution, and toxicity of mercury depend on the form in which it is introduced into the body. Mercury possesses a strong affinity for sulfhydryl, amine, phosphoryl, and carboxyl groups and inactivates a wide variety of enzymes. Mercury poisoning can be conveniently divided into four categories.

Metallic Mercury. Elemental mercury is a liquid at environmental temperatures but vaporizes with agitation as well as gentle heating. Bulk mercury is used in dental amalgams; up to 10 per cent of dental offices have been found to have excessive mercury vapor levels; and accidental spillage has occurred occasionally in homes or offices. The greatest exposure to metallic mercury is in industry. Additionally, many workers are potentially exposed because of the widespread use of mercury in electrical equipment. Heavy aerosol exposure to mercury produces chills, fever, cough, chest pain, and hemoptysis; roentgenograms show diffuse pulmonary infiltrates. Inhaled elemental mercury is readily absorbed from the alveoli; thereafter the target tissue is the brain. With mild exposure the manifestations are likely to be subtle and diagnosis difficult. Insomnia, nervousness, mild tremor, impaired judgment and coordination, decreased mental efficiency, emotional lability, headache, fatigue, loss of sexual drive, and depression are early manifestations and are often mistakenly ascribed to psychogenic causes. These symptoms have been referred to as micromercurialism. Abdominal cramps, dermatitis, and diarrhea may also occur, and the victim may complain of a metallic taste. As the poisoning becomes more severe, persistent involuntary tremors of the extremities are noted. Thereafter other signs of mercury poisoning may appear, including amblyopia, polyneuropathy, erythroderma, acrodynia, joint pains, swollen gums with a blue line around the teeth, sialorrhea, and paresthesias. The major manifestation of mercury vapor exposure may be renal damage, including the nephrotic syndrome.

Blood and urine levels may be unreliable, and clear evidence of poisoning may be documented only after administration of drugs that augment mercury excretion in the urine.

In most cases improvement occurs after removal from exposure or treatment with either dimercaprol (BAL) or *N*-acetyl penicillamine.

The effects of ingestion of even large amounts of metallic mercury range from no clinical disturbance to local gastrointestinal irritation to central nervous system damage. Aspiration of liquid mercury is also usually benign, although roentgenologic visualization of mercury globules may be evident for many years. After intravenous injection of mercury there may be no abnormalities other than roentgenologic densities or an illness ranging from mild to lethal with hepatic, renal, lung, and central nervous system dysfunction.

The wide range of clinical findings after elemental mercury exposure appears to relate in part to the rate of oxidation to mercuric salts and the rapidity of their subsequent excretion through the kidneys, saliva, and urine.

Inorganic Mercury. Exposure to $HgCl_2$ and Hg_2Cl_2 occurs primarily in industry and results from ingestion. $HgCl_2$ is far more toxic than Hg_2Cl_2. The major manifestations are renal and include proteinuria, granular casts in the urinary sediment, the nephrotic syndrome, and pyuria from tubular damage. In some cases severe oliguria, and even anuria, may occur. Additionally, diarrhea, abdominal pain, hepatic dysfunction, and lesser evidences of central nervous system disease may be found (micromercurialism). Rhabdomyolysis with striking muscle enzyme elevation and acrodynia have also been reported. In this type of mercury poisoning BAL or penicillamine is usually effective.

Organomercurials with Rapid Metabolism to Inorganic Mercury. Included are phenyl and methoxyethyl mercury salts found in diuretics and fungicides. Toxicity is limited and usually renal.

Short Chain Alkyl Mercury Compounds. Methyl mercury is far more toxic than ethyl or diethyl mercury; the latter produces primarily renal abnormalities.

Methyl mercury is well absorbed from the intestinal tract, is widely distributed in the body, and readily passes through the placenta into the fetus and also into breast milk. About 10 per cent localizes in the brain, and the ensuing damage is largely irreversible. Major epidemics have resulted from industrial contamination of water with subsequent biotransformation of elemental and inorganic mercury into methyl mercury, followed by ingestion by fish and then by man. Other epidemics have resulted from use of grains contaminated by organic mercurial pesticides or animal ingestion of seeds treated with mercury. The epidemics in the Minamata and Niigata regions of Japan and in Iraq, Guatemala, Pakistan, and the United States have resulted in a high death rate and an appalling residue of permanent brain damage. In addition to the milder symptoms listed under elemental mercury poisoning, central nervous system manifestations include severe paresthesias, dysarthria, ataxia, visual field constriction, hearing loss, blindness, microcephaly, spasticity, paralysis, and coma. Some of the children of methyl mercury–poisoned mothers show various degrees of cerebral palsy–like abnormalities and mental retardation, and some die.

Chang LW: Neurotoxic effects of mercury—a review. Environ Res 14:329, 1977. *A very useful review with good clinical-pathologic correlations.*

Elhassani SB: The many faces of methylmercury poisoning. J Toxicol Clin Toxicol 19:875, 1982–1983. *A very nice, thorough review with 133 references.*
Joselow MM, Louria DB, Browder AA: Mercurialism: Environmental and occupational aspects. Ann Intern Med 76:119, 1972. *A useful summary with 149 references.*
Magos L: Mercury and mercurials. Br Med Bull 31:241, 1975. *A concise, valuable summary of the clinical manifestations and tissue localization after exposure to different chemical forms of mercury.*

ARSENIC

ETIOLOGY. Arsenic is ubiquitous in nature; it is present in the earth's crust in concentrations of 2 to 5 parts per billion. It is found in inordinately high concentrations in some well water. It is used in the glass, pigment, and bronze-plating industries; in wood preservation; in a variety of metal alloys; in veterinary medicines; in some herbicides, insecticides, and rodenticides; in fire salts to produce multicolored flames; and by farmers and vintners. American industry uses about one half of the world's production of arsenic trioxide. Arsenic poisoning has also resulted from using certain herbal preparations, from the ingestion of illegal (moonshine) whiskey, burning of arsenate-treated wood, and administration of arsenic-containing prescription medicines.

Elemental arsenic is not toxic even if ingested in substantial amounts. There are three toxic forms of arsenic: pentavalent salts, trivalent salts, and arsine gas. The arsenic in the earth's crust and in most foods is in the pentavalent form. Trivalent arsenic, which is far more toxic, accumulates in the body more readily than the pentavalent form. Arsenic gas (arsine) is extraordinarily toxic; it is formed by the hydrolysis of metallic arsenide or by the action of acids or nascent hydrogen on arsenical compounds, especially in the refining of certain metals. Arsine is also manufactured for and used in the electronics industry. Arsine can be liberated in sewage plants, and in one small cluster of cases eight children were poisoned while cleaning out a cattle dip in Australia.

CLINICAL MANIFESTATIONS. Although there is considerable overlap in the manifestations, it seems reasonable to divide arsenical toxicity into respiratory and gastrointestinal categories.

Respiratory. Arsine gas poisoning is usually overwhelming and frequently fatal. The onset of symptoms after exposure is usually between one and 12 hours. Fever, headache, muscle pains, nausea, vomiting, epigastric pain, dysuria, and explosive diarrhea characterize the acute episode. Because arsenic preferentially binds to red blood cells, hemolytic anemia and hemoglobinuria occur early, and red cell ghosts may be seen in the peripheral blood. There may also be cyanosis and profound hypoxia. Renal failure due to acute tubular necrosis (occasionally due to cortical necrosis) occurs in the first few days after onset of symptoms. This may be accompanied by shock and encephalopathy, characterized by agitation and disorientation. Both bone marrow depression and myocardial damage may occur. Those who do not die of intractable vascular collapse often develop subacute manifestations of arsenic poisoning described below. Those who recover may develop chronic renal failure.

Gastrointestinal. Although arsine gas poisoning can be mimicked by arsenic ingestion, the latter is usually more insidious and less overwhelming. Cramping abdominal pain and diarrhea are characteristic. Other acute manifestations include nausea, vomiting, dysphagia, cyanosis, headache, hematuria, and weakness. Hyperesthesia, muscle cramps, conjunctivitis, syncope, excessive thirst, periorbital swelling, epistaxis, and tinnitus may also occur. The patient may complain of a metallic taste and there may be a garlic odor to the breath, but the latter is not pathognomonic since it also may be observed in selenium, tellurium, and phosphorus poisoning.

Leukopenia occurs frequently, but in some cases moderate leukocytosis is found and both monocytosis and eosinophilia have been described. Anemia and thrombocytopenia may supervene.

Shortly after the initial red cell binding, arsenic can be found in liver, spleen, heart, kidneys, brain, and intestinal tract. Skin, nails, and hair do not usually contain arsenic until two to four weeks after exposure, but occasionally hair accumulation can occur more rapidly.

Other manifestations that may occur in the first week include jaundice, hematuria, hepatomegaly with hepatic enzyme abnormalities; electrocardiographic abnormalities; a cardiomyopathy that can be lethal; pericarditis; pulmonary edema; evidence of encephalopathy, including headache, irritability, delusions, and hallucinations; seizures; renal dysfunction; kidney failure; and respiratory muscle paralysis. Megaloblastic changes may be seen in the bone marrow. Optic neuritis with visual field constriction has been reported after pentavalent arsenic exposure.

The most prominent manifestation after the first week of illness is symmetrical polyneuropathy. At first sensory manifestations predominate, the patient complaining of a burning sensation in a stocking-glove distribution. Motor involvement follows almost immediately with diminished or absent reflexes and severe weakness. Occasionally the neuropathy is unilateral. Prolonged encephalopathy and/or psychosis have been reported in a few instances.

In cases of subacute poisoning, Aldrich-Mees lines (transverse white bands) may be seen in the nails; like the garlic odor, these may be seen in other trace element intoxications. Erythroderma and exfoliative dermatitis may also supervene.

Chronic exposure is associated with several abnormalities. The most characteristic of these are the cutaneous lesions, particularly hyperpigmentation (arsenic melanosis) and hyperkeratoses located primarily on the palms and soles. Alopecia and so-called raindrop depigmentation may also occur. In about 5 to 10 per cent of those chronically exposed, skin cancers appear after latent periods of 5 to more than 25 years; these tend to be multiple, are situated mainly on the trunk and upper extremities, and show either intraepithelial squamous cell (Bowen's disease) or basal cell morphology on histologic examination. In the United States the most frequent cause of such skin lesions in past years was the medicinal use of Fowler's solution, an inorganic trivalent arsenical. Currently most cases arise after occupational exposure, but a small number have been ascribed to chronic exposure to well water with high arsenic content.

Epidemiologic studies on gold ore miners, vineyard workers, laborers in sheep-dip factories, and smelter workers show a clear increase in the incidence of squamous cell carcinoma of the lung, the risk of bronchogenic cancer correlating with the intensity and duration of arsenic trioxide exposure.

Several types of liver disease may occur; these include postnecrotic cirrhosis, hepatocellular carcinoma, and hemangioendothelioma. Additionally, portal fibrosis and/or sinusoidal collagenosis may be found, and this can lead to a form of noncirrhotic portal hypertension with splenomegaly and esophageal varices but normal hepatic artery wedge pressure. Like the skin cancers, the liver abnormalities may occur many years after exposure to arsenic has been discontinued, and the exposure period can have been relatively brief.

Arsenic exposure is also thought to induce chromosomal aberrations, but the significance of these abnormalities is not clear.

DIAGNOSIS. If the diagnosis is suspected, there is a qualitative urine test (Gutzeit test) employing sulfuric acid, zinc, and silver nitrate. Arsenic concentrations can be measured in blood, urine, hair, or nails by atomic absorption spectrophotometry or neutron activation techniques.

TREATMENT. The treatment of choice is dimercaprol (BAL), but it should be given within the first 24 hours after exposure. If the BAL is given later, it is less likely that improvement will be observed, and in most cases the peripheral neuropathy is refractory to treatment. Exchange transfusion or dialysis shortly after the onset of acute illness has also been reported to be beneficial.

The neuropathy and renal failure may slowly resolve completely, or there may be residual abnormalities that range from mild to severe.

Massey EW, Wold D, Heyman A: Arsenic: Homicidal intoxication. South Med J 77:848, 1984. *Four cases and a comprehensive review in four packed pages. Thirty-two references.*
Schoolmeester WL, White DR: Arsenic poisoning. South Med J 73:198, 1980. *A fine comprehensive review with 102 references. Includes ten illustrative case reports.*
Zaloga GB, Deal J, Spurling T, et al.: Case report: Unusual manifestations of arsenic intoxication. Am J Med Sci 289:210, 1985. *The case (with facial palsy and pericarditis) is interesting and the review is terrific. Twenty-eight references.*

TRACE ELEMENTS WHOSE TOXICITY IS IN LARGE PART ASSOCIATED WITH HEMODIALYSIS

ZINC. The normal adult body zinc content is 1.5 to 3.0 grams. Daily intake ranges from 5 to 35 mg. Zinc is bound to metallothioneins synthesized in the liver and is excreted by both the urine and the gastrointestinal tract. Particularly high concentrations are found in the uveal tract, choroid plexus, and prostate; substantial amounts are also found in bone, brain, skeletal muscles, and other tissues of the eye.

Zinc has a strong affinity for red cells and plasma proteins. Consequently there is no loss across dialysis membranes; instead, blood zinc concentrations may increase markedly during hemodialysis. There appear to be two well-documented zinc sources: adhesive plaster (containing zinc oxide) used to prevent dialysis coils from unwinding, and the water of the dialysis fluid. Even if water has an initially low zinc content, galvanized iron pipes or tanks may release substantial amounts. This can be prevented by using deionized or distilled water.

The manifestations of zinc toxicity do not necessarily correlate well with plasma or whole blood zinc levels. Nausea, vomiting, anorexia, lethargy, irritability, abdominal pain, and anemia are the most frequent manifestations. The mechanisms responsible for the anemia are not well understood, but in many cases the anemia may be microcytic and associated with evidence of copper deficiency. Zinc can decrease copper absorption in the gut and also promote urinary copper excretion. Fever may accompany zinc toxicity. Other manifestations may include diarrhea, muscle pain, hyperamylasemia with or without pancreatitis, intestinal bleeding, thrombocytopenia, oliguria, hypotension, and renal failure with tubular necrosis. Injection of large amounts of zinc has resulted in death. Intestinal manifestations may supervene after either orally or parenterally induced zinc intoxication.

Welders, smelter workers, and solderers are exposed to aerosolized zinc and may experience zinc fume fever, characterized by chills, fever, myalgias, a metallic taste, cough, nausea, lethargy, and occasionally hemoptysis. There may be diffuse roentgenologic infiltrates and pulmonary dysfunction. Ordinarily all manifestations disappear rapidly after cessation of exposure. If more prolonged pulmonary dysfunction occurs, it is thought to result from the effects of other metals to which the workers are simultaneously exposed.

ALUMINUM. Aluminum-induced dialysis dementia is an often fatal disease. The tap water is usually to blame. Some waters naturally contain high concentrations of aluminum. In other cases aluminum sulfate had been added to the community water supply to remove organic materials. In still other cases the dialysis fluid appeared to be less responsible than aluminum-containing gels administered by mouth to reduce phosphate levels. However, if oral aluminum hydroxide is administered to nondialyzed patients suffering from renal failure, the encephalopathy syndrome rarely occurs; young children appear to be particularly at risk. Dialysis encephalopathy occurs only after repeated dialyses, usually spanning at least several months. Use of parenteral nutrition solutions containing aluminum can also be followed by aluminum poisoning.

Early manifestations include malaise, memory loss, and a characteristic speech disturbance. As the disease progresses, dysarthria, asterixis, myoclonic twitches, dementia, somnolence, and seizures occur. The electroencephalogram shows slowing, together with bursts of delta activity and high voltage, symmetric spikes. Among those who died, aluminum levels are markedly increased in the gray matter.

Other manifestations include anemia, myalgias, proximal myopathy, and severe skeletal pain caused by profound osteodystrophy that is unresponsive to vitamin D and is followed by fractures. Aluminum is deposited at the calcified bone-osteoid junction and bone formation is impaired (Ch. 246, 249).

Although frequently lethal, in some cases the encephalopathy has regressed after intake of oral aluminum is stopped or the aluminum content of the dialysis water is reduced or following renal transplantation. Treatment with deferoxamine, which complexes with aluminum, may be beneficial. Those suffering from uremia should avoid food additives and nonprescription drugs that contain substantial amounts of aluminum.

It has been suggested that Alzheimer's disease and other types of senile dementia may be related to brain aluminum deposition, but available data are unconvincing.

Those involved in aluminum processing or manufacturing, pottery or explosive making, or welding may be exposed to aluminum aerosols. Pulmonary granulomas, fibrosis, and in some cases postfibrosis emphysema may supervene. In bauxite smelters this is known as Shaver's disease.

COPPER. Since the late 1960's, copper tubing in dialysis equipment has been known to release copper when exposed to acid water. Copper levels may also be inordinately high in the dialysis water if the water is supplied through copper plumbing. Copper is a potent red cell poison, damaging cell membranes and inhibiting a variety of red cell enzymes. Major manifestations of toxicity include hemolysis and gastrointestinal disturbances. Nausea, vomiting, diarrhea, abdominal pain, fever, chills, hemolytic anemia, jaundice, hemoglobinuria, and severe myalgias all occur frequently. Myoglobinemia, necrotizing pancreatitis, hepatic necrosis and profound leukocytosis may also occur.

Copper poisoning during dialysis is fortunately readily avoidable, since copper is no longer a component of the tubing.

Copper poisoning may also occur after intentional or accidental ingestion. There may be a metallic taste, vomiting, and abdominal pain. In more severe cases hematemesis, melena, hepatic necrosis, and shock supervene.

In Wilson's disease rapid increases in circulating copper concentrations may be followed by acute hemolytic anemia.

Those exposed to metallic copper industrially may develop transient pulmonary manifestations (metal fume fever). These disappear rapidly when exposure is stopped.

COBALT. Patients with renal failure may have elevated tissue cobalt levels. In some cases cobaltous chloride has been given by mouth to patients on maintenance hemodialysis to combat anemia. This has been associated with increased blood and myocardial cobalt levels and suggestive evidence of cardiomyopathy. In the past cobalt had been used to increase red cell production. Toxicity included nausea, vomiting, anorexia, tinnitus, peripheral neuropathy, goiter resulting from blockage of iodine uptake, neurogenic deafness, hyperlipidemia, optic atrophy, and renal tubular damage.

Cobalt was added to beer in the 1960's as a foam stabilizer. This resulted in cardiomyopathy, often accompanied by pericardial effusion. Mortality from heart failure or arrhythmias ranged from 5 to 47 per cent (see Ch. 53).

Persons exposed to cobalt industrially may also occasionally develop cardiomyopathy. Workers exposed to finely powdered cobalt may develop pulmonary interstitial fibrosis and cor pulmonale. Cobalt is often a component of alloys that are used in joint prostheses. Cases have been reported of joint pains, spontaneous dislocation of the prosthesis, and bone necrosis starting nine months to four years postoperatively, apparently caused by a reaction to the cobalt in the alloy.

OTHER METALS. In one group of dialysis patients *nickel* toxicity occurred when nickel leached from a stainless steel water heater tank into the dialysis fluid. Manifestations include nausea, vomiting, weakness, and headache. Symptoms developed within a few hours after dialysis and disappeared within 48 hours.

Tissue *tin* concentrations, especially in the liver, are increased in patients undergoing hemodialysis. However, tin levels are even higher in uremic patients who have not been dialyzed. No definite clinical disease has been associated with these increased body tin burdens.

Patients undergoing maintenance hemodialysis are often treated with *iron* for anemia. In such patients parenteral and occasionally oral iron administration may be followed by hemosiderosis and occasionally hemochromatosis. Serum ferritin concentrations exceed 500 ng per milliliter. A proximal myopathy has been described. The severity of the tissue iron overload and the likelihood of hemochromatosis may be related to the histocompatibility antigens A-3, B-7, and B-14. Iron overload has been complicated by porphyria cutanea tarda and by a variety of infections, including those due to species of *Yersinia* and *Vibrio* and to the yeast *Trichosporon cutaneum*. Treatment with deferoxamine may reduce the body iron burden.

Aggett PJ, Harrison JT: Current status of zinc in health and disease states. Arch Dis Child 54:909, 1979. *This is a superb review with 110 references. Only a small section is devoted to toxicity.*

Andreoli SP, Bergstein JM, Sherrard DJ: Aluminum intoxication from aluminum-containing phosphate binders in children with azotemia not undergoing dialysis. N Engl J Med 310:1079, 1984. *This is an important article suggesting that both dose and age are important variables in aluminum intoxication. Thirty references.*

O'Hare JA, Callaghan NM, Murnaghan DJ: Dialysis encephalopathy. Clinical, electroencephalographic and interventional aspects. Medicine 62:129, 1983. *A marvelous summary article and a careful analysis of 14 patients who developed encephalopathy 16 to 92 months after starting dialysis.*

Ott SM, Maloney NA, Klein GL, et al.: Aluminum is associated with low bone formation in patients receiving chronic parenteral nutrition. Ann Intern Med 98:910, 1983. *The toxicity of aluminum to bone is clearly shown in 14 patients receiving casein hydrolysate.*

Sandstead HH: Trace elements in uremia and hemodialysis. Am J Clin Nutr 33:1501, 1980. *A very good review article in which the author urges caution in ascribing the dialysis encephalopathy syndrome solely to aluminum.*

Simon P, Allain P, Ang KS, et al.: Prevention and treatment of aluminum intoxication in chronic renal failure. Adv Nephrol 14:439, 1985. *This is as good a review as there is, with 179 references.*

Taylor A, Marks V: Cobalt: A review. J Hum Nutr 32:165, 1978. *A nice review with 73 references.*

Webster JD, Parker TF, Alfrey A, et al.: Acute nickel intoxication by dialysis. Ann Intern Med 92:631, 1980. *Nausea, vomiting, weakness, and headache were the predominant manifestations among 37 patients. Symptoms remitted three to thirteen hours after dialysis was concluded.*

CADMIUM

ETIOLOGY. Over 10 million pounds of cadmium are used industrially every year in the United States. The metal is a component of alloys; it is used in the manufacture of electrical conductors and in electroplating; and it is present in ceramics, pigments, dental prosthetics, plastic stabilizers, and storage batteries. It is also a byproduct of zinc smelting and is used in the photographic, rubber, motor, and aircraft industries. Smelters, metal processing furnaces, and the burning of coal and oil are responsible for much of the cadmium in air.

CLINICAL MANIFESTATIONS. *Acute intoxication* by cadmium fumes produces a characteristic clinical picture. Four to ten hours after exposure dyspnea, cough, and substernal discomfort supervene, often accompanied by prominent myalgias, fatigue, headache, and vomiting. In more severe cases wheezing, hemoptysis, and progressive dyspnea caused by pulmonary edema may occur, and may be accompanied by hypotension and renal failure.

In most cases, the pulmonary manifestations resolve rapidly but pulmonary function abnormalities may not disappear for months; in these cases vital capacity is reduced and there is a restrictive defect. Occasionally pulmonary edema is lethal.

Ingestion of large amounts of cadmium results in nausea, vomiting, and abdominal pain, often accompanied by weakness, prostration, and myalgias. The onset of the gastroenteritis occurs one half to five hours after ingestion and lasts for less than 24 hours.

Chronic cadmium exposure by aerosol for at least ten years has resulted in emphysema in a small number of cases. The emphysema is not accompanied by bronchitis and may appear many years after industrial exposure has stopped. Workers exposed for at least ten years also may suffer olfactory nerve damage; in some cases this progresses to total anosmia. The most frequent long-term consequence of aerosol or oral exposure is proteinuria. After prolonged and heavy contact, cadmium urinary excretion continues for years and is associated with damage to the proximal tubule. The major urinary protein is a low molecular weight β_2 microglobulin.

On occasion the proteinuria may be accompanied by glycosuria and aminoaciduria. Only infrequently is the proteinuria and tubular damage followed by progressive renal failure. An exception to the relatively benign course of the renal damage is the disease in Japan known as itai-itai (ouch-ouch), which affected almost exclusively multiparous women of ages 40 to 70 who lived in an area contaminated by industrial cadmium waste. Manifestations included striking back and joint pains, a waddly gait, osteomalacia, bone deformities, and fractures, all presumably secondary to cadmium-induced renal tubular damage.

Some studies on workers exposed to cadmium have suggested an increased risk of lung or prostatic carcinoma, but the data are not convincing.

Brenner I: Cadmium toxicity. World Rev Nutr Diet 32:165, 1978. *Interactions with calcium, zinc, copper, and selenium are emphasized. Additionally there is a detailed analysis of the role of metallothioneins. Contains 183 references.*

Lauwery RR, Roels AA, Buchet JP, et al.: Investigations on the lung and kidney function of workers exposed to cadmium. Environ Health Persp 28:137, 1979. *Three epidemiologic studies were conducted on more than 200 workers. The kidneys were affected to a much greater extent than the lungs. Both tubular and glomerular aberrations were found, mainly in persons with substantially increased blood and urine cadmium concentrations.*

NICKEL

ETIOLOGY. Nickel is used widely industrially in various alloys, iron shell casings, ball bearings, and heart and joint prostheses. It is also used in nickel plating; as a catalyst; in magnetic tapes, dyes, and paints; and in acrylic plastics. It is found in petroleum and coal, in diesel fuels, and in soil and air. Municipal incinerators may contribute to the ambient air nickel concentrations.

Nickel is a potent contact allergen; the most frequent adverse effect for humans is nickel dermatitis, which may be both persistent and severe. Serious systemic reactions have occurred in allergic persons given fluids intravenously through a nickel-containing needle. Prosthetic joints and heart valves have failed because of a reaction to the nickel in the prosthesis. In cases of recalcitrant nickel dermatitis, restriction in dietary nickel may be helpful.

CLINICAL MANIFESTATIONS AND TREATMENT. By far the most toxic of the nickel compounds is nickel carbonyl, created by a reaction between nickel and carbon monoxide. Industrial aerosol exposure is followed immediately by headache, drowsiness, substernal pain, nausea, and vomiting. This is followed by a latent period of one to five days, after which the victim experiences fever, chills, dyspnea, a feeling of chest tightness, cough that is sometimes productive of blood-tinged sputum, muscle pains, weakness, and fatigue. Hepatic enzyme concentrations may be considerably elevated.

In severe cases cyanosis, progressive respiratory difficulties, and convulsions ensue, and death may follow in four to 23 days. At autopsy the lungs show hemorrhage, atelectasis, fibroblastic proliferation, and hyaline membrane formation. The treatment of choice is diethyl dithiocarbamate (Dithiocarb); dimercaprol (BAL) is an alternative but less effective therapeutic agent. Although overwhelming pneumonitis caused by nickel carbonyl is now rare, milder pulmonary toxicity in occupations such as welding probably occurs quite commonly and goes unrecognized under the general rubric of metal fume fever. Nickel exposure may also be followed by Löffler's syndrome.

CARCINOGENESIS. Nickel is considered a potent respiratory tract carcinogen. Studies of nickel refinery workers have shown a fivefold increase in risk of lung cancer, a 150-fold increase in the risk of nasal cancer, and a substantially increased risk of larynx cancer. Those occupations most at risk among nickel workers are roasting, smelting, and electrolysis. Workers developing lung, laryngeal, and nasal cancers have usually been exposed for at least ten years. Biopsies of nasal mucosa show potentially precancerous epithelial dysplasia in a substantial percentage of nickel workers. The cancer risk is so great that workers heavily exposed for over ten years should probably have annual nasal mucosa biopsies as well as sputum cytologic studies and roentgenologic examinations every four to six months in an attempt at secondary prevention. The incidence of respiratory tract cancer in nickel workers is dependent on both the extent of nickel exposure and the effects of cocarcinogens, in particular cigarette tobacco. Except for nickel miners and refinery workers, industrial nickel exposure has not been convincingly associated with increased risk of cancer.

Sunderman FW Jr: A review of the metabolism and toxicity of nickel. Ann Clin Lab Sci 7:377, 1977. *An excellent review by one of the world's leading authorities (with 177 references).*

Sunderman FW Sr: Efficacy of sodium diethyldithiocarbamate (Dithiocarb) in acute nickel carbonyl poisoning. Ann Clin Lab Sci 9:1, 1979. *The data presented strongly suggest that this is currently the agent of choice.*

OTHER TOXIC METALS

Thallium

ETIOLOGY AND PATHOGENESIS. Thallium is used in optical lenses, jewelry, low-temperature thermometers, semiconductors, luminescent tubes, dyes and pigments, scintillation counters, and fireworks. It forms a stainless alloy with silver, a corrosion-resistant alloy with lead, and may be a byproduct of lead and zinc production. In some areas it is still a component of rodenticides, pesticides, and insecticides. Thallium can enter the body through the respiratory tract, gastrointestinal tract, or skin. Like many other trace metals thallium has a strong affinity for sulfhydryl groups and thus interferes with many enzyme systems. Additionally, it enters the cell, exchanging for intracellular potassium.

CLINICAL MANIFESTATIONS. Poisoning can be acute and overwhelming after suicidal ingestion or it can be chronic and subtle. In acute poisoning manifestations include nausea, vomiting, headache, lethargy, abdominal pain, diarrhea that may be bloody, insomnia, myalgias, fever, hyperhidrosis, excessive thirst, delirium, seizures, coma, and respiratory failure. At least 10 per cent of acutely poisoned persons die.

Among those who survive at least a week or in those exposed to smaller amounts of thallium, the most predictable manifestations are a combined sensory and motor, often painful, peripheral neuropathy and alopecia. Although the head alopecia is total, the facial, axillary, and pubic hair are spared as is the inner one third of the eyebrows. Motor manifestations may predominate, and the ascending, predominantly motor paralysis may mimic Guillain-Barré syndrome. Abdominal colic, nausea, and vomiting occur frequently in both the acute and subacute forms of thallium toxicity and may so dominate the clinical picture that a diagnosis of acute appendicitis is made. Other manifestations of subacute intoxication include dementia, headache, fatigue, sleep disorders, intractable thirst, hallucinations, blindness caused by optic neuritis, impotence, amenorrhea, a blue discoloration of the gingivae, centrilobular hepatic necrosis, renal tubular necrosis, orthostatic hypotension, paralytic ileus and myoclonic twitches. Multiple cranial nerves may be involved, but the eighth nerve is almost always spared. The electrocardiogram may show arrhythmias and changes similar to those associated with hypokalemia.

DIAGNOSIS. Thallium can be measured in blood and urine, but blood levels are often deceptively low even during clinically apparent poisoning. Since thallium is excreted in the urine, thallium determinations on 24-hour specimens are more reliable. A qualitative urine test is available. Urine is mixed with 0.4-per-cent sodium bismuth in 20-per-cent nitric acid and 10-per-cent sodium iodide; if thallium is present, a red precipitate forms.

In some cases there is no history of occupational, environmental, or intentional exposure. Unexplained abdominal pain, neurologic abnormalities, and alopecia suggest the diagnosis.

TREATMENT. Treatment consists of hemodialysis, which can remove up to half the thallium body burden, potassium, forced diuresis, and administration of Prussian blue. Prussian blue, given by mouth, absorbs thallium so that fecal thallium concentrations increase. The half-life of thallium in the body is about one month, and repeated dialyses are usually needed. Hemoperfusion may also help. During potassium administration thallium is displaced from its intracellular site, and this may cause transient exacerbations of clinical manifestations. Barbiturates may increase the severity of the disease, and their use should be avoided.

PROGNOSIS. As many as 30 per cent of those poisoned suffer some residual effects. The neuropathy may persist for many months before resolving, and some are left with variable amounts of dementia, neuropathy, ataxia, visual impairment, alopecia, and myoclonus.

Selenium

ETIOLOGY. Selenium is well absorbed from both the gastrointestinal tract and the lungs. The amount normally ingested varies markedly, depending on the local soil selenium content and on the geographic provenance of foods consumed. Grains, pork, kidney, seafoods, garlic, mushrooms, radishes, beef, egg yolk, and chicken frequently contain substantial amounts of selenium. The element is widely used in pigment, glass, electronics, ceramics, and steel industries.

CLINICAL MANIFESTATIONS. Both deficiency and toxicity syndromes are well described in animals. Deficiency, resulting from foraging on grains grown in soil deficient of selenium, produces white muscle disease, a diffuse, often severe myopathy. Excess caused by chronic ingestion of grains containing more than 10 parts per million of selenium results in two syndromes, alkali disease and the staggers. The former is milder and is characterized by anemia, emaciation, alopecia, and hoof deformity. The staggers is manifested by visual difficulties, anemia, liver cell degeneration, paralysis, and respiratory failure. In sheep, excessive selenium intake can produce severe cardiomyopathy.

In man a *selenium deficiency syndrome* has not been clearly defined. However, in the Republic of China diffuse cardiomyopathy has been associated with low soil and blood selenium levels, and the incidence of the disease allegedly has been strikingly reduced by selenium supplementation.

Selenium toxicity syndromes in man can be divided into acute and chronic poisoning. Subjects with inordinate exposure to selenium fumes experience one or more of the following: intestinal disturbances, giddiness, apathy, lassitude, pallor, nervousness, depression, hair and nail loss, a garlic odor to the breath, and a metallic taste. Sore throat, dyspnea, and cough may also be noted. Symptoms usually disappear after removal from the occupational exposure. Among those ingesting excessive selenium the following symptoms and signs have been reported: nausea, vomiting, anorexia, fatigue, sore throat, emotional lability, a metallic taste, a garlic odor to the breath, brittle nails, brittle hair, hair loss, a bronze color to the skin, hepatic dysfunction, and diffuse dermatitis. Increased selenium burdens may be associated with an increased prevalence of dental caries.

EPIDEMIOLOGY. A most impressive epidemic of chronic selenium intoxication was observed in China in the 1960's. Subacute and chronic selenium toxicity will likely be seen with an increasing frequency because selenium is being promoted as a nonprescription supplement. Epidemiologic data suggest an inverse relationship between selenium blood levels and the incidence of certain cancers, particularly of the intestinal tract. In experimental studies oral selenium in dosage of 0.1 to 2.0 parts per million diminishes the frequency of or delays the appearance of a variety of spontaneous or induced tumors.

Manganese

Manganese toxicity occurs primarily in miners who have been exposed to manganese dioxide aerosols for prolonged periods. The manifestations, known as manganic madness, are limited to the central nervous system. The manganese is concentrated primarily in the basal ganglia and cerebellum accounting for the extrapyramidal Parkinson-like facies, the rigidity, and the difficulty in walking. Other manifestations include compulsive behavior (including singing, dancing, fighting, and running), explosive and involuntary laughter, headache, muscular weakness, tremors, somnolence, dystonia, hypotonia, retropulsion and propulsion, dementia, speech disturbances, irritability, hypersomnia, and memory defects. In some cases psychosis may be the dominant feature. There is no effective therapy. After removal from manganese exposure or following attempts to reduce the body manganese load by treatment with calcium versenate or L-dopa, the mental aberrations usually improve but the neurologic abnormalities persist. Manganese contamination of dialysates or ingestion has been associated with abdominal pain, liver dysfunction, and evidence of pancreatitis.

Barium

Barium compounds are used in printing; in the production of paints, glass, paper, leather, soap, and rubber; in ceramics, plastic, steel, oil, textile, and dye industries; as fuel additives; and in insecticides, rodenticides, and depilatories. There are two major adverse effects. After accidental or intentional ingestion of large amounts, abdominal pain, vomiting, and increased peristalsis occur. If enough is absorbed, potassium is displaced intracellularly resulting in profound hypokalemia, which in turn may produce flaccid paralysis, potentially dangerous cardiac arrhythmias, renal failure, and respiratory paralysis. Poisoning has also been described after barium chloride skin burn. Treatment consists of administration of potassium and forced diuresis to promote barium excretion.

The other adverse effect from contact with barium is a benign pneumoconiosis that may supervene after one or more years of aerosol exposure. Chest roentgenograms show extensive, very dense, bilateral nodules up to 4 to 5 mm in diameter. There is no prominent fibrosis and no clinically significant disease; the nodules often regress after occupational exposure is stopped.

Boron

There are few reports of boron toxicity. Ingestion of boric acid can result in nausea, vomiting, diarrhea, anemia, seizures, a variety of skin eruptions characterized by intense erythema, desquamation, and exfoliation, and striking alopecia. Additionally, occupational aerosol exposure to diborane (B_2H_6) in high energy fuels can produce acute pulmonary edema that resolves after the exposure is discontinued. Exposure to liquid boron hydride (B_5H_9) can produce dementia, cortical blindness, deafness, seizures, acidosis, and cardiac arrest. A subacute mild organic brain syndrome has also been observed.

Antimony

Industrial antimony toxicity is very rare, as are intentional ingestion or inadvertent poisoning from release of antimony from inexpensive enamelware. Manifestations of acute poisoning include nausea, abdominal pain, weakness, headache, vomiting, diarrhea, myalgias, and circulatory collapse. Gaseous SbH_3 (stibine) is as toxic as arsine, producing CNS toxicity and hemolysis. After antimonial injection for medicinal purposes, adverse effects include nausea, vomiting, cough, and muscle and joint pain. Hepatic dysfunction can occur, as can cardiac arrhythmias, including Adams-Stokes syndrome. Antimony is also considered one of the metals capable of causing metal fume fever.

Chromium

Chromium is used extensively in metal and galvanizing industries and in the manufacture of dyes, enamel, and paints. Chromate exposure is associated with an increased incidence of lung and certain upper respiratory tract cancers. Additionally, chromium-exposed workers may show evidence of proximal renal tubule dysfunction and may suffer nasal septum perforations.

Molybdenum

In animals, molybdenum produces diarrhea, anemia, alopecia, diminished growth, and bone and joint abnormalities. No clearly defined molybdenum toxicity syndrome has been reported in man.

Platinum

The major adverse effects observed in platinum workers are allergic pulmonary reactions, including bronchial asthma.

Plutonium

In experimental models, plutonium, because of its radioactivity, is a potent carcinogen. Workers have been generally well protected, but recent data suggest that occupational exposure may be a significant problem. Some still controversial epidemiologic studies have suggested that accidental community exposure has resulted in an increase in frequency of certain cancers and fetal malformations.

Tellurium

Used particularly in rubber, metallurgic, and electronics industries, tellurium can cause giddiness, headache, nausea, a metallic taste, and a garlic smell to the breath. In animals tellurium causes neuropathy, but this has not been convincingly demonstrated in humans.

Tin

Tin can be released into beverages or foods from tin cans; ingestion can produce nausea, vomiting, abdominal pain, and diarrhea. Such toxicity occurs infrequently. Additionally, there have been occasional reports of encephalopathy following industrial exposure to organic tin compounds; this was characterized by headache, vomiting, visual defects, and paresis. Aerosol exposure to tin may result in stannosis, a mild pneumoconiosis in which there may be dense bilateral infiltrates but usually no pulmonary dysfunction.

Vanadium

Vanadium is used in alloys and in the steel and chemical industries. Its inhalation can result in neurasthenia, anorexia, vertigo, throat pain, nasal irritation (even nasal hemorrhage), and acute bronchitis characterized by a cough that is sometimes accompanied by a whoop. The nasal mucosa of vanadium-exposed workers shows vascular hyperemia and round cell infiltration.

Bencko V, Cikrt M: Manganese: A review of occupational and environmental toxicology. J Hyg Epidem Microbiol Immunol 28:139, 1984. *All you wanted to know about manganese and then some (77 references).*

Doig AT: Baritosis: A benign pneumoconiosis. Thorax 31:130, 1976. *Nine cases are described. Despite dense infiltrates, no significant clinical disease or physiologic abnormalities occurred.*

Nordberg GF: Factors influencing metabolism and toxicity of metals: A consensus report. Environ Health Persp 25:3, 1978. *This marvelous analysis covers the toxicity and interactions with other metals of arsenic, cadmium, lead, and mercury. Highly recommended. Contains 312 references.*

Silverman JJ, Hart RP, Garrettson LK, et al.: Post-traumatic stress disorders from pentaborane intoxication. JAMA 254:2603, 1985. *Fourteen persons exposed to B_5H_9 suffered neuropsychological deficits (33 references).*

Thallium poisoning. Clinical Conferences of the Johns Hopkins Hospital. Johns Hopkins Med J 142:27, 1978. *A single case accompanied by an excellent discussion of clinical manifestations and treatment.*

Wilkinson GS, Tietjen GL, Wiggs LD, et al.: Mortality among plutonium and other radiation workers at a plutonium weapons facility. Am J Epidemiol 125:231, 1987. *Although confirmatory studies are needed, this very careful analysis of 5413 men suggests increased risks for several types of cancers.*

Yang G, Wang S, Zhou R, et al.: Endemic selenium intoxication of humans in China. Am J Clin Nutr 37:872, 1983. *This is an excellent review of selenium intoxication based on a very significant epidemic in China. Selenium-laden vegetables and coal combined with a drought that reduced the rice crop were the major culprits. Seventeen references.*

PART XXVI

LABORATORY REFERENCE RANGE VALUES OF CLINICAL IMPORTANCE

543 REFERENCE INTERVALS AND LABORATORY VALUES OF CLINICAL IMPORTANCE*

Ronald J. Elin

Reference intervals are valuable guidelines for the assessment of health and disease by the clinician, but they should not be used as absolute indicators of health and disease. For essentially every test, there is a significant overlap between the normal and diseased populations. Many factors may influence the determination of the reference interval. The method and mode of standardization are variables for the reference interval, particularly for immunologic and enzymatic tests. The selection of the "normal" population is also important since factors such as age, sex, race, diet, personal habits (alcohol consumption, smoking, etc.), and exercise may influence the reference interval for a given analyte. Lastly, the statistics chosen to define the reference interval will also be a factor. These multiple variables for the determination of the reference interval indicate why there are differences among institutions for the same analyte.

The values in this chapter are primarily for adults in the fasting state. Values for other groups, when included, are clearly identified. For convenience, this chapter is divided into the following three sections: clinical chemistry, toxicology, and serology; hematology and coagulation; and drugs—therapeutic and toxic. The list includes reference intervals for the most common tests used in the practice of internal medicine. For more information about the reference interval for a given test or a test not included in the list, I recommend *Clinical Guide to Laboratory Tests*, edited by Dr. Norbert W. Tietz. This book contains literature citations for most of the tests listed in this chapter.

All laboratory values are given in conventional and international units. If the value and units for a reference interval are the same for conventional and international units, the interval is listed only in the column for international units.

*The material in this chapter was partially extracted from Tietz NW (ed.): Clinical Guide to Laboratory Tests. Philadelphia, W.B. Saunders Company, 1983. The main contributors are RV Blanke and RA Blouin: Drugs and Toxicology; C Hougie: Coagulation; HP Lehmann: International Units; J Leonard: Endocrinology; W Mertz and RV Blanke: Trace Metals; DA Nelson: Hematology; SE Ritzmann: Proteins; and HE Sauberlich: Vitamins. The material for the section on Therapeutic Drug Concentrations was partially extracted from Tietz NW: Textbook of Clinical Chemistry. Philadelphia, W.B. Saunders Company, 1986. The main contributors to this section of the book are NW Tietz and NM Logan. Other sources are listed under references for this chapter.

The temperature for all enzyme assays listed in the chapter is 37°C. The pertinent prefixes denoting the decimal factors are listed below.

PREFIXES DENOTING DECIMAL FACTORS

Prefix	Symbol	Factor
mega	M	10^6
kilo	k	10^3
hecto	h	10^2
deka	da	10^1
deci	d	10^{-1}
centi	c	10^{-2}
milli	m	10^{-3}
micro	μ	10^{-6}
nano	n	10^{-9}
pico	p	10^{-12}
femto	f	10^{-15}

ABBREVIATIONS

AU	Arbitrary units
EU	Ehrlich unit
GD	General Diagnostics
IFA	Immunofluorescent assay
IU	International unit (of hormone activity)
RIA	Radioimmunoassay
RID	Radialimmunodiffusion
S	Substrate
U	International unit (of enzyme activity)

Beutler E: Hemolytic Anemia in Disorders of Red Cell Metabolism. New York, Plenum Publishing Company, 1978.

Brown SS, Mitchell FL, Young DS (eds.): Chemical Diagnosis of Disease. Amsterdam, Elsevier/North-Holland Biomedical Press, 1979.

Conn RB (ed.): Current Diagnosis. 7th ed. Philadelphia, W.B. Saunders Company, 1984.

Gilman AG, Goodman L, Gilman A (eds.): The Pharmacological Basis of Therapeutics. 6th ed. New York, The Macmillan Company, 1980.

Henry JB (ed.): Todd-Sanford-Davidsohn Clinical Diagnosis and Management by Laboratory Methods. 16th ed. Philadelphia, W.B. Saunders Company, 1979.

Hoeg JM, Gregg RE, Brewer HB: An approach to the management of hyperlipoproteinemia. JAMA 255:512, 1986.

Mabry C, Tietz NW: Tables of normal laboratory values. In Nelson WE, Vaughan VC, McKay JR, et al. (eds.): Nelson Textbook of Pediatrics. 23rd ed. Philadelphia, W.B. Saunders Company, 1983.

Miale JB: Laboratory Medicine: Hematology. 5th ed. St. Louis, The C.V. Mosby Company, 1977.

Tietz NW (ed.): Textbook of Clinical Chemistry. Philadelphia, W.B. Saunders Company, 1986.

Tietz NW, Blackburn RH (eds.): Reference Ranges and General Information. Clinical Laboratories, A.B. Chandler Medical Center, University of Kentucky, Lexington, Kentucky, 1984.

Tietz NW (ed.): Clinical Guide to Laboratory Tests. Philadelphia, W.B. Saunders Company, 1983.

Williams WJ, Beutler E, Erslev AJ, et al.: Hematology. 2nd ed. New York, McGraw-Hill Book Company, 1977.

CLINICAL CHEMISTRY, TOXICOLOGY, SEROLOGY

Test	Specimen	Reference Range (Conventional Units)	Reference Range (International Units)
Acetoacetate Semiquantitative	Serum or plasma (fluoride/oxalate)	Negative (<3 mg/dL)	Negative (< 0.3 mmol/L)
Acetone	Urine	Negative	Negative
Semiquantitative	Serum or plasma (fluoride/oxalate)	Negative (<1.0 mg/dL)	Negative (<0.17 mmol/L)
Quantitative		0.3–2.0 mg/dL	0.5–0.34 mmol/L
Semiquantitative	Urine	Negative	Negative
Acid phosphatase (S:p-nitrophenylphosphate)	Serum		M: 2.5–11.7 U/L F: 0.3–9.2 U/L
Adrenocorticotropic hormone (ACTH)	Plasma (heparin)	0800 h: 25–100 pg/mL 1800 h: <50 pg/mL	25–100 ng/L <50 ng/L
Alanine aminotransferase (ALT, SGPT)	Serum		5–30 U/L
Albumin			
Nephelometric, colorimetric	Serum	3.5–5.0 g/dL	35–50 g/L
Turbidimetric	CSF	15–45 mg/dL	150–450 mg/L
	Urine	<80 mg/d at rest <150 mg/d ambulatory	<80 mg/d <150 mg/d
Aldolase	Serum		1.5–12.0 U/L
Aldosterone	Plasma (heparin or EDTA) or serum	Adult, average sodium diet supine: 3–10 ng/diet upright: F 5–30 ng/dL M 6–22 ng/dL	0.08–0.28 nmol/L 0.14–0.83 nmol/L 0.17–0.61 nmol/L
Alkaline phosphatase (S:4–NPP)	Serum		Adult (>18y) F: 56–155 U/L M: 62–176 U/L
δ-Aminolevulinic acid (δ-ALA)	Serum	15–23 μg/dL	1.1–8 μmol/L
	Urine	1.3–7.0 mg/d	9.9–53.4 μmol/d
Ammonia nitrogen Resin or enzymatic	Serum or plasma (Na-heparin)	Adult 15–45 μg N/dL	11–32 μmol/L
	Urine, 24-h	140–1500 mg/d	10–107 mmol/d
Amylase (S:Beckman, defined substrate)	Serum		25–125 U/L
	Urine, timed specimen		1–17 U/h
Angiotensin I	Peripheral venous plasma (EDTA)	11–88 pg/mL	11–88 ng/L
Angiotensin II	Plasma (EDTA) Arterial blood	2.4 ± 1.2 ng/dL	24 ± 12 ng/L
Angiotensin converting enzyme	Serum		23–57 U/L
α₁-Antitrypsin (nephelometry)	Serum	78–200 mg/dl	0.78–2.00 g/L
Anion gap [Na − (Cl⁻ + HCO₃⁻)]	Plasma (heparin)	7–14 mEq/L	7–14 mmol/L
Arsenic	Whole blood (heparin)	0.2–6.2 μg/dL Chronic poisoning: 10–50 μg/dL Acute poisoning: 60–93 μg/dL	0.03–0.82 μmol/L 1.33–6.65 μmol/L 7.98–12.37 μmol/L
	Urine, 24-h	5–50 μg/d	0.067–0.665 μmol/d
Ascorbic acid (see vitamin C)			
Aspartate aminotransferase (AST, SGOT)	Serum		10–30 U/L
Base excess	Whole blood (heparin)	−2 to 3 mEq/L	−2 to 3 mmol/L
Bicarbonate	Serum	18–23 mEq/L	18–23 mmol/L
Bile acids, total	Serum, fasting	0.3–2.3 μg/mL	0.74–5.64 μmol/L
	Serum, 2-h postprandial	1.8–3.2 μg/mL	4.41–7.84 μmol/L
	Feces	120–225 mg/d	294–551 μmol/d
Bilirubin			
Total	Serum	0.2–1.0 mg/dL	3.4–17.1 μmol/L
	Urine	Negative	Negative
Conjugated (direct)	Serum	0–0.2 mg/dL	0–3.4 μmol/L
Calcium, ionized (iCa)	Serum, plasma or whole blood (heparin)	4.48–4.92 mg/dL	1.12–1.23 mmol/L
Calcium, total	Serum	8.4–10.2 mg/dL	2.10–2.55 mmol/L
	Urine, 24-h	100–300 mg/d	2.5–7.5 mmol/d
	CSF	4.2–5.4 mg/dL	1.05–1.35 mmol/L
Carbon dioxide Total (TCO₂)	Serum or plasma (heparin)	23–29 mEq/L	23–29 mmol/L
Carcinoembryonic antigen (CEA)	Serum	Nonsmokers: <2.5 ng/mL	<2.5 μg/L
β-Carotene	Serum	60–200 μg/dl	1.12–3.72 μmol/L
Catecholamines, fractionated	Urine, 24-h	Dopamine: 65–400 μg/d Epinephrine: 0–15 μg/d Norepinephrine: 0–100 μg/d	424–2612 nmol/d 0–82 nmol/d 0–590 nmol/d
	Plasma (EDTA and sodium metabisulfite)	Dopamine: <136 pg/mL Epinephrine: <88 pg/mL Norepinephrine: 104–548 pg/mL	<888 pmol/L <480 pmol/L 615–3240 pmol/L
Catecholamines, free	Urine, 24-h		<280 μg/d
Ceruloplasmin (RID)	Serum	15–60 mg/dL	150–600 mg/L

Table continued on following page

CLINICAL CHEMISTRY, TOXICOLOGY, SEROLOGY *Continued*

Test	Specimen	Reference Range (Conventional Units)	Reference Range (International Units)
Chloride	Serum or plasma (heparin)	98–106 mEq/L	98–106 mmol/L
	CSF	118–132 mEq/L	118–132 mmol/L
	Urine, 24-h	110–250 mEq/d	110–250 mmol/d
Cholesterol, total	Serum or plasma	mg/dL	mmol/L
(75th percentile from Lipid	(EDTA)	20–29 y, M: < 194	5.02
Research Clinics)		F: < 184	4.77
		20–39 y, M: < 218	5.65
		F: < 202	5.23
		40–49 y, M: < 231	5.98
		F: < 223	5.78
		≥50 y, M: < 230	5.96
		F: < 252	6.53
Chorionic gonadotropin, β-subunit (β-HCG)	Serum or plasma (EDTA)	M, & nonpregnant F: <3.0 mU/mL	<3.0 IU/L
Complement			
Total hemolytic Complement activity	Plasma (EDTA)	75–160 U/mL	75–160 kU/L
Classic pathway components:			
C1q	Serum	6.5 ± 0.7 mg/dL (1 SD)	65 ± 7 mg/L
C1r	Serum	2.5–3.8 mg/dL	25–38 mg/L
C1s (C1 esterase)	Serum	2.5–3.8 mg/dL	25–38 mg/L
C2	Serum	2.8 ± 0.6 mg/dL (1 SD)	28 ± 6 mg/L
C3 (β_1C-globulin)	Serum	80–155 mg/dL	800–1550 mg/L
C4 (β_1E-globulin)	Serum	13–37 mg/dL	130–370 mg/L
C5 (β_1F-globulin)	Serum	6.4 ± 1.3 mg/dL (1 SD)	64 ± 13 mg/L
C6	Serum	5.6 ± 0.8 mg/dL (1 SD)	56 ± 8 mg/L
C7	Serum	4.9–7.0 mg/dL	49–70 mg/L
C8	Serum	4.3–6.3 mg/dL	43–63 mg/L
C9	Serum	4.7–6.9 mg/dL	47–69 mg/L
Alternative pathway components:			
C4 binding protein	Serum	18–32 mg/dL	180–320 mg/L
Factor B (C3 proactivator)	Serum	20–45 mg/dL	200–450 mg/L
Properdin	Serum	2.8 ± 0.4 mg/dL (1 SD)	28 ± 4 mg/L
Copper	Serum	M: 70–140 µg/dL	10.99–21.98 µmol/L
		F: 80–155 µg/dL	12.56–24.34 µmol/L
	Erythrocyte (heparin)	90–150 µg/dL	14.13–23.55 µmol/L
	Urine, 24-h	15–30 µg/d	0.24–0.47 µmol/d
Coproporphyrin	Urine, 24-h	34–234 µg/d	51–351 nmol/d
	Feces, 24-h	<30 µg/g dry wt	<45 nmol/g dry wt
		400–1200 µg/d	600–1800 nmol/d
Corticobinding globulin (CBG) (see Transcortin)			
Corticosterone	Serum or plasma (heparin, EDTA, or oxalate)	0.13–2.3 µg/dL	3.75–66 nmol/L
Cortisol	Serum or plasma (heparin)	0800 h: 5–23 µg/dL	138–635 nmol/L
		1600 h: 3–15 µg/dL	82–413 nmol/L
		2000 h: ≤50% of 0800 h	Fraction of 0800 h: ≤0.50
Cortisol, free	Urine, 24-h	10–100 µg/d	27–276 nmol/d
C-Peptide	Serum	≤4.0 ng/mL	≤4.0 µg/L
C-Reactive protein	Serum	68–8200 ng/mL	68–8200 µg/L
Creatine kinase (CK)	Serum		M: 38–174 U/L
			F: 96–140 U/L
Isoenzymes	Serum	Fraction 2 (MB) <4–6% of total (method-dependent)	Fraction of total: <0.04–0.06
Creatinine	Serum or plasma	M: 0.6–1.2 mg/dL	53–106 µmol/L
Jaffe, kinetic or enzymatic		F: 0.5–1.1 mg/dL	44–97 µmol/L
	Urine, 24-h	M: 14–26 mg/kg/d	124–230 µmol/kg/d
		F: 11–20 mg/kg/d	97–177 µmol/kg/d
Creatinine clearance (endogenous)	Serum or plasma, and urine	M: 97–137 mL/min/1.73 m^2	0.93–1.32 mL/s/m^2
		F: 88–128 mL/min/1.73 m^2	0.85–1.23 mL/s/m^2
Dehydroepiandrosterone serum (DHEA)	Serum	M: 1.7–4.2 ng/mL	6–15 nmol/L
		F: 2.0–5.2 ng/mL	7–18 nmol/L
Dehydroepiandrosterone sulfate (DHEA-S)	Serum or plasma (heparin or EDTA)	M: 1.99–3.34 µg/mL	5.2–8.7 µmol/L
		F: Premenopausal 0.82–3.38 µg/mL	2.1–8.8 µmol/L
		Postmenopausal 0.11–0.61 µg/mL	0.3–1.6 µmol/L
		Pregnancy, term 0.23–1.17 µg/mL	0.6–3.0 µmol/L
11-Deoxycortisol (compound S)	Plasma (heparin, EDTA or oxalate)	Without metyrapone: <1 µg/dL	<30 nmol/L
		After metyrapone: >7 µg/dL	>200 nmol/L
Estradiol (E$_2$)	Serum or plasma (heparin or EDTA)	M: 8–36 pg/mL	29–132 pmol/L
		F: Follicular 10–90 pg/mL	37–330 pmol/L
		Midcycle 100–500 pg/mL	370–1835 pmol/L
		Luteal 50–240 pg/mL	184–880 pmol/L
		Postmenopausal 10–30 pg/mL	37–100 pmol/L
	Urine, 24-h	M: 0–6 µg/d	0–22 nmol/d
		F: Follicular 0–3 µg/d	0–11 nmol/d
		Ovulatory peak 4–14 µg/d	15–51 nmol/d
		Luteal 4–10 µg/d	15–37 nmol/d
		Postmenopausal 0–4 µg/d	0–15 nmol/d

Table continued on opposite page

CLINICAL CHEMISTRY, TOXICOLOGY, SEROLOGY *Continued*

Test	Specimen	Reference Range (Conventional Units)	Reference Range (International Units)
Estriol (E₃), total	Serum	M & nonpregnant F: <2 ng/mL	<7 nmol/L
Estrogens, total	Serum	M: 40–115 pg/mL	40–115 ng/L
		F, cycle:	
		1–10 d 61–394 pg/mL	61–394 ng/L
		11–20 d 122–437 pg/mL	122–437 ng/L
		21–30 d 156–350 pg/mL	156–350 ng/L
		Prepubertal and postmenopausal ≤40 pg/mL	≤40 ng/L
	Urine, 24-h		M: 5–25 µg/d
			F: Preovulation 4–25 µg/d
			Ovulation 28–100 µg/d
			Luteal peak 22–80 µg/d
			Pregnancy, term <45,000 µg/d
			Postmenopausal 1–7 µg/d
Estrone (E₁)	Serum	M: 30–170 pg/mL	111–630 pmol/L
		F: Follicular 20–150 pg/mL	74–555 pmol/L
	Urine, 24-h	M: 3–8 µg/d	11–30 nmol/d
		F: Ovulatory peak 11–31 µg/d	41–115 nmol/d
		Luteal 10–23 µg/d	37–85 nmol/d
		Postmenopausal 1–7 µg/d	3.7–26.0 nmol/d
Fat, fecal	Feces, 72-h	<7 g/d	
		fat-free diet: <4 g/d	
Fatty acids, nonesterified (free)	Serum or plasma (heparin)	8–25 mg/dL	0.30–0.90 mmol/L
Fatty acids, total	Serum	190–420 mg/dL	7–15 mmol/L
Ferritin	Serum	M: 15–200 ng/mL	15–200 µg/L
		F: 12–150 ng/mL	12–150 µg/L
α₁-Fetoprotein	Serum	<30 ng/mL	<30 µg/L
Fibrinogen (see Hematology and Coagulation section)			
Folate	Serum	1.8–9 ng/mL	4.1–20.4 nmol/L
	Erythrocytes (EDTA)	150–450 ng/mL packed cells	340–1020 nmol/L packed cells
Follicle-stimulating hormone (FSH)	Serum or plasma (heparin)	M: 4–25 mIU/mL	4–25 IU/L
		F: Premenopausal 4–30 mIU/mL	4–30 IU/L
		Midcycle peak 10–90 mIU/mL	10–90 IU/L
		Pregnancy low to undetectable	low to undetectable
		Postmenopausal 40–250 mIU/mL	40–250 IU/L
	Urine, 24-h	M: 4–18 U/d	4–18 IU/d
		F: 3–12 U/d	3–12 IU/d
Free thyroxine index (FT₄I)	Serum		1.2–5.0
Gastrin	Serum	<100 pg/mL	<100 ng/L
Glucose	Serum	Adult: 70–105 mg/dL	3.9–5.8 mmol/L
		>60 y: 80–115 mg/dL	4.4–6.4 mmol/L
	Whole blood (heparin)	65–95 mg/dL	3.6–5.3 mmol/L
	CSF	40–70 mg/dL	2.2–3.9 mmol/L
Quantitative, enzymatic	Urine	<0.5 g/d	<2.8 mmol/d
Qualitative	Urine		Negative
Glucose, 2-h postprandial	Serum	<120 mg/dL	<6.7 mmol/L

Glucose tolerance test (GTT), oral	Serum		mg/dL			mmol/L	
			Normal	Diabetic		Normal	Diabetic
		Fasting:	70–105	>140		3.9–5.8	>7.8
		60 min:	120–170	≥200		6.7–9.4	≥11
		90 min:	100–140	≥200		5.6–7.8	≥11
		120 min:	70–120	≥140		3.9–6.7	≥7.8

Test	Specimen	Reference Range (Conventional Units)	Reference Range (International Units)
γ-Glutamyltransferase (GGT)	Serum		M: 9–50 U/L
			F: 8–40 U/L
Glycerol, free	Plasma	0.29–1.72 mg/dl	0.032–0.187 mmol/L
Growth hormone (HGH, somatotropin)	Serum or plasma (EDTA, heparin)	Adult, M: <2 ng/mL	<2 µg/L
		F: <10 ng/mL	<10 µg/L
		>60 y, M: 0.4–10 ng/mL	0.4–10 µg/L
		F: 1–14 ng/mL	1–14 µg/L
Haptoglobin (see Hematology and Coagulation section)			
HDL-cholesterol (HDLC) (5th percentile from Lipid Research Clinics)	Serum or plasma (EDTA)	M: >29 mg/dL	>0.75 mmol/L
		F: >35 mg/dL	>0.91 mmol/L
Hemoglobin A₁c (electrophoresis)	Whole blood (heparin, EDTA or oxalate)	5.6–7.5% of total Hb	Fraction of Hb: 0.056–0.075
Homovanillic acid (HVA)	Urine, 24-h	<15 mg/d	<82 µmol/d
17-Hydroxycorticosteroids (17-OHCS)	Urine, 24-h		M: 4–12 mg/d
			F: 4–8 mg/d
5-Hydroxindole acetic acid (5-HIAA)			
Qualitative	Fresh random urine		Negative
Quanitative	Urine, 24-h	2–8 mg/d	10.4–41.6 µmol/d
17-Hydroxyprogesterone (17-OHP)	Serum	M: 0.2–1.8 ng/mL	0.6–5.4 nmol/L
		F: Follicular 0.2–0.8 ng/mL	0.6–2.4 nmol/L
		Luteal 0.8–3.0 ng/mL	2.4–9.0 nmol/L
		Postmenopausal 0.04–0.5 ng/mL	0.12–1.5 nmol/L

Table continued on following page

CLINICAL CHEMISTRY, TOXICOLOGY, SEROLOGY *Continued*

Test	Specimen	Reference Range (Conventional Units)	Reference Range (International Units)
Immunoglobulin A (IgA)	Serum	76–390 mg/dL	760–3900 mg/L
Immunoglobulin D (IgD)	Serum	0–8 mg/dL	0–80 mg/L
Immunoglobulin E (IgE)	Serum	0–380 IU/mL	0–380 kIU/L
Immunoglobulin G (IgG)	Serum	650–1500 mg/dL	6.5–15 g/L
	CSF	0.5–5 mg/dL	5–50 mg/L
Immunoglobulin M (IgM)	Serum	55–300 mg/dL	550–3000 mg/L
Insulin (12-h fasting)	Serum	6–24 μIU/mL	6–24 mIU/L
Intrinsic factor (see vitamin B_{12})			
Iron	Serum	M: 50–160 μg/dL	8.95–28.64 μmol/L
		F: 40–150 μg/dL	7.16–26.85 μmol/L
Iron-binding capacity, total (TIBC)	Serum	250–400 μg/dL	44.75–71.60 μmol/L
Iron saturation	Serum	20–55%	Fraction of iron saturation: 0.20–0.53
17-Ketogenic steroids (17-KGS)	Urine, 24-h		Adult, M: 5–23 mg/d
			F: 3–15 mg/d
			>70 y, M: 3–15 mg/d
			F: 3–13 mg/d
Ketone bodies			
Qualitative	Serum	Negative (0.5–3.0 mg/dL)	Negative (5–30 mg/L)
	Urine, random		Negative
17-Ketosteroids, total (17-KS)	Urine, 24-h	M: 18–30 y 9–22 mg/d	31–76 μmol/d
		>30 y 8–20 mg/d	28–70 μmol/d
		F: 6–15 mg/d	21–52 μmol/d
LDL-Cholesterol (LCLC)	Serum or plasma (EDTA)	mg/dL	mmol/L
(75th percentile of Lipid		20–29 y, M: <128	<3.32
Research Clinics)		F: <127	<3.29
		30–39 y, M: <149	<3.86
		F: <143	<3.70
		40–49 y, M: <160	<4.14
		F: <155	<4.01
		≥50 y, M: <166	<4.30
		F: <170	<4.40
L-Lactate	Whole blood (heparin)	Venous: 4.5–19.8 mg/dL	0.5–2.2 mmol/L
		Arterial: 4.5–14.4 mg/dL	0.5–1.6 mmol/L
Lactate dehydrogenase (LDH)	Serum		210–420 U/L
LDH Isoenzymes	Serum	%	Fraction of total:
(Electrophoresis, agarose)		Fraction 1: 14–26	0.14–0.26
		Fraction 2: 29–39	0.29–0.39
		Fraction 3: 20–26	0.20–0.26
		Fraction 4: 8–16	0.08–0.16
		Fraction 5: 6–16	0.06–0.16
Lead	Whole blood (heparin)	<40 μg/dL	<1.93 μmol/L
		Toxic: ≥100 μg/dL	≥4.83 μmol/L
	Urine, 24-h	<80 μg/L	<0.39 μmol/L
Lipase (turbidimetric)	Serum		Adult: 10–150 U/L
			>60 y: 18–180 U/L
Luteinizing hormone (LH)	Serum or plasma	M: 6–23 mIU/mL	6–23 IU/L
	(heparin)	F: Follicular phase → 5–30 mIU/mL	5–30 IU/L
		Midcycle → 75–150 mIU/mL	75–150 IU/L
		Luteal → 3–40 mIU/mL	3–40 IU/L
		Postmenopausal → 30–200 mIU/mL	30–130 IU/L
	Urine	M: 13–60 U/d	13–60 IU/d
		F: Follicular phase → 7.2–23.5 U/d	7.2–23.5 IU/d
Lysozyme	Serum, plasma	0.4–1.3 mg/dL	4–13 mg/L
Magnesium	Serum	1.3–2.1 mEq/L	0.65–1.05 mmol/L
	Urine, 24-h	6.0–10.0 mEq/d	3.00–5.00 mmol/d
Mercury	Whole blood (EDTA)	<5.0 μg/dL	<0.25 μmol/L
	Urine, 24-h	<20 μg/L	<0.1 μmol/L
		Toxic: >150 μg/L	>0.75 μmol/L
Metanephrine, total	Urine, 24-h	0.05–1.20 μg/mg creatinine	0.03–0.69 mmol/mol creatinine
Myelin basic protein	CSF		<4 ng/mL
Myoglobin	Serum		M: 49±17 μg/L (1 SD)
			F: 35±14 μg/L
	Urine, random		Negative
Osmolality	Serum		275–295 mOsmol/kg
	Urine, random		50–1400 mOsmol/kg depending on fluid intake
			After 12-h fluid restriction: >850 mOsmol/kg
	Urine, 24-h		~300–900 mOsmol/kg
Oxalate	Serum	1–2.4 μg/mL	11–27 μmol/l
		Ethylene glycol poisoning: >20 μg/mL	Ethylene glycol poisoning: >228 μmol/L
Oxygen (Po_2)	Whole blood, arterial (heparin)	83–100 mm Hg	11–14.4 kPa
Oxygen saturation	Whole blood, arterial (heparin)	95–99%	Fraction saturated: 0.95–0.99
pH (37°C)	Whole blood, arterial (heparin)		7.35–7.45

Table continued on opposite page

CLINICAL CHEMISTRY, TOXICOLOGY, SEROLOGY *Continued*

Test	Specimen	Reference Range (Conventional Units)		Reference Range (International Units)	
Phosphorus, inorganic	Serum	2.7–4.5 mg/dL		0.87–1.45 nmol/L	
		>60 y, M: 2.3–3.7 mg/dL		0.74–1.2 nmol/L	
		F: 2.8–4.1 mg/dL		0.90–1.3 nmol/L	
	Urine, 24-h	0.4–1.3 g/d		13–42 mmol/d	
Porphobilinogen (PBG)					
Quantitative	Urine, 24-h	0–2.0 mg/d		0–8.8 μmol/d	
Qualitative	Urine, fresh random			Negative	
Potassium	Serum	3.5–5.1 mEq/L		3.5–5.1 mmol/L	
	Plasma (heparin)	3.5–4.5 mEq/L		3.5–4.5 mmol/L	
	Urine, 24-h	25–125 mEq/d		25–125 mmol/d	
Pregnanediol	Urine, 24-h	M: 0.6–1.5 mg/d		1.9–4.7 μmol/d	
		F: Follicular <1.0 mg/d		<3.1 μmol/d	
		Luteal 2–7 mg/d		6.2–22 μmol/d	
		Postmenopausal 0.2–1.0 mg/d		0.6–3.1 μmol/d	
Pregnanetriol	Urine, 24-h	<2.0 mg/d		<5.9 μmol/d	
Pregnenolone	Serum	0.3–2 ng/ml		0.9–6.3 nmol/L	
Progesterone	Serum	M: 0.12–0.3 ng/mL		0.38–0.95 nmol/L	
		F: Follicular 0.02–0.9 ng/mL		0.06–2.9 nmol/L	
		Luteal 6.0–30.0 ng/mL		19–95 nmol/L	
Prolactin (hPRL)	Serum	M: <20 ng/mL		<20 μg/L	
		F: Follicular <23 ng/mL		<23 μg/L	
		Luteal 5–40 ng/mL		5–40 μg/L	
Protein					
Total	Serum	6.4–8.3 g/dL		64.0–83.0 g/L	
Electrophoresis	Serum	Albumin: 3.5–5.0 g/dL		35–50 g/L	
		α₁-Globulin: 0.1–0.3 g/dL		1–3 g/L	
		α₂-Globulin: 0.6–1.0 g/dL		6–10 g/L	
		β-Globulin: 0.7–1.1 g/dL		7–11 g/L	
		γ-Globulin: 0.8–1.6 g/dL		8–16 g/L	
Total	Urine, 24-h			50–80 mg/d at rest	
Total	CSF	Lumbar: 15–45 mg/dL		150–450 mg/L	
Protoporphyrin	Whole blood (heparin or EDTA)	<50 μg/dL RBC		<0.89 μmol/L RBC	
	Feces, 24-h	≤60 μg/g dry wt or <1500 μg/d		≤0.11 mmol/kg dry wt or <2.67 μmol/d	
Pyruvic acid	Whole blood (heparin)	0.3–0.9 mg/dL		0.03–0.10 mmol/L	
Renin (normal diet)	Plasma (EDTA)	ng/mL/h ± 1 SE		μg/L/h ± 1 SE	
		Supine: 1.6 ± 1.5		1.6 ± 1.5	
		Standing (4-h): 4.5 ± 2.9		4.5 ± 2.9	
Riboflavin (vitamin B₂)	Urine, random, fasting	80–269 μg/g creatinine		24–81 μmol/mol creatinine	
Sediment	Urine, fresh, random				
Casts				Hyaline: occasional (0–1) casts/hpf	
				RBC: not seen	
				WBC: not seen	
				Tubular epithelial: not seen	
				Transitional and squamous epithelial: not seen	
Cells				RBC: 0–2/hpf	
				WBC: M: 0–3/hpf	
				F: 0–5/hpf	
				Epithelial: few	
				Bacteria:	
				Unspun: no organisms/ oil immersion field	
				Spun: <20 organisms/hpf	
Sodium	Serum or plasma (heparin)	136–146 mEq/L		136–146 mmol/L	
	Urine, 24-h	40–220 mEq/d		40–220 mmol/d	
Specific gravity	Urine, random			1.002–1.030	
	Urine, 24-h			1.015–1.025	
Testosterone, free	Serum	ng/dl (mean ± 1 SE)	% of total	pmol/l (mean ± 1 SE)	fraction of total
		M: 7.9 ± 2.3	1.4 ± 0.3	274 ± 80	0.014 ± 0.003
		F: 0.31 ± 0.07	0.9 ± 0.2	10.8 ± 2.4	0.009 ± 0.002
Testosterone, total	Serum	M: 572 ± 135 ng/dL		19.8 ± 4.7 nmol/L	
		F: 37 ± 10 ng/dL		1.3 ± 0.3 nmol/L	
	Urine	20–50 y,			
		M: 50–135 μg/d		173–470 nmol/d	
		F: 2–12 μg/d		7–42 nmol/d	
		>50 y,			
		M: 40–60 μg/d		139–210 nmol/d	
		F: 2–8 μg/d		7–28 nmol/d	
Thiamin (vitamin B₁)	Serum	0–2 μg/dL		0–75 nmol/L	
Thyroglobulin (Tg)	Serum	<50 ng/mL		<50 μg/L	
Thyroid antibodies	Serum			<1:10	
Thyroid microsomal antibodies	Serum			Nondetectable (hemagglutination) or <1:10 (IFA)	
Thyroid-stimulating hormone (hTSH)	Serum or plasma	2–10 μIU/mL		2–10 mIU/L	
Thyrotropin-releasing hormone	Plasma	5–60 pg/mL		5–60 ng/L	
Thyroxine, free (FT₄)	Serum	0.8–2.4 ng/dL		10–31 pmol/L	

Table continued on following page

CLINICAL CHEMISTRY, TOXICOLOGY, SEROLOGY *Continued*

Test	Specimen	Reference Range (Conventional Units)	Reference Range (International Units)
Thyroxine (T$_4$), total	Serum	5–12 µg/dL	65–155 nmol/L
		>60 y, M: 5.0–10.0 µg/dL	65–129 nmol/L
		F: 5.5–10.5 µg/dL	71–135 nmol/L
Thyroxine-binding globulin (TBG)	Serum	15.0–34.0 µg/mL	15.0–34.0 mg/L
Thyroxine index, free (see Free Thyroxine Index)			
Thyroxine/TBG ratio	Serum	0.2–0.5	2.77–6.4
		T$_4$ (µg/dL)/TBG (µg/mL)	T$_4$ (nmol/L)/TBG (mg/L)
Transcortin	Serum	M: 1.5–2.0 mg/dl	15–20 mg/L
		F: Follicular 1.7–2.0 mg/dL	17–20 mg/L
		Luteal 1.6–2.1 mg/dL	16–21 mg/L
		Postmenopausal 1.7–2.5 mg/dL	17–25 mg/L
Transferrin	Serum	220–400 mg/dL	2.20–4.0 g/L
		>60 y: 180–380 mg/dL	1.80–3.80 g/L
Triglycerides (TG)	Serum, after ≥12-hr fast	29–29 y,	20–29y,
		M: 44–185 mg/dL	M: 0.50–2.09 mmol/L
		F: 40–128 mg/dL	F: 0.45–1.45 mmol/L
		30–39 y,	30–39 y,
		M: 49–284 mg/dL	M: 0.55–3.21 mmol/L
		F: 38–160 mg/dL	F: 0.43–1.81 mmol/L
		40–49 y,	40–49 y,
		M: 56–298 mg/dL	M: 0.63–3.37 mmol/L
		F: 44–186 mg/dL	F: 0.50–2.10 mmol/L
		50–59	50–59 y,
		M: 62–288 mg/dL	M: 0.70–3.25 mmol/L
		F: 55–247 mg/dL	F: 0.62–2.79 mmol/L
Tri-iodothyronine, free	Serum	230–660 pg/dL	3.54–10.16 pmol/L
Tri-iodothyronine, total (T$_3$)	Serum	120–195 ng/dL	1.85–3.00 mmol/L
		>60 y,	
		M: 105–175 ng/dl	1.62–2.69 nmol/L
		F: 108–205 ng/dl	1.66–3.16 nmol/L
Tri-iodothyronine resin uptake test (T$_3$RU)	Serum	24–34%	24–34 AU (arbitrary units)
Urea nitrogen	Serum or plasma	7–18 mg/dL	2.5–6.4 mmol/L
	Urine	12–20 g/d	0.43–0.71 mol/d
Urea nitrogen/creatinine ratio	Serum		12/1–20/1
Uric acid (uricase)	Serum	M: 3.5–7.2 mg/dL	0.21–0.42 mmol/L
		F: 2.6–6.0 mg/dL	0.15–0.35 mmol/L
	Urine, 24-h	250–750 mg/d	1.48–4.43 mmol/d
Urinary sediment (see Sediment)			
Urobilinogen	Urine, 2-h	0.1–0.8 EU	0.1–0.8 U
	Urine, 24-h	0.5–4.0 EU	0.5–4.0 U
	Feces	75–275 EU/100 g	750–2750 U/kg
		75–400 EU/d	75–400 U/d
		40–280 mg/d	67–473 µmol/d
Uroporphyrin	Urine, 24-h	<50 µg/d	<60 nmol/d
	Feces, 24-h specimen	10–40 µg/d	12–48 nmol/d
	Erythrocytes (heparin or EDTA)		Negative
Vanillylmandelic acid (vanilmandelic acid)	Urine, 24-h	2–7 mg/d	10.1–35.4 µmol/d
Viscosity	Serum		1.10–1.22 Centipoise
Vitamin A	Serum	30–65 µg/dL	1.05–2.27 µmol/L
Vitamin B$_1$ (see Thiamin)			
Vitamin B$_2$ (see Riboflavin)			
Vitamin B$_6$	Plasma (EDTA)	3.6–18 ng/mL	14.6–72.8 nmol/L
Vitamin B$_{12}$	Serum	100–700 pg/mL	74–516 pmol/L
Vitamin C	Plasma (oxalate, heparin, or EDTA)	0.6–2.0 mg/dL	34–114 µmol/L
Vitamin D$_3$, 1,25-dihydroxy	Serum	25–45 pg/mL	60–108 pmol/L
Vitamin D$_3$, 25-hydroxy	Plasma (heparin)	Summer: 15–80 ng/mL	37.4–200 nmol/L
		Winter: 14–42 ng/ml	34.9–105 nmol/L
Vitamin E	Serum	5.0–20 µg/mL	11.6–46.4 µmol/L
Zinc	Serum	70–150 µg/dL	10.7–22.9 µmol/L

HEMATOLOGY AND COAGULATION

Test	Specimen	Reference Range (Conventional Units)	Reference Range (International Units)
Activated partial thromboplastin time (APTT)	Whole blood (Na citrate)		25–35 sec
Bleeding time (BT)			
Ivy	Blood from skin		Normal: 2–7 min
			Borderline: 7–11 min
Simplate (G-D)			2.75–8 min
Blood volume	Whole blood (heparin)		M: 52–83 mL/kg
			F: 50–75 mL/kg

Table continued on opposite page

HEMATOLOGY AND COAGULATION *Continued*

Test	Specimen	Reference Range (Conventional Units)	Reference Range (International Units)
Bone marrow	Bone marrow aspirate	% (mean)	Number fraction (mean)
Differential count			
Myeloblasts		0.3–5.0 (2.0)	0.003–0.05 (0.02)
Promyelocytes		1.0–8.0 (5.0)	0.01–0.08 (0.05)
Myelocytes:			
Neutrophilic		5.0–19.0 (12.0)	0.05–0.19 (0.12)
Eosinophilic		0.5–3.0 (1.5)	0.005–0.03 (0.015)
Basophilic		0.0–0.5 (0.3)	0.00–0.005 (0.003)
Metamyelocytes		13.0–32.0 (22.0)	0.13–0.32 (0.22)
Polymorphonuclear neutrophils		7.0–30.0 (2.0)	0.07–0.30 (0.20)
Polymorphonuclear eosinophils		0.5–4.0 (2.0)	0.005–0.04 (0.02)
Polymorphonuclear basophils		0.0–0.7 (0.2)	0.0–0.007 (0.002)
Lymphocytes		3.0–17.0 (10.0)	0.03–0.17 (0.10)
Plasma cells		0.0–2.0 (0.4)	0.00–0.02 (0.004)
Monocytes		0.5–5.0 (2.0)	0.005–0.05 (0.02)
Reticulum cells		0.1–2.0 (0.2)	0.001–0.02 (0.002)
Megakaryocytes		0.03–3.0 (0.1)	0.0003–0.03 (0.001)
Pronormoblasts		1.0–8.0 (4.0)	0.01–0.08 (0.04)
Normoblasts		7.0–32.0 (18.0)	0.07–0.32 (0.18)
Clot lysis, 37°C	Whole clotted blood		48–72 h
Clot retraction screen	Whole blood (no anticoagulant)		Retraction begins at 1 h, maximum at 24 h
Clotting time, Lee-White, 37°C	Whole blood (no anticoagulant)		5–8 min
Differential count (see Bone Marrow Differential count or Leukocyte Differential count)			
Eosinophil count	Whole blood (EDTA); capillary blood	50–350 cells/μL (mm³)	50–350 × 10⁶ cells/L
Erythrocyte count (RBC count)	Whole blood (EDTA)	millions of cells/μL (mm³)	× 10¹² cells/L
		M: 4.5–5.9	4.5–5.9
		F: 4.0–5.2	4.0–5.2
Erythrocyte sedimentation rate (ESR), Wintrobe			M: 0–9 mm/h
			F: 0–20 mm/h
Ferritin (see Chemistry section)			
Fibrin degradation products (Agglutination, Thrombo-Wellco test)	Whole blood, special tube containing thrombin and proteolytic inhibitor	<10 μg/mL	<10 mg/L
	Urine: 2 mL in special tube (see above)	<0.25 μg/mL	<0.25 mg/L
Fibrinogen	Plasma (Na citrate)	200–400 mg/dL	2.00–4.00 g/L
Glucose-6-phosphate dehydrogenase (G-6-PD) in erythrocytes	Whole blood (ACD, EDTA, or heparin)	12.1 ± 2.09 U/g Hb (1 SD)	0.78 ± 0.13 MU/mol Hb (1 SD)
Haptoglobin (Hp) RID	Serum; avoid hemolysis	83–267 mg/dL	830–2670 mg/L
Hematocrit (HCT, Hct)	Whole blood (EDTA)		
Calculated from MCV and RBC (electronic displacement or laser)		M: 41–53%	0.41–0.53 volume fraction
		F: 36–46%	0.36–0.46 volume fraction
Hemoglobin (Hb)	Whole blood (EDTA)	M: 13.5–17.5 g/dL	2.09–2.71 mmol/L
		F: 12.0–16.0 g/dL	1.86–2.48 mmol/L
	Plasma (heparin, ACD)	1–4 mg/dL	0.16–0.62 μmol/L
	Urine, fresh, random		Negative
Hemoglobin electrophoresis	Whole blood (EDTA, citrate or heparin)		Mass fraction
		HbA >95%	HbA >0.95
		HbA₂ 1.5–3.5%	HbA₂ 0.015–0.035
		HbF <2%	HbF <0.02
Leukocyte count (WBC count)	Whole blood (EDTA)	4.5–11.0 × 10³ cells/μL (mm³)	4.5–11.0 × 10⁹ cells/L
	CSF	0.5 mononuclear cells/μL	0.5 × 10⁶ cells/L

Leukocyte Differential count	Whole blood (EDTA)	%	Cells/μL (mm³)	Number fraction	Cells × 10⁶/L
Myelocytes		0	0	0	0
Neutrophils—bands		3–5	150–400	0.03–0.05	150–400
Neutrophils—segmented		54–62	3000–5800	0.54–0.62	3000–5800
Lymphocytes		23–33	1500–3000	0.25–0.33	1500–3000
Monocytes		3–7	285–500	0.03–0.07	285–500
Eosinophils		1–3	50–250	0.01–0.03	50–250
Basophils		0–0.75	15–50	0–0.0075	15–50

Leukocyte Differential count	CSF	%	Number fraction
Lymphocytes		62 ± 34	0.62 ± 0.324
Monocytes (includes pia-arachnoid mesothelial cells)		36 ± 20	0.36 ± 0.20
Neutrophils		2 ± 5	0.02 ± 0.05
Histocytes			Rare
Ependymal cells			Rare
Eosinophils			Rare

Test	Specimen	Reference Range (Conventional Units)	Reference Range (International Units)
Mean corpuscular hemoglobin (MCH)	Whole blood (EDTA)	26–34 pg/cell	0.40–0.53 fmol/cell
Mean corpuscular hemoglobin concentration (MCHC)	Whole blood (EDTA)	31–37% Hb/cell or gHb/dL RBC	4.81–5.74 mmol Hb/L RBC
Mean corpuscular volume (MCV)	Whole blood (EDTA)		80–100 fL

Table continued on following page

HEMATOLOGY AND COAGULATION Continued

Test	Specimen	Reference Range (Conventional Units)	Reference Range (International Units)
Methemoglobin (MetHb)	Whole blood (EDTA, heparin, or ACD)	0.06–0.04 g/dL	9.3–37.2 µmol/L
Partial thromboplastin time (PTT)	Whole blood (Na citrate)		60–85 sec
Plasma volume	Plasma (heparin)	M: 25–43 mL/kg	0.025–0.043 L/kg
		F: 28–45 mL/kg	0.028–0.045 L/kg
Platelet count (thrombocyte count)	Whole blood (EDTA)	150–400 × 10³/µL (mm³)	150–400 × 10⁹/L
Prothrombin consumption	Whole blood (no anticoagulant)		>30 sec
Prothrombin time, two-stage modified	Whole blood (Na citrate)		18–22 sec
RBC count (see erythrocyte count)			
Red cell volume	Whole blood (heparin)	M: 20–36 mL/kg	M: 0.020–0.036 L/kg
		F: 19–31 mL/kg	F: 0.019–0.031 L/kg
Reticulocyte count	Whole blood (EDTA, heparin, or oxalate)	0.5–1.5% of erythrocytes	0.005–0.015 (number fraction)
Sulfhemoglobin	Whole blood (EDTA, heparin, or EDTA)	≤1.0% of total Hb	<0.010 of total Hb (mass fraction)
Thrombin time	Whole blood (Na citrate)		Control time ±2 when control is 9–13 sec
Thromboplastin time, activated (see Activated partial thromboplastin time [APTT])			

DRUGS—THERAPEUTIC AND TOXIC

Drug	Specimen		Reference Range (Conventional Units)	Reference Range (International Units)
Acetaminophen	Serum or plasma (hep or EDTA)	Therap:	10–30 µg/mL	66–199 µmol/L
		Toxic:	>200 µg/mL	>1324 µmol/L
Amikacin	Serum or plasma (EDTA)	Therap:		
		Peak	25–35 µg/mL	43–60 µmol/L
		Trough (severe infection):	4–8 µg/mL	6.8–13.7 µmol/
		Toxic:		
		Peak	>35 µg/mL	>60 µmol/L
		Trough	>10 µg/mL	>17 µmol/L
ε-Aminocaproic acid	Serum or plasma (hep or EDTA); trough	Therap:	>130 µg/mL	>991 µmol/L
Amitriptyline	Serum or plasma (hep or EDTA); trough (>12 h after dose)	Therap:	120–250 ng/mL	433–903 nmol/L
		Toxic:	>500 ng/mL	>1805 nmol/L
Amobarbital	Serum	Therap:	1–5 µg/mL	4–22 µmol/L
		Toxic:	>10 µg/mL	>44 µmol/L
Amphetamine	Serum or plasma (hep or EDTA)	Therap:	20–30 ng/mL	148–222 nmol/L
		Toxic:	>200 ng/mL	>1480 nmol/L
Bromide	Serum	Therap:	750–1500 µg/mL	9.4–18.7 mmol/L
		Toxic:	>1250 µg/mL	>15.6 mmol/L
Caffeine	Serum or plasma (hep or EDTA)	Therap:	3–15 µg/mL	15–77 µmol/L
		Toxic:	>50 µg/mL	>258 µmol/L
Carbamazepine	Serum or plasma (hep or EDTA); trough	Therap:	8–12 µg/mL	34–51 µmol/L
		Toxic:	>15 µg/mL	>63 µmol/L
Carbenicillin	Serum or plasma	Therap:	Dependent on minimum inhibition conc of specific organism	Same
		Toxic:	>250 µg/mL	>660 µmol/L
Chloramphenicol	Serum or plasma (hep or EDTA); trough	Therap:	10–25 µg/L	31–77 µmol/L
		Toxic:	>25 µg/mL	>77 µmol/L
Chlordiazepoxide	Serum or plasma (hep or EDTA); trough	Therap:	700–1000 ng/mL	2.34–3.34 µmol/L
		Toxic:	>5000 ng/mL	>16.7 µmol/L
Chlorpromazine	Serum or plasma (hep or EDTA); trough	Therap:	50–300 ng/mL	157–942 nmol/L
		Toxic:	>750 ng/mL	>2355 nmol/L
Cimetidine	Serum or plasma (hep or EDTA); trough	Therap:	>1.0 µg/mL	>4.0 µmol/L
Clonazepam	Serum or plasma (hep or EDTA); trough	Therap:	15–60 ng/mL	48–190 nmol/L
		Toxic:	>80 ng/mL	>254 nmol/L
Clonidine	Serum or plasma (hep or EDTA)	Therap:	1.0–2.0 ng/mL	4.4–8.7 nmol/L
Clorazepate	Serum or plasma (hep or EDTA)	As desmethyldiazepam:		
		Therap:	0.12–1.0 µg/mL	0.36–3.01 µmol/L
Cocaine	Serum or plasma (hep or EDTA); on ice	Therap:	100–500 ng/mL	330–1650 nmol/L
		Toxic:	>1000 ng/mL	>3300 nmol/L
Desipramine	Serum or plasma (hep or EDTA); trough (≥12 h after dose)	Therap:	75–160 ng/mL	281–600 nmol/L
		Toxic:	>1000 ng/mL	>3750 nmol/L
Desmethylmethsuximide	Serum	Therap:	10–40 µg/mL	53–212 µmol/L
		Toxic:	>40 µg/mL	>212 µmol/L
Diazepam	Serum or plasma (hep or EDTA); trough	Therap:	100–1000 ng/mL	0.35–3.51 µmol/L
		Toxic:	>5000 ng/mL	>17.55 µmol/L
Digitoxin	Serum or plasma (hep or EDTA); ≥6 h after dose	Therap:	20–35 ng/mL	26–46 nmol/L
		Toxic:	>45 ng/mL	>59 nmol/L
Digoxin	Serum or plasma (hep or EDTA); trough (≥12 h after dose)	Therap:	0.8–1.5 ng/mL	1.1–1.9 nmol/L
		CHF: Arrhythmias:	1.5–2.0 ng/mL	1.9–2.6 nmol/L
		Toxic:	>2.5 ng/mL	>3.2 nmol/L

Table continued on opposite page

DRUGS—THERAPEUTIC AND TOXIC *Continued*

Drug	Specimen	Reference Range (Conventional Units)		Reference Range (International Units)
Diphenylhydantoin (see Phenytoin)				
Disopyramide	Serum or plasma (hep or EDTA); trough	Therap:		
		Arrhythmias:		
		Atrial	2.8–3.2 μg/mL	8.3–9.4 μmol/L
		Ventricular	3.3–7.5 μg/mL	9.7–22 μmol/L
		Toxic:	>7 μg/mL	>20.7 μmol/L
Doxepin	Serum or plasma (hep or EDTA); trough (≥12 h after dose)	Therap:	30–150 ng/mL	107–537 nmol/L
		Toxic:	>500 ng/mL	>1790 nmol/L
Ethchlorvynol	Serum or plasma (hep or EDTA)	Therap:	2–8 μg/mL	14–55 μmol/L
		Toxic:	>20 μg/mL	>138 μmol/L
Ethosuximide	Serum or plasma (hep or EDTA); trough	Therap:	40–100 μg/mL	283–708 μmol/L
		Toxic:	>150 μg/mL	>1062 μmol/L
Fenoprofen	Plasma (EDTA)	Therap:	20–65 μg/mL	82–268 μmol/L
Furosemide	Serum (30 min after dose)	Therap:	1–2 μg/mL	3–6 μmol/L
Gentamicin	Serum or plasma (EDTA)	Therap:		
		Peak (severe infection)	8–10 μg/mL	16.7–20.9 μmol/L
		Trough (severe infection)	2–4 μg/mL	4.2–8.4 μmol/L
		Toxic:		
		Peak	>10 μg/mL	>21 μmol/L
		Trough	>4 μg/mL	>8.4 μmol/L
Glutethimide	Serum	Therap:	2–6 μg/mL	9–28 μmol/L
		Toxic:	>5 μg/mL	>23 μmol/L
Imipramine	Serum or plasma (hep or EDTA); trough (≥12 h after dose)	Therap:	125–250 ng/mL	446–893 nmol/L
		Toxic:	>500 ng/mL	>1784 nmol/L
Isoniazid	Serum or plasma (hep or EDTA)	Therap:	1–7 μg/mL	7–51 μmol/L
		Toxic:	20–710 μg/mL	146–5176 μmol/L
Kanamycin	Serum or plasma (EDTA)	Therap:		
		Peak	25–35 μg/mL	52–72 μmol/L
		Trough (severe infection)	4–8 μg/mL	8–16 μmol/L
		Toxic:		
		Peak	>35 μg/mL	>72 μmol/L
		Trough	>10 μg/mL	>21 μmol/L
Lidocaine	Serum or plasma (hep or EDTA); ≥45 min following bolus dose	Therap:	1.5–6.0 μg/mL	6.4–26 μmol/L
		Toxic:		
		CNS or cardiovascular depression	6–8 μg/mL	26–34.2 μmol/L
		Seizures, obtundation, decreased cardiac output	>8 μg/mL	>34.2 μmol/L
Lithium	Serum or plasma (hep or EDTA); (>12 h after last dose)	Therap:	0.6–1.2 mEq/L	0.6–1.2 mmol/L
		Toxic:	>2 mEq/L	>2 mmol/L
Lorazepam	Serum or plasma (hep or EDTA)	Therap:	50–240 ng/mL	156–746 nmol/L
Meperidine	Serum or plasma (hep or EDTA)	Therap:	70–500 ng/mL	283–2020 nmol/L
		Toxic:	>1 μg/mL	>4043 nmol/L
Meprobamate	Serum	Therap:	6–12 μg/mL	28–55 μmol/L
		Toxic:	>60 μg/mL	>275 μmol/L
Methadone	Serum or plasma (hep or EDTA)	Therap:	100–400 ng/mL	0.32–1.29 μmol/L
		Toxic:	>2000 ng/mL	>6.46 μmol/L
Methaqualone	Serum or plasma (hep or EDTA)	Therap:	2–3 μg/mL	8–12 μmol/L
		Toxic:	>10 μg/mL	>40 μmol/L
Methotrexate	Serum or plasma (hep or EDTA)	Therap:	variable	variable
		Toxic:		
		low-dose therapy (1–2 wk)	>9.1 ng/mL	>20 nmol/L
		high-dose therapy (48 h)	454 ng/mL	>1000 nmoll/L
Methsuximide (*N*-desmethyl methsuximide)	Serum	Therap:	10–40 μg/mL	53–212 μmol/L
		Toxic:	>40 μg/mL	>212 μmol/L
Methyldopa	Plasma (EDTA)	Therap:	1–5 μg/mL	4.7–23.7 μmol/L
		Toxic:	>7 μg/mL	>33 μmol/L
Methyprylon	Serum	Therap:	8–10 μg/mL	43–55 μmol/L
		Toxic:	>50 μg/mL	>273 μmol/L
Morphine	Serum or plasma (hep or EDTA)	Surgical anesthesia:	65–80 ng/mL	227–280 nmol/L
		Toxic:	200–5000 ng/mL	700–17,500 nmol/L
N-Acetylprocainamide	Serum or plasma (hep or EDTA); trough	Therap:	5–30 μg/mL	18–108 μmol/L
		Toxic:	>40 μg/mL	>144 μmol/L
Nitroprusside	Serum or plasma (EDTA)	As thiocyanate:		
		Therap:	6–29 μg/mL	103–499 μmol/L
Normethsuximide	Serum	Therap:	10–40 μg/mL	53–212 μmol/L
		Toxic:	>40 μg/mL	>212 μmol/L
Nortriptyline	Serum or plasma (hep or EDTA); trough (≥12 h after dose)	Therap:	50–150 ng/mL	190–570 nmol/L
		Toxic:	>500 ng/mL	>1900 nmol/L
Oxazepam	Serum or plasma (hep or EDTA)	Therap:	0.2–1.4 μg/mL	0.70–4.9 μmol/L
Paraquat	Whole blood (EDTA)	Toxic:	0.1–1.6 μg/mL	0.39–6.2 μmol/L
	Urine	Occup exp:	0.3 μg/mL	1.17 μmol/L
		Toxic:	0.9–64 μg/mL	3.50–249 μmol/L
Pentobarbital	Serum or plasma (hep or EDTA); trough	Therap:		
		Hypnotic	1–5 μg/mL	4–22 μmol/L
		Therap coma	20–50 μg/mL	88–221 μmol/L
		Toxic:	>10 μg/mL	>44 μmol/L
Phenacetin	Plasma (EDTA)	Therap:	1–20 μg/mL	6–112 μmol/L
		Toxic:	50–250 μg/mL	279–1395 μmol/L
Phencyclidine	Serum or plasma (hep or EDTA)	Toxic:	90–800 ng/mL	370–3288 nmol/L

Table continued on following page

DRUGS—THERAPEUTIC AND TOXIC Continued

Drug	Specimen	Reference Range (Conventional Units)		Reference Range (International Units)
Phenobarbital	Serum or plasma (hep or EDTA); trough	Therap:	15–40 µg/mL	65–170 µmol/L
		Toxic:		
		Slowness, ataxia, nystagmus	35–80 µg/mL	151–345 µmol/L
		Coma with reflexes	65–117 µg/mL	280–504 µmol/L
		Coma without reflexes	>100 µg/mL	>430 µmol/L
Phensuximide (both parent and N-desmethyl metabolites)	Serum or plasma (hep or EDTA)	Therap:	40–60 µg/mL	228–324 µmol/L
Phenylbutazone	Plasma (EDTA)	Therap: (not well defined)	50–100 µg/mL	162–324 µmol/L
		Toxic:	>100 µg/mL	>324 µmol/L
Phenytoin	Serum or plasma (hep or EDTA); trough	Therap:	10–20 µg/mL	40–79 µmol/L
		Toxic:	>20 µg/mL	>79 µmol/L
Primidone	Serum or plasma (hep or EDTA); trough	Therap:	5–12 µg/mL	23–55 µmol/L
		Toxic:	>15 µg/mL	>69 µmol/L
Procainamide	Serum or plasma (hep or EDTA); trough	Therap:	4–10 µg/mL	17–42 µmol/L
		Toxic:	>10–12 µg/mL	>42–51 µmol/L
		Also consider effect of metabolite, N-acetylprocainamide		
Propoxyphene	Plasma (EDTA)	Therap:	0.1–0.4 µg/mL	0.3–1.2 µmol/L
		Toxic:	>0.5 µg/mL	>1.5 µmol/L
Propranolol	Serum or plasma (hep or EDTA); trough	Therap:	50–100 ng/mL	193–386 nmol/L
Protriptyline	Serum or plasma (hep or EDTA); trough (≥12 h after dose)	Therap:	70–250 ng/mL	266–950 nmol/L
		Toxic:	>500 ng/mL	>1900 nmol/L
Quinidine	Serum or plasma (hep or EDTA); trough	Therap:	2–5 µg/mL	6–15 µmol/L
		Toxic:	>6 µg/mL	>18 µmol/L
Salicylates	Serum or plasma (hep or EDTA); trough	Therap:	150–300 µg/mL	1086–2172 µmol/L
		Toxic:	>300 µg/mL	>2172 µmol/L
Secobarbital	Serum	Therap:	1–2 µg/mL	4.2–8.4 µmol/L
		Toxic:	>5 µg/mL	>21.0 µmol/L
Theophylline	Serum or plasma (hep or EDTA)	Therap:	8–20 µg/mL	44–111 µmol/L
		Toxic:	>20 µg/mL	>110 µmol/L
Thiocyanate	Serum or plasma (EDTA)			
		Nonsmoker:	1–4 µg/mL	17–69 µmol/L
		Smoker:	3–12 µg/mL	52–206 µmol/L
		Therap, after nitroprusside infusion:	6–29 µg/mL	103–499 µmol/L
	Urine	Nonsmoker:	1–4 mg/d	17–69 µmol/d
		Smoker:	7–17 mg/d	120–292 µmol/d
Thiopental	Serum or plasma (hep or EDTA); trough	Hypnotic:	1.0–5.0 µg/mL	4.1–20.7 µmol/L
		Coma:	30–100 µg/mL	124–413 µmol/L
		Anesthesia:	7–130 µg/mL	29–536 µmol/mL
		Toxic conc:	>10 µg/mL	>41 µmol/L
Thioridazine	Serum or plasma (hep or EDTA)	Therap:	1.0–1.5 µg/mL	2.7–4.1 µmol/L
		Toxic:	>10 µg/mL	>27 µmol/L
Tobramycin	Serum or plasma (hep or EDTA)	Therap:		
		Peak (severe infection)	8–10 µg/mL	17–21 µmol/L
		Trough (severe infection)	<4 µg/mL	<9 µmol/L
		Toxic:		
		Peak	>10 µg/mL	>21 µmol/L
		Trough	>4 µg/mL	>9 µmol/L
Valproic acid	Serum or plasma (hep or EDTA); trough	Therap:	50–100 µg/mL	347–693 µmol/L
		Toxic:	>100 µg/mL	>693 µmol/L
Vancomycin	Serum or plasma (hep or EDTA); trough	Toxic: (not well established)	>80–100 µg/mL	>80–100 mg/L
Warfarin	Serum or plasma (hep or EDTA)	Therap:	1–10 µg/mL	3–32 µmol/L

INDEX

Page numbers in *Italics* refer to figures. Page numbers followed by a "t" refer to tables. For general terms such as "acute," "chronic," "idiopathic," look under the remaining portion of the term.

A polyadenylation mutation, thalassemia from, 934
A wave, in venous pulse, 176
AAV (adeno-associated virus), 1767
Abandonment, of patients, 2
Abdomen
    abscess of, 793
    discomfort in, from acute pancreatitis, 776
        from chronic hepatitis, 831
        liver disease and, 808
    distention of
        from ileus, 719
        from pneumococcal pneumonia, 1557
        from primary mesothelioma, 794
        from vomiting, 660
    flukes in, 1904
    infection of, anaerobic, 1638
        as contraindication for laparoscopy, 674
    irradiation of, 2378
    malnutrition and, 1210t
    neoplasms of, and venous thrombosis, 443, 764
    paracentesis of, for ascites, 790
    surgery of, and mesenteric venous thrombosis, 764
        mechanical ventilation after, 487
    trauma to, hepatic vein thrombosis from, 848
        intramural intestinal hemorrhage from, 764
    tuberculosis of, 1690–1691
Abdominal angina, 762
Abdominal aorta, 370
    aneurysms of, 371
        and back pain, 2250
    atheromatosis of, 633–634
Abdominal cramps
    from adenocarcinoma of duodenum, 713
    from clostridial food poisoning, 785
    from ileus, 719
    from pseudomembranous colitis, 1632
    from ulcerative colitis. treatment of, 758
    in opioid withdrawal syndrome, 57
Abdominal pain
    epigastric, from pancreatic cancer, 781
    from abdominal purpura, 1058
    from acute inflammatory autonomic neuropathy, 2262
    from acute pancreatitis, 775
    from adrenocortical insufficiency, 1351
    from alcoholic hepatitis, 843
    from bacterial peritonitis, 793
    from bile duct tumor, 871
    from cholecystitis, 865
    from chylomicronemia syndrome, 1143
    from Crohn's disease, 747
    from cryptosporidiosis, 1882
    from diabetic ketoacidosis, 1375

Abdominal pain *(Continued)*
    from free perforation of ulcer, 707
    from gastrointestinal disease, 657–658
    from hemochromatosis, 1191
    from hepatocellular carcinoma, 858
    from hookworm, 1907
    from intestinal lymphoma, 744
    from irritable bowel syndrome, 722
    from measles, 1774
    from mesenteric artery occlusion, 762
    from peritoneal disease, 790
    from polyps of large intestine, 767
    from post-streptococcal glomerulonephritis, 587
    from primary mesothelioma, 794
    from trichuriasis, 1909
    from typhoid fever, 1641
    from yersiniosis, 1664
    from Zollinger-Ellison syndrome, 708
Abducens nerve, 2115
    paralysis of, lateral sinus thrombosis and, 2185
    trauma to, 2115
Abetalipoproteinemia, 1144
    and vitamin E deficiency, 1239
    malabsorption from, 743
ABO blood groups, 948, 948t
    and von Willebrand factor, 1070
    type A, and gastric cancer, 710
Abortion
    from listeriosis, 1672
    prostaglandins and, 700
    septic, and endocarditis, 1591
        and renal failure, 637
        from *Campylobacter* infection, 1649
    spontaneous
        chromosome abnormalities and, 166
        factor XIII deficiency and, 1074
        from congenital toxoplasmosis, 1877
        from lead poisoning, 2386
        from thyrotoxicosis, 1326
        from ulcerative colitis, 760
        lupus-type inhibitors and, 1081
        systemic lupus erythematosus and, 2016
        trisomic autosomes and, 167
        ureaplasma and, 1565
    therapeutic, Lesch-Nyhan syndrome and, 1172
        severe beta thalassemia and, 935
Abruptio placentae, and kidney failure, 637
    cortical necrosis and, 636
    smoking and, 39
Abscess(es)
    abdominal, 793
    and mesenteric venous thrombosis, 764
    anorectal, 789
    chronic granulomatous disease and, 958
    computed tomography for, 83

Abscess(es) *(Continued)*
    dental, 674–675
    eosinophilic, from chronic eosinophilic pneumonia, 431
    epidural, in spine, 2186–2187
    in drug abuse, 52, 57
    in pancreatitis, 779
    in radiation enterocolitis, 806
    in spleen, 1039–1040
    metastatic, bronchiectasis and, 439
    of brain, 2181–2183, *2183*
        diagnostic imaging techniques for, 2060
        epidural, 2184
        from listeriosis, 1671
    of kidney, 628, 632
    of liver, 834–837. See also *Liver, abscess of*
    of lung, 435–438
    of skin, in opioid users, 56
    paraspinal, 1622
    Pautrier's, 1108
    pericholecystic, vs. acute cholecystitis, 865
    pericolic, from diverticulitis, 804
    perinephric, 628, 632
        pyelonephritis with, 629
    peritonsillar, from streptococcal tonsillitis, 1576
    pyogenic, of liver, 834–836
        of lungs, vs. tuberculosis, 1686
    subdiaphragmatic, and pleural pain, 468
        computed tomography for, 662
    visceral, glomerulonephritis with, 588
    vs. emphysematous cholecystitis, 867
Absence seizures, 2076, 2219–2221. See also *Seizures*
Absorption. See also *Malabsorption*
    decrease in, from drug interactions, 99
    of nutrients, normal, 733–735
    prevention of, after poisonings, 142
Acalculia, 2082
Acanthocheilonema perstans, 1919
Acanthocytes, in liver disease, 817
Acantholysis, definition of, 2329
Acanthosis nigricans, cancer and, 1112
Acatalasia, 147, 1187–1188
Acceleration injury, to brain, 2239
Accidents, 41
    adolescent deaths from, 20
    epidemiology of, 40
Acclimatization, 2382
Accommodation, definition of, 2298
Acebutolol, 137, 138t
    dosing and adverse effects of, 268t
    for angina pectoris, 327t
    for hypertension, 287t
    pharmacokinetic properties of, 266t
Acetaldehyde, in blood, from ethanol ingestion, 843

Acetaminophen, 107, 107t
  and analgesic nephropathy, 607
  chronic hepatitis from, 828
  for chronic pancreatitis, 780
  for dying patients, 32
  for fever, 1527
  for hemophiliacs, 1068
  liver disease from, 827, 828
  poisoning with, 103, 142
    N-acetylcysteine for, 143
    treatment of, 143–144
  reference intervals for, 2402t
  with narcotics for pain relief, 108
  zonal necrosis from, 827
Acetanilid, sulfhemoglobinemia from, 946
  toxicity of, to hemoglobin, 945t
Acetazolamide, 232, 535
  characteristics of, 231t, 536t
  for epilepsy, 2227
  side effects of, 2299
Acetoacetate, reference intervals for, 2395t
Acetohexamide, for diabetes mellitus, 1369,
    1370t
  metabolites of, kidney excretion of, 95
Acetone, reference intervals for, 2395t
Acetyl-beta-methylcholine, 139
Acetylcholine, 134, 139, 1282
  and control of gastric secretion, 693, 695
  in nerve terminal, 2284
  in vasodilator therapy, for pulmonary hy-
    pertension, 300
  receptors of, 137, 2284
    deficiency of, and myasthenia gravis,
      2285
    end-plate, congenital deficiency of,
      2287
Acetylcholine receptor antibody test, 2286
Acetylcholinesterase, 2284
  end-plate, congenital deficiency of, 2287
N-Acetylcysteine, as acetaminophen anti-
    dote, 103, 142, 143
  for acetaminophen-induced liver disease,
    828
Acetyldigitoxin, for heart failure, 227t
ACh. See Acetylcholine
Achalasia, 680, 684
  manometry for, 685
  radiograph of, 684
  treatment of, 686
AChE. See Acetylcholinesterase
Achilles tendon, tenosynovitis of, 1708
Achlorhydria, 712
  and ulcer disease, malignancy in, 699
  from common variable agammaglobuline-
    mia, 1943
  vitamin B₁₂ deficiency from, testing for,
    738t
Achondroplasia, 148
  of bone, 1520
AChR. See Acetylcholine, receptors of
Acid(s)
  neutralization of, for gastroesophageal re-
    flux, 683
  organic, metabolic acidosis from, 553
  poisonings with, treatment for, 144
  secretion of, and peptic ulcers, 695
    emotions and, 696
Acid phosphatase, in hairy cells, 999
  reference intervals for, 2395t
Acid-base balance
  abnormalities in, 549–558, 552
    and digitalis, 228
    and metabolic encephalopathy, 2067t
    anion patterns in, 556t
    from diuretics, 231
    from whooping cough, 1625
  calculations for, 485
  carbon dioxide and, 549–550
  in brain, and coma, 2068

Acid-base balance (Continued)
  kidneys and, 517–518, 518t
    bicarbonate processing by, 550–551
    chronic failure of, 564
  mixed metabolic disorders and, 556–557
Acid-peptic disease, endoscopy for, 669
  esophagogastroduodenoscopy for, 669
Acidemia, 549
  and right ventricular function, 475
  from oxygen therapy, 480
  isovaleric, 1159
Acidosis
  and heart contractility, 186
  and net acid excretion, 518
  and polymerization, 939
  and potassium secretion, 517
  and rhinocerebral mucormycosis, 1852
  dilutional, 553
  from blood transfusions, 950
  from chronic kidney failure, and hyper-
    kalemia, 547
  from diabetic ketoacidosis, 1375
  from hereditary fructose intolerance, 1136
  from mesenteric artery occlusion, 762
  from shock, 237, 238
    correction of, 245
  from vaso-occlusive crisis, in sickle cell
    anemia, 939
  hyperchloremic, in hyperparathyroidism,
    553
  in infants, from isovaleric acidemia, 1159
  lactic, 553–554
  metabolic, 551–555. See also Metabolic aci-
    dosis
  renal tubular, 505, 532, 623
  respiratory, 551, 557. See also Respiratory
    acidosis
  shock and, 238
  systemic, and potassium transport, 543
Aciduria, delta-aminolevulinic, 1184
  orotic, 156
Acinetobacter, and pneumonia, 1566
  and urinary tract infection, in diabetics,
    629
  penicillins for, 120
Acne, 2332–2333, 2333t
  chemical, 2375
  cystic, isotretinoin for, 2317
    retinoids for, 1238
  from chronic active hepatitis, 832
  from testosterone therapy, 1419
  systemic antibiotics for, 2317
Acoustic nerve, damage to, 2119
Acoustic neuromas, 2119
Acoustic schwannoma, 2230
  prognosis for, 2235
Acrocentric chromosomes, 163
  robertsonian translocation with, 166
Acrocephalopolysyndactyly, 1203
Acrocyanosis, 377–378
  in cold agglutinin disease, 920
  Raynaud's phenomenon vs., 376
Acrodermatitis chronica atrophicans, in
    Lyme disease, 1727
Acrodermatitis enterohepatica, 1241
Acrokeratosis paraneoplastica, 1112
Acrolein, 2365
Acromegaly, 1300, 1300–1302
  and carpal tunnel syndrome, 2268
  arthritis with, 2045
  diabetes mellitus from, 1362
  muscle in, 2280
  polyneuropathy with, 2264
ACTH. See Adrenocorticotropic hormone
ACTH/endorphin system, in sepsis, 1539
ACTH-MSH syndrome, ectopic, 1101
Actin, 2269
Actinic reticuloid, 2352
Actinomyces, lung abscess from, 436

Actinomyces muris, 1729
Actinomycetoma, 1853
Actinomycin D, for nephroblastoma, 654
  for cancer, 1125
Actinomycosis, 1673–1674
Action potentials, of Purkinje fiber, 251, 251
  slow vs. fast, 251, 252t, 252
Action tremor, 2142
Activated charcoal, for drug overdose, 2070
  for poisonings, 142
  for protoporphyria, 840
Active transport, definition of, 733
Acute phase phenomena, 1995
Acute phase proteins, 1528, 1528t
Acute phase response, 1527–1529
Acyclovir, 126
  elimination rate for, 96t
  for herpes simplex virus infection, 1783
    encephalitis from, 2195
  for herpes zoster, 2197
  for herpesvirus infections, 125, 126, 676,
    2317–2318
    genital, 2197
  for varicella, in immunosuppressed pa-
    tients, 1790
Acylcarnitines, 2278
Acyl-CoA dehydrogenase, deficiency of,
    2278
ADCC (antibody-dependent cellular cyto-
    toxicity), 1937
  in systemic lupus erythematosus, 2013
Addiction, definition of, 106
Addisonian crisis, from thyroid hormone
    replacement, 1329
Addison's disease
  ACTH immunoassay and, 1348
  and aldosterone production, 532
  and eosinophilia, 1026
  and polyglandular autoimmune disease,
    1414
  and urine sodium concentration, 524
  and water loads, 540
  autoantibodies to adrenal tissue in, 1461
  definition of, 1340
  diagnosis of, metyrapone test for, 1352
  galactorrhea in, 1450
  glucocorticosteroid therapy for, 130
  hyperkalemia in, 547
  hyperpigmentation in, 2344
  hyponatremia in, 540
  in Schmidt's syndrome, 1460
  mitochondrial antibody in, 816
  vs. ACTH deficiency, 1295
  with Hashimoto's thyroiditis, 1333
ADE (acute disseminated encephalomyeli-
    tis), 2208t, 2208–2209
  vs. multiple sclerosis, 2215
Adenematous polyps, and carcinoma of co-
    lon, 757
Adenine arabinoside, for herpesvirus, 125,
    1122, 1783, 2195
Adenine phosphoribosyltransferase, defi-
    ciency of, and kidney stones, 1172
Adenitis, mesenteric, acute, vs. appendici-
    tis, 803
Adeno-associated virus, 1767
Adenocarcinoma(s), 457
  appendicitis from, 801
  from ulcerative colitis, 757
  of lungs, 458
  of bile ducts, 871
  of colon, 768–773
    adenomas vs., 766–767
  of duodenum, 713
  of esophagus, 686
  of gallbladder, 865, 870–871
  of kidneys, 652t, 652–653, 653
    and renal vein thrombosis, 634
    solitary pulmonary nodules from, 465

Adenocarcinoma(s) (Continued)
  of large intestine, 766
  of pancreas, 781
  of peritoneum, 794
  of prostate, 1423
  of small intestine, 773
Adenohypophysis, 1290
Adenoids, enlargement of, airway obstruction from, 418
  in agammaglobulinemia, 1943
Adenoma(s), 766
  aldosterone-producing, 1350, 1358
  and colorectal cancer, 769, 770
  follicular, of thyroid, 1335
  of bile ducts, 857
  of Brunner's glands, 713
  of kidneys, 651–652
  of large intestines, 766
    vs. ulcerative colitis, 756
  of liver, 856–857
    from drugs, 828
    oral contraceptives and, 1443
  of pituitary, 1298, 2230
    and Cushing's disease, 1354
    magnetic resonance image of, 1299, 1299
  of stomach, 713
  papillary, 871
  types of, 766–767
  vs. hyperplasia, aldosteronism in, 283–284, 1350, 1359
Adenoma sebaceum, 2345
  in tuberous sclerosis, 2158
Adenomatosis, endocrine, multiple, 1458. See also Multiple endocrine neoplasia
Adenomyomatosis, 871
Adenopathy
  hilar, 463
  in Hodgkin's disease, 1015–1016
  inguinal, in chancroid, 1712
  paratracheal, from sarcoidosis, 451, 453
Adenosine deaminase
  absence of, gene therapy for, 160, 161
  deficiency of, 1172
    severe combined immunodeficiency disease with, 1946
  overproduction of, and hemolytic anemia, 917
Adenosine diphosphate, and platelet secretion, 1042
Adenosine triphosphate
  and glycolytic defects, 916
  depletion of, and heart muscle relaxation, 219
  energy of heart from, 187
  in gastrointestinal motility, 715
  in muscle function, 2269
  shock and, 242
  synthesis of, in erythrocytes, 913
Adenosylcobalamin, 902
Adenovirus(es), 1767
  disease from, 1767–1768
    vs. measles, 1774, 1775t
  immunization against, 65
  meningitis from, 2192
  pharyngitis from, 1576
  pneumonia from, 1564
Adenylate cyclase, 1258, 1259
ADH. See Antidiuretic hormone
Adhesion, of neutrophils, 957t, 957–958
  of platelets, von Willebrand factor and, 1043, 1055, 1070
Adie's tonic pupil, 2114
Adipocytes, 1222, 1223
Adipose tissue
  and caloric requirement, 1368
  in mesenteric panniculitis, 795
  regional distribution of, 1222–1223
  steroids in, 1346

Adolescence. See also Puberty
  causes of death during, 20
  cognitive development in, 17
  goiter in, 1329
  growth spurt during, in females, 1426
  immunization during, 62t
  iron deficiency in, 893
  ovulation in, 19
  pregnancy during, 20
  psychosocial development in, 16–17
  smoking during, 39
  substance abuse during, 21
  suicide during, 20–21
Adolescent medicine, 16–21
ADP (adenosine diphosphate), 1042
Adrenal(s)
  adenomas of, hirsutism from, 1446
  androgens from, measurement of, 1350
  assessment of, functional reserve of, 1349
  autoantibodies to, in Addison's disease, 1461
  autoimmune destruction of, adrenal insufficiency from, 1351
  cancer of, hirsutism from, 1446
    primary aldosteronism from, 291
  disorders of, and obesity, 1225
    anemia with, 892
  functional reserve of, assessment of, 1349
  hyperfunction of, anovulation from, 1440
  hyperplasia of. See Adrenal hyperplasia
  insufficiency of, and hyperkalemic periodic paralysis, 2281
    histoplasmosis and, 1840
    hypercalcemia from, 1503
    myopathy from, 2280
    vs. hypopituitarism, 1296
  medulla of. See Adrenal medulla
  neoplasms of
    and precocious puberty, 1428
    computed tomography for, 284
    Cushing's syndrome from, 1353
    estrogen-secreting, gynecomastia from, 1411
    renal metastasis from, 655
  steroids of. See Adrenal steroids
Adrenal cortex
  excess mineralocorticoids from, 1358–1360
  function of, laboratory evaluation of, 1348–1350
  insufficiency of, 1351–1353
    clinical features of, 1351t
    treatment of, 1352–1353, 1353t
  neoplasms of, in mothers, effects of, 1404
  structure and development of, 1340
Adrenal crisis, 1403
Adrenal hyperplasia
  bilateral, and aldosterone levels, 1350, 1358
  congenital, 1402–1404, 1403t, 1429
    and adrenal androgen excess, 1418
    and sexual precocity, 1428
    hirsutism from, 1446–1447
    in mothers, and masculinization of female infants, 1404
    lipoid, 1396–1397
    measurement of 17-hydroxyprogesterone for, 1448
    polycystic ovarian syndrome from, 1439
Adrenal hypoplasia, congenital, 1397
Adrenal medulla, 134, 1461–1467
  chromaffin cells in, 1463
Adrenal steroids, 1341–1348
  and ulcers, 696
  excessive production of, and polycythemia, 977
  for herniated disc, 2253
  for malabsorption, 741t

Adrenal steroids (Continued)
  plasma binding of, 1341–1343
  plasma concentrations of, 1341t
  secretion rates of, 1341t
  synthesis of, 1341, 1342, 1343–1344
    regulation of, 1344–1346
Adrenalectomy, bilateral, for Cushing's disease, 1357
  for metastatic breast cancer, 1457
Adrenaline, 134, 137, 1281–1282, 1462. See also Epinephrine
Adrenarche, 19
  premature, 1427
Adrenergic agents
  and mesenteric circulation, 761
  antagonists to, 137–139
  for chronic obstructive pulmonary disease, 417
  for heart failure, 235
Adrenergic function, and mood, 2096
Adrenergic inhibitors, adverse effects of, 289t
Adrenergic receptors, 134–137, 135t
  catecholamines and, 1463
  drugs interacting with, 135, 136t
    as pulmonary vasodilators, 300–301
  in shock, 247t, 247–248
  physiologic regulation of, 136–137
Adrenocorticotropic hormone
  and adrenal cortex, 1340
  and aldosterone secretion, 516, 1346
  and cancer, 1101
  and cortisol release, 1344
  as tumor marker, 1099
  circadian rhythm of, 1344
  deficiency of
    adrenocortical insufficiency from, 1352
    hypoglycemia in, 1387
    manifestations of, 1295
    treatment for, 1296
  effects of, 1291
  excess of, 1420, 1459
  for epilepsy, 2227
  for gout, 1169
  for multiple sclerosis, 2214
  from islet cell tumors, 1390
  from medullary carcinoma, 1506
  hypersecretion of, 1304–1305, 1354. See also Cushing's syndrome
  immunoassays for, 1348
  reference intervals for, 2395t
  release of, 1283
    evaluating, 1296
    feedback inhibition of, 1344–1345
  shock and, 240
  test for evaluating, 1293, 1349
  vs. glucocorticosteroid therapy, 132
Adrenogenital syndromes, 156
Adrenoleukodystrophy, 2216
Adriamycin, and hair damage, 2349
  for hepatocellular carcinoma, 859
  with radiation therapy, 1119
Adult celiac disease, 742–743. See also Nontropical sprue
Adult respiratory distress syndrome (ARDS)
  after near-drowning, 2371
  after thermal injury, 2365
  complement and, 1941
  conditions associated with, 476t
  definition of, 476, 491
  from oxygen toxicity, 496
  from pancreatitis, 469, 778
  mechanical ventilation for, 479, 492
  pulmonary capillary permeability in, 534
  pulmonary hypertension from, 293, 298
Adulterants, in drugs, reactions to, 56
Aedes aegypti mosquitoes, and dengue, 1816
  and yellow fever, 1830

Aeromonas, enterotoxins from, and secretory diarrhea, 727
Aerophagia, 718
Aerophobia, in rabies, 2201
Aerosols, abuse of, 59
  inhalation of, interstitial lung disease from, 435
  steroids as, 130
Affective disorders, 2095–2099
Afferent arc, 580
Afferent arterioles, 508
Afferent loop syndrome, after gastric surgery, 705
Afferent pupil, definition of, 2113
Afibrinogenemia, 1073
Aflatoxin(s), and cancer, 44, 1095
  hepatocellular, 858
  and food poisoning, 787
Afterload, 190, 218, *218*
  in heart, 186, 216t
  mitral regurgitation and, 348
  reduction of, by arteriolar dilators, 235
    with vasodilators, 233
    in shock, 248
Agammaglobulinemia
  acquired, 1944
  common variable, 1943
  immunization for patients with, 63
  incidence of, 1941
  replacement of gamma globulin in, 157
  testing for, 1942
  X-linked, 1942–1943
    and neoplasms, 1096t
Aganglionosis, in Hirschsprung's disease, 723
  intestinal, 170, 170t
Age
  and atherosclerosis, 320
  and body mass index, and mortality, 1221
  and bone loss, 1511
  and cardiovascular disease, 182
  and digitalis use, 229
  and encephalitis from arboviruses, 1822
  and hematocrit, 879
  and laboratory test results, 81
  and sleep patterns, 2077
Ageusia, definition of, 2110
Agglutinating antibodies, in tularemia, 1665
Aging, 21–26. See also *Elderly*
  and benign prostatic hyperplasia, 1422
  and body weight, 1220, *1221*
  and brain, 2089
  and deafness, 2119
  and dietary calcium requirements, 1472
  and glossitis, 678
  and testosterone levels, 1414
  biological theories of, 22–24
  bone loss in, and periodontal disease, 675
  clinical impact of, 24–26
  early, 1202
  exercise and, 26
  genetic aspects of, 24
  interaction of, with disease, 24–26
  of skin, by ultraviolet light, 2303
  sun and, 2306
  vs. disease, clinical medicine and, 24
Agitation, from rabies, 2201
  in psychiatric disorders, drugs for, 2094, 2094t
Agnosia, 2081, 2084, 2085
  auditory, vs. Wernicke aphasia, 2086
Agonadism, XY, 1395
Agonist drugs, 107–108
  and adrenergic receptors, 134, 136
  cholinergic, 139
Agoraphobia, definition of, 2100

Agranulocytosis, from antithyroid drugs, 1325
  from leprosy treatment, 1699
Agraphia, alexia with, 2087
AIDS (acquired immunodeficiency syndrome), 1523, 1794–1799, 1799–1808, 1881–1884, 2203–2205
  and cancer, 1095
  and lymphoma, 1008
  and tuberculosis, 1682
  appearance of, 1797
  biopsy of liver granulomas and, 838
  definition of, 1799, 1800t
  diarrhea from, 729
  disinfection precautions for, 1548
  drug abuse and, 52, 57
  enteropathy of, 729
  epidemiology of, 1800–1801
  gastroenteritis in, DHPG for, 126
  glomerular disease in, 588
  hemophilia A and, 1069
  hepatitis immunization and, 64
  human immunodeficiency virus and. See *Human immunodeficiency virus*
  immunology of, 1801–1803
  infection in, 1533
    candidiasis as, 1848
    coccidioidomycosis as, 1840
    cryptococcosis as, 1844
    cryptosporidiosis as, 1881, 1882
      treatment of, 1883
    cytomegalovirus, 1785, 2198
    disseminated histoplasmosis as, 1839
    disseminated mycobacterial, 1695
    Epstein-Barr virus, 1787
    giardiasis as, 1883
    herpes simplex virus, 1782
    mycobacterial, 1693
    mycotic, 1837
    opportunistic, 1803–1806, 1804–1805t
    protozoan, 1857
    Salmonella, 1644
    toxoplasmosis as, 1877
  Kaposi's sarcoma in, 464, 677, *678*, 790, 1110t, 1797, 1798, 1806–1807
  lymphocytopenia from, 966–967
  malabsorption in, 745
  meningitis in, 2192
  neurologic complications in, 2203, 2204t
  oral findings in, 677
  Pneumocystis carinii pneumonia in, 1803–1805, 1805t
  pneumocystosis with, 1880
  prevention of, 1798–1799
  progressive multifocal leukoencephalopathy with, 2207
  public health recommendations for, 1807–1808
  recombinant DNA vaccine for, 159
  retinitis in, DHPG for, 126
  sexually transmitted disease and, 1702
  therapy for, 1807–1808
  thrombocytopenia in, 1050
  thrush with, 2348
  thymic hypoplasia from, 1974
  transmission of, by blood transfusions, 950
    to hospital employees, 1549
  vs. Nezelof's syndrome, 1945
  vs. severe combined immunodeficiency disease, 1946
  vs. toxoplasmosis, 1878
AIDS dementia complex, 2203–2205
AIDS viruses, 1523, 1795, 1797–1799. See also *Human immunodeficiency virus*
AIDS-related complex, 1037, 1803t, 1803–1804

Air, ambient, bacteria in, 1552
Air embolism, during dialysis, 577
  from blood transfusions, 950
  in scuba divers, 2367
Air pollution, and asthma, 407
  and cancer, 1094
Airflow, resistance to, 396
  measurement of, 397
Airplane glue, abuse of, 59
Airplanes, cabin pressure in, 2366
Airway(s)
  chronic diseases of, 410–419
  management of, in acute respiratory failure, 477–478
  in coma, 2067, 2070
  in severely ill, 486–487
  narrowing of, causes of, 397
    in asthma, 403
  obstruction of
    localized, *418*, 418–419
    mechanical ventilation with, treatment for, 488
    pathophysiology of, 411, *412*
    respiratory failure from, 475
      critical care for, 490–491
  occupational disorders of, 2358–2360
Ajellomyces dermatitidis, 1842
Akathisia, from drugs, 2094, 2144
  tardive, from antipsychotic drugs, 2144
Akinesia, contralateral, 2083
  definition of, 2142
Akinetic seizures, 2076
ALA (delta-aminolevulinic acid), 1182
Alanine, as glucose precursor, 1382
Alanine aminotransferase, reference intervals for, 2395t
L-Alanine muramylamidase, 1555
Alaria americana, 1904–1905
Alastrim, 1792
Albers-Schönberg disease, 1518–1519
  myelophthisis in, 890
Albinism, 152, 153, 2344–2345t. See also *Hypoalbuminemia*
  and neoplasms, 1096t
  from melanocyte dysfunction in Chédiak-Higashi disease, 958
  oculocutaneous, 2346
Albright's disease, 2343
Albumin, 240, 1316
  as indicator of protein nutriture, 1211
  bilirubin binding to, 812
  calcium binding to, 1470
  concentration of, in viral hepatitis, 820
    with aging, 97
  distribution of, in healthy population, 80
  human biologic production of, 159
  human serum, for fluid replacement, 245
  in proteinuria, 520, 521
  reference intervals for, 2395t
  replacement of, 157
  serum concentration of, in viral hepatitis, 820
  synthesis of, in liver, 593, 810, 815
Albuminuria, in infectious mononucleosis, 1787
  in yellow fever, 1832
Alcaptonuria, 152, 1157
Alcohol
  abuse of, 48–52. See also *Alcoholics* and *Alcoholism*
  and acute gouty arthritis, 1165
  and antidiuretic hormone release, 1308
  and atrial premature depolarizations, 256
  and cancer, 44, 1093t, 1094
    breast, 1453
    esophageal, 686
    oral, 678–679
    pancreatic, 781

Alcohol (Continued)
and chylomicronemia syndrome, 1143
and gastroesophageal reflux disease, 683
and gout, 1163, 1169
and headache, 2132
and hemochromatosis, 1190
and hypertension, 285
and hypertriglyceridemia, 1143
and motor vehicle accidents, 41
and neutrophil adhesiveness, 957
and osteoporosis, 1511
and sleep, 2078
and testosterone synthesis inhibition,
    1414
and thrombocytopenia, 1048
and tinnitus, 2120
and ulcers, 696, 701
and vitamin deficiency, 1228
blackouts from, 2076
blood levels of, 48–49
consumption of, by cigarette smokers, 38
ethyl, dilated cardiomyopathy from, 353
    poisoning with, treatment for, 144
high intake of, and zinc deficiency, 1241
hypertriglyceridemia in, 320
hypoglycemia from, 1384
in diet, and atherosclerosis, 43
in drug interactions, 124t
methyl, poisoning with, 142
poisoning with, 2069t
respiratory failure from, 476
with cocaine, 54
withdrawal from, 2064, 2219
Alcohol dehydrogenase, 48
Alcohol sponging, for fever reduction, 1527
Alcoholic beverages, concentration of
    ethanol in, 48
Alcoholics. See also Alcohol and Alcoholism
cerebral atrophy in, 2138
chronic subdural hematoma in, 2244
hydrocarbon pneumonitis in, 2372
nutritional deficiency in, and anemias,
    882
polyneuropathy in, 2139
vomiting by, 658
Wernicke's encephalopathy in, 2137
Alcoholics Anonymous, 50
Alcoholism, 49–50. See also Alcohol and Al-
    coholics
acute, 48–51
addictive cycle in, 49–50
among physicians, 68
and congenital heart disease, 303
and depressive illness, 2095
and hypophosphatemia, 1193
and osteonecrosis, 1517
and pneumococcal meningitis, 1605
and pneumonia from gram-negative ba-
    cilli, 1566
and sepsis, shock from, 246
and thiamin deficiency, 1229
and vitamin B₆ deficiency, 1233
as contraindication for liver transplant,
    856
atrial flutter from, 258
blackouts in, vs. epilepsy, 2225
cardiomyopathy in, 353–354
    prognosis for, 354
chronic, in mothers, and congenital mal-
    formation, 171
    Korsakoff's dementia of, 28
gastrointestinal disease in, 656–657
genetics and, 49
hyalin in, 843
hypoglycemia in, 809
immunization for patients with, 63
in adolescents, 21

Alcoholism (Continued)
ketoacidosis in, 554, 1375, 1377
    treatment of, 555
ketosis in, 810
liver disease in, 842–844
    and bleeding from vitamin K defi-
        ciency, 1077
    genetic factors in, 843
    transaminases in, 814
    vs. hemochromatosis, 1191
myopathy in, 2282
niacin deficiency in, 1232
pancreatitis in, 775
    chronic, 779
personality disorders and, 657
prognosis in, 52
psychopathology and, 49
treatment of, 50
vitamin A deficiency in, 1237
vitamin C deficiency in, 1235
Aldolase, in hypothyroidism, 1330
in polymyositis, 2036
reference intervals for, 2395t
Aldosterone
and fluid volume depletion, 531
and kidney function, 502
and metabolic alkalosis, 518
and sodium absorption by distal convo-
    luted tubule, 502
and sodium balance, 515–516
antagonists to, 232
    characteristics of, 536t
deficiency of, 1353. See also Hypoaldoster-
    onism
excess of. See Aldosteronism
in Starling forces abnormalities, 535
measurement of, 283, 1350
metabolism of, 1341, 1343–1344
    Addison's disease and, 532
    impaired, 623
    regulation of, 1345
plasma binding of, 1343
reference intervals for, 2395t
secretion rates and plasma concentrations
    of, 1341
Aldosteronism
definition of, 1340
licorice and, 1265
primary, 1358–1359
    and hypertension, 281
    diagnosis of, 283
    screening tests for, 283t
    treatment of, 291–292
Aldrich-Mees lines, from arsenic poisoning,
    2389
Alexia, 2081, 2086–2087
    occipital lobe damage and, 2080t
ALG (antilymphocyte globulin), for aplastic
    anemias, 886, 888
Alginic acid-antacid, for gastroesophageal
    reflux, 683
Alkalemia, 549
Alkali, for distal renal tubular acidosis, 623
    poisonings with, treatment for, 144
Alkaline phosphatase, 1489
    deficiency of, and abnormal bone min-
        eralization, 1479
    in liver, disease of, 815, 820, 832, 846
        granulomas of, 837
        pyogenic abscess of, 836
    in Paget's disease, 1516
    in sclerosing cholangitis, 869
    increase in, from pancreatic cancer, 781
        from primary biliary cirrhosis, 845
        from recurrent cholestasis, 813
        hepatic neoplasms and, 858
    reference intervals for, 2395t

Alkaloids, abuse of, 59
Alkalosis
and metabolic encephalopathy, 2067t
and net acid excretion, 518
and phosphorus excretion, 518
and potassium secretion, 517
contraction, 555
from excess mineralocorticoids, 1347
from vomiting, 659
metabolic, 551, 555–556. See also Meta-
    bolic alkalosis
posthypercapneic, 556
respiratory, 551, 557–558. See also Respi-
    ratory alkalosis
systemic, and potassium transport, 543
Alkylamines, 1954t
Alkylating agents
and cancer, 1093t, 1095, 1123t, 1123–1124
for multiple myeloma, 1030
for primary thrombocythemia, 1054
sideroblastic anemia from, 900
Alkylators, for adenocarcinoma of perito-
    neum, 794
Alleles, 146, 162
for HLA complex, 1963
mutant, 147
Allergens, inhalation of, by asthmatic pa-
    tient, 405
testing for, in asthma patients, 408
Allergic reactions
alveolitis as, extrinsic, 433
angiitis as, 431, 2026, 2028
aspergillosis as, bronchopulmonary, 1850
    vs. tropical eosinophilia, 1916
asthma as, prostaglandin D₂ in, 1271
contact dermatitis as, 2318, 2373, 2374
    Langerhans' cells and, 2302
encephalomyelitis as, experimental, 2208
eosinophilia from, 1025
granulomatosis as, 599
immunoglobulin A deficiency and, 1944
interstitial disease as, acute, from penicil-
    lin, 505
interstitial nephritis as, proteinuria from,
    503
    urinalysis for, 561
purpura as, 1058–1059
thrombocytopenia in, 1052
to blood transfusions, 950
to drugs, 102–103, 103t, 1968–1972
to insulin therapy, 1372
Allergic rhinitis, 1951–1955
clinical manifestations of, 1953–1954
definition of, 1951–1952
diagnosis of, 1953–1954
etiology of, 1952
incidence and prevalence of, 1952
pathogenesis and mechanisms of, 1952,
    1952–1953
treatment of, 1954–1955
Allergic shiners, 1953
Allergic vasculitis, 431–432, 2026–2028
kidneys in, 599
vs. rat-bite fever, 1730
Alloantibodies, hemolysis from, 918
Allopurinol
and hair loss, 2349
for chronic gouty arthritis, 1169
for glycogen storage diseases, 1134
for gout, 157, 1168
for hyperuricemia, in chronic kidney fail-
    ure, 571
for leukemia, 1004
for myelofibrosis, 987
for visceral leishmaniasis, 1873
in drug interactions, 124t
interaction of, with xanthine oxidase, 101

Allopurinol (Continued)
  interstitial lung disease from, 434
  interstitial nephritis from, 605
  liver granulomas from, 828
  metabolites for, kidney excretion of, 95
  neutropenia from, 963t
  prior to tumor chemotherapy, 562
  side effects of, 1169
  site of action of, 1163
Alopecia, 2348–2349
  and polyglandular autoimmune disease,
    1414
  from thallium, 2391
  in systemic lupus erythematosus, 2015
Alopecia areata, 2348
  and nails, 2346
Alopecia neoplastica, 1108
Alpha chain disease, 1034
Alpha receptor blockers, and microcircula-
    tion, in shock, 248
Alpha toxin, from Clostridium perfringens,
    1629
Alpha-adrenergic agents, for hypertension,
    287t
Alpha-2 adrenergic agonists, and intestinal
    motility, 724
Alpha-adrenergic antagonists, 139
Alpha-adrenergic blocking agents, adverse
    effects of, 289t
  prior to surgery for pheochromocytoma,
    292
Alpha-adrenergic constrictors, and coronary
    vessels, 189
Alpha-adrenergic receptors, 134–136
3 Alpha-androstanediol glucuronide, 1406
Alpha-2-antiplasmin, 1079
  deficiency of, 1074
    testing for, 1065
Alpha-1-antiproteinase, inborn error of,
    1081
Alpha₁-antitrypsin
  deficiency of, 838–839, 1130
    and hepatocellular carcinoma, 858
    bronchiectasis from, 439t
    chronic hepatitis from, 830, 831
    emphysema from, 416
      treatment for, 417–418
    liver transplant for, 157
    vs. cryptogenic cirrhosis, 847
  inborn error of, and chronic obstructive
    pulmonary disease, 414, 415
    and clotting disorders, 1081
  normal concentration of, 838
  reference intervals for, 2395t
  synthesis of, in liver, 810
Alpha-chlorhydrin, as testicular toxin, 1416
Alpha-difluoromethylornithine, for crypto-
    sporidiosis, 1883
Alpha-fetoprotein
  as tumor marker, 1099t, 1099–1100
  embryonal cell cancer from, 1421
  hepatic neoplasms and, 858
  in blood, in ataxia-telangiectasia, 2153
  in prenatal diagnosis, 170–171
  levels of, and chromosome abnormalities,
    168
  reference intervals for, 2397t
Alpha-1,4-glucosidase, 1134
  deficiency of, 2277
Alpha-hemolytic streptococci, endocarditis
    from, 1586–1587
    treatment of, 1594t
17 Alpha-hydroxylase, deficiency of, 1397,
    1397–1398
    amenorrhea from, 1438
Alpha-interferon
  for hairy cell leukemia, 1000–1001
  for Kaposi's sarcoma, 1807

Alpha-interferon (Continued)
  for multiple myeloma, 1031, 1032
  toxic effects of, 1001
Alpha-L-iduronidase, deficiency of, 1175
Alpha-mercaptopropionylglycine, for cys-
    tinuria, 643
Alpha-methylparatyrosine, adverse effects
    of, 292
  for pheochromocytoma, 292
5 Alpha-reductase, deficiency of, 1400–
    1401, 1401, 1406
Alphaviruses, fever from, 1819
Alport's syndrome, 637–638
  kidney transplant for, 157
Alprazolam, abuse of, 53
Alprenolol, for angina pectoris, 327t
ALS. See Amyotrophic lateral sclerosis
Alström-Hallgren syndrome, and extreme
    obesity, 1289
Alström's syndrome, 1203
  hypogonadism from, 1414
Altitude
  and diffusing capacity, 400
  and hematocrit, 879
  and lung disorders, 2366–2367
  and polycythemias, 979
  and pulmonary hypertension criteria,
    293, 294t
Aluminum
  as mineralization inhibitor, 1482
  toxicity of, 2389–2390
    osteomalacia from, 1508
      treatment of, 1510
    treatment of, 1485
Aluminum acetate, in bath, for skin disor-
    ders, 2314
Aluminum hydroxide, phosphate binding
    by, 1193
Aluminum hydroxide antacids, and osteo-
    malacia, 1481
Aluminum hydroxide-magnesium hydrox-
    ide antacid, for gastroesophageal re-
    flux, 683
Alveolar hyperventilation, from pulmonary
    embolism, 443
Alveolar hypoventilation
  and hypercapnia, 484
  and right ventricular function, 475
  polycythemia from, 979
  pulmonary hypertension from, 297–298
Alveolar-capillary block syndrome, 400
Alveolar-capillary membrane, injury, in
    adult respiratory distress syndrome,
    476
Alveolitis, 423–425, 425
  allergic, extrinsic, 433, 1850–1851
  lymphocyte-macrophage, in drug-in-
    duced interstitial lung disease, 434
  measuring extent of, 428
  mononuclear phagocyte-dominant, in his-
    tiocytosis X, 430
  necrotizing, 436
Alveolus(i)
  anatomy of, 421, 421
  bacteria in, 1552–1553
  destruction of, in emphysema, 414, 415
  distortion and fibrosis of, in interstitial
    lung disease, 425
  hemorrhage of, from idiopathic pulmo-
    nary hemosiderosis, 430
  hydatid disease of, 1893
  interstitium of, 421
  proteinosis in, 432
Alzheimer's disease, 28, 29, 2083, 2089–
    2090
  aluminum and, 2390
  amyloidosis and, 1200
  and amnesia, 2084

Alzheimer's disease (Continued)
  in temporal lobe, 2081
  vs. AIDS dementia complex, 2205
  vs. brain tumors, 2234
  vs. Creutzfeldt-Jakob disease, 2206
Amanita, and food poisoning, 786–787
Amantadine
  elimination rate for, 96t
  for influenza, 126–127, 1766, 1767
  for parkinsonism, 2145
  side effects of, 2145
    antihistamines and, 127
Amastigote, 1870
Amaurosis, 2111, 2111. See also Blindness
Amaurosis fugax, 2167, 2169, 2289, 2289t
  and carotid disease, 2168
Amblyomma americanum, and Rocky Moun-
    tain spotted fever transmission, 1742
Amblyopia
  definition of, 2111
  nutritional, 2139
  tobacco-alcohol, vs. optic neuritis, 2215
  toxic, in heroin users, 57
Amblyopia ex anopia, 2114
Amebiasis, 835t, 1886–1888
  as contraindication for corticosteroid ther-
    apy, 755
  hepatic, amebic abscess from, 834
    vs. acute clonorchiasis, 1902
  metronidazole for, 121
  treatment of, 1887t, 1887–1888
  vs. gonococcal infections of rectum, 1707
  vs. ulcerative colitis, 757
  vs. ulcerative proctitis, 788
Amebic abscess, vs. echinococcosis, 1894
Amebic dysentery, vs. diverticulitis, 804
Amenorrhea, 1435–1440
  biochemical evaluation of, 1437
  causes of, 1436t
  definition of, 1435
  from adrenocortical insufficiency, 1351
  from body weight changes, 1287
  from chronic active hepatitis, 832
  from hypothalamic hypogonadism, 1287
  from methadone, 56
  from pituitary adenomas, 2232
  from prolactin-secreting tumors, 1302
  hypergonadotropic, 1437t, 1437–1438
  in 17 alpha-hydroxylase deficiency, 1398
  in anorexia nervosa, 1216
  in testicular feminization, 1399
  post-pill, 1435, 1444
Amenorrhea-galactorrhea syndrome, 1302–
    1303
Amentia, vs. dementia, 2087
American trypanosomiasis, 1865–1869. See
    also Chagas' disease
Amethasone suppression test, for Cush-
    ing's syndrome, 1349
Amethopterin, 906
Amikacin, 119, 122
  and kidney damage, 117t, 609
  dosage for, and elimination rate constant, 95
  elimination rate for, 96t
  in liver failure, 117t
  reference intervals for, 2402t
Amiloride, 232, 536
  adverse effects of, 289t
  and hyperkalemic hyperchloremic meta-
    bolic acidosis, 553
  characteristics of, 231t, 536t
  for hypertension, 286t
  for primary aldosteronism, 292
Amine(s), biogenic, from medullary carci-
    noma, 1506
Amine precursor uptake and decarboxyla-
    tion (APUD) cells, 1264–1265
  in Sipple's syndrome, 1460

Amino acid(s)
  absorption of, 734
  analogues of, synthesis of, 1253
  aromatic, in hepatic encephalopathy, 852
  branched-chain, 1159
    for hepatic encephalopathy, 853
  conversion of, to protein, insulin and, 1374
  essential, 1207
  from proteins, 733
  groups of, 619
  in acute phase response, 1529
  metabolism, 810–811
    inborn errors of, 1149–1161
      alcaptonuria as, 1157
      branched-chain aminoaciduria as, 1159–1160
      histidinemia as, 1157–1158
      homocystinuria as, 1160–1161
      hydroxyprolinemia as, 1158
      hyperphenylalaninemias as, 1155–1156
      hyperprolinemias as, 1158
      urea cycle diseases as, 1158–1159
  salts of, for metabolic alkalosis, 556
  sulfur-containing, metabolism of, 550
  transport of, 734
    and hyperaminoaciduria, 1149
Aminoacidopathies, 1150–1154t
Aminoaciduria(s), 505, 619–620, 1149
  branched-chain, 1159–1160
  hyperdibasic, 1153t
  hyperdicarboxylic, 1154t
  in pregnancy, 634
  in tubulointerstitial disease, 603
Aminoaciduriase, and degeneration of white matter, 2216
Aminoglutethimide, as inhibitor of adrenal steroid biosynthesis, 1341
  for Cushing's disease, 1356
  for metastatic breast cancer, 1456–1457
Aminoglycosides, 114, 120, 122
  action of, 113t
  and hearing loss, 2119
  and kidney damage, 117t, 559, 609
    management of, 569
  clearance of, by hemodialysis, 95
  clindamycin or lincomycin combined with, 121
  for cholangitis, 868
  for gram-negative bacilli pneumonia, 1567
  for recurrent aspiration pneumonia, 1569
  for refractory staphylococcal infections, 119
  for sepsis, 1540
  in acidic environments, 116
  in drug interactions, 124t
    with curare, 101
    with penicillins, 124
      for Pseudomonas aeruginosa, 437
  in liver failure, 117t
  peak levels of, 113
  pharmacokinetic parameters for, 89t
  pneumococci resistance to, 1555
  poor spinal fluid penetration by, 116
  resistance mechanisms to, 116t
  vertigo from, 2123
Aminophylline
  for acute asthmatic attack, 409
  for chronic respiratory failure, 480
  for pulmonary edema in heart failure, 226
  therapeutic range for, 480
Aminopterin, 906
  and folate utilization, 906
  for cancer, 1120
Aminopyrine, and asthma, 407
5-Aminosalicylate, for Crohn's disease, 751–752

Aminotransferases, 814–815. See also Transaminases
Amiodarone, 271
  and thyroid function, 1321
  chronic hepatitis from, 828, 831
  dosing and adverse effects of, 269t
  for hypertrophic cardiomyopathy, 358
  for liver disease, 843
  for recurrent ventricular tachycardia, 276
  inhibition of drug metabolism by, 100
  interaction of, with digitalis, 228
    with digoxin, 101
    with procainamide, 101
  interstitial lung disease from, 434
  pharmacokinetic properties of, 266t
Amitriptyline
  and antidiuretic hormone release, 540
  and riboflavin deficiency, 1231
  for insomnia, 2078
  for migraine, 2131
  reference intervals for, 2402t
Ammonia
  and chemical pneumonitis, 2367
  and hepatic encephalopathy, 852
  deficiency in delivery of, and renal tubular acidosis, 623
  from impaired urea cycle, 1158
  in renal acid secretion, 550
Ammonium, as buffer in acid-base balance, 564
  excretion of, 517
  in kidney stones, 638
Ammonium chloride, for metabolic alkalosis, 556
  tolerance test of, 523–524
Amnesia
  causes of, 2084
  concussion-postconcussion, 2076
  from stroke, 2166
  global, transient, 2169
  in Alzheimer's disease, 2089
  in Korsakoff's syndrome, 2138
  psychiatric, 2066
  psychogenic, 2085
  retrograde, 2084
  transient, 2085
    vs. epilepsy, 2225
  treatment of, 2085
Amniocentesis, 166, 168, 170, 173
Amniotic fluid, embolization of, defibrination syndrome after, 1079
Amobarbital, genetics in metabolism of, 102
  overdose of, and central nervous system, 2069
  reference intervals for, 2402t
Amoxicillin
  absorption of, 116
  acute interstitial nephritis from, 603
  elimination rate for, 96t
  for lung abscess, 437
  for otitis media, 1620
  for Salmonella infection, 1645
  for urinary tract infection, 630
  in drug interactions, 124t
  in kidney and liver failure, 117t
Amphetamine(s)
  abuse of, 21, 54
  and hair loss, 2349
  as analgesics, 108t, 109
    with narcotics, 108
  congenital heart disease from, 303
  for weight control, 1226–1227
  poisoning with, 2069t
  reference intervals for, 2402t
Amphotericin B
  and kidney damage, 117t, 559, 609
  elimination rate for, 96t
  for aspergillosis, 1851

Amphotericin B (Continued)
  for blastomycosis, 1843
  for Candida infection, 1849
    of esophagus, 688
  for coccidioidomycosis, 1841
  for cryptococcosis, 1845–1846
  for histoplasmosis, 1839
  for infection, with neutropenia, 966
  for mycoses, 1838
  for paracoccidioidomycosis, 1844
  for sporotrichosis, 1847
  for zygomycosis, 1852–1853
  hemolysis from, 923
  hypokalemia from, 546
  in drug interactions, 124t
  in liver failure, 117t
  poor spinal fluid penetration by, 116
Ampicillin
  acute interstitial nephritis from, 603
  allergy to, 1969
  and pseudomembranous colitis, 1632
  elimination rate for, 96t
  for acute cholecystitis, 866
  for aortic stenosis, 343
  for appendicitis, 803
  for cholangitis, 868
  for chronic bronchitis, 413
  for chronic respiratory failure, 480
  for diverticulitis, 805
  for infection in bronchiectasis, 439
  for listeriosis, 1672
  for lung abscess, 437
  for otitis media, 1620
  for pneumococcal meningitis, 1609
  for Salmonella infection, 1645
  for salpingitis, 1706
  for shigellosis, 1647
  for urinary tract infection, 630
  in drug interactions, 124t
  in kidney and liver failure, 117t
Ampulla of Vater, 775
  carcinoma of, 669
    vs. pancreatic cancer, 783
Amputation
  after electric injury, 2382
  diabetes mellitus and, 1361–1362
  for arteriosclerosis obliterans, 381
  for gas gangrene, 1630
  for thromboangiitis obliterans, 383
  for zygomycosis burn infection, 1853
  phantom limb pain after, 2137
Amrinone, 184, 235
Amyl nitrite, abuse of, 59
Amylase
  in acute pancreatitis, 776
  increase in, and jaundice, 818
    from pancreatic cancer, 781
    in acute abdomen, 802
  production of, 776
  reference intervals for, 2395t
Amyloid A protein, 1528
Amyloidosis, 359–360, 360, 1198–1202, 1199t
  and cancer, 1098–1099, 1112
    giant hypertrophic gastritis vs., 692
  and ischemic colitis, 764
  and liver disease, 840
  and skin, 2325
  autonomic insufficiency in, 2106
  bronchiectasis and, 439
  cardiac, 369–370
    endomyocardial biopsy for, 178
  diagnosis of, with biopsy, 731
  factor X deficiency in, 1078
  immunocytic, 1034–1035, 1035t
  in ankylosing spondylitis, 2007
  in Crohn's disease, 750

Amyloidosis (Continued)
   in familial Mediterranean fever, 1196,
      1197
   kidney size in, 568
   myopathy with, 2283
   neuropathy in, 2266
   purpura in, 1059
   renal, kidney transplant for, 157
   senile, 1200
   tubulointerstitial involvement in, 606
Amylophagia, 880, 896
Amyotrophic lateral sclerosis, 2156–2157,
      2157t
   and esophageal motor disorders, 683
   primary, 2154
   vs. cervical spondylosis, 2254
Anabolic steroids, for alcoholic hepatitis,
      844
   peliosis hepatitis from, 828
Anaerobic bacteria
   chloramphenicol for, 120
   clindamycin or lincomycin for, 121
   lung abscess from, 435–436
   non-spore-forming, disease from, 1637–
      1640
   penicillins for, 119
   resistance of, to tetracycline, 741–742
Anagen effluvium, 2349
Anagen phase, of hair growth, 2303
Analeptics, contraindications for, 2071
Analgesic drugs, 106–109. See also Pain
      management, drug therapy for
Analyzers, automated, in laboratories,
      79
Anaphase, in meiosis, 162
Anaphylactic shock, 240–241
Anaphylactoid purpura, 600–601. See also
      Henoch-Schönlein purpura
Anaphylaxis, 1956–1958
   acute kidney failure from, 558
   causes of, 1956
   from drugs, 103, 104, 1969, 1970t
   from insect stings, 1959
   from radiographic contrast agents, 1968
      for CT brain exam, 2058
   immunoglobulin E and, 1935
Anarthria, 2087
Anasarca. See also Edema
   from chronic lymphocytic leukemia, 995
   in heart failure, 223
Ancylostoma braziliense, 1907
Ancylostoma duodenale, 1906
Androblastoma, hormones from, 1445t
Androgen(s)
   action of, disorders of, and hypogonad-
      ism, 1412
   adrenal, measurement of, 1350
      production of, 1346
   and hair growth, 1446, 2302
   erythrocytosis from, 980
   deficiency of, 1408–1409
      and impotence, 1409
      with deficient sperm production, 1412–
         1415
   excess of, and polycythemia, 977
      hypogonadism from, 1418
      polycystic ovarian syndrome from,
         1439
   fetal exposure to, and clitoral enlarge-
      ment, 1435
      and virilization of female fetus, 1428
   for anemia, aplastic, 888
      of chronic renal insufficiency, 892
   for delayed puberty, 1418
   for functional prepubertal castrate syn-
      drome, 1414
   for hypogonadism, 1418–1419
   for myelofibrosis, 987

Androgen(s) (Continued)
   for paroxysmal nocturnal hemoglobinu-
      ria, 923
   from neoplasms, heterosexual develop-
      ment from, 1429
   function of, 1406–1407
   insensitivity to, 1399–1400
   precocious puberty from, 1420
   resistance to, 1418
   side effects of, 888
   synthesis of, 1341
      in ovaries, 1431
Androstenedione, 1433t
   and hair growth at puberty, 2303
   measurement of, 1350
   secretion rates and plasma concentrations
      of, 1341
   synthesis of, 1341
      in ovaries, 1431
Anemia(s), 878–884
   acute, 1003
      posthemorrhagic, 891t, 891–892
   after ulcer surgery, 705
   and heart, 369
   and hemorrhage in eye, 2297
   androgens for, 1419
   angina pectoris from, 324
   aplastic. See Aplastic anemias
   chronic, vs. protoporphyria, 1184
   chronic disease and, 881, 898–899
   compensation for, 879
   definition of, 878–879
   dilutional, 879
   evaluation of patient with, 879–884
   Fanconi's, 168
      and acute leukemia, 1001
   from adrenocortical insufficiency, 1351
   from alcoholic cirrhosis, 844
   from analgesic nephropathy, 607
   from bone marrow failure, 884–890
      aplastic anemias as, 885–889. See also
         Aplastic anemias
      myelophthisic anemias as, 890t, 889–
         890
   from cancer, 1098
      gastric, 711, 712
      kidney, 652
      pancreatic, 781
   from chronic kidney failure, 566
   from copper deficiency, 1242
   from dialysis, 576–577
   from drug allergy, 1971t
   from fascioliasis, 1902
   from gastrointestinal hemorrhage, 796–
      797
   from glucagonoma, 1389
   from Goodpasture's syndrome, 430
   from hereditary spherocytosis, 911
   from Hodgkin's disease, 1018
   from hookworm, 1907
   from hypopituitarism, 1295–1296
   from leptospirosis, 1731
   from leukemia, acute, 1003
      hairy cell, 999
      lymphocytic, chronic, 995
   from lung abscess, 436
   from malaria, 1858
   from medullary cystic disorders, 648
   from multiple myeloma, 1032
   from myelofibrosis, with myeloid meta-
      plasia, 986
   from pyogenic liver abscess, 836
   from rheumatoid arthritis, 2003
   from riboflavin deficiency, 1231
   from systemic lupus erythematosus, 2016
   from ulcerative colitis, treatment for, 758
   hemochromatosis from, 1192
   hemolytic. See Hemolytic anemia(s)

Anemia(s) (Continued)
   high output heart failure from, 216
   hypochromic, 892t, 892–898
      from Gaucher's disease, 1146
      red cell indices in, 892t
   in acquired immunodeficiency syndrome,
      1802
   iron deficiency, 893–898. See also Iron de-
      ficiency anemia
   laboratory tests for, 883, 884, 884t
   macrocytic, 882
   megaloblastic, 900–907. See also Megalo-
      blastic anemias
   microcytic, 881–882
      red cell indices in, 892t
   normocytic, 882
      normochromic, 890–892
         classification of, 890t
         from Waldenström's macroglobuline-
            mia, 1033
         in multiple myeloma, 1028
   of chronic renal insufficiency, 892
      management of, 570–571
   pathophysiologic classification of, 878t
   pernicious, 904–905. See also Pernicious
      anemia
   physical examination for, 881, 881t
   red cell production during, 874
   sickle cell, 149, 152, 936–942. See also
      Sickle cell anemia
   sideroblastic, 899–900
      ineffective erythropoiesis in, 895
      refractory, 1032
   thalassemias as, 147, 930–936. See also
      Thalassemia(s)
   treatment of, 884
   vitamin B_6 for, 1234
   vs. arteriosclerosis obliterans, 381
   with endocrine disorders, 892
Anemones, nonfatal envenomations from,
   1931
Anencephaly, prenatal diagnosis of, with
   ultrasonography, 173
Anesthesia
   and aspiration, 2370
   depolarizing muscle paralysis from, 548
   for pain management, 109–110, 110t
   hypertensive crisis during, pheochromo-
      cytoma and, 281
   inhalation, and malignant hyperthermia,
      2282
   local, allergy to, 1971
   pharyngeal, for upper tract endoscopy,
      668
   respiratory failure from, 476
   spinal, spinal inflammation from, 2257
   topical local, cocaine as, 55
Aneurysms
   abdominal, and back pain, 2250
   and coronary artery bypass grafts, 338
   and spontaneous intracranial hemor-
      rhage, 2173–2174
   aortic, and mesenteric artery occlusion,
      762
      dissecting, 372–374, 373. See also Dis-
         secting aneurysms, of aorta
      myocardial infarction vs., 332
      in cigarette smokers, 37
   arteriosclerotic, 380
   berry, common sites for, 2174
      in autosomal dominant polycystic kid-
         ney disease, 645
      treatment of, 2177
   carotid, hypopituitarism from, 1295
   Charcot-Bouchard, 2178
   coarctation of aorta and, 313
   congenital renal artery, 649
   definition of, 370

Aneurysms (Continued)
echocardiography for, 203
false, 334
from trauma to heart, 369
from hypertension, 277
from Marfan's syndrome, 371
functional left ventricular, 208
fusiform, 2174
giant, treatment of, 2177
in brain, diagnostic imaging techniques for, 2060
in spleen, 1039
mycotic, from endocarditis, 1590, 2186
in drug abusers, 57
of sinus of Valsalva, aortic regurgitation from, 343
congenital, 308
rupture of, 308
pathologic consequences of, 2175–2176
risk of, 371
vs. appendicitis, 802
ventricular, from myocardial infarction, 333
from sarcoidosis, 453
surgery for, 274
Angiitis
allergic, 431, 2028
leukocytoclastic, 431–432, 2026–2028
kidneys in, 599
vs. rat-bite fever, 1730
necrotizing, in drug abusers, 57
Angina, abdominal, 762
Angina pectoris
after myocardial infarction, treatment for, 335
clinical classification of, 324–325, 325t
definition of, 323
diagnosis of, 324
tests for, 325–326
from alpha antagonists, 139
from amyloidosis, 359
from anemia, 879
of gastric cancer, 711
from aortic stenosis, 188, 341
from propranolol withdrawal syndrome, 138
from sarcoidosis, 453
in cigarette smokers, 37
in diabetics, 1380
pathophysiology of, 324
stable, 324–325
treatment of, 326–328
beta-adrenergic blockers for, 138
medical vs. surgical, 337t
unstable, 325
bypass grafting for, 338
coronary arteriography for, 328
myocardial perfusion imaging and, 209
variant, 325–328, 393
verapamil for, 271
vs. esophageal colic, 684
vs. gallstones, 865
vs. heartburn, 680
vs. panic attacks, 2101
with hypothyroidism, treatment of, 1331
Angiocardiography, first-pass radionuclide, 207
for tetralogy of Fallot, 309
Angiodysplasia
and gastrointestinal vascular malformations, 765
gastrointestinal hemorrhage in, 799, 800
vs. adenocarcinoma of colon, 771
vs. ulcerative colitis, 756
Angioedema, 1948–1951, 2334
from loiasis, 1918
hereditary, 148, 1940
Angiography, 214

Angiography (Continued)
aortic, for dissecting aneurysms, 373, 373
cerebral, 2059
digital subtraction, 83, 83, 2059
for kidneys, 525
for abdominal angina, 762
for bleeding ulcers, 706
for gastrointestinal hemorrhage, 666
for ischemic colitis, 764
for mesenteric artery embolism, 763
for mesenteric artery occlusion, 762
for pulmonary hypertension, 299
for renal artery occlusion, 633
hypertensive crisis during, pheochromocytoma and, 281
indications for, 212t
pulmonary, for bullae, 420
for emboli, 296
for interstitial lung disease, 427
selective renal, 282–283
spinal, 2252
Angiokeratoma, 1145
Angiomas, in Sturge-Weber syndrome, 2159, 2174
Angioneurotic edema, hereditary, androgens for, 1419
Angiopathies, intracranial hemorrhage in, 2175
stroke from, 2165t
transient ischemic attack from, 2165t
Angioplasty
coronary, 329
percutaneous transluminal, 334, 339
for arteriosclerosis obliterans, 381
for renovascular hypertension, 288, 290
Angiosarcoma(s), 859
of liver, from vinyl chloride, 140, 828
Angiostrongyliasis, 1913
Angiostrongylus cantonensis, 1913
Angiostrongylus costaricensis, 1913
Angiotensin(s), 516
and aldosterone secretion, 516
in sarcoidosis, 456
reference intervals for, 2395t
Angiotensin II
and adrenal cortex, 1340
and fluid volume regulation, 530
and glomerular filtration rate, 531
and mesenteric circulation, 761
and mineralocorticoid production, 1345–1346
and renin release, 1345
Angiotensin III, and thirst, 530
Angiotensin converting enzyme, inhibition of, adverse effects of, 289t
reference intervals for, 2395t
Angiotensinases, 278
Angiotensinogen, 516
Anhidrosis, 2107
Anilines, and methemoglobinemia, in infants, 946
toxicity of, to hemoglobin, 945
Anion(s), of intracellular fluid, 529
Anion gap, 551–552
in metabolic acidosis, 552, 553
reference intervals for, 2395t
rise in, in chronic kidney failure, 564
Aniridia, chromosome studies for, 168
Anisakis, 1910–1911
Anisocoria, definition of, 2113
physiological, 2114
Anitschkow myocytes, 1582
Ankles, indolent ulcers of, 911
rheumatoid arthritis in, 2001
Ankylating agents, for hairy cell leukemia, 1000

Ankylosing spondylitis, 151, 473, 2005t, 2006–2007
and uveitis, 2293
aortic regurgitation from, 343
diagnosis of, human leukocyte antigens and, 1968
from Crohn's disease, 747
hereditary factors in, 2005
human leukocyte antigens and, 1966
inflammatory bowel disease with, 753, 758
interstitial lung disease with, 430
spine in, vs. in osteoarthritis, 2041
vs. Reiter's syndrome, 2008
Ankyrin, in erythrocyte skeletal membrane, 909
Annular lesions, definition of, 2307
Anonopathy, distal, 2259, 2259
Anorchia, congenital, 1408, 1413–1414
cryptorchidism in, 1415
Anorectal abscess, 789
Anorectal gonorrhea, diagnosis of, 787
Anorexia
from abdominal abscess, 793
from acute cholecystitis, 865
from adenocarcinoma of duodenum, 713
from adrenocortical insufficiency, 1351
from alcoholic hepatitis, 843
from appendicitis, 801
from ascites, 791
from bronchogenic carcinoma, 459
from chronic lymphocytic leukemia, 995
from digitalis toxicity, 229
from gastric cancer, 711
from gastric outlet obstruction, 707
from gastrointestinal disease, 656, 657
from glucocorticosteroid therapy withdrawal, 132
from hypothalamic disorders, 1289
from iron deficiency anemia, 897
from legionnaires' disease, 1571
from liver disease, 808
from opioid withdrawal syndrome, 57
from primary mesothelioma, 794
from thiamin deficiency, 1229
from viral hepatitis, 819, 824
Anorexia nervosa, 16, 657, 1215–1218
amenorrhea in, 1439
diagnostic criteria for, 1217t
emotional disturbances and, 657
neuroendocrine system in, 1289
vs. hypopituitarism, 1296
vs. superior mesenteric artery syndrome, 765
Anoscopy, for lower gastrointestinal hemorrhage, 798
Anosmia, definition of, 2110
in hypogonadotropic eunuchoidism, 1416
Anosognosia, 2082, 2125
Anovulation. See also Ovulation
and dysfunctional uterine bleeding, 1434
chronic, 1438–1440
causes of, 1438t
Anoxemia, from tricuspid atresia, 311
in neonates, transposition of great arteries and, 314
Anoxia, delirium from, 2064
epilepsia partialis continua after, 2221
jaundice from, 817
Antacids
aluminum hydroxide, and osteomalacia, 1481
and salmonellae, 1644
for acute gastritis, 689
for duodenal ulcers, 702
for gastroesophageal reflux disease, 683
for peptic ulcers, 700–701, 701t
hypercalcemia from, 1492

Antacids (Continued)
  in drug interactions, 124t
    with digitalis, 228
    with oral contraceptives, 1443
    with phosphate, 1206t
  phosphate binding, and hypophospha-
    temia, 1193
Antagonist drugs, 108, 134
  adrenergic, 136, 137–139
  aldosterone, 232
  calcium, for primary pulmonary hyper-
    tension, 301
  cholinergic, 139
Antecubital vein, as access for cardiac cath-
    eterization, 211
Anterior cerebral artery, 2160, 2160
  occlusion of, 2166
Anterior cord syndrome, 2245
Anterior pituitary, 1290–1305. See also Pituitary, anterior
Anterior uveitis, from onchocerciasis, 1917
Anthracyclines, for acute myelogenous leu-
    kemia, 1005
  for cancer, 1125
  for multiple myeloma, 1030
Anthralin, for psoriasis, 2316
Anthrax, 1667–1668
  and meningitis, 1668
  immunization against, 65
  vs. sporotrichosis, 1847
Anthropometric measurements, in nutri-
    tional assessment, 1209–1210
Antianxiety agents, drug-dependent pa-
    tients and, 60
Antiarrhythmic agents
  adverse reactions to, 102
  and heart contractility, 186
  for hypertrophic cardiomyopathy, 358
  for mitral valve prolapse, 351
  interaction of, with antiseizure medica-
    tion, 99
  neutropenia from, 963t
Antibiotic therapy
  adverse reactions to, 102
  anaphylaxis from, 1956
  and Candida infection, 1848, 1849
    oral, 677
  and hearing loss, 2119
  and photosensitivity, 2351
  and pseudomembranous colitis, 1632
  and Salmonella colonization, 1644
  and thrombotic thrombocytopenic pur-
    pura, 1052
  and vitamin deficiency, 1076, 1228
  anthracycline, for multiple myeloma,
    1030
  antitumor, 1124–1125
  avoidance of, in traveler's diarrhea, 732
  definition of, 112
  for Campylobacter, 1650
  for chronic bronchitis, 413
  for diphtheria, 1628
  for frostbite, 379
  for gram-negative bacteremia, 1660
  for infection, with neutropenia, 966
  for infective endocarditis, 1593, 1594t
  for kidney failure, 572t
  for pneumococci, 1555
    pneumonia from, 1559, 1559t
  for rheumatic fever, 1585
  for Salmonella infection, 1645
  for sepsis, 1540
  for skin disorders, 2317
    topical, 2316
  for snake bites, 1929
  for tetanus, 1635
  for tularemia, 1666
  hypokalemia from, 546

Antibiotic therapy (Continued)
  interaction of, with oral contraceptives,
    1443
  interstitial lung disease from, 434
  macrolide, cholestasis from, 827
  neutropenia from, 963t
  prophylactic
    before surgery, 1546
    for catheterized patients, 1544
    for mitral regurgitation, 349
    in multiple myeloma treatment, 1032
  topical, for skin disorders, 2316
Antibodies
  agglutinating, and tularemia diagnosis,
    1665
  and endocardial infection, 1588
  and red cell destruction, 918
  antiacetylcholine receptor, 1975
  antilymphocyte, 967
  antinuclear, in silicosis, 2362
  antisperm, 1410
  antithyroid, 1320
  deficiency disorders in, 1942–1945, 1943t
  digoxin-specific, 230
  hybridoma-derived, 1524
  hyperimmune globulins with, 1536
  in host defense, 1531, 1531t
  in systemic lupus erythematosus, 2013
  influenza infection and, 1765
  islet cell, in insulin-dependent diabetes
    mellitus, 1365
  reaginic, and inflammation, 1988
  rheumatoid factor as, 1995
  screening for, for blood transfusions, 948
  subacute endocarditis and, 1593
  to Haemophilus influenzae b meningitis,
    1618
  to thyroid antigens, and Hashimoto's
    thyroiditis, 1333
Anticancer drugs, and photosensitivity,
    2351
Anticholinergic agents
  abuse of, 59
  and intestinal motility, 724
  and toxic megacolon, 755
  constipation from, 660
  for asthma, 409
  for diffuse spasm of esophagus, 686
  for parkinsonism, 2145–2146
  for torsion dystonia, 2150
  overdoses of, treatment for, 144
  side effects of, 2146, 2150
    and eye, 2298
Anticholinesterases, 139–140
  for myasthenia gravis, 2286
Anticoagulant agents, 1080–1081
  adverse reactions to, 102
  and chronic subdural hematoma, 2244
  contraindications to, after myocardial in-
    farction, 334, 335
  in venous thrombosis, 2185
  coumarin, and vitamin K deficiency,
    1076–1077
  definition of, 1080
  for arteriosclerosis obliterans, 381
  for DC cardioversion, 273
  for deep-vein thrombosis, 387
  for emboli, after myocardial infarction,
    334
    pulmonary, 447
  for endocarditis, 1594
  for mitral stenosis, 347
  for renal vein thrombosis, 634
  for stroke prevention, 2171
  in renal artery occlusion treatment, 633
  induction of metabolism of, 99
  interaction of
    with oral contraceptives, 1443

Anticoagulant agents (Continued)
  interaction of, with oral hypoglycemics,
    99
    with sulfonylureas, 1370
    with vitamin K, 1206t
  prophylactic, for antithrombin deficiency,
    1075
  ureteral obstruction from, 613
Anticonvulsant therapy
  and osteomalacia, 1484
  aplasia from, 886
  as analgesics, 108t, 109
  congenital heart disease from, 303
  for brain tumors, 2234
  interaction of, with oral contraceptives,
    1443
    with vitamin D, 1206t, 1481, 1485
  neutropenia from, 963t
Antidepressants, and ventilation, 401
  as adjuvant analgesic, 108t
  poisoning with, 2069t
  tricyclic, 2096. See also Tricyclic antidepres-
    sants
Antidiabetic agents, aplasia from, 886
  interaction of, with oral contraceptives,
    1443
Antidiarrheal agents, for Crohn's disease,
    752
  for treating malabsorption, 741t
Antidiuretic hormone, 1305–1308
  and cortisol production, 1344
  and countercurrent system, 513
  and fluid volume, 530, 531
  and hypertension, 279
  and kidney function, 502
  and water reabsorption, 516
  as tumor marker, 1099
  biosynthesis of, 1305, 1306
  excess, and fluid volume excess, 535
    causes of, 538t, 540
  in cancer, 1103
  in heart failure, 220
  inappropriate secretion of, 538, 1288. See
    also Syndrome of inappropriate secretion of
    antidiuretic hormone
  lack of, and diabetes insipidus, 1308
  release of, 516
    pathologic alteration of, 1308, 1308t
    regulation of, 1307
    volume contraction and, 540
  secretion of, 516
Antiendotoxin antiserum, 1541
Antifolates, for cancer, 1120–1121
Antifreeze, and kidney damage, 612
Antifungal agents, for skin disorders, sys-
    temic, 2317
    topical, 2316
  in kidney and liver failure, 117t
Antigen(s), response to, acquired immuno-
    deficiency syndrome and, 1802
  senescence, 955
  T cell recognition of, 1936
Antigen-antibody complex, 1960
Antigenic drift, in influenza virus, 1762–
    1763
Antiglobin test (Coombs' test), 881, 909
  for erythrocyte immunoprotein detection,
    918
Antiglomerular basement membrane, circu-
    lating, 430
Antihistamines, 1954–1955
  and adverse reactions from amantadine,
    127
  aplasia from, 886
  as analgesics, 108t, 109
    with narcotics, 108
  classifications of, 1954t
  for skin disorders, 2316t, 2316–2317

Antihistamines (Continued)
  neutropenia from, 963t
  overdoses of, treatment for, 144
  side effects of, in elderly, 2317
Antihuman thymocyte globulin, 1040
Antihypertensive agents, adverse reactions to, 102
  for mitral regurgitation, 349
  neutropenia from, 963t
Anti-inflammatory agents. See also Nonsteroidal anti-inflammatory agents
  glucocorticosteroids as, 129
  neutropenia from, 963t
  reduction of glomerular filtration rate by, 102
Anti-insulin hormones, 1364
Antilymphocyte antibodies, 967
  with ulcerative colitis, 753
Antilymphocyte globulins, for aplastic anemia, 886, 888
Antimalarial agents
  and hemolysis, 916t
  for rheumatoid arthritis, 2003
  for skin disorders, 2317
  neutropenia from, 963t
Antimetabolites
  for adenocarcinoma of peritoneum, 794
  for chronic myelogenous leukemia, 991
  for hairy cell leukemia, 1000
  for psoriasis, 2327
Antimicrobial therapy
  action of, 113t
  administration route for, 116
  and kidney damage, 609
  aplasia from, 886
  bacteria susceptibility to, 115
  combination, 118
  drug interactions in, 123–124, 124t
  duration of, 122
  failure to respond to, 123
  for bacterial meningitis, 1609–1610
  for chronic respiratory failure, 480
  for Crohn's disease, 752
  for cystic fibrosis lung disease, 441
  for neutropenia, with sepsis, 1536t
  for whooping cough, 1625–1626
  identification of infecting agents in, 112–113
  in acute cholecystitis treatment, 866
  pharmacologic factors in, 114, 116
  resistance to, 114, 116t
  topical, 124
  toxicity to, 123, 123t
Antimony, and kidney damage, 612
  toxicity of, 2393
Antineoplastic agents, 1120–1127
  alkylating agents as, 1123–1124
  and kidney damage, 562, 610–611
  antimetabolites as, 1120–1121
  antitumor antibiotics as, 1124–1125
  aplasia from, 886t
  carcinogenicity of, 1120
  cis-platinum as, 1124
  interstitial lung disease from, 434
  neutropenia from, 961
  plant products as, 1125–1126
Antinuclear antibodies, 1996–1997
  in interstitial lung disease, 426
  in liver disease, 817
  in silicosis, 2362
Antipsychotic drugs, parkinsonism from, 2144
  sudden withdrawal of, effect of, 2149
  tardive dyskinesia from, 2149
Antipyretic therapy, 1526
  for pneumococcal pneumonia, 1559
Antipyrine, metabolism of, in cigarette smokers, 39

Antiseptics, definition of, 1547
  urinary, 122
Antithrombin(s), 1063
Antithrombin III
  deficiency of, 1075
    and recurrent thrombophlebitis, 385
  levels of, and renal vein thrombosis, 634
Antithymocyte globulins, for aplastic anemia, 886
  in immunosuppression therapy, 581
Antithyroid agents, 1324–1325
  aplasia from, 886
  cholestasis from, 827
  neutropenia from, 963t
Antitoxins, animal-derived, 61
  for diphtheria, 1628
  for tetanus, 1635
Antituberculous agents, acute interstitial nephritis from, 605
  in kidney and liver failure, 117t
  interaction of, with vitamin B$_6$, 1206t
Antiviral therapy, 124–128
  biologic agents in, 127–128
  chemotherapeutic agents in, 125
  immune globulins in, 128
  systemic, for skin disorders, 2317–2318
Autonomic fibers, disorders of, 2129
Anton's syndrome, 2113
Antral G cell hyperplasia, and postoperative recurrent ulcers, 705
  vs. peptic ulcers, 699
Antral polyps, gastric outlet obstruction from, 707
Antrectomy, truncal vagotomy with, for peptic ulcers, 703t, 704
Antrum, carcinoma of, gastric outlet obstruction from, 707
  caustic stricture of, 707
  G cell hyperplasia of, 699, 705
  of stomach, 693
Ants, stings of, 1924
Anuria, definition of, 558
Anus
  diseases of, 789–790
  epidermoid carcinomas of, 772, 789–790
  fissures of, 757, 789
  imperforate, vs. congenital megacolon, 723
  infection of, with Neisseria meningitidis, 1615
  sphincter of, dysfunction of, 790
  squamous cell carcinoma of, 766
Anxiety, 1
  and reactions to cancer chemotherapy, 1088
  and tension headache, 2132
  and tics, 2151
  chronic asthenia in, 2125
  disorders of, 2100–2101
  dyspnea from, 394
  from sedative withdrawal, 54
  from untreated pain, 106
  in heart failure, 224
  in opioid withdrawal syndrome, 57
  management of, 2078
  and sedative dependence, 53
Aorta
  abdominal, 370. See also Abdominal aorta
  aneurysms in, 370–371. See also Aortic aneurysms
  ascending, 370
  bicuspid valve of, 312, 312
    coarctation of aorta with, 313
  blood flow in, velocity of, 189
  coarctation of, 313–314
    and aortic dissection, 372
    surgical treatment for, 318
    with ventricular septal defect, 307

Aorta (Continued)
  communication with pulmonary arteries, 307–308
  disorders of, 370–374. See also Aortic aneurysms
    aortitis as, 374
    from trauma, 374
    Marfan's syndrome as, 371, 371–372
  dissection of, in hypertension, 293
  insufficiency of, 176
  involvement of, in atherosclerosis, 319
  thoracic, 370
  transposition of, with pulmonary artery, 314
Aortic aneurysms, 370–371
  and mesenteric artery occlusion, 762
  dissecting, 372–374, 373
    and stroke, 2164
    and syncope, 2074
    angiography for, 373, 373
    pain from, 393
  from syphilis, 1717
  in cigarette smokers, 37
  rupture of, and ischemic colitis, 764
  vs. appendicitis, 801
Aortic arch, anomalies of, 314
Aortic arch syndrome, 374
Aortic-pulmonary septal defect, 308
Aortic regurgitation, 343–345, 344t
  and angina pectoris, 323
  aortic aneurysm and, 370
  fragmentational hemolysis from, 924
  ventricular septal defect with, 307
Aortic root, communication with right heart, 308
Aortic stenosis, 185, 188, 215, 341–343, 342t, 350
  carotid pulse in, 176
  congenital, coarctation of aorta with, 313
  Doppler echocardiography for, 206, 206
  fragmentational hemolysis from, 924
  medical therapy for, 343
  radiograph of, 194
  subvalvular, 312–313
  supravalvular, 313
  surgery for, 343
  valvular, and aortic dissection, 372
    and sudden cardiac death, 275
  vs. mitral regurgitation, 349
Aortic valve, bicuspid, 312–313
  surgical replacement of, 345
Aortitis, 374
Aortoenteric fistula, vs. bleeding peptic ulcer, 706
Apathy, from chronic hypoxia, 477
  in chorea, 2148
  in dementias, 2088
Apatite crystal deposition disease, 2037–2038
Aperistalsis, 685
Aphasia, 2083, 2086t, 2086–2087, 2221
Aphonia, 2087
Aphthous fever, 1778
Aphthous ulcers, 675–676, 676, 2347
  in yersiniosis, 1664
  oral, in Behçet's disease, 2049
Aplasia cutis, 2349
Aplastic anemias, 885–889
  acute viral hepatitis and, 820
  bone marrow biopsy of, 888
  clinical description of, 887
  definition of, 885
  diagnosis of, 887
  etiology of, 885t, 885–886
  from chloramphenicol, 120, 123
  in liver disease, 817
  incidence of, 887
  intracranial hemorrhage in, 2175

Aplastic anemias (Continued)
management of, 887–889, 889
marrow transplants for, 1040–1041, 1041
paroxysmal nocturnal hemoglobinuria and, 922
pathogenesis of, 886–887
prognosis of, 889
Aplastic crisis, 882, 886
from hereditary spherocytosis, 911
from human papovavirus, in sickle cell anemia, 1523
Apnea
from respiratory syncytial virus, 1759
sleep, 2079
from cordotomy, 111
obesity and, 1224
Apocrine sweat glands, 2302
Apomorphine, use of, after poisonings, 142
Apoplexy, pituitary, 2135
Apoprotein B, 1138
in cholesterol-rich lipoprotein, 1139
Apoprotein CII, 1139
Appendectomy, for familial Mediterranean fever, 1197
Appendicitis
acute, 800–804
vs. acute cholecystitis, 866
and pylephlebitis, 835
computed tomography for, 662
from ascariasis, 1909
from trichuriasis, 1909
pain from, 658
surgery for, complications from, 803–804
vs. Crohn's disease, 747, 750
vs. familial Mediterranean fever, 1197
vs. omentum torsion, 796
vs. yersiniosis, 1664
Appetite
definition of, 657
loss of, in chronic kidney failure, 566
steroids and, 1346
stimulation of, neurons regulating, 1280
Apprehension, from toxemia of pregnancy, 635
Apraxia, 2082, 2087
examination for, 2054
gait, 2126
oculomotor, 2115
in ataxia-telangiectasia, 2153
APTT (activated partial thromboplastin time), 1047, 1061
evaluation of, 1065
reference intervals for, 2400t
Aqueous humor, 2290, 2291
Ara-A (Adenine arabinoside), 125, 1783, 2195
Ara-C, 1122
Arabinoside, aplasia from, 885
Arabinosyl cytosine, for chronic lymphocytic leukemia, 997
Arachidonic acid, 1271, 1986
and blood pressure decrease, 279
and brain damage, 2239
in hemostasis, 1043
metabolism of, 404, 405, 1271
by cytochrome P 450, 1274
by fatty acid cyclooxygenase, 1272
by lipoxygenase enzymes, 1273
in kidneys, 520
metabolites of, for pulmonary hypertension, 301–302
in vivo functions of, 1275–1277
stimulation of, phospholipids and, 1260
Arachnodactyly, contractural, vs. Marfan syndrome, 1178
Arachnoiditis, spinal, 2257
ARAS (ascending reticular activation system), 2061

Arboviruses, 1814–1815, 1815t
and orchitis, 1414
Colorado tick fever from, 1819–1821
dengue from, 1816–1817
encephalitis from, 1821–1829, 1822t, 2192, 2193
fevers from, 1816–1821
meningitis from, 2193
phlebotomus fever from, 1817–1818
Rift Valley fever from, 1818–1819
West Nile fever from, 1817
ARC (AIDS-related complex), 1037, 1803t, 1803–1804
Arc of Riolan, 761
Arcuate arteries, 508
Areflexia, in chronic inflammatory demyelinating polyneuropathy, 2262
Arenaviruses, hemorrhagic disease from, 1834–1835
ARF. See Rheumatic fever, acute
Argentine hemorrhagic fever, 1834–1835
Arginase, deficiency of, 1152t, 1153t, 1159
L-Arginine, to test growth hormone reserve, 1294
Arginine hydrochloride, for metabolic alkalosis, 556
Arginine vasopressin. See Antidiuretic hormone
Argininosuccinase, deficiency of, 1159
Argininosuccinate synthetase, deficiency of, 156, 1152t, 1158–1159
Argininosuccinic aciduria, 156, 1152t, 1159
Argyll Robertson pupils, 1718, 2114
from syphilis, 2188
from tabes dorsalis, 2189
in diabetic neuropathy, 2263
Armillifer armillatus, 1926
Arnold-Chiari malformation, 2258
Arrhythmias, 250–274
atrial, 256, 258, 260–262. See also Atrial arrhythmias
atrioventricular junctional, 261–262
AV junctional, 260
beta-adrenergic blockers for, 138
cardiac, from inhalant abuse, 59
in myotonic dystrophy, 1414
definition of, 252
diagnostic approaches to, 254–255
electrocardiogram for, 177
drugs for, 264–271
adverse effects of, 266t–269t
amiodarone as, 271
and sudden cardiac death, 275
bretylium tosylate as, 271
classification of, 264, 265t
disopyramide as, 270
dosages for, 266t–269t
encainide as, 270
flecainide as, 270
pharmacokinetic properties of, 266t
procainamide as, 270
propranolol as, 137, 270–271
quinidine as, 270
verapamil as, 271
from aortic stenosis, 341
from barium, 2281
from beta thalassemia, 931
from cholera, 1653
from Ebstein's anomaly of tricuspid valve, 310
from excess thyroid hormone, 369
from heart trauma, 369
from myocardial infarction, 333
from myxoma, 367
from propranolol withdrawal syndrome, 138
from toxicity, of cocaine, 55
of digitalis, 230t

Arrhythmias (Continued)
hypomagnesemia and, 1196
in shock patients, treatment of, 245–246
management of, 257t
electrical devices in, 271–273
surgery in, 274, 274t
mechanisms of, 252–254
periodic paralysis with, 2281
supraventricular. See Supraventricular arrhythmias
ventricular, 262–264. See also Ventricular arrhythmias
vs. panic attacks, 2101
Arsenic
and angiosarcoma, 859
and cancer, 458, 1093t
and cutaneous neoplasms, 2375
and kidney damage, 611–612
hemolysis from, 923
poisoning with, 141, 143, 2388–2389
reference intervals for, 2395t
Arsine, 2388
Arterial blood, pH of, and respiration modulation, 550
normal ranges for, 549
vs. pH of cerebrospinal fluid, 551
Arterial aneurysms, and spontaneous intracranial hemorrhage, 2173–2174
from hypertension, 277
in spleen, 1039
Arterial blood gas(es)
composition of, in obstructive airway disease, 297
in asthma, 407
in interstitial lung disease, 426–427
limits of, for pulmonary embolism, 444
measurement of, in severely ill, 483
monitoring of, in shock patients, 243
significance of, 403
Arterial blood gas tensions, in chest wall abnormalities, and mechanical ventilation, 490
Arterial hypertension, 276–293. See also Hypertension
Arterial pressure
and myocardial ischemia, 238
in cardiovascular physical examination, 176
monitoring of, with arterial catheterization, 244
pulmonary, and cardiac output, 293
increase in, from cocaine or amphetamines, 54
monitoring of, in critical care units, 493–494, 494, 494t
systemic, 237
and angina pectoris, 324
monitoring of, complications from, 496–497
in critical care units, 493
systolic, as afterload, 186
Arterial tachycardia, paroxysmal, anticholinesterases for, 140
Arteriography
coronary, for unstable angina pectoris, 328
to detect atherosclerosis, 326
for aneurysms, 2177
for arteriovenous malformations, 2177
for upper gastrointestinal hemorrhage diagnosis, 798
of kidneys, 525, 568–569
pulmonary, for pulmonary embolism, 444
radiocontrast agents in, and kidney damage, 609–610
Arterioles, 508
Arteriolitis, hypersensitivity, 2027

Arteriosclerosis
  and intracranial hemorrhage, 2178
  and stroke, 2163, *2163*
  aneurysms from, 370
  aortic regurgitation from, 343
  definition of, 318
  diet and, 42–43
  low output heart failure from, 216
Arteriosclerosis obliterans, 380–382
  vs. erythromelalgia, 378
  vs. thromboangiitis obliterans, 382
Arteriovenous fistula(s), 384
  congenital, of kidneys, 649
  high output heart failure from, 216
  portal hypertension from, 848
Arteriovenous malformations
  and epileptic seizures, 2219
  and spinal cord, 2257
  hemorrhage from, and acute transverse
    myelitis, 2217
    spontaneous intracranial, 2174
  in brain, diagnostic imaging techniques
    for, 2060
  prognosis for, 2177
  treatment of, 2178
Arteriovenous shunts, 240
Arteritis, 374
  aneurysms from, 370
  cranial, headache from, 2133
  giant cell, 2033–2034
    central retinal artery occlusion and,
      2298
  pulmonary, with rheumatoid arthritis, 429
  Takayasu's, 2164
Artery(ies). See also *Aorta* and under names
    of specific arteries
  abnormal communication with veins, 384
  arcuate, 508
  as access for cardiac catheterization, 211
  damage to, in immune complex disease,
    1962
  for digestive tract, 760
  gastroduodenal, 760
  in atherosclerosis, 319
  interlobar, 508
  lobar, 508
  mesenteric, inferior, 761
    superior, 760–761, *761*
  normal, 318–319
  obstruction of, cyanosis from, 378
    organic, vascular diseases from, 380–
      384
    Raynaud's phenomenon vs., 376
  occlusion of, in kidneys, 632–633, 633t
    ischemia from, 504
    sudden, 383–384
    ulcers and, 2341
  of brain, 2159–2160, *2160, 2161*
  of kidneys, multiple, 649
  pulmonary. See *Pulmonary artery (arteries)*
Arthralgia(s)
  from essential mixed cryoglobulinemia,
    601
  from familial Mediterranean fever, 1197
  from glucocorticosteroid therapy with-
    drawal, 132
  from hemochromatosis, 1191
  from mycoplasmal pneumonia, 1563
  from polyarteritis nodosa, 2029
  from polymyositis, 2035
  from rubella immunization, 64
  from systemic lupus erythematosus, 2014
  from viral hepatitis, 819, 820
Arthritis
  aortic regurgitation from, 343
  bacterial, 2009t, 2009–2010
  degenerative, in sickle cell anemia, 939
    of hip, in Paget's disease, 1517

Arthritis *(Continued)*
  from alcaptonuria, 1157
  from calcium pyrophosphate dihydrate
    crystals, 2037
  from *Campylobacter* infection, 1649
  from chronic persistent hepatitis, 831
  from congenital syphilis, 1718
  from Crohn's disease, 747
  from erysipeloid, 1673
  from familial Mediterranean fever, 1197
  from hepatitis B, 823
  from Loeffgren's syndrome, indometha-
    cin for, 457
  from mumps, 1779
  from mycoplasma pneumonia, 1563
  from sarcoidosis, 453
  from shigellosis, 1647
  from streptobacillary fever, 1729
  from systemic lupus erythematosus, 2014
  from thalassemia intermedia, 932
  from viral hepatitis, 819, 820
  fungal, 2011
  gonococcal, 2010
    treatment of, 1710
  gouty, 1165–1170. See also *Gouty arthritis*
  in agammaglobulinemia, 1943
  in Behçet's disease, 2049
  in meningococcal illness, 1615
  in Reiter's syndrome, 2007
  in yersiniosis, 1664
  infectious, 2009–2011
  juvenile chronic, 2004
  Lyme, 1726, 1727
    treatment of, 1729
  miscellaneous forms of, 2046–2047
  obesity and, 1224
  of rheumatic fever, 1582
  peripheral, in Crohn's disease, 750
    in inflammatory bowel disease, 758
    sarcoidosis with, 451
  primary biliary cirrhosis with, 845
  psoriatic, 2327
  pyogenic, in bacterial meningitis, 1608
  rheumatoid, 1998–2004, *2001*. See also
    Rheumatoid arthritis
  septic
    from disseminated gonococcal infec-
      tion, 1709
    from *Haemophilus influenzae*, 65, 1619
    staphylococcal, 1600
    vs. acute hematogenous osteomyelitis,
      1623
    vs. rheumatoid arthritis, 2000
  transient, from rubella immunization, 64
  tuberculous, 1690, 2010
  uveitis and, 2293
  viral, 2010–2011
  vs. arteriosclerosis obliterans, 381
Arthrocentesis, 1993
Arthrography, 1998
Arthropathies
  amyloid, 2042
  enteropathic, 2008
  from calcium crystal deposition, 2037–
    2038
  from hemochromatosis, 839, 1191
  juvenile chronic, 2008
  psoriatic, 2008–2009
Arthropods
  and contact dermatitis, 1926
  and viral diseases, 1814–1837. See also
    Arboviruses
  disease from, 1920–1926, 1920t
  invasive, 1925–1926
  stinging, 1924–1925
Arthroscopy, 1998
Arthus' response, 1851
Artificial heart, 235

Artificial respiration, in cardiopulmonary
    resuscitation, 500
  in critical care, complications from, 495
Artificial sweeteners, and cancer, 1096
Asbestos
  and cancer, 1093t, 1094
    lung, 458
  and primary mesothelioma, 140, 794
  exposure to, cigarette smoking with, 37,
    38
  in drinking water, and pancreatic cancer,
    781
  lung disorders from, 2362–2364
Asbestosis, 432
  and pleural disease, 469
  definition of, 2362, *2363*
  pulmonary hypertension from, 296
Ascariasis, 835t, 870, 1908
  hepatomegaly and eosinophilia from, 834
Ascaris lumbricoides, 1908
  in liver, 835t
Aschoff nodules, in rheumatic fever, 1581–
    1582, *1581*
Ascites, 790–793
  albumin gradient in, 791
  as contraindication, for laparoscopy, 674
    for liver biopsy, 817
    for percutaneous transhepatic cholan-
      giography, 863
  bloody, 791, 851, 859
  causes of, 792t
  definition of, 850
  dialysis and, 577
  formation of, factors in, 791t
  from alcoholic hepatitis, 843
  from amyloidosis, 359
  from cardiomyopathy, 352
  from chronic lymphocytic leukemia, 995
  from constrictive pericarditis, 367
  from hemochromatosis, 839
  from liver disease, 808, 809, 832
  from ovarian neoplasms, 1446
  from peritoneal disease, 790
  from portal hypertension, 847
  from tuberculous peritonitis, 1691
  in adenocarcinoma of peritoneum, 794
  from cirrhosis, 850–852
    alcoholic, 844
    cryptogenic, 847
    pathogenic factors in, 850t
  in heart failure, 223
  in liver disease, 808
  in mesenteric inflammatory disease, 795
  in primary mesothelioma, 794
  mucinous, 794
  spontaneous bacterial peritonitis with,
    793
  spur cell hemolytic anemia and, 923
  transudative vs. exudative, 791, 791t
  with portal hypertension, 674
Ascorbic acid, 1234–1236, *1234*. See also *Vi-
    tamin C*
Asherman's syndrome, 1435, 1436
Ashman phenomenon, 260, *260*
Asiatic cholera, 1651–1653. See also *Cholera*
L-Asparaginase, and drug interactions, 1118
  and pancreatitis, 775
  for cancer, 1126–1127
Aspartame, and food poisoning, 786
Aspartate aminotransferase. See also *Glu-
    tamic-oxaloacetic transaminase*
  reference intervals for, 2395t
Aspartylglucosaminuria, 1152t
Aspergillomas, 1850, 1851
Aspergillosis, 1850–1851
  allergic, vs. tropical eosinophilia, 1916
  bronchopulmonary, 432
  of central nervous system, 2182

Aspergillus, and bronchiectasis, 439
  and cancer, 44
  and chronic granulomatous disease, 958
Aspergillus flavus, and food poisoning, 787
  and hepatocellular carcinoma, 858
  and liver cancer, 1095
Aspergillus fumigatus, as central nervous system infection, in transplant recipients, 2210
Aspergillus oryzae, lactase from, 742
Aspiration
  for liver abscess, 836, *836*
  for lung abscess, 436
  needle, for amebic liver abscess, 837
  of foreign bodies, bronchiectasis vs., 439
  of hydrocarbon, 2372
  silent, 2370
  transtracheal, 1554
    contraindications to, 1554
Aspirin
  after coronary artery bypass grafts, 339
  allergy to, 104, 1971–1972
  and analgesic nephropathy, 607
  and asthma, 407
  and cardiovascular system, 1275–1276
  and hemostatic disorders, 1045
  and neutrophil adhesiveness, 957
  and platelets, 93, 1275
  and prolonged bleeding time, 1047
  and Reye's syndrome, 829, 2209
  and stroke, 1275
  and ulcers, peptic, 696, 701
    postoperative recurrent, 705
  and ventilation, 401
  as analgesic, 107, 107t
    with narcotics, 108
  as cyclooxygenase inhibitor, 1275
  as prophylaxis, for recurring myocardial infarction, 335
    for atherothrombotic stroke, 2171
  chronic hepatitis from, 828
  chronic therapy with, and influenza vaccination, 62
  contraindications to
    aplastic anemia as, 889
    coumarin anticoagulants as, 1076
    in common cold in children, 1756
  gastritis from, 689, 690
    erosive, and iron deficiency, 896
  intolerance to, and urticaria, 1950
  liver disease from, 827, 828–829
  poisoning with, 2070t
    treatment for, 143
  thromboxane A$_2$ formation inhibited by, 1271
Asplenia syndrome, 315–316
  congenital, 1039
  immunization for patients with, 63
Assays. See *Laboratory tests*
Astemizule, 1955
Astereognosia, 2082
Astereopsis, 2081
  occipital lobe damage and, 2080
Asterixis, 2143
  from hepatic encephalopathy, 853
  from metabolic encephalopathy, 2065
Asthenia, 2124–2125
  neurocirculatory, vs. hyperthyroidism, 1324
Asthma, 403–410
  acute attack of, management of, 409
  allergic, prostaglandin D$_2$ in, 1271
  allergic bronchopulmonary aspergillosis and, 1850
  and breathing control, 401
  and obstructive ventilatory disorders, 399
  arachidonic acid and, 1276
  atopic, 1850

Asthma (*Continued*)
  beta-adrenergic agonists for, 137
    tolerance to, 94
  beta blockers and, 287
  bronchial, aerosol steroids for, 130
    cor pulmonale with, 475
    pneumothorax from, 470
  cannabis for, 58
  clinical manifestations of, 407
  cough from, 391
  definition of, 411
  differential diagnosis for, 408
  extrinsic, 403
    vs. intrinsic, 403t
  from Churg-Strauss syndrome, 431
  from drug allergy, 1971t
  glucocorticosteroid therapy for, 130
    complications from, 133
  influenza vaccination for patients with, 62
  intrinsic, 403
  late-onset, 405–407, 410
  maintenance therapy for, 409–410
  occupational, 2358–2359, *2359*
    causes of, 2358
  pathology of, 403–404
  prognosis for, 410
  pulmonary embolism vs., 444
  rhinoviruses and, 1755
  sarcoidosis vs., 455
  treatment of, 408–410
Asthmatic bronchitis, 412–414
  definition of, 411
  prognosis for, 413
Astrocytomas, 2230, 2256
  treatment of, 2234
Asymmetric septal hypertrophy, and sudden cardiac death, 275
Asystole, digitalis toxic, treatment of, 257t
  prolonged, from carotid sinus pressure, 254
Ataxia(s), 2125–2126
  cerebellar, adult-onset, 2153–2154
  Freidreich's, 2152–2153
  from cannabis, 57
  from hepatic encephalopathy, 853
  from phencyclidine, 59
  from syphilis, 1717
  hereditary, 2152–2154, 2153t
  in Wernicke's encephalopathy, 2137
  locomotor, from syphilis, 2189. See also *Tabes dorsalis*
  progressive, 2152
  sensory, in acute inflammatory sensory polyneuropathy, 2262
  spinocerebellar, in Gerstmann-Straussler disease, 2206
Ataxia-telangiectasia, 168, 1947, 2153
  and acute leukemia, 1001
  and neoplasms, 1096t
  cancer and, 1113
  from thymic hypoplasia, 1974
  hypogonadism from, 1414
  thymosin fraction 5 for, 1537
Atelectasis, 419–421
  from abdominal abscess, 793
  in pulmonary embolism, 443
  lobar, in sarcoidosis, 454
Atenolol, 138, 138t
  elimination rate for, 96t
  for angina pectoris, 327t
  for hypertension, 287t
ATG (antihuman thymocyte globulin), 1040
Atherosclerosis, 318–323
  after coronary artery surgery, 328
  after kidney transplants, 581
  and angina pectoris, 323, 324
  and cardiovascular disease, 181

Atherosclerosis (*Continued*)
  and eye, 2297
  and heart, 369
  and hypertension, 281, 291, 295
  and mesenteric blood supply, 744
  and myocardial infarction, 329
  cervical, syncope from, 2074
  coarctation of aorta and, 313, 318
  coronary, and ventricular fibrillation, 264
  coronary arteriography to detect, 326
  familial combined hyperlipidemia and, 1142
  from familial hypercholesterolemia, 1140
  in arteries to intestines, 762
  in chronic kidney failure, 565
  in cigarette smokers, 37
  in diabetes, 1380
  in dysbetalipoproteinemia, 1141
  in fluoroscopy, 195
  ischemic colitis from, 764
  prevention of, 323
  radiation therapy and, 1107
  regression of, 323
  risk factors in, 319–321
Atherothrombosis, of cerebral arteries, 2165–2166
  surgery for, 2171
Athetosis, 2149, 2152
  definition of, 2142
  vs. epilepsy, 2225
Athletes, androgenic anabolic steroid use by, 1419
Ativan, abuse of, 53
Atonic seizures, 2222. See also *Drop attacks*
Atopic dermatitis, 2320
Atopic diathesis, 1949
ATP. See *Adenosine triphosphate*
ATPase, deficiency of, mitochondrial, 2279
Atresia
  biliary, 846
  of oocytes, 1425
  tricuspid, 310–311
  vs. unilateral hyperlucent lung, 420
Atrial. See also *Atrium; Cardiac...; Heart*
Atrial arrhythmias, 256, 258, 260–262
  atrial fibrillation as, 260
  atrial flutter as, 258, 260
  atrial premature depolarizations as, 256, *258*
  paroxysmal supraventricular tachycardia as, 258, *259*
  sinoatrial block as, 261
  sinus rhythm as, 256
Atrial fibrillation
  and stroke, 2163
  and surgery for mitral stenosis, 347
  carotid sinus pressure for, 255t
  DC cardioversion for, 273
  emboli from, and sudden arterial occlusion, 383
  from hypertrophic cardiomyopathy, 357
  from mitral regurgitation, 348
  from mitral stenosis, 345
  in hypertrophic cardiomyopathy, treatment for, 358
  in mitral regurgitation, digitalis for, 349
  paroxysmal, from mitral stenosis, 346
  treatment of, 257t, 270, 271, 274
Atrial flutter, 258, 260
  carotid sinus pressure for, 255t
  DC cardioversion for, 273
  procainamide for, 270
  quinidine for, 270
  treatment of, 257t
Atrial natriuretic factor, circulatory function and, 190
Atrial natriuretic peptides, 531, 1277–1278, *1278*. See also *Atriopeptin*

Atrial premature depolarizations, 256, *258*
Atrial pressures, in shock patients, 244
  right, estimation of, 186
Atrial septal defects, 304–306
  vs. mitral stenosis, 347
Atrialized right ventricle, 310
Atriopeptin, 531, 1277–1279, *1278*
  and hypertension, 279
  basal plasma levels of, 1279
  immunoreactive, 538
  in fluid volume regulation, 531
  in water repletion reaction, 1308
Atrioventricular block(s), 262
  after intra-atrial surgery, 317
  after myocardial infarction, 237, 333
  and sudden cardiac death, 275
  atropine for, 139
  complete, 316
  high-grade, treatment of, 257t
Atrioventricular canal, common, 305
  complete, 306
Atrioventricular conduction, impairment of, 360
Atrioventricular junctional arrhythmias, 261–262
  atrial fibrillation with, 260
Atrioventricular node, 184, 250
  refractory period of, digitalis and, 229
Atrium. See also *Atrial...; Cardiac...; Heart*
  dilatation of, diastolic properties of heart and, 185
  left, acute distention of, 215
    myxoma in, in echocardiogram, 346
    thrombus in, in echocardiogram, 346
  right, myxoma of, tricuspid stenosis from, 351
Atropa belladonna, toxicity of, 787
Atropine, 139
  abuse of, 59
  as insecticide antidote, 143
  diphenoxylate with, for diarrhea, 732
  for asthma, 409
  for bradycardia in shock, 245
  for cardiorespiratory arrest, 501
  for chronic bronchitis, 413
  for insecticide poisonings, 145
  overdoses of, treatment for, 144
  poisoning with, vs. botulism, 1633
  side effects of, 2299
Attention, definition of, 2083
  disorders of, metabolic encephalopathy and, 2063
Audiometry, 2118
Auditory canal, infection of, 2185
Auer rods, 1002
Aura(s), 2220
  olfactory, 2221
Auscultation, for myocardial infarction examination, 331
  for pneumococcal pneumonia, 1557
  in cardiovascular examination, 177
Austin Flint murmur, from aortic regurgitation, 344
Austrian's syndrome, 1560, 1587
Autoantibodies
  in African trypanosomiasis, 1863
  in polymyositis, 2034–2035
  in Sjögren's syndrome, 2025
  in systemic lupus erythematosus, 2013t
  to adrenal tissue, in Addison's disease, 1461
  to deoxyribonucleic acid, 1996t
  to histones, 1996t
  to nonhistone nuclear proteins, 1997t
Autocrine growth factors, from lung cancer cells, 458
Autoimmune disorders
  acute phase response to, 1528

Autoimmune disorders (*Continued*)
  and neurologic infection, 2210
  and platelet function defects, 1057
  and premature ovarian failure, 1438
  from impaired complement reaction, 1938
  polyglandular, 1414
  rheumatic fever as, 1580
Autoimmunity
  and insulin-dependent diabetes mellitus, 1365
  and Lambert-Eaton myasthenic syndrome, 2287
  and pemphigus disease, 2331
  and polymyositis, 2034
  in inflammatory myopathies, 2276
  in systemic lupus erythematosus, 2013
  primary pulmonary hypertension from, 299t
Automaticity, abnormal, in Purkinje fibers, 253
Automatisms, 2221
Autonomic nervous system
  adrenergic receptors in, 134–137, 135t
  and circulatory homeostasis, 189
  and circulatory response to oxygen consumption, 220
  and coronary artery thrombosis, 330
  cholinergic receptors in, 134–137, 135t
  disorders of, 2103–2109, 2105t
    from genital herpes, 2197
    in diabetic neuropathy, 2263–2264
  idiopathic insufficiency of, 2106–2107
  in essential hypertension, 278
  in metabolic encephalopathy, 2065
  organization and physiology of, 133–134
  peripheral, insufficiency of, 2106
    impotence from, 1410
  sympathomimetic amines in, 137
Autonomic neuropathy, inflammatory, acute, 2262
Autosomal dominant traits, pedigrees of, 147–148
Autosomal recessive disorders, 148–149
  cystic fibrosis as, 440
  polycystic kidney disease as, 644, 645t, 647
Autosomal recessive traits, pedigrees of, 148
Autosomes, metabolic disease mapped to, 156t
Autosplenectomy, 1039
AV (atrioventricular) node, 184, 250
  refractory period of, digitalis and, 229
AVM. See *Arteriovenous malformations*
AVP (arginine vasopressin). See *Antidiuretic hormone*
5–Azacytine, 1122
Azatadine maleate, 1954t
Azathioprine
  and cancer, 1095
  for autoimmune hemolytic anemia, 919
  for chronic active hepatitis, 833
  for chronic colitis, 759
  for Crohn's disease, 752
  for myasthenia gravis, 2287
  for myocarditis, 354
  for thrombocytopenic purpura, 1051
  in immunosuppression therapy, 581
  metabolism of, 101
  mutagenic potential of, 759
6–Azauridine triacetate, and homocystinuria, 1161
Azidothymidine (compound S), for AIDS, 127, 1523, 1799, 1807
  reference intervals for, 2396t
Azlocillin, 120
  in kidney and liver failure, 117t
  treatment with, 119

Azoospermia, 1416
  in Klinefelter's syndrome, 1413
  obstructive, 1410
Azotemia
  definition of, 558
  from diabetic glomerulopathy, 625
  from multiple myeloma, 1029
  in fulminant hepatic failure, 854
  in legionnaires' disease, 1571
  kidneys and, 504
  prerenal, 560
  renal vs. extrarenal causes of, 568
  urinary tract obstruction and, 507
  urine sodium concentration in, 524
AZT. See *Azidothymidine*
Aztreonam, 120, 121t
  in kidney and liver failure, 117t
Azurophil, in neutrophils, 951

B cell growth factor, 1934
B cell leukemias, human T lymphotropic retrovirus and, 1797
B cell lymphoma(s), 975
  acquired immunodeficiency syndrome and, 1798
  and Epstein-Barr virus, 1787
B cell stimulatory factor-1, 1934
B lymphocytes, 966, 971, 1932–1935
  clonal proliferation of, and hairy cell leukemia, 998
  differentiation of schema of, *996*
  helper T cells and, 1936
  immunoglobulin synthesis by, 1026
  in immune response, 1531
  monoclonal proliferation of, and chronic lymphocytic leukemia, 994
  neoplasms of, 1007
  precursors of, 874
  stimulation of, *1934*
Babesia, 1884
Babesia microti, vs. *Plasmodium falciparum*, 1860
Babesiosis, 1884–1886
  hemolytic anemia from, 924
Babinski signs, in adult-onset cerebellar ataxia, 2153
  in Friedreich's ataxia, 2152
Bacillary dysentery, 1646. See also *Shigella*
Bacillary infections, penicillins for, 120
Bacille Calmette-Guérin, 1683
  for bladder cancer, 655
Bacilli, aerobic gram-negative, pneumonia from, 1565–1568
  gram-positive non–spore-forming, 1637
Bacillus anthracis, 1667
  infection of, vs. tularemia, 1666
Bacillus cereus, food poisoning from, 784, 785
  vs. *Escherichia coli*, 1655
Bacillus stearothermophilus, sterilization and, 1548
Bacillus subtilis, sterilization and, 1548
Bacitracin, chronic kidney failure as contraindication to, 572t
Back. See also *Spine; Vertebra(e)*
  pain in, 2043–2044
    causes of, 2252t
    diagnostic imaging for, 2251–2252
    etiology of, 2043t
    from Cushing's syndrome, 1355
    from intraspinal disease, 105
    from osteoporosis, 1512
      treatment of, 1513
    from parenteral nutrition, 1250
    from spinal epidural abscess, 2186
    lower, from abdominal aortic aneurysm, 371

Back (Continued)
  pain in, management of, 2252
    occurrence of, 2247
Background diabetic retinopathy, 2297
Background radiation, 2376
Backward heart failure, 215
Backwash ileitis, vs. ileal Crohn's disease, 748
Baclofen, for multiple sclerosis, 2214
Bacteremia. See also Bacterial infections
  and spinal epidural abscess, 2186
  complications from, 1538
  from Haemophilus influenzae, 1618, 1619
  from Listeria monocytogenes, 1671
  from Salmonella, 1645
  from shigellosis, 1646
  from staphylococcal skin infection, 1599
  gonococcal, 1708
  gram-negative, and endotoxic shock, 1659–1661
  hospital-acquired, 1542, 1544–1546, 1548
  immunization against, 63
  in acute leukemia, granulocyte transfusions for, 1006
  in fulminant hepatic failure, 854
  in plague, 1662
  laboratory tests for, 1539t, 1540
  pneumococcal pneumonia and, 1556
  staphylococcal, 1602
Bacteria
  ability of, to exclude antimicrobial agents, 114
  abscess from, vs. echinococcosis, 1894
  anaerobic. See Anaerobic bacteria
  and chronic bronchitis, 412
  and ileus, 719
  arthritis from, 2009–2010, 2009t
  cystitis from, 1704
  enteric, aminoglycosides for, 122
    cephalosporins for, 120
    extraintestinal infections from, 1658–1661
  food poisoning from, 784–785
  in small intestine, normal control of, 741
  in urinary tract, 628
  infection by
    from biliary obstruction, 866
    in acquired immunodeficiency syndrome, 1805t, 1806
    in alcoholic hepatitis, 843
    systemic, and liver, 834
  introduction of, into lungs, 1551, 1551t
  mononuclear phagocytes and, 952
  nervous system infection with, 2181–2191
    parameningeal infections as, 2181–2187. See also Parameningeal infections
    syphilis as, 2187–2191. See also Neurosyphilis
  osteomyelitis from, 2257
  pharyngitis from, vs. enanthems, 1813
  prostatitis from, 1421, 1422
  protein production in, 158–159
  pyelonephritis from, 605, 606
  sexual transmission of, 1702t
  stratum corneum as barrier against, 2303
  superinfection from, influenza and, 1766
  susceptibility of, to antibiotics, 115t
  tonsillitis from, vs. enanthems, 1813
  toxins from, shock and, 237
Bacterial endocarditis, 1586. See also Infective endocarditis
Bacterial infections. See also Bacteremia
  acute phase response to, 1528
  chloramphenicol for, 120
  immunodeficiency and, 1942
  in chronic lymphocytic leukemia, 995
  neutropenia and, 963
  of mucous membrane, 2347
  of thyroid gland, 1331

Bacterial meningitis, 1604–1610
  from Haemophilus influenzae, 65, 1618
  in heroin users, 57
Bacterial overgrowth
  after gastric surgery, 705
  and toxic megacolon in ulcerative colitis, 755
  C-xylose breath test for, 739
  clinical conditions associated with, 742
  in Crohn's disease, and malabsorption, 749
  in small intestine, culture for, 739
    diarrhea from, 728
  malabsorption from, 741–742
  vitamin B₁₂ deficiency from, testing for, 738t
Bactericidal agents, definition of, 112
Bacteriostatic drugs, definition of, 112
Bacteriuria, 503
  asymptomatic, 628
    treatment for, 630
  in pregnancy, 630
  significant, 628, 629
Bacteroides, 1637
  infection with, clindamycin for, 437
  lung abscess from, 436
  resistance of, to tetracycline, 741–742
Bacteroides fragilis, 1637
  infection of,
    cefoxitin for, 120
    chloramphenicol for, 120
    clindamycin for, 121, 437
    lincomycin for, 121
    metronidazole for, 121
Bacteroides intermedius, lung abscess from, 436
Bacteroides melaninogenicus-asaccharolyticus group, 1637
BAEP (brain-stem auditory evoked potentials), 2056
BAER (brain stem auditory evoked response), 2118
Bagassosis, 1851
Bainbridge reflex, 190
Baker's cyst(s), from rheumatoid arthritis, 2001
  rupture of, vs. deep-vein thrombosis, 386
Balanitis, from Candida infection, 1848
  in Reiter's syndrome, 2007
Balantidiasis, 1889
Balantidium coli, 1889
Baldness, 150
  in myotonic dystrophy, 1414
  male pattern, 2349
Balint syndrome, 2082
Ballism, definition of, 2142
Banti's syndrome, 848, 1038
Barbital, overdose of, and central nervous system, 2069
Barbiturates
  abuse of, 53
    by adolescents, 21
  and antidiuretic hormone release, 540
  and enhanced liver metabolism of other drugs, 99
  and myocardium, 239
  coma from, 142
  poisoning with, 2069, 2069t
  respiratory failure from, 476
  side effects of, 2227
  withdrawal syndrome from, delirium from, 2064
Bardet-Biedl syndrome, 1203
  and extreme obesity, 1289
Barium
  hypokalemia from, 546
  periodic paralysis from, 2281
  spontaneous reflux of, 681

Barium (Continued)
  toxicity of, 2392
    treatment of, 2282
Barium contrast studies
  for abdominal abscess, 793
  for Crohn's disease, 748
  for peritoneal disease, 790
  for superior mesenteric artery syndrome, 765
  in esophageal cancer diagnosis, 686
    stricture evaluation with, 682
  of gastrointestinal tract, 662
Barium enema examination
  for diverticulitis, 804–805
  for ileus of colon, 719
  for lower gastrointestinal hemorrhage, 799
  for rectum, limitations of, 787
  for ulcerative colitis, 756
  severe colitis as contraindication to, 756
  toxic megacolon in ulcerative colitis from, 755
Barlow's syndrome, from mitral valve prolapse, 349
Baroreceptors
  and antidiuretic release, 1307
  high-pressure, 189–190
  in fluid volume regulation, 530
  low-pressure, 190
  shock and, 239
Barr body (X chromatin), 149, 166
  Klinefelter's syndrome and, 1412
Bartonella bacilliformis, 1681
  hemolysis from, 924
Bartonellosis, 924, 1681–1682
  and Salmonella infection, 1644
Bartter's syndrome, 505, 532, 622, 622
  aldosterone levels in, 1360
  indomethacin for, 556
  metabolic alkalosis in, 555
  potassium depletion in, 545
Basal acid output, 699
  definition of, 693
  in Zollinger-Ellison syndrome, 708
  increase in, 695
Basal ganglia
  abnormalities of, 2141–2152
  anatomy of, 2141, 2142
  calcification of, and secondary parkinsonism, 2144
Basal metabolism, definition of, 1130
  expenditure in, and obesity, 1221–1222
  rate for, and thyroid status, 1320
Basedow's disease, 1321. See also Graves' disease
Basement membrane(s), 421
  antibodies to, anti-alveolar, 430
  antiglomerular, circulating, from Goodpasture's syndrome, 430
  of glomerulus, 509
Basilar artery, 2160, 2161, 2162
  aneurysm of, and third nerve palsy, 2175
  insufficiency in, from arteritis, 374
  occlusion of, 2163
Basilar artery migraine, 2130
  vs. transient ischemic attacks, 2169
Basophilia, in myelofibrosis, with myeloid metaplasia, 986
  in paraneoplastic syndromes, 1097–1098
Basophilic stippling, prominent, 917
Basophilopenia, 966
Basophils, and inflammatory reaction, 2306
  secretion by, regulation of, 405–406, 405
Bath oil, for skin disorders, 2314
Baths, for skin disorders, 2314
Bats, and histoplasmosis, 1838
  rabies in, 2200
Battey bacillus, 1693

Battle's sign, 2066
  from skull fracture, 2241
Bayes' rule, 74–76, 75t, 75
Baze syndrome, 1112
Bazet's formula, for QT interval correction
    for heart rate, 198
BCG (bacille Calmette-Guérin), 1683
  for bladder cancer, 655
BCNU (bis-chloroethyl-nitrosourea), 2234
Becker's dystrophy, 2273
  and dilated cardiomyopathy, 354
Beclomethasone, 409, 413
Bedbugs, 1921
Bedsonia, 1732
Bedwetting, 2079
Beef, tapeworm from, 1891–1892
Bees, stings of, 1924, 1958
Behavior
  bizarre, in Wilson's disease, 1188
  changes in, abrupt, 2092
    blood alcohol levels and, 49
    nonpsychiatric disorders and, 2092t
  self-destructive, in Lesch-Nyhan syn-
      drome, 1171
Behavior modification
  for anorexia nervosa, 1218
  in hypertension therapy, 285
  in preventive medicine, 35
  in weight control, 1226
Behavioral therapy, for pain management,
    109
Behçet's disease, 1609, 2026, 2048–2049
  aphthous ulcers with, 676
  diagnostic criteria for, 2049t
  spinal inflammation from, 2257
  splenomegaly in, 1037
  ulcers in, 2342
    small intestinal, 807
  uveitis in, 2293
Bejel, 1723
Belching, 661, 897
Bell's palsy, 2266–2267
Belladonna, and intestinal motility, 724
  for peptic ulcers, 139
Belladonna-atropine drugs, and intestinal
    motility, 724
Bence Jones myeloma, 1031
Bence Jones protein(s), 1027
  and amyloid fibril deposits, 1035
  deposition of, and urinary tract obstruc-
      tion, 569
  increased concentrations of, and overflow
      proteinuria, 520
Bence Jones proteinuria, in multiple mye-
    loma, 1032
  kidney failure in, 606, 1029, 1032
  macroglobulinemia and, 1033
Bendroflumethiazide, for hypertension,
    286t
Bends, 2367
Bentiromide urinary excretion test, for mal-
    absorption, 736, 737t, 779
  in malabsorption evaluation algorithm,
    740
Bentonite flocculation test, for trichinellosis,
    1912
Benzalkonium chloride, as antibiotic, 1548
Benzathine penicillin, 119
  after contact with diphtheria patient, 62
  for rheumatic fever prevention, 1579,
    1586
Benzene
  and acute leukemia, 1002
  and cancer, 1093t
  aplastic anemia from, 886
  toxicity to, and neutropenia, 962
Benzimidazoles, for inhibiting acid secre-
    tion, 700

Benznidazole, for Chagas' disease, 1869
Benzocaine, toxicity of, to hemoglobin, 945
Benzodiazepines
  and panic attacks, 2100
  for acute manic states, 2099
  for alcohol intoxication, 49
  for anxiety, 53
  for cannabis reactions, 58
  for cocaine or amphetamine users, 55
  for delirium tremens, 51
  for panic attacks, 2100–2101
  for psychiatric syndromes, 497
  poisoning with, 2069t
  side effects of, 102, 2227
    in elderly, 26
  withdrawal syndrome for, 53
Benzopyrones, for lymphedema, 389
Benzothiadiazine diuretics, for hyperten-
    sion, 286t
Benzyl penicillin, 119. See also Penicillin G
Bereavement, 2097
Berger's disease, 584t, 588–589, 588
  vs. Alport's syndrome, 638
Beriberi, 1229
  atrial flutter from, 258
  dilated cardiomyopathy from, 354
  high output heart failure from, 216
  symptoms of, 657
Bernard-Soulier syndrome, 1055
  vs. thrombasthenia, 1057
Berry aneurysms
  and spontaneous intracranial hemor-
      rhage, 2173–2174
  common sites for, 2174
  in autosomal dominant polycystic kidney
      disease, 645
  treatment of, 2177
Berylliosis, diffusing capacity in, 400
  pulmonary sarcoidosis vs., 425–426
Beryllium, and lung cancer, 458
  disease from, 2364
  poisonings from, 141
Beta-adrenergic agents, and cellular uptake
    of potassium, 543
  for acute asthmatic attack, 409
  for chronic obstructive pulmonary dis-
      ease, 417
Beta-adrenergic agonist drugs, and myocar-
    dial contractility, 184
  for chronic bronchitis, 413
  tolerance to, 94
Beta-adrenergic antagonists, aggravation of
    heart failure by, 220
  as prophylaxis for recurring myocardial
      infarction, 335
Beta-adrenergic blocking agents, 137–139,
    138t
  adverse effects of, 289t
  and chylomicronemia syndrome, 1143
  and hair loss, 2349
  and hypertriglyceridemia, 1143
  contraindications for, 327
  for angina pectoris, 327, 327t
  for arrhythmias, 270
  for atrial flutter, 260
  for dilated cardiomyopathy, 355
  for erythromelalgia, 379
  for hypercalcemia, 1504
  for hypertension, 287, 287t
    in uremic syndrome, 570
  for hyperthyroidism, 1325
  for idiopathic restrictive cardiomyopathy,
    361
  for Marfan's syndrome, 371–372
  for migraine, 2131
  for mitral valve prolapse, 351
  for supraventricular arrhythmias in shock
      patients, 245

Beta-adrenergic blocking agents (Continued)
  induction of metabolism of, 99
  interaction of, with disopyramide, 101
  interstitial lung disease from, 434
Beta-adrenergic receptors, 134–136
  for asthma, 408
  in hyperthyroidism, 137
  on myocardial sarcolemma, 184
Beta-adrenergic stimulants, contraindica-
    tions to, 358
Beta agonists, for mast cell regulation, 406
Beta blockers. See Beta-adrenergic blocking
    agents
Beta-carotene, 1237
  as carcinogenesis inhibitor, 44
  for protoporphyria, 1184
  reference intervals for, 2395t
Beta-globin gene, structure of, 928
  abnormal, and sickle cell anemia, 936
11 Beta-hydroxylase, deficiency of, 1403–
    1404
  and virilization of female fetus, 1402
3 Beta-hydroxysteroid dehydrogenase 5–4
    isomerase deficiency, 1397, 1397
17 Beta-hydroxysteroid dehydrogenase, de-
    ficiency of, 1397, 1398
Beta-lactamases, 114
  from anaerobic organisms, 1638
  resistance mechanisms of, 116t
Beta-LPH, from anterior pituitary, 1291
Beta₂ microglobulin, 1965
  clearance of, from tubulointerstitial disor-
      ders, 521
  in multiple myeloma, 1030
Bethanechol, 139
  for gastroesophageal reflux disease, 683
Bethanidine, distribution of, 99
Bezoars, after gastric surgery, 717–718
BFU-E, 875
Bicarbonate
  absorption of, parathyroid hormone and,
    502
    proximal renal tubular acidosis and,
      505
  and mucosal integrity, 694, 694
  concentration of, kidneys and, 518
    in ileal fluid, 725
  decreased secretion of, and diminished
      mucosal defense, 695
  in fat absorption, 733
  losses of, in metabolic acidosis, 552
  processing of, by kidneys, 550–551
  reabsorption of, by proximal tubule, 512
  reference intervals for, 2395t
  replacement of, for diabetic ketoacidosis,
    1376
  wasting of, in proximal renal tubular aci-
      dosis, 552–553
Bicarbonate-carbonic acid pair, in extracellu-
    lar fluid, 549
Bicarbonaturia, in tubulointerstitial disease,
    603
Bigeminy, 262
Biguanides, as laxatives, 722
  for diabetes mellitus, 1370
Bile
  cholesterol excretion into, 1140
  composition of, 859
  concentrations of antimicrobials in, 116
  copper excretion in, 1188
  definition of, 859
  examination of, for crystals, 864
  formation of, 859–860
  impaired secretion of. See Cholestasis
  leakage of, and ascites, 792
  total daily volume of, 859
Bile acid(s)
  and diarrhea, 728

Bile acid(s) (Continued)
  and gastric ulcers, 695
  in ileus, 719
  reference intervals for, 2395t
  synthesis of, in liver, 810
Bile duct(s)
  adenomas of, 857
  blood supply to, 760
  calculi in, 661, 867–868, 868. See also Cho-
    ledocholithiasis
  carcinoma of, in Crohn's disease, 749
    in sclerosing cholangitis, 750
  common. See Common bile duct
  cystadenomas of, 857
  destruction of, in primary biliary cirrho-
    sis, 844
  dilatation of, gallstones with, 861
    ultrasonography for, 664, 863, 863
  disorders of, 859
    in viral hepatitis, 824
    parasitic, 834, 835t
    pyogenic liver abscess and, 835
    vs. peptic ulcers, 699
  fluke parasites in, 1901
  obstruction of, 818, 869–870
    as contraindication for liver biopsy,
     817
    extrahepatic, vs. primary biliary cirrho-
     sis, 845
    liver congestion from, vs. viral hepati-
     tis, 824
    pathophysiology of, 862
    secondary biliary cirrhosis from, 846
    vs. appendicitis, 802
    vs. cholestatic hepatitis syndrome, 820
  parasitic disease in, 870
  proliferation of, in acute viral hepatitis,
    819
  stricture of, 870
    jaundice from, 817
    vs. bile duct adenocarcinoma, 871
    vs. pancreatic cancer, 783
  tumors of, 871–872
Bile salts
  and pruritus, 2304
  circulation of, 733
    enterohepatic, 860
  distal ileum resection and absorption of,
    733
  gastritis from, 689
  in gastroesophageal reflux disease, 680
  increase in, from parenteral nutrition, 841
    from recurrent cholestasis, 813
  reduced concentration from, malabsorp-
    tion from, 741–742
  synthesis of, 859
Bilharziasis, 1895–1901. See also Schistosomiasis
Biliary. See also Gallbladder
Biliary atresia, secondary biliary cirrhosis
  from, 846
  vitamin E deficiency in, 1239
Biliary cirrhosis
  alcoholic hyalin in, 843
  clinical features of, 845t
  from common duct obstruction, 862
  primary, 844–846
    jaundice from, 817
    vs. bile duct carcinoma, 871
    vs. chronic active hepatitis, 832
    vs. cryptogenic cirrhosis, 847
  secondary, 846
Bilirubin
  albumin-bound, displacement of, by sul-
    fonamides, 100
  daily average production of, 811
  increase in, from abdominal abscess, 793
    from ribavirin, 127

Bilirubin (Continued)
  metabolism of, 811–814, 812
    acquired disorders of, 813–814. See also
     Hyperbilirubinemia
    inherited disorders of, 813, 813t
  reference intervals for, 2395t
Bilirubinuria, from viral hepatitis, 819
Biliverdin, 811–812
Binge eating, in bulimia, 1218
Binswanger's disease, 2168
Biofeedback therapy, for hypertension, 285
  for Raynaud's phenomenon, 377
  for seizures, 2228
Biopsies
  chorionic, 173
  endomyocardial, 178
  for esophageal cancer diagnosis, 686
  for gastric cancer, 711–712
  for leprosy diagnosis, 1699
  for oral cancer, 679
  for osteomalacia, 1484
  for prostatic cancer, 1424
  for sarcoidosis, 455, 455
  indications for, in post-streptococcal glo-
    merulonephritis, 587
  intraoperative transduodenal, for pan-
    creatic cancer, 782
  needle, for hepatic neoplasms, 859
    of pleura, 467
  of bone marrow, 887, 888
  of kidneys, 527–528, 569
    indications for, 528t
  of liver, 817
    contraindications to, 460
    for acute viral hepatitis, 824
    for alveolitis, 428
  of lung, for Wegener's granulomatosis,
    2031
  of muscle, 2272
    for polymyositis, 2034
    for trichinellosis, 1912
  of nerve, 2260
  of peritoneum, 790
  of rectum, for ulcerative colitis, 756
  of skin, 2313, 2313–2314
  of small intestines, for malabsorption
    evaluation, 737t, 739, 739, 740t
    for nontropic sprue, 743
  of thyroid, 1320
  percutaneous aspiration, for hepatic neo-
    plasms, 859
  rectal, for diarrhea, 731
Biopterin, synthesis of, defect in, 1150t
Biotin, estimated safe and adequate daily
  dietary intake of, 1206t
Bipolar disorders, 2092, 2095, 2098–2099
Birbeck granule, 2302
Birth(s). See also Delivery; Stillbirth
  live, frequency of chromosome abnormal-
    ities in, 166
Birth defects, 2355
  multiple, 1202
Bis-chloroethyl-nitrosourea, for astrocyto-
  mas, 2234
Bis (chloromethyl) ether, and cancer,
  1093t
Bismuth, and kidney damage, 612
  for acute gastritis, 689–690
  for peptic ulcers, 701
  for travelers' diarrhea, 1657
Bitot's spots, 1238
Black death, 1662
Black flies, 1922
  and onchocerciasis, 1916
Black piedra, 1854
Black water fever, 924, 1858
Black widow spider, 1923
  antivenin for, 66

Blackouts, from drugs or alcohol, 50, 2076
Bladder, 2107
  anomalies of, 650
  bacteriuria in, treatment for, 630
  calcification of, in schistosomiasis haemo-
    tobia, 1898
  cancer of
    in cigarette smokers, 38
    solitary pulmonary nodules from, 464
    transitional cell, 655
  control of, 2107–2108, 2107t
  dysfunction of
    from cordotomy, 111
    from herpes zoster, 2196
    in Ehlers-Danlos syndrome, 1179
    in multiple sclerosis, treatment of,
     2214–2215
  examination of, magnetic resonance im-
    aging for, 85, 85
  incontinence of, from syphilis, 1717
  infection of, 628. See also Cystitis
  neck obstruction of, causes of, 1423
  neoplasms of, and acute kidney failure,
    558
  neurogenic dysfunction of, 614
    management of, 617
    manifestations of, 615
  rupture of, and acute kidney failure, 558
  stones in, 638
Blast cells, 1002
  in acute leukemia, 1001
Blast crisis, in chronic myelogenous leukemia, 990
Blastomas, pulmonary, 464
Blastomyces dermatitidis, 1842
  infection of, solitary pulmonary nodules
    from, 464
Blastomycosis, 1842–1843, 2334
  diagnosis of, 1838
  South American, 1843
  vs. cutaneous leishmaniasis, 1875
Blebs, 420
  rupture of, and pneumothorax, 469
Bleeding. See also Hemorrhage
Bleeding diatheses, intramural intestinal
  hemorrhage from, 764
  systemic, and intracranial hemorrhage,
    2175
Bleeding time, determination of, 1046
  reference intervals for, 2400t
Blennorrhea, inclusion, 2293
Bleomycin
  for cancer, 1124–1125
  oral, 679
  interstitial lung disease from, 434
  with radiation therapy, 1119
Blepharoconjunctivitis, 2294
Blepharospasm, 2150–2151
Blind loop syndrome, 714, 719, 741–742
Blindness. See also Eye(s); Vision
  causes of, 2112–2113, 2112t
  color, 150
  cortical, 2113
  from diabetes mellitus, 1362, 1378
  from giant cell arteritis, 2033
  from Laurence-Moon-Bardet-Biedl syn-
    drome, 1203
  from neuromyelitis optica, 2215
  from onchocerciasis, 1917
  from optic neuritis, 2215
  from pituitary tumors, 1298
  from recurrent herpes simplex virus in-
    fection, 1782
  from trachoma, 1734
  functional, from cranial dystonia, 2150
  in malignant osteopetrosis, 1518
  in sickle cell anemia, 939
  lesion localization causing, 2111–2112, 2111

Blindness (Continued)
  Rift Valley fever and, 1818
  transient, 2167, 2169, 2289, 2289t
    and carotid disease, 2168
  vitamin A deficiency and, 1237
Blister(s), 2328–2329
Blister beetles, dermatitis from, 1926
Blister cells, definition of, 914
Bloating, 661
  epigastric, 718
  from gastric cancer, 711
  from gastric outlet obstruction, 707
Blood
  allergic drug reactions in, 1971t
  arterial, pH of, normal ranges for, 549
  bile refluxed into, 862
  carbon dioxide content of, aging and, 25
  chronic loss of, from Crohn's disease, 749
  clumps of, in cold agglutinin disease, 921
  coagulation of. See Blood coagulation
  components of, human biologic produc-
    tion of, 159
  contaminated, in blood transfusions, 949
  culture of, for infective endocarditis,
    1592–1593
    for pneumonia, 1554, 1557
  disorders of, and sinus thrombosis, 2184
  donation of, and iron loss, 880
  extracorporeal irradiation of, for chronic
    lymphocytic leukemia, 997
  flow of. See Blood flow
  in pleural fluid, 467
  in sputum, 391–392. See also Hemoptysis
  in stool, from colonic cancer, 771
    from gastrointestinal hemorrhage, 796
    from mesenteric artery occlusion, 762
  in synovial fluid, 1995
  in vomitus, from mesenteric artery occlu-
    sion, 762
  irradiation of, 950
  lead poisoning and, 2386
  loss of. See also Hemorrhage
    and anemias, 880
    reticulocytosis following, 882
  malnutrition and, 1210t
  pH of, aging and, 25
  return of, to heart, 187
  sedimentation of, 1995. See also Erythro-
    cyte sedimentation rate
  standard unit of, components of, 947
  transfusion of. See Blood transfusions
  zinc in, 1241
Blood-brain barrier, and brain tumors, 2229
  glucocorticoid penetration of, 1347
  impaired integrity of, and hepatic en-
    cephalopathy, 852
Blood cells, circulating, precursors of, 874–
  875
Blood coagulation, 1060–1065, 1062
  disorders of, 1044t, 1060–1081. See also
    names of specific coagulation disorders
    acquired, 1075–1080
    and cerebral artery thrombosis, 2164–
      2165
    and cerebral ischemia, 2165t
    and spinal epidural hematoma, 2257
    anticoagulants for, 1080–1081
    approach to, 1065–1066
    as contraindication, for laparoscopy,
      674
      for liver biopsy, 817
      for percutaneous transhepatic cho-
        langiography, 863
    from bacterial meningitis, 1608
    hematuria from, 503
    inherited, 1066
    in liver necrosis, 817
    kinin system activation, in sepsis, 1539

Blood coagulation (Continued)
  disorders of, reference intervals for,
    2400t–2402t
    Rocky Mountain spotted fever and,
      1742
    snake venom and, 1928
  dyscrasia of, primary, and marrow exam-
    ination, 883
    vs. aphthous ulcers, 676
  localization and inhibition of, 1063
  platelets and, 1043
  vitamin K and, 1240
Blood flow. See also Circulatory system
  and gastric mucosal ischemia, 695
  collateral, to brain, 2163
  coronary, regulation of, 188, 188–189
  increased portal venous, 847
  intraorgan distribution of, in shock, 240
  measurement of, in cardiac catheteriza-
    tion, 213
  pulmonary, distribution of, 400
  redistribution of, and sodium excretion,
    515
    in heart failure, 220
  through skin, 2304
  to kidneys, 508
  to stomach, and mucosal integrity, 694,
    694
Blood flukes, schistosomes as, 1895
Blood gas, arterial, significance of, 403
Blood groups, 948, 948t
  and von Willebrand factor, 1070
  group A, and gastric cancer, 710
Blood platelets, 1043–1044, 1045. See also
  Platelet(s)
Blood pressure, 189
  and renin release, 1345
  arterial. See Arterial pressure
  atriopeptin and, 1278
  classification of, 276t
  diastolic, ranges of, and treatment, 285
  genetic factors affecting, 280
  high, 276–293. See also Hypertension
  homeostasis of, 279
  in gastrointestinal hemorrhage, 796
  increase in, cigarette smoking with, 37
    from cocaine or amphetamines, 54
    from psychedelic drugs, 58
  intracranial. See Intracranial pressure
  low, 190. See also Hypotension
  maintenance of, in coma from drug over-
    dose, 2070
    in upright position, 1465
    peripheral mechanisms for, 220
  measurement of, 281
  normal, 276
  reflex control of, 190
  systolic, 281. See also Systolic blood pres-
    sure
Blood-testis barrier, 1405
Blood transfusions, 947–950
  administration of, for gastrointestinal
    hemorrhage, 797
  and bone marrow transplants, 1040
  and Chagas' disease, 1868
  and hepatitis B transmission, 822
  and marrow transplants, 1041
  before kidney transplants, 578, 580
  chemolytic reactions to, 920, 922, 948–949
  compatible blood for, 948
  contaminated, 949
  emergency, 948
  exchange, after poisoning, 143
  for acute posthemorrhagic anemia, 891
  for anemia in chronic kidney failure, 571
  for aplastic anemia, 889
  for autoimmune hemolytic anemia, 919–
    920

Blood transfusions (Continued)
  for cold agglutinin disease, 921
  for hemolytic disorders, 909
  for immunoglobulin A deficient patients,
    1944
  for paroxysmal nocturnal hemoglobinu-
    ria, 923
  for thalassemia, vs. marrow transplants,
    936
  for thalassemia major, 931
  for vaso-occlusive crises of sickle cell dis-
    ease, 941
  granulocyte, for bacteremia, in acute leu-
    kemia, 1006
  hazards of, 948–950, 949t
    acquired immunodeficiency syndrome
      transmission as, 1801
    babesiosis as, 1885
    congestive heart failure as, 879
    cytomegalovirus transmission as, 1784
    hemosiderosis as, 1189
    hepatitis as, 823
    malaria transmission as, 1858
    purpura as, 1052
    Rocky Mountain spotted fever trans-
      mission as, 1742
    syphilis as, 1713
    Trypanosoma cruzi transmission as,
      1866
  in anemia treatment, 884
  indications for, 947
  massive, thrombocytopenia from, 1054
  neutrophil, 966
  platelet, 1006, 1058
  recipients of, hepatitis immunization for,
    64
  urticaria-angioedema after, 1950
Blood urea, distribution of, in healthy population, 80
  increase in, in acute kidney failure, 559–
    560
Blood urea nitrogen
  as indicator of renal filtration, 523
  in chronic dialysis patients, 576
  in hepatic encephalopathy, 853
  in renal artery occlusion, 633
  in upper gastrointestinal hemorrhage,
    797
  levels of, in pregnancy, 634
  tetracyclines and, 609
Blood vessels. See also Artery(ies); Veins
  autoregulatory adjustment of, shock and,
    240
  damage to, in immune complex disease,
    1962
  inflammation of, 2025. See also Vasculi-
    tis(ides)
  systolic wall stress on, 186
Blood volume
  circulating, effective, 518, 529, 535
    reduction of, 503, 531, 537
  increase in, and acute kidney failure, 558
    in heart failure, 220
  reduction in, hypovolemic shock from,
    237
    reference intervals for, 2400t
    regulation of, 190
    syncope from, 2074
Bloom's syndrome, 168, 1113
  and acute leukemia, 1001
  and neoplasms, 1096t
Blue bloaters, 297, 415
Blue rubber bleb nevus syndrome, 765
Blumer's shelf, 711
Blurred vision, from atropine, 139
  from diabetes mellitus, 1378
BMR (basal metabolic rate), 1130, 1320
Body casts, and hypercalcemia, 1503

Body fluid(s)
  acid-base balance in, disturbances in,
    549–558. See also *Acid-base balance,
    abnormalities in*
    normal range for, 549
  cytologic study of, for pancreatic cancer,
    782
  human immunodeficiency virus in, 1801
  in acute kidney failure, 562
  increased ratio of solutes to water in,
    542–543
  ionic composition of, kidneys and, 510
  osmolality disturbances in, 536–543
  vascular-interstitial shifts in, 534
Body fluid volume
  nonsteroidal anti-inflammatory agents
    and, 609
  balance in, protection of, 529
  contraction of, and metabolic alkalosis,
    555
  depletion of, 531–534
    in chronic kidney failure, management
      of, 569
    vs. syndrome of inappropriate antidi-
      uretic hormone secretion, 541
  disorders of, 529–536
  excess of, 535–536, 535t
  regulation of, kidneys and, 510, 529–531,
    530
Body mass index, 1209
  age and, and mortality, 1221
  and obesity, 1219–1220, 1220
Body temperature. See also *Fever*
  basal, ovulation and, 1430, 1442
  increase in, from cocaine or ampheta-
    mines, 54
Body water, 529
Body weight, changes in, amenorrhea
    from, 1287
  set point of, 1223
  sodium retention and, 514
Boerhaave's syndrome, 688
Bohr effect, 2369
  and oxygen delivery, 927
Bohr equation, 485
Bolivian hemorrhagic fever, 1834–1835
Bombesin, for cancer, 1129
Bone(s), 1473–1476. See also *Bone marrow*
  achondroplasia of, 1520
  cancellous, examination of, magnetic res-
    onance imaging for, 85
  changes in, from growth hormone hy-
    persecretion, 1300–1301
  cortical, 1473, 1474
  demineralization of, in rheumatoid arthri-
    tis, 1991–1992
  density of, 1511
    disorders increasing, 1518–1519. See
      also *Osteosclerosis*
    in osteomalacia, 1483
    measurement of, 1513
  destruction of, by extradural tumors,
    2255
    in osteomyelitis, 1622
  diffusion of antimicrobials in, 116
  disorders of. See also names of specific
      bone disorders
    from secondary biliary cirrhosis, 846
    in uremia, 507
    inflammatory, vs. extradural tumors,
      2255
    metastatic, and hypercalciuria from net
      bone resorption, 640
  dynamics of, 1475
  enchondromatosis of, 1520
  erosion of, in midline granuloma, 2032
  fibrous dysplasia in, 1519–1520, 1520
  formation of, 1474–1475, 1474, 1510

Bone(s) *(Continued)*
  fracture of, fat embolism syndrome from,
    450
    with minimal trauma, 1180
  function of, 1473
  gumma of, 1717
  hereditary multiple exostoses in, 1520
  Hodgkin's disease and, 1016
  homeostasis of, 1469–1476
  hyperparathyroidism and, 1489
  in mastocytosis, 1973
  infarct of, and osteosarcoma, 1521
    in vaso-occlusive crisis, in sickle cell
      anemia, 939
  infection of
    anaerobic, 1639
    from congenital rubella, 1777
    mycobacteria, 1695
    quinolones for, 122
    staphylococcal, 1599–1600
    therapy duration for, 122
    with *Haemophilus influenzae*, 1619
  labeling of, with tetracycline, 1484
  lamellar, 1475
  lesions of, from congenital rubella, 1777
    in blastomycosis, 1842
    vs. gallstones, 865
  loss of, 1510
  magnesium in, 1195
  marrow of. See *Bone marrow*
  metabolic disease of
    from vitamin D deficiency, in Crohn's
      disease, 751
    osteoarthritis and, 2041
    patient evaluation in, 1475–1476
    risk factors for, 1477t
  mineralization of, 1472
    abnormal, osteomalacia or rickets from,
      1479
  necrosis of, 1517
  neoplasms of, 1521–1522
    metastatic, 1521–1522
      of bronchogenic carcinoma, 459, 462
      of colonic cancer, 771
      of renal pelvis transitional cell can-
        cers, 654
    steroids as analgesics for, 109
  osteolytic lesion in, from Langerhans cell
    granulomatosis, 1023
  osteomyelitis in, 1622–1624. See also *Os-
    teomyelitis*
  osteoporosis of, 1510–1515. See also *Os-
    teoporosis*
  pain in
    from acute leukemia, 1004
    from chronic myelogenous leukemia,
      990
    from multiple myeloma, 1029
    from myelofibrosis, with myeloid meta-
      plasia, 985
    from opioid withdrawal syndrome, 57
    from prostatic cancer, 1424
    from renal osteodystrophy, 1508
    from vitamin C deficiency, 1235
  parathyroid hormone and, 1487–1488
  periostitis of, in yaws, 1723
  remodeling of, from mycetoma, 1853
    in osteoarthritis, 2039
  resorption of, 1474–1475, 1474, 1510
    excessive, and resorptive hypercalci-
      uria, 640
    in cancer, 1102
    in inflammatory joint disease, 1984
  sarcoidosis in, 453
  sporotrichosis in, 1847
  structure of, 1473–1474, 1474
  trabecular, 1473, 1474
  tuberculosis of, 1690

Bone(s) *(Continued)*
  vitamin D in, 1478
  woven, 1475
Bone age, and sexual maturity ratings, 18
Bone hunger syndrome, 1195, 1495, 1498
  treatment of, 1499
Bone marrow
  abnormal erythroid precursors in, and
    sideroblastic anemia, 899
  allergic drug reactions in, 1971t
  anatomy of, 876–877
  and normocytic normochromic anemias,
    891
  aspiration of, for leukemia diagnosis,
    1004
  biopsy of, for Hodgkin's disease, 1019
    for myelophthisis, 890
  blood cell production in, 873, 873
  cell release from, 877
  cells of, chromosomal abnormalities in,
    and acute nonlymphocytic leukemia,
    974
  collagen deposition in, 985
  compartment of, abnormalities in, and
    neutropenia, 961–962, 962
  erythroid hyperplasia of, from hemolysis,
    909
  examination of, for neutropenia, 964
  failure of, anemia from, 884–890. See also
    Aplastic anemias
    hematopoietic progenitors and, 876
  for gene transfer, 160
  hairy cell infiltration of, 999
  heme synthesis in, 1182
  immune-mediated failure of, 886–887
  in aplastic anemia, 887
  in megaloblastosis, 901
  in myelofibrosis, with myeloid metapla-
    sia, 986
  in polycythemia vera, 982
  in visceral leishmaniasis, 1871
  infection of, and neutropenia, 962
  infectious granulomatosis of, 877
  injury to, myeloid metaplasia from, 985
  local irradiation of, 2378
  neoplasms metastatic to, myeloid meta-
    plasia from, 985
  plasmacytosis in, in multiple myeloma,
    1030
  radiation injury in, 2377, 2379t
  radiation therapy with chemotherapy
    and, 1119
  recovery of function of, reticulocytosis
    from, 882
  reference intervals for, 2400t–2401t
  replacement of, with bone, 1518
  response of, to hemolysis, 908
  suppression of
    and reticulocyte count, 882
    by drugs, 885
    from adenine arabinoside, 125
    from chemotherapy, 1020
    from immunosuppression therapy, 581
    from ribavirin, 127
    from TFT, 126
  transplants of, 1040–1042, 1536
    acyclovir after, 1537
    after whole-body radiation exposure,
      2377, 2379
    and monoclonal gammopathies, 1036
    and varicella immunization, 1790
    cytomegalovirus after, DHPG for, 126
    for adenosine deaminase deficiency,
      1173
    for aplastic anemia, 888
    for Chédiak-Higashi disease, 959
    for chronic granulomatous disease, 958
    for inborn metabolic errors, 157

Bone marrow (*Continued*)
  transplants of, for leukemia, acute lymphoblastic, 1005
      myelogenous, 992, 1005
    for myelofibrosis, 987
    for neutropenia, 964–965
    for osteopetrosis, 1518–1519
    for severe beta thalassemia, 936
    for severe combined immunodeficiency disease, 1537, 1946
    veno-occlusive disease from, 848
Bone mass, measurement of, 1476
Bone matrix, primary disorders of, and osteomalacia, 1482
Bonnevie-Ullrich syndrome, 388, 1414
  cryptorchidism in, 1415
Bordetella pertussis, 1624
Bornholm disease, 1810–1811
  vs. poliomyelitis, 2199
Boron, toxicity of, 2392–2393
Borrelia, relapsing fever from, 1724
Borrelia burgdorferi, Lyme disease from, 1726
Boston Collaborative Drug Surveillance Program, 102
Botulism, 1633–1634
  immunization against, 63t, 66
  in infants, vs. infantile spinal muscular atrophy, 2155
  vs. tick paralysis, 1923
Bouchard's nodes, 2040, *2040*
Boutonneuse fever, 1745
  clinical features of, 1738t
  epidemiologic features of, 1737t
Bowel. See *Intestine(s); Large intestine;* and *Small intestine*
Bowel disease, inflammatory. See *Inflammatory bowel disease*
Bowel habits, change in, 660
Bowen's disease of the skin, 1112–1113, 2337, 2389
Bowman's capsule, in nephron, 509
BPH (benign prostatic hyperplasia), 1422–1423
BPV (benign positional vertigo), 2123
  vs. transient ischemic attacks, 2169
Bq (Becquerel), 2375
Brachial artery, as access for cardiac catheterization, 211
Brachial neuritis, 2267
Brachydactyly, type E, as congenital malformation, 170
Brachymetacarpia, in pseudohypoparathyroidism, 1501
Bradycardia
  and cardiac output, 237
  beta blockers and, 287, 327
  from brain tumors, 2232
  from hypothyroidism, 369
  from hypoxia, 477
  sinus, atropine for, 139
Bradykinesia, definition of, 2142
  in parkinsonism, 2143
Bradykinin, from mast cells, allergic rhinitis and, 1952
  in vascular headache, 2130
  shock and, 239
Brain. See also under names of specific structures and tissues
  abscess of, 2181–2183, *2183*
    after cerebral epidural abscess, 2184
    anaerobic bacteria in, 1639
    and subdural empyema, 2184
    circulatory shunts and, 304
    diagnostic imaging techniques for, 2060
    empiric therapy for, 118t
    from listeriosis, 1671
    from *Staphylococcus aureus*, 1600–1601
    vs. viral encephalitis, 1823, 2194

Brain (*Continued*)
  AIDS dementia complex in, 2204
  and micturition abnormalities, 2107–2108
  angiography of, 2059
  arteries of, 2159–2160, *2160, 2161,* 2162
    atherosclerosis in, 319
    atherothrombosis of, 2165–2166
    occlusion of, 2166
      and multi-infarct dementia, 2090
    thrombosis of, 2164–2165
    trauma to, 2168
  as endocrine gland, 1253
  atherothrombotic disease of, surgery for, 2171
  atrophy of, in alcoholics, 2138
  berry aneurysms in, sites for, *2174*
  blood flow to, 500
    heart disease and, 2164
  cardiorespiratory arrest and, 500
  disorders of. See also *Stroke*
    and impotence, 1409
    and precocious puberty, 1427
    from alcoholism, 50
    from viral encephalitis, 2193
    metabolic, 2063–2066. See also *Metabolic encephalopathy*
    regional diagnosis of, 2080–2083
    respiratory failure from, 476
  edema of, 2080
    after near-drowning, 2371
    after stroke, 2172
    cerebral infarction with, 2162
    from bacterial meningitis, 1605, 1606
    from dialysis, 575
    from meningitis, treatment of, 1610
    from neoplasms, 1229
    from relapsing fever, 1725
    from Reye syndrome, 2209
    glucocorticosteroid therapy for, 129, 130
    in fulminant hepatic failure, 854
  ethanol and, 48
  examination of, computed tomography for, 83, *84*
    diagnostic imaging techniques for, 2058–2059, 2058t
    magnetic resonance imaging for, 85, *85*
  glucocorticoids and, 1347
  glucose consumption in, 1374
  hemorrhage in, from hypertension, *2178,* 2178–2180
  herniation in, 2062–2063
    surgical treatment to prevent, 2236
  in heart failure, 223
  in Wilson's disease, 1188
  infection of
    and epileptic seizures, 2218
    cladosporiosis as, 1855
    malaria as, 1858, 1859
      vs. rabies, 2201
    poliovirus, 2199
    toxoplasmosis as, vs. AIDS dementia complex, 2205
  inflammation of, focal, from listeriosis, 1671
    from infective endocarditis, 1590
  injury to, 2239–2240
    and secondary parkinsonism, 2144
    clinical appearance of, 2240–2241
    defibrination syndrome after, 1079
    dementia from, 28
    recovery and sequelae of, 2243, 2243t
    severe, prognosis in, 2071–2073, *2072*
  ischemia of, 2162–2173
    after head injury, 2240
    and infarction, 2175
    causes of, 2162t
    degrees of, 2162–2163

Brain (*Continued*)
  ischemia of, from anemia, from gastric cancer, 711
    from coagulation disorders, 2165t
    management of, 2170–2172
    neuropathology of, 2162
  malformation of, chronic alcoholism in mother and, 171
  mass lesions in, pathophysiology of, 2062–2063
  neoplasms of, 2229–2235, *2233*
    and diabetes insipidus, 1308
    and epilepsy, 2218–2219
    and secondary parkinsonism, 2144
    benign, 2229
    classifications and pathology of, 2229–2231, 2230t
    clinical manifestations of, 2231–2232, 2231t
    dementia from, 28
    diagnosis of, 2232, 2234
      differential, 2234
      imaging techniques for, 2059
    hemorrhage into, 2174–2175
    localization of, 2080
    pathophysiology of, 2231
    prognosis for, 2235
    treatment of, 2234, 2234t
    vs. hypercapnia, 477
    vs. Lyme disease, 1728
    vs. transient ischemic attacks, 2169
  oxygen consumption by, 500
  prophylactic irradiation of, in small cell lung cancer, 462
  sarcoidosis in, 453
  Schilder's sclerosis in, 2215
  schistosomiasis japonica in, 1900
  shrinkage of, from hypertonic disorders, 542
  structural lesions of, and secondary epilepsy, 2218
  thrombophlebitis of, vs. viral encephalitis, 1823
  thrombosis of, hyperglycemia from, 1289
  tuberculomas of, 1691
  vascular disease in, 2164, 2165t
    and seizures, 2219
    dementia from, 2090
    diagnostic imaging techniques for, 2059
  vasculitis in, from herpes zoster, 2197
  white matter in, spongy degeneration of, 2216
Brain death, 499, 2056, 2072–2073, 2073t
  from cerebral edema, in fulminant hepatic failure, 854
Brain stem
  and sleep cycle, 2077
  arteries to, 2160
  atherosclerotic cerebrovascular disease in, vs. multiple sclerosis, 2214
  capillary telangiectasias in, 2174
  cysts in, 2157
  damage to, from head trauma, 2240
  dysfunction of
    and dysconjugate eye movements, 2063
    as remote effect of cancer, 1105
    coma from, prognosis for, 2071
    sensory loss from, 2129
  infarction of, and esophageal motor disorders, 683
    vertigo from, 2124
  injury to, 2239
  lesions of, and progressive myoclonus epilepsies, 2222
    and thalamic pain, 2128
  metabolic depression of, vs. posterior fossa lesions, 2063
  poliovirus in, 2199
Branched-chain amino acids, 1159
  for hepatic encephalopathy, 853

Branched-chain aminoaciduria, 1159–1160
Branched-chain hyperaminoacidemia, 1150t
Branched-chain keto acids, for chronic liver disease with encephalopathy, 855
Branched-chain ketoaciduria, thiamin for, 1230
Branched-chain ketonuria, 1150t, 1159
thiamin for, 1230
Branchio-oto-renal syndrome, as congenital malformation, 170
Branhamella catarrhalis, pulmonary infections from, vs. meningococcal pneumonia, 1614
Branham's sign, 384
BRAO (branch retinal artery occlusion), 2298
Breast(s)
cancer of, 1452–1458
and hypercalcemia, 1502
and venous thromboembolism, 443
androgens for, 1419
combined-method therapy of, 1115t
estrogen and, 1445
male, 1457
androgen therapy contraindicated in, 1419
metastatic, 1456–1457
to bone, 888, 1522
to kidneys, 655
oral contraceptives as protection against, 1443
prognostic factors in, 1086
vs. immune system neoplasms, 1008
with pregnancy, 1457–1458
development of, 1449
disease of, 1449–1452
imaging techniques for, 1454
male, enlargement of, 1410–1411, 1450–1452, 1451. See also *Gynecomastia*
pubertal development of, 16, 18, 19t, 1426
Tanner stages for, 1436t
self-examination, 1453–1454
silicone injections in, and panniculitis, 2050
Mycobacterium fortuitum-chelonae and, 1693
traumatic panniculitis in, 2050
Breast feeding, and *Escherichia coli* infection prevention, 1655
in developing world, 1215
Breast milk, and human immunodeficiency virus transmission, 1801
glucocorticosteroids excreted in, 133
vitamin C in, 1235
Breathing, control of, 400–401
increased rate of. See *Tachypnea*
Breathing exercises, for chronic obstructive pulmonary disease, 417
Breathlessness, 185, 186, 394. See also *Dyspnea*
Bretylium
drug interactions with, 99
elimination rate for, 96t
for stabilizing ventricular fibrillation, 264
pharmacokinetic properties of, 266t
Bretylium tosylate, 271
dosing and adverse effects of, 269t
for arrhythmias in shock patients, 245
Brill-Zinsser disease, 1738, 1739
clinical features of, 1738t
epidemiologic features of, 1737t
manifestations of, 1740
Brim sign, 1516
Briquet's syndrome, 2101
Broca aphasia, 2087, 2087t
Broca's area, 2083, 2086
Brodie's abscess, 1622, 1623

Bromide, overdose of, and central nervous system, 2069
reference intervals for, 2402t
Bromocriptine
and reduction of prolactin levels, 1303
for chronic liver disease with encephalopathy, 855
for growth hormone secreting pituitary tumors, 1302
for hypoprolactinemia, 1288, 1450
for macroadenomas, 1303
for parkinsonism, 2145
for premenstrual syndrome, 1434
side effects of, 1450, 2145
to suppress lactation, 1449
Bronchi, cylindroma of, 463
obstruction of, in mechanical ventilation, 488
Bronchiectasis, 438–440
and mycobacteria infection, 1694
and obstructive ventilatory disorders, 399
atelectasis with, 419
chronic respiratory failure from, 475
cough from, 391
cylindric, 438
cystic, bronchogenic cysts vs., 420
dextrocardia and, 315
familial causes of, 439, 439t
hemoptysis from, 391
in cystic fibrosis, 440
in sarcoidosis, 454
pulmonary embolism vs., 444
saccular, 438
sputum in, 391
varicose, 438
vs. chronic bronchitis, 413
Bronchiolitis, from respiratory syncytial virus, 1759
Bronchitis, 390
and breathing control, 401
and obstructive ventilatory disorders, 399
aspergillary, 1850
asthmatic, 412–414
chronic, 410–418
and mycobacteria infection, 1694
bronchiectasis vs., 439
pulmonary hypertension from, 296, 297
vs. asthma, 408
chronic respiratory failure from, 475
exercise and, 46
from *Haemophilus influenzae*, 1619
in infants of smoking parents, 39
industrial, 2360
mucopurulent, 412
viral, 1757–1758, 1758t
vs. leptospirosis, 1732
Bronchoalveolar lavage, 427, 1554
for alveolitis, 428
Bronchoconstriction, from beta blockers, 138–139
in carcinoid syndrome, 1468
Bronchodilation, from cannabis, 57
sympathetic nervous system and, 133
Bronchodilators, for chronic bronchitis, 413
for chronic obstructive pulmonary disease, 416
for chronic respiratory failure, 480
Bronchogenic carcinoma, 457–463
and atrial flutter, 258
cough from, 391
hemoptysis from, 391
hypertrophic osteoarthropathy from, 1519
metastasis of, to bone, 462
to central nervous system, 462
pleural involvement in, 469
pulmonary embolism vs., 444
small cell vs. non-small cell, 459, 459t
solitary pulmonary nodules as, 464–465

Bronchography, 413
for bronchiectasis, 439
for unilateral hyperlucent lung, 420
Bronchopneumonia, definition of, 1556
from glanders, 1670
vs. acute paragonimiasis, 1903
Bronchoscopy
fiberoptic, 486, 1554
for solitary pulmonary nodules, 464
for atelectasis, 419
for bronchogenic carcinoma, 460
for hemoptysis, 392
for interstitial lung disease, 427
for lung abscess, 436, 437
Bronchospasm, airway narrowing from, 397
and airway obstruction, 475
Brown-Séquard syndrome, 2129, 2245, 2249
herpes zoster and, 2196
Brucellosis, 1676–1679, 1676, 1677t
splenomegaly in, 1037
vs. cat scratch disease, 1679, 1681
vs. psittacosis, 1736
vs. Q fever, 1749
vs. toxoplasmosis, 1878
vs. visceral leishmaniasis, 1872
Brudzinski's sign, from neurosyphilis, 2188
Brugia malayi, 1914
Brugia timori, 1914
Bruising, simple, 1059
Bruits
and stroke prevention, 2171–2172
from hepatocellular carcinoma, 859
in acute appendicitis, 802
internal carotid stenosis and, 2165
Brunner's glands, adenoma of, 713
Bruxism, 2079
BSF-1 (B cell stimulatory factor-1), 1934
Bubonic plague, 1661, 1662, 1662t
Buckthorn neuropathy, 2266
Budd-Chiari syndrome, 848–849
Buerger's disease, 382–383, 2026
vs. erythromelalgia, 378
Buffy-coat cells, and marrow transplants, 1041
Bulimia, 656, 1218–1219
emotional disturbances and, 657
Bulking agents, as laxatives, 722
Bullae, 420
Bullosis diabeticorum, 2332
Bullous disease, and mycobacteria infection, 1694
Bullous impetigo, 2329
Bullous pemphigoid, immunofluorescent cutaneous findings in, 2305t
in elderly, 2331
Bullous pemphigoid antigen, in dermis, 2302
Bumetanide, 232
as diuretic, for chronic kidney failure, 570
for hypertension, 286t
properties of, 231t
BUN (blood urea nitrogen) concentration, 523
Bundle branch block, electrocardiography for, 200
Buphthalmos, 2291
Buprenex, abuse of, 55
Buprenorphine, abuse of, 55
Burkitt's lymphoma, 975, 1009, 1010, 1013–1014
and Epstein-Barr virus, 1787
and Kaposi's sarcoma, 2340
appendicitis from, 801
malaria and, 1859
oncogenes in, 1092
proto-oncogenes in, 1091
Burnett's syndrome, 556, 701, 1492
hypercalcemia in, 1503
salt wasting in, 564

Burns
  acute phase response to, 1528
  and albumin degradation, 815
  and endocarditis, 1592
  and fluid volume depletion, 532
  and red cell membrane damage, 924
  and riboflavin deficiency, 1231
  and thermal injury to lungs, 2365
  aspergillosis in, 1851
  cross-infection with, 1542
  from chemicals, 2374–2375
  in elderly, 25, 25
  of esophagus, from caustic compounds,
    144
  of oral commissure, in electric injury,
    2381
  shock from, and myocardial depression,
    239
  topical antimicrobial therapy for, 124
Burow's solution, for skin disorders, 2314
Bursitis, 2047
  apatite crystals in, 2038
  vs. acute hematogenous osteomyelitis,
    1623
  vs. gout, 1168
Buruli ulcer, from *Mycobacterium ulcerans*,
  1695
Buschke-Ollendorff syndrome, 1519
Busulfan
  and infertility, 1119
  aplasia from, 885
  chronic toxicity to, 991
  for cancer, 1123
  for myelofibrosis, 987
  for polycythemia vera, 983
  hypermelanosis from, 2344
  interstitial lung disease from, 434
Butorphanol, abuse of, 55
Butyrophenones, for schizophrenia, 2094
BW509U, 127. See also *Azidothymidine*
Byssinosis, 2360

C cells, 1505–1506
C peptide, and insulin, 1366
  reference intervals for, 2396t
C-peptide suppression test, for insulinoma,
  1385, 1386
C wave, in venous pulse, 176
Cachectin (tumor necrosis factor), 957
  and acute phase response, 1528
  and bone resorption, 1102
  and endotoxin, 1538
  fever from, 1526
  in inflammatory response, 1530–1531
  production of, 158
Cachexia, diabetic neuropathic, 2263
  of malignant disease, 1097
Cadmium
  and chemical pneumonitis, 2368
  and kidney damage, 612
  as testicular toxin, 1416
  poisoning with, 786, 2390–2391
Café au lait spots, 2343, 2343
  in neurofibromatosis, 2158
Caffeine
  and atrial premature depolarizations, 256
  and panic attacks, 2100
  and tinnitus, 2120
  and ulcers, 696
  metabolism of, in cigarette smokers, 39
  reference intervals for, 2402t
Caisson disease, osteonecrosis in, 1517
Calcifediol, 1484t
Calcification
  and epilepsy, 2218
  and mesenteric disease, 795

Calcification (Continued)
  annular, mitral regurgitation from, 347
  egg-shell, in silicosis, 2362
  from phosphate therapy, 1504
  in elderly, aortic stenosis from, 341
  in hyperparathyroidism, 1489
  of gallbladder, and carcinoma, 863, 865
  of heart, fluoroscopy for, 195
  of soft tissue, in hyperparathyroidism,
    1490
    in renal osteodystrophy, 1509
  of vascular system, from renal osteodys-
    trophy, 1508
  pineal and, 1314
Calcitonin, 1505–1506
  and diarrhea from medullary carcinoma
    of thyroid, 727
  and phosphorus excretion, 518
  as tumor marker, 1099
  for osteoporosis, 1514
  for Paget's disease, 1516–1517
  from tumors, 1103
  in calcium homeostasis, 1470
  in hyperparathyroidism, 1489
  radioimmunoassay of, 1506
  therapeutic use of, 1506
Calcitriol, 1484t
  before parathyroidectomy, 1510
  for renal osteodystrophy, 1509–1510
Calcium
  absorption of, 734
    parathyroid hormone and, 502
  and renin release, 1345
  arthropathies from, 2037–2038
  circulating forms of, 1470, 1470
  control of, in renal osteodystrophy, 1509
  deficiency of, 1472. See also *Hypocalcemia*
    and abnormal bone mineralization,
      1479
    and osteomalacia, 1481–1482
    in rickets, 1484
    treatment of, 1485
  dietary requirements for, 519, 1205t,
    1472, 1482, 1514
    in hypoparathyroidism treatment, 1499
  distribution of, 1471, 1472
  excess of, 1502–1505. See also *Hypercal-
    cemia*
  heart contractions and, 216
  homeostasis of, 1469
    calcitonin in, 1505
    in erythrocytes, 910
  in extracellular fluid, parathyroid hor-
    mone and, 1486
  in kidney stones, 638
  in mediation of hormone action, 1259–
    1260, 1260
  in muscle function, 2269
  in solitary pulmonary nodules, 464
  in urine. See also *Hypercalciuria*
    normal upper limit for, 639
    increased concentrations of, and parathy-
      roid function suppression, 639
  interaction with digitalis, 1499
  intravenous, for pancreatitis, 778
  levels of, control of, in renal insuffi-
    ciency, 1507–1508
    in chronic kidney failure, 565
  loss of, in Crohn's disease, 751
  metabolism of, glucocorticoids and, 1347
    kidneys and, 518–519
  normal ranges for, 1471, 1471
  reabsorption of, by kidneys, parathyroid
    hormone and, 1487
    thiazides and, 231
  reference intervals for, 2395t
  supplements of, in hypertension therapy,
    285

Calcium (Continued)
  transport of, relationship with calci-
    otropic hormones and bone cells, 1471
  tubular reabsorption of, triazides and,
    642
Calcium antagonists
  for asthma, 409
  for idiopathic restrictive cardiomyopathy,
    361
  for primary pulmonary hypertension, 301
  for Raynaud's phenomenon, 377
Calcium blockers, for primary pulmonary
  hypertension, 301
Calcium carbonate, as antacid, 701
  for renal osteodystrophy, 1509
Calcium channel blockers
  adverse effects of, 289t
  and intestinal motility, 724
  for angina pectoris, 327, 327t–328t
  for esophageal motor disorders, 686
  for hypertrophic cardiomyopathy, 358
  for migraine, 2131
  for smooth muscle relaxation in coronary
    arteries, 189
  for supraventricular arrhythmias in shock
    patients, 245
Calcium oxalate, deposition of, in joints,
  2038
Calcium phosphate, amorphous, in bone,
  1473
Calcium pyrophosphate dihydrate, in synovial fluid, 1994
Calcium pyrophosphate dihydrate crystal
  deposition disease, 2037. See also *Pseudogout syndrome*
Calculus(i)
  and acute kidney failure, 558
  appendicitis from, 801
  diet and, 45
  from cystinuria, 619
  from gout, 1165, 1167
  hematuria from, 503
  in bile duct, 867–868, 868. See also *Choledocholithiasis*
  pain from, 615
  renal, 505–506, 638–644, 638t
    as ureteral obstruction, 507
    calcium oxalate, in homozygous aden-
      ine phosphoribosyltransferase defi-
      ciency, 157
    clinical manifestations of, 641
    diagnosis of, 641–642
    2,8-dihydroxyadenine, 1172
    ectopic kidneys and, 649
    etiology and pathogenesis of, 638–639,
      639t, 639
    from chronic myelogenous leukemia,
      990
    from Crohn's disease, 750
    from Cushing's syndrome, 1355
    from distal renal tubular acidosis, 623
    from hyperoxaluria, 1136
    from hyperparathyroidism, 1489
    in inflammatory bowel disease, 758
    in primary hyperparathyroidism, 1492
    in xanthinuria, 1170
    prophylaxis of, 642
    treatment of, 642–644
    uric acid as, 641
    vitamin C and, 1236
    vs. transitional cell cancers of renal pel-
      vis, 654
  ureteral obstruction from, 614
Calf muscles, rupture of, vs. deep-vein
  thrombosis, 386
California encephalitis, 1826–1827, 2193
CALLA (common ALL antigen), 1002
Calmodulin, 1259

Calories. See also *Energy*
average daily expenditure of, 1368
fat equivalent of, 1227
from carbohydrate, 1208
in diet, 1206–1207
in total parenteral nutrition, 1247, 1249, 1249t
intake restriction of, in hypertension therapy, 285
supplementation of, 1243–1244, 1243t, 1244
total intake of, by diabetic patient, 1368
Calymmatobacterium granulomatis, granuloma inguinale from, 1711–1712
cAMP (3′,5′-cyclic adenosine monophosphate), 1306. See also *Cyclic AMP*
Camp fever, 1739
Campylobacter, 1648
and pus in stool, 730
enteritis from, 1648–1651, 1648t
erythromycin for, 121
gastroenteritis from, vs. appendicitis, 803
infection of, Crohn's disease with, 746
vs. ulcerative colitis, 756
Campylobacter fetus, infection with, vs. colitis, 750
Campylobacter jejuni
enterotoxin from, 1649
and secretory diarrhea, 727
food poisoning by, 784
infection of, clinical presentations of, 1649t
Camurati-Engelmann disease, 1519
Canavan's disease, 2216
Cancellous bone, 1473, 1474. See also *Trabecular bone*
examination of, magnetic resonance imaging for, 85
Cancer. See also *Carcinoma(s); Neoplasm(s); Oncogenes* and names of specific neoplasms
and androgen deficiency, 1414
and anemia, 881, 899
and mycobacteria infection, 1694
and venous thromboembolism, 443
ataxia-telangiectasia and, 1947, 2153
bacterial meningitis in, 1671
death rates from, *1083*
endocrine manifestations of, 1100–1103, 1101t
epidemiology of, 1092–1096
hepatic candidiasis in, 1848
historical background of, 1082
hyperglycemia and, 1101–1102
in cigarette smokers, 37–38
monocytosis in, 970
natural inhibitors of, 44
obesity and, 1224
Candida
parenteral hyperalimentation and, 1546
superinfection of, prevention of, 1537
Candida albicans, 1847, 2322
and ulcers, 696
and urinary tract infection, in diabetics, 629
endocarditis from, 1591
endophthalmitis from, 2293
in brain abscess, 2182
superinfection with, in chronic kidney failure, 566
vaginitis from, 1704, 1705
Candida parapsilosis, endocarditis from, 1591
Candida tropicalis, endocarditis from, 1591
Candidiasis, 677, 1847–1849
chronic, in AIDS, 677
esophageal, 688
in central nervous system, of transplant recipients, 2210

Candidiasis *(Continued)*
mucocutaneous, and nails, 2347
and polyglandular autoimmune disease, 1414
chronic, 1948
polyglandular deficiency with, 1461
myeloperoxidase deficiency and, 960
oral, vs. diphtheria, 1628
vs. secondary syphilis, 1716
peritonitis from, 794
skin infection with, 2321–2322, 2334
culture for, 2313
vaginal susceptibility to, oral contraceptives and, 1443
vs. glossitis, 678
Candidosis. See *Candidiasis*
Canicola fever, 1730. See also *Leptospirosis*
Canker sores, 675. See also *Aphthous ulcers*
Cannabis, abuse of, 57–58
Canrenoate, 232
Canrenone, 232
properties of, 231t
Cantharidin, dermatitis from, 1926
CAP (carbamyl phosphate synthetase), 1152t
deficiency of, 1158
Capillaria hepatica, 1911
Capillaria philippinensis, 1911
Capillary(ies)
blood flow in, velocity of, 189
fluid transfer between, and interstitium, disorders in regulation of, 535
nutritional, 240
obstruction of, in shock, 241
pulmonary, 421, *421*
Caplan's syndrome, 2002, 2362
with rheumatoid arthritis, 429
Capnocytophaga, gum infection with, 960
Capreomycin, for tuberculosis, 1687
Capsid, 1750
Capsomeres, 1750
Capsulitis, adhesive, 2042
Captopril
and kidney damage, 596, 612
as inhibitor of converting enzyme, 1345
as vasodilator, 233, 235
for hypertension, 287, 287t
in uremic syndrome, 570
primary pulmonary, 301
Carbamate insecticides, poisonings with, treatment for, 145
Carbamazepine
and antidiuretic hormone release, 540
and enhanced liver metabolism of other drugs, 99
as analgesic, 109
for epilepsy, 2226t, 2227
for Fabry's disease, 1145
for tabes dorsalis, 2189
for trigeminal neuralgia, 2135
metabolism of, inhibited by cimetidine, 100
reference intervals for, 2402t
side effects of, 2227
Carbamyl phosphate synthetase, 1152t
deficiency of, 1158
Carbapenems, resistance mechanisms of, 116t
Carbenicillin, 119
acute interstitial nephritis from, 603
elimination rate for, 96t
for lung abscess, 437
hypokalemia from, 546
in drug interactions, 124t
in kidney and liver failure, 117t
Carbenicillin indanyl sodium, for prostatitis, 1422
Carbenoxolone, for peptic ulcers, 701

Carbohydrate(s)
absorption of, 734
and ethanol, hypoglycemia from, 1383
and hypophosphatemia, 1471
dietary requirements for, 1207
digestion of, 733
for hepatic porphyria, 1185
high molecular weight, in connective tissue, 1982
in diet, acute kidney failure and, 562
for diabetic, 1368
ingestion of, and transient hypophosphatemia, 1193
malabsorption of, osmotic diarrhea from, 726
metabolism of. See *Carbohydrate metabolism*
Carbohydrate metabolism
disorders of, 1131–1137
essential fructosuria as, 1135–1136
galactosemia as, 1131–1133
glycogen storage diseases as, 1133–1135
pentosuria as, 1135
primary hyperoxaluria as, 1136–1137
exercise and, 46
hormones and, 1262–1263
in chronic kidney failure, 567
in uremic syndrome, management of, 571
liver disease and, 809
Carbon-11, for radiolabeling, 210
Carbon dioxide
binding of, to hemoglobin, 927
diffusion of, 399
elimination of, 557
inhalation of, and panic attacks, 2100
levels of. See also *Hypercapnia*
in shock, 241
production and elimination of, 549–550
reference intervals for, 2395t
retention of, with airway obstruction, 411
transport of, by erythrocytes, 910
Carbon disulfide, and germinal epithelium damage, 1416
Carbon monoxide
exposure to, angina pectoris from, 324
poisoning from, 2365, 2369
and secondary parkinsonism, 2144
treatment for, 143, 144
Carbon tetrachloride
abuse of, 59
and kidney damage, 612
fulminant hepatic failure from, 854
zonal necrosis from, 827
Carbonic acid, in blood, P_{CO_2} and, 475
Carbonic anhydrase inhibitors, and metabolic acidosis, 553
as diuretics, 231–232
side effects of, 2299
Carboxypeptidase, and dietary protein digestion, 734
Carbuncle(s)
definition of, 2334
in diabetes mellitus, 1380
renal, 628, 632
pyelonephritis with, 629
Carcinoembryonic antigen
and pancreatic cancer, 781–782
as tumor marker, 1099t, 1100
circulating, and colonic cancer diagnosis, 772
elevation of, and metastatic disease of stomach, 712
reference intervals for, 2395t
Carcinogenesis, oncogenes and, 1092
polyunsaturated fatty acids and, 1207
Carcinoid syndrome, 773, 1467–1468
diarrhea from, 727
niacin deficiency in, 1232

Carcinoid syndrome (Continued)
  photosensitivity with, 2352
  vs. mastocytosis, 1973
Carcinoid tumors, 463
  ACTH from, 1354
  and skin reactions, 1112
  appendicitis from, 801
  asymptomatic, in small intestine, 773
  bronchial, and growth hormone secreting
    pituitary tumor, 1301
  of ileum, vs. Crohn's disease, 750
  of thymus, 1975–1976
  tricuspid stenosis from, 351
  vs. VIPoma, 1388
Carcinoma(s). See also Cancer; Oncogenes;
    Neoplasm(s) and names of specific neo-
    plasms
  adrenal, primary aldosteronism from, 291
  ampullary, in gastrointestinal tract, 669
  anorectal fistulas from, 789
  basal cell, 2336t
    from occupational skin injury, 2375
    nevoid, 1095t, 1113
    of epidermis, 2337
  bronchoalveolar, 391, 458
  bronchogenic, 457–463. See also Broncho-
    genic carcinoma
  cavitated, bronchogenic cysts vs., 420
  definition of, 1084
  eosinophilia from, 1025
  epidermoid, of anus, 789–790
  estrogen and, 1445
  from granuloma inguinale, 1712
  gastric outlet obstruction by, 716
  hepatocellular, 857–858, 858t
    alcoholic hyalin in, 843
  infiltrating, giant hypertropic gastritis vs.,
    692
  lumen-obliterating, dysphagia from, 679
  medullary. See Medullary carcinoma
  metastatic, myelophthisis from, 890
    vs. multiple myeloma, 1030
  nasopharyngeal, anaplastic, and Epstein-
    Barr virus, 1787
  radiogenic, 1094
  secondary biliary cirrhosis from, 846
  vs. colonic diverticula, 723
  vs. rectal ulcers, 788
  vs. tuberculosis of colon, 1691
Carcinoma erysipeloides, 1108
Carcinomatosis, meningeal, prognosis for,
    2235
Carcinosarcoma, 464
Cardiac. See also Heart
Cardiac catheterization, 178, 211–214
  complications from, 211, 212t
  diagnosis from, 211t
  for anomalous pulmonary venous con-
    nection, 315
  for aortic regurgitation, 345
  for aortic stenosis, 342
  for atrial septal defect, 305
  for Eisenmenger's syndrome, 317
  for heart trauma, 369
  for hypertrophic cardiomyopathy, 358
  for infective endocarditis, 1593
  for mitral regurgitation, 349
  for mitral stenosis, 347
  for mitral valve prolapse, 350–351
  for ostium primum defects, 306
  for pulmonary hypertension, 296, 299–300
  for pulmonary veno-occlusive disease,
    302
  for tetralogy of Fallot, 309
  for valvular heart disease, 341
  in pulmonic stenosis, 312
  indications for, 212t
  percutaneous, 211

Cardiac glycosides, for heart failure, 225
  interaction of, with diuretics, 101
Cardiac index, 213
  ventricular end-diastolic pressure and,
    217
Cardiac output, 216–217
  aging and, 98
  and performance assessment, 216–217
  and pulmonary arterial pressure, 294
  calculating, 485
  decreased, from gastrointestinal bleeding,
    660
  definition of, 216
  exercise and, 217
  graphing of, 186–187, 187
  impairment of, from circulatory collapse,
    534
  increased, and hypertension, 278
    in chronic anemias, 879
  measurement of, 213, 244
    in critical care units, 494
    vasodilator drugs and, 191
  peripheral mechanisms to sustain, 220
  shock and, 237
  to kidneys, 510
Cardiac tamponade, 365–366, 365
  and sudden cardiac death, 275
  echocardiography for, 178
  pericardial, 176
Cardiogenic shock
  definition of, 331
  from myocardial infarction, 333
  isoproterenol contraindicated for, 247
  management of, 244
  mechanical ventricular assistance in, 249
  mortality rates with, 336
  nitroglycerin with dopamine for, 248
  steroids contraindicated for, 246
  surgery for, 249
Cardiomegaly, 177. See also Heart, enlarge-
    ment of
Cardiomyopathies, 352–362
  alcoholic, 353–354
    prognosis for, 354
  angina pectoris from, 323
  cryptogenic cirrhosis from, 847
  definition of, 352
  dilated, 352–355
    emboli from, and sudden arterial occlu-
      sion, 383
  endomyocardial biopsy for, 178
  hypertrophic, 176, 355–359, 356
    beta-adrenergic blockers for, 138
    digitalis contraindicated for, 228
    echocardiography for, 178
    mitral prolapse vs., 351
    obstructive, 185, 356
  idiopathic restrictive, 361
  ischemic, digitalis for, 228
  low output heart failure from, 216
  muscular dystrophy with, 2273
  pathophysiologic classification of, 352t
  peripartum, 354
    prognosis of, 354
  restrictive, 359–362, 359t
  scarring from, and atrial flutter, 258
Cardiopulmonary arrest, from electric in-
    jury, 2381
  from lightning, 2382
  pathophysiology of, 499–500
Cardiopulmonary bypass, thrombocyto-
    penia in, 1053–1054
Cardiopulmonary resuscitation, 499–501
Cardiothoracic ratio, 192
Cardiovascular disease
  cannabis and, 58
  diagnostic procedures for, 177–178, 191–
    214

Cardiovascular disease (Continued)
  diagnostic procedures for, angiography
    as, 214
    cardiac catheterization as, 211–214
    echocardiography as, 201–207
    electrocardiography as, 196–201
    nuclear cardiology as, 207–211
    radiography as, 191–195
  epidemiology of, 179–183
  from android fatness, 1223
  in cigarette smokers, 37
  mortality from, 179–181, 180t, 181
  obesity and, 1224
  plasma cholesterol concentrations and,
    81t
  research in, 181–182
  risk factors in, 182–183
    smoking and oral contraceptives as, 39
  symptoms of, 175t
Cardiovascular system
  after spinal cord trauma, 2246
  arachidonic acid metabolites and, 1275–
    1276
  disorders of. See also Cardiovascular dis-
    ease
    and anti-inflammatory drug impact,
      102
    and liver, 841–842
    assessment of, 179t
    diagnosis of, 178–179
    dialysis and, 576
    estrogen and, 1445
    from alcaptonuria, 1157
    from mycoplasmal infections, 1563
    in diabetic autonomic neuropathy, 2263
    in diabetic patients, 1380
    in uremic syndrome, 565
      management of, 570
    steatorrhea from, 744
  glucocorticoids and, 1347
  growth hormone and, 1301
  hormones and, 1263
  hypermagnesemia and, 1195
  in anorexia nervosa, 1217
  in Ehlers-Danlos syndrome, 1179
  in Japanese encephalitis, 1828
  pseudoxanthoma elasticum and, 1181
  response of, to acute gastrointestinal
    bleeding, 660–661
  stabilization of, with glucocorticosteroid
    therapy, 129
  syphilis in, 1717
    treatment of, 1721
Cardioversion. See DC cardioversion
Carditis, from rheumatic fever, 1582–1583,
    1582t
  prognosis for, 1584
  nonparoxysmal atrioventricular junctional
    tachycardia and, 262
Carmustine, for multiple myeloma, 1032
Carnitine, and dilated heart failure, 354
  deficiency of, 2036, 2270, 2278–2279
Carnosinemia, 1153t
Caroli's disease, 870
Carotenoids, 1237
Carotid artery, 2159–2160, 2160
  and atherothrombotic stroke, 2163, 2163
  aneurysms of, hypopituitarism from,
    1295
  asymptomatic lesion in, 2171–2172
  atherosclerosis in, 319
  disease of, symptoms of, 2168, 2168t
  endarterectomy, 2171
  occlusion of, 2165
  spontaneous dissection of, 2164
  trauma to, 2168
Carotid sinus pressure, and chest pain, 325
  for arrhythmias, 254, 255t

Carotid sinus pressure (Continued)
  for paroxysmal supraventricular tachycardia, 258
Carotid sinus syncope, type 1, 2075
  type 2, 2075
Carotidynia, 2132
Carpal tunnel syndrome, 1695, 2047, 2264, 2267–2268
  from rheumatoid arthritis in wrist, 2001
  in acromegaly, 1301, 2045
  in amyloidosis, 2266
    from hemodialysis, 1200
  in Scheie's syndrome, 1175
  vitamin B$_6$ and, 1234
Carpenter's syndrome, 1203
Carrión's disease, 1681
Cartilage
  damage to, 1983
  degeneration of, 1978
  destruction of, in mucocutaneous leishmaniasis, 1874
    in relapsing polychondritis, 2038
  in osteoarthritis, 2039
  lubrication of, 1983
  of nose, leprosy in, 1698
  pigmentation of, in alcaptonuria, 1157
Carumonam, 120
Casal's necklace, 1232
Caseation, 1682
Casoni skin test, for echinococcosis, 1894
Castor oil, as laxative, 722
Cat(s)
  hookworm of, 1907
  tapeworm in, 1894
Cat scratch disease, 1679–1681, 1679t, 1680t
  eosinophilia in, 1025
  vs. mycobacterial lymphadenitis, 1695
  vs. sporotrichosis, 1847
  vs. toxoplasmosis, 1878
Catalase, deficiency of, in erythrocytes, 1187
Cataplexy, drop attacks from, 2127
  in narcolepsy, 2078
Cataract(s), 2289–2290
  after electric injury, 2381
  from atopic eczema, 2320
  from diabetes mellitus, 1378–1379
  from galactokinase deficiency, 1131, 1132
  from glucocorticosteroid therapy, 133, 1347
  glycosylation and, 23
  hypoparathyroidism and, 1498
  in myotonic dystrophy, 1414
  uveitis and, 2293
Catatonia, 2061t, 2093
  from phencyclidine, 59
Catechol-O-methyltransferase, and catecholamine action, 1282
  from catecholamines, 1462
Catecholamine(s), 136, 1253, 1281–1282, 1461–1462
  actions of, 1258–1262
  and myocardial contractility, 184
  and sodium reabsorption by proximal tubule, 513
  biologic roles of, 1463
  biosynthesis of, 1462, 1462
  concentrations of, pheochromocytoma and, 284, 284, 1464–1465, 1464
  degradation and elimination of, 1462–1463, 1462
  delayed afterdepolarizations from, 253
  excess of, 1462
    coronary artery thrombosis from, 330
    vs. hyperthyroidism, 1325
  for shock, 137
  heart rate increases from, and angina pectoris, 324

Catecholamine(s) (Continued)
  in cardiorespiratory arrest, 499
  in fluid volume regulation, 530
  metabolism of, 1256
    inhibition of, 101, 101t
  myonecrosis from, 354
  reference intervals for, 2395t
  synthesis of, 1253
  ventricular arrhythmias from, 271
Cathartics, ineffectiveness of, after poisonings, 142
Catheter(s)
  and bacteriuria, 630
  and Candida cystitis treatment, 1849
  arterial, for monitoring arterial pressure, 244
  balloon, 329
  in shock patients, 243
  indwelling, and peritonitis, 793
    procedures for, 1543–1544
    urinary tract infection from, 629
  infection from, 1532, 1543, 1545–1546
  intravenous, and enteric bacteria infections, 1659
    Hickman-Broviac, 1545–1546
  of heart, 211–214. See also Cardiac catheterization
  percutaneous, for direct adrenal vein sampling, 284
    for sclerosing cholangitis drainage, 870
    in diagnostic imaging of kidneys, 525
  recommendations concerning, and staphylococcal infection prevention, 1604
  sepsis from, from parenteral nutrition, 1250
  Silastic, and infection prevention, 1537
  Swan-Ganz type of, 212
  ureteral, for urinary tract obstruction treatment, 617
  urethral, for urinary tract obstruction treatment, 617
  urinary, and acute kidney failure, 558, 561–562
    for shock patients, 244
Catheterization, cardiac. See Cardiac catheterization
Cauda equina, 2248
  compression of, 2249
  pseudoclaudication of, 2254
Cauda equina syndrome, 2044
Caudate nucleus, 2141
  atrophy of, in Huntington's disease, 2148
Causalgia, 105, 2136
Caustic agents, poisonings with, treatment for, 144
Cave disease, 1838
Cavernous angiomas, spontaneous intracranial hemorrhage from, 2174
Cavernous hemangioma, 2339
  thrombocytopenia in, 1053
Cavernous sinus thrombosis, 2185
Cavitation, from coccidioidomycosis, 1840
  in legionnaires' disease, 1571
CBG (corticosteroid-binding globulin), 1341–1343
  reference intervals for, 2400t
CCNU (cyclonexyl-chloroethyl-nitrosourea), 2234
CEA. See Carcinoembryonic antigen
Cefaclor, in kidney and liver failure, 117t
Cefamandole, elimination rate for, 96t
  in drug interactions, 124t
  in kidney and liver failure, 117t
Cefazolin, 120
  elimination rate for, 96t
  for sepsis, 1540
  in kidney and liver failure, 117t
Cefmenoxime, 121t

Cefoperazone, 121t
  in drug interactions, 124t
  in kidney and liver failure, 117t
Cefotaxime, 120, 121t
  elimination rate for, 96t
  for gram-negative bacilli meningitis, 1610
  in kidney and liver failure, 117t
Cefotetan, in kidney and liver failure, 117t
Cefoxitin
  elimination rate for, 96t
  for Bacteroides fragilis, 120
  for peritonitis, 793
  for salpingitis, 1706
  in kidney and liver failure, 117t
Cefsulodin, 121t
  in kidney and liver failure, 117t
Ceftazidime, 120, 121t
  for peritonitis, 793
  in kidney and liver failure, 117t
Ceftizoxime, 121t
  in kidney and liver failure, 117t
Ceftriaxone, 120, 121t
  in kidney and liver failure, 117t
Celiac axis, 760, 761
Celiac disease
  adult, iron malabsorption in, 896
  human leukocyte antigens and, 1967
  hyposplenism from, 1039
  vitamin E deficiency in, 1239
Celiac sprue, 742–743. See also Nontropical sprue
  postvagotomy diarrhea vs., 704
  small intestinal ulceration from, 807
Cell(s)
  cholesterol content of, regulation of, 1139–1140
  division of, 162–163
  Gaucher, 1146, 1146
  hairy, 998–999, 999
  insertion of cloned genes into, 160
  Leydig, 1292
  proliferation of, proteins in regulation of, oncogenes and, 1091
  Sertoli, 1292
  transducer, 1280
Cell-mediated cytotoxicity, in organ transplants, 580
Cellophane tape test, for enterobiasis, 1910
Cellular cytotoxicity, antibody-dependent, 1937
Cellular immunity, and host defense, 1531–1532, 1531t
  depressed, 1533
  disorders of, management of, 1536–1537
Cellulitis, 2335
  crepitant, from anaerobic bacteria, 1639
  from Haemophilus influenzae, 65, 1619
  gas-forming, 1630t
  in opioid users, 56
  vs. acute hematogenous osteomyelitis, 1623
  vs. angioedema, 1951
  vs. familial Mediterranean fever, 1198
  vs. gout, 1168
Central cord syndrome, 2245, 2245
Central nervous system
  binding sites in, 136
  disorders of. See under specific disorders
  Gaucher's disease and, 1146
  Gnathostoma spinigerum in, 1911
  hormone secretion regulation by, 1255–1256, 1280–1285
  hypermagnesemia and, 1195
  irradiation of, 2378
  leukemia of, 1004–1006
  Lyme disease and, 1728
  lymphoma of, vs. AIDS dementia complex, 2205

Central nervous system (Continued)
poisoning of, 2068–2071, 2069t–2070t
radiation injury in, 2377, 2379t
regulation of hormonal secretion by, 1280–1285
stimulation of, and renin release, 1345
syphilis in, 1717–1718
treatment of, 1721
toxoplasmosis and, 1876, 1877
tuberculosis of, 1691
vasculitis of, 2026
Central venous pressure
increase in, from cocaine or amphetamines, 54
monitoring of, complications from, 497
in critical care units, 493
in shock patients, 243
Centromere, 2020
Cephalexin, elimination rate for, 96t
in kidney and liver failure, 117t
Cephaloridine, 120
nephrotoxicity of, 559
Cephalosporin(s), 119, 120, 121t
action of, 113t
and kidney damage, 609
and pseudomembranous colitis, 1632
cross-reactivity of, with penicillins, 123
in drug interactions, 124t
resistance mechanisms of, 116t
Cephalothin, 120
elimination rate for, 96t
in kidney and liver failure, 117t
Cephapirin, elimination rate for, 96t
Cephradine, elimination rate for, 96t
Cercariae, 1896
Cerebellar ataxia, 2125–2126
hereditary, 2152–2154
Cerebellar hemorrhage, 2179, 2179
Cerebellar nuclei, lesions of, and progressive myoclonus epilepsies, 2222
Cerebellopontine-angle tumors, vertigo from, 2124
Cerebellum
infarction of, vertigo from, 2124
midline dysfunction of, ataxia from, 2126
vestibular, 2121
Cerebral. See also Brain
Cerebral cortex, and epilepsy, 2217–2218
Cerebrospinal fluid
accumulation of, in cerebral ventricles, 2237. See also Hydrocephalus
breast cancer cells in, 1456
gamma globulin in, in multiple sclerosis, 2212
in bacterial meningitis diagnosis, 1606–1607
neurosyphilis and, 2190
pH of, and respiration modulation, 550
vs. pH of arterial blood, 551
rhinorrhea of, 1608–1609
sampling of, 2056
Cerebrovascular accident. See Stroke
Cerebrovascular malformations, and spontaneous intracranial hemorrhage, 2174
Ceruloplasmin, measurement of, and Wilson's disease, 832, 1188, 1189
reference intervals for, 2395t
Cerumen, and tinnitus, 2120
impacted, and hearing loss, 2118
Cervical collar, 2252
for osteoarthritis, 2041
Cervical muscle weakness, 2270
Cervical rib and thoracic outlet syndrome, 2268
Cervicitis, 1705
diagnosis of, 1704
Cervix
adenocarcinoma of, from diethylstilbestrol, 1434

Cervix (Continued)
cancer of, in cigarette smokers, 38
sexual lifestyle and, 1082
Chlamydia trachomatis in, and neonatal infection, 1735
dysplasia of, oral contraceptives and, 1443
ectopy of, vs. cervicitis, 1705
in menstrual cycle, 1430
mucus of, in menstrual cycle, 1430
Cesarean section, endometritis after, 1547
thromboembolism after, 443
Cestodes, 1890–1895
CG. See Chorionic gonadotropin
CGD (chronic granulomatous disease), 958
Chagas' disease, 352, 353, 1865–1869, 1921
and esophageal motor disorders, 684
Chagoma, 1866
Chanarin's disease, 2279
Chancre, from syphilis, 1714–1715, 1715
Chancroid, 1712–1713
ulcers of, 1715
genital, 1704, 2342
vs. granuloma inguinale, 1712
vs. lymphogranuloma venereum, 1711
Charbon, 1667
Charcoal, activated, for poisoning, 142
Charcot joints, 1379, 1717, 2046
from tabes dorsalis, 2189
Charcot-Bouchard aneurysms, 2178
Charcot-Marie-Tooth disease, 2264
vs. distal progressive muscular atrophy, 2155
Charcot's triad, 868
Chédiak-Higashi syndrome, 958–959, 959, 1057, 1113, 1534, 1536
neutrophils in, 959
vitamin C for, 1236
Cheilitis, 2348
in candidiasis, 677
Cheilosis, from riboflavin deficiency, 1231
Chelation therapy, 2387t
after poisonings, 143
for metal intoxication, 611
for thalassemia, 932
Chemoattractants, and inflammatory cell accumulation, 1987–1988, 1988
Chemodectomas, 1095t
Chemoreceptors
carotid body, and ventilatory response, 550
central medullary, and ventilatory response, 550
hypoxia and, 238
in circulatory system control, 190
shock and, 239
Chemotactic factor(s), 1530
crystal-induced, in inflammatory response, 1987
neutrophil reaction to, 951, 952
Chemotaxis, 1530
in neutrophils, abnormalities in, 958, 958t
inherited disorders of, 1534
Chemotherapy. See also under specific agents and disorders
agents for, 112
allopurinol and, for kidney failure prevention, 562
cannabis for patients undergoing, 58
combination, 1118–1119, 1119t
complications of, 462
radiation therapy with, 1119–1120
Chenodeoxycholate, 859
for gallstone dissolution, 862
Chenodeoxycholic acid, hyperbilirubinemia from, 814
Chest, closed compression of, in cardiopulmonary resuscitation, 500–501

Chest pain, 392–394. See also Angina pectoris
causes of, 324
from abdominal abscess, 793
from aortic stenosis, 341
from hypertrophic cardiomyopathy, 357
from mitral valve prolapse, 350
from myxoma, 367
from primary pulmonary hypertension, 299
in cardiovascular patient history, 175
in histiocytosis-X, 430
in pneumococcal pneumonia, 1557
manometric examination and, 685
treatment of, 393
Chest wall, 472–473
abnormalities in, respiratory failure from, critical care of, 490
disorders of, pain from, 393
respiratory failure from, 476
pain in, 175
static properties of, 395, 395
stiffness of, 485
tuberculosis of, 1689
Cheyne-Stokes respiration, in heart failure, 176, 221
Chiasm, lesions of, 2113
Chiasmata, 162, 163
Chickenpox, 1788–1790. See also Varicella
Chief cells, in stomach, 693
Chiggers, 1922
and scrub typhus transmission, 1746
Chikungunya, 1819
Chilblain, 379–380
Child(ren). See also Adolescence; Neonates
adenoviruses in, 1767
aortic stenosis vs. supra- and infravalvular lesions in, 342–343
birth defects in, 150, 170
fat content in, 18
gonorrhea in, 1708
immunization schedules for, 61t
infective endocarditis in, 1591
iron deficiency in, 893
paroxysmal supraventricular tachycardia in, 258
poisonings among, 141
polymyositis in, 2035
progressive muscular atrophy in, 2155
respiratory tract disease in, from parainfluenza viral disease, 1760
shigellosis in, 1646
stroke in, from syphilis, 2189
tuberculosis in, 1689
Child abuse, 42
insulin in, 1386
Childbirth. See Delivery
Chills, 391
from febrile transfusion reactions, 949
from hemolytic transfusion reactions, 949
in endotoxic shock, 1659
in fulminant meningococcemia, 1614
in pneumococcal pneumonia, 1557
in typhoid fever, 1641
Chinese restaurant syndrome, 786, 2132
Chironex fleckeri, 1930
Chiropsolmus quadrigatus, 1930
Chlamydia psittaci, 1732–1733
pneumonia from, vs. Legionella pneumonia, 1571
Chlamydia trachomatis, 1732–1733
acute urethral syndrome from, 628, 629
cervicitis from, 1705
lymphogranuloma venereum from, 1710
urethritis from, 1704
nongonococcal, 1702
treatment for, 630

Chlamydiae
  and Reiter's syndrome, 2007
  cultures for, 1703
  disease from, 1732–1737, 1733t
    conjunctivitis as, 2294
    in adolescents, 20
    in neonates, 1735
    psittacosis as, 1735–1737
    trachoma as, 1734–1735
    treatment of, 1733–1734
  erythromycin for, 121
    of infancy, eosinophilia and, 1025
  pneumonia, vs. pneumococcal pneumonia, 1558
  sexual transmission of, 1702t
Chloasma, from oral contraceptives, 1444
Chloracne, 2375
Chloral hydrate, for insomnia, 2078
  poisoning with, 2069t
Chlorambucil
  and infertility, 1119
  for Behçet's disease, 2049
  for cancer, 1123
  for chronic lymphocytic leukemia, 997
  for cold agglutinin disease, 921
  for focal glomerular sclerosis, 595
  for Hodgkin's disease, 1020
  for minimal change nephrotic syndrome, 594
  for polycythemia vera, 983, 984
  for Waldenström's macroglobulinemia, 1034
Chloramine, hemolysis from, 923
Chloramphenicol, 120
  action of, 113t
  and bone marrow injury, 962
  aplastic anemia from, 123, 885–886
  elimination rate for, 96t
  excretion of, 116
  liver metabolism of, 118
  marrow suppression by, 885
  penetration into spinal fluid, 116
  poisoning with, 140
  reference intervals for, 2402t
  resistance mechanisms of, 116t
Chlordiazepoxide
  and photosensitivity, 2351
  contraindications for, in chronic respiratory failure, 481
  metabolism of, inhibited by cimetidine, 100
  reference intervals for, 2402t
Chlorhexidine, as antibiotic, 1548
Chloride
  concentrations of, in ileal fluid, 725
    in stool, 725
  estimated safe and adequate daily dietary intake of, 1206t
  in urine, measurement of, 524
  levels of, in chronic kidney failure, 564–565
    in primary hyperparathyroidism, 1494
  reference intervals for, 2396t
Chloridorrhea, congenital, 726
Chlorinated hydrocarbons, and enhanced liver metabolism of other drugs, 99
Chlornaphazine, and cancer, 1093t
Chloroethylnitrosoureas, for cancer, 1123–1124
Chloromas, in acute leukemia, 1004
1–Chloro-2–nitropropane, for coccidioidomycosis prevention, 1841
Chlorophenothane, poisonings with, treatment of, 144
Chlorophenylalanine, for carcinoid syndrome, 1468
Chlorophyll, magnesium and, 1195

Chloroquine
  for amebic liver abscess, 837
  for malaria, 1550, 1860
  for porphyria cutanea tarda, 1187
  for sarcoidosis of skin, 457
  myopathy from, 2282
  side effects of, and eye, 2298
  toxicity of, to hemoglobin, 945
Chlorosis, from iron deficiency, 896
Chlorothiazide(s)
  and photosensitivity, 2351
  properties of, 231t
Chlorphenoxamine, for advanced parkinsonism, 2146
Chlorpromazine
  and cataract, 2289
  and riboflavin deficiency, 1231
  as alpha blockers, 139
  liver disease from, 829
  reference intervals for, 2402t
Chlorpropamide, and antidiuretic hormone release, 540
  for diabetes insipidus, 1312
  for diabetes mellitus, 1369, 1370t
Chlortetracycline, 121
  chronic kidney failure as contraindication for, 572t
  in kidney and liver failure, 117t
Chlorthalidone, for hypertension, 286t
  properties of, 231t
Cholangiocarcinoma, 859
  vs. pancreatic cancer, 783
Cholangiography
  dangers of, with cholangitis, 868
  for jaundice, 818
  transhepatic, 664–665, 665
    percutaneous, 863, 864, 869
Cholangiohepatitis, gallstones with, 861–862
  Oriental, 870
Cholangiopancreatography
  endoscopic retrograde, 664, 664, 671–673, 672t, 672, 779
    contraindicated for acute pancreatitis, 777
    for biliary tract, 863
    for chronic pancreatitis, 780
    for pancreatic cancer, 782, 782
    for sclerosing cholangitis, 869
Cholangitis
  from ascariasis, 1909
  in primary biliary cirrhosis, 844
  intermittent, 868
  sclerosing, 661, 869–870. See also *Sclerosing cholangitis*
  suppurative, acute, 1902
  vs. pyogenic liver abscess, 836
Cholecalciferol, 1477. See also *Vitamin D*
Cholecystectomy, 779, 856–867
  and postcholecystectomy syndrome, 872
  vs. cholecystostomy, 867
Cholecystitis
  acute, 865–867, 866
    radionuclide imaging for, 863
    technetium-labeled iminodiacetic acid scanning for, 665, 666
  chronic, definition of, 864
  emphysematous, 867
  from fascioliasis, 1902
  from obstruction of cystic duct by stones, 862
  in elderly, vs. appendicitis, 803
  liver congestion from, vs. viral hepatitis, 824
  pain from, 658
  vs. appendicitis, 801
  vs. familial Mediterranean fever, 1197

Cholecystitis *(Continued)*
  vs. myocardial infarction, 332
  vs. omentum torsion, 796
  vs. pyogenic liver abscess, 836
Cholecystography, 866
  oral, 862, 862
Cholecystokinin, and mesenteric circulation, 761
  in bile formation, 859
Cholecystokinin peptides, 657
Cholecystokinin-pancreozymin, 775
  for pseudo-obstruction, 720
  in gastrointestinal motility, 715
Cholecystolithiasis, 863–865. See also *Gallstones*
Cholecystostomy, vs. cholecystectomy, 867
Choledochal cysts, 870
Choledocholithiasis, 661, 867–868, 868. See also *Gallstones*
  endoscopic retrograde sphincterotomy for, 673
  jaundice from, 817
  vs. appendicitis, 801
  vs. postcholecystectomy syndrome, 872
Cholelithiasis, 680–682. See also *Gallstones*
Cholera, 1651–1653
  and secretory diarrhea, 727
  immunization for, 65
    before travel, 1550
  pancreatic, 1388–1389, 1389t
Cholestasis
  alpha$_1$-antitrypsin deficiency and, 838
  chronic, vitamin E deficiency in, 1239
  from drugs, 827
  from sarcoidosis, 840
  from staphylococcal exotoxins, 834
  in infants, from parenteral nutrition, 841
  in pancreatitis, 777, 779
  in suppurative cholangitis, 869
  intrahepatic, 868
    postoperative, 814
  of pregnancy, 841
    vs. primary biliary cirrhosis, 845
  pruritus from, 808
  recurrent, benign, 813
Cholesteatoma(s)
  hearing loss from, 2118
  lateral sinus thrombosis from, 2185
  prognosis for, 2235
Cholesterol, 1138
  accumulation of, in gallbladder, 871
  and coronary heart disease, 42–43
  carrying capacity of bile for, 860
  cell regulation of, 1139–1140
  conversion of, to testosterone, 1396
  crystals of, in synovial fluid, 1994
  dietary recommendations for, 1208
  excretion of, 1140
  function of, 1137
  in diet, 43
    for diabetic, 1368
  levels of
    and cardiovascular disease, 81t, 182
    changes in, 183
    control of, nicotinic acid for, 1232
    estrogen and, 1445
    excess, 1143. See also *Hypercholesterolemia*
    in hypothyroidism, 1329–1330
    low, and cancer, 44
      in polycythemia vera, 982
  prostacyclin and, 1271
  reference intervals for, 2396t
  serum reduction in, cholestyramine for, 157
  synthesis of, bile salts from, 859
    in liver, 810

Cholesterol (Continued)
transport of, lipoprotein for, 1137
Cholesterol 20, 22-desmolase, deficiency of, 1396–1397, 1397
Cholesterolosis, 871
Cholestyramine
and decreased absorption of other drugs, 99
and vitamin A deficiency, 1238
for bile acid diarrhea, 728
for diarrhea, from Clostridium difficile, 1632
for protoporphyria, 840
for pruritus, in primary biliary cirrhosis, 845
for serum cholesterol reduction in hypercholesterolemia, 157
for treating malabsorption, 741t
interaction of, with digitalis, 228
steatorrhea from, 744
Cholinergic agents, 139–140
agonist, 139
for gastroparesis diabeticorum, 718
for pseudo-obstruction, 720
Cholinergic receptors, 134–137, 135t
muscarinic, 137
Chondrocalcinosis, 2037
osteoarthritis and, 2041
vs. rheumatoid arthritis, 2000
Chondrodystrophies, 1520
Chondroitin sulfate, 1174
Chondromalacia patellae, 2040
Chondromatosis, synovial, 2048
Chondronectin, in connective tissue, 1982
Chondrosarcoma, 1521
synovial, 2048
Chordomas, 2231
Chorea(s), 2147–2149
causes of, 2147t
definition of, 2142, 2147–2148
from excessive dopamine, 2141
senile, 2149
Sydenham's, 1583, 2148
vs. epilepsy, 2225
Chorea gravidarum, 1585
Choreoathetosis, definition of, 2142
from hepatic encephalopathy, 853
Choriocarcinoma(s), 1421
and pulmonary hypertension, 295
solitary pulmonary nodules from, 464
Choriomeningitis virus, lymphocytic, 2193
Chorionic gonadotropin, 1101, 1254. See also Human chorionic gonadotropin
in cancer, 1102–1103
reference intervals for, 2396t
Chorionic villus, biopsy of, 168–169, 173
Chorioretinitis, 2293
Christmas disease, 155
Chromaffin cells, in adrenal medulla, 1463
Chromatin, 928
sex, 166–167
Chromatography, liquid, high-performance, for hormones, 1266
Chromium, 1242
and cancer, 1093t
estimated safe and adequate daily dietary intake of, 1206t
toxicity of, 2393
Chromoblastomycosis, 1854
vs. pulmonary blastomycosis, 1842
Chromogranin A, as tumor marker, 1100
Chromomycosis, 1854
Chromosome(s), 161–169
abnormalities in, 146, 165–166, 165t
and amenorrhea, 1437–1438
and chronic lymphocytic leukemia, 996
and congenital heart disease, 303
estimating risks for carriers of, 172

Chromosome(s) (Continued)
abnormalities in, frequency of, among live births, 166t
prenatal diagnosis of, 168–169
balanced reciprocal translocation in, 166, 166
breakage syndromes of, 168
heritable fragile sites for, 168
changes in, and leukemia classification, 1003
deletion of, 165, 166
disjunction in, 165
human, nomenclature for, 163, 164, 165
injury to, from ionizing radiation, 2376
inversions in, 165, 166
mapping of, 152, 153, 156t
pairing of, in meiosis, 163
preparation of, 163, 163
robertsonian translocation in, 166
sex, 162
abnormalities in, 167, 167t
clinical cytogenetics and, 167
nomenclature for, 163
translocations of, in Burkitt's lymphoma, 1013
variants in, 163
Chromosome studies, indications for, 167–168
Chubby puffer syndrome, 2079–2080
Churg-Strauss syndrome, 431, 2026, 2325
Chvostek's sign, 1497
Chylomicron(s), 734, 1138
and energy transport, 1138
in peritoneal cavity, and ascites, 792
Chylomicronemia, 1142–1144
primary, diet and, 43
vs. familial hypercholesterolemia, 1140–1141
Chylopericardium, 363
Chylothorax, 468
Chyme, control of, by stomach, 714
volume of, 725
Chymopapain, for dissolution of herniated disc, 2253
Chymotrypsin, and dietary protein digestion, 734
inhibition of, by alpha₁-antitrypsin, 838
CIE (countercurrent immunoelectrophoresis), for Haemophilus influenzae detection, 1620
in meningitis diagnosis, 1607
Cigarettes. See Smoking
Ciguatera, 1931
Ciguatera fish poisoning, 786
Cilia, immotile, 1416
Cimetidine
after head injury, 2243
and creatinine secretion, 522
and impaired iron absorption, 894
elimination rate for, 96t
gynecomastia from, 1411
inhibition of drug metabolism by, 100
interaction of, with procainamide, 101
reference intervals for, 2402t
side effects of, 700
Cimex hemipterus, 1921
Cimex lectularius, 1921
Cinchonism, from quinine, 1860
Cineangiography, coronary, 214
Cineradiography, for esophageal disorders, 684
Cinoxacin, for urinary tract infection, 630
Ciprofloxacin, 122
in kidney and liver failure, 117t
Circadian rhythms, 2077
pineal and, 1313
temperature and, 1526
Circle of Willis, aneurysm in, 2174

Circulatory system. See also Blood flow
collapse of, from diabetes insipidus, 1310
from fluid volume depletion, 532
compromise in, without external fluid losses, 534–535, 534t
disorders of, and pharmacokinetics, 97
maintenance of, after head injury, 2242
of lungs, 294
overload of, from blood transfusions, 950
peripheral, interaction of heart with, 190
regulation of, 189, 189–190
shunts of, 303–304
right to left, 304
Cirrhosis, 842–847. See also Hepatic... and Liver
and gynecomastia, 1411
and hepatocellular carcinoma, 858
anemia in, 892
ascites from, 792, 850–852
bacterial peritonitis with, 794
biliary, 844–846. See also Biliary cirrhosis
black pigment gallstones with, 861
bloody ascites from, 791
cardiac, 223, 847
causes of, 842t
cryptogenic, 846–847
focal, 857
from chronic active hepatitis, 833
gallstones in, 868
gastrointestinal hemorrhage from, 849–850
hemolysis from, 923
hepatorenal syndrome from, 852
hyponatremia in, 540
immunization for patients with, 63
in alcoholic liver disease, 842–844
in Crohn's disease, 749
pleural effusions from, 467
portal hypertension from, 847, 848
postnecrotic, vs. chronic active hepatitis, 832
subclinical encephalopathy in, 853
vs. constrictive pericarditis, 367
zinc deficiency in, 1241
Cis-platinum, 1124
administration of, 1117
and acute kidney failure, 559
and drug interactions, 1118, 1119
and kidney damage, 610
for cancer, 679, 1124
Citrobacter freundii, in intravenous infusions, 1545
Citrullinemia, 156, 1152t, 1158–1159
CJD. See Creutzfeldt-Jakob disease
CK. See Creatine kinase
Cladosporiosis, cerebral, 1855
Cladosporium bantianum, 1855
Cladosporium trichoides, 1855
Claudication
anemias and, 879
extremities' pulses and, 176
from arteriosclerosis obliterans, 380
from arteritis, 374
in cardiovascular patient history, 176
intermittent, coarctation of aorta and, 313
jaw, from giant cell arteritis, 2033
Clay, craving for, iron deficiency and, 880, 896
Cleft lip, prenatal diagnosis of, with ultrasonography, 173
Cleft palate, 170t
genetics and, 150
prenatal diagnosis of, with ultrasonography, 173
Clemastine fumarate, 1954t
Cleveland Family Study, 1754, 1768
Climacteric, definition of, 1444

Climate, and cold agglutinin disease, 921
  warm vs. cold, and chronic obstructive
    pulmonary disease, 417
Clindamycin, 121
  action of, 113t
  and pseudomembranous colitis, 1632
  diffusion of, in bone, 116
  elimination rate for, 96t
  interaction of, with curare, 101
  resistance mechanisms of, 116t
Clitoris, development of, 1392
  enlargement of, fetal exposure to andro-
    gens and, 1435
CLL. See Lymphocytic leukemia, chronic
Clofazimine, for leprosy, 1700
Clofibrate
  and antidiuretic hormone release, 540
  interaction of, with warfarin, 101
  metabolites for, kidney excretion of, 95
  protein binding by, liver or kidney dis-
    ease and, 94
Clomiphene
  for hypogonadotropic eunuchoidism,
    1417
  side effects of, 1442
  to induce ovulation, 1439, 1440, 1442
  to restore fertility, 1297
Clonazepam, for epilepsy, 2226t
  for myoclonus, 2151
  reference intervals for, 2402t
Clonidine
  absorption of, 88
  adverse effects of, 289t
  affinity of, for alpha receptors, 136
  and catecholamine levels, 1465
  and intestinal motility, 724
  and renin release, 1345
  in pheochromocytoma diagnosis, 284
  interaction of, with tricyclic antidepres-
    sants, 101
  to test growth hormone reserve, 1294
Clonorchiasis, 834, 835t, 1901–1902
Clonorchis sinensis, 1901–1902
  and bile duct carcinoma, 871
  and Oriental cholangiohepatitis, 870
  in liver, 835t
Clorazepate, for epilepsy, 2226t, 2227
  reference intervals for, 2402t
Clostridia
  disease from, 1629t, 1629–1636
    botulism as, 1633–1634
    enterotoxemias as, 1631
    myonecrosis as, 1629–1631, 1630t
    penicillin G for, 119
    pseudomembranous colitis as, 1632–
      1633
    septicemia as, 1631
    tetanus as, 1634–1636
    vs. emphysematous cholecystitis, 867
  in postoperative wounds, 1546
Clostridial myonecrosis, 1629–1631, 1630t
Clostridium botulinum, 1633
  immunization against, 66
Clostridium difficile
  and pseudomembranous colitis, 757
  Crohn's disease with infection by, 746
  enterotoxins from, and secretory diar-
    rhea, 727
  colitis from, 755
  overgrowth of, antibiotic therapy and, 123
  pseudomembranous colitis from, 1632
Clostridium perfringens, 1629
  food poisoning by, 784, 785
  vs. Escherichia coli, 1655
Clostridium tetani, 1634
Clostridium welchii, and hemolysis, 909, 923
Clostridium welchii exotoxin, red cell hemol-
    ysis from, 922

Clot lysis, reference intervals for, 2401t
Clotting factors
  deficiency of, in amyloidosis, 1200
  human biologic production of, 159
  liver-derived, elevated, and renal vein
    thrombosis, 634
  miscellaneous inhibitors of, 1081
  synthesis of, in liver, 810
Cloxacillin, 119
  in kidney and liver failure, 117t
Club foot, 170t
  and torsion dystonia, 2150
Clubbing
  of fingers and toes, 2046
    from bronchiectasis, 439
    from circulatory shunts, 304
    from infective endocarditis, 1589t
    from interstitial lung disease, 426
  of nails, 2347
Cluster headache, 2131–2132
Clutton's joints, 2011
  from congenital syphilis, 1718
CML. See Myelogenous leukemia, chronic
CMMoL (chronic myelomonocytic leuke-
    mia), 989, 991
C-MOPP chemotherapy program, for non-
    Hodgkin's lymphoma, 1011
CMV infections, 126, 1784–1786. See also
    Cytomegalovirus, infection by
Coagglutination (CoA), for Haemophilus in-
    fluenzae detection, 1620
Coagulase, from Staphylococcus aureus, 1596
Coagulation, 1060–1065. See also Blood coag-
    ulation; Hypercoagulable state
Coal tar, for psoriasis, 2316
Coarctation, reversed, 374
Coats' syndrome, in facioscapulohumeral
    dystrophy, 2274
Cobalamin. See Vitamin B₁₂
Cocaine
  abuse of, 54
    by adolescents, 21
  and catecholamine effect enhancement, 1282
  and intestinal infarction, 763
  poisoning with, 55, 2069t
  reference intervals for, 2402t
Coccidioides immitis, 1840
  infection of, in central nervous system, in
    transplant recipients, 2210
  solitary pulmonary nodules from, 464
Coccidioidin skin test, 1840
Coccidioidomycosis, 363, 1840–1841
  disseminated, 1841
  eosinophilia from, 1025
  pleural disease in, 468
  pustules from, 2334
  vs. cat scratch disease, 1681
  vs. cryptococcosis, 1845
  vs. pulmonary blastomycosis, 1842
Coccygodynia, 788
Cochlea, disorders of, and unilateral deaf-
    ness, 2119
Codeine, abuse of, 55
  as analgesic, 107t, 108
  potency of, 56
Coenurosis, 1894
Coffee
  and cancer, 44, 1096
  and hypertension, 285
  and pancreatic cancer, 781
  and thiamin deficiency, 1229
Coffin-Lowry syndrome, 170
Cognate T cell–B cell interaction, 1934
Cognition, disturbances in, in metabolic en-
    cephalopathy, 2064
Cognitive development, in adolescence, 17
Colchicine, and vitamin A deficiency, 1238
  side effects of, 1198

Cold
  and periodic paralysis, 2281
  asthma attack from, 407
  common, 1753–1757. See also Common
    cold
  disorders from, 2384–2385. See also Hypo-
    thermia
  prolonged exposure to, 379
  response to, 2304
    Raynaud's phenomenon as, 375
  urticaria-angioedema from, 1949
Cold agglutinin(s), 920–921
  Mycoplasma pneumoniae and, 1561
  testing for, 1564
Cold hemagglutinin syndrome, 1033
  and chronic lymphocytic leukemia, 996
Cold sore, 676
Colectomy, indications for, 759
Colestipol, and decreased absorption of
    other drugs, 99
  and vitamin A deficiency, 1238
  interaction of, with digitalis, 228
Colic, esophageal, 680, 684
  renal, 505
    kidney stones and, 641
Colipase, in fat absorption, 733
Colistin, 122
  action of, 113t
  elimination rate for, 96t
  in kidney and liver failure, 117t
Colitis
  acute, severe, treatment of, 758–759
  amebic, 1886
  and pus in stool, 730
  chronic, treatment of, 759
  Crohn's vs. ulcerative, 751t
  from clindamycin, 121
  fulminant, as contraindication for colon-
    oscopy, 670
  granulomatous, and colorectal cancer, 770
    monocytosis in, 970
    vs. ulcerative colitis, 671
  hemorrhagic, from Escherichia coli, 1655
    in yersiniosis, 1664
  ischemic, 763–764, 764
    hemorrhage from, 799
    in elderly, vs. ulcerative colitis, 757
    vs. adenocarcinoma of colon
    vs. diverticulitis, 804, 805, 771
  left-sided, 753. See also Ulcerative colitis
  microscopic, diagnosis of, with biopsy,
    731
    diarrhea from, 729
  pseudomembranous, 1632–1633. See also
    Pseudomembranous colitis
  ulcerative, 753–760, 787–788. See also Ul-
    cerative colitis
Colitis cystica profunda, and rectal ulcers,
    788
Collagen(s), 1043, 1981–1982, 1981
  and alveolar wall, 425
  biosynthesis of, 1982t
  excess, in dermis, 2341
  in arteries, 318
  in dermis, 2302
  metabolism of, vitamin C and, 1234
  mutation in synthesis of, 1178
  types of, 1982t
Collagen vascular disease
  and lymphoma, 1008
  and sinus thrombosis, 2184
  aneurysms with, 2174
  biopsy for, 569
  in lungs, 400, 476
  interstitial lung disease with, 429–430
  mitochondrial antibody in, 816
  pleuritis from, pulmonary embolism vs.,
    444

Collateral blood supply, 380
  checking for, 381
  to brain, 2163
  to gastrointestinal tract, 761
Collecting ducts, function of, 617
  in antidiuretic response, 537–538
  water permeability of, antidiuretic hormone and, 1306
Colles' fractures, in postmenopausal osteoporosis, 1512
Colloid, for fluid replacement, 533
  in thyroid, 1315
Colloid cyst, 2230
  prognosis for, 2235
Colon. See also *Large intestine*
  angiodysplasia of, vs. adenocarcinoma of colon, 771
  cancer of, 710, 766, 768–773
    and ischemic colitis, 764
    and monoclonal gammopathy, 1036
    as indication for surgery, 759
    clinical manifestations of, 770–771
    colonoscopy for, 671
    diagnosis of, 771
    metastases of, 771
    pathology of, 770, *770*, *771*
    prevention of, 772–773
    prognosis for, 772
    susceptibility to, 769t, 769–770
    treatment of, 771–772
    ulcerative colitis and, 755
    vs. adenomas, 766–767
    vs. appendicitis, 801
    vs. diverticulitis, 805
    with intestinal gas gangrene, 1629
  cathartic, from laxative abuse, 722
  damage to, from radiation therapy, 806
  dilatation of, 723–724
    and pseudomembranous colitis, 1632
    congenital, 170, 170t, 660
  diverticulitis of, 804–806. See also *Diverticulitis*
    vs. appendicitis, 801
  familial polyposis of, 767, *768*
    mesenteric fibromatosis in, 796
  function of, 714
  hemorrhage from, from *Campylobacter* infection, 1649
  in Chagas' disease, 1867, 1868
  infection of, vs. ischemic colitis, 764
  irrigation of, ineffectiveness of, after poisonings, 142
  motility of, disorders of, 721–724
  multiple polyposis of, genetic counseling for, 174
  muscle hypertrophy of, 771
  neoplasms of
    and occult blood with diarrhea, 730
    metastasis of, to kidneys, 655
    vs. diverticulitis, 804
    vs. ulcerative colitis, 756
  pain from, 658
  perforation of, fecal impaction and, 788
    from pseudomembranous colitis, 1632
  polyps of, colonoscopy for, 671
  strictures of, from ulcerative colitis, 757
  surgery on, aminoglycosides for prophylaxis in, 122
  toxic dilatation of, in ulcerative colitis, 755, *755*
    radiography for, 756
  transport in, 725
  tuberculosis of, 1691
Colonization, definition of, 1542
  of *Aspergillus*, 1850
Colonoscopy, 670, 671t
  for colitis, 756
  for colorectal cancer, 771

Colonoscopy (*Continued*)
  for Crohn's disease, 749
  for lower gastrointestinal hemorrhage, 799
  for polyp reomoval, 767
  preparation for, 671
Color anomia, occipital lobe damage and, 2080t
Color blindness, 150
Colorado tick fever, 1819–1821
  encephalitis from, 2193
Colorectal cancer, 768–773. See also *Colon, cancer of*
Colorimetric test, for urinary protein detection, 520
Colostomy, for colorectal cancer, 772
Coma. See also *Consciousness, altered*
  amnesia after, 2085
  causes of, 2062t
  definition of, 2061t
  emergency management of, 2067–2068
  from acute heroin reaction, 56
  from diabetes, in elderly, 26
  from drugs, depressant, 2068, 2070
    management of, 2070–2071
  from hyponatremia, 540
  from malaria, 1859
  from phencyclidine, 59
  from pontine hemorrhage, 2179
  from rabies, 2201
  from subarachnoid hemorrhage, 2176
  from treatment of diabetic ketoacidosis, 1376
  from viral encephalitis, treatment of, 2194
  Glasgow scale for, 2242t
  hepatic, 852. See also *Hepatic encephalopathy*
  hypothalamus and, 2103
  myxedema, 1329
    treatment of, 1331, 1331t
  nontraumatic, outcome from, 2071–2072, *2072*
Commissurotomy, mitral, 347
Common bile duct
  dilatation of, ultrasonography of, *863*
  distal, obstruction of, pancreatitis and, 870
  obstruction of, 862
  retained stones in, 869
  stones in, pancreatitis from, 868
Common cold, 1753–1757
  clinical manifestations of, 1755–1756, 1756t
  definition of, 1753
  diagnosis of, 1756
  enteroviruses and, 1810
  epidemiology of, 1754–1755
  etiology of, 1753t, 1753–1754
  incidence and prevalence of, 1754
  pathology of, 1755
  treatment and prevention of, 1756
  vitamin C for, 1236
  vs. allergic rhinitis, 1954
  vs. whooping cough, 1625
Communication, disorders of, after severe brain injury, 2240
  in schizophrenia, 2093
  with dying patients, 32
Communication skills, of physician, 70–71, 73
Community medicine, 7
Complement fixation test, for histoplasmosis, 1839
  for Q fever, 1749
Complement fragments, 952
  and neutrophil adhesiveness, 957
  macrophages and, 1937
Complement pathway, 918

Complement system, 1938–1941
  abnormalities of, acquired, 1940–1941
    inherited, 1940, 1940t
  activation of, by blood transfusion, 948
    in sepsis, 1539
  alternative pathway in, 1938–1939, *1939*
  and paroxysmal nocturnal hemoglobinuria, 922
  and urticaria-angioedema, 1950
  clinical measurements of, 1941
  deficiency in, 1534, 1948
    and meningococcal disease, 1613
    and systemic lupus erythematosus, 2012
    bronchiectasis from, 439
    whole fresh plasma for, 1536
  in acute interstitial nephritis, 603
  in inflammatory response, 1531, 1986–1987
  reference intervals for, 2396t
Compound nevi, 2338
Compound S (azidothymidine), for AIDS, 127, 1523, 1799, 1807
  reference intervals for, 2396t
Compression devices, external, for thromboembolism prevention, 387
Compression-entrapment neuropathy, 2267
Computers, for electrocardiography interpretation, 201
  in diagnostic imaging techniques, 87
COMT (catechol-O-methyltransferase), 1282, 1462
Concussion, amnesia following, 2076
  definition of, 2239
  labyrinthine, 2123
  to cervical cord, 2244
Condoms, and gonococcal infection prevention, 1710
Conduction disturbances, after intra-atrial surgery, 317
  after intraventricular surgery, 318
  in shock, 245
Conduction velocity, in nerves, 2057
  myelin loss and, 2212
Condyloma acuminata, 2324
  in AIDS, 677
  interferon for, 128
Congenital factors, aortic stenosis from, 341
  in acute leukemia, 1001
Congenital heart disease, 303–323
  and endocarditis, 1587, 1588t
  and pulmonary hypertension, 295
  brain abscess with, 2181
  circulatory shunts in, 303–304
  complete heart block as, 316
  counseling for, 303
  cyanotic, and brain abscess, 2182
  epidemiology of, 179
  etiology of, 303
  gout in, 1167
  malposition of heart as, 315–316
  lesions in, obstructive, 309–310
    shunt, 304–309
  surgically cured, in adults, 317–318
  transpositions as, 314–316
  uncured, adults with, 316–317
  ventricular septal defect as, 306–307, *306*
Congenital infection
  neurosyphilis as, 2189
  rubella as, 1776
    clinical manifestations of, 1777
  syphilis as, 1718
    IgM fluorescent treponemal antibody absorption test for, 1720
    treatment of, 1721
  toxoplasmosis as, 1876–1878
  with cytomegalovirus, 1784
  with herpes simplex virus, 1782
    diagnosis of, 1783

Congenital malformations, 169–171
  etiologies of, 169, 169t
  from vitamin A toxicity, 1238
  prevention of, 171
Congestive heart failure
  acute kidney failure from, 558
  and amyloidosis, 359
  and sleep interruptions, 2078
  as hypertensive complication, 293
  ascites from, 792
  atriopeptin in, 1279
  cough from, 391
  definition of, 215
  dilutional anemia from, 879
  during refeeding, 1214
  Eisenmenger's syndrome and, 317
  from anemia, from gastric cancer, 711
  from beta-blockers, 138
  from beta thalassemia, 931
  from blood transfusion, 879
  from fluid volume excess, 535
  from hypertension, 277
  from myxoma, 367
  from rheumatic fever, treatment of, 1585
  from sarcoidosis, 453
  hematuria from, 503
  hypomagnesemia in, 1196
  hyponatremia in, 540
  in radiographs, 193
  intestinal infarction from, 763
  lidocaine clearance and, 90, 97
  pleural transudates from, 467
  precipitating factors in, 224t
  proteinuria from, 503
  salt and water retention in, 190
  treatment of
    digitalis for, 228
    diuretics for, 230–233
    prazosin for, 139
  urine sodium concentration in, 524
  ventricular performance assessment and, 209
  vs. angioedema, 1951
  vs. asthma, 408
  vs. filariasis, 1915
Conidia, 1837
Conium maculatum, toxicity of, 787
Conjugate gaze, disorders of, 2116
Conjunctivae, dryness of, in vitamin A deficiency, 1238
  infection of, in Rocky Mountain spotted fever, 1742
Conjunctivitis, 2294
  from Haemophilus influenzae, 1619
  from shigellosis, 1647
  hemorrhagic, acute, 1814
  in inflammatory bowel disease, 758
  in Reiter's syndrome, 2007
  in trachoma, 1734
Conn's syndrome, 1358
Connective tissue. See under specific disorders
Connective tissue matrix, in atherosclerosis lesions, 321
Connective tissue syndrome, undifferentiated, 2021
Consanguinity, 149
  hereditary disease and, 147
Consciousness
  altered. See also Coma
    acute heroin reaction and, 56
    diagnostic approaches to, 2066–2067, 2066t
    from acute disseminated encephalomyelitis, 2209
    from herpes simplex encephalitis, 2195
    from viral encephalitis, 2193
    in complex partial seizures, 2220–2221

Consciousness (Continued)
    altered, in St. Louis encephalitis, 1826
      in subdural empyema, 2184
      neurologic examination for, 2067t
      psychiatric disorders and, 2066
      states of, 2061t
    brief loss of, 2073–2076, 2074t. See also Syncope
    definition of, 2061, 2083
    in cardiac tamponade, 366
    loss of, 2061
      from sedatives, 53
    metabolic encephalopathy and, 2063
    sustained impairments of, 2061–2066
Consolidation, in pneumococcal pneumonia, 1556
  radiograph of, 1557–1558
Constipation, 660, 721t, 721–722
  definition of, 660
Contact cheilitis, 2348
Contact dermatitis, 2318–2319, 2319t
  arthropods and, 1926
  from drugs, 1969, 1970t
  occupational, 2373–2374
  photoallergic, 2351
  steroid creams for, 130
  vs. angioedema, 1951
Contraceptives. See also Intrauterine contraceptive devices; Oral contraceptives
  after rubella vaccination, 1777
Contractures, in elderly, 30
Contrast media, for CT brain exam, anaphylaxis from, 2058
Conus medullaris, 2248–2249
Conversion disorder, 2101
Conversion reactions, 2076, 2102
  vs. epilepsy, 2225
Convulsions. See also Epilepsy(ies) and Seizures
  benign, from fever, 2218
  cannabis for, 58
  from barium, 2281
  from carotid sinus pressure, 254
  from cavernous sinus thrombosis, 2185
  from hypoparathyroidism, 1497
  from intracerebral hemorrhage, 2179
  from lateral sinus thrombosis, 2185
  from metachromatic leukodystrophy, 2216
  from opioid withdrawal syndrome, 57
  from St. Louis encephalitis, 1826
  from superior sagittal sinus thrombosis, 2185
  tonic-clonic, 2221
  vitamin B_6 for, 1234
  withdrawal, in alcoholics, 51
Cooley's anemia, 930–932
Coombs' positivity, methyldopa-induced, 103
Coombs' test, 881, 909
  direct and indirect, 918
COPD. See Obstructive pulmonary disease, chronic
Copper, 1241–1242
  accumulation of, 1188
    excessive, 839. See also Wilson's disease
    in liver, from primary biliary cirrhosis, 845
  and kidney damage, 612
  deficiency of, symptoms of, 657
  estimated safe and adequate daily dietary intake of, 1206t
  food poisoning with, 786
  hemolysis from, 923
  in urine, and Wilson's disease, 832
  reference intervals for, 2396t
  toxicity of, 2390
Copperheads, 1927

Coproporphyria, hereditary, 1184
Coproporphyrin, reference intervals for, 2396t
Cor pulmonale
  from acute respiratory failure, 475
  from chronic obstructive pulmonary disease, 415
    treatment of, 417
  from obstructive airways disease, 296
  from pulmonary embolism, 443, 444
  from sarcoidosis, 453
Cor triatriatum, 311
Coral snakes, 1927
  envenomation from, 1928, 1931
Cordotomy, for localized cancer pain, 111
  for somatic pain relief, 111
Cordylobia anthropophaga, 1925
Cornea
  inflammation of, from drying, 2296. See also Keratoconjunctivitis sicca
  Kayser-Fleischer rings in, 1188
  opacity of, in Fabry's disease, 1144
  phaeohyphomycosis of, 1854–1855
  protection of, in coma, 2068
  ulcers of, 2293
Cornification, 2301
Coronary artery(ies), 370
  angioplasty for, 329
  anomalous origin of, 308
  atherosclerosis in, 319
  bypass grafting of. See Coronary artery bypass grafts
  disorders of, 323–339. See also Coronary artery disease
    acute myocardial infarction as, 329–337
    angina pectoris as, 323–329
    prognosis for, 329
    surgery for, 337–339
    vs. intermittent cholangitis, 868
  fistula of, 308
  in hypertrophic cardiomyopathies, 355
  thrombosis of, and angina pectoris, 324
  vasoconstriction of, antidiuretic hormone and, 1307
Coronary arteriography, for unstable angina pectoris, 328
  in patient selection for coronary artery bypass grafts, 337
  to detect atherosclerosis, 326
Coronary artery bypass grafts, 337–339
  for angina pectoris, 328–329
  rejection of, cytotonic T lymphocytes and, 1965
  Y-linked inheritance and, 150
Coronary artery disease
  age-adjusted mortality rates for, 183t
  and general mortality rate, 180
  and myocardial infarction, 329, 330
  as hypertensive complication, 293
  beta-adrenergic blocking agents for, 287
  cardiac catheterization for, 211, 213
  cholesterol and, 42–43
  diet and, 1275
  digitalis and, 229
  ejection fraction and, 208
  electrocardiogram for, 177
  epidemiology of, 179
  exercise and, 46
  familial combined hyperlipidemia and, 1142
  from familial hypercholesterolemia, 1140
  genetics and, 146, 150
  in cigarette smokers, 37
  in diabetics, 1380
  mitral regurgitation from, 347, 348
  mitral valve prolapse vs., 350, 351
  mortality rates for, decline in, 36
    international, 180–181, 181

Coronary artery disease *(Continued)*
  myocardial perfusion patterns for, 209
  scarring from, and atrial flutter, 258
  shunt lesions with, 305
Coronary Artery Surgery Study, 338
Coronary heart disease. See *Coronary artery
  disease*
Coronary spasms, intermittent, angina
  from, 335
  myocardial perfusion imaging and, 209
Coronaviruses, common cold from, 1753–
  1754
  infection from, clinical manifestations of,
    1755–1756, 1756t
  seasonal occurrence of, 1755
Corpus callosum, demyelination of, 2140
  section of, for seizures, 2228
Corpus luteum, 1430, 1431
  estradiol from, 1432
Corpus striatum, 2141
Cortical bone, 1473, *1474*
  loss of, 1510
Corticoreticular epilepsy, 2218
Corticosteroid(s)
  and acute phase response, 1529
  and cancer, 1095
  and growth retardation, 749, 752
  and hair growth, 2350
  and histoplasmosis, 1838
  and lysosomes in shock, 242
  and neutrophil adhesiveness, 957
  and progressive varicella, 1790
  and prostaglandin production, 1274–1275
  and urinary tract infection, 629
  and vascular purpura, 1059
  cataract from, 2290
  cholestasis from, 827
  contraindications for, after head injury,
    2243
  erythrocytosis from, 980
  fatty liver from, 827
  for acute asthmatic attack, 409
  for alcoholic hepatitis, 844
  for aphthous ulcers, 676
  for aplastic anemia, 889
  for asthma, 408–409
  for bacteremic shock, 1616
  for brain swelling from meningitis, 1610
  for brain tumors, 2234
  for chronic active hepatitis, 832–833
  for chronic bronchitis, 413
  for chronic lymphocytic leukemia, 997
  for chronic obstructive pulmonary dis-
    ease, 416
  for chronic respiratory failure, 480
  for Crohn's disease, 752
  for drug-induced liver disease, 827
  for drug-induced thrombocytopenic pur-
    pura, 1049–1050
  for histoplasmosis, 1839
  for hypercalcemia, 1504
  for idiopathic pulmonary fibrosis, 429
  for idiopathic thrombocytopenic purpura,
    1051
  for interstitial fibrosis, 296
  for interstitial lung disease, 428
  for late-onset asthmatic response, 410
  for lipoid pneumonia, 2373
  for lymphomatoid granulomatosis, 431
  for minimal change nephrotic syndrome,
    594
  for multiple sclerosis, 2214
  for onchocerciasis, 1917
  for penicillin-induced interstitial nephri-
    tis, 604–605
  for pseudotumor cerebri, 2237
  for radiation pneumonitis, 2365
  for rheumatic fever, 1585

Corticosteroid(s) *(Continued)*
  for rheumatoid arthritis, 2004
  for sarcoidosis, 360–361, 456
  for shock, 246
  for systemic lupus erythematosus, 2017–
    2018
  for tuberculosis, 1688
  for ulcerative colitis, 759
  for ulcerative proctitis, 788
  for Wegener's granulomatosis, 2031
  in depressed patients, 2095
  in urine, measurement of, 1348
  induction of metabolism of, 99
  ineffectiveness of, for fulminant hepatic
    failure, 854
  side effects of, and eye, 2298
  systemic, for skin disorders, 2317
  therapy with, 595, 810
  topical, for allergic rhinitis, 1955
    for colitis, 759
Corticosteroid-binding globulin (transcortin), 1341–1343
  reference intervals for, 2400t
Corticosterone, reference intervals for,
  2396t
  secretion rates and plasma concentrations
    of, 1341
Corticotropin-releasing factor
  and assessment of ACTH function, 1293
  and cortisol production, 1344
  from hypothalamus, 1280
  from medullary carcinoma, 1506
  from neoplasms, 1101
  release of, 1283
  testing of, for Cushing's syndrome, 1349
Cortisol, 128, 129t, 130, 1253
  and insulin, 1374
  and sodium reabsorption, 516
  binding of, to mineralocorticoid recep-
    tors, 1257
  circadian rhythm of, 1344
  for adrenocortical insufficiency, 1296,
    1353
  for chronic respiratory failure, 480
  levels of, aging and, 25
    increased, causes of, 1348t
  metabolism of, 1343, *1343*
  methadone and, 56
  plasma binding of, 1341
  production of, regulation of, 1344
  radioimmunoassay for, 1348
  reference intervals for, 2396t
  secretion rates and plasma concentrations
    of, 1341
  sodium-retaining potency of, 129
  synthesis of, 1341
Cortisone, 129, 129t, 1343
  for ACTH deficiency, 1296
Corynebacteria, as contaminant in blood
  cultures, 113
  infection with, erythrasma from, 2321
  vancomycin for, 122
Corynebacterium diphtheriae, 1626–1627
Corynebacterium parvum, for renal cell carcinoma, 653
Corynebacterium vaginale, vaginosis from,
  1705
Coryza, from common cold, 1755
Cost-benefit analysis, 78
Co-trimoxazole, for pneumocystosis, 1880–
  1881
  for urinary tract infection, 630
Cough
  from bronchogenic carcinoma, treatment
    for, 463
  from esophageal carcinoma, 686
  from legionnaires' disease, 1571
  from mycoplasmal infections, 1562

Cough *(Continued)*
  from occupational asthma, 2359
  from pneumococcal pneumonia, 1557
  from psittacosis, 1736
  from tuberculosis, 1685
  headache from, 2132
  productive, 390–391, 420
Coumadin, in endocarditis treatment, 1594
Coumarin, and hair loss, 2349
  and vitamin K deficiency, 1076–1077
  embryopathy with, 1077
  skin necrosis from, 1075
Councilman bodies, in yellow fever, 1831
Courvoisier's law, 871
Courvoisier's sign, 661
  in pancreatic cancer, 781
  liver disease and, 809
Cowden's disease, cancer and, 1113
Cowden's multiple hamartoma syndrome,
  and neoplasms, 1096t
Coxarthrosis, 2040
Coxiella burnetii, pneumonia from, vs. *Legionella* pneumonia, 1571
  Q fever from, 1748
Coxsackieviruses, 1808, 1809t
  and thrombotic thrombocytopenic pur-
    pura, 1052
  infection from, myoglobinuria after, 2283
  vs. measles, 1774
CPM (central pontine myelinolysis), *2139,*
  2139–2140
CPPD (calcium pyrophosphate dihydrate),
  1994
Cradle cap, 2320
Cramps
  from cholera, 1652
  from cryptosporidiosis, 1882
  from ischemic colitis, 764
  from mesenteric artery embolism, 763
  from oral iron therapy, 898
  heat, 2382–2383
Cranial nerves, abnormalities in, from bac-
    terial meningitis, 1605, 1606
  and muscle weakness, 2270
  lesions of, in diabetic mononeuropathy,
    2264
Cranial neuralgias, 2135–2136
Craniopharyngiomas, 1298, 2230, 2231
  prognosis for, 2235
Craniotomy, for subdural empyema, 2184
CRAO's (central retinal artery occlusion),
  2297–2298
CRBP (cellular retinol binding protein),
  1237
C-reactive protein, 1528, 1529
  bacterial meningitis and, 1607
  in acute phase response, 1527
  in rheumatic disease, 1995
  in tularemia, 1666
  reference intervals for, 2396t
Creams, 2314
Creatine kinase, in muscle disease, 2271
  in polymyositis, 2036
  reference intervals for, 2396t
Creatine phosphokinase, 1099t, 1100
  level of, in hypothyroidism, 1329–1330
Creatinine
  clearance of, 522t
    and glomerular filtration rate, 522–523,
      523
    and initiation of dialysis, 575
    reference intervals for, 2396t
  clearance rates of, 567
  elimination of, by kidneys, 510
  in urine, and muscle mass, 1211
  levels of
    in pregnancy, 634
    in renal artery occlusion, 633

Creatinine (Continued)
  levels of, increase in, 558
    factors causing, 569t, 569–570
    in acute kidney failure, 559–560
  reference intervals for, 2396t
Crescent sign, 1517, 1850
CREST syndrome, 2341
  primary biliary cirrhosis with, 845
  vascular malformations in gastrointestinal
    tract from, 765
Cretinism
  from iodine deficiency, 1340
  from thyroid hormone deficiency, 1263
  from thyroid hormone excess, 1315
  sporadic, 1338
Creutzfeldt-Jakob disease, 2091, 2203, 2205–
    2206
  amyloidosis in, 1200
  from pituitary growth hormone therapy,
    1297
  spongiform degeneration in, 2216
  sterilization against, 1548
CRF. See Corticotropin-releasing factor
Crib death, 2079
  botulism and, 1634
  respiratory syncytial virus and, 1759
Crigler-Najjar syndrome, fasting hyperbili-
    rubinemia in, 814
  Type I, 813, 813t
  Type II, 813t
Crimean-Congo hemorrhagic fever, 1834
Critical care medicine, 482–501
Critical care units, 492–495
  attributes of, 482, 482t
  for head injury, 2242–2243
  hemodynamic monitoring in, 493–495
  hospital-acquired infections in, 1542
  oxygen therapy in, 2368
  respiratory monitoring in, 493
  staff in, 495
    psychologic consequences for, 497–498
Crohn's disease, 745, 745–752
  acute phase response to 1528
  adenocarcinoma in, 713
    of small intestine, 774
  and cancer of small intestine, 773
  and eosinophilia, 1026
  and pylephlebitis, 835
  and sphincter dysfunction, 728
  anorectal abscesses in, 789
  anorectal fistulas from, 789
  complications from, 749
  computed tomography for, 662
  definition of, 745
  demographic features of, 746t
  diagnosis of, 747–749
  epidemiology of, 745
  etiology and pathogenesis of, 746
  gastric outlet obstruction from, 707
  granulomatous peritonitis from, 795
  liver in, 841
  malabsorption in, 743
  pathology of, 746–747, 747
  polyarthritis in, 2008
  radiography of, 756
    air-contrast, 748, 748
  small intestine resection for, and mal-
    absorption, 743
  stool examination in, 730
  surgery for, 752
  total parenteral nutrition for, 1244, 1248t
  treatment of, 750–752
  vitamin E deficiency in, 1239
  vs. abdominal actinomycosis, 1674
  vs. appendicitis, 803
  vs. diverticulitis, 805
  vs. gonoccocal infection of rectum, 1707
  vs. intestinal tuberculosis, 1691

Crohn's disease (Continued)
  vs. peptic ulcers, 699
  vs. rectal ulcers, 788
  vs. ulcerative colitis, 671, 751t, 757
  vs. ulcerative proctitis, 788
  zinc deficiency in, 1241
Cromoglycate, for inhibiting intestinal se-
    cretion, 732
Cronkhite-Canada syndrome, 768
Crossed syndrome, 2166
Crossmatching, for blood transfusions, 948
Croup, from parainfluenza virus type 1,
    1761
  viral, 1757–1758, 1758t
    vs. epiglottitis, 1619
Cruveilhier-Baumgarten syndrome, 848
Cryoglobulinemia
  mixed, 2325–2326
    essential, 601
    tubulointerstitial involvement in, 606
    vasculitis in, 2027
    with hepatitis B, 820
  purpuric lesions in, 1059
Cryoprecipitate
  for dysfibrinogenemia, 1074
  for fibrinogen disorders, 1073
  for hemophilia A, 1068
  for von Willebrand disease, 1056, 1070–
    1071
Cryoprotein(s), and cold urticaria, 1949
  in synovial fluid, 1993
Cryotherapy, contraindicated for snake
    bites, 1929
Cryptococcosis, 1844–1846
  diagnosis of, 1838
  Hodgkin's disease and, 1017
Cryptococcus neoformans, 1844
  and urinary tract infection, in diabetics,
    629
  as central nervous system infection, in
    transplant recipients, 2210
Cryptorchidism, 1415–1416
  and testicular cancer, 1420
  definition of, 1404
  examination for, 1415
  unilateral, müllerian inhibiting factor de-
    ficiency and, 1395
Cryptosporidia, diarrhea from, 1523
Cryptosporidiosis, 1881–1883
Cryptosporidium, 1881, 1881–1882
  and diarrhea, 730
  in acquired immunodeficiency syndrome,
    1805–1806, 1804t
    diarrhea from, 729
    vs. Escherichia coli, 1655
Crystal(s), in synovial fluid, 1994
Crystallization, inhibitors of, concentration
    reduction of, 639
Crystalloid(s), in fluid replacement therapy,
    533
  supersaturation of, 639
CSF. See Cerebrospinal fluid
CSF-1 (macrophage colony-stimulating fac-
    tor), 876, 968
Cuirass ventilator, 486
Culex tarsalis mosquitoes, and western
    equine encephalitis, 1823
Culiseta melanura mosquitoes, and eastern
    equine encephalitis, 1824
Cullen's sign, 776
Cultures, of Haemophilus ducreyi, 1712–1713
Cupula, 2120
Curare, and urticaria, 1950
Cushing's syndrome, 708, 1304–1305, 1353–
    1357
  ACTH immunoassay and, 1348
  ACTH release in, glucocorticoids and,
    1348

Cushing's syndrome (Continued)
  and combined hyperlipidemia, 1143
  and hypercalciuria from net bone resorp-
    tion, 640
  and medullary carcinoma, 1506
  and obesity, 1225
  and testicular failure, 1417
  bilateral adrenalectomy for, and Nelson's
    syndrome, 1357
  carcinoma and, 1101
    bronchogenic, 459
  clinical features of, 1354t, 1354–1355
  corticotropin releasing factor testing for,
    1349
  cortisol in, 1266–1267
  CT scans in, 1356, 1357
  definition of, 1340, 1354
  dexamethasone suppression test for, 1349
  diabetes mellitus from, 1362
  diagnosis of, 1355, 1355–1356
  from carcinoid tumor of thymus, 1976
  galactorrhea in, 1450
  hyperpigmentation after adrenalectomy
    for, 2344
  osteoporosis from, 1513
  polycystic ovarian syndrome from, 1439
  sodium level in, 542
  tumor localization in, 1356
  vascular purpura in, 1059
C-xylose breath test, for malabsorption, 739
Cyanide-ascorbate test, and glucose-6-phos-
    phate dehydrogenase deficiency, 916
Cyanide-nitroprusside test, for cystinuria,
    619
Cyanocobalamin, 902
  chemical structure of, 903
  deficiency of, and ataxia, 2125
  for treating malabsorption, 741t
  urinary excretion test for, for malabsorp-
    tion, 737t
Cyanosis
  from absolute erythrocytosis, 977
  from hypoxia, 477
  from methemoglobinemia, 945
  from polycythemia vera, 981
  in fulminant meningococcemia, 1615
  in pneumocystosis, 1880
  in sulfhemoglobinemia, 946
  mutant hemoglobin and, 944
Cyclamate(s), and cancer, 1096
  and photosensitivity, 2351
Cyclic AMP, 1306
  and kinase activation, 1258–1259, 1259
  calcium ion and, 1259–1260
  in pseudohypoparathyroidism, 1501
  in urine, hyperparathyroidism and, 1489
  nephrogenous, in primary hyperparathy-
    roidism, 1494
Cyclocryotherapy, for glaucoma, 2291
Cyclonexyl-chloroethyl-nitrosourea, for as-
    trocytomas, 2234
Cyclooxygenase, inhibitors of, for prema-
    ture labor, 1276
  nonsteroidal antiinflammatory drugs
    as, 1275
  pathway of, 1271, 1272, 1273
Cyclopentolate, side effects of, 2299
Cyclophosphamide
  and antidiuretic hormone release, 540
  and infertility, 1119
  hypermelanosis from, 2344
  in adjuvant therapy for breast cancer,
    1457
  in immunosuppression therapy, 581
  prior to marrow transplants, 1040
  sideroblastic anemia from, 900
Cycloserine, and vitamin B_6 deficiency, 1233
  for tuberculosis, 1687

Cyclosporine
    and Epstein-Barr virus infection, 1787
    and hair growth, 2350
    for Behçet's disease, 2049
    in immunosuppression therapy, 581
    nephrotoxicity of, vs. transplant rejec-
        tion, 580
    to prevent graft-versus-host disease, 1040
Cyclothymic disorders, 2095
Cylindromas, 463
Cylindruria, 503
Cypionate, for androgen deficiency, 1419
Cyproheptadine, 1954t
    for carcinoid syndrome, 1468
    for galactorrhea, 1450
Cyst(s)
    bony, in osteoarthritis, 2041
    brain stem, 2157
    bronchogenic, 420–432
    choledochal, 870
    colloid, 2230
        prognosis for, 2235
    congenital, vs. mycobacterial lymphade-
        nitis, 1695
    epidermal inclusion, 2336t, 2337
    epidermoid, 1298
    in kidneys, 506. See also Kidney(s), cystic
        disease of
        benign vs. malignant, 645
    in spleen, 1039
    mesenteric, 795
    myxoid, 2347
    porencephalic, and epilepsy, 2218
    spinal cord, 2157
    synovial, 1998
    Toxoplasma, 1876
Cystadenocarcinomas, pseudomyxoma peri-
    tonei from, 794
Cystadenomas, of bile ducts, 857
    pseudomyxoma peritonei from, 794
Cystathionine beta-synthase, deficiency of,
    1160
Cystathioninuria, 1151t
    vitamin B6 for, 1234
Cystic duct, obstruction of, acute cholecys-
    titis from, 866
        by gallbladder stones, 862
Cystic fibrosis, 1534
    clinical manifestations of, 440t, 441t
    copper deficiency in, 1241
    diabetes mellitus from, 1362
    liver disease from, 840
    secondary biliary cirrhosis from, 846
    staphylococcal pneumonia in, 1600
    vitamin E deficiency in, 1239
Cystic medullary complex, 645t, 646, 648
Cysticerci, 1890
Cysticercosis, 1892
Cystine, in kidney stones, 638
Cystine-lysinuria, neonatal, 1153t
Cystinosis, 1154t
    Fanconi's syndrome from, 621
Cystinuria, 619–620, 734, 1153t
    and kidney stones, 641
    treatment of, 643
Cystitis, 628
    bacterial, 1704
    from Candida infection, 1848
        treatment of, 1849
    hemorrhagic, from adenovirus, 1768
        from immunosuppression therapy, 581
    vs. gonococcal infections, 1707–1708
Cytarabine, 1122. See also Cytosine arabino-
    side
Cytochrome P 450, metabolism of arachi-
    donic acid by, 1274
Cytokines, abnormality in secretion of, ac-
    quired immunodeficiency syndrome
    and, 1803

Cytomegalic inclusion disease, 1785
    and seizures, 2218
    vs. Chagas' disease, 1869
Cytomegalovirus
    acute hepatitis from, 819
    and polyclonal cold agglutinin synthesis,
        920
    and ulcers, 696
    chorioretinitis from, 2293
    infection by, 1784–1786
        in acquired immunodeficiency syn-
            drome, 1804t, 1806
        prenatal, 1785
        vs. congenital syphilis, 1718
        vs. infectious mononucleosis, 1788
        vs. toxoplasmosis, 1878
        vs. Q fever, 1749
        vs. viral hepatitis, 824
    neurologic disease from, 2198
    pharyngitis from, 1757
    transmission of, by blood transfusions,
        950
Cytopenia(s), from polycythemia vera treat-
    ment, 983
    preventing infection in, 1537
Cytoreduction, for primary thrombocy-
    themia, 1054
Cytosine arabinoside
    administration of, 1117
    and hepatic vascular lesions, 828
    aplasia from, 885
    for cancer, 1122
    for leukemia, acute myelogenous, 1005
        chronic myelogenous, 992
Cytotoxic drugs
    and spermatogenesis, 1414, 1416
    neutropenia from, 963t
    systemic, for skin disorders, 2318
    thymic hypoplasia from, 1974
Cytotoxicity, antibody-dependent cellular,
    1937
    cell-mediated, in organ transplants, 580

Dacarbazine, for cancer, 1126
    for glucagonoma, 1389
Dacryoadenitis, 2294
Dacryocystitis, 2294
Dactylitis, with periostitis, 2045
DAG (diacylglycerol), 1259
Dairy products. See also Milk
    brucellosis from, 1676
    Campylobacter infection from, 1648
    excessive ingestion of, and increased cal-
        cium absorption, 639
    listeriosis from, 1671
    vitamin D in, 1479
Dalmane, abuse of, 53
Danazol, for premenstrual syndrome, 1434
    for thrombocytopenic purpura, 1051
Dandruff, 2320
Dane particle, 821–822
Dantrolene, chronic hepatitis from, 828,
    831
    for malignant hyperthermia, 2282
Dapsone, and bone marrow injury, 962
    for skin disorders, 2317
    toxicity of, to hemoglobin, 945
Darier's sign, 1972
    cancer and, 1112
    definition of, 2313, 2335
Darmbrand, 1631
Darvon, abuse of, 55
    as analgesic, 107t
Datura stramonium, toxicity of, 787
Daunomycin, for cancer, 1125
Daunorubicin, for acute myelogenous leu-
    kemia, 1005

Davidenkow syndrome, 2274
Dawson's inclusions, in subacute sclerosing
    panencephalitis, 2206
DBP (vitamin D-binding protein), 1477
    loss of, from nephrotic syndrome, 1480
DC cardioversion, 273
    contraindication to, 230
    elective, for mitral stenosis, 347
    energy for, 273t
    for arrhythmias in shock patients, 245
    for atrial fibrillation, 260
        in hypertrophic cardiomyopathy, 358
    for atrial flutter, 260
    for ventricular tachycardia, 263
    in intermediate phase of cardiopulmo-
        nary resuscitation, 501
DCCT (Diabetes Control and Complications
    Trial), 1367
DDAVP (desmopressin), for diabetes insipi-
    dus, 1312
    for von Willebrand disease, 1056, 1071
DDS (4,4'-diaminodiphenylsulfone), 1699,
    1700
DDS syndrome, 1699
DDT, and enhanced liver metabolism of
    other drugs, 99
    poisonings with, treatment for, 144
Deafness. See also Hearing
    causes of, 2118–2119
    central, 2119
    definition of, 2119
    evaluation of, 2118
    from Alport's syndrome, 637
    from bacterial meningitis, 1606
    from congenital rubella, 1777
    from congenital syphilis, 1718
    from lightning, 2382
    from multiple sclerosis, 2213
    from mumps, 1780
    from noise, 2119, 2355–2356
    from relapsing polychondritis, 2038
    from sarcoidosis, 453
    from scrub typhus, 1747
    from typhus fever, 1740
    in malignant osteopetrosis, 1518
    mumps immunization and, 64
    pure word, vs. Wernicke aphasia, 2086
    treatment of, 2119
Death(s). See also Brain death
    accidental, due to poisonings, 140t
    sudden, from aortic stenosis, 341
        from Eisenmenger's syndrome, 317
        from pulmonary hypertension, 299
    sudden cardiac, 274–276
Debré-Sémélaigne syndrome, 2280
Debrisoquin, genetics in metabolism of,
    102
Decompression sickness, 2367
Decubitus ulcers, 2341–2342
    after spinal cord trauma, 2246
    and spinal epidural abscess, 2186
    in elderly, 30
Deer flies, and tularemia, 1664
Defibrillator, automatic implantable cardio-
    verter, for ventricular tachycardia, 273
Defibrination syndrome, 1053, 1078–1080.
    See also Disseminated intravascular coagu-
    lation
    definition of, 1078
Degenerative diseases, 2152–2159, 2153t
    definition of, 2152
    hereditary cerebellar ataxias as, 2152–2154
    hereditary spastic paraplegias as, 2154
    intrinsic motor neuron diseases as, 2154t,
        2154–2157
    of joints, 2039–2041. See also Osteo-
        arthritis
    phakomatoses as, 2158–2159
    syringomyelia as, 2157, 2157–2158

Degranulation, in neutrophil killing of microorganisms, 952, *953*
Dehydration
  from congenital hypertrophic pyloric stenosis, 717
  from diabetes insipidus, 1295
  from hemorrhagic fever, 1835
  from pseudomembranous colitis, 1632
  from vomiting, 659
  glossitis from, 678
  in diabetic ketoacidosis, 1375
  in nonketotic hyperosmolar syndrome, 1377
  in vaso-occlusive crisis, in sickle cell anemia, 939
  in western equine encephalitis, 1824
  maximal urine osmolality after, *1311*
  polycythemia from, 975
  vs. early septic shock, 1539–1540
Dehydroepiandrosterone
  increased levels of, in females, 1428
  measurement of, 1350
  reference intervals for, 2396t
  secretion rates and plasma concentrations of, 1341
  synthesis of, 1341
Deiodinase, 1316
Déjà vu, in partial seizures, 2220
Déjérine-Sottas disease, 2264
Deletion mutations, thalassemia from, 935
Delirium, 2063–2066
  definition of, 2061t
  from digitalis toxicity, 229
  from hypothalamic destruction, 2103
  from metabolic encephalopathy, 2063
  from subarachnoid hemorrhage, 2176
  neuroleptics for, 2094
  symptoms of, 2093t
  vs. dementia, 2087
Delirium tremens (DT's)
  impending, 51
  in alcohol withdrawal, 50–51
    with pneumococcal pneumonia, 1559
  Korsakoff's amnesia with, 2084
  treatment of, 51t
Delivery
  and endocarditis, 1591
  cesarean, endometritis after, 1547
    thromboembolism after, 443
  hemorrhage during, from hypopituitarism, 1295
Delta agent, hepatitis syndrome from, 819
  viral hepatitis from, 823
Delta-aminolevulinic acid, 1182, 1184
  reference intervals for, 2395t
Delusions, from amphetamine toxicity, 54
  in schizophrenia, 2092
  somatic, pain from, 105
Demeclocycline, diabetes insipidus from, 609
  in collecting tube defects, 505
  in kidney and liver failure, 117t
  vasopressin-unresponsive hyposthenuria from, 1309
Dementia(s), 2087–2092, 2188–2189
  and incontinence, 2108
  as contraindication for levodopa, 2146
  definition of, 2061t, 2087
  degenerative, apraxia in, 2087
  from cancer, 1105
  from chorea, 2148
  from Creutzfeldt-Jakob disease, 2205, 2206
  from metachromatic leukodystrophy, 2216
  from radiation therapy, 1107
  from subacute sclerosing panencephalitis, 2206

Dementia(s) *(Continued)*
  hydrocephalic, 2090
  in aged, 28–29
  multi-infarct, 2090
  neuroleptics for, 2094
  parkinsonism with, 2145
Demerol, abuse of, 55
  as analgesic, 107t
Demyelination, 2259. See also *Myelinopathy*
  and epileptic seizures, 2219
  and vision loss, 2112
  disorders causing, 2211–2217
    and internuclear ophthalmoplegia, 2116
  from acute disseminated encephalomyelitis, 2209
  from acute transverse myelitis, 2216–2217
  from multiple sclerosis, 2211–2215
  from neuromyelitis optica, 2215
  from progressive multifocal leukoencephalopathy, 2207
  in subacute sclerosing panencephalitis, 2206
  neuropathies from, 2057
    inflammatory, chronic, 2262
    large fiber loss in, 2129
  of corpus callosum, 2140
  of peripheral nervous system, in Guillain-Barré syndrome, 2261
Dendritic cells, 957, 2293
Dengue, 1816–1817
  hemorrhagic fever from, 1832–1833
  immunity to, and St. Louis encephalitis, 1825
  shock syndrome in, 1832
  vs. influenza, 1766
Dental procedures, endocarditis prophylaxis in, 1595, 1595t
  in aortic stenosis patient, 343
Dentition. See *Teeth*
Dentures, and oral candidal infection, 677
Deoxycholate, 859
2'-Deoxycoformycin, for cancer, 1123
  for hairy cell leukemia, 1001
11-Deoxycorticosterone, excess, 1359
  plasma binding of, 1343
11-Deoxycortisol, reference intervals for, 2396t
Deoxyribonucleic acid, 146
  altered structure of, and metabolic disease, 1130
  autoantibodies to, 1996t
  damage to, and lung cancer, 458
  of neoplasms, oncogenes in, 1091–1092
  random errors in, and aging, 23
  replication of, in meiosis, 162
  synthesis of, impairment of, in megaloblastosis, 901
  viral, 124
Deoxyribonucleoprotein, antibodies to, 1996
Depigmentation, from ACTH deficiency, 1295
Depolarization(s), atrioventricular junctional premature, 261–262
  of excitable cells, and sodium permeability, 545
Depressant agents
  alcohol as, 48
  poisoning with, 2069t
    coma from, 2071
    vs. brain death, 2073
  psychologic dependence on, 49
Depression
  among epileptics, 2228
  and pain, 105
  and sleep, 2079
  as neurosis, 2097t, 2097–2098
  brain stem, from acute cocaine toxicity, 55

Depression *(Continued)*
  chronic asthenia in, 2125
  definition of, 2095
  dementia vs., 28
  drugs for, 2096t
  from sedatives, 53
  from untreated pain, 106
  headache in, 2133
  in adolescents, 20–21
  in chorea, 2148
  in elderly, 28, 29
  pseudodementia from, 2088
  psychogenic, vs. metabolic encephalopathy, 2063
  symptoms of, 2093t
  vs. somatization disorders, 2102
De Quervain's syndrome, 1332, 2047
Dermacentor, and Rocky Mountain spotted fever transmission, 1742
Dermatan sulfate, 1174
Dermatitis, 2318–2322, 2319t. See also *Eczema(s)*
  and *Staphylococcus aureus* colonization, 1597
  atopic, 2320
  cercarial, 1897
  contact, 2318–2319. See also *Contact dermatitis*
  cumulative insult, 2374
  exfoliative, and albumin degradation, 815
    from drug allergy, 1970t
    from leprosy treatment, 1699
    in hypoparathyroidism, 1498
  fiberglass, 2375
  from cutaneous larva migrans, 1907
  from mites, 1922
  from poison ivy or oak, glucocorticosteroid therapy for, 131
  hyposplenism from, 1039
  perioral, 2334
  verrucous, 1854
Dermatitis herpetiformis, 2331
  sprue and, 743
Dermatoarthritis, lipoid, 2046
Dermatobia hominis, 1925
Dermatofibroma, 2336t, 2338
Dermatomyositis, 1978, 2341, 2341t
  and esophageal motor disorders, 683
  cancer and, 1106, 1112
  glucocorticosteroid therapy for, 130
  immunofluorescent cutaneous findings in, 2305t
  pulmonary hypertension from, 298
  vs. polymyositis, 2276–2277
Dermatophytes, infection of, in hair follicle, 2334
  in skin, 2321
Dermis, 2300, 2302–2303. See also *Skin*
  collagen in, 2341
Dermoepidermal junction, *2301*, 2302
  immunoreactants at, 2305
Dermographism, 1949
Dermoids, 2231
Dermopathy, diabetic, 1381
DES. See *Diethylstilbestrol*
Desensitization, 136
  for allergic rhinitis, 1955
Desferrioxamine, for aluminum intoxication, 1510
  for iron overload, 143
  in thalassemia, 932
Desipramine, reference intervals for, 2402t
Deslanoside, for heart failure, 227t
Desmethylmethsuximide, reference intervals for, 2402t
17, 20–Desmolase, deficiency of, 1398
Desmopressin, for diabetes insipidus, 1312
  for von Willebrand disease, 1056, 1071

Desmosomes, 2301
Detergents, ingestion of, and esophageal injury, 688
De Toni-Debré-Fanconi syndrome, and osteomalacia, 1481
Detoxification, 60
in liver, 811
Deuterium oxide, as testicular toxin, 1416
Devic's disease, 2215
Devil's grip, 1810–1811
vs. poliomyelitis, 2199
vs. pulmonary embolism, 444
Dexamethasone, 129, 129t
for adrenocortical insufficiency, 1353
for brain tumors, 2234
for typhoid fever, 1642
in ovulation induction, 1442
sodium-retention properties of, 130–131
suppression test for, 2095
Cushing's syndrome and, 1355
for excessive ACTH, 1293, 1304
for glucocorticoid function, 1348–1349, 1349t
Dextran, and platelet function defects, 1057
for fluid replacement, 245
for posthemorrhagic anemia, 891–892
Dextroamphetamine, abuse of, 54
as adjuvant analgesic, 109
Dextrocardia, 315
Dextropropoxyphene, for pain, in dying patients, 32
DFP (diisopropyl fluorophosphate), as cholinesterase inhibitor, 140
DGI (disseminated gonococcal infection), 1708–1709
and skin, 2325
vs. Lyme disease, 1728
DHEA. See Dehydroepiandrosterone
DHPG (9-1(1,3-dihydroxy-2-propoxymethyl) guanine), 126
DHT. See Dihydrotestosterone
Diabetes Control and Complications Trial, 1367
Diabetes insipidus, 1308–1312
after pituitary surgery, 1299
fluid volume depletion in, 531–532
from demeclocycline, 609
from Langerhans cell granulomatosis, 1023
from lithium, 611
from sarcoidosis, 453
from vasopressin deficiency, 1295
hypothalamus tumors and, 1286
nephrogenic, 505, 1309, 1310, 1312
pituitary, 1308
diagnosis of, 1310
vs. other polyuric syndromes, 1311, 1311
Diabetes mellitus, 1360–1381. See also Hyperglycemia
acute complications of, 1373–1374, 1376–1378
alcoholic hyalin in, 843
amyotrophy in, 2154–2155, 2264
and atherosclerosis, 320, 1144
and candidiasis, 1848
oral, 677
and cardiovascular disease, 182
and chylomicronemia syndrome, 1143
and corticosteroid-binding globulin, 1342
and dilated cardiomyopathy, 354
and kidneys, 624–627, 1379
and liver disease, 810, 828, 843
and melioidosis, 1669
and osteonecrosis, 1517
and periodontal disease, 675
and porphyria cutanea tarda, 1186
and sexual dysfunction, 1442

Diabetes mellitus (Continued)
and thalassemia, 931
arteriosclerosis obliterans and, 380
as contraindication for beta-blockers, 327
autonomic insufficiency in, 2106
cataract from, 2290
chronic complications of, 1378–1381
chronic interstitial nephritis in, 606–607
classification and diagnosis of, 1360–1361, 1360t
definition of, 1360
dermopathy in, 1381
diet for, 1246
elderly with, renal papillary necrosis in, 632
end-stage kidney failure from, 624
epidemiology and clinical presentation of, 1361–1362
foot ulcers in, 1379–1380, 1639
from android fatness, 1223
from glucagonoma, 1389
from glucocorticosteroid therapy, 130
from growth hormone hypersecretion, 1292
gallstones in, 863
gastroparesis diabeticorum from, 718
genetics of, 150, 1362–1363
glomerulopathy in, 624–626, 625, 626
glycosuria in, 619
human leukocyte antigens and, 1967
hypertriglyceridemia in, 1143
hypoglycemia in, from propranolol, 139
hypophosphatemia in, 1193
immunization for patients with, 63
in mothers, and congenital heart disease, 303
and congenital malformations, 171
insulin-dependent, 1360
and polyglandular autoimmune disease, 1414
clinical presentation of, 1362
in hemochromatosis, 1191
pathogenesis of, 1365–1366, 1366
vs. non–insulin-dependent diabetes, 1366
ketoacidosis in, 1373–1376. See also Diabetic ketoacidosis
kidney size in, 568
lactic acidosis in, 554
magnesium wasting in, 1195
malabsorption in, 744
metabolic bullous disease with, 2332
nephropathy in, dialysis and, 575
neuropathy in, 1379–1380, 2262–2264, 2263t
and neuropathic joint disease, 2046
and sphincter dysfunction, 728
classification of, 1379t
vs. appendicitis, 803
non–insulin-dependent, clinical presentation of, 1362
oral hypoglycemic agents for, 1370
pathogenesis of, 1364–1365
obesity and, 1224
painless infarction with, 330
pancreatic cancer and, 781
pathogenesis of, 1363–1366
peripheral vascular disease in, 110
pregnancy with, and kidney disease, 636
retinopathy in, 1378, 2297
secondary forms of, 1362
stress, 1288–1289
treatment of, 1366–1373
diet in, 1368–1369
insulin for, 1370–1373, 1372t
oral hypoglycemic agents in, 1369–1370
urinary tract infection with, 629
with chronic liver disease, 810
with cystic fibrosis, 441

Diabetic ketoacidosis, 553, 1373–1374, 1376–1377
pathophysiology of, 1375, 1375
pH of plasma and cerebrospinal fluid in, 551
rhinocerebral mucormycosis in, 1852
treatment of, 555, 1375–1377
Diacylglycerol, 1259
Diagnostic imaging techniques, 82–87. See also names of specific techniques
algorithmic approach to, 86
computers in, 87
financial considerations in, 86–87
for acute abdomen, 802
for back pain, 2044, 2251–2252
for biliary disease, 862
for breast cancer, 1454
for gastroenterology, 662–668
for neurologic disorders, 2058–2060
for pancreatic cancer, 782, 783, 783
of kidneys, 525–527
Dialysate, calcium concentration in, 1509
Dialysis, 573–577. See also Hemodialysis; Peritoneal dialysis
after poisonings, 143
and eosinophilia, 1026
and hypertriglyceridemia, 1143
and infection, 1542–1543
and pericardial disease, 363, 565–566
ascites in, 577
chronic, complications of, 576, 576–577
clinical use of, 574–576
dementia in, 577
encephalopathy in, 2389
for diabetic patients, 1379
for end-stage kidney disease, acquired renal cystic disease from, 647, 652
in diabetic patient, 627
for uremic syndrome, 507
hepatitis from, 566, 822
human immunodeficiency virus transmission by, 1801
hypersplenism from, splenectomy for, 1038
indications for, in acute kidney failure, 562
initiation of, 575–576
limitations of, 577
Mycobacterium fortuitum-chelonae infection and, 1693
routine management of, 576
technical aspects of, 573, 573–574
time-averaged clearance in, 574t
Diamines, as testicular toxin, 1416
4,4'-Diaminodiphenylsulfone, for leprosy, 1699
leprosy resistance to, 1700
Diapedesis, in hemorrhagic fever, from arenaviruses, 1835
Diaphoresis, from pheochromocytoma, 1464
from tetanus, 1635
Diaphragm, 471–472
dysfunction of, from systemic lupus erythematosus, 429
fatigue of, and cardiorespiratory arrest, 500
hernias of, 472
motion disorders of, 472
pain from irritation of, referred, 790
paralysis of, 472
pleurisy of, 392
Diaphragma sellae, 1290
Diarrhea, 660, 725–732
acute infectious, diagnosis and management of, 1650
after gastric surgery, 704–705
amebic liver abscess with, 836
and fluid volume depletion, 532

Diarrhea *(Continued)*
and riboflavin deficiency, 1231
bicarbonate wasting from, 553
chronic
and uric acid stones, 641
and vitamin K deficiency, 1076
as contraindication for gallstone dissolution therapy, 862
hypocitraturic calcium nephrolithiasis with, 643
treatment for, 758
diagnosis of, 729–731, 730t
epidemic, 1768
Giardia lamblia and, 1857
hypocitraturia from, and kidney stones, 640
of travelers, 1656–1657, 1657t. See also *Travelers' diarrhea*
osmotic, 660
overflow, from fecal impaction, 721
pathophysiology of, 726–729
potassium depletion from, 546
symptoms of, vs. Bartter's syndrome, 622
therapy for, 731–732
vs. fecal impaction, 788
watery, from polyps of large intestines, 767
Diarrheogenic syndrome, 1388–1389, 1389t
Diastematomyelia, 2258
Diastolic sounds, 177
Diazepam
abuse of, 53
contraindications to, in chronic respiratory failure, 481
for anticholinergic substance poisonings, 144
for delirium tremens, 51
for hepatic porphyria, 1185
for multiple sclerosis, 2214
for tension headache, 2132
half-life of, aging and, 98
metabolism of, inhibited by cimetidine, 100
reference intervals for, 2402t
side effects of, 2078
withdrawal syndrome for, 53
Diazoxide
for hypertensive crisis, 290t
for insulinoma, 1386
for primary pulmonary hypertension, 301
protein binding by, liver or kidney disease and, 94
Dibromochloropropane, and germinal epithelium damage, 1416
DIC. See *Disseminated intravascular coagulation*
Dichlorisoproterenol, 137
Dicloxacillin, 119
elimination rate for, 96t
in kidney and liver failure, 117t
Dicroceliasis, 1902
Dicumarol, and vitamin K, 1240
Diencephalon, compression or displacement of, and coma, 2062
lesions of, and progressive myoclonus epilepsies, 2222
Diet, 42–45
after myocardial infarction, 335
and appendicitis, 801
and cancer, 1082
colorectal, 768, 772
gastric, 710, 710t
and change in bowel habits, 660
and colonic diverticula, 723
and early reaction to radiation therapy, 806
and gout, 1169
and intestinal gas, 661

Diet *(Continued)*
and muscle disease symptoms, 2270
and peptic ulcers, 701
and primary pulmonary hypertension, 299t
assessment of, 1208–1209
bland, 1246
calcium in, 519
fiber in, 43, 1207, 1246. See also *Fiber, in diet*
folate sources in, 906
food variety in, 1204
for alcoholic hepatitis, 844
for chronic kidney failure, 571–572
for Crohn's disease, 751
for homocystinuria, 1161
for nontropic sprue, 743
for phenylketonuria, 1155–1156
for uremic syndrome, 507
for viral hepatitis, 824
in acute kidney failure, 562
in dental caries prevention, 674
in diabetes treatment, 1368–1369
in heart failure management, 225
in hypertension therapy, 285
in obesity treatment, 1225–1226
ketogenic, for seizures, 2228
liquid, 1246
magnesium in, 519, 1195
phosphorus in, 1193
protein in, hepatic encephalopathy and, 853
recommended nutrient allowances in, 1204, 1205t, 1206
restriction of, for inborn errors of metabolism, 156
restriction of macronutrient in, 1245, 1245t
sodium in, 514
supplementation of, components of, 1246, 1246t
triglyceride in, 1138
very low calorie, 1226
Dietary fiber, 43, 1207, 1246. See also *Fiber, in diet*
Diethylcarbamazine, for filariasis, 1914, 1915
for loiasis, 1918
for onchocerciasis, 1917
side effects of, 1915
Diethylstilbestrol, and adenocarcinoma of vagina or cervix, 1434
and masculinization of female fetus, 1404
for metastatic breast cancer, 1457
Diffusing capacity, in chronic obstructive pulmonary disease, 415
in sarcoidosis, 455
Diffusion
and gas exchange, 474
facilitated, definition of, 733
impaired, 401
in respiration, 399–400
passive, definition of, 733
Diflunisal, as analgesic, 107t
Difluoromethylornithine, for African trypanosomiasis, 1865
DiGeorge's syndrome, 1496, 1945
from thymic hypoplasia, 1974
thymosin fraction 5 for, 1537
Digestion, impaired, malabsorption from, 740–741
Digestive tract. See *Gastrointestinal tract*
Digibind, for digoxin poisonings, 143
Digit(s), clubbing of, 2046
from bronchiectasis, 439
cyanosis of, from Raynaud's phenomenon, 375

Digitalis. See also *Digitalis glycosides*
adverse reactions to, 102
and sinoatrial block, 261
after mitral valve replacement, 347
and amyloidosis, 360
and arrhythmias from hypokalemia, 547
and heart contractility, 184, 186
and testosterone synthesis inhibition, 1414
calcium interaction with, 1499
contraindicated, for cardiogenic shock, 248
for Wolff-Parkinson-White syndrome with atrial fibrillation, 260
delayed afterdepolarizations from, 253
drug interactions with, 228
for atrial fibrillation in mitral regurgitation, 349
for atrial premature depolarizations, 256
for heart failure, in chronic obstructive pulmonary disease, 417
for mitral stenosis, 347
gynecomastia from, 1411
magnesium deficiency and heart sensitivity to, 1196
multifocal atrial tachycardia resistance to, 261
pharmacology of, 227t
prophylactic use of, 228
sensitivity to, 228t, 228–229
serum concentrations of, 229
toxicity of, 229–230, 787
atrial tachycardia with AV block from, 258
AV junctional arrhythmias with atrial fibrillation from, 260
cardioversion contraindicated for arrhythmias from, 273
nonparoxysmal atrioventricular junctional tachycardia and, 262
treatment of, 230, 257t
ventricular premature depolarizations from, 263
Digitalis glycosides. See also *Digitalis*
electrophysiologic effects of, 226, 226t
for supraventricular arrhythmias in shock patients, 245
hemodynamic effects of, 226–227
in heart failure management, 226–230
mechanism of, 226, 226
pharmacology of, 227t, 227–228
Digitoxin
for heart failure, 228
half-life of, decrease by rifampin, 121
metabolism of, induction of, 99
inhibited by cimetidine, 100
pharmacokinetic parameters for, 89t
pharmacology of, for heart failure, 227t
protein binding by, liver or kidney disease and, 94
reference intervals for, 2402t
serum concentrations of, 229
Digoxin
adverse effects of, 266t
decreased absorption of, kaolin and, 99
distribution of, 89
dosages for, 266t
kidney disease and, 95
maintenance, 228
for atrial fibrillation, 260
for heart failure, 225, 266
in kidney disease patients, 95
interaction of, with other drugs, 101
pharmacokinetic properties of, 89t, 266t
pharmacology of, for heart failure, 227t, 227–228
poisonings with, 92

Digoxin (Continued)
poisonings with, Fab fragments for, 143
physiologic changes and, 94
reference intervals for, 2402t
Di Guglielmo's disease, 1048
Dihydrofolate reductase, 906
Dihydropteridine reductase, absence of, 1156
deficiency of, 1150t
Dihydrotachysterol, 1484t
for hypoparathyroidism, 1499
Dihydrotestosterone
and follicle-stimulating hormone inhibition, 1407
and hair growth at puberty, 2303
and luteinizing hormone inhibition, 1407
in spermatogenesis, 1400
testosterone conversion to, 1400, 1406
9-1(1,3-Dihydroxy-2-propoxymethyl) guanine (DHPG), 126
1,25-Dihydroxyvitamin D, synthesis of, and fasting hypercalciuria, 640
Diiodohydroxyquin, for amebic liver abscess, 837
Diiodotyrosine, 1253, 1315, 1316
Diisopropyl fluorophosphate (DFP), 140
Dilated cardiomyopathy, 176, 352–355. See also Cardiomyopathies
Dilation
as compensatory mechanism in heart failure, 218, 219
atrial, diastolic properties of heart and, 185
for esophageal motor disorders, 686
techniques of, for esophageal strictures, 683
Dilaudid, abuse of, 55
as analgesic, 107t
Diltiazem
adverse effects of, 269t, 289(t)
for angina pectoris, 327t, 328t
for hypertension, 287t
for hypertrophic cardiomyopathy, 358
for Raynaud's phenomenon, 377
pharmacokinetic properties of, 266t
Dimercaprol, as chelating agent after poisonings, 143
Dimethylamine, toxicity of, to hemoglobin, 945
Dimethyltryptamine (DMT), abuse of, 58
Dinitropyrroles, as testicular toxin, 1416
Dioctyl sodium sulfosuccinate, as stool softener, 722
Dipetalonema perstans, 1919
Diphenhydramine, for advanced parkinsonism, 2146
for phenothiazine-induced extrapyramidal reactions, 143
Diphenoxylate
and intestinal motility, 724
for diarrhea, from ulcerative colitis, 758
in Crohn's disease, 752
with atropine, 732
Diphenylhydantoin. See Phenytoin
2,3-Diphosphoglycerate, and hemoglobin oxygen affinity, 943
in erythrocytes, 913
2,3-Diphosphoglyceric acid, levels of, in shock, 241
Diphosphonates, for Paget's disease, 1517
Diphtheria, 1626–1628
immunization against, 61, 62, 63t
agents for, 62t, 1626
neuropathy from, 2266
vs. tick paralysis, 1923
vs. streptococcal pharyngitis, 1576

Diphtheroids, vs. Listeria monocytogenes, 1672
Diphyllobothrium latum, vitamin B$_{12}$ deficiency from, 904
Diplacusis, definition of, 2117
Diplopia, from pseudotumor cerebri, 2236
Dipylidium caninum, 1894
Dipyridamole
after coronary artery bypass grafts, 339
aspirin with, for stroke prevention, 2171
for membranoproliferative glomerulonephritis, 598
for polycythemia vera, 984
for stress perfusion imaging, 210
Dipyrroles, 880, 943
Dirofilariasis, 1919
Disaccharides, deficiency in, 742
from carbohydrates, 733
Disc, intervertebral, 2040, 2248. See also Intervertebral disc(s)
Discogenic disease, 2044
Discography, 2252
Discoid lupus erythematosus, 2340
and hair loss, 2349
immunofluorescent cutaneous findings in, 2305t
photosensitivity in, 2352
Disease. See also under names of specific diseases
alterations of drug doses in, 94–97
interaction of, with aging, 24–26
molecular, 152, 158
structural, pain from, 105
transmission of, by blood transfusions, 949–950
Disinfection, 1548
definition of, 1547
Disodium cromoglycate, for asthma, 409
for mastocytosis, 1974
glucocorticosteroid therapy and, 131
Disodium etidronate, for hypercalcemia, 1505
for Paget's disease, 1517
Disopyramide, 270
dosing and adverse effects of, 267t
hypoglycemia from, 1384
interaction of, with beta-adrenergic blockers, 101
pharmacokinetic properties of, 89t, 266t
reference intervals for, 2403t
Disorientation, from rabies, 2201
in nonketotic hyperosmolar syndrome, 1377
Dissecting aneurysms, 370
and hematocrit, 802
of aorta, 372–374, 373
and stroke, 2164
and syncope, 2074
classification of, 372, 372
mortality rate from, 374
myocardial infarction vs., 332
pain from, 393
pulmonary embolism vs., 444
Disseminated intravascular coagulation, 1053, 1078–1080, 2325
compensated, definition of, 1079
from blood transfusions, 950
from cancer, 1098
from fulminant meningococcemia, 1614
from gram-negative bacteremia, 1660
from hemolytic transfusion reactions, 949
from liver disease, 1078
from meningococcal disease, 1615
from peritoneovenous shunt, 851
from plague, 1662
from Rocky Mountain spotted fever, 1744
from sepsis, 1539, 1541

Disseminated intravascular coagulation (Continued)
from shock, 241
from Staphylococcus aureus, 1598
from thrombotic thrombocytopenic purpura, 1052
from viral hemorrhagic fevers, 1829
microthrombi from, and hemolysis, 924–925
schistocytes and, 1046
thrombocytopenia from, 1053
Distomiasis, pulmonary, 1903
Disulfiram, for alcoholics, 50, 60
in drug interactions, 124t
reactions from, metronidazole and, 121
DIT (diiodotyrosine), 1253, 1315, 1316
Diuresis
agents for. See Diuretic agents
osmotic, 532
and potassium loss, 546
hypernatremia from, 542
postobstructive, 532, 616
sodium-poor, from acute distention of left atrium, 215
solute, 532
Diuretic agents
abuse of, and hypokalemia, 547
chronic, 532
and chylomicronemia syndrome, 1143
and gout, 1161
and hyperkalemic hyperchloremic metabolic acidosis, 553
and hypertriglyceridemia, 1143
and nonketotic hyperosmolar syndrome, 1377
and plasma renin activity, 1350
and urinary potassium loss, 545
and urine sodium concentration, 524
atriopeptin as, 1279
characteristics of, 536t
combined use of, 232
complications from, 232–233
distal tubule, 535–536
for amyloidosis, 360
for ascites, 851
for chronic obstructive pulmonary disease, 416
for congestive heart failure, 230–233
for dilated cardiomyopathy, 355
for heart failure, 225
edema in, 190
in respiratory failure, 481
for hypertension, 286t
for pseudotumor cerebri, 2237
in pregnancy, 636
interaction of, 124t
with cardiac glycosides, 101
with vitamin K, 1206t
loop, 232, 234. See also Loop diuretics
neutropenia from, 963t
potassium-sparing, and hyperkalemia, 548
properties of, 231t
proximal, for fluid volume excess, 535
reactions to, vs. Bartter's syndrome, 622
thiazide, hypercalcemia from, 1502–1503
Diverticulitis, 804–806, 805
acute, 723
and pylephlebitis, 835
as contraindication to colonoscopy, 670
computed tomography for, 662
dietary fiber for, 1246
treatment of, 805
vs. appendicitis, 801, 803
vs. ischemic colitis, 764
vs. tuberculosis of colon, 1691

Diverticulosis, 723
  hemorrhage from, 799
  vs. adenocarcinoma of colon, 771
  vs. diverticulitis, 805
Diverticulum(a)
  abscess of, computed tomography of, *663*
  bleeding from, 804
  duodenal, 721
  gastric, 718
  pharyngeal, regurgitation from, 680
  ureteral, 650
  urethral, congenital, 650
  vitamin B₁₂ deficiency from, 904
Dizziness. See also *Vertigo*
  evaluation of, 2122, *2122*
  from adrenocortical insufficiency, 1351
  from spontaneous intracranial hemor-
    rhage, 2178
  from trench fever, 1748
  in cardiovascular patient history, 175
  in fulminant meningococcemia, 1614
  postural, from hemolysis, 908
DKA. See *Diabetic ketoacidosis*
DMT (dimethyltryptamine), abuse of, 58
DNA. See *Deoxyribonucleic acid*
Dobutamine
  and myocardial contractility, 184
  for ambulatory heart failure patients, 235
  for low cardiac output syndrome, after
    coronary artery bypass graft surgery,
    338
  for septic shock, 1660
  for shock, 248
  initial hemodynamic effects of, 247t
DOC (11-deoxycorticosterone), 247
  excess of, 1359
  plasma binding to, 1343
Dogs
  hookworm of, 1907
  rabies in, 2200
  tapeworm in, 1894
Döhle bodies, 969
Doll's-eye test, for progressive supranuclear
    palsy, 2145
  of vestibular function, 2121
Dolphine, 107t
Dominant traits, 147
  autosomal, pedigrees of, 147–148
  X-linked, 149
    pedigree for, 149
Domperidine, and intestinal motility, 724
Donath-Landsteiner hemolytic anemia, 921
Donors, for organ transplants, 577–578
Donovan bodies, 1712
Donovanosis, 1711. See also *Granuloma in-
    guinale*
L-Dopa
  absorption of, 99
  and vitamin B₆ deficiency, 1233
  as contraindication to vitamin B₆ therapy,
    1234
  ineffectiveness of, for fulminant hepatic
    failure, 854
  mania from, 2096
  to test growth hormone reserve, 1294
L-Dopa decarboxylase, 1100
Dopamine, 1281–1282, 1462
  and thyroid function, 1321
  as prolactin inhibitor, 1281
  as vasodilator, *234*
  biosynthesis of, 1462, *1462*
  deficiency of, in parkinsonism, 2143
  for low cardiac output syndrome, 338
  for shock, 244, 247
    septic, 1660
  in nigrostriatal pathway, 2141
  initial hemodynamic effects of, 247t
  receptors for, 136

Dopamine (Continued)
  synthesis of, 1253
  with vasodilators, for shock, 248
Doppler ultrasound, 178, *205*, 205–207, *206*
Doriden, abuse of, 53
Dorsalis pedis artery, systolic blood pres-
    sure in, 381
Dorsum sellae, 1290
Double outlet right ventricle, 314
Dowager's hump, 1513
  from osteoporosis, 1512
Down's syndrome, 167t, 170
  Alzheimer's changes in, 2089
  and acute leukemia, 1001
  and hepatitis B susceptibility, 822
  common atrioventricular canal in, 305
  heart problems in, 176, 303
  megacolon in, 723
  robertsonian translocation and, 166
Doxapram, and breathing control, 401
  as respiratory stimulant, 481
Doxepin, for inhibiting acid secretion, 700
  reference intervals for, 2403t
Doxorubicin
  and cardiotoxicity, endomyocardial bi-
    opsy for, 178
  dilated congestive cardiomyopathy from, 367
  for acute myelogenous leukemia, 1005
  for cancer, 1125
    bladder, 655
    gastric, 712
    pancreatic, 783–784
  for multiple myeloma, 1031, 1032
  for nephroblastoma, 654
  in cardiac therapy, 209
  myonecrosis from, 354
  toxicity of, and cardiomyopathy, 354–355
Doxycycline, 121
  elimination rate for, 96t
  esophageal injury from, 688
  for leptospirosis, 1732
  for prophylaxis of chloroquine-resistant
    Plasmodium falciparum, 1551
  for salpingitis, 1706
  for trachoma, 1734
  for travelers' diarrhea, 1657
  for typhus fever, 1740
  for urethritis, 630
  in kidney and liver failure, 117t
  in prostate tissue, 116
D-penicillamine. See *Penicillamine*
DPG (2,3-diphosphoglyceric acid), levels of,
    in shock, 241
Dracunculiasis, 1918–1919
Dracunculus medinensis, 1918
Dreams, 2077
Dressler's syndrome, 334, 363
  and eosinophilia, 1026
Drop attacks, 2076, 2127, 2169, 2222. See
    also *Seizures*
  causes of, 2127t
  from cerebral artery occlusion, 2166
  vs. epilepsy, 2225
Drowning, 40, 2371
Drowsiness, from chronic hypoxia, 477
  from narcotic analgesics, 109
  in metabolic encephalopathy, 2063
Drug(s). See also specific names and types
  absorption of, 87–88
    drug interactions and, 100
  abuse of. See *Drug abuse*
  accumulation of, 90–91
  acid-sensitive, delay in emptying stomach
    and, 99
  acidic, absorption of, 99
  acute urticaria from, 2334
  addiction to. See *Drug addicts; Drug de-
    pendence*

Drug(s) (Continued)
  administration route for, 108
  administration sites for, in cancer treat-
    ment, 1117
  adverse reactions to, 102–104, 1968–1972,
    1970t–1971t
    coma as, 2066
    diagnosis of, 1969
    glossitis as, 678
    in skin, 2324, *2324*, 2352–2353, 2353t
      vs. lichen planus, 2328
      vs. pityriasis rosea, 2328
    incidence and predisposing factors for,
      1968
    management of, 1969
    mechanisms of, 1968–1969
    ocular, 2298
    prevention of, 1969
    vs. aphthous ulcers, 676
    vs. measles, 1774, 1775t
    vs. staphylococcal scalded skin syn-
      drome, 1599
    vs. tropical eosinophilia, 1916
    vs. yellow fever, 1832
  affinity of, 134
  agonist, 107–108
  androgen deficiency from, 1414
  anemia from, 880t–881t
    aplastic, 885–886, 886t
  antagonist, 108
  antihypertensive, and inhibition of renin
    release, 283t
  antithyroid, 1324–1325
  binding of, to plasma proteins, 100
  blackouts from, 2076
  cholestatic jaundice from, vs. bile duct
    carcinoma, 871
  chronic intoxication from, pseudodemen-
    tia from, 2088
  clearance of, creatinine clearance and, 95
    in elderly, 98
  distribution of, aging and, 97
    drug interactions and, 100
    throughout body, 88
  diuretic, properties of, 231t
  dosages for
    adjustment of, 92
      and steady state, 91
    calculating, 95
    disease and alteration of, 94–97
    loading, 89–90, 95–96
    maintenance, 91–92
  elimination of, 90
    by kidneys, 510
    rate constant for, 95, 96t
  esophageal injury from, 688
  exaggerated responses to, 102
  fever from, 1969, 1970t
  fulminant hepatic failure from, 854
  gynecomastia from, 1411
  half-life of, 90
    aging and, 98
  hypercalcemia from, 1502–1503
  hypoglycemia from, 1384
  immune hemolysis from, 921–922
  immunologic reactions to, 103
    respiratory failure from, 475
  increased sensitivity to, liver disease and,
    811
  interaction of, 98–101
    and cancer treatment, 1118
    in antimicrobial therapy, 123–124, 124t
    pharmacokinetic, 99–101
  interference of, with laboratory tests, 80
  intermittent administration of, 92
  interstitial lung disease from, 424t, 433–
    434
  intoxication with, in elderly, 26

Drug(s) (*Continued*)
intoxication with, vs. multiple sclerosis, 2214
lipid-soluble, in elderly, 97
liver disease from, 824, 826–830
classification of, 827t, 827–828
malabsorption from, 744
metabolism of, drug interactions and, 99–100
in cigarette smokers, 39
mucous membrane reaction to, 2347
myasthenic syndromes from, 2287–2288
myopathy from, 2036
neutropenia from, 961–962, 963t
oral contraceptive interaction with, 1443
overdose of
alcoholism and deaths from, 52
and sudden cardiac death, 275
antidotes for, 2068
removal following, 92
oxidant, and glucose-6-phosphate dehydrogenase deficiency, 915, 916t
parkinsonism from, 2144
treatment of, 2146
pharmacokinetic parameters for, 89t
rash from, 2323t
reference intervals for, 2402t–2404t
resistance to, and cancer treatment, 1118
and tuberculosis treatment, 1688
retroperitoneal fibrosis from, 2051
step-down therapy with, 288
therapy with, 87–98
thrombocytopenic purpura from, 1048–1050
tinnitus from, 2120t
to enhance mucosal defense, 701
tolerance to, 94
toxic reactions to, 102–103, 103t
central nervous system in, 2068–2071, 2069t–2071t
chronic, pseudodementia from, 2088
in elderly, 26
ventricular flutter from, 264
vs. multiple sclerosis, 2214
vascular purpura from, 1059
vertigo from, 2123
water-soluble, in elderly, 97
with dose-dependent pharmacokinetics, 89t, 92
withdrawal from, and seizures, 2219
Drug abuse
among physicians, 68
and acute respiratory depression, 557
and intracerebral hemorrhage, 2175
and recurrent thromboembolism, 476
by adolescents, 21
definition of, 52
multiple use, treatment for, 54
poisonings in, treatment for, 144
recognition of, 52–53
with cannabis, 57–58
with inhalants, 59–60
with nicotine, 60
with opioids, 55–57
with psychedelics, 58–59
with sedatives, 53–54
with stimulants, 54–55
with synthetic drugs, 60
Drug addicts
acquired immunodeficiency syndrome in, 1801
and hepatitis B susceptibility, 822
endocarditis in, infective, 1590
Staphylococcus aureus, 1601
false-positive syphilis tests in, 1720
tetanus in, 1634
Drug dependence, definition of, 52
narcotics for dying patients and, 33
treatment of, 60t, 60–61

Drug therapy, 87–98
Drunkenness, ataxia from, 2126
Drusen, 2236
DSA (digital subtraction angiography), 83, 83, 2059
for kidneys, 525
DST. See *Dexamethasone, suppression test for*
DTIC (dacarbazine), for cancer, 1126
for glucagonoma, 1389
DT's. See *Delirium tremens*
Duarte variant gene, 1132, 1133
DUB (dysfunctional uterine bleeding), 1434
Dubin-Johnson syndrome, 813t
and cholestasis from oral contraceptives, 830
Duchenne dystrophy, 2272–2273
and dilated cardiomyopathy, 354
Duchenne gene, cloning of, 2275
Ductus arteriosus, patent, 307–308
echocardiography for, 205
Dumping syndrome, 717
after ulcer surgery, 704, 704, 704t
Duncan's disease, 1944
Epstein-Barr virus in, 1787
Duodenitis, endoscopy for, 669
vs. bleeding from peptic ulcers, 706
Duodenum
aortofemoral bypass graft in, fistulization of, 798
carcinoma of, vs. pancreatic cancer, 783
content reflux from, after gastric surgery, 705
diverticulum of, 721
endoscopic examination of, 668. See also
Esophagogastroduodenoscopy
mucosa of, maintenance of, 694
obstruction of, vs. peptic ulcers, 699
pain from, 658
reflux in, and chronic gastritis, 690
tumors of, 713
ulcers of. See *Peptic ulcers*
Dusts
and chronic bronchitis, 412
chemical, interstitial lung disease from, 435
inorganic, interstitial lung disease from, 423t, 432–433
lung disorders from, 2360–2362
occupational, and asthma, 407
organic, interstitial lung disease from, 424t, 433
Dwarfism
achondroplastic, 148
cartilage-hair hypoplasia and, 1947
from zinc deficiency, 1241
in Hurler's syndrome, 1175
psychosocial, 1288
Dying patients, care of, 31–34, 1089
Dynein, deficiency of, and immotile cilia, 1416
Dysarthria, cerebellar, in Friedreich's ataxia, 2152
in multiple sclerosis, 2213
vs. Broca aphasia, 2087
Dysautonomia
definition of, 2264
familial, 2106
of Riley-Day, 2265
reflex, after spinal cord trauma, 2246
Dysbetalipoproteinemia, 1140t, 1141
and atherosclerosis, 1144
vs. familial hypercholesterolemia, 1140–1141
Dyschondroplasia, 1520
Dysentery
bacillary, 1646. See also *Shigella, dysentery from*
from balantidiasis, 1889

Dysesthesia(s), definition of, 2259
in acute inflammatory sensory polyneuropathy, 2262
Dysfibrinogenemia, 1073–1074
in liver disease, 1077
Dysgammaglobulinemia, hypertriglyceridemia in, 1143
Dysgerminomas, 1394
hormones from, 1445t
Dysgeusia, definition of, 2110
Dyskinesia
definition of, 2142
oral-facial, from hepatic encephalopathy, 853
tardive, 2149
from antipsychotic drugs, 2144
vs. chorea, 2148
vs. Huntington's disease, 2149t
Dysmenorrhea, 1433
primary, during adolescence, 19
Dysmetria, ocular, 2117
Dysmyelination, from leukodystrophies, 2215
Dysosmia, 2110
Dysostosis multiplex, 1175
Dyspareunia, in menopause, 1444
Dyspepsia, 697
esophagogastroduodenoscopy for, 669
from stomach cancer, 699
functional, vs. peptic ulcers, 699
Dysphagia, 679
and iron deficiency anemia, 897
from bronchogenic carcinoma, 459
from esophageal stricture formation, 682
from esophagus motor disorders, 684
from gastric cancer, 711
from gastroesophageal reflux disease, 681
from sarcoidosis, 453
in myotonic dystrophy, 1414
in polymyositis, 2035
progressive, from esophageal carcinoma, 686
transfer, 679
Dysphasia, 2086
Dysphonia, spastic, 2150
Dysplasia
arrhythmogenic right ventricular, surgery for, 274
bronchopulmonary, from oxygen toxicity, 496
cervical, oral contraceptives and, 1443
diaphyseal, progressive, 1519
ectodermal, hereditary, 2347
fibrous, polyostotic, 2343
of colonic mucosa, and cancer, 770
olfactogenital, 1287, 1439
renal-retinal, 648
segmental, 649
total renal, 649
Dysplastic nevus syndrome, 1095t, 2339
Dyspnea, 185, 186, 394. See also names of specific disorders causing dyspnea
paroxysmal nocturnal, 394
from aortic regurgitation, 344
from dilated cardiomyopathy, 352
from heart failure, 221
Dysproteinemias, 1026. See also *Plasma cells, disorders of*
and platelet function defects, 1057
from lymphocytic interstitial pneumonitis, 431
Dysthymic disorder, 2095, 2097t, 2097–2098
Dystonia, 2142–2143, 2149–2151
action, 2143, 2150
athetotic, 2142
cranial, 2150–2151
from antipsychotic drugs, 2094, 2144
segmental, 2150

Dystonia (Continued)
  tardive, 2149
  torsion, 2142
  tremor in, 2150
Dysuria
  from appendicitis, 801
  from diverticulitis, 804
  from schistosomiasis haematobia, 1898
  from trichomoniasis, 1889
  in women, 628

E₁. See Estrone
E₂. See Estradiol
EACA. See Epsilon-aminocaproic acid
Ear(s). See also Hearing
  cartilage inflammation in, in relapsing
    polychondritis, 2038
  diphtheria infection in, 1627
  furunculosis of, pain from, 2134
  pain in, 2134
    from disease in throat, 106
Eastern equine encephalitis, 1824–1825,
    2193
Eating, disorders of, 707, 1215–1219
  excessive, 657
    and gastroesophageal reflux disease,
      683
Eaton agent, 1561
Eaton-Lambert syndrome, 459
  neuromuscular transmission studies for,
    2058
  vs. botulism, 1633
EB (epidermolysis bullosa), 2332
Ebstein's anomaly of tricuspid valve, 310,
  310
EBV. See Epstein-Barr virus
Ecchymosis, definition of, 1045
  in polycythemia vera, 981
Eccrine sweat glands, 2302
ECG (electrocardiography), 196–201. See
    also Electrocardiography
Echinococcosis, 464, 834, 835t, 1893–1894
Echinococcus, in liver, 835t
Echinostoma, 1904
Echocardiography, 201–207, 202
  two-dimensional, 202, 203, 203, 204
Echothiophate iodide, side effects of, 2299
Echoviruses, 1808, 1809t
  and orchitis, 1414
  infection by, vs. measles, 1774
Eclampsia, 634
  acute fatty liver from, 841
  hemolysis from, 925
  hypertensive encephalopathy with, 2172
ECM (erythema chronicum migrans), 1726,
  2335
ECT (electroconvulsive therapy), 2097
Ecthyma, 1578, 1659, 2342
Ectodermal dysplasia, hereditary, 2347
Ectoparasites, sexual transmission of, 1702t
Ectopic pregnancy. See Pregnancy, ectopic
Ectopy, control of, in mitral valve prolapse,
  351
Eczema(s), 2318–2322, 2319t. See also Der-
    matitis
  as contraindication to smallpox vaccina-
    tion, 1793
  atopic, 2320, 2346
    in hypoparathyroidism, 1498
  dyshidrotic, 2321
  from phenylketonuria, 1155
  immunodeficiency with, 1946–1947
  of hands, 2321
  solar, 1184
  xerotic, 2321
Eczema craquelé, 2321

Eczema herpeticum, 2329
Eczema vaccinatum, from smallpox vaccina-
    tion, 1793
Edema
  benign refeeding, 1215
  excess body fluids and, 535–536
  from arteriovenous fistula, 384
  from brain tumors, 2231
  from chronic obstructive pulmonary dis-
    ease, 415
    treatment of, 417
  from deep-vein thrombosis, 385
  from diabetic glomerulopathy, 625
  from glomerulonephritis, 584–585
    post-streptococcal, 587
  from heart failure, 223
  from hyponatremia, 541
  from liver disease, 808
  from lymphangiectasia, 744
  from nephrotic syndrome, 593
  from sepsis, 1540
  from tricuspid stenosis, 351
  from ulcerative colitis, 756
  from urticaria, 1948
  heat, 2384
  in brain, 2080. See also Brain, edema of
  in cardiovascular patient history, 176
  in children, with eastern equine encepha-
    litis, 1824
  in foot, from thromboangiitis obliterans,
    382
  malignant, 1667, 1668
  mucosal, from asthma, 403
  peripheral. See Peripheral edema
  pulmonary. See Pulmonary edema
  Starling forces and, 536
Edetate, as chelating agent after poison-
    ings, 143
Edrophonium, 139
  for myasthenia gravis diagnosis, 2286
Edwards' syndrome, 167t
EEE (eastern equine encephalitis), 1824–
    1825, 2193
EEG. See Electroencephalography
EFA (essential fatty acids), 1249–1250
Effector cells, 423
Effector sequence, in complement reaction,
    1939–1940, 1940
Effector systems, and potassium excretion,
    544
Efferent arterioles, 508
Effort syndrome, 2125
Effusion
  complicated, in gram-negative bacilli
    pneumonia, 1568
  pericardial, 364–365
    in heart failure, 223
  pleural, 222
  subdural, meningitis and, 1605
EGF. See Epidermal growth factor
Ehlers-Danlos syndrome, 153, 1178–1180,
    1179t
  and skin, 2325
  defective collagen synthesis in, 1982
  dissecting aneurysms from, 372
  osteoarthritis and, 2041
  type VI, 1131
  vitamin C for, 1236
Eicosanoids, 1271
Eisenmenger's syndrome, 306, 316–317
EIT (erythrocyte iron turnover rate), 895
Ejaculate, normal volume of, 1407
Ejaculatory ducts, development of, 1392
Ejaculatory dysfunction, 1410
Ejection fraction, 208, 214, 216
  as index of ventricular function, 186
  as measure of contractility, 218
  calcium and, 354

Ejection fraction (Continued)
  measurement of, 207
  normal, 218
  ventricular, change of, with exercise,
    325–326
Elastase, and dietary protein digestion, 734
  in lungs of smokers, 38
  inhibition of, by alpha₁-antitrypsin, 838
Elastin, in dermis, 2302
  in extracellular matrix, 1981
Elastorrhexis, systemic, 1181–1182, 1181
Elastosis, 2306
Elbow(s), pain in, 2047
  rheumatoid arthritis in, 2001
Elderly. See also Aging
  acute illness in, 28
  depression in, 28, 29, 2089
  diagnosis and management in, 28–31, 73
  diagnostic tests for, 28
  diet of, 24, 1204
  disease prevention in, 26
  drugs for, 26, 97–98
    antidepressant, 2096
    antihistamines as, side effects of, 2317
    intoxication with, 26
  long-term care of, 30
  malabsorption in, 744–745
    from bacterial overgrowth, 741
  malnutrition in, 1209, 1210
  workup of, 27–28
Electric current injury, 2380–2382, 2381
  fatalities from, 40
  ventricular flutter from, 264
Electrocardiography, 177, 196–201
  ambulatory, for arrhythmias, 254–255,
    255t
  computer interpretation of, 201
  diagnoses aided by, 198t
  false-positive exercise results for women
    in, 177
  in critical care units, 493
  interpretation of, 198
  potassium depletion and, 546–547, 547
  quality of, 198
  recording techniques for, 201, 201t
  stress test with, 20
  waveforms in, 197, 197
Electrocoagulation, for gastrointestinal
    bleeding, 670
Electroconvulsive therapy, 2097
Electrocution, 40, 2380–2382, 2381
  ventricular flutter from, 264
Electroencephalography, 2056
  changes in, from sedative withdrawal
    syndrome, 54
  for altered consciousness, 2067
  for epilepsy, 2224–2225
Electrolysis, for hirsutism, 1448
Electrolytes. See also names of specific elec-
    trolytes
  abnormalities in
    and myocardial contractility, 354
    and sudden cardiac death, 275
    dilated cardiomyopathy from, 354
    during refeeding, 1214
    from diuretics, 231
    pseudomembranous colitis and, 1632
    ventricular flutter from, 264
  absorption of, 734
  concentrations of, aging and, 25
  imbalance in, induction of, from thiazide
    diuretics, 287
  in urine, measurement of, 524
  loss of, in cholera, 1651
  nonsteroidal anti-inflammatory agents
    and, 608t
  replacement of, for diabetic ketoacidosis,
    1376

Electromyography, 2057, *2057*, 2057t, 2271–2272
  for back pain, 2252
  for myasthenia gravis diagnosis, 2286
  for polymyositis, 2036
Electron microscopy, for muscle biopsy, 2272
Electronystagmography, 2122
Elek test, 1627
Elephantiasis, 1915
  from lymphatic filariasis, 1914
Elliptocytosis, hereditary, 912t, 912–913
Emaciation, from bronchiectasis, 439
EMB. See *Ethambutol*
Embden-Meyerhof glycolytic pathway, 913, 945
Embolectomy, for sudden arterial occlusion, 383
  pulmonary, 449
Embolism
  air, from blood transfusions, 950
    in scuba divers, 2367
  and multi-infarct dementia, 2090
  arterial, and threatened stroke, 2167
    from infective endocarditis, 1589
    vs. arteriosclerosis obliterans, 381
  central retinal artery occlusion from, 2298
  distal, in lower extremities, from renal artery atheroembolization, 633
  from heart, stroke from, 2163–2164
  from mitral stenosis, 346
  paradoxical, 383
  pulmonary, 442–449. See also *Pulmonary embolism*
  risk of, in dilated cardiomyopathy, 355
  sudden arterial occlusion by, 383
  treatment of, after myocardial infarction, 334
  vs. hypertensive intracerebral hemorrhage, 2179
Embryopathy, coumarin, 1077
Emergency care, blood transfusions in, 948
  for head injury, 2242
  for heatstroke, 2383
  of spinal cord injury, 2245–2246
Emery-Dreifuss dystrophy, 2273, 2275
Emesis, induction of, after poisonings, 142
Emetine, myopathy from, 2282
EMG. See *Electromyography*
Emmonsiella capsulata, 1838
Emotion, frontal lobes and, 2082
  glucocorticoids and, 582
  in gastrointestinal disease, 657
Emphysema, 390, 410–418
  alpha$_1$-antitrypsin deficiency and, 838
  and bullae, 420
  and histoplasmosis, 1838
  and mycobacteria infection, 1694
  and obstructive ventilatory disorders, 399
  and sleep interruptions, 2078
  cadmium poisoning and, 2391
  centrilobular, 415
  chronic respiratory failure from, 475
  exercise and, 46
  in cigarette smokers, 38
  panacinar, 415
  pneumothorax from, 469
  protease-antiprotease theory of, 414
  pulmonary hypertension from, 296, 297
Empty sella syndrome, primary, 2236
  vs. pituitary tumor, 1299
Empyema, 435, 468, 865
  from acute cholecystitis, 865–866
  from anaerobic bacteria, 1638–1639
  from pneumococcal pneumonia, 1560
  lung abscess with, 435, 436
  staphylococcal, 1600

Empyema (*Continued*)
  subdural, 2183–2184. See also *Subdural empyema*
  vs. lung abscess, 436
  vs. pulmonary embolism, 444
  with gram-negative bacilli pneumonia, 1567
Enalapril, as inhibitor of converting enzyme, 1345
  for hypertension, 287, 287t
Enanthems, 1813
Encainide, 270
  dosing and adverse effects of, 268t
  pharmacokinetic properties of, 266t
Encephalitis
  after smallpox vaccination, 1793
  and secondary parkinsonism, 2144
  bulbar, cancer and, 1105
  California, 1826–1827
  cytomegalovirus, 2198
  demyelinating, 2208–2209, 2208t
    vs. multiple sclerosis, 2215
  eastern equine, 1824–1825, 2193
  from arboviruses, 1821–1829, 1822t, 2192, 2193
  from herpes simplex virus, 1782, 2195–2196
    acyclovir for, 126
    adenine arabinoside for, 125
    in temporal lobe, 2081
    IUDR ineffectiveness on, 125
  from measles immunization, 64
  from rabies, 2201
  from varicella, 1789
  hyperglycemia from, 1289
  Japanese, 1827–1828
  mumps and, 1779
  Murray Valley, 1828
  parkinsonism after, treatment for, 2146
  prognosis of, 2194
  Rocio, 1828
  St. Louis, 1825–1826
  subacute, 2203
  tick-borne, 1828–1829
  varicella-zoster virus, 2196–2197
  Venezuelan equine, 1825
  viral, 2192–2194
    frequency of, 2192t
  von Economo's, parkinsonism from, 2144
  western equine, 1823–1824
Encephalomeningitis, and diabetes insipidus, 1308
  from trichinellosis, 1912
Encephalomyelitis, 2192
  disseminated, acute, 2208t, 2208–2209
    vertigo from, 2124
    vs. multiple sclerosis, 2215
  from measles, 1774
  from rabies, 2200
  immune-mediated, 2208–2209, 2208t
  parainfectious, vertigo from, 2124
Encephalopathy
  acute, from radiation therapy to brain, 1107
  chronic liver disease with, 855
  dialysis, 2389
  from pertussis vaccine, 1626
  hepatic, 852–854
  hypertensive, 282, 2172–2173
    from accelerated hypertension, 277
  hypertonic, from diabetes insipidus, 1310
    treatment of, 1311–1312
  in alcoholic cirrhosis, 844
  in fulminant hepatic failure, 854
  metabolic, 2063–2066. See also *Metabolic encephalopathy*
  of liver, 808
  postanoxic, and amnesia, 2084

Enchondromatosis, of bone, 1520
End-plate potential, 2284–2285
End-stage kidney disease, 563. See also *Kidney(s), failure of, chronic; Uremic syndrome*
  Alport's syndrome and, 637
  atriopeptin and, 1279
  causes of, 573
  dialysis for, acquired renal cystic disease from, 647, 652
  from analgesic nephropathy, 607
  from chronic glomerulonephritis, 602
  from diabetes mellitus, 624, 1361
  from urinary tract obstruction, 616
  occurrence of, 573
Endarterectomy, carotid, 2171
Endarteritis, focal, from syphilis, 1713
  infective, 1592
Endobronchial lesions, vs. chronic bronchitis, 413
Endobronchial tuberculosis, 1689
Endocarditis
  aneurysms from, 370
  antimicrobial therapy for, 114
  bacterial
    and bacterial meningitis, 1608
    and brain, 2186
    emboli from, 2174
    prophylaxis for, 1586
    subacute, glomerulonephritis in, 587
      vs. post-streptococcal glomerulonephritis, 587
      vs. viral encephalitis, 2194
  drug abuse and, 52
  duration of therapy for, 122
  erysipeloid and, 1673
  from bacterial meningitis, 1608
  from *Candida* infection, 1848
    treatment of, 1849
  from disseminated gonococcal infection, 1709
  from enterococci, 1573
  from *Listeria monocytogenes*, 1671
  from Q fever, 1749
  infective, 1586–1596. See also *Infective endocarditis*
  Libman-Sacks, 1587
  marantic, 1587
  pneumococcal, penicillin dosage for, 113
  prophylaxis of, antibiotic, in aortic regurgitation, 345
    in asymptomatic aortic stenosis patient, 343
  prosthetic valve, antimicrobial therapy for, 119
  rifampin with penicillin for, 121
  staphylococcal, 1601–1602
  thrombotic, nonbacterial, in cancer, 1098
  vs. cytomegalovirus infection, 1785
Endocardium
  cushion defect of, 305–306
  electrical stimulation of, for arrhythmias, 255, *255*, 256t
  fibroelastosis of, 351
  fibrosis of, 1468
  ventricular, damage to, eosinophils and, 362
Endocrine, definition of, 1252
Endocrine-humoral disorders, and heart, 369
Endocrine myopathies, 2280
Endocrine neoplasia, multiple. See *Multiple endocrine neoplasia*
Endocrine system, 1252–1268. See also *Hormone(s)*
  clinical assessment of, 1265–1267
  disorders of, *1263*, 1263–1265. See also names of specific disorders

Endocrine system (Continued)
  disorders of, anemias with, 892
    dementia from, 28
    dilated cardiomyopathy from, 354
    during puberty, 19
    malabsorption in, 744
    multiple, 1265, 1458–1461
    neuropathy with, 2262–2264
    treatment of, 1267
  hyperfunction of, 1264
  hyperplasia in, 1264
  malnutrition and, 1213
  neoplasms in, 1264
  skin and, 2304–2305
Endocytosis, definition of, 733
Endometriosis, dysmenorrhea from, 1433
  from menstrual effluent, 1428–1429
Endometritis, tuberculous, 1436
Endometrium, cancer of, estrogen and, 1445
  cysts of, vs. ovarian neoplasms, 1446
  in menstrual cycle, 1430
Endomyocardium, biopsy of, 178
  disease of, Löffler's, 1025
    restrictive, 361–362
  fibrosis of, 361–362
Endophthalmitis, 2293, 2294
Endoplasmic reticulum, smooth, phenobarbital and, 157
Endorphins, 1268
  and eating, 657
  functions and known anatomic localizations of, 1270t
  in sepsis, 1539
  shock and, 240
Endoscopy
  contraindications for, 668
  for bleeding ulcers, 706
  for diagnosis of gastritis, 689
  for esophageal cancer diagnosis, 686
  for esophageal motor disorders, 685
  for esophageal reflux, 681
  for gastric cancer, 711–712
  for gastric outlet obstruction, 707
  for peptic ulcers, 697
  for pseudomembranous colitis, 1632
  for sclerosis of varices, 849
  for sphincterotomy, for choledocholithiasis, 673, 869
  gastrointestinal, 668–674
  prior to peptic ulcer surgery, 703
Endosonography, 664
Endothelial cells, 421
  damage to, in shock, 240
Endotheliosis, glomerular capillary, from toxemia of pregnancy, 635
Endothelium, 318
  capillary, pulmonary, permeability of, and pulmonary edema, 476
  injury to, and atherosclerosis, 321, 322
  from fatty acids, 450
Endotoxins, fever from, 1526
  in blood transfusions, 949
  mitochondrial damage from, 242
  shock from, 240, 1538, 1602–1603, 1659–1661
Endotracheal intubation
  for acute respiratory failure, 477
  for fulminant hepatic failure, 854
  in critical care, complications from, 495
  indications for, 487t
  obstruction of, mechanical ventilation with, treatment for, 488
  vs. tracheostomy tube, 478
Enema(s), ineffectiveness of, after poisonings, 142
  small bowel, 665
    for Crohn's disease, 748

Energy. See also Calories
  dietary requirements of, 1206–1207, 1207t
  expenditure of, in selected activities, 1226t
  intake of, and obesity, 1221
    and protein use by body, 1207
  metabolism of, magnesium in, 1195
  sources of, for parenteral nutrition, 1247
  transport of, chylomicron and, 1138
Enflurane, and malignant hyperthermia, 2282
ENG (electronystagmography), 2122
Enkephalins, and eating, 657
ENL (erythema nodosum leprosum), 1698–1699
  treatment of, 1700
Enoximone, for heart failure, 235
Entamoeba histolytica, 1886
  and pus in stool, 730
  in liver, 835t
  lung abscess from, 436, 836
Enteric bypass surgery, and liver disease, 840
Enteric fever, 1641. See also Typhoid fever
Enteritis
  eosinophilic, malabsorption from, 743
  from Campylobacter, 1648t, 1648–1651
  radiation, diarrhea from, 729
    malabsorption from, 743
  regional, 745
    in Behçet's disease, 2049
    sclerosing cholangitis with, 869
Enteritis necroticans, 1631
Enterobacteriaceae
  and pneumonia, 1566
  and urinary tract infection, 629
  growth of, in IV solution, 1545
  in spontaneous bacterial peritonitis, 851
  infection of, treatment for, 437
    cephalosporins for, 120
    vs. Campylobacter, 1648
Enterobiasis, 1910
Enterochromaffin cells, and small cell lung cancer, 458
  carcinoid tumors from, 1467
Enteroclysis, 665
  for Crohn's disease, 748
Enterococci, 1573
  infection of, treatment of, 122
  urinary tract, 629
Enterocolitis, neonatal necrotizing, and pseudomembranous colitis, 1632
  radiation, 806
  Salmonella, vs. appendicitis, 802
Enterocutaneous fistulas, total parenteral nutrition for, 1248t
Enterohepatic circulation, 860, 860
Enteropathy, AIDS, 729
  protein-losing, 1098
    and albumin degradation, 815
Enterostomy, for recurrent aspiration pneumonia, 1569
Enterotoxins
  and secretory diarrhea, 726, 727
  from Campylobacter jejuni, 1649
  from Escherichia coli, 1653, 1654
  from salmonellae, 1644
  from Staphylococcus aureus, in food poisoning, 785
  from Vibrio cholerae, 1651
Enteroviruses, 1808–1814, 1809t
  acute hemorrhagic conjunctivitis from, 1814
  encephalitis from, 2192, 2193
  meningitis from, 2192, 2193
    vs. meningococcal disease, 1615
  mucocutaneous infection from, 1813
  myocarditis from, 1811–1812

Enteroviruses (Continued)
  pericarditis from, 1811–1812
  vs. influenza, 1766
  vs. measles, 1775t
Enthesis, definition of, 1977
  spondylarthropathies and, 2004
Enthesopathy, 1977
Enuresis, 2079
  from medullary cystic disorders, 648
Environment
  and cancer, 1093, 1093t
  and colorectal cancer, 768
  and congenital heart disease, 303
  and congenital malformations, 170
  and Crohn's disease, 746
  internal, regulation of, 2103
  pollution of, 2354–2356
  temperature of, and common cold, 1755
Environmental medicine, 2355, 2356
Enzyme(s). See also names of specific enzymes
  activity amplification of, 157
  assays of, for heart trauma, 369
  changes in, myocardial infarction and, 332
  converting, 287, 291, 516, 1345
  defects of, and gout, 1167
  deficiencies in, and erythrocyte defects, 913–917
    and myopathy, 2277
  for epilepsy, 2226–2227
  in muscle disease, 2271
  in plasma, idiopathic pericarditis and, 364
  inborn errors of metabolism from specific, 154t–155t
  lysosomal, and joint destruction, 1993
    in inflammation, 1987
  pancreatic, and gastric ulcers, 695
  restriction, 158
Enzyme-linked immunosorbent assay, for AIDS, 1800
  for Haemophilus influenzae detection, 1620
  for varicella, 1790
Eosinopenia, 966
  from glucocorticosteroid therapy, 129
Eosinophil(s), 1024
  and inflammatory reaction, 2306
  granulomas from, 430, 692. See also Histiocytosis X
  in acute interstitial nephritis, 603
    drug-induced, 606
  in alveolitis, 425
  in asthma, 403
  in late-onset asthmatic response, 405
  levels of, and asthmatic bronchitis, 413
  reference intervals for, 2401t
Eosinophilia, 362, 970–971
  diseases associated with, 1025t, 1025–1026
  from adrenocortical insufficiency, 1352
  from angiostrongyliasis, 1913
  from drug allergy, 1969
  from drug-induced interstitial lung disease, 433
  from fascioliasis, 1902, 1903
  from loiasis, 1918
  from parasitic disease, 834
  from acute clonorchiasis, 1902
  from chronic myelogenous leukemia, 989
  from coccidioidomycosis, 1840
  from Hodgkin's disease, 1018
  from idiopathic thrombocytopenic purpura, 1050
  from paraneoplastic syndromes, 1097–1098
  from renal artery atheroembolization, 633
  in dialysis patients, 577
  peripheral, 692

Eosinophilia *(Continued)*
  pleural fluid from, 467
  pulmonary infiltration with, 434
  tropical, 1916
  worm infections and, 1856
Eosinophilopoietin, cancer and, 1103
EP (erythrocyte protoporphyrin), 2386
EPA (eicosapentaenoic acid), 1271
Ependymomas, 1298, 2256
  intracranial, 2230
Ephedrine, 137
  interaction of, with bretylium, 99
Ephelides, 2342
Epicondylitis, 2047
Epidermal growth factor, 322
  and regulation of cellular proliferation,
    1091
  for cancer, 1129t
  receptor of, 1258
Epidermal necrolysis, toxic, 2329
  vs. staphylococcal scalded skin syn-
    drome, 1599
Epidermis, 2300–2302
  basal layer of, 2301
  malignant tumors of, 2337
  nodules of, 2335
Epidermodysplasia verruciformis, and neo-
    plasms, 1096t
Epidermolysis bullosa, 2305t, 2332
Epidermophyton, skin infection with,
    2321
Epididymis, blockage of, and infertility,
    1410
  development of, 1392
  tuberculosis in, 1690
Epididymitis, gonococcal, 1707
Epididymo-orchitis, mumps and, 1779
Epidura, abscess of, cerebral, 2184
    in spine, 2186–2187
    Staphylococcus aureus, 1603
  blood patch of, 2238
  hematoma of, spinal, 2257
    vs. extradural tumors, 2255
  metastases to, in breast cancer, 1456
Epigastric bloating, 718
  from gastric cancer, 711
  from gastric outlet obstruction, 707
Epigastric pain, from oral iron therapy, 898
  from pancreatic cancer, 781
  postprandial, from superior mesenteric
    artery syndrome, 765
Epigastrium, cutaneous vein prominence
    in, in liver disease, 809
Epiglottis, taste buds in, 2110
Epiglottitis, 1618
  from *Haemophilus influenzae,* 65, 1618–1619
  vs. croup, 1761
Epilepsy(ies), 2217–2229. See also *Convul-
    sions* and *Seizures*
  abdominal, 2220
  catamenial, 2223
  clinical manifestations and classification
    of, 2219–2223, 2219t
  corticoreticular, 2218
  definition and prevalence of, 2217
  diagnosis of, 2223–2225
    differential, 2225–2226
  distinctive syndromes of, 2220t
  etiology of, 2218–2219, 2219t
  gelastic, 2220
  hypocalcemia and, 1497
  in tuberous sclerosis, 2158
  myoclonus, progressive, 2222
  pathogenesis of, 2217–2218
  petit mal, 2218
  photosensitive, 2223
  reflex, 2223
  rolandic, 2221

Epilepsy(ies) *(Continued)*
  seizures in, from arteriovenous malfor-
    mations, 2174
    therapeutic classification of, 2220t
  sylvian, 2218, 2221
  temporal lobe, 2081, 2081t
    vertigo from, 2124
  treatment of, 2226–2229
Epinephrine, 134, 137, 1281–1282, 1462
  and glycogenolysis, 1382
  and insulin, 1374
  and neutrophil adhesiveness, 957
  and platelet secretion, 1042
  binding of, to receptors, 1257
  biologic role of, 1463
  biosynthesis of, 1462, *1462*
  deficiency of, 1466–1467
  eosinopenia from, 966
  for adverse reaction to snake bite treat-
    ment, 1929
  for anaphylaxis, 1957
  for asthma, 408
  for erythromelalgia, 379
  for shock, 247
  in cardiopulmonary resuscitation, 501
  initial hemodynamic effects of, 247t
  interaction of, with propranolol, 101
  neutrophilia from, 969
  transitory thrombocytosis from, 1054
Epiphysis, slipped capital femoral, 19
Epipodophyllotoxins, for cancer, 1125
Episcleritis, 2296
  in inflammatory bowel disease, 758
  rheumatoid arthritis and, 2002
Episiotomy, and sphincter dysfunction, 728
Epispadias, 650
Epistaxis
  from aplastic anemia, 887
  from leeches, 1927
  from polycythemia vera, 981
  from von Willebrand disease, 1070
  from Waldenström's macroglobulinemia,
    1033
  pulmonary arteriovenous fistula and, 309
Epitaxy, 639
Epithelial cells, *421*
  in alveoli, 421
  of small intestine, damage to, from glu-
    ten, 742
  parietal, in kidneys, 509
  visceral, in kidneys, 509
Epithelium
  atrophy of, 678
  cells of. See *Epithelial cells*
  columnar, from gastroesophageal reflux
    disease, 682
    treatment of, 683
Epitopes, 1937
  T cell receptors and, *1935,* 1935–1936
Epoxygenase pathway, 1274, *1274*
EPP (end-plate potential), 2285
EPS (expressed prostatic secretions), 1421
Epsilon-aminocaproic acid
  for berry aneurysm treatment, 2177
  for hemophilia B, 1071
  for von Willebrand's disease, 1056
  in fibrinolysis, 1064
  reference intervals for, 2402t
Epstein-Barr virus
  acute hepatitis from, 819
  and Burkitt's lymphoma, 1013
  and cancer, 1095
  and rheumatoid arthritis, 1999
  antigens of, in rheumatoid arthritis, 1991
  impaired immune response to, 1944
  in AIDS, 677
  infection of, 1786–1788. See also *Mononu-
    cleosis, infectious*

Epstein-Barr virus *(Continued)*
  neurologic disease from, 2198
  pharyngitis from, 1757
  RANA and, 1997
  vs. cytomegalovirus, 1785
Equilibrium, 2120–2124
  neural pathways for, 2117
Erb-type limb-girdle dystrophy, 2273
Erect position, and syncope, 2075
Ergocalciferol, 1477, 1484t
Ergonomics, 2356
Ergonovine, as coronary vasoconstrictors,
    189
Ergot preparations, for atypical facial pain,
    2133
  for migraine, 2131
Ergotamine, for cluster headache, 2131
  toxicity to, vs. arteriosclerosis obliterans,
    381
Ergotism, side effects of, 2131
Erosive gastritis, 689
  from aspirin, and iron deficiency, 896
Erosive lichen planus, vs. aphthous ulcers,
    676
ERP (estrogen receptor proteins), 1455
Error catastrophe theory, of aging, 23
Eructation, 661, 897
Erysipelas, 1578, 2335
  vs. angioedema, 1951
Erysipeloid, 1673
Erythema
  from candidiasis, 677, *677*
  from chilblain, 379
  from ulcerative colitis, 756
  from yersiniosis, 1664
  induration from, chilblain vs., 380
  necrolytic migratory, from glucagonoma,
    1389
  in cancer, 1112
Erythema annulare, 1583, 2335
Erythema chronicum migrans, 1726,
    2335
Erythema induratum, 2050
Erythema marginatum, 2335
  in rheumatic fever, 1583–1584
  vs. Lyme disease, 1728
Erythema multiforme, 2331–2332, 2335,
    2347
  from drug allergy, 1970t
  herpes simplex virus and, 1783, 2329
  in Crohn's disease, 750
  vs. aphthous ulcers, 676
  vs. erythroplakia, 678
  vs. gingivitis, 675
  vs. Lyme disease, 1728
  vs. urticaria, 1951
Erythema multiforme major (Stevens-John-
    son syndrome), 1562–1563, 1783, 2331–
    2332
  ulcers in, vs. in Behçet's disease, 2049
  vs. toxic epidermal necrolysis, 2329
Erythema nodosum, 451, 1699, 2050, 2336t,
    2340
  chilblain vs., 380
  from Behçet's disease, 2049
  from coccidioidomycosis, 1840
  from Crohn's disease, 747, 750
  from drug allergy, 1970t
  from ulcerative colitis, 757
Erythema nodosum leprosum, 1698–1699
  treatment of, 1700
Erythermalgia, 378–379
  vs. Fabry's disease, 1145
Erythrasma, 2321
Erythroblastopenia, transient, of childhood,
    887
Erythroblastosis fetalis, immunization
    against, 63t, 65–66

Erythroblasts, development of, hemoglobin production during, 929
Erythrocyte(s), 421. See also *Red blood cell(s)*
  agglutination of, in shock, 241
  antibodies of, detection of, 918
  antibody destruction of, 918
  ATP synthesis in, 913
  characteristics of, 927–928
  cytochrome b5 reductase in, 945
  deficiency of catalase in, 1187
  drug binding to, 921
  dysfunction of, in hypophosphatemia, 1194
  for transfusion, 947t, 947–948
  fragmentation of, in hemoglobin H disease, 933
  frozen, 947t, 948
  glycosylation in, 1367, *1367*
  hemoglobin in, 925. See also *Hemoglobin(s)*
  in additive solution, 947, 947t
  in ascites fluid, 791
  in spleen, 1036
  indices for, 881–882
  iron turnover rate of, 895
  leukocyte-poor, 947, 947t
  lifespan of, 877
    in anemias of chronic disease, 899
  malaria and, 1858
  membrane of, 909–910
    in sickle cell anemia, 939
    permeability defects in, 913
    skeletal defects in, and hereditary elliptocytosis, 912
  methemoglobin-reduction system in, 926
  normal values for, 878, 878t
  nucleotide metabolic defects in, and hemolysis, 917
  packed, 947, 947t
  parasites of, hemolysis from, 924
  precursors of, 874
    megaloblastic changes in, 901
  production of, immune system and, 881
  protoporphyrin in, from lead, 2386
  reference intervals for, 2401t
  sickled, 938, *938*
  snake venom and, 1928
  spleen and, 910
  survival of, in uremic syndrome, 566
    measurement of, 907
  technetium-99m binding to, 207
  thalassemia trait and, 932
  trauma to, hemolysis from, 924–925
  volume of, maintenance of, 910
    reference intervals for, 2402t
  washed, 947, 947t
Erythrocyte sedimentation rate, 1995
  elevated
    in acute gouty arthritis, 1165
    in giant cell arteritis, 2033
    in legionnaires' disease, 1571
    in pancreatic cancer, 781
    in polymyalgia rheumatica, 2033
  in acute phase response, 1528, 1529
  in pericarditis, 364
  in rheumatoid arthritis, 2003
  in subacute thyroiditis, 1332
  in systemic lupus erythematosus, 2016
  reference intervals for, 2401t
  testing for, 1942
Erythrocytosis, 975. See also *Polycythemia*
Erythroderma, 2321, *2321*, 2327
  and thermoregulation, 2304
  from drug allergy, 1970t
  in cancer, 1111
Erythrodontia, in congenital erythropoietic porphyria, 1183

Erythroid cells, developing, destruction of, and bilirubin production, 811
  precursors of, abnormal, in marrow, and sideroblastic anemia, 899
  progenitors of, 875
Erythroid colony-forming units, 976
Erythroleukemia, 1003
Erythromelalgia, 378–379
  vs. Fabry's disease, 1145
Erythromycin, 121
  after contact with diphtheria patient, 62
  elimination rate for, 96t
  excretion of, 116
  for aortic stenosis, 343
  for chancroid, 1713
  for diphtheria, 1628
  for gram-negative bacilli pneumonia, 1567
  for legionnaires' disease, 1572
  for Lyme disease, 1729
  for mycoplasmal infections, 1561, 1564
  for prostatitis, 1422
  for relapsing fever, 1725
  for streptococcal pharyngitis, 1577
  for whooping cough, 1626
  in acidic environments, 116
  in kidney and liver failure, 117t
  in prostate tissue, 116
  liver disease from, 829
  mechanism of action of, 113t
  resistance mechanisms of, 116t
  resistance to, 114
Erythroplakia, 678
Erythropoiesis
  from androgen therapy, 1419
  ineffective
    and hyperbilirubinemia, 814
    definition of, 895
    from beta thalassemia, 930
    in megaloblastic anemia, 902
Erythropoietin, 519, 566, 875–876
  deficiency in, anemia from, 566
  estimating, 977–978
  excessive production of, and polycythemia, 977
  from neoplasms, 1103
  in uremic syndrome, management of, 571
  output of, from kidneys, 976
  production of, in uremia, 507
  recombinant human, 571
Eschar, 1745
  in rickettsialpox, 1746
  in scrub typhus, 1747
Escherichia coli, 1653
  and gastritis, 689
  and pus in stool, 730
  bacteremia from, acute suppurative cholangitis with, 1902
  cephalosporins for, 120
  colitis from, vs. ulcerative colitis, 756
  diarrhea from, secretory, 727
    travelers', 1656
  enteric infections of, 1653–1656, 1654t
  food poisoning by, 784
  in infants, 834
  in spontaneous bacterial peritonitis, 851
  infection of, hemolysis from, 923
  liver abscess from, 834
  nosocomial pneumonia from, 1544
  penicillins for, 119
  prostatitis from, 1421
  septicemia from, 246
  urinary tract infection with, 629, 630
    hospital-acquired, 1543
  vs. emphysematous cholecystitis, 867
Esophagitis
  after gastric surgery, 705
  from *Candida* infection, 1848
  hemorrhage from, 799

Esophagitis (Continued)
  reflux, endoscopy for, 669
    vs. gallstones, 864
    vs. bleeding from peptic ulcers, 706
Esophagogastroduodenoscopy, 668t, 668–670
  magnetic resonance imaging for, 85
  therapeutic applications of, 670
Esophagography, for localization of abnormal parathyroid tissue, 1494
Esophagus
  achalasic, regurgitation from, 680
  bleeding from, vs. hemoptysis, 392
  burns of, from caustic compounds, 144
  cancer of, in cigarette smokers, 38
    nitrites and, 44
    tylosis with, 1095t
  colic of, 680, 684
  disease of, 679–689. See also names of specific diseases
    clinical symptomatology of, 679–680
    gastroesophageal reflux disease as, 680–683
    motor, 683–686
    vs. intermittent cholangitis, 868
    vs. postcholecystectomy syndrome, 872
  diverticula of, 687–688
  examination of, endoscopic, 668. See also *Esophagogastroduodenoscopy*
  hypomotility of, in systemic sclerosis, 2021–2022
  in Chagas' disease, 1867, 1868, *1868*
  infections of, 688
  injury to, 688–689
  motility of, 714
  pain in, 392, 658
  pharmacologic stimulation of, 685
  reflux of, in smokers, 39
  rupture of, and pneumomediastinum, 470
    pulmonary embolism vs., 444
  spasm of, vs. gallstones, 864
  sphincters of, failure of, 684
    function of, 714
  strictures of, dilation of, with esophagogastroduodenoscopy, 670
    in gastroesophageal reflux disease, 681–682
    treatment for, 683
  tumors of, 686–687
  ulcers of, from reflux, 681
    in gastroesophageal reflux disease, 682
    treatment of, 683
  varices of
    from hemochromatosis, 839
    from portal hypertension, *848*
    hemorrhage from, 799
      and portal hypertension, 849
    in portal hypertension, 848
    vs. bleeding from peptic ulcers, 706
  web in, acquired, anemia and, 687
Espundia, 1874
ESR. See *Erythrocyte sedimentation rate*
Estradiol, 1433t
  absorption of, 88
  and follicle-stimulating hormone inhibition, 1407
  and luteinizing hormone inhibition, 1407
  conversion of estrone to, 1398
  in females, 1426, 1427t
  in menstrual cycle, 1429–1430
  in puberty, 17
  reference intervals for, 2396t
  testosterone conversion to, 1406
Estriol, reference intervals for, 2397t
Estrogen(s)
  and bone age vs. chronologic age, 1426
  and bone loss prevention, 1511

Estrogen(s) *(Continued)*
  and cancer, 1093t
    of breast, 1453
    of prostate, 1424
  and chylomicronemia syndrome, 1143
  and corticosteroid-binding globulin, 1342
  and hepatic porphyria, 1185
  and hypertriglyceridemia, 1143
  and migraine headache, 2131
  and photosensitivity, 2351
  and sodium reabsorption, 516
  and vitamin D–binding protein, 1477
  cholestasis from, 827
  decreased, and sexual dysfunction, 1442
    menopause and, 1444
  excess of, and neoplasms, 1428
    and secondary hypogonadism, 1417
  for hot flushes, 1444
  for hypercalcemia with primary hyper-
    parathyroidism, 1504
  for osteoporosis, 1514
  in puberty, 17
  increased formation of, from androgens,
    gynecomastia from, 1451
  levels of, obesity and, 1225
  receptor proteins for, in breast cancer,
    1455
  reference intervals for, 2397t
  side effects of, 1514
  synthesis of, in ovaries, 1431–1432
  synthetic, and cancer, 1094
  therapy with, 1297
    contraindications to, 1444
    for hypergonadotropic amenorrhea,
      1438
Estrone, 1433t
  conversion of, to estradiol, 1398
  in menstrual cycle, 1429–1430
  in puberty, 17
  reference intervals for, 2397t
Ethacrynic acid, 232
  and calcium excretion, 519
  and hearing loss, 2119
  and metabolic alkalosis, 555
  as diuretic after diagnosis of acute inter-
    stitial nephritis, 605
  characteristics of, 536t
  for ascites, 851
  for hypercalcemia, 1504
  for hypertension, 286t
  in drug interactions, 124t
  properties of, 231t
Ethambutol
  acute interstitial nephritis from, 605
  for tuberculosis, 1687
  in kidney and liver failure, 117t
  side effects of, ocular, 2298
Ethamivan, obsolescence of, 481
Ethanol
  abuse of, 53
    and porphyria cutanea tarda, 1186
  and carbohydrates, hypoglycemia from,
    1383
  and enhanced liver metabolism of other
    drugs, 99
  and increased porphyrin production,
    1187
  and riboflavin deficiency, 1231
  as inhibitor of drug metabolism, 101
  average daily consumption of, and cir-
    rhosis, 842
  dilated cardiomyopathy from, 353
  dose-dependent kinetics of, 89t, 92
  fatty liver from, 810, 827
  gastritis from, 689
  in body, elimination of, 48
  liver disease from, 828, 831, 842–843

Ethanol *(Continued)*
  metabolism of, 843
    genetics of, 102
  neutropenia from, 963t
  pharmacology of, 48
  toxicity of, illness from, 51t
Ethanolamines, 1954t
Ethchlorvynol, poisoning with, 2069t
  reference intervals for, 2403t
Ether, and malignant hyperthermia, 2282
Ethics, medical, 9, 12–15
Ethionamide, for tuberculosis, 1687
Ethosuximide, for epilepsy, 2226t, 2227
  reference intervals for, 2403t
Ethylene glycol
  metabolic acidosis from, 554
    treatment for, 555
  poisonings with, and kidney damage, 612
    treatment for, 145
  vs. methyl alcohol, 142
Ethylene oxide, for sterilization, 1547
Ethylenediamine, 1954t
  allergy to, 1969
  and contact dermatitis, 2319
Etidronate, 1485
  and abnormal bone mineralization, 1479
  osteomalacia from, 1482
Etretinate, for psoriasis, 2327
  for skin disorders, 2317
Eubacterium, 1637
Eukaryotes, 1837
Eumelanin, 2302
Eumycetomas, 1853
Eunuchoidism, from prepubertal testoster-
    one deficiency, 1408, *1408*
  hypogonadotropic, 1416–1417
  in Klinefelter's syndrome, 1412
European typhus, 1739
Eustachian tube blockage, in Sjögren's syn-
    drome, 2024
Evans' syndrome, in autoimmune hemo-
    lytic anemia, 919
  thrombocytopenia in, 1052
Ewing's sarcoma, 1521
  solitary pulmonary nodules from, 464
Exanthem(s), from enteroviruses, 1813
  viral, 2322–2323, 2323t
    vs. staphylococcal scalded skin syn-
      drome, 1599
Exanthem subitum, 2322
  vs. measles, 1774, 1775t
Exchange transfusions, after poisonings,
    143
  for thrombotic thrombocytopenic pur-
    pura, 1053
Exenteration, definition of, 2295
Exercise, 45–47
  aerobic, 47
  and aging process, 26
  and bone, 1514
  and congestive heart failure, 224–225
  and epileptic seizures, 2223
  and increase in high density lipoproteins,
    320
  and muscle, 2270
  and periodic paralysis, 2281
  and respiration, 403
  asthma attack from, 407
  cardiac output and, *189*, 191
  cardiovascular response to, 208
  decreased tolerance to, from dilated car-
    diomyopathy, 352
  diffusing capacity in, 400
  for angina pectoris patients, 327
  for cancer patients, 1089
  for rheumatoid arthritis, 2003
  headache from, 2132

Exercise *(Continued)*
  heart response to, 217
  in hypertension therapy, 285–286
  in myocardial perfusion imaging, 210
  in weight control, 1226, 1226t
  intermittent proteinuria from, 585
  lack of, and atherosclerosis, 321
    and cardiovascular disease, 182
  muscle cramps after, muscle phosphoryl-
    ase deficiency and, 1135
  oxygen consumption in, 400
  response to, in pulmonary hypertension,
    vasodilators and, 299
  severe, hematuria from, 503
  strenuous, and anovulation, 1439
  testing with. See *Exercise testing*
  transitory thrombocytosis from, 1054
Exercise testing
  for angina pectoris, 328
  for aortic regurgitation, 345
  for mitral stenosis, 347
  for mitral valve prolapse, 350
  for valvular heart disease, 341
Exhaustion, from heat, 2383
  from manic excitement, 2099
Exocrine, definition of, 1252
Exomphalos, prenatal diagnosis of, with ul-
    trasonography, 173
Exophthalmos, definition of, 1321
  from Graves' orbitopathy, 2295
Exostoses, multiple, and neoplasms, 1096t
Expiratory flow rate, peak, measurement
    of, in severely ill, 483
Expressivity, of genetic disorders, 148
External compression devices, for thrombo-
    embolism prevention, 387
Extracellular fluid, volume contraction of,
    prerenal kidney failure from, 560
Extrapyramidal disorder(s), 2141–2152. See
    also names of specific disorders
  vs. epilepsy, 2225
Extremities, malnutrition and, 1210t
  weakness in, in multiple sclerosis, 2213
Exudates, in nonproliferative retinopathy,
    1378
  pleural fluid, 467, 467t
Eye(s). See also *Vision*
  abnormal movements of, 2114–2115
  acute hemorrhagic conjunctivitis in, 1814
  adenovirus infection of, 1767
    TFT for, 126
  ankylosing spondylitis and, 2006
  atrophy of, 2292–2293
  cavernous sinus thrombosis and, 2185
  congenital rubella and, 1777
  Creutzfeldt-Jakob disease and, 2206
  cysticerci of, treatment of, 1895
  Cysticercus in, 1892
  disorders of, 2289–2299. See also names
    of specific disorders
    from Alport's syndrome, 637
    from diabetes mellitus, 1378–1379
    from tabes dorsalis, 1717–1718
    local glucocorticosteroid therapy for,
      130
    neoplasms of, 2295–2296
    orbital, 2295
    retrolental fibroplasia, 2297
    riboflavin deficiency and, 1231
    rosacea and, 2333
    uveitis as, 2293
    vascular, 2296–2298
  drug side effects and, 2298–2299
  dryness of, 2296. See also *Keratoconjunc-
    tivitis sicca*
  episcleritis in, 2296
  Graves' disease in, 1322–1323, *1323*

Eye(s) (Continued)
hemorrhage in, 2297
in Behçet's disease, 2049
in Graves' disease, 1324
treatment of, 1327
in Niemann-Pick disease, 1148
in systemic lupus erythematosus, 2015
infection of, 2294. See also names of specific infections
meningococcal, 1615
influenza and, 1765
larva migrans in, 1909
lens of, dislocation of, from Marfan syndrome, 1177
in homocystinuria, 1160
leprosy in, 1698
lesions in, in Fabry's disease, 1145
loiasis in, 1918
malnutrition and, 1210t
measles and, 1773
medication for, side effects of, 2299
movement of, brain stem dysfunction
and, 2063
muscles of, in myasthenia gravis, 2285
onchocerciasis in, 1917
optic disc swelling in, 2292, 2292t. See
also Papilledema
pain in, and headache, 2134–2135
pseudoxanthoma elasticum and, 1181
raccoon, from skull fracture, 2241
relapsing polychondritis in, 2038
retrolental fibroplasia of, 2297
rheumatoid arthritis and, 2002
Rift Valley fever and, 1818
sarcoidosis in, 453
scleritis in, 2296
tabes dorsalis and, 2189
topical steroids near, side effects from,
2315
toxoplasmosis and, 1877
trachoma in, 1734–1735
tuberculosis of, 1691–1692
tularemia in, 1665
voluntary movement of, 2082
Wegener's granulomatosis in, 2031

Fab fragments, purified, 230
Fabry's disease, 150, 167, 361, 1144–1145
fever in, 1525
kidney transplant for, 157
Face
abnormalities in, from cavernous sinus
thrombosis, 2185
angioedema in, 1949
angioma of, in Sturge-Weber syndrome,
2159
atypical pain in, 2133
bones of, midline granuloma and, 2032
grimacing of, from hepatic encephalopathy, 853
paralysis of, idiopathic, 2266–2267
skin disorders of, 2346t
trauma to, brain abscess from, 2181
weakness in, from Guillain-Barré syndrome, 2261
Facioscapulohumeral dystrophy, 2273–2274
Facioscapulohumeral spinal muscular atrophy, 2155–2156
Factitious disorders, 2101, 2103
fever in, 1525
Factor II, deficiency of, 1073
Factor V, deficiency of, 1073
inhibitors of, 1081
Factor VII, deficiency of, 1072
Factor VIII, and von Willebrand factor, 1070

Factor VIII concentrate, for hemophilia A,
1068
Factor VIII inhibitors, 1068–1069
as anticoagulants, 1080–1081
Factor IX, deficiency of, 1071–1072
inhibitors of, 1081
Factor X, deficiency of, 1072–1073
Factor XI, deficiency of, 1072
Factor XII, deficiency of, 1072
Factor XIII, deficiency of, 1074
FAD (flavin adenine dinucleotide), 1230
Faget's sign, in yellow fever, 1831
Fainting, 2073–2075. See also Syncope
Fallopian tubes, development of, 1392
Falls, 29, 40, 41
False aneurysms, 334, 370
from trauma to heart, 369
Familial Mediterranean fever, 147, 795,
1196–1199, 1525, 2045
Family cancer syndrome, 770
and screening for cancer, 773
Family history, in genetic counseling, 172
in hereditary disease, 147
Famotidine
for ulcers, 702
for inhibiting acid secretion, 700
for Zollinger-Ellison syndrome, 709
Fanconi's anemia, 168
and acute leukemia, 1001
and neoplasms, 1096t
Fanconi's syndrome, 505, 603, 621, 1154t
from lead poisoning, 2386
from tetracyclines, 609
glycosuria in, 619
megakaryocytic hypoplasia in, 1048
vs. galactosemia, 1133
Fansidar, for malaria, 1550–1551, 1860, 1861
side effects of, 1551
Farmer's lung, 433, 1851
Fasciculations, definition of, 2271
Fasciitis, eosinophilic, 2021
necrotizing, 1630t, 2335
from anaerobic bacteria, 1639
Fascioliasis, 834, 835t, 1902–1903
hepatomegaly and eosinophilia from, 834
Fasciolopsiasis, 1904
Fasciotomy, after electric injury, 2382
Fasting
and gastrointestinal motility, 715
and plasma amino acids, 1152t
glucose production during, 1382
hyperbilirubinemia from, 814
hypercalciuria in, 640–642
hypoglycemia in, 1382, 1384–1387
physiology of, 1373–1374, 1373
protein-supplemented modified, 1226
supervised, for insulinoma diagnosis,
1384
Fat(s)
absorption of, 733–734, 733
bile salts and, 859
assimilation of, insulin and, 1374
calorie equivalent of, 1227
digestion of, 733
fecal, reference intervals for, 2397t
in diet
and acute kidney failure, 562
and cancer, 44, 1095
colorectal, 768
pancreatic, 781
for diabetic, 1368
requirements for, 1207–1208
malabsorption of, in Zollinger-Ellison
syndrome, 708–709
reserves of, estimate of, with triceps skinfold thickness, 1209–1210, 1210t
subcutaneous, necrosis of, from chronic
pancreatitis, 779

Fat cells, in obesity, 1222, 1223
in upper vs. lower body, 1223
Fat content, in children, 18
in females, 18
Fat embolism syndrome, 450–451
Fatigability, abnormal, 2270
Fatigue, 2125
beta blockers and, 287
from adrenocortical insufficiency, 1351
from anemias, 879
from chronic myelogenous leukemia, 990
from chronic persistent hepatitis, 831
from digitalis toxicity, 229
from Ebstein's anomaly of tricuspid
valve, 310
from Gaucher's disease, 1146
from hemolysis, 908
from hypertrophic cardiomyopathy, 357
from interstitial lung disease, 425
from mitral valve prolapse, 350
from primary pulmonary hypertension,
299
from pulmonary veno-occlusive disease,
302
from systemic lupus erythematosus, 2014
from viral hepatitis, 819
from Waldenström's macroglobulinemia,
1033
in cardiovascular patient history, 175
in insulin-dependent diabetes mellitus,
1362
in legs, coarctation of aorta and, 313
in liver disease, 808
Fatty acids
deficiency of, symptoms of, 657
essential, deficiency of, in total parenteral
nutrition, 1249–1250
free, 1138. See also Free fatty acids
from fats, 733
in diabetic ketoacidosis, 1375
in hepatic encephalopathy, 852
metabolism of, disorders of, 2278
monounsaturated, 1208
omega-3, in marine fish oils, 43
polyunsaturated, 1207
radiolabeling of, 211
reference intervals for, 2397t
Fatty liver, 810
acute, of pregnancy, 841
and disseminated intravascular coagulation, 1078
from Crohn's disease, 749
from drugs, 827–828
in alcoholics, 842, 843
Fatty streak, 322, 322
in atherosclerosis, 319
regression of, 323
Fava beans, hemolysis from, glucose-6-
phosphate dehydrogenase deficiency
and, 915
Fazio-Londe syndrome, 2155
Febre maculosa, 1742
Fecal incontinence, 728, 790
Feces. See Stool
Fed state, physiology of, 1373–1374, 1373
Feeding behavior, disorders of, hypothalamus and, 2104
Feet. See Foot (feet)
Felty's syndrome, 964, 2002–2003
Female(s)
calcium intake by, 41
creatinine clearance for, 95
excess body hair on, 1446. See also Hirsutism
fat content in, 18
fetal virilization of, 1402, 1428
genital tract of. See names of specific
structures and disorders

Female(s) (Continued)
gonorrhea in, 1707–1708
lower genital tract infections in, 1704–1705
phenotypic differentiation of, 1392, 1393
pseudohermaphroditism in, 1402–1404, 1403t
smoking risks for, 38–39
urinary tract infection in, 628, 629
treatment for, 630
X-linked inheritance in, 149
Feminization, testicular, 153, 167
Femoral artery, superficial, arteriosclerosis obliterans in, 380
Femoral vein, thrombosis of, 385
Femur, shepherd's-crook deformity of, 1520
Fenfluramine, for weight control, 1226–1227
Fenoprofen
acute interstitial nephritis from, 608
as analgesic, 107t
as cyclooxygenase inhibitor, 1275
reference intervals for, 2403t
Fentanyl, abuse of, 55
FEP (free erythrocyte protoporphyrin), 897, 899
Ferritin, definition of, 894
reference intervals for, 2397t
Ferrochelatase, from protoporphyria, 840
Ferrokinetics, 895–896
Ferrous sulfate, for iron deficiency anemia, 898
Fertile eunuch syndrome, 1417
Fertility
disorders of, 1440–1441. See also Infertility
in females, peak age of, 1441
in kidney transplant patients, 582
restoration of, 1297
sperm characteristics and, 1407, 1407
Festination, definition of, 2144
Fetal alcohol syndrome, 171
Fetor hepaticus, 852
Fetoscopy, in prenatal diagnosis, 173
Fetus
development of, androgen deficiency during, 1408
female, virilization of, 1402, 1428
kidney disease in mother and, 636
of mothers age 35+, chromosome abnormalities in, 166
surgery on, 171
Fever, 391, 1525. See also names of specific fevers
and breathing variations, 401
and septic shock, 1539
as antimicrobial reaction, 123
as interferon reaction, 128
convulsions from, 2222
benign, 2218
exanthem in, vs. secondary syphilis, 1716
five-day, 1747
hemorrhagic. See Hemorrhagic fever
hypothalamic, 1526
in transplant recipients, 2210
intermittent proteinuria from, 585
manifestations of, 1526–1527
of unknown origin, 1524–1525, 1732
pathogenesis of, 1525–1527, 1526
persistence of, 123
postpartum, Mycoplasma hominis and, 1565
prolonged, in bacterial meningitis, 1608
prostaglandins and, 1276–1277
saddleback, 1820
Fever blister(s), from herpes simplex virus, 1782
in pneumococcal pneumonia, 1557
FFA. See Free fatty acids

Fiber, in diet, 43, 1207, 1246
and cancer, 44, 1095
colorectal, 768
and colonic motor function, 721
and constipation, 722
and diverticulosis coli, 723
and ulcerative colitis, 758
in diabetic diet, 1369
Fiberoptic bronchoscopy, 1554
and severely ill, 486
for solitary pulmonary nodules, 464
Fibrillation, ventricular, in cigarette smokers, 37
Fibrin, clot of, 1983
structure of, 1063, 1064
Fibrinogen, reference intervals for, 2401t
structure of, 1063, 1064
Fibrinogen binding, absence of, in thrombasthenia, 1057
Fibrinolysis, 1064
increased, with liver disease, 1077–1078
primary, 1079
system of, alterations in, and coronary artery thrombosis, 330
therapeutic, 387, 633–634, 1079
Fibroadenoma, oral contraceptives as protection against, 1443
Fibroblast(s), 421
and collagen in alveolitis, 425
growth factor of, 322
proliferation of, 985
Fibroelastosis, concentric or eccentric, 298
endocardial, tricuspid stenosis from, 351
Fibrogenesis imperfecta ossium, 1482
Fibroma(s), in kidneys, 652
in liver, 857
Fibromatosis, mesenteric, 796
Fibronectin, 955, 2302
in alveolitis, 425
in connective tissue, 1982
Fibrosarcoma(s), of kidneys, 655
of lungs, 464
of stomach, 713
Fibrosis
after shunt lesion surgery in adults, 305
atelectasis with, 419
conglomerate, pulmonary hypertension from, 297
cystic. See Cystic fibrosis
endomyocardial, 361–362
from cirrhosis, 819
from mitral stenosis, 345
from syphilis, 1713
from systemic sclerosis, 2019
interstitial
diffusing capacity in, 400
from acute interstitial nephritis, 603
from chronic eosinophilic pneumonia, 431
from chronic interstitial nephritis, 606
from irradiation restrictive cardiomyopathy, 361
in advanced kidney disease, 607
pulmonary hypertension from, 296
intimal, in coronary artery bypass grafts, 339
mediastinal, 2052
of alveolar walls, in interstitial lung disease, 425
pleural, in asbestos workers, 469
pulmonary, idiopathic, 422, 428–429. See also Pulmonary fibrosis, idiopathic
radiation, pulmonary hypertension from, 296
retroperitoneal, 2051–2052
from methysergide, 612
sclerosing cholangitis with, 869
ureteral obstruction from, 507

Fibrosis (Continued)
retroperitoneal, with Riedel's thyroiditis, 1334
Symmers', 1899
Fibrositis, 2048
Fibrous dysplasia, 1519–1520, 1520
polyostotic, 2343
vs. Paget's disease, 1515
Fibrous plaque, 322, 322
in atherosclerosis, 319, 319
reversal of, 323
Fick method, for forward stroke volume determination, 214
of cardiac blood flow measurement, 213
Fick principle, 485
Fiddleback spiders, 1923
Filarial fever, 1914–1915
Filariasis, 1913–1919, 1913t
lymphatic, 1914–1915
perstans, 1919
pulmonary hypertension from, 295
Filoviridae, 1835
Finger(s)
agnosia of, 2082
clubbing of, cancer and, 1112
congenital heart disease with, 176
from interstitial lung disease, 426
erythema of, 1673
Fingernails
atrophy or absence of, 638
dermatophytic infection of, griseofulvin for, 2317
growth rate of, 2346
iron deficiency and, 897
Fish, food poisoning from, 786, 1931
tapeworm from, 1890–1891
Fish oils, and high density lipoprotein, 320
omega-3 fatty acids in, 43
Fissures, anal, 789
Fistula(s)
after placement of vascular prostheses, 765
anorectal, 789
aortoenteric, vs. bleeding from peptic ulcers, 706
arteriovenous, 384
high output heart failure from, 216
portal hypertension from, 848
pulmonary, 308–309
hemoptysis from, 391
cholecystenteric, 865
vs. emphysematous cholecystitis, 867
coronary arterial, 308
enterocutaneous, total parenteral nutrition for, 1248t
formation of, from ulcers, 706, 707
from Crohn's disease, 747
in gallbladder, 867
in radiation enterocolitis, 806
perianal, from Crohn's disease, 749
perilymphatic, unilateral hearing loss from, 2119
rectovaginal, from ulcerative colitis, 757
to renal collecting system, in Crohn's disease, 750
tracheoesophageal, from mechanical ventilation, 489
Fits, uncinate, 2221
Fitz-Hugh-Curtis syndrome, 834, 1708
from disseminated gonococcal infection, 1709
vs. acute cholecystitis, 866
Five-day fever, 1747
Flail chest, 473, 490
and respiratory failure, 476
Flapping tremor, from hepatic encephalopathy, 809
Flashbacks, psychedelic drugs and, 59

Flat warts, 2324
Flatulence
  excessive, 661
  from cryptosporidiosis, 1882
  from iron deficiency anemia, 897
  from vitamin E deficiency, 1239
Flavivirus, and yellow fever, 1830
Flavobacterium, in intravenous infusions, 1545
Flax, and byssinosis, 2360
Fleas, 1921
  and plague, 1661
  and rickettsiae transmission, 1737
  murine typhus from, 1739, 1741
Flecainide, 270
  dosing and adverse effects of, 268t
  elimination rate for, 96t
  pharmacokinetic properties of, 266t
Flexion injury, to spine, 2244
Flichfieber, 1739
Flood fever, 1747
Floppy baby syndrome, botulism and, 1634
Flu, 1762–1767. See also *Influenza*
Flucytosine
  and diffuse ulceration of small intestine, 807
  elimination rate for, 96t
  for candidiasis, 1849
  for cryptococcosis, 1846
  for mycoses, 1838
  in kidney and liver failure, 117t
  side effects of, 1846
Fluid(s). See also *Body fluid(s)*
  accumulation of, computed tomography for, 83
  balance of, in acute respiratory failure, 479
  for tetanus, 1635
  gastrointestinal tract absorption of, mechanisms of, 725, 726
  intake of, and kidney stones, 641, 642
    for cystinuria, 620
    for gout, 1169
  physical removal of, in heart failure management, 225
  restriction of, in ascites management, 851
Fluid compartments, in heart failure, 223
Fluid therapy
  for aspiration pneumonitis, 2370
  for *Campylobacter* enteritis, 1650
  for cholera, 1652
  for dengue hemorrhagic fever, 1833
  for diabetes insipidus, 1312
  for diabetic ketoacidosis, 1376
  for diarrhea, 731
  for ileus, 719
  for *Salmonella* infection, 1645
  for shock, 244
    septic, 1660
  for viral gastroenteritis, 1771
  types of, 245
Fluid volume, regulation of, in cells, 537
Flukes, hermaphroditic, 1901–1905
Flunitrazepam, rebound insomnia from, 2078
Fluoride
  and bone formation, 1482
  estimated safe and adequate daily dietary intake of, 1206t
  for osteoporosis, 1485
  in dental caries prevention, 674
Fluoroacetamide, as testicular toxin, 1416
Fluorocarbon anesthetics, nephrogenic diabetes insipidus from, 1309
9a-Fluorocortisol, for adrenal cortex, 1353
5-Fluorodeoxyuridylate, sites of action of, 1120

Fluoropyrimidine, and drug interactions, 1118
  for cancer, 1121, 1121–1122
Fluoroscopy, digital subtraction, 83
  for heart, 195
5-Fluorouracil
  administration of, 1117
  and drug interactions, 1118
  for cancer, 1121
    breast, 1457
    colorectal, 772
    gastric, 712
    pancreatic, 783
  for glucagonoma, 1389
Fluoxymesterone, 1419
  for anemia of chronic renal insufficiency, 892
  for paroxysmal nocturnal hemoglobinuria, 923
Flurazepam, abuse of, 53
  side effects of, 2078
Flushing, cutaneous, in carcinoid syndrome, 1467
Fly larvae, tissue infestation with, 1925
FMD (foot and mouth disease), 1778
Foam cells, in Niemann-Pick disease, 1147–1148
Folacin, recommended dietary allowance for, 1205t
Folate
  deficiency of, 906
    after ulcer surgery, 705
    and macrocytosis, 882
    and megaloblastic anemia, 901t, 905–907
    neutropenia from, 962
  dietary sources of, 906
  reference intervals for, 2397t
Foley catheters, and *Candida* infection, 1849
  indwelling, infection from, 1543
Folic acid
  absorption of, 735
  chemical structure of, 905
  for hereditary spherocytosis, 912
  for malabsorption, 741t
  metabolism of, 905–906
Follicle(s), in thyroid, 1315
Follicle complex, in ovary, 1425
Follicle-stimulating hormone, 1254, 1290
  and ovarian steroid production, 1431
  and spermatogenesis, 1407
  and testicular function, 1405
  assessing function of, 1294
  deficiency of, 1295
    treatment of, 1297
  function of, 1292
  in females, 1426, 1427t
  in males, normal ranges for, 1405
    secretion of, 1405, 1406
  in menstrual cycle, 1429
  in puberty, 17
  increased, ovarian failure and, 1436
  reference intervals for, 2397t
  release of, 1283–1284
Folliculitis, 2334
  and hair loss, 2349
  chemical, 2375
Folliculogenesis, disorders of, 1440
  follicle-stimulating hormone and, 1437
Folylmonoglutamate, 906
Fonsecaea pedrosoi, 1854
Food. See also *Diet*
  additives in, and food poisoning, 786
    yellow, and asthma, 407
  allergies to, and atopic eczema, 2320
  and migraine headache, 2131
  aspiration of, and airway obstruction, 418
  and pneumonitis, 2369

Food (*Continued*)
  aspiration of, fatalities from, 40
  consumption of, changes in patterns of, 183
    energy requirements for, 1222
  enteral supplements with, 1245
  fads in, and vitamin C deficiency, 1235
  handling of, and hepatitis type A, 820
  precautions concerning, during international travel, 1549–1550
  preparation and preservation of, and cancer, 44
Food poisoning, 784–787
  and travelers' diarrhea, 1657
  and tularemia, 1664
  and typhoid fever, 1641
  bacterial, 784–785
  botulism and, 1633
  Campylobacter infection from, 1648
  chemical, 786
  Clostridium perfringens in, 1631
  definition of, 784
  Escherichia coli in, 1653
  etiology of, clinical indicators of, 784t
  from salmonellae, 1643
  staphylococcal, hypovolemic shock from, 1602
Foot (feet)
  diabetic, 1379–1380
  edema of, from thromboangiitis obliterans, 382
  fungal infection of, 2321
  Madura, 1853
  pain in, from polycythemia vera, 981
  rheumatoid arthritis in, 2001
  skin disorders of, 2346t
Foot and mouth disease, 1778
Foramen magnum, neoplasms of, vs. basilar impression, 2258
  of Bochdalek, hernias through, 472
  of Morgagni, hernias through, 472
Forced expiratory volume, 397, 397
  and chronic obstructive pulmonary disease prognosis, 416
  and dyspnea, 416
  decline of, in smokers vs. nonsmokers, 415
  in asthma, 407
  in chronic airways disease, 411
  timed, measurement of, in severely ill, 483
Fordyce's disease, vs. Fabry's disease, 1145
Foreign bodies
  and Mycobacteria infection, 1694
  and staphylococcal infection, 1598
  impaction of, and airway obstruction, 475
  in bloodstream, removal of, by mononuclear phagocyte, 955
  removal of, esophagogastroduodenoscopy for, 670
Forgetfulness, benign, 28–29, 2084
  vs. memory loss in Alzheimer's disease, 2089
Formaldehyde, for anthrax prevention, 1668
Formalin, for histoplasmosis prevention, 1840
N-Formylated oligopeptides, 952
Fort Bragg fever, 1730. See also *Leptospirosis*
Fovea, 2111
Foxes, rabies in, 2200
Foxglove, and digitalis intoxication, 787
Fractures
  compression, osteoporotic, 2043–2044
    vertebral, 2244
  from osteoporosis, 1510
  infected, 1623
  risk of, 1511, 1511
Fragile-X syndrome, 170

Framingham Heart Study, 181, 320, 321
Francisella tularensis, 1664
Frank-Starling mechanism, 185, 191, 216, 217
Freckles, 2342
Free fatty acids, 1138
    and triglyceride, 1138
    as energy source, 1374
    function of, 1137
    in liver, 810
Free radical(s), definition of, 23
    from radiation, 2375
    hydroxy, 2368
Freezing, to destroy nerve structures in pain management, 109
F-response, 2057
Friedreich's ataxia, 2152–2153
    and diabetes mellitus, 1362
    and dilated cardiomyopathy, 354
Frontal lobe(s), damage to, 2082–2083, 2082t
    disease of, gait disorders from, 2126
    neoplasms of, 2232
Frostbite, 379
Fructokinase, deficiency of, 1135
Fructose, 1135–1136
    in diabetes mellitus, 1367, *1367*
    in diabetic diet, 1369
    intolerance to
        and Fanconi's syndrome, 621
        hereditary, 1136, 1154t
        postprandial hypoglycemia with, 1384
        vs. galactosemia, 1133
Fructosemia, from hereditary fructose intolerance, 1136
Fructosuria, essential, 1135–1136
    from hereditary fructose intolerance, 1136
Fruits, consumption of, and pancreatic cancer, 781
    fresh, and hepatitis A, 825
    phototoxicity from, 2351
FSA (fetal sulfoglycoprotein antigen), 712
FSH. See *Follicle-stimulating hormone*
FTA-ABS (fluorescent treponemal antibody absorption) test, 1719
Fucosidosis, 1177
Fugue states, vs. epilepsy, 2225
Fukuyama congenital dystrophy, 2274–2275
Fumes, and asthma, 407
Function dyspepsia, vs. peptic ulcers, 699
Functional residual capacity, 395, *395*, 396, 479
    in asthma, 408
Fundus, of stomach, 693
    peritonitis from, 794
Fungi, 1837–1838
    disease from, 1837–1855. See also *Mycoses*
    sexual transmission of, 1702t
    skin examination and culture for, 2313
FUO, 1524–1525, 1732. See also *Fever, of unknown origin*
Furocoumarins, and photosensitivity, 2351
Furosemide, 232
    and calcium excretion, 519
    and hearing loss, 2119
    and hypercalcemia, 1503
    and metabolic alkalosis, 555
    as diuretic, for chronic kidney failure, 570
    characteristics of, 536t
    for ascites, 851
    for hypercalcemia, 1504
    for hypertension, 286t
    for pulmonary edema in heart failure, 226
    in drug interactions, 124t
    properties of, 231t
    reference intervals for, 2403t
Furuncle(s), and spinal epidural abscess, 2186

Furuncle(s) *(Continued)*
    definition of, 2334
    in diabetes mellitus, 1380
Furunculosis, in agammaglobulinemia, 1943
    of ear canal, pain from, 2134
    vs. sporotrichosis, 1847
Fusiform organisms, and acute gingivitis, 675
Fusobacterium, 1637
    lung abscess from, 436

GABA (gamma-aminobutyric acid), 1282
    in hepatic encephalopathy, 852
Gag reflex, absence of, from sarcoidosis, 453
    disorders of, in Guillain-Barré syndrome, 2262
GAG's. See *Glycosaminoglycans*
Gaisbock's syndrome, 976
Gait. See also *Walking ability*
    abnormalities in, acute inflammatory sensory polyneuropathy and, 2262
        in alcoholic cerebellar degeneration, 2139
        in Parkinson's disease, 2144
    apraxia of, 2126
    ataxic, from hepatic encephalopathy, 853
        in AIDS dementia complex, 2204
    hysterical, 2127
    muscle weakness and, 2271
Galactitol, and cataracts, 1132
Galactocerebroside, in globoid cell leukodystrophy, 2216
Galactokinase, and galactose metabolism, 1131
    deficiency of, 156
Galactorrhea, 1449–1450
    causes of, 1449t
    definition of, 1435
    from pituitary adenomas, 2232
    from prolactin-secreting tumors, 1302
    with hyperprolactinemia, 1439
Galactose, conversion of, to glucose, 1132
    malabsorption of, 742
Galactose-1–phosphate uridyl transferase deficiency, 156
    and galactose metabolism, 1131
    deficiency of, 156
Galactosemia, 1131–1133, 1154t
    cataract from, 2290
    children with, postprandial hypoglycemia in, 1384
    vs. hereditary fructose intolerance, 1136
Galactosyl ceramide, in globoid cell leukodystrophy, 2216
Galactosyltransferase, 1100
Galactosyltransferase isoenzyme II, and pancreatic cancer, 781–782
Gallbladder. See also *Biliary; Cholocystitis; Gallstones*
    bile in, 859, 860
    calcified, and carcinoma of gallbladder, 863, 865
    cholesterol accumulation in, 871
    disease of, familial Mediterranean fever and, 1198
        hemolytic anemia and, 880
    fistulas in, 867
    neoplasms of, 870–871
    normal, magnetic resonance of, *668*
    pain from, 658
    perforation of, 865, 867
    radionuclide imaging of, 665
    strawberry, 871
    torsion of, vs. acute cholecystitis, 865
    ultrasonography of, *663*

Gallium radioisotope scanning
    for alveolitis, 428
    for idiopathic pericarditis, 364
    for interstitial lung disease, 427
    for sarcoidosis, 456
Gallop rhythm, in left ventricular failure, 222
Gallstones
    aminotransferase level with, 818
    asymptomatic, 863–864
    cholesterol, 810
        obesity and, 1224
    dissolution of, 862
    from total parenteral nutrition, 1251
    hereditary spherocytosis and, 911
    ileus from, 867
    in cirrhosis, 868
    in Crohn's disease, 749, 750
    in protoporphyria, 1184
    in sickle cell anemia, 940
    pathophysiology of, 860–862
    pancreatitis from, 775
    predisposing factors for, 862t
    secondary biliary cirrhosis from, 846
    symptomatic, 864–865
    ultrasonography for, 663, *664*
    vs. cholestatic hepatitis syndrome, 820
    vs. pancreatic cancer, 783
Gambian sleeping sickness, 1863–1864
Gametocytes, malaria treatment and, 1860
Gamma-aminobutyric acid, 1282
    in hepatic encephalopathy, 852
Gamma chain disease, 1034
Gamma globulin. See also *Hypergammaglobulinemia; Hypogammaglobulinemia*
    for thrombocytopenic purpura, 1050, 1051
    in cerebral spinal fluid, in multiple sclerosis, 2212
    replacement of, 157
Gamma-glutamyl transpeptidase, in liver disease, 815
Gamma-glutamylcysteine synthetase, defects in, 916
Gamma-glutamyltransferase, reference intervals for, 2397t
Gamma-interferon, 1532, 1937
    and HLA class II molecule, 1965
    and macrophages, 954
    production of, 158
Gamma rays, 2375
Gamma streptococci, definition of, 1572
Gammopathies, 1026. See also *Plasma cells, disorders of*
    monoclonal, 1026
        of undetermined significance, 1035–1036
Ganglia, parasympathetic, cardiac, chronic chagasic injury to, 353
Gangliocytomas, 1286
Ganglion-blocking agents, 140
    and ileus, 719
    for hypertension, 287t
    for hypertensive crisis, 290t
    hypertensive crisis from, pheochromocytoma and, 281
    myocardial depression from, 239
Ganglioneuromas, and VIP production, 727
Gangrene
    blood pressure in dorsalis pedis or posterior tibial arteries and, 381
    from arteriosclerosis obliterans, 381
    from atherosclerosis in diabetes, 321
    from essential thrombocythemia, 987
    from frostbite, 379
    from fulminant meningococcemia, 1615
    from immersion foot, 379
    from neuropathic foot ulcer, 1380

Gangrene (Continued)
  from plague, 1662
  from Raynaud's phenomenon, 376
  from Rocky Mountain spotted fever, 1743
  from thromboangiitis obliterans, 382
  from typhus fever, 1740
  in appendices, 801
  in gallbladder, 865
  lung, 1568
  mycoplasma pneumonia with sickle cell
    disease and, 1563
  progressive synergistic, from anaerobic
    streptococci, 1574
  shock from, 1602
  streptococcal, 1630t
  synergistic, from anaerobic bacteria, 1639
  vascular, 1630t
Gardnerella vaginalis, 1621
  vaginosis from, 1705
Gardner's syndrome, 767, 769, 770, 771,
    2337
  cancer and, 1113
    of small intestine, 773
  mesenteric fibromatosis in, 796
Garrod, Archibald, 146, 152, 1157
Gas(es)
  from dietary fiber, 721
  in pleural space, 469–470. See also Pneu-
    mothorax
  intestinal, 661. See also Flatulence
    passing of, through vagina, from diver-
      ticulitis, 804
  toxic, inhalation of, 2367–2368
Gas dilution, 396
Gas exchange, 421
  adequacy of, and mechanical ventilation,
    487
  and respiratory failure, 474–475
  in respiration, 395, 401–403, 402
Gas gangrene, 1629, 1630t
Gas pain, 661
Gasoline, as inhalant, 59
    and lead poisoning, 2386
  exposure to, and pancreatic cancer, 781
Gasser's syndrome, thrombocytopenia in,
    1053, 1080
Gastrectomy
  and impaired iron absorption, 894, 896
  malabsorption following, treatment of,
    740–741
  subtotal, for duodenal ulcer disease, 703,
    703t
    for gastric cancer, 710
  vitamin B$_{12}$ deficiency from, 904
Gastric. See also Stomach
Gastric acid
  and Escherichia coli, 1654
  and gastritis, 689
  aspiration of, 2369
  in gastroesophageal reflux disease, 680
  in host defense mechanisms, 1529
  secretion of
    decreased, and acute gastritis, 689
    in chronic gastritis, 691
    measurement of, 699
    normal, 694, 695t
Gastric inhibitory polypeptide, in gastroin-
    testinal motility, 715
Gastric juice, 693, 693
Gastric lavage, after poisonings, 142
  for upper gastrointestinal hemorrhage,
    797
Gastrin
  and acid secretion, 693, 695
  and mesenteric circulation, 761
  concentrations of, in chronic gastritis, 691
  in bile formation, 859
  in gastrointestinal motility, 715

Gastrin (Continued)
  in Zollinger-Ellison syndrome, 698–699,
    698t, 708
  reference intervals for, 2397t
Gastrin-releasing peptide, as tumor marker,
    1099
Gastrinoma, 1388, 1389t. See also Zollinger-
    Ellison syndrome
Gastritis, 689–692
  acute, 689–690, 690t
  alkaline reflux, after gastric surgery, 705
  bile reflux, 692
  chronic, 690–691, 690t
    natural history of, 691
  eosinophilic, 692
    gastric outlet obstruction from, 707
  erosive, 689
    from aspirin, and iron deficiency, 896
  from Candida infection, 1848
  granulomatous, 692
  hemorrhagic, 799
    vs. bleeding from peptic ulcers, 706
  hypertrophic, 691–692
    vs. peptic ulcers, 699
  types of, 690t
  vs. acute pancreatitis, 776
Gastrocoides hominis, 1904
Gastroduodenal artery, 760
Gastroenteritis, 692
  eosinophilic, 807
    and peritoneum, 795
    vs. Crohn's disease, 750
  from Salmonella, 1644, 1645
  hemolytic uremic syndrome after, 601
  hemorrhagic, from barium, 2281
  in AIDS patients, DHPG for, 126
  infectious, acute, in children, vs. appen-
    dicitis, 803
  staphylococcal, 1598
  viral, 1768–1772. See also Viral gastroenter-
    itis
Gastroenterology, diagnostic imaging pro-
    cedures for, 662–671
Gastroesophageal reflux disease, 680–683
  diagnosis of, 681, 682
  endoscopy for, 669
  treatment of, 682–683, 682t
  vs. gallstones, 864
Gastrointestinal endoscopy, 668–674
  contraindications for, 668
Gastrointestinal hemorrhage, 660, 796–800
  and anemia, 880
  and iron deficiency, 896
  angiography for, 666
  approach to, 796
  causes of, 799t
  esophagogastroduodenoscopy for, 669,
    670
  failure to diagnose source of, 800
  from alcoholic cirrhosis, 844
  from Banti's syndrome, 1038
  from cirrhosis of liver, 849–850
  from colon, adenocarcinoma of, 770
    from Campylobacter infection, 1649
  from diverticula, 804
  from drug-induced thrombocytopenic
    purpura, 1049
  from esophageal ulcers, 682
  from fulminant hepatic failure, 854
  from gastrointestinal reflux disease, 681
  from hemophilia B, 1071
  from liver disease, 808
  from peptic ulcers, 706
  from polycythemia vera, 981, 983
  from polyps of large intestines, 767
  from renal artery atheroembolization, 633
  from ulcerative colitis, 757
    as indication for surgery, 759

Gastrointestinal hemorrhage (Continued)
  iron deficiency anemia from, 883
  lower, diagnosis of, 798–799
  magnitude of, 796
  pulmonary arteriovenous fistula and, 309
  recognition of, 796–797
  upper
    diagnosis of, 798
    endoscopy for, 798t
    therapy for, 797–798
    vs. lower, 797
Gastrointestinal sphincters, 714
Gastrointestinal syndrome, from radiation
    injury, 2377–2378
Gastrointestinal tract
  absorption in, normal physiology of, 725–
    726
  after spinal cord trauma, 2246
  and back pain, 2043
  anthrax of, 1667, 1668
  arachidonic acid metabolites and, 1276
  arsenic poisoning and, 2388–2389
  arterial blood supply to, 760
  Behçet's disease in, 2049
  bicarbonate wasting in, 553
  bleeding from, 660, 796–800. See also
    Gastrointestinal hemorrhage
  cancer of, and iron deficiency anemia,
    896
    from polycythemia vera treatment, 983
  change in, with aging, 97
  cryptosporidiosis in, 1881
  disorders of
    and osteomalacia, 1481
    and potassium depletion, 546
    emotion and stress in, 657
    from adrenocortical insufficiency, 1351
    from African hemorrhagic fever, 1836
    from diabetic autonomic neuropathy,
      2263
    from glucagonoma, 1389
    from hyperparathyroidism, 1490
    introduction to, 656–662
    non-Hodgkin's lymphoma and, 1012
    pathophysiologic basis for symptoms
      of, 657–662
    patient history for, 656–657
    physical examination for, 657
    total parenteral nutrition for, 1248
  edema of, in heart failure, 223
  evaluation of, and nutritional supplemen-
    tation, 1244
  glucocorticoids and, 1347
  gummas of, 1717
  hemorrhage of, 660, 796–800. See also
    Gastrointestinal hemorrhage
  in hypereosinophilic syndrome, 1024
  in systemic sclerosis, 2021–2022
  infection of, immunoglobulin A defi-
    ciency and, 1943
  lead poisoning and, 2386
  leeches in, 1927
  malnutrition and, 1213
  mastocytosis and, 1973
  motility of
    clinical assessment of, 716
    common disorders of, 716t
    control of, 715–716
    disorders of, 714–725
    electrical and mechanical correlates of,
      715
    normal, 714
  mucormycosis in, 1852
  normal flora in, 1658
  obesity and, 1224
  paraneoplastic syndromes in, 1098
  polyarteritis nodosa in, 2029
  shock and, 236–237

Gastrointestinal tract *(Continued)*
  Staphylococcus aureus in, antibiotics and, 1597
  systemic lupus erythematosus and, 2015
  upper, neoplasms of, malignant, endoscopy for, 669
Gastroparesis, after gastric surgery, 717–718
  idiopathic, 718
Gastrostomy, endoscopic, percutaneous, 670
  feeding, for recurrent aspiration pneumonia, 1569
  percutaneous, as feeding route, 1244
Gaucher's disease, 1145–1147
  enzyme infusions for, 157
  interstitial lung disease with, 432
  kidney transplant for, 157
  osteonecrosis in, 1517
  splenectomy for, 1038
  splenomegaly from, 1037
Gay bowel syndrome, 1646
Gaze paralysis, 2116
G CSF (granulocyte colony-stimulating factor), 876, 968
Gemfibrozil, for dysbetalipoproteinemia, 1141
  for familial hypertriglyceridemia, 1142
Gender identity, development of, 1401
Gene(s), 146
  allelic, 155
  chromosomal arrangements of, for polypeptide chains, 925, *926*
  clones of, for adenosine deaminase, 1946
    insertion of, into cells, 160
  coding portions of, 928
  defects in, and immunodeficiency, 1941
  definition of, 158
  Duarte variant, 1132, 1133
  flow of information from, to protein, 928
  frequency of, 151
  immune response of, 1966
  isolation of, 160
  mapping of, 152, 172
  nonallelic, 155
Gene splicing, 158–161
Gene therapy, 6, 159–161
  ethics of, 160–161
  in utero, 161
Generalized seizures, 2218, 2221–2222. See also *Seizures*
Genetic code, 146
Genetic compounds, 155
  and inherited metabolic diseases, 157t
Genetic counseling, 171–174
  diagnosis in, 171–172
  for hypertrophic cardiomyopathy, 358
  for sickle cell disease, 941
  prenatal diagnosis in, 173–174
Genetic disease, multifactorial, 150, *150*
  pathogenesis of, 153, 155
Genetic engineering, 158–161
Genetic heterogeneity, 155, 157t
  multifactorial inheritance vs., 151
Genetic load, 151, 166
Genetic markers, 163
Genetics, definition of, 146
Genital tract
  after spinal cord trauma, 2246
  diagnostic imaging of, 525–527
  disorders of, in diabetic autonomic neuropathy, 2263–2264
  infection of
    herpes simplex virus, 1782
    immunoglobulin A deficiency and, 1943
    in women, 1704–1705
    meningococcal, 1615
    neutropenia and, 963

Genital tract *(Continued)*
  infection of, with mycoplasma, 1564–1565
    with ureaplasma, 1564–1565
  polyarteritis nodosa in, 2029
  St. Louis encephalitis and, 1826
  tuberculosis in, 1690
  ulcers of, 1703–1704
  warts of, interferon for, 128
Genitalia
  external, ambiguous, 170
    development of, 1392
  skin disorders of, 2346t
Genitourinary tract. See *Genital tract; Urinary tract*
Gentamicin, 113, 119, 122
  and kidney damage, 609
  elimination rate for, 96t
  hypokalemia from, 546
  reference intervals for, 2403t
Geographic tongue, 2348
Geophagia, 880, 896
Geriatric medicine, 21–26
Germ cell(s), in testis, 1405
German measles, 1776–1777. See also *Rubella*
Germinal cell aplasia, 1415–1416
Germinomas, 1286
  of pineal, 1314
Gerstmann-Straussler syndrome, Creutzfeldt-Jakob disease in, 2206
GH. See *Growth hormone*
Ghon's complex, 1683
  in histoplasmosis, 1838
Giant cell(s), 954
  multinucleated, from chronic eosinophilic pneumonia, 431
Giant cell arteritis, 374, 2033–2034
  central retinal artery occlusion and, 2298
Giant cell pneumonia, from measles, 1774
Giant cell thyroiditis, 1332–1333
Giant cell tumors, of thyroid, 1336
Giant platelet syndrome, 1055
  vs. thrombasthenia, 1057
Giardia, AIDS with, diarrhea from, 729
  infection with, vs. peptic ulcers, 699
Giardia lamblia, 1883
  and diarrhea, 1857
  vs. *Escherichia coli*, 1655
Giardiasis, 1883–1884
  metronidazole for, 121
  stool examination for, 730
Gigantism, cerebral, 1288
  from growth hormone hypersecretion, 1300
Gilbert's syndrome, 813, 813t
  hyperbilirubinemia in, 814
  phenobarbital for, 157
Gilchrist's disease, 1842
Gilles de la Tourette's syndrome, 2151–2152
  vs. epilepsy, 2225
Gingiva, bleeding of, from aplastic anemia, 887
  disease of, cervicofacial actinomycosis and, 1674
Gingivitis, 675
  acute, 675, *675*
  in neutropenia, 1537
Gingivostomatitis, from herpes simplex virus, 1781–1782, 1783
  herpetic, 676, 676–677, 2347
Gitalin, pharmacology of, for heart failure, 227t
Glanders, 1670
Glans penis, development of, 1392
Glanzmann's disease, 1056–1057
Glasgow coma scale, 2242t
Glaucoma, 2112, 2290–2292
  angle-closure, 2290–2291, *2291*

Glaucoma *(Continued)*
  cannabis for, 58
  from diabetes mellitus, 1378
  from glucocorticoid therapy, 1347
  pain of, 2134
  timolol for, 138
  tonometry test for, 667
Glial tumors, 1286
Glibenclamide, for diabetes mellitus, 1370, 1370t
Glioblastoma multiforme, 2230, 2233
Gliomas, and vision loss, 2113
Glipizide, for diabetes mellitus, 1370, 1370t
Globin(s), deficient synthesis of, and thalassemias, 930
  postsynthetic modification of, 929
  stability of, mutations affecting, thalassemia from, 935
Globin gene, beta, structure of, 928
Globin RNA, 928–929
Globoid cell leukodystrophy, 2216
Globular proteins, in extracellular matrix, 1981
Globulins. See also *Gamma globulin; Immunoglobulin(s)*
  in liver disease, 815–816, 832
Globus pallidus, 2141
Glomangioma, 384
Glomerular capillary endotheliosis, from toxemia of pregnancy, 635
Glomerular disease, proteinuria from, 503
Glomerular filtration rate, 511
  accelerated, 602
  aging and, 98
  and renal plasma flow, 510
  and sodium homeostasis, 514
  and uremic symptoms, 507
  and water excretion regulation, 516
  decrease in
    causes of, 511
    from anti-inflammatory drugs, 102
    from obstructive nephropathy, 614
    from volume depletion in chronic kidney failure, 569
  elevation of, in occult diabetic glomerulopathy, 625
  in acute interstitial nephritis, 606
  in chronic kidney failure, 563
  in glomerular disorders, 584
  in heart failure, 220
  in pregnancy, 634, *635*
  loss of, with converting enzyme inhibitors, 291
  measurement of, 522–523
Glomerular immune complex, formation of, rapidly progressive glomerulonephritis from, 591
Glomerular polyanion, 511
Glomerular tubular balance, 513, 530–531
Glomerulitis
  from drug allergy, 1971t
  from immune complex, 1960
  in polyarteritis nodosa, 2029
  systemic vasculitis with, from nonsteroidal anti-inflammatory agents, 609
Glomerulocapillary sclerosis, nodular, in diabetic nephropathy, 1379
Glomerulonephritis, 504
  acute, 583–585
    and acute kidney failure, 559
      recovery from, 562
    group A streptococcal pharyngitis and, 1572
    streptococcal impetigo and, 1578
    urinalysis for, 561
  and interstitial inflammation, 605
  chronic, 602
  from endocarditis, infective, 1590
  subacute bacterial, 587

Glomerulonephritis *(Continued)*
from erythema nodosum leprosum, 1699
from essential mixed cryoglobulinemia, 601
from Goodpasture's syndrome, 430
from hepatitis, chronic, 831, 832
type B, 820, 823
from Wegener's granulomatosis, 2030
idiopathic, glucocorticosteroids for, 130
rapidly progressive, 583, 584t
renal vein thrombosis with, 634
interstitial, 504–506
membranoproliferative, 592t, *597*, 597–598
complement activation in, 1941
post-streptococcal, 584t, 585–587, *586*
urine sodium concentration in, 524
with visceral abscesses, 588
Glomerulosclerosis, focal, 592t, 593–595, *595*, 602
nodular, 625
Glomerulus, 508, 509, *509*. See also under *Glomerular*
blood flow of, 510
capillary wall of, 509
permeability of, 511, 591
disorders of, 582–602
biopsy for, 569
immunologic mechanisms of, 584
in acquired immunodeficiency syndrome, 588
in immune complex disease, 1962
filtration rate of, 511. See also *Glomerular filtration rate*
injury to, red cell casts and, 503
permeability of, and proteinuria, 521
response of, to injury, immune mechanisms and, 583
Glomus body, tumor of, 384
Glossitis, 678, 2348
from folate deficiency, 906
from riboflavin deficiency, 1231
vitamin B_{12} deficiency and, 903
Glossodynia, 2348
Glossopharyngeal neuralgia, 2135
Glossopharyngeal structures, and airway obstruction, 418
Glucagon
and glycogen homeostasis, 1364
and glycogenolysis, 1382
and insulin, 1374
and mesenteric circulation, 761
and mitochondrial fatty acid uptake, 1138
and sodium reabsorption, 516
catabolism of, in kidneys, 519
in gastrointestinal motility, 715, 724
levels of, increased, from glucagonoma, 1389
normal circulating, 1389
test of, intravenous, for insulinoma, 1385
Glucagonoma, 1112, 1389t, 1389–1390
diabetes mellitus from, 1362
Glucocerebroside, accumulation of, 1145
Glucocorticoid(s)
action of, 1346–1347
and chylomicronemia syndrome, 1143
and immune response, 1533
and mitochondrial function, 242
and phosphorus excretion, 518
and thyroid function, 1321
deficiency of. See *Addison's disease*
diabetes mellitus from, 1362
eosinopenia from, 966
excess of, 1353–1357. See also *Cushing's syndrome*
for autoimmune hemolytic anemia, 919
for gout, 1168

Glucocorticoid(s) *(Continued)*
for infectious mononucleosis, 1788
for inhibiting intestinal secretion, 732
for systemic sclerosis, 2023
function of, 1340
immunoassays for, 1348
in sepsis treatment, 1541
metabolism of, 1343
myopathy from, 2280
neutrophilia from, 969
osteoporosis from, 1514
plasma binding of, 1341–1343
production of, regulation of, 1344–1345
regulatory elements of, *1261*, 1261–1262
thymic hypoplasia from, 1974
Glucocorticoid suppression test, for hyperparathyroidism, 1494
Glucocorticosteroid therapy, 128–133
adrenocortical insufficiency after withdrawal of, 1352
alternate-day, 131–132
and growth retardation in children, 581
biochemistry and pharmacology of, 128–129
complications of, 132–133, 133t
dose and dose interval of, 131
eosinopenia from, 1024
in immunosuppression therapy, 581
mechanisms of, 129–130
preparations of, 129t
regimen design for, 130–132
side effects of, 130
vs. ACTH, 132
withdrawal syndrome from, 132
Gluconeogenesis, 1382
in liver, 809
Glucose, 1373–1374. See also *Hyperglycemia; Hypoglycemia*
concentration of, catecholamines and, 1463
consumption of, in brain, 1374
for coma, 2067–2068
galactose conversion to, 1132
homeostasis of, hormonal control of, 1382, 1382t
in cerebrospinal fluid, bacterial meningitis and, 1607
in rehydration solution, 731
in synovial fluid, 1994
intolerance to
and atherosclerosis, 319–320
definition of, 1361
from chromium deficiency, 1242
from hemochromatosis, 839
from thiazides, 231
in chronic pancreatitis, 779
in liver disease, 809–810
liver production of, in non-insulin–dependent diabetes mellitus, 1365
malabsorption of, 742
metabolism of, and congenital malformations, 171
in erythrocytes, 913–914, *914*
reference intervals for, 2397t
tolerance to, in chronic kidney failure, 567
Glucose tolerance tests, oral, for diabetes mellitus, 1361
limitations of, 1383
reference intervals for, 2397t
Glucose-6-phosphatase
deficiency of, and gout, 1167
hypoglycemia from, 1382
in glycogen storage diseases, 1134
nucleotide metabolism disorder from, 1057

Glucose-6-phosphate dehydrogenase, 914–916, *916*, 973
deficiency in, 102, 150
and HMP shunt defects, 914
and malaria treatment, 1861
and neutrophil respiratory burst, 958
and primaquine therapy, 1551
and rickettsial infection, 1742
and vitamin E deficiency, 1239
genetic counseling for, 174
hemolysis from, 909, 946
reticulocytosis from, 882
sickle cell anemia with, 939
vitamin C with, and hemolytic episodes, 1236
vs. paroxysmal nocturnal hemoglobinuria, 923
vs. unstable hemoglobin, 943
intracellular, decay of, 914, *915*
reference intervals for, 2401t
variants of, 155, 914
Glucosuria, in pregnancy, 634
Glue sniffing, 59
aplastic anemia from, 886
hydrocarbons from, and kidney damage, 612
Glutamic-oxaloacetic transaminase
in hypothyroidism, 1330
increase in, in renal artery occlusion, 633
measurement of, for myocardial infarction, 332
reference intervals for, 2395t
Glutamine, as glucose precursor, 1382
Glutathione synthetase, defects in, 916
Glutathionemia, 1152t
Gluten-sensitive enteropathy, 742–743. See also *Nontropical sprue*
small intestinal ulceration from, 807
Glutethimide
abuse of, 53
and enhanced liver metabolism of other drugs, 99
overdose of, and central nervous system, 2069
poisoning with, 2069t
reference intervals for, 2403t
L-Glycerate, in urine, 1136
L-Glyceric aciduria, 1136–1137
Glycerol, properties of, 231t
reference intervals for, 2397t
Glyceryl guaiacolate (guaifenesin), and prolonged bleeding time, 1047
Glycogen, 1133, 1373
Glycogen storage disease, 361, 1133–1135, 2277–2278
enzyme infusions for, 157
gout in, 1165, 1167
liver in, 839–840
Glycogen synthetase, deficiency of, and hypoglycemia in neonates, 1382
Glycogenolysis, 1382
in liver, 809
Glycoglycinuria, 1154t
Glycolysis, aerobic, 549
defects in, and hemolysis, 916–917
Glycoprotein(s), deficiency of, in thrombasthenia, 1057
Glycosaminoglycans, 1174–1177, 1176t, 2302
storage of, etiology of, 1174
pathologic consequences of, 1174–1175
Glycosides, cardiac, interaction of, with diuretics, 101
decreased absorption of, cholestyramine and, 99
Glycosphingolipid(s), in heart muscle, 361
Glycosphingolipidosis (Fabry's disease), 150, 167, 361, 1144–1145
fever in, 1525
kidney transplant for, 157

Glycosuria
  and phosphorus excretion, 518
  from mannitol, 542
  in tubulointerstitial disease, 603
  renal, 505, 617–619, *619*
Glycosylation, and aging, 23
  in red cells, 1367, *1367*
Glycyrrhizinic acid, 545
Glyoxylate metabolism, disorders of, 1136
Gnathostoma spinigerum, 1911
GNB. See *Gram-negative bacilli*
GnRH. See *Gonadotropin-releasing hormone*
Goblet cells, metaplasia of, in cystic fibrosis, 440
Goeckerman regimen, 2318
Goiter, 1338–1340
  adolescent, 1329
  endemic, 1316, 1339–1340
    definition of, 1338
  euthyroid, 19
  in Hashimoto's thyroiditis, 1334
  malignancy in, 1339
  multinodular, 1339
  thyroid hormone for, 156
Gold salts
  effects on kidney, 596, 611
  for rheumatoid arthritis, 2003
  for skin disorders, 2317
  interstitial lung disease from, 429, 434
  side effects of, 2003
Golfer's elbow, 2047
Gompertz equation, 1085
Gonad(s)
  atrophy of, in myotonic dystrophy, 1414
  development of, 1390–1391, *1391*
  disorders of, anemia with, 892
  dysgenesis of, 1437
    mixed, 1429
    ovarian, 167t
    pure, 1438
    reticular, 1946
    XY, 1393–1394
  function of, pituitary hormones and, 1292
  primary failure of, vs. hypopituitarism, 1296
  radiation injury in, 2377
Gonadoblastoma(s), 1394
  hormones from, 1445t
Gonadotropin, 1419–1420
  and ovarian steroid production, 1431
  deficiency of, 1295
    isolated, 1439
    prepubertal, 1417
    treatment of, 1297
  for fertility for Kallmann syndrome patients, 1417
  from pituitary tumors, 1305
  human chorionic, 1419–1420. See also
    Human chorionic gonadotropin
  in regulation of testicular function, 1406–1407
  receptors of, defects of, 1438
  secretion of, central nervous system in regulation of, 1405
    testicular feedback regulation of, 1407–1408
Gonadotropin-releasing hormone
  and ovarian regulation, 1432
  from hypothalamus, 1280
  in females, 1426
  release of, 1283, 1284
  to restore fertility, 1297, 1443
Gonioscopy, 2290
Gonococcal infections, 1706–1710. See also
  Gonorrhea
  arthritis from, 2010
    treatment of, 1710
  clinical patterns of, 1707–1709

Gonococcal infections (*Continued*)
  conjunctivitis as, 2294
  epidemiology of, 1706–1707
  laboratory diagnosis of, 1709
  of fallopian tubes, 803
  of liver, 834, 1708, 1709
  of rectum, 757
  pathogenesis of, 1708
  prevention of, 1710
  treatment of, 1708t, 1709–1710
  vs. infectious mononucleosis, 1788
Gonococcemia, transient tenosynovitis
    from, 2047
  vs. chronic meningococcemia, 1616
  vs. rat-bite fever, 1730
Gonococcus(i), and pus in stool, 730
  penicillinase-producing, 1709–1710
Gonorrhea
  anorectal, diagnosis of, 787
  in adolescents, 20
  incidence of, 1702
  proctitis from, vs. ulcerative proctitis, 788
  spectinomycin for, 122
  urethral, laboratory tests for, 1703
Goodpasture's syndrome, 584t, 589–590,
    590, 1960
  after kidney transplant for Alport's syndrome, 638
  antibody tissue destruction in, 1988
  as interstitial lung disease, 430
  hemoptysis from, 391
  kidneys in, 504
  vs. idiopathic pulmonary hemosiderosis,
    430
  vs. polyarteritis nodosa, 2030
  vs. Wegener's granulomatosis, 599, 2031
Gordon phenomenon, eosinophil and, 362
Gorlin formula, estimation of valve area
    with, 214, *214*
  for estimating pressure drop across valve,
    205
  for mitral orific size calculation, 347
Gottron's sign, 2035
Gout, 1161–1170, 1978
  acute, 1164
  and amyloidosis, 1199
  causes of death in patients with, 1166
  definition of, 1161
  diagnosis of, 1168
  from hereditary spherocytosis, 911
  heredity and, 147, 1161
  metabolic, 1163
  pathogenesis and pathology of, 1161–
    1162, 1162t
  prevalence and incidence of, 1161
  radiology for, 1997
  renal, 1163
  sarcoidosis vs., 454
  saturnine, 611, 1167
  secondary, 1167
  tophaceous, 1165–1166
    accumulation of uric acid in, 157
  treatment of, 1168–1170
  uric acid stones in, 641
  vs. arthritis from alcaptonuria, 1157
  vs. rheumatoid arthritis, 2000
  vs. sporotrichosis, 1847
  with sarcoidosis, 453
Gouty arthritis
  acute, 1165
  chronic, *1166*
    diagnosis of, 1168
    treatment of, 1169–1170
  from chronic myelogenous leukemia, 990
  from myelofibrosis, with myeloid metaplasia, 985
  hypoxanthine-guanine phosphoribosyl-
    transferase deficiency and, 1171

Gout (*Continued*)
  in glycogen storage diseases, 1134
  tophaceous, radiology for, 1997
G6PD. See *Glucose-6-phosphate dehydrogenase*
Graafian follicle(s), in ovary, 1430–1431
  rupture of, vs. appendicitis, 803
Gradenigo's syndrome, lateral sinus thrombosis and, 2185
Graft(s), bypass, coronary artery, 337–339.
    See also *Coronary artery bypass grafts*
Graft-versus-host disease
  and opportunistic infections, 2210
  from blood transfusions, 950, 1006
  from bone marrow transplants, 992, 1006,
    1040
  severe combined immunodeficiency disease and, 1946
  skin in, vs. lichen planus, 2328
  thymic hypoplasia from, 1974
Graham Steell murmurs, from pulmonic regurgitation, 351
Gram-negative bacilli
  aerobic, pneumonia from, 1565–1568
  anaerobic, 1637
  arthritis from, 2009
  bacteremia from, and endotoxic shock,
    1659–1661
  cephalosporins for, 120
  endocarditis from, 1591
  meningitis from, 1605
    cefotaxime for, 1610
    cephalosporins for, 120
  salmonellae as, 1643
  shock from, 1538
Gram-positive microorganisms, anaerobic,
    1637
  shock from, 1538
Gram's stain, 112, 113
  alternatives to, 1554
  for skin infection, 2313
Granulation tissue, brain abscess with,
    2182
Granules, lysosomal, 1987
Granulocyte(s)
  dysfunction of, and mycoses, 1837
  inflammatory response and, 1985
  life span of, 877
  precursors of, 874
    megaloblastic changes in, 901
Granulocyte colony–stimulating factor, 876,
    968
Granulocyte-macrophage colony–stimulating factor, 876, 968
Granulocyte-myeloid colony–stimulating
    factor, 1532
Granulocytopenia
  chronic kidney failure and, 566
  from drug allergy, 1971t
  from myelofibrosis, 986
  from paroxysmal nocturnal hemoglobinuria, 922
Granulocytosis, in paraneoplastic syndromes, 1097–1098
Granuloma(s)
  eosinophilic, 430, 692. See also *Histiocytosis X*
  Gnathostoma spinigerum in, 1911
  pneumothorax from, 470
  sarcoidosis vs., 454
  from activated phagocytes, 954
  from blastomycosis, 1842
  from brucellosis, 1677
  from leprosy, 1697
  from lymphocytic interstitial pneumonitis, 431
  from schistosome eggs, 1897
  from syphilis, 1714
  in liver, from drugs, 828

Granuloma(s) (Continued)
 midline, 2032–2033
  vs. zygomycosis, 1852
 necrotic, in interstitial lung disease with
  pulmonary airway disease, 432
 of skin, from chemicals, 2375
  from mycobacteria, 1695
 pyogenic, 2336t, 2340
 vs. viral encephalitis, 1823
Granuloma inguinale, 1711–1712
 and genital ulcers, 2342
 vs. chancroid, 1712
 vs. lymphogranuloma venereum, 1711
Granulomatosis
 allergic, 599
 bronchocentric, 432
 Churg-Strauss, 2026
  polyarteritis nodosa and, 2028
 in drug abusers, 57
 Langerhans cell, 1022–1024
 lymphomatoid, 431, 2026
  vs. Wegener's granulomatosis, 2031
 Wegener's, 2030–2031. See also Wegener's
  granulomatosis
Granulomatosis infantiseptica, 1672
Granulomatous disease
 and fever, 1525
 chronic, 958
 chylothorax from, 468
 hypercalcemia in, 1503
 inflammation in, 731
 lymphocytopenia in, 967
 small intestinal ulceration from, 807
Granulomatous processes, airway obstruction from, 418
Granulopoiesis, ineffective, in Chédiak-Higashi disease, 959
Granulosa cells, in ovary, 1425
Granulosa-theca cell tumor, hormones
 from, 1445t
Graphite, inhalation of, 2361
Graves' disease, 1320, 1321–1323. See also
 Hyperthyroidism; Thyrotoxicosis
 and polyglandular autoimmune disease,
  1414
 and pregnancy, 1326–1327
 hyperthyroidism of, treatment of, 1324–
  1327
 hyposplenism from, 1039
 orbitopathy of, 2295
 papilledema in, 2292
 subacute lymphocytic thyroiditis vs., 1333
 vs. gynecomastia, 1452
Grawitz' tumor, 652. See also Renal cell carcinoma
Gray syndrome, 140
Gray unit, 2375
Great arteries. See Aorta; Pulmonary artery
 (arteries)
Grey Turner's sign, 776
GRH. See Growth hormone–releasing hormone
Griseofulvin, and enhanced liver metabolism of other drugs, 99
 for skin disorders, 2317
Groin, pain in, from renal colic, 106
 skin disorders of, 2346t
Grönblad-Strandberg syndrome, 1181–1182
Groove sign, 1711
Growth
 abnormal, in sickle cell anemia, 940
  from thalassemia, 931
 hormones and, 1263
 retardation of. See Growth retardation
Growth factors, in atherosclerosis, 322
Growth hormone, 17, 1254, 1263
 and insulin, 1374
 and phosphorus excretion, 518
 and sodium reabsorption, 516

Growth hormone (Continued)
 deficiency of, 1295, 1296
  treatment of, 1297
 effect of, 1292–1293
 from somatotrophs, 1290
 hypersecretion of, 1300, 1300–1302
 in anorexia nervosa, 1217
 obesity and, 1225
 production of, 158
 reference intervals for, 2397t
 replacement therapy for, and Creutzfeldt-
  Jakob disease, 2205
 secretion of, 1284
  assessing, 1294
  from tumors, 1103
  hypothalamic disorders of, 1288
Growth hormone–releasing hormone, 657,
 1103
 from hypothalamus, 1280
 from islet cell tumors, 1390
Growth retardation
 corticosteroid therapy and, 752
 from Crohn's disease, 747, 749
  therapy for, 751
 from Lesch-Nyhan syndrome, 1171
 from medullary cystic disorders, 648
 from nephrogenic diabetes insipidus,
  1312
 from thyroid hormone deficiency, 1329
 hypothalamus tumors and, 1286
 in children, on hemodialysis, 1508
Growth spurt, adolescent, in females, 1426
GSH (reduced glutathione), for reducing
 methomoglobin, 945
 metabolism of, abnormalities in, and hemolysis, 916
GT-II (Galactosyltransferase isoenzyme II),
 781
Guaifenesin, and prolonged bleeding time,
 1047
Guanabenz, adverse effects of, 289t
 for hypertension, 137, 287t
Guanadrel, adverse effects of, 289t
 distribution of, 99
Guanethidine
 adverse effects of, 289t
 aggravation of heart failure by, 220
 distribution of, 99
 for hypertension, 287t
 hypertensive crisis from, pheochromocytoma and, 281
 interaction of, with oral contraceptives,
  1443
 myocardial depression from, 239
Guanidinosuccinic acid, in uremic platelet
 defect, 1057
Guanine, 1163
Guanylate cyclase, 406
 activation of, 1260–1261
Guillain-Barré syndrome, 2198, 2259, 2261–
 2262
 autonomic insufficiency in, 2106
 from Campylobacter infection, 1649
 from enteroviruses, 1810
 in St. Louis encephalitis, 1826
 respiratory failure from, 476
  critical care of, 489–490
 varicella and, 1789
 vs. botulism, 1633
 vs. infantile spinal muscular atrophy,
  2155
 vs. Lyme disease, 1728
 vs. poliomyelitis, 2199
 vs. rabies, 2201
 vs. tick paralysis, 1923
Guinea worm disease, 1918
Gumma, 1716–1717
 from syphilis, 2189

Gunshot wound, pericarditis from, 363
Gut lavage, after poisonings, 143
Guthrie bacterial inhibition assay, for phenylketonuria, 1155
Gutzeit test, for arsenic poisoning, 2389
Gy (gray unit), 2375
Gymnodinium breve, shellfish contamination
 with, 786
Gynecologic disorders, 1433–1442
 abnormal uterine bleeding as, 1434–1435
 amenorrhea as, 1435–1340
 during puberty, 19–20
 dysmenorrhea as, 1433
 folliculogenesis disorders as, 1440
 infertility as, 1440–1441
 premenstrual syndrome as, 1433–1434,
  1434t
 sexual dysfunction as, 1441–1442
Gynecomastia, 16, 17, 1410–1411, 1450–
 1452, 1451
 causes of, 1411t, 1451t
 from alcoholic cirrhosis, 844
 from androgen deficiency, 1409
 from cirrhosis, 842
 from Klinefelter's syndrome, 1413
 from testosterone therapy, 1419
 refeeding, 1411

H chain diseases, 1030, 1034
H₂-receptor antagonists, for inhibiting acid
 secretion, 700
 in cystic fibrosis treatment, 441
H-reflex, 2057
Habit spasms, 2151. See also Tics
Haemophilus, 1617, 1617t
 ampicillin for, 119
 infection by, 1617–1621
Haemophilus aphrophilus, 1621
Haemophilus ducreyi, chancroid from, 1712
 cultures of, 1712–1713
Haemophilus influenzae, 1617–1620
 and bronchiectasis, 439
 and chronic bronchitis, 412
 and pneumonia, 1566
 central nervous system infection from, in
  immunocompromised host, 2210
 cephalosporins for, 120
 chloramphenicol for, 112, 120
 immunization against, 65
 in acquired immunodeficiency syndrome,
  1806
 lung abscess from, 436
 meningitis from, treatment of, 1609
 penicillins for, 119
 pericarditis from, 363
 pneumonia from, vs. pneumococcal
  pneumonia, 1558
 sickle cell anemia and, 940
 trimethoprim/sulfamethoxazole combination for, 119
 vs. Listeria monocytogenes, 1672
Haemophilus parainfluenzae, 1621
Haemophilus vaginalis, 1621
 vaginosis from, 1705
Haff disease, myoglobinuria in, 2283
Hageman factor, 1531, 1950, 1987
Hailey-Hailey disease, 2331
Hair
 follicle of, 2302
  Staphylococcus aureus infection of, 2334
 growth of, 2303
  alterations in, 2348–2350
  excessive, 1446, 2349–2350. See also
   Hirsutism
  normal, 1446

Hair (Continued)
  loss of, 2348–2349. See also *Alopecia*
  malnutrition and, 1210t
Hair-pull examination, 2313
Hairy cell(s), 998–999, *999*
Hairy cell leukemia, 998–1001
  deoxycoformycin for, 1123
  human T lymphotropic retrovirus and, 1797
  marrow transplants for, 1041
  splenectomy for, 1038
  vs. chronic lymphocytic leukemia, 997
Hairy leukoplakia, in AIDS, 677, *677*
Halitosis, from esophageal carcinoma, 686
  from rumination syndrome, 1219
Hallpike maneuver, 2121
Hallucinations
  by children, 2079
  from amphetamine toxicity, 54
  from atropine, 139
  from metabolic encephalopathy, 2065
  from psychedelic drugs, 58
  from rabies, 2201
  from withdrawal of sedatives for insomnia, 2078
  in delirium, 2064–2065
  in narcolepsy, 2078
  in psychiatric disorders, 2066
  in schizophrenia, 2092
Hallucinogens, psychologic dependence on, 49
Hallucinosis, acute, in alcoholics, 51
Haloethers, and lung cancer, 458
Haloperidol
  as alpha blocker, 139
  for agitation in psychiatric disorders, 2094t
  for cocaine or amphetamine users, 55
  for psychiatric syndromes in severely ill, 497
  for tics, 2151
Halopyrimidines, and radiation therapy, 1116
Halotestin, for hairy cell leukemia, 1000
Halothane
  abuse of, 59
  and malignant hyperthermia, 2282
  fulminant hepatic failure from, 854
  liver disease from, 827, 829
  liver granulomas from, 828
Halzoun, 1903, 1927
Ham's test, 887, 909
  for paroxysmal nocturnal hemoglobinuria, 922
Hamartoma(s), 464
  and increased hypothalamic function, 1286
  hepatic, 857
  of retina, in tuberous sclerosis, 2158
Hamartoma-angiomyolipoma, 652
Hamman-Rich syndrome, 428. See also *Pulmonary fibrosis, idiopathic*
Hamman's sign, 471
Hand(s)
  abnormal sensation in, in carpal tunnel syndrome, 2267. See also *Carpal tunnel syndrome*
  blue discoloration of, from acrocyanosis, 378
  deformity of, from leprosy, treatment of, 1701
  eczema of, 2321
  erythema of, 1673
  osteoarthritis in, 2040
  rheumatoid arthritis in, 2001
  skin disorders of, 2346t
  tremor of, 2146

Hand(s) (Continued)
  washing of, and control of hospital-acquired infection, 1548
Handedness, and language dominance, 2085
Hand-foot-and-mouth disease, 1813
  vs. varicella, 1789
Hand-Schüller-Christian disease, 430, 1022, 1023
  and hypothalamus, 1286
Hangovers, 49
  headache from, 2132
Hansen's disease, 1696–1701. See also *Leprosy*
Haplotype, 1964
  analysis of, for thalassemia, 936
Haptoglobin, 907–908
  reference intervals for, 2401t
Hardy-Weinberg equation, for mutant gene distribution, 151
Harris Benedict equation, for estimating basal energy expenditure, 1206
Harrison's groove, in rickets, 1482
Hartnup disease, 619, 620, 734, 1154t
  niacin deficiency in, 1232
Hashimoto's thyroiditis, 19, 1320, 1333–1334
  pernicious anemia with, 904
  vs. Graves' disease, 1322
Hashish, abuse of, 57–58
Hashitoxicosis. See *Hashimoto's thyroiditis*
Hassall's corpuscles, 1974
Haustra, 721
Haverhill fever, 1729
Hawkinsinuria, 1150t
Hay-fever, treatment of, 1955
Hazard, definition of, 2354
Hazardous substances, labeling of, 141
Hb. See *Hemoglobin(s)*
HBLV (human B lymphotropic virus), 1798
HCA (hypothalamic chronic anovulation), 1438–1439
HCG. See *Human chorionic gonadotropin*
HDL-cholesterol, reference intervals for, 2397t
HE (hereditary elliptocytosis), 912–913, 912t
Head. See also *Skull*
  anaerobic bacteria infection in, 1639
  injury to, 2239–2244, 2239t
    amnesia from, 2084–2085
    and epilepsy, 2223
    and pneumococcal meningitis, 1605
    and recurrent bacterial meningitis, 1608
    as contraindication for thrombolytic therapy, 449
    diagnostic imaging techniques for, 2060
    epileptic seizures from, 2218
    hyperglycemia from, 1289
    management of, 2241–2243
    radiography for, 2058
    skull fracture from, 2241
  malnutrition and, 1210t
Headache, 2129–2136
  classification of, 2130t
  cluster, 2131–2132
  cough, 2132
  depressive, 2133
  diagnostic evaluation of, 2136
  exertional, 2132
  eye pain and, 2134–2135
  from alterations in intracranial pressure, 2133–2134
  from bacterial meningitis, 1606
  from brain abscess, 2182
  from brain tumors, 2231
  from cavernous sinus thrombosis, 2185
  from cerebrovascular disease, 2169

Headache (Continued)
  from chronic myelogenous leukemia, 990
  from cranial arteritis, 2133
  from digitalis toxicity, 229
  from fulminant meningococcemia, 1614
  from herpes simplex encephalitis, 2195
  from hydrocephalus, 2237
  from hypervitaminosis D, 1478
  from infectious mononucleosis, 1787
  from inflammation, 2133–2134
  from influenza, 1765
  from intracranial hypotension, 2238
  from leptospirosis, 1731
  from malaria, 1859
  from meningitis, treatment of, 2194
  from neurosyphilis, 2188
  from pheochromocytoma, 284, 1464
  from pituitary tumors, 1298
  from Pontiac fever, 1571
  from postconcussive syndrome, 2243
  from post-streptococcal glomerulonephritis, 587
  from pseudotumor cerebri, 2236
  from psittacosis, 1736
  from Rocky Mountain spotted fever, 1742
  from sarcoidosis, 453
  from spontaneous intracranial hemorrhage, 2178
  from subarachnoid hemorrhage, 2176
  from subdural empyema, 2184
  from toxemia of pregnancy, 635
  from trauma, 2133
  from trench fever, 1748
  from typhoid fever, 1641
  from typhus fever, 1739, 1740
  hangover, 2132
  hypertensive, 2132
  in transplant recipients, 2210
  migraine, 2129–2131
    oral contraceptives and, 1443
  muscle contraction, 2132–2133
  orgasmic, 2132
  sinus, 2134
  vascular, 2129–2132
Hearing, 2117–2120. See also *Ear(s)*
  disorders of, from intracranial hypotension, 2238
  examination of, 2118
  loss of, 2118–2119. See also *Deafness*
  neural pathways for, 2117
Heart. See also *Atrial; Atrium; Cardiac; Myocardial; Myocardium; Ventricle(s); Ventricular*
  abnormalities in, fragmentational hemolysis from, 924
  action potential of, potassium and, 545, *545*
  acute disease of, vs. acute cholecystitis, 866
  amyloidosis in, 1201
  anatomy of, functional, 184–185
  and peripheral circulatory system, interaction of, 190
  and syncope, 2074, 2074t
  ankylosing spondylitis in, 2006–2007
  arrhythmias of, 250–274. See also *Arrhythmias*
  artificial, 235
  as endocrine gland, 1253
  atriopeptin from, 1277–1279, *1278*
  autonomic nervous system and, 133
  average number of beats per minute by, 372
  block of. See *Heart block*
  blood flow to, determinants of, 500
    measurement of, in cardiac catheterization, 213

Heart (Continued)
bronchogenic carcinoma and, 459
cardiorespiratory arrest and, 500
catheterization of, 178, 211–214. See also
Cardiac catheterization
cellular electrophysiology in, 251–252
chamber enlargement in, solitary, 192
congenital disease of, 303–323. See also
Congenital heart disease
congenital rubella and, 1777
contractility of, 185–187, 216, 218, 349,
353
damage to, from anthracyclines, 1125
diastolic properties of, 185, 185
disease of. See also Cardiomyopathies; Endocarditis
and pulmonary hypertension, 295
and reduced cerebral blood flow, 2164
Chagas' disease and, 1866–1867
congenital, 303–323. See also Congenital
heart disease
ECG for diagnosis of, 198t
from beta thalassemia, 931
from glycosphingolipid, 1145
glycosaminoglycans in, 1175
immunization for patients with, 63
in Marfan syndrome, 1177
in Morquio's syndrome, 1176
ischemic, 275, 329
pain in arm from, 106
valvular, 340–352. See also Valvular
heart disease
venous thrombosis in, 385
electrical subsystem of, 184
electrophysiology of, 196
emboli from, stroke from, 2163–2164
endocrine system of, 1278–1279
enlargement of, 177
in leptospirosis, 1730
in spontaneous intracranial hemorrhage, 2179
left ventricular failure and, 221
examination of, magnetic resonance imaging for, 85
failure of. See Congestive heart failure;
Heart failure
fiber of, membrane responsiveness of,
252
functional anatomy of, 184–185
in Chagas' disease, 1867, 1868, 1868
in Duchenne dystrophy, 2273
in hypothermia, 2384
in pickwickian syndrome, 2079
involvement of, in systemic disease, 369–
370
ischemia of. See Myocardial ischemia
left, impaired output from, syncope
from, 2075
lesions of, and cerebral thromboembolism, 2164t
Lyme disease and, 1728
malformations of, prenatal diagnosis of,
with ultrasonography, 173
malnutrition and, 1212–1213
malposition of, 315–316
motion of, 176–177, 372
muscle of. See Heart muscle
nervous subsystem for, 184
normal, pressures and volumes for,
184
output of, 216–217. See also Cardiac output
oxygen consumption by, 500
changes in, 188
pacemakers for, 271–272. See also Pace-
maker(s)
papillary muscles of. See Papillary mus-
cle(s)

Heart (Continued)
performance assessment of, 184t, 186–
187, 216–220
and hemodynamics, 216–219
exercise testing in, 220
heart as muscle and, 219
heart in circulatory system and, 219–
220
nuclear cardiology for, 207–209, 208
performance of, influences on, 189, 190
myocardial energy expenditure and,
187–188
polyarteritis nodosa in, 2029
polymyositis and, 2035
radiation injury in, 2377, 2379t
radiography of, 191–195, 192, 193
radionuclide assessment of, 209
rate of. See Heart rate
relapsing polychondritis and, 2038
rhabdomyomas of, in tuberous sclerosis,
2158
rheumatic fever and, 1582
rheumatoid arthritis and, 2002
right, communication shunt between aortic root and, 308
failure of, cryptogenic cirrhosis from,
847
impaired filling of, syncope from,
2074–2075
rupture of, after myocardial infarction,
334
sarcoidosis in, 453
size of, in radiographs, 192, 192
stroke volume of, 216
systemic lupus erythematosus and, 2015
systemic sclerosis and, 2022
transplantation of. See Heart transplant(s)
trauma to, 368–369
tumors of, 367–368
valves of. See Prosthetic heart valves and
under names of specific valves
Wegener's granulomatosis in, 2031
Heart block
atrioventricular, 262. See also Atrioventricular block(s)
beta-adrenergic sympathomimetic amines
for, 137
complete, as congenital heart disease, 316
from myocardial infarction, 333
from beta blockers, 138
from sarcoidosis, 360, 453
Heart disease. See also Heart, disease of
congenital, 303–323. See also Congenital
heart disease
coronary. See Coronary artery disease
valvular, 340–352. See also Valvular heart
disease
Heart failure, 215–235
acute vs. chronic, 215
after stroke, 2170
and drug distribution, 97
anemias and, 879
backward vs. forward, 215
beta-adrenergic agonists for, tolerance to,
94
carotid pulse in, 176
clinical categories of, 215–216
clinical management of, 224–235, 224t
strategy for, 224–225, 225t
clinical manifestations of, 221–224
compensatory mechanisms in, 218
congestive. See Congestive heart failure
definition of, 215
from amyloidosis, 1035
from dilated cardiomyopathy, 352
from infective endocarditis, 1589
from interaction of disopyramide and
beta-adrenergic blockers, 101

Heart failure (Continued)
high vs. low output, 215–216
in aortic stenosis, 341
in left ventricle, 221–222
in radiographs, 193, 195
in respiratory failure, treatment of, 481
left vs. right, 215
liver congestion from, vs. viral hepatitis,
824
mechanisms initiating, 215
orthostatic hypotension with, 2106
refractory, 235
vasodilators for, 233–235, 233t
Heart-lung transplantation, for primary pulmonary hypertension, 302
Heart muscle, glycosphingolipids in, 361
oxygen deficiency in, angina pectoris
from, 323
self regulation by, 184
Heart rate, 186
and cardiac output, 237
and myocardial oxygen consumption, 187
beta-adrenergic sympathomimetic amines
for, 137
changes in, 191
control mechanisms and, 216
determination of, 198t
during exercise training, 47
in gastrointestinal hemorrhage, 796
increase in, and angina pectoris, 324
from cannabis, 57
from cocaine or amphetamines, 54
Heart transplants, 235
endomyocardial biopsy for, 178
for dilated cardiomyopathy, 355
painless infarction after, 330
Heartburn. See Pyrosis
Heat, disorders from, 2382–2384
in high voltage electric injury, 2380
to prevent botulism, 1634
Heat cramps, 2382–2383
Heat edema, 2384
Heat exhaustion, 2383
Heat rash, 2334
Heat stroke, 1289, 2383–2384, 2383t
Heat syncope, 2384
Heat urticaria, 1950
Heavy chain diseases, 1034
Heavy metals
and abnormal bone mineralization, 1479
poisonings with, 143
and acute kidney failure, 559
and occult blood loss with diarrhea,
730
and tubular defects, 505
vs. appendicitis, 803
Heberden's nodes, 2040, 2040
Heerfordt's syndrome, 453
Height. See also Growth retardation
metabolic bone disease and, 1476
spurt in, in puberty, 17
velocity curve for, menarche and, 19
weight and, 1209, 1209t
Heimlich maneuver, 418
Heinz bodies, 914, 942
after splenectomy, 1039
removal of, by spleen, 1036
unstable hemoglobin and, 943
Helminths, 1856–1857
infections of, vs. tropical eosinophilia,
1916
Hemagglutination, indirect, for amebic liver
abscess, 837
Hemagglutinin, in influenza virus, 1762
Hemangioblastomas, 2231
Hemangioma(s), 2336t, 2339–2340
calcified, vs. echinococcosis, 1894
cavernous, thrombocytopenia in, 1053

Hemangioma(s) *(Continued)*
choroidal, vs. intraocular melanoma, 2295
fibrinolysis of, 1079
giant, 2339
thrombocytopenia in, 1053
in kidneys, 652
in liver, 857
Hemangiomatosis, of spleen, 1039
Hemangiopericytomas, of lungs, 464
Hemarthrosis, 1045, 2046
in hemophilia A, 1067
treatment of, 1068
Hematemesis
definition of, 796
from esophageal variceal bleeding, 849
from gastritis, 689
from gastrointestinal hemorrhage, 796, 797
from pancreatic cancer, 781
in esophageal disease, 680
Hematin, for hepatic porphyria, 1185–1186, *1186*
side effects of, 1186
Hematochezia, definition of, 796
from gastrointestinal hemorrhage, 796, 797
Hematocrit
after hemorrhage, 891
aging and, 25
and acute abdomen, 802
and threatened stroke, 2170
in acute pancreatitis, 777
in anemias, 878, 879
in chronic kidney failure, 566
in cigarette smokers, 39
in Eisenmenger's syndrome, 317
in erythrocytosis, 976
in gastrointestinal hemorrhage, 796–797
in polycythemia vera, 981
in uremia, 507
reference intervals for, 2401t
secondary polycythemia and, 980
Hematologic disorders, small intestinal ulceration from, 807
Hematologic malignancies, and alveolar proteinosis, 432
Hematologic syndrome, from radiation injury, 2377
Hematology, diagnostic, 873–874
reference intervals for, 2400t–2402t
Hematoma(s)
dissecting, 370. See also *Dissecting aneurysms*
epidural, spinal, 2257
from hemophilia A, 1067
from systemic arterial pressure monitoring, 496
in brain, diagnostic imaging techniques for, 2059
intracranial, from severe brain injury, 2241
lobar, 2175
subdural, 2243–2244. See also *Subdural hematoma*
Hematopoiesis
extramedullary, in myelofibrosis with myeloid metaplasia, 985
ineffective, 962
kinetics of, 877
progenitors of, 875–876, *875*
and marrow failure, 876
regulation of, 876, *876*
therapy with, 876
stem cells in, B lymphocytes from, 1932
suppression of, by hairy cell infiltration of bone marrow, 999
in leukemia, 1003

Hematuria, 503, 522
benign recurrent, of childhood, 503
familial, benign, Alport's syndrome vs., 638
from accelerated hypertension, 277
from acquired renal cystic disease, 652
from acute glomerulonephritis, 583–584
from acute kidney failure, 559
from Alport's syndrome, 637
from autosomal dominant polycystic kidney disease, 645
from bladder cancer, 655
from congestive prostate, 1423
from kidney biopsy, 528
from legionnaires' disease, 1571
from nephroblastoma, 654
from post-streptococcal glomerulonephritis, 587
from renal cell carcinoma, 652
from schistosomiasis haemotobia, 1898
from transitional cell cancers of ureter, 655
idiopathic, 588. See also *Immunoglobulin A nephropathy*
isolated, 585
Heme, biosynthesis of, *895*, 1182, *1183*
in hemoglobin synthesis, 929
pathway of, abnormalities in, and porphyria, 2332
Heme iron, absorption of, 894
Heme synthase, deficiency of, from protoporphyria, 840
Hemiachromatopsia, occipital lobe damage and, 2080t
Hemianopia, 2111, *2111*
Hemiballism, 2148–2149
vs. epilepsy, 2225
Hemicelluloses, in dietary fiber, 721
Hemicrania, paroxysmal, chronic, 2131–2132
Hemiparesis, 2126
in viral encephalitis, 2193
Hemispherectomy, for epilepsy, 2228
Hemlock, 787
Hemobilia, 870
Hemoccult test, 883
Hemochromatosis, 150, 361, 839, 1189–1192, *1190*, 2344
and porphyria cutanea tarda, 1186
arthritis with, 2045
diabetes mellitus from, 1362
excess iron in, removal of, 157
from transfusions, 931
hypogonadotropic hypogonadism in, 1417
magnetic resonance detection of, 668
osteoarthritis and, 2041
secondary, 1192
synovial membrane in, 1995
vs. cryptogenic cirrhosis, 847
with chronic liver disease, 810
Hemoconcentration, in free perforation of peptic ulcers, 707
Hemodialysis. See also *Dialysis*
and amyloidosis, 1200
and carpal tunnel syndrome, 2268
and drug dosages, 95
and gynecomastia, 1411
and hypophosphatemia, 1193
and mineralization inhibition by aluminum, 1482
and neutrophil counts, 957–958
and subepidermal bullae, 2332
and trace metal poisoning, 2389–2390
antimicrobial therapy following, 118
children on, growth retardation in, 1508
for acute kidney failure, indications for, 576t

Hemodialysis *(Continued)*
for digitalis intoxication, 230
for drug overdose, 92, 2071
in hyperkalemia treatment, 549
patients on, hepatitis immunization for, 64
survival rate for, 577
technical aspects of, 573–574, *573*, *574*
Hemodynamic crisis, vs. cerebral ischemia, 2169–2170
Hemodynamics
and extracellular fluid volume, 529
deterioration of, in dilated cardiomyopathy, 352
monitoring of, complications of, 496–497
for shock, 243
in critical care units, 493–495
patterns of abnormalities in, in severely ill, 494, 495t
Hemofiltration, arteriovenous, continuous, 576
Hemoglobin(s)
abnormal, 943–944
biosynthesis of, and anemia, 892–893, 893t
carbon dioxide binding to, 927
denaturation of, 942, *942*
drug toxicity and, 945t, 946
electrophoresis of, for sickle cell disease, 940
reference intervals for, 2401t
fetal, hereditary persistence of, 935
function of, 926–927
high oxygen affinity, polycythemia from, 977, 979
in erythrocytes, 928
level of, in cigarette smokers, 39
oxygen-binding properties of, alteration of, 943–944, *944*
reduced affinity of, for oxygen, in anemia, 879
reference intervals for, 2397t, 2401t
structure of, 925–926, *926*
synthesis of, 927–930
genetic factors in, 928
iron accumulation and, 929
regulation of, *930*
unstable, 942–943
vs. hemolysis from drugs, 946
Hemoglobin A, oxygen binding curve for, 926–927, *927*
Hemoglobin C disease, homozygous, 942
Hemoglobin F, increased production of, mutations causing, 935
Hemoglobin Gun Hill, 942
Hemoglobin H disease, 933
Hemoglobin Kansas, 943
Hemoglobin Kempsey, 943
Hemoglobin M Hyde Park, 946
Hemoglobin Philly, 942
Hemoglobin SC disease, 149, 155
Hemoglobin-oxygen dissociation curve, 943, *944*
Hemoglobinemia, from glucose-6-phosphate dehydrogenase deficiency, 915
Hemoglobinopathies, 153
genetic counseling for, 174
hematuria from, 503
thalassemic, 934
Hemoglobinuria
from blood transfusions, 949
from glucose-6-phosphate dehydrogenase deficiency, 915
in intravascular hemolysis, 908
march, 924
paroxysmal cold, 921
and hemolysis, 909

Hemoglobinuria (Continued)
in syphilis, 1714
paroxysmal nocturnal, 887, 922–923, 1939–1940
and hemolysis, 909
and thrombosis, 848, 1074
washed red blood cells for, 947
Hemogram, 881–882
Hemolysis. See also Hemolytic
and anemia, 880
and erythrocyte appearance, 909t
causes of, 908
chronic, and gout, 1161
from paroxysmal nocturnal hemoglobinuria, 922
consequences of, 907
crisis in, 911
diagnosis of, 908
fragmentational, 924–925
from acquired erythrocyte disorders, 917–925
from chemicals, 923
from cold agglutinin disease, 920
from glucose-6–phosphate dehydrogenase deficiency, 915
from leprosy treatment, 1699
from metabolic abnormalities, 923–924
from mycoplasmal infections, 1563
from protoporphyria, 840
from rifampin, 1687
from systemic lupus erythematosus, 2016
from unstable hemoglobin, 942
from Wilson's disease, 839
hyperbilirubinemia from, 813–814
immune, mechanisms of, 917
"innocent bystander," 921–922
intramedullary, in megaloblastic anemia, 902
intravascular, 907–908
from brown spiders, 1923
neonatal, transient, 913
pathophysiology of, 907
reactive thrombocytosis from, 1054
sequestrational, 917
transfusion reaction and, 920, 922, 948–949
with acute liver disease, in Wilson's disease, 1189
without complement activation, 918
Hemolytic anemia(s)
and jaundice, 880
and vitamin E deficiency, 1239
as antimicrobial reaction, 123
autoimmune, 918–922
in cancer, 1098
in chronic lymphocytic leukemia, 995
causes of, 907t
chronic, and gout, 1167
Donath-Landsteiner, 921
from bartonellosis, 1681
from common variable agammaglobulinemia, 1943
from congenital syphilis, 1718
from homozygous hemoglobin C disease, 942
from immunodeficiency, with elevated immunoglobulin M, 1944
from malaria, 1859
from sickle cell anemia, 937, 939
from Wilson's disease, 1188
glucocorticosteroid therapy for, 130
hereditary spherocytosis as, 910–912, 911, 911t
immune, 917–918
in neonates, excessive vitamin K and, 1076
microangiopathic, in thrombotic thrombocytopenic purpura, 1052

Hemolytic anemia(s) (Continued)
mitochrondrial antibody in, 816
myeloid metaplasia from, 985
penicillin-induced, 103
pyrimidine 5'-nucleotidase deficiency in, 1173
reticulocytosis in, 882
splenectomy for, 1038
spur cell, 923
vs. acute posthemorrhagic anemia, 891
Hemolytic disorders. See also Hemolysis
black pigment gallstones with, 861
definition of, 907
extravascular destruction in, 908
in neonates, from Rh incompatibility, 948
Hemolytic-uremic syndrome, 601
and pseudomembranous colitis, 1632
from Campylobacter infection, 1649
from Escherichia coli, 1655
from shigellosis, 1646, 1647
in thrombotic thrombocytopenic purpura, 1052
thrombocytopenia in, 1053, 1080
Hemoperfusion, after poisonings, 143
for digitalis intoxication, 230
for removal of drug overdose, 92
Hemophilia, 1045
and acquired immunodeficiency syndrome, 1801
classic, 155
genetic counseling for, 174
hemarthrosis in, 2046
intracranial hemorrhage in, 2175
osteonecrosis in, 1517
replacement of factor VIII in, 157
vs. von Willebrand disease, 1070
Hemophilia A, 150, 1066–1069
prognosis for, 1069
vs. von Willebrand disease, 1069
Hemophilia B, 1071–1072
Hemophilus. See Haemophilus
Hemoptysis, 391–392
and surgery for mitral stenosis, 347
endemic, 1903
from ankylosing spondylitis, 430
from bronchiectasis, 439, 440
from bronchogenic carcinoma, 459
from cardiovascular patient history, 175
from chronic bronchitis, 412
from Eisenmenger's syndrome, 317
from Goodpasture's syndrome, 430
from heart failure, 221
from idiopathic pulmonary hemosiderosis, 431
from lymphangioleiomyomatosis, 432
from pulmonary arteriovenous fistula, 309
from pulmonary embolism, 444
from sarcoidosis, 451
from thoracic aortic aneurysms, 371
from unilateral hyperlucent lung, 420
Hemorrhage
acute, blood transfusions for, 947
acute anemia after, 891–892, 891t
adrenal destruction for, 1351
alveolar, from idiopathic pulmonary hemosiderosis, 430
and myocardial depression, 239
assessment of, 1044–1045, 1044t
capsular-putaminal, external, 2179
capsular-thalamic, internal, 2179
cerebellar, 2179, 2179
during delivery, from hypopituitarism, 1295
from acute leukemia, 1003
from arteriovenous malformation, and acute transverse myelitis, 2217
from cardiac catheterization, 211

Hemorrhage (Continued)
from essential thrombocythemia, 987
from fulminant hepatic failure, 854
from heparin therapy, 447
from hereditary connective tissue disorders, 1059
from IUDR toxicity, 125
from leptospirosis, 1730
from leukemia, chronic lymphocytic, 995
chronic myelogenous, 990
from midline granuloma, 2032
from phlebotomy with leeches, 1927
from pituitary tumors, 1298
from portal hypertension, 848
from primary thrombocythemia, 1054
from Rift Valley fever, 1818
from thrombotic agents, 449
from vitamin K deficiency, 1240
from von Willebrand disease, 1070
from warfarin with vitamin E, 1239
gastrointestinal, 660, 796–800. See also Gastrointestinal hemorrhage
hypertensive-arteriosclerotic, 2174
in eye, 2112
in subcortical white matter, 2179
interstitial lung disease vs., 423
intestinal, intramural, 764–765
intracerebral, diagnostic imaging techniques for, 2059
from hypertension, 2178–2180, 2178
vs. hypertensive encephalopathy, 2172
intracranial, 2173–2180. See also Intracranial hemorrhage
intrapituitary, hypopituitarism from, 1295
intraventricular, 2173
parenchymal, from systemic lupus erythematosus, 429
pontine, 2179, 2179
autonomic insufficiency from, 2106
postpartum, cholestasis of pregnancy and, 841
factor V deficiency and, 1073
factor X deficiency and, 1072
reactive thrombocytosis from, 1054
severe, definition of, 706
spontaneous, platelet counts in, 1047
stroke from, 2159
subarachnoid, 2173. See also Subarachnoid hemorrhage
syncope from, 2074
uterine, dysfunctional, 19
Hemorrhagic diathesis, in chronic kidney failure, 566
Hemorrhagic fever
African, 1835–1836
from arenaviruses, 1834–1835
viral, 1829–1837
with renal syndrome, 1836–1837
Hemorrhoids, 789
and sphincter dysfunction, 728
from ulcerative colitis, 757
hemorrhage from, 799
vs. adenocarcinoma of colon, 771
vs. lymphogranuloma venereum, 1711
vs. ulcerative colitis, 756
Hemosiderin, 1190
definition of, 895
Hemosiderosis, definition of, 1189
magnetic resonance detection of, 668
Hemostasis, laboratory studies of, 1045, 1046t, 1046, 1047
normal, 1042–1043, 1043
secondary, 1043
Hemothorax, 468
Hemp, and byssinosis, 2360
Henderson-Hasselbalch equation, 485, 549
Henle's loop, 510. See also Loop of Henle

Henoch-Schönlein purpura, 432, 600–601, 1058, 2027, 2046, 2325
  IgA nephropathy as form of, 588
  vs. chronic meningococcemia, 1615
Heparan sulfate, 1174
Heparin
  after myocardial infarction, 335
  and antithrombins, 1063
  and hair loss, 2349
  anticoagulant properties of, 1080
  as prophylaxis for deep-vein thrombosis, 449
  bleeding from, during dialysis, 577
  complications from, 447–448
  contraindications for, for malaria, 1861
  for cardiac catheterization, 211
  for deep-vein thrombosis, 387
  for defibrination syndrome, 1079
  for disseminated intravascular coagulation, 1098
    in meningococcemia, 1616
  for hypertrophic cardiomyopathy, 358
  for pulmonary embolism, 447
  for sudden arterial occlusion, 384
  from mast cells, 1974, 2306
  in endocarditis treatment, 1594
  in hemodialysis, 574
  partial thromboplastin time for monitoring, 1047
  thrombocytopenia from, 1049, 1075
  thrombosis from, 1075
Heparin cofactor II, deficiency of, 1075
  and recurrent thrombophlebitis, 385
Hepatic. See also Liver
Hepatic coma, 852–854
Hepatic encephalopathy, 852–854
  precipitating factors for, 853t
  spur cell hemolytic anemia and, 923
  stages of, 853t
Hepatitis
  acute, vs. acute cholecystitis, 866
  adenine arabinoside for, 125
  aggressive, 831–832
    in Crohn's disease, 749
  alcoholic, 842, 843–844
  autoimmune, 749, 831–832
  chronic, 830–833
    active, 831–832
      in Crohn's disease, 749
    causes of, 830t
    from acute viral hepatitis, 820
    lobular, 831
    persistent, 831
  cytomegalovirus infection and, 1785
  drug abuse and, 52
  from disseminated gonococcal infection, 1709
  from leprosy treatment, 1699
  from syphilis, 1716
  immunization against, 64
  in dialysis patients, 566
  infectious, 820. See also Viral hepatitis, type A
    vs. psittacosis, 1736
  isoniazid-induced, 103, 1686
  lymphocytosis from, 972
  recombinant DNA vaccine for, 159
  serum, 821, 823. See also Viral hepatitis
    transmission of, by blood transfusions, 949
  type D, prevention of, 826
  type non-A, non-B, prevention of, 826
  viral, 818–826. See also Viral hepatitis
  vs. pyogenic liver abscess, 836
  vs. typhoid fever, 1642
Hepatitis B hyperimmune globulin, ineffectiveness of, for fulminant hepatic failure, 854

Hepatitis B immune globulin, recommendations for use of, 825–826
Hepatitis B surface antigen, positive testing for, 833
Hepatization, red vs. gray, 1556
Hepatocyte poikilocytosis, 840
Hepatolenticular degeneration, 1188. See also Wilson's disease
Hepatoma, 858
Hepatorenal syndrome, 852
Hepatosplenomegaly, from congenital syphilis, 1718
Herald patch, 2327
Herald wave phenomenon, in influenza, 1764
Heredity, human, 146–152. See also Human heredity
Hermansky-Pudlak syndrome, 1057
  interstitial lung disease with, 432
Hermaphroditism, 1402
Hernia(s)
  glycosaminoglycans in, 1175
  hiatus, 680–681
  incarcerated, in elderly, vs. appendicitis, 803
  of diaphragm, 472
  vs. small intestine neoplasms, 774
Herniated disc, 2040, 2252–2253. See also Intervertebral disc(s), herniated
Herniation, in brain, 2062–2063
  transtentorial, from brain injury, 2241
    from Reye syndrome, 2210
Heroin
  abuse of, 55
    and kidney damage, 612
    by adolescents, 21
  acute reaction to, 56
  naloxone as antidote for, 143
  nephrotic syndrome from, 595
  poisoning with, 2069t
Herpangina, 1813, 2347
  with viral neurologic disease, 2194
Herpes genitalis, lesions in, TFT ineffectiveness on, 126
Herpes gestationis, 2331
  immunofluorescent cutaneous findings in, 2305t
Herpes labialis, 676, 1782
  diagnosis of, 1783
  lesions in, TFT ineffectiveness on, 126
Herpes neonatalis, acyclovir for, 126
Herpes simplex, 676, 1780–1784
  acute hepatitis from, 819
  acute proctitis from, 787
  acyclovir for, 126
  and skin, 2329
  cervicitis from, 1705
  congenital infection by, vs. cytomegalovirus, 1785–1786
  diagnosis of, 1703–1704
  encephalitis from, 2195–2196
    adenine arabinoside for, 125
    and amnesia, 2084
    in temporal lobe, 2081
  erythema multiforme from, 2332
  fulminant hepatic failure from, 854
  genital ulcers from, 1703, 2342
  in AIDS, 1805t, 1806
  in immunocompromised host, 2352
  lesions of, in malaria, 1859
  myoglobinuria after, 2283
  of oral mucosa, 2347
  reactivation of, in pneumococcal pneumonia, 1557
  skin infection by, 2329
    antiviral agents for, 2317–2318
  stomatitis from, vs. enanthems, 1813
  Tzanck smear for, 2313
    positive, 2312

Herpes-type viruses, 1780–1793
Herpes varicella-zoster virus, infection by, Reye syndrome after, 2209
Herpes virus. See also Herpes simplex; Herpes zoster
  acquired immunodeficiency syndrome with, 677
  after bone marrow transplants, 1537
  and congenital heart disease, 303
  and seizures, 2218
  and ulcers, 696
  chemotherapeutic agents for, 125
  generalized, vs. varicella, 1789
  genital, neurologic complications of, 2197
  gingivostomatitis from, 2347
  in esophagus, 688
  in nervous system, 2195–2198
  keratitis from, 2293
  keratoconjunctivitis from, vs. Chlamydia infection, 1734
  oral, 676–677
  reactivation of, in transplant recipients, 2210
  ribavirin for, 127
  stomatitis from, vs. aphthous ulcers, 676
  transmission of, in hospital employees, 1549
  ulcers of, vs. syphilis, 1715
  vs. Toxoplasma retinochoroiditis, 1878
Herpes zoster, 2196–2197
  and skin, 2330
  cancer and, 1111
  Hodgkin's disease and, 1017
  immunization against, 63t
  in immunocompromised host, 1806, 2352
  interferon for, 128
  neuralgia after, 2135, 2136
  pain of, 105
  pulmonary embolism vs., 444
  skin lesions in, 2330
    antiviral agents for, 2317
Herpetiform lesion patterns, 2310
Hetastarch, for fluid replacement, 245
Heterogeneity, genetic, 155, 157t
Heterozygotes, 146, 147
HETEs (hydroxy-eicosatetraenoic acids), 1986
Hexachlorophene, against Staphylococcus aureus colonization, 1548
  for infants, and spongiform degeneration, 2216
Hexamethonium, 140
Hexamethylmelamine, for cancer, 1126
Hexose monophosphate shunt, 913–914
  defects in, 914
HGPRT. See Hypoxanthine-guanine phosphoribosyltransferase
Hiatus hernia, and gastroesophageal reflux disease, 680–681
  symptomatic, 680. See also Gastroesophageal reflux disease
Hiccup, 472
Hickman (Silastic) catheter, 932
  and infection prevention, 1537
Hickman-Broviac intravenous catheters, 1545–1546
Hidradenitis suppurativa, 2334, 2334
High altitude, and chronic obstructive pulmonary disease, 417
  and diffusing capacity, 400
  and pulmonary edema, 2366–2367
High blood pressure, 276–293. See also Hypertension
Hilar cell tumor, hormones from, 1445t
Hip(s)
  congenital dislocation of, 170t
  degenerative arthritis of, in Paget's disease, 1517

Hip(s) *(Continued)*
disease in, knee pain from, 106
fracture of, 1510
from osteoporosis, 1476
in elderly women, 41
prevention of, 26
osteoarthritis in, 2040
prosthesis for, placement of, and osteomyelitis, *1623*
rheumatoid arthritis in, 2002
Hippocampus, and memory, 2084
damage to, 2084
Hippus, 2113
Hirschsprung's disease, 170, 170t, 660, 723–724. See also *Megacolon*
Hirsutism, 1446–1448, *1447*, 2349–2350
causes of, 1447t, 1448t
evaluation of, 1350
excess ovarian androgen synthesis and, 1431
from chronic active hepatitis, 832
from Cushing's syndrome, 1355
Hirudiniasis, 1927
His bundle, interruption of, surgery for, 274
His-Purkinje system, 184, 250, *251*
digitalis and, 229
sympathetic nerve activity in, and arrhythmias, 252
ventricular parasystole and, 263
Histamine, 1282
and acid secretion, 693, 695
and allergic rhinitis, 1953
and pruritus, 2304
and urticaria-angioedema, 1949
from mast cells, 406, 2306
allergic rhinitis and, 1952
in asthma, 404
from mastocytosis, 1973–1974
in anaphylaxis, 1956
in inflammation, 1986
in vascular headache, 2130
shock and, 239
Histamine receptor antagonists, for postoperative recurrent ulcers, 705
Histidase, decreased activity of, 1157
Histidinemia, 1157–1158
Histiocytes, definition of, 1022
Histiocytosis, and diabetes insipidus, 1308
malignant, 1109–1110
Histiocytosis X, 1022
and hypothalamus, 1286
as interstitial lung disease, 430
Histocompatibility, definition of, 578
H-Y antigen of, and testicular development, 1392
of kidney transplants, 578
restriction of, *1935*, 1936
Histones, autoantibodies to, 1996t
Histoplasma capsulatum, 1838
infection by, and solitary pulmonary nodules, 464
pericarditis from, 363
Histoplasmosis, 1838–1840
African, 1838
disseminated, 1839
recurrent, 1839
vs. cat scratch disease, 1681
vs. paracoccidioidomycosis, 1843
vs. *Toxoplasma* retinochoroiditis, 1878
vs. ulcerative colitis, 757
History taking. See *Patient history*
Histotopes, *1935*, 1936
HIV. See *Human immunodeficiency virus*
Hives, 2334
HLA system, 151, 578. See also *Human leukocyte antigen(s)*
HMSN (hereditary motor and sensory neuropathy), 2264, 2265t

Hoarseness
from bronchogenic carcinoma, 459
from primary pulmonary hypertension, 299
from sarcoidosis, 451
from thoracic aortic aneurysms, 371
Hodgkin's disease, 709, 1014–1022
ABVD drug program for, 1020
acute phase response to, 1528
amyloidosis in, 1199
and stomach, 712
clinical manifestations of, 1015–1016
diagnostic evaluation of, 1017–1019, 1017t
eosinophilia from, 1025
epidemiology of, 1015
etiology and pathogenesis of, 1014–1015
herpes zoster with, 2196
histoplasmosis with, 1838
human immunodeficiency virus infection with, 1807
lymphocytopenia in, 967
minimal change nephrotic syndrome in, 593, 594
mixed cellularity, 1015
monocytosis in, 970
myeloid metaplasia from, 985
pathology of, 1015, 1016t
patterns of spread of, 1019
prognosis for, 1021t, 1022
progressive multifocal leukoencephalopathy with, 2207
pruritus in, 1111
skin in, 1109
spread of, to kidneys, 655
staging for, 1008, 1017, 1017t
thrombocytopenia in, 1052
toxoplasmosis with, 1877
treatment of, 1019–1022, 1021t
vs. cat scratch disease, 1679
vs. infectious mononucleosis, 1787
vs. toxoplasmosis, 1878
Hodgkin's lymphoma, vs. Ewing's sarcoma, 1521
Hoechst-BUDR technique, 167
Hoesch test, for hepatic porphyria, 1185
Hoffmann's syndrome, 2280
Hollander test, for incomplete vagotomy diagnosis, 705
Holt-Oram syndrome, 176
Homans' sign, from deep-vein thrombosis, 385
Home care programs
for cancer patients, 1089
for dying patients, 34
for hemophilia A, 1068
total parenteral nutrition in, 1249
Homeostasis, *528*
impaired, in elderly, 25
kidneys and, 510
maintenance of, with extracellular substances and hormones, 1255
of bone, 1469–1476
of minerals, 1469–1476
regulation of, atriopeptin in, 1277
Homocysteine, metabolism of, abnormal, and thrombosis, 1074
Homocystinuria, 1151t, 1160–1161
pyridoxine for, 157
vitamin B₆ for, 1234
vs. Marfan syndrome, 1178
Homogentisic acid oxidase, 1157
Homosexuals
AIDS in, 1523, 1794–1808, 1881–1884, 2203–2205
amebiasis in, 1886
Campylobacter-like organisms in, 1648
hepatitis A in, 820
hepatitis B in, 826

Homosexuals *(Continued)*
hepatitis immunization for, 64
herpes simplex virus infection in, 1782
infectious proctitis in, 787
Kaposi's sarcoma in, 2340
Pneumocystis carinii pneumonia in, 1803–1805, 1805t
protocolitis in, 1648
sexually transmitted disease in, 1702
shigellosis in, 1646
syphilis in, 1714
Homovanillic acid, from dopamine, 1463
reference intervals for, 2397t
Homozygotes, 146, 147
Honey, botulism from, 1634
Honeybee, 1924
sting of, 1958
Hookworm disease, 1906–1907
Horder's spots, 1736
Hormone(s). See also *Endocrine system*
action of, 1257–1262
agonists of, definition of, 1258
altered secretion of, from central nervous system disorders, 1285–1289
and calcium regulation, 1469–1470, 1470t
and sodium reabsorption by proximal tubule, 513
antagonist to, definition of, 1258
anti-insulin, 1364
cellular sensitivity to, regulation of, 1262
counterregulatory, 1364, 1374
deficiencies in, 1263–1264
definition of, 1252
ectopic production of, by neoplasms, 1264
excess amounts of, 1264–1265
from anterior pituitary, 1291–1293, 1291t
from hypothalamus, 1282–1283
from insulinoma, 1384
from islet cell tumors, 1388
from ovarian tumors, 1445t
hyporesponsiveness to, 1264
hypothalamic and pituitary, interrelationships of, 1281–1283, *1281*
in females, 1426, 1427t
integrated responses to, 1262–1263
levels of, laboratory testing for, 1265–1267
metabolism of, 1256–1257
neurohypophyseal, 1312
production of
assessment of, 1266
excess, and hypertension, 277
human biologic, 159
regulation of, 1255–1256, *1255*
receptors of, 1257–1258, 1261, *1261*
release of, shock and, 239
secretion of, by cancers, 1101
central nervous system and, 1280–1285
steroid. See *Steroid hormones*
storage and release of, 1254
synthesis and release of, 1253–1255
therapy with. See *Hormone therapy; Steroid therapy*
transport of, 1256
types of, 1253
Hormone therapy, 1265, 1442–1444
for breast cancer, 1456
for hypopituitarism, 1296
Horner's syndrome, 2113, 2114
from bronchogenic carcinoma, 459
from cluster headache, 2131
from dissecting aortic aneurysms, 373
from idiopathic autonomic insufficiency, 2106
from internal carotid artery occlusion, 2165
from paravertebral tumors, 2254

Hornets, 1924
  stings of, 1958
Horseshoe kidneys, 649, *649*
  and renal cell carcinoma, 652
Hospice program(s), characteristics of, 31t
  for cancer patients, 1089
Hospital employees, health of, 1548–1549
Hospital-acquired infection(s), 1541–1549
  endocarditis as, 1591–1592
  high-risk locations for, 1542
  impact of, 1542t
  in bloodstream, 1544–1546
  in transplant recipients, 2210
  in urinary tract, 1543–1544
  meningitis as, 1546
  meningococcal disease as, 1612
  occurrence of, 1541
  of *Staphylococcus aureus*, 1597
    prevention of, 1604
  pneumonia as, 1544, 1566
    treatment of, 1567
  respiratory syncytial virus as, 1759
  surveillance of, 1543
    classifications for, 1543t
  varicella as, 1788, 1790
  with parainfluenza virus, 1761
Hospitalized patients
  calorie and protein requirements for,
    1244
  deep-vein thrombosis in, 384
  infection of, 1538, 1541–1549. See also
    Hospital-acquired infection(s)
  microorganism transmission to, 1542
  protein-calorie malnutrition in, causes of,
    1212, 1212t
Host cells, virus attachment to, 1750
Host defense mechanisms, 1529–1532, 1530t
  abnormalities in, 1941–1948. See also *Im-
    munodeficiency*
  against candidiasis, 1848
  anaerobiosis and, 1638
  and aspergillosis, 1850
  and *Listeria monocytogenes*, 1671
  and malaria, 1858
  and pneumonia, 1544, 1552, 1555
  and schistosomiasis, 1897
  and staphylococcal infection, 1598
  and viruses, 1751–1752
  antibodies in, 1531, 1531t
  cellular immunity and, 1531–1532, 1531t
  fever in, 1529
  inflammatory response in, 1530
Host-parasite relationship, 1856
Hot flushes, estrogen for, 1444
  in menopause, 1444
Houseflies, and salmonella infection, 1643
Howell-Jolly bodies, after splenectomy,
    1039
  removal of, by spleen, 1036
  vs. malarial parasites, 1860
HPLC (high-performance liquid chromatog-
    raphy), 1266
HPP (hereditary pyropoikilocytosis), 913
HSV. See *Herpes simplex*
HT. See *Hypothalamus*
HTLV-I (human T cell leukemia virus), 1001
HTLV-I associated adult T cell leukemia/
    lymphoma, 1010
Human chorionic gonadotropin, 1419–1420
  and malignant islet cell tumors, 1388
  as tumor marker, 1099, 1099t
  from choriocarcinoma, 1421
  from tumors, and gynecomastia, 1411
  in ovulation induction, 1442
Human heredity, 146–152. See also *Chromo-
    some(s); Congenital malformations; Metabo-
    lism, inborn errors of*
  autosomal dominant traits in, 147

Human heredity *(Continued)*
  autosomal recessive disorders in, 148–149
  family history in, 147
  gene frequency in, 151
  gene map in, 152
  mitochondrial inheritance in, 151
  monogenic disorders in, 147, 147t
  pedigree analysis in, 147, *147*
  polygenic inheritance in, *150*, 150–151
  X-linked inheritance in, 149–150
  Y-linked inheritance in, 150
Human immunodeficiency virus, 1523,
    1795, 1797–1799. See also *AIDS*
  antibodies against, measurement of, 1535
  as slow virus, 2203
  azidothymidine for, 127
  in body fluids, 1801
  infection by, detection of, 1800
    vs. infectious mononucleosis, 1788
  origin of, 1798
  receptor for, 1935
  target cells of, 1799–1800
  transmission of, 1801
Human leukocyte antigen(s), 151, 578, 1963
  and disease, 1966–1968, 1967t
  class I, *1965*, *1966*
  typing for, 1964–1966, 1965t
Human leukocyte antigen complex, nomen-
    clature and genetic organization of,
    1963–1964, *1963*, 1963t
Human milk. See *Breast milk*
Humidification, artificial airways and, 478
  in oxygen therapy, 486
Humidifier lung, 433
Humidifiers, and legionnaires' disease, 1572
Humoral disorders, management of, 1536
Hunger, definition of, 657
Hungry bone syndrome, 1195, 1495, 1498
  treatment of, 1499
Hunter's syndrome, 167, 1174, 1175, 1176t
Huntington's disease, 148, 2090–2091,
    2147–2148
  juvenile parkinsonism in, 2144
  vs. tardive dyskinesia, 2149t
Hurler-Scheie compound, 1175, 1176t
Hurler's syndrome, 155, 361, 1175, 1176t
HUS. See *Hemolytic-uremic syndrome*
Hutchinson's teeth, from congenital syphi-
    lis, 1718, 2189
HVA (homovanillic acid), from dopamine,
    1463
  reference intervals for, 2397t
H-Y histocompatibility antigen, and testicu-
    lar development, 1392
Hyalin, alcoholic, 843
Hyaline degeneration, fibrosing, lacunar in-
    farction from, 2164
Hyaline necrosis, sclerosing, acute, 843
Hyaluronic acid, concentrations of, and pri-
    mary mesothelioma, 794
  from synovium, 1986
  in synovial fluid, 1982, 1993
Hyaluronidase, 1597
Hybridoma, 1935
  antibodies derived from, 1524
Hydatid disease, 1893–1894
Hydatidiform mole, and toxemia of preg-
    nancy, 635
Hydralazine
  adverse effects of, 289t
  as arteriolar dilator, 235
  as vasodilator, 233
  for hypertension, 287t
    in uremic syndrome, 570
  for hypertensive crisis, 290t
  in primary pulmonary hypertension ther-
    apy, 300, 301t
  liver granulomas from, 828

Hydralazine *(Continued)*
  lupus syndrome from, 103
  rebound effects of, 1954
  with nitrates, for vasodilator effect, 235
Hydrarthrosis, intermittent, 2047
Hydration, for cough, 391
  in kidney failure prevention, 562
Hydrocarbon(s), and kidney damage, 612
  and pneumonitis, 2372
  poisonings with, treatment for, 144
Hydrocephalus, 2237–2238
  causes of, 2238t
  dementia from, 28, 2090
  from subarachnoid hemorrhage, 2175
  meningitis and, 1605
  otitic, 2236. See also *Pseudotumor cerebri*
  spinal cord malformation from, 2258
  subarachnoid hemorrhage with, 2176
Hydrochloric acid, loss of, from stomach,
    and metabolic alkalosis, 532
Hydrochlorothiazide, properties of, 231t
Hydrocortisone, 128, 129t, 130. See also
    Cortisol
Hydrocytosis, hereditary, 913
Hydroflumethiazide, for hypertension, 286t
Hydrogen ions, secretion of, 518
  transfer of, vitamin C and, 1234
Hydrogen peroxide, for *Mycoplasma pneumo-
    niae*, 1561
  in shock, 243
Hydrogen peroxide–saline mouth rinse, for
    candidiasis, 677
Hydromorphone
  abuse of, 55
  as analgesic, 107t, 108
  for pain in dying patients, 32
  poisoning with, 2069t
  vs. heroin, 56
Hydromyelia, 2157
Hydronephrosis, 614
  and prostatectomy, 1423
  from diverticulitis, 804
  from ureteropelvic junction obstruction,
    649, *650*
  salt wasting in, 564
  ultrasonography for, 527
Hydrophobia, in rabies, 2201
Hydrops, and Ménière syndrome, 2119
  of gallbladder, 864
Hydrops fetalis, 933
Hydroxocobalamin, 902
Hydroxyapatite, in bone, 1473
  in synovial fluid, 1994
4-Hydroxybutyric aciduria, 1153t
Hydroxychloroquine, side effects of, and
    eye, 2298
17-Hydroxycorticosteroids, reference inter-
    vals for, 2397t
18-Hydroxycorticosterone, measurement of,
    1350
Hydroxy-eicosatetraenoic acids, 1986
9-(2-Hydroxyethoxymethyl) guanine, 126.
    See also *Acyclovir*
Hydroxyethyl starch, for fluid replacement,
    245
Hydroxyhexamide, interaction of, with
    phenylbutazone, 101
5-Hydroxyindole acetic acid, increased, in
    carcinoid syndrome, 1468
  reference intervals for, 2397t
Hydroxyl radical(s), free, 2368
  in shock, 243
Hydroxylamine, toxicity of, to hemoglobin,
    945
21-Hydroxylase, and virilization of female
    fetus, 1402
  deficiency of, 1402–1403
Hydroxylysinemia, 1151t

17-Hydroxyprogesterone, measurement of, for congenital adrenal hyperplasia, 1448
reference intervals for, 2397t
secretion rates and plasma concentrations of, 1341
Hydroxyproline, 1158
in urine, osteitis fibrosa cystica and, 1489
urinary excretion of, in Paget's disease, 1516
2-Hydroxystilbamidine, for blastomycosis, 1843
5-Hydroxytryptamine. See Serotonin
Hydroxyurea
for chronic myelogenous leukemia, 992
for polycythemia vera, 983–984
for thrombocythemia, 987, 1054
prednisone with, for idiopathic hypereosinophilic syndrome, 362
Hydroxyzine, as adjuvant analgesic, 109
for nausea, in viral hepatitis, 824
Hymen, imperforate, 1429
Hymenolepis diminuta, 1894
Hymenolepis nana, 1893
Hymenoptera, 1958
Hyoscyamine, abuse of, 59
Hyperaeration, localized, 420
Hyperalaninemias, 1152t
Hyperaldosteronism
primary
hypokalemia and metabolic alkalosis from, treatment for, 556
plasma renin activity in, 1350
sodium level in, 542
secondary, 1360
Hyperalimentation, for short bowel syndrome, 743
parenteral, infection control in, 1546
Hyperaminoacidemia, branched-chain, 1150t
Hyperaminoaciduria, 1149, 1150t–1154t, 1155
mechanisms of, 1149
Hyperammonemia(s), 1152t
from ornithine transcarbamylase deficiency, 149
Hyperamylasemia, in cancer, 1098
Hyperargininemia, 1152t, 1153t, 1159
Hyper-beta-alaninemia, 1153t
Hyperbilirubinemia, 661
acquired, 813–814
from alcoholic hepatitis, 844
from blood transfusions, 949
from heart failure, 223
from hemolysis, 909
from liver granulomas, 837
from pancreatic cancer, 781
from parenteral nutrition, 841
from recurrent cholestasis, 813
phenobarbital for, 157
Hyperbradykininism, familial, orthostatic hypotension with, 2106
Hypercalcemia, 1502–1505
and bone resorption, 1102
and sudden cardiac death, 275
as contraindication for orthophosphates, 643
calcitonin for, 1506
diagnosis of, 1492
familial, benign, 1491–1492
from breast cancer, 1456
from bronchogenic carcinoma, 462
from chronic interstitial nephritis, 606
from hypernephromas, 506
from hyperparathyroidism, 1488–1490
from multiple myeloma, 1029, 1032
from prostaglandin E$_2$, 1273
from renal cell carcinoma, 652

Hypercalcemia (Continued)
from thiazide diuretic therapy, 1490
glucocorticosteroid therapy for, 129
hypocalciuric familial, 1503
in uremic patients, 1508
neoplasms and, 1102
nonparathyroid causes of, 1502–1504
treatment of, 1504–1505
vitamin A toxicity and, 1238
Hypercalciuria, and kidney stones, 639–640
treatment of, 642
parathyroid function and, 642
Hypercapnia, 294
from alveolar hypoventilation, 475
from chronic obstructive pulmonary disease, treatment for, 417
from disease of neuromuscular–chest cage system, 472
from respiratory failure, 477
in severely ill, 484
Hyperceruloplasminemia, familial, 1241
Hypercholesterolemia, 1143. See also Hyperlipidemia(s)
familial, 148, 153, 1140
and atherosclerosis, 1144
cholestyramine for, 157
homozygous, 149, 320
from nephrotic syndrome, 504
from primary biliary cirrhosis, 845
from thiazide diuretics, 287
genetics and, 150
obesity and, 1224
Hypercoagulable state
and ischemic colitis, 764
and thrombosis, 1074
mesenteric venous, 764
from cancer, 1098
from nephrotic syndrome, 593
from ulcerative colitis, 758
Hypercortisolism, in kidney transplant patients, 581
Hypercupremia, 1242
Hypercystinuria, 1153t
Hyperdipsia, 2105
Hyperemesis gravidarum, 841
and renal failure, 637
thyroid function in, 1321
Hyperemia, functional, 761
Hypereosinophilic syndrome, 1024–1025
idiopathic, 362
vs. tropical eosinophilia, 1916
Hyperesthesia, definition of, 2259
in Gambian sleeping sickness, 1864
Hypergammaglobulinemia
in infectious mononucleosis, 1787
in systemic lupus erythematosus, 2016
in Wegener's granulomatosis, 2030
polyclonal, 1494
in lepromatous leprosy, 1698
purpura from, 2325
Hypergeusia, definition of, 2110
Hyperglobulinemia, from cirrhosis, 846, 847
from viral hepatitis, 820
Hyperglobulinemic purpura, 1059
Hyperglycemia. See also Diabetes mellitus
and cancer, 1101–1102
and diabetes complications, 1366–1368
and diabetic neuropathy, 2263
causes of, 1289
from acute pancreatitis, 777
from diabetic ketoacidosis, 1375
from glucocorticoids, 1346
from nonketotic hyperosmolar syndrome, 1377
from parenteral nutrition, 1250
from thiazide diuretics, 287
of non-insulin-dependent diabetes mellitus, causes of, 1365, 1365

Hyperglycemia (Continued)
sudden, paradoxical hyperkalemia in, 548
sympathetic nervous system and, 133
treatment of. See Hypoglycemic agents
Hyperglycinemias, 1151t
Hyperhidrosis, 2107
and fluid depletion, 532
from paravertebral tumors, 2254
Hyperhistaminemia, in polycythemia vera, 981
Hyperhistidinemia, 1150t
Hyperhistidinuria, 1154t
Hyperhydroxyprolinemia, 1151t
Hyperimmunoglobulinemia E syndrome, 1947–1948
Hyperinfection syndrome, 1906
Hyperkalemia, 547–549
and bicarbonate reabsorption, 518
and electrical tissue depolarization, 545, 545
and sudden cardiac death, 275
causes of, 547t
from adrenocortical insufficiency, 1351, 1352
from blood transfusions, 950
from hyporeninemic hypoaldosteronism, 1353
from kidney failure, 560, 562, 564
from nonsteroidal anti-inflammatory agents, 609
from uremia, 507
management of, 570
in chronic dialysis patients, 576
metabolic acidosis with, 623
paradoxical, in sudden hyperglycemia, 548
periodic paralysis in, 2281–2282
treatment of, 548
Hyperkeratosis, benign, leukoplakia from, 678
Hyperketonemia, in diabetic ketoacidosis, 1375
Hyperkinesia, definition of, 2142
Hyperkinetic heart syndrome, 277. See also Hypertension, labile
Hyperlipemia, in acute pancreatitis, 777
Hyperlipidemia(s). See also Hypercholesterolemia
and atherosclerosis, 320, 1144
and myocardial infarction, 329
combined, acquired disorders and, 1143
congenital, as contraindication for oral contraceptives, 1444
familial, combined, 1140t, 1142
vs. familial Mediterranean fever, 1197
from cancer, 1098
from glucocorticoids, 1346
from lipoprotein disorders, 1137
from nephrotic syndrome, 593
inherited, fever in, 1525
pancreatitis from, 775
primary, dietary modification for, 43
Hyperlipoproteinemia(s), 1137–1144
arthritis with, 2045
clofibrate for, 157
nicotinic acid for, 1232
Hyperlordosis, 2248
Hyperlysinemia, 1151t, 1153t
Hyperlysinuria, 1153t
Hypermagnesemia, 1195
in renal osteodystrophy, 1509
vs. botulism, 1633
Hypermetabolism, from pheochromocytoma, 284
Hypermethioninemia, 1150t
Hypernatremia, 542, 1288, 2105
Hypernephroma, 506, 652. See also Renal cell carcinoma

Hyperornithinemia, 1152t
Hyperosmia, definition of, 2110
Hyperostosis, skeletal, diffuse idiopathic, 2041
Hyperoxaluria, 612
　enteric, 640–643
　from vitamin B$_6$ deficiency, 1234
　kidney stones from, 640
　primary, 1136–1137
Hyperparathyroidism
　and bone, 1480
　and cancer, 1102
　arthritis with, 2045
　as contraindication for sodium cellulose phosphate, 642
　from carcinoid tumor of thymus, 1976
　from uremia, electroencephalograms for, 566
　muscle symptoms in, 2280
　primary, 1488–1496
　　hyperchloremic acidosis in, 553
　　prognosis for, 1495–1496
　　sarcoidosis vs., 454
　secondary, and bone resorption, 1509
　　in chronic renal disease, 1507
　treatment of, 1495
Hyperphagia, in gastrointestinal disease, 657
Hyperphenylalaninemia(s), 1150t, 1155–1156
Hyperphosphatasia, hereditary, 1519
Hyperphosphatemia, 1193, 1471
　hypercalcemia with, 1494
　hypocalcemia with, in pseudohypoparathyroidism, 1501
　in hypoparathyroidism, 1496–1497
　in renal osteodystrophy, 1508
Hyperphosphaturia, in hyperparathyroidism, 1489
Hyperpigmentation
　from ACTH, 132
　from adrenocortical insufficiency, 1351
　from arsenic, 2389
　from bronchogenic carcinoma, 459
　in Nelson's syndrome, 1357
Hyperplasia, 713
　adenomyomatous, 871
　adrenal, bilateral, and aldosterone levels, 1350, 1358
　　hypertension in, spironolactone for, 291–292
　congenital, 1429
　　hirsutism from, 1446
　　lipoid, 1396–1397
　and Cushing's disease, 1354
　antral gastrin cell, 695
　　vs. peptic ulcers, 699
　benign prostatic, 1422–1423
　erythroid, of bone marrow, from hemolysis, 909
　fibromuscular, 2164
　　and mesenteric artery occlusion, 762
　focal nodular, of liver, 857
　from fascioliasis, 1902
　in endocrine glands, 1264
　lymphoid, from drug allergy, 1971t
　nodular regenerative, 857
　nodular theca-lutein, 1446
　of Peyer's patches, lymphoid, vs. Crohn's disease, 750
　of polyps, 766
　sebaceous, 2336, 2336t
　thymic, 1975
　vs. adenoma, aldosteronism in, 283–284, 1350, 1359
Hyperpnea, 394, 401
　asthma attack from, 407
　from pulmonary embolism, 443

Hyperproinsulinemia, familial, 153, 1363
Hyperprolactinemia
　galactorrhea from, 1449
　idiopathic, 1287–1288
　impotence from, 1302, 1409
　nonphysiologic, differential diagnosis of, 1302, 1303t
　testicular failure from, 1417
Hyperprolinemias, 1151t, 1153t, 1158
Hyperpyrexia, 1527
Hypersensitivity
　anaphylaxis from, 1956
　and contact dermatitis, 2318
　and fever, 1525
　animal-derived antitoxins and, 61
　delayed, 1990
　glucocorticosteroid therapy for, 130
　　dosage for, 191
　granulomatous, glucocorticosteroid therapy for, 129
　immediate, mediators of, 1972, 1973t
　Langerhans' cells and, 2302
　mast cells in, 2306
　pneumonitis of, 425, 433, 2364
　to diphtheria antitoxins, 62
　vasculitis of, 431–432, 2026–2028
　vs. sepsis, 1504
Hypersomnia(s), 2078t, 2078–2079
　definition of, 2061t
　hypothalamic lesions and, 2077
　vs. epilepsy, 2225
Hypersomnolence, 2103
Hypersplenism, 850, 917, 1038
　in thalassemia, 932
Hypertension, 276–293
　accelerated, 276–277
　adrenergic agonists for, 137
　after kidney transplants, 581
　after spinal cord injury, 2246
　and aneurysm rupture, 2174
　and aortic dissections, 372
　and atherosclerosis, 321
　and lacunar infarction, 2164
　and threatened stroke, 2170
　aortic regurgitation from, 343
　arterial, after spinal cord injury, 2246
　　pulmonary, in radiographs, 192
　autonomic nervous system in, 278
　benign, 276
　　intracranial, vs. brain tumors, 2234
　beta-adrenergic blockers for, 138
　brachydactyly type E and, 170
　cardiovascular complications of, 182, 293
　classification of, 276t
　coarctation of aorta and, 313, 318
　complicated, 277
　crisis in. See Hypertensive crisis
　diagnosis of, 276, 277t, 281–285
　dialysis and, 575
　diastolic, range of, 285
　diet and, 43–44
　encephalopathy in, 2172–2173
　erythromelalgia from, 378
　essential, 276
　　pathogenesis of, 277–280
　　vs. toxemia of pregnancy, 635
　etiology of, 277, 277t
　exercise and, 46
　extent of control of, 183
　from acute cocaine toxicity, 55
　from acute glomerulonephritis, 584
　from android fatness, 1223
　from autosomal dominant polycystic kidney disease, 645
　from barium, 2281
　from brain tumors, 2232
　from chronic kidney failure, 565
　from Cushing's syndrome, 1355

Hypertension (Continued)
　from diabetic glomerulopathy, 625
　from excess mineralocorticoids, 1347
　from hypernephromas, 506
　from hyperparathyroidism, 1490
　from kidney disorders, 504
　from nephroblastoma, 654
　from oral contraceptives, treatment for, 288, 291
　from phenylephrine solution, 2299
　from pheochromocytoma, 1463
　from polycythemia vera, 981
　from post-streptococcal glomerulonephritis, 587
　from primary aldosteronism, 1358
　from renal artery atheroembolization, 633
　from renal cell carcinoma, 652
　from uremic syndrome, management of, 570
　from urinary tract obstruction, 616
　genetics and, 146, 150
　intracranial, 2076, 2235–2236. See also *Intracranial pressure, increased*
　labile, 277
　　cardiac output in, 278
　　pheochromocytoma and, 284
　low output heart failure from, 216
　malignant, 276, 975, 2296
　obesity and, 1224
　ocular, 2290
　oral contraceptives and, 1443
　papilledema with, 2292
　pathogenesis of, 277–281
　portal. See *Portal hypertension*
　prazosin for, 139
　prevalence of, 277, 278
　primary, 276
　progressive, from chronic kidney rejection, 581
　propranolol for, 138
　proteinuria from, 503
　pulmonary, 177, 293–303. See also *Pulmonary hypertension*
　renovascular, 280–281
　　treatment of, 288, 290–291
　retinal vascular abnormalities in, 2296
　right atrial, from tricuspid stenosis, 351
　secondary, 276, 280–282
　　treatment of, 288–292
　shunt lesions with, 305
　spontaneous intracranial hemorrhage from, 2178–2180, *2178*
　systolic. See *Systolic blood pressure*
　treatment of, 285–292
　　diet in, 285
　　in atherosclerosis prevention, 323
　　pharmacologic therapy in, 286t, 287t, 286–288
　　adverse reactions to, 289t
　venous, in cardiac assessment, 219–220
　　pulmonary, 294
　　in radiographs, 192–193
　with atherosclerosis, and cardiovascular disease, 181
　with hypokalemic alkalosis, in 17 α-hydroxylase deficiency, 1398
Hypertensive crisis
　diagnosis of, 282
　drugs for, 288, 290t
　in chronic kidney failure, management of, 570
　pathogenesis of, 280
Hyperthermia
　diagnosis of, 1526
　from acute cocaine toxicity, 55
　from psychedelic drugs, 58
　hypothalamic disorders and, 2104
　in delirium, 2065

Hyperthermia (Continued)
  malignant, 2282
  vs. fever, 1525
Hyperthreoninemia, 1152t
Hyperthyroidism, 1321–1328. See also
    Graves' disease; Thyrotoxicosis
  and atrial fibrillation after DC cardiover-
      sion, 273
  and corticosteroid-binding globulin, 1342
  and digitalis, 229
  and impotence, 2109
  and myopathy, 2280
  beta receptors in, 137
  beta-adrenergic blockers for, 138
  causes of, 1321t
  definition of, 1321
  from goiter, 1339
  heart rate increases from, and angina
      pectoris, 324
  hypercalcemia from, 1503
  in Hashimoto's thyroiditis, 1334
  in multiple endocrine neoplasia, 1459
  laboratory diagnosis of, 1323–1324, 1324
  low output heart failure from, 216
  menstrual disturbances from, 1440
  muscle weakness from, 2036
  myasthenia gravis with, 2285
  of Graves' disease, treatment of, 1324–
      1327
  polycystic ovarian syndrome from, 1439
  symptoms and signs of, 1322t
  treatment of, and Graves' orbitopathy,
      2295
Hyperthyroiditis, 1332–1333, 1333
Hypertrichosis lanuginosa, acquired, 1111
Hypertriglyceridemia
  acquired disorders and, 1143
  and atherosclerosis, 320
  approach to, 1142
  beta blockers and, 287
  familial, 1140t, 1142
    and atherosclerosis, 1144
  fish oils for, 43
  from acute pancreatitis, 775
  from chronic kidney failure, 565
  from familial lipoprotein lipase defi-
      ciency, 1140
  from thiazide diuretics, 287
  from uremic syndrome, 570
  obesity and, 1224
  with hyperuricemia, 1164
Hypertrophy
  as compensatory mechanism in heart fail-
      ure, 218, 219
  asymmetric septal, and sudden cardiac
      death, 275
  beta-adrenergic blockers for, 138
  bronchial smooth muscle, from asthma,
      403
  diastolic properties of heart and, 185
  from insulin injections, 1373
  left ventricular, as hypertensive complica-
      tion, 293
  medial, pulmonary arterial pressure and,
      295
  right ventricular, from mitral stenosis,
      345
  ventricular, electrocardiography for,
      200
Hypertryptophanemias, 1151t
Hypertyrosinemias, 1150t
Hyperuricemia, 985
  and gout, 1161–1162, 1162t
  asymptomatic, treatment of, 1170
  from thiazides, 231, 287
  genetics and, 150
  in cancer patients, 1088
  in glycogen storage diseases, 1134

Hyperuricemia (Continued)
  in myelofibrosis, with myeloid metapla-
      sia, 986
  in polycythemia vera, 982
  mechanisms of, 1162–1164
Hyperuricosuria, and kidney stones, 640
    diagnosis of, 642
    treatment of, 643
  in cancer patients, 1088
Hypervalinemia, 1151t, 1159–1160
Hyperventilation, 394, 401
  alveolar, from pulmonary embolism, 443
  and petit mal absence seizures, 2223
  and syncope, 2075–2076
  in hypoparathyroidism, 1497
  in interstitial lung disease, 426–427
  in metabolic acidosis, 551, 554
  in physiologic vertigo, 2122
  with respiratory acidosis, hypophospha-
      temia from, 1193
  vs. epilepsy, 2225
  vs. pulmonary embolism, 444
Hypervitaminosis A, and hair damage, 2349
  osteosclerosis from, 1519
Hypervitaminosis D, 1478–1479
  in hypoparathyroidism treatment, 1499
Hypoaeration, localized, 419–421
Hypoalbuminemia, 1907
  ascites from, 792
  from colitis, pseudomembranous, 1632
    ulcerative, 754
  from nephrotic syndrome, 504, 593
  in secondary biliary cirrhosis, 846
  pleural effusion from, 467
  vs. hypothyroidism, 1330
Hypoaldosteronism, 553, 564, 1353
  and distal nephron dysfunction, 623
  definition of, 1340
  hyporeninemic, 532, 1353
    hyperkalemia in, 547
Hypoaminoacidemia, from glucagonoma,
    1389
Hypocalcemia
  calcitonin in, 1505
  cataract from, 2290
  from uremia, 507
  hypomagnesemia with, 1196
  in acute pancreatitis, 777
  in hypoparathyroidism, 1496–1497
  in primary biliary cirrhosis, 845
  prevention of, parathyroid hormone and,
      1486
  seizures from, 2219
  symptoms and signs of, 1497, 1497t
  vs. botulism, 1633
  with hyperphosphatemia, in pseudohy-
      poparathyroidism, 1501
Hypocalcitoninemia, 1505
Hypocapnia, from asthma, 407
Hypocarbia, from drug-induced interstitial
    lung disease, 433
Hypochloremia, from ileus, 719
Hypochlorhydria, 689
Hypochondriasis, 2101, 2102
Hypochromia, in hemoglobin H disease,
    933
Hypocitraturia, and kidney stones, 640
Hypocomplementemia, in post-streptococ-
    cal glomerulonephritis, 586
Hypocupremia, 1241
Hypoesthesia, 2259
Hypofibrinogenemia, in liver disease, 1077
Hypogammaglobulinemia
  adult-onset, gastric atrophy in, 691
  arthritis with, 2045
  chronic lymphocytic leukemia and, 995
  congenital, and cryptosporidiosis, 1883
  immunization against, 63t

Hypogammaglobulinemia (Continued)
  immunoglobulin for, 1536
  in chronic lymphocytic leukemia, treat-
      ment of, 998
  lymphocytopenia with, 967
  lymphopenic, bone marrow transplant
      for, 157
  malabsorption in, 744
  of infancy, 1943–1944
  pernicious anemia with, 904
  thymoma as, 1975
Hypogeusia, 2110
Hypoglycemia, 1381–1387
  and cancer, 1103
  and metabolic encephalopathy, 2064t
  autoimmune, 1386–1387
  cataract from, 2290
  causes of, 1382t
  clinical evaluation of, 1382–1383, 1383
  factitial, 1386, 1386
  food-deprived, 1384–1387
    definition of, 1382
  food-stimulated, 1383–1384
    definition of, 1382
  from acute suppurative cholangitis, 1902
  from adrenocortical insufficiency, 1352
  from antidiabetic therapy, 1367
  from diabetes, from propranolol, 139
  from fulminant hepatic failure, 854
  from glucagon and epinephrine defi-
      ciency, 1466
  from glucocorticosteroid therapy with-
      drawal, 132
  from heart failure, 223
  from hereditary fructose intolerance, 1136
  from insulin therapy, 1372
  from liver disease, 809
  from malaria, treatment of, 1861
  from maple syrup urine disease, 1159
  from parenteral nutrition, 1250
  from Reye syndrome, 2210
  from viral hepatitis, 820
  neurologic dysfunction from, 2076
  non–beta-cell, 1387
  physiology of, 1381–1382
  postprandial dumping syndrome from,
      704
  vs. cerebral malaria, 1859
  vs. epilepsy, 2225
  vs. galactosemia, 1133
Hypoglycemic agents
  cholestasis from, 827
  in drug interactions, 124t
    with anticoagulants, 99
  neutropenia from, 963t
  oral, 1369
    in drug interactions, 124t
Hypogonadism, 1408–1420
  and bone loss, 1511
  and delayed puberty, 1418
  from Cushing's syndrome, 1355
  from hemochromatosis, 839
  hypogonadotropic, 1412
  hypothalamic, 1287
  hypothalamus tumors and, 1286
  in females, and arm span, 1435
  in Laurence-Moon-Bardet-Biedl syn-
      drome, 1203
  infertility from, 1410
  male, causes of, 1411–1418, 1413t
  primary, in thalassemia, 931
  secondary, 1416–1418
  treatment of, 1418–1420
Hypohidrosis, in Fabry's disease, 1144
Hypokalemia, 545
  and bicarbonate reabsorption, 518, 550
  and digitalis toxicity, 228
  and excitable tissues, 545, 545

Hypokalemia (Continued)
 and metabolic alkalosis, 555
 and sudden cardiac death, 275
 and urine potassium concentrations, 524
 causes of, 545–546, 546t, 1358
 chronic, from chronic interstitial nephritis, 606
 during treatment for pernicious anemia, 905
 from barium, 2281
 from Bartter's syndrome, 622
 from diabetic ketoacidosis, 1375, 1376
 from distal renal tubular acidosis, 623
 from excess mineralocorticoids, 1347
 from fulminant hepatic failure, 854
 from primary aldosteronism, 283, 1358
 from thiazides, 231
 from VIPoma, 1388
 from vomiting, 659
 periodic paralysis in, 546, 2281–2282
 toxic megacolon in ulcerative colitis from, 755
 treatment of, 547
 ventricular flutter from, 264
 with hypomagnesemia, 1196
Hypomagnesemia, 1195t, 1195–1196
 and digitalis intoxication, 228
 and hypophosphatemia, 1193
 diagnosis of, 1498
 hypoparathyroidism from, 1486, 1496
Hyponatremia, 524, 1288
 and body fluid hypotonicity, 538
 central pontine myelinolysis after, 2140
 clinical manifestations of, 540
 from adrenocortical insufficiency, 1351
 from excess antidiuretic hormone, 540
 from fulminant hepatic failure, 854
 from hepatic porphyria, 1185
 from Starling forces disorders, 535
 hypothyroidism with, 1330
 treatment of, 541
Hypoparathyroidism, 1496–1499
 and osteomalacia, 1481
 and polyglandular autoimmune disease, 1414
 and secondary parkinsonism, 2144
Hypoperfusion syndromes, 503–504, 504t
Hypophosphatasia, 1152t
 rickets from, 1482
Hypophosphatemia, 1193–1194, 1471–1472
 after kidney transplants, 581
 and osteomalacia, 1484
 bone disease in, treatment of, 1485
 calcitonin in, 1505
 causes of, 1193, 1193t
 hemolysis from, 923–924
 in cancer, 1102
 in hyperparathyroidism, 1489
 osteomalacia from, 1508
 severe, consequences of, 1194
Hypophysectomy, after diabetes insipidus, 1310
 chemical, for pain management, 110, 110t
 for metastatic breast cancer, 1457
Hypophysiotropic hormones, secretion of, control of, 1283–1285
Hypopigmentation, 2344–2346
 from phenylketonuria, 1155
 in tuberous sclerosis, 2158
Hypopituitarism, 1294t, 1294–1297
 and anovulation, 1439
 and gonadotropin secretion impairment, 1417
 hypoglycemia in, 1387
 muscles in, 2280
Hypoplasia, 649
 adrenal, vs. congenital lipoid adrenal hyperplasia, 1397

Hypoplasia (Continued)
 as X-linked dominant trait, 149
 of thymus, 1945, 1974
Hypoproteinemia, in diabetic glomerulopathy, 625
Hypoprothrombinemia, 1073
 from cephalosporins, 120
 in primary biliary cirrhosis, 845
Hypopyon, uveitis in, 2293
Hyporeflexia, in chronic inflammatory demyelinating polyneuropathy, 2262
Hyposensitization, for allergic rhinitis, 1955
Hyposmia, definition of, 2110
 in hypogonadotropic eunuchoidism, 1416
Hypospadias, 170t, 650
Hyposplenism, 1039
Hypotension, 190
 after spinal cord injury, 2246
 and liver disease, 842
 and pharmacokinetics, 97
 antidiuresis from, 1307
 as contraindication for vasodilators in shock, 248
 during dialysis, 577
 from abdominal aortic aneurysms, 371
 from acute pancreatitis, 776
 from adrenocortical insufficiency, 1351
 from alpha antagonists, 139
 from cancer, 1098
 from cannabis, 57
 from captopril, 235
 from chlorpromazine, 139
 from dengue hemorrhagic fever, 1833
 from endotoxic shock, 1660
 from free perforation of peptic ulcers, 707
 from fulminant hepatic failure, 854
 from fulminant meningococcemia, 1614
 from gastrointestinal bleeding, 660
 from glucocorticosteroid therapy withdrawal, 132
 from mesenteric artery occlusion, 762
 from pulmonary embolism, 444
 from sedative withdrawal, 54
 from suppurative cholangitis, 869
 from trauma to heart, 368, 369
 from ulcerative colitis, 755
 from volume contraction vs. from capacitance/volume ratio increase, 534
 from vomiting, 660
 gastritis with, 689
 hemorrhagic, treatment for, 245
 intracranial, 2238
 headache from, 2134
 orthostatic, 2106–2107
 and syncope, 2075
 definition of, 2106
 from tabes dorsalis, 2189
 postural, 1466, 1466t, 2106, 2262
 recumbent, from fluid volume depletion, 532
Hypothalamic-adrenal dysfunction, 1287
Hypothalamic-lactotroph-breast axis, 1284–1285
Hypothalamic-pituitary-adrenal axis
 and adrenal cortisol and androgen production, 1344
 regulation of, 1283
 stimulation tests of, 1349
 suppression of, in glucocorticosteroid therapy, 131, 132
Hypothalamic-pituitary-gonadal axis, regulation of, 1283–1284
Hypothalamic-pituitary-ovarian axis
 and amenorrhea, 1435
 and menstrual cycle, 1429, 1431
 in puberty, 1426
Hypothalamic-pituitary-somatotroph axis, 1284

Hypothalamic-pituitary-testicular axis, and gynecomastia, 1411
Hypothalamic-pituitary-thyroid axis, regulation of, 1284
Hypothalamic releasing factors, 1255
Hypothalamus
 and circadian rhythms, 2077
 and response to cold temperature, 2304
 as neuroendocrine organ, 1252
 disorders of
 and altered hormone secretion, 1285
 and obesity, 1225
 and secondary hypogonadism, 1416–1418
 causes of, 2104t
 chronic anovulation in, 1438–1439
 etiology of, 1285t, 1285–1287
 hypogonadism as, 1287
 hypothyroidism in, 1287
 infiltrative and inflammatory, 1286
 hormones from, and pituitary hormones, 1281, 1281–1283
 mechanism of action of, 1282–1283
 in puberty, 17
 lesions of, and impotence, 2109
 neoplasms of, 1285–1286
 and Cushing's disease, 1304
 neurometabolic function of, 1280
 nonendocrine, 2103–2105, 2104t
 regulation of hormonal secretion by, 1280–1285
 thermoregulatory center in, 1525
 trauma to, 1286
Hypothermia, 2384–2385
 causes of, 2384
 from blood transfusions, 950
 hypothalamic disorders and, 2103–2104
 in delirium, 2065
 thrombocytopenia in, 1054
 ventricular flutter from, 264
Hypothyroidism, 1328–1331
 and combined hyperlipidemia, 1143
 and corticosteroid-binding globulin, 1342
 and digitalis, 229
 and esophageal motor disorders, 684
 and hair loss, 2349
 and impotence, 2109
 and polyglandular autoimmune disease, 1414
 and thalassemia, 931
 and von Willebrand factor, 1070
 causes of, 1328t
 common symptoms of, 1328–1329, 1329t
 definition of, 1328
 dementia from, 28
 elevated cholesterol levels and, 1141
 hypothalamic, 1287
 idiopathic dilated cardiomyopathy from, 369
 menstrual disturbances from, 1440
 mononeuropathy with, 2264
 muscle weakness from, 2036
 myopathy in, 2280
 polycystic ovarian syndrome from, 1439
 subclinical, 1329
 therapy for, 1330t, 1330–1331
 vs. anorexia nervosa, 1216–1217
Hypotonia, 538–541, 2143
 in maple syrup urine disease, 1159
 ipsilateral, 2126
 muscle, in rickets, 1482
Hypotonicity, apparent vs. real, 538
Hypoventilation, 401
 alveolar, and hypercapnia, 484
 polycythemia from, 979
 pulmonary hypertension from, 297–298
 and gas exchange, 474
 from oxygen therapy, 480
 hypoxemia from, 483

Hypoventilation (Continued)
in metabolic alkalosis, 551
in respiratory failure, critical care of, 490
with respiratory acidosis, mechanical
ventilation for, 487
Hypovitaminosis D, 1478. See also Vitamin
D, deficiency of
Hypovolemia, 531–534
from cholera, 1653
from coma, 2070
from gastrointestinal hemorrhage, 796,
797
from nonketotic hyperosmolar syndrome,
1377
from shock, 244
intravascular, orthostatic hypotension
with, 2106
shock in, 237–238
from adrenocortical insufficiency, 1351
from arenaviruses, 1835
Hypoxanthine, 1163
Hypoxanthine arabinoside, from adenine
arabinoside, 125
Hypoxanthine-guanine phosphoribosyltransferase, deficiency of, 1171
and gout, 1167
genetics and, 151
Hypoxemia
after spinal cord injury, 2246
arterial, 304
and medial hypertrophy, 295
and pulmonary hypertension, 295
from drug-induced interstitial lung disease, 433
polycythemia from, 979
from adult respiratory distress syndrome,
491
from aspiration pneumonitis, 2370
from asthma, 407
from atelectasis, 419
from disease of neuromuscular-chest cage
system, 472
from flail chest, 473
from fulminant hepatic failure, 854
from idiopathic pulmonary fibrosis, 428
from interstitial lung disease, 427
from near-drowning, 2371
from pulmonary embolism, 443
heart failure with, 226
mechanical ventilation for, 487
postural, polycythemia from, 979
Hypoxia
and heart contractility, 186
and metabolic encephalopathy, 2064t
arterial, definition of, 401
cellular, from ethanol, 843
from carbon monoxide, 2369
from respiratory failure, 477
from shock, correction of, 245
from tetralogy of Fallot, 309
from vaso-occlusive crisis, in sickle cell
anemia, 939
hypoventilation and, 474
intestinal infarction from, 763
shock and, 238
vs. cerebral ischemia, 2162
Hysterectomy, estrogen treatment after,
1445
Hysteria, 2101, 2102
and malingering, 2061t
vs. complex partial seizures, 2221
vs. rabies, 2201
HZ. See Herpes zoster

I band, 2269
I-cell disease, 1177
Ia antigen, 956

IASP (International Association for the
Study of Pain), 104
Ibuprofen
as analgesic, 107t
as cyclooxygenase inhibitor, 1275
with narcotics for pain relief, 108
Ice, craving for, iron deficiency and, 880, 897
Iceland disease, vs. poliomyelitis, 2199
Ichthyosis, 2326t, 2328, 2328t, 2329
etretinate for, 2317
ICP. See Intracranial pressure
ICS. See Immotile cilia syndrome
Ictal events, 2217. See also Seizures
IDDM. See Diabetes mellitus, insulin-depend-
ent
Idiopathic hypertrophic subaortic stenosis,
356
Idiotopes, 1936–1937
Idoxuridine, for herpesvirus infection, 125,
1783
IFA (indirect fluorescent antibody) test,
1878
Ig. See Immunoglobulin(s)
IGF-I (insulin-like growth factor I),1293
IH (idiopathic hyperprolactinemia), 1287–
1288
IHA (indirect hemagglutination) test, 1878,
1887
^{131}I-hippurate scan, for acute kidney failure,
561
Ileitis, from Yersinia enterocolitica infection,
746
regional, 745
Ileocolitis, 745
Ileostomy, continent, contraindications for,
759
Ileum
carcinoid of, vs. Crohn's disease, 750
disease of, steatorrhea from, 742
with hyperoxaluria, 640
fluid absorption by, 725
pain in, 658
ulcers of, sprue and, 743
Ileus, 719–720
adynamic, 719
from mesenteric artery occlusion, 762
from peritonitis, 793
gallstone, 867
in burn patients, endotoxic shock and,
1659
paralytic, anticholinesterases for, 140
from cholera, 1653
from potassium deficiency, 547
vs. pseudo-obstruction, 720
Iliac vein, thrombosis of, 385
Imaging
infarct-avid, 210
magnetic resonance, 84–86, 666–668. See
also Magnetic resonance imaging
techniques of, 82–87. See also Diagnostic
imaging techniques
thallium planar, 210
Imerslund's syndrome, 905
Imidazole, for Candida vaginitis, 1704
Iminoglycinuria, 619, 1153t
neonatal, 1153t
Imipenem, 120, 121t
in kidney and liver failure, 117t
Imipramine
and riboflavin deficiency, 1231
metabolism of, in cigarette smokers, 39
inhibited by cimetidine, 100
reference intervals for, 2403t
Immersion syndrome, 2371
Immobilization, and hypercalcemia, 1503
and hypercalciuria from net bone resorption, 640
and thrombosis, 1074

Immotile cilia syndrome, 1131, 1416
bronchiectasis from, 439t
diagnosis of, 1534
infection in, 1532, 1533
vs. chronic bronchitis, 413
Immune complex–mediated diseases, glucocorticosteroid therapy for, 130
Immune complexes
circulating
and rheumatic disease, 1997
and vasculitis, 2025
deposition of, 1961
in Wegener's granulomatosis, 2030
depletion of, and vasculitides, 2028
detection of, 1962
disease of, 1960, 1960t, 1960–1962, 1961.
See also Serum sickness
glomerular, formation of, rapidly progressive glomerulonephritis from, 591
inflammation from, 1989–1890
tissue damage from, 2026
vasculitis from, 2027
Immune response
and systemic sclerosis, 2020
genes of, 966
in Sjögren's syndrome, 2024
initiation of, 1932
macrophages in, 1937
to organ transplants, 578
Immune serum globulin, for X-linked
agammaglobulinemia, 1943
Immune system, 1932–1941
alterations in, and sarcoidosis, 451
and aging, 24
and Crohn's disease, 746
and red blood cell production, 881
and rheumatic disease, 1984
complement in, 1938
abnormalities of, 1940
deficiency of, after splenectomy, 1039
destruction of, and marrow transplants,
1040
disorders of, and chronic gastritis, 691
and interstitial nephritis, 605, 606
purine enzyme deficiencies and, 1172–
1173
Hodgkin's disease and, 1017
in primary biliary cirrhosis, 844
in ulcerative colitis, 753–754
malnutrition and, 1213
measles and, 2208
neoplasms of, 1007–1008. See also Non-
Hodgkin's lymphoma(s)
Immunity. See also Immune complexes; Immune response; Immune system
cellular, and host defense, 1531t, 1531–
1532
impaired, and nocardiosis, 1675
in ataxia-telangiectasia, 2153
specific, 1531
to malaria, 1858
to measles, 1773
to meningococcal disease, 1612–1613
Immunization, 61–66. See also Vaccination
Immunization Practices Advisory Committee, recommendations of, 1636
Immunocompromised host, 1534. See also
Host defense mechanisms; Immunodeficiency
Immunodeficiency. See also AIDS
acquired syndrome of. See AIDS
and Epstein-Barr virus, 1787
and gram-negative bacteria, 1660
and herpes simplex virus, 1782–1783
and toxoplasmosis, 1877
and varicella, 1789
bacterial peritonitis with, 793, 794
cellular disorders of, 1945, 1945t

Immunodeficiency (Continued)
diagnosis of, 1534–1535, 1535t
from multiple myeloma, 1029
infection prevention in, 1537
influenza vaccination for patients with, 62
lymphocytopenic, 966
management of, 1535–1337, 1537t
manifestations of, 1533–1534
neurologic disorders in, 2210
pathogenesis and pathology of, 1532t, 1532–1533
primary disease of, 1941–1948
antibody deficiency disorders as, 1942–1945
classification of, 1942t
severe combined disorders of, 1945–1946
suspected, approach to, 1941–1942, 1942t
varicella vaccine for patients with, 65
virus of. See Human immunodeficiency virus
Immunoelectrophoresis, 1555, 1607, 1620
Immunoglobulin(s), 1932, 1933, 1934–1935
as tumor markers, 1100
deficiency of, bronchiectasis from, 439t
deposits of, glomerulonephritis and, 583
for hypogammaglobulinemia, 1536
in acute interstitial nephritis, 603
in antiviral therapy, 128
in interstitial lung disease, 426
in lower respiratory tract, 424
in Nezelof's syndrome, 1945
in sarcoidosis, 451
in urinary protein, 520
monoclonal, disorders associated with, 1027t
in multiple myeloma, 1028–1029
on hairy cells, 999
properties of, 1934
reference intervals for, 2398t
synthesis of, by B lymphocytes, 1026
varicella zoster, 1790
Immunoglobulin A
antibodies to, 1531
deficiency of, 1533
to meningococcal polysaccharide, and susceptibility to meningococcal disease, 1612
deficiency of, selective, 1943–1944
testing for, 1942
Immunoglobulin A nephropathy, 584t, 588, 588–589
vs. Alport's syndrome, 638
Immunoglobulin E–dependent urticaria-angioedema, 1949
Immunoglobulin G antibodies, 1531
and immunity to hepatitis A virus, 821
Immunoglobulin G index, for neurosyphilis, 2190
Immunoglobulin M
deficiency of, 1944
elevated, 1944
in primary biliary cirrhosis, 845
production of, by spleen, 1036
Immunoglobulin M fluorescent treponemal antibody absorption test, for syphilis, 1719
Immunoglobulinopathies, 1026. See also Plasma cells, disorders of
Immunologic reactions, skin and, 2305, 2305t
urticaria-angioedema as, 1948
suppression of, with glucocorticoids, 1346
Immunosuppression therapy
after transplants, and infection, 1533
kidney, 581
and aspergillosis, 1850
and cancer, 1093t, 1095

Immunosuppression therapy (Continued)
and Kaposi's hemorrhagic sarcoma, 1059
and nocardiosis treatment, 1676
and oral candidal infection, 677
and skin disorders, 2352
and urinary tract infection, 629
antimicrobial therapy with, 123
as contraindication for smallpox vaccination, 1793
during rejection episode, 580
for acute leukemia, 1006
for autoimmune hemolytic anemia, 919
for Crohn's disease, 752
for increasing neutrophil count, 964
for myocarditis, 354
for renal cell carcinoma, 653
for rheumatoid arthritis, 2003–2004
glucocorticosteroids as, 129
inhalant allergen, for allergic rhinitis, 1955
lymphocytopenia from, 966
measles and, 1773
neutropenia from, 961, 963t
varicella vaccine for patients with, 65
venom, for insect sting allergy, 1959
Impedance, in cardiac performance, 216t
Impedance plethysmography, for deep-vein thrombosis, 386
Imperforate anus, vs. congenital megacolon, 723
Imperforate hymen, 1429
Impetigo, bullous, 2329
streptococcal, 1577–1578
Impotence, 1409–1410, 2108–2109
from androgen deficiency, 1409
from arteriosclerosis obliterans, 381
from diabetic autonomic neuropathy, 2264
from hemochromatosis, 1191
from hyperprolactinemia, 1302
from syphilis, 1717
from systemic sclerosis, 2023
from tabes dorsalis, 2189
genital herpes and, 2197
iron deposition in, pituitary and, 1417
Inanition, from chronic lymphocytic leukemia, 995
from hypothalamic disorders, 1289
Inclusion body myositis, 2276
Incontinence
fecal, 728, 790
in elderly, 29–30
urinary, 2107t, 2107–2108
from tabes dorsalis, 2189
in AIDS dementia complex, 2204
Incontinentia pigmenti, as X-linked dominant trait, 149
Indacrinone, properties of, 231t
Indapamide, for hypertension, 286t
properties of, 231t
Independence, development of, in adolescence, 16
Indian tick-bite typhus, 1745
Indium-111–labeled leukocytes, for abdominal abscess, 793
in radionuclide imaging, 667
Indolamines, 1282
Indomethacin
acute kidney failure from, 608
aggravation of hypertension by, 279
as cyclooxygenase inhibitor, 1275
asthma from, 104, 407
interaction of, with lithium, 101
Industrial chemicals, and transitional cell cancers, 654
Indwelling catheters, and bacteriuria, 630
and peritonitis, 793
urinary tract infection from, 629

Infantile paralysis, 2198. See also Poliomyelitis
Infarction
acute, of intestines, 762–763, 763
mortality from, 763
cerebral, diagnostic imaging techniques for, 2059
definition of, 2162
dementia from, 28
extension or expansion of, 333
in heroin users, 57
myocardial, 327–337. See also Myocardial infarction
omental, idiopathic primary, 796
watershed, 2163
Infection(s), 1523–1524. See also under names of specific infections
acute interstitial nephritis from, 605
acute leukemia and, 1003–1004
acute phase response to, 1527–1529
after splenectomy, 1039
agents of. See Infectious agents
and Crohn's disease, 746
and diarrhea, diagnosis of, 730
and fever, 1524
and gastritis, 689
and malabsorption, 743–744
and membranous nephropathy, 596
and polyclonal cold agglutinin synthesis, 920
and splenomegaly, 1037
and ulcerative colitis, 753
and ulcers, 696
aneurysms from, 370
as contraindication for kidney transplant, 578
atelectasis with, 419
cancer and, 1088
chronic, anemias of, 899
chronic granulomatous disease and, 958
congenital. See Congenital infection
defense against, malnutrition and, 1213
ectopic kidneys and, 649
eosinophilia from, 1025
from common duct obstruction, 862
from Haemophilus, 1617–1621
from induction chemotherapy, for acute myelogenous leukemia, 1006
hemolysis from, 915
Hodgkin's disease and, 1017
hospital-acquired, 1541–1549. See also Hospital-acquired infection(s)
immunosuppression therapy and, 581
in marrow space, examination for, 883
in multiple myeloma, 1032
in uremic syndrome, management of, 571
in vaso-occlusive crisis, in sickle cell anemia, 939
increased susceptibility to, complement abnormalities and, 1940
nosocomial. See Hospital-acquired infection(s)
obstructive airway disease with, oxygen therapy for, 297
of bone marrow, and neutropenia, 962
of nervous system, 2191–2207. See also Viral nervous system infections
of skin, occupational factors in, 2375
prevention of, 1541
slow, 2203
susceptibility to, in sickle cell anemia, 940
thrombocytopenia in, 1053
urinary tract obstruction with, 616
viral. See Viral infections
vs. colonization, 1542
Waldenström's macroglobulinemia and, 1033
with neutropenia, treatment of, 965–966

Infectious agents
  AIDS with, diarrhea from, 729
  and cancer, 1095
  identification of, in antimicrobial therapy,
    112–113
  interstitial lung disease after exposure to,
    435
Infectious mononucleosis, 1786–1788. See
    also Epstein-Barr virus; Mononucleosis,
    infectious
Infective endocarditis, 1586–1596
  acute bacterial endocarditis as, 1590
  and brain, 2186
  and mitral regurgitation, 347
  and skin, 2325
  bicuspid aortic valve and, 312
  clinical features of, 1589
  culture-negative, 1592
  differential diagnosis of, 1592
  echocardiography for, 203
  emboli from, 2174
  from Haemophilus parainfluenzae, 1621
  fungal endocarditis as, 1591
  gram-negative bacterial endocarditis as,
    1591
  hospital-acquired, 1591–1592
  in opioid users, 56
  microbiology of, 1586–1587, 1587t
  mitral valve prolapse and, 350
  myxoma vs. 367
  pathogenesis and pathology of, 1587,
    1587–1588
  peripheral signs of, 1589t
  prevention of, 1595t, 1595–1596
  prognosis for, 1595
  prophylaxis for, 1586
  prosthetic valve infection as, 1590–1591,
    1591t
  recurrent, 1592
  subacute, vs. chronic meningococcemia,
    1616
    vs. viral encephalitis, 2194
  susceptibility to, aortic stenosis and, 341
  treatment of, 1593–1595, 1594t
  vs. meningococcal disease, 1615
  vs. rheumatic fever, 1585
Infertility, 1440–1441. See also Fertility
  causes of, 1441t
  definition of, 1410, 1440
  from androgen deficiency, 1409
  from chemotherapy and radiation ther-
    apy, 1119–1120
  from salpingitis, 1706
    gonococcal, 1708
  from hypothalamic hypogonadism, 1287
  male, causes of, 1410
  Ureaplasma urealyticam and, 1564–1565
  varicocele and, 1416
Inflammation
  anemias of, 899
  and inhibition of eosinophil production,
    1024
  and splenomegaly, 1037
  erythrocyte sedimentation rate and, 1995
  headache from, 2133–2134
  immune system and, 1961–1962, 1984–
    1985, 1985t, 1988–1991, 1989t
  in rheumatic disease, 1977
  intra-abdominal pain from, 658
  mediators of, and Crohn's disease, 746
  of joints, 1983
  pain from, steroids for, 109
  prostaglandins and, 1276–1277
  reactive thrombocytosis from, 1054
  suppression of, with glucocorticoids,
    1346
  tissue destruction from, 1985–1986

Inflammatory bowel disease, 745–760, 800–
    807, 1199. See also Crohn's disease;
    Ulcerative colitis
  and anemia, 881
  and eosinophilia, 1026
  and mesenteric venous thrombosis, 764
  and pseudomembranous colitis, 1632
  aphthous ulcers with, 676
  arthropathy with, 2008
  colonoscopy for, 671
  hemorrhage from, 799
  incidence of, 753
  liver in, 841
  vs. amebiasis, 1886
  vs. appendicitis, 801
  vs. Campylobacter enteritis, 1650
  vs. ischemic colitis, 764
  vs. postvagotomy diarrhea, 704
  vs. tuberculosis of colon, 1691
  zinc deficiency in, 1241
Inflammatory cells
  accumulation of, 1987–1988, 1988
  in asthma, 403
  in gastritis, 689
  in lungs, 424
  in sarcoidosis, 451
Inflammatory response, 1530
  and tissue injury, 1988–1991
  from complement, 1938
  from mononuclear leukocytes, 1990–1991
  minimum circulating neutrophils for,
    1533
Influenza, 1762–1767
  amantadine for, 126–127
  and staphylococcal pneumonia, 1600
  clinical findings of, 1765–1766
  definition of, 1757, 1762
  diagnosis of, 1766
  epidemiology of, 1762–1763
  etiology of, 1762, 1762
  immunization against, 62–63
    bronchiectasis and, 439
    for COPD patients, 416
    for elderly, 62t
  myoglobinuria after, 2283
  pathogenesis and pathology of, 1764–
    1765
  Reye syndrome after, 2209
  ribavirin for, 127
  splenomegaly in, 1037
  vs. hepatitis A, 821
  vs. histoplasmosis, 1838
  vs. isoniazid toxicity, 829
  vs. leptospirosis, 1732
  vs. mycoplasmal pneumonia, 1564
  vs. psittacosis, 1736
  vs. Q fever, 1749
  vs. viral hepatitis, 819
Informed consent, 13
  adolescent cognitive development and, 17
  in defensive medicine, 8–9
Inguinal adenopathy, in chancroid, 1712
INH. See Isoniazid (isonicotinic acid hydrazide)
Inhalants, abuse of, 59–60
Inhalation, passive, of cigarette smoke, and
    lung cancer, 458
Inhalation therapy, for pain management,
    110, 110t
Inheritance, multifactorial, 150, 169, 172
Inhibin, 1284, 1405
  follicle-stimulating hormone inhibition
    by, 1408
  in menstrual cycle, 1430
Injuries
  acute phase response to, 1527–1529
  control of, 40–42
  death from, 40

Injuries (Continued)
  from falls, drug abuse and, 52
  from violence, epidemiology of, 41
INO (internuclear ophthalmoplegia), 2115–
    2116
  definition of, 2213
Inotropic agents, and myocardial contractil-
    ity, 184
  contraindicated for idiopathic restrictive
    cardiomyopathy, 361
Inotropic state, of heart, 186, 216, 216t, 218
Insect bites, hyperreactivity to, 1958–1960
  from chronic lymphocytic leukemia,
    995
  skin reactions to, 2330
  vs. varicella, 1789
Insecticides
  arsenic in, and kidney damage, 611–612
  as inhibitors of cholinesterases, 140
  as testicular toxins, 1416
  atropine as antidote for, 143
  carbamate, poisonings with, treatment
    for, 145
  organophosphate, poisonings with, treat-
    ment for, 145
  poisonings with, treatment for, 144
Insomnia(s), 2077–2078, 2078t
  hypothalamic lesions and, 2077
  in dying patients, 33
  in metabolic encephalopathy, 2063
  treatment of, and sedative dependence,
    53
Inspiratory pressure, maximal, measure-
    ment of, in severely ill, 483
Insulin
  action of, 1363–1364, 1364
    and calorie intake in diabetic, 1368
  allergy to, 1969
  and hypophosphatemia, 1471
  and mitochondrial fatty acid uptake, 1138
  and potassium transfer, 543, 546
  and sodium reabsorption, 516
  catabolism of, in kidneys, 519
  deficiency of, 1360
    in non-insulin-dependent diabetes mel-
      litus, 1364
  excess of, 1223
  hypersecretion of, in multiple endocrine
    neoplasia, 1459
  in hyperkalemia treatment, 548
  injection of, lipoatrophy from, 2051
  levels of, aging and, 25
  production of, 158, 1363
    endurance exercise training and, 46
  reference intervals for, 2398t
  resistance to. See Insulin resistance
  secretion of, regulation of, 1363
  steroids and, 1346
Insulin-dependent diabetes mellitus, 1360.
    See also Diabetes mellitus, insulin-depend-
    ent
Insulin hypoglycemia testing, 1350
  for ACTH evaluation, 1293, 1296
  for testing growth hormone, 1294
Insulin-like growth factor I, growth hor-
    mone binding to, 1293
Insulin receptor, 1258
Insulin resistance, 810, 1360, 1364
  in non-insulin-dependent diabetes melli-
    tus, 1364
  obesity and, 1223–1224
  uremia and, 567
Insulin test, for incomplete vagotomy diag-
    nosis, 705
Insulin therapy, 1370–1373
  complications of, 1372–1373
  for diabetic ketoacidosis, 1376

Insulin therapy (Continued)
for pancreatitis, 778
preparations for, 1370–1371, 1371t
Insulinoma, 1384, 1384–1386, 1385
Intellectual function, changes in, in multiple sclerosis, 2213
low, vs. metabolic encephalopathy, 2063
Intensive care. See Critical care medicine; Critical care units
Intention tremor, 2142
Interferon(s)
and acute interstitial nephritis, 605
and acute phase response, 1528
and common cold, 1756–1757
and protection against virus infection, 1752
for carcinoid syndrome, 1468
for cellular immune disorders, 1536–1537
for chronic myelogenous leukemia, 992
for herpesvirus, 125
in antiviral therapy, 127–128
in inflammation, 1987
in influenza, 1765
production of, 158
recombinant, neutropenia from, 963t
with adenine arabinoside, for hepatitis, 125
Interleukin-1, 956–957, 1937
and acute phase response, 1528
fever from, 1526
from keratinocytes, 2305
in inflammatory response, 1530–1531
Interleukin-2, 957
for cancer, 1129
for cellular immune disorders, 1536–1537
from T cells, 1935
in inflammation, 1987
production of, 158
Interleukin-4, 1934
Intermediary metabolism, definition of, 1130
glucocorticoids and, 1346, 1346
hormones and, 1262
Intermesenteric area, abscess in, 793
Intermittent claudication, coarctation of aorta and, 313
definition of, 380
Intermittent porphyria, acute, 148
vs. poliomyelitis, 2199
vs. epilepsy, 2225
Intermittent positive pressure breathing machines, 417, 479
Interstitial fibrosis
diffusing capacity in, 400
from acute interstitial nephritis, 603
from chronic eosinophilic pneumonia, 431
from chronic interstitial nephritis, 606
from irradiation restrictive cardiomyopathy, 361
in advanced kidney disease, 607
pulmonary hypertension from, 296
Interstitial fluid, pH of, normal ranges for, 549
Interstitial lung disease, 421–435
alveolar wall in, 421–422, 422
chronic eosinophilic pneumonia as, 431
clinical features of, 425–428
differential diagnosis of, 423, 424t
drug-induced, 424t, 433–434
epidemiology of, 422–423, 423t
from inhaled inorganic dusts, 423t, 432–433
from inhaled organic dusts, 424t, 433
genetic factors in, 432
Goodpasture's syndrome as, 430
histiocytosis-X as, 430

Interstitial lung disease (Continued)
idiopathic pulmonary hemosiderosis as, 430–431
idiopathic pulmonary fibrosis as, 428–429
impairment from, assessment of, 427–428
lymphangioleiomyomatosis as, 432
lymphocytic infiltrative disorders as, 431
pathogenesis of, 423–425, 425
sarcoidosis and, 429, 454
therapy for, 428
with pulmonary airway disease, 432
Interstitial nephritis, 504–506, 602. See also Tubulointerstitial disease
acute, 603–604
causes of, 603–606, 604t
clinical manifestations of, 606
from nonsteroidal anti-inflammatory agents, 608
idiopathic, 606
allergic, proteinuria from, 503
chronic, 606t, 606–607
from drug allergy, 1971t
hematuria from, 503
salt wasting in, 564
Interstitial pneumonia(s)
from congenital rubella, 1777
from respiratory syncytial virus, 1759
marrow transplants and, 1040
Interstitium, fluid transfer between capillaries and, disorders in regulation of, 535
of kidneys, 510
damage to, disorders causing, 532
Intertrigo, from Candida infection, 1848
Intervertebral disc(s), 2040, 2048
anatomy of, 2252
disease of, 2252–2254
herniated, 2040, 2252–2253
nerve root compression by, 2248
treatment of, 2044
vs. extradural tumors, 2255
pain from, 105, 2249
Intestine(s)
acute ischemic syndromes of, 762–764
aganglionosis of, 170, 170t
anaerobic streptococci as normal flora in, 1573
and calcium balance, 1472
atresia of, vs. congenital megacolon, 723
bile salt reabsorption by, 860
bilharziasis of, 1899
blood supply to, 760
bypass surgery on, necrotizing cutaneous vasculitis with, 2326
candidiasis in, 1848
carcinoma of, and hematocrit, 802
chronic ischemia syndromes of, 762
decreased absorption by, and osteomalacia or rickets, 1481
disease in, from adenovirus, 1767–1768
displacement of loop of, and mesenteric disease, 795
gangrene in, vs. appendicitis, 802
gas in, 661. See also Flatulence
hemorrhage from, in typhoid fever, 1641
hermaphroditic flukes in, 1904–1905
infarction of, 763
inflammatory diseases of, 745–760, 800–807. See also Inflammatory bowel disease
inherited polyposis syndromes of, 767–768
intramural hemorrhage of, 764–765
iron uptake from, 894
ischemia of, and pseudomembranous colitis, 1632
computed tomography for, 662
large. See Colon; Large intestine
malabsorption by, vitamin D therapy for, 1485

Intestine(s) (Continued)
motility of, agents affecting, 724–725
deranged, diarrhea from, 728
mucosa of, abnormalities in, and malabsorption, 742–743
in Crohn's disease, 747
nematodes in, 1905–1911
neoplasms of, vs. gallstones, 865
nonocclusive infarction of, 763
obstruction of
and pseudomembranous colitis, 1632
as contraindication for laparoscopy, 674
from adenocarcinoma of colon, 770
from ascariasis, 1909
from Crohn's disease, 749
in elderly, vs. appendicitis, 803
in mesenteric inflammatory disease, 795
vs. acute pancreatitis, 776
vs. familial Mediterranean fever, 1197
pain from, 656
parasites in, 1901
vs. peptic ulcers, 699
perforation of, from ascariasis, 1909
pseudo-obstruction of, 720
causes of, 720
radiation injury in, 2377, 2379t
resection of, diarrhea from, 729
for Crohn's disease, 752
response of, to vitamin D, 1478
secretion from, drugs to inhibit, 732
small. See Small intestine
spirochetosis of, diagnosis of, with biopsy, 731
structural disruption in, and diarrhea, 728t, 728–729
tuberculosis of, 1690–1691
vascular system of, diseases of, 760–765
Intimal fibrosis, in coronary artery bypass grafts, 339
Intracellular compartment, 529
as potassium reservoir, 543
metabolic disease and, 1131
potassium shift from, to extracellular compartment, 548
Intracranial hemorrhage
factor XIII deficiency and, 1074
fibrinogen disorders and, 1073
from isoimmune neonatal purpura, 1052
spontaneous, 2173–2180
etiology of, 2173–2175, 2173t
vs. hypertensive encephalopathy, 2172
Intracranial pressure
abnormally low, 2238, 2238t
alterations in, headache from, 2133–2134
disorders of, 2235–2238
increased, 2235
after near-drowning, 2371
and headache, 105, 2132, 2133–2134
and papilledema, 2292
from acute heroin reaction, 56
from aneurysm rupture, 2175
from brain abscess, 2182
from brain tumors, 2231
from head trauma, 2239–2240
from lateral sinus thrombosis, 2185
from Reye syndrome, 2209
pathogenesis of, 2236t
Intrauterine contraceptive devices
and actinomycosis in cervix, 1674
and endocarditis, 1591
and gonococcal salpingitis, 1708
and metastatic brain abscess, 2181–2182
Intravascular devices, contamination of, 1545
infection from, 1545
Intravenous fluids
and hyponatremia, 541

Intravenous fluids (Continued)
  contamination of, 1545
    infection from, 1545
  for sickle cell anemia, 941
  in management of adult respiratory distress syndrome, 488, 492
Introns, 1965
Intubation, endotracheal. See Endotracheal intubation
Intussusception, after gastric surgery, 718
  from ascariasis, 1909
Iodide, for hyperthyroidism, from Graves' disease, 1325
Iodine
  as antibiotic, 1548
    topical, 124
  deficiency of, and thyroid disease, 1339
  metabolism of, 1316
  recommended dietary allowance for, 1205t, 1316
    minimal, 1339
5-Iodo-2'-deoxyuridine (idoxuridine), 125, 1783
Ipratropium, for asthma, 409
Iridocyclitis, 2293
  in erythema nodosum leprosum, 1699
Iris lesions, definition of, 2307
Iritis, 2293
  from Crohn's disease, 747
  in inflammatory bowel disease, 758
Iron
  absorption of, 734–735, 893–894
    vitamin C and, 1234, 1236
  accumulation of, and hemoglobin synthesis, 929
  and thrombocytosis, 1054
  average intake of, 734, 893
  cellular uptake of, 894
  daily dietary requirement for, 896
  deficiency of. See also Iron deficiency anemia
    after ulcer surgery, 705
    from chronic kidney failure, 566
      management of, 571
    gastric cancer and, 711
    in elderly, 661
    pathogenesis of, 896, 896t
    symptoms of, 657
    vs. protoporphyria, 1184
    vs. thalassemia trait, 933
  distribution of, in body, 893t
  excess, in hemochromatosis, 157
  for treating malabsorption, 741t
  in diet, and increased porphyrin production, 1187
  recommended allowance for, 1205t
  in methemoglobin, 945
  intestinal absorption of, increased, 1189–1192. See also Hemochromatosis
  metabolism of, 892
  oral, in drug interactions, 124t
  overload of, 2390
    from ineffective erythropoiesis in megaloblastic anemia, 902
    from transfusions, 931
  poisoning with, 142
    desferrioxamine for, 143
  reference intervals for, 2398t
  saturation of, reference intervals for, 2398t
  storage of, 894–895
  supplements of, risks of, 884
  total body stores of, normal, 1190
  transport of, 894
Iron-binding capacity, reference intervals for, 2398t
  total, 894
Iron deficiency anemia, 893–898
  blood loss and, 880
  clinical manifestations of, 896–897

Iron deficiency anemia (Continued)
  esophageal webs from, 687
  from colonic cancer, 771
  from gastrointestinal hemorrhage, 883
  from idiopathic pulmonary hemosiderosis, 430, 431
  from ulcerative colitis, 754
  in hereditary hemorrhagic telangiectasia, 1060
  laboratory findings for, 897, 897–898
  polycythemia with, 304
  reduction of, with oral contraceptives, 1444
  treatment of, 898
  vs. pyridoxine-responsive anemia, 1234
Iron-dextran complex, 898
Iron oxide, and lung cancer, 458
Iron salts, poisonings with, treatment for, 144–145
Iron storage disease, 1189–1192, 1190. See also Hemochromatosis
Irritable bowel syndrome, 656, 660, 661, 722–723
  diagnosis of, 729, 731
  diarrhea from, 728
  dietary fiber for, 1246
  diverticula with, 723
  esophagogastroduodenoscopy for, 669
  stool examination for, 730
  vs. gallstones, 865
  vs. postcholecystectomy syndrome, 872
Ischemia
  and heart contractility, 186
  and hematocrit, 802
  and metabolic encephalopathy, 2064t
  bone necrosis from, 1517
  cellular injury and necrosis from, 327
  from arterial pressure monitoring, 496
  from arteriosclerosis obliterans, 380, 381
  from atherosclerosis, 318
  from frostbite, 379
  from occlusion, of microvasculature by sickle cells, 939
  from sudden arterial occlusion, 383
  in gastrointestinal tract, 661
    factors affecting, 761
    vs. appendicitis, 801
  in kidneys, 504
    from hypotension, 559
  intra-abdominal pain from, 658
  mitochondrial damage from, 242
  mucosal, 689
  myocardial, 208. See also Myocardial ischemia
  of brain, management of, 2170–2172
  of gastric mucosa, 695
  of gut, hemorrhage with, 730, 764
  of muscle, and myoglobinuria, 2283
  silent, 324
  stroke from, 2159
  subendocardial, in aortic stenosis, 188
  transient, anemias and, 879
  variable threshold, 177
  vascular stroke from, 2162
  ventricular, echocardiography during, 203
ISG (immune serum globulin), 1943
Islet cell antibodies, in insulin-dependent diabetes mellitus, 1365
Islet cell tumor(s), 1387–1390
  gastrinoma as, 1388, 1389t
  glucagonoma as, 1389t, 1389–1390
  insulinoma as, 1384, 1384–1386, 1385
  somatostatinoma as, 1390
  syndromes associated with, 1389t
Islets of Langerhans, 1387, 1387–1388. See also Langerhans' cell(s)
Isoetharine, 137
Isolation, of infectious patients, 1547

Isoleucine, 1159
Isoniazid (isonicotinic acid hydrazide)
  acute interstitial nephritis from, 605
  and niacin metabolism, 1232
  and vitamin B$_6$ deficiency, 1233
  chronic hepatitis from, 828, 831
  elimination rate for, 96t
  for tuberculosis, 1686
    prophylaxis of, 1683–1684
  genetics in metabolism of, 102
  in combination therapy for systemic infection, 119
  in drug interactions, 124t
  in kidney and liver failure, 117t
  interstitial lung disease from, 434
  liver disease from, 827, 829
  lupus syndrome from, 103
  penetration into spinal fluid by, 116
  reference intervals for, 2403t
  sideroblastic anemia from, 900
Isoproterenol, 137
  and infarct size, 336
  and myocardial oxygen demand, 239
  and panic attacks, 2100
  for asthma, 408
  for cardiorespiratory arrest, 501
  for muscular glycogen storage diseases, 1135
  for primary pulmonary hypertension, 300, 301t
  for shock, 247
  initial hemodynamic effects of, 247t
Isoreceptors, 136
Isosorbide dinitrate
  as vasodilator, 233
  for angina pectoris, 326, 326t
  for esophageal disorders, 686
  in primary pulmonary hypertension therapy, 300
  with hydralazine, for vasodilator effect, 235
Isospora hominis, 1889
Isosthenuria, in gout, 1166
  in sickle cell anemia, 939
Isotopes, inhalation of, 2376
Isotretinoin, for skin disorders, 2317
Itai-itai, cadmium and, 2391
Itching, 661, 2303. See also Pruritus
IUDR (idoxuridine), 125, 1783
IUD's. See Intrauterine contraceptive devices
Ivermectin, for filariasis, 1914
  for onchocerciasis, 1917
Ixodes dammini, and babesiosis transmission, 1884
Ixodes persulcatus, and encephalitis, 1828
Ixodes ricinus, and encephalitis, 1828

Jaccoud's arthritis, 1582
Jacksonian march, 2220
Jail fever, 1739
Jakob-Creutzfeldt disease. See Creutzfeldt-Jakob disease
Jamais vu, in partial seizures, 2220
Jamestown Canyon virus, encephalitis from, 1826, 1827
Janeway's lesions, definition of, 2325
  from infective endocarditis, 1589t
Japanese encephalitis, 1827–1828
  immunization for, before travel, 1550
Jargonaphasia, 2086
Jarisch-Herxheimer reactions, after treatment for relapsing fever, 1724–1725
  syphilis treatment and, 1722
Jaundice
  abnormal prothrombin time in, 816
  cholestatic, from drugs, 1969
  diagnosis of, 817–818

Jaundice (Continued)
dyserythropoietic, idiopathic, 814
Escherichia coli in infants and, 834
from acute cholecystitis, 865
from adenocarcinoma of small intestine, 713, 773
from alcoholic hepatitis, 843
from bartonellosis, 1681
from bile duct tumor, 871
from chronic persistent hepatitis, 831
from cold agglutinin disease, 921
from common duct obstruction, 862
from congenital hemolytic disorders, 908
from congenital syphilis, 1718
from gastrointestinal disease, 661–662
from glucose-6-phosphate dehydrogenase deficiency, 915
from hereditary spherocytosis, 911
from infectious mononucleosis, 1787
from liver disease, 808
from pancreatic cancer, 781
from pneumococcal pneumonia, 1557
from primary biliary cirrhosis, 845
from sclerosing cholangitis, 869
from secondary biliary cirrhosis, 846
hemolytic anemia and, 880
homologous serum, 821, 823. See also Viral hepatitis, type B
mitochondrial test for, 816
obstructive, in chronic lymphocytic leukemia, 995
postoperative, 814
spur cell hemolytic anemia and, 923
Jaw, claudication in, from giant cell arteritis, 2033
mycobacterial infection in, 1695
JC virus, and progressive multifocal leukoencephalopathy, 2207
JCA (juvenile chronic arthritis), 2004
JCAH (Joint Commission on Accreditation of Hospitals), 1543, 1547
Jejunoileal bypass, alcoholic hyalin after, 843
for obesity, 743, 1227
and liver disease, 828, 843
Jejunoileitis, chronic ulcerative, 807
nongranulomatous, vs. Crohn's disease, 750
Jejunum, pain in, 658
ulcers of, sprue and, 743
Jellyfish, 1930–1931
Jerks, myoclonic, vs. myoclonic seizures, 2222
Jet lesions, 1588
Jimson weed, toxicity of, 787
treatment for, 144
Job's syndrome, 960, 1534
and staphylococcal infection, 1598
Jodbasedow's disease, 1321, 1340
Joint(s)
aspiration of, examination of, 1993
for bacterial arthritis, 2010
bleeding into, from hemophilia B, 1071
calcium-containing crystals in, 2037
cavity of, 1983
Charcot, 2046
Clutton's, 2011
damage to, in immune complex disease, 1962
disease in, 1983–1984
dislocations of, in Ehlers-Danlos syndrome, 1179
distal interphalangeal, noninvolvement of, in rheumatoid arthritis, 2000
examination of, magnetic resonance imaging for, 85
hypermobility of, osteoarthritis and, 2041

Joints (Continued)
in disseminated coccidioidomycosis, 1841
infection of, 1978
inflammation of, 1983. See also Arthritis
systemic, 1998. See also Rheumatoid arthritis
neoplasms of, 2048
of Luschka, 2040
osteoarthritis in, 2039–2041
pain in, 105
from hyperparathyroidism, 1490
in bartonellosis, 1681
peripheral, temperature of, 1162
prosthesis for, 2004
cobalt in, 2390
proximal interphalangeal, rheumatic disease in, 2001
radiology of, 1997
sporotrichosis in, 1847
staphylococcal infection of, 1599–1600
stiffness in, in Scheie's syndrome, 1175
structure and function on, 1982–1983, 1983
Wegener's granulomatosis in, 2031
Joint Commission on Accreditation of Hospitals, 1543, 1547
Joint contractures, muscular dystrophy with, 2273
Joint National Committee on Detection, Evaluation and Treatment of High Blood Pressure, 276, 281
Judgment, impaired, in progressive dementias, 2088
Jugular veins, estimation of right atrial pressure from, 186
pulse in, 176
Junin virus, 1834
Juvenile onset diabetes, 1360. See also Diabetes mellitus, insulin-dependent
Juxtaglomerular apparatus, 510
in fluid volume regulation, 190, 530

Kaempferol, and cancer, 44
Kala-azar (visceral leishmaniasis), 835t, 1869, 1871–1873, 1872
Kaliuresis, in tubulointerstitial disease, 603
Kallikrein-kinin system, 520
and blood pressure maintenance, 278, 279
kidneys and, 503
Kallmann's syndrome, 1287, 1416–1417, 1439
LHRH for, 1420
Kanamycin, 122
decrease in use of, 119
elimination rate for, 96t
for tuberculosis, 1687
reference intervals for, 2403t
Kaolin, and decreased absorption of other drugs, 99
lung disease from, 2364
Kaopectate, interaction with digitalis, 228
Kaposi's sarcoma, 790, 1059, 2340
among homosexuals, 1082
and skin, 1110, 1110t
appendicitis from, 801
in AIDS, 464, 677, 678, 1797, 1798, 1803, 1806–1807
vs. bartonellosis, 1682
Karelian fever, 1819
Karnofsky scale, for cancer patients, 1086, 1087t
Kartagener's syndrome, 153, 1131, 1416. See also Bronchiectasis; Immotile cilia syndrome
dextrocardia and, 315

Kasabach-Merritt syndrome, 925, 2340
thrombocytopenia in, 1053
Katayama fever, 1897, 1900
Kawasaki's syndrome, 374, 2323t
rash in, 2324
retrovirus in, 1523
Kayser-Fleischer rings, in Wilson's disease, 839, 1188
examination for, 832
Kearns-Sayre syndrome, 2153t, 2279–2280
Kell antigens, 948
Keloids, 2306
Kenya tick-bite fever, 1745
Kerandel's sign, in Gambian sleeping sickness, 1864
Keratan sulfate, 1174
Keratin, 2301
in squamous tumors, granulomatous peritonitis from, 795
Keratinocytes, 2300
and immunologic reactions, 2305
Keratitis, 2294
amebic, 1888
from Herpesvirus hominis, 2293
interstitial, from congenital syphilis, 1718, 2189
punctate, from onchocerciasis, 1917
Keratoacanthomas, 2336–2337, 2336t
from occupational skin injury, 2375
Keratoconjunctivitis
epidemics of, 1768
from herpes simplex virus, 1782
vs. Chlamydia infection, 1734
with atopic eczema, 2320
Keratoconjunctivitis sicca, 2296
in Sjögren's syndrome, 2024
in systemic lupus erythematosus, 2015
in systemic sclerosis, 2023
Keratosis, actinic, 2337
seborrheic, 2336t, 2338
Kerley's B lines, 193, 195
mitral stenosis and, 346
Kernicterus, in neonates, 812
excessive vitamin K and, 1076
Kernig's sign, from neurosyphilis, 2188
in subdural empyema, 2184
Keshan disease, 1242
Keto acids, branched-chain, for chronic liver disease with encephalopathy, 855
Ketoacidosis
alcoholic, 554
diabetic, 553, 1373–1374, 1376–1377. See also Diabetic ketoacidosis
in methylmalonicaciduria, vitamin B$_{12}$ for, 157
Ketoconazole
and testosterone synthesis inhibition, 1414
for blastomycosis, 1843
for Candida infection, of esophagus, 688
for candidiasis, 677, 1849
for coccidioidomycosis, 1841
for cryptococcosis, 1845–1846
for Cushing's syndrome, 1356
for cutaneous leishmaniasis, 1875
for histoplasmosis, 1839–1840
for mycoses, 1838
for paracoccidioidomycosis, 1844
for skin disorders, 2317
for sporotrichosis, 1847
gynecomastia from, 1411
in kidney and liver failure, 117t
liver disease from, 827
17-Ketogenic steroids, reference intervals for, 2398t
Ketone bodies, 1375
reference intervals for, 2398t

Ketonemia, 522
Ketones, 1212
Ketonuria, branched-chain, 1150t, 1159
    thiamin for, 1230
Ketosis, alcoholic, 810
    from glucocorticoids, 1346
    in insulin-dependent diabetes mellitus,
        1362
17-Ketosteroids, reference intervals for,
    2398t
Key sign, in Gambian sleeping sickness,
    1864
Kidd antigens, 948
Kidney(s). See also *Glomerular; Renal; Tu-
    bule(s)*
    abnormalities in, and kidney stones, 641
    abscess of, 628, 632
    acidification capacity of, 523–524
    adenoma of, 651–652
    agenesis of, prenatal diagnosis of, 173
    allergic drug reactions in, 1971t
    allergic purpura and, 1059
    amyloidosis and, 1035, 1199, 1201
        transplant for, 157
    analgesic disease of, 607–608, 628
    and acid-base balance, 549
    and blood volume, 190
    and hyperuricemia, 1163
    and metabolic alkalosis, 556
    and phosphate balance, 1472–1473
    and sodium chloride homeostasis, 514–
        516
    angiography of, 282–283
    ankylosing spondylitis in, 2007
    anomalies of, 648–649
    arteriography of, 568–569
    as endocrine gland, 1253
    atheroembolization in, 633–634
    atriopeptin and, 1279
    bicarbonate processing in, 550–551
    biopsy of, 527–528, 569
        indications for, 528t
    blood flow to, 189, 500, 508, 510–511
        aging and, 98
        in heart failure, 220
        intraorgan, 240
        prostaglandins and, 1276
        regulation of, peptides and, 239
    calcification of, in hyperparathyroidism,
        1490
    cancer of, amyloidosis in, 1199
        in cigarette smokers, 38
    cardiorespiratory arrest and, 500
    collecting duct defects in, 505
    congenital absence of, 169–170
    cortex of, 508, 628
    cystic disease of, 147, 170, 506, 644–648
        adult, 506, 644, *646*
            and renal cell carcinoma, 644–647,
                645t, 652
            hematuria from, 503
        benign vs. malignant, 645t
        single cysts as, 644, 645t
            vs. early polycystic disease, 646t
    damage to, from aminoglycosides, 122
        urinary flow obstruction and, 507
    defective renin secretion by, hypoaldos-
        teronism from, 1353
    diagnostic imaging of, 525–527
    diminished excretion in, drug interactions
        and, 101
    disorders of. See also *Nephropathies*
        and anti-inflammatory drug effect on
            glomerular filtration rate, 102
        and blood coagulation disorders,
            1078
        and drug clearance, 94–96
        and drug dosage calculation, 97

Kidney(s) *(Continued)*
    disorders of, and drug loading doses, 95–
        96
        and drug protein binding, 94
        and gout, 1161
        and hyperkalemic periodic paralysis,
            2281
        and neuropathy, 2265
        and pericardial disease, 363
        as contraindication, for tetracyclines,
            609
            for lithium, 2099
        erythrocytosis from, 980
        from accelerated hypertension, 277
        from diabetes mellitus, 624–627, 1379
        from hyperparathyroidism, 1490
        from hypertension, 293
        from multiple myeloma, 1030
        from thrombotic thrombocytopenic
            purpura, 1052
        from Wegener's granulomatosis, 2031
        gout and, 1166–1167
        in systemic lupus erythematosus, 2013
        metabolic bullous disease with, 2332
        polycystic, 148, 506, 644–647. See also
            Polycystic kidney disease
        pregnancy with, 634–637
        presenting as acute glomerulonephritis,
            584t
        tuberculosis treatment and, 1687, 1688
        urinary manifestations of, 503
        vs. angioedema, 1951
        vs. paravertebral tumors, 2255
        vs. toxemia of pregnancy, 635
    distal tubular defects in, 505
    diuretic action in, 234
    drug elimination by, 90
        in elderly, 98
    end-stage disease of. See *End-stage kidney
        disease; Uremic syndrome*
    enlargement of, in glycogen storage dis-
        eases, 1134
        in leptospirosis, 1730
    erythropoietin-secreting function of, and
        marrow response to anemia, 892
    examination of, magnetic resonance im-
        aging for, 85
    failure of, 507–508. See also *Uremic syn-
        drome*
        acute, 506, 558–562
            causes of, 558–559, 558t
            clinical manifestations of, 559–560
            diagnosis of, 560t, 560–561
            from aminoglycosides, 609
            glomerular filtration rate in, 559
            in nephrotic syndrome, 593
            in pregnancy, 636–637
            indications for dialysis in, 576, 576t
            nonsteroidal anti-inflammatory
                agents and, 608
            pathogenesis of, 559, *559*
            postrenal, 560–561
            prerenal, 560
            prognosis for, 562
            treatment for, 561–562
            urinary indices of, 560, 560t
        and amylase level, 776
        and digitalis use, 229
        and infection, vancomycin for, 122
        as contraindication for orthophos-
            phates, 643
        bone disease from, 1507. See also *Renal
            osteodystrophy*
        chronic, 563–572. See also *Uremic syn-
            drome*
            and abnormal vitamin D metabolism,
                1480
            anemia of, 892

Kidney(s) *(Continued)*
    failure of, chronic, antibiotic dosage in,
        572t
        atriopeptin in, 1279
        diet for, 571–572
        follow-up of, 572, *572*
        hypertensive encephalopathy with,
            2172
        hyperuricemia from, and gout, 1167
        management of, 569–572
        osteomalacia in, 1483–1485
        partial hypopituitarism in, 1295
        sodium loss in, 532
        sperm and androgen production in,
            1415
        toxin retention in, 567–568
        vs. hypothyroidism, 1330
    drug dosage modification in, 116, 117t,
        118
    from acyclovir, 126
    from captopril, 235
    from dextran 40, 245
    from electric injury, 2381
    from familial Mediterranean fever, 1196
    from hypertension, 277
    from liver disease, 852
    from malaria, 1858, 1859
    from multiple myeloma, 1029, 1032
    from rifampin, 1687
    from urinary tract obstruction, 615
    from VIPoma, 1388
    gastritis with, 689
    hypercalcemia from, 1504
    hypoglycemia in, 1387
    immunization for patients with, 63
    metabolic acidosis from, 553
    oliguric, hyperkalemia from, 547
    vs. peptic ulcers, 699
    with pericardial effusion, radiograph
        for, *194*
    fluid volume regulation by, 529–531, *530*
    function of, 502–503
        and drug reactions in elderly, 26
        as endocrine organ, 503
        as endocrine receptor, 502
        deteriorating, after parathyroidectomy,
            1495
        in acid-base balance, 517–518, 518t
        in calcium metabolism, 518–519
        in elderly, 25
        in homeostasis and excretion, 511–519
        in magnesium metabolism, 519
        in mineral homeostasis, 518
        in phosphorus metabolism, 518
        in potassium balance preservation,
            516–517, 517t
        in pregnancy, 634
        in prostaglandin synthesis, 520
        in protein metabolism, 519
        in sodium chloride homeostasis, 514–
            516
        investigating, 520–528
        normal, 510t, 510–520
    gout in, 1164–1165
    hemodynamics of, proteinuria from, 522
    hereditary disorders of, 637t, 637–638
    Hodgkin's disease and, 1017
    hypoperfusion of, 503
    in Crohn's disease, 750
    in heart failure, 224, 230
    in systemic sclerosis, 2022
    in vitamin D metabolism, 1477–1478
    in yellow fever, 1831
    infarction in, hematuria from, 503
        papillary, in sickle cell anemia, 939
    infection of, 505, 628. See also *Pyelone-
        phritis*
    inhalant abuse and, 59

Kidney(s) (Continued)
interstitium of, 510
irreversible failure of, treatment of, 573–582
dialysis for, 573–577. See also Dialysis; Hemodialysis; Peritoneal dialysis
transplants for, 577–582. See also Kidney transplants
ischemia in, from occlusive disease of renal arteries, 504
isolated tubular defects of, 505
lead poisoning and, 2386
loss of mass in, with atherosclerotic disease, 291
magnesium wasting by, 1195
malnutrition and, 1213
malrotation of, 649
mass lesions in, ultrasonography for, 526–527
maximal concentrating ability of, 1307
maximum diluting capacity of, measurement of, 523
medulla of, microcystic disease of, 506
microinfarction of, from sickle cell trait, 939
medullary sponge, 645t, 646, 648
and kidney stones, 641
Caroli's disease with, 870
mineralocorticoids in, 1347
neoplasms of, 506, 650–653
benign, 651–652
classification of, 650t
diagnostic procedures for, 650–651, 651
hematuria from, 503
malignant, 652–653. See also Renal cell carcinoma
metastasized to, 655
nonsteroidal anti-inflammatory agents and, 608t
normal, vs. cystic kidney disorders, 646
paraneoplastic syndromes in, 1098
parathyroid hormone and, 1487
parenchymal syndromes of, 504t, 504–506
perfusion of, arterial blood volume drop and, 514
phosphate handling by, 1193
and osteomalacia, 1481
plasma flow to, increase in, 625
polyarteritis in, 2029
polycystic disease of, 644–647
position of, anomalies of, 649, 649
potassium handling by, 543–544, 544
potassium wasting by, 545
problems with, in male adolescent, 17
prostaglandin E_2 in, 1273
radiation injury in, 2377, 2379t
radiation therapy and, 610–611
retransplantation of, 582
sarcoidosis in, 453
sarcomas of, 655
shock and, 236
size of, as indicator of chronic kidney failure, x-rays for, 568
increase in, diabetes and, 625
sodium handling by, and hypertension, 279–280, 280
sodium retention by, and ascites, 851
structure of, 508–510
systemic lupus erythematosus and, 2016
testing for, 2017
treatment for, 2018
systemic sclerosis in, treatment of, 2023
thromboxane A_2 from, 1276
toxic injury to, 604, 607t, 607–613
common features of, 603
from radiocontrast agents, 626

Kidney(s) (Continued)
transplantation of, 577–582. See also Kidney transplants
tuberculosis in, 1690
tubular transport in, 511–514
ultrasonography of, for urinary tract obstruction, 507
vascular disorders of, 632–634, 649
Kidney stones, 505–506, 638t, 638–644. See also Calculus(i), renal
Kidney transplants, 577–582
blood transfusion before, 578, 580
clinical aspects of, 580–582
complications following, 580t
erythrocytosis from, 980
focal glomerular sclerosis in, 595
for diabetics, 1379
for end-stage kidney failure, in diabetic patient, 627, 1379
for inborn metabolic errors, 157
hypercalcemia from, 1504
idiopathic rapidly progressive glomerulonephritis in, 591
immunologic aspects of, 578, 579, 580
membranous nephropathy in, 597
minimal change nephrotic syndrome in, 593
multiple, 582
osteonecrosis after, 1517
recipients of, 578
recurrent diseases of, 582t
rejection of, 578, 580, 605
Kimmelstiel-Wilson lesions, in diabetic nephropathy, 1379
Kinase, activation of, cyclic AMP and, 1258–1259, 1259
Kinetoplast, 1870
Kinin(s), 278, 520, 1531
and sodium reabsorption, 516
formation of, 1539, 1987
shock and, 239
Kininogen, high molecular weight, deficiency in, 1072
Klatskin tumor, 871
Klebsiella
and urinary tract infection, 629
hospital-acquired, 1543
cephalosporins for, 120
enterotoxins from, and secretory diarrhea, 727
growth of, in IV solution, 1545
liver abscess from, 834
lung abscess from, 436
penicillins for, 120
pneumonia from, 1558, 1566
hospital-acquired, 1544
septicemia from, shock from, 246
Kleine-Levin syndrome, 2079
Klinefelter's syndrome, 167, 167t, 170, 1412–1413, 1413
and breast cancer, 1453
occurrence of, 1404
vs. XX males, 1402
Klippel-Feil syndrome, 2257
as congenital malformation, 170
Kluver-Bucy syndrome, 2081
Knees
degenerative joint disease of, radiology of, 1997
neoplasms of, 2048
osteoarthritis in, 2040
pain in, from hip disease, 106
rheumatoid arthritis in, 2001
Knott's technique, 1915
Koebner phenomenon, definition of, 2313
in lichen planus, 2328
in psoriasis, 2326

Koilonychia, definition of, 2346
from iron deficiency, 897
Koplik's spots, in measles, 1773, 1773
Korotkoff's sounds, in blood pressure measurement, 281
Korsakoff's syndrome, 28, 2084, 2138
Krabbe's disease, 2216
Krebs-Henseleit urea cycle, 811
Krypton-81m, for ventilation scanning, 445
Kulchitsky cells, and small cell lung cancer, 458
carcinoid tumors from, 1467
Kupffer cells, 954, 954
in viral hepatitis, 819
Kuru, 2205
Kussmaul's respiration, in diabetic ketoacidosis, 1375
in metabolic acidosis, 554
Kveim-Siltzbach test, 451
for sarcoidosis, 456
Kwashiorkor, 1213–1214
definition of, 1212
Kyasanur Forest disease, 1828, 1833–1834
Kyphoscoliosis, 473
respiratory failure from, 476
Kyphosis, 2258
from osteoporosis, 1512

LA. See Latex agglutination test
Labetalol, adverse effects of, 289t
for hypertension, 287t, 290t
for pheochromocytoma, 292
Labia majora, development of, 1392
Labia minora, development of, 1392
Labor, oxytocin and, 1313
premature, cholestasis of pregnancy and, 841
cyclooxygenase inhibitors for, 1276
Laboratory tests, 72, 75
accuracy of, 80
distribution of values in, 80–82
discontinuous, 81–82
for anemias, 883, 884, 884t
for Crohn's disease, 748
for hormone levels, 1265–1267
for patients with cardiovascular disease, 177–178
for rheumatic disease, 1979
normal range for, 81
of body fluids in poisonings, 141–142
precision of, 80
reference intervals for, 2394–2404
biologic, 81
results of, physicians and, 82
sensitivity of, 72, 75, 80
serologic, for syphilis, 1719t, 1719–1720
sources of variance in, 80
specificity of, 72, 75, 80
use and interpretation of, 79–82
Labyrinthitis, acute, 2123
Lacrimal glands, carcinomas of, 2295
Sjögren's syndrome in, 2024
LaCrosse virus, encephalitis from, 1826, 1827
Lactacidemia, mitochondrial myopathy with, 2280
Lactase, deficiency in, 742
and irritable bowel syndrome, 722
Lactation. See also Galactorrhea
absence of, postpartum, from hypopituitarism, 1295
initiation of, 1293, 1449
maintenance of, 1449
nutrient requirements for, 1204, 1205t
Lactic acidosis, 553–554
from biguanides, 1370
in cancer, 1098

Lactic acidosis (Continued)
in exertional heatstroke, 2383
thiamin for, 1230
treatment for, 555
Lactic dehydrogenase, 1100
deficiency of, and myopathy, 2278
from folate deficiency, 906
from intravascular hemolysis, 908
in polymyositis, 2036
increase in, in renal artery occlusion, 633
vitamin B₁₂ deficiency and, 903
isoenzymes of, reference intervals for, 2398t
level of, in hypothyroidism, 1330
measurement of, for myocardial infarction, 332
reference intervals for, 2398t
Lactobacillus acidophilus preparations, for pruritus ani, 789
Lactobacillus casei, and folate, 906
Lactoferrin, in host defense mechanisms, 1529
Lactogen, placental, as tumor marker, 1099
Lactoperoxidase, in host defense mechanisms, 1529
Lactose
absorption of, 734
deficiency in, postvagotomy diarrhea vs., 704
exclusion of, in irritable bowel syndrome treatment, 661
intolerance to, and diet for Crohn's disease, 751
Lactose-H₂ breath test, for lactase deficiency evaluation, 742
for malabsorption, 739
Lactosuria, vs. galactosemia, 1133
Lactotrophs, in anterior pituitary, 1290
Lactrase, for lactase deficiency, 742
Lactulose, for hepatic encephalopathy, 853
Lacunar infarction, 2164
pathogenesis of, 2167
vs. hypertensive encephalopathy, 2172–2173
Laetrile, and cyanide poisonings, 144
Lagochilascaris minor, 1911
LAK cells, for renal cell carcinoma, 653
Lambert-Eaton myasthenic syndrome, 1105, 1106, 2285, 2287
Lamina(e), 509
in arteries, 318
Lamina papyracea, Wegener's granulomatosis and, 2031
Laminectomy, indications for, 2044
Laminin, 2302
for cancer, 1129
in basement membrane, 1982
Lanatoside C, for heart failure, 227t
Langerhans' cell(s), 956, 957, 1387, 1387–1388, 2302
aging and, 2306
and immunologic reactions, 2305
in epidermis, 2301
in granulomatosis, 1022–1024
Language, 2085–2087
impairment of, and temporal lobe damage, 2081
Lanoxicaps, dosing and adverse effects of, 266t
LAP (leukocyte alkaline phosphatase), 969–970
Laparoscopy, 673–674
Laparotomy, for Zollinger-Ellison syndrome, 709
staging, for Hodgkin's disease, 1019
Laplace law, 370
Laplace relationship, for systolic wall stress, 186
in dilated heart, 219

Large intestine. See also Colon; Rectum
adenocarcinoma of, 766
carcinoma of, from ulcerative colitis, 757
inflammation of, 753. See also Ulcerative colitis
motility in, disorders of, 716t
neoplasms of, 766–773
polyps vs., 766
Laron dwarf, 1293
growth hormone and, 1301
Larva currens, from Strongyloides, 1906
Larva migrans, cutaneous, 1907
visceral, 1909
vs. acute clonorchiasis, 1902
Laryngitis, from measles, 1774
tuberculous, 1691
viral, 1757–1758, 1758t
Laryngotracheobronchitis, 1757
viral, cough from, 391
Larynx
aspiration in, from palatal weakness, 684
cancer of, in cigarette smokers, 38
edema of, airway obstruction from, 418
inflammation of, airway obstruction from, 418
injury to, from endotracheal intubation, 478
leprosy in, 1698
papillomas of, juvenile, interferon for, 128
taste buds in, 2110
Lasègue's sign, 2044
Laser, equipment for, 670
therapy with, for bleeding ulcers, 706
trabeculoplasty with, 2290
Lassa fever, 1834–1835
ribavirin for, 127
Lassitude, as interferon reaction, 128
Latex agglutination test, for Haemophilus influenzae detection, 1620
for histoplasmosis, 1839
for meningitis, 1607
Lathyrism, from Lathyrus sativus, 787
Latrodectus mactans, 1923
antivenin for, 66
Laughing, asthma attack from, 407
inappropriate, in partial seizures, 2220
Laurence-Moon-Bardet-Biedl syndrome, 1203
Laurence-Moon syndrome, and extreme obesity, 1289
LAV (lymphadenopathy virus), 1799
and cancer, 1095
Laxatives
abuse of, 656
cathartic colon from, 722
in bulimia, 1218
stool examination for, 730
and vitamin A deficiency, 1237, 1238
classes of, 722
ineffectiveness of, after poisonings, 142
reactions to, vs. Bartter's syndrome, 622
LCAT (lecithin-cholesterol-acyl-transferase), 816, 1140
deficiency of, 1144
LD bodies, 1870
LDH. See Lactic dehydrogenase
LDL (low-density lipoprotein), 1139
catabolism of, defective, 1140t, 1140–1141
LDL cholesterol, reference intervals for, 2398t
LE cell, 1996
in systemic lupus erythematosus, 2016
Lead
and kidney damage, 611
exposure to, and gout, 1167
poisoning with, 143, 2385–2387
screening tests for, 2386t

Lead (Continued)
poisoning with, sideroblastic anemia from, 900
urine in, 1183
vs. protoporphyria, 1184
reference intervals for, 2398t
Lead systems, in electrocardiography, 196t, 196, 196–197
incorrect placement of, 199
of pacemakers, placement of, 272
Learning, definition of, 2083
Leber's forms, 2113
Leber's optic atrophy, 151
vs. optic neuritis, 2215
Lecithin, for preventing arteriosclerosis, 43
Lecithin-cholesterol acyltransferase, 816, 1140
deficiency of, 1144
Leeches, 1927
Left-sidedness, bilateral, in polysplenia syndrome, 316
Leg(s)
blood pressure in, vs. in arms, coarctation of aorta and, 313
fatigue in, coarctation of aorta and, 313
paresthesia in, in diabetic neuropathy, 2263
skin disorders of, 2346t
weakness in, from tick paralysis, 1923
in AIDS dementia complex, 2204
Legionella, 1548
erythromycin for, 121
infection of, 1570–1572
interstitial lung disease after, 435
lung abscess from, 436
pneumonia from, vs. mycoplasmal pneumonia, 1564
quinolones for, 122
rifampin for, 121
Legionnaires' disease, 1570
vs. pneumococcal pneumonia, 1558
vs. psittacosis, 1736
Leigh's syndrome, 2279
thiamin for, 1230
Leiomyoma(s), in kidneys, 652
of liver, 857
of stomach, 713
Leiomyosarcoma(s)
of kidneys, 655
of lungs, 464
of small intestines, 773
of stomach, 713
Leishmania donovani, in liver, 835t
Leishmaniasis, 1869–1875, 1870t
cutaneous, 1873–1875
etiology of, 1870
immunology of, 1870–1871
parasite-host interaction in, 1870
rheumatoid factor in, 1996
visceral, 1869, 1871–1873, 1872
vs. paracoccidioidomycosis, 1843
vs. sporotrichosis, 1847
Lennox-Gastaut syndrome, 2222
electroencephalogram for, 2224
Lens, opacity of, 2289
Lentigines, actinic, 2342
Lentigo maligna melanoma, 2339, 2339
Lentigo simplex, 2342
LEOPARD syndrome, 2343
Lepromin test, 1698
Leprosy, 1696–1701
and hepatitis B susceptibility, 822
clinical manifestations of, 1698
diagnosis of, 1699
epidemiology of, 1696
etiology of, 1697
false-positive syphilis tests in, 1720
immunopathologic considerations of, 1698

Leprosy (Continued)
lepromatous, 1696–1700, 1874
pathogenesis and histopathology of, 1697, 1697t
prevention of, 1701
prognosis for, 1701
reactions in, treatment of, 1700
rheumatoid factor in, 1996
susceptibility to, 1697
transmission of, 1696–1697
treatment of, 1699–1701
vaccine for, recombinant DNA, 159
vs. streptocerciasis, 1919
Leptomeninges, metastatic neoplasms of, 2256
in breast cancer, 1456
vertigo from, 2124
viral infection of, 2192
Leptomeningitis, after cerebral epidural abscess, 2184
and subdural empyema, 2184
Leptospira interrogans, 1730
Leptospirosis, 1730–1732
vs. Q fever, 1749
vs. rat-bite fever, 1730
vs. viral hepatitis, 824
vs. yellow fever, 1832
Leriche's syndrome, 381, 1410
Lesch-Nyhan syndrome, 150, 153, 167, 1171–1172
gout in, 1165, 1167
Leser-Trélat sign, in cancer, 1112
Lesions
cutaneous, TFT ineffectiveness on, 126
from chilblain, 379
in kidneys, 527
infravalvular, aortic stenosis vs., in children, 342–343
nil, proteinuria and, 521
obstructive, in congenital heart disease, 309–314
of nerve system for pain control, 110–111
plexiform, 298
in Eisenmenger's syndrome, 316
regurgitant, in congenital heart disease, 311–314
rupial, 1716
supravalvular, aortic stenosis vs., in children, 342–343
vascular, 298
Let-down reflex, for milk, 1293
Lethargy
from glucocorticosteroid therapy withdrawal, 132
from hydrocephalus, 2237
from hypervitaminosis D, 1478
from hyponatremia, 540
from maple syrup urine disease, 1159
from metabolic encephalopathy, 2063
from uremic syndrome, 507
Letterer-Siwe disease, 430, 1022, 1023, 1024
and hypothalamus, 1286
Leucin aminopeptidase, in liver disease, 815
Leucine, 1159
Leucovorin, 1120–1121
Leukapheresis, 998
for chronic myelogenous leukemia, 992
Leukemia(s)
acute, 1001
classification of, 1002–1003, 1003t
clinical manifestations of, 1003–1004
etiology of, 1001–1002
from sideroblastic anemia, 900
incidence of, 1002
laboratory manifestations of, 1004
marrow aplasia and, 886

Leukemia(s) (Continued)
acute, paroxysmal nocturnal hemoglobinuria and, 922
pathophysiology of, 1002
polycythemia vera and, 980, 983
therapy for, 1004–1006
vs. chronic myelogenous leukemia, 991
aleukemic, 1004
and Salmonella infection, 1644
as contraindication for smallpox vaccination, 1793
B cell, human T lymphotropic retrovirus and, 1797
basophilic, 695, 991
blastic, acute, from myeloproliferative disorders, 984–985
chronic, 988–1001
hairy cell leukemia as, 998–1001. See also Hairy cell leukemia
lymphocytic, 994–998. See also Lymphocytic leukemia, chronic
myelogenous, 973–974, 988–994. See also Myelogenous leukemia, chronic
progressive multifocal leukoencephalopathy with, 2207
fever in, 1004
folate requirements in, 906
from radiation, 1094
hairy cell, 998–1001. See also Hairy cell leukemia
glucose values in, 1382
immunosuppressive therapy for, and neurologic infection, 2210
in heart, 367
intracranial hemorrhage in, 2175
lactic acidosis in, 554
lymphatic, pleural disease from, 467
lymphoblastic. See Lymphoblastic leukemia
lymphocytic. See Lymphocytic leukemia
marrow transplants for, 1041, 1041–1042
mastocytosis with, 1974
mixed lineage, 1002
myeloblastic, paroxysmal nocturnal hemoglobinuria and, 923
myelogenous. See Myelogenous leukemia
nonlymphocytic, acute, 974, 1530
and disordered neutrophil function, 1533
from radiation, 962
plasma cell, and myeloma, 1030
prolymphocytic, vs. chronic lymphocytic leukemia, 997
skin in, 1109
smoldering, 1006
splenectomy for, 1038
T cell, adult, 1009, 1795, 1796, 1797
varicella vaccine for patients with, 65
vs. aplastic anemia, 887
vs. infectious mononucleosis, 1788
with intestinal gas gangrene, 1629
Leukemia cutis, 1109
Leukemia viruses, 1795
Leukemids, 1111
Leukemoid reactions
definition of, 967
from infection, vs. chronic myelogenous leukemia, 991
in paraneoplastic syndromes, 1097–1098
neutrophilic, 970
Leukoagglutinins, respiratory failure from, 475
Leukocyte(s)
agglutination of, in shock, 241
count, 882
in cholangitis, 868
disorders of
and infection, 1533–1534
in chronic kidney failure, 566

Leukocyte(s) (Continued)
disorders of, in hypophosphatemia, 1194
management of, 1535–1536
in acute pancreatitis, 776
in ascites fluid, 791
in polycythemia vera, 981–982
labeling of, for abdominal abscess, 793
mononuclear. See Mononuclear leukocytes
polymorphonuclear, in inflammatory response, 1530, 1530t
in lung, 424
in sepsis, 1539
reference intervals for, 2401t
sodium urate crystals in, and gout, 1168, 1168
transfusion therapy with, 1536
Leukocyte endogenous mediator, 899
Leukocyte glycoprotein, deficiency in, 960
Leukocytoclasis, definition of, 2027
Leukocytosis, 967–973
definition of, 967
diabetic ketoacidosis with, 1376
eosinophilia as, 970–971
from acute clonorchiasis, 1902
from acute fascioliasis, 1902
from acute gouty arthritis, 1165
from amebic liver abscess, 836
from appendicitis, 801
from cavernous sinus thrombosis, 2185
from chronic myelogenous leukemia, 990
from congenital syphilis, 1718
from free perforation of peptic ulcers, 707
from infective endocarditis, 1592
from lymphangitis, 388
from mesenteric artery occlusion, 762
from polyarteritis nodosa, 2029
from pseudomembranous colitis, 1632
from pyogenic liver abscess, 836
from systemic lupus erythematosus, 2016
from upper gastrointestinal hemorrhage, 797
from whooping cough, 1625
lymphocytosis as, 971–973, 972, 972t
monocytosis as, 970, 971t
neutrophilia as, 968, 968–970, 970t, 971
polymorphonuclear, and acute abdomen, 802
pseudohyperkalemia in, 548
variable, in pericarditis, 364
Leukocyturia, 522
Leukoderma, chemical, 2375
Leukodystrophies, 2215–2216
Leukoencephalitis, hemorrhagic, acute, 2209
Leukoencephalopathy
diagnostic imaging techniques for, 2060
from chronic lymphocytic leukemia, 995
multifocal, progressive, 2203, 2207, 2210–2211
vs. AIDS dementia complex, 2205, 2207
Leukoerythroblastosis, 889
causes of, 968t
vs. chronic myelogenous leukemia, 991
vs. leukemoid reaction, 967–968
Leukonychia, definition of, 2346
Leukopenia, 961–967
from carbamazepine, 2227
in acquired immunodeficiency syndrome, 1802
in liver disease, 817
neutropenia as, 961–966. See also Neutropenia
severe combined immunodeficiency disease with, 1946
Leukoplakia, 678, 678
hairy, in AIDS, 677, 677
Leukostasis, in acute leukemia, 1003

Leukotriene(s), 952, 1986
  from mast cells, 2306
    allergic rhinitis and, 1952
    in asthma, 404
Levamisole, for ascariasis, 1909
  neutropenia from, 963t
Levarterenol, for upper gastrointestinal
    hemorrhage, 797
LeVeen shunt, 577. See also *Peritoneovenous
    shunting*
  and disseminated intravascular coagula-
    tion, 1078
  for ascites, 851
Levocardia, isolated, 315
Levodopa
  autoimmune hemolytic anemia from, 922
  contraindications for, 2146
  for parkinsonism, 2146
  side effects of, 2146
Levo-Dromoran, as analgesic, 107t
Levorphanol
  as analgesic, 107t, 108
  for pain in dying patients, 32–33
  half-life of, 108
  poisoning with, 2069t
Levothyroxine, for hypothyroidism, 1330
Lewy bodies, in Parkinson's disease, 2144
Leyden-Möbius type limb-girdle dystrophy,
    2273
Leydig cell(s), 1292, 1404–1405
  agenesis or dysgenesis of, 1395
  testosterone from, 1392, 1393
    impaired secretion of, 1396
  tumors of, 1421
    and precocious puberty, 1420
LGV, 1710–1711. See also *Lymphogranuloma
    venereum*
LH, 1254. See also *Luteinizing hormone*
Lhermitte's sign, 1020, 2140, 2250
  after radiation therapy, 1107
LHRH. See *Luteinizing hormone releasing hor-
    mone*
Libido
  androgens and, 1408
  central nervous system and, 1409
  diminished, from androgen deficiency,
    1409
  in liver disease, 808
Libman-Sacks endocarditis, 1587
Lice, 1920–1921
  and rickettsiae transmission, 1737
  and typhus group, 1738, 1739
  control of, 1740–1741
  lifespan of, 1724
  relapsing fever from, 1724
  trench fever transmission by, 1747
Lichen myxedematosus, monoclonal gam-
    mopathy and, 1036
Lichen planus, 2326t, 2328
  and hair loss, 2349
  and nails, 2346
  erosive, vs. aphthous ulcers, 676
  vs. erythroplakia, 678
  vs. gingivitis, 675
  vs. secondary syphilis, 1716
Lichen sclerosus, androgens for, 1419
Lichen sclerosus et atrophicus, 2341
Lichen simplex chronicus, 2320
Licorice, and primary aldosteronism, 1265
  chronic ingestion of, and hypokalemia,
    545
  for peptic ulcers, 701
Lidamidine, and intestinal motility, 724
  for inhibiting intestinal secretion, 732
Liddle's syndrome, 555
  hypokalemia in, 546
  triamterene for, 556

Lidocaine, 91–92
  accumulation and elimination of, *91*
  adverse reactions to, 102, 266t
  bioavailability of, 88
  concentrations of, after injection, *89*
  distribution of, 88, *89*
    heart failure and, 97
  dosages for, 266t
    loading, 89
  for arrhythmias, 265
    in shock patients, 245
  for digitalis intoxication, 230
  for herpesvirus infection, of esophagus,
    688
  for ventricular ectopy in cardiorespiratory
    arrest, 501
  for ventricular fibrillation, 264
  for ventricular premature depolarizations,
    263
  for ventricular tachycardia, 263
  liver clearance of, 97
  metabolism of, inhibited by cimetidine,
    100
  pharmacokinetic properties of, 89t, 266t
  reference intervals for, 2403t
  time required for elimination of, 90
  toxicity of, to hemoglobin, 945
Life expectancies, from heart failure in aor-
    tic stenosis, 341
  of patients with hypertension, 292, *292*
Life support systems, after poisonings, 142
  termination of, 499
Ligandin, and bilirubin transport, 812
Ligands, receptor, radiolabeling of, 211
Light, ultraviolet, and systemic lupus ery-
    thematosus, 2012
Light microscopy, for muscle biopsy, 2272
Light-headedness. See also *Dizziness and
    Vertigo*
  from partial seizures, 2220
  in postconcussive syndrome, 2243
  vs. vertigo, 2121
Lightning, injury from, 2382
Lignins, in dietary fiber, 721
Limb(s). See also *Leg(s)*
  arteriosclerosis obliterans in, 380
  vascular diseases of, 375–389
Limb of Henle, antidiuretic hormone and,
    1306
Limb-girdle dystrophy, 2273
  vs. acid alpha-1,4–glucosidase deficiency,
    2277
Limbic system, 2081
Limbic-autonomic system, and psychoso-
    matic disorders, 2105
Lincomycin, 121
  decreased absorption of, kaolin and, 99
  elimination rate for, 96t
  interaction of, with curare, 101
Lindane, and enhanced liver metabolism of
    other drugs, 99
  for lice, 1921
  for scabies, 1925
Linguatula serrata, 1926
Linguatuliasis, 1926–1927
Linitis plastica, 711
Link protein, 1982
Lipase, reference intervals for, 2398t
Lipemia retinalis, from chylomicronemia
    syndrome, 1143
Lipid(s). See also *Hyperlipidemia(s)*
  emulsions of, 1247
    reactions to, 1250–1251
  estrogen and, 1445
  in atherogenesis, 42
  in atherosclerosis lesions, 321
  in liver disease, 810, 816

Lipid(s) *(Continued)*
  in myelin, 2211
  in synovial fluid, 1994
  periodic acid-Schiff–positive, in alveoli,
    432
  peroxidation of, from ethanol, 843
Lipid dialysis, after poisonings, 143
Lipid mediators, in inflammation, 1986
Lipid Research Clinic Trials, 320
Lipid storage disease, 1147. See also *Nie-
    mann-Pick disease*
  myopathy in, 2278
Lipiduria, in nephrotic syndrome, 593
Lipoatrophy, 2051
Lipocortin, 129, 1274
Lipogenesis, 809, 1138
Lipohyalinosis, lacunar infarction from,
    2164
Lipoid cell tumors, hormones from, 1445t
Lipoma(s), 2336t, 2337
  of kidneys, 652
  of liver, 857
Lipopolysaccharide, and macrophages, 954
  of bacteroids, 1637
Lipoprotein(s)
  classification of, by physical and chemical
    properties, *1138*
  in liver disease, 816
  in peritoneal cavity, and ascites, 792
  low-density, 1139–1141, 1140t
    fraction of, 182
  metabolism of. See *Lipoprotein metabolism*
  remnant, catabolism of, 1139, *1139*
  structure and function of, 1137–1138
  surface catabolism in, 1140
  synthesis of, in liver, 810
  transport of, physiology of, 1137–1140
  triglyceride-rich, production of, 1138
Lipoprotein lipase, 1138, 1139
  familial deficiency of, 1140t, 1141–1142
Lipoprotein metabolism
  acquired disorders of, 1143, 1143t
  disorders of, 1137–1149
    hyperlipoproteinemias as, 1137–1144.
      See also *Hyperlipoproteinemia(s)*
    inborn errors of, 1140–1142, 1140t
Lipoprotein X, in secondary biliary cirrho-
    sis, 846
Liposarcoma, of kidneys, 655
  of stomach, 713
Lipoxygenase, inhibitors and antagonists
    for, 1275
Lipoxygenase enzymes, arachidonic acid
    metabolism by, 1273
Lipoxygenase pathway, *1273*, 1273–1274
Lips, disease of, 2348
Liquid diet, 1246
Lisinopril, for hypertension, 287
Listeria, penicillins for, 120
Listeria monocytogenes, 1670–1672
  ampicillin for, 119
  as central nervous system infection, in
    transplant recipients, 2210
  bacterial meningitis from, 1605
Lithium
  and diabetes insipidus, 1309
  and hair loss, 2349
  and kidney damage, 611
  for bipolar disorders, 2099
  for hyperthyroidism, 1325
  hypercalcemia from, 1503
  interaction of drugs with, 101
  pharmacokinetic parameters for, 89t
  poisoning with, 2070t
    and collecting duct defects, 505
  reference intervals for, 2403t
  side effects of, 2099

Lithium carbonate
  and cytotoxic therapy, 1536
  for increasing neutrophil count, 964
  for inhibiting intestinal secretion, 732
  for VIPoma, 1389
  goiter from, 1321
Lithium chloride, neutrophilia from, 969
Lithium salts, congenital heart disease
    from, 303
Lithocholate, 859
Lithotripsy, shock-wave, extracorporeal, for
    gallstone dissolution, 862
  for kidney stone treatment, 644
Livedo reticularis, 378
  in systemic lupus erythematosus, 2015
Liver. See also under Hepatic
  abnormalities of, from immunosuppres-
      sion therapy, 581
  abscess of, 834–837
    from amebiasis, 836–837, 1887
    from ascariasis, 1909
    viral hepatitis and, 824
  acute congestion of, in viral hepatitis, 824
  acute disease of, hemolysis with, in Wil-
      son's disease, 1189
  adenomas of, glycogen storage diseases
      and, 1134
  albumin synthesis by, in acute phase re-
      sponse, 1528
    normal range for, 593
  allergic drug reactions in, 1971t
  and glycogen storage diseases, 1133–1134
  and vitamin D metabolism, 1477
  angiosarcoma of, from vinyl chloride, 140
  antibiotics metabolized in, 118
  as endocrine gland, 1253
  bilirubin transport by, 812
  biopsy of, 817
    for acute viral hepatitis, 824
    for chronic active hepatitis, 832
    for hemochromatosis, 1191
    for persistent hepatitis, 831
    jaundice and, 818
  biotransformation in, 811
  blood supply to, 760
    aging and, 98
  bridging necrosis of, 819
  cancer of, from aflatoxin, 1095
    in hemochromatosis, 1191
  candidiasis in, 1848
  cellular injury to, hyperbilirubinemia
      from, 814
  change in protein synthesis by, and acute
      phase response, 1527
  chronic disease in
    and porphyria cutanea tarda, 1186
    as contraindication for gallstone disso-
        lution therapy, 862
    hypertrophic osteoarthropathy in, 1519
    megaloblastic anemia in, 906
    with encephalopathy, 855
  cirrhosis of, 842–847. See also Cirrhosis
  congenital fibrosis of, portal hypertension
      from, 848
  congestion of, from dilated cardiomyopa-
      thy, 352
    from tricuspid regurgitation, 351
  copper in, 1188
  Crohn's disease and, 749
  damage to, from acetaminophen poison-
      ings, 143
  detoxification in, 811
  disorders of. See also Hepatitis; Viral hepa-
      titis
    and abnormal vitamin D metabolism,
        1480
    and anti-inflammatory drug effect on
        glomerular filtration rate, 102

Liver (Continued)
  disorders of, and blood coagulation disor-
      ders, 1077–1078
  and corticosteroid-binding globulin, 1342
  and drug protein binding, 94
  and metabolism, 809–811
  and testicular function, 1415
  and tuberculosis treatment, 1688
  and vitamin D–binding protein, 1477
  anemia in, 892
  as contraindication for oral contracep-
      tives, 1444
  clinical approach to, 808–809
  drug metabolism and, 96–97
  drug-induced, classification of, 827t,
      827–828
  from cystic fibrosis, 840
  from inflammatory bowel disease, 758
  from parenteral nutrition, 1250
  from renal cell carcinoma, 652
  from Reye syndrome, 2209
  from thalassemia, 931
  glucocorticoid therapy for, 1344
  granulomatous, 837t, 837–838
  gynecomastia in, 1451
  hematologic tests for, 817
  hypoglycemia in, 1387
  immunization for patients with, 63
  laboratory tests for, 814–817
  laparoscopy for, 673
  malabsorption from, 741
  mycotic, 834
  porphyruria in, vs. porphyrias, 1183
  pregnancy and, 841
  rheumatoid factor in, 1996
  symptoms of, 657
  toxic and drug-induced, 826–830
  vitamin D therapy for, 1485
  vs. galactosemia, 1133
  vs. hypopituitarism, 1296
  drug clearance by, 90
    in elderly, 98
  echinococcosis in, 1893
  enlargement of
    from alcoholic hepatitis, 843
    from amyloidosis, 360, 840
    from bile duct tumor, 871
    from congenital rubella, 1777
    from constrictive pericarditis, 367
    from dengue hemorrhagic fever, 1833
    from fascioliasis, 1903
    from glycogen storage disease, 839–840
    from glycosaminoglycans, 1175
    from heart failure, in chronic respira-
        tory failure, 481
    from hemochromatosis, 361, 839, 1191
    from immunocytic amyloid, 1035
    from leptospirosis, 1730
    from liver granulomas, 837
    from myelofibrosis, with myeloid meta-
        plasia, 985
    from neoplasms, 858
    from Niemann-Pick disease, 1148
    from paracoccidioidomycosis, 1843
    from parasitic disease, 834
  enzymes of, increase in, from abdominal
      abscess, 793
  examination of, 809
    magnetic resonance imaging for, 85
  failure of
    acute kidney failure from, 558
    antimicrobial therapy in, 117t
    from primary biliary cirrhosis, 845
    from protoporphyria, 840
    from Senecio longilobus, 787
    from uridyltransferase deficiency, 1132
  fulminant, 819, 854
    from viral hepatitis, 820

Liver (Continued)
  failure of, parenteral nutrition for, 1247
    sulfonamides and tetracyclines con-
        traindicated in, 118
  fatty, 810. See also Fatty liver
  fibrosis of, Caroli's disease with, 870
  focal nodular hyperplasia of, 857
  friction rub of, from hepatocellular carci-
      noma, 859
  functioning of, 808
    in glucocorticosteroid therapy, 129
    tests for, in leptospirosis, 1731
  Gaucher's disease and, 1146
  glucose from, 1374
  glycogen stores in, 1382
  granulomas of, sarcoidosis and, 840
  heme deficiency in, 1184
  heme synthesis in, 1182
  hermaphroditic flukes in, 1901–1903
  Hodgkin's disease and, 1016–1017, 1019
  in heart failure, 223
  in heroin users, 57
  in hypereosinophilic syndrome, 1024
  in mastocytosis, 1973
  in protoporphyria, 1184
  in Q fever, 1749
  in relapsing fever, 1725
  in vaso-occlusive crisis, in sickle cell ane-
      mia, 939
  in visceral leishmaniasis, 1871
  in yellow fever, 1831
  inhalant abuse and, 59
  lymph formation in, and ascites, 850–851
  malnutrition and, 1213
  necrosis of, delirium from, 2064
    hypoglycemia in, 809
  neoplasms of, 856–859
    computed tomography for, 662
    diagnostic approach to, 858–859
    from drugs, 828
    metastatic, 859
      of bronchogenic carcinoma, 459
      of colorectal cancer, 771, 772
      of gastric cancer, 713
  of alcoholics, 48
  parasitic disease of, 834, 835t
  position of, in bilateral right-sidedness,
      315
  radiation injury to, 2377, 2379t
  radionuclide imaging of, 667
  size of, 809
  steroids in, 1346
  systemic lupus erythematosus in, 2015
  testosterone toxicity and, 1419
  transplants of, 855t, 855, 855–856
    contraindications to, 856
    for glycogen storage diseases, 1134
    for inborn metabolic errors, 157
    for sclerosing cholangitis, 870
  triglyceride synthesis in, 1138
  tuberculosis of, 1691
  veins of, thrombosis of, portal hyperten-
      sion from, 848–849
Living will, 2071
Loa loa, 1918
Lobar arteries, 508
Local anesthetics, allergy to, 1971
  topical, cocaine as, 55
Locked-in state, 2061t
  eye movement in, 2116
Locomotor ataxia, from syphilis, 2189. See
    also Tabes dorsalis
Locus ceruleus, pigmented neuron loss in,
    in parkinsonism, 2143
Loeffgren's syndrome, 451, 2045
  arthritis from, indomethacin for, 457
  fever in, 454
  remission of, 456

Lofenalac, for phenylketonuria, 1156
Löffler's endomyocardial disease, 1025
  and hypereosinophilic syndrome, 1024
Löffler's syndrome, 1909
  after nickel exposure, 2391
  vs. tropical eosinophilia, 1916
Loiasis, 1918
Loin pain–hematuria syndrome, 585
Long QT syndrome, surgery for, 274
Loop diuretics, 232, 234
  adverse effects of, 289t
  and metabolic alkalosis, 555
  characteristics of, 536t
  for fluid volume excess, 535
  for hypertension, 286t
  properties of, 231t
Loop of Henle, 509–511, 512, 513
  ascending limb of, dysfunction of, 622
  calcium reabsorption in, 519
  defects of, 505, 532, 622, 622. See also
    Bartter's syndrome
  function of, 617
  in urine formation, 502
  potassium reabsorption by, 517
Looser's zones, 1483, 1483
Loperamide
  and intestinal motility, 724
  for diarrhea, 732
    from ulcerative colitis, 758
    in Crohn's disease, 752
Lorazepam, abuse of, 53
  for agitation in psychiatric disorders,
    2094t
  reference intervals for, 2403t
Lordosis, and torsion dystonia, 2150
Lotions, 2314
Lowe's oculocerebrorenal syndrome, 1154t
LP. See Lumbar puncture
LPS (lipopolysaccharide), and macro-
    phages, 954
  of bacteroids, 1637
LPX, in liver disease, 816
LSD (lysergic acid diethylamide), abuse of, 58
  by adolescents, 21
LTB₄ (leukotriene B₄), 952, 1986
Lucio's phenomenon, in leukemia, 1698
Luder-Sheldon syndrome, 1154t
Ludwig's angina, 1639
  from dental abscess, 675
LUF (luteinized unruptured follicle syn-
    drome), 1440
Luft syndrome, 2279
Lumbar disc, disorders of, vs. arteriosclero-
    sis obliterans, 381
  pain of, vs. deep-vein thrombosis, 386
Lumbar puncture, 2056
  and intracranial hypotension, 2238
  contraindications for, 2056t, 2234
  danger from, for subdural empyema,
    2184
  for back pain, 2252
  for epilepsy, 2224
  for headache, 2136
  for meningioma, 2256
  for pseudotumor cerebri, 2237
  for spinal epidural abscess, 2186
  for subarachnoid hemorrhage, 2176
  headache from, 2134
  indications for, 2056t, 2067
  traumatic, vs. subarachnoid hemorrhage,
    2176t
Lumbosacral plexus, pain in, epidural infu-
    sions for, 110
Lumbosacral strain, 2044
Lumen, arteriosclerotic narrowing of, 380
  secretions from, airway narrowing from,
    397
    and airway obstruction, 475

Lung(s). See also Alveolus(i); Pulmonary; Res-
    piratory
  abscess of, 435–438
    amebic, 436
    bronchiectasis vs., 439
    bronchogenic cysts vs., 420
    classification of, 435t
    from anaerobic bacteria, 1638
    nocardiosis and, 1675
  aeration of, abnormalities of, 419–421
  airflow resistance in, 396–397
  allergic drug reactions in, 1971t
  and acid-base balance, 549
  ankylosing spondylitis and, 2006
  aspergillosis in, 1851
  biopsy of, contraindications for, 460
    for sarcoidosis, 455
    for Wegener's granulomatosis, 2031
  blastomas of, 464
  blastomycosis and, 1842
  blood volume of, increase in, 294
  cancer of
    and venous thromboembolism, 443
    annual death rate from, and smoking,
      38
    asbestos and, 2363
      diagnosis of, 2364
    from smoking, 37–38, 1093–1094
      involuntary, 39
      occupational, 2364
  candidiasis in, 1848
  carcinoma of, idiopathic pulmonary fibro-
    sis with, 428
  Chlamydia psittaci infection in, 1736
  chronic disease of, and pulmonic regurgi-
    tation, 351
    as contraindication for kidney trans-
      plant, 578
    from cystic fibrosis, 440
  chronic histoplasmosis of, 1839
  circulation in, resistance vessels of, 294,
    299
  coccidioidomycosis and, 1840–1841
  collagen diseases of, diffusing capacity
    in, 400
  collapse of, from pneumothorax, 469
  compliance of, 395
  cryptococcosis in, 1844, 1845
  defense against bacteria in, 1552
  diffusing capacity of, 399–400
  dirofilariasis of, 1919
  disease of
    and amylase level, 776
    and digitalis intoxication, 229
    and spinal epidural abscess, 2186
    atrial pressure in, 244
    from mycobacteria, 1694–1695
    interstitial, 421–435. See also Interstitial
      lung disease
    myocardial function in, 209
    tropical eosinophilia as, 1916
  echinococcosis in, 1893
  elastic properties of, 395, 395
  fluke parasites in, 1901
  function of, in elderly, 25
    testing for, 2357–2358
    in severely ill, 483
  gangrene of, 1568
  hemorrhage of, in Goodpasture's syn-
    drome, 590
  hereditary hemorrhagic telangiectasia
    and, 1060
  hermaphroditic flukes in, 1903–1904
  Hodgkin's disease and, 1016
  hyperinflation of, and right ventricular
    function, 475
  hyperlucent, unilateral, 420
  in Langerhans cell granulomatosis, 1023

Lung(s) (Continued)
  in Rocky Mountain spotted fever, 1743–
    1744
  in systemic sclerosis, 2022
  in Wegener's granulomatosis, 2030
  infarction of. See Pulmonary infarction
  infection of
    and alveolar proteinosis, 432
    and bloodstream infection, 1544
    and metastatic brain abscess, 2181
    from artificial airways, 496
    in amyotrophic lateral sclerosis, 2156
    in coma, prevention of, 2071
    kyphoscoliosis with, 473
    neutropenia and, 963
  inflammatory cells in, 424
  influenza in, 1766
  injury to, 2365–2373
    chemical, 2367–2369
    from adult respiratory distress syn-
      drome, 491
    from barometric pressure, 2366–2367
    radiation, 2365–2366
    thermal, 2365
  malnutrition and, 1213
  mechanics of, calculations for, 485–486
  mucormycosis in, 1852
  mycoses of, vs. tuberculosis, 1686
  necrosis of, from gram-negative bacilli
    pneumonia, 1568
  neoplasms of, 457t, 457–466
    benign, 464
    bronchogenic carcinoma as, 457–463.
      See also Bronchogenic carcinoma
    carcinoid tumors as, 463
    carcinosarcoma as, 464
    cylindromas as, 463
    metastatic, 464
      of colonic cancer, 771
      of renal pelvis transitional cell can-
        cers, 654
      to kidneys, 655
    mucoepidermoid tumors as, 463–464
    primary lymphoma as, 463
    primary sarcomas as, 464
    pulmonary blastomas as, 464
    small-cell carcinoma as, 1301
    solitary pulmonary nodule as, 464–466
  nodules of, from coccidioidomycosis,
    1840–1841
  occupational disorders of, 2356–2364
    approach to, 2357–2358
  of smokers, 38
  paracoccidioidomycosis in, 1843
  parenchyma of, brochogenic cysts in, 420
    disorders of, and respiratory failure,
      491–492
  pneumocystosis in, 1879
  polyarteritis nodosa in, 2029
  pyogenic abscess of, vs. tuberculosis,
    1686
  radiation injury to, 2377, 2379t
  residual volume in, 395–396, 408
  rheumatoid arthritis and, 2002
  rupture of, from mechanical ventilation,
    496
  sarcoidosis in, 451
  scans of, for pulmonary hypertension, 299
  stiffness of, 485
  systemic lupus erythematosus in, 2015
    lab tests for, 2017
  total capacity of, 395, 395
    in chronic obstructive pulmonary dis-
      ease, 415
  vasoconstriction in, hypoxia and, 294
  vital capacity of, 395–396, 408, 455, 483
  volume of, reduction in, 398, 399t
    variation in, 396

Lung(s) (Continued)
  weight of, and ventilation distribution, 398
Lupus band test, 2016
Lupus erythematosus
  discoid, 2340. See also Discoid lupus erythematosus
  pericarditis in, 363
  pulmonary hypertension from, 298
  systemic, 2011–2018. See also Systemic lupus erythematosus
Lupus pernio, 453
Lupus profundus, definition of, 2050
  in systemic lupus erythematosus, 2015
Lupus syndrome, drug-induced, 103
Luteal phase, dysfunction in, 1440
  of menstrual cycle, 1430
Luteinizing hormone, 1254
  and ovarian steroid production, 1431
  and spermatogenesis, 1407
  and testicular function, 1405
  and testosterone production, 1406
  assessing function of, 1294
  deficiency of, 1295, 1417
    treatment of, 1297
  from gonadotrophs, 1290
  function of, 1292
  in females, 1426, 1427t
  in puberty, 17
  methadone and, 56
  normal ranges for, in male, 1405
  reference intervals for, 2398t
  release of, 1283–1284
    in male, 1405, 1406
    in menstrual cycle, 1430
Luteinizing hormone releasing hormone, 1405
  analogues of, for prostate cancer, 1424
  defect of, and hypogonadotropic eunuchoidism, 1416
  for Kallmann's syndrome, 1420
Lutembacher's syndrome, 305
Lye, ingestion of, and esophageal injury, 688
Lyme disease, 1726–1729, 1727t
  arthritis in, 1726, 1727, 1729, 1999
  vs. viral encephalitis, 2194
Lymph formation, splanchnic, and ascites, 850
Lymph nodes
  enlarged, in bartonellosis, 1681
  peripheral, in agammaglobulinemia, 1943
  sarcoidosis in, 453
  toxoplasmosis and, 1876
  tumors of, computed tomography for, 662
Lymphadenitis
  from mycobacteria, 1695
  in erythema nodosum leprosum, 1699
  regional, acute, 1661
    from bejel, 1723
    from pinta, 1723
  staphylococcal, vs. bubonic plague, 1663
  streptococcal, vs. bubonic plague, 1663
  tuberculous, 1689–1690
Lymphadenopathy, 1799
  angioblastic, and skin, 1110
  from cat scratch disease, 1679
  from lymphogranuloma venereum, 1711
  from Waldenström's macroglobulinemia, 1033
  immune system neoplasms and, 1008
  immunoblastic, 431
    eosinophilia from, 1025
  in acquired immunodeficiency syndrome, 1803
  in filariasis, 1915
  in paracoccidioidomycosis, 1843

Lymphadenopathy (Continued)
  in scrub typhus, 1747
  in systemic lupus erythematosus, 2015
  in toxoplasmosis, 1877
Lymphangiectasia, 744, 744
Lymphangiography, for Hodgkin's disease, 1018, 1018
Lymphangioleiomyomatosis, as interstitial lung disease, 432
Lymphangitis, 388
Lymphatic system
  breast cancer metastases to, 1454
  congenital malformations of, and chylous ascites, 792
  diseases of, 388–389
  filariasis of, 1914–1915
  obstruction of, malabsorption from, 744
  sporotrichosis in, 1846
Lymphedema, 388–389
  from lymphangitis, 388
  vs. angioedema, 1951
Lymphoadenopathy-associated virus, and cancer, 1095
Lymphoblastic leukemia, acute
  marrow transplants for, 1041
  Philadelphia chromosome in, 991
  prognosis for, 1005
  treatment of, 1004–1005
Lymphocyte(s)
  and inflammatory reaction, 2306
  cytotoxic, and tumor cells, 1127
  disorders of, 1941–1948
  functioning of, in chronic kidney failure, 566
  increased destruction of, 967
  life span of, 877
  migration of, 1988
  mononuclear phagocytes and, 956, 956–957
  precursors of, 874
  vs. amebae, 1888
Lymphocyte predominance Hodgkin's disease, 1015
Lymphocyte-function–associated antigen type 1 deficiency, 1948
Lymphocytic leukemia
  acute, 975
  chronic, 974, 994–998
    autoimmune hemolytic anemia with, 881
    clinical manifestations of, 995
    clinical staging system for, 995, 995t
    deoxycoformycin for, 1123
    diagnosis of, 996–997
    etiology of, 994
    histoplasmosis with, 1838
    incidence of, 994
    laboratory abnormalities in, 995–996
    pathogenesis and mechanisms of, 994–995
    prognosis for, 998
    thrombocytopenia in, 1052
    treatment of, 997–998
    vs. hairy cell leukemia, 1000
  hemolysis from, 908
  with autoimmune hemolytic anemia, 918
Lymphocytopenia, 966–967
  causes of, 966t
  steroid-induced, 129
Lymphocytosis, 971–973, 972, 972t
  from adrenocortical insufficiency, 1352
  from chronic lymphocytic leukemia, 996
  from idiopathic thrombocytopenic purpura, 1050
  from infectious mononucleosis, 1787
  infectious, eosinophilia in, 1025
Lymphoepithelioma, 1975

Lymphogranuloma venereum, 1710–1711
  anorectal fistulas from, 789
  vs. bubonic plague, 1663
  vs. cat scratch disease, 1679, 1681
  vs. granuloma inguinale, 1712
  vs. rectal ulcers, 788
  vs. syphilis, 1715
  vs. ulcerative colitis, 757
  vs. ulcerative proctitis, 788
Lymphoid cells, 874
Lymphoid hyperplasia, and immunodeficiency, 1944
  from drug allergy, 1971t
  of Peyer's patches, benign, vs. Crohn's disease, 750
Lymphokines, 956, 1532, 1684, 1990
Lymphoma(s)
  and Epstein-Barr virus, 1787
  and human T lymphotropic retrovirus, 1797
  and Salmonella infection, 1644
  and skin, 1108–1109
  as contraindication for smallpox vaccination, 1793
  Burkitt's, 1013–1014. See also Burkitt's lymphoma
  from lymphocytic infiltrative disorders, 431
  gastric, primary, 669
  giant hypertropic gastritis vs., 692
  histiocytic, hemolytic anemia from, 920
  immunosuppressive therapy for, and neurologic infection, 2210
  in Sjögren's syndrome, 2024
  intestinal, malabsorption from, 744
  lymphoblastic, 1012
  lymphocytic, diffuse well-differentiated, vs. chronic lymphocytic leukemia, 996
  non-Hodgkins', 975, 1009–1013. See also Non-Hodgkin's lymphoma(s)
  of central nervous system, vs. AIDS dementia complex, 2205
  of small intestine, 773
    and nontropical sprue, 743
    vs. Crohn's disease, 750
  of stomach, 712–713
  of thymus, 1976
  of thyroid, 1336
    vs. Hashimoto's thyroiditis, 1334
  pleural disease from, 467
  primary, of lung, 463
  small intestinal ulceration from, 807
  spread of, to kidneys, 655
  T cell, adult, 1009, 1109
  thrombocytopenia in, 1052
  varicella vaccine for patients with, 65
  vs. chronic myelogenous leukemia, 991
  vs. hairy cell leukemia, 1000
  vs. infectious mononucleosis, 1788
  vs. mycobacterial lymphadenitis, 1695
  vs. sarcoidosis, 454, 456
  vs. toxoplasmosis, 1878
Lymphopenia, in AIDS, 1802
  in Nezelof's syndrome, 1945
Lymphoproliferative disorders, 974–975
  and hepatitis B susceptibility, 822
  and platelet function defects, 1057
  thrombocytopenia in, 1052
  X-linked, 1944–1945
    and neoplasms, 1096t
    Epstein-Barr virus in, 1787
Lymphosarcoma, of small intestines, vs. Crohn's disease, 750
Lymphotoxin, and bone resorption, 1102
Lyon hypothesis, 149, 916
Lysergic acid diethylamide (LSD), abuse of, by adolescents, 21, 58

Lysine hydrochloride, for metabolic alkalosis, 556
Lysolecithin, and gastric ulcers, 695
  in refluxed duodenal juice, 690
Lysosomal acid maltase, deficiency of, 2277
Lysosomal enzymes, and joint destruction, 1993
  in inflammation, 1987
Lysosomal theory, of shock, 242
Lysozyme(s), 1100
  definition of, 242
  in Chédiak-Higashi disease, 958
  in host defense mechanisms, 1529
  reference intervals for, 2398t
Lyssaviruses, 2200

M-component(s), from monoclonal gammopathy of unknown significance, 1035
  in myeloma, 1028
  in Waldenström's macroglobulinemia, 1033
M protein, in group A streptococcal infections, 1574
MacCallum's patch, 1582
Machado-Joseph disease, 2153
Machupo virus, 1835
Macleod's syndrome, 420
Macroadenomas, prolactin-secreting, treatment of, 1303
Macroamylasemia, 776
Macrocytosis, in liver disease, 817
Macroemboli, and renal artery occlusion, 632
Macroglobulinemia, 1059
  Waldenström's, 1033–1034. See also Waldenström's macroglobulinemia
Macromolecules, in lower respiratory tract, 424
Macrophage(s), 954, 954
  accumulation of, 1987
  and tissue damage, 1990
  and tuberculosis, 1684
  and viruses, 1751
  asbestos and, 2363
  B lymphocytes and, 957
  in immune response, 1937
  in inflammatory response, 1530–1531, 1985
  in sarcoidosis, 451
  iron in, 895
  substances secreted by, 955, 955t
  types of, 955t
Macrophage-activating factor, 954
Macrophage colony–stimulating factor, 876, 968
Macropsia, in partial seizures, 2220
Macule, 2121
  coal, 2361
Maculopapular skin disease, 2322–2326, 2323t
Madarosis, from leprosy, treatment of, 1701
Maduromycosis, 1853
Magnesium, 1242. See also Hypermagnesemia; Hypomagnesemia
  absorption of, parathyroid hormone and, 502, 1487
  and myocardial contractility, 354
  and toxic concentrations of digoxin, 94
  average levels of, 1195
  distribution of, in healthy population, 80
  excess, 1195
    in renal osteodystrophy, 1509
    vs. botulism, 1633
  excretion of, 1195

Magnesium (Continued)
  for treating malabsorption, 741t
  homeostasis of, 1473
  in body, 519
  in kidney stones, 638
  levels of, in chronic kidney failure, 565
  loss of, in Crohn's disease, 751
  metabolism of, disorders of, 1195–1196
    kidneys and, 519
  recommended dietary allowance for, 1205t
  reference intervals for, 2398t
  wasting of, aminoglycosides and, 609
    from cisplatin, 610
Magnesium citrate, in hepatic encephalopathy, 853
Magnesium salts, as laxatives, 722
Magnesium sulfate, for toxemia of pregnancy, 635–636
Magnetic fields, and pacemakers, 272
Magnetic resonance imaging, 84–86, 85, 666, 667, 667–668
  for back pain, 2251
  for bronchiectasis, 439
  for localization of tumors in Cushing's disease, 1356
  for renal cell carcinoma, 653, 653
  of brain, 2058–2059
  of kidneys, 527, 527
MAI. See Mycobacterium avium-intracellulare
Malabsorption, 732–745
  after mesenteric artery embolism, 763
  and osteomalacia, 1481
  breath tests for, 737–740
  causes of, 735, 736t
  diagnosis of, 735–740
  evaluation of, algorithm for, 740, 740
  forms of, differentiation and treatment of, 740–745
  from Crohn's disease, 749
  from giardiasis, 1884
  in acquired immunodeficiency syndrome, 745
  in elderly, 744–745
  major histocompatibility complex defects and, 1946
  of vitamin D, and osteomalacia and rickets, 1480
  radiation enteritis and, 729
  symptoms and signs of, 737t
  syndrome of. See Malabsorption syndrome
  treatment of, agents for, 741t
  zinc deficiency in, 1241
Malabsorption syndrome, 660
  and vitamin K deficiency, 816, 1076
  mastocytosis and, 1973
  stool examination for, 730
Malaise
  from cavernous sinus thrombosis, 2185
  from chronic lymphocytic leukemia, 995
  from legionnaires' disease, 1571
  from liver disease, 808
  from lung abscess, 436
  from neurosyphilis, 2188
  from viral hepatitis, 819
Malakoplakia, vs. ulcerative colitis, 757
Malaria, 835t, 1857–1861
  and false-positive syphilis tests, 1719
  and liver enlargement, 834
  and polyclonal cold agglutinin synthesis, 920
  and Salmonella infection, 1644
  and sickle cell trait, 937
  chemoprophylaxis for, international travelers and, 1550–1551
  clinical manifestations of, 1859
  complications of, 1859

Malaria (Continued)
  definition of, 1857
  diagnosis of, 1859–1860
  epidemiology of, 1858
  etiology of, 1857–1858
  falciparum, death from, sickle cell trait carriers and, 151
  hemolysis from, 924
  hyperkalemia in, and periodic paralysis, 2281
  immunity to, 1858
  innate resistance to, 1858
  pathogenesis and pathology of, 1858–1859
  prevention of, 1861
  protection from, thalassemia trait and, 933
  transmission of, by blood transfusions, 950
  treatment of, 1860–1861
  vs. typhoid fever, 1642
  vs. viral hepatitis, 824
  vs. visceral leishmaniasis, 1873
  vs. yellow fever, 1832
Male(s)
  and atherosclerosis, 320
  baldness in, 2349
  genitalia of, development of, 18, 19t
  gonorrhea in, 1707
  hypogonadism in, causes of, 1411, 1413t
  phenotypic differentiation of, 1392–1393, 1393
  sexual function of, neural control of, 2108–2109
  urologic evaluation in, 630
  with osteoporosis, treatment of, 1514
  X-linked inheritance in, 149
  XX, 1401–1402
Maleate, chronic hepatitis from, 828
Malformations, congenital, 169–171
Malignancy. See also Cancer; Carcinoma(s); Tumor(s)
  chromosome breakage syndromes and, 168
  hematologic, and alveolar proteinosis, 432
  in ulcers, 698, 702, 707
  polycythemia vera as, 980, 981
  pseudohyperparathyroidism of, and hypercalciuria from net bone resorption, 640
Malignant melanoma, 2338–2339, 2339
  as contraindication for levodopa, 2146
Malingering, 2076, 2101, 2103
Mallory body, 843
Mallory-Weiss lesion, hemorrhage from, 799
  in esophagus, 688
  vs. bleeding from peptic ulcers, 706
Malnutrition
  and ascariasis, 1909
  and bone disease, 1481
  and mortality from measles, 1772
  clinical signs of, 1210t
  diagnosis of, 1208
  evidence of, 657
  from malabsorption, 735
  hypogonadism from, 1418
  in alcoholics, 51, 843
  laboratory assessment of, 1211
  neurologic effects of, 2137–2141, 2138t
  physiologic consequences of, 1212–1213
  protein-calorie, 1212–1215. See also Protein-calorie malnutrition
  thymic hypoplasia from, 1974
  vs. hypopituitarism, 1296
Malpighian corpuscle, in nephron, 509

Malt soup extract, for pruritis ani, 789
Malum coxae senilis, 2040
Mammary artery, for coronary artery by-pass grafts, 339
Mammary gland. See *Breast(s)*
Mammography, and cancer detection, 1087
Mandelamine, 122
L-Mandelonitrile-b-glucuronic acid, and cyanide poisonings, 144
Manganese, 1242
  estimated safe and adequate daily dietary intake of, 1206t
  toxicity of, 2392
  and secondary parkinsonism, 2144
Mania, 2098t, 2099
  from L-Dopa, 2096
  symptoms of, 2093t
Manic-depressive disorders, 2092, 2095, 2098–2099
Mannitol, and danger of radiocontrast agents, 610
  properties of, 231t
Mannosidosis, 1177
Manometry, 281
  for esophageal motor function, 685, 685
Mansonella, 1919
Mantoux test, 1684
MAO. See *Monoamine oxidase*
MAOI. See *Monoamine oxidase inhibitors*
Maple bark stripper's disease, 1851
Maple syrup urine disease, 1150t, 1159
  thiamin for, 1230
Marasmus, 1214
  definition of, 1212
Marble bone disease (osteopetrosis), 1518–1519
  myelophthisis in, 890
Marboran, 126
Marburg-Ebola disease, 1835–1836
Marche à petits pas, 2126
Marchiafava-Bignami disease, 2140
Marfan's syndrome, 148, 371, 371–372, 1177–1178
  aneurysms from, 370
  aortic regurgitation from, 343
  heart problems in, 176
  mitral valve prolapse from, 350
  vs. Ehlers-Danlos syndrome, 1179
  vs. mucosal neuroma syndrome, 1460
Marijuana
  abuse of, 57–58
  gynecomastia from, 1411
  urine tests for, 58
  use of, with cocaine, 54
Marine animals, venomous vs. poisonous, 1929–1931, 1930t
Maroteaux-Lamy syndrome, 1176t, 1176–1177
Marrara's syndrome, 1927
Marrow. See *Bone marrow*
Masculinization, of brain, 1401
  of female patients, on androgens, 987
Mass lesions, in brain, pathophysiology of, 2062–2063
  in kidneys, ultrasonography for, 526–527
Mast cells, 1972, 1972
  and urticaria-angioedema, 1950
  degranulation of, drugs causing, 1974
  in asthma, 404
  in hypersensitivity reactions, 2306
  in nasal secretions, allergic rhinitis and, 1951
  in skin, 1948–1949
  products of, 1973t
  proliferation of, 1972–1974, 2335
    nasal, 1954
  prostaglandin D$_2$ from, 1271
  secretion by, regulation of, 405, 405–406

Mastectomy, and alternatives to, 1455
  prophylactic chemotherapy after, 1457
Mastocytosis, 1972–1974, 2335
  nasal, 1954
Mastoid bone, osteomyelitis of, pain from, 2134
Mastoiditis, cerebral epidural abscess with, 2184
  from scarlet fever, 1576
  lateral sinus thrombosis from, 2185
Material Safety Data Sheets, 2374
Matthews-Rumack nomogram, 142
Maupertuis, 146
May-Hegglin anomaly, 1048
Mayaro virus, 1819
Mazindol, for weight control, 1226–1227
McArdle's syndrome, 1135
  vs. arteriosclerosis obliterans, 381
  vs. polymyositis, 2036
McCune-Albright syndrome, 1428, 1460
  definition of, 1519
MCF (mononuclear cell factor), 1987
MCH. See *Mean corpuscular hemoglobin*
MCHC. See *Mean corpuscular hemoglobin concentration*
McKees-Rock mutation, 153
M-CSF (macrophage colony–stimulating factor), 876, 968
MCTD. See *Mixed connective tissue disease*
MCV. See *Mean corpuscular volume*
MDMA (5-methoxy-3,4-methylene dioxyamphetamine), abuse of, 58
2-ME (2-mercaptoethanol), in test for barcellosis, 1678
Mean corpuscular hemoglobin, 882
  reference intervals for, 2401t
Mean corpuscular hemoglobin concentration, 882
  in hereditary spherocytosis, 912
  increased, and polymerization in sickle cell anemia, 938
  reference intervals for, 2401t
Mean corpuscular volume, 881–882
  reference intervals for, 2401t
Measles, 1772–1775, 1773
  and subacute sclerosing panencephalitis, 2206
  communicability of, 1772
  differential diagnosis of, 1775t
  encephalitis after, 2208
  immunization against, 61, 63t, 64
    agents for, 62t
    before travel, 1550
  laryngitis and bronchitis from, 1757
  lymphocytopenia from, 966
  rash in, 2322
  remission of minimal change nephrotic syndrome after, 593
  vs. meningococcal disease, 1615
  vs. Rocky Mountain spotted fever, 1744
Meat, consumption of, and pancreatic cancer, 781
  contaminated, and toxoplasmosis, 1876
  preservatives in, and food poisoning, 786
Mebendazole
  for ascariasis, 1909
  for enterobiasis, 1910
  for hookworm, 1907
  for tapeworms, 1895
  for trichinellosis, 1912
  for trichuriasis, 1909
Mecamylamine, for hypertension, 287t
Mechanical ventilation, 487–489, 488t. See also *Ventilation*
  and mortality rate, 498
  complications from, 496
    as emergencies, 488–489
  decisions in, 488, 488t

Mechanical ventilation (Continued)
  endotracheal tube for, 486
  for chronic respiratory failure, 480
  for oxygen therapy, 478
  indications for, 478–479
  leaks in tubing of, treatment for, 489
  pneumothorax from, 470
  types of, 479
  weaning from, 489, 489t
    airway obstruction and, 491
    vital capacity and, 483
Mechlorethamine, 1123. See also *Nitrogen mustard*
Meckel's diverticula
  bleeding from, 800
  radionuclide imaging for, 665
  vs. appendicitis, 803
  vs. small intestine neoplasms, 774
Meclofenamate, asthma from, 104
Meconium, granulomatous peritonitis from, 795
Meconium ileus equivalent, treatment of, 441
MEDAC (multiple endocrine deficiency–autoimmune–candidiasis) syndrome, 1496
Mediastinitis, after coronary artery bypass graft surgery, 338
  fibrosing, 1838
Mediastinum, 470–471
  bronchogenic cysts in, 420
  disease of, non-Hodgkin's lymphoma and, 1012
  fibrosis of, 2052
  infections of, 471
  tumors of, 471, 471
Mediators, from mast cells, in extrinsic asthma, 404, 404t
Medicaid, 7
Medical ethics, 9, 12–15
Medical history, of patient, 71. See also *Patient history*
Medical records, 73–74
Medicare, 7, 573
Mediterranean fever, familial, 147, 795, 1196–1199, 1525, 2045
Mediterranean lymphoma, 773
Mediterranean spotted fever, 1745
Medroxyprogesterone, for osteoporosis, 1514
  for precocious puberty in females, 1428
  for renal cell carcinoma, 653
Medulla, in breathing control, 400
  of kidneys, 508
    cystic disorders of, 645t, 646, 648
    infections of, 628
    salt wasting in, 532, 564
Medullary carcinoma
  and excess calcitonin, 1505–1506
  of thyroid, 1336
    ACTH from, 1354
    diarrhea from, 727
Medullary sponge kidney, 645t, 646, 648
  and kidney stones, 641
  Caroli's disease with, 870
Medulloblastomas, 2230, 2233
Mefenamic acid, autoimmune hemolytic anemia from, 922
  for dysmenorrhea, 1433
Mefloquine, for malaria, 1860
Megacolon, 170, 170t, 660, 723–724
  and pseudomembranous colitis, 1632
  chagasic, 1868
  from lead poisoning, 2386
  myxedema, 1329
  toxic, 755, 755. See also *Toxic megacolon*
Megakaryoblasts, progenitors of, 875

Megakaryocytes, 874
   and thrombocytopenia, 1048
   in marrow, 877
   in polycythemia vera, 982
Megaloblastic anemias, 900–907
   definition of, 900
   etiology of, 900, 901t
   in orotic aciduria, 1173
   ineffective erythropoiesis in, 895
   of cobalamin deficiency, 902–904
   of folate deficiency, 905–907
   pathogenesis and pathology of, 900–902
   thiamin for, 1230
Megaloblastic crisis, from hereditary spher-
      ocytosis, 911
   of sickle cell disease, 939
Megaloblastosis, drugs and, 907
   from folate deficiency, 906
   mechanisms of, 901
Megaloureter, 650
Megalourethra, 650
Megathrombocytes, 1043
Meglumine antimonate, for visceral leish-
      maniasis, 1873
Meibomian glands, carcinomas of, 2295
Meigs's syndrome, 792, 1446, 2150–2151
   pleural effusion from, 469
   vs. tardive dyskinesia, 2149
Meiosis, 162, 162–163
Meissner's corpuscles, 2303
Melancholia, 2095
Melanin, 2300
   production of, 2302
Melanocyte(s)
   and protection against ultraviolet light,
      2303
   dysfunction of, from Chédiak-Higashi
      disease, 958
   in epidermis, 2301–2302
   loss of, aging and, 2306
Melanoma(s), 2336t
   intraocular, 2295–2296
   malignant, 2338–2339, 2339
      as contraindication for levodopa,
         2146
      in heart, 367
   of nails, 2347
   solitary pulmonary nodules from, 464
Melanosis coli, diagnosis of, with biopsy,
      731
Melanosomes, 2302
Melarsoprol, for African trypanosomiasis,
      1864
Melasma, of face, 2343, 2343
Melatonin, 1282
   from pineal, 1314
Melena
   and location of gastrointestinal hemor-
      rhage, 797
   definition of, 796
   from adenocarcinoma of duodenum, 713
   from gastritis, 689
   from gastrointestinal hemorrhage, 796
   from pancreatic cancer, 781
Melioidosis, 1669–1670
Melkersson-Rosenthal syndrome, vs. angio-
      edema, 1951
Melorheostosis, 1519
Melphalan
   for cancer, 1123
   for essential thrombocythemia, 987
   for multiple myeloma, 1031
   infertility from, 1119–1120
   sideroblastic anemia from, 900
Membrane protein, functional impairment
      of, 1131
Membrane receptors, genetic disorders of,
      148

Memory, 2083–2085
   disorders of, 2084–2085
      after mild brain injury, 2240
      and temporal lobe damage, 2081
      from hypothalamic destruction, 2103
      in AIDS dementia complex, 2204
      in delirium, 2064
      recent, from chylomicronemia syn-
         drome, 1143
         in progressive dementias, 2088
   mechanisms of, 2084
MEN syndrome. See Multiple endocrine neo-
      plasia
Menadione, 1076, 1240. See also Vitamin K
Menaquinone, 1076, 1240. See also Vitamin
      K
Menarche, 18–19
   age of, 1429
Mendel, Gregor, 146
Mendelian Inheritance in Man (McKusick),
      146
Ménétrier's disease, 691
Ménière syndrome
   deafness in, 2119
   tinnitus with, 2120
   treatment of, 2119
   vertigo in, 2123
   vs. transient ischemic attacks, 2169
Meninges
   carcinomatosis of, 2235
   infection of. See Meningitis
   leukemia of, 993
Meningioma(s), 2230, 2233, 2256
   prognosis for, 2235
   sphenoid wing, 2292
Meningismus, from rabies, 2201
Meningitis
   anthrax, 1668
   aseptic, from human immunodeficiency
      virus, 2204
   bacterial, 1604–1610. See also Bacterial
      meningitis
   chemical, 1608
   chronic, from brain tumors, 2232
      vs. multiple sclerosis, 2212
   coccidioidal, diagnosis of, 1838
   cryptococcal, 1844, 1845
      in acquired immunodeficiency syn-
         drome, 1804t, 1806
      treatment for, 1846
   definition of, 1604
   empiric therapy for, 118t
   enteric bacteria and, 1659
   from agammaglobulinemia, 1943
   from coccidioidomycosis, 1841
   from disseminated gonococcal infection,
      1709
   from genital herpes, 2197
   from herpes simplex virus, 1782
   from leptospirosis, 1731
   from Listeria monocytogenes, 1671
      in neonates, 1672
   from malignant external otitis, 2185
   from midline granuloma, 2032
   from neurosyphilis, 2188
   from sarcoidosis, 453
   from Staphylococcus aureus, 1600–1601
   from streptococci group B, 1579
   gram-negative, cephalosporins for,
      120
   granulomatous, vertigo from, 2124
   headache from, 2133
   hospital-acquired, 1546
   immunization against, 63
   manifestations of, 1613
   meningococcemia with, 1613–1614
   Mollaret's, 1609
   mumps and, 1779

Meningitis (Continued)
   pneumococcal, penicillin dosage for, 113
      predisposing factors for, 1605
   pneumococcal pneumonia with, 1560
   pyogenic, 1604
   rifampin with penicillins for, 121
   serous, 2236. See also Pseudotumor cerebri
   therapy duration for, 122
   tuberculous, 1691
   viral, 2192–2194
      frequency of, 2192t
   vs. Lyme disease, 1728
   vs. spinal epidural abscess, 2187
   vs. tetanus, 1635
   vs. tularemia, 1666
Meningococcal disease, 1611–1617
   and thrombotic thrombocytopenic pur-
      pura, 1052
   clinical manifestations, 1613–1615
   course and complications of, 1615
   diagnosis of, 1615–1616
   epidemiology of, 1611–1613
   immunity to, 65, 1612–1613
   in hospital employees, 1549
   pathogenesis and pathology of, 1613
   prevention of, 1616–1617
   prognosis for, 1617
   treatment of, 1616
Meningococcemia
   and skin, 2325
   clinical manifestations of, 1613–1614
   fulminant, 1614, 1614
   meningitis with, 1613–1614
   pathologic findings in, 1613
   vs. exanthems, from enteroviruses, 1813
   vs. rat-bite fever, 1730
   vs. Rocky Mountain spotted fever, 1744
Meningoencephalitis
   amebic, 1888
   definition of, 2192
   from Chagas' disease, 1867
   from congenital rubella, 1777
   from infective endocarditis, 1590
   from Rift Valley fever, 1818
Meningomyelitis, syphilitic, vs. vitamin B$_{12}$
      deficiency, 2140
Meningomyelocele, 170t
Menkes' disease, cytochrome C oxidase de-
      ficiency in, 2279
Menkes' kinky hair syndrome, 1241, 1242
Menometrorrhagia, differential diagnosis
      of, 20t
   in adolescents, 19
Menopause, 1444
   age of, 1429, 1444
   bone loss after, 1510, 1511, 1512
   definition of, 1444
Menorrhagia, from factor VII deficiency,
      1072
   life-threatening, factor V deficiency and,
      1073
Menstrual cycle. See also Menstruation
   and common cold susceptibility, 1755
   and estrogen secretion, 1432
   length of, 1429
   luteal phase of, hyperaldosteronism in,
      1360
   normal, 1429–1433
   synchronization of, 1284
Menstruation. See also Menstrual cycle
   and epileptic seizures, 2223
   cessation of, weight loss and, 19
   disorders of, in alcoholic cirrhosis, 844
   during menopause, 1444
   iron loss from, 896
      and anemia, 880
   life-threatening, factor X deficiency and,
      1072

Menstruation (Continued)
migraine headache during, 2131
suppression of, for aplastic anemia treatment, 889
systemic lupus erythematosus and, 2016
von Willebrand disease and, 1071
Mental competence, evaluation of, 2088, 2088t
loss of, in elderly, 28–29
in tuberous sclerosis, 2158
Mental disorders. See Psychiatric disorders
Mental retardation
androgen therapy contraindicated in, 1419
from galactosemia, 1132, 1133
from glycosaminoglycans, 1175
from homocystinuria, 1160
from isovaleric acidemia, 1159
from Laurence-Moon-Bardet-Biedl syndrome, 1203
from Lesch-Nyhan syndrome, 1171
from nephrogenic diabetes insipidus, 1312
from phenylketonuria, 1155
from pseudohypoparathyroidism, 1501
hypoparathyroidism and, 1498
risk of, as congenital malformation, 170
sex chromosome abnormalities and, 167
Mental state
altered. See also Consciousness, altered
assessment of, in elderly, 27–28
from narcotics, 108
from suppurative cholangitis, 869
from syphilis, 1718
from typhus fever, 1739, 1740
cardiorespiratory function and, 483
decline in, in hypothermia, 2384
Meperidine
abuse of, 55
as analgesic, 107t
for acute pancreatitis, 777
for esophageal motor disorders, 686
for hepatic porphyria, 1185
for pain, in dying patients, 32
in shock, 244
metabolites for, kidney excretion of, 95
multifocal myoclonus from, 109
parenteral, for pneumococcal pneumonia, 1559
poisoning with, 2069t
potency of, 56
reference intervals for, 2403t
Mephentermine, 137
Mephenytoin, for epilepsy, 2226t, 2227
genetics in metabolism of, 102
Mephobarbital, for epilepsy, 2226t, 2227
MEPPs (miniature end-plate potentials), 2284–2285
Meprobamate
abuse of, 53
poisoning with, 2069t
and central nervous system, 2069
reference intervals for, 2403t
Meralgia paresthetica, 2268
Mercaptans, and hepatic encephalopathy, 852
Mercaptobenzothiazole, and contact dermatitis, 2319
2-Mercaptoethanol, in test for brucellosis, 1678
6-Mercaptopurine
and niacin deficiency, 1232
for cancer, 1122–1123
for Crohn's disease, 752
metabolism of, 101
Mercury
and kidney damage, 611
poisonings with, 140, 141, 143, 2387–2388

Mercury (Continued)
poisonings with, dialysis after, 143
reference intervals for, 2398t
Merozoites, 1858
Merycism, 680, 1219
vs. vomiting, 658
Mesangiocapillary glomerulonephritis, 597
Mescaline, abuse of, 58
effects of, duration of, 59
Mesenteric adenitis, acute, vs. appendicitis, 803
Mesenteric arteries
embolism of, 763
inferior, 761
occlusion of, 762–763
superior, 760–761, 761
Mesenteric circulation, regulation of, 761
Mesenteric infarction, and amylase level, 776
Mesenteritis, retractile, 795
Mesentery. See also under Mesenteric
disease of, 795–796
ischemia of, appendicitis vs., 802
neoplasms of, 795
thrombosis of, 803
Mesial temporal sclerosis, and seizures, 2219
Mesocardia, 315
Mesonephric ducts, 1391–1392
Mesothelioma(s)
from asbestos poisoning, 140
of liver, 857
of pleura, 469
primary, 794
Metabolic acidosis, 551–555
acidifying salts and, 553
after hypothermia treatment, 2385
aldosterone and, 518
and metabolic encephalopathy, 2067t
and phosphorus excretion, 518
as contraindication for acetazolamide, 232
causes of, 552t
chronic, and osteomalacia, 1481
diagnosis and treatment of, 554–555
from cardiorespiratory arrest, 499
from chronic kidney failure, 564
from diabetes, 26
from fulminant liver failure, 854
from near-drowning, 2371
from nonsteroidal anti-inflammatory agents, 609
from poisoning
with aspirin, 143
with cyanide, 144
with ethylene glycol, 145
with methanol, 145
from potassium-sparing diuretics, 232
from tubulointerstitial disease, 603
hypercalciuria from, 519
in severely ill, 484
respiratory failure from airway obstruction in, mechanical ventilation with, 490–491
sodium bicarbonate loss from pancreas and, 532
with hyperkalemia, 623
Metabolic alkalosis, 551, 555–556
aldosterone and, 518
and bicarbonate synthesis, 518
and metabolic encephalopathy, 2067t
causes of, 555t
hydrochloric acid loss from stomach and, 532
in Bartter's syndrome, 622
potassium depletion in, 546
urine chloride concentrations in, 524
Metabolic data, magnetic resonance imaging for, 84

Metabolic encephalopathy, 2063–2066
acid-base disorders and, 2067t
causes of, 2064t
definition of, 2063
laboratory evaluation of, 2065t, 2066
physical examination for, 2065t
vs. viral encephalitis, 1823
Metabolic inhibitors, 157
Metabolic myopathies, 2277–2283
endocrine myopathies as, 2280
fatty acid metabolism disorders as, 2278
glycogen storage diseases as, 2277–2278
mitochondrial myopathies as, 2279t, 2279–2280
periodic paralyses as, 2281t, 2280–2282
Metabolic rate, during fever, 1527
Metabolism. See also under Metabolic
abnormalities of, and myoglobinuria, 2283
hemolysis from, 923–924
basal, definition of, 1130
carbohydrate, 1131–1137. See also Carbohydrate metabolism
definition of, 1130
disease of, acquired, 1131
and breathing variations, 401
dementia from, 28
dilated cardiomyopathy from, 354
of acid-base balance, 551
feedback regulation of, disorders in, 1131
in chronic kidney failure, management of, 570
inborn errors of, 152–158, 1130
from specific enzymes, 154t–155t
genetic compounds and, 157t
pathogenesis of, 1130–1131
treatment of, 156–158
increase in, from exercise, 45
inhibition of, by potential toxin, 142–143
intermediary, definition of, 1130
hormones and, 1262
lipoprotein, disorders of, 1137–1149. See also Lipoprotein metabolism
liver disease and, 809–811
of trace minerals, 1241–1243
Metabolites, and plasma drug concentration, 94
elimination of, by kidneys, 95
Metacarpals, sarcoidosis in, 453
Metagonimus yokogawai, 1904
Metalloproteinases, 1984
Metals. See also specific terms
allergies to, and eczema, 2318
food poisoning with, 786
heavy, and abnormal bone mineralization, 1479
trace, poisoning from, 2385–2393
Metanephrine, reference intervals for, 2398t
Metaphase, in meiosis, 162
Metaplasia, agnogenic myeloid, 973, 985
neutrophilia from, 969
Metaproterenol, 137
for asthma, 408
Metaraminol, 137
Metastatic neoplasms
in spinal column, 2255
jaundice from, 817
of bone, 1521–1522
of bone marrow, 985
of leptomeninges, 2256
of mesentery, 795
Metatarsals, sarcoidosis in, 453
Methacholine, 139
Methadone
abuse of, 55
as analgesic, 107t, 108
for opioid dependence, 60
for opioid withdrawal, 57

Methadone (Continued)
for pain in dying patients, 32
half-life of, 108
in drug interactions, 124t
poisoning with, 2069t
potency of, 56
reference intervals for, 2403t
Methamphetamine, abuse of, 54
Methane, intestinal, production of, 661
Methanol
metabolic acidosis from, 554
treatment for, 555
poisoning with, 2070t
treatment for, 145
Methaqualone
abuse of, 53
by adolescents, 21
poisoning with, 2069t
and central nervous system, 2069
reference intervals for, 2403t
Methazolamide, side effects of, 2299
Methemalbuminemia, in acute pancreatitis, 777
Methemoglobin, 896
from drugs, 945t
reference intervals for, 2402t
Methemoglobin reductase, deficiency in, 102
Methemoglobin reduction system, in erythrocyte, 926
Methemoglobinemia, 155, 945–946
from drugs, 102
methylene blue for, 143
polycythemia in, 979
recessive, 152
types of, 945t
Methenamine, for recurrent urinary tract infections, 631
Methicillin, 119
acute interstitial nephritis from, 603, 604
elimination rate for, 96t
in kidney and liver failure, 117t
marrow suppression by, 885
staphylococci resistant to, 1603
Methimazole, and kidney damage, 612
contraindicated for nursing mothers, 1327
for hyperthyroidism, from Graves' disease, 1325
Methisazone, for poxviruses, 126
Methotrexate, 906
administration of, 1117
and drug interactions, 1118
and folate utilization, 906
and kidney damage, 610
aplasia from, 885
elimination rate for, 96t
folate leucovorin for reversal of, 1120
for cancer, 1120–1121
breast, 1457
oral, 679
for prophylaxis, of central nervous system leukemia, 1005
for sarcoidosis of skin, 457
interaction of, with other drugs, 101
interstitial lung disease from, 434
sites of action of, 1120
to prevent graft-versus-host disease, 1040
with radiation therapy, 1119
Methotrimeprazine, as analgesic, 109
Methoxyflurane, and kidney damage, 612
and malignant hyperthermia, 2282
anesthesia with, nephrogenic diabetes insipidus from, 1309
5-Methoxy-3,4-methylene dioxyamphetamine (MDMA), abuse of, 58
Methsuximide, for epilepsy, 2226t, 2227
reference intervals for, 2403t
Methyclothiazide, for hypertension, 286t

Methyl isocyanate, interstitial lung disease from, 423
Methylcobalamin, 902
Methyldopa
adverse effects of, 289t
autoimmune hemolytic anemia from, 922
chronic hepatitis from, 828, 831
for hypertension, 287t, 290t
in uremic syndrome, 570
interaction with contraceptives, 1443
liver disease from, 827, 830
reference intervals for, 2403t
Methylene blue, for methemoglobinemia, 143, 946
Methylfolate trap theory, 902
1-Methylisatin-3-thiosemicarbazone, 126
Methylmalonic aciduria, from vitamin B$_{12}$ deficiency, 903, 904
ketoacidosis in, vitamin B$_{12}$ for, 157
Methylphenidate, abuse of, 54
poisoning with, 2069t
Methylprednisolone, 129t, 131
for aplastic anemia, 889
for chronic respiratory failure, 480
for pulmonary fibrosis, 429
for rapidly progressive glomerulonephritis, 591
for sepsis, 1541
sodium-retention properties of, 131
Methyl-tert-butyl, for gallstone dissolution, 862
Methyltestosterone, 1419
Methylxanthine(s)
and cancer, 44
for asthma, 408
for chronic bronchitis, 413
for mast cell regulation, 406
Methyprylon, reference intervals for, 2403t
Methysergide
for carcinoid syndrome, 1468
for cluster headache, 2131
for erythromelalgia, 379
for migraine, 2131
and retroperitoneal fibrosis, 2051
retroperitoneal fibrosis from, 612
toxicity to, vs. arteriosclerosis obliterans, 381
Metoclopramide, 99
and intestinal motility, 724
for delayed stomach emptying, after gastric surgery, 718
for gastroesophageal reflux disease, 683
for gastroparesis diabeticorum, 718
for pseudo-obstruction, 720
for VIPoma, 1389
Metolazone, 535
and metabolic alkalosis, 555
as diuretic, 231, 535
characteristics of, 536t
for hypertension, 286t
properties of, 231t
Metoprolol, 138t
for angina pectoris, 327t
for hypertension, 287t
in uremic syndrome, 570
for recurring myocardial infarction, 335
liver extraction of, 97
Metorchis conjunctus, 1904
Metrifonate, for schistosomiasis, 1901
Metronidazole, 121
action of, 113t
for amebic liver abscess, 837
for anaerobic bacteria infection, 1640
for bacterial overgrowth, with malabsorption, 742
for Crohn's disease, 752
for diverticulitis, 805
for giardiasis, 1884

Metronidazole (Continued)
in drug interactions, 124t
in kidney and liver failure, 117t
penetration into spinal fluid by, 116
penicillin with, for lung abscess, 437
Metropolitan Life Insurance Company Tables of Heights and Weights, 1219
Metyrapone
as inhibitor of adrenal steroid biosynthesis, 1341
for adrenal and pituitary functional reserve, 1349
for Cushing's disease, 1356
testing with, for Addison's disease, 1352
Mexiletine
dosing and adverse effects of, 267t
elimination rate for, 96t
for arrhythmias, 265
metabolism of, induction of, 99
pharmacokinetic properties of, 266t
Meyer's loop, 2081
Mezlocillin, 119, 120
for sepsis, 1540
in kidney and liver failure, 117t
treatment with, 119
MG, 2285–2287. See also Myasthenia gravis
MGUS (monoclonal gammopathies of undetermined significance), 1035–1036
vs. multiple myeloma, 1030
Mica, lung disease from, 2364
Micelles, 859, 860, 861
Miconazole
for Candida infection, of esophagus, 688
for meningitis, from coccidioidomycosis, 1841
for mycoses, 1838
in kidney and liver failure, 117t
Microadenomas, prolactin-secreting, treatment of, 1303
Microaggregates, in blood transfusions, 950
Microalbuminuria, 521, 625
Microaneurysms, in brain, 2178
Microangiopathy, thrombotic, 601
widespread, in diabetic glomerulopathy, 625
Microcephaly, chronic alcoholism in mothers and, 171
Microcirculation, erythrocyte polymerization and flow through, 939
in shock, 240–241
alpha receptor blockers and, 248
Microcystic kidney disease, of renal medulla, 506
Microcytosis, 882
in hemoglobin H disease, 933
Microfilaremia, asymptomatic, 1914
Microgyria, and epilepsy, 2218
Microhemagglutination assay, for T. pallidum, 1719
Microlymphocytotoxicity, 1964
Microorganisms. See also names of specific microorganisms
disease from, 1523–1524. See also Antimicrobial therapy
gram negative vs. gram positive, 1538
killing of, by mononuclear phagocytes, 955
neutrophils and, 951
reservoir for, in hospitals, 1547
Micropenis, androgens for, 1419
in hypogonadotropic eunuchoidism, 1416
Microphthalmia, prenatal diagnosis of, with ultrasonography, 173
Micropolyspora, hypersensitivity pneumonitis from, 433
Micropsia, in partial seizures, 2220
Microsporum, skin infection with, 2321
Microthrombi, and hemolysis, 924

Micturition, abnormalities in, 2107t, 2107–2108. See also *Incontinence*
syncope with, 2075
Midarm muscle area, to estimate lean body mass, 1210
Middle cerebral artery, 2160, *2160, 2161*
atheroma in, 2165–2166
Middle ear, infection of, and subdural empyema, 2184
inflammation of, 2118. See also *Otitis media*
Midges, biting, 1922
phlebotomus fever from, 1817
streptocerciasis from, 1919
Midline granuloma (midline destructive disease), 2032–2033
vs. Wegener's granulomatosis, 2031
MIF. See *Müllerian inhibitory factor*
Migraine headaches, 2129–2131
aura of, vision loss in, 2289
basilar artery, vs. transient ischemic attacks, 2169
from arteriovenous malformations, 2174
oral contraceptives and, 1443
vs. epilepsy, 2225
Miliaria, 2334, 2384
Milk. See also *Breast milk*
and galactosemia, 1133
and tick-borne encephalitis, 1828–1829
as source of supplemental phosphate, 1194
constituents of, synthesis of, 1293
intolerance to, 742
Milk-alkali syndrome, 556, 701, 1492
hypercalcemia in, 1503
salt wasting in, 564
Milk let-down reflex, 1293
Milk products. See *Dairy products*
Milkmaid's grip, in chorea, 2142
in rheumatic fever, 1583
Milkman's fractures, 1483, *1483*
Millipedes, dermatitis from, 1926
Milroy's disease, 388
Miltown, abuse of, 53
Milwaukee shoulder, 2038, 2043
Milzbrand, 1667
Minamata disease, 140
Mineral(s)
deficiency of, signs of, 657
homeostasis of, 1469–1476
kidneys and, 518
in total parenteral nutrition, 1249, 1249t
metabolism of, hormones and, 1263
Mineral oil, and vitamin A deficiency, 1237
aspiration of, lipoid pneumonia from, 2372
interstitial lung disease from, 434
Mineralization, disorders of, and osteomalacia, 1484
inhibitors of, 1482, 1485
Mineralocorticoid(s)
action of, 1347–1348
and sodium balance, 515–516
deficiency of, and urine sodium concentration, 524
excess of, 1358–1360
and fluid volume excess, 535
and potassium secretion, 545
metabolic alkalosis from, 555
function of, 1340
assessment of, 1350
metabolism of, 1343–1344
plasma binding of, 1343
production of, regulation of, 1345–1346
Minocycline, 121
elimination rate for, 96t
for meningococcal disease prophylaxis, 1549

Minocycline (*Continued*)
for prostatitis, 1422
in kidney and liver failure, 117t
in meningococcal disease prophylaxis, 1616
Minoxidil
adverse effects of, 289t
and hair growth, 2350
for hypertension, 287t
in uremic syndrome, 570
Miosis, definition of, 2113
in testing for idiopathic autonomic insufficiency, 2106
Miracidium, 1901
Mirizzi's syndrome, 865
Miscarriage, from lead poisoning, 2386
from neurosyphilis, 2189
risk of, in fetoscopy, 173
MIT (monoiodotyrosine), 1253, 1315, *1316*
Mites, 1922
and allergic rhinitis, 1952
and rickettsiae transmission, 1737
dermatitis from, 1926
rickettsialpox transmission by, 1745
scabies, 1925
Mithramycin, for hypercalcemia, 1504
for Paget's disease, 1517
side effects of, 1504
Mitochondria
antibody to, in liver disease, 816
chromosome of, 146
function of, in shock, 242
in cell survival, 241
injury to, from ethanol, 843
iron in, 894
myopathies of, 2279t, 2279–2280
respiratory chain of, defects in, 2279
Mitomycin
and kidney damage, 610
for bladder cancer, 655
for cancer, 1125
for colorectal cancer, 772
for gastric cancer, 712
for pancreatic cancer, 783
Mitosis, 162, *163*
Mitotane, as inhibitor of adrenal steroid biosynthesis, 1341
for ACTH-secreting adrenal tumors, 1356
Mitotic cells, in tumor mass, 1084
Mitotic pool, of neutrophils, 951, 961, *961*
Mitral insufficiency, and cardiac catheterization, 213
myocardial infarction and, 331
Mitral regurgitation, 347–349, 348t
and catheterization pressure measurements, 212, *213*
chronic, 188, 348
echocardiography for, 203
from Marfan's syndrome, 371
massive, from myocardial infarction, 333
Mitral stenosis, 345t, 345–347
and pulmonic regurgitation, 351
carotid pulse in, 176
congenital, 311
diagnosis of, from cardiac catheterization, 212, 213
differential, 347
Doppler echocardiography for, 206
hemoptysis from, 391
ineffectiveness of digitalis for, 228
murmurs of, from myxoma, 367
radiograph of, *194, 195*
thromboembolic stroke from, 2163
Mitral valve(s)
apparatus of, rupture of, 349
calcification of, and regurgitation, 347
calculating regurgitant stroke volume per beat across, 349

Mitral valve(s) (*Continued*)
calculation of area for, 207
calculation of orific size in, Gorlin formula for, 347
commissurotomy of, 347
disease of, emboli from, and sudden arterial occlusion, 383
insufficiency of, 213, 331
lesions of, coarctation of aorta with, 313
prolapse of, 347, 349–351, 2164
atrial septal defects and, 305
echocardiography for, 178
vs. Marfan syndrome, 1178
vs. mitral regurgitation, 349
regurgitation of, 347–349. See also *Mitral regurgitation*
replacement of, for hypertrophic cardiomyopathy, 358
rheumatic disease of, myxoma vs., 367
stenosis of, 345–347. See also *Mitral stenosis*
supravalvular ring above, 311
Mittelschmerz, 1430
Mixed connective tissue disease, 2021
immunofluorescent cutaneous findings in, 2305t
interstitial lung disease with, 430
Mixed gonadal dysgenesis, 1394–1395, 1429
Mobile spasms, 2152. See also *Athetosis*
Modeling, of bone, 1475
Mohs surgical technique, 2337
Mold spores, and allergic rhinitis, 1952
Molecular cloning, 158–161
Molecular disease, 152
Moles, 2338
hydatidiform, and toxemia of pregnancy, 635
Mollaret's meningitis, 1609
Molluscum contagiosum, 2323t, 2324
Molybdenum, estimated safe and adequate daily dietary intake of, 1206t
toxicity of, 2393
Monge's disease, 2366
polycythemia from, 979
Mongolism, 167t. See also *Down's syndrome*
Monilethrix, definition of, 2349
Monoamine(s), 1281
Monoamine oxidase, and catecholamine action, 1282
from catecholamines, 1462
Monoamine oxidase inhibitors
and hypertensive encephalopathy, 2172
as antidepressants, 2096t, 2096–2097
for panic attacks, 2100–2101
poisoning with, 2069t
Monoarthralgias, from sarcoidosis, 453
Monoblast, 954
Monoclonal antibodies, and chronic lymphocytic leukemia, 998
definition of, 1935
Monoclonal gammopathies, 1026, 1030, 1035–1036. See also *Plasma cell(s), disorder(s) of*
Monocyte(s), as precursor of mononuclear phagocyte, 954
function of, 970
in inflammatory response, 1530
Monocyte-macrophage system, acquired immunodeficiency syndrome and, 1803
Monocytopenia, 966
Monocytosis, 970, 971t
in chronic myelogenous leukemia, 989
Monod's sign, 1850
Monogenic disorders, 147
prevalence of, 147t
Monoglycerides, from fats, 733
Monoiodotyrosine, 1253, 1315, *1316*
Monokines, 956

Monolactams, 120
  for gram-negative bacilli pneumonia, 1567
Mononeuritis multiplex syndrome, rheumatoid vasculitis and, 2002
Mononeuropathy, 2057t, 2260
  in diabetics, 2264
Mononuclear cell(s), in acute interstitial nephritis, 603
  in chronic hepatitis, 831
Mononuclear leukocytes
  collections of, in typhoid fever, 1641
  effector molecules from, 1991t
  in immune complex disease, 1962
  inflammatory response from, 1990–1991
Mononuclear phagocytes, 953–957
  and liver granulomas, 837
  growth and differentiation of, 970
  structure of, 954
Mononucleosis
  acyclovir for, 126
  and splenomegaly, 1037
  chronic, 1787
  infectious, 1786–1788. See also Epstein-Barr virus
    acute hepatitis from, 819
    and cold agglutinins, 920
    and hereditary spherocytosis, 911
    and mucous membrane, 2347
    and Reed-Sternberg cells, 1015
    eosinophilia in, 1025
    lymphocytosis from, 972
    myoglobinuria after, 2283
    rash in, 2322
    vs. acute leukemia, 1004
    vs. cat scratch disease, 1681
    vs. diphtheria, 1628
    vs. Hodgkin's disease, 1008
    vs. Lyme disease, 1728
    vs. measles, 1774, 1775t
    vs. psittacosis, 1736
    vs. Q fever, 1749
    vs. rubella, 1777
    vs. scrub typhus, 1747
    vs. secondary syphilis, 1716
    vs. streptococcal pharyngitis, 1576
    vs. toxoplasmosis, 1878
    vs. viral hepatitis, 824
Mono-octanoin, to dissolve cholesterol gallstones, 869
Monosaccharides, from carbohydrates, 733
  malabsorption of, 742
Monosodium glutamate, food poisoning from, 786
  headache from, 2132
Monosodium urate, in synovial fluid, 1994
Monosynaptic reflexes, psychedelic drugs and, 58
Mood, abrupt changes in, 2092
  from hepatic porphyria, 1185
  assessment of, in elderly, 28
MOPP drug combination, for Hodgkin's disease, 1020
  and infertility, 1416
Morbidity curve, 22, 23
Morbilli, 1772–1775, 1773. See also Measles
Morbilliform exanthem, 1813
Morerastrongylus, 1913
Morphea, 2341, 2349
Morphine
  abuse of, 55
  and antidiuretic hormone release, 540
  bioavailability of, 88
  for pain, 107t, 108
    from bronchogenic carcinoma, 463
    in dying patients, 32
    in shock, 244
  for pulmonary edema in heart failure, 226
  poisoning with, 2069t

Morphine (Continued)
  potency of, 56
  reference intervals for, 2403t
  tricyclic antidepressants with, 109
Morquio's syndrome, 1176, 1176t
Mortality rates, 22, 23
  age with body mass index and, 1221
  annual, for the years 1900 and 1980, 35t
  for appendicitis, 804
  for aspiration-related lung abscess, 437
  for bladder cancer, 655
  for brain abscess, 2183
  for breast cancer, 1452
  for bronchogenic carcinoma, 457
  for cancer, 1083, 1092–1093
  for cholera, 1653
  for chronic obstructive pulmonary disease, 414
  for coronary heart disease, 36, 183t
    international, 180–181, 181
  for Crohn's disease, 752
  for delirium tremens, 50
  for dissecting aortic aneurysms, 374
  for electric injury, 2380
  for influenza, 1764, 1765
  for mushroom poisoning, 787
  for obesity, 1224, 1225t
  for pancreatic cancer, 781
  for peptic ulcers, 696, 706
  for plague, 1663
  for pulmonary embolism, 443, 449
  for renal cell carcinoma, 652
  for shigellosis, 1647
  for shock, 1541
  for snake bites, 1927
  for stroke, 2170
  for tuberculosis, 1682
  for tularemia, 1666
  for typhoid fever, 1642
  for ulcerative colitis, 760
  heart disease and, 180
  hypertension and, 292
  in critical care units, 498
  mechanical ventilation and, 498
  myocardial infarction and, 336
Mosaicism, XO/XY, 1395
Moschcowitz's syndrome, 1052–1053
Mosquitoes, 1922
  and dengue, 1816
  and encephalitis
    California, 1827
    eastern equine, 1824
    from arboviruses, 1821, 1821
    Japanese, 1827
    Venezuelan equine, 1825
  and lymphatic filariasis, 1914
  and malaria, 1857
  and West Nile fever, 1817
  and yellow fever, 1830
Mothers, age of, effect on fetus, 166
Moths, pruritic dermatitis from, 1926
Motilin, in gastrointestinal motility, 715
Motion sickness, 2122
  scopolamine for, 2124
Motivation, definition of, 2083
Motor activity, in metabolic encephalopathy, 2065
Motor function
  disorders of, 2124–2128
    asthenia as, 2124–2125
    ataxia as, 2125–2126
    fatigue as, 2125
    weakness as, 2125. See also Weakness
  episodic loss of, 2127–2128
Motor neurons, 2269
  disease of, 2057t
    early symptoms of, 2284
    intrinsic, 2154t, 2154–2157

Motor neurons (Continued)
  disease of, subacute, from cancer, 1106
    vs. inclusion body myositis, 2276
Motor neuropathy, Guillain-Barré syndrome as, 2261
  hereditary, 2264, 2265t
  proximal lower extremity, in diabetics, 2264
Motor unit, 2269
Mountain sickness, 2366
  chronic, polycythemia from, 979
Mouse (mice), and lymphocytic choriomeningitis virus transmission, 2193
  mites from, and rickettsialpox, 1746
Mouth. See Oral medicine and Teeth
  anaerobic streptococci as normal flora in, 1573
  cancer of, 678–679
  dryness of. See also Xerostomia
    malnutrition and, 1210t
  soreness in, from niacin deficiency, 1232
    riboflavin deficiency and, 1231
Movement
  control of, frontal lobes and, 2082
  disorders of, from basal ganglia abnormalities, 2141
    types of, 2142–2143
  impaired, detection of, 2080t
  involuntary, in rheumatic fever, 1583
  irregularity of, 2125. See also Ataxia(s)
Moxalactam, 120, 121t
  elimination rate for, 96t
  in drug interactions, 124t
  in kidney and liver failure, 117t
Moyamoya, 2164
MPO (myeloperoxidase), 960, 1534
MPSS (methylprednisolone sodium succinate), 429, 1541
MPTP, parkinsonism from, 60, 2144, 2145
MRNA, metabolism of, 929
  translation of, into protein, 929
    mutations affecting, and thalassemia, 934–935
MS. See Multiple sclerosis
MSG (monosodium glutamate), 786, 2132
MTT (marrow transit time), 896
Mu chain disease, 1034
Mucha-Habermann disease, 2326t, 2328
Mucin, clot of, 1983
Mucocele, and Ménière syndrome, 2119
  of gallbladder, 864
Mucolipidosis, 1177
Mucopolysaccharide storage disease, 155
Mucopolysaccharidosis, 153, 1174–1177, 1176t. See also Glycosaminoglycans
  enzyme infusions for, 157
  genetics and, 149
  type II, 267
Mucopolysacchariduria, 1175
Mucormycosis, 1852–1853
Mucosa
  as defense mechanism, 1529
    drugs to enhance, 701
  carcinoma of, 2348
  cryptococcosis and, 1845
  disorders of, 2347–2348
  edema of, airway narrowing from, 397
    and airway obstruction, 475
    from asthma, 403
  in acute gastritis, 689
  inflammation of, diagnosis of, 729
  ischemia of, 689
  nonsteroidal anti-inflammatory drugs and, 696
  of colon, dysplasia of, and cancer, 770
  of duodenum, 694
  of gastrointestinal tract, hemorrhage from, 799

Mucosa (Continued)
of intestines, abnormalities in, and malabsorption, 742–743
in Crohn's disease, 747
of large intestine, inflammation of, 753.
See also Ulcerative colitis
of stomach, 693, 693
defense by, 689
abnormalities in, 695
maintenance of, 694
prostaglandins in, 694
oropharyngeal, paracoccidioidomycosis and, 1843
polyps of, in gastrointestinal tract, 669
protection of, and infection prevention, 1537
systemic lupus erythematosus in, 2014–2015
ulceration of, and hematocrit, 802
in Crohn's disease, 748
Mucosal neuroma syndrome, 1460
Mucositis, from 5-fluorouracil, 1122
from methotrexate, 1121
Mucous glands, bronchial, mucoepidermoid tumors in, 463
enlargement of, in bronchitis, 412
Mucous patch, in syphilis, 1715, 1716
Mucus
cervical, in menstrual cycle, 1430
for protecting mucosa, 694, 694
movement of, in respiratory tract, 1552
secretion of, in allergic rhinitis, 1953
Muir's syndrome, 770, 771
Müllerian ducts, 1392
congenital malformation of, 1428–1429
Müllerian inhibiting factor, 1405
and male sexual differentiation, 1392
deficiency of, 1395–1396
from Sertoli cells, 1393
Multiple endocrine deficiency syndrome, 1460–1461, 1461t, 1496. See also Schmidt's syndrome
Multiple endocrine neoplasia, 695, 708, 727, 1095t, 1265, 1458–1460, 1459t
cancer and, 1113
hyperparathyroidism in, 1489
insulinoma in, 1384
islet cell tumors in, 1388
medullary carcinoma in, 1505
pheochromocytomas in, 1463
primary hyperparathyroidism in, 1490
Multiple myeloma, 974–975, 1027–1033
amyloidosis and, 1035
treatment of, 1201
and corticosteroid-binding globulin, 1342
and gout, 1167
and hypercalciuria from net bone resorption, 640
and skin, 1109
anemia with, 881
clinical manifestations of, 1029, 1029t
clinical staging of, 1030
diagnosis of, 1029–1030
etiology of, 1027
Gaucher's disease and, 1146
hypercalcemia from, 1502
incidence and prevalence of, 1027
kidney failure in, 606
life table survival curves for, 1029
marrow transplants for, 1041
myeloma cell mass in, 1027–1029, 1028
osteoporosis with, 1102, 1513
pathophysiology of, 1027
treatment and prognosis for, 1030–1032
vs. amyloidosis, 1200
vs. Fanconi's syndrome, 621
vs. metabolic bone disease, 1475

Multiple sclerosis
and esophageal motor disorders, 683
and sexual dysfunction, 1442
clinical manifestations of, 2213, 2213t
definition of, 2211
diagnosis of, 2213t, 2213–2214
imaging techniques for, 2060
epidemiology of, 2212
etiology of, 2211–2212
fatigue in, 2125
incidence and prevalence of, 2212
intention tremor in, 2142
laboratory abnormalities in, 2212–2213
pathology of, 2212
subacute myelopathy in, 2217
treatment of, 2214–2215
vertigo from, 2124
vs. acute disseminated encephalomyelitis, 2209
vs. AIDS dementia complex, 2205
vs. basilar impression, 2258
vs. genital herpes, 2197
vs. intradural extramedullary tumors, 2256
vs. Lyme disease, 1728
vs. spinal epidural abscess, 2187
vs. transient ischemic attacks, 2169
vs. vitamin B_{12} deficiency, 2140
Mumps, 1414, 1778–1780
immunization against, 61, 62t, 64
meningitis from, 2193
ovarian failure from, 1438
Munchausen's syndrome, 2103
Murine toxin, 1661
Murine typhus, 1739, 1739, 1741–1742
clinical features of, 1738t
epidemiologic features of, 1737t
Murmurs, 177. See also names of specific heart valves
Austin Flint, from aortic regurgitation, 344
coarctation of aorta and, 313
diagnosis of, 191
from aortic stenosis, 342
from atrial septal defect, 304
from dissecting aortic aneurysms, 373
from Ebstein's anomaly of tricuspid valve, 310
from hypertrophic cardiomyopathy, 357, 357t
from infective endocarditis, 1589
from mitral valve prolapse, 350
from patent ductus arteriosus, 307
from rheumatic fever, 1583
from tetralogy of Fallot, 309
from tricuspid stenosis, 346, 351
from valvular heart disease, diagnosis of, 340
Graham Steell, from pulmonic regurgitation, 351
holosystolic, apical, from mitral regurgitation, 348, 349
of tricuspid insufficiency, 222
pericardial friction rub vs., 363
systolic, in pneumococcal pneumonia, 1557
Murphy's sign, from acute cholecystitis, 865
Murray Valley encephalitis, 1828
Muscarinic blockers, and intestinal motility, 724
Muscarinic cholinergic receptors, 137
Muscle(s)
abnormal activity in, 2283–2284
atrophy of, 2271
in infant's spine, 2155
biopsy of, 2272
for polymyositis, 2034
for trichinellosis, 1912

Muscle(s) (Continued)
cancer and, 1106
contractures in, 2270
cramps in, 2270
during dialysis, 577
from vomiting, 660
depolarizing paralysis of, from anesthetic agents, 548
disease of, 2269–2272. See also Myopathies
fiber(s) of, congenital disproportion of, 2275
electrically silent, slow relaxation of, 2284
types of, 2269
glycogen storage diseases and, 1134–1135
hematomas of, in hemophilia, 1071
hypertrophy of, 2271
hypotonia in, in rickets, 1482
in leptospirosis, 1730–1731
inflammation of, 1978
ischemia of, and myoglobinuria, 2283
manual testing of, 2271
necrosis of, after electric injury, 2382
of calf, rupture of, vs. deep-vein thrombosis, 386
of neck, spasmodic torticollis in, 2150
of respiration, disorders of, respiratory failure from, 476
pain in, 2249, 2270
in bartonellosis, 1681
in leptospirosis, 1731
paravertebral, pain in, 2248, 2249
phorphorylase deficiency of, 1135
vs. arteriosclerosis obliterans, 381
vs. polymyositis, 2036
potassium in, in chronic kidney failure, 564
progressive atrophy of, in children, 2155
prolonged contraction of, in myotonic dystrophy, 1414
protein in, 1211
rippling, 2284
skeletal. See Skeletal muscle
spasms of, 58, 109
spinal, atrophy of, 2155–2156
strength of, clinical grading of, 2036t
stretch reflexes of, hyperactive, from hepatic encephalopathy, 853
structure and function of, 2269
sudden contractions of, 2151. See also Myoclonus
thiamin stores in, 1229
tone of, alterations in, 2143
vitamin B_6 stores in, 1233
weakness in, 2125, 2270. See also Weakness
Muscular dystrophies, 150, 2272–2275
and diabetes mellitus, 1362
and dilated cardiomyopathy, 354
classification of, 2272, 2273t
Duchenne, genetic counseling for, 174
respiratory failure in, 476
vs. muscular form of glycogen storage disease, 1134
vs. polymyositis, 2036
Musculoskeletal system
disease of, approach to, 1977–1980. See also Rheumatic disease
incidence of, 2021t
Raynaud's phenomenon in, 2020
pain in, from rheumatoid arthritis, 2000
in Paget's disease, 1515
sarcoidosis in, 453
Mushroom worker's lung, 433
Mushrooms, and cancer, 44
and food poisoning, 786–787
Music, loud, and hearing loss, 2119
Mustard gas, and cancer, 1093t, 1094

Mutagenesis, insertional, 1090
Mutation, frequency of, 148, 151
    non-sense, 153
Mutism, 2083, 2087
    in AIDS dementia complex, 2204
Myalgia(s)
    as interferon reaction, 128
    epidemic, 1810–1811
        vs. poliomyelitis, 2199
    from Colorado tick fever, 1820
    from influenza, 1765
    from opioid withdrawal syndrome, 57
    from polyarteritis nodosa, 2029
    from Pontiac fever, 1571
Myasthenia gravis, 2285–2287
    anticholinesterases for, 139–140
    cancer and, 1106
    local fatigue in, 2125
    mitochrondrial antibody in, 816
    neuromuscular transmission studies for,
        2057
    respiratory failure in, 476
        critical care of, 489–490
    strabismus in, 2115
    thymus and, 1975
    treatment of, 2286–2287
    vs. botulism, 1633
    vs. polymyositis, 2036
N-Myc, 1091
Mycetoma, 1853
Mycobacteria
    disease from, 1682–1701
        disseminated, 1692
        in AIDS, 1805t, 1806
        leprosy as, 1696–1701. See also *Leprosy*
        of lungs, and alveolar proteinosis, 432
        silicosis and, 2362
        tuberculosis as, 1682–1692. See also *Tu-*
            berculosis
            vs. coal workers' pneumoconiosis,
                2362
            vs. cutaneous leishmaniasis, 1875
            vs. toxoplasmosis, 1878
        granulomatous peritonitis from, 794
Mycobacterium avium-intracellulare, 1693–1694
    in AIDS, 729, 1805t, 1806
Mycobacterium bovis, for immunization
    against tuberculosis, 65
Mycobacterium fortuitum-chelonae, 1693
Mycobacterium kansasii, 1693–1694
Mycobacterium leprae, 1696
Mycobacterium marinum, 1693
    infection with, vs. tularemia, 1666
Mycobacterium scrofulaceum, 1693
Mycobacterium szulgai, 1694
Mycobacterium tuberculosis, 1682
    airborne transmission of, 1552
    and osteomyelitis, 1622
    erythema induratum from, 380
    immunization against, 65
    in AIDS, 1805t, 1806
    pericarditis from, 363
    streptomycin for, 122
Mycobacterium xenopi, 1693–1694
Mycoplasma(s), 1561
    and pneumonia, 1571
    and polyclonal cold agglutinin synthesis,
        920
    and Reiter's syndrome, 2007
    and thrombotic thrombocytopenic pur-
        pura, 1052
    infection with, 1561–1565. See also *Myco-*
        plasmal infections
    sexual transmission of, 1702t
Mycoplasmal infections, 1561–1565
    clinical manifestations of, 1562, *1562*
    erythromycin for, 121
    interstitial lung disease after, 435

Mycoplasmal infections (*Continued*)
    in genitals, 1564–1565
    quinolones for, 122
    pneumonia from, vs. pneumococcal
        pneumonia, 1558
        vs. psittacosis, 1736
    tetracyclines for, 121
Mycoses, 1837–1855
    aneurysms from. See *Aneurysms, mycotic*
    arthritis from, 2011
    aspergillosis as, 1850–1851
    blastomycosis as, 1842–1843
    candidiasis as, 1847–1849
    chromoblastomycosis as, 1854
    coccidioidomycosis as, 1840–1841
    cryptococcosis as, 1844–1846
    endocarditis from, 1591, 1592
    granulomatous peritonitis from, 794
    histoplasmosis as, 1838–1840
    in acquired immunodeficiency syndrome,
        1804t, 1806
    in lungs, and alveolar proteinosis, 432
    in nails, 2346–2347
    ineffectiveness of glucocorticosteroid
        therapy for, 129
    monocytosis in, 970
    mycetoma as, 1853
    of lungs, vs. tuberculosis, 1686
    paracoccidioidomycosis as, 1843–1844
    pericarditis from, 362, 363
    phaeohyphomycosis as, 1854–1855
    sporotrichosis as, 1846–1847
    vs. cervicofacial actinomycosis, 1674
    vs. cutaneous leishmaniasis, 1875
    vs. nocardiosis, 1675
    zygomycosis as, 1852–1853
Mycosis fungoides, 1010, 1109, 2326t
Mycotoxins, ergotism from, 787
Mydriasis
    definition of, 2113
    from psychedelic drugs, 58
    in testing for idiopathic autonomic insuf-
        ficiency, 2106
    sympathetic nervous system and, 133
Myelin, 2211
Myelin basic protein, 2212
    reference intervals for, 2398t
Myelinolysis, central pontine, *2139*, 2139–
    2140
Myelinopathy. See also *Demyelination*
    electrophysiologic studies of, 2057t
    in peripheral nervous system, 2259–2260,
        2260
Myelitis
    in heroin users, 57
    transverse
        from enteroviruses, 1810
        from flukes, 1903
        from systemic lupus erythematosus,
            2016
        vs. tick paralysis, 1923
Myeloblast(s), 951
Myeloblastomas, in acute leukemia, 1004
Myelodysplastic syndrome, 1006
    and neutrophil abnormalities, 958
    from radiation, 962
Myelofibrosis, 877
    acute, 987
    from chronic myelogenous leukemia, 990
    from myeloproliferative disorders, 984
    from polycythemia vera, 983
    marrow transplants for, 1041
    vs. chronic myelogenous leukemia, 991
    with myeloid metaplasia, 985–987
Myelogenous leukemia
    acute, from myeloma treatment, 1032
        prognosis for, 1006
        treatment of, 1005–1006

Myelogenous leukemia (*Continued*)
    and neutrophil abnormalities, 958
    chronic, 973–974, 988–994
        and gout, 1167
        clinical manifestations of, 990
        diagnosis of, 990–991
        etiology of, 988
        incidence and prevalence of, 988–989
        laboratory abnormalities in, 990
        neutrophilia from, 969
        pathogenesis and mechanisms of, 989–
            990
        Philadelphia chromosome–positive, 985
        physical examination for, 990
        primary thrombocythemia with, 1054
        prognosis for, 993, *993*
        proto-oncogenes in, 1091
        splenectomy for, 1038
        treatment of, 991–993
        vs. essential thrombocythemia, 987
        vs. neutrophilic leukemoid reactions,
            970, 971t
Myelography, 2059
    contrast material for, spinal inflammation
        from, 2257
    for back pain, 2251–2252
Myeloid metaplasia
    agnogenic, 973, 985
        neutrophilia from, 969
        primary thrombocythemia with, 1054
        vs. essential thrombocythemia, 987
    gout in, 1161, 1167
    myelofibrosis with, 985–987
Myeloma
    hemorrhage in, 1059
    immunization for patients with, 63
    indolent, 1032–1033
    multiple, 974–975, 1027–1033. See also
        Multiple myeloma
    solitary, 1033
Myelomatosis, 1027. See also *Multiple mye-*
    loma
Myelomeningocele, 170, 170t, 171, 173
Myelopathy, human T lymphotropic retro-
    virus-associated, 1797
Myeloperoxidase, absence of, 1534
    deficiency of, and neutrophil dysfunc-
        tion, 960
Myeloproliferative disorders, 973–974, 984–
    988
    and thrombosis, 1074
    neutrophilia from, 969
    primary thrombocythemia as, 1054
Myelosuppression
    for essential thrombocythemia, 987
    for polycythemia vera, 983, 984
    from 5-fluorouracil, 1122
    from methotrexate, 1121
Myiasis, 1925
Myoadenylate deaminase, deficiency of,
    myopathy with, 1172
Myocardial. See also *Cardiac* and *Heart*
Myocardial contractions, catecholamines
    and, 1463
    stimulation of, 184
Myocardial depressant factor, in shock, 242
Myocardial failure. See *Congestive heart fail-*
    ure; Heart failure
Myocardial infarction
    acute, 327–337
        complications of, 333–334
        differential diagnosis of, 332–333
        extension or expansion of infarct in,
            333
        life-threatening complications of, 336t
        mechanisms of, 329–330
        percutaneous transluminal coronary
            angioplasty for, 339

Myocardial infarction (Continued)
  acute, prognosis for, 336t, 336–337
    recognition of, 330–332
    vs. appendicitis, 803
    vs. sudden cardiac death syndromes, 330
  after stroke, 2170
  and mitral regurgitation, 347
  as hypertensive complication, 293
  atrial pressures in, 244
  atrioventricular block after, 237
  beta-adrenergic blockers for, 138
  coarctation of aorta and, 318
  containment of size of, 335–336, 336t
  definition of, 327
  digitalis after, 229
  electrocardiography for, 199
  emboli from, 2163
    and sudden arterial occlusion, 383
  estimation of size of, 334
  from acute cocaine toxicity, 55
  from alcaptonuria, 1157
  from cardiac catheterization, 211
  from chronic myelogenous leukemia, 990
  from dissecting aortic aneurysms, 373
  from hypertension, 277
  from propranolol withdrawal syndrome, 138
  idiopathic pulmonary fibrosis with, 428
  infarct-avid imaging for, 210
  intestinal infarction from, 763
  myocardial perfusion imaging and, 209
  nonparoxysmal atrioventricular junctional tachycardia and, 262
  pain from, 393
  pericarditis with, 363
  respiratory failure from, 476
  risk factors after, 183
  risk of, from smoking and oral contraceptives, 39
  treatment for, 334–336
  vs. pulmonary embolism, 444
  vs. sepsis, 1540
Myocardial ischemia, 208
  acute, ventricular flutter from, 264
  electrocardiogram for, 177
  pain from, 392, 393
  percutaneous transluminal coronary angioplasty for, 339
  shock and, 238
  vs. epidemic pleurodynia, 1811
Myocarditis, 364
  endomyocardial biopsy for, 178
  from Chagas' disease, 1867
  from dilated cardiomyopathy, 353
  from diphtheria, 1628
  from disseminated gonococcal infection, 1709
  from enteroviruses, 1811–1812
  from leptospirosis, 1731
  from relapsing fever, 1725
  from Rocky Mountain spotted fever, 1743
  from trichinellosis, 1912
  viral, 262
Myocardium. See also Cardiac; Heart; Myocardial
  adaptation of, to volume and pressure loads, 215
  blood supply to, 184
  calcification of, in fluoroscopy, 195
  contractility of, and right ventricular function, 475
    decrease in, and shock, 238
  depression of, from hypoxia, 477
  diseases of, 352–362. See also Cardiomyopathies
  electrical activity of, 196
  fibrosis of, from aortic stenosis, 341

Myocardium (Continued)
  function of, in lung disease, 209
  granulomatous infiltration of, 360
  in yellow fever, 1831
  injury to, from oxygen free radicals, 243
    from Trypanosoma cruzi, 353
  ischemic, protection of, 335–336
  necrosis of, infarct-avid imaging for, 210
  oxygen consumption in, and coronary blood flow, 188
    increased, shock and, 238–239
    regulation of, 187–188
  perfusion imaging of, 209–210
  perfusion in, reduction of, shock and, 237
  rupture of, echocardiography for, 203
  sarcolemma of, beta-adrenergic receptors on, 184
  stiffness in, 359
Myoclonus, 2151
  definition of, 2143
  epileptic, 2222, 2227
  from Creutzfeldt-Jakob disease, 2205, 2206
  from hepatic encephalopathy, 853
  from subacute sclerosing panencephalitis, 2206
  multifocal, from narcotic analgesics, 109
  in metabolic encephalopathy, 2065
  ocular, 2117
  palatial, 2222
  segmental, 2222
Myoedema, definition of, 2271
Myofascial pain syndrome, 2137
  vs. paravertebral tumor, 2255
Myofibrils, 2269
Myoglobin, 2282
  after electric injury, 2381
  change in, with myocardial infarction, 332
  increased concentrations of, and overflow proteinuria, 520
Myoglobinuria, 522, 2271, 2282–2283
  fatty acid metabolism disorders and, 2278
  from potassium loss by skeletal muscle, 546
  in heroin users, 57
Myoinositol, 2263
  in diabetes mellitus, 1367
Myokymia, 2284
  definition of, 2271
Myonecrosis, clostridial, 1629–1631, 1630t
  streptococcal, 1630t
Myopathies
  congenital, 2275–2276
  definition of, 2269
  diagnosis of, 2269–2271
  electrophysiologic studies of, 2057t
  examination for, 2271
  in chronic alcoholics, 2139
  in chronic kidney failure, 567
  in heroin users, 57
  in uremic syndrome, management of, 571
  infiltrative, 2283
  inflammatory, 2276t, 2276–2277
  metabolic, 2277–2283. See also Metabolic myopathies
  nutritional, 2282
  respiratory failure from, critical care of, 489–490
  symptoms in, 2270–2271
  toxic, 2282
  vs. neuropathy, 2271, 2271t
Myophosphorylase, deficiency of, and myopathy, 2278
Myositis, 1978
  inclusion body, 2276
  vs. rheumatoid arthritis, 2000

Myositis ossificans, 2277
Myotomy-myectomy, transaortic ventricular septal, 358
Myotonia, 2270
  action, definition of, 2271
Myotonia congenita, 2284
Myotonia dystrophica, and esophageal motor disorders, 683, 684
Myotonic dystrophy, 1414, 2274
  and diabetes mellitus, 1362
  cataract in, 2289
Myxedema, 1328–1331, 2341
  and ascites, 792
  and breathing control, 401
  and carpal tunnel syndrome, 2268
  and pericardial disease, 363
  coma in, 1329–1331
  definition of, 1328
  galactorrhea in, 1450
  infantile, 1338
  pretibial, in Graves' disease, 1321, 1323
    treatment of, 1327
  vs. angioedema, 1951
Myxoma(s)
  in heart, 367
  in liver, 857
  left atrial, echocardiography for, 178, 346
    vs. mitral stenosis, 347
  right atrial, tricuspid stenosis from, 351
Myxosarcoma, of stomach, 713

NADH, 945
  from EM pathway, 913
Nadolol, 138, 138t
  elimination rate for, 96t
  for hypertension, 287t
NADPH, in erythrocytes, 913
Nafcillin, 119
  acute interstitial nephritis from, 603
  elimination rate for, 96t
  for staphylococcal infection, 1603
  in kidney and liver failure, 117t
Nagana, 1862
Nail(s)
  clubbing of, 2347
  dermatophytic infection of, griseofulvin for, 2317
  disorders of, 2346–2347
  dystrophy of, in sarcoidosis, 454
  malnutrition and, 1210t
  psoriasis in, 2009, 2326
  tumor of, 2347
Nail beds, glomus tumor in, 384
Nail-patella syndrome, 638, 2347
Nairovirus, 1834
Nalbuphine, abuse of, 55
Nalidixic acid, 122
  excretion of, 113
  in drug interactions, 124t
  in kidney and liver failure, 117t
Naloxone
  abuse of, 55
  and opioids, 56
  and shock, 240
  as heroin antidote, 143
  for narcotic-induced respiratory depression, 109
  for opioid overdose, 57
  for sepsis, 1541
Naltrexone, abuse of, 55
  and opioids, 56, 60
Nandrolone decanoate, for anemia of chronic renal insufficiency, 892
  for paroxysmal nocturnal hemoglobinuria, 923

Naphthalene, and methemoglobinemia, in infants, 946
toxicity of, to hemoglobin, 945
Naphthoquinone, toxicity of, to hemoglobin, 945
Naphthylamine, poisonings from, 141
Naproxen, as analgesic, 107t
for dysmenorrhea, 1433
for gout, 1169
Narcan. See Naloxone
Narcolepsy, 2078–2079
vs. epilepsy, 2225
Narcotic agents
as analgesics, 106
for dying patients, 32–33, 32t
elderly reaction to, 26
side effects of, 109
toxic megacolon in ulcerative colitis from, 755
Nasal. See also Nose
Nasal cannulas, for oxygen therapy, 478
Nasal prongs, 486
for oxygen therapy, 478
Nasal septum, midline granuloma and, 2032
perforated, from cocaine use, 55
from drug abuse, 52
Nasogastric aspiration, for ileus, 719
Nasogastric feeding, continuous, for glycogen storage diseases, 1134
National Academy of Sciences, Food and Nutrition Board, 1204
National Cancer Institute, nutritional recommendations from, 1208
National Clearinghouse of Poison Control Centers, 141
National Diabetes Data Group, 1360
National Dialysis Registry, 563
National Heart, Lung and Blood Institute, 300
National Institutes of Health, Consensus Development Conference, 1457
Working Group on Human Gene Therapy, 161
Natriuresis, in SIADH, 539
Natriuretic factor(s), 1277–1279
and extracellular fluid volume, 516
atrial, circulatory function and, 190
Nausea
definition of, 658
from abdominal abscess, 793
from acute cholecystitis, 865
from alcoholic hepatitis, 843
from appendicitis, 801
from ascites, 791
from bacterial peritonitis, 793
from brain abscess, 2182
from brain tumors, 2232
from cannabis, 57
from cavernous sinus thrombosis, 2185
from celiac compression syndrome, 762
from chemotherapy, 1088
from digitalis toxicity, 229
from gallstones, 864
from gastric outlet obstruction, 707
from gastritis, 689
from glucocorticosteroid therapy withdrawal, 132
from hepatic porphyria, 1185
from hypervitaminosis D, 1478
from liver disease, 808
from malaria, 1859
from narcotics, 33, 108, 109
from opioid withdrawal syndrome, 57
from oral contraceptives, 1444
from oral iron therapy, 898
from partial seizures, 2220
from post-streptococcal glomerulonephritis, 587

Nausea (Continued)
from primary mesothelioma, 794
from pseudotumor cerebri, 2236
from psychedelic drugs, 58
from renal artery occlusion, 633
from sedative withdrawal, 54
from viral hepatitis, 819, 824
from vitamin E deficiency, 1239
NBT test, for neutrophil evaluation, 957
NBTE (nonbacterial thrombotic endocarditis), 1586
in cancer, 1098
NCF-A (neutrophil chemotactic factor of anaphylaxis), 1952
Near-drowning, 2371
Nebulization equipment, contaminated water in, and pneumonia, 1565
Necator americanus, 1906
Neck
anaerobic bacteria infection in, 1639
malnutrition and, 1210t
muscles of, spasmodic torticollis in, 2150
pain in, and headache, 2135
management of, 2252
rheumatoid arthritis in, 2001
stiffness in
causes of, 2066–2067
from bacterial meningitis, 1606
from pneumococcal pneumonia, 1557
from subarachnoid hemorrhage, 2176
from subdural empyema, 2184
swelling of, from Graves' disease, 1322
Necrobiosis lipoidica diabeticorum, 1380–1381
Necrosis
aseptic, after kidney transplants, 581
bridging, in chronic hepatitis, 831
of liver, 819
from atherosclerosis, 318
from frostbite, 379
ischemic, in pituitary, 1294
in shoulder, 2042
tubular, vs. allergic interstitial disease, 505
Needle(s), contaminated, and hepatitis spread, 825
use of, and Staphylococcus aureus transmittal, 1597
Neglect syndrome, 2082
Negri body, in rabies, 2200
Neisseria gonorrhoeae, 1706, 1707
cephalosporins for, 120
cervicitis from, 1705
penicillin G for, 119
Neisseria lactamica, and antibodies to Neisseria meningitidis, 1612
Neisseria meningitidis, 1611
penicillin G for, 119
Nelson's syndrome, 1304, 1357
ACTH levels in, 1348
Nematodes, 1905–1919
angiostrongyliasis from, 1913
ascariasis from, 1908
cutaneous larva migrans from, 1907
enterobiasis from, 1910
filariasis from, 1913t, 1913–1919. See also Filariasis
hookworm disease from, 1906–1907
intestinal, 1905–1911
strongyloidiasis from, 1905–1906
tissue, 1911–1919
toxocariasis from, 1908–1909
trichinellosis from 1911–1912
trichuriasis from, 1909–1910
Neomycin, 122
acute renal failure from, 609
and vitamin A deficiency, 1238
for Escherichia coli infection, in neonates, 1655

Neomycin (Continued)
for hepatic encephalopathy, 853
interaction of, with digitalis, 228
steatorrhea from, 744
Neonates
adrenal insufficiency in, 1396–1397
anoxemia in, transposition of great arteries and, 314
bacteriuria in, 629–630
bronchopulmonary dysplasia in, from oxygen toxicity, 496
Chlamydia infection in, 1735
chromosome abnormalities in, 170
cystine-lysinuria in, 1153t
Escherichia coli infection in, neomycin for, 1655
glycogen synthetase deficiency in, hypoglycemia from, 1382
gonococcal conjunctivitis in, 2294
hemolysis in, transient, 913
hepatitis B in, 822
herpes simplex virus infection in, 1782
diagnosis of, 1783
disseminated, adenine arabinoside for, 125
hyperparathyroidism in, 1504
hyperphenylalaninemia in, 1150t
hypoparathyroidism in, 1496
idiopathic thrombocytopenic purpura in, 1051
iminoglycinuria in, 1153t
isoimmune purpura in, 1052
kernicterus in, 812
malformations in, 169, 1202, 2355
meningitis in, 1546, 1605
enteric bacteria and, 1659
treatment of, 1610
myasthenia gravis in, transient, 2285–2286
myocarditis in, from enteroviruses, 1811, 1812
necrotizing enterocolitis in, 1632
nurseries for, disinfection in, 1548
of mother with Graves' disease, 1327
purpura fulminans in, protein C absence and, 1074
screening of, for hypothyroidism, 1328
seizures in, 2223
sepsis in, from streptococci group B, 1573, 1579
susceptibility of, to methemoglobinemia, 946
syphilis in, congenital, 1718
tetanus in, 1635
tyrosinemia in, 1150t
underweight, from malaria, 1859
varicella in, 1789
vernix caseosa on, 2303
vitamin K deficiency in, 1076, 1240
Neoplasm(s)
adrenal, computed tomography for, 284
after kidney transplants, 581
airway obstruction from, 418, 475
and chronic interstitial nephritis, 606
and fever, 1524
and hypercalcemia, 1102
and membranous nephropathy, 596
and osteosclerosis, 1518
and polycythemia, 977
and red cells in ascites fluid, 791
and Salmonella bacteremia, 1645
and splenomegaly, 1037
androgen-secreting, 1418
heterosexual development from, 1429
ascites from, 792
benign vs. malignant, 1084
biologic characteristics of, and treatment, 1114

Neoplasm(s) (Continued)
bronchogenic, and obstructive atelectasis, 419
carcinoid, tricuspid stenosis from, 351
cerebellopontine-angle, vertigo from, 2124
chylothorax from, 468
classification of, 1084
clonal vs. multicellular origin of, 973
computed tomography for, 83
constrictive pericarditis from, 366
disseminated, hemolysis from, 925
DNA of, oncogenes in, 1091–1092
ectopic hormone production by, 1264
eosinophilia from, 1025
erythrocytosis from, 979–980
extradural, 2255–2256
from radiation therapy, 1107
growth of, 1085, 1117
hereditary, 1095t
heterogeneity of, 1117
human immunodeficiency virus infection and, 1806–1807
hypophosphatemic osteomalacia from, 1481
in endocrine glands, 1264
in marrow space, examination for, 883
islet cell tumors. See Islet cell tumor(s)
localization of, in Cushing's disease, 1356
metastasis of. See Metastatic neoplasms
neuroectodermal, 2230
of abdomen, and mesenteric venous thrombosis, 764
of bone, 1521–1522. See also Bone(s), neoplasms of
of brain, 2229–2235. See also Brain, neoplasms of
of cerebral hemisphere, diagnostic imaging techniques for, 2059
of duodenum, 713
of esophagus, 686–687
of gallbladder, 870–871
of glomus body, 384
of heart, 367–368
echocardiography for, 203
of hypothalamus, 1285–1286
of immune system, 1007–1008. See also Non-Hodgkin's lymphoma(s)
of joints, 2048
of kidneys, 506, 650–653. See also Kidney(s), neoplasms of; Renal cell carcinoma
of large intestine, 766–773
of liver, 856–859. See also Liver, neoplasms of
of lungs, 457–466, 457t. See also Lungs, neoplasms of
of mediastinum, 471, 471
of mesentery, 795
of nails, 2347
of nerves, steroids as analgesic for, 109
of optic nerve, 2112
of pancreas, 655, 709, 1354
of peritoneum, 794–795
of pineal, 1286, 1314–1315
of pituitary, 1297–1300. See also Pituitary, neoplasms of
of pleura, 469–470
of skin, arsenic and, 2375
benign vs. malignant, 2336t
vascular, 2339–2340
of small intestine, 773–774
of spinal canal, 2254–2256, 2255
of spine, pain from, 105
vs. genital herpes, 2197
of stomach, 709–713. See also Stomach, neoplasms of
of testes, 1420–1421
of thyroid, 1334–1338

Neoplasm(s) (Continued)
of urinary tract, 654
Pancoast's, pain from, 105
paravertebral, 2254–2255
T cell, 975
thymoma as, 1975
treatment of. See also Antineoplastic agents
chemotherapy for, and kidney failure prevention, 562
urothelial, 654–655
vs. cat scratch disease, 1681
vs. granuloma inguinale, 1712
vs. multiple sclerosis, 2214
vs. splenic abscess, 1040
vs. viral encephalitis, 1823
Zollinger-Ellison syndrome with, 709
Neoplastic polyps, 766. See also Adenoma(s)
Neospinothalamic tract, 2128
Neostigmine, 139
for myasthenia gravis, 2286
Neostriatum, 2141
Nephritic syndrome, acute, 504, 583–585. See also Glomerulonephritis, acute
Nephritis
acute, hypertensive encephalopathy with, 2172
hereditary, chronic, 637–638
kidney transplant for, 157
interstitial, 504–506, 602
acute, 603–604, 606, 608
allergic, proteinuria from, 503
chronic, 606–607, 606t
from drug allergy, 1971t
hematuria from, 503
salt wasting in, 564
lupus, 599t, 599–600
shunt, vs. post-streptococcal glomerulonephritis, 587
tubulointerstitial, 602. See also Tubulointerstitial diseases
vs. leptospirosis, 1732
Nephroblastoma, 654. See also Wilms' tumor
Nephrocalcinosis, from distal renal tubular acidosis, 623
from hyperoxaluria, 1136
nephrolithiasis vs., 638
Nephrocarcinoma, 652. See also Renal cell carcinoma
Nephrogram, 525
Nephrolithiasis, 638–644. See also Calculus(i), renal
Nephroma, mesoblastic, 652
Nephron, 509–510
distal, 511, 514
diuretic action in, 234
loss of, and adaptive functional change, 508
transport process in, 512
Nephronophthisis, 645t, 646, 648
salt wasting in, 532, 564
Nephropathies
analgesic, papillary necrosis from, 628
hypokalemic, 547
IgA, 584t, 588–589, 588
in drug abusers, 57
membranous, 595–598, 596
metal, 611–612
obstructive, 614–617. See also Obstructive nephropathy
reflux, definition of, 628
toxic, 603, 604, 607–613, 607t, 626
tubular, and fluid volume depletion, 532
Nephroptosis, 649
Nephrostomy tube, for urinary tract obstruction treatment, 617
Nephrotic syndrome, 504, 591–598
and combined hyperlipidemia, 1143
and corticosteroid-binding globulin, 1342

Nephrotic syndrome (Continued)
and drug-induced acute interstitial nephritis, 605
biopsy for, 569
complications of, 593
copper deficiency in, 1241
elevated cholesterol levels and, 1141
focal glomerular sclerosis in, 594–595, 594
from cancer, 1098
from mercury vapor, 2388
from nail-patella syndrome, 638
from syphilis, 1714
from transplanted kidney, 581
glomerular permeability and, 521
Hodgkin's disease and, 1017
intermediate diabetic glomerulopathy vs., 625
minimal change, 583, 583, 592t, 593–594
osteomalacia in, 1480
pregnancy and, 636
proteinuria from, 503
renal diseases presenting as, 592t
renal vein thrombosis in, 634
vs. hypothyroidism, 1330
Nerve(s). See also Nervous system
abducens, 2115
acoustic, damage to, 2119
biopsy of, 2260
cutaneous, lateral, of thigh, 2268
herpes simplex virus latent infection of, 1781
herpes zoster infection of, pain from, 2135
in skin, as protection, 2303
peripheral, 2128–2129
tumors of, steroids as analgesic for, 109
Nerve blocks, for pain management, 110, 110t
neurolytic, 109
Nerve conduction studies, 2056–2057, 2260
Nerve roots, chronic compression of, 2249–2250, 2250–2251t
from spinal cord, 2248
inflamed, pain from, 105
Nervous system
autonomic, 133. See also Autonomic nervous system
bacterial diseases of, 2181–2191
parameningeal infections as, 2181–2187. See also Parameningeal infections
syphilis as, 2187–2191. See also Neurosyphilis
central. See Central nervous system
disorders of. See also Extrapyramidal disorder(s); Neuropathies
after near-drowning, 2371
and syncope, 2073–2074
degenerative, 2152–2159, 2153t. See also Degenerative diseases
from radiation therapy, 1107, 1107t
in immunologically compromised host, 2210
irreversible, from hepatic encephalopathy, 853
nutritional, 2137–2141, 2138t
syphilitic, 1717–1718, 2187–2191
for heart, 184
function of, vs. endocrine glands, 1252
hepatic porphyria and, 1184–1186
infection of, 2181–2207. See also Parameningeal infections; Viral nervous system infections
lead poisoning and, 2386
malnutrition and, 1210t
nonmetastatic effects of cancer on, 1104–1107, 1104t
parasympathetic, 133. See also Parasympathetic nervous system

Nervous system (Continued)
  polyarteritis nodosa in, 2029
  rheumatoid arthritis and, 2002
  sarcoidosis in, 453
  sympathetic, 133. See also Sympathetic
    nervous system
  systemic lupus erythematosus and, 2016
    testing for, 2017
  viral infections of, 2191–2207. See also
    Viral nervous system infections
  Wegener's granulomatosis in, 2031
Nervousness, from Graves' disease, 1322
  from paresis, from syphilis, 2188
Netilmicin, 119, 122
  and kidney damage, 609
  in kidney and liver failure, 117t
Neural crest, tumor of, 1465
    pheochromocytoma as, 281
Neural pathways
  for equilibrium, 2117
  for hearing, 2117
  oculomotor, 2115
  pupillary, 2113
  sensory, 2128
  visual, 2111
Neural tube defect, genetic counseling for,
  173
Neuralgia(s), cranial, 2135–2136
  glossopharyngeal, 2135
  trigeminal, in systemic sclerosis, 2023
Neuraminidase, in influenza, 1762
Neurasthenia, 2125
  in myasthenia gravis, 2286
Neuritis. See also Polyneuritis
  brachial, acute, 2267
  in erythema nodosum leprosum, 1699
  intercostal, 393
  optic, 2111, 2112, 2215. See also Optic
    neuritis
  peripheral, 2259
  retrobulbar, 2292
    definition of, 2215
  vs. spinal epidural abscess, 2186
Neuroacanthocytosis, 2148
Neuroblastoma, and skin, 1110
  vs. nephroblastoma, urine vanillylman-
    delic acid and, 654
Neurocutaneous syndromes, 2158–2159
Neurodermatitis, 2320
Neuroendocrine system, and aging, 24
  regulation of, 1280–1285
    disorders of central nervous system
      and, 1285–1289
Neuroendocrinology, 1252
Neurofibroma(s), 2256, 2336t, 2337
  in neurofibromatosis, 2158
Neurofibromatosis, 713, 2158, 2343
  and cancer, 1113
  and neoplasms, 1096t
  interstitial lung disease in, 432
  nodules in, 2337
  pheochromocytoma in, 281
Neurogenic bladder, intermittent catheters
  for, 631
Neurohormones, human biologic produc-
  tion of, 159
Neurohypophysis, 1280, 1290
  trauma to, and diabetes insipidus, 1308
Neurolabyrinthitis, viral, 2123
Neuroleptic agents, poisoning with, 2070t
  susceptibility of elderly to side effects of,
    25
Neuroleptic syndrome, malignant, 2282
Neurologic disorders. See Neuropathies
Neurologic surgery, as contraindication for
  thrombolytic therapy, 449
Neurolytic agents, in pain management,
  109–110

Neuromas, acoustic, 2119
Neuromuscular junction, animal toxins
  and, 1930
  cancer and, 1106
Neuromuscular transmission
  disorders of, 2284–2288
    classification of, 2285t
    respiratory failure from, 476–477
    safety margin of, agents affecting, 2287
    definition of, 2285
    studies of, 2057–2058
Neuromyasthenia, epidemic, vs. poliomyelitis, 2199
Neuromyelitis optica, 2215
Neuromyopathic disorders, and dilated cardiomyopathy, 354
Neuromyotonia, 2270, 2284
Neuron(s), motor, 2269. See also Motor neurons
  of neurohypophyseal system, 1280
Neuronopathy, 2260
Neuropathic joint disease, 2046
Neuropathies, 2258–2268. See also Polyneuropathy
  amyloid, 2266
  and breathing control, 401
  and ulcers, 2341
  approach to, 2053–2056
  asymmetric, 1380
  Buckthorn, 2266
  cancer and, 1106, 2266
  classification of, 2260
    anatomic, 2259–2260
  compression-entrapment, 2267
  definition of, 2259
  demyelinating, 2057
  diabetic, 1379–1380
  diagnosis of, 2054
    imaging techniques for, 2058–2060
    procedures for, 2056–2058
  diphtheritic, 2266
  entrapment, vs. paravertebral tumors,
    2255
  examination for, 2054–2055
  focal, 2259–2260
  from physical injury, 2267, 2268t
  from thallium, 2391
  hereditary, 2264–2265
  in heroin users, 57
  in uremic syndrome, management of, 571
  inflammatory polyneuropathy as, 2260–
    2262. See also Guillain-Barré syndrome
  motor. See Motor neuropathy
  optic, anterior ischemic, 2292
    compressive, from Graves' orbitopathy,
      2295
    ischemic, vs. optic neuritis, 2215
  patient history for, 2055–2056
  peripheral, in chronic renal failure, 507
    vs. erythromelalgia, 378
  respiratory failure from, 476
    critical care of, 489–490
  toxic, 2265–2266
  trigeminal, 2267
  vs. inclusion body myositis, 2276
  vs. myopathy, 2271, 2271t
  with endocrine disease, 2262–2264
Neuropeptides, and intestinal motility, 715,
  724
  human biologic production of, 159
  in hypothalamus, 1282, 1282t
Neurophysins, 1305
Neurosyphilis, 1717–1718, 2187–2191
  asymptomatic, 1717, 2188
  clinical syndromes in, 2188–2189
  congenital, 2189
  laboratory diagnosis of, 2189–2190
  pathology of, 2188

Neurosyphilis (Continued)
  treatment of, 1721, 2190–2191, 2190t
  vs. multiple sclerosis, 2212
  vs. optic neuritis, 2215
Neurotensin, and dumping syndrome, 717
Neurotoxicity, from methotrexate, 1121
Neurotransmitters, 134, 1252
  and anterior pituitary hormone secretion,
    1283t
  and hypothalamus, 1281, 1281
  catecholamines as, 1463
  human biologic production of, 159
  in depression, 2096
  radiolabeling of, 211
Neutropenia, 961–966
  and enteric bacteria infections, 1659
  and infection, 1533, 1534
  and pneumonia from gram-negative ba-
    cilli, 1566
  clinical manifestations of, 963–964
  cyclic, 1533
  definition of, 961
  diagnosis of, 964, 964, 965, 1534
  etiology and pathogenesis of, 961–963
  from autoimmune hemolytic anemia, 919
  from chronic lymphocytic leukemia, 995
  from hairy cell leukemia, 999
  gingivitis in, 1537
  infection with, treatment of, 965–966
  management of, 1535
  testing for, 1942
  treatment of, 964–966
  trimethoprim-sulfamethoxazole for, 1537
  vs. acute leukemia, 1004
  with sepsis, antimicrobial therapy for,
    1536
Neutrophil(s), 951–953
  action of, in pneumococcal pneumonia,
    1556
  adhesion of, 957t, 957–958
  and enteric bacteria infection, 1658
  and inflammatory reaction, 2306
  circulating, in acute phase response, 1528
  damage to alveolar wall by, 425
  deficiency of, bronchiectasis from, 439t
  distribution of, 961
  function of, disorders in, 957–960
    evaluation of, 957, 957t
  granules of, congenital absence of, 960
    contents of, 953t
  in acute phase response, 1529
  in idiopathic pulmonary fibrosis, 429
  in immune complex disease, and tissue
    damage, 1962
  in late-onset asthmatic response, 405
  in lungs, and pneumonia prevention,
    1552
  increase in. See Neutrophilia
  minimum circulating, for normal inflam-
    matory response, 1533
  motility of, disorders of, 960, 960t
  precursor pool for, 951, 968
  production of, 874, 874, 961
  proportions of, in idiopathic pulmonary
    fibrosis, 427
  storage pool of, 951, 961
  transfusions of, 966
  vs. mononuclear phagocyte, 955
Neutrophil chemotactic factor, 404, 1952
Neutrophilia, causes of, 970
  from steroid administration, 129
  in infective endocarditis, 1592
Nevoid basal cell carcinoma syndrome,
  1095t, 1113
Nevus(i), 2336t, 2338
  choroidal, vs. intraocular melanoma, 2295
Nevus flammeus, 2339
Newborns. See Neonates

Nezelof's syndrome, 1941, 1945
from thymic hypoplasia, 1974
NGU (nongonococcal urethritis), 1702
Niacin, 1231–1233, 1232
deficiency of, 1232, 2352
recommended dietary allowance for, 1205t, 1232
sources of, 1232
Nickel
and cancer, 1093t
lung, 458
and contact dermatitis, 2319, 2391
toxicity of, 2390, 2391
Niclosamide, for tapeworms, 1894
Nicotinamide, 1231, 1232
deficiency of, and Hartnup disease, 620
Nicotine
and antidiuretic hormone release, 1308
and tinnitus, 2120
dependence on, 60
low, in cigarettes, 39
receptors for, 137
withdrawal from, 39
Nicotinic acid, 1231, 1232
for dysbetalipoproteinemia, 1141
for inhibiting intestinal secretion, 732
NIDDM. See *Diabetes mellitus, non–insulin-dependent*
Nidinogen, in basement membrane, 1982
Nidus, in kidney stone formation, 638
Niemann-Pick disease, 1147–1149, 1148t
interstitial lung disease with, 432
splenomegaly from, 1037–1038
Nifedipine
adverse effects of, 289t
and kidney damage, 612
as vasodilator, 233
for angina pectoris, 327t, 328t
for asthma, 409
for hypertension, 287t
for hypertrophic cardiomyopathy, 358
for primary pulmonary hypertension, 301, 301t
for Raynaud's phenomenon, 377
Nifurtimox, for Chagas' disease, 1869
side effects of, 1869
Night sweats, from chronic eosinophilic pneumonia, 431
Night vision, loss of, vitamin A deficiency and, 1237, 1238
Nightmares, 2079
in metabolic encephalopathy, 2063
Nightshade, deadly, toxicity of, 787
Nigrostriatal pathway, dopamine in, 2141
Nikethamide, obsolescence of, 481
Nikolsky's sign, 1599, 2329
definition of, 2313
Nil lesion, proteinuria in, 521
Nipples, stimulation of, and oxytocin secretion, 1313
Nitrates
adverse reactions to, 102
and cancer, 44
as venous dilators, 233
contraindicated for hypertrophic cardiomyopathy, 358
for angina pectoris, 326, 326t
for mitral regurgitation, 349
with hydralazine, for vasodilator effect, 235
Nitrazepam, rebound insomnia from, 2078
Nitrites
and carcinogenesis in stomach and esophagus, 44
headache from, 2132
toxicity of, to hemoglobin, 945
with thiosulfate as antidote for cyanide, 143

Nitrobenzene, toxicity of, to hemoglobin, 945
Nitroblue tetrazolium, 957
test with, 1535
Nitrofurans, as testicular toxin, 1416
Nitrofurantoin, 122
chronic hepatitis from, 828, 831
chronic kidney failure as contraindication for, 572t
excretion of, 113
for prostatitis, 1422
for urinary tract infection, 630
genetics and reaction to, 102
in kidney and liver failure, 117t
interstitial lung disease from, 434
metabolites of, kidney excretion of, 95
Nitrogen balance, state of, 1207
Nitrogen dioxide, and chemical pneumonitis, 2367
Nitrogen mustard
for cancer, 1123
for Hodgkin's disease, 1020
hypermelanosis from, 2344
sideroblastic anemia from, 900
Nitroglycerin
absorption of, 88
and amyloidosis, 360
and cardiac output, 191
as vasodilator, 233, 248
as venous dilator, 233
deterioration of, 326
for angina pectoris, 324, 326, 326t
for diffuse spasm of esophagus, 686
for hemorrhage, from gastrointestinal varices, 799
for hyperoxaluria, 1137
for primary pulmonary hypertension, 300
for pulmonary edema in heart failure, 226
for Raynaud's phenomenon, 377
for smooth muscle relaxation in coronary arteries, 189
for variceal hemorrhage, 850
tolerance to, 94
Nitroimidazole, and radiation therapy, 1116
Nitroprusside
and cardiac output, 191
and cyanide poisonings, 144
as vasodilator, 233, 235, 248
for primary pulmonary hypertension, 300, 301t
for pulmonary edema in heart failure, 226
metabolites of, kidney excretion of, 95
reference intervals for, 2403t
Nitrosamide, and colorectal cancer, 768
Nitrosamines, and carcinoma, of stomach, 710
Nitrosourea(s)
and interstitial lung disease, 434
and kidney damage, 610
aplasia from, 885
for Hodgkin's disease, 1020
for multiple myeloma, 1030–1031
Nitrous oxide, abuse of, 59
inhalation therapy with, 110
Nits, 1920
NK (natural killer) cells, 971, 1531, 1997
and viruses, 1751, 1752
Nocardia asteroides, in transplant recipients, 2210
in brain abscess, 2182
sulfonamides for, 119
Nocardia intracellularis, 1693
Nocardiosis, 1675–1676
lung abscess from, 436
sulfonamides for, 437
vs. cervicofacial actinomycosis, 1674
Nocturia, from diabetes insipidus, 1309
in heart failure, 221

Nocturia (*Continued*)
in tubulointerstitial disease, 602
Nodules, coal, 2361–2362
of skin, 2236t, 2335–2239
Nomifensine, and catecholamine effect enhancement, 1282
Non-Hodgkin's lymphoma(s), 975, 1009–1013
and splenomegaly, 1037
classification of, 1007–1008, 1008t
definition of, 1007
diagnosis of, 1010
epidemiology of, 1009
etiology and pathogenesis of, 1009
human immunodeficiency virus infection with, 1807
lymphomas as, 1007
marrow transplants for, 1041
noninvasive studies of, 1011t
pathology and clinical features of, 1009t, 1009–1010
prognosis for, 1012, 1012–1013
skin lesions in, 1109
treatment of, 1011
vs. Ewing's sarcoma, 1521
Non-insulin-dependent diabetes mellitus, 1360. See also *Diabetes mellitus, non–insulin-dependent*
Nonsteroidal anti-inflammatory agents
acute allergic interstitial disease from, 505
acute interstitial nephritis from, 605
allergic reactions to, 1971–1972
anaphylaxis from, 1956
and minimal change nephrotic syndrome, 594
and acute kidney failure, 561
and cutaneous reactions, 2353
and diuretic action, 234
and nephrotic syndrome, 593
and peptic ulcers, 696, 701, 707
and photosensitivity, 2351
and postoperative recurrent ulcers, 705
and urticaria, 1950
as analgesics, 107
as cyclooxygenase inhibitors, 1275
contraindications for, effective circulating volume reduction as, 531
kidney disease as, 562
for ankylosing spondylitis, 2007
for gout, 1168, 1169
for pericarditis, 364
for rheumatoid arthritis, 2003
gastritis from, 689
glucocorticosteroid therapy and, 131, 132
interaction of, with loop diuretics, 232
nephropathy from, 608
prostaglandin synthesis inhibited by, 607
Nontropical sprue
biopsy of, 739, 739
lymphoma from, 744
malabsorption in, 742–743
folate, 906
iron, 896
Nonverbal communication, 72
Noonan's phenotype, 1203
Noonan's syndrome, 388, 1414
cryptorchidism in, 1415
Noradrenaline. See *Norepinephrine*
Norepinephrine, 134, 136, 137, 1281–1282, 1462
and blood pressure in upright position, 1465
and eating, 657
biologic role of, 1463
biosynthesis of, 1462, 1462
for shock, 244, 247
in hypertensive patients, 278
initial hemodynamic effects of, 247t

Norepinephrine (Continued)
  release of, and prostaglandins, 279
  with vasodilators, for shock, 248
Norfloxacin, 122
  in kidney and liver failure, 117t
Normeperidine, seizures from, 109
Normethsuximide, reference intervals for, 2403t
North African tick typhus, 1745
North American blastomycosis, 1842
North Asian tick-borne rickettsiosis, 1745
Nortriptyline, genetics in metabolism of, 102
  reference intervals for, 2403t
Norwalk virus, 1768. See also Viral gastroenteritis
Nose. See also Nasal
  allergic rhinitis and, 1951, 1953
  cartilage of, leprosy in, 1698
  congestion in, from common cold, 1755
  diphtheria infection in, 1627
  mastocytosis of, 1954
  mucosa of, dryness of, in Sjögren's syndrome, 2024
  neoplasms of, vs. zygomycosis, 1852
  regurgitation in, from palatal weakness, 684
  stuffiness in, from allergic rhinitis, 1953
    from alpha antagonists, 139
Nose drops, rebound effects of, 1954
Nosocomial infections, 1541–1549. See also Hospital-acquired infections
NREM (non–rapid eye movement) phase of sleep, 2077
Nubain, abuse of, 55
Nuclear decay, 2375
Nuclear dust, 2325
Nuclear proteins, autoantibodies to, 1997t
Nuclear tests, fallout from, 2376
Nucleocapsid, 1750
Nucleosomes, 928
5'-Nucleotidase, in liver disease, 815
Nucleotides, consensus, 929
Nucleus(i), in cancer cells, 1084
  paraventricular, 1305
  supraoptic, 1305
Null cell, 1007
Numbness, from phencyclidine, 59
  in partial seizures, 2220
Numorphan, as analgesic, 107t
Nursing mothers, malaria prevention in, 1861
  methimazole contraindicated for, 1327
Nutrients
  absorption of. See also Malabsorption
    normal, 733–735
    regions for, 733, 733t
  requirements for, 1204–1208
  serum and/or blood indices for, 1211t
Nutrition. See also Malnutrition
  abnormalities of, in ulcerative colitis, 758
  and cancer, 1088, 1095–1096
  and growth hormone secretion, 1284
  assessment of, 1208t, 1208–1211
  complications of, from Crohn's disease, 749
  myopathies from, 2282
  of elderly, 28
  parenteral, total, 1248–1250. See also Total parenteral nutrition
  respiratory failure and, 479
Nutrition therapy, enteral, 1243–1246
  for bacterial overgrowth, with malabsorption, 742
  parenteral, 1247–1251
Nystagmus, 2116–2117, 2116t
  definition of, 2115
  from cannabis, 57

Nystagmus (Continued)
  from phencyclidine, 59
  in Friedreich's ataxia, 2152
  in Wernicke's encephalopathy, 2137
  positional, 2121–2122
  vestibular, examination for, 2121
Nystatin, for Candida infection, of esophagus, 688
  of vagina, 1704

OA. See Osteoarthritis
OAF. See Osteoclast-activating factor
Oatmeal complexes, for skin disorders, 2314
Obesity, 1219–1227
  and anorexia nervosa, 1216
  and atherosclerosis, 321
  and breathing control, 401
  and cardiovascular disease, 182
  and corticosteroid-binding globulin, 1342
  and diabetes. See Diabetes mellitus
  and endocrine system, 1225
  and fatty liver, 810, 827
  and gynecomastia, 1452
  and hypertension, 285
  and hypertriglyceridemia, 1143
  and liver disease, 843
  and osteoporosis, 1511
  and plasma amino acids, 1152t
  and polycystic ovarian syndrome, 1439
  and pseudotumor cerebri, 2237
  and thrombosis, 1074
  as contraindication for kidney transplant, 578
  clinical manifestations of, 1223–1224
  definition of, 1219–1221, 1220t
  emotional disturbances and, 657
  etiology of, 1221–1222
  from Cushing's syndrome, 1355
  from hypothalamic disorders, 1289, 2104
  jejunocolic bypass surgery for, and liver disease, 840
  morbid, jejunoileal bypass for, 743
  mortality from, 1224, 1225t
  pathophysiology of, 1222–1223
  prevention of, 1227
  psychologic manifestations of, 1224
  treatment of, 1225–1227
  truncal, in Laurence-Moon-Bardet-Biedl syndrome, 1203
Obstipation, in ileus, 719
Obstructive nephropathy, 614–617
  causes of, 614t
  clinical manifestations of, 615–616, 615t
  diagnosis and evaluation of, 568, 616–617
  from chronic interstitial nephritis, 606
  from chronic kidney failure, management of, 569
  pathology and pathophysiology of, 614–615, 615t
  treatment of, 617
Obstructive pulmonary disease, 399, 399t
  and atrial fibrillation after DC cardioversion, 273
  as cause of death, 414
  beta blockers and, 287
  chronic, 399, 410
    histoplasmosis with, 1839
    influenza and, 1766
    pulmonary hypertension from, 296
  differential diagnosis of, 416
  exercise and, 46
  in cigarette smokers, 38
  mechanical ventilation contraindicated for, 480
  multifocal atrial tachycardia in, 261

Obstructive pulmonary disease (Continued)
  polycythemia from, 979
  prognosis for, 416
  treatment for, 416–418
    oxygen therapy as, 478
    potassium-sparing diuretics as, 232
  vs. panic attacks, 2101
  vs. pulmonary embolism, 446
Obtundation
  definition of, 2061t
  from Aspergillus fumigatus, in transplant recipients, 2210
  from diabetes, in elderly, 26
  from Reye syndrome, 2210
Occipital lobe(s), disorders of, 2081t, 2081–2082
  vascular, and visual field defects, 2113
Occlusion. See Stenosis
Occupational disease(s)
  asthma as, 407, 2358–2359, 2359
    causes of, 2358t
  cancer as, 1094
    lung, 458, 2364
  of skin, 2318, 2373–2375
Occupational medicine, 2354–2356, 2355
  reproductive hazards and, 2355
Ochronosis, osteoarthritis and, 2041
  synovial membrane in, 1995
Ockelbo fever, 1819
OCT (ornithine carbamyl transferase), 1158
Oculogyric crisis, from antipsychotic drugs, 2144
  from phenothiazine toxicity, vs. tetanus, 1635
Oddi, sphincter of, stenosis of, 872
Odor, anaerobic infection and, 1639
  of vomitus, 659
Odynophagia, 679
Oesophagostomum, 1911
Ofloxacin, 122
Ohara's disease, 1664
Ointment, 2314–2315
Oleander, and digitalis intoxication, 787
Olfaction, 2109–2110, 2110t
  auras in, 2221
  receptors of, 2110
Olfactogenital dysplasia, 1287, 1439
Oligoanuria, from hyperacute rejection of kidney transplant, 580
Oligodendrocyte(s), multiple sclerosis and, 2212
  myelin from, 2211
Oligodendroglioma, 2230
Oligomenorrhea, from hypothalamic hypogonadism, 1287
Oligospermia, 1409
  idiopathic, 1416
Oliguria
  anuria with, causes of, 616
  definition of, 558
  from fluid volume depletion, 532
  from gastrointestinal bleeding, 660
  in cardiac tamponade, 366
  in kidney failure, 561
    hyperkalemia from, 547
  mechanisms of, in acute kidney failure, 560
  sudden, in acute kidney failure, 506
  urine sodium concentration in, 524
Ollier's disease, 1520
Omega-3 fatty acids, in marine fish oils, 43
Omentum, 790
  disorders of, 795–796
Omeprazole, for inhibiting acid secretion, 700
  for Zollinger-Ellison syndrome, 709
Omsk hemorrhagic fever, 1828, 1833–1834
Onchocerciasis, 1916–1918

Oncocytoma, renal, 652
Oncogenes, 1089–1092
  and carcinogenesis, 1092
  in DNA of neoplasms, 1091–1092
  products of, *1091*
  recombinant DNA research on, 159
  retroviral, 1090–1091
    proteins encoded by, 1090t
  viral, 1089–1090
Oncotaxis, inflammatory, 1108
Ondine's curse, from cordotomy, 111
Onychogryphosis, definition of, 2346
Onycholysis, definition of, 2346
  in psoriasis, 2326
Onychomycosis, 1848, 2346–2347
O'nyong-nyong fever, 1819
Oocysts, *Toxoplasma*, 1876
Oocytes, 1425
  development of, 1431
  in meiosis, 162
  number of, in ovaries, by age, 1425
Operant conditioning, for seizures, 2228
Ophthalmia, gonococcal, vs. neonatal chla-
    mydial infection, 1735
Ophthalmologic surgery, as contraindica-
    tion for thrombolytic therapy, 449
Ophthalmoplegia
  in cavernous sinus thrombosis, 2185
  in progressive supranuclear palsy, 2145
  in Wernicke's encephalopathy, 2137
  internuclear, 2115–2116
    definition of, 2213
  migraine in, 2131
Opiates
  and intestinal motility, 724
  and urticaria, 1950
  in diarrhea treatment, 732
  poisoning with, 2069t
  receptors of, 1270
  respiratory failure from, 476
Opioids
  abuse of, 55–57
    treatment for, 57
  acute overdose of, 56
  adverse effects of, 56
  and eating, 657
  dependence on, methadone for, 60
  peptides of, 1268–1270, *1269*
  synthesis of, 60
  tolerance to, 56
  use of, with cocaine, 54
Opisthorchiasis, 834, 835t, 1902
Opisthotonos, from tetanus, 1635
Opitz-Frias syndrome, 170
Opium, tincture of, for diarrhea, from
    Crohn's disease, 752
    from ulcerative colitis, 758
Opsoclonus, 2117
  from cancer, 1105–1106
Opsonization, 952, *952*
Optic nerve
  aneurysms and, 2175
  atrophy of, Leber's, vs. optic neuritis,
    2215
  compression of, vs. optic neuritis, 2215
  damage to, *2111*
  demyelination of, visual evoked poten-
    tials and, 2056
  disorders of, 2215
    and vision loss, 2112
  sarcoidosis of, 453
Optic neuritis, 2111, 2112, 2215
  cryptococcosis and, 1845
  from ethambutol, 1687
  in multiple sclerosis, 2213
  in neuromyelitis optica, 2215
  papillitis as, 2292

Optic neuritis *(Continued)*
  varicella and, 1789
  vs. papilledema, 2113t
Optic tract, lesions of, 2113
Oral cavity. See also *Mouth*
  bejel in, 1723
  burns of, in electric injury, 2381
  cancer of, in cigarette smokers, 38
  candidiasis of, in AIDS, 1804t, 1806
  gangrenous lesions in, 1187
  hemorrhagic bullae of, 1049–1050
  peptostreptococci in, 1637
Oral contraceptives, 1443–1444
  and adolescent cognitive development, 17
  and cancer, 1094–1095
    breast, 1453
  and candidiasis, 1848
  and cholesterol gallstones, 860
  and colon infection, vs. ulcerative colitis,
    757
  and corticosteroid-binding globulin, 1342
  and folate deficiency, 906
  and hair growth, 2350
  and hair loss, 2349
  and hemolytic uremic-type syndrome,
    601
  and hepatocellular adenoma, 856
  and hepatocellular carcinoma, 858
  and hereditary hemorrhagic telangiecta-
    sia, 1060
  and hyperaldosteronism, 1360
  and ischemic colitis, 764
  and liver neoplasms, 828
  and loin pain–hematuria syndrome, 585
  and melasma, 2343
  and mesenteric artery occlusion, 762
  and mesenteric venous thrombosis, 764
  and migraine headache, 2131
  and sinus thrombosis, 2184
  and smoking risks, 38, 39
  and thrombotic thrombocytopenic pur-
    pura, 1052
  and vitamin C levels, 1235
  contraindications for, 1444
  for abnormal uterine bleeding, 1435
  for adolescents, 16
  for anovulation, 1439–1440
  for dysmenorrhea, 19, 1433
  for gonadotropin deficiency, 1297
  hepatic vein thrombosis from, 828, 848
  hypertension from, 280
    diagnosis of, 282
    treatment for, 288, *291*
  in drug interactions, 124t
    with folic acid, 1206t
  liver disease from, 827, 830
  metabolic effects of, 1443
  peliosis hepatitis from, 828
  side effects of, 1444
  uterine bleeding from, 1434
Oral-facial dyskinesia, from hepatic enceph-
    alopathy, 853
Oral medicine, 674–679. See also *Mouth* and
    Teeth
  acute gingivitis in, 675, *675*
  and acquired immunodeficiency syn-
    drome, 677
  aphthous ulcers in, 675–676, *676*
  cancer in, 678–679
  candidiasis in, 677
  dental abscess in, 674–675
  dental caries in, 674
  erythroplakia in, 678
  glossitis in, 678
  herpetic infections in, 676–677
  leukoplakia in, 678, *678*
  periodontal disease in, 675

Oral rehydration solution, for viral gas-
    troenteritis, 1771
  World Health Organization recommenda-
    tion for, 731
Orbit, neoplasms of, vs. zygomycosis, 1852
  pseudotumor of, 2292, 2295
  restrictive disease of, causes of, 2115
Orchiectomy, for cancer of prostate, 1424
Orchitis, in erythema nodosum leprosum,
    1699
  mumps immunization and, 64
  viral, 1414
Organ(s)
  damage of, in sickle cell anemia, 937
  failure of, from peritonitis, 793
  interdependence of, in critically ill pa-
    tient, 482
  leukemic infiltration of, 1004
  ruptures of, computed tomography in, 83
Organ transplants. See also *Heart trans-
    plants; Kidney transplants; Liver, trans-
    plants of; Transplant(s)*
  and cytomegalovirus transmission, 1784,
    1785
  central nervous system infections after,
    2210
  donors for, 577–578
  Epstein-Barr virus infection in, 1788
  for metabolic errors, 157
  human leukocyte antigens and, 1963
  immune response to, 578
  rejection of, glucocorticosteroid therapy
    for, 130, 131
  toxoplasmosis with, 1877
Organic acids, metabolic acidosis from, 553
  secretion of, in pars recta, 512
Organic anions, from dietary fiber, 721
Organic dusts, inhaled, interstitial lung dis-
    ease from, 424t, 433
Organification, 1315
Organophosphate poisonings, treatment
    for, 145
  vs. botulism, 1633
Orgasm, 1441
  and headache, 2132
Orientation, impairment of, in delirium,
    2064
Ornithine salts, for chronic liver disease
    with encephalopathy, 855
Ornithine transcarbamylase, 1152t
  deficiency of, 1158, 1173
    hyperammonemia from, as X-linked
      dominant trait, 149
Ornithosis, vs. mycoplasmal pneumonia,
    1564
Orofaciodigital syndrome, as X-linked dom-
    inant trait, 149
Oropharyngeal airway, for acute respiratory
    failure, 477
Oropharynx, muscles of, disorders of, 683
Oroya fever, 1681
Orphenadrine, for advanced parkinsonism,
    2146
ORS solution. See *Oral rehydration solution*
Orthophosphates, for hypercalciuria, 642–
    643
Orthopnea, 394
  from aortic regurgitation, 344
  from arteriovenous fistula, 384
  from dilated cardiomyopathy, 352
  in heart failure, 221
Orthostatic hypotension, 2106–2107
  and syncope, 2075
  definition of, 2106
  from tabes dorsalis, 2189
Oscillopsia, 2120, 2123
Osgood-Schlatter disease, 19

Osler-Weber-Rendu syndrome, 148, 308, 1060, 2341
  gastrointestinal hemorrhage in, 799, 800
  vascular malformations in gastrointestinal tract from, 765
  vs. petechiae, 1045
Osler's nodes, definition of, 2325
  from infective endocarditis, 1589t
Osmolality
  approximation of, 536
  balance of, in brain, and coma, 2068
  decreased maximal urinary, in tubulointerstitial disease, 602
  disturbances in, 536–543
  effective extracellular compartment, 536
  in pregnancy, 634
  of stool water, 731
  reduction of, with hyponatremia, 538
  reference intervals for, 2398t
  serum, formula for, 1377
  water balance in, 537, 537–538
Osmolar gap, 538
Osmoreceptors, 2104–2105
  in osmolality, 537
Osmotic agents, as laxatives, 722
Osmotic diuresis, 532
  and potassium loss, 546
  hypernatremia from, 542
Osmotic diuretics, 232
  properties of, 231t
Osmotic fragility test, 910, 911
  unincubated vs. incubated, 912
Osmotic pressure, colloidal, 240
Osteitis deformans, 1515–1517. See also Paget's disease of bone
Osteitis fibrosa, 566
  in renal osteodystrophy, 1507–1508
Osteitis fibrosa cystica, 1489, 1490
  radiographic sign of, 1490, 1491
Osteoarthritis, 1978, 2039–2041
  and carpal tunnel syndrome, 2268
  etiologic classification of, 2039t
  in Ehlers-Danlos syndrome, 1179
  vs. arthritis from alcaptonuria, 1157
  vs. gout, 1168
  vs. rheumatoid arthritis, 2000
Osteoarthropathy
  bronchogenic carcinoma with, 459
  hypertrophic, 1519, 2046–2047, 2347
  pulmonary, in cancer, 1098, 1112
Osteoarthrosis, 1978
Osteoblasts, 1474–1475, 1510
Osteochondroses, 1517
Osteoclast(s), 1475, 1510
  defective functioning of, osteopetrosis from, 1518
  of Paget's disease, 1515
Osteoclast-activating factor, 1502
  and bone resorption, 1102
  from myeloma cells, 1028
Osteocytes, 1475
Osteodystrophy, renal, 566, 1507–1510. See also Renal osteodystrophy
Osteoectasia, with hyperphosphatasia, 1519
Osteogenesis imperfecta, 1180t, 1180–1181, 1982
  mitral valve prolapse from, 350
  vitamin C for, 1236
Osteolysis, in multiple myeloma, 1032
Osteomalacia
  axial, 1482
  bone salt loss in chronic kidney failure and, 564
  definition of, 1479
  from Fanconi's syndrome, 621
  from hyperparathyroidism, 1489
  from primary biliary cirrhosis, 845
  from renal osteodystrophy, 1508

Osteomalacia (Continued)
  muscle symptoms in, 2280
  radiographic features of, 1509
  rickets with, 1479–1485
    diagnosis of, 1482–1484, 1483
    pathogenesis of, 1479–1482
    treatment of, 1484–1485
  vs. osteogenesis imperfecta, 1180
  vs. osteoporosis, 1513
Osteomyelitis, 1622–1624
  anaerobic, 1639
  and amyloidosis, 1199
  antimicrobial therapy for, 114
  bacterial, 2257
  cerebral epidural abscess with, 2184
  cranial, and subdural empyema, 2184
  from cervicofacial actinomycosis, 1674
  from disseminated coccidioidomycosis, 1841
  from Haemophilus influenzae, 65
  from mycobacteria infection, 1695
  from Salmonella, 1644
  from sickle cell anemia, 940
  hematogenous, from staphylococci, 1600
  multifocal, 1622
  of mastoid bone, pain from, 2134
  sternal, Mycobacterium fortuitum-chelonae and, 1693
  vertebral, and spinal epidural abscess, 2186
Osteonecrosis, 1517–1518
  after kidney transplants, 581
Osteo-onychodysplasia, 638, 2347
Osteopathia striata, 1519
Osteopenia, from Cushing's syndrome, 1355
Osteopetrosis, 1518–1519
  myelophthisis in, 890
Osteophytes, 2041
Osteopoikilosis, 1519
Osteoporosis, 41, 1510–1515
  age-related, 1512
  and decreased skeletal mass, 1475
  causes of, 1512t
  clinical considerations for, 1512–1513
  compression vertebral fractures from, 2043, 2044
  definition of, 1510
  diet for, 1246
  effects of, 1476
  etiology of, 1510–1511
  exercise and, 46
  fluoride for, 1485
  from beta thalassemia, 931
  from Crohn's disease, 750
  from glucocorticosteroid therapy, 130, 133
  from heparin, 448
  from homocystinuria, 1160
  from primary biliary cirrhosis, 845
  from sarcoidosis, 453
  in males, treatment of, 1514
  in menopause, 1444
  involutional, 1512
  juvenile, 1511–1512
  pathogenesis of, 1511
  prevention of, 1514–1515
  risk factors for, 1515
  senile, androgens for, 1419
  syndromes of, 1511–1512
  treatment of, 1513–1514
  vs. osteogenesis imperfecta, 1180
Osteosarcoma(s), 1521
  of lungs, 464
  solitary pulmonary nodules from, 464
Osteosclerosis, 1518–1519
  in Gaucher's disease, 1146
  in myelofibrosis, with myeloid metaplasia, 986

Osteosclerosis (Continued)
  in osteitis fibrosa, radiographic features of, 1509
Ostium primum defect, 305
Ostium secundum defect, 304
Otitis, in agammaglobulinemia, 1943
  malignant external, 2185–2186
Otitis media
  acute, and pneumococcal meningitis, 1605
    from Branhamella catarrhalis, 1614
    from Haemophilus influenzae, 1619
  anaerobes in, 1639
  and hearing loss, 2118
  brain abscess from, 2181
  chronic, from Langerhans cell granulomatosis, 1023
  from respiratory syncytial virus, 1759
  from scarlet fever, 1576
  immunization against, 63
  lateral sinus thrombosis from, 2185
  measles and, 1774
  pain from, 2134
  serous, allergic rhinitis in, 1953
  treatment of, 2119
  whooping cough with, 1625
Otoliths, 2121
Otomastoiditis, bacterial, chronic, vertigo from, 2123
Otorrhea, cerebrospinal fluid, from skull fracture, 2241
Otosclerosis
  hearing loss from, 2118–2119
  tinnitus with, 2120
  treatment of, 2119
  vertigo from, 2123
Ouabain, pharmacology of, for heart failure, 227t
Ovaries, 1425–1446, 1426. See also Gynecologic disorders
  breast cancer metastases to, 1456
  cysts in, and amylase level, 776
    twisted, vs. appendicitis, 803
  development of, 1391, 1391
  dysgenesis of, 167t
  embryology and anatomy of, 1425, 1426
  failure of, and polyglandular autoimmune disease, 1414
  function of, in childhood and puberty, 1425–1426
  hyperthecosis of, 1440
  in menstrual cycle, 1430–1431
  luteomas of, in mothers, and masculinization of female infants, 1404
  neoplasms of, 1445–1446
    and precocious puberty, 1428
    hirsutism from, 1446
    hormones from, 1445t
  neuroendocrine regulation of, 1432–1433
  number of oocytes in, by age, 1425
  polycystic, syndrome in, 1287, 1429. See also Polycystic ovarian syndrome
  postmenopausal, 1444
  teratoma of, and warm autoimmune hemolytic anemia, 918
  tuberculosis in, 1690
  tumor-like conditions of, vs. neoplasms, 1446
Overeating, 657, 683
Overfeeding, and obesity, 1222
Overlap syndrome, 2021
Ovulation, 1425
  absence of. See Anovulation
  in adolescents, 19
  induction of, hormone therapy for, 1442–1443
  pain at, 1430
Ovum, from meiosis, 162

Oxacillin, 119
  acute interstitial nephritis from, 603
  elimination rate for, 96t
  for staphylococcal infection, 1603
  in kidney and liver failure, 117t
  liver disease from, 827
Oxalate. See also *Hypoxia*
  and kidney damage, 612
  in kidney stones, 640
    vitamin C and, 1236
  reference intervals for, 2398t
  restricting intake of, 45
Oxalate crystal deposition disease, 2038
Oxalate disorders, urinalysis for, 561
Oxalosis, definition of, 1136
  kidney transplant for, 157
Oxamniquine, for schistosomiasis, 1901
Oxantel, for trichuriasis, 1909
Oxazepam, reference intervals for, 2403t
Oxidation-reduction potential, and anaerobic organism growth, 1636
Oxidation-reduction reactions, vitamin C and, 1234
Oxipurinol, and acute interstitial nephritis, 605
Oxprenolol, affinity of, for beta-adrenergic receptors, 138
  for angina pectoris, 327t
Oxycodone
  abuse of, 55
  as analgesic, 107t
  for pain in dying patients, 32
  poisoning with, 2069t
Oxygen
  consumption of, cardiac output and, 220, 237
    estimating, 485
    in exercise, 400
    in heart, determinants of, 219
      regulation of, 187–188
  deficiency of, in heart muscle, angina pectoris from, 323
  delivery of, metabolic acidosis and, 554
  deprivation of, and metabolic encephalopathy, 2064t
  diffusion of, 399
  dissociation curve of, 241
  for myocardial infarction, 335
  for shock, 244
  hemoglobin affinity for, shock and, 241
  hyperbaric, for sepsis, 1541
    therapeutic, 2367
  in heart failure management, 225
  inhalation of, interstitial lung disease from, 435
  reduced affinity of hemoglobin for, in anemia, 879
  reference intervals for, 2398t
  saturation of, reference intervals for, 2398t
  systemic transport of, 485
  therapy with. See *Oxygen therapy*
  toxicity of, 2368, 2368–2369
Oxygen free radicals, and myocardial depression, 239
  in shock, 243
Oxygen-hemoglobin dissociation curve, 485, *485*, 496
  in anemia, 879
  in polycythemia, 979
Oxygen therapy
  external devices for, 486
  for acute respiratory failure, 478
  for alveolar hypoventilation, 298
  for chronic obstructive pulmonary disease, 417
  for chronic respiratory failure, 479–480

Oxygen therapy (*Continued*)
  for gas gangrene, 1630
  for interstitial fibrosis, 296
  for obstructive airway disease with infection, 297
  for sepsis, 1541
  hyperbaric, therapeutic, 2367
    in critical care, complications from, 495
    toxicity in, 496
Oxygenation. See also *Hypoxemia*
  after coronary artery bypass graft surgery, 338
  equations related to, 485
  red cell mass and, 976
Oxymesterone, for paroxysmal nocturnal hemoglobinuria, 923
Oxymetazoline hydrochloride, for allergic rhinitis, 1955
Oxymetholone, for hairy cell leukemia, 1000
  for myelofibrosis, 987
Oxymorphone, as analgesic, 107t
Oxyphenbutazone, as cyclooxygenase inhibitor, 1275
  for gouty arthritis, 1169
Oxyphenisatin, chronic hepatitis from, 828, 831
Oxyphils, in thyroid tumors, 1335
Oxypurinol, elimination rate for, 96t
Oxytetracycline, 121
  elimination rate for, 96t
  in kidney and liver failure, 117t
Oxytocin, 1305, 1313
  and milk let-down reflex, 1293
  antidiuretic action of, 540
  deficiency of, 1295
  synthesis of, 1280
Oxyuris vermicularis, 1910
Ozena, definition of, 897
Ozone, and chemical pneumonitis, 2367

P cells, 250
  suppression of, 251
P waves, in electrocardiography, 197, 198
  in rhythm analysis, 254
Pacemaker(s), 271–272
  for amyloidosis, 360
  for atrioventricular block, 262
  for congenital complete heart block, 316
  for heart block from myocardial infarction, 333
  for idiopathic restrictive cardiomyopathy, 361
  for sinoatrial block, 261
  indications for, 271–272, 272t
  lead placement for, 272
  pulse generators for, 272
Pacemaker cells, 250
  suppression of, 251
Pachydermoperiostosis, 1519, 2046
  cancer and, 1112
Pacini's corpuscles, 2303
Packed red blood cells, 947, 947t
  for gastrointestinal hemorrhage, 797
  iron in, 931
  unit of, in fluid replacement therapy, 533
  volume of, in anemia, 878
PAF (platelet activating factor), 1986
Paget's disease of bone, 1515–1517
  breast cancer with, 1111
  calcitonin for, 1506
  high output heart failure from, 216
  juvenile, 1519
  osteosarcoma in, 1521
Pagophagia, 880
  definition of, 897

Pain, 104–111
  abdominal, in gastrointestinal disease, 657–658
  acute, 104–105
  after spinal cord injury, 2246
  assessment of, 105–106
  at ovulation, 1430
  at rest, in arteriosclerosis obliterans, 380
  atypical, in face, 2133
  chest, in cardiovascular patient history, 175
  chest wall, 175
  chronic, vs. hypochondriasis, 2102
  cramping, from ischemic colitis, 764
    from mesenteric artery embolism, 763
  deafferentation, 105
    neurostimulatory procedures for, 110
  definition of, 104
  endorphins and, 1270
  epigastric, postprandial, from superior mesenteric artery syndrome, 765
  etiologic characteristics of, 105
  from abdominal abscess, 793
  from aneurysms, 370
  from appendicitis, 801
  from ascites, 791
  from autosomal dominant polycystic kidney disease, 645
  from bronchogenic carcinoma, 463
  from cancer, 1089
  from celiac compression syndrome, 762
  from chronic pancreatitis, 779
    treatment for, 780
  from common duct obstruction, 862
  from deep-vein thrombosis, 385
  from dental problems, 2134
  from dissecting aortic aneurysms, 373
  from diverticulitis, 804
  from epidemic pleurodynia, 1810–1811
  from esophagus motor disorders, 684
  from Fabry's disease, 1145
  from gallstones, 864
  from gastric lymphoma, 712
  from gastritis, 689
  from hepatic porphyria, 1185
  from herniated disc, 2253
  from intermittent cholangitis, 868
  from liver disease, 808
  from nephroblastoma, 654
  from paravertebral tumors, 2254
  from peptic ulcers, 697
  from pleura, 466
  from renal artery occlusion, 633
  from shock, morphine sulfate for, 244
  from sudden arterial occlusion, 383
  from tabes dorsalis, 2189
  from thoracic aortic aneurysm, 371
  from urinary tract obstruction, 615
  from vaso-occlusive crisis, in sickle cell anemia, 939
  in abdomen, from allergic purpura, 1058
  in back, 2043–2044. See also *Back, pain in*
  in bone. See *Bone(s), pain in*
  in chest. See also *Angina pectoris*
    causes of, 324
  in dying patients, 32
  in ear, 2134
  in elbow, 2047
  in extremities, from thromboangiitis obliterans, 382
  in feet, from polycythemia vera, 981
  in head. See *Headache*
  in muscle, 2270
  in neck, and headache, 2135
  in shoulder, 2041–2043
  intensity and perception of, factors affecting, 658

Pain (Continued)
management of, 106–111. See also *Pain management*
neural pathway for, 2128
of gastrointestinal disease, 656
pericardial, 175
physiologic characteristics of, 105
pleural, 175
from lung abscess, 436
in tuberculosis, 1685
psychogenic, 106, 2101
referred, 106
in gastrointestinal disease, 658
sensitivity to, in spine, 2248, *2248*
shoulder girdle–scapular, 2267
somatic, 105
cordotomy for, 111
temporal characteristics of, 104–105
thalamic, 2128
types of, 2249
visceral, 105
Pain management, 106–111
anesthetic procedures for, 109–110, 110t
behavioral therapy for, 109
drug therapy for, 106–109
adjuvant analgesics in, 108t, 109
and hemolysis in glucose-6–phosphate dehydrogenase deficiency, 916
combinations of drugs in, 108
for hemophilia A, 1068
for pneumococcal pneumonia, 1559
narcotic analgesics in, 107t, 107–109
non-narcotic analgesics in, 107, 107t
neurolytic nerve blocks for, 109
neurosurgical procedures for, 110t, 110–111
physical therapy for, 109
placebo effects in, 106
postoperative, 108
Paint, hydrocarbons in, and kidney damage, 612
Palate, soft, taste buds in, 2110
Paleospinothalamic tract, 2128
Pallesthesia, 2128
Pallor, from pheochromocytoma, 284
Palmar erythema, from liver disease, 809
in alcoholic cirrhosis, 844
Palpation, in cardiovascular patient history, 175
Palpitations
from arteriovenous fistula, 384
from hemolysis, 908
from mitral valve prolapse, 350
from pheochromocytoma, 284, 1464
Palsy
Bell's, in sarcoidosis, 2266
pseudobulbar, 2090
supranuclear, progressive, 2145, 2153t
ulnar, 2268
Pancarditis, rheumatic, 363
Pancoast's tumor, and arm, 459
pain from, 105
Pancolitis, 753. See also *Ulcerative colitis*
Pancreas
annular, gastric outlet obstruction from, 707
artificial, 1373
ascites of, 776, 792
blood flow regulation in, peptides and, 239
cancer of, 673
celiac plexus block for pain from, 110
in cigarette smokers, 38
vs. chronic pancreatitis, 673
carcinoma of, 781–784
computed tomography for, 662
gastric outlet obstruction from, 707
symptoms of, 781t

Pancreas (Continued)
carcinoma of, vs. chronic pancreatitis, 779
disease of. See also *Pancreatitis*
and eosinophilia, 1026
lobular panniculitis with, 2050
pain from, 656
vitamin B$_{12}$ deficiency from, 904
enzymes from, gastritis from, 689
ileus from, 695
ulcers from, 695
islets of Langerhans in, 1387, *1387*
in multiple endocrine neoplasia, 1458, 1459
tumors of, 1387–1390. See also *Islet cell tumor(s)*
and growth hormone secreting pituitary tumor, 1301
and VIP production, 727
loss of sodium bicarbonate from, and metabolic acidosis, 532
neoplasms of, ACTH from, 1354
spread of, to kidneys, 655
Zollinger-Ellison syndrome and, 709
normal anatomy and physiology of, 775
pain from, 658
pseudocysts of, 468–469, 1040
transplantation of, 1373
Pancreas divisum, 775
Pancreatic cholera syndrome, 1388–1389, 1389t
diarrhea from, 727, 731
Pancreatitis, 673, 774–780
acute, 775–779, *777*
adverse prognostic signs in, 778t
complications of, 778t, 778–779
from endoscopic retrograde cholangio-pancreatography, 671
vs. acute cholecystitis, 866
vs. appendicitis, 801, 802, 803
and myocardial depression, 239
and obstruction of distal common duct, 870
ascites from, 792
chronic, 779–780, *780*
complications of, 779t
diabetes mellitus from, 1362
secondary biliary cirrhosis from, 846
vitamin B$_{12}$ deficiency from, testing for, 738t
vs. pancreatic cancer, 673, 783
with chronic liver disease, 810
classification of, 775
computed tomography for, 662, *663*
etiologic factors in, 775t
from acute viral hepatitis, 820
from ascariasis, 1909
from chylomicronemia syndrome, 1143
from clonorchiasis, 1902
from common duct stones, 868
from renal artery atheroembolization, 633
gastric outlet obstruction from, 707
mumps and, 1779
pain from, vs. gallbladder pain, 776
pleural effusion from, 468–469
total parenteral nutrition for, 1244, 1248t
vomiting from, 658
vs. familial Mediterranean fever, 1197
vs. gallstones, 864
vs. myocardial infarction, 332
vs. peptic ulcers, 699
vs. postcholecystectomy syndrome, 872
with bile duct compression, jaundice from, 817
with mumps infection, 2194
Pancytopenia
causes of, 888
definition of, 882

Pancytopenia (Continued)
from Banti's syndrome, 1038
from hairy cell leukemia, 999
from leukemia, 1004
Pandysautonomia, acute, 2106
postinfectious, 2262
Panencephalitis, rubella, progressive, 2206–2207
sclerosing, subacute, 2203, 2206–2207
vs. multiple sclerosis, 2212
Panic, from psychedelic drugs, 59
Panic disorder, 2100, 2100t
Panniculitis, lobular, 2050
mesenteric, 795
septal, 2050–2051
Panniculus adiposus, 2300
Pannus, in rheumatoid arthritis, 1999
Pantothenic acid, dietary requirements for, 1206t
Papanicolaou's smear, for herpes, 1703
Papilla of Vater, ultrasonography of, 664
Papillary muscle(s)
abnormalities in, and mitral regurgitation, 348
dysfunction in
after myocardial infarction, 333
from sarcoidosis, 360
vs. mitral regurgitation, 349
vs. mitral valve prolapse, 351
necrosis of, from analgesic nephropathy, 628
of kidneys, 632
pyelonephritis with, 629
rupture of, from myocardial infarction, 333
stenosis of, 674
Papilledema
and increased intracranial pressure, 2235
brain tumors with, 2232
causes of, 2292t
cryptococcosis and, 1845
definition of, 2292
from lateral sinus thrombosis, 2185
from pituitary tumors, 1298
from sarcoidosis, 453
malignant hypertension and, 276
vision loss from, 2113
vs. optic neuritis, 2113t
Papillitis, 2112, 2292
definition of, 2215
Papillomas, 464
of bile ducts, 871
Papillomaviruses, interferon for, 128
Pa-ping, 546
Pappataci fever, 1817
Para-aminosalicylic acid
acute interstitial nephritis from, 605
and rifampin absorption, 99
in drug interactions, 124t
toxicity of, to hemoglobin, 945
Paracentesis
abdominal, for ascites, 790, 791
in cirrhosis, 851
repeated, 851
for adenocarcinoma of peritoneum, 794
for primary mesothelioma, 794
in heart failure management, 225
Paracetamol, as cyclooxygenase inhibitor, 1275
Paracoccidioidomycosis, 1843–1844
Parafollicular cells, 1505–1506
Paragonimiasis, 1903–1904
Paragonimus westermani, lung abscess from, 436
Paraldehyde, metabolic acidosis from, 554
Paralysis
after acute hemorrhagic conjunctivitis, 1814

Paralysis (Continued)
  dialysis and, 577
  focal, frontal lobe damage and, 2082
  from amyotrophic lateral sclerosis, 2156
  from botulism, 1633
  from coxsackieviruses, 1808
  from Guillain-Barré syndrome, 2261
  from poliovirus infection, 2198–2199
  from rabies, 2201
  from severe brain injury, 2241
  from spinal epidural abscess, 2186
  from spinal epidural hematoma, 2257
  from sudden arterial occlusion, 383
  from superior sagittal sinus thrombosis,
      2185
  from tick-borne encephalitis, 1829
  from ticks, 1923
  gaze, 2116
  hypokalemic periodic, 546
  in nonpolio enteroviral infection, 1810
  of diaphragm, 472
  of the insane, 2188–2189
  of vocal cords, from dissecting aortic
      aneurysms, 373
  periodic, 2280–2282, 2281t
  respiratory, from scorpion stings, 1924
      from spinal cord trauma, 2245
  skeletal muscle permeability to potassium
      and, 545
  Todd's, after seizures, 2218
  transient focal motor, 2128, 2128t
  venous thrombosis in, 385
Paralytic ileus, anticholinesterases for, 140
  from cholera, 1653
  from potassium deficiency, 547
Paramedian incisional biopsy, 2313
Parameningeal infections, 2181–2187
  brain abscess as, 2183, 2181–2183
  cerebral epidural abscess as, 2184
  dural sinus thrombosis as, 2184–2185
  subdural empyema as, 2183–2184
  vs. bacterial meningitis, 1608
Paramesonephric ducts, 1392, 1428–1429
Paramyotonia congenita, 2281, 2284
Paramyxovirus, 1760
Paranasal sinus(es)
  aspergillosis in, 1851
  headache from, 2134
  infection of, and brain abscess, 2181
      and subdural empyema, 2183–2184
Paraneoplastic syndromes, 1097–1099
  and nervous system, 1104, 1105t
  definition of, 459, 1097
Paranoia, 2093
  from acute amphetamine toxicity, 55
Paraparesis, spastic, tropical, 1797
Paraphenylenediamine, and contact derma-
      titis, 2319
Paraplegia(s)
  and testicular function, 1416
  and testosterone levels, 1415
  from cancer, 1106
  from dissecting aortic aneurysms, 373
  from extradural tumors, 2255
  from neuromyelitis optica, 2215
  from spinal cord compression, in multi-
      ple myeloma, 1032
  spastic, hereditary, 2154
Paraproteinemias, 1026. See also Plasma
      cell(s), disorders of
  and chronic interstitial nephritis, 606
  purpura in, 1059
Parapsoriasis, chronic, 2326t
Paraquat
  and kidney damage, 612
  interstitial lung disease from, 434–435
  poisonings with, treatment for, 143, 145
  reference intervals for, 2403t

Pararotaviruses, 1769
Parasellar disorder, vs. pituitary tumor,
      1299
Parasellar neoplasms, diagnostic imaging
      techniques for, 2060
Parasites
  and diarrhea, diagnosis of, 730
  disease from, in bile ducts, 870
      peritonitis from, 794
  drugs for, in treatment of malabsorption,
      741t
  eosinophilia from, 1025
  granulomatous peritonitis from, 794
  red cell, hemolysis from, 924
  removal of, by spleen, 1036
  respiratory failure from, 475
Parasitosis, intestinal, vs. peptic ulcers, 699
Parasomnias, 2079t, 2079–2080
Paraspinal abscess, 1622
Parasympathetic nervous system, 133
  and asthma, 406
  of heart, 184
  receptors for, 137
Parasystole, ventricular, 263–264
Parathion, as cholinesterase inhibitor, 140
Parathyroid gland(s), 1252
  and hypercalciuria, 642
  hyperplasia of, in multiple endocrine
      neoplasia, 1460
  hypoplasia of, 1945
  in multiple endocrine neoplasia, 1458,
      1459
  tissue of, abnormal, preoperative localiza-
      tion of, 1494–1495
      autotransplantation of, 1510
Parathyroid hormone, 1252, 1486–1488
  action of, 1486–1487, 1487
  and calcium absorption, by intestine, 519
      by kidneys, 519
  and calcium homeostasis, 1469–1470,
      1470t
  and kidney function, 502
  and phosphate reabsorption, 1193
  and phosphorus reabsorption, 518
  and sodium reabsorption, 513, 516
  catabolism of, in kidneys, 519
  deficiency of, 1496. See also Hypoparathy-
      roidism
  hypersecretion of, and resorption hyper-
      calciuria, 640
  immunoreactive, 1487
  in chronic kidney failure, 565, 1507
  increased, and renal phosphate wasting,
      1193
  levels of, aging and, 25
  measurement of, radioimmunoassay for,
      1488
  radioimmunoassay of, 1492, 1493
  regulation of, set point for, 1508
  release of, 1486, 1486
      control of, in renal insufficiency, 1507–
          1508
      excessive, 1488. See also Hyperparathy-
          roidism
Parathyroidectomy, for renal osteodystro-
      phy, 1510
Paratracheal adenopathy, from sarcoidosis,
      451, 453
Paraventricular nuclei, 1305
Paravertebral muscles, pain in, 2248, 2249
  spasm in, 2250
Paravertebral tumors, 2254–2255
Paregoric, for diarrhea, from ulcerative coli-
      tis, 758
  in Crohn's disease, 752
Parenchymal cells
  damage to, from inflammatory cells, 425
  disease in, pleural tuberculosis from, 467

Parenchymal cells (Continued)
  disease in, uremia from, 568–569
  hemorrhage in, from systemic lupus ery-
      thematosus, 429
  infiltrates of, respiratory failure from, 475
      reticulonodular, from sarcoidosis, 451
  inflammation of, white cell casts and, 503
  iron in, 361, 1190
  renal, anomalies of, 649
Parenteral nutrition, 1247–1251
  complications of, 1250, 1250t
  infection control in, 1546
  total, 1248–1250. See also Total parenteral
      nutrition
Paresis, from syphilis, 1718, 2188–2189
Paresthesia(s), definition of, 2259
  in multiple sclerosis, 2213
  in partial seizures, 2220
Parietal cells, epithelial, 509
  in stomach, 693
Parietal epithelial cells, 509
Parietal lobe, damage to, 2081–2082, 2082t
Parinaud's syndrome, 1314, 2116
Parkinsonism, 25, 2143, 2144
  arteriosclerotic, 2144
  classification of, 2143, 2143t
  fatigue in, 2125
  from drugs, 2141
      abuse of, 55
      for schizophrenia, 2094
  from MPTP, 60
  gait of, 2126
  hyperthermic syndrome in, 2282
  hypoparathyroidism and, 1497
  in idiopathic autonomic insufficiency,
      2106
  management of, 2145
  postural hypertension and, 1466
  striatonigral degeneration in, 2145
  tremor in, 2142
  vascular, 2144–2145
  vs. essential tremor, 2146
  with dementia, 2145
Paromomycin, for tapeworms, 1895
Paronychia, 2347
  definition of, 2334
  from Candida infection, 1848
Parotid gland, enlargement of, in alcoholic
      cirrhosis, 844
  hypertrophy of, from cirrhosis, 847
  in Sjögren's syndrome, 2024
Parotitis, epidemic, 1778
Paroxysmal supraventricular tachycardia,
      258, 259
  anticholinesterases for, 140
  carotid sinus pressure for, 255t
  DC cardioversion for, 273
  encainide for, 270
  procainamide for, 270, 259
  quinidine for, 270
  surgery for, 274
  treatment of, 257t
Parrots, psittacosis from, 1735
Pars anterior, 1290
Pars distalis, 1290
Pars intermedia, 1290
Pars recta, 510, 512
Pars tuberalis, 1290
Partial seizures, 2218–2221. See also Seizures
Partial thromboplastin time, 816
  activated, 1047, 1061
      evaluation of, 1065
  reference intervals for, 2400t, 2402t
Parvovirus, 1767
  and rheumatoid arthritis, 1991
  aplastic anemia from, 886
Pastes, 2315
Pasteur, 5

Pastia's lines, 1576
Patau's syndrome, 167t
Patch tests, for allergic contact testing, 2311, 2313
Patella, hypoplasia of, 638
Patent ductus arteriosus, 307–308
  pulsed-wave Doppler echocardiography for, 205
Paternity testing, HLA typing in, 1964
Paterson-Kelly syndrome, iron deficiency anemia and, 897
Pathergy, definition of, 2313
Patient(s), 1–2
  as consumer, 8
  clinical approach to, 70–74
  clubs for, 8
  dying. See Dying patients
  education of, 2
  evaluation of, selection for, in secondary hypertension, 282
  examination of, for neurologic disorders, 2054–2055
  expectations of, 1–2
  history in. See Patient history
  ideal, qualities of, 2
  influence of, in critical care decisions, 498–499
  interview of, 71–72
  management of, 73
  medical students and, 4
  physician communication with, 2
  physicians and, 7
  preferences of, medical ethics and, 13–14
  psychologic consequences of critical care for, 497
  selection of, for coronary artery bypass grafts, 337
  understanding by, of rheumatic disease management, 1980
  with cardiovascular disease, approach to, 175–179
  with neurologic symptoms, management of, 2053
Patient history
  arrhythmias and, 254
  dermatologic, 2306–2307
  for acute myocardial infarction, 330
  for epilepsy, 2223
  for gastrointestinal disease, 656
  for occupational lung disease, 2356
  for valvular heart disease, 340
  in cardiovascular workup, 175–176
  occupational and environmental factors in, 2354–2355
  of elderly, 27
  of hypertensive patients, 282
Pattern recognition, in diagnosis, 2054
  in electrocardiography, 197, 199–201
Pautrier's abscesses, 1108
PBG (porphobilinogen), 1182
  reference intervals for, 2399t
PCO syndrome, 1287, 1429. See also Polycystic ovarian syndrome
PCP (phencyclidine), abuse of, 58
PDGF. See Platelet-derived growth factor
Peanut butter, aflatoxin in, 787
Peapicker's disease, 1730. See also Leptospirosis
Pectus excavatum, 473
Pedicels, in glomerulus, 509
Pediculosis, 1747, 1920
Pedigree analysis, 147, 147
Pel-Ebstein fever, 1016
Pelger-Huët anomaly, in myelofibrosis, with myeloid metaplasia, 986
Peliosis hepatitis, 828
Pelizaeus-Merzbacher disease, 2216

Pellagra, 1232, 2352
Pelvic brim, obstruction of, 507
Pelvic girdle, weakness of, 2270
Pelvic inflammatory disease, 1708
  acute, vs. appendicitis, 803
Pelvic organs, examination of, magnetic resonance imaging for, 85, 85
Pelvis
  abscess in, 793
  disease in, back pain from, 105, 2250
  fractures of, and fat embolism syndrome, 450
  infection of, 1639
  polymyalgia rheumatica in, 2033
Pemberton's sign, 1339
Pemphigoid, vs. aphthous ulcers, 676
  vs. erythroplakia, 678
  vs. gingivitis, 675
Pemphigus diseases, 2330–2331
  definition of, 2329
  gold salts for, 2317
  immunofluorescent cutaneous findings in, 2305t
  myasthenia gravis with, 2285
  vs. gingivitis, 675
Pendred's syndrome, 1338
Penicillamine
  adverse reactions to, 620
  and kidney damage, 612
  and membranous nephropathy, 596
  and vitamin B$_6$ deficiency, 1233
  as chelating agent after poisonings, 143
  for alcoholic hepatitis, 844
  for rheumatoid arthritis, 2003
  neutropenia from, 963t
  side effects of, 1189
Penicillin(s)
  action of, 113t
  acute allergic interstitial disease from, 505
  acute interstitial nephritis from, 603–605
  allergy to, 123, 1969, 1971
  aminoglycoside with, for Pseudomonas aeruginosa, 437
  anaphylaxis from, 103, 1957
  and decline in acute rheumatic fever, 1579
  and neutrophil destruction, 962
  antistaphylococcal, 119
  binding to erythrocytes, 921
  broad-spectrum, 119–120
  clearance of, kidney disease and, 94
  combination of, and aminoglycosides, 120
  cross-reactivity of, with cephalosporins, 123
  in bile, 116
  in kidney and liver failure, 117t
  interaction of, with aminoglycosides, 124
    with probenecid, 101
  oral desensitization protocol for, 1972t
  penetration into spinal fluid by, 116
  phenoxymethyl, 119
  pneumococci resistance to, 1555
  procaine, 119
  resistance mechanisms of, 116t
  selectivity of, 112
  serum sickness from, 103
Penicillin G, 119
  absorption of, 99
  acute interstitial nephritis from, 603
  elimination rate for, 96t
  in kidney and liver failure, 117t
  pharmacokinetic parameters for, 89t
  pneumococci resistance to, 114
Penicillin V, in kidney and liver failure, 117t
Penis, erection of, 1409
  nocturnal tumescence of, and impotence, 2109

3-Pentadecylcatechol, and contact dermatitis, 2318–2319
Pentaerythritol tetranitrate, for angina pectoris, 326t
Pentagastrin, and increased calcitonin, 1505
  in diagnosis of medullary carcinoma, 1506
Pentamidine
  as prophylactic in Gambian sleeping sickness, 1865
  for African trypanosomiasis, 1864
  for visceral leishmaniasis, 1873
  hypoglycemia from, 1384
  for pneumocystosis, 1880–1881
Pentastomiasis, 1926–1927
Pentazocine, abuse of, 55, 56
  as analgesic, 107t
Pentobarbital, overdose of, and central nervous system, 2069
  reference intervals for, 2403t
Pentolinium, in pheochromocytoma diagnosis, 284
Pentostatin, for cancer, 1123
  for hairy cell leukemia, 1001
Pentosuria, 152, 1135
Pentoxifylline, for arteriosclerosis obliterans, 381
Pepsin, in gastroesophageal reflux disease, 680
  secretion of, 694
  and peptic ulcers, 695
Peptic ulcers, 692–709
  as contraindication to gallstone dissolution therapy, 862
  belladonna alkaloids for, 139
  complications from, 706–708
  diagnostic visualization for, 697–698
  differential diagnosis for, 699
  endoscopy for, 669
  epidemiology of, 696–697
  fistula formation from, 707
  from glucocorticosteroid therapy, 130, 133
  from polycythemia vera, 983
  gastric outlet obstruction by, 716
  gastrointestinal hemorrhage from, 797, 799
  in cigarette smokers, 39
  in Zollinger-Ellison syndrome, 708
  laboratory studies for, 698–699
  long-term maintenance therapy for, 703
  medical therapy for, 700–703
  pain from, vs. pain from other causes, 699t
  pathogenesis of, 692–696
  patient abnormalities in, acid and pepsin secretion and, 695
    genetic factors in, 694–696
  perforated, and amylase level, 776
    fungal peritonitis from, 794
    in elderly, vs. appendicitis, 803
  physical examination for, 697
  surgical therapy for, 703t, 703, 703–705
    and motility disorders, 717
    complications from, 704–705
    gastritis after, 692
    ulcer recurrence after, 705
  symptoms of, 697, 697t
  treatment of, 701–703
    drugs for, 702t
  visualization of, 697, 698
  vs. acute cholecystitis, 866
  vs. adenocarcinomas of small intestine, 773
  vs. appendicitis, 801
  vs. Crohn's disease, 750
  vs. gallstones, 864
  vs. myocardial infarction, 332
  vs. pancreatic cancer, 783

Peptic ulcers (Continued)
  vs. postcholecystectomy syndrome, 872
  vs. small intestine neoplasms, 774
  with polycythemia vera, 981
Peptide(s)
  and pruritus, 2304
  atrial natriuretic, and hypertension, 279
  corticotropin-related, from anterior pituitary, 1291
  from hypothalamus, 1281
  from proteins, 733
  in inflammation, 1986–1987
  opioid, 1268–1270, 1269
Peptide hormones, and gynecomastia, 1451
  measurement of, in precocious puberty, 1428
Pepto-Bismol, for gastritis, 690
Peptococci, 1637
Peptostreptococci, 1637
  lung abscess from, 436
Perchlorate discharge test, 1338
Percodan, abuse of, 55
Percussion, for pneumococcal pneumonia, 1557
Percutaneous catheterization, for direct adrenal vein sampling, 284
  of heart, 211
  of kidneys, 525
Percutaneous transluminal angioplasty
  after myocardial infarction, 334
  for arteriosclerosis obliterans, 381
  for myocardial ischemia, 339
  for renovascular hypertension, 288, 290
Perforated viscus
  as contraindication for colonoscopy, 670
  bloody ascites from, 791
  computed tomography for, 662
  in Crohn's disease, 749
  vs. appendicitis, 801
Perforation
  from peptic ulcers, 706–707
  of appendix, 801
  of colon, from ulcerative colitis, 759
  of gallbladder, 865, 867
  of gastric cancer, 711
  of intestines. See Perforated viscus
Perfusion, in respiration, 400
Perfusion pressure, coronary, 188
  of kidneys, 510
  shock and, 238
Perhexilene, chronic hepatitis from, 828, 831
  for liver disease, 843
Perianal discomfort, from diarrhea, treatment of, 731–732
Perianal fistulas, from Crohn's disease, 749
Perianal skin, itching of, 789
  from enterobiasis, 1910
Periarteritis nodosa, 2028
  hemolysis from, 925
Periarthritis, apatite crystals in, 2038
  calcific, 1508
Pericardial effusion, 364–365
  dialysis and, 577
  echocardiography for, 203, 204
  from hypothyroidism, 369
  from sarcoidosis, 453
  in heart failure, 223
  radiographs of, 194, 195
  vs. constrictive pericarditis, 367
Pericardial friction rubs, 363, 364, 366
  and myocardial infarction, 331
Pericardial tamponade, 176
  ineffectiveness of digitalis for, 228
Pericardiocentesis, 365
  for cardiac tamponade, 366
Pericarditis
  acute, in rheumatoid arthritis, 2002

Pericarditis (Continued)
  acute viral, 363–364, 364
  and atrial fibrillation, 273
  constrictive, 366, 366–367
    cryptogenic cirrhosis from, 847
  from beta thalassemia, 931
  from chronic kidney failure, 565–566
  from enteroviruses, 1811–1812
  from Haemophilus influenzae, 65, 1619
  from meningococcal disease, 1615
  from myocardial infarction, 333–334
  from tularemia, 1666
  ineffectiveness of digitalis for, 228
  pain from, 392, 393
  recurrent, 364
  tuberculosis and, 1689
  vs. appendicitis, 803
  vs. chest pain from myocardial infarction, 335
  vs. myocardial infarction, 332
  vs. pulmonary embolism, 444
  with pericardial effusion, 364
Pericardium. See also under Pericardial
  calcification of, in fluoroscopy, 195
  constriction of, and cardiac catheterization, 212
  cysts of, 363
  diseases of, 362t, 362–367
    acute viral or idiopathic pericarditis as, 363–364, 364
    cardiac tamponade as, 365–366, 365
    etiology of, 362–363
    low output heart failure from, 216
    pericardial effusion as, 364–365
  fluid in, 178, 203
  inflammation of. See Pericarditis
  radiation injury to, vs. irradiation restrictive cardiomyopathy, 361
  tamponade of, 176
Pericholangitis, definition of, 841
  in Crohn's disease, 749
Pericholecystic abscess, vs. acute cholecystitis, 865
Pericolic abscess, from diverticulitis, 804
Peridiverticulitis, 804
Perihepatitis, gonococcal, 834, 1708
  vs. acute cholecystitis, 866
Perilymphatic fistula, unilateral hearing loss from, 2119
Perinephric abscess, 628, 632
  pyelonephritis with, 629
  vs. splenic abscess, 1040
Periodic disease, 1196. See also Familial Mediterranean fever
Periodic paralysis, 2280–2282, 2281t
Periodic peritonitis, 1196. See also Familial Mediterranean fever
Periodontal disease, 675
  and lung abscess, 436
  in AIDS, 677
Periodontitis, juvenile, 960
Periostitis, dactylitis with, 2045
  in cervicofacial actinomycosis, 1674
Peripheral blood compartment, abnormalities in, and neutropenia, 962–963, 962, 963
Peripheral edema
  from amyloidosis, 359
  from constrictive pericarditis, 367
  from Crohn's disease, 747
  from dilated cardiomyopathy, 352
  from heart failure, 215, 223
    in chronic respiratory failure, 481
  from tricuspid regurgitation, 351
Peripheral joints, temperature of, 1162
Peripheral nervous system, 2128–2129
  damage to, from arterial pressure monitoring, 496

Peripheral nervous system (Continued)
  disorders of, 2258–2268. See also Neuropathies
  in chronic kidney failure, 566
  inhalant abuse and, 59
  pain from injury to, management of, 110–111
Peripheral resistance, total, increase in, and hypertension, 278
Peripheral vascular disease
  as hypertensive complication, 293
  beta blockers and, 287
  in cigarette smokers, 37
  in heart failure, 220
Peripheral vestibulopathy, acute, 2123
Peritoneal dialysis, 562. See also Dialysis
  Candida peritonitis and, 1848
  chronic ambulatory, and phaeohyphomycosis, 1855
  continuous ambulatory, 574, 575t
  for acute kidney failure, indications for, 576t
  fungal peritonitis from, 794
  in hyperkalemia treatment, 549
  permanent access for, 575
  pleural fluid after, 467
  sclerosing peritonitis from, 795
  technical aspects of, 574
Peritoneal membrane, permeability of, 574
Peritoneoscopy, 790
Peritoneovenous shunting, for ascites, 851
  sclerosing peritonitis from, 795
Peritoneum, 790
  anatomy and physiology of, 790
  ascitic fluid reabsorption by, 851
  biopsy of, 790
  diseases of, 790–795, 792t
  excess fluid in, 850. See also Ascites
  infection of, 793–794
  neoplasms of, 794–795
Peritonitis
  acute, as contraindication for laparoscopy, 674
  and mesenteric venous thrombosis, 764
  bacterial, acute, 793, 1638, 1658
    spontaneous, 793–794, 851–852
  chylous, 792
  diffuse, vs. from appendicitis, 801, 802
  from contaminated antiseptic compounds, 1548
  from mesenteric artery occlusion, 762
  ileus with, 719
  in familial Mediterranean fever, 1196, 1197
  paroxysmal, benign, 1196. See also Familial Mediterranean fever
  periodic, 1196. See also Familial Mediterranean fever
  sclerosing, 2052
  transperitoneal fluid exchange in, 790
  tuberculous, 1691
  vs. appendicitis, 802
Peritonsillar abscess, from streptococcal tonsillitis, 1576
Perlèche, 2348
Pernicious anemia, 904–905
  and polyglandular autoimmune disease, 1414
  from common variable agammaglobulinemia, 1943
  gastric cancer and, 710, 711
  juvenile, 905
  myasthenia gravis with, 2285
  neurologic disorders in, 2140
  parietal cell antibodies in, 691
  treatment of, 691
  vitamin B$_{12}$ deficiency from, 904
    testing for, 738t

Pernicious anemia (Continued)
  vs. optic neuritis, 2215
  with Hashimoto's thyroiditis, 1333
Pernio, 379–380
Personal hygiene, and common cold prevention, 1757
Personality
  and irritable bowel syndrome, 722
  atopic dermatitis and, 2320
  change in, 2092
    from brain tumors, 2231
    in Creutzfeldt-Jakob disease, 2206
    in Parkinson's disease, 2144
Perspiration. See Sweating
Perstans filariasis, 1919
Perthes' disease, 1517
Pertussis, 1624–1626
  adenovirus and, 1767
  immunization against, 61
  lymphocytosis from, 972
Pesticides, and food poisoning, 786
  poisoning with, and muscles, 2288
Petechiae, 2324
  definition of, 1045
  from bacterial meningitis, 1606
  from fat embolism syndrome, 450
  from fulminant meningococcemia, 1614, 1615
  from infectious mononucleosis, 1787
  from infective endocarditis, 1589t
  from vitamin C deficiency, 1235
Petechial hemorrhage, from aplastic anemia, 887
Petit mal absences, 2221. See also Epilepsy(ies); Seizures
Petit mal epilepsies, 2076, 2218, 2222. See also Epilepsy(ies); Seizures
  electroencephalogram for, 2224
Petrolatum, for skin disorders, 2315
Petroleum distillates, acute poisonings with, treatment for, 144
Pets, and Campylobacter infection, 1651
  vaccination of, for rabies, 2201
Peutz-Jeghers syndrome, 767, 771
  and cancer, 1113
  and neoplasms, 1096t
  polyps of, and cancer of small intestine, 773
Peyer's patches, benign lymphoid hyperplasia of, vs. Crohn's disease, 750
PFK (phosphofructokinase), 2278
PGI₂. See Prostacyclin(s)
PGM (phosphoglycerate mutase), 2278
pH
  and urate solubility in fluid, 1162
  changes in, in severely ill, 484
  disequilibria between plasma and cerebrospinal fluid, 551
  in shock, 241
  monitoring of, in severely ill, 483
    in shock patients, 243
    of reflux, 681
  of arterial blood, equation for, 485
  of cerebrospinal fluid, and respiratory modulation, 550
  PCO_2 and, 475
  reference intervals for, 2398t
Ph¹ chromosome. See Philadelphia chromosome
Phaeohyphomycosis, 1854–1855
Phaeomelanin, 2302
Phagocytes
  and chronic granulomatous disease, 958
  in inflammatory response, 1530
  in lungs, 1552
  mononuclear, 953–957. See also Mononuclear phagocytes
  precursors of, progenitors of, 875

Phagocytic vesicle, 952
Phagocytosis, 1988, 1989
Phakomatoses, 2158–2159
Phalanges, sarcoidosis in, 453
Phalloidin, in mushrooms, 786
Phantom limb pain, 2137
Pharmacokinetics, 87, 88
Pharmacology, 87–98
Pharyngitis
  bacterial, vs. enanthems, 1813
  from group A streptococcal infection, 1574–1575
  from herpes simplex virus, 1782, 1783
  lymphonodular, acute, 1813
  streptococcal, 1575–1576
    and acute rheumatic fever, 1581
    guttate psoriasis after, 2327
    rash with, 2324
    treatment of, 1577
    vs. diphtheria, 1628
    vs. pyoderma, 1577t
  viral, 1757–1758, 1758t
Pharyngoconjunctival fever, 1767
Pharynx
  bejel in, 1723
  diphtheria infection in, 1628
  diverticulum of, regurgitation from, 680
  fascioliasis of, 1903
  gonococcal infections of, 1707
  gonorrhea of, 1706
  herpangina of, 1813
  inflammation of, airway obstruction from, 418
  taste buds in, 2110
  Zenker's diverticulum of, 687
Phenacetin
  and analgesic nephropathy, 607
  and cancer, 1093t
  in analgesics, 654
  metabolism of, in cigarette smokers, 39
  reference intervals for, 2403t
  sulfhemoglobinemia from, 946
  toxicity of, to hemoglobin, 945
Phencyclidine (PCP)
  abuse of, 58
    by adolescents, 21
  adverse reactions from, 59
  and acute kidney failure, 559
  poisonings with, treatment for, 143
  reference intervals for, 2403t
Phenformin, for diabetes mellitus, 1370
Phenindione, acute interstitial nephritis from, 605
Phenmetrazine, abuse of, 54
Phenobarbital
  and enhanced liver metabolism of other drugs, 99
  and smooth endoplasmic reticulum, 157
  and vitamin D metabolism, 1477, 1481
  for anticholinergic substance poisonings, 144
  for epilepsy, 2226t, 2227
  metabolism inhibition of, 101t
  overdose of, and central nervous system, 2069
  pharmacokinetic parameters for, 89t
  reference intervals for, 2404t
Phenol(s), in uremic platelet defect, 1057
  to destroy nerve structures in pain management, 109
Phenolphthalein, as laxative, 722
  ingestion of, diarrhea from, 730
Phenothiazine(s), 1954t
  and antidiuretic hormone release, 540
  and depression, 2096
  and distribution of other drugs, 99
  and extrapyramidal reactions, 143
  and hair growth, 2350

Phenothiazine(s) (Continued)
  and photosensitivity, 2351
  and thirst, 1308
  as analgesics, 108t, 109
  cholestasis from, 827
  constipation from, 660
  for inhibiting intestinal secretion, 732
  for schizophrenia, 2094
  interaction of, with oral contraceptives, 1443
  marrow suppression by, 885
  neutropenia from, 963t
  overdose of, treatment for, 144
  toxicity of, tetanus vs., 1365
Phenotypic differentiation, determinants of, 1392–1393
Phenoxybenzamine, 139
  as vasodilator, 233
Phensuximide, reference intervals for, 2404t
Phentolamine, 139
  affinity of, for alpha receptors, 136
  and microcirculation in shock, 248
  as vasodilator, 233
  for alpha-adrenergic receptors, 134
  for hypertensive crisis, 290t
  for primary pulmonary hypertension, 300–301, 301t
Phenylalanine, 1155
  for cancer, 1123, 1457
  for primary thrombocythemia, 1054
Phenylbutazone
  and acute leukemia, 1002
  and enhanced liver metabolism of other drugs, 99
  and thyroid function, 1321
  as cyclooxygenase inhibitor, 1275
  for ankylosing spondylitis, 2007
  for gouty arthritis, 1169
  genetics in metabolism of, 102
  interaction of
    with hydroxyhexamide, 101
    with methotrexate, 101
    with sulfonylureas, 1370
    with warfarin, 100
  liver granulomas from, 828
  reference intervals for, 2404t
Phenylephrine
  contraindications to, for allergic rhinitis, 1955
  for shock, 248
  hypertension from, 2299
  initial hemodynamic effects of, 247t
Phenylhydrazine, toxicity of, to hemoglobin, 945
Phenylketonuria, 149, 152, 153, 156, 1150t
  classic, 1155–1156
  genetics and, 149
  heredity and, 147
  hypopigmentation in, 2346
  in mothers, and congenital malformations, 171
Phenytoin
  and enhanced liver metabolism of other drugs, 99
  and folate deficiency, 906
  and hair growth, 2350
  and lymphadenopathy, 1008
  and nonketotic hyperosmolar syndrome, 1377
  and vitamin D metabolism, 1477, 1481
  as analgesic, 109
  binding of, to thyroxine-binding globulin, 1317
  chronic hepatitis from, 828, 831
  congenital heart disease from, 303
  dose-dependent kinetics of, 89t, 92
  dosing and adverse effects of, 267t
  in drug interactions, 124t

Phenytoin (Continued)
interstitial lung disease from, 434
liver disease from, 827
liver granulomas from, 828
loading dose for, 89
marrow suppression by, 885
metabolism inhibition of, 101t
by cimetidine, 100
metabolism of, genetics in, 102
osteomalacia from, 1482
pharmacokinetic properties of, 266t
protein binding by, liver or kidney disease and, 94
reference intervals for, 2404t
serum sickness from, 103
side effects of, 2227
Pheochromocytoma(s), 1463–1465
ACTH from, 1354
alpha-adrenergic antagonists for, 139
and heart, 369
beta-adrenergic blockers for, 138
diabetes mellitus from, 1362
diagnosis of, 284, 284–285, 1464t, 1464–1465
heart rate increases from, and angina pectoris, 324
hypertension from, 281
hypertensive encephalopathy with, 2172
in multiple endocrine neoplasia, 1460
treatment of, 292
vs. epilepsy, 2225
vs. hyperthyroidism, 1324
Philadelphia chromosome, 985, 1091
in acute lymphoblastic leukemia, 991
in chronic myelogenous leukemia, 970, 973, 988, 989
in eosinophilic leukemia, 1025
Phlebitis
from erythromycin, 121
from phenytoin, 265
in drug abusers, 57
septic, 385
Phlebothrombosis, 385
Phlebotomine sandflies, 1922
Phlebotomus fever, 1817–1818
Phlebotomus longipes, and cutaneous leishmaniasis, 1873
Phlebotomus papatasii, phlebotomus fever from, 1817
Phlebotomy
and urinary erythropoietin excretion, 978
diagnostic, and iron loss, 880
for chronic obstructive pulmonary disease, 417
for obstructive airway disease, 297
for polycythemia vera, 983, 984
for porphyria cutanea tarda, 1187
for secondary polycythemias, 980
Phlegmon, definition of, 778
Phobias, 2100
Phonation, abnormalities in, from poliomyelitis, 2199
Phonemic paraphasia, 2086
Phorbol ester, and cancer, 44
Phosgene, and chemical pneumonitis, 2367
Phosphatase, distribution of, in healthy population, 80
Phosphate(s). See also Hyperphosphatemia; Hypophosphatemia
absorption of, parathyroid hormone and, 502
and myocardial contractility, 354
as buffer in acid-base balance, 564
as laxative, 722
concentration of, in mesenteric artery occlusion, 762
control of, in renal osteodystrophy, 1509

Phosphate(s) (Continued)
deficiency of, and abnormal bone mineralization, 1479
depletion of, hypercalciuria from, 519
in diabetic ketoacidosis, 1376
economy of, 1472–1473
for hypercalcemia, 1504
homeostasis of, disorders of, and osteomalacia and rickets, 1481
in kidney stones, 638
in plasma, interrelationship with calcium, 1472
levels of, in chronic kidney failure, 565
in hypoparathyroidism treatment, 1498
renal leak of, and fasting hypercalciuria, 640
retention of, and secondary hyperparathyroidism, 1507
supplemental, milk as source of, 1194
wasting of, 505
Phosphaturia, in tubulointerstitial disease, 603
Phosphodiesterase inhibitor drugs, for heart failure, 235
Phosphofructokinase, deficiency of, and myopathy, 2278
Phosphofructose, muscle activity deficiency of, 1135
Phosphoglycerate mutase, deficiency of, and myopathy, 2278
Phosphoinositide turnover, stimulation of, 1260
Phospholipid(s), 1138
in hormone action, 1260
in inflammation, 1986
methylation of, stimulation of, 1260
Phospholipoprotein, in hemostasis, 1043
Phosphoribosylpyrophosphate synthetase, and gout, 1167
Phosphorus
circulating forms of, 1470, 1470
deficiency of, 1193–1194
dietary requirements for, 1472
distribution of, 1471
in healthy population, 80
function of, 1193
in plasma, 1471–1472
metabolism of, kidneys and, 518
normal distribution of, in body, 1473
normal ranges for, 1193, 1471
recommended dietary allowance for, 1205t
reference intervals for, 2399t
Phosphorylase system, defects in, 1134, 2278
Photoallergic reactions, 2351, 2351t
Photocoagulation, for proliferative diabetic retinopathy, 1378
Photodermatitis, 2319, 2319t
Photon absorptiometry, for bone evaluation, 1476
Photons, 2375
Photopatch testing, 2313
Photophobia, in Rocky Mountain spotted fever, 1742
Photosensitivity of skin, 2350–2352
from drug allergy, 1970t
from protoporphyria, 840, 1184
Phototoxic reactions, 2350–2351, 2351t
Phthalimidines, for hypertension, 286t
Phylloquinone, 1076, 1240. See also Vitamin K
Physaloptera mordens, 1911
Physical activity, 45–47. See also Exercise
Physical dependence, 52
definition of, 106
in addictive cycle, 50
on narcotic analgesics, 108

Physical examination, 72
arrhythmias and, 254
cardiovascular, 176
for anemias, 881, 881t
for gastrointestinal disease, 657
for hearing, 2118
for mitral stenosis, 346
for preventive health, 66–67, 67t
for valvular heart disease, 340
for vestibular system, 2121
of afferent visual system, 2112
of elderly, 27–28
of hypertensive patients, 282
of myocardial infarction patients, 330–332
Physical fitness, 45
Physical therapy
for chronic obstructive pulmonary disease, 417
for multiple sclerosis, 2214
for parkinsonism, 2145
in treatment for malnutrition, 1215
respiratory, 480
Physics, in medicine, 5
Physostigmine, 139
for anticholinergic substance poisonings, 144
Phytolacca americana, toxicity of, 787
Phytophotodermatitis, 2351
Piaget, Jean, and stages of cognitive development, 17, 17t
Pica, from iron deficiency anemia, 897
iron deficiency and, 880, 896
Pick's disease, 2083, 2091
Pickwickian syndrome, 477
heart in, 176, 2079
hypersomnia in, 2079
obesity and, 1224
polycythemia from, 979
Picornaviridae, 2198
Picrotoxin, obsolescence of, 481
PID (pelvic inflammatory disease), 1708
vs. appendicitis, 803
PIE (pulmonary infiltration with eosinophilia) syndrome, 434
Piebaldism, 2345
PIF (prolactin inhibiting factor), 1280
Pigbel, 1631
Pigeon breeder's disease, 1851
Pigmentation, from ACTH secretion, 1291, 1304
Pigmenturia, 943
Pili torti, definition of, 2349
Pilocarpine, side effects of, 2299
Piloerection, from psychedelic drugs, 58
in opioid withdrawal syndrome, 57
Pilosebaceous appendages, 2302–2303
Pindolol, 137, 138t
affinity of, for beta-adrenergic receptors, 138
for angina pectoris, 327t
for hypertension, 287t
Pineal, 1313–1315
neoplasms of, 1286, 1314–1315, 2230
regulation of, control system for, 1313, 1314
Pink puffers, 297, 415
Pinocytosis, 955
Pinta, 1723
Pinworms, 1910
PIP (proximal interphalangeal) joints, rheumatic disease in, 2001
Piperacillin, 119, 120
for lung abscess, 437
in kidney and liver failure, 117t
treatment with, 119
Piperazine(s), 1954t
for ascariasis, 1909

Pirenzepine, for inhibiting acid secretion, 700
Piretanide, 232
  properties of, 231t
Piroxicam, as cyclooxygenase inhibitor, 1275
PIT (plasma iron transport rate), 895
Pit vipers, 1927
  envenomation from, 1928, 1928t
Pitting, definition of, 2346
Pituitary
  adenomas of, 2230
    and Cushing's disease, 1354
    hyperprolactinemia from, and testicular failure, 1417
    in multiple endocrine neoplasia, 1459
    prolactin hypersecretion from, 2232
  anatomy of, 1290
  and amenorrhea, 1437
  and diabetes insipidus, 1308–1311
  and obesity, 1225
  anterior, 1290–1305
    cell types in, 1290–1291
    hormone function tests for, 1293–1294
    hormones from, 1291t, 1291–1293
      neurotransmitters and, 1283t
    in multiple endocrine neoplasia, 1458
    vascular supply of, 1280–1281
  apoplexy of, 1295, 1298, 2135, 2232
  assessment of functional reserve of, 1349
  CT scans of, 1356
  disorders of. See also Hypopituitarism
    and hormone deficiencies, 1417
    and secondary hypogonadism, 1416–1418
    anemia with, 892
    from Langerhans cell granulomatosis, 1023
  enlargement of, vs. tumor of, 1299
  glandular portion of, 1290
  hemorrhage in, hypopituitarism from, 1295
  hormones from, and hypothalamic hormones, 1281, 1281–1283
  hyperfunction of, 1300–1305
  in puberty, 17
  iron deposition in, and impotence, 1417
  neoplasms of, 1297–1300
    ACTH hypersecretion from, 1304–1305. See also Cushing's syndrome
    and impotence, 2109
    CT scan of, 1298–1299, 1298
    growth hormone secretion from, 1300–1305
    headache from, 2135
    magnetic resonance image of, 1299, 1299
    prognosis for, 2235
    prolactin hypersecretion from, 1302–1303
  posterior, 1305–1313
    antidiuretic hormone from, 1305–1308
    oxytocin from, 1313
Pituitary-hypothalamic axis, dysfunction of, in affective disorders, 2095–2096
Pityriasis alba, 2345
Pityriasis lichenoides et varioliformis, 2326t, 2328
Pityriasis rosea, 2326t, 2327, 2327–2328
  vs. secondary syphilis, 1716
Pityriasis rubra pilaris, 2326t, 2328
Pityrosporon orbiculare, 2323
  tinea versicolor from, 2322, 2322
PK (pyruvate kinase), 916, 917
PKU. See Phenylketonuria
PKUaid, for phenylketonuria, 1156

Placebo effect, in antiviral therapy, 125
  in pain management, 106
Placenta, immunoglobulins crossing, 1935
Placenta previa, and kidney failure, 637
  smoking and, 39
Placental lactogen, as tumor marker, 1099
Plague, 1661–1663
  immunization against, 65
    before travel, 1550
Plantar warts, 2324
Plants
  agricultural, recombinant DNA research on, 159
  alkaloids from, and food poisoning, 787
  phototoxicity from, 2351
  poisoning from, 145, 786
  products from, in cancer treatment, 1125–1126
Planum temporale, left, 2086
Plasma
  basal atriopeptin levels in, 1279
  bilirubin in, 812
  fresh frozen, for gastrointestinal hemorrhage, 797
    for hemophilia B, 1071
  in fluid replacement therapy, 533
    for thrombotic thrombocytopenic purpura, 1053
  normal, erythropoietin in, 978
    osmolality of, 1307
  vitamin B_{12} in, 903
  volume of, 529
    and polycythemia, 975
    increased, anemia and, 879
    reference intervals for, 2402t
Plasma cell(s)
  disorder(s) of, 1026–1036
    heavy chain diseases as, 1034
    immunocytic amyloidosis as, 1034–1035
    monoclonal gammopathies of undetermined significance as, 1035
    multiple myeloma as, 1027–1033. See also Multiple myeloma
    skin in, 1109
    Waldenström's macroglobulinemia as, 1033–1034. See also Waldenström's macroglobulinemia
  immunoglobulin secretion by, 1026
Plasma exchange therapy, for Goodpasture's syndrome, 590
  for idiopathic rapidly progressive glomerulonephritis, 591
Plasma oncotic pressure, abnormal Starling forces and, 535
  normal, 245
  restoration of, volume replacement for, 240
Plasma proteins
  deficiency of, genetics and, 155t
  drug binding to, 100
  hormones and, 1256
  purified, for fluid replacement, 245
Plasma renin activity, 1350
  in hypertensive patients, 278
  in primary aldosteronism, 1358–1359
Plasmacytoma, extramedullary, and skin, 1109
Plasmacytosis, in marrow, in multiple myeloma, 1030
Plasmapheresis
  for Guillain-Barré syndrome, 2261
  for hemophilia B, 1073
  for myasthenia gravis, 2287
  for porphyria cutanea tarda, 1187
  for thrombotic thrombocytopenic purpura, 1053

Plasmapheresis (Continued)
  for Waldenström's macroglobulinemia, 1033–1034
Plasmin, in fibrinolysis, 1064
Plasminogen-activating factor, and coronary artery thrombosis, 330
Plasmodium, in liver, 835t
Plasmodium falciparum
  chloroquine-resistant, 1550
  hemolysis from, 924
  in liver, 835t
  malaria from, 916, 1857, 1857t
  vs. Babesia, 1885
Plateau waves, 2076, 2236
  and drop attacks, 2127
  headache from, 2133
  in brain, 2062
Platelet(s), 1043–1044, 1045
  agglutination of, in shock, 241
  aggregation of, 1047
    coronary artery thrombosis from, 330
  and factor V, 1073
  aspirin and, 1275
  Chédiak-Higashi disease and, 958–959
  disorders of, 1044t
    drugs and, 1046t
    in hypophosphatemia, 1194
    in polycythemia vera, 982
    and myelosuppressive therapy, 984
  in spleen, 1037
  inhibition of adhesiveness of, from cephalosporins, 120
  life span of, 877
  normal count for, 1043
  precursors of, 874
  production of, decreased, thrombocytopenia from, 1048
  increased, in primary thrombocythemia, 1054
  qualitative disorders of, 1055–1058
  quantitative disorders of, 1047–1055
  release action for, abnormalities in, 1057
  secretion of, 1042
  thromboxane A_2 and, 1271
  transfusions of, 1058
    for acute leukemia, 1006
    for idiopathic thrombocytopenic purpura, 1050
Platelet activating factor, 1531
  from mast cells in asthma, 404
    allergic rhinitis and, 1952
  in immune complex disease, 1961
  in inflammation, 1986
Platelet count, 882
  and hemorrhage, 1046
  reference intervals for, 2402t
Platelet-derived growth factor, 322, 425
  and regulation of cellular proliferation, 1091
  in cancer, 1102
Platelet von Willebrand disease, 1070
Plateletpheresis, 1055
  for chronic myelogenous leukemia, 992
Platinum, toxicity of, 2393
Platybasia, 2258
Platypnea, 394
Plesiomonas, enterotoxins from, and secretory diarrhea, 727
Plethysmography, impedance, for deep-vein thrombosis, 386
Pleura, 466–470. See also Pleural space
  anatomy and physiology of, 466
  diseases of, diagnostic procedures for, 466–467
  from asbestos, 469, 2362
  respiratory failure from, 476
  rheumatoid, 2002

Pleura (Continued)
　effusions of. See Pleural effusion(s)
　infection of, and metastatic brain abscess,
　　2181
　needle biopsy of, 467
　neoplasms of, 469–470
　pain in, 175, 466. See also Pleuritic pain
　plaques in, from asbestos, 2363
　reaction of, to drugs, 1971t
Pleural effusion(s), 222, 467, 467t
　and chronic respiratory failure, 476
　culture of, for lung abscess, 436
　　for pneumonia, 1554
　from abdominal abscess, 793
　from bronchogenic carcinoma, treatment
　　for, 462
　from dissecting aortic aneurysms, 373
　from drug-induced interstitial lung dis-
　　ease, 433
　from heart failure, 223
　from Hodgkin's disease, 1016
　from hypereosinophilic syndrome, 1024
　from legionnaires' disease, 1571
　from lung abscess, 436
　from lymphangioleiomyomatosis, 432
　from pneumococcal pneumonia, 1560
　from pulmonary embolism, 445
　from pulmonary veno-occlusive disease,
　　302
　from sarcoidosis, 454
　from systemic sclerosis, 2022
　from tuberculosis, 1689
Pleural friction rub, 466
Pleural space. See also Pleura
　blood in, 468
　fluid in, 466
　gas in, 469–470. see also Pneumothorax
　pus in, 435. see also Empyema
Pleurisy, 392–393
　diaphragmatic, 392
　treatment of, 393–394
Pleuritic pain, 175, 466
　from familial Mediterranean fever, 1197
　from lung abscess, 436
　from pulmonary embolism, 444
　from tuberculosis, 1685
Pleuritis, from collagen vascular disease,
　　pulmonary embolism vs., 444
Pleurodynia, epidemic, 1810–1811
　pulmonary embolism vs., 444
　vs. poliomyelitis, 2199
Pleuropneumonia-like organisms, 1561
Plexiform lesions, 298
　in Eisenmenger's syndrome, 316
PLT (primed lymphocyte test), 1964
Plummer-Vinson syndrome, iron deficiency
　　anemia and, 897
Plummer's disease, 1339
Plutonium, inhalation of, 2376
　toxicity of, 2393
PML (polymorphous light eruption), 2352
PMNs. See Polymorphonuclear leukocytes
PMS (premenstrual syndrome), 1433–1434,
　　1434t
PMV (prolapse of mitral valve), 2164
Pneumatoceles, staphylococcal, pneumo-
　　thorax from, 470
Pneumaturia, 504
　from diverticulitis, 804
Pneumococcal pneumonia, 1554–1560
　clinical findings in, 1556–1557
　epidemiology of, 1555
　laboratory findings for, 1557
　pathogenesis of, 1555–1556
　pathology of, 1556
　penicillin dosage for, 113
　prevention of, 1560
　prognosis for, 1560

Pneumococcal pneumonia (Continued)
　roentgenography for, 1558, 1557–1558
　shock and, treatment for, 246
　sputum in, 391
　treatment of, 1558–1560
Pneumococcus(i), 1554–1555
　cephalosporins for, 120
　disease from, immunization against, 63
　　of elderly, 62t
　infection of, in acquired immunodefi-
　　ciency syndrome, 1806
　resistance of, to penicillin G, 114
Pneumoconiosis
　and mycobacterial infection, 1694
　coal workers', 2361–2362
　definition of, 432
　treatment of, 428
Pneumocystis carinii, 1879
　infection of, in acute leukemia, 1006
　interstitial pneumonitis from, vs. from
　　cytomegalovirus, 1785
　trimethoprim/sulfamethoxazole combina-
　　tion for, 119
Pneumocystis carinii pneumonia
　Hodgkin's disease and, 1017
　in AIDS, 1803–1805, 1805t
　trimethoprim-sulfamethoxazole to pre-
　　vent, in lymphocytic leukemias, 1537
　vs. Kaposi's sarcoma, 1807
Pneumocystosis, 1879–1881
Pneumomediastinum, 470–471
　from end-expiratory pressure, 479
Pneumonia(s), 1551–1554. See also names
　　of causative organisms
　and atrial flutter, 258
　and breathing control, 401
　and false-positive syphilis tests, 1719
　aspiration, 436, 1638
　bacterial, after aspiration pneumonitis,
　　2370
　　pleural inflammation in, 468
　　vs. pulmonary blastomycosis, 1842
　chlamydial, in infants, 1735
　　eosinophilia and, 1025
　chronic granulomatous disease and, 958
　clinical manifestations of, 1553–1554
　complications of, 1560
　cytomegalovirus, adenine arabinoside in-
　　effectiveness for, 125
　definition of, 1551
　differential diagnosis for, 1558
　empiric therapy for, 118t
　enteric bacteria and, 1659
　eosinophilic, chronic, as interstitial lung
　　disease, 431
　　vs. tropical eosinophilia, 1916
　from aerobic gram-negative bacilli, 1565–
　　1568
　from glanders, 1670
　from Haemophilus influenzae, 65, 1619
　from influenza, 1766
　from mycoplasmal infection, vs. pneumo-
　　coccal pneumonia, 1558
　　vs. psittacosis, 1736
　from respiratory syncytial virus, 1759
　from streptococci, 1577
　from tetanus, 1636
　from varicella, 1789
　hospital-acquired, 1544
　immunization against, 63
　in agammaglobulinemia, 1943
　in heroin users, 57
　in infants of smoking parents, 39
　in legionnaires' disease, 1570
　in nocardiosis, 1675
　interstitial, from congenital rubella, 1777
　　from respiratory syncytial virus, 1759
　　marrow transplants and, 1040

Pneumonia(s) (Continued)
　lipoid, 434, 2372–2373
　lung abscess in, 436
　measles and, 1773, 1774
　meningococcal, 1614–1615
　necrotizing, 435
　pathophysiology of, 1551
　persistent coccidioidal, 1840
　pleural effusions with, 468
　pneumococcal, 1554–1560. See also Pneu-
　　mococcal pneumonia
　Pneumocystis carinii. See Pneumocystis cari-
　　nii pneumonia
　postoperative, 1566
　primary atypical, 1561
　pulmonary embolism vs., 444
　recurrent aspiration, 1568–1569
　respiratory failure from, 475, 480
　rheumatic, 1583
　risk factors for, 1553t
　staphylococcal, 1600
　tularemia, 1666
　viral, vs. psittacosis, 1736
　vs. appendicitis, 803
　vs. epidemic pleurodynia, 1811
　vs. neonatal myocarditis from enterovi-
　　ruses, 1812
　vs. pericarditis, 364
　vs. pyogenic liver abscess, 836
　vs. tuberculosis, 1686
　whooping cough with, 1625
Pneumonic plague, 1661, 1662, 1662t
Pneumonitis
　and lung abscess, 436
　aspiration, 2369–2371
　　interstitial lung disease vs., 423
　chemical, 1544, 2367
　endocarditis in drug addicts with,
　　1590
　eosinophilic, from drug allergy, 1971t
　in ascariasis, 1909
　from amiodarone, 276
　from chronic active hepatitis, 832
　hydrocarbon, 2372
　hypersensitivity, 425, 433, 2364
　in Q fever, 1748, 1749
　in tuberculosis, 1683
　in tularemia, 1665
　interstitial, 428–429
　　cytomegalovirus, vs. from Pneumocystis
　　　carinii, 1785
　　lymphocytic, 431, 463
　myocardial infarction vs., 332
　radiation, 2365
　vs. acute cholecystitis, 866
Pneumoperitoneum, computed tomography
　　of, 663
　in free perforation of peptic ulcers, 707
Pneumothorax, 469–470
　from ankylosing spondylitis, 430
　from lymphangioleiomyomatosis, 432
　in mechanical ventilation, 488
　respiratory failure from, 476
　spontaneous, dyspnea from, 394
　　from blebs, 420
　　from end-expiratory pressure, 479
　　myocardial infarction vs., 332
　vs. pulmonary embolism, 444
Pneumovax vaccine, for COPD patients,
　　416
Pneumovirus, 1759
PNS. See Peripheral nervous system
Podagra, 1168
Podocytes, in glomerulus, 509
Podophyllotoxins, for cancer, 1126
Pogasta disease, 1819
Poikilocytosis, hepatocyte, 840
　in anemia, 883

Poikilothermia, relative, 2103–2104
POISINDEX, 141
Poison Center Network, 140
Poisoning, 140–145
  accidental, deaths due to, 140t
  and metabolic encephalopathy, 2064t
  antidotes for, 143
  diagnosis of, 141
  etiology of, 140
  fatalities from, 40
  food, 784–787
  from lead, 2385–2387
  from marine animals, 1929–1931, 1930t
  from trace metals, 2385–2393
  prevention of, 141
  toxicity rating for, 141, 142t
  treatment for, 142–145
Pokeweed, toxicity of, 787
Polar body, 1431
  nonfunctional, from meiosis, 162
Poliomyelitis, 2198–2200
  immunization against, 61, 64–65
    agents for, 62t
    before travel, 1550
    paralysis after, agammaglobulinemia
      and, 1943
  lymphocytopenia from, 966
  vs. rabies, 2201
  vs. spinal epidural abscess, 2187
  vs. tick paralysis, 1923
Pollen, and allergic rhinitis, 1952
Pollution, environmental, 2354
Polyamines, as tumor markers, 1100
Polyangiitis overlap syndrome, 2026
Polyarteritis, central retinal artery occlusion
    and, 2298
  cutaneous, 2051
Polyarteritis nodosa, 2026, 2028–2030
  and heart, 369
  aneurysms with, 2174
  from hepatitis B, 823
  Goodpasture's syndrome vs., 590
  intracranial hemorrhage with, 2175
  kidney involvement in, 598–599
  microscopic, 431–432
  neuropathy in, 2266
  small intestinal ulceration from, 807
  Wegener's granulomatosis vs., 599
Polyarthralgia(s)
  in allergic purpura, 1058
  in disseminated gonococcal infection,
    1708
  in rubella, 1776
  in sarcoidosis, 453
Polyarthritis. See also Arthritis
  cancer and, 1099
  causes of, vs. rheumatic fever, 1585
  epidemic, 1819
  in erythema nodosum leprosum, 1699
  in rubella, 1776–1777
  migratory, from rheumatic fever, 1582
Polychondritis, relapsing, 2038
  aneurysms from, 370
  dissecting, 372
  vs. midline granuloma, 2032
Polychromatophilia, in myelofibrosis, with
    myeloid metaplasia, 986
Polycyclic hydrocarbons, and cancer, 1093t,
    1094
Polycyclic lesion patterns, 2310
Polycystic kidney disease, 148, 506, 644–647
  and gout, 1167
  congenital, 170
  hematocrit in, 507
  kidney size in, 568
  prenatal diagnosis of, with ultrasonog-
    raphy, 173

Polycystic kidney disease (Continued)
  sodium loss in, 532
  ultrasonography for, 527
Polycystic ovarian syndrome, 1287, 1429
  and obesity, 1225
  anovulation from, 1439
  excess ovarian androgen synthesis and,
    1431
  hirsutism from, 1446, 1447
  testosterone levels in, 1436
Polycythemia
  absolute, 976–978
  causes of, 976–977, 977t
  clinical evaluation of, 977–978, 978
  erythromelalgia from, 378
  from circulatory shunts, 304
  from Eisenmenger's syndrome, 317
  from hypernephromas, 506
  from hypoxia, 477
  from renal cell carcinoma, 652
  from urinary tract obstruction, 616
  high affinity hemoglobin and, 944
  paraneoplastic, 1097
  primary, vs. polycythemia vera, 982
  relative, 975–976
  secondary, 979–980
    treatment of, 980
  vs. chronic myelogenous leukemia, 991
Polycythemia rubra vera, hepatic vein
    thrombosis from, 848
  neutrophilia from, 969
Polycythemia vera, 973, 980–984, 982t
  and gout, 1161, 1167
  and myelofibrosis, 986
  glucose values in, 1382
  osteonecrosis in, 1517
  primary thrombocythemia with, 1054
  pruritus in, 2304
Polycythemia Vera Study Group, 982
Polydactyly, in Laurence-Moon-Bardet-Biedl
    syndrome, 1203
  surgery for, 158
Polydipsia
  from diabetic ketoacidosis, 1375
  from insulin-dependent diabetes mellitus,
    1362
  from medullary cystic disorders, 648
  from vomiting, 660
  primary, hyponatremia in, 538
    vs. antidiuretic hormone deficiency,
      1310–1311
Polygenic disorders, 146
Polygenic inheritance, 150, 150–151
  and peptic ulcers, 695
Polymorphism, 153, 155, 156t
  balanced, 151
  restriction fragment length, linkage anal-
    ysis with, 158
Polymorphonuclear leukocytes
  accumulation of, 1987
  and Staphylococcus aureus, 1598
  and tissue damage, 1990
  disorders of, and infection, 1532
  in inflammatory response, 1530, 1530t
  in lung, 424
  in rheumatoid arthritis, 1999
  in sepsis, 1539
Polymorphonuclear leukocytosis, and acute
    abdomen, 802
Polymyalgia rheumatica, 1978, 2033
  cancer and, 1099
  in shoulder, 2042–2043
  vs. polymyositis, 2036–2037
  vs. shoulder-hand syndrome, 2042
Polymyositis, 459, 1978, 2034–2037
  cancer and, 1106
  classification of, 2034

Polymyositis (Continued)
  diagnosis of, 2036t
  glucocorticosteroid therapy for, 130
  myasthenia gravis with, 2285
  vs. acid alpha-1,4–glucosidase deficiency,
    2277
  vs. dermatomyositis, 2276–2277
  vs. inclusion body myositis, 2276
Polymyositis/dermatomyositis, interstitial
    lung disease in, 430
Polymyxin(s), 122
  in drug interactions, 124t
  poor penetration into spinal fluid by, 116
Polymyxin B
  action of, 113t
  and urticaria, 1950
  elimination rate for, 96t
  in kidney and liver failure, 117t
Polymyxin E, 122
Polyneuritis. See also Neuritis
  cranial, parainfectious, vertigo from, 2124
  from Campylobacter infection, 1649
  from cancer, 1106
  respiratory failure from, 476
Polyneuropathy, 2057t, 2259–2260. See also
    Neuropathies
  definition of, 2259
  diphtheritic, vs. tick paralysis, 1923
  distal, symmetric, 1380
  from diabetes mellitus, 1379
  in alcoholics, 2139
  in heroin users, 57
  inflammatory, 2260–2262. See also Guil-
    lain-Barré syndrome
  symmetrical. See Symmetrical polyneuropa-
    thy
Polyopsia, in partial seizures, 2220
Polyostotic fibrous dysplasia, 2343
  in McCune-Albright syndrome, 1460
Polyp(s)
  adenomatous, 713
    and gastric carcinoma, 710
    in gastrointestinal tract, 669, 713
  antral, gastric outlet obstruction from, 707
  as duodenal obstruction, vs. peptic ul-
    cers, 699
  cholesterol, 871
  definition of, 766
  from ulcerative colitis, 754, 757
  mucosal, in gastrointestinal tract, 669
  of colon, 766, 766–767
    colonoscopy for, 671
Polypectomy, colonoscopic, 767
Polypeptide(s)
  action of, 1258–1261
    mediators of, 1258t
  and receptor sensitivity, 1262
  endogenous pyrogens as, 1526
  metabolism of, 1256
  pancreatic, and eating, 657
    from islet cell tumors, 1390
  release of, 1254
  synthesis of, 1253–1254, 1254
  transport of, 1256
Polyphagia, in insulin-dependent diabetes
    mellitus, 1362
Polyposis coli, 1095t
Polyposis syndromes, inherited, of intes-
    tines, 767–768
  mesenteric fibromatosis in, 796
  multiple, genetic counseling for, 174
Polysaccharides, pneumococcal, antibodies
    against, 1536
Polyserositis, from chronic active hepatitis,
    832
  paroxysmal, familial, 1196. See also Familial
    Mediterranean fever

Polysplenia syndrome, 316
Polythiazide, for hypertension, 286t
Polyunsaturated fats, and cancer, 44
Polyunsaturated fatty acids, 1207
Polyuria
  from diabetes, 26
  from diabetes insipidus, 1309–1310
    treatment of, 1312
  from diabetic ketoacidosis, 1375
  from hypervitaminosis D, 1478
  from insulin-dependent diabetes mellitus,
    1362
  from medullary cystic disorders, 648
  from tubulointerstitial disease, 602
Polyvinyl chloride, interstitial lung disease
  from, 435
POMC (pro-opiomelanocortin), 1101, 1268
Pompe's disease, 361, 1134. See also *Glyco-*
  gen storage disease
Pompholyx, 2321
Pontiac fever, 1570
  clinical manifestations of, 1571
Pontine hemorrhage, 2179, *2179*
  autonomic insufficiency from, 2106
Popliteal artery, arteriosclerosis obliterans
  in, 380
Popliteal synovial membrane, rupture of,
  vs. deep-vein thrombosis, 386
Porcine valve, for mitral valve replacement,
  347, 349
Pork, tapeworm from, 1892
  trichinellosis from, 1912
Porphobilinogen, 1182
  reference intervals for, 2399t
Porphyria(s), 153, 1182–1187, *2332, 2332,*
  2350
  acute intermittent, 148
  autonomic insufficiency in, 2106
  classification of, 1183
  delirium from, 2064
  intermittent, acute, 1184
    vs. appendicitis, 803
    vs. poliomyelitis, 2199
    vs. epilepsy, 2225
  variegate, 1184
    vs. familial Mediterranean fever, 1198
Porphyrin, production of, 899, 1182
Porphyrinuria, vs. porphyrias, 1183
Porpoises, poisoning from, 1931
Portal hypertension
  causes of, 848t
  from cirrhosis, 845, 847–849
  from schistosomiasis, 838
  from schistosomiasis mansoni, 1899
  idiopathic, 848
  portal-systemic collaterals from, 847
Portal tract, inflammation of, from sarcoid-
  sis, 840
Portal vein pressure, measurement of, 847
Portal vein thrombosis, as contraindication
  to liver transplant, 856
Portal venous system, anatomy and phys-
  iology of, 847
Positive end-expiratory pressure, *486,* 486–
  488
Positive end-expiratory volume, 479
Positron tomography, 210–211
Postconcussion syndrome, 2123, 2243
  fatigue in, 2125
Posterior cerebral artery, 2160, *2160,* 2162
  occlusion of, 2166
Posterior cord syndrome, 2245
Posterior fossa, lesions of, 2063
Posterior pituitary, 1305–1313
  antidiuretic hormone from, 1305–1306
  oxytocin from, 1313
Postpartum fever, *Mycoplasma hominis* and,
  1565

Postpartum hemorrhage, cholestasis of
  pregnancy and, 841
  factor V deficiency and, 1073
  factor X deficiency and, 1072
Postpartum period, hypopituitarism in,
  1295
Postphlebitic syndrome, 388
Post-pill amenorrhea, 1435, 1444
Postpolio syndrome, 2199–2200
Postprandial dumping syndrome, 704
Postsurgical scarring, vs. filariasis, 1915
Post-traumatic stress disorders, 2101
Postural hypotension, 1466
  in acute inflammatory autonomic neurop-
    athy, 2262
  in idiopathic autonomic insufficiency,
    2106
Postural reflexes, disturbances of, 2143
Posture
  and renin release, 1345
  deformities in, from Parkinson's disease,
    2144
  dystonic, 2149
  upright, blood pressure maintenance in,
    1465
Potassium
  absorption of, 734
  and adrenal cortex, 1340
  and aldosterone production, 1346
  and bicarbonate reabsorption, 518
  and renin release, 1345
  and toxic concentrations of digoxin, 94
  balance of, disturbances in, 543–549
    kidneys and, 516–517, 517t
  concentrations of, in stool, 725
  daily intake of, 516, 563, 1206t
  deficiency of. See *Hypokalemia*
  excess of, 547–549. See also *Hyperkalemia*
  for digitalis intoxication, 230
  in common foods, 1246t
  in diet, acute kidney failure and, 562
  in excitable tissues, permeability of, 544
  in hemolytic transfusion reactions, 949
  in intracellular fluid, 529
  in myocardial cells, 196
  in periodic paralysis, 2280–2281
  in urine, measurement of, 524
    regulation of, 517t
  kidneys and, 543–544, *544*
  levels of, in uremic syndrome, 563–564
  movement of, in gastrointestinal tract,
    725
  plasma concentration of, and aldosterone
    secretion, 516
  reference intervals for, 2399t
  replacement of, for diabetic ketoacidosis,
    1376
  secretion of, aldosterone and, 502
    suppression of, by distal nephron di-
    uretics, 536
  supplementation of, 1246
  wasting of, aminoglycosides and, 609
Potassium citrate, for kidney stones, 643,
  643
Potassium iodide, for chronic bronchitis,
  414
  saturated solution of, for sporotrichosis,
    1847
Potassium permanganate, for skin disorders, 2314
Potassium-sparing agents, adverse effects
  of, 289t
Potassium-sparing diuretics, 232
  and hyperkalemia, 548
  for hypertension, 286t
  properties of, 231t
Potency, male. See also *Impotence*
  androgens and, 1408

Potency (*Continued*)
  of drugs, 134
Pott's disease, 1690, 2010
Poultry, salmonellae in, 1643
Powassan virus, 1828
  encephalitis from, 2193
Powders, 2314
Poxviruses, methisazone for, 126
PPLO (pleuropneumonia-like organisms),
  1561
PPNG (penicillinase-producing gonococci),
  1709–1710
PR interval, in electrocardiography, 197
PRA. See *Plasma renin activity*
Practolol, sclerosing peritonitis from, 795,
  2052
Prader-Willi syndrome, 1203
  and extreme obesity, 1289
Pralidoxime, as antidote for insecticide cholinesterase inhibitors, 140
  for insecticide poisonings, 145
Prausnitz-Küstner reaction, 1949
Praziquantel
  for clonorchiasis, 1902
  for fascioliasis, 1903
  for fasciolopsiasis, 1904
  for paragonimiasis, 1904
  for schistosomiasis, 1900–1901
  for tapeworms, 1895
  side effects of, 1901
Prazosin
  adverse effects of, 289t
  as vasodilator, 233
  for hypertension, 139, 287t
  for primary pulmonary hypertension, 301
PRC. See *Plasma renin activity*
Pre-B cell, 1932
Precordium, 176–177
Prednisolone, 129t
  sodium-retention properties of, 131
Prednisone, 129t
  for ACTH deficiency, 1296
  for acute asthmatic attack, 409
  for aphthous ulcers, 676
  for asthma, 409
  for Bell's palsy, 2267
  for chronic active hepatitis, 833
  for chronic bronchitis, 413
  for chronic obstructive pulmonary dis-
    ease, 416
  for Crohn's disease, 752
  for giant cell arteritis, 2034
  for Hodgkin's disease, 1020
  for idiopathic hypereosinophilic syn-
    drome, 362
  for leukemia, acute lymphoblastic, 1004
    chronic lymphocytic, 997
  for minimal change nephrotic syndrome,
    594
  for multiple myeloma, 1032
  for myasthenia gravis, 2286–2287
  for myocarditis, 354
  for pericarditis, 364
  for polymyalgia rheumatica, 2033
  for polymyositis, 2037
  for sarcoidosis, 456
  from interstitial lung disease, 428
  in adjuvant therapy for breast cancer,
    1457
  sodium-retention properties of, 131
  weakness from, 2280
  with radiation therapy, 1119
Preeclampsia, 634
  acute fatty liver from, 841
  and kidney failure, 637
  renal parenchymal disease vs., 636
Pregnancy
  acute kidney failure in, 636–637

Pregnancy (*Continued*)
aldosterone secretion in, 1360
and aortic dissection, 372
and carpal tunnel syndrome, 2268
and corticosteroid-binding globulin, 1342
and folate deficiency, 906
and hair loss, 2349
and liver, 841
and melasma, 2343
and mortality from non-A, non-B hepatitis, 824
and thrombotic thrombocytopenic purpura, 1052
and vitamin D–binding protein, 1477
as contraindication
to oral contraceptives, 1444
to radioiodine, 1326
to smallpox vaccination, 1793
to tetracycline, 1565
to thrombolytic therapy, 449
to warfarin, 448
bacteriuria in, 630
breast cancer with, 1457–1458
candidiasis during, 1848
cholestasis in, 830
coarctation of aorta with, 313
cocaine use during, 55
complications of
and congenital hearing loss, 2119
and hemolytic uremic-type syndrome, 601
folate deficiency and, 906
uterine bleeding from, 1434
congenital malformations in, vitamin A toxicity and, 1238
coumarin anticoagulants during, 1077
danger of death from, in Eisenmenger's syndrome, 317
diuretic use in, 636
ectopic, from salpingitis, 1706, 1708
ruptured, and amylase level, 776
vs. appendicitis, 803
epilepsy with, 2227
falciparum malaria during, 1859
familial Mediterranean fever in, 1197
glucocorticosteroid therapy during, 133
Graves' disease and, 1326–1327
hemolytic-uremic syndrome in, 1053
heroin use during, 57
herpes gestationis during, 2331
hormonally related rhinitis during, 1954
hypertrophic cardiomyopathy during, 359
immunization during, 61
hepatitis B, 826
poliomyelitis, 65
rubella, 63–64
in adolescence, 20
risk of, 16
in women with phenylketonuria, 1156
infective endocarditis during, 1591
intermittent glycosuria in, 619
iron deficiency in, 893
and anemia, 880
kidney function in, 634
listeriosis during, 1672
bacteremia from, 1671
malaria prevention during, 1861
Marfan syndrome during, 1178
mitral stenosis symptoms in, 346
multiple, after ovulation induction, 1442
nutrient requirements in, 1204, 1205t
and anemias, 882
parenchymal diseases in, 636
peripartum cardiomyopathy in, 354
progesterone secretion during, 1432
prostaglandin biosynthesis in, 1276
reflux during, 680
repeated, and iron deficiency, 896

Pregnancy (*Continued*)
risks of smoking during, 38
rubella in, 1776
salpingitis during, 1708
sickle cell anemia during, 939
transfusions for, 941
sinus thrombosis with, 2184
Sydenham's chorea with, 2148
syphilis during, treatment of, 1721
testosterone administration during, and masculinization of female infant, 1404
thrombophlebitis after, 385
thymic hypoplasia from, 1974
toxoplasmosis during, 1876, 1879
tuberculosis treatment during, 1688
ulcerative colitis and, 760
varicella during, 1789
varicose veins from, 387
Venezuelan equine encephalitis during, 1825
venous thromboembolism in, 443
viral encephalitis during, 1821
vitamin B₁₂ deficiency in, 904
vitamin C in, 1236
vomiting during, 658
von Willebrand disease in, 1071
with cystic fibrosis, 441
with kidney disease, 634–637
with multiple sclerosis, 2213
Pregnanediol, reference intervals for, 2399t
Pregnanetriol, reference intervals for, 2399t
Pregnenolone, reference intervals for, 2399t
Prehypertension, 277
cardiac output in, 278
from pheochromocytoma, 284
Prekallikrein, deficiency of, 1072
Preleukemia, 1006
marrow aplasia and, 886
marrow transplants for, 1041
Preload, *185*, 185–186, 190, 217
definition of, 237
in cardiac performance, 216t
mitral regurgitation and, 348
reduction of, with vasodilators, 233, 248
ventricular end-diastolic pressure and, 217, *217*
Preludin, abuse of, 54
Premature ejaculation, 1410
Premature ventricular contractions, from catheters for monitoring pulmonary artery pressure, 497
in hypertrophic cardiomyopathy, 358
Premature ventricular depolarizations, 262–263, *263*
procainamide for, 270
Prematurity, from congenital toxoplasmosis, 1877
measles and, 1772
retinopathy of, 2297
Premenstrual syndrome, 1433–1434, 1434t
Premenstrual tension, 1433
vitamin B₆ and, 1234
Prenatal diagnosis
in genetic counseling, 173–174
of chromosome abnormalities, 168–169
of chronic granulomatous disease, 958
of congenital malformations, 170–171
of Fabry's disease, 1145
of glycogen storage diseases, 1135
of sickle cell disease, 941–942, *942*
recombinant DNA research and, 158
Pre-proparathyroid hormone, 1486
Prepubertal castrate syndrome, functional, 1413–1414, *1408*
Prerenal azotemia, 560
from diuretics, vs. hepatorenal syndrome, 852
Prerenal syndromes, 503–504, 504t

Presbycusis, 2119
Pressure measurements, in cardiac catheterization, 212–213, *212*
Pressure sores, 2341–2342
after spinal cord trauma, 2246
in elderly, 30
Pressure urticaria-angioedema, 1949
Pressure ventilators, 479, 487
Presyncope, vs. vertigo, 2121
Pretibial myxedema, in Graves' disease, 1321, 1323
treatment of, 1327
Preventive medicine, 35–36
physical examination for, 66–67, 67t
Priapism, from chronic myelogenous leukemia, treatment of, 992
in vaso-occlusive crisis, in sickle cell anemia, 939
Prilocaine, toxicity of, to hemoglobin, 945
Primaquine, for malaria, 1861
genetics and reaction to, 102
toxicity of, to hemoglobin, 945
Primary care, 7
Primed lymphocyte test, 1964
Primidone
and enhanced liver metabolism of other drugs, 99
for epilepsy, 2226t, 2227
for essential tremor, 2146
reference intervals for, 2404t
Primordial follicle(s), in ovary, 1425, *1426*, 1430
Prinzmetal's angina, 325, 393
myocardial infarction vs., 332
treatment for, 328
Prion, 1524, 2205
Probabilities
determination of, 77
in diagnosis, 74
in genetic counseling, 172
logic and, in diagnosis, 2054
prior, in Bayes' rule, 75
Probenecid
and hair loss, 2349
for gout, 1170
genetics and reaction to, 102
hyperbilirubinemia from, 814
interaction of, with methotrexate, 101
with penicillin, 101
Problem solving, frontal lobes and, 2082
Procainamide, 270
adverse effects of, 267t–268t
and bone marrow injury, 962
arrhythmias from, 275
creatinine clearance and, 95
distribution of, heart failure and, 97
dosage for, 267t–268t
for ventricular premature depolarizations, 263
for ventricular tachycardia, 263
genetics in metabolism of, 102
interaction of, with other drugs, 101
interstitial lung disease from, vs. from systemic lupus erythematosus, 434
lupus syndrome from, 103
metabolism of, kidney disease and, 95
to acetylprocainamide, 94
pharmacokinetic properties of, 89t, 266t
reference intervals for, 2404t
steady-state concentration of, 92
Procaine, in drug interactions, 124t
Procaine penicillin, 119
for salpingitis, 1706
Procarbazine
for cancer, 1126
for Hodgkin's disease, 1020
infertility from, 1120
interstitial lung disease from, 434

Prochlorperazine, for nausea, in viral hepatitis, 824
Proctalgia fugax, 788
Proctitis, 787–788
    gonococcal, vs. ulcerative colitis, 757
    radiation, vs. ulcerative colitis, 757
    ulcerative, 753, 760. See also *Ulcerative colitis*
Proctocolitis, in homosexuals, 1648
Proctoscopy, for colonc cancer, 771
Proctosigmoiditis, 753. See also *Ulcerative colitis*
Proctosigmoidoscopy
    for Crohn's disease, 748
    for diarrhea, 730
    for ileus of colon, 719
    for lower gastrointestinal hemorrhage, 798
    for ulcerative colitis, 755
Pro-dynorphin, 1268
Pro-enkephalin, 1268
Proerythroblasts, 874
Progenitors. See also *Hematopoiesis, progenitors of*
    abnormalities of, and blood cell production, 875
Progeria, adult, 1202
Progesterone, 1433t
    and sodium reabsorption, 516
    congenital heart disease from, 303
    from corpus luteum, 1430
    receptor proteins of, in breast cancer, 1455
    reference intervals for, 2399t
    secretion rates and plasma concentrations of, 1341
    synthesis of, from ovaries, 1432
Progestin(s), and corpus luteum, 1431
    and hypogonadism, 1417
    and photosensitivity, 2351
Projectile vomiting, 717
Prokaryotes, 1837
Prokinetic drugs, and intestinal motility, 724
Prolactin, 1292
    and corpus luteum, 1431
    deficiency of, 1295
    effect of, 1293
    for lactation, 1449
    from lactotrophs, 1290
    hypersecretion of, 1302–1303
        from pituitary adenomas, 2232
    in puberty, 17
    inhibitor of, dopamine as, 1281
    levels of, amenorrhea and, 1436
    obesity and, 1225
    reference intervals for, 2399t
    secretion of, 1284–1285
        impaired, 1294
Prolactin inhibiting factor, 1280
Prolactin releasing hormone, from medullary carcinoma, 1506
Prolactinoma, and galactorrhea, 1450
Proline, 1158
Promastigote, 1870
Promegaloblasts, 901
Promonocyte, 954
Promoter mutations, thalassemia from, 934
Pro-opiomelanocortin, 1101, 1268
Propagules, 1837
Prophase, in meiosis, 162
Prophylactic shunts, for portal hypertension, 850
Propionibacterium acnes, 1637, 2333
    on skin, 1548
Propoxyphene, 107t
    abuse of, 55
    as analgesic, 108

Propoxyphene (Continued)
    metabolites for, kidney excretion of, 95
    reference intervals for, 2404t
Propranolol, 137, 138, 138t, 270–271
    aggravation of heart failure by, 220
    as prophylaxis against recurring myocardial infarction, 335
    contraindicated for cardiogenic hypotension, 248
    dosing and adverse effects of, 269t
    hyperbilirubinemia from, 814
    hypoglycemia from, 139, 1384
    interaction of, with epinephrine, 101
    liver extraction of, 97
    metabolism of, inhibited by cimetidine, 100
        to 4-hydroxypropranolol, 94
    myocardial depression from, 239
    pharmacokinetic properties of, 266t
    Raynaud's phenomenon from, 375
    reference intervals for, 2404t
    removal of, by liver, 88
    withdrawal from, 138
Proptosis, in malignant osteopetrosis, 1518
Propylthiouracil
    chronic hepatitis from, 828, 831
    for alcoholic hepatitis, 844
    for hyperthyroidism from Graves' disease, 1325
Prosody, 2085
Prosopagnosia, 2085
Prostacyclin(s), 1271
    and coronary artery thrombosis, 330
    for alveolar hypoventilation, 298
    for primary pulmonary hypertension, 300–302
    for Raynaud's phenomenon, 377
    in inflammation, 1986
    shock and, 239–240
Prostaglandin(s), 1253, 1271–1277
    and antidiuretic hormone, 1306–1307
    and corpus luteum, 1431
    and dysmenorrhea, 19
    and hypercalcemia, in cancer, 1102
    and mucosal integrity, 694
    and pruritus, 2304
    and renin release, 1345
    and sodium reabsorption, 516
    biosynthesis of, in riboflavin deficiency, 1231
    circulatory function and, 190
    deficiency of, and hypertension, 277
    drugs inhibiting production of, 608. See also *Nonsteroidal anti-inflammatory agents*
    endogenous pyrogens and, 1526
    eosinopenia from, 966
    inhibitors of, and acute gastritis, 689
        and renin release, 1345
        aspirin as, 607
    production of, kidneys and, 503, 520
        stimulation of, in obstructive nephropathy, 614
Prostaglandin D$_2$, 1271, 1273
Prostaglandin E, and thirst, 1308
    in fluid volume regulation, 531
Prostaglandin E$_1$, for arteriosclerosis obliterans, 381
Prostaglandin E$_2$, 1273
    in synovial fluid, 1994
    synthesis of, fever from, 1528
    topical, for Raynaud's phenomenon, 377
Prostaglandin F$_1$, and mesenteric circulation, 761
Prostaglandin F$_{2\alpha}$, 1273
Prostate
    antimicrobials in, 116
    benign hyperplasia of, 1422–1423
    carcinoma of, 1423–1425, 1424t, 1522

Prostate (Continued)
    carcinoma of, androgen therapy contraindicated in, 1419
        fibrinolysis of, 1079
    development of, 1392
    disease of, 1421–1425
    enlargement of, and urinary flow obstruction, 507, 568
    occurrence of, 614
    expressed secretion of, 1421
    hypertrophy of, and acute kidney failure, 558
    inflammation of, 1421–1422
    obstruction of, manifestations of, 615
        vs. irritation of, 1423
    tuberculosis in, 1690
    tumors of, and acute kidney failure, 558
Prostatectomy, for prostatic cancer, 1424
Prostatic acid phosphatase, 1100
Prostatism, 1423
Prostatitis, 1421–1422
    and acute kidney failure, 558
    enteric bacteria and, 1659
Prostatodynia, 1422
Prosthesis
    and infection, 1532
    of bone, 1622
    for reconstruction of right ventricular outflow tract, 318
    nickel in, 2391
    testicular, 1414
    vascular, fistulas after placement of, 765
Prosthetic heart valves
    Aspergillus infection of, 1851
    endocarditis of, 1586
        bacteria in, 1693
        therapy for, 119
    for mitral regurgitation, 349
    hemolysis from, 924
    infection of, 1590–1591, 1591t
    pressure gradient across, 207
Prosthetic joints, and bacterial arthritis, 2009
    infection after insertion of, 1547
    with rheumatoid arthritis, 2004
Prostration, as interferon reaction, 128
    in cavernous sinus thrombosis, 2185
Protamine, for deep-vein thrombosis, 387
    in cardiac catheterization, 211
    to counteract heparin, 1080
Protease(s), and pruritus, 2304
    from mast cells in skin, 2306
Protein(s)
    acute phase, 1528, 1528t
    altered functioning of, and metabolic disease, 1130
    amyloid, 1528
    animal, in diet, and colorectal cancer, 768
    avian, thermophilic organisms of, and hypersensitivity pneumonitis, 433
    bilirubin binding to, 812
    binding of, 116
    C-reactive, 1528, 1529
    coagulation, 1060–1061, 1061t
    cobalamin-binding, 902t
    consumption of, and gout, 1161
    conversion of amino acids to, insulin and, 1374
    deficiency of, symptoms of, 657
    degradation of, kidneys and, 503
    dietary requirements for, 1207
    digestion of, 733, 734
    distribution of, in healthy population, 80
    enteric loss of, detection of, 744
    excretion of, excessive, 591. See also *Nephrotic syndrome*
        normal, 592
        values for, 585

Protein(s) (Continued)
fibrillar, deposition of, in body tissue, 1034
in extracellular matrix, 1981
globular, in extracellular matrix, 1981
glycosylation of, and diabetes complications, 1367
in cerebrospinal fluid, bacterial meningitis and, 1607
in complement system, 1938, 1938t
in diet, acute kidney failure and, 562
and dietary calcium retention, 1511
and serum urea concentration, 571–572
in erythrocyte membrane, 909–910
in myelin, 2211
in parenteral nutrition, 1247
total, 1249, 1249t
in synovial fluid, 1983, 1993
low molecular weight, 519
metabolism of, 810
in kidneys, 519
mutant, modification of, 157
replacement of, 157
myelin basic, 2212
nephrotoxicity of, 559
production of, 158
rate of biosynthesis of, and aging, 23
recommended dietary allowance for, 1205t
reference intervals for, 2399t
requirements for, in diabetic, 1368
restriction of, for uremic syndrome, 507
secretion of, from tumor cells, 1099–1100, 1099t
sources of, 1207, 1245
structural, genetic disorders of, 148
supplements of, 1243–1245
synthesis of, 929
error in, as aging theory, 22–23
impaired by ethanol, 843
thyroid hormone regulation of, 1317
tests of, and blood coagulation disorders, 1065–1066
urinary, normal composition of, 520
normal excretion rate of, 520
van Dyke, 1305
Protein A, in Staphylococcus aureus, 1598
Protein C
deficiency of, 1074–1075
and recurrent thrombophlebitis, 385
and thrombosis, 1074
functional activities of, 1074
Protein-calorie malnutrition, 1212–1215
and fatty liver, 810
and plasma amino acids, 1152t
and reduced lymphocyte production, 966
chronic pancreatitis from, 779
diagnosis of, 1214
fatty liver from, 827
hypophosphatemia during refeeding for, 1194
in hospitalized patients, causes of, 1212, 1212t
prevention of, 1215
treatment of, 1214–1215, 1215
Protein-creatinine ratio, 520, 521
Protein kinase C, 1259
Protein-losing enteropathy, 1098
and albumin degradation, 815
from lymphangiectasia, 744
Protein S, deficiency of, and recurrent thrombophlebitis, 385
and thrombosis, 1074, 1075
Proteinosis, alveolar, as interstitial lung disease, 432
Proteinuria, 503, 520–522
and vitamin D–binding protein, 1477

Proteinuria (Continued)
Bence Jones, in multiple myeloma, 1032
kidney failure in, 606
macroglobulinemia and, 1033
from acute glomerulonephritis, 583, 584
from Alport's syndrome, 637
from amyloidosis, 1035
from analgesic nephropathy, 608
from cadmium poisoning, 2391
from chronic kidney failure, urinary tract infection and, 569
from chronic kidney rejection, 581
from diabetic glomerulopathy, 625
from diabetic nephropathy, 1379
from gout, 1166
from nephrotic syndrome, 504, 592–593
from urinary infections, 629
hematuria with, 503
isolated, 585
low molecular weight, in tubulointerstitial disease, 603
overflow, 520, 585
postural, 585
pregnancy and, 636
tubular, 521–522
types of, 521t
Proteoglycan(s)
and urate deposition in gout, 1164
in arteries, 318
in connective tissue, 1982
loss of, in cartilage damage, 1983
Proteus
and gastritis, 689
and urinary tract infection, 629
hospital-acquired, 1543
penicillins for, 119
Proteus mirabilis, cephalosporins for, 120
Proteus morgani, and scombroid fish poisoning, 786
Prothrombin, deficiency of, 1073
reference intervals for, 2402t
synthesis of, and vitamin K, 816
Prothrombin time, 816
and coagulation, 1047
in hepatitis, chronic active, 832
viral, 820
in secondary biliary cirrhosis, 846
Proto-oncogenes, 1089
Protoporphyria, 840, 1184
erythropoietic, light urticaria in, 1950
Protoporphyrin, reference intervals for, 2399t
Protozoa, 1856–1857
disease from, 1857–1889
African trypanosomiasis as, 1862, 1862t, 1862–1865
amebiasis as, 1886–1888
American trypanosomiasis as, 1865–1869
babesiosis as, 1884–1886
balantidiasis as, 1889
cryptosporidiosis as, 1881–1883
giardiasis as, 1883–1884
leishmaniasis as, 1869–1875, 1870t
malaria as, 1857–1861
pneumocystosis as, 1879–1881
sarcosporidiosis as, 1889
toxoplasmosis as, 1875–1879
trichomoniasis as, 1889
infections with, in AIDS, 1804–1805, 1804t–1805t
sexual transmission of, 1702t
Protriptyline, reference intervals for, 2404t
Prourokinase, in fibrinolysis, 1064
Provirus, 1794
Proximal tubule(s), 509, 511–513, 512
bicarbonate absorption by, 550

Proximal tubule(s) (Continued)
damage to, 603
defects of, 505
and fasting hypercalciuria, 640
in urine formation, 502
sodium absorption by, in fluid volume regulation, 530
PRP (progesterone receptor proteins), 1455
Prune-belly syndrome, 649, 650
Pruritus, 661, 2303
antihistamines for, 2316
aquagenic, 1950
from bile duct tumor, 871
from cancer, 1110–1111
from chilblain, 379
from cholestasis, 808
from chronic kidney failure, 567
management of, 571
from common duct obstruction, 862
from cutaneous larva migrans, 1907
from dialysis patients, 577
from eczemas, 2318
from Hodgkin's disease, 1016
from hyperparathyroidism, 1490
from lice bites, 1740
from onchocerciasis, 1917
from polycythemia vera, 981
from primary biliary cirrhosis, 845
from recurrent cholestasis, 813
from renal osteodystrophy, 1508
from scabies, 1925
from sclerosing cholangitis, 869
from secondary biliary cirrhosis, 846
from varicella, 1790
from viral hepatitis, 819
skin disease and, 2304t
systemic disease with, 2304t
Pruritus ani, 789
from enterobiasis, 1910
Psammoma body, 1336
Pseudobulbar palsy, 2090
Pseudochylothorax, 468
Pseudoclaudication, 2254
Pseudocoma, 2061t
Pseudocysts, 778, 778–779
ascites from, 792
pancreatic, pleural effusions from, 468–469
vs. pancreatic cancer, 783
Pseudodementia, 2088–2089
Pseudodiabetes mellitus, uremic, 567
Pseudodiverticula, 718
Pseudofractures, in osteomalacia and rickets, 1483, 1483
Pseudogout syndrome, 2037
and hyperparathyroidism, 2045
in dialysis patients, 577
vs. gout, 1168
Pseudohermaphroditism
female, 1402–1404, 1403t
causes of, 1397t
from excessive androgens, 1428
male, 1393–1404, 1394t
from androgen deficiency in fetal development, 1408
testicular feminization in, 1399
Pseudo-Hurler polydystrophy, 1177
Pseudohyperkalemia, 548
Pseudohyperparathyroidism of malignancy, and hypercalciuria from net bone resorption, 640
Pseudohypertrophy, definition of, 2271
Pseudohypoparathyroidism, 149, 1131, 1500, 1500–1501
Pseudohypophosphatasia, 1152t
Pseudoincontinence, 2108
Pseudoinfections, from contaminated antiseptic compounds, 1548

Pseudolymphoma, 431, 463, 712
  in Sjögren's syndrome, 2024
Pseudomembranous colitis, 1632–1633
  diagnosis of, 730
  from antibiotic therapy, 123
  from *Campylobacter* infection, 1649
  vs. ulcerative colitis, 757
Pseudomonas
  and pneumonia, 1566
  and urinary tract infection, 629
    hospital-acquired, 1543
  antibodies against, 1536
  disease from, 1669–1670
  resistance of, to chloramphenicol, 120
  skin infections with, examination of, 2311
Pseudomonas aeruginosa, 1565
  aminoglycosides for, 122
  and bronchiectasis, 439
  and osteomyelitis, 1622
  cephalosporins for, 120
  hot tub folliculitis from, 2334
  in auditory canal, and malignant external
    otitis, 2185
  in cystic fibrosis, 441
  infection of, after thermal injury, 2365
  lung abscess from, 436
  necrotizing alveolitis from, 436
  nosocomial pneumonia from, 1544
  penicillins for, 119
    with aminoglycoside, 437
  polymyxin or colistin for, 122
Pseudomonas cepacia, in cystic fibrosis, 441
  in intravenous infusions, 1545
Pseudomonas mallei, 1670
Pseudomonas pseudomallei, lung abscess
    from, 436
Pseudomycelia, 1847
Pseudomyxoma peritonei, 794
Pseudoneutropenia, 962
Pseudopapilledema, 2292
  definition of, 2236
Pseudoparalysis, from congenital syphilis,
    1718
Pseudopelade, and hair loss, 2349
Pseudopodagra, 1168
Pseudopolyps, 766
  in ulcerative colitis, 754
Pseudopseudohypoparathyroidism, 1500
Pseudopuberty, from ovarian tumors, 1446
  precocious, 1420
    in females, 1426
Pseudo-seizures, vs. epilepsy, 2225
Pseudosyncope, 2076
Pseudotumor, of liver, 857
  of orbit, 2292, 2295
Pseudotumor cerebri, 2236t, 2236–2237
  in galactokinase deficiency, 1132
  obesity and, 1225
  vs. brain tumors, 2234
Pseudo–von Willebrand's disease, 1056
Pseudo-Whipple's disease, 729
Pseudoxanthoma elasticum, *1181*, 1181–
    1182
Psilocybin, abuse of, 58
  duration of, 59
Psittacosis, 1735–1737
  vs. mycoplasmal pneumonia, 1564
Psoralen, with ultraviolet radiation, 2318
Psoriasis, 2326t, 2326–2327
  and amyloidosis, 1199
  and nails, 2346
  anthralin for, 2316
  coal tar for, 2316
  etretinate for, 2317
  genetic factors in, 2008
  guttate, 2327–2328
  in hypoparathyroidism, 1498
  pustular form of, 2334

Psoriasis *(Continued)*
  vs. pityriasis rubra pilaris, 2328
  vs. rash from syphilis, 1715
Psychedelics, abuse of, 58–59
  poisoning with, 2069t
Psychiatric disorders, 2091–2103
  affective disorders as, 2095–2099
  amnesia in, 2066
  and acrocyanosis, 378
  and altered consciousness, 2066
  and breathing variations, 401
  and male sexual dysfunction, 1409
  anxiety disorders as, 2100–2101
  diagnosis of, 2091–2092
  from glucocorticosteroid therapy, 130
  from infective endocarditis, 1590
  hypoparathyroidism and, 1498
  insomnia in, 2078
  neuroendocrine function in, 1289
  pancreatic cancer and, 781
  schizophrenic disorders as, 2092–2095
  somatization disorders as, 2101t, 2101–
    2103, 2102t
  thyroid function in, 1321
  vs. botulism, 1633
  vs. cryptococcosis, 1845
  vs. medical disorders, 2092
Psychic depressants, respiratory failure
    from, 476
Psychic stress, pruritus from, 2304
Psychogenic disorders, vs. multiple sclero-
    sis, 2214
  vs. vertigo, 2121
Psychologic disorders, from Cushing's syn-
    drome, 1355
  from partial seizures, 2220
  systemic lupus erythematosus and, 2016
Psychomotor activity, in metabolic encepha-
    lopathy, 2065
Psychosis
  among alcoholics, 49
  as contraindication to levodopa, 2146
  definition of, 2092
  from psychedelic drugs, 59
  in AIDS dementia complex, 2204
  symptomatic patterns of, 2093t
  syphilitic, 1718
  toxic, from metabolic encephalopathy,
    2063
    from sedative withdrawal syndrome,
      54
Psychosocial development, in adolescence,
    16–17
Psychotherapy, for alcoholics, 50
  for anorexia nervosa, 1218
  for drug abusers, 60–61
Psyllium hydrophilic colloids, for constipa-
    tion, 722
Pteroic acid, 905
Pteroylmonoglutamic acid, *905*. See also
    Folic acid
Pterygium formation, definition of, 2346
PTH, 1484–1488. See also *Parathyroid hor-
    mone*
PTU. See *Propylthiouracil*
Pubarche, premature, 1427
Puberty, 17–19. See also *Adolescence*
  and hair growth, 2303
  asynchronous development of, in fe-
    males, 1429
  delayed
    androgen therapy for, 1419
    in boys, 1418
    in females, 1427–1429
      vs. hypogonadotropic eunuchoidism,
        1417
  dentition in, 18
  endocrinology of, 17

Puberty *(Continued)*
  gynecomastia in, 1410
  health problems related to, 19–20
  heterosexual development in, 1429
  in boys, clinical indications of, 1418
  in females, 1425–1426, *1426*
    abnormalities of, 1426–1429, 1427t
    ovarian function at, 1425–1426
  physical growth during, 17–18
  precocious
    hamartomas and, 1286
    in females, 1426–1428, 1460
    in males, 1420
    pineal and, 1314
    with polyostotic fibrous dysplasia, 1520
  primary sex characteristics in, 18–19
  secondary sex characteristics in, 18
  self-concept in, 16
  sex maturity ratings for, 18
  Tanner stages for, in females, 1436t
Puestow procedure, for chronic pancreati-
    tis, 780
Puffer fish, 1931
  poisoning from, 786
  paralytic, vs. botulism, 1633
Pulmonary. See also *Lung(s)* and under *Res-
    piratory*
Pulmonary arterial pressure
  and cardiac output, 293
  diastolic, and ventricular end-diastolic
    pressure, 217
  increase in, from cocaine or ampheta-
    mines, 54
  monitoring of, complications from, 497
    in critical care units, 493–494, 494t, *494*
Pulmonary arteriography, for pulmonary
    embolism, 444, 446–447, *446*
Pulmonary arteriovenous fistula, 308–309
  hemoptysis from, 391
Pulmonary arteritis, with rheumatoid ar-
    thritis, 429
Pulmonary artery (arteries)
  bifurcation of, embolus in, 443
  communication between, and aorta, 307–
    308
  stenosis of, vs. unilateral hyperlucent
    lung, 420
  transposition of, with aorta, 314
Pulmonary aspiration, from gastroesopha-
    geal reflux disease, 682, 682t
  treatment of, 683
Pulmonary capillaries, 421, *421*
  permeability of, 476, 534
Pulmonary capillary wedge pressure, 243
Pulmonary circulation, 294
Pulmonary disease. See *Lung(s), disease of*
  and *Obstructive pulmonary disease*
Pulmonary edema
  acute, in heart failure, 221
    management of, 225–226
  after cardioversion, 273
  during refeeding, 1214
  from acute heroin reaction, 56
  from acute kidney failure, 559
  from anomalous pulmonary venous con-
    nection, 315
  from aortic regurgitation, 344
  from blood transfusions, 949
  from cholera, 1653
  from fulminant hepatic failure, 854
  from inflow obstruction to left ventricle,
    311
  from mitral regurgitation, 348
  from pulmonary embolism, 443
  from Rocky Mountain spotted fever, 1743
  from subarachnoid hemorrhage, 2176
  high-altitude, 2366–2367
  myocardial infarction with, 331

Pulmonary edema (Continued)
    pulmonary venous pressure increase and, 294
    respiratory failure from, 476, 491
    sputum in, 391
    treatment of, positive end-expiratory pressure in, 487–488
    uremic, from systemic lupus erythematosus, 429
    vs. interstitial lung disease, 423
    vs. malaria, 1859
    vs. pulmonary embolism, 444
Pulmonary embolectomy, 449
Pulmonary embolism, 442–449
    and breathing control, 401
    and pulmonic regurgitation, 351
    and syncope, 2074
    atrial pressure in, 244
    chronic obstructive pulmonary disease with, 415–416
    clinical manifestations of, 444, 444t
    dyspnea from, 394
    from deep-vein thrombosis, 384, 385
    hemoptysis from, 391
    idiopathic pulmonary fibrosis with, 428
    lung abscess from, 436
    occlusive pulmonary vascular disease from, 295
    pleural disease from, 468
    pulmonary hypertension from, 293, 296, 299t
        vs. primary pulmonary hypertension, 300
    respiratory failure from, 476
    risk factors for, 442
    therapy for, 447, 447–449, 448t
    treatment of, after myocardial infarction, 334
    vs. asthma, 408
    vs. myocardial infarction, 332
    vs. sepsis, 1540
Pulmonary fibrosis
    familial, interstitial lung disease with, 432
    from amiodarone, 276
    from asbestos, 2362–2363, 2363
    idiopathic
        alveolar structure in, 422
        alveolitis in, 423
            measurement of, 428
        as interstitial lung disease, 428–429
        familial, 432
        proportion of neutrophils in, 427
        radiography of, 426
        pneumothorax from, 470
Pulmonary function, and surgery, for bronchogenic carcinoma, 461
Pulmonary function tests
    for asthma, 407, 409
    for bronchiectasis, 439
    for cystic fibrosis, 440
    for interstitial lung disease, 426–428
        drug-induced, 434
    in left ventricular failure, 222
Pulmonary hypertension, 177, 293–302, 535
    and angina pectoris, 324
    and heart failure, 215
    and Raynaud's phenomenon, 375
    angiothrombotic, in heroin users, 57
    arterial, in radiographs, 192
    atrial pressure in, 244
    from chronic obstructive pulmonary disease, 415
    from congenital heart disease, 303
    from double outlet right ventricle, 314
    from interstitial lung disease, 425–427
    from mitral stenosis, 346
    from mixed connective tissue disease, 430

Pulmonary hypertension (Continued)
    from pulmonary embolism, 443
    from sarcoidosis, 360
    from schistosomiasis mansoni, 1899
    from systemic sclerosis, 2022
    in radiographs, 192
    in transposition of great arteries with ventricular septal defect, 314
    pain from, 393
    patent ductus arteriosus with, 307
    primary, 293, 298–302
        diagnosis of, 300
        etiologies of, 299t
        heart-lung transplantation for, 302
        prognosis for, 302
        treatment of, 300–302
    pulmonary vasculitis in, 476
    pulmonic regurgitation from, 351
    secondary, 294–298
    shunt lesions with, 305
    venous, in radiographs, 192–193
    vs. mitral stenosis, 347
Pulmonary infarction
    from emboli, 443–444
    from Swan-Ganz catheters, 497
    vs. appendicitis, 803
    vs. epidemic pleurodynia, 1811
    vs. pericarditis, 364
    vs. pneumococcal pneumonia, 1558, 1559t
Pulmonary infiltration with eosinophilia syndrome, 434
Pulmonary neoplasms, 457t, 457–466. See also Lung(s), neoplasms of
Pulmonary obstructive disease. See Obstructive pulmonary disease
Pulmonary resistance vessels, and pulmonary hypertension, 295
Pulmonary sarcoidosis, 425–429
Pulmonary thromboembolism, 273, 294
Pulmonary vascular bed, fetal, persistence of, primary pulmonary hypertension from, 299t
Pulmonary vascular diseases, 476
    and diffusing capacity, 400
    in Eisenmenger's syndrome, 316
    respiratory failure from, critical care for, 492
Pulmonary vascular resistance, 213
    and acute right heart failure, 475
    calculation of, 494
    elevation of, in Eisenmenger's syndrome, 316–317
    for assessing pulmonary circulation, 294
    in radiographs, 192–193
Pulmonary vasculitis, interstitial lung disease with, 431–432
    respiratory failure from, 476
Pulmonary vasodilators, for alveolar hypoventilation, 298
Pulmonary vein stenosis, inflow obstruction to left ventricle and, 311
Pulmonary veno-occlusive disease, pulmonary hypertension from, 302
Pulmonary venous connection, anomalous, 315
Pulmonary vessels, in radiographs, 192
Pulmonic insufficiency, aortic insufficiency vs., 346
Pulmonic regurgitation, 314, 351
Pulmonic stenosis, 311–312, 351
    acquired, 307
    double outlet right ventricle with, 314
    from tetralogy of Fallot, 309
    transposition of great arteries with, 314
    valvular, in adults, 316

Pulmonic valve, absence of, 314
    regurgitation from, 314, 351
    stenosis of, 311–312, 351. See also Pulmonic stenosis
Pulpitis, 674
Pulsation, of heart, fluoroscopy for, 195
Pulse, arterial, 176
    carotid, 176
    venous, in cardiovascular physical examination, 176
Pulse generators, for pacemakers, 272
Pulse oximeters, 493
Pulseless disease, 374, 2164
Pulsus alternans, 176
    definition of, 331
    in left ventricular failure, 222
Pulsus paradoxus, 176, 366
    in asthma, 407
    measurement of, in severely ill, 482
Pupils
    Argyll-Robertson, 1718, 2114
    dilation of
        from cocaine or amphetamines, 54
        from opioid withdrawal syndrome, 57
        from uncal herniation, 2063
        pharmacologic, and angle closure, 2290–2291
    examination of, 2113–2114
    neural control of, 2113–2114
        evaluation of, 2114
    reactivity of, disappearance of, 853
    in metabolic coma, 2065
Purging, in bulimia, 1218
Purine(s)
    and urate concentration in plasma, 1162
    biosynthesis of, 1163
    for chronic myelogenous leukemia, 992
    metabolism of, disorders of, 1170. See also Gout
    overproduction of, and uric acid stones, 641
Purine analogues, 1122–1123
Purine nucleoside phosphorylase, deficiency of, 1173, 1945
Purkinje fiber, action potentials of, 251, 251
Purkinje system, 196
Purpura, 1045, 2323t. See also Thrombocytopenic purpura
    actinic, 2325
    allergic, 1058–1059
    cocktail, 1049
    dependent nonthrombocytopenic, in Sjögren's syndrome, 2024
    from bacterial meningitis, 1606
    from immunocytic amyloid, 1035
    Henoch-Schönlein, 432, 600–601, 2027, 2046
    hyperglobulinemic, primary, 1059
    in fulminant meningococcemia, 1614, 1614
    nonpalpable, 2324–2325
    post-transfusion, 1052
    senile, 1059
    thrombocytopenic. See Thrombocytopenic purpura
    vascular, 1058t, 1058–1060
        dependent, in essential mixed cryoglobulinemia, 601
Purpura fulminans, 2325
    in defibrination syndrome, 1079
    neonatal, protein C absence and, 1074
Purpura simplex, 1059
Pustule, malignant, 1667
Putamen, 2141
PUVA, for skin disorders, 2318
PVE (prosthetic valve endocarditis), 1586
    antimicrobial therapy for, 119
    Mycobacterium fortuitum-thelonae and, 1693

Pyelography
  antegrade, 525
  intravenous, 282, 525, 560
    for acute kidney failure, 561
  retrograde, 525
Pyelonephritis, 505, 628
  acute, kidney failure from, in liver disease, 852
  bacterial, 505
    candidiasis as, 1848
    chronic, 606
  chronic, 628
  clinical manifestations of, 629
  enteric bacteria and, 1658–1659
  from renal calculus, 505
  in hyperparathyroidism, 1489
  in pregnancy, 630
  salt wasting in, 564
  transplant, 581
  treatment for, 630
  vs. acute cholecystitis, 866
  vs. appendicitis, 803
Pyknodysostosis, 1519
Pyloric stenosis, 170t, 707, 716–717
Pyloroplasty, truncal vagotomy with, for peptic ulcers, 703–704, 703t
Pyoderma(s), 2342
  from group A streptococci, 1577
  from ulcerative colitis, 757
  in Crohn's disease, 750
  lice and, 1920
  streptococcal, 1575
  systemic antibiotics for, 2317
  vs. streptococcal pharyngitis, 1577
Pyomyositis, staphylococcal, 1603
  tropical, myositis from, 2036
Pyopneumothorax, 469
Pyrantel pamoate
  for ascariasis, 1909
  for enterobiasis, 1910
  for hookworm, 1907
  for trichinellosis, 1912
Pyrazinamide, for tuberculosis, 1687
Pyrethrum, inhalation of, interstitial lung disease from, 435
Pyrexia, from renal cell carcinoma, 652
  in erythema nodosum leprosum, 1699
Pyridostigmine, 139
  for myasthenia gravis, 2286
Pyridoxal, 1233
Pyridoxamine, 1233
Pyridoxine, 1233, 1233–1234. See also Vitamin B₆
Pyrimethamine, for toxoplasmosis, 1879
Pyrimidine, antagonists to, for chronic myelogenous leukemia, 992
  dimers of, production of, by ultraviolet radiation, 2376
  metabolism of, disorders of, 1173
  nucleotides of, 917, 1173
Pyrogens, endogenous, 1526
  exogenous, fever from, 1526
Pyropoikilocytosis, hereditary, 913
Pyrosis
  from ascites, 791
  from esophageal disease, 680
  from gastroesophageal reflux disease, 681
  from iron deficiency anemia, 897
  veno-occlusive disease from, 848
Pyruvate kinase, deficiency in, and hemolysis, 916, 917
Pyruvic acid, reference intervals for, 2399t
Pyrvinium pamoate, for enterobiasis, 1910
Pyuria, definition of, 629
  from diverticulitis, 804
  in chronic kidney failure, urinary tract infection and, 569
PZA (pyrazinamide), 1687

Q fever, 1738t, 1748–1749
  clinical features of, 1738t
  epidemiologic features of, 1737t
  vs. mycoplasmal pneumonia, 1564
  vs. psittacosis, 1736
  vs. viral hepatitis, 824
Q wave, in electrocardiography, 197
QRS complex, in electrocardiography, 197, 198
QS wave, in electrocardiography, 197
QT interval, correction of, for heart rate, 198
  in electrocardiography, 197
Quaalude, abuse of, 53
Quadriplegia, from hepatic porphyria, 1185
  from spinal cord trauma, 2245
Queensland tick typhus, 1745
Quellung reaction, 1555
Quercetin, and cancer, 44
Quinacrine hydrochloride, for giardiasis, 1884
Quinazoline, for hypertension, 286t, 301
Quinethazone, for hypertension, 286t
Quinidine, 270
  and photosensitivity, 2351
  arrhythmias from, 275
  distribution of, heart failure and, 97
  dosing and adverse effects of, 268t
  esophageal injury from, 688
  for digitalis intoxication, 230
  for malaria, 1861
  for mitral stenosis, 347
  genetics and reaction to, 102
  induction of metabolism of, 99
  interaction of, with curare, 101
    with digitalis, 228
    with digoxin, 101
  liver granulomas from, 828
  metabolism of, inhibited by cimetidine, 100
  pharmacokinetic properties of, 89t, 266t
  reference intervals for, 2404t
  thrombocytopenia from, 1049
  ventricular premature depolarizations from, 263
Quinine
  and photosensitivity, 2351
  for babesiosis, 1886
  for malaria, 1860–1861
  genetics and reaction to, 102
  hemolytic anemia from, 103
  heroin with, 56
  hypoglycemia from, 1384
  interaction of, with curare, 101
  side effects of, and eye, 2298
  thrombocytopenia from, 103
Quinolones, 122
  action of, 113t
  in drug interactions, 124t
  in kidney and liver failure, 117t
  resistance mechanisms of, 116t
Quinsy, from streptococcal tonsillitis, 1576
Quintan fever, 1747

R state, of hemoglobin, 943
R wave, in electrocardiography, 197
RA, 1998–2004. See also Rheumatoid arthritis
Rabbits, and tularemia, 1664, 1665
Rabies, 2200–2202
  central nervous system infection with, 2191
  immunization against, 62t, 63, 63t
    before travel, 1550
  in raccoons, 2200
  postexposure prophylaxis for, 2201–2202, 2202

Raccoon eyes, 2066
  from skull fracture, 2241
Race, and anemias, 880
  and hirsutism, 2349
  and hypertension, 277
Radiation. See also under Radioactive
  dose specification for, 2375, 2376t
  injury from, 2375–2380. See also Radiation injury
  ionizing, 2375
    and cancer, 1094
    and thyroid tumors, 1335
    biology of, 2376
  low-level, delayed effects of, 2378
  of testis, 1416
    effect of, 1415
  therapy with. See Radiation therapy
Radiation dose, 2375
Radiation enteritis, diarrhea from, 729
  malabsorption from, 743
Radiation enterocolitis, 806
Radiation fibrosis, pulmonary hypertension from, 296
Radiation injury, 2375–2380
  and acute leukemia, 1001
  and bone marrow injury, 962
  and breast cancer, 1453
  and cancer, 1093t, 1094
  and chronic myelogenous leukemia, 988
  and epidermal neoplasms, 2337
  constrictive pericarditis from, 366
  clinical manifestations of, 2377–2378
  definition of, 2375
  diagnosis of, 2378–2379
  epidemiology of, 2376–2377
  etiology of, 2376
  incidence and prevalence of, 2376–2377
  interstitial lung disease from, 435
  lymphocytopenia from, 966
  nephritis from, 610
  organ damage from, 2379t
  pathogenesis of, 2377
  pericarditis from, 363
  prevention of, 2380
  prognosis for, 2380
  symptoms, therapy and prognosis after, 2378t
  to bone, and osteosarcoma, 1521
  to intestines, stool examination for, 730
  to lungs, 2365–2366
  treatment of, 2379–2380
Radiation proctitis, vs. ulcerative colitis, 757
  vs. ulcerative proctitis, 788
Radiation therapy, 2376
  and eosinophilia, 1026
  and hair damage, 2349
  and hypothalamic dysfunction, 1286–1287
  and premature ovarian failure, 1438
  anorectal fistulas from, 789
  for cancer, 1088, 1115, 1115–1116
    bronchogenic, 461, 462
    colorectal, 772
    gastric, 712
    pancreatic, 784
    small cell lung, 462
  for chronic lymphocytic leukemia, 997
  for Cushing's disease, 1304–1305, 1356
  for Hodgkin's disease, 1019–1020
  for Langerhans cell granulomatosis, 1023
  for low-grade non-Hodgkin's lymphoma, 1011
  for midline granuloma, 2032
  for neoplasms
    extradural, 2256
    of brain, 2234, 2235
    of esophagus, 687
    pineal, 1315
    pituitary, 1299–1300

Radiation therapy (Continued)
for neoplasms, pituitary, growth hormone secreting, 1301–1302
thyroid, 1338
for nephroblastoma, 654
hypopituitarism from, 1295
infertility from, 1119–1120
injury to nervous system from, 1107, 1107t
normal tissue tolerance to, 1116t
of spleen, for chronic myelogenous leukemia, 992
side effects of, 1020
with chemotherapy, 1119–1120
Radicals, 2376
Radicular pain, 2249, 2250
from herniated disc, 2253
Radiculopathy, 2057t
electrophysiologic studies of, 2057t
Radioactive iodine
for hyperthyroidism, 1326
with goiter, 1339
for thyroid neoplasms, 1338
pregnancy as contraindication for, 1326
uptake of, and thyroid function, 1319
Radioactive phosphorus, for polycythemia vera, 983
Radioactive thallium, scanning with, 178
Radioallergosorbent test, 408, 1951
Radiocontrast agents
allergic reaction to, 104, 526, 1968, 1971
anaphylaxis from, 1956
and kidney damage, 559, 561, 609–610
glomerulopathy and, 626
management of, 570
and urticaria, 1950
as osmotic diuretics, 232
for roentgenograms of kidneys, 525
toxic reactions to, 526
Radiography
chest
for anomalous origin of left coronary artery, 308
for atrial septal defect, 305
for cardiovascular disease patients, 177–178
for left ventricular failure, 222
for ostium primum defects, 306
for patent ductus arteriosus, 307
for preventive health, 66
for tetralogy of Fallot, 309
for acute pancreatitis, 777
for amyloidosis, 360
for anomalous pulmonary venous connection, 315
for aortic regurgitation, 344
for aortic stenosis, 342
for back pain, 2251
for biliary disease, 862
for bone age determination, 18
for bronchogenic carcinoma, 460
for coarctation of aorta, 313
for constrictive pericarditis, 367
for Crohn's disease, 747–748, 748
for dilated cardiomyopathy, 353
for diverticulitis, 804
for Ebstein's anomaly of tricuspid valve, 310
for Eisenmenger's syndrome, 317
for esophageal disorders, 684
for gallstones, 866
for gastric cancer diagnosis, 711
for hypertrophic cardiomyopathy, 357
for ileus, 719
for infective endocarditis, 1593
for interstitial lung disease, 426, 426
for kidney stones, 641

Radiography (Continued)
for localization of pain, 106
for lymphoma, of stomach, 712
for mediastinal disorders, 470, 471
for mitral regurgitation, 349
for mitral stenosis, 346
for mitral valve prolapse, 350
for peptic ulcers, 697
for pulmonary hypertension, 299
for pulmonic stenosis, 311, 312
for sarcoidosis, 454, 454
for tricuspid atresia, 311
for ulcerative colitis, 756, 756
for valvular heart disease, 341
limits of, for pulmonary embolism, 445
of dead vs. living bone, 1517
of kidneys, 525
Radioimmunoassay
of calcitonin, 1506
of hormones, 1265–1266
of parathyroid hormone, 1488, 1492, 1493
Radioisotope(s)
for adenocarcinoma of peritoneum, 794
in joint radiology, 1997
injection of, 207
systemic exposure to, diagnosis of, 2379
Radioligand binding studies, to measure adrenergic receptors, 136
Radiology, 82–87. See also Diagnostic imaging techniques
and urinary tract, 629
for Hodgkin's disease, 1018
for malabsorption diagnosis, 740
for pyogenic liver abscess, 836
pleural fluid in, 466
Radionuclide(s), systemic exposure to, 2378
treatment with, 2379–2380
Radionuclide scanning
before coronary artery bypass grafts, 337
computed tomography vs., 284
for acute abdomen, 803
for cardiovascular disease patients, 178
for gallstones, 866
for localization of pain, 106
for lower gastrointestinal hemorrhage, 798
for pyogenic liver abscess, 836
for valvular heart disease, 341
of biliary tree, 863
of bone, for back pain, 2251
of gastrointestinal system, 665–667, 665
Radioreceptor assays, 1266
Radium, ingested, 2376
Radon, and cancer, 458, 1094
Ragpicker's disease, 1667
Ragweed, and allergic rhinitis, 1952
Ramazzini, Bernardino, 1092
Ramsay Hunt syndrome, 2222
herpes zoster and, 2196
vertigo from, 2124
RANA, and Epstein-Barr virus, 1997
Ranitidine
elimination rate for, 96t
for acute gastritis, 690
for duodenal ulcers, 702
for gastric ulcers, 702
for inhibiting acid secretion, 700
for Zollinger-Ellison syndrome, 709
RAP (rheumatoid arthritis precipitin), 1991
Rapaport-Luebering shunt, 913, 914
Rapid eye movement phase of sleep, 2077
Rapid plasma reagin test, 1719
for syphilis, 2190
Rapidly progressive glomerulonephritis, 589t, 589, 589–591
idiopathic, 583, 584t, 591
Rash
from chronic meningococcemia, 1614

Rash (Continued)
from drug allergy, 1970t, 2352
from herpes zoster, 2196
from hypereosinophilic syndrome, 1024
from infectious mononucleosis, 1787
from measles, 1773
from murine typhus, 1741
from onchocerciasis, 1917
from polymyositis, 2035
from Rocky Mountain spotted fever, 1742–1743, 1744
from rubella, 1776
immunization for, 64
from scrub typhus, 1747
from streptobacillary fever, 1729
from syphilis, 1715
from systemic lupus erythematosus, 2014–2015
from typhoid fever, 1641
from typhus fever, 1739, 1740
with viral neurologic disease, 2194
Raspberry tongue, 1576
RAST (radioallergosorbent test), 408, 1951
Rat(s), and plague, 1661
poisons for, coumarin compounds in, 1077
Rat-bite fevers, 1729–1730
Rate-responsive pacing, 272
Rathke's pouch, 1290
Rattlesnakes, 1927
Rauwolfia alkaloids, adverse effects of, 289t
for hypertension, 287t
Raynaud's disease, 375
vs. secondary Raynaud's phenomenon, 376
Raynaud's phenomenon, 369, 375–377
causes of, 375t
from thromboangiitis obliterans, 382
in essential mixed cryoglobulinemia, 601
in musculoskeletal disease, 2020t
in mycoplasmal infections, 1563
in systemic lupus erythematosus, 2015
in systemic sclerosis, 2019
management of, 2023
M-components and, 1028
Raynaud's sign, in polymyositis, 2035
Reaction time, delayed, from chronic hypoxia, 477
Reaginic antibodies, and inflammation, 1988
Rebound tenderness, from diffuse peritonitis, 801
Rebuck skin window test, 960
for neutrophil evaluation, 957
Receptor(s)
for hormones, 1253
abnormalities in, 1264
opiate, 1270
sensory, 2128–2129
Receptor cross-linkage-dependent activation, 1934
Receptor ligands, radiolabeling of, 211
Receptor-apotransferrin complex, 929
Receptor-mediated endocytosis, 955
Recessive disorder(s), autosomal, 148–149
cystic fibrosis as, 440
frequency of, 151
Recessive methemoglobinemia, 152
Recessive traits, 147
autosomal, pedigree of, 148
X-linked, 150
Reciprocal translocation, in chromosomes, 165, 166, 166
Recombinant deoxyribonucleic acid technology, 158–161, 1524
Recombinant human erythropoietin, 571
Recommended dietary allowances, 1204, 1205t, 1206

Recruitment, from sensorineural lesions, 2117
  measurement of, 2118
Rectosigmoid cancer, screening for, 773
Rectovaginal fistulas, from ulcerative colitis, 757
Rectum
  biopsy of, for diarrhea, 731
    for ulcerative colitis, 756
  bleeding from
    as contraindication for proctosigmoidoscopy, 755
    from ischemic colitis, 764
    from radiation therapy, 806
    from ulcerative colitis, 754
  chancre of, 1715
  disease of, 787–788
  examination of, magnetic resonance imaging for, 85, 85
  gonococcal infections in, 1707
  infection of, vs. ulcerative proctitis, 788
  ischemia of, 788
  lacerations of, vs. gonococcal infections of rectum, 1707
  prolapse of, from shigellosis, 1646
    from trichuriasis, 1909
    from ulcerative colitis, 757
  scarring of, from lymphogranuloma venereum, 1711
  solitary ulcer in, 788
  tumors of, magnetic resonance of, 667
  ulcerative colitis in, 760. See also Ulcerative colitis
Red blood cell(s), 421. See also Erythrocyte(s)
  aplasia(s) of, in cancer, 1098
    pure, autoimmunity in, 887
      treatment of, 889
  casts of, and glomerular injury, 503
    hematuria with, in acute glomerulonephritis, 584
  counts of, depressions in, from ribavirin, 127
    in polycythemia vera, 981
  frozen, 942t, 948
  mass of
    and polycythemia, 975
    normal averages for, 976
    reduction in, and anemia, 878–879
    regulation of, 976
    by kidneys, 519
  packed, 947. See also Packed red blood cells
Reed-Sternberg cell, in Hodgkin's disease, 1007, 1014, 1015, 1015
Refeeding, complications of, 1214–1215
  gynecomastia from, 1411
Reference intervals, 81, 2394t-2404t
Referred pain, 2249, 2250
  in back, 2043
  in gastrointestinal disease, 658
Reflex(es)
  deep tendon, 2271
    in periodic paralysis, 2281
    loss of, in Friedreich's ataxia, 2152
    in amyotrophic lateral sclerosis, 2156
    increased, in adult-onset cerebellar ataxia, 2153
  loss of peripheral, from syphilis, 1717
  monosynaptic, psychedelic drugs and, 58
  postural, disturbances in, 2143
  primitive, in Parkinson's disease, 2144
Reflex sympathetic dystrophies, 2136
  nerve blocks for pain in, 110
Reflux
  diagnosis of, 682
  odynophagia in, 679
  of duodenal juice, and chronic gastritis, 690
  ureteral, 649–650

Refractoriness, 251–252
Regan isozyme, 815
Regional enteritis, 745, 747. See also Crohn's disease; Ulcerative colitis
  in Behçet's disease, 2049
  sclerosing cholangitis with, 869
Regional ileitis, 745
Regurgitation
  from esophageal disease, 680
  from gastroesophageal reflux disease, 681
  in congenital heart disease, 311–314
  nasal, from palatal weakness, 684
  pulmonic, 314, 351
  tricuspid, 351
Rehabilitation, after oral cancer treatment, 679
  after stroke, 2172
Reifenstein's syndrome, 1399, 1418
  cryptorchidism in, 1415
  gynecomastia in, 1451
Reiter's syndrome, 151, 2005t, 2007–2008, 2326t
  aortic regurgitation from, 343
  diagnosis of, human leukocyte antigens and, 1968
  from Campylobacter infection, 1649
  from shigellosis, 1647
  ulcers in, vs. ulcers in Behçet's disease, 2049
  uveitis in, 2293
  vs. disseminated gonococcal infection, 1709
  vs. Lyme disease, 1728
  vs. psoriasis, 2327
Rejection, of transplants, 578–579
Relapsing fever, 1724–1725
Relaxation techniques, for hypertension, 278, 285
REM (rapid eye movement) phase of sleep, 2077
Remnant removal disease, 1140t, 1141
  and atherosclerosis, 1144
  vs. familial hypercholesterolemia, 1140–1141
Remodeling, in wound healing, 2306
  of bone, 1475
Renal. See also Kidney(s) and under Glomerular
Renal adenocarcinoma. See Renal cell carcinoma
Renal agenesis, bilateral, 170
Renal calculi, 505–506, 638t, 638–644. See also Calculi, renal
Renal carbuncle, pyelonephritis with, 629
Renal cell carcinoma, 506, 652t, 652–653, 653
  and renal vein thrombosis, 634
  solitary pulmonary nodules from, 465
Renal colic, 505
  from transitional cell cancers of ureter, 655
  kidney stones and, 641
  pain in groin and testicle from, 106
Renal columns of Bertin, 508
Renal failure. See Kidney(s), failure of
Renal Medicare Program, 573
Renal osteodystrophy, 566, 1507–1510
  and osteosclerosis, 1518
  biochemical features of, 1508–1509
  bone salt loss in chronic kidney failure and, 564
  clinical manifestations of, 1508
  components of, 1507t
  in chronic renal failure, 507
  management of, 571
  radiographic features of, 1509
  renal tubular acidosis and, 623
  treatment of, 1509t, 1509–1510

Renal pelvis, 508
  transitional cell cancers of, 506, 654, 654–655
  tumors of, urinary cytology for, 503
Renal syndrome, hemorrhagic fever with, 1836–1837
Renal tubular acidosis, 532, 621t
  distal, 505
    classic, 622–624
    defects of, 505
    diuretics for, 535–536
    flow rate of, 517
    hypokalemia in, 546
    metabolic acidosis in, 553
    treatment of, 554
  from nephrocalcinosis, 606
  hypocitraturia from, and kidney stones, 640
  of glomerular insufficiency, 623
  primary biliary cirrhosis with, 845
  proximal, 620, 620–621
  type IV, 532, 564
  vs. polymyositis, 2036
Renal vein thrombosis, 634
  causes of, 634t
  in membranous nephropathy, 597
Renal-retinal dysplasia, 648
Rendu-Osler-Weber syndrome, 308. See also Osler-Weber-Rendu syndrome
Renin, 503, 516
  and mineralocorticoid production, 1345
  arachidonic acid metabolites and, 1276
  assessment of, 1350
  in Starling force abnormalities, 535
  measurement of, and renovascular hypertension, 283
  reference intervals for, 2399t
  release of, antihypertensive agents inhibiting, 283t
    by kidney, in fluid volume regulation, 530
  stimulation of, 283
  secretion of, and hypertension, 277
  suppression of, in primary aldosteronism, 1358
Renin-angiotensin system, 190, 220, 1345
  and hypertension, 278, 279
  in chronic kidney failure, and hypertension, 565
  in heart failure, 230
  shock and, 239
  suppression of, in primary aldosteronism, 1358
Renin-angiotensin-aldosterone, and sodium balance, 515–516
Renovascular hypertension, 280–281
  diagnosis of, 282
  treatment for, 288, 290–291
Replacement therapy
  for blood coagulation disorders, 1066
  for hemophilia A, 1068
  for hemophilia B, 1071
  for hormones, 1265
  for hypophosphatemia, 1194
  for magnesium deficiency, 1196
  for von Willebrand disease, 1070
Repolarization, of excitable cells, 545
Reproducibility, of laboratory tests, 80
Reproductive functions, hormones and, 1263
Reproductive system, arachidonic acid metabolites and, 1276
RES. See Reticuloendothelial system
Research, 5
  patients used for, 14
Reserpine
  adverse effects of, 289t

Reserpine (Continued)
  aggravation of heart failure by, 220
  and catecholamine depletion, 1282
  and depression, 2096
  derivatives of, rebound effects of, 1954
  for Huntington's disease, 2148
  for hypertension, 287t
  for Raynaud's phenomenon, 377
  myocardial depression from, 239
  parkinsonism from, 2144
Reservoir masks, for oxygen therapy, 478
Resistance, combination antimicrobial therapy and, 118
Resorcinol(s), for asthma, 408
  toxicity of, to hemoglobin, 945
Respiration, 395–403. See also Lung(s) and under Pulmonary and Respiratory
  Cheyne-Stokes, in heart failure, 176
  control of breathing in, 400–401
  definition of, 390, 395
  depression of, narcotics and, 109
  diffusion in, 399–400
  disorders of. See Respiratory disorders
  exercise and, 403
  failure of. See Respiratory failure
  gas exchange in, 401–403, 402
  modulation of, 550
  muscles of, disorders of, respiratory failure from, 476
  perfusion in, 400
  stimulants of, 481
  techniques for supporting, 486–489
  ventilation in, 395, 395–399
Respiratory acidosis, 551, 557
  acute, and transient hypophosphatemia, 1193
  and metabolic encephalopathy, 2067t
  and phosphorus excretion, 518
  heart failure with, 226
  hypoventilation with, mechanical ventilation for, 487
Respiratory alkalosis, 551, 557–558
  and bicarbonate synthesis, 518
  and hypophosphatemia, 1471
  and metabolic encephalopathy, 2067t
  from aspirin poisonings, 143
  in fulminant hepatic failure, 854
  in interstitial lung disease, 426
Respiratory burst, absence of, in chronic granulomatous disease, 958
  in neutrophil killing of microorganisms, 952–953, 954
Respiratory care equipment, and infection, 1544
  for shock patients, 245
Respiratory disorders
  acute, 390
  chronic, 390
  of acid-base balance, 551
  pulmonary hypertension from, 296
Respiratory distress syndrome
  adult. See Adult respiratory distress syndrome (ARDS)
  fat embolism syndrome and, 450
  from acute heroin reaction, 56
  from ascites, 791
  in neonates, glucocorticoids and, 1347
Respiratory failure, 473–481
  acute, monitoring progress in, 479
    treatment of, 477–479
    vs. chronic respiratory failure, 474
  causes of, 475–477
  chronic, surgery and, 481
    treatment of, 479–481
  clinical manifestations of, 477
  critical care for, 489–492
  definition of, 473
  differential diagnosis of, 2277

Respiratory failure (Continued)
  gastritis with, 689
  in anaphylaxis, 1957
  pathophysiology of, 474–475
Respiratory muscles, cardiorespiratory arrest and, 500
  paralysis of, from scorpion stings, 1924
    from spinal cord trauma, 2245
Respiratory rate, measurement of, in severely ill, 482
Respiratory syncytial virus, 1758–1760
  ribavirin for, 127
Respiratory system
  arachidonic acid metabolites and, 1276
  arsenic poisoning and, 2388
  compliance of, 485
  disorders of, acute hemorrhagic leukoencephalitis after, 2209
    from Mycoplasma pneumoniae, 1561–1564
    from progressive muscular atrophy, 2155
    vs. panic attacks, 2101
  gummas of, 1717
  hormones and, 1263
  in Duchenne dystrophy, 2272–2273
  in Japanese encephalitis, 1828
  infection of
    anaerobic, 1638
    and asthma, 407
    chronic, in immotile cilia syndrome, 1416
    hemolytic uremic syndrome after, 601
    immunoglobulin A deficiency and, 1943
    quinolones for, 122
    vs. whooping cough, 1625
  injury to, from aspiration, 2369–2373
  leeches in, 1927
  lower. See also Interstitial lung disease
    anatomy of, 421, 421–422
    immunoglobulins in, 424
    macromolecules in, 424
  monitoring of, in critical care units, 493
  obesity and, 1224
  severe dysfunction of, assessment of, 482–486
    calculations for, 484–486
  upper, Haemophilus in, 1617
    meningococcal infection of, 1614
  viral infection of, 1753–1768
    common cold as, 1753–1757
    from adenovirus, 1767–1768
    immunodeficiency and, 1942
    influenza as, 1762–1767
    parainfluenza, 1760–1761
Rest, for angina pectoris, 324
  for systemic lupus erythematosus, 2017
  response to, in pulmonary hypertension, vasodilators and, 299
Restless leg syndrome, 567
  in hyperparathyroidism, 1490
Restlessness
  from drugs for schizophrenia, 2094
  from metabolic encephalopathy, 2063
  from opioid withdrawal syndrome, 57
  from psychiatric disorders vs. organic encephalopathies, 2092
  from sedative withdrawal, 54
  from tetanus, 1635
Restriction enzyme(s), 158
  polymorphisms of, and prenatal diagnosis of thalassemia, 935–936
Restriction fragment length polymorphism, 974
  linkage analysis with, 158
Resuscitation, cardiopulmonary, 499–501
  for gastrointestinal hemorrhage, 797

Retained antrum syndrome, 695
  and postoperative recurrent ulcers, 705
  vs. peptic ulcers, 699
Retching, definition of, 658
Reticular dysgenesis, 1946
  from thymic hypoplasia, 1974
Reticular fibers, in kidneys, 510
Reticulocyte, conditioning of, in spleen, 1036–1037
  definition of, 882
  iron receptors in, 894
Reticulocyte count, 882–883
  reference intervals for, 2402t
Reticulocyte index, 908
Reticulocytopenia, from riboflavin deficiency, 1231
Reticulocytosis
  after hemorrhagic episode, 891
  from hemolysis, 909
  from hemolytic anemia, 882
  from normocytic normochromic anemias, 890
Reticuloendothelial system, 884
  in inflammatory response, 1531
  tumors of, spread of, to kidneys, 655
Reticuloendotheliosis, leukemic, 998. See also Hairy cell leukemia
Reticulohistiocytosis, multicentric, 2046
Reticuloid, actinic, 2352
Reticulonodularity, in sarcoidosis, 451, 454, 454
Reticulosis, malignant midline, vs. midline granuloma, 2032, 2032t
Reticulum, sarcoplasmic, 184
Retina, 2111
  appearance of, and threatened stroke, 2167
  Bruch's membrane of, defects in, 1516
  detachment of, in sickle cell anemia, 939
  dystrophy of, in Laurence-Moon-Bardet-Biedl syndrome, 1203
  hamartomas of, in tuberous sclerosis, 2158
  hemorrhage of, from aplastic anemia, 887
  malignancy of, 2295
  pigmentary degeneration of, in adult-onset cerebellar ataxia, 2153
  tears and detachment in, 2112
  vitamin E deficiency and, 2140
Retinal artery, branch, occlusion of, 2298
  central occlusion of, 2297–2298
Retinal vein, occlusion of, 2298
Retinitis, in AIDS patients, DHPG for, 126
Retinitis pigmentosa, 2236
  and optic atrophy, 2292–2293
Retinoblastoma, 1095t, 2295
  chromosome studies for, 168
Retinochoroiditis, from toxoplasmosis, 1877
  differential diagnosis of, 1878
Retinoic acid, 1237
Retinoids, and hair damage, 2349
  for skin disorders, 2317
  side effects of, 2317
Retinol, 1236. See also Vitamin A
Retinopathy, diabetic, 1378, 2297
  Kimmelstiel-Wilson, 277
  of prematurity, 2297
Retrocollis, 2150
Retrolental fibroplasia, 2297
Retroperitoneal fibrosis, 2051–2052
  from methysergide, 612
  sclerosing cholangitis with, 869
  ureteral obstruction from, 507
  with Riedel's thyroiditis, 1334
Retropulsion, 2127
Retrovir (azidothymidine), 127, 1523, 1799, 1807
  reference intervals for, 2396t

Retroviral oncogenes, pathogenic mechanisms of, 1090–1091
  proteins encoded by, 1090t
Retroviruses, 1794. See also *RNA viruses*
  classification of, 1794
  disadvantages of, 161
  disease from, 1794–1807
    acquired immunodeficiency syndrome as, 1799–1808. See also *AIDS*
    acute leukemia as, 1001
    double infection with, 1799
  effects of, 1794
  human, features of, 1795, 1795t, *1796*
  life cycle of, 1090, *1090, 1794*
  vectors of, 160
Rewarming shock, 2384, 2385
Reye's syndrome, 2209–2210
  after varicella, 1789
  aspirin and, 829, 1756
  from adenovirus infection, 1767
  hypoglycemia in, 809
  influenza and, 1766
  vs. fulminant hepatic failure, 854
Rh blood group, 948
Rhabdomyolysis, 1472
  exertional, vs. polymyositis, 2036
  fatty acid metabolism disorders and, 2278
  from heatstroke, 2383
  from hypokalemia, 548
  from hypophosphatemia, 1194
  from potassium loss by skeletal muscle, 546
  in heroin users, 57
  myoglobinuria and, 2282
Rhabdomyoma(s), in heart, 367
  in tuberous sclerosis, 2158
Rhabdomyosarcoma, 2295
  of kidneys, 655
  solitary pulmonary nodules from, 464
Rheumatic disease
  approach to, 1977–1980
  categories of, 1978t
  diagnostic procedures in, 1993–1998
  healing period for, 1979
  inflammation in, 1984–1992
  laboratory tests in, 1979
  location of, *1978*
  long-term outcome of, planning for, 1979–1980
  of heart. See *Rheumatic heart disease*
  mediators of inflammation in, 1986–1987
  tissue destruction in, 1984–1992
Rheumatic fever, 11, 1580–1586
  acute, after streptococcal infection, 1575
    decline in, 1579
    group A streptococcal pharyngitis and, 1572
    nonparoxysmal atrioventricular junctional tachycardia and, 262
    pathology of, 1581–1582
    vs. gout, 1168
  aortic regurgitation from, 343
  aortic stenosis from, 341
  average age for, 345
  chronic, 1584
  clinical manifestations of, 1582–1584
  course and prognosis for, 1584
  diagnosis of, 1584–1585
    Jones criteria for, 1584t, 1584–1585
  epidemiology of, 1581
  glucocorticosteroid therapy for, 130
  group A streptococci and, 1574
  laboratory findings for, 1584
  mitral stenosis from, 345
  pathogenesis of, 1580–1581
  penicillin for, 119
  prevention of, 1586

Rheumatic fever (*Continued*)
  recurrence of, 1579, 1581
    preventing, 1586
  Sydenham's chorea with, 2148
  treatment of, 1585
  tricuspid stenosis from, 351
  vs. chronic meningococcemia, 1616
  vs. Fabry's disease, 1145
  vs. Lyme disease, 1728
  vs. sarcoidosis, 454
  vs. systemic lupus erythematosus, 2017
Rheumatic heart disease
  cryptogenic cirrhosis from, 847
  epidemiology of, 179
  mitral regurgitation from, 347
  pancarditis, 363
  scarring from, and atrial flutter, 258
Rheumatism, nonarticular, 2047–2048
  palindromic, 2047
Rheumatoid arthritis, 1998–2004, *2001*
  acute phase response to, 1528
  and amyloidosis, 1199
  and anemia, 881
  and carpal tunnel syndrome, 2268
  and warm autoimmune hemolytic anemia, 918
  anemias of, 899
  aortic regurgitation from, 343
  articular manifestations of, 2001
  clinical features of, 2000
  diagnosis of, 1979
    criteria for, 1999
    differential, 2000–2001
  etiology of, 1999
  excess copper in, 1242
  extra-articular manifestations of, 2002–2003
  genetics and, 146
  glucocorticosteroid therapy for, 130
  interstitial lung disease and, 429
  juvenile
    and uveitis, 2293
    human leukocyte antigens and, 1967
    skin lesions in, 2335
    vs. acute leukemia, 1004
    vs. systemic lupus erythematosus, 2017
  laboratory findings for, 2003
  myasthenia gravis with, 2285
  neuropathy in, 2266
  pathogenesis of, 2000
  pathology of, 1999–2000
  pericarditis in, 363
  pernicious anemia with, 905
  pleuritis from, 468
  prostaglandin E₂ in, 1273
  radiology for, 1997
  remission criteria for, 2000
  Sjögren's syndrome in, 2296
  small intestinal ulceration from, 807
  solitary pulmonary nodules from, 464
  splenomegaly in, 1037
  synovial membrane in, 1995
  synovitis in, 1984
  therapeutic management of, 2003–2004
  tissue destruction in, 1991–1992, *1992*
  vasculitis in, 2027
  vs. ankylosing spondylitis, 2006
  vs. arthritis from alcaptonuria, 1157
  vs. gout, 1168
  vs. Lyme disease, 1728
  vs. multicentric reticulohistiocytosis, 2046
  vs. osteoarthritis, 2041
  vs. polymyalgia rheumatica, 2033
  vs. pseudogout syndrome, 2037
  vs. shoulder-hand syndrome, 2042
  vs. sporotrichosis, 1847
  with systemic sclerosis, 2021

Rheumatoid arthritis precipitin, 1991
Rheumatoid factor, 1995–1996, 1999
  in interstitial lung disease, 426
  in Sjögren's syndrome, 2025
  in synovial fluid, 1993
  in Wegener's granulomatosis, 2030
Rheumatoid nodules, 2336t, 2340
Rhinitis
  allergic, 1951–1955. See also *Allergic rhinitis*
  from congenital syphilis, 1718
  from occupational asthma, 2359
Rhinitis medicamentosa, 1954, 1955
Rhinophyma, 2333, *2333*
Rhinorrhea
  cerebrospinal fluid, 1608–1609
    from skull fracture, 2241
  from common cold, 1755
  in opioid withdrawal syndrome, 57
Rhinoscleroma, vs. zygomycosis, 1852
Rhinoviruses
  common cold from, 1753
  infection of, clinical manifestations of, 1755–1756, 1756t
  interferon for, 128
  transmission of, 1754
Rhipicephalus sanguineus, and Rocky Mountain spotted fever transmission, 1742
Rhodesian sleeping sickness, 1864
Rib(s), fractures of, from cough, 391
  pulmonary embolism vs., 444
  respiratory failure from, critical care of, 490
Ribavirin, for respiratory syncytial virus, 127, 1760
Ribbing disease, 1519
Riboflavin, *1230*, 1230–1231. See also *Vitamin B₂*
Ribonucleic acid, in erythroblasts, 929
  viral, 124
  xenogeneic immune, for renal cell carcinoma, 653
Richter's syndrome, chronic lymphocytic leukemia and, 996
Rickets, 1479–1485, 1480t. See also *Osteomalacia*
  definition of, 1479
  from Fanconi's syndrome, 621
  vitamin D–dependent, 1154t
    type I, 1480–1481
    type II, 1481
  vitamin D–resistant, 153
    as X-linked dominant trait, 149
    vs. hypophosphatemia in cancer, 1102
    vs. osteogenesis imperfecta, 1180
Rickettsia(e)
  disease from, 1737t, 1737–1749, 1738t
    chloramphenicol for, 120
    Q fever as, 1748–1749
    rickettsialpox as, 1745–1746
    Rocky Mountain spotted fever as, 1742–1744, *1743*
    scrub typhus as, 1746–1747
    tetracyclines for, 121
    trench fever as, 1747–1748
    typhus group in, 1738–1742
    vs. rat-bite fever, 1730
    vs. viral encephalitis, 2194
  fever from, vs. yellow fever, 1832
  hemolysis from, 925
Rickettsia akari, 1745
Rickettsia australis, 1745
Rickettsia canada, 1739
Rickettsia conorii, 1745
Rickettsia prowazekii, in typhus fever, 1738, 1739
Rickettsia rickettsii, and Rocky Mountain spotted fever, 1742

Rickettsia siberica, 1745
Rickettsia tsutsugamushi, 1746
Rickettsia typhi, 1741
Rickettsialpox, 1745–1746
   clinical features of, 1738t
   epidemiologic features of, 1737t
   vs. varicella, 1789
Rickettsiosis, vs. leptospirosis, 1732
Riedel's thyroiditis, 1334
   sclerosing cholangitis with, 869
Rifampin, 121
   action of, 113t
   acute interstitial nephritis from, 605
   and enhanced liver metabolism of other
      drugs, 99
   elimination rate for, 96t
   for brucellosis, 1678
   for endocarditis, 114
   for legionnaires' disease, 1572
   for leprosy, 1699–1700
   for meningococcal disease prophylaxis,
      1549
   for osteomyelitis, 114
   for refractory staphylococcal infections,
      119
   for tuberculosis, 1686–1687
   hyperbilirubinemia from, 814
   in drug interactions, 124t
   in *Haemophilus influenzae* prophylaxis,
      1620
   in kidney and liver failure, 117t
   in meningococcal disease prophylaxis,
      1616
   liver disease from, 829–830
   penetration into spinal fluid by, 116
   reduced absorption of, para-aminosali-
      cylic acid and, 99
Rift Valley fever, 1818–1819
Right-sidedness, bilateral, in asplenia syn-
      drome, 315
Rigid-spine syndrome, 2274
Rigidity, 2143
Riley-Day dysautonomia, 2265
Riley-Day syndrome, 2106
Rimantadine, 127
   for influenza, 1766
RIND (reversible ischemic neurologic dis-
      ability), 2162
Ring(s), formation of, in brain abscess, 2183
   in esophagus, 687
Ringed sideroblasts, 899
Ringer's lactate solution, 245
Ringworm, vs. pityriasis rosea, 2327
Riolan, arc of, 761
Risk modification, in preventive medicine,
      35
Ristocetin, for von Willebrand disease diag-
      nosis, 1070
Ritalin, abuse of, 54
River blindness, 1916–1918
River fever, 1747
RMP. See *Rifampin*
RMSF. See *Rocky Mountain spotted fever*
RNA. See *Ribonucleic acid*
RNA viruses, acute leukemia from, 1001
   and cancer, 1095
Robertsonian translocation, in chromo-
      somes, 165, 166
Rochalimaea quintana, trench fever from,
      1747
Rocio encephalitis, 1828
Rocky Mountain spotted fever, 1737, 1742–
      1744, 1743
   clinical features of, 1738t
   epidemiologic features of, 1737t
   immunization against, 65
   rash in, 2325

Rocky Mountain spotted fever *(Continued)*
   splenomegaly in, 1037
   vs. Colorado tick fever, 1820
   vs. meningococcal disease, 1615
   vs. murine typhus, 1741
Rod myopathy, 2275
Rodent ulcer, 2337, 2337
Rodenticides, as testicular toxins, 1416
Rodents, and hemorrhagic fever with renal
      syndrome, 1836
Roentgenograms. See *Radiography*
Rolandic epilepsy, 2221
Romana's sign, in Chagas' disease, 1867
Romberg test, for elderly, 27
Rombergism, 2125
Romberg's sign, definition of, 2189
   in diabetic neuropathy, 2263
   in tabes dorsalis, 2189
Rosacea, 2333, 2333t
Rose spots, in typhoid fever, 1641
Rosenbach, erysipeloid of, 1673
Roseoliform exanthems, 1813
Ross River fever, 1819
Ross River virus, arthritis from, 1999
Rotator cuff tears, 2042
Rotavirus, 1769, 1769. See also *Viral gas-
      troenteritis*
   and diarrhea, 729
   gastroenteritis from, 1769–1770
Rothmann-Makai syndrome, 2050
Roth's spots, definition of, 2297
   from infective endocarditis, 1589t
Rotor's syndrome, 813t
Rous, Peyton, 1082
Roussy-Levy syndrome, 2264
Rowley-Rosenberg syndrome, 1154t
RPR (rapid plasma reagin) test, 1719, 2190
RSV (respiratory syncytial virus), 1758–1760
   ribavirin for, 127
Rubella, 1776–1777
   acute hepatitis from, 819
   and arthritis, 2010
   and cataract, 2289
   and congenital heart disease, 303
   and seizures, 2218
   congenital infection of, vs. cytomegalovi-
      rus, 1785–1786
   immunization against, 61, 63t, 63–64
      agents for, 62t
   intrauterine, megakaryocytic hypoplasia
      from, 1048
   panencephalitis in, progressive, 2206–
      2207
   rash in, 2322
   vs. congenital syphilis, 1718
   vs. exanthems, from enteroviruses, 1813
   vs. measles, 1774, 1775t
   vs. rat-bite fever, 1730
Rubeola, 1772–1775, 1773. See also *Measles*
Rule of thirds, for body fluid compart-
      ments, 529
Rumination, 680, 1219
   vomiting vs., 658
Rumpel-Leed test, 1235, 1576
Russell's viper venom, 1072
   response to, 1073

S wave, in electrocardiography, 197
SA (sinoatrial) node, 184
Saber shins, from congenital syphilis, 2189
Sabin-Feldman dye test, for toxoplasmosis,
      1878
Saccharin, and cancer, 1096
Saccharopinuria, 1151t
Saccule, 2120

Sacroiliitis, in ankylosing spondylitis, 2006
   in inflammatory bowel disease, 758
Sacrum, pain in, epidural infusions for, 110
Saddle nose, from congenital syphilis, 2189
Saddleback fever, 1820
Safety caps, and poisoning prevention, 141
St. Anthony's fire, 1578, 2335
   vs. angioedema, 1951
St. Louis encephalitis, 1825–1826, 2193
St. Vitus' dance, 1583, 2148. See also *Syden-
      ham's chorea*
Salbutamol, 137
Salicylates
   and aspirin hepatotoxicity, 828
   and hearing loss, 2119
   as cyclooxygenase inhibitor, 1275
   binding of, to thyroxine-binding globulin,
      1317
   contraindications for, in varicella, 1790
   displacement of bilirubin by, 100
   dose-dependent kinetics of, 89t, 92
   for chronic pancreatitis, 780
   for gout, 1170
   for rheumatoid arthritis, 2003
   genetics in metabolism of, 102
   hypoglycemia from, 1384
   interaction of, with methotrexate, 101
   metabolic acidosis from, treatment for,
      555
   poisoning with, 142, 2070t
      treatment for, 143
   reference intervals for, 2404t
Salicylic acid, protein binding by, liver or
      kidney disease and, 94
Salicylism, 554
Saline load tests, for gastric outlet obstruc-
      tion, 707, 708
   for motility assessment, 716
Saline solution, isotonic, 245
Salivary glands
   blood flow regulation in, peptides and,
      239
   enlargement of, in acromegaly, 1301
   inflammation of, and amylase level, 776
   mumps and, 1779
   Sjögren's syndrome in, 2024
Salmonella
   enterotoxins from, and secretory diar-
      rhea, 727
   infection with, 1643–1645
      ampicillin for, 119
      and osteomyelitis, 1622
      and pus in stool, 730
      and Reiter's syndrome, 151
      cephalosporin antibiotics for, 113
      enterocolitis from, vs. appendicitis, 802
      gastroenteritis from, 784
         vs. appendicitis, 803
      in acquired immunodeficiency syn-
         drome, 1805t, 1806
         diarrhea from, 729
      penicillins for, 119
      reactive arthropathy from, 2008
      vs. ulcerative colitis, 756
      vs. viral hepatitis, 824
   vs. *Campylobacter*, 1649
Salmonella typhi, typhoid fever from, 1641
Salmonella typhosa, acalculous cholecystitis
      from, 865
Salpingitis, 1639, 1705–1706
   from gonorrhea, 1708
   gonococcal, vs. appendicitis, 803
   treatment of, 1710
   tuberculous, 1690
Salt(s). See also *Sodium*
   absorption of, by limb of Henle, antidi-
      uretic hormone and, 1306

Salt(s) (Continued)
  acidifying, metabolic acidosis from, 553
  amino acid, for metabolic alkalosis, 556
  craving for, from adrenocortical insufficiency, 1351
  depletion of, in heat exhaustion, 2383
  intake of, and hypertension, 43
  retention of, from chronic distention of left atrium, 215
    in heart failure, 190, 220
  wasting of, diagnosis and treatment of, 624
    from distal nephron dysfunction, 623
Salt depletion heat exhaustion, 2383
San Joaquin Valley, California, pericarditis in, 363
Sand, industrial uses of, and silicosis, 2361–2362
Sandflies, and bartonellosis, 924, 1681
  and leishmaniasis, 1870
  phlebotomine, 1922
Sandfly fever, 1817
Sanfilippo's syndrome, 1175–1176, 1176t
Santorini, duct of, 775
Sao Paulo typhus, 1742
Sarcocystis hominis, 1889
Sarcoidosis, 360–361, 451–457, 452
  activity of, 456, 456t
  alveolar wall in, 421–422, 422
  alveolitis in, 423
    measurement of, 428
  and acute interstitial nephritis, 605
  and diabetes insipidus, 1308
  and fever, 1525
  and increased calcium absorption, 639
  and liver, 840
  arthritis with, 2045
  as interstitial lung disease, 429
  clinical presentation of, 451, 452, 453
  collecting duct defects in, 505
  diagnosis of, 455t, 455–456
    differential, 454
  diffusing capacity in, 400
  glucocorticosteroid therapy for, 130
  granulomatous peritonitis from, 795
  hypercalcemia in, 1503
  immunopathology of, 451, 452
  in hypothalamus, 1286
  monocytosis in, 970
  myasthenia gravis with, 2285
  neuropathy in, 2266
  physical findings in, 453–454
  portal hypertension from, 848
  pulmonary, 425–429
  pulmonary hypertension from, 296, 298
  radiography for, 454, 454
  therapy for, 456–457
  thrombocytopenia in, 1052
  vs. cat scratch disease, 1679, 1681
  vs. cutaneous leishmaniasis, 1875
  vs. midline granuloma, 2032
  vs. multiple sclerosis, 2214
  vs. sporotrichosis, 1847
  vs. toxoplasmosis, 1878
  vs. tuberculosis, 1686
Sarcolemma, ionic channels in, antiarrhythmic drugs and, 264
  of cardiac cells, 251
Sarcoma(s)
  definition of, 1084
  eosinophilia from, 1025
  in heart, 367
  Kaposi's, 790, 1059, 1797, 1798, 2340. See also Kaposi's sarcoma
  of kidneys, 655
  osteogenic, 19
Sarcomeres, 2269

Sarcoplasmic reticulum, 184
Sarcoptes scabiei, 1925
Sarcosinemia, 1151t
Sarcosporidiosis, 1889
Sassafras, and cancer, 44
Satiety, early, from ascites, 791
  from gastric cancer, 711
  neurons regulating, 1280
Saturated fat, in diet, 43
Savage syndrome, 1438
Saxitoxin, from shellfish, 1931
SBE (subacute bacterial endocarditis), 1586, 1594, 1601
SBT (serum bacterial titer), 1593
Scabies, 1925
  vs. secondary syphilis, 1716
Scalded skin syndrome, staphylococcal, 1598, 1599, 2329
Scalp, disorders of, 2346t
Scapuloperoneal syndrome, 2274
Scar, formation of, in porphyria cutanea tarda, 1186
  hypertrophic, 2306
Scarlet fever, 1575, 1576–1577, 2323t
  erythrogenic toxins in, 1574
  rash in, 2324
  vs. measles, 1774, 1775t
  vs. rubella, 1777
Scarpa's ganglion, 2121
Scatchard equation, 1257
Scavengers, mononuclear phagocytes as, 955
Schamberg's disease, and skin, 2325
Schatzki's ring, 687, 687
Scheie's syndrome, 155, 1175, 1176t
Schick test, for diphtheria susceptibility, 1628
Schilder's cerebral sclerosis, 2215
Schilling test, 691, 692, 905
  for vitamin B_{12} absorption, 738
Schirmer test, for Sjögren's syndrome, 2024
Schistocytes, and disseminated intravascular coagulation, 1046
Schistosomiasis, 834, 835t, 1644, 1895–1901
  acute, 1897
  appendicitis from, 801
  control of, 1897–1898
  definition of, 1895
  diagnosis of, with biopsy, 731
  epidemiology of, 1896
  etiology of, 1895–1896
  hepatomegaly and eosinophilia from, 834
  management of, 1897, 1900–1901
  occlusive pulmonary vascular disease from, 295
  pathogenesis of, 1896–1897
  portal hypertension from, 838, 848
  recurrent thromboembolism in, 476
  vs. visceral leishmaniasis, 1873
Schistosomula, 1896
Schizont, 1858
Schizophrenic disorders, 2092–2095
  cannabis and, 58
  clinical symptoms of, 2092–2093, 2093t
  drugs for, 2094, 2094t
  genetics and, 150
  symptoms of, 2093t
  vs. AIDS dementia complex, 2205
  vs. manic episode, 2098
Schlichter test, in endocarditis management, 1593
Schmidt's syndrome, 1265, 1333, 1351, 1460–1461, 1461t
  hypothyroidism with, 1330
Schmorl's nodes, 1513
Schönlein syndrome, vs. urticaria, 1951
Schöffner's dots, 1860

Schwann cell, myelinopathy and, 2259
Schwannomas, acoustic, 2230
  prognosis for, 2235
  in neurofibromatosis, 2158
Schwartz-Jampel syndrome, 2284
SCID (severe combined immunodeficiency disorders), 1945–1946
  from thymic hypoplasia, 1974
Scientific method, 3, 7, 72–73
Scintigraphy, for interstitial lung disease, 427
  for myocardial infarction, 332
Scintillation, in classic migraine, 2130
Scleral icterus, from viral hepatitis, 819
Scleritis, 2296
Sclerodactyly, 2021
Scleroderma, 2018, 2341. See also Systemic sclerosis
  and acute kidney failure, 559
  diverticula with, 687
  heart problems in, 176, 361, 369
  kidney size in, 568
  of esophagus, manometry for, 685
  primary biliary cirrhosis with, 845
  pulmonary hypertension from, 298
  pulmonary vasculitis in, 476
  Raynaud's phenomenon and, 375
  treatment of, 686
  vs. leprosy, 1699
  vs. other inflammatory myopathies, 2277
  vs. superior mesenteric artery syndrome, 765
Sclerosing cholangitis, 661, 869–870
  in Crohn's disease, 749–750
  jaundice from, 817
  percutaneous transhepatic cholangiogram of, 864
  secondary biliary cirrhosis from, 846
  small duct, 841
  vs. adenocarcinoma of bile ducts, 871
  with Riedel's thyroiditis, 1334
Sclerosis
  and esophageal motor disorders, 683
  arteriolar, and threatened stroke, 2168
  cerebral, Schilder's, 2215
  diffuse, 2215
  focal glomerular, from chronic glomerulonephritis, 602
    in minimal change nephrotic syndrome, 593–594
  glomerulocapillary, nodular, in diabetic nephropathy, 1379
  lateral, amyotrophic, 2156–2157, 2157t
    and esophageal motor disorders, 683
    vs. cervical spondylosis, 2254
    primary, 2154
  mesial temporal, and seizures, 2219
  multiple. See Multiple sclerosis
  of varices, endoscopy for, 849
  systemic, 2018–2023. See also Systemic sclerosis
    and heart, 369
    and warm autoimmune hemolytic anemia, 918
    immunofluorescent cutaneous findings in, 2305t
    progressive, interstitial lung disease with, 429
  transitional, 2215
  tuberous, 2158–2159, 2344, 2345
    and neoplasms, 1096t
    interstitial lung disease in, 432
Sclerotic bodies, 1854
Scoliosis, 2258
  and chest wall deformity, 473
  and torsion dystonia, 2150
  from Marfan syndrome, 1177

Scoliosis (Continued)
idiopathic, 19
in progressive muscular atrophy, 2155
in syringomyelia, 2157
Scombroid fish poisoning, 786
Scopolamine, 139
absorption of, 88
abuse of, 59
for cough, from bronchogenic carcinoma,
463
for motion sickness, 2124
side effects of, 2299
Scopolamine-atropine, poisoning with,
2069t
Scorpions, stings of, 1924–1925
Scotomas, 2111, 2111
fortification, in classic migraine, 2130
Scrapie, 2203, 2205
Scribner shunt, for dialysis, 575
Scrofula, 1689, 1693
Scrotum, development of, 1392
Scrub typhus, 1738t, 1746–1747
clinical features of, 1738t
epidemiologic features of, 1737t
Scuba divers, air embolism in, 2367
Scurvy, 1235
as inborn error of metabolism, 146
hemorrhage in, 1059
symptoms of, 657
Sea snakes, 1930
Seafood, and Vibrio parahaemolyticus food
poisoning, 785
cholera from, 1651
Seals, poisoning from, 1931
Seattle Heart Watch study, 274
Sebaceous cells, 2302
Sebaceous glands, aging and, 2306
hyperplasia of, 2336t, 2336
Seborrheic dermatitis, 2320–2321
and hair loss, 2349
Seborrheic keratosis, 2336t, 2338
Sebum, 2302
production of, and acne, 2333
Secobarbital, overdose of, and central nervous system, 2069
reference intervals for, 2404t
Secondary hypertension, 276
evaluation for, selection of patients for,
282
pathogenesis of, 280–281
pulmonary, 294–298
treatment for, 288–292
Secondary tear, in aortic dissection, 372
Secondary thrombocytosis, 1054
Secretin, from pancreas, 775
in bile formation, 859
in gastrointestinal motility, 715
Secretin test, for impaired pancreatic function, 736, 737t
for Zollinger-Ellison syndrome, 709
in malabsorption evaluation algorithm,
740
Sedatives
and breathing control, 401
and peptic ulcers, 701
aplasia from, 886
contraindications for, in chronic respiratory failure, 481
drug-dependent patients and, 60
for hemoptysis, 392
for hypothyroid patients, coma from,
1331
for insomnia, 2078
narcotic analgesics as, 108, 109
overdose of, 53–54
and central nervous system, 2069
treatment for, 54

Sedatives (Continued)
respiratory failure from, 476
use of, with cocaine, 54
withdrawal syndrome from, 53–54
Sediment, reference intervals for, 2399t
Segmental dysplasia, 649
Segmental dystonia, 2150
Segmental myoclonus, 2222
Segregation (heredity), 146
Segregation ratios, 172
Segregational load, 151
Seizures. See also Convulsions; Epilepsy(ies)
absence, 2076, 2219–2223
akinetic, 2076
atonic, 2222. See also Drop attacks
epileptic, from arteriovenous malformations, 2174
from acute cocaine toxicity, 55
from acute disseminated encephalomyelitis, 2209
from acute heroin reaction, 56
from adenine arabinoside, 125
from Aspergillus fumigatus, in transplant
recipients, 2210
from bacterial meningitis, 1606
treatment of, 1610
from brain abscess, 2182
from brain tumors, 2231–2232
from digitalis toxicity, 229
from epilepsy, 2217
from hepatic porphyria, 1185
from metabolic encephalopathy, 2065
from phenylketonuria, 1155
from rabies, 2201
from Reye syndrome, 2210
from sarcoidosis, 453
from sedative withdrawal syndrome, 54
from systemic lupus erythematosus, 2016
from viral encephalitis, 2193
treatment of, 2194
from vitamin B₆ deficiency, 1233
generalized, 2218, 2221–2222
in neonates, 2223
myoclonic, 2221–2222
partial, 2218–2221
syncope and, 2076
tonic, 2222
treatment for, 2068, 2227
vs. panic attacks, 2101
Seldinger technique, for cardiac catheterization, 211
Selectivity, of antimicrobics, 112
Selenium, 1239, 1242, 2392
as carcinogenesis inhibitor, 44
deficiency of, 2392
estimated safe and adequate daily dietary
intake of, 1206t
Self-concept, in adolescence, 16
Self-destructive behavior, in Lesch-Nyhan
syndrome, 1171
Self-esteem, in anorexia nervosa, 1216
of dying patients, 31
Sella turcica, 1290
neoplasms of, diagnostic imaging tech-
niques for, 2060
Semi-Fowler's position, 2252
Semilente insulin, 1373
Seminal fluid, analysis of, 1407
Seminal vesicles, development of, 1392
tuberculosis in, 1690
Seminiferous tubules, 1404
damage to, 1415
evaluation of, 1407
Semmelweis, Ignaz, 1541
Senecio longilobus, liver failure from, 787
Senescence antigen, 955
Senna, as laxative, 722, 727

Sensation
disorders of, 2128–2137
headache as, 2129–2136. See also Headache
in diabetic neuropathy, 2263
in Guillain-Barré syndrome, 2261
symptoms of, 2128t, 2128–2129
in Friedreich's ataxia, 2152
itch as, 2303. See also Pruritus
loss of, in cancer, 1106
in syringomyelia, 2157
in viral encephalitis, 2193
Senses, 2109–2124
hearing as, 2117–2120. See also Hearing
smell as, 2109–2110
taste as, 2109–2110
vision as, 2111–2117. See also Vision
Sensory ataxia, 2125
in acute inflammatory sensory polyneuropathy, 2262
Sensory evoked potentials, 2056
Sensory neurons, peripheral, disorders of,
2264–2265
Sensory neuropathy, 2262–2264
Sensory receptors, 2128–2129
SEP (somatosensory evoked potentials),
2056
Sepsis
acute kidney failure from, 558
atrial pressures in, 244
bacterial, vs. congenital syphilis, 1718
vs. cytomegalovirus infection, 1785
vs. neonatal myocarditis from enteroviruses, 1812
catheter-related, from parenteral nutrition, 1250
clinical manifestations of, 1539t, 1539–
1540
complications of, 1539
treatment of, 1540
definition of, 1538
diagnosis of, 1540
disseminated, in viral hepatitis, 824
from Haemophilus influenzae, 65
from peritoneovenous shunt, 851
gastritis with, 689
hematuria from, 503
hypovolemia with, 534
shock syndromes from, 1538t, 1538–1541
treatment for, 246
treatment for, 1540–1541
with suppurative cholangitis, 869
Septal defects
aortic-pulmonary, 308
atrial, 304–306
intraventricular, myocardial infarction
and, 331
pulsed wave Doppler echocardiography
for, 205
secundum atrial, 307
ventricular, 306, 306–307
echocardiography for, 203
myocardial infarction and, 331
Septal panniculitis, definition of, 2050
without vasculitis, 2050–2051
Septic arthritis. See Arthritis, septic
Septic shock
definition of, 1538
from lipopolysaccharide of Fusobacterium
nucleatum, 1637
from Staphylococcus aureus, 1598, 1602
isoproterenol contraindicated for, 247
treatment of, 246, 1540–1541, 1660
glucocorticosteroids in, dosages for,
131
Septicemia(s)
and multiple organ failure, 1539

Septicemia(s) (Continued)
  and myocardial depression, 239
  and pustules, 2334
  and subdural empyema, 2184
  empiric therapy for, 118t
  from clostridia, 1630
  from peritonitis, 793
  in agammaglobulinemia, 1943
  in opioid users, 56
Sequestrum, 1622
Serology, reference intervals for, 2395t–2400t
Seros…
Serosiitis, in dialysis patients, 577
Serotonin, 1282
  and angina pectoris, 324
  and carcinoid syndrome, 1467
    diarrhea in, 727
  and coronary artery thrombosis, 330
  and dumping syndrome, 717
  biosynthesis and degradation of, 1467, 1467
  in asthma, 404–405
  in inflammation, 1986
  in vascular headache, 2130
  shock and, 239
Serpiginous lesion patterns, 2310
Serpiginous ulcer, 1712
Serratia, growth of, in IV solution, 1545
Serratia marcescens, and urinary tract infection, in diabetics, 629
Sertoli cells, 1292
  follicle-stimulating hormone regulation of, 1407
  in testis, 1405
  müllerian inhibiting factor from, 1393
  tumors of, 1421
Sertoli cell-only syndrome, 1415–1416
Serum hepatitis, 821, 823. See also Viral hepatitis, type B; Viral hepatitis, type non-A, non-B
Serum sickness, 1585, 1960–1962, 1960, 1960t, 1961
  and tissue damage, 1990
  as antimicrobial reaction, 123
  from antivenom, 1929
  from toxic drug reactions, 103, 1970t
  hypersensitivity and, 2027
  urticaria in, 1950
  vs. Lyme disease, 1728
Set point, for body weight, 1223
  for parathyroid hormone regulation, 1508
Severe combined immunodeficiency disorders, 1945–1946
  from thymic hypoplasia, 1974
Sex (gender)
  and cardiovascular disease, 182
  and hematocrit, 879
  and hypertension, 277
  influence of, on laboratory tests, 81
Sex characteristics, primary, in puberty, 18–19
  secondary, in puberty, 18
Sex chromatin, 166–167
Sex chromosomes, 162
  abnormalities in, 167, 167t
  absence of, in Turner's syndrome, 1437
  clinical cytogenetics and, 167
  nomenclature for, 163
Sex hormone binding globulin, and testosterone transport, 1406
Sex steroid hormones
  concentrations of, in blood, 1433t
  from ovaries, 1425, 1431–1432, 1432, 1433t
  ingestion of, and precocious puberty, 1427
  metabolic clearance rates for, 1433t

Sex steroid hormones (Continued)
  ovarian secretion rates for, 1433t
  production rates for, 1433t
Sexual differentiation
  abnormalities of, 1393–1404
    androgen-dependent target area, dysfunction at, 1399–1401, 1399
    female pseudohermaphroditism as, 1402–1404, 1403t
    testicular differentiation and development disorders as, 1393–1395, 1394
    XX males as, 1401–1402
  disorders of, testicular function disorders as, 1395–1399
  normal, 1390–1393, 1391
Sexual dysfunction, beta blockers and, 287
Sexual experimentation, in adolescents, 20
Sexual function and dysfunction, 1441–1442. See also Impotence
  male, neural control of, 2108–2109
  methadone and, 56
Sexual identity, in adolescence, 16
Sexual maturation, delay in, from Crohn's disease, 749
Sexual precocity, from pineal tumors, 1314
Sexually transmitted disease, 1701–1722, 1702t
  acquired immunodeficiency syndrome as, 1801
  and rectum, 787
  asymptomatic, 1702
  cervicitis from, 1705
  chancroid as, 1712–1713
  definition of, 1701
  epidemiologic considerations of, 1701–1702
  genital ulcer syndrome in, 1703
  gonococcal infection as, 1706–1710
  granuloma inguinale as, 1711–1712
  in adolescents, 20
  in homosexual males, 1702
  incidence of, 1702
  lymphogranuloma venereum as, 1710–1711
  salpingitis as, 1705–1706
  syphilis as, 1713–1722
  urethritis in, 1702–1703, 1703
  vaginitis from, 1704–1705, 1704t
Sézary's syndrome, 1109
  vs. chronic lymphocytic leukemia, 997
SGOT. See Glutamic-oxaloacetic transaminase
Sham feeding, for incomplete vagotomy diagnosis, 705
Shave biopsy, 2313
Shaver's disease, 2390
Shaving, for hirsutism, 1448
SHBG (sex hormone binding globulin), 1406
Shellfish
  and hepatitis A, 825
  poisoning from, 786, 1931
    paralytic, vs. botulism, 1633
Shepherd's-crook deformity, of femur, 1520
Shift reticulocytes, 882
Shift work, health effects of, 2356
Shigella, 1646
  and pus in stool, 730
  dysentery from, 784
    colitis from, vs. ulcerative colitis, 756
    vs. diverticulitis, 804
    vs. ulcerative proctitis, 788
  enterotoxins from, and secretory diarrhea, 727
  infection of, 1646–1648, 1647t
    and Reiter's syndrome, 151
    penicillins for, 119
    vs. gonococcal infections of rectum, 1707

Shigella (Continued)
  vs. Campylobacter, 1649
Shin(s), pain in, from trench fever, 1748
  saber, from congenital syphilis, 2189
Shin spots, 1381
Shin-bone fever, 1747
Shingles, 2196–2197. See also Herpes zoster
Ship fever, 1739
Shock, 236–249
  anaphylactic, 240–241
  and drug distribution, 97
  and microcirculation, 240–241
  biochemical factors in, 241–243
  cardiogenic, 331. See also Cardiogenic shock
  causes of, 236t
  cellular factors in, 241–243
  circulatory control in, 237–241
  clinical presentation of, 236
  complement activation in, 242–243
  definition of, 236
  endotoxic, 240, 1538
    from staphylococci, 1602–1603
    gram-negative bacteria and, 1659–1661
  from abdominal aortic aneurysm, 371
  from bacterial meningitis, 1608
  from bacterial peritonitis, 793
  from cholera, 1652
  from hypoxia, 477
  from peritonitis, 793
  from sepsis, 1538t, 1538–1541
  from ulcerative colitis, 755
  hemorrhagic, and lungs, 241
    fluid therapy for, 891
  hypotensive, anaphylaxis and, 1957
  hypovolemic, 237–238
    from adrenocortical insufficiency, 1351
    from arenaviruses, 1835
  in dengue hemorrhagic fever, 1833
  intestinal infarction from, 763
  irreversible, 236–237
  liver clearance of lidocaine in, 97
  pathophysiology and stages of, 236t, 236–237, 237
  septic, 1538. See also Septic shock
  sympathomimetic amines for, 246–248
  toxic. See Toxic shock syndrome
  treatment of, 243–249
    catecholamines for, 137
    corticosteroids for, 129, 246
    vasodilators for, 248
  vascular factors in, 239–240
Shock lung syndrome, 240, 241, 245
Shock syndromes, from sepsis, 1538t, 1538–1541
Short bowel syndrome, 718, 729
  and liver disease from total parenteral nutrition, 841
  avoidance of, in surgery for mesenteric artery occlusion, 763
  malabsorption from, 743
  total parenteral nutrition for, 1244
Shoulder
  frozen, 2042
  pain in, 2041–2043
  polymyalgia rheumatica in, 2033
  rheumatoid arthritis in, 2001–2002
Shoulder girdle-scapular pain, 2267
Shoulder-hand syndrome, 334, 2042
Shunts
  arteriovenous, 240
  between aortic root and right heart, 308
  circulatory, 303–304
  detection of, with first-pass radionuclide angiocardiogram, 209
  for portal hypertension, 850
  from total airway collapse, 419

Shunts (Continued)
hyperbilirubinemia from, 814
hypoxemia from, in severely ill, 483, 483–484
in congenital heart disease, 304–309
intracardiac, 205
pulsed wave Doppler echocardiography for, 205, 206
left ventricular-right atrial, ventricular septal defect with, 307
LeVeen, for dialysis, 577
nephritis from, vs. post-streptococcal glomerulonephritis, 587
pathways for, 725
peritoneovenous, for ascites, 851
sclerosing peritonitis from, 795
right-to-left, and gas exchange, 474–475
and hypoxemia, calculations for, 485
causes of, 474
hypoxia from, 402–403
Scribner, for dialysis, 575
volume of, determination of, 305
Shy-Drager syndrome, 1466, 2106–2107, 2153t
Sia test, 1033
SIADH, 535. See also Syndrome of inappropriate secretion of antidiuretic hormone
Sialic acid, in complement activation, 1939
Sialidoses, 1177
Sialometaplasia, necrotizing, vs. midline granuloma, 2032
Sialorrhea, in eastern equine encephalitis, 1824
Siberian ulcer, 1667
Sick sinus syndrome, 252, 261
after intra-atrial surgery, 317
and sudden cardiac death, 275
cardioversion and, 273
treatment of, 257t
Sickle cell anemia, 149, 152, 936–942
and meningitis, 1605
and retinopathy, 2297
and Salmonella infections, 1644
and testosterone levels, 1415
and ulcers, 2341
and vitamin E deficiency, 1239
aplastic crisis in, from human papovavirus, 1523
arthritis with, 2045
as recessive trait, 147
chronic interstitial nephritis in, 606–607
clinical manifestations of, 939–940
definition of, 936–937
diagnosis of, 940
differential, 938t
frequency of, 151
heredity and, 147
immunization for patients with, 63
modification of mutant protein in, 157
mycoplasmal pneumonia with, 1563
osteonecrosis in, 1517
pathophysiology, 937–939
prevalence of, 937
prevention of, 941
prognosis for, 941
recurrent thromboembolism in, 476
treatment of, 941
vs. appendicitis, 803
vs. rheumatic fever, 1585
zinc deficiency in, 1241
Sickle cell trait and malaria resistancy, 1858
clinical manifestations of, 939
Sideroblastic anemias, 899–900
ineffective erythropoiesis in, 895
refractory, chronic, from myeloma treatment, 1032
Sideroblasts, ringed, 899

Siderocytes, vs. malarial parasites, 1860
Siderosis, hepatic, porphyria cutanea tarda with, 1187
Sievert, 2376
Sigmoidoscopy, flexible, 670–671, 671t
for colorectal cancer, 771
for ischemic colitis, 764
Silastic (Hickman) catheters, 932
and infection prevention, 1537
Silicon, and kidney damage, 612
Silicosis, 425, 432, 2360, 2360–2361, 2361
and alveolar proteinosis, 432
sarcoidosis vs., 454
Silk surgical sutures, and postoperative recurrent ulcers, 705
Silo-filler's disease, 2367
Silver nitrate, for skin disorders, 2314
to prevent gonorrhea in infants, 1708
Silver sulfadiazine, for skin disorders, 2316
Silver-Russell syndrome, 1428
Simultanagnosia, 2081, 2082
Single photon absorptiometry, for bone mass measurement, 1476
Single photon emission computed tomography (SPECT), 210
for liver scans, 667
Single ventricle, congenital, 311
Singultus, 472
Sinoatrial block, as atrial arrhythmias, 261
Sinoatrial node, 184
Sinus(es)
paranasal, aspergillosis in, 1851
headache from, 2134
infection of, and brain abscess, 2181
and subdural empyema, 2183–2184
thrombophlebitis of, after cerebral epidural abscess, 2184
Sinus bradycardia, atropine for, 139
Sinus headache, 2134
Sinus node, 250
rate of firing in, and arrhythmias, 252
Sinus of Valsalva
aneurysm of, 370
aortic regurgitation from, 343
congenital, 308
ruptured, fragmentational hemolysis from, 924
Sinus rate, digitalis and, 229
Sinus rhythm, as atrial arrhythmia, 256
Sinus tachycardia, carotid sinus pressure for, 255t
Sinus thrombosis, 2184–2185
Sinus venosus defect, 304
Sinusitis
anaerobes and, 1639
chronic, from allergic rhinitis, 1953
dextrocardia and, 315
from drug abuse, 52
in agammaglobulinemia, 1943
paranasal, cerebral epidural abscess with, 2184
perinasal, from scarlet fever, 1576
phaeohyphomycosis and, 1855
pneumococcal, and pneumococcal meningitis, 1605
with bronchiectasis, 439
Sinuvertebral nerves, and pain transmission, 2248
Sipple's syndrome, 1095t, 1460. See also Multiple endocrine neoplasia
Sitophobia, from gastric outlet obstruction, 707
Sjögren's syndrome, 2024–2025
antibodies in, 1996
chronic interstitial nephritis in, 606
clinical presentation of, 2024
collecting duct defects in, 505

Sjögren's syndrome (Continued)
definition of, 2296
from chronic active hepatitis, 832
human leukocyte antigens in, 1967
interstitial lung disease with, 430
lymphocytic interstitial pneumonitis with, 431
myasthenia gravis with, 2285
necrotizing venulitis in, 1950
primary biliary cirrhosis with, 845
rheumatoid arthritis and, 2002
with Hashimoto's thyroiditis, 1333
Skeletal muscle
estimating mass of, 1210
myoadenylate deaminase in, 1172
polymyositis in, 2034
rate of contraction and relaxation of, and thyroid status, 1320
Skeletal system
deformities of, in Paget's disease, 1515
in thalassemia major, 931
in uremia, 566. See also Renal osteodystrophy
problems of, during puberty, 19
Skin. See also Dermatitis; Rash
abscesses of, in opioid users, 56
aging of, by ultraviolet light, 2303
and vitamin A toxicity, 1238
angioedema of, 1948
appendages of, 2302
as defense mechanism, 1529
atrophy of, from Cushing's syndrome, 1355
biopsy of, 2313, 2313–2314
with fetoscopy, 173
blistering of light-exposed, 1186
blood flow through, 2304
cancer of, from polycythemia vera treatment, 983
metastatic, 1108, 1108t
solar radiation and, 1094
care of, after spinal cord trauma, 2246
charring of, from electric injury, 2380, 2381
cosmetic importance of, 2306
cryptococcosis and, 1845
cyanosis of, 377–378
in cold agglutinin disease, 920
Raynaud's phenomenon vs., 376
desquamation of, from glucocorticosteroid withdrawal, 132
diagnostic tests of, 2310–2311, 2313–2314
disease of, 2300–2353
cellulitis as, 2335
classification of, 2311t
eczemas as, 2318–2322, 2319t
eosinophilia from, 1025
figurate erythemas as, 2335
immunosuppression and, 2352
maculopapular, 2322–2326, 2323t
occupational, 2373–2375
papulosquamous, 2326t, 2326–2328
prevalence of, 2300t
pustular, 2332–2334, 2333t
regional diagnosis of, 2346t, 2346–2350
treatment of, 2314–2318
urticaria as, 1948, 2334–2335, 2335t. See also Urticaria
vesiculobullous, 2328–2332, 2330t
drug reactions in, 1970–1971t, 2352–2353, 2353t
examination of, 2306–2314
flushing of, in carcinoid syndrome, 1467
function of, 2303–2306
granulomas of, from chemicals, 2375
hyperpigmentation of, 2342t, 2342–2344
hypoparathyroidism and, 1498

Skin (Continued)
  hypopigmentation of, 2342t
  in adult T cell leukemia, 1797
  in anaphylaxis, 1957
  in Behçet's disease, 2049
  in Ehlers-Danlos syndrome, 1179
  in hypopituitarism, 1295
  in systemic sclerosis, 2020, 2021
  indurations of, 2341
  infection of
    anaerobic, 1639
    and bloodstream infection, 1544
    and spread of diphtheria, 1627
    anthrax as, 1667
    bacterial, in varicella, 1789
    blastomycosis as, 1842
    candidiasis as, 1848
    fungal, vs. eczema, 2321–2322
    Gram's stain for, 2313
    leishmaniasis as, 1873–1875
      diffuse, 1871
      visceral, 1871–1872
    mycobacterial, 1695
    neutropenia and, 963
    occupational factors in, 2375
    staphylococcal, 1599
    streptococcal, 1577–1578
    viral, vesicles from, 2329
  infestation of, with fleas, 1926
  inflammatory reactions in, 2305–2306
  internal malignancy and, 1107–1113
  larva migrans of, 1907
  leprosy and, 1697
  lesions of, 2307–2310. See also Skin, ulcers
    of
    from familial Mediterranean fever, 1197
    from viral infections, 1772–1780
    in bartonellosis, 1682
    in diabetes mellitus, 1380–1381
    in tuberous sclerosis, 2158
  lupus erythematosus in, 2014–2015
  malnutrition and, 1210t
  mastocytosis in, 1972
  mechanobullous conditions of, 2332
  microorganisms on, 1548, 2303
  mucormycosis of, 1852
  neoplasms of, arsenic and, 2375
    benign vs. malignant, 2336
    vascular, 2339–2340
  neurofibromatosis and, 2158
  nodules of, 2335–2339
    inflammatory, 2340
  obesity and, 1224
  onchocerciasis in, 1917
  paraneoplastic syndromes in, 1098
  phaeohyphomycosis of, 1854–1855
  photosensitivity of, 2350–2352
    in protoporphyria, 1184
  physical examination of, 2307, 2310
  pigmentation of
    café-au-lait, in McCune-Albright syndrome, 1460
    hyper-, 2342t, 2342–2344
    hypo-, 2342t
    in hemochromatosis, 839, 1190, 1191
    melanocytes and, 2301–2302
  polyarteritis in, 2029, 2051
  pseudoxanthoma elasticum and, 1181, 1181
  radiation injury to, 2377, 2379t
    treatment of, 2379
  rashes of, in chronic active hepatitis, 832
  rheumatoid arthritis and, 2002
  sarcoidosis in, 451, 453
    treatment of, 457
  scarring of, 2340–2341
  sporotrichosis in, 1846

Skin (Continued)
  structure and function of, 2300–2306, 2301t
  systemic lupus erythematosus in, 2014–2015
  temperature of, rise in, and erythromelalgia, 378
  tests of
    for allergic rhinitis, 1953–1954
    for coccidioidomycosis, 1840
    for drug allergy, 1969
    for echinococcosis, 1894
    for mycoses, 1838
  tuberculosis of, 1692
  ulcers of, 2341–2342
    from chemicals, 2375
    from nonsyphilitic treponematoses, 1723
    in sickle cell anemia, 939
  urticaria of, 1948, 2334–2335, 2335t. See
    also Urticaria
  vascular tumors of, 2339–2340
  vitamin D₃ production in, 1477
  wound healing in, 2306
Skull. See also Head
  diagnostic imaging techniques for, 2058t, 2058–2059
  fractures of, 2066, 2241
    immunization for patients with, 63
  in Paget's disease, 1516, 1516
  lesions of, in Paget's disease, 1515
  trauma to, brain abscess from, 2181
  wounds of, and subdural empyema, 2184
Skunks, rabies in, 2200
Sleep, 2077, 2077
  complaints concerning, 2077, 2078t
  disorders of, classification of, 2077–2078
    hypothalamus and, 2103
    vs. epilepsy, 2225
  from cannabis, 57
  patterns of, in liver disease, 808
  periodic movements of, 2151
Sleep apnea, 298, 476–477, 2079
  from testosterone, 1419
  obesity and, 1224
Sleep paralysis, 2078
Sleep talking, 2079
Sleep walking, 2079
Sleepiness, from melatonin, 1314
Sleeping sickness (African trypanosomiasis), 1282, 1282t, 1862–1865
Sliding filament hypothesis, of heart muscle
  contraction, 216
Slow-channel syndrome, 2287
Slow-reacting substance of anaphylaxis,
  from mast cells in asthma, 404
SM. See Streptomycin
Small airways disease, 411
Small bowel enema, 665. See also Enteroclysis
Small cell lung cancer, 459, 459t
  Kulchitsky's cell and, 458
  staging of, 460, 461t
  treatment of, 462
Small intestine. See also Duodenum; Ileum;
    Jejunum
  amoxicillin absorption by, 116
  bacteria within, normal control of, 741
  biopsy of, for malabsorption evaluation,
    737t, 739, 739, 740t
    for nontropic sprue, 743
  chyme movement through, 714
  culture of, 737t, 739
  damage to, from radiation therapy, 806
  disease of, vs. postcholecystectomy syndrome, 872
  diverticula of, 721

Small intestine (Continued)
  epithelial cells of, damage to, from gluten, 742
  examination of, 665
  hemangiomas of, 765
  infarction of, resection for, and malabsorption, 743
  lesions of, radiographic studies of, 800
  lymphoma of, and nontropic sprue, 743
    vs. Crohn's disease, 750
  motility disorders of, 716t, 718–721
    and gas pain, 661
    hypo-, in systemic sclerosis, 2022
  neoplasms of, 773–774
  normal secretion by, 726
  obstruction of, vs. appendicitis, 801, 802
  trauma to, resection for, and malabsorption, 743
  ulceration of, 807
Smallpox, 1792–1793
  eradication of, 1791–1792
  immunization against, 65
    before travel, 1550
    complications from, 126
  methisazone for, 126
  recurrence of, potential for, 1792
Smell, 2109–2110. See also Nasal; Nose
  loss of, causes of, 2110, 2110t
Smoke, and lung injury, 2365
Smoked foods, and cancer, 44
Smoking
  and atherosclerosis, 319–321
  and atrial premature depolarization, 256
  and cancer, 1093t, 1093–1094
    of kidneys, 652
    of lungs, 457–458
    of pancreas, 781
    oral, 678–679
    squamous cell, of esophagus, 686
    transitional cell, 654
  and cardiovascular disease, 182
  and chronic bronchitis, 412, 413
  and chronic obstructive pulmonary disease, 414
  and familial hypercholesterolemia, 1141
  and gastroesophageal reflux disease, 683
  and gingivitis, 675
  and histiocytosis-X, 430
  and hypertension, 285
  and myocardial infarction, 335
  and occupational lung disease, 2356
  and osteoporosis, 1511
  and pneumoconiosis, 433
  and thromboangiitis obliterans, 382, 383
  and ulcers, 696
    peptic, 701
  and vitamin A intake, 1238
  and vitamin C levels, 1235
  by adolescents, 21
  by physicians, 68
  carbon monoxide in, 2369
  cessation of, 40
  changes in, 183
  chronic, and enhanced liver metabolism
    of other drugs, 99
  cigar, 39
  contraindicated, for arteriosclerosis obliterans, 381
    for Raynaud's phenomenon, 377
  decrease in, and high density lipoprotein, 320
  increased health risks from, 36t
  interaction of, with other risks, 37
  involuntary, 39
  oral contraceptives with, and thromboembolism, 1443
  pipe, 39

Smooth endoplasmic reticulum, phenobarbital and, 157
Smooth muscle(s)
  antibodies to, in liver disease, 817
  autonomic nervous system and, 133
  bronchial, prostaglandin E₂ in, 1273
  dilation of, prostacyclin and, 1271
  in arteries, 318
  in atherosclerosis lesions, 321
  in intestinal pseudo-obstruction, 720
  in system venous bed, dilators for, 233, 235
  migration of, into intima, 322
  oxytocin and, 1313
  tracheobronchial, hyper-responsiveness of, in asthma, 403
  vascular, abnormal responses of, 375–379
    tone of, 239
Snails, and schistosomiasis, 1896
Snake bites, 1927–1929, 1927t
  antivenin for, 66
  disseminated intravascular coagulation from, 1080
  immunization against, 63t
Snake venom, lipolytic toxins from, hemolysis from, 923
  poisoning from, shock from, 240–241
  red cell hemolysins from, 922
Sneezing, from allergic rhinitis, 1953
  from common cold, 1755
  in opioid withdrawal syndrome, 57
Snow Mountain virus, 1768
Snuff, 39
Social behavior, disturbances of, 2083
  frontal lobes and, 2082
SOD (superoxide dismutase), 1638, 1952, 2368
Sodium, 529. See also Salt(s)
  absorption of, 734
    aldosterone and, 502
    by proximal tubule, 530
  and aldosterone, 1360
  and atrial natriuretic peptides, 279
  balance of, control of, 230–231
  concentrations of, in stool, 725
  deficiency of, 524, 1288. See also Hyponatremia
  drug interaction with, 101
  excess, in blood, 542, 1288, 2105
  in chronic kidney failure, 564
  in common foods, 1246t
  in diet
    acute kidney failure and, 562
    and hypertension, 277
    recommendations for, 1206t, 1208
    restriction of, 230
      and heart failure, 225
      in ascites management, 851
      in hypertension therapy, 285
  in hypernatremia, 2105
  in myocardial cells, 196
  in uremic syndrome, management of, 570
  in urine, measurement of, 524
  plasma concentration of, and aldosterone secretion, 516
  reabsorption of, and potassium excretion, 517
    by proximal tubule, 512, 513
  reduction of, in hypotonic disorders, 538–539
  reference intervals for, 2399t
  retention of
    by kidneys, and fluid volume excess, 535
    from excess mineralocorticoids, 1347
    in pregnancy, 634
    in primary aldosteronism, 1358

Sodium (Continued)
  retention of, nonsteroidal anti-inflammatory agents and, 609
  serum concentrations of, dangers of rapidly increasing, 541
  solutions containing, in fluid replacement therapy, 533
  tubular reabsorption of, 514–516, 515
  wasting of, in Addison's disease, 532
    in chronic kidney failure, 564
    in tubulointerstitial disease, 603
Sodium bicarbonate
  as antacid, 701
  for acidosis in shock patients, 245
  in cystic fibrosis treatment, 441
  in hyperkalemia treatment, 548
  loss of, from pancreas, and metabolic acidosis, 532
Sodium chloride
  for hypercalcemia, 1504
  homeostasis of, kidneys and, 514–516
  in diarrhea treatment, 731
  inefficient excretion of, and hypertension, 43
  reabsorption of, in distal convoluted tubule, 514
Sodium fluoride, for osteoporosis, 1514
  side effects of, 1514
Sodium nitroprusside, for dissecting aortic aneurysm, 374
  for hypertensive crisis, 288, 290t
  for hypertensive encephalopathy, 2173
Sodium-potassium ATPase system, and energy requirements, 1212
Sodoku, 1729–1730
Soft tissue
  bleeding from, and iron loss, 880
  calcification of, in renal osteodystrophy, 1509
  infection of, 1630t
    anaerobic, 1639
    mycobacterial, 1695
Sohval-Soffer syndrome, hypogonadism from, 1414
Solar radiation, and skin cancer, 1094
Solar urticaria, 1184
  photosensitivity in, 2352
Somatic cells, gene therapy for, 160
Somatic pain, 105
  chronic, cordotomy for, 111
Somatization disorders, 2101t, 2101–2103, 2102t
Somatomammotropic hormones, 1292–1293
Somatomedin(s), 1263
Somatomedin-C, growth hormone binding to, 1293
  in puberty, 17
Somatosensory evoked potentials, 2056
Somatostatin
  action of, 1282–1283
  and intestinal motility, 724
  for glucagonoma, 1389
  for variceal hemorrhage, 850
  for VIPoma, 1389
  infusion of, effect of, 1390
  inhibition of TSH release by, 1318
Somatostatinoma, 1389t, 1390
  vs. VIPoma, 1388
Somatostatinoma syndrome, 459
Somatotrophs, in anterior pituitary, 1290
Somatotropin release inhibiting factor, from hypothalamus, 1280
Somnambulism, 2079
Somnolence, from hyponatremia, 540
  from vitamin B₁₂ deficiency, 904
  from vomiting, 660
Somogyi phenomenon, 1372

Sonofluoroscopy, for kidneys, 526
Sonography, for acute abdomen, 802
Sorbitol, accumulation of, in diabetic neuropathy, 2263
  in diabetes mellitus, 1367, 1367
Sore throat, 1575. See also Pharyngitis, streptococcal
  from common cold, 1755
Sotalol, for angina pectoris, 327t
South American blastomycosis, 1843
Space sickness, 2122
Sparganosis, 1891
Spasms
  habit, 2151–2152
    definition of, 2143
  in ataxia, 2126
  in paraparesis, 1797
  in paraplegia, 2154
  infantile, 2222–2223
  mobile, 2152. See also Athetosis
  torsion, 2149–2150
Spasticity, after spinal cord trauma, 2246
  vs. rigidity, 2143
Spatial processing, defects in, 2082
Specific gravity, reference intervals for, 2399t
SPECT (single photon emission computed tomography), 210
  for liver scans, 667
Spectinomycin, 122
  for mycoplasmas, 1565
  for ureaplasma, 1565
  in kidney and liver failure, 117t
Spectrin, deficiency in, in hereditary spherocytosis, 910
  in erythrocyte skeletal membrane, 909
Spectroscopy, magnetic resonance, 668
Speech
  disorders of, from arteritis, 374
  in delirium, 2065
  slurred, from hepatic encephalopathy, 853
  from phencyclidine, 59
Speech discrimination test, 2118
Speech reception threshold, 2118
Sperm
  appearance of, at puberty, 18
  deficiency of, with deficient androgen production, 1412–1415
  from meiosis, 162
  normal concentrations of, in ejaculate, 1407, 1407
  production of, isolated deficiency in, 1409, 1412, 1415–1416
Spermatids, in meiosis, 162
Spermatocytes, in meiosis, 162
Spermatogenesis
  dihydrotestosterone in, 1400
  hormonal control of, 1407
  testosterone and, 1400, 1405
Spermatogenic tissue, damage to, from DHPG, 126
Spherocytes, 910
Spherocytosis, hereditary, 148, 910–912, 911t, 911
  splenectomy for, 157–158, 1038
Spherulin skin test, for coccidioidomycosis, 1840
Sphincter(s)
  anal, dysfunction of, 790
  gastrointestinal, 714
  of esophagus, 680, 683
    function of, 714
  of Oddi, stenosis of, 872
  precapillary, 240
Sphincterotomy, endoscopic retrograde, for choledocholithiasis, 673

Sphingolipidoses, 153
Sphygmomanometers, 244
Spider bites, 1923
    antivenin for, 66
    immunization against, 63t
    lipolytic toxins from, hemolysis from, 923
Spike wave stupor, 2223
Spina bifida, 170, 170t
    chronic alcoholism in mothers and, 171
    prenatal diagnosis of, with ultrasonography, 173
Spina bifida occulta, 2257
Spinal canal, inflammation of, 2256–2257
    neoplasms of, 2254–2256, 2255
    vascular disorders of, 2257
Spinal cord, 2248
    AIDS dementia complex in, 2204
    cancer and, 1106
    cervical, compression of, 2214, 2249
    compression of
        acute transverse myelitis from, 2217
        and bladder function, 2108
        from thalassemia intermedia, 932
        in ankylosing spondylitis, 2006
        in breast cancer, 1456
        in Hodgkin's disease, 1016
        in Morquio's syndrome, 1176
        in multiple myeloma, 1032
        indications of, 2250
    cysts in, 2157
    disorders of
        acute transverse myelitis from, 2216
        and impotence, 1409
        autonomic insufficiency from, 2106
        respiratory failure from, 476
        sensory loss from, 2129
    examination of, magnetic resonance imaging for, 85
    injury to, 2244
        respiratory failure from, critical care of, 489–490
    lumbar, lesions of, 2249
    metastasis of bronchogenic carcinoma to, 459
    neoplasms of, vs. vitamin B$_{12}$ deficiency, 2140
    subacute combined system disease of, from vitamin B$_{12}$ deficiency, 904
    transection of, and gastrointestinal motility, 724
Spinal fluid, penetration of antimicrobials into, 116
Spinal shock, definition of, 2245
Spine. See also Back; Vertebrae
    anatomy and physiology of, 2247–2248
    angiography of, 2252
    ankylosing spondylitis in, 2006
    cervical, trauma to, 2244, 2246
    compression fractures of, from osteoporosis, 2043, 2044
    congenital malformations of, 2257–2258
    diagnostic imaging techniques for, 2059, 2060, 2060t
    disorders of, approach to, 2250–2252
    epidural abscess in, 2186–2187
    examination of, computed tomography for, 83
    hematogenous osteomyelitis of, 1622
    injury to, 2244–2247
    lesions of, vs. gallstones, 865
    lumbar. See under Lumbar
    muscular atrophy of, 2155–2156
        in infants, 2155
    neoplasms of, vs. genital herpes, 2197
    osteoarthritis in, 2040–2041
    osteoporosis of, in homocystinuria, 1160
    stenosis of, pain in, 2249
    subdural empyema of, 2187

Spine (Continued)
    thoracic, trauma to, 2244
    tuberculosis of, 1690
Spinocerebellar degeneration, vs. multiple sclerosis, 2214
Spinocerebellar disorders, ataxia from, 2126, 2206
Spiramycin, for cryptosporidiosis, in acquired immunodeficiency syndrome, 1883
Spirillary fever, 1729–1730
Spirillum minor, 1729
Spirochete organisms, and acute gingivitis, 675
Spirochetosis, intestinal, diagnosis of, with biopsy, 731
Spironolactone, 232, 234, 536
    adverse effects of, 289t, 292
    and hyperkalemia, 548
    and hyperkalemic hyperchloremic metabolic acidosis, 553
    as predictor of adrenalectomy success, 291
    characteristics of, 536t
    for ascites, 851
    for Cushing's disease, 1356
    for hypertension, 286t
    gynecomastia from, 1411
    properties of, 231t
    testosterone synthesis inhibited by, 1414
Spleen
    abscess in, 1039–1040
    absence of, 315
        and penicillin prophylaxis, 1560
        congenital, 1039
    and erythrocytes, 910
    arterial aneurysms of, 1039
    blood supply to, 760
    cords of Billroth in, 1036
    cysts in, 1039
    disease of, 1036–1040
    enlargement of, 1037–1038, 1037t
        anemia from, 879
        chronic congestive, 848, 1038
        from amyloidosis, 840
        from chronic malaria, 924
        from chronic meningococcemia, 1614
        from chronic myelogenous leukemia, 990
        from congenital erythropoietic porphyria, 1183
        from congenital rubella, 1777
        from cryptogenic cirrhosis, 847
        from glycolytic defects, 916
        from hairy cell leukemia, 999
        from hereditary spherocytosis, 911
        from hypereosinophilic syndrome, 1024
        from infectious mononucleosis, 1787
        from infective endocarditis, 1589
        from myelofibrosis, 985, 986
        from Niemann-Pick disease, 1148
        from paracoccidioidomycosis, 1843
        from polycythemia vera, 981
        from portal hypertension, 847, 848
        from primary thrombocythemia, 1054
        from psittacosis, 1736
        from systemic lupus erythematosus, 2015
        from viral hepatitis, 819
        portal hypertension from, 848
        spur cell hemolytic anemia and, 923
        thrombocytopenia from, 1054
    evaluation of, 1037
    Gaucher's disease and, 1146, 1147
    hemangiomatosis of, 1039
    in histoplasmosis, 1838
    in Hodgkin's disease, 1019
    in iron deficiency anemia, 897

Spleen (Continued)
    in relapsing fever, 1725
    in sickle cell anemia, 939
    in visceral leishmaniasis, 1871
    infarction of, 1039
        from chronic myelogenous leukemia, 990
            treatment of, 992
        vs. splenic abscess, 1040
    malaria and, 1859
    multiple masses of, 316
    physiology and functions of, 1036–1037, 1036
    radiation of, for chronic myelogenous leukemia, 992
    rupture of, 1039
    sarcoidosis in, 453
Splenectomy
    alternatives to, 1038–1039
    and anemia, 883
    babesiosis after, 1885
    central nervous system infection after, 2210
    consequences of, 1039
    contraindicated for essential thrombocythemia, 987
    for autoimmune hemolytic anemia, 919
    for Gaucher's disease, 1147
    for hairy cell leukemia, 1000
    for hereditary spherocytosis, 157–158, 912
    for idiopathic thrombocytopenic purpura, 1050, 1051
    for increasing neutrophil count, 964
    for myelofibrosis, 987
    for thalassemia, 932
    indications for, 1038–1039
    infection after, 1532
    pneumococcal vaccine before, 1537
    reactive thrombocytosis after, 1054
Splenic fever, 1667
Splenic flexure syndrome, 722
Splenic vein thrombosis, portal hypertension from, 848
Splenomegaly, 1037–1038, 1037t. See also Spleen, enlargement of
Splenomegaly syndrome, tropical, 1859
Splinter hemorrhages, definition of, 2325
    from infective endocarditis, 1589t
    in nails, 2347
Spondylarthritis, 2008
Spondylarthropathies, 2004–2009
    ankylosing spondylitis as, 2005t, 2006–2007
    comparison of, 2005t
    enteropathic arthropathy as, 2008
    enteropathic spondylitis as, 2005t
    etiologic factors in, 2005–2006
    hereditary factors in, 2005
    juvenile arthropathy as, 2005t, 2008
    psoriatic arthropathy as, 2005t, 2008–2009
    reactive arthropathy as, 2005t, 2008
    Reiter's syndrome as, 2005t, 2007–2008
    types of, 2005, 2005
Spondylitis
    ankylosing, 151, 473, 2005t, 2006–2007. See also Ankylosing spondylitis
    in Crohn's disease, 750
    psoriatic, 2009
    tuberculous, 1690
Spondylolisthesis, 2044, 2257
Spondylosis, 2253–2254
    cervical, 2168
        vs. vitamin B$_{12}$ deficiency, 2140
        vs. extradural tumors, 2255
Sponge(s), nonfatal envenomations from, 1931
Spongiosis, 2329
    definition of, 2318

Spontaneous abortion. See *Abortion, spontaneous*

Spontaneous hemorrhage
intracranial, 2173–2180
causes of, 2173t
etiology of, 2173–2175
platelet counts and, 1047

Spontaneous pneumothorax. See *Pneumothorax, spontaneous*

Spores, 1837

Sporotrichosis, 1846–1847, 2334
vs. cat scratch disease, 1681
vs. cutaneous leishmaniasis, 1875
vs. paracoccidioidomycosis, 1843
vs. tularemia, 1666

Sporozoites, 1858

Sprays, 2315

Sprue, diarrhea from, 729

Spur cells, in liver disease, 817

Sputum
blood in, 391–392. See also *Hemoptysis*
culture of, for bronchiectasis, 439
for chronic lung disease, 480
from lung abscess, 436
Gram-stained, for pneumococcal pneumonia, 1557
in diagnosis, 391
in pneumonia, 1553–1554
in respiratory failure, control of, 480
of asthma patients, 407
study of, for bronchogenic carcinoma, 460

Squamous cell carcinoma, 2336t, 2338
from occupational skin injury, 2375
of anal canal, 766
of epidermis, 2337
of lungs, 457, 458
vs. erythroplakia, 678

Square wave jerks, 2117

Squatting maneuver, and murmur from mitral valve prolapse, 350
by children with hypoxemia, 309

SRIF (somatotropin release inhibiting factor), 1280

SRT (speech reception threshold), 2118

SSc. See *Systemic sclerosis*

SSSS (staphylococcal scalded skin syndrome), 1598, 1599, 2329

ST segment, in electrocardiography, 197, 198

STA (standard tube agglutination) test, 1678

Stadol, abuse of, 55

Stagnant loop syndrome, 741–742

Standard tube agglutination (STA) test, for brucellosis, 1678

Staphylococcal scalded skin syndrome, 1598, 1599, 2329

Staphylococcus(i)
abscess from, in hyperimmunoglobulinemia E syndrome, 1947
and gastritis, 689
and urinary tract infection, 629
antimicrobial therapy for, 114
cephalosporins for, 120
coagulase-producing, penicillin G contraindicated for, 119
exotoxins from, cholestasis from, 834
food poisoning from, 784–785
infections of, 1596–1604
and mucous membrane, 2347
bacteremia from, 1602
clinical manifestations of, 1598–1603
diagnosis of, 1603
endocarditis from, 1601–1602
epidemiology of, 1597
erythromycin for, 121

Staphylococcus(i) *(Continued)*
pathogenesis of, 1597–1598
treatment of, 1603–1604
vs. tularemia, 1666
lymphadenitis from, vs. bubonic plague, 1663
pericarditis from, 362
pneumatoceles from, pneumothorax from, 470
pneumonia from, vs. pneumococcal pneumonia, 1558
rifampin for, 121
septic shock syndrome from, 1602

Staphylococcus aureus, 1596
access infections from, in dialysis patients, 577
acute endocarditis from, 1590
and cavernous sinus thrombosis, 2185
and chronic granulomatous disease, 958
and spinal epidural abscess, 2186
arthritis from, 2009
capsule of, 1598
carrier state of, 1597
cellulitis from, 2335
cephalosporins for, 120
endocarditis from, 1587
treatment of, 1594
enterotoxins from, and secretory diarrhea, 727
food poisoning by, 784–785
in cystic fibrosis, 441
in postoperative wounds, 1546
in spinal subdural empyema, 2187
infection of, 1532
after thermal injury, 2365
cutaneous, 2317
immunosuppression and, 2352
hemolysis from, 923
hospital-acquired, 1542
pneumonia from, 1544
in hair follicle, 2334
lung abscess from, vancomycin for, 437
shock from, treatment for, 246
urinary tract, 1601
liver abscess from, 834
lung abscess from, 436
lymphangitis from, 388
meningitis from, 1605
treatment of, 1609–1610
opioids and, 56
osteomyelitis from, 1622
sickle cell anemia and, 940
subacute bacterial endocarditis with glomerulonephritis from, 587
toxins from, 1597–1598
vancomycin for, 122
vs. *Escherichia coli*, 1655

Staphylococcus epidermidis, 119
and hospital-acquired infections, 1542
as contaminant in blood cultures, 113
bloodstream infection of, catheters and, 1545
meningitis from, 1601
on skin, 1548
osteomyelitis from, 1622, 1623
prosthetic valve infection from, 1591
vancomycin for, 122

Staphylococcus faecalis, endocarditis from, treatment of, 1594
vancomycin, for, 122

Staphylococcus saprophyticus, 1596
urinary tract infections from, 629, 1601

Staphylococcus viridans, subacute bacterial endocarditis with glomerulonephritis from, 587

Starch, absorption of, 734
craving for, iron deficiency and, 880, 896

Stark-Kaeser syndrome, 2274

Starling equation, 529

Starling forces, disturbances in, and fluid volume excess, 535

Starvation
and alcoholic ketoacidosis, 1377
gynecomastia in, 1451
hyponatremia in, 539
hypophosphatemia during refeeding for, 1194
metabolic acidosis in, 554
preservation of body protein during, 1212

Stasis syndrome, 741

Status asthmaticus, 403

Status epilepticus, 2223
electroencephalogram for, 2225
major motor, emergency treatment of, 2228, 2228t

Status thymolymphaticus, 1975

Stauffer's syndrome, 652–653, 2098

STD's, 1701–1722. See also *Sexually transmitted disease*

Steal syndromes, in dialysis patients, 577

Steatorrhea
and malabsorption diagnosis, 735
diagnosis of, 729
from ileal disease, 742
from intestinal lymphoma, 744
from secondary biliary cirrhosis, 846
in mesenteric inflammatory disease, 795
in Zollinger-Ellison syndrome, 708–709

Steeple sign, 1761

Stein-Leventhal syndrome, 1287

Stem cells
circulating, 985
defective, and aplastic anemias, 886
hierarchy of, 984
leukemic, 989
pluripotent, 875
residual normal, in chronic myelogenous leukemia, 974

Stenosis
aortic, 341–343, 342t. See also *Aortic stenosis*
aortic valve, radiograph of, *194*
hypertrophic pyloric, gastric outlet obstruction from, 707
meatal, 650
mitral, 345–347, 345t. See also *Mitral stenosis*
of carotid artery, 2165
of renal arteries, 632–633, 633t
papillary, 674
pulmonic, 311–312, 351
acquired, 307
pyloric, 170t, 716–717
spinal, pain of, 2249
subaortic, idiopathic hypertrophic, 356
tracheal, from tracheostomy, 496
tricuspid, 351. See also *Tricuspid stenosis*

Stepped-care regimen, for drug therapy, 286–287, *288*

Stereoanesthesia, 2128

Sterility, definition of, 1440
from chemotherapy, 1020

Sterilization, 1547–1548
definition of, 1547
from radiation injury, 2377

Sternum, congenital deformity of, 473
steering wheel injuries to, 369

Steroid hormones. See also *Hormone(s)*
actions of, 1261–1262, *1261*
measurement of, in precocious puberty, 1428

Steroid hormones (Continued)
  metabolism of, 1254, 1256–1257
  responses to, 1262
  transport of, 1256
Steroid therapy. See also Glucocorticosteroid therapy
  and cancer, 1093t
  as adjuvant analgesic, 108t
  as analgesics, 109
  for paroxysmal nocturnal hemoglobinuria, 923
  for VIPoma, 1389
  half-life of, decreased by rifampin, 121
  in drug interactions, 124t
  lobular panniculitis after, 2050
  myopathy from, vs. polymyositis, 2036
  nonketotic hyperosmolar syndrome from, 1377
  spinal inflammation from, 2257
  systemic, for skin disorders, 2317
  topical, for skin disorders, 2315–2316, 2315t
    side effects of, 2315
Stethoscope, and infection, 1547
  use of, in cardiovascular physical examination, 177
Stevens-Johnson syndrome, 1562–1563, 1783, 2331–2332
  ulcers in, vs. in Behçet's disease, 2049
  vs. toxic epidermal necrolysis, 2329
Stewart-Treves syndrome, 1111
Stickler syndrome, vs. Marfan syndrome, 1178
Stiff-man syndrome, 2270, 2284
Stiffness, in rheumatoid arthritis, 2000
  myocardial vs. chamber, 359
Still's disease, 2004, 2008
  vs. rat-bite fever, 1730
Stillbirth
  alpha thalassemia and, 933
  chromosome abnormalities and, 166
  from Campylobacter infection, 1649
  from congenital toxoplasmosis, 1877
  from listeriosis, 1672
  from malaria, 1859
  from measles, 1772
  from syphilis, 1718, 2189
Stimulants, abuse of, 54–55, 2069t
  psychologic dependence on, 49
Stingrays, 1930
Stokes-Adams attack, 2164
Stomach
  acidity of, and cholera prevention, 1651
    drugs to reduce, 700–701, 700
  acute dilatation of, 718
  adenomas of, 713
  aspiration of contents of, pneumonitis from, 1544
  atrophy of, 690
    from common variable agammaglobulinemia, 1943
  bleeding from, vs. hemoptysis, 392
  blood supply to, 760
    and mucosal integrity, 694, 694
  cancer of
    amyloidosis in, 1199
    in cigarette smokers, 38
    nitrites and, 44
    pernicious anemia with, 905
    vs. pancreatic cancer, 783
    vs. peptic ulcers, 699
  decompression of, 708
  diverticula of, 718
  emptying, after drug overdose, 2070
    delayed, and ulcer disease, 696
  endoscopic examination of, 688t, 668–670
  function of, 714

Stomach (Continued)
  hydrochloric acid loss from, and metabolic alkalosis, 532
  hypomotility of, in systemic sclerosis, 2022
  irradiation of, in gastroesophageal reflux disease treatment, 683
  metoclopramide and, 99
  motility disorders of, 716t
    vomiting from, 658
  mucosa of, inflammation of, 689–692. See also Gastritis
    maintenance of, 694
  neoplasms of, 709–713
    carcinoma as, 710–712, 710
    leiomyosarcoma as, 713
    lymphoma as, 712–713
    metastasized to kidneys, 655
    vs. bleeding from peptic ulcers, 706
  outlet obstruction of, 170t, 716–717
    from peptic ulcers, 707–708
    vomiting from, 658
    vs. appendicitis, 802
    vs. peptic ulcers, 699
  pain from, 658
  prostaglandin E$_2$ in, 1273
  structure of, 693, 693
  surgery on, for obesity, 1227
    gastritis after, 692
  ulcers of. See also Peptic ulcers
    and cancer, 710
    benign, and chronic gastritis, 691
    endoscopy for, 669
    fistula formation from, 707
    treatment of, 702
      drugs for, 702t
      surgical, 704
    visualization of, 698, 698
  varices of, hemorrhage from, 799
  volvulus of, 718
Stomatitis
  angular, from iron deficiency, 896–897
    from riboflavin deficiency, 1231
  aphthous, 675–676, 676, 2347
    Behçet's disease and, 2049
  epizootic, 1778
  herpetic, vs. aphthous ulcers, 676
  in inflammatory bowel disease, 758
Stomatocytosis, hereditary, 913
Stonefish, stings from, 1930
Stool
  analysis of, for fat content, 731
  bacteria in, 1658
  blood in, from colonic cancer, 771
    from gastrointestinal hemorrhage, 796
    from mesenteric artery occlusion, 762
    occult, gastric cancer and, 711
  chemical analysis of fat in, and steatorrhea, 735
  color of, from viral hepatitis, 819
    liver disease and, 808
  culture of, for cholera, 1652
  daily normal weight of, 725
  examination of, 730
    for acute abdomen, 802
    for Campylobacter, 1649
    for liver disease, 817
    for shigellosis, 1647
    microscopic, and malabsorption, 736, 738
  hepatitis A virus shedding in, 821
  impaction of, 788
  loose, from adenocarcinoma of colon, 770
  passing of, through vagina, from diverticulitis, 804
  silver-colored, from pancreatic cancer, 781

Stool (Continued)
  testing of, for occult blood, 883
  twenty-four-hour volume, and diagnosis of diarrheal cause, 731
Stool softeners, 722
Strabismus, causes of, 2115, 2116
  definition of, 2114
Stratum corneum, 2300
  and chemical photosensitivity, 2374
  protection by, 2303
Stratum germinativum, 2300
Stratum spinosum cells, 2301
Streptobacillary fever, 1729
Streptocerciasis, 1919
Streptococcus(i), 1572
  aerobic, and lung abscess, 436
  and gastritis, 689
  bacteremia from, shock from, 246
  cephalosporins for, 120
  classification of, 1572–1574, 1573t
  disease from, 1572–1580
  gangrene from, 1630t
  group A, 1573
    beta-hemolytic, in postoperative wounds, 1546
    cellulitis from, 2335
    endocarditis from, treatment of, 1594
    infections of, 1574–1577
      penicillin for, 114
      preventing, 1578–1579
      skin, immunosuppression and, 2352
    rheumatic fever from, 1580
  group B, 1573
    and neonatal meningitis, 1605
    infections with, 1579–1580
  group D, 1573
  impetigo from, 1577–1578
  in brain abscess, 2182
  in subdural empyema, 2184
  infection of
    and post-streptococcal glomerulonephritis, 585
    erythromycin for, 121
    skin, 1577–1578
    vs. emphysematous cholecystitis, 867
    vs. infectious mononucleosis, 1788
  lung abscess from, 436
  lymphadenitis from, vs. bubonic plague, 1663
  lymphangitis from, 388
  myonecrosis from, 1630t
  pharyngitis from, guttate psoriasis after, 2327
    rash with, 2324
    vs. diphtheria, 1628
  pneumonia from, 1577
  vs. Listeria monocytogenes, 1672
Streptococcus bovis, endocarditis from, treatment of, 1594t
Streptococcus faecalis, and folate, 906
  penicillin G for, 112
Streptococcus milleri, lung abscess from, 436
Streptococcus mutans, 1573
Streptococcus pneumoniae
  and bronchiectasis, 439
  and chronic bronchitis, 412
  central nervous system infection from, in immunocompromised host, 2210
  hemolysis from, 923
  in spontaneous bacterial peritonitis, 851
  lung abscess from, 436
  penicillin G for, 119
  pneumococcal pneumonia from, 1554
  sickle cell anemia and, 940
Streptococcus pyogenes, infection with, 1532
  penicillin G for, 119
    skin, 2317

Streptococcus pyogenes (Continued)
lung abscess from, 436
Streptococcus viridans, in spontaneous bacterial peritonitis, 851
infection of, penicillin G for, 119
Streptokinase
for myocardial infarction, 334
for pulmonary embolism, 448
for sudden arterial occlusion, 383
in fibrinolysis, 1064, 1079
thrombolysis with, 387
Streptolysin O, 1574
Streptomycin, 122
decrease in use of, 119
elimination rate for, 96t
for plague, 1663
for tuberculosis, 1687
for tularemia, 1666
nephrotoxicity of, 559, 609
resistance to, 114
Streptothrix muris ratti, 1729
Streptozocin
and acute kidney failure, 559
and kidney damage, 610
for glucagonoma, 1389
for pancreatic cancer, 783
Streptozyme test, for post-streptococcal glomerulonephritis, 587
Stress
and alopecia, 2349
and atherosclerosis, 320
and cortisol secretion, 1344
and diabetes, 1288–1289
and irritable bowel syndrome, 722
and tics, 2151
cardiovascular evaluation during, 208
emotional, and asthma, 407
endorphins and, 1270
exercise and, 46
gastritis with, 799
glucocorticoids and, 1347, 1417
hormonal response to, glucocorticosteroid therapy and, 132
in gastrointestinal disease, 657
reduction of, in hypertension therapy, 285
response to, adrenocortical insufficiency and, 1351
with hypertension, 278
thymic hypoplasia from, 1974
with ACTH deficiency, 1295
Stress disorders, after trauma, 2101
Stress testing, electrocardiography, 201
for mitral valve prolapse, 350
Stretch receptors, 190
and antidiuretic release, 1307
Striations, 2141
definition of, 2346
Striatonigral degeneration, in parkinsonism, 2145
Strictures
esophageal, esophagogastroduodenoscopy for dilation of, 670
in gastroesophageal reflux disease, 681–682
treatment for, 683
from active peptic esophagitis, dysphagia from, 679
secondary biliary cirrhosis from, 846
vs. small intestine neoplasms, 774
Stridor, 391
definition of, 475
in localized airway obstruction, 418
Strobila, 1890
Stroke, 2159
amnesia from, 2166
apraxia with, 2087
as contraindication for thrombolytic therapy, 449

Stroke (Continued)
as hypertensive complication, 293
atherothrombotic, 2163
by arterial territories, 2165–2166
coarctation of aorta and, 318
completed
course of, 2170, 2170t
definition of, 2163
prognosis of, 2170
treatment of, 2172
death from, 180
epidemiology of, 179
epilepsia partialis continua after, 2221
evolving, 2163
from angiopathies, 2165t
from bacterial endocarditis, 2186
from cardiac catheterization, 211
from carotid sinus pressure, 254
from dissecting aortic aneurysms, 373
from emboli from heart, 2163–2164
from hypertension, 277
from infective endocarditis, 1590
hemiballism after, 2148
in children, from syphilis, 2189
in cigarette smokers, 37
in vaso-occlusive crisis, in sickle cell anemia, 939
lacunar, 2166, 2167t
management of, 2170
nonprogressing, partial, 2163
paralysis from, and venous thromboembolism, 443
rehabilitation after, 2172
spontaneous intracranial hemorrhage as, 2173–2180
threatened, pathogenesis of, 2166–2168, 2167t
prognosis of, 2170
treatment of, 2170–2171
vs. botulism, 1633
vs. brain abscess, 2182
vs. brain tumors, 2234
vs. viral encephalitis, 1823
Stroke volume, 216
shock and, 237–238
Stroke work, 185
Strokelike episodes, with mitochondrial myopathy, 2280
Stromal cells, 970
Strongyloides
AIDS with, diarrhea from, 729
infection with, 835t, 1905–1906
hepatomegaly and eosinophilia from, 834
vs. peptic ulcers, 699
Structural disease, pain from, 105
Struma ovarii, 1327
Strumpell's disease, 2154
Struvite, in kidney stones, 638
and urinary tract infection, 641
diagnosis of, 642
treatment of, 643–644
Strychnine, poisoning from, vs. tetanus, 1635
Stupor
brain wave in, 2223
causes of, 2062t
definition of, 2061t
from depressant drug poisoning, 2068, 2070
Sturge-Weber syndrome, 2159
venous angiomas in, 2174
Subaortic stenosis, idiopathic hypertrophic, 356
Subarachnoid hemorrhage, 2173
arteriography for, 2177
clinical features of, 2176
headache from, 2133
hydrocephalus from, 2175

Subarachnoid hemorrhage (Continued)
laboratory investigation of, 2176
prognosis in, 2177
risk of, from smoking and oral contraceptives, 39
spinal, 2257
treatment of, 2177
unconsciousness from, 2076
vs. orgasmic headache, 2132
vs. tetanus, 1635
vs. traumatic lumbar puncture, 2176
Subclavian artery, occlusion of, 2166
Subclavian vein, thrombosis of, 385
Subcutaneous tissue, 2050, 2300
loss of, 2051
Subdural effusions, meningitis and, 1605
Subdural empyema, 2183–2184
after cerebral epidural abscess, 2184
from anaerobes, 1639
of spine, 2187
vs. viral encephalitis, 1823
Subdural hematoma
chronic, 2243–2244
infection of, and subdural empyema, 2184
speed of treatment for, and prognosis, 2241
vs. brain tumors, 2234
vs. transient ischemic attacks, 2169
Submetacentric chromosomes, 163
Subphrenic abscess, 793, 1040
Substance abuse. See *Drug abuse*
Substance P, in vascular headache, 2130
Substantia nigra, 2141
dopamine content of, aging and, 25
pigmented neuron loss in, in parkinsonism, 2143
Substrate transfer, inhibition of, and hyperaminoaciduria, 1149
Subtentorial lesions, 2062
coma from, 2063
Subthalamic nucleus, 2141
Succinic acid, and iron absorption, 898
Succinylcholine, and malignant hyperthermia, 2282
myasthenia from, 2287
Suckling, and oxytocin secretion, 1313
Sucralfate
and warfarin absorption, 99
for acute gastritis, 690
for duodenal ulcers, 702
for peptic ulcers, 701
Sucrose, absorption of, 734
in diet, for diabetic, 1368–1369
Sucrose hemolysis test, 887, 922
Sudan stain, for fat, in diarrhea, 730
Sudden death
cardiac death, 274–276
definition of, 274
prevention of, 275–276
vs. acute myocardial infarction, 330
from amyloidosis, 360
from aortic stenosis, 341
from dilated cardiomyopathy, 352
from hypertrophic cardiomyopathy, 357
from pulmonary hypertension, 299
Sudden infant death syndrome, 2079
botulism and, 1634
respiratory syncytial virus and, 1759
Suffocation, flukes and, 1903
Suicide, 2097–2098
alcoholism and, 52
among epileptics, 2228
among physicians, 68
anorexia nervosa and, 1218
attempts at, with antifreeze ingestion, 612
with drugs, 2071
bulimia and, 1218

Suicide (Continued)
　by adolescents, 20–21
　from poisonings, 141
　Huntington's disease and, 2091
　insulin in, 1386
　psychedelic drugs and, 59
　with digitalis overdose, 229–230
Sulfadiazine, for toxoplasmosis, 1879
　in kidney and liver failure, 117t
Sulfamethoxazole
　elimination rate for, 96t
　for prostatitis, 1422
　hypoglycemia from, 1384
　in kidney and liver failure, 117t
　trimethoprim with, for bacterial infec-
　　　tions, 119
　　for urinary tract infection in women,
　　　630
Sulfamethoxazole-trimethoprim, for chronic
　　　bronchitis, 413
Sulfanilamide, toxicity of, to hemoglobin,
　　　945
Sulfasalazine
　adverse reactions to, 759
　for inflammatory bowel disease, 751
　for ulcerative colitis, 759
　for ulcerative proctitis, 788
Sulfates, as laxatives, 722
Sulfhemoglobin, from drugs, 945
　reference intervals for, 2402t
Sulfhemoglobinemia, 946–947
Sulfhydryl compounds, and radiation ther-
　　　apy, 1116
Sulfinpyrazone, as cyclooxygenase inhibi-
　　　tor, 1275
　for gout, 1170
　interaction of, with warfarin, 100
Sulfisoxazole, for lymphogranuloma vener-
　　　eum, 1711
　in kidney and liver failure, 117t
Sulfite oxidase, deficiency of, with xanthine
　　　oxidase deficiency, 1170
Sulfonamides, 119
　action of, 113t
　acute interstitial nephritis from, 605
　and hemolysis in glucose-6-phosphate
　　　dehydrogenase deficiency, 916
　and kidney damage, 612
　and photosensitivity, 2351
　chronic hepatitis from, 828
　displacement of bilirubin by, 100
　for Nocardia infection, 437, 1675–1676
　for paracoccidioidomycosis, 1844
　for streptococcal pharyngitis, 1577
　for streptococci A prophylaxis, 1579
　for urinary tract infection, 630
　genetics and reaction to, 102
　in drug interactions, 124t
　in kidney failure, 117t
　in prostate tissue, 116
　liver disease from, 117t, 827
　liver metabolism of, 118
　meningococci resistance to, 1616
　penetration into spinal fluid by, 116
　protein binding by, 94
　resistance mechanisms of, 116t
　selectivity of, 112
　serum sickness from, 103
　shillae resistance to, 1647
　toxic reactions to, 123
Sulfones, and hemolysis in glucose-6-phos-
　　　phate dehydrogenase deficiency, 916
　genetics and reaction to, 102
Sulfonylurea(s)
　and photosensitivity, 2351
　and thyroid function, 1321
　for diabetes mellitus, 1369, 1370t
　half-life of, decreased by rifampin, 121

Sulfur dioxide, and chemical pneumonitis,
　　　2367
Sulindac, as cyclooxygenase inhibitor, 1275
Sun, and skin aging process, 2306
　reduced exposure to, and osteomalacia
　　　and rickets, 1479
　ultraviolet radiation from, 2350
Sunburn, 2350
　extensive, prednisone for, 2317
Sunflower cataract, 2289
Sunscreens, 2316
Superinfection, 114
　bacterial, influenza and, 1766
　from IUDR toxicity, 125
　gram-negative bacilli pneumonia and,
　　　1568
Superior mesenteric artery, 760–761, 761
Superior mesenteric artery syndrome, 765
Superior mesenteric vein, thrombosis of,
　　　764
Superior sagittal sinus thrombosis, 2185
Superior sulcus tumor, and arm, 459
　pain from, 105
Superior vena cava, obstruction of, Hodg-
　　　kin's disease and, 1016
　mediastinal fibrosis and, 2052
　thrombosis of, 385
Superior vena cava syndrome, from bron-
　　　chogenic carcinoma, 459
　from dissecting aortic aneurysms, 373
Superoxide, 2368
Superoxide anion, in shock, 243
Superoxide dismutase, 2368
　from anaerobic organisms, 1638
　from mast cells, allergic rhinitis and, 1952
Suppressor T lymphocytes, 1932, 1936
Supranuclear palsy, progressive, 2145,
　　　2153t
Supraoptic nuclei, 1305
Supratentorial lesions, stupor or coma
　　　from, 2062
Supraventricular arrhythmias
　after intra-atrial surgery, 317
　atrial septal defect and, 305
　in shock, treatment for, 245
　phenytoin for, 265
　propranolol for, 271
　surgery for, 274
　verapamil for, 271
Suramin
　for African trypanosomiasis, 1864
　for filariasis, 1914
　for onchocerciasis, 1917
　side effects of, 1864
Surfactant, 241, 395, 421
　synthesis of, 400
Surgery
　abdominal, and mesenteric venous
　　　thrombosis, 764
　and acute gouty arthritis, 1165
　and riboflavin deficiency, 1231
　bleeding after, in hemophilia A, 1067
　chronic respiratory failure and, 481
　emergency, for bleeding ulcers, 706
　for achalasia, 686
　for adenocarcinoma of colon, 771–772
　for adrenocortical insufficient patients,
　　　steroid coverage for, 1353
　for aortic regurgitation, 345
　for aortic stenosis, 343
　for appendicitis, 803
　for arteriosclerosis obliterans, 381
　for bile duct carcinoma, 872
　for brain abscess, 2183
　for brain tumors, 2234
　for bronchiectasis, 439–440
　for bronchogenic carcinoma, 461
　for cancer, 1088, 1115

Surgery (Continued)
　for cancer, gastric, 712
　　lymphedema from, 388
　　of esophagus, 687
　for cardiogenic shock, 249
　for cerebral aneurysms, 2177
　for cerebral atherothrombotic disease,
　　　2171
　for chronic obstructive pulmonary dis-
　　　ease, 417
　for chronic pancreatitis, 780
　for constrictive pericarditis, 367
　for Cushing's disease, 1304, 1356
　for dissecting aortic aneurysm, 374
　for diverticulitis, 805
　for endocarditis, 1594
　for epilepsy, 2228
　for gallstones, 865
　for gastroesophageal reflux disease, 683
　for hemoptysis, 392
　for herniated disc, 2253
　for hyperparathyroidism, 1495
　for hyperthyroidism, 1326
　for hypertrophic cardiomyopathy, 358
　for insulinoma, 1385
　for kidney stone removal, 644
　for lung abscess, 437
　for metastatic lung tumors, 464
　for mitral regurgitation, 349
　for mitral stenosis, 347
　for myxoma, 367
　for obesity, 1227
　for patent ductus arteriosus, 308
　for perforated peptic ulcers, 707
　for pheochromocytoma, 1465
　for pituitary tumors, 1299
　　growth hormone secreting, 1301
　for portal hypertension, 850
　for pulmonic stenosis, 312
　for renal artery occlusion, 633
　for renal cell carcinoma, 653
　for renovascular hypertension, 290–291
　for shunt lesions, 305
　for simple transposition of great arteries,
　　　314
　for sudden arterial occlusion, 383
　for suppurative cholangitis, 869
　for tetralogy of Fallot, 310
　for toxic megacolon, 758–759
　for tuberculosis, 1689
　for ulcerative colitis, 759–760
　for urinary tract obstruction, 617
　fungal peritonitis from, 794
　gastrointestinal motility disorders from,
　　　717
　granulomatous peritonitis after, from
　　　contaminants, 795
　hyperbilirubinemia following, 814
　intra-atrial, 317
　intraventricular, 317–318
　mechanical ventilation after, 487
　mycobacteria infections after, 1695
　on coronary arteries, for angina pectoris,
　　　328–329
　on neck, and hypoparathyroidism, 1496
　pancreatitis after, 775
　pulmonary embolism after, 442
　wounds from, and gas gangrene, 1629
Sutures, silk, and postoperative recurrent
　　　ulcers, 705
Swallowing
　bolus arrest during, 679. See also Dys-
　　　phagia
　disorders of
　　and recurrent aspiration pneumonia,
　　　1568–1569
　　from poliomyelitis, 2199
　　from rabies, 2201

Swallowing (Continued)
  disorders of, in Guillain-Barré syndrome, 2262
  in pneumonia prevention, 1552
  pain from, 679
Swan-Ganz catheter, 212
  for shock patients, 243–244
  for ventricular function evaluation, 334
  intrapulmonary complications from, 497
  pulmonary capillary wedge pressure measurement with, 533
Sweat, sodium in, heart failure and, 220
Sweat glands, 2302
  aging and, 2306
  in cystic fibrosis, 440
Sweat test, for cystic fibrosis, 441
Sweating
  abnormalities of, 2107
  and thermoregulation, 2304
  excessive, and fluid volume depletion, 532
    from paravertebral tumors, 2254
  from pheochromocytoma, 284
  in opioid withdrawal syndrome, 57
Sweeteners, artificial, and cancer, 1096
Sweet's syndrome, cancer and, 1113
Swelling. See Edema
Swimmers, lung injury in, from barometric pressure, 2367
Swimmer's itch, 1897
Swimming, as exercise, 47
  during international travel, 1550
Swimming pool granuloma, 1695
Swyer-James syndrome, 420
Sydenham's chorea, 2148
  in rheumatic fever, 1583
Sylvest's disease, 1810–1811
Sylvian fissure, language and, 2086
Symmers' fibrosis, 1899
Symmetrel, 126. See also Amantadine
Symmetrical polyneuropathy
  definition of, 2259
  distal, 1380
  from arsenic poisoning, 2389
  generalized, 2259–2260
  in diabetes mellitus, 2262–2264
Sympathectomy, preganglionic, for Raynaud's phenomenon, 377
  lumbar, for arteriosclerosis obliterans, 382
Sympathetic blocks, for hypertensive crisis, 290t
  for pain management, 109
Sympathetic nervous system, 133
  and gastrointestinal motility, 715
  and heart contractility, 218
  and kidney blood flow, 510–511
  and metabolic regulation disturbances, 1288–1289
  and Raynaud's phenomenon, 375
  for heart, 184
  in kidneys, and sodium homeostasis, 516
  increased activity by, and hypertension, 277
  regulation of mesenteric circulation by, 761
Sympathetic-parasympathetic dysfunction, 2106
Sympathoadrenal system, 134
Sympathochromaffin system, 1461
  physiology of, 1462–1463
Sympathomimetic amines, 137
  and distribution of other drugs, 99
  for shock, 246–248
Sympathomimetic drugs, for asthma, 408
  for chronic respiratory failure, 480
Synapsis, in meiosis, 162

Syncope, 2073–2075, 2074t
  cause and frequency of, 2073t
  definition of, 2061t
  from aortic stenosis, 341
  from arteritis, 374
  from brain injury, 2240
  from carotid sinus pressure, 254
  from congenital complete heart block, 316
  from cough, 391
  from dissecting aortic aneurysms, 373
  from Eisenmenger's syndrome, 317
  from myxoma, 367
  from primary pulmonary hypertension, 299
  heat, 2384
  in cardiovascular patient history, 175
  vasodepressor, orthostatic hypotension with, 2106
  vs. epilepsy, 2225
Syndrome of inappropriate secretion of antidiuretic hormone, 535, 1103, 1288, 1308
  after head injury, 2242–2243
  causes of, 539t
  characteristics of, 539t
  hyponatremia in, 539–540, 539
    treatment for, 541
  in St. Louis encephalitis, 1826
  legionnaires' disease and, 1571
Synechiae, posterior, 2293
Synovial fluid
  analysis of, 1993–1995, 1994t
  for rheumatoid arthritis, 2003
  in inflammatory joint disease, 1984
  in joint cavity, 1983
  Mycobacterium tuberculosis in, 2010
Synoviocytes, 1986
Synoviography, 1998
Synovioma, 2048
Synovitis, 1977
  crystal-induced, 1978
  from immune complex, 1960
  granulomatous sarcoid, chronic, 2045
  in rheumatoid arthritis, 1991
  polyarticular, in systemic sclerosis, 2022
  rheumatoid, 1985–1986
  villonodular, pigmented, 2048
    vs. sporotrichosis, 1847
Synovium, 1982
  cysts of, 1998
  membrane of, 1982, 1995
    inflammation in, 1977. See also Synovitis
  normal, 1985–1986, 1985
  tumors of, 2048
Syntenic chromosomes, 162
Syphilis, 11, 1713–1722
  and seizures, 2218
  aneurysms from, 370
  aortic regurgitation from, 343
  cardiovascular, 1717
  clinical manifestations of, 1714–1718
  congenital, 1718
    treatment of, 1721
    vs. cytomegalovirus, 1785–1786
  diagnosis of, 1718–1720
  epidemiologic investigation and treatment for, 1722
  epidemiology of, 1714
  etiology of, 1713
  false-positive test results for, leprosy and, 1698
  follow-up examinations for, 1721–1722, 1722t
  genital ulcers from, 1703, 2342
  hair loss in, 2349

Syphilis (Continued)
  hepatitis from, 834
  in central nervous system, 1717–1718, 2187–2191. See also Neurosyphilis
  joint disease in, 2011
  late, 1716–1718, 1716t
  latent, 1716
    treatment of, 1721
  meningovascular, 1717
  paroxysmal cold hemoglobinuria in, 921
  pathogenesis and host response for, 1713
  penicillin for, 119
  prevention of, 1722
  psychosis in, 1718
  relapsing, 1716
  secondary, 2326t
    vs. pityriasis rosea, 2328
  splenomegaly in, 1037
  tabes dorsalis in, and neuropathic joint disease, 2046
  transmission of, by blood transfusions, 950
  treatment of, 1720–1722, 1720t
  untreated, natural course of, 1714
  vs. bubonic plague, 1663
  vs. cat scratch disease, 1681
  vs. Chagas' disease, 1869
  vs. cutaneous leishmaniasis, 1875
  vs. gonococcal infections of rectum, 1707
  vs. granuloma inguinale, 1712
  vs. lymphogranuloma venereum, 1711
  vs. measles, 1774
  vs. paracoccidioidomycosis, 1843
  vs. peptic ulcers, 699
  vs. sporotrichosis, 1847
  vs. Toxoplasma retinochoroiditis, 1878
  vs. viral hepatitis, 824
  vs. zygomycosis, 1852
Syringomyelia, 2157–2158, 2157
Systemic arterial pressure. See Arterial pressure
Systemic disease, and musculoskeletal disease, 1979
  pruritus with, 2304t
Systemic infection, and central nervous system disorders, 2208–2211
  isoniazid in combination with other agents for, 119
  with Haemophilus influenzae, 1618
Systemic lupus erythematosus, 2011–2018
  and false-positive syphilis tests, 1720
  and hair loss, 2349
  and heart, 369
  and membranous nephropathy, 596
  and occlusive pulmonary vascular disease, 295
  and peritoneum, 795
  and porphyria cutanea tarda, 1186
  and skin, 2340–2341
  autoantibodies in, 2013t
  autoimmune hemolytic anemia with, 881, 918
  autoimmunity and disease in, 2013
  bullous, immunofluorescent cutaneous findings in, 2305t
  cancer and, 1099
  circulating anticoagulant in, 1081
  classification of, 2011t
  clinical manifestations of, 2014–2016, 2015t
  complement system in, 1940
  diagnosis of, 2017
  dilated cardiomyopathy from, 353
  drug-induced, 103, 1970t
  endocarditis in, 1587
  etiology of, 2012

Systemic lupus erythematosus (Continued)
  glucocorticosteroid therapy for, 130, 131
  hemolysis from, 908
  human leukocyte antigens in, 1967
  hypertriglyceridemia in, 1143
  hyposplenism from, 1039
  immunofluorescent cutaneous findings in, 2305t
  in mothers, and AV block in infants, 316
  incidence of, 2012
  infection susceptibility in, glucocorticosteroid therapy and, 133
  inflammation from immune complexes in, 1990
  initiation and perpetuation of, 2012
  interstitial lung disease with, 429–430
    vs. from hydralazine or procainamide, 434
  interstitial nephritis in, 605
  intracranial hemorrhage in, 2175
  kidneys in, 504, 599–600, 599t
  laboratory findings for, 2016–2017
  LE cell and, 1996
  light urticaria in, 1950
  myasthenia gravis with, 2285
  necrotizing venulitis in, 1950
  neuropathy in, 2266
  pathogenesis of, 2013–2014
  pathology of, 2014
  photosensitivity in, 2352
  pleuritis from, 468
  pregnancy and, 636
  retinopathies in, 2297
  small intestinal ulceration from, 807
  splenomegaly in, 1037
  synovial membrane in, 1995
  therapy for, 2017–2018
  thrombocytopenia in, 1052
  vasculitis in, 2027
  vs. Goodpasture's syndrome, 590
  vs. idiopathic pulmonary hemosiderosis, 430
  vs. leprosy, 1699
  vs. Lyme disease, 1728
  vs. multiple sclerosis, 2214
  vs. post-streptococcal glomerulonephritis, 587
  vs. rheumatic fever, 1585
  vs. rheumatoid arthritis, 2000
  vs. syphilis, 1716
  with Hashimoto's thyroiditis, 1333
  with systemic sclerosis, 2021
Systemic sclerosis, 2018–2023
  and heart, 369
  and warm autoimmune hemolytic anemia, 918
  clinical manifestations of, 2021–2023
  cumulative survival rate for, 2020
  definition of, 2019
  diagnosis of, 2020–2021
    differential, 2019t, 2021
  diffuse, 2020
  limited cutaneous, 2020
  pathogenesis and pathology of, 2019–2020
  progressive, interstitial lung disease with, 429
  subsets of, 2019t
  treatment of, 2023
Systolic blood pressure
  and myocardial oxygen consumption, 187
  as afterload, 186
  bleeding from peptic ulcers and, 706
  development of, and angina pectoris, 323
  in dorsalis pedis, 381
  in elderly, 287
  in posterior tibial arteries, 381

Systolic blood pressure (Continued)
  in septic shock, 1538
  measurement of, 281
  ventricular, calculation of, 207
Systolic sounds, 177

T antigen, and group A streptococci, 1574
T cell growth factor, 957. See also Interleukin 2
T cell leukemia, adult, 1795, 1796, 1797
T cell lymphomas, cutaneous, 1108–1109, 1109t, 2375
T lymphocytes, 250, 966, 971, 1935–1936
  cytotoxic, 1936, 1936, 1965
    and tumor cells, 1127
    and viruses, 1751
  defects in, 1942
  donor, and graft-versus-host disease, 1040
  functioning of, assessment of, 1942
  helper, 451, 1932–1936
  in acute interstitial nephritis, 603
  in Chédiak-Higashi disease, 959
  in hypersensitivity pneumonitis, 433
  in immune response, 1531, 1932
  mononuclear phagocytes and, 956
  neoplasms of, 975, 1007
  precursors of, 874
  proportions of, in pulmonary sarcoidosis, 427
T wave, in electrocardiography, 197, 198, 199, 200, 201
TA-AB (teichoic acid antibody) assay, 1603
Tabardillo, 1739
Tabes dorsalis, 1717–1718
  autonomic insufficiency in, 2106
  from syphilis, 2189
  pain from, 2136
  vs. appendicitis, 803
Taboparesis, 2189
Tache noire, 1745
Tachyarrhythmias, digitalis glycosides and, 226
  ventricular, from carotid sinus pressure, 254
Tachycardia
  and cardiac output, 237
  as compensatory mechanism in heart failure, 218
  carotid sinus pressure for, 255t
  compensatory, 352
  from abdominal abscess, 793
  from acute cocaine toxicity, 55
  from acute pancreatitis, 776
  from alpha antagonists, 139
  from bacterial peritonitis, 793
  from hepatic porphyria, 1185
  from hypoxia, 477
  from increased stretch of atrial receptors, 190
  from mesenteric artery occlusion, 762
  from psychedelic drugs, 58
  from ulcerative colitis, 755
  in cavernous sinus thrombosis, 2185
  in Colorado tick fever, 1820
  in free perforation of peptic ulcers, 707
  paroxysmal, atrial, 258, 259
    anticholinesterases for, 140
    supraventricular, 258, 259. See also Paroxysmal supraventricular tachycardia
  postural, from fluid volume depletion, 532
  sinus, carotid sinus pressure for, 255t
  sympathetic nervous system and, 133
  treatment of, 257t

Tachycardia (Continued)
  ventricular, 259, 263, 263
    after intraventricular surgery, 318
    isoproterenol for, 248
Tachyphylaxis, 2316
Tachypnea
  from diabetic ketoacidosis, 1375
  from fat embolism syndrome, 450
  from left ventricular failure, 221
  from pneumocystosis, 1880
  from pulmonary emboli, 296, 444
  from respiratory syncytial virus, 1759
Tactoids, 937
Taenia, 1891–1892
Taipan venom, 1073
Takahara's disease, 1187
Takayasu's arteritis, 374, 2026, 2164
Takayasu's syndrome, aneurysms from, 370
Talcosis, 425, 2364
Talking, in sleep, 2079
Tamm-Horsfall glycoprotein, in urinary casts, 503
Tamoxifen, for carcinoid syndrome, 1468
  for metastatic breast cancer, 1456, 1457
Tamponade, cardiac, 365–366, 365
  and sudden death, 275
  echocardiography for assessment of, 178
  pericardial, 176
Tangier disease, 1144
Tanning, 2350
Tapeworms, 1890–1895. See also Cestodes
Tar, in cigarette smoke, 37, 39
Tar bath preparations, for skin disorders, 2314
Tardive akathisia, from antipsychotic drugs, 2144
Tardive dyskinesia, 2149
  from antipsychotic drugs, 2094, 2144
  vs. chorea, 2142, 2148
  vs. Huntington's disease, 2149t
Tardive dystonia, 2149
Target cells, 910
  of human immunodeficiency virus, 1799–1800
  sensitivity of, evaluating, 1267
  to hormones, 1252, 1262, 1265
Tartrazine yellow, and asthma, 407
Taste, 2109–2110. See also Mouth; Oral medicine
  loss of, causes of, 2110, 2110t
  perception of, in oral cancer, zinc for, 679
Tat protein, 1795
Tay-Sachs disease, 149
  enzyme infusions for, 157
  genetic counseling for, 174
  heredity and, 147
TBG. See Thyroxine-binding globulin
Tea(s), home-brewed, and digitalis intoxication, 787
  and cancer, 44
Tearing, from allergic rhinitis, 1953
Technetium-99m, binding of, to erythrocytes, 207
  for nuclear cardiology, 207
Technetium-labeled iminodiacetic acid, in radionuclide imaging, 665
Technetium-99m diethylene triamine pentaacetate, for ventilation scanning, 445
Technetium-99m diphosphonate, 1997–1998
Technetium-99m pertechnetate, labeling red blood cells with, for angina pectoris testing, 325
Technetium-99m stannous pyrophosphate, for infarct-avid imaging, 210
  in scintigraphy for myocardial infarction, 332

Teeth
abscess of, 674–675
care of, hemophilia A and, 1068
poor, and taste distortions, 2110
decay in, 674
cervicofacial actinomycosis and, 1674
in Sjögren's syndrome, 2024
plaque and, 674
Streptococci mutans and, 1573
development of, hypoparathyroidism and, 1498
in puberty, 18
in rickets, 1482
infection in, and spinal epidural abscess, 2186
loose, from Langerhans cell granulomatosis, 1023
metastatic brain abscess from, 2181
pain in, 2134
rumination syndrome and, 1219
Teichoic acid antibody assay, for staphylococcal infection, 1603
Telangiectasia(s), hemorrhagic, hereditary, 308, 1060, 2341. See also Osler-Weber-Rendu syndrome
in carcinoid syndrome, 1467
in Fabry's disease, 1145
spider, in liver disease, 808
Telecanthus-hypospadias syndrome, 170
Tellurium, toxicity of, 2393
Telogen effluvium, 2349
Telogen phase, of hair growth, 2303
Temazepam, rebound insomnia from, 2078
Temperature
and urate solubility in fluid, 1162
cold, and common cold, 1755
in endotoxic shock, 1659
neural pathway for, 2128
of peripheral joints, 1162
regulation of, disorders of, and metabolic encephalopathy, 2064t
Temporal lobe, bilateral medial resection of, and antegrade amnesia, 2084
damage to, 2081, 2081t
neoplasm of, 2232
Temporomandibular joint syndrome, headache from, 2132–2133
TEN (toxic epidermal necrolysis), 2329
vs. staphylococcal scalded skin syndrome, 1599
Tendinitis, in shoulder, 2042
vs. gout, 1168
Tennis elbow, 2047
Tenosynovitis, 2047
in dialysis patients, 577
in disseminated gonococcal infection, 1708
Tension, headache from, 105, 2132–2133
premenstrual, 1433
Tepanil, abuse of, 54
Teratomas, 2231
hormones from, 1445t
of liver, 857
of testis, 1421
Terbutaline, 137
for asthma, 408
Terfenadine, 1954t, 1955
Terminal hair, 2303
definition of, 1446
Ternides deminutus, 1911
Tertiary care, 8
Testicular feminization syndrome, 153, 167, 1264
and gynecomastia, 1451
Testis (testes), 1404–1421
atrophy of, from cirrhosis, 844, 847
development of, 1391, 1391
differentiation of, 1392

Testis (testes) (Continued)
disorders of, 1395–1399
from viral orchitis, 1414
hypogonadism as, 1408–1420. See also Hypogonadism
in cryptorchidism, 1415
ectopic, 1415
estrogen-secreting tumor of, gynecomastia from, 1411
function of, 1404
gonadotropin regulation of, 1406–1407
irradiation of, effect of, 1415
leprosy in, 1698
leukemia relapse in, 1005
mumps and, 1779
neoplasms of, 1420–1421
normal descent of, 1415
pain in, from renal colic, 106
precocious puberty and, 1420
regression of, 1395
retractile, 1415
structure and physiology of, 1404–1408, 1405
trauma to, 1416
Testosterone, 1433t
administration of, during pregnancy, and masculinization of female infant, 1404
and follicle-stimulating hormone inhibition, 1407
and hair growth at puberty, 2303
and luteinizing hormone inhibition, 1407
and male sexual differentiation, 1392, 1408
and spermatogenesis, 1405
conversion of, to dihydrotestosterone, 1400, 1400
erythrocytosis from, 980
for androgen deficiency, 1419
for myelofibrosis, 987
for osteoporosis, 1514
in females, high levels of, 1428
normal levels of, 1448
in puberty, 17
in spermatogenesis, 1400
increased concentrations of, 1447
methadone and, 56
peripheral metabolism of, 1406
reference intervals for, 2399t
replacement therapy with, 1297
secretion of, normal levels of, 1406
plasma concentrations of, 1341
synthesis of, 1341
deficiency of, 1396–1398, 1398t
in ovaries, 1431
transport of, 1406
Testotoxicosis, and precocious puberty, 1420
Tetanospasmin, 1634
Tetanus, 1633–1636
antitoxin for, in wound management, 1636
dracunculiasis and, 1918
immunization against, 61–62, 62t, 63t, 1626
in heroin users, 57
vs. epilepsy, 2225
vs. rabies, 2201
Tetanus-diphtheria-toxoid booster, before travel, 1550
Tetanus immunoglobulin, 1635
Tetany, 2270
in hypoparathyroidism, 1497
treatment for, 1499
Tetracyclines, 121
action of, 113t
anaerobe resistance to, 741–742
and kidney damage, 117t, 609
as antidepressant, 2096t

Tetracyclines (Continued)
bone labeling with, 1484
decreased absorption of, 99
diffusion of, in bone, 116
elimination rate for, 96t
esophageal injury from, 688
fatty liver from, 828
for bronchiectasis, 439
for brucellosis, 1678
for cholera, 1652
for chronic bronchitis, 413
for chronic respiratory failure, 480
for Crohn's disease, 752
for leptospirosis, 1732
for Lyme disease, 1729
for lymphogranuloma venereum, 1711
for malignant pleural effusion, 469
for murine typhus, 1741
for mycoplasmal infections, 1561, 1565
pneumonia from, 1564
for plague, 1663
for psittacosis, 1736
for relapsing fever, 1725
for Rocky Mountain spotted fever, 1744
for tularemia, 1666
for typhus fever, 1740
for ureaplasma, 1565
for urethritis, 630
for urinary tract infection, 630
in bile, 116
in drug interactions, 124t
in kidney failure, 117t
liver disease from, 117t, 827
liver metabolism of, 118
resistance mechanisms of, 116t
streptococci resistance to, 1577, 1580
Tetrad forms, in blood smears, and babesiosis, 1885
Tetradecanoylphorbol acetate, 1260
Tetrahydrobiopterin, 1156
Tetrahydrocannabinol, in cannabis, 57
Tetralogy of Fallot, 309–310, 310
absence of pulmonic valve in, 314
acyanotic, 309
beta-adrenergic blockers for, 138
radiographs for, 192
surgery for, 274
Tetrodotoxin, from toad fish and puffer fish, 1931
in octopus venom, 1930
TFT (trifluridine), 125–126
Tg. See Thyroglobulin
TgAb's (thyroglobulin antibodies), 1320
TGF-alpha (transforming growth factor alpha), 1102
TGF-beta (transforming growth factor beta), 322, 1102, 1987
Thalamic pain, 2128
Thalamic syndrome, 2129
Thalamus, disorders of, sensory loss from, 2129
Thalassemia(s), 147, 930–936
alpha, genetics of, 933
clinical classification of, 930t
globin genes of, 928
ineffective erythropoiesis in, 895
intermedia, 932
major, splenectomy for, 1038
molecular genetics of, 933–935
prenatal diagnosis of, 935–936
severe beta, 930–932
silent carrier in, 933
Thalassemia trait, 930, 932–933
and malaria protection, 933
Thalidomide, for erythema nodosum leprosum, 1700
Thallium, 209–210
and kidney damage, 612

Thallium (Continued)
for perfusion imaging, for myocardial infarction, 332
in testing for angina pectoris, 325
radioactive, scanning with, 178
toxicity of, 2391–2392
THBR (thyroid hormone-binding ratio), 1318
Theca cells, in ovary, 1425
Thelarche, premature, 1427
Theophylline
adverse reactions to, 102
clearance of, by hemodialysis, 95
distribution of, 97
for acute asthmatic attack, 409
for chronic obstructive pulmonary disease, 417
in drug interactions, 124t
metabolism of, in cigarette smokers, 39
induction of, 99
inhibition of, 101t
by cimetidine, 100
pharmacokinetic parameters for, 89t
poisoning with, treatment for, 145
reference intervals for, 2404t
Thermal injury, to lungs, 2365
to testes, 1416
Thermoactinomyces, lung disease from, 433
Thermodilution method, for cardiac output measurement, 213
Thermogenesis, 1221
Thermography, liquid crystal, for deep-vein thrombosis, 386
Thermoregulation, 2382
by skin, 2304
hypothalamic center of, 1525
sweat glands and, 2302
Thiabendazole
for cutaneous larva migrans, 1907
for strongyloidiasis, 1906
for toxocariasis, 1909
for trichinellosis, 1912
Thiamin, 1229, 1229–1230
deficiency of, 1229. See also Beriberi
dietary sources of, 1229
for coma, 2068
for maple syrup urine disease, 1159
for Wernicke's encephalopathy, 2138
recommended dietary allowance for, 1205t, 1229
reference intervals for, 2399t
Thiazide(s), 535
adverse effects of, 289t
and hypocalciuria, 519
and tubular calcium reabsorption, 642
as diuretics, 231
diabetes mellitus from, 1362
for diabetes insipidus, 1312
for hypertension, 287
hypercalcemia from, 1502–1503
vs. from hyperparathyroidism, 1490
in hypoparathyroidism treatment, 1499
for ascites, 851
for hypertension, 286t
hypercalcemia from, 1492
properties of, 231t, 536t
Thigh, lateral cutaneous nerve of, 2268
Thioctic acid, for mushroom poisoning, 787
Thiocyanate, reference intervals for, 2404t
6–Thioguanine, and hepatic vascular lesions, 828
for cancer, 1122–1123
Thiopental, reference intervals for, 2404t
Thioridazine, reference intervals for, 2404t
side effects of, and eye, 2298
Thiosemicarbazone, 126

Thiosulfate, nitrites with, as antidote for cyanide, 143
Thiotepa, for bladder cancer, 655
Thiothixene, and antidiuretic hormone release, 540
for agitation in psychiatric disorders, 2094t
Thiouracil, and hair loss, 2349
marrow suppression by, 885
serum sickness from, 103
Thiourea compounds, 1315
Thiozanthenes, for schizophrenia, 2094
Third space phenomenon, 535
Thirst
angiotensin III and, 530
center of, 537
from cholera, 1652
hypothalamus and, 2104
receptors for, 2104–2105
regulation of, 1308
Thiuram, and contact dermatitis, 2319
Thomsen-Friedenreich antigen, skin test reactivity to, 782
Thomsen's disease, 2284
Thoracentesis, 466–467
for pulmonary embolism, 445
in heart failure management, 225
Thoracic aorta, 370
aneurysms of, 371
Thoracic surgery, mechanical ventilation after, 487
Thoracotomy, 471
chronic pain after, 2255
Thorax, irradiation of, 2378
malnutrition and, 1210t
tuberculosis of, 1689
Thorn apple, toxicity of, 787
Thorotrast, and angiosarcoma, 859
and hepatocellular carcinoma, 858
Throat, disease in, pain in ear from, 106
Thrombasthenia, 1056–1057
Thrombin, and platelet secretion, 1042
in coagulation, 1061
in hemostasis, 1043
Thrombin time, 1047
reference intervals for, 2402t
Thromboangiitis obliterans, 382–383, 2026
vs. erythromelalgia, 378
Thrombocythemia
essential, 973, 987–988
primary, 1054
hyposplenism from, 1039
vs. polycythemia vera, 985
Thrombocytopenia, 1047–1054
and hemorrhage in eye, 2297
autoimmune, secondary, 1052
bleeding from, in heparin therapy, 447–448
causes of, 1047t
definition of, 1047
evaluation of, 1048
from acquired immunodeficiency syndrome, 1802, 1804
from autoimmune hemolytic anemia, 919
from congenital syphilis, 1718
from dengue hemorrhagic fever, 1833
from drug allergy, 1971t
from gram-negative bacteremia, 1660
from heparin, 1075, 1080
from leukemia, lymphocytic, chronic, 995
myelogenous, chronic, 990
from paroxysmal nocturnal hemoglobinuria, 922
from quinine, 103
from rifampin, 1687
from Rocky Mountain spotted fever, 1744

Thrombocytopenia (Continued)
from rubella, 1777
immunodeficiency with, 1946–1947
with elevated immunoglobulin M, 1944
microangiopathic, 1080
definition of, 1079
sarcoidosis with, 453
splenectomy for, 1038
Thrombocytopenic purpura
autoimmune, 1050
from blood transfusions, 949
from congenital rubella, 1777
from drugs, 1048–1050, 1049t
idiopathic, 1050–1051
immune globulin for, 66
immunization against, 63t
in cancer, 1098
refractory, 1051
with Hashimoto's thyroiditis, 1333
intracranial hemorrhage in, 2175
thrombotic, 925, 1052–1053
hemolytic uremic syndrome with, 601
microangiopathic thrombocytopenia from, 1080
splenectomy for, 1038
vs. paroxysmal nocturnal hemoglobinuria, 923
Thrombocytopoiesis, ineffective, 1048
Thrombocytosis, 1054
after splenectomy, 1039
and renal vein thrombosis, 634
cerebral and retinal ischemia from, 2165
essential, neutrophilia from, 969
in chronic myelogenous leukemia, 990
in Hodgkin's disease, 1018
pseudohyperkalemia in, 548
Thromboembolism. See also Thrombosis; Thrombus
after mitral valve replacement, 347, 349
and surgery for mitral stenosis, 347
from hemophilia B treatment, 1071
in homocystinuria, 1160
of cerebral arteries, 2165–2166
oral contraceptives and, 1443, 1444
prevention of, 386–387, 386t
pulmonary, 273, 294
recurrent, respiratory failure from, 476
relative erythrocytosis and, 976
Thrombolysis, 1079
agents for, 334
contraindications to, 449
for pulmonary embolism, 447, 448–449
for sudden arterial occlusion, 383
human biologic production of, 159
myocardial perfusion imaging and, 210
with fibrinolytic agents, 387
Thrombophlebitis, 384–387
as contraindication for oral contraceptives, 1444
cerebral, vs. viral encephalitis, 1823
from chronic myelogenous leukemia, 990
treatment of, 992
from major antithrombin deficiency, 1075
from parenteral nutrition, 1250
in opioid users, 56
in thromboangiitis obliterans, 382
lymphatic filariasis with, 1915
migratory, in cancer, 1098
of cortical veins, from subdural empyema, 2184
pancreatic cancer and, 781
panniculitis with, 2051
suppurative, from catheters, 1545
vs. angioedema, 1951
vs. familial Mediterranean fever, 1198
vs. gout, 1168

Thrombophlebitis (Continued)
vs. herniated disc, 2253
vs. ruptured synovial cysts, 1998
Thromboplastin, 442
Thromboplastin time, partial, 816, 1047
reference intervals for, 2402t
Thrombosis. See also Thromboembolism;
Thrombus(i)
cerebral, hyperglycemia from, 1289
coronary artery, and angina pectoris, 324
deep-vein, 384
from heparin, 1075
in polycythemia vera, 980, 983
inherited tendencies toward, 1074–1075
intravascular, risk of, in shunts, 304
mesenteric, in elderly, vs. appendicitis,
803
of cerebral arteries, 2164
of cortical veins, from subdural empyema, 2184
of hepatic veins, portal hypertension
from, 848–849
renal vein, 634
in membranous nephropathy, 597
risk of, during catheterization, 211
sudden arterial occlusion by, 383
venous. See also Venous thrombosis
vs. hypertensive intracerebral hemorrhage, 2179
Thrombosis in situ, and renal artery occlusion, 632
Thromboxane(s), 1271
and angina pectoris, 324
and coronary artery thrombosis, 330
aspirin and, 1275
from mast cells, allergic rhinitis and, 1952
in inflammation, 1986
shock and, 239–240
Thrombus(i). See also Thromboembolism;
Thrombosis
and myocardial infarction, 330
dissolution of, 387
formation of, in nephrotic syndrome, 593
in left atrium, in echocardiogram, 346
mural, echocardiography for, 203
Thrush, 2348
from Candida infection, 1848
in acquired immunodeficiency syndrome,
1084t, 1086
vs. secondary syphilis, 1716
Thymectomy, effects of, 1975
for myasthenia gravis, 2286
Thymidylate, impaired synthesis of, 901
from folate deficiency, 906
Thymolipoma, 1975
Thymoma(s), 1975
ACTH from, 1354
immunodeficiency with, 1947
in myasthenia gravis, 2285
Thymosin fraction 5, for immune defects,
1537
Thymus, 1974
and myasthenia gravis, 1975
carcinoid tumor of, 1975–1976
disease of, 1974–1976
hyperplasia of, 1975
in myasthenia gravis, 2285
hypoplasia of, 1945
in Nezelof's syndrome, 1945
T cell differentiation in, 1935, 1935
Thyroglobulin, antibodies to, in Hashimoto's disease, 1320
normal serum concentration of, 1320
reference intervals for, 2399t
Thyroid disease, and digitalis use, 229
heart problems in, 176, 369
Thyroid gland, 1315–1340
anatomic evaluation of, 1320

Thyroid gland (Continued)
chronic, 1333–1334
disorders of. See also Goiter; Hyperthyroidism; Hypothyroidism; Thyroiditis
and impotence, 1409
and obesity, 1225
and TSH secretion, 1267
anemia with, 892
testing for, 1318
vs. zygomycosis, 1852
embryology and anatomy of, 1315
enlargement of, 1318
function of
direct tests of, 1318–1319
drugs and, 1317, 1321
illness and, 1321
regulation of, 1317–1318, 1318
testing of, 1320–1321
thyroid storm and, 138, 1327, 1327t
myopathy during, 2280
hyperfunction of, 1321–1328. See also Hyperthyroidism
hypofunction of, 1328–1331. See also Hypothyroidism
medullary carcinoma of, 1505
ACTH from, 1354
diarrhea from, 727
in multiple endocrine neoplasia, 1460
neoplasms of, 1334–1338
benign, 1335–1336
diagnosis of, 1336–1338, 1337
malignant, 1336–1338
physical examination of, 1318
physiology of, 1315–1317
regulation of, tests of, 1319–1320
status of, metabolic indices of, 1320
Thyroid hormone(s), 1261, 1262, 1315–1319
action of, 1317–1318
antibodies to, reference intervals for,
2399t
autoantibodies to, in primary biliary cirrhosis, 845
deficiency of, and cretinism, 1263
and delayed puberty, 1418
for goiter, 156
from adenomas, 1335
radioimmunoassays of, 1318
replacement of, 1330, 1330t
serum concentrations of, 1318t
synthesis of, 1256, 1315–1316, 1316
disorders of, and hypothyroidism from
goiter, 1338
transport of, 1256
Thyroid hormone–binding proteins, 1316
Thyroid hormone–binding ratio, 1318
Thyroid storm, 138, 1327, 1327t
myopathy during, 2280
Thyroid-stimulating hormone, 1254
and thyroid tumors, 1335
assay for, 1292
deficiency of, 1295
treatment of, 1296–1297
from anterior pituitary, 1292
from pituitary tumors, 1305
from thyrotrophs, 1290
function of, evaluating, 1296
hypersecretion of, and goiter, 1338
normal serum concentration of, 1319
reference intervals for, 2399t
response to, 2095
secretion of, 1284
impairment of, 1293–1294
Thyroiditis, 1331–1334, 1333
acute, 1331
from chronic active hepatitis, 832
Hashimoto's, 19, 1320, 1333–1334
pernicious anemia with, 904
vs. Graves' disease, 1322

Thyroiditis (Continued)
lymphocytic, 1332–1333, 1333, 1460
mitochondrial antibody in, 816
subacute, 1332–1333
Thyrotoxicosis. See also Graves' disease; Hyperthyroidism
and hypercalciuria from net bone resorption, 640
atrial flutter from, 258
causes of, 1321t
factitious, vs. Graves' disease, 1324
gynecomastia in, 1451
paroxysmal supraventricular tachycardia
in, 258
pernicious anemia with, 904
T₃, 1319
Thyrotoxicosis factitia, 1321
Thyrotrophs, in anterior pituitary, 1290
Thyrotropin-releasing hormone, 1317
from hypothalamus, 1280
infusion test of, 1319–1320, 1320
reference intervals for, 2399t
secretion of, 1284
Thyrotropin-releasing hormone infusion
test, 1319–1320, 1320
Thyroxine
decreased absorption of, cholestyramine
and, 99
for hypothyroidism in goiter, 1339
for thyroid-stimulating hormone deficiency, 1296–1297
from thyroid, 1315
levels of, aging and, 25
reference intervals for, 2399t–2400t
Thyroxine-binding globulin, 1316
circulating concentration of, changes in,
1317t
normal, 1319
reference intervals for, 2400t
Thyroxine-binding prealbumin, 1237, 1316
Thyroxine index, reference intervals for,
2400t
Thyroxine/TBG ratio, reference intervals
for, 2400t
TIA. See Transient ischemic attack
TIBC (total iron-binding capacity), 894, 1211
Tibial arteries, posterior, systolic blood
pressure in, 381
Tic(s), 2151–2152
definition of, 2143
vs. epilepsy, 2225
Tic douloureux, 2135
in systemic sclerosis, 2023
Ticarcillin
elimination rate for, 96t
for sepsis, 1540
in drug interactions, 124t
in kidney and liver failure, 117t
treatment with, 119
Tick(s), 1922–1923
avoidance of, 1886
babesiosis from, 1884
Colorado tick fever from, 1819–1821
encephalitis from, 1828–1829
flavivirus fever transmission by, 1833
Lyme disease from, 1726
Q fever from, 1748
relapsing fever from, 1724
rickettsioses from, 1737, 1745
Rocky Mountain spotted fever from,
1742, 1744
tularemia from, 1664, 1666
Tick paralysis, 1923
vs. botulism, 1633
Tidal volume, 395, 395
Tietze's syndrome, 393, 2047–2048
Tifus exantematico, 1739
TIG (tetanus immunoglobulin), 1635

Timolol, 138t
affinity of, for beta-adrenergic receptors, 138
for angina pectoris, 327t
for hypertension, 287t
for recurring myocardial infarction, 335
Tin, food poisoning with, 786
toxicity of, 2390, 2393
Tinea capitis, vs. alopecia, 2348
Tinea corporis, vs. pityriasis rosea, 2328
Tinea nigra, 1854
Tinea versicolor, 2322, 2322
Tinel's sign, 2047
Tinnitus, 2119–2120, 2120
definition of, 2117
from drugs, 2120t
from pseudotumor cerebri, 2236
from sarcoidosis, 453
from typhus fever, 1740
Tissue
accumulation of stored materials in, metabolic errors and, 157
damage to, and acute phase phenomena, 1995
inflammatory response and, 1988–1991
excitable, 544–545
necrosis of, anaerobic infection and, 1639
inflammation and, 1985–1986
oxygen delivery to, 485
penetration of, antimicrobial therapy and, 116
perfusion determinants of, in shock, 237–241, 238t
Tissue chemistry, magnetic resonance imaging for, 84
Tissue factor, and extrinsic pathway, 1062
in coagulation, 1061
Tissue plasminogen activator, 339, 1064
fibrinolysis from, 1079
for myocardial infarction, 334
Tissue typing, for kidney transplants, 578
T-M (time-motion) echocardiography, 202, 203
TMAb (thyroid microsomal antibody), 1320
TNM staging system, for cancer, 1086, 1086t
Toad fish, 1931
Tobacco, 36–40. See also Smoking
and cancer, 1082
Tobramycin, 113, 119, 122
and kidney damage, 117t, 609
elimination rate for, 96t
in liver failure, 117t
reference intervals for, 2404t
Tocainide
dosing and adverse effects of, 267t
elimination rate for, 96t
for arrhythmias, 265
pharmacokinetic properties of, 266t
Tocopherols, 1238
as carcinogenesis inhibitor, 44
Tocotrienols, 1238
Todd's paralysis, after seizures, 2218
vs. transient ischemic attacks, 2169
Toenails, dermatophytic infection of, griseofulvin for, 2317
growth rate of, 2346
Tokyo-Yokohama asthma, 407
Tolazamide, for diabetes mellitus, 1369, 1370t
Tolbutamide, for diabetes mellitus, 1369, 1370t
metabolism inhibition of, 101t
Tolbutamide test, for insulinoma, 1385, 1385
Tolerance
definition of, 106
drug abuse and, 49–50, 52
to antimicrobial agents, 114

Tolerance (Continued)
to drugs, 94
to narcotic analgesics, 108, 109
Tolerance intervals, 81
Tolmetin, as cyclooxygenase inhibitor, 1275
Tolosa-Hunt syndrome, 2295
Toluene, abuse of, 59
inhalation of, interstitial lung disease from, 435
Tone decay, from sensorineural lesions, 2117
Tongue
disorders of, 2348
enlargement of, from immunocytic amyloid, 1035
inflammation of, 678. See also Glossitis
taste buds in, 2110
Tongue worms, 1926
Tonic-clonic convulsions, 2221, 2222
generalized, first aid for, 2228
Tonic seizures, 2222
Tonsil(s), diphtheria infection in, 1627
enlargement of, airway obstruction from, 418
in agammaglobulinemia, 1943
Tonsillectomy, and common respiratory illness, 1756
Tonsillitis, bacterial, vs. enanthems, 1813
streptococcal, 1574–1475
rash with, 2324
Tooth. See Teeth
Tophi, in gout, 1161, 1164–1166, 1166, 1168
development of, 1165
Topical therapy, 2314–2316, 2315t
antibiotic, 124, 2316
antifungal, 2316
antiparasitic, 2316
corticosteroids for, 2315–2316, 2315t
for colitis, 759
side effects of, 2315
local anesthetic, cocaine as, 55
TORCH syndrome, splenomegaly in, 1037
Torre's syndrome, 770
cancer and, 1113
Torsades de pointes, 253, 264, 264
from antiarrhythmic agents, 275
isoproterenol for, 248
Torticollis, and torsion dystonia, 2150
spasmodic, 2150
Tortipelvis, and torsion dystonia, 2150
Total parenteral nutrition, 1248–1250
after head injury, 2243
and liver disease, 841
for Crohn's disease, 751
vs. forced enteral feeding, 1244
Touch, neural pathway for, 2128
Tourette's syndrome, 2151–2152. See also Tic(s)
vs. epilepsy, 2225
Toxemia, laboratory tests for, 1539t, 1540
Toxemia of pregnancy, 634–636
and hydropic infants, 933
Toxic megacolon, 755, 755
from Campylobacter infection, 1649
from pseudomembranous colitis, 1632
radiography for, 756
treatment of, 758–759
Toxic shock syndrome, 1598, 2323t
cholestasis from, 834
in adolescents, 20
rash in, 2324
Toxicity, definition of, 2354
to drugs, 102–103, 103t
to vitamins, 1228
Toxicology, reference intervals for, 2395t–2400t
Toxin(s)
bacterial, shock and, 237
elimination of, by kidneys, 510

Toxins (Continued)
enteric, in hepatic encephalopathy, therapy to reduce, 853
environmental, aplastic anemia from, 886, 886t
from Bordetella pertussis, 1624
from clostridia, 1629
from Clostridium botulinum, 1633
from Corynebacterium diphtheriae, 1627
from Staphylococcus aureus, disease from, 1598–1599
in chronic kidney failure, management of, 570
retention of, 567–568
liver injury from, 824
murine, 1661
reactions to, vs. yellow fever, 1832
screening for, in encephalopathy, 853
Toxocariasis, 834, 835t, 1908–1909
hepatomegaly and eosinophilia from, 834
Toxoplasma gondii, 1875–1876
and polymyositis, 2035
as central nervous system infection, in transplant recipients, 2210
in acquired immunodeficiency syndrome, 1805, 1805t
in liver, 835t
Toxoplasmosis, 835t, 1875–1879
and seizures, 2218
chorioretinitis in, 2293
congenital, vs. Chagas' disease, 1869
vs. cytomegalovirus, 1785–1786
vs. cat scratch disease, 1681
vs. congenital syphilis, 1718
vs. infectious mononucleosis, 1788
vs. Q fever, 1749
vs. viral hepatitis, 824
TPA. See Tissue plasminogen activator
TPA (tetradecanoylphorbol acetate), 1260
TPHA (treponemal hemagglutination test), 2190
TPI (treponemal immobilization) test, 2190
TPN. See Total parenteral nutrition
Trabecular bone, 1473, 1474
loss of, 1510
osteosclerosis of, 1518
Trabeculoplasty, laser, 2290
Trace elements
deficiency of, dilated cardiomyopathy from, 354
from Crohn's disease, 751
symptoms of, 657
in total parenteral nutrition, 1249, 1249t
metabolism of, 1241–1243
poisoning from, 2385–2393
Trachea
cylindroma of, 463
inflammation of, airway obstruction from, 418
injury to, from endotracheal intubation, 478
obstruction of, in mechanical ventilation, 488
stenosis of, from tracheostomy, 496
Tracheobronchitis, from oxygen toxicity, 496
Tracheoesophageal fistula, from endotracheal tubes, 495
from mechanical ventilation, 489
Tracheostomy
complications from, 495–496
for acute respiratory failure, 477–478
for recurrent aspiration pneumonia, 1569
in severely ill, 486, 487
tube for, obstruction of, 488
Trachoma, 2294
Trachoma-inclusion conjunctivitis agents, 1732

Tranquilizers, abuse of, by adolescents, 21
  aplasia from, 886
Transaminase(s)
  in bile duct obstruction, 817
  in hepatitis, 820, 832
  in liver disease, 814–815
  in liver granulomas, 837
  in polymyositis, 2036
  increase in, hepatic neoplasms and, 858
  unexpected increase of, 833
Transamination, of amino acids, 810
Transcobalamin, 903
Transcortin, 1341–1343
  reference intervals for, 2400t
Transcriptase, reverse, 1794
Transducer cells, 1280
Transferrin, 929
  iron binding to, 893, 894
  levels of, in hemochromatosis, 1191
  reference intervals for, 2400t
  saturation of, and hemochromatosis, 839
  synthesis of, in liver, 810
Transforming growth factor alpha, in cancer, 1102
Transforming growth factor beta, 322, 1987
  in cancer, 1102
Transfusions, 947–950. See also *Blood transfusions*
Transient ischemic attack(s)
  and transient paralysis, 2128
  anemias and, 879
  definition of, 2162
  differential diagnosis of, 2169–2170
  from angiopathies, 2165t
  from arteritis, 374
  management of, 2170
  vs. epilepsy, 2225
Transillumination, in skin examination, 2311
Transitional cell(s), 250. See also *T lymphocytes*
Transitional cell cancer, of urinary tract, 654–655
Transitional cell tumors, of renal pelvis, 506
Transplant(s). See also under names of specific organs
  and cytomegalovirus transmission, 1784, 1785
  central nervous system infections after, 2210
  donors for, 577–578
  Epstein-Barr virus infection in, 1788
  for metabolic errors, 157
  heart-lung, for primary pulmonary hypertension, 302
  human leukocyte antigens and, 1963
  immune response to, 578
  rejection of, glucocorticosteroid therapy for, 130, 131
  risk of skin cancer after, 2352
  toxoplasmosis with, 1877
Transthyretin, 1237, 1316
Transudates, pleural fluid, 467, 467t
Transverse myelitis
  acute, 2216–2217, 2216t
    vs. poliomyelitis, 2199
    vs. spinal epidural abscess, 2187
  from enteroviruses, 1810
  from flukes, 1903
  from systemic lupus erythematosus, 2016
  varicella and, 1789
Trauma
  acute gouty arthritis from, 1165
  acute gouty attack from, 1164
  acute phase response to, 1527–1529
  airway obstruction from, 418

Trauma *(Continued)*
  and riboflavin deficiency, 1231
  aneurysms from, 370
  aortic disease from, 374
  atrial pressures in, 244
  bloody ascites from, 791
  chylothorax from, 468
  coma from, prognosis for, 2072
  diaphragmatic hernias of, 472
  dissecting aneurysms from, 372
  dissection of vertebral artery from, 2164
  fungal peritonitis from, 794
  headache from, 2133
  hematuria from, 503
  hypothalamic disorders from, 1286
  lobular panniculitis from, 2050
  pericarditis from, 363
  pneumothorax from, 469
  secondary lymphedema from, 388
  small intestinal ulceration from, 807
  stress disorders after, 2101
  sudden arterial occlusion from, 383
  to abducens nerve, 2115
  to cerebral arteries, 2168
  to erythrocytes, hemolysis from, 924–925
  to esophagus, 688–689
  to eye, and secondary glaucoma, 2291
  to face, brain abscess from, 2181
  to head, diagnostic imaging techniques for, 2060
    epileptic seizures from, 2218
    radiography for, 2058
  to heart, 368–369
  to muscle, and myoglobinuria, 2283
  to neurohypophysis, and diabetes insipidus, 1308
  to skull, brain abscess from, 2181
  vertigo from, 2123
  vs. filariasis, 1915
  wounds from, and gas gangrene, 1629
Travelers
  advice to, 1549–1551
  amebiasis in, 1886
  and disease prevention
    of hepatitis, 64
    of shigellosis, 1647–1648
    of typhoid fever, 1642
    of typhus fever, 1741
  diarrhea of, 1656–1657. See also *Travelers' diarrhea*
  giardiasis in, 1883–1884
  rickettsial infection in, 1738
Travelers' diarrhea, 1656–1657, 1657t
  avoidance of antibiotics for, 732
  from *Escherichia coli*, 1654
  Norwalk virus infections and, 1769
  pus in stool in, 730
  tetracyclines for, 121
Trazodone, as antidepressant, 2096
Treadmill exercise testing, to provoke angina pectoris, 325
Trematodes, 1895–1905
  schistosomiasis from, 1895–1901
Tremor(s)
  classification of, 2142t
  definition of, 2142
  dystonic, 2150
  essential, 2146
    and torsion dystonia, 2150
  flapping, from hepatic encephalopathy, 809
  from adenine arabinoside, 125
  from AIDS dementia complex, 2204
  from cannabis, 57
  from hepatic encephalopathy, 853
  from metabolic encephalopathy, 2065

Tremor(s) *(Continued)*
  from paresis, from syphilis, 2188
  from phenylketonuria, 1155
  in infants, from isovaleric acidemia, 1159
Tremulousness, from sedative withdrawal, 54
Trench fever, 1738t, 1747–1748
  epidemiologic features of, 1737t
Trench foot, 379
Trendelenburg test, 388
Treponema carateum, 1723
Treponema pallidum, 2187
  in liver, 834
  syphilis from, 1713
Treponema pertenue, 1723
Treponemal antibody test, for syphilis, 1719
Treponemal hemagglutination test, for syphilis, 2190
Treponemal immobilization test, for syphilis, 2190
Treponematoses, nonsyphilitic, 1723
Trepopnea, 394
Trexan, abuse of, 55
TRH. See *Thyrotropin-releasing hormone*
Triamcinolone, 129t, 1169, 2316
Triamterene, 232, 536
  adverse effects of, 289t
  and hyperkalemia, 548
  and hyperkalemic hyperchloremic metabolic acidosis, 553
  characteristics of, 231t, 536t
  for ascites, 851
  for hypertension, 286t
Triazolam, abuse of, 53
  rebound insomnia from, 2078
TRIC agents, 1732
Tricarboxylic acid cycle, 810
Triceps skinfold thickness, 1209–1210, 1210t
Trichinella spiralis, 1911
Trichinosis (trichinellosis), 1911–1912
  myositis from, 2036
  vs. botulism, 1633
Trichlormethiazide, for hypertension, 286t
  properties of, 231t
Trichomonas vaginalis, 1704, 1705, 1889
Trichomoniasis, 1889
  metronidazole for, 121
Trichophyton, skin infection with, 2321
Trichopoliodystrophy, cytochrome C oxidase deficiency in, 2279
Trichorrhexis nodosa, definition of, 2349
Trichostrongylus, 1910
Trichotillomania, definition of, 2348
Trichuriasis, 1909–1910
Tricuspid regurgitation, 351
  from Marfan's syndrome, 371
  vs. mitral regurgitation, 349
Tricuspid stenosis, 351
  murmur of, 346
  with mitral stenosis, 346
Tricuspid valve
  atresia of, 310–311
  Ebstein's anomaly of, 310, *310*
  insufficiency of, 351
    diagnosis of, from cardiac catheterization, 212
    murmur of, 222
    myocardial infarction and, 331
  prolapse of, 350–351
  regurgitation of. See also *Tricuspid regurgitation*
  stenosis of. See *Tricuspid stenosis*
Tricyclic antidepressants, 2096
  and catecholamine effect enhancement, 1282
  and distribution of other drugs, 99

Tricyclic antidepressants *(Continued)*
as analgesics, 109
clearance of, 92
for panic attacks, 2100–2101
for parkinsonism, 2146
interaction of, with clonidine, 101
poisoning with, 2069t
treatment for, 144
ventricular premature depolarizations from, 263
Trientine, for Wilson's disease, 1189
Trifluoperazine, for VIPoma, 1389
Trifluridine (trifluorothymidine), 125–126
for herpesvirus, 125–126, 1783
Trigeminal nerve, herpes zoster in, 2196
treatment of, 2197
lateral sinus thrombosis and, 2185
Trigeminal neuralgia, 2135
in systemic sclerosis, 2023
Trigeminal neuropathy, 2267
Trigeminy, 263
Trigger point injections, 109
for pain management, 110t
Trigger points, 2255
and pain, 2137, 2249
Triglyceride(s)
accumulation of, in liver, 810
and increases in very low density lipoproteins, 320
catabolism of, 1138–1139
digestion of, 733
failure of, in chronic pancreatitis, 779
for treating malabsorption, 741t
level of, control of, nicotinic acid for, 1232
in hypothyroidism, 1329–1330
reference intervals for, 2400t
transport of, lipoprotein for, 1137
3,5,3'-Triiodothyronine
circulating, 1316–1317
from thyroid, 1315
reference intervals for, 2400t
suppression test for, 1320
vs. 3,5,3',5'-tetraiodothyronine, 1317
Tri-iodothyronine resin uptake test, reference intervals for, 2400t
Trimazosin, as vasodilator, 233
Trimethadione, and kidney damage, 612
congenital heart disease from, 303
for epilepsy, 2226t, 2227
Trimethaphan, 140, 290t
Trimethobenzamide, for nausea, in viral hepatitis, 824
Trimethoprim
and creatinine secretion, 522
elimination rate for, 96t
for Crohn's disease, 752
for prostatitis, 1422
for urinary tract infection, 630
hypoglycemia from, 1384
in kidney and liver failure, 117t
in prostate tissue, 116
resistance mechanisms of, 116t
Trimethoprim-sulfamethoxazole
for bacterial infections, 119
for chronic granulomatous disease, 958
for chronic respiratory failure, 480
for infection in bronchiectasis, 439
for *Pneumocystis carinii* pneumonia prevention, 1537
for shigellosis, 1647
for travelers' diarrhea, 1657
Trimipramine, for inhibiting acid secretion, 700
Trinitrotoluene, toxicity of, to hemoglobin, 945
Tripotassium dicitrato-bismuthate, for peptic ulcers, 701

Trismus, from tetanus, 1635
Trisomy, 21, 167t, 170. See also *Down's syndrome*
Trisomy X, 1438
Trombiculid mites, larva of, and scrub typhus transmission, 1746
Trophozoites, 1858, 1875–1876
Tropical sprue, malabsorption from, 743
Tropomyosin, 2269
Troponin, 1259, 2269
Trousseau's sign, 1497, *1497*
Trousseau's syndrome, 711, 1079
in cancer, 1098
Truncal muscle, weakness in, 2270
Truncal vagotomy, with antrectomy, 703t, 704
with pyloroplasty, 703–704, 703t
Truncus arteriosus, 308
Trypanosoma brucei, 1862
in liver, 835t
life cycle of, *1863*
Trypanosoma cruzi, 1865. See also *Chagas' disease*
in liver, 835t
life cycle of, 1865–1866, *1866*
myocardial injury from, 353
Trypanosoma gambiense, in liver, 835t
Trypanosoma rhodesiense, in liver, 835t
Trypanosomes, 1856
Trypanosomiasis, 835t
African, 1862–1865, 1862t, *1862*
American, 352, 353, 1865–1869
and esophageal motor disorders, 684
from triatomine kissing bugs, 1921
and polyclonal cold agglutinin synthesis, 920
Trypsin, and dietary protein digestion, 734
and pruritus, 2304
levels of, in malabsorption evaluation algorithm, 740
Tryptophan, as precursor of serotonin, 1282
Tryptophanemia, 1151t
Tsetse flies, and African trypanosomiasis, 1862
TSH. See *Thyroid-stimulating hormone*
TSS. See *Toxic shock syndrome*
Tsutsugamushi disease, epidemiologic features of, 1737t
TTP. See *Thrombocytopenic purpura, thrombotic*
Tubercle, 1682
Tuberculin skin test, 1684–1685, 1686
Tuberculosis, 11, 1682–1692
adrenal insufficiency from, 1351
and amyloidosis, 1199
and diabetes insipidus, 1308
and mycobacteria infection, 1694
anorectal fistulas from, 789
arthritis in, 1690, 2010
ascites from, 791, 792
bronchiectasis vs., 439
clinical description of, 1685–1686
congenital, 1685
control of, 1683–1684
cough from, 391
cryptic, 1692
dialysis and, 577
disseminated, 1692
drug resistance in, 1688
endobronchial, 1689
endometriosis in, 1436
epidemiology of, 1683–1684
etiology of, 1682
extrapulmonary disease in, 1689–1692
glucocorticosteroid therapy for, ineffectiveness of, 129
hemoptysis from, 391
ileocecal, vs. Crohn's disease, 750

Tuberculosis *(Continued)*
immunization against, 65
immunology of, 1684–1685
in heroin users, 57
in hospital employees, 1548
incidence of, 1682
lymphadenitis in, 1689–1690
miliary, 1692
vs. psittacosis, 1736
monocytosis in, 970
myelofibrosis with, 986
myeloid metaplasia from, 985
nonreactive, 1692
of pleura, 467–468
onset of, 1685
pathology and pathogenesis of, 1682–1683
pericarditis in, 363
peritonitis in, 794, 1691
pulmonary, 1685
reactivation, 1685
recombinant DNA vaccine for, 159
recurrence of, 1685
relapse of, 1688
renal, 606
retreatment of, 1688
rheumatoid factor in, 1996
rifampin for, 121
salpingitis in, 1690
skeletal, 1690
spondylitis in, 1690
splenomegaly in, 1037
stages in, 1683
synovial membrane in, 1995
treatment of, 1686–1689
vertebral, 2256
vs. abdominal actinomycosis, 1674
vs. AIDS dementia complex, 2205
vs. cat scratch disease, 1679, 1681
vs. cervicofacial actinomycosis, 1674
vs. chronic lymphocytic leukemia, 996
vs. coccidioidomycosis, 1841
vs. cryptococcosis, 1845
vs. flukes, 1904
vs. mycobacterial lymphadenitis, 1695
vs. nocardiosis, 1675
vs. paracoccidioidomycosis, 1843
vs. peptic ulcers, 699
vs. psittacosis, 1736
vs. pulmonary blastomycosis, 1842
vs. sarcoidosis, 454
vs. *Toxoplasma* retinochoroiditis, 1878
vs. zygomycosis, 1852
Tuberculum sellae, 1290
Tuberous sclerosis, 2158–2159, *2344, 2345*
and neoplasms, 1096t
biologic fitness of, 148
hamartoma-angiomyolipoma in, 652
interstitial lung disease in, 432
Tubocurarine, and urticaria, 1950
Tubular necrosis, acute, vs. transplant rejection, 580
vs. allergic interstitial disease, 505
Tubule(s), 509–510
calcium reabsorption by, impaired, and renal hypercalciuria, 640
triazides and, 642
disorders of, 617–624, 618t
and urinary tract obstruction, 616
injury to, acute, urinalysis for, 561
acute kidney failure from, 562
obstruction of, by uric acid, 611
occlusion of, and acute kidney failure, 559
and regulation of water excretion, 516
Tubulointerstitial disease
and medullary cystic disease, 648
biopsy for, 569

Tubulointerstitial disease (Continued)
chronic, 505
common features of, 602–603
toxic nephropathy and, 603
Tubulointerstitial system, of kidneys, damage to, 504
Tularemia, 1664–1666
vs. bubonic plague, 1663
vs. cat scratch disease, 1679, 1681
vs. psittacosis, 1736
vs. sporotrichosis, 1847
vs. toxoplasmosis, 1878
Tumor(s). See Neoplasm(s) and names of specific body parts
Tumor cachexia, 1097
Tumor lysis syndrome, acute kidney failure from, 611
in chronic myelogenous leukemia, 992
non-Hodgkin's lymphoma and, 1012
Tumor markers, 1099–1100, 1099t
Tumor necrosis factor, 957, 1987. See also Cachectin
Tunga penetrans, 1926
Tungiasis, 1926
Tuning fork tests, 2118
Turcot's syndrome, 767
Turner's syndrome, 167, 167t, 170, 1392, 1437
and diabetes mellitus, 1362
and Duchenne dystrophy, 2273
coarctation of aorta in, 313
congenital heart disease in, 303
heart problems in, 176
in mixed gonadal dysgenesis, 1394
male, 388, 1414
cryptorchidism in, 1415
Turtles, salmonella from, 1643
TWAR agent, 1733, 1736
Twins, life expectancy of, 24
Two-point discrimination, 2128
Tylosis, with esophageal carcinoma, 1095t
Tympanum, rupture of, pain from, 2134
Typhlitis, 1659
Typhoid fever, 1641–1642, 1642t
chloramphenicol for, 120
immunization from, 65
before travel, 1550
Salmonella and, 1644
vs. psittacosis, 1736
vs. Q fever, 1749
vs. rabies, 2201
vs. visceral leishmaniasis, 1872
Typhus exanthematique, 1739
Typhus fever, 1738–1742
epidemic, 1739–1741
epidemiologic features of, 1737t
scrub, 1746–1747
tick-borne, 1742
vs. typhoid fever, 1642
Tyramine, metabolic inhibition of, 101, 101t
Tyrosinase, in albinism, 2346
Tyrosine, 1253
as precursor for catecholamines, 1281
from phenylalanine metabolism, 1155
Tyrosine kinase, activation of, 1260
Tyrosinemia
hereditary, 1154t
neonatal, 1150t
vitamin C for, 1236
vs. hereditary fructose intolerance, 1136
Tyrosinosis, 1150t
Tzanck smear
for herpes virus, 1704, 2312, 2313
for varicella, 1790

U wave, electrocardiography, 197
UCTS (undifferentiated connective tissue syndrome), 2021

Ulcer(s)
aphthous, in yersiniosis, 1664
as malignancy, 669
black, from rickettsia, 1745
Buruli, from Mycobacterium ulcerans, 1695
colonic, from balantidiasis, 1889
cutaneous, 2341–2342
from chemicals, 2375
decubitus, and spinal epidural abscess, 2186
definition of, 692
duodenal, vs. small intestine neoplasms, 774
from arteriosclerosis obliterans, 381
from chilblain, 379
from thromboangiitis obliterans, 382
from tularemia, 1666
mucosal, in Crohn's disease, 748
of ankles, from hereditary spherocytosis, 911
of chancroid, 1715
of cornea, 2293
of esophagus, from infection, 688
from reflux, 681
of ileum, sprue and, 743
of jejunum, sprue and, 743
of mucous membrane, 2347
of small intestines, 807
pain from, 656
peptic, 692–709. See also Peptic ulcers
pressure, in elderly, 30
serpiginous, 1712
Siberian, 1667
solitary, in rectum, 788
stercoral, from fecal impaction, 721
in rectum, 788
Ulcerative colitis, 753–760, 787–788
age of onset of, 753
and colorectal cancer, 769, 769–770, 773
and eosinophilia, 1026
and pregnancy, 760
and warm autoimmune hemolysis, 919
as contraindication to opiates in diarrhea treatment, 732
chronic, liver in, 841
clinical manifestations of, 754–755
complications of, 757–758
definition of, 745
diagnosis of, 755–756
differential, 756–757
emotion in, 657
from chronic active hepatitis, 832
glucocorticosteroid therapy for, 130
hyposplenism from, 1039
in Behçet's disease, 2049
monocytosis in, 970
myasthenia gravis with, 2285
pathology of, 754, 754
polyarthritis in, 2008
prognosis for, 760
sclerosing cholangitis with, 869
total parenteral nutrition for, 1244, 1248t
treatment of, 758–760
glucocorticosteroids for, 130
vs. abdominal actinomycosis, 1674
vs. adenocarcinoma of colon, 771
vs. amebiasis, 1886
vs. Crohn's colitis, 751t
vs. diverticulitis, 804
vs. gonococcal infections of rectum, 1707
vs. shigellosis, 1647
Ulnar palsy, 2268
Ultimobranchial cells, 1505–1506
Ultrasonography, 83–84, 84
for abdominal abscess, 793
for biliary disease, 863
for deep-vein thrombosis, 386
for gallstones, 864, 866
for gastrointestinal system, 663–664, 664

Ultrasonography (Continued)
for kidneys, 526
polycystic disease in, 647
tumors of, 650
for liver disease, 818
for localization of abnormal parathyroid tissue, 1494
for peritoneal disease, 790
for prenatal diagnosis of congenital malformations, 170, 173
for pyogenic liver abscess, 836
for renovascular hypertension diagnosis, 282
pulsed reflexed, 201, 203, 205. See also Echocardiology
Ultraviolet radiation, 2375
and skin cancer, 1093t, 1094
and skin reactions, 2319
and systemic lupus erythematosus, 2012
and vitamin D_3 production, 1477
biology of, 2376
from sun, 2350
in skin disorder treatment, 2318
protection of skin against, 2316
skin as protection against, 2300
Umbilical stump, delayed separation of, 960
oozing from, fibrinogen disorders and, 1073
Umbilicus, cutaneous vein prominence around, in liver disease, 809
Uncinate fits, 2221
Unconsciousness, 2073–2075, 2074t. See also Coma; Consciousness; Syncope
Undifferentiated connective tissue syndrome, 2021
Unintended injuries, 41
epidemiology of, 40
Unipolar depressive illness, 2095
U.S. Army Medical Research Institute of Infectious Diseases, 1666
U.S. Food and Drug Administration, licensing of biologic production by, 158
U.S. Occupational Safety and Health Administration, 2356
U.S. Public Health Service, 8
Advisory Committee on Immunization Practices, Collective Immunization Recommendations of, 61
Unverricht-Lundborg progressive myoclonus epilepsy, 2222
Uranium, and kidney damage, 612
and lung cancer, 458
interaction with cigarette smoking, 38
Urate, in plasma, solubility of, and gout, 1162t, 1162
levels of, hormonal factors and, 1164
normal serum values for, 1162
Urate crystals, and acute gouty attack, 1164
Urate disorders, urinalysis for, 561
Urea
clearance of, by kidneys, 510
in peritoneal dialysis vs. hemodialysis, 575
rates for, 567
in chronic kidney failure, 567–568
in uremic platelet defect, 1057
Urea cycle, diseases of, 1158–1159
Urea nitrogen, level of, increase in, 558. See also Azotemia
reference intervals for, 2400t
Urea nitrogen/creatinine ratio, reference intervals for, 2400t
Ureaplasma, 1561
infections by, in genitals, 1564–1565
nongonococcal urethritis from, 1702
tests for, 1703
Uremic syndrome, 507–508, 563, 563t. See also End-stage kidney disease
and platelet function defects, 1057

Uremic syndrome (Continued)
  and pseudomembranous colitis, 1632
  approach to, 568–569
  blood coagulation disorders in, 1078
  chronic, hypertriglyceridemia in, 1143
  complications of, 570–571
  component(s) of, 563–567
    acid-base balance in, 564
    carbohydrate metabolism in, 567
    cardiovascular abnormalities as, 565
    electrolyte metabolism in, 563–565
    gastrointestinal disorders in, 566
    hematologic abnormalities as, 566
    infections as, 566
    myopathy as, 567
    neuropathy as, 566–567, 2265
    osteodystrophy in, 566
    pruritus as, 567
    uric acid in, 567
    water metabolism in, 563–565
  definition of, 502
  delirium from, 2064
  development of, in acute kidney failure,
      560
  from hemorrhagic fever, from arenavi-
      ruses, 1835
  hemolytic, microangiopathic thrombocy-
      topenia from, 1080
    with thrombotic thrombocytopenia pur-
        pura, 601
  pleural effusion from, 469
  vomiting from, 658
  vs. hypertensive encephalopathy, 2172
Ureter(s)
  diverticuli of, 650
  duplication of, 649
  obstruction of, and acute kidney failure,
      558, 560
    from anticoagulant therapy, 613
    vs. appendicitis, 801, 802
  retrocaval, 650
  retroperitoneal fibrosis and, 2052
  transitional cell cancers of, 655
  tumors of, urinary cytology for, 503
Ureteral catheters, for pyelonephritis, 629
  for urinary tract obstruction treatment,
      617
Ureteral reflux, 649–650
Ureteral valves, 650
Ureterocele, 650
Ureteropelvic junction, obstruction of, 507,
    649, 650
Ureterosigmoidostomy, metabolic acidosis
    from, 553
Ureterovesical junction, obstruction of, 507
Urethra
  anomalies of, 650
  bacteriuria in, treatment for, 630
  congenital strictures of, 650
  diverticuli of, 650
  obstruction of, manifestations of, 615
Urethral catheters, for urinary tract obstruc-
    tion treatment, 617
Urethral syndrome, acute, 628
  in women, 629, 1704
Urethritis, 1702–1703, 1703
  from Chlamydia trachomatis, treatment for,
      630
  from shigellosis, 1647
  in Reiter's syndrome, 2007
Uric acid. See also Hyperuricemia
  accumulation of, in tophaceous gout, 157
  crystals of, deposition of, and urinary
      tract obstruction, 569
  distribution of, in healthy population, 80
  elimination of, by kidneys, 510
    in gout, 1168

Uric acid (Continued)
  in chronic kidney failure, management
      of, 571
  in kidney stones, 638
  increased production of, in Lesch-Nyhan
      syndrome, 1171
    in polycythemia vera, 981
  levels of, in chronic kidney failure, 567
  obstruction of tubules by, 611
  reference intervals for, 2400t
  synthesis of, pathway for, 1163
Uric acid nephropathy, vs. urate nephropa-
    thy, 1167
Uric acid stones, 640, 641
  diagnosis of, 642
  in Crohn's disease, 750
  in gout, 1165
  treatment of, 643
Uridine diphosphate-4-epimerase, and ga-
    lactose metabolism, 1131
Uridyltransferase, deficiency of, in infants,
    1132
Urinalysis
  for acute abdominal pain, 802
  for acute kidney failure, 561
  for analgesic nephropathy, 608
  for appendicitis, 801
  for infective endocarditis, 1592
  for post-streptococcal glomerulonephritis,
      587
Urinary antiseptics, 122
Urinary bilharziasis, 1898
Urinary casts, tubular, presence of, 503
Urinary catheters, and acute kidney failure,
    558, 561–562
  for shock patients, 244
Urinary cytology, 503
Urinary D-xylose test, for malabsorption,
    736, 737t
Urinary glucose, measurement of, 1371
Urinary incontinence, 2107t, 2107–2108. See
    also Incontinence, urinary
Urinary protein, 520
Urinary retention
  cholinergic agonists for, 139
  from atropine, 139
  from tabes dorsalis, 2189
  genital herpes and, 2197
  postoperative, anticholinesterases for, 140
Urinary tract
  after spinal cord trauma, 2246
  anomalies of, 648–650
  bacteria in, 628
  diagnostic imaging of, 525–527
  disorders of, in diabetic autonomic neu-
      ropathy, 2263–2264
    in multiple sclerosis, 2213
  infection of, 628–632
    and back pain, 2250
    and kidney stones, 641
    and spinal epidural abscess, 2186
    bloodstream infection from, 1544
    by Mycoplasma and Ureaplasma, 1564
    by streptococci group B, 1579–1580
    clinical manifestations of, 628–629
    complications from, 632
      treatment of, 631
    diagnosis of, 629
    definition of, 628
    epidemiology and natural history of,
        629–630
    hospital-acquired, 1542, 1543–1544
    hypocitraturia from, 640
    immunoglobulin A deficiency and,
        1943
    in women, 1704
    neutropenia and, 963

Urinary tract (Continued)
  infection of, recurrent, 631
    and prostatectomy, 1423
    staphylococcal, 1601
    treatment for, 630–631, 631
      in chronic kidney failure, 569–570
      quinolones for, 122
      tetracyclines for, 121
  lower, irritation of, differential diagnosis
      for, 1422
  neoplasms of, 654
  obstruction of, 614–617. See also Obstruc-
      tive nephropathy
  polyarteritis nodosa in, 2029
  St. Louis encephalitis and, 1826
  transitional cell carcinoma of, analgesic
      nephropathy and, 608
  tuberculosis in, 1690
Urinary xylose test, in malabsorption evalu-
    ation algorithm, 740
Urination, pain from, and vesicoureteral re-
    flux, 615
Urine
  air in, 504, 804
  aldosterone in, 1359
  amylase in, 776
  calcium in, measurement of, in hypercal-
      cemia, 1494
    normal upper limit for, 639
  color of
    brown, 2282
    hemolytic anemia and, 880
    in porphyria cutanea tarda, 1186
    liver disease and, 808
    pink, in congenital erythropoietic por-
        phyria, 1183
    smoky, from post-streptococcal glomer-
        ulonephritis, 587
  copper in, and Wilson's disease, 832
  corticosteroids in, measurement of, 1348
  creatinine in, and muscle mass, 1211
  daily volume of, 516
  electrolytes in, measurement of, 524
  erythropoietin in, phlebotomy in, 978
  examination of, for liver disease, 817
  fecal matter in, from fistulas from
      Crohn's disease, 750
  flow of, cessation of, 506
    obstruction of, 507
  formation of, 502, 510–511
  glycolate in, 1136
  hormone measurements in, 1267
  hypertonic, antidiuretic hormone and,
      1306
  impedance of crystallization in, 638
  in diabetes insipidus, 1310
  in leptospirosis, 1731
  increased volume of, from atriopeptin,
      1279
  L-glycerate in, 1136
  odor of, in maple syrup urine disease,
      1159
  osmolality of, 523
    maximal, 513, 1311
  outflow obstruction of, from prostatic
      cancer, 1424
  output of, in endotoxic shock, 1660
  pH of, during gout treatment, 1170
  retention of, and prostatectomy, 1423
  solute concentration of, measurement of,
      523
  specific gravity of, measurement of, 523
Urine ascites, 792
Urine cultures, 630
Urobilinogen, reference intervals for, 2400t
Urogenital tract. See Genital tract; Urinary
    tract

Urograms, excretory, 525, 650
Urography, adverse effects of, 526
  radiocontrast agents in, and kidney damage, 609–610
Urokinase
  fibrinolysis from, 1079
  for myocardial infarction, 334
  for pulmonary embolism, 448
  for sudden arterial occlusion, 383
  in fibrinolysis, 1064
  thrombolysis with, 387
Urolithiasis. See Calculus(i)
Uroporphyrin, reference intervals for, 2400t
Uroporphyrinogen III synthetase, 1186
Ursodeoxycholate, for gallstone dissolution, 862
  in bile, 859
Urticaria, 1948–1951, 2334–2335, 2335t
  from blood transfusions, 950
  from chemicals, 2375
  from viral hepatitis, 819, 820, 823
  prednisone for, 2317
  solar, 1184
Urticaria pigmentosa, 2335
  cancer and, 1112
  from mastocytosis, 1972, 1973
  vs. urticaria, 1951
Urticaria-angioedema, classification of, 1949t
  in systemic lupus erythematosus, 2015
Uterus
  development of, 1392
  dysfunctional bleeding from, 1434–1435
    in adolescents, 19
  tuberculosis in, 1690
Utricle, 2120
Uveitis, 2293
  anterior, from onchocerciasis, 1917
  from Crohn's disease, 747
  sarcoidosis with, 451
Uveomeningitis, 2293
Uvula, taste buds in, 2110

V wave, in venous pulse, 176
Vaccination, 61–66
  absence of antibodies after, 1946
  and atypical measles, 1774
  after splenectomy, 912
  central nervous system disorders from, 2208–2211
  for AIDS, 1523
  for diphtheria, 1626, 1628
  for enteroviruses, 1809
  for Francisella tularensis, 1666
  for Haemophilus influenzae, 1620
  for hepatitis B, 824–825, 826
    for hospital employees, 1548
  for influenza, 1766–1767
  for international travel, 1550
  for Japanese encephalitis, 1828
  for measles, 1775
  for meningococcal disease, 1616–1617
  for mumps, 1780
  for mycoplasmal infections, 1564
  for plague, 1663
  for poliomyelitis, 2200
  for Q fever, 1749
  for rabies, 2202
    acute disseminated encephalomyelitis after, 2208
  for rubella, 1776, 1777
    arthritis after, 2011
  for smallpox, 1791, 1793
  for tetanus, 1626, 1635
  for typhoid fever, 1642
  for whooping cough, 1625, 1626
  for yellow fever, 1832

Vaccination (Continued)
  human biologic production of, 159
  live virus, contraindications for, in immunodeficient patients, 1537
  of bacille Calmette-Guérin, for tuberculosis, 1683
  of physicians, 69
  polyvalent pneumococcal, 1560
  splenectomy and, 912, 1039
Vaccinia gangrenosa, 1793
Vagabonds' disease, 1920
Vagina
  adenocarcinoma of, from diethylstilbestrol, 1434
  anaerobic streptococci as normal flora in, 1573
  bleeding from, before puberty, causes of, 1428
  candidiasis of, in diabetes mellitus, 1380
    oral contraceptives and, 1443
  development of, 1392
  discharge from, from trichomoniasis, 1889
  in menstrual cycle, 1430
  lubrication of, 1441
  passing of gas or stool through, from diverticulitis, 804
  staphylococcal infection in, 1598
Vaginal deliveries, endometritis after, 1547
Vaginitis, 1704t, 1704–1705
  from Gardnerella vaginalis, 1621
Vaginosis, 1705
Vagotomy, incomplete, and postoperative recurrent ulcers, 705
  proximal gastric, for peptic ulcers, 704
  truncal, with pyloroplasty, for peptic ulcers, 703–704, 703t
Vagovagal attacks, 2075
Valine, 1159
Valium, abuse of, 53
Valley fever, 1840
Valproate, for myoclonus, 2151
Valproic acid
  fatty liver from, 828
  for epilepsy, 2226t, 2227
  liver disease from, 827
  protein binding by, liver or kidney disease and, 94
  reference intervals for, 2404t
Valsalva, sinus of. See Sinus of Valsalva
Valsalva maneuver, 191, 220
  and chest pain, 325
  and murmur from mitral valve prolapse, 350
  definition of, 359
  for paroxysmal supraventricular tachycardia, 258
  radiography during, 191
Valves. See also under names of specific valves
  aortic, pressure drop across, 205
  calcification of, 195
  estimation of area of, with Gorlin formula, 214, 214
  obstruction of, and right ventricular outflow, 311
  prosthetic, pressure gradient across, 207
  ureteral, 650
Valvular heart disease, 340–352
  aortic regurgitation as, 343–345, 344t
  aortic stenosis as, 341–343, 342t
  digitalis for, 228
  low output heart failure from, 216
  mitral regurgitation as, 347–348, 348t
  mitral stenosis as, 345t, 345–347
  mitral valve prolapse as, 349–351
  pulmonic regurgitation as, 351
  pulmonic stenosis as, 316, 351

Valvular heart disease (Continued)
  radionuclide assessment of, 209
  tricuspid insufficiency as, 351
  tricuspid stenosis as, 351
  volume work of heart in, 188
  vs. chronic kidney failure with sodium retention, 564
Valvuloplasty, balloon, for severe pulmonic stenosis, 312
  for mitral stenosis, 347
Van Dyke protein, 1305
Vanadium, 1242–1243
  toxicity of, 2393
Vancomycin, 119, 122
  action of, 113t
  elimination rate for, 96t
  for pseudomembranous colitis, 1632–1633
  for staphylococcal infection, 437, 1603
  in kidney and liver failure, 117t
  penetration into spinal fluid by, 116
  reference intervals for, 2404t
Vanillylmandelic acid, reference intervals for, 2400t
Variant angina pectoris, 325, 393
  calcium channel antagonists for, 327
  myocardial infarction vs., 332
  treatment for, 328
Varicella, 1788–1790
  and skin, 2330
  immunization against, 63t, 65
  interferon for, 128
  vs. enanthems, 1813
  vs. rickettsialpox, 1746
Varicella zoster, acyclovir for, 126
  in acute leukemia, 1006
  lymphocytopenia from, 966
Varicella zoster immune globulin, 1790
Varices, spur-cell hemolytic anemia and, 923
Varicocele, 1409
  definition of, 1416
Varicose veins, 387–388
  arteriovenous fistula and, 384
  obesity and, 1224
  thrombophlebitis and, 385
Variola, 1792–1793. See also Smallpox
Vas deferens, blockage of, and infertility, 1410
  development of, 1392
Vasa recta, 508
Vascular abnormality, 170
Vascular anomalies, gastrointestinal hemorrhage from, 800
Vascular capacitance, increase in, circulatory collapse from, 534
Vascular diseases
  and syncope, 2074
  hemorrhage with, 2175
  of limbs, 375–389
    from abnormal communication between arteries and veins, 384
    from abnormal responses of smooth muscle, 375–379
    from damage by cold, 379–380
    from organic arterial obstruction, 380–384
    in lymphatic vessels, 388–389
    in veins, 384–388
  peripheral, in cigarette smokers, 37
  pulmonary, respiratory failure from, critical care for, 492
  small intestinal ulceration from, 807
Vascular gangrene, 1630t
Vascular headache, 2129–2132
Vascular-interstitial fluid shifts, 534
Vascular lesions, 298
  hemolysis from, 925
  in liver, from drugs, 828

Vascular necrosis, vs. appendicitis, 802
Vascular occlusions, in polycythemia vera, 983
Vascular prostheses, fistulas after placement of, 765
Vascular resistance, 213, 237
  calculation of, 239
  in kidneys, 510
  pulmonary, calculation of, 494
    elevation of, in Eisenmenger's syndrome, 316–317
    for assessing pulmonary circulation, 294
  systemic, calculation of, 494
  total peripheral, 189
Vascular rings, 314
Vascular system
  anomalies of, gastrointestinal hemorrhage from, 800
    vs. small intestine neoplasms, 774
  calcification of, from renal osteodystrophy, 1508
  disorders of, 1044t
  injury to, from immersion foot, 379
  insufficiency of, and pancreatitis, 775
    vertigo from, 2123–2124
  peripheral, in systemic sclerosis, 2021
Vasculitic syndromes, 2025–2028
  classification of, 2026, 2026t
Vasculitis(ides)
  acute kidney failure from, recovery from, 562
  allergic. See Allergic vasculitis
  and ischemic colitis, 764
  and mesenteric blood supply, 744
  and skin, 2325
  aneurysms with, 2174
  cerebral, from herpes zoster, 2197
  definition of, 2025
  from hepatitis, chronic, 831, 832
    type B, 820, 823
  from drug allergy, 1970t
  glucocorticosteroid therapy for, 130
  hypersensitivity, 431–432, 2026–2028
    kidneys in, 599
    vs. rat-bite fever, 1730
  hypocomplementemic, and skin, 2325
  in leprosy, 1698
  in murine typhus, 1741
  in typhus fever, 1740
  intracranial, from acute cocaine toxicity, 55
  intramural intestinal hemorrhage from, 764
  lobular panniculitis with, 2050
  mesenteric, 763
  nodular, 2050
  pulmonary, interstitial lung disease with, 431–432
    respiratory failure from, 476
  rheumatoid, 2002
  systemic, mesenteric artery occlusion from, 562
    with glomerulitis, from nonsteroidal anti-inflammatory agents, 609
  vs. chronic meningococcemia, 1616
  vs. pulmonary hemosiderosis, 430
  Wegener's granulomatosis as, 2030. See also Wegener's granulomatosis
Vasectomy, to induce infertility, 1410
Vasoactive drugs, for threatened stroke, 2171
Vasoactive intestinal polypeptide, and diarrhea, 731
  in gastrointestinal motility, 715
  in pancreatic cholera syndrome, 727
Vasoconstriction
  catecholamines and, 1463

Vasoconstriction (Continued)
  from chemoreceptor stimulation, 190
  in endotoxic shock, 1660
  peripheral, as compensatory mechanism in heart failure, 220
  sustained, and primary pulmonary hypertension, 299t
  sympathetic nervous system and, 133
Vasoconstrictive agents, for erythromelalgia, 379
  ischemic tubular injury from, 559
Vasodilation, in sepsis, 1538–1539
Vasodilators
  adverse effects of, 289t
  and cardiac output, 191
  and circulatory collapse from increased vascular resistance, 534
  and migraine headache, 2131
  and response to exercise or rest in pulmonary hypertension, 299
  contraindicated for arteriosclerosis obliterans, 381
  deficiency in, and hypertension, 277
  for dilated cardiomyopathy, 355
  for heart failure, 233t, 233–235
  for hypertension, 287t
  for hypertensive crisis, 290t
  for pulmonary hypertension, primary, 301t, 300–302
    secondary, 297
  for shock, 248
  for thromboangiitis obliterans, 382
  prostaglandins as, 531
Vasomotor center, shock and, 239
Vasomotor instability, in menopause, 1444
Vaso-occlusive crisis, in sickle cell anemia, 939
Vasopressin
  and atriopeptin, 1279
  and mesenteric circulation, 761
  and renin release, 1345
  and urine osmolality, 1311
  as coronary vasoconstrictors, 189
  deficiency of, 1295
  for hemorrhage, from gastrointestinal varices, 799
  for variceal hemorrhage, 849–850
  hypothalamus and, 2104
  in cancer, 1103
  shock and, 239
  synthesis of, 1280, 1305
Vater, ampulla of, 775
  papilla of, ultrasonography of, 664
VDRL (Venereal Disease Research Laboratory) test, 1719, 2190
Vectorcardiograms, 201
Vegetable oil, aspiration of, lipoid pneumonia from, 2372
Vegetables, consumption of, and pancreatic cancer, 781
  fresh, and hepatitis A, 825
  phototoxicity from, 2351
Vegetarians, fats in diet of, 43
  vitamin B$_{12}$ deficiency in, 738
    testing for, 738t
Vegetative state, definition of, 2061t
Veins
  abnormal communication between, and arteries, 384
  angiomas of, in Sturge-Weber syndrome, 2174
  as access for cardiac catheterization, 211
  blood volume in, 189
  catheters in, for central venous pressure monitoring, 243
  congestion of, systemic, in heart failure, 215
  dilators of, 233, 235

Veins (Continued)
  disease of, vs. arteriosclerosis obliterans, 381
  flow in, increased resistance to, and portal hypertension, 847
  insufficiency of, and ulcers, 2341
  occlusion of, liver congestion from, vs. viral hepatitis, 824
  of intestines, 761
  of kidneys, 508
  of limbs, disease of, 384–388
  of liver, thrombosis of, from oral contraceptives, 828
  portal, anatomy and physiology of, 847
Vellus hair, 2303
  definition of, 1446
Vena cava, interruption of, in pulmonary embolism treatment, 449
Venereal disease, 1701–1722, 1702t. See also Sexually transmitted disease
Venereal Disease Research Laboratory test, 1719, 2190
Venereal warts, 2324
  in AIDS, 677
  interferon for, 128
Venezuelan encephalitis, 1825, 2193
Venography, for deep-vein thrombosis, 385
  of kidneys, 525
Venom
  from blue-ringed octopus, 1930
  from box jellyfish, 1930
  from cone shells, 1930
  from marine animals, 1929–1931, 1930t
  from snakes, 1927–1928
    biochemistry of, 1928t
  immunotherapy with, for insect sting allergy, 1959
Venous infarction, intracranial, hemorrhage with, 2175
Venous pressure
  central, monitoring of, in critical care units, 493
  in cardiac tamponade, 366
  in cardiovascular physical examination, 176, 176
  increase in, from heart failure, in chronic respiratory failure, 481
Venous return, 186–187
  changes in, 191
Venous stasis, 385
  from immobilization, 442
  obesity and, 1224
Venous thrombosis
  deep-vein, 384
    and pulmonary embolism, 385
    prophylaxis for, 449
    therapy for, 387
  from venous stasis, 442
  mesenteric, 764
  pulmonary embolism from, 442
  risk factors for, 442t
  vs. hypertensive intracerebral hemorrhage, 2179
  vs. right-to-left shunt, 402–403
Ventilation
  abnormalities of, 398–399
  after head injury, 2242, 2243
  artificial, devices for, 486
    in cardiopulmonary resuscitation, 500
  distribution of, 397–398
  equations related to, 484–485
  in Guillain-Barré syndrome treatment, 2261
  in respiration, 395, 395–399
  mechanical, 487–489. See also Mechanical ventilation
  positive-pressure, for aspiration pneumonitis, 2370

Ventilation (Continued)
  stimulation of, from pulmonary embolism, 443
Ventilation-perfusion lung scans, 444, 445, 445, 445t, 446
  for bullae, 420
Ventilation-perfusion mismatch
  for bronchiectasis, 439
  hypoxemia from, in severely ill, 483, 483–484
  hypoxia from, 402, 474, 474
  in chronic airways disease, 411, 415
  in interstitial lung disease, 427
  in kyphoscoliosis, 473
  in pulmonary embolism, 443
Ventricle(s), 184. See also Cardiac; Heart; Ventricular
  aneurysms of. See Ventricular aneurysms
  arrhythmias of, 262–264. See also Ventricular arrhythmias
  diastolic filling of, 219
    abnormality in, 359
  dilated, angina pectoris from, 323
  function of, ejection fraction as index of, 186
    evaluation of, after myocardial infarction, 334
  hypertrophy of, 200, 323
  in cardiogenic shock, mechanical assistance for, 249
  interaction of, 216
  inversion of, with transposition of great arteries, 315
  ischemia of, 203
  left
    diastolic blood flow obstruction to, from mitral stenosis, 345
    filling pressure of, monitoring, 243
    heart failure in, 221–222
    hypertrophy of, 355
    increase in internal dimension of, 352
    inflow obstruction to, 311
    outflow obstruction to, 312–313
      angina pectoris from, 323
    reservoir of blood for, 400
    severe dilation of, and mitral regurgitation, 348
    volume overload on, from aortic regurgitation, 343
  performance of, 185
    and congestive heart failure, 209
  right
    atrialized, 310
    double outlet, 314
    enlargement of, electrocardiogram and, 297
      in pulmonary hypertension, 297
    failure of, 222–224
      and pulmonary hypertension, 294
    hypertrophy of, from tetralogy of Fallot, 309
    infarction of, from myocardial infarction, 333
    obstruction to outflow of, 311
    reconstruction of outflow tract for, 318
    septal defect of, 170t, 306, 306–307. See also Ventricular septal defect
    single, 311
    tachycardia of, 259, 263, 263. See also Ventricular tachycardia
    volume overload of, and angina pectoris, 324
Ventricular aneurysms
  from myocardial infarction, 333
  from sarcoidosis, 453
  functional left, 208
  surgery for, 274
Ventricular arrhythmias, 262–264
  and sudden cardiac death, 275

Ventricular arrhythmias (Continued)
  bretylium for, 271
  from catheters, 497
  in cardiomyopathy, dilated, 355
    hypertrophic, treatment for, 358
  lidocaine for, 265
  malignant, amiodarone for, 271
  mexiletine for, 265
  prognostic classification of, 265t
  tocainide for, 265
Ventricular ectopy, after myocardial infarction, 334
Ventricular ejection fraction, change of, with exercise, 325–326
Ventricular end-diastolic pressure, and preload, 217, 217
Ventricular end-diastolic volume, as preload indicator, 185
Ventricular fibrillation, 263, 264
  DC cardioversion for, 273
  in cigarette smokers, 37
  prophylaxis of, bretylium for, 271
  treatment of, 257t
Ventricular filling pressure, as preload indicator, 185
Ventricular flutter, 264
Ventricular function curve, 185, 185–186, 186, 217, 217
Ventricular infarction, 208
Ventricular parasystole, 263–264
Ventricular premature beats, and myocardial infarction, 331, 333
  and sudden cardiac death, 275
Ventricular premature depolarizations, 262–263, 263
  flecainide for, 270
  symptomatic, treatment of, 257t
Ventricular septal defect, 170t, 306, 306–307
  absence of pulmonic valve in, 314
  coarctation of aorta with, 313
  echocardiography for, 203
  from myocardial infarction, 331, 333
  from tetralogy of Fallot, 309
  in adults, 316
  surgery for, 338
  transposition of great arteries with, 314
  vs. double outlet right ventricle, 314
  vs. mitral regurgitation, 349
Ventricular systolic pressure, calculation of, 207
Ventricular tachycardia, 259, 263, 263
  after intraventricular surgery, 318
  automatic implantable cardioverter defibrillator for, 273
  carotid sinus pressure for, 255t
  DC cardioversion for, 273
  flecainide for, 270
  isoproterenol for, 248
  procainamide for, 270
  recurrent, amiodarone for, 276
  sustained, surgery for, 274
Ventricular volume curve, 207
Ventriculitis, in bacterial meningitis, 1605
Ventriculography, 214
  left, for mitral regurgitation, 349
  radionuclide, 178
    for myxoma, 367
Venturi mask, 486
  for oxygen therapy, 478
Venturi nebulizers, infection from, 1544
Venulitis, hypersensitivity, 2027
  necrotizing, 1950
VEP (visual evoked potentials), 2056
Verapamil, 271
  adverse effects of, 269t, 289t
  contraindicated for Wolff-Parkinson-White syndrome with atrial fibrillation, 260
  dosing of, 269t

Verapamil (Continued)
  for angina pectoris, 327t, 328t
  for asthma, 409
  for atrial flutter, 260
  for cardiomyopathy, hypertrophic, 358
    idiopathic restrictive, 361
  for hypertension, 287t
  for multifocal atrial tachycardia, 261
  for paroxysmal supraventricular tachycardia, 258
  interaction of, with digitalis, 228
    with digoxin, 101
  pharmacokinetic properties of, 266t
Vermiculite, lung disease from, 2364
Verner-Morrison syndrome, 727, 1388
Vernix caseosa, 2303
Verruca peruana, 1681
Verruca vulgaris, 2323t, 2324
Vertebra(e). See also Back; Spine
  anomalies of, chronic alcoholism in mothers and, 171
  bone density of, measurement of, 1513
  fractures of, compression, from cough, 391
    crush, in metabolic bone disease, 1476
    in osteoporosis, 1512
  mineral content of, measurement of, 1476
  osteomyelitis of, 2186
  radiograph of, osteoporosis in, 1513
  transitional, 2257
  tuberculosis of, 2256
Vertebral artery, 2159–2160, 2160, 2161
  occlusion of, 2163, 2166
  trauma to, 2168
Vertebral canal, size of, 2248
Vertebrobasilar artery, disease of, symptoms of, 2168–2169, 2168t, 2169t
  insufficiency of, vertigo with, 2124
  spontaneous dissection of, 2164
Vertigo, 2120. See also Dizziness
  causes of, 2121, 2122–2124
  definition of, 2122
  from multiple sclerosis, 2213
  from pseudotumor cerebri, 2236
  from relapsing polychondritis, 2038
  from sarcoidosis, 453
  from typhus fever, 1740
  posture, benign, vs. transient ischemic attacks, 2169
  treatment of, 2124
  vs. epilepsy, 2225
Vesicoureteral reflux, pain from urination and, 615
Vesiculobullous diseases, 2328–2332, 2330t
Vespids, stings of, 1958
Vestibular system, 2120–2124
  anatomy and physiology of, 2120–2121
  and drop attacks, 2127
  examination of, 2121
Vestibulo-ocular reflex, testing of, 2121
Vestibulopathy, peripheral, acute, 2123
Veterans Administration Cooperative Study, 339
Vibrio, vs. Campylobacter, 1649
  vs. Escherichia coli, 1655
Vibrio cholerae, 1651
  food poisoning by, 784
Vibrio parahaemolyticus, food poisoning by, 784, 785
Vidarabine, for herpes simplex infection, 125, 1783, 2195
Vinblastine, for cancer, 1125–1126
  for Hodgkin's disease, 1020
  for renal cell carcinoma, 653
Vinca alkaloids, for cancer, 1125–1126
Vincent's angina, vs. diphtheria, 1628
  vs. streptococcal pharyngitis, 1576
Vincent's infection, 675, 675

Vincristine
and antidiuretic hormone release, 540
as postoperative therapy, for nephroblastoma, 654
for acute lymphoblastic leukemia, 1004
for cancer, 1125–1126
for Hodgkin's disease, 1020
for multiple myeloma, 1031, 1032
for thrombocytopenic purpura, 1051
in adjuvant therapy for breast cancer, 1457
Vinyl chloride, exposure to, and angiosarcoma, 140, 828, 859
and cancer, 1093t, 1094
interstitial lung disease from, 435
Violence, adolescents and, 20–21
alcohol and, 49
implications of, for medical practice, 41–42
VIP, 727. See also Vasoactive intestinal polypeptide
VIPoma, 1388–1389, 1389t
diarrhea from, 727, 731
Vira-A (adenine arabinoside), 125, 1783, 2195
Viral exanthems, 2322–2323, 2323t
Viral gastroenteritis, 1768–1772
clinical manifestations of, 1770
diagnosis of, 1770–1771
diarrhea from, 728–729
epidemiology of, 1769–1770
etiology of, 1768–1769
pathology and pathogenesis of, 1770
prevention of, 1771–1772
stool examination for, 730
treatment of, 1771
Viral hepatitis, 818–826, 822
acute, 818–826
definition of, 818
diagnosis of, 824
in drug abusers, 57
liver biopsy for, 824
vs. clonorchiasis, 1901
and jaundice, 818
and plasma amino acids, 1152t
aplastic anemia from, 886
chronic, and eosinophilia, 1026
Niemann-Pick disease and, 1148
vs. cryptogenic cirrhosis, 847
complications of, 820
during pregnancy, 841
etiology of, 818–819, 819t
from hemophilia B treatment, 1071
fulminant hepatic failure from, 854
immunization for, before travel, 1550
in drug abusers, 57
in hospital employees, 1548
manifestations of, 819–820
pathology of, 819
predisposing factors for, 808
prevention of, 824–826
serologic tests in, 821
splenomegaly in, 1037
type A, 820–821, 821
immunization against, 63t
preventing spread of, 825
testing for, 824
type B, 821–823
and cancer, 1095
arthritis in, 2010
vs. rat-bite fever, 1730
chronic, corticosteroid therapy contraindicated for, 832
chronic persistent hepatitis from, 831
cryptogenic cirrhosis with, 847
dialysis patients as chronic carriers of, 1542
immunization against, 62t, 63t

Viral hepatitis (Continued)
type B, necrotizing cutaneous vasculitis with, 2326
necrotizing venulitis in, 1950
polyarteritis with, 2028
preventing spread of, 825–826
risk of, with dialysis, 575
vaccine for, 824–826, 1524
vs. Lyme disease, 1728
type D, 823
type non-A, non-B, 823–824
vs. infectious mononucleosis, 1788
vs. leptospirosis, 1732
vs. Wilson's disease, 1188
vs. yellow fever, 1832
Viral infections. See also Retroviruses
and inflammatory rheumatic syndromes, 1999
arthropods and, 1814–1837. See also Arboviruses
colitis from, vs. ulcerative colitis, 756
cutaneous lesions from, 1772–1780
laryngotracheobronchitis from, cough from, 391
lymphocytosis from, 972
meningitis from, vs. amebic meningoencephalitis, 1888
myocarditis from, 262
of nervous system, 2191–2207. See also Viral nervous system infections
of respiratory system, vs. streptococcal infection, 1576
orchitis from, 1414
and germ cell damage, 1416
paroxysmal cold hemoglobinuria in, 921
pericarditis from, 362–364, 364
pneumonia from, vs. psittacosis, 1736
remission of minimal change nephrotic syndrome after, 593
vs. chronic lymphocytic leukemia, 996
vs. leptospirosis, 1732
vs. rheumatoid arthritis, 2000
Viral nervous system infections, 2191–2207
acute transverse myelitis from, 2216
causes of, 2192t
encephalitis as, 2192–2194
meningitis as, 2192–2194
poliomyelitis as, 2198–2200
rabies as, 2200–2202
slow, 2203t, 2203–2207
with herpesvirus, 2195–2198
Virazole (ribavirin), 127, 1760
Virchow's node, 711
Viridans, 1573
Virilism, excess ovarian androgen synthesis and, 1431
Virions, 1750
Viroptic (trifluridine), 125–126
Viruses, 124. See also Antiviral therapy
AIDS, 1795
characteristics of, 1750–1751
classification of, 1750t
definition of, 1750
disease from, 1752t
in respiratory tract, 1753–1768. See also Respiratory system, viral infection of
prevention and control of, 1753
hemorrhagic fever from, 1829–1837
herpes-type, infection of, 1780–1793
host defenses and, 1751
infection of, and taste and smell disorders, 2110
in acquired immunodeficiency syndrome, 1805t, 1806
leukemia, 1795
lymphocytopenia from, 966
pathogenesis of, 1752–1753
sexual transmission of, 1702t

Viruses (Continued)
slow spongiform encephalopathy, 2205
Visceral abscesses, glomerulonephritis with, 588
Visceral pain, 105
in gastrointestinal disease, 658
Visceral reflex syncope, 2075
Viscus, perforated
as contraindication for colonoscopy, 670
bloody ascites from, 791
computed tomography for, 662
vs. appendicitis, 801, 802
Vision. See also Eye(s)
abnormalities in, in viral encephalitis, 2193
agnosia of, 2080t, 2085
blurred, from atropine, 139
from diabetes mellitus, 1378
brain processing of, 2080
disorders of, cerebral artery disease and, 2168
from arteritis, 374
from pseudotumor cerebri, 2236, 2237
from subacute sclerosing panencephalitis, 2206
from syphilis, 2189
from toxemia of pregnancy, 635
from Waldenström's macroglobulinemia, 1033
evaluating field of, in pituitary tumor diagnosis, 1299
examination for, 2112
field defects of, 2111
loss of. See Blindness
neural pathways for, anatomy of, 2111
neurologic basis for, 2111–2117
vitamin A and, 1237
Visna, 2203
Visual association cortex, ischemia of, 2166
Visual disorientation, 2082
Visual evoked potentials, 2056
Visual evoked response, 1299
measurement of, for multiple sclerosis, 2212
Visual field, defects of, from pituitary adenomas, 2232
definition of, 2111, 2111
Vital capacity, 395–396, 395
in asthma, 408
in sarcoidosis, 455
measurement of, in severely ill, 483
Vitamin(s)
body's capacity to store, 1228
deficiency of, causes of, 1228
signs of, 657
dialysis and, 576
fat-soluble, absorption of, 734
for treatment of malabsorption, 741t
malabsorption of, from Crohn's disease, 749
for chronic kidney failure, 572
in total parenteral nutrition, 1249, 1249t
metabolism of, disorders of, 1228–1241
supplements of, 1228
synthesis of, 1228
Vitamin A, 1236, 1236–1238
as carcinogenesis inhibitor, 44
deficiency of, symptoms of, 657
dietary sources of, 1237
for treatment of malabsorption, 741t
hypercalcemia from, 1503
intoxication with, and hair damage, 2349
osteosclerosis from, 1519
recommended dietary allowance for, 1205t, 1237
reference intervals for, 2400t

Vitamin B complex, deficiency of, symptoms of, 657
for treatment of malabsorption, 741t
Vitamin B₁, *1229*, 1229–1230. See also *Thiamin*
Vitamin B₂, *1230*, 1230–1231
  deficiency of, 1231
  for methemoglobinemia, 946
  recommended dietary allowance for, 1205t, 1231
  reference intervals for, 2399t
  sources of, 1231
Vitamin B₆, *1233*, 1233–1234
  deficiency of, 1233
    and kidney stones, 640
    seizures from, 2219
  for galactorrhea, 1450
  for hyperoxaluria, 1137
  for premenstrual syndrome, 1434
  for sideroblastic anemia, 900
  recommended dietary allowance for, 1205t, 1233
  reference intervals for, 2400t
  sources of, 1233
Vitamin B₁₂
  absorption of, 735, *735*
    tests for, 691, 737t, 738, 738t
  average daily intake of, 902
  binding proteins of, as tumor markers, 1100
  deficiency of, 903–904
    after ulcer surgery, 705
    and macrocytosis, 882
    and megaloblastic anemia, 901t, 902–904
    dementia from, 28
    neurologic disorders from, 2140–2141
    neutropenia from, 962
    symptoms of, 657
    vs. Friedreich's ataxia, 2153
    vs. multiple sclerosis, 2214
  distal ileum resection and absorption of, 733
  for ketoacidosis in methylmalonicaciduria, 157
  for pernicious anemia, 884
  for treatment of malabsorption, 741t
  in myelofibrosis, with myeloid metaplasia, 986
  malabsorption of, from ileitis, 749
    in chronic pancreatitis, 779
  metabolism of, 902–903
  molecule of, 902, *903*
  protein binding of, 902t
  recommended dietary allowance for, 1205t
  reference intervals for, 2400t
  therapy with, and potassium shifts, 546
    indications for, 905
Vitamin C, *1234*, 1234–1236
  and cancer, 44, 1095
    of stomach, 710
  and common cold, 1756
  and iron absorption, 898
  and iron removal in thalassemia, 932
  deficiency of, 657. See also *Scurvy*
  dietary sources of, 1235
  esophageal injury from, 688
  excess, and kidney stones, 640
  for Chédiak-Higashi disease, 959
  for methemoglobinemia, 945, 946
  recommended dietary allowance for, 1205t, 1235
  reference intervals for, 2400t
Vitamin D, *1477*, 1477–1479
  absorption of, 734
  and bone, 1476, 1508
  and calcium absorption by intestine, 519

Vitamin D (*Continued*)
  and hypercalcemia, 1492, 1503
  and parathyroid hormone, 1489
  and phosphorus reabsorption, 518
  binding protein of, 1477
    loss of, from nephrotic syndrome, 1480
  deficiency of, 1478
    and abnormal bone mineralization, 1479
    in osteomalacia, 1483
    in rickets, 153, 1154t, 1483
    metabolic bone disease from, in Crohn's disease, 751
    symptoms of, 657
    treatment of, 1484
  excess of, and increased calcium absorption, 639
  for hypoparathyroidism, 1499
  for osteoporosis, 1514
  for renal osteodystrophy, 1509
  for treating malabsorption, 741t
  in calcium homeostasis, 1470
  measurement of, 1478
  metabolism of, alternations in, and renal osteodystrophy, 1507
    kidneys and, 518
  metabolites of, 1477, 1478t
    for osteomalacia and rickets, 1484t
  recommended dietary allowance for, 1205t
  reference intervals for, 2400t
  toxicity of, 1478–1479
    in hypoparathyroidism treatment, 1499
Vitamin D endocrine system, and osteomalacia and rickets, 1479–1481
Vitamin D₃, parathyroid hormone and, 502
  production of, in skin, 1477
Vitamin E, 1238–1239, *1239*
  deficiency of, and myopathy, 2282
    neurologic syndrome with, 2140
    vs. Friedreich's ataxia, 2153
  dietary allowance for, 1239
  recommended dietary allowance for, 1205t
  reference intervals for, 2400t
Vitamin K, *1240*, 1240–1241
  and methemoglobinemia, in infants, 946
  and prothrombin synthesis, 816
  daily dietary intake of, 1076, 1206t
  deficiency of, and bleeding in alcoholic liver disease, 1077
    and blood coagulation disorders, 1076–1077
    symptoms of, 657
  dietary sources of, 1240
  for primary biliary cirrhosis, 845
  for treating malabsorption, 741t
  genetics and reaction to, 102
  interaction of, with warfarin, 101
  metabolism and function of, 1076
    abnormality in, and hemorrhage, 1073
  toxicity of, to hemoglobin, 945
Vitamin K₁, for deep-vein thrombosis, 387
Vitiligo, 2344–2345
  and polyglandular autoimmune disease, 1414
  pernicious anemia with, 905
  vs. chemical leukoderma, 2375
  synthesis of, *1138*
Vocal cords
  injury to, from endotracheal intubation, 478
  paralysis of, airway obstruction from, 418
    from dissecting aortic aneurysms, 373
    from sarcoidosis, 453
Vocalization, as tic, 2151
Vogt-Koyanagi-Harada syndrome, 2293
Voiding, act of, 2107

Volhynia fever, 1747
Volume overload, in heart failure, 215
Volume receptors, in hypothalamus, 2105
Volume ventilators, 479
Volume work, of heart, oxygen cost of, 187
Volvulus, from ascariasis, 1909
  gastric, 718
  vs. small intestine neoplasms, 774
Vomiting
  and fluid volume regulation, 532
  by infants, from isovaleric acidemia, 1159
  definition of, 658
  esophageal injury from, 688
  forced, 656
  from abdominal abscess, 793
  from acute pancreatitis, 776
  from adenocarcinoma of duodenum, 713
  from alcoholic hepatitis, 843
  from bacterial meningitis, 1606
  from bacterial peritonitis, 793
  from brain abscess, 2182
  from brain tumors, 2232
  from bulimia, 1218
  from cannabis, 57
  from celiac compression syndrome, 762
  from chemotherapy, 1088
  from cholecystitis, 865
  from cholera, 1652
  from cough, 391
  from digitalis toxicity, 229
  from febrile transfusion reactions, 949
  from gallstones, 864
  from gastric cancer, 711
  from gastric outlet obstruction, 707
  from gastritis, 689
  from gastrointestinal disease, 658–660, 659t
  from hepatic porphyria, 1185
  from ileus, 719
  from infectious mononucleosis, 1787
  from ischemic colitis, 764
  from liver disease, 808
  from narcotics, 33, 108, 109
  from neurosyphilis, 2188
  from opioid withdrawal syndrome, 57
  from oral contraceptives, 1444
  from pancreatic cancer, 781
  from post-streptococcal glomerulonephritis, 587
  from primary mesothelioma, 794
  from pseudotumor cerebri, 2236
  from psychedelic drugs, 58
  from renal artery occlusion, 633
  from Reye syndrome, 2209
  from sedative withdrawal, 54
  from subdural empyema, 2184
  from viral hepatitis, 819
  from whooping cough, 1625
  metabolic consequences of, *659*
  potassium depletion from, 546
  psychogenic, 718
  symptoms from, vs. Bartter's syndrome, 622
Vomitus, blood in, from mesenteric artery occlusion, 762
von Economo's encephalitis, parkinsonism from, 2144
von Gierke's disease, 152, 1133–1134
  and gout, 1167
  hypoglycemia from, 1382
von Hippel-Lindau syndrome, 2231
  and renal cell carcinoma, 652
  and neoplasms, 1096t
von Recklinghausen's disease, 713, 2158, 2343. See also *Neurofibromatosis*
von Willebrand factor, function of, 1069–1070
  inhibitors in, 1081

von Willebrand's disease, 1055–1056, 1056t, 1069–1071
  platelet aggregation in, 1047
  uterine bleeding from, 1434
  vs. hemophilia A, 1067
Vulvovaginitis, from *Candida* infection, 1848

Waardenburg's syndrome, 2345
Wade-Fite stain method, for leprosy, 1699
WAIS (Wechsler Adult Intelligence Scale), 2088
Waldenström's macroglobulinemia, 975, 1033–1034
  and skin, 1109
  tubulointerstitial involvement in, 606
  vs. leukemia, chronic lymphocytic, 996–997
    hairy cell, 1000
Walking, after stroke, 2172
  as exercise, 47
  disorders of, and lumbar spondylosis, 2254
Walking ability. See also *Gait*
  in hereditary spastic paraplegias, 2154
  loss of, in adult-onset cerebellar ataxia, 2153
    in Duchenne dystrophy, 2272
    in Friedreich's ataxia, 2152
Wallenberg's syndrome, 2129, 2166
Walruses, poisoning from, 1931
War fever, 1739
Warfarin, 1075
  absorption of, sucralfate and, 99
  and vitamin K, 1076–1077, 1240
  congenital heart disease from, 303
  decreased absorption of, cholestyramine and, 99
  drugs and response to, 1077t
  effects of, metronidazole and, 121
  for deep-vein thrombosis, 387
  for pulmonary embolism, 448
  genetics in metabolism of, 102
  in drug interactions, 124t
  induction of metabolism of, 99
  interaction of, with clofibrate, 101
    with phenylbutazone or sulfinpyrazone, 100
    with vitamin K, 101
  metabolism inhibition of, 101t
    by cimetidine, 100
  pregnancy as contraindication for, 448
  reference intervals for, 2404t
  vitamin E with, hemorrhage from, 1239
Warts, 2324, 2335–2336, 2336t
  genital, interferon for, 128
  in immunocompromised host, 2352
  vs. calluses, 2313
Wasps, stings of, 1924, 1958
Wassermann test, for syphilis, 1719
Water
  absorption of, 734
  and solute balance, external, alterations in, 529
  barometric pressure under, 2367
  contaminated
    and tularemia, 1664
    and typhoid fever, 1641
    Campylobacter from, 1648
    cholera from, 1651
    Escherichia coli from, 1653
  daily requirements of, 1206
  deprivation of, in diabetes insipidus, 1310
  excess loss of, and hypernatremia, 542
  excretion of, kidneys and, 516
  inadequate intake of, and hypernatremia, 542
    and urolithiasis, 45

Water (*Continued*)
  movement of, in gastrointestinal tract, 725
  reabsorption of, by proximal tubule, 512
  regulation of, central nervous system disorders of, 1288
  retention of
    from chronic distention of left atrium, 215
    in acute kidney failure, 559
    in congestive heart failure, 190
    in heart failure, 220
    in pregnancy, 634
  schistosomiasis from, 1898
  self-induced intoxication with, 2105
  skin contact with, and urticaria, 1950
Water balance, hypothalamus and, 2104–2105
Water lily sign, 1894
Water loss heat exhaustion, 2383
Water metabolism, hormones and, 1263
Water moccasins, 1927
Water repletion reaction, 1308
Water sponging, for fever reduction, 1527
Water supply, and giardiasis, 1883
  chloramine in, hemolysis from, 923
Water-borne hepatitis, type A hepatitis as, 820
Water-soluble drugs, in elderly, 97
Waterhouse-Friderichsen syndrome, 1613
  in defibrination syndrome, 1079
Watershed infarction, 2163
Watery diarrhea–hypokalemia–hypochlorhydria syndrome, 727, 731, 1388–1389
Watson-Schwartz test, for hepatic porphyria, 1185
Weakness, 2125, 2270
  from adrenocortical insufficiency, 1351
  from alcoholic-nutritional neuropathy, 2139
  from bronchogenic carcinoma, 459, 462
  from cardiovascular patient history, 175
  from chronic kidney failure, 567
  from essential mixed cryoglobulinemia, 601
  from fluid volume depletion, 532
  from glucocorticosteroid therapy withdrawal, 132
  from hemochromatosis, 1191
  from hypervitaminosis D, 1478
  from hyponatremia, 540
  from legionnaires' disease, 1571
  from multiple myeloma, 1029
  from polymyositis, 2035
  from potassium depletion, 546
  from primary pulmonary hypertension, 299
  from relapsing fever, 1725
  from renal osteodystrophy, 1508
  from sedative withdrawal, 54
  from sudden atrial occlusion, 383
  from trench fever, 1748
  from vomiting, 660
  from Waldenström's macroglobulinemia, 1033
  in face, from Guillain-Barré syndrome, 2261
Weber test, for hearing, 2118
Weber-Christian disease, 2050
Wechsler Adult Intelligence Scale, 2088
WEE (western equine encephalitis), 1823–1824, 2193
Wegener's granulomatosis, 431, 2030–2031
  Goodpasture's syndrome vs., 590
  hemolysis from, 925
  kidneys in, 599
  solitary pulmonary nodules from, 464
  vs. idiopathic pulmonary hemosiderosis, 430

Wegener's granulomatosis (*Continued*)
  vs. midline granuloma, 2032, 2032t
  vs. orbital pseudotumor, 2295
  vs. polyarteritis nodosa, 2030
Weight. See also *Obesity*
  and height, 1209, 1209t
  control of, exercise and, 46
  dry, definition of, 575
  during acute malnutrition, 1212
  loss of. See *Weight loss*
  spurt in, during puberty, 18
  velocity curve for, menarche and, 19
Weight loss, 391
  after gastric surgery, 705
  amphetamines for, 54
  and hyperglycemia improvement, 1368
  and malnutrition, 1209
  from adenocarcinoma, of duodenum, 713
    of peritoneum, 794
  from adrenocortical insufficiency, 1351
  from bile duct tumor, 871
  from carcinoma
    bronchogenic, 459, 462
    esophageal, 686
    hepatocellular, 858
  from chronic eosinophilic pneumonia, 431
  from chronic lymphocytic leukemia, 995
  from chronic pancreatitis, 779
  from Crohn's disease, 747
  from cryptosporidiosis, 1882
  from gastric cancer, 711
  from gastrointestinal disease, 656
  from giardiasis, 1884
  from glucagonoma, 1389
  from glucocorticosteroid therapy withdrawal, 132
  from Graves' disease, 1322
  from insulin-dependent diabetes mellitus, 1362
  from liver disease, 808
  from lung abscess, 436
  from malabsorption, 660, 735
  from malnutrition, 1212, 1214
  from pancreatic cancer, 781
  from pheochromocytoma, 284
  from systemic lupus erythematosus, 2014
  from thiamin deficiency, 1229
  from ulcerative colitis, 754
  from Waldenström's macroglobulinemia, 1033
  in treatment for non–insulin-dependent diabetes mellitus, 1368
  maintenance of, 1227
  self-induced, 1215
  with uremia, 507
Weil's disease, 1730, 1731. See also *Leptospirosis*
Weil-Felix reaction, for rickettsioses, 1745, 1746
  for Rocky Mountain spotted fever, 1744
Weinstein syndrome, hypogonadism from, 1414
Wenckebach block, from myocardial infarction, 333
Werdnig-Hoffman disease, 2155
Wermer's syndrome, 1095t, 1458–1460, 1459t. See also *Multiple endocrine neoplasia*
Werner's syndrome, 1202
  and neoplasms, 1096t
  hypogonadism from, 1414
Wernicke aphasia, 2086, 2086t
Wernicke's area, language and, 2086
Wernicke's disease, autonomic insufficiency in, 2106
Wernicke's encephalopathy, 2137–2138
  Korsakoff's amnesia with, 2084
  predisposing conditions for, 2138

Wernicke-Korsakoff syndrome, 2137–2138
  from thiamin deficiency, 1229
West Nile fever, 1817
West's syndrome, 2223
Westergren sedimentation rate, 1995
Western equine encephalitis, 1823–1824,
  2193
Whales, poisoning from, 1931
Wheezing, 391
  from asthma, 403
    occupational, 2359
  from obstruction of intrathoracic airway,
    475
Whipple's disease
  and malabsorption, 743–744
  and peritoneum, 795
  arthritis with, 2046
  diagnosis of, with biopsy, 731
Whipple's resection, for pancreatic cancer,
  783
Whipple's triad, 1383
  in insulinoma, 1384, 1385
Whirlpool, for skin disorders, 2314
White blood cell(s), in expressed prostatic
    secretions, 1421
  in stool, 730
White blood cell count
  in alcoholic hepatitis, 844
  in myelofibrosis, with myeloid metapla-
    sia, 986
  in renal artery occlusion, 633
  in synovial fluid, 1993
  peripheral, normal, 961
White cell casts, and parenchymal inflam-
    mation, 503
White matter, disease of, diagnostic imag-
    ing techniques for, 2060
  spongy degeneration of, 2216
  subcortical, hemorrhage in, 2179
White muscle disease, selenium and, 2392
Whitlow, 1549
  herpetic, 1782
Whole-body radiation syndrome, 2377
  diagnosis of, 2379
  treatment of, 2379
Whooping cough, 1624–1626. See also Per-
    tussis
Wickham's striae, 2328
Widal test, for agglutinating antibodies,
  1641
Wildlife, rabies in, 2200
Will, living, 2071
Williams syndrome, supravalvular aortic
    stenosis in, 313
Williams-Campbell syndrome, bronchiec-
    tasis from, 439t
Wilms' tumor, 654
  chromosome studies for, 168
  solitary pulmonary nodules from, 464
  vs. mesoblastic nephroma, 652
Wilson, Frank N., 196
Wilson's disease, 1154t, 1188–1189
  alcoholic hyalin in, 843
  and proximal tubular defects, 505
  cataract in, 2289
  chronic hepatitis from, 830, 831
  copper in, 2390
  genetic counseling for, 174
  hemolysis in, 923
  jaundice from, 817
  juvenile parkinsonism in, 2144
  liver in, 839
  liver transplant for, 157
  penicillamine for, 157
  tests for, 832
  vs. cryptogenic cirrhosis, 847
  vs. fulminant hepatic failure, 854
  vs. viral hepatitis, 824
Winter vomiting disease, 1768

Winterbottom's sign, 1864
Wirsung, duct of, 775
Wiskott-Aldrich syndrome, 1048, 1057,
    1942, 1946–1947
  and neoplasms, 1096t
  bone marrow transplant for, 157
  cancer and, 1113
Withdrawal syndrome, 52
  acute, in alcoholics, 50–51
  from cigarette smoking, 39
  from cocaine, 54
  from glucocorticosteroid therapy, 132
  from opioids, 57
  from sedatives, 53–54, 2069
  in alcoholics, 50
    convulsions in, 51
  naloxone for opioid overdose and, 57
  vs. hangover, 49
  vs. panic attacks, 2101
Wohlfahrtia, 1925
Wolff-Chaikoff effect, 1328
Wolff-Parkinson-White syndrome
  and sudden cardiac death, 275
  arrhythmias in, disopyramide for, 270
  atrial fibrillation from, 260
  atrial septal defect and, 305
  cardiac catheterization for, 178
  digitalis contraindicated for, 228
  in Ebstein's anomaly of tricuspid valve,
    310
  paroxysmal supraventricular tachycardia
    in, encainide for, 258, 270
  with atrial fibrillation, surgery for, 274
Wolffian ducts, 1391–1392
Women. See Female(s)
Wood's light, in skin examination, 2311
Woolsorter's disease, 1667
Workplace
  deaths from, 2354
  evaluation of, 2358
  human error in, 2356
  standards for, 2356–2357
Work-related disorders, 2354–2358. See also
    Occupational disease(s)
World Health Organization
  and smallpox eradication, 1791
  Cancer Pain Relief Program, 111
  diabetes standards from, 1360
  leprosy treatment recommendations
    from, 1700
  oral rehydration solution recommenda-
    tions from, 731, 1771
Wounds
  healing of, 2306
    malnutrition and, 1213
    vitamin C deficiency and, 1235
  infection of
    with botulism, 1634
    with clostridia, 1629
    with Mycobacterium fortuitum-chelonae,
      1693
    with tetanus, 1635
  management of, tetanus prophylaxis in,
    62, 1636t
  of skull, and subdural empyema, 2184
  postoperative, infection of, 1546
    and bloodstream infection, 1544
  puncture, and mycobacteria infection,
    1694
  slow healing of, from Cushing's syn-
    drome, 1355
Wrist, rheumatoid arthritis in, 2001
Writer's cramp, and torsion dystonia, 2150
Wuchereria bancrofti, 1914

X body, 1023
X chromatin (Barr body), 166
  Klinefelter's syndrome and, 1412

X chromosomes, late-replicating, identifica-
    tion of, 167
X descent, in venous pulse, 176
X-inactivation, 149
X-linked diseases. See under name of spe-
    cific disease
X-linked traits, 149–150
  dominant, 149
  recessive, 150
  vs. sex-influenced autosomal dominant
    inheritance, 150
X-ray(s), 2375. See also Radiography
  and skin, 2341
  thymic hypoplasia from, 1974
Xanax, abuse of, 53
Xanthelasma, from liver disease, 809, 846
Xanthine, in kidney stones, 638
Xanthine oxidase, deficiency of, 1170
  interaction of, with allopurinol, 101
Xanthinuria, 1170–1171
Xanthomas, 2336t, 2340
  eruptive, from chylomicronemia syn-
    drome, 1143
  from liver disease, 809
  from secondary biliary cirrhosis, 846
  in dysbetalipoproteinemia, 1141
Xenon-133, for ventilation scanning, 445
Xeongeneic immune ribonucleic acid, for
    renal cell carcinoma, 653
Xerocytosis, hereditary, 913
Xeroderma pigmentosum, 2343–2344
  and neoplasms, 1096t
Xerostomia
  and oral candidal infection, 677
  from cannabis, 57
  glossitis from, 678
  in AIDS, 677
  in oral cancer, 679
  in systemic sclerosis, 2023
Xg(a+) blood group, as X-linked dominant
    trait, 149
XO/XY mosaicism, 1395
Xovirax, 126. See also Acyclovir
XX males, 1401–1402
XY agonadism, 1395
XY gonadal dysgenesis, 1393–1394
Xylohypha bantiana, 1855
L-Xylulose, in urine, pentosuria and, 1135

Y chromatin bodies, 166
Y chromosome, and testicular differentia-
    tion, 1392, 1392
Y-linked inheritance, 150
Yato-byo, 1664
Yawning, in opioid withdrawal syndrome,
    57
Yaws, 1723
  vs. paracoccidioidomycosis, 1843
Yeast infection, vaginitis from, 1704, 1705
Yellow fever, 1830t, 1830–1832
  acute hepatitis from, 819
  immunization for, before travel, 1550
  vs. viral hepatitis, 824
Yellow nail syndrome, 2347
Yellowjackets, 1924
  stings of, 1958
Yersinia, infection of, 1661–1664
  and Reiter's syndrome, 151
  plague as, 1661–1663
  reactive arthropathy from, 2008
Yersinia enterocolitica, 1663–1664
  Crohn's disease with infection of, 746
  enterotoxins from, and secretory diar-
    rhea, 727
  gastroenteritis from, vs. appendicitis, 803
  infection with, vs. Crohn's disease, 750,
    756–757
  vs. Campylobacter, 1649

Yersinia pseudotuberculosis, 1663–1664
Yohimbine, affinity of, for alpha receptors, 136
  and panic attacks, 2100
Yttrium aluminum garnet laser, for electro-coagulation, 670

Zebrafish, stings from, 1930
Zenker's diverticulum, 684, 687
Zerostomia, in oral cancer, 679
Zidovudine, 127. See also *Azidothymidine*
Ziehl-Neelsen stain, for leprosy, 1699

Zinc, 1241
  deficiency of, from Crohn's disease, 751
    symptoms of, 657
  food poisoning with, 786
  for improved taste perception, in oral cancer, 679
  for Wilson's disease, 1189
  recommended dietary allowance for, 1205t
  reference intervals for, 2400t
  toxicity of, 2389
Zollinger-Ellison syndrome, 695, 708–709
  and postoperative recurrent ulcers, 705
  diarrhea from, 727–728

Zollinger-Ellison syndrome *(Continued)*
  gastrin levels and, 698–699, 698t
    in multiple endocrine neoplasia, 1459
  malabsorption from, 741
  ulcers in, 692
  vs. Crohn's disease, 750
  vs. giant hypertrophic gastritis, 692
  vs. VIPoma, 1338
Zona fasciculata, 1340
Zona glomerulosa, 1340
Zona reticularis, 1340
Zoster sine herpete, 2196
Zosteriform, definition of, 2307
Zygomycosis, 1852–1853

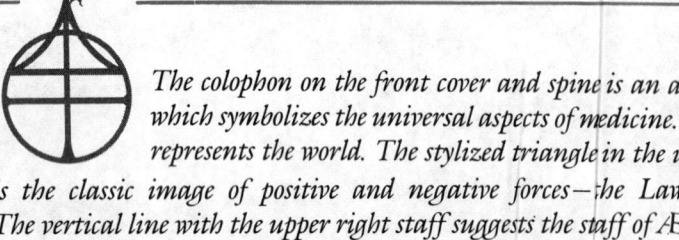

The colophon on the front cover and spine is an abstraction which symbolizes the universal aspects of medicine. The circle represents the world. The stylized triangle in the upper area is the classic image of positive and negative forces—the Law of Life. The vertical line with the upper right staff suggests the staff of Æsculapius and Hermes, and the horizontal bar connects all three symbols into the total summation of medicine as Art and Science.